LiveAdvise

Medical-Surgical Nursing

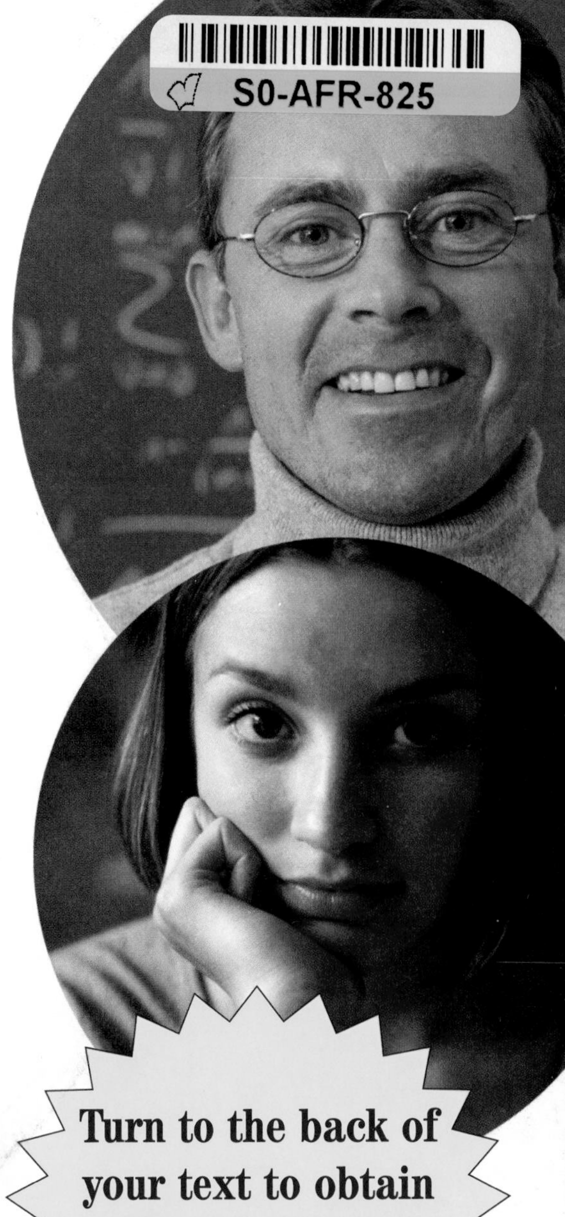

Turn to the back of your text to obtain your access code and instructions!

Lippincott Williams & Wilkins

offers online teaching advice and student tutoring with this textbook!

Students—have you ever needed:

...help studying for a test at a time your instructor was not available?

...questions answered outside of class?

...feedback on assignments before turning them in?

Instructors—have you ever wanted to:

...get help generating classroom activities or discussion ideas from an expert in your discipline?

...ask questions about the content of your adopted textbook or ancillary package, and have someone get back to you right away?

...have your lesson plans evaluated?

If so, LiveAdvise: Medical-Surgical Nursing is the service you need!

Our tutors are handpicked educators that we train to help you. They are very familiar with the textbook you are using in class and the text's ancillary package. You can connect live to a tutor during certain hours of the week, or send e-mail style messages to which the tutor will respond quickly – often within 24 hours.

And the best part—the service is free with the purchase of your textbook!

Instructors—to use this service, please visit **http://thePoint.LWW.com/LiveAdvise**

Students—see the codebook inside the front cover of this book for more details.
In it you'll find instructions for using this great service, along with your own personal code to log on and get started.

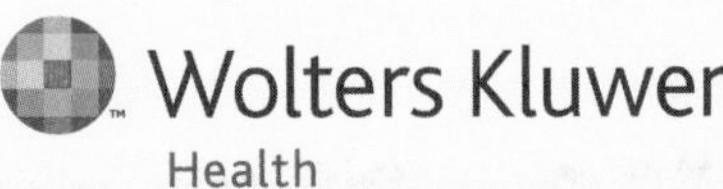

Lippincott
Williams & Wilkins

Brunner & Suddarth's

Textbook of Medical-Surgical Nursing

Eleventh Edition

Suzanne C. Smeltzer, EdD, RN, FAAN
Professor and Director, Center for Nursing Research
Villanova University College of Nursing
Villanova, Pennsylvania

Brenda G. Bare, RN, MSN
Consultant, Inova Health System
Fairfax, Virginia

Janice L. Hinkle, PhD, RN, CNRN
Senior Research Fellow, Acute Stroke Programme
Oxford Brookes University and John Radcliffe Hospital
Oxford, United Kingdom

Kerry H. Cheever, PhD, RN
Professor and Chairperson
St. Luke's Hospital School of Nursing at Moravian College
Assistant Vice President
St. Luke's Hospital & Health Network
Bethlehem, Pennsylvania

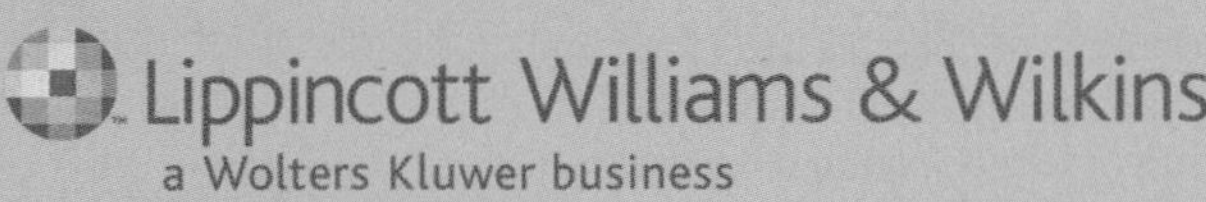
Lippincott Williams & Wilkins
a Wolters Kluwer business
Philadelphia • Baltimore • New York • London
Buenos Aires • Hong Kong • Sydney • Tokyo

Acquisitions Editor: Pete Darcy
Development Editor: Melanie Cann
Senior Production Editor: Marian A. Bellus/Tom Gibbons
Director of Nursing Production: Helen Ewan
Senior Managing Editor / Production: Erika Kors
Art Director, Design: Joan Wendt
Art Director, Illustration: Brett MacNaughton
Senior Manufacturing Manager: William Alberti
Manufacturing Coordinator: Karin Duffield
Indexer: Maria Coughlin
Compositor: Circle Graphics
Printer: R. R. Donnelley-Willard

Eleventh Edition

9 8 7 6 5 4 3 2 1

Library of Congress Cataloging-in-Publication Data

Brunner & Suddarth's textbook of medical-surgical nursing. — 11th ed. / [edited by] Suzanne C. Smeltzer . . . [et al.].
p. ; cm.
Includes bibliographical references and index.
ISBN-13: 978-0-7817-5978-6 (one-volume ed. : alk. paper)
ISBN-10: 0-7817-5978-1 (one-volume ed. : alk. paper)
ISBN-13: 978-0-7817-6695-1 (two-volume ed. : alk. paper)
ISBN-10: 0-7817-6695-8 (two-volume ed. : alk. paper) 1. Nursing. 2. Surgical nursing. I. Brunner, Lillian Sholtis. II. Smeltzer, Suzanne C. O'Connell. III. Title: Brunner and Suddarth's textbook of medical-surgical nursing. IV. Title: Textbook of medical-surgical nursing.
[DNLM: 1. Nursing Care. 2. Perioperative Nursing. WY 150 B8972 2007]

RT41.T46 2007
610.73—dc22

2006026479

LWW.com

Contributors

Roberta H. Baron, RN, MSN, AOCN
Clinical Nurse Specialist
Memorial Sloan Kettering Cancer Center
New York, New York
Chapter 48: Assessment and Management of Patients With Breast Disorders

Lisa Bowman, RN, MSN, CNRN, CRNP
Nurse Practitioner
Thomas Jefferson University Hospital
Philadelphia, Pennsylvania
Chapter 62: Management of Patients With Cerebrovascular Disorders

Jo Ann Brooks, DNS, RN, FAAN, FCCP
Vice President, Quality
Clarian Health Partners Inc.
Indianapolis, Indiana
Chapter 23: Management of Patients With Chest and Lower Respiratory Tract Disorders
Chapter 24: Management of Patients With Chronic Obstructive Pulmonary Disease

Kim Cantwell-Gab, BSN, RN, CVN, RVT, RDMS
Clinical Nurse Specialist, Vascular Surgery
University of Washington
Seattle, Washington
Chapter 31: Assessment and Management of Patients With Vascular Disorders and Problems of Peripheral Circulation

Patricia E. Casey, RN, MSN
Director, Clinical Content, Care Management Group
Quality Department
Kaiser Permanente Mid-Atlantic States
Rockville, Maryland
Chapter 27: Management of Patients With Dysrhythmias and Conduction Problems

Jill Cash, MSN, APRN, BC
Family Nurse Practitioner
Southern Illinois OB-GYN Associates, SC
Carbondale, Illinois
Chapter 59: Assessment and Management of Patients With Hearing and Balance Disorders

Kerry H. Cheever, PhD, RN
Professor and Chairperson
St. Luke's Hospital School of Nursing at Moravian College
Assistant Vice President
St. Luke's Hospital & Health Network
Bethlehem, Pennsylvania
Chapter 66: Assessment of Musculoskeletal Function
Chapter 69: Management of Patients With Musculoskeletal Trauma

JoAnn Coleman, RN, MS, ACNP, AOCN
Acute Care Nurse Practitioner
Gastrointestinal Surgical Oncology
Johns Hopkins Hospital
Baltimore, Maryland
Chapter 37: Management of Patients With Gastric and Duodenal Disorders

Linda Carman Copel, PhD, APRN, BC, DAPA
Associate Professor
Villanova University College of Nursing
Villanova, Pennsylvania
Chapter 4: Health Education and Health Promotion
Chapter 6: Homeostasis, Stress and Adaptation
Chapter 7: Individual and Family Considerations Related to Illness

Susanna L. Cunningham, PhD, RN, FAAN
Professor
University of Washington School of Nursing
Department of Biobehavioral Nursing and Health Systems
Seattle, Washington
Chapter 32: Assessment and Management of Patients With Hypertension

Nancy E. Donegan, RN, BSN, MPH
Director—Infection Control
Washington Hospital Center
Washington, District of Columbia
Chapter 70: Management of Patients With Infectious Diseases

Diane Dressler, RN, MSN, CCRN
Clinical Assistant Professor
Marquette University College of Nursing
Milwaukee, Wisconsin
Chapter 28: Management of Patients With Coronary Vascular Disorders
Chapter 30: Management of Patients With Complications From Heart Disease

Phyllis Dubendorf, RN, MSN, CS-ACNP
Lecturer, Acute Care Nurse Practitioner Program
University of Pennsylvania, School of Nursing
Philadelphia, Pennsylvania
Chapter 61: Neurologic Dysfunction

Linda S. Ehrlich-Jones, PhD, RN, CS
Clinical Research Coordinator
Rehabilitation Institute of Chicago
Chicago, Illinois
Chapter 54: Management of the Patient With Rheumatic Disorders

Susan M. Fallone, RN, MS, CNN
Clinical Nurse Specialist, Adult and Pediatric Dialysis
Albany Medical Center
Albany, New York
Chapter 43: Assessment of Renal and Urinary Tract Function
Chapter 44: Management of Patients With Kidney Disorders
Chapter 45: Management of Patients With Urinary Disorders

Catharine Farnan, RN, MS, CRRN, ONC
Member
American Spinal Injury Association; Association of American Spinal Cord Injury Nurses; Association of Rehabilitation Nurses
Philadelphia, Pennsylvania
Chapter 11: Principles and Practices of Rehabilitation

Eleanor Fitzpatrick, RN, MSN, CCRN
Clinical Nurse Specialist
Thomas Jefferson University Hospital
Philadelphia, Pennsylvania
Chapter 39: Assessment and Management of Patients With Hepatic Disorders
Chapter 40: Assessment and Management of Patients With Biliary Disorders

Virginia M. Fitzsimons, RNC, EdD, FAAN
Professor
Kean University, Department of Nursing
Union, New Jersey
Chapter 38: Management of Patients With Intestinal and Rectal Disorders

Kathleen K. Furniss, RNC, MSN, DMH
Coordinator, Women's Imaging
Mountainside Hospital
Montclair, New Jersey
Nurse Practitioner, Health Service
Drew University
Madison, New Jersey
Chapter 46: Assessment and Management of Problems Related to Female Physiologic Processes
Chapter 47: Management of Patients With Female Reproductive Disorders

Margaret J. Griffiths, RN, MSN, AOCN, CNE
Professor
Thomas Jefferson University
Philadelphia, Pennsylvania
Chapter 50: Assessment of Immune Function
Chapter 51: Management of Patients With Immunodeficiency

Janice L. Hinkle, PhD, RN, CNRN
Senior Research Fellow, Acute Stroke Programme
Oxford Brookes University and John Radcliffe Hospital
Oxford, United Kingdom
Chapter 5: Health Assessment
Chapter 60: Assessment of Neurologic Function
Chapter 63: Management of Patients With Neurologic Trauma
Chapter 65: Management of Patients With Oncologic or Degenerative Neurologic Disorders

Joyce Y. Johnson, PhD, RN, CCRN
Dean
College of Health Professions/Department of Nursing
Albany State University
Albany, Georgia
Chapter 1: Health Care Delivery and Nursing Practice
Chapter 2: Community-Based Nursing Practice
Chapter 3: Critical Thinking, Ethical Decision Making, and the Nursing Process
Chapter 8: Perspectives in Transcultural Nursing

Elizabeth Keech, PhD, RN
Assistant Professor
Villanova University College of Nursing
Villanova, Pennsylvania
Chapter 12: Health Care of the Older Adult

Dale Halsey Lea, RN, MPH, CGC, APGN, FAAN
Assistant Director
Southern Maine Regional Genetics Services
Scarborough, Maine
Chapter 9: Genetics Perspectives in Nursing

Mary Beth Flynn Makic, RN, MS CNS, CCNS, CCRN
Clinical Nurse Specialist/Senior Instructor
University of Colorado Hospital
Denver, Colorado
Chapter 15: Shock and Multisystem Failure

Barbara J. Maschak-Carey, RN, MSN, CDE
Clinical Nurse Specialist
University of Pennsylvania
Philadelphia, Pennsylvania
Chapter 41: Assessment and Management of Patients With Diabetes Mellitus

Agnes Masny, RN, MPH, MSN, CRNP
Research Associate/Nurse Practitioner
Population Science Division, Family Risk Assessment Program
Fox Chase Cancer Center
Philadelphia, Pennsylvania
Chapter 9: Genetics Perspectives in Nursing

LouAnn McGinty, RN, MSN
Part-Time Instructor
Villanova University College of Nursing
Villanova, Pennsylvania
Chapter 64: Management of Patients With Neurologic Infections, Autoimmune Disorders, and Neuropathies

Carol Gullo Mest, PhD, APRN, BC
Associate Professor
DeSales University, Department of Nursing and Health
Center Valley, Pennsylvania
Chapter 68: Management of Patients With Musculoskeletal Disorders

Barbara A. Moyer, RN, EdD
Assistant Professor
DeSales University, Department of Nursing and Health
Center Valley, Pennsylvania
Chapter 67: Musculoskeletal Care Modalities

Martha A. Mulvey, MS, RN, CNS, C
Advanced Practice Nurse, Neurology
University Hospital
University of Medicine and Dentistry of New Jersey
Newark, New Jersey
Chapter 14: Fluid and Electrolytes: Balance and Disturbances

Victoria Navarro, RN, MAS, MSN
Director of Nursing
The Wilmer Eye Institute at Johns Hopkins
Baltimore, Maryland
Chapter 58: Assessment and Management of Patients With Eye and Vision Disorders

Donna Nayduch, RN, MSN, ACNP, CCRN
Trauma Consultant
K-Force
Evans, Colorado
Chapter 71: Emergency Nursing
Chapter 72: Terrorism, Mass Casualty, and Disaster Nursing

Kathleen Nokes, PhD, RN, FAAN
Professor
Hunter College
New York, New York
Chapter 52: Management of Patients With HIV Infection and AIDS

Janet A. Parkosewich, RN, MSN, CCRN, FAHA
Cardiac Clinical Nurse Specialist
Yale-New Haven Hospital
New Haven, Connecticut
Chapter 26: Assessment of Cardiovascular Function

Jana Perun, ARNP, AOCN
Formerly, Nurse Practitioner
M. D. Anderson Cancer Center Orlando
Orlando, Florida
Chapter 22: Management of Patients With Upper Respiratory Tract Disorders
Chapter 49: Assessment and Management of Problems Related to Male Reproductive Processes

Kimberly L. Quinn, RN, MSN, CCRN, ACNP, ANP
Nurse Practitioner—Thoracic Surgery
Union Memorial Hospital
Baltimore, Maryland
Chapter 35: Management of Patients With Oral and Esophageal Disorders

Patricia S. Regojo, RN, MSN
Nurse Manager—Burn Unit
Temple University Hospital
Philadelphia, Pennsylvania
Chapter 57: Management of Patients With Burn Injury

JoAnne Reifsnyder, PhD, APRN, BC-PCM
Senior Vice President, Research
excelleRx, Inc.
Philadelphia, Pennsylvania
Chapter 17: End-of-Life Care

Judith L. Reishtein, PhD, RN
Assistant Professor
College of Nursing and Health Professions
Drexel University
Philadelphia, Pennsylvania
Chapter 25: Respiratory Care Modalities

Susan Rokita, CRNP, MS
Nurse Practitioner/Hematology Oncology
Milton S. Hershey Medical Center
Hershey, Pennsylvania
Chapter 16: Oncology: Nursing Management in Cancer Care

Catherine Sackett, RN, BS, CANP
Ophthalmic Research Nurse Practitioner
Wilmer Eye Institute
Retinal Vascular Center
The Johns Hopkins Medical Institutions
Baltimore, Maryland
Chapter 58: Assessment and Management of Patients With Eye and Vision Disorders

Linda Schakenbach, MSN, RN, CNS, CCRN, CWCN, APRN, BC
Clinical Nurse Specialist, Medical Cardiology
Inova Fairfax Hospital—Inova Heart and Vascular Institute
Falls Church, Virginia
Chapter 29: Management of Patients With Structural, Infectious, and Inflammatory Cardiac Disorders

Suzanne C. Smeltzer, EdD, RN, FAAN
Professor and Director, Center for Nursing Research
Villanova University College of Nursing
Villanova, Pennsylvania
Chapter 10: Chronic Illness and Disability
Chapter 21: Assessment of Respiratory Function
Chapter 53: Assessment and Management of Patients With Allergic Disorders

Cathy Stanfield, MS, CRNP
Acute Care Nurse Practitioner
Gastro-Intestinal Surgery Service
The John Hopkins Medical Institutions
Baltimore, Maryland
Chapter 34: Assessment of Digestive and Gastrointestinal Function

Cindy Stern, RN, MSN
Cancer Network Coordinator
University of Pennsylvania Cancer Center
University of Pennsylvania Health System
Philadelphia, Pennsylvania
Chapter 16: Oncology: Nursing Management in Cancer Care

Caroline Steward, RN, MSN, APN C, CCRN, CNN
Case Manager
Renaissance Health Care, Fresenius Medical Care North America
Broomfield, Colorado
Chapter 43: Assessment of Renal and Urinary Tract Function
Chapter 44: Management of Patients With Kidney Disorders
Chapter 45: Management of Patients With Urinary Disorders

Christine Tea, RN, MSN
Service Line Director
Main OR Perioperative Services
Inova Fairfax Hospital
Falls Church, Virginia
Chapter 18: Preoperative Nursing Management
Chapter 19: Intraoperative Nursing Management
Chapter 20: Postoperative Nursing Management

Jean Smith Temple, DNS, RN
Assistant Dean and Associate Professor
College of Nursing
Valdosta State University
Valdosta, Georgia
Chapter 1: Health Care Delivery and Nursing Practice

Chapter 2: Community-Based Nursing Practice
Chapter 3: Critical Thinking, Ethical Decision Making, and the Nursing Process
Chapter 8: Perspectives in Transcultural Nursing

Mary Laudon Thomas, RN, MS, AOCN
Hematology Clinical Nurse Specialist
Veterans Affairs Palo Alto Health Care System
Palo Alto, California
Chapter 33: Assessment and Management of Patients With Hematologic Disorders

Renay D. Tyler, RN, MSN, ACNP, CNSN
Acute Care Nurse Practitioner
The Johns Hopkins Hospital
Department of Surgical Nursing
Baltimore, Maryland
Chapter 36: Gastrointestinal Intubation and Special Nutritional Modalities

Joan M. Webb, RN, MSN
Instructor
Widener University, College of Nursing
Chester, Pennsylvania
Chapter 42: Assessment and Management of Patients With Endocrine Disorders

Joyce S. Willens, PhD, RN, C
Assistant Professor
Villanova University College of Nursing
Villanova, Pennsylvania
Chapter 13: Pain Management

Iris Woodard, RN-CS, ANP
Dermatology Nurse Practitioner
Kaiser Permanente
Springfield, Virginia
Chapter 55: Assessment of Integumentary Function
Chapter 56: Management of Patients With Dermatologic Problems

Preface

As we complete the first half of the first decade of the 21st century, nursing continues to be influenced by the expansion of science and technology and by a myriad of social, cultural, economic, and environmental changes throughout the world. At the same time, today's nurses are faced with the many challenges that result from the acute shortage of nurses throughout health care settings. This worldwide nursing shortage has resulted in the need for nurses to have increasingly high levels of nursing knowledge and skills in meeting the acute care, long-term care, and health promotion needs of individuals and groups. Nurses must be particularly skilled in critical thinking and clinical decision-making as well as in consulting and collaborating with other members of the multidisciplinary health care team.

Along with the challenges that today's nurses confront, there are many opportunities for them to provide skilled, compassionate nursing care in a variety of health care settings, for patients in the various stages of illness, and for patients across the age continuum. At the same time, there are significant opportunities for fostering health promotion activities for individuals and groups; this is an integral part of providing nursing care.

This eleventh edition of *Brunner & Suddarth's Textbook of Medical-Surgical Nursing* is designed to assist nurses in preparing for their roles and responsibilities within the complex health care system. A goal of the textbook is to provide balanced attention to the art and science of adult medical-surgical nursing. The textbook focuses on physiologic, pathophysiologic, and psychosocial concepts as they relate to nursing care, and emphasis is placed on integrating a variety of concepts from other disciplines such as nutrition, pharmacology, and gerontology. Throughout the textbook particular emphasis has been placed on addressing the nursing care and health care needs of people with disabilities, identified in 2005 by the U.S. Surgeon General as a priority for the education and training of tomorrow's health care professionals. In addition, content relative to nursing research findings and evidence-based practice has been expanded to provide opportunities for the nurse to refine clinical decision-making skills.

ORGANIZATION

Brunner & Suddarth's Textbook of Medical-Surgical Nursing, 11th edition, is organized into 16 units. Units 1 through 4 cover core concepts related to medical-surgical nursing practice. Units 5 through 16 discuss adult health conditions that are treated medically or surgically. Each unit covering adult health conditions is structured in the following way, to facilitate understanding:

- The first chapter in the unit covers assessment and includes a review of normal anatomy and physiology of the body system being discussed.
- The subsequent chapters in the unit cover management of specific disorders. Pathophysiology, clinical manifestations, assessment and diagnostic findings, medical management, and nursing management are presented. Special "Nursing Process" sections, provided for selected conditions, clarify and expand on the nurse's role in caring for patients with these conditions.

FEATURES

Practice-Oriented Features

Nurses assume many different roles when caring for patients. Many of the features in this textbook have been developed to help nurses fulfill these varied roles.

The Nurse as Practitioner

One of the central roles of the nurse is to provide holistic care to patients and their families, both independently and through collaboration with other health care professionals. Many features in *Brunner & Suddarth's Textbook of Medical-Surgical Nursing* are designed to assist students with clinical practice.

Nursing Process sections. The nursing process is the basis for all nursing practice. Special sections throughout the text, organized according to the nursing process framework, clarify the nurse's responsibilities in caring for patients with selected disorders.

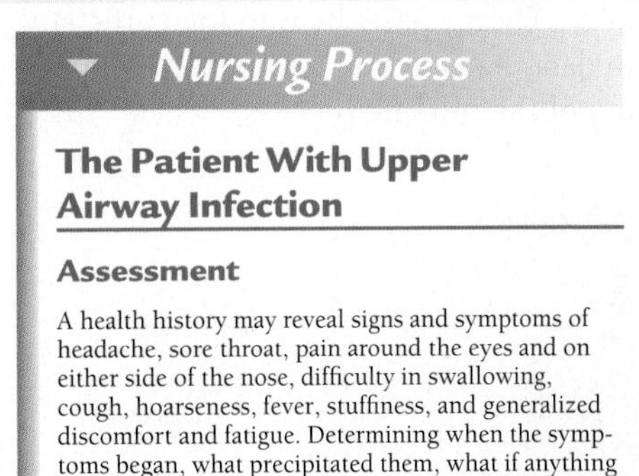

Nursing Process

The Patient With Upper Airway Infection

Assessment

A health history may reveal signs and symptoms of headache, sore throat, pain around the eyes and on either side of the nose, difficulty in swallowing, cough, hoarseness, fever, stuffiness, and generalized discomfort and fatigue. Determining when the symptoms began, what precipitated them, what if anything relieves them, and what aggravates them is part of the

Plans of Nursing Care. These plans, provided for selected disorders, illustrate how the nursing process is applied to meet the person's health care and nursing needs.

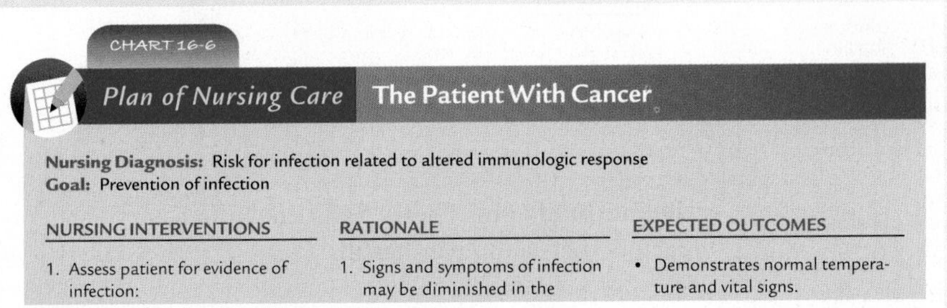

CHART 16-6

Plan of Nursing Care **The Patient With Cancer**

Nursing Diagnosis: Risk for infection related to altered immunologic response
Goal: Prevention of infection

NURSING INTERVENTIONS	RATIONALE	EXPECTED OUTCOMES
1. Assess patient for evidence of infection:	1. Signs and symptoms of infection may be diminished in the	• Demonstrates normal temperature and vital signs.

Applying Concepts from NANDA, NIC, and NOC. Each unit begins with a case study and a chart presenting examples of NANDA, NIC, and NOC terminologies related to the case study. Concept maps, which provide a visual representation of the NANDA, NIC, and NOC chart for each case study, are found in Appendix C. This feature introduces the student to the NIC and NOC language and classifications and brings them to life in graphic form.

Nursing Classifications and Languages

NANDA Nursing Diagnoses	NIC Nursing Interventions	NOC Nursing Outcomes Return to functional baseline status, stabilization of, or improvement in:
Chronic Pain—Unpleasant sensory and emotional experience arising from actual or potential tissue damage or described in terms of such damage; sudden or slow onset of any intensity from mild to severe, constant or recurring, without an anticipated or predictable end and a duration of greater than 6 months	**Pain Management**—Alleviation of pain or reduction in pain to a level of comfort that is acceptable to the patient	**Pain Level**—Severity of observed or reported pain
Risk for Powerlessness—At risk for perceived lack of control over a situation and/or one's ability to significantly affect an outcome	**Medication Management**—Facilitation of safe and effective use of prescribed or over-the-counter medicine	**Comfort Level**—Extent of positive perception of physical and psychological ease
	Simple Relaxation Therapy—Use of techniques to encourage and elicit relaxation for the purpose of decreasing undesirable signs and symptoms such as pain, muscle tension, or anxiety	**Pain Control**—Personal actions to control pain
	Simple Guided Imagery—Purposeful use of imagination to achieve relaxation and/or direct attention away from undesirable sensations	**Pain: Disruptive Effects**—Severity of observed or reported disruptive effects of chronic pain on daily functioning
	Emotional Support—Provision of reassurance, acceptance, and encouragement during times of stress	**Pain: Adverse Psychological Response**—Severity of observed or reported adverse responses to physical pain
	Self-Esteem Enhancement—Assisting a patient to increase his or her personal judgment of self-worth	

NANDA International (2005). *Nursing diagnoses: Definitions & classification 2005–2006.* Philadelphia: North American Nursing Diagnosis Association.
Dochterman, J. M. & Bulechek, G. M. (2004). *Nursing interventions classification (NIC)* (4th ed.). St. Louis: Mosby.
Iowa Outcomes Project (2004). In Moorhead, S., Johnson, M. & Maas, M. (2004). *Nursing outcomes classification (NOC)* (3rd ed.). St. Louis: Mosby.
Dochterman, J. M. & Jones, D. A. (2003). *Unifying nursing languages: The harmonization of NANDA, NIC, and NOC.* Washington, D.C.: American Nurses Association.

Assessment charts. These charts help to focus the student's attention on data that should be collected as part of the assessment step of the nursing process.

CHART 17-8

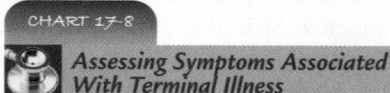

Assessing Symptoms Associated With Terminal Illness

- How is this symptom affecting the patient's life?
- What is the meaning of the symptom to the patient? To the family?
- How does the symptom affect physical functioning, mobility, comfort, sleep, nutritional status, elimination, activity level, and relationships with others?
- What makes the symptom better?
- What makes it worse?
- Is it worse at any particular time of the day?
- What are the patient's expectations and goals for managing the symptom? The family's?
- How is the patient coping with the symptom?
- What is the economic effect of the symptom and its management?

Adapted from Jacox, A., Carr, D. B., & Payne, R. (1994). *Management of cancer pain*. Rockville, MD: AHCPR.

CHART 23-3

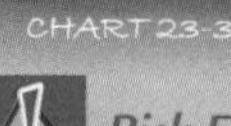

Risk Factors for Tuberculosis

- Close contact with someone who has active TB. Inhalation of airborne nuclei from an infected person is proportional to the amount of time spent in the same air space, the proximity of the person, and the degree of ventilation.
- Immunocompromised status (eg, those with HIV infection, cancer, transplanted organs, and prolonged high-dose corticosteroid therapy)
- Substance abuse (IV/injection drug users and alcoholics)
- Any person without adequate health care (the homeless; impoverished; minorities, particularly children under age 15 y and young adults between ages 15 and 44 y)
- Preexisting medical conditions or special treatment (eg, diabetes, chronic renal failure, malnourishment, selected malignancies, hemodialysis, transplanted organ, gastrectomy, jejunoileal bypass)
- Immigration from countries with a high prevalence of TB (southeastern Asia, Africa, Latin America, Caribbean)
- Institutionalization (eg, long-term care facilities, psychiatric institutions, prisons)
- Living in overcrowded, substandard housing
- Being a health care worker performing high-risk activities: administration of aerosolized pentamidine and other medications, sputum induction procedures,

Risk Factor charts. These charts draw the student's attention to factors that can impair health.

CHART 25-9 **Guidelines for Care of the Patient With a Tracheostomy Tube**

ACTIONS	RATIONALE
1. Gather the needed equipment, including sterile gloves, hydrogen peroxide, normal saline solution or sterile water, cotton-tipped applicators, dressing and twill tape (and the type of tube prescribed, if the tube is to be changed).	Everything needed to care for a tracheostomy should be readily on hand for the most effective care.
A cuffed tube (air injected into cuff) is required during mechanical ventilation. A low-pressure cuff is most commonly used.	A cuffed tube prevents air from leaking during positive-pressure ventilation and also prevents tracheal aspiration of gastric contents. An adequate seal is indicated by the disappearance of any air leakage from the mouth or tracheostomy or by the disappearance of the harsh, gurgling sound of air coming from the throat.
Patients requiring long-term use of a tracheostomy tube and who can breathe spontaneously commonly	Low-pressure cuffs exert minimal pressure on the tracheal mucosa and thus reduce the danger of tracheal

Guidelines charts. These charts review key nursing interventions, and the rationales for those interventions, for specific patient care situations.

Pharmacology charts and tables. Pharmacology charts and tables remind the student of important considerations relative to administering medications and monitoring drug therapy.

℞ TABLE 16-6 Antineoplastic Agents

Drug Class and Examples	Mechanism of Action	Cell Cycle Specificity	Common Side Effects
Alkylating Agents			
Busulfan, carboplatin, chlorambucil, cisplatin, cyclophosphamide, dacarbazine, hexamethyl melamine, ifosfamide, melphalan, nitrogen mustard, oxaliplatin, thiotepa	Alter DNA structure by misreading DNA code, initiating breaks in the DNA molecule, cross-linking DNA strands	Cell cycle–nonspecific	Bone marrow suppression, nausea, vomiting, cystitis (cyclophosphamide, ifosfamide), stomatitis, alopecia, gonadal suppression, renal toxicity (cisplatin)
Nitrosureas			
Carmustine (BCNU), lomustine (CCNU), semustine (methyl CCNU), streptozocin	Similar to the alkylating agents; cross the blood–brain barrier	Cell cycle–nonspecific	Delayed and cumulative myelosuppression, especially thrombocytopenia; nausea, vomiting
Topoisomerase I Inhibitors			
Irinotecan, topotecan	Induce breaks in the DNA	Cell cycle–specific	Bone marrow suppression,

NURSING ALERT

Because of the prolonged clotting time, only essential arterial punctures or venipunctures are performed, and manual pressure is applied to any puncture site

Nursing Alerts. These special sections offer brief tips for clinical practice and red-flag warnings to help students avoid common mistakes.

CHART 11-2

Concerns of Older Adults Facing Disability

- Loss of independence, which is a source of self-respect and dignity
- Increased potential for discrimination or abuse
- Increased social isolation
- Added burden on spouse, who may also have impaired health
- Less access to community services and health care
- Less access to religious institutions
- Increased vulnerability to declining health secondary to other disorders, reduced physiologic reserve, or preexisting impairments of mobility and balance
- Fears and doubts about ability to learn or relearn

Gerontologic Considerations. In the United States, older adults comprise the fastest-growing segment of the population. This icon is applied to headings, charts, and tables as appropriate to highlight information that pertains specifically to the care of the older adult patient.

Genetics in Nursing Practice charts. These charts summarize and highlight the role that genetics play in many disorders.

GENETICS IN NURSING PRACTICE

Concepts and Challenges in Management of the Patient with Cancer

Cancer is a genetic disease. Every phase of carcinogenesis is affected by multiple gene mutations. Some of these mutations are inherited (present in germ-line cells), but most (90%) are somatic mutations that are acquired mutations in specific cells. Examples of cancers influenced by genetics include

- Cowden syndrome
- Familial adenomatous polyposis
- Familial melanoma syndrome
- Hereditary breast and ovarian cancer
- Hereditary non-polyposis colon cancer
- Neurofibromatosis type 1
- Retinoblastoma

NURSING ASSESSMENTS

Family History Assessment

- Obtain information about both maternal and paternal sides of family.

MANAGEMENT ISSUES SPECIFIC TO GENETICS

- Assess patient's understanding of genetics factors related to his or her cancer.
- Refer for cancer risk assessment when a hereditary cancer syndrome is suspected so that patient and family can discuss inheritance risk with other family members and availability of genetic testing.
- Offer appropriate genetics information and resources.
- Assess patient's understanding of genetics information.
- Provide support to patients and families with known genetic test results for hereditary cancer syndromes.
- Participate in the management and coordination of risk-reduction measures for those with known gene mutations.

GENETICS RESOURCES

American Cancer Society www.cancer.org—offers general information about cancer and support resources for families

Gene Clinics www.geneclinics.org—a listing of common genetic disorders with up-to-date clinical summaries, genetic counseling, and testing information

National Organization of Rare Disorders www.rarediseases.org—a directory of support groups and information for patients and families with rare genetic disorders

National Cancer Institute www.cancernet.nci.nih.gov—a listing of cancers with clinical summaries and treatment reviews, information on genetic risks for cancer, listing of cancer centers providing genetic cancer risk assessment services

Genetic Alliance www.geneticalliance.org—a directory of support groups for patients and families with

Physiology/Pathophysiology

↓ Blood volume
↑ Serum osmolality
Stimulates
Concentrated urine excreted
(↑ Thirst and water intake) ECF volume deficit
Stimulates
↑ ADH production in hypothalamus (osmoreceptors)
↓ Arterial B/P (stimulates baroreceptors)
↑ Sympathetic discharge
↓ Renal perfusion
Inhibits
Diuresis results
↓ H_2O and Na^+ filtered by kidney
Renin release (↓ GFR) (promotes peripheral vasoconstriction)
↑ ADH release into bloodstream from storage in posterior pituitary
↑ Angiotensin I and II
↑ Aldosterone by adrenal cortex
↑ Blood volume
↓ Serum osmolality
↑ Reabsorption of H_2O by distal tubule of kidneys
↓ Na^+ and H_2O excretion by kidneys
↑ Blood pressure
↓ Urine excretion

Physiology/Pathophysiology figures. These illustrations and algorithms help students to understand normal physiologic and pathophysiologic processes.

The Nurse as Educator

Health education is a primary responsibility of the nursing profession. Nursing care is directed toward promoting, maintaining, and restoring health; preventing illness; and helping patients and families adapt to the residual effects of illness. Teaching, in the form of patient education and health promotion, is central to all of these nursing activities.

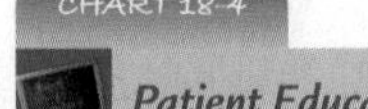

CHART 18-4

Patient Education

Preoperative Instructions to Prevent Postoperative Complications

DIAPHRAGMATIC BREATHING

Diaphragmatic breathing refers to a flattening of the dome of the diaphragm during inspiration, with resultant enlargement of the upper abdomen as air rushes in. During expiration, the abdominal muscles contract.

1. Practice in the same position you would assume in bed after surgery: a semi-Fowler's position, propped in bed with the back and shoulders well supported with pillows.
2. With your hands in a loose-fist position, allow the hands to rest lightly on the front of the lower ribs, with your fingertips against lower chest to feel the movement.

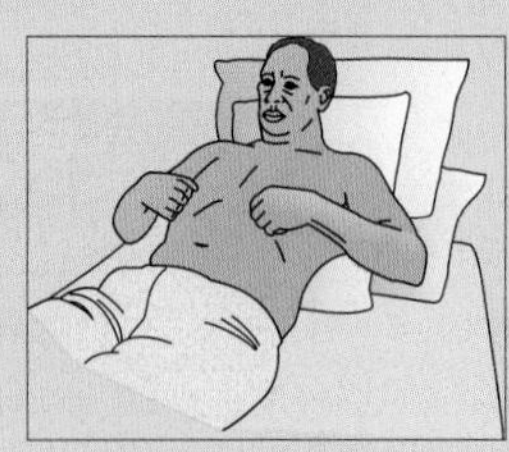

Diaphragmatic breathing

2. Breathe with the diaphragm as described under "Diaphragmatic Breathing."
3. With your mouth slightly open, breathe in fully.
4. "Hack" out sharply for three short breaths.
5. Then, keeping your mouth open, take in a quick deep breath and immediately give a strong cough once or twice. This helps clear secretions from your chest. It may cause some discomfort but will not harm your incision.

LEG EXERCISES

1. Lie in a semi-Fowler's position and perform the following simple exercises to improve circulation.
2. Bend your knee and raise your foot—hold it a few seconds, then extend the leg and lower it to the bed.

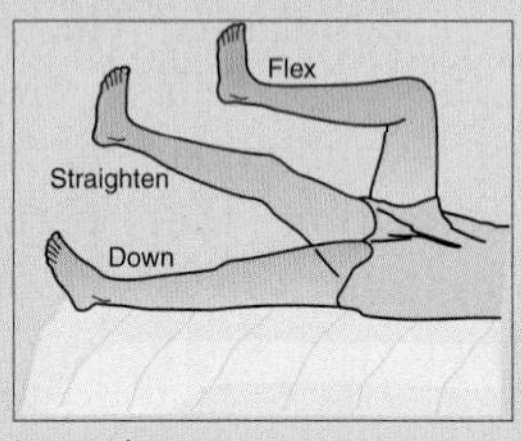

Leg exercises

Patient Education charts. These charts help the nurse to prepare the patient and family for procedures, assist them with understanding the patient's condition, and explain to them how to provide for self-care after discharge from the health care facility.

CHART 23-8

HOME CARE CHECKLIST • **Prevention of Recurrent Pulmonary Embolism**

At the completion of the home care instruction, the patient or caregiver will be able to:	Patient	Caregiver
• Describe the underlying process leading to pulmonary embolism.	✔	✔
• Describe the need for continued anticoagulant therapy after the initial embolism.	✔	✔
• Name the anticoagulant prescribed and identify dosage and schedule of administration.	✔	✔
• Describe potential side effects of coagulation such as bruising and bleeding and identify ways to prevent bleeding.	✔	✔
• Avoid the use of sharps (razors, knives, etc.) to prevent cuts; shave with an electric shaver.		
• Use a toothbrush with soft bristles to prevent gum injury.		
• Do not take aspirin or antihistamines while taking warfarin sodium (Coumadin).		

Home Care checklists. These checklists review points that should be covered as part of patient education prior to discharge from the health care facility.

Health Promotion charts. These charts review important points that the nurse should discuss with the patient to prevent common health problems from developing.

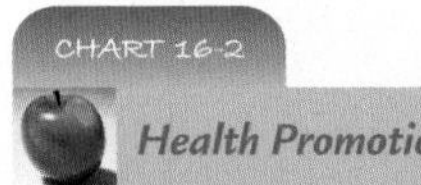

CHART 16-2

Health Promotion

Reducing Cancer Risk

- Encourage patients to increase consumption of fresh vegetables (especially those of the cabbage family) because studies indicate that roughage and vitamin-rich foods help to prevent certain kinds of cancer.
- Encourage increased fiber intake because high-fiber diets may reduce the risk for certain cancers (eg, breast, prostate, and colon).
- Recommend increased intake of vitamin A, which reduces the risk for esophageal, laryngeal, and lung cancers.
- Recommend increased intake of foods rich in vitamin C, such as citrus fruits and broccoli, which are thought to protect against stomach and esophageal
- Advise patients to reduce intake of dietary fat because a high-fat diet increases the risk for breast, colon, and prostate cancers.
- Recommend moderation in consumption of salt-cured, smoked, and nitrate-cured foods; these have been linked to esophageal and gastric cancers.
- Advise patients to stop smoking cigarettes and cigars, which are carcinogens.
- Advise patients to reduce alcohol intake because drinking large amounts of alcohol increases the risk of liver cancer. (*Note:* People who drink heavily and smoke are at greater risk for cancers of the mouth, throat, larynx, and esophagus.)

The Nurse as Patient Advocate

Nurses advocate for patients by protecting their rights (including the right to health care) and assisting patients and their families to make informed decisions about health care.

Ethics and Related Issues charts. These charts present a scenario, a description of potential ethical dilemmas that could arise as a result of the scenario, and a list of questions about the scenario to stimulate thought and discussion.

CHART 11-1

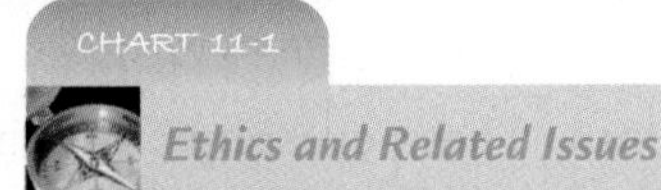
Ethics and Related Issues

Are All Persons Entitled to Rehabilitation?

SITUATION

You work in an area where many illegal aliens and uninsured residents live. Community violence often creates life-threatening and disabling conditions in members of the population. After a victim of violence has been saved and stabilized, the health care team identifies rehabilitation needs. You are concerned about your patient's inability to perform self-care and to demonstrate safe mobility skills.

DILEMMA

As a health care provider, you are concerned about the community as a whole; costs to the community, and the values of the community. You are also aware of client fiduciary responsibility; you recognize costs to your patient when treatment is provided or not provided.

DISCUSSION

The Nurse as Researcher

Nurses identify potential research problems and questions to increase nursing knowledge and improve patient care. Use and evaluation of research findings in nursing practice are essential to further the science of nursing.

Nursing Research Profiles. These charts identify the implications and applications of nursing research findings for nursing practice.

NURSING RESEARCH PROFILE

The Effect of Preoperative Teaching on Outcomes

Oetker-Black, S. L., Jones, S., Estok, P., et al. (2003). Preoperative teaching and hysterectomy outcomes. *AORN Journal, 77*(6), 1215–1231.

Purpose

This study used a theoretical model of self-efficacy to determine whether an efficacy-enhancing teaching protocol was effective in improving immediate post-operative behaviors and selected short- and long-term health outcomes in women who underwent abdominal hysterectomy.

Design

A sample of 108 women admitted to a 486-bed teaching hospital in the Midwest for total abdominal hysterectomy was obtained by convenience sampling. Data collectors used the operating room schedule to identify potential participants based on pre-determined criteria (eg, age, able to read English, alert and oriented). Those willing to participate in the 6-month study were randomly assigned to one of the study groups and received either the usual care protocol or the efficacy-enhancing teaching protocol. The efficacy-enhancing group received enhanced preoperative teaching. Sessions stressed the importance of early ambulation, included a detailed demonstration of the effective way to get out of bed, and required that participants demonstrate how to get out of bed.

Findings

There were no significant differences found between groups except in ambulation. Patients who received the efficacy-enhancing teaching ambulated significantly longer than those in the usual care group (330 seconds compared to a mean of 56 seconds).

Nursing Implications

The most common postoperative complications of hysterectomy or any major abdominal surgery are atelectasis, pneumonia, paralytic ileus, and deep vein thrombosis. Studies have previously shown that postoperative ambulation decreases or prevents all these complications. By incorporating enhanced preoperative patient instruction with return demonstrations, perioperative nurses can improve patients' postoperative ambulation.

Evidence-Based Practice (EBP) questions. This icon [ebp] appears next to critical thinking exercises that encourage the student to think about the evidence base for specific nursing interventions. A journals supplement (new to the 11th edition) offers students free on-line access to over 70 journal articles that relate to the evidence-based practice questions in the text.

Critical Thinking Exercises

1. An 80-year-old patient with Parkinson's disease is scheduled for surgery to replace a fractured hip. Identify the considerations and associated responsibilities of the OR nurse for safe intraoperative care of this patient.
2. [ebp] A patient has a large open lower-extremity wound caused by a motorcycle accident and is undergoing emergency surgery. What resources would you use to identify the current guidelines for surgical asepsis? What is the evidence base for current patient and environmental surgical asepsis practices? Identify the criteria used to evaluate the strength of the evidence for these practices.
3. A patient develops a temperature of 38°C (100°F) and becomes tachycardic halfway through an abdominal surgery. Five minutes later, the patient's temperature is 42°C (104°F). Describe the protocol you would follow and the medication you would administer for this condition.
4. [ebp] A patient with an infected wound is undergoing an incision and drainage in the OR. Develop an evidence-based plan of care that will reduce the risk of contamination and infection.

Pedagogical Features

Learning Objectives. Each chapter begins with a list of learning objectives. These give the student an overview of the chapter and help to focus his or her reading.

Glossaries. Glossaries provided at the beginning of each chapter let the student review vocabulary words before reading the chapter, and also serve as a useful reference tool while reading.

Critical Thinking Exercises. These questions, which appear at the end of each chapter, foster critical thinking by challenging the student to apply textbook knowledge to clinical scenarios.

References and Selected Readings. A list of current references cited and a bibliography are given at the end of each chapter.

Resources. A resource list at the end of each chapter directs the reader to sources of additional information, websites, agencies, and patient education materials.

A COMPREHENSIVE PACKAGE FOR TEACHING AND LEARNING

To further facilitate teaching and learning, a carefully designed ancillary package is available. In addition to the usual print resources, we are pleased to present multimedia tools that have been developed in conjunction with the text.

Resources for Students

Interactive CD-ROM. Packaged with the textbook at no additional charge, this CD helps students test their knowledge and enhance their understanding of medical-surgical nursing. This CD includes:

- 500 self-study questions organized by unit
- 3000 bonus NCLEX-style cross-disciplinary questions
- **CONCEPTS** in action **ANIMATION** Concepts in Action™ Animations
- Nursing in Action™ Video: Performing a Physical Examination
- Clinical Simulations
- Bonus Tutorials on fluids and electrolytes and NCLEX alternate-format items
- Spanish-English Audioglossary

Study Guide to Accompany Smeltzer, Bare, Hinkle & Cheever: Brunner & Suddarth's Textbook of Medical-Surgical Nursing, 11th edition. Available at student bookstores or at www.LWW.com, this study guide presents a variety of exercises to reinforce the textbook content and enhance learning.

Handbook to Accompany Smeltzer, Bare, Hinkle & Cheever: Brunner & Suddarth's Textbook of Medical-Surgical Nursing, 11th edition. Available at student bookstores or at www.LWW.com, this clinical reference presents need-to-know information on nearly 200 commonly encountered disorders in an easy-to-use alphabetized outline format.

Resources for Instructors

Instructor's Resource CD-ROM. The instructor's resource CD contains the following items:

- A thoroughly revised and augmented test generator, containing 2100 NCLEX-style questions
- Sample syllabi for 1-semester, 2-semester, and 3-semester courses
- Strategies for effective teaching
- PowerPoint™ lectures, guided lecture notes, and prelecture quizzes
- An image bank
- Discussion topics and assignments

Partners in Education. This service is available to assist with faculty development, technology training, curriculum development, and more.

Resources for Students and Instructors

thePoint **ThePoint*** (http://thepoint.lww.com) is a web-based course and content management system that provides every resource instructors and students need in one easy-to-use site. Advanced technology and superior content combine at thePoint to allow instructors to design and deliver on-line and off-line courses, maintain grades and class rosters, and communicate with students. Students can visit thePoint to access supplemental multimedia resources to enhance their learning experience, check the course syllabus, download content, upload assignments, and join an on-line study group. ThePoint . . . where teaching, learning, and technology click!

LiveAdvise Student Online Tutorial Service. This service, powered by Smarthinking™, provides on-line tutoring and assistance for students and instructors. Med-Surg instructors are available Sunday through Thursday, 8:30 P.M. to 11:30 P.M., to assist with questions.

MyPowerLearning is a learning styles assessment and assistance service for instructors and students.

It is with pleasure that we introduce these resources—the textbook and the ancillary package—to you. One of our primary goals in creating these resources has been to help prepare nursing students to provide quality care to patients and families across health care settings and in the home. We hope that we have succeeded in that goal, and we welcome feedback from our readers.

Suzanne C. O'Connell Smeltzer, EdD, RN, FAAN
Brenda G. Bare, RN, MSN
Janice L. Hinkle, PhD, RN, CNRN
Kerry H. Cheever, PhD, RN

*thePoint is a trademark of Wolters Kluwer Health.

Reviewers

Elizabeth A. (Libby) Archer, EdD, RN
Associate Professor
Baptist College of Health Sciences
Memphis, Tennessee

Liz Aycock, RN, BSN, MSN
Associate Professor of Nursing
Middle Georgia College
Cochran, Georgia

Roberta P. Bartee, MS, RNc
Assistant Professor, Charity School of Nursing
Delgado Community College
New Orleans, Louisiana

Barbara J. Bloink, RN, BSN, MSN
Professor
St. Clair County Community College
Port Huron, Michigan

Diane M. Breckenridge, PhD, RN
Associate Professor
LaSalle University
Philadelphia, Pennsylvania
Associate Research Director
Abington Memorial Hospital
Abington, Pennsylvania

Sandra Drozdz Burke, PhD, APRN, CDE, BC-ADM
BroMenn Assistant Professor
Illinois State University
Mennonite College of Nursing
Normal, Illinois

Lisa Burkhart, MPH, PhD, RN
Assistant Professor
Marcella Niehoff School of Nursing
Loyola University Chicago
Chicago, Illinois

Susan E. Caulkins, MSN, CS, FNP
ADN Nursing Instructor
Central Carolina Technical College
Sumter, South Carolina

Joy Churchill, RN, MSN
Associate Professor of Nursing
Northern Kentucky University
Highland Heights, Kentucky

Pattie Clark, RN, MSN
Associate Professor and Nursing Outreach Coordinator
Abraham Baldwin College
Tifton, Georgia

John D. Colbath, MSN, MBA, RNC
Professor of Nursing and Department Chairman
New Hampshire Community Technical College
Berlin, New Hampshire

Lora Crowe, RN, MSN, FNP
Assistant Professor
Macon State College
Macon, Georgia

Jan Fletcher, RN, MNSc, CEN
Assistant Professor of Nursing
Arkansas Tech University
Russellville, Arkansas

Mary Catherine Gebhardt, RN, PhD, CRRN
Assistant Professor
Byrdine F. Lewis School of Nursing at Georgia State University
Atlanta, Georgia

Bonnie Higgins, EdD, MS, BS, RN, CMSRN
Professor
Tarrant County College
Fort Worth, Texas

Jane Hook, RN, BSN, MSN
Lecturer/Coordinator Medical Surgical Faculty
California State University, Los Angeles
Los Angeles, California

Sara M. Howell, RN, MSN
Assistant Professor of Nursing, ASN Program
Mississippi University for Woman
Columbus, Mississippi

Brenda Jordan, RN, MSN
Instructor in Associate Degree Nursing
South Plains College
Levelland, Texas

Eileen Kaslatas, BSN, MSN, RN
Professor
Macomb County Community College
Clinton Township, Michigan

Colleen Kiberd, RN, BN, MEd, MN
Assistant Professor
Dalhousie University
School of Nursing
Halifax, Nova Scotia

Mary F. King, RN, BSN, MS
Level Coordinator, Associate Degree Instructor
Phillips Community College of the University of Arkansas
West Helena, Arkansas

Cathy MacDonald, MN
Assistant Professor
Saint Francis Xavier University
Antigonish, Nova Scotia

Rosemary Macy, RN, MS
Assistant Professor
Boise State University
Boise, Idaho

Cecilia Jane Maier, MS, RN, CCRN
Assistant Professor
Mount Carmel College of Nursing
Columbus, Ohio

Ann Powers-Prather, PhD, RN
Faculty, Coordinator Research and Evaluation
El Centro College
Dallas, Texas

Miley O. Pulliam, RN, MSN
Associate Degree Nursing Instructor
McLennan Community College
Waco, Texas

Diane Reynolds, RN, MS, OCN, CNE
Assistant Professor of Nursing
Long Island University
Brooklyn, New York

Mattie L. Rhodes, PhD, RN
Clinical Associate Professor, Nursing
State University New York at Buffalo
Buffalo, New York

Buckie Sasser, RN, MSN
Assistant Professor of Nursing
South Georgia College
Douglas, Georgia

Katherine Saulnier, BScN, RN, CCNP
Clinical Associate
Saint Francis Xavier University
Antigonish, Nova Scotia

Donna Schutte, RN, DNSc
Associate Professor, Nursing
Riverside Community College
Riverside, California

Debra P. Shelton, MSN, RN, CAN, OCN
Assistant Professor
Northwestern State University College of Nursing
Shreveport, Louisiana

Mary B. Wiese, RN, MSEd
Associate Professor
Ivy Tech State College
Lafayette, Indiana

Regina L. Wright, MSN, RN, CEN
Clinical Assistant Professor
Drexel University
Philadelphia, Pennsylvania

Contents

UNIT 6

Cardiovascular, Circulatory, and Hematologic Function 778

UNIT 1

Basic Concepts in Nursing

Case Study

Applying Concepts from NANDA, NIC, and NOC

The Community with an Identified Health Problem

A nurse working in an urgent care clinic that serves an economically depressed urban area notes a high incidence of elderly patients with dehydration and heatstroke in the summer months. The nurse verifies the observations by accessing data about hospital admissions for dehydration and heatstroke. The nurse determines that many of the admitted patients live in the area served by the clinic and that many of the patients live alone and have other chronic illnesses. The nurse sees the need for a plan that includes a community response to this problem. The plan includes arranging an education program about the prevention of dehydration; a community support buddy system in which neighbors or volunteers call or visit homebound elders during critical periods in the summer; and economic support to air condition the senior citizens' center.

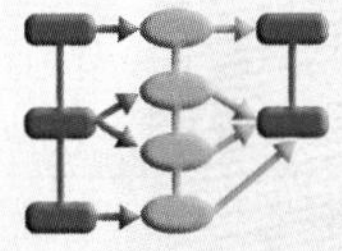

Turn to Appendix C to see a concept map that illustrates the relationships that exist between the nursing diagnoses, interventions, and outcomes for the community's identified health problem.

Nursing Classifications and Languages

NANDA Nursing Diagnoses	NIC Nursing Interventions	NOC Nursing Outcomes Return to functional baseline status, stabilization of, or improvement in:
Ineffective Community Therapeutic Regimen Management—Pattern of regulating and integrating into community processes programs for treatment of illness and the sequelae of illness that are unsatisfactory for meeting health-related goals	**Community Health Development**—Assisting members of a community to identify a community's health concerns, mobilize resources, and implement solutions **Program Development**—Planning, implementing, and evaluating a coordinated set of activities designed to enhance wellness, or to prevent, reduce or eliminate one or more health problems for a group or community	**Community Competence**—Capacity of a community to collectively problem solve to achieve community goals
Ineffective Community Coping—Pattern of community activities (for adaptation and problem solving) that is unsatisfactory for meeting the demands or needs of the community	**Surveillance: Community**—Purposeful and ongoing acquisition, interpretation, and synthesis of data for decision making in the community	**Community Health Status**—The general state of well-being of a community or population
Readiness for Enhanced Community Coping—Pattern of community activities for adaptation and problem solving that is satisfactory for meeting the demands or needs of the community but can be improved for management of current and future problems/stressors	**Environmental Risk Protection**—Preventing and detecting disease and injury in populations at risk from environmental hazards	

NANDA International (2005). *Nursing diagnoses: Definitions & Classification 2005–2006.* Philadelphia: North American Nursing Diagnosis Association.
Dochterman, J. M., & Bulechek, G. M. (2004). *Nursing interventions classification (NIC)* (4th ed.). St. Louis: Mosby.
Iowa Outcomes Project (2004). In Moorhead, S., Johnson, M. & Maas, M. (2004). *Nursing outcomes classification (NOC)* (3rd ed.). St. Louis: Mosby.
Dochterman, J. M. & Jones, D. A. (2003). *Unifying nursing languages: The harmonization of NANDA, NIC, and NOC.* Washington D.C.: American Nurses Association.

CHAPTER 1

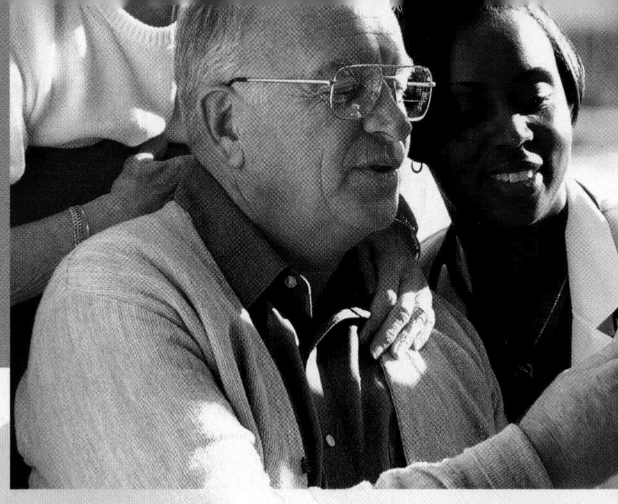

Health Care Delivery and Nursing Practice

Learning Objectives

On completion of this chapter, the learner will be able to:

1. Define health and wellness.
2. Describe factors causing significant changes in the health care delivery system and their impact on the health care field and the nursing profession.
3. Describe the practitioner, leadership, and research roles of nurses.
4. Describe nursing care delivery models.
5. Discuss expanded nursing roles.

Health care in the United States has undergone profound changes during the past several decades. Nursing, as a health care profession and a major component of the health care system, has been significantly affected by these changes. Nursing has played an important role in affecting the health care system and will continue to do so.

The Health Care Industry and the Nursing Profession

Nursing Defined

Since the time of Florence Nightingale, who wrote in 1858 that the goal of nursing was "to put the patient in the best condition for nature to act upon him," nursing leaders have described nursing as both an art and a science. However, the definition of nursing has evolved over time. In its Social Policy Statement (2003), the American Nurses Association (ANA) defined nursing as the diagnosis and treatment of human responses to health and illness. The ANA provides the following list of phenomena that are the focus for nursing care and research:

- Self-care processes
- Physiologic and pathophysiologic processes such as rest, sleep, respiration, circulation, reproduction, activity, nutrition, elimination, skin, sexuality, and communication
- Comfort, pain, and discomfort
- Emotions related to health and illness
- Meanings ascribed to health and illnesses
- Decision making and ability to make choices
- Perceptual orientations such as self-image and control over one's body and environments
- Transitions across the life span, such as birth, growth, development, and death
- Affiliative relationships, including freedom from oppression and abuse
- Environmental systems

Nurses have a responsibility to carry out their role as described in the Social Policy Statement, to comply with the nurse practice act of the state in which they practice, and to comply with the Code for Nurses as spelled out by the International Council of Nurses and the ANA. To obtain a foundation for examining the delivery of nursing care, it is necessary to understand the needs of health care consumers and the health care delivery system, including the forces that affect nursing and health care delivery.

The Patient/Client: Consumer of Nursing and Health Care

The central figure in health care services is, of course, the patient. The term *patient,* which is derived from a Latin verb meaning "to suffer," has traditionally been used to describe those who are recipients of care. The connotation commonly attached to the word is one of dependence. For this reason, many nurses prefer to use the term *client,* which is derived from a Latin verb meaning "to lean," connoting alliance and interdependence. The term *patient* is used throughout this book, with the understanding that either term is acceptable.

The patient who seeks care for a health problem or problems (increasing numbers of people have multiple health problems) is also an individual person, a member of a family, and a citizen of the community. Patients' needs vary depending on their problems, associated circumstances, and past experiences. Among the nurse's important functions in health care delivery is identifying the patient's immediate needs and taking measures to address them.

The Patient's Basic Needs

Certain needs are basic to all people. Some of these needs are more important than others. Once an essential need is met, people often experience a need on a higher level of priority. Addressing needs by priority reflects Maslow's hierarchy of needs (Fig. 1-1).

Maslow's Hierarchy

Maslow ranked human needs as follows: physiologic needs; safety and security; sense of belonging and affection; esteem and self-respect; and self-actualization, which includes self-fulfillment, desire to know and understand, and aesthetic needs. Lower-level needs always remain, but a person's ability to pursue higher-level needs indicates movement toward psychological health and well-being. Such a hierarchy of needs is a useful framework that can be applied to the various nursing models for assessment of a patient's strengths, limitations, and need for nursing interventions.

Health Care in Transition

Changes occurring in health care delivery and nursing are the result of societal, economic, technological, scientific,

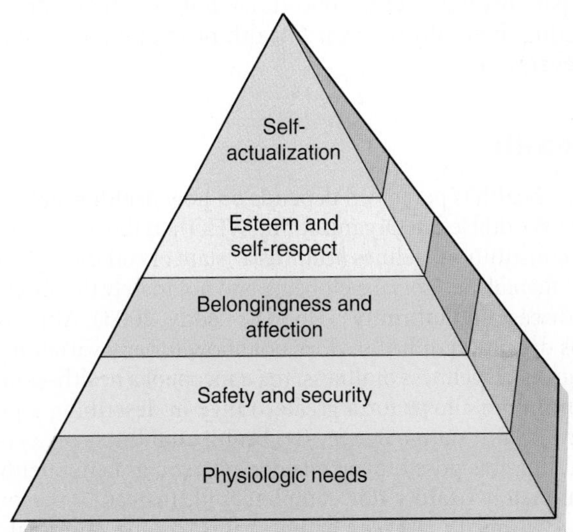

FIGURE 1-1. This scheme of Maslow's hierarchy of human needs shows how a person moves from fulfillment of basic needs to higher levels of needs, with the ultimate goal being integrated human functioning and health.

and political forces that have evolved throughout the 20th and into the 21st century. Among the most significant changes are shifts in population demographics, particularly the increase in the aging population and the cultural diversity of the population; changing patterns of diseases; increased technology; increased consumer expectations; higher costs of health care and changes in health care financing; and other health care reform efforts. These changes have led to institutional restructuring, staff downsizing, increased outpatient care services, decreased lengths of hospital stay, and increased health care in community and home settings. Such changes have dramatically influenced where nurses practice. These changes have influenced society's view of health and illness and affected the focus of nursing and health care.

As the proportion of the population reaching age 65 years has increased, and with the shift from acute illnesses to chronic illnesses, the traditional disease management and care focus of the health care professions has expanded. There is increasing concern about emerging infectious diseases, trauma, obesity, and bioterrorism. Thus, health care must focus more on disease prevention, health promotion, and management of chronic conditions than in previous times. This shift in focus coincides with a nationwide emphasis on cost control and resource management directed toward providing cost-efficient and cost-effective health care services to the population as a whole.

Health, Wellness, and Health Promotion

The health care system of the United States, which traditionally has been disease-oriented, is placing increasing emphasis on health and its promotion. Similarly, a significant portion of nurses were formerly focused on the care of patients with acute conditions, but now many are directing their efforts toward health promotion and illness prevention.

Health

How health is perceived depends on how health is defined. The World Health Organization (WHO), in the preamble to its constitution, defines *health* as a "state of complete physical, mental, and social well-being and not merely the absence of disease and infirmity" (Hood & Leddy, 2003). Although this definition of health does not allow for any variation in degrees of wellness or illness, the concept of a health–illness continuum allows for a greater range in describing a person's health status. By viewing health and illness on a continuum, it is possible to consider a person as being neither completely healthy nor completely ill. Instead, a person's state of health is ever-changing and has the potential to range from high-level wellness to extremely poor health and imminent death. Use of the health–illness continuum makes it possible to view a person as simultaneously possessing degrees of both health and illness.

The limitations of the WHO definition of health are clear in relation to chronic illness and disability. Chronically ill people do not meet the standards of health as established by the WHO definition. However, when viewed from the perspective of the health–illness continuum, people with a chronic illness or disability may be viewed as having the potential to attain a high level of wellness if they are successful in meeting their health potential within the limits of their chronic illness or disability.

Wellness

Wellness has been defined as being equivalent to health. Wellness involves being proactive and involving people in efforts toward a state of physical, psychological, and spiritual well-being in which they look and feel their best (Stone, 2003). Hood and Leddy (2003) consider that wellness has four components: (1) the capacity to perform to the best of his or her ability, (2) the ability to adjust and adapt to varying situations, (3) a reported feeling of well-being, and (4) a feeling that "everything is together" and harmonious. With this in mind, it becomes evident that the goal of health care providers is to promote positive changes that are directed toward health and well-being. The sense of wellness has a subjective aspect that emphasizes the importance of recognizing and responding to patient individuality and diversity in health care and nursing.

Health Promotion

Today, increasing emphasis is placed on health, health promotion, wellness, and self-care. Health is seen as resulting from a lifestyle oriented toward wellness. The result has been the evolution of a wide range of health promotion strategies, including multiphasic screening, genetic testing, lifetime health monitoring, environmental and mental health programs, risk reduction, and nutrition and health education. A growing interest in self-care skills is evidenced by the large number of health-related publications, conferences, and workshops designed for the lay public.

People are increasingly knowledgeable about their health and take more interest in and responsibility for their health and well-being. Organized self-care education programs emphasize health promotion, disease prevention, management of illness, self-care, and judicious use of the professional health care system. In addition, well over 500,000 self-help groups and numerous websites and chat groups promote sharing of experiences and information about self-care with others who have similar conditions, chronic diseases, or disabling conditions.

Special efforts are being made by health care professionals to reach and motivate members of various cultural and socioeconomic groups about lifestyle and health practices. Stress, improper diet, lack of exercise, smoking, use of drugs, high-risk behaviors (including risky sexual practices), and poor hygiene are all lifestyle behaviors known to affect health negatively. Health care professionals are concerned with encouraging behavior that promotes health. The goal is to motivate people to make improvements in the way they live, to modify risky behaviors, and to adopt healthy behaviors.

Influences on Health Care Delivery

The health care delivery system is rapidly changing as the population and its health care needs and expectations change. The shifting demographics of the population, the increase in chronic illnesses and disability, the greater emphasis on health care costs, and technologic advances have resulted in changing emphases in health care delivery and in nursing.

Population Demographics

Changes in the population in general are affecting the need for and the delivery of health care. The 2000 U.S. census data indicated that there were 281,421,906 people in the country (U.S. Bureau of the Census, 2000). Population growth is attributed in part to improved public health services and improved nutrition.

Not only is the population increasing, but the composition of the population is also changing. The decline in birth rate and the increase in life span due to improved health care have resulted in fewer school-age children and more senior citizens, most of whom are women. Much of the population resides in highly congested urban areas, with a steady migration of members of ethnic minorities to the inner cities and a migration of members of the middle class to suburban areas. The number of homeless people, including entire families, has increased significantly. The population has become more culturally diverse as increasing numbers of people from different national backgrounds enter the country.

Because of such population changes, the need for health care for specific age groups, for women, and for diverse groups of people in specific geographic locations is altering the effectiveness of traditional means of providing health care. As a result, far-reaching changes in the overall health care delivery system are necessary.

Aging Population

The elderly population in the United States has increased significantly and will continue to grow in future years. In 2000, the 34.5 million adults who are older than 65 years of age constituted 12.7% of the U.S. population. By the year 2030, 20% of the U.S. population is expected to be older than 65 years of age. According to the U.S. Bureau of the Census (2000), the number of people 65 to 74 years of age was 8 times larger in 1999 than in 1900, and the number of people 75 to 84 years of age was 16 times larger. In addition, people 85 years of age and older constitute one of the fastest-growing segments of the population; the number was 34 times larger in 1999 than in 1900.

The health care needs of older adults are complex and demand significant investments, both professional and financial, by the health care industry. Many elderly people suffer from multiple chronic conditions that are exacerbated by acute episodes. In particular, elderly women, whose conditions are frequently underdiagnosed and undertreated, are of concern. There are approximately three women for every two men in the older population, and elderly women are expected to continue to outnumber elderly men.

Cultural Diversity

An appreciation for the diverse characteristics and needs of people from varied ethnic and cultural backgrounds is important in health care and nursing. Some projections indicate that by 2030, racial and ethnic minority groups will constitute 40% of the population of the United States (Baldwin, 2004). With increased immigration, both legal and illegal, this figure could easily increase to more than 50% by the year 2030. As the cultural composition of the population changes, it is increasingly important to address cultural considerations in the delivery of health care. Patients from diverse sociocultural groups not only bring various health care beliefs, values, and practices to the health care setting, but they also have a variety of risk factors for some disease conditions and unique reactions to treatment. These factors significantly affect an individual's responses to health care problems or illnesses, to caregivers, and to the care itself. Unless these factors are understood and respected by health care providers, the care delivered may be ineffective, and health care outcomes may be negatively affected.

Culture is defined as learned patterns of behavior, beliefs, and values that are shared by a particular group of people. Included among the many characteristics that distinguish cultural groups are the manner of dress, language spoken, values, rules or norms of behavior, gender-specific practices, economics, politics, law and social control, artifacts, technology, dietary practices, and health beliefs and practices. Health promotion, illness prevention, causes of sickness, treatment, coping, caring, dying, and death are part of the health-related component of every culture. Every person has a unique belief and value system that has been shaped at least in part by his or her cultural environment. This belief and value system guides the person's thinking, decisions, and actions. It provides direction for interpreting and responding to illness and disability and to health care.

To promote an effective nurse–patient relationship and positive outcomes of care, nursing care must be culturally competent, appropriate, and sensitive to cultural differences. All attempts should be made to help each person retain his or her unique cultural characteristics. Providing special foods that have significance and arranging for special religious observances may enable a patient to maintain a feeling of wholeness at a time when he or she may feel isolated from family and community (Campinha-Bacote, 2003).

Knowing the cultural and social significance that particular situations have for each patient helps the nurse avoid imposing a personal value system when the patient has a different point of view. In most cases, cooperation with the plan of care is greatest when communication among the nurse, the patient, and the patient's family is directed toward understanding the situation or the problem and respecting each other's goals.

Changing Patterns of Disease

During the past 50 years, the health problems of the American people have changed significantly. Although many infectious diseases have been controlled or eradicated, others, such as tuberculosis, acquired immunodeficiency syndrome (AIDS), and sexually transmitted diseases/infections, are on the rise. An increasing number of infectious agents are becoming resistant to antibiotic therapy as a result of widespread inappropriate use of antibiotics. Obesity has become a major health concern, and the multiple comorbidities that accompany it, such as hypertension, heart disease, diabetes, and cancer, add significantly to its associated mortality.

Conditions that were once easily treated have become more complex and life-threatening. The prevalence of chronic illnesses and disability is increasing because of the lengthening life span of Americans and the advances in care and treatment options for conditions such as cancer, human immunodeficiency virus (HIV) infection, and spina bifida. In addition, improvements in care for trauma and other serious acute health problems have meant that many people with these conditions live decades longer than in the past. People with chronic illness are the largest group of health care consumers in the United States (Harrison, 2003). Because the majority of health problems seen today are chronic in nature, many people are learning to maximize their health within the constraints of chronic illness and disability.

As chronic conditions increase, health care broadens from a focus on cure and eradication of disease to include the prevention or rapid treatment of exacerbations of chronic conditions. Nursing, which has always encouraged patients to take control of their conditions, plays a prominent role in the current focus on management of chronic illness and disability.

Advances in Technology and Genetics

Advances in technology and genetics have occurred with greater frequency during the past several decades than in all other periods of civilization. Sophisticated techniques and devices have revolutionized surgery and diagnostic testing, making it possible to perform many procedures and tests on an outpatient basis. Increased knowledge and understanding of genetics have resulted in expanded screening, diagnostic testing, and treatments for a variety of conditions. The sophisticated communication systems that connect most parts of the world, with the capability of rapid storage, retrieval, and dissemination of information, have stimulated brisk change as well as swift obsolescence in health care delivery strategies. Advances in genetics and technology have resulted in many ethical issues for the health care system, health care providers, patients, families, and society.

Economic Changes

The belief that comprehensive, quality health care should be provided for all citizens prompted governmental concern about rising health care costs and wide variations in charges among providers. In 1983, the U.S. Congress passed the most significant health legislation since the Medicare program was enacted in 1965. The federal government was no longer able to afford to reimburse hospitals for patient care that was delivered without any defined limits on costs. Therefore, it approved a prospective payment system (PPS) for hospital inpatient services. Based on diagnosis-related groups (DRGs), a PPS sets the reimbursement rates for Medicare payments for hospital services. Hospitals receive payment at a fixed rate for patients with diagnoses that fall into a specific DRG. A fixed payment has been predetermined for more than 470 possible diagnostic categories, covering the majority of medical diagnoses of patients admitted to the hospital. Hospitals receive the same payment for every patient with a given diagnosis, or DRG. If the cost of the patient's care is lower than the payment, the hospital makes a profit; if the cost is higher, the hospital incurs a loss. As a result, hospitals are placing greater emphasis on reducing costs, utilization of services, and length of patient stay.

In addition, the Balanced Budget Act of 1997 added new rate requirements for ambulatory payment classifications (APCs) to hospitals and other providers of ambulatory care services.

To qualify for Medicare reimbursement, care providers and hospitals must contract with peer review organizations (PROs) to perform quality and utilization review with the goals of cost-effectiveness and reduced costs. The PROs monitor admission patterns, lengths of stay, transfers, and quality of services, and they also validate the DRG coding. The DRG system has provided an incentive to cut costs and discharge patients as quickly as possible.

Nurses in hospitals now care for patients who are older and sicker and require more nursing services; nurses in the community are caring for patients who have been discharged earlier and need high-technology acute care services as well as long-term care. The importance of effective discharge planning, along with utilization review and quality improvement, cannot be overstated. Nurses in acute care settings must work with other health care team members to maintain quality care while facing pressures to discharge patients and decrease staffing costs. They must also work with nurses and others in community settings to ensure continuity of care.

Demand for Quality Health Care

The general public has become increasingly interested in and knowledgeable about health care and health promotion through television, newspapers, magazines, and other communications media. Health care has become a topic of political debate. The public has also become more health conscious and subscribes to the belief that health and quality health care constitute a basic right, rather than a privilege for a chosen few.

Quality Improvement and Evidence-Based Practice

In the 1980s, hospitals and other health care agencies implemented ongoing quality assurance (QA) programs. These programs were required for reimbursement for services and for accreditation by the Joint Commission on Accreditation of Healthcare Organizations (JCAHO). QA programs sought to establish accountability to society on the part of the health professions for the quality, appropriateness, and cost of health services provided.

In the early 1990s, it was recognized that quality of care as defined by regulatory agencies continued to be difficult to measure. QA criteria were identified as measures to ensure minimal expectations only; they did not provide mechanisms for identifying causes of problems or for determining systems or processes that needed improvement. Continuous quality improvement (CQI) was identified as a more effective mechanism for improving the quality of health care. In 1992, the revised standards of the JCAHO mandated that health care organizations implement a CQI program. Recent amendments to JCAHO standards have specified that patients have the right to health care that is considerate and preserves dignity; that respects cultural, psychosocial, and spiritual values; and that is age-specific (Krozok & Scoggins, 2002). Quality improvement efforts have focused on ensuring that the care provided meets or exceeds JCAHO standards.

Unlike QA, which focuses on individual incidents or errors and minimal expectations, CQI focuses on the processes used to provide care, with the aim of improving quality by assessing and improving those interrelated processes that most affect patient care outcomes and patient satisfaction. CQI involves analyzing, understanding, and improving clinical, financial, and operational processes. Problems that occur as more than isolated events are subject to examination, and all issues that may affect patient outcome are studied. Nurses directly involved in the delivery of care are engaged in analyzing data and refining the processes used in CQI. Their knowledge of the processes and conditions that affect patient care is critical in designing changes to improve the quality of the care provided.

As health care agencies continue to implement CQI, nurses have many opportunities to be involved in quality improvement. One such opportunity is through facilitation of evidence-based practice, which involves identifying and evaluating current literature and research, as well as incorporating the findings into care guidelines. This process has been designated as a means of ensuring quality care. Evidence-based practice includes the use of outcome assessment and standardized plans of care such as clinical guidelines, clinical pathways, or algorithms. Many of these measures are being implemented by nurses, particularly by nurse managers and advanced practice nurses, often in collaboration with other health care professionals.

Clinical Pathways and Care Mapping

Many hospitals, managed care facilities, and home health services nationwide use clinical pathways or care mapping to coordinate care for caseloads of patients (Kinsman, 2004; Kinsman, James, & Ham, 2004). Clinical pathways are tools for tracking a patient's progress toward achieving positive outcomes within specified time frames. Clinical pathways based on current literature and clinical expertise have been developed for patients with certain DRGs (eg, open heart surgery, pneumonia with comorbidity, fractured hip), for high-risk patients (eg, those receiving chemotherapy), and for patients with certain common health problems (eg, diabetes, chronic pain). The pathways indicate key events, such as diagnostic tests, treatments, activities, medications, consultation, and education, that must occur within specified times for patients to achieve the desired and timely outcomes.

A case manager often facilitates and coordinates interventions to ensure that the patient progresses through the key events and achieves the desired outcomes. Nurses who provide direct care play an important role in the development and use of clinical pathways through their participation in researching the literature and then developing, piloting, implementing, and revising clinical pathways. In addition, nurses monitor outcome achievement and document and analyze variances. Examples of clinical pathways can be found in Appendix A.

Other evidence-based practice tools used for planning patient care are care mapping, multidisciplinary action plans (MAPs), clinical guidelines, and algorithms. These tools are used to move patients toward predetermined outcome markers. Algorithms are used more often in acute situations to determine a particular treatment based on patient information or response. Care maps, clinical guidelines, and MAPs (the most detailed of these tools) provide coordination of care and education throughout hospitalization and after discharge.

Because care mapping and guidelines are used for conditions in which a patient's progression often defies prediction, specific time frames for achieving outcomes are excluded. A patient with a highly complex condition or multiple underlying illnesses may benefit more from care mapping or guidelines than from clinical pathways, because the use of outcome markers (rather than specific time frames) is more realistic.

Through case management and the use of clinical pathways or care mapping, patients and the care they receive are continually assessed from preadmission to discharge—and in many cases after discharge in the home care and community settings. These tools are used in hospitals and other health care settings to facilitate the effective and efficient care of large groups of patients. Continuity of care, effective utilization of services, and cost containment are expected to be major benefits for society and for the health care system.

Alternative Health Care Delivery Systems

The rising cost of health care over the past few decades has led to the use of managed health care and alternative health care delivery systems, including health maintenance organizations (HMOs) and preferred provider organizations (PPOs).

Managed Care

Managed care is an important trend in health care. The failure of the efforts of past decades to reduce costs and the escalation of health care costs to 15% to 22% of the gross domestic product have prompted business, labor, and government to assume greater control over the financing and delivery of health care. The common features that characterize managed care include prenegotiated payment rates, mandatory precertification, utilization review, limited choice of providers, and fixed-price reimbursement. The scope of managed care has expanded from in-hospital services to HMOs or variations such as PPOs; ambulatory, long-term, and home care services; and related diagnostic and therapeutic services.

Managed care has contributed to a dramatic reduction in inpatient hospital days, continuing expansion of ambulatory care, fierce competition, and marketing strategies that appeal to consumers as well as to insurers and regulators. Hospitals are faced with declining revenues, a declining number of patients, more severely ill patients with shorter lengths of stay, and a need for cost-effective outpatient or ambulatory care services. As patients return to the community, they have more health care needs, many of which are complex. The demand for home care and community-based services is escalating. Despite their successes, managed care organizations are faced with the challenge of providing quality services under resource constraints. Case management is a strategy used by many organizations to meet this challenge.

Case Management

Case management is a system of coordinating health care services to ensure cost-effectiveness, accountability, and quality care. It dates back to the public health programs of the early 1900s, in which public health nursing played a dominant role. The premise of case management is that the responsibility for meeting patient needs rests with one person or team whose goals are to provide the patient and family with access to required services, to ensure coordination of these services, and to evaluate how effectively these services are delivered.

Case management has gained such prominence because of decreased costs of care associated with decreased lengths of hospital stays coupled with rapid and frequent inter-unit transfers from specialty to standard care units. The case manager role, instead of focusing on direct patient care, focuses on managing the care of an entire caseload of patients and collaborating with nurses and other health care personnel who care for patients. In some settings, particularly the community setting, the focus of the nurse case manager is on managing the treatment plan of the patient with complex conditions (Schifalacqua, Ulch, & Schmidt, 2004). The caseload is usually limited in scope to patients with similar diagnoses, needs, and therapies. Case managers are experts in their specialty areas, and they coordinate the inpatient and outpatient services needed by patients. The goals of case management are quality, appropriateness, and timeliness of services as well as cost reduction. The case manager follows the patient throughout hospitalization and at home after discharge in an effort to coordinate health care services that will avert or delay rehospitalization. Evidence-based pathways or similar plans are often used in case management of similar patient populations.

Roles of the Nurse

As stated previously, nursing is the diagnosis and treatment of human responses to health and illness and therefore focuses on a broad array of phenomena. Professional nurses who work in institutional, community-oriented, or community-based settings play three major roles: the practitioner role, which includes teaching and collaborating; the leadership role; and the research role. Although each role carries specific responsibilities, these roles are characteristic of all nursing positions and relate to one another. These roles are designed to meet the immediate and future needs of consumers who are the recipients of nursing care. Often, nurses act in a combination of roles to provide comprehensive patient care.

Practitioner Role

The practitioner role involves those actions taken by nurses to meet the health care and nursing needs of individual patients, their families, and significant others. This role is the dominant role of nurses in primary, secondary, and tertiary health care settings and in home care and community nursing. It is achieved through use of the nursing process, the basis of all nursing practice. Nurses help patients meet their needs through direct intervention, by teaching patients and family members to perform care, and by coordinating and collaborating with other disciplines to provide needed services.

Leadership Role

The leadership role is often perceived as a specialized role assumed by nurses who have titles that suggest leadership and who are the leaders of large groups of nurses or related health care professionals. However, because of the constant fluctuation of health care delivery demands and consumers, a broader definition of nursing leadership, one that identifies the leadership role as inherent within all nursing positions, is required. The leadership role involves those actions that nurses execute when they assume responsibility for the actions of others directed toward determining and achieving patient care goals.

Nursing leadership involves four components: decision making, relating, influencing, and facilitating. Each of these components promotes change and the ultimate outcome of goal achievement. Basic to the entire process is effective communication, which determines the success of the process and achievement of goals. Leadership in nursing is a process in which nurses use interpersonal skills to effect change in the behavior of others. The components of the leadership process are appropriate during all phases of the nursing process and in all settings.

Research Role

The primary task of nursing research is to contribute to the scientific base of nursing practice. Studies are needed to determine the effectiveness of nursing interventions and nursing care. The science of nursing grows through research, leading to the generation of a scientifically based rationale for nursing practice and patient care. This process is the basis of evidence-based practice, with a resultant increase in the quality of patient care.

The research role is considered to be a responsibility of *all* nurses in clinical practice. Nurses must constantly be alert for nursing problems and important issues related to patient care that can serve as a basis for the identification of researchable questions. Nurses with a background in research methods can use their research knowledge and skills to initiate and implement timely, relevant studies.

Nurses directly involved in patient care are often in the best position to identify potential research problems and questions, and their clinical insights are invaluable. Nurses also have a responsibility to become actively involved in ongoing research studies. This may involve facilitating the data collection process, or it may include actual collection of data. Explaining the study to patients and their families and to other health care professionals is often of invaluable assistance to the researcher who is conducting the study.

Above all, nurses must use research findings in their nursing practice; the use, validation, replication, dissemination, and evaluation of research findings further the science of nursing. As stated previously, evidence-based practice requires the use of valid research. Nurses must continually be aware of studies that are directly related to their own area of clinical practice and critically analyze those studies to determine the applicability of their implications for specific patient populations. Relevant conclusions and implications can be used to improve patient care.

Models of Nursing Care Delivery

Several organizational methods or models that vary greatly from one facility to another and from one set of patient circumstances to another may be used to carry out nursing care. These methods and models have changed over the years and have included functional nursing, team nursing, and, more recently, primary nursing.

Primary Nursing

Primary nursing (not to be confused with primary health care, which pertains to first-contact general health care) refers to comprehensive, individualized care provided by the same nurse throughout the period of care. This type of nursing care allows the nurse to give direct patient care rather than manage and supervise the functions of others who care for a particular patient. This care method is too costly for many institutions because a smaller patient–nurse ratio, with a larger professional staff, is needed. However, primary nursing may provide a foundation for transition to case management in some institutions.

The primary nurse is responsible for directly involving the patient and family in all facets of care. The primary nurse accepts total 24-hour responsibility for a patient's nursing care, which is directed toward meeting the individualized needs of that patient. To promote continuity of care and collaboration directed toward quality patient care, the primary nurse communicates with other members of the health care team regarding the patient's health.

When a particular primary nurse is not working, an associate nurse or co-nurse assists in overseeing the delivery of care. This nurse implements the nursing plan of care and provides feedback to the primary nurse for evaluating the plan of care. The primary nurse retains responsibility for making appropriate referrals and for ensuring that all relevant information is provided to people involved in the patient's continuing care, including family members.

The long-term survival of primary nursing is uncertain. Although primary nursing continues to be used in many health care agencies, many variations have been developed to meet the needs of the particular agency. As cost-containment measures continue and patient acuity increases, staffing ratios of patients to nurses are increasing. Many nursing service departments and agencies are meeting the increased workload demands by modifying their approach to primary nursing or by reverting to team or functional systems of care. Others are changing their staffing mix and redesigning their practice models to accommodate nonprofessional staff. Still others are changing to more innovative systems such as case management.

Community-Based Nursing and Community-Oriented/ Public Health Nursing

Community-based care and community-oriented/public health nursing are not new concepts in nursing. Nursing has played a vital role in the community since the middle to late 1800s, when visiting nurses provided care to the sick and poor in their homes and communities and educated patients and families. Although community health nursing, public health nursing, community-based nursing, and home health nursing may be discussed together and aspects of care in each type do overlap, these terms are distinct from one another. Confusion exists regarding the differences, and the similar settings may blur these distinctions (Stanhope & Lancaster, 2004). The central idea of community-oriented nursing practice is that nursing intervention can promote wellness, reduce the spread of illness, and improve the health status of groups of citizens or the community at large. Its emphasis is on primary, secondary, and tertiary prevention. Nurses in these settings have traditionally focused on health promotion, maternal and child health, and chronic care.

Community-based nursing occurs in a variety of settings within the community and is directed toward individuals and families (Stanhope & Lancaster, 2004). It includes home health care nursing. Most community-based and home health care is directed toward specific patient groups with identified needs, which usually relate to illness, injury, or disability, resulting most often from advanced age or chronic illness. However, both community-based and community-oriented nurses are now meeting the needs of groups of patients with a variety of problems and needs. Home health care is a major aspect of community-based care discussed throughout this text. Home health care services are provided by community-based programs and agencies for specific populations (eg, the elderly, ventilator-dependent patients), as well as by home health care agencies, hospices, independent professional nursing practices, and freestanding health care agencies.

As shortened hospital stays and increased use of outpatient health care services continue, the need for nursing care in the home and community setting increases. Because nursing services are provided outside as well as inside the hospital, nurses have a choice of practicing in a variety of health care delivery settings. These settings include acute care medical centers, ambulatory care settings, clinics, urgent care centers, outpatient departments, neighborhood health centers, home health care agencies, independent or group nursing centers, and managed care agencies.

Community nursing centers, which have emerged in the past few decades, are nurse-managed and provide primary care services such as ambulatory and outpatient care, immunizations, health assessment and screening services, and patient and family education and counseling. These centers serve varied populations that typically include a high proportion of patients who are rural, very young, very old, poor, or members of racial minorities—groups that are generally underserved.

The numbers and kinds of agencies that provide care in the home and community have increased because of the expanding needs of patients requiring care. Home health care nurses are challenged because patients are discharged from acute care institutions to their homes and communities early in the recovery process and with more complex needs. Many are elderly, and many have multiple medical and nursing diagnoses and multisystem health problems that require acute and intensive nursing care. Medical technologies such as ventilatory support and intravenous or parenteral nutrition therapy, once limited to the acute care setting, have been adapted to the home care setting.

As a result, the community-based care setting is becoming one of the largest practice areas for nursing. Home care nursing is now a specialty area that requires advanced knowledge and skills in general nursing practice, with emphasis on community health and acute medical-surgical nursing. Also required are high-level assessment skills, critical thinking, and decision-making skills in a setting where other health care professionals are not available to validate observations, conclusions, and decisions.

Home care nurses often function as acute care nurses in the home, providing "high-tech, high-touch" services to patients with acute health care needs. In addition, they are responsible for patient and family teaching and for contacting community resources and coordinating the continuing care of patients. For these reasons, the scope of medical-surgical nursing encompasses not only the acute care setting within the hospital but also the acute care setting as it expands into the community and the home. Throughout this textbook, the home health care needs of patients are addressed, with particular attention given to the teaching, self-care management, and health maintenance needs of patients and their families.

Expanded Nursing Roles

Professional nursing is adapting to meet changing health needs and expectations. The role of the nurse has expanded in response to the need to improve the distribution of health care services and to decrease the cost of health care. Nurse practitioners (NPs), clinical nurse specialists (CNSs), certified nurse-midwives, and certified registered nurse anesthetists (CRNAs) are identified as advanced practice nurses. Nurses who function in these roles provide direct care to patients through independent practice, practice within a health care agency, or collaboration with a physician. Specialization in nursing has evolved as a result of the recent explosion of technology and knowledge.

Nurses may receive advanced education in such specialties as family care, critical care, coronary care, respiratory care, oncologic care, maternal and child health care, neonatal intensive care, rehabilitation, trauma, rural health, and gerontologic nursing. Various titles have emerged to specify the functions as well as educational preparation. In medical-surgical nursing, the most significant of these titles are *nurse practitioner* (NP) and *clinical nurse specialist* (CNS), and the more recent title of *advanced practice nurse* (APN), which encompasses both nurse practitioners and clinical nurse specialists. Most states require both nurse practitioners and clinical nurse specialists to have graduate-level education.

Nurse practitioners are prepared as generalists (eg, pediatric, geriatric) or specialists. They define their role in terms of direct provision of a broad range of primary health care services to patients and families. The focus is on providing primary health care to patients and collaborating with other health professionals. Nurse practitioners practice in both acute and non-acute care settings. The 1997 Balanced Budget Act provided for nurse practitioners to receive direct Medicare reimbursement. In addition, in some states nurse practitioners have prescriptive authority (Hales, 2002).

Clinical nurse specialists, on the other hand, are prepared as specialists who practice within a circumscribed area of care (eg, cardiovascular, oncology). They define their role as having five major components: clinical practice, education, management, consultation, and research. Studies have shown that in reality clinical nurse specialists often focus on their education and consultation roles, which involve education and counseling of patients and families, as well as education, counseling, and consultation with nursing staff. Some states have granted clinical nurse specialists prescriptive authority if they have the required educational preparation. Clinical nurse specialists practice in a variety of settings, including the community and the home, although most practice in acute care settings. Recently, clinical nurse specialists have been identified by many nursing leaders as ideal case managers. They have the educational background and the clinical expertise to organize and coordinate services and resources to meet the patient's health care needs in a cost-effective and efficient manner. The expanding role of the nurse case manager has contributed to the designation of the advanced practice nurse case manager as an advanced practice role (Hamric, Spross, & Hanson, 2005).

With advanced practice roles has come a continuing effort by professional nursing organizations to define more clearly the practice of nursing. Nurse practice acts have been amended to give nurses the authority to perform functions that were previously restricted to the practice of medicine. These functions include diagnosis (nursing), treatment, performance of selected invasive procedures, and prescription of medications and treatments. The board of nursing in each state stipulates regulations regarding these functions. In addition, the board defines the education and experience required and determines the clinical situations in which a nurse may perform these functions.

In general, initial care, ambulatory health care, palliative care, and anticipatory guidance are all becoming increasingly important in nursing practice. Advanced practice roles enable nurses to function interdependently with other health care professionals and to establish a more collegial relationship with physicians. As changes in health care continue, the role of advanced practice nurses is expected to increase in terms of scope, responsibility, and recognition.

Collaborative Practice

This chapter has explored the changing role of nursing. Many references have been made to the significance of nurses as members of the health care team. As the unique competencies of nurses are becoming more clearly articulated, there is increasing evidence that nurses provide certain health care services distinct to the profession. However, nursing continues to recognize the importance of collaboration with other health care disciplines in meeting the needs of patients.

Some institutions use the collaborative practice model (Fig. 1-2). Nurses, physicians, and ancillary health personnel function within a decentralized organizational structure, collaboratively making clinical decisions. A joint practice committee, with representation from all care providers, may function at the unit level to monitor, support, and foster collaboration. Collaborative practice is further enhanced with integration of the health or medical record and with joint patient care record reviews.

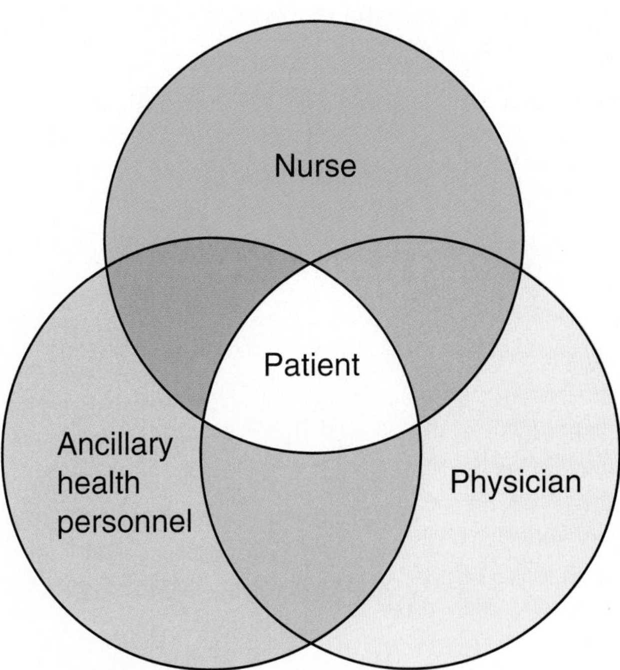

FIGURE 1-2. Collaborative practice model.

The collaborative model, or a variation of it, should be a primary goal for nursing—a venture that promotes shared participation, responsibility, and accountability in a health care environment that is striving to meet the complex health care needs of the public.

Critical Thinking Exercises

1 Your clinical assignment is on a rehabilitation nursing unit. Identify a patient care issue (eg, discharge planning) that could be improved. Describe the mechanism that is available within a clinical facility to address such quality improvement issues.

2 You are planning the discharge of an elderly patient who has several chronic medical conditions. A case manager has been assigned to this patient. How would you explain the role of the case manager to the patient and her husband?

3 ebp You are assigned to care for a hospitalized patient who is obese and newly diagnosed with diabetes. There is a diabetes clinical nurse specialist on staff at the hospital. Identify the evidence that supports the effectiveness of clinical nurse specialists in providing education to patients and promoting positive patient outcomes. What is the strength of the evidence? How might this specific patient's care be affected?

REFERENCES AND SELECTED READINGS

BOOKS

American Nurses Association. (2003). *Nursing's social policy statement* (2nd ed.). Washington, DC: Author.

American Nurses Association. (1992). *Nursing's agenda for health care reform.* Kansas City, MO: Author.

Hamric, A. B., Spross, J. A., & Hanson, C. M. (2005). *Advanced practice nursing: An integrative approach* (5th ed.). St. Louis: Elsevier.

Hood, L., & Leddy, S. K. (2003). *Leddy & Pepper's conceptual bases of professional nursing* (5th ed.). Philadelphia: Lippincott Williams & Wilkins.

Joel, L. A. (2004). *Advanced practice nursing: Essentials for role development.* Philadelphia: F. A. Davis.

Krozok, C., & Scoggins, A. (2002). *Patient rights . . . amended to comply with 2002 JCAHO standards.* Glendale, CA: CINAHL Information Systems.

Melnyk, B. M., & Fineout-Overholt, E. (2005). *Evidence-based practice in nursing & healthcare.* Philadelphia: Lippincott Williams & Wilkins.

Stanhope, M., & Lancaster, J. (2004). *Community & public health nursing.* St. Louis: Mosby-Year Book.

Stanley, J. M. (2005). *Advanced practice nursing* (2nd ed.). Philadelphia: F. A. Davis.

U.S. Bureau of the Census. (Internet release date: Jan. 13, 2000). *Profile of older Americans: 2000. Population projections of the United States by age, sex, race, and Hispanic origin: 1995–2050.* Current Population Reports, P25-1130. Washington, DC: Author.

JOURNALS

Abrams, R. B. (2002). Rights and responsibilities for nurses: Another look. *HealthLeaders.com*, July 10, 2002.

Baldwin, D. (2003). Disparities in health and health care: Focusing efforts to eliminate unequal burdens. *Online Journal of Issues in Nursing, 8*(1). http://www.nursingworld.org/ojin/topic20/tpc20_1.htm

Campinha-Bacote, J. (2003). Many faces: Addressing diversity in health care. *Online Journal of Issues in Nursing, 8*(1).

Charlebois, D., & Wilmoth, D. (2004). Critical care of patients with obesity. *Critical Care Nurse, 24*(4), 19–27.

Hales, A. (2002). Perspectives on prescribing: Pioneer's narratives and advice. *Perspectives in Psychiatric Care, 38*(3), 79–88.

Harrison, T. (2003). Women aging with childhood onset disability: A holistic approach using the life course paradigm. *Journal of Holistic Nursing, 21*(3), 242–259.

Kinsman, L. (2004). Clinical pathway compliance and quality improvement. *Nursing Standard, 18*(18), 33–35.

Kinsman, L., James, E., & Ham, J. (2004). An interdisciplinary, evidence-based process of clinical pathway implementation increases pathway usage. *Lippincott's Case Management: Managing the Process of Patient Care,* 9(4), 184–196.

Lein, C., Collins, C., Lyles, J. S., et al. (2004). Building research relationships with managed care organizations: Issues and strategies. *Family Systems & Health, 21*(2), 205–214.

Reid Ponte, P. (2004). The American health care system at a crossroads: An overview of the American Organization of Nurse Executives Monograph. *Online Journal of Issues in Nursing,* 9(2), Manuscript 2. Available at http://www.nursingworld.org/ojin/topic24/tpc24_2.htm.

Schifalacqua, M. M., Ulch, P. O., & Schmidt, M. (2004). How to make a difference in the health care of a population, one person at a time. *Nursing Administration Quarterly, 28*(1), 29–35.

Stone, P. (September/October 2003). Wellness care for the athlete. *Today's Chiropractic,* 64–67.

Young, H. (2003). Challenges and solutions for care of frail older adults. *Online Journal of Issues in Nursing,* 8(2), Manuscript 4. Available at: http://www.nursingworld.org/ojin/topic21/tpc21_4.htm.

CHAPTER 2

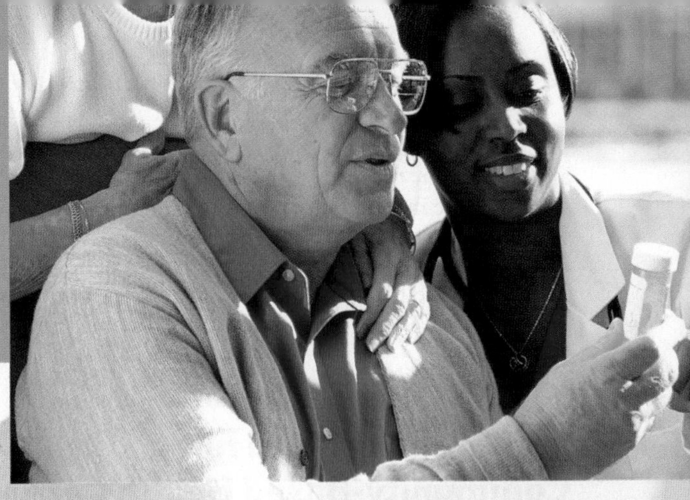

Community-Based Nursing Practice

Learning Objectives

On completion of this chapter, the learner will be able to:

1. Discuss the changes in the health care system that have increased the need for medical-surgical nurses to practice in community-based settings.
2. Compare the differences and similarities between community-based and hospital nursing.
3. Describe the discharge planning process in relation to home care preparation.
4. Explain methods for identifying community resources and making referrals.
5. Discuss how to prepare for a home health care visit and how to conduct the visit.
6. Identify personal safety precautions a home care nurse should take when making home visits.
7. Describe the various types of nursing functions provided in ambulatory care facilities, in occupational health and school nursing programs, in community nurse-managed centers, in hospice care settings, and to the homeless.

The changes that have occurred in the health care system and society in the past two decades have increased the need for care in ambulatory settings and in the home. The demand for registered nurses in ambulatory settings is likely to continue to increase, creating a demand for highly skilled and well-prepared nurses to provide community-based care (Centers for Disease Control and Prevention [CDC], 2003).

The Growing Need for Community-Based Health Care

As described in Chapter 1, the shift in the settings for health care delivery is a result of several factors, including new population trends. The growing number of older adults in the United States increases the demand for medical and social services within the public health system. Increased life expectancy is coupled with the need for more attention to people with chronic conditions, such as hypertension, which affects more than 50 million Americans (Chobanian, Bakris, Black, et al., 2003), and decreased quality of life (Goulding, Rogers, & Smith, 2003). Increases in chronic health problems such as diabetes and obesity are at an all-time high, mandating an increased need for community health care services.

Other factors, such as changes in federal legislation, tighter insurance regulations, decreasing hospital revenues, and alternative health care delivery systems, also have affected the ways in which health care is delivered. As a result of federal legislation passed in 1983 and 1997, hospitals and other health care providers are now reimbursed at a fixed rate for patients who have the same diagnosis as defined by diagnosis-related groups (DRGs). Under this system, hospitals and other health care providers can reduce costs and earn income by carefully monitoring the types of services they provide and discharging patients as soon as possible. Consequently, patients are being discharged from acute care facilities to their homes or to residential or long-term care facilities at much earlier stages of recovery than in the past. Complex technical equipment, such as dialysis machines, intravenous lines, and ventilators, is often part of home health care (Stanhope & Lancaster, 2004). Nurses play a role in evaluating the safety and cost of technology in the home setting. In addition, "tele-health" is an emerging trend in home care that facilitates exchange of information via telephone lines between patients and nurses regarding health information such as blood glucose readings, vital signs, and cardiac parameters (Stanhope & Lancaster, 2004).

Health care systems, such as health maintenance organizations, preferred provider organizations, and managed health care systems, have also contributed to the drive to control costs and the availability of health care services. As described in Chapter 1, managed care has dramatically reduced the length of hospital stay and has led to patients being treated more frequently in ambulatory care settings and at home.

The largest group of health care professionals practicing in public health are nurses (CDC, 2003). As more health care delivery shifts into the community, more nurses are working in a variety of public health and community-based settings. These settings include public health departments, ambulatory health clinics, long-term care facilities, prenatal and well-baby clinics, hospice agencies, industrial settings (as occupational nurses), homeless shelters and clinics, nursing centers, home health agencies, urgent care centers, same-day surgical centers, short-stay facilities, and patients' homes. In these settings, nurses often deliver care without direct on-site supervision or support of other health care personnel. They must be self-directed, flexible, adaptable, and tolerant of various lifestyles and living conditions. To function effectively in community-based settings, nurses must have expertise in independent decision making, critical thinking, assessment, health education, and competence in basic nursing care (Stanhope & Lancaster, 2004).

In addition, nurses in community settings must be culturally competent. Green-Hernandez, Quinn, Denman-Vitale, et al. (2004, p. 216) underscore that "health care is the practice of care that is ethically and culturally appropriate." In working with patients and families, culture plays a role in the assignment of value priorities to health (ie, the priorities given to various aspects of health and illness from a cultural perspective) (Locsin, 2003).

Community-Based Care

Community-based nursing is a philosophy of care of people and families in which the care is provided as patients and their families move among various service providers outside of hospitals (Stanhope & Lancaster, 2004). This nursing practice focuses on promoting and maintaining the health of individuals and families, preventing and minimizing the progression of disease, and improving quality of life (Stanhope & Lancaster, 2004). The actions of community health nurses may include providing direct care to patients and families as well as political advocacy to secure resources for aggregate populations (eg, the aged population). Community health nurses have many roles, including epidemiologist, case manager for a group of patients, coordinator of services provided to a group of patients, occupational health nurse, school nurse, visiting nurse, or parish nurse. (In parish nursing, the members of the religious community—the parish—are the recipients of care.) These roles have one element in common: a focus on community needs as well as on the needs of individual patients. Community-based care is generally focused on individuals or their families, although efforts may be undertaken to improve the health of the entire community (Fig. 2-1).

The primary concepts of community-based nursing care are self-care and preventive care within the context of culture and community. Two other important concepts are continuity of care and collaboration. Some community-based areas of nursing have become specialties in their own right, such as school health nursing and home health nursing.

Primary, secondary, and tertiary levels of preventive care are used by nurses in community-based practice. The focus of primary prevention is on health promotion and prevention of illness or disease, including interventions such as teaching about healthy lifestyles. Secondary prevention centers on health maintenance and is aimed at early detection and prompt intervention to prevent or minimize loss of

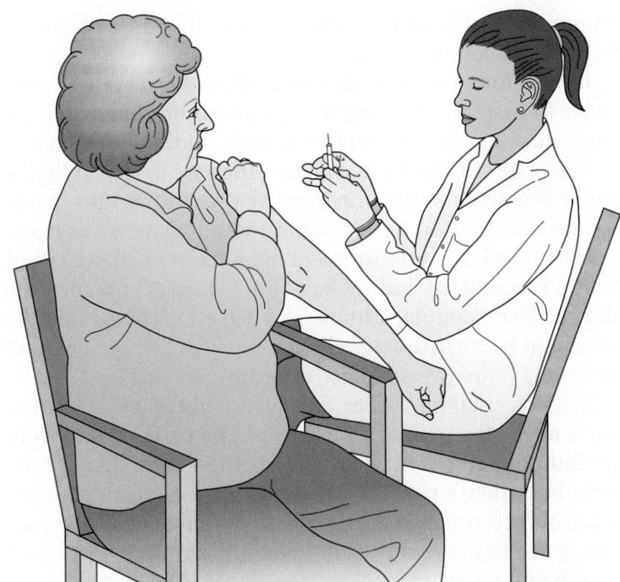

FIGURE 2-1. Community-based nursing takes many forms and focuses. Here the nursing focus is on wellness and the nursing setting is industry. When enlightened employers offer flu vaccines or other health services, the whole community benefits.

function and independence, including interventions such as health screening and health risk appraisal. Tertiary prevention focuses on minimizing deterioration and improving quality of life, including rehabilitation to assist patients in achieving their maximum potential by working through their physical or psychological challenges.

Home Health Care

Home health care is becoming one of the largest practice areas for nurses. Because of the high acuity level of patients, nurses with acute care and high-technology experience are in demand in this field. Tertiary preventive nursing care, which focuses on rehabilitation and restoring maximum health function, is a major goal for home care nurses, although primary and secondary prevention are also included. Health care visits may be intermittent or periodic, and telephonic case management may be used to promote communication with home care consumers.

Home care nursing is a unique component of community-based nursing. Home care visits are made by nurses who work for home care agencies, public health agencies, and visiting nurse associations; by nurses who are employed by hospitals; and by parish nurses who voluntarily work with the members of their religious communities to promote health. Such visits may also be part of the responsibilities of school nurses, clinic nurses, or occupational health nurses. The type of nursing services provided to patients in their homes varies from agency to agency. Nurses from home care or hospice agencies make home visits to provide skilled nursing care, follow-up care, and teaching to promote health and prevent complications. Hospice nursing has become a specialty area of nursing practice in which nurses provide palliative care in patients' homes, thus promoting comfort, peace, and dignity to patients who are dying. Clinic nurses may conduct home visits as part of patient follow-up. Public health, parish, and school nurses may make visits to provide anticipatory guidance to high-risk families and follow-up care to patients with communicable diseases. Many home care patients are acutely ill, and many have chronic health problems and disabilities, requiring that nurses provide more education and monitoring to patients and families to facilitate compliance.

Holistic care is provided in the home through the collaboration of an interdisciplinary team that includes professional nurses; home health aides; social workers; physical, speech, and occupational therapists; and physicians. An interdisciplinary approach is used to provide health and social services with oversight of the total health care plan by a case manager, clinical nurse specialist, or nurse practitioner. Interdisciplinary collaboration is required if a home health agency is to receive Medicare certification (Stanhope & Lancaster, 2004).

Health care services are provided by official, publicly funded agencies; nonprofit agencies; private businesses; proprietary chains; and hospital-based agencies. Some agencies specialize in high-technology services. Most agencies are reimbursed from a variety of sources, including Medicare and Medicaid programs, private insurance, and direct patient payment. Many home health care expenditures are financed by Medicare and are affected by provisions of the Balanced Budget Act of 1997. Each funding source has its own requirements for services rendered, number of visits allowed, and amount of reimbursement the agency receives.

The elderly are the most frequent users of home care services. To be eligible for service, the patient must be acutely ill, homebound, and in need of skilled nursing services. Nursing care includes skilled assessment of the patient's physical, psychological, social, and environmental status. Nursing interventions may include IV therapy and injections (Fig. 2-2), parenteral nutrition, venipuncture, catheter

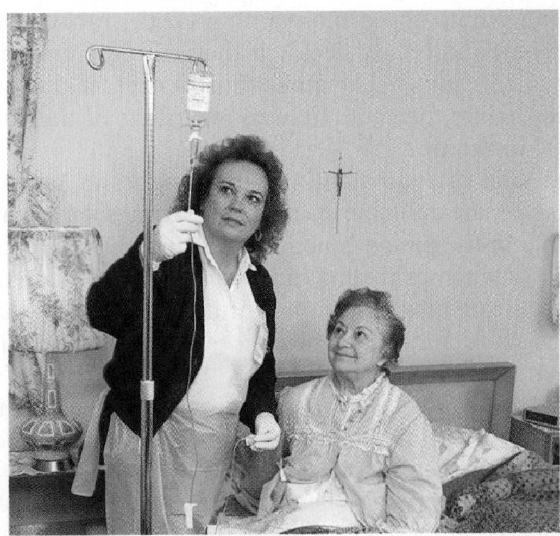

FIGURE 2-2. Intravenous therapy is one of many types of skilled nursing care that may be provided in the home. Courtesy Good Samaritan Certified Home Health Agency, Babylon, NY.

insertion, pressure ulcer treatment, wound care, ostomy care, and patient and family teaching. The nurse instructs the patient and family in skills and self-care strategies and in health maintenance and promotion activities (eg, nutritional counseling, exercise programs, stress management).

Medicare allows nurses to manage and evaluate patient care for seriously ill patients who have complex, labile conditions and are at high risk for rehospitalization. Nurses serve as case managers and monitor the delivery of care provided to patients in their homes.

Community-Based Nursing

Providing nursing care in a patient's home is different from providing care in a hospital. Patients must sign a release form to stay and receive treatment in a hospital, where they have little control over what happens to them and to their environment. They are expected to comply with the hospital's rules, regulations, and schedule of activities, and they are given care, treatments, baths, and medications at times that are usually determined by institutional schedules rather than patient preference. Although hospitalized patients may select meals from a daily menu, there are limited choices in the type of food they are offered. Family members and friends may visit only during visiting hours.

In contrast, the home care nurse is considered a guest in the patient's home and must have permission to visit and give care. The nurse has minimal control over the lifestyle, living situation, and health practices of the patients he or she visits. This lack of full decision-making authority can create a conflict for the nurse and lead to problems in the nurse–patient relationship. To work successfully with patients in any setting, the nurse must be nonjudgmental and convey respect for the patient's beliefs, even if they differ sharply from the nurse's. This can be difficult when a patient's lifestyle involves activities that a nurse considers harmful or unacceptable, such as smoking, use of alcohol, drug abuse, or overeating.

The cleanliness of a patient's home may not meet the standards of a hospital. Although the nurse can provide teaching points about maintaining clean surroundings, the patient and family decide if they will implement the nurse's suggestions. The nurse must accept this possibility and deliver the care required regardless of the conditions of the setting.

The kind of equipment and the supplies or resources that usually are available in acute care settings are often unavailable in the patient's home. The nurse has to learn to improvise when providing care, such as when changing a dressing or catheterizing a patient in a regular bed that is not adjustable and lacks a bedside table (Smith-Temple & Johnson, 2005).

Infection control is as important in the home as it is in the hospital, but it can be more challenging in the home and requires creative approaches. As in any situation, it is important to clean one's hands before and after giving direct patient care, even in a home that does not have running water. If aseptic technique is required, the nurse must have a plan for implementing this technique before going to the home. This applies also to standard precautions, transmission-based precautions, and disposal of bodily secretions and excretions.

If injections are given, the nurse should use a closed container to dispose of syringes. Injectable and other medications must be kept out of the reach of children during visits and must be stored in a safe place if they are to remain in the house. Nurses who perform invasive procedures must be up to date with their immunizations, including hepatitis B and tetanus. The home environment often has more distractions than a hospital, including background noise, people, and objects. For example, a nurse may have to request that the television be turned down during the visit or that a patient move to a more private place to be interviewed.

Friends, neighbors, or family members may ask the nurse about the patient's condition. The patient has a right to confidentiality, and information should be shared only with the patient's permission. If the nurse carries a patient's medical record into a house, he or she must put it in a secure place to prevent it from being picked up by others or from being misplaced.

Discharge Planning for Home Care

Discharge planning is an important part of making the transition from the acute to the home care setting. It is required for reimbursement from Medicare (Birmingham, 2004). Discharge planning begins with the patient's admission to prepare for early hospital discharge and the possible need for follow-up home care. Several different personnel or agencies may be involved in the planning process. In hospitals, nurses or social workers may serve as the discharge planners. Some home care agencies have liaison nurses who work with discharge planners to ensure that the patient's needs are met upon discharge from the hospital. Professionals in ambulatory health care settings may refer patients for home care services to prevent hospitalization. Public health nurses care for patients referred for anticipatory guidance with high-risk families, for case finding, and for follow-up treatment (eg, patients with communicable diseases). Parish nurses may have patients referred, or they may be contacted directly by members of the parish community who need guidance or referrals related to physical or psychosocial health needs (Carson & Koenig, 2002).

The development of a comprehensive discharge plan requires collaboration with professionals at both the referring agency and the home care agency, public health agency, or other community resource. The process involves identifying the patient's needs and developing a thorough plan to meet them. Communication with and cooperation of the patient and family are essential.

Community Resources and Referrals

As case managers, community-based nurses may make referrals to other team members, such as home health aides and social workers. These nurses work collaboratively with the health team and the referring agency or person. Continuous coordinated care among all health care providers involved in a patient's care is essential to avoid duplication of effort by the various personnel caring for the patient.

A community-based nurse must be knowledgeable about community resources available to patients as well as services provided by local agencies, eligibility requirements, and any possible charges for the services. Most communities have directories of health and social service agencies that the nurse can consult. These directories must be continually updated as resources change. If a community does not have a resource booklet, an agency may develop one for its staff. It should include the commonly used community resources that patients need, as well as the costs of the services and eligibility requirements. The telephone book is often useful in helping patients identify the locations of grocery and drug stores, banks, health care facilities, ambulances, physicians, dentists, pharmacists, social service agencies, and senior citizens' programs. In addition, a patient's place of worship or parish may be an important resource for services.

The community-based nurse is responsible for informing the patient and family about the community resources available to meet their needs. During initial and subsequent home visits, the nurse helps the patient and family identify these community services and encourages them to contact the appropriate agencies. When appropriate, nurses may make the initial contact.

Home Health Visits

Preparing for a Home Visit

Most agencies have a policy manual that states the agency's philosophy and procedures and defines the services provided. Becoming familiar with these policies is essential before initiating a home visit. It is also important to know the agency's policies and the state law regarding what actions to take if the nurse finds a patient dead, encounters an abusive situation in the family, determines that a patient cannot safely remain at home, or observes a situation that possibly indicates malicious harm to the community at large.

Before making a home visit, the nurse should review the patient's referral form and other pertinent data concerning the patient. It may be necessary to contact the referring agency if the purpose for the referral is unclear or if important information is missing. The first step is to call the patient to obtain permission to visit, schedule a time for the visit, and verify the address. This initial phone conversation provides an opportunity to introduce oneself, identify the agency, and explain the reason for the visit. If the patient does not have a telephone, the nurse should see if the people who made the referral have a number where a phone message can be left for the patient. If an unannounced visit to a patient's home must be made, the nurse should ask permission to come in before entering the house. Explaining the purpose of the referral at the outset and setting up the times for future visits before leaving are also recommended.

Most agencies provide nurses with bags that contain standard supplies and equipment needed during home visits. It is important to keep the bag properly supplied and to bring any additional items that might be needed for the visit. Patients rarely have the medical supplies needed for treatment.

Conducting a Home Visit

Personal Safety Precautions

Community nurses must pay particular attention to personal safety, because their practice settings are often in unknown environments. Based on the principle of due diligence, agencies must inform employees of at-risk working environments. Agencies have policies and procedures concerning the promotion of safety for clinical staff, and training is provided to facilitate personal safety. Environments must be carefully assessed, and proactive measures must be taken by the individual nurse as well as the agency (Skillen, Olson, & Gilbert, 2003).

Whenever a nurse makes a home visit, the agency should know the nurse's schedule and the locations of the visits. The nurse should learn about the neighborhood and obtain directions to the destination. A plan of action should always be established in case of emergencies. If a dangerous situation is encountered during the visit, the nurse should return to the agency and contact his or her supervisor or law enforcement officials, or both. Suggested precautions to take when making a home visit are presented in Chart 2-1.

Initial Home Visit

The first visit sets the tone for subsequent visits and is crucial in establishing the nurse–patient relationship. The situations encountered depend on numerous factors. Patients may be in pain and unable to care for themselves. Family members may be overwhelmed and doubt their ability to care for their loved ones. They may not understand why the patient was sent home from the hospital before being totally rehabilitated. They may not comprehend what home care is or why they cannot have 24-hour nursing services. It is critical that the nurse conveys an understanding of what patients and families are experiencing and how the illness is affecting their lives.

During the initial home visit, which usually lasts less than an hour, the individual patient is evaluated and a plan of care is established to be followed or modified on subsequent visits. The nurse informs the patient of the agency's practices, policies, and hours of operation. If the agency is to be reimbursed for the visit, the nurse asks for insurance information, such as a Medicare or Medicaid card.

The initial assessment includes evaluating the patient, the home environment, the patient's self-care abilities or the family's ability to provide care, and the patient's need for additional resources. Identification of possible hazards, such as cluttered walk areas, potential fire risks, air or water pollution, or inadequate sanitation facilities, is also part of the initial assessment.

Documentation considerations for home visits follow fairly specific regulations. The patient's needs and the nursing care provided are documented to ensure that the agency qualifies for payment for the visit. Medicare, Medicaid, and third-party payers require documentation of the patient's homebound status and the need for skilled professional

CHART 2-1

Safety Precautions in Home Health Care

- Learn or preprogram a cellular phone with the telephone numbers of the agency and police and emergency services.
- Let the agency know your daily schedule and the telephone numbers of your patients so that you can be located if you do not return when expected.
- Know where the patient lives before leaving to make the visit and carry a map for quick referral.
- Keep your car in good working order and have sufficient gas in the tank.
- Park the car near the patient's home and lock it during the visit.
- Do not drive an expensive car or wear expensive jewelry when making visits.
- Know the regular bus schedule and know the routes when using public transportation or walking to the patient's house.
- Carry agency identification and have enough change to make telephone calls in case you get lost or have problems. Most agencies provide cellular phones for their nurses so that the agency can contact the nurse, and so that the nurse can contact the agency in case of an emergency or unexpected situation.
- When making visits in high-crime areas, visit with another person rather than alone.
- Schedule visits only during daylight hours.
- Never walk into a patient's home uninvited.
- If you do not feel safe entering a patient's home, leave the area.
- Become familiar with the layout of the house, including exits from the house.
- If a patient or family member is intoxicated, hostile, or obnoxious, reschedule the visit and leave.
- If a family is having a serious argument or abusing the patient or anyone else in the household, reschedule the visit, contact your supervisor, and report the abuse to the appropriate authorities.

nursing care. The medical diagnosis and specific detailed information on the functional limitations of the patient are usually part of the documentation. The goals and the actions appropriate for attaining them must be identified. Expected outcomes of the nursing interventions must be stated in terms of patient behaviors and must be realistic and measurable. They must reflect the nursing diagnosis or the patient's problems and must specify those actions that address the patient's problems. If the documentation is inadequate, the agency may not be paid for the visit (Scala-Foley, Caruso, Ramos, et al., 2004).

Determining the Need for Future Visits

While conducting an assessment of a patient's situation, the home care nurse evaluates the need for future visits and the frequency with which those visits may need to be made. To make these judgments, the nurse should consider the questions listed in Chart 2-2. With each subsequent visit, these

CHART 2-2

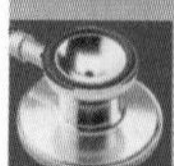

Assessing the Need for Home Visits

CURRENT HEALTH STATUS
- How well is the patient progressing?
- How serious are the present signs and symptoms?
- Has the patient shown signs of progressing as expected, or does it seem that recovery will be delayed?

HOME ENVIRONMENT
- Are worrisome safety factors apparent?
- Are family or friends available to provide care, or is the patient alone?

LEVEL OF SELF-CARE ABILITY
- Is the patient capable of self-care?
- What is the patient's level of independence?
- Is the patient ambulatory or bedridden?
- Does the patient have sufficient energy, or is he or she frail and easily fatigued?

LEVEL OF NURSING CARE NEEDED
- What level of nursing care does the patient require?
- Does the care require basic skills or more complex interventions?

PROGNOSIS
- What is the expectation for recovery in this particular instance?
- What are the chances that complications may develop if nursing care is not provided?

EDUCATIONAL NEEDS
- How well has the patient or family grasped the teaching points made?
- Is there a need for further follow-up and retraining?
- What level of proficiency does the patient or family show in carrying out the necessary care?

MENTAL STATUS
- How alert is the patient?
- Are there signs of confusion or thinking difficulties?
- Does the patient tend to be forgetful or have a limited attention span?

LEVEL OF ADHERENCE
- Is the patient following the instructions provided?
- Does the patient seem capable of following the instructions?
- Are the family members helpful, or are they unwilling or unable to assist in caring for the patient as expected?

same factors are evaluated to determine the continuing health needs of the patient. As progress is made and the patient, with or without the help of significant others, becomes more capable of self-care and more independent, the need for home visits may decline.

Ending the Visit

As the visit comes to a close, it is important to summarize the main points of the visit for the patient and family and to identify expectations for future visits or patient achievements. The following points should be considered at the end of each visit:

- What are the main points the patient or family should remember from the visit?
- What positive attributes have been noted about the patient and the family that will give them a sense of accomplishment?
- What were the main points of the teaching plan or the treatments needed to ensure that the patient and family understand what they must do? A written set of instructions should be left with the patient or family, provided they can read and see (alternative formats include video or audio recordings). Printed material should be in the patient's primary language and in large print when indicated.
- Whom should the patient or family call if they need to contact someone immediately? Are current emergency telephone numbers readily available? Is telephone service available, or can an emergency cellular phone service be provided?
- What signs of complications should be reported immediately?
- How frequently will visits be made? How long will they last (approximately)?
- What is the day and time of the next visit? Will a different nurse make the visit?

Other Community-Based Health Care Settings

Ambulatory Settings

Ambulatory health care is provided for patients in community or hospital-based settings. The types of agencies that provide such care are medical clinics, ambulatory care units, urgent care centers, cardiac rehabilitation programs, mental health centers, student health centers, community outreach programs, and nursing centers. Some ambulatory centers provide care to a specific population, such as migrant workers or Native Americans. Neighborhood health centers provide services to patients who live in a geographically defined area. The centers may operate in freestanding buildings, storefronts, or mobile units. Agencies may provide ambulatory health care in addition to other services, such as an adult day care or health program. The kinds of services offered and the patients served depend on the agency's mission.

Nursing responsibilities in ambulatory health care settings include providing direct patient care, conducting patient intake screenings, treating patients with acute or chronic illnesses or emergency conditions, referring patients to other agencies for additional services, teaching patients self-care activities, and offering health education programs that promote health maintenance. A useful tool for community-based nurses might be the classification scheme developed by the Visiting Nurses Association of Omaha, which contains patient-focused problems in one of four domains: environmental, psychosocial, physiologic, and health-related behaviors (Barton, Clark, & Baramee, 2004).

Nurses also work as clinic managers, direct the operation of clinics, and supervise other health team members. Nurse practitioners, educated in primary care, often practice in ambulatory care settings that focus on gerontology, pediatrics, family or adult health, or women's health. Constraints imposed by federal legislation and ambulatory payment classifications require efficient and effective management of patients in ambulatory settings. Nurses can play an important part in facilitating the function of ambulatory care facilities.

Occupational Health Programs

Federal legislation, especially the Occupational Safety and Health Act (OSHA), has had a major impact on health conditions in the workplace, with a goal of safe and healthy work conditions. It is in an employer's interest to provide a safe working environment, because decreased employee absenteeism, hospitalization, and disability are associated with reduced costs.

Occupational nurses may work in solo units in industrial settings, or they may serve as consultants on a limited or part-time basis. They may be members of an interdisciplinary team composed of a variety of personnel such as nurses, physicians, exercise physiologists, health educators, counselors, nutritionists, safety engineers, and industrial hygienists. Occupational health nurses may:

- Provide direct care to employees who become ill or injured
- Conduct health education programs for company staff members
- Set up health programs aimed at establishing specific health behaviors, such as eating properly and getting enough exercise
- Monitor employees' hearing, vision, blood pressure, or blood glucose
- Track exposure to radiation, infectious diseases, and toxic substances, reporting results to government agencies as necessary

Occupational health nurses must be knowledgeable about federal regulations pertaining to occupational health and familiar with other pertinent legislation, such as the Americans with Disabilities Act.

School Health Programs

School health programs provide services to students and may also serve the school's community. School-age children and adolescents with health problems are at major risk for underachieving or failing in school. The leading health problems of elementary school children are injuries, infections (including influenza and pneumonia), malnutrition, dental disease, and cancer. The leading problems of high school students are alcohol and drug abuse, injuries, homicide, pregnancy, eating disorders, sexually transmitted diseases/infections, sports injuries, dental disease, and mental and emotional problems.

Ideally, school health programs have an interdisciplinary health team consisting of physicians, nurses, dentists, social workers, counselors, school administrators, parents, and students. The school may serve as the site for a family health clinic that offers primary health and mental health services to children and adolescents as well as to all family members in the community. School nurses with baccalaureate and advanced degrees are ideally suited to provide primary care in these settings. Physical examinations are performed by advanced practice nurses, who then diagnose and treat students and families for acute and chronic illnesses. These clinics are cost-effective and benefit students from low-income families who lack access to traditional health care or have no health insurance.

School nurses play a number of roles, including care provider, health educator, consultant, and counselor. They collaborate with students, parents, administrators, and other health and social service professionals regarding student health problems. School nurses perform health screenings, provide basic care for minor injuries and complaints, administer medications, monitor the immunization status of students and families, and identify children with health problems. They need to be knowledgeable about state and local regulations affecting school-age children, such as ordinances for excluding students from school because of communicable diseases or parasites such as lice or scabies.

School nurses are also health education consultants for teachers. In addition to providing information on health practices, teaching health classes, or participating in the development of the health education curriculum, school nurses educate teachers and classes when one of the students has a special problem, a disability, or a disease such as hemophilia, human immunodeficiency virus (HIV) infection, or acquired immunodeficiency syndrome (AIDS).

Community Nurse–Managed Centers

Community nurse–managed centers are a relatively new concept in community-based nursing, having appeared only in the past 25 years. Frequently sponsored by academic centers, these centers typically are designed for the delivery of primary health care. Their services are geared toward serving people and groups who are vulnerable, uninsured, and without access to health services. Typically, community nurse–managed centers are run by advanced practice nurses and serve a large number of patients who are poor, members of minority groups, women, elderly, or homeless. The nurses provide health teaching, wellness and illness care, case management services, and psychosocial counseling (Neff, Mahama, Mohar, et al., 2003).

Care for the Homeless

No exact figures exist on the number of homeless people in the United States, but in any given year an estimated 3.5 million people, 1.35 million of them children, are homeless (National Coalition for the Homeless, 2002; Urban Institute, 2000). Homelessness is a growing problem, and the homeless population includes growing numbers of women with children (often victims of abuse) and elderly people. The homeless are a heterogeneous group, including members of dysfunctional families, the unemployed, and those who cannot find affordable housing. A large number of homeless people are chronically mentally ill or abuse alcohol or other drugs (National Coalition for the Homeless, 2004). Some are temporarily homeless as a result of catastrophic natural disasters.

Homeless people often have limited or no access to health care. Because of numerous barriers, they seek health care late in the course of a disease and deteriorate more quickly than other patients. Many of their health problems are related in large part to their living situation. Street life exposes people to the extremes of hot and cold environments and compounds their health risks. Homeless people have high rates of trauma, tuberculosis, upper respiratory tract infections, poor nutrition and anemia, lice, scabies, peripheral vascular problems, sexually transmitted diseases/infections, dental problems, arthritis, hypothermia, skin disorders, and foot problems. Common chronic health problems also include diabetes, hypertension, heart disease, AIDS, and mental illness. These problems are made more difficult by living on the streets or being discharged to a transitory, homeless situation in which follow-up care is unlikely. Shelters frequently are overcrowded and unventilated, promoting the spread of communicable diseases such as tuberculosis.

Community-based nurses who work with homeless people must be nonjudgmental, patient, and understanding. They must be skilled in dealing with people who have a wide variety of health problems and needs and must recognize that individualized treatment strategies are required in highly unpredictable environments (Bailey, 2004). Nursing interventions are aimed at evaluating the health care needs of people who live in shelters and attempting to obtain health care services for all homeless people.

Critical Thinking Exercises

1 You are assisting with discharge of a homeless 20-year-old woman who has a healthy newborn 8-pound boy. What processes are needed to secure resources for follow-up care for the mother and child? What problems do you anticipate in trying to secure the services? How can you facilitate the use of community resources by this woman?

2 ebp An elderly man with diabetes is being referred for home care after discharge from the hospital, and he will need glucose monitoring and teaching. He has no family at home; his wife died 3 years ago, and his only daughter lives several hundred miles away. During the nurse's initial visit to the man's home, the nurse learns that he has difficulty seeing and therefore cannot read. What is the evidence base for conducting a safety assessment of the home environment for elderly patients and for patients with visual limitations? Evaluate the strength of the evidence. What assessment criteria would you use to assess the needs of the patient's home care situation?

REFERENCES AND SELECTED READINGS

BOOKS

Carson, V. B., & Koenig, H. G. (2002). *Parish nursing.* Radnor, PA: Templeton Foundation Press.

Clark, M. J. (2003). *Community health nursing: Caring for populations* (4th ed). Upper Saddle River, NJ: Prentice-Hall/Pearson Education, Inc.

Smith-Temple, A. J., & Johnson, J. Y. (2005). *Nurses' guide to clinical procedures.* Philadelphia: Lippincott Williams & Wilkins.

Stanhope, M., & Lancaster, J. (2004). *Community and public health nursing* (6th ed). St. Louis: Mosby.

JOURNALS

Bailey, S. (2004). Nursing knowledge in integrated care. *Nursing Standard, 18*(44), 38–41.

Barton, A. J., Clark, L., & Baramee J. (2004). Tracking outcomes in community-based care. *Home Health Care Management & Practice, 16*(3), 171–176.

Birmingham, J. (2004). Discharge planning: A collaboration between provider and payer case managers using Medicare's conditions of participation. *Lippincott's Case Management, 9*(3), 147–151.

Chobanian, A. V., Bakris, G. L., Black, H. R., et al. (2003). Seventh Report of the Joint National Committee on Prevention, Detection, Evaluation, and Treatment of High Blood Pressure. *Hypertension, 42*(6), 1206–1252.

Goulding, M. R., Rogers, M. E., & Smith, S. M. (2003). Public health and aging: Trends in aging, United States and worldwide. *Journal of American Medical Association, 289*(11), 1371–1373.

Green-Hernandez, C., Quinn, A., Denman-Vitale, S., et al. (2004). Making nursing care culturally competent. *Holistic Nursing Practice, 18*(4), 215–218.

Kovner, C., & Harrington, C. (2001). Counting nurses: What is community health-public health nursing? *American Journal of Nursing, 101*(1), 59–60.

Locsin, R. (2003). The integration of family health, culture, and nursing: Prescriptions and practices. *Holistic Nursing Practice, 17*(1), 8–10.

Mezey, M. (2001). CH-PH nursing and older adults. *American Journal of Nursing, 101*(1), 60–61.

Milone-Nuzzo, P. (2003). Clinical nurse specialists in home care. *Clinical Nurse Specialist, 17*(5), 234–235.

National Association for Home Care and Hospice (2004). Basic statistics about home care. Available at: http://www.nahc.org/NAHC/Research/04HPC_stats.pdf. Accessed May 3, 2006.

National Association for Home Care and Hospice (2002). Hospice facts and statistics. Available at: http://www.nahc.org/NAHC/Research/04HPC_stats.pdf. Accessed May 3, 2006.

National Coalition for the Homeless (September 2002). How many people experience homelessness? (Fact sheet #2). Available at http://www.nationalhomeless.org/numbers.html. Retrieved Sept. 29, 2004.

National Coalition for the Homeless (May 2004). Who is homeless? (Fact sheet #3). Available at: http://www.nationalhomeless.org/who.html. Retrieved Sept. 29, 2004.

Neff, D. F., Mahama, N., Mohar, D., & Kinion, E. (2003). Nursing care delivered at academic community-based nurse-managed center. *Outcomes Management, 7*(2), 84–89.

Scala-Foley, M., Caruso, J., Ramos, R., & Reinhard, S. (2004). Medicare eligibility, enrollment, and coverage: Understanding the basics of a complicated system. *American Journal of Nursing, 104*(2), 81–83.

Skillen, D. L., Olson, J. K., & Gilbert, J. A. (2003). Promoting personal safety in community health: Four educational strategies. *Nurse Educator, 28*(2), 89–94.

Urban Institute. A new look at homelessness in America. Available at: http://www.urban.org. Retrieved Sept. 29, 2004.

Centers for Disease Control and Prevention. CDC/ADSTR strategic plan for public health workforce development. Available at: http://www.phppo.cdc.gov. Accessed May 1, 2006.

RESOURCES

Case Management Society of America (CMSA), 8201 Cantrell Road, Suite 230, Little Rock, AR 72227; 1-501-225-2229; http://www.cmsa.org. Accessed June 5, 2006.

Centers for Disease Control and Prevention (CDC), 1600 Clifton Road, Atlanta, GA 30333; 1-800-311-3435; http://www.cdc.gov. Accessed June 5, 2006.

Centers for Medicare and Medicaid Services (CMS), 7500 Security Boulevard, Baltimore, MD 21244-1850; 1-877-267-2323; http://www.cms.hhs.gov. Accessed June 5, 2006.

Joint Commission on Accreditation of Healthcare Organizations (JCAHO), One Renaissance Blvd., Oakbrook Terrace, IL 60181; 1-630-792-5000; http://www.jcaho.org. Accessed June 5, 2006.

National Association for Home Care, 228 7th Street, SE, Washington, DC 20003; 1-202-547-7424.

National Association of School Nurses, Inc., Eastern Office, P.O. Box 1300, Scarborough, ME 04070-1300; 1-877-627-6476; http://www.nasn.org. Accessed June 5, 2006.

National Guideline Clearing House (NGC): http://www.guideline.gov. Accessed June 5, 2006.

NurseLinx.com (MDLinx Inc.), 1025 Vermont Avenue, NW, Suite 810, Washington, DC 20005; 1-202-543-6544; http://www.nurselinx.com. Accessed June 5, 2006.

Urban Institute, 2100 M Street, NW, Washington, DC 20037.

CHAPTER 3

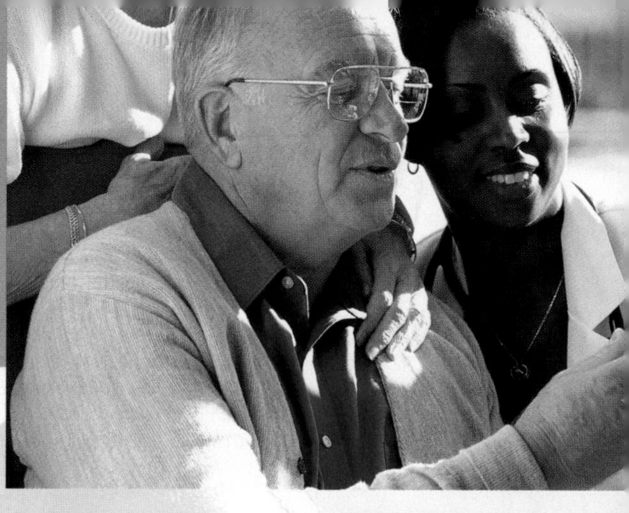

Critical Thinking, Ethical Decision Making, and the Nursing Process

Learning Objectives

On completion of this chapter, the learner will be able to:

1. Define the characteristics of critical thinking and critical thinkers.
2. Describe the critical thinking process.
3. Define ethics and nursing ethics.
4. Identify several ethical dilemmas common to the medical-surgical area of nursing practice.
5. Specify strategies that can be helpful to nurses in ethical decision making.
6. Describe the components of the nursing process.
7. Describe the nursing process.
8. Develop a plan of nursing care for a patient using strategies of critical thinking.

In today's health care arena, nurses are faced with increasingly complex issues and situations resulting from advanced technology, greater acuity of patients in hospital and community settings, an aging population, and complex disease processes, as well as ethical issues and cultural factors. Traditionally, nurses have used a problem-solving approach in planning and providing nursing care. Today, the decision-making part of problem solving has become increasingly complex and requires critical thinking.

Critical Thinking

Definition

Critical thinking is a multidimensional skill, a cognitive or mental process or set of procedures. It involves reasoning and purposeful, systematic, reflective, rational, outcome-directed thinking based on a body of knowledge, as well as examination and analysis of all available information and ideas. Critical thinking leads to the formulation of conclusions and alternatives that are the most appropriate for the situation. Although many definitions of critical thinking have been offered in various disciplines, some consistent themes within those definitions are (1) a strong formal and informal foundation of knowledge; (2) willingness to pursue or ask questions; and (3) ability to develop solutions that are new, even those that do not fit the standard or current state of knowledge or attitudes. Willingness and openness to various viewpoints are inherent in critical thinking, and it is important to question the current state of a situation or knowledge (Jackson, 2004). Critical thinking includes metacognition, the examination of one's own reasoning or thought processes, to help refine thinking skills (Wilkinson, 2001). Independent judgments and decisions evolve from a sound knowledge base and the ability to synthesize information within the context in which it is presented. Nursing practice in today's society requires the use of high-level critical thinking skills within the nursing process. Critical thinking enhances clinical decision making, helping to identify patient needs and to determine the best nursing actions that will assist patients in meeting those needs.

As indicated previously, critical thinking is a conscious, outcome-oriented activity. Critical thinking is not erratic but rather is systematic and organized. Critical thinking and critical thinkers have distinctive characteristics. People who engage in critical thinking are inquisitive truth seekers who are open to the alternative solutions that might surface. Alfaro-LeFevre (2003) identified critical thinkers as individuals with the following ideal characteristics: active thinker, fair-minded, open-minded, persistent, empathic, independent in thought, good communicator, honest, organized and systematic, proactive, flexible, realistic, humble, cognizant of the rules of logic, curious and insightful, and creative and committed to excellence. The skills involved in critical thinking are developed over time, through effort, practice, and experience.

Rationality and Insight

Skills needed in critical thinking include interpretation, analysis, evaluation, inference, explanation, and self-regulation. Critical thinking requires background knowledge and knowledge of key concepts as well as standards of logical thinking. Nurses use this disciplined process to validate the accuracy of data and the reliability of any assumptions they have made, and they then carefully evaluate the effectiveness of what they have identified as the necessary actions to take (Jackson, 2004). Nurses also evaluate the reliability of sources, being mindful of and questioning inconsistencies. Nurses use interpretation to determine the significance of data that are gathered, analysis to identify patient problems suggested by the data, and inference to draw conclusions. Explanation is the justification of actions or interventions used to address patient problems and to help patients move toward desired outcomes. Evaluation is the process of determining whether outcomes have been or are being met. Self-regulation is the process of examining the care provided and adjusting the interventions as needed.

Critical thinking is also reflective, involving metacognition, active evaluation, and refinement of the thinking process. Nurses engaged in critical thinking consider the possibility of personal bias when interpreting data and determining appropriate actions. Critical thinkers must be insightful and have a sense of fairness and integrity; the courage to question personal ethics; and the perseverance to strive continuously to minimize the effects of egocentricity, ethnocentricity, and other biases on the decision-making process (Alfaro-LeFevre, 2003).

Components of Critical Thinking

Certain cognitive or mental activities are key components of critical thinking. Critical thinkers:

- Ask questions to determine why certain developments have occurred and to see whether more information is needed to understand the situation accurately
- Gather as much relevant information as possible to consider as many factors as possible
- Validate the information presented to make sure that it is accurate (not just supposition or opinion), that it makes sense, and that it is based on fact and evidence
- Analyze the information to determine what it means and to see whether it forms clusters or patterns that point to certain conclusions
- Draw on past clinical experience and knowledge to explain what is happening and to anticipate what might happen next, acknowledging personal bias and cultural influences
- Maintain a flexible attitude that allows the facts to guide thinking and takes into account all possibilities
- Consider available options and examine each in terms of its advantages and disadvantages
- Formulate decisions that reflect creativity and independent decision making

Critical thinking requires going beyond basic problem solving into a realm of inquisitive exploration, looking for all relevant factors that affect the issue, and being an "out-of-the-box" thinker. It includes questioning all findings until a comprehensive picture emerges that explains the phenomenon, possible solutions, and creative methods for proceeding (Wilkinson, 2001). Critical thinking in nursing practice results in a comprehensive plan of care with maximized potential for success.

Critical Thinking in Nursing Practice

Critical thinking and decision making have been associated with improved clinical expertise (Martin, 2002). Critical thinking is at the center of the process of clinical reasoning and clinical judgment (Jackson, 2004). Using critical thinking to develop a plan of nursing care requires considering the human factors that might influence the plan. Nurses interact with patients, families, and other health care providers in the process of providing appropriate, individualized nursing care. The culture, attitude, and thought processes of nurses, patients, and others affect the critical thinking process from the data-gathering stage through the decision-making stage; therefore, aspects of the nurse–patient interaction must be considered (Wilkinson, 2001).

Nurses must use critical thinking skills in all practice settings—acute care, ambulatory care, extended care, and the home and community. Regardless of the setting, each patient situation is viewed as unique and dynamic. Key components of critical thinking behavior are withholding judgment and being open to options and explanations from one patient to another in similar circumstances (Jackson, 2004). The unique factors that patients and nurses bring to the health care situation are considered, studied, analyzed, and interpreted. Interpretation of the information then allows nurses to focus on those factors that are most relevant and most significant to the clinical situation. Decisions about what to do and how to do it are then developed into a plan of action.

In decision making related to the nursing process, nurses use intellectual skills in critical thinking. These skills include systematic and comprehensive assessment, recognition of assumptions and inconsistencies, verification of reliability and accuracy, identification of missing information, distinguishing relevant from irrelevant information, support of the evidence with facts and conclusions, priority setting with timely decision making, determination of patient-specific outcomes, and reassessment of responses and outcomes (Alfaro-LeFevre, 2003).

Because developing the skill of critical thinking takes time and practice, critical thinking exercises are offered throughout this book as a means of honing one's ability to think critically. Some of the exercises include questions that stimulate the reader to seek information about evidence-based practice relative to the clinical situation described. Additional exercises may be found in the study guide that accompanies the text. The questions listed in Chart 3-1 can serve as a guide in working through the exercises, although it is important to remember that each situation is unique and calls for an approach that fits the particular circumstances described.

In addition, much emphasis is placed on nurses basing their clinical actions on research, using evidence-based practice. Critical thinking has been associated with the

CHART 3-1

The Inquiring Mind: Critical Thinking in Action

Throughout the critical thinking process, a continuous flow of questions evolves in the thinker's mind. Although the questions will vary according to the particular clinical situation, certain general inquiries can serve as a basis for reaching conclusions and determining a course of action.

When faced with a patient situation, it is often helpful to seek answers to some or all of the following questions in an attempt to determine those actions that are most appropriate:

- What relevant assessment information do I need, and how do I interpret this information? What does this information tell me?
- To what problems does this information point? Have I identified the most important ones? Does the information point to any other problems that I should consider?
- Have I gathered all the information I need (signs and symptoms, laboratory values, medication history, emotional factors, mental status)? Is anything missing?
- Is there anything that needs to be reported immediately? Do I need to seek additional assistance?
- Does this patient have any special risk factors? Which ones are most significant? What must I do to minimize these risks?
- What possible complications must I anticipate?
- What are the most important problems in this situation? Do the patient and the patient's family recognize the same problems?
- What are the desired outcomes for this patient? Which have the highest priority? Do the patient and I agree on these points?
- What is going to be my first action in this situation?
- How can I construct a plan of care to achieve the goals?
- Are there any age-related factors involved, and will they require some special approach? Will I need to make some change in the plan of care to take these factors into account?
- How do the family dynamics affect this situation, and will they have an effect on my actions or the plan of care?
- Are there cultural factors that I must address and consider?
- Am I dealing with an ethical issue here? If so, how am I going to resolve it?
- Has any nursing research been conducted on this subject? What are the nursing implications of this research for care of this patient?

use of research findings (Profetto-McGrath, Hesketh, Lang, et al., 2003).

Ethical Nursing Care

In the complex modern world, we are surrounded by ethical issues in all facets of our lives. Consequently, there has been a heightened interest in the field of ethics in an attempt to gain a better understanding of how these issues influence us. Specifically, the focus on ethics in health care has intensified in response to controversial developments, including advances in technology and genetics, as well as diminished health care and financial resources.

Today, sophisticated technology can prolong life well beyond the time when death would have occurred in the past. Expensive experimental procedures, medications, equipment, and devices are available for attempting to preserve life, even when such attempts are likely to fail. The development of technologic support has influenced patients at all stages of life and also contributed to an increase in average life expectancy. For example, the prenatal period has been influenced by genetic screening, in vitro fertilization, the harvesting and freezing of embryos, and prenatal surgery. Premature infants who once would have died early in life now may survive because of technical advances. Children and adults who would have died of organ failure are living longer because of organ transplantation.

These advances in technology have been a mixed blessing. Questions have been raised about whether it is appropriate to use such technology, and if so, under what circumstances. Although many patients do achieve a better quality of life, others face extended suffering as a result of efforts to prolong life, usually at great expense. Ethical issues also surround those practices or policies that seem to allocate health care resources unjustly on the basis of age, race, gender, disability, or social mores.

The ethical dilemmas nurses may encounter in the medical-surgical nursing arena are numerous and diverse and occur in all settings. An awareness of underlying philosophical concepts helps nurses use reason to work through these dilemmas. Basic concepts related to moral philosophy, such as ethics and its terminology, theories, and approaches, are included in this chapter. Understanding the role of the professional nurse in ethical decision making helps nurses articulate their ethical positions and develop the skills needed to make ethical decisions.

Ethics Versus Morality

The terms *ethics* and *morality* are used to describe beliefs about right and wrong and to suggest appropriate guidelines for action. In essence, ethics is the formal, systematic study of moral beliefs, whereas morality is the adherence to informal personal values. Because the distinction between the *ethics* and *morality* is slight, the two terms are often used interchangeably.

Ethics Theories

One classic theory in ethics is teleologic theory or consequentialism, which focuses on the ends or consequences of actions. The best-known form of this theory, utilitarianism, is based on the concept of "the greatest good for the greatest number." The choice of action is clear under this theory, because the action that maximizes good over bad is the correct one. The theory poses difficulty when one must judge intrinsic values and determine whose good is the greatest. In addition, it is important to ask whether good consequences can justify any amoral actions that might be used to achieve them.

Another theory in ethics is the deontologic or formalist theory, which argues that ethical standards or principles exist independently of the ends or consequences. In a given situation, one or more ethical principles may apply. Nurses have a duty to act based on the one relevant principle, or the most relevant of several ethical principles. Problems arise with this theory when personal and cultural biases influence the choice of the most primary ethical principle.

Approaches to Ethics

Two approaches to ethics are meta-ethics and applied ethics. An example of meta-ethics (understanding the concepts and linguistic terminology used in ethics) in the health care environment is analysis of the concept of informed consent. Nurses are aware that patients must give consent before surgery, but sometimes a question arises as to whether a patient is truly informed. Delving more deeply into the concept of informed consent would be a meta-ethical inquiry.

An example of applied ethics is for a specific discipline to identify ethical problems within that discipline's practice. Various disciplines use the frameworks of general ethical theories and principles and apply them to specific problems within their domain. Common ethical principles that apply in nursing include autonomy, beneficence, confidentiality, double effect, fidelity, justice, nonmaleficence, paternalism, respect for people, sanctity of life, and veracity. Brief definitions of these important principles can be found in Chart 3-2.

Nursing ethics may be considered a form of applied ethics because it addresses moral situations that are specific to the nursing profession and patient care. Some ethical problems that affect nursing may also apply to the broader area of bioethics and health care ethics. However, the nursing profession is a "caring" rather than a predominantly "curing" profession; therefore, it is imperative that one not equate nursing ethics solely with medical ethics, because the medical profession has a "cure" focus. Nursing has its own professional code of ethics.

Moral Situations

Many situations exist in which ethical analysis is needed. Some are *moral dilemmas,* situations in which a clear conflict exists between two or more moral principles or competing moral claims, and nurses must choose the lesser of two evils. Other situations represent *moral problems,* in which there may be competing moral claims or principles, but one claim or principle is clearly dominant. Some situations result in *moral uncertainty,* when one cannot accurately define what the moral situation is or what moral principles apply but has a strong feeling that something is not right. Still other situations may result in *moral distress,* in which one is aware of the correct course of action but institutional constraints stand in the way of pursuing the correct action.

CHART 3-2

Common Ethical Principles

The following common ethical principles may be used to validate moral claims.

AUTONOMY

This word is derived from the Greek words *autos* ("self") and *nomos* ("rule" or "law"), and therefore refers to self-rule. In contemporary discourse it has broad meanings, including individual rights, privacy, and choice. Autonomy entails the ability to make a choice free from external constraints.

BENEFICENCE

Beneficence is the duty to do good and the active promotion of benevolent acts (eg, goodness, kindness, charity). It may also include the injunction not to inflict harm (see nonmaleficence).

CONFIDENTIALITY

Confidentiality relates to the concept of privacy. Information obtained from an individual will not be disclosed to another unless it will benefit the person or there is a direct threat to the social good.

DOUBLE EFFECT

This is a principle that may morally justify some actions that produce both good and evil effects.

All four of the following criteria must be fulfilled:

1. The action itself is good or morally neutral.
2. The agent sincerely intends the good and not the evil effect (the evil effect may be foreseen but is not intended).
3. The good effect is not achieved by means of the evil effect.
4. There is proportionate or favorable balance of good over evil.

FIDELITY

Fidelity is promise keeping; the duty to be faithful to one's commitments. It includes both explicit and implicit promises to another person.

JUSTICE

From a broad perspective, justice states that like cases should be treated alike. A more restricted version of justice is *distributive justice,* which refers to the distribution of social benefits and burdens based on various criteria that may include the following:

- Equality
- Individual need
- Individual effort
- Societal contribution
- Individual merit
- Legal entitlement

Retributive justice is concerned with the distribution of punishment.

NONMALEFICENCE

This is the duty not to inflict harm as well as to prevent and remove harm. Nonmaleficence may be included within the principle of beneficence, in which case nonmaleficence would be more binding.

PATERNALISM

Paternalism is the intentional limitation of another's autonomy, justified by an appeal to beneficence or the welfare or needs of another. Under this principle, the prevention of evil or harm takes precedence over any potential evil caused by interference with the individual's autonomy or liberty.

RESPECT FOR PERSONS

Respect for persons is frequently used synonymously with *autonomy*. However, it goes beyond accepting the notion or attitude that people have autonomous choices, to treating others in such a way that enables them to make choices.

SANCTITY OF LIFE

This is the perspective that life is the highest good. Therefore, all forms of life, including mere biologic existence, should take precedence over external criteria for judging quality of life.

VERACITY

Veracity is the obligation to tell the truth and not to lie or deceive others.

For example, a patient tells a nurse that if he is dying, he wants all possible measures taken to save his life. However, the surgeon and family have made the decision not to tell the patient that he is terminally ill and not to resuscitate him if he stops breathing. From an ethical perspective, the patient should be told the truth about his diagnosis and should have the opportunity to make decisions about treatment. Ideally, this information should come from the physician, with the nurse present to assist the patient in understanding the terminology and to provide further support, if necessary. A moral problem exists because of the competing moral claims of the family and physician, who wish to spare the patient distress, and the nurse, who wishes to be truthful with the patient as the patient has requested. If the patient's competency were questionable, a moral dilemma would exist because no dominant principle would be evident. The nurse could experience moral distress if the hospital threatened disciplinary action or job termination because the information is disclosed to the patient without the agreement of the physician or the family, or both.

It is essential that nurses freely engage in dialogue concerning moral situations, even though such dialogue is difficult for everyone involved. Improved interdisciplinary communication is supported when all members of the health care team can voice their concerns and come to an understanding of the moral situation. The use of an ethics consultant or consultation team could be helpful to assist the health care team, patient, and family to identify the moral dilemma and possible approaches to the dilemma. Nurses should be familiar with agency policy supporting patient self-determination and resolution of ethical issues.

Types of Ethical Problems in Nursing

As a profession, nursing is accountable to society. This accountability is spelled out in the American Hospital Association's Patient Care Partnership (Chart 3-3), which reflects social beliefs about health and health care. In addition to accepting this document as one measure of accountability, nursing has further defined its standards of accountability through a formal code of ethics that explicitly states the profession's values and goals. The code (Chart 3-4), established by the American Nurses Association (ANA), consists of ethical standards, each with its own interpretive statements (ANA, 2001). The interpretive statements provide guidance to address and resolve ethical dilemmas by incorporating universal moral principles (ANA's Code of Ethics Project Task Force, 2000). The code is an ideal framework for nurses to use in ethical decision making.

Ethical issues have always affected the role of professional nurses. The accepted definition of professional nursing has inspired a new advocacy role for nurses. The ANA, in *Nursing's Social Policy Statement* (2003, p. 6), defines nursing as "the protection, promotion, and optimization of health and abilities, prevention of illness and injury, alleviation of suffering through the diagnosis and treatment of human response, and advocacy in the care of individuals, families, communities, and populations." This definition supports the claim that nurses must be actively involved in the decision-making process regarding ethical concerns surrounding health care and human responses. Efforts to enact this standard may cause conflict in health care settings in which the traditional roles of nurses are delineated within a bureaucratic structure. However, if nurses learn to present ethical conflicts within a logical, systematic framework, struggles over jurisdictional boundaries may decrease. Health care settings in which nurses are valued members of the team promote interdisciplinary communication and may enhance patient care. To practice effectively in these settings, nurses must be aware of ethical issues and assist patients in voicing their moral concerns.

A basic ethical framework of the nursing profession is the phenomenon of human caring. Nursing theories that incorporate the biopsychosocial–spiritual dimensions emphasize a holistic viewpoint, with humanism or caring as the core. As the nursing profession strives to delineate its own theory of ethics, caring is often cited as the moral foundation. For nurses to embrace this professional ethos, they must be aware not only of major ethical dilemmas but also of those daily interactions with health care consumers that frequently give rise to less easily identifiable ethical challenges. Although technologic advances and diminished resources have been instrumental in raising numerous ethical questions and controversies, including life-and-death issues, nurses should not ignore the many routine sit-

CHART 3-3

The Patient Care Partnership: Understanding Expectations, Rights, and Responsibilities

When you need hospital care, your doctor and the nurses and other professionals at our hospital are committed to working with you and your family to meet your health care needs. Our dedicated doctors and staff serve the community in all its ethnic, religious, and economic diversity. Our goal is for you and your family to have the same care and attention we would want for our families and ourselves.

The sections below explain some of the basics about how you can expect to be treated during your hospital stay. They also cover what we will need from you to care for you better. If you have questions at any time, please ask them. Unasked or unanswered questions can add to the stress of being in the hospital. Your comfort and confidence in your care are very important to us.

What to Expect During Your Hospital Stay

High quality hospital care. Our first priority is to provide you the care you need, when you need it, with skill, compassion, and respect. Tell your caregivers if you have concerns about your care or if you have pain. You have the right to know the identity of doctors, nurses, and others involved in your care, as well as when they are students, residents, or other trainees.

A clean and safe environment. Our hospital works hard to keep you safe. We use special policies and procedures to avoid mistakes in your care and keep you free from abuse or neglect. If anything unexpected and significant happens during your hospital stay, you will be told what happened and any resulting changes in your care will be discussed with you.

Involvement in your care. You and your doctor often make decisions about your care before you go to the hospital. Other times, especially in emergencies, those decisions are made during your hospital stay. When they take place, making decisions should include:

- *Discussing your medical condition and information about medically appropriate treatment choices.* To make informed

continued >

CHART 3-3 *The Patient Care Partnership: Understanding Expectations, Rights, and Responsibilities, continued*

decisions with your doctor, you need to understand several things:
- The benefits and risks of each treatment.
- Whether it is experimental or part of a research study.
- What you can reasonably expect from your treatment and any long-term effects it might have on your quality of life.
- What you and your family will need to do after you leave the hospital.
- The financial consequences of using uncovered services or out-of-network providers.

Please tell your caregivers if you need more information about treatment choices.

- *Discussing your treatment plan.* When you enter the hospital, you sign a general consent to treatment. In some cases, such as surgery or experimental treatment, you may be asked to confirm in writing that you understand what is planned and agree to it. This process protects your right to consent to or refuse a treatment. Your doctor will explain the medical consequences of refusing recommended treatment. It also protects your right to decide if you want to participate in a research study.
- *Getting information from you.* Your caregivers need complete and correct information about your health and coverage so that they can make good decisions about your care. That includes:
  - Past illnesses, surgeries, or hospital stays.
  - Past allergic reactions.
  - Any medicines or diet supplements (such as vitamins and herbs) that you are taking.
  - Any network or admission requirements under your health plan.
- *Understanding your health care goals and values.* You may have health care goals and values or spiritual beliefs that are important to your well-being. They will be taken into account as much as possible throughout your hospital stay. Make sure your doctor, your family, and your care team know your wishes.
- *Understanding who should make decisions when you cannot.* If you have signed a health care power of attorney stating who should speak for you if you become unable to make health care decisions for yourself, or a "living will" or "advance directive" that states your wishes about end-of-life care, give copies to your doctor, your family, and your care team. If you or your family need help making difficult decisions, counselors, chaplains, and others are available to help.

Protection of your privacy. We respect the confidentiality of your relationship with your doctor and other caregivers, and the sensitive information about your health and health care that are part of that relationship. State and federal laws and hospital operating policies protect the privacy of your medical information. You will receive a Notice of Privacy Practices that describes the ways that we use, disclose and safeguard patient information and that explains how you can obtain a copy of information from our records about your care.

Help preparing you and your family for when you leave the hospital. Your doctor works with hospital staff and professionals in your community. You and your family also play an important role. The success of your treatment often depends on your efforts to follow medication, diet and therapy plans. Your family may need to help care for you at home.

You can expect us to help you identify sources of follow-up care and to let you know if our hospital has a financial interest in any referrals. As long as you agree we can share information about your care with them, we will coordinate our activities with your caregivers outside the hospital. You can also expect to receive information and, where possible, training about the self-care you will need when you go home.

Help with your bill and filing insurance claims. Our staff will file claims for you with health care insurers or other programs such as Medicare and Medicaid. They will also help your doctor with needed documentation. Hospital bills and insurance coverage are often confusing. If you have questions about your bill, contact our business office. If you need help understanding your insurance coverage or health plan, start with your insurance company or health benefits manager. If you do not have health coverage, we will try to help you and your family find financial help or make other arrangements. We need your help with collecting needed information and other requirements to obtain coverage or assistance.

While you are here, you will receive more detailed notices about some of the rights you have as a hospital patient and how to exercise them. We are always interested in improving. If you have questions, comments, or concerns, please contact ________________.

CHART 3-4

American Nurses Association Code of Ethics for Nurses

1. The nurse, in all professional relationships, practices with compassion and respect for the inherent dignity, worth, and uniqueness of every individual, unrestricted by considerations of social or economic status, personal attributes, or the nature of health problems.
2. The nurse's primary commitment is to the patient, whether an individual, family, group, or community.
3. The nurse promotes, advocates for, and strives to protect the health, safety, and rights of the patient.
4. The nurse is responsible and accountable for individual nursing practice and determines the appropriate delegation of tasks consistent with the nurse's obligation to provide optimum patient care.
5. The nurse owes the same duties to self as to others, including the responsibility to preserve integrity and safety, to maintain competence, and to continue personal and professional growth.
6. The nurse participates in establishing, maintaining, and improving health care environments and conditions of employment conducive to the provision of quality health care and consistent with the values of the profession through individual and collective action.
7. The nurse participates in the advancement of the profession through contributions to practice, education, administration, and knowledge development.
8. The nurse collaborates with other health professionals and the public in promoting community, national, and international efforts to meet health needs.
9. The profession of nursing, as represented by associations and their members, is responsible for articulating nursing values, for maintaining the integrity of the profession and its practice, and for shaping social policy.

uations that involve ethical considerations. Some of the most common issues faced by nurses today include confidentiality, use of restraints, trust, refusing care, and end-of-life concerns.

Confidentiality

All nurses should be aware of the confidential nature of information obtained in daily practice. If information is not pertinent, they should question whether it is prudent to record it in a patient's chart. In the practice setting, discussion of patients with other members of the health care team is often necessary. However, these discussions should occur in a private area where it is unlikely that the conversation will be overheard. Nurses should also be aware that the use of family members as interpreters for patients who are not fluent in the English language or who are deaf violates a patient's rights of confidentiality. Translation services should be provided for non–English-speaking patients and interpreters should be provided for those who use sign language.

Another threat to confidentiality is the widespread use of computers and the easy access people have to them. This may increase the potential for misuse of information. Because of these possibilities of maleficence (see Chart 3-2), sensitivity to the principle of confidentiality is essential.

Restraints

The use of restraints (including physical and pharmacologic measures) is another issue with ethical overtones. It is important to weigh carefully the risks of limiting a person's autonomy and increasing the risk of injury by using restraints against the risks of not using restraints. Before restraints are used, other strategies, such as asking family members to sit with the patient, should be tried. The Joint Commission on Accreditation of Healthcare Organizations (JCAHO) and the Centers for Medicare and Medicaid Services (CMS) have designated standards for use in care of patients with restraints; these standards are available on the website listed at the end of this chapter (JCAHO, 2003).

Trust Issues

Telling the truth (veracity) is one of the basic principles of our culture. Two ethical dilemmas in clinical practice that can directly conflict with this principle are the use of placebos (nonactive substances used to treat symptoms) and not revealing a diagnosis to a patient. Both involve the issue of trust, which is an essential element in the nurse–patient relationship. Placebos may be used in experimental research, in which a patient is involved in the decision-making process and is aware that placebos are being used in the treatment regimen. However, the use of a placebo as a substitute for an active drug to show that a patient does not have actual symptoms is deceptive, and this practice may severely undermine the nurse–patient relationship.

Informing a patient of his or her diagnosis when the family and physician have chosen to withhold information is a common ethical situation in nursing practice. The nursing staff may often use evasive comments with the patient as a means of maintaining professional relationships with other health practitioners. This area is indeed complex, because it challenges a nurse's integrity. Strategies nurses could consider include the following:

- Not lying to the patient
- Providing all information related to nursing procedures and diagnoses
- Communicating the patient's requests for information to the family and physician. The family is often unaware of the patient's repeated questions to a nurse. With a better understanding of the situation, the family members may change their perspective.

Finally, although providing the information may be the morally appropriate behavior, the manner in which the patient is told is important. Nurses must be compassionate and caring while informing patients; disclosure of information merely for the sake of patient autonomy does not convey respect for others.

Refusing to Provide Care

Any nurse who feels compelled to refuse to provide care for a particular type of patient faces an ethical dilemma. The reasons given for refusal range from a conflict of personal values to fear of personal injury. The ethical obligation to care for all patients is clearly identified in the first statement of the Code of Ethics for Nurses. To avoid facing these moral situations, nurses can follow certain strategies. For example, when applying for a job, a nurse should ask questions regarding the patient population. If a nurse is uncomfortable with a particular situation, then not accepting the position would be an option. Denial of care, or providing substandard nursing care to some members of society, is not acceptable nursing practice.

End-of-Life Issues

Dilemmas that center on death and dying are prevalent in medical-surgical nursing practice and frequently initiate moral discussion. Curing is paramount in health care, and this compounds the dilemmas. With advanced technology, it may be difficult to accept the fact that nothing more can be done to prolong life, or that technology may prolong life but at the expense of comfort and quality of life. Nurses are being faced with increasingly controversial dilemmas concerning patient desires to avoid prolongation of life. Many people who are terminally ill seek legal options for a peaceful and dignified death. Nurses may be in a quandary: they must choose between respect for the patient's autonomy and preservation of life (Valente, 2004).

End-of-life issues shift the focus from curative care to palliative and end-of-life care. Focusing on the caring as well as the curing role may help nurses deal with these difficult moral situations. Needs of patients and families require holistic and interdisciplinary approaches. In end-of-life care, nurses play the roles of clinician, advocate, and guide for patients and families (Norlander, 2001). End-of life issues are discussed in detail in Chapter 17.

PAIN CONTROL

The intent or goal of nursing interventions is to alleviate pain and suffering while promoting comfort. The administration of analgesia should be governed by the patient's needs. Patients in excruciating pain may require large doses of analgesics, and the use of opioids to alleviate the pain may present a dilemma for nurses. Fear of respiratory depression or unwarranted fear of addiction should not prevent nurses from attempting to alleviate pain in a dying patient or in a patient experiencing an episode of acute pain. For example, in the case of the terminally ill patient, the actions may be justified by the principle of double effect (see Chart 3-2). Induction of respiratory depression is not the intent of the actions and should not be used as a reason for withholding analgesia. However, the patient's respiratory status should be carefully monitored, and any signs of respiratory depression should be reported to the physician.

"DO-NOT-RESUSCITATE" ORDERS

The "do not resuscitate" (DNR) order can result in controversy. When a patient is competent to make decisions and chooses a DNR order, this choice should be honored, according to the principles of autonomy or respect for the person. However, a DNR order is sometimes interpreted to mean that patients require less nursing care, when actually these patients may have significant medical and nursing needs, all of which demand attention. Ethically, all patients deserve and should receive appropriate nursing care, regardless of their resuscitation status.

LIFE SUPPORT

It is important to consider the contrasting situation, in which a DNR decision has not been made by or for a dying patient. Nurses may be put in the uncomfortable position of initiating life-support measures when, because of a patient's physical condition, they appear futile. This frequently occurs when a patient is not competent to make the decision and the family (or surrogate decision maker) refuses to consider a DNR order as an option. In such cases, nurses may be told to perform a "slow code" (ie, not to rush to resuscitate the patient) or may be given a verbal order not to resuscitate the patient; both are unacceptable.

In such a situation, the best recourse for the nurse is to be aware of hospital policy related to the Patient Self-Determination Act (see the section on preventive ethics in this chapter, as well as Chapter 17) and execution of advance directives. The nurse should communicate with the physician. Discussion of the issue with the physician may lead to further communication with the family and to a reconsideration of the decision, especially if family members are afraid to let a loved one die with no further efforts at resuscitation. Finally, the nurse may find that when working with colleagues who are confronting such difficult situations, it helps to talk and listen to their concerns as a way of providing support.

FOOD AND FLUID

In addition to requesting that no heroic measures be taken to prolong life, dying patients may request that no more food or fluid be administered. Many people think that food and hydration are basic human needs, not "invasive measures," and therefore should always be maintained. However, some consider food and hydration as means of prolonging suffering. When evaluating this issue, the nurse must take into consideration the potential harm as well as the benefit to the patient of either administering or withdrawing sustenance.

Evaluation of harm requires a careful review of the reasons a person has requested the withdrawal of food and hydration. Although the principle of autonomy has considerable merit and is supported by the Code of Ethics for Nurses, there may be situations when the request for withdrawal of food and hydration cannot be upheld. For patients with decreased decision-making capacity, the issues are more complex. Some of these cases have reached courts of law, and different states have different case law precedents forbidding withdrawal of sustenance. Although an advance directive may provide some answers, at present there are no firm guidelines to assist nurses in this area.

Preventive Ethics

When a nurse is faced with two conflicting alternatives, it is his or her moral decision to choose the lesser of the two evils. Various preventive strategies are available to help nurses anticipate or avoid certain kinds of ethical dilemmas.

Frequently, dilemmas occur when health care practitioners are unsure of the patient's wishes because the patient is unconscious or too cognitively impaired to communicate directly. One famous court case in this area of clinical ethics is that of Nancy Cruzan, a young woman who was involved in a car crash, after which she remained in a persistent vegetative state. Her family endured a 3-year legal battle to have her feeding tube removed so that she could be allowed to die. The U.S. Supreme Court decided that a state could require "clear and convincing evidence" of the patient's wishes before withdrawing life support. This ruling and the public response to it served as an impetus for legislation concerning advance directives, entitled the Patient Self-Determination Act, which became effective in December 1991. The intent of this legislation is to encourage people to prepare advance directives in which they indicate their wishes concerning the degree of supportive care to be provided if they become incapacitated. The regulatory language is quite broad and allows different institutions latitude in implementing a person's directives. This legislation does not require a patient to have an advance directive, but it does require that the patient be informed about advance directives by the staff of the health care facility. Consequently, this is an area in which nursing can play a significant role in patient education.

In 2005, the highly publicized case of Terri Schiavo focused national attention on the importance of advance directives. Schiavo was a young woman who suffered severe brain damage in 1990 after her heart stopped because of a chemical imbalance that was believed to have been caused by an eating disorder. Court-appointed physicians ruled she was in a persistent vegetative state with no real consciousness or chance of recovery. She left no living will or advance directive. Her husband requested that her feeding tube be removed to allow her to die, but her parents opposed this for 7 years. They involved the courts, Congress, and the President. Terri Schiavo died in 2005 after the courts ruled that her feeding tube could be removed and not replaced. This case represents an area in which nurses can play a significant role in patient education about the significance of advance directives.

Advance Directives

Advance directives are legal documents that specify a person's wishes before hospitalization and provide valuable information that may assist health care providers in decision making. A living will is one type of advance directive. In most situations, living wills are limited to situations in which the patient's medical condition is deemed terminal. Because it is difficult to define "terminal" accurately, living wills are not always honored. Another potential drawback is that living wills are frequently written while people are in good health. It is not unusual for people to change their minds as their illness progresses; therefore, patients retain the option to nullify these documents.

Durable power of attorney for health care, in which one person identifies another person to make health care decisions on his or her behalf, is another type of advance directive. Patients may have clarified their wishes concerning a variety of medical situations. As such, the power of attorney for health care is a less restrictive type of advance directive. Laws concerning advance directives vary among state jurisdictions. However, even in states where these documents are not legally binding, they provide helpful information to determine the patient's prior expressed wishes in situations in which this information can no longer be obtained directly.

Ethics Committees

Institutional ethics committees, which exist in many hospitals to assist practitioners with ethical dilemmas, also aid in preventive ethics. The purpose of these multidisciplinary committees varies among institutions. In some hospitals, the committees exist solely for the purpose of developing policies, whereas in others, they may have a strong educational or consultation focus. Because these committees usually are composed of people with some advanced training in ethics, they are important resources for the health care team, patient, and family. Nurses with a particular interest or expertise in the area of ethics are valuable members of ethics committees and can serve as valuable resources for staff nurses.

The heightened interest in ethical decision making has resulted in many continuing education programs, ranging from small seminars or workshops to full-semester courses offered by local colleges or professional organizations. In addition, nursing and medical journals contain articles on ethical issues, and numerous textbooks on clinical ethics or nursing ethics are available. These are valuable resources because they discuss ethical theory and dilemmas of practice in greater depth. ANA publications also assist nurses with ethical decision making.

Ethical Decision Making

As noted in the preceding discussions, ethical dilemmas are common and diverse in nursing practice. Situations vary, and experience indicates that there are no clear solutions to these dilemmas. However, the fundamental philosophical principles are the same, and the process of moral reflection helps nurses justify their actions. The approach to ethical decision making can follow the steps of the nursing process. Chart 3-5 outlines the steps of an ethical analysis.

CHART 3-5

Steps of an Ethical Analysis

The following are guidelines to assist nurses in ethical decision making. These guidelines reflect an active process in decision making, similar to the nursing process detailed in this chapter.

ASSESSMENT

1. Assess the ethical/moral situations of the problem. This step entails recognition of the ethical, legal, and professional dimensions involved.
   a. Does the situation entail substantive moral problems (conflicts among ethical principles or professional obligations)?
   b. Are there procedural conflicts? (For example, who should make the decisions? Any conflicts among the patient, health care providers, family and guardians?)
   c. Identify the significant people involved and those affected by the decision.

PLANNING

2. Collect information.
   a. Include the following information: the medical facts, treatment options, nursing diagnoses, legal data, and the values, beliefs, and religious components.
   b. Make a distinction between the factual information and the values/beliefs.
   c. Validate the patient's capacity, or lack of capacity, to make decisions.
   d. Identify any other relevant information that should be elicited.
   e. Identify the ethical/moral issues and the competing claims.

IMPLEMENTATION

3. List the alternatives. Compare alternatives with applicable ethical principles and professional code of ethics. Choose either of the frameworks below, or other frameworks, and compare outcomes.
   a. *Utilitarian approach*: Predict the consequences of the alternatives; assign a positive or negative value to each consequence; choose the consequence that predicts the highest positive value or "the greatest good for the greatest number."
   b. *Deontological approach:* Identify the relevant moral principles; compare alternatives with moral principles; appeal to the "higher-level" moral principle if there is a conflict.

EVALUATION

4. Decide and evaluate the decision.
   a. What is the best or morally correct action?
   b. Give the ethical reasons for your decision.
   c. What are the ethical reasons against your decision?
   d. How do you respond to the reasons against your decision?

The Nursing Process

Definition

The nursing process is a deliberate problem-solving approach for meeting people's health care and nursing needs. Although the steps of the nursing process have been stated in various ways by different writers, the common components cited are assessment, diagnosis, planning, implementation, and evaluation. ANA's *Standards of Clinical Nursing Practice* (1998) includes an additional component entitled "outcome identification" and established the sequence of steps in the following order: assessment, diagnosis, outcome identification, planning, implementation, and evaluation. For the purposes of this text, the nursing process is based on the traditional five steps and delineates two components in the diagnosis step: nursing diagnoses and collaborative problems. After the diagnoses or problems have been determined, the desired outcomes are often evident. The traditional steps are defined as follows:

1. *Assessment:* The systematic collection of data to determine the patient's health status and any actual or potential health problems. (Analysis of data is included as part of the assessment. Analysis may also be identified as a separate step of the nursing process.)
2. *Diagnosis:* Identification of the following two types of patient problems:
   - *Nursing diagnoses:* Actual or potential health problems that can be managed by independent nursing interventions
   - *Collaborative problems:* "Certain physiologic complications that nurses monitor to detect onset or changes in status. Nurses manage collaborative problems using physician-prescribed and nursing-prescribed interventions to minimize the complications of the events" (Carpenito-Moyet, 2004).
3. *Planning:* Development of goals and outcomes, as well as a plan of care designed to assist the patient in resolving the diagnosed problems and achieving the identified goals and desired outcomes
4. *Implementation:* Actualization of the plan of care through nursing interventions
5. *Evaluation:* Determination of the patient's responses to the nursing interventions and the extent to which the outcomes have been achieved

Dividing the nursing process into distinct steps serves to emphasize the essential nursing actions that must be taken to address the patient's nursing diagnoses and manage any collaborative problems or complications. However, dividing the process into separate steps is artificial: the process functions as an integrated whole, with the steps being interrelated, interdependent, and recurrent (Fig. 3-1). Chart 3-6 presents an overview of the nursing activities involved in applying the nursing process.

Using the Nursing Process

Assessment

Assessment data are gathered through the health history and the physical assessment. In addition, ongoing monitoring is crucial to remain aware of changing patient needs and the effectiveness of nursing care.

HEALTH HISTORY

The health history is conducted to determine a person's state of wellness or illness and is best accomplished as part of a planned interview. The interview is a personal dialogue between a patient and a nurse that is conducted to obtain information. The nurse's approach to the patient largely determines the amount and quality of the information that is received. To achieve a relationship of mutual trust and respect, the nurse must have the ability to communicate a sincere interest in the patient. Examples of effective therapeutic communication techniques that can be used to achieve this goal are found in Table 3-1.

The use of a health history guide may help in obtaining pertinent information and in directing the course of the interview. A variety of health history formats designed to guide the interview are available, but they must be adapted to the responses, problems, and needs of the person. See Chapter 5 for further information about the health history.

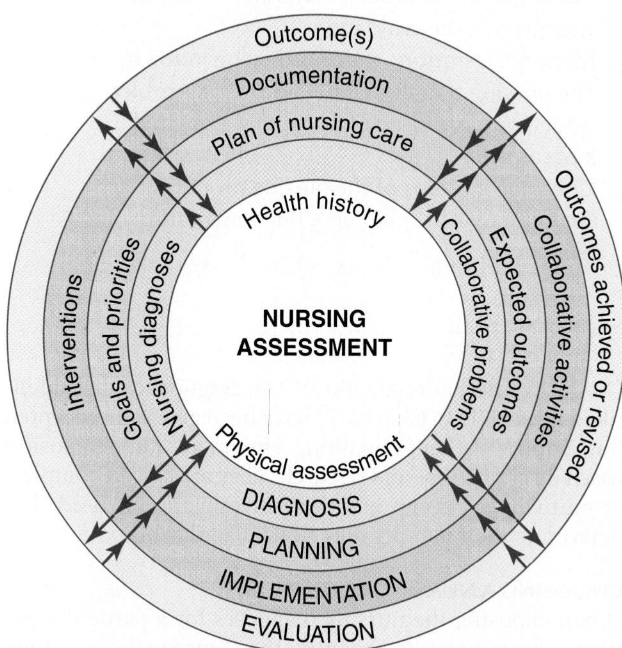

FIGURE 3-1. The nursing process is depicted schematically in this circle. Starting from the innermost circle, nursing assessment, the process moves outward through the formulation of nursing diagnoses and collaborative problems; planning, with setting of goals and priorities in the nursing plan of care; implementation and documentation; and, finally, the ongoing process of evaluation and outcomes.

PHYSICAL ASSESSMENT

A physical assessment may be carried out before, during, or after the health history, depending on a patient's physical and emotional status and the immediate priorities of the situation. The purpose of the physical assessment is to identify those aspects of a patient's physical, psychological, and emotional state that indicate a need for nursing care. It requires the use of sight, hearing, touch, and smell, as well as the appropriate interview skills and techniques. Physical examination techniques as well as techniques and strategies for assessing behaviors and role changes are presented in Chapters 5 and 7 and in each unit of this book.

OTHER COMPONENTS OF THE ASSESSMENT

Additional relevant information should be obtained from the patient's family or significant others, from other members of the health team, and from the patient's health record or chart. Depending on the patient's immediate needs, this information may have been completed before the health history and the physical assessment were obtained. Whatever the sequence of events, it is important to use all available sources of pertinent data to complete the nursing assessment.

RECORDING THE DATA

After the health history and physical assessment are completed, the information obtained is recorded in the patient's permanent record. This record provides a means of communication among members of the health care team and facilitates coordinated planning and continuity of care. The record fulfills other functions as well:

- It serves as the legal and business record for a health care agency and for the professional staff members who are responsible for the patient's care. A variety of systems are used for documenting patient care, and each health care agency selects the system that best meets its needs.
- It serves as a basis for evaluating the quality and appropriateness of care and for reviewing the effective use of patient care services.
- It provides data that are useful in research, education, and short- and long-range planning.

Diagnosis

The assessment component of the nursing process serves as the basis for identifying nursing diagnoses and collaborative problems. Soon after the completion of the health history and the physical assessment, nurses organize, analyze, synthesize, and summarize the data collected and determine the patient's need for nursing care.

CHART 3-6

Steps of the Nursing Process

ASSESSMENT
1. Conduct the health history.
2. Perform the physical assessment.
3. Interview the patient's family or significant others.
4. Study the health record.
5. Organize, analyze, synthesize, and summarize the collected data.

DIAGNOSIS

Nursing Diagnosis
1. Identify the patient's nursing problems.
2. Identify the defining characteristics of the nursing problems.
3. Identify the etiology of the nursing problems.
4. State nursing diagnoses concisely and precisely.

Collaborative Problems
1. Identify potential problems or complications that require collaborative interventions.
2. Identify health team members with whom collaboration is essential.

PLANNING
1. Assign priority to the nursing diagnoses.
2. Specify the goals.
   a. Develop immediate, intermediate, and long-term goals.
   b. State the goals in realistic and measurable terms.
3. Identify nursing interventions appropriate for goal attainment.
4. Establish expected outcomes.
   a. Make sure that the outcomes are realistic and measurable.
   b. Identify critical times for the attainment of outcomes.
5. Develop the written plan of nursing care.
   a. Include nursing diagnoses, goals, nursing interventions, expected outcomes, and critical times.
   b. Write all entries precisely, concisely, and systematically.
   c. Keep the plan current and flexible to meet the patient's changing problems and needs.
6. Involve the patient, family or significant others, nursing team members, and other health team members in all aspects of planning.

IMPLEMENTATION
1. Put the plan of nursing care into action.
2. Coordinate the activities of the patient, family or significant others, nursing team members, and other health team members.
3. Record the patient's responses to the nursing actions.

EVALUATION
1. Collect data.
2. Compare the patient's actual outcomes with the expected outcomes. Determine the extent to which the expected outcomes were achieved.
3. Include the patient, family or significant others, nursing team members, and other health care team members in the evaluation.
4. Identify alterations that need to be made in the nursing diagnoses, collaborative problems, goals, nursing interventions, and expected outcomes.
5. Continue all steps of the nursing process: assessment, diagnosis, planning, implementation, and evaluation.

NURSING DIAGNOSIS

Nursing, unlike medicine, does not yet have a complete taxonomy, or classification system, of diagnostic labels. Nursing diagnoses, the first taxonomy created in nursing, have fostered the development of autonomy and accountability in nursing and have helped to delineate the scope of practice. Many state nurse practice acts include nursing diagnosis as a nursing function, and nursing diagnosis is included in the ANA's *Standards of Clinical Nursing Practice* and the standards of many nursing specialty organizations.

NANDA International (founded in 1982 as the North American Nursing Diagnosis Association) is the official organization that has assumed responsibility for developing the taxonomy of nursing diagnoses and formulating nursing diagnoses acceptable for study. The most commonly selected nursing diagnoses are compiled and categorized by NANDA in a taxonomy that is updated at least every 2 years (NANDA International, 2005). The diagnostic labels identified by NANDA (Chart 3-7) have been generally accepted but require further validation, refinement, and expansion based on clinical use and research. They are not yet complete or mutually exclusive, and more investigation is needed to determine their validity and clinical applicability.

CHOOSING A NURSING DIAGNOSIS

When choosing the nursing diagnoses for a particular patient, nurses must first identify the commonalities among the assessment data collected. These common features lead to the categorization of related data that reveal the existence of a problem and the need for nursing intervention. The identified problems are then defined as specific nursing diagnoses (see Chart 3-7). Nursing diagnoses represent actual or potential health problems that can be managed by independent nursing actions.

TABLE 3-1 Therapeutic Communication Techniques

Technique	Definition	Therapeutic Value
Listening	Active process of receiving information and examining one's reactions to the messages received	Nonverbally communicates nurse's interest in patient
Silence	Periods of no verbal communication among participants for therapeutic reasons	Gives patient time to think and gain insights, slows the pace of the interaction, and encourages the patient to initiate conversation, while conveying the nurse's support, understanding, and acceptance
Restating	Repeating to the patient what the nurse believes is the main thought or idea expressed	Demonstrates that the nurse is listening and validates, reinforces, or calls attention to something important that has been said
Reflection	Directing back to the patient his or her feelings, ideas, questions, or content	Validates the nurse's understanding of what the patient is saying and signifies empathy, interest, and respect for the patient
Clarification	Asking the patient to explain what he or she means or attempting to verbalize vague ideas or unclear thoughts of the patient to enhance the nurse's understanding	Helps to clarify the patient's feelings, ideas, and perceptions and to provide an explicit correlation between them and the patient's actions
Focusing	Questions or statements to help the patient develop or expand an idea	Allows the patient to discuss central issues and keeps communication goal-directed
Broad openings	Encouraging the patient to select topics for discussion	Indicates acceptance by the nurse and the value of the patient's initiative
Humor	Discharge of energy through the comic enjoyment of the imperfect	Promotes insight by bringing repressed material to consciousness, resolving paradoxes, tempering aggression, and revealing new options; a socially acceptable form of sublimation
Informing	Providing information	Helpful in health teaching or patient education about relevant aspects of patient's well-being and self-care
Sharing perceptions	Asking the patient to verify the nurse's understanding of what the patient is thinking or feeling	Conveys the nurse's understanding to the patient and has the potential to clarify confusing communication
Theme identification	Underlying issues or problems experienced by the patient that emerge repeatedly during the course of the nurse–patient relationship	Allows the nurse to best promote the patient's exploration and understanding of important problems
Suggesting	Presentation of alternative ideas for the patient's consideration relative to problem solving	Increases the patient's perceived options or choices

Adapted from Stuart, G. W., & Laraia, M. T. (2004). *Stuart and Sundeen's principles and practice of psychiatric nursing* (8th ed.). St Louis: CV Mosby.

It is important to remember that nursing diagnoses are not medical diagnoses; they are not medical treatments prescribed by the physician, and they are not diagnostic studies. Nursing diagnoses are not the equipment used to implement medical therapy, and they are not the problems that nurses experience while caring for patients. Nursing diagnoses are succinct statements in terms of specific patient problems that guide nurses in the development of the nursing plan of care.

To give additional meaning to the nursing diagnosis, the characteristics and the etiology of the problem are identified and included as part of the diagnosis. For example, the nursing diagnoses and their defining characteristics and etiology for a patient who has anemia may include the following:

- Activity intolerance related to weakness and fatigue
- Ineffective tissue perfusion related to inadequate blood volume
- Imbalanced nutrition: Less than body requirements related to fatigue and inadequate intake of essential nutrients

COLLABORATIVE PROBLEMS

In addition to nursing diagnoses and their related nursing interventions, nursing practice involves certain situations and interventions that do not fall within the definition of nursing diagnoses. These activities pertain to potential problems or complications that are medical in origin and require collaborative interventions with the physician and other members of the health care team.

CHART 3-7

NANDA-Approved Nursing Diagnoses 2005–2006

This list represents the NANDA-approved nursing diagnoses for clinical use and testing.

Activity Intolerance
Activity Intolerance, Risk for
Adjustment, Impaired
Airway Clearance, Ineffective
Allergy Response, Latex
Allergy Response, Risk for Latex
Anxiety
Anxiety, Death
Aspiration, Risk for
Attachment, Risk for Impaired Parent/Infant/Child
Autonomic Dysreflexia
Autonomic Dysreflexia, Risk for
Body Image, Disturbed
Body Temperature, Risk for Imbalanced
Bowel Incontinence
Breastfeeding, Effective
Breastfeeding, Ineffective
Breastfeeding, Interrupted
Breathing Pattern, Ineffective
Cardiac Output, Decreased
Caregiver Role Strain
Caregiver Role Strain, Risk for
Communication, Impaired Verbal
Communication, Readiness for Enhanced
Conflict, Decisional (Specify)
Conflict, Parental Role
Confusion, Acute
Confusion, Chronic
Constipation
Constipation, Perceived
Constipation, Risk for
Coping, Ineffective
Coping, Defensive
Coping, Readiness for Enhanced
Coping, Ineffective Community
Coping, Readiness for Enhanced Community
Coping, Compromised Family
Coping, Disabled Family
Coping, Readiness for Enhanced Family
Death Syndrome, Risk for Sudden Infant
Denial, Ineffective
Dentition, Impaired
Development, Risk for Delayed
Diarrhea
Disuse Syndrome, Risk for
Diversional Activity, Deficient
Energy Field, Disturbed
Environmental Interpretation Syndrome, Impaired
Failure to Thrive, Adult
Falls, Risk for
Family Processes, Dysfunctional: Alcoholism
Family Processes, Interrupted
Family Processes, Readiness for Enhanced
Fatigue
Fear
Fluid Balance, Readiness for Enhanced
Fluid Volume, Deficient
Fluid Volume, Excess
Fluid Volume, Risk for Deficient
Fluid Volume, Risk for Imbalanced
Gas Exchange, Impaired
Grieving, Anticipatory
Grieving, Dysfunctional
Grieving, Risk for Dysfunctional
Growth and Development, Delayed
Growth, Risk for Disproportionate
Health Maintenance, Ineffective
Health-Seeking Behaviors (Specify)
Home Maintenance, Impaired
Hopelessness
Hyperthermia
Hypothermia
Identity, Disturbed Personal
Incontinence, Functional Urinary
Incontinence, Reflex Urinary
Incontinence, Stress Urinary
Incontinence, Total Urinary
Incontinence, Urge Urinary
Incontinence, Risk for Urge Urinary
Infant Behavior, Disorganized
Infant Behavior, Risk for Disorganized
Infant Behavior, Readiness for Enhanced Organized
Infant Feeding Pattern, Ineffective
Infection, Risk for
Injury, Risk for
Injury, Risk for Perioperative-Positioning
Intracranial Adaptive Capacity, Decreased
Knowledge, Deficient (Specify)
Knowledge, Readiness for Enhanced (Specify)
Lifestyle, Sedentary
Loneliness, Risk for
Memory, Impaired
Mobility, Impaired Bed
Mobility, Impaired Physical
Mobility, Impaired Wheelchair
Nausea
Neglect, Unilateral
Noncompliance
Nutrition, Imbalanced: Less Than Body Requirements

CHART 3-7 NANDA-Approved Nursing Diagnoses 2005–2006, continued

Nutrition, Imbalanced: More Than Body Requirements
Nutrition, Readiness for Enhanced
Nutrition, Risk for Imbalanced: More Than Body Requirements
Oral Mucous Membrane, Impaired
Pain, Acute
Pain, Chronic
Parenting, Readiness for Enhanced
Parenting, Impaired
Parenting, Risk for Impaired
Peripheral Neurovascular Dysfunction, Risk for
Poisoning, Risk for
Post-Trauma Syndrome
Post-Trauma Syndrome, Risk for
Powerlessness
Powerlessness, Risk for
Protection, Ineffective
Rape-Trauma Syndrome
Rape-Trauma Syndrome: Compound Reaction
Rape-trauma Syndrome: Silent Reaction
Religiosity, Impaired
Religiosity, Readiness for Enhanced
Religiosity, Risk for Impaired
Relocation Stress Syndrome
Relocation Stress Syndrome, Risk for
Role Performance, Ineffective
Self-Care Deficit, Bathing/Hygiene
Self-Care Deficit, Dressing/Grooming
Self-Care Deficit, Feeding
Self-Care Deficit, Toileting
Self-Concept, Readiness for Enhanced
Self-Esteem, Chronic Low
Self-Esteem, Situational Low
Self-Esteem, Risk for Situational Low
Self-Mutilation
Self-Mutilation, Risk for
Sensory Perception, Disturbed (Specify: Visual, Auditory, Kinesthetic, Gustatory, Tactile, Olfactory)
Sexual Dysfunction
Sexuality Pattern, Ineffective
Skin Integrity, Impaired
Skin Integrity, Risk for Impaired
Sleep Deprivation
Sleep Pattern, Disturbed
Sleep, Readiness for Enhanced
Social Interaction, Impaired
Social Isolation
Sorrow, Chronic
Spiritual Distress
Spiritual Distress, Risk for
Spiritual Well-Being, Readiness for Enhanced
Suffocation, Risk for
Suicide, Risk for
Surgical Recovery, Delayed
Swallowing, Impaired
Therapeutic Regimen Management, Effective
Therapeutic Regimen Management, Ineffective
Therapeutic Regimen Management, Readiness for Enhanced
Therapeutic Regimen Management, Ineffective Community
Therapeutic Regimen Management, Ineffective Family
Thermoregulation, Ineffective
Thought Processes, Disturbed
Tissue Integrity, Impaired
Tissue Perfusion, Ineffective (Specify Type: Renal, Cerebral, Cardiopulmonary, Gastrointestinal, Peripheral)
Transfer Ability, Impaired
Trauma, Risk for
Urinary Elimination, Impaired
Urinary Elimination, Readiness for Enhanced
Urinary Retention
Ventilation, Impaired Spontaneous
Ventilatory Weaning Response, Dysfunctional
Violence, Risk for Other-Directed
Violence, Risk for Self-Directed
Walking, Impaired
Wandering

NANDA International (2005). *Nursing diagnoses: Definitions & classification 2005–2006*. Philadelphia: Author.

The term *collaborative problem* is used to identify these situations.

Collaborative problems are certain physiologic complications that nurses monitor to detect changes in status or onset of complications. Nurses manage collaborative problems using physician-prescribed and nursing-prescribed interventions to minimize complications (Carpenito-Moyet, 2004). When treating collaborative problems, a primary nursing focus is monitoring patients for the onset of complications or changes in the status of existing complications. The complications are usually related to the disease process, treatments, medications, or diagnostic studies. The nurse recommends nursing interventions that are appropriate for managing the complications and implements the treatments prescribed by the physician. The algorithm in Figure 3-2 depicts the differences between nursing diagnoses and collaborative problems. After the nursing diagnoses and collaborative problems have been identified, they are recorded on the plan of nursing care.

Planning

Once the nursing diagnoses have been identified, the planning component of the nursing process begins. This phase involves the following steps:

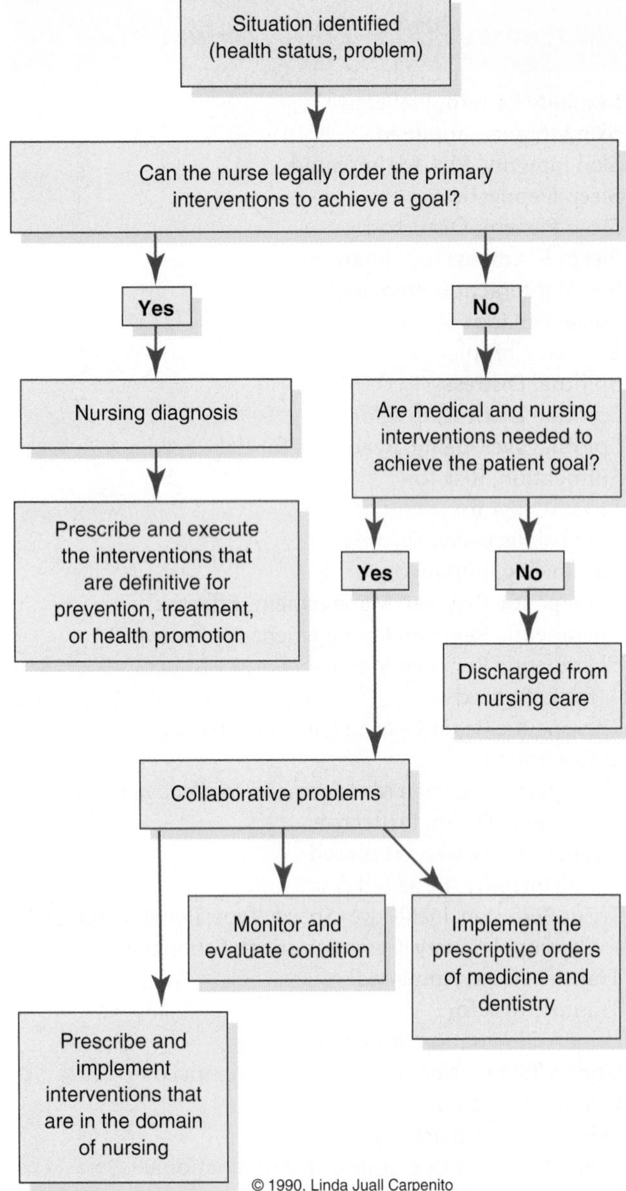

FIGURE 3-2. Differentiating nursing diagnoses and collaborative problems. From Carpenito-Moyet, L. J. (2004). *Nursing diagnosis: Application to clinical practice* (10th ed.). Philadelphia: Lippincott Williams & Wilkins.

1. Assigning priorities to the nursing diagnoses and collaborative problems
2. Specifying expected outcomes
3. Specifying the immediate, intermediate, and long-term goals of nursing action
4. Identifying specific nursing interventions appropriate for attaining the outcomes
5. Identifying interdependent interventions
6. Documenting the nursing diagnoses, collaborative problems, expected outcomes, nursing goals, and nursing interventions on the plan of nursing care
7. Communicating to appropriate personnel any assessment data that point to health care needs that can best be met by other members of the health care team

SETTING PRIORITIES

Assigning priorities to the nursing diagnoses and collaborative problems is a joint effort by the nurse and the patient or family members. Any disagreement about priorities is resolved in a way that is mutually acceptable. Consideration must be given to the urgency of the problems, with the most critical problems receiving the highest priority. The Maslow hierarchy of needs provides a useful framework for prioritizing problems, with importance being given first to physical needs; once those basic needs are met, higher-level needs can be addressed.

ESTABLISHING EXPECTED OUTCOMES

Expected outcomes of the nursing interventions are expressed in terms of the patient's behaviors and the time period in which the outcomes are to be achieved, as well as any special circumstances related to achieving the outcome (Smith-Temple & Johnson, 2005). These outcomes must be realistic and measurable. Resources for identifying appropriate expected outcomes include the Nursing-Sensitive Outcomes Classification (NOC) (Chart 3-8) and standard outcome criteria established by health care agencies for people with specific health problems. These outcomes can be associated with nursing diagnoses and interventions and can be used when appropriate. However, the NOC may need to be adapted to establish realistic criteria for the specific patient involved.

The expected outcomes that define the desired behavior of the patient are used to measure the progress made toward resolving the problem. The expected outcomes also serve as the basis for evaluating the effectiveness of the nursing interventions and for deciding whether additional nursing care is needed or whether the plan of care needs to be revised.

ESTABLISHING GOALS

After the priorities of the nursing diagnoses and expected outcomes have been established, goals (immediate, intermediate, and long-term) and the nursing actions appropriate for attaining the goals are identified. The patient and family are included in establishing goals for the nursing actions. Immediate goals are those that can be attained within a short period. Intermediate and long-term goals require a longer time to be achieved and usually involve preventing complications and other health problems and promoting self-care and rehabilitation. For example, goals for a patient with a nursing diagnosis of impaired physical mobility related to pain and edema following total knee replacement may be stated as follows:

- Immediate goal: Stands at bedside 6 to 12 hours after surgery
- Intermediate goal: Ambulates with walker or crutches in hospital and home
- Long-term goal: Ambulates independently 1 to 2 miles each day

DETERMINING NURSING ACTIONS

In planning appropriate nursing actions to achieve the desired goals and outcomes, the nurse, with input from the patient and significant others, identifies individualized interventions based on the patient's circumstances and

CHART 3-8

Nursing-Sensitive Outcomes Classification (NOC)

The NOC is a classification of patient outcomes sensitive to nursing interventions. Each outcome is a neutral statement about a variable patient condition, behavior, or perception, coupled with a rating scale. The outcome statement and scale can be used to identify baseline functioning, expected outcomes, and actual outcomes for individual patients. The following table is an example of a nursing-sensitive outcome.

Respiratory Status: Airway Patency (0410)

Domain—Physiologic Health (II)
Class—Cardiopulmonary (E)
Scale(s)—Severely compromised to Not compromised (a) and Severe to None (n)
Definition Open, clear tracheobronchial passages for air exchange
OUTCOME TARGET RATING: Maintain at ____ Increase to ___

Respiratory Status: Airway Patency Overall Rating		Severely Compromised 1	Substantially Compromised 2	Moderately Compromised 3	Mildly Compromised 4	Not Compromised 5	
INDICATORS:							
041009	Ease of breathing	1	2	3	4	5	NA
041004	Respiratory rate	1	2	3	4	5	NA
041005	Respiratory rhythm	1	2	3	4	5	NA
041006	Moves sputum out of airway	1	2	3	4	5	NA
041010	Moves blockage out of airway	1	2	3	4	5	NA
		Severe	**Substantial**	**Moderate**	**Mild**	**None**	
041002	Anxiety	1	2	3	4	5	NA
041011	Fear	1	2	3	4	5	NA
041003	Choking	1	2	3	4	5	NA
041007	Adventitious breath sounds	1	2	3	4	5	NA

With permission from Moorhead, S., Johnson, M., & Maas, M. (Eds.). (2004). *Nursing outcomes classification [NOC]: Iowa Outcomes Project* (3rd ed.). St. Louis: Mosby-Year Book.

preferences that address each outcome. Interventions should identify the activities needed and who will implement them. Determination of interdisciplinary activities is made in collaboration with other health care providers as needed.

The nurse identifies and plans patient teaching and return demonstration as needed to assist the patient in learning certain self-care activities. Planned interventions should be ethical and appropriate to the patient's culture, age, and gender. Standardized interventions, such as those found on institutional care plans or in the Nursing Interventions Classification (NIC) (Dochterman & Bulechek, 2004) can be used. Chart 3-9 describes the NIC system and provides an example of an NIC system intervention. It is important to individualize prewritten interventions to promote optimal effectiveness for each patient. Actions of nurses should be based on established standards.

Implementation

The implementation phase of the nursing process involves carrying out the proposed plan of nursing care. The nurse assumes responsibility for the implementation and coordinates the activities of all those involved in implementation, including the patient and family, other members of the nursing team, and other members of the health care team, so that the schedule of activities facilitates the patient's recovery.

CHART 3-9

Nursing Interventions Classification (NIC)

The NIC is a standardized classification of nursing treatments (interventions) that includes independent and collaborative interventions. Intervention labels are terms such as hemorrhage control, medication administration, or pain management. Listed under each intervention are multiple discrete nursing actions that together constitute a comprehensive approach to the treatment of a particular condition. Not all actions are applicable to every patient; nursing judgment will determine which actions to implement. The following is an example of a nursing intervention:

CHEST PHYSIOTHERAPY

Definition

Assisting the patient to move airway secretions from peripheral airways to more central airways for expectoration and/or suctioning

Activities

Determine presence of contraindications for use of chest physical therapy.

Determine which lung segment(s) needs to be drained.

Position patient with the lung segment to be drained in uppermost position.

Use pillows to support patient in designated position.

Use percussion with postural drainage by cupping hands and clapping the chest wall in rapid succession to produce a series of hollow sounds.

Use chest vibration in combination with postural drainage, as appropriate.

Use an ultrasonic nebulizer, as appropriate.

Use aerosol therapy, as appropriate.

Administer bronchodilators, as appropriate.

Monitor amount and type of sputum expectoration.

Encourage coughing during and after postural drainage.

Monitor patient tolerance by means of SaO_2, respiratory rhythm and rate, cardiac rhythm and rate, and comfort levels.

With permission from Dochterman, G. M., & Bulechek, G. M. (Eds.). (2004). *Nursing interventions classification (NIC)* (4th ed.). St. Louis: Mosby.

The plan of nursing care serves as the basis for implementation, as described below:

- The immediate, intermediate, and long-term goals are used as a focus for the implementation of the designated nursing interventions.
- While implementing nursing care, the nurse continually assesses the patient and his or her response to the nursing care.
- Revisions are made in the plan of care as the patient's condition, problems, and responses change and when reordering of priorities is required.

Implementation includes direct or indirect execution of the planned interventions. It is focused on resolving the patient's nursing diagnoses and collaborative problems and achieving expected outcomes, thus meeting the patient's health needs. Examples of nursing interventions are assisting with hygiene care; promoting physical and psychological comfort; supporting respiratory and elimination functions; facilitating the ingestion of food, fluids, and nutrients; managing the patient's immediate surroundings; providing health teaching; promoting a therapeutic relationship; and carrying out a variety of therapeutic nursing activities. Judgment, critical thinking, and good decision-making skills are essential in the selection of appropriate evidence-based and ethical nursing interventions. All nursing interventions are patient-focused and outcome-directed and are implemented with compassion, confidence, and a willingness to accept and understand the patient's responses.

Although many nursing actions are independent, others are interdependent, such as carrying out prescribed treatments, administering medications and therapies, and collaborating with other health care team members to accomplish specific expected outcomes and to monitor and manage potential complications. Such interdependent functioning is just that—interdependent. Requests or orders from other health care team members should not be followed blindly but should be assessed critically and questioned when necessary. The implementation phase of the nursing process ends when the nursing interventions have been completed.

Evaluation

Evaluation, the final step of the nursing process, allows the nurse to determine the patient's response to the nursing interventions and the extent to which the objectives have been achieved. The plan of nursing care is the basis for evaluation. The nursing diagnoses, collaborative problems, priorities, nursing interventions, and expected outcomes provide the specific guidelines that dictate the focus of the evaluation. Through evaluation, the nurse can answer the following questions:

- Were the nursing diagnoses and collaborative problems accurate?
- Did the patient achieve the expected outcomes within the critical time periods?
- Have the patient's nursing diagnoses been resolved?

- Have the collaborative problems been resolved?
- Do priorities need to be reordered?
- Have the patient's nursing needs been met?
- Should the nursing interventions be continued, revised, or discontinued?
- Have new problems evolved for which nursing interventions have not been planned or implemented?
- What factors influenced the achievement or lack of achievement of the objectives?
- Should changes be made in the expected outcomes and outcome criteria?

Objective data that provide answers to these questions are collected from all available sources (eg, patients, families, significant others, health care team members). These data are included in patients' records and must be substantiated by direct patient observation before the outcomes are documented.

Documentation of Outcomes and Revision of Plan

Outcomes are documented concisely and objectively. Documentation should relate outcomes to the nursing diagnoses and collaborative problems, describe the patient's responses to the interventions, indicate whether the outcomes were met, and include any additional pertinent data. An example of an individualized plan of nursing care is given in Chart 3-10.

The plan of care is subject to change as a patient's needs change, as the priorities of needs shift, as needs are resolved, and as additional information about a patient's state of health is collected. As the nursing interventions are implemented, the patient's responses are evaluated and documented, and the plan of care is revised accordingly. A well-developed, continuously updated plan of care is the greatest assurance that the patient's nursing diagnoses and collaborative problems are addressed and his or her basic needs are met.

Framework for a Common Nursing Language: Combining NANDA, NIC, and NOC

Various frameworks or taxonomies can be used for determining nursing diagnoses (eg, NANDA), establishing outcomes (eg, NOC), and designing interventions (eg, NIC). Ultimately a framework that uses a language common to all aspects of nursing, regardless of the classification system, is desirable. Although still controversial and in its infancy, significant efforts have been made toward accomplishing this goal of unifying the language of nursing. In 2001, a Taxonomy of Nursing Practice was developed for

CHART 3-10

Example of an Individualized Plan of Nursing Care

Mrs. Wilma Bryer, a 52-year-old court stenographer, was admitted to the nursing unit from her physician's office. She had had a gnawing pain on her right side radiating to her back for 3 days. She now describes her pain as "excruciating after eating or drinking." In the past 48 hours she has been vomiting about 2 to 3 hours after she eats. She has not had anything to eat or drink for the past 12 hours.

Mrs. Bryer stated that she had not been successful in adhering to the weight reduction diet that had been prescribed by her physician and that she had rapidly lost, then regained, weight several times in the past year and a half. She stated, "My life is just too busy—I work late hours in the court system and have to buy my meals out a lot." She indicated that in addition to her work, she and her husband share the responsibility for raising their two teenage daughters

Admission physical examination revealed BP 138/88, P 102, R 24, T 99.9°F, height 5′7″, weight 270 lbs, skin warm, no jaundice. She stated that her urine has been "a strange dark-golden color" and her stools were "like putty and grayish." She was admitted with the diagnosis of acute cholecystitis. The physician's orders on admission included: monitor vital signs every 4 hours; IV of D_5 Ringer's lactate 125 mL per hour; 1500-calorie, low-fat liquid diet and progress to low-fat soft diet if no pain in 16 hours; morphine sulfate 2 mg IV every 2 hours as needed; notify physician for sudden increase in frequency or intensity of pain; promethazine 12.5 mg IV every 4 hours as needed for nausea or vomiting.

Nursing Diagnoses

- Acute pain related to distended cystic duct and inflamed or infected gallbladder
- Risk for deficient fluid volume related to vomiting and decreased intake
- Ineffective coping related to role and responsibilities at work and home
- Imbalanced nutrition: More than body requirements, related to knowledge deficit about sedentary lifestyle, poor food choices and eating pattern

continued >

CHART 3-10 Example of an Individualized Plan of Nursing Care, continued

Collaborative Problems
- Risk for cystic duct necrosis or perforation
- Obesity

Goals

Immediate:
- Relief of pain
- Prevent fluid volume deficit and electrolyte imbalance
- Promote rest
- Early detection of any complications

Intermediate:
- Initiation of lifestyle alterations to decrease stress and facilitate rest

Long-term:
- Alteration of lifestyle to reduce emotional and environmental stressors
- Compliance with dietary regimen
- Weight reduction

NURSING INTERVENTIONS	EXPECTED OUTCOMES	OUTCOMES
1. Monitor BP, pulse, temperature, and respirations every 4 hours.	1. Vital signs within normal limits	1. BP range 110/62–128/78 with pain relief measures; temperature 98°–98.8°F; pulse range 74–88; respirations 18–22
2. Monitor pain status with accompanying abdominal assessment every 2 hours, or more frequently, as needed. a. Assess pain characteristics every 2 hours or as needed. b. Assess abdomen every 2 hours or with pain assessment. c. Use nonpharmacologic measures (pillows, repositioning, etc.) as desired and tolerated by patient for pain relief. d. Administer analgesic at regular intervals as needed, and assess response.	2. Experiences pain relief; abdominal assessment within normal limits	2. Verbalized decrease in pain from severe (8) to low (2) intensity within 10 minutes after morphine administered; no pain radiation to back Abdomen soft and nontender
3. Monitor and support fluid and electrolyte status: a. Monitor weight. b. I&O c. Monitor skin turgor and temperature. d. Monitor serum electrolytes. e. Monitor color and consistency of urine and stool output. f. Encourage low-fat liquid intake if pain-free. g. Administer promethazine as prescribed to control or relieve vomiting.	3. Fluid balance maintained; electrolytes within normal limits	3. Weight 270 on admission and 269 after 2-day period Urinary output adequate in relation to oral and IV intake Skin warm and supple, good recoil Electrolytes in normal range Urine dark amber in color, no sediment; stools soft, formed, light brown No vomiting reported

CHART 3-10 *Example of an Individualized Plan of Nursing Care, continued*

NURSING INTERVENTIONS	EXPECTED OUTCOMES	OUTCOMES
4. Promote atmosphere conducive to physical and mental rest: a. Encourage alternation of rest and activity. b. Encourage limitation of visitors and interactions that are stress-producing.	4. Alternates periods of rest and activity Limits visitors to family in the evenings Avoids stress-producing interactions	4. Rests in bed 2 hr in morning and 2 hr in afternoon; disconnects phone during rest periods. 8 hours uninterrupted sleep at night; husband and daughters visit 2 hours in evening; patient calm and relaxed after visits Accurately described relationship between stress, sedentary lifestyle, and obesity
5. Assist patient to alter lifestyle to decrease stress: a. Discuss relationship between emotional stress and physiologic function. b. Encourage patient to identify stress-producing stimuli. c. Encourage patient to identify adjustments necessary to reduce stress relative to the home and work setting.	5. Describes stress, sedentary lifestyle, and obesity as precursors to alteration in physiologic functioning Identifies lifestyle factors that produce stress	5. Identified the following stressors: Demands of job Excessive involvement in daughters' school and recreational activities
6. Encourage patient to identify sedentary lifestyle, obesity, and repetitive weight loss and gain as physiologic and emotional stressors; request consultation with dietitian and reinforce instructions given.	6. Identifies lifestyle adjustments necessary to reduce stress Discusses lifestyle adjustments with family	6. Identified need to decrease work hours to maximum of 8 hr per day Consulted with husband and daughters; will alternate with husband in attending daughters' activities; all family members supportive
7. Teach importance of maintaining low-fat liquid diet and progression toward long-term low-fat diet. Teach food and menu choices low in fat.	7. Identifies harmful effects of obesity and high-fat foods Makes plans for losing weight Makes plans for pre-planned meals Identifies foods/menu choices low in fat	7. Accurately described effects of obesity and intake of high-fat foods on overall physical health and well-being Plans to attend Weight Watchers; has had success with this program in the past Identified that preparing low-fat lunches at home the night before work is a good preplanning option

the harmonization of NANDA, NIC, and NOC. This three-part combination links nursing diagnoses, accompanying interventions, and outcomes, organizing them in the same way. Such organization of concepts in a common language may facilitate the process of critical thinking, because interventions and outcomes are more accurately matched with appropriately developed nursing diagnoses (Dochterman & Jones, 2003). The final taxonomic scheme identifies four clinical domains (functional, physiological, psychosocial, and environmental), which contain the 28 classes of diagnoses, outcomes, and interventions. Chart 3-11 presents the taxonomy of nursing practice.

CHART 3-11

Hierarchy of Taxonomy in Nursing Practice: A Unified Structure of Nursing Language

I. The **functional domain** is defined as the diagnoses, outcomes, and interventions that promote basic needs and includes the following eight classes:

Activity/exercise: physical activity, including energy, conservation, and expenditure

Comfort: a sense of emotional, physical, and spiritual well-being and relative freedom from distress

Growth and development: physical, emotional, and social growth and developmental milestones

Nutrition: processes related to taking in, assimilating, and using nutrients

Self-care: ability to accomplish basic and instrumental activities of daily living

Sexuality: maintenance or modification of sexual identity and patterns

Sleep/rest: the quantity and quality of sleep, rest, and relaxation patterns

Values/beliefs: ideas, goals, perceptions, spiritual, and other beliefs that influence choices or decisions

II. The **physiological domain** is defined as the diagnoses, outcomes, and interventions to promote optimal biophysical health and includes the following ten classes:

Cardiac function: cardiac mechanisms used to maintain tissue perfusion

Elimination: processes related to secretion and excretion of body wastes

Fluid and electrolyte: regulation of fluid/electrolytes and acid-base balance

Neurocognition: mechanisms related to the nervous system and neurocognitive functioning, including memory, thinking, and judgment

Pharmacological function: effects (therapeutic or adverse) of medications or drugs and other pharmacologically active products

Physical regulation: body temperature, endocrine, and immune system responses to regulate cellular processes.

Reproduction: processes related to human procreation and birth

Respiratory function: ventilation adequate to maintain arterial blood gases within normal limits

Sensation/perception: intake and interpretation of information through the senses, including seeing, hearing, touching, tasting, and smelling

Tissue integrity: skin and mucous membrane protection to support secretion, excretion, and healing

III. The **psychosocial domain** is defined as the diagnoses, outcomes, and interventions to promote optimal mental and emotional health and social functioning and includes the following seven classes:

Behavior: actions that promote, maintain, or restore health

Communication: receiving, interpreting, and expressing spoken, written, and nonverbal messages

Coping: adjusting or adapting to stressful events

Emotional: a mental state of feeling that may influence perception of the world

Knowledge: understanding and skill in applying information to promote, maintain, and restore health

Roles/relationships: maintenance and/or modification of expected social behaviors and emotional connectedness with others

Self-perception: awareness of one's body and personal identity

IV. The **environmental domain** is defined as the diagnoses, outcomes, and interventions that promote and protect the environmental health and safety of individuals, systems, and communities and includes the following three classes:

Health care system: social, political, and economic structures and processes for delivery of health care services

Populations: aggregates of individuals or communities having characteristics in common

Risk management: avoidance or control of identifiable health threats

From: Dochterman, J. M., & Jones, D. A. (Eds.). (2003). *Unifying nursing languages: The harmonization of NANDA, NIC, and NOC.* Washington, DC: NurseBooks.org.

Critical Thinking Exercises

1 A patient who is in end-stage multisystem failure has just been admitted to your unit. What processes would you use to prioritize his care needs, even though he has an end-stage diagnosis? What resources facilitate critical thinking in this situation?

2 You are at the bedside of a patient who has advance directives for no resuscitation. When she codes, her son yells, "Help, save her!" What actions could be taken in this situation? What ethical and legal dilemmas exist? What other health professionals could be helpful in resolving any issues?

3 ebp Two patients are admitted with cardiac pain to the telemetry observation unit. One has had no pain for 2 days and is asymptomatic, and the other has had at least four episodes of pain today. How would the individualized plans of care differ for these two patients? What is the evidence base for the differences in these patients' plans of care? What criteria would you use to evaluate the strength of the evidence?

REFERENCES AND SELECTED READINGS

BOOKS

Alfaro-LeFevre, R. (2003). *Critical thinking in nursing: A practical approach* (3rd ed.). Philadelphia: Saunders.

American Nurses Association. (1998). *Standards of clinical nursing practice* (2nd ed.). Washington, DC: Author.

American Nurses Association. (2001). *Code of ethics for nurses with interpretive statements.* Washington, DC: American Nurses Publishing.

American Nurses Association. (2003). *Nursing's social policy statement* (2nd ed). Washington, DC: Author.

Bickley, L. S., & Fiona, R. (2004). *Bates' guide to physical examination and history taking* (8th ed.). Philadelphia: Lippincott Williams & Wilkins.

Carpenito-Moyet, L. J. (2004). *Nursing care plans and documentation* (4th ed). Philadelphia: Lippincott Williams & Wilkins.

Carpenito-Moyet, L. J. (2004). *Nursing diagnosis: Application to clinical practice* (10th ed.). Philadelphia: Lippincott Williams & Wilkins.

Dochterman, J. M., & Bulechek, G. M. (Eds.) (2004). *Nursing interventions classification (NIC).* (4th ed.). St. Louis: Mosby-Year Book.

Dochterman, J. M., & Jones, D. A. (Eds.) (2003). *Unifying nursing languages: The harmonization of NANDA, NIC, and NOC.* Washington, DC: NursesBooks.org.

Jackson, M. (2004). Defining the concept of critical thinking. In M. Jackson, D. Ignatavicius, & B. Case (Eds.), *Conversations in critical thinking and clinical judgment* (pp. 3–17; 33–47). Pensacola, FL: Pohl Publishing.

Jameton, A. (1984). *Nursing practice: The ethical issues.* Englewood Cliffs, NJ: Prentice-Hall.

Joint Commission for Accreditation of Hospital Organizations (JCAHO). (2003). *2003 Hospital accreditation standards.* Oakbrook Terrace, IL: Author.

Moorhead, S., Johnson, M., & Maas, M. (Eds.). (2004). *Nursing outcomes classification (NOC): Iowa Outcomes Project* (3rd ed.). St. Louis: Mosby-Year Book.

NANDA International. (2005). *Nursing diagnoses: Definitions & classification 2005–2006.* Philadelphia: NANDA International.

Norlander, N. (2001). *To comfort always: A nurse's guide to end-of-life care.* Washington, DC: American Nurses Association.

Smith-Temple, J., & Johnson, J. Y. (2005). *Nurses' guide to clinical procedures* (5th ed.). Philadelphia: Lippincott Williams & Wilkins.

Stuart, G. W., & Laraia, M. T. (2004). *Stuart and Sundeen's principles and practice of psychiatric nursing* (8th ed.). St. Louis: Mosby.

Wilkinson, J. M. (2001). *Nursing process and critical thinking.* New Jersey: Prentice-Hall.

JOURNALS

American Nurses Association's Code of Ethics Project Task Force. (2000). A code of ethics for nurses. *American Journal of Nursing, 100*(7), 69–72.

Aquilino, M. L., & Keenan, G. (2000). Having our say: Nursing's standardized nomenclatures. *American Journal of Nursing, 100*(7), 33–38.

Cody, W. K. (2002). Theoretical concerns. Critical thinking and nursing science: Judgment, or vision? *Nursing Science Quarterly, 15*(3), 184–189.

Croke, E. (2003). Nurses, negligence, and malpractice. *American Journal of Nursing, 103*(9), 54–63.

Jackson, L., & Gleason, J. (2004). Proactive management breaks the fall cycle. *Nursing Management, 35*(6), 37–38.

Kirschling, J., & Lentz, J. (2004). Infusion nurses' role in care at the end of life. *Journal of Infusion Nursing, 27*(2), 112–117.

Lunney, M. (2003). Critical thinking and accuracy of nurses' diagnoses. *International Journal of Nursing Terminologies and Classifications, 14*(3), 96–100.

Martin, C. (2002). The theory of critical thinking of nursing, *Nursing Education Perspectives, 23*(5), 243–247.

Pitorak, E. F. (2003). Care at the time of death: How nurses can make the last hours of life a richer, more comfortable experience. *American Journal of Nursing, 103*(7), 42–52.

Profetto-McGrath, J., Hesketh, K. L., Lang, S., et al. (2003). A study of critical thinking and research utilization among nurses. *Western Journal of Nursing Research, 25*(3), 322–337.

Sheehan, D. K., & Schirm, V. (2003). End-of-life care of older adults: Debunking some common misconceptions about dying in old age. *American Journal of Nursing, 103*(11), 48–58.

Trammelleo, A. D. (2000). Protecting patients' end-of-life choices. *RN, 63*(8), 75–79.

Truong, R. D., Alexandra, F., M., Brackett, S. E., et al. (2001). Recommendations for end-of-life care in the intensive care unit: The Ethics Committee of the Society of Critical Care Medicine. *Critical Care Medicine, 29*(12), 2332–2348.

Valente, S. M. (2004). End-of-life challenges: Honoring autonomy. *Cancer Nursing, 27*(4), 314–319.

RESOURCES AND WEBSITES

American Nurses Association, Center for Ethics and Human Rights. 8515 Georgia Avenue, Suite 400; Silver Spring, MD 20910; 301-628-5000; http://www.nursingworld.org/ethics. Accessed June 5, 2006.

Centers for Medicare & Medicaid Services (CMS), 7500 Security Boulevard, Baltimore, MD 21244-1850; 877-267-2323; http://www.cms.hhs.gov. Accessed June 5, 2006.

Joint Commission on Accreditation of Healthcare Organizations (JCAHO), One Renaissance Blvd., Oakbrook Terrace, IL 60181; 630-792-5000; http://www.jcaho.org. Accessed June 5, 2006.

NANDA International, 1211 Locust St., Philadelphia, PA 19107; 215-545-8107; http://www.nanda.org. Accessed June 5, 2006.

CHAPTER 4

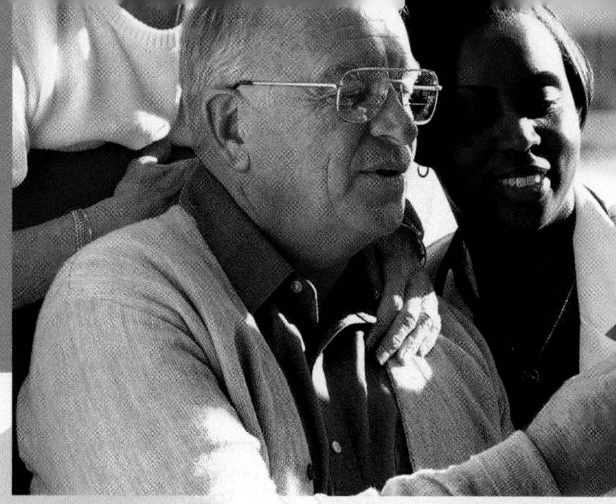

Health Education and Health Promotion

Learning Objectives

On completion of this chapter, the learner will be able to:

1. Describe the purposes and significance of health education.
2. Describe the concept of adherence to a therapeutic regimen.
3. Identify variables influencing the elderly person's adherence to a therapeutic regimen.
4. Distinguish the variables that affect learning readiness.
5. Describe strategies that facilitate elderly adults' learning abilities.
6. Describe the relationship of the teaching–learning process to the nursing process.
7. Develop a teaching plan for a patient.
8. Identify modifications indicated when teaching patients with disabilities.
9. Define the concepts of health, wellness, and health promotion.
10. Discuss major health promotion theories.
11. Describe the components of health promotion: self-responsibility, nutritional awareness, stress reduction and management, and physical fitness.
12. Specify the variables that affect health promotion activities for children, young and middle-aged adults, and elderly adults.
13. Describe the role of the nurse in health promotion.

Effective **health education** lays a solid foundation for individual and **community** wellness. Teaching is an integral tool that all nurses use to assist patients and families in developing effective health behaviors and in altering lifestyle patterns that predispose people to health risks. Health education is an influential factor directly related to positive patient care outcomes.

Health Education Today

The changes in today's health care environment mandate the use of an organized approach to health education so that patients can meet their specific health care needs. Significant factors for nurses to consider when planning patient education include the availability of health care outside the hospital setting, the use of diverse health care providers to accomplish care management goals, and the increased use of alternative strategies rather than traditional approaches to care. Careful consideration of these factors can provide patients with the comprehensive information that is essential for making informed decisions about health care. Demands from consumers for comprehensive information about their health issues throughout the life cycle accentuate the need for holistic health education to occur in every patient–nurse encounter.

Teaching, as a function of nursing, is included in all state nurse practice acts and in the *Standards of Clinical Nursing Practice* of the American Nurses Association (ANA, 2004). Health education is an independent function of nursing practice and is a primary nursing responsibility. All nursing care is directed toward promoting, maintaining, and restoring health; preventing illness; and helping people adapt to the residual effects of illness. Many of these nursing activities are accomplished through health education or patient teaching. Nurses who serve as teachers are challenged to focus on the educational needs of communities as well as to provide specific patient and family education. Health education is important to nursing care because it affects the abilities of people and families to perform important self-care activities.

Every contact an individual nurse has with a health care consumer, whether or not that person is ill, should be considered an opportunity for health teaching. Although people have a right to decide whether or not to learn, nurses have the responsibility to present information that motivates people to recognize the need to learn. Therefore, nurses must use opportunities in all health care settings to promote **wellness.** Educational environments may include homes, hospitals, community health centers, schools, places of business, service agencies, shelters, and consumer action or support groups.

Purpose of Health Education

This emphasis on health education stems in part from the public's right to comprehensive health care, which includes up-to-date health information. It also reflects the emergence of an informed public that is asking more significant questions about health and health care. Because of the importance American society places on health and the responsibility each person has to maintain and promote his or her own health, members of the health care team, specifically nurses, are obligated to make health education consistently available. Without adequate knowledge and training in self-care skills, consumers cannot make informed decisions about their health.

People with chronic illnesses and disabilities are among those most in need of health education. As the life span of the population increases, the number of people with such illnesses also increases. People with chronic illness need health care information to participate actively in and assume responsibility for much of their own care. Health education can help those with chronic illness adapt to their illness, prevent complications, carry out prescribed therapy, and solve problems when confronted with new situations. It can also prevent crisis situations and reduce the potential for rehospitalization resulting from inadequate information about self-care. The goal of health education is to teach people to live life to its healthiest—that is, to strive toward achieving their maximum health potential.

Glossary

adherence: the process of faithfully following guidelines or directions

community: an interacting population of individuals living together within a larger society

feedback: the return of information about the results of input given to a person or a system

health education: a variety of learning experiences designed to promote behaviors that facilitate health

health promotion: the art and science of assisting people to change their lifestyle toward a higher state of wellness

learning: the act of gaining knowledge and skill

learning readiness: the optimum time for learning to occur; usually corresponds to the learner's perceived need and desire to obtain specific knowledge

nutrition: the science that deals with food and nourishment in humans

physical fitness: the condition of being physically healthy as a result of proper exercise and nutrition

reinforcement: the process of strengthening a given response or behavior to increase the likelihood that the behavior will continue

self-responsibility: personal accountability for one's actions or behavior

stress management: behaviors and techniques used to strengthen a person's resources against stress

teaching: the imparting of knowledge

therapeutic regimen: a routine that promotes health and healing

wellness: a condition of good physical and emotional health sustained by a healthy lifestyle

In addition to the public's right to and desire for health education, patient education is also a strategy for promoting self-care at home and in the community, reducing health care costs by preventing illness, avoiding expensive medical treatments, decreasing lengths of hospital stays, and facilitating earlier discharge. For health care agencies, offering community wellness programs is a public relations tool for increasing patient satisfaction and for developing a positive image of the institution. Patient education is also a cost-avoidance strategy for those who believe that positive staff–patient relationships avert malpractice suits.

Adherence to the Therapeutic Regimen

One of the goals of patient education is to encourage people to adhere to their **therapeutic regimen. Adherence** to treatment usually requires that a person make one or more lifestyle changes to carry out specific activities that promote and maintain health. Common examples of behaviors facilitating health include taking prescribed medications, maintaining a healthy diet, increasing daily activities and exercise, self-monitoring for signs and symptoms of illness, practicing specific hygiene measures, seeking recommended health evaluations and screening, and performing other therapeutic and preventive measures.

Many people do not adhere to their prescribed regimens; rates of adherence are generally low, especially when the regimens are complex or of long duration. Nonadherence to prescribed therapy has been the subject of many studies. For the most part, findings have been inconclusive, and no one predominant causative factor has been identified. Instead, a wide range of variables appears to influence the degree of adherence, including the following:

- Demographic variables, such as age, gender, race, socioeconomic status, and level of education
- Illness variables, such as the severity of the illness and the relief of symptoms afforded by the therapy
- Therapeutic regimen variables, such as the complexity of the regimen and uncomfortable side effects
- Psychosocial variables, such as intelligence, availability of significant and supportive people (especially family members), attitudes toward health professionals, acceptance or denial of illness, and religious or cultural beliefs
- Financial variables, especially the direct and indirect costs associated with a prescribed regimen

Nurses' success with health education is determined by ongoing assessment of the variables that affect patients' ability to adopt specific behaviors, to obtain resources, and to maintain a helpful social environment (Murray & Zentner, 2001). Teaching programs are more likely to succeed if the variables affecting patient adherence are identified and considered in the teaching plan.

The problem of nonadherence to therapeutic regimens is a substantial one that must be addressed before patients can achieve their maximum health potential. Surprisingly, patients' need for knowledge has not been found to be a sufficient stimulus for acquiring knowledge and thereby enabling complete adherence to a health regimen. Teaching directed toward stimulating patient motivation results in varying degrees of adherence. The variables of choice, establishment of mutual goals, and the quality of the patient–provider relationship directly influence the behavioral changes that can result from patient education (Rankin & Stallings, 2004). These factors are directly linked to motivation for learning.

Using a learning contract or agreement can also be a motivator for learning. Such a contract is based on assessment of patient needs; health care data; and specific, measurable goals (Redman, 2004). A well-designed learning contract is realistic and positive; it includes measurable goals, with a specific time frame and reward system for goal achievement. The learning contract is recorded in writing and contains methods for ongoing evaluation.

The value of the contract lies in its clarity, its specific description of what is to be accomplished, and its usefulness for evaluating behavioral change. In a typical learning contract, a series of goals is established, beginning with small, easily attainable objectives and progressing to more advanced goals. Frequent, positive **reinforcement** is provided as the person moves from one goal to the next. For example, incremental goals such as weight loss of 1 to 2 pounds per week are more appropriate in a weight reduction program than a general goal such as a 30-pound weight loss.

Gerontologic Considerations

Nonadherence to therapeutic regimens is a significant problem for elderly people, leading to increased morbidity, mortality, and cost of treatment (U.S. Public Health Service, 2000). Many admissions to nursing homes and hospitals are associated with nonadherence.

Elderly people frequently have one or more chronic illnesses that are managed with numerous medications and complicated by periodic acute episodes. Elderly people may also have other problems that affect adherence to therapeutic regimens, such as increased sensitivity to medications and their side effects, difficulty in adjusting to change and stress, financial constraints, forgetfulness, inadequate support systems, lifetime habits of self-treatment with over-the-counter medications, visual and hearing impairments, and mobility limitations. To promote adherence among the elderly, all variables that may affect health behavior should be assessed (Fig. 4-1). Nurses must also consider that cognitive impairment may be manifested by the elderly person's inability to draw inferences, apply information, or understand the major teaching points (Eliopoulos, 2004). The person's strengths and limitations must be assessed to encourage use of existing strengths to compensate for limitations. Above all, health care professionals must work together to provide continuous, coordinated care; otherwise, the efforts of one health care professional may be negated by those of another.

The Nature of Teaching and Learning

Learning can be defined as acquiring knowledge, attitudes, or skills. **Teaching** is defined as helping another person learn. These definitions indicate that the teaching–learning process is an active one, requiring the involvement of both

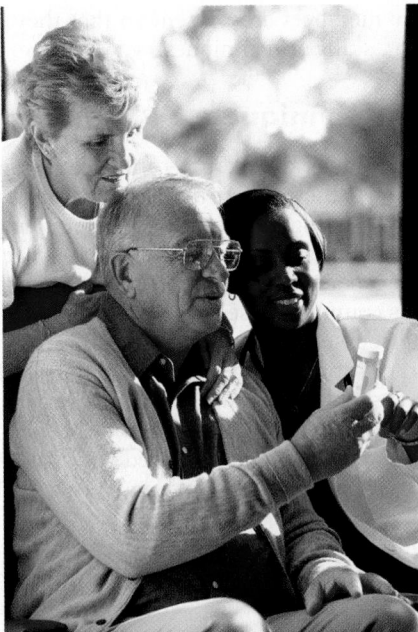

FIGURE 4-1. Taking time to teach patients about their medication and treatment program promotes interest and cooperation. Older adults who are actively involved in learning about their medication and treatment program and the expected effects may be more likely to adhere to the therapeutic regimen.

CHART 4-1

Cultural Assessment Components to Consider When Formulating a Teaching Plan

When formulating a teaching plan, consider the patient's beliefs about

- Body size, shape, boundaries, and functions
- Beauty and strength
- Value of the mind or brain
- Nature and function of blood
- Diet and nutrition
- Communication
- Gender
- Family and social support
- Physical health and illness
- Mental health and illness
- Age-related changes
- Pain
- Medicine, herbs, and talismans
- Spirituality or religion

teacher and learner in the effort to reach the desired outcome, a change in behavior. The teacher does not simply give knowledge to the learner, but instead serves as a facilitator of learning.

In general, there is no definitive theory about how learning occurs and how it is affected by teaching. However, learning can be affected by factors such as readiness to learn, the learning environment, and the teaching techniques used (Bastable, 2003; Kreuter, Lezin, Kreuter, et al., 2003).

Learning Readiness

One of the most significant factors influencing learning is a person's **learning readiness.** For adults, readiness is based on culture, personal values, physical and emotional status, and past experiences in learning. The "teachable moment" occurs when the content and skills being taught are congruent with the task to be accomplished (Redman, 2004).

Culture encompasses values, ideals, and behaviors, and the traditions within each culture provide the framework for solving the issues and concerns of daily living. Because people with different cultural backgrounds have different values and lifestyles, choices about health care vary. Culture is a major variable influencing readiness to learn because it affects how people learn and what information can be learned. Sometimes people do not accept health teaching because it conflicts with culturally mediated values. Before beginning health teaching, nurses must conduct an individual cultural assessment instead of relying only on generalized assumptions about a particular culture. A patient's social and cultural patterns must be appropriately incorporated into the teaching–learning interaction. Chart 4-1 describes cultural assessment components to consider when formulating a teaching plan.

A person's values include beliefs about behaviors that are desirable and undesirable. The nurses must know what value the patient places on health and health care. In clinical situations, patients express their values through their actions and the level of knowledge pursued (Andrews & Boyle, 2002). When the nurse is unaware of the patient's cultural values, misunderstanding, lack of cooperation, and negative health outcomes may occur (Leininger, 2001). A person's values and behaviors can be either an asset or a deficit to the readiness to learn. Therefore, patients are unlikely to accept health education unless their values and beliefs about health and illness are respected (Giger & Davidhizar, 2004).

Physical readiness is of vital importance, because until the person is physically capable of learning, attempts at teaching and learning may be both futile and frustrating. For example, a person in acute pain is unable to focus attention away from the pain long enough to concentrate on learning. Likewise, a person who is short of breath concentrates on breathing rather than on learning.

Emotional readiness also affects the motivation to learn. A person who has not accepted an existing illness or the threat of illness is not motivated to learn. A person who does not accept a therapeutic regimen, or who views it as conflicting with his or her present lifestyle, may consciously avoid learning about it. Until the person recognizes the need to learn and demonstrates an ability to learn, teaching efforts may be thwarted. However, it is not always wise to wait for the person to become emotionally ready to learn, because that time may never come unless the nurse makes an effort to stimulate the person's motivation.

Illness and the threat of illness are usually accompanied by anxiety and stress. Nurses who recognize such reactions can use simple explanations and instructions to alleviate these anxieties and provide further motivation to learn. Because learning involves behavior change, it often produces mild anxiety, which can be a useful motivating factor.

Emotional readiness can be promoted by creating a warm, accepting, positive atmosphere and by establishing realistic learning goals. When learners achieve success and a feeling of accomplishment, they are often motivated to participate in additional learning opportunities.

Feedback about progress also motivates learning. Such feedback should be presented in the form of positive reinforcement when the learner is successful, and in the form of constructive suggestions for improvement when he or she is unsuccessful.

Experiential readiness refers to past experiences that influence a person's ability to learn. Previous educational experiences and life experiences in general are significant determinants of a person's approach to learning. People with little or no formal education may not be able to understand the instructional materials presented. People who have had difficulty learning in the past may be hesitant to try again. Many behaviors required for reaching maximum health potential require knowledge, physical skills, and positive attitudes. In their absence, learning may be very difficult and very slow. For example, a person who does not understand the basics of normal nutrition may not be able to understand the restrictions of a specific diet. A person who does not view the desired learning as personally meaningful may reject teaching efforts. A person who is not future-oriented may be unable to appreciate many aspects of preventive health teaching. Experiential readiness is closely related to emotional readiness, because motivation tends to be stimulated by an appreciation for the need to learn and by those learning tasks that are familiar, interesting, and meaningful.

Before initiating a teaching–learning program, it is important to assess the person's physical and emotional readiness to learn, as well as his or her ability to learn what is being taught. This information then becomes the basis for establishing goals that can motivate the person. Involving learners in establishing mutually acceptable goals serves the purpose of encouraging active involvement in the learning process and shared responsibility for learning.

The Learning Environment

Although learning can take place without teachers, most people who are attempting to learn new or altered health behaviors benefit from the services of nurses. The interpersonal interaction between the person and the nurse who is attempting to meet the person's learning needs may be formal or informal, depending on the method and techniques of teaching.

Learning may be optimized by minimizing factors that interfere with the learning process. For example, the room temperature, lighting, noise levels, and other environmental conditions should be appropriate to the learning situation. In addition, the time selected for teaching should be suited to the needs of the individual person. Scheduling a teaching session at a time of day when a patient is fatigued, uncomfortable, or anxious about a pending diagnostic or therapeutic procedure, or when visitors are present, is not conducive to learning. However, if the family is to participate in providing care, the sessions should be scheduled when family members are present so that they can learn any necessary skills or techniques.

Teaching Techniques

Teaching techniques and methods enhance learning if they are appropriate to the patient's needs. Numerous techniques are available, including lectures, group teaching, and demonstrations, all of which can be enhanced with specially prepared teaching materials. The lecture or explanation method of teaching is commonly used but should always be accompanied by discussion. Discussion is important because it affords learners opportunities to express their feelings and concerns, to ask questions, and to receive clarification.

Group teaching is appropriate for some people because it allows them not only to receive needed information but also to feel secure as members of a group. People with similar problems or learning needs have the opportunity to identify with each other and gain moral support and encouragement. However, not everyone relates or learns well in groups or benefits from such experiences. Also, if group teaching is used, assessment and follow-up are imperative to ensure that each person has gained sufficient knowledge and skills.

Demonstration and practice are essential ingredients of a teaching program, especially when teaching skills. It is best to demonstrate the skill and then give the learner ample opportunity for practice. When special equipment is involved, such as syringes, colostomy bags, dialysis equipment, dressings, or suction apparatus, it is important to teach with the same equipment that will be used in the home setting. Learning to perform a skill with one kind of equipment and then having to change to a different kind may lead to confusion, frustration, and mistakes.

Teaching aids used to enhance learning include books, pamphlets, pictures, films, slides, audio and video tapes, models, programmed instruction, CD-ROMs, and computer-assisted learning modules. These are made available as needed for home, clinic, or hospital use, and they allow review and reinforcement of content and enhanced visual and auditory learning. Such teaching aids are invaluable when used appropriately and can save a significant amount of personnel time and related cost. However, all such aids should be reviewed before use to ensure that they meet the person's learning needs. Human interaction and discussion cannot be replaced by teaching technologies but may be enhanced by them.

Reinforcement and follow-up are important because learning takes time. Allowing ample time to learn and reinforcing what is learned are important teaching strategies; a single teaching session is rarely adequate. Follow-up sessions are imperative to promote the learner's confidence in his or her abilities and to plan for additional teaching sessions. For hospitalized patients who may not be able to transfer what they have learned in the hospital to the home setting, follow-up after discharge is essential to ensure that they have realized the full benefits of a teaching program.

Teaching People With Disabilities

When providing health information to people with disabilities, the individual needs of each person must be assessed and incorporated into the teaching plan. Teaching techniques and the imparting of information may need to be altered. When teaching specific groups of people with physical disabilities, emotional disabilities, hearing and visual impairments, learning disabilities, and developmental disabilities, the nurse must be aware of their health promotion needs and institute new or modified approaches to teach them about their health. Table 4-1 outlines some of the teaching strategies to use when teaching people with disabilities.

Gerontologic Considerations

Nurses caring for elderly people must be aware of how the normal changes that occur with aging affect learning abilities and how they can help elderly people adjust to these changes. Above all, it is important to recognize that just because a person is elderly does not mean that he or she cannot learn. Studies have shown that older adults *can* learn and remember if information is paced appropriately, relevant, and followed by the appropriate feedback strategies that apply to all learners (Rankin & Stallings, 2004). Because changes associated with aging vary significantly among elderly people, the nurse should conduct a thorough assessment of each person's level of physiologic and psychological functioning before beginning teaching.

Changes in cognition with age may include slowed mental functioning; decreased short-term memory, abstract thinking, and concentration; and slowed reaction time.

TABLE 4-1 Teaching People with Disabilities

Type of Disability	Teaching Strategy
Physical, Emotional, or Cognitive Disability	Adapt information to accommodate the person's cognitive, perceptual, and behavioral disabilities. Give clear written and oral information. Highlight significant information for easy reference. Avoid medical terminology.
Hearing Impairment	Use slow, directed, deliberate speech. Use sign language or interpreter services if appropriate. Position yourself so that the person can see your mouth if speech reading. Use telecommunication devices (TTY or TDD) for the hearing impaired. Use written materials and visual aids, such as models and diagrams. Use captioned videos, films, and computer-generated materials. Teach on the side of the "good ear" if unilateral deafness is present.
Visual Impairment	Use optical devices such as a magnifying lens. Use proper lighting and proper contrast of colors on materials and equipment. Use large-print materials. Use Braille materials if appropriate. Convert information to auditory and tactile formats. Obtain audiotapes and talking books. Explain noises associated with procedures, equipment, and treatments. Arrange materials in clockwise pattern.
Learning Disabilities	
Input disability	If visual perceptual disorder: • Explain information verbally, repeat, and reinforce frequently. • Use audiotapes. • Encourage learner to verbalize information received. If auditory perceptual disorder: • Speak slowly with as few words as possible, repeat, and reinforce frequently. • Use direct eye contact to focus person on task. • Use demonstration and return demonstration such as modeling, role playing, and hands-on experiences. • Use visual tools, written materials, and computers.
Output disability	Use all senses as appropriate. Use written, audiotape, and computer information. Review information and give time to interact and ask questions. Use hand gestures and motions.
Developmental disability	Base information and teaching on developmental stage, not chronologic age. Use nonverbal cues, gestures, signing, and symbols as needed. Use simple explanations and concrete examples with repetition. Encourage active participation. Demonstrate information and have the person perform return demonstrations.

These changes are often accentuated by the health problems that cause the elderly person to seek health care in the first place. Effective teaching strategies include a slow-paced presentation of small amounts of material at a time; frequent repetition of information; and the use of reinforcement techniques, such as audiovisual and written materials and repeated practice sessions. Distracting stimuli should be minimized as much as possible in the teaching environment.

Sensory changes associated with aging also affect teaching and learning. Teaching strategies to accommodate decreased visual acuity include large-print and easy-to-read materials printed on nonglare paper. Because color discrimination is often impaired, the use of color-coded or highlighted materials may not be effective. To maximize hearing, teachers must speak distinctly with a normal or lowered pitch, facing the person so that speech reading can occur as needed. Visual cues often help to reinforce verbal teaching.

Family members should be involved in teaching sessions when possible. They provide another source for reinforcement of material and can help the elderly person recall instructions later. Family members can also provide valuable assessment information about the person's living situation and related learning needs.

When nurses, families, and other involved health care professionals work collaboratively to facilitate the elderly person's learning, chances of success are maximized. Successful learning for the elderly should result in improved self-care management skills, enhanced self-esteem, confidence, and a willingness to learn in the future.

The Nursing Process in Patient Teaching

The steps of the nursing process—assessment, diagnosis, planning, implementation, and evaluation—are used when constructing a teaching plan to meet people's teaching and learning needs (Chart 4-2).

Assessment

Assessment in the teaching–learning process is directed toward the systematic collection of data about the person's learning needs and readiness to learn, as well as the family's learning needs. All internal and external variables that affect the patient's readiness to learn are identified. A learning assessment guide may be used for this purpose. Some of the available guides are very general and are directed toward the collection of general health information, whereas others are specific to common medication regimens or disease processes. Such guides facilitate the assessment but must be adapted to the responses, problems, and needs of each person. As soon as possible after completing the assessment, the nurse organizes, analyzes, synthesizes, and summarizes the data collected and determines the patient's need for teaching.

Nursing Diagnosis

The process of formulating nursing diagnoses makes educational goals and evaluations of progress more specific and meaningful. Teaching is an integral intervention implied by all nursing diagnoses, and for some diagnoses, education is the primary intervention. Examples of nursing diagnoses that help in planning for educational needs are Ineffective therapeutic regimen management, Ineffective home maintenance, Health-seeking behaviors, and Decisional conflict. The diagnosis "Deficient knowledge" should be used cautiously, because knowledge deficit is not a human response but a factor relating to or causing the diagnosis (eg, "Ineffective therapeutic regimen management related to a deficiency of information about wound care" is a more appropriate nursing diagnosis than "Deficient knowledge") (Carpenito-Moyet, 2003). A nursing diagnosis that relates specifically to a patient's and family's learning needs serves as a guide in the development of the teaching plan.

Planning

Once the nursing diagnoses have been identified, the planning component of the teaching–learning process is established in accordance with the steps of the nursing process:

1. Assigning priorities to the diagnoses
2. Specifying the immediate, intermediate, and long-term goals of learning
3. Identifying specific teaching strategies appropriate for attaining goals
4. Specifying the expected outcomes
5. Documenting the diagnoses, goals, teaching strategies, and expected outcomes of the teaching plan

As in the nursing process, the assignment of priorities to the diagnoses should be a joint effort by the nurse and the patient or family members. Consideration must be given to the urgency of the patient's learning needs; the most critical needs should receive the highest priority.

After the diagnostic priorities have been established, it is important to identify the immediate and long-term goals and the teaching strategies appropriate for attaining the goals. Teaching is most effective when the objectives of both the patient and nurse are in agreement (Bastable, 2003). Learning begins with the establishment of goals that are appropriate to the situation and realistic in terms of the patient's ability and desire to achieve them. Involving the patient and family in establishing goals and in planning teaching strategies promotes their cooperation in the implementation of the teaching plan.

Expected outcomes of teaching strategies can be stated in terms of behaviors of patients, families, or both. Outcomes should be realistic and measurable, and the critical time periods for attaining them should also be identified. The desired outcomes and the critical time periods serve as a basis for evaluating the effectiveness of the teaching strategies.

During the planning phase, the nurse must consider the sequence in which the subject matter is presented in each of the teaching strategies. Critical information (eg, survival skills for a patient with diabetes) and material that the person or family identifies to be of particular importance receive high priority. An outline is often helpful for arranging the subject matter and for ensuring that all necessary information is included. In addition, appropriate teaching aids to be used in implementing teaching strategies are prepared or selected at this time.

CHART 4-2

A Guide to Patient Education

ASSESSMENT

1. Assess the person's readiness for health education.
   a. What are the person's health beliefs and behaviors?
   b. What physical and psychosocial adaptations does the person need to make?
   c. Is the learner ready to learn?
   d. Is the person able to learn these behaviors?
   e. What additional information about the person is needed?
   f. Are there any variables (eg, hearing or visual impairment, cognitive issues, literacy issues) that will affect the choice of teaching strategy or approach?
   g. What are the person's expectations?
   h. What does the person want to learn?
2. Organize, analyze, synthesize, and summarize the collected data.

NURSING DIAGNOSIS

1. Formulate the nursing diagnoses that relate to the person's learning needs.
2. Identify the learning needs, their characteristics, and their etiology.
3. State nursing diagnoses concisely and precisely.

PLANNING AND GOALS

1. Assign priority to the nursing diagnoses that relate to the individual's learning needs.
2. Specify the immediate, intermediate, and long-term learning goals established by teacher and learner together.
3. Identify teaching strategies appropriate for goal attainment.
4. Establish expected outcomes.
5. Develop the written teaching plan.
   a. Include diagnoses, goals, teaching strategies, and expected outcomes.
   b. Put the information to be taught in logical sequence.
   c. Write down the key points.
   d. Select appropriate teaching aids.
   e. Keep the plan current and flexible to meet the person's changing learning needs.
6. Involve the learner, family or significant others, nursing team members, and other health care team members in all aspects of planning.

IMPLEMENTATION

1. Put the teaching plan into action.
2. Use language the person can understand.
3. Use appropriate teaching aids and provide Internet resources if appropriate.
4. Use the same equipment that the person will use after discharge.
5. Encourage the person to participate actively in learning.
6. Record the learner's responses to the teaching actions.
7. Provide feedback.

EVALUATION

1. Collect objective data.
   a. Observe the person.
   b. Ask questions to determine whether the person understands.
   c. Use rating scales, checklists, anecdotal notes, and written tests when appropriate.
2. Compare the person's behavioral responses with the expected outcomes. Determine the extent to which the goals were achieved.
3. Include the person, family or significant others, nursing team members, and other health care team members in the evaluation.
4. Identify alterations that need to be made in the teaching plan.
5. Make referrals to appropriate sources or agencies for reinforcement of learning after discharge.
6. Continue all steps of the teaching process: assessment, diagnosis, planning, implementation, and evaluation.

The entire planning phase of the teaching–learning process concludes with the formulation of the teaching plan. This teaching plan communicates the following information to all members of the nursing team:

- The nursing diagnoses that specifically relate to the patient's learning needs and the priorities of these diagnoses
- The goals of the teaching strategies
- The teaching strategies, expressed in the form of teaching orders
- The expected outcomes, which identify the desired behavioral responses of the learner
- The critical time period within which each outcome is expected to be met
- The patient's behavioral responses (which are documented on the teaching plan)

The same rules that apply to writing and revising the plan of nursing care apply to the teaching plan.

Implementation

In the implementation phase of the teaching–learning process, the patient, the family, and other members of the nursing and health care team carry out the activities outlined in the teaching plan. The nurse coordinates these activities.

Flexibility during the implementation phase of the teaching–learning process and ongoing assessment of patient responses to the teaching strategies support modification of the teaching plan as necessary. Creativity in promoting and sustaining the patient's motivation to learn is essential. New learning needs that may arise after discharge from the hospital or after home care visits have ended should also be taken into account.

The implementation phase ends when the teaching strategies have been completed and when the patient's responses to the actions have been recorded. This record serves as the basis for evaluating how well the defined goals and expected outcomes have been achieved.

Evaluation

Evaluation of the teaching–learning process determines how effectively the patient has responded to teaching and to what extent the goals have been achieved. An evaluation must be made to determine what was effective and what needs to be changed or reinforced. It cannot be assumed that patients have learned just because teaching has occurred; learning does not automatically follow teaching. An important part of the evaluation phase addresses the question, "What can be done to improve teaching and enhance learning?" Answers to this question direct the changes to be made in the teaching plan.

A variety of measurement techniques can be used to identify changes in patient behavior as evidence that learning has taken place. These techniques include directly observing the behavior; using rating scales, checklists, or anecdotal notes to document the behavior; and indirectly measuring results using oral questioning and written tests. All direct measurements should be supplemented with indirect measurements whenever possible. Using more than one measuring technique enhances the reliability of the resulting data and decreases the potential for error from a measurement strategy.

In many situations, measurement of actual behavior is the most accurate and appropriate technique. Nurses often perform comparative analyses using patient admission data as the baseline: selected data points observed when nursing care is given and self-care is initiated are compared with the patient's baseline data. In other cases, indirect measurement may be used. Some examples of indirect measurement are patient satisfaction surveys, attitude surveys, and instruments that evaluate specific health status variables.

However, measurement is only the beginning of evaluation, which must be followed by data interpretation and value judgments about learning and teaching. These aspects of evaluation should be conducted periodically throughout the teaching–learning program, at its conclusion, and at varying periods after the teaching has ended.

Evaluation of learning after hospitalization is highly desirable, because the analysis of teaching outcomes must extend into home care. With shortened lengths of hospital stay and with short-stay and same-day surgical procedures, follow-up evaluation in the home is especially important. Coordination of efforts and sharing of information between hospital-based and community-based nursing personnel facilitate postdischarge teaching and home care evaluation.

Evaluation is not the final step in the teaching–learning process, but the beginning of a new patient assessment. The information gathered during evaluation should be used to redirect teaching actions, with the goal of improving the patient's responses and outcomes.

Health Promotion

Health teaching and **health promotion** are linked by a common goal—to encourage people to achieve as high a level of wellness as possible so that they can live maximally healthy lives and avoid preventable illnesses. The call for health promotion has become a cornerstone in health policy because of the need to control costs and reduce unnecessary sickness and death.

The nation's first public health agenda was established in 1979 and set goals for improving the health of all Americans. Additional goals defined as the "1990 Health Objectives" identified improvements to be made in health status, risk reduction, public awareness, health services, and protective measures (U.S. Public Health Service, 2000).

Health goals for the nation were also established in the publication *Healthy People 2000*. The priorities from this initiative were identified as health promotion, health protection, and the use of preventive services. The most recent publication, *Healthy People 2010*, defines the current national health promotion and disease prevention initiative for the nation. The two essential goals from this report are (1) to increase the quality and years of healthy life for people and (2) to eliminate health disparities among various segments of the population (U.S. Public Health Service, 2000) (Chart 4-3).

Definition

Health promotion may be defined as those activities that assist people in developing resources that maintain or enhance well-being and improve their quality of life. These

CHART 4-3

Leading Health Indicators to be Used to Measure the Health of the Nation

1. Physical activity
2. Overweight and obesity
3. Tobacco use
4. Substance abuse
5. Responsible sexual behavior
6. Mental health
7. Injury and violence
8. Environmental quality
9. Immunization
10. Access to health care

From U.S. Department of Health & Human Services (2000). *Healthy People 2010*. Washington, DC: U.S. Government Printing Office.

activities involve people's efforts to remain healthy in the absence of symptoms and do not require the assistance of a health care team member.

The purpose of health promotion is to focus on the person's potential for wellness and to encourage appropriate alterations in personal habits, lifestyle, and environment in ways that reduce risks and enhance health and well-being. Health promotion is an active process; that is, it is not something that can be prescribed or dictated. It is up to each person to decide whether to make changes to promote a higher level of wellness. Only the individual can make these choices.

The concepts of health, wellness, health promotion, and disease prevention have been a topic of extensive discussion in the lay literature and news media as well as in professional journals. As a result, public demand for health information has increased, and health care professionals and agencies have responded by providing this information. Health promotion programs, once limited to hospital settings, have now moved into community settings such as clinics, schools, churches, and the workplace. As employers strive to reduce costs associated with absenteeism, health insurance, hospitalization, disability, excessive turnover of personnel, and premature death, the workplace has become an important site for health promotion programs.

Health and Wellness

The concept of health promotion has evolved because of a changing definition of health and an awareness that wellness exists at many levels of functioning. Health is viewed as a dynamic, ever-changing condition that enables people to function at an optimal potential at any given time. The ideal health status is one in which people are successful in achieving their full potential, regardless of any limitations they might have.

Wellness, as a reflection of health, involves a conscious and deliberate attempt to maximize one's health. Wellness does not just happen; it requires planning and conscious commitment and is the result of adopting lifestyle behaviors for the purpose of attaining one's highest potential for well-being. Wellness is not the same for every person. The person with a chronic illness or disability may still be able to achieve a desirable level of wellness. The key to wellness is to function at the highest potential within the limitations over which there is no control.

A significant amount of research has shown that people, by virtue of what they do or fail to do, influence their own health. Today, many of the major causes of illness are chronic diseases that have been closely related to lifestyle behaviors (eg, heart disease, lung and colon cancer, chronic obstructive pulmonary diseases, hypertension, cirrhosis, traumatic injury, human immunodeficiency virus [HIV] infection, or acquired immunodeficiency syndrome [AIDS]). To a large extent, a person's health status may be reflective of his or her lifestyle.

Health Promotion Models

Since the 1950s, many health promotion models have been constructed to identify health-protecting behaviors and to help explain what makes people engage in these preventive behaviors. A health-protecting behavior is defined as any behavior performed by people, regardless of their actual or perceived health condition, for the purpose of promoting or maintaining their health, whether or not the behavior produces the desired outcome (Downie, Fyfe, & Tannahill, 1996). One model, the health belief model, was designed to foster understanding of why some healthy people choose actions to prevent illness, whereas others refuse to engage in these protective recommendations (Becker, 1974). Another model, the resource model of preventive health behavior, addresses the ways in which people use resources to promote health (Downie, Fyfe, & Tannahill, 1996). Nurse educators can use this model to assess how demographic variables, health behaviors, and social and health resources influence health promotion.

The Canadian health promotion initiative, Achieving Health for All, builds on Lalonde's work in the 1970s, in which four determinants of health—human biology, environment, lifestyle, and the health care delivery system—were identified. Determinants of health were defined as factors and conditions that have an influence on the health of individuals and communities (Lalonde, 1977). Since the 1970s a total of 12 determinants have been identified, and this number will continue to increase as population health research progresses. Determinants of health provide a framework for assessing and evaluating the population's health.

The health promotion model developed by Becker and colleagues (1993) is based on the premise that four variables influence the selection and use of health promotion behaviors. Demographic and disease factors, the first variable, include patient characteristics such as age, gender, education, employment, severity of illness or disability, and length of illness. Barriers, the second variable, are defined as factors leading to unavailability or difficulty in gaining access to a specific health promotion alternative. Resources, the third variable, encompass such items as financial and social support. Perceptual factors, the fourth variable, consist of how the person views his or her health status, self-efficacy, and the perceived demands of the illness. Becker and colleagues demonstrated that these four variables have a positive correlation with a person's quality of life.

The health promotion model developed by Pender (2005) is based on social learning theory and emphasizes the importance of motivational factors in acquiring and sustaining health promotion behaviors. This model explores how cognitive-perceptual factors affect the person's view of the importance of health. It also examines perceived control of health, self-efficacy, health status, and the benefits and barriers to health-promoting behaviors.

These models of health promotion, along with others that can be found in the health promotion literature, can serve as an organizing framework for clinical work and research that supports the enhancement of health. Studies aim to increase understanding of the health promotion behaviors of families and communities (eg, Epple, Wright, Joish, et al., 2003; Javo, Alapack, Keyerdall, et al., 2003).

Components of Health Promotion

There are several components of health promotion as an active process: self-responsibility, nutritional awareness, stress reduction and management, and physical fitness.

Self-Responsibility

Taking responsibility for oneself is the key to successful health promotion. The concept of **self-responsibility** is based on the understanding that the individual controls his or her life. Each person alone must make the choices that determine how healthy his or her lifestyle is. As more people recognize that lifestyle and behavior significantly affect health, they may assume responsibility for avoiding high-risk behaviors such as smoking, alcohol and drug abuse, overeating, driving while intoxicated, risky sexual practices, and other unhealthy habits. They may also assume responsibility for adopting routines that have been found to have a positive influence on health, such as engaging in regular exercise, wearing seat belts, and eating a healthy diet.

A variety of different techniques have been used to encourage people to accept responsibility for their health, ranging from extensive educational programs to reward systems. No one technique has been found to be superior to any other. Instead, self-responsibility for health promotion is very individualized and depends on a person's desires and inner motivations. Health promotion programs are important tools for encouraging people to assume responsibility for their health and to develop behaviors that improve health.

Nutritional Awareness

Nutrition as a component of health promotion has become the focus of considerable attention and publicity. A vast array of books and magazine articles address the topics of special diets; natural foods; and the hazards associated with certain substances, such as sugar, salt, cholesterol, trans fats, carbohydrates, artificial colors, and food additives. It has been suggested that good nutrition is the single most significant factor in determining health status and longevity.

Nutritional awareness involves an understanding of the importance of a healthy diet that supplies all of the essential nutrients. Understanding the relationship between diet and disease is an important facet of a person's self-care. Some clinicians believe that a healthy diet is one that substitutes "natural" foods for processed and refined ones and reduces the intake of sugar, salt, fat, cholesterol, caffeine, alcohol, food additives, and preservatives.

Chapter 5 contains further information about the assessment of a person's nutritional status. It describes the physical signs indicating nutritional status, assessment of food intake (food record, 24-hour recall), the dietary guidelines presented in the MyPyramid plan, and calculation of ideal body weight.

Stress Reduction and Management

Stress management and stress reduction are important aspects of health promotion. Studies have shown the negative effects of stress on health and a cause-and-effect relationship between stress and infectious diseases, traumatic injuries (eg, motor vehicle crashes), and some chronic illnesses. Stress has become inevitable in contemporary societies in which demands for productivity have become excessive. More and more emphasis is placed on encouraging people to manage stress appropriately and to reduce stress that is counterproductive. Techniques such as relaxation training, exercise, and modification of stressful situations are often included in health promotion programs dealing with stress. Further information on stress management, including health risk appraisal and stress reduction methods such as biofeedback and the relaxation response, can be found in Chapter 6.

Physical Fitness

Physical fitness is another important component of health promotion. Clinicians and researchers (Anspaugh, Hamrick, & Rosato, 2003; Leifer & Hartston, 2004; U.S. Department of Health & Human Services, 2002) who have examined the relationship between health and physical fitness have found that a regular exercise program can promote health in the following ways:

- Improve the function of the circulatory system and the lungs
- Decrease cholesterol and low-density lipoprotein levels
- Decrease body weight by increasing calorie expenditure
- Delay degenerative changes such as osteoporosis
- Improve flexibility and overall muscle strength and endurance

An appropriate exercise program can have a significantly positive effect on a person's performance capacity, appearance, and general state of physical and emotional health. An exercise program should be designed specifically for a given person, with consideration given to age, physical condition, and any known cardiovascular or other risk factors. Exercise can be harmful if it is not started gradually and increased slowly in accordance with a person's response.

Health Promotion Throughout the Life Span

Health promotion is a concept and a process that extends throughout the life span. Studies have shown that the health of a child can be affected either positively or negatively by the health practices of the mother during the prenatal period. Therefore, health promotion starts before birth and extends through childhood, adolescence, adulthood, and old age.

Health promotion includes health screening. The American Academy of Family Physicians has developed recommendations for periodic health examinations that identify the age groups for which specific screening interventions are appropriate. Table 4-2 presents general population guidelines. Specific population standards and guidelines have also been recommended.

Children and Adolescents

Health screening has traditionally been an important aspect of childhood health care. The goal has been to detect health problems at an early age so that they can be treated early in life. Today, health promotion goes beyond the mere screening of children for disabilities and includes extensive efforts

TABLE 4-2 Routine Health Promotion Screening for Adults

Type of Screening	Suggested Time Frame
Routine health examination	Yearly
Blood chemistry profile	Baseline at age 20, then as mutually determined by patient and clinician
Complete blood count	Baseline at age 20, then as mutually determined by patient and clinician
Lipid profile	Baseline at age 20, then as mutually determined by patient and clinician
Hemoccult screening	Yearly after age 50
Electrocardiogram	Baseline at age 40, then as mutually determined by patient and clinician
Blood pressure	Yearly, then as mutually determined by patient and clinician
Tuberculosis skin test	Every 2 years or as mutually determined by patient and clinician
Chest x-ray film	For positive PPD results
Breast self-examination	Monthly
Mammogram	Yearly for women over 40, or earlier or more often if indicated
Clinical breast examination	Yearly
Gynecologic examination	Yearly
Pap test	Yearly
Bone density screening	Based on identification of primary and secondary risk factors (prior to onset of menopause, if indicated)
Nutritional screening	As mutually determined by patient and clinician
Digital rectal examination	Yearly
Colonoscopy	Every 3–5 years after age 50 or as mutually determined by patient and clinician
Prostate examination	Yearly
Prostate-specific antigen	Every 1–2 years after age 50
Testicular examination	Monthly
Skin examination	Yearly or as mutually determined by patient and clinician
Vision screening	Every 2–3 years
Glaucoma	Baseline at age 40, then every 2–3 years until age 70, then yearly
Dental screening	Every 6 months
Hearing screening	As needed
Health risk appraisal	As needed
Adult Immunizations	
Tetanus	Boosters every 10 years
Diphtheria	Boosters every 10 years
Rubella	Given to women of childbearing age if not previously given or if titer is low
Pneumococcal vaccine	Given one time at age 65 or younger if chronic illness or disability is present
Hepatitis B (if not received as a child)	Series of three doses (now, 1 month later, then 5 months after the second date)
Influenza vaccine	Yearly
Lyme disease vaccine, if at risk	Series of three doses (now, 1 month later, and 11 months after the second dose)

Note: Any of these screenings may be performed more frequently if deemed necessary by the patient or recommended by the health care provider.

to promote positive health practices at a very young age. Because health habits and practices are formed early in life, children should be encouraged to develop positive health attitudes. For this reason, more and more programs are being offered to school-age children and to adolescents to help them develop good health habits. Although the negative results of practices such as smoking, risky sexual activities, alcohol and drug abuse, and poor nutrition are explained in these educational programs, emphasis is also placed on values training, self-esteem, and healthy lifestyle practices. The projects are designed to appeal to a particular age group, with emphasis on learning experiences that are fun, interesting, and relevant.

Young and Middle-Aged Adults

Young and middle-aged adults represent an age group that not only expresses an interest in health and health promotion but also responds enthusiastically to suggestions that show how lifestyle practices can improve health. Adults are frequently motivated to change their lifestyles in ways that are believed to enhance their health and wellness. Many adults who wish to improve their health turn to health promotion programs to help them make the desired changes in their lifestyles. Many have responded to programs that focus on topics such as general wellness, smoking cessation, exercise, physical conditioning, weight control, conflict resolution, and stress management. Because of the nationwide emphasis on health during the reproductive years, young adults actively seek programs that address prenatal health, parenting, family planning, and women's health issues.

Programs that provide health screening, such as those that screen for cancer, high cholesterol, hypertension, diabetes, abdominal aneurysm, and visual and hearing impairments, are quite popular with young and middle-aged adults. Programs that involve health promotion for people with specific chronic illnesses such as cancer, diabetes, heart disease, and pulmonary disease are also popular. It is becoming more evident that chronic disease and disability do not preclude health and wellness; rather, positive health attitudes and practices can promote optimal health for people who must live with the limitations imposed by their chronic illnesses and disabilities.

Health promotion programs can be offered almost anywhere in the community. Common sites include local clinics, elementary and high schools, community colleges, recreation centers, churches, and even private homes. Health fairs are frequently held in civic centers and shopping malls. The outreach idea for health promotion programs has served to meet the needs of many adults who otherwise would not avail themselves of opportunities to strive toward a healthier lifestyle.

The workplace has become a center for health promotion activity for several reasons. Employers have become increasingly concerned about the rising costs of health care insurance to treat illnesses related to lifestyle behaviors, and they are also concerned about increased absenteeism and lost productivity. Some employers use health promotion specialists to develop and implement these programs, and others purchase packaged programs that have already been developed by health care agencies or private health promotion corporations.

Programs offered at the workplace usually include employee health screening and counseling, physical fitness, nutritional awareness, work safety, and stress management and stress reduction. In addition, efforts are made to promote a safe and healthy work environment. Many large businesses provide exercise facilities for their employees and offer their health promotion programs to retirees. If employers can show cost-containment benefits from such programs, their dollars will be considered well spent, and more businesses will provide health promotion programs as a benefit of employment.

Gerontologic Considerations

Health promotion is as important for the elderly as it is for other adults and children. Although 80% of people older than 65 years have one or more chronic illnesses and many are limited in their activity, the elderly as a group experience significant gains from health promotion. The elderly are very health-conscious, and most view their health positively and are willing to adopt practices that will improve their health and well-being (Ebersole, Hess, & Luggen, 2004). Although their chronic illnesses and disabilities cannot be eliminated, these adults can benefit from activities that help them maintain independence and achieve an optimal level of health.

Various health promotion programs have been developed to meet the needs of older Americans. Both public and private organizations continue to be responsive to health promotion, and more programs that serve the elderly are

NURSING RESEARCH PROFILE

Health Promotion in the Elderly

McPhee, S. D., Johnson, T. R., & Dietrich, M. S. (2004). Comparing health status with healthy habits in elderly assisted-living residents. *Family and Community Health, 27*(2), 158–170.

Purpose

The purpose of this study was to determine the relationship between seven healthy lifestyle habits, as identified by the Health Generation Survey, and the health status of adults living in assisted-living residences. The habits studied were water consumption, tobacco use, alcohol use, hours of sleep per night, breakfast eating, healthy snack eating, and engagement in physical activity. The practice of healthy lifestyle habits and their relationships to the five most common medical conditions (arthritis, heart disease, stroke, cancer, diabetes) seen in residents of assisted-living facilities were examined.

Design

The Health Generation Survey was distributed to the residents of several assisted-living facilities in the southeastern part of the United States. There were 1,079 adults who completed the survey within the first 6 weeks of their entrance to the facilities. This particular study was a secondary data analysis of the original data collected.

Findings

The findings of this study revealed that older adults with a greater number of current physical health problems reported that they had more healthy lifestyle habits than older adults without health problems. People began to incorporate a greater number of healthy habits into their lifestyle after they were determined to have certain specific health problems. In addition, the study also found that residents who engaged in physical exercise and recreational activities reported a greater overall participation in other healthy lifestyle habits.

Nursing Implications

Because older adults in assisted-living facilities tend to experience more health-related problems than older adults living within the community, nurses need to focus on the health habits examined in this study and be in a position to assess and implement strategies for healthy living. The development of appropriate educational programs and individual reinforcement of healthy habits with the residents may further increase their participation in health promotion activities.

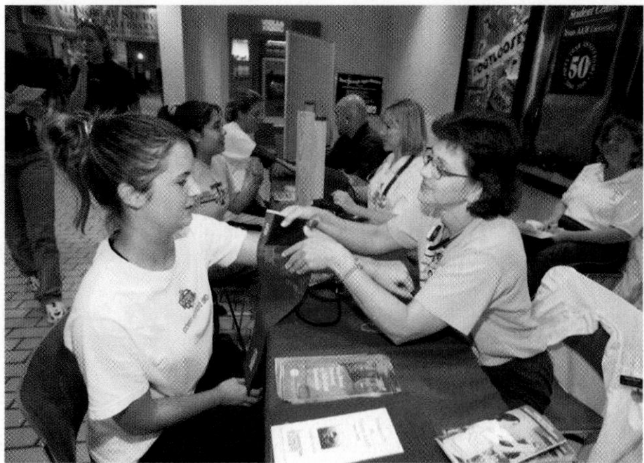

FIGURE 4-2. Health promotion programs are held in community settings such as clinics, schools, churches, and the workplace. Nurses play a vital role in organizing and providing wellness services to the general public. Here, a nurse takes a student's blood pressure at a health fair held on a college campus. (Cushing Memorial Library and Archives, Texas A&M University.)

emerging. Many of these programs are offered by health care agencies, churches, community centers, senior citizen residences, and a variety of other organizations. The activities directed toward health promotion for the elderly are the same as those for other age groups: physical fitness and exercise, nutrition, safety, and stress management.

Nursing Implications

By virtue of their expertise in health and health care and their long-established credibility with consumers, nurses play a vital role in health promotion. In many instances, they have initiated health promotion and health screening programs or have participated with other health care personnel in developing and providing wellness services in a variety of settings (Fig. 4-2).

As health care professionals, nurses have a responsibility to promote activities that foster well-being, self-actualization, and personal fulfillment. Every interaction with consumers of health care must be viewed as an opportunity to promote positive health attitudes and behaviors.

Critical Thinking Exercises

1 A nurse is designing a patient teaching plan for a 57-year-old woman with a history of gastrointestinal problems. This woman has been diagnosed with osteoporosis, and her physician has recommended that she begin taking alendronate sodium (Fosamax). Describe the health promotion strategies you would develop for this patient. Determine what variables may influence her willingness to follow the recommended therapy.

2 A home health nurse is instructing a 55-year-old man with cardiovascular disease about healthy eating habits. He has recently been widowed, and his service animal (seeing-eye dog) of 15 years died last month. What physiologic and psychosocial variables would be relevant to understanding this patient's needs? How would a teaching plan be constructed to promote adequate nutrition? How would you modify the teaching plan, knowing that the patient is visually impaired?

3 ebp A 72-year-old man is informed by an advanced practice nurse about a health fair being held at the local community center across the street from his home. He declines to attend, saying, "I am too old and it is too late to be concerned about health promotion. The damage to my body has already been done." What resources would you use to identify evidence of the effectiveness of health promotion activities for the elderly? Discuss the strength of the evidence. Identify the criteria used to evaluate the strength of the evidence. What information would you then include in a discussion with the patient about promoting health in the elderly?

REFERENCES AND SELECTED READINGS

BOOKS

Alfaro-LeFevre, R. (2004). *Critical thinking and clinical judgment.* Philadelphia: Saunders.

American Nurses Association. (2004). *Standards of clinical nursing practice.* Washington, DC: Author.

Andrews, M. M., & Boyle, J. S. (2002). *Transcultural concepts in nursing care* (4th ed.). Philadelphia: Lippincott Williams & Wilkins.

Anspaugh, D. J., Hamrick, M. H., & Rosato, F. D. (2003). *Wellness: Concepts and applications* (5th ed.). St. Louis: Mosby.

Bastable, S. B. (Ed.). (2003). *Nurse as educator: Principles of teaching and learning.* Boston: Jones & Bartlett.

Becker, M. H. (Ed.). (1974). *The health belief model and personal health behavior.* Thorofare, NJ: Charles B. Slack.

Carpenito-Moyet, L. J. (2003). *Nursing diagnosis: Application to clinical practice* (10th ed.). Philadelphia: Lippincott Williams & Wilkins.

Downie, R. S., Fyfe, C., & Tannahill, A. (1996). *Health promotion: Models and values* (2nd ed.). New York: Oxford University Press.

Doyle, E., & Ward, S. (2001). *The process of community health education and promotion.* Palo Alto, CA: Mayfield Publishing.

Ebersole, P., Hess, P. & Luggen, A. (2004). *Toward health aging: Human needs and nursing responses* (6th ed.). St. Louis: Mosby.

Eliopoulos, C. (2004). *Gerontological nursing* (6th ed.). Philadelphia: Lippincott Williams & Wilkins.

Giger, J. N., & Davidhizar, R. E. (2004). *Transcultural nursing: Assessment and intervention* (4th ed.). St. Louis: Mosby.

Glouberman, S. (2001). *Towards a new perspective on health policy.* Ottawa, Ontario: Commission on the Future of Health in Canada.

Kreuter, M. W., Lezin, M. A., Kreuter, M. W., & Green, L. W. (2003). Community health promotion ideas that work (2nd ed.). Sudburg, MA: Jones & Bartlett.

Insel, P. M., & Roth, W. T. (2000). *Core concepts in health.* Palo Alto, CA: Mayfield Publishing.

Lalonde, M. (1977). *New perspectives on the health of Canadians: A working document.* Ottawa, Canada: Minister of Supply and Services.

Leifer, G., & Hartston, H. (2004). Growth and Development Across the Lifespan: A Health Promotion Focus: St. Louis: Elsevier.

Leininger, M. M. (2001). *Culture care diversity and universality: A theory of nursing.* Boston: Jones & Bartlett.

Murray, R. B., & Zentner, J. P. (2001). *Nursing assessment and health promotion through the life span* (7th ed.). Englewood Cliffs, NJ: Prentice-Hall.

O'Donnell, M. P. (2001). *Health promotion in the workplace.* Albany, NY: Delmar Publishing.

Pender, N. J., Murdaugh, C., & Parsons, M. A. (2005). *Health promotion in nursing practice* (5th ed.). Upper Saddle River, NJ: Prentice-Hall Health, Inc.

Rankin, S. H., & Stallings, K. D. (2004). *Patient education in health and illness* (5th ed.). Philadelphia: Lippincott Williams & Wilkins.

Redman, B. (2004). *Advances in patient education.* New York: Springer Publishing Company.

U.S. Department of Health & Human Services (2002). *Physical activity fundamental to preventing disease.* Atlanta: U.S. Department of Health and Human Services, Centers for Disease Control and Prevention, National Center for Chronic Disease Prevention and Health Promotion.

U.S. Public Health Service. (1990). *Healthy people 2000.* Washington, DC: U.S. Government Printing Office.

U.S. Public Health Service. (1995). *Healthy people 2000: Midcourse review and 1995 revision.* Washington, DC: U.S. Government Printing Office.

U.S. Public Health Service. (2000). *Healthy people 2010: Understanding and improving health.* Washington, DC: U.S. Government Printing Office.

Whitman, T. L. (Ed.). (1999). *Life-span perspectives on health and illness.* Mahwah, NJ: Lawrence Erlbaum Associates.

Woolf, S. H., Jonas, S., & Lawrence, R. S. (1996). *Health promotion and disease prevention in clinical practice.* Baltimore: Williams & Wilkins.

JOURNALS

Asterisks indicate nursing research articles.

Becker, H. A., Stuifbergen, A. K., Oh, H., et al. (1993). The self-rated abilities for health practices scale: A health self-efficacy measure. *Health Values, 17,* 42–50.

Britton, J. (2003). The use of emollients and their correct application. *Journal of Community Nursing, 17*(9), 22–25.

Cox, R. H., Carpenter, J. P., Bruce, F. A., et al. (2004). Characteristics of low-income African Americans and Caucasian adults that are important in self-management of type 2 diabetes. *Journal of Community Health, 29*(2), 155–170.

Daniel, B. T., Damato, K. L., & Johnson, J. (2004). Educational issues in oral care. *Seminars in Oncology Nursing, 20*(1), 48–52.

Duman, M., & Clark, A. (2004). Patient information: Part 4. Content and presentation. *Professional Nurse, 19*(6), 354–355.

*Enriquez, M., Gore, P. A., O'Connor, M. C., et al. (2004). Assessment of readiness for adherence by HIV-positive males who had previously failed treatment. *Journal of the Association of Nurses in AIDS Care, 15*(1), 42–49.

Epple, C., Wright, A. L., Joish, V. N., et al. (2003). The role of active family nutritional support in Navajos' type 2 diabetes mellitus control. *Diabetes Care, 26*(10), 2829–2834.

Glouberman, S. & Miller, J. (2003). Evolution of the determinants of health, health policy, and health information systems. *American Journal of Public Health, 93*(3), 388–392.

*Gyurcsik, N. C., Bray, S. R., & Brittain, D. R. (2004). Coping with barriers to vigorous physical activity during transition to university. *Family and Community Health, 27*(2), 130–143.

Hong, S., Friedman, J., & Alt, S. (2003). Modifiable risk factors for the primary prevention of heart disease in women. *Journal of the American Medical Women's Association, 58*(4), 278–284.

Javo, C., Alapack, R., Heyerdall, S., et al. (2003). Parental values and ethnic identity in indigenous Sami families: A qualitative study. *Family Process, 42*(1), 151–162.

*Jones, E. D., Kennedy-Malone, L., & Wideman, L. (2004). Early detection of type 2 diabetes among older African Americans. *Geriatric Nursing, 25*(1), 24–28.

Lai, S. C., & Cohen, M. N. (1999). Promoting lifestyle changes. *American Journal of Nursing, 99*(4), 63–67.

*Lev, E. L., & Owen, S. V. (1996). A measure of self-care self-efficacy: Strategies used by people to promote health. *Research in Nursing and Health, 19*(5), 421–429.

*Linfante, A. H., Allan, R., Smith, S. C., & Mosca, L. (2003). Psychosocial factors predict coronary heart disease, but what predicts psychosocial risk in women? *Journal of the American Medical Women's Association, 58*(4), 248–253.

Lucas, J. A., Orshan, S. A., & Cook, F. (2000). Determinants of health-promoting behaviors among women ages 65 and above living in the community. *Scholarly Inquiry for Nursing Practice, 14*(1), 77–109.

*McPhee, S. D., Johnson, T. R., & Dietrich, M. S. (2004). Comparing health status with healthy habits in elderly assisted-living residents. *Family and Community Health, 27*(2), 158–170.

*Murray, E., Lo, B., Pollack, L., Donelan, K., et al. (2003). The impact of health information on the internet on the physician–patient relationship: Patient perceptions. *Archives of Internal Medicine, 163*(14), 1727–1738.

Roberts, K. (2004). Simplify, simplify: Tackling health literacy by addressing reading literacy. *American Journal of Nursing, 104*(3), 118–119.

Robinson, A. W., & Sloan, H. L. (2000). Healthy People 2000: Heart health and old women. *Journal of Gerontological Nursing, 26*(5), 38–45.

Schank, M. J. (1999). Educational innovations—Self-health appraisal: Learning the difficulties of lifestyle change. *Journal of Nursing Education, 38*(1), 10–12.

Smeltzer, S. C., Zimmerman, V., DeSilets, L. D., et al. (2003). Accessible online health promotion information for persons with disabilities. *Online Journal of Issues in Nursing, 9*(1), 11. Available at: http://www.nursingworld.org/ojin/topic16/tpc16_5.htm.

RESOURCES AND WEBSITES

Centers for Disease Control and Prevention, 1600 Clifton Road, Atlanta, GA 30333; 404-639-3311; http://www.cdc.gov. Accessed June 6, 2006.

Health Education Resources Exchange, Washington State Department of Health, Office of Health Promotion, P.O. Box 47833, Olympia, WA 98504; 800-525-0127; http://www.doh.wa.gov/here/Default.html. Accessed June 6, 2006.

Health Promotion for Women With Disabilities, Villanova University College of Nursing, 800 Lancaster Avenue, Villanova, PA 19085; 610-519-4900; http://www.nurseweb.villanova.edu/WomenWithDisabilities//welcom.htm. Accessed June 6, 2006.

U.S. Army Center for Health Promotion and Preventive Medicine (USACHPPM), 5158 Blackhawk Road, Aberdeen Proving Ground, MD 21010; 800-222-9698; chppm-www.apgea.army.mil/. Accessed June 6, 2006.

U.S. Department of Health and Human Services, National Institutes of Health: http://www.nih.gov/icd/. Accessed June 6, 2006.

U.S. Department of Health and Human Services, Office of Disease Prevention and Health Promotion, 1101 Wooton Parkway, Suite LL100, Rockville, MD 20852; http://www.odphp.osophs.dhhs.gov. Accessed June 6, 2006.

World Health Organization, Avenue Appia 20, 1211 Geneva 27, Switzerland; telephone: (+41 22) 791 21 11; http://www.who.int/hpr/. Accessed June 6, 2006.

CHAPTER 5

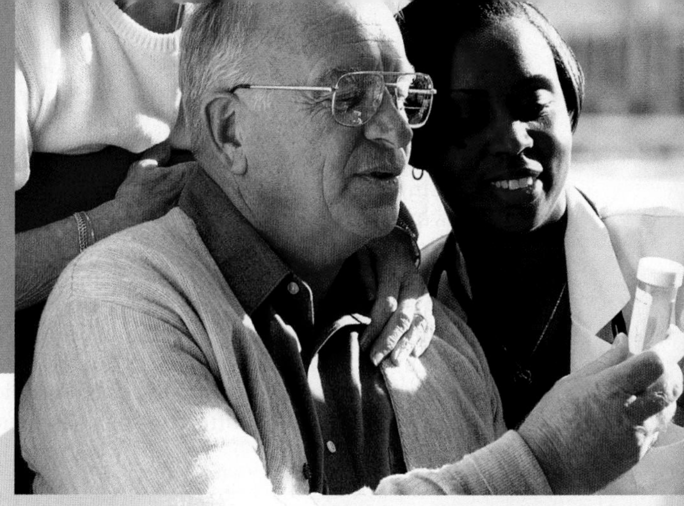

Health Assessment

Learning Objectives

On completion of this chapter, the learner will be able to:

1. Describe the components of the health history.
2. Apply culturally sensitive interviewing skills and techniques to conduct a successful health history, physical examination, and nutritional assessment.
3. Identify modifications needed to obtain a health history and conduct a physical assessment for a person with a disability.
4. Identify genetic aspects nurses should incorporate into the health history and physical assessment.
5. Describe the physical examination techniques of inspection, palpation, percussion, and auscultation.
6. Apply the techniques of inspection, palpation, percussion, and auscultation to perform physical assessment of the major body systems of a person.
7. Discuss the techniques of measurement of body mass index, biochemical assessment, clinical examination, and assessment of food intake to assess a person's nutritional status.
8. Identify ethical considerations necessary for protecting a person's rights related to data collected in the health history and physical examination.
9. Describe factors that may contribute to altered nutritional status in high-risk groups such as adolescents and the elderly.
10. Conduct a health history and physical and nutritional assessment of a person at home.

The ability to assess patients is one of the most important skills of nursing, regardless of the practice setting. In all settings in which nurses interact with patients and provide care, eliciting a complete health history and using appropriate assessment skills are critical to identifying physical and psychological problems and concerns experienced by the patient. As the first step in the nursing process, patient assessment is necessary to obtain data that enable the nurse to make a nursing diagnosis, identify and implement nursing interventions, and assess their effectiveness.

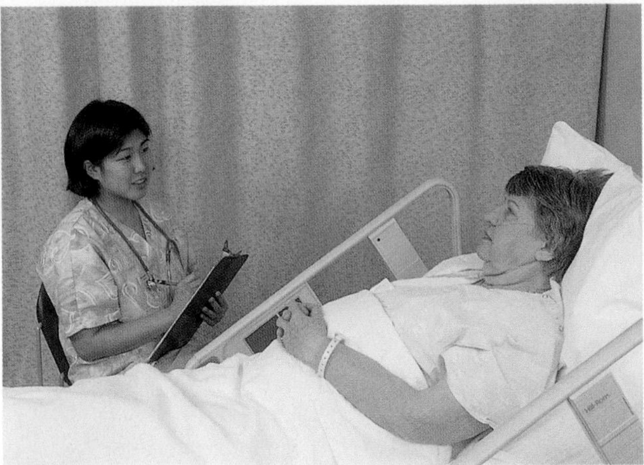

FIGURE 5-1. A comfortable, relaxed atmosphere and an attentive interviewer are essential for a successful clinical interview. Photo © B. Proud.

The Role of the Nurse in Health Assessment

In health assessment, the nurse obtains the patient's health history and performs a physical assessment, which can be carried out in a variety of settings, including the acute care setting, clinic or outpatient office, school, long-term care facility, or the home. A growing list of nursing diagnoses is used by nurses to identify and categorize patient problems that nurses have the knowledge, skills, and responsibility to treat independently (NANDA International, 2005) (see also Chapter 3, Chart 3-7). All members of the health care team—physicians, nurses, nutritionists, social workers, and others—use their unique skills and knowledge to contribute to the resolution of patient problems by first obtaining a health history and physical examination (Rasmor & Brown, 2003; Sanchez, Schreiber, Glynn, et al., 2003). Because the focus of each member of the health care team is unique, a variety of health history and physical examination formats have been developed. Regardless of the format, the information obtained by the nurse complements the data obtained by other members of the health care team and focuses on nursing's unique concerns for the patient.

Basic Guidelines for Conducting a Health Assessment

People who seek health care for a specific problem often feel anxious. Their anxiety may be increased by fear about potential diagnoses, possible disruption of lifestyle, and other concerns. With this in mind, the nurse attempts to establish rapport, put the patient at ease, encourage honest communication, make eye contact, and listen carefully to the patient's responses to questions about health issues (Fig. 5-1).

When obtaining a health history or performing a physical examination, the nurse must be aware of his or her own nonverbal communication, as well as that of the patient. The nurse should take into consideration the patient's educational and cultural background (Flowers, 2004) as well as language proficiency. Questions and instructions to the patient are phrased in a way that is easily understandable. Technical terms and medical jargon are avoided. In addition, the nurse must take into consideration the patient's disabilities or impairments (hearing, vision, cognitive, and physical limitations). At the end of the assessment, the nurse may summarize and clarify the information obtained and ask the patient if he or she has any questions; this gives the nurse the opportunity to correct misinformation and add facts that may have been omitted.

Ethical Use of History or Physical Examination Data

Whenever information is elicited from a person through a health history or physical examination, the person has the right to know why the information is sought and how it will be used. For this reason, it is important to explain what the history and physical examination are, how the information will be obtained, and how it will be used (Sanchez et al., 2003). It is also important that the person be aware that the decision to participate is voluntary. A private setting for the history interview and physical examination promotes trust and encourages open, honest communication. After the history and examination are completed, the nurse selectively records the data pertinent to the patient's health status. This written record of the patient's history and physical examination findings is then maintained in a secure place and made available only to those health professionals directly involved in the care of the patient. This protects confidentiality and promotes professional conduct.

Increasing Use of Technology

The use of technology to augment the information-gathering process has become an increasingly important aspect of obtaining a health history and physical examination. Computerization of medical records is becoming more common in private health care providers' offices as well as in medical centers. Electronic health records are thought to improve the quality of care, reduce medical errors, and help reduce health care costs. Computerized needs assessments are being used to gather family health histories (Kinzie, Cohn, Julian, et al., 2002), screen blood donors (Sanchez et al., 2003), and screen for intimate partner violence (Rhodes, Lauderdale, He, et al., 2002). Assessments can be completed and multiple aspects of health can be researched online (Eng, 2001). Nurses must be sensitive to the needs of the elderly and others who may not be comfortable with the new technology, and they may need to allow extra time and provide detailed instructions.

The Health History

Throughout assessment, and particularly when obtaining the history, attention is focused on the impact of psychosocial, ethnic, and cultural background on a person's health, illness, and health promotion behaviors. The interpersonal and physical environments, as well as the person's lifestyle and activities of daily living, are explored in depth. Many nurses are responsible for obtaining a detailed history of the person's current health problems, past medical history, and family history and a review of the person's functional status. This results in a total health profile that focuses on health as well as illness and is more appropriately called a health history rather than a medical or a nursing history.

The format of the health history traditionally combines the medical history and the nursing assessment, although formats based on nursing frameworks, such as functional health patterns, have also become a standard. Both the review of systems and the patient profile are expanded to include individual and family relationships, lifestyle patterns, health practices, and coping strategies. These components of the health history are the basis of nursing assessment and can be easily adapted to address the needs of any patient population in any setting, institution, or agency (Rasmor & Brown, 2003). Combining the information obtained by the physician and the nurse into one health history prevents duplication of information and minimizes efforts on the part of the patient to provide this information repeatedly. This also encourages collaboration among members of the health care team who share in the collection and interpretation of the data.

Special considerations when obtaining a health history from an older adult are given in Chart 5-1.

The Informant

The informant, or the person providing the health history, may not always be the patient, as in the case of a developmentally delayed, mentally impaired, disoriented, confused, unconscious, or comatose patient. The interviewer assesses the reliability of the informant and the usefulness of the information provided. For example, a disoriented patient is often unable to provide reliable information; people who use illicit drugs and alcohol often deny using these substances. The interviewer must make a clinical judgment about the reliability of the information (based on the context of the entire interview) and include this assessment in the record.

CHART 5-1

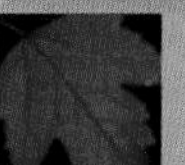

Health Assessment in the Older Adult

A health history should be obtained from elderly patients in a calm, unrushed manner. Because of the increased incidence of impaired hearing and vision in the elderly, lighting should be adequate but not glaring, and distracting noises should be kept to a minimum. The interviewer should assume a position that enables the person to read lips and facial expressions. People who normally use a hearing aid are asked to use it during the interview. The interviewer should also recognize that there is wide diversity among the elderly and that differences exist in health practices, gender, income, and functional status (Loeb, 2004; Yarcheski, Mahon, Yarcheski, et al., 2004).

Elderly people often assume that new physical problems are a result of age rather than a treatable illness. In addition, the signs and symptoms of illness in the elderly are often more subtle than those in younger people and may go unreported. Therefore, the interviewer inquires about subtle physical symptoms and recent changes in function and well-being. Special care is taken in obtaining a complete history of medications used, because many elderly people take many different kinds of prescription and over-the-counter (OTC) medications. Although elderly people may experience a decline in mental function, it should not be assumed that they are unable to provide an adequate history (Stotts & Deitrich, 2004). Nevertheless, including a member of the family in the interview process (eg, spouse, adult child, sibling, caretaker) may validate information and provide missing details. However, this should be done after obtaining the patient's permission. Further details about assessment of the older adult are provided in Chapter 12.

Cultural Considerations

When obtaining the health history, the person's cultural background (Weber & Kelley, 2003) is taken into account. Cultural attitudes and beliefs about health, illness, health care, hospitalization, the use of medications, and use of complementary and alternative therapies, which are derived from personal experiences (Flowers, 2004), vary according to ethnic and cultural background. A person from another culture may have different views of personal health practices from those of the health care practitioner.

Similarly, people from some ethnic and cultural backgrounds will not complain of pain, even when it is severe, because outward expressions of pain are considered unacceptable. In some instances, they may refuse to take analgesics. Other cultures have their own folklore and beliefs about the treatment of illnesses. All such differences in outlook must be taken into account and accepted when caring for members of other cultures. Attitudes and beliefs about family relationships and the roles of women and elderly members of a family must be respected, even if they conflict with those of the interviewer.

Content of the Health History

When a patient is seen for the first time by a member of the health care team, the first requirement is that baseline information be obtained (except in emergency situations). The sequence and format of obtaining data about a patient may vary, but the content, regardless of format, usually addresses the same general topics. A traditional approach includes the following:

- Biographical data
- Chief complaint
- Present health concern (or present illness)
- Past history
- Family history
- Review of systems
- Patient profile

Biographical Data

Biographical information puts the patient's health history into context. This information includes the person's name, address, age, gender, marital status, occupation, and ethnic origins. Some interviewers prefer to ask more personal questions at this part of the interview, whereas others wait until more trust and confidence have been established or until a patient's immediate or urgent needs are first addressed. A patient who is in severe pain or has another urgent problem is unlikely to have a great deal of patience for an interviewer who is more concerned about marital or occupational status than with quickly addressing the problem at hand.

Chief Complaint

The chief complaint is the issue that brings a person to the attention of the health care provider. Questions such as, "Why have you come to the health center today?" or "Why were you admitted to the hospital?" usually elicit the chief complaint. In the home setting, the initial question might be, "What is bothering you most today?" When a problem is identified, the person's exact words are usually recorded in quotation marks (Orient, 2005). However, a statement such as, "My doctor sent me," should be followed up with a question that identifies the probable reason why the person is seeking health care; this reason is then identified as the chief complaint.

Present Health Concern or Illness

The history of the present health concern or illness is the single most important factor in helping the health care team arrive at a diagnosis or determine the patient's needs. The physical examination is helpful but often only validates the information obtained from the history. A careful history assists in correct selection of appropriate diagnostic tests. Although diagnostic test results can be helpful, they often support rather than establish the diagnosis.

If the present illness is only one episode in a series of episodes, the entire sequence of events is recorded. For example, a history from a patient whose chief complaint is an episode of insulin shock describes the entire course of the diabetes to put the current episode in context. The details of the health concern or present illness are described from onset until the time of contact with the health care team. These facts are recorded in chronologic order, beginning with, for example, "The patient was in good health until . . ." or "The patient first experienced abdominal pain 2 months prior to seeking help."

The history of the present illness or problem includes such information as the date and manner (sudden or gradual) in which the problem occurred, the setting in which the problem occurred (at home, at work, after an argument, after exercise), manifestations of the problem, and the course of the illness or problem. This includes self-treatment (including complementary and alternative therapies), medical interventions, progress and effects of treatment, and the patient's perceptions of the cause or meaning of the problem.

Specific symptoms (pain, headache, fever, change in bowel habits) are described in detail, along with the location and radiation (if pain), quality, severity, and duration. The interviewer also asks whether the problem is persistent or intermittent, what factors aggravate or alleviate it, and whether any associated manifestations exist.

Associated manifestations are symptoms that occur simultaneously with the chief complaint. The presence or absence of such symptoms may shed light on the origin or extent of the problem, as well as on the diagnosis. These symptoms are referred to as significant positive or negative findings and are obtained from a review of systems directly related to the chief complaint. For example, if a patient reports a vague symptom such as fatigue or weight loss, all body systems are reviewed and included in this section of the history. If, on the other hand, a patient's chief complaint is chest pain, only the cardiopulmonary and gastrointestinal systems may be included in the history of the present illness. In either situation, both positive and negative findings are recorded to define the problem further.

Past Health History

A detailed summary of a person's past health is an important part of the health history. After determining the general health status, the interviewer should inquire about immunization status according to the recommendations of the adult immunization schedule and record the dates of immunization (if known). The Advisory Committee on Immunization Practices (ACIP), which approved the first adult immunization schedule in 2002, updates the schedule each year (ACIP, 2005). Research suggests that the health history is an economical alternative to serotesting for measles, mumps, and rubella in military recruits (Burnham, Thompson & Jackson, 2002). The interviewer should also inquire about any known allergies to medications or other substances, along with the type of allergy and adverse reactions. Other relevant material includes information, if known, about the patient's last physical examination, chest x-ray, electrocardiogram, eye examination, hearing test, dental checkup, Papanicolaou (Pap) smear and mammogram (if female), digital rectal examination of the prostate gland (if male), bone density testing, colon cancer screening, and any other pertinent tests. The interviewer then discusses previous illnesses and records negative as well as positive responses to a list of specific diseases. Dates of illness, or the age of the patient at the time, as well as the names of the primary health care provider and hospital, the diagnosis, and the treatment are noted. The interviewer elicits a history of the following areas:

- Childhood illnesses—rubeola, rubella, polio, whooping cough, mumps, measles, chickenpox, scarlet fever, rheumatic fever, strep throat
- Adult illnesses
- Psychiatric illnesses
- Injuries—burns, fractures, head injuries
- Hospitalizations
- Surgical and diagnostic procedures
- Current medications—prescription, over-the-counter (OTC), home remedies, complementary therapies
- Use of alcohol and other drugs

If a particular hospitalization or major medical intervention is related to the present illness, the account of it is not repeated; rather, the report refers to the appropriate part of the record, such as "See history of present illness" or "See HPI," on the data sheet.

Family History

To identify diseases that may be genetic (Guttmacher, Collins & Carmona, 2004), communicable, or possibly environmental in origin, the interviewer asks about the age and health status, or the age and cause of death, of first-order relatives (parents, siblings, spouse, children) and second-order relatives (grandparents, cousins). In general, it is necessary to include the following diseases: cancer, hypertension, heart disease, diabetes, epilepsy, mental illness, tuberculosis, kidney disease, arthritis, allergies, asthma, alcoholism, and obesity. One of the easiest methods of recording such data is by using the family tree or genogram (Fig. 5-2). The results of genetic testing or screening, if known, are recorded. See Chapter 9 for a detailed discussion of genetics.

Review of Systems

The review of systems includes an overview of general health as well as symptoms related to each body system. Questions are asked about each of the major body systems in terms of past or present symptoms. Reviewing each body system helps reveal any relevant data. Negative as well as positive answers are recorded. If a patient responds positively to questions about a particular system, the information is analyzed carefully. If any illnesses were previously mentioned or recorded, it is not necessary to repeat them in this part of the history. Instead, reference is made to the appropriate place in the health history where the information can be found.

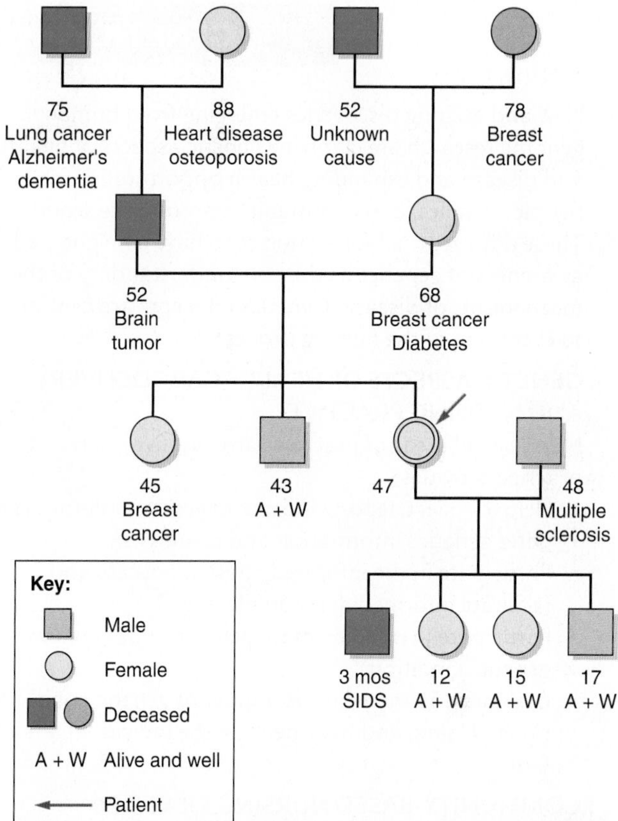

FIGURE 5-2. Diagram (called a genogram) used to record history of family members, including their age and cause of death or, if living, their current health status.

A review of systems can be organized in a formal checklist, which becomes a part of the health history. One advantage of a checklist is that it can be easily audited and is less subject to error than a system that relies heavily on the interviewer's memory.

Patient Profile

In the patient profile, more biographical information is gathered. A complete composite, or profile, of the patient is critical to analysis of the chief complaint and of the person's ability to deal with the problem. A complete patient profile is summarized in Chart 5-2.

At this point in the interview, the information elicited is highly personal and subjective. People are encouraged to express feelings honestly and to discuss personal experiences. It is best to begin with general, open-ended questions and to move to direct questioning when specific facts are needed. Interviews that progress from information that is less personal (birthplace, occupation, education) to information that is more personal (sexuality, body image, coping abilities) often reduce anxiety.

A general patient profile consists of the following content areas:

- Past life events related to health
- Education and occupation

GENETICS IN NURSING PRACTICE

New and exciting discoveries emerging from human genome research are clarifying genetic aspects of health and disease and expanding health opportunities for people, families, and communities around the world. These advances call for all nurses to have a heightened awareness of genetics as the core understanding of the mechanisms of disease. Genetics concepts are central to every step of the nursing process.

GENETIC ASPECTS OF HEALTH CARE DELIVERY AND NURSING PRACTICE

Nurses in all areas of practice carry out five main practice activities:

- Help to collect, report, and record genetics information
- Offer genetics information and resources
- Participate in the informed consent process and facilitate informed decision making
- Participate in ongoing management of patients with genetic conditions
- Evaluate and monitor the impact of genetic conditions, testing, and treatment on the individual and family

COMMUNITY-BASED NURSING PRACTICE

Nurses providing community-based care:

- Participate in genetic screening (eg, prenatal screening and newborn screening)
- Provide health care regarding genetic risk factors and management of genetically related disorders in a way that respects the beliefs and concerns of specific ethnic communities
- Educate the public about the contribution of genetics to health and disease
- Engage in dialogue with the public about ethical, legal, and social issues related to genetics discoveries

CRITICAL THINKING AND DECISION MAKING

Nurses use these skills in providing genetics-related health care when they:

- Assess and analyze family history data for genetic risk factors
- Identify those individuals and families in need of referral for genetic testing or counseling
- Ensure the privacy and confidentiality of genetics information

HEALTH EDUCATION AND PROMOTION

Nurses in all settings should be prepared to:

- Inquire about patients' and families' desired health outcomes with regard to genetics-related conditions or risk factors
- Refer patients for genetics services when indicated
- Identify barriers to accessing genetics-related health services
- Offer appropriate genetics information and resources

HEALTH ASSESSMENT

Nurses incorporate a genetics focus into the following health assessments:

- Family history—assess for genetics-related risk factors
- Cultural, social, and spiritual assessment—assess for individual and family perceptions and beliefs around genetics topics
- Physical assessment—assess for clinical features that may suggest a genetic condition is present (eg, unusually tall stature—Marfan syndrome)
- Ethnic background—since many conditions are more common in specific ethnic populations, the nurse gathers information about ethnic background (eg, Tay-Sachs disease in Ashkenazi Jewish populations or thalassemia in Southeast Asian populations)

GENETICS RESOURCES FOR NURSES AND PATIENTS ON THE WEB

Genetic Alliance, www.geneticalliance.org—a directory of support groups for patients and families with genetic conditions

Gene Clinics, www.geneclinics.org—a listing of common genetic disorders with up-to-date clinical summaries, genetic counseling and testing information

National Organization of Rare Disorders, www.rarediseases.org—a directory of support groups and information for patients and families with rare genetic disorders

OMIM: Online Mendelian Inheritance in Man, www.ncbi.nlm.nih.gov/Omim/mimstats.html—a complete listing of inherited genetic conditions

- Environment (physical, spiritual, cultural, interpersonal)
- Lifestyle (patterns and habits)
- Presence of a physical or mental disability
- Self-concept
- Sexuality
- Risk for abuse
- Stress and coping response

PAST LIFE EVENTS RELATED TO HEALTH

The patient profile begins with a brief life history. Questions about place of birth and past places of residence help focus attention on the earlier years of life. Personal experiences during childhood or adolescence that have special significance may be elicited by asking a question such as, "Was there anything that you experienced as a child or

CHART 5-2

Patient Profile

PAST EVENTS RELATED TO HEALTH
Place of birth
Places lived
Significant childhood/adolescent experiences

EDUCATION AND OCCUPATION
Jobs held in past
Current position/job
Length of time at position
Educational preparation
Work satisfaction and career goals

FINANCIAL RESOURCES
Income
Insurance coverage

ENVIRONMENT
Physical—living arrangements (type of housing, neighborhood, presence of hazards)
Spiritual—extent to which religion is a part of individual's life; religious beliefs related to perception of health and illness; religious practices
Interpersonal—ethnic background (language spoken, customs and values held, folk practices used to maintain health or to cure illness); family relationships (family structure, roles, communication patterns, support system); friendships (quality of relationship)

LIFESTYLE PATTERNS
Sleep (time person retires, hours per night, comfort measures, awakens rested)
Exercise (type, frequency, time spent)
Nutrition (24-hour diet recall, idiosyncrasies, restrictions)
Recreation (type of activity, time spent)
Caffeine (coffee, tea, cola, chocolate)—kind, amount
Smoking (cigarette, pipe, cigar, marijuana)—kind, amount per day, number of years, desire to quit
Alcohol—kind, amount, pattern over past year
Drugs—kind, amount, route of administration

PHYSICAL OR MENTAL DISABILITY
Presence of a disability (physical or mental)
Effect of disability on function and health access
Accommodations needed to support functioning

SELF-CONCEPT
View of self in present
View of self in future
Body image (level of satisfaction, concerns)

SEXUALITY
Perception of self as a man or woman
Quality of sexual relationships
Concerns related to sexuality or sexual functioning

RISK FOR ABUSE
Physical injury in past
Afraid of partner, caregiver, or family member
Refusal of caregiver to provide necessary equipment or assistance

STRESS AND COPING RESPONSE
Major concerns or problems at present
Daily "hassles"
Past experiences with similar problems
Past coping patterns and outcomes
Present coping strategies and anticipated outcomes
Individual's expectations of family/friends and health care team in problem resolution

adolescent that would be helpful for me to know about?" The interviewer's intent is to encourage the patient to make a quick review of his or her earlier life, highlighting information of particular significance. Although many patients may not recall anything significant, others may share information such as a personal achievement, a failure, a developmental crisis, or an instance of physical, emotional, or sexual abuse.

EDUCATION AND OCCUPATION

Inquiring about current occupation can reveal much about a person's economic status and educational preparation. A statement such as, "Tell me about your job," often elicits information about role, job tasks, and satisfaction with the position. Direct questions about past employment and career goals may be asked if the person does not provide this information.

It is important to learn about a person's educational background. Asking a person what kind of educational requirements were necessary to attain his or her present job is a more sensitive approach than asking whether he or she graduated from high school. Information about the patient's general financial status may be obtained by questions such as, "Do you have any financial concerns at this time?" or "Sometimes there just doesn't seem to be enough money to make ends meet. Are you finding this true?" Inquiries about the person's insurance coverage and plans for health care payment are also appropriate.

ENVIRONMENT

The concept of environment includes a person's physical environment and its potential hazards, spiritual awareness, cultural background, interpersonal relationships, and support system.

Physical Environment. Information is elicited about the type of housing (apartment, duplex, single-family) in which the person lives, its location, the level of safety and comfort within the home and neighborhood, and the presence of environmental hazards (eg, isolation, potential fire risks, inadequate sanitation). If the patient is homeless or living in a homeless shelter or has a disability, the patient's environment assumes special importance.

Spiritual Environment. The term "spiritual environment" refers to the degree to which a person thinks about or contemplates his or her existence, accepts challenges in life, and seeks and finds answers to personal questions. Spirituality may be expressed through identification with a particular religion. Spiritual values and beliefs often direct a person's behavior and approach to health problems and can influence responses to sickness. Illness may create a spiritual crisis and can place considerable stress on a person's internal resources and beliefs. Inquiring about spirituality can identify possible support systems as well as beliefs and customs that need to be considered in planning care. Information is gathered about the following three areas:

- The extent to which religion is a part of the person's life
- Religious beliefs related to the person's perception of health and illness
- Religious practices related to health and illness

A spiritual assessment may involve asking the following questions:

- Is religion or God important to you?
- If yes, in what way?
- If no, what is the most important thing in your life?
- Are there any religious practices that are important to you?
- Do you have any spiritual concerns because of your present health problem?

Interpersonal and Cultural Environment. Cultural influences, relationships with family and friends, and the presence or absence of a support system are all part of a patient's interpersonal environment. The beliefs and practices that have been shared from generation to generation are known as cultural or ethnic patterns. They are expressed through language, dress, dietary choices, and role behaviors; in perceptions of health and illness; and in health-related behaviors. The influence of these beliefs and customs on how a person reacts to health problems and interacts with health care providers cannot be underestimated. For this reason, the health history includes information about ethnic identity (cultural and social) and racial identity (biologic) (Judd, Griffith & Faustman, 2004). The following questions may assist in obtaining relevant information:

- Where did your parents or ancestors come from? When?
- What language do you speak at home?
- Are there certain customs or values that are important to you?
- Is there anything special you do to keep in good health?
- Do you have any specific practices for treating illness?

Family Relationships and Support System. An assessment of family structure (members, ages, and roles), patterns of communication, and the presence or absence of a support system is an integral part of the patient profile. Although the traditional family is recognized as a mother, a father, and children, many different types of living arrangements exist within our society. "Family" may mean two or more people bound by emotional ties or commitments. Live-in companions, roommates, and close friends can all play a significant role in a person's support system.

LIFESTYLE

The lifestyle section of the patient profile provides information about health-related behaviors. These behaviors include patterns of sleep, exercise, nutrition, and recreation, as well as personal habits such as smoking and the use of illicit drugs, alcohol, and caffeine. Although most people readily describe their exercise patterns or recreational activities, many are unwilling to report their smoking, alcohol use, and illicit drug use, and many deny or understate the degree to which they use such substances (Bridevaux, Bradley, Bryson, et al., 2004; Finfgeld-Connett, 2004). Questions such as, "What kind of alcohol do you enjoy drinking at a party?" may elicit more accurate information than, "Do you drink?" The specific type of alcohol (eg, wine, liquor, beer) and the amount ingested per day or per week (eg, 1 pint of whiskey daily for 2 years) are described.

If alcohol abuse is suspected, additional information may be obtained by using common alcohol screening questionnaires such as the CAGE (*C*utting down, *A*nnoyance by criticism, *G*uilty feelings, and *E*ye-openers), AUDIT (*A*lcohol *U*se *D*isorders *I*dentification *T*est), TWEAK (*T*olerance, *W*orry, *E*ye-opener, *A*mnesia, *K*ut down), or SMAST (*S*hort *M*ichigan *A*lcoholism *S*creening *T*est). Chart 5-3 shows the CAGE Questions Adapted to Include Drugs (CAGEAID).

CHART 5-3

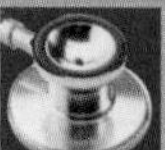

Assessing for Alcohol or Drug Use

CAGE Questions Adapted to Include Drugs (CAGEAID)*

Have you felt you ought to cut down on your drinking *(or drug use)*?

_____Yes _____No

Have people annoyed you by criticizing your drinking *(or drug use)*?

_____Yes _____No

Have you felt bad or guilty about your drinking *(or drug use)*?

_____Yes _____No

Have you ever had a drink *(or used drugs)* first thing in the morning to steady your nerves or get rid of a hangover *(or to get the day started)*?

_____Yes _____No

* Boldface text shows the original CAGE questions; boldface italic text shows modifications of the CAGE questions used to screen for drug disorders. In a general population, two or more positive answers indicate a need for more in-depth assessment.

From Fleming, M. F., & Barry, K. L. (1992). *Addictive Disorders*. St. Louis: Mosby; and Ewing, J. A. (1984). Detecting alcoholism: The CAGE questionnaire. *Journal of the American Medical Association, 252*(14), 1905–1907.

The MAST has also been recently updated to include drug use (Westermeyer, Yargic & Thuras, 2004).

Similar questions can be used to elicit information about smoking and caffeine consumption. Questions about illicit drug use follow naturally after questions about smoking, caffeine consumption, and alcohol use. A nonjudgmental approach makes it easier for a person to respond truthfully and factually. If street names or unfamiliar terms are used to describe drugs, the person is asked to define the terms used (Bridevaux et al., 2004; Finfgeld-Connett, 2004).

Investigation of lifestyle should also include questions about complementary and alternative therapies. It is estimated that as many as 40% of Americans use some type of complementary or alternative therapies, including special diets, prayer, visualization or guided imagery, massage, meditation, herbal products, and many others (Capriotti, 2004). Marijuana is used for management of symptoms, especially pain, in a number of chronic conditions (Steinbrook, 2004).

PHYSICAL OR MENTAL DISABILITY

The general patient profile also needs to contain questions about any hearing, vision, cognitive, or physical disability (Stotts & Deitrich, 2004). The presence of an obvious physical limitation (eg, using crutches to walk or using a wheelchair to get around) necessitates further investigation. The etiology of the disability should be elicited, and the length of time the patient has had the disability and the impact on function and health access are important to assess. Chart 5-4 presents specific issues that the nurse should consider when obtaining health histories and conducting physical assessments of patients with disabilities.

SELF-CONCEPT

Self-concept refers to a person's view of himself or herself, an image that has developed over many years. To assess self-concept, the interviewer might ask how a person views life, using a question such as, "How do you feel about your life in general?" A person's self-concept can be threatened very easily by changes in physical function or appearance or other threats to health. The impact of certain medical conditions or surgical interventions, such as a colostomy or a mastectomy, can threaten body image. The question, "Do you have any particular concerns about your body?" may elicit useful information about self-image.

SEXUALITY

No area of assessment is more personal than the sexual history. Interviewers are frequently uncomfortable with such questions and ignore this area of the patient profile or conduct a very cursory interview about this subject. Lack of knowledge about sexuality and anxiety about one's own sexuality may hamper the interviewer's effectiveness in dealing with this subject (Nusbaum & Hamilton, 2002).

Sexual assessment can be approached at the end of the interview, at the time interpersonal or lifestyle factors are assessed, or it may be easier to discuss sexuality as a part of the genitourinary history within the review of systems. In female patients, a discussion of sexuality would follow questions about menstruation. In male patients, a similar discussion would follow questions about the urinary system.

NURSING RESEARCH PROFILE

Predictors of Positive Health

Yarcheski, A., Mahon, N. E., Yarcheski, T. J., et al. (2004). A meta-analysis of predictors of positive health practices. *Journal of Nursing Scholarship, 36*(2) 102–108.

Purpose

This study was designed to identify predictors of positive health practices based on previous investigations in which the Personal Lifestyle Questionnaire (PLQ) had been used. Positive health practices were defined as exercise and relaxation activities.

Design

The PLQ, a 24-item, 4-point scale, has been available for more than 20 years and has proved reliable and valid for use in adolescents and adults. Quantitative meta-analysis was used to synthesize the findings of 37 studies that measured positive health practices with the PLQ. Meta-analysis was conducted on 14 predictors.

Results

Eight predictors had a moderate (0.30) effect size: loneliness, social support, perceived health status, self-efficacy, future time perspective, self-esteem, hope, and depression. Six predictors had a small (0.10) effect size: stress, education, marital status, age, income, and gender. Sex and income were not useful variables in predicting positive health practices.

Nursing Implications

During health assessment, the nurse should be aware that positive predictors of the use of exercise and relaxation involve many factors. Loneliness has a negative influence on the practice of positive health behaviors. Social support appears to influence positive health practices by increasing the information available on how to take care of oneself and prevent disease. People who take responsibility for their personal self-management and have a view toward the future also tend to practice more positive health behaviors. Further testing of these predictors is recommended.

CHART 5-4

Health Assessment of People with Disabilities

OVERVIEW

People with disabilities are entitled to the same level of health assessment and physical examination as people without disabilities. The nurse needs to be aware of the patient's disabilities or impairments (hearing, vision, cognitive, and physical limitations) and take these into consideration when obtaining a health history and conducting a physical assessment. It is appropriate to ask the patient what assistance he or she needs rather than assuming that help is needed for all activities or that, if assistance is needed, the patient will ask for it.

HEALTH HISTORY

Communication between the nurse and the patient is essential. To ensure that the patient is able to respond to assessment questions and provide needed information, interpreters, assistive listening devices, or other alternate formats (eg, Braille, large-print forms) may be required.

When interpreters are needed, interpretation services should be arranged. Health care facilities have a responsibility to provide these services without charge to the patient. Family members (especially children) should *not* be used as interpreters, because doing so violates the patient's right to privacy and confidentiality.

The nurse should speak directly to the patient and not to family members or others who have accompanied the patient. If the patient has vision or hearing loss, normal tone and volume of the voice should be used when conducting the assessment. The patient should be able to see the nurse's face clearly during the health history, so that speech reading and nonverbal clues can be used to aid communication.

The health history should address general health issues that are important to all patients, including sexual history and risk for abuse. It should also address the impact of the patient's disability on health issues and access to care and the effect of the patient's current health problem on his or her disability.

The nurse should verify what the patient has said; if the patient has difficulty communicating verbally, the nurse should ask for clarification rather than assume that it is too difficult for the patient to do so. Most people would rather be asked to explain again than run the risk of being misunderstood.

PHYSICAL EXAMINATION

Inaccessible facilities remain a major barrier to health care for people with disabilities. Barriers include lack of ramps and grab bars, inaccessible restrooms, small examination rooms, and examination tables that cannot be lowered to allow the patient to move himself or herself onto, or be transferred easily and safely to, the examination table. The patient may need help getting undressed for the physical examination (and dressed again), moving on and off the examination table, and maintaining positions usually required during physical examination maneuvers. It is important to ask the patient what assistance is needed.

If the patient has impaired sensory function (eg, lack of sensation, hearing or vision loss), it is important to inform the patient that you will be touching him or her. Furthermore, it is important to explain all procedures and maneuvers.

Gynecologic examinations should *not* be deferred because a patient has a disability or is assumed to be sexually inactive. Explanations of the examination are important for all women, and even more so for women with disabilities, because they may have had previous negative experiences. Slow, gentle moving and positioning of the patient for the gynecologic examination and warming the speculum before attempting insertion often minimize spasticity in women with neurologically related disabilities.

HEALTH SCREENING AND TESTING

Many people with disabilities report that they have not been weighed for years or even decades because they are unable to stand for this measurement. Alternative methods (eg, use of wheelchair scales) are needed to monitor weight and body mass index. This is particularly important because of the increased incidence of obesity and its effects on health status and transfer of persons with disabilities (Sharts-Hopko & Sullivan, 2003).

Patients with disabilities may require special assistance if urine specimens are to be obtained as part of the visit. They are often able to suggest strategies to obtain urine specimens based on previous experience.

If it is necessary for the nurse to wear a mask during a procedure or if the patient is unable to see the face of the nurse during a procedure, it is important to explain the procedure and the expected role of the patient ahead of time. If the patient is unable to hear or is unable to communicate with the nurse or other health care provider verbally during an examination or diagnostic test, a method of communication (eg, signaling the patient by tapping his or her arm, signaling the nurse by using a bell) should be established beforehand.

Inaccessible facilities have resulted in decreased participation of people with disabilities in recommended preventive screening, including gynecologic examinations, mammograms, and bone density testing (Smeltzer, Zimmerman & Capriotti, 2005; Iezzoni, O'Day, Killeen, et al., 2001). Therefore, it is important to ask about health screening and recommendations for screening. In addition, people with disabilities should be asked about their participation in health promotion activities, because inaccessible environments may limit their participation in exercise, health programs, and other health promotion efforts.

Obtaining the sexual history provides an opportunity to discuss sexual matters openly and gives the person permission to express sexual concerns to an informed professional. The interviewer must be nonjudgmental and must use language appropriate to the patient's age and background (Nusbaum & Hamilton, 2002). The assessment begins with an orienting sentence such as, "Next, I would like to ask about your sexual health and practices." Such an opening may lead to a discussion of concerns related to sexual expression or the quality of a relationship, or to questions about contraception, risky sexual behaviors, and safer sex practices. Examples of other questions are, "Do you have one or more sexual partners?" and "Are you satisfied with your sexual relationships?"

Determining whether a person is sexually active should precede any attempts to explore issues related to sexuality and sexual function. Care should be taken to initiate conversations about sexuality with elderly patients and patients with disabilities and not to treat them as asexual people (Stotts & Deitrich, 2004). Questions are worded in such a way that the person feels free to discuss his or her sexuality regardless of marital status or sexual preference. Direct questions are usually less threatening when prefaced with such statements as, "Most people feel that . . ." or "Many people worry about. . . ." This suggests the normalcy of such feelings or behavior and encourages the person to share information that might otherwise be omitted from fear of seeming "different."

If a person answers abruptly or does not wish to carry the discussion any further, then the interviewer should move to the next topic. However, introducing the subject of sexuality indicates to the person that a discussion of sexual concerns is acceptable and can be approached again in the future if so desired. Further discussion of the sexual history is presented in Chapters 46 and 49.

RISK FOR ABUSE

Physical, sexual, and psychological abuse is a topic of growing importance in today's society. Such abuse occurs to people of both genders, of all ages, and from all socioeconomic, ethnic, and cultural groups. However, few patients discuss this topic unless they are asked specifically about it. In fact, one study revealed that among women currently in an abusive relationship, 92% had never told a health care provider (Rhodes et al., 2002). Therefore, it is important to ask direct questions, such as

- Is anyone physically hurting you or forcing you to have sexual activities?
- Has anyone ever hurt you physically or threatened to do so?
- Are you ever afraid of anyone close to you (your partner, caregiver, or other family members)?

Patients who are elderly or have disabilities are at increased risk for abuse and should be asked about it as a routine part of assessment. However, when elderly patients are questioned directly, they rarely admit to abuse (Fulmer, 2003). Health care professionals should assess for risk factors, such as high levels of stress or alcoholism in caregivers, evidence of violence, and emotional outbursts, as well as financial, emotional, or physical dependency.

Two additional questions have been found to be effective in uncovering specific types of abuse that may occur only in people with disabilities (McFarlane, Hughes, Nosek, et al., 2001):

- Does anyone prevent you from using a wheelchair, cane, respirator, or other assistive device?
- Does anyone you depend on refuse to help you with an important personal need, such as taking your medicine, getting to the bathroom, getting in or out of bed, bathing, dressing, or getting food or drink?

If a person's response indicates that abuse is a risk, further assessment is warranted, and efforts are made to ensure the patient's safety and provide access to appropriate community and professional resources and support systems (McFarlane et al., 2001). Further discussion of domestic violence and abuse is presented in Chapter 46.

STRESS AND COPING RESPONSES

Each person handles stress differently. How well people adapt depends on their ability to cope. During a health history, past coping patterns and perceptions of current stresses and anticipated outcomes are explored to identify the person's overall ability to handle stress. It is especially important to identify expectations that a person may have of family, friends, and caregivers in providing financial, emotional, or physical support.

Other Health History Formats

The health history format discussed in this chapter is only one possible design that is useful in obtaining and organizing information about a person's health status. Some experts consider this traditional format to be inappropriate for nurses, because it does not focus exclusively on the assessment of human responses to actual or potential health problems. Several attempts have been made to develop an assessment format and database with this focus in mind. One example is the nursing database prototype based on the Unitary Person Framework of the North American Nursing Diagnosis Association and its nine human response patterns: exchanging, communicating, relating, valuing, choosing, moving, perceiving, knowing, and feeling (NANDA International, 2005). Although there is support in nursing for using this approach, no consensus for its use has been reached.

The National Center for Health Services Research of the U.S. Department of Health and Human Services (USDHHS) and other groups from the public and private sectors have focused on assessing not only biologic health but also other dimensions of health. These dimensions include physical, functional, emotional, mental, and social health. Modern efforts to assess health status have focused on the manner in which disease or disability affects a patient's functional status—that is, the ability of the person to function normally and perform his or her usual physical, mental, and social activities. An emphasis on functional assessment is viewed as more holistic than the traditional health or medical history. Instruments to assess health status in these ways may be used by nurses along with their own clinical assessment skills to determine the impact of illness, disease, disability, and health problems on functional status.

Health concerns that are not complex (eg, earache, sinusitis) and can be resolved in a short period usually do not require the depth or detail that is necessary when a person is experiencing a major illness or health problem (Stotts & Deitrich, 2004). Additional assessments that go beyond the general patient profile may be used if the patient's health problems are acute and complex or if the illness is chronic (Rosenthal & Kavic, 2004). The person should be asked about continuing health promotion and screening practices. If the person has not been involved in these practices in the past, he or she should be educated about their importance and referred to appropriate health care providers.

Regardless of the assessment format used, the focus of nurses during data collection is different from that of physicians and other health team members. However, the nursing focus complements these other approaches and encourages collaboration among the health care providers, with each member bringing his or her own expertise and focus to the situation.

Physical Assessment

Physical assessment, or the physical examination, is an integral part of nursing assessment. The basic techniques and tools used in performing a physical examination are described in general in this chapter. The examinations of specific systems, including special maneuvers, are described in the appropriate chapters throughout the book. Because a patient's nutritional status is an important factor in overall health and well-being, a section on nutritional assessment is included in this chapter.

The physical examination is usually performed after the health history is obtained. It is carried out in a well-lighted, warm area. The patient is asked to (or helped to) undress and is draped appropriately so that only the area to be examined is exposed. The person's physical and psychological comfort are considered at all times. It is necessary to describe procedures to the patient and explain what sensations to expect before each part of the examination. The examiner's hands are washed before and immediately after the examination. Fingernails are kept short to avoid injuring the patient. If there is a possibility of coming into contact with blood or other body secretions during the physical examination, gloves should be worn.

An organized and systematic examination is the key to obtaining appropriate data in the shortest time. Such an approach encourages cooperation and trust on the part of the patient. The person's health history provides the examiner with a health profile that guides all aspects of the physical examination. Although the sequence of physical examination depends on the circumstances and on the patient's reason for seeking health care, the complete examination usually proceeds as follows:

- Skin
- Head and neck
- Thorax and lungs
- Breasts
- Cardiovascular system
- Abdomen
- Rectum
- Genitalia
- Neurologic system
- Musculoskeletal system

In clinical practice, all relevant body systems are tested throughout the physical examination, not necessarily in the sequence described (Weber & Kelley, 2003). For example, when the face is examined, it is appropriate to check for facial asymmetry and, thus, for the integrity of the fifth and seventh cranial nerves; the examiner does not need to repeat this as part of a neurologic examination. (See Chapter 60 for a full description of assessment of the cranial nerves.) When systems are combined in this manner, the patient does not need to change positions repeatedly, which can be exhausting and time-consuming.

A "complete" physical examination is not routine. Many of the body systems are selectively assessed on the basis of the presenting problem. For example, if a healthy 20-year-old college student requires an examination to play basketball and reports no history of neurologic abnormality, the neurologic assessment is brief. Conversely, a history of transient numbness and diplopia (double vision) usually necessitates a complete neurologic investigation (see Chapter 60). Similarly, a patient with chest pain receives a much more intensive examination of the chest and heart than one with an earache. In general, the health history guides the examiner in obtaining additional data for a complete picture of the patient's health.

The process of learning to perform a physical examination requires repetition and reinforcement in a clinical setting. Only after basic physical assessment techniques are mastered can the examiner tailor the routine screening examination to include thorough assessments of particular systems, including special maneuvers.

The basic tools of the physical examination are vision, hearing, touch, and smell. These human senses may be augmented by special tools (eg, stethoscope, ophthalmoscope, reflex hammer) that are extensions of the human senses; they are simple tools that anyone can learn to use well. Expertise comes with practice, and sophistication comes with the interpretation of what is seen and heard. The four fundamental techniques used in the physical examination are inspection, palpation, percussion, and auscultation (Rasmor & Brown, 2003).

Inspection

The first fundamental technique is inspection or observation. General inspection begins with the first contact with the patient. Introducing oneself and shaking hands provide opportunities for making initial observations: Is the person old or young? How old? How young? Does the person appear to be his or her stated age? Is the person thin or obese? Does the person appear anxious or depressed? Is the person's body structure normal or abnormal? In what way, and how different from normal? It is essential to pay attention to the details in observation. Vague, general statements are not a substitute for specific descriptions based on careful observation. Consider the following examples:

- "The person appears sick." In what way does he or she appear sick? Is the skin clammy, pale, jaundiced, or cyanotic? Is the person grimacing in pain or having difficulty breathing? Does he or she have edema? What specific physical features or behavioral manifestations indicate that the person is "sick"?
- "The person appears chronically ill." In what way does he or she appear chronically ill? Does the person appear to have lost weight? People who lose weight secondary to muscle-wasting diseases (eg, acquired immunodeficiency syndrome [AIDS], malignancy) have a different appearance than those who are merely thin, and weight loss may be accompanied by loss of muscle mass or atrophy. Does the skin have the appearance of chronic illness (ie, is it pale, or does it give the appearance of dehydration or loss of subcutaneous tissue)?

These important specific observations are documented in the patient's chart or health record. Among general observations that should be noted in the initial examination of the patient are posture and stature, body movements, nutritional status, speech pattern, and vital signs.

Posture

The posture that a person assumes often provides valuable information. Patients who have breathing difficulties (dyspnea) secondary to cardiac disease prefer to sit and may report feeling short of breath when lying flat for even a brief time. Patients with obstructive pulmonary disease not only sit upright but also may thrust their arms forward and laterally onto the edge of the bed (tripod position) to place accessory respiratory muscles at an optimal mechanical advantage. Patients with abdominal pain due to peritonitis prefer to lie perfectly still; even slight jarring of the bed causes agonizing pain. In contrast, patients with abdominal pain due to renal or biliary colic are often restless and may pace the room. Patients with meningeal irritation may experience head or neck pain on bending the head or flexing the knees.

Body Movements

Abnormalities of body movement are of two kinds: generalized disruption of voluntary or involuntary movement and asymmetry of movement. The first category includes tremors of a wide variety; some tremors may occur at rest (Parkinson's disease), whereas others occur only on voluntary movement (cerebellar ataxia). Other tremors may exist during both rest and activity (alcohol withdrawal syndrome, thyrotoxicosis). Some voluntary or involuntary movements are fine, and others are quite coarse. At the extreme are the convulsive movements of epilepsy or tetanus and the choreiform (involuntary and irregular) movements of patients with rheumatic fever or Huntington's disease. Other aspects of body movement that are noted on inspection include spasticity, muscle spasms, and an abnormal gait.

Asymmetry of movement, in which only one side of the body is affected, may occur with disorders of the central nervous system (CNS), principally in those patients who have had a cerebrovascular accident (stroke). Patients may have drooping of one side of the face, weakness or paralysis of the extremities on one side of the body, and a foot-dragging gait. Spasticity (increased muscle tone) may also be present, particularly in patients with multiple sclerosis.

Nutritional Status

Nutritional status is important to note. Obesity may be generalized as a result of excessive intake of calories, or it may be specifically localized to the trunk in patients who have an endocrine disorder (Cushing's disease) or who have been taking corticosteroids for long periods. Loss of weight may be generalized as a result of inadequate caloric intake, or it may be seen in loss of muscle mass with disorders that affect protein synthesis. Nutritional assessment is discussed in more detail later in this chapter.

Speech Pattern

Speech may be slurred because of CNS disease or because of damage to cranial nerves. Recurrent damage to the laryngeal nerve results in hoarseness, as do disorders that produce edema or swelling of the vocal cords. Speech may be halting, slurred, or interrupted in flow in patients with some CNS disorders (eg, multiple sclerosis, stroke).

Vital Signs

The recording of vital signs is a part of every physical examination (Bickley & Szilagyi, 2003). Blood pressure, pulse rate, respiratory rate, and body temperature measurements are obtained and recorded. Acute changes and trends over time are documented, and unexpected changes and values that deviate significantly from a patient's normal values are brought to the attention of the patient's primary health care provider. The "fifth vital sign," pain, is also assessed and documented, if indicated.

Fever is an increase in body temperature above normal. On average, a normal oral temperature for most people is 37.0°C (98.6°F); however, some variation is normal. Some people's temperatures are quite normal at 36.6°C (98°F) or 37.3°C (99°F). There is a normal diurnal variation of a degree or two in body temperature throughout the day; temperature is usually lowest in the morning and increases during the day to between 37.3° and 37.5°C (99° to 99.5°F), and it then decreases during the night.

Palpation

Palpation is a vital part of the physical examination (Rasmor & Brown, 2003). Many structures of the body, although not visible, may be assessed through the techniques of light and deep palpation (Fig. 5-3). Examples include the super-

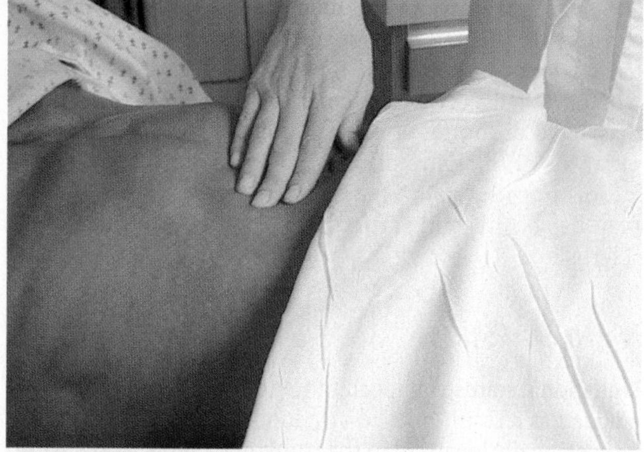

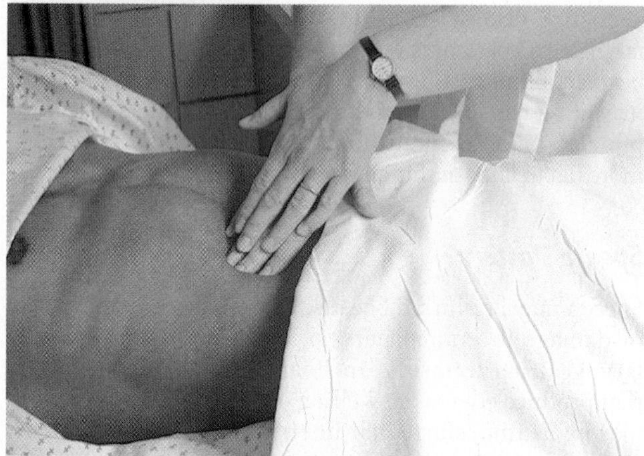

FIGURE 5-3. Light palpation technique (*top*) and deep palpation (*bottom*). Photo © Ken Kasper.

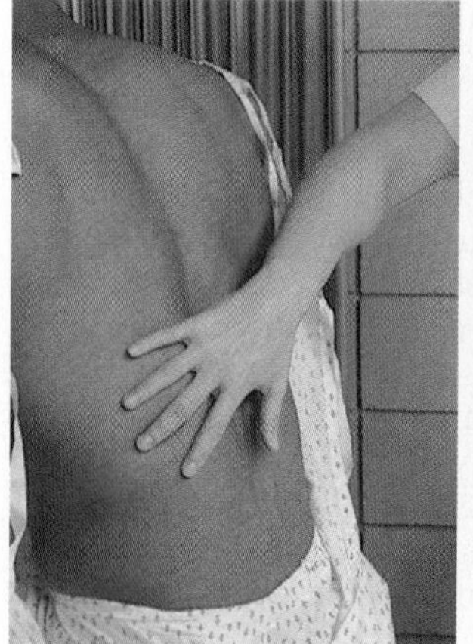

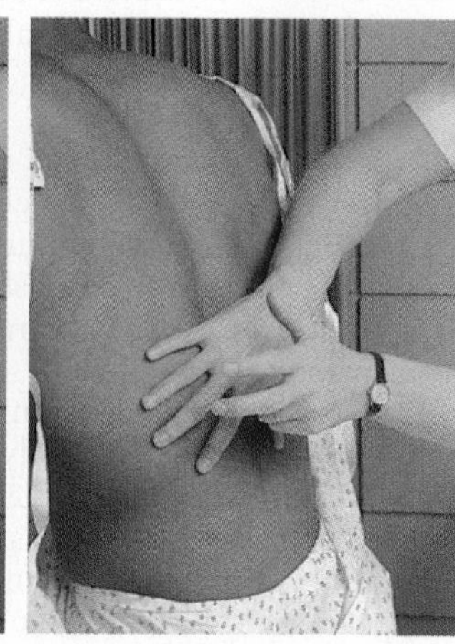

FIGURE 5-4. Percussion technique. The middle finger of one hand strikes the terminal phalanx of the middle finger of the other hand, which is placed firmly against the body. If the action is performed sharply, a brief, resonant tone will be produced. The clarity of the tone depends on the brevity of the action. The intensity of the tone varies with the force used. Photo © Ken Kasper.

ficial blood vessels, lymph nodes, thyroid gland, organs of the abdomen and pelvis, and rectum. When the abdomen is examined, auscultation is performed before palpation and percussion to avoid altering bowel sounds (Bickley & Szilagyi, 2003).

Sounds generated within the body, if within specified frequency ranges, also may be detected through touch. For example, certain murmurs generated in the heart or within blood vessels (thrills) may be detected. Thrills cause a sensation to the hand much like the purring of a cat. Voice sounds are transmitted along the bronchi to the periphery of the lung. These may be perceived by touch and may be altered by disorders affecting the lungs. The phenomenon is called *tactile fremitus* and is useful in assessing diseases of the chest. The significance of these findings is discussed in Chapters 21 and 26.

Percussion

The technique of percussion (Fig. 5-4) translates the application of physical force into sound. It is a skill requiring practice that yields much information about disease processes in the chest and abdomen (Bickley & Szilagyi, 2003). The principle is to set the chest wall or abdominal wall into vibration by striking it with a firm object. The sound produced reflects the density of the underlying structure. Certain densities produce sounds as percussion notes. These sounds, listed in a sequence that proceeds from the least to the most dense, are tympany, hyperresonance, resonance, dullness, and flatness. Tympany is the drumlike sound produced by percussing the air-filled stomach. Hyperresonance is audible when one percusses over inflated lung tissue in a person with emphysema. Resonance is the sound elicited over air-filled lungs. Percussion of the liver produces a dull sound, whereas percussion of the thigh produces a flat sound.

Percussion allows the examiner to assess such normal anatomic details as the borders of the heart and the movement of the diaphragm during inspiration. It is also possible to determine the level of a pleural effusion (fluid in the pleural cavity) and the location of a consolidated area caused by pneumonia or atelectasis (collapse of alveoli). The use of percussion is described further with disorders of the thorax and abdomen (see Chapters 21 and 34).

Auscultation

Auscultation is the skill of listening to sounds produced within the body created by the movement of air or fluid. Examples include breath sounds, the spoken voice, bowel sounds, heart sounds, and cardiac murmurs. Physiologic sounds may be normal (eg, first and second heart sounds) or pathologic (eg, heart murmurs in diastole, crackles in the lung). Some normal sounds may be distorted by abnormalities of structures through which the sound must travel (eg, changes in the character of breath sounds as they travel through the consolidated lung of a patient with lobar pneumonia).

Sound produced within the body, if of sufficient amplitude, may be detected with the stethoscope, which functions as an extension of the human ear and channels sound. Two end-pieces are available for the stethoscope: the bell and the diaphragm. The bell is used to assess very-low-frequency sounds such as diastolic heart murmurs. The entire surface of the bell's disk is placed lightly on the skin surface to avoid flattening the skin and reducing audible vibratory sensations. The diaphragm, the larger disk, is used to assess high-frequency sounds such as heart and lung sounds and is held in firm contact with the skin surface (Fig. 5-5). Touching the tubing or rubbing other surfaces (hair, clothing) during auscultation is avoided to minimize extraneous noises.

Sound produced by the body, like any other sound, is characterized by intensity, frequency, and quality. The *intensity,* or loudness, associated with physiologic sound is low; therefore, the use of the stethoscope is needed. The *frequency,* or pitch, of physiologic sound is in reality "noise," in that most sounds consist of a frequency spectrum, as opposed to the single-frequency sounds that we associate with music or a tuning fork. The frequency spectrum may be quite low, yielding a rumbling noise, or comparatively high, producing a harsh or blowing sound. *Quality* of sound relates to overtones that allow one to distinguish among various sounds. Sound quality enables the examiner to distinguish between the musical quality of high-pitched wheezing and the low-pitched rumbling of a diastolic murmur.

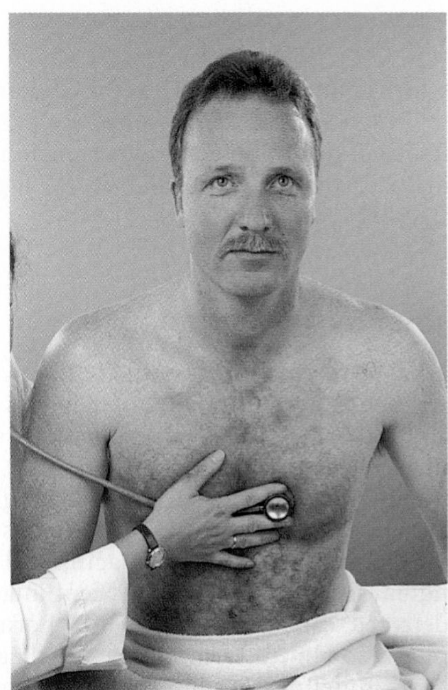

FIGURE 5-5. Technique for auscultating the heart. Photo © B. Proud.

Nutritional Assessment

Nutrition is important to maintain health and to prevent disease and death (Worthington, 2004). When illness or injury occurs, optimal nutrition is an essential factor in promoting healing and resisting infection and other complications. An in-depth nutritional assessment is often integrated into the health history and physical examination. Assessment of the patient's nutritional status provides information about obesity, weight loss, undernutrition, malnutrition, deficiencies in specific nutrients, metabolic abnormalities, the effects of medications on nutrition, and special problems affecting patients both in hospitals and in the home and other community settings.

Disorders caused by nutritional deficiency, overeating, or eating unhealthy meals are among the leading causes of illness and death in the United States today. The three leading causes of death—heart disease, cancer, and stroke—are related, in part, to consequences of unhealthy nutrition. A recent study of the fourth leading cause of death, chronic obstructive pulmonary disease (COPD), suggested that body mass index (BMI) is an important predictor of death in patients with COPD (Celli, Cote, Marin, et al., 2004). Other examples of health problems associated with poor nutrition include obesity, osteoporosis, cirrhosis, diverticulitis, and eating disorders.

Certain signs and symptoms that suggest possible nutritional deficiency, such as muscle wasting, poor skin integrity, loss of subcutaneous tissue, and obesity, are easy to note because they are specific; these should be pursued further. Other physical signs may be subtle and must be carefully assessed and pursued further (Worthington, 2004). For example, certain signs that appear to indicate nutritional deficiency may actually reflect other systemic conditions (eg, endocrine disorders, infectious disease). Others may result from impaired digestion, absorption, excretion, or storage of nutrients in the body.

The sequence of assessment of parameters may vary, but evaluation of nutritional status includes one or more of the following methods: measurement of BMI and waist circumference, biochemical measurements, clinical examination findings, and dietary data. The first two methods are discussed in this chapter.

Special considerations for nutritional assessment in the older adult are given in Chart 5-5.

Body Mass Index

BMI is a ratio based on body weight and height. The obtained value is compared to the established standards; however, trends or changes in values over time are considered more useful than isolated or one-time measurements. BMI (Fig. 5-6) is highly correlated with body fat, but increased lean body mass or a large body frame can also increase the BMI. People who have a BMI lower than 24 (or who are 80% or less of their desirable body weight for height) are at increased risk for problems associated with poor nutritional status. In addition, a low BMI is associated with a higher mortality rate among hospitalized patients and

CHART 5-5

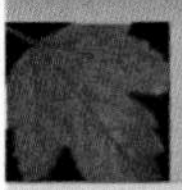

Nutritional Assessment in the Older Adult

Nutritional screening in the elderly is a first step in maintaining adequate nutrition and replacing nutrient losses to maintain the individual's health and well being. In the United States, about 40% of hospitalized patients and 85% of those in nursing homes are estimated to be malnourished (Hogan, 2004). Elderly people who are malnourished tend to have longer and more expensive hospital stays than those who are adequately nourished; the risk of costly complications is also increased in malnourished patients (Dudek, 2006).

Inadequate dietary intake in the elderly may result from physiologic changes in the gastrointestinal tract, social and economic factors, drug interactions, disease, excessive use of alcohol, and poor dentition or missing teeth. Malnutrition is a common consequence of these factors and in turn leads to illness and frailty of the elderly. Important aspects of care of the elderly in the hospital, home, outpatient setting, or extended care facility include recognizing risk factors and identifying those who are at risk for inadequate nutrition (Sabol, 2004).

Many elderly people take excessive and inappropriate medications; this is referred to as polypharmacy. The number of adverse reactions increases proportionately with the number of prescribed and over-the-counter medications taken. Age-related physiologic and pathophysiologic changes may alter the metabolism and elimination of many medications. Medications can influence food intake by producing side effects such as nausea, vomiting, decreased appetite, and changes in sensorium. They may also interfere with the distribution, utilization, and storage of nutrients. Disorders affecting any part of the gastrointestinal tract can alter nutritional requirements and health status in people of any age; however, they are likely to occur more quickly and more frequently in the elderly.

Nutritional problems in the elderly often occur or are precipitated by such illnesses as pneumonia and urinary tract infections. Acute and chronic diseases may affect the metabolism and utilization of nutrients, which already are altered by the aging process. Influenza and pneumonia immunizations, prompt treatment of bacterial infections, and social programs such as Meals on Wheels may reduce the risk of illness-associated malnutrition. Alcohol and substance abuse are potential factors in the elderly population that should not be overlooked (Finfgeld-Connett, 2004; Bridevaux, et al., 2004). Even the well elderly may be nutritionally at risk because of decreased odor perception, poor dental health, limited ability to shop and cook, financial hardship, and the fact that they often eat alone. Also, reduction in exercise with age without concomitant changes in carbohydrate intake places the elderly at risk for obesity.

community-dwelling elderly. Those who have a BMI of 25 to 29 are considered overweight; those with a BMI of 30 to 39, obese; and those with a BMI greater than 40, extremely obese (Dudek, 2006). In analyzing BMI, the nurse must be aware that cutoff scores for normal, overweight, and obese may differ for different ethnic groups (Wildman, Gu, Reynolds, et al., 2004).

It is important to assess for usual body weight and height and to compare these values with ideal weight (Chart 5-6). Current weight does not provide information about recent changes in weight; therefore, patients are asked about their usual body weight. Loss of height may be due to osteoporosis, an important problem related to nutrition, especially in postmenopausal women (USDHHS Public Health Service, 2004). A loss of 2 or 3 inches of height may indicate osteoporosis.

In addition to the calculation of BMI, waist circumference measurement is particularly useful for adult patients who are categorized as being of normal weight or overweight (Dudek, 2006). To measure waist circumference, a tape measure is placed in a horizontal plane around the abdomen at the level of the iliac crest. A waist circumference greater than 40 inches for men or 35 inches for women indicates excess abdominal fat. Those with a high waist circumference are at increased risk for diabetes, dyslipidemias, hypertension, cardiovascular disease, and atrial fibrillation (Wang, Parise, Levy, et al., 2004).

Biochemical Assessment

Biochemical assessment reflects both the tissue level of a given nutrient and any abnormality of metabolism in the utilization of nutrients. These determinations are made from studies of serum (albumin and globulin, transferrin, retinol-binding protein, electrolytes, hemoglobin, vitamin A, carotene, and vitamin C) and studies of urine (creatinine, thiamine, riboflavin, niacin, and iodine). Some of these tests, while reflecting recent intake of the elements detected, can also identify below-normal levels when there are no clinical symptoms of deficiency. See Table 5-1 for guidelines for interpreting albumin and prealbumin levels.

Low serum albumin and prealbumin levels are most often used as measures of protein deficit in adults (Dudek,

Body Mass Index

The body mass index (BMI) is used to determine who is overweight.

$$\text{BMI} = \frac{703 \times \text{weight in pounds}}{(\text{height in inches})^2} \quad \text{OR} \quad \frac{\text{weight in kilograms}}{(\text{height in meters})^2}$$

BMI score is at the intersection of height and weight. A body mass index score of 25 or more is considered overweight and 30 or more is considered obese.

25 Overweight Limit   Overweight

Weight / Height	100	105	110	115	120	125	130	135	140	145	150	155	160	165	170	175	180	185	190	195	200	205
5′0″	20	21	21	22	23	24	25	26	27	28	29	30	31	32	33	34	35	36	37	38	39	40
5′1″	19	20	21	22	23	24	25	26	26	27	28	29	30	31	32	33	34	35	36	37	38	39
5′2″	18	19	20	21	22	23	24	25	26	27	27	28	29	30	31	32	33	34	35	36	37	37
5′3″	18	19	19	20	21	22	23	24	25	26	27	27	28	29	30	31	32	33	34	35	35	36
5′4″	17	18	19	20	21	21	22	23	24	25	26	27	27	28	29	30	31	32	33	33	34	35
5′5″	17	17	18	19	20	21	22	22	23	24	25	26	27	27	28	29	30	31	32	32	33	34
5′6″	16	17	18	19	19	20	21	22	23	23	24	25	26	27	27	28	29	30	31	31	32	33
5′7″	16	16	17	18	19	20	20	21	22	23	23	24	25	26	27	27	28	29	30	31	31	32
5′8″	15	16	17	17	18	19	20	21	21	22	23	24	24	25	26	27	27	28	29	30	30	31
5′9″	15	16	16	17	18	18	19	20	21	21	22	23	24	24	25	26	27	27	28	29	30	30
5′10″	14	15	16	17	17	18	19	19	20	21	22	22	23	24	24	25	26	27	27	28	29	29
5′11″	14	15	15	16	17	17	18	19	20	20	21	22	22	23	24	24	25	26	26	27	28	29
6′0″	14	14	15	16	16	17	18	18	19	20	20	21	22	22	23	24	24	25	26	26	27	28
6′1″	13	14	15	15	16	16	17	18	18	19	20	20	21	22	22	23	24	24	25	26	26	27
6′2″	13	13	14	15	15	16	17	17	18	19	19	20	21	21	22	22	23	24	24	25	26	26
6′3″	12	13	14	14	15	16	16	17	17	18	19	19	20	21	21	22	22	23	24	24	25	26
6′4″	12	13	13	14	15	15	16	16	17	18	18	19	19	20	21	21	22	23	23	24	24	25

Source: Shape Up America. National Institutes of Health

FIGURE 5-6. Body mass index.

CHART 5-6

Calculating Ideal Body Weight

WOMEN

- Allow 100 lb for 5 feet of height.
- Add 5 lb for each additional inch over 5 feet.
- Subtract 10% for small frame; add 10% for large frame.

MEN

- Allow 106 lb for 5 feet of height.
- Add 6 lb for each additional inch over 5 feet.
- Subtract 10% for small frame, add 10% for large frame.

Example: Ideal body weight for a 5′6″ adult is

	Female	Male
5′ of height	100 lb	106 lb
Per additional inch	6″ × 5 lb/inch = 30 lb	6″ × 6 lb/inch = 36 lb
Ideal body weight	130 lb ± 13 lb depending on frame size	142 lb ± 14 lb depending on frame size

2006; Worthington, 2004). Albumin synthesis depends on normal liver function and an adequate supply of amino acids. Because the body stores a large amount of albumin, the serum albumin level may not decrease until malnutrition is severe; therefore, its usefulness in detecting recent protein depletion is limited. Decreased albumin levels may be caused by overhydration, liver or renal disease, or excessive protein loss due to burns, major surgery, infection, or cancer. Serial measurements of prealbumin levels are also used to assess the results of nutritional therapy (Worthington, 2004). Prealbumin, also called thyroxin-binding protein, is

TABLE 5-1 General Guidelines for Interpreting Albumin and Prealbumin Levels

Interpretation	Albumin (g/dL)	Prealbumin (mg/dL)
Normal	3.5–5.5	23–43
Mild depletion	2.8–3.4	10–15
Moderate depletion	2.1–2.7	5–9
Severe depletion	<2.1	<5

From Dudek, S. G. (2006). *Nutrition essentials for nursing practice* (5th ed.). Philadelphia: Lippincott Williams & Wilkins.

a more sensitive indicator of protein status than albumin, but the test is more expensive and therefore less frequently ordered (Dudek, 2006).

Additional laboratory data, such as levels of transferrin and retinol-binding protein, anergy panels, lymphocyte and electrolyte counts, are used in many institutions (Sabol, 2004). Transferrin is a protein that binds and carries iron from the intestine through the serum. Because of its short half-life, transferrin levels decrease more quickly than albumin levels in response to protein depletion. Although measurement of retinol-binding protein is not available from many laboratories, it may be a useful means of monitoring acute, short-term changes in protein status. The total lymphocyte count may be reduced in people who are acutely malnourished as a result of stress and low-calorie feeding and in those with impaired cellular immunity. Anergy, the absence of an immune response to injection of small concentrations of recall antigen under the skin, may also indicate malnutrition because of delayed antibody synthesis and response. Serum electrolyte levels provide information about fluid and electrolyte balance and kidney function. The creatinine/height index calculated over a 24-hour period assesses the metabolically active tissue and indicates the degree of protein depletion, comparing expected body mass for height with actual body cell mass. A 24-hour urine sample is obtained, and the amount of creatinine is measured and compared to normal ranges based on the patient's height and gender. Values lower than normal may indicate loss of lean body mass and protein malnutrition.

Clinical Examination

The state of nutrition is often reflected in a person's appearance. Although the most obvious physical sign of good nutrition is a normal body weight with respect to height, body frame, and age, other tissues can serve as indicators of general nutritional status and adequate intake of specific nutrients; these include the hair, skin, teeth, gums, mucous membranes, mouth and tongue, skeletal muscles, abdomen, lower extremities, and thyroid gland (Table 5-2). Specific aspects of clinical examination that are useful in identifying nutritional deficits include oral examination and assessment of skin for turgor, edema, elasticity, dryness, subcutaneous tone, poorly healing wounds and ulcers, purpura, and bruises (Roth & Townsend, 2003; Worthington, 2004). The musculoskeletal examination also provides information about muscle wasting and weakness.

Dietary Data

Commonly used methods of determining individual eating patterns include the food record and the 24-hour food recall, which help estimate whether food intake is adequate

TABLE 5-2 Physical Indicators of Nutritional Status

Indicator	Signs of Good Nutrition	Signs of Poor Nutrition
General appearance	Alert, responsive	Listless, appears acutely or chronically ill
Hair	Shiny, lustrous; firm, healthy scalp	Dull and dry, brittle, depigmented, easily plucked; thin and sparse
Face	Skin color uniform; healthy appearance	Skin dark over cheeks and under eyes, skin flaky, face swollen or hollow/sunken cheeks
Eyes	Bright, clear, moist	Eye membranes pale, dry (xerophthalmia); increased vascularity, cornea soft (keratomalacia)
Lips	Good color (pink), smooth	Swollen and puffy; angular lesion at corners of mouth (cheilosis)
Tongue	Deep red in appearance; surface papillae present	Smooth appearance, swollen, beefy-red, sores, atrophic papillae
Teeth	Straight, no crowding, no dental caries, bright	Dental caries, mottled appearance (fluorosis), malpositioned
Gums	Firm, good color (pink)	Spongy, bleed easily, marginal redness, recession
Thyroid	No enlargement of the thyroid	Thyroid enlargement (simple goiter)
Skin	Smooth, good color, moist	Rough, dry, flaky, swollen, pale, pigmented; lack of fat under skin
Nails	Firm, pink	Spoon-shaped, ridged, brittle
Skeleton	Good posture, no malformation	Poor posture, beading of ribs, bowed legs or knock knees
Muscles	Well developed, firm	Flaccid, poor tone, wasted, underdeveloped
Extremities	No tenderness	Weak and tender; edematous
Abdomen	Flat	Swollen
Nervous system	Normal reflexes	Decreased or absent ankle and knee reflexes
Weight	Normal for height, age, and body build	Overweight or underweight

and appropriate. If these methods are used to obtain the dietary history, instructions must be given to the patient about measuring and recording food intake.

Food Record

The food record is used most often in nutritional status studies. A person is instructed to keep a record of food actually consumed over a period of time, varying from 3 to 7 days, and to accurately estimate and describe the specific foods consumed. Food records are fairly accurate if the person is willing to provide factual information and able to estimate food quantities.

24-Hour Recall

As the name implies, the 24-hour recall method is a recall of food intake over a 24-hour period. A person is asked to recall all foods eaten during the previous day and to estimate the quantities of each food consumed. Because information does not always represent usual intake, at the end of the interview the patient is asked whether the previous day's food intake was typical. To obtain supplementary information about the typical diet, it is also necessary to ask how frequently the person eats foods from the major food groups.

Conducting the Dietary Interview

The success of the interviewer in obtaining information for dietary assessment depends on effective communication, which requires that good rapport be established to promote respect and trust. The interviewer explains the purpose of the interview. The interview is conducted in a nondirective and exploratory way, allowing the respondent to express feelings and thoughts while encouraging him or her to answer specific questions. The manner in which questions are asked influences the respondent's cooperation. The interviewer must be nonjudgmental and avoid expressing disapproval, either by verbal comments or by facial expression.

CHARACTER OF GENERAL INTAKE

Several questions may be necessary to elicit the information needed. When attempting to elicit information about the type and quantity of food eaten at a particular time, leading questions such as, "Do you use sugar or cream in your coffee?" should be avoided. In addition, assumptions are not made about the size of servings; instead, questions are phrased so that quantities are more clearly determined. For example, to help determine the size of one hamburger, the patient may be asked, "How many servings were prepared with the pound of meat you bought?" Another approach to determining quantities is to use food models of known sizes in estimating portions of meat, cake, or pie, or to record quantities in common measurements, such as cups or spoonfuls (or the size of containers, when discussing intake of bottled beverages).

In recording a particular combination dish, such as a casserole, it is useful to ask about the ingredients, recording the largest quantities first. When recording quantities of ingredients, the interviewer notes whether the food item was raw or cooked and the number of servings provided by the recipe. When a patient lists the foods for the recall questionnaire, it may help to read back the list of foods and ask whether anything was forgotten, such as fruit, cake, candy, between-meal snacks, or alcoholic beverages.

Additional information obtained during the interview should include methods of preparing food, sources available for food (including donated foods and food stamps), food-buying practices, use of vitamin and mineral supplements, and income range.

CULTURAL AND RELIGIOUS CONSIDERATIONS

An individual's culture determines to a large extent which foods are eaten and how they are prepared and served. Culture and religious practices together often determine whether certain foods are prohibited and whether certain foods and spices are eaten on certain holidays or at specific family gatherings. Because of the importance of culture and religious beliefs to many individuals, it is important to be sensitive to these factors when obtaining a dietary history. It is, however, equally important not to stereotype individuals and assume that, because they are from a certain culture or religious group, they adhere to specific dietary customs. One particular area of consideration is the presence of fish and shellfish in the diet and their methods of collection and preparation. These methods may put certain populations at risk for toxicity due to contaminants (Judd, Griffith & Faustman, 2004). Culturally sensitive materials, such as the food pagoda and the Mediterranean Pyramid, are available for making appropriate dietary recommendations (U.S. Department of Agriculture, 2005; Worthington, 2004).

EVALUATING DIETARY INFORMATION

After obtaining basic dietary information, the nurse evaluates the patient's dietary intake and communicates the information to the dietitian and the rest of the health care team for more detailed assessment and for clinical nutrition intervention. If the goal is to determine whether the patient generally eats a healthful diet, his or her food intake may be compared with the dietary guidelines outlined in the U.S. Department of Agriculture's Food Guide Pyramid (Fig. 5-7). The pyramid divides foods into five major groups (grains, vegetables, fruits, milk products, and meat and beans), plus fats and oils. Recommendations are provided for variety in the diet, proportion of food from each food group, and moderation in eating fats, oils, and sweets. A person's food intake is compared with recommendations based on various food groups for various age levels (Roth & Townsend, 2003; Stotts & Deitrich, 2004).

If nurses or dietitians are interested in knowing about the intake of specific nutrients, such as vitamin A, iron, or calcium, the patient's food intake is analyzed by consulting

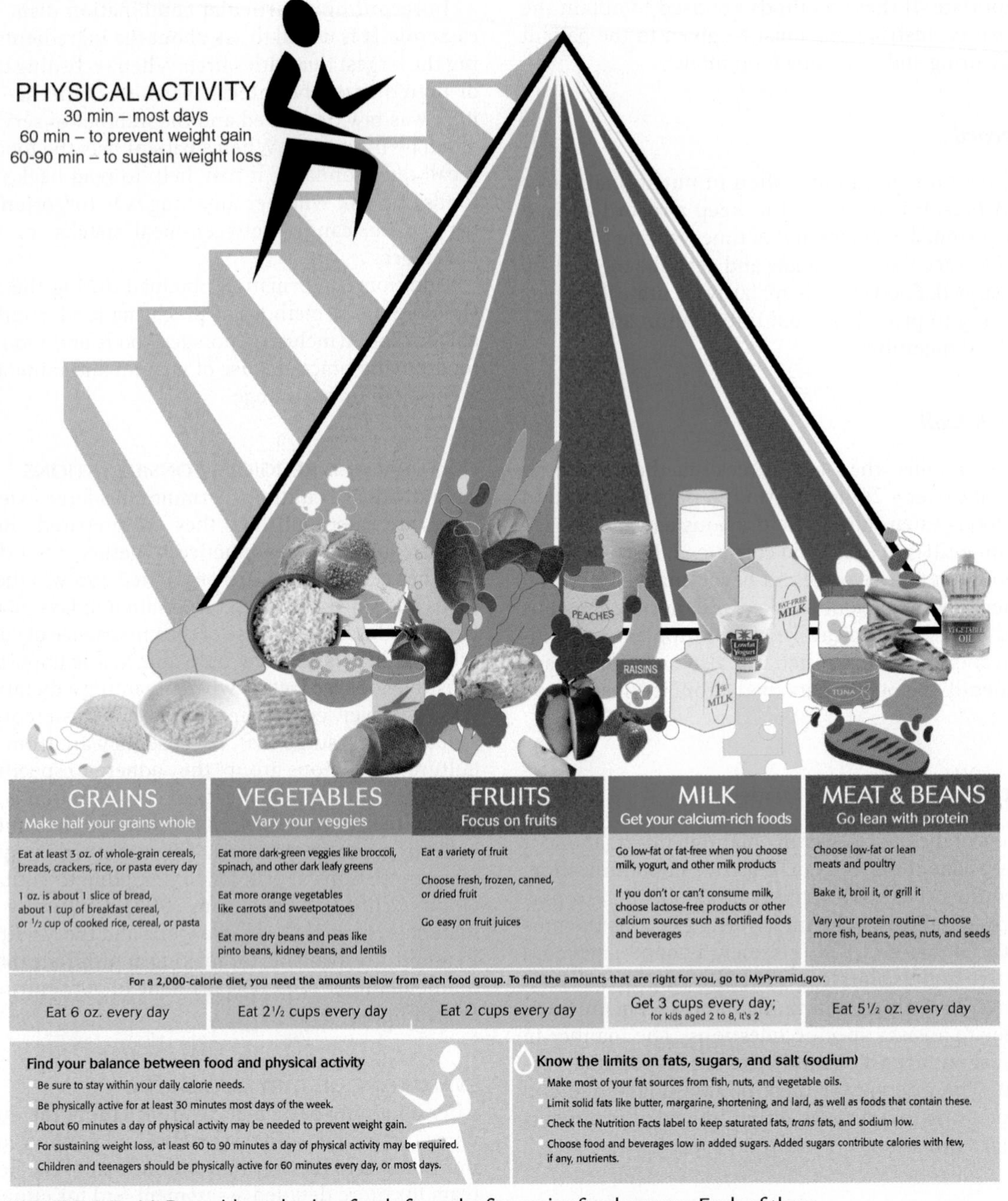

PHYSICAL ACTIVITY
30 min – most days
60 min – to prevent weight gain
60-90 min – to sustain weight loss
PEACHES
RAISINS
FAT-FREE MILK
1% MILK
TUNA
GRAINS
Make half your grains whole
Eat at least 3 oz. of whole-grain cereals, breads, crackers, rice, or pasta every day
1 oz. is about 1 slice of bread, about 1 cup of breakfast cereal, or 1/2 cup of cooked rice, cereal, or pasta
VEGETABLES
Vary your veggies
Eat more dark-green veggies like broccoli, spinach, and other dark leafy greens
Eat more orange vegetables like carrots and sweetpotatoes
Eat more dry beans and peas like pinto beans, kidney beans, and lentils
FRUITS
Focus on fruits
Eat a variety of fruit
Choose fresh, frozen, canned, or dried fruit
Go easy on fruit juices
MILK
Get your calcium-rich foods
Go low-fat or fat-free when you choose milk, yogurt, and other milk products
If you don't or can't consume milk, choose lactose-free products or other calcium sources such as fortified foods and beverages
MEAT & BEANS
Go lean with protein
Choose low-fat or lean meats and poultry
Bake it, broil it, or grill it
Vary your protein routine – choose more fish, beans, peas, nuts, and seeds
For a 2,000-calorie diet, you need the amounts below from each food group. To find the amounts that are right for you, go to MyPyramid.gov.
Eat 6 oz. every day
Eat 2 1/2 cups every day
Eat 2 cups every day
Get 3 cups every day; for kids aged 2 to 8, it's 2
Eat 5 1/2 oz. every day
Find your balance between food and physical activity
Be sure to stay within your daily calorie needs.
Be physically active for at least 30 minutes most days of the week.
About 60 minutes a day of physical activity may be needed to prevent weight gain.
For sustaining weight loss, at least 60 to 90 minutes a day of physical activity may be required.
Children and teenagers should be physically active for 60 minutes every day, or most days.
Know the limits on fats, sugars, and salt (sodium)
Make most of your fat sources from fish, nuts, and vegetable oils.
Limit solid fats like butter, margarine, shortening, and lard, as well as foods that contain these.
Check the Nutrition Facts label to keep saturated fats, *trans* fats, and sodium low.
Choose food and beverages low in added sugars. Added sugars contribute calories with few, if any, nutrients.

FIGURE 5-7. MyPyramid emphasizes foods from the five major food groups. Each of these food groups provides some, but not all, of the nutrients an adult needs. Foods in one group cannot replace those in another. No one of these major food groups is more important than another. (Source: U.S. Department of Agriculture & U.S. Department of Health and Human Services, 2005.)

a list of foods and their composition and nutrient content (Roth & Townsend, 2003). The diet is analyzed in terms of grams and milligrams of specific nutrients. The total nutritive value is then compared with the recommended dietary allowances specific for the patient's age category, gender, and special circumstances such as pregnancy or lactation (Worthington, 2004).

Fat intake and cholesterol levels are additional aspects of the nutritional assessment. Trans fats are produced when hydrogen atoms are added to monounsaturated or polyunsaturated fats to produce a semisolid product, such as margarine (Roth & Townsend, 2003). Trans fats, which are contained in many baked goods and restaurant foods, are a concern, because increased amounts of trans fats have been associated with increased risk for heart disease and stroke (Satchithanandam, Oles, Spease, et al., 2004). Effective January 2006, the Food and Drug Administration has amended food labeling regulations to require the inclusion of trans fats information on food labels (Satchithanandam et al., 2004).

Factors Influencing Nutritional Status in Various Situations

One sensitive indicator of the body's gain or loss of protein is its nitrogen balance. An adult is said to be in nitrogen equilibrium when the nitrogen intake (from food) equals the nitrogen output (in urine, feces, and perspiration); it is a sign of health. A positive nitrogen balance exists when nitrogen intake exceeds nitrogen output and indicates tissue growth, such as occurs during pregnancy, childhood, recovery from surgery, and rebuilding of wasted tissue. A negative nitrogen balance indicates that tissue is breaking down faster than it is being replaced. In the absence of an adequate intake of protein, the body converts protein to glucose for energy. This can occur with fever, starvation, surgery, burns, and debilitating diseases. Each gram of nitrogen loss in excess of intake represents the depletion of 6.25 g of protein or 25 g of muscle tissue. Therefore, a negative nitrogen balance of 10 g/day for 10 days could mean the wasting of 2.5 kg (5.5 lb) of muscle tissue as it is converted to glucose for energy.

When conditions that result in negative nitrogen balance are combined with anorexia (loss of appetite), they can lead to malnutrition. Malnutrition interferes with wound healing, increases susceptibility to infection, and contributes to an increased incidence of complications, longer hospital stays, and prolonged confinement of patients to bed (Roth & Townsend, 2003).

Patients who are hospitalized may have an inadequate dietary intake because of the illness or disorder that necessitated the hospital stay or because the hospital's food is unfamiliar or unappealing (Worthington, 2004). Patients who are cared for at home may feel too sick or fatigued to shop and prepare food, or they may be unable to eat because of other physical problems or limitations. Limited or fixed incomes or the high costs of medications may result in insufficient money to buy nutritious foods. Patients with inadequate housing or inadequate cooking facilities are unlikely to have an adequate nutritional intake. Because complex treatments (eg, ventilators, intravenous infusions, chemotherapy), once used only in the hospital setting, are now being provided in the home and outpatient settings, nutritional assessment of patients in these settings is an important aspect of home and community-based care (Sabol, 2004; Worthington, 2004).

Many medications influence nutritional status by suppressing the appetite, irritating the oral or gastric mucosa, or causing nausea and vomiting. Others may influence bacterial flora in the intestine or directly affect nutrient absorption so that secondary malnutrition results. People who must take many medications in a single day often report feeling too full to eat. A patient's use of prescription and OTC medications and their effects on appetite and dietary intake are assessed. Many of the factors that contribute to poor nutritional status are identified in Table 5-3.

Analysis of Nutritional Status

Physical measurements (BMI, waist circumference) and biochemical, clinical, and dietary data are used in combination to determine a patient's nutritional status. Often, these data provide more information about the patient's nutritional status than the clinical examination, which

TABLE 5-3 Factors Associated With Potential Nutritional Deficits

Factor	Possible Consequences
Dental and oral problems (missing teeth, ill-fitting dentures, impaired swallowing or chewing)	Inadequate intake of high-fiber foods
NPO for diagnostic testing	Inadequate caloric and protein intake; dehydration
Prolonged use of glucose and saline IV fluids	Inadequate caloric and protein intake
Nausea and vomiting	Inadequate caloric and protein intake; loss of fluid, electrolytes, and minerals
Stress of illness, surgery, and/or hospitalization	Increased protein and caloric requirement; increased catabolism
Wound drainage	Loss of protein, fluid, electrolytes, and minerals
Pain	Loss of appetite; inability to shop, cook, eat
Fever	Increased caloric and fluid requirement; increased catabolism
Gastrointestinal intubation	Loss of protein, fluid, and minerals
Tube feedings	Inadequate amounts; various nutrients in each formula
Gastrointestinal disease	Inadequate intake and malabsorption of nutrients
Alcoholism	Inadequate intake of nutrients; increased consumption of calories without other nutrients; vitamin deficiencies
Depression	Loss of appetite; inability to shop, cook, eat
Eating disorders (anorexia, bulimia)	Inadequate caloric and protein intake; loss of fluid, electrolytes, and minerals
Medications	Inadequate intake due to medication side effects, such as dry mouth, loss of appetite, decreased taste perception, difficulty swallowing, nausea and vomiting, physical problems that limit shopping, cooking, eating; malabsorption of nutrients
Restricted ambulation or disability	Inability to help self to food, liquids, other nutrients

may not detect subclinical deficiencies unless they become so advanced that overt signs develop. A low intake of nutrients over a long period may lead to low biochemical levels and, without nutritional intervention, may result in characteristic and observable signs and symptoms (see Table 5-2). A plan of action for nutritional intervention is based on the results of the dietary assessment and the patient's clinical profile. To be effective, the plan must meet the patient's need for a healthy diet, maintain (or control) weight, and compensate for increased nutritional needs.

Considerations in Adolescents

Adolescence is a time of critical growth and acquisition of lifelong eating habits, and therefore nutritional assessment and analysis are critical. In the past two decades, the percentage of adolescents who are overweight has almost tripled (USDHHS, 2001). Total milk consumption has decreased by 36% compared to prior years (Cavadini, Siega-Riz & Popkin, 2000), and fruit and vegetable consumption is also lower than the recommended five servings per day.

Adolescent girls are at particular nutritional risk, because iron, folate, and calcium intakes are below recommended levels. Adolescents with other nutritional disorders, such as anorexia and bulimia, have a better chance of recovery if these disorders are identified in the adolescent years rather than in adulthood (USDHHS, 2001).

Assessment in the Home and Community

Assessment of people in community settings, including the home, consists of collecting information specific to existing health problems, including data on the patient's physiologic and emotional status, the community and home environment, the adequacy of support systems or care given by family and other care providers, and the availability of needed resources. In addition, it is important to evaluate the ability of the individual and family to cope with and address their respective needs. The physi-

CHART 5-7

Assessing the Home Environment

PHYSICAL FACILITIES (check all that apply)

Exterior

- ☐ steps________
- ☐ unsafe steps________
- ☐ porch________
- ☐ litter________
- ☐ noise________
- ☐ inadequate lighting________
- ☐ other________

Interior

- ☐ accessible bathroom________
- ☐ level, safe floor surface________
- ☐ number of rooms________
- ☐ privacy________
- ☐ sleeping arrangements________
- ☐ refrigeration________
- ☐ trash management________
- ☐ animals________
- ☐ adequate lighting________
- ☐ steps/stairs________
- ☐ other________

SAFETY HAZARDS found in the patient's current residence (check all that apply)

- ☐ none
- ☐ inadequate floor, roof, or windows
- ☐ inadequate lighting
- ☐ unsafe gas/electric appliances
- ☐ inadequate heating
- ☐ inadequate cooling
- ☐ lack of fire safety devices
- ☐ unsafe floor coverings
- ☐ inadequate stair rails
- ☐ lead-based paint
- ☐ improperly stored hazardous material
- ☐ improper wiring/electrical cords
- ☐ other________

SAFETY FACTORS (check all that apply)

- ☐ fire/smoke detectors________
- ☐ telephone________
- ☐ placement of electrical cords________
- ☐ emergency plan________
- ☐ emergency phone numbers displayed________
- ☐ safe portable heaters________
- ☐ obstacle-free paths________
- ☐ other________

cal assessment in the community and home consists of the same techniques used in the hospital, outpatient clinic, or office setting. Privacy is provided, and the person is made as comfortable as possible.

Before the first home visit, the nurse usually calls the patient's home to let the patient know when to expect the home care nurse; this also gives the patient's primary caregiver the opportunity to be available. During the home visit, assessment is not limited to physical assessment of the patient. Other aspects of assessment include the home environment, safety factors (eg, smoke alarms, obstacles, safety bars in the bathroom, emergency evacuation plans), adequacy of facilities required for the patient's care and recovery, accessibility if the patient has a disability, food preparation and storage facilities, bathroom facilities, access to a telephone, and the availability of family and community supports (Chart 5-7). The patient may have no family members available to assist him or her and may live alone in substandard housing or in a shelter for the homeless. Therefore the nurse must be aware of resources available in the community and methods of obtaining those resources for the patient.

Critical Thinking Exercises

1 Identify the approach and techniques you would use to perform an admission assessment on a 58-year-old woman with metastatic lung cancer. How would your approach and technique differ if the patient has metastatic lesions to the brain and is disoriented? If the patient is disoriented and blind or hard of hearing? If the patient is from a culture with very different values from yours?

2 Your health history and physical examination of a young adult female patient with cognitive impairment alerts you to the possibility of sexual abuse. Explain how you would pursue this. What assessments are available to assist in a more comprehensive evaluation? How would you modify your assessment to evaluate the patient for other forms of abuse?

3 ebp You are conducting a health history on a middle-aged patient and inquire about immunizations. What resources would you use to identify the current adult immunization schedule? What is the evidence base for the use of health history questionnaires versus serotesting for immunization status? Discuss the strength of the evidence for the method you think is most effective in identifying immunization status. Identify the criteria used to evaluate the strength of the evidence for this practice.

4 ebp Your health assessment of a male college freshman reveals that he has a high fat intake, has minimal calcium intake, and gets little exercise. What recommendations would you make for this patient? If the patient is a vegetarian, what dietary instructions would you develop for him? What is the evidence base for the type of instructional method to use with an adolescent patient? Identify the criteria used to evaluate the strength of the evidence for this practice.

5 How would you modify your health history and physical assessment technique if your patient has the following disabilities: (1) paraplegia due to spinal cord injury, (2) profound hearing loss, (3) blindness, or (4) impaired communication due to aphasia secondary to stroke?

6 You have received a referral for home care for a 75-year-old patient who has recently had a stroke and who lives alone in a trailer. What physical and environmental factors are important to assess on the initial home visit? Identify the elements in the home that would be safety hazards and those that would be safety factors to assess.

REFERENCES AND SELECTED READINGS

BOOKS

Advisory Committee on Immunization Practices (ACIP). (2005). *Recommended adult immunization schedule, United States, October 2004–September 2005.* U.S. Department of Health and Human Services, Centers for Disease Control and Prevention. Available at: www.cdc.gov/nip/recs/adult-schedule.pdf (accessed May 4, 2006).

Bickley, L. S. & Szilagyi, P. G. (2003). *Bates' guide to physical examination and history taking* (8th ed.). Philadelphia: Lippincott Williams & Wilkins.

Dudek, S. G. (2006). *Nutrition essentials for nursing practice* (5th ed.). Philadelphia: Lippincott Williams & Wilkins.

Eng, T. (2001). *The eHealth landscape: A terrain map of emerging information and communication technologies in health and health care.* Princeton, NJ: Robert Wood Johnson Foundation.

Food and Nutrition Board, Institutes of Medicine. (2002). *Dietary reference intakes for energy, carbohydrates, fiber, fat, protein and amino acids (macronutrients): A report of the Panel on Micronutrients, Subcommittees on Upper Reference Levels of Nutrients and Interpretation and Uses of Dietary Reference Intakes, and the Standing Committee on the Scientific Evaluation of Dietary Reference Intakes.* Washington, DC: National Academy Press.

Klimis-Zaras, D. & Wolinsky, I. (2004). *Nutritional concerns for women* (2nd ed.). New York: CRC Press.

Melnyk, B. M. & Fineout-Overholt, E. (2005). *Evidence-based practice in nursing and healthcare: A guide to best practices.* Philadelphia: Lippincott Williams & Wilkins.

NANDA International. (2005). *Nursing diagnoses: Definitions and classification 2005–2006.* Philadelphia: North American Nursing Diagnosis Association.

Orient, J. (2005). *Sapira's art and science of bedside diagnosis* (3rd ed.). Philadelphia: Lippincott Williams & Wilkins.

Porth, C. M. (2005). *Pathophysiology: Concepts of altered health states* (7th ed.). Philadelphia: Lippincott Williams & Wilkins.

Roth, R. & Townsend, C. E. (2003). *Nutrition & diet therapy* (8th ed.). Clifton Park: Delmar Learning.

Stanley, M., Blair, K. A. & Beare, P. G. (2005). *Gerontological nursing: Promoting successful aging with older adults* (3rd ed). Philadelphia: F. A. Davis.

U.S. Department of Agriculture, Center for Nutrition Policy and Promotion. (2005). *My Pyramid: Steps to a healthier you*. April 2005. Available at: http://www.mypyramid.gov/ (accessed March 5, 2006).

U.S. Department of Agriculture & U.S. Department of Health and Human Services. (2005). *Dietary guidelines for Americans* (5th ed). Available at: http://www.healthierus.gov/dietaryguidelines/index.html (accessed March 5, 2006).

U.S. Department of Health and Human Services. (2004). *Bone health and osteoporosis: A report of the Surgeon General*. Rockville, MD: USDHHS.

U.S. Department of Health and Human Services Centers for Disease Control and Prevention. (2003). *A public health action plan to prevent heart disease and stroke*. Atlanta: USDHHS.

U.S. Department of Health and Human Services Public Health Service. (2001). *The Surgeon General's call to action to prevent and decrease overweight and obesity*. Rockville, MD: USDHHS.

Weber, J. & Kelley, J. (2003). *Health assessment in nursing* (2nd ed.). Philadelphia: Lippincott Williams & Wilkins.

Worthington, P. H. (2004). *Practical aspects of nutritional support*. Philadelphia: Saunders.

JOURNALS

**An asterisk indicates a nursing research article.*

General Assessment

Bridevaux, I. P., Bradley, K. A., Bryson, C. L., et al. (2004). Alcohol screening results in elderly male veterans: Association with health status and mortality. *Journal of the American Geriatrics Society, 52*(9), 1510–1517.

Burnham, B. R., Thompson, D. F. & Jackson, W. G. (2002). Positive predictive value of a health history questionnaire. *Military Medicine, 167*(8), 639–642.

Capriotti, T. (2004). Any science behind the hype of natural dietary supplements? *MedSurg Nursing, 13*(5), 339–347.

Fiellin, D. A., Reid, M. C. & O'Connor, P. G. (2000). Screening for alcohol problems in primary care: A systematic review. *Archives of Internal Medicine, 160*(13), 1977–1989.

Finfgeld-Connett, D. (2004). Treatment of substance misuse in older women. *Journal of Gerontological Nursing, 30*(8), 30–37.

Flowers, D. L. (2004). Culturally competent nursing care: A challenge for the 21st century. *Critical Care Nurse, 24*(4), 48–52.

Fulmer, T. (2003). Elder abuse and neglect assessment. *Journal of Gerontological Nursing, 29*(1), 8–9.

Guttmacher, A. E., Collins, F. S. & Carmona, R. H. (2004). The family history: More important than ever. *New England Journal of Medicine, 351*(22), 2333–2336.

Iezzoni, L. I., O'Day, B. L., Killeen, M., et al. (2004). Communicating about health care: Observations from persons who are deaf or hard of hearing. *Annals of Internal Medicine, 140*(5), 356–362.

Judd, N. L., Griffith, W. C. & Faustman, E. M. (2004). Consideration of cultural and lifestyle factors in defining susceptible populations for environmental disease. *Toxicology, 198*(1–3), 121–133.

Kinzie, M. B., Cohn, W., Julian, M. F., et al. (2002). A user-centered model for web site design: Needs assessment, user interface design, and rapid prototyping. *Journal of the American Medical Informatics Association, 9*(4), 320–330.

*Loeb, S. (2004). Older men's health. *Nursing Research, 53*(3), 198–206.

McFarlane, J., Hughes, R. B., Nosek, M. A., et al. (2001). Abuse Assessment Screen—Disability (AAS-D): Measuring frequency, type, and perpetrator of abuse toward women with physical disabilities. *Journal of Women's Health and Gender-Based Medicine, 10*(9), 861–866.

Nusbaum, M. R. H. & Hamilton, C. D. (2002). The proactive sexual health history. *American Family Physician, 66*(9), 1705–1712.

Rasmor, M. & Brown, C. M. (2003). Physical examination for the occupational health nurse. *AAOHN Journal, 51*(9), 390–401.

Rhodes, K. V., Lauderdale, D., He, T., Howes, D. S. & Levinson, W. (2002). "Between me and the computer": Increased detection of intimate partner violence using a computer questionnaire. *Annals of Emergency Medicine, 40*(5), 476–484.

Rosenthal, R. A. & Kavic, S. M. (2004). Assessment and management of the geriatric patient. *Critical Care Medicine, 32*(4), S92–S105.

Sanchez, A. M., Schreiber, G., Glynn, S., et al. (2003). Blood-donor perceptions of health history screening with a computer-assisted self-administered interview. *Transfusion, 43*(2), 165–172.

Smeltzer, S. C., Zimmerman, V. & Capriotti, T. (2005). Bone mineral density and osteoporosis risks in women with disabilities. *Archives of Physical Medicine and Rehabilitation, 86*(3), 582–586.

Smeltzer, S. C., Zimmerman, V., DeSilets, L. D., et al. (2003). Accessible online health promotion information for persons with disabilities. *Online Journal of Issues in Nursing, 9*(1), 11. Available at: http://nursingworld.org/ojin/topic16/tpc16_5.htm (accessed May 5, 2006).

Steinbrook, R. (2004). Medical marijuana, physician-assisted suicide, and the Controlled Substances Act. *New England Journal of Medicine, 351*(14), 1380–1383.

Stotts, N. A. & Deitrich, C. E. (2004). The challenge to come: The care of older adults. *American Journal of Nursing, 104*(8), 40–47.

Westermeyer, J., Yargic, I. & Thuras, P. (2004). Michigan Assessment Screening Test for Alcohol and Drugs (MAST/AD): Evaluation in a clinical sample. *American Journal on Addictions, 13*(2), 151–162.

*Yarcheski, A., Mahon, N. E., Yarcheski, T. J., et al. (2004). A meta-analysis of predictors of positive health practices. *Journal of Nursing Scholarship, 36*(2), 102–108.

Nutritional Assessment

Celli, B. R., Cote, C. G., Marin, J. M., et al. (2004). The body-mass index, airflow obstruction, dyspnea, and exercise capacity index in chronic obstructive pulmonary disease. *New England Journal of Medicine, 350*(10), 1005–1012.

Cavadini, C., Siega-Riz, A. M. & Popkin, B. M. (2000). US adolescent food intake trends from 1965 to 1996. *Archives of Disease in Childhood, 83*(1), 18–24.

Hogan, S. L. (2004). How to help wounds heal. *RN, 67*(8), 26–31.

Sabol, V. (2004). Nutritional assessment of the critically ill adult. *AACN Clinical Issues, 15*(4), 595–606.

Satchithanandam, S., Oles, C. J., Spease, C. J., et al. (2004). Trans, saturated, and unsaturated fat in foods in the United States prior to mandatory trans-fat labeling. *Lipids, 39*(1), 11–18.

Sharts-Hopko, N. C. & Sullivan, M. P. (2003). Obesity as a confounding health factor among women with mobility impairment. *Journal of the American Academy of Nurse Practitioners, 15*(10), 438–443.

Wang, T. J., Parise, H., Levy, D., et al. (2004). Obesity and the risk of new-onset atrial fibrillation. *JAMA, 292*(20), 2471–2477.

Wildman, R. P., Gu, D., Reynolds, K., et al. (2004). Appropriate body mass index and waist circumference cutoffs for categorization of overweight and central adiposity among Chinese adults. *American Journal of Clinical Nutrition, 80*(5), 1129–1136.

RESOURCES

Advisory Committee on Immunization Practices (ACIP), Centers for Disease Control and Prevention, National Immunization Program, Division of Epidemiology and Surveillance, Mail Stop E61, 1600 Clifton Road, NE Atlanta, GA 30333; 404-639-3311; Public Inquiries: 404-639-3534 or 800-311-3435; http://www.cdc.gov/nip/recs/adult-schedule.pdf. Accessed March 5, 2006.

Alliance of Cannabis Therapeutics, P.O. Box 21210, Kalorama Station, Washington, DC 20009; 202-483-8595; http://marijuana-as-medicine.org/alliance.htm. Accessed March 5, 2006.

American Dietetic Association, 216 W. Jackson Blvd., Suite 800, Chicago, IL 60606; Consumer Nutrition Hotline: 800-366-1655; http://www.eatright.org. Accessed March 5, 2006.

American Heart Association, 7320 Greenville Ave., Dallas, TX 75231; National Center: 214-373-6300; Nutrition Information: 214-706-1179; http://www.americanheart.org. Accessed March 5, 2006.

Medical Records Institute, 425 Boylston Street, 4th Floor, Boston, MA 02116; 617-964-3923; fax 617-964-3926; http://www.medrecinst.com. Accessed March 5, 2006.

National Cancer Institute, Cancer Information Service, 9000 Rockville Pike, Bldg. 31, Room 10A-24, Bethesda, MD 20892; 1-800-4-CANCER; http://www.nci.nih.gov or http://www.cancer.gov. Accessed March 5, 2006.

Pennsylvania State Nutrition Center, The Pennsylvania State University, Ruth Building, 417 E. Calder Way, University Park, PA 16802; 814-865-6323.

UNIT 2

Biophysical and Psychosocial Concepts in Nursing Practice

Case Study

Applying Concepts from NANDA, NIC, and NOC

A Patient with Fear Accompanied By Somatic Complaints Unsubstantiated By Physical Findings

Mr. Roberts is a 40-year-old man who comes to the emergency department (ED) for treatment of high blood pressure. On his previous visit to the ED he reported chest pressure, feelings of numbness and tingling in his arms, and extreme fearfulness that he was having a heart attack. Even though a myocardial infarction was ruled out and subsequent testing revealed that he had no heart disease, Mr. Roberts continues to have feelings of chest pressure and fear that he is having a heart attack. The only abnormal finding has been an elevation of blood pressure (158/88 mm Hg). The nurse interviews Mr. Roberts, who reveals he is under intense financial pressure. The nurse assesses his compliance with his antihypertensive therapy and suggests interventions to help with Mr. Robert's anxiety.

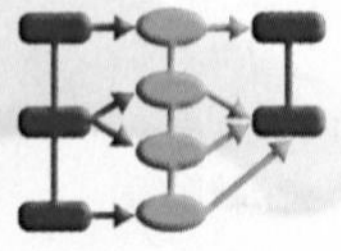

Turn to Appendix C to see a concept map that illustrates the relationships that exist between the nursing diagnoses, interventions, and outcomes for the patient's clinical problems.

Nursing Classifications and Languages

NANDA Nursing Diagnoses	NIC Nursing Interventions	NOC Nursing Outcomes Return to functional baseline status, stabilization of, or improvement in:
Anxiety—Vague uneasy feeling of discomfort or dread accompanied by an autonomic response (the source often nonspecific or unknown to the individual); a feeling of apprehension caused by anticipation of danger. It is an alerting signal that warns of impending danger and enables the individual to take measures to deal with threat.	**Anxiety Reduction**—Minimizing apprehension, dread, foreboding, or uneasiness related to unidentified source of anticipated danger	**Anxiety Self-Control**—Personal actions to eliminate or reduce feelings of apprehension, tension, or uneasiness from an unidentifiable source
Ineffective Coping—Inability to form a valid appraisal of the stressors, inadequate choices of practiced responses, and/or inability to use available resources	**Coping Enhancement**—Assisting a patient to adapt to perceived stressors, changes, or threats that interfere with meeting life demands and roles **Counseling**—Use of an interactive helping process focusing on the needs, problems, or feelings of the patient and significant others to enhance or support coping, problem-solving, and interpersonal relationships **Support System Enhancement**—Facilitation of support to patient by family, friends, and community	**Coping**—Personal actions to manage stressors that tax an individual's resources

NANDA International (2005). *Nursing diagnoses: Definitions & Classification 2005–2006.* Philadelphia: North American Nursing Diagnosis Association.
Dochterman, J. M. & Bulechek, G. M. (2004). *Nursing interventions classification (NIC)* (4th ed.). St. Louis: Mosby.
Iowa Outcomes Project (2004). In Moorhead, S., Johnson, M. & Maas, M. (2004). *Nursing outcomes classification (NOC)* (3rd ed.). St. Louis: Mosby.
Dochterman, J. M. & Jones, D. A. (2003). *Unifying nursing languages: The harmonization of NANDA, NIC, and NOC.* Washington D.C.: American Nurses Association.

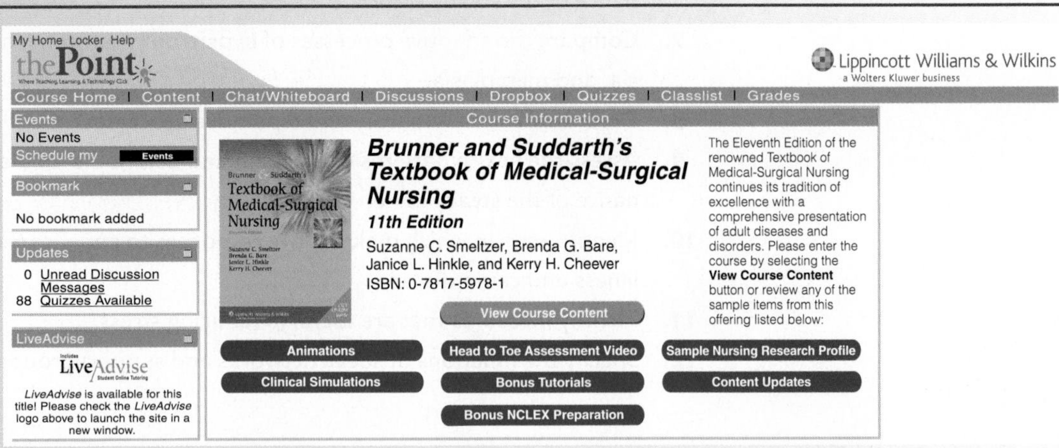

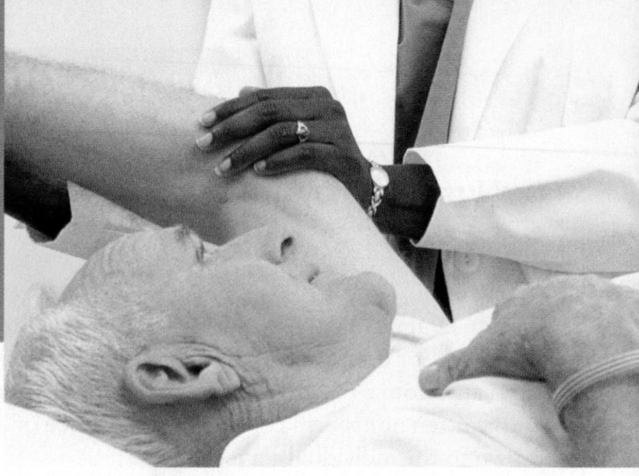

CHAPTER 6

Homeostasis, Stress, and Adaptation

Learning Objectives

On completion of this chapter, the learner will be able to:

1. Relate the principles of internal constancy, homeostasis, stress, and adaptation to the concept of steady state.
2. Identify the significance of the body's compensatory mechanisms in promoting adaptation and maintaining the steady state.
3. Identify physiologic and psychosocial stressors.
4. Compare the sympathetic-adrenal-medullary response to stress to the hypothalamic-pituitary response to stress.
5. Describe the general adaptation syndrome as a theory of adaptation to biologic stress.
6. Describe the relationship of the process of negative feedback to the maintenance of the steady state.
7. Compare the adaptive processes of hypertrophy, atrophy, hyperplasia, dysplasia, and metaplasia.
8. Describe the inflammatory and reparative processes.
9. Assess the health patterns of a person and determine their effects on maintenance of the steady state.
10. Identify ways in which maladaptive responses to stress can increase the risk of illness and cause disease.
11. Identify measures that are useful in reducing stress.
12. Specify the functions of social networks and support groups in reducing stress.

When the body is threatened or suffers an injury, its response may involve functional and structural changes; these changes may be adaptive (having a positive effect) or maladaptive (having a negative effect). The defense mechanisms that the body uses determine the difference between adaptation and maladaptation—health and disease.

Stress and Function

Each body system performs specific functions to sustain optimal life for an organism. Mechanisms for adjusting internal conditions promote the normal steady state of the organism and ultimately its survival. These mechanisms are compensatory in nature and work to restore balance in the body. An example of this restorative effort is the development of rapid breathing (hyperpnea) after intense exercise in an attempt to compensate for an oxygen deficit and excess lactic acid accumulated in the muscle tissue.

Pathophysiologic processes result when cellular injury occurs at such a rapid rate that the body's compensatory mechanisms can no longer make the adaptive changes necessary to remain healthy. An example of a pathophysiologic change is the development of heart failure; the body reacts by retaining sodium and water and increasing venous pressure, which worsens the condition. These pathophysiologic responses give rise to symptoms that are reported by patients or signs that are observed by patients or nurses or other health care providers. These observations, plus a sound knowledge of physiologic and pathophysiologic processes, can assist in determining the existence of a problem and can guide nurses in planning the appropriate course of action.

Dynamic Balance: The Steady State

Physiologic mechanisms must be understood in the context of the body as a whole. Each person, as a living system, has both an internal and an external environment, between which information and matter are continuously exchanged. Within the internal environment, each organ, tissue, and cell is also a system or subsystem of the whole, each with its own internal and external environment, each exchanging information and matter (Fig. 6-1). The goal of the interaction of the body's subsystems is to produce a dynamic balance or **steady state** (even in the presence of change), so that all subsystems are in harmony with each other. Four concepts—constancy, homeostasis, stress, and adaptation—are key to the understanding of steady state.

Claude Bernard, a 19th-century French physiologist, developed the biologic principle that for life there must be a constancy or "fixity of the internal milieu" despite changes

Glossary

adaptation: a change or alteration designed to assist in adapting to a new situation or environment

adrenocorticotropic hormone (ACTH): a hormone produced by the anterior lobe of the pituitary gland that stimulates the secretion of cortisone and other hormones by the adrenal cortex

antidiuretic hormone (ADH): a hormone secreted by the posterior lobe of the pituitary gland that constricts blood vessels, elevates blood pressure, and reduces the excretion of urine

catecholamines: any of the group of amines (such as epinephrine, norepinephrine, or dopamine) that serve as neurotransmitters

coping: the cognitive and behavioral strategies used to manage the stressors that tax a person's resources

dysplasia: a change in the appearance of a cell after exposure to chronic irritation

glucocorticoids: the group of steroid hormones, such as cortisol, that are produced by the adrenal cortex; they are involved in carbohydrate, protein, and fat metabolism and have anti-inflammatory properties

gluconeogenesis: the formation of glucose, especially by the liver from noncarbohydrate sources such as amino acids and the glycerol portion of fats

guided imagery: the mindful use of a word, phrase, or visual image to achieve relaxation or direct attention away from uncomfortable sensations or situations

homeostasis: a steady state within the body; the stability of the internal environment

hyperplasia: an increase in the number of new cells

hypoxia: inadequate supply of oxygen to the cell

infectious agents: biologic agents, such as viruses, bacteria, rickettsiae, mycoplasmas, fungi, protozoa, and nematodes, that cause disease in people

inflammation: a localized, protective reaction of tissue to injury, irritation, or infection, manifested by pain, redness, heat, swelling, and sometimes loss of function

metabolic rate: the speed at which some substances are broken down to yield energy for bodily processes and other substances are synthesized

metaplasia: a cell transformation in which a highly specialized cell changes to a less specialized cell

negative feedback: feedback that decreases the output of a system

positive feedback: feedback that increases the output of a system

primary intention healing: healing by fibrous adhesion, without suppuration or granulation tissue formation

secondary intention healing: delayed closure of two granulating surfaces

steady state: a stable condition that does not change over time, or when change in one direction is balanced by change in an opposite direction

stress: a disruptive condition that occurs in response to adverse influences from the internal or external environments

vasoconstriction: the narrowing of a blood vessel

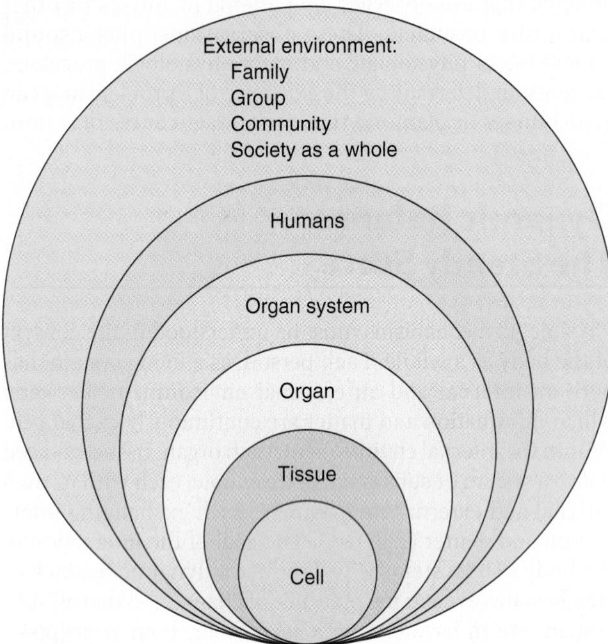

FIGURE 6-1. Constellation of systems. Each system is a subsystem of the larger system (suprasystem) of which it is a part. In this figure the cells represent the smallest system and are a subsystem of all other systems.

in the external environment. The internal milieu was the fluid that bathed the cells, and the constancy was the balanced internal state maintained by physiologic and biochemical processes. His principle implied a static process.

Later, Walter Cannon used the term *homeostasis* to describe the stability of the internal environment, which, he said, was coordinated by homeostatic or compensatory processes that responded to changes in the internal environment. Any change within the internal environment initiated a "righting" response to minimize the change. These biologic processes sought physiologic and chemical balance and were under involuntary control.

Rene Jules Dubos (1965) provided further insight into the dynamic nature of the internal environment with his theory that two complementary concepts, homeostasis and adaptation, were necessary for balance. Homeostatic processes occurred quickly in response to stress, rapidly making the adjustments necessary to maintain the internal environment. Adaptive processes resulted in structural or functional changes over time. Dubos also emphasized that acceptable ranges of response to stimuli existed and that these responses varied for different individuals: "absolute constancy is only a concept of the ideal." Homeostasis and adaptation were both necessary for survival in a changing world.

Homeostasis, then, refers to a steady state within the body. When a change or stress occurs that causes a body function to deviate from its stable range, processes are initiated to restore and maintain the dynamic balance. When these adjustment processes or compensatory mechanisms are not adequate, the steady state is threatened, function becomes disordered, and dysfunctional responses occur. This can lead to disease and may be active during disease, which is a threat to the steady state. Disease is an abnormal variation in the structure or function of any part of the body. It disrupts function and therefore limits freedom of action.

Stress and Adaptation

Stress is a state produced by a change in the environment that is perceived as challenging, threatening, or damaging to a person's dynamic balance or equilibrium. The person is, or feels, unable to meet the demands of the new situation. The change or stimulus that evokes this state is the stressor. The nature of the stressor is variable; an event or change that is stressful for one person may not be stressful for another, and an event that produces stress at one time and place may not do so at another time and place. A person appraises and copes with changing situations. The desired goal is **adaptation**, or adjustment to the change so that the person is again in equilibrium and has the energy and ability to meet new demands. This is the process of **coping** with the stress, a compensatory process with physiologic and psychological components.

Adaptation is a constant, ongoing process that requires a change in structure, function, or behavior so that a person is better suited to the environment; it involves an interaction between the person and the environment. The outcome depends on the degree of "fit" between the skills and capacities of the person, the type of social support available, and the various challenges or stressors encountered. As such, adaptation is an individual process: each person has varying abilities to cope or respond. As new challenges are met, this ability to cope and adapt can change, thereby providing the person with a wide range of adaptive ability. Adaptation occurs throughout the lifespan as the person encounters many developmental and situational challenges, especially related to health and illness. The goal of these encounters is to promote adaptation. In situations of health and illness, this goal is realized by optimal wellness.

Because both stress and adaptation may exist at different levels of a system, it is possible to study these reactions at the cellular, tissue, and organ levels. Biologists are concerned mainly with subcellular components or with subsystems of the total body. Behavioral scientists, including many nurse researchers, study stress and adaptation in individuals, families, groups, and societies; they focus on how a group's organizational features are modified to meet the requirements of the social and physical environment in which the group exists. In any system, the desired goals of adaptation are survival, growth, and reproduction.

Stress: Threats to the Steady State

Types of Stressors

Each person operates at a certain level of adaptation and regularly encounters a certain amount of change. Such change is expected; it contributes to growth and enhances life. A stressor can upset this equilibrium. A stressor may be defined as an internal or external event or situation that creates the potential for physiologic, emotional, cognitive, or behavioral changes in an individual.

Stressors exist in many forms and categories. They may be described as physical, physiologic, or psychosocial. Physical stressors include cold, heat, and chemical agents; physiologic stressors include pain and fatigue. Examples of psychosocial stressors are fear of failing an examination, losing a job, and waiting for a diagnostic test result. Stressors can also occur as normal life transitions that require some adjustment, such as going from childhood into puberty, getting married, or giving birth.

Stressors have also been classified as (1) day-to-day frustrations or hassles; (2) major complex occurrences involving large groups, even entire nations; and (3) stressors that occur less frequently and involve fewer people. The first group, the day-to-day stressors, includes such common occurrences as getting caught in a traffic jam, experiencing computer downtime, and having an argument with a spouse or roommate. These experiences vary in effect. For example, encountering a rainstorm while you are vacationing at the beach will most likely evoke a more negative response than it might at another time. These less dramatic, frustrating, and irritating events—daily hassles—have been shown to have a greater health impact than major life events because of the cumulative effect they have over time. They can lead to high blood pressure, palpitations, or other physiologic problems (Rice, 1999).

The second group of stressors influences larger groups of people, possibly even entire nations. These include events of history, such as terrorism and war, which are threatening situations when experienced either directly, in the war zone, or indirectly, through live news coverage. The demographic, economic, and technologic changes occurring in society also serve as stressors. The tension produced by any stressor is sometimes a result not only of the change itself but also of the speed with which the change occurs.

The third group of stressors has been studied most extensively and concerns relatively infrequent situations that directly affect people. This category includes the influence of life events such as death, birth, marriage, divorce, and retirement. It also includes the psychosocial crises described by Erikson as occurring in the life cycle stages of the human experience. More enduring chronic stressors have also been placed in this category and may include having a permanent functional disability or coping with the difficulties of providing long-term care to a frail elderly parent.

Duration may also be used to categorize stressors, as in the following list:

- An acute, time-limited stressor, such as studying for final examinations
- A stressor sequence—a series of stressful events that result from an initial event such as job loss or divorce
- A chronic intermittent stressor, such as daily hassles
- A chronic enduring stressor that persists over time, such as chronic illness, a disability, or poverty

Stress as a Stimulus for Disease

Relating life events to illness (the theoretical approach that defines stress as a stimulus) has been a major focus of psychosocial studies. This can be traced to Adolph Meyer, who in the 1930s observed a link between illnesses and critical life events in "life charts" of his patients. Subsequent research revealed that people under constant stress have a high incidence of psychosomatic disease.

Holmes and Rahe (1967) developed life events scales that assign numerical values, called life-change units, to typical life events. Because the items in the scales reflect events that require a change in a person's life pattern, and stress is defined as an accumulation of changes in one's life that require psychological adaptation, one can theoretically predict the likelihood of illness by checking off the number of recent events and deriving a total score. The Recent Life Changes Questionnaire (Tausig, 1982) contains 118 items such as death, birth, marriage, divorce, promotions, serious arguments, and vacations. The items include both desirable and undesirable events.

Sources of stress for patients have been well researched (Elder, Wollin, Hartel, et al., 2003; Erlandsson & Eklund, 2003). People typically experience distress related to alterations in their physical and emotional health status, changes in their level of daily functioning, and decreased social support or the loss of significant others. Fears of immobilization, isolation, loneliness, sensory changes, financial problems, and death or disability increase a person's anxiety level. Loss of one's role or perceived purpose in life can cause intense discomfort. Any of these identified variables, plus a myriad of other conditions or overwhelming demands, are likely to cause ineffective coping, and a lack of necessary coping skills is often a source of additional distress for the person. When a person endures prolonged or unrelenting suffering, the outcome is frequently the development of a stress-related illness. Nurses possess the skills to assist people to alter their distressing circumstances and manage their responses to stress.

Psychological Responses to Stress

After recognizing a stressor, a person consciously or unconsciously reacts to manage the situation. This is termed the mediating process. A theory developed by Lazarus (1991a) emphasizes cognitive appraisal and coping as important mediators of stress. Appraisal and coping are influenced by antecedent variables, including the internal and external resources of the individual person.

Appraisal of the Stressful Event

Cognitive appraisal (Lazarus, 1991a; Lazarus & Folkman, 1984) is a process by which an event is evaluated with respect to what is at stake (primary appraisal) and what might and can be done (secondary appraisal). What a person sees as being at stake is influenced by his or her personal goals, commitments, or motivations. Important factors include how important or relevant the event is to the person, whether the event conflicts with what he or she wants or desires, and whether the situation threatens the person's own sense of strength and ego identity.

Primary appraisal results in the situation being identified as either nonstressful or stressful. A nonstressful situation is irrelevant or benign (positive). A stressful situation may be one of three kinds: (1) one in which harm or loss has occurred; (2) one that is threatening, in that harm or loss is anticipated; and (3) one that is challenging, in that some opportunity or gain is anticipated.

Secondary appraisal is an evaluation of what might and can be done about the situation. Actions include assigning blame to the person responsible for a frustrating event; thinking about whether it is possible to do something about the situation (coping potential); and determining future expectancy, or whether things are likely to change for better or worse (Lazarus, 1991a, 1991c). A comparison of what is at stake and what can be done about it (a type of risk–benefit analysis) determines the degree of stress.

Reappraisal, a change of opinion based on new information, also occurs. The appraisal process is not necessarily sequential; primary and secondary appraisal and reappraisal may occur simultaneously. Information learned from an adaptational encounter can be stored, so that when a similar situation is encountered again, the entire process does not need to be repeated.

The appraisal process contributes to the development of an emotion. Negative emotions such as fear and anger accompany harm/loss appraisals, and positive emotions accompany challenge. In addition to the subjective component or feeling that accompanies a particular emotion, each emotion also includes a tendency to act in a certain way. For example, unprepared students may view an unexpected quiz as threatening. They might feel fear, anger, and resentment and might express these emotions through hostile behavior or comments.

Lazarus (1991a) expanded his former ideas about stress, appraisal, and coping into a more complex model relating emotion to adaptation. He called this model a "cognitive-motivational-relational theory," with the term *relational* "standing for a focus on negotiation with a physical and social world" (p. 13). A theory of emotion was proposed as the bridge to connect psychology, physiology, and sociology: "More than any other arena of psychological thought, emotion is an integrative, organismic concept that subsumes psychological stress and coping within itself and unites motivation, cognition, and adaptation in a complex configuration" (p. 40).

Coping With the Stressful Event

Coping, according to Lazarus, consists of the cognitive and behavioral efforts made to manage the specific external or internal demands that tax a person's resources and may be emotion-focused or problem-focused. Coping that is emotion-focused seeks to make the person feel better by lessening the emotional distress. Problem-focused coping aims to make direct changes in the environment so that the situation can be managed more effectively. Both types of coping usually occur in a stressful situation. Even if the situation is viewed as challenging or beneficial, coping efforts may be required to develop and sustain the challenge—that is, to maintain the positive benefits of the challenge and to ward off any threats. In harmful or threatening situations, successful coping reduces or eliminates the source of stress and relieves the emotion it generated.

Appraisal and coping are affected by internal characteristics such as health, energy, personal belief systems, commitments or life goals, self-esteem, control, mastery, knowledge, problem-solving skills, and social skills. The characteristics that have been studied most often in nursing research are health-promoting lifestyles and hardiness. A health-promoting lifestyle buffers the effect of stressors. From a nursing practice standpoint, this outcome—buffering the effect of stressors—supports nursing's goal of promoting health. In many circumstances, promoting a healthy lifestyle is more achievable than altering the stressors.

Hardiness is the name given to a general quality that comes from having rich, varied, and rewarding experiences. It is a personality characteristic composed of control, commitment, and challenge. Hardy people perceive stressors as something they can change and therefore control. To them, potentially stressful situations are interesting and meaningful; change and new situations are viewed as challenging opportunities for growth. Some positive support has been found for hardiness as a significant variable that positively influences rehabilitation and overall improvement after an onset of an acute or chronic illness (Brooks, 2003; Ptacek & Pierce, 2003).

Physiologic Response to Stress

The physiologic response to a stressor, whether it is physical or psychological, is a protective and adaptive mechanism to maintain the homeostatic balance of the body. When a stress response occurs, it triggers a series of neurologic and hormonal processes to be activated within the brain and body systems. The duration and intensity of the stress can cause both short-term and long-term effects. A stressor can disrupt homeostasis to the point where adaptation to the stressor fails, and a disease process results.

Selye's Theory of Adaptation

Hans Selye developed a theory of adaptation that profoundly influenced the scientific study of stress. In 1936, Selye first described a syndrome consisting of enlargement of the adrenal cortex; shrinkage of the thymus, spleen, lymph nodes, and other lymphatic structures; and the appearance of deep, bleeding ulcers in the stomach and duodenum. He identified this as a nonspecific response to diverse, noxious stimuli.

GENERAL ADAPTATION SYNDROME

Selye then developed a theory of adaptation to biologic stress that he named the general adaptation syndrome, which has three phases: alarm, resistance, and exhaustion. During the alarm phase, the sympathetic "fight-or-flight" response is activated with release of **catecholamines** and the onset of the **adrenocorticotropic hormone** (ACTH)–adrenal cortical response. The alarm reaction is defensive and anti-inflammatory but self-limited. Because living in a continuous state of alarm would result in death, people move into the second stage, resistance. During the resistance stage, adaptation to the noxious stressor occurs, and cortisol activity is still increased. If exposure to the stressor is prolonged, the third stage, exhaustion, occurs. During the exhaustion stage, endocrine activity increases, and this has negative effects on the body systems (especially the circulatory, digestive, and immune systems) that can lead to death. Stages one and two of this syndrome are repeated, in different degrees, throughout life as the person encounters stressors.

Selye compared the general adaptation syndrome with the life process. During childhood, too few encounters with stress occur to promote the development of adaptive functioning, and children are vulnerable. During adulthood, a number of stressful events occur, and people develop resistance or adaptation. During the later years, the accumulation of life's stressors and wear and tear on the organism again decrease people's ability to adapt, resistance falls, and eventually death occurs.

LOCAL ADAPTATION SYNDROME

According to Selye, a local adaptation syndrome also occurs. This syndrome includes the inflammatory response and repair processes that occur at the local site of tissue injury. The local adaptation syndrome occurs in small, topical injuries, such as contact dermatitis. If the local injury is severe enough, the general adaptation syndrome is activated as well.

Selye emphasized that stress is the nonspecific response common to all stressors, regardless of whether they are physiologic, psychological, or social. The many conditioning factors in each person's environment account for why different demands are experienced by different people as stressors. Conditioning factors also account for differences in the tolerance of different people for stress: some people may develop diseases of adaptation, such as hypertension and migraine headaches, whereas others are unaffected.

Interpretation of Stressful Stimuli by the Brain

Physiologic responses to stress are mediated by the brain through a complex network of chemical and electrical messages. The neural and hormonal actions that maintain homeostatic balance are integrated by the hypothalamus, which is located in the center of the brain, surrounded by the limbic system and the cerebral hemispheres. The hypothalamus is made up of a number of nuclei and integrates autonomic nervous system mechanisms that maintain the chemical constancy of the internal environment of the body. Together with the limbic system, which contains the amygdala, hippocampus, and septal nuclei, along with other structures, the hypothalamus regulates emotions and many visceral behaviors necessary for survival (eg, eating, drinking, temperature control, reproduction, defense, aggression).

Each of these structures responds differently to stimuli, and each has its own characteristic response (Furman & Gallo, 2000). The cerebral hemispheres are concerned with cognitive functions: thought processes, learning, and memory. The limbic system has connections with both the cerebral hemispheres and the brainstem. In addition, the reticular activating system (RAS), a network of cells that forms a two-way communication system, extends from the brain stem into the midbrain and limbic system. This network controls the alert or waking state of the body.

In the stress response, afferent impulses are carried from sensory organs (eye, ear, nose, skin) and internal sensors (baroreceptors, chemoreceptors) to nerve centers in the brain. The response to the perception of stress is integrated in the hypothalamus, which coordinates the adjustments necessary to return to homeostatic balance. The degree and duration of the response varies; major stress evokes both sympathetic and pituitary adrenal responses.

Neural and neuroendocrine pathways under the control of the hypothalamus are also activated in the stress response. Initially, there is a sympathetic nervous system discharge, followed by a sympathetic-adrenal-medullary discharge. If the stress persists, the hypothalamic-pituitary system is activated (Fig. 6-2).

SYMPATHETIC NERVOUS SYSTEM RESPONSE

The sympathetic nervous system response is rapid and short-lived. Norepinephrine is released at nerve endings that are in direct contact with their respective end organs to cause an increase in function of the vital organs and a state of general body arousal. The heart rate is increased and peripheral **vasoconstriction** occurs, raising the blood pressure. Blood is also shunted away from abdominal organs. The purpose of these responses is to provide better perfusion of vital organs (brain, heart, skeletal muscles). Blood glucose is increased, supplying more readily available energy. The pupils are dilated, and mental activity is increased; a greater sense of awareness exists. Constriction of the blood vessels of the skin limits bleeding in the event of trauma. The person is likely to experience cold feet, clammy skin and hands, chills, palpitations, and "knots" in the stomach. Typically, the person appears tense, with the muscles of the neck, upper back, and shoulders tightened; respirations may be rapid and shallow, with the diaphragm tense.

SYMPATHETIC-ADRENAL-MEDULLARY RESPONSE

In addition to its direct effect on major end organs, the sympathetic nervous system also stimulates the medulla of the adrenal gland to release the hormones epinephrine and norepinephrine into the bloodstream. The action of these hormones is similar to that of the sympathetic nervous system and has the effect of sustaining and prolonging its actions. Epinephrine and norepinephrine are catecholamines that stimulate the nervous system and produce metabolic effects that increase the blood glucose level and increase the **metabolic rate.** The effect of the sympathetic-adrenal-medullary responses is summarized in Table 6-1. This effect is called the "fight-or-flight" reaction.

HYPOTHALAMIC-PITUITARY RESPONSE

The longest-acting phase of the physiologic response, which is more likely to occur in persistent stress, involves the hypothalamic-pituitary pathway. The hypothalamus secretes corticotropin-releasing factor, which stimulates the anterior pituitary to produce ACTH, which in turn stimulates the adrenal cortex to produce **glucocorticoids**, primarily cortisol. Cortisol stimulates protein catabolism, releasing amino acids; stimulates liver uptake of amino acids and their conversion to glucose (**gluconeogenesis**); and inhibits glucose uptake (anti-insulin action) by many body cells but not those of the brain and heart. These cortisol-induced metabolic effects provide the body with a ready source of energy during a stressful situation. This effect has some important implications. For example, a person with diabetes who is under stress, such as that caused by an infection, needs more insulin than usual. Any patient who is under stress (eg, illness, surgery, trauma, or prolonged psychological stress) catabolizes body protein and needs

Physiology/Pathophysiology

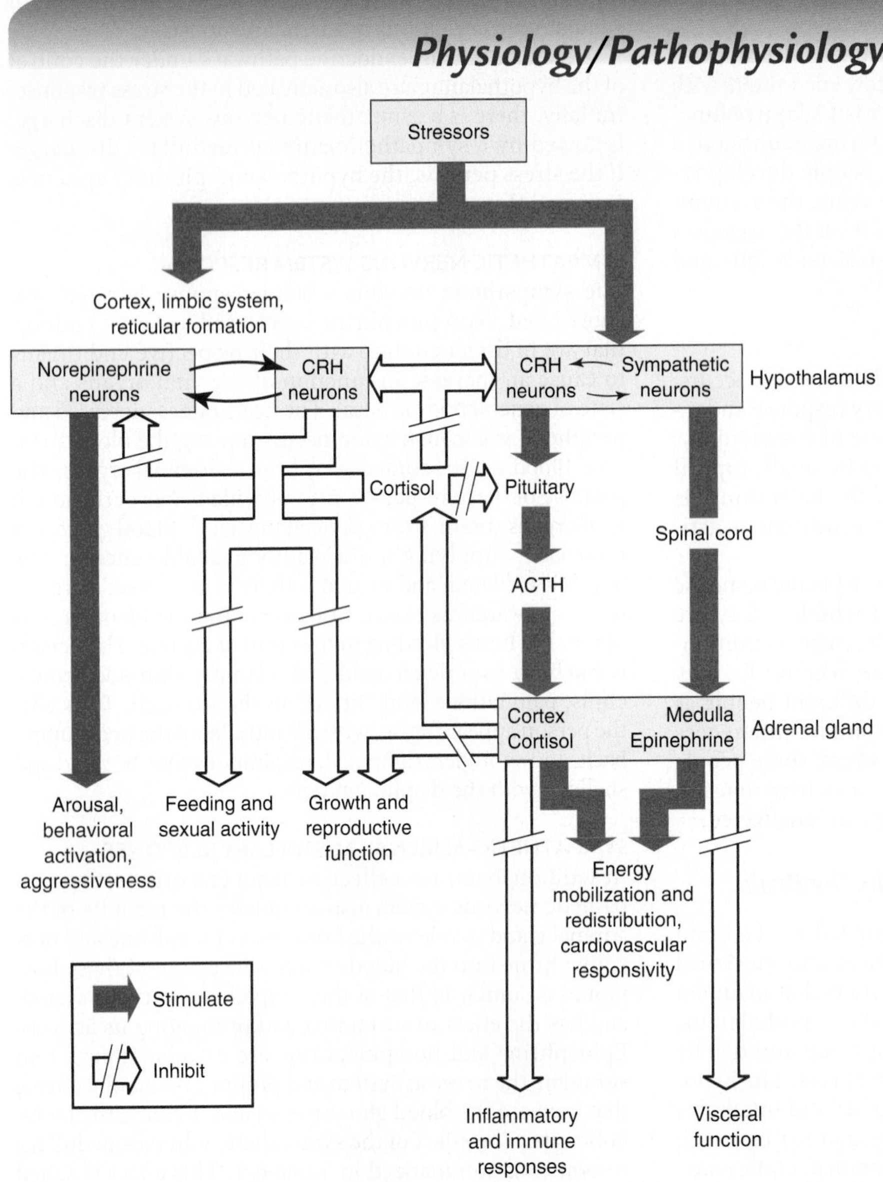

FIGURE 6-2. Integrated responses to stress mediated by the sympathetic nervous system and the hypothalamic–pituitary–adrenocortical axis. The responses are mutually reinforcing at both the central and peripheral levels. Negative feedback by cortisol also can limit an overresponse that might be harmful to the individual. *Colored arrows* represent stimulation, *open arrows,* inhibition. CRH, corticotropin-releasing hormone; ACTH, adrenocorticotropic hormone. Reproduced with permission from Berne, R. M., & Levy, M. N. (2003). *Physiology.* St. Louis: C. V. Mosby.

supplements. Growth is retarded in a child who has been subjected to severe stress.

The actions of the catecholamines (epinephrine and norepinephrine) and cortisol are the most important in the general response to stress. Other hormones that play a role are **antidiuretic hormone** (ADH) released from the posterior pituitary and aldosterone released from the adrenal cortex. ADH and aldosterone promote sodium and water retention, which is an adaptive mechanism in the event of hemorrhage or loss of fluids through excessive perspiration. ADH has also been shown to influence learning and may thus facilitate coping in new and threatening situations. Secretion of growth hormone and glucagon stimulates the uptake of amino acids by cells, helping to mobilize energy resources. Endorphins, which are endogenous opiates, increase during stress and enhance the threshold for tolerance of painful stimuli. They may also affect mood and have been implicated in the so-called high that long-distance runners experience. The secretion of other hormones is also affected, but their adaptive function is less clear.

IMMUNOLOGIC RESPONSE

Research findings show that the immune system is connected to the neuroendocrine and autonomic systems. Lymphoid tissue is richly supplied by autonomic nerves capable of releasing a number of different neuropeptides that can have a direct effect on leukocyte regulation and the inflammatory response. Neuroendocrine hormones released by the central nervous system and endocrine tissues can inhibit or stimulate leukocyte function. The wide variety of stressors a person experiences may result in different alterations in autonomic activity and subtle variations in neurohormone and neuropeptide synthesis. All of these possible autonomic and neuroendocrine responses can interact to initiate, weaken, enhance, or terminate an immune response (Chiorazzi, 2003).

TABLE 6-1 Sympathetic–Adrenal–Medullary Response to Stress

Effect	Purpose	Mechanism
Increased heart rate and blood pressure	Better perfusion of vital organs	Increased cardiac output due to increased myocardial contractility and heart rate; increased venous return (peripheral vasoconstriction)
Increased blood glucose level	Increased available energy	Increased liver and muscle glycogen breakdown; increased breakdown of adipose tissue triglycerides
Mental acuity	Alert state	Increase in amount of blood shunted to the brain from the abdominal viscera and skin
Dilated pupils	Increased awareness	Contraction of radial muscle of iris
Increased tension of skeletal muscles	Preparedness for activity, decreased fatigue	Excitation of muscles; increase in amount of blood shunted to the muscles from the abdominal viscera and skin
Increased ventilation (may be rapid and shallow)	Provision of oxygen for energy	Stimulation of respiratory center in medulla; bronchodilation
Increased coagulability of blood	Prevention of hemorrhage in event of trauma	Vasoconstriction of surface vessels

The study of the relationships among the neuroendocrine system, the central and autonomic nervous systems, and the immune system and the effects of these relationships on overall health outcomes is called *psychoneuroimmunology*. Because one's perception of events and one's coping styles determine whether, and to what extent, an event activates the stress response system, and because the stress response affects immune activity, one's perceptions, ideas, and thoughts can have profound neurochemical and immunologic consequences. Multiple studies have demonstrated alteration of immune function in people who are under stress (Constantino, Secula, Rabin, et al., 2000; Norman, 2003; Robinson, Matthews, & Witek-Janusek, 2000). Other studies have identified certain personality traits, such as optimism and active coping, as having positive effects on health (Brissette, Leventhal, & Leventhal, 2003; Kennedy, 2000; Whitty, 2003). As research continues, this new field of study will likely uncover to what extent and by what mechanisms people can consciously influence their immunity.

Maladaptive Responses to Stress

The stress response, which, as indicated earlier, facilitates adaptation to threatening situations, has been retained from humans' evolutionary past. The "fight-or-flight" response, for example, is an anticipatory response that mobilized the bodily resources of our ancestors to deal with predators and other harsh factors in their environment. This same mobilization comes into play in response to emotional stimuli unrelated to danger. For example, a person may get an "adrenaline rush" when competing over a decisive point in a ball game, or when excited about attending a party.

When the responses to stress are ineffective, they are referred to as *maladaptive*. Maladaptive responses are chronic, recurrent responses or patterns of response over time that do not promote the goals of adaptation. The goals of adaptation are somatic or physical health (optimal wellness); psychological health or having a sense of well-being (happiness, satisfaction with life, morale); and enhanced social functioning, which includes work, social life, and family (positive relationships). Maladaptive responses that threaten these goals include faulty appraisals and inappropriate coping (Lazarus, 1991a).

The frequency, intensity, and duration of stressful situations contribute to the development of negative emotions and subsequent patterns of neurochemical discharge. By appraising situations more adequately and coping more appropriately, it is possible to anticipate and defuse some of these situations. For example, frequent potentially stressful encounters (eg, marital discord) might be avoided with better communication and problem solving, or a pattern of procrastination (eg, delaying work on tasks) could be corrected to reduce stress when deadlines approach.

Coping processes that include the use of alcohol or drugs to reduce stress increase the risk of illness. Other inappropriate coping patterns may increase the risk of illness less directly. For example, people who demonstrate "type A" behaviors such as impatience, competitiveness, and achievement orientation and have an underlying hostile approach to life are more prone than others to develop stress-related illnesses. Type A behaviors increase the output of catecholamines, the adrenal-medullary hormones, with their attendant effects on the body.

Other forms of inappropriate coping include denial, avoidance, and distancing. Denial may be illustrated by the woman who feels a lump in her breast but downplays its seriousness and delays seeking medical attention. The intent of denial is to control the threat, but it may also endanger life.

Models of illness frequently cite stress and maladaptation as precursors to disease. A general model of illness, based on Selye's theory, suggests that any stressor elicits a state of disturbed physiologic equilibrium. If this state is prolonged or the response is excessive, it increases the susceptibility of the person to illness. This susceptibility, coupled with a predisposition in the person (from genetic traits, health, or age), leads to illness. If the sympathetic adrenal-medullary response is prolonged or excessive, a state of chronic arousal develops that may lead to high blood pressure, arteriosclerotic changes, and cardiovascular disease. If the production of ACTH is prolonged or excessive, behavior patterns of withdrawal and depression are seen. In addition, the immune response is decreased, and infections and tumors may develop.

Selye (1976) proposed a list of disorders that he called diseases of maladaptation: high blood pressure, diseases of the heart and blood vessels, diseases of the kidney, hypertension of pregnancy, rheumatic and rheumatoid arthritis, inflammatory diseases of the skin and eyes, infections, allergic and hypersensitivity diseases, nervous and mental diseases, sexual dysfunction, digestive diseases, metabolic diseases, and cancer.

Indicators of Stress

Indicators of stress and the stress response include both subjective and objective measures. Chart 6-1 lists signs and symptoms that may be observed directly or reported by a person. They are psychological, physiologic, or behavioral and reflect social behaviors and thought processes. Some of these reactions may be coping behaviors. Over time, each person tends to develop a characteristic pattern of behavior during stress to warn that the system is out of balance.

Laboratory measurements of indicators of stress have helped in understanding this complex process. Blood and urine analyses can be used to demonstrate changes in hormonal levels and hormonal breakdown products. Blood levels of catecholamines, glucocorticoids, ACTH, and eosinophils are reliable measures of stress. Serum cholesterol and free fatty acid levels can also be used to measure stress. When the body experiences distress, it automatically produces adrenal hormones such as cortisol and aldosterone. As the levels of these chemicals increase, there is a simultaneous release of additional cholesterol into the general circulation. Both physical and psychological distress can trigger an elevated cholesterol level. In addition, the results of immunoglobulin assays are increased when a person is exposed to a variety of stressors, especially infections and immunodeficiency conditions. With greater attention to the field of neuroimmunology, improved laboratory measures are likely to follow.

In addition to using laboratory tests, researchers have developed questionnaires to identify and assess stressors, stress, and coping strategies. Some of these questionnaires are referenced in the work of Rice (1999), which is a compilation of information gained from research on stress, coping, and health. Some examples of the research instruments that nurses commonly use to measure levels of client distress and client functioning can be found in a variety of research reports (Cutler, Fishbain, Steele-Rosomoff, et al., 2003; Olofsson, Bengtsson, & Brink, 2003; Shapley, Jordan, & Croft, 2003). Miller and Smith (1993) provided a stress audit and a stress profile measurement tool that is available in the popular lay literature.

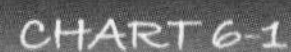

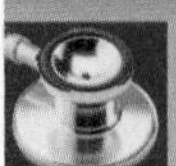

Assessing for Stress

Be on the alert for the following signs and symptoms:

- Restlessness
- Depression
- Dry mouth
- Overpowering urge to act out
- Fatigue
- Loss of interest in life activities
- Intense periods of anxiety
- Strong startle response
- Hyperactivity
- Gastrointestinal distress
- Diarrhea
- Nausea or vomiting
- Changes in menstrual cycle
- Change in appetite
- Injury-prone
- Palpitations
- Impulsive behaviors
- Emotional lability
- Concentration difficulties
- Feeling weak or dizzy
- Increased body tension
- Tremors
- Nervous habits
- Nervous laughter
- Bruxism (grinding of teeth)
- Difficulty sleeping
- Excessive perspiration
- Urinary frequency
- Headaches
- Pain in back, neck, or other parts of the body
- Increased use of tobacco
- Substance use or abuse

Nursing Implications

It is important for nurses to realize that the optimal point of intervention to promote health is during the stage when a person's own compensatory processes are still functioning effectively. A major role of nurses is the early identification of both physiologic and psychological stressors. Nurses should be able to relate the presenting signs and symptoms of distress to the physiology they represent and identify a person's position on the continuum of function, from health and compensation to pathophysiology and disease.

For example, if an anxious middle-aged woman presented for a checkup and was found to be overweight and have a blood pressure of 150/85 mm Hg, the nurse would counsel her with respect to diet, stress management, and activity. The nurse would also encourage weight loss and discuss the woman's intake of salt (which affects fluid balance) and caffeine (which provides a stimulant effect). The patient and the nurse would identify both individual and environmental stressors and discuss strategies to decrease her lifestyle stress, with the ultimate goal being to create a healthy lifestyle and prevent hypertension and its sequelae.

Stress at the Cellular Level

Pathologic processes may occur at all levels of the biologic organism. If the cell is considered the smallest unit or subsystem (tissues being aggregates of cells, organs aggregates of tissues, and so on), the processes of health and disease or adaptation and maladaptation can all occur at the cellular level. Indeed, pathologic processes are often described by scientists at the subcellular or molecular level.

The cell exists on a continuum of function and structure, ranging from the normal cell, to the adapted cell, to the injured or diseased cell, to the dead cell (Fig. 6-3). Changes from one state to another may occur rapidly and may not be readily detectable, because each state does not have discrete boundaries, and disease represents disruption of normal processes. The earliest changes occur at the molecular or subcellular level and are not perceptible until steady-state functions or structures are altered. With cell injury, some changes may be reversible; in other instances, the injuries are lethal. For example, tanning of the skin is an adaptive, morphologic response to exposure to the rays of the sun. However, if the exposure is continued, sunburn and injury occur, and some cells may die, as evidenced by desquamation ("peeling").

Different cells and tissues respond to stimuli with different patterns and rates of response, and some cells are more vulnerable to one type of stimulus or stressor than others. The cell involved, its ability to adapt, and its physiologic state are determinants of the response. For example, cardiac muscle cells respond to **hypoxia** (inadequate oxygenation) more quickly than do smooth muscle cells.

Other determinants of cellular response are the type or nature of the stimulus, its duration, and its severity. For example, neurons that control respiration can develop a tolerance to regular, small amounts of a barbiturate, but one large dose may result in respiratory depression and death.

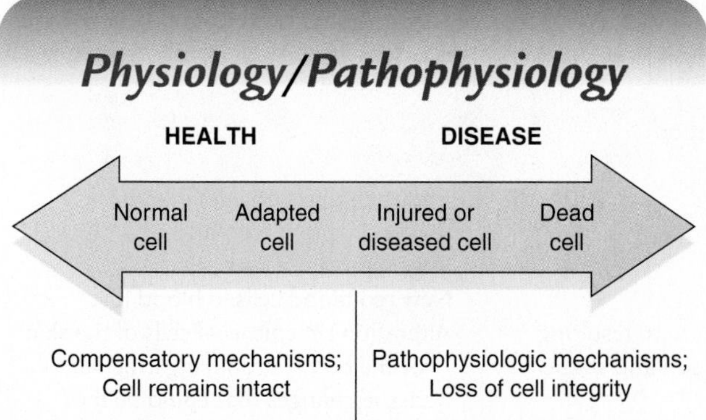

FIGURE 6-3. The cell on a continuum of function and structure. Changes in the cell are not as easily discerned as the diagram depicts, and the point at which compensation subsides and pathophysiology begins is not clearly defined.

Control of the Steady State

The concept of the cell as existing on a continuum of function and structure includes the relationship of the cell to compensatory mechanisms, which occur continuously in the body to maintain the steady state. Compensatory processes are regulated primarily by the autonomic nervous system and the endocrine system, with control achieved through negative feedback.

Negative Feedback

Negative feedback mechanisms throughout the body monitor the internal environment and restore homeostasis when conditions shift out of the normal range. These mechanisms work by sensing deviations from a predetermined set point or range of adaptability and triggering a response aimed at offsetting the deviation. Blood pressure, acid–base balance, blood glucose level, body temperature, and fluid and electrolyte balance are examples of functions regulated through such compensatory mechanisms.

Most of the human body's control systems are integrated by the brain and influenced by the nervous and endocrine systems. Control activities involve detecting deviations from the predetermined reference point and stimulating compensatory responses in the muscles and glands of the body. The major organs affected are the heart, lungs, kidneys, liver, gastrointestinal tract, and skin. When stimulated, these organs alter their rate of activity or the amount of secretions they produce. Because of this, they have been called the "organs of homeostasis or adjustment."

In addition to the responses controlled by the nervous and endocrine systems, local responses consisting of small feedback loops in a group of cells or tissues are possible. The cells detect a change in their immediate environment and initiate an action to counteract its effect. For example, the accumulation of lactic acid in an exercised muscle stimulates dilation of blood vessels in the area to increase blood flow and improve the delivery of oxygen and removal of waste products.

The net result of the activities of feedback loops is homeostasis. A steady state is achieved by the continuous, variable action of the organs involved in making the adjustments and by the continuous small exchanges of chemical substances among cells, interstitial fluid, and blood. For example, an increase in the carbon dioxide concentration of the extracellular fluid leads to increased pulmonary ventilation, which decreases the carbon dioxide level. On a cellular level, increased carbon dioxide raises the hydrogen ion concentration of the blood. This is detected by chemosensitive receptors in the respiratory control center of the medulla of the brain. The chemoreceptors stimulate an increase in the rate of discharge of the neurons that innervate the diaphragm and intercostal muscles, which increases the rate of respiration. Excess carbon dioxide is exhaled, the hydrogen ion concentration returns to normal, and the chemically sensitive neurons are no longer stimulated (Porth, 2005).

Positive Feedback

Another type of feedback, **positive feedback**, perpetuates the chain of events set in motion by the original disturbance instead of compensating for it. As the system becomes more unbalanced, disorder and disintegration occur. There are some exceptions to this; blood clotting in humans, for example, is an important positive feedback mechanism.

Cellular Adaptation

Cells are complex units that dynamically respond to the changing demands and stresses of daily life. They possess a maintenance function and a specialized function. The maintenance function refers to the activities that the cell must perform with respect to itself; specialized functions are those that the cell performs in relation to the tissues and organs of which it is a part. Individual cells may cease to function without posing a threat to the organism. However, as the number of dead cells increases, the specialized functions of the tissues are altered, and health is threatened.

Cells can adapt to environmental stress through structural and functional changes. Some of these adaptations are hypertrophy, atrophy, hyperplasia, dysplasia, and metaplasia (Table 6-2). These adaptations reflect changes in the normal cell in response to stress. If the stress is unrelenting, cellular injury and death may occur.

Hypertrophy and atrophy lead to changes in the size of cells and hence the size of the organs they form. Compensatory hypertrophy is the result of an enlarged muscle mass and commonly occurs in skeletal and cardiac muscle that experiences a prolonged, increased workload. One example is the bulging muscles of the athlete who engages in body building.

Atrophy can be the consequence of a disease or of decreased use, decreased blood supply, loss of nerve supply, or inadequate nutrition. Disuse of a body part is often associated with the aging process and immobilization. Cell size and organ size decrease, and the structures principally affected are the skeletal muscles, the secondary sex organs, the heart, and the brain.

Hyperplasia is an increase in the number of new cells in an organ or tissue. As cells multiply and are subjected to increased stimulation, the tissue mass enlarges. This mitotic response (a change occurring with mitosis) is reversible when the stimulus is removed. This distinguishes hyperplasia from neoplasia or malignant growth, which continues after the stimulus is removed. Hyperplasia may be hormonally induced. An example is the increased size of the thyroid gland caused by thyroid-stimulating hormone (secreted from the pituitary gland) when a deficit in thyroid hormone occurs.

Dysplasia is the change in the appearance of cells after they have been subjected to chronic irritation. Dysplastic cells have a tendency to become malignant; dysplasia is seen commonly in epithelial cells in the bronchi of smokers.

Metaplasia is a cell transformation in which highly specialized cells change to less specialized cells. This serves a protective function, because less specialized cells are more resistant to the stress that stimulated the change. For example, the ciliated columnar epithelium lining the bronchi of smokers is replaced by squamous epithelium. The squamous cells can survive; loss of the cilia and protective mucus, however, can have damaging consequences.

TABLE 6-2 Cellular Adaptation to Stressors

Adaptation	Stimulus	Example
Hypertrophy—increase in cell size leading to increase in organ size	Increased workload	Leg muscles of runner Arm muscles in tennis player Cardiac muscle in person with hypertension
Atrophy—shrinkage in size of cell, leading to decrease in organ size	Decrease in: Use Blood supply Nutrition Hormonal stimulation Innervation	Secondary sex organs in aging person Extremity immobilized in cast
Hyperplasia—increase in number of new cells (increase in mitosis)	Hormonal influence	Breast changes of a girl in puberty or of a pregnant woman Regeneration of liver cells New red blood cells in blood loss
Dysplasia—change in the appearance of cells after they have been subjected to chronic irritation	Reproduction of cells with resulting alteration of their size and shape	Alterations in epithelial cells of the skin or the cervix, producing irregular tissue changes that could be the precursors of a malignancy
Metaplasia—transformation of one adult cell type to another (reversible)	Stress applied to highly specialized cell	Changes in epithelial cells lining bronchi in response to smoke irritation (cells become less specialized)

Cellular Injury

Injury is defined as a disorder in steady-state regulation. Any stressor that alters the ability of the cell or system to maintain optimal balance of its adjustment processes leads to injury. Structural and functional damage then occurs, which may be reversible (permitting recovery) or irreversible (leading to disability or death). Homeostatic adjustments are concerned with the small changes within the body's systems. With adaptive changes, compensation occurs and a steady state is achieved, although it may be a new level. With injury, steady-state regulation is lost, and changes in functioning ensue.

Causes of disorder and injury in the system (cell, tissue, organ, body) may arise from the external or internal environment (Fig. 6-4) and include hypoxia, nutritional imbalance, physical agents, chemical agents, infectious agents, immune mechanisms, genetic defects, and psychogenic factors. The most common causes are hypoxia (oxygen deficiency), chemical injury, and infectious agents. In addition, the presence of one injury makes the system more susceptible to another injury. For example, inadequate oxygenation and nutritional deficiencies make the system vulnerable to infection. These agents act at the cellular level by damaging or destroying:

- The integrity of the cell membrane, necessary for ionic balance
- The ability of the cell to transform energy (aerobic respiration, production of adenosine triphosphate)
- The ability of the cell to synthesize enzymes and other necessary proteins
- The ability of the cell to grow and reproduce (genetic integrity)

Hypoxia

Inadequate cellular oxygenation (hypoxia) interferes with the cell's ability to transform energy. Hypoxia may be caused by:

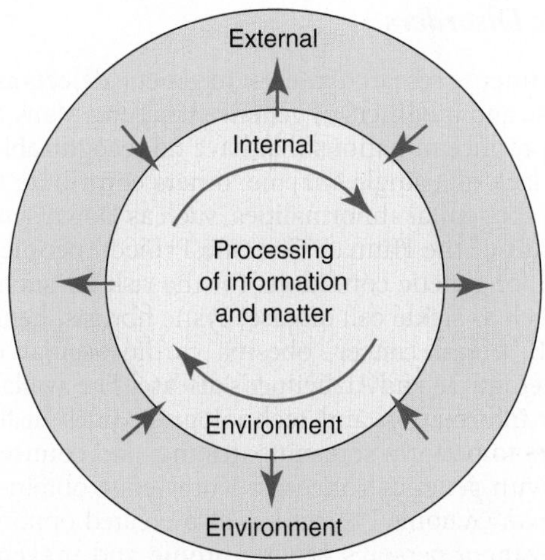

FIGURE 6-4. Influences leading to disorder may arise from the internal environment and the external environment of the system. Excesses or deficits of information and matter may occur, or there may be faulty regulation of processing.

- A decrease in blood supply to an area
- A decrease in the oxygen-carrying capacity of the blood (decreased hemoglobin)
- A ventilation/perfusion or respiratory problem that reduces the amount of oxygen available in the blood
- A problem in the cell's enzyme system that makes it unable to use the oxygen delivered to it

The usual cause of hypoxia is ischemia, or deficient blood supply. Ischemia is commonly seen in myocardial cell injury in which arterial blood flow is decreased because of atherosclerotic narrowing of blood vessels. Ischemia also results from intravascular clots (thrombi or emboli) that may form and interfere with blood supply. Thrombi and emboli are common causes of cerebrovascular accidents (strokes, brain attacks). The length of time different tissues can survive without oxygen varies. For example, brain cells may succumb in 3 to 6 minutes, depending on the situation. If the condition leading to hypoxia is slow and progressive, collateral circulation may develop, whereby blood is supplied by other blood vessels in the area. However, this mechanism is not highly reliable.

Nutritional Imbalance

Nutritional imbalance refers to a relative or absolute deficiency or excess of one or more essential nutrients. This may be manifested as undernutrition (inadequate consumption of food or calories) or overnutrition (caloric excess). Caloric excess to the point of obesity overloads cells in the body with lipids. By requiring more energy to maintain the extra tissue, obesity places a strain on the body and has been associated with the development of disease, especially pulmonary and cardiovascular disease.

Specific deficiencies arise when an essential nutrient is deficient or when there is an imbalance of nutrients. Protein deficiencies and avitaminosis (deficiency of vitamins) are typical examples. An energy deficit leading to cell injury can occur if there is insufficient glucose, or insufficient oxygen to transform the glucose into energy. A lack of insulin, or the inability to use insulin, may also prevent glucose from entering the cell from the blood. This occurs in diabetes mellitus, a metabolic disorder that can lead to nutritional deficiency.

Physical Agents

Physical agents, including temperature extremes, radiation, electrical shock, and mechanical trauma, can cause injury to the cells or to the entire body. The duration of exposure and the intensity of the stressor determine the severity of damage.

TEMPERATURE

When a person's temperature is elevated, hypermetabolism occurs and the respiratory rate, heart rate, and basal metabolic rate all increase. With fever induced by infections, the hypothalamic thermostat may be reset at a higher temperature and then return to normal when the fever abates. The increase in body temperature is achieved through physiologic mechanisms. Body temperatures greater than 41°C (106°F) indicate hyperthermia, because the physiologic function of the thermoregulatory center breaks down and the temperature soars. This physiologic condition occurs in people who have heat stroke. Eventually, the high temperature causes coagulation of cell proteins, and cells die. The body must be cooled rapidly to prevent brain damage.

The local response to thermal or burn injury is similar. There is an increase in metabolic activity, and, as heat increases, protein is coagulated, enzyme systems are destroyed, and, in the extreme, charring or carbonization occurs. Burns of the epithelium are classified as partial-thickness burns if epithelializing elements remain to support healing. Full-thickness burn wounds lack such elements and must be grafted for healing. The amount of body surface involved determines the patient's prognosis. If the injury is severe or extensive, the entire body becomes involved, and hypermetabolism develops as a pathophysiologic response.

Extremes of low temperature, or cold, cause vasoconstriction. Blood flow becomes sluggish and clots form, leading to ischemic damage in the involved tissues. With still lower temperatures, ice crystals may form, and cells may burst.

RADIATION AND ELECTRICAL SHOCK

Radiation is used for diagnosis and treatment of diseases. Ionizing forms of radiation may cause injury by their destructive action. Radiation decreases the protective inflammatory response of the cell, creating a favorable environment for opportunistic infections. Electrical shock produces burns as a result of the heat generated when electrical current travels through the body. It may also abnormally stimulate nerves, leading, for example, to fibrillation of the heart.

MECHANICAL TRAUMA

Mechanical trauma can result in wounds that disrupt the cells and tissues of the body. The severity of the wound, the amount of blood loss, and the extent of nerve damage are significant factors in the outcome.

Chemical Agents

Chemical injuries are caused by poisons, such as lye, which have a corrosive action on epithelial tissue, or by heavy metals, such as mercury, arsenic, and lead, each of which has its own specific destructive action. Many other chemicals are toxic in certain amounts, in certain people, and in specific tissues. Excessive secretion of hydrochloric acid can damage the stomach lining; large amounts of glucose can cause osmotic shifts, affecting the fluid and electrolyte balance; and too much insulin can cause subnormal levels of glucose in the blood (hypoglycemia) and can lead to coma.

Drugs, including prescribed medications, can also cause chemical poisoning. Some people are less tolerant of medications than others and manifest toxic reactions at the usual or customary dosages. Aging tends to decrease tolerance to medications. Polypharmacy (taking many medications at one time) also occurs frequently in the aging population and is a problem because of the unpredictable effects of the resulting medication interactions.

Alcohol (ethanol) is also a chemical irritant. In the body, alcohol is broken down into acetaldehyde, which has a direct toxic effect on liver cells that leads to a variety of liver abnormalities, including cirrhosis in susceptible people. Disordered liver cell function leads to complications in other organs of the body.

Infectious Agents

Biologic agents known to cause disease in humans are viruses, bacteria, rickettsiae, mycoplasmas, fungi, protozoa, and nematodes. The severity of the infectious disease depends on the number of microorganisms entering the body, their virulence, and the host's defenses (eg, health, age, immune responses).

Some bacteria, such as those that cause tetanus and diphtheria, produce exotoxins that circulate and create cell damage. Others, such as gram-negative bacteria, produce endotoxins when they die. Tubercle bacilli induce an immune reaction.

Viruses, the smallest living organisms known, survive as parasites of the living cells they invade. Viruses infect specific cells. Through a complex mechanism, viruses replicate within cells and then invade other cells, where they continue to replicate. An immune response is mounted by the body to eliminate the viruses, and the cells harboring the viruses can be injured in the process. Typically, an inflammatory response and immune reaction are the physiologic responses of the body to viral infection.

Disordered Immune Responses

The immune system is an exceedingly complex system, the purpose of which is to defend the body from invasion by any foreign object or foreign cell type, such as cancerous cells. This is a steady-state mechanism, but like other adjustment processes it can become disordered, and cell injury occurs. The immune response detects foreign bodies by distinguishing non-self substances from self substances and destroying the non-self entities. The entrance of an antigen (foreign substance) into the body evokes the production of antibodies that attack and destroy the antigen (antigen–antibody reaction).

The immune system may function normally or it may be hypoactive or hyperactive. When it is hypoactive, immunodeficiency diseases occur; when it is hyperactive, hypersensitivity disorders occur. A disorder of the immune system itself can result in damage to the body's own tissues. Such disorders are labeled autoimmune diseases (see Unit 11).

Genetic Disorders

There is intense research interest in genetic defects as causes of disease and modifiers of genetic structure. Many of these defects produce mutations that have no recognizable effect, such as lack of a single enzyme; others contribute to more obvious congenital abnormalities, such as Down syndrome. As a result of the Human Genome Project, people can be assessed for genetic conditions (or the risk for such conditions) such as sickle cell disease, cystic fibrosis, hemophilia A and B, breast cancer, obesity, cardiovascular disease, phenylketonuria, and Alzheimer's disease. The availability of genetics information and technology enables health care providers to perform screening, testing, and counseling for people with genetics concerns. Knowledge obtained from the Human Genome Project has also created opportunities for assessing a person's genetic profile and preventing or treating diseases. Diagnostic genetics and gene therapy have the potential to identify and modify genes before they begin to express traits that would lead to disease or disability. (For further information, see Chapter 9.)

Cellular Response to Injury: Inflammation

Cells or tissues of the body may be injured or killed by any of the agents (physical, chemical, infectious) described earlier. When this happens, an inflammatory response (or inflammation) naturally occurs in the healthy tissues adjacent to the site of injury. **Inflammation** is a defensive reaction intended to neutralize, control, or eliminate the offending agent and to prepare the site for repair. It is a nonspecific response (not dependent on a particular cause) that is meant to serve a protective function. For example, inflammation may be observed at the site of a bee sting, in a sore throat, in a surgical incision, and at the site of a burn. Inflammation also occurs in cell injury events, such as strokes and myocardial infarctions.

Inflammation is not the same as infection. An infectious agent is only one of several agents that may trigger an inflammatory response. An infection exists when the infectious agent is living, growing, and multiplying in the tissues and is able to overcome the body's normal defenses.

Regardless of the cause, a general sequence of events occurs in the local inflammatory response. This sequence involves changes in the microcirculation, including vasodilation, increased vascular permeability, and leukocytic cellular infiltration (Fig. 6-5). As these changes take place, five cardinal signs of inflammation are produced: redness, heat, swelling, pain, and loss of function.

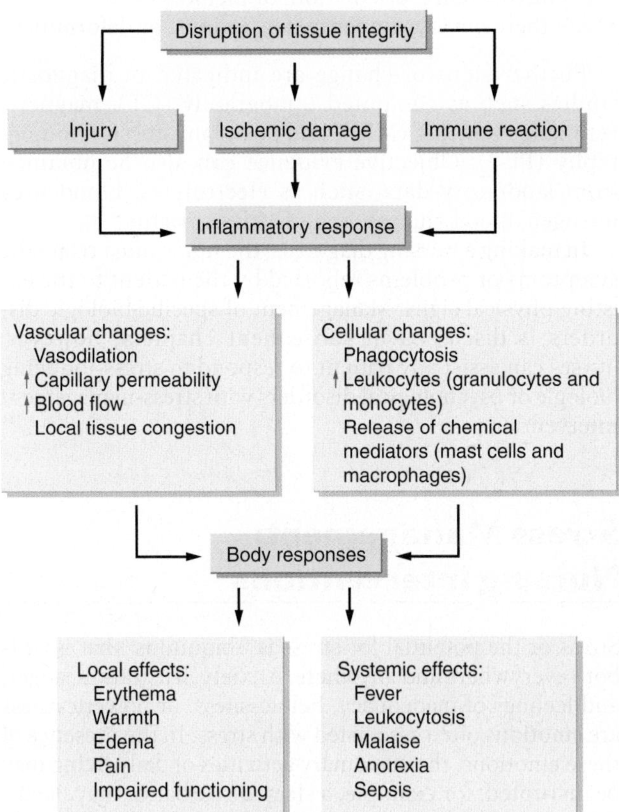

FIGURE 6-5. Inflammatory response.

The transient vasoconstriction that occurs immediately after injury is followed by vasodilation and an increased rate of blood flow through the microcirculation to the area of tissue damage. Local heat and redness result. Next, the structure of the microvascular system changes to accommodate the movement of plasma protein from the blood into the tissues. Following this increase in vascular permeability, plasma fluids (including proteins and solutes) leak into the inflamed tissues, producing swelling. Leukocytes migrate through the endothelium and accumulate in the tissue at the site of the injury. The pain that occurs is attributed to the pressure of fluids or swelling on nerve endings and to the irritation of nerve endings by chemical mediators released at the site. Bradykinin is one of the chemical mediators suspected of causing pain. Loss of function is most likely related to the pain and swelling, but the exact mechanism is not completely known.

As blood flow increases and fluid leaks into the surrounding tissues, the formed elements (red blood cells, white blood cells, and platelets) remain in the blood, causing it to become more viscous. Leukocytes (white blood cells) collect in the vessels, exit, and migrate to the site of injury to engulf offending organisms and to remove cellular debris in a process called phagocytosis. Fibrinogen in the leaked plasma fluid coagulates, forming fibrin for clot formation, which serves to wall off the injured area and prevent the spread of infection.

Chemical Mediators of Inflammation

Injury initiates the inflammatory response, but chemical substances released at the site induce the vascular changes. Foremost among these chemicals are histamine and kinins. Histamine is present in many tissues of the body but is concentrated in the mast cells. It is released when injury occurs and is responsible for the early changes in vasodilation and vascular permeability. Kinins increase vasodilation and vascular permeability, and they also attract neutrophils to the area. Prostaglandins, another group of chemical substances, are also suspected of causing increased permeability (Porth, 2005).

Systemic Response to Inflammation

The inflammatory response is often confined to the site, causing only local signs and symptoms. However, systemic responses can also occur. Fever is the most common sign of a systemic response to injury, and it is most likely caused by endogenous pyrogens (internal substances that cause fever) released from neutrophils and macrophages (specialized forms of leukocytes). These substances reset the hypothalamic thermostat, which controls body temperature, and produce fever. Leukocytosis, an increase in the synthesis and release of neutrophils from bone marrow, may occur to provide the body with greater ability to fight infection. During this process, general, nonspecific symptoms develop, including malaise, loss of appetite, aching, and weakness.

Types of Inflammation

Inflammation is categorized primarily by its duration and the type of exudate produced. It may be acute, subacute, or chronic. Acute inflammation is characterized by the local vascular and exudative changes described earlier and usually lasts less than 2 weeks. An acute inflammatory response is immediate and serves a protective function. After the injurious agent is removed, the inflammation subsides and healing takes place with the return of normal or near-normal structure and function.

Chronic inflammation develops if the injurious agent persists and the acute response is perpetuated. Symptoms are present for many months or years. Chronic inflammation may also begin insidiously and never have an acute phase. The chronic response does not serve a beneficial and protective function; on the contrary, it is debilitating and can produce long-lasting effects. As the inflammation becomes chronic, changes occur at the site of injury and the nature of the exudate becomes proliferative. A cycle of cellular infiltration, necrosis, and fibrosis begins, with repair and breakdown occurring simultaneously. Considerable scarring may occur, resulting in permanent tissue damage.

Subacute inflammation falls between acute and chronic inflammation. It includes elements of the active exudative phase of the acute response as well as elements of repair, as in the chronic phase. The term "subacute inflammation" is not widely used.

Cellular Healing

The reparative process begins at approximately the same time as the injury and is interwoven with inflammation. Healing proceeds after the inflammatory debris has been removed. Healing may occur by regeneration, in which gradual repair of the defect occurs by proliferation of cells of the same type as those destroyed, or by replacement, in which cells of another type, usually connective tissue, fill in the tissue defect and result in scar formation.

Regeneration

The ability of cells to regenerate depends on whether they are labile, permanent, or stable. Labile cells multiply constantly to replace cells worn out by normal physiologic processes; these include epithelial cells of the skin and those lining the gastrointestinal tract. Permanent cells include neurons—the nerve cell bodies, not their axons. Destruction of neurons is permanent, but axons may regenerate. If normal activity is to return, tissue regeneration must occur in a functional pattern, especially in the growth of several axons. Stable cells have a latent ability to regenerate. Under normal physiologic processes, they are not shed and do not need replacement, but if they are damaged or destroyed, they are able to regenerate. These include functional cells of the kidney, liver, and pancreas.

Replacement

Depending on the extent of damage, tissue healing may occur by primary intention or by secondary intention. In **primary intention healing**, the wound is clean and dry and the edges are approximated, as in a surgical wound. Little scar formation occurs, and the wound healing usually occurs in a week. In **secondary intention healing**, the wound or defect is larger and gaping and has necrotic or dead material. The wound fills with granulation tissue from the bottom upward. The process of repair takes longer and results in more scar formation, with loss of specialized function. For example, people who have recovered from myocardial infarction have abnormal electrocardiographic tracings because the electrical signal cannot be conducted through the connective tissue that has replaced the infarcted area.

The condition of the host, the environment, and the nature and severity of the injury affect the processes of inflammation and repair. Any of the injuries previously discussed can lead to cell death. Essentially, the cell membrane becomes impaired, resulting in a nonrestricted flow of ions. Sodium and calcium enter the cell, followed by water, which leads to edema, and energy transformation ceases. Nerve impulses are no longer transmitted; muscles no longer contract. As the cell ruptures, lysosomal enzymes that destroy tissues escape, and cell death and necrosis occur.

Nursing Implications

In the assessment of people who seek health care, both objective signs and subjective symptoms are the primary indicators of existing physiologic processes. The following questions are addressed:

- Are the heart rate, respiratory rate, and temperature normal?
- What emotional distress may be contributing to the patient's health problems?
- Are there other indicators of steady-state deviation?
- What are the patient's blood pressure, height, and weight?
- Are there any problems in movement or sensation?
- Are there any problems with affect, behavior, speech, cognitive ability, orientation, or memory?
- Are there obvious impairments, lesions, or deformities?

Further signs of change are indicated in diagnostic studies such as computed tomography (CT), magnetic resonance imaging (MRI), and positron emission tomography (PET). Objective evidence can also be obtained from laboratory data, such as electrolytes, blood urea nitrogen, blood glucose, and urinalysis results.

In making a nursing diagnosis, the nurse must relate the symptoms or problems reported by the patient to the existing physical signs. Management of specific biologic disorders is discussed in subsequent chapters; however, nurses can assist any patient to respond to stress-inducing biologic or psychological disorders with stress-management interventions.

Stress Management: Nursing Interventions

Stress or the potential for stress is ubiquitous; that is, it is both everywhere and anywhere. Anxiety, frustration, anger, and feelings of inadequacy, helplessness, or powerlessness are emotions often associated with stress. In the presence of these emotions, the customary activities of daily living may be disrupted; for example, a sleep disturbance may occur, eating and activity patterns may be altered, and family processes or role performance may be disrupted.

Many nursing diagnoses are possible for patients suffering from stress. One nursing diagnosis related to stress is Anxiety, which is defined as a vague, uneasy feeling, the source of which may be nonspecific or not known to the person. Stress may also be manifested as ineffective coping patterns, impaired thought processes, or disrupted relationships. These human responses are reflected in the nursing diagnoses of Impaired adjustment, Ineffective coping, Defensive coping, and Ineffective denial, all of which indicate poor adaptive responses. Other possible nursing diagnoses include Social isolation, Risk for impaired parenting, Risk for spiritual distress, Readiness for enhanced family coping, Decisional conflict, Situational low self-esteem, and Risk for powerlessness, among others. Because human responses to stress are varied, as are the sources of stress, arriving at an accurate diagnosis allows interventions and goals to be more specific and leads to improved outcomes.

Stress management is directed toward reducing and controlling stress and improving coping. Nurses might use these methods not only with their patients but also in their own lives. The need to prevent illness, improve the quality of life, and decrease the cost of health care makes efforts to promote health essential, and stress control is a significant health promotion goal. Stress reduction methods and coping enhancements can derive from either internal or external sources. For example, healthy eating habits and relaxation techniques are internal resources that help reduce stress, and a broad social network is an external resource that helps reduce stress. Goods and services that can be purchased are also external resources for stress management. It is much easier for people with adequate financial resources to cope with constraints in the environment, because their sense of vulnerability to threat is decreased.

Promoting a Healthy Lifestyle

A health-promoting lifestyle provides internal resources that aid in coping, and it buffers or cushions the impact of stressors. Lifestyles or habits that contribute to the risk of illness can be identified through a health risk appraisal, an assessment method designed to promote health by examining a person's habits and recommending changes when a health risk is identified.

Health risk appraisals involve the use of health risk questionnaires that estimate the likelihood that people with a given set of characteristics will become ill. It is hoped that if people are provided with this information, they will alter their activities (eg, stop smoking, have periodic screening examinations) to improve their health. Questionnaires typically address the information presented in Chart 6-2.

The personal information is compared with average population risk data, and the risk factors are identified and weighted. From this analysis, the person's risks and major health hazards are identified. Further comparisons with population data can estimate how many years will be added to a person's lifespan if the suggested changes are made. However, research has not yet demonstrated that providing people with such information ensures that they will change their habits. The single most important factor for determining health status is social class, and within a social class the research suggests that the major factor influencing health is level of education (Bastable, 2003).

CHART 6-2

Information Addressed in Health Risk Questionnaires

Demographic data: age, gender, race, ethnic background
Personal and family history of diseases and health problems
Lifestyle choices
- Eating, sleeping, exercise, smoking, drinking, sexual activity, and driving habits
- Stressors at home and on the job
- Role relationships and associated stressors

Physical measurements
- Blood pressure
- Height, weight, body mass index (BMI)
- Laboratory analyses of blood and urine

Participation in high-risk behaviors

Enhancing Coping Strategies

Dochterman and Bulechek (2004, p. 264) identified "coping enhancement" as a nursing intervention and defined it as "assisting a patient to adapt to perceived stressors, changes, or threats that interfere with meeting life demands and roles" (Chart 6-3). The nurse can build on the patient's existing coping strategies, as identified in the health appraisal, or teach new strategies for coping if necessary.

The five predominant ways of coping with illness identified in a review of 57 nursing research studies were as follows (Jalowiec, 1993):

- Trying to be optimistic about the outcome
- Using social support
- Using spiritual resources
- Trying to maintain control either over the situation or over feelings
- Trying to accept the situation

Other ways of coping included seeking information, reprioritizing needs and roles, lowering expectations, making compromises, comparing oneself to others, planning activities to conserve energy, taking things one step at a time, listening to one's body, and using self-talk for encouragement.

Teaching Relaxation Techniques

Relaxation techniques are a major method used to relieve stress. Commonly used techniques include progressive muscle relaxation, the Benson Relaxation Response, and relaxation with guided imagery. The goal of relaxation training is to produce a response that counters the stress response. When this goal is achieved, the action of the hypothalamus adjusts and decreases the activity of the sympathetic and parasympathetic nervous systems. The sequence of physiologic effects and their signs and symptoms are interrupted, and psychological stress is reduced. This is a learned response and requires practice to achieve.

CHART 6-3

Coping Enhancement: Nursing Interventions

DEFINITION

Assisting a patient to adapt to perceived stressors, changes, or threats that interfere with meeting life demands and roles

ACTIVITIES

Appraise a patient's adjustment to changes in body image as indicated.
Appraise the impact of the patient's life situation on roles and relationships.
Encourage the patient to identify a realistic description of change in role.
Appraise the patient's understanding of the disease process.
Appraise and discuss alternative responses to the situation.
Use a calm, reassuring approach.
Provide an atmosphere of acceptance.
Assist the patient in developing an objective appraisal of the event.
Help the patient to identify the information that he or she is most interested in obtaining.
Provide factual information concerning diagnosis, treatment, and prognosis.
Provide the patient with realistic choices about certain aspects of care.
Encourage an attitude of realistic hope as a way of dealing with feelings of helplessness.
Evaluate the patient's decision-making ability.
Seek to understand the patient's perspective of a stressful situation.
Discourage decision making when the patient is under severe stress.
Encourage gradual mastery of the situation.
Encourage patience in developing relationships.
Encourage relationships with persons who have common interests and goals.
Encourage social and community activities.
Encourage the acceptance of limitations in others.
Acknowledge the patient's spiritual/cultural background.
Encourage the use of spiritual resources if desired.
Explore the patient's previous achievements.
Explore the patient's reasons for self-criticism.
Confront the patient's ambivalent (angry or depressed) feelings.
Foster constructive outlets for anger and hostility.
Arrange situations that encourage the patient's autonomy.
Assist the patient in identifying positive responses from others.
Encourage the identification of specific life values.
Explore with the patient previous methods of dealing with life problems.
Introduce the patient to persons (or groups) who have successfully undergone the same experience.
Support the use of appropriate defense mechanisms.
Encourage verbalization of feelings, perceptions, and fears.
Discuss the consequences of not dealing with guilt and shame.
Encourage the patient to identify his or her own strengths and abilities.
Assist the patient in identifying appropriate short- and long-term goals.
Assist the patient in breaking down complex goals into small, manageable steps.
Assist the patient in examining available resources to meet the goals.
Reduce stimuli in the environment that could be misinterpreted as threatening.
Appraise the patient's needs and desires for social support.
Assist the patient to identify available support systems.
Determine the risk of the patient's inflicting self-harm.
Encourage family involvement as appropriate.
Encourage the family to verbalize their feelings about the ill family member.
Provide appropriate social skills training.
Assist the patient to identify positive strategies to deal with limitations and manage needed lifestyle or role changes.
Assist the patient to solve problems in a constructive manner.
Instruct the patient in the use of relaxation techniques as needed.
Assist the patient to grieve and to work through the losses of chronic illness and/or disability if appropriate.
Assist the patient to clarify misconceptions.
Encourage the patient to evaluate his or her own behavior.

The different relaxation techniques share four similar elements: (1) a quiet environment, (2) a comfortable position, (3) a passive attitude, and (4) a mental device (something on which to focus one's attention, such as a word, phrase, or sound).

Progressive Muscle Relaxation

Progressive muscle relaxation involves tensing and releasing the muscles of the body in sequence and sensing the difference in feeling. It is best if the person lies on a soft cushion, in a quiet room, breathing easily. Someone usually reads the instructions in a low tone in a slow and relaxed manner, or a recording of the instructions may be played. The person tenses the muscles in the entire body (one muscle group at a time), holds, senses the tension, and then relaxes. As each muscle group is tensed, the person keeps the rest of the body relaxed. Each time the focus is on feeling the tension and relaxation. When the exercise is completed, the entire body should be relaxed (Benson, 1993; Benson & Stark, 1996).

Benson's Relaxation Response

Benson (1993) describes the following steps of the Benson Relaxation Response:

1. Pick a brief phrase or word that reflects your basic belief system.
2. Choose a comfortable position.
3. Close your eyes.
4. Relax your muscles.
5. Become aware of your breathing, and start using your selected focus word.
6. Maintain a passive demeanor.
7. Continue for a set period of time.
8. Practice the technique twice daily.

This response combines meditation with relaxation. Along with the repeated word or phrase, a passive demeanor is essential. If other thoughts or distractions (noises, pain) occur, Benson recommends not fighting the distraction but simply continuing to repeat the focus phrase. Time of day is not important, but the exercise works best on an empty stomach.

Relaxation With Guided Imagery

Simple **guided imagery** is the mindful use of a word, phrase, or visual image for the purpose of distracting oneself from distressing situations or consciously taking time to relax or reenergize. A nurse can help a person select a pleasant scene or experience, such as watching the ocean or dabbling the feet in a cool stream. This image serves as the mental device in this technique. As the person sits comfortably and quietly, the nurse guides the person to review the scene, trying to feel and relive the imagery with all of the senses. A recording may be made of the description of the image, or commercial recordings for guided imagery and relaxation can be used. Other relaxation techniques include meditation, breathing techniques, massage, Reiki, music therapy, biofeedback, and the use of humor.

Educating About Stress Management

Two commonly prescribed nursing educational interventions—providing sensory information and providing procedural information (eg, preoperative teaching)—have the goal of reducing stress and improving the patient's coping ability. This preparatory education includes giving structured content, such as a lesson in childbirth preparation to expectant parents, a review of cardiovascular anatomy to a cardiac patient, or a description of sensations a patient will experience during cardiac catheterization. These techniques may alter the person–environment relationship such that something that might have been viewed as harmful or a threat will now be perceived more positively. Giving patients information also reduces the emotional response so that they can concentrate and solve problems more effectively (Loo, Espinosa, Tyler, et al., 2003; Millio & Sullivan, 2000).

Enhancing Social Support

The nature of social support and its influence on coping have been studied extensively. Social support has been demonstrated to be an effective moderator of life stress. Social support has been found to provide people with several different types of emotional information (Ben-Ari, 2004; Heitzman & Kaplan, 1998). The first type of information leads people to believe that they are cared for and loved. This emotional support appears most often in a relationship between two people in which mutual trust and attachment are expressed by helping one another meet their emotional needs. The second type of information leads people to believe that they are esteemed and valued. This is most effective when there is recognition demonstrating a person's favorable position in the group. Known as esteem support, this elevates the person's sense of self-worth. The third type of information leads people to feel that they belong to a network of communication and mutual obligation. Members of this network share information and make goods and services available to the members as needed.

Social support also facilitates a person's coping behaviors; however, this depends on the nature of the social support. People can have extensive relationships and interact frequently, but the necessary support comes only when there is a deep level of involvement and concern, not when people merely touch the surface of each other's lives. The critical qualities within a social network are the exchange of intimate communications and the presence of solidarity and trust.

Emotional support from family and significant others provides love and a sense of sharing the burden. The emotions that accompany stress are unpleasant and often increase in a spiraling fashion if relief is not provided. Being able to talk with someone and express feelings openly may help a person gain mastery of the situation. Nurses can provide this support; however, it is important to identify the person's social support system and encourage its use. People who are "loners," who are isolated, or who withdraw in times of stress have a high risk of coping failure.

Because anxiety can also distort a person's ability to process information, it helps to seek information and advice from others who can assist with analyzing the threat and developing a strategy to manage it. Again, this use of others helps people maintain mastery of a situation and self-esteem.

Thus, social networks assist with management of stress by providing people with:

- A positive social identity
- Emotional support
- Material aid and tangible services
- Access to information
- Access to new social contacts and new social roles

Recommending Support and Therapy Groups

Support groups exist especially for people in similar stressful situations. Groups have been formed by parents of children with leukemia; people with ostomies; women who have had mastectomies; and people with other kinds of cancer or other serious diseases, chronic illnesses, and disabilities. There are groups for single parents, substance abusers and their family members, and victims of child abuse. Professional, civic, and religious support groups are active in many communities. There are also encounter groups, assertiveness training programs, and consciousness-raising groups to help people modify their usual behaviors in their transactions with their environment. Being a member of a group with similar problems or goals has a releasing effect on a person that promotes freedom of expression and exchange of ideas.

As previously noted, a person's psychological and biologic health, internal and external sources of stress management, and relationships with the environment are predictors of health outcomes. These factors are directly related to the person's health patterns. The nurse has a significant role and responsibility in identifying the health patterns of the patient receiving care. If those patterns are not achieving physiologic, psychological, and social balance, the nurse is obligated, with the assistance and agreement of the patient, to seek ways to promote balance.

Although this chapter has presented some physiologic mechanisms and perspectives on health and disease, the way that one copes with stress, the way one relates to others, and the values and goals held are also interwoven into those physiologic patterns. To evaluate a patient's health patterns and to intervene if a problem exists requires a total assessment of the person. Specific problems and their nursing management are addressed in greater depth in other chapters.

Critical Thinking Exercises

1 A female patient was carjacked, raped, and left on the shoulder of the road, where she was hit by a car. She is hospitalized with injuries related to her sexual assault and hit-and-run vehicle crash. Describe the physiologic and psychological trauma she has experienced. Prioritize her needs and identify appropriate nursing interventions to alleviate the major stressors.

2 A 50-year-old woman had a myocardial infarction after being diagnosed as HIV-positive. For the past 6 months, she has been working 7 days a week to buy her immunosuppressive medications. The nurse evaluates the woman's coping style. What indications would the nurse note in her interactions and follow-up care that demonstrate that the woman uses problem-focused coping or emotion-focused coping?

3 A patient experiences a severe hemorrhage of the leg after being involved in a boating crash. Describe the manner in which homeostasis has been disrupted and the compensatory mechanisms that are evident. How does the patient's medical treatment support the compensatory mechanisms? How do you determine the nursing interventions that are appropriate for promoting the healing process?

4 ebp A 90-year-old man recently moved to an assisted living community, where he maintains himself on an independent and supervised unit. A nurse practitioner assesses this patient's health promotion needs. The family's health history reveals that his mother had type 2 diabetes and thyroid disease and that his father had coronary artery disease. This client has ample resources for making necessary lifestyle changes. What suggestions would the nurse practitioner initiate to promote a healthy lifestyle? What is the evidence base that supports the relationship between lifestyle and health status? Describe the strength of the evidence regarding the effectiveness of lifestyle changes in promoting health. Identify the criteria used to evaluate the strength of the evidence.

REFERENCES AND SELECTED READINGS

BOOKS

Bastable, S. B. (Ed.). (2003). *Nurse as educator: Principles of teaching and learning.* Boston: Jones & Bartlett.

Benson, H. (1993). The relaxation response. In D. Goleman & J. Gurin (Eds.), *Mind-body medicine: How to use your mind for better health.* Yonkers, NY: Consumer Reports Books.

Benson, H., & Proctor, W. (1984). *Beyond the relaxation response.* New York: Berkley Books.

Benson, H., & Stark, M. (1996). *Timeless healing.* New York: Scribner.

Chiorazzi, N. (2003). *Immune mechanisms and disease.* New York: New York Academy of Science.

Copel, L. C. (2000). *Nurse's clinical guide: Psychiatric and mental health care* (2nd ed.). Springhouse, PA: Springhouse.

Dochterman, J. C., & Bulechek, G. M. (Eds.). (2004). *Nursing interventions classification (NIC)* (4th ed.). St. Louis: Mosby.

Dubos, R. (1965). *Man adapting.* New Haven, CT: Yale University Press.

Evans, P., Hucklebridge, F., & Clow, A. (2000). *Mind, immunity, and health: The science of psychoimmunology.* New York: Free Association Books.

Fauci, A. (Ed.). (2001). *Harrison's principles of internal medicine* (15th ed.). New York: McGraw-Hill.

Furman, M. E., & Gallo, F. (2000). *The neurophysics of human behavior: Explorations at the interface of the brain, mind, behavior, and information.* Boca Raton, FL: CRC Press.

Guyton, A. C., & Hall, J. E. (2001). *Textbook of medical physiology* (10th ed.). Philadelphia: W. B. Saunders.

Guyton, A. C., Hall, J. E., & Schmitt, W. (1997). *Human physiology and mechanisms of disease* (6th ed.). Philadelphia: W. B. Saunders.

Jalowiec, A. (1993). Coping with illness: Synthesis and critique of the nursing literature from 1980–1990. In J. D. Barnfather & B. L. Lyon (Eds.), *Stress and coping: State of the science and implications for nursing theory, research, and practice.* Indianapolis: Sigma Theta Tau International.

Lazarus, R. S. (1991a). *Emotion and adaptation.* New York: Oxford University Press.

Lazarus, R. S. (1993). Why we should think of stress as a subset of emotion. In L. Goldberger & S. Breznitz (Eds.), *Handbook of stress: Theoretical and clinical aspects* (2nd ed.). New York: The Free Press.

Lazarus, R. S., & Folkman, S. (1984). *Stress, appraisal, and coping.* New York: Springer Publishing Co.

McPhee, S. J., Lingrappa, V. R., & Ganong, W. F. (2003). *Pathophysiology of disease: An introduction to clinical medicine* (4th ed.). New York: McGraw-Hill.

Mickler, M. (1997). *Community organizing and community building for health.* New Brunswick, NJ: Rutgers University Press.

Miller, L. H., & Smith, A. D. (1993). *The stress solution.* New York: Pocket Books.

North American Nursing Diagnosis Association. (2002). *NANDA nursing diagnoses: Definitions and classifications 2003–2004.* Philadelphia: Author.

Pearsall, P. (2003). *The Beethoven factor: The new positive psychology of hardiness, happiness, healing, and hope.* Charlottesville, VA: Hampton Roads Publishing Company.

Porth, C. M. (2005). *Pathophysiology. Concepts of altered health status.* Philadelphia: Lippincott Williams & Wilkins.

Rice, V. (1999). *Handbook of stress, coping, and health: Implications for nursing research, theory, and practice.* Thousand Oaks, CA: Sage.

Selye, H. (1976). *The stress of life.* (Rev. ed.). New York: McGraw-Hill.

Slikker, W., Andrews, R., & Trembly, B. (2003). *Neuroprotective agents.* New York: New York Academy of Science.

Sternberg, E. M., Haour, F. G., & Smith, C. C. (Eds.). (2003). *Neuroendocrine and neural regulation of autoimmune and inflammatory disease: Molecular, systems, and clinical insights.* New York: New York Academy of Science.

Zautra, A. J. (2003). *Emotions, stress, and health.* Oxford & New York: Oxford University Press.

JOURNALS

**Asterisks indicate nursing research articles.*

*al-Absi, M., Hatsukami, D., Davis, G. L., et al. (2004). Prospective examination of effects of smoking abstinence on cortisol and withdrawal symptoms of early smoking relapse. *Drug and Alcohol Dependence, 73*(3), 267–278.

*Ben-Ari, A. (2004). Sources of social support and attachment styles among Israeli-Arab students. *International Social Work, 47*(2), 187–201.

*Brissette, I., Leventhal, H., & Leventhal, E. A. (2003). Observer ratings of health and sickness: Can other people tell us anything about our health that we don't already know? *Health Psychology, 22*(5), 471–478.

Brooks, M. V. (2003). Health-related hardiness and chronic illness: A synthesis of current research. *Nursing Forum, 38*(3), 11–19.

Carter-Snell, C., & Hegadoren, K. (2003). Stress disorders and gender: Implications for theory and research. *Canadian Journal of Nursing Research, 35*(2), 35–55.

Clark, A. M. (2003). "It's like an explosion in your life"—lay perspectives on stress and myocardial infarction. *Journal of Clinical Nursing, 12*(4), 544–553.

*Constantino, R. E., Sekula, L. K., Rabin, B., et al. (2000). Negative life experiences, depression, and immune function in abused and nonabused women. *Biological Research in Nursing, 1*(3), 190–198.

Cooper, M. A., Pommering, T. L., & Koranyi, K. (2003). Primary immunodeficiencies. *American Family Physician, 68*(10), 2001–2011.

Cutler, R. B., Fishbain, D. A., Steele-Rosomoff, R., et al. (2003). Relationships between functional capacity measures and baseline psychological measures in chronic pain patients. *Journal of Occupational Rehabilitation, 13*(4), 249–258.

Donnelly, G. (2004). From surviving to thriving: The Beethoven factor. *Holistic Nursing Practice, 18*(2), 51–52.

Dosani, S. (2003). Review: Stress is a problem for mental health nurses but research on interventions is insufficient. *Evidence-Based Mental Health, 6*(4), 126.

Edwards, D., & Burnard, P. (2003). A systematic review of stress and stress management interventions for mental health nurses. *Journal of Advanced Nursing, 42*(2), 169–200.

*Elder, R., Wollin, J., Hartel, C., et al. (2003). Hassles and uplifts associated with caring for people with cognitive impairment in community settings. *International Journal of Mental Health Nursing, 12*(4), 271–278.

*Erlandsson, L., & Eklund, M. (2003). Women's experiences of hassles and uplifts in their everyday patterns of occupations. *Occupational Therapy International, 10*(2), 95–114.

*Gross, R., Brammli-Greenberg, S., & Bentur, N. (2003). Women caring for disabled parents and other relatives: Implications for social workers in the health services. *Social Work in Health Care, 37*(4), 19–37.

Hausmann, O. N. (2003). Post-traumatic inflammation following spinal cord injury. *Spinal Cord, 41*(7), 369–378.

Heitzman, C. A., & Kaplan, R. M. (1998). Assessment of methods for measuring social support. *Health Psychology, 7,* 75–109.

Holmes, T. H., & Rahe, R. H. (1967). The social readjustment rating scale. *Journal of Psychosomatic Research, 11,* 213–218.

*Kennedy, J. W. (2000). Women's inner balance: A comparison of stressors, personality traits, and health problems by age groups. *Journal of Advanced Nursing, 31*(3), 639–650.

*Kincy, J., Pratt, D., Slater, R., et al. (2003). A survey of patterns and sources of stress among medical and nursing staff in an intensive care unit setting. *Care of the Critically Ill, 19*(3), 83–87.

Lazarus, R. S. (1991b). Cognition and motivation in emotion. *American Psychologist, 46*(4), 352–367.

Lazarus, R. S. (1991c). Progress on a cognitive-motivational-relational theory of emotion. *American Psychologist, 46*(8), 819–834.

Loo, K. K., Espinosa, M., Tyler, R., et al. (2003). Using knowledge to cope with stress in the NICU: How parents integrate learning to read the physiologic and behavioral cues of the infant. *Neonatal Network: Journal of Neonatal Nursing, 22*(1), 31–37.

*Millio, M. E., & Sullivan, K. (2000). Patients with operable esophageal cancer: Their experience of information giving in a regional thoracic unit. *Journal of Clinical Nursing, 9*(2), 236–246.

Mortzer, S. A., & Hertig, V. (2004). Stress, stress response, and health. *Nursing Clinics of North America, 39*(3), 1–17.

Norman, D. (2003). The effects of stress on wound healing and leg ulceration. *British Journal of Nursing, 12*(21), 1256–1263.

*Olofsson, B., Bengtsson, C., & Brink, E. (2003). Absence of response: A study of nurses' experience of stress in the workplace. *Journal of Nursing Management, 11*(5), 351–358.

Pike, J. L., Smith, T. L., Hauger, R. L., et al. (1997). Chronic life stress alters sympathetic, neuroendocrine, and immune responsivity to an acute psychological stressor in humans. *Psychosomatic Medicine, 59*(4), 447–457.

Ptacek, J. T., & Pierce, G. R. (2003). Issues in the study of stress and coping in rehabilitation settings. *Rehabilitation Psychology, 48*(2), 113–124.

Rankin, J. A. (2004). Biological mediators of acute inflammation. *AACN Clinical Issues: Advanced Practice in Acute and Critical Care, 15*(1), 3–17.

Rider, S. H. (2004). Psychological distress: Concept analysis. *Journal of Advanced Nursing, 45*(5), 536–545.

Robinson, F. P., Matthews, H. L., & Witek-Janusek, L. (2000). Stress reduction and HIV disease: A review of intervention studies using a psychoimmunology framework. *Journal of the Association of Nurses in AIDS Care, 11*(2), 87–96.

Sansovich, D. (2003). Harm reduction, substance use and the immune system. *HIV Clinician 15*(2), 13–15.

Shapley, M., Jordan, K., & Croft, P. R. (2003). Increased vaginal bleeding and psychological distress: A longitudinal study of their relationship in the community. *International Journal of Obstetrics and Gynecology, 110*(6), 548–554.

*Tausig, M. (1982). Measuring life events. *Journal of Health and Social Behavior, 23*(1), 52–64.

*Vines, S. W., Gupta, S., Whiteside, T., et al. (2003). The relationship between chronic pain, immune function, depression, and health behaviors. *Biological Research for Nursing, 5*(1), 18–29.

Whitty, M. T. (2003). Coping and defending: Age differences in maturity of defense mechanisms and coping strategies. *Aging and Mental Health, 7*(2), 123–132.

CHAPTER 7

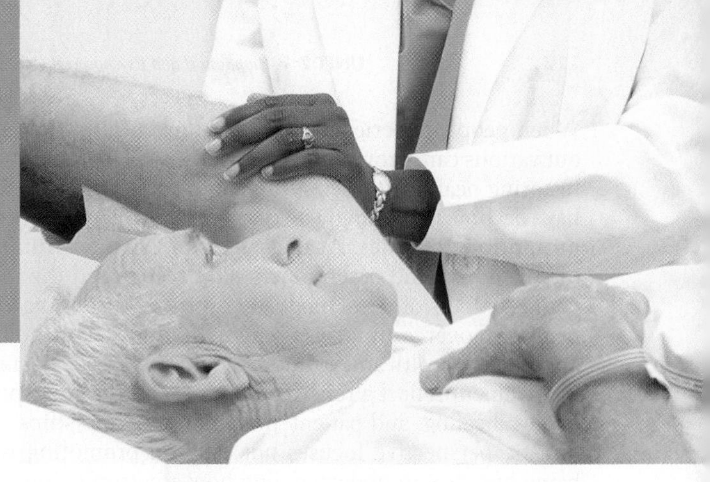

Individual and Family Considerations Related to Illness

Learning Objectives

On completion of this chapter, the learner will be able to:

1. Describe the holistic approach to sustaining health and well-being.
2. Discuss the concepts of emotional well-being and emotional distress.
3. Identify variables that influence the ability to cope with stress and that are antecedents to emotional disorders.
4. Explain the concepts of anxiety, posttraumatic stress disorder, depression, loss, and grief.
5. Assess the impact of illness on the patient's family and on family functioning.
6. Determine the role of the nurse in identifying substance abuse problems and in helping families to cope.
7. Explore the concept of spirituality and address the spiritual needs of patients.
8. Identify nursing actions that promote effective coping for both patients and families.

When people experience threats to their health, they seek out various care providers for the purpose of maintaining or restoring health. In recent years, both patients and families have become increasingly involved in health care and health promotion activities. At the same time, greater numbers of consumers and practitioners have recognized the interconnectedness of mind, body, and spirit in sustaining well-being and overcoming or coping with illness. This holistic approach to health and wellness and the increased consumer involvement reflect a renewed emphasis on the concepts of choice, healing, and patient–practitioner partnerships. The holistic perspective focuses not only on promoting well-being but also on understanding how a person's emotional state contributes to health and illness. By using this knowledge, people are better able to prevent the recurrence or exacerbation of health problems and to develop strategies to improve their future health status.

CHART 7-1

Common Complementary and Alternative Therapies

- Alternative medical systems including acupuncture, Ayurveda, homeopathic medicine, and naturopathic medicine
- Mind-body interventions including meditation, certain uses of hypnosis, dance, music, art therapy, and prayer
- Biologically based therapies including herbal, special dietary, orthomolecular, and individual biological therapies
- Manipulative and body-based methods including chiropractic and osteopathy
- Energy therapies including Qi gong, Reiki, and therapeutic touch

Reprinted with permission from Dossey, B. M., Guzzetta, C., & Keegan, L. (2002). *Holistic nursing: A handbook for practice.* Gaithersburg, MD: Aspen Publications.

Holistic Approach to Health and Health Care

Since the 1980s, holistic therapies have more frequently accompanied traditional health care. It is estimated that approximately 35% to 45% of consumers in the United States follow **holistic health** practices. More than 50% of people supplement traditional health care treatments with **complementary and alternative therapies.** In an ambulatory care setting in which human immunodeficiency virus (HIV) and acquired immunodeficiency syndrome (AIDS) are treated, 51% of patients reported discussing their complementary therapies with their health care providers (Chang, Van Servellen, & Lombardi, 2003). In all settings, it is imperative that during clinical assessments the use of these adjunct therapies be assessed. Some of the most commonly used complementary therapies are listed in Chart 7-1.

For some people, the holistic approach is viewed as a way to capitalize on personal strengths and recultivate the values and beliefs about health that were common before the age of technological innovations and the sophistication of biomedical science. A lack of focus on individual patients, families, and their environments by some health care providers has created feelings of disillusionment and depersonalization in many people. The cost of illness, especially care for chronic disease, continues to escalate and accounts for an increasing percentage of health care dollars. At the same time, patient satisfaction with health care has decreased.

Active participation by patients and families in health promotion supports the self-care model historically embraced by the nursing profession. This model is congruent with the philosophy that seeks to balance and integrate the use of crisis medicine and advanced technology with the

Glossary

anxiety: an emotional state characterized by feelings of apprehension, discomfort, restlessness, or worry

bereavement: feelings, thoughts, and responses that occur after a loss

complementary therapies: used as an adjunct to traditional health modalities; they typically influence the effects of stress, anxiety, depression, and other physical and emotional states

depression: state in which a person feels sad, distressed, and hopeless, with little to no energy for normal activities

faith: belief and trust in a God or higher power

family: a group whose members are related by reciprocal caring, mutual responsibilities, and loyalties

grief: a universal response to any loss

holistic health: promotion of the total health of mind, body, and spirit

homeopathic medicine: a system of medicine that promotes healing of the whole person by stimulating the natural healing processes within the person

mental disorder: a state in which a person has deficits in functioning, has a distorted sense of self or the world, is unable to sustain relationships, or cannot handle stress or conflict effectively

mental health: a state in which a person can meet basic needs, assume responsibilities, sustain relationships, resolve conflicts, and grow throughout life

posttraumatic stress disorder (PTSD): the development of severe anxiety-type symptoms after the experience of a traumatic life event

substance abuse: a maladaptive pattern of drug use that causes physical and emotional harm with the potential for disruption of daily life

influence of the mind and spirit on healing. A holistic approach to health reconnects the traditionally separate approaches to mind and body. Factors such as the physical environment, economic conditions, sociocultural issues, emotional state, interpersonal relationships, and support systems can work together or alone to influence health. The connections among physical health, emotional health, and spiritual well-being must be understood and considered when providing health care. It is the nurse's conceptual integration of the physiologic health condition with the emotional and social context, along with the tasks and developments of the patient's life stage, that allows for the development of a holistic plan of nursing care.

The Brain and Physical and Emotional Health

Research on brain structure and function, neurochemical messenger systems (neurotransmitters), and brain–body connections suggests fundamental, delicate, two-way relationships between the brain's environment and mood, behavior, and resistance to disease. One focus of brain research has been to identify and integrate traditional medical and psychiatric knowledge with new psychobiologic and psychoneuroimmunologic data. Researchers in the field of psychobiology study the biologic basis of mental disturbances and have identified some relationships between mental disorders and changes in the structure and function of the brain. Researchers in the field of psychoneuroimmunology study the connections between the emotions, the central nervous system, the neuroendocrine system, and the immune system and have established compelling evidence that psychosocial variables can affect the functioning of the immune system.

As this neuroscientific research continues, data about neurotransmitters and the functioning of the brain will augment existing understanding of emotions, intelligence, memory, and many aspects of general body functioning. In the future, an accepted definition of mental illness may well include biologic information. By enhancing the biologic knowledge base about the brain and nervous system, scientists have established the foundation for breakthroughs in the treatment of both symptoms and illnesses.

These findings suggest that the health care community should place as much emphasis on emotional health as it places on physiologic health and should recognize how biologic, emotional, and societal problems combine to affect individual patients, families, and communities. Some problems that nurses and other health care providers must address include **substance abuse**, homelessness, family violence, eating disorders, trauma, and chronic **mental health** conditions such as anxiety and depression. To focus attention on these and other mental health problems, the U.S. Department of Health and Human Services initiated a mental health agenda for the nation in *Healthy People 2010* (U.S. Public Health Service, 2000). The objectives identified are summarized in Chart 7-2. Nurses in all settings encounter patients with mental health problems and can play an integral role in helping to achieve the national goals by recognizing and relieving emotional distress and promoting emotional health.

CHART 7-2

Major Mental Health Objectives for Healthy People in the Year 2010

- Reduce the proportion of children and adolescents with disabilities who are reported to be sad, unhappy, or depressed.
- Reduce the proportion of adults with disabilities who report feelings such as sadness, unhappiness, or depression that prevent them from being active.
- Increase the proportion of adults with disabilities reporting sufficient emotional support.
- Increase the proportion of adults with disabilities reporting satisfaction with life.
- Reduce the suicide rate.
- Reduce the rate of suicide attempts by adolescents.
- Reduce the proportion of homeless adults who have serious mental illness.
- Increase the proportion of persons with serious mental illness who are employed.
- Reduce the relapse rates for persons with eating disorders including anorexia nervosa and bulimia nervosa.
- Increase the number of persons in primary care who receive mental health screening and assessment.
- Increase the proportion of children with mental health problems who receive treatment.
- Increase the proportion of juvenile justice facilities that screen admissions for mental health problems.
- Increase the proportion of adults with mental disorders who receive treatment.
- Increase the proportion of persons with co-occurring substance abuse and mental disorders who receive treatment for both disorders.
- Increase the number of states and the District of Columbia that track consumer satisfaction with the mental health services they receive.
- Increase the number of states, territories, and the District of Columbia with an operational mental health plan that addresses cultural competence.

U.S. Public Health Service. (2000). *Healthy people 2010: Understanding and improving health*. Washington, DC: U.S. Government Printing Office.

Emotional Health and Emotional Distress

Emotional health involves the ability to function as comfortably and productively as possible. Typically, people who are mentally healthy are satisfied with themselves and their life situations. In the usual course of living, emotionally healthy people focus on activities geared to meet their needs and attempt to accomplish personal goals while concurrently managing everyday challenges and problems. Often, people must work hard to balance their feelings, thoughts, and behaviors to alleviate emotional distress, and much energy is used to change, adapt, or manage the obstacles inherent in daily living. A mentally healthy person accepts reality and has a positive sense of self. Emotional health is also manifested by having moral and humanistic values and beliefs, having satisfying interpersonal relationships, doing productive work, and maintaining a realistic sense of hope (Chart 7-3).

When people have unmet emotional needs or distress, they experience an overall feeling of unhappiness. As tension escalates, security and survival are threatened. How different people respond to these troublesome situations reflects their level of coping and maturity. Emotionally healthy people endeavor to meet the demands of distressing situations while still coping with the typical issues that emerge in their lives. The ways in which people respond to uncomfortable stimuli reflect their exposure to various biologic, emotional, and sociocultural experiences.

When stress interferes with a person's ability to function comfortably and inhibits the effective management of personal needs, that person is at risk for emotional problems. The use of ineffective and unhealthy methods of coping is manifested by dysfunctional behaviors, thoughts, and feelings. These behaviors are aimed at relieving the overwhelming stress, even though they may cause further problems.

Coping ability is strongly influenced by biologic or genetic factors, physical and emotional growth and development, family and childhood experiences, and learning. Typically, people revert to the strategies observed early in life that were used by family members, caregivers, and others to resolve conflicts. If these strategies were not adaptive, the person exhibits a range of painful and nonproductive behaviors. Dysfunctional behavior in one person not only seriously affects that person's emotional health but can also put others at risk for injury or death. As these destructive behaviors are repeated, a cyclic pattern becomes evident: impaired thinking, negative feelings, and more dysfunctional actions that prevent the person from meeting the demands of daily living (Chart 7-4).

No universally accepted definition of what constitutes an emotional disorder exists, but many views and theories share the idea that a number of variables can interfere with emotional growth and development and impede successful adaptation to the environment. Most clinicians have adopted the statement from the American Psychiatric Association's *Diagnostic and Statistical Manual of Mental Disorders (DSM-IV-TR)*, which defines the term **mental disorder** as a group of behavioral or psychological symptoms or a pattern that manifests itself in significant distress, impaired functioning, or accentuated risk of enduring severe suffering or possible death (American Psychiatric Association, 2000). Risk factors for mental health problems are listed in Chart 7-5.

Patients seen in medical-surgical settings often struggle with psychosocial issues of anxiety, depression, loss, and grief. Abuse, addiction, chemical dependency, body image disturbances, and eating disorders are a few examples of health situations that require extensive physical and emotional care to restore optimal functioning. The dual challenge for the health care team is to understand how the patient's emotions influence current physiologic conditions and to

CHART 7-3

Characteristics Associated With Mental Health

- Positive sense of self
- Satisfying interpersonal relationships
- Wide range of appropriate emotions
- Love and care for self and others
- Realistic and responsible behavior
- Effective coping skills
- Ability to negotiate and resolve conflict
- Cooperative and interdependent in working with others
- Engagement in rewarding, productive work
- Adaptable to the daily challenges of life
- Finds meaning and purpose in life
- Has hopes and dreams
- Knowledge of personal strengths and areas needing improvement
- Sense of humor
- Respect for the rights and differences of others

CHART 7-4

Characteristics Associated With Mental Disorders

- Severe anxiety
- Severe depression
- Ineffective coping mechanisms
- Extreme feelings of helplessness or powerlessness
- Maladaptive ways of dealing with stress
- Uncomfortable with self and others
- Lack of pleasure from living
- Extreme negative thoughts, feelings, and behaviors
- Disorganized or disturbed thoughts
- Inability to accept reality
- Personality traits that contribute to dysfunctional behaviors
- Desire to hurt self or others
- History of traumatic experience
- Inability to satisfy basic needs
- Lack of a support system
- Physiologic problems resulting from severe, unrelenting stress

CHART 7-5

Risk Factors for Mental Health Problems

Nonmodifiable Risk Factors

- Age
- Gender
- Genetic background
- Family history

Modifiable Risk Factors

- Marital status
- Family environment
- Housing problems
- Poverty or economic difficulties
- Physical health
- Nutritional status
- Stress level
- Social environment and activities
- Exposure to trauma
- Alcohol and drug use
- Environmental toxins or other pollutants
- Availability, accessibility, and cost of health services

identify the best care for the patient experiencing underlying emotional and spiritual distress.

CHART 7-6

Adult Developmental Tasks

Developmental stage and associated tasks can have an impact on how individuals cope with illness.

Young Adult

- Establish independence
- Establish lifestyle
- Develop career
- Develop intimate relationships
- Marry and start a family

Middle Adult

- Establish financial security
- Prepare for retirement
- Launch children
- Refocus on marital/family relationship
- Support growing children and aging parents

Older Adult

- Adapt to retirement and alteration in role
- Adapt to declining physical stamina
- Review life's accomplishments
- Prepare for death

Family Health and Distress

The **family** plays a central role in the life of the patient and is a major part of the context of the patient's life. It is within families that people grow, are nurtured, acquire a sense of self, develop beliefs and values about life, and progress through life's developmental stages (Chart 7-6). Families are also the first source for socialization and teaching about health and illness. Families prepare people with strategies for balancing closeness with separateness and togetherness with individuality. A major role of families is to provide physical and emotional resources to maintain health and a system of support in times of crises, such as in periods of illness. Educating families has been shown to add to their resiliency, adaptation, and adjustment to life stressors (Friedman, Bowden, & Jones, 2003).

Health problems often affect the family's ability to function. Five family functions described by Wright and Leahey (2000) are viewed as essential to the growth of individuals and families. The first function, management, involves the use of power, decision making about resources, establishment of rules, provision of finances, and future planning—responsibilities assumed by the adults of the family. The second function, boundary setting, makes clear distinctions between the generations and the roles of adults and children within the family structure. The third function, communication, is important to individual and family growth; healthy families have a full range of clear, direct, and meaningful communication among their members. The fourth function consists of education and support, which are interrelated. Education involves modeling skills for living a physically, emotionally, and socially healthy life. Support is manifested by actions that tell family members they are cared about and loved; it promotes health and is seen as a critical factor in coping with crises and illness situations. The fifth function, socialization, involves families' transmission of culture and the acceptable behaviors needed to perform adequately in the home and in the world.

Nursing Implications

When a family member becomes ill, injured, or disabled, all members of the family are affected. Depending on the nature of the health problem, family members may need to modify their existing lifestyles or even restructure their lives.

There are many degrees of family functioning. Nurses assess family functioning to determine how the particular family will cope with the impact of the health condition. If the family is chaotic or disorganized, promoting coping skills becomes a priority in the plan of care. The family with preexisting problems may require additional assistance before participating fully in the current health situation. In performing a family assessment, the nurse must evaluate the present family structure and function. Areas of appraisal include demographic data, developmental information (keeping in mind that different family members can be in different developmental stages simultaneously), family structure, family functioning, and coping abilities. The role that the environment plays in family health is also assessed.

Interventions with family members are based on strengthening coping skills through direct care, communication skills, and education. Healthy family communication has a strong influence on the quality of family life and can help the family make appropriate choices, consider alternative strategies, or persevere through complex circumstances. Within a family system, for example, a particular patient may be undergoing extensive surgery for cancer while the partner has cardiac disease, an adolescent has type 1 diabetes mellitus, and a child has a fractured arm. In this situation, there are multiple health concerns along with competing developmental tasks and needs. Despite the obvious concerns of the family members, both individually and collectively, a crisis may or may not be present. The family may be coping effectively, or it may be in crisis or unable to handle the situation. Ideally, the health care team conducts a careful and comprehensive family assessment, develops interventions tailored to handle the stressors, implements the specified treatment protocols, and facilitates the construction of social support systems.

The use of existing family strengths, resources, and education is augmented by therapeutic family interventions. The primary goals of the nurse are to maintain and improve the patient's present level of health and to prevent physical and emotional deterioration. Next, the nurse intervenes in the cycle that the illness creates: patient illness, stress for other family members, new illness in other family members, and additional patient stress.

Helping the family members handle the myriad stressors that bombard them daily involves working with family members to develop coping skills. Burr and associates (Burr, Klein, Burr, et al., 1984) identified seven traits that enhance coping of family members under stress. Communication skills and spirituality were the most useful traits. Cognitive abilities, emotional strengths, relationship capabilities, willingness to use community resources, and individual strengths and talents were also associated with effective coping. As nurses work with families, they must not underestimate the impact that their therapeutic interactions, educational information, positive role modeling, provision of direct care, and corrective teaching have on promoting health.

Without the active support of the family members and the health care team, the potential for maladaptive coping increases. Often, denial and blaming of individuals occur. Sometimes, physiologic illness, emotional withdrawal, and physical distancing are the results of severe family conflict, violent behavior, or addiction to drugs and alcohol. Substance abuse may develop in family members who feel unable to cope or solve problems. Frequently, people engage in these dysfunctional behaviors when faced with difficult or problematic situations.

Anxiety

All people experience some degree of **anxiety** (a tense emotional state) as they face new, challenging, or threatening life situations. In clinical settings, fear of the unknown, unexpected news about one's health, and any impairment of bodily functions engenders anxiety. Although a mild level of anxiety can mobilize a person to take a position, act on the task that needs to be done, or learn to alter lifestyle habits, more severe anxiety can be paralyzing. Anxiety that escalates to a near panic state can be incapacitating. When patients receive unwelcome news about results of diagnostic studies, they are certain to experience anxiety. Different patients manifest physiologic, emotional, and behavioral signs and symptoms of anxiety in different ways.

Nursing Implications

Early clinical observations of guilt or anxiety are an essential component of nursing care (Chart 7-7). A high level of anxiety in a patient will probably exacerbate physiologic distress. For example, a postoperative patient who is in pain may discover that anxiety intensifies the sensation of pain. A patient newly diagnosed with type 1 diabetes mellitus may be worried and fearful and therefore unable to focus on or complete essential self-care activities. Somatic symptoms may occur in any patient with moderate to severe anxiety.

The *DSM-IV-TR* (2000) lists general medical conditions that cause anxiety. They include endocrine diseases, such as hypothyroidism, hyperthyroidism, hypoglycemia, and hyperadrenocorticism; cardiovascular conditions, such as cardiac dysrhythmia, heart failure, and pulmonary emboli; respiratory disorders, such as pneumonia and chronic obstructive pulmonary disease; and neurologic disorders, such as multiple sclerosis, encephalitis, and neoplasms.

All nurses must be vigilant about patients who worry excessively and deteriorate in emotional, social, or occupational functioning. If participation in the therapeutic regimen (eg, administration of insulin) becomes a problem because of extreme anxiety, nursing interventions must be immediately initiated. Caring strategies emphasize ways for the patient to verbalize feelings and fears and to identify sources of anxiety. The need to teach and promote effective coping abilities and the use of relaxation techniques are the priorities of care. In some cases, antianxiety medication may be prescribed. Chart 7-8 provides a list of basic nursing principles that are useful for assisting patients to manage severe anxiety. Chapter 6 presents additional information about stress and the relaxation response.

Posttraumatic Stress Disorder

In medical-surgical settings, especially in emergency departments, burn units, and rehabilitation centers, nurses care for extremely anxious patients who have experienced overwhelming events that are considered to be outside the range of normal human experience. Many of these patients suffer from **posttraumatic stress disorder** (PTSD), a condition that generates waves of anxiety, anger, aggression, depression, and suspicion; threatens a person's sense of self; and interferes with daily functioning. Specific examples of events that place people at risk for PTSD are rape, family violence, torture, terrorist attacks, fire, earthquake, and military combat. Patients who have experienced a traumatic event are often frequent users of the health care system, seeking treatment for the overall emotional and physical trauma that they experienced.

The physiologic responses noted in people who have been severely traumatized include increased activity of the sympa-

NURSING RESEARCH PROFILE

Anxiety and Coping Behaviors

Clark, A. M. (2003). "It's like an explosion in your life": Lay perspectives on stress and myocardial infarction. *Journal of Clinical Nursing, 12*(4), 544–553.

Purpose

Different people manifest the physiologic, emotional, and behavioral signs and symptoms of stress and anxiety in different ways. This research study explored patient reports about the nature and complexities of emotional disturbances after myocardial infarction (MI). Patients who had an MI described their views of how stress affects functioning and the relationship of stress to their MI.

Design

This qualitative study used a semistructured interview technique to encourage investigation of stress from patients' perspectives. Fourteen patients (eight men and six women) from a hospital in Glasgow, Scotland, participated in the study. Criteria for inclusion in the study were first MI diagnosis, conscious and not intubated, stable vital signs, no pain, and no invasive procedure other than blood work for at least 8 hours prior to data collection.

Findings

The participants expressed their feelings and responses related to the experience of having an MI. An example of a participant's explanation was, "It's like an explosion in your life. Everything changes, everything." Patients reflected on their emotional conceptions of the situation and focused on everyday stress as playing a major role in the development of their MI. They used words such as "worry," "fright," "anger," "panic," and "sweats." Overall, stress was conceptualized as a cause of the MI, a societal norm, a personal trait, a response to major life events, and a response to daily life events. This study confirmed that both similarities and differences exist between how laypeople and health care professionals communicate about stress related to coronary artery disease.

Nursing Implications

Nurses must understand patient views of stress, because this understanding can shape beneficial nursing interventions. Nurses must recognize that the word "stress" is used by patients to denote conditions ranging from the stress of daily living to the response to major life events; nurses must focus on the language that patients use and the meaning of such language. In addition, nurses must be careful not to make assumptions about patient stress. If patients view stress as beyond their control, nursing interventions to reduce stress may not be viewed as practical. If nurses have limited or inadequate knowledge about patients' perspectives of stress, nursing interventions will be less effective.

---

thetic nervous system, increased plasma catecholamine levels, and increased urinary epinephrine and norepinephrine levels. It has been postulated (Loseke, Gelles, & Cavanaugh, 2004) that people with PTSD lose the ability to control their response to stimuli. The resulting excessive arousal can increase overall body metabolism and trigger emotional reactivity. In this situation, nurses observe that patients have difficulty sleeping, have an exaggerated startle response, and are excessively vigilant.

Symptoms of PTSD can occur hours to years after the trauma is experienced. Acute PTSD is defined as the experience of symptoms for less than a 3-month period. Chronic PTSD is defined as the experience of symptoms lasting longer than 3 months. In the case of delayed PTSD, up to 6 months may elapse between the trauma and the manifestation of symptoms (American Psychiatric Association, 2000). For more information, see Chart 7-9.

Nursing Implications

It is often thought that the incidence of PTSD is very low in the overall population. However, when high-risk groups are studied, the results indicate that more than 50% of study participants have PTSD (Cathersall, 2004). Therefore, it is important that nurses consider which of their patients are at risk for PTSD and be knowledgeable about the common symptoms associated with it. Older people are more susceptible to the physical effects of trauma and the effects of PTSD because of the neural inactivation associated with aging. It has also been speculated that people who have a preexisting tendency to become extremely anxious have an increased vulnerability for PTSD (Sharhabani-Ary, Amir, Kotler, et al., 2003).

The sensitivity and caring of the nurse creates the interpersonal relationship necessary to work with patients who have PTSD. These patients are physically compromised and are struggling emotionally with situations that are not considered part of normal human experience—situations that violate the commonly held perceptions of human social justice. Treatment of patients with PTSD includes several essential components: establishing a trusting relationship, addressing and working through the trauma experience, and providing education about the coping skills needed for recovery and self-care. The patient's progress can be influenced by the ability to cope with the various aspects of both the physical and the emotional distress.

CHART 7-7

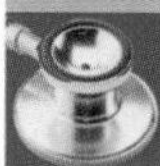

Assessing for Anxiety

Be on the alert for the following signs and symptoms:

Physiologic Indicators

- Appetite change
- Headaches
- Muscle tension
- Fatigue or lethargy
- Weight change
- Cold and flu symptoms
- Digestive upsets
- Grinding teeth
- Palpitations
- Hypertension
- Restlessness
- Difficulty sleeping
- Skin irritations
- Injury prone
- Increased use of any alcohol or drugs

Emotional Indicators

- Forgetfulness
- Low productivity
- Feeling dull
- Poor concentration
- Negative attitude
- Confusion
- Whirling mind
- No new ideas
- Boredom
- Negative self-talk
- Anxiety
- Frustration
- Depression
- Crying periods
- Irritability
- Worrying
- Feeling discouraged
- Nervous laughter

Relational Indicators

- Isolation
- Intolerance
- Resentment
- Loneliness
- Lashing out
- "Clamming up"
- Nagging
- Distrust
- Few friends
- No intimacy
- Using people

Spiritual Indicators

- Emptiness
- Loss of meaning
- Doubt
- Unforgiving attitude
- Martyrdom
- Loss of direction
- Cynicism
- Apathy

CHART 7-8

Managing Anxiety

- Listen actively and focus on having the patient discuss personal feelings.
- Use positive remarks and focus on the positive aspects of life in the "here and now."
- Use appropriate touch (with patient permission) to demonstrate support.
- Discuss the importance of safety and the patient's overall sense of well-being.
- Explain all procedures, policies, diagnostic studies, medications, treatments, or protocols for care.
- Explore coping strategies and work with the patient to practice and use them effectively (eg, breathing, progressive relaxation, visualization, imagery).
- Use distraction as indicated to relax and prevent self from being overwhelmed.

Depression

Depression is a common response to health problems and is an often underdiagnosed problem in the patient population. People may become depressed as a result of injury or illness; may be suffering from an earlier loss that is compounded by a new health problem; or may seek health care for somatic manifestations of depression.

Clinical depression is distinguished from everyday feelings of sadness by its duration and severity. Most people occasionally feel down or depressed, but these feelings are short-lived and do not result in impaired functioning. Clinically depressed people usually have had signs of a depressed mood or a decreased interest in pleasurable activities for at least a 2-week period. An obvious impairment in social, occupational, and overall daily functioning occurs in some people. Others function appropriately in their interactions with the outside world by exerting great effort and forcing themselves to mask their distress. Sometimes they are successful at hiding their depression for months or years and astonish family members and others when they finally admit that they are seriously depressed.

Many people experience depression but seek treatment for somatic complaints. The leading somatic complaints of patients struggling with depression are headache, backache, abdominal pain, fatigue, malaise, anxiety, and decreased desire or problems with sexual functioning (Varcarolis, 2004). These sensations are frequently manifestations of depression. The depression is undiagnosed about half of the time and masquerades as physical health problems (Townsend, 2003). People with depression also exhibit poor functioning and frequent absences from work and school.

Specific symptoms of clinical depression include feelings of sadness, worthlessness, fatigue, guilt, and difficulty concentrating or making decisions. Changes in appetite, weight gain or loss, sleep disturbances, and psychomotor retardation or agitation are also common. Often, patients have recurrent thoughts about death or suicide or have made suicide attempts. A diagnosis of clinical depression is made when a person presents with at least five of nine diagnostic criteria for depression (Chart 7-10). Unfortunately, only one of three depressed people is properly diagnosed and appropriately treated (American Psychiatric Association, 2000).

Nursing Implications

Because any loss in function, change in role, or alteration in body image is a possible antecedent to depression, nurses in all settings encounter patients who are depressed or who have thought about suicide. Depression is suspected if changes in the patient's thoughts or feelings and a loss of self-esteem are noted. Chart 7-11 lists risk factors for depression. Depression can occur at any age, and it is diagnosed more frequently in women than in men. In elderly patients, nurses should be aware that decreased mental

CHART 7-9

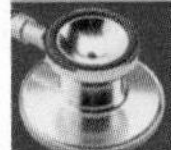

Assessing for Posttraumatic Stress Disorder (PTSD)

Be on the alert for the following signs and symptoms:

Physiologic Indicators

- Dilated pupils
- Headaches
- Sleep pattern disturbances
- Tremors
- Elevated blood pressure
- Tachycardia or palpitations
- Diaphoresis with cold, clammy skin
- Hyperventilation
- Dyspnea
- Smothering or choking sensation
- Nausea, vomiting, or diarrhea
- Stomach ulcers
- Dry mouth
- Abdominal pain
- Muscle tension or soreness
- Exhaustion

Psychological Indicators

- Anxiety
- Anger
- Depression
- Fears or phobias
- Survivor guilt
- Hypervigilance
- Nightmares or flashbacks
- Intrusive thoughts about the trauma
- Impaired memory
- Dissociative states
- Restlessness or irritability
- Strong startle response
- Substance abuse
- Self-hatred
- Feelings of estrangement
- Feelings of helplessness, hopelessness, or powerlessness
- Lack of interest in life
- Inability to concentrate
- Difficulty communicating, caring, and expressing love
- Problems with relationships
- Sexual problems ranging from acting out to impotence
- Difficulty with intimacy
- Inability to trust
- Lack of impulse control
- Aggressive, abusive, or violent behavior, including suicide
- Thrill-seeking behaviors

Copel, L. C. (2000). *Nurse's clinical guide: Psychiatric and mental health care* (2nd ed.). Springhouse, PA: Springhouse.

CHART 7-10

Diagnostic Criteria for Depression Based on the DSM-IV-TR

A person experiences at least five out of nine characteristics, with one of the first two symptoms present most of the time:

1. Depressed mood
2. Loss of pleasure or interest
3. Weight gain or loss
4. Sleeping difficulties
5. Psychomotor agitation or retardation
6. Fatigue
7. Feeling worthless
8. Inability to concentrate
9. Thoughts of suicide or death

American Psychiatric Association. (2000). *Diagnostic and statistical manual of mental disorders (DSM-IV-TR)* (4th ed.). Washington, DC: Author.

alertness and withdrawal-type responses may be indicative of depression. Consultation with a psychiatric liaison nurse to assess and differentiate between dementia-like symptoms and depression is often helpful.

Talking with the patient about his or her fears, frustration, anger, and despair can help alleviate a sense of helplessness and lead to necessary treatment. Helping the patient learn to cope effectively with conflict, interpersonal problems, and grief and encouraging the patient to discuss actual and potential losses may hasten his or her recovery from depression. It may also be possible to help the patient identify and decrease negative self-talk and unrealistic expectations and show how these contribute to depression. The nurse should monitor the patient for the onset of new problems, because depression adversely affects physical health and self-care activities. All patients with depression should be evaluated to determine if they would benefit from antidepressant therapy.

CHART 7-11

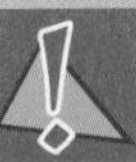

Risk Factors for Depression

- Family history
- Stressful situations
- Female gender
- Prior episodes of depression
- Onset before age 40 years
- Medical comorbidity
- Past suicide attempts
- Lack of support systems
- History of physical or sexual abuse
- Current substance abuse

In addition to the measures previously listed, psychoeducational programs, establishment of support systems, and counseling can reduce anxiety- and depression-related distress (Mirowsky & Ross, 2003). Psychoeducational programs can help patients and their families understand depression, treatment options, and coping strategies. (In crisis situations, it is imperative that patients be referred to psychiatrists, psychiatric nurse specialists, or crisis centers.) Explaining to patients that depression is a medical illness and not a sign of personal weakness, and that effective treatment will allow them to feel better and stay emotionally healthy, is an important aspect of care (Varcarolis, 2004).

In the United States, about 15% of severely depressed people commit suicide, and two thirds of patients who have committed suicide had been seen by health care practitioners during the month before their death (U.S. Preventive Service Task Force Agency for Healthcare Research and Quality, 2004). When patients make statements that are self-deprecating, express feelings of failure, or are convinced that things are hopeless and will not improve, they may be at risk for suicide. Risk factors for suicide are listed in Chart 7-12.

Substance Abuse

Some people use mood-altering substances in an attempt to cope with life's challenges. People who abuse substances use illegally obtained drugs, prescribed or over-the-counter medications, and alcohol alone or in combination with other drugs in ineffective attempts to cope with the pressures, strains, and burdens of life. They are unable to make healthy decisions and to solve problems effectively. Typically, they are also unable to identify and implement adaptive behaviors. Some people may respond to personal illness or the illness of a loved one by using substances to decrease emotional pain. Over time, physiologic, emotional, cognitive, and behavioral problems develop as a result of continuous substance use. These problems cause distress for people, their families, and their communities.

Nursing Implications

Substance abuse is encountered in all clinical settings. Intoxication and withdrawal are two common substance abuse problems. Often, nurses see patients who have experienced trauma as a result of intoxication. Other patients who are active substance abusers enter the primary care setting with a diagnosis other than that of substance abuse. Many do not disclose the extent of their substance use. The patient's use of denial or lack of knowledge about the harmful effects of psychoactive substances can be detected by the nurse who performs a substance use assessment. Nurses can incorporate tools into the assessment to detect drug use. Examples of such instruments are the CAGE Questionnaire (Ewing, 1984), the Michigan Alcohol Screening Test (Selzer, 1971), and the Addiction Severity Index (McLellan, Kushner, Metzger, et al., 1992). The CAGE Questions Adapted to Include Drugs (CAGEAID) instrument is presented in Chapter 5, Chart 5-3. Information that is commonly addressed in substance abuse questionnaires is summarized in Chart 7-13.

Health professionals are in pivotal positions to identify substance abuse problems, institute treatment protocols, and make referrals. Because substance abuse severely affects families, nurses can help family members confront the situation, decrease enabling behaviors, and motivate the person with the substance abuse problem to obtain treatment.

Caring for codependent family members is another nursing priority. Codependent people tend to manifest unhealthy patterns in relationships with others. Codependents struggle with a need to be needed, an urge to control others, and a willingness to remain involved and suffer with a person who has a drug problem.

Families may approach the health care team to help set limits on the dysfunctional behavior of people who abuse substances. At these times, a therapeutic intervention is organized for the purpose of confronting the patient about substance use and the need to obtain drug or alcohol treatment. Nurses or other skilled addiction counselors help fam-

CHART 7-12

Risk Factors for Suicide

- Age younger than 20 or older than 45 years, especially older than 65 years
- Gender—women make more attempts, men are more successful
- Dysfunctional family—members have experienced cumulative multiple losses and possess limited coping skills
- Family history of suicide
- Severe depression
- Severe, intractable pain
- Chronic, debilitating medical problems
- Substance abuse
- Severe anxiety
- Overwhelming problems
- Severe alteration in self-esteem or body image
- Lethal suicide plan

CHART 7-13

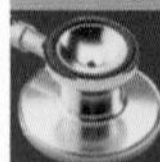

Assessing for Substance Abuse

- Past and recurrent use of the substance
- Patient's view of substance use as a problem
- Age when substance was first used and last used
- Length and duration of use of substance
- Preferred method of use of substance
- Amount of substance used
- How substance is procured
- Effect of or reaction to substance
- Previous attempts to cease or decrease substance use

ilies present the addicted person with a realistic perspective about the problem, their concerns about and caring for the person, and a specific plan for treatment. This therapeutic intervention works on the premise that honest and caring confrontation can break through a person's denial of the addiction. If a person refuses to participate in the designed plan, the family members define the consequences and state their commitment to follow through with them. This intervention is empowering to the family and usually provides the structure needed to secure treatment.

However, even with treatment, the patient may experience relapse. The nurse works with the patient and family to prevent relapse and to be prepared if relapse occurs. Relapse is considered a part of the illness process and therefore must be viewed and addressed in the same way that chronic illness is treated.

Nurses who work with patients and families struggling with addiction must dispel the myth that addiction is a defect in character or a moral fault. Views on substance abuse vary within society. A person's background may help determine whether he or she uses drugs, what drugs are used, and when they are used (Copel, 2000). The combination of variables, such as values and beliefs, family and personal norms, spiritual convictions, and conditions of the current social environment, predisposes a person to the possibility of drug use, motivation for treatment, and continual recovery (Copel, 2000). It has also been said that a person's attitude, especially toward alcohol, reflects the overall beliefs and attitudes of that person's culture (Giger & Davidhizar, 2004).

Loss and Grief

Loss is a part of the life cycle. All people experience loss in the form of change, growth, and transition. The experience of loss is painful, frightening, and lonely, and it triggers an array of emotional responses (Chart 7-14). People may vacillate between denial, shock, disbelief, anger, inertia, intense yearning, loneliness, sadness, loss of control, depression, and spiritual despair (Walsh & McGoldrick, 2004).

In addition to normal losses associated with life cycle stages, there are the potential losses of health, a body part, self-image, self-esteem, and even one's life. When loss is not acknowledged or there are multiple losses, anxiety, depression, and health problems may occur. Likewise, people with physical health problems, such as diabetes mellitus, HIV infection/AIDS, cardiac disorders, gastrointestinal disorders, disabilities, and neurologic impairments, tend to respond to these conditions with feelings of **grief**.

People grieve in different ways, and there is no timeline for completing the **bereavement** process. The time of griev-

NURSING RESEARCH PROFILE

Substance Abuse

Zakrzewski, R. F., & Hector, M. A. (2004). The lived experience of alcohol addiction: Men of Alcoholics Anonymous. *Issues in Mental Health Nursing, 25*(1), 61–77.

Purpose

Alcohol is the most widely used drug in the United States, and alcohol addiction is one of the most common psychiatric disorders among the general population. Alcoholics Anonymous (AA) is the largest self-help group for alcoholics. This research study identified themes and commonalities in the experiences of alcohol addiction of male members of AA.

Design

An existential phenomenologic methodology was chosen for the study. The researchers sought to gain an in-depth understanding of the subjects' experiences with alcohol addiction through the use of nondirective interviews. The sample consisted of seven men who had addiction to alcohol. All participants were between 32 and 65 years of age, sober for a period of 1 to 25 years, and AA members.

Findings

The subjects reflected about times before, during, and after their addiction to alcohol. They spoke about their childhoods, when they started drinking, their drinking years, turning points in their lives, treatment, and the period after attaining sobriety. Four themes were identified from the men's experiences: emotions, control, awareness of others, and turning points. Telling their stories had a therapeutic effect. All the men spoke of the "high" that alcohol provided and about their perceptions that drinking was fun. They said that they drank to mask negative feelings about themselves. For these men, challenges included relearning how to live after achieving sobriety and coping with problems previously dealt with by alcohol use.

Nursing Implications

Nurses must recognize that people recovering from alcoholism need to understand their feelings about alcohol use and have opportunities to discuss in their own words their experiences with alcohol. Strategies are needed to assist people recovering from alcoholism to find healthy outlets for achieving positive feelings and to identify ways to have fun without using alcohol. People recovering from alcohol addiction must handle their feelings of boredom related to sobriety and develop strategies for enjoying life. Mental health professionals can help teach them ways to cope with everyday stressors and feelings that previously led to the use of alcohol.

CHART 7-14

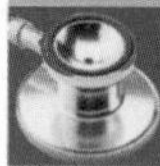

Assessing for Grieving

Be on the alert for the following signs and symptoms:

Physiologic Indicators

- Heart rate changes
- Blood pressure alterations
- Gastrointestinal disturbances
- Chest discomfort
- Shortness of breath
- Weakness
- Appetite changes
- Sleep problems
- Vague, but distressing, physical symptoms

Emotional Indicators

- Sadness
- Depression
- Anger
- Social withdrawal
- Loneliness
- Apathy
- Longing for who or what was lost
- Blaming of self or others
- Questioning of beliefs

Behavioral Indicators

- Slow movements
- Forgetfulness
- Purposeless activity
- Crying
- Sighing
- Lack of interest
- Easily distracted from tasks

ing often depends on the significance of the loss, the anticipation of or preparation for the loss, the person's emotional stability and maturity, and the person's coping ability (Arnold & Boggs, 2003).

Regardless of the duration of the grieving process, there are two basic goals: (1) healing the self and (2) recovering from the loss. Other factors that influence grieving are the type of loss, life experiences with various changes and transitions, religious beliefs, cultural background, and personality type (Walsh & McGoldrick, 2004). Some patients may resort to abuse of prescription medications, illegal drugs, or alcohol if they find it difficult to cope with the loss; the grief process is then complicated by the use of addictive substances.

Nursing Implications

Nurses identify patients and family members who are grieving and work with them to accomplish the four major tasks of the grief process: (1) acceptance of the loss, (2) acknowledgment of the intensity of the pain of the loss, (3) adaptation to life after the loss, and (4) cultivation of new relationships and activities (Worden, 2001). Nurses also assess and differentiate between grief and depression by knowing the common thoughts, feelings, physical or bodily reactions, and behaviors associated with grief compared with depression.

The physical response to grief includes the sensation of somatic distress, a tightness in the throat followed by a choking sensation or shortness of breath, the need to sigh, an empty feeling inside the abdomen, a lack of muscle power, and intense disabling distress. Grief can further debilitate already compromised patients and can have a strong impact on family functioning.

Death and Dying

Coping with the death of a loved one or with anticipation of one's own death is considered the ultimate challenge. The idea of death is threatening and anxiety-provoking to many people. Kubler-Ross (1975, p. 1) stated, "The key to the question of death unlocks the door of life. . . . For those who seek to understand it, death is a highly creative force." Common fears of dying people are fear of the unknown, pain, suffering, loneliness, loss of the body, and loss of personal control.

In recent years, the experience of dying has changed as advances have been made in the care of chronically and terminally ill patients. Technologic innovations and modern therapeutic treatments have prolonged the life span, and many deaths are now the result of chronic illnesses that result in physiologic deterioration and subsequent multisystem failure. For more information on end-of-life care and death and dying, see Chapter 17.

Spirituality and Spiritual Distress

Spirituality is defined as connectedness with self, others, a life force, or God that allows people to experience self-transcendence and find meaning in life. Spirituality helps people discover a purpose in life, understand the ever-changing qualities of life, and develop their relationship with God or a higher power. Within the framework of spirituality, people may discover truths about the self, about the world, and about concepts such as love, compassion, wisdom, honesty, commitment, imagination, reverence, and morality. Sacred texts for the major religious traditions offer guidelines for personal conduct and social and spiritual behavior. It is important that the spiritual beliefs of people and families be acknowledged, valued, and respected for the comfort and guidance they provide.

Often, spiritual behavior is expressed through sacrifice, self-discipline, and spending time in activities that focus on the inner self or the soul. Although religion and nature are two vehicles that people use to connect themselves with God or a higher power, bonds to religious institutions, beliefs, or dogma are not required to experience the spiritual sense of self. **Faith**, considered the foundation of spirituality, is a belief in something that a person cannot see. The spiritual part of a person views life as a mystery that unfolds over the lifetime, encompassing questions about meaning, hope, relatedness to God, acceptance or forgiveness, and transcendence (Hawks, 2004; Wright, 2004).

A strong sense of spirituality or religious faith can have a positive impact on health (Dunn & Horgas, 2000; Kendrick & Robinson, 2000; Phillips, 2003). Spirituality is also a component of hope, and, especially during chronic, serious, or terminal illness, patients and their families often find comfort and emotional strength in their religious traditions or spiritual beliefs. At other times, illness and loss can cause a loss of faith or meaning in life and a spiritual crisis. The nursing diagnosis of Spiritual distress is applicable to those who have a disturbance in the belief or value system that provides strength, hope, and meaning in life.

Nursing Implications

Spiritually distressed patients (or family members) may show despair, discouragement, ambivalence, detachment, anger, resentment, or fear. They may question the meaning of suffering, life, and death and express a sense of emptiness. The nurse assesses spiritual strength by inquiring about the person's sense of spiritual well-being, hope, and peacefulness. The nurse assesses whether spiritual beliefs and values have changed in response to illness or loss. The nurse also assesses current and past participation in religious or spiritual practices and notes the patient's responses to questions about spiritual needs—grief, anger, guilt, depression, doubt, anxiety, or calmness—to help determine the patient's need for spiritual care. Another simple assessment technique is to inquire about the patient's and family's desire for spiritual support.

For nurses to provide spiritual care, they must be open to being present and supportive when patients experience doubt, fearfulness, suffering, despair, or other difficult psychological states of being. Interventions that foster spiritual growth or reconciliation include being fully present; listening actively; conveying a sense of caring, respect, and acceptance; using therapeutic communication techniques to encourage expression; suggesting the use of prayer, meditation, or imagery; and facilitating contact with spiritual leaders or performance of spiritual rituals (Hawks, 2004).

Patients with serious, chronic, or terminal illnesses face physical and emotional losses that threaten their spiritual integrity. During acute and chronic illness, rehabilitation, or the dying process, spiritual support can stimulate patients to regain or strengthen their connections with their inner selves, their loved ones, and God or a higher power to transcend suffering and find meaning. Nurses can alleviate distress and suffering and enhance wellness by meeting their patients' spiritual needs.

Critical Thinking Exercises

1 A 55-year-old man in a hospital clinic tells the nurse that he does not want to suffer and will obtain medication for his pain when he has a colon biopsy. He states, "I am nervous about this procedure. I know that biopsies are painful, despite what the surgeon says. I'm going to get some medicine to decrease my pain and my nervousness, aren't I?" How does the nurse handle this situation? What assessment data should be collected to determine measures that will most likely allay this patient's anxiety? What complementary or alternative methods might be helpful to this patient?

2 ebp The night before a patient's surgery, the nurse is approached by the man's daughter. She fears that her father's daily use of alcohol may have untoward postoperative outcomes. What would you tell her? How would you approach the patient? What strategies would be useful for this patient and for the entire family? What is the evidence base for use of these strategies? Discuss the strength of the evidence. Identify the criteria used to evaluate the strength of the evidence for the strategies.

REFERENCES AND SELECTED READINGS

BOOKS

Aiken, L. (2000). *Dying, death, and bereavement* (4th ed.). Mahwah, NJ: Lawrence Erlbaum.

American Psychiatric Association. (2000). *Diagnostic and statistical manual of mental disorders (DSM-IV-TR)* (4th ed.). Washington, DC: Author.

Arnold, E., & Boggs, K. (2003). *Interpersonal relationships: Professional communication skills for nurses* (3rd ed.). Philadelphia: W. B. Saunders.

Boss, P., & Mulligan, C. (2003). *Family stress: Classic and contemporary readings*. Thousand Oaks, CA: Sage.

Boyd-Franklin, N., & Bry, B. H. (2001). *Reaching out in family therapy*. New York: Guilford Press.

Burr, W., Klein, S., Burr, R., et al. (1994). *Reexamining family stress: New theory and research*. Thousand Oaks, CA: Sage.

Cathersall, D. R. (2004). *The handbook of stress, trauma, and family*. New York: Brunner-Routledge.

Copel, L. C. (2000). *Nurse's clinical guide: Psychiatric and mental health care* (2nd ed.). Springhouse, PA: Springhouse.

DiClemente, C. S. (2003). *Addiction and change: How addiction develops and addicted people recover*. NY: Guilford Press.

Feldman, R. S. (2002). *Development across the life span* (3rd ed.). Upper Saddle River, NJ: Prentice Hall.

Freeman, S. (2004). *Grief and loss: Understanding the journey*. Pacific Grove, CA: Brooks/Cole.

Friedman, M. M., Bowden, V. R., & Jones, E. G. (2003). *Family nursing: Research, theory, and practice* (5th ed.). Upper Saddle River, NJ: Prentice Hall.

Gelles, R. J. (1997). *Intimate violence in families*. Thousands Oaks, CA: Sage.

Giger, J. N., & Davidhizar, R. E. (2004). *Transcultural nursing: Assessment and intervention* (4th ed.). St. Louis: C. V. Mosby.

Jeffreys, J. S. (2004). *Helping grieving people*. New York: Brunner/Routledge.

Johnson, J. (2004). *Fundamentals of substance abuse.* Pacific Grove, CA: Brooks/Cole.

Kail, R. V., & Cavanaugh, R. C. (2004). *Human development: A life span view* (3rd ed.). Pacific Grove, CA: Brooks/Cole.

Keegan, L. (2001). *Healing with complementary and alternative therapies.* Albany, NY: Delmar.

Kubler-Ross, E. (1975). *Death: The final stage of growth.* Englewood Cliffs, NJ: Prentice-Hall.

Kuhn, M. A. (1999). *Complementary therapies for health care providers.* Philadelphia: Lippincott Williams & Wilkins.

Lattanzi-Licht, M., & Doka, K. J. (2003). *Living with grief.* New York: Brunner/Routledge.

Loseke, D. R., Gelles, R. J., & Cavanaugh, M. M. (Eds.). (2004). *Current controversies on family violence.* Newbury Park, CA: Sage.

Martocchio, B. C. (1982). *Living while dying.* Bowie, MD: Robert J. Brady.

Matthews, D. A., & Larson, D. B. (1995). *The faith factor: An annotated bibliography of clinical research on spiritual subjects* (Vol. 3). Rockville, MD: National Institute for Health Care Research.

Mirowsky, J., & Ross, C. E. (2003). *Social causes of psychological distress* (2nd ed.). New York: Aldine De Gruyter.

Munoz, C., & Luckmann, J. (2005). *Transcultural communication in nursing.* Albany, NY: Delmar.

Murray, R. B., & Zentner, J. P. (2001). *Health assessment and promotion strategies through the life span* (7th ed.). Stamford, CT: Appleton & Lange.

Nowinski, J. K. (1998). *Family recovery and substance abuse.* Thousand Oaks, CA: Sage.

Palmer, S., Cooper, C., & Thomas, K. (2003). *Creating a balance: Managing stress.* London: British Library Publishing.

Rice, F. P. (2001). *Human development: A lifespan approach* (4th ed.). Upper Saddle River, NJ: Prentice Hall.

Rice, V. H. (Ed.). (2000). *Handbook of stress, coping, and health: Implications for nursing research, theory, and practice.* Thousand Oaks, CA: Sage.

Scott, M. J. (2003). *Trauma and posttraumatic stress disorder.* Thousand Oaks, CA: Sage.

Stanhope, M., & Lancaster, J. (2004). *Community and public health nursing* (6th ed.). St. Louis: C. V. Mosby.

Suls, J., & Wallston, K. (2003). *Social psychological foundations of health and illness.* Malden, MA: Blackwell Publishing.

Townsend, M. C. (2003). *Psychiatric mental health nursing: Concepts of care.* Philadelphia: F. A. Davis.

U.S. Preventive Service Task Force Agency for Healthcare Research and Quality. (2004). *Guide to clinical prevention services* (3rd ed.). (AHRQ Publication No. 04-IP003). Rockville, MD: U.S. Government Printing Office.

U.S. Public Health Service. (2000). *Healthy people 2010: Understanding and improving health.* Washington, DC: U.S. Government Printing Office.

Varcarolis, E. M. (2004). *Foundations of psychiatric mental health nursing: A clinical approach* (4th ed.). Philadelphia: Saunders.

Walsh, F., & McGoldrick, M. (2004). *Living beyond loss.* New York: Norton.

Worden, J. W. (2001). *Grief counseling and grief therapy: A handbook for the mental health practitioner* (3rd ed.). New York: Springer Publishing.

Wright, L. M. (2004). *Spirituality, suffering, and illness: Ideas for healing.* Philadelphia: Davis.

Wright, L. M., & Leahey, M. (2000). *Nurses and families: A guide to family assessment and intervention.* Philadelphia: Davis.

JOURNALS

**Asterisks indicate nursing research articles.*

General

Hansen, A. M., Kaergaard, A., Andersen, J. H., et al. (2003). Associations between repetitive work and endocrinological indicators of stress. *Work and Stress, 17*(3), 264–276.

Litsey, T. (2003). Acupuncture vs. cancer: Re-engaging the body's immune system. *Acupuncture Today, 4*(10), 1–21.

*Marquis, R., Freegard, H., & Hoogland, L. (2004). Influences on positive family involvement in aged care: An ethnographic view. *Contemporary Nurse, 16*(3), 178–186.

Mitchell, E., & Moore, K. (2004). Stroke: Holistic care and management. *Nursing Standard, 18*(33), 43–56.

*Montbriand, M. J. (2004). Seniors' life histories and perceptions of illness. *Western Journal of Nursing Research, 26*(2), 242–260.

Robinson, F. P., Matthews, H. L., Witek-Janusek, L. (2003). Psycho-endocrine-immune response to mindfulness-based stress reduction in individuals infected with the human immunodeficiency virus: A quasi-experimental study. *Journal of Alternative and Complementary Medicine, 9*(5), 683–694.

Tower, K. D. (2003). Disability through the lens of culture. *Journal of Social Work in Disability and Rehabilitation, 2*(2/3), 5–22.

Complementary or Alternative Therapies

Burman, M. E. (2003). Complementary and alternative medicine: Core competencies for family nurse practitioners. *Journal of Nursing Education, 42*(1), 28–35.

*Chang, B. L., Van Servellen, G., & Lombardi, E. (2003). Factors associated with complementary therapy use in people living with HIV/AIDS receiving antiretroviral therapy. *Journal of Alternative and Complementary Medicine, 9*(5), 695–710.

Dorcas, A., & Yung, P. (2003). Qigong: Harmonizing the breath, the body and the mind. *Complementary Therapies in Nursing and Midwifery, 9*(4), 198–202.

*Richardson, T. (2003). Health status and health behaviors of inner city older African-Americans: Health disparities in Wellness Center participants. *Journal of Multicultural Nursing and Health, 9*(3), 62–67.

*Tsai, J., Wang, W., Chan, P., et al. (2003). The beneficial effects of Tai Chi Chuan on blood pressure and lipid profile and anxiety status in a randomized controlled trial. *Journal of Alternative and Complementary Medicine, 9*(5), 747–754.

Coping

*Clark, A. M. (2003). "It's like an explosion in your life": Lay perspectives on stress and myocardial infarction. *Journal of Clinical Nursing, 12*(4), 544–553.

DalMonte, J., Finlayson, M., & Helfrich, C. (2003). In their own words: Coping processes among women aging with multiple sclerosis. *Occupational Therapy in Health Care, 17*(3/4), 115–137.

Diamond, H., & Precin, P. (2003). Disabled and experiencing disaster: Personal and professional accounts. *Occupational Therapy in Mental Health, 19*(3/4), 27–41.

*Diokno, A. C., Burgio, K., Fultz, N. H., et al. (2004). Medical and self-care practices reported by women with urinary incontinence. *American Journal of Managed Care, 10*(Part 1), 69–78.

Johnson, D. M., Sheahan, T. C., & Chard, K. M. (2003). Personality disorders, coping strategies, and posttraumatic stress disorder in women with histories of childhood sexual abuse. *Journal of Child Sexual Abuse, 12*(2), 19–39.

Lee, S. (2003). Effects of using a nursing crisis intervention program on psychosocial responses and coping strategies of infertile women during in vitro fertilization. *Journal of Nursing Research, 11*(3), 197–207.

*Moser, D. K., Chung, M. L., McKinley, S., et al. (2003). Critical care nursing practice regarding patient anxiety assessment and management. *Intensive and Critical Care Nursing, 19*(5), 276–288.

*Rustoen, T., Wahl, A. K., Hanestad, B. R., et al. (2004). Expression of hope in cystic fibrosis patients: A comparison with the general population. *Heart and Lung, 33*(2), 111–118.

Scott, A. (2004). Managing anxiety in ICU patients: The role of pre-operative information provision. *Nursing in Critical Care, 9*(2), 72–79.

Sears, S. R., Stanton, A. L., & Danoff-Burg, S. (2003). The Yellow Brick Road and the Emerald City: Benefit finding, positive reappraisal coping, and posttraumatic growth in women with early-stage breast cancer. *Health Psychology, 22*(5), 487–497.

Stuban, S. L. (2004). Living, not dying with ALS: Confounding the predictions of Lou Gehrig disease. *American Journal of Nursing, 104*(5), 72–76.

Depression

*Bruce, M. L., Ten-Have, T. R., Reynolds, C. F., et al. (2004). Reducing suicidal ideation and depressive symptoms in depressed older primary care patients: A randomized controlled trial. *Journal of the American Medical Association, 291*(9), 1081–1091.

*Carpenter, J. S., Elam, J. L., Ridner, S. H., et al. (2004). Sleep, fatigue, and depressive symptoms in breast cancer survivors and matched healthy women experiencing hot flashes. *Oncology Nursing Forum, 31*(3), 591–598.

*Coleman, C. L. (2004). The contribution of religious and existential well-being to depression among African American heterosexuals with infection. *Issues in Mental Heath Nursing, 25*(1), 103–110.

*Kubik, M. Y., Lytle, L. A., Birnbaum, A. S., et al. (2003). Prevalence and correlates of depressive symptoms in young adolescents. *American Journal of Health Behavior, 27*(5), 546–553.

Nelson, R. (2004). Suicide rates rise among soldiers in Iraq. *Lancet, 363*(9405), 300.

Putnam, K., & McKibben, L. (2004). Managing workplace depression: An untapped opportunity for occupational health professionals. *Journal of the American Association of Occupational Health Nursing, 52*(3), 122–131.

Grief

Finlayson, M., & van Denend, T. (2003). Experiencing the loss of mobility: Perspectives of older adults with MS. *Disability and Rehabilitation, 25*(20), 1168–1180.

Leichtling, B. (2004). Leadership and management: Dealing with dying, death, and grief. *Caring, 23*(1), 38–39.

Murphy, M. (2003). A model to help nurses caring for patients who are terminally ill. *Professional Nurse, 19*(4), 213–215.

*Mystakidou, K., Tsilika, E., Parpa, E., et al. (2003). Greek perspective on concepts of death and expression of grief, with implications for practice. *International Journal of Palliative Care, 9*(12), 534–537.

*Rabow, M., W., Schanche, K., Petersen, J., et al. (2003). Patient perceptions of an outpatient palliative care intervention: "It had been on my mind before, but I did not know how to start talking about death . . ." *Journal of Pain and Symptom Management, 26*(5), 1010–1015.

Ramsey, A. (2003). Monitoring the dying patient in ITC: A personalized discussion. *Nursing in Critical Care, 8*(5), 209–211.

Posttraumatic Stress Disorder

Otis, J. D., Keane, T. M., & Kerns, R. D. (2003). An examination of the relationship between chronic pain and posttraumatic stress disorder. *Journal of Rehabilitation Research and Development, 40*(5), 397–405.

*Pulcino, T., Galea, S., Ahern, J., et al. (2003). Posttraumatic stress in women after the September 11 attacks in New York City. *Journal of Women's Health, 12*(8), 809–820.

Seo, D., & Torabi, M. R. (2004). National study of emotional and perceptual changes since September 11. *American Journal of Health Education 35*(1), 37–45.

*Sharhabani-Arzy, R., Amir, M., Kotler, M., et al. (2003). The toll of domestic violence: PTSD among battered women in an Israeli sample. *Journal of Interpersonal Violence 18*(11), 1335–1346.

*Sorenson, D. S. (2003). Healing traumatizing provider interactions among women through short-term group therapy. *Archives of Psychiatric Nursing, 17*(6), 259–269.

Spirituality

Dunn, K. S., & Horgas, A. L. (2000). The prevalence of prayer as a spiritual self-care modality in elders. *Journal of Holistic Nursing, 18*(4), 337–351.

Hawks, S. (2004). Spiritual wellness, holistic health, and the practice of health education. *American Journal of Health Education, 35*(1), 11–16.

Kendrick, K. D., & Robinson, S. (2000). Spirituality: Its relevance and purpose for clinical nursing in a new millennium. *Journal of Clinical Nursing, 9*(5), 701–705.

Lloyd, M., (2003). Innovations in care: Challenging depression: Taking a spiritually enhanced approach. *Geriaction, 21*(4), 26–29.

*Musgrave, C. F., & McFarlane, E. A. (2004). Israeli oncology nurses' religiosity, spiritual well-being, and attitudes toward spiritual care: A path analysis. *Oncology Nursing Forum, 31*(2), 321–327.

Phillips, I. (2003). Infusing spirituality into geriatric health care: Practical applications from the literature. *Topics in Geriatric Rehabilitation, 19*(4), 249–256.

Substance Abuse

*Boyd, M. R., Phillips, K., & Dorsey, C. J. (2003). Alcohol and other drug disorders, comorbidity, and violence: Comparison of rural African American and Caucasian women. *Archives of Psychiatric Nursing, 17*(6), 249–258.

deWit, H., Soderpalm, A. H. V., Nikolayev, L., et al. (2003). Effects of acute social stress on alcohol consumption in healthy subjects. *Alcoholism: Clinical and Experimental Research, 27*(8), 1270–1277.

Ewing, J. A. (1984). Detecting alcoholism: The CAGE questionnaire. *Journal of the American Medical Association, 252*(14), 1906.

Hugh, T. (2003). Research reviews: Prevalence of alcohol. *Journal of Addictions Nursing, 14*(3), 165–167.

McLellan, A. T., Kushner, H., Metzger, D., et al. (1992). The fifth edition of the Addiction Severity Index. *Journal of Substance Abuse Treatment, 9*(3), 199–213.

Sansovich, D. (2003). HIV and substance use: Pain and the drug-seeking patient. *HIV Clinician, 15*(1), 15–16.

Selzer, M. L. (1971). The Michigan alcoholism screening test: The quest for a new diagnostic instrument. *American Journal of Psychiatry, 127*, 1653–1658.

*Tarrier, N., & Sommerfield, C. (2003). Alcohol and substance use in civilian chronic PTSD patients seeking psychological treatment. *Journal of Substance Use, 8*(4), 197–204.

*Zakrzewski, R. F., & Hector, M. A. (2004). The lived experience of alcohol addiction: Men of Alcoholics Anonymous. *Issues in Mental Health Nursing, 25*(1), 61–77.

RESOURCES

AGENCIES

American Holistic Nurses Association (AHNA), P.O. Box 2130, Flagstaff, AZ 86003-2130; 1-800-278-AHNA; http://www.ahna.org. Accessed June 6, 2006.

Grief Recovery Institute Education Foundation, Inc. (GRIEF), P.O. Box 6061-382, Sherman Oaks, CA 91413; 1-818-907-9600; 1-800-445-4808 (hotline); http://www.grief.net. Accessed June 6, 2006.

National Hospice and Palliative Care Organization (NHO), 1901 North Moore Street, Suite 901, Arlington, VA 22209; 1-703-243-5900; http://www.nhpco.org. Accessed June 6, 2006.

Aging

American Association of Retired Persons (AARP), 601 "E" Street NW, Washington, DC 20049-0001; 1-202-434-2277; 1-800-424-3410; http://www.aarp.org. Accessed July 6, 2006.

Children of Aging Parents, P.O. Box 167, Richboro, PA 18954; 1-800-227-7294; www.caps4caregivers.org. Accessed July 6, 2006.

National Association for Families Caring for their Elders—Eldercare America, 1141 Loxford Terrace, Silver Spring, MD 20901-1130; 1-301-593-1621

National Council on Aging, 409 3rd Street SW, Washington, DC 20024; 1-202-424-1200; 1-800-424-9046; http://www.ncoa.org. Accessed June 6, 2006.

National Office of the Gray Panthers, P.O. Box 214777, Washington, DC 20009; 1-202-466-3132; 1-800-280-5362; http://www.graypanthers.org. Accessed June 6, 2006.

Anxiety

Anxiety Disorders Association of America, 11900 Parklawn Drive #100, Rockville, MD 20852-2624; 1-301-231-9350; http://www.adaa.org. Accessed July 6, 2006.

Bereavement

Compassionate Friends, P.O. Box 3696, Oak Brook, IL 60522-3696; 1-630-990-0010; nationaloffice@compassionatefriends.org; http://www.compassionatefriends.org. Accessed June 6, 2006.

They Help Each Other Spiritually (THEOS), 322 Boulevard of the Allies #105, Pittsburgh, PA 15222-1919; 1-412-471-7779

Widowed Persons Service, 601 "E" Street NW, Washington, DC 20049-0001; 1-202-434-2260

Depression

Depression Awareness, Recognition, and Treatment (D/ART), NIMH, 5600 Fishers Lane Room 10-85, Rockville, MD 20857; 1-800-421-4211; 1-301-443-4140; http://www.nmha.org. Accessed July 6, 2006.

National Alliance for the Mentally Ill, 200 N. Grebe Road #1015, Arlington, VA 22201-3062; 1-703-524-7600; 1-800-950-NAMI; http://www.nami.org. Accessed June 6, 2006.

National Mental Health Association, 1021 Prince Street, Alexandria, VA 22314-2971; 1-703-684-7722; 1-800-969-6642; 1-800-433-5959; http://www.nmha.org. Accessed June 6, 2006.

Eating Disorders

American Anorexia Bulimia Association Inc., 293 Central Park West, New York, NY 10024; 1-212-501-8351

National Eating Disorders Association (NEDA), 603 Stewart St., Suite 803, Seattle, WA 98101;1-206-382-3587; http://www.nationaleatingdisorders.org. Accessed June 6, 2006.

Posttraumatic Stress Disorder

National Center for PTSD, VA Medical Center (116D), White River Junction, VT 05009; 1-802-296-5132; http://www.ncptsd.org. Accessed June 6, 2006.

Substance Abuse

Adult Children of Alcoholics, P.O. Box 3216, Torrence, CA 90510; 1-310-534-1815; http://www.adultchildren.org. Accessed June 6, 2006.

Alanon and Alateen Family Group Headquarters Inc., 1600 Corporate Landing Parkway, Virginia Beach, VA 23454-5617; 1-888-4AL-ANON (888-425-2666); http://www.al-anon.alateen.org. Accessed June 6, 2006.

Alcoholics Anonymous, Grand Central Station, P.O. Box 459, New York, NY 10163; 1-212-870-3400; http://www.aa.org. Accessed June 6, 2006.

Center for Substance Abuse Prevention Workplace, 800-WORKPLACE (1-800-967-5752)

Center for Substance Abuse Treatment, 800-662-HELP (1-800-662-4357)

Children of Alcoholics Foundation, 164 West 74th Street, New York, NY 10115; 1-800-359-2623

Co-Anon Family Groups, P.O. Box 64742-66, Los Angeles, CA 90064; 1-818-377-4317; http://www.co-anon.org. Accessed June 6, 2006.

Cocaine Anonymous, 3740 Overland Avenue Suite G, Los Angeles, CA 90034; 1-800-347-8998; http://www.ca.org. Accessed June 6, 2006.

Dual Recovery Anonymous World Services, P.O. Box 8107, Prairie Village, KS 66208; 877-883-2332; http://www.draonline.org. Accessed June 6, 2006.

Narcotics Anonymous, P.O. Box 9999, Van Nuys, CA 91409; 1-818-773-9999; http://www.na.org. Accessed June 6, 2006.

National Alcohol Hotline, Helpline: 1-800-NCA-CALL (1-800-622-2255)

National Cocaine Hotline, 1-800-COCAINE (1-800-262-2463)

Rational Recovery Systems, Box 800, Lotus, CA 95651; 1-530-621-4374; http://www.rational.org. Accessed June 6, 2006.

Secular Organizations for Sobriety (SOS), The Center for Inquiry, 5521 Grosvenor Boulevard, Los Angeles, CA 90066; 1-310-821-8430; http://www.secularhumanism.org. Accessed June 6, 2006.

CHAPTER 8

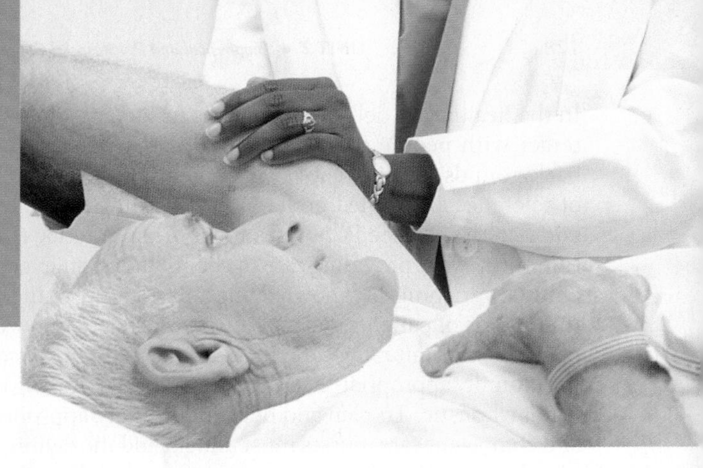

Perspectives in Transcultural Nursing

Learning Objectives

On completion of this chapter, the learner will be able to:

1. Identify key components of cultural assessment.
2. Apply transcultural nursing principles, concepts, and theories when providing nursing care to people, families, groups, and communities.
3. Develop strategies for planning, providing, and evaluating culturally competent nursing care for patients from diverse backgrounds.
4. Critically analyze the influence of culture on nursing care decisions and actions for patients.
5. Discuss the impact of diversity and health care disparities on health care delivery.

In the health care delivery system, as in society, nurses interact with people of similar as well as diverse cultural backgrounds. People may have similar or different frames of reference and varied preferences regarding their health and health care needs. Nurses must often practice *transcultural nursing,* providing care to clients and families across cultural variations. Acknowledging and adapting to the cultural needs of patients and significant others are important components of nursing care. In addition, facilitating access to culturally appropriate health care is critical if nursing care is to be holistic. To plan and deliver culturally appropriate and competent care, nurses must understand the definitions of culture, culturally appropriate care, and cultural competence and the various aspects of culture that should be explored for each patient.

Cultural Concepts

The concept of culture and its relationship to the health care beliefs and practices of the patient and his or her family and friends provide the foundation for transcultural nursing. This awareness of culture in the delivery of nursing care has been described in different terms and phrases, including respect for cultural diversity, culturally sensitive or comprehensive care, and culturally competent or appropriate nursing care (Giger & Davidhizar, 2004; Spector, 2004), or culturally congruent nursing care (Leininger, 2001). Two commonly discussed concepts are cultural diversity and culturally competent care.

The term *culture* was initially defined by the British anthropologist Sir Edward Tylor in 1871 as the knowledge, belief, art, morals, laws, customs, and any other capabilities and habits acquired by humans as members of society (Campinha-Bacote, 2003). During the past century, and especially during recent decades, hundreds of definitions of culture have been offered that integrate the themes stated by Tylor and the themes of ethnic variations of a population based on race, nationality, religion, language, physical characteristics, and geography (Spector, 2004). To fully appreciate the broad impact of culture, factors such as disabilities, gender, social class, physical appearance (eg, weight, height), ideologies (political views), or sexual orientation must be integrated into the definition of culture as well (Green-Hernandez, Quinn, Denman-Vitale, et al., 2004).

Madeleine Leininger, founder of the specialty called transcultural nursing, writes that culture involves learned and transmitted knowledge about values, beliefs, rules of behavior, and lifestyle practices that guide designated groups in their thinking and actions in patterned ways (2001). Giger and Davidhizar (2004) define transcultural nursing as a research-focused, client-based practice field of culturally competent nursing. Transcultural nursing addresses the differences and similarities among cultures in relation to health, health care, and illness, with consideration of patient values, beliefs, and practices. Culture develops over time as a result of exposure to social and religious structures and intellectual and artistic manifestations, and each individual person, including each nurse, is culturally unique (Giger & Davidhizar, 2004).

The concept of ethnic culture has four basic characteristics:

- It is learned from birth through language and socialization.
- It is shared by members of the same cultural group, and it includes an internal sense and external perception of distinctiveness.
- It is influenced by specific conditions related to environmental and technical factors and to the availability of resources.
- It is dynamic and ever-changing.

With the exception of the first characteristic, cultures related to age, physical appearance, lifestyle, and other less frequently acknowledged aspects also share the above characteristics.

Cultural diversity has also been defined in a number of ways. Often, differences in skin color, religion, and geographic area are the only elements used to identify diversity, with ethnic minorities being considered the primary sources of cultural diversity. However, there are many other possible sources of cultural diversity. To truly acknowledge the cultural differences that may influence health care delivery, the nurse must confront self-deception and bias and recognize the influence of his or her own culture and cultural heritage (Swanson, 2004).

Culturally competent nursing care has been defined as effective, individualized care that demonstrates respect for the dignity, personal rights, preferences, beliefs, and practices of the person receiving care, while acknowledging the biases of the caregiver and preventing these biases from interfering with the care provided. Culturally competent nursing care is a dynamic process that requires comprehensive knowledge of culture-specific information and an awareness of, and sensitivity to, the effect that culture has on the care situation. It requires that the nurse integrate cultural knowledge, awareness of his or her own cultural perspective, and the patient's cultural perspectives when preparing a plan of care (Giger & Davidhizar, 2004). Exploring one's own cultural beliefs and how they might conflict with the beliefs of the patients being cared for is a first step toward becoming culturally competent. Understanding the diversity within cultures, such as subcultures, is also important. In addition, culturally competent care involves facilitating patient access to culturally appropriate resources (Green-Hernandez et al., 2004).

Subcultures

Although culture is a universal phenomenon, it takes on specific and distinctive features for a particular group because it encompasses all of the knowledge, beliefs, customs, and skills acquired by the members of that group. When such groups function within a larger cultural group, they are referred to as subcultures.

The term *subculture* is used for relatively large groups of people who share characteristics that enable them to be identified as a distinct entity. Examples of American subcultures based on ethnicity (ie, subcultures with common traits such as physical characteristics, language, or ancestry) include African Americans, Hispanic/Latino Americans, Asian/Pacific Islanders, and Native Americans. Each of these subcultures may be further divided; for example, Native Americans consist of American Indians and Alaska Natives, who represent more than 500 federally and state-recognized tribes in addition to an unknown number of tribes that receive no official recognition.

Subcultures may also be based on religion (more than 1,200 religions exist in the United States), occupation (eg, nurses, physicians, other members of the health care team), or disability (eg, the Deaf community) or illness. In addition, subcultures may be based on age (eg, infants, children, adolescents, adults, older adults), gender (eg, male, female), sexual orientation (eg, homosexual, bisexual, heterosexual), or geographic location (eg, Texan, Southern, Appalachian).

Nurses should also be sensitive to the interracial applications of cultural competence. Tensions between subcultures within a designated group could add to the complexity of planning culturally competent care. Some members of one ethnic subculture may be offended or angered if they are mistaken for members of a different subculture. Similarly, if the attributes of one subculture are mistakenly generalized to patients who belong to a different subculture, extreme offense could result, as well as inappropriate care planning and implementation (Flowers, 2004). Nurses must refrain from culturally stereotyping patients in an attempt to be culturally competent. Instead, patients or significant others should be consulted regarding personal values, beliefs, preferences, and cultural identification. This strategy is also applicable for members of nonethnic subcultures.

Minorities

The term *minority* refers to a group of people whose physical or cultural characteristics differ from the majority of people in a society. At times, minorities may be singled out or isolated from others in society or treated in different or unequal ways. Although there are four generally identified minority groups—Blacks/African Americans, Hispanics, Asian/Pacific Islanders, and Native Americans (Baldwin, 2004; Sullivan Commission, 2004)—the concept of "minority" varies widely and must be understood in a cultural context. For example, men may be considered a minority within the nursing profession, but they constitute a majority within the field of medicine. In addition, Caucasians may be in the minority in some communities in the United States, but they are currently the majority group in the country (although it has been projected that by the middle to late 21st century, Caucasians will be in the minority in the United States). Because at times the term *minority* connotes inferiority, members of many racial and ethnic groups object to being identified as minorities.

Transcultural Nursing

Transcultural nursing, a term sometimes used interchangeably with cross-cultural, intercultural, or multicultural nursing, refers to a research-focused practice field that focuses on patient-centered, culturally competent nursing. Transcultural nursing incorporates the care (caring) values, beliefs, and practices of people and groups from a particular culture without imposing the nurse's cultural perspective on the patient (Giger & Davidhizar, 2004). The underlying focus of transcultural nursing is to provide culture-specific and culture-universal care that promotes the well-being or health of individuals, families, groups, communities, and institutions (Giger & Davidhizar, 2004; Leininger, 2001). All people as well as the community or institution at large benefit when culturally competent care is provided. When the care is delivered beyond a nurse's national boundaries, the term *international* or *transnational nursing* is often used.

Although many nurses, anthropologists, and others have written about the cultural aspects of nursing and health care, Leininger (2001) developed a comprehensive research-based theory called Culture Care Diversity and Universality to promote culturally congruent nursing for people of different or similar cultures. This means promoting recovery from illness, preventing conditions that would limit the patient's health or well-being, or facilitating a peaceful death in ways that are culturally meaningful and appropriate. Nursing care needs to be tailored to fit the patient's cultural values, beliefs, and lifestyles.

Leininger's theory stresses the importance of providing culturally congruent nursing care (meaningful and beneficial health care tailored to fit the patient's cultural values) through culture care accommodation and culture care restructuring (Fig. 8-1). *Culture care accommodation* refers to professional actions and decisions that nurses make in their care to help people of a designated culture achieve a beneficial or satisfying health outcome. *Culture care restructuring* or repatterning refers to professional actions and decisions that help patients reorder, change, or modify their lifestyles toward new, different, or more beneficial health care patterns. At the same time, the patient's cultural values and beliefs are respected, and a better or healthier lifestyle is provided. Other terms and definitions that provide further insight into culture and health care include the following:

- *Acculturation:* the process by which members of a cultural group adapt to or learn how to take on the behaviors of another group
- *Cultural blindness:* the inability of people to recognize their own values, beliefs, and practices and those of others because of strong ethnocentric tendencies (the tendency to view one's own culture as superior to others)
- *Cultural imposition:* the tendency to impose one's cultural beliefs, values, and patterns of behavior on a person or people from a different culture
- *Cultural taboos:* activities or behaviors that are avoided, forbidden, or prohibited by a particular cultural group

Culturally Competent Nursing Care

Culturally competent or *culturally congruent nursing care* refers to the delivery of interventions within the cultural context of the patient (Campinha-Bacote, 2003). It involves a complex integration of attitudes, knowledge, and skills (including assessment, decision making, judgments, critical thinking, and evaluation) that enables nurses to provide care in a culturally sensitive and appropriate manner. Agency policies are important to achieve culturally competent care. Policies that promote culturally competent care establish flexible regulations pertaining to visitors (number, frequency, and length of visits), provide translation services

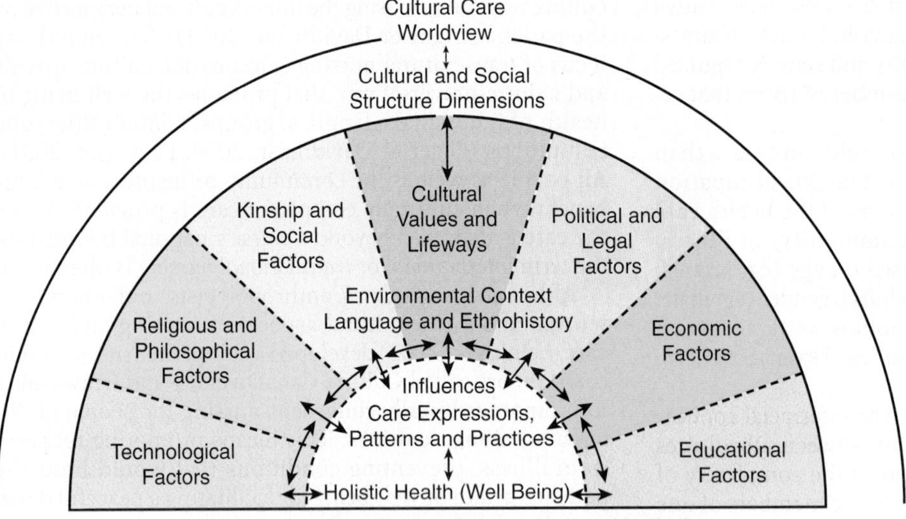

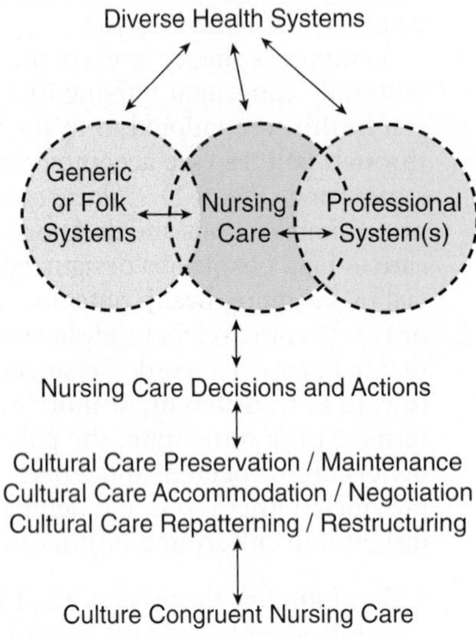

FIGURE 8-1. Leininger's Sunrise Model depicts her theory of cultural care diversity and universality. From Leininger, M. M. (Ed.). (2001). *Culture care diversity and university: A theory of nursing.* New York: National League for Nursing Press.

for non–English-speaking patients, and train staff to provide care for patients with different cultural values (Simpson, 2004). Culturally competent policies are developed to promote an environment in which the traditional healing, spiritual, and religious practices of patients are respected and encouraged and to recognize the special dietary practices of patients from selected cultural groups (Green-Hernandez et al., 2004).

Giger and Davidhizar (2004) created an assessment model to guide nurses in exploring cultural phenomena that might affect nursing care. They identified communication, space, time orientation, social organization, environmental control, and biologic variations as relevant phenomena. This model has been used in various patient care settings to provide data essential to the provision of culturally competent care.

Cross-Cultural Communication

Establishment of an environment of culturally congruent care and respect begins with effective communication, which occurs not only through words, but also through body language and other cues, such as voice, tone, and loudness. Nurse–patient interactions, as well as communications among members of a multicultural health care team, are dependent on the ability to understand and be understood.

Approximately 150 different languages are spoken in the United States, with Spanish accounting for the largest percentage after English. Obviously, nurses cannot become fluent in all languages, but certain strategies for fostering effective cross-cultural communication are necessary when providing care for patients who are not fluent in English. Cultural needs should be considered when choosing an interpreter; for instance, fluency in varied dialects is beneficial (Simpson, 2004). The interpreter's voice quality, pronunciation, use of silence, use of touch, and use of nonverbal communication should also be considered (Giger & Davidhizar, 2004).

During illness, patients of all ages tend to regress, and the regression often involves language skills. Chart 8-1 summarizes suggested strategies for overcoming language

CHART 8-1

Overcoming Language Barriers

- Greet the patient using the last or complete name. Avoid being too casual or familiar. Point to yourself and say your name. Smile.
- Proceed in an unhurried manner. Pay attention to any effort by the patient or family to communicate.
- Speak in a low, moderate voice. Avoid talking loudly. Remember that there is a tendency to raise the volume and pitch of your voice when the listener appears not to understand. The listener may perceive that you are shouting and/or angry.
- Organize your thoughts. Repeat and summarize frequently. Use audiovisual aids when feasible.
- Use short, simple sentence structure and speak in the active voice.
- Use simple words, such as "pain" rather than "discomfort." Avoid medical jargon, idioms, and slang. Avoid using contractions, such as don't, can't, won't.
- Use nouns repeatedly instead of pronouns. *Example:* Do not say: "He has been taking his medicine, hasn't he?" Do say: "Does Juan take medicine?"
- Pantomime words (use gestures) and simple actions while verbalizing them.
- Give instructions in the proper sequence. *Example:* Do not say: "Before you rinse the bottle, sterilize it." Do say: "First, wash the bottle. Second, rinse the bottle."
- Discuss one topic at a time, and avoid giving too much information in a single conversation. Avoid using conjunctions. *Example:* Do not say: "Are you cold and in pain?" Do say (while pantomiming/gesturing): "Are you cold?" "Are you in pain?"
- Talk directly to the patient rather than to the person who accompanied him or her.
- Validate whether the person understands by having him or her repeat instructions, demonstrate the procedure, or act out the meaning.
- Use any words you know in the person's language. This indicates that you are aware of and respect the patient's primary means of communicating.
- Try a third language. Many Indo-Chinese speak French. Europeans often know three or four languages. Try Latin words or phrases, if you are familiar with the language.
- Be aware of culturally based gender and age differences and diverse socioeconomic, educational, and tribal/regional differences when choosing an interpreter.
- Obtain phrase books from a library or bookstore, make or purchase flash cards, contact hospitals for a list of interpreters, and use both formal and informal networking to locate a suitable interpreter. Although they are costly, some telecommunication companies provide translation services.

barriers. Nurses should also assess how well patients and families have understood what has been said. The following cues may signify lack of effective communication:

- Efforts to change the subject: This could indicate that the listener does not understand what you are saying and is attempting to talk about something more familiar.
- Absence of questions: Paradoxically, this often means that the listener is not grasping the message and therefore has difficulty formulating questions to ask.
- Inappropriate laughter: A self-conscious giggle may signal poor comprehension and may be an attempt to disguise embarrassment.
- Nonverbal cues: A blank expression may signal poor understanding. However, among some Asian Americans, it may reflect a desire to avoid overt expression of emotion. Similarly, avoidance of eye contact may be a cultural expression of respect for the speaker in some Native Americans and Asian Americans.

Culturally Mediated Characteristics

Nurses should be aware that patients act and behave in a variety of ways, in part because of the influence of culture on behaviors and attitudes. However, although certain attributes and attitudes are frequently associated with particular cultural groups, as described in the following pages, it is important to remember that not all people from the same cultural background share the same behaviors and views. Although nurses who fail to consider patients' cultural preferences and beliefs are considered insensitive and possibly indifferent, nurses who assume that all members of any one culture act and behave in the same way run the risk of stereotyping people. As previously stated, the best way to avoid stereotyping is to view each patient as an individual and to find out the patient's cultural preferences. A thorough culture assessment using a culture assessment tool or questionnaire (see later discussion) is very beneficial.

Many aspects of care may be influenced by the diverse cultural perspectives held by health care providers, patients, families, or significant others. One example is the issue of informed consent and full disclosure. In general, nurses may argue that patients have the right to full disclosure concerning their disease and prognosis and may believe that advocacy means working to provide that disclosure. However, family members in some cultural backgrounds may believe it is their responsibility to protect and spare the patient (their loved one) knowledge about a terminal illness. Similarly, patients may in fact not want to know about their condition and may expect their family members to "take the burden" of that knowledge and related decision making. Nurses should not decide that a family or patient is simply wrong or that a patient must know all details of his or her illness regardless of the patient's preference. Similar concerns may be noted when patients refuse pain medication or treatment because of cultural beliefs regarding pain or beliefs in divine intervention or faith healing.

Determining the most appropriate and ethical approach to patient care requires an exploration of the cultural aspects of these situations. Self-examination and recognition of one's own cultural bias and world view, as discussed earlier, play a major part in helping the nurse resolve cultural and ethical conflicts. Nurses must promote open dialogue and work with patients, families, physicians, and other health care providers to reach the culturally appropriate solution for the individual patient.

Space and Distance

People tend to regard the space in their immediate vicinity as an extension of themselves. The amount of space they need between themselves and others to feel comfortable is a culturally determined phenomenon.

Because nurses and patients usually are not consciously aware of their personal space requirements, they frequently have difficulty understanding different behaviors in this regard. For example, one patient may perceive the nurse sitting close to him or her as an expression of warmth and care; another patient may perceive the nurse's act as a threatening invasion of personal space. Research reveals that people from the United States, Canada, and Great Britain require the most personal space between themselves and others, whereas those from Latin America, Japan, and the Middle East need the least amount of space and feel comfortable standing close to others (Giger & Davidhizar, 2004).

If the patient appears to position himself or herself too close or too far away, the nurse should consider cultural preferences for space and distance. Ideally, the patient should be permitted to assume a position that is comfortable to him or her in terms of personal space and distance. The nurse should be aware that the wheelchair of a person with a disability is considered an extension of the person; therefore, the nurse should ask the person's permission before moving or touching the wheelchair. Because a significant amount of communication during nursing care requires close physical contact, the nurse should be aware of these important cultural differences and consider them when providing care (Simpson, 2004).

Eye Contact

Eye contact is also a culturally determined behavior. Although most nurses have been taught to maintain eye contact when speaking with patients, some people from certain cultural backgrounds may interpret this behavior differently. For example, some Asians, Native Americans, Indo-Chinese, Arabs, and Appalachians may consider direct eye contact impolite or aggressive, and they may avert their own eyes when talking with nurses and others whom they perceive to be in positions of authority. Some Native Americans stare at the floor during conversations, a cultural behavior conveying respect and indicating that the listener is paying close attention to the speaker. Some Hispanic patients maintain downcast eyes as a sign of appropriate deferential behavior toward others on the basis of age, gender, social position, economic status, and position of authority (Giger & Davidhizar, 2004). If the nurse is aware that eye contact may be culturally determined, he or she can better understand the patient's behavior and provide an atmosphere in which the patient can feel comfortable.

Time

Attitudes about time vary widely among cultures and can be a barrier to effective communication between nurses and patients. Views about punctuality and the use of time are culturally determined, as is the concept of waiting. Symbols of time, such as watches, sunrises, and sunsets, represent methods for measuring the duration and passage of time (Giger & Davidhizar, 2004; Spector, 2004).

For most health care providers, time and promptness are extremely important. For example, nurses frequently expect patients to arrive at an exact time for an appointment, although patients are often kept waiting by health care providers who are running late. Health care providers are likely to function according to an appointment system in which there are short intervals of perhaps only a few minutes. However, for patients from some cultures, time is a relative phenomenon, with little attention paid to the exact hour or minute. For example, some Hispanic people consider time in a wider frame of reference and make the primary distinction between day and night. Time may also be determined according to traditional times for meals, sleep, and other activities or events. For people from some cultures, the present is of the greatest importance, and time is viewed in broad ranges rather than in terms of a fixed hour. Being flexible in regard to schedules is the best way to accommodate these differences.

Value differences also may influence a person's sense of priority when it comes to time. For example, responding to a family matter may be more important to a patient than meeting a scheduled health care appointment. Allowing for these different views is essential in maintaining an effective nurse–patient relationship. Scolding or acting annoyed at patients for being late undermines their confidence and may result in further missed appointments or indifference to health care suggestions.

Touch

The meaning people associate with touching is culturally determined to a great degree. In some cultures (eg, Hispanic, Arab), male health care providers may be prohibited from touching or examining certain parts of the female body. Similarly, it may be inappropriate for females to care for males. Among many Asian Americans, it is impolite to touch a person's head because the spirit is believed to reside there. Therefore, assessment of the head or evaluation of a head injury requires permission of the patient or a family member, if the patient is not able to give permission.

The patient's culturally defined sense of modesty must also be considered when providing nursing care. For example, some Jewish and Islamic women believe that modesty requires covering their head, arms, and legs with clothing.

Observance of Holidays

People from all cultures observe certain civil and religious holidays. Nurses should familiarize themselves with major observances for members of the cultural groups they serve. Information about these observances is available from various sources, including religious organizations, hospital chaplains, and patients themselves. Routine health appointments, diagnostic tests, surgery, and other major procedures should be scheduled to avoid observances patients identify as significant. If not contraindicated, efforts should also be made to accommodate patients and families or significant others who wish to perform cultural and religious rituals in the health care setting.

Diet

The cultural meanings associated with food vary widely but usually include one or more of the following: relief of hunger; promotion of health and healing; prevention of disease or illness; expression of caring for another; promotion of interpersonal closeness among individual people, families, groups, communities, or nations; and promotion of kinship and family alliances. Food may also be associated with solidification of social ties; celebration of life events (eg, birthdays, marriages, funerals); expression of gratitude or appreciation; recognition of achievement or accomplishment; validation of social, cultural, or religious ceremonial functions; facilitation of business negotiations; and expression of affluence, wealth, or social status.

Culture determines which foods are served and when they are served, the number and frequency of meals, who eats with whom, and who is given the choicest portions. Culture also determines how foods are prepared and served, how they are eaten (with chopsticks, hands, or fork, knife, and spoon), and where people shop (eg, ethnic grocery stores, specialty food markets). Culture also determines the impact of excess weight and obesity on self-esteem and social standing. In some cultures, physical bulk is viewed as a sign of affluence and health (eg, a healthy baby is a chubby baby).

Religious practices may include fasting (eg, Mormons, Catholics, Buddhists, Jews, Muslims), abstaining from selected foods at particular times (eg, Catholics abstain from meat on Ash Wednesday and on Fridays during Lent), and considerations for medication use (eg, Muslims may prefer to use non–pork-derived insulin). Practices may also include the ritualistic use of food and beverages (eg, Passover dinner, consumption of bread and wine during religious ceremonies). Chart 8-2 summarizes some dietary practices of selected religious groups.

Many groups tend to feast, often in the company of family and friends, on selected holidays. For example, many Christians eat large dinners on Christmas and Easter and consume other traditional high-calorie, high-fat foods, such as seasonal cookies, pastries, and candies. These culturally based dietary practices are especially significant in the care of patients with diabetes, hypertension, gastrointestinal disorders, obesity, and other conditions in which diet plays a key role in the treatment and health maintenance regimen.

CHART 8-2

Prohibited Foods and Beverages of Selected Religious Groups

Hinduism

All meats
Animal shortenings

Islam

Pork
Alcoholic products and beverages (including extracts, such as vanilla and lemon)
Animal shortenings
Gelatin made with pork, marshmallow, and other confections made with gelatin

Judaism

Pork
Predatory fowl
Shellfish and scavenger fish (eg, shrimp, crab, lobster, escargot, catfish). Fish with fins and scales are permissible.
Mixing milk and meat dishes at same meal
Blood by ingestion (eg, blood sausage, raw meat). Blood by transfusion is acceptable.
Note: Packaged foods will contain labels identifying kosher ("properly preserved" or "fitting") and pareve (made without meat or milk) items.

Mormonism (Church of Jesus Christ of Latter-Day Saints)

Alcohol
Tobacco
Beverages containing caffeine stimulants (coffee, tea, colas, and selected carbonated soft drinks)

Seventh-Day Adventism

Pork
Certain seafood, including shellfish
Fermented beverages
Note: Optional vegetarianism is encouraged.

Biologic Variations

Along with psychosocial adaptations, nurses must also consider the physiologic impact of culture on patients' response to treatment, particularly medications. Data have been collected for many years regarding differences in the effect some medications have on people of diverse ethnic or cultural origins. Genetic predispositions to different rates of metabolism cause some patients to be prone to overdose reactions to the standard dose of a medication, whereas other patients are likely to experience a greatly reduced benefit from the standard dose of the medication. For example, an antihypertensive agent may work well for a white man within a 4-week time span but may take much longer to work or not work at all for an African-American man with hypertension. General polymorphism—biologic variation in response to medications resulting from patient age, gender, size, and body composition—has long been acknowledged by the health care community. Nurses must be aware that ethnicity and related factors such as values and beliefs regarding the use of herbal supplements, dietary intake, and genetic factors can affect the effectiveness of treatment and compliance with the treatment regimen (Giger & Davidhizar, 2004; Green-Hernandez et al., 2004).

Complementary and Alternative Therapies

Interventions for alterations in health and wellness vary among cultures. Interventions most commonly used in the United States have been labeled as *conventional medicine* by the National Institutes of Health (NCCAM, 2004). Other names for conventional medicine are allopathy, Western medicine, regular medicine, mainstream medicine, and biomedicine. Alternative therapy used to supplement conventional medicine may be referred to as *complementary therapy*. Interest in interventions that are not an integral part of conventional medicine prompted the National Institutes of Health to create the Office of Alternative Medicine in 1992, and then to establish the National Center for Complementary and Alternative Medicine (NCCAM) in 1999.

According to a nationwide survey, 36% of adults in the United States use some form of complementary and alternative medicine. This value increases to 75% when prayer specifically for health reasons is included in the definition. Complementary and alternative interventions are classified into five main categories: alternative medical systems, mind–body interventions, biologically based therapies, manipulative and body-based methods, and energy therapies (NCCAM, 2004):

- *Alternative medical systems* are defined as complete systems of theory and practice that are different from conventional medicine. Some examples are traditional Eastern medicine (including acupuncture, herbal medicine, Oriental massage, and Qi gong); India's traditional medicine, Ayurveda (including diet, exercise, meditation, herbal medicine, massage, exposure to sunlight, and controlled breathing to restore harmony of a person's body, mind, and spirit); homeopathic medicine (including herbal medicine and minerals); and naturopathic medicine (including diet, acupuncture, herbal medicine, hydrotherapy, spinal and soft-tissue manipulation, electrical currents, ultrasound and light therapy, therapeutic counseling, and pharmacology).
- *Mind–body interventions* are defined as techniques to facilitate the mind's ability to affect symptoms and bodily functions. Some examples are meditation, dance, music, art therapy, prayer, and mental healing.
- *Biologically based therapies* are defined as natural and biologically based practices, interventions, and products. Some examples are herbal therapies (an herb is a plant or plant part that produces and contains chemical substances that act on the body), special diet therapies (such as those of Drs. Atkins, Ornish, and Pritikin), orthomolecular therapies (magnesium, melatonin, megadoses of vitamins), and biologic therapies (shark cartilage, bee pollen).
- *Manipulative and body-based methods* are defined as interventions based on body movement. Some examples are chiropractic (primarily manipulation of the spine), osteopathic manipulation, massage therapy (soft-tissue manipulation), and reflexology.
- *Energy therapies* are defined as interventions that focus on energy fields within the body (biofields) or externally (electromagnetic fields). Some examples are Qi gong, Reiki, therapeutic touch, pulsed electromagnetic fields, magnetic fields, alternating electrical current, and direct electrical current.

Patients may choose to seek an alternative to conventional medical or surgical therapies. Many of these alternative therapies are becoming widely accepted as feasible treatment options. Therapies such as acupuncture and herbal treatments may be recommended by physicians to address aspects of a condition that are unresponsive to conventional medical treatment or to minimize the side effects associated with conventional medical therapy. Physicians and advanced practice nurses may work in collaboration with herbalists or with spiritualists or shamans to provide a comprehensive treatment plan. Out of respect for the way of life and beliefs of patients from different cultures, it is often necessary that the healers and health care providers respect the strengths of each approach (NCCAM, 2004).

Complementary therapy is becoming more common as health care consumers learn what information is available in printed media and on the Internet. As patients become more informed, they are more likely to participate in a variety of therapies in conjunction with their conventional medical treatments (Barnes, Powell-Griner, McFann, et al., 2004). Nurses must assess all patients for use of complementary therapies, be alert to the danger of herb–drug interactions or conflicting treatments, and be prepared to provide information to patients about treatments that may be harmful. However, nurses must be accepting of patients' beliefs and right to control their own care. As patient advocates, nurses facilitate the integration of conventional medical, complementary, and alternative therapies.

Causes of Illness

Three major views, or paradigms, attempt to explain the causes of disease and illness: the biomedical or scientific view, the naturalistic or holistic perspective, and the magico-religious view.

Biomedical or Scientific

The biomedical or scientific world view prevails in most health care settings and is embraced by most nurses and other health care providers. The basic assumptions underlying the biomedical perspective are that all events in life have a cause and effect, that the human body functions much like a machine, and that all of reality can be observed and measured (eg, blood pressures, PaO_2 levels, intelligence tests). One example of the biomedical or scientific view is the bacterial or viral explanation of communicable diseases.

Naturalistic or Holistic

The second way that some cultures explain the cause of illness is through the naturalistic or holistic perspective, a viewpoint that is found among many Native Americans, Asians, and others. According to this view, the forces of nature must be kept in natural balance or harmony.

One example of a naturalistic belief, held by many Asian groups, is the yin/yang theory, in which health is believed to exist when all aspects of a person are in perfect balance or harmony. Rooted in the ancient Chinese philosophy of Taoism (which translates as "The Way"), the yin/yang theory proposes that all organisms and objects in the universe consist of yin and yang energy. The seat of the energy forces is within the autonomic nervous system, where balance between the opposing forces is maintained during health. Yin energy represents the female and negative forces, such as emptiness, darkness, and cold, whereas the yang forces are male and positive, emitting warmth and fullness. Foods are classified as cold (yin) or hot (yang) in this theory and are transformed into yin and yang energy when metabolized by the body. Cold foods are eaten when a person has a hot illness (eg, fever, rash, sore throat, ulcer, infection), and hot foods are eaten when a person has a cold illness (eg, cancer, headache, stomach cramps, "cold"). The yin/yang theory is the basis for Eastern or Chinese medicine and is embraced by some Asian Americans.

Many Hispanic, African-American, and Arab groups also embrace the hot/cold theory of health and illness. The four humors of the body—blood, phlegm, black bile, and yellow bile—regulate basic bodily functions and are described in terms of temperature and moisture. The treatment of disease consists of adding or subtracting cold, heat, dryness, or wetness to restore the balance of these humors. Beverages, foods, herbs, medicines, and diseases are classified as hot or cold according to their perceived effects on the body, not their physical characteristics. According to the hot/cold theory, the person as a whole, not just a particular ailment, is significant. People who embrace the hot/cold theory maintain that health consists of a positive state of total well-being, including physical, psychological, spiritual, and social aspects of the person.

According to the naturalistic world view, breaking the laws of nature creates imbalances, chaos, and disease. People who embrace the naturalistic paradigm use metaphors such as "the healing power of nature." For example, from the perspective of many Chinese people, illness is viewed not as an intruding agent but as a part of life's rhythmic course and an outward sign of disharmony within.

Magico-Religious

The third major way in which people view the world and explain the causes of illness is the magico-religious world view. This view's basic premise is that the world is an arena in which supernatural forces dominate and that the fate of the world and those in it depends on the action of supernatural forces for good or evil. Examples of magical causes of illness include belief in voodoo or witchcraft among some African Americans and people from Caribbean countries. Faith healing is based on religious beliefs and is most prevalent among selected Christian religions, including Christian Science, whereas various healing rituals may be found in many other religions, such as Roman Catholicism and Mormonism (Church of Jesus Christ of Latter-Day Saints).

Of course, it is possible to hold a combination of world views, and many patients offer more than one explanation for the cause of their illness. As a profession, nursing largely embraces the scientific or biomedical world view, but some aspects of holism have begun to gain popularity, including a wide variety of techniques for managing chronic pain, such as hypnosis, therapeutic touch, and biofeedback. Belief in spiritual power is also held by many nurses who credit supernatural forces with various unexplained phenomena related to patients' health and illness states. Regardless of the view held and whether the nurse agrees with the patient's beliefs in this regard, it is important to be aware of how the person views illness and health and to work within this framework to promote patient care and well-being.

Folk Healers

People of some cultures believe in folk or indigenous healers. For example, nurses may find that some Hispanic patients may seek help from a *curandero* or *curandera, espiritualista* (spiritualist), *yerbo* (herbalist), or *sabador* (healer who manipulates bones and muscles). Some African-American patients may seek assistance from a *hougan* (voodoo priest or priestess), spiritualist, root doctor (usually a woman who uses magic rituals to treat diseases), or "old lady" (an older woman who has successfully raised a family and who specializes in child care and folk remedies). Native American patients may seek assistance from a shaman or medicine man or woman. Asian patients may mention that they have visited herbalists, acupuncturists, or bone setters. Several cultures have their own healers, most of whom speak the native tongue of that culture, make house calls, and cost significantly less than healers practicing in the conventional medical health care system.

People seeking complementary and alternative therapies have expanded the practices of folk healers beyond their traditional populations, so the nurse should ask the patient about use of folk healers regardless of the patient's cultural background. It is best not to disregard the patient's belief in folk healers or try to undermine trust in the healers. To do so may alienate the patient and drive him or her away from receiving the prescribed care. Nurses should make an effort to accommodate the patient's beliefs while also advocating the treatment proposed by health science.

Cultural Assessment

Cultural nursing assessment refers to a systematic appraisal or examination of individuals, families, groups, and communities in terms of their cultural beliefs, values, and practices. The purpose of such an assessment is to provide culturally competent care (Giger & Davidhizar, 2004). In an effort to establish a database for determining a patient's cultural background, nurses have developed cultural assessment tools or modified existing assessment tools (Leininger, 2001; Spector, 2004) to ensure that transcultural considerations are included in the plan of care. Giger and Davidhizar's model has been used to design nursing care from health promotion to nursing skills activities (Giger & Davidhizar, 2004; Smith-Temple & Johnson, 2005). The information presented in this chapter and the general guidelines presented in Chart 8-3 can be used to direct nursing assessment of culture and its influence on a patient's health beliefs and practices.

Additional Cultural Considerations: Know Thyself

Because the nurse–patient interaction is the focal point of nursing, nurses should consider their own cultural orientation when conducting assessments of patients and their families and friends. The following guidelines may prove useful to nurses wishing to provide culturally appropriate care:

- Know your own cultural attitudes, values, beliefs, and practices.
- Regardless of "good intentions," everyone has cultural "baggage" that ultimately results in ethnocentrism.
- In general, it is easier to understand those whose cultural heritage is similar to your own, while viewing those who are unlike you as strange and different.
- Maintain a broad, open attitude. Expect the unexpected. Enjoy surprises.
- Avoid seeing all people as alike; that is, avoid cultural stereotypes, such as "all Chinese like rice" or "all Italians eat spaghetti."
- Try to understand the reasons for any behavior by discussing commonalities and differences.
- If a patient has said or done something that you do not understand, ask for clarification. Be a good listener. Most patients will respond positively to questions that arise from a genuine concern for and interest in them.
- If at all possible, speak the patient's language (even simple greetings and social courtesies are appreciated). Avoid feigning an accent or using words that are ordinarily not part of your vocabulary.
- Be yourself. There are no right or wrong ways to learn about cultural diversity.

CHART 8-3

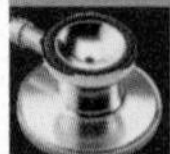

Assessing for Patients' Cultural Beliefs

- What is the patient's country of origin? How long has the patient lived in this country? What is the patient's primary language and literacy level?
- What is the patient's ethnic background? Does he or she identify strongly with others from the same cultural background?
- What is the patient's religion, and how important is it to his or her daily life?
- Does the patient participate in cultural activities such as dressing in traditional clothing and observing traditional holidays and festivals?
- Are there any food preferences or restrictions?
- What are the patient's communication styles? Is eye contact avoided? How much physical distance is maintained? Is the patient open and verbal about symptoms?
- Who is the head of the family, and is he or she involved in decision making about the patient?
- What does the patient do to maintain his or her health?
- What does the patient think caused the current problem?
- Has the advice of traditional healers been sought?
- Have complementary and alternative therapies been used?
- What kind of treatment does the patient think will help? What are the most important results he or she hopes to get from this treatment?
- Are there cultural or religious rituals related to health, sickness, or death that the patient observes?

Health Disparities

Health disparities—higher rates of morbidity, mortality, and burden of disease in a population or community than found in the overall population—are significant in ethnic and racial minorities. Key health indicators in the United States reveal a significant gap in health status between the overall American population and people of specific ethnic backgrounds (Keltner, Kelley, & Smith, 2004). Ethnic and racial minorities are disproportionately burdened with cancer, heart disease, diabetes, human immunodeficiency virus (HIV) infection/acquired immunodeficiency syndrome (AIDS), and other conditions. They receive a lower quality of health care than non-minorities and are at a greater risk for declining health. Many reasons are cited for these disparities, including low socioeconomic status; health behaviors; limited access to health care because of poverty or disability; environmental factors; and direct and indirect manifestations of discrimination. Other causes include lack of health insurance; overdependence on publicly funded facilities; and barriers to health care such as insufficient transportation, geographic location (not enough providers in an area), cost of services, and the low numbers of minority health care providers (Baldwin, 2004; Beal, 2004; Institute of Medicine, 2003).

The Future of Transcultural Nursing Care

By the middle of the 21st century, the average American patient will trace his or her ancestry to Africa, Asia, the Pacific Islands, or the Hispanic or Arab worlds, rather than to Europe (Giger & Davidhizar, 2004). As indicated previously, the concept of culturally competent care applies to health care institutions, which must develop culturally sensitive policies and provide a climate that fosters the provision of culturally competent care by nurses. Nurses, who reflect the multicultural complexion of our society, must learn to acknowledge and adapt to diversity among their colleagues in the workplace (Simpson, 2004).

As the population becomes more culturally diverse, efforts to increase the number of ethnic minority nurses must continue and accelerate (Sullivan Commission, 2004). Today more than 88% of all nurses are Caucasian. Progress in increasing the percentage of culturally diverse nurses has been significantly slower than the increasing percentage of ethnic minorities in the United States (Washington, Erickson, & Ditomasi, 2004). Greater efforts must be made to facilitate the recruitment and program completion of nursing students who are members of ethnic minorities. In addition, educational institutions must prepare nurses to deliver culturally competent care and must work to increase the number of ethnic minority providers in the nursing workforce. Nursing programs are exploring creative ways to promote cultural competence in nursing students, including offering multicultural health studies in their curricula (Spector, 2004).

Cultural diversity remains one of the foremost issues in health care today. With increasing frequency, nurses will be expected to provide culturally competent care for patients. Nurses must work effectively with the increasing number of patients, other nurses, and other health care team members whose ancestry reflects the multicultural complexion of contemporary society.

Critical Thinking Exercises

1. ebp You are assigned to care for a hospitalized patient whose cultural background is very different from yours. What is the evidence base for use of a cultural assessment tool to ensure that cultural considerations are included in the nursing plan of care? What is the strength of that evidence? What resources are available to you to promote culturally competent care? Explain why it is important to examine your own feelings about each patient's cultural beliefs and practices.
2. An elderly Asian woman who does not speak English is hospitalized with heart failure. Her immediate family members insist on staying with her around the clock, and many extended family members visit each day, staying late into the night. They share all their meals in the waiting room. Some staff members have complained that the family members are not adhering to the hospital's established visiting hours and are disturbing other patients and visitors. How can you help the nursing staff explore the meaning of the family's behavior and understand their own negative feelings about this behavior? Devise a strategy that will help resolve this situation.
3. You have been caring for an elderly patient who does not speak English. Her family members speak only limited English. You are unable to communicate well enough with the patient and the family to provide the necessary discharge teaching. What resources would you use to assist you in providing the discharge teaching? What aspects of the patient's and family's background would you want to assess to determine the need for referral to a home health care agency?

REFERENCES AND SELECTED READINGS

BOOKS

American Academy of Nursing, Subpanel on Cultural Competence in Nursing. (1995). *Promoting cultural competence in and through nursing education*. New York: Author.

American Association of Colleges of Nursing. (1996). *Diversity Task Force Report, October 1996*. Washington, DC: Author.

Andrews, M. M., & Boyle, J. S. (2002). *Transcultural concepts in nursing care* (4th ed.). Philadelphia: J. B. Lippincott.

Giger, J. N., & Davidhizar, R. E. (2004). *Transcultural nursing: Assessment and intervention* (4th ed.). St. Louis: C. V. Mosby.

Institute of Medicine. (2003). *Unequal treatment: Confronting racial and ethnic disparities in healthcare*. Smedley, B. D., Stith, A. Y., & Nelson, A. R. (Eds.). Washington, DC: National Academy Press.

Leininger, M. M. (Ed.). (2001). *Culture care diversity and universality: A theory of nursing*. New York: National League for Nursing Press.

Smith-Temple, J., & Johnson, J. Y. (2005). *Nurse's guide to clinical procedures* (5th ed.). Philadelphia: Lippincott Williams & Wilkins.

Spector, R. E. (2004). *Cultural diversity in health and illness* (6th ed.). New Jersey: Prentice-Hall.

JOURNALS

Baldwin, D. M. (2004). Disparities in health and health care: Focusing efforts to eliminate unequal burdens. *Online Journal of Issues in Nursing. 8*(1), Manuscript 1. Available at: nursingworld.org/ojin/topic20/tpc20_1.htm

Barnes, P. M., Powell-Griner, E., McFann, K., et al. (May 27, 2004). Complementary and alternative medicine use among adults: United States, 2002. *Advance Data from Vital and Health Statistics, 343*.

Beal, A. (2004). Perspective: Policies to reduce racial and ethnic disparities in child health and health care. *Health Affairs, 23*(5), 171–179.

Betancourt, S. R. (2004). Cultural competence—marginal or mainstream movement? *New England Journal of Medicine, 351*(10), 953–954.

Campinha-Bacote, J. (2003). Many faces: Addressing diversity in health care. *Online Journal of Issues in Nursing, 8*(1). Available at http://www.nursingworld.org/ojin/topics20/tpc20_2.htm

Flowers, D. (2004). Culturally competent nursing care: A challenge for the 21st century. *Critical Care Nurse, 24*(4), 48–52.

Green-Hernandez, C., Quinn, A. A., Denman-Vitale, S., et al. (2004). Making nursing care culturally competent. *Holistic Nursing Practice, 29*(4), 215–218.

Keltner, B., Kelley, F., & Smith, D. (2004). Leadership to reduce health disparities. *Nursing Administration Quarterly, 28*(3), 181–190.

Leininger, M. M. (1988). Leininger's theory of nursing: Cultural care diversity and universality. *Nursing Science Quarterly, 1*(4), 152–159.

National Institutes of Health, National Center for Complementary and Alternative Medicine (NCCAM). *Major domains of complementary and alternative medicine*. http://nccam.nih.gov (Accessed May 5, 2006).

Simpson, R. (2004). Recruit, retain, assess technology's role in diversity. *Nursing Administration Quarterly, 28*(3), 217–220.

Swanson, J. W. (2004). Diversity: Creating an environment of inclusiveness. *Nursing Administration Quarterly, 28*(3), 145–169.

Washington, D., Erikson, J. I., & Ditomassi, M. (2004). Mentoring the minority nurse leader of tomorrow. *Nursing Administration Quarterly, 28*(3), 165–169.

Watts, R. (2003). Race consciousness and the health of African Americans. *Online Journal of Issues in Nursing, 8*(1), Manuscript 3. Available at: http://nursingworld.org/ojin/topic20/tpc20_3.htm. Accessed May 5, 2006.

RESOURCES

ORGANIZATIONS

Asian & Pacific Islander Nurses Association, 400 N. Ingalls, Suite 3160, Ann Arbor, MI 48109; 734-998-1030

Council on Nursing and Anthropology, c/o Dr. Mildred Roberson, Nursing and Health Sciences, Salisbury State University, Salisbury, MD 21801

Language Line Services; 1-877-886-3885; http://www.languageline.com/. Accessed July 6, 2006. (Provides written and oral translation in 140 languages.)

National Black Nurses Association, 8630 Fenton St., Suite 330, Silver Spring, MD 20910; 301-589-3200; http://www.nbna.org. Accessed June 6, 2006.

National Institutes of Health, National Center for Complementary and Alternative Medicine, 6707 Democracy Blvd., Suite 2000, Bethesda, MD 20892; 1-888-644-6226; fax 1-866-464-3616; http://nccam.nih.gov. Accessed June 6, 2006.

Office of Minority Health, U.S. Department of Health and Human Services, 5600 Fisher's Lane, Room 10-49, Rockville, MD 20857; 301-443-5084; http://www.omhrc.gov. Accessed June 6, 2006.

Transcultural Nursing Society, c/o Madonna University College of Nursing and Health, 36600 Schoolcraft Road, Livonia MI 48150; 888-432-5470; http://www.tcns.org. Accessed June 6, 2006.

CHAPTER 9

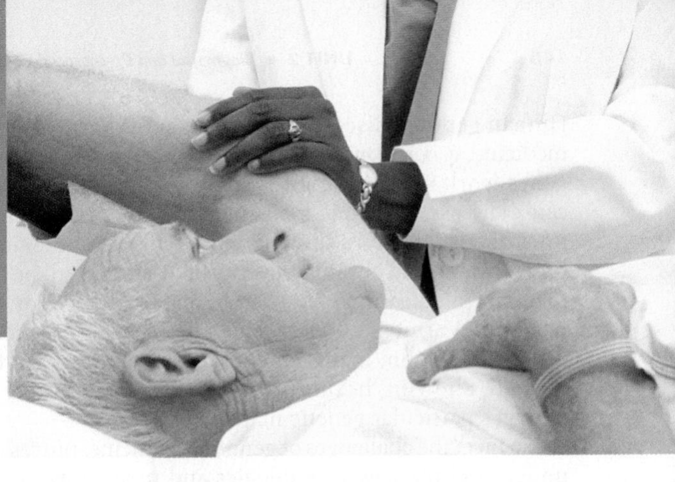

Genetics Perspectives in Nursing

Learning Objectives

On completion of this chapter, the learner will be able to:

1. Describe the role of the nurse in integrating genetics in nursing care.
2. Conduct a genetics-based assessment.
3. Identify the common patterns of inheritance of genetic disorders.
4. Identify ethical issues in nursing related to genetics.

Human **genome** discoveries have ushered in a new era of medicine, *genomic medicine,* which recognizes that multiple genes work in concert with environmental influences to cause disease. Genomic medicine aims to improve predictions about a person's susceptibility to diseases; the time of onset, extent, and eventual severity of diseases; and the treatments or medications likely to be most effective or most harmful (Varmus, 2004). New gene-based strategies for disease detection, management, and treatment have been created, allowing health professionals to tailor care to a person's particular genetic makeup.

To meet the challenges of genomic medicine, nurses must understand the new technologies and treatments of gene-based health care. Nurses also must recognize that they are a vital link between the patient and health care services; patients often turn to nurses first with questions about a family history of risk factors, genetics information, and genetic tests and interpretations. The incorporation of genetics into nursing means bringing a genetic framework to health assessments, planning, and interventions that supports identification of and response to the changing genetics-related health needs of people (Lea & Monsen, 2003).

When obtaining family and health histories, nurses must learn to recognize patterns of inheritance and understand when it is appropriate to consider new gene-based testing and treatment options. This chapter offers a foundation for the clinical application of genetics principles in medical and surgical nursing, outlines the nurse's role in genetic coun-

Glossary

allele: any one of two or more alternate forms of a gene at the same location. An allele for each gene is inherited from each parent.

autosome: a single chromosome from any of the 22 pairs of chromosomes not involved in sex determination (XX or XY)

carrier: person who is heterozygous; possessing two different alleles of a gene pair

chromosome: microscopic structures in the cell nucleus that contain genetic information and are constant in number in a species (eg, humans have 46 chromosomes)

deoxyribonucleic acid (DNA): the primary genetic material in humans consisting of nitrogenous bases, a sugar group, and phosphate combined into a double helix

diploid: the number of chromosomes normally present in somatic cells. For humans, that number is 46

dominant: a genetic trait that is normally expressed when a person has a gene mutation on one of a pair of chromosomes and the "normal" form of the gene is on the other chromosome

genetics: the scientific study of heredity; how specific traits or predispositions are transmitted from parents to offspring

genome: the total genetic complement of an individual genotype

genomics: the study of the human genome, including gene sequencing, mapping, and function

genotype: the genes and the variations therein that a person inherits from his or her parents

haploid: the number of chromosomes present in egg or sperm (gametes); in humans, this is 23

Human Genome Project: an international research effort aimed at identifying and characterizing the order of every base in the human genome

meiosis: the reduction division of diploid egg or sperm (germ cells) resulting in haploid gametes (having 23 chromosomes each)

mitosis: cell division occurring in somatic cells that normally results in daughter cells with the same number of chromosomes—46 (diploid)

monosomy: missing one of a chromosome pair in normally diploid cells (for example, 45,X females have only one X chromosome)

mutation: a heritable alteration in the genetic material

nondisjunction: the failure of a chromosome pair to separate appropriately during meiosis, resulting in abnormal chromosome numbers in reproductive cells (gametes)

nucleotide: a nucleic acid "building block" composed of a nitrogenous base, a five-carbon sugar, and a phosphate group

pedigree: a diagrammatic representation of a family history

penetrance: the percentage of individuals known to carry the gene for a trait who actually manifest the condition. For example, a trait with 90% penetrance will not be manifested by 10% of persons possessing the gene.

phenotype: a person's entire physical, biochemical, and physiologic makeup, as determined by the person's genotype and environmental factors

polymorphism: a genetic variation with two or more alleles that is maintained in a population

population screening: the application of a test or inquiry to a group to determine if persons in the group have an increased likelihood of a genetic condition or a mutation in a specific gene (eg, cholesterol screening for hypercholesterolemia)

predisposition testing: testing that is used to determine the likelihood that a healthy person with or without a family history of a condition will develop the disorder. Having the gene mutation would indicate that the person has an increased susceptibility to the disorder, but this is not a diagnosis. One example is DNA mutation testing for hereditary breast/ovarian cancer.

prenatal screening: testing that is used to identify whether a fetus is at risk for a birth defect such as Down syndrome or spina bifida (eg, multiple marker maternal serum screening in pregnancy)

presymptomatic testing: genetic testing that is used to determine whether persons with a family history of a disorder, but no current symptoms, have the gene mutation. An example of this would be Huntington disease.

recessive: a genetic trait that is expressed only when a person has two copies of a mutant autosomal gene or a single copy of a mutant X-linked gene in the absence of another X chromosome

transcription: the process of transforming information from DNA into new strands of messenger RNA

trisomy: the presence of one extra chromosome in an otherwise diploid chromosome complement—for example, trisomy 21 (Down syndrome)

variable expression: variation in the degree to which a trait is manifested; clinical severity

X-linked: located on the X chromosome

seling and evaluation, addresses important ethical issues, and provides genetics resources for nurses and patients.

Framework for Integrating Genetics Into Nursing Practice

The unique contribution of nursing to genomic medicine is its philosophy of holism. Nurses are ideally positioned to incorporate genetics into the care of patients at all ages and stages of life and in all settings. The holistic view that characterizes nursing takes into account each person's intellectual, physical, spiritual, social, cultural, biopsychologic, ethical, and esthetic experiences while addressing genetic information, gene-based testing, diagnosis, and treatment. Thus, knowledge of genetics is basic to nursing practice (Olsen, Feetham, Jenkins, et al., 2003).

A framework for integrating genetics into nursing practice includes a philosophy of care that recognizes when genetic factors are playing a role or could play a role in a person's health. This means using family history and the results of genetic tests effectively, informing patients about genetics concepts, understanding the personal and societal impact of genetics information, and valuing the privacy and confidentiality of genetics information.

A person's response to genetics information, genetic testing, or genetics-related conditions may be either empowering or disabling. Genetics information may stigmatize people if it affects how they view themselves or how others view them. Nurses can help individuals and families learn how genetic traits and conditions are passed on within families and how genetic and environmental factors influence health and disease (Greco, 2003).

Nurses facilitate communication among family members, the health care system, and community resources, and they offer valuable support by virtue of their continuity of care with patients and families. All nurses should be able to recognize when a patient is asking a question related to genetics information and should know how to obtain genetics information by gathering family and health histories and conducting physical and developmental assessments. Being able to recognize a genetics concern allows nurses to provide appropriate genetics resources and support to patients and families (Lea & Monsen, 2003).

Essential to a genetic framework in nursing is the awareness of one's attitudes, experience, and assumptions about genetics concepts and how these are manifested in one's own practice. Chart 9-1 offers insights on how nurses can conduct periodic self-assessments.

Genetics Concepts

Scientists and philosophers have long speculated about heredity and developed theories to explain how traits are transmitted to offspring. Developments in technology and research have increased understanding of genetics, resulting in better understanding of relatively rare diseases such as phenylketonuria (PKU) or hemophilia that are related to mutations of a single gene inherited in families. New technologies and tools allow scientists to characterize inherited metabolic variations that interact over time and lead to common diseases such as cancer, heart disease, and dementia. This transition from **genetics** to **genomics** highlights how understanding of single genes and their individual functions has evolved to understanding how multiple genes act and control biologic processes. Most health conditions are now believed to be the result of a combination of genetic and environmental influences (Guttmacher & Collins, 2004).

Genes and Their Role in Human Variation

Genes are central components of human health and disease. Work on the **Human Genome Project** (an international research effort to map and sequence the human genome) has shown how basic human genetics is to human development, health, and disease. Knowledge that specific genes are associated with specific genetic conditions makes diagnosis possible, even in the unborn. Research demonstrates that many common conditions have genetic causes. Many more associations between genetics, health, and disease are likely be identified with refinement of human genome mapping and sequencing.

Genes and Chromosomes

A person's unique genetic constitution, called a **genotype**, is made up of some 30,000 to 40,000 genes (Guttmacher & Collins, 2004). A person's **phenotype**, the observable characteristics of his or her genotype, includes physical appearance and other biologic, physiologic, and molecular traits. Environmental influences modify every person's phenotype, even phenotypes with a major genetic component.

Human growth, development, and disease occur as a result of both genetic and environmental influences and interactions. The contribution of genetic factors may be large or small. For example, in a person with cystic fibrosis or PKU, the genetic contribution is significant. In contrast, the genetic contribution underlying a person's response to infection may be less important.

A single gene is conceptualized as a unit of heredity. A gene is composed of a segment of **deoxyribonucleic acid (DNA)** that contains a specific set of instructions for making the protein or proteins needed by body cells for proper functioning. Genes regulate both the types of proteins made and the rate at which proteins are produced. The structure of the DNA molecule is referred to as the double helix. The essential components of the DNA molecule are sugar–phosphate molecules and pairs of nitrogenous bases. Each **nucleotide** contains a sugar (deoxyribose), a phosphate group, and one of four nitrogenous bases: adenine (A), cytosine (C), guanine (G), and thymine (T). DNA is composed of two paired strands, each made up of a number of nucleotides. The strands are held together by hydrogen bonds between pairs of bases (Fig. 9-1).

Genes are packaged and arranged in a linear order within **chromosomes**, which are located in the cell nucleus. In humans, 46 chromosomes occur in pairs in all body cells except oocytes (eggs) and sperm, which each contain only 23 chromosomes. Twenty-two pairs of chromosomes, called **autosomes**, are the same in females and males.

CHART 9-1

Examining Our Own Attitudes, Experiences, and Assumptions

Self-knowledge is one of the cornerstones to providing quality nursing care, and as practitioners, our attitudes and experiences have an impact on clinical practice. These attitudes emerge from social, cultural, and religious experiences in one's personal life. Awareness of our own values, beliefs, and cultural perceptions not only is important to the nurse–patient relationship but is also the first step in developing a genetics framework.

Periodic self-assessment can help maintain an effective framework as nurses update genetics knowledge and practice. Nurses can develop an awareness of their own attitudes, experiences, and assumptions about genetics concepts by considering the following:

- *One's family's beliefs or values about health.* What are your family, religious, or cultural beliefs about the cause of illness? How have your values or biases influenced your understanding of genetics conditions?
- *One's philosophical, theologic, cultural, and ethical perspectives related to health.* How would these attitudes influence your own use of genetics information or services? What experiences have you had with people from different social, cultural, religious, or ethnic groups? How would you deliver genetics information to individuals from different social, cultural, or ethnic groups? Can you recognize when personal values or biases may affect or interfere with the delivery of genetics information?
- *One's level of genetics expertise.* Can you recognize the limitations of your own experience in genetics and know when to refer patients for further genetic workup?
- *One's experience with birth defects, chronic illnesses, and genetic conditions.* Do you have a family member or friend who has a genetic condition or disorder? Has your experience been that genetic disorders are disabling or empowering? Do you view a parent as being "at fault" for having a baby born with a birth defect or genetic condition? Do you advocate for fair access and other rights for individuals who have birth defects, genetic conditions, or other disabilities?
- *One's view of DNA (the most basic concept of who we are, since our genetic makeup is unlike that of any other person except an identical twin).* What are your assumptions about DNA? For example, do you assume that the genetic component of "the self" is a defective self? As another example, healthy carriers of genetic alterations that predispose them to develop certain diseases in the future now belong to a new class of "at risk" individuals. A person who is "at risk" is not ill at present but may not remain well as long as the "average" person. Is it good to know that you are "at risk", or is this information that should not be identified or revealed because of the risk of potential discrimination?
- *One's beliefs about reproductive options.* What are your beliefs regarding reproductive options such as prenatal diagnosis and pregnancy termination? How might these influence your care of a patient who holds different beliefs?
- *One's view of genetic testing and engineering.* Do you see genetic testing and engineering—the ability to eliminate or enhance certain traits—as a way to create an "ideal genetic self"?
- *One's approach to patients with disabilities.* How are your attitudes made apparent in your practice and practice settings? For example, do you have access to TTY machines and/or interpreters for those who have hearing impairment? Are your intake procedures adapted to meet the needs of an individual with disabilities?

Adapted from National Coalition of Health Professional Education in Genetics. (2001). *Core competencies*; http://www.nchpeg.org; Kenan, R. (1996). The at-risk health status and technology: A diagnostic invitation and the gift of knowing. *Social Science and Medicine, 42*(11), 1545–1553; Peters, J. A., Djurdjinovic, L. & Baker, D. (1999). The genetic self: The Human Genome Project, genetic counseling and family therapy. *Families, Systems & Health, 17*(1), 5–25.

The 23rd pair is referred to as the sex chromosomes. A female has two X chromosomes, whereas a male has one X and one Y chromosome. At conception, each parent normally gives one chromosome of each pair to his or her children. As a result, children receive half of their chromosomes from their father and half from their mother (Fig. 9-2).

Careful examination of DNA sequences from many people shows that these sequences have multiple versions in a population. These different versions, or sequence variations, are called **alleles.** Sequences found in many forms are said to be polymorphic, meaning that there are at least two common forms of a particular gene.

Cell Division

The human body grows and develops as a result of the process of cell division. Mitosis and meiosis are two distinctly different types of cell division.

Mitosis is involved in cell growth, differentiation, and repair. During mitosis, the chromosomes of each cell du-

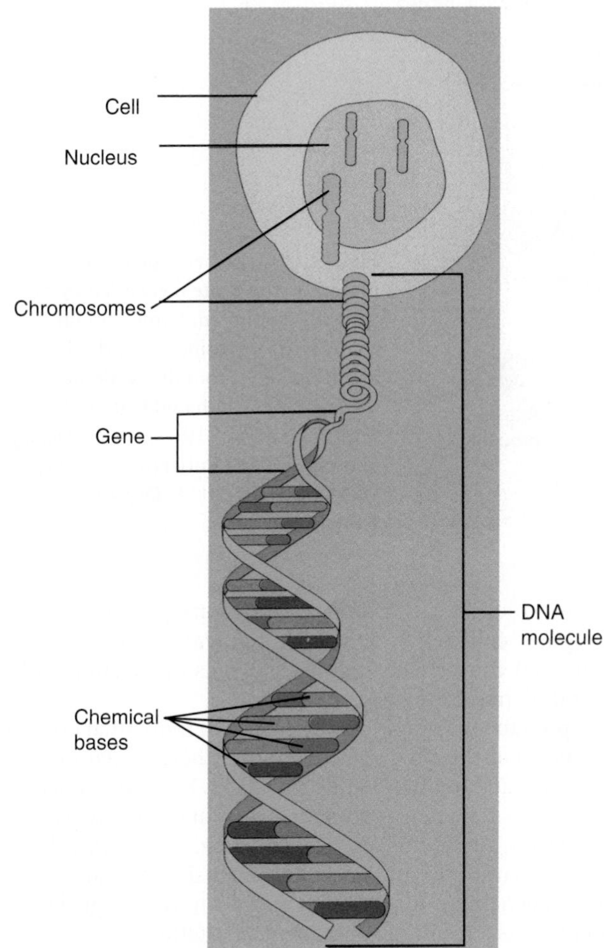

FIGURE 9-1. DNA carrying the instructions that allows cells to make proteins is made up of four chemical bases. Tightly coiled strands of DNA are packaged in units called chromosomes, which are housed in the cell's nucleus. Working subunits of DNA are known as genes. (From the National Institutes of Health and National Cancer Institute. [1995]. *Understanding gene testing* [NIH Pub. No. 96-3905]. Washington, DC: U.S. Department of Human Services.)

plicate. The result is two cells, called daughter cells, which each contain the same number of chromosomes as the parent cell. The daughter cells are said to be **diploid** because they contain 46 chromosomes in 23 pairs. Mitosis occurs in all cells of the body except oocytes (eggs) and sperm.

Meiosis, in contrast, occurs only in reproductive cells and is the process by which oocytes and sperm are formed. During meiosis, a reduction in the number of chromosomes takes place, resulting in oocytes or sperm that contain half the usual number, or 23 chromosomes. Oocytes and sperm are referred to as **haploid** because they contain a single copy of each chromosome, compared to the usual two copies in all other body cells. During the initial phase of meiosis, as the paired chromosomes come together in preparation for cell division, portions cross over, and an exchange of genetic material occurs before the chromosomes separate. This event, called recombination, creates greater diversity in the makeup of oocytes and sperm.

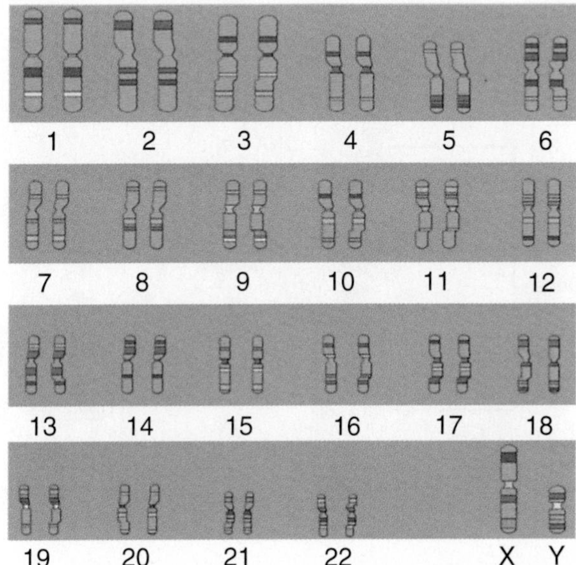

FIGURE 9-2. Each human cell contains 23 pairs of chromosomes, which can be distinguished by size and by their unique banding patterns. This set is from a male, because it contains a Y chromosome. Females have two X chromosomes. (From the National Institutes of Health and National Cancer Institute. [1995]. *Understanding gene testing* [NIH Pub. No. 96-3905]. Washington, DC: U.S. Department of Human Services.)

During meiosis, a pair of chromosomes may fail to separate completely, creating a sperm or oocyte that contains either two copies or no copy of a particular chromosome. This sporadic event, called **nondisjunction**, can lead to either a trisomy or a monosomy. Down syndrome is an example of **trisomy**. People with Down syndrome have three copies of chromosome number 21. Turner syndrome is an example of **monosomy**. Girls with Turner syndrome usually have a single X chromosome, causing them to have short stature and infertility (Rimoin, Connor, Pyeritz, et al., 2002).

Gene Mutations

Within each cell, many intricate and complex interactions regulate and express human genes. Gene structure and function, **transcription** and translation, and protein synthesis are all involved. Alterations in gene structure and function and the process of protein synthesis may influence a person's health. Changes in gene structure, called **mutations**, permanently change the sequence of DNA, which in turn can alter the nature and type of proteins made (Fig. 9-3).

Some gene mutations have no significant effect on the protein product, whereas others cause partial or complete changes. How a protein is altered and its importance to proper body functioning determine the impact of the mutation. Gene mutations may occur in hormones, enzymes, or other important protein products, with significant implications for health and disease. Sickle cell anemia is an example of a genetic condition caused by a small gene mutation that affects protein structure, producing hemoglobin S. A person who inherits two copies of the hemoglobin S gene

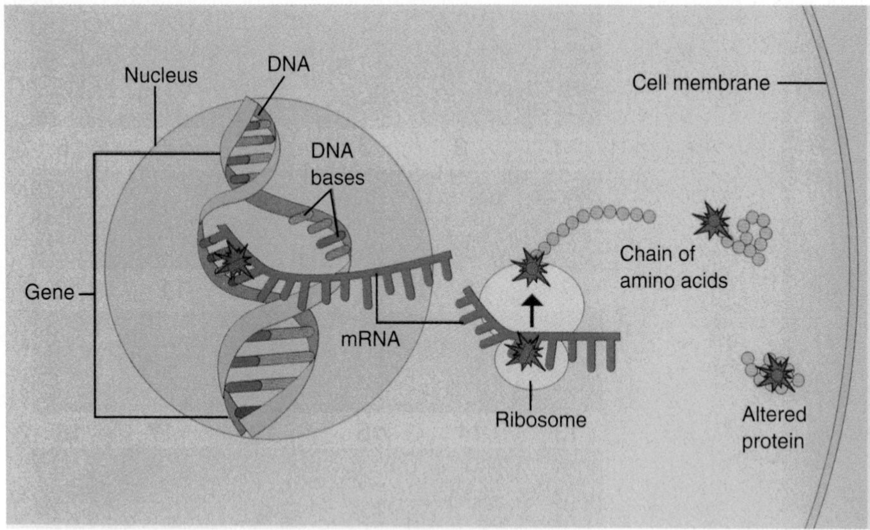

FIGURE 9-3. When a gene contains a mutation, the protein encoded by that gene will be altered. Some protein changes are insignificant, and others are disabling. (From the National Institutes of Health and National Cancer Institute. [1995]. *Understanding gene testing* [NIH Pub. No. 96-3905]. Washington, DC: U.S. Department of Human Services.)

mutation has sickle cell anemia and experiences the symptoms of severe anemia and thrombotic organ damage resulting from hypoxia (Rimoin et al., 2002).

Other gene mutations may be larger, such as a deletion (loss), insertion (addition), duplication (multiplication), or rearrangement (translocation) of a longer DNA segment. Duchenne muscular dystrophy, an inherited form of muscular dystrophy, is an example of a genetic disorder caused by structural gene mutations such as deletions or duplications in the dystrophin gene. Another type of gene mutation, called a triplet or trinucleotide repeat, involves expansion to more than the usual number of copies of a triplet repeat sequence within a gene. Myotonic dystrophy, Huntington disease, and fragile X syndrome are examples of conditions caused by this type of gene mutation.

Gene mutations may be inherited or acquired. Inherited or germline gene mutations are present in the DNA of all body cells and are passed on in reproductive cells from parent to child. Germline mutations are passed on to all daughter cells when body cells replicate (Fig. 9-4). The gene that causes Huntington disease is one example of a germline mutation.

Spontaneous mutations take place in individual oocytes or sperm at the time of conception. These mutations are not inherited in other family members. However, a person who carries the new "spontaneous" mutation may pass on the mutation to his or her children. Achondroplasia, Marfan syndrome, and neurofibromatosis type 1 are examples of genetic conditions that may occur in a single family member as a result of spontaneous mutation.

Acquired mutations take place in somatic cells and involve changes in DNA that occur after conception, during a person's lifetime. Acquired mutations develop as a result of cumulative changes in body cells other than reproductive cells (Fig. 9-5). Somatic gene mutations are passed on to the daughter cells derived from that particular cell line.

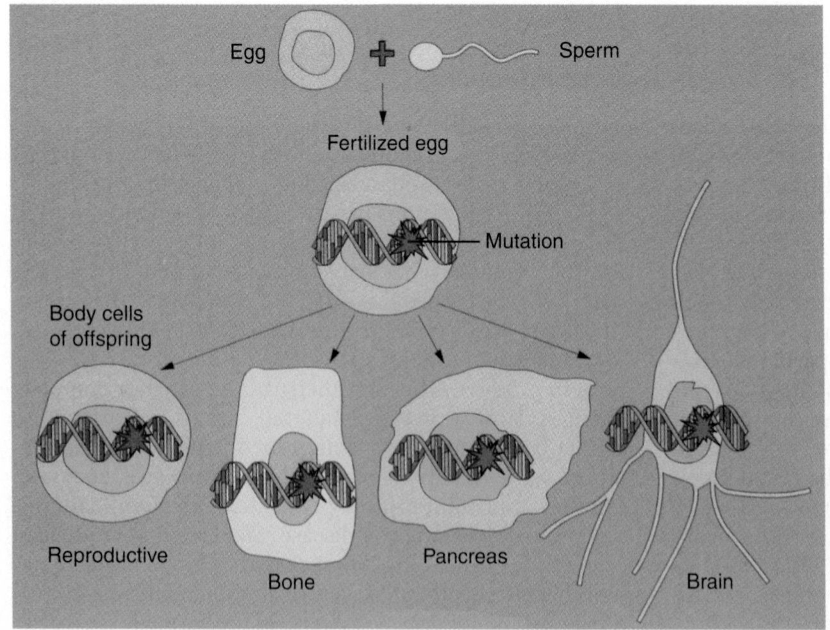

FIGURE 9-4. Hereditary mutations are carried in the DNA of the reproductive cells. When reproductive cells containing mutations combine to produce offspring, the mutation is present in all of the offspring's body cells. (From the National Institutes of Health and National Cancer Institute. [1995]. *Understanding gene testing* [NIH Pub. No. 96-3905]. Washington, DC: U.S. Department of Human Services.)

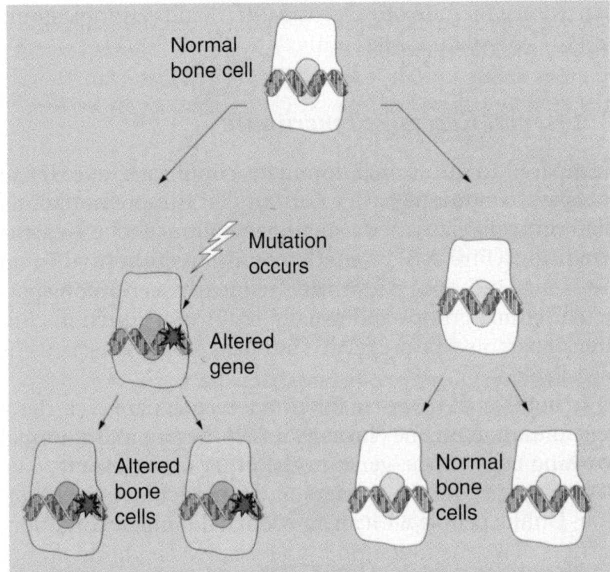

FIGURE 9-5. Acquired mutations develop in DNA during a person's lifetime. If the mutation arises in a body cell, copies of the mutation will exist only in the descendants of that particular cell. (From the National Institutes of Health and National Cancer Institute. [1995]. *Understanding gene testing* [NIH Pub. No. 96-3905]. Washington, DC: U.S. Department of Human Services.)

Gene mutations occur in the human body all the time. Cells have built-in mechanisms by which they can recognize mutations in DNA, and in most situations they correct the changes before they are passed on by cell division. However, over time, body cells may lose their ability to repair damage from gene mutations, causing an accumulation of genetic changes that may ultimately result in diseases such as cancer and possibly other conditions of aging, such as Alzheimer disease (Lea, 2000).

Genetic Variation

Research is ongoing to sort out the genetic components of complex conditions (eg, heart disease, diabetes, common cancers, psychiatric disorders) that result from the interaction of environment, lifestyle, and genetic effects. New studies of genetic variation in humans are underway to develop a map of common DNA variants. Genetic variations occur among people of all populations. **Polymorphisms** and single nucleotide polymorphisms (SNPs, or "snips") are the terms used for common genetic variations that occur most frequently throughout the human genome. Some SNPs may contribute directly to a trait or disease expression by altering function. SNPs are becoming increasingly important for the discovery of DNA sequence variations that affect biologic function. Such knowledge allows clinicians to subclassify diseases and adapt therapies to individual patients (Collins & McKusick, 2001; Guttmacher & Collins, 2004). For example, a polymorphism or SNP can alter protein or enzyme activity, and thereby affect drug efficacy and safety, if it occurs in proteins that are targets of medication regimens or that are involved in drug transport or drug metabolism (Evans & McLeod, 2003).

Inheritance Patterns

Nursing assessment of the patient's health includes obtaining and recording family history information. Evaluation of family history in the form of a **pedigree** is a first step in establishing the pattern of inheritance. Nurses must be familiar with mendelian patterns of inheritance and pedigree construction and analysis to help identify patients and families who may benefit from further genetic counseling, testing, and treatment (Jenkins & Lea, 2004).

Mendelian conditions, named after Gregor Mendel, are genetic conditions that are inherited in fixed proportions among generations. They result from gene mutations that are present on one or both chromosomes of a pair. A single gene inherited from one or both parents can cause a mendelian condition. Mendelian conditions are classified according to their pattern of inheritance: autosomal dominant, autosomal recessive, and **X-linked.** The terms **dominant** and **recessive** refer to the trait, genetic condition, or phenotype but not to the genes or alleles that cause the observable characteristics (Nussbaum, McGinnis & Willard, 2001).

Autosomal Dominant Inheritance

Autosomal dominant inherited conditions affect female and male family members equally and follow a vertical pattern of inheritance in families (Fig. 9-6). A person who has an autosomal dominant inherited condition carries a gene mutation for that condition on one chromosome of a pair. Each of that person's offspring has a 50% chance of inheriting the gene mutation for the condition and a 50% chance of inheriting the normal version of the gene (Fig. 9-7). Offspring who do not inherit the gene mutation for the dominant condition do not develop the condition and do not have an increased chance for having children with the same condition. Table 9-1 presents characteristics and examples of different patterns of inherited conditions.

Autosomal dominant conditions often manifest with varying degrees of severity among affected people. Some may have significant symptoms, whereas others may have only mild ones. This characteristic is referred to as **variable**

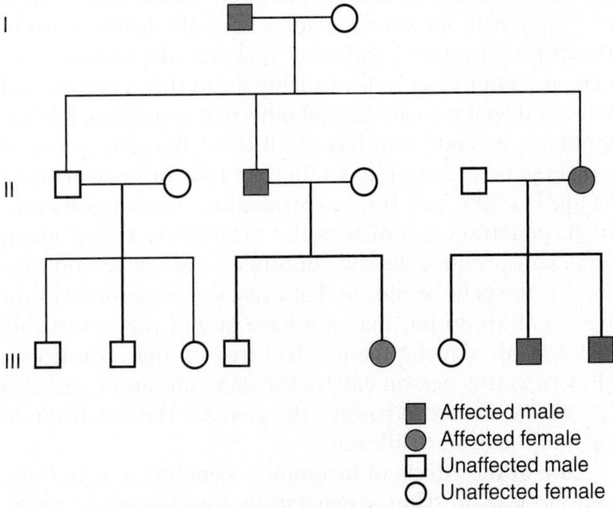

FIGURE 9-6. Three-generation pedigree illustrating autosomal dominant inheritance.

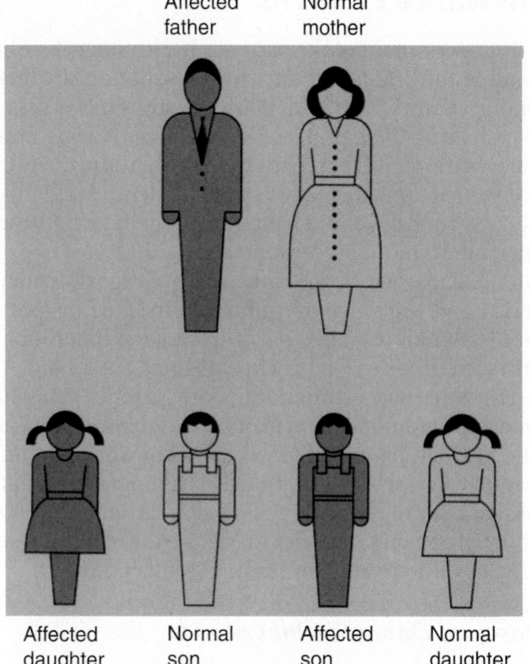

FIGURE 9-7. In dominant genetic disorders, if one affected parent has a disease-causing allele that dominates its normal counterpart, each child in the family has a 50% chance of inheriting the disease allele and the disorder. (From the National Institutes of Health and National Cancer Institute. [1995]. *Understanding gene testing* [NIH Pub. No. 96-3905]. Washington, DC: U.S. Department of Human Services.)

expression; it results from the influences of genetic and environmental factors on clinical presentation.

Another phenomenon observed in autosomal dominant inheritance is **penetrance**, or the percentage of persons known to have a particular gene mutation who actually show the trait. Almost complete penetrance is observed in conditions such as achondroplasia, in which nearly 100% of people with the gene mutation typically display traits of the disease. In some conditions, however, the presence of a gene mutation does not invariably mean that a person will have or develop an autosomal inherited condition. For example, a woman who has the BRCA1 hereditary breast cancer gene mutation has a lifetime risk for breast cancer as high as 80%, not 100%. This quality, known as incomplete penetrance, indicates the probability that a given gene will produce disease. In other words, a person may inherit the gene mutation that causes an autosomal dominant condition but may not have any of the observable physical or developmental features of that condition. However, this person carries the gene mutation and still has a 50% chance of passing the gene for the condition to each of his or her children.

One of the effects of incomplete penetrance is that the gene appears to "skip" a generation, thus leading to errors in interpreting family history and in genetic counseling. Examples of other genetic conditions with incomplete penetrance include otosclerosis (40%) and retinoblastoma (80%) (Nussbaum, McGinnis & Willard, 2001).

Autosomal Recessive Inheritance

Compared to autosomal dominant conditions, autosomal recessive conditions have a pattern that is more horizontal than vertical; relatives of a single generation tend to have the condition (Fig. 9-8). Genetic conditions inherited in an autosomal recessive pattern are frequently seen among particular ethnic groups and usually occur more often in children of parents who are related by blood, such as first cousins (see Table 9-1).

In autosomal recessive inheritance, each parent carries a gene mutation on one chromosome of the pair and a normal working copy of the gene on the other chromosome. The parents are said to be **carriers** of the particular gene mutation. Unlike people with an autosomal dominant condition, carriers of a gene mutation for a recessive condition do not have symptoms of the genetic condition. When carriers have children together, there is a 25% chance that each child may inherit the gene mutation from both parents and have the condition (Fig. 9-9). Gaucher's disease is one example of a condition inherited in an autosomal recessive manner (Enderlin, Vogel & Conway, 2003). Other examples include cystic fibrosis, sickle cell anemia, and PKU.

X-Linked Inheritance

X-linked conditions may be inherited in recessive or dominant patterns (see Table 9-1). In both, the gene mutation is located on the X chromosome. All males inherit an X chromosome from their mothers and a Y chromosome from their fathers for a normal sex constitution of 46,XY. Because males have only one X chromosome, they do not have a counterpart for its genes, as do females. This means that a gene mutation on the X chromosome of a male is expressed even though it is present in only one copy. Females, on the other hand, inherit one X chromosome from each parent for a normal sex constitution of 46,XX. A female may be an unaffected carrier of a gene mutation, or she may be affected if the condition results from a gene mutation causing a X-linked dominant condition. Either the X chromosome that she received from her mother or the X chromosome she received from her father may be passed on to each of her offspring, and this is a random occurrence.

The most common pattern of X-linked inheritance is that in which a female is a carrier for a gene mutation on one of her X chromosomes. This is referred to as X-linked recessive inheritance. In X-linked recessive conditions, a female carrier has a 50% chance of passing on the gene mutation to a son, who would be affected, or to a daughter, who would be a carrier like her mother (Fig. 9-10). Examples of X-linked recessive conditions include factor VIII and factor IX hemophilia, severe combined immunodeficiency, and Duchenne muscular dystrophy.

Nontraditional Inheritance

Although mendelian conditions manifest with a specific pattern of inheritance in some families, many diseases

TABLE 9-1 Patterns of Mendelian Inheritance

Characteristics	Examples
Autosomal Dominant Inherited Conditions	
Vertical transmission in families Males and females equally affected Variable expression among family members and others with condition Reduced penetrance (in some conditions) Advanced paternal age associated with sporadic cases	Hereditary breast/ovarian cancer syndrome Familial hypercholesterolemia Hereditary non-polyposis colorectal cancer Huntington disease Marfan syndrome Neurofibromatosis
Autosomal Recessive Inherited Conditions	
Horizontal pattern of transmission seen in families Males and females equally affected Associated with consanguinity (genetic relatedness) Associated with particular ethnic groups	Cystic fibrosis Galactosemia Phenylketonuria Sickle cell anemia Tay-Sachs disease Canavan disease
X-Linked Recessive Inherited Conditions	
Vertical transmission in families Males predominantly affected	Duchenne muscular dystrophy Hemophilia A and B Wiscott-Aldrich syndrome Protan and Deutran forms of color blindness
Multifactorial Inherited Conditions	
Occur as a result of combination of genetic and environmental factors May recur in families Inheritance pattern does not demonstrate characteristic pattern of inheritance seen with other mendelian conditions	Congenital heart defects Cleft lip and/or palate Neural tube defects (anencephaly and spina bifida) Diabetes mellitus Osteoarthritis High blood pressure

Adapted from Lea, D. H., Jenkins, J. F., & Francomano, C. A. (1998). *Genetics in clinical practice: New directions for nursing and health care.* Sudbury, MA: Jones & Bartlett; Lea, D. H. (2002). Genetics. In Maher, A. B., Salmond, S. W., & Pellino, T. A. (Eds.) *Orthopaedic nursing.* Philadelphia: W. B. Saunders.

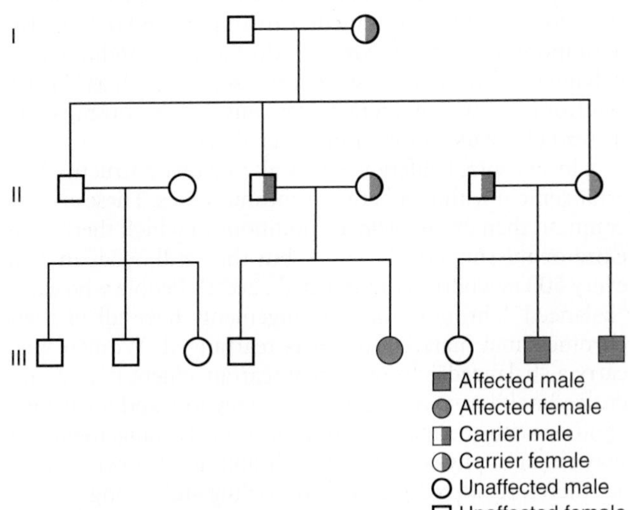

FIGURE 9-8. Three-generation pedigree illustrating autosomal recessive inheritance.

and traits do not follow these simple patterns. A variety of factors influence how a gene performs and is expressed. Different mutations in the same gene can produce variable symptoms in different people, as in cystic fibrosis. Different mutations in several genes can lead to identical outcomes, as in Alzheimer disease. Some traits involve simultaneous mutation in two or more genes. A recently observed phenomenon, imprinting, can determine which of a pair of genes (the mother's or the father's) is silenced or activated. This form of inheritance has been observed in Angelman syndrome, a severe form of mental retardation and ataxia (Nussbaum, McGinnis & Willard, 2001).

Multifactorial Inheritance and Complex Genetic Conditions

Many birth defects and common health conditions such as heart disease, high blood pressure, cancer, osteoarthritis, and diabetes occur as a result of interactions of multiple gene mutations and environmental influences. Thus, they are called multifactorial or complex conditions (see Table 9-1). Other examples of multifactorial genetic conditions include

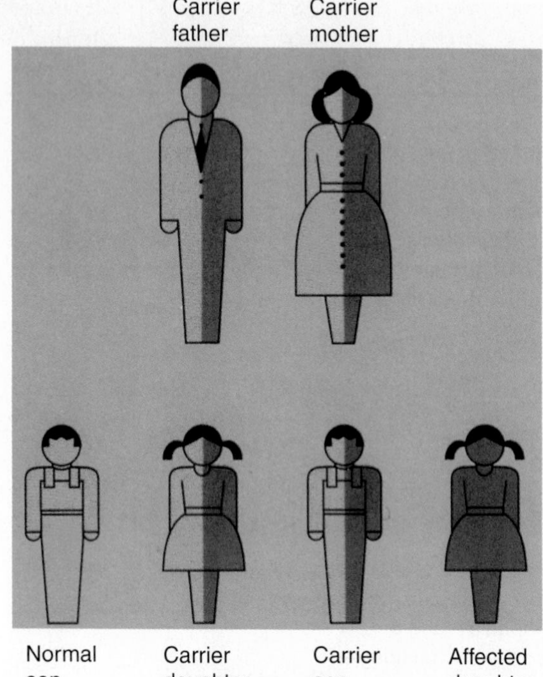

FIGURE 9-9. In diseases associated with altered recessive genes, both parents—although disease-free themselves—carry one normal allele and one altered allele. Each child has one chance in four of inheriting two abnormal alleles and developing the disorder; one chance in four of inheriting two normal alleles; and two chances in four of inheriting one normal and one altered allele, and therefore being a carrier like both parents.

neural tube defects such as spina bifida and anencephaly. Multifactorial conditions may cluster in families, but they do not always result in the characteristic pattern of inheritance seen in families who have mendelian inherited conditions (Fig. 9-11).

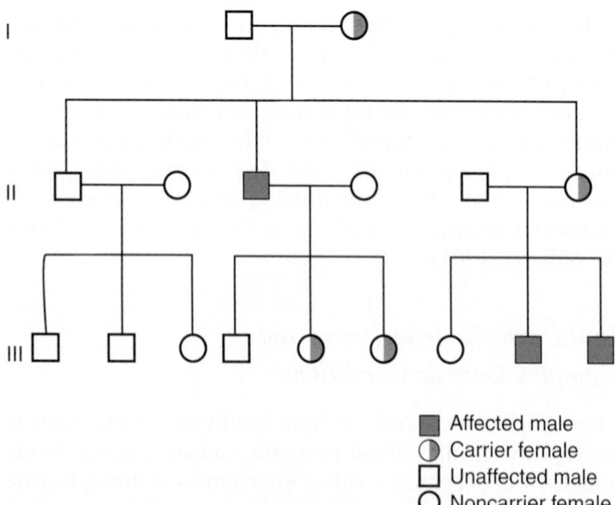

FIGURE 9-10. Three-generation pedigree illustrating X-linked recessive inheritance.

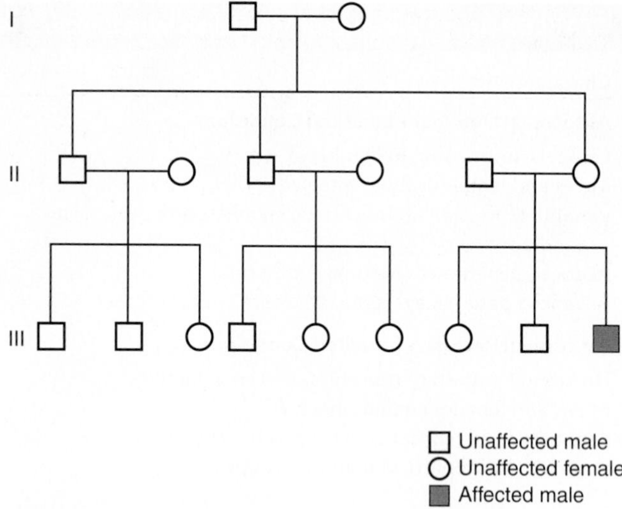

FIGURE 9-11. Three-generation pedigree illustrating multifactorial conditions.

Chromosomal Differences and Genetic Conditions

Differences in the number or structure of chromosomes are a major cause of birth defects, mental retardation, and malignancies. Chromosomal differences are present in approximately 1 of every 160 liveborn infants and are the cause of greater than 50% of all spontaneous first-trimester pregnancy losses (Rimoin et al., 2002). Chromosomal differences most commonly involve an extra or missing chromosome; this is called aneuploidy. Whenever there is an extra or missing chromosome, there is always associated mental or physical disability to some degree.

Down syndrome, or trisomy 21, is a common chromosomal condition that occurs with greater frequency in pregnancies of women who are 35 years of age or older. A person who has trisomy 21 Down syndrome has a complete extra chromosome 21, which causes a particular facial appearance and increased risk for congenital heart defects, thyroid and vision problems, and mental retardation. Other examples of chromosomal differences include trisomy 13 and trisomy 18, both more severe than Down syndrome, and conditions involving extra or missing sex chromosomes, such as Turner syndrome, in which a female has only one X chromosome instead of the usual two (Rimoin et al., 2002).

Chromosomal differences may also involve a structural rearrangement within or between chromosomes. These are less common than chromosomal conditions in which there is an extra or missing chromosome, but they still occur in 1 of every 500 newborns (Rimoin et al., 2002). People who carry "balanced" chromosome rearrangements have all of their chromosomal material, but it is rearranged. Women who carry a "balanced" chromosomal rearrangement have an increased risk for spontaneous pregnancy loss and for having children with an unbalanced chromosomal arrangement that may result in physical or mental disabilities. Known carriers are therefore offered prenatal counseling and testing.

Chromosome studies may be needed at any age, depending on the indication. Two common indications are a suspected diagnosis such as Down syndrome and a history of two or more unexplained pregnancy losses. Chromosome studies are accomplished by obtaining a tissue sample (eg, blood, skin, amniotic fluid), preparing and staining the chromosomes, and analyzing them under a microscope. The microscopic study of chromosomes, called cytogenetics, is an area that is rapidly evolving. Today, cytogenetics is used with new molecular techniques such as fluorescent in situ hybridization (FISH), which permits more detailed examination of chromosomes. FISH is useful to detect small abnormalities and to characterize chromosomal rearrangements (Rimoin et al., 2002).

Clinical Applications of Genetics

One of the most immediate applications of new genetic discoveries is the development of genetic tests that can be used to detect a trait, diagnose a genetic condition, and identify people who have a genetic predisposition to a disease such as cancer or heart disease. Another emerging application is pharmacogenetics, which involves the use of genetic testing to identify genetic variations that relate to the safety and efficacy of medications and gene-based treatments, so that individualized treatment and management plans can be developed. Future applications may include the use of gene chips to map a person's individual genome for genetic variations that may lead to disease. Nurses will be involved in caring for patients who are undergoing genetic testing and gene-based treatments. Knowledge of the clinical applications of modern genetic technologies will prepare nurses to inform and support patients and to provide high-quality genetics-related health care.

Genetic Testing

Genetic tests provide information leading to the diagnosis of inherited conditions or other conditions with a known genetic contribution. Genetic testing involves the use of specific laboratory analyses of chromosomes, genes, or gene products (eg, enzymes, proteins) to learn whether a genetic alteration related to a specific disease or condition is present. This testing may be DNA-based, chromosomal, or biochemical.

Genetic testing can be used for a variety of purposes in prenatal, pediatric, and adult populations (Burke, 2004). Prenatal testing is widely used for **prenatal screening** and diagnosis of such conditions as Down syndrome. Carrier testing is used to determine carrier status—that is, to discover whether a person carries a recessive allele for an inherited condition (eg, cystic fibrosis, sickle cell anemia, Tay-Sachs disease) and therefore risks passing it on to his or her children. Genetic testing is also used widely in newborn screening. In the United States, it is made available for an increasing number of genetic conditions (eg, PKU, galactosemia). Diagnostic testing is used to detect the presence or absence of a particular genetic alteration or allele to identify or confirm a diagnosis of a disease or condition (eg, myotonic dystrophy, fragile X syndrome). Increasingly, genetic tests are being used to predict drug response and to design specific and individualized treatment and management plans. For example, genetic testing is used to identify specific gene variants that can predict therapeutic success of treatments for human immunodeficiency virus (HIV) infection and the use of tacrine for Alzheimer disease (Weinshilboum, 2004). Examples of current uses of genetic tests are shown in Table 9-2.

Nurses are increasingly participating in genetic testing, especially in the area of patient education. In addition, they contribute by ensuring informed health choices and consent, advocating for privacy and confidentiality with regard to genetic test results, and helping patients understand the complex issues involved (Lea & Williams, 2002).

Genetic Screening

Genetic screening, in contrast to genetic testing, is a broader concept and applies to testing of populations or groups independent of a positive family history or symptom manifestation. Genetic screening, as defined in 1975 by the Committee for the Study of Inborn Errors of Metabolism of the National Academy of Sciences (Secretary's Advisory Committee on Genetic Testing, 2000), has several major aims. The first aim is to improve management—that is, to identify people with treatable genetic conditions that could prove dangerous to their health if left untreated. For example, newborns are screened for an increasing number of conditions, including PKU, congenital hypothyroidism, and galactosemia. The second aim is to provide reproductive options to people with a high probability of having children with severe, untreatable diseases and for whom genetic counseling, prenatal diagnosis, and other reproductive options could be helpful and of interest. For example, people of Ashkenazi Jewish descent are screened for conditions such as Tay-Sachs disease and Canavan disease. The third aim is to screen pregnant women using multiple marker screening to detect birth defects such as neural tube defects and Down syndrome. Genetic screening may also be used for public health purposes to determine the incidence and prevalence of a birth defect or to investigate the feasibility and value of new genetic testing methods.

Most commonly, genetic screening occurs in prenatal and newborn programs that involve nurses in various roles and settings. In the future, population-based (widespread) genetic screening will be used to help identify people who are predisposed to conditions such as breast and colon cancer, diabetes, and heart disease. Nurses will be expected to participate in explaining risk and genetic predisposition, supporting informed health decisions and opportunities for prevention and early intervention, and protecting patients' privacy (Lea & Williams, 2002). Table 9-3 gives examples of genetic screening.

Testing and Screening for Adult-Onset Conditions

Adult-onset conditions are disorders with a genetic basis that are manifested in later life. Often clinical signs or symptoms occur only in late adolescence or adulthood, and disease is clearly observed to run in families. Some of these conditions are attributed to specific genetic mutations and follow either an autosomal dominant or an autosomal recessive inheritance pattern. However, the majority of adult-onset condi-

TABLE 9-2 Genetic Tests: Examples of Current Uses

Purpose of Genetic Test	Type of Genetic Test
Carrier Testing	
Cystic fibrosis	DNA analysis
Tay-Sachs disease	Hexosaminidase A activity testing and DNA analysis
Canavan disease	DNA analysis
Sickle cell anemia	Hemoglobin electrophoresis
Thalassemia	Complete blood count and hemoglobin electrophoresis
Prenatal Diagnosis—amniocentesis is often performed when there is a risk for a chromosomal or genetic disorder:	
Risk for Down syndrome	Chromosomal analysis
Risk for cystic fibrosis	DNA analysis
Risk for Tay-Sachs disease	Hexosaminidase A activity testing and/or DNA analysis
Risk for open neural tube defect	Protein analysis
Diagnosis	
Down syndrome	Chromosomal analysis
Fragile X syndrome	DNA analysis
Myotonic dystrophy	DNA analysis
Presymptomatic Testing	
Huntington disease	DNA analysis
Myotonic dystrophy	DNA analysis
Susceptibility Testing	
Hereditary breast/ovarian cancer	DNA analysis
Hereditary non-polyposis colorectal cancer	DNA analysis

tions are considered to be multifactorial (polygenetic); examples include heart disease, diabetes, and arthritis. Multifactorial influences involve the interactions among several genes (gene–gene interaction) and between genes and the environment (gene–environment interactions) (Guttmacher & Collins, 2004).

Nursing assessment for adult-onset conditions is based on family history, personal and medical risk factors, and identification of associated diseases or clinical manifestations. Knowledge of adult-onset conditions and their genetic bases (ie, mendelian versus multifactorial conditions) influences the nursing considerations for genetic testing and health promotion. Table 9-4 describes selected adult-onset conditions, their age of onset, pattern of inheritance, and risk factors, both genetic and environmental.

If a single gene accounts for an adult-onset condition in a symptomatic person, diagnostic testing is used to confirm a diagnosis to assist in the plan of care and management. Diagnostic testing for adult-onset conditions is most frequently used with autosomal dominant conditions, such

TABLE 9-3 Applications for Genetic Screening

Timing of Screening	Purpose	Examples
Preconception screening	For autosomal recessive inherited genetic conditions that occur with greater frequency among individuals of certain ethnic groups	Cystic fibrosis—all couples, but especially Northern European Caucasian, and Ashkenazi Jewish Tay-Sachs disease—Ashkenazi Jewish Sickle cell anemia—African American, Puerto Rican, Mediterranean, Middle Eastern Alpha-thalassemia—Southeast Asian, African American
Prenatal screening	For genetic conditions that are common and for which prenatal diagnosis is available when a pregnancy is identified at increased risk	Neural tube defects—spina bifida, anencephaly Down syndrome Other chromosomal abnormalities—trisomy 18
Newborn screening	For genetic conditions for which there is specific treatment	Phenylketonuria (PKU) Galactosemia Homocystinuria Biotinidase deficiency

TABLE 9-4 Adult-Onset Disorders

Clinical Description	Age of Onset (y)	Inheritance	Risk Factors
Neurologic Conditions			
Early-Onset Familial Alzheimer Disease			
Progressive dementia, memory failure, personality disturbance, loss of intellectual functioning associated with cerebral cortical atrophy, beta-amyloid plaque formation, intraneuronal neurofibrillary tangles	<60–65 and often before 55	A.D. <2%	Mutations on preslin 1, preslin 2 and/or beta-amyloid precursor protein Carriers of apolipoprotein E4
Late-Onset Familial Alzheimer Disease			
Progressive dementia, cognitive decline	>60–65	A.D. ~25% M.F. ~75%	Gene-gene interactions Diabetes Hypercholesterolemia Cerebrovascular or cardiovascular disease
Huntington Disease			
Widespread degenerative brain change with progressive motor loss, both voluntary and involuntary disability, cognitive decline, chorea (involuntary movements) at later stage, psychiatric disturbances	35–44 (mean)	A.D. 100%	*HD* gene
Hematologic Conditions			
Hereditary Hemochromatosis (HHC)			
High absorption of iron by gastrointestinal mucosa, resulting in excessive iron storage in liver, skin, pancreas, heart, joints, and testes Early symptoms of abdominal pain, weakness, lethargy, weight loss Possible pigmentation, diabetes mellitus, hepatic fibrosis or cirrhosis, heart failure, and arrhythmias or arthritis in untreated people	40–60 in males; after menopause in females	A.R. ~60–90% M.F. ~10–30%	Carrier or sibling of carrier of *HFE* gene mutations Liver disease such as alcoholic liver disease, acute viral hepatitis, or chronic hepatitis C Iron overload resulting from ingested iron in foods, cookware, and medicines, as well as parenteral iron from iron injections or transfusions for a chronic anemia such as beta-thalassemia or sickle cell disease
Factor V Leiden Thrombophilia			
Poor anticoagulant response to activated protein C with increased risk for venous thrombosis and risk for increased fetal loss during pregnancy	30s; during pregnancy in females	A.D.	Carriers or relatives of individuals known to have factor V Leiden mutations Families with high rates of venous thromboembolism, deep venous thrombosis, or pulmonary embolism, especially if age <50 y Women with recurrent pregnancy loss or venous thromboembolism during pregnancy or who use oral contraceptives
Diabetes Mellitus Type 2			
Insulin resistance, impaired glucose tolerance	Variable onset; most often >30	M.F.	Gene-gene interactions Obesity Hypertension Hyperlipidemia High intake of refined carbohydrates

continued >

TABLE 9-4 Adult-Onset Disorders (Continued)

Clinical Description	Age of Onset (y)	Inheritance	Risk Factors
Cardiovascular Disease			
Familial hypercholesterolemia Elevated LDL levels leading to coronary artery disease, xanthomas, and corneal arcus	35–50	A.D.	Family or personal history of coronary heart disease at <45 y in women or <40 y in men Elevated LDL
Oncology Conditions			
Multiple Endocrine Neoplasia			
Familial medullary thyroid cancer, pheochromocytoma, and parathyroid abnormalities	Early adulthood; 40–50 y	A.D.	Carrier or relative of carrier of a *RET* mutation Family history of medullary thyroid cancer, pheochromocytoma, and parathyroid abnormalities
Breast Cancer			
BRCA1 and BRCA2 hereditary breast/ovarian cancer Breast, ovarian, and prostate (BRCA1) Breast, ovarian, and other cancer (BRCA2)	30–70; often <50	A.D. ~5–10% of breast and ovarian cancers	Mutations in BRCA1, BRCA2
		M.F. >75%	Older age Early menses (<11 y) Nulliparity Family history Breast biopsies
Hereditary Non-polyposis Colorectal Cancer (HNPCC)			
Colorectal, ovarian, endometrial, bladder, gastric, biliary, and renal cell cancers	<50	A.D. ~1–3% of colorectal colon cancer; ~1% of endometrial cancers	Mutations in family of repair genes
		M.F. >75%	Older age Personal or family history of colon cancer or adenomas High-fat, low-fiber diet Inflammatory bowel disease

A.D., autosomal dominant; A.R., autosomal recessive; LDL, low-density lipoprotein; M.F., multifactorial.

From Brandi, M. L., Gagel, R. F., Angeli, A., et al. (2001). Guidelines for diagnosis and therapy of MEN type 1 and type 2. *Journal of Clinical Endocrinology and Metabolism, 86:*5658–5671; Burt, M. J., George, P. M., Upton, J. D., et al. (1998). The significance of haemochromatosis gene mutations in the general population: Implications for screening. *Gut, 43,* 830–836; Campion, D., Dumanchin, C., Hannequin, D., et al. (1999). Early-onset autosomal dominant Alzheimer disease: prevalence, genetic heterogeneity, and mutation spectrum. *American Journal of Human Genetics, 65*(3), 664–670; Colditz, G. A., Rosner, B. A. & Speizer, F. E. (1996). Risk factors for breast cancer according to family history of breast cancer. For the Nurses' Health Study Research Group. *Journal of the National Cancer Institute, 88*(6), 365–371; Cunningham, J. M., Kim, C. Y., Christensen, E. R., et al. (2001). The frequency of hereditary defective mismatch repair in a prospective series of unselected colorectal carcinomas. *American Journal of Human Genetics, 69,* 780–790; Grody, W. W., Griffin, J. H., Taylor, A. K., et al. (2001). American College of Medical Genetics Consensus statement on factor V Leiden mutation testing. *Genetics in Medicine, 3*(2), 139–148.

as Huntington disease or factor V Leiden thrombophilia, and with autosomal recessive conditions such as hemochromatosis. In families with known adult-onset conditions or with a confirmed genetic mutation in an affected family member, **presymptomatic testing** provides asymptomatic people with information about the presence of a genetic mutation and about the likelihood of developing the disease. Huntington disease has served as the model for presymptomatic testing because the presence of the genetic mutation predicts disease onset and progression. Although preventive measures are not yet available for Huntington disease, the genetics information enables health care providers to develop a clinical, supportive, and psychological plan of care. Presymptomatic testing is considered for people in families with a known adult-onset condition in which either a positive or a negative test result indicates an increased or reduced risk for developing the disease, affects medical management, or allows earlier treatment of a condition.

The foremost factor that may influence the development and severity of disease is a person's genetic makeup. However, in the absence of a single disease-causing gene, it is thought that multiple genes and other environmental factors are related to the onset of most adult diseases. For some diseases, the interactions among several genes and other environmental or metabolic events affect disease onset and progression. Specific gene–gene interactions or SNPs can confer susceptibility to disease. Most susceptibility testing is conducted in the research setting to identify candidate genes for diseases such as Alzheimer disease, psychiatric conditions, heart disease, hypertension, and hypercholesterolemia. Susceptibility testing helps distinguish variations within the same disease or response to treatment. For example, no single gene is associated with osteoporosis. Several polymorphisms on candidate genes related to the vitamin D receptor, estrogen and androgen receptors, and cytokine production and its associated stimulation of osteoclasts are under study to predict bone mineral density and fracture risk (Ralston, 2004). Some susceptibility genes may predict treatment response. For example, people may present with similar clinical signs and symptoms of asthma but have different responses to treatment. Susceptibility testing helps classify people with asthma as sensitive or resistant to treatment with corticosteroids (Cookson, 2002).

Population screening, the use of genetic testing for large groups or whole populations, to identify late-onset conditions is under development. For a test to be considered for population screening, there must be (1) sufficient information about gene distribution within populations, (2) accurate prediction about the development and progression of disease, and (3) appropriate medical management for asymptomatic people with a mutation (Burke, Coughlin, Lee, et al., 2001). Currently, population screening is offered in some ethnic groups to identify cancer-predisposing genes. For example, Ashkenazi Jews (Jews of Eastern European origin) have a greater chance of having a specific genetic mutation in the BRCA1 or BRCA2 gene. People with one of these BRCA mutations have approximately an 80% risk for breast cancer, a 40% to 65% risk for ovarian cancer (BRCA1 carriers), a 20% risk for ovarian cancer (BRCA2 carriers) (King, Marks, Mandell, et al., 2003), and a 16% risk for prostate cancer (Kirchhoff, Kauff, Mitra, et al., 2004). The identification of one of these mutations gives patients options for cancer screening as well as chemoprevention or prophylactic mastectomy or oophorectomy in carriers. Population screening is being explored for other adult-onset conditions such as type 2 diabetes and hereditary hemochromatosis (iron overload disorder).

Nurses must be alert for family histories indicating that multiple generations (autosomal dominant inheritance) or multiple siblings (autosomal recessive inheritance) are affected with the same condition or that onset of disease is earlier than expected (eg, multiple generations with early-onset hyperlipidemia). Possible adult-onset conditions are discussed with other members of the health care team for appropriate resources and referral. When a family history of disease is identified, the nurse must be responsible for making the patient aware that this is a risk factor for disease. Regardless of whether a particular patient pursues a genetic testing workup, risk information for the disease should be explained. For example, if a 45-year-old woman presents for her annual gynecology visit and has a family history showing colon cancer in multiple paternal relatives, including her father, the nurse discusses the family history with the gynecologist. In addition, the woman is alerted to the risk for colon cancer based on the family history, and she is given information about possible genetic testing and referral for a colonoscopy.

If the existence of a mutation for an adult-onset condition in a family is identified, at-risk family members can be referred for **predisposition testing.** If the patient is found to be a carrier of the mutation, the nurse provides him or her with information about the risk to other family members. In that discussion, the nurse assures the patient that the test results are private and confidential and will not be shared with others, including family members, without the patient's permission. If the patient is an unaffected family member, the nurse discusses inheritance and the risk for developing the disease, provides support for the decision-making process, and offers referral for genetics services.

Individualizing Genetic Profiles and Pharmacogenetics

Information about genes and their variations is helping researchers identify genetic differences that predispose certain people or groups to disease and affect their responses to treatment. The use of individualized genetics data to predict predisposition to common diseases will take considerable time to develop. Genetic tests that identify the role of genetic variations in drug response are currently under study. Drug metabolism involves genetically controlled enzyme activity for absorption, distribution, drug–cell interaction, inactivation, and excretion. Polymorphisms (genetic variations in populations) most often affect enzyme activity in the drug metabolism pathways. Pharmacogenetics, the study of the role of genetic variation in drug response and toxicity, involves methods that rapidly identify which genetic variations influence a drug's effect (Goetz, Ames, & Weinshilboum, 2004).

Variations in genes activated for enzyme activity can cause either decreased or increased drug metabolism. Genetic testing for these variations is providing a genetic profile, classifying patients according to their drug metabolism. Four classes of metabolic variations have been identified: (1) poor metabolizers, who lack enzyme function; (2) intermediate metabolizers, who have reduced enzyme activity; (3) extensive metabolizers, who have normal or expected enzyme activity; and (4) ultrarapid metabolizers, who have increased enzyme activity. The cytochrome P450 (CYP) family of enzymes has long been known for its involvement in drug metabolism. Three CYP enzymes—CYP2C9, CYP2C19, and CYP2D6—are active in about 40% of CYP-mediated drug responses (Ingelman-Sundberg, 2004). People with genetic variations in these enzymes are more likely to experience adverse drug reactions or poor response. Table 9-5 shows examples of differences in drug response for poor versus ultrarapid metabolizers. Reduced enzyme activity in poor metabolizers results in higher blood levels of active drug, predisposing them to adverse drug reactions. Ultrarapid metabolizers have increased enzyme activity with rapid breakdown and excretion of drug compounds, which results in lower blood levels of active drug and poor treatment response.

Nurses have traditionally monitored and reported drug response and drug adverse effects. In the near future, pharmacogenetic testing for CYP activity will give patients more

TABLE 9-5 Clinical Effects of Cytochrome P450 Enzyme Variations

Enzyme	Drug	Effects	
		Poor metabolizer	**Ultrarapid metabolizer**
CYP2C9	Warfarin	Bleeding	Longer treatment time to achieve stable dosing
	Phenytoin	Ataxia	
	Tolbutamide	Hypoglycemia	
CYP2C19	Diazepam	Sedation	Poor response
CYP2D6	Tricyclic antidepressants	Cardiotoxicity	No response to recommended dose; need 10-fold increase in dose
	Selective serotonin reuptake inhibitors	Nausea	
	Antipsychotics	Parkinson-like effects	Longer treatment time and higher drug costs

From Ingelman-Sundberg, M. (2004). Pharmacogenetics of cytochrome P450 and its applications in drug therapy: The past, present and future. *Trends in Pharmacological Science, 25*(4), 193–200.

information about drug dosage, time to achieve response, and risk for adverse effects. Nurses will be expected to provide education about a particular patient's profile for drug metabolism and explain the rationale for the recommended dosage and likelihood of adverse effects. Although genetic profiles will add to individualized drug treatment plans, nurses will continue to incorporate information about gender differences, food interactions, and drug compliance into patient education (Nicol, 2003; Prows & Prows, 2004).

Applications of Genetics in Nursing Practice

Nurses in genetics-related health care blend the principles of human genetics with nursing care in collaboration with other professionals, including genetic specialists, to foster improvement, maintenance, and restoration of patients' health. In all nursing practice settings, nurses have five main tasks: (1) help collect and interpret relevant family and medical histories, (2) identify patients and families who need further genetics evaluation and counseling and refer them to appropriate genetics services, (3) offer genetics information and resources to patients and families, (4) collaborate with genetics specialists, and (5) participate in the management and coordination of care of patients with genetic conditions. Genetics-related nursing practice involves the care of people who have genetic conditions, those who may be predisposed to develop or pass on genetic conditions, and those who are seeking genetics information and referral for additional genetics services (Jenkins & Lea, 2004).

Nurses support patients and families with genetics-related health concerns by ensuring that their health choices are informed ones and by advocating for the privacy and confidentiality of genetics information and for equal access to genetic testing and treatments. *The Scope and Standards of Genetics Clinical Nursing Practice,* developed by the International Society of Nurses in Genetics (ISONG, 1998) and published by the American Nurses Association, delineates roles and responsibilities for nurses in providing genetics-related health care.

Genetics and Health Assessment

Assessment of a person's genetics-related health status is an ongoing process. Nurses collect information that can help identify individuals and families who have actual or potential genetics-related health concerns or who may benefit from further genetics information, counseling, testing, and treatment. This process can begin before conception and continue throughout the lifespan. Nurses evaluate family and past medical histories, including prenatal history, childhood illnesses, developmental history, adult-onset conditions (in adults), past surgeries, treatments, and medications; this information may relate to the genetic condition at hand or to a condition being considered. (See Chapter 5 for more information on assessing past medical history.) Nurses also identify the patient's ethnic background and conduct a physical assessment to gather pertinent genetics information. The assessment also includes information about culture, spiritual beliefs, and ancestry. Genetics-related health assessment always includes determining a patient's or family's understanding of actual or potential genetics-related health concerns and awareness of how these issues are communicated within a family (ISONG, 1998; Jenkins & Lea, 2004; Williams & Lea, 2003).

Family History Assessment

Nurses in any practice setting continuously assess families' genetics histories to identify the presence of a genetic trait, inherited condition, or predisposition. Targeted questions are used to identify genetic conditions for which further information, education, testing, or treatment can be offered (Chart 9-2). In consultation and collaboration with other health care providers and specialists, nurses can then determine whether further genetic testing and evaluation should be offered for the trait or condition in question. A well-documented family history is a tool used by the health care team to make a diagnosis, identify testing strategies, and establish a pattern of inheritance. The family history should include at least three generations, as well as information about the current and past health status of all family members, including the age at onset of any illnesses, cause of death, and age at death. Nurses also inquire about medical conditions that are known to have a heritable com-

CHART 9-2

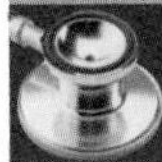

Genetics Family History: An Essential Tool for All Nurses

A well-documented family history is a tool for
- Making a medical diagnosis
- Deciding on testing strategies
- Establishing pattern of inheritance
- Identifying family members at increased risk
- Calculating risks
- Determining reproductive options
- Distinguishing genetic from other risk factors
- Making decisions about management or surveillance
- Developing patient rapport
- Educating patients

Key questions to ask about each family member include
- What is the current age or what was the age at death?
- What is the ethnic background (some genetic conditions are more common in certain ethnic groups)?
- Is there a history of
  - multiple pregnancy losses/stillbirths?
  - unexplained infertility?
  - birth defects?
  - medical problems in children whose parents are closely related (second cousins or closer)?
  - developmental delay/mental retardation?
  - learning disabilities or behavioral problems?
  - congenital or juvenile blindness, cataracts, hearing loss/deafness?
  - very short or very tall stature?
  - several close relatives with the same or related conditions (eg, breast cancer, colon cancer)?
  - occurrence of a common condition with earlier age at onset than is typical (eg, breast cancer, colon cancer, hearing loss, dementia, heart disease)?

From American Medical Association (2004). Family Medical History in Disease Prevention. Available at: www.ama-assn.org/ama/pub/category/2380.html (accessed March 3, 2006).

ponent and for which genetic testing may be available. Nurses obtain information about the presence of birth defects, mental retardation, familial traits, or similarly affected family members (Williams & Lea, 2003).

Nurses also consider the presence of genetic relatedness (consanguinity) among family members when assessing the risk for genetic conditions in couples or families. For example, when obtaining a preconception or prenatal family history, the nurse asks if the prospective parents have common ancestors (ie, are they first cousins?). This is important to know, because people who are related have more genes in common than those who are unrelated, thus increasing their chance for having children with an autosomal recessive inherited condition such as cystic fibrosis. The number of shared genes depends on the degree of relationship. For example, a parent and child share one half of their genes, whereas first cousins share one eighth of their genes. Ascertaining genetic relatedness gives nurses the opportunity to offer additional genetic counseling and evaluation. It may also serve as an explanation for parents who have a child with a rare autosomal recessive inherited condition or for a person who is similarly affected.

When the assessment of family history reveals that a patient has been adopted, genetics-based health assessment becomes more challenging. The nurse and the health care team should make all efforts to help the patient obtain as much information as possible about his or her biologic parents, including their ethnic backgrounds.

Questions regarding reproductive history (eg, history of miscarriage or stillbirth) are included in genetics family history health assessments to identify possible chromosomal conditions. Nurses also inquire about any history of family members with inherited conditions or birth defects; maternal health conditions such as type 1 diabetes, seizure disorders, or PKU, which may increase the risk for birth defects in children, and about exposure to alcohol or other drugs during pregnancy. Maternal age is also noted; women who are 35 years of age or older who are considering pregnancy and childbearing or who are already pregnant should be offered prenatal diagnosis (eg, testing through amniocentesis) because of the association between advanced maternal age and chromosomal abnormalities such as Down syndrome (Williams & Lea, 2003).

Physical Assessment

Physical assessment may provide clues that a particular genetic condition is present in a person and family. Family history assessment may offer initial guidance regarding the particular area for physical assessment. For example, a family history of familial hypercholesterolemia would alert the nurse to assess family members for symptoms of hyperlipidemias (xanthomas, corneal arcus, abdominal pain of unexplained origin). As another example, a family history of neurofibromatosis type 1, an inherited condition involving tumors of the central nervous system, would prompt the nurse to carry out a detailed assessment of closely related family members. Skin findings such as *café-au-lait* spots, axillary freckling, or tumors of the skin (neurofibromas) would warrant referral for further evaluation, including genetic evaluation and counseling (Lea & Smith, 2003).

If a genetic condition is suspected as a result of a family history or physical assessment, the nurse, in collaboration with the health care team, may initiate further discussion and evaluation. Providing genetics information, offering and discussing genetic tests, and suggesting a referral to a geneticist are part of the nurse's role (Chart 9-3).

Ancestry, Cultural, Social, and Spiritual Assessment

When collecting and discussing genetics information, nurses assess the ancestry of patients and families, as well as their ethnic, cultural, social, and spiritual orientation. Assessment of ancestry and ethnicity helps identify individual patients and groups who could benefit from genetic testing for carrier identification, prenatal diagnosis, and

CHART 9-3

Indications for Making a Genetics Referral

PREPREGNANCY AND PRENATAL

- Maternal age of 35 years or greater at expected time of delivery
- Previous child with a chromosome problem
- Positive alpha-fetoprotein profile screening test
- Previous child with a birth defect or family history of birth defects
- Pregnancy history of two or more unexplained miscarriages
- Maternal conditions such as diabetes, epilepsy, or alcoholism
- Exposures to certain medications or drugs during pregnancy
- Family history of mental retardation

PEDIATRIC

- Positive newborn screening test
- One or more major birth defects
- Unusual (dysmorphic) facial features
- Developmental delay/mental retardation
- Suspicion of a metabolic disorder
- Unusually tall or short stature, or growth delays
- Known chromosomal abnormality

ADULT

- Mental retardation without a known cause
- Unexplained infertility or multiple pregnancy losses
- A personal or family history of thrombotic events
- Adult-onset conditions such as hemochromatosis, hearing loss, visual impairment
- Family history of an adult-onset neurodegenerative disorder (eg, Huntington disease)
- Features of a genetic condition such as neurofibromatosis (*café-au-lait* spots, neurofibromas on the skin), Marfan syndrome (unusually tall stature, dilation of the aortic root), others

CANCER HISTORY

- A personal or family history of cancer with a known or suspected inherited predisposition (eg, early-onset breast cancer, colon cancer, ovarian cancer, retinoblastoma)
- Several family members affected by cancer
- A family member with cancer at an unusually young age
- A family member with an unusual type of cancer

susceptibility testing. For example, carrier testing for sickle cell anemia is routinely offered to people of African American descent, and carrier testing for Tay-Sachs disease and Canavan disease is offered to people of Ashkenazi Jewish descent. Professional organizations such as the American College of Obstetrics and Gynecology (ACOG) recommend that members of at-risk racial and ethnic populations be offered carrier testing (ACOG, 2001). ACOG and the American College of Medical Genetics (ACMG) recommend that all couples, particularly those of Northern European and Ashkenazi Jewish ancestry, be offered carrier screening for cystic fibrosis (ACOG, 2001). Ideally, carrier testing is offered before conception to allow people who are carriers to make decisions about reproduction. Prenatal diagnosis is offered and discussed when both partners of a couple are found to be carriers.

It is also important to inquire about the patient's ethnic backgrounds when assessing for susceptibilities to adult-onset conditions such as hereditary breast or ovarian cancer. For example, a BRCA1 cancer-predisposing gene mutation seems to occur more frequently in women of Ashkenazi Jewish descent. Therefore, asking about ethnicity can help identify people with an increased risk for cancer gene mutations (American Medical Association, 2004).

The nurse also should consider the patient's views about the significance of a genetic condition and its effect on self-concept, as well as the patient's perception of the role of genetics in health and illness, reproduction, and disability. The patient's social and cultural backgrounds determine his or her interpretations and values about information obtained from genetic testing and evaluation and thus influence his or her perceptions of health, illness, and risk. Family structure and decision making and educational background contribute in the same way (Jenkins & Lea, 2004; Lea & Smith, 2003).

Assessment of the patient's beliefs, values, and expectations regarding genetic testing and genetics information helps the nurse provide appropriate information about the specific genetics topic. For example, in some cultures, people believe that health means the absence of symptoms and that the cause of illness is supernatural. Patients with these beliefs may initially reject suggestions for presymptomatic or carrier testing. However, by including resources such as family, cultural, and religious community leaders when providing genetics-related health care, nurses can help ensure that patients receive information in a way that transcends social, cultural, and economic barriers (Tranin, Masny & Jenkins, 2003).

Psychosocial Assessment

Psychosocial assessment is an essential nursing component of the genetics health assessment (Chart 9-4). After conducting an initial psychosocial assessment, nurses become aware of the potential impact of new genetics information on the patient and family and how they may cope with this information.

Genetic Counseling and Evaluation Services

People seek genetic counseling for a variety of reasons and at different stages of life. Some are seeking preconception or prenatal information, others are referred after the birth of a child with a birth defect or suspected genetic condition, and still others are seeking information for themselves or their families because of the presence of, or a family history

CHART 9-4

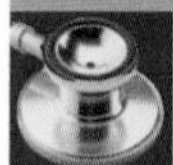

Assessing for Psychosocial Genetics Health

The nurse assesses:

- Educational level and understanding of the genetic condition or concern in the family.
- Desired goals and health outcomes in relation to genetic condition or concern.
- Family rules regarding disclosure of medical information (eg, some families may not reveal a history of diseases such as cancer or mental illness during the family history assessment).
- Family rules, boundaries, and cultural practices as well as personal preferences about knowing medical information.
- Past coping mechanisms and social support.
- Ability to make an informed decision (eg, is the patient under stress from family situations, acute or chronic illness, or medications that may impair the ability to make an informed decision)

of, a genetic condition. Regardless of the timing or setting, genetic counseling is offered to all people who have questions about genetics and their health. In collaboration with the health care team, nurses consider referral for genetic counseling for any patient who belongs to a family with a hereditary condition and who asks questions such as, "What are my chances for having this condition? Is there a genetic test that will tell me? Is there a gene-based treatment or cure? What are my options?" (Lea & Smith, 2003).

As the contribution of genetics to the health–illness continuum is recognized, the process of genetic counseling is expected to become a responsibility of all health care professionals in clinical practice. Nurses are obvious and natural providers of genetics services because they are often aware of the patient's personal and family history. Nurses assess the patient's health and make referrals for specialized diagnosis and treatment. They offer anticipatory guidance by explaining the purpose and goals of a referral. They collaborate with primary healthcare providers and specialists in giving supportive and follow-up counseling. They coordinate follow-up and case management.

Genetics Services

Genetics services provide genetic information, education, and support to patients and families with genetics-related health concerns. Genetics professionals, including medical geneticists, genetics counselors, and advanced practice nurses in genetics, provide specific genetics services to patients and families who are referred by their primary health care providers. A team approach is often used by genetics specialists to obtain and interpret complex family history information, evaluate and diagnose genetic conditions, interpret and discuss complicated genetic test results, support patients throughout the evaluation process, and offer resources for additional professional and family support. Patients participate as team members and decision-makers throughout the process. Overall, genetics services are an evaluation and communication process by which patients and their families come to learn and understand relevant aspects of genetics, to make informed health decisions, and to receive support as they integrate personal and family genetics information into daily living (Tranin et al., 2003).

Genetic counseling may take place over an extended period and may entail more than one counseling session, which may include other family members. This allows patients and families to learn and understand genetics information, to receive support and guidance in decision-making, and to obtain comprehensive and coordinated care if they have specific genetic conditions or concerns. The components of genetic counseling are outlined in Chart 9-5. Although genetic counseling may be offered at any point during the lifespan, counseling issues are often relevant to the life stage in which counseling is sought. Some examples are presented in Chart 9-6 (Lea & Smith, 2003).

Nursing Care and Interventions in Genetic Counseling

The process of genetic counseling and evaluation often involves additional genetic testing and procedures as well as decisions by patients and families with regard to reproduction, fertility, testing of children, and management options such as prophylactic surgery. Nurses have responsibilities in each of these areas for assessment and for providing psychosocial interventions and accurate information as family members consider their genetic testing and treatment options. In all of these areas, nurses consider individual patients in the context of the family.

When patients or family members are considering genetic testing, nurses provide accurate information as patients consider their options. For prenatal testing, this includes information and support for subsequent decisions regarding the pregnancy in the event of diagnosis of a genetic condition in the fetus. When a diagnosis such as Down syndrome or hereditary breast or ovarian cancer is made, families need information about the range and severity of potential problems, the proportion of people with milder aspects of the condition, management options, support organizations, and current understanding of the long-term prognosis (Williams & Lea, 2003).

Decision-making support is an important nursing intervention in many genetic counseling situations. Examples include consideration of pregnancy termination, presymptomatic testing for conditions such as Huntington disease, or predisposition testing for a hereditary cancer. Nurses help patients and families acquire information about options, identify the "pros" and "cons" of each option, and explore their values and beliefs. In addition, nurses help patients respect each person's right to receive or not to receive information and help them explain their decision to others (Dochterman & Bulechek, 2004).

Other essential components of nursing care and genetic counseling include teaching and an intervention known as "coping enhancement." For example, teaching is needed

CHART 9-5

Components of Genetic Counseling

INFORMATION AND ASSESSMENT SOURCES
- Reason for referral
- Family history
- Medical history/records
- Relevant test results and other medical evaluations
- Social and emotional concerns
- Relevant cultural, educational, and financial factors

ANALYSIS OF DATA
- Family history
- Physical examination as needed
- Additional laboratory testing and procedures (eg, echocardiogram, ophthalmology or neurologic examination)

COMMUNICATION OF GENETIC FINDING
- Natural history of disorder
- Pattern of inheritance
- Reproductive and family health issues and options
- Testing options
- Management and treatment issues

COUNSELING AND SUPPORT
- Identify individual and family questions and concerns
- Identify existing support systems
- Provide emotional and social support
- Refer for additional support and counseling as indicated

FOLLOW-UP
- Written summary to referring primary care providers and family
- Coordination of care with primary care providers and specialists
- Additional discussions of test results or diagnosis

From Lea, D. H., Jenkins, J. F., & Francomano, C. A. (1998). *Genetics in clinical practice: New directions for nursing and health care*. Sudbury, MA: Jones & Bartlett.

when a new genetics diagnosis is made. Patients and families need information about the range of possible health outcomes, treatment options, and, in the case of prenatal diagnosis of a genetic condition, management options regarding continuing or ending the pregnancy. Coping enhancement involves helping people adapt to perceived stressors or changes that interfere with daily living and functioning (Dochterman & Bulechek, 2004). Coping enhancement is essential throughout the entire genetic counseling, evaluation, and testing process. Indicators of patient knowledge, decision making, and coping outcomes have been developed (Dochterman & Bulechek, 2004), and nurses can use these indicators when documenting nursing care provided to families and its effectiveness.

Specific Nursing Roles in Genetic Counseling

Nurses refer patients, collaborate with genetics specialists, and participate in genetic counseling when they carry out the following activities:

- Provide appropriate genetics information before, during, and in follow-up to genetic counseling
- Help gather relevant family and medical history information
- Offer support to patients and families throughout the genetic counseling process
- Coordinate genetics-related health care with relevant community and national support resources

These activities are carried out in collaboration with patients and families and help ensure that they receive the most benefit from genetic counseling (Lea & Monsen, 2003).

RESPECTING PATIENTS' RIGHTS

Respecting the patient's right to self-determination—that is, supporting decisions that reflect the patient's personal beliefs, values, and interests—is a central principle directing how nurses provide genetics information and counseling. Genetics specialists and nurses participating in genetic counseling make every attempt to respect the patient's ability to make autonomous decisions. A first step in providing such nondirective counseling is recognizing one's own values (see Chart 9-1) and how communication of genetics information may be influenced by those values.

Confidentiality of genetics information and respect for privacy are other essential principles underlying genetic counseling. Patients have the right to have testing without having the results divulged to anyone, including insurers or physicians. Some patients pay for testing themselves so that insurers will not learn of the test, and others use a different name for testing to protect their privacy. The Health Insurance Portability and Accountability Act (HIPAA) of 1996 prohibits the use of genetics information to establish insurance eligibility. However, HIPAA does not prohibit group plans from increasing premiums, excluding coverage for a specific condition, or imposing a lifetime cap on benefits. The National Human Genome Research Institute, Policy and Public Affairs and Legislative Activities Branch has a summary of each state's legislation on employment and insurance discrimination (see the resources list at the end of this chapter).

All genetics specialists, including nurses who participate in the genetic counseling process and those with access to people's genetics information, must honor a patient's desire for confidentiality. Genetics information should be kept from family members, insurance companies, employers,

CHART 9-6

Genetic Counseling Across the Lifespan

PRENATAL ISSUES
- Understanding prenatal screening and diagnosis testing
- Implications of reproductive choices
- Potential for anxiety and emotional distress
- Effects on partnership, family, and parental–fetal bonding

NEWBORN ISSUES
- Understanding newborn screening results
- Potential for disrupted parent–newborn relationship on diagnosis of a genetic condition
- Parental guilt
- Implications for siblings and other family members
- Coordination and continuity of care

PEDIATRIC ISSUES
- Caring for children with complex medical needs
- Coordination of care
- Potential for impaired parent–child relationship
- Potential for social stigmatization

ADOLESCENT ISSUES
- Potential for impaired self-image and decreased self-esteem
- Potential for altered perception of family
- Implications for lifestyle and family planning

ADULT ISSUES
- Potential for ambiguous test results
- Identification of a genetic susceptibility or diagnosis without an existing cure ("therapeutic gap")
- Effect on marriage, reproduction, parenting, and lifestyle
- Potential impact on insurability and employability

From Lea, D. H., Jenkins, J. F., & Francomano, C. A. (1998). *Genetics in clinical practice: New directions for nursing and health care.* Sudbury, MA: Jones & Bartlett.

and schools if the patient so desires, even if keeping the information confidential is difficult. A nurse may want to disclose genetics information to family members who could experience significant harm if they do not know such information. However, the patient may have other views and may wish to keep this information from the family, resulting in an ethical dilemma for both patient and nurse. The nurse must honor the patient's wishes, while explaining to the patient the potential benefit this information may have for other family members (ISONG, 2002).

PROVIDING PRECOUNSELING INFORMATION

Preparing the patient and family, promoting informed decision making, and obtaining informed consent are essential in genetic counseling. Nurses assess the patient's capacity and ability to give voluntary consent. This includes assessment of factors that may interfere with informed consent, such as hearing loss, language differences, cognitive impairment, and the effects of medication. Nurses make sure that a person's decision to undergo testing is not affected by coercion, persuasion, or manipulation. Because information may need to be repeated over time, nurses offer follow-up discussion as needed (Tranin et al., 2003).

The genetics service to which a nurse refers a patient or family for genetic counseling will ask the nurse to provide background information for evaluation. Genetics specialists need to know the reason for referral, the patient's or family's reason for seeking genetic counseling, and potential genetics-related health concerns. For example, a nurse may refer a family with a new diagnosis of hereditary breast or ovarian cancer to obtain more information or counseling or to discuss the likelihood of developing the disease and the implications for other family members. The family may have concerns about confidentiality and privacy. Using the nursing assessment, the genetics specialist tailors the genetic counseling to respond to these concerns.

With the patient's permission, nurses may also provide genetics specialists with the relevant test results and medical evaluations. Nurses need to obtain permission from the patient and, if applicable, from other family members to retrieve, review, and transfer medical records that document the genetic condition of concern. In some situations, evaluation of more than one family member may be necessary to establish a diagnosis of a genetic disorder. Nurses can prepare the family for this assessment by explaining that the medical information and evaluation are necessary to ensure that appropriate information and counseling (including risk interpretation) are provided.

Nurses will be asked to provide information about the emotional and social status of the patient and family. Genetics specialists will want to know the coping skills of patients and families who have recently learned of the diagnosis of a genetic disorder and will want to know what type of genetics information is being sought. Nurses help identify cultural and other issues that may influence how information is provided and by whom. For example, for patients with hearing loss, a sign interpreter's services may have to be arranged. For those with vision loss, alternative forms of communication may be necessary. Genetics professionals prepare for the genetic counseling and evaluation with these relevant issues in mind (Lea & Smith, 2003).

PREPARING PATIENTS FOR GENETICS EVALUATION

Before a genetic counseling appointment, the nurse discusses with the patient and family the type and nature of family history information that will be collected during the consultation. Family history collection and analysis are comprehensive and focus on information that may be relevant to the genetics-related concern in question. Although targeted to each genetic counseling situation, such analysis always includes assessment for any other potentially inherited conditions for which testing and preventive and treatment measures may be available.

A physical examination performed by the medical geneticist may be needed to identify specific clinical features that are diagnostic of a genetic condition. The examination also helps determine whether additional laboratory tests are needed to clarify the diagnosis of a genetic disorder. The detailed physical examination generally involves assessment of all body systems, with a focus on specific physical characteristics considered for diagnosis. The nurse describes the diagnostic evaluations that are part of a genetics consultation and explains their purposes (Lea & Smith, 2003).

COMMUNICATING GENETICS INFORMATION TO PATIENTS

After the family history and physical examination are completed, the genetics team reviews the information gathered before beginning genetic counseling with the patient and family. The genetics specialists meet with the patient and family to discuss their findings. If information from family and medical histories and examination confirms the presence of a genetic condition in a family, genetics specialists discuss with the patient the natural history of the condition, the pattern of inheritance, and the implications of the condition for reproductive and general health. When appropriate, the specialists also discuss relevant testing and management options. The nurse assesses the patient's understanding of the genetics consultation and clarifies information given by specialists.

PROVIDING SUPPORT

The genetics team provides support throughout the counseling session and makes every effort to elicit personal and family concerns. Genetics specialists use principles of active listening to interpret patient concerns and emotions, seek and provide feedback, and demonstrate understanding of those concerns. When necessary, genetics specialists suggest referral for additional social and emotional support. Genetics specialists discuss pertinent patient and family concerns and needs with nurses and primary health care teams so that they can provide additional support and guidance (Lea & Smith, 2003). The nurse assesses the patient's understanding of the information given during the counseling session, clarifies information, answers questions, assesses patient reactions, and identifies support systems.

Follow-Up After Genetic Evaluation

As follow-up to genetic evaluation and counseling, genetics specialists prepare a written summary of the evaluation and counseling session and, with the patient's permission, send this summary to the primary health care provider as well as all other providers and participants in the patient's care, as identified by the family. The consultation summary outlines the results of the family history and physical and laboratory assessments, provides a discussion of the specific diagnosis (if made), reviews the inheritance and associated risk of recurrence for the patient and family, presents reproductive and general health options, and makes recommendations for further testing and management. The summary is also sent to the patient, and a copy is retained in the patient's medical records. The nurse plays an important role in reviewing the summary with the patient and family and identifying information, education, and counseling for which follow-up genetic counseling may be useful (Lea & Smith, 2003; Lea & Williams, 2002).

Follow-up genetic counseling is always offered to patients and families, because some people may need more time to understand and discuss the specifics of a genetic test or diagnosis, or they may wish to review reproductive options again later, when pregnancy is being considered. Follow-up genetic counseling is also offered to patients when further evaluation and counseling of extended family members is recommended (Lea & Smith, 2003).

As part of follow-up, nurses can educate patients about where to find information about genetics issues. Some resources that provide the most up-to-date and reliable genetics information are available on the Internet; several of these are listed at the end of this chapter.

Ethical Issues

With the recent advances in genetics, nurses must consider their responsibilities in handling genetics information and potential ethical issues such as informed decision-making, privacy and confidentiality of genetics information, and access to and justice in health care. The ethical principles of autonomy, fidelity, and veracity are also important (American Nurses Association, 2001).

Ethical questions relating to genetics occur in various settings and at all levels of nursing practice. At the level of direct patient care, nurses participate in providing genetics information, testing, and gene-based therapeutics. They offer patient care based on the values of self-determination and personal autonomy. The American Nurses Association (2001) states that patients should be as fully involved as possible in the planning and implementation of their own health care. To do so, patients need appropriate, accurate, and complete information given at such a level and in such a form that they and their families can make well-informed personal, medical, and reproductive health decisions. Nurses, as the most accessible health care professionals, are invaluable in the informed consent process. They can help patients clarify values and goals, assess understanding of information, protect patients' rights, and support their decisions. Nurses can advocate for patient autonomy in health decisions. ISONG's position statements, "Informed Decision-Making and Consent" (2000) and "Genetic Counseling of Vulnerable Populations" (2002), support and guide nurses who help patients considering genetic counseling and testing. Other nursing societies have also issued position statements to guide nursing practice in genetic counseling and testing. Chart 9-7 provides a list of position statements of selected genetics professional societies.

Nurses need to ensure the privacy and confidentiality of genetics information derived from such sources as the family history, genetic tests, and other genetics-based interventions. Many Americans are increasingly concerned about threats to their personal privacy. Nurses must be aware of the potential ethical issues related to the privacy and confidentiality of genetics information, including conflicts between the patient's privacy and the family's need for genetics information. ISONG's position statement, "Privacy and Confidentiality of Genetic Information" (2005), is a useful resource.

An ethical foundation provides nurses with a holistic framework for handling ethical issues with integrity. It also supplies the basis for communicating genetics information

CHART 9-7

Genetics Resources for Nurses

INTERNATIONAL SOCIETY OF NURSES IN GENETICS, INC. (ISONG)

Web site: www.isong.org

ISONG is an international nursing specialty organization dedicated to fostering the scientific and professional growth of nurses in human genetics. ISONG members represent the United States, Australia, Canada, England, Japan, Israel, Korea, Ireland, and New Zealand. Members practice in diverse health care settings, including reproductive, prenatal, pediatric, and adult settings. ISONG serves as a forum for education and support for nurses who provide genetics-related health care, and promotes integration of the nursing process into the delivery of genetics-related health care services. Major goals of ISONG are incorporation of the principles of human genetics into all levels of nursing education, promotion of the development of standards of practice for nurses in human genetics, and advancement of nursing research in human genetics.

Documents created by ISONG

- *Scope and Standards of Genetics Clinical Nursing Practice* (published in 1998 and currently being revised): developed, written, and published in conjunction with the American Nurses Association. This document delineates competencies expected for nurses practicing at the basic level, as well as enhanced competencies for nurses practicing at the advanced level.

Position statements (available on the Web site)

- Informed Decision-Making and Consent: The Role of Nursing (approved September 30, 2000; revised April 4, 2005)
- Privacy and Confidentiality of Genetic Information: The Role of the Nurse (approved August 8, 2005)
- Genetic Counseling for Vulnerable Populations: The Role of Nursing (approved October 10, 2002)
- Access to Genomic Healthcare: The Role of the Nurse (approved September 9, 2003).

ONCOLOGY NURSING SOCIETY (ONS)

Web site: www.ons.org

ONS is a professional organization of more than 30,000 registered nurses and other health care providers dedicated to excellence in patient care, education, research, and administration in oncology nursing. It is the largest professional oncology association in the world.

Position statements (available on the Web site)

- Cancer Predisposition Genetic Testing and Risk Assessment Counseling
- The Role of the Oncology Nurse in Cancer Genetic Counseling

Cancer genetics resources

- ONS Genetics Short Course for Cancer Nurses
- ONS Genetics and Cancer Care Tool Kit (available on the Web site)
- Internet Resources in Genetics for Cancer Nurses (includes evidence-based practice resource center available on the Web site)
- Tranin, A., Masny, A. & Jenkins, J. (2003). *Genetics in Oncology Practice: Cancer Risk Assessment.* PA: Oncology Nursing Press.

ASSOCIATION OF WOMEN'S HEALTH AND NEONATAL NURSES (AWHONN)

Web site: www.awhonn.org

AWHONN is the leading professional association for nurses who specialize in the care of women and newborns. Members include neonatal nurses, advanced practice nurses, women's health nurses, obstetrics/gynecology and labor and delivery nurses, nurse scientists, nurse executives and managers, childbirth educators, and nurse practitioners.

Position statements

- The Role of the Registered Nurse as Related to Genetic Testing (available on the Web site)

AMERICAN NURSES ASSOCIATION (ANA)

Web site: www.ana.org

Online Journal of Issues in Nursing: The Genetic Revolution: What, Why, How? (Available at: nursingworld.org/ojin/admin/topics.htm) (accessed March 3, 2006).

to a patient, a family, other care providers, community agencies and organizations, and society as a whole. In addition, it provides support for nurses facing clinical situations that involve ethical dilemmas. Principle-based ethics offers moral guidelines that nurses can use to justify their nursing practice. The emphasis is on ethical principles of beneficence (to do good) and nonmaleficence (to do no harm), as well as autonomy, justice, fidelity, and veracity, to help solve ethical dilemmas that may arise in clinical care. Respect for people is the ethical principle underlying all nursing care. Using an ethical foundation based on these principles that incorporates the values of caring, nurses can promote the kind of thoughtful discussions that are useful when patients and families are facing genetics-related health and reproductive decisions and consequences (ISONG, 2000; Tranin et al., 2003).

Critical Thinking Exercises

1 A 42-year-old man has just been diagnosed with colon cancer. He tells you that he is not surprised, because his father died from colon cancer when he was 45 years of age, and he has a paternal aunt who died in her late 40s from colon cancer. A paternal uncle was treated for colon cancer when he was 39 years of age, and the patient's maternal grandmother died from uterine cancer. What pattern of inheritance is suggested in this family? What genetics information would you provide to this patient?

2 ebp A 28-year-old woman is admitted to the medical unit with deep venous thrombosis (DVT). Your nursing assessment reveals that she has had three miscarriages, and her only child was born prematurely due to placental problems. Her mother had DVT at 32 years of age when she was pregnant with your patient. A maternal uncle had a pulmonary embolism when he was 45 years of age. What adult-onset condition does this history suggest? What nursing actions would you take? What is the evidence base for the nursing actions that you have identified? Explain how you would determine the strength of the evidence.

3 A 45-year-old woman has been admitted to your nursing unit with a new diagnosis of type 2 diabetes mellitus. She has a history of obesity and hypertension. In obtaining her family history, you learn that her 50-year-old sister and 70-year-old mother also have type 2 diabetes mellitus. Your patient has three daughters, and her 15-year-old daughter has a history of obesity. Your patient tells you, "I was afraid that I would get the diabetes, and now I have. I am so worried about my daughters. What is causing this in our family? What can we do?" How might you respond to the patient? What are the counseling issues that are important for this family? What other clinical resources could you make available to them?

REFERENCES AND SELECTED READINGS

BOOKS

American College of Obstetricians and Gynecologists (ACOG). (2001). *Preconception and prenatal carrier screening for cystic fibrosis: Clinical and laboratory guidelines.* Washington, DC: Author.

American Medical Association. (2001). *Identifying and managing hereditary risk for breast and ovarian cancer.* Chicago: Author.

American Nurses Association. (2001). *Code for nurses with interpretive statements.* Washington, DC: Author.

Burke, W. (2004). Genetic testing. In Guttmacher, A. E., Collins F. S. & Drazen, J. M. (Eds.). *Articles from the New England Journal of Medicine: Genomic medicine.* Baltimore, MD: The Johns Hopkins University Press.

Dochterman, J. M. & Bulechek, G. M. (Eds.). (2004). *Nursing interventions classification (NIC): Iowa Intervention Project* (4th ed.). St. Louis: C. V. Mosby.

Gardiner, R. R. M. & Sutherland, G. R. (1996). *Chromosome abnormalities and genetic counseling* (2nd ed.). New York: Oxford University Press.

Guttmacher, A. E. & Collins, F. S. (2004). Genomic medicine: A primer. In Guttmacher, A. E., Collins, F. S. & Drazen, J. M. (Eds.). *Articles from the New England Journal of Medicine: Genomic medicine.* Baltimore, MD: The Johns Hopkins University Press.

International Society of Nurses in Genetics (ISONG). (1998). *Statement on the scope and standards of genetics clinical nursing practice.* Washington, DC: American Nurses Association.

Jenkins, J. & Lea, D. H. (2004). *Nursing care in the genomic era: A case-based approach.* Sudbury, MA: Jones & Bartlett.

Lea, D. H. (2002). Genetics. In Maher, A. B., Salmond, S. W. & Pellino, T. A. (Eds.). *Orthopaedic nursing.* Philadelphia: W. B. Saunders.

Lea, D. H., Jenkins, J. F. & Francomano, C. A. (1998). *Genetics in clinical practice: New directions for nursing and health care.* Sudbury, MA: Jones & Bartlett.

Lea, D. H. & Smith, R. S. (2003). *The genetics resource guide: A handy reference for public health nurses.* Scarborough, ME: Foundation for Blood Research.

Moorhead, S., Johnson, M. & Maas, M. L. (Eds.). (2004). *Nursing interventions classification* (2nd ed.) St. Louis: C. V. Mosby.

NANDA International. (2005). *Nursing diagnoses: Definitions and classification 2005–2006* (5th ed.). Philadelphia: North American Nursing Diagnosis Association.

National Academy of Sciences, Committee for the Study of Inborn Errors of Metabolism. (1975). *Genetic screening.* Washington, DC: National Academy of Sciences.

National Institutes of Health, National Cancer Institute. (1995). *Understanding gene testing.* NIH Pub. No. 9603905. Washington, DC: U.S. Department of Health and Human Services.

Nussbaum, R. L., McInnes, R. R. & Willard, H. F. (2001). *Thompson and Thompson's genetics in medicine* (6th ed.). Philadelphia: W. B. Saunders.

Rimoin, D. L., Connor, M. J., Pyeritz, R. E., et al. (2002). *Emery and Rimoin's principles and practice of medical genetics* (4th ed.). London: Churchill Livingstone.

Roesser, K. A. & Mullineaux, L. G. (2005). *Genetic testing and hereditary cancer: Implications for nurses.* Pittsburgh, PA: Oncology Education Services.

Secretary's Advisory Committee on Genetic Testing (SACGT). (2000). *A public consultation of oversight of genetic tests.* Bethesda, MD: National Institutes of Health. Available at: www4.od.nih.gov/oba/sacgt.htm (accessed March 5, 2006).

Tranin, A. S., Masny, A. & Jenkins, J. (Eds.). (2003). *Genetics in oncology practice: Cancer risk assessment.* Pittsburgh, PA: Oncology Nursing Society.

U.S. Preventive Services Task Force. (2004). *Guide to clinical preventive services.* Baltimore: Williams & Wilkins.

Varmus, H. (2004). Getting ready for gene-based medicine. In Guttmacher, A. E., Collins, F. S. & Drazen, J. M. (Eds.). *Articles from the New England Journal of Medicine: Genomic medicine.* Baltimore, MD: The Johns Hopkins University Press.

Weinshilboum, R. (2004). Genomic medicine: Inheritance and drug response. In Guttmacher, A. E., Collins, F. S. & Drazen, J. M. (Eds.). *Articles from the New England Journal of Medicine: Genomic medicine.* Baltimore, MD: The Johns Hopkins University Press.

Williams, J. K. & Lea, D. H. (2003). *Genetic issues for perinatal nurses* (2nd ed.). White Plains, NY: March of Dimes.

JOURNALS

American Academy of Pediatrics, Committee on Genetics. (1999). Folic acid for the prevention of neural tube defects. *Pediatrics, 104*(2 Pt 1), 325–327.

American College of Medical Genetics/American Society of Human Genetics Huntington Disease Genetic Testing Working Group. (1998). ACMG/ASHG statement: Laboratory guidelines for Huntington disease genetic testing. *American Journal of Human Genetics, 62*(5), 1243–1247.

American College of Obstetrics and Gynecology, Committee on Genetics. (1996). Screening for Tay-Sachs disease. *International Journal of Gynaecology and Obstetrics, 52*(3), 311–312.

American College of Obstetrics and Gynecology, Committee on Genetics. (1999). Screening for Canavan disease. *International Journal of Gynaecology and Obstetrics, 65*(1), 91–92.

American College of Obstetrics and Gynecology, Committee on Genetics. (2001). Genetic screening for hemoglobinopathies. *International Journal of Gynaecology and Obstetrics, 74*(3), 309–310.

American Medical Association (2004). *Family medical history in disease prevention*. Es26:03-503:25M:6/04. Available at: www.ama-assn.org/go/genetics (accessed March 5, 2006).

American Society of Clinical Oncology. (2003). Policy statement update: Genetic testing for cancer susceptibility. *Journal of Clinical Oncology, 21*(12), 2397–2406.

Anderson, G., Monsen, R. B., Prows, C. A., et al. (2000). Preparing the nursing profession for participation in a genetic paradigm in health care. *Nursing Outlook, 48*(1), 23–27.

Bartsch, H., Nair, U., Risch, A., et al. (2000). Genetic polymorphism of CYP genes, alone or in combination, as a risk modifier of tobacco-related cancers. *Cancer Epidemiology, Biomarkers and Prevention, 9*(1), 3–28.

Billings, P. R. (2000). Applying advances in genetic medicine: Where do we go from here? *Healthplan, 41*(6), 32–35.

Brookes, A. J. (1999). The essence of SNPs. *Gene, 234*(2), 177–186.

Burke, W., Coughlin, S. S., Lee, N. C., et al. (2001). Applications of population screening principles to genetic screening for adult-onset conditions. *Genetic Testing, 5*(3), 201–211.

Burke, W., Thomson, E., Khoury, M. J., et al. (1998). Hereditary hemochromatosis: Gene discovery and its implications for population-based screening. *Journal of American Medical Association, 280*(2), 172–178.

Cashion, A. (2002). Genetics in transplantation. *MedSurg Nursing 11*(2), 91–94.

Collins, F. S. (1999). Medical and societal consequences of the Human Genome Project. *New England Journal of Medicine, 341*(1), 28–37.

Collins, F. S., & McKusick, V. A. (2001). Implications of the Human Genome Project for medical science. *Journal of American Medical Association, 285*(5), 540–544.

Conley, Y. P. & Gorin, M. B. (2003). The genetics of age-related macular degeneration. *MedSurg Nursing 12*(4), 238–241, 259.

Cookson, W. O. (2002). Asthma genetics. *Chest, 121*(Suppl), 7S–13S.

Cox, N. J., Frigge, M., Nicolae, D. L., et al. (1999). Loci on chromosomes 2 (NIDDM1) and 15 interact to increase susceptibility to diabetes in Mexican Americans. *Nature Genetics, 21*(2), 213–215.

Enderlin, C., Vogel, R. & Conaway, P. (2003). Gaucher disease. *American Journal of Nursing 102*(12), 50–60.

Evans, W. E. & McLeod, H. L. (2003). Drug therapy: Pharmacogenomics—Drug disposition, drug targets, and side effects. *New England Journal of Medicine, 348*(6), 538–549.

Evans, W. E. & Relling, M. V. (1999). Pharmacogenomics: Translating functional genomics into rational therapeutics. *Science, 286*(5439), 487–491.

Feetham, S. (1999). Families and the genetic revolution: Implications for primary healthcare, education, and research. *Families, Systems and Health, 17*(1), 27–43.

FitzGerald, M. G., MacDonald, D. J., Krainer, M., et al. (1996). Germ-line BRCA1 mutations in Jewish and non-Jewish women with early-onset breast cancer. *New England Journal of Medicine, 334*(3), 143–149.

Fleisher, L. K. & Cole, J. (2001). Health Insurance Portability and Accountability Act is here: What price privacy? *Genetics in Medicine, 3*(4), 286–289.

Ghosh, S., Watanabe, R. M., Valle, T. T., et al. (2000). The Finland-United States Investigation of Non-insulin-dependent Diabetes Mellitus Genetics (FUSION) Study. I. An autosomal genome scan for genes that predispose to type 2 diabetes. *American Journal of Human Genetics, 67*(5), 1174–1185.

Glassford, B. (2003). A case study in caring: Trisomy 18 syndrome. *American Journal of Nursing 103*(7), 81–83.

Goetz, M. P., Ames, M. M., & Weinshilboum, R. M. (2004). Primer on medical genomics. Part XII. Pharmacogenomics—General principles with cancer as a model. *Mayo Clinic Proceedings, 79*(3), 376–384.

Greco, K. E. (2003). Nursing in the genomic era: Nurturing our genetic nature. *MedSurg Nursing, 12*(5), 307–312.

Hetteberg, C. & Prows, C. A. (2004). A checklist to assist in the integration of genetics into nursing curricula. *Nursing Outlook 52*(2), 85–88.

Horner, S. D., Abel, E., Taylor, K., et al. (2004). Using theory to guide the diffusion of genetics content in nursing curricula. *Nursing Outlook 52*(2), 80–84.

Houfek, J. F. & Atwood, J. R. (2003). Genetic susceptibility to lung cancer: Implications for smoking cessation. *MedSurg Nursing 12*(1), 45–49.

Ingelman-Sundberg, M. (2004). Pharmacogenetics of cytochrome P450 and its applications in drug therapy: The past, present and future. *Trends in Pharmacological Sciences, 25*(4), 193–200.

International Society of Nurses in Genetics (ISONG). (2000). Position statement. Informed decision-making and consent: The role of nursing. *International Society of Nurses in Genetics Newsletter, 11*(3), 7–8. Available at: www.isong.org/about/ps_consent.cfm (accessed March 3, 2006).

International Society of Nurses in Genetics (ISONG). (2002). Position statement. Genetic counseling for vulnerable populations: The role of nursing. *MedSurg Nursing, 11*(6), 305. Available at: www.isong.org/about/ps_vulnerable.cfm (accessed March 3, 2006).

International Society of Nurses in Genetics. (2003). Position statement. Access to genomic healthcare: The role of the nurse. Available at: www.isong.org/abut/ps_genomic.cfm (accessed March 7, 2006).

International Society of Nurses in Genetics (ISONG). (2005). Position statement. Privacy and confidentiality of genetic information: The role of the nurse. *MedSurg Nursing, 11*(2), *103*. Available at: www.isong.org/about/ps_privacy.cfm (accessed March 3, 2006).

Khoury, M. J. & Jones, S. L. (2004). The confluence of two clinical specialties: Genetics and assisted reproductive technologies. *MedSurg Nursing, 13*(2), 114–121.

King, M. C., Marks, J. H., Mandell, J. B. & New York Breast Cancer Study Group. (2003). Breast and ovarian cancer risks due to inherited mutations in BRCA1 and BRCA2. *Science, 302*(5645), 643–646.

Kirchhoff, T., Kauff, N. D., Mitra, N., et al. (2004). BRCA mutations and risk of prostate cancer in Ashkenazi Jews. *Clinical Cancer Research, 10*(9), 2918–2921.

Lea, D. H. (2000). A clinician's primer in human genetics: What nurses need to know. *Nursing Clinics of North America, 35*(3), 583–614.

Lea, D. H., Anderson, G., & Monsen, R. B. (1998). A multiplicity of roles for genetic nursing: Building toward holistic practice. *Holistic Nursing Practice, 12*(3), 77–87.

Lea, D. H. & Monsen, R. B. (2003). Preparing nurses for a 21st century role in genomics-based health care. *Nursing Education Perspectives, 24*(2), 75–80.

Lea, D. H. & Williams, J. K. (2002). Genetic testing and screening. *American Journal of Nursing, 102*(7), 36–50.

Lea, D. H., Williams, J. K., Jenkins, J., et al. (2000). Genetic health care: Creating interdisciplinary partnerships with nursing in clinical practice. *National Academies of Practice Forum, 2*(3), 177–186.

McCabe, L. L., & McCabe, E. R. B. (2003). Population screening in the age of genomic medicine. *New England Journal of Medicine, 348*(1), 50–58.

McCarthy, J. J. & Hilfiker, R. (2000). The use of single-nucleotide polymorphism maps in pharmacogenomics. *Nature Biotechnology, 18*(5), 505–508.

McKinnon, W. C., Baty, B. J., Bennett, R. L., et al. (1997). Predisposition genetic testing for late-onset disorders in adults. A position paper of the National Society of Genetic Counselors. *Journal of the American Medical Association, 278*(15), 1217–1220.

Nebert, D. W. & Dieter, M. Z. (2000). The evolution of drug metabolism. *Pharmacology, 61*(3), 124–135.

Nicol, M. J. (2003). The variation of response to pharmacotherapy: Pharmacogenetics—A new perspective to "the right drug for the right person." *MedSurg Nursing, 12*(4), 242–249.

Norton, R. M. (2001). Clinical pharmacogenomics: Applications in pharmaceutical R&D. *Drug Discovery Today, 6*(4), 180–185.

Olsen, S. J., Feetham, S. L., Jenkins, J., et al. (2003). Creating a nursing vision for leadership in genetics. *MedSurg Nursing, 12*(3), 177–183.

Parker, A., Meyer, J., Lewitzky, S., et al. (2001). A gene conferring susceptibility to type 2 diabetes in conjunction with obesity is located on chromosome 18p11. *Diabetes, 50*(3), 675–680.

Pasacreta, J. V., Jacobs, L. & Cataldo, J. K. (2002). Genetic testing for breast and ovarian cancer risk: The psychosocial issues. *American Journal of Nursing, 102*(12), 40–47.

Phillips, M. (2003). Genetics of hearing loss. *MedSurg Nursing, 12*(6), 386–390, 411.

Prows, C. A. & Prows, D. R. (2004). Medication selection by genotype. *American Journal of Nursing, 104*(5), 60–70.

Peters, J. L., Djurdjinovic, L. & Baker, D. (1999). The genetic self: The Human Genome Project, genetic counseling and family therapy. *Families, Systems and Health, 17*(1), 5–25.

Ralston, S. (2004). Genetic control of susceptibility to osteoporosis. *Journal of Clinical Endocrinology and Metabolism, 87*(6), 2460–2466.

Sachidanandam, R., Weissman, D., Schmidt, S. C., et al. (2001). A map of human genome sequence variation containing 1.42 million single nucleotide polymorphisms. *Nature, 409*(6822), 928–933.

Struewing, J. P., Abeliovich, D., Peretz, T. et al. (1996). The carrier frequency of the BRCA1 185delAG mutation is approximately 1 percent in Ashkenazi Jewish individuals. *Nature Genetics, 12*(1), 198–200.

Subramanian, G., Adams, D., Venter, C., et al. (2001). Implications of the Human Genome for understanding human biology and medicine. *Journal of the American Medical Association, 286*(18), 2296–2307.

Williams, J. K., Tripp-Reimer, T., Schutte, D., et al. (2004). Advancing genetic nursing knowledge. *Nursing Outlook 52*(2), 73–79.

Wung, S.-F. (2002). Genetic advances in coronary artery disease. *MedSurg Nursing, 11*(6), 296–300.

RESOURCES

Association of Women's Health, Obstetric and Neonatal Nurses, 2000 L. Street NW, Suite 740, Washington, DC 20036; 202-261-2400 or 800-673-8499; fax 202-728-0575; http://www.awhonn.org. Accessed March 3, 2006.

Gene Tests, Children's Hospital and Regional Medical Center, P.O. Box 5371, Seattle, WA 98105; 206-527-5742; fax 206-527-5743; e-mail: genetests@genetests.org.

Genetic Alliance, Inc., 4301 Connecticut Ave. NW, Suite 404, Washington, DC 20008; 202-966-5557; e-mail: info@geneticalliance.org; http://www.geneticalliance.org. Accessed March 3, 2006.

Genetic and Rare Diseases Information Center; P.O. Box 8126, Gaithersburg, MD 20898; 888-205-2311; fax 240-632-9164; e-mail: GARDinfo@nih.gov; http://www.genome.gov/Health/GARD. Accessed May 2, 2006.

Genetics Nursing Credentialing Commission. http://www.geneticnurse.org/. Accessed March 5, 2006.

International Society of Nurses in Genetics, Inc. (ISONG), 2593 W. 15th Street, Newton, IA 50208; 641-831-9230; fax 956-581-3108; http://www.isong.org. Accessed March 3, 2006.

National Cancer Institute (NCI), Public Inquiries Office, Building 31, Room 10A03, 31 Center Drive, MSC 2580, Bethesda, MD 20892-2580; 301-435-3848; http://www.nci.nih.gov. Accessed March 5, 2006.

National Coalition for Health Professional Education in Genetics (NCHPEG), 2630 W. Joppa Rd., Suite 320, Lutherville, MD 21093; 410-583-0600; http://www.nchpeg.org. Accessed March 5, 2006.

National Human Genome Research Institute, Policy and Public Affairs and Legislative Activities Branch [summary of each state's legislation on employment and insurance discrimination], http://www.genome.gov/PolicyEthics/LegDatabase/pubsearch.cfm. Accessed May 2, 2006.

National Organization for Rare Disorders, Inc. (NORD), 55 Kenosia Avenue, PO Box 1968, Danbury, CT 06813; 203-744-0100; voicemail 800-999-6673, TDD 203-797-9590, fax 203-798-2291; e-mail: orphan@rarediseases.org; http://www.rarediseases.org. Accessed March 3, 2006.

Online Mendelian Inheritance in Man (OMIM), National Center for Biotechnology Information, National Library of Medicine, Building 38A, Room 8N805, Bethesda, MD 20894; 301-496-2475; fax 301-480-9241; http://www.ncbi.nlm.nih.gov/Omim. Accessed March 3, 2006.

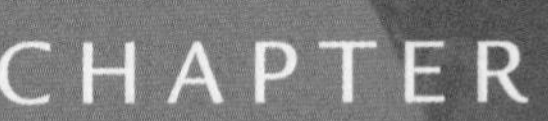

10

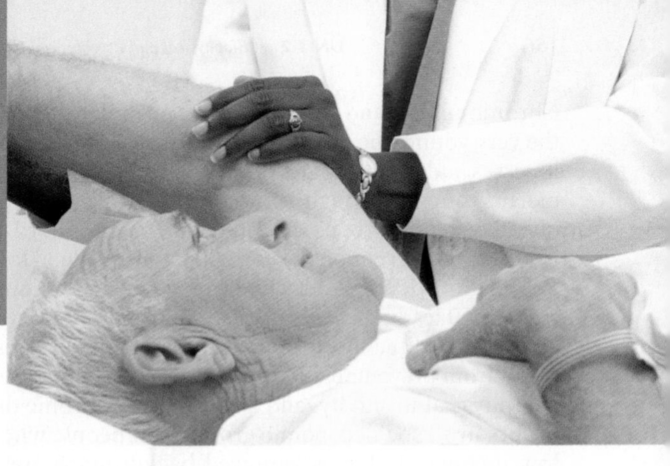

Chronic Illness and Disability

Learning Objectives

On completion of this chapter, the learner will be able to:

1. Define "chronic conditions."
2. Identify factors related to the increasing incidence of chronic conditions.
3. Describe characteristics of chronic conditions and implications for people with chronic conditions and for their families.
4. Describe advantages and disadvantages of various models of disability.
5. Describe implications of disability for nursing practice.

Chronic illness and disability affect people of all ages—the very young, the middle-aged, and the very old. Chronic illnesses and disability are found in all ethnic, cultural, and racial groups, although some disorders occur more frequently in some groups than in others (Centers for Disease Control and Prevention [CDC], 2004; Robert Wood Johnson Foundation [RWJF], 2001). Chronic diseases account for 7 of the 10 leading causes of death in the United States, including the three most frequently occurring diseases that result from preventable causes (tobacco use, improper diet and physical inactivity, and alcohol use). Chronic disease occurs in all socioeconomic groups, but people who have low incomes and disadvantaged backgrounds are more likely to report poor health (RWJF, 2001). Factors such as poverty and inadequate health insurance decrease the likelihood that people with chronic illness or disability receive health care and health screening measures such as mammography, cholesterol testing, and routine checkups (United States Department of Health and Human Services [USDHHS], 2005).

Many people with chronic health conditions and disability function independently with only minor inconvenience to their everyday lives; others require frequent and close monitoring or placement in long-term care facilities. Certain conditions require advanced technology for survival, as in the late stages of amyotrophic lateral sclerosis or end-stage renal disease, or intensive care for periods of weeks or months. People with disorders such as these have been described as chronically critically ill (Carson & Bach, 2002). Some chronic conditions have little effect on quality of life, but others have a considerable effect because they result in disability. However, not all disabilities are a result of chronic illness, and not all chronic illnesses cause disability. In this chapter, chronic illness is discussed, followed by a discussion of disability and the implications for nursing practice.

Overview of Chronicity

Although each chronic condition has its own specific physiologic characteristics, chronic conditions do share common features. Many chronic conditions, for example, have pain and fatigue as associated symptoms. Some degree of disability is usually present in severe or advanced chronic illness, limiting the patient's participation in many activities. Many chronic conditions require therapeutic regimens to keep them under control. Unlike the term "acute," which implies a curable and relatively short disease course, the term "chronic" describes a long disease course and conditions that may be incurable. This often makes managing chronic conditions difficult for those who must live with them.

Psychological and emotional reactions of patients to acute and chronic conditions and changes in their health status are described in detail in Chapter 7. People who develop chronic conditions or disabilities may react with shock, disbelief, depression, anger, resentment, or a number of other emotions. How people react to and cope with chronic illness is usually similar to how they react to other events in their lives, depending, in part, on their understanding of the condition and their perceptions of its potential impact on their own and their family's lives. Adjustment to chronic illness (and disability) is affected by various factors:

- Suddenness, extent, and duration of lifestyle changes necessitated by the illness
- Family and individual resources for dealing with stress
- Stages of individual/family life cycle
- Previous experience with illness and crises
- Underlying personality characteristics
- Unresolved anger or grief from the past

Psychological, emotional, and cognitive reactions to chronic conditions are likely to occur at their onset and to recur if symptoms worsen or recur after a period of remission. Symptoms associated with chronic health conditions are often unpredictable and may be perceived as crisis events by patients and their families, who must contend with both the uncertainty of chronic illness and the changes it brings to their lives. These possible effects of chronic conditions can guide nursing assessment and interventions for the patient who has a chronic illness.

Definition of Chronic Conditions

Chronic conditions are often defined as medical conditions or health problems with associated symptoms or disabilities that require long-term management (3 months or longer). Chronic conditions can also be defined as illnesses or diseases that have a prolonged course, that do not resolve spontaneously, and for which complete cures are rare (McKenna, Taylor, Marks, et al., 1998). The specific condition may be a result of illness, genetic factors, or injury; it may be a consequence of conditions or unhealthy behaviors that began

Glossary

chronic conditions: medical or health problems with associated symptoms or disabilities that require long-term management (3 months or longer)

disability: restriction or lack of ability to perform an activity in a normal manner; the consequences of impairment in terms of an individual's functional performance and activity. Disabilities represent disturbances at the level of the person (eg, bathing, dressing, communication, walking, grooming).

impairment: loss or abnormality of psychological, physiologic, or anatomic structure or function at the organ level (eg, dysphagia, hemiparesis); an abnormality of body structure, appearance, and organ or system function resulting from any cause.

secondary conditions or disorders: preventable physical, mental, or social disorders resulting directly or indirectly from an initial disabling condition during childhood and young adulthood. Management of chronic conditions includes learning to live with symptoms or disabilities and coming to terms with identity changes resulting from having a chronic condition. It also consists of carrying out the lifestyle changes and regimens designed to control symptoms and to prevent complications. Although some people assume what might be called a "sick role" identity, most people with chronic conditions do not consider themselves to be sick or ill and try to live as normal a life as possible. Only when complications develop or symptoms interfere with activities of daily living (ADLs) do most people with chronic health conditions think of themselves as being sick or disabled (Nijhof, 1998).

Prevalence and Causes of Chronic Conditions

Chronic conditions occur in people of every age group, socioeconomic level, and culture. In 1995, an estimated 99 million people in the United States had chronic conditions, and it has been projected that by the year 2050, about 167 million people will be affected (RWJF, 2001). As the incidence of chronic illnesses increases, the costs associated with these illnesses (ie, hospital costs, equipment, medications, supportive services) also increase. Expenditures for health care for people with chronic conditions exceed billions of dollars every year (Table 10-1). Chronic disease is associated with 70% of health care costs in the United States (CDC, 2004).

Although some chronic health conditions cause little or no inconvenience, others are severe enough to cause major activity limitations. When people with activity limitations are unable to meet their needs for health care and personal services, they may be unable to carry out their therapeutic regimens or have their prescriptions filled on time, may miss appointments and office visits with their health care providers, and may be unable to carry out their ADLs.

Chronic disease is a global issue that affects both rich and poor nations (Mascie-Taylor & Karim, 2003). Chronic conditions have become the major cause of health-related problems in developed countries and are increasing in incidence in the developing countries, which are also trying to cope with new and emerging infectious diseases. Causes of the increasing number of people with chronic conditions include the following:

- A decrease in mortality from infectious diseases, such as smallpox, diphtheria, and other serious conditions
- Longer lifespans because of advances in technology and pharmacology, improved nutrition, safer working conditions, and greater access (for some people) to health care
- Improved screening and diagnostic procedures, enabling early detection and treatment of diseases
- Prompt and aggressive management of acute conditions, such as myocardial infarction and acquired immunodeficiency syndrome (AIDS)–related infections
- The tendency to develop chronic illnesses with advancing age
- Lifestyle factors, such as smoking, chronic stress, and sedentary lifestyle, that increase the risk for chronic health problems such as respiratory disease, hypertension, cardiovascular disease, and obesity

Consequences of unhealthy lifestyles include an alarming increase in the incidence of diabetes, hypertension, obesity, and cardiac and chronic respiratory disorders (Juarbe, 1998; McKenna et al., 1998; USDHHS, 2001; Wing, Goldstein, Acton, et al., 2001). Physiologic changes in the body often occur before the appearance of symptoms of chronic disease. Therefore, the goal of emphasizing healthy lifestyles early in life is to improve overall health status and slow the development of such disorders.

Characteristics of Chronic Conditions

Sometimes it is difficult for people who are disease-free to understand the often profound effect of chronic illness on the lives of patients and their families. It is easy for health professionals to focus on the illness or disability itself while overlooking the person who has the disorder. In all illnesses, but even more so with chronic conditions, the illness cannot be separated from the person. People with chronic illness must contend with it daily. To relate to what people must cope with or to plan effective interventions, nurses must understand what it means to have a chronic illness (Cumbie, Conley & Burman, 2004). Characteristics of chronic illness include the following:

- Managing chronic illness involves more than managing medical problems. Associated psychological and social problems must also be addressed, because living for long periods with illness symptoms and disability can threaten identity, bring about role changes, alter body image, and disrupt lifestyles. These changes require continuous adaptation and accommodation, depending on age and situation in life. Each decline in functional ability requires physical, emotional, and social adaptation for patients and

TABLE 10-1 Estimated Number of People and Direct Medical Costs for People With Chronic Conditions, Selected Years, 1995–2050

	1995	2000	2005	2010	2020	2030	2040	2050
People (millions)	99	105	112	120	134	148	158	167
Dollar costs (billions)	$470	$503	$539	$582	$685	$798	$864	$906

With permission from Robert Wood Johnson Foundation. (1996). *Chronic care in America: A 21st century challenge.* Princeton, NJ: Robert Wood Johnson Foundation.

their families (Corbin, 2003; Williams, Williams, Graff, et al., 2002).

- Chronic conditions usually involve many different phases over the course of a person's lifetime. There can be acute periods, stable and unstable periods, flare-ups, and remissions. Each phase brings its own set of physical, psychological, and social problems, and each requires its own regimens and types of management.
- Keeping chronic conditions under control requires persistent adherence to therapeutic regimens. Failing to adhere to a treatment plan or to do so consistently increases the risks of developing complications and accelerating the disease process. However, the realities of daily life, including the impact of culture, values, and socioeconomic factors, affect the degree to which people adhere to a treatment regimen. Managing a chronic illness takes time, requires knowledge and planning, and can be uncomfortable and inconvenient. It is not unusual for patients to stop taking medications or alter dosages because of side effects that are more disturbing or disruptive than symptoms of the illness, or to cut back on regimens they consider overly time-consuming, fatiguing, or costly (Corbin, 2003).
- One chronic disease can lead to the development of other chronic conditions. Diabetes, for example, can eventually lead to neurologic and vascular changes that may result in visual, cardiac, and kidney disease and erectile dysfunction (CDC, 2004). The presence of a chronic illness also contributes to a higher risk of morbidity and mortality in patients admitted to the intensive care unit with acute health conditions (Johnston, Wagner, Timmons, et al., 2002).
- Chronic illness affects the entire family. Family life can be dramatically altered as a result of role reversals, unfilled roles, loss of income, time required to manage the illness, decreases in family socialization activities, and the costs of treatment. Stress and caretaker fatigue are common with severe chronic conditions, and the entire family rather than just the patient may need care (Fisher & Weiks, 2000). However, some families are able to master the treatment regimen and changes that accompany chronic illness as well as make the treatment regimen a routine part of life. Furthermore, they are able to keep the chronic illness from becoming the focal point of family life (Knafl & Gilliss, 2002).
- The day-to-day management of illness is largely the responsibility of people with chronic disorders and their families. As a result, the home, rather than the hospital, is the center of care in chronic conditions. Hospitals, clinics, physicians' offices, nursing homes, nursing centers, and community agencies (home care services, social services, and disease-specific associations and societies) are considered adjuncts or backup services to daily home management.
- The management of chronic conditions is a process of discovery. People can be taught how to manage their conditions. However, each person must discover how his or her own body reacts under varying circumstances—for example, what it is like to be hypoglycemic, what activities are likely to bring on angina, and how these or other conditions can best be prevented and managed.
- Managing chronic conditions must be a collaborative process that involves many different health care professionals working together with patients and their families to provide the full range of services that are often needed for management at home. The medical, social, and psychological aspects of chronic health problems are often complex, especially in severe conditions.
- The management of chronic conditions is expensive (see Table 10-1). Many of the expenses incurred by an individual patient (eg, costs for hospital stays, diagnostic tests, equipment, medications, supportive services) may be covered by health insurance and by federal and state agencies. However, the cost increases affect society as a whole as insurance premiums increase to cover these costs. Cost increases at the government level decrease resources that might benefit society. In addition, many out-of-pocket expenses are not reimbursed. Many people with chronic disorders, including the elderly and people who are working, are uninsured or underinsured and may be unable to afford the high costs of care often associated with chronic illnesses (Mold, Fryer, & Thomas, 2004). Absence from work because of chronic disorders may jeopardize job security and income.
- Chronic conditions raise difficult ethical issues for patients, health care professionals, and society. Problematic questions include how to establish cost controls, how to allocate scarce resources (eg, organs for transplantation), and what constitutes quality of life and when life support should be withdrawn.
- Living with chronic illness means living with uncertainty (Bailey, Mishel, Belyea, et al., 2004; Mishel, 1999; Mishel, Germino, Belyea, et al., 2003). Although health care providers may be aware of the usual progression of a chronic disease such as Parkinson's disease, no one can predict with certainty a person's illness course because of individual variation. Even when a patient is in remission or symptom-free, he or she often fears that the illness will reappear.

Implications of Managing Chronic Conditions

Chronic conditions have implications for everyday living and management for people and their families as well as for society at large. Most importantly, individual efforts should be directed at preventing chronic conditions, because many chronic illnesses or disorders are linked to unhealthy lifestyles or behaviors such as smoking and overeating. Therefore, changes in lifestyle can prevent some chronic disorders, or at least delay onset until a later age. Because most people resist change, bringing about alterations in people's lifestyles is a major challenge for nurses today.

Once a chronic condition has occurred, the focus shifts to managing symptoms, avoiding complications (eg, eye complications in a person with diabetes), and avoiding the development of other acute illnesses (eg, pneumonia in a person with chronic obstructive lung disease). Quality of life, often overlooked by health professionals in their approach to people with chronic conditions, is also important. Health-promoting behaviors, such as exercise, are essential to quality of life even in people who have chronic illnesses and disabilities, because they help to maintain functional status (Stuifbergen & Rogers, 1997).

Although coworkers, extended family, and health care professionals are affected by chronic illnesses, the problems of living with chronic conditions are most acutely experienced by patients and their immediate families. They experience the greatest impact, with lifestyle changes that directly affect quality of life. Nurses provide direct care, especially during acute episodes, but they also provide the teaching and secure the resources and other supports that enable people to integrate their illness into their lives and to have an acceptable quality of life despite the illness. To understand what nursing care is needed, it is important to recognize and appreciate the issues that people with chronic illness and their families contend with and manage, often on a daily basis. The challenges of living with chronic conditions include the need to accomplish the following:

- Alleviate and manage symptoms
- Psychologically adjust to and physically accommodate disabilities
- Prevent and manage crises and complications
- Carry out regimens as prescribed
- Validate individual self-worth and family functioning
- Manage threats to identity
- Normalize personal and family life as much as possible
- Live with altered time, social isolation, and loneliness
- Establish the networks of support and resources that can enhance quality of life
- Return to a satisfactory way of life after an acute debilitating episode (eg, another myocardial infarction or stroke) or reactivation of a chronic condition
- Die with dignity and comfort

Many people with chronic illness must face an additional challenge: the need to deal with more than one chronic illness at a time. The symptoms or treatment of a second chronic condition may aggravate the first chronic condition (Bayliss, Steiner, Fernald, et al., 2003). Patients need to be able to deal with their various chronic conditions separately as well as in combination. Some Medicare beneficiaries have five or more chronic conditions, see an average of 13 physicians per year, and fill an average of 50 prescriptions per year (Anderson, 2005). Furthermore, the effects of increasing longevity among Americans are likely to increase health care costs in the future (Rice & Fineman, 2004).

Even more challenging for many people with chronic illness is the need to hire and oversee caregivers who come into their homes to assist with ADLs and instrumental activities of daily living (IADLs). It is difficult for many people to be in a position of hiring, supervising, and sometimes firing people who may provide them with intimate physical care. The need to balance the role of recipient of care and oversight of the person providing care may lead to blurring of role boundaries (Allen & Ciambrone, 2003).

The challenges of living with and managing a chronic illness are well known, and people with chronic illnesses often report receiving inadequate care, information, services, and counseling (Chart 10-1). This provides an opportunity for nurses to assume a more active role in addressing many of the issues experienced, coordinating care, and serving as an advocate for patients who need additional assistance to manage their illness while maintaining a quality of life that is acceptable to them.

Phases of Chronic Conditions

Chronic conditions can pass through different phases, as described in Table 10-2. However, this course may be too uncertain to predict with any degree of accuracy. The course of an illness can be thought of as a trajectory that can be managed or shaped over time, to some extent, through proper illness management strategies (Corbin, 1998; Robinson, Bevil, Arcangelo, et al., 2001). It is important to keep in mind that not all phases occur in all patients; some phases do not occur at all, and some phases may recur. Each phase is characterized by different medical and psychosocial issues. For example, the needs of a patient with a stroke who is a good candidate for rehabilitation are very different from those of a patient with terminal cancer. By thinking in terms of phases and individual patients within a phase, nurses can target their care more specifically to each person. Not every chronic condition is necessarily life-threatening, and not every patient passes through each possible phase of a chronic condition in the same order.

Using the trajectory model enables the nurse to put the present situation into the context of what might have happened to the patient in the past—that is, the life factors and understandings that might have contributed to the present state of the illness. In this way, the nurse can more readily address the underlying issues and problems.

Nursing Care of Patients With Chronic Conditions

Nursing care of patients with chronic conditions is varied and occurs in a variety of settings. Care may be direct or supportive. Direct care may be provided in the clinic or physician's office, the hospital, or the patient's home, depending on the status of the illness. Examples of direct care include assessing the patient's physical status, providing wound care, managing and overseeing medication regimens, and performing other technical tasks. The availability of this type of nursing care may allow the patient to remain at home and return to a more normal life after an acute episode of illness.

Because much of the day-to-day responsibility for managing chronic conditions rests with the patient and family, nurses often provide supportive care at home. Supportive care may include ongoing monitoring, teaching, counseling, serving as an advocate for the patient, making referrals, and case-managing. Giving supportive care is just as important as giving technical care. For example, through ongoing monitoring either in the home or in a clinic, a nurse might detect early signs of impending complications and make a referral (ie, contact the physician or consult the medical protocol in a clinic) for medical evaluation, thereby preventing a lengthy and costly hospitalization.

Working with people with chronic illness or disability requires not just dealing with the medical aspects of their dis-

CHART 10-1

Characteristics of Patients With Chronic Illness in America, 2001

A representative sample of 24,053 people with one of six chronic health conditions (arthritis, asthma, hypertension, cardiovascular disease, depression, type 2 diabetes) or family caregivers of people with chronic illness were invited to participate in an online survey.

A total of 6,447 people (4013 patients and 2434 family caregivers) completed the online survey. The findings reveal that people with chronic illnesses

- Experience greater gaps in economic and cultural access to the health care system than those without chronic illness
- Report having increasing difficulty affording health care
- Have high rates of unmet needs for support services, including home care and transportation, rehabilitation services, referral, and counseling
- Lack financial access to health care and to insurance coverage and affordability, as well as physical access
- Report poorer quality of life, fewer visits to health care providers, less knowledge about how to manage their illness, poorer relationships with their physicians, and less complete benefit from modern standards of care if they are uninsured or underinsured when compared with those who have adequate insurance
- Do not receive the information and services needed to manage their illness successfully
- Are infrequently advised by their physicians to make healthy behavior choices
- Do not receive recommended condition-specific tests and treatments about one half of the time
- Are at high risk for having unmet health-related needs
- Are less likely to receive appropriate levels of care, information, and attention from their physicians if they are members of minority groups, especially Hispanics, are poor, or are younger than 25 years of age
- Report that they do not receive adequate information and counseling about self-care from their physician, including information about medication therapy needed to avoid complications
- Report being confused about self-care activities even if they receive counseling about self-care from their physicians
- Report that treatment options and their pros and cons are not discussed with them by their physicians
- Report that their preferences regarding treatment are not taken into account and they do not feel that their physicians collaborate with them about management of their illness
- Do not feel fully involved in decisions about their own care and do not feel a sense of confidence about managing their illness
- Report that they were never advised or are confused about how to manage their illness
- Report having little sense of control over their lives and their illness
- Report infrequently receiving information or recommendations from their physicians about healthy behaviors (eg, exercise, weight control, smoking avoidance, misuse of alcohol, healthy eating)

Adapted from Robert Wood Johnson Foundation. (2001). *A portrait of the chronically ill in America, 2001.* Report from the Robert Wood Johnson Foundation National Strategic Indicator Survey. Princeton, NJ: Robert Wood Johnson Foundation.

order, but also working with the whole person—physically, emotionally, and socially. This holistic approach to care requires nurses to draw on their knowledge and skills, including knowledge from the social sciences and psychology in particular. People often respond to illness, health teaching, and regimens in ways that differ from the expectations of health care providers. Although quality of life is usually affected by chronic illness, especially if the illness is severe, patients' perceptions of what constitutes quality of life often drive their management behaviors or affect how they view advice about health care. Nurses and other health care professionals need to recognize this, even though it may be difficult to see patients make unwise choices and decisions about lifestyles and disease management. People have the right to receive care without fearing ridicule or refusal of treatment, even if their behaviors (eg, smoking, substance abuse, overeating, failure to follow health care providers' recommendations) may have contributed to their chronic disorder.

Applying the Nursing Process Using the Phases of the Chronic Illness System

The focus of care for patients with chronic conditions is determined largely by the phase of the illness and is directed by the nursing process, which includes assessment, diagnosis, planning, implementation, and evaluation.

Step 1: Identifying Specific Problems and the Trajectory Phase

The first step is assessment of the patient to determine the specific problems identified by the patient, family, nurse, and other health care providers. Assessment enables the nurse to identify the specific medical, social, and psychological problems likely to be encountered in a phase. For instance, the problems of a patient with an acute myocardial infarction are very different from those likely to occur with

TABLE 10-2 Phases in the Trajectory Model of Chronic Illness

Phase	Description	Focus of Nursing Care
Pretrajectory	Genetic factors or lifestyle behaviors that place a person or community at risk for a chronic condition	Refer for genetic testing and counseling if indicated; provide education about prevention of modifiable risk factors and behaviors
Trajectory onset	Appearance or onset of noticeable symptoms associated with a chronic disorder; includes period of diagnostic workup and announcement of diagnosis; may be accompanied by uncertainty as patient awaits a diagnosis and begins to discover and cope with implications of diagnosis	Provide explanations of diagnostic tests and procedures and reinforce information and explanations given by primary health care provider; provide emotional support to patient and family
Stable	Illness course and symptoms are under control as symptoms, resulting disability and everyday life activities are being managed within limitations of illness; illness management centered in the home	Reinforce positive behaviors and offer ongoing monitoring; provide education about health promotion and encourage participation in health promoting activities and health screening
Unstable	Characterized by an exacerbation of illness symptoms, development of complications, or reactivation of an illness in remission Period of inability to keep symptoms under control or reactivation of illness; difficulty in carrying out everyday life activities May require more diagnostic testing and trial of new treatment regimens or adjustment of current regimen, with care usually taking place at home	Provide guidance and support; reinforce previous teaching
Acute	Severe and unrelieved symptoms or the development of illness complications necessitating hospitalization, bed rest, or interruption of the person's usual activities to bring illness course under control	Provide direct care and emotional support to the patient and family members
Crisis	Critical or life-threatening situation requiring emergency treatment or care and suspension of everyday life activities until the crisis has passed	Provide direct care, collaborate with other health care team members to stabilize patient's condition
Comeback	Gradual recovery after an acute period and learning to live with or to overcome disabilities and return to an acceptable way of life within the limitations imposed by the chronic condition or disability; involves physical healing, limitations stretching through rehabilitative procedures, psychosocial coming-to-terms, and biographical reengagement with adjustments in everyday life activities	Assist in coordination of care; rehabilitative focus may require care from other health care providers; provide positive reinforcement for goals identified and accomplished
Downward	Illness course characterized by rapid or gradual worsening of a condition; physical decline accompanied by increasing disability or difficulty in controlling symptoms; requires biographical adjustment and alterations in everyday life activities with each major downward step	Provide home care and other community-based care to help patient and family adjust to changes and come to terms with these changes; assist patient and family to integrate new treatment and management strategies; encourage identification of end-of-life preferences and planning
Dying	Final days or weeks before death; characterized by gradual or rapid shutting down of body processes, biographical disengagement and closure, and relinquishment of everyday life interests and activities	Provide direct and supportive care to patients and their families through hospice programs

Adapted from Corbin, J. M. (1998). The Corbin and Strauss Chronic Illness Trajectory Model: An update. *Scholarly Inquiry for Nursing Practice, 12*(1), 33–41.

the same patient, 10 years later, dying at home of heart failure. The types of direct care, referrals, teaching, and emotional support needed in each situation are different as well. Because complementary and alternative therapies are often used by people with chronic illness, it is important to determine whether a patient with a chronic illness is using these regimens.

Step 2: Establishing and Prioritizing Goals

Once the phase of illness has been identified for a specific patient, along with the specific medical problems and related social and psychological problems, the nurse helps prioritize problems and establish the goals of care. Identification of goals must be a collaborative effort, with the patient, family, and nurse working together, and the goals must be consistent with the abilities, desires, motivations, and resources of those involved.

Step 3: Defining the Plan of Action to Achieve Desired Outcomes

Once goals have been established, it is necessary to identify a realistic and mutually agreed-on plan for achieving them, including specific criteria that will be used to assess the patient's progress. The identification of the person responsible for each task in the action plan is also essential.

In addition, identification of the environmental, social, and psychological factors that might interfere with or facilitate achieving the desired outcome is an important part of planning.

Step 4: Implementing the Plan and Interventions

This step addresses implementation of the plan. Possible nursing interventions include providing direct care, serving as an advocate for the patient, teaching, counseling, making referrals, and case-managing (eg, arranging for resources). Nurses can help patients implement the actions that allow patients to live with the symptoms and therapies associated with chronic conditions, thus helping them to gain independence. The nurse works with each patient and family to identify the best ways to integrate treatment regimens into their ADLs to accomplish two tasks: (1) adhering to regimens to control symptoms and keep the illness stable, and (2) dealing with the psychosocial issues that can hinder illness management and affect quality of life. Helping patients and their families to understand and implement regimens and to carry out ADLs within the limits of the chronic illness or disability is an important aspect of nursing care for patients with chronic disorders and disabilities and their families.

Step 5: Following Up and Evaluating Outcomes

The final step involves following up to determine if the problem is resolving or being managed and if the patient and family are adhering to the plan. This follow-up may uncover the existence of new problems resulting from the intervention, problems that interfere with the ability of the patient and family to carry out the plan, or previously unexpected problems. Maintaining the stability of the chronic condition while preserving the patient's control over his or her life and the patient's sense of identity and accomplishment is a primary goal. Based on the follow-up and evaluation, consideration of alternative strategies or revision of the initial plan may be warranted.

Helping the patient and family to integrate changes into their lifestyle is an important part of the process. Change takes time, patience, and creativity and often requires encouragement from the nurse. Validation by the nurse for each small increment toward goal accomplishment is important for enhancing self-esteem and reinforcing behaviors. Success may be defined as making some progress toward a goal when a patient is unable to implement rapid and dramatic changes in his or her life. If no progress is made, or if progress toward goals seems too slow, it may be necessary to redefine the goals, the intervention, or the time frame. The nurse must realize and accept that some people will not change. Patients share responsibility for management of their conditions, and outcomes are as much related to their ability to accommodate the illness and carry out regimens as they are to nursing intervention.

Home and Community-Based Care

Teaching Patients Self-Care

Because chronic conditions are so costly to people, families, and society, one of the major goals of nursing today should be the prevention of chronic conditions and the care of people with them. This requires promoting healthy lifestyles and encouraging the use of safety and disease-prevention measures, such as wearing seat belts and obtaining immunizations. Prevention should also begin early in life and continue throughout life. Self-care teaching may need to address interactions among the patient's chronic conditions as well as skills necessary to care for the individual diseases and their interactive effects (Bayliss et al., 2003).

Patient and family teaching is an important nursing role that may make the difference in the ability of the patient and family to adapt to chronic conditions. Well-informed, educated patients are more likely than uninformed patients to be concerned about their health and to do what is necessary to maintain it. They are also more likely to manage symptoms, recognize the onset of complications, and seek health care early. Knowledge is the key to making informed choices and decisions during all phases of the chronic illness trajectory.

Despite the importance of teaching the patient and family, the nurse must recognize that patients recently diagnosed with serious chronic conditions and their families may need time to understand the significance of their condition and its effect on their lives. Teaching must be planned carefully so that it is not overwhelming. Furthermore, it is important to assess the impact of a new diagnosis of chronic illness on a patient's life and the meaning of self-management to the patient (Kralik, Koch, Price, et al., 2004).

The nurse who cares for patients with chronic conditions in the hospital, clinic, or home should assess each patient's knowledge about his or her illness and its management; the nurse cannot assume that a patient with a long-standing chronic condition has the knowledge necessary to manage the condition. Learning needs change as the trajectory phase and the patient's personal situation changes. The nurse must also recognize that patients may know how their body responds under certain conditions and how best to manage their symptoms (Gallo & Knafl, 1998). Contact with patients in the hospital, clinic, home, or long-term care facility offers nurses the ideal opportunity to reassess patients' learning needs and to provide additional teaching about an illness and its management.

Teaching strategies and teaching materials should be adapted to the individual patient, so that the patient and family can understand and follow recommendations from health care providers. For instance, teaching materials should be tailored for people with low literacy levels and available

NURSING RESEARCH PROFILE

Chronic Illness Self-Management: The Patient's Perspective

Kralik, D., Koch, T., Price, K., et al. (2004). Chronic illness self-management: Taking action to create order. *Journal of Clinical Nursing, 13*(2), 259–267.

Purpose

Although self-management is widely considered essential to successful coping with chronic illness, what self-management means to people with chronic illness is not well described. The purpose of this study was to explore the ways in which people who live with chronic illness view the notion of self-management. Participants in this study had arthritis, but the focus was on the meaning of self-management rather than the experience of living with the symptoms of arthritis.

Design

Nine community-dwelling adults with arthritis participated in this qualitative study. The sample included six women and three men between 48 years and 75 years of age (mean, 60 years) who had lived with arthritis for 4 years to 52 years (mean, 17 years). Those who agreed to participate were asked to record or write an autobiography about their lives and experiences of coping with a chronic illness. Two telephone interviews were conducted with each participant. The first interview introduced the study and provided an opportunity for participants to ask questions. The second interview was conducted using probing questions and lasted for an average of 85 minutes. Examples of questions used included the following: What have you experienced when you sought medical help? How do you live with arthritis? How has life changed for you (since diagnosis)? One participant requested a face-to-face interview that was conducted in the person's home. Notes were taken during the interviews and transcribed as soon as possible. After preliminary analysis of the data, the participants and their partners attended a dinner meeting to discuss and provide feedback on the preliminary research findings. The discussion was recorded and transcribed.

Findings

The constant-comparative method of analysis of the three sources of data (autobiography, telephone interview transcripts, and group discussion transcripts) revealed that self-management is a complex, multidimensional process that people use to create order from the disorder imposed by illness. The researchers identified four themes:

- *Recognizing and monitoring boundaries.* Boundaries are created by pain and by the disorder and disruption it creates. The existence of pain serves as a constant reminder of the boundaries and dependencies created by illness.
- *Mobilizing resources.* This involves identifying, understanding, and making the most of the psychological, physical, and material resources available to help people live well. The desire to maintain independence influences use of available resources, and the availability of resources also influences the desire to maintain independence. Use of resources involves balancing self-protective behaviors without burdening others.
- *Managing the shift in self-identify.* The experience of learning to live with chronic illness involves a process of shifts in self-identity as a result of disruption in work and family relationships and future plans. Some participants experience a profound loss of self and shifts in identity.
- *Balancing, pacing, planning, and prioritizing.* Daily activities need to be paced so that patients are able to tolerate pain or not aggravate it and to balance the undesired side effects of medication against the benefits of pain reduction.

At times, self-management is predictable and certain, and at other times it requires management of a crisis. Planning and prioritizing are closely linked to accepting and managing the action needed for change and determining what is most important to the participant.

Nursing Implications

The findings of this study revealed that self-management is perceived by people with chronic illness in ways that differ from the views of health care providers. Nurses must consider that self-management is not perceived as involving education about the illness or adherence to medical treatment regimens. Self-management should be viewed from the perspective of the person who is living with the chronic illness. The illness as well as its consequences and self-management are both a structure and a process. Although self-management interventions have been identified for chronic illness, these have often been developed from the viewpoint of the health care provider or health care system rather than from an understanding of what it is like to live with and cope with a chronic illness. Strategies to empower and support people to manage chronic illness successfully are essential for effective nursing care.

in several languages and in various alternative formats (eg, Braille, large print, audiotapes). It may be necessary to provide sign interpreters.

Continuing Care

Chronic illness management is a collaborative process between the patient, family, nurse, and other health care providers. Collaboration extends to all settings and throughout the illness trajectory (Corbin & Cherry, 2001). Keeping an illness stable over time requires careful monitoring of symptoms and attention to management regimens. Detecting problems early and helping patients develop appropriate management strategies can make a significant difference in outcomes.

Most chronic conditions are managed in the home. Therefore, care and teaching during hospitalization should focus on essential information about the condition so that management can continue once the patient is discharged home. Nurses in all settings should be aware of the resources and services available in a community and should make the arrangements (before hospital discharge, if the patient is hospitalized) that are necessary to secure those resources and services. When appropriate, home care services are contacted directly. The home care nurse reassesses how the patient and family are adapting to the chronic condition and its treatment and continues or revises the plan of care accordingly.

Because chronic conditions occur worldwide and the world is increasingly interconnected, nurses should think beyond the personal level to the community and global levels. In terms of illness prevention and health promotion, this entails wide-ranging efforts to assess people for risks of chronic illness (eg, blood pressure and diabetes screening, stroke risk assessments) and group teaching related to illness prevention and management.

In addition, nurses should also remind patients with chronic illnesses or disabilities and their families about the need for ongoing health promotion and screening recommended for all people, because chronic illness and disability are often considered the main concern while other health-related issues are ignored.

Nursing Care for Special Populations With Chronic Illness

When providing care and teaching, the nurse must consider a variety of factors (eg, age, gender, culture and ethnicity, cognitive status, the presence of physical and sensory limitations) that influence susceptibility to chronic illness and the ways patients respond to chronic disorders. Certain populations, for example, tend to be more susceptible to certain chronic conditions. Populations at high risk for specific conditions can be targeted for special teaching and monitoring programs. People of different cultures and genders tend to respond to illness differently, and being aware of these differences is essential (Bates, Rankin-Hill & Sanchez-Ayendez, 1997; Becker, Beyene, Newsom, et al., 1998; Thorne, McCormick & Carty, 1997). For cultures in which patients rely heavily on the support of their families, families must be involved and made part of the nursing care plan. As the United States becomes more multicultural and ethnically diverse, and as the general population ages, nurses need to be aware of how a person's culture and age affect chronic illness management and prepared to adapt their care accordingly (Becker et al., 1998; Jennings, 1999; Rehm, 1999).

It is also important to consider the effect of a preexisting disability, or a disability associated with recurrence of a chronic condition, on the patient's ability to manage ADLs, self-care, and the therapeutic regimen. These issues are discussed in the following section.

Overview of Disability

Definitions of Disability

A person is considered to have a disability such as a limitation in performance or function in everyday activities if he or she has difficulty talking, hearing, seeing, walking, climbing stairs, lifting or carrying objects, performing ADLs, doing school work, or working at a job. A severe disability is present if a person is unable to perform one or more activities, uses an assistive device for mobility, or needs help from another person to accomplish basic activities. People are also considered severely disabled if they receive federal benefits because of an inability to work.

The World Health Organization (WHO) once defined a disability as a limitation in a person's abilities (eg, mobility, personal care, communication, behavior), an **impairment** as a body system or function affected (eg, neurologic, respiratory, urologic), and a **handicap** as a disadvantage experienced by a person in his or her environment (eg, workplace, economic sufficiency, independence) (Lollar & Crews, 2003; WHO, 1980). In an effort to change the focus from a classification based on *disease* to one based on *health,* these definitions were revised in 2001. According to the WHO, *disability* is an umbrella term for impairments, activity limitations, participation restrictions, and environmental factors, and *impairment* is a loss or abnormality in body structure or physiologic function, including mental function. A person's functioning or disability is viewed as a dynamic interaction between health conditions (ie, diseases, disorders, injuries, trauma) and contextual factors (ie, personal and environmental factors).

The term "handicap" is no longer included in the revised WHO classification system: *International Classification of Functioning, Disability and Health—ICF* (WHO, 2001). The term was used previously to identify those circumstances in which the environment played a role in limiting the participation of people with disabilities in activities. The term *societal participation* is used in the revised WHO classification system in place of handicap, to acknowledge the fact that the environment is always interacting with people to either assist or hinder participation in life activities. The revision of the classification system acknowledges that the environment may have a greater impact on the ability of an individual to participate in life activities than does the physical, mental, or emotional condition (Lollar & Crews, 2003).

Federal legislation uses more than 50 definitions of disability, which illustrates how difficult it is to define the term

(Lollar & Crews, 2003). However, the Americans With Disabilities Act of 1990 (ADA; discussed later) defines a person with a **disability** as one who (1) has a physical or mental impairment that substantially limits one or more major life activities, (2) has a record of such an impairment, or (3) is regarded as having such an impairment. Other terms that are used to describe people with disability but are not universally accepted or understood are "people who are physically challenged," and "people with special needs."

Another approach to disability is described by Lutz and Bowers (2005), who stated that none of the existing definitions adequately addresses disability in everyday life. They defined disability as a multifaceted, complex experience that is integrated into the lives of people with disabilities. The degree of the integration is influenced by three disability-related factors: (1) the effects of the disabling condition, (2) others' perceptions of disability, and (3) the need for and use of resources by the person with a disability.

Prevalence of Disability

It is estimated that there are 54 to 60 million people in the United States with disabilities (U.S. Census Bureau, 2003). This number is expected to increase over time as people with early-onset disabilities, chronic disorders, and severe trauma survive and have normal or near-normal lifespans (Vandenakker & Glass, 2001). In addition, changes in the demographic profile are resulting in an increased number of older people with chronic illnesses and disabilities. As the population ages, the prevalence of disability is expected to increase. Although disability is often perceived as being associated only with old age, national data demonstrate that disability occurs across the lifespan; however, its incidence increases with age (U.S. Census Bureau, 2003; USDHHS, 2005).

The most recent United States Census, conducted in 2000, indicates that 20% of people have a disability and 10% have a severe disability. More than 46% of people with one disability have other disabilities. More than 50% of people with a disability are women. Although the prevalence of disability is higher in males than in females for people younger than 65 years of age, the prevalence is higher in women than in men for people older than 65 years of age. Among people 65 years of age and older, almost 60% of those with disabilities are women (U.S. Census Bureau, 2003).

Currently, more than 10 million people need personal assistance with one or more ADLs, which include bathing, dressing, feeding, and toileting, or IADLs, which include grocery shopping, meal preparation, housekeeping, transportation, and managing finances. In addition, more than 9.3 million people have sensory disabilities that affect hearing or vision. About 5 million people use a cane, more than 2 million use a wheelchair, and at least 1 million use crutches or a walker.

Among all people 21 to 64 years of age (the prime employable years), approximately 33% of people with a severe disability and 77% of those with a nonsevere disability are employed, compared with 82% of people without a disability. However, employed people with a disability earn less money than people without disabilities (U.S. Census Bureau, 2003). Furthermore, 17.5% of people with disabilities live in poverty. Many people with disabilities who are unemployed want to work; however, they are often unable to do so because of the limited access to work settings, lack of accommodations in the workplace, reluctance of employers to hire them, and financial risk if their income exceeds eligibility limits to qualify for disability benefits.

Characteristics of Disability

Categories and Types of Disability

Disabilities can be categorized as developmental disabilities, acquired disabilities, and age-associated disabilities. Developmental disabilities are those that occur any time from birth to 22 years of age and result in impairment of physical or mental health, cognition, speech, language, or self-care. Examples of developmental disabilities are spina bifida, cerebral palsy, Down syndrome, and muscular dystrophy. Acquired disabilities may occur as a result of an acute and sudden injury (eg, traumatic brain injury, spinal cord injury, traumatic amputation), acute nontraumatic disorders (eg, stroke, myocardial infarction), or progression of a chronic disorder (eg, arthritis, multiple sclerosis, chronic obstructive pulmonary disease, blindness due to diabetic retinopathy). Age-related disabilities are those that occur in the elderly population and are thought to be due to the aging process. Examples of age-related disabilities include osteoarthritis, osteoporosis, and hearing loss. Because people with disabilities, including those with severe developmental disabilities, are surviving longer than ever before, there is a growing number of young, middle-aged, and elderly adults with disabilities, including developmental disabilities.

Types of disability include sensory disabilities that affect hearing or vision; learning disabilities that affect the ability to learn, remember, or concentrate; disabilities that affect the ability to speak or communicate; and disabilities that affect the ability to work, shop, care for oneself or obtain health care (U.S. Census Bureau, 2003). Many disabilities are visible, but invisible disabilities are often as disabling as those that can be seen. Some disabilities affect only IADLs, whereas others affect ADLs. People can be temporarily disabled because of an injury or acute exacerbation of an chronic disorder but later return to full functioning; this definition of disability may not apply for legal purposes.

Although different impairments may result from different types of disabilities, there are some similarities across disabilities. People with disabilities are often considered by society to be dependent and needing to be cared for by others; however, many people with disabilities are highly functioning, independent, productive people who are capable of caring for themselves and others, having children and raising families, holding a full-time job, and making significant and major contributions to society (Fig. 10-1). Like other people, those with disabilities often prefer to live in their own homes with family members. Most people with disabilities are able to live at home independently. Some patients live alone in their own homes and use home care services. However, alternative living arrangements may be necessary; these include assisted living facilities, long-term care facilities, and group homes.

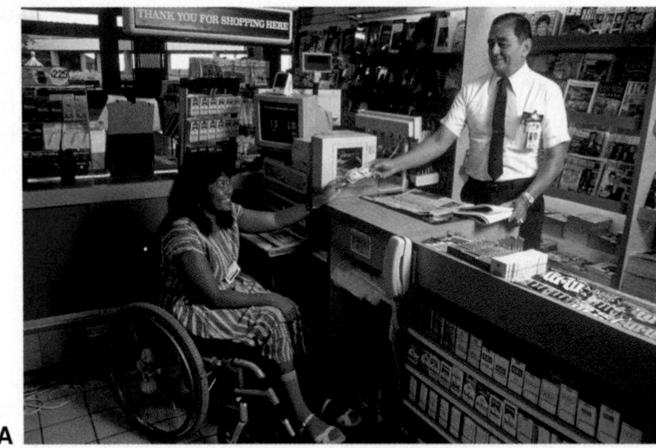

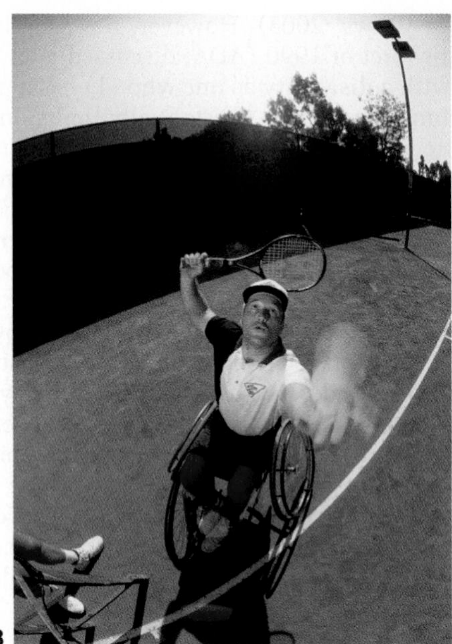

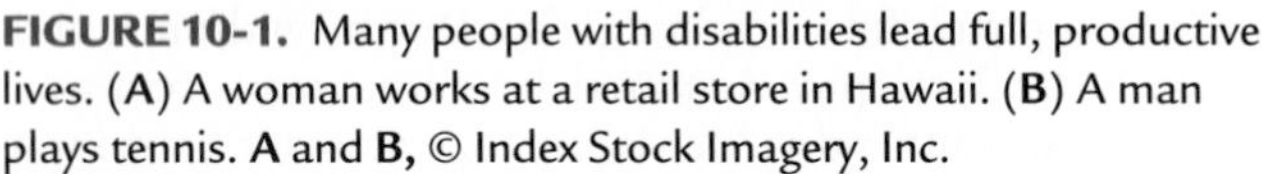

FIGURE 10-1. Many people with disabilities lead full, productive lives. (**A**) A woman works at a retail store in Hawaii. (**B**) A man plays tennis. **A** and **B,** © Index Stock Imagery, Inc.

Models of Disability

Several models of disability have been used to address or explain the issues encountered by people with disabilities (Lollar & Crews, 2003). These include the medical and rehabilitation models, the social model, the biopsychosocial model, and the interface model. Chart 10-2 briefly describes these models of disability. Of these, the interface model (Goodall, 1995) may be the most appropriate for use by nurses to provide care that is empowering rather than care that promotes dependency. The interface model does not ignore the disabling condition or its disabling effects; instead, it promotes the view that people with disabilities are capable, responsible people who are able to function effectively despite having a disability. The interface model can serve as a basis for the role of nurses as advocates for removal of barriers to health care and for examination of how society and health care professionals contribute to discrimination by viewing disability as an abnormal state.

Disability Versus Disabling Disorders

Regardless of which definition or model of disability is adopted, it is important to realize that it is possible to understand the pathophysiology of a disabling condition or injury or be very knowledgeable about the physical changes resulting from a disorder without understanding the concept of disability. The nurse caring for patients with preexisting disabilities or new disabilities must recognize the implications of the existence of a disability on current and future health and well-being, ability to participate in self-care or self-management, and ability to obtain required health care and health screening. Nursing management, from assessment through evaluation of the effectiveness of nursing interventions, must be examined to determine whether appropriate modifications have been made to ensure that people with disabilities receive health care equal to that of people without disabilities. Furthermore, nurses as well as other health care providers need to examine their facilities and procedures to ensure that the needs of people with a variety of disabilities can be adequately addressed. Although the health care needs of people with disabilities generally do not differ from those of the general population, some disabilities create special needs and necessitate the use of special accommodations. Chart 10-3 reviews specific areas of assessment when caring for people with disabilities.

Federal Legislation

Because of widespread discrimination against people with disabilities, the United States Congress has enacted legislation to address health care disparities in this population. This legislation includes the Rehabilitation Act of 1973 and the ADA. Health care in people with disabilities has received further national attention through the first-time inclusion of specific national objectives that address health care for people with disabilities in *Healthy People 2010* (USDHHS, 2000). In 2005, the United States Surgeon General called for action to improve the health and wellness of people with disabilities (USDHHS, 2005).

The Rehabilitation Act of 1973 is a law that protects people from discrimination based on their disability. The act applies to employers and organizations that receive financial assistance from any federal department or agency; this includes many hospitals, long-term care facilities, mental health centers, and human service programs. It forbids organizations from excluding or denying people with disabilities equal access to program benefits and services. It also prohibits discrimination related to availability, accessibility, and delivery of services, including health care services.

The ADA, passed by the U.S. Congress in 1990, took effect in 1992. It mandates that people with disabilities have access to job opportunities and to the community. According to the ADA, employers must evaluate an applicant's ability to perform the job and not discriminate on the basis of a disability. The act stipulates that communities must provide public transportation that is accessible to people

CHART 10-2

Models of Disability

MEDICAL MODEL

This model equates disabled people with their disabilities and views disability as a problem of the person, directly caused by disease, trauma, or other health condition, which requires medical care provided in the form of individual treatment by professionals. Health care providers, rather than people with disabilities, are viewed as the experts or authorities. Management of the disability is aimed at cure or the person's adjustment and behavior change. The model is viewed as promoting passivity and dependency. People with disabilities are viewed as tragic (Goodall, 1995; Scullion, 1999b, 2000; World Health Organization, 2001; Lollar & Crews, 2003).

REHABILITATION MODEL

The rehabilitation model emerged from the medical model. It regards disability as a deficiency that requires a rehabilitation specialist or other helping professional to fix the problem. People with disabilities are often perceived as having failed if they do not overcome the disability (Lollar & Crews, 2003).

SOCIAL MODEL

The social model, which is also referred to as the barriers or disability model, views disability as socially constructed and as a political issue that is a result of social and physical barriers in the environment. Its perspective is that disability can be overcome by removal of these barriers (French, 1992; Richardson, 1997; Shakespeare & Watson, 1997; World Health Organization, 2001).

BIOPSYCHOSOCIAL MODEL

The biopsychosocial model integrates the medical and social models to address perspectives of health from a biologic, individual, and social perspective (World Health Organization, 2001; USDHHS, 2005). Critiques of this model have suggested that the disabling condition, rather than the person and the experience of the person with a disability, remains the defining construct of the biopsychosocial model (Lutz & Bowers, 2005).

INTERFACE MODEL

The interface model is based on the life experience of the person with a disability and views disability at the intersection (ie, interface) of the medical diagnosis of a disability and environmental barriers. It considers rather than ignores the diagnosis. The person with a disability, rather than others, defines the problems and seeks or directs solutions (Goodall, 1995).

with disabilities. The law requires that "reasonable accommodations" be provided to facilitate employment of a person with a disability. Facilities used by the public must be accessible and accommodate those with disabilities. Examples of reasonable accommodations in health care settings include accessible facilities and equipment (eg, adjustable examination tables, access ramps, grab bars, elevated toilet seats) and alternative communication methods (eg, telecommunication devices and sign interpreters for use by people who are deaf).

Although the ADA was enacted in 1992, compliance has been slow because the provisions mandating reasonable accommodation "without undue hardship" have enabled facilities to continue with inaccessible conditions. However, all new construction and modifications of public facilities must address access for people with disabilities. Examples of modifications that should be considered if one is to provide equal access to health care to people with disabilities are identified in Chart 10-3.

Right of Access to Health Care

People with disabilities have the right of access to health care that is equal in quality to that of other people. For years, people with disabilities have been discriminated against in employment, public accommodations, and public and private services, including health care. The needs of the people with disabilities in health care settings produce many challenges to health care providers: how to communicate effectively if there are communication deficits, the additional physical requirements for mobility, and time required to provide assistance with self-care routines during hospitalization. Health care providers, including nurses, may not be aware of the specific needs of people with disabilities and may fail to provide appropriate care and services for them. However, it is essential that health care providers, including nurses, realize that people with disabilities have a legally mandated right to accessible health care facilities for all medical care and screening procedures. Furthermore, people with disabilities have the right to health care provided by professionals who are knowledgeable about and sensitive to the effects of disability on access to health care, including care that addresses their reproductive issues and sexuality. Reasonable accommodations are mandated by law and are the financial responsibility of the health care provider or facility. People with disabilities should not be expected to provide their own accommodations (eg, sign interpreters, assistants). Family members should not be expected to serve as interpreters because of concern for the patient's privacy and confidentiality and the risk for errors in interpreting information by either the patient or the health care provider. Chart 10-4 identifies strategies to communicate effectively with people with disabilities.

(text continues on page 182)

CHART 10-3

Strategies to Ensure Quality Health Care for People With Disabilities

COMMUNICATION STRATEGIES

- Does the patient with a disability require or prefer accommodations (eg, a sign interpreter) to ensure full participation in conversations about his or her own health care?
- Are accommodations made to communicate with the patient?
- Are efforts made to direct all conversations to the patient rather than to others who have accompanied the patient to the health care facility?

ACCESSIBILITY OF THE HEALTH CARE FACILITY

- Are clinics, hospital rooms, offices, restrooms, and laboratories accessible to people with disabilities, as legally required by the Americans with Disabilities Act and Rehabilitation Act?
- Has accessibility been verified by a person with a disability?
- Is a sign interpreter other than family member available to assist in obtaining a patient's health history and in conducting a physical assessment?
- Does the facility include appropriate equipment to permit people with disabilities to obtain health care (including mammography, gynecologic examination and care, dental care) in a dignified and safe manner?

ASSESSMENT

Usual Health Considerations

- Does the health history address the same issues that would be included when obtaining a history from a person without disabilities, including sexuality, sexual function, and reproductive health issues?

Disability-Related Considerations

- Does the health history address the patient's specific disability and the effect of disability on the patient's ability to obtain health care, manage self-care activities, and obtain preventive health screening and follow-up care?
- What physical modifications and positioning are needed to ensure a thorough physical examination, including pelvic or testicular and rectal examination?

Abuse

- Is the increased risk for abuse (physical, emotional, financial, and sexual) by a variety of people (family, paid care providers, strangers) addressed in the assessment?
- If abuse is detected, are men and women with disabilities who are survivors of abuse directed to appropriate resources, including accessible shelters and hotlines?

Depression

- Is the patient experiencing depression? If so, is treatment offered just as it would be to a patient without a disability, without assuming that depression is normal and a result of having a disability?

Aging

- What concerns does the patient have about aging with a preexisting disability?
- What effect has aging had on the patient's disability and what effect has the disability had on the patient's aging?

Secondary Conditions

- Does the patient have secondary conditions related to his or her disability or its treatment?
- Are strategies in place to reduce the risk for secondary conditions or to treat existing secondary conditions?

Accommodations in the Home

- What accommodations does the patient have at home to encourage or permit self-care?
- What additional accommodations does the patient need at home to encourage or permit self-care?

COGNITIVE STATUS

- Is it assumed that the patient is able to participate in discussion and conversation rather than assuming that he or she is unable to do so because of a disability?
- Are appropriate modifications made in written and verbal communication strategies?

MODIFICATIONS IN NURSING CARE

- Are modifications made during hospital stays, acute illness or injury, and other health care encounters to enable a patient with disability to be as independent as he or she prefers?
- Is "person-first language" used in referring to a patient with disability, and do nurses and other staff talk directly to the patient rather than to those who accompanied the patient?
- Are all staff informed about the activities of daily living (ADLs) for which the patient will require assistance?
- Are accommodations made to enable the patient to use his or her assistive devices (hearing/visual aids, prostheses, limb support devices, ventilators, service animals)?
- If a patient with disability is immobilized because of surgery, illness, injury, or treatments, are risks of immobility addressed and strategies implemented to minimize those risks?

CHART 10-3 Strategies to Ensure Quality Health Care for People With Disabilities, continued

- Is the patient with a disability assessed for other illnesses and health issues (eg, other acute or chronic illness, depression, psychiatric/mental health and cognitive disorders) not related to his or her primary disability?

PATIENT TEACHING

- Are accommodations and alternative formats of teaching materials (large print, Braille, visual materials, audiotapes) provided for patients with disabilities?
- Does patient teaching address the modifications (eg, use of assistive devices) needed by patients with disabilities to enable them to adhere to recommendations?
- Are modifications made in teaching strategies to address learning needs, cognitive changes, and communication impairment?

HEALTH PROMOTION AND DISEASE PREVENTION

- Are health promotion strategies discussed with people with disabilities along with their potential benefits: improving quality of life and preventing secondary conditions (health problems that result because of preexisting disability)?
- Are patients aware of accessible community-based facilities (eg, health care facilities, imaging centers, public exercise settings, transportation) to enable them to participate in health promotion?

INDEPENDENCE VERSUS DEPENDENCE

- Is independence, rather than dependence, of the person with a disability the focus of nursing care and interaction?
- Are care and interaction with the patient focused on empowerment rather than promoting dependence of the patient?

INSURANCE COVERAGE

- Does the patient have access to the health insurance coverage and other services for which he or she qualifies?
- Is the patient aware of various insurance and other available programs?
- Would the patient benefit from talking to a social worker about eligibility for Medicaid, Medicare, Disability Insurance, and other services?

CHART 10-4 Interacting and Communicating With People With Disabilities

Patients will feel most comfortable receiving health care if you consider the following suggestions.

GENERAL CONSIDERATIONS

- Do not be afraid to make a mistake when interacting and communicating with someone with a disability or chronic medical condition. Keep in mind that a person with a disability is a person first, and is entitled to the dignity, consideration, respect, and rights you expect for yourself.
- Treat adults as adults. Address people with disabilities by their first names only if extending the same familiarity to all others present. Never patronize people by patting them on the head or shoulder.
- Relax. If you do not know what to do, allow the person who has a disability to identify how you may be of assistance and to put you at ease.
- If you offer assistance and the person declines, do not insist. If your offer is accepted, ask how you can best help, and follow directions. Do not take over.
- If someone with a disability is accompanied by another individual, address the person with a disability directly rather than speaking through the accompanying companion.
- Be considerate of the extra time it might take for a person with a disability to get things done or said. Let the person set the pace.
- Do not be embarrassed to use common expressions such as, "See you later," or "Got to be running," that seem to relate to the person's disability.
- Use person-first language: refer to "a person with a disability" rather than "a disabled person," and avoid referring to people by the disability they have (eg, "the diabetic").

MOBILITY LIMITATIONS

- Do not make assumptions about what a person can and cannot do.
- Do not push a person's wheelchair or grab the arm of someone walking with difficulty without first ask-

continued >

CHART 10-4 Interacting and Communicating With People With Disabilities, continued

ing if you can be of assistance and how you can assist. Personal space includes a person's wheelchair, scooter, crutches, walker, cane, or other mobility aid.

- Never move someone's wheelchair, scooter, crutches, walker, cane, or other mobility aid without permission.
- When speaking for more than a few minutes to a person who is seated in a wheelchair, try to find a seat for yourself, so that the two of you are at eye level.
- When giving directions to people with mobility limitations, consider distance, weather conditions, and physical obstacles such as stairs, curbs, and steep hills.
- It is appropriate to shake hands when introduced to a person with a disability. People who have limited hand use or who wear an artificial limb do shake hands.

VISION LOSS (LOW VISION AND BLINDNESS)

- Identify yourself when you approach a person who has low vision or blindness. If a new person approaches, introduce him or her.
- It is appropriate to touch the person's arm lightly when you speak so that he or she knows to whom you are speaking before you begin.
- Face the person and speak directly to him or her. Use a normal tone of voice.
- Do not leave without saying you are leaving.
- If you are offering directions, be as specific as possible, and point out obstacles in the path of travel. Use specifics such as, "Left about twenty feet," or "Right two yards." Use clock cues, such as, "The door is at 10 o'clock."
- When you offer to assist someone with vision loss, allow the person to take your arm. This will help you to guide rather than propel or lead the person. When offering seating, place the person's hand on the back or arm of the seat.
- Alert people with low vision or blindness to posted information.
- Never pet or otherwise distract a canine companion or service animal unless the owner has given you permission.

HEARING LOSS (HARD OF HEARING, DEAF, DEAF-BLIND)

- Ask the person how he or she prefers to communicate.
- If you are speaking through a sign language interpreter, remember that the interpreter may lag a few words behind—especially if there are names or technical terms to be fingerspelled—so pause occasionally to allow the interpreter time to translate completely and accurately.
- Talk directly to the person who has hearing loss, not to the interpreter. However, although it may seem awkward to you, the person who has hearing loss will look at the interpreter and may not make eye contact with you during the conversation.
- Before you start to speak, make sure you have the attention of the person you are addressing. A wave, a light touch on the arm or shoulder, or other visual or tactile signals are appropriate ways of getting the person's attention.
- Speak in a clear, expressive manner. Do not overenunciate or exaggerate words. Unless you are specifically requested to do so, do not raise your voice. Speak in a normal tone; do not shout.
- To facilitate lip reading, face the person and keep your hands and other objects away from your mouth. Maintain eye contact. Do not turn your back or walk around while talking. If you look away, the person might assume the conversation is over.
- Avoid talking while you are writing a message for someone with hearing loss, because the person cannot read your note and your lips at the same time.
- Try to eliminate background noise.
- Encourage feedback to assess clear understanding.
- If you do not understand something that is said, ask the person to repeat it or to write it down. The goal is communication; do not pretend to understand if you do not.
- If you know any sign language, try using it. It may help you communicate, and it will at least demonstrate your interest in communicating and your willingness to try.

SPEECH DISABILITIES OR SPEECH DIFFICULTIES

- Talk to people with speech disabilities as you would talk to anyone else.
- Be friendly; start up a conversation.
- Be patient; it may take the person a while to answer. Allow extra time for communication. Do not speak for the person.
- Give the person your undivided attention.
- Ask the person for help in communicating with him or her. If the person uses a communication device such as a manual or electronic communication board, ask the person how best to use it.
- Speak in your regular tone of voice.
- Tell the person if you do not understand what he or she is trying to say. Ask the person to repeat the message, spell it, tell you in a different way, or write it down. Use hand gestures and notes.
- Repeat what you understand. The person's reactions will clue you in and guide you to understanding.
- To obtain information quickly, ask short questions that require brief answers or a head nod. However,

CHART 10-4 Interacting and Communicating With People With Disabilities, continued

try not to insult the person's intelligence with oversimplification.
- Keep your manner encouraging rather than correcting.

INTELLECTUAL/COGNITIVE DISABILITIES

- Treat adults with intellectual/cognitive disabilities as adults.
- Try to be alert to the individual's responses so that you can adjust your method of communication as necessary. For example, some people may benefit from simple, direct sentences or from supplementary visual forms of communication, such as gestures, diagrams, or demonstrations.
- Use concrete rather than abstract language. Be specific, without being too simplistic. When possible, use words that relate to things you both can see. Avoid using directional terms such as right, left, east, or west.
- Be prepared to give the person the same information more than once in different ways.
- When asking questions, phrase them to elicit accurate information. People with intellectual/cognitive disabilities may be eager to please and may tell you what they think you want to hear. Verify responses by repeating the question in a different way.
- Give exact instructions. For example, "Be back for lab work at 4:30," not "Be back in 15 minutes."
- Too many directions at one time may be confusing.
- The person may prefer information provided in written or verbal form. Ask the person how you can best relay the information.
- Using humor is fine, but do not interpret a lack of response as rudeness. Some people may not grasp the meaning of sarcasm or other subtleties of language.
- People with brain injuries may have short-term memory deficits and may repeat themselves or require information to be repeated.
- People with auditory perceptual problems may need to have directions repeated and may take notes to help them remember directions or the sequence of tasks. They may benefit from watching a task demonstrated.
- People with perceptual or "sensory overload" problems may become disoriented or confused if there is too much to absorb at once. Provide information gradually and clearly. Reduce background noise if possible.
- Repeat information using different wording or a different communication approach if necessary. Allow time for the information to be fully understood.
- Do not pretend to understand if you do not. Ask the person to repeat what was said. Be patient, flexible, and supportive.
- Some people who have an intellectual disability are easily distracted. Try not to interpret distraction as rudeness.
- Do not expect all people to be able to read well. Some people may not read at all.

PSYCHIATRIC DISABILITIES

- Speak directly to the person. Use clear, simple communication.
- Offer to shake hands when introduced. Use the same good manners in interacting with a person who has a psychiatric disability that you would with anyone else.
- Make eye contact and be aware of your own body language. Like others, people with psychiatric disabilities will sense your discomfort.
- Listen attentively and wait for the person to finish speaking. If needed, clarify what the person has said. Never pretend to understand.
- Treat adults as adults. Do not patronize, condescend, or threaten. Do not make decisions for the person or assume that you know the person's preferences.
- Do not give unsolicited advice or assistance. Do not panic or summon an ambulance or the police if a person appears to be experiencing a mental health crisis. Calmly ask the person how you can help.
- Do not blame the person. A person with a psychiatric disability has a complex, biomedical condition that is sometimes difficult to control. They cannot just "shape up." It is rude, insensitive, and ineffective to tell or expect a person to do so.
- Question the accuracy of media stereotypes of psychiatric disabilities: movies and media often sensationalize psychiatric disabilities. Most people never experience symptoms that include violent behavior.
- Relax. Be yourself. Do not be embarrassed if you happen to use common expressions that seem to relate to a psychiatric disability.
- Recognize that beneath the symptoms and behaviors of psychiatric disabilities is a person who has many of the same wants, needs, dreams, and desires as anyone else. If you are afraid, learn more about psychiatric disabilities.

This material is adapted and based in part on *Achieving Physical and Communication Accessibility,* a publication of the National Center for Access Unlimited; *Community Access Facts,* an Adaptive Environments Center publication; and *The Ten Commandments of Interacting with People with Mental Health Disabilities,* a publication of The Ability Center of Greater Toledo.

Barriers to Health Care

Many people with disabilities encounter barriers to full participation in life, including health care, health screening, and health promotion (Becker & Stuifbergen, 2004). Some of these barriers are structural and make certain facilities inaccessible. Examples of structural barriers include stairs, lack of ramps, narrow doorways that do not permit entry of a wheelchair, and restroom facilities that cannot be used by people with disabilities (eg, restrooms that lack grab bars and larger restroom stalls designed for people using wheelchairs).

Structural barriers to accessibility are most easily identified and eliminated. Other, less visible barriers include negative and stereotypic attitudes (eg, believing that all people with disabilities have a poor quality of life and are dependent and nonproductive) on the part of the public. Health care providers with similar negative attitudes make it difficult for people with disabilities to obtain health care equal in quality to that of people without disabilities. The Rehabilitation Act and the ADA were enacted more than 30 and 15 years ago, respectively, to ensure equal access to people with disabilities, but people with disabilities continue to encounter and report multiple barriers to health care facilities and providers (Nosek & Center for Research on Women with Disabilities, 2004). This legislation and the United States Surgeon General's call to improve the health and wellness of people with disabilities (USDHHS, 2005) are examples of efforts to eliminate barriers encountered by people with disabilities.

People with disabilities have reported that they often encounter barriers that prevent them from obtaining recommended health care screening and care. They have also reported lack of access to information, transportation difficulties, inability to pay because of limited income, difficulty finding a health care provider knowledgeable about their particular disability, previous negative health care encounters, reliance on caretakers, and the demands of coping with the disability itself (Nosek, Howland, Rintala, et al., 1997). These issues affect both men and women with severe disabilities; however, women appear to be at higher risk for receiving a lower level of health care than men. Women with disabilities are significantly less likely to receive pelvic examinations than women without disabilities; the more severe the disability, the less frequent the examination. In particular, minority women and older women with disabilities are less likely to have regular pelvic examinations and Papanicolaou (Pap) tests. Reasons given by women for not having regular pelvic examinations are difficulty transferring onto the examination table, belief that they do not need pelvic examinations because of their disability, difficulty in accessing the office or clinic, and difficulty finding transportation (Coyle & Santiago, 2002; Odette, Yoshida, Israel, et al., 2003; Schopp, Sanford, Hagglund, et al., 2002). Health care providers may underestimate the effect of disabilities on women's ability to access health care, including health screening and health promotion, and may focus on women's disabilities while ignoring their general health issues and concerns. Furthermore, women with disabilities have also reported lack of knowledge about disability and insensitivity on the part of health care providers (Nosek et al., 1997).

Because of the persistence of these barriers, it is essential that nurses and other health care providers take steps to ensure that clinics, offices, hospitals, and other health care facilities are accessible to people with disabilities. This includes removal of structural barriers by the addition of ramps, designation of accessible parking spaces, and modification of restrooms to make them usable by people with disabilities. Alternative communication methods (eg, sign interpreters, TTY devices, assistive listening devices) and types of patient education (eg, audiotapes, large print, Braille) are essential to provision of appropriate health-related information to people with disabilities (Fig. 10-2). These reasonable accommodations are mandated by the ADA, which requires their provision without cost to the patient.

Federal Assistance Programs

Lack of financial resources, including health insurance, is an important barrier to health care for people with chronic illness and disabilities. However, several federal assistance programs provide financial assistance for health-related expenses for people with some chronic illnesses, acquired disabling acute and chronic diseases, and disabilities from childhood (Mold et al., 2004).

Medicare is a federal health insurance program that is available to most people 65 years of age and older, people with permanent renal failure, and qualified people with disabilities. Title II of the Social Security Disability Insurance program pays benefits to those people who meet medical criteria for disability, who have worked long enough (40 quarters of covered employment) to qualify, and who have paid Social Security taxes. Title II also provides benefits to people disabled since childhood (younger than 22 years of age) who are dependents of a deceased insured parent or a parent entitled to disability or retirement benefits, and disabled widows or widowers, 50 years to 60 years of age, if their de-

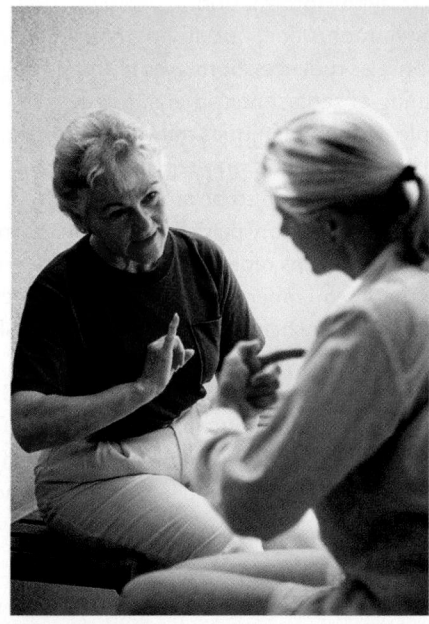

FIGURE 10-2. Alternative communication methods and types of patient education are essential to provision of appropriate health-related information to people with disabilities. © Will & Deni McIntyre/Photo Researchers, Inc.

ceased spouse was insured under Social Security. Title XVI of the Social Security Disability Insurance program provides supplemental security income (SSI) payments to people who are disabled and have limited income and resources.

Medicaid provides home and community-based services to people with disabilities and long-term illnesses to enable them to lead meaningful lives in their families and communities (USDHHS, 2005). (See Resources at the end of the chapter for more information about these benefits.)

Despite the availability of these federal programs, people with disabilities often have health-related costs and other expenses related to disability that result in low incomes. Furthermore, people must undergo a disability determination process to establish eligibility for benefits, and the process can be prolonged and cumbersome for those who may need assistance in establishing their eligibility.

Nursing Care of Patients With Disabilities

As active members of society, people with disabilities are no longer an invisible minority. An increased awareness of the needs of people with disabilities will bring about changes to improve their access and accommodate their needs. Modification of the physical environment permits access to public and private facilities and services, including health care, and nurses can serve as advocates for people with disabilities to eliminate discriminatory practices (Clingerman, Stuifbergen & Becker, 2004).

Nursing Considerations During Hospitalization

During hospitalization, as well as during periods of acute illness or injury or while recovering from surgery, patients with preexisting disabilities may require assistance with carrying out ADLs that they could otherwise manage at home independently and easily. Patients should be asked preferences about approaches to carrying out their ADLs, and assistive devices they require should be readily available. Careful planning with patients to ensure that the hospital room is arranged with their input enables them to manage as independently as possible. For example, patients who have paraplegia may be able to transfer independently from bed to wheelchair; however, if the bed is left in an elevated position, they may be unable to do so. If patients usually use service animals to assist them with ADLs, it is necessary to make arrangements for the accommodation of these animals. When patients with hearing loss or communication impairments are hospitalized, it is essential to establish effective communication strategies. Alternative methods for these patients to communicate with the health care team must be put in place and used, and all staff members must be aware that some patients are not able to respond to the intercom or telephone.

Health Promotion and Prevention

Health care providers often neglect health promotion concerns of people with disabilities, who may be unaware of these concerns. For example, people who have had hearing loss since childhood may lack exposure to information about AIDS through radio and television. People with lifelong disabilities may not have received information about general health issues as children, and people with new-onset as well as lifelong disabilities may not receive encouragement to participate in health promotion activities. Therefore, nurses should take every opportunity to emphasize the importance of participation, both in health promotion activities (eg, healthy diet, exercise, social interactions) and in preventive health screening.

The management of some disabilities increases the risk for illness, and in some people, health screening (eg, bone density testing, gynecologic examinations, mammography) may be required earlier in life or more frequently (Smeltzer, 2006; Smeltzer & Sharts-Hopko, 2005). Referrals by nurses to accessible sites for screening may be needed, because many imaging centers are inaccessible. In addition, nursing consultation with physical therapists may be needed to identify creative ways of enabling people with disabilities to exercise safely, because exercise facilities are also often inaccessible for people with disabilities.

General health promotion strategies and health screening recommendations for all men and women also apply to those with disabilities. Although physical limitations, cognitive impairments, and structural and attitudinal barriers existing in clinical facilities may make it difficult for some men and women to obtain health care and preventive health screening, the presence of a disability should not be used as a reason or excuse to defer recommended screening. Rather, the presence of a disability may increase the risk for **secondary conditions** that require screening and follow-up. Just as people without disabilities should have regular screening tests, such as mammography or testicular and prostate examinations, so should people with disabilities (Kinne, Patrick & Doyle, 2003; USDHHS, 2005). Nurses are often in a position to influence decisions about how equipment and procedures can be adapted to meet the special needs of their patients, whether these needs are cognitive, motor, or communicative.

The effect of the disabling condition on health risks should be considered. For example, the risk for osteoporosis may be increased in women and men whose disabilities limit their ability to participate in weight-bearing exercise or who use medications that contribute to bone loss (Smeltzer, Zimmerman & Capriotti, 2005). Although people with disabilities have an increased risk for osteoporosis at a younger age than people without disabilities, little attention is given to prevention, detection, and treatment of osteoporosis, despite the increased risk for falls associated with disabling disorders (Smeltzer, 2006).

Nurses can provide expert health promotion education classes that are targeted to people with disabilities and refer them to accessible online resources (Smeltzer, Zimmerman, DeSilets, et al., 2003). Classes on nutrition and weight management are extremely important to people who are wheelchair users and need assistance with transfers. Safer sex classes are needed by adolescents and young adults who have spinal cord injury, traumatic brain injury, or developmental disabilities, because the threats of sexually transmitted diseases (STDs) and unplanned pregnancy exist for these populations just as they do for the population in general.

Other healthy behaviors about which people with neurologic disabilities need education include avoiding alcohol and nonprescription medications while taking antispasmodic and antiseizure medications.

Significance of "People-First" Language

It is important to all people, both those with and those without disabilities, that they not be equated with their illness or physical condition. Therefore, it is important to refer to all people using "people-first" language. Using "people-first" language means referring to the person first: "the patient with diabetes" rather than "the diabetic" or "the diabetic patient"; "the person with a disability" rather than the "disabled person"; "women with disabilities" rather than "disabled women"; and "people who are wheelchair users" rather than "the wheelchair-bound." This simple use of language conveys the message that the person, rather than the illness or disability, is of greater importance to the nurse.

Gerontologic Considerations

Stereotypical thinking often leads to the conclusion that disability is associated only with being elderly. However, aging is an important issue that affects people with preexisting disabilities. In addition, the process of aging has been described as accelerated in people with disabilities, because they often develop changes associated with aging at a younger age than do those without disabilities (Harrison, 2003; Klingbeil, Baer & Wilson, 2004). Therefore, it is important that the nurse consider the effects of aging on a preexisting disability and in turn the effects of disability on aging. The following examples may be useful.

- People who use crutches for ambulation because of polio often experience muscle problems as they age because of long-time overuse of the upper extremities; symptoms may not occur for many years but may cause discomfort and interfere with the person's ability to perform ADLs.
- People who experienced respiratory compromise with the onset of polio decades earlier may experience increasing respiratory symptoms with aging (Bartels & Omura, 2005).
- Women with long-standing mobility limitations and lack of weight-bearing exercise may experience bone loss and osteoporosis prior to menopause (Smeltzer et al., 2005). Therefore, people with preexisting disability should be evaluated for early onset of changes related to aging.

Concern about what the future holds is common in elderly people with disabilities, who may have questions about what physical, financial, and emotional supports they will have as they age (Nosek, 2000). If their disability becomes more severe in the future, they may be concerned about placement in an assisted living facility or a long-term care facility. The nurse should recognize the concerns of people with disabilities about their future and encourage them to make suitable plans, which may relieve some of their fears and concerns about what will happen to them as they age.

Parents of adult children with developmental disabilities often fear what will happen when they are no longer available and able to care for their children. The nurse should assess the concerns and arrangements made by aging parents of adult children with disabilities to help reduce some of their fears about their children's futures.

Disability in Medical-Surgical Nursing Practice

Disability is often considered an issue that is specific or confined to rehabilitation nursing or to gerontologic nursing. However, as noted previously, disability can occur across the lifespan, and it is encountered in all settings. Patients with preexisting disabilities due to conditions that have been present from birth or due to illnesses or injuries experienced as an adolescent or young adult often require health care and nursing care in medical-surgical settings. Although in the past many people with lifelong disabilities or adult onset of severe disabilities may have had shortened lifespans, today most can expect to have a normal or near-normal lifespan and to live a productive and meaningful life (Vandenakker & Glass, 2001). They are also at risk for the same acute and chronic illnesses that affect all people.

Because of unfavorable interactions with health care providers, including negative attitudes, insensitivity, and lack of knowledge, people with disabilities may avoid seeking medical intervention or health care services. For this reason, and because the number of people with disabilities is increasing, nurses must acquire knowledge and skills and be accessible to assist these people in maintaining a high level of wellness. Nurses are in key positions to influence the architectural design of health care settings and the selection of equipment that promotes ease of access and health. Padded examination tables that can be raised or lowered make transfers easier for people with disabilities. Birthing chairs benefit women with disability during yearly pelvic examinations and Pap smears and during urologic evaluations. Ramps, grab bars, and raised and padded toilet seats benefit many people who have neurologic or musculoskeletal disabilities and need routine physical examination and monitoring (eg, bone density measurements). When a patient is admitted to the hospital, the patient's needs for these modifications should be assessed and addressed.

Men and women with disabilities may be encountered in hospitals, clinics, offices, and nursing centers when they seek health care to address a problem related to their disability. However, they may also be encountered in these settings when they seek care for a health problem that is not related in any way to their disability. For example, a woman with spina bifida or polio might seek health care related to a gynecologic issue, such as vaginal bleeding. Although her disability should be considered in the course of assessment and delivery of health and nursing care, it should not become the overriding focus or exclusive focus of the assessment or the care that she receives. Furthermore, neither a severe physical disability that affects a woman's ability to transfer to an examination table for a gynecologic examination nor a cognitive disability should be a reason to defer a complete health assessment and physical examination, including a pelvic examination. Health care, including preventive health screening, is essential to enable people with disabilities to live the highest quality of life within the limitations imposed by their disabling conditions. Men and women with disabilities have the same needs and same rights for health care and preventive health screening as others, although in some cases, the consequences of their disability increase rather than decrease their need for health screening and for participation in health-promoting activities (Smeltzer & Sharts-Hopko, 2005). Therefore, it is essential that medical-surgical nurses be knowledgeable about disability and how it affects people across the lifespan and how to provide sensitive and quality nursing care for patients with preexisting as well as new-onset disability. In an effort to address these issues, specific information on health care of people with disabilities has been included throughout this book.

Home and Community-Based Care

Teaching Patients Self-Care

A major and often overlooked issue in teaching patients about a health problem, a treatment regimen, or health promotion strategies is the need for alternative formats to accommodate people with a variety of disabilities. Patients with disabilities are in need of the same information as other patients; however, they often require large print, Braille, audiotapes, or the assistance of a sign interpreter. Materials may be obtained from a variety of sources for patients who need these teaching strategies and for patients with cognitive impairments due to developmental disabilities or newly acquired disabilities.

Nurses should ensure that all people, whether or not they have disabilities, recognize the warning signs and symptoms of stroke, heart attack, and cancer, as well as how to access help. In addition, nurses should teach all patients who are stroke survivors and those with diabetes how to monitor their own blood pressure or glucose levels.

Continuing Care

When caring for patients with disabilities and helping them plan for discharge and continuing care in the home, it is important to consider how a particular disability affects a patient's ability to adhere to recommended treatment regimens and to keep follow-up appointments. Furthermore, it is important to consider how the health issue or treatment regimen affects the disability. Although many people with disabilities are independent and able to make decisions, arrangements for transportation, and appointments to accessible facilities, others may have difficulty doing so, particularly if they are experiencing a health problem. The nurse should recognize the effect that the disability has on the patient's ability to follow-up. The nurse should ask the patient whether he or she anticipates having any difficulties arranging for follow-up care. It is important for the nurse to assist the patient with disabilities to identify unmet needs and to find and use resources (community and social resources, financial and transportation services) that enable the patient to obtain needed services while remaining in his or her home, if preferred. The nurse should have a list of accessible sites and services available and share those resources with the patient and family. In collaboration with other health care providers (occupational and physical therapists, speech therapists), the nurse can identify needed home modifications, including those that are simple and inexpensive that will enable the patient to participate in self-care at home.

Critical Thinking Exercises

1 A 65-year-old hard-working attorney experiences a mild stroke during coronary artery bypass surgery. Assessment reveals that his neurologic function is about 68% of normal. He has been transferred to a rehabilitation center. During his stay, the nurse discusses lifestyle changes with him to reduce his risk of subsequent myocardial infarction and stroke. The patient is impatient with efforts to teach him about risks and lifestyle changes, saying that he is unlikely to have subsequent cardiac problems because his heart problem has been fixed. Develop a teaching plan for this patient with rationale for including specific content and plans to use specific teaching approaches.

2 A 28-year-old woman with two children younger than 3 years of age has recently been diagnosed with type 1 diabetes. She is very active in her community and church and states that she cannot fit learning about diabetes, treatments, or blood glucose testing into her busy life. Identify approaches you would use to establish a plan of care with her. Link your teaching to the trajectory onset phase of chronic illness. How would your teaching plan change in the acute and crisis stages of chronic illness?

3 A 40-year-old woman with spina bifida is admitted to the hospital for a pneumonectomy to treat lung cancer. What modifications are needed to make sure that this patient's needs are addressed throughout her hospital stay? What planning is needed to prepare her for hospital discharge?

4 ebp A 43-year-old woman experienced a spinal cord injury 4 years ago as a result of a diving mishap. She has been admitted to the hospital for treatment of a grade IV pressure ulcer. The health history reveals that the patient has not been under close care of a health care provider for the past 3 years and that she has not been following recommendations for skin care and other healthy practices, including health screening. However, she indicates that she is ready to begin to take a more active role in self-care to avoid development of further pressure ulcers. What recommendations would you make to her for self-care to prevent secondary conditions and disabilities and for health screening? What is the evidence base for your recommendations? What criteria would you use to evaluate the strength of the evidence? Develop an evidence-based plan of care for her.

REFERENCES AND SELECTED READINGS

BOOKS

Corbin, J. & Cherry, J. (2001). Epilogue: A proactive model of health care. In Hyman, R. & Corbin, J. (Eds.). *Chronic illness: Research and theory for nursing practice*. New York: Springer.

DePoy, E. & Gilson, S. F. (2004). *Rethinking disability: Principles for professional and social change*. Belmont, CA: Thomson/Brooks/Cole.

Falvo, D. R. (2005). *Medical and psychosocial aspects of chronic illness and disability*. Sudbury, MA: Jones & Bartlett.

Jans, L. & Stoddard, S. (1999). *Chartbook on women and disability in the United States*. Washington, DC: U.S. Department of Education, National Institutes on Disability and Rehabilitation Research.

Krahn, G. (2003). *Changing concepts of health and disability*. Portland, OR: Rehabilitation Research and Training Center, Health and Wellness Consortium.

Lubkin, I. M. (1997). *Chronic illness: Impact and interventions*. Boston: Jones & Bartlett.

McKenna, M. T., Taylor, W. R., Marks, J. S., et al. (1998). Current issues and challenges in chronic disease control. In Brownson, R. C., Remington, P. L. & Davis, J. R. (Eds.). *Chronic disease epidemiology and control*. Washington, DC: American Public Health Association.

National Center for Law and Deafness. (n.d.) *ADA questions and answers for health care providers*. Washington, DC: Gallaudet University.

Neal, L. J. & Guillett, S. E. (2004) *Care of the adults with a chronic illness or disability: A team approach*. St. Louis: Mosby.

Nehring, W. M. (2205). *Core curriculum for specializing in intellectual and developmental disability: A resource for nurses and other health care professionals*. Sudbury, MA: Jones & Bartlett.

Nosek, M. & Center for Research on Women with Disabilities (CROWD). (2004). *Improving the health and wellness of women with disabilities: A symposium to establish a research agenda (Executive summary)*. Houston: Center for Research on Women with Disabilities.

Nosek, M. A., Howland, C. A., Rintala, D. H., et al. (1997). *National study of women with physical disabilities: Final report*. Houston: Center for Research on Women with Disabilities.

Robert Wood Johnson Foundation. (1996). *Chronic care in America: A 21st century challenge*. Princeton, NJ: Author.

Robert Wood Johnson Foundation. (2001). *A portrait of the chronically ill in America, 2001*. Princeton, NJ: Author.

Robinson, L., Bevil, C., Arcangelo, V., et al. (2001). Operationalizing the Corbin and Strauss Trajectory Model for elderly clients with chronic illness. In Hyman, R. & Corbin, J. (Eds.). *Chronic illness: Research and theory for nursing practice*. New York: Springer.

Rogers, J. (2006). The disabled woman's guide to pregnancy and birth. New York: Demos Publications.

Sipski, M. & Alexander, C. (1997). Sexual function in people with disability and chronic illness: A health professional's guide. Gaithersburg, MD: Aspen.

Smeltzer, S. C. (1992). Use of the trajectory model of nursing in multiple sclerosis. In Woog, P. (Ed.). *The chronic illness trajectory framework*. New York: Springer.

Smeltzer, S. C. & Sharts-Hopko, N. C. (2005). *A provider's guide for the care of women with physical disabilities and chronic health conditions*. Chapel Hill, NC: North Carolina Office on Disability and Health.

Social Security Administration (2005). *Disability evaluation under Social Security*. SSA Pub. No. 64-039 ICN 468600. Washington, DC: Social Security Administration, Office of Disability Programs.

United Spinal Association. (2004). *Understanding the Americans with Disabilities Act (ADA)*. Jackson Heights, NY: United Spinal Association. Available at: www.unitedspinal.org (accessed March 10, 2006).

U.S. Census Bureau. (2003). *Disability status, 2000*. Washington, DC: U.S. Department of Commerce.

U.S. Department of Health and Human Services. (2000). *Healthy People 2010*. U.S. Washington, DC: Author.

U.S. Department of Health and Human Services. (2001). *Surgeon General's call to action to prevent and decrease overweight and obesity 2001*. Rockville, MD: Public Health Service, Office of the Surgeon General.

U.S. Department of Health and Human Services. (2005). *Surgeon General's call to action to improve the health and wellness of people with disabilities*. Rockville, MD: Public Health Service, Office of the Surgeon General.

Welner, S. L. & Haseltine, F. (2004). *Welner's guide to the care of women with disabilities*. Philadelphia: Lippincott Williams & Wilkins.

Welner, S. L. & Temple, B. (2004). General health concerns and the physical examination. In Welner, S. L. & Haseltine, F. (Eds.). *Welner's guide to the care of women with disabilities*. Philadelphia: Lippincott Williams & Wilkins.

World Health Organization. (1980). *International classification of impairments, disabilities, and handicaps*. Geneva: WHO.

World Health Organization. (2001). *International classification of functioning, disability and health. Short version*. Geneva: WHO.

JOURNALS

**An asterisk indicates a nursing research article.*

Bates, M. S., Rankin-Hill, L. & Sanchez-Ayendez, M. (1997). The effects of the cultural context of health care on treatment of and response to chronic pain and illness. *Social Science in Medicine, 45*(9), 1333–1347.

Becker, G., Beyene, Y., Newsom, E. M. & Rodgers, D. V. (1998). Knowledge and care of chronic illness in three ethnic minority groups. *Family Medicine, 30*(3), 173–178.

Gallo, A. M. & Knafl, K. A. (1998). Parents' reports of "tricks of the trade" for managing childhood chronic illness. *Journal of the Society of Pediatric Nurses, 3*(3), 93–100.

Jennings, A. (1999). The use of available social support networks by older blacks. *Journal of National Black Nurses Association, 10*(2), 4–13.

Juarbe, T. C. (1998). Risk factors for cardiovascular disease in Latina women. *Progress in Cardiovascular Nursing, 13*(2), 17–27.

Mishel, M. H. (1999). Uncertainty in chronic illness. *Annual Review of Nursing Research, 17:* 269–294.

Nijhof, G. (1998). Heterogeneity in the interpretation of epilepsy. *Qualitative Health Research, 8*(1), 95–105.

*Rehm, R. S. (1999). Religious faith in Mexican-American families dealing with chronic childhood illness. *Image: Journal of Nursing Scholarship, 31*(1), 33–38.

*Thorne, S., McCormick, J. & Carty, E. (1997). Deconstructing the gender neutrality of chronic illness and disability. *Health Care Women International, 18*(1), 1–16.

Wing, R., Goldstein, M., Acton, K., et al. (2001). Behavioral science research in diabetes: Lifestyle changes related to obesity, eating behavior, and physical activity. *Diabetes Care,* 24(1), 117–123.

Chronic Illness

Anderson, G. F. (2003). Physician, public, and policymaker perspectives on chronic conditions. *Archives of Internal Medicine, 163*(4), 437–442.

Anderson, G. F. (2005). Medicare and chronic conditions. *New England Journal of Medicine, 353*(3), 305–309.

Anonymous. (2002). Many working age people with chronic conditions are among the uninsured. *Healthcare Leadership and Management Report, 10*(2),12.

*Arthur, V. & Clifford, C. (2004). Rheumatology: The expectations and preferences of patients for their follow-up monitoring care. A qualitative study to determine the dimensions of patient satisfaction. *Journal of Clinical Nursing, 13*(2), 234–242.

*Bailey, D. E., Mishel, M. H., Belyea, M., et al. (2004). Uncertainty intervention for watchful waiting in prostate cancer. *Cancer Nursing, 27*(5), 339–346.

Bayliss, E. A., Steiner, J. F., Fernald, D. H., et al. (2003). Descriptions of barriers to self-care by people with comorbid chronic diseases. *Annals of Family Medicine, 1*(1), 15–21.

*Becker, H. & Stuifbergen, A. (2004). What makes it so hard? Barriers to health promotion experienced by people with multiple sclerosis and polio. *Family and Community Health, 27*(1), 75–85.

*Brooks, M. V. (2003). Health-related hardiness and chronic illness: A synthesis of current research. *Nursing Forum, 38*(3), 11–20.

Carasa, M. & Nespoli, G. (2002). Nursing the chronically critically ill patient. *Critical Care Clinics, 18*(3), 493–507.

Carson, S. S. & Bach, P. B. (2002). The epidemiology and costs of chronic critical illness. *Critical Care Clinics, 18*(3), 461–476.

Centers for Disease Control and Prevention (CDC). (2004). Indicators for chronic disease surveillance. *Morbidity and Mortality Weekly Report: Recommendations and Reports, 53*(RR-11), 1–6.

*Clingerman, E., Stuifbergen, A. & Becker, H. (2004). The influence of resources on perceived functional limitations among women with multiple sclerosis. *Journal of Neuroscience Nursing, 36*(6), 312–321.

Corbin, J. M. (1998). The Corbin and Strauss chronic illness trajectory model: An update. *Scholarly Inquiry for Nursing Practice, 12*(1), 33–41.

Corbin, J. M. (2003). The body in health and illness. *Qualitative Health Research, 13*(2), 256–267.

Cumbie, S. A., Conley, V. M. & Burman, M. E. (2004). Advanced practice nursing model for comprehensive care with chronic illness: Model for promoting process engagement. *Advances in Nursing Science, 27*(1), 70–80.

Denny, C. H., Holtzman, D., Goins, T., et al. (2005). Disparities in chronic disease risk factors and health status between American Indian/Alaska Native and white elders: Findings from a telephone survey, 2001 and 2002. *American Journal of Public Health, 95*(5), 825–827.

*Dingley, C. & Roux, G. (2003). Inner strength in older Hispanic women with chronic illness. *Journal of Cultural Diversity, 10*(1), 11–22.

Fisher, L. & Weiks, K. L. (2000). Can addressing family relationships improve outcomes in chronic disease? Report of the National Working Group on Family-Based Interventions in Chronic Disease. *Journal of Family Practice, 49*(6), 561–566.

Frich, L. M. (2003). Nursing interventions for patients with chronic conditions. *Journal of Advanced Nursing, 44*(2), 137–153.

Goertzel, R. Z., Hawkins, K., Ozminkowski, R. J., et al. (2003). The health and productivity cost burden of the "top 10" physical and mental health conditions affecting six large U.S. employers in 1999. *Journal of Occupational and Environmental Medicine, 45*(1), 5–14.

Johnston, J. A., Wagner, D. P., Timmons, S., et al. (2002). Impact of different measures of comorbid disease on predicted mortality of intensive care unit patients. *Medical Care, 40*(10), 929–940.

*Knafl, K. A. & Gillis, C. L. (2002). Families and chronic illness: A synthesis of current research. *Journal of Family Nursing, 8*(3), 178–198.

*Kralik, D., Koch, T., Price K., et al. (2004). Chronic illness self-management: Taking action to create order. *Journal of Clinical Nursing, 13*(2), 259–267.

*Loeb, S. J., Penrod, J., Falkenstern, S., et al. (2003). Supporting older adults living with multiple chronic conditions. *Western Journal of Nursing Research, 25*(1), 8–23; discussion 23–29.

*Lorig, K. R., Ritter, P. L. & Gonzalez, V. M. (2003). Hispanic chronic disease self-management: A randomized community-based outcome trial. *Nursing Research, 52*(6), 361–369.

Mack, K. A. & Ahluwalia, I. B. (2003). Observations from the CDC: Monitoring women's health in the United States—Selected chronic disease indicators, 1991–2001 BRFSS. *Journal of Women's Health, 12*(4), 309–314.

Marshall, J. G. (2004). Cancer screening in women with chronic illness: The unanswered questions. *MedSurg Nursing, 13*(2), 110–113.

Mascie-Taylor, C. G. & Karim, E. (2003). The burden of chronic disease. *Science, 302*(5652), 1921–1922.

Michels, K. B. (2003). Early life predictors of chronic disease. *Journal of Women's Health, 12*(2), 157–161.

*Mishel, M. H., Germino, B. B., Belyea, M., et al. (2003). Moderators of an uncertainty management intervention: For men with localized prostate cancer. *Nursing Research, 52*(2), 89–97.

Mold, J. W., Fryer, G. E. & Thomas, C. H. (2004). Who are the uninsured elderly in the United States? *Journal of the American Geriatrics Society, 52*(4), 601–606.

*Öhman, M., Söderberg, S. & Lundman, B. (2003). Hovering between suffering and enduring: The meaning of living with serious chronic illness. *Qualitative Health Research, 13*(4), 528–542.

Rice, D. P. & Fineman, N. (2004). Economic implications of increased longevity in the United States. *Annual Review of Public Health, 25*, 457–473.

*Stuifbergen, A. K. & Becker, H. (2001). Health promotion practices in women with multiple sclerosis: Increasing quality and years of healthy life. *Physical Medicine and Rehabilitation Clinics of North America, 12*(1), 9–22.

*Stuifbergen, A. K., Harrison, T. C., Becker, H., et al. (2004). Adaptation of a wellness intervention for women with chronic disabling conditions. *Journal of Holistic Nursing, 22*(1), 12–31.

Stuifbergen, A. K. & Rogers, S. (1997). Health promotion: An essential component of rehabilitation for persons with chronic disabling conditions. *Advances in Nursing Science, 19*(4), 1–20.

*Stuifbergen, A. K., Seraphine, A., Harrison, T., et al. (2005). An explanatory model of health promotion and quality of life for people with post-polio syndrome. *Social Science and Medicine, 60*(2), 383–393.

*Sullivan, T., Weinert, C. & Cudney, S. (2002). Management of chronic illness: Voices of rural women. *Journal of Advanced Nursing, 44*(6), 566–574.

*Williams, A. (2004). Patients with comorbidities: Perceptions of acute care services. *Journal of Advanced Nursing, 46*(1), 13–22.

Williams, P. D., Williams, A. R., Graff, J. C., et al. (2002). Interrelationships among variables affecting well siblings and mothers in families of children with a chronic illness or disability. *Journal of Behavioral Medicine, 25*(5), 411–424.

Disabilities

Allen, S. M. & Ciambrone, D. (2003). Community care for people with disability: Blurring boundaries between formal and informal caregivers. *Qualitative Health Research, 13*(2), 207–226.

Bartels, M. N. & Omura, A. (2005). Aging in polio. *Physical Medicine and Rehabilitation Clinics of North America, 16*(1), 197–218.

Brown, A. A. & Gill, C. J. (2002). Women with developmental disabilities: Health and aging. *Current Women's Health Reports, 2*(3), 219–225.

Campbell, M. L., Sheets, D. & Strong, P. S. (1999). Secondary health conditions among middle-aged people with chronic physical disabilities: Implications for unmet needs for services. *Assistive Technology, 11*(2), 105–122.

Carson, A. R. & Hieber, K. V. (2001). Adult pediatric patients. *American Journal of Nursing, 101*(3), 46–54.

Coyle, C. P. & Santiago, M. C. (2002). Healthcare utilization among women with physical disabilities. *Medscape Women's Health eJournal, 7*(4), 2.

French, S. (1992). Simulation exercises in disability awareness training. *Disability, Handicap and Society, 7*(3), 257–266.

Goodall, C. J. (1995). Is disability any business of nurse education? *Nurse Education Today, 15*(5), 323–327.

Hahn, J. E. & Marks, B. A. (Eds.) (2003). Intellectual and developmental disabilities. *Nursing Clinics in North America, 38*(2), 185–393.

*Harrison, T. (2003). Women aging with childhood onset disability. *Journal of Holistic Nursing, 21*(3), 242–259.

*Harrison, T. & Stuifbergen, A. (2001). Barriers that further disablement: A study of survivors of polio. *Journal of Neuroscience Nursing, 33*(3), 160–166.

Honeycutt, A., Dunlap, L., Chen, H., et al. (2004). Economic costs associated with mental retardation, cerebral palsy, hearing loss, and vision impairment. *MMWR Morbidity and Mortality Weekly Report, 53*(03), 57–69.

Kinne, S., Patrick, D. L. & Doyle, D. L. (2003). Prevalence of secondary conditions among people with disabilities. *American Journal of Public Health, 94*(3), 443–445.

Klingbeil, H., Baer, H. R. & Wilson, P. E. (2004). Aging with a disability. *Archives of Physical Medicine and Rehabilitation, 85*(Suppl 3), S68–S73.

Lollar, D. J. & Crews, J. E. (2003). Redefining the role of public health in disability. *Annual Review of Public Health, 24,* 195–208.

Long, S. K. & Coughlin, T. A. & Kendall, S. J. (2002). Access to care among disabled adults on Medicaid. *Health Care Financing Review, 23*(4), 159–173.

*Lutz, B. J. & Bowers, B. J. (2005). Disability in everyday life. *Qualitative Health Research, 15*(8), 1037–1054.

*McFarlane, J., Hughes, R. B., Nosek, M. A., et al. (2001). Abuse Assessment Screen—Disability (AAS-D): Measuring frequency, type, and perpetrator of abuse toward women with physical disabilities. *Journal of Women's Health and Gender-Based Medicine, 10*(9), 861–866.

Nosek, M. A. (2000). Overcoming the odds: The health of women with physical disabilities in the United States. *Archives of Physical Medicine and Rehabilitation, 81*(2), 135–138.

Odette, F., Yoshida, K. K., Israel, P., et al. (2003). Barriers to wellness activities for Canadian women with physical disabilities. *Health Care for Women International, 24*(2), 125–134.

Richardson, M. (1997). Addressing barriers: Disabled rights and the implications for nursing of the social construct of disability. *Journal of Advanced Nursing, 25*(6), 1269–1275.

Schopp, L. H., Sanford, T. C., Hagglund, K. J., et al. (2002). Removing service barriers for women with physical disabilities: Promoting accessibility in the gynecologic care setting. *Journal of Midwifery and Women's Health, 47*(2), 74–79.

Scullion, P. (1999a). Challenging discrimination against disabled patients. *Nursing Standard, 13*(8), 37–40.

*Scullion, P. (1999b). Conceptualizing disability in nursing: Some evidence from students and their teachers. *Journal of Advanced Nursing, 29*(3), 648–657.

Scullion, P. (2000). Enabling disabled people: Responsibilities of nurse education. *British Journal of Nursing, 9*(15), 1010–1015.

Shakespeare, T. & Watson, N. (1997). Defending the social model. *Disability and Society, 12*(2), 293–300.

*Smeltzer, S. C. (2002). Reproductive decision making in women with multiple sclerosis. *Journal of Neuroscience Nursing, 34*(3), 145–157.

Smeltzer, S. C. (2006). Preventive health screening for breast and cervical cancer and osteoporosis in women with physical disabilities *Family and Community Health, 29*(1 Suppl.), 35S–43S.

*Smeltzer, S. C. & Zimmerman, V. (2005). Health promotion interests of women with disabilities. *Journal of Neuroscience Nursing, 37*(2), 80–86.

*Smeltzer, S. C., Zimmerman, V. & Capriotti, T. (2005). Osteoporosis risk and low bone mineral density in women with disabilities. *Archives of Physical Medicine and Rehabilitation, 86*(3), 582–586.

Smeltzer, S. C., Zimmerman, V., DeSilets, L. D., et al. (2003). Accessible online health promotion information for people with disabilities. *Online Journal of Issues in Nursing, 9*(1), 11. Available at: nursingworld.org/ojin/topic16/tpc16_5.htm (accessed May 6, 2006).

Vandenakker, C. B. & Glass, D. D. (2001). Menopause and aging with disability. *Physical Medicine and Rehabilitation Clinics of North America, 12*(1), 133–151.

RESOURCES

Abledata, 8630 Fenton Street, Suite 930, Silver Spring, MD 20910; 800-227-0216; http://abledata.com. Accessed ***.

American Association of the Deaf-Blind, 8630 Fenton Street, Suite 121, Silver Spring, MD 20910; 301-495-4403; TTY: 301-495-4402; http://www.aadb.org. Accessed March 10, 2006.

American Association on Mental Retardation, 444 North Capitol Street, Suite 846, Washington, DC 20001; 800-424-3688; http://www.aamr.org. Accessed March 10, 2006.

American Foundation for the Blind, 11 Penn Plaza, Suite 300, New York, NY 10001; 800-232-5463; http://www.afb.org. Accessed March 10, 2006.

Americans With Disabilities Act Information Technology Center, 451 Hungerford Drive, Suite 607, Rockville, MD 20850; 800-949-4232; http://www.adainfo.org or http://www.adata.org/. Accessed March 10, 2006.

American Speech-Language-Hearing Association, 10801 Rockville Pike, Rockville, MD 20852; 800-498-2072, fax 301-571-0457, TTY 301-897-5700; http://www.asha.org. Accessed March 10, 2006.

Arc of the United States, 1010 Wayne Avenue, Suite 650, Silver Spring, MD 20910; 301-656-3842, fax 301-565-3843; http://www.thearc.org. Accessed March 10, 2006.

Association of Late Deafened Adults, 8038 Macintosh Lane, Rockford, IL 61107, 866-402-2532, TTY 866-402-2532; http://www.alda.org. Accessed March 10, 2006.

Centers for Medicare and Medicaid Services, 7500 Security Boulevard, Baltimore, MD 21244; 800-633-4227 or 800-MEDICARE; http://www.cms.hhs.gov. Accessed March 10, 2006.

Center for Research on Women with Disabilities (CROWD), 3440 Richmond Avenue, Houston, TX 77046; 713-960-0505; http://www.bcm.edu/crowd. Accessed March 10, 2006.

ChronicNet, http://www.chronicnet.org/chronnet/project.htm. Accessed March 10, 2006. This website provides local and national data on chronic care issues and populations.

National Aphasia Association, 7 Dey Street, Suite 600, New York, NY 10007; 800-922-4622; http://www.aphasia.org. Accessed March 10, 2006.

National Center for Learning Disabilities, 381 Park Avenue South, Suite 1401, New York, NY 10016; 212-545-7510 or toll-free 888-575-7373, fax 212-545-9665; http://www.ncld.org. Accessed March 10, 2006.

North Carolina Office on Disability and Health, Division of Public Health, 1928 Mail Service Center, Raleigh, NC 27699; 919-707-5672; http://www.fpg.unc.edu/~ncodh or http://www.wch.dhhs.state.nc.us/cay.htm. Accessed March 10, 2006.

Robert Wood Johnson Foundation, http://www.rwjf.org. Accessed March 10, 2006. This website has information about health care in the United States, including proceedings of "Patient Education and Consumer Activation in Chronic Disease," July 7, 2000.

Through the Looking Glass, 2198 Sixth Street, Suite 100, Berkeley, CA 94710; 800-644-2666, TTY 800-804-1616; http://www.lookingglass.org. Accessed March 10, 2006.

United Cerebral Palsy, 1660 L Street NW, Suite 700, Washington, DC 20036; 800-872-5827; http://www.ucp.org. Accessed March 10, 2006.

United Spinal Association, 75-20 Astoria Boulevard, Jackson Heights, NY 11370; 718-803-3782, fax 718-803-0414; http://www.unitedspinal.org. Accessed March 10, 2006.

Villanova University Health Promotion for Women with Disabilities Project, Villanova University College of Nursing, 800 Lancaster Avenue, Villanova, PA 19085; http://www.villanova.nursing.edu/WomenWithDisabilities. Accessed April 30, 2006.

CHAPTER 11

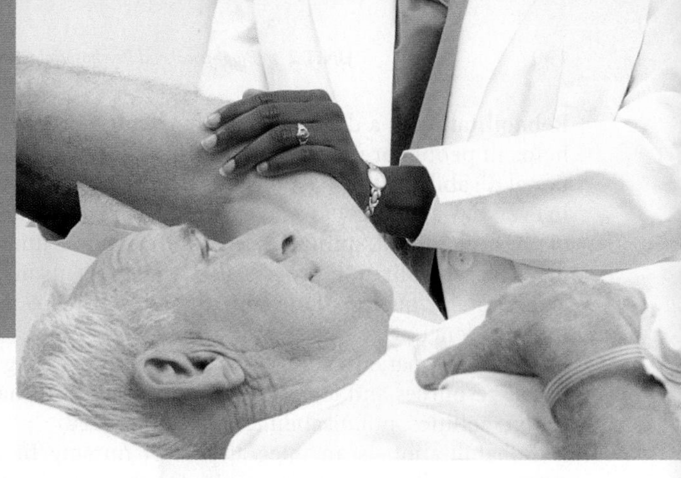

Principles and Practices of Rehabilitation

Learning Objectives

On completion of this chapter, the learner will be able to:

1. Describe the goals of rehabilitation.
2. Discuss the interdisciplinary approach to rehabilitation.
3. Identify emotional reactions exhibited by patients with disabilities.
4. Use the nursing process as a framework for care of patients with self-care deficits, impaired physical mobility, impaired skin integrity, and altered patterns of elimination.
5. Describe nursing strategies appropriate for promoting self-care through activities of daily living.
6. Describe nursing strategies appropriate for promoting mobility and ambulation and the use of assistive devices.
7. Describe risk factors and related nursing measures to prevent development of pressure ulcers.
8. Incorporate bladder training and bowel training into the plan of care for patients with bladder and bowel problems.
9. Describe the significance of continuity of care and community re-entry from the health care facility to the home or extended care facility for patients who need rehabilitative assistance and services.

Rehabilitation is a dynamic, health-oriented process that helps ill people or people with physical, mental, or emotional **disabilities** (restrictions in performance or function in everyday activities) to achieve the greatest possible level of physical, mental, spiritual, social, and economic functioning. The rehabilitation process also helps patients achieve an acceptable quality of life with dignity, self-respect, and independence. During rehabilitation—sometimes called habilitation—patients adjust to disabilities by learning how to use resources and focus on existing abilities. In **habilitation**, abilities, not disabilities, are emphasized.

Rehabilitation is an integral part of nursing because every major illness or injury carries the threat of disability or **impairment**, which involves a loss of function or an abnormality. The principles of rehabilitation are basic to the care of all patients, and rehabilitation efforts should begin during the initial contact with a patient. The goal of rehabilitation is to restore the patient's ability to function independently or at a preillness or preinjury level of functioning as quickly as possible. If this is not possible, the aims of rehabilitation are to maximize independence and prevent secondary disability as well as to promote a quality of life acceptable to the patient. Realistic goals based on individual patient assessment are established with each patient to guide the rehabilitation program.

Rehabilitation services are required by more people than ever before because of advances in technology that save or prolong the lives of seriously ill and injured patients and patients with disabilities. Increasing numbers of patients who are recovering from serious illnesses or injuries are returning to their homes and communities with ongoing needs. All patients, regardless of age, gender, ethnic group, socioeconomic status, or diagnosis, have a right to rehabilitation services (Chart 11-1).

CHART 11-1

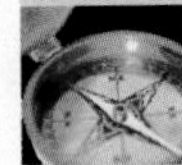

Ethics and Related Issues

Are All Persons Entitled to Rehabilitation?

SITUATION

You work in an area where many illegal aliens and uninsured residents live. Community violence often creates life-threatening and disabling conditions in members of the population. After a victim of violence has been saved and stabilized, the health care team identifies rehabilitation needs. You are concerned about your patient's inability to perform self-care and to demonstrate safe mobility skills.

DILEMMA

As a health care provider, you are concerned about the community as a whole; costs to the community, and the values of the community. You are also aware of client fiduciary responsibility; you recognize costs to your patient when treatment is provided or not provided.

DISCUSSION

1. Who determines the length of stay and level of care?
2. Who will take care of patients who need rehabilitation but who are unable to pay? Is rehabilitation a basic health care need?

A person is considered to have a disability, such as a restriction in performance or function in everyday activities, if he or she has difficulty talking, hearing, seeing, walking,

Glossary

activities of daily living (ADLs): self-care activities including bathing, grooming, dressing, eating, toileting, and bowel and bladder care

adaptive device: a type of assistive technology that is used to change the environment or help the person to modify the environment (eg, a ramp that can be used in place of steps for someone in a wheelchair)

assistive device: a type of assistive technology that helps people with disabilities perform a given task (eg, a lap board with pictures that is used to assist a person who cannot talk to communicate)

assistive technology: any item, piece of equipment, or product system—whether acquired commercially, off the shelf, modified, or customized—that is used to improve the functional capabilities of individuals with disabilities. This term encompasses both assistive devices and adaptive devices.

disability: restriction or lack of ability to perform an activity in a normal manner; the consequences of impairment in terms of an individual's functional performance and activity. Disabilities represent disturbances at the level of the person (eg, bathing, dressing, communication, walking, grooming).

habilitation: making able; learning new skills and abilities to meet maximum potential.

impairment: loss or abnormality of psychological, physiologic, or anatomic structure or function at the organ level (eg, dysphagia, hemiparesis); an abnormality of body structure, appearance, and organ or system function resulting from any cause.

instrumental activities of daily living (IADLs): complex aspects of independence including meal preparation, grocery shopping, household management, finances, and transportation.

pressure ulcers: breakdown of the skin due to prolonged pressure and insufficient blood supply, usually at bony prominences.

rehabilitation: making able again; relearning skills or abilities or adjusting existing functions.

climbing stairs, lifting or carrying objects, performing activities of daily living, doing schoolwork, or working at a job. The disability is severe if the person cannot perform one or more activities or use an assistive device for mobility, or needs help from another person to accomplish basic activities. The goal of **assistive devices** and **adaptive devices** is to maximize independence and thereby promote access. A person is also considered severely disabled if he or she receives federal benefits because of an inability to work.

Approximately 1 in 5 Americans has some form of disability, and 1 in 10 has a severe disability (U.S. Census Bureau, 2000). Approximately 60 million are affected by some form of disability, and this number is expected to increase in the coming decades due to the aging of the population. More than half of the people with disability are women, and women with disability outnumber men in all age groups except for those 15 to 24 years of age (Jans & Stoddard, 1999). One third of women 75 years of age and older need personal assistance. Currently, more than 10 million people need personal assistance with one or more **activities of daily living** (ADLs), which include bathing, dressing, feeding, and toileting, or **instrumental activities of daily living** (IADLs), which include grocery shopping, meal preparation, housekeeping, transportation, and managing finances. About 5 million people use a cane, more than 2 million use a wheelchair, and at least 1 million use crutches or a walker. Use of these devices and other types of **assistive technology** has increased dramatically due to the aging of the population, technologic advances, public policy initiatives, and changes in the delivery and financing of health care (U.S. Census Bureau, 2000).

Americans With Disabilities Act

For years, people with disabilities have been discriminated against in employment, public accommodations, and public and private services, including health care. In 1990, the U.S. Congress passed the Americans With Disabilities Act (ADA) (PL 101-336), which is civil rights legislation designed to provide people with disabilities with access to job opportunities and to the community. See Chapter 10 for discussion of the ADA, access to health care and health promotion, and special issues that should be addressed in providing health care to people with disabilities.

Patients' Reactions to Disability

Disability can occur at any age and may result from an acute incident, such as stroke or trauma, or from the progression of a chronic condition, such as arthritis or multiple sclerosis. People with disabilities experience many losses, including loss of function, independence, social role, status, and income. The patient and family experience a range of emotional reactions to these losses that may progress from disorganization and confusion to denial of the disability, grief over the lost function or body part, depression, anger, and, finally, acceptance of the disability. The reactions may subside over time and may recur at a later time, especially if chronic illness is progressive and results in increasing losses. Not all patients experience all of the stages, although most do exhibit grief. Patients who exhibit grief should not be dismissed and encouraged to "cheer up." The nurse should show a willingness to listen to the patient talk about the disability and should understand that grief, anger, regret, resentment, and acceptance are all part of the healing process. Chart 11-2 lists concerns unique to older adults.

The patient's preexisting coping abilities play an important role in the adaptation process. One patient may be particularly independent and determined, whereas another may be dependent and feel powerless. One goal of rehabilitation is to help the patient gain a positive self-image through effective coping. The nurse must recognize different coping abilities and identify when a patient is not coping well or not adjusting to the disability. The patient and family may benefit from participating in a support group or talking with a mental health professional to achieve this goal. Refer to Chapter 6 for a detailed discussion of adaptive and maladaptive responses to illness.

The Rehabilitation Team

Rehabilitation is a creative, dynamic process that requires a team of professionals working together with patients and families. The team members represent a variety of disciplines, with each health professional making a unique contribution. Each health professional assesses the patient and identifies the patient's needs within his or her discipline's domain. Rehabilitative goals are set. Team members hold frequent group sessions to collaborate, evaluate progress, and modify goals as needed to facilitate rehabilitation and to promote independence, self-respect, and an acceptable quality of life for the patient.

The patient is a key member of the rehabilitation team. The patient is the focus of the team's effort and the one who

CHART 11-2

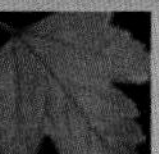

Concerns of Older Adults Facing Disability

- Loss of independence, which is a source of self-respect and dignity
- Increased potential for discrimination or abuse
- Increased social isolation
- Added burden on spouse, who may also have impaired health
- Less access to community services and health care
- Less access to religious institutions
- Increased vulnerability to declining health secondary to other disorders, reduced physiologic reserve, or preexisting impairments of mobility and balance
- Fears and doubts about ability to learn or relearn self-care activities, exercises, and transfer and independent mobility techniques
- Inadequate support system for successful rehabilitation

determines the final outcomes of the process. The patient participates in goal setting, in learning to function using remaining abilities, and in adjusting to living with disabilities.

The patient's family is also incorporated into the team. Families are dynamic systems; therefore, the disability of one member affects other family members. Only by incorporating the family into the rehabilitation process can the family system adapt to the change in one of its members. The family provides ongoing support, participates in problem solving, and learns to provide necessary ongoing care.

The nurse develops a therapeutic and supportive relationship with the patient and family. The nurse emphasizes the patient's assets and strengths, positively reinforcing the patient's efforts to improve self-concept and self-care abilities. During nurse–patient interactions, the nurse actively listens, encourages, and shares the patient's successes.

Using the nursing process, the nurse develops a plan of care designed to facilitate rehabilitation, restore and maintain optimal health, and prevent complications. The nurse helps the patient identify strengths and past successes and develop new goals. Coping with the disability, self-care, mobility limitations, skin care, and bowel and bladder management are areas that frequently require nursing interventions. The nurse acts as a caregiver, teacher, counselor, patient advocate, case manager, and consultant. The nurse is often responsible for coordinating the total rehabilitative plan and collaborating with and coordinating the services provided by all members of the health care team, including home care nurses, who are responsible for directing patient care after the patient returns home.

Other members of the rehabilitation team may include physicians, nurse practitioners, physiatrists, physical therapists, occupational therapists, recreational therapists, speech-language therapists, psychologists, psychiatric liaison nurses, social workers, vocational counselors, orthotists or prosthetists, and sex counselors.

Areas of Specialty Rehabilitation

Although rehabilitation must be a component of every patient's care, specialty rehabilitation programs have been established in general hospitals, free-standing rehabilitation hospitals, and outpatient facilities. The Commission for the Accreditation of Rehabilitation Facilities (CARF) sets standards for these programs and monitors compliance with the standards.

- *Stroke recovery programs* and *traumatic brain injury rehabilitation* emphasize cognitive remediation, helping patients compensate for memory, perceptual, judgment, and safety deficits as well as teaching self-care and mobility skills. Other goals include helping patients swallow food safely and communicate effectively. Neurologic disorders treated in addition to stroke and brain injury include multiple sclerosis, Parkinson's disease, amyotrophic lateral sclerosis, and nervous system tumors.
- *Spinal cord injury rehabilitation* programs have increased in number since World War II. Integral components of the programs include understanding the effects and complications of spinal cord injury; neurogenic bowel and bladder management; sexuality and fertility enhancement; self-care, including prevention of skin breakdown; bed mobility and transfers; and driving with adaptive equipment. The programs also focus on vocational assessment, training, and reentry into employment and the community. Currently, there are 16 federally funded designated spinal cord injury centers in the United States.
- *Orthopedic rehabilitation programs* provide comprehensive services to patients with traumatic or nontraumatic amputation, patients undergoing joint replacements, and patients with arthritis. Learning to be independent with a prosthesis or a new joint is a major goal of these programs. Other goals include pain management, energy conservation, and joint protection.
- *Cardiac rehabilitation* for patients who have had myocardial infarction begins during the acute hospitalization and continues on an outpatient basis. Emphasis is placed on monitored, progressive exercise; nutritional counseling; stress management; sexuality; and risk reduction.
- *Pulmonary rehabilitation* programs may be appropriate for patients with restrictive or chronic obstructive pulmonary disease or ventilator dependency. Respiratory therapists help patients achieve more effective breathing patterns. The programs also teach energy conservation techniques, self-medication, and home ventilatory management.
- *Comprehensive pain management programs* are available for people with chronic pain, especially low back pain. These programs focus on alternative pain treatment modalities, exercise, supportive counseling, and vocational evaluation.
- *Comprehensive burn rehabilitation programs* may serve as step-down units from intensive care burn units. Although rehabilitation strategies are implemented immediately in acute care, a program focused on progressive joint mobility, self-care, and ongoing counseling is imperative for burn patients.
- *Pediatric rehabilitation programs* meet the needs of children with developmental and acquired disabilities, including cerebral palsy, spina bifida, traumatic brain injuries, and spinal cord injuries.

As in all areas of nursing practice, nurses practicing in the area of rehabilitation must be skilled and knowledgeable about the care of patients with substance abuse. For all people with disabilities, including adolescents, nurses must assess actual or potential substance abuse. Almost 15 million Americans use illicit drugs, approximately 58 million engage in binge or heavy drinking of alcohol, and about 34% of the population uses tobacco products. Parental alcoholism is one of the strongest predictors of substance abuse. Alcohol abuse rates for people with disabilities may be twice as high as in the general population. Fifty percent of spinal cord injuries are related to substance abuse, and approximately 50% of all patients with traumatic brain injury were intoxicated at the time of injury (U.S. Department of Health and Human Services, 2003).

Substance abuse is a critical issue in rehabilitation, especially for people with disabilities who are attempting to gain employment via vocational rehabilitation. Treatment for alcoholism and drug dependencies includes a thorough physical and psychosocial evaluation; detoxification; counseling; medical treatment; psychological assistance for patients and families; treatment of any coexisting psychiatric illness; and referral to community resources for social, legal, spiritual, or vocational assistance. The length of treatment and the rehabilitation process depends on the patient's needs. Self-help groups are also encouraged, although attendance at meetings of such groups (eg, Alcoholics Anonymous, Narcotics Anonymous) poses various challenges for people who have neurologic disorders, are permanent wheelchair users, or must adapt to encounters with nondisabled attendees who may not understand disability. All specialty areas of rehabilitation require implementation of the nursing process as described in this chapter.

Assessment of Functional Ability

Comprehensive assessment of functional capacity is the basis for developing a rehabilitation program. Functional capacity is a person's ability to perform ADLs and IADLs. ADLs include activities performed to meet basic needs, such as personal hygiene, dressing, toileting, eating, and moving. IADLs include activities that are necessary for independent living, such as the ability to shop for and prepare meals, use the telephone, clean, manage finances, and travel.

The nurse observes the patient performing specific activities (eg, eating, dressing) and notes the degree of independence; the time taken; the patient's mobility, coordination, and endurance; and the amount of assistance required. The nurse also carefully assesses joint motion, muscle strength, cardiovascular reserve, and neurologic function, because functional ability depends on these factors as well. Observations are recorded on a functional assessment tool. These tools provide a way to standardize assessment parameters and include a scale or score against which improvements may be measured. They also clearly communicate the patient's level of functioning to all members of the rehabilitation team. Rehabilitation staff members use these tools to provide an initial assessment of the patient's abilities and to monitor the patient's progress in achieving independence.

One of the most frequently used tools to assess the patient's level of independence is the Functional Independence Measure (FIM™). The FIM™ is a minimum data set, measuring 18 items. The self-care items measured are eating, bathing, grooming, dressing upper body, dressing lower body, toileting, bladder management, and bowel management. The FIM™ addresses transfers and the ability to ambulate and climb stairs and also includes communication and social cognition items. A WeeFIM instrument is used for children. For both children and adults, scoring is based on a seven-point scale, with items used to assess the patient's level of independence.

Other tools used to assess the patient's functional ability include the following:

- The PULSES profile is used to assess physical condition (eg, health/illness status), upper extremity functions (eg, eating, bathing), lower extremity functions (eg, transfer, ambulation), sensory function (eg, vision, hearing, speech), bowel and bladder function (ie, control of bowel or bladder), and situational factors (eg, social and financial support). Each of these areas is rated on a scale from one (independent) to four (greatest dependency).
- The Barthel Index is used to measure the patient's level of independence in ADLs (feeding, bathing, dressing, grooming), continence, toileting, transfers, and ambulation (or wheelchair mobility). This scale does not address communicative or cognitive abilities.
- The Patient Evaluation Conference System (PECS) contains 15 categories. This comprehensive assessment scale includes such areas as medications, pain, nutrition, use of assistive devices, psychological status, vocation, and recreation.

In addition to the detailed functional assessment, the nurse assesses the patient's physical, mental, emotional, spiritual, social, and economic status. Secondary problems related to the patient's disability, such as muscle atrophy and deconditioning, are assessed, as are residual strengths unaffected by disease or disability. Other areas that require nursing assessment include potential for altered skin integrity, altered bowel and bladder control, and sexual dysfunction. Many other assessment tools are designed to evaluate function in people with specific disabling conditions.

Nursing Process

The Patient With Self-Care Deficits in Activities of Daily Living

ADLs are those self-care activities that the patient must accomplish each day to meet personal needs. ADLs include personal hygiene/bathing, dressing/grooming, feeding, and toileting. Many patients cannot perform such activities easily. An ADL program is started as soon as the rehabilitation process begins, because the ability to perform ADLs is frequently the key to independence, return to the home, and reentry into the community.

Assessment

The nurse must observe and assess the patient's ability to perform ADLs to determine the level of independence in self-care and the need for nursing intervention. The activity of bathing requires obtaining bath water and items used for bathing (eg, soap, washcloth), washing, and drying the body after bathing. Dressing requires getting clothes from the closet, putting on and taking off clothing, and fastening the clothing. Self-feeding requires using utensils to bring food to the mouth, and chewing and swallowing the food. The activity of toileting includes removing clothing to use the toilet, cleansing oneself, and readjusting clothing. Grooming activities include combing hair, brushing one's teeth, shaving or applying makeup, and handwashing. Patients who can sit up and raise their hands to their head can begin self-care activities. Assistive devices are often essential in achieving some level of independence in ADL.

In addition, the nurse should be aware of the patient's medical conditions or other health problems, the effect that they have on the ability to perform ADLs, and the family's involvement in the patient's ADLs. This information is valuable in setting goals and developing the plan of care to maximize self-care.

Nursing Diagnosis

Based on the assessment data, major nursing diagnoses may include the following:

- Self-care deficit: bathing/hygiene, dressing/grooming, feeding, toileting

Planning and Goals

The major goals include bathing/hygiene independently or with assistance, using adaptive or assistive devices as appropriate; dressing/grooming independently or with assistance, using adaptive or assistive devices as appropriate; feeding independently or with assistance, using adaptive or assistive devices as appropriate; and toileting independently or with assistance, using adaptive or assistive devices as appropriate. Another goal is patient expression of satisfaction with the extent of independence in self-care activities.

Nursing Interventions

Fostering Self-Care Abilities

To learn methods of self-care effectively, the patient must be motivated. An "I'd rather do it myself" attitude is encouraged. The nurse must also help the patient identify the safe limits of independent activity; knowing when to ask for assistance is particularly important.

The nurse teaches, guides, and supports the patient who is learning or relearning how to perform self-care activities. Consistency in instructions and assistance given by health care providers facilitates the learning process. Recording the patient's performance provides data for evaluating progress and may be used as a source for motivation and morale building. Guidelines for teaching about ADLs are given in Chart 11-3.

Often, a simple maneuver requires concentration and the exertion of considerable effort on the part of the patient with a disability; therefore, self-care techniques need to be adapted to accommodate the lifestyle of individual patients. There is usually more than one way to accomplish a self-care activity, and common sense and a little ingenuity may promote increased independence. For example, a person who cannot quite reach his or her head may be able to do so by leaning forward. Encouraging the patient to participate in a support group may also help the patient discover creative solutions to self-care problems.

Recommending Assistive and Adaptive Devices

If the patient has difficulty performing an ADL, an adaptive or assistive device (self-help device) may be useful. A large variety of adaptive devices are available commercially or can be constructed by the nurse, occupational therapist, patient, or family. The nurse

CHART 11-3

Teaching About Activities of Daily Living

1. Define the goal of the activity with the patient. Be realistic. Set short-term goals that can be accomplished in the near future.
2. Identify several approaches to accomplish the task (eg, there are several ways to put on a given garment).
3. Select the approach most likely to succeed.
4. Specify the approach on the patient's plan of care and the patient's level of accomplishment on the progress notes.
5. Identify the motions necessary to accomplish the activity (eg, to pick up a glass, extend arm with hand open; place open hand next to glass; flex fingers around glass; move arm and hand holding glass vertically; flex arm toward body).
6. Focus on gross functional movements initially, and gradually include activities that use finer motions (eg, buttoning clothes, eating with a fork).
7. Encourage the patient to perform the activity up to maximal capacity within the limitations of the disability.
8. Monitor the patient's tolerance.
9. Minimize frustration and fatigue.
10. Support the patient by giving appropriate praise for effort put forth and for acts accomplished.
11. Assist the patient to perform and practice the activity in real-life situations and in a safe environment.

should be alert to "gadgets" coming on the market and evaluate their potential usefulness. The nurse must exercise professional judgment and caution in recommending devices, because in the past, unscrupulous vendors have marketed unnecessary, overly expensive, or useless items to patients.

A wide selection of computerized devices is available, or devices can be designed to help individual patients with severe disabilities to function more independently. The ABLEDATA project (see Resources list at the end of this chapter) offers a computerized listing of commercially available aids and equipment for patients with disabilities.

Helping Patients Accept Limitations

If the patient has a severe disability, independent self-care may be an unrealistic goal; in this situation, the nurse teaches the patient how to direct his or her own care. The patient may require a personal attendant to perform ADLs. Family members may not be appropriate for providing bathing/hygiene, dressing/grooming, feeding, and toileting assistance, and spouses may have difficulty providing bowel and bladder care for patients and maintaining the role of sexual partners. If a personal caregiver is necessary, the patient and family members must learn how to manage an employee effectively. The nurse helps the patient accept self-care dependency. Independence in other areas, such as social interaction, should be emphasized to promote positive self-concept.

Evaluation

Expected Patient Outcomes

Expected patient outcomes may include:

1. Demonstrates independent self-care in bathing/hygiene or with assistance, using adaptive devices as appropriate
    a. Bathes self at maximal level of independence
    b. Uses adaptive devices effectively
    c. Reports satisfaction with level of independence in bathing/hygiene
2. Demonstrates independent self-care in dressing/grooming or with assistance, using adaptive devices as appropriate
    a. Dresses/grooms self at maximal level of independence
    b. Uses adaptive devices effectively
    c. Reports satisfaction with level of independence in dressing/grooming
    d. Demonstrates increased interest in appearance
3. Demonstrates independent self-care in feeding or with assistance, using adaptive and assistive devices as appropriate
    a. Feeds self at maximal level of independence
    b. Uses adaptive and assistive devices effectively
    c. Demonstrates increased interest in eating
    d. Maintains adequate nutritional intake
4. Demonstrates independent self-care in toileting or with assistance, using adaptive and assistive devices as appropriate
    a. Toilets self at maximal level of independence
    b. Uses adaptive and assistive devices effectively
    c. Indicates positive feelings regarding level of toileting independence
    d. Experiences adequate frequency of bowel and bladder elimination
    e. Does not experience incontinence, constipation, urinary tract infection, or other complications

Nursing Process

The Patient With Impaired Physical Mobility

Problems commonly associated with immobility include weakened muscles, joint contracture, and deformity. Each joint of the body has a normal range of motion; if the range is limited, the functions of the joint and of the muscles that move the joint are impaired, and painful deformities may develop. The nurse must identify patients at risk for such complications. The nurse needs to assess, plan, and intervene to prevent complications of immobility.

Another problem frequently seen in rehabilitation nursing is an altered ambulatory/mobility pattern. Patients with disabilities may be either temporarily or permanently unable to walk independently and unaided. The nurse assesses the mobility of the patient and designs care that promotes independent mobility within the prescribed therapeutic limits.

If a person cannot exercise and move his or her joints through their full range of motion, contractures may develop. A contracture is a shortening of the muscle and tendon that leads to deformity and limits joint mobility. When the contracted joint is moved, the patient experiences pain; in addition, more energy is required to move when joints are contracted.

Assessment

At times, mobility is restricted because of pain, paralysis, loss of muscle strength, systemic disease, an immobilizing device (eg, cast, brace), or prescribed limits to promote healing. Assessment of mobility includes positioning, ability to move, muscle strength and tone, joint function, and the prescribed mobility limits. The nurse may need to collaborate with physical therapists or other team members to assess mobility.

During position change, transfer, and ambulation activities, the nurse assesses the patient's abilities, the extent of disability, and residual capacity for physiologic adaptation. The nurse observes for orthostatic hypotension, pallor, diaphoresis, nausea, tachycardia, and fatigue.

In addition, the nurse assesses the patient's ability to use various assistive devices that promote mobility. If the patient cannot ambulate without assistance, the nurse assesses the patient's ability to balance, transfer, and use assistive devices (eg, crutches, walker). Crutch walking requires high energy expenditure and produces considerable cardiovascular stress; therefore, people with reduced exercise capacity, decreased arm strength, and problems with balance because of aging or multiple diseases may be unable to use them. A walker is more stable and may be a better choice for such patients. If the patient uses an orthosis (an external appliance that provides support, prevents or corrects joint deformities, and improves function), the nurse monitors the patient for effective use and potential problems associated with its use.

Nursing Diagnosis

Based on the assessment data, major nursing diagnoses may include the following:

- Impaired physical mobility
- Activity intolerance
- Risk for injury
- Risk for disuse syndrome
- Impaired walking
- Impaired wheelchair mobility
- Impaired bed mobility

Planning and Goals

The major goals may include absence of contracture and deformity, maintenance of muscle strength and joint mobility, independent mobility, increased activity tolerance, and prevention of further disability.

Nursing Interventions

Positioning to Prevent Musculoskeletal Complications

Deformities and contractures can often be prevented by proper positioning. Maintaining correct body alignment when the patient is in bed is essential regardless of the position selected. During each patient contact, the nurse evaluates the patient's position and assists the patient to achieve and maintain proper positioning and alignment. The most common positions that patients assume in bed are supine (dorsal), side-lying (lateral), and prone. The nurse helps the patient assume these positions and uses pillows to support the body in correct alignment (Chart 11-4). At times, a splint (eg, wrist or hand splint) may be made by the occupational therapist to support a joint and prevent deformity. The nurse must ensure proper use of the splint and provide skin care.

PREVENTING EXTERNAL ROTATION OF THE HIP

The patient who is in bed for an extended period of time may develop external rotation deformity of the hip because the ball-and-socket joint of the hip tends to rotate outward when the patient lies on his or her back. A trochanter roll extending from the crest of the ilium to the midthigh prevents this deformity; with correct placement, it serves as a mechanical wedge under the projection of the greater trochanter.

PREVENTING FOOTDROP

Footdrop is a deformity in which the foot is plantarflexed (the ankle bends in the direction of the sole of the foot). If the condition continues without correction, the patient will not be able to hold the foot in a normal position and will be able to walk only on his or her toes, without touching the ground with the heel of the foot. The deformity is caused by contracture of both the gastrocnemius and soleus muscles. Damage to the peroneal nerve or loss of flexibility of the Achilles tendon may also result in footdrop.

NURSING ALERT

Prolonged bed rest, lack of exercise, incorrect positioning in bed, and the weight of bedding that forces the toes into plantar flexion contribute to footdrop.

To prevent this disabling deformity, the patient is positioned to sit at 90 degrees in a wheelchair with his or her feet on the footrests or flat on the floor. When the patient is supine in bed, padded splints or protective boots are used to keep the patient's feet at right angles to the legs. Frequent skin inspection of the feet must also be performed to determine whether positioning devices have created any unwanted pressure areas.

The patient is encouraged to perform the following ankle exercises several times each hour: dorsiflexion and plantar flexion of the feet, flexion and extension (curl and stretch) of the toes, and eversion and inversion of the feet at the ankles. The nurse provides frequent passive range-of-motion exercises if the patient cannot perform active exercises.

Maintaining Muscle Strength and Joint Mobility

Optimal function depends on the strength of the muscles and joint motion, and active participation in ADLs promotes maintenance of muscle strength and joint mobility. Range-of-motion exercises and specific therapeutic exercises may be included in the nursing plan of care.

PERFORMING RANGE-OF-MOTION EXERCISES

Range of motion involves moving a joint through its full range in all appropriate planes (Chart 11-5). To maintain or increase the motion of a joint, range-of-motion exercises are initiated as soon as the patient's

CHART 11-4

Positioning a Patient in Bed

Supine (Dorsal) Position

1. Align the head with the spine, both laterally and anteroposteriorly.
2. Position the trunk to minimize hip flexion.
3. Flex the arms at the elbow and rest the hands against the abdomen.
4. Extend the legs with a small, firm support under the popliteal area.
5. Support the heels off the mattress with a small pillow or towel roll at the ankles.
6. Point the toes straight up using protective boots to prevent footdrop.
7. Place trochanter rolls under the greater trochanters to prevent external rotation of the hip.

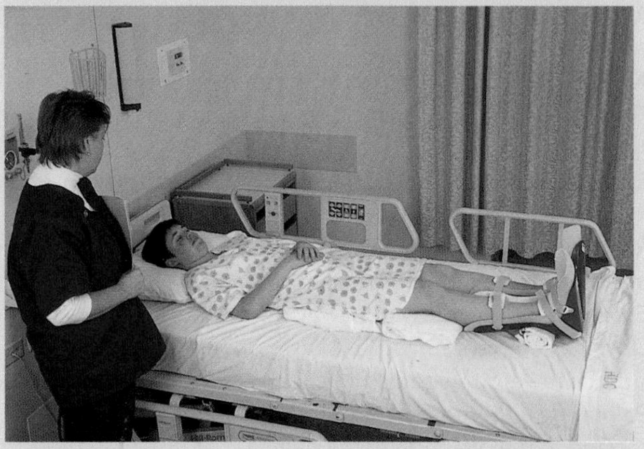

Side-Lying (Lateral Position)

1. Align the head with the spine, and support it with a pillow.
2. Properly align the body; avoid twisting at the shoulders, waist, or hips.
3. Flex shoulders and elbows and support the upper arm with a pillow.
4. Position the uppermost hip joint slightly forward and support the leg in a position of slight abduction by a pillow.
5. Place and support the feet in neutral dorsiflexion.
6. Support the back with a pillow.

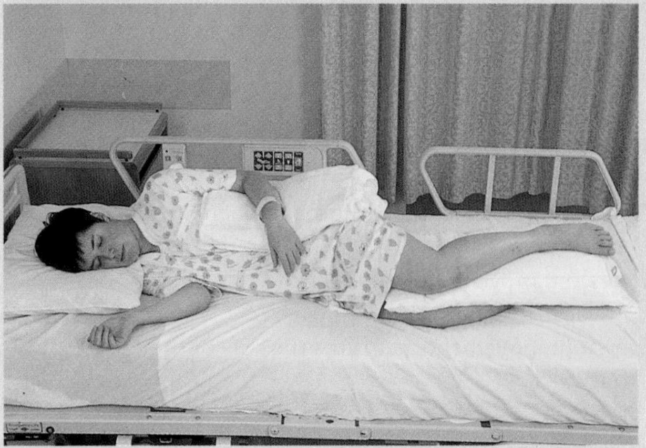

Prone (on Abdomen) Position

1. Turn the head laterally and align it with the rest of the body.
2. Abduct and externally rotate the arms at the shoulder joint; flex the elbows.
3. Place a small, flat support under the pelvis, extending from the level of the umbilicus to the upper third of the thigh.
4. Maintain the lower extremities in a neutral position.
5. Suspend the toes over the edge of the mattress.

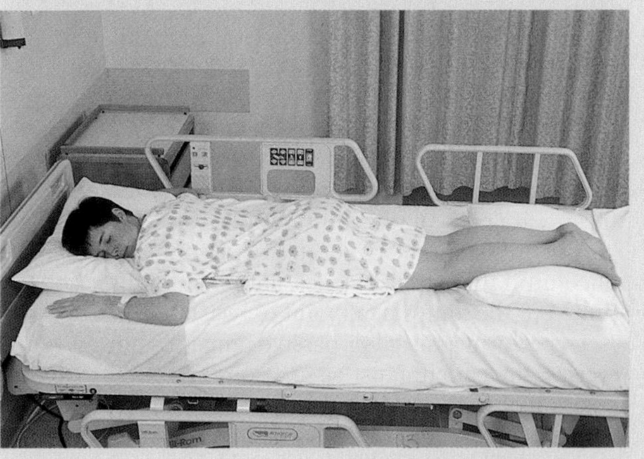

Note: Side rails of bed are down for photographic purposes; they should remain raised if the patient is at risk for falling.

condition permits. The exercises are planned for individual patients to accommodate the wide variation in the degrees of motion that people of varying body builds and age groups can attain (Chart 11-6).

Range-of-motion exercises may be active (performed by the patient under the supervision of the nurse), assisted (with the nurse helping if the patient cannot do the exercise independently), or passive (performed by the nurse). Unless otherwise prescribed, a joint should be moved through its range of motion three times, at least twice a day. The joint to be exercised is supported, the bones above the joint are stabilized, and the body part distal to the joint is moved through the range of motion of the joint. For

CHART 11-5

Range-of-Motion Terminology

Abduction: movement away from the midline of the body
Adduction: movement toward the midline of the body
Flexion: bending of a joint so that the angle of the joint diminishes
Extension: the return movement from flexion; the joint angle is increased
Rotation: turning or movement of a part around its axis
Internal: turning inward, toward the center
External: turning outward, away from the center
Dorsiflexion: movement that flexes or bends the hand back toward the body or the foot toward the leg
Palmar flexion: movement that flexes or bends the hand in the direction of the palm
Plantar flexion: movement that flexes or bends the foot in the direction of the sole
Pronation: rotation of the forearm so that the palm of the hand is down
Supination: rotation of the forearm so that the palm of the hand is up
Opposition: touching the thumb to each fingertip on same hand
Inversion: movement that turns the sole of the foot inward
Eversion: movement that turns the sole of the foot outward

example, the humerus must be stabilized while the radius and ulna are moved through their range of motion at the elbow joint.

A joint should not be moved beyond its free range of motion; the joint is moved to the point of resistance and stopped at the point of pain. If muscle spasms are present, the joint is moved slowly to the point of resistance. Gentle, steady pressure is then applied until the muscle relaxes, and the motion is continued to the joint's final point of resistance.

To perform assisted or passive range-of-motion exercises, the patient must be in a comfortable supine position with the arms at the sides and the knees extended. Good body posture is maintained during the exercises. The nurse also uses good body mechanics during the exercise session.

PERFORMING THERAPEUTIC EXERCISES

Therapeutic exercises are prescribed by the physician and performed with the assistance and guidance of the physical therapist or nurse. The patient should have a clear understanding of the goal of the prescribed exercise. Written instructions about the frequency, duration, and number of repetitions, as well as simple line drawings of the exercise, help ensure adherence to the exercise program. Return demonstration of the exercises also helps the patient and family to follow the instructions correctly.

When performed correctly, exercise assists in maintaining and building muscle strength, maintaining joint function, preventing deformity, stimulating circulation, developing endurance, and promoting relaxation. Exercise is also valuable in helping restore motivation and the well-being of the patient. Weight-bearing exercises may slow the bone loss that occurs with disability. There are five types of exercise: passive, active-assistive, active, resistive, and isometric. The description, purpose, and action of each of these exercises are summarized in Table 11-1.

Promoting Independent Mobility

When the patient's condition stabilizes and his or her physical condition permits, the patient is assisted to sit up on the side of the bed and then to stand. Tolerance of this activity is assessed. Orthostatic (postural) hypotension may develop when the patient assumes a vertical position. Because of inadequate vasomotor reflexes, blood pools in the splanchnic (visceral) area and in the legs, resulting in inadequate cerebral circulation. If indicators of orthostatic hypotension (eg, drop in blood pressure, pallor, diaphoresis, nausea, tachycardia, dizziness) are present, the activity is stopped, and the patient is assisted to a supine position in bed.

Some disabilities, such as spinal cord injury, acute brain injury, and other conditions that require extended periods in the recumbent position, prevent the patient from assuming an upright position at the bedside. Several strategies can be used to help the patient assume a 90-degree sitting position. A reclining wheelchair with elevating leg rests allows a slow and controlled progression from a supine position to a 90-degree sitting position. A tilt table (a board that can be tilted in 5- to 10-degree increments from a horizontal to a vertical position) may also be used. The tilt table promotes vasomotor adjustment to positional changes and helps patients with limited standing balance and limited weight-bearing activities avoid the decalcification of bones and low bone mass associated with disuse syndrome and lack of weight-bearing exercise. Physical therapists may use a tilt table for patients who have not been upright due to illness or disability. Gradual elevation of the head of the bed may help. When getting patients with spinal cord injury out of bed, it is important to gradually raise the head of the bed to a 90-degree angle; this may take approximately 10 to 15 minutes.

Elastic compression stockings are used to prevent venous stasis. For some patients, a compression garment (leotard) or snug-fitting abdominal binder and elastic compression bandaging of the legs are needed to prevent venous stasis and orthostatic hypotension. When the patient is standing, the feet are protected with a pair of properly fitted shoes. Extended periods of standing are avoided because of venous pooling

CHART 11-6

Performing Range-of-Motion Exercises

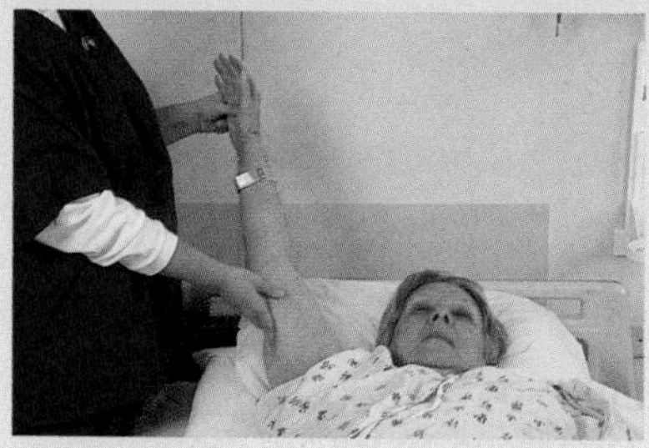

Abduction of shoulder. Move arm from side of body to above the head, then return arm to side of body or neutral position (adduction).

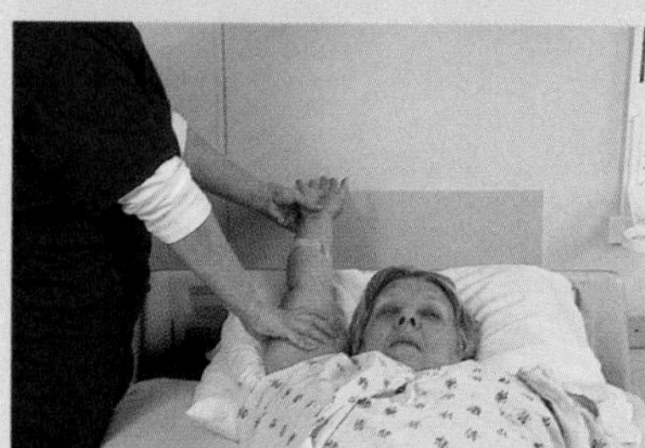

Forward flexion of shoulder. Move arm forward and upward until it is alongside of head.

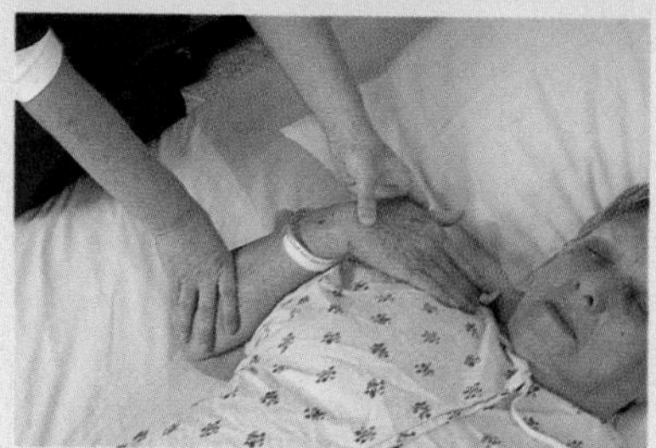

Flexion of elbow. Bend elbow, bringing forearm and hand toward shoulder, then return forearm and hand to neutral position (arm straight).

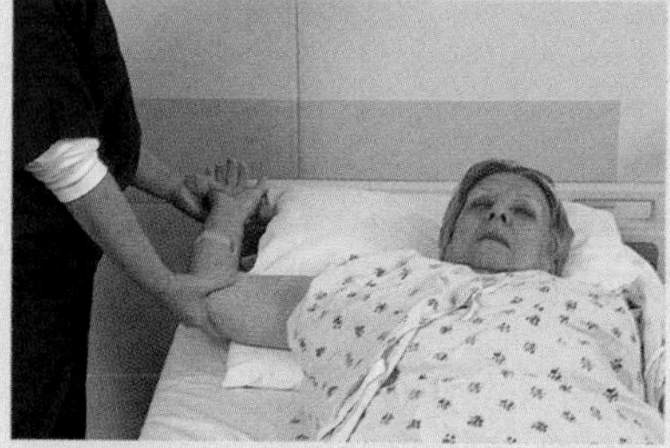

Internal rotation of shoulder. With arm at shoulder height, elbow bent at a 90-degree angle, and palm toward feet, turn upper arm until palm and forearm point backward.

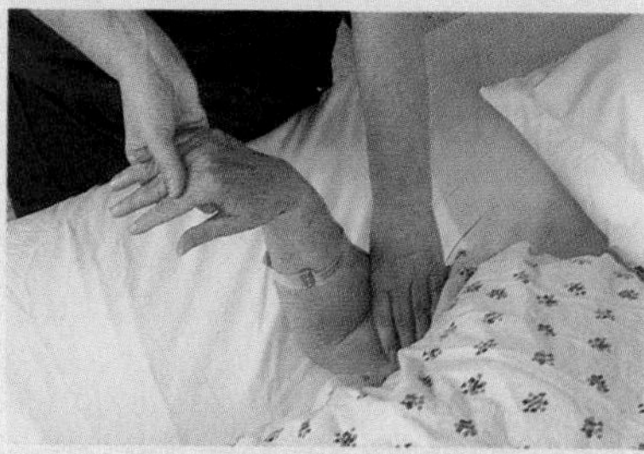

Pronation of forearm. With elbow at waist and bent at a 90-degree angle, turn hand so that palm is facing down.

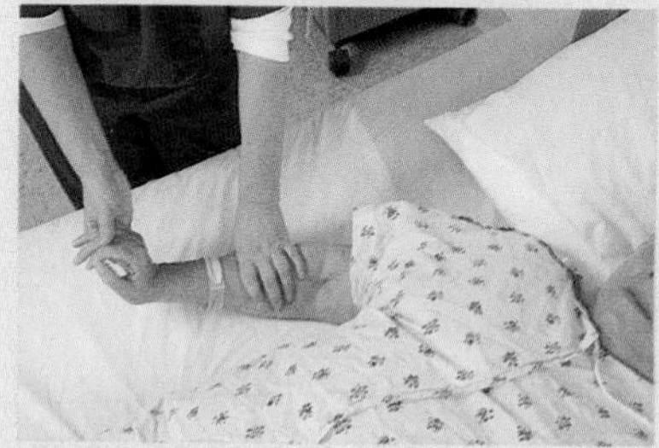

Wrist extension.

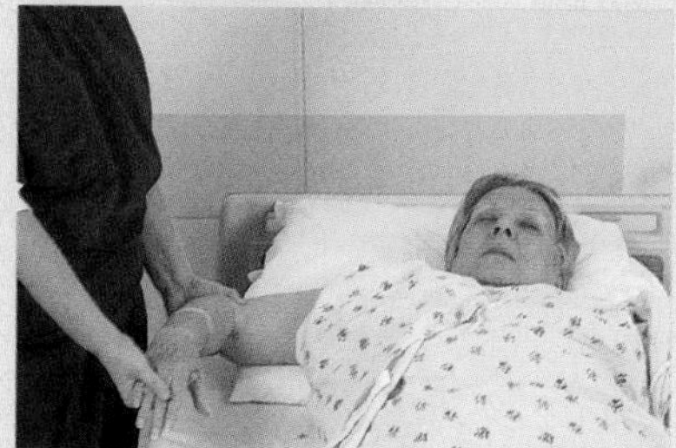

External rotation of shoulder. With arm at shoulder height, elbow bent at a 90-degree angle, and palm toward feet, turn upper arm until the palm and forearm point forward.

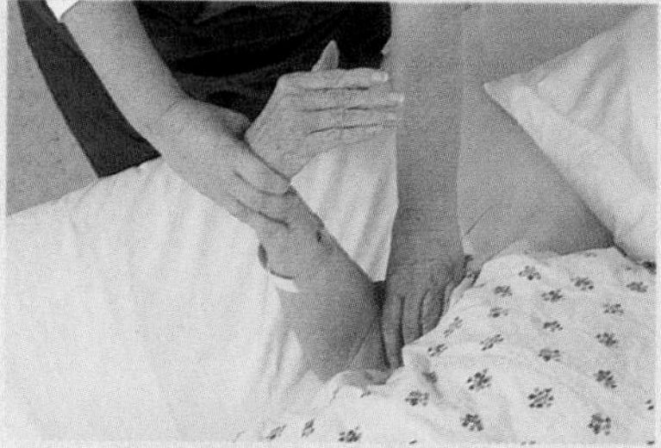

Supination of forearm. With elbow at waist and arm bent at a 90-degree angle, turn hand so that palm is facing up.

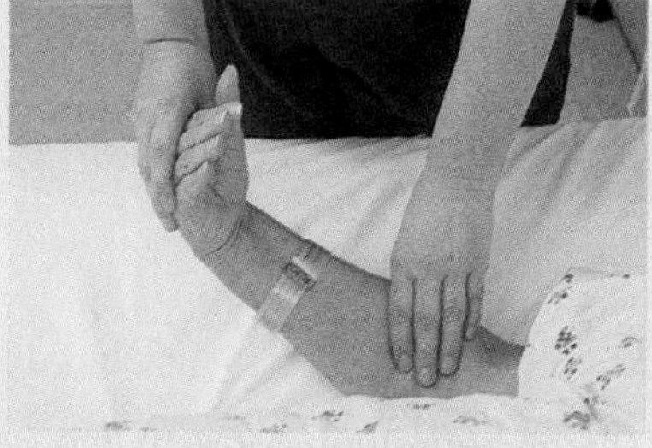

Flexion of wrist. Bend wrist so that palm is toward forearm. Straighten to a neutral position.

continued >

CHART 11-6 Performing Range-of-Motion Exercises, continued

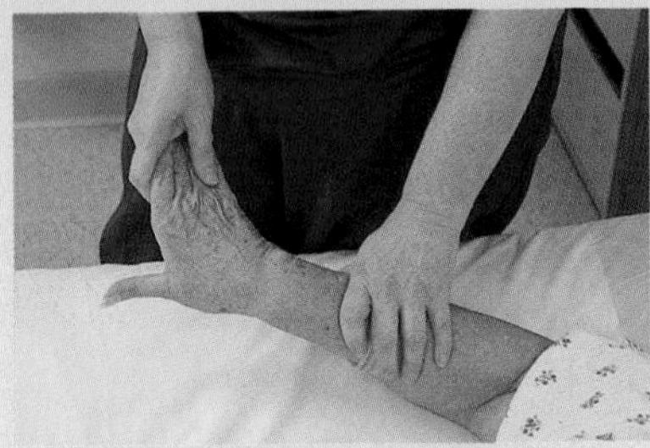

Ulnar deviation. Move hand sideways so that the side of hand on which the little finger is located moves toward forearm.

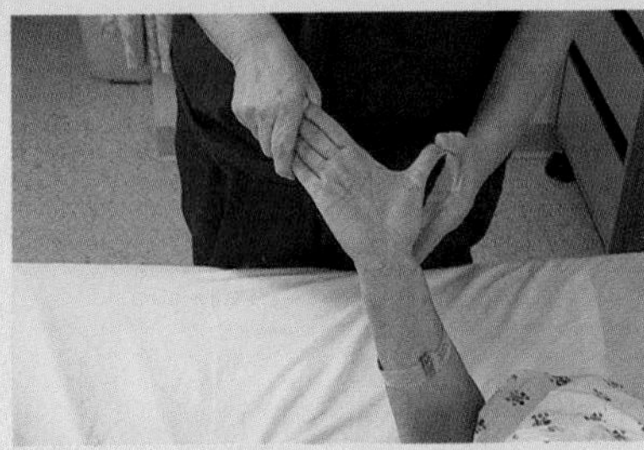

Extension of fingers.

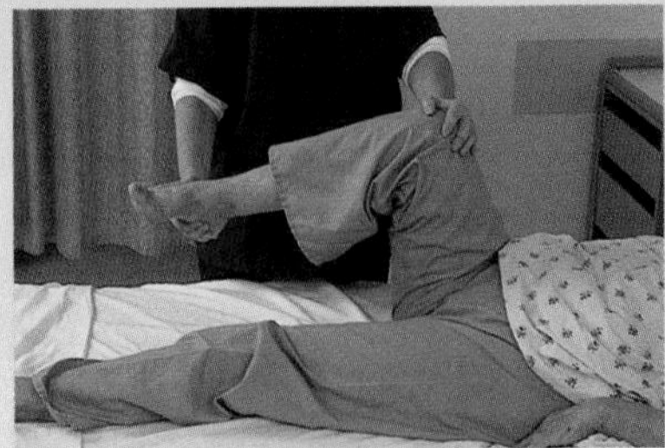

Internal-external rotation of hip. Turn leg in an inward motion so that toes point in. Turn leg in an outward motion so that toes point out.

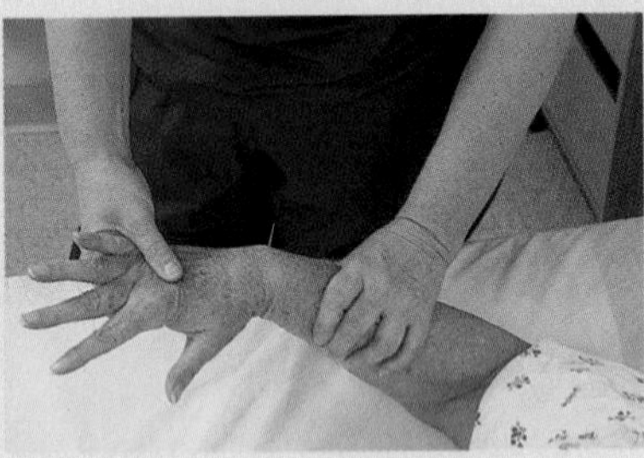

Radial deviation. Move hand sideways so that side of hand on which thumb is located moves toward forearm.

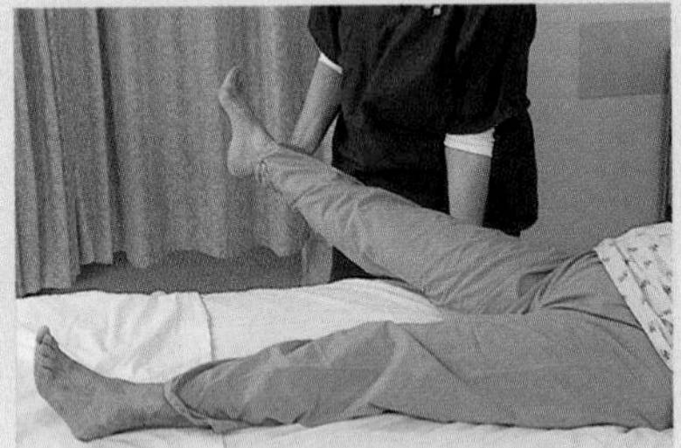

To perform abduction-adduction of hip, move leg outward from the body as far as possible, as shown. Return leg from abducted position to neutral position and across the other leg as far as possible.

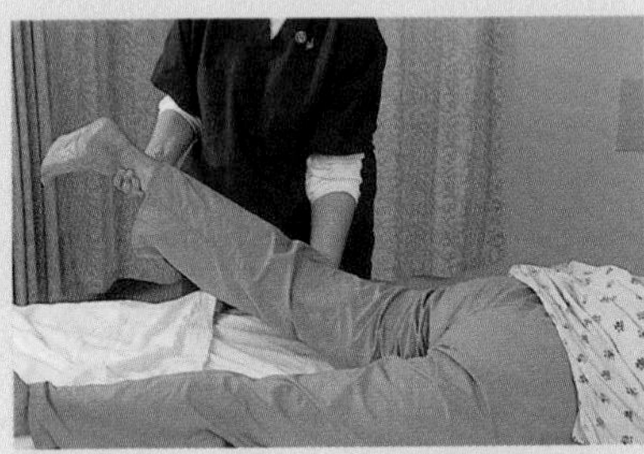

Hyperextension of hip. Place the patient in a prone position, and move leg backward from the body as far as possible.

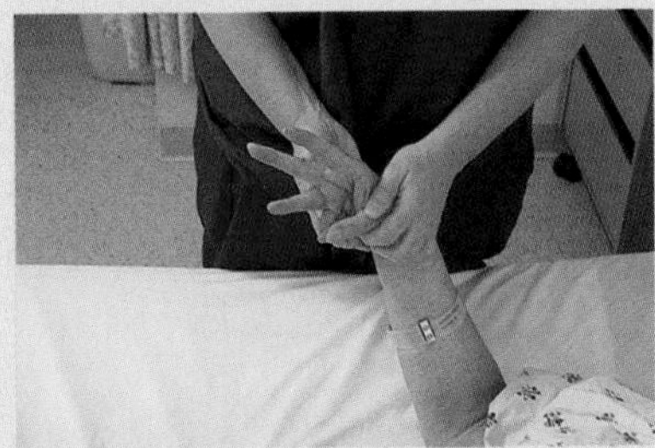

Thumb opposition. Move thumb out and around to touch little finger.

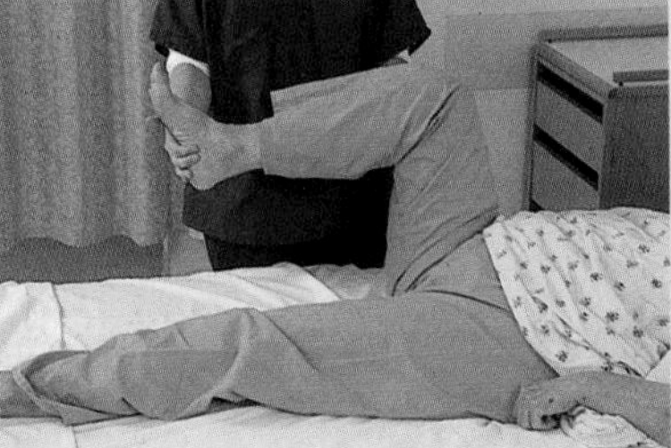

Flexion of the hip and the knee. Bend hip by moving the leg forward as far as possible. Return leg from the flexed position to the neutral position.

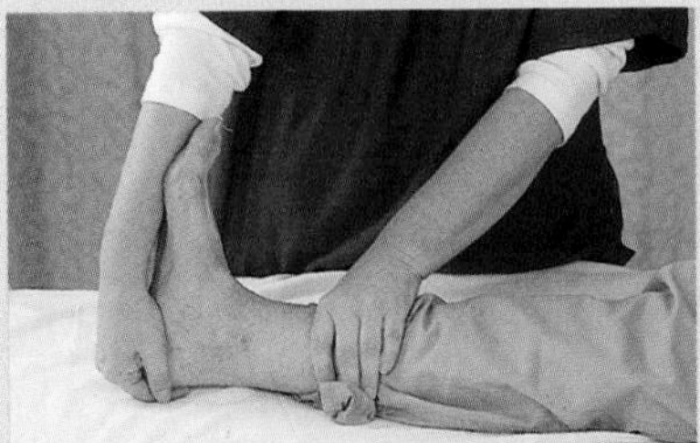

Dorsiflexion of foot. Move foot up and toward the leg. Then move the foot down and away from the leg (plantar flexion).

CHART 11-6 Performing Range-of-Motion Exercises, continued

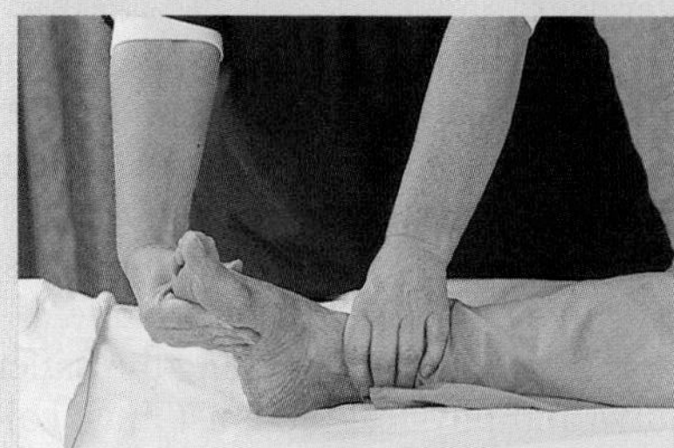

Inversion and eversion of foot. Move foot so that sole is facing outward (eversion). Then move foot so that sole is facing inward (inversion).

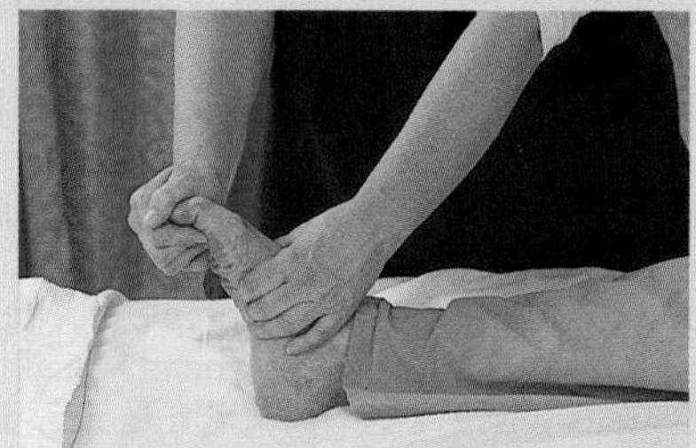

Flexion of toes. Bend the toes toward the ball of foot.

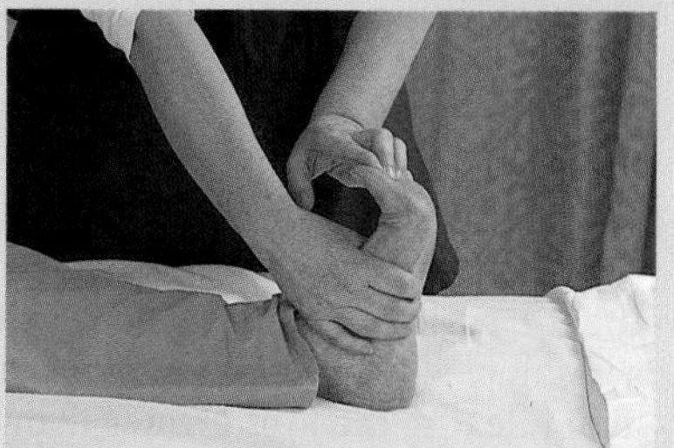

Extension of toes. Straighten toes and pull them toward the leg as far as possible.

and pressure on the soles of the feet. The nurse monitors the patient's blood pressure and pulse and observes for signs and symptoms of orthostatic hypotension and cerebral insufficiency (eg, the patient reports feeling faint and weak), which suggest intolerance of the upright position. If the patient does not tolerate the upright position, the nurse should return the patient to the reclining position and elevate his or her legs.

ASSISTING PATIENTS WITH TRANSFER

A transfer is movement of the patient from one place to another (eg, bed to chair, chair to commode, wheelchair to tub). As soon as the patient is permitted out

TABLE 11-1 Therapeutic Exercises

	Description	Purposes	Action
Passive	An exercise carried out by the therapist or the nurse without assistance from the patient	To retain as much joint range of motion as possible; to maintain circulation	Stabilize the proximal joint and support the distal part; move the joint smoothly, slowly, and gently through its full range of motion; avoid producing pain.
Active-assistive	An exercise carried out by the patient with the assistance of the therapist or the nurse	To encourage normal muscle function	Support the distal part, and encourage the patient to take the joint actively through its range of motion; give no more assistance than is necessary to accomplish the action; short periods of activity should be followed by adequate rest periods.
Active	An exercise accomplished by the patient without assistance; activities include turning from side to side and from back to abdomen and moving up and down in bed	To increase muscle strength	When possible, active exercise should be performed against gravity; the joint is moved through full range of motion without assistance; make sure that the patient does not substitute another joint movement for the one intended.
Resistive	An active exercise carried out by the patient working against resistance produced by either manual or mechanical means	To provide resistance to increase muscle power	The patient moves the joint through its range of motion while the therapist resists slightly at first and then with progressively increasing resistance; sandbags and weights can be used and are applied at the distal point of the involved joint; the movements should be performed smoothly.
Isometric or muscle setting	Alternately contracting and relaxing a muscle while keeping the part in a fixed position; this exercise is performed by the patient	To maintain strength when a joint is immobilized	Contract or tighten the muscle as much as possible without moving the joint, hold for several seconds, then let go and relax; breathe deeply.

of bed, transfer activities are started. The nurse assesses the patient's ability to participate actively in the transfer and determines, in conjunction with occupational therapists or physical therapists, the adaptive equipment required to promote independence and safety. A lightweight wheelchair with brake extensions, removable and detachable arm rests, and leg rests minimizes structural obstacles during the transfer. Tub seats or benches make transfers in and out of the tub easier and safer. Raised, padded commode seats may also be warranted for patients who must avoid flexing the hips greater than 90 degrees when transferring to a toilet. It is important that the nurse teach the patient hip precautions (ie, no adduction past the midline, no flexion greater than 90 degrees, and no internal rotation); abduction pillows can be used to keep the hip in correct alignment if precautions are warranted.

It is important that the patient maintain muscle strength and, if possible, perform push-up exercises to strengthen the arm and shoulder extensor muscles. The push-up exercise requires the patient to sit upright in bed; a book is placed under each of the patient's hands to provide a hard surface, and the patient is instructed to push down on the book, raising the body. The nurse should encourage the patient to raise and move the body in different directions by means of these push-up exercises.

The nurse or physical therapist teaches the patient how to transfer. There are several methods of transferring from the bed to the wheelchair when the patient cannot stand, and the technique chosen should take into account the patient's abilities and disabilities. It is helpful for the nurse to demonstrate the technique. If the physical therapist is involved in teaching the patient to transfer, the nurse and physical therapist must collaborate so that consistent instructions are given to the patient. During transfer, the nurse assists and coaches the patient. Figure 11-1 shows weight-bearing and non–weight-bearing transfer.

If the patient's muscles are not strong enough to overcome the resistance of body weight, a polished lightweight board (transfer board, sliding board) may be used to bridge the gap between the bed and the chair. The patient slides across on the board with or without assistance from a caregiver. This board may also be used to transfer the patient from the chair to the toilet or bathtub bench. It is important to avoid

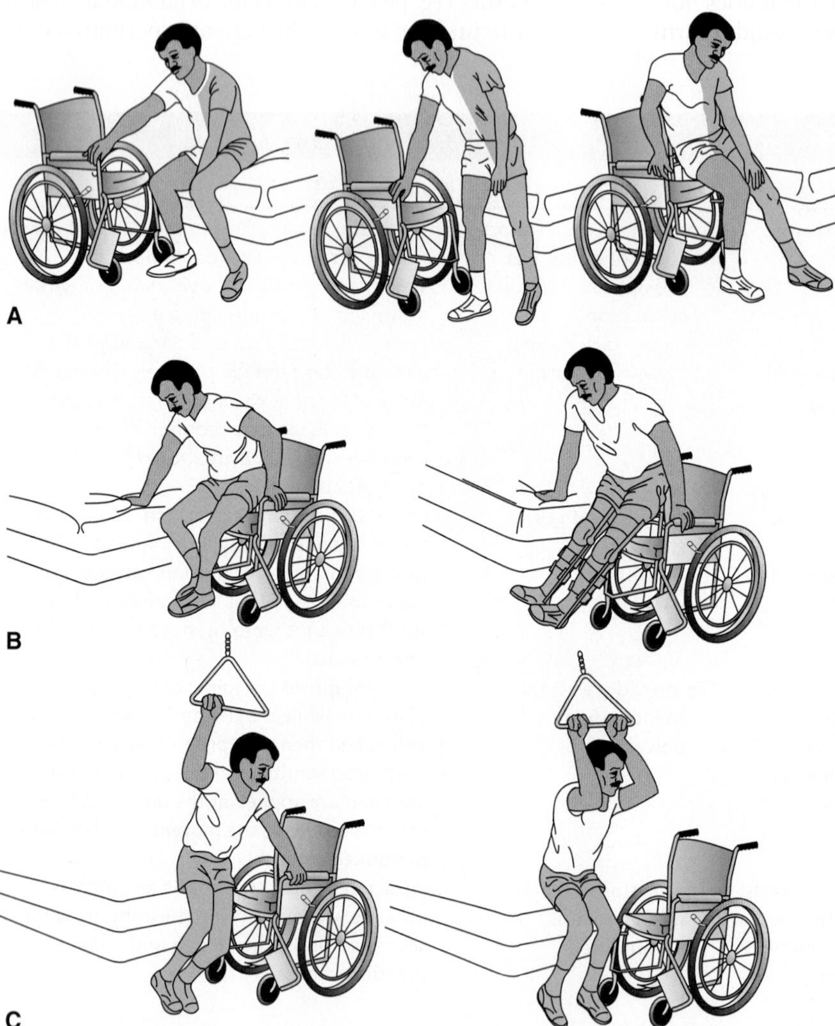

FIGURE 11-1. Methods of patient transfer from the bed to a wheelchair. The wheelchair is in a locked position. Colored areas indicate non–weight-bearing body parts. (**A**) Weight-bearing transfer from bed to chair. The patient stands up, pivots until his back is opposite the new seat, and sits down. (**B**) (*Left*) Non–weight-bearing transfer from chair to bed. (*Right*) With legs braced. (**C**) (*Left*) Non–weight-bearing transfer, combined method. (*Right*) Non–weight-bearing transfer, pull-up method. One of the wheelchair arms is removed to make getting in and out of the chair easier.

the effects of shear on the patient's skin while sliding across the board. The nurse should make sure that the patient's fingers do not curl around the edge of the board during the transfer, because the patient's body weight can crush his or her fingers as he or she moves across the board. Safety is a primary concern during a transfer, and the following guidelines are recommended:

- Wheelchairs and beds must be locked before transfer begins.
- Detachable arm and foot rests are removed to make getting in and out of the chair easier.
- One end of the transfer board is placed under the buttocks and the other end on the surface to which the transfer is being made (eg, the chair).
- The patient is instructed to lean forward, push up with his or her hands, and then slide across the board to the other surface.

Nurses frequently assist weak and incapacitated patients out of bed. The nurse supports and gently assists the patient during position changes, protecting the patient from injury. The nurse avoids pulling on a weak or paralyzed upper extremity to prevent dislocation of the shoulder. The patient is assisted to move toward the stronger side (Chart 11-7).

In the home setting, getting in and out of bed and performing chair, toilet, and tub transfers are difficult for patients with weak muscles and loss of hip, knee, and ankle motion. A rope attached to the headboard of the bed enables the patient to pull himself or herself toward the center of the bed, and the use of a rope attached to the footboard facilitates getting in and out of bed. The height of a chair can be raised with cushions on the seat or with hollowed-out blocks placed under the chair legs. Grab bars can be attached to the wall near the toilet and tub to provide leverage and stability.

PREPARING FOR AMBULATION

Regaining the ability to walk is a prime morale builder. However, to be prepared for ambulation—whether with brace, walker, cane, or crutches—the patient must strengthen the muscles required. Therefore, exercise is the foundation of preparation. The nurse and physical therapist instruct and supervise the patient in these exercises.

For ambulation, the quadriceps muscles, which stabilize the knee joint, and the gluteal muscles are strengthened. To perform quadriceps-setting exercises, the patient contracts the quadriceps muscle by attempting to push the popliteal area against the mattress and at the same time raising the heel. The patient maintains the muscle contraction for a count of five and relaxes for a count of five. The exercise is repeated 10 to 15 times hourly. Exercising the quadriceps muscles prevents flexion contractures of the knee.

In gluteal setting, the patient contracts or "pinches" the buttocks together for a count of five, relaxes for a count of five; the exercise is repeated 10 to 15 times hourly. If assistive devices (ie, walker, cane, crutches) will be used, the muscles of the upper extremities are exercised and strengthened. Push-up exercises are especially useful. While in a sitting position, the patient raises the body by pushing the hands against the chair seat or mattress. The patient should be encouraged to do push-up exercises while in a prone position also.

CHART 11-7

Assisting the Patient Out of Bed

Technique for Moving the Patient to the Edge of the Bed

1. Move head and shoulders of patient toward the edge of the bed.
2. Move feet and legs to the edge of the bed. (The patient is now in a crescent position, which gives good range of motion to the lateral trunk muscles.)
3. Place both arms well under the patient's hips. Next, tighten (set) the muscles of your back and abdomen.
4. Straighten your back while moving the patient toward you.

Technique for Sitting Patient on the Edge of the Bed

1. Place arm and hand under the patient's shoulders.
2. Instruct the patient to push into the bed with the elbow while you lift the patient's shoulders with one arm and swing the legs over the edge of the bed with the other. (Gravity pulls the legs downward, which aids in raising the patient's trunk.)

Technique for Assisting Patient to Stand

1. Position the patient's feet so that they will be well grounded.
2. Face the patient while firmly grasping each side of the patient's rib cage with your hands.
3. Push your knee against one knee of the patient.
4. Rock the patient forward to a standing position. (Your knee is pushed against the patient's knee as he or she comes to the standing position.)
5. Ensure that the patient's knees are "locked" (in full extension) while standing. ("Locking" the patient's knees is a safety measure for those who are weak or have been in bed for some time.)
6. Give the patient enough time to establish balance.
7. Pivot the patient into a sitting position in the chair.

Pull-up exercises done on a trapeze while lifting the body are also effective for conditioning. The patient is taught to raise the arms above the head and then lower them in a slow, rhythmic manner while holding weights. Gradually, the weight is increased. The hands are strengthened by squeezing a rubber ball.

Typically, the physical therapist designs exercises to help the patient develop the sitting and standing balance, stability, and coordination needed for ambulation. After sitting and standing balance is achieved, the patient is able to use parallel bars. Under the supervision of the physical therapist, the patient practices shifting weight from side to side, lifting one leg while supporting weight on the other, and then walking between the parallel bars.

A patient who is ready to begin ambulation must be fitted with the appropriate assistive device, instructed about the prescribed weight-bearing limits (eg, non–weight-bearing, partial weight-bearing ambulation), and taught how to use the device safely. The nurse continually assesses the patient for stability and adherence to weight-bearing precautions and protects the patient from falling. The nurse provides contact guarding by holding on to a gait belt that the patient wears around the waist. The patient should wear sturdy, well-fitting shoes and be advised of the dangers of wet or highly polished floors and throw rugs. The patient should also learn how to ambulate on inclines, uneven surfaces, and stairs.

Ambulating With Crutches

A patient who is prescribed partial weight-bearing or non–weight-bearing ambulation may use crutches. The nurse or physical therapist should determine whether crutches are appropriate for the patient, because good balance, adequate cardiovascular reserve, strong upper extremities, and erect posture are essential for crutch walking. Ambulating a functional distance (at least the length of a room or house) or maneuvering stairs on crutches requires significant arm strength, because the arms must bear the patient's weight. Muscle groups important for crutch walking include the following:

- Shoulder depressors—to stabilize the upper extremity and prevent shoulder hiking
- Shoulder adductors—to hold the crutch top against the chest wall
- Arm flexors, extensors, and abductors (at the shoulder)—to move crutches forward, backward, and sideways
- Forearm extensors—to prevent flexion or buckling; important in raising the body for swinging gait
- Wrist extensors—to enable weight bearing on the hand-piece
- Finger and thumb flexors—to grasp the hand-piece

PREPARING PATIENTS TO WALK WITH CRUTCHES

Preparatory exercises are prescribed to strengthen the shoulder girdle and upper extremity muscles. Meanwhile, crutches need to be adjusted for the patient before he or she begins ambulating. To determine the approximate crutch length, the patient is measured standing or lying down. Standing patients are positioned against the wall with the feet slightly apart and away from the wall. Then a distance of 5 cm (2 inches) is marked on the floor, out to the side from the tip of the toe; 15 cm (6 inches) is measured straight ahead from the first mark, and this point is marked on the floor. Next, 5 cm (2 inches) is measured below the axilla to the second mark for the approximate crutch length.

If the patient must be measured while lying down, he or she is measured from the anterior fold of the axilla to the sole of the foot, and then 5 cm (2 inches) are added. If the patient's height is used, 40 cm (16 inches) is subtracted to obtain the approximate crutch length. The hand-piece should be adjusted to allow 20 to 30 degrees of flexion at the elbow. The wrist should be extended and the hand dorsiflexed. A foam rubber pad on the underarm piece is used to relieve the pressure of the crutch on the upper arm and thoracic cage. For safety, crutches should have large rubber tips, and the patient should wear firm-soled shoes that fit well.

TEACHING CRUTCH WALKING

The nurse or physical therapist explains and demonstrates to the patient how to use the crutches. The patient learns standing balance by standing on the unaffected leg by a chair. To help the patient maintain balance, the nurse holds the patient near the waist or uses a transfer belt.

The patient is taught to support his or her weight on the hand-pieces. (For patients who cannot support their weight through the wrist and hand because of arthritis or fracture, platform crutches that support the forearm and allow the weight to be borne through the elbow are available.) If weight is borne on the axilla, the pressure of the crutch can damage the brachial plexus nerves, producing "crutch paralysis."

For maximum stability, the patient first assumes the tripod position by placing the crutches about 20 to 25 cm (8 to 10 inches) in front and to the side of his or her toes (Fig. 11-2). (This base of support is adjusted according to the height of the patient; a tall person requires a broader base of support than does a short person.) In this position, the patient learns how to shift weight and maintain balance. Before teaching crutch walking, the nurse or therapist determines which gait is best for the patient. The more common gaits are the four-point, the three-point, the two-point, and the swinging-to and swinging-through gaits. The sequence of movements for each of these gaits is depicted in Chart 11-8.

The selection of crutch gait depends on the type and severity of the patient's disability and on the patient's physical condition, arm and trunk strength, and body balance. The patient should be taught two gaits so that he or she can change from one to another. Shifting crutch gaits relieves fatigue, because each gait requires the use of a different combination of muscles (if a muscle is forced to contract steadily

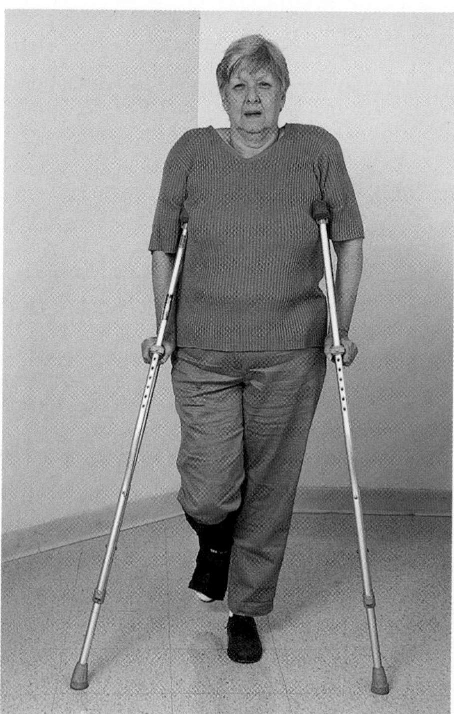

FIGURE 11-2. Crutch walking. The tripod position for basic crutch stance.

without relaxing, the circulation of the blood to that part is decreased). A faster gait can be used when walking an uninterrupted distance, and a slower gait can be used for short distances or in crowded places.

The nurse walks with the patient who is just learning how to ambulate with crutches, holding the patient at the waist as needed for balance. During this time, the nurse protects the patient from falls and continually assesses the patient's stability and stamina, because prolonged periods of bed rest and inactivity affect strength and endurance. Sweating and shortness of breath are indications that crutch-walking practice should be stopped and the patient permitted to rest.

TEACHING MANEUVERING TECHNIQUES

Before the patient is considered to be independent in crutch walking, he or she should learn to sit in a chair, stand from sitting, and go up and down stairs using the crutches.

To sit down:

1. Grasp the crutches at the hand-pieces for control.
2. Bend forward slightly while assuming a sitting position.
3. Place the affected leg forward to prevent weight bearing and flexion.

To stand up:

1. Move forward to the edge of the chair with the strong leg slightly under the seat.
2. Place both crutches in the hand on the side of the affected extremity.
3. Push down on the hand-piece while raising the body to a standing position.

To go down stairs:

1. Walk forward as far as possible on the step.
2. Advance crutches to the lower step. The weaker leg is advanced first and then the stronger one. In this way, the stronger extremity shares with the arms the work of raising and lowering the body weight.

To go up stairs:

1. Advance the stronger leg first up to the next step.
2. Advance the crutches and the weaker extremity. Note that the strong leg goes up first and comes down last. A memory device for patients is, "Up with the good, down with the bad."

Ambulating With a Walker

A walker provides more support and stability than a cane or crutches. There are two types of walkers: pick-up walkers and rolling walkers. A pick-up walker (one that has to be picked up and moved with each step forward) does not permit a natural walking pattern and is useful for patients who have poor balance or limited cardiovascular reserve or who cannot use crutches. A rolling walker allows automatic walking and is used by patients who cannot lift or who inappropriately carry a pick-up walker. The height of the walker is adjusted to the individual patient. The patient's arms should exhibit 20 to 30 degrees of flexion at the elbows when his or her hands are resting on the walker's hand grips. The patient should wear sturdy, well-fitting shoes. The nurse walks with the patient, holds him or her at the waist as needed for balance, continually assesses the patient's stability, and protects the patient from falls.

Patients are instructed to ambulate with a pick-up walker as follows:

1. Push off a chair or bed to come to a standing position. Never pull yourself up using the walker.
2. Hold the walker on the hand grips for stability.
3. Lift the walker, placing it in front of you while leaning your body slightly forward.
4. Walk into the walker, supporting your body weight on your hands when advancing your weaker leg, permitting partial weight bearing or non–weight bearing as prescribed.
5. Balance yourself on your feet.
6. Lift the walker, and place it in front of you again. Continue this pattern of walking.
7. Remember to look up as you walk.

Ambulating With a Cane

A cane helps the patient walk with greater balance and support and relieves the pressure on weight-bearing joints by redistributing weight. Quad canes (four-footed canes) provide more stability than straight canes. To fit a patient for a cane, the patient is instructed to flex the elbow at a 30-degree angle, hold

CHART 11-8

Crutch Gaits

Shaded areas are weight-bearing. Arrow indicates advance of foot or crutch. (Read chart from bottom, starting with beginning stance.)

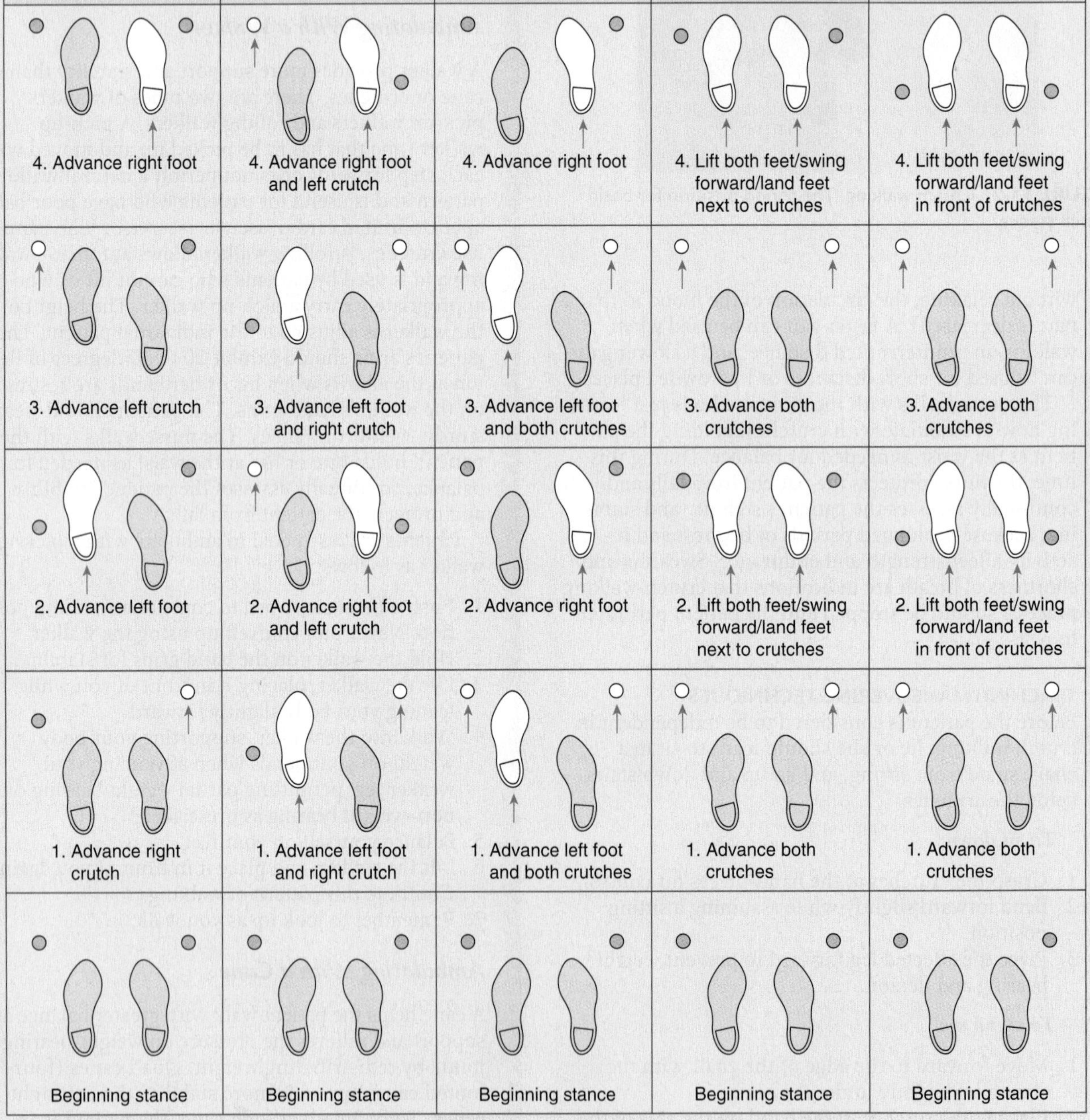

4-POINT GAIT	2-POINT GAIT	3-POINT GAIT	SWING-TO	SWING-THROUGH
• Partial weight bearing both feet • Maximal support provided • Requires constant shift of weight	• Partial weight bearing both feet • Provides less support • Faster than a 4 point gait	• Non-weight bearing • Requires good balance • Requires arm strength • Faster gait • Can use with walker	• Weight bearing both feet • Provides stability • Requires arm strength • Can use with walker	• Weight bearing • Requires arm strength • Requires coordination/ balance • Most advanced gait
4. Advance right foot	4. Advance right foot and left crutch	4. Advance right foot	4. Lift both feet/swing forward/land feet next to crutches	4. Lift both feet/swing forward/land feet in front of crutches
3. Advance left crutch	3. Advance left foot and right crutch	3. Advance left foot and both crutches	3. Advance both crutches	3. Advance both crutches
2. Advance left foot	2. Advance right foot and left crutch	2. Advance right foot	2. Lift both feet/swing forward/land feet next to crutches	2. Lift both feet/swing forward/land feet in front of crutches
1. Advance right crutch	1. Advance left foot and right crutch	1. Advance left foot and both crutches	1. Advance both crutches	1. Advance both crutches
Beginning stance	Beginning stance	Beginning stance	Beginning stance	Beginning stance

the handle of the cane about level with the greater trochanter, and place the tip of the cane 15 cm (6 inches) lateral to the base of the fifth toe. Adjustable canes make individualization easy. The cane should be fitted with a gently flaring tip that has flexible, concentric rings; the tip with its concentric rings provides optimal stability, functions as a shock absorber, and enables the patient to walk with greater speed and less fatigue.

The cane is held in the hand opposite the affected extremity. In normal walking, the opposite leg and arm move together (reciprocal motion); this motion is to be carried through in walking with a cane. Patients are taught to ambulate with a cane as follows:

Cane–foot sequence:

1. Hold the cane in the hand opposite the affected extremity to widen the base of support and to reduce the stress on the involved extremity. If the patient cannot use the cane in the opposite hand for some reason, the cane may be used on the same side.
2. Advance the cane at the same time the affected leg is moved forward.
3. Keep the cane fairly close to the body to prevent leaning.
4. Bear down on the cane when the unaffected extremity begins the swing phase.

To go up and down stairs using the cane:

1. Step up on the unaffected extremity.
2. Place the cane and affected extremity up on the step.
3. Reverse this procedure for descending steps ("up with the good, down with the bad").

As with all patients beginning ambulation with an assistive device, the nurse continually assesses the patient's stability and protects the patient from falls. The nurse accompanies the patient, holding him or her at the waist as needed for balance. The patient is assessed for tolerance of walking, and rest periods are provided as needed.

Assisting Patients with an Orthosis or Prosthesis

Orthoses and prostheses are designed to facilitate mobilization and to maximize the patient's quality of life. An orthosis is an external appliance that provides support, prevents or corrects deformities, and improves function. Orthoses include braces, splints, collars, corsets, and supports that are designed and fitted by orthotists or prosthetists. Static orthoses (no moving parts) are used to stabilize joints and prevent contractures. Dynamic orthoses are flexible and are used to improve function by assisting weak muscles. A prosthesis is an artificial body part; it may be internal, such as an artificial knee or hip joint, or external, such as an artificial leg or arm.

In addition to learning how to apply and remove the orthosis and maneuver the affected body part correctly, rehabilitation patients must learn how to properly care for the skin that comes in contact with the appliance. Skin problems or **pressure ulcers** may develop if the device is applied too tightly or too loosely, or if it is adjusted improperly. The nurse instructs the patient to clean and inspect the skin daily, to make sure the brace fits snugly without being too tight, to check that the padding distributes pressure evenly, and to wear a cotton garment without seams between the orthosis and the skin.

If the patient has had an amputation, the nurse promotes tissue healing, uses compression dressings to promote residual limb shaping, and minimizes contracture formation. A permanent prosthetic limb cannot be fitted until the tissue has healed completely and the residual limb shape is stable and free of edema. The nurse also helps the patient cope with the emotional issues surrounding loss of a limb and encourages acceptance of the prosthesis. The prosthetist, nurse, and physician collaborate to provide instructions related to skin care and care of the prosthesis.

Evaluation

Expected Patient Outcomes

Expected patient outcomes may include:

1. Demonstrates improved physical mobility
   a. Maintains muscle strength and joint mobility
   b. Does not develop contractures
   c. Participates in exercise program
2. Transfers safely
   a. Demonstrates assisted transfers
   b. Performs independent transfers
3. Ambulates with maximum independence
   a. Uses ambulatory aid safely
   b. Adheres to weight-bearing prescription
   c. Requests assistance as needed
4. Demonstrates increased activity tolerance
   a. Does not experience episodes of orthostatic hypotension
   b. Reports absence of fatigue with ambulatory efforts
   c. Gradually increases distance and speed of ambulation

Nursing Process

The Patient With Impaired Skin Integrity

An estimated 1.5 to 3 million patients develop pressure ulcers annually (Morrison, 2001). Both prevention and treatment of pressure ulcers are costly in terms of health care dollars and quality of life for patients at risk. All possible efforts to prevent skin breakdown should be made.

Pressure ulcers are localized areas of infarcted soft tissue that occur when pressure applied to the skin over time is greater than normal capillary closure pressure, which is about 32 mm Hg. Critically ill patients have a lower capillary closure pressure and a greater risk of pressure ulcers. Patients confined to bed for long periods, those with motor or sensory dysfunction, and those who experience muscular atrophy and reduction of padding between the overlying skin and the underlying bone are prone to pressure ulcers. The initial sign of pressure is erythema (redness of the skin) caused by reactive hyperemia, which normally resolves in less than 1 hour. Unrelieved pressure results in tissue ischemia or anoxia. The cutaneous tissues become broken or destroyed, leading to progressive destruction and necrosis of underlying soft tissue, and the resulting pressure ulcer is painful and slow to heal.

Assessment

Immobility, impaired sensory perception or cognition, decreased tissue perfusion, decreased nutritional status, friction and shear forces, increased moisture, and age-related skin changes all contribute to the development of pressure ulcers.

Immobility

When a person is immobile and inactive, pressure is exerted on the skin and subcutaneous tissue by objects on which the person rests, such as a mattress, chair seat, or cast. The development of pressure ulcers is directly related to the duration of immobility: if pressure continues long enough, small vessel thrombosis and tissue necrosis occur, and a pressure ulcer results. Weight-bearing bony prominences are most susceptible to pressure ulcer development because they are covered only by skin and small amounts of subcutaneous tissue. Susceptible areas include the sacrum and coccygeal areas, ischial tuberosities (especially in people who sit for prolonged periods), greater trochanter, heel, knee, malleolus, medial condyle of the tibia, fibular head, scapula, and elbow (Fig. 11-3).

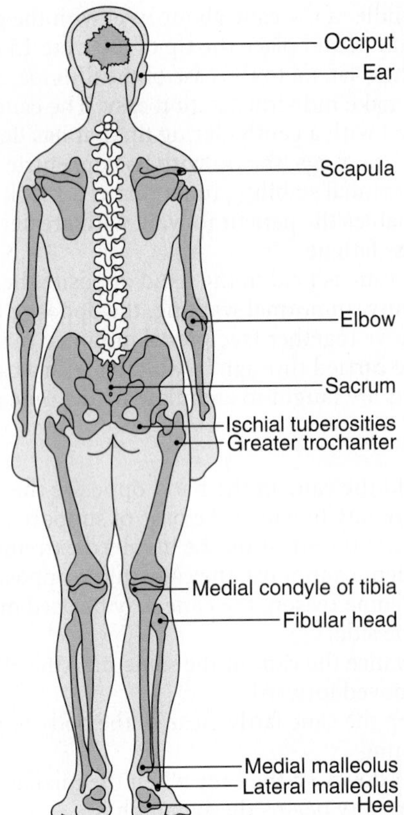

FIGURE 11-3. Areas susceptible to pressure ulcers.

Impaired Sensory Perception or Cognition

Patients with sensory loss, impaired level of consciousness, or paralysis may not be aware of the discomfort associated with prolonged pressure on the skin and therefore may not change their position themselves to relieve the pressure. This prolonged pressure impedes blood flow, reducing nourishment of the skin and underlying tissues. A pressure ulcer may develop in a short period of time.

Decreased Tissue Perfusion

Any condition that reduces the circulation and nourishment of the skin and subcutaneous tissue (altered peripheral tissue perfusion) increases the risk of pressure ulcer development. Patients with diabetes mellitus experience an alteration in microcirculation. Similarly, patients with edema have impaired circulation and poor nourishment of the skin tissue. Obese patients have large amounts of poorly vascularized adipose tissue, which is susceptible to breakdown.

Decreased Nutritional Status

Nutritional deficiencies, anemias, and metabolic disorders also contribute to development of pressure ulcers. Anemia, regardless of its cause, decreases the blood's oxygen-carrying ability and predisposes the patient to pressure ulcers. Patients who have low protein levels or who are in a negative nitrogen balance experience tissue wasting and inhibited tissue repair. Serum albumin is a sensitive indicator of protein deficiency; serum albumin levels of less than 3 g per mL are associated with hypoalbuminemic tissue edema and increased risk of pressure ulcers. The nurse should assess the patient's prealbumin and albumin values and electrolyte panel. Specific nutrients, such as vitamin C and trace minerals, are needed for tissue maintenance and repair.

Friction and Shear

Mechanical forces also contribute to the development of pressure ulcers. Friction is the resistance to movement that occurs when two surfaces are moved across each other. Shear is created by the interplay of gravitational forces (forces that push the body down) and friction. When shear occurs, tissue layers slide over one another, blood vessels stretch and twist, and the microcirculation of the skin and subcutaneous tissue is disrupted. Evidence of deep tissue damage may be slow to develop and may present through the development of a sinus tract. The sacrum and heels are most susceptible to the effects of shear. Pressure ulcers from friction and shear occur when the patient slides down in bed (Fig. 11-4) or when the patient is positioned or moved improperly (eg, dragged up in bed). Spastic muscles and paralysis increase the patient's vulnerability to pressure ulcers related to friction and shear.

Increased Moisture

Prolonged contact with moisture from perspiration, urine, feces, or drainage produces maceration (softening) of the skin. The skin reacts to the caustic substances in the excreta or drainage and becomes irritated. Moist, irritated skin is more vulnerable to pressure breakdown. Once the skin breaks, the area is invaded by microorganisms (eg, streptococci, staphylococci, *Pseudomonas aeruginosa, Escherichia coli*), and infection occurs. Foul-smelling infectious drainage is present. The lesion may enlarge and allow a continuous loss of serum, which may further deplete the body of essential protein needed for tissue repair and maintenance. The lesion may continue to enlarge and extend deep into the fascia, muscle, and bone, with multiple sinus tracts radiating from the pressure ulcer. With extensive pressure ulcers, life-threatening infections and sepsis may develop, frequently from gram-negative organisms.

Gerontologic Considerations

In older adults, the skin has diminished epidermal thickness, dermal collagen, and tissue elasticity. The skin is drier as a result of diminished sebaceous and sweat gland activity. Cardiovascular changes result in decreased tissue perfusion. Muscles atrophy, and bone structures become prominent. Diminished sensory perception and reduced ability to reposition oneself contribute to prolonged pressure on the skin. Therefore, older adults are more susceptible to pressure ulcers, which cause pain and suffering and reduce quality of life.

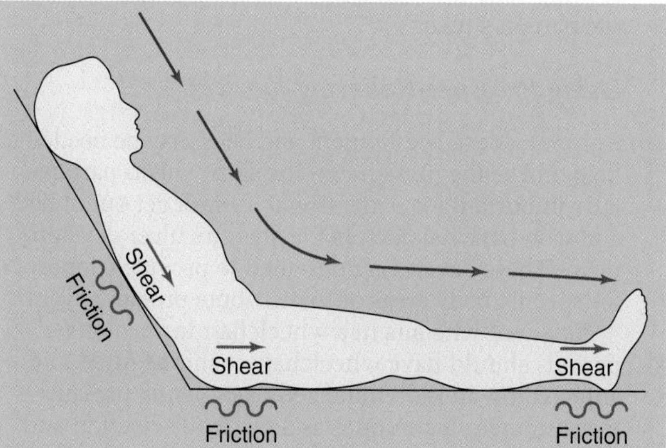

FIGURE 11-4. Mechanical forces contribute to pressure ulcer development. As the person slides down or is improperly pulled up in bed, *friction* resists this movement. *Shear* occurs when one layer of tissue slides over another, disrupting microcirculation of skin and subcutaneous tissue.

Nursing Actions Related to Assessment

In assessing patients for potential risk for pressure ulcer development, the nurse assesses the patient's mobility, sensory perception, cognitive abilities, tissue perfusion, nutritional status, friction and shear forces, sources of moisture on the skin, and age. Nursing actions include the following:

- Assess total skin condition at least twice a day.
- Inspect each pressure site for erythema.
- Assess areas of erythema for blanching response.
- Palpate the skin for increased warmth.
- Inspect for dry skin, moist skin, breaks in skin.
- Note drainage and odor.
- Evaluate level of mobility.
- Note safety and assistive devices (eg, restraints, splints).
- Evaluate circulatory status (eg, peripheral pulses, edema).
- Assess neurovascular status.
- Determine presence of incontinence.
- Evaluate nutritional and hydration status.
- Review the patient's record for laboratory studies, including hematocrit, hemoglobin, electrolytes, albumin, transferrin, and creatinine.
- Note present health problems.
- Review current medications.

Scales such as the Braden or Norton scale may be used to facilitate systematic assessment and quantification of a patient's risk for pressure ulcer, although the nurse should recognize that the reliability of these scales is not well established for all patient populations. Chart 11-9 lists risk factors for pressure ulcers. If a pressure area is noted, the nurse notes its size and location and uses a grading system to describe its severity (Chart 11-10).

Generally, a stage I pressure ulcer is an area of nonblanchable erythema, tissue swelling, and congestion. The patient complains of discomfort. The skin temperature is elevated because of the increased vasodilation. The redness progresses to a dusky, cyanotic blue-gray appearance, which is the result of skin capillary occlusion and subcutaneous weakening.

A stage II pressure ulcer is a break in the skin that extends through the epidermis or the dermis. An abrasion, blister, or shallow crater may be seen. Necrosis occurs along with venous sludging and thrombosis and edema with cellular extravasation and infiltration.

A stage III pressure ulcer extends into the subcutaneous tissues or fascia. Clinically, a deep crater with or without undermining of adjacent tissues is noted.

CHART 11-9

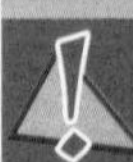

Risk Factors for Pressure Ulcers

- Prolonged pressure on tissue
- Immobility, compromised mobility
- Loss of protective reflexes, sensory deficit/loss
- Poor skin perfusion, edema
- Malnutrition, hypoproteinemia, anemia, vitamin deficiency
- Friction, shearing forces, trauma
- Incontinence of urine or feces
- Altered skin moisture: excessively dry, excessively moist
- Advanced age, debilitation
- Equipment: casts, traction, restraints

A stage IV pressure ulcer extends into the underlying structures, including the muscle and possibly the bone. The skin lesion may appear insignificant when, in reality, beneath the small surface ulcer is a large undermined area of necrotic tissue.

The appearance of purulent drainage or foul odor suggests an infection. With an extensive pressure ulcer, deep pockets of infection are often present. Drying and crusting of exudate may be present. Infection of a pressure ulcer may advance to osteomyelitis, pyarthrosis (pus formation within a joint cavity), sepsis, and septic shock.

Nursing Diagnosis

Based on the assessment data, the nursing diagnoses may include the following:

- Risk for impaired skin integrity
- Impaired skin integrity (related to immobility, decreased sensory perception, decreased tissue perfusion, decreased nutritional status, friction and shear forces, excessive moisture, or advanced age)

Planning and Goals

The major goals may include relief of pressure, improved mobility, improved sensory perception, improved tissue perfusion, improved nutritional status, minimized friction and shear forces, dry surfaces in contact with skin, and healing of pressure ulcer, if present.

Nursing Interventions

Relieving Pressure

Frequent changes of position are needed to relieve and redistribute the pressure on the patient's skin and to prevent prolonged reduced blood flow to the skin and subcutaneous tissues. This can be accomplished by teaching the patient to change position or by turning and repositioning the patient. The patient's family members should be taught how to position and turn the patient at home to prevent pressure ulcers. Shifting weight allows the blood to flow into the ischemic areas and helps tissues recover from the effects of pressure. Thus, the patient should be cared for as follows:

- Turned and repositioned at 1- to 2-hour intervals
- Encouraged to shift weight actively every 15 minutes

Positioning the Patient

The patient should be positioned laterally, prone, and dorsally in sequence unless a position is not tolerated or is contraindicated. The recumbent position is preferred to the semi-Fowler's position because of increased supporting body surface area in this position. In addition to regular turning, there should be small shifts of body weight, such as repositioning of an ankle, elbow, or shoulder. The skin is inspected at each position change and assessed for temperature elevation. If redness or heat is noted or if the patient complains of discomfort, pressure on the area must be relieved.

Another way to relieve pressure over bony prominences is the bridging technique, accomplished through the correct positioning of pillows. Just as a bridge is supported on pillars to allow traffic to move underneath, the body can be supported by pillows to allow for space between bony prominences and the mattress. A pillow or commercial heel protector may be used to support the heels off the bed when the patient is supine. Placing pillows superior and inferior to the sacrum relieves sacral pressure. Supporting the patient in a 30-degree side-lying position avoids pressure on the trochanter. In aging patients, frequent small shifts of body weight may be effective. Placing a small rolled towel or sheepskin under a shoulder or hip allows a return of blood flow to the skin in the area on which the patient is sitting or lying. The towel or sheepskin is moved around the patient's pressure points in a clockwise fashion. A turning schedule can help the family keep track of the patient's turns.

Using Pressure-Relieving Devices

At times, special equipment and beds may be needed to help relieve the pressure on the skin. This is particularly important for patients who cannot get out of bed and who have risk factors for pressure ulcer development. These devices are designed to provide support for specific body areas or to distribute pressure evenly.

A patient who sits in a wheelchair for prolonged periods should have wheelchair cushions fitted and adjusted on an individualized basis, using pressure measurement techniques as a guide to selection and fitting. The aim is to redistribute pressure away from areas at risk for ulcers, but no cushion can eliminate excessive pressure completely. The patient should be reminded to shift weight frequently and to rise for a few seconds every 15 minutes while sitting in a chair (Fig. 11-5).

CHART 11-10

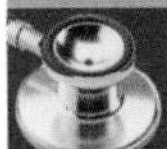

Assessing for Pressure Ulcer Stages

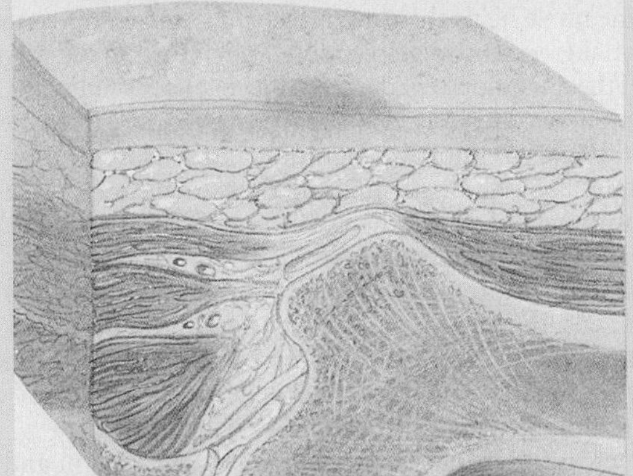

Stage I

- Area of erythema
- Erythema does not blanch with pressure
- Skin temperature elevated
- Tissue swollen and congested
- Patient complains of discomfort
- Erythema progresses to dusky blue-gray

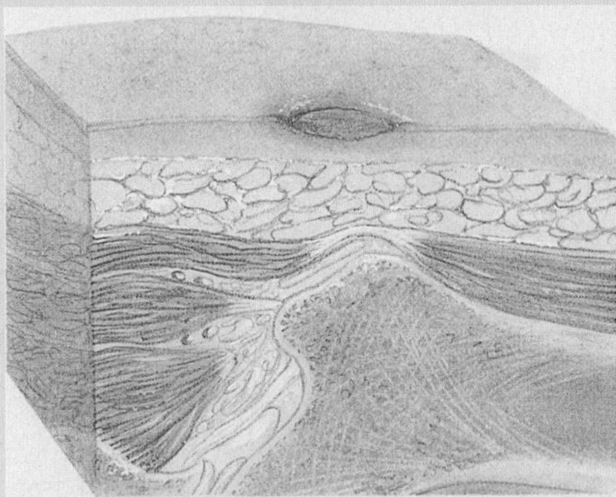

Stage II

- Skin breaks
- Abrasion, blister, or shallow crater
- Edema persists
- Ulcer drains
- Infection may develop
- Partial-thickness wound

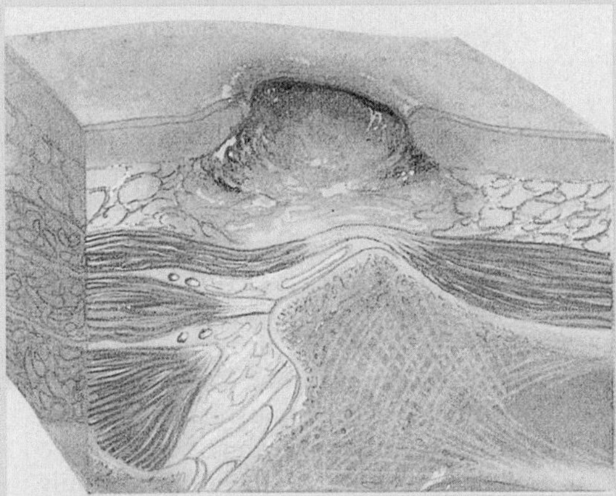

Stage III

- Ulcer extends into subcutaneous tissue
- Necrosis and drainage continue
- Infection develops
- Full-thickness wound

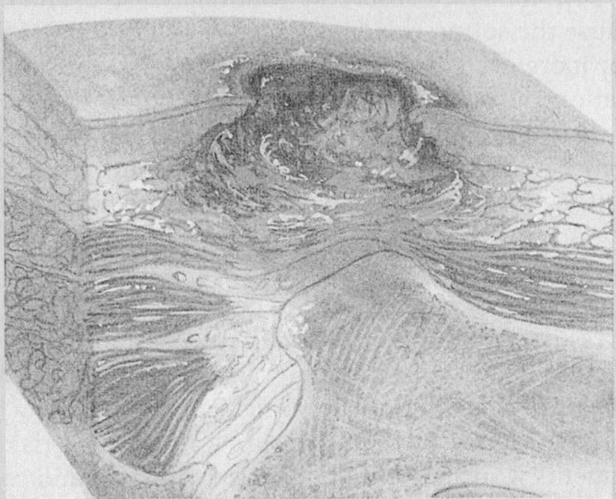

Stage IV

- Ulcer extends to underlying muscle and bone
- Deep pockets of infection develop
- Necrosis and drainage continue
- Full-thickness wound

From Weber, J. W., & Kelley, J. (2003). *Health assessment in nursing* (2nd ed.). Philadelphia: Lippincott Williams & Wilkins.

Static support devices (such as high-density foam, air, or liquid mattress overlays) distribute pressure evenly by bringing more of the patient's body surface into contact with the supporting surface. Gel-type flotation pads and air-fluidized beds reduce pressure. The weight of a body floating on a fluid system is evenly distributed over the entire supporting surface (according to Pascal's law). Therefore, as the body sinks into the fluid, additional surface becomes available for weight bearing, body weight per unit area is decreased, and there is less pressure on the body parts.

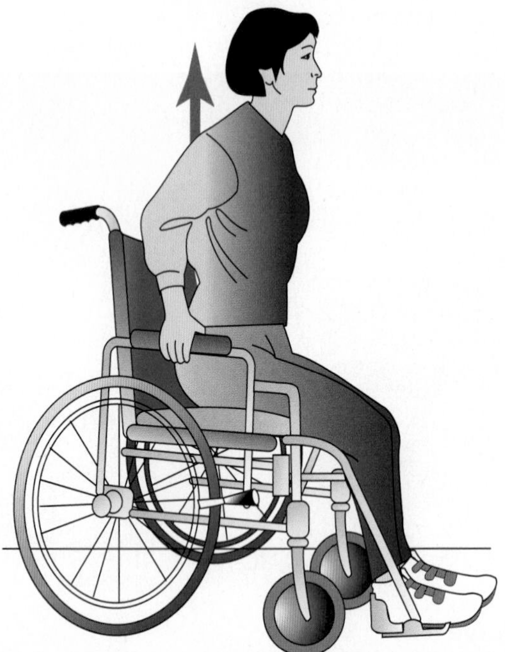

FIGURE 11-5. Wheelchair push-up to prevent ischial pressure ulcers. These push-ups should become an automatic routine (every 15 minutes) for the person with paraplegia. The person should stay up, out of contact with the seat for several seconds. The wheels are kept in the locked position during the exercise.

Soft, moisture-absorbing padding is also useful because the softness and resilience of padding provide for more even distribution of pressure and the dissipation and absorption of moisture, along with freedom from wrinkles and friction. Bony prominences may be protected by gel pads, sheepskin padding, or soft foam rubber beneath the sacrum, the trochanters, heels, elbows, scapulae, and back of the head when there is pressure on these sites.

Specialized beds have been designed to prevent pressure on the skin. Air-fluidized beds allow the patient to float. Dynamic support surfaces, such as low air-loss pockets, alternately inflate and deflate sections to change support pressure for very high-risk patients who are critically ill and debilitated and cannot be repositioned to relieve pressure. Oscillating or kinetic beds change pressure by means of rocking movements of the bed that redistribute the patient's weight and stimulate circulation. These beds are frequently used with patients who have injuries due to multiple trauma.

Improving Mobility

The patient is encouraged to remain active and is ambulated whenever possible. When sitting, the patient is reminded to change positions frequently to redistribute weight. Active and passive exercises increase muscular, skin, and vascular tone. Activity stimulates circulation, which relieves tissue ischemia, the forerunner of pressure ulcers. For patients at risk for pressure ulcers, turning and exercise schedules are essential: repositioning must occur around the clock.

Improving Sensory Perception

The nurse helps the patient recognize and compensate for altered sensory perception. Depending on the origin of the alteration (eg, decreased level of consciousness, spinal cord lesion), specific interventions are selected. Strategies to improve cognition and sensory perception may include stimulating the patient to increase awareness of self in the environment, encouraging the patient to participate in self-care, or supporting the patient's efforts toward active compensation for loss of sensation (eg, a patient with paraplegia lifting up from the sitting position every 15 minutes). A patient with quadriplegia should be weight-shifted every 30 minutes while sitting in a wheelchair. When decreased sensory perception exists, the patient and caregivers are taught to inspect potential pressure areas visually every morning and evening, using a mirror if necessary, for evidence of pressure ulcer development.

Improving Tissue Perfusion

Exercise and repositioning improve tissue perfusion. Massage of erythematous areas is avoided because damage to the capillaries and deep tissue may occur.

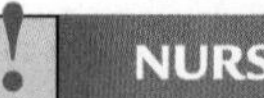

NURSING ALERT

Avoid massaging reddened areas, because this may increase the damage to already traumatized skin and tissue.

In patients who have evidence of compromised peripheral circulation (eg, edema), positioning and elevation of the edematous body part to promote venous return and diminish congestion improve tissue perfusion. In addition, the nurse or family must be alert to environmental factors (eg, wrinkles in sheets, pressure of tubes) that may contribute to pressure on the skin and diminished circulation and remove the source of pressure.

Improving Nutritional Status

The patient's nutritional status must be adequate and a positive nitrogen balance must be maintained because pressure ulcers develop more quickly and are more resistant to treatment in patients with nutritional disorders. A high-protein diet with protein supplements may be helpful. Iron preparations may be necessary to raise the hemoglobin concentration so that tissue oxygen levels can be maintained within acceptable limits. Ascorbic acid (vitamin C) is necessary for tissue healing. Other nutrients associated with healthy skin include vitamin A, B vitamins, zinc, and sulfur. With balanced nutrition and hydration, the skin can remain healthy and damaged tissues can be repaired (Table 11-2).

To assess the patient's nutritional status in response to therapeutic strategies, the nurse monitors the patient's hemoglobin, prealbumin level, and body weight weekly. Nutritional assessment is described in further detail in Chapter 5.

Reducing Friction and Shear

Shear occurs when patients are pulled, allowed to slump, or move by digging heels or elbows into the mattress. Raising the head of the bed by even a few centimeters increases the shearing force over the sacral area; therefore, the semireclining position is avoided in patients at risk. Proper positioning with adequate support is also important when the patient is sitting in a chair. Polyester sheepskin pads are thought to reduce shear and friction and may be used with at-risk patients.

NURSING ALERT

To avoid shearing forces when repositioning patients, nurses must lift and must avoid dragging patients across a surface.

Minimizing Irritating Moisture

Continuous moisture on the skin must be prevented by meticulous hygiene measures. Perspiration, urine, stool, and drainage must be removed from the skin promptly. The soiled skin should be washed immediately with mild soap and water and blotted dry with a soft towel. The skin may be lubricated with a bland lotion to keep it soft and pliable. Drying agents and powders are avoided. Topical barrier ointments (eg, petroleum jelly) may be helpful in protecting the skin of patients who are incontinent.

Absorbent pads that wick moisture away from the body should be used to absorb drainage. Patients who are incontinent need to be checked regularly and have their wet incontinence pads and linens changed promptly. Their skin needs to be cleansed and dried promptly.

Promoting Pressure Ulcer Healing

Regardless of the stage of the pressure ulcer, the pressure on the area must be eliminated, because the ulcer will not heal until all pressure is removed. The patient must not lie or sit on the pressure ulcer, even for a few minutes. Individualized positioning and turning schedules must be written in the plan of nursing care and followed meticulously.

In addition, inadequate nutritional status and fluid and electrolyte abnormalities must be corrected to promote healing. Wounds from which body fluids and protein drain place the patient in a catabolic state and predispose to hypoproteinemia and serious secondary infections. Protein deficiency must be corrected to heal the pressure ulcer. Carbohydrates are necessary to "spare" the protein and to provide an energy source. Vitamin C and trace elements, especially zinc, are necessary for collagen formation and wound healing.

STAGE I PRESSURE ULCERS

To permit healing of stage I pressure ulcers, the pressure is removed to allow increased tissue perfusion, nutritional and fluid and electrolyte balance are maintained, friction and shear are reduced, and moisture to the skin is avoided.

TABLE 11-2 Nutritional Requirements to Promote Healing of Pressure Ulcers

Nutrient	Rationale	Recommended Amount
Protein	Tissue repair	1.25–1.50 g/kg/day
Calories	Spare protein Restore normal weight	30–35 calories/kg/day
Water	Maintain homeostasis	1 mL/calorie fed or 30 mL/kg/day
Multivitamin	Promote collagen formation	1 daily
Vitamin C	Promote collagen synthesis Support integrity of capillary wall	500–1000 mg daily
Zinc sulfate	Cofactor for collagen formation and protein synthesis Normal lymphocyte and phagocyte response	220 mg daily
Vitamin A	Stimulate epithelial cells Stimulate immune response *Caution:* An excess can cause an excessive inflammatory response that could impair healing	—

STAGE II PRESSURE ULCERS

Stage II pressure ulcers have broken skin. In addition to measures listed for stage I pressure ulcers, a moist environment, in which migration of epidermal cells over the ulcer surface occurs more rapidly, should be provided to aid wound healing. The ulcer is gently cleansed with sterile saline solution. Use of a heat lamp to dry the open wound is avoided, as is use of antiseptic solutions that damage healthy tissues and delay wound healing. Semipermeable occlusive dressings, hydrocolloid wafers, or wet saline dressings are helpful in providing a moist environment for healing and in minimizing the loss of fluids and proteins from the body.

STAGE III AND IV PRESSURE ULCERS

Stage III and IV pressure ulcers are characterized by extensive tissue damage. In addition to the measures listed for stage I, these advanced draining, necrotic pressure ulcers must be cleaned (débrided) to create an area that will heal. Necrotic, devitalized tissue favors bacterial growth, delays granulation, and inhibits healing. Wound cleaning and dressing are uncomfortable; therefore, the nurse must prepare the patient for the procedure by explaining what will occur and administering prescribed analgesia.

Débridement may be accomplished by wet-to-damp dressing changes, mechanical flushing of necrotic and infective exudate, application of prescribed enzyme preparations that dissolve necrotic tissue, or surgical dissection. If an eschar covers the ulcer, it is removed surgically to ensure a clean, vitalized wound. Exudate may be absorbed by dressings or special hydrophilic powders, beads, or gels. Cultures of infected pressure ulcers are obtained to guide the selection of antibiotic therapy.

After the pressure ulcer is clean, a topical treatment is prescribed to promote granulation. New granulation tissue must be protected from reinfection, drying, and damage, and care should be taken to prevent pressure and further trauma to the area. Dressings, solutions, and ointments applied to the ulcer should not disrupt the healing process. Multiple agents and protocols are used to treat pressure ulcers, but consistency is an important key to success. Objective evaluation of the pressure ulcer (eg, measurement of the size and depth of the pressure ulcer, inspection for granulation tissue) for response to the treatment protocol must be made every 4 to 6 days. Taking photographs at weekly intervals is a reliable strategy for monitoring the healing process, which may take weeks to months.

Surgical intervention is necessary when the ulcer is extensive, when complications (eg, fistula) exist, and when the ulcer does not respond to treatment. Surgical procedures include débridement, incision and drainage, bone resection, and skin grafting. Osteomyelitis is a common complication of wounds of stage IV depth. See Chapter 68 for more information on osteomyelitis.

Preventing Recurrence

Recurrence of pressure ulcers should be anticipated; therefore, active, preventive intervention and frequent continuing assessments are essential. The patient's tolerance for sitting or lying on the healed pressure area is increased gradually by increasing the time that pressure is allowed on the area in 5- to 15-minute increments. The patient is taught to increase mobility and to follow a regimen of turning, weight-shifting, and repositioning. The patient teaching plan includes strategies to reduce the risk of pressure ulcers and methods to detect, inspect, and minimize pressure areas. Early recognition and intervention are keys to long-term management of potential impaired skin integrity.

Evaluation

Expected Patient Outcomes

Expected patient outcomes may include:

1. Maintains intact skin
   a. Exhibits no areas of nonblanchable erythema at bony prominences
   b. Avoids massage of bony prominences
   c. Exhibits no breaks in skin
2. Limits pressure on bony prominences
   a. Changes position every 1 to 2 hours
   b. Uses bridging techniques to reduce pressure
   c. Uses special equipment as appropriate
   d. Raises self from seat of wheelchair every 15 minutes
3. Increases mobility
   a. Performs range-of-motion exercises
   b. Adheres to turning schedule
   c. Advances sitting time as tolerated
4. Sensory and cognitive ability improved
   a. Demonstrates improved level of consciousness
   b. Remembers to inspect potential pressure ulcer areas every morning and evening
5. Demonstrates improved tissue perfusion
   a. Exercises to increase circulation
   b. Elevates body parts susceptible to edema
6. Attains and maintains adequate nutritional status
   a. Verbalizes the importance of protein and vitamin C in diet
   b. Eats diet high in protein and vitamin C
   c. Exhibits hemoglobin, electrolyte, prealbumin, transferrin, and creatinine levels at acceptable levels
7. Avoids friction and shear
   a. Avoids semireclining position
   b. Uses sheepskin pad and heel protectors when appropriate
   c. Lifts body instead of sliding across surfaces
8. Maintains clean, dry skin
   a. Avoids prolonged contact with wet or soiled surfaces
   b. Keeps skin clean and dry
   c. Uses lotion to keep skin lubricated

Nursing Process

The Patient With Altered Elimination Patterns

Urinary and bowel incontinence or constipation and impaction are problems that often occur in patients with disabilities. Incontinence curtails the person's independence, causing embarrassment and isolation. It occurs in as much as 15% of the community-based elderly population, and nearly 50% of nursing home residents have bowel or bladder incontinence or both. In addition, constipation may be a problem in patients with disabilities. Complete and predictable evacuation of the bowel is the goal. If a bowel routine is not established, the patient may experience abdominal distention; small, frequent oozing of stool; or impaction.

Assessment

Urinary incontinence may result from multiple causes, including urinary tract infection, detrusor instability, bladder outlet obstruction or incompetence, neurologic impairment, bladder spasm or contracture, and inability to reach the toilet in time. Urinary incontinence can be classified as urge, reflex, stress, functional, or total:

- *Urge incontinence:* involuntary elimination of urine associated with a strong perceived need to void
- *Reflex (neurogenic) incontinence:* associated with a spinal cord lesion that interrupts cerebral control, resulting in no sensory awareness of the need to void
- *Stress incontinence:* associated with weakened perineal muscles that permit leakage of urine when intra-abdominal pressure is increased (eg, with coughing or sneezing)
- *Functional incontinence:* incontinence in patients with intact urinary physiology who experience mobility impairment, environmental barriers, or cognitive problems and cannot reach and use the toilet before soiling themselves
- *Total incontinence:* occurs in patients who cannot control excreta because of physiologic or psychological impairment; management of the excreta is an essential focus of nursing care.

The health history is used to explore bladder and bowel function, symptoms associated with dysfunction, physiologic risk factors for elimination problems, perception of micturition and defecation cues, and functional toileting abilities. Previous and current fluid intake and voiding patterns may be helpful in designing the plan of nursing care. A record of times of voiding and amounts voided is kept for at least 48 hours. In addition, episodes of incontinence and associated activity (eg, coughing, sneezing, lifting), fluid intake time and amount, and medications are recorded. This record is analyzed and used to determine patterns and relationships of incontinence to other activities and factors.

The ability to get to the bathroom, manipulate clothing, and use the toilet are important functional factors that may be related to incontinence. Related cognitive functioning (perception of need to void, verbalization of need to void, and ability to learn to control urination) must also be assessed. In addition, the nurse reviews the results of the diagnostic studies (eg, urinalysis, urodynamic tests, postvoiding residual volumes). Chart 11-11 presents the factors that affect elimination in older adults.

Bowel incontinence and constipation may result from multiple causes, such as diminished or absent sphincter control, cognitive or perceptual impairment, neurogenic factors, diet, and immobility. The origin of the bowel problem must be determined. The nurse assesses the patient's normal bowel patterns, nutritional patterns, use of laxatives, gastrointestinal problems (eg, colitis), bowel sounds, anal reflex and tone, and functional abilities. The character and frequency of bowel movements are recorded and analyzed.

Nursing Diagnosis

Based on the assessment data, major nursing diagnoses may include the following:

- Impaired bowel elimination
- Impaired urinary elimination

Planning and Goals

The major goals may include control of urinary incontinence or urinary retention, control of bowel incontinence, and regular elimination patterns.

CHART 11-11

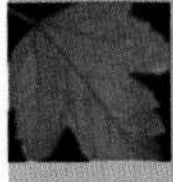

Factors That Alter Urinary Elimination Patterns in the Older Adult

- Decreased bladder capacity
- Decreased muscle tone
- Increased residual volumes
- Delayed perception of elimination cues
- Use of medications that alter elimination patterns, such as diuretics (increase volume of urine produced), sedatives (alter bladder sensitivity to cues), and adrenergics or anticholinergics (cause urinary retention)
- Functional immobility
- Sedentary lifestyle

Nursing Interventions

Promoting Urinary Continence

After the nature of the urinary incontinence has been identified, a nursing plan of care is developed based on analysis of the assessment data. Various approaches to promote urinary continence have been developed. Most approaches attempt to condition the body to control urination or to minimize the occurrence of unscheduled urination. Selection of the approach depends on the cause and type of the incontinence. For the program to be successful, participation by the patient and a desire to avoid incontinence episodes are crucial; an optimistic attitude with positive feedback for even slight gains is essential for success. Accurate recording of intake and output and of the patient's response to selected strategies is essential for evaluation.

At no time should the fluid intake be restricted to decrease the frequency of urination. Sufficient fluid intake (2,000 to 3,000 mL per day, according to patient needs) must be ensured. To optimize the likelihood of voiding as scheduled, measured amounts of fluids may be administered about 30 minutes before voiding attempts. In addition, most of the fluids should be consumed before evening to minimize the need to void frequently during the night.

The goal of bladder training is to restore the bladder to normal function. Bladder training can be used with cognitively intact patients experiencing urge incontinence. A voiding and toileting schedule is formulated based on analysis of the assessment data. The schedule specifies times for the patient to try to empty the bladder using a bedpan, toilet, or commode. Privacy should be provided during voiding efforts. The interval between voiding times in the early phase of the bladder training period is short (90 to 120 minutes). The patient is encouraged not to void until the specified voiding time. Voiding success and episodes of incontinence are recorded. As the patient's bladder capacity and control increase, the interval is lengthened. Usually, there is a temporal relationship between drinking, eating, exercising, and voiding. Alert patients can participate in recording intake, activity, and voiding and can plan the schedule to achieve maximum continence. Barrier-free access to the toilet and modification of clothing can help patients with functional incontinence achieve self-care in toileting and continence.

Habit training is used to try to keep patients dry by strict adherence to a toileting schedule and may be successful with stress, urge, or functional incontinence. If the patient is confused, caregivers take the patient to the toilet according to the schedule before involuntary voiding occurs. Simple cuing and consistency promote success. Periods of continence and successful voidings are positively reinforced.

Biofeedback is a system through which patients learn consciously to contract urinary sphincters and control voiding cues. Cognitively intact patients who have stress or urge incontinence may gain bladder control through biofeedback.

Pelvic floor exercises (Kegel exercises) strengthen the pubococcygeus muscle. The patient is instructed to tighten the pelvic floor muscles for 4 seconds ten times, and this is repeated four to six times a day. Stopping and starting the stream during urination is recommended to increase control. Daily practice is essential. These exercises are helpful for cognitively intact women who experience stress incontinence.

Suprapubic tapping or stroking of the inner thigh may produce voiding by stimulating the voiding reflex arc in patients with reflex incontinence. However, this method is not always effective, because of detrusor–sphincter dyssynergy. As the bladder reflexively contracts to expel urine, the bladder sphincter reflexively closes, producing a high residual urine volume and an increased incidence of urinary tract infection.

Intermittent self-catheterization is an appropriate alternative for managing reflex incontinence, urinary retention, and overflow incontinence due to an overdistended bladder. The emphasis of patient teaching is on regular emptying of the bladder rather than sterility. Patients with disabilities may reuse and clean catheters with bleach or hydrogen peroxide solutions or soap and water and may use a microwave oven to sterilize catheters. Aseptic intermittent catheterization technique is required in health care institutions because of the potential for bladder infection from resistant organisms. Intermittent self-catheterization may be difficult for patients with limited mobility, dexterity, or vision; however, family members can be taught the procedure.

Indwelling catheters are avoided if at all possible because of the high incidence of urinary tract infections with their use. Short-term use may be needed during treatment of severe skin breakdown due to continued incontinence. Patients with disabilities who cannot perform intermittent self-catheterization may elect to use suprapubic catheters for long-term bladder management. Suprapubic catheters are easier to maintain than indwelling catheters. A daily fluid intake of 3000 mL is encouraged.

External catheters (condom catheters) and leg bags to collect spontaneous voidings are useful for male patients with reflex or total incontinence. The appropriate design and size must be chosen for maximal success, and the patient or caregiver must be taught how to apply the condom catheter and how to provide daily hygiene, including skin inspection. Instruction on emptying the leg bag must also be provided, and modifications can be made for patients with limited hand dexterity.

Incontinence pads (briefs) may be useful at times for patients with stress or total incontinence to protect clothing, but they should be avoided whenever possible. Incontinence pads only manage, rather than solve, the incontinence problem. Also, they have a negative psychological effect on patients, because many people think of the pads as diapers. Every effort should be made to reduce the incidence of incontinence episodes through the other methods that have been described. When incontinence pads are used, they should wick moisture away from the body to minimize contact of moisture and excreta with the skin. Wet incontinence pads must be changed promptly, the skin cleansed, and a moisture

NURSING RESEARCH PROFILE

Satisfaction with Urinary Management Following Spinal Cord Injury

Brillhart, B. (2004). Studying the quality of life and life satisfaction among persons with spinal cord injury undergoing urinary management. *Rehabilitation Nursing, 29*(4), 122–126.

Purpose

Patients with spinal cord injury (SCI) have needs related to urinary management and the prevention of urinary complications. The purpose of this study was to investigate quality of life and life satisfaction of patients with SCI who require different types of urinary management, including reflex voiding, indwelling catheter, suprapubic catheter, intermittent catheterization, external catheter, or a combination of intermittent catheterization and external catheter.

Design

From a nationwide survey of people with SCI, a sample of 230 people were selected to participate in the study. The mean age of the subjects was 44.6 years, and 75 percent of the subjects were male. The Quality of Life Index (QLI) and a Satisfaction with Life Scale (SWLS) were used as assessment tools to measure quality of life in these patients.

Findings

Results of the study revealed no significant differences in QLI and SWLS when comparing patients with the different types of urinary management ($p = .945$) and when comparing patients with different levels (cervical 1–4, cervical 5–7, thoracic 1–12, lumbar 1–4) of SCI ($p = .157$). However, the QLI and SWLS scores were significantly higher ($p = .002$, $p = .001$ and $p = .003$, respectively) for subjects who had greater ability to work, were attending school, and who participated in activities. Subjects who had not experienced skin complications related to urinary dysfunction had significantly higher QLI scores than those who had experienced such complications.

Nursing Implications

When caring for patients with SCI, nurses should help these patients focus on self-management of their urinary condition and resolution of any problems related to urinary management. Their plans of care should be individualized to promote maximum activity and function and should be flexible to meet their changing needs. Further studies are needed to determine common factors among SCI patients that promote self-care decision making and activities.

barrier applied to protect the skin. It is important for the patient's self-esteem to avoid use of the term "diapers."

Promoting Bowel Continence

The goals of a bowel training program are to develop regular bowel habits and to prevent uninhibited bowel elimination. Regular, complete emptying of the lower bowel results in bowel continence. A bowel-training program takes advantage of the patient's natural reflexes. Regularity, timing, nutrition and fluids, exercise, and correct positioning promote predictable defecation.

The nurse records defecation time, character of stool, nutritional intake, cognitive abilities, and functional self-care toileting abilities for 5 to 7 days. Analysis of this record is helpful when designing a bowel program for patients with fecal incontinence.

Consistency in implementing the plan is essential. A regular time for defecation is established, and attempts at evacuation should be made within 15 minutes of the designated time daily. Natural gastrocolic and duodenocolic reflexes occur about 30 minutes after a meal; therefore, after breakfast is one of the best times to plan for bowel evacuation. However, if the patient had a previously established habit pattern at a different time of day, it should be followed.

The anorectal reflex may be stimulated by a rectal suppository (eg, glycerin) or by mechanical stimulation (eg, digital stimulation with a lubricated gloved finger or anal dilator). Mechanical stimulation should be used only in patients with a disability who have no voluntary motor function and no sensation as a result of injuries above the sacral segments of the spinal cord, such as patients with quadriplegia, high paraplegia, or severe brain injuries. The technique is not effective in patients who do not have an intact sacral reflex arc (eg, those with flaccid paralysis). Mechanical stimulation, suppository insertion, or both should be initiated about 30 minutes before the scheduled bowel elimination time, and the interval between stimulation and defecation is noted for subsequent modification of the bowel program. Once the bowel routine is well established, stimulation with a suppository may not be necessary.

The patient should assume the normal squatting position and be in a private bathroom for defecation if at all possible, although a padded commode chair or bedside toilet is an alternative. An elevated toilet seat is a simple modification that may make use of the toilet easier for the patient with a disability.

Seating time is limited in patients who are at risk for skin breakdown. Bedpans should be avoided. A patient with a disability who cannot sit on a toilet should be positioned on the left side with legs flexed and the head of the bed elevated 30 to 45 degrees to increase intra-abdominal pressure. Protective padding is placed behind the buttocks. When possible, the patient is instructed to bear down and to contract the abdominal muscles. Massaging the abdomen from right to left facilitates movement of feces in the lower tract.

Preventing Constipation

The record of bowel elimination, character of stool, food and fluid intake, level of activity, bowel sounds, medications, and other assessment data are reviewed to develop the plan of care. Multiple approaches may be used to prevent constipation. The diet should be well balanced and should include adequate intake of high-fiber foods (vegetables, fruits, bran) to prevent hard stools and to stimulate peristalsis. Daily fluid intake should be 2 to 3 L unless contraindicated. Prune juice or fig juice (120 mL) taken 30 minutes before a meal once daily is helpful in some cases when constipation is a problem. Physical activity and exercise are encouraged, as is self-care in toileting. Patients are encouraged to respond to the natural urge to defecate. Privacy during toileting is provided. Stool softeners, bulk-forming agents, mild stimulants, and suppositories may be prescribed to stimulate defecation and to prevent constipation.

Evaluation

Expected Patient Outcomes

Expected patient outcomes may include:

1. Demonstrates control of bowel and bladder function
   a. Experiences no episodes of incontinence
   b. Avoids constipation
   c. Achieves independence in toileting
   d. Expresses satisfaction with level of bowel and bladder control
2. Achieves urinary continence
   a. Uses therapeutic approach that is appropriate to type of incontinence
   b. Maintains adequate fluid intake
   c. Washes and dries skin after episodes of incontinence
3. Achieves bowel continence
   a. Participates in bowel program
   b. Verbalizes need for regular time for bowel evacuation
   c. Modifies diet to promote continence
   d. Uses bowel stimulants as prescribed and needed
4. Experiences relief of constipation
   a. Uses high-fiber diet, fluids, and exercise to promote defecation
   b. Responds to urge to defecate

Disability and Sexuality Issues

An important issue confronting patients with disabilities, and a vital component of self-concept, is sexuality. Sexuality involves not only biologic sexual activity but also one's concept of masculinity or femininity. It affects the way people react to others and are perceived by them, and it is expressed not only by physical intimacy but also by caring and emotional intimacy.

Sexuality problems experienced by patients with disabilities include limited access to information about sexuality, lack of opportunity to form friendships and loving relationships, impaired self-image, and low self-esteem. People with disabilities may have physical and emotional difficulties that interfere with sexual activities. For example, diabetes and spinal cord injury may affect the ability of men to have erections. Patients who have suffered a heart attack or stroke may fear having a life-threatening event (eg, another heart attack or stroke) during sexual activity. Some patients may fear loss of bowel or bladder control during intimate moments. Changes in desire for sex and in the quality of sexual activities can occur for the patient and his or her partner, who may be too involved as a caregiver to have the desire and energy for sexual activities.

Unfortunately, society and some health care providers contribute to these problems by ignoring the patient's sexuality and by viewing people with disabilities as asexual. Health care providers' own discomfort and lack of knowledge related to sexuality issues prevent them from providing patients with disabilities and their partners with interventions that promote healthy intimacy. Nurses caring for people with disabilities must recognize and address sexual issues to promote feelings of self-worth. The nurse should give the patient "permission" to discuss sexuality concerns and show a willingness to listen and help the patient overcome these concerns. The nurse also plays a key role in providing appropriate patient education about how specific disabilities affect sexual function. For example, arthritis produces fatigue and morning stiffness, making planned afternoon sex a better alternative; spinal cord injury impairs erections and ejaculations; and traumatic brain injury may produce an increased or decreased interest in sexual behavior. Classes, books, movies, and support groups are useful tools to help patients learn about sexuality and disability. When open discussion and education about disability and sexuality do not result in the patient achieving his or her sexuality goals, the nurse should refer the patient for ongoing counseling with a sex counselor or therapist. The patient may need training in communication and in social and assertiveness skills to develop desired relationships.

Fatigue

People with disabilities frequently experience fatigue. Physical and emotional weariness may be caused by discomfort and pain associated with a chronic health problem, deconditioning associated with prolonged periods of bed rest and immobility, impaired motor function requiring excessive expenditure of energy to ambulate, and the frustrations of performing ADLs. Ineffective coping with the disability, unresolved grief, disordered sleep patterns, and depression can also contribute to fatigue. The patient is encouraged to use coping strategies to manage the psychological impact of the disability and pain management techniques to control the associated discomforts (see Chapter 13 for a discussion of pain management). In addition, the nurse can teach the patient to manage fatigue through priority setting and energy-conserving techniques (Chart 11-12).

Complementary and Alternative Therapies

People with disabilities may seek a variety of different therapies. For some people, therapeutic horseback riding influences the entire body and has a profound effect on all body systems. Instructors are certified through the North American Riding for the Handicapped Association. Pet therapy and canine companion programs have reduced stress and promoted coping for many people with disabilities. Some animals, including simian monkeys, can pick up the phone, retrieve small assistive devices, assist with drinking beverages, or assist with activating emergency calls. The "working" animals provide companionship as well as physical assistance for elderly people and people with disability who may live alone.

Nurses can also encourage people with disabilities to take advantage of community programs. T'ai chi classes improve muscle strength, balance, and coordination and can help to prevent falls in the elderly. People with disabilities, including wheelchair users, can participate in T'ai chi classes for improved balance, coordination, muscle strength and control, and a sense of well-being.

Daily journal writing has helped depressed people and their families overcome many emotionally draining reactions to adverse circumstances. Nurses are instrumental in teaching patients and family members this cost-effective technique. Relaxation exercises can also be taught by the nurse and encouraged in all settings, including the hospital, rehabilitation setting, outpatient areas, and the home.

CHART 11-12

Learning to Cope With Disabilities

Take Control of Your Life

- Face the reality of your disability.
- Emphasize areas of strength.
- Remain outward looking.
- Seek inventive ways to tackle problems.
- Share concerns and frustrations.
- Maintain and improve general health.
- Plan for recreation.

Have Well-Defined Goals and Priorities

- Keep priorities in order; eliminate nonessential activities.
- Plan and pace your activities.

Organize Your Life

- Plan each day.
- Organize work.
- Perform tasks in steps.
- Distribute heavy work throughout the day or week.

Conserve Energy

- Rest before undertaking difficult tasks.
- Stop the activity before fatigue occurs.
- Continue with an exercise conditioning program to strengthen muscles.

Control Your Environment

- Try to be well organized.
- Keep possessions in the same place, so that they can be found with a minimum of effort.
- Store equipment (personal care, crafts, work) in a box or basket.
- Use energy-conservation and work-simplification techniques.
- Keep work within easy reach and in front of you.
- Use adaptive equipment, self-help aids, and labor-saving devices.
- Recruit assistance from others; delegate when necessary.
- Take safety precautions.

Promoting Home and Community-Based Care

An important goal of rehabilitation is to assist the patient to return to the home environment after learning to manage the disability. A referral system maintains continuity of care when the patient is transferred to the home or to an extended care facility. The plan for discharge is formulated when the patient is first admitted to the hospital, and discharge plans are made with the patient's functional potential in mind.

Teaching Patients Self-Care

The patient's support system (family, friends) is assessed. The attitudes of family and friends toward the patient, his or her disability, and the return home are important in making a successful transition to home. Not all families can carry out the arduous programs of exercise, physical therapy, and personal care that the patient may need. They may not have the resources or stability to care for family members with a severe disability. Even a stable family may be overwhelmed by the physical, emotional, economic, and energy strains of a disabling condition. Members of the rehabilitation team must not judge the family but rather should provide supportive interventions that help the family to attain its highest level of function.

The family members need to know as much as possible about the patient's condition and care so that they do not fear the patient's return home. The nurse develops methods to help the patient and family cope with problems that may arise. A skill checklist individualized for the patient and family can be developed to make certain that the family is proficient in assisting the patient with certain tasks (Chart 11-13).

CHART 11-13

HOME CARE CHECKLIST • Managing the Therapeutic Regimen at Home

At the completion of the home care instruction, the patient or caregiver will be able to:	Patient	Caregiver
• State the impact of disability on physiologic functioning.	✔	✔
• State changes in lifestyle necessary to maintain health.	✔	✔
• State the name, dose, side effects, frequency, and schedule for all medications.	✔	✔
• State how to obtain medical supplies after discharge.	✔	✔
• Identify durable medical equipment needs, proper usage, and maintenance necessary for safe utilization: [ ] Wheelchair—manual/power [ ] Cushion [ ] Grab bars [ ] Sliding board [ ] Mechanical lift [ ] Raised padded commode seat [ ] Padded commode wheelchair [ ] Bedside toilet [ ] Crutches [ ] Walker [ ] Prosthesis [ ] Orthosis [ ] Specialty bed	✔	✔
• Demonstrate usage of adaptive equipment for activities of daily living: [ ] Long-handled sponge [ ] Reacher [ ] Universal cuff [ ] Plate mat and guard [ ] Rocker-knife, spork, weighted utensils [ ] Special closures for clothing [ ] Other	✔	✔
• Demonstrate mobility skills: [ ] Transfers: bed to chair; in and out of toilet and tub; in and out of car [ ] Negotiate ramps, curbs, stairs [ ] Assume sitting from supine position [ ] Turn side to side in bed [ ] Maneuver wheelchair; manage arm and leg rests; lock brakes [ ] Ambulate safely using assistive devices [ ] Perform range-of-motion exercises [ ] Perform muscle-strengthening exercises	✔	✔
• Demonstrate skin care: [ ] Inspect bony prominences every morning and evening [ ] Identify stage I pressure ulcer and actions to take if present [ ] Change dressings for stage II to IV pressure ulcers [ ] State dietary requirements to promote healing of pressure ulcers [ ] Demonstrate pressure relief at prescribed intervals [ ] State sitting schedule and demonstrate weight lifts in wheelchair [ ] Demonstrate adherence to bed turning schedule, bed positioning, and use of bridging techniques [ ] Apply and wear protective boots at prescribed times [ ] Demonstrate correct wheelchair sitting posture [ ] Demonstrate techniques to avoid friction and shear in bed [ ] Demonstrate proper hygiene to maintain skin integrity	✔	✔
• Demonstrate bladder care: [ ] State schedule for voiding, toileting, and catheterization [ ] Identify relationship of fluid intake to voiding and catheterization schedule [ ] State how to perform pelvic floor exercises [ ] Demonstrate clean self-intermittent catheterization and care of catheterization equipment [ ] Demonstrate indwelling catheter care [ ] Demonstrate application of external condom catheter [ ] Demonstrate application, emptying, and cleaning of urinary drainage bag	✔	✔

CHART 11-13 **HOME CARE CHECKLIST** • **Managing the Therapeutic Regimen at Home, continued**

	Patient	Caregiver
[ ] Demonstrate application of incontinence pads and performing perineal hygiene [ ] State signs and symptoms of urinary tract infection		
• Demonstrate bowel care [ ] State optimum dietary intake to promote evacuation [ ] Identify schedule for optimum bowel evacuation [ ] Demonstrate techniques to increase intra-abdominal pressure; Valsalva maneuver; abdominal massage; leaning forward [ ] Demonstrate techniques to stimulate bowel movements: ingesting warm liquids; digital stimulation; insertion of suppositories [ ] Demonstrate optimum position for bowel evacuation: on toilet with knees higher than hips; left side in bed with knees flexed and head slightly elevated [ ] Identify complications and corrective strategies for bowel retraining: constipation, impaction, diarrhea, hemorrhoids, rectal bleeding, anal tears	✔	✔
• Identify community resources for peer and family support [ ] Identify phone numbers of support groups for people with disabilities [ ] State meeting locations and times	✔	✔
• Demonstrate how to access transportation [ ] Identify locations of wheelchair accessibility for public buses or trains [ ] Identify phone numbers for private wheelchair van [ ] Contact Division of Motor Vehicles for handicapped parking permit [ ] Contact Division of Motor Vehicles for driving test when appropriate [ ] Identify resources for adapting private vehicle with hand controls or wheelchair lift	✔	✔
• Identify vocational rehabilitation resources [ ] State name and phone number of vocational rehabilitation counselor [ ] Identify educational opportunities that may lead to future employment	✔	✔
• Identify community resources for recreation [ ] State local recreation centers that offer programs for people with disabilities [ ] Identify leisure activities that can be pursued in the community	✔	✔
• Identify the need for health promotion and screening activities	✔	✔

Continuing Care

A home care nurse may visit the patient in the hospital, interview the patient and the family, and review the ADL sheet to learn which activities the patient can perform. This helps ensure that continuity of care is provided and that the patient does not regress, but instead maintains the independence gained while in the hospital or rehabilitation setting. The family may need to purchase, borrow, or improvise needed equipment, such as safety rails, a raised toilet seat or commode, or a tub bench. Ramps may need to be built or doorways widened to allow full access.

Family members are taught how to use equipment and are given a copy of the equipment manufacturer's instruction booklet, the names of resource people, lists of equipment-related supplies, and locations where they may be obtained. A written summary of the care plan is included in family teaching. The patient and family members are reminded about the importance of routine health screening and other health promotion strategies.

A network of support services and communication systems may be required to enhance opportunities for independent living. The nurse uses collaborative, administrative skills to coordinate these activities and to pull together the network of care. The nurse also provides skilled care, initiates additional referrals when indicated, and serves as a patient advocate and counselor when obstacles are encountered. The nurse continues to reinforce prior teaching and helps the patient to set and achieve attainable goals. The degree to which the patient adapts to the home and community environment depends on the confidence and self-esteem developed during the rehabilitation process and on the acceptance, support, and reactions of family members, employers, and community members.

There is a growing trend toward independent living by people with severe disabilities, either alone or in groups that share resources. Preparation for independent living should include training in managing a household and working with personal care attendants as well as training in mobility. The goal is integration into the community—living and working in the community with accessible housing, employment, public buildings, transportation, and recreation.

State rehabilitation administration agencies provide services to assist people with disabilities in obtaining the help they need to engage in gainful employment. These services include diagnostic, medical, and mental health services. Counseling, training, placement, and follow-up services are available to help people with disabilities select and obtain jobs.

If the patient is transferred to an extended care facility, the transition is planned to promote continued progress. Independence gained continues to be supported, and progress is fostered. Adjustment to the extended care facility is promoted through communication. Family members are encouraged to visit, to be involved, and to take the patient home on weekends and holidays if possible.

Critical Thinking Exercises

1 A 62-year-old man who is recovering from a heart transplant has just been admitted to your nursing unit. He is very weak and deconditioned as a result of years of debilitating heart disease and the recent surgery. In discussing the patient's level of functioning with the physical rehabilitation team, describe the kinds of self-care activities that you would include in your rehabilitation plan for the patient. How does a functional assessment tool help determine the patient's level of functioning?

2 ebp A 22-year-old man who sustained a spinal cord injury with resulting paraplegia is being discharged to his home. He will be cared for by family and will continue physical and occupational therapy as an outpatient. Family members are particularly concerned about what they can do to prevent pressure ulcers. Describe the instructions you would give the patient and the family about prevention of pressure ulcers. What is the evidence base that supports the appropriateness of these instructions, and how strong is this evidence? What criteria did you use to determine the strength of the evidence for interventions that assist in the prevention of pressure ulcers?

3 The patient described in the preceding question has had bowel and bladder training. He and his family have been taught to perform intermittent catheterization to manage his reflex urinary incontinence. As the home care nurse for this patient, what assessment parameters would you use to determine the patient's needs relative to bowel and bladder functioning? What aspects of the home care environment would you assess? What instructions would you provide for the patient and his family?

REFERENCES AND SELECTED READINGS

BOOKS

Agency for Health Care Policy and Research, Public Health Service, U.S. Department of Health and Human Services. Panel for the Prediction and Prevention of Pressure Ulcers in Adults. (1992). *Pressure ulcers in adults: Prediction and prevention.* Clinical Practice Guideline Number 3. AHCPR Publication No. 92-0050. Rockville, MD: Author.

Agency for Health Care Policy and Research, Public Health Service, U.S. Department of Health and Human Services. (1994). *Treatment of pressure ulcers.* Clinical Practice Guideline Number 15. AHCPR Publication No. 95-0653. Rockville, MD: Author.

Association of Rehabilitation Nurses. (1995). *Twenty-one rehabilitation nursing diagnoses: A guide to interventions and outcomes.* Glenview, IL: Author.

Association of Rehabilitation Nurses. (1996). *Scope and standards of advanced clinical practice in rehabilitation nursing.* Glenview, IL: Author.

Association of Rehabilitation Nurses. (1997). *Advanced practice in rehabilitation nursing: A core curriculum.* Glenview, IL: Author.

Association of Rehabilitation Nurses. (2000). *Standards and scope of rehabilitation nursing practice.* Glenview, IL: Author.

Association of Rehabilitation Nurses. (2000). *The specialty practice of rehabilitation nursing: A core curriculum* (4th ed.). Skokie, IL: Author.

Centers for Disease Control and Prevention (2004). *Key resources on traumatic brain injury (TBI).* Atlanta, GA, June 3, 2004.

Cuddigan, J., Ayello, E. A., & Sussman, C. (2001). Pressure ulcers in America: Prevalence, incidence & implications for the future. Reston, VA: National Pressure Ulcer Advisory Panel.

Derstine, J., & Hargrove, S. (2001). *Comprehensive rehabilitation nursing.* St. Louis, MO: W. B. Saunders.

Hess, C. T. (2000). *Nurse's clinical guide to wound care.* Springhouse, PA: Springhouse.

Jans, L., & Stoddard, S. (1999). *Chartbook on women and disability in the United States.* Washington, DC: U.S. National Institute on Disability and Rehabilitation Research.

McCrory, D. C., Pompeii, L. A., & Skeen, M. B. (2004). *Criteria to determine disability related to multiple sclerosis.* (Rep. No. AHRQ Publication No. 04-E019-1). Rockville, MD: Agency for Healthcare Research and Quality.

Morrison, M. (2001). *The prevention and treatment of pressure ulcers.* St. Louis, MO: Mosby.

National Science Database (2004). *Spinal cord injury facts and figures at a glance.* www.spinal-injury.net. Accessed May 4, 2006.

U.S. Census Bureau (2000). *Disability statistics.* Available at www.census.gov

U.S. Department of Health and Human Services (2003). *HHS Fact Sheet. Substance abuse: A national challenge: Prevention, treatment and research at HHS.* Washington, DC: U.S. Government Printing Office.

JOURNALS

Asterisks indicate nursing research articles.

Adedokun, A. O., & Wilson, M. M. (2004). Urinary incontinence: Historical, global, and epidemiologic perspectives. *Clinical Geriatric Medicine, 20*(3), 399–407.

Bodenheimer, C. F., Roig, R. L., Worsowicz, G. M., et al. (2004). Geriatric rehabilitation. 5. The societal aspects of disability in the older adult. *Archives of Physical Medicine and Rehabilitation, 85*(7), S23–S26.

Bogey, R. A., Elovic, E. P., Bryant, P. R., et al. (2004). Rehabilitation of movement disorders. *Archives of Physical Medicine and Rehabilitation, 85*(3), S41–S45.

Bogey, R. A., Geis, C. C., Bryant, P. R., et al. (2004). Stroke and neurodegenerative disorders. 3. Stroke: rehabilitation management. *Archives of Physical Medicine and Rehabilitation, 85*(3), S15–S20.

Bolton, L., McNees, P., van Rijswijk, L., et al. (2004). Wound-healing outcomes using standardized assessment and care in clinical practice. *Journal of Wound Ostomy Continence Nursing, 31*(3), 65–71.

Braden, B. J., & Maklebust, J. (2005). Preventing pressure ulcers with the Braden scale. *American Journal of Nursing, 105*(6), 70–72.

Brem, H., & Lyder, C. (2004). Protocol for the successful treatment of pressure ulcers. *American Journal of Surgery, 188*(1A), 9–17.

*Brillhart, B. (2004). Studying the quality of life and life satisfaction among persons with spinal cord injury undergoing urinary management. *Rehabilitation Nursing, 29*(4), 122–126.

Bryant, P. R., Geis, C. C., Moroz, A., et al. (2004). Stroke and neurodegenerative disorders. 4. Neurodegenerative disorders. *Archives of Physical Medicine and Rehabilitation, 85*(3), S21–S33.

Chaudhuri, A., & Behan, P. O. (2004). Fatigue in neurological disorders. *Lancet, 363*(9413), 978–988.

Cullum, N., McInnes, E., Bell-Syer, S. E., et al. (2004). Support surfaces for pressure ulcer prevention. *Cochrane Database System Reviews,* CD001735.

DeGroot, M. H., Phillips, S. J., & Eskes, G. A. (2003). Fatigue associated with stroke and other neurologic conditions: Implications for stroke rehabilitation. *Archives of Physical Medicine and Rehabilitation, 84*(6), 1714–1720.

Dement, J. M., Pompeii, L. A., Ostbye, T., et al. (2004). An integrated comprehensive occupational surveillance system for health care workers. *American Journal of Industrial Medicine, 45*(6), 528–538.

Doloresco, L. (2001). CARF: Symbol of rehabilitation excellence. *SCI Nursing, 18*(11), 165, 172.

Hackett, M. L., Anderson, C. S., & House, A. O. (2004). Interventions for treating depression after stroke. *Cochrane Database System Reviews,* CD003437.

Horrocks, J. A., Hackett, M. L., Anderson, C. S., et al. (2004). Pharmaceutical interventions for emotionalism after stroke. *Stroke, 35*(11), 2610–2611.

Kelly, A., & Dowling, M. (2004). Reducing the likelihood of falls in older people. *Nursing Standard, 18*(5), 33–40.

*Lutz, B. J. (2004). Determinants of discharge destination for stroke patients. *Rehabilitation Nursing, 29*(5), 154–163.

MacKenzie, A. E., & Change, A. M. (2002). Predictors of quality of life following stroke. *Disability and Rehabilitation, 24*(5), 259–265.

Mechanick, J. I. (2004). Practical aspects of nutritional support for wound-healing patients. *American Journal of Surgery, 188,* 52–56.

*Missik, E. (2001). Women and cardiac rehabilitation: Accessibility issues and policy recommendations. *Rehabilitation Nursing, 26*(4), 141–147.

Moroz, A., Bogey, R. A., Bryant, P. R., et al. (2004). Stroke and neurodegenerative disorders. 2. Stroke: Comorbidities and complications. *Archives of Physical Medicine and Rehabilitation, 85*(3), S11–S14.

O'Neill, B. J., Geis, C. C., Bogey, R. A., et al. (2004). Stroke and neurodegenerative disorders. 1. Acute stroke evaluation, management, risks, prevention, and prognosis. *Archives of Physical Medicine and Rehabilitation, 85*(3), S3–S10.

Olkin, R. (2002). Could you hold the door for me? Including disability in diversity. *Cultural Diversity and Ethnic Minority Psychology,* 8(2), 130–137.

Ostaszkiewicz, J., Johnston, L., & Roe, B. (2004). Habit retraining for the management of urinary incontinence in adults. *Cochrane Database System Reviews,* CD002802.

Ostaszkiewicz, J., Johnston, L., & Roe, B. (2004). Timed voiding for the management of urinary incontinence in adults. *Cochrane Database System Reviews,* CD002802.

Palmer, S. & Wegener, S. T. (2003). Rehabilitation psychology. Overview and key concepts. *Maryland Medical Journal,* 4(2), 20–22.

Phillips, E. M., Bodenheimer, C. F., Roig, R. L., et al. (2004). Geriatric rehabilitation. 4. Physical medicine and rehabilitation interventions for common age-related disorders and geriatric syndromes. *Archives of Physical Medicine and Rehabilitation, 85*(5), S18–S22.

Pompeii, L. A. (1998). Inferential and advanced analysis of research data. *AAOHN Journal, 46*(10), 514–516.

Roig, R. L., Worsowicz, G. M., Stewart, D. G., et al. (2004). Geriatric rehabilitation. 3. Physical medicine and rehabilitation interventions for common disabling disorders. *Archives of Physical Medicine and Rehabilitation, 85*(7), S12–S17.

Saunders, D. H., Greig, C. A., Young, A., et al. (2004). Physical fitness training for stroke patients. *Stroke, 35*(9), 2235.

Siegert, R. J., McPherson, K. M., & Taylor, W. J. (2004). Toward a cognitive-affective model of goal-setting in rehabilitation: Is self-regulation theory a key step? *Disability and Rehabilitation, 26*(20), 1175–1183.

Sipski, M. L., Jackson, A. B., Gomez-Marin, O., et al. (2004). Effects of gender on neurologic and functional recovery after spinal cord injury. *Archives of Physical Medicine and Rehabilitation, 85*(11), 1826–1836.

Smeltzer, S. C. (2000). Viewpoint: Double jeopardy. The health care system slights women with disabilities. *American Journal of Nursing, 100*(8), 11.

Sorensen, J. L., Jorgensen, B., & Gottrup, F. (2004). Surgical treatment of pressure ulcers. *American Journal of Surgery, 188*(1A), 42–51.

Stein, J. (2004). Motor recovery strategies after stroke. *Topics in Stroke Rehabilitation, 11*(1), 12–22.

Stewart, D. G., Phillips, E. M., Bodenheimer, C. F., et al. (2004). Geriatric rehabilitation. 2. Physiatric approach to the older adult. *Archives of Physical Medicine and Rehabilitation, 85*(7), S7–11.

Storey, K. (2003). A review of research on natural support interventions in the workplace for people with disabilities. *International Journal of Rehabilitation Research, 26*(8), 79–84.

Tate, D. G., Roller, S., & Riley, B. (2001). Quality of life for women with physical disabilities. *Physical Medicine and Rehabilitation Clinics of North America, 12*(11), 23–37.

Walsh, N. E. (2004). The Walter J. Zeiter lecture. Global initiatives in rehabilitation medicine. *Archives of Physical Medicine and Rehabilitation, 85*(9), 1395–1402.

Worsowicz, G. M., Stewart, D. G., Phillips, E. M., et al. (2004). Geriatric rehabilitation. 1. Social and economic implications of aging. *Archives of Physical Medicine and Rehabilitation, 85*(7), S3–S6.

Zehr, E. P., & Duysens, J. (2004). Regulation of arm and leg movement during human locomotion. *Neuroscientist, 10*(4), 347–361.

RESOURCES

ABLEDATA, 8401 Colesville Road, Suite 200, Silver Spring, MD 20910; 1-800-227-0216; http://www.abledata.com. Accessed June 6, 2006.

Agency for Healthcare Research and Quality, 2101 East Jefferson Street, Suite 501, Rockville, MD 20852; 1-800-358-9295; http://www.ahrq.gov. Accessed June 6, 2006.

American Society of Addiction Medicine, 4601 North Park Avenue, Arcade Suite 101, Chevy Chase, MD 20815; 1-301-656-3920; http://www.asam.org. Accessed June 6, 2006.

Assistive Technology Industry Association, 526 Davis Street, Suite 217, Evanston, IL 60201; 1-877-687-2842/847-969-1282; http://www.atia.org. Accessed June 6, 2006.

Association of Rehabilitation Nurses, 4700 W. Lake Avenue, Glenview, IL 60025; 1-800-229-7530; fax 1-847-375-4710; http://www.rehabnurse.org. Accessed June 6, 2006.

Canine Companions for Independence, PO Box 446, Santa Rosa, CA 95402; 1-800-572-2275; www.caninecompanions.org. Accessed June 6, 2006.

Council for Disability Rights, 205 West Randolph, Suite 1650, Chicago, IL 60606; 1-312-444-9484; www.disabilityrights.org. Accessed June 6, 2006.

National Center for the Dissemination of Disability Research 2004–2005; 1-800-266-1832; http://www.ncddr.org. Accessed June 6, 2006.

National Center for Health Statistics, Division of Data Services, Hyattsville, MD 20782; 1-301-458-4636; http://www.cdc.gov/nchs. Accessed June 6, 2006.

National Council on Alcoholism and Drug Dependence, Inc., 20 Exchange Place, Suite 2902, New York, NY 10005; 1-212-269-7797; http://www.ncadd.org. Accessed June 6, 2006.

National Council on Disability, 1331 F Street, NW, Suite 1050, Washington, DC 20004; 1-202-272-2004; http://www.ncd.gov. Accessed June 6, 2006.

National Rehabilitation Information Center (NARIC), 1010 Wayne Avenue, Suite 800, Silver Spring, MD 20910; 1-800-346-2742; http://www.naric.com. Accessed June 6, 2006.

Sexuality and Information and Education Council of the U.S. (SIECUS), 130 West 42nd Street, Suite 350, New York, NY 10036; 1-212-819-9770; http://www.siecus.org. Accessed June 6, 2006.

Substance Abuse Resources and Disability Issues, Wright State University School of Medicine, Dayton, OH 45435; 1-937-775-1484; http://www.med.wright.edu. Accessed June 6, 2006.

U.S. Census Bureau, 4700 Silver Hill Road, Suitland, MD 20746; http://www.census.gov. Accessed June 6, 2006.

U.S. Department of Health and Human Services, 200 Independence Avenue SW, Washington, DC 20201; http://www.hhs.gov. Accessed July 6, 2006.

CHAPTER 12

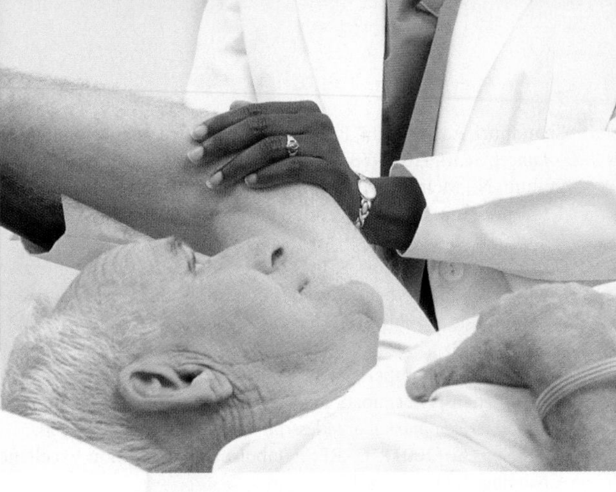

Health Care of the Older Adult

Learning Objectives

On completion of this chapter, the learner will be able to:

1. Describe the aging American population based on demographic trends and statistical data.
2. Describe the significance of preventive health care and health promotion for the elderly.
3. Compare and contrast the physiologic aspects of aging in older adults with those of middle-aged adults.
4. Identify the important physical and mental health problems of aging and their effects on the functioning of older people and their families.
5. Specify nursing implications related to medication therapy in older people.
6. Examine the concerns of older people and their families in the home and community, in the acute care setting, and in the long-term care facility.
7. Identify the resources available to allow older adults to receive medical and nursing services in their own homes.
8. Discuss the potential economic effect on health care of the large aging population in America.
9. Identify ethical and legal issues relevant to the care of older people.

Aging, the normal process of time-related change, begins with birth and continues throughout life. Americans are living longer than ever before, and the number of older Americans is growing more rapidly than the rest of the population. This chapter discusses the theories of aging, normal age-related changes, health problems associated with aging, and how nurses can address the health issues of older adults.

Overview of Aging

Demographics of Aging

Life expectancy, the average number of years that a person can be expected to live, has risen dramatically in the past 100 years. The proportion of Americans 65 years of age and older has tripled in that time (4.1% in 1900 and 12.3% in 2002). By 2030, it is estimated that 20% of Americans will be 65 years of age or older (Fig. 12-1). In 1900, average life expectancy was 47 years, but by 2001 that figure had increased to 77.2 years. According to data from the National Vital Statistics System, in 2001, a Caucasian 65-year-old could be expected to live until the age of 83.2 years and an African-American 65-year-old could be expected to live until the age of 81.4 years (National Center for Health Statistics, 2004). As the older population increases, the number of people who live to a very old age also increases: in 2002, 50,564 people were 100 years of age or older, an increase of 35% from 1990 (Administration on Aging, 2003).

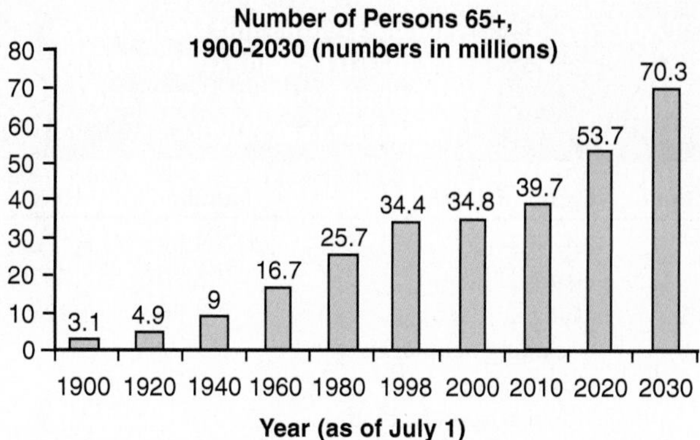

FIGURE 12-1. Profile of Americans age 65 and older based on data from the U.S. Bureau of the Census. Data from 1900 to the present is used to predict the millions of Americans aged 65 and older in the year 2030 (www.aoa.gov/aoa/stats/profile/default.htm).

The older population will also become more diverse, reflecting the changing demographics in the United States. Although the older population will increase in all racial and

Glossary

advance directive: a formal, legally endorsed document that provides instructions for care ("living will")

ageism: a bias that discriminates, stigmatizes, and disadvantages older people based solely on their chronologic age

delirium: an acute, confused state that begins with disorientation but, if not immediately evaluated and treated, can progress to changes in level of consciousness, irreversible brain damage, and sometimes death

dementia: broad term for a syndrome characterized by a general decline in higher brain functioning, such as reasoning, with a pattern of eventual decline in ability to perform even basic activities of daily living, such as toileting and eating

depression: the most common affective (mood) disorder of old age; results from changes in reuptake of the neurochemical serotonin in response to chronic illness and emotional stresses related to the physical and social changes associated with the aging process

durable power of attorney: a formal, legally endorsed document that identifies a proxy decision maker who can make decisions if the signer becomes incapacitated

elder abuse: the physical, emotional, or financial harm to an elderly person by one or more of the individual's children, caregivers, or others; includes neglect

geriatrics: the study of old age that includes the physiology, pathology, diagnosis, and management of the disorders and diseases of older adults

gerontologic/geriatric nursing: the field of nursing that relates to the assessment, nursing diagnosis, planning, implementation, and evaluation of older adults in all environments, including acute, intermediate, and skilled care as well as within the community

gerontology: the combined biologic, psychological, and sociologic study of older adults within their environment

life expectancy: the average number of years that a person is expected to live

lifespan: the maximum number of years an individual can be expected to live in the absence of disease or life-threatening trauma

orientation: a person's ability to recognize who and where he or she is in a time continuum; used to evaluate an individual's basic cognitive status

polypharmacy: the administration of multiple medications at the same time; common in older persons with several chronic illnesses

presbycusis: the decreased ability to hear high-pitched tones that naturally begins in midlife as a result of irreversible inner ear changes

presbyopia: the decrease in visual accommodation that occurs with advancing age

sundowning: increased confusion at night

urinary incontinence: the unplanned loss of urine, which affects up to 50% of community-residing older adults and approximately 75% to 85% of nursing home residents

TABLE 12-1 Annual Deaths and Death Rates for the 10 Leading Causes of Death in People 65 Years and Older For Year 2000

Rank	Cause of death	Number	Rate†
	All causes	1,799,825	5,176.4
1	Heart diseases	593,707	1,707.2
2	Malignant neoplasms, including neoplasms of lymphatic and hematopoietic tissues	392,966	1,128.2
3	Cerebrovascular diseases	148,045	425.7
4	Chronic obstructive pulmonary diseases and allied conditions	106,375	305.9
5	Pneumonia and influenza	58,557	168.4
6	Diabetes mellitus	52,414	150.7
7	Alzheimer's disease	48,993	140.9
8	Nephritis, nephrotic syndrome, and nephrosis	31,225	89.8
9	Accidents (unintentional injuries)	31,061	89.8
10	Septicemia	24,796	89.3
	All other causes (residual)	312,906	898.0

National Vital Statistics Report, Vol. 50, No. 16, Sept. 16, 2002. Available at: www.cdc.gov/nchs/fastats/pdf/nvbr50 lbtl.pdf

ethnic groups, the rate of growth is projected to be fastest in the Hispanic population, in which it will increase from 2 million in 2000 to 13 million in 2050. By 2028, the older Latino population is expected to outnumber the older African-American population (Older Americans, 2000).

Although most older adults enjoy good health, in national surveys as many as 20% of adults 65 years of age and older report a chronic disability. Chronic disease is the major cause of disability, and between 1980 and 2001, heart disease, cancer, and stroke continued to be the three leading causes of death in people 65 years of age and older in the United States (Table 12-1). In 2002, Alzheimer's disease ranked eighth as a cause of disease and accounted for more than 58,000 deaths (National Center for Health Statistics, 2004).

Health Status of the Older Adult

The vast majority of deaths (75%) in the United States occur in people 65 years of age and older, and more than half of these are caused by chronic illnesses such as heart disease and cancer. However, improvements in the prevention and early detection and treatment of diseases have had a noticeable impact on the health of people 65 years of age and older. In the past 50 years, there has been a decline in overall deaths (30%) and disability. During the 1990s deaths from heart disease and stroke declined 17.0%. Death from cancer, the second leading cause of death, rose until 1995, when it decreased slightly. Chronic obstructive pulmonary disease, the fourth leading cause of death, has been increasing since 1980, reflecting the effects of smoking. Diabetes, the sixth leading cause of death, is also identified on death certificates as a contributor to diseases such as heart disease, kidney disease, and stroke (Health, United States, 2003b).

From 1994 to 1996, 72% of older Americans reported their health to be good, very good, or excellent. Men and women reported comparable levels of health status; however, positive health reports declined with advancing age, and a greater number of African-American men and women as well as Hispanic men were less likely to report good health. The proportion of older Americans with a limitation in activities of daily living (ADLs) declined from 6.7% in 1997 to 6.4% in 2001. Similar declines in limitations in instrumental activities of daily living (IADLs) were also reported: 13.7% in 1997 and 12.6% in 2001 (Health, United States, 2003b). These declines in limitations reflect recent trends in health promotion and disease prevention activities, such as improved nutrition, decreased smoking, increased exercise, and early detection and treatment of risk factors such as hypertension and increased serum cholesterol levels.

Many chronic conditions commonly found among older people can be managed, limited, and even prevented. Older people are more likely to maintain good health and functional independence if encouraged to do so and if appropriate community-based support services are available. Nurses are challenged to promote positive lifelong health behaviors among all populations, because the impact of unhealthy behaviors and choices results in many of the chronic diseases seen among the elderly.

Nursing Care of the Older Adult

Gerontology, the scientific study of the aging process, is a multidisciplinary field that draws from the biologic, psychological, and sociologic sciences. Because aging is a normal occurrence, care for the elderly cannot be limited to one discipline but is best provided through a cooperative effort. An interdisciplinary team can combine expertise and resources to provide insight into all aspects of the aging process through comprehensive geriatric assessment and intervention. Nurses collaborate with the team to obtain non-nursing services for patients and provide a holistic approach to care.

Gerontologic or **geriatric nursing** is the field of nursing that specializes in the care of the elderly. The *Standards and Scope of Gerontological Nursing Practice* was originally developed in 1969 by the American Nurses Association and was revised in 1976 and again in 1987. The nurse gerontologist can be either a specialist or a generalist offering comprehensive nursing care to older people by combining the basic nursing process of assessment, diagnosis, planning, implementation, and evaluation with a specialized knowledge of aging. Gerontologic nursing is provided in acute care, skilled and assisted living, community, and home settings. Its goals include promoting and maintaining functional status and helping older adults identify and use their strengths to achieve optimal independence.

Nurses who are certified in gerontologic nursing have specialized knowledge of the acute and chronic changes specific to older people. The use of advanced practice nurses (APNs) in long-term care has proved to be very effective; when APNs using current scientific knowledge about clinical problems collaborate with nursing home staff, significantly less deterioration in the overall health issues of patients has been demonstrated (Ryden, Snyder, Gross, et al., 2000).

Nurses who work in all areas of adult medical-surgical nursing encounter elderly patients. They must be knowledgeable about geriatric nursing and skilled in meeting the needs of older patients. It is important that nurses and caregivers who work with older patients understand that aging is not synonymous with disease and that the effects of the aging process alone are not the primary contributors to disability and disease (Fryer, 2001). As research and scientific knowledge increase, it is becoming apparent that aging is a highly complex and varied process.

Functional assessment is a common framework for assessing elderly, dependent people. Age-related changes, as well as additional risk factors such as disease and the effects of medications, can result in functional consequences that have a negative impact on a particular person. However, with nursing interventions that focus on facilitating the highest level of function or quality of life, negative functional consequences can be turned into positive consequences. For example, it is possible to compensate for normal age-related changes in vision by increasing the light for reading or wearing sunglasses to reduce glare. These actions result in increased safety and quality of life (Miller, 2004). Assessing the functional consequences of aging and proposing practical interventions is significant to maintaining and even improving the health of the elderly. The goal is to help older people maintain maximum autonomy and dignity despite physical, social, and psychological losses. Early intervention can prevent further complications and help maximize the quality of life.

Theories of Aging

Aging has been defined chronologically by the passing of time—subjectively, as in how a person feels, and functionally, as in changes in physical or mental capabilities. Each theory of aging attempts to provide a framework in which to understand aging from different perspectives. Scientists examine the aging process from the biologic and cellular level. Social scientists and psychologists examine the aging process from developmental and experiential models. Each theory is useful to the clinician because a framework and insight into the differences among elderly patients are provided.

Biologic Theories

It is useful to consider the biologic theories of aging because they help distinguish normal aging from disease. Normal aging is intrinsic aging (from within a person) and refers to those changes caused by the normal aging process that are genetically programmed and essentially universal and irreversible within a species. Universality is the major criterion used to distinguish normal from abnormal aging. Chronologic age is often less predictive of obvious aging characteristics than other factors such as genetics and lifestyle practices.

Many biologic theories of aging are being explored. Much of the current research into biologic aging is at the cellular level. The "wear-and-tear theory" suggests that with use the body, similar to a machine, eventually wears out. The autoimmune theory proposes that over time the body's immune system becomes defective and can no longer recognize and attack foreign invaders. The noticeable changes in the body's collagen that lead to wrinkles as a person ages has led to the "cross-linkage" and "free radical" theories, which suggest that the body accumulates cross-linking compounds or gathers byproducts (free radicals) that eventually impede cell function. It has been suggested that DNA has a genetic "clock" that recognizes a limited **lifespan** or limits cellular reproduction, because cells of older people replicate fewer times than cells of younger people.

Developmental Theories

Erikson (1963) theorized that a person's life consists of eight stages, each representing a crucial turning point in life stretching from birth to death, with its own developmental conflict to be resolved. According to Erikson, the major developmental task of old age is either to achieve ego integrity or to suffer despair. Achieving ego integrity requires accepting one's lifestyle, believing that one's choices were the best that could be made at a particular time, and being in control of one's life. Despair results when the older person feels dissatisfied and disappointed with his or her life and would live differently if given another chance.

Havighurst (1968) also proposed developmental tasks that occur at certain times in a person's life. The tasks of older people include adjusting to retirement after a lifetime of employment with a possible reduction of income, adjusting to decreases in physical strength and health, adjusting to the death of a spouse, establishing affiliation with one's age group, adapting to new social roles in a flexible way, and establishing satisfactory physical living arrangements.

By combining the concepts of both Erikson and Havighurst, it is possible to identify the following developmental tasks for older adults: (1) maintenance of self-worth, (2) conflict resolution, (3) adjustment to the loss of dominant roles, (4) adjustment to the deaths of significant others, (5) environmental adaptation, and (6) maintenance of optimal levels of wellness. Nurses can facilitate reflection and reminiscence as useful experiences for elderly patients.

Sociologic Theories

Sociologic theories of aging attempt to predict and explain the social interactions and roles that contribute to successful adjustment to old age in older adults. Older theories include the activity theory, which proposes that life satisfaction in normal aging requires maintaining the active lifestyle of middle age (Havighurst, 1968), and the continuity theory, which proposes that successful adjustment to old age requires continuing life patterns across a lifetime (Atchley, 1989; Neugarten, 1961). Continuity and a connection to the past are maintained through a continuation of well-established habits, values, and interests that are integral to a person's present lifestyle. Other theories suggest that people move through their lives as cohort groups experiencing major life events together, such as war or economic depression, and that these events mold their lives in similar ways. The person-environment fit theory considers the interrelationship between people and their environment (Lawton, 1982). All of these theories provide a framework in which gerontologic nurses can appreciate individual patients within the context of their lives. The theories emphasize the importance of environmental and psychosocial factors in the development and current functioning of the patient.

Nursing Theory

Miller (2004) has developed the functional consequences theory, which challenges nurses to consider while planning care the effects of normal age-related changes as well as the damage incurred through disease or environmental and behavioral risk factors. Miller suggests that nurses can alter the outcome for patients through nursing interventions that address the consequences of these changes. The functional consequences theory postulates that

> [O]lder adults experience functional consequences because of age-related changes and additional risk factors. Without interventions, many functional consequences are negative; with them, however, functional consequences can be positive. The role of the gerontologic nurse is to identify the factors that cause negative functional consequences and to initiate interventions that will result in positive ones. (p. 59)

According to Miller's theory, normal age-related changes and risk factors may negatively interfere with patient outcomes and actually impair patient activity and quality of life. For example, normal age-related changes in vision may increase sensitivity to glare. Alterations in the environment that reduce glare may enhance patient comfort and safety. In contrast, the development of cataracts, which is not a normal age-related change, also may increase sensitivity to glare. The nurse must differentiate between normal age-related changes that cannot be reversed and risk factors that can be modified. Doing so is useful in designing appropriate nursing interventions that have a positive impact on patient outcomes for the elderly—most importantly, for quality of life.

Age-Related Changes

The well-being of older people depends on physical, mental, social, economic, and environmental factors. A total assessment includes an evaluation of all major body systems, social and mental status, and the ability of a person to function independently despite having a chronic illness or disability.

Psychosocial Aspects of Aging

Successful psychological aging is reflected in the ability of older people to adapt to physical, social, and emotional losses and to achieve contentment, serenity, and life satisfaction. Because changes in life patterns are inevitable over a lifetime, older people need resiliency and coping skills when confronting stresses and change. A positive self-image enhances risk taking and participation in new, untested roles.

Although attitudes toward older people differ in ethnic subcultures, a subtle theme of **ageism**—prejudice or discrimination against older people—predominates in our society, and many myths surround aging. Ageism is based on stereotypes, simplified and often untrue beliefs that reinforce society's negative image of older people. Although older people make up an extremely heterogeneous and increasingly a racially and ethnically diverse group, negative stereotypes are attributed to all of them.

Fear of aging and the inability of many to confront their own aging process may trigger ageist beliefs. Retirement and perceived nonproductivity are also responsible for negative feelings, because a younger working person may see an older person as someone who is not contributing to society and who is draining economic resources. Concern about the large numbers of elderly leaving the work force (baby boomers begin to turn age 65 in 2011) is fueling this debate.

Many negative images are so common in society that the elderly themselves often believe and perpetuate them. Only through an understanding of the aging process and respect for each person as an individual can the myths of aging be dispelled. If the elderly are treated with dignity and encouraged to maintain autonomy, the quality of their lives will improve.

Stress and Coping in the Older Adult

Coping patterns and the ability to adapt to stress develop over the course of a lifetime and remain consistent later in life. Experiencing success in younger adulthood helps a person develop a positive self-image that remains solid through the adversities of old age. A person's abilities to adapt to changes, make decisions, and respond predictably are also determined by past experiences. A flexible, well-functioning person will probably continue as such. However, losses may accumulate within a short period of time and may become overwhelming. The older person will often have fewer choices and diminished resources to deal with stressful events. Common stressors of old age include normal aging changes that impair physical function, activities, and appearance; disabilities from chronic illness; social and environmental losses related to loss of income and decreased ability to perform previous roles and activities; and the deaths of significant others. Many older adults rely strongly on their spiritual beliefs for comfort during stressful times.

Living Arrangements

More than 95% of the elderly live in the community, and more than 78% own their homes. In 2003, 58.5% of elderly people were living alone. Of the elderly people who live alone in the community, widowed women predominate. In 2003, 71% of men ages 65 to 74 were married compared to 41% of women in the same age group. Among those aged 85 or older, about 50% of the men were married compared to only 13% of the women. This difference in marital status is a result of several factors: women have a longer life expectancy than men do; women tend to marry older men; and women tend to remain widowed, whereas men often remarry (Older Americans 2000, 2005; Administration on Aging, 2004).

Older people often do best in their own environment and can successfully remain at home for many years. Furthermore, the family home and familiar community may have strong emotional significance for them, and this should not be ignored. With advanced age and increasing disability, adjustments to the environment may be required to allow older adults to remain in their own homes or apartments. Additional family support or more formal support such as Meals on Wheels or transportation services may be necessary to compensate for declining function and mobility.

Many elderly people have more-than-adequate financial resources and good health even until very late in life; therefore, they have many housing options. Older people tend to relocate in response to changes in their lives such as retirement or widowhood, a significant deterioration in health, or disability. The type of housing they choose depends on their reason for moving (Hooyman & Kiyak, 2002). For example, there has been a significant increase in the elderly population in the "Sun Belt"—in the states of Florida, California, Texas, and Arizona—as relatively young older adults (60 to 74 years of age) and recent retirees move to warmer climates and retirement communities. With increasing disability and illness, elderly people may move to retirement facilities or assisted living communities that provide some support such as meals, transportation, and housekeeping but allow them to live somewhat independently. If they develop a serious illness or disability and can no longer live independently or semi-independently, they may need to move to a setting where additional support is available. Older people may move in with a relative or to a nursing home or an assisted living setting nearer a child's home. For this reason, while Florida has the largest population of the elderly, it ranks only 24th in the percentage of very old people (Falgoust, 2004).

There are many implications when elderly people choose to remain in their own home. For example, the person tends to be living on a fixed income, which may have been adequate when the person first retired but is no longer sufficient to pay maintenance expenses or taxes and utilities. Creative solutions are available, such as reverse mortgages that lend the older person money via a credit line on his or her mortgage. This is available to elderly people who have little or no mortgage debt and allows them to use the assets of the home to finance daily needs. In addition, house sharing programs with family members or even strangers, although difficult to plan and arrange, can be successful and benefit both the older person and the individual or family sharing the home. Many communities have planned senior housing, much of which may be subsidized for low-income elderly people; some elderly adults who have "downsized" from larger homes and moved into apartment buildings find that they are "aging in place" with other elderly people in similar circumstances.

Sometimes older adults or couples agree to move in with adult children. This can be a rewarding experience as the children, their parents, and the grandchildren interact and share household responsibilities. It can also be stressful, depending on family dynamics. Adult children and their older parents may also choose to pool their financial resources by moving into a house that has an attached "in-law suite." This arrangement provides security for the older adult along with privacy for both families.

Unfortunately, many elderly people and their adult children make housing decisions in times of crisis, such as a serious illness or the death of a spouse. Older people and their families often are unaware of all of the ramifications of shared housing and assuming care for an increasingly dependent person. Families can be helped by anticipatory guidance and long-term planning before a crisis occurs. Older adults should participate in decisions that affect them as much as possible.

CONTINUING CARE RETIREMENT COMMUNITIES

Continuing care retirement communities (CCRCs), retirement communities that provide three levels of living arrangements and care, are becoming more popular as the first baby boomers enter their retirement years. CCRCs consist of independent single-dwelling houses or apartments for people who can manage all of their day-to-day needs; assisted living apartments for those who need limited assistance with their daily living needs; and skilled nursing services when continuous nursing assistance is required. CCRCs usually contract for a large down payment before the resident moves into the community. This payment gives a person or couple the option to reside in the community from the time of total independence through the need for assisted or skilled nursing care. Decisions about living arrangements and health care can be made before any decline in health status occurs. CCRCs also provide continuity at a time in an older adult's life when many other factors, such as health status, income, and availability of friends and family members, may be changing.

ASSISTED LIVING FACILITIES

Assisted living facilities are an option when an older person's physical or cognitive changes necessitate at least minimal supervision or assistance. Assisted living allows for a degree of independence while providing minimal nursing assistance (eg, administration of medication and assistance with ADLs or chronic health care needs). Other services, such as laundry, cleaning, and meals, may also be included.

NURSING HOMES

Skilled nursing facilities offer continuous nursing care. Contrary to the myth of family abandonment and the fear of "ending up in a nursing home," the actual percentage of long-term nursing home residents has declined, from 5.4% in 1985 to 4.5% in 1997 (Older Americans, 2000). However, the actual number of elderly people who reside in nursing homes has risen due to the large increase in the aging population and the multiple uses of nursing homes today for short-term rehabilitation.

Short-term nursing home care is often reimbursed by Medicare if the patient is recovering from an acute illness such as a stroke, myocardial infarction, or cancer and requires skilled nursing care or therapy for recuperation. Usually, if an older adult suffers a major health event and is hospitalized and then goes to a nursing home, Medicare covers the cost of the first 30 to 90 days in a skilled nursing facility if ongoing therapy is needed. The requirement for continued Medicare coverage during this time is documentation of persistent improvement in the condition that requires therapy, most often physical therapy, occupational therapy, respiratory therapy, and cognitive therapy. Some adults choose to have long-term care insurance as a means of paying, at least in part, for the cost of these services should they become necessary. For elderly people who are living in nursing homes and who generally have multiple chronic and debilitating health concerns, costs are primarily paid "out-of-pocket" by the patient. Family members are not responsible for nursing home costs. When a person's financial resources become exhausted as a result of prolonged nursing home care, the patient, the institution, or both may apply for Medicaid reimbursement.

An increasing number of skilled nursing facilities offer subacute care. This area of the facility offers a high level of nursing care that may either prevent the need for a resident to be transferred to a hospital from the nursing home or allow a hospitalized patient to be transferred back to the nursing facility sooner.

The Role of the Family

Planning for care and understanding the psychosocial issues confronting older people must be accomplished within the context of the family. If dependency needs occur, the spouse often assumes the role of primary caregiver. In the absence of the surviving spouse, an adult child usually assumes caregiver responsibilities and may eventually need help in providing or arranging for care and support. Approximately 81% of elderly people have living children. Of elderly people who live alone, two thirds have at least one child living within 30 minutes of their home, and 62% see at least one adult child weekly (Administration on Aging, 2004).

Two common myths in American society are that adult children and their aged parents are socially alienated and that adult children abandon their parents when health and other dependency problems arise. Extensive research refutes both of these beliefs (Markson, 2003). More than 70% of elderly people receive most of their care from informal caregivers. The family has been and continues to be an important source of support for older people; similarly, older family members provide a great deal of support to younger family members (Fig. 12-2).

Although adult children are not financially responsible for their older parents, social attitudes and cultural values often dictate that adult children should provide services and assume the burden of care if their aged parents cannot care for themselves. In the United States, 70% to 80% of community-based caregiving is provided to the elderly by informal caregivers, predominately by family, friends, and neighbors. This caregiving, which may continue for many years, can become a source of family stress. For prolonged periods, it is not uncommon for caregivers to neglect their own emotional and health needs (Myers, 2003). In addition, because many of the baby boomers (those born between 1946 and 1964) tended to have children later in life, these children face the competing demands of caring for their aging parents while caring for their own dependent children (Spillman, 2001). Furthermore, because of smaller family sizes, future generations of families will have to contend with fewer numbers of siblings to help with parental care issues. If community agencies or adult children cannot provide care, elders are at high risk for institutionalization.

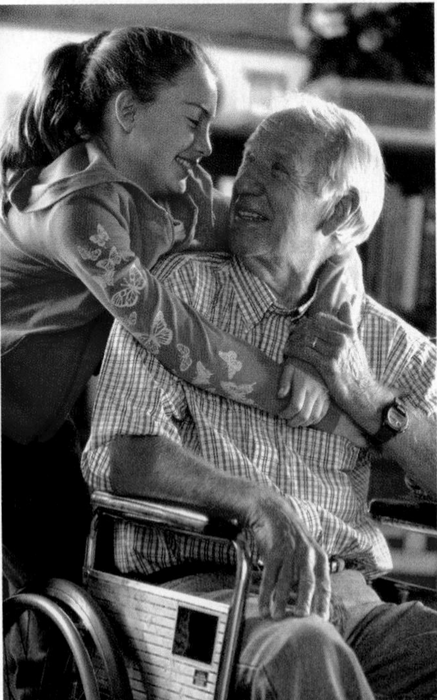

FIGURE 12-2. Families are an important source of psychosocial and physical support for elderly people and youngsters alike. Caring interaction among grandchildren, grandparents, and other family members typically contributes to the health of all.

Physical Aspects of Aging

As previously mentioned, intrinsic aging (from within the person) refers to those changes caused by the normal aging process that are genetically programmed and essentially universal within a species. Universality is the major criterion used to distinguish normal aging from pathologic changes associated with illness. However, people age quite differently and at different rates, so chronologic age is often less predictive of obvious aging characteristics than other factors, such as genetics and lifestyle. For example, extrinsic aging results from influences outside the person. Air pollution and excessive exposure to sunlight are examples of extrinsic factors that may hasten the aging process and that can be eliminated or reduced.

Cellular and extracellular changes of old age cause a change in physical appearance and a decline in function. Measurable changes in shape and body makeup occur. The body's ability to maintain homeostasis becomes increasingly diminished with cellular aging, and organ systems cannot function at full efficiency because of cellular and tissue deficits. Cells become less able to replace themselves, and they accumulate a pigment known as lipofuscin. A degradation of elastin and collagen causes connective tissue to become stiffer and less elastic. All of this results in diminished capacity for organ function and increased vulnerability to disease and stress.

Table 12-2 summarizes the signs and symptoms of age-related changes in the functioning of body systems. More in-depth information about age-related changes can be found in the chapters pertaining to each organ system. Specifics of diseases, medical and surgical management, as well as nursing interventions are also presented in the related chapters.

Cardiovascular System

Heart disease is the leading cause of death in the elderly. Heart failure is the leading cause of hospitalization among Medicare recipients, and it is also a major cause of morbidity and mortality among the elderly population in the United States. Age-related changes reduce the efficiency of the heart and contribute to decreased compliance of the heart muscle.

TABLE 12-2 Age-Related Changes in Body Systems and Health Promotion Strategies

Changes	Subjective and Objective Findings	Health Promotion Strategies
Cardiovascular System		
Decreased cardiac output; diminished ability to respond to stress; heart rate and stroke volume do not increase with maximum demand; slower heart recovery rate; increased blood pressure	Complaints of fatigue with increased activity Increased heart rate recovery time Normal BP ≤140/90 mm Hg	Exercise regularly; pace activities; avoid smoking; eat a low-fat, low-salt diet; participate in stress-reduction activities; check blood pressure regularly; medication compliance; weight control
Respiratory System		
Increase in residual lung volume; decrease in vital capacity; decreased gas exchange and diffusing capacity; decreased cough efficiency	Fatigue and breathlessness with sustained activity; impaired healing of tissues as a result of decreased oxygenation; difficulty coughing up secretions	Exercise regularly; avoid smoking; take adequate fluids to liquefy secretions; receive yearly influenza immunization; avoid exposure to upper respiratory tract infections
Integumentary System		
Decreased protection against trauma and sun exposure; decreased protection against temperature extremes; diminished secretion of natural oils and perspiration	Skin appears thin and wrinkled; complaints of injuries, bruises, and sunburn; complaints of intolerance to heat; bone structure is prominent; dry skin	Avoid solar exposure (clothing, sunscreen, stay indoors); dress appropriately for temperature; maintain a safe indoor temperature; shower preferable to tub bath; lubricate skin
Reproductive System		
Female: Vaginal narrowing and decreased elasticity; decreased vaginal secretions *Male:* Decreased size of penis and testes *Male and Female:* Slower sexual response	*Female:* Painful intercourse; vaginal bleeding following intercourse; vaginal itching and irritation; delayed orgasm *Male:* Delayed erection and achievement of orgasm	May require vaginal estrogen replacement; gynecology/urology follow-up; use a lubricant with intercourse
Musculoskeletal System		
Loss of bone density; loss of muscle strength and size; degenerated joint cartilage	Height loss; prone to fractures; kyphosis; back pain; loss of strength, flexibility, and endurance; joint pain	Exercise regularly; eat a high-calcium diet; limit phosphorus intake; take calcium and vitamin D supplements as prescribed
Genitourinary System		
Male: Benign prostatic hyperplasia	Urinary retention; irritative voiding symptoms including frequency, feeling of incomplete bladder emptying, multiple nighttime voidings	Seek referral to urology specialist; have ready access to toilet; wear easily manipulated clothing; drink adequate fluids; avoid bladder irritants (eg, caffeinated beverages, alcohol, artificial sweeteners); pelvic floor muscle exercises, preferably learned via biofeedback; consider urologic workup
Female: Relaxed perineal muscles, detrusor instability (urge incontinence), urethral dysfunction (stress urinary incontinence)	Urgency/frequency syndrome, decreased "warning time," bathroom mapping; drops of urine lost with cough, laugh, position change	Wear easily manipulated clothing; drink adequate fluids; avoid bladder irritants (eg, caffeinated beverages, alcohol, artificial sweeteners); pelvic floor muscle exercises, preferably learned via biofeedback; consider urologic workup
Gastrointestinal System		
Decreased salivation; difficulty swallowing food; delayed esophageal and gastric emptying; reduced gastrointestinal motility	Complaints of dry mouth; complaints of fullness, heartburn, and indigestion; constipation, flatulence, and abdominal discomfort	Use ice chips, mouthwash; brush, floss, and massage gums daily; receive regular dental care; eat small, frequent meals; sit up and avoid heavy activity after eating; limit antacids; eat a high-fiber, low-fat diet; limit laxatives; toilet regularly; drink adequate fluids

continued >

TABLE 12-2 Age-Related Changes in Body Systems and Health Promotion Strategies (Continued)

Changes	Subjective and Objective Findings	Health Promotion Strategies
Nervous System		
Reduced speed in nerve conduction; increased confusion with physical illness and loss of environmental cues; reduced cerebral circulation (becomes faint, loses balance)	Slower to respond and react; learning takes longer; becomes confused with hospital admission; faintness; frequent falls	Pace teaching; with hospitalization, encourage visitors; enhance sensory stimulation; with sudden confusion, look for cause; encourage slow rising from a resting position
Special Senses		
Vision: Diminished ability to focus on close objects; inability to tolerate glare; difficulty adjusting to changes of light intensity; decreased ability to distinguish colors	Holds objects far away from face; complains of glare; poor night vision; confuses colors	Wear eyeglasses, use sunglasses outdoors; avoid abrupt changes from dark to light; use adequate indoor lighting with area lights and nightlights; use large-print books; use magnifier for reading; avoid night driving; use contrasting colors for color coding; avoid glare of shiny surfaces and direct sunlight
Hearing: Decreased ability to hear high-frequency sounds	Gives inappropriate responses; asks people to repeat words; strains forward to hear	Recommend a hearing examination; reduce background noise; face person; enunciate clearly; speak with a low-pitched voice; use nonverbal cues
Taste and smell: Decreased ability to taste and smell	Uses excessive sugar and salt	Encourage use of lemon, spices, herbs

These changes include sclerosis of the endocardium, fibrosis of the valves, increased myocardial stiffness, decreased muscle fibers, and reduced myocardial strength (Maas et al., 2001). As a result, the heart valves become thicker and stiffer, and the heart muscle and arteries lose their elasticity. Calcium and fat deposits accumulate within arterial walls, and veins become increasingly tortuous.

It is difficult to differentiate between age- and disease-related changes in cardiovascular function because of the significant influence of behavioral factors on cardiovascular health. When cross-cultural studies are conducted, cardiovascular changes that in the past were thought to be age-related do not consistently appear. For example, the higher blood pressure found in older adults in Western societies does not occur in less developed societies and may be a result of different lifestyle behaviors rather than normal age-related changes (Miller, 2004). Under normal circumstances, the cardiovascular system can adapt to the normal age-related changes, and an older person is unaware of any significant decline in cardiovascular performance. However, when challenged, the cardiovascular system of an older person is less efficient under conditions of stress and exercise and when life-sustaining activities are needed.

Careful assessment of older people is necessary because they often present with different symptoms than those seen in younger patients. Older people are more likely to have dyspnea or neurologic symptoms associated with heart disease, and they may experience mental status changes or report vague symptoms such as fatigue, nausea, and syncope. Rather than the typical substernal chest pain associated with myocardial ischemia, older patients may report burning or sharp pain or discomfort in an area of the upper body. Complicating the assessment is the fact that many elderly patients have more than one underlying disease. When a patient complains about symptoms related to digestion and breathing and upper extremity pain, cardiac disease must be considered (Miller, 2004). The absence of chest pain in an older patient is not a good indicator of the absence of heart disease.

Hypotension may be a concern. The risk for orthostatic and postprandial hypotension increases significantly after 75 years of age (Miller, 2004). A patient experiencing hypotension should be counseled to rise slowly (from a lying, to a sitting, to a standing position), to avoid straining when having a bowel movement, and to consider having five or six small meals each day, rather than three, to minimize the hypotension that can occur after a large meal. Extremes in temperature, including hot showers and whirlpool baths, should be avoided.

Respiratory System

The respiratory system is the one system that seems to be the most able to compensate for the functional changes of aging. In general, healthy, nonsmoking, older adults show very little decline in respiratory function; however, there are substantial individual variations. The age-related changes that do occur are subtle and gradual, and healthy older adults are able to compensate for these changes (Miller, 2004). Diminished respiratory efficiency as well as reduced maximal inspiratory and expiratory force may occur as a result of calcification and weakening of the muscles of the chest wall. The alveoli within the lungs enlarge and become thinner, increasing the amount of anatomic dead space.

Conditions of stress, such as illness, may increase the demand for oxygen and affect the overall function of other systems. Like cardiovascular diseases, respiratory diseases manifest more subtly in older adults than in younger adults and do not necessarily follow the typical pattern of cough, chills, and fever. Older adults may exhibit headache, weakness, lethargy, anorexia, dehydration, and mental status changes (Miller, 2004).

Smoking is the most significant risk factor for respiratory and other diseases. Therefore, a major focus of health promotion activities should be on smoking cessation and avoidance of environmental smoke. Pneumonia and influenza together are the fifth leading cause of death in people older than 65 years of age. Education to promote the use of pneumonia and influenza vaccines is an essential nursing intervention. A pneumococcal vaccine that prevents 85% to 90% of all cases of pneumonia is available, and it is effective in preventing 75% of cases in people older than 65 years of age. Influenza vaccination is less effective in preventing influenza in the elderly than in the younger population, but it reduces influenza-related deaths, hospitalizations, and other complications (Miller, 2004).

Activities that help elderly people maintain adequate respiratory function include regular exercise, appropriate fluid intake, pneumococcal vaccination, yearly influenza immunizations, and avoidance of people who are ill. Hospitalized older adults should be frequently reminded to cough and take deep breaths, particularly postoperatively, because their decreased lung capacity and decreased cough efficiency predispose them to atelectasis and respiratory infections.

Integumentary System

The functions of the skin include protection, temperature regulation, sensation, and excretion. With aging, changes occur that affect the function and appearance of the skin. There is a decrease of epidermal proliferation, and the dermis becomes thinner. Elastic fibers are reduced in number, and collagen becomes stiffer. Subcutaneous fat diminishes, particularly in the extremities. Decreased numbers of capillaries in the skin result in diminished blood supply. These changes cause a loss of resiliency and wrinkling and sagging of the skin. The skin becomes drier and susceptible to burns, injury, and infection. Hair pigmentation may change, and balding may occur; genetic factors strongly influence these changes. These changes in the integument reduce tolerance to temperature extremes and sun exposure.

Lifestyle practices are likely to have a large impact on skin changes. Therefore, strategies to promote healthy skin function include not smoking, avoiding exposure to the sun, using a sun protection factor (SPF) of 15 or higher, using emollient skin cream containing petrolatum or mineral oil, avoiding hot soaks in the bathtub, and maintaining optimal nutrition and hydration. Older adults should be encouraged to have any suspicious changes in the skin examined, because early detection and treatment of precancerous or cancerous lesions are essential to prevent serious negative consequences.

Reproductive System

Sexuality is no longer considered pertinent only to the young. However, research about sexuality among the elderly, especially in women, has not been extensive. Ovarian production of estrogen and progesterone ceases with menopause. Changes occurring in the female reproductive system include thinning of the vaginal wall, along with a narrowing in size and a loss of elasticity; decreased vaginal secretions, resulting in vaginal dryness, itching, and decreased acidity; involution (atrophy) of the uterus and ovaries; and decreased pubococcygeal muscle tone, resulting in a relaxed vagina and perineum. Without the use of water-soluble lubricants, these changes may contribute to vaginal bleeding and painful intercourse.

In older men, the penis and testes decrease in size, and levels of androgens diminish. Decreased libido and erectile dysfunction may develop but are more likely to be associated with factors other than age-related changes. These risk factors include cardiovascular disease; neurologic disorders; diabetes; respiratory disease; pain; and medications such as cardiac drugs, vasodilators, antihypertensive agents, and tricyclic antidepressants.

Although there is a less intense response to sexual stimulation and a decline in sexual activity with increasing age, sexual desire does not disappear. Men may experience a decline in sexual function related to health conditions or interference from medications. Women may lose their partner; the absence of a partner is often a primary factor causing lack of sexual activity. Many couples are unaware of the causes of decreased libido or erectile dysfunction and are often reluctant to discuss decreased sexual function, and a thorough assessment is important. There are many methods of improving the quality of sexual interactions, but the assessment and communication require sensitivity and expert knowledge in the field of sexual dysfunction. If sexual dysfunction is present, referral to a gynecologist, urologist, or sex therapist is warranted.

Genitourinary System

The genitourinary system continues to function adequately in older people, although there is a decrease in kidney mass, primarily because of a loss of nephrons. Changes in kidney function vary widely; about one third of elderly people show no decrease in renal function (Miller, 2004). Therefore, changes in renal function may be a combination of aging and pathologic conditions such as hypertension. The changes most commonly seen include a decreased filtration rate, diminished tubular function with less efficiency in resorbing and concentrating the urine, and a slower restoration of acid–base balance in response to stress. Older adults who take medications may experience serious consequences due to decline in renal function because of impaired absorption, decreased ability to maintain fluid and electrolyte balance, and decreased ability to concentrate urine.

Certain genitourinary disorders are more common in older adults than the general population. Approximately 13 million people in the United States suffer from **urinary incontinence.** About 85% of people with incontinence are women, and this condition is often mistakenly viewed as a normal consequence of aging. It is costly and embarrassing and should be evaluated because in most cases it is reversible or can be treated (Maas et al., 2001) Urinary incontinence is discussed in more detail in Chapter 45. Benign prostatic hyperplasia (enlarged prostate gland), a common finding in older men, causes a gradual increase in urine retention and overflow incontinence. Prostate cancer, a slow-growing cancer, is most often seen in men older than 70 years of age. Kidney and bladder cancers are most frequently seen in people older than 50 years of age. Smoking is known to be a primary factor in these carcinomas.

Adequate consumption of fluids is important to reduce the risk of bladder infections and urinary incontinence.

Gastrointestinal System

Digestion of food is less influenced by age-related changes than by the risk for poor nutrition. Older people can adjust to the age-related changes but often have more difficulty in purchasing, preparing, and enjoying their meals. The sense of smell diminishes as a result of neurologic changes and environmental factors such as smoking, medications, and vitamin B_{12} deficiencies. The ability to recognize sweet, sour, bitter, or salty foods diminishes over time, altering satisfaction with food. Salivary flow does not decrease in healthy adults, but about 30% of older people may experience a dry mouth as a result of medications and diseases (Miller, 2004). Difficulties with chewing and swallowing are generally associated with disease.

Experts disagree on the extent of gastric changes that occur as a result of normal aging. However, there does appear to be a modest slowing of gastric motility, which results in delayed emptying of stomach contents and early satiation (feeling of fullness). Diminished secretion of gastric acid and pepsin, seemingly the result of pathologic conditions rather than normal aging, reduces the absorption of iron, calcium, and vitamin B_{12}. Absorption of nutrients in the small intestine, particularly calcium and vitamin D, appears to diminish with age. The function of the liver, gallbladder, and pancreas is generally maintained, although absorption and tolerance to fat may decrease. The incidence of gallstones and common bile duct stones increases progressively with advancing years.

Difficulty in swallowing, or dysphagia, affects 1 in 17 people, including 6.2 million Americans older than 60 years of age, with 300,000 to 600,000 new cases diagnosed each year. This serious condition can be life-threatening. It is caused by interruption or dysfunction of neural pathways, such as can occur with stroke. It may also result from dysfunction of the striated and smooth muscles of the gastrointestinal tract in as many as 50% of patients with Parkinson's disease and in patients with conditions such as multiple sclerosis, poliomyelitis, and amyotrophic lateral sclerosis (Lou Gehrig's disease). Aspiration of food or fluid is the most serious complication and can occur in the absence of coughing or choking (Galvan, 2001).

Constipation is a common pathologic condition that affects as many as 80% of institutionalized and 45% of community-dwelling elderly people (Miller, 2004). Symptoms of mild constipation are abdominal discomfort and flatulence, and more serious constipation leads to fecal impaction that contributes to diarrhea around the impaction, fecal incontinence, and obstruction. Predisposing factors for constipation include lack of dietary bulk, prolonged use of laxatives, use of some medications, inactivity, insufficient fluid intake, and excessive dietary fat. Ignoring the urge to defecate may also be a contributing factor.

Practices that promote gastrointestinal health include regular tooth brushing and flossing; receiving regular dental care; eating small, frequent meals; avoiding heavy activity after eating; eating a high-fiber, low-fat diet; drinking enough fluids; and avoiding the use of laxatives and antacids. Understanding that there is a direct correlation between loss of smell and taste perception and food intake helps caregivers to intervene to maintain elderly patients' nutritional health.

Nutritional Health

The social, psychological, and physiologic functions of eating influence the dietary habits of older people. Increasing age alters nutrient requirements; the elderly require fewer calories and a more nutrient-rich, healthy diet in response to alterations in body mass and a more sedentary lifestyle. Recommendations include reducing fat intake while getting enough protein, vitamins, minerals, and dietary fiber for health and disease prevention. Decreased physical activity and a slower metabolic rate reduce the number of calories needed by older adults to maintain an ideal weight. As previously stated, age-related changes that alter pleasure in eating include a decrease in taste and smell. Older people are likely to maintain a taste for sweetness but require more sugar to achieve a sweet flavor. They also may lose the ability to differentiate sour, salty, and bitter tastes. Apathy, immobility, depression, loneliness, poverty, inadequate knowledge, and poor oral health also contribute to suboptimal nutrient intake. Budgetary constraints and physical limitations may interfere with food shopping and meal preparation.

Health promotion includes encouraging a diet that is low in sodium and saturated fats and high in vegetables, fruits, and fish. Education regarding healthy foods versus foods with inadequate nutrients is helpful. Sixty-nine percent of older Americans were considered overweight or obese in 2002, and among those 65 to 74 years of age, the percentage rose from 57% to 73% in just two decades (National Center for Health Statistics, 2004).

Older adults require a variety of foods to maintain healthy nutrition. No more than 20% to 25% of dietary calories should be consumed as fat. Reducing salt intake is also advocated, because sodium reduction has been shown to correct hypertension in some people. Protein intake should be increased in later adulthood to maintain adequate nitrogen equilibrium (Chernoff, 2002). Carbohydrates, a major source of energy, should supply 55% to 60% of the daily calories. Simple sugars should be avoided and complex carbohydrates should be encouraged. Potatoes, whole grains, brown rice, and fruit are sources of minerals, vitamins, and fiber and should be encouraged. Drinking 8 to 10 eight-ounce glasses of water per day is recommended unless contraindicated by a medical condition. A multivitamin each day helps maintain daily nutritional needs. Adults older than 65 years of age should increase their daily calcium intake to 1200 g. In addition, whereas adequate vitamin D can be obtained by 10 to 15 minutes of sun exposure two or three times a week, homebound or institutionalized elderly may need 400 to 800 IU of vitamin D to avoid bone loss (National Osteoporosis Foundation, 2004).

Callen (2004) reports that as many as 50% of surgical patients and 44% of medical patients are malnourished. Furthermore, many people are unaware of dietary deficits. Nurses are in an ideal position to identify nutritional problems among their patients and to work within the patient's own framework of knowledge of his or her health status to improve health behaviors.

Sleep

Sleep disturbances affect more than 50% of adults 65 years of age or older. The elderly tend to take longer to fall asleep, awaken more easily and frequently, and spend less time in deep sleep. Consequently, they may feel that their sleep is less satisfactory (Miller, 2004). Although older adults require as much sleep as younger people, they may experience variations in their normal sleep–wake cycles, and the lack of quality sleep at night often creates the need for napping during the day. Older people are more likely to awaken because of environmental factors such as noise, pain, or nocturia.

Sleep apnea (a sleep disorder characterized by brief periods in which respirations are absent) increases with age. As many as 24% of those over 65 years of age have been diagnosed with obstructive sleep apnea (Mezey, Fulmer, Abraham, et al., 2002). Sleep apnea is discussed in more detail in Chapter 22.

The nurse is the one caregiver who observes patients while they are sleeping. The nurse can observe problems and also recommend prudent sleep hygiene behaviors such as avoiding use of the bed for activities other than sleeping (or sex), maintaining a consistent bedtime routine, avoiding or limiting daytime napping, limiting alcohol intake to less than three drinks a day, and avoiding caffeine and nicotine after noon.

Musculoskeletal System

Intact musculoskeletal and neurologic systems are essential for the maintenance of safe mobility and performance of ADLs and IADLs, which allows older adults to remain independent and live in the community. Age-related changes that affect mobility include alterations in bone remodeling, leading to decreased bone density, loss of muscle mass, deterioration of muscle fibers and cell membranes, and degeneration in the function and efficiency of joints. These factors are discussed in detail in Unit 15.

Without exercise, a gradual, progressive decrease in bone mass begins before 40 years of age. The cartilage of joints also progressively deteriorates in middle age. Degenerative joint disease is found in all adults older than 70 years, and weight-bearing joint and back pain is a common complaint. Excessive loss of bone density results in osteoporosis, which leads to potentially life-altering hip and vertebral fractures. Osteoporosis is now considered preventable, but there is concern about the future for today's young people, who are not getting enough exercise and are not consuming adequate calcium and vitamin D, even as children.

The axiom "use it or lose it" is very relevant to the physical capacity of older adults. Nurses play an important role by encouraging older adults to participate in a regular exercise program. The benefits of regular exercise cannot be overstated. Aerobic exercises are the foundation of programs of cardiovascular conditioning, but strength training and flexibility exercises are essential components of an exercise program. *Promoting Exercise and Behavior Change in Older*

NURSING RESEARCH PROFILE

Nutritional Health in Older Adults

Callen, B. (2004) Understanding nutritional health in older adults: A pilot study. *Journal of Gerontological Nursing, 30*(1), 36–42.

Purpose

This study examined the nutritional health of community-dwelling older adults admitted to a hospital for acute care who were identified as being at nutritional risk. This study solicited patients' perceptions of their nutritional health and asked patients how they could improve their nutritional status.

Design

This cross-sectional descriptive pilot study used a convenience sample of 10 community-dwelling patients 65 years of age and older who were identified as at nutritional risk by a hospital dietitian. Upon consent, researchers conducted a two-part interview and a nutritional assessment using two tools for comparison. To elicit patients' perception of their nutritional status and recommendations about how to improve their diets, researchers used an open-ended questionnaire.

Findings

Although all 10 participants were identified as at nutritional risk, none believed he or she was at risk. Consequently, no participants had suggestions regarding how they could improve their nutritional status. In most cases, the nutritional decline occurred over a long time period, suggesting that if participants had had early nutritional intervention, their state of nutrition could have improved prior to their hospitalization.

Nursing Implications

Differences between patients' perceptions of their nutritional health and those identified by the screening tools have important implications for nurses, who are ideally positioned to assess nutritional status. Patients often do not understand the negative effects of their own nutritional practices. It may be necessary to design interventions that are tailored to patients' basic knowledge level and their perceptions of their own nutritional needs.

Adults (Burbank & Reibe, 2002) is an excellent reference for designing exercise strategies for the elderly.

Even late in life, it is generally believed that exercise has the benefits of increasing strength, aerobic capacity, and flexibility. One study (Keysor & Jette, 2001) found an 88% increase in strength in older patients who participated in an exercise program compared with those who did not exercise. Even those who are very old benefit from exercise: in an early study, Fiatarone et al. (1990) reported that a group of nursing home residents 90 years of age and older who participated in a high-intensity resistance program showed significant growth in muscle strength and size and in mobility.

Nervous System

The structure and function of the nervous system change with advanced age, and a reduction in cerebral blood flow accompanies nervous system changes. The loss of nerve cells contributes to a progressive loss of brain mass, and the synthesis and metabolism of the major neurotransmitters are also reduced. Because nerve impulses are conducted more slowly, older people take longer to respond and react. The autonomic nervous system performs less efficiently, and postural hypotension, which causes people to lose consciousness or feel lightheaded when standing up quickly, may occur. Neurologic changes can affect gait and balance, which may interfere with mobility and safety. Nurses advise elderly people to allow a longer time to respond to a stimulus and to move more deliberately. Homeostasis is more difficult to maintain, but in the absence of pathologic changes, older people function adequately and retain their cognitive and intellectual abilities.

This slowed reaction time puts older people at risk for falls and injuries, including driving errors. The per-mile fatality rate for drivers 70 years of age and older is nine times that for drivers 25 to 69 years of age. Elderly people who are driving unsafely should receive a driving fitness evaluation. This is often administered by an occupational therapist in conjunction with a neuropsychologist, who conducts more detailed cognitive testing (Dolinar, McQuillen, & Ranseen, 2001).

Mental function is threatened by physical or emotional stresses. A sudden onset of confusion may be the first symptom of an infection or change in physical condition (eg, pneumonia, urinary tract infection, medication interactions, dehydration).

Sensory System

People interact with the world through their senses. Sensory losses associated with old age affect all sensory organs, and it can be devastating not to be able to see to read or watch television, hear conversation well enough to communicate, or discriminate taste well enough to enjoy food. In 2002, nearly half of older men and one third of older women reported difficulty hearing without a hearing aid. Sixteen percent of older men and 19% of older women reported difficulty seeing, even with corrective lenses (Older Americans, 2005). An uncompensated alteration in a sensory loss negatively affects the functional ability and quality of life of the older adult.

SENSORY LOSS VERSUS SENSORY DEPRIVATION

Sensory loss can often be compensated for by assistive devices such as glasses and hearing aids. In contrast, sensory deprivation is the absence of stimuli in the environment or the inability to interpret existing stimuli (perhaps as a result of a sensory loss). Sensory deprivation can lead to boredom, confusion, irritability, disorientation, and anxiety. A decline in sensory input can mimic a decline in cognition that is in fact not present. Meaningful sensory stimulation offered to the older person is often helpful in correcting this problem. One sense can substitute for another in observing and interpreting stimuli. Nurses can enhance sensory stimulation in the environment with colors, pictures, textures, tastes, smells, and sounds. The stimuli are most meaningful if they are interpreted to older people and if the stimuli are changed often. Cognitively impaired people tend to respond well to touch and to familiar music.

VISION

As new cells form on the outside surface of the lens of the eye, the older central cells accumulate and become yellow, rigid, dense, and cloudy, leaving only the outer portion of the lens elastic enough to change shape (accommodate) and focus at near and far distances. As the lens becomes less flexible, the near point of focus gets farther away. This condition, **presbyopia**, usually begins in the fifth decade of life and requires the person to wear reading glasses to magnify objects. In addition, the yellowing, cloudy lens causes light to scatter and makes the older person sensitive to glare. The ability to discern blue from green decreases. The pupil dilates slowly and less completely because of increased stiffness of the muscles of the iris, so the older person takes more time to adjust when going to and from light and dark settings and needs brighter light for close vision. Pathologic visual conditions are not a part of normal aging, but the incidence of eye disease (most commonly cataracts, glaucoma, diabetic retinopathy, and age-related macular degeneration) increases in older people.

Age-related macular degeneration is the primary cause of vision loss in the elderly. More than 25% of people older than 75 years of age have some signs of this disease, and 6% to 8% have advanced disease associated with severe vision loss. Macular degeneration does not affect peripheral vision, which means that it does not cause blindness. However, it affects central vision, color perception, and fine detail, greatly affecting common visual skills such as reading, driving, and seeing faces. Risk factors include sunlight exposure, cigarette smoking, and heredity, and people with fair skin and blue eyes may be at increased risk. Sunglasses and hats with visors provide some protection, and stopping smoking is paramount in preventing the disease. Although there is no definitive treatment and no cure that restores vision, several treatment options are available, depending on factors such as the location of the abnormal blood vessels. Photodynamic therapy, a "cool laser" therapy, is the mainstay of treatment for the wet type of acute macular degeneration (*Harvard Health Letter*, 2003). The earlier this condition is diagnosed, the greater the chances of preserving sight.

HEARING

Auditory changes begin to be noticed at about 40 years of age. Environmental factors, such as exposure to noise, medications, and infections, as well as genetics, may contribute to hearing loss as much as age-related changes. **Presbycusis** is a gradual, sensorineural loss that progresses from the loss of the ability to hear high-frequency tones to a generalized loss of hearing. It is attributed to irreversible inner ear changes. Older people often cannot follow conversation because tones of high-frequency consonants (the sounds *f, s, th, ch, sh, b, t, p*) all sound alike. Hearing loss may cause older people to respond inappropriately, misunderstand conversation, and avoid social interaction. This behavior may be erroneously interpreted as confusion. Wax buildup or other correctable problems may also be responsible for hearing difficulties. A properly prescribed and fitted hearing aid may be useful in reducing some types of hearing deficits.

TASTE AND SMELL

Of the four basic tastes (sweet, sour, salty, and bitter), sweet tastes are particularly dulled in older people. Blunted taste may contribute to the preference for salty, highly seasoned foods, but herbs, onions, garlic, and lemon can be used as substitutes for salt to flavor food.

Changes in the sense of smell are related to cell loss in the nasal passages and in the olfactory bulb in the brain. Environmental factors such as long-term exposure to toxins (eg, dust, pollen, and smoke) contribute to the cellular damage.

Cognitive Aspects of Aging

Cognition can be affected by many variables, including sensory impairment, physiologic health, environment, and psychosocial influences. Older adults may experience temporary changes in cognitive function when hospitalized or admitted to skilled nursing facilities, rehabilitation centers, or long-term care facilities. These changes are related to differences in the environment or in medical therapy, or to alteration in role performance. In 2002, the proportion of people with moderate to severe memory impairment ranged from approximately 5% among people ages 65 to 69 years to 32% among people 85 years and older (Older Americans, 2005).

Intelligence

When intelligence test scores from people of all ages are compared, test scores for older adults show a progressive decline beginning in midlife. However, research has shown that environment and health have a considerable influence on scores and that certain types of intelligence (eg, spatial perceptions and retention of nonintellectual information) decline, whereas others (eg, problem-solving ability based on past experiences, verbal comprehension, mathematical ability) do not. Cardiovascular health, a stimulating environment, high levels of education, occupational status, and income all appear to have a positive effect on intelligence scores in later life.

Learning and Memory

According to Hooyman and Kiyak (2002, p. 271), "significant age-related declines in intelligence, learning, and memory appear not to be inevitable." These authors summarized the major studies on cognitive function in later years and provided the following overview.

Many factors affect the ability of older people to learn and remember and to perform well in testing situations. Older adults who have higher levels of education, good sensory function, good nutrition, and jobs that require complex problem-solving skills continue to demonstrate intelligence, memory, and the capacity for learning. Part of the problem in testing older adults is determining what is actually being tested (eg, speed of response) and whether the test results are indicative of a normal age-related change, a sensory deficit, or poor health. However, age differences continue to emerge even with untimed tests and when the tests are controlled for variations in motor and sensory function. In general, there is a decline in fluid intelligence, the biologically determined intelligence used for flexibility in thinking and problem solving. Crystallized intelligence, that gained through education and lifelong experiences (eg, verbal skills), remains intact. This is termed the classic aging pattern of intelligence. Despite these slight declines, many older people continue to learn and participate in varied educational experiences.

Good health and motivation are important influences on learning. Nurses can support the process by which older adults learn by using the following strategies:

- Supplying mnemonics to enhance recall of related data
- Encouraging ongoing learning
- Linking new information with familiar information
- Using visual, auditory, and other sensory cues
- Encouraging learners to wear prescription glasses and hearing aids
- Providing glare-free lighting
- Providing a quiet, nondistracting environment
- Setting short-term goals with input from the learner
- Keeping teaching periods short
- Pacing learning tasks according to the endurance of the learner
- Encouraging verbal participation by learners
- Reinforcing successful learning in a positive manner

Pharmacologic Aspects of Aging

Older people use more medications than any other age group. Although they represent only 12.6% of the total population, they use 30% of all prescribed medications and 40% of all over-the-counter medications (Mezey, Fulmer, & Abraham, 2003). Medications improve the health and well-being of older people by relieving pain and discomfort, treating chronic illnesses, and curing infectious processes. However, adverse drug reactions are common because of medication interactions, multiple medication effects, incorrect dosages, and the use of multiple medications (**polypharmacy**). The potential for drug–drug interactions increases with increased drug use; such interactions are responsible for numerous emergency department and physician visits, which cost billions of dollars annually (Delafuente, 2003; Mezey et al., 2003).

Certain types of medications that carry high risks for older patients are often inappropriately prescribed. A study matching explicit criteria for appropriate prescription against a comprehensive drug benefit plan for elderly patients found that significant percentages of patients could be considered to be taking certain medications inappropriately (38% of patients taking antidepressants, 19% taking oral hypoglycemic agents, 18% taking sedative-hypnotics, and 13% taking nonsteroidal anti-inflammatory drugs [NSAIDs]) (Anderson, Beers, & Kerluke, 1997).

Any medication is capable of altering nutritional status, and the nutritional health of the elderly person may already be compromised by a marginal diet or by chronic disease and its treatment. Medications can affect the appetite, cause nausea and vomiting, irritate the stomach, cause constipation or diarrhea, and decrease absorption of nutrients. In addition, these medications may alter electrolyte balance as well as carbohydrate and fat metabolism. For example, antacids cause thiamine deficiency; cathartics diminish absorption; antibiotics and phenytoin (Dilantin) reduce utilization of folic acid; and phenothiazines, estrogens, and corticosteroids increase food intake and cause weight gain.

Combining multiple medications with alcohol, as well as with over-the-counter and herbal medications, complicates the problem. For example, St. John's wort, a common herbal supplement used for mild depression, decreases the anticoagulant effect of warfarin (Coumadin) and interacts with many other medications metabolized in the liver (Lam, 2000).

Altered Pharmacokinetics

Alterations in absorption, metabolism, distribution, and excretion occur as a result of normal aging and may also result from drug and food interactions. Absorption may be affected by changes in gastric pH and a decrease in gastrointestinal motility. Drug distribution may be altered as a result of decrease in body water and increase in body fat. Normal age-related changes and diseases that alter blood flow, liver and renal function, or cardiac output may affect distribution and metabolism (Mezey et al., 2003) (Table 12-3).

Nursing Implications

Prescription principles that have been identified for older patients include "start low and go slow" and "keep the medication regimen as simple as possible" (Mezey et al., 2003). A comprehensive assessment that begins with a thorough medication history, including use of alcohol, recreational drugs, and over-the-counter and herbal medications, is essential. It is best to ask the patient or reliable informants to provide all medications for review. Ascertaining the patient's understanding of when and how to take each medication as well as the purpose of each medication allows the nurse to assess the patient's knowledge about and compliance with the medication regimen. The patient's beliefs and concerns about the medications are identified. It is also helpful to know whether patients believe that a given medication is helpful.

Noncompliance leads to significant morbidity and mortality among the elderly. Among people 60 years of age and older, reports of noncompliance with medication regimens range from 26% to 59% (van Eijken, Tsang, Wensing, et al., 2003). The many contributing factors include the number of medications prescribed, the complexity of the regimen, difficulty opening containers, inadequate patient education, financial cost, and the disease or medication interfering with the patient's life. Furthermore, visual and hearing problems may make it difficult to read or to hear directions.

Multifaceted interventions tailored to the individual patient are the most effective strategies in improving compliance (van Eijken et al., 2003). The following steps can help patients manage their medications and improve compliance:

- Explain the purpose, adverse effects, and dosage of each medication.
- Provide the medication schedule in writing.
- Encourage the use of standard containers without safety lids (if there are no children in the household).
- Suggest the use of a multiple-day, multiple-dose medication dispenser to help the patient adhere to the medication schedule (Fig. 12-3).
- Destroy or remove old, unused medications.
- Encourage the patient to inform the primary health care provider about the use of over-the-counter medications and herbal agents, alcohol, and recreational drugs.
- Encourage the patient to keep a list of all medications, including over-the-counter and herbal medications, in his or her purse or wallet to share with the primary care provider at each visit and in case of an emergency.
- Review the medication schedule periodically and update it as necessary.
- Recommend using one supplier for prescriptions; pharmacies frequently track patients and are likely to notice a prescription problem such as duplication or contraindications in the medication regimen.
- If the patient's competence is doubtful, identify a reliable family member or friend who might monitor the patient for compliance.

Mental Health Problems in the Older Adult

Changes in cognitive ability, excessive forgetfulness, and mood swings are not a part of normal aging. These symptoms should not be dismissed as age-related changes; a thorough assessment may reveal a treatable, reversible physical or mental condition. Changes in mental status may be related to many factors, such as alterations in diet and fluid and electrolyte balance, fever, or low oxygen levels associated with many cardiovascular and pulmonary diseases. Cognitive changes may be reversible when the underlying condition is identified and treated. However, the incidence of dementia and susceptibility to depression and delirium increase with age. Older adults are less likely than younger people to seek treatment for mental health symptoms. Therefore, health professionals must recognize, assess, refer, collaborate, treat, and support older adults who exhibit noticeable changes in intellect or affect.

Depression

Depression is the most common affective or mood disorder of old age. About 15% of older Americans suffer from significant depression (Burke & Laramie, 2004). The incidence of depression is significant among the hospitalized elderly

TABLE 12-3 Altered Drug Responses in Older People

Age-Related Changes	Effect of Age-Related Change	Applicable Medications
Absorption		
Reduced gastric acid; increased pH (less acid)	Rate of drug absorption—possibly delayed	Vitamins
Reduced gastrointestinal motility; prolonged gastric emptying	Extent of drug absorption—not affected	Calcium
Distribution		
Decreased albumin sites	Serious alterations in drug binding to plasma proteins (the unbound drug gives the pharmacologic response); highly protein-bound medications have fewer binding sites, leading to increased effects and accelerated metabolism and excretion	Selected highly protein-binding medications: Oral anticoagulants (warfarin) Oral hypoglycemic agents (sulfonylureas) Barbiturates Calcium channel blockers Furosemide (Lasix) Nonsteroidal anti-inflammatory drugs (NSAIDs) Sulfonamides Quinidine Phenytoin (Dilantin)
Reduced cardiac output	Decreased perfusion of many bodily organs	
Impaired peripheral blood flow	Decreased perfusion	
Increased percentage of body fat	Proportion of body fat increases with age, resulting in increased ability to store fat-soluble medications; this causes drug accumulation, prolonged storage, and delayed excretion	Selected fat-soluble medications: Barbiturates Diazepam (Valium) Lidocaine Phenothiazines (antipsychotics) Ethanol Morphine
Decreased lean body mass	Decreased body volume allows higher peak levels of medications	
Metabolism		
Decreased cardiac output and decreased perfusion of the liver	Decreased metabolism and delay of breakdown of medications, resulting in prolonged duration of action, accumulation, and drug toxicity	All medications metabolized by the liver
Excretion		
Decreased renal blood flow; loss of functioning nephrons; decreased renal efficiency	Decreased rates of elimination and increased duration of action; danger of accumulation and drug toxicity	Selected medications with prolonged action: Aminoglycoside antibiotics Cimetidine (Tagamet) Chlorpropamide (Diabinase) Digoxin Lithium Procainamide

(12%) and increases to 30% among nursing home residents. Depression among the elderly often follows a major precipitating event or loss but may also be secondary to a medication interaction or an undiagnosed physical condition. Signs of depression include feelings of sadness, fatigue, diminished memory and concentration, feelings of guilt or worthlessness, sleep disturbances, appetite disturbances with excessive weight loss or gain, restlessness, impaired attention span, and suicidal ideation. Depression disrupts quality of life and increases the risk for suicide, especially among elderly Caucasian and Asian-American men (Kennedy-Malone, Fletcher, & Plank, 2004).

Geriatric depression may be confused with dementia. However, the cognitive impairment resulting from depression is a result of apathy rather than decline in brain function. When depression and medical illnesses coexist, as they often

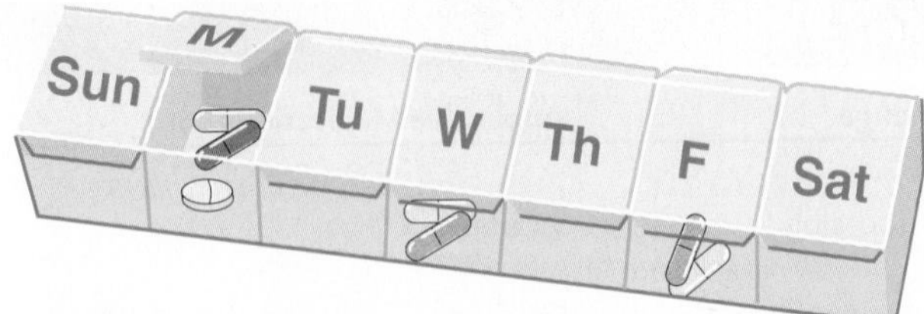

FIGURE 12-3. Commercially available, multiple-dose, multiple-day medication dispensers such as this one help older people to follow complex medication regimens safely at home.

do, neglect of the depression can retard physical recovery. Assessing the patient's mental status, including depression, is vital and must not be overlooked (Charts 12-1 and 12-2).

Depression is responsive to treatment but is often overlooked and therefore is undertreated. Initial management involves evaluation of the patient's medication regimen and eliminating or changing any medications that contribute to depression. Furthermore, treatment of underlying medical conditions that may produce depressive symptoms may alleviate the depression. Both antidepressants and short-term psychotherapy, particularly in combination, are effective in treating late-life depression. Newer atypical antidepressants, such as bupropion (Wellbutrin), venlafaxine (Effexor), mirtazapine (Remeron), and nefazodone (Serzone), and selective serotonin reuptake inhibitors, such as paroxetine (Paxil), may be used (Kennedy-Malone et al., 2004). It is recommended that the initial dose of antidepressants be low. The following factors also should be considered: age, coexisting conditions, adverse effects, and prior response to these medications. Tricyclic antidepressants are also clinically effective for depression. However, those with anticholinergic, cardiac, and orthostatic adverse effects, as well as interactions with other medications, should be used with care to avoid medication toxicity. It may take 4 to 6 weeks for symptoms to diminish, and during this period, nurses should offer explanations and encouragement.

Alcohol and Drug Abuse

Alcohol and drug abuse may be related to depression, and its incidence is significant in the elderly population. In people between 65 and 84 years of age, 35% to 38% of men and 21% to 32% of women have reported drinking moderately (one drink or less a day). Heavy drinking (more than one drink a day) is reportedly between 9% and 10% for men and between 2.2% and 2.6% for women (Breslow, Faden, & Smothers, 2003). Among 565 geriatric veteran inpatients studied, 4% were diagnosed with nonalcoholic substance disorders, 3% had prescription drug use disorders, and 1% had illegal drug use disorders (Widlitz & Marin, 2002).

Alcohol abuse is especially dangerous in older people because of changes in renal and liver function as well as the probability of interactions with prescription medications and the resultant adverse effects. Alcohol- and drug-related problems in older people often remain hidden because many older adults deny their habit when questioned.

CHART 12-1

Mini-Mental State Examination

Maximum Score	
ORIENTATION	
5	What is the (year) (season) (date) (day) (month)?
5	Where are we (state) (county) (city) (hospital) (floor)?
REGISTRATION	
3	Name three objects: One second to say each. Then ask the patient all three after you have said them. Give one point for each correct answer. Repeat them until he learns all three. Count trials and record number. Number of trials: _____.
ATTENTION AND CALCULATION	
5	Begin with 100 and count backwards by 7 (stop after five answers). Alternatively, spell "world" backwards.
RECALL	
3	Ask for the three objects repeated above. Give one point for each correct answer.
LANGUAGE	
2	Show a pencil and a watch, and ask subject to name them.
1	Repeat the following: "No 'if's,' 'and's,' or 'but's.' "
3	A three-stage command: "Take a paper in your right hand; fold it in half, and put it on the floor."
1	Read and obey the following: (Show subject the written item.) CLOSE YOUR EYES.
1	Write a sentence.
1	Copy a design (complex polygon as in Bender-Gestalt).
30	**Total score possible**

Reprinted from Folstein, M. F., Folstein, S., & McHugh, P. R. (1975). Mini-mental state: A practical method for grading the cognitive state of patients for the clinician. *Journal of Psychiatric Research*, *12*, 189–198. With permission from Pergamon Press Ltd, Headington Hill Hall, Oxford OX3 OBW, UK.

Delirium

Delirium, often called acute confusional state, begins with confusion and progresses to disorientation. Delirium affects an estimated 2.3 million elderly people and accounts for more than 17.5 annual hospital days at a cost of more than $4 billion a year; as many as 10% to 16% of elderly patients are delirious on admission to the hospital (Kennedy-Malone et al., 2004). Delirium is the most frequent complication of

CHART 12-2

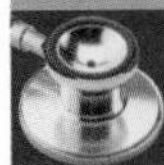

Geriatric Depression Scale

Choose the best answer for how you felt this past week.

*1.	Are you basically satisfied with your life?	YES	NO
2.	Have you dropped many of your activities and interests?	YES	NO
3.	Do you feel that your life is empty?	YES	NO
4.	Do you often get bored?	YES	NO
*5.	Are you hopeful about the future?	YES	NO
6.	Are you bothered by thoughts you can't get out of your head?	YES	NO
*7.	Are you in good spirits most of the time?	YES	NO
8.	Are you afraid that something bad is going to happen to you?	YES	NO
*9.	Do you feel happy most of the time?	YES	NO
10.	Do you often feel helpless?	YES	NO
11.	Do you often get restless and fidgety?	YES	NO
12.	Do you prefer to stay at home, rather than going out and doing new things?	YES	NO
13.	Do you frequently worry about the future?	YES	NO
14.	Do you feel you have more problems with memory than most?	YES	NO
*15.	Do you think it is wonderful to be alive now?	YES	NO
16.	Do you often feel downhearted and blue?	YES	NO
17.	Do you feel pretty worthless the way you are now?	YES	NO
18.	Do you worry a lot about the past?	YES	NO
*19.	Do you find life very exciting?	YES	NO
20.	Is it hard for you to get started on new projects?	YES	NO
*21.	Do you feel full of energy?	YES	NO
22.	Do you feel that your situation is hopeless?	YES	NO
23.	Do you think that most people are better off than you are?	YES	NO
24.	Do you frequently get upset over little things?	YES	NO
25.	Do you frequently feel like crying?	YES	NO
26.	Do you have trouble concentrating?	YES	NO
*27.	Do you enjoy getting up in the morning?	YES	NO
28.	Do you prefer to avoid social gatherings?	YES	NO
*29.	Is it easy for you to make decisions?	YES	NO
*30.	Is your mind as clear as it used to be?	YES	NO

Score: _____ (*Number of "depressed" answers*)

NORMS

Normal: 5 ± 4

Mildly depressed: 15 ± 6

Very depressed: 23 ± 5

* Appropriate (nondepressed) answers = yes; all others = no.

Yesavage, J., et al. (1983). Development and validation of a geriatric screening scale: A preliminary report. *Journal of Psychiatric Research, 17* (1), 37–49. Reprinted with permission from Pergamon Press Ltd., Headington Hill Hall, Oxford OX3 OBW, UK.

hospitalization. Patients may experience an altered level of consciousness, ranging from stupor to excessive activity. Thinking is disorganized and the attention span is short. Hallucinations, delusions, fear, anxiety, and paranoia may also be evident.

Delirium occurs secondary to a number of causes, including physical illness, medication or alcohol toxicity, dehydration, fecal impaction, malnutrition, infection, head trauma, lack of environmental cues, and sensory deprivation or overload. Older adults are particularly vulnerable to acute confusion because of their decreased biologic reserve and the large number of medications they may take. Nurses must recognize the grave implications of the acute symptoms and report them immediately. Because of the acute and unexpected onset of symptoms and the unknown underlying cause, delirium is a medical emergency. If the delirium goes unrecognized and the underlying cause is not treated, permanent, irreversible brain damage or death can follow. Attentive clinical assessment is essential, because delirium is sometimes mistaken for dementia; Table 12-4 compares

TABLE 12-4 Summary of Differences Between Dementia and Delirium

	Dementia		
	Alzheimer's Disease (AD)	***Vascular (Multi-Infarct) Dementia***	**Delirium**
Etiology	Familial (genetic [chromosomes 14, 19, 21]) Sporadic	Cardiovascular (CV) disease Cerebrovascular disease Hypertension	Drug toxicity and interactions; acute disease; trauma; chronic disease exacerbation Fluid and electrolyte disorder
Risk factors	Advanced age; genetics	Preexisting CV disease	Preexisting cognitive impairment
Occurrence	50%–60% of dementias	20% of dementias	20% of hospitalized older people
Onset	Slow	Often abrupt Follows a stroke or transient ischemic attack	Rapid, acute onset A harbinger of acute medical illness
Age of onset (yr)	Early onset AD: 30s–65 Late onset AD: 65+ Most commonly: 85+	Most commonly 50–70 yr	Any age, but predominantly in older persons
Gender	Males and females equally	Predominantly males	Males and females equally
Course	Chronic, irreversible; progressive, regular, downhill	Chronic, irreversible Fluctuating, stepwise progression	Acute
Duration	2–20 yr	Variable; years	Lasts 1 day to 1 month
Symptom progress	Onset insidious. *Early*—mild and subtle *Middle and late*—intensified Progression to death (infection or malnutrition)	Depends on location of infarct and success of treatment; death due to underlying CV disease	Symptoms are fully reversible with adequate treatment; can progress to chronicity or death if underlying condition is ignored
Mood	Early depression (30%)	Labile: mood swings	Variable
Speech/language	Speech remains intact until late in disease *Early*—mild anomia (cannot name objects); deficits progress until speech lacks meaning; echoes and repeats words and sounds; mutism.	May have speech deficit/aphasia depending on location of lesion	Fluctuating; often cannot concentrate long enough to speak
Physical signs	*Early*—no motor deficits *Middle*—apraxia (70%) (cannot perform purposeful movement) *Late*—Dysarthria (impaired speech) *End stage*—loss of all voluntary activity; positive neurologic signs	According to location of lesion: focal neurologic signs, seizures Commonly exhibits motor deficits	Signs and symptoms of underlying disease
Orientation	Becomes lost in familiar places (topographic disorientation) Has difficulty drawing three-dimensional objects (visual and spatial disorientation) Disorientation to time, place, and person—with disease progression		May fluctuate between lucidity and complete disorientation to time, place, and person
Memory	Loss is an early sign of dementia; loss of recent memory is soon followed by progressive decline in recent and remote memory		Impaired recent and remote memory; may fluctuate between lucidity and confusion
Personality	Apathy, indifference, irritability *Early disease*—social behavior intact; hides cognitive deficits *Advanced disease*—disengages from activity and relationships; suspicious; paranoid delusions caused by memory loss; aggressive; catastrophic reactions		Fluctuating; cannot focus attention to converse; alarmed by symptoms (when lucid); hallucinations; paranoid
Functional status, activities of daily living	Poor judgment in everyday activities; has progressive decline in ability to handle money, use telephone, function in home and workplace		Impaired
Attention span	Distractable; short attention span		Highly impaired; cannot maintain or shift attention

TABLE 12-4 Summary of Differences Between Dementia and Delirium (Continued)

	Dementia		
	Alzheimer's Disease (AD)	*Vascular (Multi-Infarct) Dementia*	**Delirium**
Psychomotor activity	Wandering, hyperactivity, pacing, restlessness, agitation		Variable; alternates between high agitation, hyperactivity, restlessness, and lethargy
Sleep-wake cycle	Often impaired; wandering and agitation at nighttime		Takes brief naps throughout day and night

dementia and delirium. It helps to know an individual patient's mental status prior to hospitalization and whether the changes noted are long term or are abrupt in onset.

In the management of delirium, treatment of the underlying cause is most important, and therapeutic interventions vary depending on the cause. Delirium increases the risk of falls; therefore, management of patient safety and behavioral problems is essential. Because medication interactions and toxicity are often implicated, nonessential medications should be discontinued. Nutritional and fluid intake should be supervised and monitored. The environment should be quiet and calm. To increase function and comfort, the nurse provides familiar environmental cues and encourages family members or friends to touch and talk to the patient. Ongoing mental status assessments using prior mental cognitive status as baseline are helpful in evaluating responses to treatment and to the admission to a hospital or extended-care facility. If the underlying problem is adequately treated, the patient often returns to baseline within several days.

Dementia

Dementia reportedly affects 3% to 11% of community-residing adults older than 65 years of age and about half of community-residing adults older than 85 years of age. Many of those suffering from dementia who are older than 85 reside in institutional settings. Almost 60% of adults 100 years of age and older demonstrate dementia. Despite this high incidence, clinicians fail to detect dementia in 21% to 72% of patients. For a diagnosis of dementia to be made, at least two domains of function must be altered—memory and at least one of the following: language, perception, visuospatial function, calculation, judgment, abstraction, and problem-solving (Mayo Foundation for Medical Education and Research [Mayo], 2001).

Symptoms of dementia are usually subtle in onset and often progress slowly until they are obvious and devastating. The characteristic changes fall into three general categories—cognitive, functional, and behavioral—and they eventually destroy a person's ability to function. The two most common types of dementia are Alzheimer's disease (AD), which accounts for 50% to 60% of cases, and vascular or multi-infarct dementia, which accounts for 10% to 20% of cases. Other non-Alzheimer dementias include Parkinson's disease, acquired immunodeficiency syndrome (AIDS)-related dementia, and Pick's disease; these types of dementia account for fewer than 15% of cases (National Institute of Neurological Disorders and Stroke, 2006).

Alzheimer's Disease

AD is a progressive, irreversible, degenerative neurologic disease that begins insidiously and is characterized by gradual losses of cognitive function and disturbances in behavior and affect. Although AD can occur in people as young as 40, it is uncommon before age 65. The prevalence of AD increases dramatically with increasing age, affecting 30% of those 85 and older (Harvard Men's Health Watch, 2002). There are numerous theories about the cause of age-related cognitive decline. Although the greatest risk for AD is increasing age, many environmental, dietary, and inflammatory factors also may affect whether a person suffers from this cognitive disease. AD is a form of dementia, a complex brain disorder caused by a combination of various factors (McDonald, 2002). These factors may include genes, neurotransmitter changes, vascular abnormalities, stress hormones, circadian changes, head trauma, and seizures.

AD can be classified into two types: familial or early-onset AD and sporadic or late-onset AD. Familial AD is rare, accounting for only 5% to 10% of all cases, and is frequently associated with genetic mutations. It occurs in middle-aged adults. If family members have at least one other relative with AD, then there is a familial component, which nonspecifically includes both environmental triggers and genetic determinants. Sporadic AD generally occurs in people older than 65 years of age (Marin, Sewell, & Schlechter, 2002), and it has no obvious pattern of inheritance.

Since 1995, molecular biologists have discovered specific genetic information about the various forms of AD, including genetic differences between early- and late-onset AD. These genetic differences help pinpoint risk factors associated with the disease, although the genetic indicators are not specific enough to be used as reliable diagnostic markers (Mayo, 2001).

PATHOPHYSIOLOGY

Specific neuropathologic and biochemical changes are found in patients with AD. These include neurofibrillary tangles (tangled masses of nonfunctioning neurons) and senile or neuritic plaques (deposits of amyloid protein, part of a larger protein called amyloid precursor protein [APP]) in the brain. The neuronal damage occurs primarily in the cerebral cortex and results in decreased brain size. Similar changes are found in the normal brain tissue of older adults, but to a lesser extent. Cells that use the neurotransmitter acetylcholine are those principally affected by AD. Biochemically, the enzyme active in producing acetylcholine, which is specifically involved in memory processing, is decreased.

Several theories are being tested to explain what predisposes people to develop the plaques and neurotangles that can be seen at autopsy in the brains of patients with AD (Mayo, 2001). Scientists continue to increase their understanding of the complex ways in which aging and genetic and nongenetic factors affect and damage brain cells over time, eventually leading to AD. Researchers have recently discovered how amyloid plaques form and cause neuronal death, as well as the possible relationship between various forms of tau protein and impaired function, which leads to neuronal death. (The major role of tau protein is to regulate the assembly and stability of neurons.) Researchers are also beginning to discover the roles of inflammation and oxidative stress and the contribution of brain infarctions to the disease (Iqbal & Grundke-Iqbal, 2004).

CLINICAL MANIFESTATIONS

In the early stages of AD, forgetfulness and subtle memory loss occur. Patients may experience small difficulties in work or social activities but have adequate cognitive function to hide the loss and function independently. Depression may occur. With further progression of AD, the deficits can no longer be concealed. Forgetfulness is manifested in many daily actions; patients may lose their ability to recognize familiar faces, places, and objects, and they may become lost in a familiar environment. They may repeat the same stories because they forget that they have already told them. Trying to reason with people with AD and using reality **orientation** only increases their anxiety without increasing function. Conversation becomes difficult, and word-finding difficulties occur. The ability to formulate concepts and think abstractly disappears; for example, a patient can interpret a proverb only in concrete terms. Patients are often unable to recognize the consequences of their actions and will therefore exhibit impulsive behavior. For example, on a hot day, a patient may decide to wade in the city fountain fully clothed. Patients have difficulty with everyday activities, such as operating simple appliances and handling money.

Personality changes are also usually evident. Patients may become depressed, suspicious, paranoid, hostile, and even combative. Progression of the disease intensifies the symptoms: speaking skills deteriorate to nonsense syllables, agitation and physical activity increase, and patients may wander at night. Eventually, assistance is needed for most ADLs, including eating and toileting, because dysphagia and incontinence develop. The terminal stage, in which patients are usually immobile and require total care, may last months or years. Occasionally, patients may recognize family members or caregivers. Death occurs as a result of complications such as pneumonia, malnutrition, or dehydration.

ASSESSMENT AND DIAGNOSTIC FINDINGS

A definitive diagnosis of AD can be made only at autopsy, but an accurate clinical diagnosis can be made in about 90% of cases. The most important goal is to rule out other causes of dementia or reversible causes of confusion, such as other types of dementia, depression, delirium, alcohol or drug abuse, or inappropriate drug dosage or drug toxicity (Marin et al., 2002).

The health history—including medical history, family history, social and cultural history, and medication history—and the physical examination, including functional and mental health status, are essential to the diagnosis of probable AD. Diagnostic tests, including complete blood count, chemistry profile, and vitamin B_{12} and thyroid hormone levels, as well as screening with electroencephalography, computed tomography (CT), magnetic resonance imaging (MRI), and examination of the cerebrospinal fluid may all refute or support a diagnosis of probable AD.

Depression can closely mimic early-stage AD and coexists in many patients. A depression scale is helpful in screening for underlying depression. Tests of cognitive function such as the Mini-Mental State Examination (see Chart 12-1) and the clock-drawing test are useful for screening. CT and MRI scans of the brain are useful for excluding hematoma, brain tumor, stroke, normal-pressure hydrocephalus, and atrophy but are not reliable in making a definitive diagnosis of AD. Infections, physiologic disturbances such as hypothyroidism, Parkinson's disease, and vitamin B_{12} deficiency can cause cognitive impairment that may be misdiagnosed as AD. Biochemical abnormalities can be excluded through examination of the blood and cerebrospinal fluid, but the findings are not sufficiently specific to make the diagnosis. AD is a diagnosis of exclusion, and a diagnosis of probable AD is made when the medical history, physical examination, and laboratory tests have excluded all known causes of other dementias.

MEDICAL MANAGEMENT

The primary goal in the medical management of AD is to manage the cognitive and behavioral symptoms. There is no cure and no way to slow the progression of the disease. Cholinesterase inhibitors such as donepezil hydrochloride (Aricept), rivastigmine tartrate (Exelon), and galantamine hydrobromide (Reminyl) enhance acetylcholine uptake in the brain, thus maintaining memory skills for a period of time. The drug memantine (Namenda), which is reported to reduce the clinical deterioration in moderate to severe AD, was recently approved for use in the United States (*Mental Health Weekly Digest,* 2004). One clinical trial demonstrated that use of donepezil in combination with memantine increases cognitive function in patients with AD (National Institute of Neurological Disorders and Stroke, 2003). Cognitive ability improves within 6 to 12 months of therapy, but cessation of the medications results in cognitive decline commensurate with disease progression. It is recommended that treatment continue at least through the moderate stage of the illness. Ancillary treatment with an NSAID or vitamin E may be considered; however, research supporting such treatment is limited (Marin et al., 2002).

Behavioral problems such as agitation and psychosis can be managed by behavioral and psychosocial therapies. Associated depression and behavioral problems can also be treated with antidepressants and the newer atypical neuroleptics, which are replacing the typical neuroleptics such as haloperidol (Haldol); the newer drugs have fewer adverse effects. Other atypical neuroleptics include olanzapine (Zyprexa), quetiapine fumarate (Seroquel), and risperidone (Risperdal) (Cohen, 2002).

NURSING MANAGEMENT

Nursing interventions for dementia are aimed at promoting patient function and independence for as long as possible.

Other important goals include promoting the patient's physical safety, promoting independence in self-care activities, reducing anxiety and agitation, improving communication, providing for socialization and intimacy, promoting adequate nutrition, promoting balanced activity and rest, and supporting and educating family caregivers. Nursing interventions apply to all patients with dementia, regardless of the cause.

Supporting Cognitive Function. Because dementia of any type is degenerative and progressive, patients display a decline in cognitive function over time. In the early phase of dementia, minimal cueing and guidance may be all that are needed for the patient to function fairly independently for a number of years. However, as the patient's cognitive ability declines, family members must provide more and more assistance and supervision. A calm, predictable environment helps people with AD interpret their surroundings and activities. Environmental stimuli are limited, and a regular routine is established. A quiet, pleasant manner of speaking, clear and simple explanations, and use of memory aids and cues help minimize confusion and disorientation and give patients a sense of security. Prominently displayed clocks and calendars may enhance orientation to time. Color-coding the doorway may help patients who have difficulty locating their room. Active participation may help patients maintain cognitive, functional, and social interaction abilities for a longer period. Physical activity and communication have also been demonstrated to slow some of the cognitive decline of AD (Tappen, Roach, Applegate, et al., 2000).

Promoting Physical Safety. A safe home environment allows the patient to move about as freely as possible and relieves the family of constant worry about safety. To prevent falls and other injuries, all obvious hazards are removed and hand rails are installed. A hazard-free environment allows the patient maximum independence and a sense of autonomy. Adequate lighting, especially in halls, stairs, and bathrooms, is necessary. Nightlights are helpful, particularly if the patient has increased confusion at night (**sundowning**). Driving is prohibited, and smoking is allowed only with supervision. The patient may have a short attention span and be forgetful. Wandering behavior can often be reduced by gentle persuasion or distraction. Restraints should be avoided, because they increase agitation. Doors leading from the house must be secured. Outside the home, all activities must be supervised to protect the patient, and the patient should wear an identification bracelet or neck chain in case he or she becomes separated from the caregiver.

Promoting Independence in Self-Care Activities. Pathophysiologic changes in the brain make it difficult for people with AD to maintain physical independence. Patients should be assisted to remain functionally independent for as long as possible. One way to do this is to simplify daily activities by organizing them into short, achievable steps so that the patient experiences a sense of accomplishment. Frequently, occupational therapists can suggest ways to simplify tasks or recommend adaptive equipment. Direct patient supervision is sometimes necessary, but maintaining personal dignity and autonomy is important for people with AD, who should be encouraged to make choices when appropriate and to participate in self-care activities as much as possible.

Reducing Anxiety and Agitation. Despite profound cognitive losses, patients are sometimes aware of their diminishing abilities. Patients need constant emotional support that reinforces a positive self-image. When losses of skills occur, goals are adjusted to fit the patient's declining ability.

The environment should be kept familiar and noise-free. Excitement and confusion can be upsetting and may precipitate a combative, agitated state known as a catastrophic reaction (overreaction to excessive stimulation). The patient may respond by screaming, crying, or becoming abusive (physically or verbally); this may be the person's only way of expressing an inability to cope with the environment. When this occurs, it is important to remain calm and unhurried. Forcing the patient to proceed with the activity only increases the agitation. It is better to postpone the activity until later, even to another day. Frequently, the patient quickly forgets what triggered the reaction. Measures such as moving to a familiar environment, listening to music, stroking, rocking, or distraction may quiet the patient. Structuring activity is also helpful. Becoming familiar with a particular patient's predicted responses to certain stressors helps caregivers avoid similar situations.

Many older people with dementia who have progressed to the late stages of the disease typically reside in nursing homes and are predominantly cared for by nurses' aides. Dementia education for caregivers is essential to minimize patient agitation and can be effectively taught by advanced practice nurses.

Improving Communication. To promote the patient's interpretation of messages, the nurse should remain unhurried and reduce noises and distractions. Use of clear, easy-to-understand sentences to convey messages is essential, because patients frequently forget the meaning of words or have difficulty organizing and expressing thoughts. In the earlier stages of dementia, lists and simple written instructions that serve as reminders may be helpful. In later stages, the patient may be able to point to an object or use nonverbal language to communicate. Tactile stimuli, such as hugs or hand pats, are usually interpreted as signs of affection, concern, and security.

Providing for Socialization and Intimacy Needs. Because socialization with friends can be comforting, visits, letters, and phone calls are encouraged. Visits should be brief and nonstressful; limiting visitors to one or two at a time helps reduce overstimulation. Recreation is important, and people with dementia are encouraged to enjoy simple activities. Realistic goals for activities that provide satisfaction are appropriate. Hobbies and activities such as walking, exercising, and socializing can improve the quality of life. The nonjudgmental friendliness of a pet may provide stimulation, comfort, and contentment. Care of plants or of a pet can also be satisfying and an outlet for energy.

AD does not eliminate the need for intimacy. Patients and their spouses may continue to enjoy sexual activity. Spouses should be encouraged to talk about any sexual concerns, and sexual counseling may be necessary. Simple expressions of love, such as touching and holding, are often meaningful.

Promoting Adequate Nutrition. Mealtime can be a pleasant social occasion or a time of upset and distress, and it should be kept simple and calm, without confrontations. Patients prefer familiar foods that look appetizing and taste good. To avoid any "playing" with food, one dish is offered at a time. Food is cut into small pieces to prevent choking. Liquids may be easier to swallow if they are converted to gelatin. Hot food and beverages are served warm, and the temperature of the foods should be checked to prevent burns.

When lack of coordination interferes with self-feeding, adaptive equipment is helpful. Some patients may do well eating with a spoon or with their fingers. If this is the case, an apron or a smock, rather than a bib, is used to protect clothing. As deficits progress, it may be necessary to feed the patient. Forgetfulness, disinterest, dental problems, lack of coordination, overstimulation, and choking may all serve as barriers to good nutrition and hydration.

Promoting Balanced Activity and Rest. Many patients with dementia exhibit sleep disturbances, wandering, and behaviors that may be considered inappropriate. These behaviors are most likely to occur when there are unmet underlying physical or psychological needs. Caregivers must identify the needs of patients who are exhibiting these behaviors because further health decline may occur if the source of the problem is not corrected. Adequate sleep and physical exercise are essential. If sleep is interrupted or the patient cannot fall asleep, music, warm milk, or a back rub may help the patient to relax. During the day, patients should be encouraged to participate in exercise because a regular pattern of activity and rest enhances nighttime sleep. Long periods of daytime sleeping are discouraged.

Supporting Home and Community-Based Care. The emotional burden on the families of patients with AD is enormous. The physical health of the patient is often very stable, and the mental degeneration is gradual. Family members may cling to the hope that the diagnosis is incorrect and that their relative will improve with greater effort. Family members are faced with numerous difficult decisions (eg, when the patient should stop driving, when to assume responsibility for the patient's financial affairs). Aggression and hostility exhibited by the patient are often misunderstood by families or caregivers, who feel unappreciated, frustrated, and angry. Feelings of guilt, nervousness, and worry contribute to caregiver fatigue, depression, and family dysfunction.

In some cases, caregivers themselves can become so fatigued as a result of the stress of caregiving that self-neglect or neglect or abuse of the patient can occur. This has been documented in home situations as well as in institutions. If neglect or abuse of any kind—including physical, emotional, sexual, or financial abuse—is suspected, the local adult protective services agency must be notified. The role of the nurse is to report the suspected abuse, not to prove it.

The Alzheimer's Disease and Related Disorders Association is a coalition of family members and professionals who share the goals of family support and service, education, research, and advocacy. This national organization has addressed the multiple needs of family caregivers. Family support groups, respite (relief) care, and adult day care may be available through different community resources, such as the Area Agency on Aging or the Alzheimer's Disease and Related Disorders Association, in which concerned volunteers are trained to provide structure to caregiver support groups. Respite care is a commonly provided service in which caregivers can get away from the home for short periods while someone else tends to the needs of the patient.

Vascular Dementia

Vascular or multi-infarct dementia is associated with hypertension and cardiovascular disease. It is sometimes confused with AD, paranoia, or delirium because of its unpredictable clinical course. Vascular dementia tends to have a more abrupt onset than AD, and it is characterized by an uneven, stepwise downward decline in mental function associated with a vascular incident such as a subclinical stroke. Diagnosis may be even more difficult if a patient has both AD and vascular dementia.

Because vascular dementia is associated with hypertension and cardiovascular disease, risk factors (eg, hypercholesterolemia, history of smoking, diabetes mellitus) are similar. Prevention and management are also similar. Therefore, therapy to decrease blood pressure and lower cholesterol levels may prevent future mini-infarcts. In addition, clinical trials have shown that giving donepezil hydrochloride (Aricept) to patients with vascular dementia enhances cognitive function (*Chemist and Druggist*, 2003).

Common Health Issues of the Older Adult

To widely varying extents, elderly people tend to acquire multiple problems and illnesses as they age. The decline of physical function leads to a loss of independence and increasing frailty as well as to susceptibility to both acute and chronic health problems, which generally result from several factors rather than from a single cause. When combined with a decrease in host resistance, these factors can lead to illness or injury. Although the problems may develop slowly, the onset of symptoms is often acute. Furthermore, the presenting symptoms may appear in other body systems before becoming apparent in the affected system.

The term "frail" is used to describe elderly people who are at highest risk for adverse health outcomes. According to the most widely accepted definition, people who are frail tend to be 85 or older, suffer from multiple chronic diseases, and have difficulty performing IADLs or ADLs independently. However, there are no standard clinical criteria for frailty.

Impaired Mobility

The causes of decreased mobility are many and varied. Common causes are Parkinson's disease, diabetic neuropathy, cardiovascular compromise, osteoarthritis, osteoporosis, and sensory deficits. Environmental barriers and iatrogenic factors are also significant. Elderly patients should be encouraged to stay as active as possible to avoid the downward spiral of immobility. During illness, bed rest should be kept to a minimum, because even brief periods of bed rest quickly lead to deconditioning and, consequently, to a wide range of complications. When bed rest cannot be avoided, patients should perform active range-of-motion and strengthening exercises with the unaffected extremities, and nurses or family caregivers should perform passive range-of-motion exercises on the affected extremities. Frequent position changes help offset the hazards of immobility. Both the health care staff and the patient's family can assist in maintaining the current level of mobility (Tappen et al., 2000).

Dizziness

Older people frequently seek help for dizziness, which presents a particular challenge because there are so many possible internal and external causes. For many, the problem is complicated by an inability to differentiate between true dizziness (a sensation of disorientation in relation to position) and vertigo (a spinning sensation). Other similar sensations include near-syncope and disequilibrium. The causes for these sensations range in severity from minor (eg, buildup of ear wax) to severe (eg, dysfunction of the cerebral cortex, cerebellum, brainstem, proprioceptive receptors, or vestibular system). Even a minor reversible cause, such as ear wax impaction, can result in a loss of balance and a subsequent fall and injury. Because dizziness has many predisposing factors, nurses should seek to identify any potentially treatable factors related to the condition. This preventive strategy may reduce the vulnerability of older people to injury (Tinetti, Williams, & Gill, 2000).

Falls and Falling

Injuries rank seventh as a cause of death for older people, and falls are the leading cause of injury in the elderly, accounting for 62% of all nonfatal injuries treated in emergency departments in 2001 (Public Health and Aging, 2003). Between 35% and 40% of community-dwelling elderly people and 60% of nursing home residents fall annually, and about half fall multiple times. The incidence of falls rises with increasing age and tends to be highest in those 80 and older.

Although most falls by elderly adults do not result in injury, between 5% and 10% of elderly people who fall sustain serious injury. The most common fracture occurring from falls is hip fracture, which results from both osteoporosis and the situation that provoked the fall. Of the estimated 1% of elderly adults who fall and sustain a hip fracture, 20% to 30% die within 1 year of the fracture (Tideiksaar, 2003). Overall, elderly women who fall sustain a greater degree of injury than elderly men.

Causes of falls are multifactorial. Both extrinsic factors such as changes in the environment or poor lighting and intrinsic factors such as physical illness, neurologic changes, or sensory impairment play a role. Use of many medications, medication interactions, and use of alcohol precipitate falls by causing drowsiness, decreased coordination, and postural hypotension. Falls have physical dangers as well as serious psychological and social consequences. It is not uncommon for an older person who has experienced a fall to become fearful and lose self-confidence (Public Health and Aging, 2003; Tideiksaar, 2003).

Nurses can encourage older adults and their families to make lifestyle and environmental changes to prevent falls. Adequate lighting with minimal glare and shadow can be achieved through the use of small area lamps, indirect lighting, sheer curtains to diffuse direct sunlight, dull rather than shiny surfaces, and nightlights. Sharply contrasting colors can be used to mark the edges of stairs. Grab bars by the bathtub, shower, and toilet are useful. Loose clothing, improperly fitting shoes, scatter rugs, small objects, and pets create hazards and increase the risk for falls. Older adults function best in familiar settings when the arrangement of furniture and objects remains unchanged, if safely possible.

In institutionalized elderly people, physical restraints (lap belts; geriatric chairs; vest, waist, and jacket restraints) and chemical restraints (medications) precipitate many of the injuries they were meant to prevent. Documented injuries and deaths resulting from these restraints include strangulation, vascular and neurologic damage, pressure ulcers, skin tears, fractures, increased confusion, and significant emotional trauma. The time required to supervise restrained patients adequately is better used addressing the unmet need that provoked the behavior that resulted in the use of restraint. Because of the overwhelming negative consequences of restraint use, accrediting agencies of nursing homes and acute care facilities now maintain stringent guidelines concerning their use (Capezuti, Strumpf, Evans, et al., 1999).

Urinary Incontinence

Urinary incontinence may be acute, occurring during an illness, or it may develop chronically over a period of years. Older patients often do not report this very common problem unless specifically asked. Transient causes may be attributed to *d*elirium and *d*ehydration; *r*estricted mobility and restraints; *i*nflammation, *i*nfection, and *i*mpaction; and *p*harmaceuticals and *p*olyuria (the acronym *drip* may be used to remember them). Once identified, the causative factor can be eliminated. Incontinence may also be a result of neurologic or structural abnormalities. Urinary incontinence has been associated with depression and low self-esteem and may reduce the patient's quality of life by causing restriction in social activities.

The pelvic floor serves as the supporting mechanism or "hammock" for the bladder, uterus, and rectum. It may have become weakened as a result of pregnancy, labor and delivery, prior pelvic surgeries, or activities that required prolonged standing or lifting. Dysfunction of the pelvic floor can be greatly improved with Kegel exercises. Other measures that help prevent episodes of incontinence include having quick access to toilet facilities and wearing clothing that can be unfastened easily.

Patients with incontinence should be urged to seek help from appropriate health care providers, because incontinence can be both emotionally devastating and physically debilitating. Nurses who specialize in behavioral approaches to urinary incontinence management can assist patients to regain full continence or to significantly improve the level of continence. Although medications such as anticholinergics may decrease some of the symptoms of urge incontinence (detrusor instability), the adverse effects of these drugs (dry mouth, slowed gastrointestinal motility, and confusion) may make them inappropriate choices for the elderly. Various surgical procedures are also used to manage urinary incontinence, particularly stress urinary incontinence.

Detrusor hyperactivity with impaired contractility is a type of urge incontinence that is seen predominantly in the elderly population. In this variation of urge incontinence, patients have no warning that they are about to urinate. They often void only a small volume of urine or none at all and then experience a large volume of incontinence after leaving the bathroom. The nursing staff should be familiar with this form of incontinence and should not show disapproval when it occurs. Many patients with dementia suffer from this type of incontinence, because both incontinence and dementia are a result of dysfunction in similar areas of the brain. Prompted, timed voiding can be of assistance in these patients, although clean intermittent catheterization may be necessary because of postvoid residual urine.

Increased Susceptibility to Infection

Infectious diseases present a significant threat of morbidity and mortality to older people, in part because of the blunted response of host defenses caused by a reduction in both cell-mediated and humoral immunity (see Chapters 50 and 51). Age-related loss of physiologic reserve and chronic illnesses also contribute to increased susceptibility. Pneumonia, urinary tract infections, tuberculosis (TB), gastrointestinal infections, and skin infections are some of the common infections in older people.

The effects of influenza and pneumococcal infections on older people are also significant. An estimated 10% to 20% of Americans have influenza each year; an average of 114,000 are hospitalized with influenza-related complications, and 36,000 die (CDC, 2004). Hospital-acquired pneumonia is responsible for 300,000 deaths annually in the United States, making it the second most common nosocomial infection (after urinary tract infection) and the leading cause of death from hospital-acquired infection. Many of these deaths involve older adults because of their increased vulnerability to infection (Smith-Sims, 2001).

The influenza vaccine is prepared yearly to adjust for the specific immunologic characteristics of the influenza viruses at that time. This inactivated preparation should be administered annually in the fall. The pneumococcal vaccine has 23 type-specific capsular polysaccharides. Protection lasts 4 years or longer, and revaccination is recommended every 5 years. Both of these injections can be received at the same time in separate injection sites. Nurses should urge older people to be vaccinated. All health care providers working with older people or high-risk chronically ill people should also be immunized.

TB affects a significant number of older adults. Case rates for TB are highest among those who are 65 or older, with the exception of people with human immunodeficiency virus (HIV) infection. Nursing home residents account for the majority of the cases of TB in older adults. Much of the infection rate is attributed to reactivation of old infection. Pulmonary TB and extrapulmonary TB often have subtle, nonspecific symptoms. This is of particular concern in nursing homes, because an active case of TB places patients and staff at risk for infection.

The Centers for Disease Control and Prevention (CDC) guidelines suggest that all patients newly admitted to nursing homes have a Mantoux (purified protein derivative [PPD]) test unless there is a history of TB or a previous positive response. All patients whose tests are negative (a positive test is indicated by induration of more than 10 mm at 48 to 72 hours) should have a second test in 1 to 2 weeks. The first PPD serves to boost the suppressed immune response that may occur in older people. Chest x-rays and possibly sputum studies should be used to follow up on PPD-positive responders and converters. For positive converters, a course of preventive therapy for 6 to 9 months with isoniazid (INH) is effective in eliminating active disease. All patients who test negative should be periodically retested (CDC, 2004).

AIDS is no longer only a disease of young people. It is increasingly recognized that AIDS does not spare the older segment of society. According to the CDC, between 1981 and 1989, more than 10% of all AIDS patients nationwide were 50 or older at the time of diagnosis, and about 3% were 60 or older. In that report, male homosexual contact and blood transfusions were the predominant modes of transmission among older patients. Transmission by contaminated blood products has declined in recent years, and the predominant mode of transmission in older people now is by sexual contact. The most common AIDS-indicator disease in older people is *Pneumocystis* pneumonia (PCP). Wasting syndrome and HIV encephalopathy are also common in older HIV-infected people.

Altered Pain and Febrile Responses

Many altered physical, emotional, and systemic reactions to disease are attributed to age-related changes in older people. Physical indicators of illness that are useful and reliable in young and middle-aged people cannot be relied on for the diagnosis of potential life-threatening problems in older adults. The response to pain in older people may be lessened because of reduced acuity of touch, alterations in neural pathways, and diminished processing of sensory data.

Research has demonstrated that many older adults experiencing a myocardial infarction do not have chest pain. Hiatal hernia or upper gastrointestinal distress is often responsible for chest pain in elderly people. Acute abdominal conditions may go unrecognized in elderly people because of atypical signs and absence of pain.

The baseline body temperature for older people is about 1°F lower than it is for younger people. In the event of illness, therefore, the body temperature of an older person may not be high enough to qualify as a traditionally defined "fever." A temperature of 37.8°C (100°F), in combination with systemic symptoms, may signal infection. A temperature of 38.3°C (101°F) almost certainly indicates a serious infection that needs prompt attention. A blunted fever in the face of an infection often indicates a poor prognosis. Temperatures rarely exceed 39.5°C (103°F). Nurses must be alert to other subtle signs of infection, such as mental confusion, increased respirations, tachycardia, and changed facial appearance and color.

Altered Emotional Impact

The emotional component of illness in older people may differ from that in younger people. Many elderly people equate good health with the absence of old age and believe "you are as old as you feel." An illness that requires hospitalization or a change in lifestyle is an imminent threat to well-being. Admission to the hospital is often feared and actively avoided. Older people admitted to the hospital are at high risk for disorientation, confusion, change in level of consciousness, and other symptoms of delirium, as well as anxiety and fear. In addition, economic concerns and fear of becoming a burden to families often lead to high anxiety in older people. Nurses must recognize the implications of fear, anxiety, and dependency in elderly patients. They should encourage autonomy and independent decision making. A positive and confident demeanor in nurses and family members promotes a positive mental outlook in elderly patients.

Altered Systemic Response

In an elderly person, illness has far-reaching repercussions. The decline in organ function that occurs in every system of the aging body eventually depletes the body's ability to respond at full capacity. Illness places new demands on body systems that have little or no reserve to meet the crisis. Homeostasis, the ability of the body to maintain an internal balance of function and chemical composition, is jeopardized. Older people may be unable to respond effectively to an acute illness or, if a chronic health condition is present, they may be unable to sustain appropriate responses over a long period. Furthermore, their ability to respond to definitive treatment is impaired. The altered responses of older adults reinforce the need for nurses to monitor all body system functions closely, being alert to signs of impending systemic complication.

Other Aspects of Health Care of the Older Adult

Elder Neglect and Abuse

Older adults who live in communities and institutions are at risk for abuse and neglect, and studies indicate that the prevalence rate is 3% to 5% (about 5 million older Americans). Elder neglect and abuse are believed to be underreported and more widespread than previously thought; one study estimated that 84% of cases are not reported. Both victims and perpetrators are reluctant to report the abuse, and clinicians seemingly are unaware of the frequency of the problems (Levine, 2003).

Neglect is the most common type of abuse, and self-neglect constitutes almost 50% of the caseload of workers in Adult Protective Services. Other forms of abuse are physical, emotional, sexual, and financial abuse. Contributing factors include a family history of violence, mental illness, and drug or alcohol abuse, as well as financial dependency on the older person. In addition, diminished cognitive and physical function or disruptive and abusive behavior on the part of the older person can lead to caregiver strain and emotional exhaustion. Elderly people with disabilities of all types are at increased risk for abuse from family members and paid caregivers (Levine, 2003).

Nurses should be alert to possible **elder abuse** and neglect. During the health history, the elderly person should be asked about abuse during a private portion of the interview. Most states require that care providers, including nurses, report suspected abuse. Preventive action should be taken when caregiver strain is evident, before elder abuse occurs. Early detection and intervention may provide sufficient resources to the family or person at risk to ensure patient safety. Interdisciplinary team members, including the psychologist, social worker, or chaplain, can be enlisted to help the caregiver develop self-awareness, increased insight, and an understanding of the disease or aging process. Community resources also may be useful for both the elderly person and the caregiver (Geldmacher, Heck, & O'Toole, 2001).

Social Services

Since the 1960s, many programs have been instituted for older Americans, including Medicare, Medicaid, the Older Americans Act, Supplemental Security Income (SSI), Social Security amendments, Section 202 housing, and Title XX social services legislation. These federal programs have dramatically increased health care options and financial support for elderly Americans. The Older Americans Act mandated creation of a federal aging network, resulting in the establishment of the Area Agencies on Aging (AAAs), a national system of social services and network for the elderly. Many community services for the elderly are available through the more than 700 AAAs. Each state has an advisory network that is charged with overseeing statewide planning and advocacy for the elderly throughout the state. Among the services provided by the AAAs are assessment of need, information and referral, case management, transportation, outreach, homemaker services, day care, nutritional education and congregate meals, legal services, respite care, senior centers, and part-time community work. The AAAs target low-income, ethnic minority, rural-living, and frail elders who are at risk for institutionalization; however, the assessment and information services are available to all elderly people (Hooyman & Kiyak, 2002). Similar services such as homemaker, home health aide, and chore services can be obtained at an hourly rate through these agencies or through local community nursing services if the family does not meet the low-income criteria. Informal sources of help, such as family, friends, mail carriers, church members, and neighbors, can all keep an informal watch on community-dwelling senior citizens.

Other community support services are available to help older people outside the home. Senior centers have social and health promotion activities, and some provide a nutritious noontime meal. Adult day care facilities offer daily nursing care and social opportunities for elderly people who cannot be left alone. Adult day care services, although expensive, provide respite and enable family members to carry on daily activities while the older person is at the day care center.

Health Care Costs of Aging

Health care is a major expenditure for the elderly, especially for those with chronic illness and limited financial resources. The elderly, who make up about 13% of the population, consume more than 33% of health care costs, particularly in the last year of life (Hoover et al., 2002). They occupy about half of the adult hospital beds, use more than two thirds of the available health care services, and spend 3 times as many days in hospitals and 30 times as many days in long-term care facilities than younger people (Miller, 2004). Therefore, whenever nurses work with an adult population, they are likely to encounter a majority of elderly patients.

The two major programs that finance health in the United States are Medicare and Medicaid, both of which are overseen by the Centers for Medicaid and Medicare Services (CMS).

Medicare is funded by the federal government, whereas Medicaid is funded jointly by the federal and state governments to provide health care for the poor. Medicare is the source of payment for acute health care for most older Americans. The services covered under Medicare have changed over the past decade, but principally it covers acute care needs such as inpatient hospitalization, physician care, outpatient care, home health services, and skilled nursing care in a nursing facility. In 2001, Medicare funding covered slightly more than half (54%) of the health care costs for those older than 65 years of age. Medicaid covered 10% of health care costs for older Americans and 46% of nursing home costs. Older Americans paid 15% out of pocket for their health care costs and 48% of their nursing home costs (National Center for Health Statistics, 2004).

In 1996, 1% of Medicare beneficiaries who were 65 or older incurred 13% of health care expenditures in that age group, and the top 5% of beneficiaries with the highest expenditures incurred 37% of all health expenditures (Older Americans, 2003). Medicare pays for only about 55% of all personal health costs, requiring the patient to pay the balance (Liu et al., 2002). For older adults with limited incomes, even with the support of Medicare, paying out-of-pocket expenses can be a hardship that at times they are unable to afford. Despite the recent additional Medicare prescription benefit plan, out-of-pocket expenditures and prescription costs are burdensome.

Use of home care services and skilled nursing home care increases markedly with age (Older Americans, 2003). Eligibility and costs for Medicaid services vary from state to state. As more and more people in the United States become eligible for publicly funded health programs in the future, there are serious concerns about whether sufficient health services will be available.

Home Health Care

Because of the rapidly growing elderly population and the availability of Medicare funding for acute care, including home care, home health care in the United States rapidly expanded in the 1990s. By the end of the 1990s, home health care had come to represent almost 10% of the total Medicare budget. Home health care, or visiting nursing, is the specialty practice of nursing applied in the home to patients with a wide range of illnesses and chronic conditions. Although people of all ages receive home care, 70% of home care patients are 65 and older (Administration on Aging, 2004). Medicare is a primary payer of home care services.

Home care involves the individual patient, the family, and caregivers. Home care nurses are generally considered skilled generalists who are holistic in their approach to care. In addition to providing skilled nursing care, home care nurses also consider the needs of the family and the impact of the environment and community on the patient situation, and they identify areas for collaboration and referral. Care is episodic (periodic short visits). Home care agencies generally offer several services, including skilled nursing; hospice care; physical, occupational, and speech therapy; and home health aide and homemaker services. Consultation with specialists in nutrition, cardiac, diabetic, and wound care is available. As hospital stays have shortened, the acuity level of home care patients has risen dramatically. "High-tech" therapies such as infusion therapy are frequently available. The primary goal is to promote optimal health and independent function in the home for both patients and their families.

Hospice Services

Hospice is a program of supportive and palliative services for terminally ill patients and their families that includes physical, psychological, social, and spiritual care. In most cases, patients are not expected to live longer than 6 months. The goal of hospice is to improve the quality of life by focusing on symptom management, pain control, and emotional support. Under Medicare and Medicaid, all needed medical and nursing services are provided to keep patients as pain-free and comfortable as possible. Hospice services may be incorporated into the care of residents in long-term care facilities and include care for end-stage dementia.

Home care and hospice nurses are in a unique position to facilitate discussions about a patient's wishes and goals at the end of life. Too often, discussion regarding end-of-life care is postponed until a crisis occurs, making it difficult or impossible for the patient to be an active participant in the discussion. Home health nurses can assist patients and families by identifying options and initiating conversation about preparing an end-of-life plan. For an in-depth discussion of hospice care, see Chapter 17.

Aging With a Disability

As the life expectancy of people with all types of physical, cognitive, and mental disabilities has increased, individuals must deal with the normal changes associated with aging in addition to their pre-existing disabilities. There are still large gaps in our understanding of the interaction between disabilities and aging, including how this interaction varies depending on the type and degree of disability and other factors such as socioeconomics and gender. For adults without disabilities, the changes associated with aging may be minor inconveniences. For adults with disorders such as polio, multiple sclerosis, and cerebral palsy, aging may lead to greater disability. In addition, many people with disabilities are greatly concerned and fearful about what will happen to them as they age and whether assistance will be available when they need care.

Minkler and Fadem (2002) support a "new paradigm of disability," which was first suggested by Bleecker (2000). Under this paradigm, a person with a disability should be viewed as someone who needs an accommodation to function rather than as someone who cannot function because of an impairment. Use of this functional approach would encourage public policies that support full participation of all citizens, such as personal assistants and accessible and affordable transportation. Therefore, research and public policy must focus on supports and interventions that allow people with preexisting disabilities who are aging to increase or maintain function within their personal environment as well as in the outside community. Important questions include the following: Who will provide the care? How will it be financed? Qualitative research would be particularly helpful in providing insight into the lives and therefore the needs of older people with disabilities.

Today, children born with intellectual and physical disabilities and those who acquire them early in life are also living into middle and older age. Often, their care has been provided by the family, primarily by the parents. As the parents age and can no longer provide the needed care, they are seeking additional help with the care or long-term care alternatives for their children. However, few services are available at present to support a smooth transition between caregiving by parents and then by others (Bigby, Ozanne, & Gordon, 2002). Again, further research is needed to identify the needs and to guide policy makers who design services and resources for this population of aging adults.

Ethical and Legal Issues Affecting the Older Adult

Nurses play an important role in supporting and informing patients and families when making treatment decisions. This nursing role becomes even more important in the care of aging patients who are facing serious, life-altering, and possibly end-of-life decisions. There is the potential for loss of rights, victimization, and other serious problems if a patient has made no plans for personal and property management in the event of disability or death. As advocates, nurses can encourage end-of-life decision making and educate older people to prepare advance care planning for future decision making in the event of incapacitation (Plotkin & Roche, 2000).

An **advance directive** is a formal, legally endorsed document that provides instructions for care (living will) or names a proxy decision maker (**durable power of attorney**). It is to be implemented if the signer becomes incapacitated. This written document must be signed by the person and by two witnesses, and a copy should be given to the physician and placed in the medical record. The person must understand that the advance directive is not meant to be used only when certain (or all) types of medical treatment are withheld; rather, it allows for a detailed description of all health care preferences, including full use of all available medical interventions. The health care proxy has the authority to interpret the patient's wishes on the basis of medical circumstances and is not restricted to the decisions or situations stated in the living will, such as whether life-sustaining treatment can be withdrawn or withheld.

When such serious decisions are made, possibilities exist for significant conflict of values among patients, family members, health care providers, and the legal establishment. Autonomy and self-determination are Western concepts, and people from different cultures may view advance directives as a method for denial of care. Elderly people from some cultures may be unwilling to consider the future, or they may wish to protect relatives and not want them to be informed about a serious illness. Nurses can facilitate the decision-making process by being sensitive to the complexity of patients' values and respecting that decision making is a process that occurs over time. Directives must be focused on the wishes of the patient, not those of the family or the designated proxy (Mezey et al., 2003) (Chart 12-3).

CHART 12-3

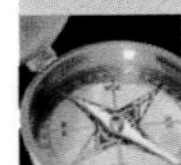

Ethics and Related Issues

Should an Elderly Person be Allowed to Refuse a Feeding Tube When the Primary Care Practitioner Believes it Would Enhance the Person's Quality of Life?

SITUATION

This patient is an 82-year-old retired office worker who has never married and who has a close relationship with her many nieces and nephews. Until suffering several small strokes following her 80th birthday, she lived independently, drove, and participated in many family and community functions. She appeared to recover from the strokes, and for the next year she continued to drive and engaged in social activities. One year prior to her admission to the nursing home, she suffered another stroke and required a gastric tube for long-term feeding. Gradually, she recovered sufficiently to have the tube removed; however, she continued to experience difficulty swallowing and ate only puddings and ice cream. She was cognitively intact but slowly becoming weaker.

Eight months later, the patient's primary care practitioner recommended reinserting the gastric tube to improve her nutritional status. She refused placement of the gastric tube. The nursing staff and family members disagreed about what should be done about her refusal and can make a case for both positions.

DILEMMA

Several ethical issues were relevant to the resolution of the situation. The obligation to respect the patient's autonomy in the decision to refuse gastric feedings affects her nutritional status and may even have put her life at risk. She had had a gastric tube in the past and understood what it is and the purpose of the gastric feedings. The nurses who care for her watched her deteriorate and realized that there was a possible medical solution. However, not all the nurses and family members were in agreement about what to do.

DISCUSSION

1. What arguments would you offer *against* reinsertion of the gastric tube?
2. What arguments would you offer *in favor* of reinsertion of the gastric tube?
3. What arguments would you offer *against* and *in favor of* supporting the patient in her decision to refuse the feeding tube?

If no advance arrangement has been made and the older person appears unable to make decisions, anyone can petition the court for a competency hearing. Mezey et al. (2003) report that anecdotally, about 30% of the elderly do not have a relative, friend, or guardian who could make health care decisions for them. If the court rules that an elderly person is incompetent, the judge will appoint a guardian—a third party who is given powers by the court to assume responsibility for making financial or personal decisions for that person.

People with communication difficulties or mild dementia may be viewed as incapable of self-determination. Most people with mild dementia have sufficient cognitive capability to make some, but perhaps not all, decisions. For example, a patient may be able to identify a proxy decision maker yet be unable to select specific treatment options (Mezey et al., 2003). People with mild dementia may be competent to understand the nature and significance of such decisions.

In 1990, the Patient Self-Determination Act (PSDA), a federal law, was enacted to require patient education about advance directives at the time of hospital admission, as well as documentation of this education. Nursing homes are also mandated by PSDA to enhance residents' autonomy by increasing their involvement in health care decision making. A growing body of research indicates that nursing homes implement the PSDA more vigorously than hospitals. However, in both settings, the documentation and placement of advance directives in the medical record and the education of patients about advance directives vary considerably from facility to facility. Processes for fulfilling the requirements of the law are continuously being revised in many facilities to promote compliance. The PSDA provides no guidelines regarding how often the advance directives of nursing home residents should be reviewed. Continuing quality improvement programs that establish guidelines for review are more likely to exist in nursing homes that have ethics committees.

Critical Thinking Exercises

1 You recently have accepted a position as staff educator at a local hospital. You have met with a group of newly hired nurses and overheard several of them saying that they hoped they would not be assigned to the skilled nursing facility at the hospital, where many of the patients are elderly. One comment was, "That would be the lowest level of nursing—more like babysitting." You realize you need to plan a program for these new nurses to address their misconceptions about care for the elderly. What would be important for these nurses to learn? What issues would you discuss? What recommendations would you make?

2 You are a community health nurse assigned to a neighborhood senior center that provides lunch and activities for 50 to 75 seniors a day. You are concerned about the many medications the seniors report taking and would like to provide a "brown bag medication review." To initiate this program, you ask each senior to bring all of the medications he or she takes to the senior center the following week. What information would you also provide to the seniors in preparation for the review to make the review as useful as possible? What health care providers would you ask to participate in this review? During the review, what information would you seek from each senior and what information would you provide?

3 ebp You are a charge nurse in an emergency department when a 75-year-old man with late-stage Alzheimer's disease is admitted with "mental status changes." His vital signs are stable. He is generally pleasant but confused and at times becomes easily agitated. What is the evidence base that indicates how elderly people respond to acute illnesses? What is the strength of the evidence? Based on the evidence-based information that you have found, what assessment parameters would you evaluate? What laboratory and clinical studies would you expect to be ordered? What information would you obtain from the patient's caregiver? What plan of action would you initiate?

REFERENCES AND SELECTED READINGS

BOOKS

Administration on Aging (2005). A profile of older Americans: 2005. Available at: http://www.aoa.gov/prof/Statistics/profile/2005/2.asp. Accessed May 11, 2006.

Administration on Aging (2004). A profile of older Americans: 2003. Available at: http://www.aoa.gov/prof/Statistics/profile/2003/2_pf.asp. Accessed May 11, 2006.

Albert, S. M. (2004). *Public health and aging: An introduction to maximizing function and well-being.* New York: Springer.

Bales, C. W., & Ritchie, C. S. (2003). *Handbook of clinical nutrition and aging.* Totowa, NJ: Humana Press.

Blass, J., Halter, J., Hazzard, W., et al. (2003). *Principles of geriatric medicine and gerontology.* New York: McGraw-Hill.

Beers, M. H. (2004). *Merck manual of health and aging.* Whitehouse Station, NJ: Merck & Co.

Beers, M. H., & Berkow, R. (2000). *Merck manual of geriatrics* (3rd ed.). Whitehouse Station, NJ: Merck & Co.

Burbank, P. M., & Reibe, D. (Eds.). (2002). *Promoting exercise and behavior change in older adults.* New York: Springer.

Burke, M. M., & Laramie, J. A. (2004). *Primary care of the older adult* (2nd ed.). St. Louis: Mosby.

CDC (2004). Key facts about influenza and the influenza vaccine. Available at: http://www.cdc.gov/flu/keyfacts.htm. Accessed May 11, 2006.

Centers for Medicare and Medicaid Services. (2002). *Home health PPS.* Baltimore: Author. Available at: http://www.cms.hhs.gov/HomeHealthPPS. Accessed May 11, 2006.

Division of Tuberculosis Elimination. Available at: http://www.cdc.gov/nchstp/tb/faqs/qa_latenttbinf.htm#Infection3. Accessed May 11, 2003.

Ebersole, P. R., Hess, P., & Luggen, A. S. (2004). *Toward healthy aging: Human needs & nursing response* (6th ed.). Philadelphia: Mosby.

Eliopoulos, C. (2005). *Gerontological nursing* (6th ed.). Philadelphia: Lippincott Williams & Wilkins.

Erikson, E. H. (1963). *Childhood and society* (2nd ed.). New York: W. W. Norton.

Fryer, G. (2001). Normal changes with aging. In M. L. Mass (Ed.), *Nursing care of older adults: Diagnoses, outcomes, & interventions.* Philadelphia: Mosby.

Gallo, J. J., Fulmer, T., Paveza, G. J., et al. (2000). *Handbook of geriatric assessment* (3rd ed.). Gaithersburg, MD: Aspen.

Ham, R. J., & Warshaw G. (2001). *Primary care geriatrics: A case-based approach* (4th ed.). St. Louis: Mosby–Year Book.

Health Services Research on Aging. (2000, January). *Building on biomedical and clinical research. Translating research into practice fact sheet.* (AHRQ Publication No. 00-P012). Rockville, MD: Agency for Healthcare Research and Quality. Available at: http://www.ahrq.gov/research/tripage.htm. Accessed May 11, 2006.

Health, United States (2003a). Chartbook on trends in the health of Americans. National Centers for Health Statistics. Available at: http://www.cdc.gov/nchs/data/hus/hus03cht.pdf. Accessed May 11, 2006.

Health, United States (2003b). Chartbook on trends in the health of Americans. National Centers for Health Statistics. Available at: http://www.cdc.gov/nchs/data/hus/tables/2003/03hus056.pdf. Accessed May 11, 2006.

Hogstel, M. O. (2001). *Gerontology: Nursing care of the older adult.* Albany: Delmar Publishing.

Holmes, D., Teresi, J. A., & Ory, M. (2000). *Special care units: Research and practice in Alzheimer disease,* Vol. 4. New York: Springer.

Hooyman, N. R., & Kiyak, H. A. (2002). *Social gerontology: A multidisciplinary perspective* (6th ed.). Boston: Allyn & Bacon.

Kane, R. L. (2004). *Essentials of clinical geriatrics* (5th ed.). New York: McGraw-Hill.

Kennedy-Malone, L., Fletcher, K. R., & Plank, L. M. (2004). *Management guidelines for nurse practitioners* working with older adults. Philadelphia: F. A. Davis.

Lawton, M. P. (1982). Competence, environmental press, and the adaptation of older people. In M. P. Lawton, P. G., Windley & T. O. Byerts (Eds.), *Aging and the environment: Theoretical approaches.* New York: Springer.

Liu, H., Ginsberg, C. Olin, G., et al. (2002). *Health and health care of the Medicare population: Data from the 1996 Medicare current beneficiary survey.* Rockville, MD: West.

Lueckenotte, A. G. (2000). *Gerontologic nursing* (2nd ed.). St. Louis: Mosby–Year Book.

Maas, M. L., Buckwalter, K. C., Hardy, M. D., et al. (2001). *Nursing care of older adults: Diagnosis, outcomes, & interventions.* St. Louis: Mosby.

Markson, E. W. (2003). *Social gerontology today: An introduction.* Los Angeles: Roxbury Publishing Co.

Mayo Foundation for Medical Education and Research. (2001). *Dementia: Epidemiology.* Available at: http://www.mayo.edu/geriatrics-rst/Dementia.I.html.

Mezey, M., Fulmer, T., Abraham, I., et al. (2002). *Geriatric nursing protocols for best practice* (2nd ed.). New York: Springer.

Mezey, M. D., Berkman, B. J., & Callahan, C. (2000). *The encyclopedia of elder care: The comprehensive resource on geriatric and social care.* New York: Springer.

Miller, C. A. (2004). *Nursing for wellness in older adults: Theory and practice* (4th ed.). Philadelphia: Lippincott Williams & Wilkins.

National Center for Health Statistics (2004). Available at: http://www.cdc.gov/nchs/fastats/pdf/nvbr50_btl.pdf. Accessed May 11, 2006.

National Institute of Neurological Disorders and Stroke (reviewed January 24, 2006). *NINDS Pick's disease information page.* Available at: http://www.ninds.nih.gov/disorders/Niemann/Niemann.htm

National Institute of Neurological Disorders and Stroke (2006). *NINDS Alzheimer disease information page.* Available at: http://www.ninds.nih.gov/health_and_medical/disorders/alzheimersdisease_doc.htm. Accessed May 4, 2006.

National Osteoporosis Foundation (2004). *Prevention, Calcium & Vitamin D.* Available at: http://www.nof.org/prevention/calcium.htm. Accessed May 11, 2006.

Neugarten, B. L. (1961). *Personality in middle and late life.* New York: Atherton Press.

Noelker, L. S., & Harel, Z. (2000). *Linking quality of long term care and quality of life.* New York: Springer.

Older Americans 2000 (2005). *Key indicators of well-being.* Available at: http://www.agingstats.gov/. Accessed May 11, 2006.

Schmidt Luggen, A., Meiner, S. E., & National Gerontological Nursing Association (2000). *NGNA: Core curriculum for gerontological nursing* (2nd ed.). St. Louis: Mosby.

Silin, P. S. (2001). *Nursing homes: The family's journey.* Baltimore: Johns Hopkins University Press.

Strumpf, N. E., Evans, L. K., Wagner, J., et al. (1992). *Reducing restraints: Individualized approaches to behavior. A teaching guide.* Huntingdon Valley, PA: Geriatric Research and Training Center.

JOURNALS

**Asterisks indicate nursing research articles.*

Adams, W., Atkinson, R., Ganz, S. B., et al. (2000). Alcohol problems in the elderly. *Patient Care for the Nurse Practitioner, 10*(3), 68–89.

Anderson, G. M., Beers, M. H., & Kerluke, K. (1997). Auditing prescription practice using explicit criteria and computerized drug benefit claims data. *Journal of Evaluation in Clinical Practice,* (4)3, 283.

Atchley, R. C. (1989). Continuity theory of normal aging. *Gerontologist, 29*(2), 183–190.

Bigby, C., Ozanne, E., & Gordon, M. (2002). Facilitating transition: Elements of successful case management practice for older parents of adults with intellectual disability. *Journal of Gerontological Social Work, 37*(i3–4), 25.

Bleecker, T. (2000). The new paradigm of disability: Implications for research and policy. *Consumer Choice, 4,* 1, 3.

Breslow, R. A., Faden, V. B., & Smothers, B. (2003). Alcohol consumption by elderly Americans. *Journal of Studies on Alcohol, (64)6,* 884.

*Callen, B. (2004) Understanding nutritional health in older adults: A pilot study. *Journal of Gerontological Nursing, 30*(1), 36.

*Capezuti, E. (2000). Preventing falls and injuries while reducing side rail use. *Annals of Long Term Care, 8*(6), 57–63.

*Capezuti, E., Strumpf, N., Evans, L. K., et al. (1999). Outcomes of nighttime physical restraint removal for severely impaired nursing home residents. *American Journal of Alzheimer Disease, 14*(1), 157–164.

*Capezuti, E., Strumpf, N. E., Evans, L. K., et al. (1998). The relationship between physical restraint removal and falls and injuries among nursing home residents. *Journal of Gerontology, Series A, 53*(1), M47.

Chemist and Druggist (Aug. 30, 2003). Donezepil helps vascular dementia, p. 16.

Chernoff, R. (2002). Health promotion for older women: Benefits of nutrition and exercise programs. *Topics in Geriatric Rehabilitation, 1*(18), 59.

Cohen, G. D. (2002). Alzheimer disease: Managing behavioral problems in patients with progressive dementia. *Geriatrics,* 2(57), 53–54.

Delafuente, J. C. (2003). Understanding and preventing drug interactions in elderly patients. *Critical Reviews in Oncology/Hematology,* 2(48), 133.

DiMaria-Ghadili, R. A., & Amello, E. (2005). Nutrition in older adults. *American Journal of Nursing, 105*(3), 40–51.

Dolinar, T. M., McQuillen, A. D., Ranseen, J. D., et al. (2001). Health, safety, and the older driver. *Patient Care, 35*(4), 22–34.

Edwards, N. (2003). Differentiating the three D's: Delirium, dementia, and depression. *MEDSURG Nursing, 12*(6), 347–357.

Falgoust, M. (2004). United States 85 and over population by state. Communication with Mark Falgoust, Statistical Analyst II, PA Department of Health, Aug. 31, 2004.

Fiatarone, M. A., Marks, E. C., Ryan, N. D., et al. (1990). High-intensity strength training in nonagenarians: Effects on skeletal muscle. *Journal of American Medical Association, 263*(8), 3029.

*Forbes, D. A. (2001). Enhancing mastery and sense of coherence: Important determinants of health in older adults. *Geriatric Nursing, 22*(1), 29–32.

*Galvan, T. J. (2001). Dysphagia: Going down and staying down. *American Journal of Nursing, 101*(1), 37–42.

Geldmacher, D. S., Heck, E., & O'Toole, E. (2001). Providing for the caregiver. *Patient Care for the Nurse Practitioner, 4*(2), 36–48.

Goldrick, B. A. (2005). Infection in the older adult. *American Journal of Nursing, 105*(6), 31–34.

Harvard Health Letter (2003). The latest on macular degeneration, *28*(7).

Harvard Men's Health Watch (June 6, 2002). Lest we forget, II: Alzheimer disease. Issue 11.

Havighurst, R. J. (1968). Personality and patterns of aging. *Gerontologist, 8,* 20–23.

Heidrich, S. M., & Wells, T. J. (2004) Effects of urinary incontinence: Psychological well-being and distress in older community dwelling women. *Journal of Gerontological Nursing, 30*(5), 47–54.

Hoban, S., & Kearney, K. (2000). Elder abuse and neglect: It takes many forms—If you're not looking, you may miss it. *American Journal of Nursing, 100*(1), 49–50.

Hofmann, M. T., & Nahass, D. (2001). Case report: The use of an ethics committee regarding the case of an elderly female with blood loss after hip surgery. *Annals of Long-Term Care, 9*(3), 55–59.

Hoover, D. R., Crystal, S., Kumar, R., et al. (2002). Medical expenditures during the last year of life: Findings from the 1992–1996 Medicare current beneficiary survey. *Health Services Research, 37*(6), 1625–1642.

Iqbal, K., & Grundke-Iqbal, I., (2004). Inhibition of neurofibrilary degeneration: A promising approach to Alzheimer disease and other taupathies. *Current Drug Targets, 5*(6), 495–501.

Keysor, J. J., & Jette, A. M. (2001). Have we over-sold the benefit of late-life exercise? *Journal of Gerontology, Series B, (51)3,* S150.

Kiely, D. K., Simon, S. E., Jones, R. N., et al. (2000). The protective effect of social engagement on mortality in long-term care. *Journal of the American Geriatrics Society, 48*(11), 1367–1372.

Lam, Y. W. F. (2000). Warfarin, St. John's Wort effect on P-450 enzymes. *Psychopharmacology Update, 5*(11), 2.

Levine, J. M. (2003). Elder neglect and abuse: A primer for primary care physicians. *Geriatrics, 58(10),* 37.

Marin, D. B., Sewell, M. C. & Schlechter, A. (2002). Alzheimer disease: Accurate and early diagnosis in the primary care setting. *Geriatrics, 57*(2), 36–40.

McDonald, R. J. (2002). Multiple combinations of co-factors produce variants of age-related cognitive decline: A theory. *Canadian Journal of Experimental Psychology, 56*(3), 221–239.

Mental Health Weekly Digest (July 26, 2004). Mechanisms of memantine activity determined. Via NewsRx.com and NewsRx.net, p. 9.

Mezey, M., Mitty, E., & Ramsey, G. (1997). Assessment of decision making capacity: Nurses' role. *Journal of Gerontological Nursing, 23*(3), 28–35.

Miles, S. H., & Irvine, P. (1992). Deaths caused by physical restraints. *Gerontologist, 32*(6), 762–766.

Minkler, M., & Fadem, P. (2002). "Successful aging:" A disability perspective. *Journal of Disability Policy Studies, 12*(4), 229–235.

Myers, J. E. (2003). Coping with caregiver stress: A wellness-oriented, strengths-based approach for family counselors. *Family Journal, 11*(2), 153–161.

*Naylor, M., Brooten, D., Campbell, R., et al. (1999). Comprehensive discharge planning and home follow-up of hospitalized elders. *Journal of American Medical Association, 281*(7), 613–620.

Naylor, M. D., Stephens, C., Bowles, K. H., et al. (2005). Cognitively impaired older adults: From hospital to home. *American Journal of Nursing, 105*(2), 52–61.

*Norlander, L., & McSteen, K. (2000). The kitchen table discussion: A creative way to discuss end-of-life issues. *Home Healthcare Nurse, 18*(8), 532–540.

Nusbaum, N. J. (2000). Issues in home rehabilitative care. *Annals of Long-Term Care, 8*(11), 43–48.

Patient Self-Determination Act (PSDA). (1990). *Omnibus Budget Reconciliation Act.* Title IV, Sec. 4206. *Congressional Record,* 12368, ct 26.

Peterson, J. A. (2001). Osteoporosis overview. *Geriatric Nursing, 22*(5), 17–23.

*Plotkin, K., & Roche, J. (2000). The future of home and hospice care: Linking interventions to outcomes in home health care. *Home Healthcare Nurse, 18*(8), 442–450.

Public health and aging: Non-fatal injuries among older adults treated in hospital emergency departments, United States, 2001. (2003). *Journal of American Medical Association, 290*(20), 2657–2658.

*Resnick, B. (2001). Promoting health in older adults: A four-year analysis. *Journal of the American Academy of Nurse Practitioners, 13*(1), 23–33.

Ruckenstein, M. J. (2001). The dizzy patient: How you can help. *Consultant, 41,* 29–34.

*Ryden, M. B., Snyder, M., Gross, C. R., et al. (2000). Value-added outcomes: The lure of advanced practice nurses in long-term care facilities. *Gerontologist, 40*(6), 654–662.

*Schafer, S. L. (2001). Prescribing for seniors: It's a balancing act. *Journal of American Academy of Nurse Practitioners, 13,* 108–112.

Shugrue, D. T., & Larocque, K. L. (1996). Reducing restraint use in the acute care setting. *Nursing Management, 25*(10), 32H.

Silverstein, M., & Lablotsky, D. L. (1996) Health and social precursors of late life retirement-community migration. *Journal of Gerontology, Series B, (51)3,* S150.

*Smith-Sims, K. (2001). Hospital-acquired pneumonia. *American Journal of Nursing, 101*(1), 24AA–24EE.

Specht, J. K. P. (2005). Myths of incontinence in older adults. *American Journal of Nursing, 105*(6), 58–69.

Spillman, B. (2001). A conversation with Brenda Spillman, Ph.D.: Interface interview. *Long-Term Care Interface, 2,* 27–29.

*Tappen, R., Roach, K., Applegate, E. B., et al. (2000). Effect of a combined walking and conversation intervention on functional mobility of nursing home residents with Alzheimer disease. *Alzheimer Disease and Associated Disorders, 14*(4), 196–201.

Tideiksaar, R. (2003). Best practice approach to fall prevention in community living elders. *Topics in Geriatric Rehabilitation, 19*(3), 199–205.

Tinetti, M. E., Williams, C. S., & Gill, T. M. (2000). Dizziness among older adults: A possible geriatric syndrome. *Annals of Internal Medicine, 132,* 337–344.

Tumolo, J. (2000). Caregivers who hurt: The tragedy of elder abuse. *Advance for Nurse Practitioners, 8*(9), 63–65.

Van Eijken, M., Tsang, S., Wensing, M., et al. (2003). Interventions to improve medication compliance on older patients living in the community: A systematic review of the literature. *Drugs & Aging, 20*(3), 229–240.

Wagner, L. S., & Wagner, T. H. (2003). The effect of age on the use of health and self-care information: Confronting the stereotype. *Gerontologist, 43*(3), 318–324.

Widlitz, M., & Marin, D. B. (2002). Substance in older adults: an overview. *Geriatrics, 57*(12), 29–34.

RESOURCES

Administration on Aging, 1 Massachusetts Avenue, Suites 4100 & 5100, Washington, DC 20201; 202-619-0724; http://www.aoa.dhhs.gov. Accessed May 13, 2006.

Alzheimer's Disease and Related Disorders Association, Inc., 225 N. Michigan Avenue, 17th floor, Chicago, IL 60601; 800-272-3900; http://www.alz.org. Accessed May 13, 2006.

American Association for Geriatric Psychiatry (AAGP), 7910 Woodmont Ave., Suite 1050, Bethesda, MD 20814; 301-654-7850; http://www.aagpgpa.org. Accessed May 13, 2006.

American Association of Homes and Services for the Aging, 2519 Connecticut Avenue NW, Washington, DC 20008; 1-202-783-2242; http://www.aahsa.org. Accessed May 13, 2006.

American Association of Retired Persons, 601 E Street NW, Washington, DC 20049; 888-687-2277; http://www.aarp.org. Accessed May 13, 2006.

American Federation for Aging Research (AFAR), 70 West 40th Street, 11th Floor, New York, NY 10018; 212-703-9977, 888-582-2327; http://www.afar.org. Accessed May 13, 2006.

American Foundation for the Blind, 15 West 16th Street, New York, NY 10011; 212-620-2000; http://www.afb.org. Accessed May 13, 2006.

American Geriatrics Society, Empire State Building, 350 Fifth Ave, Suite 801, New York, NY 10118; 212-308-1414; http://www.americangeriatrics.org. Accessed May 13, 2006.

Association for Gerontology in Higher Education (AGHE), 1030 15th Street, NW, Suite 240, Washington, DC 20005; 202-289-9806; 202-289-9824 (fax); http://www.aghe.org. Accessed May 13, 2006.

Children of Aging Parents (CAPS), PO Box 167, Richboro, PA 18954; 800-227-7294; http://www.caps4caregivers.org. Accessed May 13, 2006.

Elderhostel, 877-426-8056; http://www.elderhostel.org. Accessed May 13, 2006).

Family Caregiver Alliance (FCA), 690 Market St., San Francisco, CA 94104; 800-445-8106; http://www.caregiver.org. Accessed May 13, 2006.

Gerontological Society of America (GSA), 1030 15th Street NW, Suite 250, Washington, DC 20005; 202-842-1275; http://www.geron.org. Accessed May 13, 2006.

Legal Services for the Elderly, 17th Floor, 130 West 42nd Street, New York, NY 10036; 212-391-0120

National Association of State Units on Aging, 1201 15th Street NW, Suite 350, Washington, DC 20005; 1-202-898-2586; http://www.nasua.org. Accessed May 13, 2006.

National Caucus and Center on Black Aged, Inc., Suite 500, 1424 K Street NW, Washington, DC 20005; 202-637-8400

National Council on the Aging, Inc., 202-479-1200; http://www.ncoa.org. Accessed May 13, 2006.

National Gerontological Nursing Association, 7794 Grow Drive, Pensacola, FL 32514; 800-723-0560; http://www.ngna.org. Accessed May 13, 2006).

Nurse Competence in Aging Initiative; http://www.geronurseonline.org. Accessed May 13, 2006.

Safe Return (program for locating lost patients), Box A-3956, Chicago, IL 60690; 800-572-1122 (to report a lost patient).

UNIT 3

Concepts and Challenges in Patient Management

Case Study

Applying Concepts from NANDA, NIC, and NOC

A Patient With Debilitating Pain

Mr. Southers is a 48-year-old man who sustained a back injury in a work-related incident. He reports severe shooting pains in his lower back and both buttocks. Mr. Southers is not a candidate for surgery and has undergone physical therapy with little improvement in his pain. He reports that the pain makes it impossible for him to return to his former job, work around the house, or obtain enjoyment from leisure activities. He has been referred to a pain clinic for management.

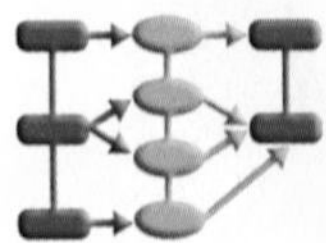

Turn to Appendix C to see a concept map that illustrates the relationships that exist between the nursing diagnoses, interventions, and outcomes for the patient's clinical problems.

Nursing Classifications and Languages

NANDA Nursing Diagnoses	NIC Nursing Interventions	NOC Nursing Outcomes Return to functional baseline status, stabilization of, or improvement in:
Chronic Pain—Unpleasant sensory and emotional experience arising from actual or potential tissue damage or described in terms of such damage; sudden or slow onset of any intensity from mild to severe, constant or recurring, without an anticipated or predictable end and a duration of greater than 6 months	**Pain Management**—Alleviation of pain or reduction in pain to a level of comfort that is acceptable to the patient	**Pain Level**—Severity of observed or reported pain
Risk for Powerlessness—At risk for perceived lack of control over a situation and/or one's ability to significantly affect an outcome	**Medication Management**—Facilitation of safe and effective use of prescribed or over-the-counter medicine	**Comfort Level**—Extent of positive perception of physical and psychological ease
	Simple Relaxation Therapy—Use of techniques to encourage and elicit relaxation for the purpose of decreasing undesirable signs and symptoms such as pain, muscle tension, or anxiety	**Pain Control**—Personal actions to control pain
	Simple Guided Imagery—Purposeful use of imagination to achieve relaxation and/or direct attention away from undesirable sensations	**Pain: Disruptive Effects**—Severity of observed or reported disruptive effects of chronic pain on daily functioning
	Emotional Support—Provision of reassurance, acceptance, and encouragement during times of stress	**Pain: Adverse Psychological Response**—Severity of observed or reported adverse responses to physical pain
	Self-Esteem Enhancement—Assisting a patient to increase his or her personal judgment of self-worth	

NANDA International (2005). *Nursing diagnoses: Definitions & classification 2005–2006.* Philadelphia: North American Nursing Diagnosis Association.

Dochterman, J. M. & Bulechek, G. M. (2004). *Nursing interventions classification (NIC)* (4th ed.). St. Louis: Mosby.

Iowa Outcomes Project (2004). In Moorhead, S., Johnson, M. & Maas, M. (2004). *Nursing outcomes classification (NOC)* (3rd ed.). St. Louis: Mosby.

Dochterman, J. M. & Jones, D. A. (2003). *Unifying nursing languages: The harmonization of NANDA, NIC, and NOC.* Washington, D.C.: American Nurses Association.

CHAPTER 13

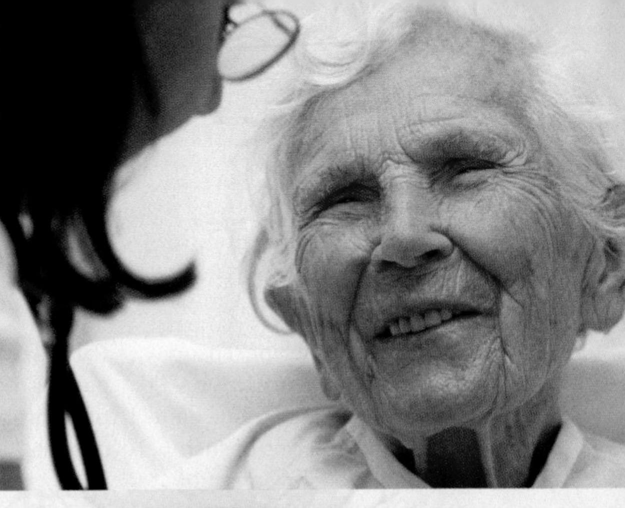

Pain Management

Learning Objectives

On completion of this chapter, the learner will be able to:

1. Compare characteristics of acute pain, chronic (persistent) pain, and cancer pain.
2. Describe the negative consequences of pain.
3. Describe the pathophysiology of pain.
4. Describe factors that can alter the perception of pain.
5. Demonstrate appropriate use of pain measurement instruments.
6. Explain the physiologic basis of pain relief interventions.
7. Explain the impact of aging on pain.
8. Discuss when opioid tolerance may be a problem.
9. Identify appropriate pain relief interventions for selected groups of patients.
10. Compare the various types of neurosurgical procedures used to treat intractable pain.
11. Develop a plan to prevent and treat the adverse effects of analgesic agents.
12. Use the nursing process as a framework for the care of patients with pain.

Pain has been defined as an unpleasant sensory and emotional experience associated with actual or potential tissue damage (Merskey & Bogduk, 1994). It is the most common reason for seeking health care. It occurs as the result of many disorders, diagnostic tests, and treatments. It disables and distresses more people than any single disease. Because nurses spend more time with patients in pain than other health care providers do, nurses need to understand the pathophysiology of pain, the physiologic and psychological consequences of acute and chronic (persistent) pain, and the methods used to treat pain. Nurses encounter patients in pain in a variety of settings, including acute care, outpatient, and long-term care settings, as well as in the home. Therefore, they must have the knowledge and skills to assess pain, to implement pain relief strategies, and to evaluate the effectiveness of these strategies, regardless of setting.

Pain: The Fifth Vital Sign

Pain management is considered such an important part of care that the American Pain Society (2003) refers to pain as "the fifth vital sign" to emphasize its significance and to increase the awareness among health care professionals of the importance of effective pain management. Documentation of pain assessment is now as prominent as documentation of the "traditional" vital signs. Pain assessment and management are also mandated by the Joint Commission on the Accreditation of Healthcare Organizations (JCAHO) (2005).

Identifying pain as the fifth vital sign suggests that the assessment of pain should be as automatic as taking a patient's blood pressure and pulse. The JCAHO (2005) has incorporated pain assessment and management into its standards. JCAHO's standards state that "pain is assessed in all patients" and that "patients have the right to appropriate assessment and management of pain." Most institutions require the nurse to document assessment of the patient's pain in the medical record (Arnstein, 2003).

These standards reflect the importance of pain management. The American Pain Foundation developed the Pain Care Bill of Rights, which addresses the importance of pain management (Chart 13-1). To date, California is the only state to have enacted a Pain Patient's Bill of Rights. In addition, the United States Congress identified 2000 to 2010 as the Decade of Pain Control and Research. In 2003, Congress passed the National Pain Care Policy Act (NPCPA), the first comprehensive and proactive pain care legislation. This Act established a White House Conference on Pain Care to educate the public that pain is a significant health problem. In addition, the NPCPA authorized a National Center for Pain and Palliative Care Research within the National Institutes of Health (headaches.about.com/cs/advocacy/a/npcpa_call.htm; accessed March 12, 2006).

Glossary

addiction: a behavioral pattern of substance use characterized by a compulsion to take the substance (drug or alcohol) primarily to experience its psychic effects

agonist: a substance that when combined with the receptor produces the drug effect or desired effect. Endorphins and morphine are agonists on the opioid receptors.

algogenic: causing pain

antagonist: a substance that blocks or reverses the effects of the agonist by occupying the receptor site without producing the drug effect. Naloxone (Narcan) is an opioid antagonist.

balanced analgesia: using more than one form of analgesia concurrently to obtain more pain relief with fewer side effects

breakthrough pain: a sudden and temporary increase in pain occurring in a patient being managed with opioid analgesia

endorphins and enkephalins: morphine-like substances produced by the body. Primarily found in the central nervous system, they have the potential to reduce pain.

dependence: occurs when a patient who has been taking opioids experiences a withdrawal syndrome when the opioids are discontinued; often occurs with opioid tolerance and does not indicate an addiction

nociception: activation of sensory transduction in nerves by thermal, mechanical, or chemical energy impinging on specialized nerve endings. The nerves involved convey information about tissue damage to the central nervous system.

nociceptor: a receptor preferentially sensitive to a noxious stimulus

non-nociceptor: nerve fiber that usually does not transmit pain

opioid: a morphine-like compound that produces bodily effects including pain relief, sedation, constipation, and respiratory depression. This term is preferred over narcotic.

pain: an unpleasant sensory and emotional experience resulting from actual or potential tissue damage

pain threshold: the point at which a stimulus is perceived as painful

pain tolerance: the maximum intensity or duration of pain that a person is willing to endure

patient-controlled analgesia (PCA): self-administration of analgesic agents by a patient instructed about the procedure

placebo effect: analgesia that results from the expectation that a substance will work, not from the actual substance itself

prostaglandins: chemical substances that increase the sensitivity of pain receptors by enhancing the pain-provoking effect of bradykinin

referred pain: pain perceived as coming from an area different from that in which the pathology is occurring. An example would be the perception of left arm or jaw pain in a person having a myocardial infarction.

sensitization: a heightened response seen after exposure to a noxious stimulus. Response to the same stimulus is to feel more pain.

tolerance: occurs when a person who has been taking opioids becomes less sensitive to their analgesic properties (and usually side effects). Characterized by the need for increasing doses to maintain the same level of pain relief.

CHART 13-1

Pain Care Bill of Rights

Although not always required by law, these are the rights you should expect, and if necessary demand, for your pain care.

As a person with pain, you have the right to

- Have your report of pain taken seriously and be treated with dignity and respect by doctors, nurses, pharmacists, and other health care professionals.
- Have your pain thoroughly assessed and promptly treated.
- Be informed by your health care provider about what may be causing the pain, possible treatments, and the benefits, risks, and cost of each.
- Participate actively in decisions about how to manage your pain.
- Have your pain reassessed regularly and your treatment adjusted if your pain has not been eased.
- Be referred to a pain specialist if your pain persists.
- Get clear and prompt answers to your questions, take time to make decisions, and refuse a particular type of treatment if you choose.

Courtesy of the American Pain Foundation, 201 N. Charles Street, Suite 710, Baltimore, MD 21201, *www.painfoundation.org*

The role of primary health care providers is to assess and relieve pain by administering medications and other treatments. Nurses collaborate with other health care professionals while administering most pain relief interventions, evaluating their effectiveness, and serving as patient advocates when the intervention is ineffective. In addition, nurses serve as educators to patients and families, teaching them to manage the pain relief regimen themselves when appropriate.

The definition of pain of the International Association for the Study of Pain identified at the beginning of this chapter encompasses the multidimensional nature of pain (Merskey & Bogduk, 1994). A broad definition of pain is, "whatever the person says it is, existing whenever the experiencing person says it does" (McCaffery & Pasero, 1999). This definition emphasizes the highly subjective nature of pain and pain management. Patients are the best authority on the existence of pain. Therefore, validation of the existence of pain is based on the patient's report that it exists.

Although it is important to believe patients who report pain, it is equally important to be alert to patients who deny pain in situations where pain would be expected. A nurse who suspects pain in a patient who denies it should explore with the patient the reason for suspecting pain, such as the fact that the disorder or procedure is usually painful or that the patient grimaces when moving or avoids movement. It may also be helpful to explore why the patient may be denying that he or she is in pain. Some people deny pain because they fear the treatment that may result if they report or admit pain. Others deny pain for fear of becoming addicted to **opioids** (previously referred to as narcotics) if these medications are prescribed.

Types of Pain

Pain is categorized according to its duration, location, and etiology. Three basic categories of pain are generally recognized: acute pain, chronic (persistent, nonmalignant) pain, and cancer-related pain. To further clarify pain terminology and treatment, many pain specialists now refer to chronic pain as persistent pain (ie, pain that is not relieved by many different interventions (American Geriatrics Society [AGS] Guidelines, 2002).

Acute Pain

Usually of recent onset and commonly associated with a specific injury, acute pain indicates that damage or injury has occurred. Pain is significant in that it draws attention to its existence and teaches people to avoid similar potentially painful situations. If no lasting damage occurs and no systemic disease exists, acute pain usually decreases as healing occurs. For purposes of definition, acute pain can be described as lasting from seconds to 6 months. However, the 6-month time frame has been criticized (Brookoff, 2000) as inaccurate, because many acute injuries heal within a few weeks and most heal by 6 weeks. In a situation in which healing is expected in 3 weeks and a patient continues to be in pain, the pain should be considered persistent, and appropriate treatment should be used.

Chronic Pain

Chronic pain is constant or intermittent pain that persists beyond the expected healing time and that can seldom be attributed to a specific cause or injury. It may have a poorly defined onset, and it is often difficult to treat because the cause or origin may be unclear. Although acute pain may be a useful signal that something is wrong, chronic or persistent pain usually becomes a problem in its own right.

Chronic pain may be defined as pain that lasts for 6 months or longer, although 6 months is an arbitrary period for differentiating between acute and chronic pain. An episode of pain may assume the characteristics of chronic pain before 6 months have elapsed, or some types of pain may remain primarily acute in nature for longer than 6 months. Nevertheless, after 6 months, most pain experiences are accompanied by problems related to the pain itself. Chronic pain serves no useful purpose. If it continues, it may become a patient's primary disorder.

Nurses may come in contact with patients with chronic pain when these patients are admitted to the hospital for treatment or when they are seen out of the hospital for home care. Frequently, nurses are called on in community-based settings to assist patients in managing pain. For more information about common pain syndromes, see Chart 13-2.

CHART 13-2

Pain Syndromes and Unusual Severe Pain Problems

COMPLEX REGIONAL PAIN SYNDROME

Complex regional pain syndrome (CRPS) refers to a group of conditions previously described as causalgia, reflex sympathetic dystrophy (RSD), and other diagnoses. Complex regional pain syndrome describes a variety of painful conditions that often follow an injury. The magnitude and duration of the pain far exceed the expected duration and often result in significant impairment of motor function. There are two categories of CRPS: type I and type II. CRPS type I, the most common type, is characterized by unexplained diffuse burning pain, usually in the periphery of an extremity. RSD is categorized as CRPS type I and occurs after a relatively minor trauma (St. Marie, 2003). Pain is accompanied by weakness, a change in skin color and temperature relative to the other extremity, limited range of motion, hyperesthesia, hypoesthesia, edema, altered hair growth, and sweating.

Pain, which worsens with movement, cutaneous stimulation, or stress, often occurs after surgery or trauma to the extremity but is not limited to the area of surgery or trauma. CRPS type I is usually managed through a pain clinic. Currently, regional sympathetic blockade and regional intravenous (IV) bretylium offer promise for relief. Tricyclic antidepressants may be tried as well.

CRPS type II refers to causalgia. Type II is more likely to develop after trauma with detectable peripheral nerve lesions (Janig, 2001). The pain is characterized as burning and hyperpathia in an extremity after partial injury to a nerve or one of its major branches.

POSTMASTECTOMY PAIN SYNDROME (PMP)

Postmastectomy pain syndrome (PMP) occurs after mastectomy with node dissection but is not necessarily related to the continuation of disease. Characterized by the sensation of constriction accompanied by a burning, prickling, or numbness in the posterior arm, axilla, or chest wall, PMP is often aggravated by movement of the shoulder, resulting in a frozen shoulder from immobilization (Smith, Bourne, Squair, et al., 1999).

FIBROMYALGIA (FIBROSITIS)

Fibromyalgia, a chronic pain syndrome characterized by generalized musculoskeletal pain, trigger points, stiffness, fatigability, and sleep disturbances, is aggravated by stress and overexertion. Treatment consists of nonsteroidal anti-inflammatory drugs (NSAIDs), trigger point injections with local anesthetics, tricyclic antidepressants, stress reduction, and regular exercise (Gevirtz, 2004).

HEMIPLEGIA-ASSOCIATED SHOULDER PAIN

Hemiplegia-associated shoulder pain is a pain syndrome that affects as many as 80% of stroke patients. It may result from stretching of the shoulder joint due to the uncompensated pull of gravity on the impaired arm. It may be preventable with functional electrical stimulation of involved shoulder muscles.

PAIN ASSOCIATED WITH SICKLE CELL DISEASE

Pain experienced by patients with sickle cell disease results from venous occlusion caused by the sickle shape of the blood cells, impaired circulation to a muscle or organ, ischemia, and infarction. Acute pain may be managed with IV opioid analgesics administered according to a schedule or by a patient-controlled analgesia (PCA) pump and NSAIDs. Warm soaks and elevating the affected body part may help as well. Meperidine (Demerol) therapy is not recommended in patients with compromised renal function, nor is cold therapy. Patients with sickle cell disease may have a long history of chronic pain. Some issues related to their history include tolerance, possible long-term dependence, racial prejudice, and inadequate pain treatment (Jacob, 2001).

AIDS-RELATED PAIN

As AIDS progresses, so do problems that produce increasing amounts of pain, such as neuropathy, esophagitis, headaches, postherpetic pain, and abdominal, back, bone, and joint pain (Marcus, Kerns, Rosenfeld & Breithart, 2000). Pain relief interventions are individualized and may consist of NSAIDs, long-lasting opioids, such as fentanyl patches, and topical lidocaine. Tricyclic antidepressants may provide comfort in neuropathic and postherpetic pain.

BURN PAIN

Possibly the most severe pain, burn pain requires accurate assessment by all health care professionals to effectively manage pain. Besides administration of IV opioid analgesic agents, current therapies to relieve or control pain in burn patients include débridement under general anesthesia; anxiety reduction; intervention with PCA devices, such as a handheld nitrous oxide delivery system; and cognitive techniques, particularly hypnosis.

GUILLAIN-BARRÉ SYNDROME AND PAIN

A progressive, inflammatory disorder of the peripheral nervous system, Guillain-Barré syndrome is characterized by flaccid paralysis accompanied by paresthesia and pain—muscle pain and severe, unrelenting, burning pain. Complaints of severe pain may be difficult to

continued >

CHART 13-2 Pain Syndromes and Unusual Severe Pain Problems, continued

accept in the face of the characteristic flaccid facial response; therefore, the nurse must be sensitive and learn to disregard nonverbal cues that contradict the verbal report of pain. Treatment interventions include NSAIDs for muscle pain and opioids if NSAIDs are ineffective. Causalgia and neurogenic pain may be relieved by systemic or epidural opioids or, possibly, antiseizure agents or tricyclic antidepressants. To relieve the burning, some patients beg to have windows opened and clothing removed, even in cold weather. This suggests that gentle ice massage may help. Research is needed, however, to test its effectiveness.

OPIOID TOLERANCE

Opioid tolerance is common among patients treated for chronic pain, especially patients being treated by multiple health care providers. Opioid tolerance should be suspected if a patient (1) complains of significantly more pain than is usually associated with the condition, (2) requires unusually high doses of opioids to achieve pain relief, or (3) experiences an unusually low incidence and severity of side effects from opioids. Cancer patients also often develop a tolerance to opioids, requiring larger and larger doses of medication to obtain pain relief. In such cases, the nurse must recognize the signs of tolerance, seek additional information from the patient or family, and then obtain additional prescriptions for analgesics or an alternative intervention. In patients undergoing surgery, epidural local anesthetic agents provide excellent postoperative analgesia, but the problem of opioid tolerance must be elicited from the patient preoperatively.

A patient recovering from heroin addiction may be seen in an acute pain situation (surgery or trauma). This patient may be undergoing treatment with naltrexone (Trexan), a long-acting form of the opioid antagonist naloxone (Narcan). Both the short-acting naloxone and the long-acting naltrexone act by binding to the opioid receptors, so opioids cannot be effective. If surgery is planned, the naltrexone should be discontinued a few days before the procedure. If a patient receiving naltrexone is in immediate need of pain relief, very high doses of opioids may be necessary. Alternative methods of pain relief (local or regional blockade and NSAIDs) should be incorporated in the pain management plan.

Cancer-Related Pain

Pain associated with cancer may be acute or chronic. Pain resulting from cancer is so ubiquitous that when cancer patients are asked about possible outcomes, pain is reported to be the most feared outcome (Sutton, Porter & Keefe, 2002). Pain in patients with cancer can be directly associated with the cancer (eg, bony infiltration with tumor cells or nerve compression), a result of cancer treatment (eg, surgery or radiation), or not associated with the cancer (eg, trauma). However, most pain associated with cancer is a direct result of tumor involvement. An approach to cancer pain management is illustrated in Figure 13-1. This three-step approach illustrates the types of analgesic medications used for various levels of pain. A cancer pain algorithm developed as a set of analgesic guiding principles is given in Figure 13-2.

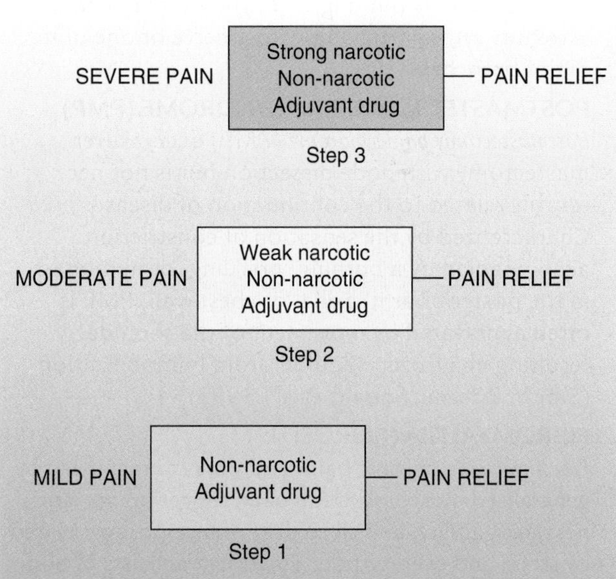

FIGURE 13-1. The World Health Organization three-step ladder approach to relieving cancer pain. Analgesic regimens are based on pain reported as ranging from mild to moderate to severe. Various opioid (narcotic) and nonopioid medications may be combined with other medications to control pain.

Pain Classified by Location

The previous discussion of acute and chronic pain is an example of the categorization of pain according to duration. Pain can also be categorized according to location (eg, pelvic pain, headache, chest pain). This type of categorization aids in communication about and treatment of the pain. For example, chest pain suggests angina or a myocardial infarction and indicates the need for diagnostic evaluation and treatment according to cardiac care standards as appropriate.

Pain Classified by Etiology

Pain can also be categorized according to etiology. Burn pain and postherpetic neuralgia are examples of pain de-

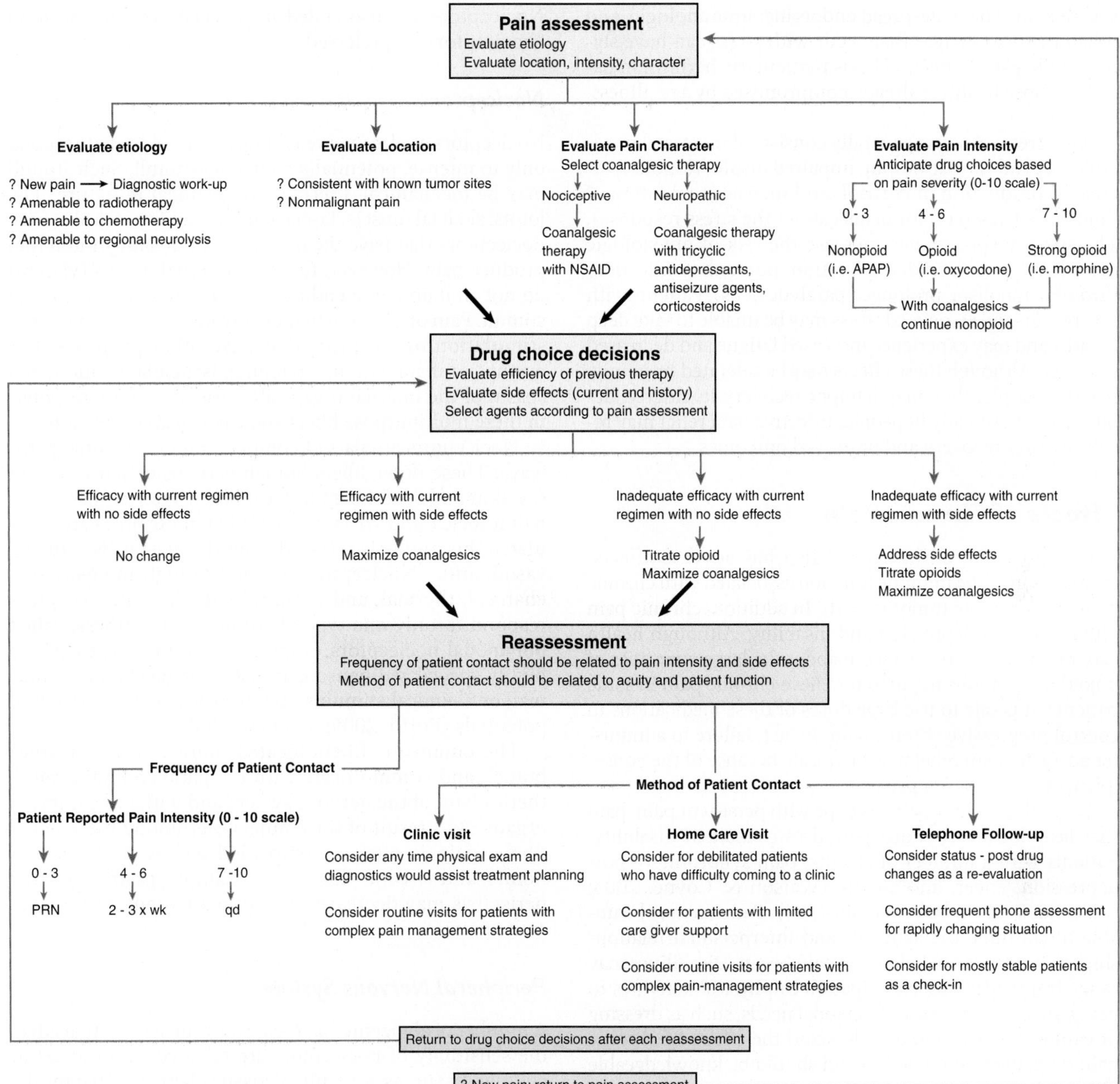

FIGURE 13-2. The cancer pain algorithm (highest-level view) is a decision-tree model for pain treatment that was developed as an interpretation of the AHCPR Guideline for Cancer Pain, 1994. Reproduced with permission from DuPen, A. R., DuPen, S., Hansberry, J., et al. (2000). An educational implementation of a cancer pain algorithm for ambulatory care. *Pain Management Nursing, 1*(4), 118.

scribed in terms of their cause. Clinicians often can predict the course of pain and plan effective treatment using this categorization.

Harmful Effects of Pain

Regardless of its nature, pattern, or cause, pain that is inadequately treated has harmful effects beyond the suffering it causes. For example, unrelieved pain is associated with sleep alterations. Sleep deprivation affects the pain experience. Kunderman, Kreig, Schreiber, et al. (2004) noted that sleep deprivation produces hyperalgesic changes in which patients report greater pain from the same stimulus when they are sleep deprived. Analgesics may also be less effective if patients experience sleep deprivation.

Effects of Acute Pain

Unrelieved acute pain can affect the pulmonary, cardiovascular, gastrointestinal, endocrine, and immune systems. The stress response ("neuroendocrine response to stress") that occurs with trauma also occurs with other causes of severe pain. The widespread endocrine, immunologic, and inflammatory changes that occur with stress can have significant negative effects. This is particularly harmful in patients whose health is already compromised by age, illness, or injury.

The stress response generally consists of increased metabolic rate and cardiac output, impaired insulin response, increased production of cortisol, and increased retention of fluids (see Chapter 6 for details about the stress response). The stress response may increase the risk of physiologic disorders (eg, myocardial infarction, pulmonary infection, thromboembolism, prolonged paralytic ileus). Patients with severe pain and associated stress may be unable to take deep breaths and may experience increased fatigue and decreased mobility. Although these effects may be tolerated by young, healthy people, they may hamper recovery in elderly, debilitated, or critically ill people. Effective pain relief may result in faster recovery and improved outcomes.

Effects of Chronic Pain

Like acute pain, chronic pain also has adverse effects. Suppression of the immune function associated with chronic pain may promote tumor growth. In addition, chronic pain often results in depression and disability. Although health care providers express concern about the large quantities of opioid medications required to relieve chronic pain in some patients, it is safe to use large doses of these medications to control progressive chronic pain. In fact, failure to administer adequate pain relief may be unsafe because of the consequences of unrelieved pain.

Regardless of how patients cope with persistent pain, pain that lasts for an extended period can result in disability. Patients with a number of chronic pain syndromes report depression, anger, and fatigue (Watson & Coyne, 2003; Yezierski, Radison & Vanderah, 2004). Patients may be unable to continue the activities and interpersonal relationships they engaged in before the pain began. Disabilities may range from curtailing participation in physical activities to being unable to take care of personal needs, such as dressing or eating. Nurses should understand the effects of chronic pain on patients and families and should be knowledgeable about pain relief strategies and appropriate resources to assist effectively with pain management.

Pathophysiology of Pain

The sensory experience of pain depends on the interaction between the nervous system and the environment. The processing of noxious stimuli and the resulting perception of pain involve the peripheral and central nervous systems.

Pain Transmission

Among the nerve mechanisms and structures involved in the transmission of pain perceptions to and from the area of the brain that interprets pain are nociceptors, or pain receptors, and chemical mediators. **Nociceptors** are receptors that are preferentially sensitive to a noxious stimulus. Nociceptors are also called pain receptors, but the term "nociceptors" is preferred.

Nociceptors

Nociceptors are free nerve endings in the skin that respond only to intense, potentially damaging stimuli. Such stimuli may be mechanical, thermal, or chemical in nature. The joints, skeletal muscle, fascia, tendons, and cornea also have nociceptors that have the potential to transmit stimuli that produce pain. However, the large internal organs (viscera) do not contain nerve endings that respond only to painful stimuli. Pain originating in these organs results from intense stimulation of receptors that have other purposes. For example, inflammation, stretching, ischemia, dilation, and spasm of the internal organs all cause an intense response in these multipurpose fibers and can cause severe pain.

Nociceptors are part of complex multidirectional pathways. These nerve fibers branch very near their origin in the skin and send fibers to local blood vessels, mast cells, hair follicles, and sweat glands. When these fibers are stimulated, histamine is released from the mast cells, causing vasodilation. Nociceptors respond to high-intensity mechanical, thermal, and chemical stimuli. Some receptors respond to only one type of stimulus, and others, called polymodal nociceptors, respond to all three types. These highly specialized neurons transfer the mechanical, thermal, or chemical stimulus into electrical activity or action potentials (Porth, 2005; Summers, 2000).

The cutaneous fibers located more centrally further branch and communicate with the paravertebral sympathetic chain of the nervous system and with large internal organs. As a result of the connections among these nerve fibers, pain is often accompanied by vasomotor, autonomic, and visceral effects. For example, gastrointestinal peristalsis may decrease or stop in a patient with severe acute pain.

Peripheral Nervous System

A number of **algogenic** (pain-causing) substances that affect the sensitivity of nociceptors are released into the extracellular tissue as a result of tissue damage. Histamine, bradykinin, acetylcholine, serotonin, and substance P are chemicals that increase the transmission of pain. The transmission of pain is also referred to as **nociception. Prostaglandins** are chemical substances that are believed to increase the sensitivity of pain receptors by enhancing the pain-provoking effect of bradykinin. These chemical mediators also cause vasodilation and increased vascular permeability, resulting in redness, warmth, and swelling of the injured area.

Once nociception is initiated, the nociceptive action potentials are transmitted by the peripheral nervous system. The first-order neurons travel from the periphery (skin, cornea, visceral organs) to the spinal cord via the dorsal horn. There are two main types of fibers involved in the transmission of nociception. Smaller, myelinated Aδ (A delta) fibers transmit nociception rapidly, which produces the initial "fast pain." Type C fibers are larger, unmyelinated fibers that transmit what is called "second pain." This type of pain has dull, aching, or burning qualities that last longer than the initial fast pain. The type and concentration of nerve fibers to transmit pain vary by tissue type.

If there is repeated C fiber input, a greater response is noted in dorsal horn neurons, causing the person to perceive more pain. In other words, the same noxious stimulus produces hyperalgesia, and the person reports greater pain than was felt at the first stimulus. For this reason, it is important to treat patients with analgesic agents when they first feel pain. Patients require less medication and experience more effective pain relief if analgesia is administered before they become sensitized to the pain.

Chemicals that reduce or inhibit the transmission or perception of pain include **endorphins** and **enkephalins.** These morphine-like neurotransmitters are endogenous (produced by the body). They are examples of substances that reduce nociceptive transmission when applied to certain nerve fibers. The term "endorphin" is a combination of two words: endogenous and morphine. Endorphins and enkephalins are found in heavy concentrations in the central nervous system (CNS), particularly the spinal and medullary dorsal horn, periaqueductal gray matter, hypothalamus, and amygdala. Morphine and other opioid medications act at receptor sites to suppress the excitation initiated by noxious stimuli. The binding of opioids to receptor sites is responsible for the effects noted after their administration. Each receptor (mu, kappa, delta) responds differently when activated (Porth, 2005). Table 13-1 summarizes the classification and action of opioid receptors.

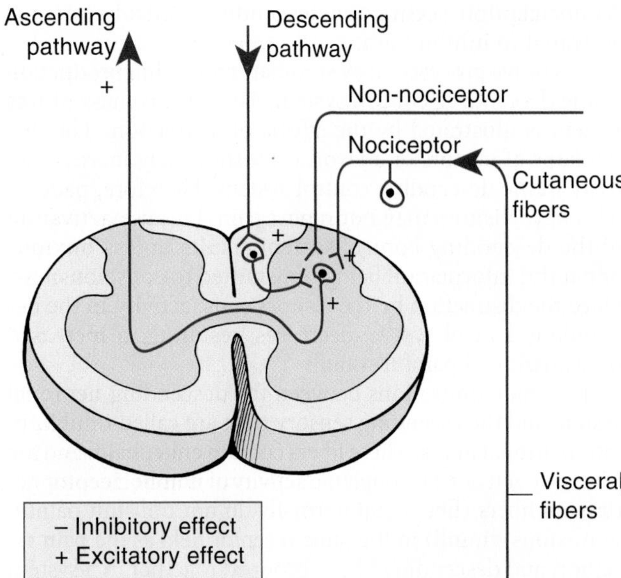

FIGURE 13-3. Representative nociception system, showing ascending and descending sensory pathways of the dorsal horn.

Central Nervous System

After tissue injury occurs, nociception (the neurologic transmission of pain impulses) to the spinal cord via the Aδ and C fibers continues. The fibers enter the dorsal horn, which is divided into laminae based on cell type. The laminae II cell type is commonly referred to as the substantia gelatinosa. In the substantia gelatinosa are projections that relay nociception to other parts of the spinal cord (Fig. 13-3).

Nociception continues from the spinal cord to the reticular formation, thalamus, limbic system, and cerebral cortex. Here nociception is localized, and its characteristics become apparent, including the intensity. The involvement of the reticular formation, limbic, and reticular activating systems is responsible for the individual variations in the perception of noxious stimuli. People may report the same stimulus differently based on their anxiety, past experiences, and expectations. This is a result of the conscious perception of pain.

For pain to be consciously perceived, neurons in the ascending system must be activated. Activation occurs as a result of input from the nociceptors located in the skin and internal organs. Once activated, the inhibitory interneuronal fibers in the dorsal horn inhibit or turn off the transmission of noxious stimulating information in the ascending pathway.

Descending Control System

The descending control system is a system of fibers that originate in the lower and midportion of the brain (specifically, in the periaqueductal gray matter) and terminate on the inhibitory interneuronal fibers in the dorsal horn of the spinal cord. This system is probably always somewhat active; it prevents continuous transmission of stimuli as painful, partly through the action of the endorphins.

℞ **TABLE 13-1 Opioid Classification and Action**

Organ Effect	μ	κ	δ
Eye: Pupil	Miosis	Miosis	Mydriasis
Lung: Respiratory rate	Stimulation, then depression	No change	Stimulation
Heart: Rate	Bradycardia	No change	Tachycardia
Body: Temperature	Hypothermia	No change	Unknown
Affect	Indifference	Sedation	Dysphoria
Gastrointestinal system	Constipation	No effects	Nausea

μ = mu; κ = kappa; δ = delta

From Willens, J. S. (1994). Pain management in the trauma patient. In V. D. Cardona, P. D. Hurn, P. J. B. Mason, A. M. Scanlon, & S. W. Veise-Berry (Eds.), *Trauma nursing from resuscitation through rehabilitation* (2nd ed., pp 325–362). Philadelphia: W. B. Saunders.

As nociception occurs, the descending control system is activated to inhibit pain.

Cognitive processes may stimulate endorphin production in the descending control system. The effectiveness of this system is illustrated by the effects of distraction. The distractions of visitors or a favorite TV show may increase activity in the descending control system. Therefore, patients who have visitors may not report pain, because activation of the descending control system results in less noxious or painful information being transmitted to consciousness. Once the distraction by the visitors ends, activity in the descending control system decreases, resulting in increased transmission of painful stimuli.

The interconnections between the descending neuronal system and the ascending sensory tract are called inhibitory interneuronal fibers. These fibers contain enkephalin and are primarily activated through the activity of **non-nociceptor** peripheral fibers (fibers that normally do not transmit painful or noxious stimuli) in the same receptor field as the pain receptor, and descending fibers, grouped together in a system called descending control. The enkephalins and endorphins are thought to inhibit pain impulses by stimulating the inhibitory interneuronal fibers, which in turn reduce the transmission of noxious impulses via the ascending system (Hudspith & Munglani, 2003; Porth, 2005).

The classic gate control theory of pain, described by Melzack and Wall in 1965, was the first to articulate the existence of a pain-modulating system clearly (Melzack, 1996). This theory proposed that stimulation of the skin evokes nervous impulses that are then transmitted by three systems located in the spinal cord. The substantia gelatinosa in the dorsal horn, the dorsal column fibers, and the central transmission cells act to influence nociceptive impulses. The noxious impulses are influenced by a "gating mechanism." Melzack and Wall proposed that stimulation of the large-diameter fibers inhibits the transmission of pain, thus "closing the gate." Conversely, when smaller fibers are stimulated, the gate is opened. The gating mechanism is influenced by nerve impulses that descend from the brain. This theory proposes a specialized system of large-diameter fibers that activate selective cognitive processes via the modulating properties of the spinal gate. Figure 13-4 shows a schematic representation of a gate control system and nociceptive pathways.

The gate control theory was the first theory to suggest that psychological factors play a role in the perception of pain. The theory guided research toward the cognitive-behavioral approaches to pain management. This theory helps explain how interventions such as distraction and music therapy relieve pain.

Melzack (1996) extended the gate control theory after studying phantom limb pain. He proposed that a large, widespread network of neurons exists that consists of loops between the thalamus and cortex and between the cortex and the limbic system. Melzack labeled this network the neuromatrix. As information is processed in the neuromatrix, a characteristic pattern emerges. This pattern, referred to as the neurosignature, is a continuous outflow from the neuromatrix. Ultimately, the neurosignature output, with a constant stream of input and varying patterns, produces the feelings of the whole body with constantly changing qualities.

Melzack (1996) theorized that, in the absence of modulating inputs from the missing limb, the active neuromatrix produces a neurosignature pattern that is perceived as pain. The neuromatrix theory highlights the role of the brain in sustaining the experience of pain. Research to support the theory has been conducted. Andre, Martinet, Paysant, et al. (2001) studied the effects of vestibular caloric stimulation (cold water placed in the ear canal) on people who had an amputation. They noted that vestibular caloric stimulation produced a temporary perception of a normal phantom limb in 16 of 17 of those who previously did not experience phantom limb pain.

Factors Influencing Pain Response

Several factors, including past experiences with pain, anxiety, culture, age, gender, genetics, and expectations about pain relief, influence a person's experience of pain. These factors may increase or decrease perception of pain, increase or decrease tolerance for pain, and affect responses to pain.

Past Experience

It is tempting to expect that people who have had multiple or prolonged experiences with pain will be less anxious and more tolerant of pain than those who have had little experience with pain. However, this is not true for most people. Often, the more experience a person has had with pain, the more frightened he or she is about subsequent painful events. The person may be less able to tolerate pain; that is, he or she wants relief from pain sooner, before it becomes severe. This reaction is more likely to occur if the person has received inadequate pain relief in the past. A person with repeated pain experiences may have learned to fear the escalation of pain and its inadequate treatment. Once a person experiences severe pain, he or she knows just how severe it can be. Conversely, a person who has never had severe pain may have no fear of such pain.

The way a person responds to pain is a result of many separate painful events during a lifetime. For some, past pain may have been constant and unrelenting, as in chronic pain. Such people may become irritable, withdrawn, and depressed.

The undesirable effects that may result from previous experience point to the need for the nurse to be aware of the patient's past experiences with pain. If pain is relieved promptly and adequately, the person may be less fearful of future pain and better able to tolerate it.

Anxiety and Depression

Although it is commonly believed that anxiety increases pain, this is not necessarily true. Postoperative anxiety is most related to preoperative anxiety and postoperative complications. However, anxiety that is relevant or related to the pain may increase the patient's perception of pain. For example, the patient who was treated 2 years ago for breast cancer and now has hip pain may fear that the pain indicates metastasis. In this case, the anxiety may result in increased pain. Anxiety that is unrelated to the pain may distract the patient and may actually decrease the percep-

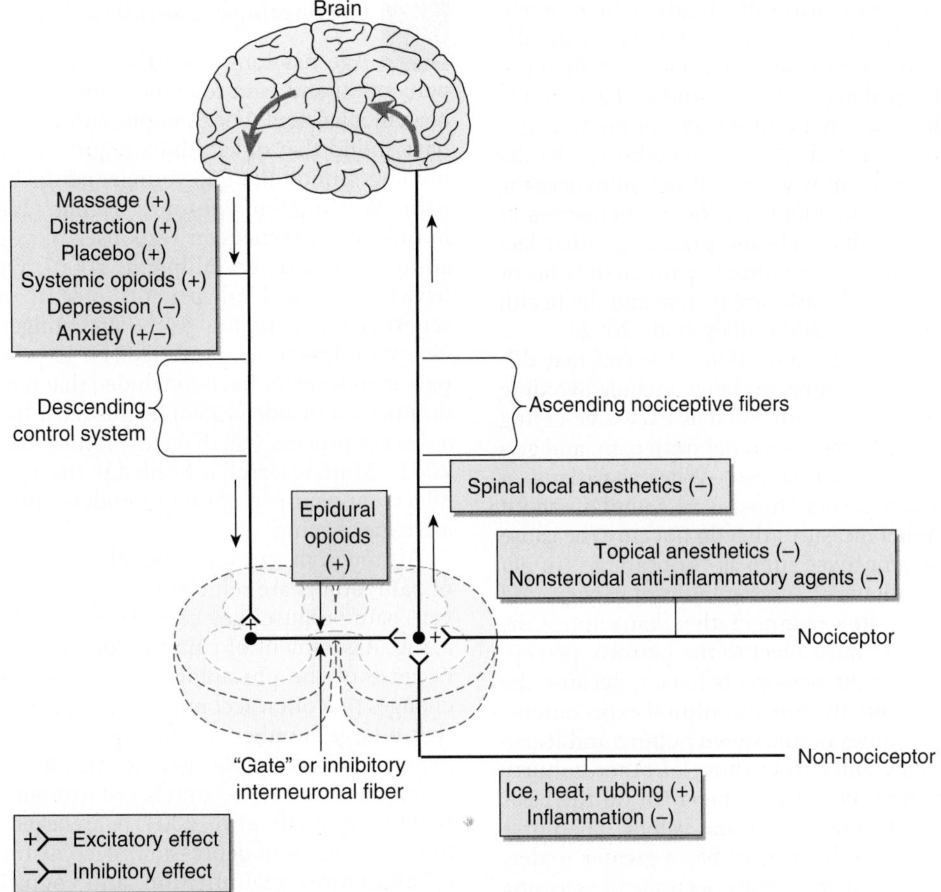

FIGURE 13-4. A schematic representation of the gate control system and aspects of the nociceptive system. The nervous system is made up of stimulatory and inhibitory fibers. For example, stimulation of the nociceptor results in the transmission of an impulse that will be interpreted as pain. When it is stimulated, it will stimulate transmission at the next fiber junction (represented as +≻–). The interneuronal fiber is an inhibitory neuron (–≻–). When it is stimulated, it, in turn, inhibits or shuts off transmission at the next junction. So a placebo has a (+) stimulatory effect on the descending control system, which has a stimulatory effect (+) on the interneuronal fiber, which has an inhibitory effect (–) on the ascending control system. A topical anesthetic has an inhibitory effect (–) on nerve transmission at the nociceptor level, and a spinal anesthetic has the same impact (–) on the ascending nociceptive fibers.

tion of pain. For example, a mother who is hospitalized with complications from abdominal surgery and is anxious about her children may perceive less pain as her anxiety about her children increases.

The routine use of antianxiety medications to treat anxiety in patients with pain may prevent patients from reporting pain because of sedation and may impair their ability to take deep breaths, get out of bed, and cooperate with the treatment plan. The most effective way to relieve pain is by directing the treatment at the pain rather than at the anxiety.

Just as anxiety is associated with pain because of concerns and fears about the underlying disease, depression is associated with chronic pain and unrelieved cancer pain. In cases of chronic pain, the incidence of depression is increased (Bair, Robinson, Katon, et al., 2003). Depression is associated with major life changes caused by the limiting effects of persistent pain, specifically unemployment. Unrelieved cancer pain drastically interferes with the patient's quality of life, and relieving the pain may go a long way toward treating the depression.

Culture

Beliefs about pain and how to respond to it differ from one culture to the next. Early in childhood, people learn from those around them what responses to pain are acceptable or unacceptable. For example, a child may learn that a sports injury is not expected to hurt as much as a comparable injury caused by a motor vehicle crash. The child also learns what stimuli are expected to be painful and what behavioral responses are acceptable. These beliefs vary from one culture to another; therefore, people from different cultures who experience the same intensity of pain may not report it or respond to it in the same ways.

Cultural factors must be taken into account to manage pain effectively. Many studies have examined the cultural aspects of pain. Inconsistent results, methodologic weaknesses or flaws, and failure of many researchers to carefully distinguish ethnicity, culture, and race make it difficult to interpret the findings of many of these studies. Factors that help explain differences in a cultural group include age, gender, education level, and income. In addition, the degree to which patients identify with a culture influences the degree to which they will adopt new health behaviors or rely on traditional health beliefs and practices. Other factors that affect the patient's response to pain include his or her interactions with the health care system and the health care provider (Green et al., 2003; Riley et al., 2002).

The cultural expectations and values of nurses may differ from those of other cultures and may include avoiding exaggerated expressions of pain, such as excessive crying and moaning; seeking immediate relief from pain; and giving complete descriptions of the pain. Whereas patients of one cultural background may moan and complain about pain, refuse pain relief measures that do not cure the cause of the pain, or use adjectives such as "unbearable" in describing the pain, patients of another cultural background may behave in a quiet, stoic manner rather than express the pain loudly. The nurse must react to the person's perception of pain and not to the person's behavior, because the behavior may differ from the nurse's cultural expectations.

Recognizing the values of one's own culture and learning how these values differ from those of other cultures helps avoid evaluating the patient's behavior on the basis of one's own cultural expectations and values. The nurse who recognizes cultural differences has a greater understanding of the patient's pain, is more accurate in assessing pain and behavioral responses to pain, and is more effective at relieving pain.

The main issues to consider when caring for patients of a different culture are

- What does the illness mean to the patient?
- Are there culturally based stigmas related to this illness or pain?
- What is the role of the family in health care decisions?
- Are traditional pain-relief remedies used?
- What is the role of stoicism in the patient's culture?
- Are there culturally determined ways of expressing and communicating pain?
- Does the patient have any fears about the pain?
- Has the patient seen or does the patient want to see a traditional healer?

Regardless of the patient's culture, the nurse should learn about that particular culture and be aware of power and communication issues that affect care outcomes (Watt-Watson, Stevens, Garfinkel, et al., 2001). The nurse should avoid stereotyping the patient by culture and provide individualized care rather than assuming that a patient of a specific culture will exhibit more or less pain. In addition to avoiding stereotyping, health care providers should individualize the amount of medications or therapy according to the information provided by the patient. The nurse should recognize that stereotypes exist and become sensitive to how stereotypes negatively affect care. In turn, patients must be instructed about how and what to communicate about their pain.

Gerontologic Considerations

Age has long been the focus of research on pain perception and pain tolerance, and again the results have been inconsistent. For example, although some researchers have found that older adults require a higher intensity of noxious stimuli than do younger adults before they report pain (Washington, Gibson & Helme, 2000), others have found no differences in responses of younger and older adults (Edwards & Fillingim, 2000). Other researchers have found that elderly patients (older than 65 years of age) report significantly less pain than younger patients do (Li, Greenwald, Gennis, et al., 2001). Experts in the field of pain management have concluded that if pain perception is diminished in elderly people, it is most likely secondary to a disease process (eg, diabetes) rather than to aging (AGS, 2002). More research is needed in the area of aging and its effects on pain perception to understand what the elderly are experiencing.

Although many elderly people seek health care because of pain, others are reluctant to seek help even when in severe pain because they consider pain to be part of normal aging. Assessment of pain in older adults may be difficult because of the physiologic, psychosocial, and cognitive changes that often accompany aging. Research has revealed that a large number of nursing home residents reported being in pain daily; this pain is often described as excruciating and often persists unrelieved without treatment (Teno, Kabumoto, Wetle, et al., 2004). Unrelieved pain contributes to the problems of depression, sleep disturbances, delayed rehabilitation, malnutrition, and cognitive dysfunction (Miaskowski, 2000).

The way older people respond to pain may differ from the way younger people respond. Because elderly people have a slower metabolism and a greater ratio of body fat to muscle mass than younger people do, small doses of analgesic agents may be sufficient to relieve pain, and these doses may be effective longer. Elderly patients deal with pain according to their lifestyle, personality, and cultural background, as do younger adults. Many elderly people are fearful of addiction and, as a result, do not report that they are in pain or ask for medication to relieve pain. Others fail to seek care because they fear that the pain may indicate serious illness or that pain relief will be associated with a loss of independence.

Elderly patients must receive adequate pain relief after surgery or trauma. When an elderly person becomes confused after surgery or trauma, the confusion is often attributed to medications, which are then discontinued. However, confusion in the elderly may be a result of untreated and unrelieved pain. In some cases, postoperative confusion clears once the pain is relieved. Judgments about pain and the adequacy of treatment should be based on the patient's report of pain and pain relief rather than on age.

Gender

Researchers have compared pain intensity, pain unpleasantness, and pain-related emotions (depression, anxiety, frustration, fear, and anger) in men and women who were asked to rate their experiences with chronic pain. However, the results of studies of gender in regard to pain levels and response to pain have been inconsistent. A recent study demonstrated that women report significantly greater pain intensity than men in a laboratory setting, but when the level of anxiety and stereotypes about willingness to report pain are taken into account, gender is not a significant predictor of pain. In other studies, women have consistently reported higher pain intensity, pain unpleasantness, frustration, and fear, compared to men (Wise, Price, Myers, et al., 2002). Men and women are thought to be socialized to respond differently and differ in their expectations relative to pain perception. The pharmacokinetics and pharmacodynamics of opioids differ in men and women and have been attributed to hepatic metabolism, where the microsomal enzyme activity differs (Miaskowski, Gear & Levine, 2000).

Genetics

Genetics factors play a role in the varied responses to nonsteroidal anti-inflammatory drugs (NSAIDs) and opioids seen in patients (Desmeules, Piguet, Ehret, et al., 2004). African Americans reported greater levels of pain than Caucasians for many different types of pain, including migraines, postoperative pain, and myofascial pain. Studying the physiologic responses and clinical pain in combination with subjects with chronic pain, Edwards and colleagues (2001) found that African Americans had higher levels of clinical pain, greater pain-related disability, and less pain tolerance compared with Caucasians. Because African Americans are a genetically mixed population (Collins-Schramm, Phillips, Operario, et al., 2002), these findings may serve as a basis for further study into the potential genetics-based causes of the different responses to analgesics.

The most extensively studied genetics variation in humans is in the metabolism of codeine. Drug metabolism involves genetically controlled enzyme activity for absorption, distribution, inactivation, and excretion. In both experimental and clinical pain, a polymorphism (DNA proteins with variant alleles) in CYP2D6 (encoding cytochrome P450) results both in poor metabolism and poor analgesic efficacy. People who are "poor metabolizers" do not demethylate codeine to morphine; therefore, they do not experience its analgesic effects. See Chapter 9 for further discussion.

Placebo Effect

A **placebo effect** occurs when a person responds to the medication or other treatment because of an expectation that the treatment will work rather than because it actually does so. Simply receiving a medication or treatment may produce positive effects. The placebo effect results from natural (endogenous) production of endorphins in the descending control system. It is a true physiologic response that can be reversed by naloxone, an opioid antagonist (Wall & Melzack, 1999).

A patient's positive expectations about treatment may increase the effectiveness of a medication or other intervention. Often, the more cues the patient receives about the intervention's effectiveness, the more effective it is. Patients who are told that a medication is expected to relieve pain are more likely to experience pain relief than those who are told that a medication is unlikely to have any effect.

Researchers have shown that different verbal instructions given to patients about therapies affect patient behavior and affect opioid intake significantly. Pollo et al. (2001) studied the effect of information and expectations in patients who had undergone thoracotomy. Patients in three groups were given an intravenous (IV) infusion of normal saline solution and could receive a dose of buprenorphine (Buprenex) on request. The first group was given no information about the analgesic effect of the regimen; the second group was informed that the infusion received could be an analgesic or a placebo; and the third group was told that the infusion was a powerful analgesic. Although subjects in the three groups did not differ in reported level of pain, those in the group told that the infusion was a powerful analgesic used less opioid than patients in the other groups.

Two analyses of multiple published research studies examined the placebo effect in clinical trials and had similar results (Hrobjartsson & Gotzsche, 2001, 2004). Although other clinical conditions were studied, including obesity, asthma, hypertension, insomnia, and anxiety, pain was the only condition in which a placebo effect was demonstrated.

The American Society for Pain Management Nurses (2005) contends that placebos (tablets or injections with no active ingredients) should not be used to assess or manage pain in any patient, regardless of age or diagnosis. Furthermore, the group recommends that all health care institutions have policies in place prohibiting the use of placebos for this purpose. Educational programs should be conducted to educate nurses and other health care providers about effective pain management, and ethics committees should assist in developing and disseminating these policies (Chart 13-3).

CHART 13-3

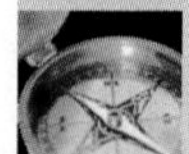

Ethics and Related Issues

Administration of Placebos

Because of misperceptions about placebos and the placebo effect, it is important to keep in mind some specific principles and guidelines:

- A placebo effect is not an indication that the person does not have pain; rather, it is a true physiologic response.
- Placebos (tablets or injections with no active ingredients) should never be used to test the person's truthfulness about pain or as the first line of treatment.
- A positive response to a placebo (eg, reduction in pain) should never be interpreted as an indication that the person's pain is not real.
- A patient should never be given a placebo as a substitute for an analgesic medication. Although a placebo can produce analgesia, patients receiving a placebo may report that their pain is relieved or that they feel better simply to avoid disappointing the nurse.

Nursing Assessment of Pain

The highly subjective nature of pain means that pain assessment and management present challenges for all clinicians. The report of pain is a social transaction; therefore, assessment and management of pain require a good rapport with the person in pain. In assessing a patient with pain, the nurse reviews the patient's description of the pain and other factors that may influence pain (eg, previous experience, anxiety, age), as well as the patient's response to pain relief strategies. Documentation of the pain level as rated on a pain scale becomes part of the patient's medical record, as does the record of the pain relief obtained from interventions.

Pain assessment includes determining what level of pain relief the acutely ill patient believes is needed to recover quickly or improve function, or what level of relief the chronically or terminally ill patient requires to maintain comfort (Chart 13-4). Part of a thorough pain assessment is understanding the patient's expectations and misconceptions about pain (Chart 13-5). People who understand that pain relief not only contributes to comfort but also hastens recovery are more likely to request or self-administer treatment appropriately.

Characteristics of Pain

The factors to consider in a complete pain assessment are the intensity, timing, location, quality, and personal meaning of pain; aggravating and alleviating factors; and pain behaviors. Pain assessment begins by careful patient observation, noting overall posture and presence or absence of overt pain behaviors. In addition, it is essential to ask the patient to describe, in his or her own words, the specifics of the pain. The words used to describe the pain may point toward the cause. For example, the classic description of chest pain that results from a myocardial infarction includes pressure or squeezing on the chest. A detailed history should follow the initial description of pain.

Intensity

The intensity of pain ranges from none to mild discomfort to excruciating. There is no correlation between reported intensity and the stimulus that produced it. The reported intensity is influenced by the person's **pain threshold** and **pain tolerance.** Pain threshold is the smallest stimulus for which a person reports pain, and pain tolerance is the maximum amount of pain a person can tolerate. To understand variations, the nurse can ask about the present pain intensity as well as the least and the worst pain intensity. Various scales and surveys are helpful to patients trying to describe pain intensity. Examples of pain scales appear in Figure 13-5.

Timing

Sometimes the cause of pain can be determined when time aspects are known. Therefore, the nurse inquires about the onset, duration, relationship between time and intensity (eg, at what time is the pain worst), and changes in rhythmic patterns. The patient is asked if the pain began suddenly or increased gradually. Sudden pain that rapidly reaches maximum intensity is indicative of tissue rupture, and immediate intervention is necessary. Pain from ischemia gradually increases and becomes intense over a longer time. The chronic (or persistent) pain of arthritis illustrates the usefulness of determining the relationship between time and intensity, because people with arthritis usually report that pain is worse in the morning.

Location

The location of pain is best determined by having the patient point to the area of the body involved. Some general assessment forms include drawings of human figures, on which the patient is asked to shade in the area involved. This is especially helpful if the pain radiates (**referred pain**). The shaded figures are helpful in determining the effectiveness of treatment or change in the location of pain over time.

Quality

The nurse asks the patient to describe the pain in his or her own words without offering clues. For example, the nurse asks the patient to describe what the pain feels like. The nurse must give the patient sufficient time to describe the pain, and the nurse must record all words in the answer. If the patient cannot describe the quality of the pain, the nurse can suggest words such as burning, aching, throbbing, or stabbing. It is important to document the exact words used by the patient to describe the pain and which words were suggested by the nurse conducting the assessment.

Personal Meaning

Pain means different things to different people; as a result, patients experience pain differently. The meaning of the pain experience helps the clinician understand how the patient is affected and assists in planning treatment. It is important to ask how the pain affects the person's daily life. Some people with pain can continue to work or study, whereas others may be disabled by their pain. The pain may affect family finances. For some patients, the recurrence of pain may mean worsening of disease, such as the spread of cancer.

Aggravating and Alleviating Factors

The nurse asks the patient what, if anything, makes the pain worse and what makes it better and asks specifically about the relationship between activity and pain. This helps detect factors associated with pain. For example, in a patient with advanced metastatic cancer, pain with coughing may signal spinal cord compression. The nurse ascertains whether environmental factors influence pain, because they may easily be changed to help the patient. For example, making the room warmer may help a patient relax and may decrease the person's pain. Finally, the nurse asks the patient whether the pain is influenced by or affects the quality of sleep or anxiety. Both can significantly affect pain intensity and the quality of life.

Knowledge of alleviating factors assists the nurse in developing a treatment plan. Therefore, it is important to ask about the patient's use of medications (prescribed and over-the-counter [OTC]), including amount and frequency. In addition, the nurse asks if herbal remedies, nonpharmaco-

CHART 13-4

Pain at the End of Life

Pain is one of the most feared symptoms at the end of life. Most patients experience pain as a terminal illness progresses. The inadequate treatment of cancer pain has been well documented. In the Study to Understand Prognoses and Preferences for Outcomes and Risks of Treatments (SUPPORT) (1995), investigators noted that nearly 40% of severely chronically ill and older patients who died in hospitals suffered moderate to severe pain in the last 3 days of life. The suffering caused by unrelieved pain touches all aspects of quality of life (activity, appetite, sleep) and can weaken an already fatigued person. Psychologically, unrelieved pain can create anxiety and depression, negatively affect relationships, and promote thoughts of suicide.

The Joint Commission on Accreditation of Health Care Organizations (JCAHO) implemented pain standards in January 2001. These standards present a unique opportunity to improve care for hospitalized patients. Even though hospices and palliative care agencies are not subject to JCAHO review, many patients with chronic illness who are receiving palliative care may be hospitalized at various times. The standards emphasize pain assessment, patient and family education, continuity of care for symptom management, and evaluation of interventions.

Current barriers to pain management include lack of education, lack of access to opioids, fear of addiction, and legislative issues.

Lack of Education

Strategies to increase knowledge about pain, pain assessment, and pain management in general and at the end of life are needed to ensure that a patient's pain is effectively addressed. Many studies have increased what is known about pain and pain management. However, the information from these studies must be disseminated to health care providers to be translated into evidence-based practice. Health care professionals, including nurses, must remain current about the pharmacokinetics and pharmacodynamics of analgesics and about new technologies to deliver analgesic medications. Continuing education (CE), which can be accessed in many ways, is one option available to improve knowledge about pain and pain management. CE can be provided through conferences, journal articles, and online programs. Chapters of the American Society for Pain Management Nurses provide opportunities for CE about pain assessment and management. National pain organizations list the dates and locations of their CE programs and conferences on the Web sites. Studies are needed to evaluate the effect that educational interventions have on health care providers' knowledge about pain and their ability to manage pain effectively (Gunnarsdottir, Donovan & Ward, 2003).

ACCESSIBILITY

The lack of access to opioids is another barrier to adequate pain relief. Patients may have difficulty affording medications. Some pharmacists, fearing crime, paperwork, and regulatory oversight, may not stock opioids or may keep limited quantities on hand. Some insurance companies limit the types of medications they will reimburse and the amount and frequency of renewal of analgesics.

ADDICTION FEARS

The fear of addiction plays a role even at the end of life. Family members may be hesitant to assist the patient in pain management for fear of the social stigma of addiction. This causes needless pain and suffering. Some health care providers continue to have unfounded fears of contributing to a patient's risk for addiction when administering opioids.

LEGAL BARRIERS

Legislative issues play a role in the inadequate management of pain. Many states are enacting Intractable Pain Statutes. These laws are aimed at reducing physicians' fear of civil or criminal liability or disciplinary action for aggressively managing pain. The tracking system by the Drug Enforcement Agency acts as a deterrent since opioids prescribed by physicians can be tracked. Some physicians fear that prescribing "too many" opioids could be interpreted as treating an addicted patient.

OTHER ISSUES

Pain management at the end of life differs little from general pain management. Patients still require comprehensive pain assessment and pain management, even though assessment may be hampered by confusion, delirium, or unconsciousness. Caregivers are taught to observe for signs of restlessness or facial expressions as a "proxy" indicator of pain.

Analgesic agents should be titrated to find the most effective dose and the best tolerated route. The nurse and family members should assess the effectiveness of the current pain therapy. If the pain is not relieved, a larger dose of medication may be necessary. If the pain continues, another medication may be needed or the patient should be given a different analgesic. The titration process requires frequent assessment to effectively manage pain. The analgesic agent or treatment should be appropriate for the type of pain. For example,

continued >

CHART 13-4 Pain at the End of Life, continued

neuropathic pain, usually described as burning, tingling, numbness, shooting, stabbing, or electric, requires a different treatment approach than acute pain.

Nonpharmacologic approaches, such as guided imagery and relaxation, can be used to decrease pain and help the patient cope. Careful patient positioning and environmental control are other methods to increase patient comfort.

Respiratory depression should be assessed because over time, the patient's risk for this side effect increases. The rate, depth, and level of consciousness should be monitored to determine whether respiratory depression is occurring and requires treatment. A respiratory rate of 6 per minute or greater is usually adequate. If respiratory depression is suspected, a decrease in the opioid dose may be indicated. Frequent stimulation to encourage deep breathing may be required until the opioid is metabolized. In the last few days of life the patient may become restless, which is an indicator of pain. The need to increase the opioid to provide pain relief and the respiratory effects of opioids are considered in decision making. However, comfort should be a priority in the case of a person who clearly is at the end of life, where cure is no longer the goal.

Side effects from analgesics must be managed as in other painful conditions. Tolerance to constipation is rare. Therefore, a careful bowel regimen involving diet, bowel stimulants, stool softeners, and/or osmotic agents must be instituted. Vigilance in the assessment, management, and treatment of other side effects is similar to that included in previous discussions.

Careful assessment and management of pain at the end of life can make a "good" death possible. Education of health care providers and the family can help patients realize the goal of adequate pain relief throughout the dying process.

logic interventions, or alternative therapies have been used with success. This information assists the nurse in determining teaching needs.

Pain Behaviors

When experiencing pain, people express pain through many different behaviors. These nonverbal and behavioral expressions of pain are not consistent or reliable indicators of the quality or intensity of pain, and they should not be used to determine the presence of or the severity of pain experienced. A patient may grimace, cry, rub the affected area, guard the affected area, or immobilize it. Others may moan, groan, grunt, or sigh. Not all patients exhibit the same behaviors, and there may be different meanings associated with the same behavior.

CHART 13-5 Common Concerns and Misconceptions About Pain and Analgesia

- Complaining about pain will distract my doctor from his primary responsibility—curing my illness.
- Pain is a natural part of aging.
- I don't want to bother the nurse—he/she is busy with other patients.
- Pain medicine can't really control pain.
- People get addicted to pain medicine easily.
- It is easier to put up with pain than with the side effects that come from pain medicine.
- Good patients avoid talking about pain.
- Pain medicine should be saved in case the pain gets worse.
- Pain builds character. It's good for you.
- Patients should expect to have pain; it's part of almost every hospitalization.

Adapted with permission from Gordon, D. B., & Ward, S. E. (1995). Correcting patient misconceptions about pain. *American Journal of Nursing, 95*(7):43–45.

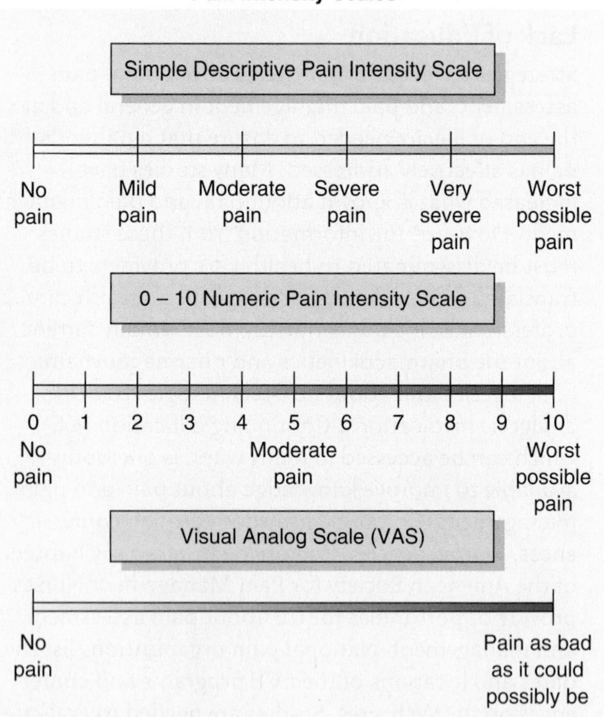

FIGURE 13-5. Examples of pain intensity scales.

Sometimes in nonverbal patients, pain behaviors are used as a proxy to assess pain. It is unwise to make judgments and formulate treatment plans based on behaviors that may or may not indicate pain. In unconscious patients, pain should be assumed to be present and treated. All patients have a right to adequate pain management.

Physiologic responses to pain, such as tachycardia, hypertension, tachypnea, pallor, diaphoresis, mydriasis, hypervigilance, and increased muscle tone, are related to stimulation of the autonomic nervous system. These responses are short-lived as the body adapts to the stress. These physiologic signs could be the result of a change in the patient's condition, such as the onset of hypovolemia. Use of physiologic signs to indicate pain is unreliable. Although it is important to observe for any and all pain behaviors, the absence of these behaviors does not indicate an absence of pain.

Instruments for Assessing the Perception of Pain

Only the patient can accurately describe and assess his or her pain. Clinicians consistently underestimate patients' levels of pain (McCaffery, Ferrell & Pasero, 2000). Therefore, a number of pain assessment tools have been developed to assist in the assessment of the patient's perception of pain (see Fig. 13-5). Such tools may be used to document the need for intervention, to evaluate the effectiveness of the intervention, and to identify the need for alternative or additional interventions if the initial intervention is ineffective in relieving the pain. For a pain assessment tool to be useful, it must require little effort on the part of the patient, be easy to understand and use, be easily scored, and be sensitive to small changes in the characteristic being measured. Figure 13-6 shows a pain assessment pathway that can be used at the time of assessment to direct clinical decisions for pain management.

Visual Analogue Scales

Visual analogue scales (VAS; see Fig. 13-5) are useful in assessing the intensity of pain. One version of the scale includes a horizontal 10-cm line, with anchors (ends) indicating the extremes of pain. The patient is asked to place a mark indicating where the current pain lies on the line. The left anchor usually represents "none" or "no pain," whereas the right anchor usually represents "severe" or "worst possible pain." To score the results, a ruler is placed along the line, and the distance the patient marked from the left or low end is measured and reported in millimeters or centimeters.

Some patients (eg, children, elderly patients, visually or cognitively impaired patients) may find it difficult to use an unmarked VAS. In those circumstances, ordinal scales, such as a simple descriptive pain intensity scale or a 0-to-10 numeric pain intensity scale, may be used.

NURSING RESEARCH PROFILE

Pain Assessment by Nurses Compared With Patients

Puntillo, K., Neighbor, M., O'Neil, N. & Nixon, R. (2004). Accuracy of emergency nurses in assessment of patients' pain. *Pain Management Nursing, 4*(4): 171–175.

Purpose

Pain is one of the most common reasons for patients' visits to the emergency department (ED). To manage pain effectively, it must be assessed accurately, treated, and then reassessed to determine treatment efficacy. This study sought to determine if there is a difference between patients' ratings of pain intensity and triage nurses' ratings of patients' pain in the emergency department. The researchers also investigated whether patients' chief complaints influence pain ratings by both nurses and patients.

Design

This prospective, descriptive study included a convenience sample of triage nurses, non-triage ED nurses, and patients who presented to a Level 1 trauma center. A horizontal 0-to-10 numeric rating scale was used to measure pain intensity. Research assistants in the triage area asked patients to rate their pain intensity. Nurses who were blinded to the patients' responses were then asked to rate the same patients' pain intensity.

Findings

A total of 156 patients and 37 nurses participated in the study. Significant differences ($p = .001$) were found between triage nurses' ratings (mean = 5.1 ± 2.4) and patients' ratings (mean = 7.5 ± 2.2). Significant differences ($p = .001$) were also found between the non-triage nurses' and patients' intensity ratings. The mean pain intensity scores of non-triage nurses and patients were 4.2 ± 2.3 and 7.7 ± 2.2, respectively.

To determine what factors may contribute to these discrepancies in ratings, the researchers examined pain intensity ratings between patients and nurses based on patients' chief complaints. The greatest differences in pain intensity ratings occurred in patients with musculoskeletal disorders, abdominal pain, and cellulitis/abscesses. The least differences in pain intensity ratings occurred in patients with headaches, fractures, and radiculopathies.

Nursing Implications

The results of this study indicate that nurses continue to underestimate the intensity of patients' pain. Because pain management is based on nurses' assessments of patients' pain intensity, nurses should ask patients to rate their own pain rather than using assessments based on nurses' own assumptions and biases.

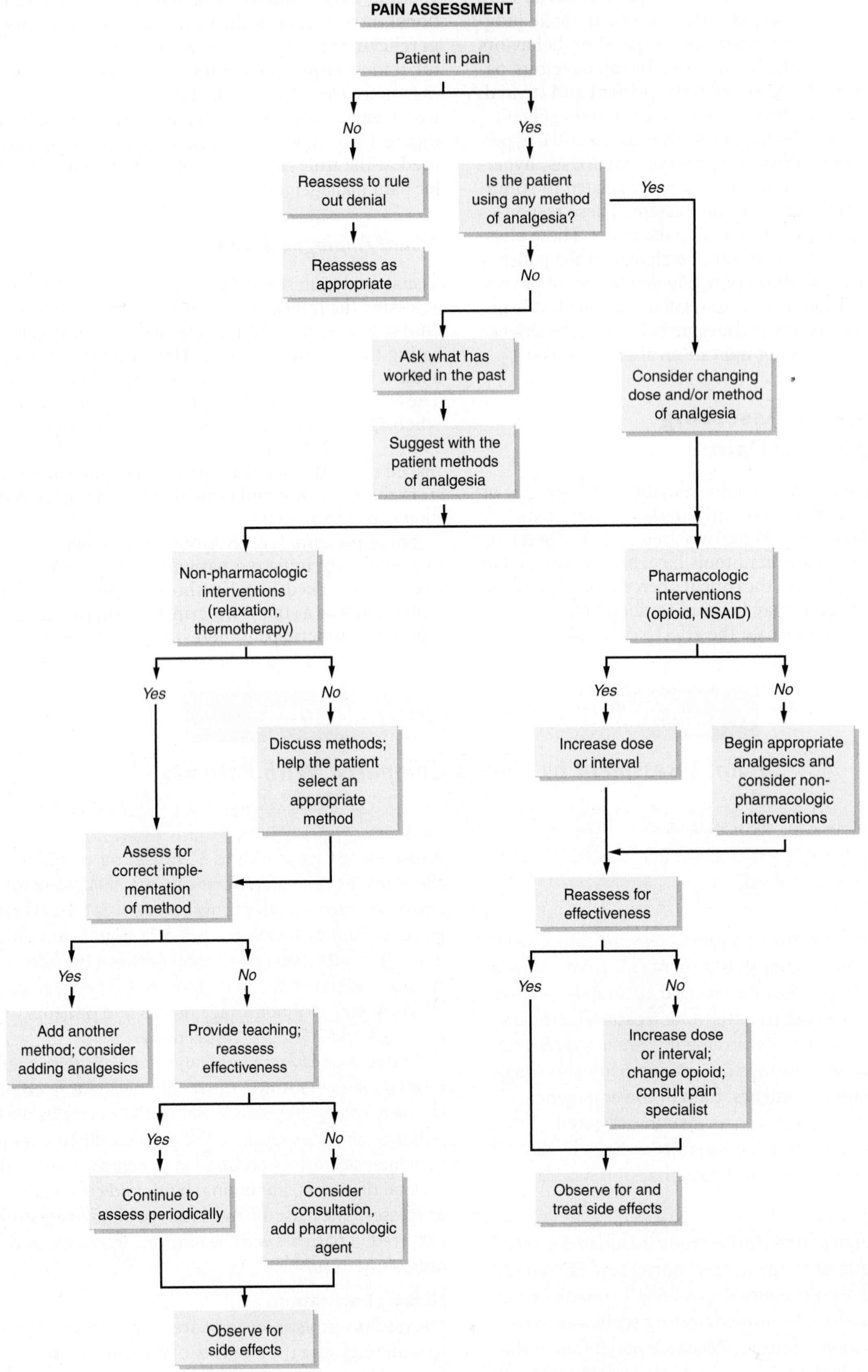

FIGURE 13-6. Pain assessment pathway.

Faces Pain Scale–Revised

This instrument has six faces depicting expressions that range from contented to obvious distress (Fig. 13-7). The patient is asked to point to the face that most closely resembles the intensity of his or her pain. Evidence of reliability and validity of this scale has been established (Hicks, von Baeyer, Spafford, et al., 2001).

Guidelines for Using Pain Assessment Scales

Using a written scale to assess pain may not be possible if a person is seriously ill, is in severe pain, or has just returned from surgery. In these cases, the nurse can ask the patient, "On a scale of 0 to 10, 0 being no pain and 10 being pain as bad as it can be, how bad is your pain now?" For patients who have difficulty with a 0 to 10 scale, a 0 to 5 scale may be tried. Whichever scale is used, it should be used consistently. Most patients usually can respond without difficulty. Ideally, the nurse teaches the patient how to use the pain scale before the pain occurs (eg, before surgery). The patient's numerical rating is documented and used to assess the effectiveness of pain relief interventions.

If a particular patient does not speak English or cannot clearly communicate information needed to manage pain, an interpreter, translator, or family member familiar with the person's method of communication should be consulted and a method established for pain assessment. Often a chart can be constructed with English words on one side and the foreign language on the other. The patient can then point to the corresponding word to tell the nurse about the pain.

When people with pain are cared for at home by family caregivers or home care nurses, a pain scale may help assess the effectiveness of the interventions if the scale is used before and after the interventions are implemented. The patient and family caregivers can be taught to use a pain assessment scale to assess and manage the patient's pain. Scales that address the location and pattern of pain may be useful in identifying new sources or sites of pain in chronically or terminally ill patients and in monitoring changes in the patient's level of pain. For example, a home care nurse who sees a patient only at intervals may benefit from consulting the patient's or family's written record of the pain scores to evaluate how effective the pain management strategies have been over time.

On occasion, a person will deny having pain when most people in similar circumstances would report significant pain. For example, it is not uncommon for a patient recovering from a total joint replacement to deny feeling "pain," but on further questioning he or she will readily admit to having a "terrible ache, but I wouldn't call it pain." From then on, when evaluating this person's pain, the nurse would use the patient's words rather than the word "pain."

Guidelines for Assessing Pain in Patients With Disabilities

Alternative forms of communication may be necessary for people with sensory impairments or other disabilities.

- For people who are blind and who know how to read Braille, pain assessment instruments can be obtained in Braille. In addition, there is now computer software that allows written documents to be scanned and converted into Braille. If these programs are not available, agencies that provide services for people who are blind may be able to assist in developing Braille versions.
- For people who are deaf or hard of hearing, outside interpreters (ie, not family members) should be used. Other useful communication strategies may include sign language, written notes, or pictures. When writing notes on a "magic slate" or making written notes, it is necessary to make every effort to guard the patient's privacy and confidentiality.
- For people with disabilities that result in communication impairment, computer-generated speech may be useful.

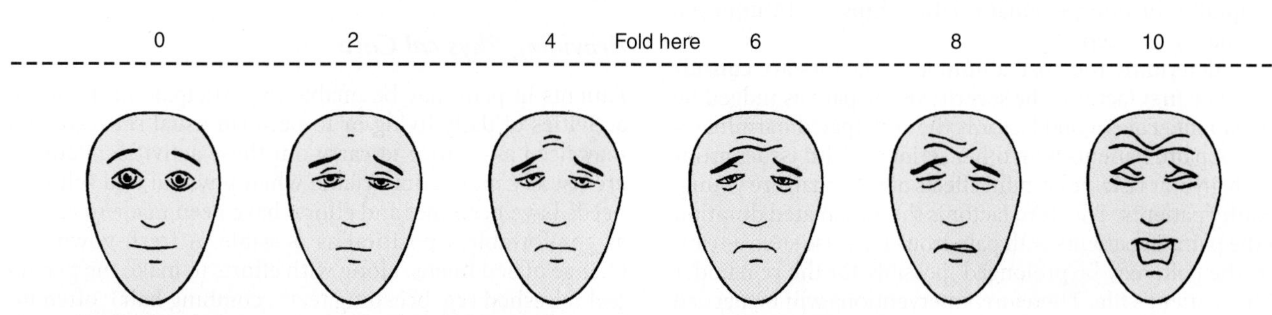

FIGURE 13-7. Faces Pain Scale–Revised. This pain scale is especially suited for helping children describe pain. Instructions for using this scale follow: "These faces show how much something can hurt. This face (*point to left-most face*) shows *no pain.* The faces show more and more pain (*point to each from left to right*) up to this one (*point to right-most face*). It shows *very much pain.* Point to the face that shows how much you hurt (right now)." Score the chosen face 0, 2, 4, 6, 8, or 10, counting left to right, so 0 = no pain and 10 = very much pain. Do not use words like "happy" or "sad." This scale is intended to measure how children feel inside, not how their face looks. (From the *Pediatric Pain Sourcebook.* Original copyright © 2001. Used with permission of the International Association for the Study of Pain and the Pain Research Unit, Sydney Children's Hospital, Randwick NSW 2031, Australia.)

The Nurse's Role in Pain Management

Before discussing what the nurse can do to intervene in the patient's pain, it is necessary to review the role of the nurse in pain management. The nurse helps relieve pain by administering pain-relieving interventions (including both pharmacologic and nonpharmacologic approaches), assessing the effectiveness of those interventions, monitoring for adverse effects, and serving as an advocate for the patient when the prescribed intervention is ineffective in relieving pain. It is important to assess the patient's past medical history and family history for response to analgesics (eg, codeine). It is also critical to assess the patient's ethnic and racial background, because there appears to be a higher frequency of poor drug metabolizers among Caucasian people compared with Asian American and African American people. For example, when assessing a patient's lack of response to codeine, it may be appropriate to consider a genetics cause and obtain a prescription for a different opioid. In addition, the nurse provides education to the patient and family to enable them to manage the prescribed intervention themselves when appropriate.

Identifying Goals for Pain Management

The information the nurse obtains from the pain assessment is used to identify goals for managing pain. These goals are shared and validated with the patient. For a few patients, the goal may be complete elimination of the pain. However, this expectation may be unrealistic. Other goals may include a decrease in the intensity, duration, or frequency of pain and a decrease in the negative effects of the pain. For example, pain may have a negative effect by interfering with sleep and thereby hampering recovery from an acute illness or decreasing appetite. In such instances, the goals might be to sleep soundly and to take adequate nutrition. Chronic pain may affect the patient's quality of life by interfering with work, interpersonal relationships, or sleep (Call-Schmidt & Richardson, 2003). Therefore, a goal might be to decrease time lost from work, to increase the quality of interpersonal relationships, or to improve the quality of sleep.

To determine the goal, a number of factors are considered. The first factor is the severity of the pain as judged by the patient. The second factor is the anticipated harmful effects of pain. Patients with other serious health issues are at much greater risk for harmful effects of pain than are young, healthy patients. The third factor is the anticipated duration of the pain. In patients with pain from a disease such as cancer, the pain may be prolonged, possibly for the remainder of the patient's life. Therefore, interventions will be needed for some time and should not detract from the patient's quality of life. A different set of interventions is required if the pain is likely to last for only a few days or weeks.

In patients receiving palliative care who had pain when they were conscious, it should be assumed that the pain persists even if the patient cannot communicate. Often family members can be taught what behaviors to look for to assess for pain: a furrowed brow, stiffening of a part of the body, or moaning.

The goals for the patient may be accomplished by pharmacologic or nonpharmacologic means, but most success is achieved with a combination of these methods. In the acute stages of illness, the patient may be unable to participate actively in relief measures, but when sufficient mental and physical energy is present, the patient may learn self-management techniques to relieve the pain. Therefore, as the patient progresses through the stages of recovery, increased patient use of self-management pain relief measures may be a goal.

Establishing the Nurse–Patient Relationship and Teaching

A positive nurse–patient relationship and teaching are key to managing analgesia in patients with pain, because open communication and patient cooperation are essential to success. A positive nurse–patient relationship characterized by trust is essential. By conveying to the patient the belief that he or she has pain, the nurse often helps reduce the patient's anxiety. Saying to the patient, "I know that you have pain," often eases the patient's mind. Occasionally, a patient who fears that no one believes that he or she has pain feels relieved to know that the nurse can be trusted to believe that the pain exists.

Teaching is equally important, because the patient or family may be responsible for managing the pain at home and preventing or managing side effects. Teaching the patient about pain and strategies to relieve it may reduce pain in the absence of other pain relief measures and may enhance the effectiveness of the pain relief measures used.

The nurse also provides information by explaining how pain can be controlled. For example, the patient should be informed that pain should be reported in the early stages. When the patient waits too long to report pain, **sensitization** may occur, and the pain may be so intense that it is difficult to relieve. The phenomenon of sensitization is important in effective pain management. A heightened response is seen after exposure to a noxious stimulus; as a result, the response to that stimulus is greater, causing the person to feel more pain. When health care providers assess and treat pain before it becomes severe, sensitization is diminished or avoided, and less medication is needed.

Providing Physical Care

Patients in pain may be unable to participate in the usual activities of daily living or to perform usual self-care and may need assistance to carry out these activities. Patients are usually more comfortable when physical and self-care needs have been met and efforts have been made to ensure as comfortable a position as possible. A fresh gown and change of bed linens, along with efforts to make the person feel refreshed (eg, brushing teeth, combing hair), often increase the level of comfort and improve the effectiveness of the pain relief measures.

In acute, long-term, and home settings, the nurse who provides physical care to patients also has the opportunity to perform complete assessments and to identify problems that may contribute to the patient's discomfort and pain. Appropriate and gentle physical touch during care may be reassuring and comforting. If topical treatments such as fentanyl (an opioid analgesic) patches or intravenous or intraspinal catheters are used, the skin around the patch or catheter should be assessed for integrity during physical care.

Managing Anxiety Related to Pain

Anxiety may affect the patient's response to pain. A patient who anticipates pain may become increasingly anxious. Teaching the patient about the nature of the impending painful experience and the ways to reduce pain often decreases anxiety; people who experience pain use previously learned strategies to reduce anxiety and pain. Learning about measures to relieve pain may lessen the threat of pain and give the patient a sense of control. The patient's anxiety may be reduced by explanations that point out the degree of pain relief that can be expected from each measure. For example, a patient who is informed that an intervention may not eliminate pain completely is less likely to become anxious when a certain amount of pain persists.

A patient who is anxious about pain may be less tolerant of the pain, which in turn may increase his or her anxiety level. To prevent the pain and anxiety from escalating, the anxiety-producing cycle must be interrupted. Pain relief measures should be used before pain becomes severe. Many patients believe that they should not request pain relief measures until they cannot tolerate the pain, making it difficult for medications to provide relief. It is important to explain to all patients that pain relief or control is more successful if such measures begin before the pain becomes unbearable.

Pain Management Strategies

Reducing pain to a "tolerable" level was once considered the goal of pain management. However, even patients who have described pain relief as adequate often report disturbed sleep and marked distress because of pain. In view of the harmful effects of pain and inadequate pain management, the goal of tolerable pain has been replaced by the goal of relieving the pain. Pain management strategies include both pharmacologic and nonpharmacologic approaches. These approaches are selected on the basis of the requirements and goals of particular patients. Appropriate analgesic medications are used as prescribed. They are not considered a last resort to be used only when other pain relief measures fail. As previously discussed, any intervention is most successful if it is initiated before pain sensitization occurs, and the greatest success is usually achieved if several interventions are applied simultaneously.

Pharmacologic Interventions

Pharmacologic management of pain is accomplished in collaboration with physicians, patients, and often families. A physician or nurse practitioner prescribes specific medications for pain or may insert an IV line for administration of analgesic medications. Alternatively, an anesthesiologist or nurse anesthetist may insert an epidural catheter for administration of such analgesic agents. However, it is the nurse who maintains the analgesia, assesses its effectiveness, and reports whether the intervention is ineffective or produces side effects (Table 13-2).

Close collaboration and effective communication among health care providers is necessary. In the home setting, the family often manages the patient's pain and assesses the effectiveness of pharmacologic interventions, and the home care nurse evaluates the adequacy of pain relief strategies and the ability of the family to manage the pain. Home care nurses reinforce teaching and ensure communication among patients, family care providers, physicians, pharmacists, and other health care providers involved in the care of patients.

Premedication Assessment

Before administering any medication, the nurse should ask the patient about allergies to medications and the nature of any previous allergic responses. True allergic or anaphylactic responses to opioids are rare, but it is not uncommon for patients to report an allergy to one of the opioids. On further questioning, the nurse often learns that the extent of the allergy is "itching" or "nausea and vomiting." These responses are not allergies; rather, they are side effects that can be managed while the patient's pain is relieved. The patient's description of responses or reactions should be documented and reported before medication is administered.

The nurse obtains the patient's medication history (eg, current, usual, or recent use of prescription or OTC medications or herbal agents), along with a history of health disorders. Certain medications or conditions may affect the

TABLE 13-2 Adverse Interactions of Herbal Substances or Foods With Analgesics

Analgesic	Herb or Food	Effect
NSAIDs	Ginkgo, garlic, ginger, bilberry, dongquai, feverfew, ginseng, turmeric, meadowsweet, willow	Enhanced risk of bleeding
Acetaminophen	Ginkgo and possibly some of the above-mentioned herbs	Enhanced risk of bleeding
	Echinacea, kava, willow, meadowsweet	Increased potential for hepatotoxicity and nephrotoxicity
Opioids	Valerian, kava, chamomile	Increased central nervous system depression
	Ginseng	Inhibits analgesic effects
Alfentanil, fentanyl, sufentanil	Grapefruit juice	Inhibits the cytochrome P450 3A4 enzyme in the liver, blocking metabolism of the drug

NSAID, nonsteroidal anti-inflammatory drugs.

From Abebe, W. (2002). Herbal medication: Potential for adverse interactions with analgesic drugs. *Journal of Clinical Pharmacologic Therapies, 27*(6), 391–401; and Karch, A. (2004). The grapefruit challenge. *American Journal of Nursing, 104*(12), 33–35.

analgesic medication's effectiveness or its metabolism and excretion. Before administering analgesic agents, the nurse should assess the patient's pain status, including the intensity of current pain, changes in pain intensity after the previous dose of medication, and side effects of the medication.

Gerontologic Considerations

Physiologic changes in older adults require that analgesic agents be administered with caution. Drug interactions are more likely to occur in older adults because of the higher incidence of chronic illness and the increased use of prescription and OTC medications. Although the elderly population is an extremely heterogeneous group, differences in response to pain or medications by patients over this 40-year span (60 to 100 years) are more likely to be due to chronic illness or other individual factors than to age. Before administering opioid and nonopioid analgesic agents to elderly patients, the nurse should obtain a careful medication history to identify potential drug interactions (see Table 13-2).

Elderly patients are more sensitive to medications and at an increased risk for drug toxicity (American Geriatrics Society [AGS], 2002). Liver, renal, and gastrointestinal functions are decreased in elderly patients, resulting in changes in the absorption and metabolism of medications. In addition, changes in body weight, protein stores, and distribution of body fluid alter the distribution of medications in the body. Consequently, medications are not metabolized as quickly, and blood levels of the medications remain higher for a longer period.

Opioid and nonopioid analgesic medications can be administered to elderly patients but must be used cautiously because of the increased susceptibility to depression of both the nervous and the respiratory systems. Although there is no reason to avoid opioids in patients simply because they are elderly, meperidine should be avoided because its active and neurotoxic metabolite, normeperidine, is more likely to accumulate and cause CNS excitation and seizures. In addition, because of decreased binding of meperidine by plasma proteins, blood concentrations of the medication twice those found in younger patients may occur.

In many cases, the initial dose of analgesic medication prescribed for elderly patients is the same as that for younger patients, or slightly smaller than the normal dose, but because of slowed metabolism and excretion related to aging, the safe interval for subsequent doses may be longer (or prolonged). The AGS (2002) has published clinical practice guidelines for managing persistent pain in elderly patients. As always, the best guide to pain management and administration of analgesic agents in all patients, regardless of age, is what the individual patient says. Elderly patients may obtain more pain relief for a longer time than younger patients do from the same dose. As a result, smaller and less frequent doses of analgesics may be required.

Approaches for Using Analgesic Agents

Medications are most effective when the dose and interval between doses are individualized to meet the needs of a particular patient. The only safe and effective way to administer analgesic medications is by asking the patient to rate the pain and by observing the response to medications.

BALANCED ANALGESIA

Pharmacologic interventions are most effective when a multimodal or balanced analgesia approach is used. **Balanced analgesia** refers to the use of more than one form of analgesia concurrently to obtain more pain relief with fewer side effects. The three general categories of analgesic agents are opioids, NSAIDs, and local anesthetics. These agents work by different mechanisms. Using two or three types of agents simultaneously can maximize pain relief while minimizing the potentially toxic effects of any one agent. When one agent is used alone, it usually must be used in a higher dose to be effective. In other words, although it might require 15 mg morphine to relieve a certain pain, it may take only 8 mg morphine plus 30 mg ketorolac (an NSAID) to relieve the same pain.

PRO RE NATA

In the past, the standard approach was to administer the analgesic *pro re nata* (PRN), or "as needed." The standard practice was for the nurse to wait for the patient to complain of pain and then administer analgesia. As a result, many patients remained in pain because they did not know they needed to ask for medication or waited until the pain became intolerable.

By its very nature, the PRN approach to analgesia leaves patients sedated or in severe pain much of the time. To receive pain relief from an opioid analgesic, the serum level of that opioid must be maintained at a minimum therapeutic level (Fig. 13-8). By the time the patient complains of pain, the serum opioid concentration is below the therapeutic level. From the time the patient requests pain medication until the nurse administers it, the patient's serum levels continue to decrease. The lower the serum opioid level, the more difficult it is to achieve the therapeutic level with the next dose. Using this method, the only way to ensure significant periods of analgesia is to give doses large enough to produce periodic sedation.

PREVENTIVE APPROACH

Currently, a preventive approach to relieving pain by administering analgesic agents is considered the most effective strategy, because a therapeutic serum level of medication is maintained. With the preventive approach, analgesic agents are administered at set intervals so that the medication acts before the pain becomes severe and before the serum opioid level decreases to a subtherapeutic level.

Administering analgesic medication on a time basis, rather than on the basis of a patient's report of pain, prevents the serum drug level from falling to subtherapeutic levels. For example, a patient takes prescribed morphine or a prescribed NSAID (eg, ibuprofen) every 4 hours rather than waiting until the pain is severe. If the pain is likely to occur around the clock or for a substantial portion of a 24-hour period, a regular around-the-clock schedule of administering analgesia may be indicated. Even if the analgesic is prescribed PRN, it can be administered on a preventive basis before the patient is in severe pain, as long as the prescribed interval between doses is observed. The preventive approach reduces the peaks and troughs in the serum level and provides more pain relief with fewer adverse effects.

Smaller doses of medication are needed with the preventive approach, because the pain does not escalate to a level

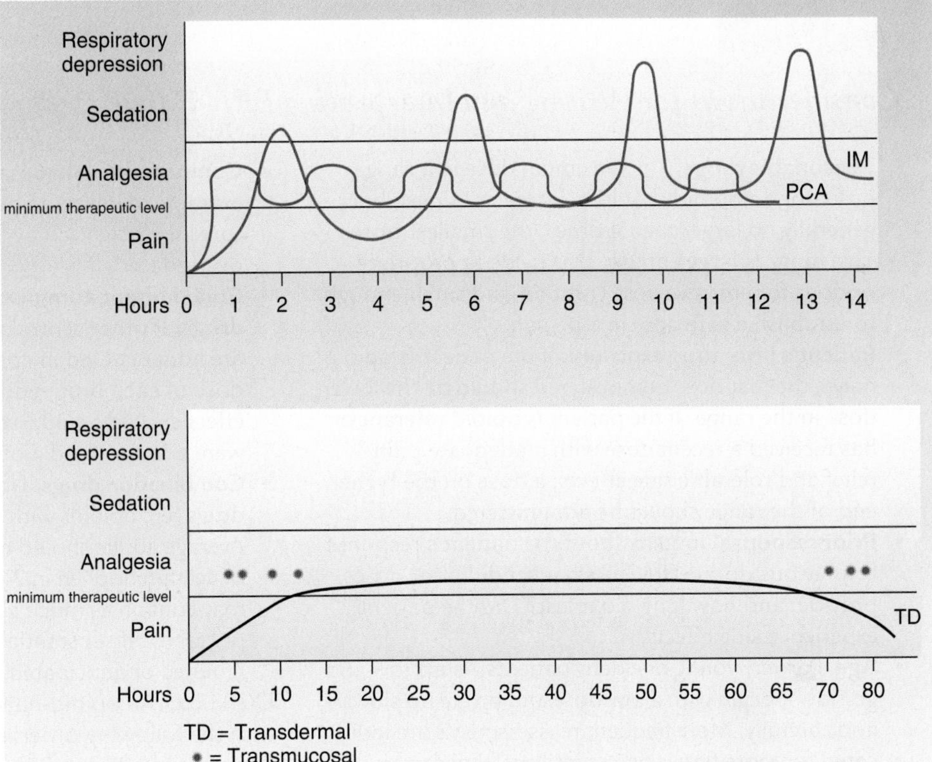

FIGURE 13-8. Relationship of mode of delivery of analgesia to serum analgesic level. *Top:* intramuscular (IM) and intravenous (IV) patient-controlled analgesia (PCA). *Bottom:* transdermal (TD) and transmucosal (•) delivery.

of severe intensity. Therefore, a preventive approach may result in the administration of less medication over a 24-hour period, helping prevent tolerance to analgesic agents and decreasing the severity of side effects (eg, sedation, constipation). Better pain control can be achieved with a preventive approach, reducing the amount of time patients are in pain.

In using the preventive approach, the nurse assesses the patient for sedation before administering the next dose. The goal is to provide analgesia before the pain becomes severe. It is not safe to medicate the patient with opioids repeatedly if the patient is sedated or not in pain. It may be necessary to decrease the dosage of the opioid analgesic so that the patient receives pain relief with less sedation.

USE OF "AS NEEDED" RANGE ORDERS FOR OPIOID ANALGESICS

Because of individual variation in patients' needs and responses to analgesics, PRN range doses have been used to relieve pain. Physicians have prescribed opioids with orders that allow the nurse to determine doses of medication to be administered and intervals between doses based on the nurse's assessment of the patient. Because of concern about patient safety with this method of prescribing analgesics, JCAHO established a policy in 2003 requiring specificity (eg, drug name, dose, route) when prescribing medications or a maximal allowable difference between the high and low dose no more than four times the lowest dose. In response, the American Society for Pain Management Nurses and the American Pain Society developed a consensus statement on as-needed range orders for opioids (Gordon et al., 2004). Chart 13-6 provides further information about as-needed range orders for opioids.

INDIVIDUALIZED DOSAGE

The dosage and the interval between doses should be based on the patient's requirements rather than on an inflexible standard or routine. People metabolize and absorb medications at different rates and experience different levels of pain. Therefore, a certain dose of an opioid medication given at specified intervals may be effective for one patient but ineffective for another.

Because of the fear of promoting addiction or causing respiratory depression, health care providers tend to prescribe and administer inadequate dosages of opioid agents to treat acute pain or persistent pain, particularly in terminally ill patients (Chart 13-7). However, even prolonged administration of opioid agents is associated with an extremely low incidence of addiction (less than 1%). Furthermore, small doses are not necessarily safe doses. For example, some patients receiving a relatively small dose (25 to 50 mg) of meperidine (Demerol) intramuscularly have experienced respiratory depression, whereas other patients have not exhibited any sedation or respiratory depression with very large doses of opioids.

Therefore, the effects of opioid analgesic medications must be monitored, especially when the first dose is given or when the dose is changed or given more frequently. The time, date, patient's pain rating (scale of 0 to 10), analgesic agent, other pain relief measures, side effects, and patient activity are recorded. For example, when the first dose of an analgesic is administered, the nurse should record a pain rating score, blood pressure, and respiratory and pulse rates (all of which are considered "vital signs"). If the pain has not decreased in 30 minutes (sooner if an IV route is used) and the patient is reasonably alert and has a satisfactory respiratory status, blood pressure, and pulse rate, then some change in analgesia is indicated. Although the dose

CHART 13-6

Considerations for Writing and Interpreting PRN Range Orders for Opioid Analgesics

- **Reasonable range.** The maximum dose in a range order for an opioid should be at least 2 times, but generally no larger than 4 times, the smallest dose. This range is large enough to provide appropriate options for effective dose titration and small enough to establish a safe dose in a person.
- **Patient's prior drug exposure.** If the patient is opioid naïve, the first dose administered should be the lower dose in the range. If the patient is opioid tolerant or has received a recent dose with inadequate pain relief and tolerable side effects, a dose on the higher end of the range should be administered.
- **Prior response.** Inquire about the patient's response to previous doses. How much relief did prior doses provide, and how long did it last? Did the patient experience side effects?
- **Age.** For very young or elderly patients, "start low and go slow"; begin with a low dose and titrate up slowly and carefully. More frequent reassessments are indicated for more fragile or less resilient patients.
- **Hepatic and renal function.** If the patient has hepatic or renal insufficiency, anticipate a more pronounced peak effect and a longer duration of action.
- **Kinetics.** Know the onset, peak, and duration of action for the specific drug prescribed. Doses of short-acting opioids can be increased at each specified dosing interval, unlike scheduled long-acting opioid formulations.
- **Comorbidities that may affect patient response.** For example, debilitated patients and those with respiratory insufficiency may be at more risk for hypoxia if oversedated.
- **Concomitant administration of other sedating drugs.** If other central nervous system depressants are administered in combination with opioids, the dose of each drug required to achieve the desired effect should be 30% to 50% less than if either drug were administered alone.
- **Combination drugs.** Limit doses of combination drugs (eg, opioids with acetaminophen or an NSAID). Average adults should not receive more than 4000 mg of acetaminophen in 24 hours. Combination drugs may contain as much as 750 mg of acetaminophen per tablet. If substantial upward dose titration is required or anticipated, use opioid-only preparations.

EXAMPLE: An opioid-naïve patient arrives on the unit with the following order: morphine sulfate 2 mg to 6 mg IV every 2 hour PRN for pain.

- Give 2 mg for the first dose. Assess effects after 5 to 15 minutes. If the patient experiences adequate relief, reassess in 1 to 2 hours.
- If the patient experiences no side effects but inadequate relief, give additional 4 mg at time of peak effect from first dose.
- Total dose is 6 mg in a 2-hour period.

NSAID, nonsteroidal anti-inflammatory drug; PRN, "as required."

of analgesic medication is safe for this patient, it is ineffective in relieving the pain. Therefore, another dose of medication may be indicated. In such instances, the nurse consults with the physician to determine what further action is warranted.

PATIENT-CONTROLLED ANALGESIA

Used to manage postoperative pain as well as persistent pain, **patient-controlled analgesia** (PCA) allows patients to control the administration of their own medication within predetermined safety limits. This approach can be used with oral analgesic agents as well as with continuous infusions of opioid analgesic agents by IV, subcutaneous, or epidural routes. PCA can be used in hospitals or in home settings (Pasero & McCaffery, 2005).

The PCA pump permits the patient to self-administer continuous infusions of medication (basal rates) safely and to administer extra medication (bolus doses) with episodes of increased pain or painful activities. A PCA pump is electronically controlled by a timing device. A patient experiencing pain can administer small amounts of medication directly into his or her IV, subcutaneous, or epidural catheter by pressing a button. The pump then delivers a preset amount of medication.

The PCA pump also can be programmed to deliver a constant, background infusion of medication or basal rate and still allow the patient to administer additional bolus doses as needed. The timer can be programmed to prevent additional doses from being administered until a specified time period has elapsed (lock-out time) and until the first dose has had time to exert its maximal effect. Even if the patient pushes the button multiple times in rapid succession, no additional doses are released. If another dose is required at the end of the delay period, the button must be pushed again to receive the dose. Patients who are controlling their own opioid administration usually become sedated and stop pushing the button before any significant respiratory depression occurs. Nevertheless, assessment of respiratory status remains a major nursing role.

To initiate PCA or any analgesia used at home or in the hospital, it is important to avoid playing "catch-up." Pain should be brought under control before PCA starts, often by the use of an initial, larger bolus dose or loading dose. Then, after control is achieved, the pump is programmed to deliver small doses of medication at a time. If a patient with severe pain has a low serum level of opioid analgesic because of an inadequate basal rate, it is difficult to regain control with the small doses available by pump. Before the

CHART 13-7

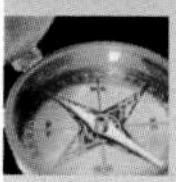

Ethics and Related Issues

Inadequate Pain Management

SITUATION

When taking over the care of ethnic minority patients at the change of shift from a particular colleague, you usually find these patients to be in a great deal of pain. Your nonsystematic observations have led you to conclude that these patients receive only a small portion of the analgesia prescribed for them. You have heard a nurse colleague state a belief that people of certain ethnic groups have "no pain tolerance" and are "just looking for drugs."

DILEMMA

Racial biases are difficult to deal with and change. To confront this nurse may not alter the behavior but will certainly disrupt the working relationships on the unit. It would be easier to look the other way. On the other hand, you believe that the nurse is giving inadequate and unethical care to selected patients and placing them at greater risk for postoperative complications.

DISCUSSION

- What information would you need to collect before acting?
- From whom could you seek counsel?
- Are the two aspects of the dilemma equally important?

PCA pump is used, repeated bolus doses of an IV opioid may be administered as prescribed over a short period until the pain is relieved. Then PCA is initiated. If pain control is not achieved with the maximal dose of medication prescribed, further prescriptions are obtained. The goal is to achieve a minimum therapeutic level of analgesia and to allow the patient to maintain that level by using the PCA pump. The patient is instructed not to wait until the pain is severe before pushing the button to obtain a bolus dose. The patient is also reminded not to become so distracted by an activity or visitor that he or she forgets to self-administer a prescribed dose of medication. One potential drawback to distraction is that the patient who is using a PCA pump may not self-administer any analgesia during the time of effective distraction. When distraction ends suddenly (eg, a movie ends, visitors leave), the patient may be left without a therapeutic serum opioid level. When intermittent distraction is used for pain relief, a continuous low-level background infusion of opioid through the PCA pump may be prescribed so that, after the distraction ends, it will not be necessary to try to "catch up."

A continuous infusion plus bolus doses may be effective with cancer patients who require large doses of analgesia and with postsurgical patients. Although this allows more uninterrupted sleep, the risk of sedation increases, especially when the patient has minimal or decreasing pain.

Patients who use PCA achieve better pain relief and often require less pain medication than those who are treated in the standard PRN fashion (Colwell, 2004). Because the patient can maintain a near-constant level of medication, the periods of severe pain and sedation that occur with the traditional PRN regimen are avoided.

If PCA is to be used in the patient's home, the patient and family are taught about the operation of the pump as well as the side effects of the medication and strategies to manage them (Pasero & McCaffery, 2005).

NURSING ALERT

Family members are cautioned not to push the button for a patient, especially if the patient is asleep, because this overrides some of the safety features of the PCA system.

Local Anesthetic Agents

Local anesthetics work by blocking nerve conduction when applied directly to the nerve fibers. They can be applied directly to the site of injury (eg, a topical anesthetic spray for sunburn) or directly to nerve fibers by injection or at the time of surgery. They can also be administered through an epidural catheter.

TOPICAL APPLICATION

Local anesthetic agents have been successful in reducing the pain associated with thoracic or upper abdominal surgery when injected by the surgeon intercostally. Local anesthetic agents are rapidly absorbed into the bloodstream, resulting in decreased availability at the surgical or injury site and an increased anesthetic level in the blood, increasing the risk of toxicity. Therefore, a vasoconstrictive agent (eg, epinephrine or phenylephrine) is added to the anesthetic agent to decrease its systemic absorption and maintain its concentration at the surgical or injury site.

A topical anesthetic agent known as eutectic mixture or emulsion of local anesthetics, or EMLA cream, has been effective in preventing the pain associated with invasive procedures such as lumbar puncture or the insertion of intravenous lines. To be effective, EMLA must be applied to the site 60 to 90 minutes before the procedure.

A lidocaine 5% (Lidoderm) patch, which has been on the market since 1999, has been shown to be effective in postherpetic neuralgia (Meier, Wasner, Kuntzer, et al., 2003). Currently, this is the only use approved by the U.S. Food and Drug Administration. The patch acts locally by targeting damaged nerves responsible for discharging pain impulses. Because the lidocaine 5% patch does not cause sensory block in the area of application, it has a wide margin of safety. The recommended dose is one to three patches at a time applied for 12 hours daily.

INTRASPINAL ADMINISTRATION

Intermittent or continuous administration of local anesthetic agents through an epidural catheter has been used for years to produce anesthesia during surgery. Although the administration of local anesthetic agents in the spinal canal is still largely confined to acute pain, such as postoperative pain and pain associated with labor and delivery, the epidural administration of local anesthetic agents for pain management is increasing.

A local anesthetic agent administered through an epidural catheter is applied directly to the nerve root. The anesthetic agent can be administered continuously in low doses, intermittently on a schedule, or on demand as the patient requires it, and it is often combined with the epidural administration of opioids. Surgical patients treated with this combination experience fewer complications after surgery, ambulate sooner, and have shorter hospital stays than patients who receive standard therapy (Correll, Viscusi, Grunwald, et al., 2001).

Opioid Analgesic Agents

The goal of administering opioids is to relieve pain and improve quality of life; therefore, the route of administration, dose, and frequency of administration are determined on an individual basis. Factors that are considered in determining the route, dose, and frequency of medication include the characteristics of the pain (eg, its expected duration and severity), the overall status of the patient, the patient's response to analgesic medications, and the patient's report of pain. Opioids can be administered by various routes—oral, IV, subcutaneous, intraspinal, intranasal, rectal, and transdermal. Although the oral route is usually preferred for opioid administration, oral opioids must be given frequently enough and in large enough doses to be effective. Opioid analgesic agents given orally may provide a more consistent serum level than those given intramuscularly.

If the patient is expected to require opioid analgesic agents at home, the clinician should consider the ability of the patient and family to administer opioids as prescribed at the planning stages and should take steps to ensure that the required medications will be available to the patient. Many pharmacies, especially those in smaller rural areas or inner cities, may be reluctant to stock large amounts of opioids. Therefore, arrangements for obtaining these prescription medications must be made ahead of time.

With the administration of opioids by any route, side effects must be considered and anticipated. Clinicians who take steps to minimize the side effects increase the likelihood that the patient will receive adequate pain relief without interrupting therapy to treat the effects.

RESPIRATORY DEPRESSION AND SEDATION

Respiratory depression is the most serious adverse effect of opioid analgesic agents administered by IV, subcutaneous, or epidural routes. However, it is relatively rare because doses administered through these routes are small, and tolerance to respiratory depressant effects increases if the dose is increased slowly. The risk of respiratory depression increases with age and with the concomitant use of other opioids or other CNS depressants. The risk of respiratory depression also increases when the epidural catheter is placed in the thoracic area and when the intra-abdominal or intrathoracic pressure is increased.

A patient who receives opioids by any route must be assessed frequently for changes in respiratory status. Specific notable changes are shallow respirations and decreasing respiratory rate. Despite the risks associated with their use, IV and epidural opioids are considered safe, with the risks related to epidural administration no greater than those related to IV or other systemic routes of administration. Sedation, which may occur with any method of administering opioids, is likely to occur when opioid doses are increased. However, patients often develop tolerance quickly, so that in a short time they are no longer sedated by the dose that initially caused sedation. Increasing the time between doses or reducing the dose temporarily, as prescribed, usually prevents deep sedation from occurring. Patients at risk for sedation must be monitored closely for changes in respiratory status. Patients are also at risk for problems associated with sedation and immobility. The nurse must initiate strategies to prevent problems such as skin breakdown.

NAUSEA AND VOMITING

Nausea and vomiting frequently occur with opioid use. Usually these effects occur some hours after the initial injection. Patients, especially postoperative patients, may not think to tell the nurse that they are nauseated, particularly if the nausea is mild. However, a patient receiving opioids should be assessed for nausea and vomiting, which may be triggered by a position change and may be prevented by having the patient change positions slowly. Adequate hydration and the administration of antiemetic agents may also decrease the incidence of nausea. Opioid-induced nausea and vomiting often subside within a few days.

CONSTIPATION

Constipation, a common side effect of opioid use, may become so severe that the patient is forced to choose between relief of pain and relief of constipation. This situation can occur in patients after surgery and in patients receiving large doses of opioids to treat cancer-related pain. Preventing constipation must be a high priority in all patients receiving opioids. Whenever a patient receives opioids, a bowel regimen should begin at the same time. Tolerance to this side effect does not occur; rather, constipation persists even with long-term use of opioids.

Several strategies may help prevent and treat opioid-related constipation. Mild laxatives and a high intake of fluid and fiber may be effective in managing mild constipation. Unless contraindicated, a mild laxative and a stool softener should be administered on a regular schedule. However, continued severe constipation often requires the use of a stimulating cathartic agent, such as senna derivatives (Senokot) or bisacodyl (Dulcolax). Oral laxatives and stool softeners may prevent constipation. If oral agents fail, rectal suppositories may be used (Plaisance & Ellis, 2002).

INADEQUATE PAIN RELIEF

One factor commonly associated with ineffective pain relief is an inadequate dose of opioid. This is most likely to occur when the caregiver underestimates the patient's pain or fails to consider differences in absorption and action after a change in the route of administration. Consequently, the patient receives doses that are too small to be effective and, possibly, too infrequent to relieve pain. For example, if opioid delivery is changed from the IV route to the oral route, the oral dose must be approximately three times greater than that given parenterally to provide relief. Because of differences in absorption of orally administered opioids among individuals, patients must be assessed carefully to ensure that the pain is relieved.

Table 13-3 lists opioids and dosages that are equivalent to morphine. It serves only as a guide; the doses listed are

TABLE 13-3 Selected Opioid Analgesics Commonly Used for Moderate and Severe Pain in Adults

	Starting Dose (milligrams)			
Name	***Moderate Pain***	***Severe Pain***	**Comments**	**Precautions and Contraindications**
Morphine	–	30–60 (oral) 10 (parenteral)	Acts as an agonist at specific opioid receptors in the CNS to produce analgesia, euphoria, and sedation.	Use with caution, especially in elderly patients, very ill patients, and those with respiratory impairment. Major risks include respiratory depression, apnea, circulatory depression, and respiratory arrest, shock, and cardiac arrest. Obtain history of hypersensitivity to opioids. Monitor patient closely. If prescribed in correct dose, oral preparations (MS Contin) are effective in treating moderate and severe pain.
Codeine	15–30 (oral)	60 (oral) up to 360/24 hr	Acts as an agonist at specific opioid receptors in the CNS to produce analgesia, euphoria, and sedation. Is also an antitussive. 10% of people lack the enzyme needed to make codeine active. Codeine may cause more nausea and constipation per unit of analgesia than other mu agonist opioids.	Many preparations of codeine and the other opioids in this table are combinations with nonopioid analgesics. Caution must be used in patients with impaired ventilation, bronchial asthma, increased intracranial pressure, or impaired liver function and in elderly and very ill patients.
Oxycodone (OxyContin)	5 (oral)	10–20 (oral)	Acts as an agonist at specific opioid receptors in the CNS to produce analgesia, euphoria, and sedation.	Caution must be used in patients with impaired ventilation, bronchial asthma, increased intracranial pressure, or impaired liver function and in elderly and very ill patients.
Meperidine (Demerol)	50 (oral)	300 (oral) 75 (parenteral)	Acts as an agonist at specific opioid receptors in the CNS to produce analgesia, euphoria, and sedation. Shorter acting than morphine. Meperidine is biotransformed to normeperidine, a toxic metabolite.	Normeperidine, a toxic metabolic of meperidine, accumulates with repetitive dosing, causing CNS excitation. High risk for seizures. Should be avoided in patients with impaired renal function who are receiving MAO inhibitors. Is irritating to tissues with repeated intramuscular injections. Chronic use should be avoided. Should not be used for more than 1 or 2 days.
Propoxyphene (Darvon)	65–130 (oral)	–	Weak analgesic; acts as an agonist at specific opioid receptors in the CNS to produce analgesia, euphoria, and sedation. Many preparations include nonopioid analgesics; biotransformed to potentially toxic metabolite (norpropoxphene).	Accumulation of propoxyphene and toxic metabolites occurs with repetitive dosing. Overdose is complicated by seizures. Propoxyphene is not recommended for older adults or patients with renal impairment.
Hydrocodone (Vicodin)	5–10 (oral)	–	–	Most preparations are combined with nonopioid analgesics.
Tramadol (Ultram)	50–100 (oral)	–	Unique mechanism; analgesia results from the synergy of two mechanisms. Maximum dose is 400 mg/day.	Most common side effects are dizziness, nausea, constipation, and somnolence. Lowers seizure threshold.

CNS, central nervous system; MAO, monoamine oxidase.

Adapted from American Pain Society. (2003). *Principles of analgesic use in the treatment of acute pain and cancer pain* (5th ed.). Glenview, IL: American Pain Society; and Karch, A. M. (2005). *Lippincott's nursing drug guide.* Philadelphia: Lippincott Williams & Wilkins.

not necessarily the most appropriate doses for all patients. However, the table does give clinicians some idea of equivalency between two different opioids. After administering the first dose of an opioid, clinicians should perform a complete pain assessment to determine the efficacy of that dose. In general, no recalculation needs to be done when changing from one brand of an agent to another brand of the same medication, with the exception of extended-release oral morphine. Currently, three brands of extended-release morphine (MS Contin, Oramorph, Kadian) are commonly used by cancer patients. Although these agents come in the same dosage form and contain the same drug, they are not considered therapeutically equivalent because they use different release mechanisms. Patients who need to change brands should be monitored carefully both for overdose and for inadequate pain relief.

OTHER EFFECTS OF OPIOIDS

When asked about drug allergies, patients with previous hospital experience (especially for surgery) may report that they are "allergic" to morphine. This report should be thoroughly investigated. Commonly, this "allergy" is described as itching only. Pruritus (itching) is a frequent side effect of opioids administered by any route, but it is not an allergic reaction. It can be relieved by administering prescribed antihistamines. Epidurally administered opioids may also cause urinary retention or pruritus. The patient should be monitored and may require urinary catheterization. Small doses of naloxone may be prescribed to relieve these problems in patients who are receiving epidural opioids for the relief of acute postoperative pain.

A number of factors may influence the safety and effectiveness of opioid administration. Opioid analgesic agents are primarily metabolized by the liver and excreted by the kidney. Therefore, metabolism and excretion of analgesic medications are impaired in patients with liver or kidney disease, increasing the risk of cumulative or toxic effects. In addition, normeperidine, a metabolite of meperidine, may rapidly or unexpectedly accumulate to toxic levels. This is more likely to occur in patients with impaired kidney function and may result in seizures in susceptible patients. Many institutions no longer stock meperidine because of the risks associated with the metabolite normeperidine and because most physicians do not prescribe a high enough dose for it to be effective.

Patients with untreated hypothyroidism are more susceptible to the analgesic effects and side effects of opioids. In contrast, patients with hyperthyroidism may require larger doses for pain relief. Patients with a decreased respiratory reserve from disease or aging may be more susceptible to the depressant effects of opioids and must be carefully monitored for respiratory depression.

Patients who are dehydrated are at increased risk for the hypotensive effects of opioids. Patients who become hypotensive after the administration of an opioid should be kept recumbent and rehydrated unless fluids are contraindicated. Patients who are dehydrated are also more likely to experience nausea and vomiting with opioid use. Rehydration usually relieves these symptoms.

Patients receiving certain other medications, such as monoamine oxidase inhibitors, phenothiazines, or tricyclic antidepressants, may have an exaggerated response to the depressant effects of opioids. Patients taking these medications should receive small doses of opioids and must be monitored closely. Continued pain in these patients indicates that a therapeutic level of the analgesic has not been achieved. Patients must be monitored for sedation even if an analgesic effect has not been obtained.

TOLERANCE AND ADDICTION

There is no maximum safe dosage of opioids, nor is there any easily identifiable therapeutic serum level. Both the maximal safe dosage and the therapeutic serum level are relative and individual. **Tolerance** (the need for increasing doses of opioids to achieve the same therapeutic effect) develops in almost all patients taking opioids for extended periods. Patients requiring opioids over a long term, especially cancer patients, need increasing doses to relieve pain. After the first few weeks of therapy, their dosing requirements usually level off. Patients who become tolerant to the analgesic effects of large doses of morphine may obtain pain relief by changing to a different opioid. Symptoms of physical dependence may occur when the opioids are discontinued; dependence often occurs with opioid tolerance and does not indicate an addiction. It is an expected physiologic response that will occur in all people exposed to continuous opioid administration (Compton & Athanos, 2003).

> **NURSING ALERT**
>
> **Although patients may need increasing levels of opioids, they are not addicted. Physical tolerance usually occurs in the absence of addiction. Tolerance to opioids is common and becomes a problem primarily in terms of delivering or administering the medication (eg, how to administer very large doses of morphine to a patient). On the other hand, addiction is rare and should not be the primary concern of nurses caring for patients in pain.**

Addiction is a behavioral pattern of substance use characterized by a compulsion to take the substance (drug or alcohol) primarily to experience its psychic effects. Fear that patients will become addicted or dependent on opioids has contributed to inadequate treatment of pain. This fear is commonly expressed by health care providers as well as patients and results from lack of knowledge about the low risk of addiction.

Addiction after therapeutic opioid administration is so negligible that it should not be a consideration when caring for patients in pain. Therefore, patients and health care providers should be dissuaded from withholding opioid analgesics because of concerns about addiction.

When caring for people with a known history of addiction, nurses should consider that each individual person has the right to be treated for pain. The American Society for Pain Management Nurses (2002) developed a position paper on pain management of patients with addictive disease. It stressed education, communication about methods for pain management, and methods to discontinue opioids in this patient population. The opioids should be tapered slowly to prevent withdrawal symptoms (Nichols, 2003).

Nonsteroidal Anti-inflammatory Drugs

NSAIDs are thought to decrease pain by inhibiting cyclooxygenase (COX), the rate-limiting enzyme involved in the production of prostaglandin from traumatized or inflamed tissues. There are two types of COX, COX-1 and COX-2.

COX-1 mediates prostaglandin formation involved in the maintenance of physiologic functions. Some of the physiologic functions of COX-1 include platelet aggregation through the provision of thromboxane precursors and increased gastric mucosal blood flow. This prevents ischemia and promotes mucosal integrity. Inhibition of COX-1 results in gastric ulceration, bleeding, and renal damage.

COX-2 mediates prostaglandin formation that results in symptoms of pain, inflammation, and fever. Therefore, inhibition of COX-2 is desirable. Celecoxib (Celebrex), rofecoxib (Vioxx), and valdecoxib (Bextra) are examples of COX-2 inhibitors. Evidence of increased cardiovascular risk for people taking rofecoxib (Vioxx) for longer than 18 months prompted its manufacturer to withdraw it from the market. The manufacturer noted that there was an increased incidence of cardiovascular events (stroke and myocardial infarction) associated with its use (Shaya & Suwannaprom, 2005). The U.S. Food and Drug Administration then mandated that a warning be added to the label of all COX-2 inhibitors about these risks. The pharmaceutical company that makes valdecoxib (Bextra) withdrew it from the market. Shaya and Suwannaprom (2005) stated that the findings of studies on the cardiovascular effects of COX-2 inhibitors should be interpreted with caution, because if no data were collected about cardiovascular status of patients, researchers cannot conclude that cardiovascular events are or are not related to these medications.

Ibuprofen (Advil, Motrin), another NSAID, blocks both COX-1 and COX-2, is effective in relieving mild to moderate pain, and has a low incidence of adverse effects. Aspirin, the oldest NSAID, also blocks COX-1 as well as COX-2; however, because it causes frequent and severe side effects, aspirin is infrequently used to treat significant acute or persistent pain.

NSAIDs are very helpful in treating arthritic diseases and may be especially powerful in treating cancer-related bone pain. They have been effectively combined with opioids to treat postoperative and other severe pain. The use of NSAIDs in combination with opioids relieves pain more effectively than opioids alone. In such cases, patients may obtain pain relief with decreased doses of opioid and with fewer side effects. In addition, intraoperative administration of NSAIDs reportedly improves postoperative pain control after abdominal hysterectomy surgery (Karamanlioglu, Turan, Memis, et al., 2004). A regimen of a fixed-dose, time-contingent NSAID (eg, every 4 hours) and a separately administered fluctuating dose of opioid may be effective in managing moderate to severe cancer pain. In more severe pain, the opioid dose is also fixed, with an additional fluctuating dose as needed for **breakthrough pain** (a sudden increase in pain despite the administration of pain-relieving medications). These regimens result in better pain relief with fewer opioid-related side effects.

Most patients tolerate NSAIDs well. However, those with impaired kidney function may require a smaller dose and must be monitored closely for side effects. Patients taking NSAIDs bruise easily because the agents have some anticoagulant effect. Furthermore, NSAIDs may displace other medications, such as warfarin (Coumadin), from serum proteins and increase their effects. High doses or prolonged use can irritate the stomach and in some cases result in gastrointestinal bleeding as well. For this reason, monitoring for gastrointestinal bleeding is indicated (Gordon, 2003).

Tricyclic Antidepressant Agents and Anticonvulsant Medications

Pain of neurologic origin (eg, causalgia, tumor impingement on a nerve, postherpetic neuralgia) is difficult to treat and in general is not responsive to opioid therapy. If these pain syndromes are accompanied by dysesthesia (burning or cutting pain), they may be responsive to a tricyclic antidepressant or an antiseizure agent. When indicated, tricyclic antidepressant agents, such as amitriptyline (Elavil) or imipramine (Tofranil), are prescribed in doses considerably smaller than those generally used for depression. Patients need to know that a therapeutic effect may not occur until they have taken the medication for 3 weeks. Antiseizure medications such as phenytoin (Dilantin) or carbamazepine (Tegretol) also are used in doses lower than those prescribed for seizure disorders. Because a variety of medications can be tried, nurses should be familiar with the possible side effects and should teach patients and families how to recognize these effects.

Routes of Administration

The route selected for administration of an analgesic agent (Table 13-4) depends on the condition of the individual patient and the desired effect of the medication. Analgesic agents can be administered by parenteral, oral, rectal, transdermal, transmucosal, intraspinal, or epidural routes. Each method of administration has advantages and disadvantages. The route chosen should be based on patient need.

Parenteral Route

Parenteral administration (intramuscular, IV, or subcutaneous) of the analgesic medication produces effects more rapidly than oral administration does, but these effects are of shorter duration. Parenteral administration may be indicated if the patient is not permitted oral intake or is vomiting.

℞ TABLE 13-4 Administration Routes for Analgesics

Route	Site
Parenteral	Intramuscular (IM) Intravenous (IV) Subcutaneous (SC)
Gastrointestinal	Oral (PO) Rectal (PR)
Transdermal	Skin
Transmucosal	Oral mucosa Intranasal mucosa Bronchial mucosa
Topical	Skin or mucosa
Epidural	Epidural space
Intraspinal	Spinal canal

Medication administered by the intramuscular route enters the bloodstream more slowly than medication given IV and is metabolized slowly. The rate of absorption may be erratic; it depends on the site selected and the amount of body fat.

The IV route is an alternative to intramuscular injection for many but not all analgesic medications. The IV route is the preferred parenteral route in most acute care situations because it is much more comfortable for patients. In addition, peak serum levels and pain relief occur more rapidly and more reliably. Because the action of the opioid peaks rapidly (usually within minutes) and it is metabolized quickly, an appropriate IV dose is smaller and is prescribed at shorter intervals than an intramuscular dose.

Intravenous opioids may be administered by intravenous push or slow push (eg, over a 5- to 10-minute period) or by continuous infusion with a pump. Continuous infusion provides a steady level of analgesia and is indicated when pain occurs over a 24-hour period, such as after surgery for the first day or so, or in a patient with prolonged cancer pain who cannot take medication by other routes. The dose of analgesic agent is calculated carefully to relieve pain without producing respiratory depression and other side effects.

The subcutaneous route for infusion of opioid analgesic agents is used for patients with severe pain such as cancer pain. In addition, it is particularly useful for patients with limited intravenous access who cannot take oral medications and for patients who are managing their pain at home. The subcutaneous route is often an effective and convenient way to manage pain, but the dose of opioid that can be infused through this route is limited because of the small volume that can be administered at one time into the subcutaneous tissue.

Oral Route

Oral administration is preferred over parenteral administration if the patient can take medication by mouth, because it is easy, noninvasive, and not painful. Severe pain can be relieved with oral opioids if the doses are high enough (see Table 13-3). In terminally ill patients with prolonged pain, doses may gradually be increased as the disease progresses and causes more pain or as the patient builds up a tolerance to the medication. If these higher doses are increased gradually, they usually provide additional pain relief without producing respiratory depression or sedation. If the route of administration is changed from a parenteral route to the oral route at a dose that is not equivalent in strength (equianalgesic), the smaller oral dose may result in a withdrawal reaction and recurrence of pain.

Rectal Route

The rectal route may be indicated in patients who cannot take medications by any other route. The rectal route may also be indicated for patients with bleeding problems, such as hemophilia. The onset of action of opioids administered rectally is unclear but is delayed compared with other routes of administration. Similarly, the duration of action is prolonged.

Transdermal Route

The transdermal route is used to achieve a consistent opioid serum level through absorption of the medication via the skin. It is most often used in cancer patients at home or in hospice care who take oral sustained-release morphine. The only commercially available transdermal opioids are fentanyl (Duragesic) and buprenorphine (Buprenex), which are marketed as patches consisting of a reservoir containing the medication and a porous membrane.

Fentanyl was the first commercially available transdermal opioid (Chart 13-8). When the fentanyl transdermal system is first applied to the skin, fentanyl, which is fat-soluble, binds to the skin and fat layers. Then it is slowly and systemically absorbed. Therefore, there is a delay in effect while the dermal layer is being saturated. A drug reservoir actually forms in the upper layer of skin. This results in a slowly rising serum level and a slow tapering of the serum level once the patch is removed (see Fig. 13-8). Because it takes 12 to 24 hours for the fentanyl levels to gradually increase from the first patch, the last dose of sustained-release morphine should be administered at the same time the first patch is applied (D'Arcy, 2005a, 2005b; Pasero, 2005). Transdermal fentanyl is associated with slightly less constipation than oral opioids are. Absorption is increased in febrile patients. A heating pad should never be applied to the area where the patch is applied. Transdermal fentanyl is much more expensive than sustained-release morphine, but it is less costly than methods that deliver parenteral opioids.

Buprenorphine, the second transdermal system to be approved, is available in three strengths. It has many of the same advantages as fentanyl and has been shown in limited clinical studies to be associated with a high level of patient adherence and improved quality of life (Bohme, 2002).

CHART 13-8

Safe Use of Transdermal Fentanyl

The U.S. Food and Drug Administration issued a public health advisory in 2005 about the use of fentanyl skin patches and warned patients and health care providers about the need for the patches to be used as intended. The advisory also included precautions about safe storage and disposal of fentanyl skin patches:

- Fentanyl skin patches are very strong opioids and should always be prescribed at the lowest dose needed for pain relief. They should be used only for patients with chronic pain that is not well controlled with shorter-acting opioids.
- Patients should be cautioned that a sudden and possibly dangerous rise in the level of fentanyl in their blood can occur with use of alcohol or other medications that affect brain function; an increase in body temperature or exposure to heat; or use of other medicines that affect the metabolism of fentanyl.
- Patients should be informed about signs and symptoms of fentanyl overdose (ie, shallow or difficult breathing; fatigue, extreme sleepiness, or sedation; inability to think, talk, or walk normally; and feeling faint, dizzy, or confused).

Once it is determined that switching from other routes of morphine administration to a transdermal system is appropriate, the correct dosage or strength for the patch must be calculated. If the patient uses an opioid other than morphine, conversion to milligrams of oral morphine is the first step. After determining how many milligrams of morphine (or morphine equivalents) the patient has been using over 24 hours, an initial dose of transdermal fentanyl or buprenorphine is calculated (Skaer, 2004). Patients switched from morphine to transdermal patches of either fentanyl or buprenorphine should be assessed not only for pain and potential side effects but also for dependence, reflected by withdrawal symptoms, which may consist of shivering, a feeling of coldness, sweating, headache, and paresthesia (Gordon & Dahl, 2003). Patients may require short-acting opioids for breakthrough pain before the systemic opioid delivered through the transdermal system reaches a therapeutic level.

NURSING ALERT

Conversion tables available for the transdermal systems should be used only to establish the initial dose of the transdermal fentanyl or buprenorphine when patients switch from oral morphine to the transdermal route of delivery (and not vice versa). If these tables are inappropriately used to determine the dosages of oral morphine for patients who have been receiving transdermal fentanyl or buprenorphine, many patients will not achieve satisfactory analgesia and will require an increase in their opioid dose to treat breakthrough pain.

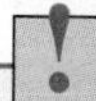

NURSING ALERT

If the conversion table or equation is used incorrectly to calculate a morphine dose, there is a risk of overdose. If a patient requires a change from transdermal fentanyl or buprenorphine back to oral or intravenous morphine (as in the case of surgery), the patch should be removed and intravenous morphine administered on an as-needed basis. Before a new patch is applied, the patient should be carefully checked for any older, forgotten patches, which should be removed and discarded. Patches should be replaced every 72 hours.

Transmucosal Route

People with cancer pain who are being cared for at home may be receiving continuous opioids using sustained-release morphine, hydromorphone, oxycodone, transdermal fentanyl or buprenorphine, or other medications. These patients often experience short episodes of severe pain (eg, after coughing or moving), or they may experience sudden increases in their baseline pain resulting from a change in their condition. These periods, called breakthrough pain, can be well managed with an oral dose of a short-acting transmucosal opioid that has a rapid onset of action. Available transmucosal opioids are fentanyl, buprenorphine, sufentanil, and methadone.

Currently, butorphanol (Stadol) and fentanyl (Duragesic, Sublimaze), sufentanil (Sufenta), and morphine are the only approved transmucosal opioid analgesic agents commercially available in the form of nasal sprays. Butorphanol is a complex medication that simultaneously acts to induce or promote (**agonist**) and inhibit or reverse (**antagonist**) opioid effects. It works like an opioid agonist and an opioid antagonist at the same time. Butorphanol in any form cannot be combined with other opioids (eg, for cancer breakthrough pain), because the antagonist component blocks the action of the opioids the patient is already receiving. The principal use of this agent is for brief, moderate to severe pain, such as migraine headaches.

Intranasal morphine is useful in cancer-related breakthrough pain. When it is given in this form, analgesia is achieved within 5 to 10 minutes, resulting in significant decreases in pain intensity and high patient satisfaction (Fitzgibbon, Morgan, Docketer, et al., 2003).

Intraspinal and Epidural Routes

Infusion of opioids or local anesthetic agents into the subarachnoid space (intrathecal space or spinal canal) or epidural space has been used for effective control of pain in postoperative patients and those with chronic pain unrelieved by other methods. A catheter is inserted into the subarachnoid or the epidural space at the thoracic or lumbar level for administration of opioid or anesthetic agents (Fig. 13-9). With intrathecal administration, medication infuses directly into the subarachnoid space and cerebrospinal fluid, which surrounds the spinal cord. With epidural administration, medication is deposited in the dura of the spinal canal and diffuses into the subarachnoid space. It is believed that pain relief from intraspinal administration of opioids is based on the existence of opioid receptors in the spinal cord.

Infusion of opioids and local anesthetic agents through an intrathecal or epidural catheter results in pain relief with fewer side effects, including sedation, than with systemic analgesia. Adverse effects associated with intraspinal administration include spinal headache resulting from loss of spinal fluid when the dura is punctured. This is more likely to occur in younger patients (less than 40 years of age). The dura must be punctured with the intrathecal route, and dural puncture may occur inadvertently with the epidural route. If dural puncture inadvertently occurs, spinal fluid seeps out of the spinal canal. The resultant headache is likely to be more severe with an epidural needle because it is larger than a spinal needle, and therefore more spinal fluid escapes.

Respiratory depression generally peaks 6 to 12 hours after epidural opioids are administered, but it can occur earlier or up to 24 hours after the first injection. Depending on the lipophilicity (affinity for body fat) of the opioid injected, the time frame for respiratory depression can be short or long. Morphine is hydrophilic, and the time for

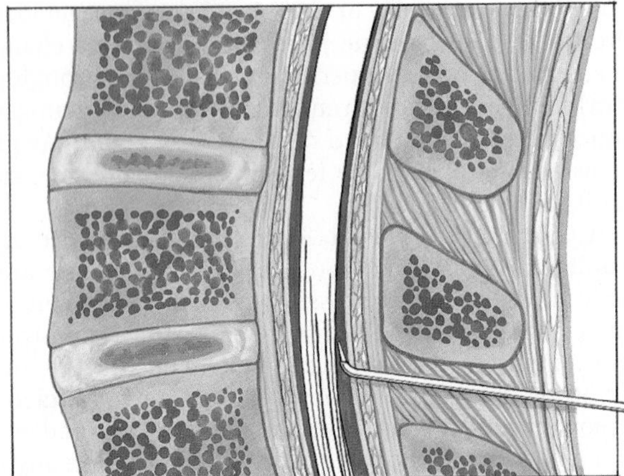

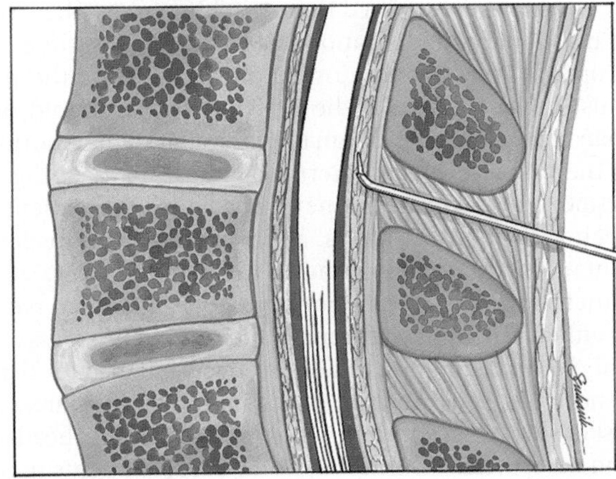

FIGURE 13-9. Placement of intraspinal catheters for administration of analgesic medications: (**A**) intrathecal route, (**B**) epidural route.

peak effect is longer than that of fentanyl, which is lipophilic. The patient should be monitored closely for at least 24 hours after the first injection and longer if changes in respiratory status or level of consciousness occur. Opioid antagonist agents such as naloxone must be available for IV use if respiratory depression occurs.

The patient is also observed for urinary retention, pruritus, nausea, vomiting, and dizziness. Precautions must be taken to avoid infection at the catheter site and catheter displacement. Only medications without preservatives should be administered into the subarachnoid or epidural space because of the potential neurotoxic effects of preservatives.

During surgery, intrathecal opioids are used almost exclusively after a spinal anesthetic agent is administered. For patients undergoing large abdominal surgical procedures, especially those at risk for postoperative complications, a combination of a general inhaled anesthetic agent administered before surgery and a local epidural anesthetic agent and epidural opioids administered after surgery results in excellent pain control with fewer postoperative complications.

For patients who have persistent, severe pain that fails to respond to other treatments, or who obtain pain relief only with the risk of serious side effects, medication administered by a long-term intrathecal or epidural catheter may be effective. After the physician tunnels the catheter through the subcutaneous tissue and places the inlet (or port) under the skin, the medication is injected through the skin into the inlet and catheter, which delivers the medication directly into the epidural space. It may be necessary to inject the medication several times a day to maintain an adequate level of pain relief.

For patients who require more frequent doses or continuous infusions of opioid analgesic agents to relieve pain, an implantable infusion device or pump may be used to administer the medication continuously. The medication is administered at a small, constant dose at a preset rate into the epidural or subarachnoid space. The reservoir of the infusion device stores the medication for slow release and needs to be refilled every 1 or 2 months, depending on the patient's needs. This eliminates the need for repeated injections through the skin.

A new delivery method of epidural morphine has been developed that provides effective analgesia for patients who have undergone major surgical procedures. A single-dose extended-release epidural morphine (Depodur) is administered into the epidural space at the lumbar level immediately prior to surgery. The morphine is released slowly from microvesicular liposomes. One dose of 5 to 15 mg is absorbed around the epidural space and systemically. Depodur has been shown to provide up to 48 hours of postoperative analgesia. Although supplemental analgesic agents may be needed, patients who have received Depodur tend to report less intense pain and greater satisfaction with pain relief (Gambling, Hughes, Martin, et al., 2005). Side effects are similar to those of other epidural opioids (ie, nausea, vomiting, pruritus, and hypotension); its use is contraindicated in patients with allergy to morphine, respiratory depression, severe asthma or upper airway obstruction, and circulatory shock.

NURSING ALERT

Epidural catheters inserted for pain control are usually managed by nurses. Baseline information necessary to provide safe and effective pain control includes the level or site of catheter insertion, the medications (eg, local anesthetic agents, opioids) that have been administered, and the medications anticipated in the future. The infusion rate is increased with caution when anesthetic agents are combined with opioids. Sensory deficits can occur, and patients must be assessed frequently. An infusion with a lower concentration of anesthetic agent allows for administration of a greater concentration of opioid with a lower risk of sensory deficits.

NURSING MANAGEMENT OF SIDE EFFECTS

Headache resulting from spinal fluid loss may be delayed. Therefore, the nurse needs to assess regularly for headache after either type of catheter is placed. If headache develops, the patient should remain flat in bed and should be given large amounts of fluids (provided the medical condition allows), and the physician should be notified. An epidural blood patch may be performed to reduce leakage of spinal fluid.

Cardiovascular effects (hypotension and decreased heart rate) may result from relaxation of the vasculature in the lower extremities. Therefore, the nurse should assess frequently for decreases in blood pressure, pulse rate, and urine output.

Urinary retention and pruritus may develop, and the physician may prescribe small doses of naloxone to combat these effects. The nurse administers these doses in continuous IV infusions that are small enough to reverse the side effects of the opioids without reversing the analgesic effects. Diphenhydramine (Benadryl) may also be used to relieve opioid-related pruritus.

PROMOTING HOME AND COMMUNITY-BASED CARE

Patients who receive epidural analgesic agents at home and their families must be taught how to administer the prescribed medication using sterile technique and how to assess for infection. Patients and families also need to learn how to recognize side effects and what to do about them. Respiratory depression is uncommon, but urinary retention may be a problem, and patients and families must be prepared to deal with it if it occurs. Implanted analgesic delivery systems can be safely and confidently used at home only if health care personnel are available for consultation and, possibly, intervention on short notice.

Nonpharmacologic Interventions

Analgesic medication is the most powerful tool for pain relief that is available, but it is not the only one. Nonpharmacologic nursing activities can assist in pain relief, usually with low risk to the patient. Although such measures are not a substitute for medication, they may be all that is necessary or appropriate to relieve episodes of pain lasting only seconds or minutes. In instances of severe pain that lasts for hours or days, combining nonpharmacologic interventions with medications may be the most effective way to relieve pain. Several of these interventions are used, but the evidence base for many of them is sparse (Rakel & Barr, 2003); further studies of their effectiveness are needed.

Cutaneous Stimulation and Massage

The gate control theory of pain proposes that stimulation of fibers that transmit nonpainful sensations can block or decrease the transmission of pain impulses. Several nonpharmacologic pain relief strategies, including rubbing the skin and using heat and cold, are based on this theory.

Massage, which is generalized cutaneous stimulation of the body, often concentrates on the back and shoulders. A massage does not specifically stimulate the nonpain receptors in the same receptor field as the pain receptors, but it may have an impact through the descending control system (see previous discussion). Massage also promotes comfort because it produces muscle relaxation (Rakel & Barr, 2003).

Thermal Therapies

Ice and heat therapies may be effective pain relief strategies in some circumstances; however, their effectiveness and mechanisms of action need further study. Proponents believe that ice and heat stimulate the nonpain receptors in the same receptor field as the injury.

For greatest effect, ice should be placed on the injury site immediately after injury or surgery. Ice therapy after joint surgery can significantly reduce the amount of analgesic medication required. Ice therapy may also relieve pain if applied later. Care must be taken to assess the skin before treatment and to protect the skin from direct application of the ice. Ice should be applied to an area for no longer than 15 to 20 minutes at a time and should be avoided in patients with compromised circulation (Porth, 2005). Long applications of ice may result in frostbite or nerve injury.

Application of heat increases blood flow to an area and contributes to pain reduction by speeding healing. Both dry and moist heat may provide some analgesia, but their mechanisms of action are not well understood.

Both ice and heat therapy must be applied carefully and monitored closely to avoid injuring the skin. Neither therapy should be applied to areas with impaired circulation or used in patients with impaired sensation.

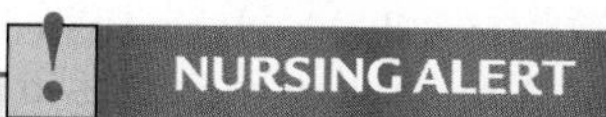

Heat should not be applied to a painful area that is the site of acute untreated infection (eg, mastitis, tooth abscess), because it may cause increased pain with increased blood flow to the site.

Transcutaneous Electrical Nerve Stimulation

Transcutaneous electrical nerve stimulation (TENS) uses a battery-operated unit with electrodes applied to the skin to produce a tingling, vibrating, or buzzing sensation in the area of pain. It has been used in both acute and chronic pain relief and is thought to decrease pain by stimulating the nonpain receptors in the same area as the fibers that transmit the pain. This mechanism is consistent with the gate control theory of pain and explains the effectiveness of cutaneous stimulation when applied in the same area as an injury. For example, when TENS is used in a postoperative patient, the electrodes are placed around the surgical wound. Other possible explanations for the effectiveness of TENS are the placebo effect (the patient expects it to be effective) (Porth, 2005) and release of endorphins and enkephalins (Rakel & Barr, 2003).

Distraction

Distraction helps relieve both acute and chronic pain (Porth, 2005). Distraction, which involves focusing the patient's attention on something other than the pain, may be the mechanism responsible for other effective cognitive techniques. Distraction is thought to reduce the perception of pain by stimulating the descending control system, resulting in fewer painful stimuli being transmitted to the brain. The effectiveness of distraction depends on the patient's ability to receive and create sensory input other than pain. Distraction techniques may range from simple activities, such as watching TV or listening to music, to highly complex physical and mental exercises. Pain relief generally increases in direct proportion to the patient's active participation, the number of sensory modalities used, and interest in the stimuli. Therefore, the stimulation of sight, sound, and touch is likely to be more effective in reducing pain than is the stimulation of a single sense.

Visits from family and friends are effective in relieving pain. Watching an action-packed movie on a large screen with "Surround Sound" through headphones may be effective (provided the patient finds it acceptable). Others may benefit from games and activities (eg, chess, crossword puzzles) that require concentration. Not all patients obtain pain relief with distraction, especially those in severe pain. Severe pain may prevent patients from concentrating well enough to participate in complex physical or mental activities.

Relaxation Techniques

Skeletal muscle relaxation is believed to reduce pain by relaxing tense muscles that contribute to the pain. Recent research findings support the use of relaxation in relieving postoperative pain. In a study of pain in patients who had undergone abdominal surgery, Roykulcharoen and Good (2004) reported that fewer participants who used relaxation techniques requested opioids compared with those in the control group. Almost all participants in the relaxation group reported a decrease in pain and an increase in sense of control.

A simple relaxation technique consists of abdominal breathing at a slow, rhythmic rate. The patient may close both eyes and breathe slowly and comfortably. A constant rhythm can be maintained by counting silently and slowly with each inhalation ("in, two, three") and exhalation ("out, two, three"). When teaching this technique, the nurse may count out loud with the patient at first. Slow, rhythmic breathing may also be used as a distraction technique. Relaxation techniques, as well as other noninvasive pain relief measures, may require practice before the patient becomes skilled in using them. Patients who already know a relaxation technique may need to be reminded to use it to reduce or prevent increased pain.

Almost all people with persistent pain can benefit from some method of relaxation. Regular relaxation periods may help combat the fatigue and muscle tension that occur with and increase chronic pain.

Guided Imagery

Guided imagery is using one's imagination in a special way to achieve a specific positive effect. Guided imagery for relaxation and pain relief may consist of combining slow, rhythmic breathing with a mental image of relaxation and comfort (Antall & Kresevic, 2004). The nurse instructs the patient to close his or her eyes and breathe slowly in and out. With each slowly exhaled breath, the patient imagines muscle tension and discomfort being breathed out, carrying away pain and tension and leaving behind a relaxed and comfortable body. With each inhaled breath, the patient imagines healing energy flowing to the area of discomfort.

If guided imagery is to be effective, it requires a considerable amount of time to explain the technique and time for the patient to practice it. Usually, the patient is asked to practice guided imagery for about 5 minutes, three times a day. Several days of practice may be needed before the intensity of pain is reduced. Many patients begin to experience the relaxing effects of guided imagery the first time they try it. Pain relief can continue for hours after the imagery is used. Patients should be informed that guided imagery may work only for some people. Guided imagery should be used only in combination with all other forms of treatment that have demonstrated effectiveness.

Hypnosis

Hypnosis, which has been effective in relieving pain or decreasing the amount of analgesic agents required in patients with acute and chronic pain, may promote pain relief in particularly difficult situations (eg, burns). The mechanism by which hypnosis acts is unclear. Its effectiveness depends on the hypnotic susceptibility of the individual (DePascalis, Bellusci, Gallo, et al., 2004). In some cases, hypnosis may be effective in the first session, with effectiveness increasing in additional sessions. In other cases, hypnosis does not work at all. Usually, hypnosis must be induced by specially skilled people (a psychologist or a nurse with specialized training in hypnosis). Some patients may learn to perform self-hypnosis.

Music Therapy

Music therapy is an inexpensive and effective therapy for the reduction of pain and anxiety. Research has shown that it significantly decreases pain as measured by the short-form McGill questionnaire and VAS in elderly patients with chronic osteoarthritis (McCaffery & Freeman, 2003). The investigators compared the pain of patients who sat quietly for 20 minutes a day for 2 weeks (standard care) to that of similar patients who listened to music 20 minutes daily for the same period. Pain from osteoarthritis was consistently significantly lower in the group who listened to music. Another group of researchers (Nilsson, Rawal & Unosson, 2003) compared two groups of patients undergoing inguinal hernia repair or varicose vein surgery; one group listened to music intraoperatively or postoperatively, and the control group listened to "white" noise. Patients exposed to music reported significantly lower pain intensity at 1 and 2 hours after surgery.

Alternative Therapies

People suffering chronic, debilitating pain are often desperate. Often they will try anything, recommended by anyone, at any price. Information about an array of potential therapies can be found on the Internet and in the self-help section of many bookstores. Therapies specifically recommended for pain from these sources include, but are not limited to, chelation, therapeutic touch, herbal therapy, reflexology, magnetic therapy, electrotherapy, polarity therapy, acupressure, emu oil, pectin therapy, aromatherapy, homeopathy, and macrobiotic dieting. Many of these "therapies" (with the exception of macrobiotic dieting) are probably not harmful. However, they have yet to be proved effective by the standards used to evaluate the effectiveness of medical and nursing interventions. The National Institutes of Health has established an office to examine the effectiveness of complementary and alternative therapies.

Despite the lack of scientific evidence that these alternative therapies are effective, patients may find any one of them helpful via the placebo response. Problems arise when patients do not find relief but are deprived of conventional therapy because the alternative therapy "should be helping," or when patients abandon conventional therapy for alternative therapy. In addition, few alternative therapies are free. Desperate patients may risk financial ruin seeking alternative therapies that are ineffective.

It is important when caring for patients who are using or considering using untested therapies (often referred to as alternative therapies) not to diminish the patient's hope and the potential placebo response. This must be weighed against the nurse's responsibility to protect the patient from costly and potentially harmful and dangerous therapies that the patient is not in a position to evaluate scientifically.

Nurses should help patients and families understand scientific research and how it differs from anecdotal evidence. Without diminishing the placebo effects that may occur, the nurse encourages the patient to assess the effectiveness of the therapy, continually using standard pain assessment techniques. In addition, the nurse encourages the patient to combine alternative therapies with conventional therapies and to discuss this with their physicians.

Neurologic and Neurosurgical Approaches to Pain Management

In some situations, especially with long-term and severe intractable pain, usual pharmacologic and nonpharmacologic methods of pain relief are ineffective. In those situations, neurologic and neurosurgical approaches to pain management may be considered. Intractable pain refers to pain that cannot be relieved satisfactorily by the usual approaches, including medications. Such pain often is the result of malignancy (especially of the cervix, bladder, prostate, and lower bowel), but it may occur in other conditions, such as postherpetic neuralgia, trigeminal neuralgia, spinal cord arachnoiditis, and uncontrollable ischemia and other forms of tissue destruction.

Neurologic and neurosurgical methods available for pain relief include (1) stimulation procedures (intermittent electrical stimulation of a tract or center to inhibit the transmission of pain impulses), (2) administration of intraspinal opioids (see previous discussion), and (3) interruption of the tracts conducting the pain impulse from the periphery to cerebral integration centers. Stimulation of nerves with minute amounts of electricity is used if other pharmacologic and nonpharmacologic treatments fail to provide adequate relief. These treatments are reversible. If they need to be discontinued, the nervous system continues to function. However, methods that involve interruption of the tracts are destructive or ablative procedures. They are used only after other methods of pain relief have failed, because their effects are permanent.

Stimulation Procedures

Electrical stimulation, or neuromodulation, is a method of suppressing pain by applying controlled low-voltage electrical pulses to the different parts of the nervous system. Electrical stimulation is thought to relieve pain by blocking painful stimuli (the gate control theory). This pain-modulating technique is administered by many modes. TENS (discussed earlier) and dorsal spinal cord stimulation are the most common types of electrical stimulation used. There are also brain-stimulating techniques, in which electrodes are implanted in the periventricular area of the posterior third ventricle, allowing the patient to stimulate this area to produce analgesia.

Spinal cord stimulation is a technique used for the relief of persistent, intractable pain, ischemic pain, and pain from angina. A surgically implanted device allows the patient to apply pulsed electrical stimulation to the dorsal aspect of the spinal cord to block pain impulses (Linderoth & Meyerson, 2002). (The largest accumulation of afferent fibers is found in the dorsal column of the spinal cord.) The dorsal column stimulation unit consists of a radiofrequency stimulation transmitter, a transmitter antenna, a radiofrequency receiver, and a stimulation electrode. The battery-powered transmitter and antenna are worn externally; the receiver and electrode are implanted. A laminectomy is performed above the highest level of pain input, and the electrode is placed in the epidural space over the posterior column of the spinal cord. (The placement of the stimulating systems varies.) A subcutaneous pocket is created over the clavicular area or at some other site for placement of the receiver. The two are connected through a subcutaneous tunnel. Careful patient selection is necessary, and not all patients receive total pain relief.

Deep brain stimulation is performed for special pain problems if there is no response to the usual techniques of pain control. Under local anesthesia, electrodes are introduced through a burr hole in the skull and inserted into a selected site in the brain, depending on the location or type of pain. After the effectiveness of stimulation is confirmed, the implanted electrode is connected to a radiofrequency device or pulse-generator system operated by external telemetry. It is used for patients with neuropathic pain that may be caused by damage or injury from a stroke, brain or spinal cord injuries, or phantom limb pain. Use of deep brain stimulation is effective for chronic cluster headaches (Ekbom & Waldenlind, 2004; Leone, 2004).

Interruption of Pain Pathways

Pain-conducting fibers can be interrupted at any point from their origin to the cerebral cortex. Some part of the nervous system is destroyed, resulting in varying amounts of neurologic deficit and incapacity. In time, pain usually returns as a result of either regeneration of axonal fibers or the development of alternative pain pathways. Destructive procedures used to interrupt the transmission of pain include cordotomy and rhizotomy. These procedures are offered if it is thought that the patient is near the end of life and the procedure will result in an improved quality of life (Linderoth & Meyerson, 2002). Often these procedures can provide pain relief for the duration of the patient's life. The use of other methods to interrupt pain transmission is decreasing, because intraspinal therapies and newer pain management treatments are available.

CORDOTOMY

Cordotomy is the division of certain tracts of the spinal cord (Fig. 13-10). It may be performed percutaneously, by the open method after laminectomy, or by other techniques. Cordotomy is performed to interrupt the transmission of pain (Hodge & Christensen, 2002). Care must be taken to destroy only the sensation of pain, leaving motor functions intact.

RHIZOTOMY

Sensory nerve roots are destroyed where they enter the spinal cord. A lesion is made in the dorsal root to destroy neuronal dysfunction and reduce nociceptive input. With the advent of microsurgical techniques, the complications are few, with mild sensory deficits and mild weakness (Fig. 13-11).

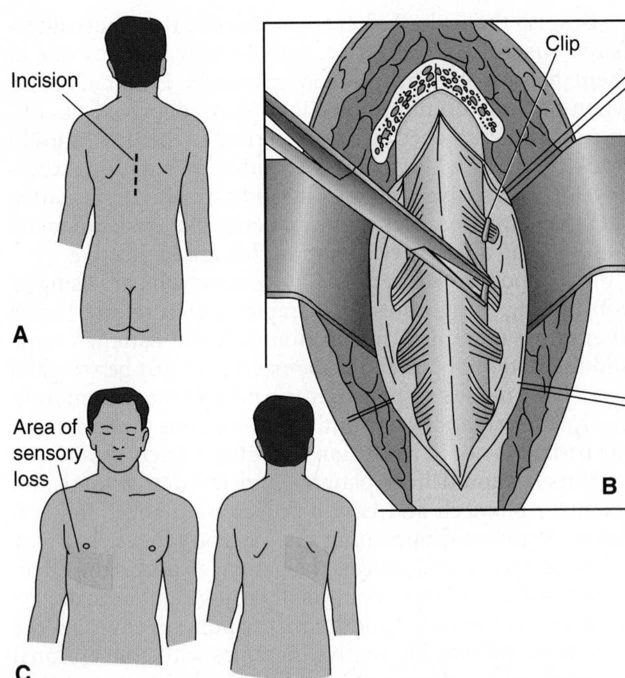

FIGURE 13-11. A rhizotomy may be performed surgically, percutaneously, or chemically, depending on a patient's condition and needs. The procedure is usually performed to relieve severe chest pain, for example, from lung cancer. In a surgical rhizotomy (**A**), the spinal roots (**B**) are divided and banded with a clip to form a lesion and produce subsequent loss of sensation (**C**). Adapted with permission from Loeser, J. D. (Ed.) (2000). *Bonica's management of pain* (3rd ed.). Philadelphia: Lippincott Williams & Wilkins.

Nursing Interventions

With each of these procedures, the patient is provided with written and verbal instructions about the intervention's expected effect on pain and on possible untoward consequences. The patient is monitored for specific effects of each method of pain intervention, both positive and negative. The specific nursing care of patients who undergo neurologic and neurosurgical procedures for the relief of chronic pain depends on the type of procedure performed, its effectiveness in relieving the pain, and the changes in neurologic function that accompany the procedure. After the procedure, the patient's pain level and neurologic function are assessed. Other nursing interventions that may be indicated include positioning, turning and skin care, bowel and bladder management, and interventions to promote patient safety. Pain management remains an important aspect of nursing care with each of these procedures.

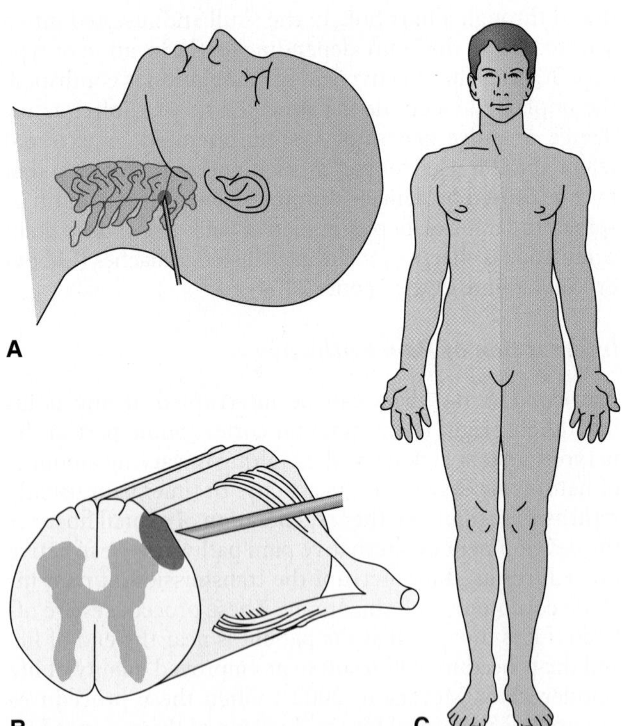

FIGURE 13-10. (**A**) Site of percutaneous C1–C2 cordotomy. (**B**) Lesion produced by percutaneous C1–C2 cordotomy. (**C**) Extent of analgesia produced by left C1–C2 percutaneous cordotomy.

Promoting Home and Community-Based Care

In preparing the patient and family to manage pain at home, the patient and family should be taught and guided about what type of pain or discomfort to expect, how long the pain is expected to last, and when the pain indicates a problem that should be reported. People who have experienced pain as a result of injury, illness, a medical procedure, or surgery will probably receive one or more prescriptions for analgesic medication for use at home.

Teaching Patients Self-Care

The patient and family must understand the purpose of each medication, the appropriate time to use it, the associated side effects, and the strategies that can be used to prevent these problems. The patient and family often need reassurance that pain can be successfully managed at home.

Inadequate control of pain at home is a common reason people seek health care or are readmitted to the hospital. When persistent pain exists, anxiety and fear are often intensified at the time the patient is about to return home. The patient and family are instructed about the techniques for assessing pain, using pain assessment tools, and administering medications to relieve pain. These instructions are given verbally and in writing (Chart 13-9).

Opportunities are provided for the patient and family members to practice administering the medication until they are comfortable and confident with the procedure. They are instructed about the risks of respiratory and CNS depression associated with opioids and ways to assess for these complications. If the medications cause other predictable effects, such as constipation, the instructions include measures for preventing and treating the problem, as previously described. Steps are taken to ensure that the needed medications are available from the local pharmacy so that the patient receives the medication when required.

Education for patients and families must stress the need for keeping analgesic agents away from children, who might mistake them for candy. Elderly patients may become lax about this because no children live in the home, but visiting children can be placed at risk. Analgesic agents must also be kept away from other family members who

CHART 13-9

Patient Education

At-Home Pain Management Plan

Pain control plan for

____

At home, I will take the following medicines for pain control:

Medicine	How to take	How many	How often	Comments

Medicines that I may take to help treat side effects:

Side effect	Medicine	How to take	How many	How often	Comments

Constipation is a very common problem when taking opioid medications. When this occurs, do the following:

- Increase fluid intake (8 to 10 glasses of fluid).
- Exercise regularly.
- Increase fiber in the diet (bran, fresh fruits, vegetables).
- Use a mild laxative, such as milk of magnesia, if no bowel movement in 3 days.
- Take __________ every day at __________ (time) with a full glass of water.
- Use a glycerin suppository every morning (this may help make a bowel movement less painful).

Nondrug pain control methods:

____

____

Additional instructions:

____

____

____

Important phone numbers:

Your doctor ____________________ Your nurse ____________________

Your pharmacy ____________________ Emergencies ____________________

Call your doctor or nurse immediately if your pain increases or if you have a new pain. Also call your doctor early for refill of pain medicines. Do not let your medicines get below 3 or 4 days' supply.

From Agency for Health Care Policy and Research. (1994). Management of cancer pain. Clinical Practice Guidelines. Rockville, MD: Agency for Health Care Policy and Research, Public Health Service, U.S. Department of Health and Human Services.

CHART 13-10

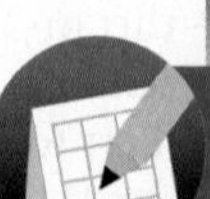

Plan of Nursing Care — Care of the Patient With Pain

Nursing Diagnosis: Pain
Goal: Relief of pain or decrease in intensity of pain

NURSING INTERVENTIONS	RATIONALE
1. Reassure patient that you know pain is real and will assist him or her in dealing with it.	1. Fear that pain will not be accepted as real increases tension and anxiety and decreases pain tolerance.
2. Use pain assessment scale to identify intensity of pain.	2. Provides baseline for assessing changes in pain level and evaluating interventions
3. Assess and record pain and its characteristics: location, quality, frequency, and duration.	3. Data assist in evaluating pain and pain relief and identifying multiple sources and types of pain.
4. Administer balanced analgesics as prescribed to promote optimal pain relief.	4. Analgesics are more effective if administered early in pain cycle. Simultaneous use of analgesics that work on different portions of the nociceptive system will provide greater pain relief with fewer side effects.
5. Readminister pain assessment scale.	5. Permits assessment of effectiveness of analgesia and identifies need for further action if ineffective
6. Document severity of patient's pain on chart.	6. Assists in demonstrating need for additional analgesic or alternative approach to pain management
7. Obtain additional prescriptions as needed.	7. Inadequate pain relief results in an increased stress response, suffering, and prolonged hospitalizations.
8. Identify and encourage patient to use strategies that have been successful with previous pain.	8. Encourages use of pain relief strategies familiar to and accepted by patient
9. Teach patient additional strategies to relieve pain and discomfort: distraction, relaxation, cutaneous stimulation, etc.	9. Use of these strategies along with analgesia may produce more effective pain relief.
10. Instruct patient and family about potential side effects of analgesics and their prevention and management.	10. Anticipating and preventing side effects enable the patient to continue analgesia without interruption because of side effects.

EXPECTED OUTCOMES

- Reports relief that pain is accepted as real and that he or she will receive assistance in pain relief
- Reports lower intensity of pain and discomfort after interventions implemented
- Reports less disruption from pain and discomfort after use of intervention
- Uses pain medication as prescribed
- Identifies effective pain relief strategies
- Demonstrates use of new strategies to relieve pain and reports their effectiveness
- Experiences minimal side effects of analgesia without interruption to treat side effects
- Increases interactions with family and friends

CHART 13-11

Expected Patient Outcomes for the Patient With Pain

Relief of pain, evidenced when the patient
- Rates pain at a lower intensity (on a scale of 0 to 10) after intervention
- Rates pain at a lower intensity for longer periods

Correct administration of prescribed analgesic medications, evidenced when the patient or family
- States correct dose of medication
- Administers correct dose using correct procedure
- Identifies side effects of medication
- Describes actions taken to prevent or correct side effects

Use of nonpharmacologic pain strategies as recommended, evidenced when the patient:
- Reports practice of nonpharmacologic strategies
- Describes expected outcomes of nonpharmacologic strategies

Minimal effects of pain and minimal side effects of interventions, evidenced when the patient:
- Participates in activities important to recovery (eg, drinking fluids, coughing, ambulating)
- Participates in activities important to self and to family (eg, family activities, interpersonal relationships, parenting, social interaction, recreation, work)
- Reports adequate sleep and absence of fatigue and constipation

may take them inadvertently. In addition, analgesic medications should be stored safely in their original containers and clearly labeled. They should be stored out of sight to prevent others from taking them for their own use or diverting them to others.

Continuing Care

If a patient is to receive parenteral or intraspinal analgesia at home, he or she should be referred to a home care nurse. This nurse will make a home visit to assess the patient, and to determine whether the pain management program is being implemented and the technique for injecting or infusing the analgesic agent is being carried out safely and effectively. If the patient has an implanted infusion pump in place, the nurse examines the condition of the pump or injection site and may refill the reservoir with medication as prescribed or may supervise family members in this procedure. The nurse assesses for any change in the patient's need for analgesic medications, and, in collaboration with the physician, the nurse may assist the patient and family in modifying the medication dose. These efforts enable the patient to obtain adequate pain relief while remaining at home and with family.

As tolerance develops with chronic pain or cancer pain, ever-increasing amounts of opioids are needed. It is important to reassure the patient and family that slowly increasing doses will not increase the risk for respiratory depression and CNS depression, because the patient will become tolerant to these effects also. However, the patient will not become tolerant to the constipating effects of opioids, and increased efforts to prevent constipation will be necessary.

Evaluating Pain Management Strategies

An important aspect of caring for patients in pain is reassessing the pain after the intervention has been implemented. The measure's effectiveness is based on the patient's assessment of pain, as reflected in pain assessment tools. If the intervention was ineffective, the nurse should consider other measures. If these are ineffective, pain relief goals need to be reassessed in collaboration with the physician. The nurse serves as the patient's advocate in obtaining additional pain relief.

After interventions have had a chance to work, the nurse asks the patient to rate the intensity of pain. The nurse repeats this assessment at appropriate intervals after the intervention and compares the result with the previous rating. These assessments indicate the effectiveness of the pain relief measures and provide a basis for continuing or modifying the plan of care. A plan of nursing care for a patient with pain is given in Chart 13-10. Expected patient outcomes are given in Chart 13-11.

Critical Thinking Exercises

1. A 65-year-old Hispanic woman is admitted to the hospital with advanced cancer of the left breast with metastasis. She speaks little English, and three of her adult children are with her. Her health history indicates that she initially refused surgery after noticing a lump in her breast, because she believes that the breast is where the soul resides, but finally consented to a left mastectomy. After undergoing surgery, she was transferred from the postanesthesia care unit to a surgical unit. There she is moaning and appears to be writhing in pain. Ten minutes ago, she was given 8 mg of morphine sulfate intravenously. What cultural factors need to be considered in the care of this woman? Identify methods that can be used to communicate with her. How would the nurse assess the patient's pain intensity and the effectiveness of pain management strategies? What level of involvement is appropriate for the family in the assessment and management of her pain? Explain your reasoning.
2. A 27-year-old man is readmitted to a medical center because of severe pain one day after his discharge following an open reduction of his left humerus with internal fixation. He was discharged with a prescription for oxycodone (Percocet), one tablet every 4 hours as needed (total of 20 tablets). He rates his pain intensity as an 11 on a scale of 0 to 10. When the pain escalated at home, he

increased the dose and subsequently ran out of the Percocet. His physician decides to change the analgesic to long-acting morphine in an effort to relieve his pain. How would the nurse determine what prescribed dose of the long-acting morphine to administer? What concerns should the nurse have about the amount of Percocet the patient consumed? What medication should be on hand and what assessments, including laboratory tests, should be performed?

3 A 35-year-old man who is a recovering heroin addict is admitted to the hospital for an emergency appendectomy. During surgery the appendix ruptures, and the patient remains hospitalized for several days for intravenous antibiotics. He tells the nurse that he has been "clean" for the past 3 months. He complains of pain (7 on a 0-to-10 scale) and refuses to use the patient-controlled analgesia that is prescribed for him. He states, "I don't want to get hooked again." Describe how you would address pain relief in this patient, and give the rationale for your actions. How would you address his fears? Who would you consult to help with this patient's pain management?

4 A 76-year-old man with a history of angina and peripheral vascular disease collapses in the street after suffering a massive heart attack and is rushed to a major hospital center. Despite his medical history, he has continued to smoke about one pack of cigarettes a day. He is intubated and placed on a ventilator to provide adequate oxygenation. He is able to report his pain intensity by holding up the number of fingers to correspond to a 0-to-10 rating scale. At first he rates the pain as a 9, but after receiving morphine he rates the pain as a 2. Discuss how morphine works to decrease the intensity of the patient's pain. Identify other interventions, including other medications, that would contribute to decreasing his pain.

5 ebp A 48-year-old woman has severe chronic pain secondary to cancer due to metastasis to the bone. She is reluctant to take opioids because she wants to remain alert to enjoy being around her family. Furthermore, she is concerned about having opioids around the house because of the presence of young children in the home. Identify pharmacologic alternatives and nonpharmacologic interventions that might be appropriate. Identify the evidence base and the strength of the evidence for the use of the nonpharmacologic interventions.

REFERENCES AND SELECTED READINGS

BOOKS

American Cancer Society. (2001). *American Cancer Society's guide to pain control: Powerful methods to overcome cancer pain.* Atlanta: American Cancer Society.

American Pain Society. (2003). *Principles of analgesic use in the treatment of acute pain and chronic cancer pain* (5th ed.). Skokie, IL: Author.

American Society for Pain Management Nurses. (2002). *Core curriculum for pain management nursing.* Philadelphia: Saunders.

Bonica, J. J. (2000). *The management of pain* (3rd ed.). Philadelphia: Lea & Febiger.

Desmeules, J. A., Piguet, V., Ehret, G. B., et al. (2004). Pharmacogenetics, pharmacokinetics, and analgesia. In Mogil, J. S. (Ed.). *The genetics of pain* (pp. 211–237). Seattle: IASP Press.

Fillingim, R. B. (2000). *Progress in pain research and management: Vol. 17. Sex, gender, and pain.* Seattle: IASP Press.

Freeman, L. W. & Lawlis, G. F. (2001). *Mosby's complementary and alternative medicine: A research-based approach.* St. Louis: Mosby.

Harden, R. N., Baron, R. & Janig, W. (2001). *Progress in pain research and management: Vol. 22. Complex regional pain syndrome.* Seattle: IASP Press.

Hodge, C. J., & Christensen, M. (2002). Anterolateral cordotomy. In K. J. Burchiel (Ed.). *Surgical management of pain.* New York: Thieme.

Hudspith, M. & Munglani, R. (2003). Sites of analgesic action. In Bountra, C., Munglani, R. & Schmidt, W. K. (Eds.). *Pain: Current understanding, emerging therapies, and novel approaches to drug discovery.* New York: Marcel-Dekker.

Janig, W. (2001). CRPS-I and CRPS-II: A strategic view. In Harden, R. N., Baron, R., & Janig, W. (Eds.). *Progress in pain research and management: Vol. 22. Complex regional pain syndrome.* Seattle: IASP Press.

Joint Commission on Accreditation of Healthcare Organizations. (2005). *2005 Hospital accreditation standards.* Oakbrook Terrace, IL: JCAHO.

Kuhn, M. A. (1999). *Complementary therapies for health care providers.* Philadelphia: Lippincott Williams & Wilkins.

Linderoth, B. & Meyerson, B. A. (2002). Spinal cord stimulation: Mechanisms of action. In Burchiel, K. (Ed.). *Surgical management of pain.* New York: Thieme.

MacGregor, A. J. (2004). The heritability of pain in humans. In Mogil, J. S. (Ed.). *Progress in pain research and management: Vol. 28. The genetics of pain.* Seattle: IASP Press.

McCaffery, M. & Pasero, C. (1999). *Pain: Clinical manual* (2nd ed.). St. Louis: Mosby.

Merskey, H. & Bogduk, N. (1994). *Classification of Chronic Pain,* 2nd ed. International Association for the Study of Pain (IASP) Task Force on Taxonomy. Seattle, WA: IASP Press.

Mogil, J. S. (Ed.). (2004). *Progress in pain research and management: Vol. 28. The genetics of pain.* Seattle: IASP Press.

National Institutes of Health. (1995). *Integration of behavioral and relaxation approaches into the treatment of chronic pain and insomnia.* NIH Technology Assessment Statement, Oct. 16–18, 1995. http://consensus.nih.gov/1995/1995BehaviorRelaxPainInsomniata017html.htm. Accessed May 24, 2006.

Porth, C. M. (2005). *Pathophysiology: Concepts of altered health status,* 7th ed. Philadelphia: Lippincott Williams & Wilkins.

Rezai, A. R. & Lozano, A. M. (2002). Deep brain stimulation for chronic pain. In Burchiel, K. J. (Ed.). *Surgical management of pain.* New York: Thieme.

Wall, P. D. & Melzack, R. (Eds). (1999). *Textbook of pain* (4th ed.). New York: Churchill Livingstone.

JOURNALS

**Asterisks indicate nursing research articles.*

American Geriatrics Society Panel on Persistent Pain in Older Persons. (2002). The management of persistent pain in older persons. *Journal of the American Geriatrics Society, 50*(6S), 205–224.

American Society of Pain Management Nurses. (2005). ASPMN position statement: Use of placebos in pain management. Available at: http//www.aspmn.org/html/Psplacebo.htm. Accessed June 7, 2005. http//www.aspmn.org/Organization/position_papers.htm. Accessed May 22, 2006.

Anderson, R., Saiers, J. H., Abram, S. & Schlicht, C. (2001). Accuracy in equianalgesic dosing: Conversion dilemmas. *Journal of Pain and Symptom Management, 21*(5), 397–406.

Andre, J. M., Martinet, N., Paysant, J., et al. (2001). Temporary phantom limbs evoked by vestibular caloric stimulation in amputees. *Neuropsychiatry Neuropsychology Behavioral Neurology, 14*(3), 190–196.

Antall, G. F. & Kresevic, D. (2004). The use of guided imagery to manage pain in an elderly orthopaedic population. *Orthopaedic Nursing, 23*(5), 335–340.

Arnstein, P. (2003). Comprehensive analysis and management of chronic pain. *Nursing Clinics of North America, 38*(1), 403–417.

Bair, M. J., Robinson, R. L., Katon, W., et al. (2003). Depression and pain comorbidity: A literature review. *Archives of Internal Medicine, 163*(20), 2433–2445.

Bohme, K. (2002). Buprenorphine in a transdermal therapeutic system. A new option. *Clinical Rheumatology, 21* (Suppl.), S13–S16.

Brookoff, D. (2000). Chronic pain: 1. A new disease? *Hospital Practice, 35*(7), 42–59.

California Pain Patients' Bill of Rights. Available at: www.paincare.org/pain_management/advocacy/ca_bill.html (accessed March 12, 2006).

*Call-Schmidt, T. A. & Richardson, S. J. (2003). Prevalence of sleep disturbance and its relationship to pain in adults with chronic pain. *Pain Management Nursing, 4*(3), 124–133.

Collins-Schramm, H. E., Phillips, C. M., Operario, D. J., et al. (2002). Ethnic-difference markers for use in mapping by admixture linkage disequilibrium. *American Journal of Human Genetics, 70*(3), 737–750.

Colwell, C. W. (2004). The use of the pain pump and patient-controlled analgesia in joint reconstruction. *American Journal of Orthopedics, 33*(5S), 10–12.

Compton, P., & Athanos, P. (2003). Chronic pain, substance abuse and addiction. *Nursing Clinics of North America, 38*(1), 525–537.

Correll, D. J., Viscusi, E. R., Grunwald, Z., et al. (2001). Epidural analgesia compared with intravenous morphine patient-controlled analgesia: Postoperative outcome measures after mastectomy with immediate TRAM flap breast reconstruction. *Regional Anesthesia Pain Medicine, 26*(5), 444–449.

Dalton, J. A. & Coyne, P. (2003). Cognitive-behavioral therapy: Tailored to the individual. *Nursing Clinics of North America, 38*(1), 465–476.

D'Arcy, Y. (2005a). What you need to know about fentanyl patches. *Nursing, 35*(8), 73.

D'Arcy, Y. (2005b). Patching together transdermal pain control options. *Nursing, 35*(9), 17

DePascalis, V., Bellusci, A., Gallo, C., et al. (2004). Pain reduction strategies in hypnotic context and hypnosis: ERPs and SCRs during a secondary auditory task. *International Journal of Clinical Experimental Hypnosis, 52*(4), 343–363.

*DuPen, A. R., DuPen, S., Hansberry, J., et al. (2000). An educational implementation of a cancer pain algorithm for ambulatory care. *Pain Management Nursing, 1*(4), 116–128.

*Dysvik, E., Lindstrom, T. C., Eikland, O., et al. (2004). Health-related quality of life and pain beliefs among people suffering from chronic pain. *Pain Management Nursing, 5*(2), 66–74.

Edwards, R., Augustson, E. M., & Fillingim, R. (2000). Sex-specific effects of pain related anxiety on adjustment to chronic pain. *Clinical Journal of Pain, 16*(1), 46–53.

Edwards, R. R., & Fillingim, R. B. (2000). Age-associated differences in responses to noxious stimuli. *Journal of Gerontology Series A: Biological Science and Medical Science, 56*(3), M180–M185.

Ekbom, K. & Waldenlind, E. (2004). Cluster headache: The history of the Cluster Club and a review of clinical research. *Functional Neurology, 19*(2), 73–81.

Fischer, L. M., Schlienger, R. G., Matter, C. M., et al. (2004). Discontinuation of nonsteroidal anti-inflammatory drug therapy and risk of acute myocardial infarction. *Archives of Internal Medicine, 164*(22), 2472–2476.

Fitzgibbon, D., Morgan, D. Dockter, D., et al. (2003). Initial pharmacokinetic, safety and efficacy evaluation of nasal morphine gluconate for breakthrough pain in cancer patients. *Pain, 106*(3), 309–315.

Furlan, A. D., Sandoval, J. A., Mailis-Gagnon, A. et al. (2006). Opioids for chronic noncancer pain: a meta-analysis of effectiveness and side effects. *Canadian Medical Association Journal, 174*(11), 1589–1594.

Gambling, D., Hughes, T., Martin, G., et al. (2005). A comparison of Depodur, a novel, single-dose extended-release epidural morphine, with standard epidural morphine for pain relief after lower abdominal surgery. *Anesthesia & Analgesia, 100*(4), 1065–1074.

Gammaitoni, A. R., Fine, P., Alvarez, N., et al. (2003). Clinical application of opioid equianalgesic data. *Clinical Journal of Pain, 19*(5), 286–297.

Gevirtz, C. (2003). Anesthesia-assisted opiate detoxification. *International Anesthesiology Clinic, 41*(2), 79–93.

Gilron, I., Bailey, J. M., Dongsheng, T., et al. (2005). Morphine, gabapentin, or their combination for neuropathic pain. *New England Journal of Medicine, 352*(13), 1324–1334.

Gordon, D. B. (2003). Nonopioid and adjuvant analgesics in chronic pain management: strategies for effective use. *Nursing Clinics of North America, 38*(1), 447–464.

Gordon, D. & Dahl, J. (2003) Fast facts and concepts #95: Opioid withdrawal. End-of-life/Palliative Education Resource Center. Available at: http://www.eperc.mcw.edu/fastFact/ff_95.htm (accessed March 12, 2006).

Gordon, D. B., Dahl, J., Phillips, P., et al. (2004). The use of "as-needed" range orders for opioid analgesics in the management of acute pain: A consensus statement of the American Society for Pain Management Nurses and the American Pain Society. *Pain Management Nursing, 5*(2), 53–58.

Gordon, D. B. & Ward, S. E. (1995). Correcting patient misconceptions about pain. *American Journal of Nursing, 95*(7), 43–45.

Green, C. R., Anderson, K. O., Baker, T. A., et al. (2003). The unequal burden of pain: Confronting racial and ethnic disparities in pain. *Pain Medicine, 4*(3), 277–294.

Gunnarsdottir, S., Donovan, H. & Ward, S. (2003). Interventions to overcome clinician- and patient-related barriers to pain management. *Nursing Clinics of North America, 38*(1), 419–434.

Holleran, R. S. (2002). The problem of pain in emergency care. *Nursing Clinics of North America, 37*(1), 67–78.

Hicks, C. L., von Baeyer, C. L., Spafford, P. A., et al. (2001). The Faces Pain Scale–Revised: Toward a common metric in pediatric pain measurement. *Pain, 93*(2), 173–183.

*Horgas, A. L. & Dunn, K. (2001). Pain in nursing home residents: Comparison of residents' self-report and nursing assistants' perceptions. Incongruencies exist in resident and caregiver reports of pain; therefore, pain management education is needed to prevent suffering. *Journal of Gerontological Nursing, 27*(3), 44–53.

Hrobjartsson, A. & Gotzsche, P. C. (2001). Is placebo powerless? An analysis of clinical trials comparing placebo with no treatment. *New England Journal of Medicine, 344*(21), 1594–1602.

Hrobjartsson, A. & Gotzsche, P. C. (2004). Is the placebo powerless? Update of a systematic review with 52 new randomized trials comparing placebo with no treatment. *Journal of Internal Medicine, 256*(2), 91–100.

Hunter, M., McDowell, L., Hennessy, R., et al. (2000). An evaluation of the Faces Pain Scale with young children. *Journal of Pain and Symptom Management, 20*(2), 122–129.

Jacob, E. (2001). The pain experience of patients with sickle cell anemia. *Pain Management Nursing, 2*(3), 74–83.

Karamanlioglu, B., Turan, A., Memis, D., et al. (2004). Preoperative oral rofecoxib reduces postoperative pain and tramadol consumption in patients after abdominal hysterectomy. *Anesthesia Analgesia, 98*(4), 1039–1043.

Keefe, F. J., Rumble, M. E., Scipio, C. D., et al. (2004). Psychological aspects of persistent pain: Current state of the science. *Journal of Pain, 5*(4), 195–211.

Kundermann, B., Krieg, J. C., Schreiber, W., et al. (2004). The effect of sleep deprivation on pain. *Pain Research Management, 9*(1), 25–32.

*Lasch, K., Greenhill, K., Wilkes, G., et al. (2002). Why study pain? A qualitative analysis of medical and nursing faculty and students' knowledge of and attitudes to cancer pain management. *Journal of Palliative Medicine, 5*(1), 57–71.

Leone, M. (2004). Chronic cluster headache: New and emerging treatment options. *Current Pain Headache Report, 8*(5), 347–352.

Li, S. F., Greenwald, P. W., Gennis, P., et al. (2001). Effect of age on acute pain perception of a standardized stimulus in the emergency department. *Annals of Emergency Medicine, 38*(6), 644–647.

Marcus, K. S., Kerns, R. D., Rosenfeld, B., et al. (2002). HIV/AIDS-related pain as a chronic pain condition: Implication of a biopsychosocial model for comprehensive assessment and effective management. *Pain Medicine, 1*(3), 260–273.

Mayer, D. M., Torma, L., Byock, I., et al. (2001). Speaking the language of pain. *American Journal of Nursing, 101*(2), 44–49.

McCaffery, M. (2002). What is the role of nondrug methods in the nursing care of patients with acute pain? *Pain Management Nursing, 3*(3), 77–80.

McCaffery, M. (2003). Switching from i.v. to p.o. *American Journal of Nursing, 103*(5), 62–63.

*McCaffery, M., Ferrell, B. R., & Pasero, C. (2000). Nurses' personal opinions about patients' pain and their effect on recorded assessments and titration of opioid doses. *Pain Management Nursing, 1*(3), 79–87.

*McCaffery, R. & Freeman, W. (2003). Effect of music on chronic osteoarthritis pain in older people. *Journal of Advanced Nursing, 44*(5), 517–524.

McCaffery, M., & Pasero, C. (2001). Stigmatizing patients as addicts. *American Journal of Nursing, 101*(5), 77–79.

McCaffery, M., & Pasero, C. (2003). Breakthrough pain. *American Journal of Nursing, 103*(4), 83–84,86.

*McNeill, J. A., Sherwood, G. D., Starck, P. L., et al. (2001). Pain management outcomes for hospitalized Hispanic patients. *Pain Management Nursing, 2*(4), 25–36.

Meier, T., Wasner, G., Kuntzer, T., et al. (2003). Efficacy of lidocaine patch 5% in the treatment of focal peripheral neuropathic pain syndromes: A randomized, double-blind, placebo-controlled study. *Pain, 106*(1–2), 151–158.

Melzack, R. (1996). Gate control theory: On the evolution of pain concepts. *Pain Forum, 5*(1), 128–138.

*Miaskowski, C. (2000). The impact of age on a patient's perception of pain and ways it can be managed. *Pain Management Nursing, 1*(3), S1,S2–S7.

Miaskowski, C. (2004). Psychoeducational interventions for cancer pain serve as a model for behavioral research. *Communicating Nursing Research, 37*, 51,53–71.

Miaskowski, C. (2005). Patient-controlled modalities for acute postoperative pain management. *Journal of Perianesthesia Nursing, 20*(4), 255–267.

*Miaskowski, C., Dodd, M., West, C., et al. (2004). Randomized clinical trial of the effectiveness of a self-care intervention to improve cancer pain management. *Journal of Clinical Oncology, 22*(9), 1713–1720.

Miaskowski, C., Gear, R. W. & Levine, J. D. (2000). Sex-related differences in analgesic responses. In Sex, gender and pain. *Progress in Pain Research and Management, 17*, 209–230.

Nichols, R. (2003). Pain management in patients with addictive disease. *American Journal of Nursing, 103*(3), 87–89.

Nilsson, U., Rawal, N., & Unosson, M. (2003). A comparison of intraoperative or postoperative exposure to music: A controlled trial of the effects on postoperative pain. *Anaesthesia, 58*(7), 699–703.

Panke, J. T. (2002). Difficulties in managing pain at the end of life. *American Journal of Nursing, 102*(7), 26–33.

Pasero, C. (2002a). Subcutaneous opioid infusion. *American Journal of Nursing, 102*(7), 61–62.

Pasero, C. (2002b). The challenge of pain assessment in the PACU. *Journal of Perianesthesia Nursing, 17*(5), 348–350.

Pasero, C. (2003a). Epidural analgesia for postoperative pain. *American Journal of Nursing, 103*(10), 62–64.

Pasero, C. (2003b). Epidural analgesia for postoperative pain: Part 2. *American Journal of Nursing, 103*(11), 43–45.

Pasero, C. (2003c). Lidocaine patch 5%. *American Journal of Nursing, 103*(9),75, 77–78.

Pasero, C. (2003d). Multimodal balanced analgesia in the PACU. *Journal of Perianesthesia Nursing, 18*(4), 265–268.

Pasero, C. (2003e). Pain in the critically ill patient. *Journal of Perianesthesia Nursing, 18*(6), 422–425.

Pasero, C. (2003f). Pain in the emergency department. *American Journal of Nursing, 103*(7), 73–74.

Pasero, C. (2004a). Pain and comfort issues. *Journal of Perianesthesia Nursing, 19*(3), 135–137.

Pasero, C. (2004b). Perineural local anesthetic infusion. *American Journal of Nursing, 104*(7), 89–93.

Pasero, C. (2005). Fentanyl for acute pain management. *Journal of Perianesthesia Nursing, 20*(4), 279–284.

Pasero, C. & McCaffery, M. (2002). Monitoring sedation. *American Journal of Nursing, 102*(2), 67–69.

Pasero, C. & McCaffery, M. (2003). Accountability for pain relief: Use of comfort-function goals. *Journal of Perianesthesia Nursing, 18*(1), 50–52.

Pasero, C. & McCaffery, M. (2004a). Comfort-function goals: A way to establish accountability for pain relief. *American Journal of Nursing, 104*(9), 77–78,81.

Pasero, C. & McCaffery, M. (2004b). Controlled-release oxycodone. *American Journal of Nursing, 104*(1), 30–32.

Pasero, C. & McCaffery, M. (2004c). Safe use of a continuous infusion with i.v. PCA. *Journal of Perianesthesia Nursing, 19*(1), 42–45.

Pasero, C. & McCaffery, M. (2005). Authorized and unauthorized use of PCA pumps. *American Journal of Nursing, 105*(7), 30–31,33.

Pasero, C. & Montgomery, R. (2002). Intravenous fentanyl: Out of the operating room and gaining in popularity. *American Journal of Nursing, 102*(4), 73,75,76.

Perez, R. S. G. M., Kwakkel, G., Zuurmond, W. W. A., et al. (2001). Treatment of reflex sympathetic dystrophy (CRPS type I): A research synthesis of 21 randomized clinical trials. *Journal of Pain and Symptom Management, 21*(6), 511–526.

Perin, M. L. (2000). Corticosteroids for cancer pain. *American Journal of Nursing, 100*(4), 15–16.

Plaisance, L. & Ellis, J. A. (2002). Opioid-induced constipation. *American Journal of Nursing, 102*(3), 72–73.

Pollo, A., Amanzio, M., Arslanina, A., et al. (2001). Response expectancies in placebo analgesia and their clinical relevance. *Pain, 93*(1), 77–84.

*Puntillo, K., Neighbor, M., O'Neil, N., et al. (2004). Accuracy of emergency nurses in assessment of patient's pain. *Pain Management Nursing, 4*(4), 171–175.

*Puntillo, K. A., Stannard, D., Miaskowski, C., et al. (2002). Use of a pain assessment and intervention notation (P.A.I.N.) tool in critical care nursing practice: Nurses' evaluations. *Heart & Lung, 31*(4), 303–314.

Rakel, B., & Barr, J. O. (2003). Physical modalities in chronic pain management. *Nursing Clinics of North America, 38*(1), 477–494.

Rakel, B. & Herr, K. (2004). Assessment and treatment of postoperative pain in older adults. *Journal of Perianesthesia Nursing, 19*(3), 194–208.

Riley, J. L., 3rd, Wade, J. B., Myers, C. D., et al. (2002). Racial/ethnic differences in the experience of chronic pain. *Pain, 100*(3), 291–298.

Robinson, M. E., Wise, E. A., Gagnon, C., et al. (2004). Influences of gender role and anxiety on sex differences in temporal summation of pain. *Journal of Pain, 5*(2), 77–82.

*Roykulcharoen, V., & Good, M. (2004). Systematic relaxation to relieve postoperative pain. *Journal of Advanced Nursing, 48*(2), 140–148.

*Schumacher, K. L., Koresawa, S., West, C., et al. (2002). Putting cancer pain management regimens into practice at home. *Journal of Pain and Symptom Management, 23*(5), 369–382.

Shaya, F. T., & Suwannaprom, P. (2005). Cyclooxygenase-2 inhibitors and cardiovascular risk: How can the evidence guide prescribing decisions? *Topics in Pain Management, 20*(10), 1–7.

Skaer, T. L. (2004). Practice guidelines for transdermal opioids in malignant pain. *Drugs, 64*(23), 2629–2638.

Slaughter, A., Pasaro, C., & Manworren, R. (2002). Unacceptable pain levels. *American Journal of Nursing, 102*(5), 75–77.

Smith, W. C., Bourne, D., Squair, J., et al., (1999). A retrospective cohort study of post mastectomy pain syndrome. *Pain, 83*(1), 91–95.

Snyder, M. & Wieland, J. (2003). Complementary and alternative therapies: What is their place in the management of chronic pain? *Nursing Clinics of North America, 38*(1), 495–508.

St. Marie, B. (2003). The complex patient: Interventional treatment and nursing issues. *Nursing Clinics of North America, 38*(1), 539–554.

*Stotts, N. A., Puntillo, K., Morris, A. B., et al. (2004). Wound care pain in hospitalized adult patients. *Heart & Lung, 33*(5), 321–332.

Summers, S. (2000). Evidence-based practice part 1: Pain definitions, pathophysiologic mechanisms and theories. *Journal of Perianesthesia Nursing, 15*(5), 357–365.

The SUPPORT Principal Investigators. (1995). A controlled trial to improve care for seriously ill hospitalized patients. The study to understand prognoses and preferences for outcomes and risks of treatments (SUPPORT). *Journal of American Medical Association, 274*(20), 1591–1598.

Sutton, L. M., Porter, L. S. & Keefe, F. J. (2002). Cancer pain at the end of life: A biopsychosocial perspective. *Pain, 99*(9), 1–2,5–10.

Teno, J. M., Kabumoto, G., Wetle, T., et al. (2004). Daily pain that was excruciating at some time in the previous week: Prevalence, characteristics, and outcomes in nursing home residents. *Journal of American Geriatrics Society, 52*(5), 762–767.

Vallerand, A. H. (2003). The use of long-acting opioids in chronic pain management. *Nursing Clinics of North America, 38*(1), 435–445.

Walker, B., Shafer, M., Henzi, I., et al. (2002). Efficacy and safety of patient-controlled opioid analgesia for postoperative pain: A quantitative systematic review. *Acta Anaesthesiology Scandinavia, 45*(7), 795–804.

*Wang, H. L. & Keck, J. F. (2004). Foot and hand massage as an intervention for postoperative pain. *Pain Management Nursing, 5*(2), 59–65.

Washington, L. L., Gibson, S. J. & Helme, R. D. (2000). Age-related differences in endogenous analgesic response to repeated cold water immersion in human volunteers. *Pain, 89*(1), 89–96.

Watson, A. C. & Coyne, P. (2003). Recognizing the faces of cancer pain. *Nursing, 33*(4), 32hn1–32hn8. Available at: http://www.nursingworld.com. Accessed May 24, 2006.

*Watt-Watson, J., Chung, F., Chan, V. W., et al. (2004). Pain management following discharge after ambulatory same-day surgery. *Journal of Nursing Management, 12*(3), 153–161.

Watt-Watson, J., Stevens, B., Garfinkel, P., et al. (2001). Relationship between nurses' pain knowledge and pain management outcomes for their postoperative cardiac patients. *Journal of Advanced Nursing, 36*(4), 535–545.

*Watt-Watson, J., Stevens, B., Katz, J., et al. (2004). Impact of preoperative education on pain outcomes after coronary artery bypass graft surgery. *Pain, 109*(1–2), 73–85.

Weiner, D. K. (2004). Pain in nursing home residents: What does it really mean, and how can we help? *Journal of the American Geriatrics Society, 52*(6), 1020–1022.

Westley, C. (2004). Pain: Geriatric self-learning module. *Med Surg Nursing, 13*(6), 399–404.

*Wilkes, G., Lasch, K. E., Lee, J. C., et al. (2003). Evaluation of a cancer pain education module. *Oncology Nursing Forum Online, 30*(6), 1037–1043.

Wise, E. A., Price, D. D., Myers, C. D., et al. (2002). Gender role expectations of pain: Relationship to experimental pain perception. *Pain, 96*(3), 335–342.

Yezierski, R. P., Radson, E. & Vanderah, T. W. (2004). Understanding chronic pain. *Nursing, 34*(4), 22–23.

Zeppetella, G. (2000). An assessment of the safety, efficacy, and acceptability of intranasal fentanyl citrate in the management of breakthrough pain: A pilot study. *Journal of Pain and Symptom Management, 20*(4), 253–258.

RESOURCES

American Academy of Pain Management, 13947 Mono Way #A, Sonora, CA 95370; 209-533-9744; http://www.aapainmanage.org. Accessed March 12, 2006.

American Chronic Pain Association, P.O. Box 850, Rocklin, CA 95677; 800-533-3231; http://www.theacpa.org. Accessed March 12, 2006.

American Pain Foundation, 201 N. Charles Street, Suite 710, Baltimore, MD 21201; 888-615-7246; http://www.painfoundation.org. Accessed March 3, 2006.

American Pain Society, 4700 W. Lake Street, Glenview, IL 60025; (847) 375-4715; http://www.ampainsoc.org. Accessed March 12, 2006.

American Society for Pain Management Nurses, 7794 Grow Drive, Pensacola, FL 32514; 222-34ASPMN; fax 850-484-8762; http://www.aspmn.org. Accessed March 12, 2006.

National Hospice Organization, Suite 901, 1901 N. Moore St., Arlington, VA 22209; 703-243-5900; http://www.nho.org. Accessed March 12, 2006.

Mendelian Inheritance in Man. A complete listing of inherited genetic conditions. http://www.ncbi.nlm.nih.gov/Omim/mimstats/html. Accessed March 3, 2006.

"Pain Control," a monthly column in *American Journal of Nursing*; http://www.ajnonline.com.

Reflex Sympathetic Dystrophy Syndrome Association, P.O. Box 502, Milford, CN 06460; 203-877-3790 or 877-662-7737; http://www.rsds.org. Accessed March 12, 2006.

CHAPTER 14

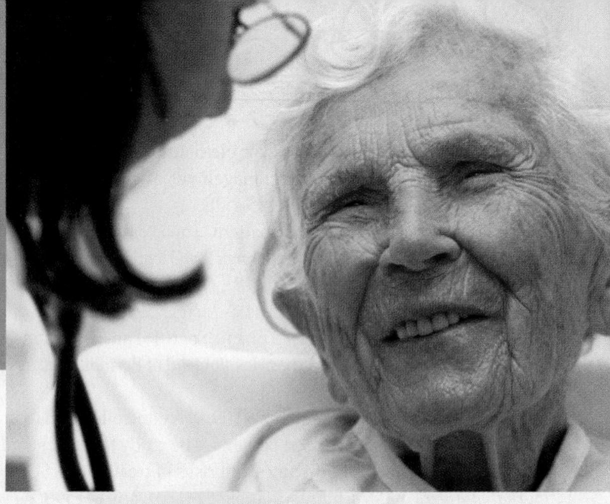

Fluid and Electrolytes: Balance and Disturbances

Learning Objectives

On completion of this chapter, the learner will be able to:

1. Differentiate between osmosis, diffusion, filtration, and active transport.
2. Describe the role of the kidneys, lungs, and endocrine glands in regulating the body's fluid composition and volume.
3. Identify the effects of aging on fluid and electrolyte regulation.
4. Plan effective care of patients with the following imbalances: fluid volume deficit and fluid volume excess; sodium deficit (hyponatremia) and sodium excess (hypernatremia); potassium deficit (hypokalemia) and potassium excess (hyperkalemia).
5. Describe the cause, clinical manifestations, management, and nursing interventions for the following imbalances: calcium deficit (hypocalcemia) and calcium excess (hypercalcemia); magnesium deficit (hypomagnesemia) and magnesium excess (hypermagnesemia); phosphorus deficit (hypophosphatemia) and phosphorus excess (hyperphosphatemia); chloride deficit (hypochloremia) and chloride excess (hyperchloremia).
6. Explain the roles of the lungs, kidneys, and chemical buffers in maintaining acid–base balance.
7. Compare metabolic acidosis and alkalosis with regard to causes, clinical manifestations, diagnosis, and management.
8. Compare respiratory acidosis and alkalosis with regard to causes, clinical manifestations, diagnosis, and management.
9. Interpret arterial blood gas measurements.
10. Demonstrate a safe and effective procedure of venipuncture.
11. Describe measures used for preventing complications of intravenous therapy.

Fluid and electrolyte balance is a dynamic process that is crucial for life and **homeostasis.** Potential and actual disorders of fluid and electrolyte balance occur in every setting, with every disorder, and with a variety of changes that affect healthy people (eg, increased fluid and sodium loss with strenuous exercise and high environmental temperature, inadequate intake of fluid and electrolytes) as well as those who are ill.

Fundamental Concepts

Nurses need to understand the physiology of fluid and electrolyte balance and acid–base balance to anticipate, identify, and respond to possible imbalances in each. Nurses also must use effective teaching and communication skills to help prevent and treat various fluid and electrolyte disturbances.

Amount and Composition of Body Fluids

Approximately 60% of the weight of a typical adult consists of fluid (water and electrolytes). Factors that influence the amount of body fluid are age, gender, and body fat. In general, younger people have a higher percentage of body fluid than older people, and men have proportionately more body fluid than women. People who are obese have less fluid than those who are thin, because fat cells contain little water. The skeleton also has a low water content. Muscle, skin, and blood have the highest amount of water.

Body fluid is located in two fluid compartments: the intracellular space (fluid in the cells) and the extracellular space (fluid outside the cells). Approximately two thirds of body fluid is in the intracellular fluid (ICF) compartment and is located primarily in the skeletal muscle mass. Approximately one third is in the extracellular fluid (ECF) compartment.

The ECF compartment is further divided into the intravascular, interstitial, and transcellular fluid spaces. The intravascular space (the fluid within the blood vessels) contains plasma. Approximately 3 L of the average 6 L of blood volume is made up of plasma. The remaining 3 L is made up of erythrocytes, leukocytes, and thrombocytes. The interstitial space contains the fluid that surrounds the cell and totals about 11 to 12 L in an adult. Lymph is an interstitial fluid. The transcellular space is the smallest division of the ECF compartment and contains approximately 1 L. Examples of transcellular fluids are cerebrospinal, pericardial, synovial, intraocular, and pleural fluids; sweat; and digestive secretions.

Body fluid normally shifts between the two major compartments or spaces in an effort to maintain an equilibrium between the spaces. Loss of fluid from the body can disrupt this equilibrium. Sometimes fluid is not lost from the body but is unavailable for use by either the ICF or ECF. Loss of ECF into a space that does not contribute to equilibrium between the ICF and the ECF is referred to as a third-space fluid shift, or "third spacing" for short.

Glossary

acidosis: an acid–base imbalance characterized by an increase in H^+ concentration (decreased blood pH). A low arterial pH due to reduced bicarbonate concentration is called metabolic acidosis; a low arterial pH due to increased PCO_2 is respiratory acidosis

active transport: physiologic pump that moves fluid from an area of lower concentration to one of higher concentration; active transport requires adenosine triphosphate (ATP) for energy

alkalosis: an acid–base imbalance characterized by a reduction in H^+ concentration (increased blood pH). A high arterial pH with increased bicarbonate concentration is called metabolic alkalosis; a high arterial pH due to reduced PCO_2 is respiratory alkalosis

diffusion: the process by which solutes move from an area of higher concentration to one of lower concentration; does not require expenditure of energy

hemostasis: a dynamic process that involves the cessation of bleeding from an injured vessel, which requires activity of blood vessels, platelets, coagulation and fibrinolytic systems

homeostasis: maintenance of a constant internal equilibrium in a biological system that involves positive and negative feedback mechanisms

hydrostatic pressure: the pressure created by the weight of fluid against the wall that contains it. In the body, hydrostatic pressure in blood vessels results from the weight of fluid itself and the force resulting from cardiac contraction

hypertonic solution: a solution with an osmolality higher than that of serum

hypotonic solution: a solution with an osmolality lower than that of serum

isotonic solution: a solution with the same osmolality as serum and other body fluids. Osmolality falls within normal range for serum (280–300 mOsm/kg).

osmolality: the number of osmoles (the standard unit of osmotic pressure) per kilogram of solution. Expressed as mOsm/kg. Used more often in clinical practice than the term osmolarity to evaluate serum and urine. In addition to urea and glucose, sodium contributes the largest number of particles to osmolality.

osmolarity: the number of osmoles, the standard unit of osmotic pressure per liter of solution. It is expressed as milliosmoles per liter (mOsm/L); describes the concentration of solutes or dissolved particles.

osmosis: the process by which fluid moves across a semipermeable membrane from an area of low solute concentration to an area of high solute concentration; the process continues until the solute concentrations are equal on both sides of the membrane.

tonicity: the measurement of the osmotic pressure of a solution; another term for osmolality

Early evidence of a third-space fluid shift is a decrease in urine output despite adequate fluid intake. Urine output decreases because fluid shifts out of the intravascular space; the kidneys then receive less blood and attempt to compensate by decreasing urine output. Other signs and symptoms of third spacing that indicate an intravascular fluid volume deficit include increased heart rate, decreased blood pressure, decreased central venous pressure, edema, increased body weight, and imbalances in fluid intake and output (I&O). Third-space shifts occur in ascites, burns, peritonitis, bowel obstruction, and massive bleeding into a joint or body cavity. Fluid shifts may also occur with stress associated with undergoing surgery (van Wissen & Breton, 2004).

Electrolytes

Electrolytes in body fluids are active chemicals (cations that carry positive charges and anions that carry negative charges). The major cations in body fluid are sodium, potassium, calcium, magnesium, and hydrogen ions. The major anions are chloride, bicarbonate, phosphate, sulfate, and proteinate ions.

These chemicals unite in varying combinations. Therefore, electrolyte concentration in the body is expressed in terms of milliequivalents (mEq) per liter, a measure of chemical activity, rather than in terms of milligrams (mg), a unit of weight. More specifically, a milliequivalent is defined as being equivalent to the electrochemical activity of 1 mg of hydrogen. In a solution, cations and anions are equal in milliequivalents per liter.

Electrolyte concentrations in the ICF differ from those in the ECF, as reflected in Table 14-1. Because special techniques are required to measure electrolyte concentrations in the ICF, it is customary to measure the electrolytes in the most accessible portion of the ECF, namely the plasma.

Sodium ions, which are positively charged, far outnumber the other cations in the ECF. Because sodium concentration affects the overall concentration of the ECF, sodium is important in regulating the volume of body fluid. Retention of sodium is associated with fluid retention, and excessive loss of sodium is usually associated with decreased volume of body fluid.

As shown in Table 14-1, the major electrolytes in the ICF are potassium and phosphate. The ECF has a low concentration of potassium and can tolerate only small changes in potassium concentrations. Therefore, release of large stores of intracellular potassium, typically caused by trauma to the cells and tissues, can be extremely dangerous.

The body expends a great deal of energy maintaining the high extracellular concentration of sodium and the high intracellular concentration of potassium. It does so by means of cell membrane pumps that exchange sodium and potassium ions. Normal movement of fluids through the capillary wall into the tissues depends on **hydrostatic pressure** (the pressure exerted by the fluid on the walls of the blood vessel) at both the arterial and the venous ends of the vessel and the osmotic pressure exerted by the protein of plasma. The direction of fluid movement depends on the differences in these two opposing forces (hydrostatic versus osmotic pressure).

TABLE 14-1 Approximate Major Electrolyte Content in Body Fluid

Electrolytes	mEq/L
Extracellular Fluid (Plasma)	
Cations	
Sodium (Na)	142
Potassium (K)	5
Calcium (Ca^{++})	5
Magnesium (Mg^{++})	2
Total cations	154
Anions	
Chloride (Cl^-)	103
Bicarbonate (HCO_3^-)	26
Phosphate (HPO_4^-)	2
Sulfate (SO_4^-)	1
Organic acids	5
Proteinate	17
Total anions	154
Intracellular Fluid	
Cations	
Potassium (K^+)	150
Magnesium (Mg^{++})	40
Sodium (Na^+)	10
Total cations	200
Anions	
Phosphates and sulfates	150
Bicarbonate (HCO_3^-)	10
Proteinate	40
Total anions	200

In addition to electrolytes, the ECF transports other substances, such as enzymes and hormones. It also carries blood components, such as red and white blood cells, throughout the body.

Regulation of Body Fluid Compartments

Osmosis and Osmolality

When two different solutions are separated by a membrane that is impermeable to the dissolved substances, fluid shifts through the membrane from the region of low solute concentration to the region of high solute concentration until the solutions are of equal concentration. This diffusion of water caused by a fluid concentration gradient is known as **osmosis** (Fig. 14-1A). The magnitude of this force depends on the number of particles dissolved in the solutions, not on their weights. The number of dissolved particles contained in a unit of fluid determines the osmolality of a solution, which influences the movement of fluid between the fluid compartments. **Tonicity** is the ability of all the solutes to cause an osmotic driving force that promotes water movement from one compartment to another (Porth, 2005). The control of tonicity determines the normal state of cellular hydration and cell size. Sodium, mannitol, glucose, and

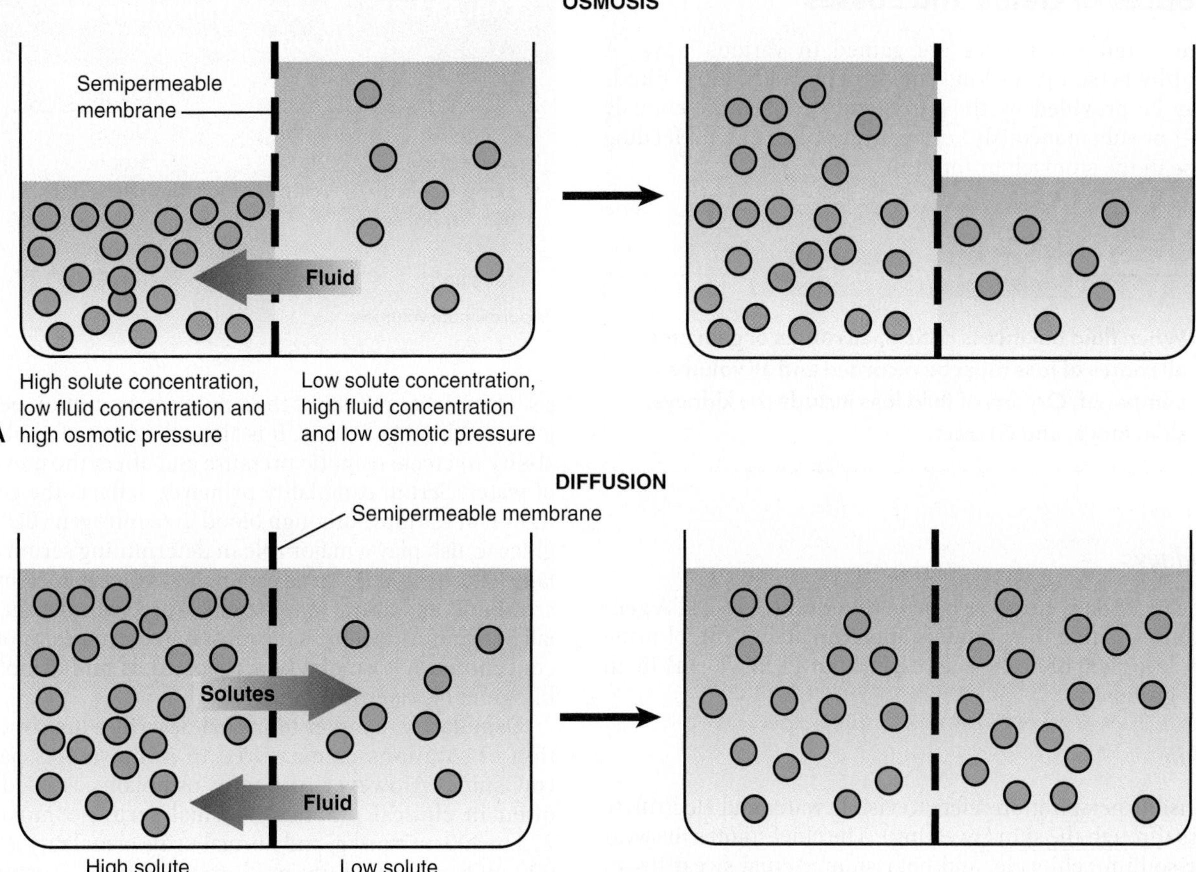

FIGURE 14-1 (**A**) Osmosis: movement of fluid from an area of lower solute concentration to an area of higher solute concentration with eventual equalization of the solute concentrations. (**B**) Diffusion: movement of solutes from an area of greater concentration to an area of lesser concentration, leading ultimately to equalization of the solute concentrations.

sorbitol are effective osmoles (capable of affecting water movement). Three other terms are associated with osmosis: osmotic pressure, oncotic pressure, and osmotic diuresis.

- Osmotic pressure is the amount of hydrostatic pressure needed to stop the flow of water by osmosis. It is primarily determined by the concentration of solutes.
- Oncotic pressure is the osmotic pressure exerted by proteins (eg, albumin).
- Osmotic diuresis is the increase in urine output caused by the excretion of substances such as glucose, mannitol, or contrast agents in the urine.

Diffusion

Diffusion is the natural tendency of a substance to move from an area of higher concentration to one of lower concentration (see Fig. 14-1B). It occurs through the random movement of ions and molecules (Porth, 2005). Examples of diffusion are the exchange of oxygen and carbon dioxide between the pulmonary capillaries and alveoli and the tendency of sodium to move from the ECF compartment, where the sodium concentration is high, to the ICF, where its concentration is low.

Filtration

Hydrostatic pressure in the capillaries tends to filter fluid out of the intravascular compartment into the interstitial fluid. Movement of water and solutes occurs from an area of high hydrostatic pressure to an area of low hydrostatic pressure. Filtration allows the kidneys to filter 180 L of plasma per day. Another example of filtration is the passage of water and electrolytes from the arterial capillary bed to the interstitial fluid; in this instance, the hydrostatic pressure is furnished by the pumping action of the heart.

Sodium–Potassium Pump

As previously stated, the sodium concentration is greater in the ECF than in the ICF, and because of this, sodium tends to enter the cell by diffusion. This tendency is offset by the sodium–potassium pump, which is located in the cell membrane and actively moves sodium from the cell into the ECF. Conversely, the high intracellular potassium concentration is maintained by pumping potassium into the cell. By definition, **active transport** implies that energy must be expended for the movement to occur against a concentration gradient.

Routes of Gains and Losses

Water and electrolytes are gained in various ways. A healthy person gains fluids by drinking and eating. Fluids may be provided by the parenteral route (intravenously [IV] or subcutaneously) or by means of an enteral feeding tube in the stomach or intestine.

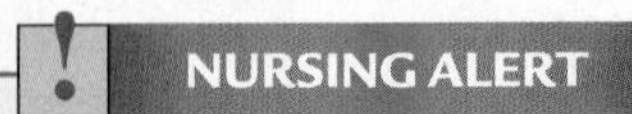

NURSING ALERT

When fluid balance is critical, all routes of gain and all routes of loss must be recorded and all volumes compared. Organs of fluid loss include the kidneys, skin, lungs, and GI tract.

Kidneys

The usual daily urine volume in the adult is 1 to 2 L. A general rule is that the output is approximately 1 mL of urine per kilogram of body weight per hour (1 mL/kg/h) in all age groups.

Skin

Sensible perspiration refers to visible water and electrolyte loss through the skin (sweating). The chief solutes in sweat are sodium, chloride, and potassium. Actual sweat losses can vary from 0 to 1000 mL or more every hour, depending on the environmental temperature. Continuous water loss by evaporation (approximately 600 mL/day) occurs through the skin as insensible perspiration, a nonvisible form of water loss. Fever greatly increases insensible water loss through the lungs and the skin, as does loss of the natural skin barrier (eg, through major burns).

Lungs

The lungs normally eliminate water vapor (insensible loss) at a rate of approximately 400 mL every day. The loss is much greater with increased respiratory rate or depth, or in a dry climate.

Gastrointestinal Tract

The usual loss through the gastrointestinal (GI) tract is only 100 to 200 mL daily, even though approximately 8 L of fluid circulates through the GI system every 24 hours (called the GI circulation). Because the bulk of fluid is normally reabsorbed in the small intestine, diarrhea and fistulas cause large losses. In healthy people, the daily average intake and output of water are approximately equal (Table 14-2).

TABLE 14-2 Average Daily Intake and Output in an Adult

Intake (mL)		Output (mL)	
Oral liquids	1300	Urine	1500
Water in food	1000	Stool	200
Water produced by metabolism	300	Insensible	
		Lungs	300
		Skin	600
Total gain*	2600	Total loss*	2600

*Approximate volumes

Laboratory Tests for Evaluating Fluid Status

Osmolality is the concentration of fluid that affects the movement of water between fluid compartments by osmosis. Osmolality measures the solute concentration per kilogram in blood and urine. It is also a measure of a solution's ability to create osmotic pressure and affect the movement of water. Serum osmolality primarily reflects the concentration of sodium, although blood urea nitrogen (BUN) and glucose also play a major role in determining serum osmolality (Porth, 2005). Urine osmolality is determined by urea, creatinine, and uric acid. When measured with serum osmolality, urine osmolality is the most reliable indicator of urine concentration. Osmolality is reported as milliosmoles per kilogram of water (mOsm/kg).

Osmolarity, another term that describes the concentration of solutions, is measured in milliosmoles per liter (mOsm/L). However, the term osmolality is used more often in clinical practice. Normal serum osmolality is 275 to 300 mOsm/kg, and normal urine osmolality is 250 to 900 mOsm/kg. Sodium predominates in ECF osmolality and holds water in this compartment.

Factors that increase and decrease serum and urine osmolality are identified in Chart 14-1. Serum osmolality may be measured directly through laboratory tests or estimated at the bedside by doubling the serum sodium level or by using the following formula:

$$Na^+ \times 2 = \frac{\text{Glucose}}{18} + \frac{\text{BUN}}{3}$$

$$= \text{Approximate value of serum osmolality}$$

The calculated value usually is within 10 mOsm of the measured osmolality.

Urine specific gravity measures the kidneys' ability to excrete or conserve water. The specific gravity of urine is compared to the weight of distilled water, which has a specific gravity of 1.000. The normal range of urine specific gravity is 1.010 to 1.025. Urine specific gravity can be measured at the bedside by placing a calibrated hydrometer or urinometer in a cylinder of approximately 20 mL of urine. Specific gravity can also be assessed with a refractometer or dipstick with a reagent for this purpose. Specific gravity varies inversely with urine volume; normally, the larger the volume of urine, the lower the specific gravity. Specific gravity is a less reliable indicator of concentration than urine osmolality; increased glucose or protein in urine can cause a falsely elevated specific gravity. Factors that increase or decrease urine osmolality are the same as those for urine specific gravity.

CHART 14-1

Factors Affecting Serum and Urine Osmolality

FLUID	FACTORS INCREASING OSMOLALITY	FACTORS DECREASING OSMOLALITY
Serum (275–300 mOsm/kg water)	• Severe dehydration • Free water loss • Diabetes insipidus • Hypernatremia • Hyperglycemia • Stroke or head injury • Renal tubular necrosis • Consumption of methanol or ethylene glycol (antifreeze)	• Fluid volume excess • Syndrome of inappropriate antidiuretic hormone (SIADH) • Renal failure • Diuretic use • Adrenal insufficiency • Hyponatremia • Overhydration • Paraneoplastic syndrome associated with lung cancer
Urine (250–900 mOsm/kg water)	• Fluid volume deficit • SIADH • Congestive heart failure • Acidosis	• Fluid volume excess • Diabetes insipidus • Hyponatremia • Aldosteronism • Pyelonephritis

BUN is made up of urea, which is an end product of the metabolism of protein (from both muscle and dietary intake) by the liver. Amino acid breakdown produces large amounts of ammonia molecules, which are absorbed into the bloodstream. Ammonia molecules are converted to urea and excreted in the urine. The normal BUN is 10 to 20 mg/dL (3.6 to 7.2 mmol/L). The BUN level varies with urine output. Factors that increase BUN include decreased renal function, GI bleeding, dehydration, increased protein intake, fever, and sepsis. Those that decrease BUN include end-stage liver disease, a low-protein diet, starvation, and any condition that results in expanded fluid volume (eg, pregnancy).

Creatinine is the end product of muscle metabolism. It is a better indicator of renal function than BUN because it does not vary with protein intake and metabolic state. The normal serum creatinine is approximately 0.7 to 1.4 mg/dL (62 to 124 mmol/L); however, its concentration depends on lean body mass and varies from person to person. Serum creatinine levels increase when renal function decreases.

Hematocrit measures the volume percentage of red blood cells (erythrocytes) in whole blood and normally ranges from 42% to 52% for males and 35% to 47% for females. Conditions that increase the hematocrit value are dehydration and polycythemia, and those that decrease hematocrit are overhydration and anemia.

Urine sodium values change with sodium intake and the status of fluid volume: as sodium intake increases, excretion increases; as the circulating fluid volume decreases, sodium is conserved. Normal urine sodium levels range from 75 to 200 mEq/24 h (75 to 200 mmol/24 h). A random specimen usually contains more than 40 mEq/L of sodium. Urine sodium levels are used to assess volume status and are useful in the diagnosis of hyponatremia and acute renal failure.

Homeostatic Mechanisms

The body is equipped with remarkable homeostatic mechanisms to keep the composition and volume of body fluid within narrow limits of normal. Organs involved in homeostasis include the kidneys, lungs, heart, adrenal glands, parathyroid glands, and pituitary gland (Porth, 2005).

Kidney Functions

Vital to the regulation of fluid and electrolyte balance, the kidneys normally filter 170 L of plasma every day in the adult, while excreting only 1.5 L of urine. They act both autonomously and in response to bloodborne messengers, such as aldosterone and antidiuretic hormone (ADH) (Porth, 2005). Major functions of the kidneys in maintaining normal fluid balance include the following:

- Regulation of ECF volume and osmolality by selective retention and excretion of body fluids
- Regulation of electrolyte levels in the ECF by selective retention of needed substances and excretion of unneeded substances
- Regulation of pH of the ECF by retention of hydrogen ions
- Excretion of metabolic wastes and toxic substances

Given these functions, it is readily apparent that renal failure results in multiple fluid and electrolyte abnormalities. Renal function declines with advanced age, as do muscle mass and daily exogenous creatinine production. Therefore, high-normal and minimally elevated serum creatinine values may indicate substantially reduced renal function in the elderly.

Heart and Blood Vessel Functions

The pumping action of the heart circulates blood through the kidneys under sufficient pressure to allow for urine formation. Failure of this pumping action interferes with renal perfusion and thus with water and electrolyte regulation.

Lung Functions

The lungs are also vital in maintaining homeostasis. Through exhalation, the lungs remove approximately 300 mL of water daily in the normal adult. Abnormal conditions, such as hyperpnea (abnormally deep respiration) or continuous coughing, increase this loss; mechanical ventilation with excessive moisture decreases it. The lungs also play a major role in maintaining acid–base balance. Normal aging results in decreased respiratory function, causing increased difficulty in pH regulation in older adults with major illness or trauma.

Pituitary Functions

The hypothalamus manufactures ADH, which is stored in the posterior pituitary gland and released as needed. ADH is sometimes called the water-conserving hormone because it causes the body to retain water. Functions of ADH include maintaining the osmotic pressure of the cells by controlling the retention or excretion of water by the kidneys and by regulating blood volume (Fig. 14-2).

Adrenal Functions

Aldosterone, a mineralocorticoid secreted by the zona glomerulosa (outer zone) of the adrenal cortex, has a profound effect on fluid balance. Increased secretion of aldosterone causes sodium retention (and thus water retention) and potassium loss. Conversely, decreased secretion of aldosterone causes sodium and water loss and potassium retention.

Cortisol, another adrenocortical hormone, has only a fraction of the mineralocorticoid potency of aldosterone. However, when secreted in large quantities (or administered as corticosteroid therapy), it can also produce sodium and fluid retention.

Parathyroid Functions

The parathyroid glands, embedded in the thyroid gland, regulate calcium and phosphate balance by means of parathyroid hormone (PTH). PTH influences bone resorption, calcium absorption from the intestines, and calcium reabsorption from the renal tubules.

Other Mechanisms

Changes in the volume of the interstitial compartment within the ECF can occur without affecting body function. However, the vascular compartment cannot tolerate change as readily and must be carefully maintained to ensure that tissues receive adequate nutrients.

BARORECEPTORS

The baroreceptors are small nerve receptors that detect changes in pressure within blood vessels and transmit this information to the central nervous system. They are responsible for monitoring the circulating volume, and they regulate sympathetic and parasympathetic neural activity as well as endocrine activities. They are categorized as either low-pressure or high-pressure baroreceptors. Low-pressure baroreceptors are in the cardiac atria, particularly the left atrium. High-pressure baroreceptors are nerve endings in the aortic arch and the carotid sinus, as well as in the afferent arteriole of the juxtaglomerular apparatus of the nephron.

As arterial pressure decreases, baroreceptors transmit fewer impulses from the carotid sinuses and the aortic arch to the vasomotor center. A decrease in impulses stimulates the sympathetic nervous system and inhibits the parasympathetic nervous system. The outcome is an increase in cardiac rate, conduction, and contractility and an increase in circulating blood volume. Sympathetic stimulation constricts renal arterioles; this increases the release of aldosterone, decreases glomerular filtration, and increases sodium and water reabsorption.

RENIN–ANGIOTENSIN–ALDOSTERONE SYSTEM

Renin is an enzyme that converts angiotensinogen, an inactive substance formed by the liver, into angiotensin I (Porth, 2005). Renin is released by the juxtaglomerular cells of the kidneys in response to decreased renal perfusion. Angiotensin-converting enzyme (ACE) converts angiotensin I to angiotensin II. Angiotensin II, with its vasoconstrictor properties, increases arterial perfusion pressure and stimulates thirst. As the sympathetic nervous system is stimulated, aldosterone is released in response to an increased release of renin. Aldosterone is a volume regulator and is also released as serum potassium increases, serum sodium decreases, or adrenocorticotropic hormone (ACTH) increases.

ANTIDIURETIC HORMONE AND THIRST

ADH and the thirst mechanism have important roles in maintaining sodium concentration and oral intake of fluids. Oral intake is controlled by the thirst center located in the hypothalamus (Porth, 2005). As serum concentration or osmolality increases or blood volume decreases, neurons in the hypothalamus are stimulated by intracellular dehydration; thirst then occurs, and the person increases his or her intake of oral fluids. Water excretion is controlled by ADH, aldosterone, and baroreceptors, as mentioned previously. The presence or absence of ADH is the most significant factor in determining whether the urine that is excreted is concentrated or dilute.

OSMORECEPTORS

Located on the surface of the hypothalamus, osmoreceptors sense changes in sodium concentration. As osmotic pressure increases, the neurons become dehydrated and quickly release impulses to the posterior pituitary, which increases the release of ADH. The ADH then travels in the blood to the kidneys, where it alters permeability to water, causing increased reabsorption of water and decreased urine output. The retained water dilutes the ECF and returns its concentration to normal. Restoration of normal osmotic pressure provides feedback to the osmoreceptors to inhibit further ADH release (see Fig. 14-2).

Physiology/Pathophysiology

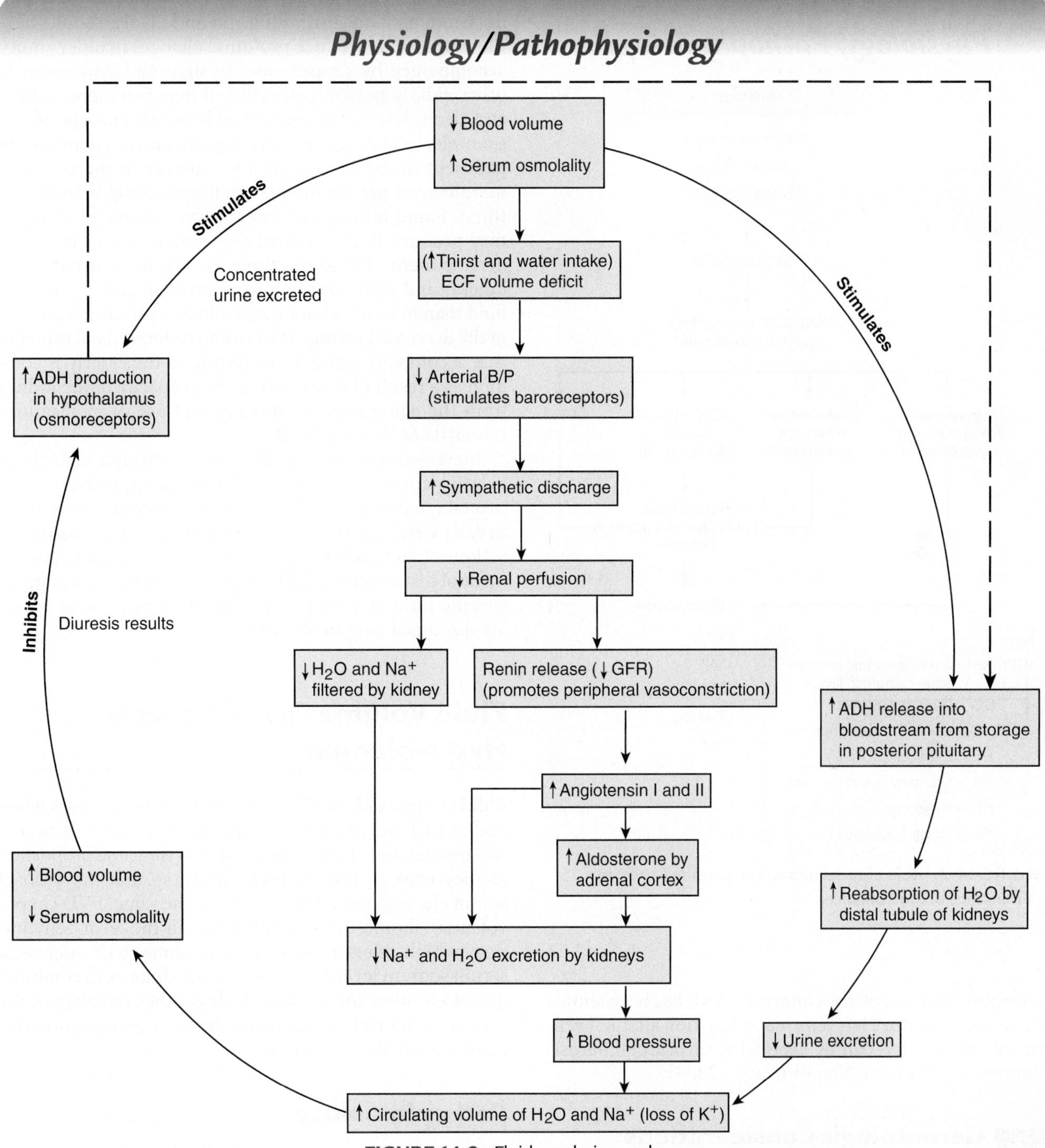

FIGURE 14-2. Fluid regulation cycle.

RELEASE OF ATRIAL NATRIURETIC PEPTIDE

Atrial natriuretic peptide (ANP), also called atrial natriuretic factor, is a 28-amino-acid peptide that is synthesized, stored, and released by muscle cells of the atria of the heart in response to several factors. These factors include increased atrial pressure, angiotensin II stimulation, endothelin (a powerful vasoconstrictor of vascular smooth muscle peptide released from damaged endothelial cells in the kidneys or other tissues), and sympathetic stimulation (Porth, 2005). In addition, any condition that results in volume expansion (exercise, pregnancy), hypoxia, or increased cardiac filling pressures (eg, high sodium intake, heart failure, chronic renal failure, atrial tachycardia, or use of vasoconstrictor agents such as epinephrine) increases the release of ANP. The action of ANP is the direct opposite of the renin–angiotensin–aldosterone system; ANP decreases blood pressure and volume (Fig. 14-3). The ANP measured in plasma is normally 20 to 77 pg/mL (20 to 77 ng/L). This level increases in acute heart failure, paroxysmal atrial tachycardia, hyperthyroidism, subarachnoid hemorrhage, and small cell lung cancer. The level decreases in chronic heart failure and with the use of medications such as urea

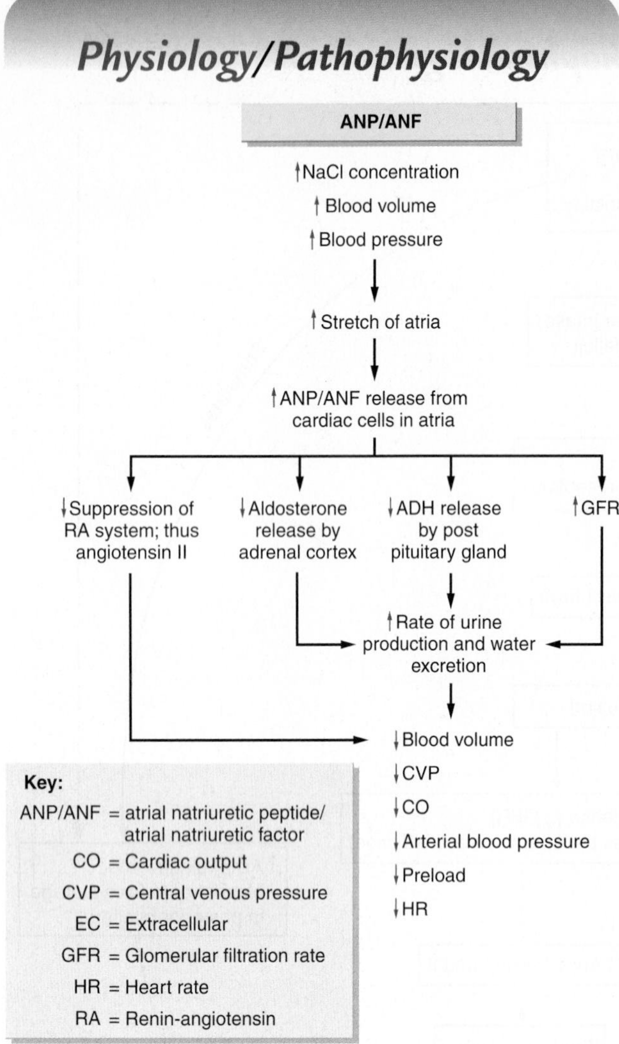

FIGURE 14-3. Role of atrial natriuretic peptide (ANP) in maintenance of fluid balance.

(Ureaphil) and prazosin (Minipress). ANP has been shown in studies to improve left ventricular function after left ventricular aneurysm repair by decreasing myocardial fibrosis (Tsuneyoshi, Nishina, Nomoto, et al., 2004).

Gerontologic Considerations

Normal physiologic changes of aging, including reduced cardiac, renal, and respiratory function and reserve and alterations in the ratio of body fluids to muscle mass, may alter the responses of elderly people to fluid and electrolyte changes and acid–base disturbances. In addition, the frequent use of medications in the older adult can affect renal and cardiac function and fluid balance, thereby increasing the likelihood of fluid and electrolyte disturbances. Routine procedures, such as the vigorous administration of laxatives before colon x-ray studies, may produce a serious fluid volume deficit, necessitating the use of intravenous (IV) fluids to prevent hypotension and other effects of hypovolemia.

Alterations in fluid and electrolyte balance that may produce minor changes in young and middle-aged adults have the potential to produce profound changes in older adults, accompanied by a rapid onset of signs and symptoms. In other elderly patients, the clinical manifestations of fluid and electrolyte disturbances may be subtle or atypical. For example, fluid deficit may cause confusion or cognitive impairment in the elderly person, whereas in the young or middle-aged person the first sign commonly is increased thirst. Rapid infusion of an excessive volume of IV fluids may produce fluid overload and cardiac failure in the elderly patient. These reactions are likely to occur more quickly and with the administration of smaller volumes of fluid than in healthy young and middle-aged adults because of the decreased cardiac reserve and reduced renal function that accompany aging. Dehydration in the elderly is common as a result of decreased reserve capacity of the kidney from the aging process, disease, and use of medications (Suhayda & Walton, 2002).

Increased sensitivity to fluid and electrolyte changes in elderly patients requires careful assessment, with attention to intake and output of fluids from all sources and to changes in daily weight; careful monitoring of side effects and interactions of medications; and prompt reporting and management of disturbances. Additional considerations relating to specific fluid and electrolyte disturbances in older adults are discussed later in this chapter.

Fluid Volume Disturbances: Hypovolemia

Fluid volume deficit (FVD), or hypovolemia, occurs when loss of ECF volume exceeds the intake of fluid. It occurs when water and electrolytes are lost in the same proportion as they exist in normal body fluids, so that the ratio of serum electrolytes to water remains the same. FVD (hypovolemia) should not be confused with the term dehydration, which refers to loss of water alone, with increased serum sodium levels. FVD may occur alone or in combination with other imbalances. Unless other imbalances are present concurrently, serum electrolyte concentrations remain essentially unchanged.

Pathophysiology

FVD results from loss of body fluids and occurs more rapidly when coupled with decreased fluid intake. FVD can develop from inadequate intake alone if the decreased intake is prolonged. Causes of FVD include abnormal fluid losses, such as those resulting from vomiting, diarrhea, GI suctioning, and sweating, and decreased intake, as in nausea or inability to gain access to fluids (Heitz & Horne, 2005).

Additional risk factors include diabetes insipidus, adrenal insufficiency, osmotic diuresis, hemorrhage, and coma. Third-space fluid shifts, or the movement of fluid from the vascular system to other body spaces (eg, with edema formation in burns, ascites with liver dysfunction), also cause FVD.

NURSING RESEARCH PROFILE

Bowel Cleansing for Colonoscopy

Hayes, A., Buffum, M. & Fuller, D. (2003). Bowel preparation comparison: Flavored versus unflavored colyte. *Gastroenterology Nursing, 26*(3), 106–109.

Purpose

Inadequate bowel cleansing prior to colonoscopy often necessitates repeated colon lavage and a second attempt at colonoscopy. Patients who have poorly cleansed bowels often complain about the taste of colon lavage solutions they were required to consume in preparation for colonoscopy. This study was conducted to determine whether flavoring in lavage solutions had an effect on bowel cleansing in preparation for colonoscopy.

Design

A randomized clinical trial was conducted with 130 patients, who received either flavored or unflavored lavage solution. The health care staff who assessed the effectiveness of bowel cleansing were blinded to group assignment of patients to the type of lavage solution received. Questionnaires were used to determine patients' opinions about the taste of the solution, the amount consumed, and their willingness to drink the solution again if necessary. A colon preparation rating scale completed by the endoscopist and endoscopy nurse was used to rate the adequacy of bowel cleansing in preparation for the colonoscopy.

Findings

Chi square analysis revealed no significant difference in bowel cleansing between the patients who consumed flavored solution and those who consumed unflavored solution. Although both groups reported disliking the flavor of the solution, there was no difference in their adherence to instructions. The authors concluded that taste of the solution did not affect bowel cleansing.

Nursing Implications

No differences were detected in the effect of flavoring of colon lavage solution on the adequacy of bowel cleansing in preparation for colonoscopy. Therefore, other factors must be involved. Further research is needed to identify factors that affect adequacy of bowel cleansing with the goals of decreasing the likelihood that patients may have to undergo repeated efforts to cleanse the bowel and increasing the likelihood of successful colonoscopy. Because of the importance of colonoscopy in early detection of colon cancer, efforts are needed to improve the effectiveness of bowel cleansing and to reduce the discomfort and cost associated with ineffective cleansing and potential fluid and electrolyte disturbances associated with repeated doses.

Clinical Manifestations

FVD can develop rapidly and can be mild, moderate, or severe, depending on the degree of fluid loss. Important characteristics include acute weight loss; decreased skin turgor; oliguria; concentrated urine; postural hypotension; a weak, rapid heart rate; flattened neck veins; increased temperature; decreased central venous pressure; cool, clammy skin related to peripheral vasoconstriction; thirst; anorexia; nausea; lassitude; muscle weakness; and cramps.

Assessment and Diagnostic Findings

Laboratory data useful in evaluating fluid volume status include BUN and its relation to serum creatinine concentration. A volume-depleted patient has a BUN elevated out of proportion to the serum creatinine (ratio greater than 20:1). The cause of hypovolemia may be determined through the health history and physical examination. The BUN can be elevated because of dehydration or decreased renal perfusion and function. Also, the hematocrit level is greater than normal because the red blood cells become suspended in a decreased plasma volume.

Serum electrolyte changes may also exist. Potassium and sodium levels can be reduced (hypokalemia, hyponatremia) or elevated (hyperkalemia, hypernatremia).

- Hypokalemia occurs with GI and renal losses.
- Hyperkalemia occurs with adrenal insufficiency.
- Hyponatremia occurs with increased thirst and ADH release.
- Hypernatremia results from increased insensible losses and diabetes insipidus.

Urine specific gravity is increased in relation to the kidneys' attempt to conserve water and decreased with diabetes insipidus. Urine osmolality is greater than 450 mOsm/kg, because the kidneys try to compensate by conserving water. Normal values for these tests are listed in Table 14-3.

Gerontologic Considerations

Elderly patients have special nursing care needs because of their propensity for developing fluid and electrolyte imbalances (Zwicker, 2003). Fluid balance in many elderly patients is often marginal at best because of certain physiologic changes associated with the aging process. Some of these changes include reduction in total body water (associated with increased body fat content and decreased muscle mass); reduction in renal function, resulting in decreased ability to concentrate urine; decreased cardiovascular and respiratory function; and disturbances in hormonal regulatory functions. Although these changes are often viewed as

TABLE 14-3 Laboratory Values Used In Evaluating Fluid and Electrolyte Status in Adults

Test	Usual Reference Range	SI Units
Serum sodium	135–145 mEq/L	135–145 mmol/L
Serum potassium	3.5–5.0 mEq/L	3.5–5.0 mmol/L
Total serum calcium	8.6–10.2 mg/dL	2.15–2.55 mmol/L
Ionized calcium	4.5–5.0 mg/dL	1.05–1.30 mmol/L
Serum magnesium	1.3–2.5 mEq/L	0.65–1.25 mmol/L
Serum phosphorus	2.5–4.5 mg/dL	0.87–1.45 mmol/L
Serum chloride	97–107 mEq/L	97–107 mmol/L
Carbon dioxide content	24–32 mEq/L	24–32 mmol/L
Serum osmolality	275–300 mOsm/kg	275–300 mmol/kg
Blood urea nitrogen (BUN)	10–20 mg/dL	3.6–7.2 mmol/L
Serum creatinine	0.7–1.4 mg/dL	62–124 μmol/L
BUN to creatinine ratio	10:1–20:1	—
Hematocrit	Males: 42–52% Females: 35–47%	Volume fraction: 0.42–0.52 Volume fraction: 0.35–0.47
Serum glucose	60–110 mg/dL	3.3–6.05 mmol/L
Serum albumin	3.5–5.0 g/dL	3.5–5.0 g/L
Urinary sodium	75–200 mEq/day	75–200 mmol/day
Urinary potassium (intake-dependent)	26–123 mEq/day	26–123 mmol/day
Urinary chloride	110–250 mEq/24 h	110–250 mmol/24 h
Urine specific gravity	1.003–1.030	1.002–1.030
Urine osmolality	250–900 mOsm/kg	250–900 mmol/kg
Urinary pH	Random: 4.5–8.0 Typical urine <5–6	4.5–8.0 <5–6

a normal part of the aging process, they must be considered when elderly people become ill, because age-related changes predispose people to fluid and electrolyte imbalances. These physiologic changes must be considered during assessment of elderly patients as well as before initiating treatment for fluid and electrolyte imbalances.

Assessment of elderly patients should be modified somewhat from that of younger adults. For example, in an elderly patient, assessment of skin turgor is less valid because the skin has lost some of its elasticity due to the decreased number of papillae and collagen fibers; therefore, other assessment measures (eg, slowness in filling of veins of the hands and feet) become more useful in detecting FVD. In elderly patients, skin turgor is best tested over the forehead or the sternum, because alterations in skin elasticity are less marked in these areas. As in all patients, skin turgor should be monitored serially to detect subtle changes.

The nurse should perform a functional assessment of the ability of the elderly patient to determine fluid and food needs and to obtain adequate intake. For example, is the patient mentally clear? Is the patient able to ambulate and to use both arms and hands to reach fluids and foods? Is the patient able to swallow? All of these questions have a direct bearing on how the patient will be able to meet his or her own need for fluids and foods. During an elderly patient's hospital stay, the nurse provides fluids for the patient if he or she is unable to carry out self-care activities.

Another concern is that some elderly patients deliberately restrict their fluid intake to avoid embarrassing episodes of incontinence. In this situation, the nurse also identifies interventions to deal with the incontinence, such as encouraging the patient to wear protective clothing or devices, to carry a urinal in the car, or to pace fluid intake to allow access to toilet facilities during the day. Elderly people without cardiovascular or renal dysfunction should be reminded to drink adequate fluids, particularly in very warm or humid weather.

Medical Management

When planning the correction of fluid loss for the patient with FVD, the health care provider considers the usual maintenance requirements of the patient and other factors (eg, fever) that can influence fluid needs. If the deficit is not severe, the oral route is preferred, provided the patient can drink. However, if fluid losses are acute or severe, the IV route is required. Isotonic electrolyte solutions (eg, lactated Ringer's solution, 0.9% sodium chloride) are frequently used to treat the hypotensive patient with FVD because they expand plasma volume. As soon as the patient becomes normotensive, a hypotonic electrolyte solution (eg, 0.45% sodium chloride) is often used to provide both electrolytes and water for renal excretion of metabolic wastes. These and additional fluids are listed in Table 14-4.

Accurate and frequent assessments of I&O, weight, vital signs, central venous pressure, level of consciousness, breath sounds, and skin color should be performed to determine when therapy should be slowed to avoid volume overload. The rate of fluid administration is based on the severity of loss and the patient's hemodynamic response to volume replacement (Suhayda & Walton, 2002).

If the patient with severe FVD is not excreting enough urine and is therefore oliguric, the health care provider needs to determine whether the depressed renal function is caused by reduced renal blood flow secondary to FVD (prerenal azotemia) or, more seriously, by acute tubular necro-

TABLE 14-4 Selected Water and Electrolyte Solutions

Solution	Comments
Isotonic Solutions	
0.9% NaCl (isotonic, also called normal saline [NS]) Na^+ 154 mEq/L Cl^- 154 mEq/L (308 mOsm/L) Also available with varying concentrations of dextrose (the most frequently used is a 5% dextrose concentration)	• An isotonic solution that expands the extracellular fluid (ECF) volume, used in hypovolemic states, resuscitative efforts, shock, diabetic ketoacidosis, metabolic alkalosis, hypercalcemia, mild Na^+ deficit • Supplies an excess of Na^+ and Cl^-; can cause fluid volume excess and hyperchloremic acidosis if used in excessive volumes, particularly in patients with compromised renal function, heart failure, or edema • Not desirable as a routine maintenance solution, as it provides only Na^+ and Cl^- (and these are provided in excessive amounts) • When mixed with 5% dextrose, the resulting solution becomes hypertonic in relation to plasma and, in addition to the above described electrolytes, provides 170 cal/L • Only solution that may be administered with blood products
Lactated Ringer's solution (Hartmann's solution) Na^+ 130 mEq/L K^+ 4 mEq/L Ca^{++} 3 mEq/L Cl^- 109 mEq/L Lactate (metabolized to bicarbonate) 28 mEq/L (274 mOsm/L) Also available with varying concentrations of dextrose (the most common is 5% dextrose)	• An isotonic solution that contains multiple electrolytes in roughly the same concentration as found in plasma (note that solution is lacking in Mg^{++}): provides 9 cal/L • Used in the treatment of hypovolemia, burns, fluid lost as bile or diarrhea, and for acute blood loss replacement • Lactate is rapidly metabolized into HCO_3^- in the body. Lactated Ringer's solution should not be used in lactic acidosis because the ability to convert lactate into HCO_3^- is impaired in this disorder. • Not to be given with a pH > 7.5 because bicarbonate is formed as lactate breaks down, causing alkalosis • Should not be used in renal failure because it contains potassium and can cause hyperkalemia • Similar to plasma
5% dextrose in water (D_5W) No electrolytes 50 g of dextrose	• An isotonic solution that supplies 170 cal/L and free water to aid in renal excretion of solutes • Used in treatment of hypernatremia, fluid loss, and dehydration • Should not be used in excessive volumes in the early postoperative period (when anti-diuretic hormone secretion is increased due to stress reaction) • Should not be used solely in treatment of fluid volume deficit, because it dilutes plasma electrolyte concentrations • Contraindicated in head injury because it may cause increased intracranial pressure • Should not be used for fluid resuscitation because it can cause hyperglycemia • Should be used with caution in patients with renal or cardiac disease because of risk of fluid overload • Electrolyte-free solutions may cause peripheral circulatory collapse, anuria in patients with sodium deficiency, and increased body fluid loss. • Converts to hypotonic solution as dextrose is metabolized by body. Over time, D_5W without NaCl can cause water intoxication (intracellular fluid volume excess [FVE]) because the solution is hypotonic.
Hypotonic Solutions	
0.45% NaCl (half-strength saline) Na^+ 77 mEq/L Cl^- 77 mEq/L (154 mOsm/L) Also available with varying concentrations of dextrose (the most common is a 5% concentration)	• Provides Na^+, Cl^-, and free water • Free water is desirable to aid the kidneys in elimination of solute. • Lacking in electrolytes other than Na^+ and Cl^- • When mixed with 5% dextrose, the solution becomes slightly hypertonic to plasma and in addition to the above-described electrolytes provides 170 cal/L. • Used to treat hypertonic dehydration, Na^+ and Cl^- depletion, and gastric fluid loss • Not indicated for third-space fluid shifts or increased intracranial pressure • Administer cautiously, because it can cause fluid shifts from vascular system into cells, resulting in cardiovascular collapse and increased intracranial pressure.

continued >

TABLE 14-4 Selected Water and Electrolyte Solutions (Continued)

Solution	Comments
Hypertonic Solutions	
3% NaCl (hypertonic saline) Na^+ 513 mEq/L Cl^- 513 mEq/L (1026 mOsm/L)	• Used to increase ECF volume, decrease cellular swelling • Highly hypertonic solution used only in critical situations to treat hyponatremia • Must be administered slowly and cautiously, because it can cause intravascular volume overload and pulmonary edema • Supplies no calories • Assists in removing intracellular fluid excess
5% NaCL (hypertonic solution) Na^+ 855 mEq/L Cl^- 855 mEq/L (1710 mOsm/L)	• Highly hypertonic solution used to treat symptomatic hyponatremia • Administered slowly and cautiously, because it can cause intravascular volume overload and pulmonary edema • Supplies no calories
Colloid Solutions	
Dextran in NS or 5% D_5W Available in low-molecular-weight (Dextran 40) and high-molecular-weight (Dextran 70) forms	• Colloid solution used as volume/plasma expander for intravascular part of ECF • Affects clotting by coating platelets and decreasing ability to clot • Remains in circulatory system up to 24 hours • Used to treat hypovolemia in early shock to increase pulse pressure, cardiac output, and arterial blood pressure • Improves microcirculation by decreasing red blood cell aggregation • Contraindicated in hemorrhage, thrombocytopenia, renal disease, and severe dehydration • Not a substitute for blood or blood products

sis from prolonged FVD. The test used in this situation is referred to as a fluid challenge test. During a fluid challenge test, volumes of fluid are administered at specific rates and intervals while the patient's hemodynamic response to this treatment is monitored (ie, vital signs, breath sounds, sensorium, central venous pressure, urine output).

A typical example of a fluid challenge involves administering 100 to 200 mL of normal saline solution over 15 minutes. The goal is to provide fluids rapidly enough to attain adequate tissue perfusion without compromising the cardiovascular system. The response by a patient with FVD but normal renal function is increased urine output and an increase in blood pressure and central venous pressure.

Shock can occur when the volume of fluid lost exceeds 25% of the intravascular volume, or when fluid loss is rapid. Shock and its causes and treatment are discussed in detail in Chapter 15.

Nursing Management

To assess for FVD, the nurse monitors and measures fluid I&O at least every 8 hours, and sometimes hourly. As FVD develops, body fluid losses exceed fluid intake. This loss may be in the form of excessive urination (polyuria), diarrhea, vomiting, and so on. Later, after FVD fully develops, the kidneys attempt to conserve needed body fluids, leading to a urine output of less than 30 mL/h in an adult. Urine in this instance is concentrated and represents a healthy renal response. Daily body weights are monitored; an acute loss of 0.5 kg (1 lb) represents a fluid loss of approximately 500 mL. (One liter of fluid weighs approximately 1 kg, or 2.2 lb.)

Vital signs are closely monitored. The nurse observes for a weak, rapid pulse and postural hypotension (ie, a decrease in systolic pressure exceeding 15 mm Hg when the patient moves from a lying to a sitting position). A decrease in body temperature often accompanies FVD, unless there is a concurrent infection.

Skin and tongue turgor is monitored on a regular basis. In a healthy person, pinched skin immediately returns to its normal position when released. This elastic property, referred to as turgor, is partially dependent on interstitial fluid volume. In a person with FVD, the skin flattens more slowly after the pinch is released. In a person with severe FVD, the skin may remain elevated for many seconds. Tissue turgor is best measured by pinching the skin over the sternum, inner aspects of the thighs, or forehead.

NURSING ALERT

The skin turgor test is not as valid in elderly people as in younger people because skin elasticity decreases with age; therefore, other assessment parameters must be considered.

Evaluating tongue turgor, which is not affected by age, may be more valid than evaluating skin turgor. In a normal person, the tongue has one longitudinal furrow. In the person with FVD, there are additional longitudinal furrows and the tongue is smaller, because of fluid loss. The degree of oral mucous membrane moisture is also assessed; a dry mouth may indicate either FVD or mouth breathing.

Urine concentration is monitored by measuring the urine specific gravity. In a volume-depleted patient, the urine specific gravity should be greater than 1.020, indicating healthy renal conservation of fluid.

Mental function is eventually affected in severe FVD as a result of decreasing cerebral perfusion. Decreased peripheral perfusion can result in cold extremities. In patients with relatively normal cardiopulmonary function, a low central venous pressure is indicative of hypovolemia. Patients with acute cardiopulmonary decompensation require more extensive hemodynamic monitoring of pressures in both sides of the heart to determine if hypovolemia exists.

Preventing Fluid Volume Deficit

To prevent FVD, the nurse identifies patients at risk and takes measures to minimize fluid losses. For example, if the patient has diarrhea, diarrhea control measures should be implemented and replacement fluids administered. These measures may include administering antidiarrheal medications and small volumes of oral fluids at frequent intervals.

Correcting Fluid Volume Deficit

When possible, oral fluids are administered to help correct FVD, with consideration given to the patient's likes and dislikes. The type of fluid the patient has lost is also considered, and attempts are made to select fluids most likely to replace the lost electrolytes. If the patient is reluctant to drink because of oral discomfort, the nurse assists with frequent mouth care and provides nonirritating fluids. The patient may be offered small volumes of oral rehydration solutions (eg, Rehydralyte, Elete, Cytomax). These solutions provide fluid, glucose, and electrolytes in concentrations that are easily absorbed. If nausea is present, antiemetics may be needed before oral fluid replacement can be tolerated.

If the patient cannot eat and drink, fluid may need to be administered by an alternative route (enteral or parenteral) until adequate circulating blood volume and renal perfusion are achieved (Suhayda & Walton, 2002). Isotonic fluids are prescribed to increase ECF volume.

Fluid Volume Disturbances: Hypervolemia

Fluid volume excess (FVE), or hypervolemia, refers to an isotonic expansion of the ECF caused by the abnormal retention of water and sodium in approximately the same proportions in which they normally exist in the ECF. It is always secondary to an increase in the total body sodium content, which, in turn, leads to an increase in total body water. Because there is isotonic retention of body substances, the serum sodium concentration remains essentially normal.

Pathophysiology

FVE may be related to simple fluid overload or diminished function of the homeostatic mechanisms responsible for regulating fluid balance. Contributing factors can include heart failure, renal failure, and cirrhosis of the liver. Another contributing factor is consumption of excessive amounts of table or other sodium salts. Excessive administration of sodium-containing fluids in a patient with impaired regulatory mechanisms may predispose him or her to a serious FVE as well (Heitz & Horne, 2005).

Clinical Manifestations

Clinical manifestations of FVE stem from expansion of the ECF and include edema, distended neck veins, and crackles (abnormal lung sounds). Other manifestations include tachycardia; increased blood pressure, pulse pressure, and central venous pressure; increased weight; increased urine output; and shortness of breath and wheezing.

Assessment and Diagnostic Findings

Laboratory data useful in diagnosing FVE include BUN and hematocrit levels. In FVE, both of these values may be decreased because of plasma dilution. Other causes of abnormalities in these values include low protein intake and anemia. In chronic renal failure, both serum osmolality and the sodium level are decreased due to excessive retention of water. The urine sodium level is increased if the kidneys are attempting to excrete excess volume. Chest x-rays may reveal pulmonary congestion. Hypervolemia occurs when aldosterone is chronically stimulated (ie, cirrhosis, heart failure, and nephrotic syndrome). Therefore, the urine sodium level does not increase in these conditions.

Medical Management

Management of FVE is directed at the causes. If the fluid excess is related to excessive administration of sodium-containing fluids, discontinuing the infusion may be all that is needed. Symptomatic treatment consists of administering diuretics and restricting fluids and sodium.

Pharmacologic Therapy

Diuretics are prescribed when dietary restriction of sodium alone is insufficient to reduce edema by inhibiting the reabsorption of sodium and water by the kidneys. The choice of diuretic is based on the severity of the hypervolemic state, the degree of impairment of renal function, and the potency of the diuretic. Thiazide diuretics block sodium reabsorption in the distal tubule, where only 5% to 10% of filtered sodium is reabsorbed. Loop diuretics, such as furosemide (Lasix), bumetanide (Bumex), or torsemide (Demadex), can cause a greater loss of both sodium and water because they block sodium reabsorption in the ascending limb of the loop of Henle, where 20% to 30% of filtered sodium is normally reabsorbed. Generally, thiazide diuretics, such as hydrochlorothiazide (HydroDIURIL) or metolazone (Mykrox, Zaroxolyn), are prescribed for mild to moderate hypervolemia and loop diuretics for severe hypervolemia.

Electrolyte imbalances may result from the effect of the diuretic. Hypokalemia can occur with all diuretics except those that work in the last distal tubule of the nephrons (eg, spironolactone). Potassium supplements can be prescribed to avoid this complication. Hyperkalemia can occur with diuretics that work in the last distal tubule, especially in patients with decreased renal function. Hyponatremia occurs with diuresis due to increased release of ADH secondary to reduction in circulating volume. Decreased magnesium levels occur with administration of loop and thiazide diuretics due to decreased reabsorption and increased excretion of magnesium by the kidney.

Azotemia (increased nitrogen levels in the blood) can occur with FVE when urea and creatinine are not excreted due to decreased perfusion by the kidneys and decreased excretion of wastes. High uric acid levels (hyperuricemia) can also occur from increased reabsorption and decreased excretion of uric acid by the kidneys.

Hemodialysis

If renal function is so severely impaired that pharmacologic agents cannot act efficiently, other modalities are considered to remove sodium and fluid from the body. Hemodialysis or peritoneal dialysis may be used to remove nitrogenous wastes and control potassium and acid–base balance, and to remove sodium and fluid. Continuous renal replacement therapy may also be required. See Chapter 44 for discussion of these treatment modalities.

Nutritional Therapy

Treatment of FVE usually involves dietary restriction of sodium. An average daily diet not restricted in sodium contains 6 to 15 g of salt, whereas low-sodium diets can range from a mild restriction to as little as 250 mg of sodium per day, depending on the patient's needs. A mild sodium-restricted diet allows only light salting of food (about half the usual amount) in cooking and at the table, and no addition of salt to commercially prepared foods that are already seasoned. Of course, foods high in sodium must be avoided. It is the sodium salt, sodium chloride, rather than sodium itself that contributes to edema. Therefore, patients are instructed to read food labels carefully to determine salt content.

Because about half of ingested sodium is in the form of seasoning, seasoning substitutes can play a major role in decreasing sodium intake. Lemon juice, onions, and garlic are excellent substitute flavorings, although some patients prefer salt substitutes. Most salt substitutes contain potassium and must therefore be used cautiously by patients taking potassium-sparing diuretics (eg, spironolactone, triamterene, amiloride). They should not be used at all in conditions associated with potassium retention, such as advanced renal disease. Salt substitutes containing ammonium chloride can be harmful to patients with liver damage.

In some communities, the drinking water may contain too much sodium for a sodium-restricted diet. Depending on its source, water may contain as little as 1 mg or more than 1500 mg per quart. Patients may need to use distilled water if the local water supply is very high in sodium. Bottled water can have a sodium content from 0 to 1200 mg/L; therefore, if sodium is restricted, the label must be carefully examined for sodium content before purchasing and drinking bottled water. Also, patients on sodium-restricted diets should be cautioned to avoid water softeners that add sodium to water in exchange for other ions, such as calcium. Protein intake may be increased in patients who are malnourished or who have low serum protein levels in an effort to increase capillary oncotic pressure and pull fluid out of the tissues into vessels for excretion by the kidneys.

Nursing Management

To assess for FVE, the nurse measures I&O at regular intervals to identify excessive fluid retention. The patient is weighed daily, and acute weight gain is noted. An acute weight gain of 2.2 lb (1 kg) is equivalent to a gain of approximately 1 L of fluid. The nurse also needs to assess breath sounds at regular intervals in at-risk patients, particularly if parenteral fluids are being administered. The nurse monitors the degree of edema in the most dependent parts of the body, such as the feet and ankles in ambulatory patients and the sacral region in patients confined to bed. The degree of pitting edema is assessed, and the extent of peripheral edema is monitored by measuring the circumference of the extremity with a tape marked in millimeters.

Preventing Fluid Volume Excess

Specific interventions vary somewhat with the underlying condition and the degree of FVE. However, most patients require sodium-restricted diets in some form, and adherence to the prescribed diet is encouraged. Patients are instructed to avoid over-the-counter medications without first checking with a health care provider, because these substances may contain sodium. If fluid retention persists despite adherence to a prescribed diet, hidden sources of sodium, such as the water supply or use of water softeners, should be considered.

Detecting and Controlling Fluid Volume Excess

It is important to detect FVE before the condition becomes critical. Interventions include promoting rest, restricting sodium intake, monitoring parenteral fluid therapy, and administering appropriate medications.

Regular rest periods may be beneficial, because bed rest favors diuresis of edema fluid. The mechanism is probably related to diminished venous pooling and the subsequent increase in effective circulating blood volume and renal perfusion. Sodium and fluid restriction should be instituted as indicated. Because most patients with FVE require diuretics, the patient's response to these agents is monitored. The rate of parenteral fluids and the patient's response to these fluids are also closely monitored. If dyspnea or orthopnea is present, the patient is placed in a semi-Fowler's position to promote lung expansion. The patient is turned and positioned at regular intervals because edematous tissue is more prone to skin breakdown than normal tissue. Because conditions predisposing to FVE are likely to be chronic, patients are taught to monitor their response to therapy by documenting fluid intake and output and body weight changes. The importance of adhering to the treatment regimen is emphasized.

Teaching Patients About Edema

Because edema is a common manifestation of FVE, patients need to recognize its symptoms and understand its importance. The nurse gives special attention to edema when teaching the patient with FVE. Edema can occur as a result of increased capillary fluid pressure, decreased capillary oncotic pressure, or increased interstitial oncotic pressure, causing expansion of the interstitial fluid compartment (Porth, 2005). Edema can be localized (eg, in the ankle, as in rheumatoid arthritis) or generalized (as in cardiac and renal failure). Severe generalized edema is called *anasarca*.

Edema occurs when there is a change in the capillary membrane, increasing the formation of interstitial fluid or decreasing the removal of interstitial fluid. Sodium retention is a frequent cause of the increased ECF volume. Burns and infection are examples of conditions associated with increased interstitial fluid volume. Obstruction to lymphatic outflow, a plasma albumin level less than 1.5 to 2 g/dL, or a decrease in plasma oncotic pressure contributes to increased interstitial fluid volume. The kidneys retain sodium and water when there is decreased ECF volume as a result of decreased cardiac output from heart failure. A thorough medication history is necessary to identify any medications that could cause edema, such as nonsteroidal anti-inflammatory drugs (NSAIDs), estrogens, corticosteroids, and antihypertensive agents.

Ascites is a form of edema in which fluid accumulates in the peritoneal cavity; it results from nephrotic syndrome, cirrhosis, and some malignant tumors. The patient commonly reports shortness of breath and a sense of pressure because of pressure on the diaphragm.

Edema usually affects dependent areas. It can be seen in the ankles, sacrum, scrotum, or the periorbital region of the face. Pitting edema is so named because a pit forms after a finger is pressed into edematous tissue. In pulmonary edema, the amount of fluid in the pulmonary interstitium and the alveoli increases. Manifestations include shortness of breath, increased respiratory rate, diaphoresis, and crackles and wheezing on auscultation of the lungs. Decreased hematocrit resulting from hemodilution, arterial blood gas results indicative of respiratory **alkalosis** and hypoxemia, and decreased serum sodium and osmolality from retention of fluid may occur with edema. BUN and creatinine levels increase, urine specific gravity decreases as the kidneys attempt to excrete excess water, and the urine sodium level decreases because of increased aldosterone production.

The goal of treatment is to preserve or restore the circulating intravascular fluid volume. In addition to treating the cause, other treatments may include diuretic therapy, restriction of fluids and sodium, elevation of the extremities, application of elastic compression stockings, paracentesis, dialysis, and continuous renal replacement therapy in cases of renal failure or life-threatening fluid volume overload (See Chapter 44).

Electrolyte Imbalances

Disturbances in electrolyte balances are common in clinical practice and must be corrected for the patient's health and safety. Table 14-5 summarizes the major fluid and electrolyte imbalances that are described in this chapter. An example of an electrolyte imbalance is an altered sodium balance.

Sodium Imbalances

Sodium is the most abundant electrolyte in the ECF; its concentration ranges from 135 to 145 mEq/L (135 to 145 mmol/L). Consequently, sodium is the primary determinant of ECF osmolality. Decreased sodium is associated with parallel changes in osmolality. Sodium has a major role in controlling water distribution throughout the body, because it does not easily cross the cell wall membrane and because of its abundance and high concentration in the body. Sodium is regulated by ADH, thirst, and the renin–angiotensin–aldosterone system. It is the primary regulator of ECF volume. A loss or gain of sodium is usually accompanied by a loss or gain of water. Sodium also functions in establishing the electrochemical state necessary for muscle contraction and the transmission of nerve impulses.

Sodium imbalance occurs frequently in clinical practice and can develop under simple or complex circumstances. The two most common sodium imbalances are sodium deficit and sodium excess.

Sodium Deficit (Hyponatremia)

Hyponatremia refers to a serum sodium level that is below normal (less than 135 mEq/L [135 mmol/L]). Plasma sodium concentration represents the ratio of total body sodium to total body water. A decrease in this ratio can occur because of a low quantity of total body sodium with a lesser reduction in total body water, normal total body sodium content with excess total body water, or an excess of total body sodium with an even greater excess of total body water. However, a hyponatremic state can be superimposed on an existing FVD or FVE.

Sodium may be lost by way of vomiting, diarrhea, fistulas, or sweating, or it may be lost as the result of the use of diuretics, particularly in combination with a low-salt diet. A deficiency of aldosterone, as occurs in adrenal insufficiency, also predisposes to sodium deficiency.

In dilutional hyponatremia (water intoxication), the patient's serum sodium level is diluted by an increase in the ratio of water to sodium. Dilutional hyponatremia, therefore, results from an increased extracellular fluid volume and a normal or increased total body sodium. Predisposing conditions for this type of hyponatremia include syndrome of inappropriate secretion of antidiuretic hormone (SIADH); hyperglycemia; and increased water intake through the administration of electrolyte-poor parenteral fluids, the use of tap-water enemas, or the irrigation of nasogastric tubes with water instead of normal saline solution. Water may be gained abnormally by the excessive parenteral administration of dextrose and water solutions, particularly during periods of stress. It may also be gained by compulsive water drinking (psychogenic polydipsia).

The basic physiologic disturbances in SIADH are excessive ADH activity, with water retention and dilutional hy-

(text continues on page 318)

TABLE 14-5 Major Fluid and Electrolyte Imbalances

Imbalance	Contributing Factors	Signs/Symptoms and Laboratory Findings
Fluid volume deficit (hypovolemia)	Loss of water and electrolytes, as in vomiting, diarrhea, fistulas, fever, excess sweating, burns, blood loss, gastrointestinal suction, and third-space fluid shifts; and decreased intake, as in anorexia, nausea, and inability to gain access to fluid. Diabetes insipidus and uncontrolled diabetes mellitus also contribute to a depletion of extracellular fluid volume.	Acute weight loss, decreased skin turgor, oliguria, concentrated urine, weak rapid pulse, capillary filling time prolonged, low CVP, ↓ blood pressure, flattened neck veins, dizziness, weakness, thirst and confusion, ↑ pulse, muscle cramps, sunken eyes *Labs indicate:* ↑ hemoglobin and hematocrit, ↑ serum and urine osmolality and specific gravity, ↓ urine sodium, ↑ BUN and creatinine, ↑ urine specific gravity and osmolality
Fluid volume excess (hypervolemia)	Compromised regulatory mechanisms, such as renal failure, heart failure, and cirrhosis; overzealous administration of sodium-containing fluids; and fluid shifts (ie, treatment of burns). Prolonged corticosteroid therapy, severe stress, and hyperaldosteronism augment fluid volume excess.	Acute weight gain, peripheral edema and ascites, distended jugular veins, crackles, and elevated CVP, shortness of breath, ↑ blood pressure, bounding pulse and cough, ↑ respiratory rate *Labs indicate:* ↓ hemoglobin and hematocrit, ↓ serum and urine osmolality, ↓ urine sodium and specific gravity
Sodium deficit (hyponatremia) Serum sodium <135 mEq/L	Loss of sodium, as in use of diuretics, loss of GI fluids, renal disease, and adrenal insufficiency. Gain of water, as in excessive administration of D_5W and water supplements for patients receiving hypotonic tube feedings; disease states associated with SIADH such as head trauma and oat-cell lung tumor; medications associated with water retention (oxytocin and certain tranquilizers); and psychogenic polydipsia. Hyperglycemia and heart failure cause a loss of sodium.	Anorexia, nausea and vomiting, headache, lethargy, dizziness, confusion, muscle cramps and weakness, muscular twitching, seizures, papilledema, dry skin, ↑ pulse, ↓ BP, weight gain, edema *Labs indicate:* ↓ serum and urine sodium, ↓ urine specific gravity and osmolality
Sodium excess (hypernatremia) Serum sodium >145 mEq/L	Water deprivation in patients unable to drink at will, hypertonic tube feedings without adequate water supplements, diabetes insipidus, heatstroke, hyperventilation, watery diarrhea, burns, and diaphoresis. Excess corticosteroid, sodium bicarbonate, and sodium chloride administration, and salt water near-drowning victims.	Thirst, elevated body temperature, swollen dry tongue and sticky mucous membranes, hallucinations, lethargy, restlessness, irritability, focal or grand mal seizures, pulmonary edema, hyperreflexia, twitching, nausea, vomiting, anorexia, ↑ pulse, and ↑ BP. *Labs indicate.* ↑ serum sodium, ↓ urine sodium, ↑ urine specific gravity and osmolality, ↓ CVP
Potassium deficit (hypokalemia) Serum potassium <3.5 mEq/L	Diarrhea, vomiting, gastric suction, corticosteroid administration, hyperaldosteronism, carbenicillin, amphotericin B, bulimia, osmotic diuresis, alkalosis, starvation, diuretics, and digoxin toxicity	Fatigue, anorexia, nausea and vomiting, muscle weakness, polyuria, decreased bowel motility, ventricular asystole or fibrillation, paresthesias, leg cramps, ↓ BP, ileus, abdominal distention, hypoactive reflexes. *ECG:* flattened T waves, prominent U waves, ST depression, prolonged PR interval.
Potassium excess (hyperkalemia) Serum potassium >5.0 mEq/L	Pseudohyperkalemia, oliguric renal failure, use of potassium-conserving diuretics in patients with renal insufficiency, metabolic acidosis, Addison's disease, crush injury, burns, stored bank blood transfusions, and rapid IV administration of potassium	Vague muscular weakness, tachycardia → bradycardia, dysrhythmias, flaccid paralysis, paresthesias, intestinal colic, cramps, irritability, anxiety. *ECG:* tall tented T waves, prolonged PR interval and QRS duration, absent P waves, ST depression.
Calcium deficit (hypocalcemia) Serum calcium <8.5 mg/dL	Hypoparathyroidism (may follow thyroid surgery or radical neck dissection), malabsorption, pancreatitis, alkalosis, vitamin D deficiency, massive subcutaneous infection, generalized peritonitis, massive transfusion of citrated blood, chronic diarrhea, decreased parathyroid hormone, diuretic phase of renal failure, ↑ PO_4, fistulas, burns	Numbness, tingling of fingers, toes, and circumoral region; positive Trousseau's sign and Chvostek's sign; seizures, carpopedal spasms, hyperactive deep tendon reflexes, irritability, bronchospasm, anxiety, impaired clotting time, ↓ prothrombin. *ECG:* prolonged QT interval and lengthened ST. *Labs indicate.* ↓ Mg^{++}

TABLE 14-5 Major Fluid and Electrolyte Imbalances (Continued)

Imbalance	Contributing Factors	Signs/Symptoms and Laboratory Findings
Calcium excess (hypercalcemia) Serum calcium >10.5 mg/dL	Hyperparathyroidism, malignant neoplastic disease, prolonged immobilization, overuse of calcium supplements, vitamin D excess, oliguric phase of renal failure, acidosis, corticosteroid therapy, thiazide diuretic use, increased parathyroid hormone, and digoxin toxicity	Muscular weakness, constipation, anorexia, nausea and vomiting, polyuria and polydipsia, dehydration, hypoactive deep tendon reflexes, lethargy, deep bone pain, pathologic fractures, flank pain, and calcium stones. *ECG:* shortened ST segment and QT interval, bradycardia, heart blocks.
Magnesium deficit (hypomagnesemia) Serum magnesium <1.8 mg/dL	Chronic alcoholism, hyperparathyroidism, hyperaldosteronism, diuretic phase of renal failure, malabsorptive disorders, diabetic ketoacidosis, refeeding after starvation, parenteral nutrition, chronic laxative use, diarrhea, acute myocardial infarction, heart failure, decreased serum K^+ and Ca^{++} and certain pharmacologic agents (such as gentamicin, cisplatin, and cyclosporine)	Neuromuscular irritability, positive Trousseau's and Chvostek's signs, insomnia, mood changes, anorexia, vomiting, increased tendon reflexes, and ↑ BP. *ECG:* PVCs, flat or inverted T waves, depressed ST segment, prolonged PR interval and widened QRS
Magnesium excess (hypermagnesemia) Serum magnesium >2.7 mg/dL	Oliguric phase of renal failure (particularly when magnesium-containing medications are administered), adrenal insufficiency, excessive IV magnesium administration, DKA, and hypothyroidism	Flushing, hypotension, drowsiness, hypoactive reflexes, depressed respirations, cardiac arrest and coma, diaphoresis. *ECG:* tachycardia → bradycardia, prolonged PR interval and QRS.
Phosphorus deficit (hypophosphatemia) Serum phosphorus <2.5 mg/dL	Refeeding after starvation, alcohol withdrawal, diabetic ketoacidosis, respiratory alkalosis, ↓ magnesium, ↓ potassium, hyperparathyroidism, vomiting, diarrhea, hyperventilation, vitamin D deficiency associated with malabsorptive disorders, burns, acid–base disorders, parenteral nutrition, and diuretic and antacid use	Paresthesias, muscle weakness, bone pain and tenderness, chest pain, confusion, cardiomyopathy, respiratory failure, seizures, tissue hypoxia, and increased susceptibility to infection, nystagmus
Phosphorus excess (hyperphosphatemia) Serum phosphorus >4.5 mg/dL	Acute and chronic renal failure, excessive intake of phosphorus, vitamin D excess, respiratory acidosis, hypoparathyroidism, volume depletion, leukemia/lymphoma treated with cytotoxic agents, increased tissue breakdown, rhabdomyolysis	Tetany, tachycardia, anorexia, nausea and vomiting, muscle weakness, signs and symptoms of hypocalcemia; hyperactive reflexes; soft tissue calcifications in lungs, heart, kidneys, and cornea
Chloride deficit (hypochloremia) Serum chloride <96 mEq/L	Addison's disease, reduced chloride intake or absorption, untreated diabetic ketoacidosis, chronic respiratory acidosis, excessive sweating, vomiting, gastric suction, diarrhea, sodium and potassium deficiency, metabolic alkalosis; loop, osmotic, or thiazide diuretic use; overuse of bicarbonate, rapid removal of ascitic fluid with a high sodium content, intravenous fluids that lack chloride (dextrose and water), draining fistulas and ileostomies, heart failure, cystic fibrosis	Agitation, irritability, tremors, muscle cramps, hyperactive deep tendon reflexes, hypertonicity, tetany, slow shallow respirations, seizures, dysrhythmias, coma *Labs indicate:* ↓ serum chloride, ↓ serum sodium, ↑ pH, ↑ serum bicarbonate, ↑ total carbon dioxide content, ↓ urine chloride level, ↓ serum potassium
Chloride excess (hyperchloremia) Serum chloride >108 mEq/L	Excessive sodium chloride infusions with water loss, head injury (sodium retention), hypernatremia, renal failure, corticosteroid use, dehydration, severe diarrhea (loss of bicarbonate), respiratory alkalosis, administration of diuretics, overdose of salicylates, Kayexalate, acetazolamide, phenylbutazone and ammonium chloride use, hyperparathyroidism, metabolic acidosis	Tachypnea, lethargy, weakness, deep rapid respirations, decline in cognitive status, decreased cardiac output, dyspnea, tachycardia, pitting edema, dysrhythmias, coma *Labs indicate:* ↑ serum chloride, ↑ serum potassium and sodium, ↓ serum pH, ↓ serum bicarbonate, normal anion gap, ↑ urinary chloride level

↑ increased; ↓ decreased; BP, blood pressure; BUN, blood urea nitrogen; CVP, central venous pressure; DKA, diabetic ketoacidosis; GI, gastrointestinal; IV, intravenous; PVCs, premature ventricular contractions; SIADH, syndrome of inappropriate secretion of antidiuretic hormone.

ponatremia, and inappropriate urinary excretion of sodium in the presence of hyponatremia. SIADH can be the result of either sustained secretion of ADH by the hypothalamus or production of an ADH-like substance from a tumor (aberrant ADH production). Conditions associated with SIADH include oat-cell lung tumors; head injuries; endocrine and pulmonary disorders; physical or psychological stress; and the use of medications such as oxytocin, cyclophosphamide, vincristine, thioridazine, and amitriptyline. SIADH is discussed in more detail in Chapter 42.

Clinical Manifestations

Clinical manifestations of hyponatremia depend on the cause, magnitude, and speed with which the deficit occurs. Poor skin turgor, dry mucosa, headache, decreased saliva production, orthostatic fall in blood pressure, nausea, and abdominal cramping occur. Neurologic changes, including altered mental status, status epilepticus, coma, and obtundation, are probably related to the cellular swelling and cerebral edema associated with hyponatremia. As the extracellular sodium level decreases, the cellular fluid becomes relatively more concentrated and pulls water into the cells (Fig. 14-4). In general, patients with an acute decrease in serum sodium levels have more cerebral edema and higher mortality rates than do those with more slowly developing hyponatremia. Acute decreases in sodium, developing in less than 48 hours, may be associated with brain herniation and compression of midbrain structures. Chronic decreases in sodium, developing over 48 hours or more, can occur in status epilepticus and cerebral pontine myelinolysis.

Features of hyponatremia associated with sodium loss and water gain include anorexia, muscle cramps, and a feeling of exhaustion. The severity of symptoms increases with the degree of hyponatremia and the speed with which it develops. When the serum sodium level decreases to less than 115 mEq/L (115 mmol/L), signs of increasing intracranial pressure, such as lethargy, confusion, muscle twitching, focal weakness, hemiparesis, papilledema, and seizures, may occur.

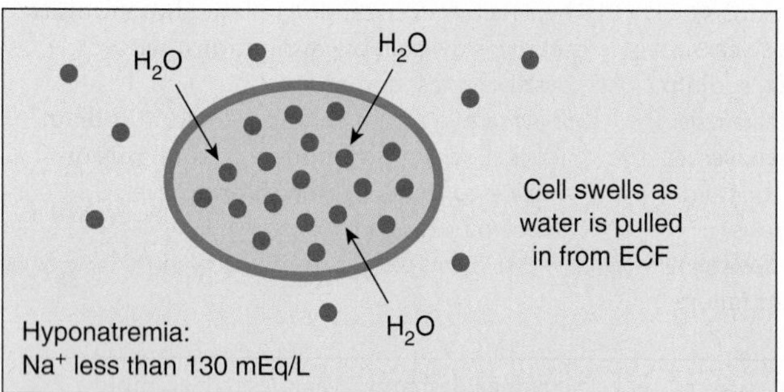

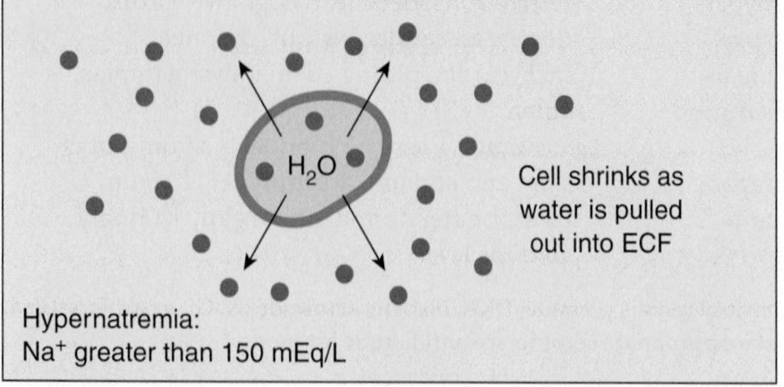

FIGURE 14-4. Effect of extracellular sodium level on cell size.

Assessment and Diagnostic Findings

Regardless of the cause of hyponatremia, the serum sodium level is less than 135 mEq/L; in SIADH it may be as low as 100 mEq/L (100 mmol/L) or even less. Serum osmolality is also decreased, except in azotemia or ingestion of toxins. When hyponatremia is due primarily to sodium loss, the urinary sodium content is less than 20 mEq/L (20 mmol/L), suggesting increased proximal reabsorption of sodium secondary to ECF volume depletion, and the specific gravity is low (1.002 to 1.004). However, when hyponatremia is due to SIADH, the urinary sodium content is greater than 20 mEq/L, and the urine specific gravity is usually greater than 1.012. Although the patient with SIADH retains water abnormally and therefore gains body weight, there is no peripheral edema; instead, fluid accumulates inside the cells. This phenomenon is sometimes manifested as "fingerprinting" when the finger is pressed over a bony prominence, such as the sternum.

Medical Management

The key to treating hyponatremia is assessment; this includes assessment of the speed with which hyponatremia occurred, as well as assessment of the patient's actual serum sodium value (Elgart, 2004).

SODIUM REPLACEMENT

The obvious treatment for hyponatremia is careful administration of sodium by mouth, nasogastric tube, or a parenteral route. For patients who can eat and drink, sodium is easily replaced, because sodium is consumed abundantly in a normal diet. For those who cannot consume sodium, lactated Ringer's solution or isotonic saline (0.9% sodium chloride) solution may be prescribed. Serum sodium must not be increased by more than 12 mEq/L in 24 hours, to avoid neurologic damage due to osmotic demyelination. This condition may occur when the serum sodium concentration is overcorrected (exceeding 140 mEq/L) too rapidly or in the presence of hypoxia or anoxia (Lin, Hsu & Chiu, 2003). It may produce lesions in the pons that cause paraparesis, dysarthria, dysphagia, and coma. The usual daily sodium requirement in adults is approximately 100 mEq, provided there are no abnormal losses. Selected water and electrolyte solutions are described in Table 14-4.

In SIADH, the administration of hypertonic saline solution alone cannot change the plasma sodium concentration. Excess sodium would be excreted rapidly in a highly concentrated urine. With the addition of the diuretic furosemide (Lasix), urine is not concentrated and isotonic urine is excreted to effect a change in water balance. In patients with SIADH, in whom water restriction is difficult, lithium or demeclocycline can antagonize the osmotic effect of ADH on the medullary collecting tubule.

WATER RESTRICTION

In a patient with normal or excess fluid volume, hyponatremia is treated by restricting fluid to a total of 800 mL in 24 hours. This is far safer than sodium administration and is usually effective. However, if neurologic symptoms are present, it may be necessary to administer small volumes of a hypertonic sodium solution, such as 3% or 5% sodium chloride. Incorrect use of these fluids is extremely dangerous, because 1 L of 3% sodium chloride solution contains 513 mEq of sodium and 1 L of 5% sodium chloride solution contains 855 mEq of sodium. If edema exists alone, sodium is restricted; if edema and hyponatremia occur together, both sodium and water are restricted.

NURSING ALERT

Highly hypertonic sodium solutions (3% and 5% sodium chloride) should be administered only in intensive care settings under close observation, because only small volumes are needed to elevate the serum sodium concentration from a dangerously low level. These fluids are administered slowly and in small volumes, and the patient is monitored closely for fluid overload. The purpose is to relieve acute manifestations of cerebral edema and to prevent neurologic complications rather than to specifically correct the sodium concentration. Along with the sodium solution, the patient may receive a loop diuretic to prevent ECF volume overload and to increase water excretion.

Nursing Management

The nurse needs to identify patients at risk of hyponatremia so that they can be monitored. Early detection and treatment of this disorder are necessary to prevent serious consequences. For patients at risk, the nurse monitors fluid I&O as well as daily body weight. It is also necessary to note abnormal losses of sodium or gains of water, as well as GI manifestations such as anorexia, nausea, vomiting, and abdominal cramping. The nurse must be particularly alert for central nervous system changes, such as lethargy, confusion, muscle twitching, and seizures. In general, more severe neurologic signs are associated with very low sodium levels that have fallen rapidly because of fluid overloading. Serum sodium is monitored very closely in patients who are at risk for hyponatremia; when indicated, urine sodium and specific gravity are also monitored.

Hyponatremia is a frequently overlooked cause of confusion in elderly patients, who have an increased risk for hyponatremia because of changes in renal function and subsequent decreased ability to excrete excessive water loads. Administration of medications causing sodium loss or water retention is a predisposing factor.

DETECTING AND CONTROLLING HYPONATREMIA

For a patient who is experiencing abnormal losses of sodium and can consume a general diet, the nurse encourages foods and fluids with a high sodium content. For example, broth made with one beef cube contains approximately 900 mg of sodium; 8 oz of tomato juice contains approximately 700 mg of sodium. The nurse also needs to be familiar with the sodium content of parenteral fluids (see Table 14-4).

NURSING ALERT

When administering fluids to patients with cardiovascular disease, the nurse assesses for signs of circulatory overload (eg, cough, dyspnea, puffy eyelids, dependent edema, weight gain in 24 hours). The lungs are auscultated for crackles. Extreme care is taken when administering highly hypertonic sodium fluids (eg, 3% or 5% sodium chloride), because these fluids can be lethal if infused carelessly.

For the patient taking lithium, the nurse observes for lithium toxicity, particularly when sodium is lost by an abnormal route. In such instances, supplemental salt and fluid are administered. Because diuretics promote sodium loss, the patient taking lithium is instructed not to use diuretics without close medical supervision. For all patients on lithium therapy, adequate salt intake should be ensured.

Excess water supplements are avoided in patients receiving isotonic or hypotonic enteral feedings, particularly if abnormal sodium loss occurs or water is being abnormally retained (as in SIADH). Actual fluid needs are determined by evaluating fluid I&O, urine specific gravity, and serum sodium levels.

RETURNING THE SODIUM LEVEL TO NORMAL

If the primary problem is water retention, it is safer to restrict fluid intake than to administer sodium. Administering sodium to a patient with normovolemia or hypervolemia predisposes the patient to fluid volume overload. As stated previously, the nurse must monitor the patient with cardiovascular disease very closely.

In severe hyponatremia, the aim of therapy is to elevate the serum sodium level only enough to alleviate neurologic signs and symptoms. It is generally recommended that the serum sodium concentration be increased to no greater than 125 mEq/L (125 mmol/L) with a hypertonic saline solution.

Sodium Excess (Hypernatremia)

Hypernatremia is a higher-than-normal serum sodium level (exceeding 145 mEq/L [145 mmol/L]) (Kee, Paulanka & Purnell, 2004). It can be caused by a gain of sodium in excess of water or by a loss of water in excess of sodium. It can occur in patients with normal fluid volume or in those with FVD or FVE. With a water loss, the patient loses more water than sodium; as a result, the serum sodium concentration increases and the increased concentration pulls fluid out of the cell. This is both an extracellular and an intracellular FVD. In sodium excess, the patient ingests or retains more sodium than water.

A common cause of hypernatremia is fluid deprivation in unconscious patients who cannot perceive, respond to, or communicate their thirst (Porth, 2005). Most often affected are very old, very young, and cognitively impaired patients. Administration of hypertonic enteral feedings without adequate water supplements leads to hypernatremia, as does watery diarrhea and greatly increased insensible water loss (eg, hyperventilation, denuding effects of burns).

Diabetes insipidus, a deficiency of ADH from the posterior pituitary gland, leads to hypernatremia if the patient does not experience, or cannot respond to, thirst, or if fluids are excessively restricted. Neurogenic or nephrogenic causes of diabetes insipidus should be considered in the assessment (Olson, Meek & Lynch, 2004).

Less common causes of hypernatremia are heat stroke, near-drowning in sea water (which contains a sodium concentration of approximately 500 mEq/L), and malfunction of either hemodialysis or peritoneal dialysis proportioning systems. IV administration of hypertonic saline or excessive use of sodium bicarbonate also causes hypernatremia (Porth, 2005).

Clinical Manifestations

The clinical manifestations of hypernatremia are primarily neurologic and are the consequence of increased plasma osmolality caused by an increase in plasma sodium concentration. Water moves out of the cell into the ECF, resulting in cellular dehydration (Rose & Post, 2000). Hypernatremia leads to a relatively concentrated ECF (see Fig. 14-4). Clinically, these changes may be manifested by restlessness and weakness in moderate hypernatremia and by disorientation, delusions, and hallucinations in severe hypernatremia. Dehydration (resulting in hypernatremia) is often overlooked as the primary reason for behavioral changes in elderly patients. If hypernatremia is severe, permanent brain damage can occur (especially in children). Brain damage is apparently due to subarachnoid hemorrhages that result from brain contraction.

A primary characteristic of hypernatremia is thirst. Thirst is such a strong *defender* of serum sodium levels in healthy people that hypernatremia never occurs unless the person is unconscious or does not have access to water. However, ill people may have an impaired thirst mechanism. Other signs include a dry, swollen tongue and sticky mucous membranes. Flushed skin, peripheral and pulmonary edema, postural hypotension, and increased muscle tone and deep tendon reflexes are additional signs and symptoms of hypernatremia. Body temperature may increase mildly, but it returns to normal after the hypernatremia is corrected.

Assessment and Diagnostic Findings

In hypernatremia, the serum sodium level exceeds 145 mEq/L (145 mmol/L) and the serum osmolality exceeds 300 mOsm/kg (300 mmol/L). The urine specific gravity and urine osmolality are increased as the kidneys attempt to conserve water (provided the water loss is from a route other than the kidneys) (Rose & Post, 2000).

Medical Management

Treatment of hypernatremia consists of a gradual lowering of the serum sodium level by the infusion of a hypotonic electrolyte solution (eg, 0.3% sodium chloride) or an isotonic nonsaline solution (eg, dextrose 5% in water [D_5W]). D_5W is indicated when water needs to be replaced without sodium. Many clinicians consider a hypotonic sodium solution to be safer than D_5W because it allows a gradual reduction in the serum sodium level, thereby decreasing the risk of cerebral edema. It is the solution of choice in severe hyperglycemia with hypernatremia. A rapid reduction in the serum sodium level temporarily decreases the plasma osmolality below that of the fluid in the brain tissue, causing dangerous cerebral edema. Diuretics also may be prescribed to treat the sodium gain.

There is no consensus about the exact rate at which serum sodium levels should be reduced. As a general rule, the serum sodium level is reduced at a rate no faster than 0.5 to 1 mEq/L per hour to allow sufficient time for readjustment through diffusion across fluid compartments. Desmopressin acetate (DDAVP), a synthetic antidiuretic hormone, may be prescribed to treat diabetes insipidus if it is the cause of hypernatremia (Porth, 2005).

Nursing Management

As in hyponatremia, fluid losses and gains are carefully monitored in patients who are at risk for hypernatremia. The nurse should assess for abnormal losses of water or low water intake and for large gains of sodium, as might occur with ingestion of over-the-counter medications that have a high sodium content (eg, Alka-Seltzer). In addition, the nurse obtains a medication history, because some prescription medications have a high sodium content. The nurse also notes the patient's thirst or elevated body temperature and evaluates it in relation to other clinical signs. The nurse monitors for changes in behavior, such as restlessness, disorientation, and lethargy.

PREVENTING HYPERNATREMIA

The nurse attempts to prevent hypernatremia by offering fluids at regular intervals, particularly in debilitated or unconscious patients who are unable to perceive or respond to thirst. If fluid intake remains inadequate, the nurse consults with the physician to plan an alternative route for intake, either by enteral feedings or by the parenteral route. If enteral feedings are used, sufficient water should be administered to keep the serum sodium and BUN within normal limits. As a rule, the higher the osmolality of the enteral feeding, the greater the need for water supplementation.

For patients with diabetes insipidus, adequate water intake must be ensured. If the patient is alert and has an intact thirst mechanism, merely providing access to water may be sufficient. If the patient has a decreased level of consciousness or other disability interfering with adequate fluid intake, parenteral fluid replacement may be prescribed. This therapy can be anticipated in patients with neurologic disorders, particularly in the early postoperative period.

CORRECTING HYPERNATREMIA

When parenteral fluids are necessary for managing hypernatremia, the nurse monitors the patient's response to the fluids by reviewing serial serum sodium levels and by observing for changes in neurologic signs. With a gradual decrease in the serum sodium level, the neurologic signs should improve. As stated in the discussion on management, too-rapid reduction in the serum sodium level renders the plasma temporarily hypo-osmotic to the fluid in the brain tissue, causing movement of fluid into brain cells and dangerous cerebral edema (Hankins, Lonsway-Waldman, Hedrick, et al., 2001).

Potassium Imbalances

Potassium is the major intracellular electrolyte; in fact, 98% of the body's potassium is inside the cells. The remaining 2% is in the ECF, and it is this 2% that is important in neuromuscular function. Potassium influences both skeletal and cardiac muscle activity. For example, alterations in its concentration change myocardial irritability and rhythm. Under the influence of the sodium–potassium pump and based on the body's needs, potassium is constantly moving in and out of cells. The normal serum potassium concentration ranges from 3.5 to 5.0 mEq/L (3.5 to 5 mmol/L), and even minor variations are significant. Potassium imbalances are commonly associated with various diseases, injuries, medications (diuretics, laxatives, antibiotics), and special treatments, such as parenteral nutrition and chemotherapy (Hogan & Wane, 2003).

To maintain potassium balance, the renal system must function, because 80% of the potassium excreted daily leaves the body by way of the kidneys; the other 20% is lost through the bowel and in sweat. The kidneys are the primary regulators of potassium balance; they accomplish this by adjusting the amount of potassium that is excreted in the urine. As serum potassium levels increase, so does the potassium level in the renal tubular cell. A concentration gradient occurs, favoring the movement of potassium into the renal tubule, with subsequent loss of potassium in the urine. Aldosterone also increases the excretion of potassium by the kidney. Because the kidneys do not conserve potassium as well as they conserve sodium, potassium may still be lost in urine in the presence of a potassium deficit.

Potassium Deficit (Hypokalemia)

Hypokalemia (below-normal serum potassium concentration) usually indicates an actual deficit in total potassium stores. However, it may occur in patients with normal potassium stores: when alkalosis is present, a temporary shift of serum potassium into the cells occurs (see later discussion).

As previously stated, hypokalemia is a common imbalance, especially with the use of diuretics. GI loss of potassium is probably the most common cause of potassium depletion (Burger, 2004b). Vomiting and gastric suction frequently lead to hypokalemia, partly because potassium is actually lost when gastric fluid is lost, but more so because potassium is lost through the kidneys in association with metabolic alkalosis. Because relatively large amounts of potassium are contained in intestinal fluids, potassium deficit occurs frequently with diarrhea. Intestinal fluid may contain as much potassium as 30 mEq/L. Potassium deficit also occurs from prolonged intestinal suctioning, recent ileostomy, and villous adenoma (a tumor of the intestinal tract characterized by excretion of potassium-rich mucus).

Alterations in acid–base balance have a significant effect on potassium distribution. The mechanism involves shifts of hydrogen and potassium ions between the cells and the ECF. Hypokalemia can cause alkalosis, and in turn alkalosis can cause hypokalemia (Burger, 2004b). For example, hydrogen ions move out of the cells in alkalotic states to help correct the high pH, and potassium ions move in to maintain an electrically neutral state (see later discussion of acid–base balance).

Hyperaldosteronism increases renal potassium wasting and can lead to severe potassium depletion. Primary hyperaldosteronism is seen in patients with adrenal adenomas. Secondary hyperaldosteronism occurs in patients with cirrhosis, nephrotic syndrome, heart failure, or malignant hypertension (Heitz & Horne, 2005).

Potassium-losing diuretics, such as the thiazides (eg, chlorothiazide [Diuril] and polythiazide [Renese]), can induce hypokalemia, particularly when administered in large doses to patients with inadequate potassium intake (Burger, 2004b). Other medications that can lead to hypokalemia include corticosteroids, sodium penicillin, carbenicillin, and amphotericin B.

Because insulin promotes the entry of potassium into skeletal muscle and hepatic cells, patients with persistent insulin hypersecretion may experience hypokalemia, which is often the case in patients receiving high-carbohydrate parenteral fluids (as in parenteral nutrition).

Patients who are unable or unwilling to eat a normal diet for a prolonged period are at risk for hypokalemia. This may occur in debilitated elderly people, patients with alcoholism, and patients with anorexia nervosa. In addition to poor intake, people with bulimia frequently suffer increased potassium loss through self-induced vomiting and laxative and diuretic abuse (Burger, 2004b).

Magnesium depletion causes renal potassium loss and must be corrected first; otherwise, urine loss of potassium will continue. Penicillins may produce renal potassium loss by acting as poorly reabsorbable anions and thereby increasing distal sodium delivery and sodium–potassium loss.

Clinical Manifestations

Potassium deficiency can result in widespread derangements in physiologic function. Severe hypokalemia can cause death through cardiac or respiratory arrest. Clinical signs rarely develop before the serum potassium level has decreased to less than 3 mEq/L (3 mmol/L) unless the rate of decline has been rapid. Manifestations of hypokalemia include fatigue, anorexia, nausea, vomiting, muscle weakness, leg cramps, decreased bowel motility, paresthesias (numbness and tingling), dysrhythmias, and increased sensitivity to digitalis. If prolonged, hypokalemia can lead to an inability of the kidneys to concentrate urine, causing dilute urine (resulting in polyuria, nocturia) and excessive thirst. Potassium depletion depresses the release of insulin and results in glucose intolerance. Decreased muscle strength and tendon reflexes can be found on physical assessment.

Assessment and Diagnostic Findings

In hypokalemia, the serum potassium concentration is less than the lower limit of normal. Electrocardiographic (ECG) changes can include flat T waves or inverted T waves or both, suggesting ischemia, and depressed ST segments (Fig. 14-5). An elevated U wave is specific to hypokalemia. Hypokalemia increases sensitivity to digitalis, predisposing the patient to digitalis toxicity at lower digitalis levels.

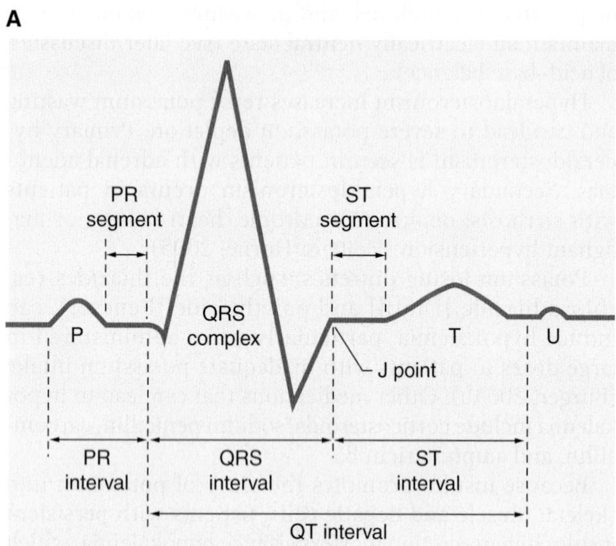

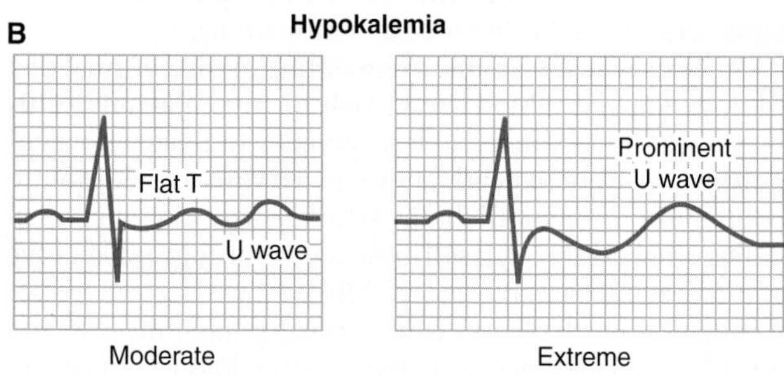

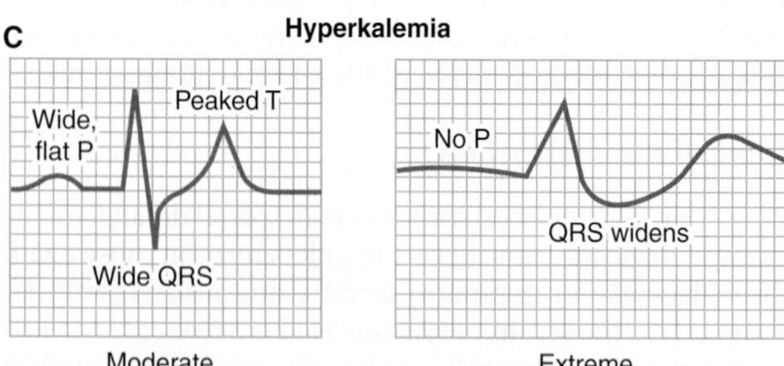

FIGURE 14-5. Effect of potassium on the electrocardiogram (ECG). **(A)** Normal tracing. **(B)** Hypokalemia: serum potassium level below normal. *Left,* flattening of the T wave and the appearance of a U wave. *Right,* further flattening with prominent U wave. **(C)** Hyperkalemia: serum potassium level above normal. *Left,* moderate elevation with wide, flat P wave, wide QRS complex, and peaked T wave. *Right,* ECG changes seen with extreme potassium elevation: widening of QRS complex and absence of P wave.

Metabolic alkalosis is commonly associated with hypokalemia (Burger, 2004b). This is discussed further in the section on acid–base disturbances.

The source of the potassium loss is usually evident from a careful history. However, if the cause of the loss is unclear, a 24-hour urinary potassium excretion test can be performed to distinguish between renal and extrarenal loss. Urinary potassium excretion exceeding 20 mEq/24 h with hypokalemia suggests that renal potassium loss is the cause.

Medical Management

If hypokalemia cannot be prevented by conventional measures such as increased intake in the daily diet, it is treated with oral or IV replacement therapy (Kee et al., 2004). Potassium loss must be corrected daily; administration of 40 to 80 mEq/day of potassium is adequate in the adult if there are no abnormal losses of potassium.

For patients who are at risk for hypokalemia, a diet containing sufficient potassium should be provided. Dietary intake of potassium in the average adult is 50 to 100 mEq/day. Foods high in potassium include most fruits and vegetables, legumes, whole grains, milk, and meat.

If dietary intake is inadequate for any reason, the physician may prescribe oral or IV potassium supplements (Kee et al., 2004). Many salt substitutes contain 50 to 60 mEq of potassium per teaspoon and may be sufficient to prevent hypokalemia.

> **NURSING ALERT**
>
> **Oral potassium supplements can produce small-bowel lesions; therefore, the patient must be assessed for and cautioned about abdominal distention, pain, or GI bleeding.**

If oral administration of potassium is not feasible, the IV route is indicated. The IV route is mandatory for patients with severe hypokalemia (eg, serum level of 2 mEq/L). Although potassium chloride is usually used to correct potassium deficits, potassium acetate or potassium phosphate may be prescribed.

Nursing Management

Because hypokalemia can be life-threatening, the nurse needs to monitor for its early presence in patients who are at risk. Fatigue, anorexia, muscle weakness, decreased bowel motility, paresthesias, and dysrhythmias are signals that warrant assessing the serum potassium concentration. When available, the ECG may provide useful information. For example, patients receiving digitalis who are at risk for potassium deficiency should be monitored closely for signs of digitalis toxicity, because hypokalemia potentiates the action of digitalis. Most physicians prefer to keep the serum potassium level greater than 3.5 mEq/L (3.5 mmol/L) in patients receiving digitalis medications such as digoxin.

PREVENTING HYPOKALEMIA

Measures are taken to prevent hypokalemia when possible (Kee et al., 2004). Prevention may involve encouraging the patient at risk to eat foods rich in potassium (when the diet allows). Sources of potassium include fruit and fruit juices (bananas, melon, citrus fruit), fresh and frozen vegetables, fresh meats, milk, and processed foods. If the hypokalemia is caused by abuse of laxatives or diuretics, patient education may help alleviate the problem. Part of the health history and assessment should be directed at identifying problems that are amenable to prevention through education. Careful monitoring of fluid intake and output is necessary, because 40 mEq of potassium is lost for every liter of urine output. The ECG is monitored for changes, and arterial blood gas values are checked for elevated bicarbonate and pH levels.

CORRECTING HYPOKALEMIA

Great care should be exercised when administering potassium, particularly in older adults, who have lower lean body mass and total body potassium levels and therefore lower potassium requirements. In addition, because of the physiologic loss of renal function with advancing years, potassium may be retained more readily in older than in younger people.

ADMINISTERING INTRAVENOUS POTASSIUM

Potassium should be administered only after adequate urine flow has been established. A decrease in urine volume to less than 20 mL/h for 2 consecutive hours is an indication to stop the potassium infusion until the situation is evaluated. Potassium is primarily excreted by the kidneys; therefore, when oliguria occurs, potassium administration can cause the serum potassium concentration to rise dangerously (Burger, 2004b).

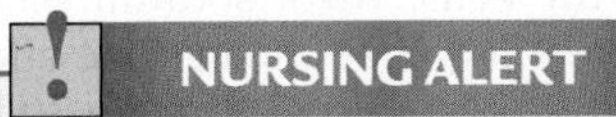

NURSING ALERT

Potassium is *never* administered by IV push or intramuscularly to avoid replacing potassium too quickly. IV potassium must be administered using an infusion pump.

Each health care facility has its own standard of care for the administration of potassium, which should be consulted; however, the maximum concentration of potassium that should be administered on a medical-surgical unit through a peripheral IV line is 20 mEq/100 mL and the rate no faster than 10 to 20 mEq/h. Concentrations of potassium greater than 20 mEq/100 mL should be administered through a central IV catheter using an infusion pump with the patient monitored by ECG. Caution must be used when selecting the correct premixed solution of IV fluid containing potassium chloride as the concentrations range from 10 to 40 mEq/100 mL. IV bags of 1000 mL of fluid containing potassium are also available with 20 to 40 mEq/L. Renal function should be monitored through BUN and creatinine levels and urine output if the patient is receiving potassium replacement (Morton, Fontaine, Hudak et al., 2005).

Potassium Excess (Hyperkalemia)

Hyperkalemia (greater-than-normal serum potassium concentration) seldom occurs in patients with normal renal function. Like hypokalemia, hyperkalemia is often caused by iatrogenic (treatment-induced) causes. Although hyperkalemia is less common than hypokalemia, it is usually more dangerous, because cardiac arrest is more frequently associated with high serum potassium levels.

Pseudohyperkalemia (a variation of hyperkalemia) has a number of causes. The most common causes are the use of a tight tourniquet around an exercising extremity while drawing a blood sample and hemolysis of the sample before analysis. Other causes include marked leukocytosis (white blood cell count exceeding 200,000) or thrombocytosis (platelet count exceeding 1 million); drawing blood above a site where potassium is infusing; and familial pseudohyperkalemia; in which potassium leaks out of the red blood cells while the blood is awaiting analysis. Failure to be aware of these causes of pseudohyperkalemia can lead to aggressive treatment of a nonexistent hyperkalemia, resulting in serious lowering of serum potassium levels. Therefore, measurements of grossly elevated levels should be verified by retesting.

The major cause of hyperkalemia is decreased renal excretion of potassium (Burger, 2004a). For this reason, significant hyperkalemia is commonly seen in patients with untreated renal failure, particularly those in whom potassium levels increase as a result of infection or excessive intake of potassium in food or medications. In addition, patients with hypoaldosteronism or Addison's disease are at risk for hyperkalemia, because these conditions are characterized by deficient adrenal hormones, leading to sodium loss and potassium retention.

Medications have been identified as a probable contributing factor in more than 60% of hyperkalemic episodes. Medications commonly implicated are potassium chloride, heparin, ACE inhibitors, captopril, NSAIDs, and potassium-sparing diuretics (Palmer, 2004). In most such cases, potassium regulation is compromised by renal insufficiency (Burger, 2004a).

Although a high intake of potassium can cause severe hyperkalemia in patients with impaired renal function, hyperkalemia rarely occurs in people with normal renal function. However, improper use of potassium supplements predisposes all patients to hyperkalemia, especially if salt substitutes are used. Not all patients receiving potassium-losing diuretics require potassium supplements, and patients receiving potassium-conserving diuretics should not receive supplements.

NURSING ALERT

Potassium supplements are extremely dangerous for patients who have impaired renal function and thus decreased ability to excrete potassium. Even more dangerous is the IV administration of potassium to such patients, because serum levels can rise very quickly. Aged (stored) blood should not be administered to patients with impaired renal function, because the serum potassium concentration of stored blood increases as the storage time increases, a result of red blood cell deterioration. It is possible to exceed the renal tolerance of any patient with rapid IV potassium administration, as well as when large amounts of oral potassium supplements are ingested.

In **acidosis**, potassium moves out of the cells and into the ECF. This occurs as hydrogen ions enter the cells, a process that buffers the pH of the ECF (see later discussion). An elevated ECF potassium level should be anticipated when extensive tissue trauma has occurred, as in burns, crushing injuries, or severe infections. Similarly, it can occur with lysis of malignant cells after chemotherapy.

Clinical Manifestations

The most important consequence of hyperkalemia is its effect on the myocardium. Cardiac effects of elevated serum potassium are usually not significant when the level is less than 7 mEq/L (7 mmol/L), but they are almost always present when the level is 8 mEq/L (8 mmol/L) or greater. As the plasma potassium level rises, disturbances in cardiac conduction occur. The earliest changes, often occurring at a serum potassium level greater than 6 mEq/L (6 mmol/L), are peaked, narrow T waves; ST-segment depression; and a shortened QT interval. If the serum potassium level continues to increase, the PR interval becomes prolonged and is followed by disappearance of the P waves. Finally, there is decomposition and prolongation of the QRS complex (see Fig. 14-5). Ventricular dysrhythmias and cardiac arrest may occur at any point in this progression.

Severe hyperkalemia causes skeletal muscle weakness and even paralysis, related to a depolarization block in muscle. Similarly, ventricular conduction is slowed. Although hyperkalemia has marked effects on the peripheral nervous system, it has little effect on the central nervous system. Rapidly ascending muscular weakness leading to flaccid quadriplegia has been reported in patients with very high serum potassium levels. Paralysis of respiratory and speech muscles can also occur. In addition, GI manifestations, such as nausea, intermittent intestinal colic, and diarrhea, may occur in hyperkalemic patients.

Assessment and Diagnostic Findings

Serum potassium levels and ECG changes are crucial to the diagnosis of hyperkalemia, as discussed previously. Arterial blood gas analysis may reveal metabolic acidosis; in many cases, hyperkalemia occurs with acidosis (Burger, 2004a).

Medical Management

An immediate ECG should be obtained to detect changes. Shortened repolarization and peaked T waves are seen initially. To verify results, it is also prudent to obtain a repeat serum potassium level from a vein without an IV infusing a potassium-containing solution.

In nonacute situations, restriction of dietary potassium and potassium-containing medications may suffice. For example, eliminating the use of potassium-containing salt substitutes in a patient who is taking a potassium-conserving diuretic may be all that is needed to deal with mild hyperkalemia.

Prevention of serious hyperkalemia by the administration, either orally or by retention enema, of cation exchange resins (eg, Kayexalate) may be necessary in patients with renal impairment. Cation exchange resins cannot be used if the patient has a paralytic ileus, because intestinal perforation can occur. Kayexalate can bind with other cations in the GI tract and contribute to the development of hypomagnesemia and hypocalcemia; it may also cause sodium retention and fluid overload (Rose & Post, 2000).

EMERGENCY PHARMACOLOGIC THERAPY

If serum potassium levels are dangerously elevated, it may be necessary to administer IV calcium gluconate. Within minutes after administration, calcium antagonizes the action of hyperkalemia on the heart. Infusion of calcium does not reduce the serum potassium concentration, but it immediately antagonizes the adverse cardiac conduction abnormalities. Calcium chloride and calcium gluconate are not interchangeable: calcium gluconate contains 4.5 mEq of calcium and calcium chloride contains 13.6 mEq of calcium; therefore, caution must be used.

Monitoring the blood pressure is essential to detect hypotension, which may result from the rapid IV administration of calcium gluconate. The ECG should be continuously monitored during administration; the appearance of bradycardia is an indication to stop the infusion. The myocardial protective effects of calcium are transient, lasting about 30 minutes. Extra caution is required if the patient has been "digitalized" (ie, has received accelerated dosages of a digitalis-based cardiac glycoside to reach a desired serum digitalis level rapidly), because parenteral administration of calcium sensitizes the heart to digitalis and may precipitate digitalis toxicity.

IV administration of sodium bicarbonate may be necessary to alkalinize the plasma and cause a temporary shift of potassium into the cells. Also, sodium bicarbonate furnishes sodium to antagonize the cardiac effects of potassium. Effects of this therapy begin within 30 to 60 minutes and may persist for hours; however, they are temporary.

IV administration of regular insulin and a hypertonic dextrose solution causes a temporary shift of potassium into the cells. Glucose and insulin therapy has an onset of action within 30 minutes and lasts for several hours. Loop diuretics, such as furosemide (Lasix), increase excretion of water by inhibiting sodium, potassium, and chloride reabsorption in the ascending loop of Henle and distal renal tubule.

Beta-2 agonists, such as albuterol (Proventil, Ventolin), are highly effective in decreasing potassium but remain controversial, because they can cause tachycardia and chest discomfort (Porth, 2005). Beta-2 agonists also move potassium into the cells and may be used in the absence of ischemic cardiac disease. Administration of these medications is a stopgap measure that only temporarily protects the patient from hyperkalemia. If the hyperkalemic condition is not transient, actual removal of potassium from the body is required; this may be accomplished by using cation exchange resins, peritoneal dialysis, hemodialysis, or other forms of renal replacement therapy.

Nursing Management

Patients at risk for potassium excess (eg, those with renal failure) should be identified so they can be monitored closely for signs of hyperkalemia. The nurse observes for signs of muscle weakness and dysrhythmias. The presence of paresthesias and GI symptoms such as nausea and intestinal colic are noted. For patients at risk, serum potassium levels are measured periodically (Burger, 2004a).

Because measurements of elevated serum potassium levels may be erroneous, highly abnormal levels should always be verified by repeating the test. To avoid false reports of hyperkalemia, prolonged use of a tourniquet while drawing the blood sample is avoided, and the patient is cautioned not to exercise the extremity immediately before the blood sample is obtained. The blood sample is delivered to the laboratory as soon as possible, because hemolysis of the sample results in a falsely elevated serum potassium level.

PREVENTING HYPERKALEMIA

Measures are taken to prevent hyperkalemia in patients at risk, when possible, by encouraging the patient to adhere to the prescribed potassium restriction. Potassium-rich foods to be avoided include many fruits and vegetables, legumes, whole-grain breads, meat, milk, eggs, coffee, tea, and cocoa (Dudek, 2006). Conversely, foods with minimal potassium content include butter, margarine, cranberry juice or sauce, ginger ale, gumdrops or jellybeans, hard candy, root beer, sugar, and honey.

CORRECTING HYPERKALEMIA

As previously stated, it is possible to exceed the tolerance for potassium in any person if it is administered rapidly by the IV route. Therefore, great care should be taken to administer and monitor potassium solutions closely, paying close attention to the solution's concentration and rate of administration. When potassium is added to parenteral solutions, the potassium is mixed with the fluid by inverting the bottle several times. Potassium chloride should never be added to a hanging bottle, because the potassium might be administered as a bolus (potassium chloride is heavy and settles to the bottom of the container).

It is important to caution patients to use salt substitutes sparingly if they are taking other supplementary forms of potassium or potassium-conserving diuretics. Also, potassium-conserving diuretics, such as spironolactone (Aldactone), triamterene (Dyrenium), and amiloride (Midamor); potassium supplements; and salt substitutes should not be administered to patients with renal dysfunction. Most salt substitutes contain approximately 50 to 60 mEq of potassium per teaspoon.

Calcium Imbalances

More than 99% of the body's calcium is located in the skeletal system; calcium is a major component of bones and teeth. About 1% of skeletal calcium is rapidly exchangeable with blood calcium, and the rest is more stable and only slowly exchanged. The small amount of calcium located outside the bone circulates in the serum, partly bound to protein and partly ionized. Calcium plays a major role in transmitting nerve impulses and helps regulate muscle contraction and relaxation, including cardiac muscle. Calcium is instrumental in activating enzymes that stimulate many essential chemical reactions in the body, and it also plays a role in blood coagulation. Because many factors affect calcium regulation, both hypocalcemia and hypercalcemia are relatively common disturbances.

The normal total serum calcium level is 8.6 to 10.2 mg/dL (2.2 to 2.6 mmol/L). Calcium exists in plasma in three forms: ionized, bound, and complexed. About 50% of the serum calcium exists in a physiologically active ionized form that is important for neuromuscular activity and blood coagulation; this is the only physiologically and clinically significant form. The normal ionized serum calcium level is 4.5 to 5.1 mg/dL (1.1 to 1.3 mmol/L). Less than half of the plasma calcium is bound to serum proteins, primarily albumin. The remainder is combined with nonprotein anions: phosphate, citrate, and carbonate.

Calcium is absorbed from foods in the presence of normal gastric acidity and vitamin D. Calcium is excreted primarily in the feces, with the remainder excreted in the urine. The serum calcium level is controlled by PTH and calcitonin. As ionized serum calcium decreases, the parathyroid glands secrete PTH. This, in turn, increases calcium absorption from the GI tract, increases calcium reabsorption from the renal tubule, and releases calcium from the bone. The increase in calcium ion concentration suppresses PTH secretion. When calcium increases excessively, the thyroid gland secretes calcitonin. It briefly inhibits calcium reabsorption from bone and decreases the serum calcium concentration.

Calcium Deficit (Hypocalcemia)

Hypocalcemia (lower-than-normal serum concentration of calcium) occurs in a variety of clinical situations. A patient may have a total body calcium deficit (as in osteoporosis) but a normal serum calcium level. Elderly people with osteoporosis who spend an increased amount of time in bed have an increased risk for hypocalcemia, because bed rest increases bone resorption.

Several factors can cause hypocalcemia, including primary hypoparathyroidism and surgical hypoparathyroidism. The latter is far more common. Not only is hypocalcemia associated with thyroid and parathyroid surgery, but it can also occur after radical neck dissection and is most likely in the first 24 to 48 hours after surgery. Transient hypocalcemia can occur with massive administration of citrated blood (as in exchange transfusions in newborns or for adults who experience massive hemorrhage and shock), because citrate can combine with ionized calcium and temporarily remove it from the circulation.

Inflammation of the pancreas causes the breakdown of proteins and lipids. It is thought that calcium ions combine with the fatty acids released by lipolysis, forming soaps. As a result of this process, hypocalcemia occurs and is common in pancreatitis. It has also been suggested that hypocalcemia might be related to excessive secretion of glucagon from the inflamed pancreas, which results in increased secretion of calcitonin (a hormone that lowers serum calcium).

Hypocalcemia is common in patients with renal failure, because these patients frequently have elevated serum phosphate levels. Hyperphosphatemia usually causes a reciprocal drop in the serum calcium level. Other causes of hypocalcemia include inadequate vitamin D consumption, magnesium deficiency, medullary thyroid carcinoma, low serum albumin levels, alkalosis, and alcohol abuse. Medications predisposing to hypocalcemia include aluminum-containing antacids, aminoglycosides, caffeine, cisplatin, corticosteroids, mithramycin, phosphates, isoniazid, and loop diuretics.

Clinical Manifestations

Tetany is the most characteristic manifestation of hypocalcemia and hypomagnesemia. Tetany refers to the entire symptom complex induced by increased neural excitability. These symptoms are caused by spontaneous discharges of both sensory and motor fibers in peripheral nerves. Sensations of tingling may occur in the tips of the fingers, around the mouth, and, less commonly, in the feet. Spasms of the muscles of the extremities and face may occur. Pain may develop as a result of these spasms. These clinical signs indicate tetany and hyperactive deep tendon reflexes.

Trousseau's sign (Fig. 14-6) can be elicited by inflating a blood pressure cuff on the upper arm to about 20 mm Hg above systolic pressure; within 2 to 5 minutes, carpal spasm (an adducted thumb, flexed wrist and metacarpophalangeal joints, extended interphalangeal joints with fingers together) will occur as ischemia of the ulnar nerve develops. Chvostek's sign consists of twitching of muscles supplied by the facial nerve when the nerve is tapped about 2 cm anterior to the earlobe, just below the zygomatic arch.

Seizures may occur because hypocalcemia increases irritability of the central nervous system as well as of the peripheral nerves. Other changes associated with hypocalcemia include mental changes such as depression, impaired memory, confusion, delirium, and even hallucinations. A prolonged QT interval is seen on the ECG due to prolongation of the ST segment, and a form of ventricular tachycardia called torsades de pointes may occur. Respiratory effects with decreasing calcium include dyspnea and laryngospasm. Signs and symptoms of chronic hypocalcemia include hyperactive bowel sounds, dry and brittle hair and nails, and abnormal clotting.

Osteoporosis is associated with prolonged low intake of calcium and represents a total body calcium deficit, even though serum calcium levels are usually normal. This disorder occurs in millions of Americans and is most common in postmenopausal women. It is characterized by loss of bone mass, which causes bones to become porous and brittle and therefore susceptible to fracture. See Chapter 68 for further discussion of osteoporosis.

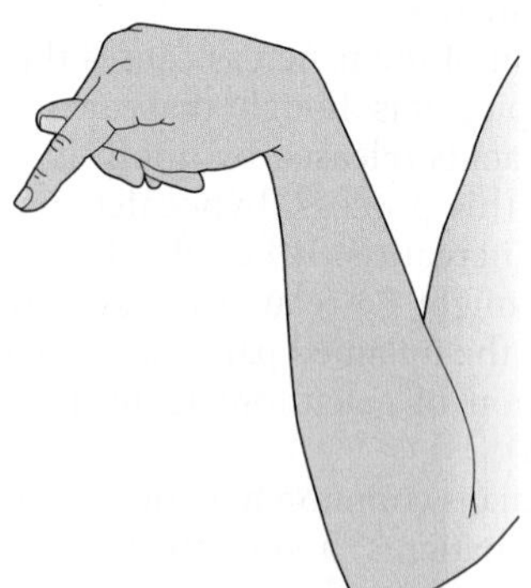

FIGURE 14-6. Trousseau's sign. Ischemia-induced carpal spasm can occur with hypocalcemia or hypomagnesemia. Occluding the brachial artery with a blood pressure cuff for 3 minutes can produce carpal spasm that mimics the spasm that occurs with hypocalcemia or hypomagnesemia.

Assessment and Diagnostic Findings

When evaluating serum calcium levels, one must consider several other variables, such as the serum albumin level and the arterial pH. Because abnormalities in serum albumin levels may affect interpretation of the serum calcium level, it may be necessary to calculate the corrected serum calcium if the serum albumin level is abnormal. For every decrease in serum albumin of 1 g/dL below 4 g/dL, the total serum calcium level is underestimated by approximately 0.8 mg/dL. The following is a quick method to calculate the corrected serum calcium level:

$$\text{Measured total serum Ca}^{++}\text{ level}\left(\text{mg/dL}\right) + 0.8$$
$$\times\left(4.0 - \text{Measured albumin level }\left[\text{g/dL}\right]\right)$$
$$= \text{Corrected total calcium concentration }\left(\text{mg/dL}\right)$$

An example of the calculations needed to obtain the corrected total serum calcium level is as follows:

A patient's reported serum albumin level is 2.5 g/dL; the reported serum calcium level is 10.5 mg/dL. First, the decrease in serum albumin level from normal (ie, the difference from the normal albumin concentration of 4 g/dL) is calculated: 4 g/dL – 2.5 g/dL = 1.5 g/dL. Next, the following ratio is calculated:

$$0.8\ \text{mg/dL} : 1\,\text{g/dL} = \text{X mg/dL} : 1.5\,\text{mg/dL}$$
$$\text{X} = 0.8 \times 1.5\,\text{mg/dL}$$
$$\text{X} = 1.2\,\text{mg/dL calcium}$$

Finally, 1.2 mg/dL is added to 10.5 mg/dL (the reported serum calcium level) to obtain the corrected total serum calcium level: 1.2 mg/dL + 10.5 mg/dL = 11.7 mg/dL

Clinicians often discount a low serum calcium level in the presence of a similarly low serum albumin level. The ionized calcium level is usually normal in patients with reduced total serum calcium levels and concomitant hypoalbuminemia. When the arterial pH increases (alkalosis), more calcium becomes bound to protein. As a result, the ionized portion decreases. Symptoms of hypocalcemia may occur with alkalosis. Acidosis (low pH) has the opposite effect; that is, less calcium is bound to protein and therefore more exists in the ionized form. However, relatively small changes in serum calcium levels occur in these acid–base abnormalities.

Ideally, the ionized level of calcium should be measured in the laboratory. However, in many laboratories, only the total calcium level is reported; therefore, the concentration of the ionized fraction must be estimated by simultaneous measurement of the serum albumin level. PTH levels are decreased in hypoparathyroidism. Magnesium and phosphorus levels need to be assessed to identify possible causes of decreased calcium.

Medical Management

Acute symptomatic hypocalcemia is life-threatening and requires prompt treatment with IV administration of calcium (Kee et al., 2004). Parenteral calcium salts include calcium gluconate, calcium chloride, and calcium gluceptate. Although calcium chloride produces a significantly higher ionized calcium level than calcium gluconate does, it is not used as often because it is more irritating and can cause sloughing of tissue if it infiltrates. Too-rapid IV administration of calcium can cause cardiac arrest, preceded by bradycardia. IV administration of calcium is particularly dangerous in patients receiving digitalis-derived medications, because calcium ions exert an effect similar to that of digitalis and can cause digitalis toxicity, with adverse cardiac effects. Therefore, calcium should be diluted in D_5W and administered as a slow IV bolus or a slow IV infusion using a volumetric infusion pump. The IV site must be observed often for any evidence of infiltration because of the risk of extravasation and resultant cellulitis or necrosis. A 0.9% sodium chloride solution should not be used with calcium because it increases renal calcium loss. Solutions containing phosphates or bicarbonate should not be used with calcium because they cause precipitation when calcium is added. The nurse must clarify with the physician which calcium salt to administer, because calcium gluconate yields 4.5 mEq of calcium and calcium chloride provides 13.6 mEq of calcium. Calcium can cause postural hypotension; therefore, the patient is kept in bed during IV replacement, and blood pressure is monitored.

Vitamin D therapy may be instituted to increase calcium absorption from the GI tract. Aluminum hydroxide, calcium acetate, or calcium carbonate antacids may be prescribed to decrease elevated phosphorus levels before treating hypocalcemia in the patient with chronic renal failure. Increasing the dietary intake of calcium to at least 1000 to 1500 mg/day in the adult is recommended; calcium-containing foods include milk products; green, leafy vegetables; canned salmon; sardines; and fresh oysters. Hypomagnesemia can also cause tetany; if the tetany responds to IV calcium, then a low magnesium level is considered as a possible cause in chronic renal failure.

Nursing Management

It is important to observe for hypocalcemia in patients at risk. Seizure precautions are initiated if hypocalcemia is severe. The status of the airway is closely monitored, because laryngeal stridor can occur. Safety precautions are taken, as indicated, if confusion is present.

People who have a high risk for osteoporosis are instructed about the need for adequate dietary calcium intake; it is important to teach the patient what foods are rich in calcium. The nurse must also advise the patient to consider calcium supplements if sufficient calcium is not consumed in the diet. Such supplements should be taken in divided doses with meals. In addition, the value of regular weight-bearing exercise in decreasing bone loss should be emphasized, as well as the effect of medications on calcium balance. For example, alcohol and caffeine in high doses inhibit calcium absorption, and moderate cigarette smoking increases urinary calcium excretion. Additional teaching includes discussion of medications such as alendronate (Fosamax), risedronate (Actonel), raloxifene (Evista), calcitonin, and ibandronate (Boniva), a once-a-month bisphosphonate to reduce the rate of bone loss. Teaching also includes strategies to reduce the risk of falls. The patient is also cautioned to avoid the overuse of laxatives and antacids that contain phosphorus, because their use decreases calcium absorption.

Calcium Excess (Hypercalcemia)

Hypercalcemia (excess of calcium in the plasma) is a dangerous imbalance when severe; in fact, hypercalcemic crisis has a mortality rate as high as 50% if not treated promptly.

The most common causes of hypercalcemia are malignancies and hyperparathyroidism. Malignant tumors can produce hypercalcemia by a variety of mechanisms (Stewart, 2005). The excessive PTH secretion associated with hyperparathyroidism causes increased release of calcium from the bones and increased intestinal and renal absorption of calcium. Calcifications of soft tissue occur when the calcium–phosphorus product (serum calcium × serum phosphorus) exceeds 70 mg/dL (Rose & Post, 2000).

Bone mineral is lost during immobilization, and sometimes this causes elevation of total (and especially ionized) calcium in the bloodstream. However, symptomatic hypercalcemia from immobilization is rare; when it does occur, it is virtually limited to people with high calcium turnover rates (eg, adolescents during a growth spurt). Most cases of hypercalcemia secondary to immobility occur after severe or multiple fractures or spinal cord injury.

Thiazide diuretics can cause a slight elevation in serum calcium levels because they potentiate the action of PTH on the kidneys, reducing urinary calcium excretion. The milk-alkali syndrome has occurred in patients with peptic ulcer treated previously for a prolonged period with milk and alkaline antacids, particularly calcium carbonate. Vitamin A and D intoxication, as well as the use of lithium, can cause calcium excess. Calcium levels are inversely related to phosphorus levels.

Clinical Manifestations

As a rule, the symptoms of hypercalcemia are proportional to the degree of elevation of the serum calcium level. Hypercalcemia reduces neuromuscular excitability because it suppresses activity at the myoneural junction. Symptoms such as muscle weakness, incoordination, anorexia, and constipation may be caused by decreased tone in smooth and striated muscle. Cardiac standstill can occur when the serum calcium level is about 18 mg/dL (4.5 mmol/L). The inotropic effect of digitalis is enhanced by calcium; therefore, digitalis toxicity is aggravated by hypercalcemia.

Anorexia, nausea, vomiting, and constipation are common symptoms of hypercalcemia. Dehydration occurs with nausea, vomiting, anorexia, and calcium reabsorption at the proximal renal tubule. Abdominal and bone pain may also be present. Abdominal distention and paralytic ileus may complicate severe hypercalcemic crisis. Excessive urination due to disturbed renal tubular function produced by hypercalcemia may occur. Severe thirst may occur secondary to the polyuria caused by the high solute (calcium) load.

Patients with chronic hypercalcemia may develop symptoms similar to those of peptic ulcer because hypercalcemia increases the secretion of acid and pepsin by the stomach.

Confusion, impaired memory, slurred speech, lethargy, acute psychotic behavior, or coma may occur (Stewart, 2005). The more severe symptoms tend to appear when the serum calcium level is approximately 16 mg/dL (4 mmol/L) or higher. However, some patients become profoundly disturbed with serum calcium levels of only 12 mg/dL (3 mmol/L). These symptoms resolve as serum calcium levels return to normal after treatment.

Hypercalcemic crisis refers to an acute rise in the serum calcium level to 17 mg/dL (4.3 mmol/L) or higher. Severe thirst and polyuria are often present. Other findings may include muscle weakness, intractable nausea, abdominal cramps, obstipation (very severe constipation) or diarrhea, peptic ulcer symptoms, and bone pain. Lethargy, confusion, and coma may also occur. This condition is very dangerous and may result in cardiac arrest.

Assessment and Diagnostic Findings

The serum calcium level is greater than 10.2 mg/dL (2.6 mmol/L). Cardiovascular changes may include a variety of dysrhythmias (ie, heart blocks) and shortening of the QT interval and ST segment. The PR interval is sometimes prolonged. The double-antibody PTH test may be used to differentiate between primary hyperparathyroidism and malignancy as a cause of hypercalcemia: PTH levels are increased in primary or secondary hyperparathyroidism and suppressed in malignancy. X-rays may reveal the presence of osteoporosis if the patient has hypercalcemia secondary to a malignancy, bone cavitation, or urinary calculi. The Sulkowitch urine test analyzes the amount of calcium in the urine; in hypercalcemia, dense precipitation is observed due to hypercalciuria.

Medical Management

Therapeutic aims in hypercalcemia include decreasing the serum calcium level and reversing the process causing hypercalcemia. Treating the underlying cause (eg, chemotherapy for a malignancy, partial parathyroidectomy for hyperparathyroidism) is essential.

PHARMACOLOGIC THERAPY

General measures include administering fluids to dilute serum calcium and promote its excretion by the kidneys, mobilizing the patient, and restricting dietary calcium intake. IV administration of 0.9% sodium chloride solution temporarily dilutes the serum calcium level and increases urinary calcium excretion by inhibiting tubular reabsorption of calcium. Administering IV phosphate can cause a reciprocal drop in serum calcium. Furosemide (Lasix) is often used in conjunction with administration of a saline solution; in addition to causing diuresis, furosemide increases calcium excretion. Although it is an often-overlooked measure, fluids and medications that contain calcium and dietary sources of calcium should be halted (Stewart, 2005).

Calcitonin can be used to lower the serum calcium level and is particularly useful for patients with heart disease or renal failure who cannot tolerate large sodium loads. Calcitonin reduces bone resorption, increases the depositing of calcium and phosphorus in the bones, and increases urinary excretion of calcium and phosphorus (Karch, 2006). Although several forms are available, calcitonin derived from salmon is commonly used. Skin testing for allergy to salmon calcitonin is necessary before the hormone is administered. Systemic allergic reactions are possible because this hormone is a protein; resistance to the medication may develop later because of antibody formation. Calcitonin is administered by intramuscular injection rather than subcutaneously, because patients with hypercalcemia have poor perfusion of subcutaneous tissue.

For patients with cancer, treatment is directed at controlling the condition by surgery, chemotherapy, or radiation therapy. Corticosteroids may be used to decrease bone turnover and tubular reabsorption for patients with sarcoidosis, myelomas, lymphomas, and leukemias; patients with solid tumors are less responsive. The bisphosphonates inhibit osteoclast activity. Pamidronate (Aredia) is a potent form and is administered intravenously; it causes a transient, mild pyrexia, decreased white blood cell count, and myalgia. Etidronate (Didronel) is another bisphosphonate that is given by IV, but its action is slower. Mithramycin, a cytotoxic antibiotic, inhibits bone resorption and thus lowers the serum calcium level. This agent must be used cautiously because it has significant side effects, including thrombocytopenia, nephrotoxicity, rebound hypercalcemia when discontinued, and hepatotoxicity. Inorganic phosphate salts can be administered orally or by nasogastric tube (in the form of Phospho-Soda or Neutra-Phos), rectally (as retention enemas), or intravenously. IV phosphate therapy is used with extreme caution in the treatment of hypercalcemia, because it can cause severe calcification in various tissues, hypotension, tetany, and acute renal failure.

Nursing Management

It is important to monitor for hypercalcemia in patients who are at risk. Interventions such as increasing patient mobility and encouraging fluids can help prevent hypercalcemia, or at least minimize its severity. Hospitalized patients who are at risk for hypercalcemia are encouraged to ambulate as soon as possible; outpatients and those cared for in their homes are informed of the importance of frequent ambulation.

When encouraging oral fluids, the nurse considers the patient's likes and dislikes. Fluids containing sodium should be administered unless contraindicated, because sodium favors calcium excretion. Patients are encouraged to drink 3 to 4 quarts of fluid daily. Adequate fiber should be provided in the diet to offset the tendency for constipation. Safety precautions are implemented, as necessary, when mental symptoms of hypercalcemia are present. The patient and family are informed that these mental changes are reversible with treatment. Increased calcium potentiates the effects of digitalis; therefore, the patient is assessed for signs and symptoms of digitalis toxicity. Because ECG changes (premature ventricular contractions, paroxysmal atrial tachycardia, and heart block) can occur, the cardiac rate and rhythm are monitored for any abnormalities.

Magnesium Imbalances

Magnesium is the most abundant intracellular cation after potassium. It acts as an activator for many intracellular enzyme systems and plays a role in both carbohydrate and protein metabolism. The normal serum magnesium level is 1.3 to 2.3 mEq/L (1.8 to 3.0 mg/dL; 0.8 to 1.2 mmol/L). Approximately one third of serum magnesium is bound to protein; the remaining two thirds exists as free cations—the active component (Mg^{++}). Magnesium balance is important in neuromuscular function. Because magnesium acts directly on the myoneural junction, variations in the serum concentration of magnesium affect neuromuscular irritability and contractility. For example, an excess of magnesium diminishes the excitability of the muscle cells, whereas a deficit increases neuromuscular irritability and contractility. Magnesium produces its sedative effect at the neuromuscular junction, probably by inhibiting the release of the neurotransmitter acetylcholine. It also increases the stimulus threshold in nerve fibers.

Magnesium exerts effects on the cardiovascular system, acting peripherally to produce vasodilation. Magnesium is thought to have a direct effect on peripheral arteries and arterioles, which results in a decreased total peripheral resistance. Magnesium is predominantly found in bone and soft tissues. It is primarily eliminated by the kidneys.

Magnesium Deficit (Hypomagnesemia)

Hypomagnesemia refers to a below-normal serum magnesium concentration (1.3 to 2.3 mEq/L; 1.8 to 3.0 mg/dL; 0.8 to 1.2 mmol/L). Magnesium is similar to calcium in two aspects: (1) it is the ionized fraction of magnesium that is primarily involved in neuromuscular activity and other physiologic processes, and (2) magnesium levels should be evaluated in combination with albumin levels. Low serum albumin levels decrease total magnesium.

Hypomagnesemia is a common yet often overlooked imbalance in acutely and critically ill patients. It may occur with withdrawal from alcohol and administration of tube feedings or parenteral nutrition.

An important route of magnesium loss is the GI tract. Loss of magnesium from the GI tract may occur with nasogastric suction, diarrhea, or fistulas. Because fluid from the lower GI tract has a higher concentration of magnesium (10 to 14 mEq/L) than fluid from the upper tract (1 to 2 mEq/L), losses from diarrhea and intestinal fistulas are more likely to induce magnesium deficit than are those from gastric suction. Although magnesium losses are relatively small in nasogastric suction, hypomagnesemia will occur if losses are prolonged and magnesium is not replaced through IV infusion. Because the distal small bowel is the major site of magnesium absorption, any disruption in small bowel function, as in intestinal resection or inflammatory bowel disease, can lead to hypomagnesemia.

Alcoholism is currently the most common cause of symptomatic hypomagnesemia in the United States. Hypomagnesemia is particularly troublesome during treatment of alcohol withdrawal. Therefore, the serum magnesium level should be measured at least every 2 or 3 days in patients undergoing withdrawal from alcohol. The serum magnesium level may be normal on admission but may decrease as a result of metabolic changes, such as the intracellular shift of magnesium associated with IV glucose administration.

During nutritional replacement, the major cellular electrolytes move from the serum to newly synthesized cells. Therefore, if the enteral or parenteral feeding formula is deficient in magnesium content, serious hypomagnesemia will occur. Because of this, serum magnesium levels should be measured at regular intervals in patients who are receiving parenteral nutrition and enteral feedings, especially those who have undergone a period of starvation. Other causes of hypomagnesemia include the administration of aminoglycosides, cyclosporine, cisplatin, diuretics, digitalis, and amphotericin and the rapid administration of citrated blood, especially to patients with renal or hepatic disease. Magnesium deficiency often occurs in diabetic ketoacidosis, secondary to increased renal excretion during osmotic diuresis and shifting of magnesium into the cells with insulin therapy. Other contributing causes are sepsis, burns, and hypothermia.

Clinical Manifestations

Clinical manifestations of hypomagnesemia are largely confined to the neuromuscular system. Some of the effects are due directly to the low serum magnesium level; others are due to secondary changes in potassium and calcium metabolism. Symptoms do not usually occur until the serum magnesium level has dropped to less than 1 mEq/L (0.5 mmol/L).

Among the neuromuscular changes are hyperexcitability with muscle weakness, tremors, and athetoid movements (slow, involuntary twisting and writhing). Others include tetany, generalized tonic–clonic or focal seizures, laryngeal stridor, and positive Chvostek's and Trousseau's signs (see earlier discussion), which occur, in part, because of accompanying hypocalcemia.

Magnesium deficiency can disturb the ECG by prolonging the QRS, depressing the ST segment, and predisposing to cardiac dysrhythmias, such as premature ventricular contractions, supraventricular tachycardia, torsades de pointes (a form of ventricular tachycardia), and ventricular fibrillation. Increased susceptibility to digitalis toxicity is associated with low serum magnesium levels. This is important, because patients receiving digoxin are also likely to be receiving diuretic therapy, predisposing them to renal loss of magnesium.

Hypomagnesemia may be accompanied by marked alterations in mood. Apathy, depression, apprehension, and extreme agitation have been noted, as well as ataxia, dizziness, insomnia, and confusion. At times, delirium, auditory or visual hallucinations, and frank psychoses may occur.

Assessment and Diagnostic Findings

On laboratory analysis, the serum magnesium level is less than 1.3 mEq/L or 1.8 mg/dL (0.75 mmol/L). Hypomagnesemia is frequently associated with hypokalemia and hypocalcemia. About 25% of magnesium is protein-bound, principally to albumin. A decreased serum albumin level can, therefore, reduce the measured total magnesium concentration; however, it does not reduce the ionized plasma magnesium concentration. ECG evaluations reflect magnesium, calcium, and potassium deficiencies, tachydysrhythmias, prolonged PR and QT intervals, widening QRS, ST-segment depression, flattened T waves, and a prominent U wave. Torsades de pointes is associated with a low magnesium level. Premature ventricular contractions, paroxysmal atrial tachycardia, and heart block may also occur. Urine magnesium levels may be helpful in identifying causes of magnesium depletion and are measured after a loading dose of magnesium sulfate is administered. Two newer diagnostic techniques (nuclear magnetic resonance spectroscopy and the ion-selective electrode) are sensitive and direct means of measuring ionized serum magnesium levels.

Medical Management

Mild magnesium deficiency can be corrected by diet alone. Principal dietary sources of magnesium, which is a component of chlorophyll, are green leafy vegetables, nuts, seeds, legumes, whole grains, and seafood. Magnesium is also plentiful in peanut butter and cocoa.

If necessary, magnesium salts can be administered orally in an oxide or gluconate form to replace continuous excessive losses. Diarrhea is a common complication of excessive ingestion of magnesium. Patients receiving parenteral nutrition require magnesium in the IV solution to prevent hypomagnesemia. Magnesium sulfate must be administered intravenously by an infusion pump and at a rate not to exceed 150 mg/min, or 67 mEq over 8 hours. A bolus dose of magnesium sulfate given too rapidly can produce alterations in cardiac conduction leading to heart block or asystole. Vital signs must be assessed frequently during magnesium administration to detect changes in cardiac rate or rhythm, hypotension, and respiratory distress. Monitoring urine output is essential before, during, and after magnesium administration; the physician is notified if urine volume decreases to less than 100 mL over 4 hours. Calcium gluconate must be readily available to treat hypocalcemic tetany or hypermagnesemia.

Overt symptoms of hypomagnesemia are treated with parenteral administration of magnesium. Magnesium sulfate is the most commonly used magnesium salt. Serial measurements of serum magnesium levels can be used to regulate the dosage.

Nursing Management

The nurse should be aware of patients who are at risk for hypomagnesemia and observe them for its signs and symptoms. Patients receiving digitalis are monitored closely, because a deficit of magnesium can predispose them to digitalis toxicity. If hypomagnesemia is severe, seizure precautions are implemented. Other safety precautions are instituted, as indicated, if confusion is observed.

Because difficulty in swallowing (dysphagia) may occur in magnesium-depleted patients, the ability to swallow should be tested with water before oral medications or foods are offered. Dysphagia is probably related to the athetoid or choreiform (rapid, involuntary, and irregular jerking) movements associated with magnesium deficit. To determine neuromuscular irritability, the nurse needs to assess and grade deep tendon reflexes (see Chapter 60).

Teaching plays a major role in treating magnesium deficit, particularly that resulting from abuse of diuretic or laxative medications. In such cases, the nurse instructs the patient about the need to consume magnesium-rich foods. For patients experiencing hypomagnesemia from abuse of alcohol, the nurse provides teaching, counseling, support, and possible referral to alcohol abstinence programs or other professional help.

Magnesium Excess (Hypermagnesemia)

Hypermagnesemia is a rare electrolyte abnormality, because the kidneys are efficient in excreting magnesium. A serum magnesium level can appear falsely elevated if blood specimens are allowed to hemolyze or are drawn from an extremity with a tourniquet that was applied too tightly.

By far the most common cause of hypermagnesemia is renal failure. In fact, most patients with advanced renal failure have at least a slight elevation in serum magnesium levels. This condition is aggravated when such patients receive magnesium to control seizures or inadvertently take one of the many commercial antacids that contain magnesium salts.

Hypermagnesemia can occur in a patient with untreated diabetic ketoacidosis when catabolism causes the release of cellular magnesium that cannot be excreted because of profound fluid volume depletion and resulting oliguria. An excess of magnesium can also result from excessive magnesium administered to treat hypertension of pregnancy or to treat low hypomagnesemia. Increased serum magnesium levels can also occur in adrenocortical insufficiency, Addison's disease, or hypothermia. Excessive use of antacids (eg, Maalox, Riopan, Mylanta); laxatives (Milk of Magnesia); and medications that decrease GI motility, including opioids and anticholinergics, can also increase serum magnesium levels. Decreased elimination of magnesium or its increased absorption due to intestinal hypomotility from any cause can contribute to hypermagnesemia. Lithium intoxication can also cause an increase in serum magnesium levels.

Clinical Manifestations

Acute elevation of the serum magnesium level depresses the central nervous system as well as the peripheral neuromuscular junction. At mildly increased levels, there is a tendency for lowered blood pressure because of peripheral vasodilation. Nausea, vomiting, weakness, soft tissue calcifications, facial flushing, and sensations of warmth may also occur. At higher magnesium concentrations, lethargy, difficulty speaking (dysarthria), and drowsiness can occur. Deep tendon reflexes are lost, and muscle weakness and paralysis may develop. The respiratory center is depressed when serum magnesium levels exceed 10 mEq/L (5 mmol/L). Coma, atrioventricular heart block, and cardiac arrest can occur when the serum magnesium level is greatly elevated and not treated. High levels of magnesium also result in platelet clumping and delayed thrombin formation (Chernecky & Berger, 2004).

Assessment and Diagnostic Findings

On laboratory analysis, the serum magnesium level is greater than 2.5 mEq/L or 3.0 mg/dL (1.25 mmol/L). Increased potassium and calcium are present concurrently. As creatinine clearance decreases to less than 3.0 mL/min, the serum magnesium levels increase (Hogan & Wane, 2003). ECG findings may include a prolonged PR interval, tall T waves, a widened QRS, and a prolonged QT interval, as well as an atrioventricular block.

Medical Management

Hypermagnesemia can be prevented by avoiding the administration of magnesium to patients with renal failure and by carefully monitoring seriously ill patients who are receiving magnesium salts. In patients with severe hypermagnesemia, all parenteral and oral magnesium salts are discontinued. In emergencies, such as respiratory depression or defective cardiac conduction, ventilatory support and IV calcium gluconate are indicated. In addition, hemodialysis with a magnesium-free dialysate can reduce the serum magnesium to a safe level within hours. Administration of loop diuretics (Lasix) and sodium chloride or lactated Ringer's IV solution enhances magnesium excretion in patients with adequate renal function. IV calcium gluconate antagonizes the cardiovascular and neuromuscular effects of magnesium.

Nursing Management

Patients at risk for hypermagnesemia are identified and assessed. If hypermagnesemia is suspected, the nurse monitors the vital signs, noting hypotension and shallow respirations. The nurse also observes for decreased patellar reflexes and changes in the level of consciousness. Medications that contain magnesium are not administered to patients with renal failure or compromised renal function, and patients with renal failure are cautioned to check with their health care providers before taking over-the-counter medications. Caution is essential when preparing and administering magnesium-containing fluids parenterally, because available parenteral magnesium solutions (eg, 2-mL ampules, 50-mL vials) differ in concentration.

Phosphorus Imbalances

Phosphorus is a critical constituent of all the body's tissues. It is essential to the function of muscle and red blood cells, the formation of adenosine triphosphate (ATP) and of 2,3-diphosphoglycerate, which facilitates release of oxygen from hemoglobin, and the maintenance of acid–base balance, as well as to the nervous system and the intermediary metabolism of carbohydrate, protein, and fat. It provides structural support to bones and teeth. Phosphorus is the primary anion of the ICF. About 85% of phosphorus is located in bones and teeth, 14% in soft tissue, and less than 1% in the ECF. The normal serum phosphorus level is 2.5 to 4.5 mg/dL (0.8 to 1.45 mmol/L) and may be as high as 6 mg/dL (1.94 mmol/L) in infants and children. Serum phosphorus levels are greater in children presumably because of the high rate of skeletal growth; the levels decrease with age.

Phosphorus Deficit (Hypophosphatemia)

Hypophosphatemia is a below-normal serum concentration of inorganic phosphorus. Although it often indicates phosphorus deficiency, hypophosphatemia may occur under a variety of circumstances in which total body phosphorus stores are normal. Conversely, phosphorus deficiency is an abnormally low content of phosphorus in lean tissues that may exist in the absence of hypophosphatemia. It can be caused by an intracellular shift of potassium from serum into cells, by increased urinary excretion of potassium, or by decreased intestinal absorption of potassium.

Hypophosphatemia may occur during the administration of calories to patients with severe protein–calorie malnutrition. It is most likely to occur with overzealous intake or administration of simple carbohydrates. This syndrome can be induced in anyone with severe protein–calorie malnutrition (eg, patients with anorexia nervosa or alcoholism, elderly debilitated patients who are unable to eat). As many as 50% of patients hospitalized because of chronic alcoholism have hypophosphatemia.

Marked hypophosphatemia may develop in malnourished patients who receive parenteral nutrition if the phosphorus loss is not adequately corrected. Other causes of hypophosphatemia include pain, heat stroke, prolonged intense hyperventilation, alcohol withdrawal, poor dietary intake, diabetic ketoacidosis, hepatic encephalopathy, and major thermal burns. Low magnesium levels, low potassium levels, and hyperparathyroidism related to increased urinary losses of phosphorus contribute to hypophosphatemia. Loss of phosphorus through the kidneys also occurs with acute volume expansion, osmotic diuresis, use of carbonic anhydrase inhibitors (acetazolamide [Diamox]), and some malignancies. Respiratory alkalosis can cause a decrease in phosphorus because of an intracellular shift of phosphorus, which often stimulates intracellular glycolysis.

Excess phosphorus binding by antacids containing magnesium, calcium, or albumin may decrease the phosphorus available from the diet to an amount lower than required to maintain serum phosphorus balance. The degree of hypophosphatemia depends on the amount of phosphorus in the diet compared to the dose of antacid. Phosphate can occur with chronic diarrhea or through severe potassium restriction. Vitamin D regulates intestinal ion absorption; therefore, a deficiency of vitamin D may cause decreased calcium and phosphorus levels, which may lead to osteomalacia (softened, brittle bones).

Clinical Manifestations

Most of the signs and symptoms of phosphorus deficiency appear to result from a deficiency of ATP, 2,3-diphosphoglycerate, or both. ATP deficiency impairs cellular energy resources; diphosphoglycerate deficiency impairs oxygen delivery to tissues.

A wide range of neurologic symptoms, such as irritability, fatigue, apprehension, weakness, numbness, paresthesias, dysarthria, dysphagia, diplopia, confusion, seizures, and coma, may occur. Low levels of diphosphoglycerate may reduce the delivery of oxygen to peripheral tissues, resulting in tissue anoxia. Hypoxia then leads to an increase in respiratory rate and respiratory alkalosis, causing phosphorus to move into the cells and potentiating hypophosphatemia. Hemolytic anemia may lead to pale skin and conjunctivae.

It is thought that hypophosphatemia predisposes a person to infection. In laboratory animals, hypophosphatemia is associated with depression of the chemotactic, phagocytic, and bacterial activity of granulocytes.

Muscle damage may develop as the ATP level in the muscle tissue declines. Clinical manifestations are muscle weakness, which may be subtle or profound and may affect any muscle group, muscle pain, and at times acute rhabdomyolysis (disintegration of striated muscle). Weakness of respiratory muscles may greatly impair ventilation. Hypophosphatemia also may predispose a person to insulin resistance and thus hyperglycemia. Chronic loss of phosphorus can cause bruising and bleeding from platelet dysfunction.

Assessment and Diagnostic Findings

On laboratory analysis, the serum phosphorus level is less than 2.5 mg/dL (0.80 mmol/L) in adults. When reviewing laboratory results, the nurse should keep in mind that glucose or insulin administration causes a slight decrease in the serum phosphorus level. PTH levels are increased in hyperparathyroidism. Serum magnesium may decrease due to increased urinary excretion of magnesium. Alkaline phosphatase is increased with osteoblastic activity. X-rays may show skeletal changes of osteomalacia or rickets.

Medical Management

Prevention of hypophosphatemia is the goal. In patients at risk for hypophosphatemia, serum phosphate levels should be closely monitored and correction initiated before deficits become severe. Adequate amounts of phosphorus should be added to parenteral solutions, and attention should be paid to the phosphorus levels in enteral feeding solutions.

Severe hypophosphatemia is dangerous and requires prompt attention. Aggressive IV phosphorus correction is usually limited to the patient whose serum phosphorus levels decrease to less than 1 mg/dL (0.3 mmol/L) and whose GI tract is not functioning. Possible dangers of IV administration of phosphorus include tetany from hypocalcemia and calcifications in tissues (blood vessels, heart, lung, kidney, eyes) from hyperphosphatemia. IV preparations of phosphorus are available as sodium or potassium phosphate. The rate of phosphorus administration should not exceed 10 mEq/h, and the site should be carefully monitored because tissue sloughing and necrosis can occur with infiltration. In less acute situations, oral phosphorus replacement is usually adequate.

Nursing Management

The nurse identifies patients who are at risk for hypophosphatemia and monitors them. Because malnourished patients receiving parenteral nutrition are at risk when calories are introduced too aggressively, preventive measures involve gradually introducing the solution to avoid rapid shifts of phosphorus into the cells.

For patients with documented hypophosphatemia, careful attention is given to preventing infection, because hypophosphatemia may alter the granulocytes. In patients requiring correction of phosphorus losses, the nurse frequently monitors serum phosphorus levels and documents and reports early signs of hypophosphatemia (apprehension, confusion, change in level of consciousness). If the patient experiences mild hypophosphatemia, foods such as milk and milk products, organ meats, nuts, fish, poultry, and whole grains should be encouraged. With moderate hypophosphatemia, supplements such as Neutra-Phos capsules (250 mg phosphorus/capsule) or Fleet's Phospho-Soda (815 mg phosphorus/5 mL) may be prescribed.

Phosphorus Excess (Hyperphosphatemia)

Hyperphosphatemia is a serum phosphorus level that exceeds normal. Various conditions can lead to this imbalance, but the most common is renal failure. Other causes include increased intake, decreased output, or a shift from the intracellular to extracellular space. Other causes include chemotherapy for neoplastic disease, hypoparathyroidism, metabolic or respiratory acidosis, diabetic ketoacidosis, acute hemolysis, high phosphate intake, profound muscle necrosis, and increased phosphorus absorption. The primary complication of increased phosphorus is metastatic calcification (soft tissue, joints, and arteries), which occurs when the calcium–magnesium product (calcium × magnesium) exceeds 70 mg/dL.

Clinical Manifestations

An increased serum phosphorus level causes few symptoms. Symptoms that do occur usually result from decreased calcium levels and soft tissue calcifications. The most important short-term consequence is tetany. Because of the reciprocal relationship between phosphorus and calcium, a high serum phosphorus level tends to cause a low serum calcium concentration. Tetany can result, causing tingling sensations in the fingertips and around the mouth. Anorexia, nausea, vomiting, bone and joint pain, muscle weakness, hyperreflexia, and tachycardia may occur.

The major long-term consequence is soft tissue calcification, which occurs mainly in patients with a reduced glomerular filtration rate. High serum levels of inorganic phosphorus promote precipitation of calcium phosphate in nonosseous sites, decreasing urine output, impairing vision, and producing palpitations.

Assessment and Diagnostic Findings

On laboratory analysis, the serum phosphorus level exceeds 4.5 mg/dL (1.5 mmol/L) in adults. Serum phosphorus levels are normally higher in children, presumably because of the high rate of skeletal growth. The serum calcium level is useful also for diagnosing the primary disorder and assessing the effects of treatments. X-ray studies may show skeletal changes with abnormal bone development. PTH levels are decreased in hypoparathyroidism. BUN and creatinine levels are used to assess renal function. Renal ultrasonography may be indicated as part of the diagnostic assessment for renal failure; bone studies and coronary calcification studies also provide information about the chronicity and prognosis of renal failure.

Medical Management

When possible, treatment is directed at the underlying disorder. For example, hyperphosphatemia may be related to volume depletion or respiratory or metabolic acidosis. In renal failure, elevated PTH production contributes to a high phosphorus level and bone disease. Measures to decrease the serum phosphate level in these patients include vitamin D preparations, such as calcitriol, which is available in both oral (Rocaltrol) and parenteral (Calcijex, paricalcitol [Zemplar]) forms. IV administration of calcitriol does not increase the serum calcium unless its dose is excessive, thus permitting more aggressive treatment of hyperphosphatemia with calcium-binding antacids (calcium carbonate or calcium citrate), phosphate-binding gels or antacids, restriction of dietary phosphate, forced diuresis with a loop diuretic, volume repletion with saline, and dialysis. Surgery may be indicated for removal of large calcium–phosphorus deposits.

Nursing Management

The nurse monitors patients at risk for hyperphosphatemia. if a low-phosphorus diet is prescribed, the patient is instructed to avoid phosphorus-rich foods such as hard cheese, cream, nuts, meats, whole-grain cereals, dried fruits, dried vegetables, kidneys, sardines, sweetbreads, and foods made with milk. When appropriate, the nurse instructs the patient to avoid phosphate-containing substances such as laxatives and enemas. The nurse also teaches the patient to recognize the signs of impending hypocalcemia and to monitor for changes in urine output.

Chloride Imbalances

Chloride, the major anion of the ECF, is found more in interstitial and lymph fluid compartments than in blood. Chloride is also contained in gastric and pancreatic juices, sweat, bile, and saliva. Sodium and chloride in water make up the composition of the ECF and assist in determining osmotic pressure.

The normal serum chloride level is 97 to 107 mEq/L (96 to 106 mmol/L). Inside the cell, the chloride level is 4 mEq/L. The serum level of chloride reflects a change in dilution or concentration of the ECF and does so in direct proportion to the sodium concentration. Serum osmolality parallels chloride levels as well. Aldosterone secretion increases sodium reabsorption, thereby increasing chloride reabsorption. The choroid plexus, where cerebrospinal fluid forms in the brain, depends on sodium and chloride to attract water to form the fluid portion of the cerebrospinal fluid. Bicarbonate has an inverse relationship with chloride. As chloride moves from plasma into the red blood cells (called the chloride shift), bicarbonate moves back into the plasma. Hydrogen ions are formed, which then help release oxygen from hemoglobin. When the level of one of these three electrolytes (sodium, bicarbonate, or chloride) is disturbed, the other two are also affected. Chloride assists in maintaining acid–base balance and works as a buffer in the exchange of oxygen and carbon dioxide in red blood cells. Chloride is primarily obtained from the diet as table salt.

Chloride Deficit (Hypochloremia)

Chloride control depends on the intake of chloride and the excretion and reabsorption of its ions in the kidneys. Chloride is produced in the stomach, where it combines with hydrogen to form hydrochloric acid. A small amount of chloride is lost in the feces. GI tube drainage and severe vomiting and diarrhea are risk factors for hypochloremia. Administration of chloride-deficient formulas, low sodium intake, decreased serum sodium levels, metabolic alkalosis, prolonged therapy with IV dextrose, diuretic therapy, burns, and fever may also cause hypochloremia. Administration of aldosterone, ACTH, corticosteroids, bicarbonate, or laxatives decreases serum chloride levels as well. As chloride decreases (usually because of volume depletion), sodium and bicarbonate ions are retained by the kidney to balance the loss. Bicarbonate accumulates in the ECF, which raises the pH and leads to hypochloremic metabolic alkalosis.

Clinical Manifestations

The signs and symptoms of hypochloremia are those of acid–base and electrolyte imbalances. The signs and symptoms of hyponatremia, hypokalemia, and metabolic alkalosis may also be present. Metabolic alkalosis is a disorder that results in a high pH and a high serum bicarbonate level as a result of excess alkali intake or loss of hydrogen ions. With compensation, the partial pressure of carbon dioxide in arterial blood ($PaCO_2$) increases to 50 mm Hg. Hyperexcitability of muscles, tetany, hyperactive deep tendon reflexes, weakness, twitching, and muscle cramps may result. Hypokalemia can cause hypochloremia, resulting in cardiac dysrhythmias. In addition, because low chloride levels parallel low sodium levels, a water excess may occur. Hyponatremia can cause seizures and coma.

Assessment and Diagnostic Findings

In addition to the chloride level, sodium and potassium levels are also evaluated, because these electrolytes are lost along with chloride. Arterial blood gas analysis identifies the acid–base imbalance, which is usually metabolic alkalosis. The urine chloride level, which is also measured, decreases in hypochloremia.

Medical Management

Treatment involves correcting the cause of hypochloremia and the contributing electrolyte and acid–base imbalances. Normal saline (0.9% sodium chloride) or half-strength saline (0.45% sodium chloride) solution is administered by IV to replace the chloride. The physician may reevaluate whether the patient receiving a diuretic (loop, osmotic, or thiazide) should discontinue the medications or change to another diuretic.

Foods high in chloride are provided; these include tomato juice, bananas, dates, eggs, cheese, milk, salty broth, canned vegetables, and processed meats. A patient who drinks free water (water without electrolytes) or bottled water excretes large amounts of chloride; therefore, the patient is instructed to avoid this kind of water. Ammonium chloride, an acidifying agent, may be prescribed to treat metabolic alkalosis; the dosage depends on the patient's weight and serum chloride level. This agent is metabolized by the liver, and its effects last for about 3 days. Its use should be avoided in patients with impaired liver or renal function.

Nursing Management

The nurse monitors the patient's I&O, arterial blood gas values, and serum electrolyte levels, as well as level of consciousness and muscle strength and movement. Changes are reported to the physician promptly. Vital signs are monitored, and respiratory assessment is carried out frequently. The nurse teaches the patient about foods with high chloride content.

Chloride Excess (Hyperchloremia)

Hyperchloremia exists when the serum level of chloride exceeds 107 mEq/L (107 mmol/L). Hypernatremia, bicarbonate loss, and metabolic acidosis can occur with high chloride levels. Hyperchloremic metabolic acidosis is also known as normal anion gap acidosis (see later discussion). It is usually caused by the loss of bicarbonate ions via the kidney or the GI tract with a corresponding increase in chloride ions. Chloride ions in the form of acidifying salts accumulate and acidosis occurs with a decrease in bicarbonate ions. Head trauma, increased perspiration, excess adrenocortical hormone production, and decreased glomerular filtration can lead to a high serum chloride level.

Clinical Manifestations

The signs and symptoms of hyperchloremia are the same as those of metabolic acidosis, hypervolemia, and hypernatremia. Tachypnea; weakness; lethargy; deep, rapid respirations; diminished cognitive ability; and hypertension occur. If untreated, hyperchloremia can lead to a decrease in cardiac output, dysrhythmias, and coma. A high chloride level is accompanied by a high sodium level and fluid retention.

Assessment and Diagnostic Findings

The serum chloride level is 108 mEq/L (108 mmol/L) or greater, the serum sodium level is greater than 145 mEq/L (145 mmol/L), the serum pH is less than 7.35, the serum bicarbonate level is less than 22 mEq/L (22 mmol/L), and there is a normal anion gap of 8 to 12 mEq/L (8 to 12 mmol/L). Urine chloride excretion increases. Increased chloride sweat levels are present in cystic fibrosis, diabetes insipidus, glucose-6-phosphate deficiency, hypothyroidism, malnutrition, and acute renal failure.

Calculation of the serum anion gap is important in analyzing acid–base disorders. The sum of all negatively charged electrolytes (anions) equals the sum of all positively charged electrolytes (cations) with several anions that are not routinely measured leading to an anion gap. It is based primarily on three electrolytes: sodium, chloride, and bicarbonate or serum carbon dioxide (CO_2). A low anion gap may be attributed to hypoproteinemia, whereas an elevated anion gap can be due to metabolic acidosis.

Medical Management

Correcting the underlying cause of hyperchloremia and restoring electrolyte, fluid, and acid–base balance are essential. Hypotonic IV solutions may be given to restore balance. Lactated Ringer's solution may be prescribed to convert lactate to bicarbonate in the liver, which increases the base bicarbonate level and corrects the acidosis. IV sodium bicarbonate may be administered to increase bicarbonate levels, which leads to the renal excretion of chloride ions as bicarbonate and chloride compete for combination with sodium. Diuretics may be administered to eliminate chloride as well. Sodium, chloride, and fluids are restricted.

Nursing Management

Monitoring vital signs, arterial blood gas values, and I&O is important to assess the patient's status and the effectiveness of treatment. Assessment findings related to respiratory, neurologic, and cardiac systems are documented, and changes discussed with the physician. The nurse teaches the patient about the diet that should be followed to manage hyperchloremia and maintain adequate hydration.

Acid–Base Disturbances

Acid–base disturbances are commonly encountered in clinical practice. Identification of the specific acid–base imbalance is important in identifying the underlying cause of the disorder and determining appropriate treatment.

Plasma pH is an indicator of hydrogen ion (H^+) concentration. Homeostatic mechanisms keep pH within a normal range (7.35 to 7.45). These mechanisms consist of buffer systems, the kidneys, and the lungs. The H^+ concentration is extremely important: the greater the concentration, the more acidic the solution and the lower the pH; the lower the H^+ concentration, the more alkaline the solution and the higher the pH. The pH range compatible with life (6.8 to 7.8) represents a tenfold difference in H^+ concentration in plasma.

Buffer systems prevent major changes in the pH of body fluids by removing or releasing H^+; they can act quickly to prevent excessive changes in H^+ concentration. Hydrogen ions are buffered by both intracellular and extracellular buffers. The body's major extracellular buffer system is the bicarbonate–carbonic acid buffer system, which is assessed when arterial blood gases are measured. Normally, there are 20 parts of bicarbonate (HCO_3^-) to one part of carbonic acid (H_2CO_3). If this ratio is altered, the pH will change. It is the ratio of HCO_3^- to H_2CO_3 that is important in maintaining pH, not absolute values. CO_2 is a potential acid; when dissolved in water, it becomes carbonic acid ($CO_2 + H_2O = H_2CO_3$). Therefore, when CO_2 is increased, the carbonic acid content is also increased, and vice versa. If either bicarbonate or carbonic acid is increased or decreased so that the 20:1 ratio is no longer maintained, acid–base imbalance results.

Less important buffer systems in the ECF include the inorganic phosphates and the plasma proteins. Intracellular buffers include proteins, organic and inorganic phosphates, and, in red blood cells, hemoglobin.

The kidneys regulate the bicarbonate level in the ECF; they can regenerate bicarbonate ions as well as reabsorb them from the renal tubular cells. In respiratory acidosis and most cases of metabolic acidosis, the kidneys excrete hydrogen ions and conserve bicarbonate ions to help restore balance. In respiratory and metabolic alkalosis, the kidneys retain hydrogen ions and excrete bicarbonate ions to help restore balance. The kidneys obviously cannot compensate for the metabolic acidosis created by renal failure. Renal compensation for imbalances is relatively slow (a matter of hours or days).

The lungs, under the control of the medulla, control the CO_2 and thus the carbonic acid content of the ECF. They do so by adjusting ventilation in response to the amount of CO_2 in the blood. A rise in the partial pressure of CO_2 in arterial blood ($PaCO_2$) is a powerful stimulant to respiration. Of course, the partial pressure of oxygen in arterial blood (PaO_2) also influences respiration. However, its effect is not as marked as that produced by the $PaCO_2$.

In metabolic acidosis, the respiratory rate increases, causing greater elimination of CO_2 (to reduce the acid load). In metabolic alkalosis, the respiratory rate decreases, causing CO_2 to be retained (to increase the acid load).

Acute and Chronic Metabolic Acidosis (Base Bicarbonate Deficit)

Metabolic acidosis is a clinical disturbance characterized by a low pH (increased H^+ concentration) and a low plasma bicarbonate concentration. It can be produced by a gain of hydrogen ion or a loss of bicarbonate (Whittier & Rutecki, 2004). It can be divided clinically into two forms, according to the values of the serum anion gap: high anion gap acidosis and normal anion gap acidosis. The anion gap reflects normally unmeasured anions (phosphates, sulfates, and proteins) in plasma. Measuring the anion gap is essential in analyzing acid–base disorders correctly. The anion gap can be calculated by either one of the following equations:

$$\text{Anion gap} = Na^+ + K^+ - (Cl^- + HCO_3^-)$$

$$\text{Anion gap} = Na^+ - (Cl^- + HCO_3^-)$$

Potassium is often omitted from the equation because of its low level in the plasma; therefore, the second equation is used more often than the first.

The normal value for an anion gap is 8 to 12 mEq/L (8 to 12 mmol/L) without potassium in the equation. If potassium is included in the equation, the normal value for the anion gap is 12 to 16 mEq/L (12 to 16 mmol/L). The unmeasured anions in the serum normally account for less than 16 mEq/L of the anion production. An anion gap greater than 16 mEq (16 mmol/L) suggests excessive accumulation of unmeasured anions. An anion gap occurs because not all electrolytes are measured. More anions are left unmeasured than cations.

Normal anion gap acidosis results from the direct loss of bicarbonate, as in diarrhea, lower intestinal fistulas, ureterostomies, and use of diuretics; early renal insufficiency; excessive administration of chloride; and the administration of parenteral nutrition without bicarbonate or bicarbonate-producing solutes (eg, lactate). Normal anion gap acidosis is also referred to as hyperchloremic acidosis. A reduced or negative anion gap is primarily caused by hypoproteinemia. Disorders that cause a decreased or negative anion gap are rare compared to those related to an increased or high anion gap (Rose & Post, 2000).

High anion gap acidosis results from excessive accumulation of fixed acid. If it is increased to 30 mEq/L (30 mmol/L) or more, then a high anion gap metabolic acidosis is present regardless of what the pH and the HCO_3^- are. High ion gap occurs in ketoacidosis, lactic acidosis, the late phase of salicylate poisoning, uremia, methanol or ethylene glycol toxicity, and ketoacidosis with starvation. The hydrogen is buffered by HCO_3^-, causing the bicarbonate concentration to fall. In all of these instances, abnormally high levels of anions flood the system, increasing the anion gap above normal limits.

Clinical Manifestations

Signs and symptoms of metabolic acidosis vary with the severity of the acidosis. They may include headache, confusion, drowsiness, increased respiratory rate and depth, nausea, and vomiting. Peripheral vasodilation and decreased cardiac output occur when the pH drops to less than 7. Additional physical assessment findings include decreased blood pressure, cold and clammy skin, dysrhythmias, and shock (Whittier & Rutecki, 2004). Chronic metabolic acidosis is usually seen with chronic renal failure. The bicarbonate and pH decrease slowly, and the patient is asymptomatic until the bicarbonate is approximately 15 mEq/L or less.

Assessment and Diagnostic Findings

Arterial blood gas measurements are valuable in diagnosing metabolic acidosis (Kee et al., 2004). Expected blood gas changes include a low bicarbonate level (less than 22 mEq/L) and a low pH (less than 7.35). The cardinal feature of metabolic acidosis is a decrease in the serum bicarbonate level. Hyperkalemia may accompany metabolic acidosis as a result of the shift of potassium out of the cells. Later, as the acidosis is corrected, potassium moves back into the cells and hypokalemia may occur. Hyperventilation decreases the CO_2 level as a compensatory action. As stated previously, calculation of the anion gap is helpful in determining the cause of metabolic acidosis. An ECG detects dysrhythmias caused by the increased potassium.

Medical Management

Treatment is directed at correcting the metabolic defect (Kee et al., 2004). If the problem results from excessive intake of chloride, treatment is aimed at eliminating the source of the chloride. When necessary, bicarbonate is administered if the pH is less than 7.1 and the serum bicarbonate level is less than 10 mEq/L. Although hyperkalemia occurs with acidosis, hypokalemia may occur with reversal of the acidosis and subsequent movement of potassium back into the cells. Therefore, the serum potassium level is monitored closely, and hypokalemia is corrected as acidosis is reversed.

In chronic metabolic acidosis, low serum calcium levels are treated before the chronic metabolic acidosis is treated, to avoid tetany resulting from an increase in pH and a decrease in ionized calcium. Alkalizing agents may be administered if the serum bicarbonate level is less than 12 mEq/L. Treatment modalities may also include hemodialysis or peritoneal dialysis.

Acute and Chronic Metabolic Alkalosis (Base Bicarbonate Excess)

Metabolic alkalosis is a clinical disturbance characterized by a high pH (decreased H^+ concentration) and a high plasma bicarbonate concentration. It can be produced by a gain of bicarbonate or a loss of H^+ (Porth, 2005).

Probably the most common cause of metabolic alkalosis is vomiting or gastric suction with loss of hydrogen and chloride ions. The disorder also occurs in pyloric stenosis, in which only gastric fluid is lost. Gastric fluid has an acid pH (usually 1 to 3), and loss of this highly acidic fluid increases the alkalinity of body fluids. Other situations predisposing to metabolic alkalosis include those associated with loss of potassium, such as diuretic therapy that promotes excretion of potassium (eg, thiazides, furosemide), and excessive adrenocorticoid hormones (as in hyperaldosteronism and Cushing's syndrome).

Hypokalemia produces alkalosis in two ways: (1) the kidneys conserve potassium, and therefore H^+ excretion increases; and (2) cellular potassium moves out of the cells into the ECF in an attempt to maintain near-normal serum levels (as potassium ions leave the cells, hydrogen ions must enter to maintain electroneutrality). Excessive alkali ingestion from antacids containing bicarbonate or from use of sodium bicarbonate during cardiopulmonary resuscitation can also cause metabolic alkalosis.

Chronic metabolic alkalosis can occur with long-term diuretic therapy (thiazides or furosemide), villous adenoma, external drainage of gastric fluids, significant potassium depletion, cystic fibrosis, and the chronic ingestion of milk and calcium carbonate.

Clinical Manifestations

Alkalosis is primarily manifested by symptoms related to decreased calcium ionization, such as tingling of the fingers and toes, dizziness, and hypertonic muscles. The ionized fraction of serum calcium decreases in alkalosis as more calcium combines with serum proteins. Because it is the ionized fraction of calcium that influences neuromuscular activity, symptoms of hypocalcemia are often the predominant symptoms of alkalosis. Respirations are depressed as a compensatory action by the lungs. Atrial tachycardia may occur. As the pH increases to greater than 7.6 and hypokalemia develops, ventricular disturbances may occur. Decreased motility and paralytic ileus may also occur.

Symptoms of chronic metabolic alkalosis are the same as for acute metabolic alkalosis, and as potassium decreases, frequent premature ventricular contractions or U waves are seen on the ECG.

Assessment and Diagnostic Findings

Evaluation of arterial blood gases reveals a pH greater than 7.45 and a serum bicarbonate concentration greater than 26 mEq/L. The $PaCO_2$ increases as the lungs attempt to compensate for the excess bicarbonate by retaining CO_2. This hypoventilation is more pronounced in semiconscious, unconscious, or debilitated patients than in alert patients. The former may develop marked hypoxemia as a result of hypoventilation. Hypokalemia may accompany metabolic alkalosis.

Urine chloride levels may help identify the cause of metabolic alkalosis if the patient's history provides inadequate information. Metabolic alkalosis is the setting in which urine chloride concentration may be a more accurate estimate of volume than the urine sodium concentration. Urine chloride concentrations help to differentiate between vomiting, diuretic therapy, and excessive adrenocorticosteroid secretion as the cause of the metabolic alkalosis. In patients with vomiting or cystic fibrosis, those receiving nutritional repletion, and those receiving diuretic therapy, hypovolemia and hypochloremia produce urine chloride concentrations lower than 25 mEq/L. Signs of hypovolemia are not present, and the urine chloride concentration exceeds 40 mEq/L in patients with mineralocorticoid excess or alkali loading; these patients usually have expanded fluid volume. The urine chloride concentration should be less than 15 mEq/L when decreased chloride levels and hypovolemia occur.

Medical Management

Treatment of both acute and chronic metabolic alkalosis is aimed at correcting the underlying acid–base disorder (Hogan & Wane, 2003). Because of volume depletion from GI loss, the patient's fluid I&O must be monitored carefully.

Sufficient chloride must be supplied for the kidney to absorb sodium with chloride (allowing the excretion of excess bicarbonate). Treatment also includes restoring normal fluid volume by administering sodium chloride fluids (because continued volume depletion serves to maintain the alkalosis). In patients with hypokalemia, potassium is administered as KCl to replace both K^+ and Cl^- losses. H_2 receptor antagonists, such as cimetidine (Tagamet), reduce the production of gastric HCl, thereby decreasing the metabolic alkalosis associated with gastric suction. Carbonic anhydrase inhibitors are useful in treating metabolic alkalosis in patients who cannot tolerate rapid volume expansion (eg, patients with heart failure).

Acute and Chronic Respiratory Acidosis (Carbonic Acid Excess)

Respiratory acidosis is a clinical disorder in which the pH is less than 7.35 and the $PaCO_2$ is greater than 42 mm Hg. It may be either acute or chronic.

Respiratory acidosis is always due to inadequate excretion of CO_2 with inadequate ventilation, resulting in elevated plasma CO_2 concentrations and, consequently, increased levels of carbonic acid (Morton, Fontaine, Hudak et al., 2005). In addition to an elevated $PaCO_2$, hypoventilation usually causes a decrease in PaO_2. Acute respiratory acidosis occurs in emergency situations, such as acute pulmonary edema, aspiration of a foreign object, atelectasis, pneumothorax, overdose of sedatives, sleep apnea syndrome, administration of oxygen to a patient with chronic hypercapnia (excessive CO_2 in the blood), severe pneumonia, and acute respiratory distress syndrome. Respiratory acidosis can also occur in diseases that impair respiratory muscles, such as muscular dystrophy, myasthenia gravis, and Guillain-Barré syndrome.

Mechanical ventilation may be associated with hypercapnia if the rate of effective alveolar ventilation is inadequate. Ventilation is fixed, and CO_2 may be retained if the rate of CO_2 production is increased.

Clinical Manifestations

Clinical signs in acute and chronic respiratory acidosis vary. Sudden hypercapnia (elevated $PaCO_2$) can cause increased pulse and respiratory rate, increased blood pressure, mental cloudiness, and a feeling of fullness in the head. An elevated $PaCO_2$ causes cerebrovascular vasodilation and increased cerebral blood flow, particularly when it is greater than 60 mm Hg. Ventricular fibrillation may be the first sign of respiratory acidosis in anesthetized patients.

If respiratory acidosis is severe, intracranial pressure may increase, resulting in papilledema and dilated conjunctival blood vessels. Hyperkalemia may result as the hydrogen concentration overwhelms the compensatory mechanisms and H^+ moves into cells, causing a shift of potassium out of the cell.

Chronic respiratory acidosis occurs with pulmonary diseases such as chronic emphysema and bronchitis, obstructive sleep apnea, and obesity. As long as the $PaCO_2$ does not exceed the body's ability to compensate, the patient will be asymptomatic. However, if the $PaCO_2$ increases rapidly, cerebral vasodilation will increase the intracranial pressure, and cyanosis and tachypnea will develop. Patients with chronic obstructive pulmonary disease (COPD) who gradually accumulate CO_2 over a prolonged period (days to months) may not develop symptoms of hypercapnia because compensatory renal changes have had time to occur.

NURSING ALERT

If the $PaCO_2$ is chronically higher than 50 mm Hg, the respiratory center becomes relatively insensitive to CO_2 as a respiratory stimulant, leaving hypoxemia as the major drive for respiration. Oxygen administration may remove the stimulus of hypoxemia, and the patient develops "carbon dioxide narcosis" unless the situation is quickly reversed. Therefore, oxygen is administered only with extreme caution.

Assessment and Diagnostic Findings

Arterial blood gas analysis reveals a pH lower than 7.35, a $PaCO_2$ greater than 42 mm Hg, and a variation in the bicarbonate level, depending on the duration of the acute respiratory acidosis. When compensation (renal retention of bicarbonate) has fully occurred, the arterial pH may be within the lower limits of normal. Depending on the cause of respiratory acidosis, other diagnostic measures would include monitoring of serum electrolyte levels, chest x-ray for determining any respiratory disease, and a drug screen if an overdose is suspected. An ECG to identify any cardiac involvement as a result of COPD may be indicated as well.

Medical Management

Treatment is directed at improving ventilation; exact measures vary with the cause of inadequate ventilation (Hogan & Wane, 2003). Pharmacologic agents are used as indicated. For example, bronchodilators help reduce bronchial spasm, antibiotics are used for respiratory infections, and thrombolytics or anticoagulants are used for pulmonary emboli.

Pulmonary hygiene measures are initiated, when necessary, to clear the respiratory tract of mucus and purulent drainage. Adequate hydration (2 to 3 L/day) is indicated to keep the mucous membranes moist and thereby facilitate the removal of secretions. Supplemental oxygen is administered as necessary.

Mechanical ventilation, used appropriately, may improve pulmonary ventilation. Inappropriate mechanical ventilation (eg, increased dead space, insufficient rate or volume settings, high fraction of inspired oxygen [FiO_2] with excessive CO_2 production) may cause such rapid excretion of CO_2 that the kidneys are unable to eliminate excess bicarbonate quickly enough to prevent alkalosis and seizures. For this reason, the elevated $PaCO_2$ must be decreased slowly. Placing the patient in a semi-Fowler's position facilitates expansion of the chest wall. Treatment of chronic respiratory acidosis is the same as for acute respiratory acidosis.

Acute and Chronic Respiratory Alkalosis (Carbonic Acid Deficit)

Respiratory alkalosis is a clinical condition in which the arterial pH is greater than 7.45 and the $PaCO_2$ is less than 38 mm Hg. As with respiratory acidosis, acute and chronic conditions can occur.

Respiratory alkalosis is always caused by hyperventilation, which causes excessive "blowing off" of CO_2 and, hence, a decrease in the plasma carbonic acid concentration. Causes can include extreme anxiety, hypoxemia, the early phase of salicylate intoxication, gram-negative bacteremia, and inappropriate ventilator settings that do not match the patient's requirements.

Chronic respiratory alkalosis results from chronic hypocapnia, and decreased serum bicarbonate levels are the consequence. Chronic hepatic insufficiency and cerebral tumors are predisposing factors.

Clinical Manifestations

Clinical signs consist of lightheadedness due to vasoconstriction and decreased cerebral blood flow, inability to concentrate, numbness and tingling from decreased calcium ionization, tinnitus, and sometimes loss of consciousness. Cardiac effects of respiratory alkalosis include tachycardia and ventricular and atrial dysrhythmias (Heitz & Horne, 2005).

Assessment and Diagnostic Findings

Analysis of arterial blood gases assists in the diagnosis of respiratory alkalosis. In the acute state, the pH is elevated above normal as a result of a low $PaCO_2$ and a normal bicarbonate level. (The kidneys cannot alter the bicarbonate level quickly.) In the compensated state, the kidneys have had sufficient time to lower the bicarbonate level to a near-normal level. Evaluation of serum electrolytes is indicated to identify any decrease in potassium as hydrogen is pulled out of the cells in exchange for potassium; decreased calcium, as severe alkalosis inhibits calcium ionization, resulting in carpopedal spasms and tetany; or decreased phosphate due to alkalosis, causing an increased uptake of phosphate by the cells. A toxicology screen should be performed to rule out salicylate intoxication.

Patients with chronic respiratory alkalosis are usually asymptomatic, and the diagnostic evaluation and plan of care are the same as for acute respiratory alkalosis.

Medical Management

Treatment depends on the underlying cause of respiratory alkalosis. If the cause is anxiety, the patient is instructed to breathe more slowly to allow CO_2 to accumulate or to breathe into a closed system (such as a paper bag). A sedative may be required to relieve hyperventilation in very anxious patients. Treatment of other causes of respiratory alkalosis is directed at correcting the underlying problem.

Mixed Acid–Base Disorders

Patients can simultaneously experience two or more independent acid–base disorders. A normal pH in the presence of changes in the $PaCO_2$ and plasma HCO_3^- concentration immediately suggests a mixed disorder. The only mixed disorder that cannot occur is a mixed respiratory acidosis and alkalosis, because it is impossible to have alveolar hypoventilation and hyperventilation at the same time. An example of a mixed disorder is the simultaneous occurrence of metabolic acidosis and respiratory acidosis during respiratory and cardiac arrest.

Compensation

Generally, the pulmonary and renal systems compensate for each other to return the pH to normal. In a single acid–base disorder, the system not causing the problem will try to compensate by returning the ratio of bicarbonate to carbonic acid to the normal 20:1. The lungs compensate for metabolic disturbances by changing CO_2 excretion. The kidneys compensate for respiratory disturbances by altering bicarbonate retention and H^+ secretion.

In respiratory acidosis, excess hydrogen is excreted in the urine in exchange for bicarbonate ions. In respiratory alkalosis, the renal excretion of bicarbonate increases, and hydrogen ions are retained. In metabolic acidosis, the compensatory mechanisms increase the ventilation rate and the renal retention of bicarbonate.

In metabolic alkalosis, the respiratory system compensates by decreasing ventilation to conserve CO_2 and increase the $PaCO_2$. Because the lungs respond to acid–base disorders within minutes, compensation for metabolic imbalances occurs faster than compensation for respiratory imbalances. Table 14-6 summarizes compensation effects.

Blood Gas Analysis

Blood gas analysis is often used to identify the specific acid–base disturbance and the degree of compensation that has occurred. The analysis is usually based on an arterial blood sample, but if an arterial sample cannot be obtained, a mixed venous sample may be used. Results of arterial blood gas analysis provide information about alveolar ventilation, oxygenation, and acid–base balance. It is necessary to evaluate the concentrations of serum electrolytes (sodium, potassium, and chloride) and carbon dioxide along with arterial blood gas data, because they are often the first sign of an acid–base disorder. The health history, physical examination, previous blood gas results, and serum electrolytes should always be part of the assessment used to determine the cause of the acid–base disorder (Porth, 2005). Treatment of the underlying condition usually corrects most acid–base disorders. Table 14-7 compares normal ranges of venous and arterial blood gas values. See also Chart 14-2.

Parenteral Fluid Therapy

When no other route of administration is available, fluids are administered intravenously in hospitals, outpatient di-

TABLE 14-6 Acid–Base Disturbances and Compensation

Disorder	Initial Event	Compensation
Respiratory acidosis	↓ pH, ↑ or normal HCO_3^-, ↑ $PaCO_2$	↑ Renal acid excretion and ↑ serum HCO_3^-
Respiratory alkalosis	↑ pH, ↓ or normal HCO_3^-, ↓ $PaCO_2$	↓ Renal acid excretion and ↓ serum HCO_3^-
Metabolic acidosis	↓ pH, ↓ HCO_3^-, ↓ or normal $PaCO_2$	Hyperventilation with resulting ↓ PaCO (conserves HCO_3^-)
Metabolic alkalosis	↑ pH, ↑ HCO_3^-, ↑ or normal $PaCO_2$	Hypoventilation with resulting ↑ $PaCO_2$

TABLE 14-7 Normal Values for Arterial and Mixed Venous Blood

Parameter	Arterial Blood	Mixed Venous Blood
pH	7.35–7.45	7.33–7.41
$PaCO_2$	35–45 mm Hg	41–51 mm Hg
PaO_2*	80–100 mm Hg	35–40 mm Hg
HCO_3^-	22–26 mEq/L	22–26 mEq/L
Base excess/deficit	± 2 mEq/L	± 2 mEq/L
Oxygen saturation	> 94%	75%

*At altitudes of 3,000 feet and higher, the values for oxygen are decreased.

agnostic and surgical settings, clinics, and homes to replace fluids, administer medications, and provide nutrients.

Purpose

The choice of an IV solution depends on the purpose of its administration. Generally, IV fluids are administered to achieve one or more of the following goals:

- To provide water, electrolytes, and nutrients to meet daily requirements
- To replace water and correct electrolyte deficits
- To administer medications and blood products

IV solutions contain dextrose or electrolytes mixed in various proportions with water. Pure, electrolyte-free water can never be administered IV because it rapidly enters red blood cells and causes them to rupture.

Types of Intravenous Solutions

Solutions are often categorized as **isotonic**, **hypotonic**, or **hypertonic**, according to whether their total osmolality is the same as, less than, or greater than that of blood (see earlier discussion of osmolality).

Electrolyte solutions are considered isotonic if the total electrolyte content (anions + cations) is approximately 310 mEq/L, hypotonic if the total electrolyte content is less than 250 mEq/L, and hypertonic if the total electrolyte content is greater than 375 mEq/L. The nurse must also consider a solution's osmolality, keeping in mind that the osmolality of plasma is approximately 300 mOsm/L (300 mmol/L). For example, a 10% dextrose solution has an osmolality of approximately 505 mOsm/L.

When administering parenteral fluids, the nurse monitors the patient's response to the fluids, considering the fluid volume, the content of the fluid, and the patient's clinical status.

Isotonic Fluids

Fluids that are classified as isotonic have a total osmolality close to that of the ECF and do not cause red blood cells to shrink or swell. The composition of these fluids may or may not approximate that of the ECF. Isotonic fluids expand the ECF volume. One liter of isotonic fluid expands the ECF by 1 L; however, it expands the plasma by only 0.25 L because it is a crystalloid fluid and diffuses quickly into the ECF compartment. For the same reason, 3 L of isotonic fluid is needed to replace 1 L of blood loss. Because these fluids expand the intravascular space, patients with hypertension and heart failure should be carefully monitored for signs of fluid overload.

D_5W

A solution of D_5W has a serum osmolality of 252 mOsm/L. Once administered, the glucose is rapidly metabolized, and this initially isotonic solution then disperses as a hypotonic fluid, one-third extracellular and two-thirds intracellular. It is essential to consider this action of D_5W, especially if the patient is at risk for increased intracranial pressure. During fluid resuscitation, this solution should not be used, because it can cause hyperglycemia. Therefore, D_5W is used mainly to supply water and to correct an increased serum osmolality. About 1 L of D_5W provides fewer than 200 kcal and is a minor source of the body's daily caloric requirements.

NORMAL SALINE SOLUTION

Normal saline (0.9% sodium chloride) solution has a total osmolality of 308 mOsm/L. Because the osmolality is entirely contributed by electrolytes, the solution remains within the ECF. For this reason, normal saline solution is often used to correct an extracellular volume deficit. Although referred to as "normal," it contains only sodium and chloride and does not actually simulate the ECF. It is used with administration of blood transfusions and to replace large sodium losses, as in burn injuries. It is not used for heart failure, pulmonary edema, renal impairment, or sodium retention. Normal saline does not supply calories.

OTHER ISOTONIC SOLUTIONS

Several other solutions contain ions in addition to sodium and chloride and are somewhat similar to the ECF in composition. Lactated Ringer's solution contains potassium and calcium in addition to sodium chloride. It is used to correct dehydration and sodium depletion and replace GI losses. Lactated Ringer's solution contains bicarbonate precursors as well. These solutions are marketed, with slight variations, under various trade names.

Hypotonic Fluids

One purpose of hypotonic solutions is to replace cellular fluid, because it is hypotonic compared with plasma. Another is to provide free water for excretion of body wastes. At times, hypotonic sodium solutions are used to treat hypernatremia and other hyperosmolar conditions. Half-strength saline (0.45% sodium chloride) solution, with an osmolality of 154 mOsm/L, is frequently used. Multiple-electrolyte solutions are also available. Excessive infusions of hypotonic solutions can lead to intravascular fluid depletion, decreased blood pressure, cellular edema, and cell damage. These solutions exert less osmotic pressure than the ECF.

Hypertonic Fluids

When normal saline solution or lactated Ringer's solution contains 5% dextrose, the total osmolality exceeds that of the ECF. However, the dextrose is quickly metabolized, and only the isotonic solution remains. Therefore, any effect on the intracellular compartment is temporary.

CHART 14-2

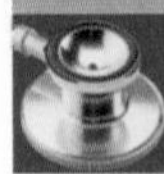

Assessing for Arterial Blood Gases

The following steps are recommended to evaluate arterial blood gas values. They are based on the assumption that the average values are:

pH = 7.4
$PaCO_2$ = 40 mm Hg
HCO_3^- = 24 mEq/L

1. *First, note the pH.* It can be high, low, or normal, as follows:
   pH > 7.4 (alkalosis)
   pH < 7.4 (acidosis)
   pH = 7.4 (normal)

   A normal pH may indicate perfectly normal blood gases, *or* it may be an indication of a *compensated* imbalance. A compensated imbalance is one in which the body has been able to correct the pH by either respiratory or metabolic changes (depending on the primary problem). For example, a patient with primary metabolic acidosis starts out with a low bicarbonate level but a normal CO_2 level. Soon afterward, the lungs try to compensate for the imbalance by exhaling large amounts of CO_2 (hyperventilation). As another example, a patient with primary respiratory acidosis starts out with a high CO_2 level; soon afterward, the kidneys attempt to compensate by retaining bicarbonate. If the compensatory mechanism is able to restore the bicarbonate to carbonic acid ratio back to 20:1, full compensation (and thus normal pH) will be achieved.
2. The next step is to determine the primary cause of the disturbance. This is done by evaluating the $PaCO_2$ and HCO_3^- in relation to the pH.

   Example: pH > 7.4 (alkalosis)

   a. If the $PaCO_2$ is < 40 mm Hg, the primary disturbance is respiratory alkalosis. (This situation occurs when a patient hyperventilates and "blows off" too much CO_2. Recall that CO_2 dissolved in water becomes carbonic acid, the acid side of the "carbonic acid–bicarbonate buffer system.")

   b. If the HCO_3^- is >24 mEq/L, the primary disturbance is metabolic alkalosis. (This situation occurs when the body gains too much bicarbonate, an alkaline substance. Bicarbonate is the basic or alkaline side of the "carbonic acid–bicarbonate buffer system.")

   Example: pH < 7.4 (acidosis)

   a. If the $PaCO_2$ is >40 mm Hg, the primary disturbance is respiratory acidosis. (This situation occurs when a patient hypoventilates and thus retains too much CO_2, an acidic substance.)

   b. If the HCO_3^- is <24 mEq/L, the primary disturbance is metabolic acidosis. (This situation occurs when the body's bicarbonate level drops, either because of direct bicarbonate loss or because of gains of acids such as lactic acid or ketones.)
3. The next step involves determining if compensation has begun. This is done by looking at the value other than the primary disorder. If it is moving in the same direction as the primary value, compensation is underway. Consider the following gases:

pH	$PaCO_2$	HCO_3^-
(1) 7.2	60 mm Hg	24 mEq/L
(2) 7.4	60 mm Hg	37 mEq/L

   The first set (1) indicates acute respiratory acidosis without compensation (the $PaCO_2$ is high, the HCO_3^- is normal). The second set (2) indicates chronic respiratory acidosis. Note that compensation has take place; that is, the HCO_3^- has elevated to an appropriate level to balance the high $PaCO_2$ and produce a normal pH.
4. Two distinct acid–base disturbances may occur simultaneously. These can be identified when the pH does not explain one of the changes.

   Example: Metabolic and respiratory acidosis

a. pH	7.2	decreased acid
b. $PaCO_2$	52	increased acid
c. HCO_3	13	decreased acid

   This is an example of metabolic and respiratory acidosis.

Similarly, with hypotonic multiple-electrolyte solutions containing 5% dextrose, once the dextrose is metabolized, these solutions disperse as hypotonic fluids.

Higher concentrations of dextrose, such as 50% dextrose in water, are administered to help meet caloric requirements. These solutions are strongly hypertonic and must be administered into central veins so that they can be diluted by rapid blood flow.

Saline solutions are also available in osmolar concentrations greater than that of the ECF. These solutions draw water from the ICF to the ECF and cause cells to shrink. If administered rapidly or in large quantity, they may cause an extracellular volume excess and precipitate circulatory overload and dehydration. As a result, these solutions must be administered cautiously and usually only when the serum osmolality has decreased to dangerously low levels. Hypertonic solutions exert an osmotic pressure greater than that of the ECF.

Other Intravenous Substances

When the patient's GI tract is unable to tolerate food, nutritional requirements are often met using the IV route. Parenteral solutions may include high concentrations of glucose, protein, or fat to meet nutritional requirements (see Chapter 36). The parenteral route may also be used to administer colloids, plasma expanders, and blood products. Examples of blood products include whole blood, packed red blood cells, albumin, and cryoprecipitate; these are discussed in more detail in Chapter 33.

Many medications are also delivered by the IV route, either by infusion or directly into the vein. Because IV medications enter the circulation rapidly, administration by this route is potentially very hazardous. All medications can produce adverse reactions; however, medications administered by the IV route can cause these reactions within 15 minutes after administration, because the medications are delivered directly into the bloodstream. Administration rates and recommended dilutions for individual medications are available in specialized texts pertaining to IV medications and in manufacturers' package inserts; these should be consulted to ensure safe IV administration of medications.

NURSING ALERT

The nurse must assess the patient for a history of allergic reactions to medications. Although this is important when any medication is to be administered, it is even more important with IV administration, because the medication is delivered directly into the bloodstream.

Nursing Management of the Patient Receiving Intravenous Therapy

CONCEPTS in action ANIMATION

The ability to perform venipuncture to gain access to the venous system for administering fluids and medication is an expected nursing skill in many settings. This responsibility includes selecting the appropriate venipuncture site and type of cannula and being proficient in the technique of vein entry.

Preparing to Administer Intravenous Therapy

Before performing venipuncture, the nurse carries out hand hygiene, applies gloves, and informs the patient about the procedure. Next, the nurse selects the most appropriate insertion site and type of cannula for a particular patient. Factors influencing these choices include the type of solution to be administered, the expected duration of IV therapy, the patient's general condition, and the availability of veins. The skill of the person initiating the infusion is also an important consideration.

Choosing an Intravenous Site

Many sites can be used for IV therapy, but ease of access and potential hazards vary. Veins of the extremities are designated as peripheral locations and are ordinarily the only sites used by nurses. Because they are relatively safe and easy to enter, arm veins are most commonly used (Fig. 14-7). The metacarpal, cephalic, basilic, and median veins and their branches are recommended sites because of their size and ease of access. More distal sites should be used first, with more proximal sites used subsequently. Leg veins should rarely, if ever, be used because of the high risk of thromboembolism. Additional sites to avoid include veins distal to a previous IV infiltration or phlebitic area, sclerosed or thrombosed veins, an arm with an arteriovenous shunt or fistula, and an arm affected by edema, infection, blood clot, or skin breakdown. The arm on the side of a mastectomy is avoided because of impaired lymphatic flow.

Central veins commonly used by physicians include the subclavian and internal jugular veins. It is possible to gain access to (or cannulate) these larger vessels even when peripheral sites have collapsed, and they allow for the administration of hyperosmolar solutions. However, the potential hazards are much greater and include inadvertent entry into an artery or the pleural space.

Ideally, both arms and hands are carefully inspected before a specific venipuncture site that does not interfere with

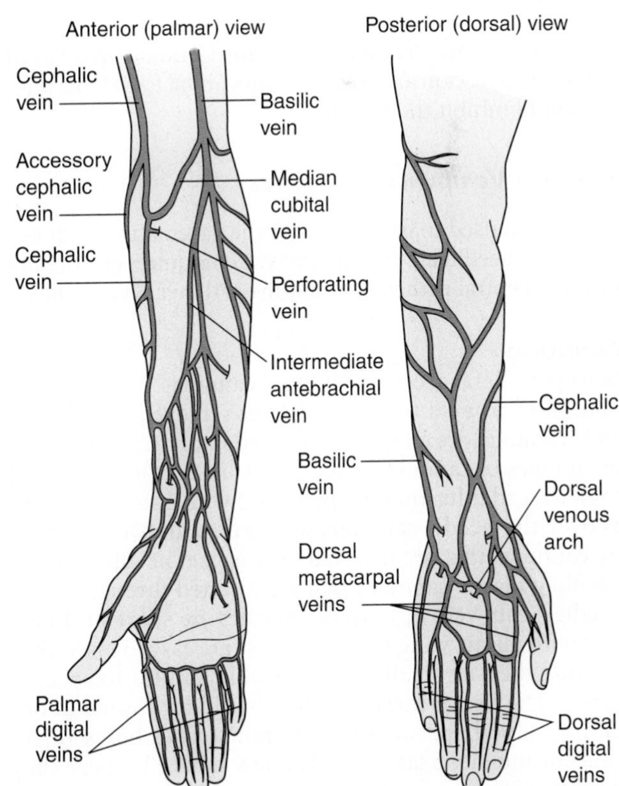

FIGURE 14-7. Site selection for peripheral cannulation of veins: anterior (palmar) veins at *left*, posterior (dorsal) veins at *right*. Adapted from Agur, A. M. R., Lee, M. J. & Boileau Grant, M. J. (1999). *Grant's atlas of anatomy* (10th ed.). Philadelphia: Lippincott Williams & Wilkins.

mobility is chosen. For this reason, the antecubital fossa is avoided, except as a last resort. The most distal site of the arm or hand is generally used first, so that subsequent IV access sites can be moved progressively upward. The following factors should be considered when selecting a site for venipuncture:

- Condition of the vein
- Type of fluid or medication to be infused
- Duration of therapy
- Patient's age and size
- Whether the patient is right- or left-handed
- Patient's medical history and current health status
- Skill of the person performing the venipuncture

After applying a tourniquet, the nurse palpates and inspects the vein. The vein should feel firm, elastic, engorged, and round—not hard, flat, or bumpy. Because arteries lie close to veins in the antecubital fossa, the vessel should be palpated for arterial pulsation (even with a tourniquet on), and cannulation of pulsating vessels should be avoided. General guidelines for selecting a cannula include the following:

- Length: 0.75 to 1.25 inches long
- Diameter: narrow diameter of the cannula to occupy minimal space within the vein
- Gauge: 20 to 22 gauge for most IV fluids; a larger gauge for caustic or viscous solutions; 14 to 18 gauge for blood administration and for trauma patients and those undergoing surgery

Hand veins are easiest to cannulate. Cannula tips should not rest in a flexion area (eg, the antecubital fossa), because this could inhibit the IV flow.

Selecting Venipuncture Devices

Equipment used to gain access to the vasculature includes cannulas, needleless IV delivery systems, and peripherally inserted central catheter or midline catheter access lines.

CANNULAS

Most peripheral access devices are cannulas. They have an obturator inside a tube that is later removed. "Catheter" and "cannula" are terms that are used interchangeably. The main types of cannula devices available are those referred to as winged infusion sets (butterfly) with a steel needle or as over-the-needle catheters with wings; indwelling plastic cannulas that are inserted over a steel needle; and indwelling plastic cannulas that are inserted through a steel needle. Scalp vein or butterfly needles are short steel needles with plastic wing handles. These are easy to insert, but because they are small and nonpliable, infiltration occurs easily. The use of these needles should be limited to obtaining blood specimens or administering bolus injections or infusions lasting only a few hours, because they increase the risk of vein injury and infiltration. Insertion of an over-the-needle catheter requires the additional step of advancing the catheter into the vein after venipuncture. Because these devices are less likely to cause infiltration, they are frequently preferred over winged infusion sets.

Plastic cannulas inserted through a hollow needle are usually called intracatheters. They are available in long lengths and are well suited for placement in central locations. Because insertion requires threading the cannula through the vein for a relatively long distance, these can be difficult to insert. The most commonly used infusion device is the over-the-needle catheter. A hollow metal stylet is preinserted into the catheter and extends through the distal tip of the catheter to allow puncture of the vessel, in an effort to guide the catheter as the venipuncture is performed. The vein is punctured and a flashback of blood appears in the closed chamber behind the catheter hub. The catheter is threaded through the stylet into the vein and the stylet is then removed. Many safety over-the-needle catheter designs with retracting stylets are available to protect health care workers from needlestick injuries.

Many types of cannulas are available for IV therapy. Some of the variations in these cannulas include the thickness of the cannula wall (affects rate of flow), the sharpness of the insertion needles (determines needle insertion technique), the softening properties of the cannula (influences the length of time the cannula can remain in place), safety features (minimizes risk of needlestick injuries and bloodborne exposure), and the number of lumens (determines the number of solutions that can be infused simultaneously). Cannula systems that help prevent needlesticks and transmission of bloodborne diseases are discussed later in this chapter. Most standard peripheral catheters are composed of some form of plastic. Teflon (polytetrafluoroethylene)–coated catheters have fewer thrombogenic properties and are less inflammatory than those coated with polyurethane or polyvinyl chloride (PVC). Catheters for steel needles can range from 3/8 inch to 1.5 inches in length and can be 27 to 13 gauge in size. Plastic catheters can range in length from 5/8 inch to 2 inches or as long as 12 inches and range in size from 27 to 12 gauge.

To select the ideal product for use, consideration should be given to which product provides the greatest patient satisfaction and offers quality, cost-effective infusion care. All devices should be radiopaque to determine catheter location by x-ray, if necessary. All catheters are thrombogenic and differ only in the incidence of thrombus occurrence. Biocompatibility, another characteristic of a catheter, ensures that inflammation and irritation do not occur. Silicone catheters are the most bioinert catheters available today.

Needleless Intravenous Delivery Systems. The federal Needlestick Safety and Prevention Act, which was signed into law in November of 2000, requires needleless systems. In an effort to decrease needlestick injuries and exposure to human immunodeficiency virus (HIV), hepatitis, and other bloodborne pathogens, agencies have implemented needleless IV delivery systems. These systems have built-in protection against needlestick injuries and provide a safe means of using and disposing of an IV administration set (which consists of tubing, an area for inserting the tubing into the container of IV fluid, and an adapter for connecting the tubing to the needle). Numerous companies produce needleless components. IV line connectors allow the simultaneous infusion of IV medications and other intermittent medications (known as a piggyback delivery) without the use of needles (Fig. 14-8). Technology is advancing and moving away from use of the traditional stylet. An

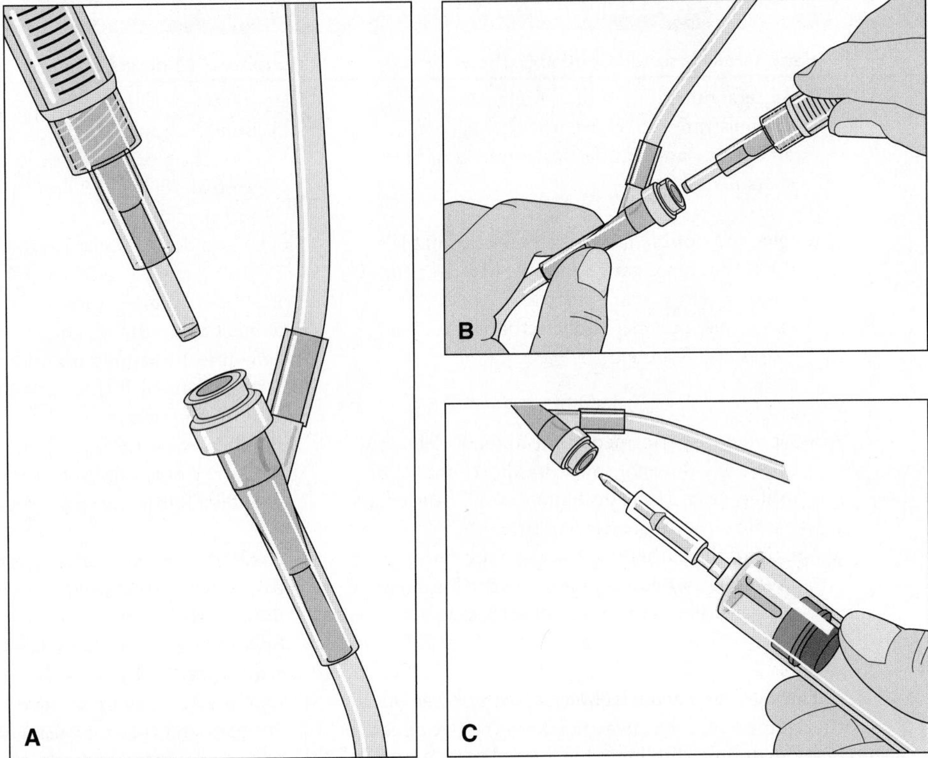

FIGURE 14-8. One example of a needleless intravenous access device. The Clearink Access System (Baxter Healthcare Corp., Becton Dickinson Division, Franklin Lakes, NJ) (**A**) is designed to prevent needlesticks and other accidents. After drawing medication into a syringe according to the manufacturer's guidelines and swabbing the Y-site intersection with antiseptic, the nurse can insert the syringe-cannula apparatus into the Y site (**B**) and deliver bolus dose medications. If a blood tube holder (**C**) is attached to the cannula, blood can be withdrawn safely without fear of contact or spills.

example is a self-sheathing stylet that is recessed into a rigid chamber at the hub of the catheter when its insertion is complete. Other designs have placed the stylet at the end of a flexible wire to avoid needlesticks.

Many examples of these devices are on the market. Each institution must evaluate products to determine its own needs based on Occupational Safety and Health Administration (OSHA) guidelines and the institution's policies and procedures.

Peripherally Inserted Central Catheter or Peripheral-Midline Catheter Access Lines. Patients who need moderate- to long-term parenteral therapy often receive a peripherally inserted central catheter or a peripheral-midline catheter. These catheters are also used for patients with limited peripheral access (eg, obese or emaciated patients, IV/injection drug users) who require IV antibiotics, blood, and parenteral nutrition. For these devices to be used, the median cephalic, basilic, and cephalic veins must be pliable (not sclerosed or hardened) and not subject to repeated puncture. If these veins are damaged, then central venous access via the subclavian or internal jugular vein, or surgical placement of an implanted port or a vascular access device, must be considered as an alternative. Table 14-8 compares peripherally inserted central and peripheral-midline catheters.

The principles for inserting these lines are much the same as those for inserting peripheral catheters; however, their insertion should be undertaken only by practitioners who are experienced and specially skilled in inserting IV lines.

The physician prescribes the line and the solution to be infused. Insertion of either catheter requires sterile technique. The size of the catheter lumen chosen is based on the type of solution, the patient's body size, and the vein to be used. The patient's consent is obtained before use of these catheters. Use of the dominant arm is recommended as the site for inserting the cannula into the superior vena cava to ensure adequate arm movement, which encourages blood flow and reduces the risk of dependent edema.

Teaching the Patient

Except in emergency situations, a patient should be prepared in advance for an IV infusion. The venipuncture, the expected length of infusion, and activity restrictions are explained. If the patient requires alternative formats (eg, interpreter, large-print written materials) to understand the procedure, these should be provided. Then the patient should have an opportunity to ask questions and express concerns. For example, some patients believe that they will die if small bubbles in the tubing enter their veins. After acknowledging this fear, the nurse can explain that usually only relatively large volumes of air administered rapidly are dangerous.

TABLE 14-8 Comparison of Peripherally Inserted Central and Peripheral-Midline Catheters

	Peripherally Inserted Central Catheter	Peripheral-Midline Catheter
Indications	Parenteral nutrition; IV fluid replacement; administration of chemotherapy agents, analgesics, and antibiotics; removal of blood specimens	Parenteral nutrition; IV fluid replacement; administration of analgesics and antibiotics (no solution or medications with a pH <5 or >9 or osmolarity >500 mOsm/L); removal of blood specimens
Features	Single- and double-lumen catheters available 40–60 cm long; gauge variable (16–24 gauge)	Single- and double-lumen catheters available (16–24 gauge) 7.5–20 cm in length. Can increase two gauges in size as it softens
Material	Radiopaque, polymer (polyurethane), Silastic materials. Flexible.	Silicone, polyurethane, and their derivatives; available impregnated with heparin to ↓ thrombogenicity (radiopaque or clear, with radiopaque strip)
Insertion sites	Venipuncture performed in the antecubital fossa, above or below it into the basilic, cephalic, or axillary veins of the dominant arm. The median basilic is the ideal insertion site.	Venipuncture performed 1½ inches above or below the antecubital fossa through the cephalic, basilic, or median cubital vein.
Catheter placement	The tip of the catheter lies in the superior vena cava. The catheter is placed via the basilic or cephalic vein at the antecubital fossa.	Between the antecubital area and the head of the clavicle (tip in axilla region). The tip terminates in the proximal portion of the extremity below axilla and proximal to central veins and is advanced 3–10 inches.
Insertion method	Through-the-needle technique, with or without a guidewire, breakaway needle with introducer or cannula with introducer (peelaway sheath). (A peripherally inserted central catheter can also be used as a midline catheter.) Insertion can be accomplished at the bedside using sterile technique. Arm to be used should be positioned in abduction to 90-degree angle. Consent is required. Catheter may stay in place for up to 12 months or as long as required without complications.	No separate guidewire or introducer is needed. Stiff catheter is passed using the catheter advancement tab. Insertion can be accomplished at the bedside using sterile technique. Arm to be used should be positioned in abduction to 45-degree angle. Consent is required. Catheter may stay in place for 2–4 weeks.
Potential complications	Malposition, pneumothorax, hemothorax, hydrothorax, dysrhythmias, nerve or tendon damage, respiratory distress, catheter embolism, thrombophlebitis, or catheter occlusion. Compared with centrally placed catheters, venipuncture in the antecubital space reduces risk of insertion complications.	Thrombosis, phlebitis, air embolism, infection, vascular perforation, bleeding, catheter transection, occlusion
Contraindications	Dermatitis, cellulitis, burns, high fluid volume infusions, rapid bolus injections, hemodialysis, and venous thrombosis. No clamping of this catheter or splinting of the arm permitted. No blood pressure or tourniquets to be used on extremity where peripherally inserted central catheter is inserted.	Dermatitis, cellulitis, burns, high fluid volume infusions, rapid bolus injection, hemodialysis, and venous thrombosis. No blood pressure or tourniquet to be used on extremity where midline catheter is placed.
Catheter maintenance	Sterile dressing changes according to agency policy and procedures. Generally, dressing is changed 2 or 3 ×/week or when wet, soiled, or nonocclusive. Line is flushed every 12 hours with 3 mL normal saline followed by heparin 3 mL (100 U/mL) per lumen.	Sterile dressing changes according to policy and procedures. Generally, dressing is changed 2 or 3 ×/week or when wet, soiled, or nonocclusive. Line is flushed after each infusion or every 12 hours with 5–10 mL normal saline followed by 1 mL of heparin (100 U/mL). Catheter must be anchored securely to prevent its dislodgment.
Postplacement	Chest x-ray needed to confirm placement of catheter tip.	Chest x-ray to assess placement may be obtained if unable to flush catheter, if no free flow blood return, if difficulty with catheter advancement, or if guidewire difficult to remove or bent on removal.

TABLE 14-8 Comparison of Peripherally Inserted Central and Peripheral-Midline Catheters (Continued)

	Peripherally Inserted Central Catheter	Peripheral-Midline Catheter
Assessment	Daily measurement of arm circumference (4″ above insertion site) and length of exposed catheter	Daily measurement of arm circumference (4″ above insertion site) and length of exposed catheter
Removal	Catheter should be removed when no longer indicated for use, if contaminated, or if complications occur. Arm is abducted during removal. Patient should be in a dorsal recumbent position with head of bed flat and should perform the Valsalva maneuver while catheter is withdrawn. Pressure is applied on removal with a sterile dressing and antiseptic ointment to site. Dressing is changed every 24 hours until epithelialization occurs.	Catheter should be removed when no longer indicated for use, if contaminated, or if complications occur. Arm is abducted during removal. Pressure is applied on removal with a sterile dressing and antiseptic ointment to site. Dressing is changed every 24 hours until epithelialization occurs.
Advantages	Reduces cost and avoids repeated venipunctures compared with centrally placed catheters. Decreases incidence of catheter-related infections.	Reduces cost and avoids repeated venipunctures compared with centrally placed catheters. Decreases incidence of catheter-related infections.

Preparing the Intravenous Site

Before preparing the skin, the nurse should ask the patient whether he or she is allergic to latex or iodine, products commonly used in preparing for IV therapy. Excessive hair at the selected site may be removed by clipping to increase the visibility of the veins and to facilitate insertion of the cannula and adherence of dressings to the IV insertion site. Because infection can be a major complication of IV therapy, the IV device, the fluid, the container, and the tubing must be sterile. The insertion site is scrubbed with a sterile pad soaked in 10% povidone–iodine (Betadine) or chlorhexidine gluconate solution for 30 seconds, working from the center of the area to the periphery and allowing the area to air dry for approximately 2 minutes. The site should not be wiped with 70% alcohol, because the alcohol negates the effect of the disinfecting solution. (Alcohol pledgets are used for 30 seconds instead, only if the patient is allergic to iodine.) The nurse must perform hand hygiene and put on gloves. Gloves (nonsterile, disposable) must be worn during the venipuncture procedure because of the likelihood of coming into contact with the patient's blood.

Performing Venipuncture

Guidelines and a suggested sequence for venipuncture are presented in Chart 14-3. For veins that are very small or particularly fragile, modifications in the technique may be necessary. Alternative methods can be found in journal articles or in specialized textbooks of IV therapy. Institutional policies and procedures determine whether all nurses must be certified to perform venipuncture. A nurse certified in IV therapy or an IV team can be consulted to assist with initiating IV therapy.

Maintaining Therapy

Maintaining an existing IV infusion is a nursing responsibility that demands knowledge of the solutions being administered and the principles of flow. In addition, patients must be assessed carefully for both local and systemic complications.

Factors Affecting Flow

The flow of an IV infusion is governed by the same principles that govern fluid movement in general:

- Flow is directly proportional to the height of the liquid column. Raising the height of the infusion container may improve a sluggish flow.
- Flow is directly proportional to the diameter of the tubing. The clamp on IV tubing regulates the flow by changing the tubing diameter. In addition, the flow is faster through large-gauge rather than small-gauge cannulas.
- Flow is inversely proportional to the length of the tubing. Adding extension tubing to an IV line decreases the flow.
- Flow is inversely proportional to the viscosity of a fluid. Viscous IV solutions, such as blood, require a larger cannula than do water or saline solutions.

Monitoring Flow

Because so many factors influence gravity flow, a solution does not necessarily continue to run at the speed originally set. Therefore, the nurse monitors IV infusions frequently to make sure that the fluid is flowing at the intended rate. The IV container should be marked with tape to indicate at a glance whether the correct amount has infused. The flow rate is calculated when the solution is originally started and then monitored at least hourly. To calculate the flow rate, the nurse determines the number of drops delivered per milliliter; this varies with equipment and is usually printed on the administration set packaging. A formula that can be used to calculate the drop rate is

$$\text{gtt/mL of infusion set}/60(\text{min in 1 hr}) \times \text{total hourly volume} = \text{gtt/min}$$

CHART 14-3

Guidelines for Starting an Intravenous Infusion

NURSING ACTION	RATIONALE
Preparation	
1. Verify prescription for IV therapy, check solution label, and identify patient.	1. Serious errors can be avoided by careful checking.
2. Explain procedure to patient.	2. Knowledge increases patient comfort and cooperation.
3. Carry out hand hygiene and put on disposable non-latex gloves.	3. Asepsis is essential to prevent infection. Use of non-latex gloves prevents exposure of nurse to patient's blood and of patient and nurse to latex.
4. Apply a tourniquet 4–6 inches above the site and identify a suitable vein.	4. This will distend the veins and allow them to be visualized.
5. Choose site. Use distal veins of hands and arms first.	5. Careful site selection will increase likelihood of successful venipuncture and preservation of vein. Using distal sites first preserves sites proximal to the previously cannulated site for subsequent venipunctures. Veins of feet and lower extremity should be avoided due to risk of thrombophlebitis. (In consultation with the physician, the saphenous vein of the ankle or dorsum of the foot may occasionally be used.)
6. Choose IV cannula or catheter.	6. Length and gauge of cannula should be appropriate for both site and purpose of infusion. The shortest gauge and length needed to deliver prescribed therapy should be used.
7. Connect infusion bag and tubing, and run solution through tubing to displace air; cover end of tubing.	7. Prevents delay; equipment must be ready to connect immediately after successful venipuncture to prevent clotting
8. Raise bed to comfortable working height and position for patient; adjust lighting. Position patient's arm below heart level to encourage capillary filling. Place protective pad on bed under patient's arm.	8. Proper positioning will increase likelihood of success and provide comfort for patient.
Procedure	
1. Depending on agency policy and procedure, lidocaine 1% (without epinephrine) 0.1–0.2 mL may be injected locally to the IV site or a transdermal analgesic cream (EMLA) may be applied to the site 60 minutes before IV placement or blood withdrawal. Alternatively, topical application of lidocaine (Numby Stuff) via an iontophoretic drug delivery system (iontophoresis) may be used to numb the skin up to a depth of 10 mm; it takes 10 minutes to work. Intradermal injection of bacteriostatic 0.9% sodium chloride may also have a local anesthetic effect.	1. Reduces pain locally from procedure and decreases anxiety about pain
2. Question the patient carefully about sensitivity to latex; use blood-pressure cuff rather than latex tourniquet if there is possibility of sensitivity.	2. Reduces risk of allergic reaction
3. Apply a new tourniquet for each patient or a blood pressure cuff 15 to 20 cm (6–8 in) above injection site. Palpate for a pulse distal to the tourniquet. Ask patient to open and close fist several times or position patient's arm in a dependent position to distend a vein.	3. The tourniquet distends the vein and makes it easier to enter; it should never be tight enough to occlude arterial flow. If a radial pulse cannot be palpated distal to the tourniquet, it is too tight. A new tourniquet should be used for each patient to prevent the transmission of microorganisms. A blood pressure cuff may be used for elderly patients to avoid

CHART 14-3 Guidelines for Starting an Intravenous Infusion, continued

NURSING ACTION	RATIONALE
	rupture of the veins. A clenched fist encourages the vein to become round and turgid. Positioning the arm below the level of the patient's heart promotes capillary filling. Warm packs applied for 10–20 min. prior to venipuncture can promote vasodilation. Bedside ultrasound-guided visualization of vein location and assessment of venous pathway and flow using ultrasonic waves may also be used.
4. Ascertain if the patient is allergic to iodine. Prepare site by scrubbing with chlorhexidine gluconate or povidone–iodine swabs for 2–3 min in circular motion, moving outward from injection site. Allow to dry.	4. Strict asepsis and careful site preparation are essential to prevent infection.
a. If the site selected is excessively hairy, clip hair. (Check agency's policy and procedure about this practice.)	
b. 70% isopropyl alcohol is an alternative solution that may be used.	
5. With hand not holding the venous access device, steady patient's arm and use finger or thumb to pull skin taut over vessel.	5. Applying traction to the vein helps to stabilize it.
6. Holding needle bevel up and at 5–25° angle, depending on the depth of the vein, pierce skin to reach but not penetrate vein.	6. Bevel down technique is necessary for small veins to prevent extravasation. One-step method of catheter insertion directly into vein with immediate thrust through the skin is excellent for large veins but may cause a hematoma if used in small veins.
7. Decrease angle of needle further until nearly parallel with skin, then enter vein either directly above or from the side in one quick motion.	7. Two-stage procedure decreases chance of thrusting needle through posterior wall of vein as skin is entered. No attempt should be made to reinsert the stylet because of risk of severing or puncturing the catheter.
8. If backflow of blood is visible, straighten angle and advance needle. Additional steps for catheter inserted over needle:	8. Backflow may not occur if vein is small; this position decreases chance of puncturing posterior wall of vein.
a. Advance needle 0.6 cm (¼–½ in) after successful venipuncture.	a. Advancing the needle slightly makes certain the plastic catheter has entered the vein.
b. Hold needle hub, and slide catheter over the needle into the vein. Never reinsert needle into a plastic catheter or pull the catheter back into the needle.	b. Reinsertion of the needle or pulling the catheter back can sever the catheter, causing catheter embolism.
c. Remove needle while pressing lightly on the skin over the catheter tip; hold catheter hub in place.	c. Slight pressure prevents bleeding before tubing is attached.
9. Release tourniquet and attach infusion tubing; open clamp enough to allow drip.	9. Infusion must be attached promptly to prevent clotting of blood in cannula. After two unsuccessful attempts at venipuncture, assistance by a more experienced health care provider is recommended to avoid unnecessary trauma to the patient and the possibility of limiting future sites for vascular access.
10. Slip a sterile 2-in × 2-in gauze pad under the catheter hub.	10. The gauze acts as a sterile field.
11. Anchor needle firmly in place with tape.	11. A stable needle is less likely to become dislodged or to irritate the vein.

continued >

CHART 14-3 Guidelines for Starting an Intravenous Infusion, continued

NURSING ACTION	RATIONALE
12. Cover the insertion site with a transparent dressing, bandage, or sterile gauze; tape in place with nonallergenic tape but do not encircle extremity.	12. Tape encircling extremity can act as a tourniquet and impede blood flow and infusion of fluid.
13. Tape a small loop of IV tubing onto dressing.	13. The loop decreases the chance of inadvertent cannula removal if the tubing is pulled.
14. Cover the insertion site with a dressing according to hospital policy and procedure. A gauze or transparent dressing may be used.	14. Transparent dressings allow assessment of the insertion site for phlebitis, infiltration, and infection without removing the dressing.
15. Label dressing with type and length of cannula, date, time, and initials.	15. Labeling facilitates assessment and safe discontinuation.
16. A padded, appropriate-length arm board may be applied to an area of flexion (neurovascular checks should be performed frequently).	16. Secures cannula placement and allows correct flow rate (neurovascular checks assess nerve, muscle, and vascular function to be sure function is not affected by immobilization)
17. Calculate infusion rate and regulate flow of infusion. For hourly IV rate use the following formula: gtt/mL of infusion set/60 (min in hr) × total hourly vol = gtt/min	17. Infusion must be regulated carefully to prevent overinfusion or underinfusion. Calculation of the IV rate is essential for the safe delivery of fluids. Safe administration requires knowledge of the volume of fluid to be infused, total infusion time, and the calibration of the administration set (found on the IV tubing package; 10, 12, 15, or 60 drops to deliver 1 mL of fluid).
18. Document date and time therapy initiated; type and amount of solution; additives and dosages; flow rate; gauge, length, and type of vascular access device; catheter insertion site; patient response to procedure; and name and title of the health care provider who inserted the catheter.	18. Documentation is essential to promote continuity of care.
19. Discard needles, stylets, or guidewires into a puncture-resistant needle container that meets OSHA guidelines.	19. Proper disposal of sharps decreases risk of needlesticks.

Flushing of a vascular device is performed to ensure patency and to prevent the mixing of incompatible medications or solutions. This procedure should be carried out at established intervals, according to hospital policy and procedure, especially for intermittently used catheters. Most manufacturers and researchers suggest the use of saline for flushing (Hankins et al., 2001). The volume of the flush solution should be at least twice the volume capacity of the catheter. The catheter should be clamped before the syringe is completely empty and withdrawn to prevent reflux of blood into the lumen, which could cause catheter clotting.

A variety of electronic infusion devices are available to assist in IV fluid delivery. These devices allow more accurate administration of fluids and medications than is possible with routine gravity-flow setups. A pump is a positive-pressure device that uses pressure to infuse fluid at a pressure of 10 psi; newer models use a pressure of 5 psi. The pressure exerted by the pump overrides vascular resistance (increased tubing length, low height of the IV container).

Volumetric pumps calculate the volume delivered by measuring the volume in a reservoir that is part of the set and is calibrated in milliliters per hour (mL/h). A controller is an infusion assist device that relies on gravity for infusion; the volume is calibrated in drops (gtt) per minute. A controller uses a drop sensor to monitor the flow. Factors essential for the safe use of pumps include alarms to signify the presence of air in the IV line or an occlusion. The standard for the accurate delivery of fluid or medication via an electronic IV infusion pump is plus or minus 5%. The manufacturer's directions must be read carefully before use of any infusion pump or controller, because there are many variations in available models. Use of these devices does not eliminate the need for the nurse to monitor the infusion and the patient frequently.

Discontinuing an Infusion

The removal of an IV catheter is associated with two possible dangers: bleeding and catheter embolism. To prevent excessive bleeding, a dry, sterile pressure dressing should be held over the site as the catheter is removed. Firm pressure is applied until hemostasis occurs.

If a plastic IV catheter is severed, the loose fragment can travel to the right ventricle and block blood flow. To detect this complication when the catheter is removed, the nurse compares the expected length of the catheter with its actual length. Plastic catheters should be withdrawn carefully and their length measured to make certain that no fragment has broken off in the vein.

Great care must be exercised when using scissors around the dressing site. If the catheter clearly has been severed, the nurse can attempt to occlude the vein above the site by applying a tourniquet to prevent the catheter from entering the central circulation (until surgical removal is possible). However, as always, it is better to prevent a potentially fatal problem than to deal with it after it has occurred. Fortunately, catheter embolism can be prevented easily by following simple rules:

- Avoid using scissors near the catheter.
- Avoid withdrawing the catheter through the insertion needle.
- Follow the manufacturer's guidelines carefully (eg, cover the needle point with the bevel shield to prevent severance of the catheter).

Managing Systemic Complications

IV therapy predisposes the patient to numerous hazards, including both local and systemic complications. Systemic complications occur less frequently but are usually more serious than local complications. They include circulatory overload, air embolism, febrile reaction, and infection.

FLUID OVERLOAD. Overloading the circulatory system with excessive IV fluids causes increased blood pressure and central venous pressure. Signs and symptoms of fluid overload include moist crackles on auscultation of the lungs, edema, weight gain, dyspnea, and respirations that are shallow and have an increased rate. Possible causes include rapid infusion of an IV solution or hepatic, cardiac, or renal disease. The risk of fluid overload and subsequent pulmonary edema is especially increased in elderly patients with cardiac disease; this is referred to as circulatory overload.

The treatment for circulatory overload is decreasing the IV rate, monitoring vital signs frequently, assessing breath sounds, and placing the patient in a high Fowler's position. The physician is contacted immediately. This complication can be avoided by using an infusion pump for infusions and by carefully monitoring all infusions. Complications of circulatory overload include heart failure and pulmonary edema.

AIR EMBOLISM. The risk of air embolism is rare but ever-present. It is most often associated with cannulation of central veins. Manifestations of air embolism include dyspnea and cyanosis; hypotension; weak, rapid pulse; loss of consciousness; and chest, shoulder, and low back pain. Treatment calls for immediately clamping the cannula and replacing a leaking or open infusion system, placing the patient on the left side in the Trendelenburg position, assessing vital signs and breath sounds, and administering oxygen. Air embolism can be prevented by using a Luer-Lok adapter on all lines, filling all tubing completely with solution, and using an air detection alarm on an IV pump. Complications of air embolism include shock and death. The amount of air necessary to induce death in humans is not known; however, the rate of entry is probably as important as the actual volume of air.

SEPTICEMIA AND OTHER INFECTION. Pyrogenic substances in either the infusion solution or the IV administration set can induce a febrile reaction and septicemia. Signs and symptoms include an abrupt temperature elevation shortly after the infusion is started, backache, headache, increased pulse and respiratory rate, nausea and vomiting, diarrhea, chills and shaking, and general malaise. In severe septicemia, vascular collapse and septic shock may occur. Causes of septicemia include contamination of the IV product or a break in aseptic technique, especially in immunocompromised patients. Treatment is symptomatic and includes culturing of the IV cannula, tubing, or solution if it is suspect and establishing a new IV site for medication or fluid administration. See Chapter 15 for a discussion of septic shock.

Infection ranges in severity from local involvement of the insertion site to systemic dissemination of organisms through the bloodstream, as in septicemia. Measures to prevent infection are essential at the time the IV line is inserted and throughout the entire infusion. Prevention includes the following:

- Careful hand hygiene before every contact with any part of the infusion system or the patient
- Examining the IV containers for cracks, leaks, or cloudiness, which may indicate a contaminated solution
- Using strict aseptic technique
- Firmly anchoring the IV cannula to prevent to-and-fro motion
- Inspecting the IV site daily and replacing a soiled or wet dressing with a dry sterile dressing. (Antimicrobial agents that should be used for site care include 2% tincture of iodine, 10% povidone–iodine, alcohol, or chlorhexidine gluconate, used alone or in combination.)
- Disinfecting injection/access ports with antimicrobial solution before use
- Removing the IV cannula at the first sign of local inflammation, contamination, or complication
- Replacing the peripheral IV cannula every 48 to 72 hours, or as indicated
- Replacing the IV cannula inserted during emergency conditions (with questionable asepsis) as soon as possible
- Using a 0.2-μm air-eliminating and bacteria/particulate retentive filter with non–lipid-containing solutions that require filtration. The filter can be added to the proximal or distal end of the administration set. If added to the proximal end between the fluid container and the tubing spike, the filter ensures sterility and particulate removal from the infusate container and prevents inadvertent infusion of air. If added to the distal end of the administration set, it filters air particles and contaminants introduced from add-on devices, secondary administration sets, or interruptions to the primary system.
- Replacing the solution bag and administration set in accordance with agency policy and procedure
- Infusing or discarding medication or solution within 24 hours of its addition to an administration set
- Changing primary and secondary continuous administration sets every 72 hours, or immediately if contamination is suspected
- Changing primary intermittent administration sets every 24 hours, or immediately if contamination is suspected

Managing Local Complications

Local complications of IV therapy include infiltration and extravasation, phlebitis, thrombophlebitis, hematoma, and clotting of the needle.

INFILTRATION AND EXTRAVASATION. Infiltration is the unintentional administration of a nonvesicant solution or medication into surrounding tissue. This can occur when the IV cannula dislodges or perforates the wall of the vein. Infiltration is characterized by edema around the insertion site, leakage of IV fluid from the insertion site, discomfort and coolness in the area of infiltration, and a significant decrease in the flow rate. When the solution is particularly irritating, sloughing of tissue may result. Close monitoring of the insertion site is necessary to detect infiltration before it becomes severe.

Infiltration is usually easily recognized if the insertion area is larger than the same site of the opposite extremity; however, it is not always so obvious. A common misconception is that a backflow of blood into the tubing proves that the catheter is properly placed within the vein. However, if the catheter tip has pierced the wall of the vessel, IV fluid will seep into tissues as well as flow into the vein. Although blood return occurs, infiltration has occurred as well. A more reliable means of confirming infiltration is to apply a tourniquet above (or proximal to) the infusion site and tighten it enough to restrict venous flow. If the infusion continues to drip despite the venous obstruction, infiltration is present.

As soon as the nurse notes infiltration, the infusion should be stopped, the IV discontinued, and a sterile dressing applied to the site after careful inspection to determine the extent of infiltration. The infiltration of any amount of blood product, irritant, or vesicant is considered the most severe.

The IV infusion should be started in a new site or proximal to the infiltration if the same extremity must be used again. A warm compress may be applied to the site if small volumes of noncaustic solutions have infiltrated over a long period, or if the solution was isotonic with a normal pH; the affected extremity should be elevated to promote the absorption of fluid. If the infiltration is recent and the solution was hypertonic or had an increased pH, a cold compress may be applied to the area. Infiltration can be detected and treated early by inspecting the site every hour for redness, pain, edema, blood return, coolness at the site, and IV fluid leaking from the IV site. Using the appropriate size and type of cannula for the vein prevents this complication. The Infusion Nursing Standards of Practice state that a standardized infiltration scale should be used to document the infiltration (Alexander, 2000) (Chart 14-4).

Extravasation is similar to infiltration, with an inadvertent administration of vesicant or irritant solution or medication into the surrounding tissue. Medications such as dopamine, calcium preparations, and chemotherapeutic agents can cause pain, burning, and redness at the site. Blistering, inflammation, and necrosis of tissues can occur. The extent of tissue damage is determined by the concentration of the medication, the quantity that extravasated, the location of the infusion site, the tissue response, and the duration of the process of extravasation.

CHART 14-4

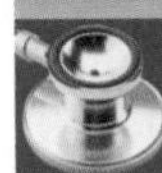

Assessing for Infiltration

GRADE	CLINICAL CRITERIA
0	No clinical symptoms
1	Skin blanched, edema less than 1 inch in any direction, cool to touch, with or without pain
2	Skin blanched, edema 1 to 6 inches in any direction, cool to touch, with or without pain
3	Skin blanched, translucent, gross edema greater than 6 inches in any direction, cool to touch, mild to moderate pain, possible numbness
4	Skin blanched, translucent, skin tight, leaking, skin discolored, bruised, swollen, gross edema greater than 6 inches in any direction, deep pitting tissue edema, circulatory impairment, moderate to severe pain, infiltration of any amount of blood products, irritant, or vesicant

The infusion must be stopped and the physician notified promptly. The agency's protocol to treat extravasation is initiated; the protocol may specify specific treatments, including antidotes specific to the medication that extravasated, and may indicate whether the IV line should remain in place or be removed before treatment. The protocol often specifies infiltration of the infusion site with an antidote prescribed after assessment by the physician, removal of the cannula; and application of warm compresses to sites of extravasation from vinca alkaloids or cold compresses to sites of extravasation from alkylating and antibiotic vesicants (Hankins et al., 2001). The affected extremity should not be used for further cannula placement. Thorough neurovascular assessments of the affected extremity must be performed frequently.

Reviewing the institution's IV policy and procedures and incompatibility charts and checking with the pharmacist before administering any IV medication, whether given peripherally or centrally, is a prudent way to determine incompatibilities and vesicant potential to prevent extravasation. Careful, frequent monitoring of the IV site, avoiding insertion of IV devices in areas of flexion, securing the IV line, and using the smallest catheter possible that accommodates the vein help minimize the incidence and severity of this complication. In addition, when vesicant medication is administered by IV push, it should be given through a side port of an infusing IV solution to dilute the medication and decrease the severity of tissue damage if extravasation occurs. Extravasation should always be rated as a grade 4 on the infiltration scale.

PHLEBITIS. Phlebitis is defined as inflammation of a vein, which can be categorized as chemical, mechanical, or bacterial; however, two or more of these types of irritation often occur simultaneously. Chemical phlebitis can be caused by an irritating medication or solution (increased pH or high osmolality of a solution), rapid infusion rates, and medication incompatibilities. Mechanical phlebitis results from long periods of cannulation, catheters in flexed areas, catheter gauges larger than the vein lumen, and poorly secured catheters. Bacterial phlebitis can develop from poor hand hygiene, lack of aseptic technique, failure to check all equipment before use, and failure to recognize early signs and symptoms of phlebitis. Other factors include poor venipuncture technique, catheter in place for a prolonged period, and failure to adequately secure the catheter. Phlebitis is characterized by a reddened, warm area around the insertion site or along the path of the vein, pain or tenderness at the site or along the vein, and swelling. The incidence of phlebitis increases with the length of time the IV line is in place, the composition of the fluid or medication infused (especially its pH and tonicity), the size and site of the cannula inserted, ineffective filtration, inadequate anchoring of the line, and the introduction of microorganisms at the time of insertion. The Intravenous Nursing Society has identified specific standards for assessing phlebitis (Alexander, 2000); these appear in Chart 14-5. Phlebitis should be graded according to the most severe presenting indication.

Treatment consists of discontinuing the IV and restarting it in another site, and applying a warm, moist compress to the affected site. Phlebitis can be prevented by using aseptic technique during insertion, using the appropriate-size cannula or needle for the vein, considering the composition of fluids and medications when selecting a site, observing the site hourly for any complications, anchoring the cannula or needle well, and changing the IV site according to agency policy and procedures.

CHART 14-5

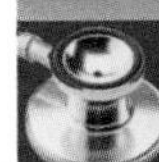

Assessing for Phlebitis

GRADE	CLINICAL CRITERIA
0	No clinical symptoms
1	Erythema at access site with or without pain
2	Pain at access site Erythema, edema, or both
3	Pain at access site Erythema, edema, or both Streak formation Palpable venous cord (1 inch or shorter)
4	Pain at access site with erythema Streak formation Palpable venous cord (longer than 1 inch) Purulent drainage

Note: If this scale is not being used in an institution, then the description associated with the number can be used to describe the assessment.

From Infusion Nursing Standards of Practice (2000). *Journal of Intravenous Nursing, 23*(6S), S56–S69.

THROMBOPHLEBITIS. Thrombophlebitis refers to the presence of a clot plus inflammation in the vein. It is evidenced by localized pain, redness, warmth, and swelling around the insertion site or along the path of the vein, immobility of the extremity because of discomfort and swelling, sluggish flow rate, fever, malaise, and leukocytosis.

Treatment includes discontinuing the IV infusion; applying a cold compress first, to decrease the flow of blood and increase platelet aggregation, followed by a warm compress; elevating the extremity; and restarting the line in the opposite extremity. If the patient has signs and symptoms of thrombophlebitis, the IV line should not be flushed (although flushing may be indicated in the absence of phlebitis to ensure cannula patency and to prevent mixing of incompatible medications and solutions). The catheter should be cultured after the skin around the catheter is cleaned with alcohol. If purulent drainage exists, the site is cultured before the skin is cleaned.

Thrombophlebitis can be prevented by avoiding trauma to the vein at the time the IV is inserted, observing the site every hour, and checking medication additives for compatibility.

HEMATOMA. Hematoma results when blood leaks into tissues surrounding the IV insertion site. Leakage can result if the opposite vein wall is perforated during venipuncture, the needle slips out of the vein, or insufficient pressure is applied to the site after removal of the needle or cannula. The signs of a hematoma include ecchymosis, immediate swelling at the site, and leakage of blood at the insertion site.

Treatment includes removing the needle or cannula and applying light pressure with a sterile, dry dressing; applying ice for 24 hours to the site to avoid extension of the hematoma; elevating the extremity; assessing the extremity for any circulatory, neurologic, or motor dysfunction; and restarting the line in the other extremity if indicated. A hematoma can be prevented by carefully inserting the needle and by using diligent care with patients who have a bleeding disorder, are taking anticoagulant medication, or have advanced liver disease.

CLOTTING AND OBSTRUCTION. Blood clots may form in the IV line as a result of kinked IV tubing, a very slow infusion rate, an empty IV bag, or failure to flush the IV line after intermittent medication or solution administrations. The signs are decreased flow rate and blood backflow into the IV tubing.

If blood clots in the IV line, the infusion must be discontinued and restarted in another site with a new cannula and administration set. The tubing should not be irrigated or milked. Neither the infusion rate nor the solution container should be raised, and the clot should not be aspirated from the tubing. Clotting of the needle or cannula may be prevented by not allowing the IV solution bag to run dry, taping the tubing to prevent kinking and maintain patency, maintaining an adequate flow rate, and flushing the line after intermittent medication or other solution administration. In some cases, a specially trained nurse or physician may inject a thrombolytic agent into the catheter to clear an occlusion resulting from fibrin or clotted blood.

Promoting Home and Community-Based Care

TEACHING PATIENTS SELF-CARE. At times, IV therapy must be administered in the home setting, in which case much of the daily management rests with the patient and family. Teaching becomes essential to ensure that the patient and family can manage the IV fluid and infusion correctly and avoid complications. Written instructions as well as demonstration and return demonstration help reinforce the key points for all these functions.

CONTINUING CARE. Home infusion therapies cover a wide range of treatments, including antibiotic, analgesic, and antineoplastic medications; blood or blood component therapy; and parenteral nutrition. When direct nursing care is necessary, arrangements are made to have an infusion nurse visit the home and administer the IV therapy as prescribed. In addition to implementing and monitoring the IV therapy, the nurse carries out a comprehensive assessment of the patient's condition and continues to teach the patient and family about the skills involved in overseeing the IV therapy setup. Any dietary changes that may be necessary because of fluid or electrolyte imbalances are explained or reinforced during such sessions.

Periodic laboratory testing may be necessary to assess the effects of IV therapy and the patient's progress. Blood specimens may be obtained by a laboratory near the patient's home, or a home visit may be arranged to obtain blood specimens for analysis.

The nurse collaborates with the case manager in assessing the patient, family, and home environment; developing a plan of care in accordance with the patient's treatment plan and level of ability; and arranging for appropriate referral and follow-up if necessary. Any necessary equipment may be provided by the agency or purchased by the patient, depending on the terms of the home care arrangements. Appropriate documentation is necessary to assist in obtaining third-party payment for the service provided.

Critical Thinking Exercises

1 A 28-year-old man with a history of diabetes mellitus has an open fracture of the tibia as the result of a motorcycle crash. In the emergency department, his temperature is 103°F. His laboratory test results are as follows: blood glucose, 450 mg/dL; BUN, 35 mg/dL; sodium, 140 mEq/L; potassium, 4.1 mEq/L; pH, 7.1; PCO_2, 10 mm Hg; and HCO_3^-, 12 mEq/L. His urine ketones are 3+. What fluid and electrolyte or acid–base disorders is the patient experiencing? What IV fluids would you anticipate being prescribed? Give the rationale for their use. What treatments would address the patient's fluid and electrolyte or acid–base disorders?

2 A 30-year-old woman comes to the emergency department with nausea, confusion, dehydration, and oliguria. Her mother reports that she has been depressed after losing her job as a bank executive. An empty bottle of aspirin was found in her bathroom sink. Her laboratory values are as follows: pH, 7.35; $PaCO_2$, 16 mm Hg; PaO_2, 130 mm Hg; and HCO_3^-, 15 mEq/L. What acid–base disorder does this patient have? What treatments and relevant nursing actions related to the underlying disorder and its treatment should the nurse anticipate?

3 A 58-year-old woman is vomiting bright red blood. She is hypotensive. Her pulse rate is 38 bpm, and her pulse is weak and thready. Her arterial blood gases results are as follows: pH, 7.34; $PaCO_2$, 35 mm Hg; PaO_2, 69 mm Hg; and HCO_3^-, 20 mEq/L. Her hemoglobin is 4 g/dL. How do you interpret the patient's blood gas values? What treatment would you anticipate?

4 ebp A female patient with a developmental delay and cognitive impairment requires frequent and repeated venipunctures and IV infusions for several weeks as part of treatment for osteomyelitis. She becomes very distressed in anticipation of the venipunctures. A nurse on the IV team has suggested the use of the local anesthetic EMLA to decrease her discomfort and distress related to venipuncture. What is the evidence for use of a local anesthetic agent in this case? What criteria would you use to assess the strength of the evidence for the use of the anesthetic? How would you use it in this patient's case?

5 ebp A patient is receiving long-term parenteral fluids to treat recurrent dehydration secondary to GI losses. In an effort to ensure the patency of the IV catheter, the nurse considers irrigating the line with heparin. Do research findings support the use of heparin to keep the IV line open? What is the evidence base to determine whether heparin or saline irrigation is more effective? What are the benefits and risks of irrigation of the IV line with heparin versus saline?

6 ebp A patient who has been receiving IV fluids for more than a week complains of pain and discomfort in the arm in which the fluids are being infused. The nurse assesses the IV insertion site and concludes that the patient has developed phlebitis at the site. The nurse decides to remove the IV catheter and restart the infusion in the patient's other arm. The nurse also applies warm compresses to the site. Identify the evidence that supports the use of warm compresses and evaluate the strength of the evidence. What criteria would you use to determine the strength of the evidence for or against use of warm compresses?

REFERENCES AND SELECTED READINGS

BOOKS

Alexander, M. & Corrigan, A. (2004). *Core curriculum for infusion nursing* (4th ed.). Philadelphia: Lippincott Williams & Wilkins.

Baumberger-Henry, M. (2004). *Quick look nursing: Fluid and electrolytes.* Thorofare, NJ: Slack.

Chernecky, C. C. & Berger, B. J. (2004). *Laboratory tests and diagnostic procedures* (3rd ed.). Philadelphia: W. B. Saunders.

Dudek, S. G. (2006). *Nutrition essentials for nursing practice* (5th ed.). Philadelphia: Lippincott Williams & Wilkins.

Hankins, J., Lonsway-Waldman, R., Hedrick, C., et al. (2001). *Infusion therapy in clinical practice* (2nd ed.). Philadelphia: W. B. Saunders.

Heitz, U. & Horne, M. (2005). *Guide to fluid, electrolyte, and acid-base balance* (4th ed.). St. Louis: Mosby.

Hogan, M. & Wane, D. (2003). *Fluids, electrolytes and acid-base balance* (5th ed.). Upper Saddle River, NJ: Pearson Education, Inc. Prentice-Hall.

Holmes, N. H. (2001). *Handbook of pathophysiology*. Philadelphia: Lippincott Williams & Wilkins.

Infusion Nurses Society. (2004). *Policies and procedures for infusion nursing of the older adult*. Norwood, MA: Author.

Infusion Nurses Society. (2006). *Infusion nursing standards of practice*. Norwood, MA: Author.

Karch, A. M. (2006). *Lippincott's nursing drug guide*. Philadelphia: Lippincott Williams & Wilkins.

Kee, J., Paulanka, B. & Purnell, L. (2004). *Handbook of fluids and electrolytes and acid-base imbalances*. Albany, NY: Delmar.

Martin, L. (1999). *All you really need to know how to interpret arterial blood gases* (2nd ed.). Philadelphia: Lippincott Williams & Wilkins.

Metheny, N. M. (2000). *Fluid and electrolyte balance: Nursing considerations* (4th ed.). Philadelphia: Lippincott Williams & Wilkins.

Morton, P. G., Fontaine, D. K., Hudak, C. M., et al. (2005). *Critical care nursing: A holistic approach*. Philadelphia: Lippincott Williams & Wilkins.

Otto, S. E. (2001). *Pocket guide to intravenous therapy* (4th ed.). St. Louis: Mosby.

Porth, C. M. (2005). *Pathophysiology: Concepts of altered health states* (6th ed.). Philadelphia: Lippincott Williams & Wilkins.

Price, S. A., & Wilson, L. M. (2002). *Pathophysiology: Clinical concepts of disease processes* (6th ed.). St. Louis: Mosby–Year Book.

Rose, B. & Post, T. (2000). *Clinical physiology of acid–base disorders* (5th ed.). New York: McGraw-Hill.

Speakman, E. & Weldy, N. J. (2001). *Body fluids and electrolytes: A programmed presentation* (8th ed.). Philadelphia: Elsevier Science Publishers.

Weinstein, S. (2006). *Plumer's principles and practice of intravenous therapy* (8th ed.). Philadelphia: Lippincott Williams & Wilkins.

JOURNALS

**Asterisks indicate nursing research articles.*

Fluid and Electrolyte Balances and Imbalances

Allison, S. P., & Lobo, D. N. (2004). Fluid and electrolytes in the elderly. *Current Opinion in Clinical Nutrition and Metabolic Care, 7*(1), 27–33.

American Heart Association. (2005). 2005 guidelines for cardiopulmonary resuscitation and emergency cardiovascular care. *Circulation*. Available at: www.americanheart.org/presenter.jhtml?identifier=3035517 (accessed May 26, 2006).

Burger, C. M. (2004a). Hyperkalemia. *American Journal of Nursing, 104*(10), 66–70.

Burger, C. M. (2004b). Hypokalemia. *American Journal of Nursing, 104*(11), 61–65.

Byrd, R. (2003). Magnesium: Its proven clinical significance. *Southern Medical Journal, 96*(1), 104–105.

Eaton, J. (2003). Detection of hyponatremia in the PACU. *Journal of Perianesthesia Nursing, 18*(6), 392–397.

Elgart, H. N. (2004). Assessment of fluids and electrolytes. *AACN Clinical Issues, 15*(4), 607–621.

*Hayes, A., Buffum, M. & Fuller, D. (2003). Bowel preparation comparison: Flavored versus unflavored colyte. *Gastroenterology Nursing, 26*(3), 106–109.

Inzucchi, S. (2004a). Management of hypercalcemia: Diagnostic work up, therapeutic options for hyperparathyroidism and other common causes. *Postgraduate Medicine, 115*(5), 27–36.

Inzucchi, S. (2004b). Understanding hypercalcemia: Its metabolic basis, signs, and symptoms. *Postgraduate Medicine, 115*(4), 69–70, 73–76.

Lin, S. H., Hsu, Y. J., Chiu, J. S., et al. (2003). Osmotic demyelination syndrome: A potentially avoidable disaster. *Quarterly Journal of Medicine, 96*(12), 935–947.

Lobo, D. N. (2004). Fluid, electrolytes and nutrition: Physiological and clinical aspects. *Proceedings of the Nutrition Society, 63*(3), 453–466.

Luckey, A. E. & Parsa, C. J. (2003). Fluid and electrolytes in the aged. *Archives of Surgery, 138*(10), 1055–1060.

Olson, D. M., Meek, L. G., & Lynch, J. R. (2004). Accurate patient history contributes to differentiating diabetes insipidus: A case study. *Journal of Neuroscience Nursing, 36*(4), 228–230.

Palmer, B. F. (2004). Managing hyperkalemia caused by inhibitors of the rennin-angitensin-aldosterone system. *New England Journal of Medicine, 351*(6), 585–592.

Pirzada, N. A. & Ali, I. I. (2001). Central pontine myelinolysis. *Mayo Clinic Proceedings, 76*(5), 559–562.

Ryland, B. & Thomas, R. (2003). Magnesium: Its proven and potential clinical significance. *Southern Medical Journal, 96*(1), 104.

SAFE Study Investigators. (2004). A comparison of albumin and saline for fluid resuscitation in the intensive care unit. *New England Journal of Medicine, 350*(22), 2247–2256.

Suhayda, R. & Walton, J. C. (2002). Preventing and managing dehydration. *MedSurg Nursing, 11*(6), 267–278.

Stewart, A. F. (2005). Hypercalcemia associated with cancer. *New England Journal of Medicine, 352*(4), 373–379.

Tsuneyoshi, H., Nishina, T., Nomoto, T., et al. (2004). Atrial natriuretic peptide helps prevent late remodeling after left ventricular aneurysm repair. *Circulation, 110*(11 Suppl 1), II174–II179.

van Wissen, L. & Breton, C. (2004). Perioperative influences on fluid distribution. *MedSurg Nursing, 13*(5), 304–311.

Weiss-Guillet, E. M., Takala, J. & Jakob, S. M. (2003). Diagnosis and management of electrolyte emergencies. *Best Practice and Research Clinical Endocrinology and Metabolism, 17*(4), 623–651.

Zwicker, C. D. (2003). The older adult at risk. *Journal of Infusion Nursing, 26*(3), 137–143.

Acid–Base Balance

Bartlett, D. (2005). Understanding the anion and osmolal gaps laboratory values: What they are and how to use them. *Journal of Emergency Nursing, 31*(1), 109–111.

Herd, A. M. (2005). An approach to complex acid-base problems: Keeping it simple. *Canadian Family Physician, 51*, 226–232.

Kellum, J. A. (2005). Determinants of plasma acid-base balance. *Critical Care Clinics, 21*(2), 329–346.

Kraut, J. A. & Madias, N. E. (2001). Approach to patients with acid-base disorders. *Respiratory Care, 46*(4), 392–403.

Lafrance, J. P., & Leblanc, M. (2005). Metabolic, electrolytes, and nutritional concerns in critical illness. *Critical Care Clinics, 21*(2), 305–327.

Lynes, D. (2003). An introduction to blood gas analysis. *Nursing Times, 99*(11), 54–55.

Whittier, W. L. & Rutecki, G. W. (2004). Primer on clinical acid-base problem solving. *Disease-a-Month, 50*(3), 122–162.

Yucha, C. (2004). Renal regulation of acid-base balance. *Nephrology Nursing Journal, 31*(2), 201–208.

Intravenous Administration

Alexander, M. (2000). Infusion nursing standards of practice. *Journal of Intravenous Nursing, 23*(6 Suppl), S5–S88.

Anderson, R. N. (2004). Midline catheters. *Journal of Infusion Nursing, 27*(5), 313–321.

*Brown, J. (2003). Using lidocaine for peripheral IV insertions: Patients' preferences and pain experiences. *MedSurg Nursing, 12*(2), 95–100.

*Fetzer, S. J. (2002). Reducing venipuncture and intravenous insertion pain with eutectic mixture of local anesthetic: A meta-analysis. *Nursing Research, 51*(2), 119–124.

Foley, M. (2004). Update on needlestick and sharps injuries: The Needlestick Safety and Prevention Act of 2000. *American Journal of Nursing, 104*(8), 96–97.

Fry, C. & Ahold, D. (2001). Local anesthesia prior to the insertion of peripherally inserted central catheters. *Journal of Infusion Nursing, 24*(6), 404–408.

Gorski, L. A. & Czaplewski, L. M. (2004). Peripherally inserted central catheters and midline catheters for the homecare nurse. *Journal of Infusion Nursing, 27*(6), 399–409.

Haire, W. D. & Herbst, S. (2000). Highlights bulletin: Consensus conference on the use of Alteplase (t-PA) for the management of thrombotic catheter dysfunction. *Journal of Vascular Access Devices, 5*(2), 28–36.

Intravenous Nurses Society. (1997). Position paper: Midline and midclavicular catheters. *Journal of Intravenous Nursing, 20*(4), 175–178.

Intravenous Nurses Society. (1997). Position paper: Peripherally inserted central catheters. *Journal of Intravenous Nursing, 20*(4), 172–174.

Macklin, D. (2003). Phlebitis. *American Journal of Nursing, 103*(2), 55–58.

Macklin, D. (2000). Removing PICC. *American Journal of Nursing, 100*(1), 52–54.

McKnight, S. (2004). Nurse's guide to understanding and treating thrombotic occlusion of central venous access devices. *MedSurg Nursing, 13*(6), 377–382.

O'Grady, N. P., Alexander, M., Dellinger, E. P., et al. (2002). Guidelines for the prevention of intravascular catheter-related infections. Centers for Disease Control and Prevention. *Morbidity and Mortality Weekly Report Recommendations and Reports, 51*(RR-10), 1–29.

Penny-Timmons, E. & Sevedge, S. (2004). Outcome data for peripherally inserted central catheters used in an acute care setting. *Journal of Infusion Nursing, 27*(6), 431–436.

Peter, D. A. & Saxman, C. (2003). Preventing air embolism when removing CVCs: An evidence-based approach to changing practice. *MedSurg Nursing, 12*(4), 223–228.

Shafiee, M. A., Bohn, D., Hoorn, E. J., et al. (2003). How to select optimal maintenance intravenous fluid therapy. *QJM 96*(8), 601–610.

*Snelling, R., Jones, G., Figueredo, A., et al. (2001). Central venous catheters for infusion therapy in gastrointestinal cancer: A comparative study of tunnelled centrally placed catheters and peripherally inserted central catheters. *Journal of Intravenous Nursing, 24*(1), 38–47.

RESOURCES

Infusion Nurses Society, 220 Norwood Park South, Norwood, MA 02062; 781-440-9408; http://www.ins1.org. Accessed May 25, 2006.

CHAPTER 15

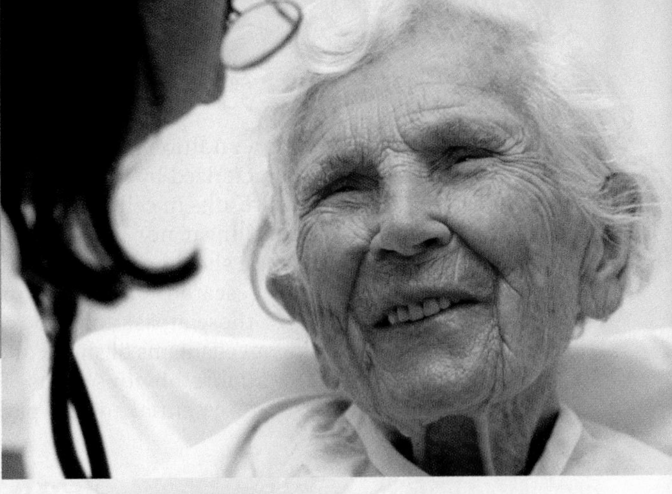

Shock and Multisystem Failure

Learning Objectives

On completion of this chapter, the learner will be able to:

1. Describe shock and its underlying pathophysiology.
2. Compare clinical findings of the compensatory, progressive, and irreversible stages of shock.
3. Describe organ damage that may occur with shock.
4. Describe similarities and differences in shock due to hypovolemic, cardiogenic, neurogenic, anaphylactic, and septic shock states.
5. Identify medical and nursing management priorities in treating patients in shock.
6. Identify vasoactive medications used in treating shock, and describe nursing implications associated with their use.
7. Discuss the importance of nutritional support in all forms of shock.
8. Discuss the role of nurses in psychosocial support of patients experiencing shock and their families.
9. Discuss multiple organ dysfunction syndrome.

Shock is a life-threatening condition with a variety of underlying causes. It is characterized by inadequate tissue perfusion that, if untreated, results in cell death. The progression of shock is neither linear nor predictable, and shock states, especially septic shock, comprise a current area of aggressive clinical research. Nurses caring for patients with shock and for those at risk for shock must understand the underlying mechanisms of shock and recognize its subtle as well as more obvious signs. Rapid assessment and response are essential to the patient's recovery.

Shock and Its Significance

Shock can best be defined as a condition in which tissue perfusion is inadequate to deliver oxygen and nutrients to support vital organs and cellular function (Hameed, Aird, & Cohn, 2003). Adequate blood flow to the tissues and cells requires the following components: adequate cardiac pump, effective vasculature or circulatory system, and sufficient blood volume. If one component is impaired, perfusion to the tissues is threatened or compromised. Without treatment, inadequate blood flow to the tissues results in poor delivery of oxygen and nutrients to the cells, cellular starvation, cell death, organ dysfunction progressing to organ failure, and eventual death.

Shock affects all body systems. It may develop rapidly or slowly, depending on the underlying cause. During shock, the body struggles to survive, calling on all its homeostatic mechanisms to restore blood flow. Any insult to the body can create a cascade of events resulting in poor tissue perfusion. Therefore, almost any patient with any disease state may be at risk for developing shock.

Nursing care of patients with shock requires ongoing systematic assessment. Many of the interventions required in caring for patients with shock call for close collaboration with other members of the health care team and rapid implementation of physicians' orders. Nurses must anticipate orders, because these orders need to be executed with speed and accuracy.

Conditions Precipitating Shock

Classification of Shock

Conventionally, the primary underlying pathophysiologic process and the underlying disorder are used to classify the shock state. Several definitions of shock states are found in the literature. In this chapter, the following shock states will be described:

- **Hypovolemic shock**, which occurs when there is a decrease in the intravascular volume
- **Cardiogenic shock**, which occurs when the heart has an impaired pumping ability; it may be of coronary or noncoronary event origin
- **Septic shock**, which is caused by an infection
- **Neurogenic shock**, which is caused by alterations in vascular smooth muscle tone, caused by either nervous system injury or complications associated with medications such as epidural anesthesia
- **Anaphylactic shock**, which is caused by a hypersensitivity reaction

Shock states that are caused by a loss of vascular tone, including septic, neurogenic, and anaphylactic shock, are discussed later in this chapter as **circulatory shock** (also termed distributive or vasoactive shock). In addition, traumatic shock has been described in the literature (Kellum & Pinsky, 2002).

Regardless of the initial cause of shock, researchers have gradually concluded that certain physiologic responses are common to all types of shock. These physiologic responses are hypoperfusion of the tissues, hypermetabolism, and activation of the inflammatory response. The body responds to shock states by activating the sympathetic nervous system and mounting a hypermetabolic and inflammatory re-

Glossary

anaphylactic shock: circulatory shock state resulting from a severe allergic reaction producing an overwhelming systemic vasodilation and relative hypovolemia

biochemical mediators: messenger substances that may be released by a cell to create an action at that site or be carried by the bloodstream to a distant site before being activated; also called cytokines

cardiogenic shock: shock state resulting from impairment or failure of the myocardium

colloids: intravenous solutions that contain molecules that are too large to pass through capillary membranes

crystalloids: electrolyte solutions that move freely between the intravascular compartment and interstitial spaces

circulatory shock: shock state resulting from displacement of blood volume creating a relative hypovolemia and inadequate delivery of oxygen to the cells; also called distributive shock

hypovolemic shock: shock state resulting from decreased intravascular volume due to fluid loss

neurogenic shock: shock state resulting from loss of sympathetic tone causing relative hypovolemia

septic shock: circulatory shock state resulting from overwhelming infection causing relative hypovolemia

shock: physiologic state in which there is inadequate blood flow to tissues and cells of the body

systemic inflammatory response syndrome (SIRS): overwhelming inflammatory response in the absence of infection causing relative hypovolemia and decreased tissue perfusion

sponse. A derangement in the compensatory mechanisms to effectively restore physiologic balance is the final pathway of all shock states (Ahrens & Vollman, 2003; Hameed et al., 2003; Kleinpell, 2003). Once shock develops, the patient's survival may have more to do with the body's response than with the initial cause of shock (Kleinpell, 2003). The final common pathway of all forms of shock is inadequate perfusion to the cells that results in cellular hypoxia, end organ damage, and ultimately death.

Normal Cellular Function

Energy metabolism occurs within the cell, where nutrients are chemically broken down and stored in the form of adenosine triphosphate (ATP). Cells use this stored energy to perform necessary functions, such as active transport, muscle contraction, and biochemical synthesis, as well as specialized cellular functions, such as the conduction of electrical impulses. ATP can be synthesized aerobically (in the presence of oxygen) or anaerobically (in the absence of oxygen). Aerobic metabolism yields far greater amounts of ATP per mole of glucose than does anaerobic metabolism; therefore, it is a more efficient and effective means of producing energy. In addition, anaerobic metabolism results in the accumulation of the toxic end product, lactic acid, which must be removed from the cell and transported to the liver for conversion into glucose and glycogen.

Pathophysiology

In shock, the cells lack an adequate blood supply and are deprived of oxygen and nutrients; therefore, they must produce energy through anaerobic metabolism. This results in low energy yields from nutrients and an acidotic intracellular environment. Because of these changes, normal cell function ceases (Fig. 15-1). The cell swells and the cell membrane becomes more permeable, allowing electrolytes and fluids to seep out of and into the cell. The sodium–potassium pump becomes impaired; cell structures, primarily the mitochondria, are damaged; and death of the cell results.

Glucose is the primary substrate required for the production of cellular energy in the form of ATP. In stress states, catecholamines, cortisol, glucagons, and inflammatory cytokines and mediators are released, causing hyperglycemia and insulin resistance to mobilize glucose for cellular metabolism. Activation of these substances promotes gluconeogenesis, which is the formation of glucose from noncarbohydrate sources such as proteins and fats. Glycogen that has been stored in the liver is also converted to glucose through glycogenolysis, increasing the amount of glucose in the bloodstream. The net result is hyperglycemia to meet increased metabolic demands.

Continued activation of the stress response by shock states causes a depletion of glycogen stores, resulting in increased proteolysis and eventual organ failure (Baldwin & Morris, 2002; Flynn, 2004). The inability of the body to have enough nutrients and oxygen for normal cellular metabolism causes a buildup of metabolic end products in the cells and interstitial spaces. Cellular metabolism is impaired, and a vicious cycle of negative feedback is initiated.

Vascular Responses

Oxygen attaches to the hemoglobin molecule in red blood cells, and the blood carries it to body cells. The amount of

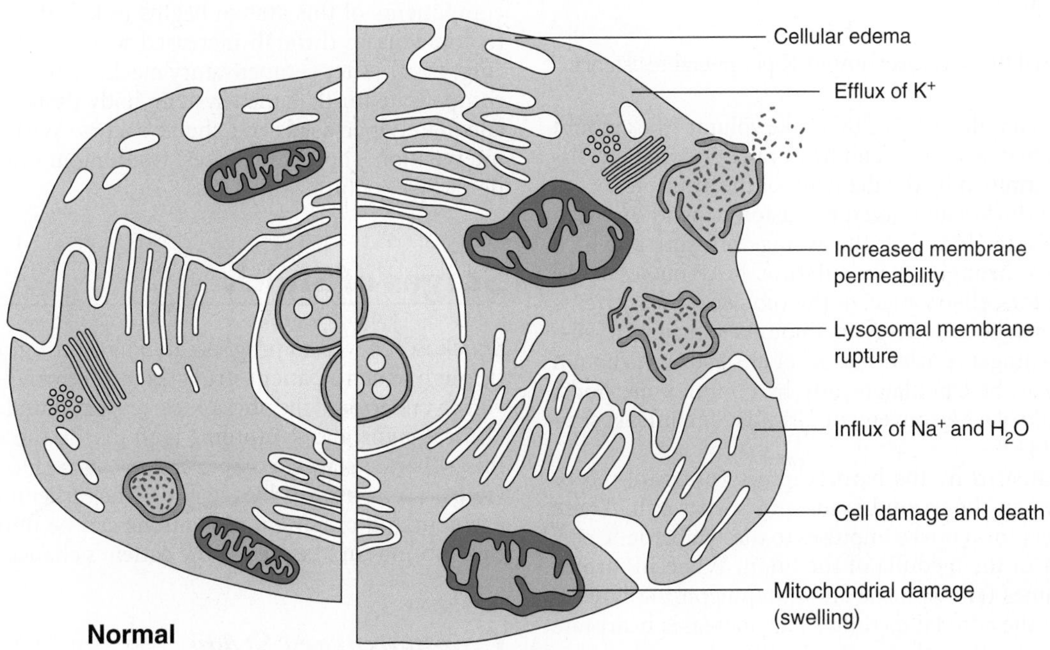

FIGURE 15-1. Cellular effects of shock. The cell swells and the cell membrane becomes more permeable; fluids and electrolytes seep from and into the cell. Mitochondria and lysosomes are damaged, and the cell dies.

oxygen that is delivered to cells depends both on blood flow to a specific area and on blood oxygen concentration. Blood is continuously recycled through the lungs to be reoxygenated and to eliminate end products of cellular metabolism, such as carbon dioxide. The heart muscle is the pump that propels the freshly oxygenated blood out to the body tissues. This process of circulation is facilitated through an elaborate and dynamic vasculature consisting of arteries, arterioles, capillaries, venules, and veins. The vasculature can dilate or constrict based on central and local regulatory mechanisms. Central regulatory mechanisms stimulate dilation or constriction of the vasculature to maintain an adequate blood pressure (BP). Local regulatory mechanisms, referred to as autoregulation, stimulate vasodilation or vasoconstriction in response to biochemical mediators (cytokines) released by the cell, communicating its need for oxygen and nutrients (Hameed et al., 2003; Kellum & Pinsky, 2002). A biochemical mediator is a substance released by a cell or immune cells such as monocytes and macrophages; the substance triggers an action at a cell site or travels in the bloodstream to a distant site, where it triggers action. Researchers are learning more every day about the physiologic actions of the more than 100 cytokines (Sommers, 2003).

Blood Pressure Regulation

Three major components of the circulatory system—blood volume, the cardiac pump, and the vasculature—must respond effectively to complex neural, chemical, and hormonal feedback systems to maintain an adequate BP and ultimately perfuse body tissues. BP is regulated through a complex interaction of neural, chemical, and hormonal feedback systems affecting both cardiac output and peripheral resistance. This relationship is expressed in the following equation:

$$\text{Mean arterial BP} = \text{cardiac output} \times \text{peripheral resistance}$$

Cardiac output is determined by stroke volume (the amount of blood ejected at systole) and heart rate. Peripheral resistance is determined by the diameter of the arterioles.

Tissue perfusion and organ perfusion depend on mean arterial pressure (MAP), or the average pressure at which blood moves through the vasculature. MAP must exceed 65 mm Hg for cells to receive the oxygen and nutrients needed to metabolize energy in amounts sufficient to sustain life (Dellinger, Carlet, Masur, et al., 2004). Although true MAP can be calculated only by complex methods, Chart 15-1 displays a convenient formula for clinical use in estimating MAP.

BP is regulated by the baroreceptors (pressure receptors) located in the carotid sinus and aortic arch. These pressure receptors convey impulses to the sympathetic nervous center in the medulla of the brain. When BP drops, catecholamines (epinephrine and norepinephrine) are released from the adrenal medulla. This increases heart rate and vasoconstriction, thus restoring BP. Chemoreceptors, also located in the aortic arch and carotid arteries, regulate BP and respiratory rate using much the same mechanism in response to changes in oxygen and carbon dioxide concentrations in the blood. These primary regulatory mechanisms can respond to changes in BP on a moment-to-moment basis.

CHART 15-1

Formula for Estimating Mean Arterial Pressure (MAP)

$$\text{MAP} = \frac{\text{systolic BP} + 2\ (\text{diastolic BP})}{3}$$

Example: patient's BP = 125/75 mm Hg

$$\text{MAP} = \frac{125 + (2 \times 75)}{3}$$

MAP = 92 (rounded to nearest 1/10)

The kidneys also play an important role in BP regulation. They regulate BP by releasing renin, an enzyme needed for the conversion of angiotensin I to angiotensin II, a potent vasoconstrictor. This stimulation of the renin–angiotensin mechanism and the resulting vasoconstriction indirectly lead to the release of aldosterone from the adrenal cortex, which promotes the retention of sodium and water. The increased concentration of sodium in the blood then stimulates the release of antidiuretic hormone (ADH) by the pituitary gland. ADH causes the kidneys to retain water further in an effort to raise blood volume and BP. These secondary regulatory mechanisms may take hours or days to respond to changes in BP.

To summarize, adequate blood volume, an effective cardiac pump, and an effective vasculature are necessary to maintain BP and tissue perfusion. When one of the three components of this system begins to fail, the body is able to compensate through increased work by the other two (Fig. 15-2). After compensatory mechanisms can no longer compensate for the failed system, body tissues become inadequately perfused, and shock occurs. Without prompt intervention, shock progresses, resulting in organ dysfunction, organ failure, and death.

Stages of Shock

Shock is believed to progress along a continuum of stages through which a patient struggles to survive. A convenient way to understand the physiologic responses and subsequent clinical signs and symptoms is to divide the continuum into separate stages: compensatory (stage 1), progressive (stage 2), and irreversible (stage 3). The earlier medical management and nursing interventions can be initiated along this continuum, the greater the patient's chance of survival.

Compensatory Stage

In the compensatory stage of shock, the BP remains within normal limits. Vasoconstriction, increased heart rate, and increased contractility of the heart contribute to maintain-

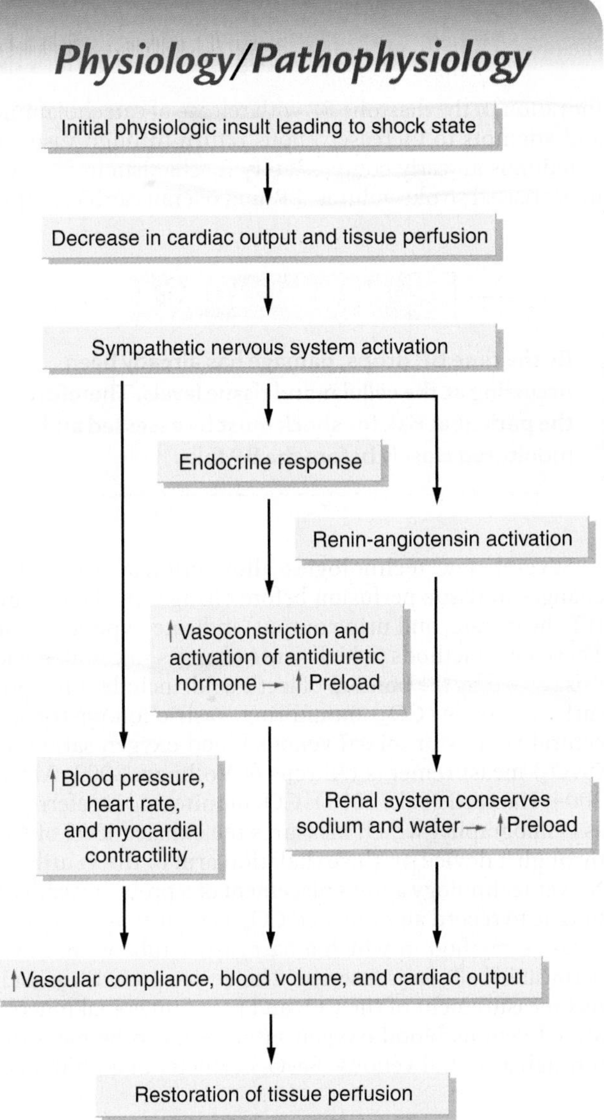

FIGURE 15-2. Compensatory mechanisms in shock. Adapted with permission from Jones, K. (1996). Shock. In Clochesy, J. M., Breu, C., Cardin, S., et al. (Eds.). *Critical care nursing* (2nd ed.) Philadelphia: W. B. Saunders.

ing adequate cardiac output. This results from stimulation of the sympathetic nervous system and subsequent release of catecholamines (epinephrine and norepinephrine). Patients display the often-described "fight or flight" response. The body shunts blood from organs such as the skin, kidneys, and gastrointestinal tract to the brain and heart to ensure adequate blood supply to these vital organs. As a result, the skin is cool and clammy, bowel sounds are hypoactive, and urine output decreases in response to the release of aldosterone and ADH.

Clinical Manifestations

Despite a normal BP, the patient shows numerous clinical signs indicating inadequate organ perfusion (Table 15-1). The result of inadequate perfusion is anaerobic metabolism and a buildup of lactic acid, producing metabolic acidosis. The respiratory rate increases in response to metabolic acidosis. This rapid respiratory rate facilitates removal of excess carbon dioxide but raises the blood pH and often causes a compensatory respiratory alkalosis. The alkalotic state causes mental status changes, such as confusion or combativeness, as well as arteriolar dilation. If treatment begins in this stage of shock, the prognosis for the patient is good.

Medical Management

Medical treatment is directed toward identifying the cause of the shock, correcting the underlying disorder so that shock does not progress, and supporting those physiologic processes that thus far have responded successfully to the threat. Because compensation cannot be effectively maintained indefinitely, measures such as fluid replacement and medication therapy must be initiated to maintain an adequate BP and reestablish and maintain adequate tissue perfusion.

Nursing Management

Early intervention along the continuum of shock is the key to improving the patient's prognosis. Therefore, the nurse must assess the patient at risk for shock systematically to recognize the subtle clinical signs of the compensatory stage before the patient's BP drops. Special considerations related

TABLE 15-1 Clinical Findings in Stages of Shock

	Stage		
Finding	***Compensatory***	***Progressive***	***Irreversible***
Blood pressure	Normal	Systolic <80–90 mm Hg	Requires mechanical or pharmacologic support
Heart rate	>100 bpm	>150 bpm	Erratic or asystole
Respiratory status	>20 breaths/min	Rapid, shallow respirations; crackles	Requires intubation
Skin	Cold, clammy	Mottled, petechiae	Jaundice
Urinary output	Decreased	0.5 mL/kg/h	Anuric, requires dialysis
Mentation	Confusion	Lethargy	Unconscious
Acid-base balance	Respiratory alkalosis	Metabolic acidosis	Profound acidosis

to recognizing early signs of shock in the elderly patient are given in Chart 15-2.

Monitoring Tissue Perfusion

In assessing tissue perfusion, the nurse observes for changes in level of consciousness, vital signs (including pulse pressure), urinary output, skin, and laboratory values (base deficit and lactic acid levels). In the compensatory stage of shock, serum sodium and blood glucose levels are elevated in response to the release of aldosterone and catecholamines.

The roles of the nurse at the compensatory stage of shock are to monitor the patient's hemodynamic status and promptly report deviations to the physician, to assist in identifying and treating the underlying disorder by continuous in-depth assessment of the patient, to administer prescribed fluids and medications, and to promote patient safety. Vital signs are key indicators of hemodynamic status; however, BP is an indirect method of monitoring tissue hypoxia. The nurse should report a systolic BP lower than 90 mm Hg or a drop in systolic BP of 40 mm Hg.

Pulse pressure correlates well with stroke volume, or the amount of blood ejected from the heart with systole. Pulse pressure is calculated by subtracting the diastolic measurement from the systolic measurement; the difference is the pulse pressure (Porth, 2005). Normally, the pulse pressure is 30 to 40 mm Hg. Narrowing or decreased pulse pressure is an earlier indicator of shock than a drop in systolic BP. Decreased or narrowing pulse pressure, an early indication of decreased stroke volume, is illustrated in the following example:

Systolic BP − Diastolic BP = Pulse pressure

Normal pulse pressure:

120 mg Hg − 80 mm Hg = 40 mm Hg

Narrowing of pulse pressure:

90 mm Hg − 70 mm Hg = 20 mm Hg

Elevation in the diastolic BP with release of catecholamines and attempts to increase venous return through vasoconstriction is an early compensatory mechanism in response to decreased stroke volume, BP, and overall cardiac output.

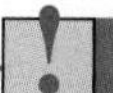

NURSING ALERT

By the time BP drops, damage has already been occurring at the cellular and tissue levels. Therefore, the patient at risk for shock must be assessed and monitored closely before the BP falls.

Several new technologies allow clinicians to detect changes in tissue perfusion before changes in classic signs (BP, heart rate, and urine output) indicate hypoperfusion. These new methods, which sense changes in cellular acidosis caused by the buildup of lactic acid, include sublingual carbon dioxide (CO_2) monitoring, gastric tonometry, and central venous or mixed venous blood oxygen saturation ($S\bar{v}O_2$) measurements (Ahrens & Vollman, 2003; Ahrns, 2004; Hameed et al., 2003). CO_2 monitoring is referred to as capnography, which measures the exhaled level of CO_2 through a device on the exhalation arm of the ventilator. Newer technology allows placement of a probe beneath the tongue to record an estimated CO_2. Gastric tonometry is an invasive method in which a nasogastric tube with a CO_2-permeable balloon is inserted. The device provides an indirect measurement of the CO_2 and pH of intestinal mucosa. Mixed venous blood oxygen saturation can be measured through a central venous ($Sc\bar{v}O_2$) catheter or a pulmonary

CHART 15-2

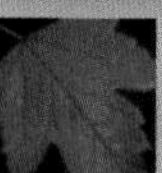

Recognizing Shock in Older Patients

The physiologic changes associated with aging, coupled with pathologic and chronic disease states, place older people at increased risk for developing a state of shock and possibly multiple organ dysfunction syndrome (MODS). Elderly people can recover from shock if it is detected and treated early with aggressive and supportive therapies. Nurses play an essential role in assessing and interpreting subtle changes in older patients' responses to illness.

- Medications such as beta-blocking agents (metoprolol [Lopressor]) used to treat hypertension may mask tachycardia, a primary compensatory mechanism to increase cardiac output, during hypovolemic states.
- The aging immune system may not mount a truly febrile response (temperature more than 40°C or 104°F), but an increasing trend in body temperature should be addressed.
- The heart does not function well in hypoxemic states, and the aging heart may respond to decreased myocardial oxygenation with dysrhythmias that may be misinterpreted as a normal part of the aging process.
- Changes in mentation may be inappropriately misinterpreted as dementia. Older people with a sudden change in mentation should be aggressively treated for the presence of infection and organ hypoperfusion.

artery catheter ($S\bar{v}O_2$) that has a sensor imbedded in the device. The sensor detects changes in saturation of hemoglobin and calculates the venous oxygen saturation.

Although treatments are prescribed and initiated by the physician, the nurse usually implements them, operates and troubleshoots equipment used in treatment, monitors the patient's status during treatment, and assesses the immediate effects of treatment. In addition, the nurse assesses the response of the patient and family to the crisis and its treatment.

Reducing Anxiety

Patients often become anxious and apprehensive when they face a major threat to health and well-being and are the focus of attention of many health care providers. Providing brief explanations about the diagnostic and treatment procedures, supporting the patient during these procedures, and providing information about their outcomes are usually effective in reducing stress and anxiety and thus promoting the patient's physical and mental well-being. Speaking in a calm, reassuring voice and using gentle touch also help ease the patient's concerns. These actions may provide solace and comfort for critically ill, frightened patients (Benner, 2004).

Promoting Safety

Another nursing intervention is monitoring potential threats to the patient's safety, because a high anxiety level and altered mental status typically impair judgment. In this stage of shock, patients who were previously cooperative and followed instructions may now disrupt intravenous (IV) lines and catheters and complicate their condition. Therefore, close monitoring and frequent reorientation interventions are essential.

Progressive Stage

In the second stage of shock, the mechanisms that regulate BP can no longer compensate, and the MAP falls below normal limits. Patients are clinically hypotensive; this is defined as a systolic BP of less than 90 mm Hg or a decrease in systolic BP of 40 mm Hg (Kleinpell, 2003).

Pathophysiology

Although all organ systems suffer from hypoperfusion at this stage, several events perpetuate the shock syndrome. First, the overworked heart becomes dysfunctional; the body's inability to meet increased oxygen requirements produces ischemia; and biochemical mediators cause myocardial depression (Delling, 2003; Kellum & Pinsky, 2002). This leads to failure of the cardiac pump, even if the underlying cause of the shock is not of cardiac origin. Second, the autoregulatory function of the microcirculation fails in response to the numerous biochemical cytokines and mediators released by the cells, resulting in increased capillary permeability, with areas of arteriolar and venous constriction further compromising cellular perfusion (Ahrens & Vollman, 2003; Ahrns, 2004; Fishel, Are, & Barbul, 2003). At this stage, the prognosis worsens. The relaxation of precapillary sphincters causes fluid to leak from the capillaries, creating interstitial edema and return of less fluid to the heart. In addition, the inflammatory response to injury is activated, and proinflammatory and anti-inflammatory cytokines and mediators are released, which in turn activate the coagulation system in an effort to reestablish homeostasis (Kleinpell, 2003; Sommers, 2003). The body mobilizes energy stores and increases oxygen consumption to meet the increased metabolic needs of the underperfused tissues and cells.

Even if the underlying cause of the shock is reversed, the sequence of compensatory responses to the decrease in tissue perfusion perpetuates the shock state, and a vicious circle ensues. The cellular reactions that occur during the progressive stage of shock are an active area of clinical research. It is believed that the body's response to shock or lack of response in this stage of shock may be the primary factor determining the patient's survival.

Assessment and Diagnostic Findings

Chances of survival depend on the patient's general health before the shock state as well as the amount of time it takes to restore tissue perfusion. As shock progresses, organ systems decompensate.

Respiratory Effects

The lungs, which become compromised early in shock, are affected at this stage. Subsequent decompensation of the lungs increases the likelihood that mechanical ventilation will be needed. Respirations are rapid and shallow. Crackles are heard over the lung fields. Decreased pulmonary blood flow causes arterial oxygen levels to decrease and carbon dioxide levels to increase. Hypoxemia and biochemical mediators cause an intense inflammatory response and pulmonary vasoconstriction, perpetuating the pulmonary capillary hypoperfusion and hypoxemia. The hypoperfused alveoli stop producing surfactant and subsequently collapse. Pulmonary capillaries begin to leak, spilling their contents, thus causing pulmonary edema, diffusion abnormalities (shunting), and additional alveolar collapse. Interstitial inflammation and fibrosis are common as the pulmonary damage progresses (Berry & Pinard, 2003). This condition is sometimes referred to as acute respiratory distress syndrome (ARDS), acute lung injury, shock lung, or noncardiogenic pulmonary edema. Further explanation of ARDS, as well as its nursing management, can be found in Chapter 23.

Cardiovascular Effects

A lack of adequate blood supply leads to dysrhythmias and ischemia. The heart rate is rapid, sometimes exceeding 150 bpm. The patient may complain of chest pain and even suffer a myocardial infarction. Levels of cardiac enzymes (eg, lactate dehydrogenase [LDH], creatine phosphokinase myocardium and muscle [CPK-MB], cardiac troponin [cTn-I]) increase. In addition, myocardial depression and ventricular dilation may further impair the heart's ability to pump enough blood to the tissues to meet oxygen requirements.

New laboratory markers also can be used to assess the function of the heart. B-type natriuretic peptide (BNP) is one of these markers. BNP is increased when the ventricle is overdistended; therefore, elevations in BNP can be used to assess ventricular function of patients in shock states (Dellinger, 2003; Hachey & Smith, 2003).

Neurologic Effects

As blood flow to the brain becomes impaired, mental status deteriorates. Changes in mental status occur with decreased cerebral perfusion and hypoxia. Initially, the patient may exhibit a subtle change in behavior or agitation and confusion. Subsequently, lethargy increases, and the patient begins to lose consciousness.

Renal Effects

When the MAP falls below 70 mm Hg (Huether, 2002), the glomerular filtration rate of the kidneys cannot be maintained, and drastic changes in renal function occur. Acute renal failure (ARF) may develop. ARF is characterized by an increase in blood urea nitrogen (BUN) and serum creatinine levels, fluid and electrolyte shifts, acid–base imbalances, and a loss of the renal-hormonal regulation of BP. Urinary output usually decreases to less than 0.5/mL/kg per hour (or less than 30 mL/h) but may vary depending on the phase of ARF. For further information about ARF, see Chapter 44.

Hepatic Effects

Decreased blood flow to the liver impairs the ability of liver cells to perform metabolic and phagocytic functions. Consequently, the patient is less able to metabolize medications and metabolic waste products, such as ammonia and lactic acid. Metabolic activities of the liver, including gluconeogenesis and glycogenolysis, are impaired. The patient becomes more susceptible to infection as the liver fails to filter bacteria from the blood. Liver enzymes (aspartate aminotransferase [AST], alanine aminotransferase [ALT], lactate dehydrogenase [LDH]) and bilirubin levels are elevated, and the patient appears jaundiced.

Gastrointestinal Effects

Gastrointestinal ischemia can cause stress ulcers in the stomach, putting the patient at risk for gastrointestinal bleeding. In the small intestine, the mucosa can become necrotic and slough off, causing bloody diarrhea. Beyond the local effects of impaired perfusion, gastrointestinal ischemia leads to bacterial toxin translocation, in which bacterial toxins enter the bloodstream through the lymph system. In addition to causing infection, bacterial toxins can cause cardiac depression, vasodilation, increased capillary permeability, and an intense inflammatory response with activation of additional biochemical mediators. The net result is interference with healthy cells and their ability to metabolize nutrients (Ceppa, Fuh, & Bulkey, 2003).

Hematologic Effects

The combination of hypotension, sluggish blood flow, metabolic acidosis, coagulation system imbalance, and generalized hypoxemia can interfere with normal hemostatic mechanisms. In shock states, the inflammatory cytokines activate the clotting cascade, causing deposition of microthrombi in multiple areas of the body and consumption of clotting factors. The alterations of the hematologic system, including imbalance of the clotting cascade, are linked to the overactivation of the inflammatory response of injury (Ahrens & Vollman, 2003). Disseminated intravascular coagulation (DIC) may occur either as a cause or as a complication of shock. In this condition, widespread clotting and bleeding occur simultaneously. Bruises (ecchymoses) and bleeding (petechiae) may appear in the skin. Coagulation times (prothrombin time, partial thromboplastin time) are prolonged. Clotting factors and platelets are consumed and require replacement therapy to achieve hemostasis. Further discussion of DIC appears in Chapter 33.

Medical Management

Specific medical management in the progressive stage of shock depends on the type of shock and its underlying cause. It is also based on the degree of decompensation in the organ systems. Medical management specific to each type of shock is discussed later in this chapter. Although there are several differences in medical management by type of shock, some medical interventions are common to all types. These include the use of appropriate IV fluids and medications to restore tissue perfusion by the following methods:

- Optimizing intravascular volume
- Supporting the pumping action of the heart
- Improving the competence of the vascular system
- Supporting the respiratory system

Other aspects of management may include early enteral nutritional support, aggressive hyperglycemic control with IV insulin (van den Berghe, Wouters, & Weekers, 2001), and use of antacids, histamine-2 (H_2) blockers, or antipeptic agents to reduce the risk of gastrointestinal ulceration and bleeding.

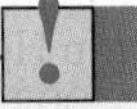

NURSING ALERT

Tight glycemic control (blood glucose, 80 to 110 mg/dL) has been shown to reduce morbidity and mortality of acutely ill patients.

Nursing Management

Nursing care of patients in the progressive stage of shock requires expertise in assessing and understanding shock and the significance of changes in assessment data. Early interventions are essential to the survival of patients in shock; therefore, suspecting that a patient may be in shock and reporting subtle changes in assessment are imperative. Patients in the progressive stage of shock are often cared for in the intensive care setting to facilitate close monitoring (hemodynamic monitoring, electrocardiographic [ECG] monitoring, arterial blood gases, serum electrolyte levels, physical and mental status changes); rapid and frequent administration of various prescribed medications and fluids; and possibly interventions with supportive technologies, such as mechanical ventilation, dialysis, and intra-aortic balloon pump.

Working closely with other members of the health care team, the nurse carefully documents treatments, medications, and fluids that are administered by members of the team, recording the time, dosage or volume, and patient response. In addition, the nurse coordinates both the scheduling of diagnostic procedures that may be carried out at the bedside and the flow of health care personnel involved in care of patients.

Preventing Complications

If supportive technologies are used, the nurse helps reduce the risk of related complications and monitors the patient for early signs of complications. Monitoring includes evaluating blood levels of medications, observing invasive vascular lines for signs of infection, and checking neurovascular status if arterial lines are inserted, especially in the lower extremities. Simultaneously, the nurse promotes the patient's safety and comfort by ensuring that all procedures, including invasive procedures and arterial and venous punctures, are carried out using correct aseptic techniques and that venous and arterial puncture and infusion sites are maintained with the goal of preventing infection. Nursing interventions that reduce the incidence of ventilator-associated pneumonias must also be implemented. These include frequent oral care, aseptic suction technique, turning, and elevating the head of the bed to prevent aspiration (Rello, Ollendorf, Oster, et al., 2002). Positioning and repositioning of the patient to promote comfort and maintain skin integrity are essential.

Promoting Rest and Comfort

Efforts are made to minimize the cardiac workload by reducing the patient's physical activity and fear or anxiety. Promoting patient rest and comfort is a priority. To ensure that the patient obtains as much uninterrupted rest as possible, the nurse performs only essential nursing activities. To conserve the patient's energy, the nurse should protect the patient from temperature extremes (excessive warmth or shivering cold), which can increase the metabolic rate and thus the cardiac workload. The patient should not be warmed too quickly, and warming blankets should not be applied, because they can cause vasodilation and a subsequent drop in BP.

Supporting Family Members

Because patients in shock are the object of intense attention by the health care team, families may be overwhelmed and frightened. Family members may be reluctant to ask questions or seek information for fear that they will be in the way or will interfere with the attention given to the patient. The nurse should make sure that the family is comfortably situated and kept informed about the patient's status. Often, families need advice from the health care team to get some rest; family members are more likely to take this advice if they feel that the patient is being well cared for and that they will be notified of any significant changes in the patient's status. A visit from the hospital chaplain may be comforting and provides some attention to the family while the nurse concentrates on the patient.

Irreversible Stage

The irreversible (or refractory) stage of shock represents the point along the shock continuum at which organ damage is so severe that the patient does not respond to treatment and cannot survive. Despite treatment, BP remains low. Renal and liver failure, compounded by the release of necrotic tissue toxins, creates an overwhelming metabolic acidosis. Anaerobic metabolism contributes to a worsening lactic acidosis. Reserves of ATP are almost totally depleted, and mechanisms for storing new supplies of energy have been destroyed. Respiratory system failure prevents adequate oxygenation and ventilation despite mechanical ventilatory support, and the cardiovascular system is ineffective in maintaining an adequate MAP for tissue perfusion. Multiple organ dysfunction progressing to complete organ failure has occurred, and death is imminent. Multiple organ dysfunction can occur as a progression along the shock continuum or as a syndrome unto itself and is described in more detail later in this chapter.

Medical Management

Medical management during the irreversible stage of shock is usually the same as for the progressive stage. Although the patient may have progressed from the progressive to the irreversible stage, the judgment that the shock is irreversible can be made only retrospectively on the basis of the patient's failure to respond to treatment. Strategies that may be experimental (ie, investigational medications, such as antibiotic agents and immunomodulation therapy) may be tried to reduce or reverse the severity of shock.

Nursing Management

As in the progressive stage of shock, the nurse focuses on carrying out prescribed treatments, monitoring the patient, preventing complications, protecting the patient from injury, and providing comfort. Offering brief explanations to the patient about what is happening is essential even if there is no certainty that the patient hears or understands what is being said. Simple comfort measures, including reassuring touches, should continue to be provided despite the patient's nonresponsiveness to verbal stimuli (Benner, 2004).

As it becomes obvious that the patient is unlikely to survive, the family must be informed about the prognosis and likely outcome. Opportunities should be provided, throughout the patient's care, for the family to see, touch, and talk to the patient. Close family friends or spiritual advisors may be of comfort to the family members in dealing with the inevitable death of their loved one. Whenever possible and appropriate, the patient's family should be approached regarding any living wills, advance directives, or other written or verbal wishes the patient may have shared in the event that he or she became unable to participate in end-of-life decisions. In some cases, ethics committees may assist families and health care teams in making difficult decisions.

During this stage of shock, the family may misinterpret the actions of the health care team. They have been told that nothing has been effective in reversing the shock and that the patient's survival is very unlikely, yet they find physicians and nurses continuing to work feverishly on the patient. Distraught, grieving families may interpret this as a chance for recovery when none exists, and family members may become angry when the patient dies. Conferences with all members of the health care team and the family promote better understanding by the family of the patient's prognosis and the purpose for management measures. During these conferences, it is essential to explain that the equipment and treatments being provided are intended for patient comfort and do not suggest that the patient will recover. Family members should be encouraged to express their wishes concerning the use of life-support measures.

Overall Management Strategies in Shock

As described previously and in the discussion of types of shock to follow, management in all types and all phases of shock includes the following:

- Fluid replacement to restore intravascular volume
- Vasoactive medications to restore vasomotor tone and improve cardiac function
- Nutritional support to address the metabolic requirements that are often dramatically increased in shock

Therapies described in this section require collaboration among all members of the health care team to ensure that the manifestations of shock are quickly identified and that adequate and timely treatment is instituted to achieve the best outcome possible.

Fluid Replacement

Fluid replacement is administered in all types of shock. The type of fluids administered and the speed of delivery vary, but fluids are administered to improve cardiac and tissue oxygenation, which in part depends on flow. The fluids administered may include **crystalloids** (electrolyte solutions that move freely between intravascular and interstitial spaces), **colloids** (large-molecule IV solutions), and blood components.

Crystalloid and Colloid Solutions

The best fluid to treat shock remains controversial. In emergencies, the "best" fluid is often the fluid that is readily available. Fluid resuscitation should be initiated early in shock to maximize intravascular volume. Both crystalloids and colloids, as described later, can be administered to restore intravascular volume. There is no consensus regarding whether crystalloids or colloids should be used; however, with crystalloids, more fluid is necessary to restore intravascular volume (Vincent, 2003). Blood component therapy is used most frequently in hypovolemic shock that is caused by blood loss.

Crystalloids are electrolyte solutions that move freely between the intravascular compartment and the interstitial spaces. Isotonic crystalloid solutions are often selected because they contain the same concentration of electrolytes as the extracellular fluid and therefore can be given without altering the concentrations of electrolytes in the plasma.

Common IV fluids used for resuscitation in hypovolemic shock include 0.9% sodium chloride solution (normal saline) and lactated Ringer's solution (Revell, Greaves, & Porter, 2003). Ringer's lactate is an electrolyte solution containing the lactate ion, which should not be confused with lactic acid. The lactate ion is converted to bicarbonate, which helps buffer the overall acidosis that occurs in shock.

A disadvantage of using isotonic crystalloid solutions is that three parts of the volume are lost to the interstitial compartment for every one part that remains in the intravascular compartment. This occurs in response to mechanisms that store extracellular body fluid. Diffusion of crystalloids into the interstitial space means that more fluid must be administered than the amount lost (Revell et al., 2003; Vincent, 2003).

Care must be taken when rapidly administering isotonic crystalloids to avoid causing excessive edema, particularly pulmonary edema. For this reason, and depending on the cause of the hypovolemia, a hypertonic crystalloid solution, such as 3% sodium chloride, is sometimes administered in hypovolemic shock. Hypertonic solutions produce a large osmotic force that pulls fluid from the intracellular space to the extracellular space to achieve a fluid balance (Ahrns, 2004; Vincent, 2003). The osmotic effect of hypertonic solutions results in fewer fluids being administered to restore intravascular volume. Complications associated with use of hypertonic saline solution include excessive serum osmolality, hypernatremia, hypokalemia, and altered thermoregulation.

Generally, IV colloidal solutions are considered to be plasma proteins, which are molecules that are too large to pass through capillary membranes. Colloids expand intravascular volume by exerting oncotic pressure, thereby pulling fluid into the intravascular space. Colloidal solutions have the same effect as hypertonic solutions in increasing intravascular volume, but less volume of fluid is required than with crystalloids. In addition, colloids have a longer duration of action than crystalloids, because the molecules remain within the intravascular compartment longer.

An albumin solution is commonly used to treat hypovolemic shock. Albumin is a plasma protein; an albumin solution is prepared from human plasma and is heated during production to reduce its potential to transmit disease. The disadvantage of albumin is its high cost. Synthetic colloid preparations, such as hetastarch and dextran solution, are now widely used. However, dextran may interfere with platelet aggregation and therefore is not indicated if hemorrhage is the cause of the hypovolemic shock or if the patient has a coagulation disorder (coagulopathy).

NURSING ALERT

With all colloidal solutions, side effects include the rare occurrence of anaphylactic reactions, for which nurses must monitor patients closely.

Complications of Fluid Administration

Close monitoring of the patient during fluid replacement is necessary to identify side effects and complications. The most common and serious side effects of fluid replacement are cardiovascular overload and pulmonary edema.

The patient receiving fluid replacement must be monitored frequently for adequate urinary output, changes in mental status, skin perfusion, and changes in vital signs. Lung sounds are auscultated frequently to detect signs of fluid accumulation. Adventitious lung sounds, such as crackles, may indicate pulmonary edema.

Often a right atrial pressure line (also known as a central venous pressure [CVP] line) is inserted. In addition to physical assessment, the right atrial pressure value helps in monitoring the patient's response to fluid replacement. A normal right atrial pressure value or CVP is 4 to 12 mm Hg or cm H_2O. Several readings are obtained to determine a range, and fluid replacement is continued to achieve a CVP of 8 to 12 mm Hg (Dellinger et al., 2004). With newer technologies, right atrial catheters can be placed that allow the monitoring of intravascular pressures and venous oxygen levels. Assessment of venous oxygenation ($S\bar{v}O_2$, or $Sc\bar{v}O_2$ with a CVP line) is helpful in evaluating the adequacy of intravascular volume (Ahrens & Vollman, 2003; Ahrns, 2004; Kleinpell, 2003). Hemodynamic monitoring with arterial and pulmonary artery lines may be implemented to allow close monitoring of the patient's perfusion and cardiac status as well as response to therapy. For additional information about hemodynamic monitoring, see Chapter 26.

Vasoactive Medication Therapy

Vasoactive medications are administered in all forms of shock to improve the patient's hemodynamic stability when fluid therapy alone cannot maintain adequate MAP. Specific medications are selected to correct the particular hemodynamic alteration that is impeding cardiac output. Specific vasoactive medications are prescribed for patients in shock because they can support the patient's hemodynamic status. These medications help increase the strength of myocardial contractility, regulate the heart rate, reduce myocardial resistance, and initiate vasoconstriction.

Vasoactive medications are selected for their action on receptors of the sympathetic nervous system. These receptors are known as alpha-adrenergic and beta-adrenergic receptors. Beta-adrenergic receptors are further classified as beta-1 and beta-2 adrenergic receptors. When alpha-adrenergic receptors are stimulated, blood vessels constrict in the cardiorespiratory and gastrointestinal systems, skin, and kidneys. When beta-1 adrenergic receptors are stimulated, heart rate and myocardial contraction increase. When beta-2 adrenergic receptors are stimulated, vasodilation occurs in the heart and skeletal muscles, and the bronchioles relax. The medications used in treating shock consist of various combinations of vasoactive medications to maximize tissue perfusion by stimulating or blocking the alpha- and beta-adrenergic receptors.

When vasoactive medications are administered, vital signs must be monitored frequently (at least every 15 minutes until stable, or more often if indicated). Vasoactive medications should be administered through a central venous line, because infiltration and extravasation of some vasoactive medications can cause tissue necrosis and sloughing. An IV pump or controller should be used to ensure that the medications are delivered safely and accurately.

Individual medication dosages are usually titrated by the nurse, who adjusts drip rates based on the prescribed dose and the patient's response. Dosages are changed to maintain the MAP at a physiologic level that ensures adequate tissue perfusion (usually greater than 65 mm Hg).

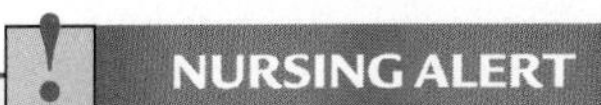

Vasoactive medications should never be stopped abruptly, because this could cause severe hemodynamic instability, perpetuating the shock state.

Dosages of vasoactive medications should be tapered, and the patient should be weaned from medication with frequent monitoring of BP (every 15 minutes). Table 15-2 presents some of the commonly prescribed vasoactive medications used in treating shock. Occasionally, the patient does not respond as expected to vasoactive medications. A current topic of active research is evaluation of patients' adrenal function. Several recent studies have suggested that critically ill patients should be evaluated for corticosteroid insufficiency, and, if this condition is present, corticosteroid replacement should be initiated (Cooper & Stewart, 2003; Marik & Zaloga, 2003).

Nutritional Support

Nutritional support is an important aspect of care for patients with shock. Increased metabolic rates during shock increase energy requirements and therefore caloric requirements. Patients in shock may require more than 3000 calories daily.

The release of catecholamines early in the shock continuum causes depletion of glycogen stores in about 8 to 10 hours. Nutritional energy requirements are then met by breaking down lean body mass. In this catabolic process, skeletal muscle mass is broken down even when the patient has large stores of fat or adipose tissue. Loss of skeletal muscle greatly prolongs the patient's recovery time. Parenteral or enteral nutritional support should be initiated as soon as possible, with some form of enteral nutrition always administered. The integrity of the gastrointestinal system depends on direct exposure to nutrients. In addition, glutamine (an essential amino acid during stress) is important in the immunologic function of the gastro-

TABLE 15-2 Vasoactive Agents Used in Treating Shock

Medication	Desired Action in Shock	Disadvantages
Sympathomimetics Amrinone (Inocor) Dobutamine (Dobutrex) Dopamine (Intropin) Epinephrine (Adrenalin) Milrinone (Primacor)	Improve contractility, increase stroke volume, increase cardiac output	Increase oxygen demand of the heart
Vasodilators Nitroglycerine (Tridil) Nitroprusside (Nipride)	Reduce preload and afterload, reduce oxygen demand of heart	Cause hypotension
Vasoconstrictors Norepinephrine (Levophed) Phenylephrine (Neo-Synephrine) Vasopressin (Pitressin)	Increase blood pressure by vasoconstriction	Increase afterload, thereby increasing cardiac workload; compromise perfusion to skin, kidneys, lungs, gastrointestinal tract

intestinal tract, providing a fuel source for lymphocytes and macrophages. Glutamine can be administered through enteral nutrition (DeLegge, 2001; Flynn, 2004).

Stress ulcers occur frequently in acutely ill patients because of the compromised blood supply to the gastrointestinal tract. Therefore, antacids, H_2 blockers (eg, famotidine [Pepcid], ranitidine [Zantac]), and proton pump inhibitors (eg, lansoprazole [Prevacid]) are prescribed to prevent ulcer formation by inhibiting gastric acid secretion or increasing gastric pH.

Hypovolemic Shock

Nurses who care for patients in the different stages of shock must tailor interventions to the type of shock, whether hypovolemic, cardiogenic, or circulatory shock. Hypovolemic shock, the most common type of shock, is characterized by a decreased intravascular volume. Body fluid is contained in the intracellular and extracellular compartments. Intracellular fluid accounts for about two thirds of the total body water. The extracellular body fluid is found in one of two compartments: intravascular (inside blood vessels) or interstitial (surrounding tissues). The volume of interstitial fluid is about three to four times that of intravascular fluid. Hypovolemic shock occurs when there is a reduction in intravascular volume by 15% to 25%, which represents a loss of 750 to 1300 mL of blood in a 70-kg (154-lb) person.

Pathophysiology

Hypovolemic shock can be caused by external fluid losses, as in traumatic blood loss, or by internal fluid shifts, as in severe dehydration, severe edema, or ascites (Chart 15-3). Intravascular volume can be reduced both by fluid loss and by fluid shifting between the intravascular and interstitial compartments.

The sequence of events in hypovolemic shock begins with a decrease in the intravascular volume. This results in decreased venous return of blood to the heart and subsequent decreased ventricular filling. Decreased ventricular filling results in decreased stroke volume (amount of blood ejected from the heart) and decreased cardiac output. When cardiac output drops, BP drops and tissues cannot be adequately perfused (Fig. 15-3).

Medical Management

Major goals in the treatment of hypovolemic shock are (1) to restore intravascular volume to reverse the sequence of events leading to inadequate tissue perfusion, (2) to redistribute fluid volume, and (3) to correct the underlying cause of the fluid loss as quickly as possible. Depending on the severity of shock and the patient's condition, it is likely that efforts will be made to address all three goals simultaneously.

Treatment of the Underlying Cause

If the patient is hemorrhaging, efforts are made to stop the bleeding. This may involve applying pressure to the bleeding site or surgery to stop internal bleeding. If the cause of the hypovolemia is diarrhea or vomiting, medications to treat diarrhea and vomiting are administered while efforts

CHART 15-3

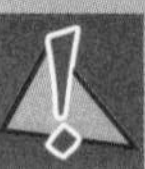

Risk Factors for Hypovolemic Shock

EXTERNAL: FLUID LOSSES
- Trauma
- Surgery
- Vomiting
- Diarrhea
- Diuresis
- Diabetes insipidus

INTERNAL: FLUID SHIFTS
- Hemorrhage
- Burns
- Ascites
- Peritonitis
- Dehydration

Physiology/Pathophysiology

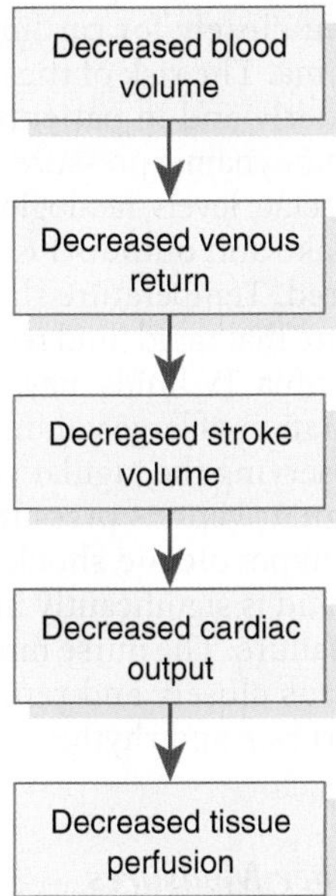

FIGURE 15-3. Pathophysiologic sequence of events in hypovolemic shock.

are made to identify and treat the cause. In elderly patients, dehydration may be the cause of hypovolemic shock.

Fluid and Blood Replacement

Beyond reversing the primary cause of the decreased intravascular volume, fluid replacement (also referred to as fluid resuscitation) is of primary concern. At least two large-gauge IV lines are inserted to establish access for fluid administration. Two IV lines allow simultaneous administration of fluid, medications, and blood component therapy if required. Because the goal of the fluid replacement is to restore intravascular volume, it is necessary to administer fluids that will remain in the intravascular compartment, to avoid fluid shifts from the intravascular compartment into the intracellular compartment. Table 15-3 summarizes the fluids commonly used in the treatment of shock.

Lactated Ringer's solution and 0.9% sodium chloride solution are isotonic crystalloid fluids commonly used in hypovolemic shock (Revell et al., 2003; Stern & Bobek, 2001). Large amounts of fluid must be administered to restore intravascular volume, because isotonic crystalloid solutions move freely between the fluid compartments of the body and do not remain in the vascular system.

Colloids (eg, albumin, hetastarch, and dextran) may also be used. Dextran is not indicated if the cause of the hypovolemic shock is hemorrhage, because it interferes with platelet aggregation.

Blood products, which are also colloids, may need to be administered, particularly if the cause of the hypovolemic shock is hemorrhage. However, there is a risk of transmitting bloodborne viruses, as well as scarcity of blood products; therefore, these products are used only if other alternatives are unavailable or blood loss is extensive and rapid. Packed red blood cells are administered to replenish the patient's oxygen-carrying capacity in conjunction with other fluids that will expand volume. Currently, the need for transfusions is based on the patient's oxygenation needs, which are determined by vital signs, blood gas values, and clinical appearance rather than an arbitrary laboratory value. An area of active research is the development of synthetic forms of blood (ie, compounds capable of carrying oxygen in the same way that blood does) as potential alternatives to blood component therapy.

Redistribution of Fluid

In addition to administering fluids to restore intravascular volume, positioning the patient properly assists fluid redistribution. A modified Trendelenburg position (Fig. 15-4) is recommended in hypovolemic shock. Elevation of the legs promotes the return of venous blood. It is not recom-

TABLE 15-3 Fluid Replacement in Shock

Fluids	Advantages	Disadvantages
Crystalloids		
0.9% sodium chloride (normal saline solution)	Widely available, inexpensive	Requires large volume of infusion; can cause pulmonary edema
Lactated Ringer's	Lactate ion helps buffer metabolic acidosis	Requires large volume of infusion; can cause pulmonary edema
Hypertonic saline (3%, 5%, 7.5%)	Small volume needed to restore intravascular volume	Danger of hypernatremia
Colloids		
Albumin (5%, 25%)	Rapidly expands plasma volume	Expensive; requires human donors; limited supply; can cause heart failure
Dextran (40, 70)	Synthetic plasma expander	Interferes with platelet aggregation; not recommended for hemorrhagic shock
Hetastarch	Synthetic; less expensive than albumin; effect lasts up to 36 h	Prolongs bleeding and clotting times

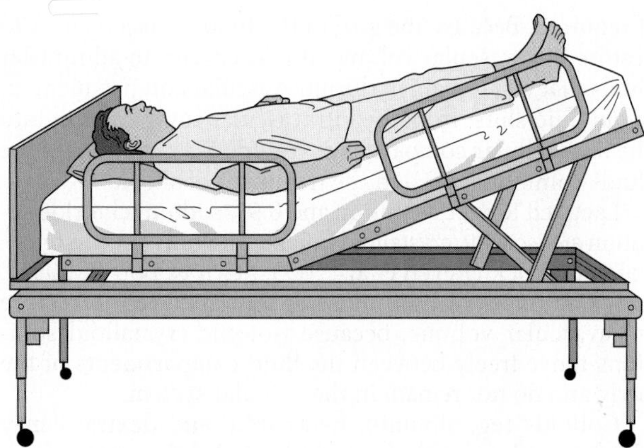

FIGURE 15-4. Proper positioning (modified Trendelenburg) for the patient who shows signs of shock. The lower extremities are elevated to an angle of about 20 degrees; the knees are straight, the trunk is horizontal, and the head is slightly elevated.

mended that patients be put in a full Trendelenburg position, because this makes breathing difficult.

Pharmacologic Therapy

If fluid administration fails to reverse hypovolemic shock, then the same medications given in cardiogenic shock are used, because unreversed hypovolemic shock progresses to cardiogenic failure (the vicious circle).

If the underlying cause of the hypovolemia is dehydration, medications are also administered to reverse the cause of the dehydration. For example, insulin is administered if dehydration is secondary to hyperglycemia, desmopressin (DDAVP) is administered for diabetes insipidus, antidiarrheal agents for diarrhea, and antiemetic medications for vomiting.

Nursing Management

Primary prevention of shock is an essential focus of nursing care. Hypovolemic shock can be prevented in some instances by closely monitoring patients who are at risk for fluid deficits and assisting with fluid replacement before intravascular volume is depleted. In other circumstances, nursing care focuses on assisting with treatment targeted at the cause of the shock and restoring intravascular volume.

General nursing measures include ensuring safe administration of prescribed fluids and medications and documenting their administration and effects. Another important nursing role is monitoring for signs of complications and side effects of treatment and reporting these signs early in treatment.

Administering Blood and Fluids Safely

Administering blood transfusions safely is a vital nursing role. In emergency situations, it is important to acquire blood specimens quickly, to obtain a baseline complete blood count and to type and cross-match the blood in anticipation of blood transfusions. A patient who receives a transfusion of blood products must be monitored closely for adverse effects (see Chapter 33).

Fluid replacement complications can occur, often when large volumes are administered rapidly. Therefore, the nurse monitors the patient closely for cardiovascular overload and pulmonary edema. The risk of these complications is increased in the elderly and in patients with preexisting cardiac disease. Hemodynamic pressure, vital signs, arterial blood gases, serum lactate levels, hemoglobin and hematocrit levels, and fluid intake and output (I & O) are among the parameters monitored. Temperature should also be monitored closely to ensure that rapid fluid resuscitation does not precipitate hypothermia. IV fluids may need to be warmed during the administration of large volumes. Physical assessment focuses on observing the jugular veins for distention and monitoring jugular venous pressure. Jugular venous pressure is low in hypovolemic shock; it increases with effective treatment and is significantly increased with fluid overload and heart failure. The nurse must monitor cardiac and respiratory status closely and report changes in BP, pulse pressure, heart rate and rhythm, and lung sounds to the physician.

Implementing Other Measures

Oxygen is administered to increase the amount of oxygen carried by available hemoglobin in the blood. A patient who is confused may feel apprehensive with an oxygen mask or cannula in place, and frequent explanations about the need for the mask may reduce some of the patient's fear and anxiety. Simultaneously, the nurse must direct efforts to the safety and comfort of the patient.

Cardiogenic Shock

Cardiogenic shock occurs when the heart's ability to contract and to pump blood is impaired and the supply of oxygen is inadequate for the heart and tissues. The causes of cardiogenic shock are known as either coronary or noncoronary. Coronary cardiogenic shock is more common than noncoronary cardiogenic shock and is seen most often in patients with myocardial infarction. Coronary cardiogenic shock occurs when a significant amount of the left ventricular myocardium has been damaged (Hochman, 2003). Patients who experience an anterior wall myocardial infarction are at greatest risk for cardiogenic shock because of the potentially extensive damage to the left ventricle caused by occlusion of the left anterior descending coronary artery. Noncoronary causes of cardiogenic shock are related to conditions that stress the myocardium (eg, severe hypoxemia, acidosis, hypoglycemia, hypocalcemia, and tension pneumothorax) as well as conditions that result in ineffective myocardial function (eg, cardiomyopathies, valvular damage, cardiac tamponade, dysrhythmias).

Pathophysiology

In cardiogenic shock, cardiac output, which is a function of both stroke volume and heart rate, is compromised. When stroke volume and heart rate decrease or become erratic,

BP falls, and tissue perfusion is compromised. Blood supply for tissues and organs and for the heart muscle itself is inadequate, resulting in impaired tissue perfusion. Because impaired tissue perfusion weakens the heart and impairs its ability to pump blood forward, the ventricle does not fully eject its volume of blood at systole. As a result, fluid accumulates in the lungs. This sequence of events can occur rapidly or over a period of days (Fig. 15-5).

Clinical Manifestations

Patients in cardiogenic shock may experience the pain of angina and develop dysrhythmias and hemodynamic instability.

Medical Management

The goals of medical management in cardiogenic shock are (1) to limit further myocardial damage and preserve the healthy myocardium and (2) to improve the cardiac function by increasing cardiac contractility, decreasing ventricular afterload, or both (Hochman, 2003). In general, these goals are achieved by increasing oxygen supply to the heart muscle while reducing oxygen demands.

Correction of Underlying Causes

As with all forms of shock, the underlying cause of cardiogenic shock must be corrected. It is necessary first to treat the oxygenation needs of the heart muscle to ensure its continued ability to pump blood to other organs. In the case of coronary cardiogenic shock, the patient may require thrombolytic therapy, angioplasty, coronary artery bypass graft surgery, intra-aortic balloon pump therapy, or some combination of these treatments. In the case of noncoronary cardiogenic shock, interventions focus on correcting the underlying cause, such as replacement of a faulty cardiac valve, correction of a dysrhythmia, correction of acidosis and electrolyte disturbances, or treatment of the tension pneumothorax.

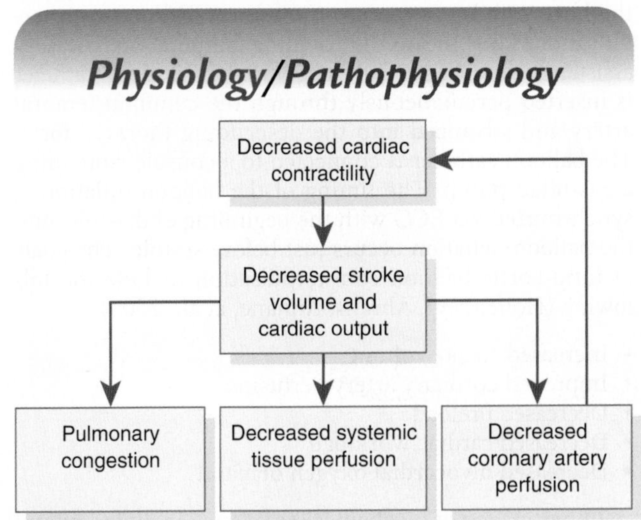

FIGURE 15-5. Pathophysiologic sequence of events in cardiogenic shock.

Initiation of First-Line Treatment

First-line treatment of cardiogenic shock involves the following actions:

- Supplying supplemental oxygen
- Controlling chest pain
- Providing selected fluid support
- Administering vasoactive medications
- Controlling heart rate with medication or by implementation of a transthoracic or IV pacemaker
- Implementing mechanical cardiac support (intra-aortic balloon counterpulsation therapy, ventricular assist systems, or extracorporeal cardiopulmonary bypass [CPB])

OXYGENATION

In the early stages of shock, supplemental oxygen is administered by nasal cannula at a rate of 2 to 6 L/min to achieve an oxygen saturation exceeding 90%. Monitoring of arterial blood gas values and pulse oximetry values helps determine whether the patient requires a more aggressive method of oxygen delivery.

PAIN CONTROL

If a patient experiences chest pain, IV morphine sulfate is administered for pain relief. In addition to relieving pain, morphine dilates the blood vessels. This reduces the workload of the heart by both decreasing the cardiac filling pressure (preload) and reducing the pressure against which the heart muscle has to eject blood (afterload). Morphine also decreases the patient's anxiety.

HEMODYNAMIC MONITORING

Hemodynamic monitoring is initiated to assess the patient's response to treatment. In many institutions, this is performed in the intensive care unit (ICU), where an arterial line can be inserted. The arterial line enables accurate and continuous monitoring of BP and provides a port from which to obtain frequent arterial blood samples without having to perform repeated arterial punctures. A multi-lumen pulmonary artery catheter is inserted to allow measurement of the pulmonary artery pressures, myocardial filling pressures, cardiac output, and pulmonary and systemic resistance. For more information, see Chapter 30.

LABORATORY MARKER MONITORING

Laboratory markers for ventricular dysfunction (BNP) and cardiac enzyme levels (CPK-MB and cTn-I) are measured, and serial 12-lead ECGs are obtained to assess the degree of myocardial damage.

Pharmacologic Therapy

Vasoactive medication therapy consists of multiple pharmacologic strategies to restore and maintain adequate cardiac output. In coronary cardiogenic shock, the aims of vasoactive medication therapy are improved cardiac contractility, decreased preload and afterload, and stabilized heart rate and rhythm.

Because improving contractility and decreasing cardiac workload are opposing pharmacologic actions, two types of medications may be administered in combination:

sympathomimetic agents and vasodilators. Sympathomimetic medications increase cardiac output by mimicking the action of the sympathetic nervous system through vasoconstriction, resulting in increased preload, and through increasing myocardial contractility (inotropic action) or increasing the heart rate (chronotropic action). Vasodilators are used to decrease preload and afterload, thus reducing the workload of the heart and the oxygen demand. Medications commonly combined to treat cardiogenic shock include dobutamine, dopamine, and nitroglycerin (see Table 15-2).

DOBUTAMINE

Dobutamine (Dobutrex) produces inotropic effects by stimulating myocardial beta-receptors, increasing the strength of myocardial activity and improving cardiac output. Myocardial alpha-adrenergic receptors are also stimulated, resulting in decreased pulmonary and systemic vascular resistance (decreased afterload). Dobutamine enhances the strength of cardiac contraction, improving stroke volume ejection and overall cardiac output (Hochman, 2003; Kellum & Pinsky, 2002).

NITROGLYCERIN

IV nitroglycerin (Tridil) in low doses acts as a venous vasodilator and therefore reduces preload. At higher doses, nitroglycerin causes arterial vasodilation and therefore reduces afterload as well. These actions, in combination with dobutamine, increase cardiac output while minimizing cardiac workload. In addition, vasodilation enhances blood flow to the myocardium, improving oxygen delivery to the weakened heart muscle (Hochman, 2003).

DOPAMINE

Dopamine (Intropin) is a sympathomimetic agent that has varying vasoactive effects depending on the dosage. It may be used with dobutamine and nitroglycerin to improve tissue perfusion. Low-dose dopamine (0.5 to 3.0 μg/kg/min) is believed to increase renal and mesenteric blood flow, thereby preventing ischemia of these organs, because shock causes blood to be shunted away from the kidneys and the mesentery. However, this dosage does not improve cardiac output. Medium-dose dopamine (4 to 8 μg/kg/min) has sympathomimetic properties, improves contractility (inotropic action), and slightly increases the heart rate (chronotropic action). At this dosage, dopamine may increase cardiac output. High-dose dopamine (8 to 20 μg/kg/min) predominantly causes vasoconstriction, which increases afterload and thus increases cardiac workload. Because this effect is undesirable in patients with cardiogenic shock, dopamine dosages must be carefully titrated. In severe metabolic acidosis, which occurs in the later stages of shock, the effectiveness of dopamine is diminished. To maximize the effectiveness of any vasoactive agent, metabolic acidosis must first be corrected. Physicians often prescribe IV sodium bicarbonate to treat the acidosis (Dellinger et al., 2004).

OTHER VASOACTIVE MEDICATIONS

Additional vasoactive agents that may be used in managing cardiogenic shock include norepinephrine (Levophed), epinephrine (Adrenalin), milrinone (Primacor), amrinone (Inocor), vasopressin (Pitressin), and phenylephrine (Neo-Synephrine). Each of these medications stimulates different receptors of the sympathetic nervous system. A combination of these medications may be prescribed, depending on the patient's response to treatment. All vasoactive medications have adverse effects, making specific medications more useful than others at different stages of shock. Diuretics such as furosemide (Lasix) may be administered to reduce the workload of the heart by reducing fluid accumulation (see Table 15-2).

ANTIARRHYTHMIC MEDICATIONS

Multiple factors, such as hypoxemia, electrolyte imbalances, and acid–base imbalances, contribute to serious cardiac dysrhythmias in all patients with shock. In addition, as a compensatory response to decreased cardiac output and BP, the heart rate increases beyond normal limits. This impedes cardiac output further by shortening diastole and thereby decreasing the time for ventricular filling. Consequently, antiarrhythmic medications are required to stabilize the heart rate. For a full discussion of cardiac dysrhythmias as well as commonly prescribed medications, see Chapter 27. General principles regarding the administration of vasoactive medications are discussed later in this chapter.

FLUID THERAPY

Appropriate fluid administration is also necessary in the treatment of cardiogenic shock. Administration of fluids must be monitored closely to detect signs of fluid overload. Incremental IV fluid boluses are cautiously administered to determine optimal filling pressures for improving cardiac output. A fluid bolus should never be given rapidly, because rapid fluid administration in patients with cardiac failure may result in acute pulmonary edema.

Mechanical Assistive Devices

If cardiac output does not improve despite supplemental oxygen, vasoactive medications, and fluid boluses, mechanical assistive devices are used temporarily to improve the heart's ability to pump. Intra-aortic balloon counterpulsation is one means of providing temporary circulatory assistance (see Chapter 30). A polyurethane balloon catheter is inserted percutaneously through the common femoral artery and advanced into the descending thoracic aorta. The balloon catheter is connected to a console containing a gas-filled pump. The timing of the balloon inflation is synchronized via ECG with the beginning of diastole, and the balloon deflation occurs just before systole. The goals of intra-aortic balloon counterpulsation include the following (Hollenberg, Ahrens, Annane, et al., 2004):

- Increased stroke volume
- Improved coronary artery perfusion
- Decreased preload
- Decreased cardiac workload
- Decreased myocardial oxygen demand

Other means of mechanical assistance include left and right ventricular assist devices and total temporary artificial hearts. These devices are electrical pumps or pumps driven by air. They assist or replace the ventricular pumping action of the heart. Human heart transplantation may be the only option remaining for a patient who has cardiogenic shock and who cannot be weaned from mechanical assistive devices. (Mechanical assistive devices and heart transplantation are discussed in Chapters 29 and 30.)

Another short-term means of providing cardiac or pulmonary support to the patient in cardiogenic shock is through an extracorporeal device similar to the cardiopulmonary bypass (CPB) system used in open-heart surgery. The CPB system requires systemic anticoagulation; arterial and venous cannulation of the femoral artery and vein; and connection to a centrifugal, oxygenated pump. The catheter tip is advanced into the right atrium. This system lowers left and right ventricular pressures, reducing the workload and oxygen needs of the heart. Complications of CPB include coagulopathies, myocardial ischemia, infection, and thromboembolism. CPB is used only in emergency situations until definitive treatment, such as heart transplantation, can be initiated.

Nursing Management

Preventing Cardiogenic Shock

In some circumstances, identifying at-risk patients early, promoting adequate oxygenation of the heart muscle, and decreasing cardiac workload can prevent cardiogenic shock. This can be accomplished by conserving the patient's energy, promptly relieving angina, and administering supplemental oxygen. Often, however, cardiogenic shock cannot be prevented. In such instances, nursing management includes working with other members of the health care team to prevent shock from progressing and to restore adequate cardiac function and tissue perfusion.

Monitoring Hemodynamic Status

A major role of the nurse is monitoring the patient's hemodynamic and cardiac status. Arterial lines and ECG monitoring equipment must be well maintained and functioning properly. The nurse anticipates the medications, IV fluids, and equipment that might be used and is ready to assist in implementing these measures. Changes in hemodynamic, cardiac, and pulmonary status and laboratory values are documented and reported promptly. In addition, adventitious breath sounds, changes in cardiac rhythm, and other abnormal physical assessment findings are reported immediately.

Administering Medications and Intravenous Fluids

The nurse plays a critical role in the safe and accurate administration of IV fluids and medications. Fluid overload and pulmonary edema are risks because of ineffective cardiac function and accumulation of blood and fluid in the pulmonary tissues. The nurse documents and records medications and treatments that are administered as well as the patient's response to treatment.

The nurse must be knowledgeable about the desired effects as well as the side effects of medications. For example, it is important to monitor the patient for decreased BP after administering morphine or nitroglycerin. Patients receiving thrombolytic therapy must be monitored for bleeding. Arterial and venous puncture sites must be observed for bleeding, and pressure must be applied at the sites if bleeding occurs. Neurologic assessment is essential after the administration of thrombolytic therapy to assess for the potential complication of cerebral hemorrhage associated with the therapy. IV infusions must be observed closely because tissue necrosis and sloughing may occur if vasopressor medications infiltrate the tissues. Urine output, BUN, and serum creatinine levels are monitored to detect decreased renal function secondary to the effects of cardiogenic shock or its treatment.

Maintaining Intra-aortic Balloon Counterpulsation

The nurse plays a critical role in caring for the patient receiving intra-aortic balloon counterpulsation (see Chapter 30). The nurse makes ongoing timing adjustments of the balloon pump to maximize its effectiveness by synchronizing it with the cardiac cycle. The patient is at great risk of circulatory compromise to the leg on the side where the catheter for the balloon has been placed; therefore, the nurse must check the neurovascular status of the lower extremities frequently.

Enhancing Safety and Comfort

Throughout care, the nurse must take an active role in safeguarding the patient, enhancing comfort, and reducing anxiety. This includes administering medication to relieve chest pain, preventing infection at the multiple arterial and venous line insertion sites, protecting the skin, and monitoring respiratory and renal function. Proper positioning of the patient promotes effective breathing without decreasing BP and may also increase patient comfort while reducing anxiety.

Brief explanations about procedures that are being performed and the use of comforting touch often provide reassurance to the patient and family. The family is usually anxious and benefits from opportunities to see and talk to the patient. Explanations of treatments and the patient's responses are often comforting to family members.

Circulatory Shock

Circulatory shock occurs when blood volume is abnormally displaced in the vasculature (eg, when blood volume pools in peripheral blood vessels). The displacement of blood volume causes a relative hypovolemia because not enough blood returns to the heart, which leads to subsequent inadequate tissue perfusion. The ability of the blood vessels to constrict helps return the blood to the heart. The vascular tone is determined both by central regulatory mechanisms, as in BP regulation, and by local regulatory mechanisms, as in tissue demands for oxygen and nutrients. Therefore, circulatory shock can be caused either by a loss of sympathetic tone or by release of biochemical mediators from cells.

The varied mechanisms leading to the initial vasodilation in circulatory shock further subdivide this classification of shock into three types: (1) **septic shock,** (2) **neurogenic shock,** and (3) **anaphylactic shock.**

The different types of circulatory shock cause variations in the pathophysiologic chain of events and are explained here separately. In all types of circulatory shock, massive arterial and venous dilation allows blood to pool peripherally. Arterial dilation reduces systemic vascular resistance. Initially, cardiac output can be high, both from the reduction in afterload (systemic vascular resistance) and from the heart muscle's increased effort to maintain perfusion despite the incompetent vasculature secondary to arterial dilation. Pooling of blood in the periphery results in decreased venous return. Decreased venous return results in decreased stroke volume and decreased cardiac output. Decreased cardiac output, in turn, causes decreased BP and ultimately decreased tissue perfusion. Figure 15-6 presents the pathophysiologic sequence of events in circulatory shock.

CHART 15-4

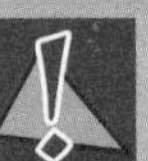

Risk Factors for Circulatory Shock

SEPTIC SHOCK
- Immunosuppression
- Extremes of age (<1 yr and >65 yr)
- Malnourishment
- Chronic illness
- Invasive procedures

NEUROGENIC SHOCK
- Spinal cord injury
- Spinal anesthesia
- Depressant action of medications
- Glucose deficiency

ANAPHYLACTIC SHOCK
- Penicillin sensitivity
- Transfusion reaction
- Bee sting allergy
- Latex sensitivity
- Severe allergy to some foods or medications

Septic Shock

Septic shock, the most common type of circulatory shock, is caused by widespread infection (Chart 15-4). Despite the increased sophistication of antibiotic therapy, the incidence of septic shock has continued to rise during the past 60 years. It is the most common cause of death in noncoronary ICUs in the United States; annually, an estimated 215,000 deaths are due to severe sepsis (Aird, 2003). Finding and aggressively treating the source of infection is an important determinant of the clinical outcome.

Nosocomial infections (infections occurring in the hospital) in critically ill patients that may progress to septic shock most frequently originate in the bloodstream, lungs, and urinary tract (in decreasing order of frequency) (Ahrens & Vollman, 2003; Kleinpell, 2003; Sommers, 2003). Other infections include intra-abdominal infections, wound infections, and bacteremia associated with intravascular catheters (Eggimann & Pittet, 2001) and indwelling urinary catheters (urosepsis). Additional risk factors that contribute to the growing incidence of septic shock are increased awareness and identification of the condition; the increased number of immunocompromised patients (due to malnutrition, alcoholism, malignancy, diabetes mellitus, and AIDS); the increased use of invasive procedures and indwelling medical devices; the increased number of resistant microorganisms; and the increasingly older population (Ahrens & Vollman, 2003; Kleinpell, 2003). The incidence of septic shock can be reduced by débriding wounds to remove necrotic tissue; carrying out infection control practices, including the use of meticulous aseptic technique; properly cleaning and maintaining equipment; and using thorough hand-hygiene techniques (Dellinger et al., 2004).

Elderly patients continue to be at particular risk for sepsis because of decreased physiologic reserves and an aging immune system (Kleinpell, 2003; Sommers, 2003). Other patients at risk are those undergoing surgical and other invasive procedures; those with malnutrition or immunosuppression; and those with chronic illness such as diabetes mellitus, hepatitis, chronic renal failure, and immunodeficiency disorders (Kleinpell, 2003).

A significant body of research has been conducted in the past decade in an effort aimed at reducing the morbidity and mortality caused by septic shock. In 1991, the American College of Chest Physicians and the Society of Critical Care Medicine convened a consensus conference to clarify the

Physiology/Pathophysiology

Precipitating event
↓
Vasodilation
↓
Activation of inflammatory response
↓
Maldistribution of blood volume
↓
Decreased venous return
↓
Decreased cardiac output
↓
Decreased tissue perfusion

FIGURE 15-6. Pathophysiologic sequence of events in circulatory shock.

understanding of sepsis and related disorders (Sommers, 2003). In 2002, the Society of Critical Care Medicine further defined the definitions to promote recognition and earlier treatment of patients with sepsis (Chart 15-5). Research efforts continued to define further the physiologic mystery of sepsis progressing to multisystem organ dysfunction and potential treatments. In March 2003, critical care experts and infectious disease experts evaluated the research and provided evidence-based recommendations for the acute management of patients with sepsis and septic shock (Dellinger et al., 2004).

Pathophysiology

The most common causative microorganisms of septic shock are the gram-negative bacteria. However, there is also an increased incidence of gram-positive bacterial infections. Currently, gram-positive bacteria are responsible for 50% of bacteremic events (Houghton, 2002). Other infectious agents, such as viruses and fungi, also can cause septic shock. However, it is estimated that 20% to 30% of patients with severe sepsis may never have an identifiable site of infection (Sommers, 2003).

When microorganisms invade body tissues, patients exhibit an immune response. This immune response provokes the activation of biochemical cytokines and mediators associated with an inflammatory response and produces a complex cascade of physiologic events that leads to poor tissue perfusion. Increased capillary permeability, which leads to fluid seeping from the capillaries, and vasodilation are two such effects that interrupt the ability of the body to provide adequate perfusion, oxygen, and nutrients to the tissues and cells. In addition, proinflammatory and anti-inflammatory cytokines released during the inflammatory response activate the coagulation system, which begins to form clots in areas where a clot may or may not be needed, further compromising tissue perfusion. The imbalance of the inflammatory response and the clotting and fibrinolysis

CHART 15-5

Definitions to Promote Recognition and Earlier Treatment of Patients With Sepsis

Bacteremia: the presence of bacteria in the blood

Infection: the presence of microorganisms that trigger an inflammatory response

Hypotension: a systolic blood pressure <90 mm Hg or a drop in systolic blood pressure of >40 mm Hg from the patient's baseline blood pressure

Sepsis: a systemic response to *infection;* may occur after a burn, surgery, or serious illness and is manifested by two or more clinical signs and symptoms:

- Temperature >38°C or <36°C
- Heart rate >90 bpm
- Respiratory rate >30 breaths/min
- $PaCO_2$ <32 mm Hg
- WBC count >12,000 cells/mm^3, <4000 cells/mm^3, or >10% immature WBC (bands)
- Hyperglycemia and abnormal clotting and bleeding

***PIRO* model:** a method useful in recognizing and trending patients with sepsis

- **P**atient genetic predisposition and response to infection
- **I**nfection
- **R**esponse to infection
- **O**rgan dysfunction associated with infectious response

Severe sepsis: the presence of signs and symptoms of sepsis-related organ dysfunction, hypotension, and/or hypoperfusion; clinical signs and symptoms include those of sepsis as well as

- Lactic acidosis
- Oliguria
- Altered level of consciousness
- Thrombocytopenia
- Alternated level of consciousness

Septic shock: shock associated with sepsis; characterized by symptoms of sepsis plus hypotension and hypoperfusion despite adequate fluid volume replacement

Systemic inflammatory response syndrome (SIRS): a syndrome resulting from a *severe clinical insult* that initiates an overwhelming inflammatory response by the body; clinical signs and symptoms may include

- Temperature >38°C or <36°C (>100.4°F or < 96.8°F)
- Heart rate >90 bpm
- Respiratory rate >30 breaths/min
- $PaCO_2$ <32 mm Hg
- WBC count >12,000 cells/mm^3, <4000 cells/mm^3, or >10% immature WBC (bands)

Multiple organ dysfunction syndrome: the presence of altered function of one or more organs in an acutely ill patient requiring intervention and support of the organs to achieve physiologic functioning required for homeostasis; clinical signs and symptoms may be

- Cardiovascular: hypotension and hypoperfusion
- Respiratory: hypoxemia, hypercarbia, adventitious breath sounds
- Renal: increased creatinine, decreased urine output
- Hematologic: thrombocytopenia, bleeding
- Metabolic: lactic acidemia, metabolic acidosis
- Neurologic: altered level of consciousness
- Hepatic: elevated liver function tests

Adapted from Sommers, M. S. (2003). The cellular basis of septic shock. *Critical Care Nursing Clinics of North America, 15*(1), 13–26.

cascades are considered critical elements of the devastating physiologic progression that is present in patients with severe sepsis.

Sepsis is an evolving process, with neither clearly definable clinical signs and symptoms nor predictable progression. In the past, septic shock has been described as having two phases, a hyperdynamic and a hypodynamic phase. Although the division into phases may promote understanding of sepsis, its actual progression into severe sepsis and septic shock is not always easy to recognize clinically. Initially, a hyperdynamic response occurs; it is characterized by a high cardiac output with systemic vasodilation. The BP may remain within normal limits, or the patient may be hypotensive but responsive to fluids. The heart rate increases, progressing to tachycardia. Hyperthermia and fever, with warm, flushed skin and bounding pulses, is evident. The respiratory rate is elevated. Urinary output may remain at normal levels or decrease. Gastrointestinal status may be compromised, as evidenced by nausea, vomiting, diarrhea, or decreased bowel sounds. Signs of hypermetabolism include increased serum glucose and insulin resistance. Subtle changes in mental status, such as confusion or agitation, may be present.

As the sepsis progresses, tissues become more underperfused and acidotic, compensation begins to fail, and the patient becomes more hypodynamic. The cardiovascular system also begins to fail, the BP does not respond to vasoactive agents and fluid resuscitation, and signs of end-organ damage are visible (eg, renal failure, pulmonary failure, hepatic failure). As sepsis progresses to septic shock, the BP drops, and the skin becomes cool and pale. Temperature may be normal or below normal. Heart and respiratory rates remain rapid. Urine production no longer occurs, and multiple organ dysfunction progressing to failure develops.

Systemic inflammatory response syndrome (SIRS) presents clinically like sepsis. The only difference between SIRS and sepsis is that there is no identifiable source of infection. SIRS stimulates an overwhelming inflammatory immunologic and hormonal response similar to that seen in septic patients. Any overwhelming insult stimulates SIRS and may progress to sepsis. Therefore, despite an absence of infection, antibiotic agents may still be administered because of the possibility of unrecognized infection. Additional therapies directed to support patients with SIRS are similar to those for sepsis. If the inflammatory process progresses, septic shock may develop.

Medical Management

Current treatment of septic shock involves identification and elimination of the cause of infection. Specimens of blood, sputum, urine, wound drainage, and tips of invasive catheters are collected for culture using aseptic technique.

Any potential routes of infection must be eliminated. IV lines are removed and reinserted at other body sites. Antibiotic-coated IV central lines may be inserted to decrease the risk of invasive line-related bacteremia in high-risk patients, such as the elderly (Eggimann & Pittet, 2001). If possible, urinary catheters are removed. Any abscesses are drained, and necrotic areas are débrided.

Fluid replacement must be instituted to correct the hypovolemia that results from the incompetent vasculature and the inflammatory response. Crystalloids, colloids, and blood products may be administered to increase intravascular volume.

Pharmacologic Therapy

If the infecting organism is unknown, broad-spectrum antibiotic agents are started until culture and sensitivity reports are received (Houghton, 2002). A third-generation cephalosporin plus an aminoglycoside may be prescribed initially. This combination works against most gram-negative and some gram-positive organisms. When culture and sensitivity reports become available, the antibiotic agents may be changed to agents that are more specific to the infecting organism and less toxic to the patient.

Research efforts show promise for improving the outcomes of septic shock. Although past treatments focused on destroying the infectious organism, emphasis is now on altering the patient's immune response to the organism as well as modulating the inflammatory and coagulation response to infection. Current research focuses on the development of medications that adjust the effects of biochemical cytokines and mediator responses.

Studies have recently demonstrated that recombinant human activated protein C (rhAPC) reduces mortality in patients with severe sepsis (Ahrens & Vollman, 2003; Angus, Zinde-Zwirble, Clermont, et al., 2003; Kleinpell, 2003). The U.S. Food and Drug Administration has approved its use for treatment of adults with severe sepsis and resulting acute organ dysfunction who are at high risk for death. rhAPC acts as an antithrombotic, anti-inflammatory, and profibrinolytic agent. In sepsis, an imbalance in proinflammatory mediators activates the coagulation cascade and deposits microthrombi that alter tissue perfusion. rhAPC is an anti-inflammatory cytokine that stimulates fibrinolysis, restoring balance in the coagulation–anticoagulation homeostatic process of the body's inflammatory response to injury and infection.

APC, available as drotrecogin alfa (Xigris), has provided a significant breakthrough in the successful pharmacologic treatment of patients with sepsis. However, the medication should be administered as early as possible in the sequence of pathophysiologic events of sepsis. Nurses are critical in the identification of patients in the early stage of sepsis for treatment with drotrecogin alfa (Kleinpell, 2003). The medication is not without side effects, bleeding being the most common serious effect. Stopping the medication reduces the risk of bleeding. The patient should be evaluated with regard to the relative risk of bleeding versus the potential benefit from the medication. Drotrecogin alfa is contraindicated in patients with active internal bleeding, recent hemorrhagic stroke, intracranial surgery, or head injury.

Nutritional Therapy

Aggressive nutritional supplementation is critical in the management of septic shock, because malnutrition further impairs the patient's resistance to infection. Nutritional supplementation should be initiated within the first 24 hours after ICU admission (DeLegge, 2001), and continuous infusions of insulin should be used to control hyperglycemia (Dellinger et al., 2004). Enteral feedings are preferred to the parenteral route because of the increased risk of iatrogenic infection associated with IV catheters; however, enteral feedings may not be possible if decreased perfusion to the gastrointestinal tract reduces peristalsis and impairs absorption.

Nursing Management

Nurses caring for patients in any setting must keep in mind the risks of sepsis and the high mortality rate associated with sepsis, severe sepsis, and septic shock. All invasive procedures must be carried out with aseptic technique after careful hand hygiene. In addition, IV lines, arterial and venous puncture sites, surgical incisions, traumatic wounds, urinary catheters, and pressure ulcers must be monitored for signs of infection in all patients. Nurses identify patients who are at particular risk for sepsis and septic shock (ie, elderly and immunosuppressed patients and those with extensive trauma, burns, or diabetes), keeping in mind that these high-risk patients may not develop typical or classic signs of infection and sepsis. For example, confusion may be the first sign of infection and sepsis in elderly patients.

When caring for a patient with septic shock, the nurse collaborates with other members of the health care team to identify the site and source of sepsis and the specific organisms involved. Appropriate specimens for culture and sensitivity are often obtained by the nurse.

Elevated body temperature (hyperthermia) is common with sepsis and raises the patient's metabolic rate and oxygen consumption. Fever is one of the body's natural mechanisms for fighting infections. Therefore, elevated temperatures may not be treated unless they reach dangerous levels (more than 40°C [104°F]) or unless the patient is uncomfortable. Efforts may be made to reduce the temperature by administering acetaminophen or applying a hypothermia blanket. During these therapies, the nurse monitors the patient closely for shivering, which increases oxygen consumption. Efforts to increase comfort are important if the patient experiences fever, chills, or shivering.

The nurse administers prescribed IV fluids and medications, including antibiotic agents and vasoactive medications, to restore vascular volume. Because of decreased perfusion to the kidneys and liver, serum concentrations of antibiotic agents that are normally cleared by these organs may increase and produce toxic effects. Therefore, the nurse monitors blood levels (antibiotic agent, BUN, creatinine, white blood cell count, hemoglobin, hematocrit, platelet levels, coagulation studies) and reports changes to the physician. As with other types of shock, the nurse monitors the patient's hemodynamic status, fluid intake and output, and nutritional status. Daily weights and close monitoring of serum albumin levels help determine the patient's protein requirements.

Neurogenic Shock

In neurogenic shock, vasodilation occurs as a result of a loss of balance between parasympathetic and sympathetic stimulation. Sympathetic stimulation causes vascular smooth muscle to constrict, and parasympathetic stimulation causes the vascular smooth muscle to relax or dilate. The patient experiences a predominant parasympathetic stimulation that causes vasodilation lasting for an extended period, leading to a relative hypovolemic state. However, blood volume is adequate, because the vasculature is dilated; the blood volume is displaced, producing a hypotensive (low BP) state. The overriding parasympathetic stimulation that occurs with neurogenic shock causes a drastic decrease in the patient's systemic vascular resistance and bradycardia. Inadequate BP results in the insufficient perfusion of tissues and cells that is common to all shock states.

Neurogenic shock can be caused by spinal cord injury, spinal anesthesia, or nervous system damage. It may also result from the depressant action of medications or from lack of glucose (eg, insulin reaction or shock). Neurogenic shock may have a prolonged course (spinal cord injury) or a short one (syncope or fainting). Normally, during states of stress, the sympathetic stimulation causes the BP and heart rate to increase. In neurogenic shock, the sympathetic system is not able to respond to body stressors. Therefore, the clinical characteristics of neurogenic shock are signs of parasympathetic stimulation. It is characterized by dry, warm skin rather than the cool, moist skin seen in hypovolemic shock. Another characteristic is hypotension with bradycardia, rather than the tachycardia that characterizes other forms of shock.

Medical Management

Treatment of neurogenic shock involves restoring sympathetic tone, either through the stabilization of a spinal cord injury or, in the instance of spinal anesthesia, by positioning the patient properly. Specific treatment depends on cause of the shock. Further discussion of management of patients with a spinal cord injury is presented in Chapter 63. If hypoglycemia (insulin shock) is the cause, glucose is rapidly administered. Hypoglycemia and the insulin reaction are described further in Chapter 41.

Nursing Management

It is important to elevate and maintain the head of the bed at least 30 degrees to prevent neurogenic shock when a patient receives spinal or epidural anesthesia. Elevation of the head helps prevent the spread of the anesthetic agent up the spinal cord. In suspected spinal cord injury, neurogenic shock may be prevented by carefully immobilizing the patient to prevent further damage to the spinal cord.

Nursing interventions are directed toward supporting cardiovascular and neurologic function until the usually transient episode of neurogenic shock resolves. Applying elastic compression stockings and elevating the foot of the bed may minimize pooling of blood in the legs. Pooled blood increases the risk for thrombus formation. Therefore, the nurse must check the patient daily for any lower-extremity pain, redness, tenderness, and warmth of the calves. If the patient complains of pain and objective assessment of the calf is suspicious, the patient should be evaluated for deep vein thrombosis.

Administration of heparin or low-molecular-weight heparin (Lovenox) as prescribed, application of elastic compression stockings, or use of pneumatic compression of the legs may prevent thrombus formation. Passive range of motion of the immobile extremities helps promote circulation.

A patient who has experienced a spinal cord injury may not report pain caused by internal injuries. Therefore, in the immediate postinjury period, the nurse must monitor the patient closely for signs of internal bleeding that could lead to hypovolemic shock.

Anaphylactic Shock

Anaphylactic shock occurs rapidly and is life-threatening. Because anaphylactic shock occurs in patients already exposed to an antigen and who have developed antibodies to it, it can often be prevented. Patients with known allergies should understand the consequences of subsequent exposure to the antigen and should wear medical identification that lists their sensitivities. This could prevent inadvertent administration of a medication that would lead to anaphylactic shock. In addition, patients and families need instruction about emergency use of medications for treatment of anaphylaxis.

Anaphylactic shock is caused by a severe allergic reaction when patients who have already produced antibodies to a foreign substance (antigen) develop a systemic antigen–antibody reaction. This process requires that the patient has previously been exposed to the substance. An antigen–antibody reaction provokes mast cells to release potent vasoactive substances, such as histamine or bradykinin, causing widespread vasodilation and capillary permeability.

Medical Management

Treatment of anaphylactic shock requires removing the causative antigen (eg, discontinuing an antibiotic agent), administering medications that restore vascular tone, and providing emergency support of basic life functions. Epinephrine is given for its vasoconstrictive action. Diphenhydramine (Benadryl) is administered to reverse the effects of histamine, thereby reducing capillary permeability. These medications are given intravenously. Nebulized medications, such as albuterol (Proventil), may be given to reverse histamine-induced bronchospasm.

If cardiac arrest and respiratory arrest are imminent or have occurred, cardiopulmonary resuscitation is performed. Endotracheal intubation or tracheotomy may be necessary to establish an airway. IV lines are inserted to provide access for administering fluids and medications. Anaphylaxis and specific chemical mediators are discussed further in Chapter 53.

Nursing Management

The nurse has an important role in preventing anaphylactic shock. The nurse must assess all patients for allergies or previous reactions to antigens (eg, medications, blood products, foods, contrast agents, latex) and communicate the existence of these allergies or reactions to others. In addition, the nurse assesses the patient's understanding of previous reactions and steps taken by the patient and family to prevent further exposure to antigens. When new allergies are identified, the nurse advises the patient to wear or carry identification that names the specific allergen or antigen.

When administering any new medication, the nurse observes all patients for allergic reactions. This is especially important with IV medications. Allergy to penicillin is one of the most common causes of anaphylactic shock. Patients who have a penicillin allergy may also develop an allergy to similar medications. For example, they may react to cefazolin sodium (Ancef) because it has a similar antimicrobial action of attaching to the penicillin-binding proteins found on the walls of infectious organisms. Previous adverse drug reactions increase the risk that the patient will develop an undesirable reaction to a new medication. If the patient reports an allergy to a medication, the nurse must be aware of the risks involved in the administration of similar medications.

In the hospital and outpatient diagnostic testing sites, the nurse must identify patients who are at risk for anaphylactic reactions to the contrast agents (radiopaque, dye-like substances that may contain iodine) that are used for diagnostic tests. These include patients with a known allergy to iodine or fish and those who have had previous allergic reactions to contrast agents. This information must be conveyed to the staff at the diagnostic testing site, including x-ray personnel.

The nurse must be knowledgeable about the clinical signs of anaphylaxis, must take immediate action if signs and symptoms occur, and must be prepared to begin cardiopulmonary resuscitation if cardiorespiratory arrest occurs. In addition to monitoring the patient's response to treatment, the nurse assists with intubation if needed, monitors the hemodynamic status, ensures IV access for administration of medications, administers prescribed medications and fluids, and documents treatments and their effects.

Community health and home care nurses who administer medications, including antibiotic agents, in the patient's home or other settings, must be prepared to administer epinephrine subcutaneously or intramuscularly in the event of an anaphylactic reaction.

After recovery from anaphylaxis, the patient and family require an explanation of the event. Furthermore, the nurse provides instruction about avoiding future exposure to antigens and administering emergency medications to treat anaphylaxis (see Chapter 53).

Multiple Organ Dysfunction Syndrome

Multiple organ dysfunction syndrome (MODS) is altered organ function in acutely ill patients that requires medical intervention to support continued organ function. It is another phase in the progression of shock states. The actual incidence of MODS is difficult to determine, because it develops with acute illnesses that compromise tissue perfusion. In addition, there is a lack of consistent definitions to describe the organ failure that is found in MODS (Vincent et al., 2002). It is estimated that MODS has an associated mortality rate as high as 75% (Schulman, 2003).

Pathophysiology

MODS can be classified as primary or secondary. Primary MODS is the result of direct tissue insult, which then leads to impaired perfusion or ischemia. Secondary MODS is most often a complication of SIRS and sepsis. However, MODS may be a complication of any form of shock because of inadequate tissue perfusion. As previously described, in shock, all organ systems suffer damage from a lack of adequate perfusion that can result in organ failure. Sequential organ failure has been further observed. The exact triggering mechanism is unknown.

Various causes of MODS have been identified, including dead or injured tissue, infection, and perfusion deficits. However, it is not possible as yet to predict which patients will develop MODS, partly because much of the organ damage occurs at the cellular level and therefore cannot be directly observed or measured. The organ failure usually begins in the lungs and is followed by failure of the liver, gastrointestinal system, and kidneys (Vincent et al., 2002). Advanced age, malnutrition, and coexisting diseases appear to increase the risk of MODS in acutely ill patients.

Clinical Manifestations

In both primary and secondary MODS, an initial event results in low BP. After treatment for the cause of the decrease in BP, the patient appears to respond.

In primary MODS, which occurs most often when the initiating event is a pulmonary one such as lung injury, the patient experiences respiratory compromise that necessitates intubation. This usually occurs within 72 hours after the initiating event. Respiratory failure leads rapidly to MODS, resulting in a mortality rate of 30% to 75% (Fein & Calalang-Colucci, 2000).

In secondary MODS, which occurs most often in patients with septic shock, the pattern is more insidious and progressively unfolds over about 1 month. Patients also experience respiratory failure and require intubation. They remain hemodynamically stable for about 7 to 14 days. Despite this apparent stability, they exhibit a hypermetabolic state that is characterized by hyperglycemia (elevated blood glucose level), hyperlacticacidemia (excess of lactic acid in the blood), and polyuria (excessive urinary output). The metabolic rate is 1.5 to 2 times the basal metabolic rate. Infection is usually present, and skin breakdown begins. During this stage, there is a severe loss of skeletal muscle mass (autocatabolism). If the hypermetabolic phase can be reversed, the patient may survive with some damage to affected organ systems (DeLegge, 2001). If the hypermetabolic process cannot be halted and cells do not receive adequate oxygen and nutrients, the patient has irreversible organ failure and dies.

If the hypermetabolic phase cannot be reversed, MODS progresses and is characterized by jaundice, hyperbilirubinemia (liver failure), and oliguria progressing to anuria (renal failure) often requiring dialysis. Patients become less hemodynamically stable and begin to require vasoactive medications and fluid support. The onset of organ dysfunction is an ominous prognostic sign; the more organs that fail, the worse the outcome.

Medical Management

Prevention remains the top priority in managing MODS. Elderly patients are at increased risk for MODS because of the lack of physiologic reserve associated with aging and the natural degenerative process, especially immune compromise (Schulman, 2003; Vincent et al., 2002). Early detection and documentation of initial signs of infection are essential in managing MODS in elderly patients. Subtle changes in mentation and a gradual rise in temperature are early warning signs. Other patients at risk for MODS are those with chronic illness, malnutrition, immunosuppression, or surgical or traumatic wounds.

If preventive measures fail, treatment measures to reverse MODS are aimed at (1) controlling the initiating event, (2) promoting adequate organ perfusion, and (3) providing nutritional support.

Nursing Management

The general plan of nursing care for patients with MODS is the same as that for patients in septic shock. Primary nursing interventions are aimed at supporting the patient and monitoring organ perfusion until primary organ insults are halted. Providing information and support to family members is a critical role of the nurse. It is important that the health care team address end-of-life decisions to ensure that supportive therapies are congruent with the patient's wishes (see Chapter 17).

Promoting Communication

Nurses encourage frequent and open communication about treatment modalities and options to ensure that the patient's wishes regarding medical management are met. For patients who survive MODS, it is essential that they be informed about the goals of rehabilitation and expectations for progress toward these goals, because the massive loss of skeletal muscle mass makes rehabilitation a long, slow process. A strong nurse–patient relationship built on effective communication provides needed encouragement during this phase of recovery.

Promoting Home and Community-Based Care

Teaching Patients Self-Care

Patients who experience and survive shock may have been unable to get out of bed for an extended period of time and are likely to have a slow, prolonged recovery. The patient and family are instructed about strategies to prevent further episodes of shock by identifying the factors implicated in the initial episode. In addition, the patient and family require instruction about assessments needed to identify the complications that may occur after the patient is discharged from the hospital. Depending on the type of shock and its management, the patient or family may require instruction about treatment modalities such as emergency administration of medications, IV therapy, parenteral nutrition, skin care, exercise, and ambulation. The patient and family are also instructed about the need for gradual increases in ambulation and other activity. The need for adequate nutrition is another crucial aspect of teaching.

Continuing Care

Because of the physical toll associated with recovery from shock, patients may be cared for in an extended care facility or rehabilitation setting after hospital discharge. Alternatively, a referral may be made for home care. The home care nurse assesses the patient's physical status and monitors recovery. The nurse also assesses the adequacy of treatments that are continued at home and the ability of the patient and family to cope with these treatments. The patient is likely to require close medical supervision until complete recovery occurs. The home care nurse reinforces the importance of continuing medical care and helps the patient and family identify and mobilize community resources.

Critical Thinking Exercises

1 You administer an antibiotic to a patient before he goes to surgery. The patient's chart states that he has no known drug allergies. After 15 minutes, the patient complains of anxiety, shortness of breath, and chest discomfort. He is flushed and visibly uncomfortable. What are your nursing priorities in providing care to this patient? What assessment data do you need to obtain to determine if this patient is experiencing cardiogenic or anaphylactic shock? What nursing interventions and medical treatments would you anticipate for cardiogenic shock? In terms of anaphylactic shock, what nursing interventions and medical treatments would you anticipate?

2 ebp An elderly man with a 10-year history of Alzheimer's disease was admitted with sudden, increasing confusion and combative behavior. You know that changes in mental status may be an early sign of sepsis in the elderly. How would you assess this patient for the possibility of sepsis? What risk factors place an older patient at higher risk for sepsis? What is the evidence base for these risk factors? How would you evaluate the strength of the evidence on these risk factors and for strategies to reduce the patient's risks? How would the management of the elderly patient differ from that of a younger patient?

3 While driving, you witness a car hit a man riding a bicycle. You call 911 and stop to help. The rider of the bicycle has been thrown approximately 25 feet from his bike and appears to be seriously injured. As you approach, you notice that his leg is severely deformed with an open fracture and that he is bleeding profusely. He is unconscious and blood is escaping from under his bike helmet. Describe the type of shock this patient is at greatest risk for developing. What actions would you take at the scene to prevent shock or prevent it from progressing?

4 A patient who has used a wheelchair for the last 10 years because of a spinal cord injury is burned when her clothing catches fire as she prepares dinner. Her burns are extensive but limited to her upper body. What types of shock are possible in this patient? What therapy directed at prevention or treatment of shock would you anticipate? Describe the rationale for the therapies that you have identified. How would this patient's disability affect management? How would you expect required treatments, in turn, to affect her disability?

REFERENCES AND SELECTED READINGS

BOOKS

Baldwin, K. M. & Morris, S. E. (2002). Shock, multiple organ dysfunction syndrome, and burns in adults. In McCance, K. L. & Heuther, S. E. (Eds.). *Pathophysiology: The biologic basis for disease in adults and children* (4th ed.). St. Louis: Mosby.

Huether, S. E. (2002). Alterations of renal and urinary tract function. In McCance, K. L. & Heuther, S. E. (Eds.). *Pathophysiology: The biologic basis for disease in adults and children* (4th ed.). St. Louis: Mosby.

McCance, K. L. & Heuther, S. E. (Eds.). *Pathophysiology: The biologic basis for disease in adults and children* (4th ed.). St. Louis: Mosby.

Morton, P. G., Fontaine, D. K., Hudak, C. M., et al. (2005). *Critical care nursing: A holistic approach.* Philadelphia: Lippincott Williams & Wilkins.

Porth, C. M. (2005). *Pathophysiology: Concepts of altered health states* (7th ed.). Philadelphia: Lippincott Williams & Wilkins.

Stern, S. A. & Bobek, E. M. (2001). Resuscitation: Management of shock. In Ferrera, P. C., Colucciello, S. A., Marx, J. A., et al. (Eds): *Trauma management: An emergency medicine approach.* St. Louis: Mosby.

Vincent, J. L. (2003). Correcting the deficit: Fluids, pressors and RBCs in resuscitation. In Levy, M. M. & Vincent, J. L. (Eds.). *Sepsis: Pathophysiologic insights and current management.* Chicago: Society of Critical Care Medicine.

JOURNALS

Ahrns, K. S. (2004). Trends in burn resuscitation. *Critical Care Nursing Clinics of North America, 16*(1), 75–98.

Ahrens, T. & Vollman, K. (2003). Severe sepsis management: Are we doing enough? *Critical Care Nurse, 23*(5), S2–S15.

Aird, W. C. (2003). The role of the endothelium in severe sepsis and multiple organ dysfunction syndrome. *Blood, 101*(10), 3765–3777.

Angus, D. C., Linde-Zwirble, W. T., Lidicker, J., et al. (2001). Epidemiology of severe sepsis in the United States: Analysis of incidence, outcome and associated costs of care. *Critical Care Medicine, 29*(7), 1303–1310.

Angus, D. C., Linde-Zwirble, W. T., Clermont, G., et al. (2003). Cost-effectiveness of drotrecogin alfa (activated) in treatment of severe sepsis. *Critical Care Medicine, 31*(1), 1–11.

Benner, P. (2004). Relational ethics of comfort, touch, and solace: Endangered arts? *American Journal of Critical Care, 13*(4), 346–349.

Bernard, G. R., Vincent, J. L., Laterre, R. F., et al. (2001). Efficacy and safety of recombinant human activated protein C for severe sepsis. *New England Journal of Medicine, 344*(10), 699–707.

Berry, B. E. & Pinard, A. E. (2003). Assessing tissue oxygenation. *Critical Care Nurse, 22*(3), 22–42.

Ceppa, E. P., Fuh, C. & Bulkley, G. B. (2003). Mesenteric hemodynamic response to circulatory shock. *Current Opinion in Critical Care, 9*(2), 127–123.

Cooper, M. S. & Stewart, P. M. (2003). Corticosteroid insufficiency in acutely ill patients. *New England Journal of Medicine, 348*(8), 727–734.

Dellinger, R. P. (2003). Cardiovascular management of septic shock. *Critical Care Medicine, 31*(3), 946–955.

Dellinger, R. P., Carlet, J. M., Masur, H., et al. (2004). Surviving Sepsis Campaign guidelines for management of severe sepsis and septic shock. *Critical Care Medicine, 32*(3), 858–873.

DeLegge, M. (2001). Enteral access: The foundation of feeding. *Journal of Parenteral and Enteral Nutrition, 25*(2), S8–S13.

Eggimann, P. & Pittet, D. (2001). Catheter-related infections in intensive care units: An overview with special emphasis on prevention. *Advances in Sepsis, 1*(1), 2–13.

Fein, A. M., & Calalang-Colucci, M. G. (2000). Acute lung injury and acute respiratory distress syndrome in sepsis and septic shock. *Critical Care Clinics, 16*(2), 289–313.

Fishel, R. S., Are, C. & Barbul, A. (2003). Vessel injury and capillary leak. *Critical Care Medicine, 31*(8), S502–S511.

Flynn, M. B. (2004). Nutritional support of the burn-injured patient. *Critical Care Nursing Clinics of North America, 16*(1), 139–144.

Hachey, D. M. & Smith, T. (2003). Use of nesiritide to treat acute decompensated heart failure. *Critical Care Nurse, 23*(1), 53–58.

Hameed, S. M., Aird, W. C., & Cohn, S. M. (2003). Oxygen delivery. *Critical Care Medicine, 31*(12), S658–S667.

Hochman, J. (2003). Cardiogenic shock complicating acute myocardial infarction: Expanding the paradigm. *Circulation, 107*(24), 2998–3002.

Hollenberg, S. M., Ahrens, T. S., Annane, D., et al. (2004). Practice parameters for hemodynamic support of sepsis in adult patients: 2004 update. *Critical Care Medicine, 32*(9), 1928–1949.

Hotchkiss, R. S., & Karl, I. E. (2003). The pathophysiology and treatment of sepsis. *New England Journal of Medicine, 348*(2), 138–149.

Houghton, D. (2002). Antimicrobial resistance in the intensive care unit: Understanding the problem. *AACN Clinical Issues, 13*(2), 410–420.

Kellum, J. A. & Pinsky, M. R. (2002). Use of vasopressor agents in critically ill patients. *Current Opinion in Critical Care, 8*(3), 236–241.

Kleinpell, R. (2003). Advances in treating patients with severe sepsis. *Critical Care Nurse, 23*(3), 16–29.

Marik, P. E. & Zaloga, G. P. (2003). Adrenal insufficiency during septic shock. *Critical Care Medicine, 31*(1), 141–145.

Mikhail, J. (1999). Resuscitation endpoints in trauma. *AACN Clinical Issues, 10*(1), 10–21.

Rello, J., Ollendorf, D. A., Oster, G., et al. (2002). Epidemiology and outcomes of ventilator-associated pneumonia in a large US database. *Chest, 122*(6), 2115–2121.

Revell, M., Greaves, I. & Porter, K. (2003). Endpoints for fluid resuscitation in hemorrhagic shock. *Journal of Trauma, 54*(5), S63–S67.

SAFE Study Investigators. (2005). A comparison of albumin and saline for fluid resuscitation in the intensive care unit. *New England Journal of Medicine, 350*(22), 2247–2256.

Schulman, C. S. (2003). New thoughts on sepsis. *Dimensions in Critical Care Nursing, 22*(1), 20–30.

Sommers, M. S. (2003). The cellular basis of septic shock. *Critical Care Nursing Clinics of North America, 15*(1), 13–26.

Van den Berghe, G., Wouters, P., Weekers, F., et al. (2001). Intensive insulin therapy in critically ill patients. *New England Journal of Medicine, 345*(19), 1359–1367.

Vincent, J. L, Abraham, E., Annane, D., et al. (2002). Reducing mortality in sepsis: New directions. *Critical Care, 6*(3S), S1–S18.

CHAPTER 16

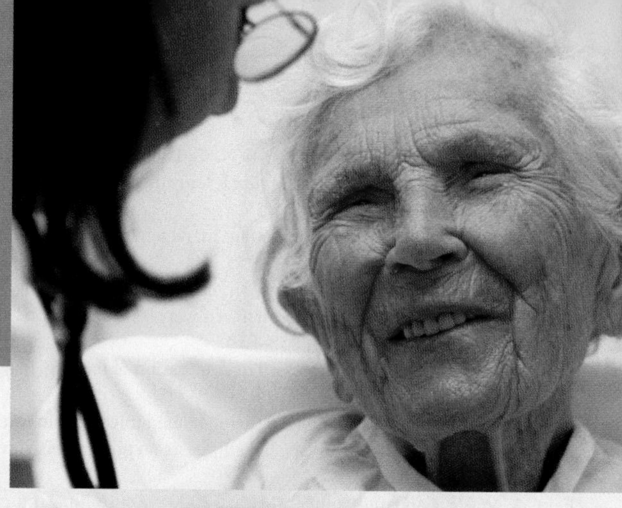

Oncology: Nursing Management in Cancer Care

Learning Objectives

On completion of this chapter, the learner will be able to:

1. Compare the structure and function of the normal cell and the cancer cell.
2. Differentiate between benign and malignant tumors.
3. Identify agents and factors that have been found to be carcinogenic.
4. Describe the significance of health education and preventive care in decreasing the incidence of cancer.
5. Differentiate among the purposes of surgical procedures used in cancer treatment, diagnosis, prophylaxis, palliation, and reconstruction.
6. Describe the roles of surgery, radiation therapy, chemotherapy, bone marrow transplantation, and other therapies in treating cancer.
7. Describe the special nursing needs of patients receiving chemotherapy.
8. Describe common nursing diagnoses and collaborative problems of patients with cancer.
9. Use the nursing process as a framework for care of patients with cancer.
10. Describe the concept of hospice in providing care for patients with advanced cancer.
11. Discuss the role of the nurse in assessment and management of common oncologic emergencies.

Cancer is not a single disease with a single cause; rather, it is a group of distinct diseases with different causes, manifestations, treatments, and prognoses. Cancer nursing practice covers all age groups and nursing specialties and is carried out in a variety of health care settings, including the home, community, acute care institutions, and rehabilitation centers. The scope, responsibilities, and goals of cancer nursing, also called **oncology** nursing, are as diverse and complex as those of any nursing specialty. Because many people associate cancer with pain and death, nurses need to identify their own reactions to cancer and set realistic goals to meet the challenges inherent in caring for patients with cancer.

In addition, cancer nurses must be prepared to support patients and families through a wide range of physical, emotional, social, cultural, and spiritual crises. Chart 16-1 identifies major areas of responsibility for nurses caring for patients with cancer.

Epidemiology of Cancer

Although cancer affects people of all ages, most cancers occur in people older than 65 years of age. Overall, the incidence of cancer is higher in men than in women and higher in industrialized sectors and nations.

More than 1.3 million Americans are diagnosed each year with a cancer affecting one of various body sites (Fig. 16-1). Cancer is second only to cardiovascular disease as a leading cause of death in the United States. More than 560,000 Americans die from a malignant process each year. The leading causes of cancer death in the United States, in order of frequency, are lung, prostate, and colorectal cancer in men and lung, breast, and colorectal cancer in women (Jemal, Murray, Ward, et al., 2005).

Relative 5-year survival rates for African Americans compared to whites are lower for cancer at every site. In the United States, cancer mortality in African Americans is

Glossary

alopecia: hair loss

anaplasia: cells that lack normal cellular characteristics and differ in shape and organization with respect to their cells of origin; usually, anaplastic cells are malignant

apoptosis: programmed cell death

biologic response modifier (BRM) therapy: use of agents or treatment methods that can alter the immunologic relationship between the tumor and the host to provide a therapeutic benefit

biopsy: a diagnostic procedure to remove a small sample of tissue to be examined microscopically to detect malignant cells

brachytherapy: delivery of radiation therapy through internal implants

cancer: a disease process whereby cells proliferate abnormally, ignoring growth-regulating signals in the environment surrounding the cells

carcinogenesis: process of transforming normal cells into malignant cells

chemotherapy: use of medications to kill tumor cells by interfering with cellular functions and reproduction

control: containment of the growth of cancer cells

cure: prolonged survival and disappearance of all evidence of disease so that the patient has the same life expectancy as anyone else in his or her age group

cytokines: substances produced by cells of the immune system to enhance production and functioning of components of the immune system

dysplasia: bizarre cell growth resulting in cells that differ in size, shape, or arrangement from other cells of the same type of tissue

extravasation: leakage of medication from the veins into the subcutaneous tissues

grading: identification of the type of tissue from which the tumor originated and the degree to which the tumor cells retain the functional and structural characteristics of the tissue of origin

graft-versus-host disease (GVHD): an immune response initiated by T lymphocytes of donor tissue against the recipient's tissues (skin, gastrointestinal tract, liver); an undesirable response

graft-versus-disease effect: the donor cell response against the malignancy; a desirable response

hyperplasia: increase in the number of cells of a tissue; most often associated with periods of rapid body growth

malignant: having cells or processes that are characteristic of cancer

metaplasia: conversion of one type of mature cell into another type of cell

metastasis: spread of cancer cells from the primary tumor to distant sites

myelosuppression: suppression of the blood cell-producing function of the bone marrow

nadir: lowest point of white blood cell depression after therapy that has toxic effects on the bone marrow

neoplasia: uncontrolled cell growth that follows no physiologic demand

neutropenia: abnormally low absolute neutrophil count

oncology: field or study of cancer

palliation: relief of symptoms associated with cancer

radiation therapy: use of ionizing radiation to interrupt the growth of malignant cells

stomatitis: inflammation of the oral tissues, often associated with some chemotherapeutic agents

staging: process of determining the size and spread, or metastasis, of a tumor

targeted therapies: cancer treatments that seek to minimize the negative effects on healthy tissues by disrupting specific cancer cell functions such as malignant transformation, communication pathways, processes for growth and metastasis, and genetic coding

thrombocytopenia: decrease in the number of circulating platelets; associated with the potential for bleeding

tumor-specific antigen (TSA): protein on the membrane of cancer cells that distinguishes the malignant cell from a benign cell of the same tissue type

vesicant: substance that can cause tissue necrosis and damage, particularly when extravasated

xerostomia: dry oral cavity resulting from decreased function of salivary glands

CHART 16-1

Responsibilities of the Nurse in Cancer Care

- Support the idea that cancer is a chronic illness that has acute exacerbations rather than one that is synonymous with death and suffering.
- Assess own level of knowledge relative to the pathophysiology of the disease process.
- Make use of current research findings and practices in the care of the patient with cancer and his or her family.
- Identify patients at high risk for cancer.
- Participate in primary and secondary prevention efforts.
- Assess the nursing care needs of the patient with cancer.
- Assess the learning needs, desires, and capabilities of the patient with cancer.
- Identify nursing problems of the patient and the family.
- Assess the social support networks available to the patient.
- Plan appropriate interventions with the patient and the family.
- Assist the patient to identify strengths and limitations.
- Assist the patient to design short-term and long-term goals for care.
- Implement a nursing care plan that interfaces with the medical care regimen and that is consistent with the established goals.
- Collaborate with members of a multidisciplinary team to foster continuity of care.
- Evaluate the goals and resultant outcomes of care with the patient, the family, and members of the multidisciplinary team.
- Reassess and redesign the direction of the care as determined by the evaluation.

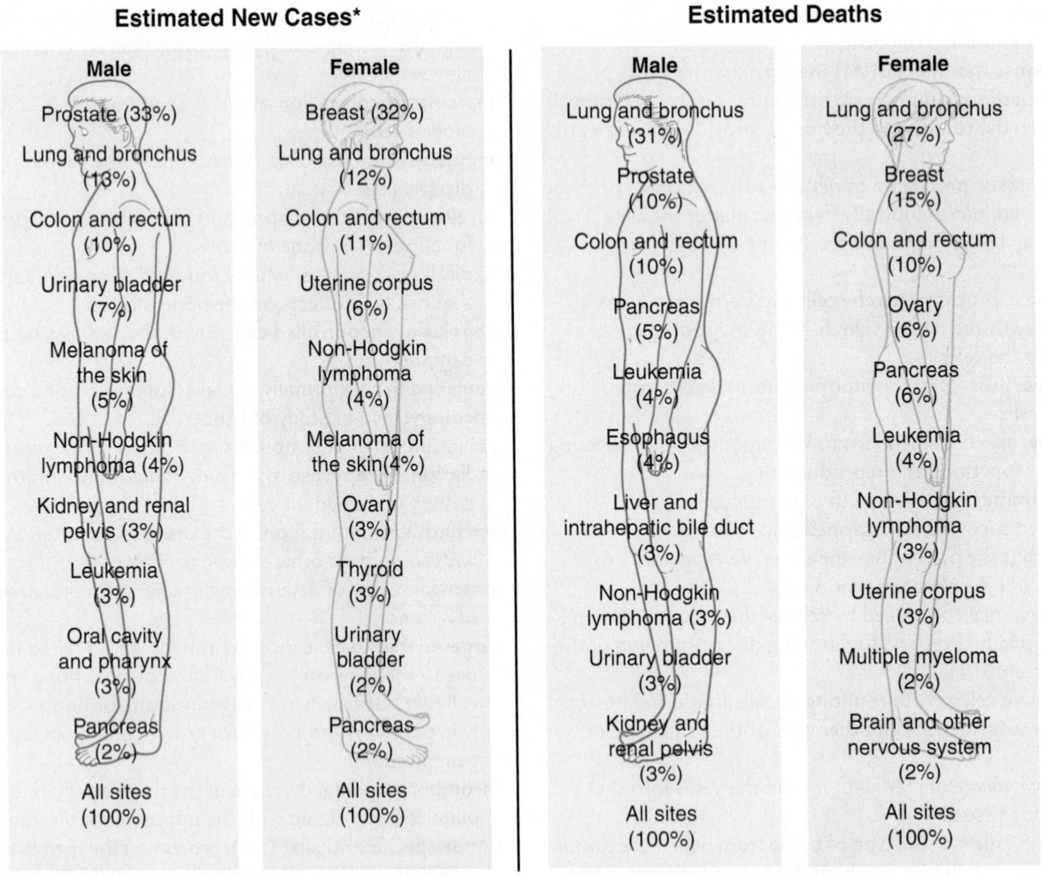

FIGURE 16-1. Ten leading types of cancer by gender determined on the bases of estimated new cancer cases and deaths in the United States in 2004. *Excludes basal and squamous cell skin cancers and in situ carcinomas except urinary bladder. Note: Percentages may not total 100 because of rounding. From the American Cancer Society. (2004). Surveillance research, 2004. *CA: A Cancer Journal for Clinicians, 54*[1], 8–29.

higher than in any other racial group. This finding is related to the higher incidence and later stage of diagnosis among African Americans. The increased cancer morbidity and mortality in this group are largely a result of economic factors, education, and access to health care rather than racial characteristics (Ward, Jemal, Cokkinides, et al., 2004).

Pathophysiology of the Malignant Process

Cancer is a disease process that begins when an abnormal cell is transformed by the genetic mutation of the cellular DNA. This abnormal cell forms a clone and begins to proliferate abnormally, ignoring growth-regulating signals in the environment surrounding the cell. The cells acquire invasive characteristics, and changes occur in surrounding tissues. The cells infiltrate these tissues and gain access to lymph and blood vessels, which carry the cells to other areas of the body. This phenomenon is called **metastasis** (cancer spread to other parts of the body).

Proliferative Patterns

During the lifespan, various body tissues normally undergo periods of rapid or proliferative growth that must be distinguished from malignant growth activity. Several patterns of cell growth exist: **hyperplasia, metaplasia, dysplasia, anaplasia,** and **neoplasia.**

Cancerous cells are described as **malignant** neoplasms. They demonstrate uncontrolled cell growth that follows no physiologic demand. Benign and malignant growths are classified and named by tissue of origin, as described in Table 16-1. Benign and malignant cells differ in many cellular growth characteristics, including the method and rate of growth, ability to metastasize or spread, general effects, destruction of tissue, and ability to cause death. These differences are summarized in Table 16-2. The degree of anaplasia ultimately determines the malignant potential.

TABLE 16-1 Names of Selected Benign and Malignant Tumors According to Tissue Types

Tissue Type	Benign Tumors	Malignant Tumors
Epithelial		
Surface	Papilloma	Squamous cell carcinoma
Glandular	Adenoma	Adenocarcinoma
Connective		
Fibrous	Fibroma	Fibrosarcoma
Adipose	Lipoma	Liposarcoma
Cartilage	Chondroma	Chondrosarcoma
Bone	Osteoma	Osteosarcoma
Blood vessels	Hemangioma	Hemangiosarcoma
Lymph vessels	Lymphangioma	Lymphangiosarcoma
Lymph tissue		Lymphosarcoma
Muscle		
Smooth	Leiomyoma	Leiomyosarcoma
Striated	Rhabdomyoma	Rhabdomyosarcoma
Neural Tissue		
Nerve cell	Neuroma	Neuroblastoma
Glial tissue	Glioma (benign)	Glioblastoma, astrocytoma, medulloblastoma, oligodendroglioma
Nerve sheaths	Neurilemmoma	Neurilemmal sarcoma
Meninges	Meningioma	Meningeal sarcoma
Hematologic		
Granulocytic		Myelocytic leukemia
Erythrocytic		Erythrocytic leukemia
Plasma cells		Multiple myeloma
Lymphocytic		Lymphocytic leukemia or lymphoma
Monocytic		Monocytic leukemia
Endothelial Tissue		
Blood vessels	Hemangioma	Hemangiosarcoma
Lymph vessels	Lymphangioma	Lymphangiosarcoma
Endothelial lining		Ewing's sarcoma

Reproduced with permission from Porth, C. M. (2005). *Pathophysiology: Concepts of altered health states* (7th ed.). Philadelphia: Lippincott Williams & Wilkins.

TABLE 16-2 Characteristics of Benign and Malignant Neoplasms

Characteristics	Benign	Malignant
Cell characteristics	Well-differentiated cells that resemble normal cells of the tissue from which the tumor originated	Cells are undifferentiated and often bear little resemblance to the normal cells of the tissue from which they arose
Mode of growth	Tumor grows by expansion and does not infiltrate the surrounding tissues; usually encapsulated	Grows at the periphery and sends out processes that infiltrate and destroy the surrounding tissues
Rate of growth	Rate of growth is usually slow	Rate of growth is variable and depends on level of differentiation; the more anaplastic the tumor, the faster its growth
Metastasis	Does not spread by metastasis	Gains access to the blood and lymphatic channels and metastasizes to other areas of the body
General effects	Is usually a localized phenomenon that does not cause generalized effects unless its location interferes with vital functions	Often causes generalized effects, such as anemia, weakness, and weight loss
Tissue destruction	Does not usually cause tissue damage unless its location interferes with blood flow	Often causes extensive tissue damage as the tumor outgrows its blood supply or encroaches on blood flow to the area; may also produce substances that cause cell damage
Ability to cause death	Does not usually cause death unless its location interferes with vital functions	Usually causes death unless growth can be controlled

Reproduced with permission from Porth, C. M. (2005). *Pathophysiology: Concepts of altered health states* (7th ed.). Philadelphia: Lippincott Williams & Wilkins.

Characteristics of Malignant Cells

Despite their individual differences, all cancer cells share some common cellular characteristics in relation to the cell membrane, special proteins, the nuclei, chromosomal abnormalities, and the rate of mitosis and growth. The cell membranes are altered in cancer cells, which affects fluid movement in and out of the cell. The cell membrane of malignant cells also contains proteins called **tumor-specific antigens** (eg, carcinoembryonic antigen [CEA] and prostate-specific antigen [PSA]), which develop as they become less differentiated (mature) over time. These proteins distinguish the malignant cell from a benign cell of the same tissue type. They may be useful in measuring the extent of disease in a person and in tracking the course of illness during treatment or relapse. Malignant cellular membranes also contain less fibronectin, a cellular cement. They are therefore less cohesive and do not adhere to adjacent cells readily.

Typically, nuclei of cancer cells are large and irregularly shaped (pleomorphism). Nucleoli, structures within the nucleus that house ribonucleic acid (RNA), are larger and more numerous in malignant cells, perhaps because of increased RNA synthesis. Chromosomal abnormalities (translocations, deletions, additions) and fragility of chromosomes are commonly found when cancer cells are analyzed.

Mitosis (cell division) occurs more frequently in malignant cells than in normal cells. As the cells grow and divide, more glucose and oxygen are needed. If glucose and oxygen are unavailable, malignant cells use anaerobic metabolic channels to produce energy, which makes the cells less dependent on the availability of a constant oxygen supply.

Invasion and Metastasis

Malignant disease processes have the ability to allow the spread or transfer of cancerous cells from one organ or body part to another by invasion and metastasis. Patterns of metastasis can be partially explained by circulatory patterns and by specific affinity for certain malignant cells to bind to molecules in specific body tissue.

Invasion, which refers to the growth of the primary tumor into the surrounding host tissues, occurs in several ways. Mechanical pressure exerted by rapidly proliferating neoplasms may force fingerlike projections of tumor cells into surrounding tissue and interstitial spaces. Malignant cells are less adherent and may break off from the primary tumor and invade adjacent structures. Malignant cells are thought to possess or produce specific destructive enzymes (proteinases), such as collagenases (specific to collagen), plasminogen activators (specific to plasma), and lysosomal hydrolyses. These enzymes are thought to destroy surrounding tissue, including the structural tissues of the vascular basement membrane, facilitating invasion of malignant cells. The mechanical pressure of a rapidly growing tumor may enhance this process.

Metastasis is the dissemination or spread of malignant cells from the primary tumor to distant sites by direct spread of tumor cells to body cavities or through lymphatic and blood circulation. Tumors growing in or penetrating body cavities may shed cells or emboli that travel within the body cavity and seed the surfaces of other organs. This can occur in ovarian cancer when malignant cells enter the peritoneal cavity and seed the peritoneal surfaces of such abdominal organs as the liver or pancreas.

Mechanisms of Metastasis

Lymph and blood are key mechanisms by which cancer cells spread. Angiogenesis, a mechanism by which the tumor cells are ensured a blood supply, is another important process.

LYMPHATIC SPREAD

Lymphatic spread (the transport of tumor cells through the lymphatic circulation) is the most common mechanism of metastasis. Tumor emboli enter the lymph channels by way of the interstitial fluid, which communicates with lymphatic fluid. Malignant cells also may penetrate lymphatic vessels by invasion. After entering the lymphatic circulation, malignant cells either lodge in the lymph nodes or pass between the lymphatic and venous circulations. Tumors arising in areas of the body with rapid and extensive lymphatic circulation are at high risk for metastasis through lymphatic channels. Breast tumors frequently metastasize in this manner through axillary, clavicular, and thoracic lymph channels.

HEMATOGENOUS SPREAD

Hematogenous spread is the dissemination of malignant cells via the bloodstream. Hematogenous spread is directly related to the vascularity of the tumor. Few malignant cells can survive the turbulence of arterial circulation, insufficient oxygenation, or destruction by the body's immune system. In addition, the structure of most arteries and arterioles is far too secure to permit malignant invasion. Those malignant cells that do survive this hostile environment are able to attach to endothelium and attract fibrin, platelets, and clotting factors to seal themselves from immune system surveillance. The endothelium retracts, allowing the malignant cells to enter the basement membrane and secrete lysosomal enzymes. These enzymes destroy surrounding body tissues and thereby allow implantation.

ANGIOGENESIS

Angiogenesis is the growth of new capillaries from the host tissue by the release of growth factors and enzymes such as vascular endothelial growth factor (VEGF). These proteins rapidly stimulate formation of new blood vessels, which helps malignant cells obtain the necessary nutrients and oxygen. It is also through this vascular network that tumor emboli can enter the systemic circulation and travel to distant sites. Large tumor emboli that become trapped in the microcirculation of distant sites may further metastasize to other sites. Therapies that target VEGF or its receptors are being used to treat many cancers effectively.

Carcinogenesis

Malignant transformation, or **carcinogenesis**, is thought to be at least a three-step cellular process, involving initiation, promotion, and progression.

During *initiation,* initiators (carcinogens), such as chemicals, physical factors, and biologic agents, escape normal enzymatic mechanisms and alter the genetic structure of the cellular DNA. Normally, these alterations are reversed by DNA repair mechanisms, or the changes initiate programmed cellular death (apoptosis). Occasionally, cells escape these protective mechanisms, and permanent cellular mutations occur. These mutations usually are not significant to cells until the second step of carcinogenesis.

During *promotion,* repeated exposure to promoting agents (cocarcinogens) causes the expression of abnormal or mutant genetics information even after long latency periods. Latency periods for the promotion of cellular mutations vary with the type of agent and the dosage of the promoter as well as the innate characteristics of the target cell.

Cellular oncogenes, which exist in all mammalian systems, are responsible for the vital cellular functions of growth and differentiation. Cellular proto-oncogenes act as an "on switch" for cellular growth. Proto-oncogenes are influenced by multiple growth factors that stimulate cell proliferation, such as epidermal growth factor (EGF) and transforming growth factor alpha. Another proto-oncogene that plays an important role in cancer development is the *k-ras (KRAS2)* oncogene located on chromosome 12.

Just as proto-oncogenes "turn on" cellular growth, cancer suppressor genes "turn off," or regulate, unneeded cellular proliferation. When suppressor genes become mutated, rearranged, or amplified or lose their regulatory capabilities, malignant cells are allowed to reproduce. The *p53 (TP53)* gene is a tumor suppressor gene that is frequently mutated in many human cancers. This gene determines whether cells will live or die after their DNA is damaged. Apoptosis is the innate cellular process of programmed cell death. Alterations in *TP53* may decrease apoptotic signals, thus decreasing mutant cell death, giving rise to a survival advantage for mutant cell populations. Mutant *TP53* is associated with a poor prognosis and may be associated with determining response to treatment. Once this genetic expression occurs in cells, the cells begin to produce mutant cell populations that are different from their original cellular ancestors.

During *progression,* the cellular changes formed during initiation and promotion exhibit increased malignant behavior. These cells have a propensity to invade adjacent tissues and to metastasize. Agents that initiate or promote cellular transformation are referred to as carcinogens.

Etiology

Categories of agents or factors implicated in carcinogenesis include viruses and bacteria, physical agents, chemical agents, genetic or familial factors, dietary factors, and hormonal agents.

Viruses and Bacteria

Viruses are difficult to evaluate as a cause of human cancers because they are difficult to isolate. However, infectious causes are considered or suspected when specific cancers appear in clusters. Viruses are thought to incorporate themselves in the genetic structure of cells, thus altering future generations of that cell population—perhaps leading to cancer. For example, the Epstein-Barr virus is highly suspect as a cause in Burkitt lymphoma, nasopharyngeal cancers, and some types of non-Hodgkin lymphoma and Hodgkin disease.

Herpes simplex virus type II, cytomegalovirus, and human papillomavirus types 16, 18, 31, and 33 are associated with dysplasia and cancer of the cervix. The hepatitis B and hepatitis C viruses are implicated in cancer of the liver; the human T-cell lymphotropic virus may be a cause of some lymphocytic leukemias and lymphomas; and the human immunodeficiency virus (HIV) is associated with Kaposi's sarcoma. The bacterium *Helicobacter pylori* has been associated with an increased incidence of gastric malignancy, perhaps secondary to inflammation and injury to gastric cells.

Physical Agents

Physical factors associated with carcinogenesis include exposure to sunlight or radiation, chronic irritation or inflammation, and tobacco use.

Excessive exposure to the ultraviolet rays of the sun, especially in fair-skinned, blue- or green-eyed people, increases the risk of skin cancers. Factors such as clothing styles (sleeveless shirts or shorts); use of sunscreens; occupation; recreational habits; and environmental variables, including humidity, altitude, and latitude, all play a role in the amount of exposure to ultraviolet light.

Exposure to ionizing radiation can occur with repeated diagnostic x-ray procedures or with radiation therapy used to treat disease. Fortunately, improved x-ray equipment appropriately minimizes the risk of extensive radiation exposure. Radiation therapy used in disease treatment and exposure to radioactive materials at nuclear weapon manufacturing sites or nuclear power plants are associated with a higher incidence of leukemias, multiple myeloma, and cancers of the lung, bone, breast, thyroid, and other tissues. Background radiation from the natural decay processes that produce radon has also been associated with lung cancer. Homes with high levels of trapped radon should be ventilated to allow the gas to disperse into the atmosphere.

Chemical Agents

About 75% of all cancers are thought to be related to the environment. Tobacco smoke, thought to be the single most lethal chemical carcinogen, accounts for at least 30% of cancer deaths (Casciato, 2004). Smoking is strongly associated with cancers of the lung, head and neck, esophagus, pancreas, cervix, and bladder. Tobacco may also act synergistically with other substances, such as alcohol, asbestos, uranium, and viruses, to promote cancer development.

Chewing tobacco is associated with cancers of the oral cavity, which primarily occurs in men younger than 40 years of age. Many chemical substances found in the workplace have proved to be carcinogens or cocarcinogens. The extensive list of suspected chemical substances continues to grow and includes aromatic amines and aniline dyes; pesticides and formaldehydes; arsenic, soot, and tars; asbestos; benzene; betel nut and lime; cadmium; chromium compounds; nickel and zinc ores; wood dust; beryllium compounds; and polyvinyl chloride.

Most hazardous chemicals produce their toxic effects by altering DNA structure in body sites distant from chemical exposure. The liver, lungs, and kidneys are the organ systems most often affected, presumably because of their roles in detoxifying chemicals.

Genetics and Familial Factors

Almost every cancer type has been shown to run in families. This may be due to genetics, shared environments, cultural or lifestyle factors, or chance alone. Genetic factors play a role in cancer cell development. Abnormal chromosomal patterns and cancer have been associated with extra chromosomes, too few chromosomes, or translocated chromosomes. Specific cancers with underlying genetic abnormalities include Burkitt lymphoma, chronic myelogenous leukemia, meningiomas, acute leukemias, retinoblastomas, Wilms tumor, and skin cancers, including malignant melanoma.

Approximately 5% of cancers of adults display a familial predisposition. The hallmarks of families with a hereditary cancer syndrome include cancer in two or more relatives, cancer in family members younger than 50 years of age, the same type of cancer in several family members, family members with more than one type of cancer, and a rare cancer in one or more family members (Sifri, Gangadharappa & Acheson, 2004). Cancers associated with familial inheritance include retinoblastomas, nephroblastomas, pheochromocytomas, malignant neurofibromatosis, and breast, ovarian, colorectal, stomach, prostate, and lung cancers. In the 1990s, the *BRCA1* and *BRCA2* genes were identified and linked to breast and ovarian cancer syndrome. Mutations in *BRCA1* are associated with an 80 to 90% risk of breast cancer and a 40 to 65% risk of ovarian cancer by 70 years of age (Hutson, 2003).

Dietary Factors

Dietary factors are also linked to environmental cancers. Dietary substances can be proactive (protective), carcinogenic, or cocarcinogenic. The risk of cancer increases with long-term ingestion of carcinogens or cocarcinogens or chronic absence of protective substances in the diet.

Dietary substances that appear to increase the risk of cancer include fats, alcohol, salt-cured or smoked meats, and nitrate- and nitrite-containing foods. A high caloric dietary intake is also associated with an increased cancer risk. Consumption of high-fiber foods (such as fruits, vegetables, and whole grain cereals) and cruciferous vegetables (such as cabbage, broccoli, cauliflower, Brussels sprouts, and kohlrabi) appears to decrease the risk of cancer. Obesity is associated with endometrial cancer and postmenopausal breast cancers (Casciato, 2004).

Hormonal Agents

Tumor growth may be promoted by disturbances in hormonal balance, either by the body's own (endogenous) hormone production or by administration of exogenous hormones. Cancers of the breast, prostate, and uterus are thought to depend on endogenous hormonal levels for growth. Diethylstilbestrol (DES) has long been recognized as a cause of vaginal carcinomas. Oral contraceptives and prolonged estrogen replacement therapy are associated with an increased incidence of hepatocellular, endometrial, and breast cancers, but they decrease the risk of ovarian cancer. The combination of estrogen and progesterone appears safer than estrogen alone in decreasing the risk of endometrial cancers; however, the Women's Health Initiative studies support discontinuing hormonal therapy with estrogens and progestins because of the increased risk of breast cancer, coronary heart disease, stroke, and blood clots (National Institutes of Health, 2004).

GENETICS IN NURSING PRACTICE

Concepts and Challenges in Management of the Patient with Cancer

Cancer is a genetic disease. Every phase of carcinogenesis is affected by multiple gene mutations. Some of these mutations are inherited (present in germ-line cells), but most (90%) are somatic mutations that are acquired mutations in specific cells. Examples of cancers influenced by genetics include

- Cowden syndrome
- Familial adenomatous polyposis
- Familial melanoma syndrome
- Hereditary breast and ovarian cancer
- Hereditary non-polyposis colon cancer
- Neurofibromatosis type 1
- Retinoblastoma

NURSING ASSESSMENTS

Family History Assessment

- Obtain information about both maternal and paternal sides of family.
- Obtain cancer history of at least three generations.
- Look for clustering of cancers that occur at young ages, multiple primary cancers in one individual, cancer in paired organs, and two or more close relatives with the same type of cancer suggestive of hereditary cancer syndromes.

Patient Assessment

- Physical findings that may predispose the patient to cancer, such as multiple colon polyps, suggestive of a polyposis syndrome
- Skin findings, such as atypical moles, that may be related to familial melanoma syndrome
- Multiple *café au lait* spots, axillary freckling, and two or more neurofibromas associated with neurofibromatosis type 1
- Facial trichilemmomas, mucosal papillomatosis, multinodular thyroid goiter or thyroid adenomas, macrocephaly, fibrocystic breasts and other fibromas or lipomas related to Cowden syndrome

MANAGEMENT ISSUES SPECIFIC TO GENETICS

- Assess patient's understanding of genetics factors related to his or her cancer.
- Refer for cancer risk assessment when a hereditary cancer syndrome is suspected so that patient and family can discuss inheritance risk with other family members and availability of genetic testing.
- Offer appropriate genetics information and resources.
- Assess patient's understanding of genetics information.
- Provide support to patients and families with known genetic test results for hereditary cancer syndromes.
- Participate in the management and coordination of risk-reduction measures for those with known gene mutations.

GENETICS RESOURCES

American Cancer Society, www.cancer.org—offers general information about cancer and support resources for families

Gene Clinics, www.geneclinics.org—a listing of common genetic disorders with up-to-date clinical summaries, genetic counseling, and testing information

National Organization of Rare Disorders, www.rarediseases.org—a directory of support groups and information for patients and families with rare genetic disorders

National Cancer Institute, www.cancernet.nci.nih.gov—a listing of cancers with clinical summaries and treatment reviews, information on genetic risks for cancer, listing of cancer centers providing genetic cancer risk assessment services

Genetic Alliance, www.geneticalliance.org—a directory of support groups for patients and families with genetic conditions

OMIM: Online Mendelian Inheritance in Man, www.ncbi.nlm.nih.gov/Omim/mimstats.html—a complete listing of known inherited genetic conditions

Hormonal changes with reproduction are also associated with cancer incidence. Increased numbers of pregnancies are associated with a decreased incidence of breast, endometrial, and ovarian cancers.

Role of the Immune System

In humans, malignant cells are capable of developing on a regular basis. However, some evidence indicates that the immune system can detect the development of malignant cells and destroy them before cell growth becomes uncontrolled. When the immune system fails to identify and stop the growth of malignant cells, clinical cancer develops.

Patients who are immunoincompetent have been shown to have an increased incidence of cancer. Organ transplant recipients who receive immunosuppressive therapy to prevent rejection of the transplanted organ have an increased incidence of lymphoma, Kaposi's sarcoma, squamous cell cancer of the skin, and cervical and anogenital cancers. Patients with immunodeficiency diseases, such as acquired immunodeficiency syndrome (AIDS), have an increased incidence of Kaposi's sarcoma, lymphoma, and rectal and head and neck cancers. Some patients who have received alkylating chemotherapeutic agents to treat Hodgkin disease have an increased incidence of secondary malignancies. Autoimmune diseases, such as rheumatoid arthritis and Sjögren syndrome, are associated with increased cancer development. Finally, age-related changes, such as declining organ function, increased incidence of chronic diseases, and diminished immunocompetence, may contribute to an increased incidence of cancer in older people.

Normal Immune Responses

Normally, an intact immune system has the ability to combat cancer cells in several ways. Usually, the immune system recognizes as foreign certain antigens on the cell membranes of many cancer cells. These antigens, known as tumor-associated antigens (also called tumor cell antigens), are capable of stimulating both cellular and humoral immune responses.

Along with the macrophages, T lymphocytes, the soldiers of the cellular immune response, are responsible for recognizing tumor-associated antigens. When T lymphocytes recognize tumor antigens, other T lymphocytes that are toxic to the tumor cells are stimulated. These lymphocytes proliferate and are released into the circulation. In addition to possessing cytotoxic (cell-killing) properties, T lymphocytes can stimulate other components of the immune system to rid the body of malignant cells.

Certain lymphokines, which are substances produced by lymphocytes, are capable of killing or damaging various types of malignant cells. Other lymphokines can mobilize other cells, such as macrophages, that disrupt cancer cells. Interferon, a substance produced by the body in response to viral infection, also possesses some antitumor properties. Antibodies produced by B lymphocytes, associated with the humoral immune response, also defend the body against malignant cells. These antibodies act either alone or in combination with the complement system or the cellular immune system.

Natural killer (NK) cells are a major component of the body's defense against cancer. NK cells are a subpopulation of lymphocytes that act by directly destroying cancer cells or by producing lymphokines and enzymes that assist in cell destruction.

Immune System Failure

How is it, then, that malignant cells can survive and proliferate despite the elaborate immune system defense mechanisms? Several theories suggest how tumor cells can evade an apparently intact immune system. If the body fails to recognize the malignant cell as different from "self" (ie, as non-self or foreign), the immune response may not be stimulated. When tumors do not possess tumor-associated antigens that label them as foreign, the immune response is not alerted. The failure of the immune system to respond promptly to the malignant cells allows the tumor to grow too large to be managed by normal immune mechanisms.

Tumor antigens may combine with the antibodies produced by the immune system and hide or disguise themselves from normal immune defense mechanisms. These tumor antigen–antibody complexes can suppress further production of antibodies. Tumors are also capable of changing their appearance or producing substances that impair usual immune responses. These substances not only promote tumor growth but also increase the patient's susceptibility to infection by various pathogenic organisms. As a result of prolonged contact with a tumor antigen, the body may be depleted of the specific lymphocytes and no longer be able to mount an appropriate immune response.

Abnormal concentrations of host suppressor T lymphocytes may play a role in cancer development. Suppressor T lymphocytes normally assist in regulating antibody production and diminishing immune responses when they are no longer required. Low levels of serum antibodies and high levels of suppressor cells have been found in patients with multiple myeloma, a cancer associated with hypogammaglobulinemia (low amounts of serum antibodies). Carcinogens, such as viruses and certain chemicals, including chemotherapeutic agents, may weaken the immune system and ultimately enhance tumor growth.

Detection and Prevention of Cancer

Nurses and physicians have traditionally been involved with tertiary prevention, the care and rehabilitation of patients after cancer diagnosis and treatment. However, in recent years, the American Cancer Society, the National Cancer Institute, clinicians, and researchers have placed greater emphasis on primary and secondary prevention of cancer. Primary prevention is concerned with reducing the risks of cancer in healthy people. Secondary prevention involves detection and screening to achieve early diagnosis and prompt intervention to halt the cancer process.

Primary Prevention

By acquiring the knowledge and skills necessary to educate the community about cancer risk, nurses in all settings play a key role in cancer prevention. One way to reduce the risk of cancer is to help patients avoid known carcinogens. Another way involves encouraging patients to make dietary and various lifestyle changes that epidemiologic and laboratory studies show influence the risk for cancer. Nurses can use their teaching and counseling skills to encourage patients to participate in cancer prevention programs and to adopt healthful lifestyles. Several clinical trials have been conducted to identify medications that may help reduce the incidence of certain types of cancer. For example, an important breast cancer prevention study supported by the National Cancer Institute was conducted at multiple medical centers throughout the country. The results of this study indicated that the medication tamoxifen can reduce the incidence of breast cancer by 49% in postmenopausal women identified as being at high risk for breast cancer (Fisher, 1998). Additional trials exploring chemoprevention agents in breast cancer, such as raloxifene, are ongoing (Dunn, Wickerham & Ford, 2005; Goss & Strasser-Weippl, 2004).

Secondary Prevention

The evolving understanding of the role of genetics in cancer cell development has contributed to prevention and screening efforts. People with specific gene mutations have an increased susceptibility to cancer. For example, people who have the gene for familial adenomatosis polyposis have an increased risk for colon cancer. Women in whom the *BRCA1* and *BRCA2* genes have been identified have an increased risk for breast and ovarian cancer. To provide individualized education and recommendations for continued surveillance and care in high-risk populations, nurses should be familiar with ongoing developments in the field of genetics and cancer (Calzone & Masny, 2004). Many centers across the country are offering innovative cancer risk evaluation programs that provide in-depth screening and follow-up for people who are found to be at high risk for cancer.

Nurses must be aware of factors such as race, cultural influences, access to care, physician–patient relationship, level of education, income, and age, which influence the knowledge, attitudes, and beliefs people have about cancer. These factors also may affect health-promoting behaviors people practice.

Public awareness about health-promoting behaviors can be increased in a variety of ways. Health education and health maintenance programs are sponsored by community organizations such as churches, senior citizen groups, and parent–teacher associations. Although primary prevention programs may focus on the hazards of tobacco use or the importance of nutrition, secondary prevention programs may promote breast and testicular self-examination and Papanicolaou (Pap) tests. Many organizations conduct cancer screening events that focus on cancers with the highest incidence rates or those that have improved survival rates if diagnosed early, such as breast or prostate cancers. These events offer education and examinations such as mammograms, digital rectal examinations, and PSA blood tests for minimal or no cost. These programs are often targeted to people who lack access to health care or cannot afford to participate on their own. In developing these programs, nurses must use strategies that are culturally sensitive to foster participation (Woods, Montgomery & Herring, 2004).

Similarly, nurses in all settings can develop programs that identify risks for patients and families and that incorporate teaching and counseling into all educational efforts, particularly for patients and families with a high incidence of cancer. Nurses support public education campaigns that guide patients and families in taking steps to reduce cancer risks (Chart 16-2). Nurses and physicians can encourage people to comply with detection efforts as suggested by the American Cancer Society (Table 16-3).

Diagnosis of Cancer and Related Nursing Considerations

A cancer diagnosis is based on assessment for physiologic and functional changes and results of the diagnostic evaluation. Patients with suspected cancer undergo extensive testing to (1) determine the presence of tumor and its extent, (2) identify possible spread (metastasis) of disease or invasion of other body tissues, (3) evaluate the function of involved and uninvolved body systems and organs, and (4) obtain tissue and cells for analysis, including evaluation of tumor stage and grade. The diagnostic evaluation is guided by information

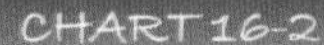

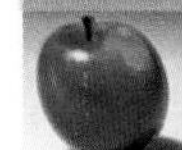

Health Promotion

Reducing Cancer Risk

- Encourage patients to increase consumption of fresh vegetables (especially those of the cabbage family) because studies indicate that roughage and vitamin-rich foods help to prevent certain kinds of cancer.
- Encourage increased fiber intake because high-fiber diets may reduce the risk for certain cancers (eg, breast, prostate, and colon).
- Recommend increased intake of vitamin A, which reduces the risk for esophageal, laryngeal, and lung cancers.
- Recommend increased intake of foods rich in vitamin C, such as citrus fruits and broccoli, which are thought to protect against stomach and esophageal cancers.
- Advise patients to practice weight control because obesity is linked to cancers of the uterus, gallbladder, breast, and colon.
- Advise patients to reduce intake of dietary fat because a high-fat diet increases the risk for breast, colon, and prostate cancers.
- Recommend moderation in consumption of salt-cured, smoked, and nitrate-cured foods; these have been linked to esophageal and gastric cancers.
- Advise patients to stop smoking cigarettes and cigars, which are carcinogens.
- Advise patients to reduce alcohol intake because drinking large amounts of alcohol increases the risk of liver cancer. (*Note:* People who drink heavily and smoke are at greater risk for cancers of the mouth, throat, larynx, and esophagus.)
- Advise patients to avoid overexposure to the sun, wear protective clothing, and use a sunscreen to prevent skin damage from ultraviolet rays that increase the risk of skin cancer.

Adapted from the "Taking Control" program of the American Cancer Society.

TABLE 16-3 American Cancer Society Recommendations for Early Detection of Cancer in Asymptomatic, Average Risk People

Site	Gender	Age (y)	Evaluation	Frequency
Breast	F	20–39	Clinical breast examination (CBE)	Every 3 years
			Self breast examination (SBE)	Every month
		≥40	CBE	Every year
			SBE	Every month
			Mammogram	Every year
Colon/rectum	F/M	≥50	Fecal occult blood test *and*	Every year
			Flexible sigmoidoscopy *or*	Every 5 years
			Colonoscopy *or*	Every 10 years
			Double-contrast barium enema	Every 5 years
Prostate	M	≥50 (or 40–45 if at high risk)	Prostate-specific antigen and digital rectal examination	Every year
Cervix	F	≥21 or within 3 y after starting to have intercourse	Papanicolaou (Pap) test*	Every year if regular Pap; every 2 years if liquid Pap test
			Pelvic examination	Every year
Cancer-related checkups	M/F	≥20–39	Examination for cancers of the thyroid, testicles, ovaries, lymph nodes, oral cavity, and skin as well as counseling about health practices and risk factors	Every 3 years
		40+	Same as for 20–39	Every year

*At age 30 after three or more consecutive normal examinations, the Pap test may be performed every 2–3 years at the discretion of the physician; human papillomavirus (HPV) test should be included at that time

Adapted from American Cancer Society (2004). ACS cancer detection guidelines. Available at: www.cancer.org.

obtained through a complete history and physical examination. Knowledge of suspicious symptoms and of the behavior of particular types of cancer assists in determining which diagnostic tests are most appropriate (Table 16-4).

Patients undergoing extensive testing are usually fearful of the procedures and anxious about the possible test results. The nurse can help relieve the patient's fear and anxiety by explaining the tests to be performed, the sensations likely to be experienced, and the patient's role in the test procedures. The nurse encourages the patient and family to voice their fears about the test results, supports the patient and family throughout the test period, and reinforces and clarifies information conveyed by the physician. The nurse also encourages the patient and family to communicate and share their concerns and to discuss their questions and concerns with each other.

Tumor Staging and Grading

A complete diagnostic evaluation includes identifying the stage and grade of the tumor. This is accomplished before treatment begins to provide baseline data for evaluating outcomes of therapy and to maintain a systematic and consistent approach to ongoing diagnosis and treatment. Treatment options and prognosis are determined on the basis of staging and grading.

Staging determines the size of the tumor and the existence of metastasis. Several systems exist for classifying the anatomic extent of disease. The TNM system is frequently used (Green et al., 2002). In this system, "T" refers to the extent of the primary tumor, "N" refers to lymph node involvement, and "M" refers to the extent of metastasis (Chart 16-3). A variety of other staging systems are used to describe the extent of cancers, such as central nervous system (CNS) cancers, hematologic cancers, and malignant melanoma, that are not well described by the TNM system. Staging systems also provide a convenient shorthand notation that condenses lengthy descriptions into manageable terms for comparisons of treatments and prognoses.

Grading refers to the classification of the tumor cells. Grading systems seek to define the type of tissue from which the tumor originated and the degree to which the tumor cells retain the functional and histologic characteristics of the tissue of origin. Samples of cells to be used to establish the grade of a tumor may be obtained through cytology (examination of cells from tissue scrapings, body fluids, secretions, or washings), biopsy, or surgical excision.

This information helps the health care team predict the behavior and prognosis of various tumors. The tumor is assigned a numeric value ranging from I to IV. Grade I tumors, also known as well-differentiated tumors, closely resemble the tissue of origin in structure and function. Tumors that do not clearly resemble the tissue of origin in structure or function are described as poorly differentiated or undifferentiated and are assigned grade IV. These tu-

TABLE 16-4 Diagnostic Aids Used to Detect Cancer

Test	Description	Diagnostic Uses
Tumor marker identification	Analysis of substances found in blood or other body fluids that are made by the tumor or by the body in response to the tumor	Breast, colon, lung, ovarian, testicular, prostate cancers
Magnetic resonance imaging (MRI)	Use of magnetic fields and radiofrequency signals to create sectioned images of various body structures	Neurologic, pelvic, abdominal, thoracic cancers
Computed tomography (CT)	Use of narrow-beam x-ray to scan successive layers of tissue for a cross-sectional view	Neurologic, pelvic, skeletal, abdominal, thoracic cancers
Fluoroscopy	Use of x-rays that identify contrasts in body tissue densities; may involve the use of contrast agents	Skeletal, lung, gastrointestinal cancers
Ultrasonography (ultrasound)	High-frequency sound waves echoing off body tissues are converted electronically into images; used to assess tissues deep within the body	Abdominal and pelvic cancers
Endoscopy	Direct visualization of a body cavity or passageway by insertion of an endoscope into a body cavity or opening; allows tissue biopsy, fluid aspiration, and excision of small tumors; both diagnostic and therapeutic	Bronchial, gastrointestinal cancers
Nuclear medicine imaging	Uses intravenous injection or ingestion of radioisotope substances followed by imaging of tissues that have concentrated the radioisotopes	Bone, liver, kidney, spleen, brain, thyroid cancers
Positron emission tomography (PET)	Through the use of a tracer; provides black and white or color-coded images of the biologic activity of a particular area, rather than its structure; used in detection of cancer or its response to treatment	Lung, colon, liver, pancreatic, head and neck cancers; Hodgkin and non-Hodgkin lymphoma and melanoma
PET fusion	Use of a PET scanner and a CT scanner in one machine to provide an image combining anatomic detail, spatial resolution, and functional metabolic abnormalities	See PET
Radioimmunoconjugates	Monoclonal antibodies are labeled with a radioisotope and injected intravenously into the patient; the antibodies that aggregate at the tumor site are visualized with scanners	Colorectal, breast, ovarian, head and neck cancers; lymphoma and melanoma

mors tend to be more aggressive and less responsive to treatment than well-differentiated tumors.

Management of Cancer

Treatment options offered to cancer patients should be based on realistic and achievable goals for each specific type of cancer. The range of possible treatment goals may include complete eradication of malignant disease (**cure**), prolonged survival and containment of cancer cell growth (**control**), or relief of symptoms associated with the disease (**palliation**).

The health care team, the patient, and the patient's family must have a clear understanding of the treatment options and goals. Open communication and support are vital as the patient and family periodically reassess treatment plans and goals when complications of therapy develop or disease progresses.

Multiple modalities are commonly used in cancer treatment. A variety of approaches, including surgery, radiation therapy, chemotherapy, and targeted therapies, may be used at various times throughout treatment. Understanding the principles of each and how they interrelate is important in understanding the rationale and goals of treatment.

Surgery

Surgical removal of the entire cancer remains the ideal and most frequently used treatment method. However, the specific surgical approach may vary for several reasons. Diagnostic surgery is the definitive method of identifying the cellular characteristics that influence all treatment decisions. Surgery may be the primary method of treatment, or it may be prophylactic, palliative, or reconstructive.

Diagnostic Surgery

Diagnostic surgery, such as a **biopsy**, is usually performed to obtain a tissue sample for analysis of cells suspected to be malignant. In most instances, the biopsy is taken from the actual tumor, but in some situations, it is necessary to biopsy lymph nodes near the suspicious tumor. It is well known that many cancers can metastasize from the primary site to other areas of the body through the lymphatic circulation. Knowing whether adjacent lymph nodes contain tumor cells helps physicians plan for systemic therapies instead of or in addition to surgery, to combat tumor cells that have gone beyond the primary tumor site. The use of injectable dyes and nuclear medicine imaging can help the

CHART 16-3

TNM Classification System

T The extent of the primary tumor
N The absence or presence and extent of regional lymph node metastasis
M The absence or presence of distant metastasis

The use of numerical subsets of the TNM components indicates the progressive extent of the malignant disease.

PRIMARY TUMOR (T)

Tx Primary tumor cannot be assessed
T0 No evidence of primary tumor
Tis Carcinoma in situ
T1, T2, T3, T4 Increasing size and/or local extent of the primary tumor

REGIONAL LYMPH NODES (N)

Nx Regional lymph nodes cannot be assessed
N0 No regional lymph node metastasis
N1, N2, N3 Increasing involvement of regional lymph nodes

DISTANT METASTASIS (M)

Mx Distant metastasis cannot be assessed
M0 No distant metastasis
M1 Distant metastasis

From Green, F., et al. (Eds) (2002). *AJCC cancer staging manual* (6th ed.). New York: Springer-Verlag.

surgeon identify lymph nodes (sentinel nodes) that process lymphatic drainage for the involved area. This procedure has been accepted as the standard of care for melanoma and is rapidly becoming the standard of care for breast cancer. Sentinel node biopsy is still considered investigational for gastrointestinal malignancies and tumors of the vulva (Jakub, Pendas & Reintgen, 2003).

CHOICE OF BIOPSY METHOD

The choice of biopsy method is based on many factors. Of greatest importance is the type of treatment anticipated if the cancer diagnosis is confirmed. Definitive surgical approaches include excision of the original biopsy site so that any cells disseminated during the biopsy are excised at the time of surgery. Nutrition and hematologic, respiratory, renal, and hepatic function are considered in determining the method of treatment as well. If the biopsy requires general anesthesia and if subsequent surgery is likely, the effects of prolonged anesthesia on the patient are considered.

The patient and family are given the opportunity to discuss the options before definitive plans are made. The nurse, as the patient's advocate, serves as a liaison between the patient and physician to facilitate this process. Time should be set aside to minimize interruptions and distractions. The patient should have time to ask questions and to think through all that has been discussed.

BIOPSY TYPES

The three most common biopsy methods are the excisional, incisional, and needle methods (Abeloff, Armitage, Niederhuber, et al., 2004).

Excisional biopsy is most frequently used for easily accessible tumors of the skin, breast, upper and lower gastrointestinal tract, and upper respiratory tract. In many cases, the surgeon can remove the entire tumor and surrounding marginal tissues as well. This removal of normal tissue beyond the tumor area decreases the possibility that residual microscopic disease cells may lead to a recurrence of the tumor. This approach not only provides the pathologist, who stages and grades the cells, with the entire tissue specimen but also decreases the chance of seeding the tumor (disseminating cancer cells through surrounding tissues).

Incisional biopsy is performed if the tumor mass is too large to be removed. In this case, a wedge of tissue from the tumor is removed for analysis. The cells of the tissue wedge must be representative of the tumor mass so that the pathologist can provide an accurate diagnosis. If the specimen does not contain representative tissue and cells, negative biopsy results do not guarantee the absence of cancer.

Excisional and incisional approaches are often performed through endoscopy. However, surgical incision may be required to determine the anatomic extent or stage of the tumor. For example, a diagnostic or staging laparotomy (the surgical opening of the abdomen to assess malignant abdominal disease) may be necessary to assess malignancies such as gastric cancer.

Needle biopsies are performed to sample suspicious masses that are easily accessible, such as some growths in the breasts, thyroid, lung, liver, and kidney. Needle biopsies are fast, relatively inexpensive, and easy to perform and usually require only local anesthesia. In general, the patient experiences slight and temporary physical discomfort. In addition, the surrounding tissues are disturbed only minimally, thus decreasing the likelihood of seeding cancer cells. Needle aspiration biopsy involves aspirating tissue fragments through a needle guided into an area suspected of bearing disease. Occasionally, x-ray, computed tomography (CT) scanning, ultrasonography, or magnetic resonance imaging (MRI) is used to help locate the suspicious area and guide the placement of the needle. In some instances, the aspiration biopsy does not yield enough tissue to permit accurate diagnosis. A needle core biopsy uses a specially designed needle to obtain a small core of tissue. Most often, this specimen is sufficient to permit accurate diagnosis.

Surgery as Primary Treatment

When surgery is the primary approach in treating cancer, the goal is to remove the entire tumor or as much as is feasible (a procedure sometimes called debulking) and any involved surrounding tissue, including regional lymph nodes.

Two common surgical approaches used for treating primary tumors are local and wide excisions. Local excision is warranted when the mass is small. It includes removal of the mass and a small margin of normal tissue that is easily accessible. Wide or radical excisions (en bloc dissections) include removal of the primary tumor, lymph nodes, adjacent involved structures, and surrounding tissues that may be at high risk for tumor spread (Kufe, Pollock, Wechselbaum, et al., 2003). This surgical method can result in disfigurement and altered functioning. However, wide excisions are considered if the tumor can be removed completely and the chances of cure or control are good.

In some situations, video-assisted endoscopic surgery is replacing surgery associated with long incisions and extended recovery periods. In this procedure, an endoscope with intense lighting and an attached multichip minicamera is inserted into the body through a small incision. The surgical instruments are inserted into the surgical field through one or two additional small incisions, each about 3 cm in length. The camera transmits the image of the involved area to a monitor so the surgeon can manipulate the instruments to perform the necessary procedure. Video-assisted endoscopic surgery is now being used for many thoracic and abdominal surgeries.

Salvage surgery is an additional treatment option that uses an extensive surgical approach to treat the local recurrence of a cancer after the use of a less extensive primary approach. A mastectomy to treat recurrent breast cancer after primary lumpectomy and radiation is an example of salvage surgery.

In addition to surgery that uses surgical blades or scalpels to excise the mass and surrounding tissues, several other types of surgical techniques are available. Electrosurgery makes use of electrical current to destroy the tumor cells. Cryosurgery uses liquid nitrogen or a very cold probe to freeze tissue to cause cell destruction. Chemosurgery uses chemicals applied to tissues to facilitate their removal. Laser surgery (*l*ight *a*mplification by *s*timulated *e*mission of *r*adiation) makes use of light and energy aimed at an exact tissue location and depth to vaporize cancer cells. Laser surgery is also referred to as *photocoagulation or photoablation.* Stereotactic radiosurgery is a single and highly precise administration of high-dose radiation therapy used in some types of brain and head and neck cancers. This type of radiation has such a dramatic effect on the target area that the changes are considered to be comparable to more traditional surgical approaches even though no incision is actually made (Law, Mangarin & Kelvin, 2003; Witt, Haas, Marrinan et al., 2003). (Radiation therapy is discussed later in this chapter.)

A multidisciplinary approach to patient care is essential during and after any type of surgery. The effects of surgery on the patient's body image, self-esteem, and functional abilities are addressed. If necessary, a plan for postoperative rehabilitation is made before the surgery is performed.

The growth and dissemination of cancer cells may have produced distant micrometastases by the time the patient seeks treatment. Therefore, attempting to remove wide margins of tissue in the hope of "getting all the cancer cells" may not be feasible. This reality substantiates the need for a coordinated multidisciplinary approach to cancer therapy (Abeloff et al., 2004). Once the surgery has been completed, one or more additional (or adjuvant) modalities may be chosen to increase the likelihood of destroying the remaining cancer cells. However, some cancers that are treated surgically in the very early stages are considered to be curable (eg, skin cancers, testicular cancers).

Prophylactic Surgery

Prophylactic surgery involves removing nonvital tissues or organs that are likely to develop cancer. The following factors are considered when physicians and patients discuss possible prophylactic surgery:

- Family history and genetic predisposition
- Presence or absence of symptoms
- Potential risks and benefits
- Ability to detect cancer at an early stage
- The patient's acceptance of the postoperative outcome

Colectomy, mastectomy, and oophorectomy are examples of prophylactic surgeries. Recent developments in the ability to identify genetic markers indicative of a predisposition to develop some types of cancer may play a role in decisions concerning prophylactic surgeries. However, what is adequate justification for prophylactic surgery is controversial. For example, several factors are considered when deciding to proceed with a prophylactic mastectomy, including a strong family history of breast cancer; positive *BRCA1* or *BRCA2* findings; an abnormal physical finding on breast examination, such as progressive nodularity and cystic disease; a proven history of breast cancer in the opposite breast; abnormal mammography findings; and abnormal biopsy results.

Because the long-term physiologic and psychological effects are unknown, prophylactic surgery is offered selectively to patients and discussed thoroughly with patients and families. Preoperative teaching and counseling, as well as long-term follow-up, are provided.

Palliative Surgery

When cure is not possible, the goals of treatment are to make the patient as comfortable as possible and to promote a satisfying and productive life for as long as possible. Whether the period is extremely brief or lengthy, the major goal is a high quality of life—with quality defined by the patient and his or her family. Palliative surgery is performed in an attempt to relieve complications of cancer, such as ulcerations, obstructions, hemorrhage, pain, and malignant effusions (Table 16-5). Honest and informative communication with the patient and family about the goal of surgery is essential to avoid false hope and disappointment.

Reconstructive Surgery

Reconstructive surgery may follow curative or radical surgery and is carried out in an attempt to improve function or obtain a more desirable cosmetic effect. It may be performed in one operation or in stages. The surgeon who will perform the surgery discusses possible reconstructive surgical options with the patient before the primary surgery is performed. Reconstructive surgery may be indicated for breast, head and neck, and skin cancers.

The nurse must recognize the patient's needs and the impact that altered functioning and altered body image may have on quality of life. It is imperative for the nurse to provide the patient and family with opportunities to discuss these issues. The individual needs of the patient undergoing reconstructive surgery must be accurately assessed and addressed.

Nursing Management in Cancer Surgery

Patients undergoing surgery for cancer require general perioperative nursing care, as described in Unit 4 of this text,

TABLE 16-5 Indications for Pallative Surgical Procedures

Procedure	Indications
Pleural drainage tube placement	Pleural effusion
Peritoneal drainage tube placement (Tenckoff catheter)	Ascites
Abdominal shunt placement (Levine shunt)	Ascites
Pericardial drainage tube placement	Pericardial effusion
Colostomy or ileostomy	Bowel obstruction
Gastrostomy, jejunostomy tube placement	Upper gastrointestinal tract obstruction
Biliary stent placement	Biliary obstruction
Ureteral stent placement	Ureteral obstruction
Nerve block	Pain
Cordotomy	Pain
Venous access device placement (for administering parenteral analgesics)	Pain
Epidural catheter placement (for administering epidural analgesics)	Pain
Hormone manipulation (removal of ovaries, testes, adrenals, pituitary)	Tumors that depend on hormones for growth

along with specific care related to age, organ impairment, nutritional deficits, disorders of coagulation, and altered immunity that may increase the risk of postoperative complications. Combining other treatment methods, such as radiation and chemotherapy, with surgery also contributes to postoperative complications, such as infection, impaired wound healing, altered pulmonary or renal function, and the development of deep vein thrombosis. In these situations, the nurse completes a thorough preoperative assessment for factors that may affect the patient undergoing the surgical procedure.

Patients who are undergoing surgery for the diagnosis or treatment of cancer are often anxious about the surgical procedure, possible findings, postoperative limitations, changes in normal body functions, and prognosis. The patient and family require time and assistance to deal with the possible changes and outcomes resulting from the surgery.

The nurse provides education and emotional support by assessing the needs of the patient and family and by discussing their fears and coping mechanisms with them. The nurse encourages the patient and family to take an active role in decision making when possible. If the patient or family ask about the results of diagnostic testing and surgical procedures, the nurse's response is guided by the information the physician has previously conveyed to the patient and family. The patient and family may also ask the nurse to explain and clarify information that the physician initially provided but that they did not grasp because they were anxious at the time. It is important that the nurse communicate frequently with the physician and other members of the health care team to be certain that the information provided is consistent.

After surgery, the nurse assesses the patient's responses to the surgery and monitors the patient for possible complications, such as infection, bleeding, thrombophlebitis, wound dehiscence, fluid and electrolyte imbalance, and organ dysfunction (Morris & Ward, 2003). The nurse also provides for the patient's comfort. Postoperative teaching addresses wound care, activity, nutrition, and medication information.

Plans for discharge, follow-up and home care, and treatment are initiated as early as possible to ensure continuity of care from hospital to home or from a cancer referral center to the patient's local hospital and health care provider. Patients and families are also encouraged to use community resources such as the American Cancer Society for support and information.

Radiation Therapy

In **radiation therapy**, ionizing radiation is used to interrupt cellular growth. More than half of patients with cancer receive a form of radiation therapy at some point during treatment. Radiation may be used to cure the cancer, as in Hodgkin disease, testicular seminomas, thyroid carcinomas, localized cancers of the head and neck, and cancers of the uterine cervix. Radiation therapy may also be used to control malignant disease when a tumor cannot be removed surgically or when local nodal metastasis is present, or it can be used prophylactically to prevent leukemic infiltration to the brain or spinal cord.

Palliative radiation therapy is used to relieve the symptoms of metastatic disease, especially when the cancer has spread to brain, bone, or soft tissue, or to treat oncologic emergencies, such as superior vena cava syndrome or spinal cord compression.

Two types of ionizing radiation—electromagnetic rays (x-rays and gamma rays) and particles (electrons [beta particles], protons, neutrons, and alpha particles)—can lead to tissue disruption. The most harmful tissue disruption is the alteration of the DNA molecule within the cells of the tissue. Ionizing radiation breaks the strands of the DNA helix, leading to cell death. Ionizing radiation can also ionize constituents of body fluids, especially water, leading to the formation of free radicals and irreversibly damaging DNA. If the DNA is incapable of repair, the cell may die immediately, or it may initiate cellular suicide (apoptosis), a genetically programmed cell death (Abeloff et al., 2004; Casciato, 2004).

Cells are most vulnerable to the disruptive effects of radiation during DNA synthesis and mitosis (early S, G_2, and M phases of the cell cycle). Therefore, those body tissues that undergo frequent cell division are most sensitive to radiation therapy. These tissues include bone marrow, lymphatic tissue, epithelium of the gastrointestinal tract, hair cells, and gonads. Slower-growing tissues and tissues at rest are relatively radioresistant (less sensitive to the effects of radiation). Such tissues include muscle, cartilage, and connective tissues.

A radiosensitive tumor is one that can be destroyed by a dose of radiation that still allows for cell regeneration in the normal tissue. Tumors that are well oxygenated also appear to be more sensitive to radiation. In theory, therefore, radiation therapy may be enhanced if more oxygen can be delivered to tumors. In addition, if the radiation is delivered when most tumor cells are cycling through the cell cycle, the number of cancer cells destroyed (cell kill) is maximal (Abeloff et al., 2004; Casciato, 2004).

Certain chemicals, including chemotherapy agents, act as radiosensitizers and sensitize more hypoxic (oxygen-poor) tumors to the effects of radiation therapy. Radiation is delivered to tumor sites by external or internal means.

External Radiation

If external radiation therapy is used, one of several delivery methods may be chosen, depending on the depth of the tumor. Depending on the amount of energy they contain, x-rays can be used to destroy cancerous cells at the skin surface or deeper in the body. The higher the energy, the deeper the penetration into the body. Kilovoltage therapy devices deliver the maximal radiation dose to superficial lesions, such as lesions of the skin and breast, whereas linear accelerators and betatron machines produce higher-energy x-rays and deliver their dosage to deeper structures with less harm to the skin and less scattering of radiation within the body tissues. Gamma rays are another form of energy used in radiation therapy. This energy is produced from the spontaneous decay of naturally occurring radioactive elements such as cobalt-60. The gamma rays also deliver this radiation dose beneath the skin surface, sparing skin tissue from adverse effects.

Some centers nationwide treat more hypoxic, radiation-resistant tumors with particle-beam radiation therapy. This type of therapy accelerates subatomic particles (neutrons, photons) through body tissue. This therapy, which is also known as high linear energy transfer radiation, damages target cells as well as other cells in its path (Abeloff et al., 2004; Casciato, 2004).

Internal Radiation

Internal radiation implantation, or **brachytherapy**, delivers a high dose of radiation to a localized area. The specific radioisotope for implantation is selected on the basis of its half-life, which is the time it takes for half of its radioactivity to decay. This internal radiation can be implanted by means of needles, seeds, beads, or catheters into body cavities (vagina, abdomen, pleura) or interstitial compartments (breast). Brachytherapy may also be administered orally, as with the isotope iodine-131, which is used to treat thyroid carcinomas (Abeloff et al., 2004, Casciato, 2004; Gordils-Perez, Rawlins-Duell & Kelvin, 2003).

Intracavitary radioisotopes are frequently used to treat gynecologic cancers. In these malignancies, the radioisotopes are inserted into specially positioned applicators after the position is verified by x-ray. These radioisotopes remain in place for a prescribed period and then are removed. The patient is maintained on bed rest and log-rolled to prevent displacement of the intracavitary delivery device. An indwelling urinary catheter is inserted to ensure that the bladder remains empty. Low-residue diets and antidiarrheal agents, such as diphenoxylate (Lomotil), are provided to prevent bowel movements during therapy to prevent displacement of the radioisotopes.

Interstitial implants, used in treating such malignancies as prostate, pancreatic, or breast cancer, may be temporary or permanent, depending on the radioisotopes used. These implants usually consist of seeds, needles, wires, or small catheters positioned to provide a local radiation source and are less frequently dislodged. With internal radiation therapy, the farther the tissue is from the radiation source, the lower the dosage. This spares the noncancerous tissue from the radiation dose.

Because patients receiving internal radiation emit radiation while the implant is in place, contacts with the health care team are guided by principles of time, distance, and shielding to minimize exposure of personnel to radiation. Safety precautions used in caring for a patient receiving brachytherapy include assigning the patient to a private room, posting appropriate notices about radiation safety precautions, having staff members wear dosimeter badges, making sure that pregnant staff members are not assigned to the patient's care, prohibiting visits by children or pregnant visitors, limiting visits from others to 30 minutes daily, and seeing that visitors maintain a 6-foot distance from the radiation source. Patients with seed implants may be able to return home; radiation exposure to others is minimal. Information about any precautions, if needed, is provided to the patient and family members to ensure safety.

Radiation Dosage

The radiation dosage is dependent on the sensitivity of the target tissues to radiation and on the tumor size. The lethal tumor dose is defined as that dose that will eradicate 95% of the tumor yet preserve normal tissue. The total radiation dose is delivered over several weeks to allow healthy tissue to repair and to achieve greater cell kill by exposing more cells to the radiation as they begin active cell division. Repeated radiation treatments over time (fractionated doses) also allow for the periphery of the tumor to be reoxygenated repeatedly, because tumors shrink from the outside inward. This increases the radiosensitivity of the tumor, thereby increasing tumor cell death (Abeloff et al., 2004; Casciato, 2004).

Toxicity

Toxicity of radiation therapy is localized to the region being irradiated. Toxicity may be increased if concomitant chemotherapy is administered. Acute local reactions occur when normal cells in the treatment area are also destroyed and cellular death exceeds cellular regeneration. Body tissues most affected are those that normally proliferate rapidly, such as the skin; the epithelial lining of the gastrointestinal tract, including the oral cavity; and the bone marrow. Altered skin integrity is a common effect and can include alopecia (hair loss), erythema, and shedding of skin (desquamation). Reepithelialization occurs after treatments have been completed.

Alterations in oral mucosa secondary to radiation therapy include stomatitis, **xerostomia** (dryness of the mouth), change and loss of taste, and decreased salivation. The entire gastrointestinal mucosa may be involved, and esophageal irritation with chest pain and dysphagia may result. Anorexia, nausea, vomiting, and diarrhea may occur if the stomach or colon is in the irradiated field. Symptoms subside and gastrointestinal reepithelialization occurs after treatments have been completed.

Bone marrow cells proliferate rapidly, and if sites containing bone marrow (e.g., the iliac crest, sternum) are included in the radiation field, anemia, leukopenia (decreased white blood cells [WBCs]), and **thrombocytopenia** (a decrease in platelets) may result. The patient is then at increased risk for infection and bleeding until blood cell counts return to normal. Chronic anemia may occur (Abeloff et al., 2004; Casciato, 2004).

Research to develop cytoprotective agents that can protect normal tissue from radiation damage continues. The most commonly used cytoprotectant is amifostine (Ethyol), which is a scavenger of free radicals that prevents damage to DNA (Wilkes & Barton-Burke, 2004).

Certain systemic side effects are also commonly experienced by patients receiving radiation therapy. These manifestations, which are generalized, include fatigue, malaise, and anorexia. This syndrome may be secondary to substances released when tumor cells break down. The effects are temporary and subside with the cessation of treatment.

Late effects of radiation therapy may also occur in various body tissues. These effects are chronic, usually produce fibrotic changes secondary to a decreased vascular supply, and are irreversible. These late effects can be most severe when they involve vital organs such as the lungs, heart, CNS, and bladder. Toxicities may intensify when radiation is combined with other treatment modalities.

Nursing Management in Radiation Therapy

Patients receiving radiation therapy and their families often have questions and concerns about its safety. To answer questions and allay fears about the effects of radiation on the tumor and on the patient's normal tissues and organs, the nurses can explain the procedure for delivering radiation and describe the equipment, the duration of the procedure (often minutes only), the possible need for immobilizing the patient during the procedure, and the absence of new sensations, including pain, during the procedure. If a radioactive implant is used, the nurse informs the patient and family about the restrictions placed on visitors and health care personnel and other radiation precautions. The patient also should understand his or her own role before, during, and after the procedure. See Chapter 47 for further discussion of radiation treatment for gynecologic cancers.

PROTECTING SKIN AND ORAL MUCOSA

The nurse assesses the patient's skin, nutritional status, and general feeling of well-being. The nurse assesses the skin

---

NURSING RESEARCH PROFILE

Patients' Need for Information About Cancer Therapy

Skalla, K. A., Bakitas, M., Furstenberg, C. T., et al. (2004). Patients' need for information about cancer therapy. *Oncology Nursing Forum, 31*(2), 313–319.

Purpose

Treatment of cancer is a difficult and stressful experience. Research continues to show that patients want information, yet they do not perceive that they are receiving the information they need for successful coping. The purpose of this study was to obtain detailed information about the preferences of patients with cancer and their need for information about side effects of cancer treatment, with the goal of designing an interactive multimedia education program.

Design

Data were gathered from focus groups of 51 patients who had undergone chemotherapy, radiation therapy, or combined modality treatment in the past year; the study group included 14 spouses. The questions addressed at each focus group by a trained facilitator were designed to encourage discussion about the nature of the symptoms experienced and patients' informational needs about treatment and management of treatment-related side effects. Each focus group was audiotaped for later discussion and analysis. Participants' comments were reviewed, coded, and organized into categories. A qualitative software program was used to organize data analysis. Categories of themes were developed based on participants' comments.

Findings

Results indicated that patients reported that they did not receive the information they wanted or needed to enhance coping. Most patients wanted as much information as possible about treatment and treatment-related side effects. Patients desired individualized, practical information about how the treatments would affect their daily lives, identified as increasingly important because treatment is often being performed on an outpatient basis. Patients reported that it was difficult to absorb and retain information given to them. They often experienced informational overload with traditional teaching methods.

Nursing Implications

This study shows that nurses must tailor educational programs to better meet the informational demands of patients with cancer. Interactive multimedia technology (audio, text, graphics, video) offers an innovative approach to patient education that can overcome many educational barriers by allowing patients to control the pace of information. Multimedia technology offers advantages to meet patients' needs, but these tools need to be developed to meet changing educational expectations of patients.

and oral mucosa frequently for changes (particularly if radiation therapy is directed to these areas). The skin is protected from irritation, and the patient is instructed to avoid using ointments, lotions, or powders on the area.

Gentle oral hygiene is essential to remove debris, prevent irritation, and promote healing. If systemic symptoms, such as weakness and fatigue, occur, the patient may need assistance with activities of daily living and personal hygiene. In addition, the nurse offers reassurance by explaining that these symptoms are a result of the treatment and do not represent deterioration or progression of the disease.

PROTECTING CAREGIVERS

When the patient has a radioactive implant in place, the nurse and other health care providers need to protect themselves as well as the patient from the effects of radiation. Specific instructions are usually provided by the radiation safety officer from the x-ray department. The instructions identify the maximum time that can be spent safely in the patient's room, the shielding equipment to be used, and special precautions and actions to be taken if the implant is dislodged. The nurse should explain the rationale for these precautions to keep the patient from feeling unduly isolated.

Chemotherapy

In **chemotherapy**, antineoplastic agents are used in an attempt to destroy tumor cells by interfering with cellular functions, including replication. Chemotherapy is used primarily to treat systemic disease rather than localized lesions that are amenable to surgery or radiation. Chemotherapy may be combined with surgery, radiation therapy, or both, to reduce tumor size preoperatively, to destroy any remaining tumor cells postoperatively, or to treat some forms of leukemia. The goals of chemotherapy (cure, control, palliation), must be realistic because they will define the medications to be used and the aggressiveness of the treatment plan.

Cell Kill and the Cell Cycle

CONCEPTS in action **ANIMATION**

Each time a tumor is exposed to a chemotherapeutic agent, a percentage of tumor cells (20% to 99%, depending on dosage) is destroyed. Repeated doses of chemotherapy are necessary over a prolonged period to achieve regression of the tumor. Eradication of 100% of the tumor is almost impossible. Instead, the goal of treatment is eradication of enough of the tumor so that the remaining tumor cells can be destroyed by the body's immune system.

Actively proliferating cells within a tumor are the most sensitive to chemotherapeutic agents (the ratio of dividing cells to resting cells is referred to as the growth fraction). Nondividing cells capable of future proliferation are the least sensitive to antineoplastic medications and consequently are potentially dangerous. However, the nondividing cells must be destroyed to eradicate a cancer. Repeated cycles of chemotherapy are used to kill more tumor cells by destroying these nondividing cells as they begin active cell division.

Reproduction of both healthy and malignant cells follows the cell cycle pattern (Fig. 16-2). The cell cycle time is the time required for one tissue cell to divide and reproduce two identical daughter cells. The cell cycle of any cell has four distinct phases, each with a vital underlying function:

1. G_1 phase—RNA and protein synthesis occur
2. S phase—DNA synthesis occurs
3. G_2 phase—premitotic phase; DNA synthesis is complete, mitotic spindle forms
4. Mitosis—cell division occurs

The G_0 phase, the resting or dormant phase of cells, can occur after mitosis and during the G_1 phase. In the G_0 phase are those dangerous cells that are not actively dividing but have the potential for replicating. The administration of certain chemotherapeutic agents (as well as some other forms of therapy) is coordinated with the cell cycle.

Classification of Chemotherapeutic Agents

Chemotherapeutic agents may be classified by their relationship to the cell cycle. Certain chemotherapeutic agents that are specific to certain phases of the cell cycle are termed cell cycle–specific agents. These agents destroy cells that are actively reproducing by means of the cell cycle; most affect cells in the S phase by interfering with DNA and RNA synthesis. Other agents, such as the vinca or plant alkaloids, are specific to the M phase, where they halt mitotic spindle formation. Chemotherapeutic agents that act independently of the cell cycle phases are termed

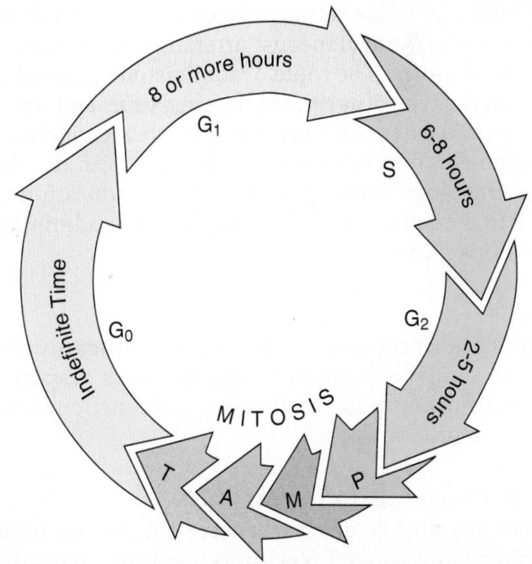

FIGURE 16-2. Phases of the cell cycle extend over the interval between the midpoint of mitosis and the subsequent end point in mitosis in a daughter cell. G_1 is the postmitotic phase during which ribonucleic acid (RNA) and protein syntheses are increased and cell growth occurs. G_0 is the resting, or dormant, phase of the cell cycle. In the S phase, nucleic acids are synthesized and chromosomes are replicated in preparation for cell mitosis. During G_2, RNA and protein synthesis occur as in G_1. P, prophase; M, metaphase; A, anaphase; T, telophase. From Porth, C. M. (2002). *Pathophysiology: Concepts of altered health states* (6th ed.). Philadelphia: Lippincott Williams & Wilkins.

cell cycle–nonspecific agents. These agents usually have a prolonged effect on cells, leading to cellular damage or death. Many treatment plans combine cell cycle–specific and cell cycle–nonspecific agents to increase the number of vulnerable tumor cells killed during a treatment period (Abeloff et al., 2004; Casciato, 2004; Wilkes & Barton-Burke, 2004).

Chemotherapeutic agents are also classified by chemical group, each with a different mechanism of action. These include the alkylating agents, nitrosoureas, antimetabolites, antitumor antibiotics, plant alkaloids, hormonal agents, and miscellaneous agents. The classification, mechanism of action, common drugs, cell cycle specificity, and common side effects of antineoplastic agents are listed in Table 16-6.

Chemotherapeutic agents from every category may be used to enhance tumor cell kill during therapy by creating multiple cellular lesions. Combined medication therapy relies on agents of differing toxicities and with synergistic actions. Use of combination therapy also prevents the development of drug-resistant mechanisms.

Combining older medications with other agents, such as levamisole, leucovorin, hormones, or interferons, has shown some benefit in combating resistance of cells to chemotherapeutic agents. Newer investigational agents are being studied for effectiveness in resistant tumor lines. For more information about investigational agents, see Chart 16-4.

Administration of Chemotherapeutic Agents

Chemotherapeutic agents may be administered in the hospital, clinic, or home setting by topical, oral, intravenous, intramuscular, subcutaneous, arterial, intracavitary, and intrathecal routes. The route of administration usually depends on the type of agent; the required dose; and the type, location, and extent of tumor being treated. Guidelines for the administration of chemotherapy have been developed by the Oncology Nursing Society. Patient education is essential to maximize safety if chemotherapy is administered in the home (Chart 16-5).

DOSAGE

Dosage of antineoplastic agents is based primarily on the patient's total body surface area, previous response to chemotherapy or radiation therapy, and function of major organ systems.

SPECIAL PROBLEMS: EXTRAVASATION

Special care must be taken whenever intravenous vesicant agents are administered. **Vesicants** are those agents that, if deposited into the subcutaneous tissue (**extravasation**), cause tissue necrosis and damage to underlying tendons, nerves, and blood vessels. Although the complete mechanism of tissue destruction is unclear, it is known that the pH of many antineoplastic drugs is responsible for the severe inflammatory reaction as well as the ability of these drugs to bind to tissue DNA. Sloughing and ulceration of the tissue may be so severe that skin grafting may be necessary. The full extent of tissue damage may take several weeks to become apparent. Medications classified as vesicants include dactinomycin, daunorubicin, doxorubicin (Adriamycin), nitrogen mustard, mitomycin, vinblastine, vincristine, and vindesine.

Only specially trained physicians and nurses should administer vesicants. Careful selection of peripheral veins, skilled venipuncture, and careful administration of medications are essential. Indications of extravasation during administration of vesicant agents include the following:

- Absence of blood return from the intravenous catheter
- Resistance to flow of intravenous fluid
- Swelling, pain, or redness at the site

If extravasation is suspected, the medication administration is stopped immediately, and ice is applied to the site (unless the extravasated vesicant is a vinca alkaloid). The physician may aspirate any infiltrated medication from the tissues and inject a neutralizing solution into the area to reduce tissue damage. Selection of the neutralizing solution depends on the extravasated agent. Examples of neutralizing solutions include sodium thiosulfate, hyaluronidase, and sodium bicarbonate. Recommendations and guidelines for managing vesicant extravasation have been issued by individual medication manufacturers, pharmacies, and the Oncology Nursing Society, and they differ from one medication to the next.

If frequent, prolonged administration of antineoplastic vesicants is anticipated, right atrial Silastic catheters or venous access devices may be inserted to promote safety during medication administration and reduce problems with access to the circulatory system (Figs. 16-3 and 16-4). Complications associated with their use include infection and thrombosis.

TOXICITY

Toxicity associated with chemotherapy can be acute or chronic. Cells with rapid growth rates (eg, epithelium, bone marrow, hair follicles, sperm) are very susceptible to damage, and various body systems may be affected as well.

Gastrointestinal System. Nausea and vomiting are the most common side effects of chemotherapy and may persist for as long as 24–48 hours after its administration. Delayed nausea and vomiting may persist for as long as 1 week after chemotherapy. The vomiting centers in the brain are stimulated by the following mechanisms (Marek, 2003):

- Activation of the receptors found in the chemoreceptor trigger zone (CTZ) of the medulla by serotonin, substance P, and other neurotransmitters such as dopamine
- Stimulation of peripheral autonomic pathways (gastrointestinal tract and pharynx)
- Stimulation of the vestibular pathways (inner ear imbalances, labyrinth input)
- Cognitive stimulation (CNS disease, anticipatory nausea, and vomiting)
- A combination of these factors

Medications that can decrease nausea and vomiting include serotonin blockers, such as ondansetron, granisetron, dolasetron, and palonosetron, which block serotonin receptors of the gastrointestinal tract and CTZ, and dopaminergic blockers, such as metoclopramide (Reglan), which block dopamine receptors of the CTZ. Newer agents include neurokinin-1 receptor antagonists (eg, aprepitant

TABLE 16-6 Antineoplastic Agents

Drug Class and Examples	Mechanism of Action	Cell Cycle Specificity	Common Side Effects
Alkylating Agents			
Busulfan, carboplatin, chlorambucil, cisplatin, cyclophosphamide, dacarbazine, hexamethyl melamine, ifosfamide, melphalan, nitrogen mustard, oxaliplatin, thiotepa	Alter DNA structure by misreading DNA code, initiating breaks in the DNA molecule, cross-linking DNA strands	Cell cycle–nonspecific	Bone marrow suppression, nausea, vomiting, cystitis (cyclophosphamide, ifosfamide), stomatitis, alopecia, gonadal suppression, renal toxicity (cisplatin)
Nitrosureas			
Carmustine (BCNU), lomustine (CCNU), semustine (methyl CCNU), streptozocin	Similar to the alkylating agents; cross the blood–brain barrier	Cell cycle–nonspecific	Delayed and cumulative myelosuppression, especially thrombocytopenia; nausea, vomiting
Topoisomerase I Inhibitors			
Irinotecan, topotecan	Induce breaks in the DNA strand by binding to enzyme topoisomerase I, preventing cells from dividing	Cell cycle–specific (S phase)	Bone marrow suppression, diarrhea, nausea, vomiting, hepatotoxicity
Antimetabolites			
5-Azacytadine, capecitabine (Xeloda), cytarabine, edatrexate fludarabine, 5-fluorouracil (5-FU), FUDR, gemcitabine, hydroxyurea, leustatin, 6-mercaptopurine, methotrexate, pentostatin, 6-thioguanine	Interfere with the biosynthesis of metabolites or nucleic acids necessary for RNA and DNA synthesis	Cell cycle–specific (S phase)	Nausea, vomiting, diarrhea, bone marrow suppression, proctitis, stomatitis, renal toxicity (methotrexate), hepatotoxicity
Antitumor Antibiotics			
Bleomycin, dactinomycin, daunorubicin, doxorubicin (Adriamycin), idarubicin, mitomycin, mitoxantrone, plicamycin	Interfere with DNA synthesis by binding DNA; prevent RNA synthesis	Cell cycle–nonspecific	Bone marrow suppression, nausea, vomiting, alopecia, anorexia, cardiac toxicity (daunorubicin, doxorubicin)
Mitotic Spindle Poisons			
Plant alkaloids: etoposide, teniposide, vinblastine, vincristine (VCR), vindesine, vinorelbine	Arrest metaphase by inhibiting mitotic tubular formation (spindle); inhibit DNA and protein synthesis	Cell cycle–specific (M phase)	Bone marrow suppression (mild with VCR), neuropathies (VCR), stomatitis
Taxanes: paclitaxel, docetaxel	Arrest metaphase by inhibiting tubulin depolymerization	Cell cycle–specific (M phase)	Bradycardia, hypersensitivity reactions, bone marrow suppression, alopecia, neuropathies
Hormonal Agents			
Androgens and antiandrogens, estrogens and antiestrogens, progestins and antiprogestins, aromatase inhibitors, luteinizing hormone–releasing hormone analogues, steroids	Bind to hormone receptor sites that alter cellular growth; block binding of estrogens to receptor sites (antiestrogens); inhibit RNA synthesis; suppress aromatase of P450 system, which decreases estrogen level	Cell cycle–nonspecific	Hypercalcemia, jaundice, increased appetite, masculinization, feminization, sodium and fluid retention, nausea, vomiting, hot flashes, vaginal dryness
Miscellaneous Agents			
Asparaginase, procarbazine	Unknown or too complex to categorize	Varies	Anorexia, nausea, vomiting, bone marrow suppression, hepatotoxicity, anaphylaxis, hypotension, altered glucose metabolism

CHART 16-4

℞ PHARMACOLOGY • Investigational Antineoplastic Therapies and Clinical Trials

Evaluation of the effectiveness and toxic potential of promising new modalities for preventing, diagnosing, and treating cancer is accomplished through clinical trials. Before new chemotherapy agents are approved for clinical use, they are subjected to rigorous and lengthy evaluations to identify beneficial effects, adverse effects, and safety.

- *Phase I* clinical trials determine optimal dosing, scheduling, and toxicity.
- *Phase II* trials determine effectiveness with specific tumor types and further define toxicities. Participants in these early trials are most often those who have not responded to standard forms of treatment. Because phase I and II trials may be viewed as last-chance efforts, patients and families are fully informed about the experimental nature of the trial therapies. Although it is hoped that investigational therapy will effectively treat the disease, the purpose of early phase trials is to gather information concerning maximal tolerated doses, adverse effects, and effects of the antineoplastic agents on tumor growth.
- *Phase III* clinical trials establish the effectiveness of new medications or procedures as compared with conventional approaches. Nurses may assist in the recruitment, consent, and education processes for patients who participate. In many cases, nurses are instrumental in monitoring adherence, assisting patients to adhere to the parameters of the trial, and documenting data describing patients' responses. The physical and emotional needs of patients in clinical trials are addressed in much the same way as those of patients who receive standard forms of cancer treatment.
- *Phase IV* testing further investigates medications in terms of new uses, dosing schedule, and toxicities.

[Emend]), which block the activity of substance P, another potent neurotransmitter involved in stimulating nausea and vomiting (Flemm, 2004).

Nausea and vomiting involve multiple pathways; therefore, corticosteroids, phenothiazines, sedatives, and histamines are helpful, especially when used in combination with serotonin blockers to provide improved antiemetic protection. Delayed nausea and vomiting that occur longer than 48 to 72 hours after chemotherapy are troublesome for some patients. To minimize discomfort, some antiemetic medications are necessary for the first week at home after chemotherapy. Relaxation techniques and imagery can also help decrease stimuli contributing to symptoms. Small frequent meals, bland foods, and comfort foods may reduce the frequency or severity of these symptoms.

Although the epithelium that lines the oral cavity quickly renews itself, its rapid rate of proliferation makes it susceptible to the effects of chemotherapy. As a result, stomatitis and anorexia are common. The entire gastrointestinal tract is susceptible to mucositis (inflammation of the mucosal lining), and diarrhea is a common result. Antimetabolites and antitumor antibiotics are the major culprits in mucositis and other gastrointestinal symptoms. Irinotecan is responsible for causing diarrhea, which can be severe in some patients.

Hematopoietic System. Most chemotherapeutic agents cause **myelosuppression** (depression of bone marrow

CHART 16-5

HOME CARE CHECKLIST • Chemotherapy Administration

At the completion of the home care instruction, the patient or caregiver will be able to:	Patient	Caregiver
• Demonstrate how to administer the chemotherapy agent in the home.	✔	✔
• Demonstrate safe disposal of needles, syringes, IV supplies, or unused chemotherapy medications.	✔	✔
• List possible side effects of chemotherapeutic agents.	✔	✔
• List complications of medications necessitating a call to the nurse or physician.	✔	✔
• List complications of medications necessitating a visit to the emergency department.	✔	✔
• List names and telephone numbers of resource personnel involved in care (ie, home care nurse, infusion services, IV vendor, equipment company).	✔	✔
• Explain treatment plan (protocol) and importance of upcoming visits to physician.	✔	✔

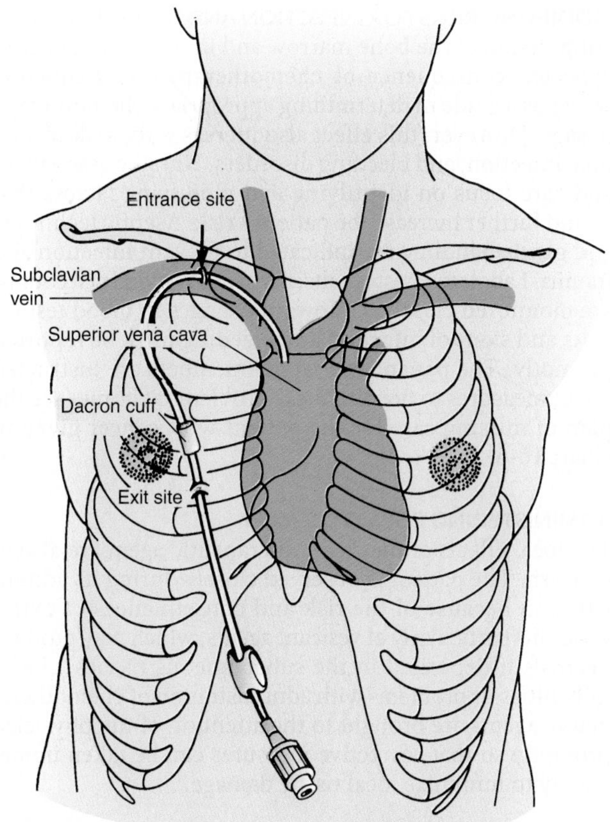

FIGURE 16-3. Right atrial catheter. The right atrial catheter is inserted into the subclavian vein and advanced until its tip lies in the superior vena cava just above the right atrium. The proximal end is then tunneled from the entry site through the subcutaneous tissue of the chest wall and brought out through an exit site on the chest. The Dacron cuff anchors the catheter in place and serves as a barrier to infection.

function), resulting in decreased production of blood cells. Myelosuppression decreases the number of WBCs (leukopenia), red blood cells (RBCs) (anemia), and platelets (thrombocytopenia) and increases the risk of infection and bleeding. Depression of these cells is the usual reason for limiting the dose of the chemotherapeutic agents. Monitoring blood cell counts frequently is essential, because it allows strategies to be implemented to protect patients from infection and injury, particularly while blood cell counts are depressed.

Other agents, called colony-stimulating factors (granulocyte colony-stimulating factor [G-CSF], granulocyte-macrophage colony-stimulating factor [GM-CSF], and erythropoietin [EPO]), can be administered after chemotherapy. G-CSF and GM-CSF stimulate the bone marrow to produce WBCs, especially neutrophils, at an accelerated rate, thus decreasing the duration of neutropenia. The colony-stimulating factors decrease the episodes of infection and the need for antibiotics and allow for more timely cycling of chemotherapy with less need to reduce the dosage. EPO stimulates RBC production, thus decreasing the symptoms of chronic anemia and reducing the need for blood transfusions (Bedell, 2003b; Cappozzo, 2004; Gillespie, 2003).

Renal System. Chemotherapeutic agents can damage the kidneys because of their direct effects during excretion and the accumulation of end products after cell lysis. Cisplatin, methotrexate, and mitomycin are particularly toxic to the kidneys. Rapid tumor cell lysis after chemotherapy results in increased urinary excretion of uric acid, which can cause renal damage. In addition, intracellular contents are released into the circulation, resulting in excessive levels of potassium and phosphates (hyperkalemia and hyperphosphatemia) and diminished levels of calcium (hypocalcemia). (See later discussion of tumor lysis syndrome.)

Monitoring blood urea nitrogen (BUN), serum creatinine, creatinine clearance, and serum electrolyte levels is

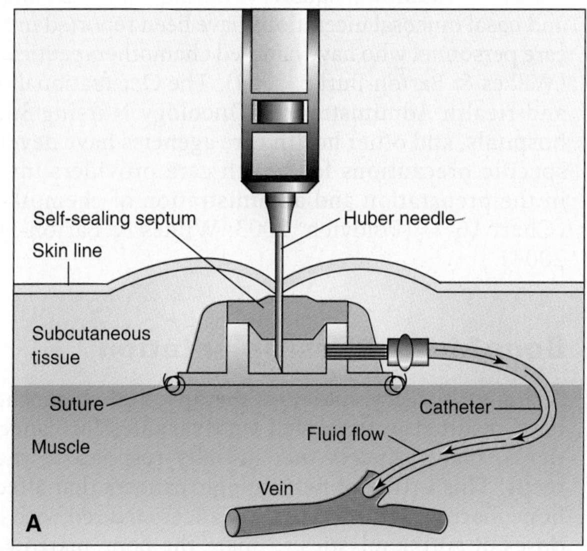

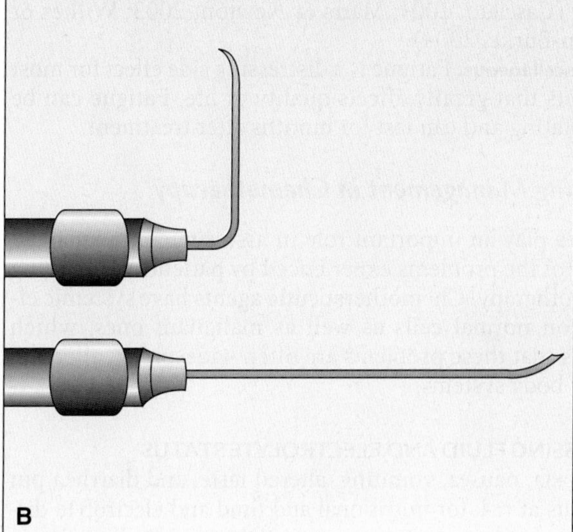

FIGURE 16-4. Implanted vascular access device. (**A**) A schematic diagram of an implanted vascular access device used for administration of medications, fluids, blood products, and nutrition. The self-sealing septum permits repeated puncture by Huber needles without damage or leakage. (**B**) Two Huber needles used to enter the implanted vascular port. The 90-degree needle is used for top-entry ports for continuous infusions.

essential. Adequate hydration, alkalinization of the urine to prevent formation of uric acid crystals, and the use of allopurinol are frequently indicated to prevent these side effects (Richerson, 2004).

Cardiopulmonary System. Antitumor antibiotics (daunorubicin and doxorubicin) are known to cause irreversible cumulative cardiac toxicities, especially when total dosage reaches 550 mg/m^2. Cardiac ejection fraction (volume of blood ejected from the heart with each beat) and signs of heart failure must be monitored closely. Bleomycin, carmustine (BCNU), and busulfan are known for their cumulative toxic effects on lung function. Pulmonary fibrosis can be a long-term effect of prolonged dosage with these agents. Therefore, patients are monitored closely for changes in pulmonary function, including pulmonary function test results. Total cumulative doses of bleomycin are not to exceed 400 units.

Reproductive System. Testicular and ovarian function can be affected by chemotherapeutic agents, resulting in possible sterility. Normal ovulation, early menopause, or permanent sterility may occur. In men, temporary or permanent azoospermia (absence of spermatozoa) may develop. Reproductive cells may be damaged during treatment, resulting in chromosomal abnormalities in offspring. Banking of sperm is recommended for men before treatments are initiated to protect against sterility or any mutagenic damage to sperm.

Patients and their partners need to be informed about potential changes in reproductive function resulting from chemotherapy. They are advised to use reliable methods of birth control while receiving chemotherapy and not to assume that sterility has resulted.

Neurologic System. The taxanes and plant alkaloids, especially vincristine, can cause neurologic damage with repeated doses. Peripheral neuropathies, loss of deep tendon reflexes, and paralytic ileus may occur. These side effects are usually reversible and disappear after completion of chemotherapy. Cisplatin is also responsible for peripheral neuropathies, and hearing loss due to damage to the acoustic nerve can also occur (Casciato, 2004; Marrs & Newton, 2003; Wilkes & Barton-Burke, 2004).

Miscellaneous. Fatigue is a distressing side effect for most patients that greatly affects quality of life. Fatigue can be debilitating and can last for months after treatment.

Nursing Management in Chemotherapy

Nurses play an important role in assessing and managing many of the problems experienced by patients undergoing chemotherapy. Chemotherapeutic agents have systemic effects on normal cells as well as malignant ones, which means that these problems are often widespread, affecting many body systems.

ASSESSING FLUID AND ELECTROLYTE STATUS

Anorexia, nausea, vomiting, altered taste, and diarrhea put patients at risk for nutritional and fluid and electrolyte disturbances. Changes in the mucosa of the gastrointestinal tract may lead to irritation of the oral cavity and intestinal tract, further threatening the patient's nutritional status. Therefore, it is important for the nurse to assess the patient's nutritional and fluid and electrolyte status frequently and to use creative ways to encourage an adequate fluid and dietary intake.

MODIFYING RISKS FOR INFECTION AND BLEEDING

Suppression of the bone marrow and immune system is an expected consequence of chemotherapy and frequently serves as a guide in determining appropriate chemotherapy dosage. However, this effect also increases the risk of anemia, infection, and bleeding disorders. Nursing assessment and care focus on identifying and modifying factors that would further increase the patient's risk. Aseptic technique and gentle handling are indicated to prevent infection and trauma. Laboratory test results, particularly blood cell counts, are monitored closely. Untoward changes in blood test results and signs of infection and bleeding must be reported promptly. The patient and family members are instructed about measures to prevent these problems at home (see the plan of nursing care for the patient with cancer given in Chart 16-6).

ADMINISTERING CHEMOTHERAPY

The local effects of the chemotherapeutic agent are also of concern. The patient is observed closely during its administration because of the risk and consequences of extravasation (particularly of vesicant agents, which may produce necrosis if deposited in the subcutaneous tissues). Local difficulties or problems with administration of chemotherapeutic agents are brought to the attention of the physician promptly so that corrective measures can be taken immediately to minimize local tissue damage.

PROTECTING CAREGIVERS

Nurses involved in handling chemotherapeutic agents may be exposed to low doses of the agents by direct contact, inhalation, or ingestion. Urinalyses of personnel repeatedly exposed to cytotoxic agents have demonstrated mutagenic activity. Although long-term studies of nurses who handle chemotherapeutic agents have not been conducted, it is known that chemotherapeutic agents are associated with secondary formation of cancers and chromosome abnormalities. In addition, nausea, vomiting, dizziness, alopecia, and nasal mucosal ulcerations have been reported in health care personnel who have handled chemotherapeutic agents (Wilkes & Barton-Burke, 2004). The Occupational Safety and Health Administration, Oncology Nursing Society, hospitals, and other health care agencies have developed specific precautions for health care providers involved in the preparation and administration of chemotherapy (Chart 16-7) (Polovich, 2003; Wilkes & Barton-Burke, 2004).

Bone Marrow Transplantation

Although surgery, radiation therapy, and chemotherapy have resulted in improved survival rates for cancer patients, many cancers that initially respond to therapy recur. This is true of hematologic cancers that affect the bone marrow and solid tumor cancers treated with lower doses of antineoplastics to spare the bone marrow from larger, ablative doses of chemotherapy or radiation therapy. The role of bone marrow transplantation (BMT) for malignant and some nonmalignant diseases continues to grow.

(text continues on page 415)

CHART 16-6

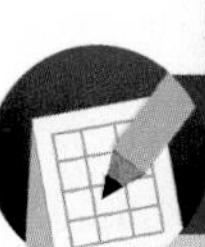

Plan of Nursing Care The Patient With Cancer

Nursing Diagnosis: Risk for infection related to altered immunologic response
Goal: Prevention of infection

NURSING INTERVENTIONS	RATIONALE	EXPECTED OUTCOMES
1. Assess patient for evidence of infection: a. Check vital signs every 4 hours. b. Monitor WBC count and differential each day. c. Inspect all sites that may serve as entry ports for pathogens (intravenous sites, wounds, skin folds, bony prominences, perineum, and oral cavity).	1. Signs and symptoms of infection may be diminished in the immunocompromised host. Prompt recognition of infection and subsequent initiation of therapy will reduce morbidity and mortality associated with infection.	• Demonstrates normal temperature and vital signs. • Exhibits absence of signs of inflammation: local edema, erythema, pain, and warmth. • Exhibits normal breath sounds on auscultation. • Takes deep breaths and coughs every 2 hours to prevent respiratory dysfunction and infection.
2. Report fever ≥38.3°C (101°F), chills, diaphoresis, swelling, heat, pain, erythema, exudate on any body surfaces. Also report change in respiratory or mental status, urinary frequency or burning, malaise, myalgias, arthralgias, rash, or diarrhea.	2. Early detection of infection facilitates early intervention.	• Exhibits absence of pathologic bacteria on cultures. • Avoids contact with others with infections. • Avoids crowds. • All personnel carry out hand hygiene after each voiding and bowel movement.
3. Obtain cultures and sensitivities as indicated before initiation of antimicrobial treatment (wound exudate, sputum, urine, stool, blood).	3. These tests identify the organism and indicate the most appropriate antimicrobial therapy. Use of inappropriate antibiotics enhances proliferation of additional flora and encourages growth of antibiotic-resistant organisms.	• Excoriation and trauma of skin are avoided. • Trauma to mucous membranes is avoided (avoidance of rectal thermometers, suppositories, vaginal tampons, perianal trauma).
4. Initiate measures to minimize infection.	4. Exposure to infection is reduced.	• Uses recommended procedures and techniques if participating in management of invasive lines or catheters.
a. Discuss with patient and family (1) Placing patient in private room if absolute WBC count <1,000/mm^3 (2) Importance of patient avoiding contact with people who have known or recent infection or recent vaccination	a. Preventing contact with pathogens helps prevent infection.	• Uses electric razor. • Is free of skin breakdown and stasis of secretions. • Adheres to dietary and environmental restrictions. • Exhibits no signs of septicemia or septic shock.
b. Instruct all personnel in careful hand hygiene before and after entering room.	b. Hands are significant source of contamination.	• Exhibits normal vital signs, cardiac output, and arterial pressures when monitored.
c. Avoid rectal or vaginal procedures (rectal temperatures, examinations, suppositories; vaginal tampons).	c. Incidence of rectal and perianal abscesses and subsequent systemic infection is high. Manipulation may cause disruption of mem-	• Demonstrates ability to administer colony-stimulating factor.

continued >

CHART 16-6

Plan of Nursing Care — The Patient With Cancer (Continued)

NURSING INTERVENTIONS	RATIONALE	EXPECTED OUTCOMES
	brane integrity and enhance progression of infection.	
d. Use stool softeners to prevent constipation and straining.	d. This minimizes trauma to tissues.	
e. Assist patient in practice of meticulous personal hygiene.	e. This prevents skin irritation.	
f. Instruct patient to use electric razor.	f. Minimizes skin trauma.	
g. Encourage patient to ambulate in room unless contraindicated.	g. Minimizes chance of skin breakdown and stasis of pulmonary secretions.	
h. Avoid fresh fruits, raw meat, fish, and vegetables if absolute WBC count <1,000/mm^3; remove fresh flowers and potted plants.	h. Fresh fruits and vegetables harbor bacteria not removed by ordinary washing. Flowers and potted plants are sources of organisms.	
i. Each day: change water pitcher, denture cleaning fluids, and respiratory equipment containing water.	i. Stagnant water is a source of infection.	
5. Assess intravenous sites every day for evidence of infection:	5. Nosocomial staphylococcal septicemia is closely associated with intravenous catheters.	
a. Change intravenous sites every other day.	a. Incidence of infection is increased when catheter is in place >72 hr.	
b. Cleanse skin with povidone-iodine before arterial puncture or venipuncture.	b. Povidone-iodine is effective against many gram-positive and gram-negative pathogens.	
c. Change central venous catheter dressings every 48 hours.	c. Allows observation of site and removes source of contamination.	
d. Change all solutions and infusion sets every 48 hours.	d. Once introduced into the system, microorganisms are capable of growing in infusion sets despite replacement of container and high flow rates.	
6. Avoid intramuscular injections.	6. Reduces risk for skin abscesses.	
7. Avoid insertion of urinary catheters; if catheters are necessary, use strict aseptic technique.	7. Rates of infection greatly increase after urinary catheterization.	
8. Teach patient or family member to administer granulocyte (or granulocyte-macrophage) colony-stimulating factor when prescribed.	8. Granulocyte colony-stimulating factor decreases the duration of neutropenia and the potential for infection.	

CHART 16-6

Plan of Nursing Care The Patient With Cancer (Continued)

Nursing Diagnosis: Impaired skin integrity: erythematous and wet desquamation reactions to radiation therapy
Goal: Maintenance of skin integrity

NURSING INTERVENTIONS

1. In erythematous areas:
   a. Avoid the use of soaps, cosmetics, perfumes, powders, lotions and ointments, deodorants.
   b. Use only lukewarm water to bathe the area.
   c. Avoid rubbing or scratching the area.
   d. Avoid shaving the area with a straight-edged razor.
   e. Avoid applying hot-water bottles, heating pads, ice, and adhesive tape to the area.
   f. Avoid exposing the area to sunlight or cold weather.
   g. Avoid tight clothing in the area. Use cotton clothing.
   h. Apply vitamin A&D ointment to the area.
2. If wet desquamation occurs:
   a. Do not disrupt any blisters that have formed.
   b. Avoid frequent washing of the area.
   c. Report any blistering.
   d. Use *prescribed* creams or ointments.
   e. If area weeps, apply a thin layer of gauze dressing.

RATIONALE

1. Care to the affected areas must focus on preventing further skin irritation, drying, and damage
   g. Allows air circulation to affected area.
   h. Aids healing.
2. Open weeping areas are susceptible to bacterial infection. Care must be taken to prevent introduction of pathogens.
   d. Decreases irritation and inflammation of the area.
   e. Enhances drying.

EXPECTED OUTCOMES

- Avoids use of soaps, powders, and other cosmetics on site of radiation therapy.
- States rationale for special care of skin.
- Exhibits minimal change in skin.
- Avoids trauma to affected skin region (avoids shaving, constricting and irritating clothing, extremes of temperature, and use of adhesive tape).
- Reports change in skin promptly.
- Demonstrates proper care of blistered or open areas.
- Exhibits absence of infection of blistered and opened areas.

Nursing Diagnosis: Impaired oral mucous membrane: stomatitis
Goal: Maintenance of intact oral mucous membranes

NURSING INTERVENTIONS

1. Assess oral cavity daily.
2. Instruct patient to report oral burning, pain, areas of redness, open lesions on the lips, pain associated with swallowing, or decreased tolerance to temperature extremes of food.

RATIONALE

1. Provides baseline for later evaluation.
2. Identification of initial stages of stomatitis will facilitate prompt interventions, including modification of treatment as prescribed by physician.

EXPECTED OUTCOMES

- States rationale for frequent oral assessment and hygiene.
- Identifies signs and symptoms of stomatitis to report to nurse or physician.
- Participates in recommended oral hygiene regimen.
- Avoids mouthwashes with alcohol.

continued >

CHART 16-6

Plan of Nursing Care The Patient With Cancer (Continued)

NURSING INTERVENTIONS	RATIONALE
3. Encourage and assist in oral hygiene.	
Preventive	
a. Avoid commercial mouthwashes.	a. Alcohol content of mouthwashes will dry oral tissues and potentiate breakdown.
b. Brush with soft toothbrush; use non-abrasive toothpaste after meals and bedtime; floss every 24 h unless painful or platelet count falls below 40,000 cu/mm.	b. Limits trauma and removes debris.
Mild stomatitis (generalized erythema, limited ulcerations, small white patches: *Candida*)	
c. Use normal saline mouth rinses every 2 h while awake; every 6 h at night.	c. Assists in removing debris, thick secretions, and bacteria.
d. Use soft toothbrush or toothette.	d. Minimizes trauma.
e. Remove dentures except for meals; be certain dentures fit well.	e. Minimizes friction and discomfort.
f. Apply lip lubricant.	f. Promotes comfort.
g. Avoid foods that are spicy or hard to chew and those with extremes of temperature.	g. Prevents local trauma.
Severe stomatitis (confluent ulcerations with bleeding and white patches covering more than 25% of oral mucosa)	
h. Obtain tissue samples for culture and sensitivity tests of areas of infection.	h. Assists in identifying need for anti-microbial therapy.
i. Assess ability to chew and swallow; assess gag reflex.	i. Patient may be in danger of aspiration.
j. Use oral rinses (may combine in solution saline, anti-*Candida* agent, such as Mycostatin, and topical anesthetic agent as described below) as prescribed or place patient on side and irrigate mouth; have suction available.	j. Facilitates cleansing, provides for safety and comfort.
k. Remove dentures.	k. Prevents trauma from ill-fitting dentures.

EXPECTED OUTCOMES

- Brushes teeth and mouth with soft toothbrush.
- Uses lubricant to keep lips soft and non-irritated.
- Avoids hard-to-chew, spicy, and hot foods.
- Exhibits clean, intact oral mucosa.
- Exhibits no ulcerations or infections of oral cavity.
- Exhibits no evidence of bleeding.
- Reports absent or decreased oral pain.
- Reports no difficulty swallowing.
- Exhibits healing (reepithelialization) of oral mucosa within 5 to 7 days (mild stomatitis).
- Exhibits healing of oral tissues within 10 to 14 days (severe stomatitis).
- Exhibits no bleeding or oral ulceration.
- Consumes adequate fluid and food.
- Exhibits absence of dehydration and weight loss.

CHART 16-6

Plan of Nursing Care The Patient With Cancer (Continued)

NURSING INTERVENTIONS	RATIONALE	EXPECTED OUTCOMES
l. Use toothette or gauze soaked with solution for cleansing.	l. Limits trauma, promotes comfort.	
m. Use lip lubricant.	m. Promotes comfort.	
n. Provide liquid or pureed diet.	n. Ensures intake of easily digestible foods.	
o. Monitor for dehydration.	o. Decreased oral intake and ulcerations potentiate fluid deficits.	
4. Minimize discomfort.		
a. Consult physician for use of topical anesthetic, such as dyclonine and diphenhydramine, or viscous lidocaine.	a. Alleviates pain and increases sense of well-being; promotes participation in oral hygiene and nutritional intake.	
b. Administer systemic analgesics as prescribed.		
c. Perform mouth care as described.	c. Promotes removal of debris, healing, and comfort.	

Nursing Diagnosis: Impaired tissue integrity: alopecia
Goal: Maintenance of tissue integrity; coping with hair loss

NURSING INTERVENTIONS	RATIONALE	EXPECTED OUTCOMES
1. Discuss potential hair loss and regrowth with patient and family.	1. Provides information so patient and family can begin to prepare cognitively and emotionally for loss.	• Identifies alopecia as potential side effect of treatment. • Identifies positive and negative feelings and threats to self-image.
2. Explore potential impact of hair loss on self-image, interpersonal relationships, and sexuality.	2. Facilitates coping.	• Verbalizes meaning that hair and possible hair loss have for him or her.
3. Prevent or minimize hair loss through the following:	3. Retains hair as long as possible.	• States rationale for modifications in hair care and treatment.
a. Use scalp hypothermia and scalp tourniquets, if appropriate.	a. Decreases hair follicle uptake of chemotherapy (not used for patients with leukemia or lymphoma because tumor cells may be present in blood vessels or scalp tissue).	• Uses mild shampoo and conditioner and shampoos hair only when necessary. • Avoids hair dryer, curlers, sprays, and other stresses on hair and scalp.
b. Cut long hair before treatment. c. Use mild shampoo and conditioner, gently pat dry, and avoid excessive shampooing. d. Avoid electric curlers, curling irons, dryers, clips, barrettes, hair sprays, hair dyes, and permanent waves. e. Avoid excessive combing or brushing; use wide-toothed comb.	b–e. Minimizes hair loss due to the weight and manipulation of hair.	• Wears hat or scarf over hair when exposed to sun. • Takes steps to deal with possible hair loss before it occurs; purchases wig or hairpiece. • Maintains hygiene and grooming. • Interacts and socializes with others. • States that hair loss and necessity of wig are temporary.

continued >

CHART 16-6

Plan of Nursing Care The Patient With Cancer (Continued)

NURSING INTERVENTIONS	RATIONALE	EXPECTED OUTCOMES
4. Prevent trauma to scalp.	4. Preserves tissue integrity.	
a. Lubricate scalp with vitamin A&D ointment to decrease itching.	a. Assists in maintaining skin integrity.	
b. Have patient use sunscreen or wear hat when in the sun.	b. Prevents ultraviolet light exposure.	
5. Suggest ways to assist in coping with hair loss:	5. Minimizes change in appearance.	
a. Purchase wig or hairpiece before hair loss.	a. Wig that closely resembles hair color and style is more easily selected if hair loss has not begun.	
b. If hair loss has occurred, take photograph to wig shop to assist in selection.	b. Facilitates adjustment.	
c. Begin to wear wig before hair loss.		
d. Contact the American Cancer Society for donated wigs, or a store that specializes in this product.		
e. Wear hat, scarf, or turban.	e. Conceals loss.	
6. Encourage patient to wear own clothes and retain social contacts.	6. Assists in maintaining personal identity.	
7. Explain that hair growth usually begins again once therapy is completed.	7. Reassures patient that hair loss is usually temporary.	

Nursing Diagnosis: Imbalanced nutrition, less than body requirements, related to nausea and vomiting
Goal: Fewer episodes of nausea and vomiting before, during, and after chemotherapy

NURSING INTERVENTIONS	RATIONALE	EXPECTED OUTCOMES
1. Assess the patient's previous experiences and expectations of nausea and vomiting, including causes and interventions used.	1. Identifies patient concerns, misinformation, potential strategies for intervention. Also gives patient sense of empowerment and control.	• Identifies previous triggers of nausea and vomiting. • Exhibits decreased apprehension and anxiety. • Identifies previously used successful interventions for nausea and vomiting.
2. Adjust diet before and after drug administration according to patient preference and tolerance.	2. Each patient responds differently to food after chemotherapy. A diet containing foods that relieve the patient's nausea or vomiting is most helpful.	• Reports decrease in nausea. • Reports decrease in incidence of vomiting.
3. Prevent unpleasant sights, odors, and sounds in the environment.	3. Unpleasant sensations can stimulate the nausea and vomiting center.	• Consumes adequate fluid and food when nausea subsides.

CHART 16-6

Plan of Nursing Care — The Patient With Cancer (Continued)

NURSING INTERVENTIONS	RATIONALE	EXPECTED OUTCOMES
4. Use distraction, music therapy, biofeedback, self-hypnosis, relaxation techniques, and guided imagery before, during, and after chemotherapy.	4. Decreases anxiety, which can contribute to nausea and vomiting. Psychological conditioning may also be decreased.	• Demonstrates use of distraction, relaxation, and imagery when indicated. • Exhibits normal skin turgor and moist mucous membranes. • Reports no additional weight loss.
5. Administer prescribed antiemetics, sedatives, and corticosteroids before chemotherapy and afterward as needed.	5. Administration of antiemetic regimen before onset of nausea and vomiting limits the adverse experience and facilitates control. Combination drug therapy reduces nausea and vomiting through various triggering mechanisms.	
6. Ensure adequate fluid hydration before, during, and after drug administration; assess intake and output.	6. Adequate fluid volume dilutes drug levels, decreasing stimulation of vomiting receptors.	
7. Encourage frequent oral hygiene.	7. Reduces unpleasant taste sensations.	
8. Provide pain relief measures, if necessary.	8. Increased comfort increases physical tolerance of symptoms.	
9. Assess other causes of nausea and vomiting, such as constipation, gastrointestinal irritation, electrolyte imbalance, radiation therapy, medications, and central nervous system metastasis.	9. Multiple factors may cause nausea and vomiting.	

Nursing Diagnosis: Imbalanced nutrition: less than body requirements, related to anorexia, cachexia, or malabsorption
Goal: Maintenance of nutritional status and of weight within 10% of pretreatment weight

NURSING INTERVENTIONS	RATIONALE	EXPECTED OUTCOMES
1. Teach patient to avoid unpleasant sights, odors, sounds in the environment during mealtime.	1. Anorexia can be stimulated or increased with noxious stimuli.	• Exhibits weight loss no greater than 10% of pretreatment weight. • Reports decreasing anorexia and increased interest in eating. • Demonstrates normal skin turgor. • Identifies rationale for dietary modifications. • Participates in calorie counts and diet histories. • Uses appropriate relaxation and imagery before meals.
2. Suggest foods that are preferred and well tolerated by the patient, preferably high-calorie and high-protein foods. Respect ethnic and cultural food preferences.	2. Foods preferred, well tolerated, and high in calories and protein maintain nutritional status during periods of increased metabolic demand.	
3. Encourage adequate fluid intake, but limit fluids at mealtime.	3. Fluids are necessary to eliminate wastes and prevent dehydration. Increased fluids with meals can lead to early satiety.	

continued >

CHART 16-6

Plan of Nursing Care — The Patient With Cancer (Continued)

NURSING INTERVENTIONS	RATIONALE	EXPECTED OUTCOMES
4. Suggest smaller, more frequent meals.	4. Smaller, more frequent meals are better tolerated because early satiety does not occur.	• Exhibits laboratory and clinical findings indicative of adequate nutritional intake: normal serum protein and transferrin levels; normal serum iron levels; normal hemoglobin, hematocrit, and lymphocyte levels; normal urinary creatinine levels.
5. Promote relaxed, quiet environment during mealtime with increased social interaction as desired.	5. A quiet environment promotes relaxation. Social interaction at mealtime increases appetite.	• Consumes diet high in required nutrients.
6. If possible, serve wine at mealtime with foods.	6. Wine often stimulates appetite and adds calories.	• Carries out oral hygiene before meals.
7. Consider cold foods, if desired.	7. Cold, high-protein foods are often more tolerable and less odorous than hot foods.	• Reports that pain does not interfere with meals.
8. Encourage nutritional supplements and high-protein foods between meals.	8. Supplements and snacks add protein and calories to meet nutritional requirements.	• Reports decreasing episodes of nausea and vomiting.
9. Encourage frequent oral hygiene.	9. Oral hygiene stimulates appetite and increases saliva production.	• Participates in increasing levels of activity.
10. Provide pain relief measures.	10. Pain impairs appetite.	• States rationale for use of tube feedings or parenteral nutrition.
11. Provide control of nausea and vomiting.	11. Nausea and vomiting increase anorexia.	• Participates in management of tube feedings or parenteral nutrition, if prescribed.
12. Increase activity level as tolerated.	12. Increased activity promotes appetite.	
13. Decrease anxiety by encouraging verbalization of fears, concerns; use of relaxation techniques; imagery at mealtime.	13. Relief of anxiety may increase appetite.	
14. Position patient properly at mealtime.	14. Proper body position and alignment are necessary to aid chewing and swallowing.	
15. For collaborative management, provide enteral tube feedings of commercial liquid diets, elemental diets, or blenderized foods as prescribed.	15. Tube feedings may be necessary in the severely debilitated patient who has a functioning gastrointestinal system.	
16. Provide parenteral nutrition with lipid supplements as prescribed.	16. Parenteral nutrition with supplemental fats supplies needed calories and proteins to meet nutritional demands, especially in the nonfunctional gastrointestinal system.	
17. Administer appetite stimulants as prescribed by physician.	17. Although the mechanism is unclear, medications such as megestrol acetate (Megace) have been noted to improve appetite in patients with cancer and HIV infection.	

CHART 16-6

Plan of Nursing Care — The Patient With Cancer (Continued)

Nursing Diagnosis: Fatigue
Goal: Increased activity tolerance and decreased fatigue level

NURSING INTERVENTIONS	RATIONALE	EXPECTED OUTCOMES
1. Encourage several rest periods during the day, especially before and after physical exertion.	1. During rest, energy is conserved and levels are replenished. Several shorter rest periods may be more beneficial than one longer rest period.	• Reports decreasing levels of fatigue. • Increases participation in activities gradually. • Rests when fatigued. • Reports restful sleep. • Requests assistance with activities appropriately. • Reports adequate energy to participate in activities important to him or her (eg, visiting with family, hobbies). • Consumes diet with recommended protein and caloric intake. • Uses relaxation exercises and imagery to decrease anxiety and promote rest. • Participates in planned exercise program gradually. • Reports no breathlessness during activities. • Exhibits acceptable hemoglobin and hematocrit levels. • Exhibits normal fluid and electrolyte balance. • Reports decreased discomfort. • Exhibits improved mobility.
2. Increase total hours of nighttime sleep.	2. Sleep helps to restore energy levels.	
3. Rearrange daily schedule and organize activities to conserve energy expenditure.	3. Reorganization of activities can reduce energy losses and stressors.	
4. Encourage patient to ask for others' assistance with necessary chores, such as housework, child care, shopping, cooking.	4. Conserves energy.	
5. Encourage reduced job workload, if possible, by reducing number of hours worked per week.	5. Reducing workload decreases physical and psychological stress and increases periods of rest and relaxation.	
6. Encourage adequate protein and calorie intake.	6. Protein and calorie depletion decreases activity tolerance.	
7. Encourage use of relaxation techniques, mental imagery.	7. Promotion of relaxation and psychological rest decreases physical fatigue.	
8. Encourage participation in planned exercise programs.	8. Proper exercise programs increase endurance and stamina.	
9. For collaborative management, administer blood products as prescribed.	9. Lowered hemoglobin and hematocrit predispose patient to fatigue due to decreased oxygen availability.	
10. Assess for fluid and electrolyte disturbances.	10. May contribute to altered nerve transmission and muscle function.	
11. Assess for sources of discomfort.	11. Coping with discomfort requires energy expenditure.	
12. Provide strategies to facilitate mobility.	12. Impaired mobility requires increased energy expenditure.	

Nursing Diagnosis: Chronic pain
Goal: Relief of pain and discomfort

NURSING INTERVENTIONS	RATIONALE	EXPECTED OUTCOMES
1. Use pain scale to assess pain and discomfort characteristics: location, quality, frequency, duration, etc.	1. Provides baseline for assessing changes in pain level and evaluation of interventions.	• Reports decreased level of pain and discomfort on pain scale. • Reports less disruption from pain and discomfort.

continued >

CHART 16-6

Plan of Nursing Care — The Patient With Cancer (Continued)

NURSING INTERVENTIONS	RATIONALE	EXPECTED OUTCOMES
2. Assure patient that you know that pain is real and will assist him or her in reducing it.	2. Fear that pain will not be considered real increases anxiety and reduces pain tolerance.	• Explains how fatigue, fear, anger, etc., contribute to severity of pain and discomfort.
3. Assess other factors contributing to patient's pain: fear, fatigue, anger, etc.	3. Provides data about factors that decrease patient's ability to tolerate pain and increase pain level.	• Accepts analgesia as prescribed.
4. Administer analgesics to promote optimum pain relief within limits of physician's prescription.	4. Analgesics tend to be more effective when administered early in pain cycle.	• Exhibits decreased physical and behavioral signs of pain and discomfort in acute pain (no grimacing, crying, moaning; displays interest in surroundings and activities around him).
5. Assess patient's behavioral responses to pain and pain experience.	5. Provides additional information about patient's pain.	• Takes an active role in administration of analgesia.
6. Collaborate with patient, physician, and other health care team members when changes in pain management are necessary.	6. New methods of administering analgesia must be acceptable to patient, physician, and health care team to be effective; patient's participation decreases the sense of powerlessness.	• Identifies additional effective pain relief strategies. • Uses alternative pain relief strategies appropriately. • Reports effective use of new pain relief strategies and decrease in pain intensity.
7. Encourage strategies of pain relief that patient has used successfully in previous pain experience.	7. Encourages success of pain relief strategies accepted by patient and family.	• Reports that decreased level of pain permits participation in other activities and events.
8. Teach patient new strategies to relieve pain and discomfort: distraction, imagery, relaxation, cutaneous stimulation, etc.	8. Increases number of options and strategies available to patient.	

Nursing Diagnosis: Anticipatory grieving related to loss; altered role functioning
Goal: Appropriate progression through grieving process

NURSING INTERVENTIONS	RATIONALE	EXPECTED OUTCOMES
1. Encourage verbalization of fears, concerns, and questions regarding disease, treatment, and future implications.	1. An increased and accurate knowledge base decreases anxiety and dispels misconceptions.	• The patient and family progress through the phases of grief as evidenced by increased verbalization and expression of grief.
2. Encourage active participation of patient or family in care and treatment decisions.	2. Active participation maintains patient independence and control.	• The patient and family identify resources available to aid coping strategies during grieving.
3. Visit family frequently to establish and maintain relationships and physical closeness.	3. Frequent contacts promote trust and security and reduce feelings of fear and isolation.	• The patient and family use resources and supports appropriately.
4. Encourage ventilation of negative feelings, including projected anger and hostility, within acceptable limits.	4. This allows for emotional expression without loss of self-esteem.	• The patient and family discuss the future openly with each other.
5. Allow for periods of crying and expression of sadness.	5. These feelings are necessary for separation and detachment to occur.	• The patient and family discuss concerns and feelings openly with each other.

CHART 16-6

Plan of Nursing Care — The Patient With Cancer (Continued)

NURSING INTERVENTIONS	RATIONALE	EXPECTED OUTCOMES
6. Involve spiritual advisor as desired by the patient and family.	6. This facilitates the grief process and spiritual care.	• The patient and family use nonverbal expressions of concern for each other.
7. Advise professional counseling as indicated for patient or family to alleviate pathologic grieving.	7. This facilitates the grief process.	
8. Allow for progression through the grieving process at the individual pace of the patient and family.	8. Grief work is variable. Not every person uses every phase of the grief process, and the time spent in dealing with each phase varies with every person. To complete grief work, this variability must be allowed.	

Nursing Diagnosis: Disturbed body image and situational low self-esteem related to changes in appearance, function, and roles
Goal: Improved body image and self-esteem

NURSING INTERVENTIONS	RATIONALE	EXPECTED OUTCOMES
1. Assess patient's feelings about body image and level of self-esteem.	1. Provides baseline assessment for evaluating changes and assessing effectiveness of interventions.	• Identifies concerns of importance. • Takes active role in activities. • Maintains previous role in decision making. • Verbalizes feelings and reactions to losses or threatened losses. • Participates in self-care activities. • Permits others to assist in care when he or she is unable to be independent. • Exhibits interest in appearance and uses aids (cosmetics, scarves, etc.) appropriately. • Participates with others in conversations and social events and activities. • Verbalizes concern about sexual partner and/or significant others. • Explores alternative ways of expressing concern and affection.
2. Identify potential threats to patient's self-esteem (eg, altered appearance, decreased sexual function, hair loss, decreased energy, role changes). Validate concerns with patient.	2. Anticipates changes and permits patient to identify importance of these areas to him or her.	
3. Encourage continued participation in activities and decision making.	3. Encourages and permits continued control of events and self.	
4. Encourage patient to verbalize concerns.	4. Identifying concerns is an important step in coping with them.	
5. Individualize care for the patient.	5. Prevents or reduces depersonalization and emphasizes patient's self-worth.	
6. Assist patient in self-care when fatigue, lethargy, nausea, vomiting, and other symptoms prevent independence.	6. Physical well-being improves self-esteem.	
7. Assist patient in selecting and using cosmetics, scarves, hair pieces, and clothing that increase his or her sense of attractiveness.	7. Promotes positive body image.	
8. Encourage patient and partner to share concerns about altered sexuality and sexual function and to explore alternatives to their usual sexual expression.	8. Provides opportunity for expressing concern, affection, and acceptance.	

continued >

CHART 16-6

Plan of Nursing Care — The Patient With Cancer (Continued)

Collaborative Problem: Potential complication: risk for bleeding problems
Goal: Prevention of bleeding

NURSING INTERVENTIONS	RATIONALE
1. Assess for potential for bleeding: monitor platelet count.	1. Mild risk: 50,000–100,000/mm^3 (0.05–0.1 × 10^{12}/L) Moderate risk: 20,000–50,000/mm^3 (0.02–0.05 × 10^{12}/L) Severe risk: less than 20,000/mm^3 (0.02 × 10^{12}/L)
2. Assess for bleeding:	2. Early detection promotes early intervention.
a. Petechiae or ecchymosis	a. Indicates injury to microcirculation and larger vessels.
b. Decrease in hemoglobin or hematocrit	b–e. Indicates blood loss.
c. Prolonged bleeding from invasive procedures, venipunctures, minor cuts or scratches	
d. Frank or occult blood in any body excretion, emesis, sputum	
e. Bleeding from any body orifice	
f. Altered mental status	f. Indicates neurologic involvement.
3. Instruct patient and family about ways to minimize bleeding:	3. Patient can participate in self-protection.
a. Use soft toothbrush or toothette for mouth care.	a. Prevents trauma to oral tissues.
b. Avoid commercial mouthwashes.	b. Contain high alcohol content that will dry oral tissues.
c. Use electric razor for shaving.	c. Prevents trauma to skin.
d. Use emery board for nail care.	d. Reduces risk of trauma to nailbeds.
e. Avoid foods that are difficult to chew.	e. Prevents oral tissue trauma.
4. Initiate measures to minimize bleeding.	4. Preserves circulating blood volume.
a. Draw all blood for lab work with one daily venipuncture.	a. Minimizes trauma and blood loss.
b. Avoid taking temperature rectally or administering suppositories and enemas.	b. Prevents trauma to rectal mucosa.
c. Avoid intramuscular injections; use smallest needle possible.	c. Prevents intramuscular bleeding.

EXPECTED OUTCOMES

- Signs and symptoms of bleeding are identified.
- Exhibits no blood in feces, urine, or emesis.
- Exhibits no bleeding of gums or of injection or venipuncture sites.
- Exhibits no ecchymosis (bruising).
- Patient and family identify ways to prevent bleeding.
- Uses recommended measures to reduce risk of bleeding (uses soft toothbrush, shaves with electric razor only).
- Exhibits normal vital signs.
- Reports that environmental hazards have been reduced or removed.
- Consumes adequate fluid.
- Reports absence of constipation.
- Avoids substances interfering with clotting.
- Absence of tissue destruction.
- Exhibits normal mental status and absence of signs of intracranial bleeding.
- Avoids medications that interfere with clotting (eg, aspirin).
- Absence of epistaxis and cerebral bleeding.

CHART 16-6

Plan of Nursing Care — The Patient With Cancer (Continued)

NURSING INTERVENTIONS	RATIONALE	EXPECTED OUTCOMES
d. Apply direct pressure to injection and venipuncture sites for at least 5 min.	d. Minimizes blood loss.	
e. Lubricate lips with petrolatum.	e. Prevents skin from drying.	
f. Avoid bladder catheterizations; use smallest catheter if catheterization is necessary.	f. Prevents trauma to urethra.	
g. Maintain fluid intake of at least 3 L/24 h unless contraindicated.	g. Hydration helps to prevent skin drying.	
h. Use stool softeners or increase bulk in diet.	h. Prevents constipation and straining that may injure rectal tissue.	
i. Avoid medications that will interfere with clotting (eg, aspirin).	i. Minimizes risk of bleeding.	
j. Recommend use of water-based lubricant before sexual intercourse.	j. Prevents friction and tissue trauma.	
5. When platelet count is less than 20,000/mm^3, institute the following:	5. Platelet count of less than 20,000/mm^3 (0.02×10^{12}/L) is associated with increased risk of spontaneous bleeding.	
a. Bed rest with padded side rails	a. Reduces risk of injury	
b. Avoidance of strenuous activity	b. Increases intracranial pressure and risk of cerebral hemorrhage.	
c. Platelet transfusions as prescribed; administer prescribed diphenhydramine hydrochloride (Benadryl) or hydrocortisone sodium succinate (Solu-Cortef) to prevent reaction to platelet transfusion.	c. Allergic reactions to blood products are associated with antigen–antibody reaction that causes platelet destruction.	
d. Supervise activity when out of bed.	d. Reduces risk of falls.	
e. Caution against forceful nose blowing.	e. Prevents trauma to nasal mucosa and increased intracranial pressure.	

The process of obtaining donor cells has evolved over the years. Donor cells can be obtained by the traditional harvesting of large amounts of bone marrow tissue under general anesthesia in the operating room. A second method, referred to as peripheral blood stem cell transplantation (PBSCT), has also gained widespread use. This method of collection uses apheresis of the donor to collect peripheral blood stem cells (PBSCs) for reinfusion. It is a safe and cost-effective means of collection rather than the traditional harvesting of marrow.

Types of BMT based on the source of donor cells include:

- Allogeneic (from a donor other than the patient): either a related donor (ie, family member) or a matched unrelated donor (national bone marrow registry, cord blood registry)

CHART 16-7

Safety in Administering Chemotherapy

Safety recommendations from the Occupational Safety and Health Administration (OSHA), Oncology Nursing Society (ONS), hospitals, and other health care agencies for the preparation and handling of antineoplastic agents follow:

- Use a biologic safety cabinet for the preparation of all chemotherapy agents.
- Wear surgical gloves when handling antineoplastic agents and the excretions of patients who received chemotherapy.
- Wear disposable, long-sleeved gowns when preparing and administering chemotherapy agents.
- Use Luer-Lok fittings on all intravenous tubing used to deliver chemotherapy.
- Dispose of all equipment used in chemotherapy preparation and administration in appropriate, leak-proof, puncture-proof containers.
- Dispose of all chemotherapy wastes as hazardous materials.

When followed, these precautions greatly minimize the risk of exposure to chemotherapy agents.

- Autologous (from patient)
- Syngeneic (from an identical twin)

Allogeneic BMT, used primarily for disease of the bone marrow, depends on the availability of a human leukocyte antigen–matched donor. This greatly limits the number of possible transplants. An advantage of allogeneic BMT is that the transplanted cells should not be immunologically tolerant of a patient's malignancy and should cause a lethal **graft-versus-disease effect** in the malignant cells. Allogeneic BMT may involve either ablative (high-dose) or nonablative ("mini"-dose) chemotherapy. In ablative allogeneic BMT, the recipient must undergo ablative doses of chemotherapy and possibly total body irradiation to destroy all existing bone marrow and malignant disease. The harvested donor marrow or PBSCs are infused intravenously into the recipients, and they travel to sites in the body where they produce bone marrow and establish themselves. Once engraftment is complete (2 to 4 weeks, sometimes longer), the new bone marrow becomes functional and begins producing RBCs, WBCs, and platelets. In nonablative allogeneic BMT, the chemotherapy doses are lower and are aimed at suppressing the recipient's immune system to allow engraftment of donor bone marrow or PBSCs. The lower doses of chemotherapy create less organ toxicity and thus can be offered to older patients or those with underlying organ dysfunction, for whom high-dose chemotherapy would be prohibitive. After engraftment, it is hoped that the donor cells will create a graft-versus-disease effect (Ezzone, 2004).

Before engraftment, patients are at high risk for infection, sepsis, and bleeding. Side effects of the high-dose chemotherapy and total body irradiation can be acute and chronic. Acute side effects include alopecia, hemorrhagic cystitis, nausea, vomiting, diarrhea, and severe stomatitis. Chronic side effects include sterility, pulmonary dysfunction, cardiac dysfunction, and liver disease.

To prevent **graft-versus-host disease (GVHD)**, patients receive immunosuppressant drugs, such as cyclosporine (Neoral), tacrolimus (FK 506, Prograf), or sirolimus (Rapamune). In allogeneic transplant recipients, GVHD occurs when the T lymphocytes proliferating from the transplanted donor marrow or PBSCs become activated and mount an immune response against the recipient's tissues (skin, gastrointestinal tract, liver). T lymphocytes respond in this manner because they view the recipient's tissue as "foreign," immunologically different from what they recognize as "self" in the donor. GVHD may occur acutely or chronically.

The first 100 days or so after allogeneic BMT are crucial for patients; the immune system and blood-making capacity (hematopoiesis) must recover sufficiently to prevent infection and hemorrhage. Most acute side effects, such as nausea, vomiting, and mucositis, also resolve in the initial 100 days after transplantation. Patients are also at risk for venous occlusive disease (VOD), a vascular injury to the liver caused by high-dose chemotherapy, in the first 30 days or so after BMT. VOD can lead to acute liver failure and death (Ezzone, 2004).

Autologous BMT is considered for patients with disease of the bone marrow who do not have a suitable donor for allogeneic BMT and for patients who have healthy bone marrow but require bone marrow–ablative doses of chemotherapy to cure an aggressive malignancy. Stem cells are collected from the patient and preserved for reinfusion; if necessary, they are treated to kill any malignant cells within the marrow. The patient is then treated with ablative chemotherapy and, possibly, total body irradiation to eradicate any remaining tumor. Stem cells are then reinfused and engraft. Until engraftment occurs in the bone marrow sites of the body, there is a high risk of infection, sepsis, and bleeding. Acute and chronic toxicities from chemotherapy and radiation therapy may be severe. The risk of VOD is also present after autologous transplantation. No immunosuppressant medications are necessary after autologous BMT, because the patient does not receive foreign tissue. A disadvantage of autologous transplantation is the risk that viable tumor cells may remain in the bone marrow despite high-dose chemotherapy (conditioning regimens) (Ezzone, 2004).

Syngeneic transplants use an identical twin as the marrow donor. Syngeneic transplants result in less incidence of GVHD and graft rejection; however, there is also less graft-versus-tumor effect to fight the malignancy. For this reason, even when an identical twin is available for marrow donation, another matched sibling or even an unrelated donor may be the most suitable donor to combat an aggressive malignancy.

Nursing Management in Bone Marrow Transplantation

Nursing care of patients undergoing BMT is complex and demands a high level of skill. Transplantation nursing can be extremely rewarding yet extremely stressful. The success of BMT is greatly influenced by nursing care throughout the transplantation process.

IMPLEMENTING PRETRANSPLANTATION CARE

All patients must undergo extensive pretransplantation evaluations to assess the current clinical status of the disease. Nutritional assessments, extensive physical examinations and organ function tests, and psychological evaluations are conducted. Blood work includes assessing past antigen exposure (eg, hepatitis virus, cytomegalovirus, herpes simplex virus, HIV, and syphilis). The patient's social support systems and financial and insurance resources are also evaluated. Informed consent and patient teaching about the procedure and pretransplantation and posttransplantation care are vital.

PROVIDING CARE DURING TREATMENT

Skilled nursing care is required during the treatment phase of BMT when high-dose chemotherapy (conditioning regimen) and total body irradiation are administered. The acute toxicities of nausea, diarrhea, mucositis, and hemorrhagic cystitis require close monitoring and constant attention by the nurse.

Nursing management during the bone marrow or stem cell infusions consists of monitoring the patient's vital signs and blood oxygen saturation; assessing for adverse effects, such as fever, chills, shortness of breath, chest pain, cutaneous reactions, nausea, vomiting, hypotension or hypertension, tachycardia, anxiety, and taste changes; and providing ongoing support and patient teaching.

Throughout the period of bone marrow aplasia until engraftment of the new marrow occurs, the patient is at high risk for death from sepsis and bleeding. The patient requires support with blood products and hemopoietic growth factors. Potential infections may be bacterial, viral, fungal, or protozoan in origin. Renal complications arise from the nephrotoxic chemotherapy agents used in the conditioning regimen or those used to treat infection (amphotericin B, aminoglycosides). Tumor lysis syndrome and acute tubular necrosis are also risks after BMT.

GVHD requires skillful nursing assessment to detect early effects on the skin, liver, and gastrointestinal tract. VOD resulting from the conditioning regimens used in BMT can result in fluid retention, jaundice, abdominal pain, ascites, tender and enlarged liver, and encephalopathy. Pulmonary complications, such as pulmonary edema, interstitial pneumonia, and other pneumonias, often complicate the recovery after BMT (Ezonne, 2004).

PROVIDING POSTTRANSPLANTATION CARE

Caring for Recipients. Ongoing nursing assessment in follow-up visits is essential to detect late effects of therapy after BMT, which occur 100 days or more after the procedure. Late effects include infections (eg, varicella zoster infection), restrictive pulmonary abnormalities, and recurrent pneumonias. Sterility often results. Chronic GVHD involves the skin, liver, intestine, esophagus, eyes, lungs, joints, and vaginal mucosa. Cataracts may also develop after total body irradiation.

Psychosocial assessments by nursing staff must be ongoing. In addition to the stressors affecting patients at each phase of the transplantation experience, marrow donors and family members also have psychosocial needs that must be addressed.

Caring for Donors. Like BMT recipients, donors also require nursing care. They commonly experience mood alterations, decreased self-esteem, and guilt from feelings of failure if the transplantation fails. Family members must be educated and supported to reduce anxiety and promote coping during this difficult time. In addition, they must also be assisted to maintain realistic expectations of themselves as well as of the patient. As BMT becomes more prevalent, many moral and ethical issues become apparent, including those related to informed consent, allocation of resources, and quality of life.

Hyperthermia

Hyperthermia (thermal therapy), the generation of temperatures greater than physiologic fever range (greater than 41.5°C [106.7°F]), has been used for many years to destroy tumors in human cancers. Malignant cells may be more sensitive than normal cells to the harmful effects of high temperatures for several reasons. Malignant cells lack the mechanisms necessary to repair damage caused by elevated temperatures. Most tumor cells lack an adequate blood supply to provide needed oxygen during periods of increased cellular demand, such as during hyperthermia. Cancerous tumors lack blood vessels of adequate size for dissipation of heat. In addition, the body's immune system may be indirectly stimulated when hyperthermia is used.

Hyperthermia is most effective when combined with radiation therapy, chemotherapy, or biologic therapy. Hyperthermia and radiation therapy are thought to work well together because hypoxic tumor cells and cells in the S phase of the cell cycle are more sensitive to heat than radiation; the addition of heat damages tumor cells so that they cannot repair themselves after radiation therapy. Hyperthermia is thought to alter cellular membrane permeability when used with chemotherapy, allowing for an increased uptake of the chemotherapeutic agent. Hyperthermia may enhance the function of immune system cells, such as macrophages and T cells, which are stimulated by many biologic agents.

Heat can be produced by using radiowaves, ultrasound, microwaves, magnetic waves, hot-water baths, or even hot-wax immersions. Hyperthermia may be local or regional, or it may include the whole body. Local or regional hyperthermia may be delivered to a cancerous extremity (for malignant melanoma) by regional perfusion, in which the affected extremity is isolated by a tourniquet and an extracorporeal circulator heats the blood flowing through the affected part. Hyperthermia probes may also be inserted around a tumor in a local area and attached to a heat source during treatment. Chemotherapeutic agents, such as melphalan (Alkeran), may also be heated and instilled into the region's circulating blood. Local or regional hyperthermia may also include infusion of heated solutions into cancerous body organs. Whole-body hyperthermia to treat disseminated disease may be achieved by extracorporeal circulation, immersion of the patient in heated water or paraffin, or enclosure in a heated suit.

Side effects of hyperthermic treatments include skin burns and tissue damage, fatigue, hypotension, peripheral neuropathies, thrombophlebitis, nausea, vomiting, diarrhea, and electrolyte imbalances. Resistance to hyperthermia may develop during the treatment because cells adapt to repeated thermal insult. Research into the effectiveness of hyperthermia, methods of delivery, and side effects is ongoing.

Nursing Management in Hyperthermia

Although hyperthermia has been used for many years, many patients and their families are unfamiliar with this cancer treatment. Consequently, they need explanations about the procedure, its goals, and its effects. The nurse assesses the patient for adverse effects and acts to reduce the occurrence and severity of adverse effects. Local skin care at the site of the implanted hyperthermic probes is necessary.

Targeted Therapies

Recent advances in the fields of molecular biology, biochemistry, immunology, and genetics have lead to an improved understanding of cancer development. Traditional therapies such as chemotherapy and radiation are nonspecific, affecting all actively proliferating cells. As a result, both healthy cells and malignant cells are subject to harmful systemic effects of treatment. **Targeted therapies** seek to minimize the negative effects on healthy tissues by disrupting specific cancer cell functions such as malignant transformation, communication pathways, processes for growth and metastasis and genetic coding (Capriotti, 2004; Gemmill & Idell, 2003). Mechanisms of action of targeted therapies include stimulation or augmentation of immune responses through the use of biologic response modifiers, targeting of cancer cell growth factors, promotion of apoptosis (programmed cell death), and genetic manipulation through gene therapy (Gale, 2003; Gemmill & Idell, 2003; Lui, 2003).

Biologic Response Modifiers

Biologic response modifier (BRM) therapy involves the use of naturally occurring or recombinant (reproduced through genetic engineering) agents or treatment methods that can alter the immunologic relationship between the tumor and the cancer patient (host) to provide a therapeutic benefit. Although the mechanisms of action vary with each type of BRM, the goal is to destroy or stop the malignant growth. The basis of BRM treatment lies in the restoration, modification, stimulation, or augmentation of the body's natural immune defenses against cancer (Gemmill & Idell, 2003).

NONSPECIFIC BIOLOGIC RESPONSE MODIFIERS

Some of the early investigations of the stimulation of the immune system involved nonspecific agents such as bacille Calmette-Guérin (BCG) and *Corynebacterium parvum*. When injected into the patient, these agents serve as antigens that stimulate an immune response. The hope is that the stimulated immune system will then eradicate malignant cells. Extensive animal and human investigations with BCG have shown promising results, especially in treating localized malignant melanoma. In addition, BCG is considered to be a standard form of treatment for localized bladder cancer. However, use of nonspecific agents in advanced cancer remains limited, and research is continuing in an effort to identify other uses and other agents (Abeloff et al., 2004).

MONOCLONAL ANTIBODIES

Monoclonal antibodies (MoAbs), another type of BRM, have become available through technologic advances, enabling investigators to grow and produce targeted antibodies for specific malignant cells. Theoretically, this type of specificity allows MoAbs to destroy the cancer cells and spare normal cells.

The production of MoAbs involves injecting tumor cells that act as antigens into mice (murine models). Antibodies made in response to injected antigens can be found in the spleen of the mouse. Antibody-producing spleen cells are combined with a cancer cell that has the ability to grow indefinitely in culture medium and continue producing more antibodies. The combination of spleen cells and the cancer cells is referred to as a hybridoma. From hybridomas that continue to grow in the culture medium, the desired antibodies are harvested, purified, and prepared for diagnostic or therapeutic use (Fig. 16-5). Recent advances in genetic engineering have led to the production of MoAbs with combinations of mouse and human components (*chimeric MoAbs*) or all-human components (*humanized MoAbs*). MoAbs made with human genes have greater immunologic properties and are less likely to cause allergic reactions (Schmidt & Wood, 2003).

MoAbs are being used as aids in diagnostic evaluation. By attaching radioactive substances to MoAbs, physicians can detect both primary and metastatic tumors through radiologic techniques. This process is referred to as radioimmunodetection. OncoScint (Cytogen Corp., Princeton, NJ) is a U.S. Food and Drug Administration (FDA)–approved MoAb that is used to assist in diagnosing ovarian and colorectal cancers. The use of MoAbs in detecting breast, gastric, and prostate cancers and lymphoma is under investigation. MoAbs are also used in purging residual tumor cells from the bone marrow or peripheral blood of patients who are undergoing BMT or peripheral stem cell rescue after high-dose cytotoxic therapy.

Several MoAbs have been approved for treatment in cancer (Table 16-7). Some of the MoAbs are used alone, whereas others are used in combination with agents that facilitate their antitumor actions. Gemtuzumab ozogamicin (Mylotarg) is a combination of a MoAb and the antitumor antibiotic calicheamicin, which is used for the treatment of a specific type of acute myeloid leukemia (Schmidt & Wood, 2003). Gemtuzumab ozogamicin is an example of immunoconjugate therapy or a "magic bullet" that transports cancer-killing substances to the cancer cells. Ibritumomab-tiuxetan (Zevalin) and tositumomab (Bexxar) are forms of immunoconjugate therapy that combine a monoclonal antibody and a radioactive source for the treatment of specific types of non-Hodgkin lymphoma. The monoclonal antibody delivers the radioactive source to the malignant cells, causing the cells to be destroyed by both radioactivity and normal immune responses (Schmidt & Wood, 2003). Researchers are continuing to explore the development and use of other MoAbs, either alone or in combination with other substances such as radioactive materials, chemotherapeutic agents, toxins, hormones, or other BRMs. Some specific targets for MoAbs under investigation include malignant cell growth factors, cell proteins, and substances that stimulate tumors to develop blood vessels (angiogenesis factors).

CYTOKINES

Cytokines, substances produced by cells of the immune system to enhance the production and functioning of com-

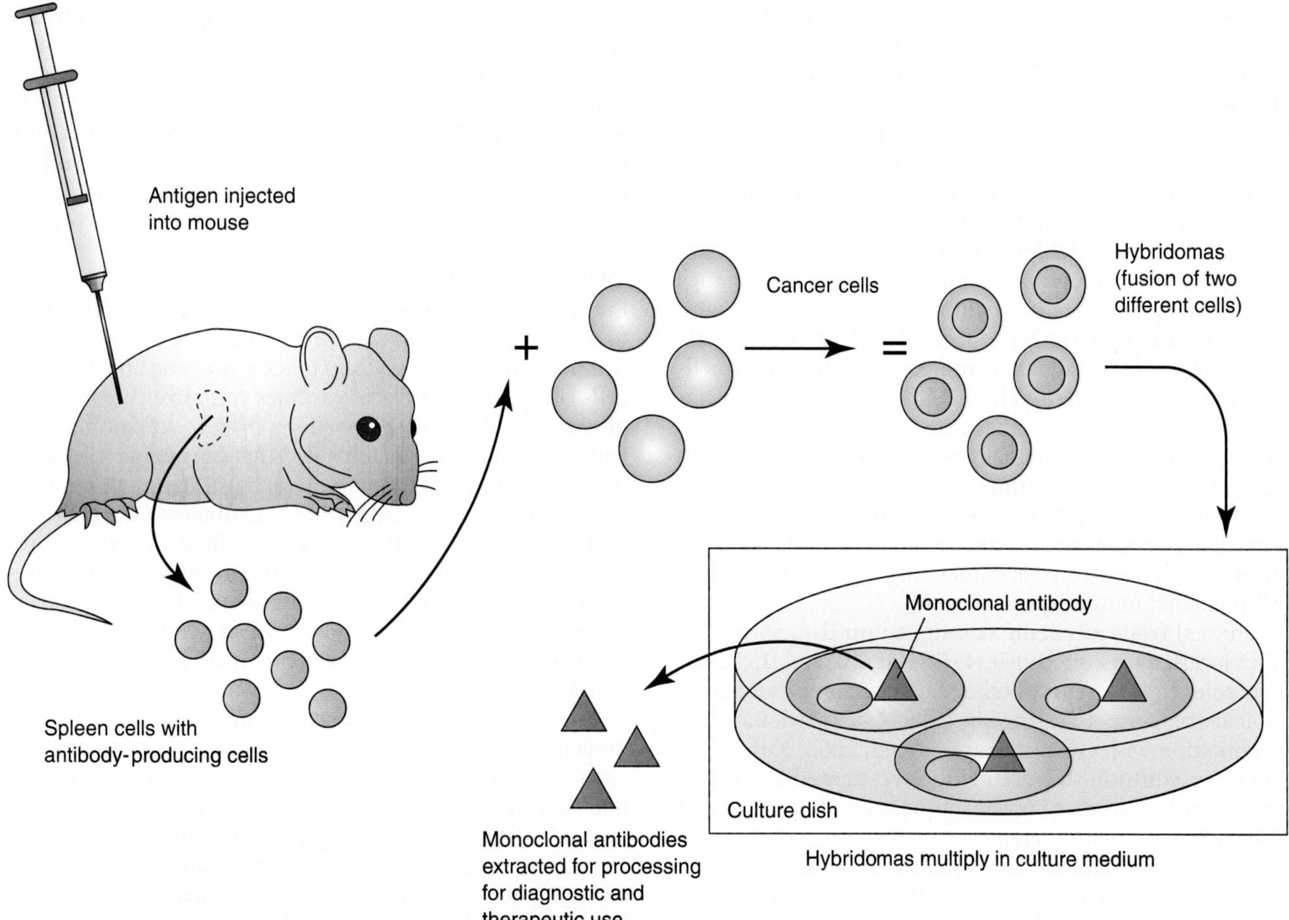

FIGURE 16-5. Antibody-producing spleen cells are fused with cancer cells. This process produces cells called hybridomas. These cells, which can grow indefinitely in a culture medium, produce antibodies that are harvested, purified, and prepared for diagnostic or treatment purposes.

ponents of the immune system, are also the focus of cancer treatment research (Janeway, Travers, Walport, et al., 2005). Cytokines are grouped into families, such as interferons, interleukins, colony-stimulating factors, and tumor necrosis factors.

Interferons. Interferons (IFNs) are examples of cytokines with both antiviral and antitumor properties. When stimulated, all nucleated cells are capable of producing these glycoproteins, which are classified according to their biologic and chemical properties: IFN-α is produced by leukocytes, IFN-β is produced by fibroblasts, and IFN-γ is produced by lymphocytes.

Multiple antitumor effects of IFNs, which have been identified in a variety of malignancies, include antiangiogenesis, direct destruction of tumor cells, inhibition of growth factors, and disruption of the cell cycle (Kufe et al., 2003). IFN-α has been approved by the FDA for treatment of hairy-cell leukemia, Kaposi's sarcoma, chronic myelogenous leuke-

℞ TABLE 16-7 Food and Drug Administration–Approved Therapeutic Monoclonal Antibodies

Monoclonal Antibody	Indication	Target
Alemtuzumab (Campath)	Chronic lymphocytic leukemia	Marker on cell membrane of lymphocytes, monocytes, and macrophages
Bevacizumab (Avastin)	Metastatic colorectal cancer	Vascular endothelial growth factor
Cetuximab (Erbitux)	Metastatic colorectal cancer	Epidermal growth factor
Gemtuzumab ozogamicin (Mylotarg)	Acute leukemia	Marker on cell membrane of leukemic cells
Ibritumomab-tiuxetan (Zevalin)	Non-Hodgkin lymphoma	Marker on cell membrane of lymphocytes
Rituximab (Rituxan)	Non-Hodgkin lymphoma	Marker on cell membrane of lymphocytes
Tositumomab (Bexxar)	Non-Hodgkin lymphoma	Marker on cell membrane of lymphocytes
Trastuzumab (Herceptin)	Breast cancer	Growth factor protein on cell membrane

mia, high-grade non-Hodgkin lymphoma, renal cell cancer, cutaneous T-cell lymphoma, and melanoma. (IFN-α, IFN-β, and IFN-γ have been approved by the FDA for the treatment of several nonmalignant diseases, such as multiple sclerosis.) IFN is administered by subcutaneous, intramuscular, intravenous, and intracavitary routes. Efforts are underway to establish the effectiveness of IFN in combination with other treatment regimens for treatment of various malignancies.

Interleukins. Interleukins (ILs) are a subgroup of cytokines known as lymphokines and monokines because they are primarily produced by lymphocytes and monocytes. About 25 different ILs have been identified (Kufe et al., 2003). They act by signaling and coordinating other cells of the immune system. The FDA has approved IL-2 as a treatment option for renal cell cancer and metastatic melanoma in adults. Originally referred to as T-cell growth factor, IL-2 is known to stimulate the production and activation of several different types of lymphocytes. In addition, IL-2 enhances the production of other types of cytokines and plays a role in influencing both humoral and cell-mediated immunity.

Clinical trials are being conducted on IL-2 as well as other interleukins, such as IL-1, IL-4, IL-10, and IL-12, for their roles in treatment of other cancers. Some early-stage clinical trials are assessing the effects of interleukins in combination with chemotherapy (Breed, 2003; Kufe et al., 2003). In addition, ILs are being investigated as growth factors for treatment of myelosuppression after the use of some forms of chemotherapy.

Hematopoietic Growth Factors (Colony-Stimulating Factors). Hematopoietic growth factors, also known as colony-stimulating factors, are hormone-like substances naturally produced by cells within the immune system. Hematopoietic growth factors of different types regulate the production of all cells in the blood, including neutrophils, macrophages, monocytes, RBCs, and platelets. Use of GM-CSF, G-CSF, IL-11, and EPO, all of which are FDA-approved, has contributed significantly to the supportive care of patients with cancer (Bedell, 2003b; Cappozzo, 2004; Mock & Olsen, 2003).

Although these agents do not treat the underlying malignancy, they do target the effects of myelotoxic cancer therapies (ie, those that adversely affect the bone marrow), such as radiation and chemotherapy. Previously, the myelotoxic or bone marrow suppressive effects of chemotherapy had imposed limits on some chemotherapy agents and contributed to the development of life-threatening infections.

GM-CSF is used to treat the **neutropenia** (decreased numbers of neutrophils in the blood) associated with BMT. G-CSF is used to treat neutropenia associated with chemotherapy for solid tumor malignancies. IL-11 is used to prevent severe thrombocytopenia and reduce the need for platelet transfusions after myelosuppressive therapy for nonmyeloid cancers, but its use has been limited because of toxicities such as fatigue, edema, dysrhythmias, and syncope (Capo & Waltzman, 2004). EPO is used to treat anemia in patients with cancer as well as in those with chronic renal disease and in those with HIV infection and zidovudine-induced anemia.

RETINOIDS

Retinoids are vitamin A derivatives (retinol, all-*trans*-retinoic acid, and 13-*cis*-retinoic acid) that play a role in growth, reproduction, programmed cell death (*apoptosis*), epithelial cell differentiation, and immune function. All-*trans*-retinoic acid (tretinoin) is used in treating acute promyelocytic leukemia, a rare form of leukemia, and cutaneous T-cell lymphoma. Retinoids are being tested for treatment of both hematologic cancers and solid tumors and for prevention of a variety of cancers such as prostate and brain cancers (Galsky & Kelly, 2003; Kristal, 2004).

CANCER VACCINES

Like viral and bacterial vaccines, cancer vaccines are given to mobilize the body's immune response. Cancer vaccines stimulate the immune system to recognize and attack cancer cells (King, 2004). Cancer vaccines contain either portions of cancer cells alone or portions of cells in combination with other substances (adjuvants) that can augment or boost immune responses. *Autologous* vaccines are made from the patient's own cancer cells, which are obtained during diagnostic biopsy or surgery. The cancer cells are killed and prepared for injection back into the patient. *Allogeneic* vaccines are made from cancer cells that are obtained from other people who have a specific type of cancer. These cancer cells are grown in a laboratory and eventually killed and prepared for injection.

Prophylactic vaccines, such as polio vaccine, are given to prevent people from developing a disease. *Therapeutic* vaccines are given to kill existing cancer cells and to provide long-lasting immunity against further cancer development. Multiple clinical trials are being conducted to develop therapeutic vaccines for cancers of the prostate, breast, kidney, and lung, as well as for melanoma, myeloma, and lymphoma (King, 2004). A vaccine that prevents cervical cancer due to two types of human papillomavirus (HPV) is the first to be shown to be effective in prevention of cancer. If widespread use of the vaccine is adopted, it is predicted that the incidence of cervical cancer in vaccinated populations will decrease significantly (National Cancer Institute, 2006).

NURSING MANAGEMENT IN BIOLOGIC RESPONSE MODIFIER THERAPY

Patients receiving BRM therapy have many of the same needs as cancer patients undergoing other treatment approaches. However, some BRM therapies are still investigational and are considered a last-chance effort by many patients who have not responded to standard treatments. Consequently, it is essential for the nurse to assess the need for education, support, and guidance for both the patient and the family and assist in planning and evaluating patient care.

Monitoring Therapeutic and Adverse Effects. The nurse should be familiar with each agent given and its potential effects (Table 16-8). Adverse effects, such as fever, myalgia, nausea, and vomiting, as seen with IFN therapy, may not be life-threatening. However, the nurse must be aware of the impact of these side effects on the patient's quality of life. Other life-threatening adverse effects (eg, capillary leak syndrome, pulmonary edema, hypotension) may occur with IL-2 therapy. The nurse must work closely with the physician to assess and manage potential toxicities of BRM therapy. Because of the investigational nature of many of these agents, the nurse often administers them in a research setting. Accurate observations and careful documentation

TABLE 16-8 Side Effects of FDA-Approved Biologic Response

Agent	Selected Side Effects
Monoclonal Antibodies	
Alemtuzumab	Allergic/anaphylactic reactions; fever; chills; rash; hives; itching; sweating; nausea; vomiting; diarrhea; stomatitis; abdominal pain; indigestion; infection; headache; dizziness; muscle pain; insomnia; dyspnea; cough; bronchitis/pneumonitis; pharyngitis; fatigue; skeletal pain; anorexia; weakness; peripheral edema; decreased white blood cell (WBC), platelet, and red blood cell (RBC) counts
Bevacizumab	Weakness; abdominal pain; deep vein thrombosis; hypertension; syncope; diarrhea; constipation; decreased WBC count; hemorrhage; gastrointestinal perforation; proteinuria; congestive heart failure
Cetuximab	Allergic/anaphylactic reactions; fever; chills; rash; hives; itching; acne-like rash; lung inflammation; sepsis; pulmonary embolus; kidney failure; malaise; weakness; diarrhea; nausea; abdominal pain; vomiting; anorexia; constipation; insomnia
Gemtuzumab	Allergic/anaphylactic reactions; fever; chills; weakness; abdominal pain; headache; dyspnea; epistaxis; cough; tachycardia; hemorrhage; local skin reaction; rash; petechiae; peripheral edema; nausea; vomiting; diarrhea; anorexia; stomatitis; constipation; indigestion; dizziness; decreased platelet, WBC and RBC counts; increased bilirubin, potassium, and lactate dehydrogenase (LDH) values
Ibritumomab	Decreased platelets, WBC and RBC counts; weakness; chills; abdominal pain; fever; difficulty breathing; nausea and vomiting
Rituximab	Allergic/anaphylactic reactions; fever; chills; nausea; headache; abdominal pain; decreased lymphocyte, WBC, platelet, and RBC counts; back pain; night sweats; itching; cough; infection
Tositumomab	Allergic/anaphylactic reactions; fever chills, rash, hives, itching; anemia; decreased WBC count; bone marrow impairment; hypothyroidism; infection; nausea; vomiting; abdominal pain; diarrhea; difficulty breathing; headache; weakness; myalgias; arthralgias
Trastuzumab	Allergic/anaphylactic reactions; hypotension; fever; chills; heart failure; stroke; diarrhea; infection; rash; nausea; vomiting; anorexia; insomnia; dizziness; headache; chills; back pain; weakness; rhinitis; pharyngitis; cough
Cytokines	
Interferon alfa	Flu-like symptoms (fever, chills, weakness, muscle and joint pain, headaches); fatigue; anorexia; mental status changes; rash; pruritus; hair loss; abdominal pain; nausea; constipation; diarrhea; irritation at the injection site; depression; irritability; insomnia; cough; decreased WBC, RBC, and platelet counts; abnormal liver function values
Interleukin-2	Flu-like symptoms (fever, chills, weakness, muscle and joint pain, headaches); fatigue; anorexia; nausea; vomiting; diarrhea; capillary leak syndrome; edema and fluid retention; hypotension; tachycardia; skin rash; erythema; desquamation; irritation at the injection site; weight gain during therapy due to fluid retention; weight loss after therapy related to anorexia with long-term therapy; decreased WBC, RBC, and platelet counts; abnormal liver function values
Filgrastim (granulocyte growth factor)	Bone pain, malaise, fever, fatigue, headache, skin rash, weakness
Sargranstim (granulocyte-macrophage growth factor)	Allergic/anaphylactic reaction with first dose; bone pain; fever; fatigue; headache; weakness; chills; skin rash; infection
Epoetin alfa (erythrocyte growth factor)	Fever; fatigue; weakness; bone pain; diarrhea; dizziness; nausea; edema; shortness of breath
Oprelvekin (platelet growth factor)	Edema; fever; headache; rash; chills; bone pain; fatigue; nausea; vomiting; abdominal pain; constipation; rhinitis; cough; arrhythmia; skin discoloration; bleeding; dehydration; amblyopia; dermatitis
Retinoids	
Retinoic acid	Headache; fever; skin and mucous membrane dryness; bone pain; nausea and vomiting; dyspnea; pleural and pericardial effusions; malaise; chills; bleeding; heart failure; mental status changes; depression; abnormal liver function tests

are essential components of patient assessment and data collection.

Promoting Home and Community-Based Care. The nurse teaches patients self-care and assists in providing for continuing care. Some BRMs, such as IFN, EPO, and G-CSF, can be administered by the patient or family members at home. As needed, the nurse teaches the patient and family how to administer these agents through subcutaneous injections. The nurse also provides instructions about side effects and helps the patient and family identify strategies to manage many of the common side effects of BRM therapy, such as fatigue, anorexia, and flu-like symptoms.

Referral for home care is usually indicated to monitor the patient's responses to treatment and to continue and reinforce patient and family teaching. During home visits, the nurse assesses the patient's and family members' technique in administering medications. The nurse collaborates with physicians, third-party payors, and pharmaceutical companies to help the patient obtain reimbursement for home administration of BRM therapies. The nurse also reminds the patient about the importance of keeping follow-up appointments with the physician and assesses the patient's need for changes in care.

Gene Therapy

As early as 1914, the somatic mutation theory of cancer suggested that cancer develops as a result of inherited or acquired genetic mutations that lead to a disturbance in the normal chromosomal balance regulating cell growth and reproduction. Technologic advances and information gained through intense study of genetics have helped researchers and clinicians predict, diagnose, and treat cancer. Gene therapy includes approaches that correct genetic defects or manipulate genes to induce tumor cell destruction in the hope of preventing or combating disease.

Three general approaches have been used in the development of gene therapies.

- *Tumor-directed therapy* is introduction of a therapeutic gene (suicide gene) into tumor cells in an attempt to destroy them. This approach is very challenging, because it is difficult to identify which gene would be the most beneficial. In addition, patients with widespread disease would require multiple injections to treat every site of disease.
- *Active immunotherapy* is the administration of genes that will invoke the antitumor responses of the immune system (Lui, 2003).
- *Adoptive immunotherapy* is the administration of genetically altered lymphocytes that are programmed to cause tumor destruction.

Although gene therapy is currently investigational, researchers predict that it will have a profound impact on health care in the 21st century. More than 150 clinical trials in various stages are exploring gene therapy as a treatment for cancer. Tumor-directed gene therapy is being investigated as a treatment for brain, colorectal, and prostate cancers (Lui, 2003); active immunotherapy has been investigated in the treatment of malignant melanoma (Lui, 2003); and adoptive immunotherapy is being explored in the treatment of ovarian, renal, and brain cancers. For more information about investigational therapies, see Chart 16-4.

Growth Factors

The secretion of growth factors permits cancer cells to avoid apoptosis (normal cell destruction) and grow in an uncontrolled fashion. In addition, growth factors enable cancer cells to develop their own blood supply (angiogenesis), allowing them to continue growing and metastasize to distant sites. Many of the new targeted therapy agents are directed at promoting apoptosis or inhibiting growth factor production and actions (Gemmill & Idell, 2003). Bortezomib (Velcade), which has been approved for the treatment of myeloma, induces cancer cell destruction (Colson, Doss, Swift, et al., 2004). Gefitinib (Iressa), used in the treatment of lung cancer, is an oral agent that targets a specific cancer cell growth factor referred to as epidermal growth factor (Gale, 2003). Many other agents are currently in clinical trials to determine their efficacy in preventing tumor growth and angiogenesis (Gale, 2003).

Photodynamic Therapy

Photodynamic therapy, or phototherapy, is a cancer treatment that uses photosensitizing agents, such as porfimer (Photofrin). When administered intravenously, these agents are retained in higher concentrations in malignant tissue than in normal tissue. They are then activated by a light source, usually laser light, which penetrates body tissue. The light-activated agent creates activated singlet oxygen molecules that are cytotoxic or harmful to body tissue cells. Because most of the photosensitizing agent has been retained in malignant tissue, a selective cytotoxicity can be achieved with minimal destruction to normal tissues.

Cancers treated with phototherapy include esophageal cancers, lung tumors, and precancerous lesions of the esophagus called Barrett esophagus. The major side effect of therapy is photosensitivity for 4 to 6 weeks after treatment. Patients must protect themselves from direct and indirect sunlight to prevent skin burns. In addition, local reactions are observed in the area treated (Ernst & LoCicero, 2004).

Unproven and Unconventional Therapies

A diagnosis of cancer evokes many emotions in patients and families, including feelings of fear, frustration, and loss of control. Despite increasing 5-year survival rates with the use of traditional methods of treatment, a significant number of patients use or seriously consider using some form of unconventional treatment. Hopelessness, desperation, unmet needs, lack of factual information, and family or social pressures are major factors that motivate patients to seek unconventional methods of treatment and allow them to fall prey to deceptive practices and quackery.

Unconventional treatments have not demonstrated scientifically—in an objective, reproducible method—the ability to cure or control cancer. In addition to being ineffective, some unconventional treatments may also be harmful to the patient and may cost thousands of dollars. Although research is scant and accuracy of reports may be questionable, it is estimated that as many as 64% of patients with cancer use complementary or alternative methods of treatment (Abeloff et al., 2004).

Caring for patients who choose unconventional methods may place members of the health care team in difficult situations professionally, legally, and ethically. The nurse must keep in mind ethical principles that help guide professional practice, such as autonomy, beneficence, nonmaleficence, and justice.

Machines and Devices

Electrical gadgets and devices are commonly reputed to cure cancers. Most are operated by people with questionable training who report unrealistic and unlikely success stories. Such machines are often decorated with elaborate lights and dials and produce vibrations or other sensations.

Drugs and Biologic Agents

Medicinal agents, herbs, proteins (eg, shark cartilage), megavitamins (including vitamin C), immune therapy, vaccines, enzymes, hydrogen peroxide, and sera have been frequent components of fraudulent cancer therapies. These agents have included oral, intravenous, and external medications derived from weeds, flowers, and herbs, as well as from the blood and urine of patients and animals. Many of these agents, especially in megadoses, can be toxic and can have untoward interactions with concomitant medications. Herbs commonly used by people with cancer include echinacea, essiac, ginseng, green tea, pau d'arco, and hoxsey (Montbriand, 2004). Many of these treatments are very costly.

Metabolic and Dietary Regimens

Metabolic and dietary regimens emphasize the ingestion of only natural substances to purify the body and retard cancerous growth. These regimens include the grape diet; the carrot juice diet; and intake of garlic, onions, various teas, coffee enemas, and raw liver. Laetrile (vitamin B, amygdalin), one of the best-known substances in cancer quackery, was advocated as an agent to kill tumor cells by releasing cyanide, which is especially toxic to malignant cells. The National Cancer Institute, in response to public demand, investigated the effects of laetrile and reported no therapeutic benefits with its use; indeed, many toxic effects (cyanide poisoning, fever, rash, headache, vomiting, diarrhea, and hypotension) were reported. Macrobiotic diets have also been advocated as a cancer treatment to reestablish balance between the major forces in the universe, yin and yang. People who adhere to macrobiotic diets tend to develop vitamin, mineral, and protein deficiencies; experience additional weight loss due to decreased calorie intake; and receive no therapeutic benefits from the diet.

Mystical and Spiritual Approaches

Traditional Chinese medicine attempts to balance chi forces in order to heal the body. Mystical or spiritual approaches to cancer therapy include such techniques as psychic surgery, faith healing, "laying on of hands," prayer groups, and invocation of mystical universal powers to kill cancerous growths. These techniques are difficult to disclaim because they are based on faith (Abeloff et al., 2004).

Nursing Management in Unconventional Therapies

The most effective way to protect patients and families from fraudulent therapies and questionable cancer cures is to establish a trusting relationship, provide supportive care, and promote hope. Truthful responses given in a nonjudgmental manner to questions and inquiries about unproven methods of cancer treatments may alleviate the fear and guilt on the part of the patient and family that they are not "doing everything we can" to obtain a cure. The nurse may inform the patient and family of the characteristics common to fraudulent therapies so that they will be informed and cautious when evaluating other forms of "therapy." The nurse also should encourage patients who use unconventional therapies to inform their physicians about such use. This knowledge can help prevent interactions with medications and other therapies that may be prescribed and avoid attributing the side effects of unconventional therapies to prescribed medications.

Nursing Process

The Patient With Cancer

The outlook for patients with cancer has greatly improved because of scientific and technologic advances. However, as a result of the underlying disease or various treatment modalities, patients with cancer may experience a variety of secondary problems, such as infection, reduced WBC counts, bleeding, skin problems, nutritional problems, pain, fatigue, and psychological stress.

Assessment

Regardless of the type of cancer treatment or prognosis, many patients with cancer are susceptible to the following problems and complications. An important role of nurses on oncology teams is to assess patients for these problems and complications.

Infection

For patients in all stages of cancer, the nurse assesses factors that can promote infection. Infection is the leading cause of death in cancer patients. Factors predisposing patients to infection are summarized in Table 16-9. The nurse monitors laboratory studies to detect early changes in WBC counts. Common sites of infection, such as the pharynx, skin, perianal area, urinary tract, and respiratory tract, are assessed frequently. However, the typical signs of infection

TABLE 16-9 Factors Predisposing Cancer Patients to Infection

Factors	Underlying Mechanisms
Impaired skin and mucous membrane integrity	Loss of body's first line of defense against invading organisms.
Chemotherapy	Many agents cause suppression of bone marrow, resulting in decreased production and function of white blood cells. Chemotherapy agents that cause mucositis impair skin and mucous membrane integrity. Organ damage associated with certain agents may also predispose patients to infection. Organ damage such as pulmonary fibrosis or cardiomyopathy that is associated with certain agents may also predispose patients to infection.
Radiation therapy	Radiation involving sites of bone marrow production may result in bone marrow suppression. May also lead to impaired tissue integrity.
Biologic response modifiers	Some biologic response modifiers may cause bone marrow suppression and organ dysfunction.
Malignancy	Malignant cells may infiltrate the bone marrow and interfere with production of white blood cells and lymphocytes. Hematologic malignancies (leukemias and lymphomas) are associated with impaired function and production of blood cells.
Malnutrition	Results in impaired production and function of cells of the immune response. May contribute to impaired skin integrity.
Medications	Antibiotics disturb the balance of normal flora, allowing them to become pathogenic. This process occurs most commonly in the gastrointestinal tract. Corticosteroids and nonsteroidal anti-inflammatory drugs (NSAIDs) mask inflammatory responses.
Urinary catheter	Creates port and mechanism of entry for organisms.
Intravenous catheter	Results in impaired skin integrity and site of entry for organisms.
Other invasive procedures (surgery, paracentesis, thoracentesis, drainage tubes, endoscopy, mechanical ventilation)	Create port of entry and possible introduction of exogenous organisms into the system.
Contaminated equipment	Environmental objects such as stagnant water in oxygen equipment are associated with growth of microorganisms.
Age	Increasing age is associated with declining organ function and decreased production and functioning of the cells of the immune system.
Chronic illness	Associated with impaired organ function and altered immune responses.
Prolonged hospitalization	Allows increased exposure to nosocomial infection and colonization by new organisms.

(swelling, redness, drainage, and pain) may not occur in immunosuppressed patients because of a diminished local inflammatory response. Fever may be the only sign of infection. The nurse also monitors the patient for sepsis, particularly if invasive catheters or infusion lines are in place.

WBC function is often impaired in patients with cancer. There are three types of WBCs: neutrophils (granulocytes), basophils, and eosinophils. The neutrophils, totaling 60% to 70% of all the body's WBCs, play a major role in combating infection by engulfing and destroying infective agents in a process called phagocytosis. Both the total WBC count and the concentration of neutrophils are important in determining the patient's ability to fight infection. A decrease in circulating WBCs is referred to as leukopenia. Granulocytopenia is a decrease in neutrophils.

A differential WBC count identifies the relative numbers of WBCs and permits tabulation of polymorphonuclear neutrophils (mature neutrophils, reported as "polys," PMNs, or "segs") and immature forms of neutrophils (reported as bands, metamyelocytes, and "stabs"). These numbers are compiled and reported as the absolute neutrophil count (ANC). The ANC is calculated by the following formula:

$$\text{ANC} = \frac{(\text{Total WBC count} \times [\%\ \text{segmented neutrophils} + \%\ \text{bands}])}{100}$$

For example, if the total WBC count is 6000 cells/mm^3, with segmented neutrophils 25% and bands 25%, the ANC is 3000 cells/mm^3.

Neutropenia, an abnormally low ANC, is associated with an increased risk for infection. The risk for infection rises as the ANC decreases and persists. An ANC of less than 1000 cells/mm^3 reflects a severe risk of infection. **Nadir** is the lowest ANC after myelosuppressive chemotherapy or radiation therapy. Therapies that suppress bone marrow function are called myelosuppressive. Febrile patients who are neutropenic are assessed for infection through cultures of blood, sputum, urine, stool, catheter, or wounds, if appropriate. In addition, a chest x-ray is often included to assess for pulmonary infections.

Bleeding

The nurse assesses the patient with cancer for factors that may contribute to bleeding. These include bone marrow suppression from radiation, chemotherapy, and other medications that interfere with coagulation and platelet functioning, such as aspirin, dipyridamole (Persantine), heparin, or warfarin (Coumadin). Common bleeding sites include skin and mucous membranes; the intestinal, urinary, and respiratory tracts; and the brain. Gross hemorrhage, as well as blood in the stools, urine, sputum, or vomitus (melena, hematuria, hemoptysis, hematemesis); oozing at injection sites; bruising (ecchymosis); petechiae; and changes in mental status, are monitored and reported.

Skin Problems

The nurse assesses the patient with cancer for any skin problems. Maintaining integrity of skin and tissue poses a problem for patients with cancer because of the effects of chemotherapy, radiation therapy, surgery, and invasive procedures carried out for diagnosis and therapy. As part of the assessment, the nurse identifies which of these predisposing factors are present and assesses the patient for other risk factors, including nutritional deficits, bowel and bladder incontinence, immobility, immunosuppression, multiple skin folds, and changes related to aging. The nurse notes the presence of skin lesions or ulcerations secondary to the tumor. Alterations in tissue integrity throughout the gastrointestinal tract are particularly bothersome to patients. The nurse notes the presence of any lesions of the oral mucous membranes and whether they affect the patient's nutritional status and comfort level.

Hair Loss

The nurse notes the presence of **alopecia** (hair loss), which is another form of tissue disruption common in patients with cancer who receive radiation therapy or chemotherapy. In addition, the nurse assesses the psychological impact of this side effect on the patient and family.

Nutritional Concerns

Assessment of the patient's nutritional status is an important nursing role. Impaired nutritional status may contribute to disease progression, decreased survival, immune incompetence, increased incidence of infection, delayed tissue repair, diminished functional ability, decreased capacity to continue antineoplastic therapy, increased length of hospital stay, and impaired psychosocial functioning. Altered nutritional status, weight loss, and cachexia (muscle wasting, emaciation) may be secondary to decreased protein and caloric intake, metabolic or mechanical effects of the cancer, systemic disease, side effects of the treatment, or the patient's emotional status.

The patient's weight and caloric intake are monitored on a consistent basis. Other information obtained by assessment includes diet history, any episodes of anorexia, changes in appetite, situations and foods that aggravate or relieve anorexia, and medication history. Difficulty in chewing or swallowing is identified, and the presence of nausea, vomiting, or diarrhea is noted.

Clinical and laboratory data useful in assessing nutritional status include anthropometric measurements (triceps skin fold and middle-upper arm circumference), serum protein levels (albumin and transferrin), serum electrolytes, lymphocyte count, skin response to intradermal injection of antigens, hemoglobin levels, hematocrit, urinary creatinine levels, and serum iron levels.

Pain

The nurse assesses the patient with cancer for the source and site of pain. In cancer, pain and discomfort may be related to underlying disease, pressure exerted by the tumor, diagnostic procedures, or the cancer treatment itself. As in any other situation involving pain, cancer pain is affected by both physical and psychosocial influences.

The nurse also assesses those factors that increase the patient's perception of pain, such as fear and apprehension, fatigue, anger, and social isolation. Pain assessment scales (see Chapter 13) are useful for assessing the patient's pain before pain-relieving interventions are instituted and for evaluating the effectiveness of these interventions.

Fatigue

To make an accurate assessment, the nurse must distinguish between acute fatigue, which occurs after an energy-demanding experience, and chronic fatigue, which is often overwhelming, excessive, and not responsive to rest. Acute fatigue serves a protective function, whereas chronic fatigue does not. Chronic fatigue seriously affects quality of life. Fatigue is the most commonly reported side effect in patients who receive chemotherapy and radiation therapy. The nurse assesses for feelings of weariness, weakness, lack of energy, inability to carry out necessary and valued daily functions, lack of motivation, and inability to concentrate. The patient may become less verbal and may appear pale, with relaxed facial musculature. The nurse assesses physiologic and psychological stressors that can contribute to fatigue, including pain, nausea, dyspnea, constipation, fear, and anxiety.

Psychosocial Status

Nursing assessment also focuses on the patient's psychological and mental status as the patient and family face this life-threatening experience, unpleasant diagnostic tests and treatment modalities, and progression of disease. The nurse assesses the patient's mood and emotional reaction to the results of diagnostic testing and prognosis and looks for evidence that the patient is progressing through the stages of grief and can talk about the diagnosis and prognosis with family members.

Body Image

The nurse identifies potential threats to the patient's body image and assesses the patient's ability to cope with the many assaults to body image he or she experiences throughout the course of disease and treatment. Entry into the health care system is often accompanied by depersonalization. Threats to self-concept are enormous as the patient faces the realization of illness, disfigurement, possible disability, and death. To accommodate treatments or because of the disease, many patients with cancer are forced to alter their lifestyles. Priorities and values change when body image is threatened. Disfiguring surgery, hair loss, cachexia, skin changes, altered communication patterns, and sexual dysfunction are some of the devastating results of cancer and its treatment that threaten the patients' self-esteem and body image.

Diagnosis

Nursing Diagnoses

Based on the assessment data, nursing diagnoses for the patient with cancer may include the following:

- Impaired oral mucous membrane
- Impaired tissue integrity
- Impaired tissue integrity: alopecia
- Impaired tissue integrity: malignant skin lesions
- Imbalanced nutrition, less than body requirements
- Anorexia
- Malabsorption
- Cachexia
- Chronic pain
- Fatigue
- Disturbed body image
- Anticipatory grieving

Collaborative Problems/ Potential Complications

Based on the assessment data, potential complications include the following:

- Infection and sepsis
- Hemorrhage
- Superior vena cava syndrome (SVCS)
- Spinal cord compression
- Hypercalcemia
- Pericardial effusion
- Disseminated intravascular coagulation (DIC)
- Syndrome of inappropriate secretion of antidiuretic hormone (SIADH)
- Tumor lysis syndrome

See the section on oncologic emergencies for more information.

Planning and Goal

The major goals for the patient may include management of stomatitis, maintenance of tissue integrity, maintenance of nutrition, relief of pain, relief of fatigue, improved body image, effective progression through the grieving process, and absence of complications.

Nursing Interventions

Patients with cancer are at risk for various adverse effects of therapy and complications. Nurses in all health care settings, including the home, help patients and families manage these problems.

Managing Stomatitis

Mucositis is a common side effect of radiation and some types of chemotherapy that may lead to inflammation and ulceration of any portion of the gastrointestinal tract from the oral cavity throughout the alimentary canal. One form of mucositis, **stomatitis**, is an inflammatory response of the oral tissues that is characterized by mild redness (erythema) and edema or, if severe, by painful ulcerations, bleeding, and secondary infection. Stomatitis commonly develops 5 to 14 days after patients receive certain chemotherapeutic agents, such as doxorubicin and 5-fluorouracil, and BRMs, such as IL-2 and IFN. As many as 40% of patients receiving chemotherapy experience some degree of stomatitis during treatment. Patients receiving dose-intensive chemotherapy (considerably higher doses than conventional dosing), such as those undergoing BMT, are at increased risk for stomatitis. Stomatitis may also occur after radiation treatments to the head and neck.

As a result of normal everyday wear and tear, the epithelial cells that line the oral cavity undergo rapid turnover and slough off routinely. Until recently, stomatitis was thought to occur because chemotherapy and radiation interfered with this process. Recent molecular studies have improved our understanding of the processes involved. Both chemotherapy and radiation generate chemical substances that lead to the destruction of cells in the mucosa of the epithelium, connective tissue, and blood vessels in the oral cavity (McGuire & Peterson, 2004). This initiates the inflammatory process, leading to further tissue damage. The end result is ulceration and impaired oral tissues. Normal flora of the oral cavity invade the ulcerations and cause additional damage. Poor oral hygiene, existing dental disease, use of other medications that dry mucous membranes, advanced age, smoking, previous cancer treatment, diminished renal function, and impaired nutritional status all contribute to morbidity associated with stomatitis. Radiation-induced xerostomia (dry mouth) associated with decreased function of the salivary glands may contribute to stomatitis in patients who have received radiation to the head and neck.

Myelosuppression (bone marrow depression), resulting from underlying disease or its treatment, predisposes the patient to oral bleeding and infection. Severe pain associated with ulcerated oral tissues can significantly interfere with nutritional intake, speech, and a willingness to maintain oral hygiene. Advanced stomatitis may cause or prolong hospitalizations. In addition, stomatitis may lead to interruptions in chemotherapy and radiation administration or decreases in the intended dosing until the inflammation subsides. Further, it may significantly reduce the patient's quality of life (Garfunkel, 2004).

Although multiple studies on stomatitis have been published, the optimal prevention and treatment approaches have not been identified. Future studies will focus on addressing the cascade of inflammatory events and release of chemical substances that lead to the cellular and tissue destruction underlying stomatitis. At this time, most clinicians agree that good oral hygiene, including brushing, flossing, and rinsing, is necessary to minimize the risk of oral complications associated with cancer therapies. Soft-bristled toothbrushes and nonabrasive toothpaste prevent or reduce trauma to the oral mucosa. Oral swabs with spongelike applicators may be used in place of a toothbrush for painful oral tissues. Flossing may be performed unless it causes pain or unless platelet levels are less than $40{,}000/mm^3$ ($0.04 \times 10^{12}/L$). Oral rinses with saline solution or tap water may be necessary for patients who cannot tolerate toothbrushing. Products that irritate oral tissues or impair healing, such as alcohol-based mouth rinses, are avoided. Foods that are difficult to chew or are hot or spicy are avoided to minimize further trauma. The patient's lips are lubricated to keep them from becoming dry and cracked. Topical anti-inflammatory and anesthetic agents may be prescribed to promote healing and minimize discomfort. Products that coat or protect oral mucosa are used to promote comfort and prevent further trauma. Patients who experience severe pain and discomfort with stomatitis require systemic analgesics.

Adequate fluid and food intake is encouraged. In some instances, parenteral hydration and nutrition are necessary. Topical or systemic antifungal and antibiotic medications are prescribed to treat local or systemic infections.

Palifermin (Kepivance), a synthetic form of human keratinocyte growth factor, is an intravenous medication approved in 2005 by the FDA for treatment of mucositis in patients with cancer who are undergoing chemotherapy and radiation prior to BMT. Palifermin appears to promote more rapid replacement of cells in the mouth and gastrointestinal tract (Spielberger, Stiff, Bensinger, et al., 2004). It has not yet been tested in other patients with cancer. Careful timing of administration and monitoring are essential for maximum effectiveness and to detect adverse effects.

Maintaining Tissue Integrity

Some of the most frequently encountered disturbances of tissue integrity, in addition to stomatitis, include skin and tissue reactions to radiation therapy, alopecia, and metastatic skin lesions. Patients with skin and tissue reactions to radiation therapy require careful skin care to prevent further skin irritation, drying, and damage. The skin over the affected area is handled gently; rubbing and use of hot or cold water, soaps, powders, lotions, and cosmetics are avoided. Patients may avoid tissue injury by wearing loose-fitting clothes and avoiding clothes that constrict, irritate, or rub the affected area. If blistering occurs, care is taken not to disrupt the blisters, thus reducing the risk of introducing bacteria. Moisture- and vapor-permeable dressings, such as hydrocolloids and hydrogels, are helpful in promoting healing and reducing pain. Aseptic wound care is indicated to minimize the risk for infection and sepsis. Topical antibiotics, such as 1% silver sulfadiazine cream (Silvadene), may be prescribed for use on areas of moist desquamation (painful, red, moist skin).

Helping Patients Cope With Alopecia

The temporary or permanent thinning or complete loss of hair is a potential adverse effect of various radiation therapies and chemotherapeutic agents. The extent of alopecia depends on the dose and duration of therapy. These treatments cause alopecia by damaging stem cells and hair follicles. As a result, the hair is brittle and may fall out or break off at the surface of the scalp. Loss of other body hair is less frequent. Hair loss usually begins 2 to 3 weeks after the initiation of treatment; regrowth begins within 8 weeks after the last treatment. Some patients who undergo radiation to the head may sustain permanent hair loss. Many health care providers view hair loss as a minor problem when compared with the potentially life-threatening consequences of cancer. However, for many patients, hair loss is a major assault on body image, resulting in depression, anxiety, anger, rejection, and isolation. To patients and families, hair loss can serve as a constant reminder of the challenges cancer places on their coping abilities, interpersonal relationships, and sexuality.

The nurse provides information about alopecia and supports the patient and family in coping with disturbing effects of therapy, such as hair loss and changes in body image. The patient is encouraged to acquire a wig or hairpiece before hair loss occurs so that the replacement matches the patient's own hair.

Use of attractive scarves and hats may make the patient feel less conspicuous. The nurse can refer the patient to supportive programs, such as "Look Good, Feel Better," offered by the American Cancer Society. Knowledge that hair usually begins to regrow after therapy is completed may comfort some patients, although the color and texture of the new hair may be different.

Managing Malignant Skin Lesions

Skin lesions may occur with local extension of the tumor or embolization of the tumor into the epithelium and its surrounding lymph and blood vessels. Secondary growth of cancer cells into the skin may result in redness (erythematous areas), or it may progress to wounds involving tissue necrosis and infection. The most extensive lesions tend to disintegrate and are purulent and malodorous. In addition, these lesions are a source of considerable pain and discomfort. Although this type of lesion is most often associated with breast cancer and head and neck cancers, it can also occur with lymphoma, leukemia, melanoma, and cancers of the lung, uterus, kidney, colon, and bladder. The development of severe skin lesions is usually associated with a poor prognosis for extended survival.

Ulcerating skin lesions usually indicate widely disseminated disease that is unlikely to be eradicated. Managing these lesions becomes a nursing priority. Nursing care includes carefully assessing and cleansing the skin, reducing superficial bacteria, controlling bleeding, reducing odor, protecting the skin from further trauma, and relieving pain. The patient and family require assistance and guidance to care for these skin lesions at home. Referral for home care is indicated.

Promoting Nutrition

Most patients with cancer experience some weight loss during their illness. Anorexia, malabsorption, and cachexia are examples of nutritional problems that commonly occur in patients with cancer; special attention is needed to prevent weight loss and promote nutrition.

ANOREXIA

Among the many causes of anorexia in patients with cancer are alterations in taste, manifested by increased salty, sour, and metallic taste sensations, and altered responses to sweet and bitter flavors; these changes lead to decreased appetite, decreased nutritional intake, and protein–calorie malnutrition. Taste alterations may result from mineral (eg, zinc) deficiencies, increases in circulating amino acids and cellular metabolites, or the administration of chemotherapeutic agents. Patients undergoing radiation therapy to the head and neck may experience "mouth blindness," which is a severe impairment of taste.

Alterations in the sense of smell also alter taste; this is a common experience of patients with head and neck cancers. Anorexia may occur because people feel full after eating only a small amount of food. This sense of fullness occurs secondary to a decrease in digestive enzymes, abnormalities in the metabolism of glucose and triglycerides, and prolonged stimulation of gastric volume receptors, which convey the feeling of being full. Psychological distress (eg, fear, pain, depression, and isolation) throughout illness may also have a negative impact on appetite. Patients may develop an aversion to food because of nausea and vomiting after treatment.

MALABSORPTION

Many patients with cancer are unable to absorb nutrients from the gastrointestinal system as a result of tumor activity and cancer treatment. Tumors can affect the gastrointestinal activity in several ways. They may impair enzyme production or produce fistulas. They secrete hormones and enzymes, such as gastrin; this leads to increased gastrointestinal irritation, peptic ulcer disease, and decreased fat digestion. They also interfere with protein digestion.

Chemotherapy and radiation can irritate and damage mucosal cells of the bowel, inhibiting absorption. Radiation therapy can cause sclerosis of the blood vessels in the bowel and fibrotic changes in the gastrointestinal tissue. Surgical intervention may change peristaltic patterns, alter gastrointestinal secretions, and reduce the absorptive surfaces of the gastrointestinal mucosa, all leading to malabsorption.

CACHEXIA

Cachexia is common in patients with cancer, especially in advanced disease. Cancer cachexia is related to inadequate nutritional intake along with increasing metabolic demand, increased energy expenditure due to anaerobic metabolism of the tumor, impaired glucose metabolism, competition of the tumor cells for nutrients, altered lipid metabolism, and a suppressed appetite. In addition, current literature suggests that cachexia in cancer may be related to a cytokine-induced inflammatory response (Holder, 2003; MacDonald, 2003). Cachexia is characterized by loss of body weight, adipose tissue, visceral protein, and skeletal muscle. Patients with cachexia complain of loss of appetite, early satiety, and fatigue. As a result of protein losses, they often have anemia and peripheral edema.

GENERAL NUTRITIONAL CONSIDERATIONS

Whenever possible, every effort is used to maintain adequate nutrition through the oral route. Food should be prepared in ways that make it appealing. Unpleasant smells and unappetizing-looking foods are avoided. Family members are included in the plan of care to encourage adequate food intake. The patient's preferences, as well as physiologic and metabolic requirements, are considered when selecting foods. Small, frequent meals are provided, with supplements between meals. Patients often tolerate larger amounts of food earlier in the day rather than later, so meals can be planned accordingly. To avoid early satiety, the patient should avoid drinking fluids while eating. Oral hygiene before mealtime often makes meals more pleasant. It is important to assess and manage pain, nausea, and other symptoms that may interfere with nutrition. Medications such as corticosteroids or progestational agents such as megestrol acetate have been used successfully as appetite stimulants. Prokinetic agents such as metoclopramide are used to increase gastric emptying in patients with early satiety and delayed gastric emptying. A variety of other agents and approaches are currently being investigated as supportive care for patients with anorexia and cachexia (MacDonald, 2003).

If adequate nutrition cannot be maintained by oral intake, nutritional support via the enteral route may be necessary. Short-term nutritional supplementation may be provided through a nasogastric tube. However, if nutritional support is needed for longer than several weeks, a gastrostomy or jejunostomy tube may be inserted. The patient and family are taught to administer enteral nutrition in the home.

If malabsorption is a problem, enzyme and vitamin replacement may be instituted. Additional strategies include changing the feeding schedule, using simple diets, and relieving diarrhea. If malabsorption is severe, parenteral nutrition may be necessary. Parenteral nutrition can be administered in several ways: by a long-term venous access device (eg, right atrial catheter), by an implanted venous port, or by a peripherally inserted central catheter (PICC) (Fig. 16-6). The nurse teaches the patient and family to care for venous access devices and to administer parenteral nutrition. Home care nurses may assist with or supervise parenteral nutrition administration in the home.

Interventions to reduce cachexia usually do not prolong survival or improve nutritional status significantly. Further study is needed to assess the effects of nutritional intervention on disease status and the patient's quality of life (MacDonald, 2003). Before invasive nutritional strategies are instituted, the nurse should assess the patient carefully and discuss options with the patient and family. Creative dietary therapies, enteral (tube) feedings, or parenteral nutrition may be necessary to ensure adequate nutrition. Nursing care is also directed toward preventing trauma, infection, and other complications that increase metabolic demands.

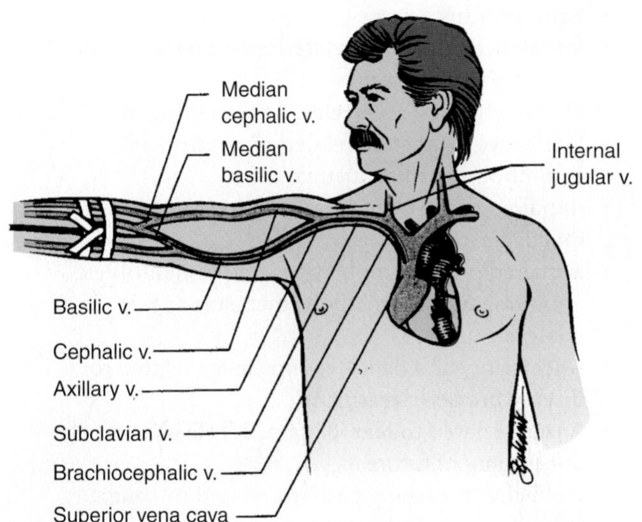

FIGURE 16-6. A peripherally inserted central catheter (PICC) is advanced through the cephalic or basilic vein to the axillary, subclavian, or brachiocephalic vein or the superior vena cava.

Relieving Pain

Of all patients with progressive cancer, it is estimated that at least 80% experience pain (Saunders & Booth, 2003). Although the pain may be acute, it is more frequently characterized as chronic. (For more information on cancer-related pain, see Chapter 13.) As in other situations involving pain, the experience of cancer pain is influenced by both physical and psychosocial factors.

Cancer can cause pain in various ways (Table 16-10). Pain is also associated with various cancer treatments. Acute pain is linked with trauma from surgery. Occasionally, chronic pain syndromes, such as postsurgical neuropathies (pain related to nerve tissue injury), occur. Some chemotherapeutic agents cause tissue necrosis, peripheral neuropathies, and stomatitis—all potential sources of pain—whereas radiation therapy can cause pain secondary to skin or organ inflammation. Cancer patients may have other sources of pain, such as arthritis or migraine headaches, that are unrelated to the underlying cancer or its treatment.

In today's society, most people expect pain to disappear or resolve quickly, and in fact it usually does. Although it is controllable, cancer pain is commonly irreversible and not quickly resolved. For many patients, pain is a signal that the tumor is growing and that death is approaching. As patients anticipate the pain and their anxiety increases, pain perception heightens, producing fear and further pain. Chronic cancer pain, then, can be best described as a cycle progressing from pain to anxiety to fear and back to pain.

Pain tolerance, the point past which pain can no longer be tolerated, varies among people. Pain tolerance is decreased by fatigue, anxiety, fear of death, anger, powerlessness, social isolation, changes in role identity, loss of independence, and past experiences. Adequate rest and sleep, diversion, mood elevation, empathy, and medications such as antidepressants, antianxiety agents, and analgesics enhance tolerance to pain.

Inadequate pain management is most often the result of misconceptions and insufficient knowledge about pain assessment and pharmacologic interventions on the part of patients, families, and health care providers. Successful management of cancer pain is based on thorough and objective pain assessment that examines physical, psychosocial, environmental, and spiritual factors. A multidisciplinary team approach is essential to determine optimal management of the patient's pain. Unlike instances of chronic nonmalignant pain, systemic analgesics play a central role in managing cancer pain.

TABLE 16-10 Examples of Sources of Cancer Pain

Source	Descriptions	Underlying Cancer
Bone metastasis	Throbbing, aching	Breast, prostate, myeloma
Nerve compression, infiltration	Burning, sharp, tingling	Breast, prostate, lymphoma
Lymphatic or venous obstruction	Dull, aching, tightness	Lymphoma, breast, Kaposi's sarcoma
Ischemia	Sharp, throbbing	Kaposi's sarcoma
Organ obstruction	Dull, crampy, gnawing	Colon, gastric
Organ infiltration	Distention, crampy	Liver, pancreatic
Skin inflammation, ulceration, infection, necrosis	Burning, sharp	Breast, head and neck, Kaposi's sarcoma

The World Health Organization (Hough & Portenoy, 2004) advocates a three-step approach to treat cancer pain (see Chapter 13). Analgesics are administered based on the patient's level of pain. Nonopioid analgesics (eg, acetaminophen) are used for mild pain; weak opioid analgesics (eg, codeine) are used for moderate pain; and strong opioid analgesics (eg, morphine) are used for severe pain. If the pain escalates, the strength of the analgesic medication is increased until the pain is controlled. Adjuvant medications are also administered to enhance the effectiveness of analgesics and to manage other symptoms that may contribute to the pain experience. Examples of adjuvant medications include antiemetics, antidepressants, anxiolytics, antiseizure agents, stimulants, local anesthetics, radiopharmaceuticals (radioactive agents that may be used to treat painful bone tumors), and corticosteroids.

Preventing and reducing pain help to decrease anxiety and break the pain cycle. This can be accomplished best by administering analgesics on a regularly scheduled basis as prescribed (the preventive approach to pain management), with additional analgesics administered for breakthrough pain as needed and as prescribed.

Various pharmacologic and nonpharmacologic approaches offer the best methods of managing cancer pain. No reasonable approaches, even those that may be invasive, should be overlooked because of a poor or terminal prognosis. The nurse helps the patient and family take an active role in managing pain. The nurse provides education and support to correct fears and misconceptions about opioid use. Inadequate pain control leads to suffering, anxiety, fear, immobility, isolation, and depression. Improving the patient's quality of life is as important as preventing a painful death.

Decreasing Fatigue

In recent years, fatigue has been recognized as one of the most significant and frequent symptoms experienced by patients receiving cancer therapy. The nurse helps the patient and family understand that fatigue is usually an expected and temporary side effect of the cancer process and of many treatments used. Fatigue also stems from the stress of coping with cancer. It does not always signify that the cancer is advancing or that the treatment is failing. Potential sources of fatigue are summarized in Chart 16-8.

Nursing strategies are implemented to minimize fatigue or help the patient cope with existing fatigue. Helping the patient identify sources of fatigue aids in selecting appropriate and individualized interventions. Ways to conserve energy are developed to help the patient plan daily activities. Alternating periods of rest and activity are beneficial. Regular, light exercise may decrease fatigue and facilitate coping, whereas lack of physical activity and "too much rest" can actually contribute to deconditioning and associated fatigue.

The patient is encouraged to maintain as normal a lifestyle as possible by continuing with activities that he or she values and enjoys. Prioritizing necessary and valued activities can help the patient plan for each day. The patient and family are encouraged to plan to reallocate responsibilities, such as attending to child care, cleaning, and preparing meals. Patients who are employed full-time may need to reduce the number of hours worked each day or week. The nurse

CHART 16-8

Sources of Fatigue in Cancer Patients

- Pain, pruritus
- Imbalanced nutrition related to anorexia, nausea, vomiting, cachexia
- Electrolyte imbalance related to vomiting, diarrhea
- Ineffective protection related to neutropenia, thrombocytopenia, anemia
- Impaired tissue integrity related to stomatitis, mucositis
- Impaired physical mobility related to neurologic impairments, surgery, bone metastasis, pain, and analgesic use
- Uncertainty and deficient knowledge related to disease process, treatment
- Anxiety related to fear, diagnosis, role changes, uncertainty of future
- Ineffective breathing patterns related to cough, shortness of breath, and dyspnea
- Disturbed sleep pattern related to cancer therapies, anxiety, and pain

helps the patient and family cope with these changing roles and responsibilities.

The nurse also addresses factors that contribute to fatigue and implements pharmacologic and nonpharmacologic strategies to manage pain. The nurse provides nutrition counseling to patients who are not eating enough calories or protein. Small, frequent meals require less energy for digestion. The nurse monitors the patient for deficiencies in serum hemoglobin and hematocrit and administers blood products or EPO as prescribed. In addition, the nurse monitors the patient for alterations in oxygenation and electrolyte balances. Physical therapy and assistive devices are beneficial for patients with impaired mobility.

Improving Body Image and Self-Esteem

A positive approach is essential when caring for patients with altered body image. To help the patient retain control and positive self-esteem, it is important to encourage independence and continued participation in self-care and decision making. The patient is assisted to assume those tasks and participate in those activities that are personally of most value. Any negative feelings that the patient has or threats to body image should be identified and discussed. The nurse serves as a listener and counselor to both the patient and the family. Referral to a support group can provide the patient with additional assistance in coping with the changes resulting from cancer or its treatment. In many cases, cosmetologists can provide ideas about hair or wig styling, makeup, and the use of scarves and turbans to help with body image concerns.

Patients who experience alterations in sexuality and sexual function are encouraged to discuss concerns openly with their partners. Alternative forms of sexual expression are explored with patients and their partners to promote positive self-worth and acceptance. Nurses who identify serious physiologic, psychological, or communication difficulties related to sexuality or sexual function are in a key position to help patients and partners seek further counseling if necessary.

Assisting in the Grieving Process

A cancer diagnosis need not indicate a fatal outcome. Many forms of cancer are curable; others may be cured if treated early. Despite these facts, many patients and their families view cancer as a fatal disease that is inevitably accompanied by pain, suffering, debility, and emaciation. Grieving is a normal response to these fears and to the losses anticipated or experienced by patients with cancer. These may include loss of health, normal sensations, body image, social interaction, sexuality, and intimacy. Patients, families, and friends may grieve for the loss of quality time to spend with others, the loss of future and unfulfilled plans, and the loss of control over the patient's body and emotional reactions.

Patients and their families who have just been informed of a cancer diagnosis frequently respond with shock, numbness, and disbelief. It is often during this stage that the patient and family are called on to make important initial decisions about treatment. They require the support of physicians, nurses, and all members of the health care team to make these decisions. The nurse plays an important role in answering any questions the patient and family have and clarifying information provided by physicians.

In addition to assessing the response of the patient and family to the diagnosis and planned treatment, the nurse helps to clarify and present the patient's and family's questions and concerns, identify available resources and support people (eg, spiritual advisor, counselor), and communicate their concerns with each other. Support groups for patients and families are available through hospitals and various community organizations. These groups provide direct assistance, advice, and emotional support.

As the patient and family progress through the grieving process, they may express anger, frustration, and depression. During this time, the nurse encourages the patient and family members to verbalize their feelings in an atmosphere of trust and support. The nurse continues to assess the patient's and family members' reactions and provides assistance and support as the patient and family confront and learn to deal with new problems.

If the patient enters the terminal phase of disease, the nurse may realize that the patient and family members are at different stages of grief. In such cases, the nurse helps the patient and family to acknowledge and cope with their reactions and feelings. The nurse also helps the patient and family to explore preferences for issues related to end-of-life care, such as withdrawal of active disease treatment, desire for the use of life-support measures, and symptom management. Support, which can be as simple as holding a patient's hand or just being with a patient at home or at the bedside, often contributes to peace of mind. After the death of a patient with cancer, maintaining contact with surviving family members may help them work through their feelings of loss and grief. See Chapter 17 for further discussion of end-of-life issues.

Monitoring and Managing Potential Complications

Despite advances in cancer care, infection remains a common problem for patients with cancer. Defense against infection is compromised in many different ways. The integrity of the skin and mucous membranes, the body's first line of defense, is challenged by multiple invasive diagnostic and therapeutic procedures, by adverse effects of radiation and chemotherapy, and by the detrimental effects of immobility.

Impaired nutrition resulting from anorexia, nausea, vomiting, diarrhea, and the underlying disease alters the body's ability to combat invading organisms. Medications such as antibiotics disturb the balance of normal flora, allowing the overgrowth of pathogenic organisms. Other medications can also alter the immune response (see Chapter 50). Cancer itself may be immunosuppressive. Cancers such as leukemia and lymphoma are often associated with defects in cellular and humoral immunity. Advanced cancer can lead to obstruction by the tumor of the hollow viscera (eg, intestines), blood vessels, and lymphatic vessels, creating a favorable environment for proliferation of pathogenic organisms. In some patients, tumor cells infiltrate bone marrow and prevent normal production of WBCs. However, most often, a decrease in WBCs is a result of bone marrow suppression after chemotherapy or radiation therapy.

The use of the hematopoietic growth factors, also called colony-stimulating factors (see previous discussion), has reduced the severity and duration of neutropenia associated with myelosuppressive chemotherapy and radiation therapy. The administration of these factors assists in reducing the risk for infection and, possibly, in maintaining treatment schedules, drug dosages, treatment effectiveness, and quality of life.

INFECTION

Gram-positive bacteria (*Streptococcus* and *Staphylococcus* species) and gram-negative organisms (*Escherichia coli, Klebsiella pneumoniae,* and *Pseudomonas aeruginosa*) are the most frequently isolated causes of infection. Fungal organisms, such as *Candida albicans,* also contribute to the incidence of serious infection. Viral infections in immunocompromised patients are caused mostly by herpesviruses and respiratory viruses.

Fever is probably the most important sign of infection in immunocompromised patients. Although fever may be related to a variety of noninfectious conditions, including the underlying cancer, any temperature of 38.3°C (101°F) or higher is reported and dealt with promptly.

Antibiotics may be prescribed to treat infections after cultures of wound drainage, exudate, sputum, urine, stool, or blood are obtained. Patients with neutropenia are treated with broad-spectrum antibiotics before the infecting organism is identified because of the high incidence of mortality associated with untreated infection. Broad-spectrum antibiotic coverage or empiric therapy most often includes a combination of medications to defend the body against the major pathogenic organisms. It is important for the nurse to administer these medications promptly according to the prescribed schedule to achieve adequate blood levels of the medications.

Strict asepsis is essential when handling IV lines, catheters, and other invasive equipment. Exposure of the patient to others with active infections and to crowds is avoided. Patients with profound immunosuppression, such as BMT recipients, may need to be placed in a protective environment where the room and its contents are sterilized and the air is filtered. These patients may also receive low-bacteria diets, avoiding fresh fruits and vegetables. Hand hygiene and appropriate general hygiene are necessary to reduce exposure to potentially harmful bacteria and to eliminate environmental contaminants. Invasive procedures, such as injections, vaginal or rectal examinations, rectal temperatures, and surgery, are avoided. The patient is encouraged to cough and to perform deep-breathing exercises frequently to prevent atelectasis and other respiratory problems. Prophylactic antimicrobial therapy may be used for patients who are expected to be profoundly immunosuppressed and at risk for certain infections. The nurse teaches the patient and family to recognize signs and symptoms of infection to report, perform effective hand hygiene, use antipyretics, maintain skin integrity, and administer hematopoietic growth factors when indicated.

SEPTIC SHOCK

The nurse assesses the patient frequently for infection and inflammation throughout the course of the disease. Septicemia and septic shock are life-threatening complications that must be prevented or detected and treated promptly. Patients with signs and symptoms of impending sepsis and septic shock require immediate hospitalization and aggressive treatment.

Signs and symptoms of septic shock (see Chapter 15) include altered mental status, either subnormal or elevated temperature, cool and clammy skin, decreased urine output, hypotension, dysrhythmias, electrolyte imbalances, and abnormal arterial blood gas values. Patients and family members are instructed about signs of septicemia, methods for preventing infection, and actions to take if infection or septicemia occurs.

Septic shock is most often associated with overwhelming gram-negative bacterial infections. In a patient with shock, the nurse monitors blood pressure, pulse rate, respirations, and temperature every 15 to 30 minutes. Neurologic assessments are carried out to detect changes in orientation and responsiveness. Fluid and electrolyte status is monitored by measuring fluid intake and output and serum electrolytes. Arterial blood gas values and pulse oximetry are monitored to determine tissue oxygenation. Nurses administer IV fluids, blood products, and vasopressors as prescribed to maintain blood pressure and tissue perfusion, as well as broad-spectrum antibiotics, which may be prescribed to combat the underlying infection (see Chapter 15). Supplemental oxygen is often necessary.

BLEEDING AND HEMORRHAGE

Platelets are essential for normal blood clotting and coagulation (hemostasis). Thrombocytopenia, a decrease in the circulating platelet count, is the most common cause of bleeding in patients with cancer and is usually defined as a platelet count of less than 100,000/mm^3 (0.1×10^{12}/L). When the platelet count decreases to between 20,000 and 50,000/mm^3 (0.02 to 0.05×10^{12}/L), the risk of bleeding increases. Platelet counts lower than 20,000/mm^3 (0.02×10^{12}/L) are associated with an increased risk for spontaneous bleeding, for which patients require a platelet transfusion.

Thrombocytopenia often results from bone marrow depression after certain types of chemotherapy and radiation therapy. Tumor infiltration of the bone marrow can also impair the normal production of platelets. In some cases, platelet destruction is associated with an enlarged spleen (hypersplenism) and abnormal antibody function, which occur with leukemia and lymphoma.

In addition to monitoring laboratory values, the nurse continues to assess the patient for bleeding. The nurse also takes steps to prevent trauma and minimize the risk of bleeding by encouraging the patient to use a soft, not stiff, toothbrush and an electric, not straight-edged, razor. In addition, the nurse avoids unnecessary invasive procedures (eg, rectal temperatures, intramuscular injections, catheterization) and helps the patient and family identify and remove environmental hazards that may lead to falls or other trauma. Soft foods, increased fluid intake, and stool softeners, if prescribed, may be indicated to reduce trauma to the gastrointestinal tract. The joints and extremities are handled and moved gently to minimize the risk of spontaneous bleeding. In limited circumstances, the nurse may administer IL-11, which has been approved by the FDA to prevent severe thrombocytopenia and to reduce the need for platelet transfusions after myelosuppressive chemotherapy in patients with nonmyeloid malignancies (Abehoff et al., 2003). In some instances, the nurse teaches the patient or family members to administer IL-11 in the home.

Hemorrhage may be related to various underlying abnormalities, such as thrombocytopenia and coagulation disorders. These clinical situations are often associated with the cancer itself or with the adverse effects of cancer treatments. Sites of hemorrhage may include the gastrointestinal, respiratory, and genitourinary tracts and the brain. When a hospitalized patient experiences bleeding, the nurse monitors blood pressure and pulse and respiratory rates every 15 to 30 minutes.

Serum hemoglobin and hematocrit are monitored carefully for changes indicating blood loss. The nurse tests all urine, stool, and emesis for occult blood. Neurologic assessments are performed to detect changes in orientation and behavior. The nurse administers fluids and blood products as prescribed to replace any losses. Vasopressor agents may be prescribed to maintain blood pressure and ensure tissue oxygenation. Supplemental oxygen may be necessary.

Promoting Home and Community-Based Care

TEACHING PATIENTS SELF-CARE

Patients with cancer usually return home from acute care facilities or receive treatment in the home or outpatient area rather than acute care facilities. The shift from the acute care setting also shifts the responsibility for care to the patient and family. As a result, family members and friends must assume increased involvement in patient care, which requires teaching that enables them to provide care. Teaching initially focuses on providing information needed by the patient and family to address the most immediate care needs likely to be encountered at home.

Side effects of treatments and changes in the patient's status that should be reported are reviewed verbally and reinforced with written information. Strategies to deal with side effects of treatment are discussed with the patient and family. Other learning needs are identified based on the priorities conveyed by the patient and family as well as on the complexity of care provided in the home.

Technologic advances allow home administration of chemotherapy, parenteral nutrition, blood products, parenteral antibiotics, and parenteral analgesics, as well as management of symptoms and care of vascular access devices. Although home care nurses provide care and support for patients receiving this advanced technical care, patients and families need instruction and ongoing support that allow them to feel comfortable and proficient in managing these treatments at home. Follow-up visits and telephone calls from the nurse are often reassuring and increase the patient's and family's comfort in dealing with complex and new aspects of care. Continued contact facilitates evaluation of the patient's progress and assessment of the ongoing needs of the patient and family.

CONTINUING CARE

Referral for home care is often indicated for patients with cancer. The responsibilities of the home care nurse include assessing the home environment, suggesting modifications in the home or in care to help the patient and family address the patient's physical needs, providing physical care, and assessing the psychological and emotional impact of the illness on the patient and family.

Assessing changes in the patient's physical status and reporting relevant changes to the physician help ensure that appropriate and timely modifications in therapy are made. The home care nurse also assesses the adequacy of pain management and the effectiveness of other strategies to prevent or manage the side effects of treatment modalities.

It is necessary to assess the patient's and family's understanding of the treatment plan and management strategies and to reinforce previous teaching. The nurse often facilitates coordination of patient care by maintaining close communication with all involved health care providers. The nurse may make referrals and coordinate available community resources (eg, local office of the American Cancer Society, home aides, church groups, parish nurses, support groups) to assist patients and caregivers.

Evaluation

Expected Patient Outcomes

For specific patient outcomes, see the plan of nursing care (Chart 16-6). Expected patient outcomes may include the following:

1. Maintains integrity of oral mucous membranes
2. Maintains adequate tissue integrity
3. Maintains adequate nutritional status
4. Achieves relief of pain and discomfort
5. Demonstrates increased activity tolerance and decreased fatigue
6. Exhibits improved body image and self-esteem
7. Progresses through the grieving process
8. Experiences no complications, such as infection, or sepsis, and no episodes of bleeding or hemorrhage

Cancer Rehabilitation

Many patients with cancer, including those who receive primary surgical treatment and adjuvant chemotherapy or radiation therapy, return to work and their usual activities of daily living. These patients may encounter a variety of problems, including changes in their functional abilities and in the attitudes of employers, coworkers, and family members who still view cancer as a terminal, debilitating disease.

Nurses play an important role in the rehabilitation of patients with cancer. Both the patient and family are included as part of any rehabilitation effort, because cancer affects not only the patient but also the family members. In addition, with the shift away from inpatient care, many families are caring for patients at home. To maximize beneficial outcomes, evaluation of the patient's needs related to cancer rehabilitation begins early in cancer treatment (Table 16-11). Depending on the patient's functional abilities, the nurse works with the multidisciplinary health care team to encourage the patient to participate in some form of exercise program to facilitate activity tolerance and quality of life (Young-McCaughan, Mays, Arzola et al., 2003).

Assessment for body image changes as a result of disfiguring treatments is necessary to facilitate the patient's adjustment to changes in appearance or functional abilities. The nurse can refer the patient and family to a variety of support groups sponsored by the American Cancer Society, such as those for people who have had laryngectomies or mastectomies. The nurse also collaborates with physical, occupational, and enterostomal therapists (wound care specialists) in improving the patient's abilities in the use of prosthetic and assistive devices and in altering the home environment as needed.

Patients often experience distress (eg, pain, nausea) related to the underlying cancer or treatments. These symptoms may interfere with work and quality of life. The nurse assesses for these problems and helps the patient identify strategies for coping with them. For patients with gastrointestinal disturbances after chemotherapy, altering work hours or receiving treatments in the evenings may prove helpful. Collaboration with physicians and pharmacists is helpful in identifying appropriate interventions.

TABLE 16-11 Assessing Patient Needs for Cancer Rehabilitation

Area of Need	Factors to Assess
Functional	
Activities of daily living	Mobility Cognitive impairment Sensory impairments Communication barriers Preexisting disabilities
Physiologic	
Nutrition	Need for enteral or parenteral nutrition
Elimination	Alterations in bowel and bladder function
Symptoms related to disease or treatment	Pain Nausea, vomiting, diarrhea Dyspnea, fatigue Skin impairment, alopecia
Psychosocial Resources	
Family	Availability of caregiver, home physical environment
Community	Availability of private transportation; affordability of transportation
Personal	Availability of public transportation; affordability of transportation Availability and access to community organizations for assistance and support Spiritual concerns Family relationships Body image Coping abilities Sexuality
Financial	Job security for patient and family members Need for vocational training

The nurse collaborates with the dietitian to help the patient plan meals that will be acceptable and meet nutritional requirements. The nurse is also involved in the ongoing assessment of the patient to detect any long-term consequences of cancer treatment.

Although the Americans With Disabilities Act of 1990 was intended to protect patients with disabling disorders against discrimination, recovering cancer patients have reported instances of unfair practices and discrimination in the workplace. Some employers do not understand that different kinds of cancers have different prognoses and different effects on functional ability. As a result, employers may hesitate to hire or continue to employ people with cancer, especially if ongoing treatment regimens require adjustments in work schedules. Employers, coworkers, and families may continue to view the person as "sick" despite

NURSING RESEARCH PROFILE

Effects of Exercise in Cancer Rehabilitation

Young-McCaughan, S., Mays, M. Z., Arozola, S. M., et al. (2003). Change in exercise tolerance, activity and sleep patterns, and quality of life in patients with cancer participating in a structured exercise program. *Oncology Nursing Forum, 30*(3), 441–452.

Purpose

Multiple studies have shown that physical activity in patients with cancer can lead to improvements in functional capacity, levels of fatigue, and quality of life. The purpose of this study was to investigate the feasibility of an exercise intervention program modeled to improve selected physical and psychological parameters of health in patients with cancer. Changes in exercise tolerance, activity, sleep patterns, and quality of life were assessed. In addition, the authors examined whether certain demographic, cancer-related, treatment-related, physical, and psychological variables either encouraged or prevented patients with cancer from participating in the rehabilitation program.

Design

The Roy Adaptation Model was used as the conceptual framework for this prospective, repeated-measures study. Subjects were recruited from oncology clinics at two major military medical centers in the southwestern United States. To be eligible for the study, participants had to have a biopsy-proven cancer diagnosis within the previous 2 years, be at least 18 years of age, speak and read English, and have a statement from the primary care physician or medical oncologist that participation in the exercise program was not contraindicated. Patients with bone or joint destruction that could have been aggravated by the exercise and patients with severe cognitive impairment were excluded from participation. Of the 323 patients who were approached about the study, 62 (19%) consented to participate.

Patients participated in a 12-week exercise program that included classes on exercise, nutrition, stress management, cancer therapies, drug reviews, sleep, spiritual health, quality of life, and health evaluation and assessment. Exercise tolerance was measured before and after participation in the program by assessing the maximal oxygen uptake. This value was converted into metabolic equivalents (METs), which reflect exercise capacity. Activity and sleep patterns were collected from a wrist-worn actigraph that measured movement in three dimensions. This information was collected at baseline and during weeks 4, 8, and 12 of the study. Quality of life was measured using the Cancer Rehabilitation Evaluation System–Short Form (CARES-SF) at the same four time points.

Findings

Analysis of data revealed a significant improvement in METs among subjects who completed the exercise program, reflecting improvements in exercise capacity ($p < .001$). In addition, there was a significant improvement in both duration and intensity of exercise between baseline and week 12 testing ($p < .001$). For subjects who completed the exercise program, there was a significant improvement in self-report of energy ($p = .004$), although there was no reported significant change in activity level or percentage of napping. Despite a lack of significant improvement in objective measures of sleep during the course of the rehabilitation program, the subjects' self-reports of difficulty sleeping did show significant improvement ($p = .03$). Analysis of quality-of-life data revealed significant improvement for global scores ($p = .03$), as well as for physical ($p = .002$) and psychological ($p = .09$) subscales.

The authors reported that patients who had completed their cancer treatment were more likely to complete the exercise program than those still in active treatment ($p = .001$). Subjects with early-stage cancer had higher completion rates than those with late stages of cancer ($p = .003$). Some patients reported that the structured program enhanced their return to normal routines.

Nursing Implications

The findings of this study demonstrate that patients with various types and stages of cancer can benefit from exercise using a cardiac rehabilitation model. Improvements in exercise tolerance, activity, sleep patterns and quality of life are possible for this population. In addition, exercise facilitates both physical and psychological adaptation. Patients with cancer may have limitations based on personal and lifestyle factors and their disease and responses to treatment; however, nurses can collaborate with the multidisciplinary team to assess these limitations and offer individualized cancer rehabilitation through structured exercise programs.

ongoing recovery or completion of treatment. Attitudes of coworkers can be a problem when the patient has a communication impairment, as may occur in some head and neck cancers. Patients may benefit from vocational rehabilitation services of the American Cancer Society or other agencies.

Nurses can participate in efforts to educate employers and the public in general to ensure that the rights of patients with cancer are maintained. Whenever possible, the nurse assists the patient and family to resume preexisting roles. Psychologists and clergy or spiritual advisors are consulted to assist with psychosocial and spiritual concerns. Rehabilitation shifts the focus from what has been lost to what can be done with existing strengths and abilities. In that spirit, the nurse encourages the patient to regain the highest level of function and independence possible.

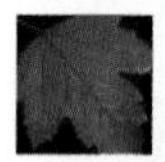

Gerontologic Considerations

As a result of an increased life expectancy and an increased risk of cancer with age, nurses are providing cancer-related care for growing numbers of elderly patients. More than 58% of all cancers occur in people older than 65 years of age, and about two thirds of all cancer deaths occur in people 65 years of age and older. Nursing care of this population addresses special needs, including physical, psychosocial, and financial concerns.

Oncology nurses working with the elderly population must understand the normal physiologic changes that occur with aging. These changes include decreased skin elasticity; decreased skeletal mass, structure, and strength; decreased organ function and structure; impaired immune system mechanisms; alterations in neurologic and sensory functions; and altered drug absorption, distribution, metabolism, and elimination. These changes ultimately influence the ability of elderly patients to tolerate cancer treatment. In addition, many elderly patients have other chronic diseases and associated treatments that may limit tolerance to cancer treatments (Table 16-12).

Potential chemotherapy-related toxicities, such as renal impairment, myelosuppression, fatigue, and cardiomyopathy, may increase as a result of declining organ function and diminished physiologic reserves. The recovery of normal tissues after radiation therapy may be delayed, and older patients may experience more severe adverse effects, such as mucositis, nausea and vomiting, and myelosuppression. Because of decreased tissue healing capacity and declining pulmonary and cardiovascular functioning, older patients are slower to recover from surgery. Elderly patients are also at increased risk for complications such as atelectasis, pneumonia, and wound infections.

Access to cancer care for elderly patients may be limited by discriminatory or fatalistic attitudes of health care providers, caregivers, and patients themselves. Issues such as the gradual loss of supportive resources, declining health

TABLE 16-12 Age-Related Changes and Their Effects on Patients with Cancer

Age-Related Changes	Implications
Impaired immune system	Use special precautions to avoid infection; monitor for atypical signs and symptoms of infection.
Altered drug absorption, distribution, metabolism, and elimination	Mandates careful calculation of chemotherapy and frequent assessment for drug response and side effects; dose adjustments may be necessary.
Increased prevalence of other chronic diseases	Monitor for effect of cancer or its treatment on patient's other chronic diseases; monitor patient's tolerance for cancer treatment; monitor for interactions with medications used to treat chronic diseases.
Diminished renal, respiratory, and cardiac reserve	Be proactive in prevention of decreased renal function, atelectasis, pneumonia, and cardiovascular compromise; monitor for side effects of cancer treatment.
Decreased skin and tissue integrity; reduction in body mass; delayed healing	Prevent pressure ulcers secondary to immobility; monitor skin and mucous membranes for changes related to radiation or chemotherapy; monitor nutritional status.
Decreased musculoskeletal strength	Prevent falls; assess support for performing activities of daily living in home setting; encourage safe use of assistive mobility devices
Decreased neurosensory functioning: loss of vision, hearing, and distal extremity tactile senses	Provide teaching and instructions modified for patient's hearing and vision changes; provide instruction concerning safety and skin care for distal extremities; assess home for safety.
Altered social and economic resources	Assess for financial concerns, living conditions, and resources for support
Potential changes in cognitive and emotional capacity	Provide teaching and support modified for patient's level of functioning and safety

or loss of a spouse, and unavailability of relatives or friends may result in limited access to care and unmet needs for assistance with activities of daily living. In addition, the economic impact of health care may be difficult for those living on fixed incomes.

Nurses must be aware of the special needs of the aging population. Cancer prevention, detection, and screening efforts are directed toward the elderly as well as the younger population. Nurses carefully monitor elderly patients receiving cancer treatments for signs and symptoms of adverse effects. In addition, elderly patients are instructed to report all symptoms to the physician. It is not uncommon for elderly patients to delay reporting symptoms, attributing them to "old age." Many elderly people do not want to report illness for fear of losing their independence or financial security. Sensory losses (eg, hearing and visual losses) and memory deficits are considered when planning patient education, because they may affect the patient's ability to process and retain information. In such cases, the nurse acts as a patient advocate, encouraging independence and identifying resources for support when indicated.

Care of the Patient With Advanced Cancer

Patients with advanced cancer are likely to experience many of the problems previously described, but all to a greater degree. Symptoms of gastrointestinal disturbances, nutritional problems, weight loss, and cachexia make patients more susceptible to skin breakdown, fluid and electrolyte problems, and infection.

Although not all cancer patients experience pain, those who do commonly fear that it will not be adequately treated. Although treatment at this stage of illness is likely to be palliative rather than curative, prevention and appropriate management of problems can improve the patient's quality of life considerably. For example, use of analgesia at set intervals rather than on an "as needed" basis usually breaks the cycle of tension and anxiety associated with waiting until pain becomes so severe that pain relief is inadequate once the analgesic is given. Working with the patient and family as well as with other health care providers on a pain-management program based on the patient's requirements frequently increases the patient's comfort and sense of control. In addition, the dose of opioid analgesic required is often reduced as pain becomes more manageable and other medications (eg, sedatives, tranquilizers, muscle relaxants) are added to assist in relieving pain.

If the patient is a candidate for radiation therapy or surgical intervention to relieve severe pain, the consequences of these procedures (eg, percutaneous nerve block, cordotomy) are explained to the patient and family. Measures are taken to prevent complications resulting from altered sensation, immobility, and changes in bowel and bladder function.

With the appearance of each new symptom, patients may experience dread and fear that the disease is progressing. However, one cannot assume that all symptoms are related to the cancer. The new symptoms and problems are evaluated and treated aggressively if possible to increase the patient's comfort and improve quality of life.

Weakness, immobility, fatigue, and inactivity typically occur in the advanced stages of cancer as a result of the tumor, treatment, inadequate nutritional intake, or shortness of breath. The nurse works with the patient to set realistic goals and to provide rest balanced with planned activities and exercise. Other measures include helping the patient identify energy-conserving methods for accomplishing tasks and promoting activities that the patient values most.

Efforts are made throughout the course of the disease to provide the patient with as much control and independence as desired but with assurance that support and assistance are available when needed. In addition, health care teams work with the patient and family to ascertain and comply with the patient's wishes about treatment methods and care as the terminal phase of illness and death approach.

Hospice

For many years, society was unable to cope appropriately with patients in the most advanced stages of cancer, and patients died in acute care settings rather than at home or in facilities designed to meet their needs. The needs of patients with terminal illnesses are best met by a comprehensive multidisciplinary program that focuses on quality of life, palliation of symptoms, and provision of psychosocial and spiritual support for patients and families when cure and control of the disease are no longer possible. The concept of hospice, which originated in Great Britain, best addresses these needs. Most important, the focus of care is on the family, not just the patient. Hospice care can be provided in several settings: free-standing, hospital-based, and community or home-based settings.

Because of the high costs associated with maintaining free-standing hospices, care is often delivered through coordination of services provided by hospitals and the community. Although physicians, social workers, clergy, dietitians, pharmacists, physical therapists, and volunteers are involved in patient care, nurses are most often the coordinators of all hospice activities. It is essential that home care and hospice nurses possess advanced skills in assessing and managing pain, nutrition, dyspnea, bowel dysfunction, and skin impairments.

In addition, hospice programs facilitate clear communication among family members and health care providers. Most patients and families are informed of the prognosis and are encouraged to participate in decisions regarding pursuing or terminating cancer treatment. Through collaboration with other support disciplines, the nurse helps the patient and family cope with changes in role identity, family structure, grief, and loss. Hospice nurses are actively involved in bereavement counseling. In many instances, family support for survivors continues for about 1 year. See Chapter 17 for detailed discussion of end-of-life care.

Oncologic Emergencies

For information about these emergencies, see Table 16-13.

(text continues on page 442)

TABLE 16-13 Oncologic Emergencies: Manifestations and Management

Emergency	Clinical Manifestations and Diagnostic Findings	Management
Superior Vena Cava Syndrome (SVCS) Compression or invasion of the superior vena cava by tumor, enlarged lymph nodes, intraluminal thrombus that obstructs venous circulation, or drainage of the head, neck, arms, and thorax. Typically associated with lung cancer, SVCS can also occur with breast cancer, Kaposi's sarcoma, thymoma, lymphoma and mediastinal metastases (Flounders, 2003a). If untreated, SVCS may lead to cerebral anoxia (because not enough oxygen reaches the brain), laryngeal edema, bronchial obstruction, and death.	***Clinical*** Gradually or suddenly impaired venous drainage giving rise to • Progressive shortness of breath (dyspnea), cough, hoarseness, chest pain, and facial swelling • Edema of the neck, arms, hands, and thorax and reported sensation of skin tightness and difficulty swallowing • Possibly engorged and distended jugular, temporal, and arm veins • Dilated thoracic vessels causing prominent venous patterns on the chest wall • Increased intracranial pressure, associated visual disturbances, headache, and altered mental status ***Diagnostic*** Diagnosis is confirmed by • Clinical findings • Chest x-ray • Thoracic computed tomography (CT) scan • Thoracic magnetic resonance imaging (MRI) Intraluminal thrombosis is identified by venogram.	***Medical*** • Radiation therapy to shrink tumor size and relieve symptoms • Chemotherapy for chemosensitive cancers (eg, lymphoma, small cell lung cancer) or when the mediastinum has been irradiated to maximum tolerance (Flounders, 2003a) • Anticoagulant or thrombolytic therapy for intraluminal thrombosis • Surgery (less common), such as vena cava bypass graft (synthetic or autologous), to redirect blood flow around the obstruction • Supportive measures such as oxygen therapy, corticosteroids, and diuretics ***Nursing*** • Identify patients at risk for SVCS. • Monitor and report clinical manifestations of SVCS. • Monitor cardiopulmonary and neurologic status. • Avoid upper extremity venipuncture and blood pressure measurement (Flounders, 2003a). • Facilitate breathing by positioning the patient properly. This helps to promote comfort and reduce anxiety produced by difficulty breathing resulting from progressive edema. • Promote energy conservation to minimize shortness of breath. • Monitor the patient's fluid volume status and administer fluids cautiously to minimize edema. • Assess for thoracic radiation-related problems such as dysphagia (difficulty swallowing) and esophagitis. • Monitor for chemotherapy-related problems, such as myelosuppression. • Provide postoperative care as appropriate.
Spinal Cord Compression Potentially leading to permanent neurologic impairment and associated morbidity and mortality, compression of the cord and its nerve roots may result from tumor, lymphomas, intervertebral collapse, or interruption of blood supply to the nerve tissues (Flounders, 2003a). The prognosis depends on the severity and rapidity of onset. About 60% of compressions occur at the thoracic level, 30% in the lumbosacral level, and 10% in the cervical region (Abrahm, 2004). Metastatic cancers (breast, lung, kidney, prostate, myeloma, lymphoma) and related bone erosion are associated with spinal cord compression (Flounders, 2003a).	***Clinical*** • Local inflammation, edema, venous stasis, and impaired blood supply to nervous tissues • Local or radicular back or neck pain along the dermatomal areas innervated by the affected nerve root (Flounders, 2003a) (eg, thoracic radicular pain extends in a band around the chest or abdomen) • Pain exacerbated by movement, supine recumbent position, coughing, sneezing, or the Valsalva maneuver • Neurologic dysfunction, and related motor and sensory deficits (numbness, tingling, feelings of coldness in the affected area, inability to detect vibration, loss of positional sense)	***Medical*** • Radiation therapy to reduce tumor size to halt progression and corticosteroid therapy to decrease inflammation and swelling at the compression site • Surgery if symptoms progress despite radiation therapy or if vertebral fracture leads to additional nerve damage; surgery is also an option when the tumor is not radiosensitive or is located in an area that was previously irradiated (Flounders, 2003a). • Chemotherapy as adjuvant to radiation therapy for patients with lymphoma or small cell lung cancer • *Note:* Despite treatment, patients with poor neurologic function before treatment are less likely to regain complete motor and sensory function; patients who develop complete paralysis usually do not regain all neurologic function (Abrahm, 2004).

TABLE 16-13 Oncologic Emergencies: Manifestations and Management (Continued)

Emergency	Clinical Manifestations and Diagnostic Findings	Management
	• Motor loss ranging from subtle weakness to flaccid paralysis • Bladder and/or bowel dysfunction depending on level of compression (above S2, overflow incontinence; from S3 to S5, flaccid sphincter tone and bowel incontinence) ***Diagnostic*** • Percussion tenderness at the level of compression • Abnormal reflexes • Sensory and motor abnormalities • MRI, myelogram, spinal cord x-rays, bone scans, and CT scan	***Nursing*** • Perform ongoing assessment of neurologic function to identify existing and progressing dysfunction. • Control pain with pharmacologic and non-pharmacologic measures. • Prevent complications of immobility resulting from pain and decreased function (eg, skin breakdown, urinary stasis, thrombophlebitis, decreased clearance of pulmonary secretions). • Maintain muscle tone by assisting with range-of-motion exercises in collaboration with physical and occupational therapists. • Institute intermittent urinary catheterization and bowel training programs for patients with bladder or bowel dysfunction. • Provide encouragement and support to patient and family coping with pain and altered functioning, lifestyle, roles, and independence.
Hypercalcemia In patients with cancer, hypercalcemia is a potentially life-threatening metabolic abnormality resulting when the calcium released from the bones is more than the kidneys can excrete or the bones can reabsorb. It may result from • Bone destruction by tumor cells and subsequent release of calcium • Production of prostaglandins and osteoclast-activating factor, which stimulate bone breakdown and calcium release (Shuey, 2004) • Tumors that produce parathyroid-like substances that promote calcium release (Shuey, 2004) • Excessive use of vitamins and minerals and conditions unrelated to cancer, such as dehydration, renal impairment, primary hyperparathyroidism, thyrotoxicosis, thiazide diuretics, and hormone therapy	***Clinical*** Fatigue, weakness, confusion, decreased level of responsiveness, hyporeflexia, nausea, vomiting, constipation, polyuria (excessive urination), polydipsia (excessive thirst), dehydration, and dysrhythmias (Shuey & Brant, 2004) ***Diagnostic*** Serum calcium level exceeding 11 mg/dL (2.74 mmol/L)	***Medical*** See Chapter 14. ***Nursing*** • Identify patients at risk for hypercalcemia and assess for signs and symptoms of hypercalcemia. • Educate patient and family; prevention and early detection can prevent fatality. • Teach at-risk patients to recognize and report signs and symptoms of hypercalcemia. • Encourage patients to consume 2–3 L of fluid daily unless contraindicated by existing renal or cardiac disease. • Explain the use of dietary and pharmacologic interventions such as stool softeners and laxatives for constipation. • Advise patients to maintain nutritional intake without restricting normal calcium intake. • Discuss antiemetic therapy if nausea and vomiting occur. • Promote mobility by emphasizing its importance in preventing demineralization and breakdown of bones (Shuey & Brant, 2004).
Pericardial Effusion and Cardiac Tamponade Cardiac tamponade is an accumulation of fluid in the pericardial space. The accumulation compresses the heart and thereby impedes expansion of	***Clinical*** • Neck vein distention during inspiration (Kussmaul's sign) • Pulsus paradoxus (systolic blood pressure decrease exceeding 10 mm Hg during inspiration; pulse gets stronger on expiration)	***Medical*** • Pericardiocentesis (the aspiration or withdrawal of pericardial fluid by a large-bore needle inserted into the pericardial space). In malignant effusions, pericardiocentesis provides only temporary relief; fluid usually reaccumulates. Windows or openings in the pericardium can be created surgically as a palliative

continued >

TABLE 16-13 Oncologic Emergencies: Manifestations and Management (Continued)

Emergency	Clinical Manifestations and Diagnostic Findings	Management
the ventricles and cardiac filling during diastole. As ventricular volume and cardiac output fall, the heart pump fails, and circulatory collapse develops. With gradual onset, fluid accumulates gradually, and the outer layer of the pericardial space stretches to compensate for rising pressure. Large amounts of fluid accumulate before symptoms of heart failure occur. With rapid onset, pressures rise too quickly for the pericardial space to compensate. Cancerous tumors, particularly from adjacent thoracic tumors (lung, esophagus, breast cancers), and cancer treatment are the most common causes of cardiac tamponade. Radiation therapy of 4000 cGy or more to the mediastinal area has also been implicated in pericardial fibrosis, pericarditis, and resultant cardiac tamponade. Untreated pericardial effusion and cardiac tamponade lead to circulatory collapse and cardiac arrest (Flounders, 2003a).	• Distant heart sounds, rubs and gallops, cardiac dullness • Compensatory tachycardia (heart beats faster to compensate for decreased cardiac output) • Increased venous and vascular pressures ***Diagnostic*** • Electrocardiography (ECG) helps diagnose pericardial effusion • In small effusion, chest x-rays show small amounts of fluid in the pericardium; in large effusions, x-ray films disclose "water-bottle" heart (obliteration of vessel contour and cardiac chambers) • CT scans help diagnose pleural effusions and evaluate effect of treatment • Narrow pulse pressure • Shortness of breath and tachypnea • Weakness, chest pain, orthopnea, anxiety, diaphoresis, lethargy, and altered consciousness from decreased cerebral perfusion (Flounders, 2003a; Casciato, 2004)	measure to drain fluid into the pleural space. Catheters may also be placed in the pericardial space and sclerosing agents (such as tetracycline, talc, bleomycin, 5-fluorouracil, or thiotepa) injected to prevent fluid from reaccumulating. • Radiation therapy or antineoplastic agents, depending on how sensitive the primary tumor is to these treatments. In mild effusions, prednisone and diuretic medications may be prescribed and the patient's status carefully monitored. ***Nursing*** • Monitor vital signs and oxygen saturation frequently. • Assess for pulsus paradoxus. • Monitor ECG tracings. • Assess heart and lung sounds, neck vein filling, level of consciousness, respiratory status, and skin color and temperature. • Monitor and record intake and output. • Review laboratory findings (eg, arterial blood gas and electrolyte levels). • Elevate the head of the patient's bed to ease breathing. • Minimize patient's physical activity to reduce oxygen requirements; administer supplemental oxygen as prescribed. • Provide frequent oral hygiene. • Reposition and encourage the patient to cough and take deep breaths every 2 h. • As needed, maintain patent IV access, reorient the patient, and provide supportive measures and appropriate patient instruction (Flounders, 2003a; Casciato, 2004).
Disseminated Intravascular Coagulation (DIC, also called consumption coagulopathy) Complex disorder of coagulation or fibrinolysis (destruction of clots), which results in thrombosis or bleeding. DIC is most commonly associated with hematologic cancers (leukemia); cancer of prostate, gastrointestinal (GI) tract, and lungs; chemotherapy (methotrexate, prednisone, l-asparaginase, vincristine, and 6-mercaptopurine); and disease processes such as sepsis, hepatic failure, and anaphylaxis. Blood clots form when normal coagulation mechanisms are triggered. Once activated, the clotting cascade continues to consume clotting factors and	***Clinical*** *Chronic DIC:* Few or no observable symptoms or easy bruising, prolonged bleeding from venipuncture and injection sites, bleeding of the gums, and slow GI bleeding *Acute DIC:* life-threatening hemorrhage and infarction; clinical symptoms of this syndrome are varied and depend on the organ system involved in thrombus and infarction or bleeding episodes ***Diagnostic*** • Prolonged prothrombin time (PT or protime) • Prolonged partial thromboplastin time (PTT) • Prolonged thrombin time (TT) • Decreased fibrinogen level • Decreased platelet level • Decrease in clotting factors	***Medical*** • Chemotherapy, biologic response modifier therapy, radiation therapy, or surgery is used to treat the underlying cancer. • Antibiotic therapy is used for sepsis. • Anticoagulants, such as heparin or antithrombin III, decrease the stimulation of the coagulation pathways. • Transfusion of fresh-frozen plasma or cryoprecipitates (which contain clotting factors and fibrinogen), packed red blood cells, and platelets may be used as replacement therapy to prevent or control bleeding. • Although controversial, antifibrinolytic agents such as aminocaproic acid (Amicar), which is associated with increased thrombus formation, may be used. ***Nursing*** • Monitor vital signs. • Measure and document intake and output. • Assess skin color and temperature; lung, heart, and bowel sounds; level of consciousness, headache, visual disturbances, chest pain, decreased urine output, and abdominal tenderness. • Inspect all body orifices, tube insertion sites, incisions, and bodily excretions for bleeding.

TABLE 16-13 Oncologic Emergencies: Manifestations and Management (Continued)

Emergency	Clinical Manifestations and Diagnostic Findings	Management
platelets faster than the body can replace them. Clots are deposited in the microvasculature, placing the patient at great risk for impaired circulation, tissue hypoxia, and necrosis. In addition, fibrinolysis occurs, breaking down clots and increasing the circulating levels of anticoagulant substances, thereby placing the patient at risk for hemorrhage (Casciato, 2004).	• Decreased hemoglobin • Decreased hematocrit • Elevated fibrin split products • Positive protamine sulfate precipitation test (thrombin activation test) (Krimmel, 2003)	• Review laboratory test results. • Minimize physical activity to decrease injury risks and oxygen requirements. • Prevent bleeding; apply pressure to all venipuncture sites, and avoid nonessential invasive procedures; provide electric rather than straight-edged razors; avoid tape on the skin and advise gentle but adequate oral hygiene. • Assist the patient to turn, cough, and take deep breaths every 2 h. • Reorient the patient, if needed; maintain a safe environment; and provide appropriate patient education and supportive measures.
Syndrome of Inappropriate Secretion of Antidiuretic Hormone (SIADH) The continuous, uncontrolled release of antidiuretic hormone (ADH), produced by tumor cells or by the abnormal stimulation of the hypothalamic–pituitary network, leads to increased extracellular fluid volume, water intoxication, hyponatremia, and increased excretion of urinary sodium. As fluid volume increases, stretch receptors in the right atrium respond by releasing a second hormone, atrial natriuretic factor (ANF). The release of ANF causes increased renal excretion of sodium, which worsens hyponatremia. The most common cause of SIADH is cancer, especially small cell cancers of the lung. Antineoplastics—vincristine, vinblastine, cisplatin, and cyclophosphamide—and morphine also stimulate ADH secretion, which promotes conservation and reabsorption of water by the kidneys. As more fluid is absorbed, the circulatory volume increases, ANF is released, and sodium is actively excreted by the kidneys in compensation (Flounders, 2003a; Casciato, 2004).	***Clinical*** *Serum sodium levels lower than 120 mEq/L* (120 mmol/L): symptoms of hyponatremia including personality changes, irritability, nausea, anorexia, vomiting, weight gain, fatigue, muscular pain (myalgia), headache, lethargy, and confusion (Langfeldt & Cooley, 2003). *Serum sodium levels lower than 110 mEq/L* (110 mmol/L): seizure, abnormal reflexes, papilledema, coma, and death. Edema is rare. ***Diagnostic*** • Decreased serum sodium level • Increased urine osmolality • Increased urinary sodium level • Decreased blood urea nitrogen (BUN), creatinine, and serum albumin levels secondary to dilution • Abnormal water load test results	***Medical*** Fluid intake range limited to 500–1000 mL/day to increase the serum sodium level and decrease fluid overload. If water restriction alone is not effective in correcting or controlling serum sodium levels, demeclocycline is often prescribed to interfere with the antidiuretic action of ADH and ANF. If neurologic symptoms are severe, parenteral sodium replacement and diuretic therapy are indicated. Electrolyte levels are monitored carefully to detect secondary magnesium, potassium, and calcium imbalances. After the symptoms of SIADH are controlled, the underlying cancer is treated. If water excess continues despite treatment, pharmacologic intervention (urea and furosemide) may be indicated (Flounders, 2003a; Casciato, 2004). ***Nursing*** • Maintain intake and output measurements. • Assess level of consciousness, lung and heart sounds, vital signs, daily weight, and urine specific gravity; also assess for nausea, vomiting, anorexia, edema, fatigue, and lethargy. • Monitor laboratory test results, including serum electrolyte levels, osmolality, and BUN, creatinine, and urinary sodium levels. • Minimize the patient's activity; provide appropriate oral hygiene; maintain environmental safety; and restrict fluid intake if necessary. • Reorient the patient and provide instruction and encouragement as needed (Langfeldt & Cooley, 2003).

continued >

TABLE 16-13 Oncologic Emergencies: Manifestations and Management (Continued)

Emergency	Clinical Manifestations and Diagnostic Findings	Management
Tumor Lysis Syndrome Potentially fatal complication associated with radiation- or chemotherapy-induced cell destruction of large or rapidly growing cancers such as leukemia, lymphoma, and small cell lung cancer (Cope, 2004). The release of intracellular contents from the tumor cells leads to electrolyte imbalances—hyperkalemia, hypocalcemia, hyperphosphatemia, and hyperuricemia—because the kidneys can no longer excrete large volumes of the released intracellular metabolites.	***Clinical*** Clinical manifestations depend on the extent of metabolic abnormalities. • Neurologic: fatigue, weakness, memory loss, altered mental status, muscle cramps, tetany, paresthesias (numbness and tingling), seizures • Cardiac: elevated blood pressure, shortened QT complexes, widened QRS waves, dysrhythmias, cardiac arrest • GI: anorexia, nausea, vomiting, abdominal cramps, diarrhea • Renal: flank pain, oliguria, anuria, renal failure, acidic urine pH ***Diagnostic*** Electrolyte imbalances identified by laboratory test results (Casciato, 2004)	***Medical*** • To prevent renal failure and restore electrolyte balance, aggressive fluid hydration is initiated 48 hours before and after the initiation of cytotoxic therapy to increase urine volume and eliminate uric acid and electrolytes. Urine is alkalinized by adding sodium bicarbonate to IV fluid to maintain a urine pH of 7 or higher; this prevents renal failure secondary to uric acid precipitation in the kidneys. • Diuretic therapy, with a carbonic anhydrase inhibitor or acetazolamide, to alkalinize the urine • Allopurinol therapy to inhibit the conversion of nucleic acids to uric acid (Cope, 2004) • Administration of a cation-exchange resin, such as sodium polystyrene sulfonate (Kayexalate) to treat hyperkalemia by binding and eliminating potassium through the bowel • Administration of hypertonic dextrose and regular insulin temporarily shifts potassium into cells and lowers serum potassium levels. • Administration of phosphate-binding gels, such as aluminum hydroxide, to treat hyperphosphatemia by promoting phosphate excretion in the feces. • Hemodialysis when patients are unresponsive to the standard approaches for managing uric acid and electrolyte abnormalities (Casciato, 2004) ***Nursing*** • Identify at-risk patients, including those in whom tumor lysis syndrome may develop up to 1 week after therapy has been completed. • Institute essential preventive measures (eg, fluid hydration, allopurinol). • Assess patient for signs and symptoms of electrolyte imbalances. • Assess urine pH to confirm alkalization. • Monitor serum electrolyte and uric acid levels for evidence of fluid volume overload secondary to aggressive hydration. • Instruct patients to report symptoms indicating electrolyte disturbances.

Critical Thinking Exercises

1 ebp Your patient has been receiving high doses of chemotherapy to treat leukemia. She reports that she wants to stop the chemotherapy because of the oral ulcerations and pain that have developed since she started on the chemotherapy. What would your response be to her? What evidence-based nursing interventions would you implement to relieve the ulcers and her pain? What is the evidence for the interventions you identified? How strong is that evidence, and what criteria did you use to assess the strength of that evidence?

2 A 74-year-old patient with prostate cancer and metastasis to the bone is to begin a continuous subcutaneous infusion of analgesia through an ambulatory infusion pump to relieve his severe pain. The patient's wife is afraid that he will become addicted, and his adult children state that his pain remains unrelieved. As a home care nurse, what assessments would be of highest priority to you during your initial visit to this patient? What nursing interventions and teaching would be indicated in this situation? How would you modify your interventions if the patient is receiving fentanyl by transdermal patch and still reporting severe pain?

3 A 45-year-old woman of Ashkenazi Jewish descent has presented to the cancer center for treatment of advanced

breast cancer. Her evaluation revealed that she is positive for the *BRCA1* gene. In reviewing her family history, you note that her mother and older sister (who are both deceased) had metastatic breast cancer. You also note that she has two younger sisters. What information about the *BRCA1* gene will guide you as you plan to assess the screening needs for this woman, her sisters, and her children? What type of referral would be appropriate for this woman and her family?

4 Your 68-year-old patient with lung cancer has been admitted for emergent radiation therapy for the diagnosis of superior vena cava syndrome. Describe the underlying pathology that can lead to the signs and symptoms of superior vena cava syndrome. What patient monitoring will be essential during this patient's course of care? Describe the medical and nursing management strategies that will be used for this patient.

5 A patient with colon cancer who has undergone a successful resection of her bowel has been referred to the medical oncologist for participation in an adjuvant therapy clinical trial involving investigational chemotherapy. After the physician reviews the trial and consent form with the patient, she leaves the room for the patient to consider enrollment into the trial. The patient tells you that she is afraid of being a "guinea pig." Describe the role and the importance of clinical trials in oncology care. What would you tell the patient regarding safeguards that are in place to protect patients who participate in human research. How would you support this patient in her decision-making process regarding participation in a clinical trial?

REFERENCES AND SELECTED READINGS

BOOKS

Abeloff, M. D., Armitage, J. D., Niederhuber, J. E., et al. (Eds). (2004). *Clinical oncology* (3rd ed.). Philadelphia: Elsevier/Churchill Livingstone.

Boik, J. (1995). *Cancer and natural medicine: A textbook of basic science and clinical research.* Princeton, MN: Oregon Medical Press.

Casciato, D. A. (Ed.). (2004). *Manual of clinical oncology* (5th ed.). Philadelphia: Lippincott Williams & Wilkins.

Ellis, L. E., Curley, S. A. & Tanabe, K. K. (Eds.) (2004). *Radiofrequency ablation for cancer: Current indications, techniques and outcomes.* New York: Springer-Verlag.

Ezzone, S. (Ed.) (2004). *Hematopoietic stem cell transplantation: A manual for nursing practice.* Pittsburgh: Oncology Nursing Society.

Govindan, R. (Ed.). (2002). *The Washington manual of oncology.* Philadelphia: Lippincott Williams & Wilkins.

Green, F., Page, D. L., Fleming, I. D., et al. (Eds.). (2002). *AJCC cancer staging manual* (6th ed.). New York: Springer-Verlag.

Higginson, I. J., Hearn, J. & Addington-Hall, J. (2003). Epidemiology of cancer pain. In Sykes, N., Fallon, M. T. & Patt, R. B. (Eds.) *Cancer pain.* New York: Oxford University Press.

Hough, S. W. & Kanner, R. M. (2004). Cancer pain syndromes. In Warfield, C. A. & Bajwa, Z. H. (Eds.) *Principles and practice of pain medicine* (2nd ed.). New York: McGraw-Hill.

Hough, S. W. & Portenoy, R. K. (2004). Medical management of cancer pain. In Warfield, C. A. & Bajwa, Z. H. (Eds.) *Principles and practice of pain medicine* (2nd ed.). New York: McGraw-Hill.

Janeway, C. A., Travers, P., Walport, M., et al. (2005). *Immunobiology: The immune system in health and disease* (6th ed.). New York: Garland Science.

Kufe, D. W., Pollock, R. E., Wechselbaum, R. R., et al. (Eds.) (2003). *Cancer medicine* (6th ed.). Hamilton, Ontario: B. C. Decker.

Lenhard, R. E., Osteen, R. T., & Gansler, T. (Eds.). (2001). *Clinical oncology.* Atlanta: American Cancer Society.

Morris, D. & Ward, K. (2003). Perioperative nursing. In Booker, C. & Nicol, M. J. (Eds.). *Nursing adults: The practice of caring.* Edinburgh: Mosby/Elsevier.

Overcash, J. & Balducci, L. (Eds.). (2003). *The older cancer patient.* New York: Springer.

Pazdur, R., Coia, L. R., Hoskins, H. S., et al. (Eds.). (2003). *Cancer management: A multidisciplinary approach* (7th ed.). New York: The Oncology Group.

Polovich, M. (Ed.). (2003). *Safe handling of hazardous drugs.* Pittsburgh: Oncology Nursing Society.

Ratain, M. J., Tempero, M., & Skosey, C. (2001). *Outline of oncology therapeutics.* Philadelphia: Saunders.

Richerson, M. T. (2004). Electrolyte imbalances. In Yarbro, C. H., Frogge, M. H., & Goodman, M. (Eds.). *Cancer symptom management* (3rd ed.). Boston: Jones and Bartlett.

Saunders, M. & Booth, S. (2003). Cancer pain therapy. In Munglani, C. R. & Schmidt, W. R. (Eds.). *Pain: Current understanding, emerging therapies and novel approaches to drug discovery.* New York: Marcel Dekker.

Vogel, W. H., Wilson, M. A. & Melvin, M. S. (2004). *Advanced practice oncology and palliative care guidelines.* Philadelphia: Lippincott Williams & Wilkins.

Wilkes, G. M. & Barton-Burke, M. (Eds.). (2004). *2004 oncology nursing handbook.* Sudbury, Massachusetts: Jones & Bartlett.

Yarbro, C. H., Frogge, M. H., & Goodman, M. (Eds.). (2004). *Cancer symptom management* (3rd ed.). Boston: Jones & Bartlett.

JOURNALS

**Asterisks indicate nursing research articles.*

General

American Cancer Society. (2004a). ACS cancer detection guidelines. Available at: www.cancer.org (accessed March 5, 2006).

American Cancer Society. (2004b). Surgery. Available at: www.cancer.org (accessed March 12, 2006).

Anonymous. (2003). Clinical trials in supportive care: Cancer cachexia and anorexia. *Journal of Supportive Oncology, 1*(4), 294–295.

Berger, A. (2003). Treating fatigue in cancer patients. *The Oncologist, 8*(Suppl 1), 10–14.

Braccia, D. P. & Hoffernan, N. (2003). Surgical and ablative modalities for the treatment of colorectal cancer with liver metastasis. *Clinical Journal of Oncology Nursing, 7*(2), 178–184.

Brown, J. K., Byers, T., Doyle, C., et al. (2003). Nutrition and physical activity during and after cancer treatment: An American Cancer Society guide for informed choices. *CA: A Cancer Journal for Clinicians, 53*(5), 268–291.

Bruce, S. D. (2004). Radiation-induced xerostomia: How dry is your patient? *Clinical Journal of Oncology Nursing, 8*(1), 61–67.

Calzone, K. A. & Masny, A. (2004). Genetics and oncology nursing. *Seminars in Oncology Nursing, 20*(3), 178–185.

Coyne, P. (2003). When the Word Health Organization analgesic therapies ladder fails: The role of invasive analgesic therapies. *Oncology Nursing Forum, 30*(5), 777–783.

Dunn, B. N. K., Wickerham, D. L. & Ford, L. G. (2005). Prevention of hormone-related cancers: Breast cancer. *Journal of Clinical Oncology, 23*(2), 357–367.

Ernst, A., Feller-Kopman, D., Becker, H. D., et al. (2004). Central airway obstruction. *American Journal of Respiratory and Critical Care Medicine, 169*(12), 1278–1297.

Fisher, J. P. (1998). Tamoxifen for prevention of breast cancer: Report of the National Surgical Adjuvant Breast and Bowel Project P-1 study. *Journal of National Cancer Institute, 90*(18), 1371–1388.

Garfunkel, A. A. (2004). Oral mucositis: The search for a solution. *New England Journal of Medicine, 351*(25), 2649–2651.

Gillespie, T. W. (2003). Anemia in cancer. *Cancer Nursing, 26*(2), 119–128.

Goodwin, J. A. & Coleman, E. A. (2003). Exploring measures of functional dependence in the older adult with cancer. *MedSurg Nursing, 12*(6), 359–365.

Gordils-Perez, J., Rawlins-Duell, R. & Kelvin, J. F. (2003). Advances in radiation treatment of patients with breast cancer. *Clinical Journal of Oncology Nursing, 7*(6), 629–636.

Goss, P. E., & Strasser-Weippl, K. (2004). Prevention strategies with aromatase inhibitors. *Clinical Cancer Research, 10*(1 Pt 2), 372S–379S.

Haughney, A. (2004). Nausea and vomiting in end-stage cancer. *American Journal of Nursing, 104*(11), 40–48.

Holder, H. (2003). Nursing management of nutrition in cancer and palliative care. *British Journal of Nursing, 12*(11), 667–668,670, 672–674.

Hood, L. E. (2003). Chemotherapy in the elderly: Supportive measures for chemotherapy induced myelotoxicity. *Clinical Journal of Oncology Nursing, 7*(2), 185–190.

Hutson, S. P. (2003). Attitudes and psychological impact of genetic testing, genetic counseling, and breast cancer risk assessment among women at increased risk. *Oncology Nursing Forum, 30*(2), 241–246.

Jakub, J. W., Pendas, S. & Reintgen, D. S. (2003). Current status of sentinel lymph node mapping and biopsy: Facts and controversies. *The Oncologist, 8*(1), 59–68.

Jemal, A., Murray, T., Ward, E., et al. (2005). Cancer statistics. *CA Cancer Journal for Clinicians, 55*(1), 10–30.

Jemal, A., Tiwari, R. C., Murray, T., et al. (2004). Cancer statistics, 2004, *CA Cancer Journal for Clinicians, 54*(1), 8–29.

Law, E., Mangarin, E. & Kelvin, J. F. (2003). Nursing management of patients receiving stereotactic radiosurgery. *Clinical Journal of Oncology Nursing, 7*(4), 387–392.

Leather, A., Bushell, L. & Gillespie, L. (2003, November). The provision of nutritional support for people with cancer. *Nursing Times, 99*(46), 18–24,53–55.

Leon, T. G. & Pase, M. (2004). Essential oncology facts for the float nurse. *MedSurg Nursing, 13*(3), 165–171.

Lobrano, M. B. & Singha, P. (2003). Positron emission tomography in oncology. *Clinical Journal of Oncology Nursing, 7*(4), 379–385.

MacDonald, N. (2003). Is there evidence for earlier intervention in cancer-associated weight loss? *Journal of Supportive Oncology, 1*(4), 279–286.

McGuire, D. B. & Peterson, D. E. (eds.) (2004). Mucositis. *Seminars in Oncology Nursing, 20*(1), 1–68.

Mahon, S. M. (2003). Patient education regarding cancer screening guidelines. *Clinical Journal of Oncology Nursing, 7*(5), 581–585.

Marrs, J. & Newton, S. (2003). Updating your peripheral neuropathy "know-how." *Clinical Journal of Oncology Nursing, 7*(3), 299–303.

Mock, V. (2003). Clinical excellence through evidence-based practice: Fatigue management as a model. *Oncology Nursing Forum, 30*(5), 787–795.

Mock, V. & Olsen, M. (2003). Current management of fatigue and anemia in patients with cancer. *Seminars in Oncology Nursing, 19*(4 Suppl 2), 36–41.

Montbriand, M. J. (1999). Past and present herbs used to treat cancer: Medicine, magic, or poison? *Oncology Nursing Forum, 26*(1), 49–59.

Montbriand, M. (2004). Herbs or natural products that decrease cancer growth (part one of four).*Oncology Nursing Forum, 31*(4), E75–E90.

National Cancer Institute. (2006). Vaccine protects against virus linked to half of all cervical cancers. Available at: http://www.cancer.gov/clinicaltrials/results/cervical-cancer-vaccine1102 (accessed May 25, 2006).

Sadler, G. R., Wasserman, L., Fullerton, J. T., et al. (2004). Supporting patients through genetic screening for cancer risk. *MedSurg Nursing, 13*(4), 233–246.

*Schreier, A. M. & Williams, S. A. (2004). Anxiety and quality of life of women who receive radiation or chemotherapy for breast cancer. *Oncology Nursing Forum, 31*(1), 127–130.

Shelton, B. K. (2003). Evidence-based care for the neutropenic patient with leukemia. *Seminars in Oncology Nursing, 19*(2), 133–141.

Sifri, R., Gangadharappa, S., & Acheson, L. S. (2004). Identifying and testing for hereditary susceptibility to common cancers. *CA Cancer Journal for Clinicians, 54*(6), 309–326.

*Skalla, K. A., Bakitas, M., Furstenberg, C. T., et al. (2004). Patients' need for information about cancer therapy. *Oncology Nursing Forum, 31*(2), 313–319.

Sparber, A., Bauer, L., Curt, G., et al. (2000). Use of complementary medicine by adult patients participating in cancer clinical trials. *Oncology Nursing Forum, 27*(4), 623–630.

Sterman, E, Gauker, S. & Krieger, J. (2003). A comprehensive approach to improving cancer pain management and patient satisfaction. *Oncology Nursing Forum, 30*(5), 857–864.

Stiff, P. J., Erder, H., Bensinger, W. I., et al. (2006). Reliability and validity of a patient self-administered daily questionnaire to assess impact of oral mucositis (OM) on pain and daily functioning in patients undergoing autologous hematopoietic stem cell transplantation (HSCT). *Bone Marrow Transplant, 37*(4), 393–401.

*Thome, B., Dykes, A. K., Gunnars, B., et al. (2003). The experiences of older people living with cancer. *Cancer Nursing, 26*(2), 85–96.

Vickers, A. (2004). Alternative cancer cures: "Unproven" or "disproven"? *CA Cancer Journal for Clinicians, 54*(2), 110–118.

Ward, E., Jemal, A., Cokkinides, V., et al. (2004). Cancer disparities by race/ethnicity and socioeconomic status. *CA Cancer Journal for Clinicians, 544*(2), 78–93.

Whiteside, T. L. (2003). Immune responses to malignancies. *Journal of Allergy and Clinical Immunology, 111*(2 Suppl), S677–S686.

Wickline, M. M. (2004). Prevention and treatment of acute radiation dermatitis: A literature review. *Oncology Nursing Forum, 31*(2), 237–244.

Wohlschlaeger, A. (2004). Prevention and treatment of mucositis: A guide for nurses. *Journal of Pediatric Oncology Nursing, 21*(5), 281–287.

*Woods, D. V., Montgomery, S. B., & Herring, R. P. (2004). Recruiting Black/African American men for research on prostate cancer prevention. *Cancer, 100*(5), 1017–1025.

*Young-McCaughan, S., Mays, M. Z., Arzola, S. M., et al. (2003). Change in exercise tolerance, activity and sleep patterns, and quality of life in patients with cancer participating in a structured exercise program. *Oncology Nursing Forum, 30*(3), 441–452.

Bone Marrow Transplantation

DeMeyer, D. H. (2003). Hematopoietic cell transplantation in the treatment of leukemia. *Seminars in Oncology Nursing, 19*(2), 118–132.

Hacker, E. D. (2003). Quantitative measurement of quality of life in adult patients undergoing bone marrow transplant or peripheral blood stem cell transplant: A decade in review. *Oncology Nursing Forum, 30*(4), 613–629.

Latchford, T. & Shelton, B. K. (2004). Respiratory syncytial virus in blood and marrow transplant recipients. *Clinical Journal of Oncology Nursing, 7*(4), 418–422.

Moore, S. L. (2003). Bronchiolitis obliterans organizing pneumonia: A late complication of stem cell transplantation. *Clinical Journal of Oncology Nursing, 7*(6), 659–662.

Tierney, D. K. (2004). Sexuality following hematopoietic cell transplantation. *Clinical Journal of Oncology Nursing, 8*(1), 43–47.

West, F. & Mitchell, S. A. (2004). Evidence-based guidelines for the management of neutropenia following outpatient hematopoietic stem cell transplantation. *Clinical Journal of Oncology Nursing, 8*(6), 601–613.

Carcinogenesis and Risk Factors

Likes, W. M. & Itano, J. (2003). Human papillomavirus and cervical cancer: Not just a sexually transmitted disease. *Clinical Journal of Oncology Nursing, 7*(3), 271–276.

National Institutes of Health, NIH News. (2004). WHI study finds no heart disease benefit, increased stroke risk with estrogen alone. Available at: http://www.nhlbi.nih.gov/new/press/04-04-13.htm (accessed March 15, 2006).

Tsao, A. S., Kim, E. S. & Hong, W. K. (2004). Chemoprevention of cancer. *CA Cancer Journal for Clinicians, 54*(3), 150–180.

Chemotherapy

Capriotti, T. (2002). Gleevec: Zeroing in on cancer. *MedSurg Nursing, 11*(6), 301–304.

Bedell, C. M. (2003a). A changing paradigm for cancer treatment: The advent of new oral chemotherapy agents. *Clinical Journal of Oncology Nursing, 7*(6 Suppl), 5–9.

Birner, A. (2003). Pharmacology of oral chemotherapy agents. *Clinical Journal of Oncology Nursing, 7*(6 Suppl), 11–19.

Flemm, L. A. (2004). Aprepitant for chemotherapy-induced nausea and vomiting. *Clinical Journal of Oncology Nursing, 8*(3), 303–306.

Green, J. M. & Hacker, E. D. (2004). Chemotherapy in the geriatric population. *Clinical Journal of Oncology Nursing, 8*(6), 591–597.

Griffin, E. (2003). Safety considerations and safe handling of oral chemotherapy agents. *Clinical Journal of Oncology Nursing, 7*(6 Suppl), 25–29.

Harris, D. J. & Knobf, M. T. (2004). Assessing and managing chemotherapy-induced mucositis pain. *Clinical Journal of Oncology Nursing, 8*(6), 622–628.

Marek, C. (2003). Antiemetic therapy in patients receiving cancer chemotherapy. *Oncology Nursing Forum, 30*(2), 259–269.

Rittenberg, C. N. (2004). The next generation of chemotherapy-induced nausea and vomiting prevention and control: A new 5-HT3 antagonist arrives. *Clinical Journal of Oncology Nursing,* 8(3), 307–308.

Sadler, G. R., Stoudt, A., Fullerton, J. T., et al. (2003). Managing the oral sequelae of cancer therapy. *MedSurg Nursing, 12*(1), 28–36.

Sorich, J., Taubes, B., Wagner, A., et al. (2004). Oxaliplatin: Practical guidelines for administration. *Clinical Journal of Oncology Nursing, 8*(3), 251–256.

Spielberger, R., Stiff, P., Bensinger, W. et al. (2004). Palifermin for oral mucositis after intensive therapy for hematologic cancers. *New England Journal of Medicine, 351*(25), 2590–2598.

Oncologic Emergencies

Abrahm, J. L. (2004). Assessment and treatment of patients with spinal cord compression. *Journal of Supportive Oncology, 2*(5), 377–401.

Cantril, C. A. & Haylock, P. J. (2004). Tumor lysis syndrome. *American Journal of Nursing, 104*(4), 49–52.

Cope, D. (2004). Tumor lysis syndrome. *Clinical Journal of Oncology Nursing, 8*(4), 415–416.

Flounders, J. A. (2003a). Cardiovascular emergencies: Pericardial effusion and cardiac tamponade. *Oncology Nursing Forum, 30*(2), E48–E55.

Flounders, J. A. (2003b). Superior vena cava syndrome. [Online exclusive.] *Oncology Nursing Forum, 30*(4), E84–E90.

Flounders, J. A. (2003c). Syndrome of inappropriate antidiuretic hormone. *Oncology Nursing Forum, 30*(3), E63–E68.

Flounders, J. A. & Ott, B. B. (2003). Oncologic emergency modules: Spinal cord compression. [Online exclusive.] *Oncology Nursing Forum, 30*(1), E17–E23.

Krimmel, T. (2003). Disseminated intravascular coagulation. *Clinical Journal of Oncology Nursing, 7*(4), 479.

Langfeldt, L. A. & Cooley, M. E. (2003). Syndrome of inappropriate antidiuretic hormone secretion in malignancy: Review and implications for nursing management. *Clinical Journal of Oncology Nursing, 7*(4), 425–430.

Shuey, K. M. (2004). Hypercalcemia of malignancy: Part I. *Clinical Journal of Oncology Nursing, 8*(2), 209–210.

Shuey, K. M. & Brant, J., M. (2004). Hypercalcemia of malignancy: Part II. *Clinical Journal of Oncology Nursing, 8*(3), 321–323.

Viale, P. H. & Yamamoto, D. S. (2003). Biphosphonates: Expanded roles in the treatment of patients with cancer. *Clinical Journal of Oncology Nursing, 7*(4), 393–401.

Radiation Therapy

Abel, L., Dafoe-Lambie, J., Butler, W. M., et al. (2003). Treatment outcomes and quality-of-life issues for patients treated with prostate brachytherapy. *Clinical Journal of Oncology Nursing, 7*(1), 48–54.

Estes, J. M. & Clapp, K. J. (2004). Radioimmunotherapy with tositumomab and iodine-131 tositumomab for low-grade non-Hodgkin lymphoma: Nursing implications. *Oncology Nursing Forum, 31*(6), 1119–1126.

Hogle, W. P., Quinn, A. E., & Heron, D. E. (2003). Advances in brachytherapy: New approaches to target breast cancer. *Clinical Journal of Oncology Nursing, 7*(3), 324–328.

Iwamoto, R. R., & Maher, K. E. (2001). Radiation therapy for prostate cancer. *Seminars in Oncology Nursing, 17*(2), 90–100.

Stajduhar, K. I., Neithercut, J., Chu, E., et al. (2000). Thyroid cancer patients' experiences of receiving iodine-131 therapy. *Oncology Nursing Forum, 27*(8), 1213–1218.

Wickline, M. M. (2004). Prevention and treatment of acute radiation dermatitis: A literature review. *Oncology Nursing Forum, 31*(2), 237–244.

Witt, M. E., Haas, M., Marrinan, M. A., et al. (2003). Understanding stereotactic radiosurgery for intracranial tumors; seed implants for prostate cancer; and intravascular brachytherapy for cardiac restenosis. *Cancer Nursing, 26*(6), 494–502.

Targeted Therapies

Bedell, C. M. (2003b). Pegfilgrastin for chemotherapy-induced neutropenia. *Clinical Journal of Oncology Nursing, 7*(1), 55–58.

Breed, C. D. (2003). Diagnosis, treatment and nursing care of patients with chronic leukemia. *Seminars in Oncology Nursing, 19*(3), 109–117.

Capo, G. & Waltzman, R. (2004). Managing hematologic toxicities. *Journal of Supportive Oncology, 2*(1), 65–77.

Cappozzo, C. (2004). Optimal use of granulocyte-colony stimulating factor in patients with cancer who are at risk for chemotherapy-induced neutropenia. *Oncology Nursing Forum, 31*(3), 569–574.

Capriotti, T. (2004). New oncology strategy: Molecular targeting of cancer cells. *MedSurg Nursing,* 13(3), 191–195.

Colson, K., Doss, D. S., Swift, R., et al. (2004). Bortezomib, a newly approved proteasome inhibitor for the treatment of multiple myeloma: Nursing implications. *Clinical Journal of Oncology Nursing, 8*(5), 473–480.

Gale, D. M. (2003). Molecular targets in cancer therapy. *Seminars in Oncology Nursing, 19*(2), 193–205.

Galsky, M. & Kelly, W. K. (2003). The development of differentiation agents for the treatment of prostate cancer. *Seminars in Oncology, 30*(5), 689–697.

Gemmill, R. & Idell, C. S. (2003). Biological advances for new treatment approaches. *Seminars in Oncology Nursing, 19*(2), 162–168.

King, S. E. (2004). Therapeutic cancer vaccines: An emerging treatment option. *Clinical Journal of Oncology Nursing, 8*(3), 271–278.

Kristal, A. R. (2004). Vitamin A, retinoids and carotenoids as chemoprevention agents for prostate cancer. *Journal of Urology, 17*(2, part 2 of 2), S54–S58.

Krozely, P. (2004). Epidermal growth factor receptor tyrosine kinase inhibitors: Evolving role of the treatment of solid tumors. *Clinical Journal of Oncology Nursing, 8*(2), 163–168.

Lui, K. (2003). Breakthroughs in cancer gene therapy. *Seminars in Oncology Nursing, 19*(2), 217–226.

Schmidt, K. V. & Wood, B. A. (2003). Trends in cancer therapy: Role of monoclonal antibodies. *Seminars in Oncology Nursing, 19*(2), 169–179.

Stull, D. M. (2003). Targeted therapies for treatment of leukemia. *Seminars in Oncology Nursing, 19*(2), 90–97.

Yarbro, C. H. (Ed.). (2004). Yttrium 90 ibritumamab tiuxetan (Zevalin) radioimmunotherapy for B-cell non-Hodgkin's lymphoma. *Seminars in Oncology Nursing, 20*(1 Suppl 1), 1–25.

RESOURCES

PROFESSIONAL ORGANIZATIONS

American Society of Clinical Oncology (ASCO), 1900 Duke Street, Suite 200, Alexandria, VA 22314; 703-299-0150, fax 703-299-1044; http://www.asco.org. Accessed March 15, 2006.

National Comprehensive Cancer Network, 500 Old York Road, Suite 250, Jenkintown, PA 9046; 215-690-0360, fax 215-728-3877, 888-909-NCCN, 888-909-6226; http://www.nccn.org. Accessed March 15, 2006.

Oncology Nursing Society (ONS), 125 Enterprise Drive, RIDC Part West, Pittsburgh, PA 15275-1214; 866-257-4ONS, fax 877-369-5497; http://www.ons.org. Accessed March 15, 2006.

PATIENT/FAMILY SUPPORT AND EDUCATION

American Brain Tumor Association, 2720 River Road, Des Plaines, IL 60018; 800-886-2282, fax 847-827-9918, Patient line: 800-886-2282; http://www.abta.org. Accessed March 15, 2006.

American Cancer Society. ACS), 800-ACS-2345 (check your local directory for the unit of division nearest you); http://www.cancer.org. Accessed March 15, 2006.

Cancer Care, Inc., National Office, 275 Seventh Ave., New York, NY 10001; Services: 212-302-2400, 800-813-HOPE (×4673); http://www.cancercare.org. Accessed March 15, 2006.

Make Today Count, 1235 East Cherokee Street, Springfield, MO 85804; 407-885-3324 or 800-432-2273.

The National Cancer Institute, Building, 31, Room 10A31, 31 Center Drive, MSC 2580, Bethesda, MD 20892-2580; (800)-4-CANCER; http://www.nci.nih.gov. Accessed March 15, 2006.

National Coalition for Cancer Survivorship, 1010 Wayne Avenue, Suite 770, Silver Spring, MD 20910-5600; 301-650-9127 or 877-NCCS-YES (877-622-7937); fax: 301-565-9670; http://www.canceradvocacy.org. Accessed March 15, 2006.

The National Hospice and Palliative Care Organization, 1700 Diagonal Road, Suite 300, Alexandria, VA 22314; 703-837-1500; http://www.nhpco.org. Accessed March 15, 2006.

Oncolink, the University of Pennsylvania Cancer Center, 3400 Spruce St., Philadelphia, PA 19104; http://www.oncolink.upenn.edu. Accessed March 15, 2006.

The Wellness Community, 919 18th Street NW, Suite 54, Washington, DC 2006, 202-659-9709, fax 202-659-9801, 888-793-WELL; http://www.wellness-community.org. Accessed March 15, 2006.

CHAPTER 17

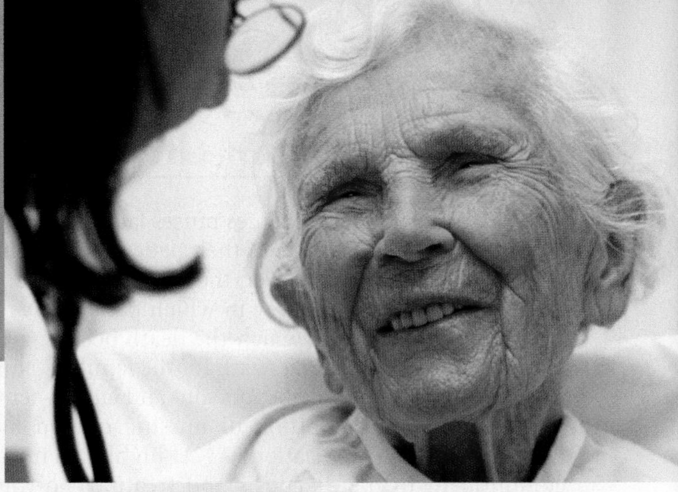

End-of-Life Care

Learning Objectives

On completion of this chapter, the learner will be able to:

1. Discuss the historical, legal, and sociocultural perspectives of palliative and end-of-life care in the United States.
2. Define palliative care.
3. Compare and contrast the settings where palliative care and end-of-life care are provided.
4. Describe the principles and components of hospice care.
5. Identify barriers to improving care at the end of life.
6. Reflect on personal experience with and attitudes toward death and dying.
7. Apply skills for communicating with terminally ill patients and their families.
8. Provide culturally and spiritually sensitive care to terminally ill patients and their families.
9. Implement nursing measures to manage physiologic responses to terminal illness.
10. Support actively dying patients and their families.
11. Identify components of uncomplicated grief and mourning and implement nursing measures to support patients and families.

Nursing and End-of-Life Care

One of the most difficult realities nurses face is that, despite their very best efforts, some of their patients die. Although nurses cannot change this fact, they can have a significant and lasting effect on the way in which patients live until they die, the manner in which the death occurs, and the enduring memories of that death for the families. Nursing has a long history of holistic, person- and family-centered care. Indeed, the definition of nursing offered by the American Nurses Association (ANA) highlights nursing's commitment to the diagnosis and treatment of human responses to illness (ANA, 2003). There is perhaps no setting or circumstance in which nursing care—that is, attention to human responses—is more important than in caring for dying patients.

Knowledge about end-of-life decisions and principles of care is essential to supporting patients during decision making and in end-of-life closure in ways that recognize patients' unique responses to illness and that support their values and goals. Education, clinical practice, and research concerning end-of-life care are evolving, and the need to prepare nurses and other health care professionals to care for the dying has emerged as a priority. At no time in nursing's history has there been a greater opportunity to bring research, education, and practice together to change the culture of dying, bringing much-needed improvement to care that is relevant across practice settings, age groups, cultural backgrounds, and illnesses. The National Institute for Nursing Research has taken the lead in coordinating research related to end-of-life care within the National Institutes of Health and has included end-of-life care in its strategic plan for the 21st century (see Resources).

The Context of Death and Dying in America

In the past three to four decades, there has been a surge of interest in the care of the dying, with an emphasis on the settings in which death occurs, the technologies used to sustain life, and the challenges of trying to improve end-of-life care. The focus on care of the dying has been motivated by the aging of the population, the prevalence of and publicity surrounding life-threatening illnesses such as cancer and acquired immunodeficiency syndrome (AIDS), and the efforts of health care providers to build a continuum of service that spans the lifetime from birth until death (Jennings, Ryndes, D'Onofrio, et al., 2003). Although there are more opportunities than ever before to allow peaceful death, the knowledge and technologies available to health care providers have made the process of dying anything but peaceful. According to Callahan (1993), Americans view death as what happens when medicine fails, and this attitude often places the study of death and improvement of the dying process outside the focus of modern medicine and health care. Numerous initiatives aimed at improving end-of-life care have been launched in recent years, spurred by a widespread call for substantive change in the way Americans deal with death.

The Palliative Care Task Force of the Last Acts Campaign (Last Acts, 1997) identified the following as precepts or principles underlying a more comprehensive and humane approach to care of the dying:

- Respecting patients' goals, preferences, and choices
- Attending to the medical, emotional, social, and spiritual needs of dying people

Glossary

assisted suicide: use of pharmacologic agents to hasten the death of a terminally ill patient; illegal in most states

autonomy: self-determination; in the health care context, the right of the individual to make choices about the use and discontinuation of medical treatment

bereavement: period during which mourning for a loss takes place

euthanasia: Greek for "good death;" has evolved to mean the intentional killing by act or omission of a dependent human being for his or her alleged benefit

grief: the personal feelings that accompany an anticipated or actual loss

hospice: a coordinated program of interdisciplinary care and services provided primarily in the home to terminally ill patients and their families

interdisciplinary collaboration: communication and cooperation among members of diverse health care disciplines jointly to plan, implement, and evaluate care

Medicare Hospice Benefit: a Medicare entitlement that provides for comprehensive, interdisciplinary palliative care and services for eligible beneficiaries who have a terminal illness and a life expectancy of less than 6 months

mourning: individual, family, group, and cultural expressions of grief and associated behaviors

palliative care: comprehensive care for patients whose disease is not responsive to cure; care also extends to patients' families

palliative sedation: use of pharmacologic agents, at the request of the terminally ill patient, to induce sedation when symptoms have not responded to other management measures. The purpose is not to hasten the patient's death but to relieve intractable symptoms.

spirituality: personal belief systems that focus on a search for meaning and purpose in life, intangible elements that impart meaning and vitality to life, and a connectedness to a higher or transcendent dimension

terminal illness: progressive, irreversible illness that despite cure-focused medical treatment will result in the patient's death

- Using strengths of interdisciplinary resources
- Acknowledging and addressing caregiver concerns
- Building mechanisms and systems of support

Technology and End-of-Life Care

In the last century, chronic, degenerative diseases replaced communicable diseases as the major causes of death. Although technologic advances in health care have extended and improved the quality of life for many people, the ability of technologies to prolong life beyond the point that some people would consider meaningful has raised troubling ethical issues. In particular, the use of technology to sustain life has raised perplexing issues with regard to quality of life, prolongation of dying, adequacy of pain relief and symptom management, and allocation of scarce resources. The major ethical question that has emerged concerning the use of technology to extend life is this: Because medical professionals can prolong life through a particular intervention, does it necessarily follow that they must do so? In the latter half of the 20th century, a "technologic imperative" practice pattern among health care professionals emerged, along with an expectation among patients and families that every available means to extend life must be tried.

Decisions to apply every available technology to extend life have contributed to the shift in the place of death from the home to the hospital or extended care facility. In the earlier part of the 20th century, most deaths occurred at home. Because of this, most families had direct experience with death, providing care to family members at the end of life, and mourning for the loss of loved ones. As the place of death shifted to hospitals, families became increasingly distanced from the death experience. By the early 1970s, when hospice care was just beginning in this country, technology had become the expected companion of the critically and terminally ill (Waller & Caroline, 2000). The implications of technologic intervention at the end of life continue to be profound, affecting a societal view of death that influences how clinicians care for the dying, how family and friends participate in care, how patients and families understand and choose among end-of-life care options, how families prepare for **terminal illness** and death, and how they heal after the death of a loved one.

Sociocultural Context

Although each person experiences terminal illness uniquely, such illness is also shaped substantially by the social and cultural contexts in which it occurs. In the United States, life-threatening illness, life-sustaining treatment decisions, dying, and death occur in a social environment in which illness is largely considered a foe and battles are either lost or won (Benoliel, 1993). A care/cure dichotomy has emerged, in which health care providers may view cure as the ultimate good and care as second best, a good only when cure is no longer possible. In such a model of health or medical care, alleviating suffering is not as valued as curing disease, and patients who cannot be cured feel distanced from the health care team, concluding that, when treatment has failed, they too have failed. Patients and families who have internalized the socially constructed meaning of care as second-best may fear that any shift from curative goals in the direction of comfort-focused care will result in no care or lower-quality care, and that the clinicians on whom they have come to rely will abandon them if they withdraw from the battle for cure.

The reduction of patients to their diseases is exemplified in the frequently relayed message in late-stage illness that "nothing more can be done." This all-too-frequently used statement communicates the belief of many clinicians that there is nothing of value to offer patients who are beyond cure. In a care-focused perspective, mind, body, and spirit are inextricable, and treating the body without attending to the other components is considered inadequate to evoke true healing. This expanded notion of healing as care, along with and beyond cure, implies that healing can take place throughout life and outside the boundaries of contemporary medicine. In this expanded definition, there continue to be opportunities for physical, spiritual, emotional, and social healing, even as body systems begin to fail at the end of life.

Clinicians' Attitudes Toward Death

Clinicians' attitudes toward the terminally ill and dying remain the greatest barrier to improving care at the end of life. Kübler-Ross illuminated the concerns of the seriously ill and dying in her seminal work, *On Death and Dying*, published in 1969. At that time, it was common for patients to be kept uninformed about life-threatening diagnoses, particularly cancer, and for physicians and nurses to avoid open discussion of death and dying with their patients (Krisman-Scott, 2000). Kübler-Ross taught the health care community that having open discussion about life and death issues did not harm patients, and that the patients in fact welcomed such openness. She was plainly critical of what she called "a new but depersonalized science in the service of prolonging life rather than diminishing human suffering" (Kübler-Ross, 1969). She taught the health care community that healing could not take place in a conspiracy of silence, and that as clinicians break the silence and enter the patient's world, they too can be healed by their struggles and strengths. Her work revealed that, given adequate time and some help in working through the process, patients could reach a stage of acceptance in which they were neither angry nor depressed about their fate (Kübler-Ross, 1969).

Clinicians' reluctance to discuss disease and death openly with patients stems from their own anxieties about death as well as misconceptions about what and how much patients want to know about their illnesses. In an early study of care of the dying in hospital settings, sociologists Glaser and Strauss (1965) discovered that health care professionals in hospital settings avoided direct communication about dying in hopes that the patient would discover it on his or her own. They identified four "awareness contexts," described as the patient's, physician's, family's, and other health care professionals' awareness of the patient's status and their recognition of each other's awareness (Glaser & Strauss, 1965):

1. *Closed awareness:* The patient is unaware of his or her terminal state, whereas others are aware. Closed awareness may be characterized as a conspiracy between the family and health care professionals to guard the "secret," fearing that the patient not be able to cope with full disclosure about his or her status, and the patient's

acceptance of others' accounts of his or her "future biography" as long as the others give him or her no reason to be suspicious.
2. *Suspected awareness:* The patient suspects what others know and attempts to find out details about his or her condition. Suspected awareness may be triggered by inconsistencies in the family's and the clinician's communication and behavior, discrepancies between clinicians' accounts of the seriousness of the patient's illness, or a decline in the patient's condition or other environmental cues.
3. *Mutual pretense awareness:* The patient, the family, and the health care professionals are aware that the patient is dying but all pretend otherwise.
4. *Open awareness:* The patient, the family, and the health care professionals are aware that the patient is dying and openly acknowledge that reality.

Glaser and Strauss (1965) also identified a pattern of clinician behavior in which those clinicians who feared or were uncomfortable discussing death developed and substituted "personal mythologies" for appraisals of what level of disclosure patients actually wanted. For example, clinicians avoided direct communication with patients about the seriousness of their illness based on their beliefs that (1) patients already knew the truth or would ask if they wanted to know, or (2) patients would subsequently lose all hope, give up, or be psychologically harmed by disclosure.

Glaser and Strauss' findings were published more than 40 years ago, yet their observations remain valid today. Although a growing number of health care providers are becoming comfortable with assessing patients' and families' information needs and disclosing honest information about the seriousness of illness, many still avoid the topic of death in hopes that the patient will ask or find out on his or her own. Despite progress on many health care fronts, those who work with dying patients have identified the persistence of a "conspiracy of silence" about dying (Stanley, 2000, p. 34).

Patient and Family Denial

Denial on the part of the patient and family about the seriousness of terminal illness also has been cited as a barrier to discussion about end-of-life treatment options. Kübler-Ross (1969) was one of the first to examine patient denial and expose it as a useful coping mechanism that enables the patient to gain temporary emotional distance from something that is too painful to contemplate fully. Patients who are characterized as being in denial may be using that strategy to preserve important interpersonal relationships, to protect others from the emotional effects of their illness, or to protect themselves because of fears of abandonment.

Connor (1992) studied a small group of terminally ill cancer patients who were characterized by their use of denial as a coping mechanism. Participants in the experimental group were questioned in structured interviews about their perceptions of the most difficult aspects of having cancer and those actions that they or others take that make these difficulties easier or more difficult to bear. They were offered psychosocial intervention that consisted largely of therapeutic communication followed by a postintervention assessment of their use of denial as a defense mechanism. The use of denial by patients in a control group was also assessed, but these patients did not receive the psychosocial intervention. The researcher concluded that terminally ill patients using denial respond favorably to sensitive psychosocial intervention, as indicated by decreased scores on an instrument to measure denial. However, Connor acknowledged the need for additional research to gauge the timing of such interventions according to some measure of patient readiness.

In a more recent study, researchers reported that, although the majority of a sample of 200 patients with advanced cancer were completely aware of their medical prognosis in their final weeks of life, 26.5% were either unaware or only partially aware (Chochinov, Tataryn, Wilson, et al., 2000). Depression was almost three times greater in patients who were unaware of their prognosis. The researchers concluded that patients with underlying psychological or emotional distress are more likely to deny their prognosis. Similarly, Chow and colleagues (2001) reported that many patients surveyed about their understanding of palliative radiation therapy for advanced cancer believed that their disease was curable, that the radiation therapy would cure their cancer, or that the therapy would prolong their lives. Importantly, most also reported that they were unfamiliar with the concept of radiation therapy, were not given information, or were not satisfied with the information their physicians had provided. Clearly, further research is needed to examine the complex interactions between patients' misconceptions about advanced illness, their underlying psychological states, and clinicians' persistent lack of explanations of treatment expectations and prognosis.

The question of how to communicate with patients in a way that acknowledges where they are on the continuum of acceptance, while providing them with unambiguous information, remains a challenge. Zerwekh (1994) analyzed stories from 32 hospice nurses and concluded that nurses in a hospice setting were adept at interventions deemed important in care of the dying, namely truth telling and encouraging patient **autonomy** (Chart 17-1). Although Zerwekh acknowledged that each person views "truth" differently, she observed that hospice nurses deliberately spoke about sensitive matters that were usually avoided and gave patients and families truthful representations of their status when patients were in transition from curative to palliative care. Timing of sensitive questions takes experience, but speaking the truth can be a relief to patients and families, enhancing their autonomy by making way for truly informed consent as the basis for decision making (Pitorak, 2003a).

Assisted Suicide

The assisted suicide debate has aimed a spotlight on the adequacy and quality of end-of-life care in the United States. **Assisted suicide** refers to providing another person the means to end his or her own life. Physician-assisted suicide involves the prescription by a physician of a lethal dose of medication for the purpose of ending someone's life (not to be confused with the ethically and legally supported practice of withholding or withdrawing medical treatment in accordance with the wishes of the terminally ill person).

CHART 17-1

Dying Person's Bill of Rights

- I have the right to be treated as a living human being until I die.
- I have the right to maintain a sense of hopefulness, however changing its focus may be.
- I have the right to be cared for by those who can maintain a sense of hopefulness, however changing this may be.
- I have the right to express my feelings and emotions and my approaching death in my own way.
- I have the right to participate in decisions concerning my care.
- I have the right to expect continuing medical and nursing attention, even though "cure" goals must be changed to "comfort" goals.
- I have the right not to die alone.
- I have the right to be free from pain.
- I have the right to have my questions answered honestly.
- I have the right not to be deceived.
- I have the right to have help from and for my family in accepting my death.
- I have the right to die in peace and dignity.
- I have the right to retain my individuality and not be judged by my decisions, which may be contrary to the beliefs of others.
- I have the right to discuss and enlarge my religious and/or spiritual experiences, regardless of what they mean to others.
- I have the right to expect that the sanctity of the human body will be respected after death.
- I have the right to be cared for by caring, sensitive, knowledgeable people who will attempt to understand my needs and will be able to gain some satisfaction in helping me face my death.

Although the preference to take one's own life instead of awaiting death has been evident through the ages, these recent efforts to legalize assisted suicide underscore the need for changes in the ways people with terminal illnesses are cared for and treated at the end of their lives. This is further emphasized by the efforts of groups such as the Hemlock Society to have physician-assisted suicide legalized and the Hemlock Society's publication of information describing methods for ending one's own life when such assistance from a physician is not available.

Although assisted suicide is expressly prohibited under statutory or common law in all states but Oregon, the calls for legalized assisted suicide have highlighted inadequacies in the care of the dying. In 1990, Dr. Jack Kevorkian, a retired pathologist, assisted a 54-year-old woman with early Alzheimer's disease to end her life using a device that allowed her to control the infusion of a lethal dose of potassium chloride. In 1999, after 130 deaths and nine trials, Kevorkian was convicted on second-degree murder charges in the death of a 52-year-old man with amyotrophic lateral sclerosis and received a 10- to 25-year prison sentence.

Meanwhile, public support for physician-assisted suicide has resulted in a number of state ballot initiatives. In 1994, Oregon voters approved the Oregon Death With Dignity Act, the first—and to date, only—such legislative initiative to pass. This law provides for access to physician-assisted suicide by terminally ill patients under very controlled circumstances. After numerous challenges, a majority of Oregonians voted against an attempted repeal, and the law was enacted in 1997. The most recent challenges to the law, both unsuccessful, were the 1999 federal Pain Relief Promotion Act, a bill designed to derail the implementation of the Oregon law by prohibiting the use of federally controlled substances for physician-assisted suicide, and a 2001 directive from the U.S. Attorney General to the Drug Enforcement Agency to track and prosecute physicians who prescribe under the Oregon law. Oregon subsequently filed a lawsuit in 2001, and a U.S. district court issued a temporary restraining order against Attorney General Ashcroft's ruling. In 2002, the Death with Dignity Act was upheld in U.S. district court and Attorney General Ashcroft filed an appeal. The appeal was denied. After several additional requests by the Attorney General and denials, the U.S. Supreme Court affirmed the lower court's decision on January 6, 2006, allowing the Death with Dignity Act to remain in effect (Oregon Department of Human Services, 2006). Since 1997, the number of Oregonians who have self-administered physician-prescribed lethal medication has remained small, growing from 15 persons in 1999 to 42 persons in 2003, then decreasing to 37 in 2004 and 38 in 2005 (Oregon Department of Human Services, 2006).

Although Oregon is currently the only state with a statute legalizing physician-assisted suicide, it is likely that the issue will be pursued in the courts and through ballot measures in other states. Proponents of physician-assisted suicide argue that terminally ill people should have a legally sanctioned right to make independent decisions about the value of their lives and the timing and circumstances of their deaths, and its opponents argue for greater access to symptom management and psychosocial support for people approaching the end of life. Numerous ethical and legal issues have been raised, including voluntariness and authenticity of requests in relation to the mental competence and decision-making capacity of patients who request physician-assisted suicide, the existence of underlying untreated clinical depression or other suffering, and issues of overt or perceived coercion. Assisted suicide is opposed by nursing and medical organizations as a violation of the ethical traditions of nursing and medicine (Chart 17-2). The ANA Position Statement on Assisted Suicide acknowledges the complexity of the assisted suicide debate but clearly states that nursing participation in assisted suicide is a violation of the Code for Nurses. The ANA Position Statement further stresses the important role of the nurse in supporting effective symptom management, contributing to the creation of environments for care that honor the patient's and family's wishes, and ascertaining and addressing their concerns and fears (ANA, 1994).

CHART 17-2

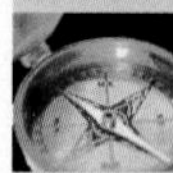

Ethics and Related Issues

"What If a Patient Asks You to Help Him End His Life?"

SITUATION

You are a hospice nurse visiting a coworker's patients. A 72-year-old man with end-stage congestive heart failure and dyspnea at rest has two-pillow orthopnea while receiving continuous oxygen at 4 L/min by nasal cannula. When compared to the findings reported in your colleague's notes from previous visits, the patient's condition appears to be declining. After you have completed your physical examination, you sit in a chair next to the patient's bed and ask him how he feels he is doing. He sighs and tells you that he thinks he is "getting close to the end" and will "soon be ready for that pill." When you inquire about the pill, the patient says that "John [the name of the usual hospice nurse] knows and is going to help, so don't worry." At this point, the patient says that he is tired and does not want to talk any more today.

DILEMMA

The patient's autonomy conflicts with the nurse's obligation to respect and protect human life, to promote comfort and relieve suffering, and to "do no harm."

DISCUSSION

1. What should your follow-up consist of?
2. Should you discuss the patient's request with his wife before you end the visit that day? Discuss the moral basis for your decision.
3. What is the position of the American Nurses Association (ANA) on assisted suicide, and how does the ANA position relate to your understanding of your moral obligation?
4. How should you follow up with John?
5. With another student, role play your discussion with John.
6. What would you do next if John will not discuss the patient's request with you?
7. Who are the other stakeholders in this situation, and what is your ethical responsibility to each?

Settings for End-of-Life Care: Palliative Care Programs and Hospice

Palliative Care

As concerns have grown about the poor quality of life patients experience during progressive illness, broadening of the concept of palliative care beyond the hospice has begun to take hold in health care settings across the country. **Palliative care** is an approach to care for the seriously ill that has long been a part of cancer care. Both palliative care and hospice care have been recognized as important bridges between a medical bias in the direction of cure-oriented treatment and the needs of the terminally ill patients and their families for comprehensive care in the final years, months, or weeks of life (Hallenbeck, 2003). Advocates for improved care for the dying have stated that acceptance, management, and understanding of death should become fully integrated concepts in mainstream health care. Increasingly, palliative care is being offered to patients with noncancer chronic illnesses, where comprehensive symptom management and psychosocial and spiritual support can enhance the patient's and family's quality of life.

Although hospice care is considered by many to be the "gold standard" for palliative care, the term **hospice** is generally associated with palliative care that is delivered at home or in special facilities to patients who are approaching the end of life. Palliative care is conceptually broader than hospice care, and is defined as the active, total care of patients whose disease is not responsive to treatment (World Health Organization, 1990). When palliative care coexists with disease-oriented treatment, patients and their families benefit from more comprehensive management of the illness experience (Abrahm, 2000).

Palliative care emphasizes management of psychological, social, and spiritual problems in addition to control of pain and other physical symptoms. As the definition suggests, palliative care is not care that begins when cure-focused treatment ends. The goal of palliative care is to improve the patient's and family's quality of life, and many aspects of this type of comprehensive, comfort-focused approach to care are applicable earlier in the process of life-threatening disease, in conjunction with cure-focused treatment. However, definitions of palliative care, the services that are part of it, and the clinicians who provide it are evolving steadily.

Some would argue that palliative care is no different from comprehensive nursing, medical, social, and spiritual care and that patients should not have to be labeled as "dying" to receive person-focused care and symptom management. In addition to a focus on the multiple dimensions of the illness experience for both patients and their families, palliative care emphasizes the interdisciplinary collaboration that is necessary to bring about the desired outcomes for patients and their families. **Interdisciplinary collaboration** is distinguished from multidisciplinary practice in that the former is based on communication and cooperation among the various disciplines, each member of the team contributing to a single integrated care plan that addresses the needs of the patient and family. Multidisciplinary care refers to participation of clinicians with varied backgrounds and skill sets but without coordination and integration.

Palliative Care at the End of Life

As previously discussed, palliative care is broadly conceptualized as comprehensive, person- and family-centered care when disease is not responsive to treatment. The broadening of the concept of palliative care actually followed the development of hospice services in the United States. Hospice care

NURSING RESEARCH PROFILE

Nurses' Responses to Their Patients' Requests for Assisted Dying

Schwarz, J. K. (2003). Understanding and responding to patients' requests for assistance in dying. *Journal of Nursing Scholarship, 35*(4), 377–384.

Purpose

Nurses have reported increasing numbers of requests from patients or their family members for assistance in dying. Little is known about how nurses have interpreted and responded to such requests. This study explored how nurses understand the meaning of being asked by people competent to make decisions for assistance in dying and how they determine what their response will be.

Design

The researcher used interpretive phenomenology to structure and carry out this qualitative study. The research question that guided the study was, "What is the nature of the experience of being asked to help someone die?" Participating nurses self-identified having had an experience when a competent patient asked them for help to die. Participants practiced in settings that included hospice ($n = 4$), with AIDS patients ($n = 3$), in critical care ($n = 2$), and with patients who had spinal cord injuries ($n = 1$). Nine of the 10 participants were interviewed in their homes, one was interviewed by telephone, and all but one received a follow-up interview to react to the researcher's analysis of the data. The researcher began each initial interview by asking the participant to tell her "about a time when a patient asked you for help in dying." As the researcher coded and re-coded interview transcripts, themes and subthemes were identified in the participants' stories.

Findings

The researcher identified four major themes: (1) being open to hear and hearing, (2) interpreting and responding to the meaning, (3) responding to persistent requests for assistance in dying, and (4) reflections. Nurses experienced considerable difficulty in dealing with requests. Few directly agreed or refused to participate in assisting patients to die. Instead, they responded by providing supportive end-of-life care and remaining present during difficult times. Participants described "unspoken understandings and covert agreements with family members and collusion with physician colleagues." The participants struggled with identifying a "reliable moral line" for providing palliative interventions that might intentionally or inadvertently hasten death.

Nursing Implications

Nurses who care for patients at the end of life witness considerable suffering among the patients and family members for whom they care. Often, they practice in settings in which they are isolated from immediate support from colleagues, such as in home hospice care. Nurses need time with supportive colleagues to reflect on their feelings about morally problematic situations and to determine an ethically and emotionally satisfactory resolution.

is in fact palliative care. The difference is that hospice care is associated with the end of life, and although it focuses on quality of life, hospice care by necessity usually includes realistic emotional, social, spiritual, and financial preparation for death. In the mid-1970s, when hospice care was introduced in the United States, it was more broadly conceived as care that addressed the entire person—physical, social, emotional, and spiritual—and was available to patients earlier in the process of life-threatening illness. After hospice care was recognized as a distinct program of services under Medicare in the early 1980s, organizations providing hospice care were able to receive Medicare reimbursement if they could demonstrate that the hospice program met the Medicare "conditions of participation," or regulations, for hospice providers.

Medicare reimbursement resulted in new rules for hospices, and it also defined when Medicare beneficiaries were able to use their **Medicare Hospice Benefit.** In most programs, the Medicare definitions for patient eligibility are used to guide all enrollment decisions. According to Medicare, the patient who wishes to use his or her Medicare Hospice Benefit must be certified by a physician as terminally ill, with a life expectancy of 6 months or less if the disease follows its natural course. Thus, hospice has come to be defined as care provided to terminally ill persons and their families in the last 6 months of the patient's life. Because of additional Medicare rules concerning completion of all cure-focused medical treatment before the Medicare Hospice Benefit may be accessed, many patients delay enrollment in hospice programs until very close to the end of life. Hospice programs are reaching out to patients with very advanced illness and seeking ways to provide them with hospice services while they are completing courses of treatment that many programs previously defined as "life-prolonging," such as certain types of chemotherapy.

The reasons for late referral to hospice and underuse of hospice services are complex. They include values and attitudes of health care providers, inadequate dissemination of existing knowledge about pain and symptom management, health care providers' difficulties in effectively communicating with terminally ill patients, insufficient attention to palliative care concepts in health care providers' education and training, and confusion about eligibility criteria for hospice services.

Hospices provide care for approximately 29% of patients who are eligible (National Hospice and Palliative Care Organization [NHPCO], 2003). For the most part, the remainder of terminally ill patients die in hospitals and long-term care facilities. It is clear that better care for the dying is urgently needed in hospitals, long-term care facilities, home care agencies, and outpatient settings. At the same time, many chronic diseases do not have a predictable "end stage" that fits hospice eligibility criteria, meaning that many patients die after a long, slow, and often painful decline, without the benefit of the coordinated palliative care that is unique to hospice programs. The palliative approach to care could benefit many more patients if it were available across care settings and earlier in the disease process. In an attempt to make this valuable approach to care more widely available, palliative care programs are being developed in other settings for patients who are either not eligible for hospice or who are "not ready" to enroll in a formal hospice program. As yet, there is no dedicated reimbursement to providers for palliative care services when they are delivered outside the hospice setting, making the sustainability of such programs challenging.

Palliative Care in the Hospital Setting

Since the advent of diagnosis-related groups (DRGs) as the basis for prospective payment for hospital services in the 1980s, hospitals have a financial incentive to transfer patients with terminal illnesses who are no longer in need of acute care to other settings, such as long-term care facilities and home, to receive care (Field & Cassel, 1997). Despite the economic and human costs associated with death in the hospital setting, as many as 50% of all deaths occur in acute care settings (Hogan, Lynn, Gabel, et al., 2000). The landmark Study to Understand Prognoses and Preferences for Outcomes and Risks of Treatments (SUPPORT Principal Investigators, 1995) documented troubling deficiencies in the care of the dying in hospital settings:

- Many patients received unwanted care at the end of life.
- Clinicians were not aware of patient preferences for life-sustaining treatment, even when preferences were documented in the clinical record.
- Pain was often poorly controlled at the end of life.
- Efforts to enhance communication were ineffective.

It is clear that many patients will continue to opt for hospital care or will by default find themselves in hospital settings at the end of life. Increasingly, hospitals are conducting system-wide assessments of end-of-life care practices and outcomes and are developing innovative models for delivering high-quality, person-centered care to patients approaching the end of life. Hospitals cite considerable financial barriers to providing high-quality palliative care in acute care settings (Cassel, Ludden & Moon, 2000). Public policy changes have been called for that would provide reimbursement to hospitals for care delivered via designated hospital-wide palliative care beds, clustered palliative care units, or palliative care consultation services in acute care settings.

Palliative Care in Long-Term Care Facilities

Although the total number of nursing home residents declined between 1985 and 1999, the number of residents older than 65 years of age has been increasing due to aging of the population (Federal Interagency Forum on Aging-Related Statistics, 2004). As a result, the likely place of death for a growing number of Americans after age 65 will be the long-term care facility. As many as one third of all Medicare beneficiaries who die in any given year spend all or part of their last year of life in a long-term care facility (Hogan et al., 2000). The trend favoring care of dying patients in long-term care facilities will continue as the population ages and as managed care payers pressure health care providers to minimize costs (Field & Cassel, 1997).

Yet residents of long-term care facilities typically have poor access to high-quality palliative care. Regulations that govern how care in these facilities is organized and reimbursed tend to emphasize restorative measures and serve as a disincentive to palliative care (Zerzan, Stearns & Hanson, 2000). Since 1986, home hospice programs have been permitted to enroll long-term care facility residents in hospice programs and to provide interdisciplinary services to residents who qualify for hospice care. However, The Office of the Inspector General (1997), an oversight arm of the federal government, has questioned whether such services are an unnecessary duplication of services already provided by long-term care facility staff. At the same time, long-term care facilities of all types are under increasing public pressure to improve care of the dying and are beginning to develop palliative care units or services; contract with home hospice programs to provide hospice care in the facilities; and educate staff, residents, and their families about pain and symptom management and end-of-life care.

Hospice Care

Hospice in the United States is not a place, but a concept of care in which the end of life is viewed as a developmental stage. The root of the word hospice is *hospes,* meaning "host." Historically, hospice referred to a shelter or way station for weary travelers on a pilgrimage. In the years that followed Kübler-Ross's groundbreaking work, the concept of hospice care as an alternative to depersonalized death in institutions began as a grassroots movement. Her work, and the development of the concept of hospice in England by Dr. Cicely Saunders, resulted in recognition of gaps in the existing system of care for the terminally ill (Amenta, 1986). Hospice care began in response to "noticeable gaps . . . (1) between treating the disease and treating the person, (2) between technological research and psychosocial support, and (3) between the general denial of the fact of death in our society and the acceptance of death by those who face it" (Wentzel, 1981, p. 11). According to Saunders, who founded the world-renowned St. Christopher's Hospice in London, the principles underlying hospice are as follows:

- Death must be accepted.
- The patient's total care is best managed by an interdisciplinary team whose members communicate regularly with each other.

- Pain and other symptoms of terminal illness must be managed.
- The patient and family should be viewed as a single unit of care.
- Home care of the dying is necessary.
- Bereavement care must be provided to family members.
- Research and education should be ongoing.

Hospice Care in the United States

Although the concept dates to ancient times, hospice as a way of caring for those at the end of life did not emerge in the United States until the 1960s (Hospice Association of America, 2002). The hospice movement in the United States is based on the belief that meaningful living is achievable during terminal illness and that it is best supported in the home, free from technologic interventions to prolong physiologic dying. After the first hospice in the United States was founded in 1974 in Connecticut, the concept quickly spread, and the number of hospice programs in the United States increased dramatically. In the years between 1984 and 1996, after the creation of the Medicare Hospice Benefit, there was a 73-fold increase in the number of hospices participating in Medicare (Hospice Association of America, 2002). By 2003, there were 3300 hospice programs in operation, serving almost 1 million patients (NHPCO, 2003).

Despite more than 30 years of existence in the United States, hospice remains an option for end-of-life care that has not been fully integrated into mainstream health care. Although hospice care is available to people with any life-limiting condition, it has primarily been used by patients with advanced cancer, in which the disease staging and trajectory lend themselves to more reliable prediction about the end of life (Boling & Lynn, 1998; Christakis & Lamont, 2000). Many reasons have been suggested to explain the reluctance of physicians to refer patients to hospice and the reluctance of patients to accept this form of care. These include the difficulties in making a terminal prognosis, the strong association of hospice with death, advances in "curative" treatment options in late-stage illness, and financial pressures on health care providers that may cause them to retain rather than refer hospice-eligible patients. The result is that patients who could benefit from the comprehensive, interdisciplinary support offered by hospice programs frequently do not enter hospice care until their final days (or hours) of life (Christakis & Lamont, 2000).

Hospice is a coordinated program of interdisciplinary services provided by professional caregivers and trained volunteers to patients with serious, progressive illnesses that are not responsive to cure. In hospice settings, the patient and family make up the unit of care. The goal of hospice care is to enable the patient to remain at home, surrounded by the people and objects that have been important to him or her throughout life. Hospice care does not seek to hasten death, nor does it encourage the prolongation of life through artificial means. Hospice care hinges on the competent patient's full or "open" awareness of dying; it embraces a realism about death and helps patients and families understand the dying process so that they can live each moment as fully as possible.

Although most hospice care is provided in the patient's own home, some hospice programs have developed inpatient facilities or residences where terminally ill patients without family support and those who desire inpatient care may receive hospice services.

Eligibility criteria for hospice vary depending on the hospice program, but generally patients must have a progressive, irreversible illness and limited life expectancy and must have opted for palliative care rather than cure-focused treatment. Although hospices have historically served cancer patients, patients with any life-limiting illness are eligible.

Medicare Hospice Benefit

In 1983, the Medicare Hospice Benefit was implemented to cover hospice care for Medicare beneficiaries. State Medical Assistance (Medicaid) also provides coverage for hospice care, as do most commercial insurers. Federal reimbursement for hospice care ushered in a new era in hospice, in which program standards developed and published by the federal government codified what had formerly been a grassroots, loosely organized, and somewhat undefined ideal for care at the end of life. To receive Medicare dollars for hospice services, programs are required to comply with conditions of participation promulgated by the Centers for Medicare and Medicaid Services. In many aspects, Medicare standards have come to largely define hospice philosophy and services.

Eligibility criteria for hospice coverage under the Medicare Hospice Benefit are presented in Chart 17-3. Federal rules for hospices require that patients' eligibility be reviewed

CHART 17-3

Eligibility Criteria for Hospice Care

GENERAL

- Serious, progressive illness
- Limited life expectancy
- Informed choice of palliative care over cure-focused treatment

HOSPICE-SPECIFIC

- Presence of a family member or other caregiver continuously in the home when the patient is no longer able to safely care for him/herself (some hospices have created special services within their programs for patients who live alone, but this varies widely)

MEDICARE AND MEDICAID HOSPICE BENEFITS

- Medicare Part A; Medical Assistance eligibility
- Waiver of traditional Medicare/Medicaid benefits for the terminal illness
- Life expectancy of 6 months or less
- Physician certification of terminal illness
- Care must be provided by a Medicare-certified hospice program

periodically. There is no limit to the length of time that eligible patients may continue to receive hospice care. Patients who live longer than 6 months under hospice care are not discharged if their physician and the hospice medical director continue to certify that the patient is terminally ill with a life expectancy of 6 months or less, assuming that the disease continues its expected course. The hospice certification and review process and the open-ended benefit structure are intended to address the difficulty physicians face in predicting how long a patient will live, so that patients are not restricted to a lifetime limit on the number of hospice days they may receive.

To use hospice benefits under Medicare or Medicaid, patients must meet eligibility criteria and "elect" to use the hospice benefit in place of traditional Medicare or Medicaid benefits for the terminal illness. Once a patient elects the benefit, the Medicare-certified hospice program assumes responsibility for providing and paying for the care and treatment related to the underlying illness for which hospice care was elected. The Medicare-certified hospice is paid a predetermined dollar amount for each day of hospice care each patient receives. Four levels of hospice care are covered under Medicare and Medicaid hospice benefits:

- *Routine home care:* All services provided are included in the daily rate to the hospice.
- *Inpatient respite care:* A 5-day inpatient stay, provided on an occasional basis to relieve the family caregivers.
- *Continuous care:* Continuous nursing care is provided in the home for management of a medical crisis. Care reverts to the routine home care level after the crisis is resolved. (For example, seizure activity develops, and a nurse is placed in the home continuously to monitor the patient and administer medications. After 72 hours, the seizure activity is under control, the family has been instructed how to care for the patient, and the continuous nursing care is stopped.)
- *General inpatient care:* Inpatient stay for symptom management that cannot be provided in the home. This is not subject to the guidelines for a standard hospital inpatient stay.

Most hospice care is provided at the "routine home care" level and includes the services depicted in Chart 17-4. According to federal guidelines, hospices may provide no more than 20% of the aggregate annual patient days at the inpatient level. Patients may "revoke" their hospice benefits at any time, resuming traditional coverage under Medicare or Medicaid for the terminal illness. They may also reelect to use their hospice benefits at a later time after reassessment for eligibility according to these criteria.

The Medicare Act of 2003 included new provisions for the coverage of hospice services. Effective January 1, 2004, the cost of a consultation visit with the hospice medical director or physicians employed by a hospice are now covered by Medicare. The consultation visit can be provided for pain and symptom management or for counseling regarding end-of-life care options and advance care planning. This provision allows hospice programs to extend their expertise to patients who are terminally ill but have not yet enrolled in a hospice program.

CHART 17-4

Home Hospice Services Covered Under the Medicare / Medicaid Hospice Benefit Routine Home Care Level

- Nursing care provided by or under the supervision of a registered nurse, available 24 hours a day
- Medical social services
- Physician's services
- Counseling services, including dietary counseling
- Home health aide/homemaker
- Physical/occupational/speech therapists
- Volunteers
- Bereavement follow-up (for up to 13 months after the death of the patient)
- Medical supplies for the palliation of the terminal illness
- Medical equipment for the palliation of the terminal illness
- Medications for the palliation of the terminal illness

Nursing Care of Terminally Ill Patients

Many patients suffer unnecessarily when they do not receive adequate attention for the symptoms accompanying serious illness. Careful evaluation of the patient should include not only the physical problems but also the psychosocial and spiritual dimensions of the patient's and family's experience of serious illness. This approach contributes to a more comprehensive understanding of how the patient's and family's life has been affected by illness and leads to nursing care that addresses the needs in every dimension.

Psychosocial Issues

Nurses are responsible for educating patients about the possibilities and probabilities inherent in their illness and their life with the illness, and for supporting them as they conduct life review, values clarification, treatment decision making, and end-of-life closure. The only way to do this effectively is to try to appreciate and understand the illness from the patient's perspective.

Kübler-Ross's (1969) work revealed that patients in the final stages of life can and will talk openly about their experiences, exposing as a myth the view that patients are harmed by honest discussion with their caregivers about death. Despite the continued reluctance of health care providers to engage in open discussion about end-of-life issues, studies have confirmed that patients want information about their illness and end-of-life choices and that they are not harmed by open discussion about death (Bailey, 2003).

At the same time, nurses should be both culturally aware and sensitive in their approaches to communication with patients and families about death. Attitudes toward open disclosure about terminal illness vary widely among different cultures, and direct communication with patients about such matters may be viewed as harmful (Blackhall, Murphy, Frank, et al., 1995). To provide effective patient- and family-centered care at the end of life, nurses must be willing to set aside their own assumptions and attitudes so that they can discover what type and amount of disclosure is most meaningful to each patient and family within their unique belief systems.

The social and legal evolution of advance directive documents represents some progress in people's willingness to both contemplate and communicate their wishes surrounding the end of life (Chart 17-5). Now legally sanctioned in every state and federally sanctioned through the Patient Self-Determination Act of 1990, advance directives are written documents that allow competent people to document their preferences regarding the use or nonuse of medical treatment at the end of life, specify their preferred setting for care, and communicate other valuable insights into their values and beliefs. The addition of a proxy directive (the appointment and authorization of another person to make medical decisions on behalf of the person who created the advance directive when he or she can no longer speak for himself or herself) is an important addition to the "living will" or medical directive that specifies the signer's preferences. Although these documents are widely available from health care providers, community organizations, bookstores, and the Internet, their underuse reflects society's continued discomfort with openly confronting the subject of death. Furthermore, the existence of a properly executed advance directive does not reduce the complexity of end-of-life decisions. The advance directive should not be considered a substitute for ongoing communication among the health care provider, patient, and family as the end of life approaches (Wenger & Rosenfeld, 2001).

CHART 17-5

Methods of Stating End-of-Life Preferences

Advance directives—written documents that allow the individual of sound mind to document preferences regarding end-of-life care that should be followed when the signer is terminally ill and unable to verbally communicate his/her wishes. The documents are generally completed in advance of serious illness, but may be completed after a diagnosis of serious illness if the signer is still of sound mind. The most common types are the durable power of attorney for health care and the living will.

Durable power of attorney for health care—a legal document through which the signer appoints and authorizes another individual to make medical decisions on his/her behalf when he/she is no longer able to speak for him/herself. This is also known as a health care power of attorney or a proxy directive.

Living will—a type of advance directive in which the individual documents treatment preferences. It provides instructions for care in the event that the signer is terminally ill and not able to communicate his/her wishes directly and often is accompanied by a durable power of attorney for health care. This is also known as a medical directive or treatment directive.

Information about the advance care planning and state-specific advance directive documents and instructions are available at www.caringinfo.org.

Communication

As previously discussed, remarkable strides have been made in the ability to prolong life, but attention to care for the dying lags behind. On one level, this comes as no surprise. Each of us will eventually face death, and most would agree that one's own demise is a subject he or she would prefer not to contemplate. Indeed, Glaser and Strauss (1965) noted that unwillingness in our culture to talk about the process of dying is tied to our discomfort with the notion of particular deaths—those of our patients and our own—rather than death in the abstract. Finucane (2002) observed that our struggle to stay alive is a prerequisite to being human. Confronting death in our patients uncovers our own deeply rooted fears.

To develop a level of comfort and expertise in communicating with seriously and terminally ill patients and their families, nurses and other clinicians should first consider their own experiences with and values concerning illness and death. Reflection, reading, and talking with family members, friends, and colleagues can help nurses examine beliefs about death and dying. Talking with people from different cultural backgrounds can help nurses view personally held beliefs through a different lens and can help nurses become sensitive to death-related beliefs and practices in other cultures. Discussion with nursing and non-nursing colleagues can also be useful; it may reveal the values shared by many health care professionals and identify diversity in the values of patients in their care. Values clarification and personal death awareness exercises can provide a starting point for self-discovery and discussion.

Skills for Communicating With the Seriously Ill

Nurses need to develop skill and comfort in assessing patients' and families' responses to serious illness and planning interventions that will support their values and choices throughout the continuum of care. Patients and families need ongoing assistance: telling a patient something once is not teaching, and hearing the patient's words is not the same as active listening. Throughout the course of a serious illness, patients and their families encounter complicated treatment decisions, bad news about disease progression, and recurring emotional responses. In addition to the time of initial diagnosis, lack of response to the treatment course, decisions to continue or withdraw particular interventions, and decisions about hospice care are examples of critical points on the treatment continuum that demand patience, empathy, and honesty from nurses. Discussing sensitive issues such as serious illness, hopes for survival, and fears associated with death is never easy. However, the art of therapeutic communication can be learned and, like other skills, must be practiced to gain expertise. Similar to other skills, communication should be practiced in a "safe" setting, such as a classroom or clinical skills laboratory with other students or clinicians.

Although communication with each patient and family should be tailored to their particular level of understanding and values concerning disclosure, general guidelines for nurses include the following (Addington, 1991):

- Deliver and interpret the technical information necessary for making decisions without hiding behind medical terminology.
- Realize that the best time for the patient to talk may be when it is least convenient for you.
- Being fully present during any opportunity for communication is often the most helpful form of communication.
- Allow the patient and family to set the agenda regarding the depth of the conversation.

Nursing Interventions When Patients and Families Receive Bad News

Communicating about a life-threatening diagnosis or about disease progression is best accomplished by the interdisciplinary team in any setting: a physician, nurse, and social worker should be present whenever possible to provide information, facilitate discussion, and address concerns. Most importantly, the presence of the team conveys caring and respect for the patient and family. If the patient wishes to have family present for the discussion, arrangements should be made to have the discussion at a time that is best for everyone (Griffie, Nelson-Marten, & Muchka, 2004). Creating the right setting is particularly important. A quiet area with a minimum of disturbances should be used. All clinicians present should turn off beepers, cell phones, and other communication devices for the duration of the meeting and should allow sufficient time for the patient and family to absorb and respond to the news. Finally, the space in which the meeting takes place should be conducive to seating all participants at eye level. It is difficult enough for the patient and family to be the recipients of bad news without having an array of clinicians standing uncomfortably over them at the foot of the patient's bed.

After the initial discussion of a life-threatening illness or progression of a disease, the patient and family have many questions and may need to be reminded of factual information. Coping with news about a serious diagnosis or poor prognosis is an ongoing process. The nurse should be sensitive to these ongoing needs and may need to repeat previously provided information or simply be present while the patient and family react emotionally. The most important intervention the nurse can provide is listening empathetically. Seriously ill patients and their families need time and support to cope with the changes brought about by serious illness and the prospect of impending death. The nurse who is able to sit comfortably with another's suffering, time and time again, without judgment and without the need to solve the patient's and family's problems, provides an intervention that is a gift beyond measure. Keys to effective listening include the following:

- Resist the impulse to fill the "empty space" in communication with talk.
- Allow the patient and family sufficient time to reflect and respond after asking a question.
- Prompt gently: "Do you need more time to think about this?"
- Avoid distractions (noise, interruptions).
- Avoid the impulse to give advice.
- Avoid canned responses: "I know just how you feel."
- Ask questions.
- Assess understanding—your own and the patient's—by restating, summarizing, and reviewing.

Responding With Sensitivity to Difficult Questions

Patients often direct questions or concerns to nurses before they have been able to fully discuss the details of their diagnosis and prognosis with their physicians or the entire health care team. Using open-ended questions allows the nurse to elicit the patient's and family's concerns, explore misconceptions and needs for information, and form the basis for collaboration with physicians and other team members.

In one case, a seriously ill patient may ask the nurse, "Am I dying?" The nurse should avoid making unhelpful responses that dismiss the patient's real concerns or defer the issue to another care provider. Nursing assessment and intervention are always possible, even when a need for further discussion with a physician is clearly indicated. Whenever possible, discussions in response to a patient's concerns should occur when the patient expresses a need, although that may be the least convenient time for the nurse. Creating an uninterrupted space of just 5 minutes can do much to identify the source of the concern, allay anxieties, and plan for follow-up.

In another case, in response to the question, "Am I dying?," the nurse could establish eye contact and follow with a statement acknowledging the patient's fears ("This must be very difficult for you") and an open-ended statement or question ("Tell me more about what is on your mind."). The nurse then needs to listen intently, ask additional questions for clarification, and provide reassurance only when it is realistic. In this example, the nurse might quickly ascertain that the patient's question emanates from a need for specific information—about diagnosis and prognosis from the physician, about the physiology of the dying process from the nurse, or perhaps about financial implications for the family from the social worker. The chaplain may also be called to talk with the patient about existential concerns.

As a member of the interdisciplinary team caring for the patient at the end of life, the nurse plays an important role in facilitating the team's understanding of the patient's values and preferences, family dynamics concerning decision making, and the patient's and family's response to treatment and changing health status. Many dilemmas in patient care at the end of life are related to poor communication between team members and the patient and family, as well as to failure of team members to communicate with each other effectively. Regardless of the care setting, the nurse can ensure a proactive approach to the psychosocial care of the patient and family. Periodic, structured assessments provide an opportunity for all parties to consider their priorities and plan for an uncertain future. The nurses can help the patient and family clarify their values and preferences concerning end-of-life care by using a structured approach. Sufficient time must be devoted to each step, so that the patient and family have time to process new information, formulate questions, and consider their options. Nurses may need to plan several meetings to accomplish the four steps described in Table 17-1.

Providing Culturally Sensitive Care at the End of Life

Although death, grief, and mourning are universally accepted aspects of living, values, expectations, and practices during serious illness, as death approaches, and after death are culturally bound and expressed. Health care providers may share very similar values concerning end-of-life care and may find that they are inadequately prepared to assess for and implement care plans that support culturally diverse perspectives. Historical mistrust of the health care system and unequal access to even basic medical care may underlie the beliefs and attitudes among ethnically diverse populations (West & Levi, 2004). In addition, lack of education or knowledge about end-of-life care treatment options and language barriers influence decisions among many socioeconomically disadvantaged groups.

Much of the formal structure concerning health care decisions in the United States is rooted in the Western notions of autonomy, truth telling, and the acceptability of withdrawing or withholding life-prolonging medical treatment

TABLE 17-1 Discussing End-of-Life Care

Steps	Actions
1. Initiate discussion	• Establish a supportive relationship with patient and family • State the purposes of the patient/family–health care team conference: • To ensure that the plan of care is consistent with patient and family values and preferences • To find out how best to support this patient and family • Inquire if the patient or family have questions or concerns that they want to express • Elicit values and preferences concerning • Patient and family decision-making roles • How have major decisions been made in the past? • How have treatment/care decisions been made during the course of the illness? • Has the patient appointed a surrogate? • Formal (Durable Power of Attorney) • Informal • How does the patient/family want decisions to be structured from this point on? • Setting for receiving care at the end of life • Home • Home with hospice care • Assisted living or long-term care with/without hospice • Disposition when unable to care for self independently (plan for how and where the patient prefers to receive care when he/she can no longer live independently) • Family involvement in care provision
2. Clarify understanding of the medical treatment plan and prognosis	• Identify what the patient and family understand • Identify gaps in knowledge, need for consultation with other members of the health care team • Use simple, everyday language
3. Identify end-of-life priorities	• Facilitate open discussion about priorities • "What is most important to you now?" • "How can (I/we) best help you to meet your goals?" • Allow sufficient time for emotional response
4. Contribute to the interdisciplinary care plan	• Provide guidance and/or referral for understanding medical options • Make recommendations for referrals to other disciplines or services (eg, spiritual care, support groups, community resources) • Identify need for patient/family teaching • Develop a plan for follow-up: • Schedule (frequency, time, place) • Participants • Tasks/assignments • Communication that needs to occur before the next meeting • Family member responsible for coordination

Adapted with permission from Balaban, R. B. (2000). A physician's guide to talking about end-of-life care. *Journal of General Internal Medicine, 15*(3), 195–200. Oxford: Blackwell Science Ltd.

at the end of life. In many cultures, however, interdependence is valued over autonomy, leading to communication styles that favor relinquishment of decision making to family members or to perceived authority figures, such as physicians (Crawley, Marshall, Lo, et al., 2002). In addition, there is variation in preference regarding the use of life-prolonging medical treatments such as cardiopulmonary resuscitation and artificially provided nutrition and hydration at the end of life; some groups are less likely to agree with withholding or withdrawing such life supports from the patient with a terminal illness (Caralis, Davis, Wright et al., 1993).

The nurse's role is to assess the values, preferences, and practices of every patient, regardless of ethnicity, socioeconomic status, or background. The nurse can share knowledge about a patient's and family's cultural beliefs and practices with the health care team and facilitate the adaptation of the care plan to accommodate these practices. For example, a nurse may find that a male patient prefers to have his eldest son make all of his care decisions. Institutional practices and laws governing informed consent are also rooted in the Western notion of autonomous decision making and informed consent. If a patient wishes to defer decisions to his son, the nurse can work with the team to negotiate informed consent, respecting the patient's right not to participate in decision making and honoring his family's cultural practices (Kagawa-Singer & Blackhall, 2001).

The nurse should assess and document the patient's and family's specific beliefs, preferences, and practices regarding end-of-life care, preparation for death, and after-death rituals. Chart 17-6 identifies topics that the nurse should cover and questions that the nurse may use to elicit the information.

CHART 17-6

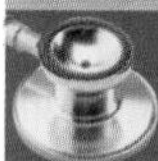

Assessing End-of-Life Care Beliefs, Preferences, and Practices

Disclosure/truth telling: "Tell me how you/your family talk about very sensitive or serious matters."

- Content: "Are there any topics that you or your family are uncomfortable discussing?"
- Person responsible for disclosure: "Is there one person in the family who assumes responsibility for obtaining and sharing information?"
- Disclosure practices regarding children: "What kind of information may be shared with children in your family, and who is responsible for communicating with the children?"
- Sharing of information within the family or community group: "What kind/how much information should be shared with your immediate family? Your extended family? Others in the community (for example, members of a religious community)?"

Decision-making style: "How are decisions made in your family? Who would you like to be involved in decisions about your treatment or care?"

- Individual
- Family-centered
- Family elder or patriarch/matriarch
- Deference to authority (such as the physician)

Symptom management: "How would you like us to help you to manage the physical effects of your illness?"

- Acceptability of medications used for symptom relief
- Beliefs regarding expression of pain and other symptoms
- Degree of symptom management desired

Life-sustaining treatment expectations: "Have you thought about what type of medical treatment you or your loved one would want as the end of life is nearing? Do you have an advance directive (living will and/or durable power of attorney)?"

- Nutrition/hydration at the end of life
- Cardiopulmonary resuscitation
- Ventilator
- Dialysis
- Antibiotics
- Medications to treat infection

Desired location of dying: "Do you have a preference about being at home or in some other location when you die?"

- Desired role for family members in providing care: "Who do you want to be involved in caring for you at the end of life?"
- Gender-specific prohibitions: "Are you uncomfortable having either males or females provide your care or your loved one's personal care?"

Spiritual/religious practices and rituals: "Is there anything that we should know about your spiritual or religious beliefs about death? Are there any practices that you would like us to observe as death is nearing?"

Care of the body after the death: "Is there anything that we should know about how a body/your body should be treated after death?"

Expression of grief: "What types of losses have you and your family experienced? How do you and your family express grief?"

Funeral and burial practices: "Are there any rituals or practices associated with funerals or burial that are especially important to you?"

Mourning practices: "How have you and your family carried on after a loss in the past? Are their particular behaviors or practices that are expected or required?"

The nurse must use judgment and discretion about the timing and setting for eliciting this information. Some patients may wish to have a family member speak for them or may be unable to provide information because of advanced illness. The nurse should give the patient and family a context for the discussion, such as, "It is very important to us to provide care that addresses your needs and the needs of your family. We want to honor and support your wishes, and want you to feel free to tell us how we are doing, and what we could do to better meet your needs. I'd like to ask you some questions; what you tell me will help me to understand and support what is most important to you at this time. You don't need to answer anything that makes you uncomfortable. Is it all right to ask some questions?" The assessment of end-of-life beliefs, preferences, and practices probably should be carried out in short segments over a period of time (for example, across multiple days of an inpatient hospital stay or in conjunction with multiple patient visits to an outpatient setting). The discomfort of novice nurses with asking questions and discussing this type of sensitive content can be reduced by prior practice in a classroom or clinical skills laboratory, observation of interviews conducted by experienced nurses, and partnering with experienced nurses during the first few assessments.

Goal Setting in Palliative Care at the End of Life

As treatment goals begin to shift in the direction of comfort care over aggressive disease-focused treatment, symptom relief and patient/family-defined quality of life assume greater prominence in treatment decision making. Patients, families, and clinicians may all be accustomed to an almost automatic tendency to pursue exhaustive diagnostic testing to locate and treat the source of patients' illnesses or symptoms. Each decision to withdraw treatment or discontinue diagnostic testing is an extremely emotional one for the patient and family. They may fear that the support from health care providers on which they have come to rely will be withdrawn along with the treatment.

Throughout the course of the illness, and especially as the patient's functional status and symptoms indicate approaching death, the clinician should help the patient and family weigh the benefits of continued diagnostic testing and disease-focused medical treatment against the burdens of those activities. The patient and family may be extremely reluctant to forego monitoring that has become routine throughout the illness (eg, blood testing, x-rays) but that may contribute little to a primary focus on comfort. Likewise, health care providers from other disciplines may have difficulty discontinuing such diagnostic testing or medical treatment.

Specifically, the nurse should collaborate with other members of the interdisciplinary team to share assessment findings and develop a coordinated plan of care (Fig. 17-1). In addition, the nurse should help the patient and family clarify their goals, expected outcomes, and values as they consider treatment options (Chart 17-7). The nurse should work with interdisciplinary colleagues to ensure that the patient and family are referred for continuing psychosocial support, symptom management, and assistance with other care-related challenges (eg, arrangements for home care or hospice support, referrals for financial assistance).

Spiritual Care

Attention to the spiritual component of the illness experienced by the patient and family is not new within the context of nursing care, yet many nurses lack the comfort or skills to assess and intervene in this dimension. **Spirituality** contains features of religiosity, but the two concepts are not interchangeable (Highfield, 2000). Spirituality involves the "search for meaning and purpose in life and relatedness to a transcendent dimension" (Hermann, 2001). For most people, contemplating one's own death raises many issues, such as the meaning of existence, the purpose of suffering, and the existence of an afterlife. In a national survey on spiritual beliefs and the dying process conducted by Gallup for the Nathan Cummings Foundation and the Fetzer Institute in 1996 (George H. Gallup International Institute, 1997), respondents' greatest worries about death included the following:

- The medical matter of greatest worry was the possibility of being vegetable-like for some period of time (73%).
- The emotional matter of greatest worry was not having the chance to say goodbye to someone (73%) or the possibility of having great physical pain before death (67%).
- The practical matter of greatest worry was how family or loved ones will be cared for (65%) or thinking that death will be a cause of inconvenience and stress for those who love them (64%).
- The spiritual matter of greatest worry was not being forgiven by God (56%) or dying when removed or cut off from God or a higher power (51%).

The spiritual assessment is a key component of comprehensive nursing assessment for terminally ill patients and their families. Although the nursing assessment should include religious affiliation, spiritual assessment is conceptually much broader than religion and therefore is relevant regardless of a patient's expression of religious preference or affiliation. In addition to assessment of the role of religious faith and practices, important religious rituals, and connection to a religious community, the nurse should further explore

- The harmony or discord between the patient's and the family's beliefs
- Other sources of meaning, hope, and comfort
- The presence or absence of a sense of peace of mind and purpose in life
- Spiritually or religiously based beliefs about illness, medical treatment, and care of the sick

Maugans (1996) created the useful mnemonic "SPIRIT" to assist health care professionals to include spiritual assessment in their practice:

- *S*piritual belief system
- *P*ersonal spirituality
- *I*ntegration and involvement with others in a spiritual community

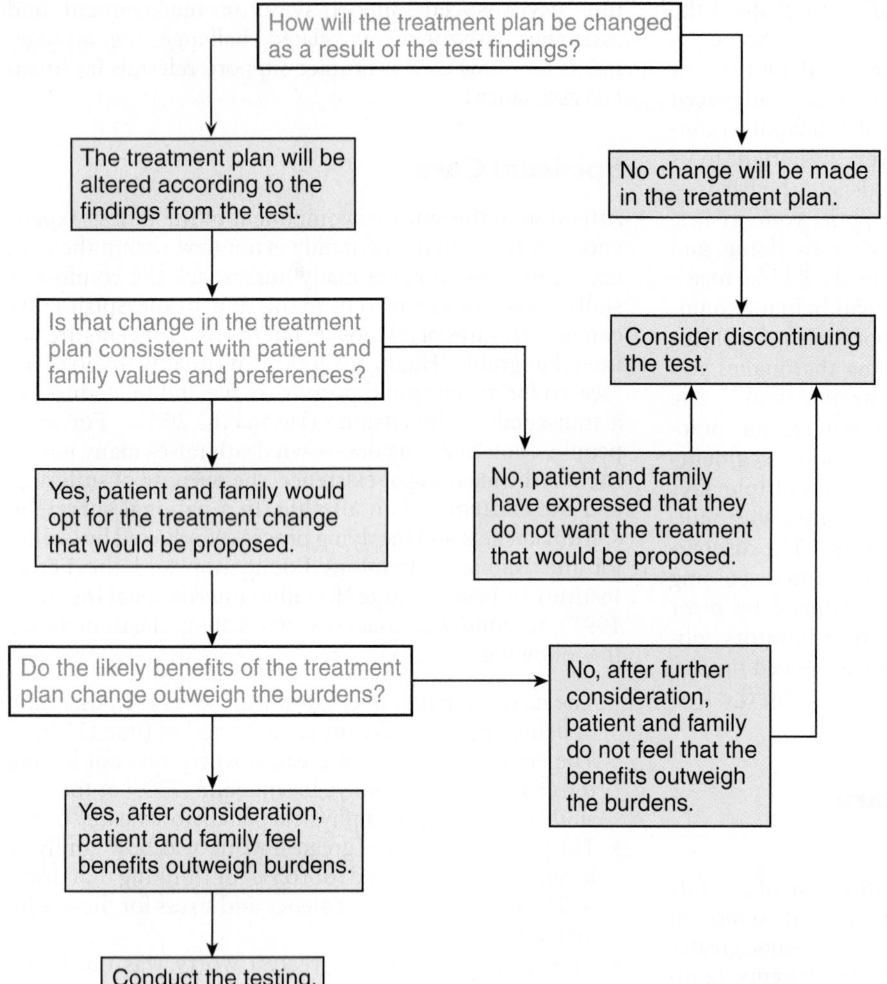

FIGURE 17-1. An algorithm for decision making about diagnostic testing at the end of life.

- *R*itualized practices and restrictions
- *I*mplications for medical care
- *T*erminal events planning

Hope

Kübler-Ross maintained that hope persists across every stage of terminal illness, noting that "even the most accepting, the most realistic patients left the possibility open for some cure, for the discovery of a new drug, or the 'last-minute success in a research project' " (1969, p 139). Viktor Frankl (1984), a survivor of the Holocaust, described a human capacity for optimism that can be maintained in spite of the possibility or even the certainty of pain and death. In terminal illness, hope represents the patient's imagined future, forming the basis of a positive, accepting attitude and providing the patient's life with meaning, direction, and optimism (O'Gorman, 2002). When hope is viewed in this way, it is not limited to cure of the disease; instead, it focuses on what is achievable in the time remaining. Many patients find hope in working on important relationships and creating legacies. Terminally ill patients can be extremely resilient, reconceptualizing hope repeatedly as they approach the end of life.

The concept of hope has been delineated and studied by numerous nurse researchers, and its presence has been related to concepts such as spirituality, quality of life, and transcendence. Morse and Doberneck (1995) defined hope as a multidimensional construct that provides comfort as one endures life threats and personal challenges. These authors identified seven universal components of hope from their study of patients who had survived serious illness:

- Realistic initial assessment of the threat
- Envisioning alternatives and setting goals
- Bracing for negative outcomes
- Realistic assessment of resources
- Solicitation of mutually supportive relationships
- Continuous evaluation for signs reinforcing the goals
- Determination to endure

Nurses can support the patient and family by using effective listening and communication skills and encouraging realistic hope that is specific to the patient's and family's needs for information, expectations for the future, and values and preferences concerning the end of life. It is important for the nurse to engage in self-reflection and to identify his or her own biases and fears concerning illness, life, and death. As the nurse becomes more skilled in working with seriously ill patients, he or she can become less determined to "fix" and more willing to listen; more comfortable with silence, grief, anger, and sadness; and more fully present with patients and their families.

CHART 17-7

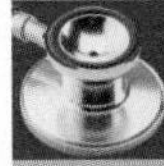

Assessing the Patient and Family Perspective: Goal Setting in Palliative Care

Patient and family

- **Awareness of diagnosis, illness stage, and prognosis:** "Tell me your understanding of your illness right now."
- **Values:** "Tell me what is most important to you as you are thinking about the treatment options available to you/your loved one."
- **Preferences:** "You've said that being comfortable and pain-free is most important to you right now. Where would you like to receive care (home, hospital, long-term care facility, doctor's office), and how can I help?"
- **Expected/desired outcomes:** "What are your hopes and expectations for this (diagnostic test [eg, CT scan] or treatment)?"
- **Benefits and burdens:** "Is there a point at which you would say that the testing or treatment is outweighed by the burdens it is causing you (eg, getting from home to the hospital, pain, nausea, fatigue, interference with other important activities)?"

Nursing interventions for enabling and supporting hope include the following:

- Listening attentively
- Encouraging sharing of feelings
- Providing accurate information
- Encouraging and supporting the patient's control over his or her circumstances, choices, and environment whenever possible
- Assisting patients to explore ways for finding meaning in their lives
- Encouraging realistic goals
- Facilitating effective communication within families
- Making referrals for psychosocial and spiritual counseling
- Assisting with the development of supports in the home or community when none exist

Managing Physiologic Responses to Terminal Illness

Patients approaching the end of life experience many of the same symptoms, regardless of their underlying disease processes. Symptoms in terminal illness may be caused by the disease, either directly (eg, dyspnea due to chronic obstructive lung disease) or indirectly (eg, nausea and vomiting related to pressure in the gastric area); by the treatment for the disease; or by a coexisting disorder that is unrelated to the disease. Chapter 13 presents assessment principles for pain that include identifying the effect of the pain on the patient's life, the importance of believing the patient's report of the pain and its effect, and the importance of systematic assessment of pain. Similarly, symptoms such as dyspnea, nausea, weakness, and anxiety should also be carefully and systematically assessed and managed. Questions that guide the assessment of symptoms are listed in Chart 17-8.

The patient's goals should guide symptom management. Medical interventions may be aimed at treating the underlying causes of the symptoms or reducing the impact of symptoms. For example, a medical intervention such as thoracentesis (an invasive procedure in which fluid is drained from the pleural space) may be performed to temporarily relieve dyspnea in a patient with pleural effusion secondary to lung cancer. Pharmacologic and nonpharmacologic methods for symptom management may be used in combination with medical interventions to modify the physiologic causes of symptoms. In addition, pharmacologic management with low-dose oral morphine is very effective in relieving dyspnea, and guided relaxation may reduce the anxiety associated with the sensation of breathlessness. As is true with pain, the principles of pharmacologic symptom management are use of the smallest dose of the medication to achieve the desired effect, avoidance of polypharmacy, anticipation and management of medical side effects, and creation of a therapeutic regimen that is acceptable to the patient based on his or her goals for maximizing quality of life.

The patient's goals take precedence over the clinicians' goals to relieve all symptoms at all costs. Although clinicians may believe that symptoms must be completely relieved whenever possible, the patient might choose instead to decrease symptoms to a tolerable level rather than to relieve them completely if the side effects of medications are unacceptable to him or her. This often allows the patient to have greater independence, mobility, and alertness, and to

CHART 17-8

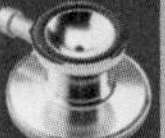

Assessing Symptoms Associated With Terminal Illness

- How is this symptom affecting the patient's life?
- What is the meaning of the symptom to the patient? To the family?
- How does the symptom affect physical functioning, mobility, comfort, sleep, nutritional status, elimination, activity level, and relationships with others?
- What makes the symptom better?
- What makes it worse?
- Is it worse at any particular time of the day?
- What are the patient's expectations and goals for managing the symptom? The family's?
- How is the patient coping with the symptom?
- What is the economic effect of the symptom and its management?

Adapted from Jacox, A., Carr, D. B., & Payne, R. (1994). *Management of cancer pain*. Rockville, MD: AHCPR.

NURSING RESEARCH PROFILE

Assessing Symptoms at the End of Life

McMillan, S. C. & Moody, L. E. (2003). Hospice patient and caregiver congruence in reporting patients' symptom intensity. *Cancer Nursing, 26*(2), 113–118.

Purpose

Increasingly, care is provided to patients with advanced illness in their homes, where family members assume responsibility for myriad complex tasks that nurses and others previously performed when the patients were hospitalized. Family members frequently administer medications to a very ill loved one and often must assess the ill family member's symptoms before giving a dose of a medication. This study assessed how well primary caregivers (family members) report the symptom intensity of a family member with cancer.

Design

The subjects in this study were participants in a larger, National Institutes of Health–funded clinical trial that examined symptom management and quality of life. Patients had been admitted to hospice within the previous 48 hours and had one of three symptoms (pain, dyspnea, or constipation). Patients were excluded if they were cognitively unable to respond or were close to death. More than 260 patients and their caregivers completed demographic questionnaires, numeric rating scales for pain and dyspnea (providing a rating of 0 to 10 to describe the intensity of a symptom), and the Constipation Assessment Scale. Patients and caregivers completed the instruments independently. The researchers used paired *t* tests to test for significant differences in patient and caregiver mean ratings for each symptom and Pearson correlations to examine the relationship between scores of patients and caregivers.

Findings

For each symptom, caregivers reported higher intensity than did the patients ($p = .000$). Patient and caregiver scores were weakly to moderately correlated ($r = .399$ to $.512$; $p < .000$), which accounted for 16% to 26% of the variance in responses.

Nursing Implications

The findings of this study suggest that family members overestimate the intensity of pain, dyspnea, and constipation compared to the patients. Hospice nurses frequently rely on family members' assessments of symptoms, which, according to this study, are generally unreliable. Whenever possible, patients' self-reports should guide treatment. However, patients' declining conditions in combination with other factors, such as language barriers, often require that family members assess and report symptoms. There is a need for better teaching of family members to enable them to accomplish this task more accurately.

devote attention to issues he or she considers of higher priority and greater importance.

Anticipating and planning interventions for symptoms that have not yet occurred is a cornerstone of end-of-life care. Both patients and family members cope more effectively with new symptoms and exacerbations of existing symptoms when they know what to expect and how to manage it. Hospice programs typically provide "emergency kits" containing ready-to-administer doses of a variety of medications that are useful to treat symptoms in advanced illness. For example, a kit might contain small doses of oral morphine liquid for pain or shortness of breath, a benzodiazepine for restlessness, and an acetaminophen suppository for fever. Family members can be instructed to administer a prescribed dose from the emergency kit, often avoiding prolonged suffering for the patient as well as rehospitalization for symptom management.

Pain

Numerous studies have shown that patients with advanced illness, particularly cancer, experience considerable pain (Field & Cassel, 1997; Jacox, Carr, & Payne, 1994). Pain is a significant symptom for many cancer patients throughout their treatment and disease course; it results from both the disease and the modalities used to treat it. It is estimated that this is true in as many as 70% of patients with advanced cancer (Jacox et al., 1994; World Health Organization, 1990). Pain and suffering are among the most feared consequences of cancer (Waller & Caroline, 2000). Although the means to relieve pain have existed for many years, the continued, pervasive undertreatment of pain has been well documented (American Pain Society, 2003). Poorly managed pain affects the psychological, emotional, social, and financial well-being of patients. Despite studies demonstrating the negative effects of inadequate pain management, practice has been slow to change (Spross, 1992).

Patients who are taking an established regimen of analgesics should continue to receive those medications as they approach the end of life. Inability to communicate pain should not be equated with the absence of pain. Although most pain can be managed effectively using the oral route, as the end of life nears, patients may be less able to swallow oral medications due to somnolence or nausea. Patients who have been receiving opioids should continue to receive equianalgesic doses via rectal or sublingual routes. Concentrated morphine solution can be very effectively delivered by the sublingual route, because the small liquid volume is well tolerated even if swallowing is not possible. As long as the patient continues to receive opioids, a regimen to combat constipation must be implemented. If the patient cannot swallow laxatives or stool softeners, rectal suppositories or enemas may be necessary.

The nurse should teach the family about continuation of comfort measures as the patient approaches the end of life, how to administer analgesics via alternative routes, and how to assess for pain when the patient cannot verbally report pain intensity. Because the analgesics administered orally or rectally are short-acting, typically scheduled as frequently as every 3 to 4 hours around the clock, there is always a strong possibility that a patient approaching the end of life will die in close proximity to the time of analgesic administration. If the patient is at home, family members administering analgesics should be prepared for this possibility. They need reassurance that they did not "cause" the death of the patient by administering a dose of analgesic medication (see Chart 13-4 in Chapter 13).

Dyspnea

Dyspnea is an uncomfortable awareness of breathing that is common in patients approaching the end of life (Brant, 1998). Dyspnea is a highly subjective symptom that often is not associated with visible signs of distress, such as tachypnea, diaphoresis, or cyanosis. Patients with primary lung tumors, lung metastases, pleural effusion, or restrictive lung disease may experience significant dyspnea. Although the underlying cause of the dyspnea can be identified and treated in some cases, the burdens of additional diagnostic evaluation and treatment aimed at the physiologic problem may outweigh the benefits. The treatment of dyspnea varies depending on the patient's general physical condition and imminence of death. For example, a blood transfusion may provide temporary symptom relief for a patient with anemia earlier in the disease process; however, as the patient approaches the end of life, the benefits are typically short-lived or absent.

NURSING ASSESSMENT AND INTERVENTION

As with assessment and management of pain, reports of dyspnea by patients must be believed. As is true for physical pain, what dyspnea means to an individual patient may increase his or her suffering. For example, the patient may interpret increasing dyspnea as a sign that death is approaching. For some patients, sensations of breathlessness may invoke frightening images of drowning or suffocation, and the resulting cycle of fear and anxiety may increase the sensation of breathlessness. Therefore, the nurse should conduct a careful assessment of the psychosocial and spiritual components of the dyspnea. Physical assessment parameters include

- Symptom intensity, distress, and interference with activities (scale of 0 to 10)
- Auscultation of lung sounds
- Assessment of fluid balance
- Measurement of dependent edema (circumference of lower extremities)
- Measurement of abdominal girth
- Temperature
- Skin color
- Sputum quantity and character
- Cough

To determine the intensity of dyspnea and its interference with daily activities, the patient can be asked to report the severity of the dyspnea using a scale of 0 to 10, where 0 is no dyspnea and 10 is the worst imaginable dyspnea. The patient's baseline rating before treatment and subsequent measurements taken during exacerbation of the symptom, periodically during treatment, and whenever the treatment plan changes provide ongoing objective evidence for the efficacy of the treatment plan. In addition, physical assessment findings may assist in locating the source of the dyspnea and selecting nursing interventions to relieve the symptom. The components of the assessment change as the patient's condition changes. For example, when the patient who has been on daily weights can no longer get out of bed, the goal of comfort may outweigh the benefit of continued weights. Like other symptoms at the end of life, dyspnea can be managed effectively in the absence of assessment and diagnostic data (ie, arterial blood gases) that are standard when a patient's illness or symptom is reversible.

Nursing management of dyspnea at the end of life is directed toward administering medical treatment for the underlying pathology, monitoring the patient's response to treatment, helping the patient and family manage anxiety (which exacerbates dyspnea), altering the perception of the symptom, and conserving energy (Chart 17-9). Pharmacologic intervention is aimed at modifying lung physiology and improving performance as well as altering the perception of the symptom. Bronchodilators and corticosteroids are examples of medications used to treat underlying obstructive pathology, thereby improving overall lung function. Low doses of opioids are very effective in relieving dyspnea, although the mechanism of relief is not entirely clear. Although dyspnea in terminal illness is typically not associated with diminished blood oxygen saturation, low-flow oxygen often provides psychological comfort to both patients and families, particularly in the home setting.

As previously mentioned, dyspnea may be exacerbated by anxiety, and anxiety may trigger episodes of dyspnea, setting off a respiratory crisis in which the patient and family may panic. For patients receiving care at home, patient and family instruction should include anticipation and management of crisis situations and a clearly communicated emergency plan. The patient and family should be instructed about medication administration, condition changes that should be reported to the physician and nurse, and strategies for coping with diminished reserves and increasing symptomatology as the disease progresses. The patient and family need reassurance that the symptom can be effectively managed at home without the need for activation of the emergency medical services or hospitalization and that a nurse will be available at all times via telephone or to make a visit.

Nutrition and Hydration at the End of Life

ANOREXIA

Anorexia and cachexia are common problems in the seriously ill. The profound changes in the patient's appearance and the concomitant lack of interest in the socially important rituals of mealtime are particularly disturbing to families. The approach to the problem varies depending on the patient's stage of illness, level of disability associated with the illness, and desires. The anorexia–cachexia syndrome is characterized by disturbances in carbohydrate, protein,

CHART 17-9

Palliative Nursing Interventions for Dyspnea

DECREASE ANXIETY

- Administer prescribed anxiolytic medications as indicated for anxiety or panic associated with dyspnea.
- Assist with relaxation techniques, guided imagery.
- Provide patient with a means to call for assistance (call bell/light within reach in a hospital or long-term care facility; handheld bell or other device for home).

TREAT UNDERLYING PATHOLOGY

- Administer prescribed bronchodilators and corticosteroids (obstructive pathology).
- Administer blood products, erythropoietin as prescribed (typically not beneficial in advanced disease).
- Administer prescribed diuretics and monitor fluid balance.

ALTER PERCEPTION OF BREATHLESSNESS

- Administer prescribed oxygen therapy via nasal cannula, if tolerated; masks may not be well tolerated.
- Administer prescribed low-dose opioids via oral route (morphine sulfate is used most commonly).
- Provide air movement in the patient's environment with a portable fan.

REDUCE RESPIRATORY DEMAND

- Teach patient and family to implement energy conservation measures.
- Place needed equipment, supplies, and nourishment within reach.
- For home or hospice care, offer bedside commode, electric bed (with head that elevates).

and fat metabolism; endocrine dysfunction; and anemia. The syndrome results in severe asthenia (loss of energy).

Although causes of anorexia may be controlled for a period of time, progressive anorexia is an expected and natural part of the dying process. Anorexia may be related to or exacerbated by situational variables (eg, the ability to have meals with the family versus eating alone in the "sick room"), progression of the disease, treatment for the disease, or psychological distress. The patient and family should be instructed in strategies to manage the variables associated with anorexia (Table 17-2).

Use of Pharmacologic Agents to Stimulate Appetite. A number of pharmacologic agents are commonly used to stimulate appetite in anorectic patients. Commonly used medications for appetite stimulation include dexamethasone (Decadron), megestrol acetate (Megace), and dronabinol (Marinol). Although several of these agents may result in temporary weight gain, their use is not associated with an increase in lean body mass in the terminally ill patient. Therapy should be tapered or discontinued after 4 to 8 weeks if there is no response (Wrede-Seaman, 1999).

Dexamethasone initially increases appetite and may provide short-term weight gain in some patients. However, therapy may need to be discontinued in patients with a longer life expectancy, because after 3 to 4 weeks corticosteroids interfere with the synthesis of muscle protein.

Megestrol acetate produces temporary weight gain of primarily fatty tissue, with little effect on protein balance. Because of the time required to see any effect from this agent, therapy should not be initiated if life expectancy is less than 30 days.

Dronabinol is a psychoactive compound found in cannabis that may be helpful in reducing nausea and vomiting, appetite loss, pain, and anxiety, thereby improving food and fluid intake in some patients. However, dronabinol is not as effective as the other agents for appetite stimulation in most patients.

CACHEXIA

Cachexia refers to severe muscle wasting and weight loss associated with illness. Although anorexia may exacerbate cachexia, it is not the primary cause. Cachexia is associated with changes in metabolism that include hypertriglyceridemia, lipolysis, and accelerated protein turnover, leading to depletion of fat and protein stores (Inui, 2002). However, the pathophysiology of cachexia in terminal illness is not well understood. In terminal illness, the severity of tissue wasting is greater than would be expected from reduced food intake alone, and typically increasing appetite or food intake does not reverse cachexia in the terminally ill.

Anorexia and cachexia differ from starvation (simple food deprivation) in several important ways. Appetite is lost early in the process, the body becomes catabolic in a dysfunctional way, and supplementation by gastric feeding (tube feeding) or parenteral nutrition in advanced disease does not replenish lean body mass that has been lost. At one time it was believed that cancer patients with rapidly growing tumors developed cachexia because the tumor created an excessive nutritional demand and diverted nutrients from the rest of the body. Research links cytokines produced by the body in response to a tumor to a complex inflammatory-immune response present in patients whose tumors have metastasized, leading to anorexia, weight loss, and altered metabolism. An increase in cytokines occurs not only in cancer but also in AIDS and many other chronic diseases (Inui, 2002).

ARTIFICIAL NUTRITION AND HYDRATION

Along with breathing, eating and drinking are essential to survival throughout life. Near the end of life, the body's nutritional needs change, and the desire for food and fluid may diminish. People may no longer be able to use, eliminate, or store nutrients and fluids adequately. Eating and sharing meals are important social activities in families and communities, and food preparation and enjoyment are linked to happy memories, strong emotions, and hopes for survival. For patients with serious illness, food preparation and mealtimes often become battlegrounds in which well-meaning family members argue, plead, and cajole to encourage ill people to eat. It is not unusual for seriously ill patients to lose their appetites entirely, to develop strong aversions for foods they have enjoyed in the past, or to crave a particular food to the exclusion of all other foods.

Although nutritional supplementation may be an important part of the treatment plan in early or chronic illness, unintended weight loss and dehydration are expected sequelae of progressive illness. As illness progresses, patients, families, and clinicians may believe that, without artificial nutrition and hydration, terminally ill patients will "starve," causing

TABLE 17-2 Measures for Managing Anorexia

Nursing Interventions	Patient and Family Teaching Tips
Initiate measures to ensure adequate dietary intake without adding stress to the patient at mealtimes.	Reduce the focus on "balanced" meals; offer the same food as often as the patient desires it.
Assess the impact of medications (eg, chemotherapy, antiretrovirals) or other therapies (radiation therapy, dialysis) that are being used to treat the underlying illness.	Increase the nutritional value of meals. For example, add dry milk powder to milk, and use this fortified milk to prepare cream soups, milkshakes, and gravies.
Administer and monitor effects of prescribed treatment for nausea, vomiting, and delayed gastric emptying.	
Encourage patient to eat when effects of medications have subsided.	Allow and encourage the patient to eat when hungry, regardless of usual meal times.
Assess and modify environment to eliminate unpleasant odors and other factors that cause nausea, vomiting, and anorexia.	Eliminate or reduce noxious cooking odors, pet odors, or other odors that may precipitate nausea, vomiting, or anorexia.
Remove items that may reduce appetite (soiled tissues, bedpans, emesis basins, clutter).	Keep patient's environment clean, uncluttered, and comfortable.
Assess and manage anxiety and depression to the extent possible.	Make mealtime a shared experience away from the "sick" room whenever possible. Reduce stress at mealtimes. Avoid confrontations about the amount of food consumed. Reduce or eliminate routine weighing of the patient.
Position to enhance gastric emptying.	Encourage patient to eat in a sitting position; elevate the head of the patient's bed. Plan meals (food selection and portion size) that the patient desires. Provide small frequent meals if they are easier for patient to eat.
Assess for constipation and/or intestinal obstruction.	Ensure that patient and family understand that prevention of constipation is essential, even when the patient's intake is minimal.
Prevent and manage constipation on an ongoing basis, even when the patient's intake is minimal.	Encourage adequate fluid intake, dietary fiber, and use of bowel program to prevent constipation.
Provide frequent mouth care, particularly following nourishment.	Assist the patient to rinse after every meal. Avoid mouthwashes that contain alcohol or glycerine, which dry mucous membranes.
Ensure that dentures fit properly.	Weight loss may cause dentures to loosen and cause irritation. Remove them to inspect the gums and to provide oral care.
Administer and monitor effects of topical and systemic treatment for oropharyngeal pain.	The patient's comfort may be enhanced if medications for pain relief given on an as-needed basis for breakthrough pain are administered before mealtimes.

profound suffering and hastened death. However, starvation should not be viewed as the failure to implant tubes for nutritional supplementation or hydration of terminally ill patients with irreversible progression of disease. Studies have demonstrated that terminally ill patients who were hydrated had neither improved biochemical parameters nor improved states of consciousness (Waller, Hershkowitz & Adunsky, 1994). Similarly, survival was not increased when terminally ill patients with advanced dementia received enteral feeding (Meier, Ahronheim, Morris, et al., 2001). Furthermore, in patients who are close to death, there are beneficial effects to withholding or withdrawing artificial nutrition and hydration, such as decreased urine output and incontinence, decreased gastric fluids and emesis, decreased pulmonary secretions and respiratory distress, decreased edema, and decreased discomfort from pressure associated with accumulated fluids in the tissues (Zerwekh, 1987).

As the patient approaches the end of life, the family and health care providers should offer the patient what he or she prefers and can most easily tolerate. The nurse should instruct the family how to separate feeding from caring, demonstrating love, sharing, and caring by being with the loved one in other ways. Preoccupation with appetite, feeding, and weight loss diverts energy and time that the patient and family could use in other meaningful activities. The following are tips to promote nutrition for terminally ill patients:

- Offer small portions of favorite foods.
- Do not be overly concerned about a "balanced" diet.
- Cool foods may be better tolerated than hot foods.
- Offer cheese, eggs, peanut butter, mild fish, chicken, or turkey. Meat (especially beef) may taste bitter and unpleasant.
- Add milkshakes, "Instant Breakfast" drinks, or other liquid supplements.
- Add dry milk powder to milkshakes and cream soups to increase protein and calorie content.
- Place nutritious foods at the bedside (fruit juices, milkshakes in insulated drink containers with straws).
- Schedule meals when family members can be present to provide company and stimulation.
- Avoid arguments at mealtime.
- Help the patient to maintain a schedule of oral care. Rinse the mouth after each meal or snack. Avoid mouthwashes

that contain alcohol. Use a soft toothbrush. Treat oral ulcers or lesions. Make sure dentures fit well.
- Treat pain and other symptoms.
- Offer ice chips made from frozen fruit juices.
- Allow the patient to refuse foods and fluids.

Delirium

Many patients remain alert, arousable, and able to communicate until very close to death. Others sleep for long intervals and awaken only intermittently, with eventual somnolence until death. Delirium refers to concurrent disturbances in level of consciousness, psychomotor behavior, memory, thinking, attention, and sleep–wake cycle (Lawlor, Gagnon, Mancini, et al., 2000). In some patients, a period of agitated delirium precedes death, sometimes causing families to be hopeful that suddenly active patients may be getting better. Confusion may be related to underlying, treatable conditions such as medication side effects or interactions, pain or discomfort, hypoxia or dyspnea, or a full bladder or impacted stool. In patients with cancer, confusion may be secondary to brain metastases. Delirium may also be related to metabolic changes, infection, and organ failure.

Patients with delirium may become hypoactive or hyperactive, restless, irritable, and fearful. Sleep deprivation and hallucinations may occur. If treatment of the underlying factors contributing to these symptoms brings no relief, a combination of pharmacologic intervention with neuroleptics or benzodiazepines may be effective in decreasing distressing symptoms. Haloperidol (Haldol) may reduce hallucinations and agitation. Benzodiazepines (eg, lorazepam [Ativan]) can reduce anxiety but do not clear the sensorium and may contribute to worsening cognitive impairment if used alone.

Nursing interventions are aimed at identifying the underlying causes of delirium; acknowledging the family's distress over its occurrence; reassuring family members about what is normal; teaching family members how to interact with and ensure safety for the patient with delirium; and monitoring the effects of medications used to treat severe agitation, paranoia, and fear. Confusion may mask the patient's unmet spiritual needs and fears about dying. Spiritual intervention, music therapy, gentle massage, and therapeutic touch may provide some relief. Reduction of environmental stimuli, avoidance of harsh lighting or very dim lighting (which may produce disturbing shadows), presence of familiar faces, and gentle reorientation and reassurance are also helpful.

Depression

Clinical depression should not be accepted as an inevitable consequence of dying, nor should it be confused with sadness and anticipatory grieving, which are normal reactions to the losses associated with impending death. Emotional and spiritual support and control of disturbing physical symptoms are appropriate interventions for situational depression associated with terminal illness. Researchers have linked the psychological sequelae of cancer pain to suicidal thought and, less frequently, to carrying out a planned suicide (Ripamonti, Filiberti, Totis, et al., 1999). Cancer patients with advanced disease are especially vulnerable to delirium, depression, suicidal ideation, and severe anxiety. Higher levels of debilitation predict higher levels of pain and depressive symptoms, and the presence of pain doubles the likelihood of developing major psychiatric complications of illness (Roth & Breitbart, 1996). Patients and their families must be given space and time to experience sadness and to grieve, but patients should not have to endure untreated depression at the end of their lives. An effective combined approach to clinical depression includes relief of physical symptoms, attention to emotional and spiritual distress, and pharmacologic intervention with psychostimulants, selective serotonin reuptake inhibitors, and tricyclic antidepressants (Block, 2000).

Palliative Sedation at the End of Life

Effective control of symptoms can be achieved under most conditions, but some patients may experience distressing, intractable symptoms. Although **palliative sedation** remains controversial, it is offered in some settings to patients who are close to death or who have symptoms that do not respond to conventional pharmacologic and nonpharmacologic approaches, resulting in unrelieved suffering. Palliative sedation is distinguished from **euthanasia** or physician-assisted suicide in that the intent of palliative sedation is to relieve symptoms, not to hasten death. Palliative sedation is most commonly used when the patient exhibits intractable pain, dyspnea, seizures, or delirium, and it is generally considered appropriate in only the most difficult situations. Before implementing palliative sedation, the health care team should assess for the presence of underlying and treatable causes of suffering, such as depression or spiritual pain. Finally, the patient and family should be fully informed about the use of this treatment and alternatives.

Palliative sedation is accomplished through infusion of a benzodiazepine or barbiturate in doses adequate to induce sleep and eliminate signs of discomfort (Quill & Byock, 2000). Nurses act as collaborating members of the interdisciplinary health care team, providing emotional support to patients and families, facilitating clarification of values and preferences, and providing comfort-focused physical care. Once sedation has been induced, the nurse should continue to comfort the patient, monitor the physiologic effects of the sedation, support the family during the final hours or days of their loved one's life, and ensure communication within the health care team and between the team and family.

Nursing Care of Patients Who Are Close to Death

Providing care to patients who are close to death and being present at the time of death can be one of the most rewarding experiences a nurse can have. Patients and their families are understandably fearful of the unknown, and the approach of death may prompt new concerns or cause previous fears or issues to resurface. It has often been said that as we age and as we approach death, we do not become different people, just more like ourselves. Family members who have always had difficulty communicating or who are part of families in which there are old resentments and hurts may experience heightened difficulty as their loved ones near death. In contrast, the time at the end of life can also afford opportunities to resolve old hurts and learn new ways of being a family. Regardless of the setting, skilled practitioners can make the dying patient comfortable, make space for their loved ones to remain present when they wish, and can give family members the opportunity to experience growth and healing. Likewise, regardless of setting, the patient and family may be less apprehensive near the time of death if they know what to expect and how to respond.

Expected Physiologic Changes

As death approaches and organ systems begin to fail, observable, expected changes in the body take place. Nursing care measures aimed at patient comfort should be continued: pain medications (administered rectally or sublingually), turning, mouth care, eye care, positioning to facilitate draining of secretions, and measures to protect the skin from urine or feces (if the patient is incontinent) should be continued. The nurse should consult with the physician about discontinuing measures that no longer contribute to patient comfort, such as drawing blood, administering tube feedings, suctioning (in most cases), and invasive monitoring. The nurse should prepare the family for the normal, expected changes that accompany the period immediately preceding death. Although the exact time of death cannot be predicted, it is often possible to identify when the patient is very close to death. Hospice programs frequently provide written information for families so they know what to expect and what to do as death nears (Chart 17-10).

If family members have been prepared for the time of death, they are less likely to panic and are better able to be with their loved ones in a meaningful way. Noisy, gurgling breathing or moaning is generally most distressing to family members. In most cases, the sounds of breathing at the end of life are related to oropharyngeal relaxation and diminished awareness. Family members may have difficulty believing that the patient is not in pain or that the patient's breathing could not be improved by suctioning secretions. Patient positioning and family reassurance are the most helpful responses to these symptoms.

When death is imminent, patients may become increasingly somnolent and unable to clear sputum or oral secretions, which may lead to further impairment of breathing from pooled or dried and crusted secretions. The sound ("terminal bubbling") and appearance of the secretions are often more distressing to family members than is the presence of the secretions to the patient. Family distress over the changes in the patient's condition may be eased by supportive nursing care. Continuation of comfort-focused interventions and reassurance that the patient is not in any distress can do much to ease family concerns. Gentle mouth care with a moistened swab or very soft toothbrush helps maintain the integrity of the patient's mucous membranes. In addition, gentle oral suctioning, positioning to enhance drainage of secretions, and sublingual or transdermal administration of anticholinergic drugs (Table 17-3) reduces the production of secretions and provides comfort to the patient and support to the family. Deeper suctioning may cause significant discomfort to the dying patient and is rarely of any benefit, because secretions reaccumulate rapidly.

The Death Vigil

Although every death is unique, it is often possible for experienced clinicians to assess that the patient is "actively" or imminently dying and to prepare the family in the final days or hours leading to death. As death nears, the patient may withdraw, sleep for longer intervals, or become somnolent. Family members should be encouraged to be with the patient, to speak and reassure the patient of their presence, to stroke or touch the patient, or to lie alongside the patient (even in the hospital or long-term care facility) if the family members are comfortable with this degree of closeness and can do so without causing discomfort to the patient.

The family may have gone to great lengths to ensure that their loved one will not die alone. However, despite the best intentions and efforts of the family and clinicians, the patient may die at a time when no one is present. In any setting, it is unrealistic for family members to be at the patient's bedside 24 hours a day, and it is not unusual for a patient to die when family members have stepped away from the bedside just briefly. Experienced hospice clinicians have observed and reported that some patients appear to "wait" until family members are away from the bedside to die, perhaps to spare their loved ones the pain of being present at the time of death. Nurses can reassure family members throughout the death vigil by being present intermittently or continuously, modeling behaviors (such as touching and speaking to the patient), providing encouragement in relation to family caregiving, providing reassurance about normal physiologic changes, and encouraging family rest breaks. If a patient dies while family members are away from the bedside, they may express feelings of guilt and profound grief and may need emotional support.

After-Death Care

The time of death is generally preceded by a period of gradual diminishment of bodily functions in which increasing intervals between respirations, a weakened and irregular pulse, diminishing blood pressure, and skin color changes or mottling may occur. For patients who have received adequate management of symptoms and for families who have received adequate preparation and support, the actual time of death is commonly peaceful and occurs without struggle. Nurses may or may not be present at the time of a patient's death. In many states, nurses may be authorized to make the pronouncement of death and sign the death certificate. The determination of death is made through a physical examination that includes auscultation for the absence of breathing and heart sounds. Home care or hospice programs in which nurses make the time-of-death visit and pronouncement of death have polices and procedures to guide the nurse's actions during this visit. Immediately on cessation of vital functions, the body begins to change. It becomes dusky or bluish, waxen-appearing, and cool; blood darkens and pools in dependent areas of the body (eg, the back and sacrum if the body is in a supine position); and urine and stool may be evacuated.

Immediately after death, family members should be allowed and encouraged to spend time with the deceased. Normal responses of family members at the time of death vary widely and range from quiet expressions of grief to overt expressions that include wailing and prostration. The family's desire for privacy during their time with the deceased should be honored. Family members may wish to independently manage or assist with care of the body after death. If the death occurs in a long-term care facility, nurses follow the facility's procedure for preparation of the body and transportation to the facility's morgue. However, the needs of families to remain with the deceased, to wait until other family

CHART 17-10

Patient Education

Signs of Approaching Death

The person will show less interest in eating and drinking. For many patients, refusal of food is an indication that they are ready to die. Fluid intake may be limited to that which will keep their mouths from feeling too dry.

- What you can do: Offer, but do not force, fluids and medication. Sometimes, pain or other symptoms that have required medication in the past may no longer be present. For most patients, pain medications will still be needed, and can be provided by concentrated oral solutions placed under the tongue or by rectal suppository.

Urinary output may decrease in amount and frequency.

- What you can do: No response is needed unless the patient expresses a desire to urinate and cannot. Call the hospice nurse for advice if you are not sure.

As the body weakens, the patient will sleep more and begin to detach from the environment. He or she may refuse your attempts to provide comfort.

- What you can do: Allow your loved one to sleep. You may wish to sit with him or her, play soft music, or hold hands. Your loved one's withdrawal is normal and is not a rejection of your love.

Mental confusion may become apparent, as less oxygen is available to supply the brain. The patient may report strange dreams or visions.

- What you can do: As he or she awakens from sleep, remind him or her of the day and time, where he or she is, and who is present. This is best done in a casual, conversational way.

Vision and hearing may become somewhat impaired, and speech may be difficult to understand.

- What you can do: Speak clearly but no more loudly than necessary. Keep the room as light as the patient wishes, even at night. Carry on all conversations as if they can be heard, because hearing may be the last of the senses to cease functioning.
- Many patients are able to talk until minutes before death and are reassured by the exchange of a few words with a loved one.

Secretions may collect in the back of the throat and rattle or gurgle as the patient breathes though the mouth. He or she may try to cough, and his or her mouth may become dry and encrusted with secretions.

- What you can do: if the patient is trying to cough up secretions and is experiencing choking or vomiting, call the hospice nurse for assistance.
- Secretions may drain from the mouth if you place the patient on his/her side and provide support with pillows.
- Cleansing the mouth with moistened mouth swabs will help to relieve the dryness that occurs with mouth breathing.
- Offer water in small amounts to keep the mouth moist. A straw with one finger placed over the end can be used to transfer sips of water to the patient's mouth.

Breathing may become irregular with periods of no breathing (apnea). The patient may be working very hard to breathe and may make a moaning sound with each breath. As the time of death nears, the breathing remains irregular and may become more shallow and mechanical.

- What you can do: Raising the head of the bed may help the patient to breathe more easily. The moaning sound does not mean that the patient is in pain or other distress; it is the sound of air passing over very relaxed vocal cords.

As the oxygen supply to the brain decreases, the patient may become restless. It is not unusual to pull at the bed linens, to have visual hallucinations, or even to try to get out of bed at this point.

- What you can do: Reassure the patient in a calm voice that you are there. Prevent him or her from falling by trying to get out of bed. Soft music or a back rub may be soothing.

The patient may feel hot one moment and cold the next as the body loses its ability to control the temperature. As circulation slows, the arms and legs may become cool and bluish. The underside of the body may darken. It may be difficult to feel a pulse at the wrist.

- What you can do: Provide and remove blankets as needed. Avoid using electric blankets, which may cause burns because the patient cannot tell you if he or she is too warm.
- Sponge the patient's head with a cool cloth if this provides comfort.

Loss of bladder and bowel control may occur around the time of death.

- What you can do: Protect the mattress with waterproof padding and change the padding as needed to keep the patient comfortable.

As people approach death, many times they report seeing gardens, libraries, or family or friends who have died. They may ask you to pack their bags and find tickets or a passport. Sometimes they may become insistent and attempt to do these chores themselves. They may try getting out of bed (even if they have been confined to bed for a long time) so that they can "leave."

- What you can do: Reassure the patient that it is all right; he or she can "go" without getting out of bed. Stay close, share stories, and be present.

TABLE 17-3 Pharmacologic Management of Excess Oral/Respiratory Secretions When Death is Imminent

Medication	Dose
Atropine sulfate drops 1%	1 or 2 drops 1% oral/sublingual q4–6h prn or around the clock (ATC) up to 12 drops/d
Atropine injection	0.4–0.6 mg intravenous/subcutaneous/intramuscular q4–6h prn or ATC (if oral therapy is ineffective)
Glycopyrrolate (Robinul)	1–2 mg oral/rectal/sublingual TID prn or ATC (maximum dose 6 mg/d)
Hyoscyamine (Levsin)	0.125–0.25 mg oral/sublingual q4–6h prn or ATC (maximum dose 1.5 mg/d)
Scopolamine (Transderm Scop)	1–3 patches q3d (maximum dose 3 patches every 72 h)

Reprinted with permission from ExcelleRx, Inc. (2004). *Hospice pharmacia pharmaceutical care tool kit* (6th ed.). Philadelphia: Author.

members arrive before the body is moved, and to perform after-death rituals should be honored. When an expected death occurs in the home setting, the funeral director often transports the body directly to the funeral home.

Grief, Mourning, and Bereavement

A wide range of feelings and behaviors are normal, adaptive, and healthy reactions to the loss of a loved one. **Grief** refers to the personal feelings that accompany an anticipated or actual loss. **Mourning** refers to individual, family, group, and cultural expressions of grief and associated behaviors. **Bereavement** refers to the period of time during which mourning takes place. Both grief reactions and mourning behaviors change over time as people learn to live with the loss. Although the pain of the loss may be tempered by the passage of time, loss is an ongoing developmental process, and time does not heal the bereaved individual completely (Silverman, 2002). That is, the bereaved do not get over a loss entirely, nor do they return to who they were before the loss. Rather, they develop a new sense of who they are and where they fit in a world that has changed dramatically and permanently.

Anticipatory Grief and Mourning

Denial, sadness, anger, fear, and anxiety are normal grief reactions in people with life-threatening illness and those close to them. Kübler-Ross (1969) described five common emotional reactions to dying that are applicable to the experience of any loss (Table 17-4). Although the stages that Kübler-Ross described are useful in understanding the overall experience of the dying process, they have been misinterpreted as following a linear, expected trajectory. Not every patient or family member experiences every stage; many patients never reach a stage of acceptance, and patients and families fluctuate on a sometimes daily basis in their emotional responses. Furthermore, although impending loss stresses the patient, people who are close to him or her, and the functioning of the family unit, awareness of dying also provides a unique opportunity for family members to reminisce, resolve relationships, plan for the future, and say goodbye.

Individual and family coping with the anticipation of death is complicated by the varied and conflicting trajectories that grief and mourning may assume in families. For example, although the patient may be experiencing sadness while contemplating role changes that have been brought about by the illness, the patient's spouse or partner may be expressing or suppressing feelings of anger about the current changes in role and impending loss of the relationship. Others in the family may be engaged in denial (eg, "Dad will get better; he just needs to eat more"), fear ("Who will take care of us?" or "Will I get sick too?"), or profound sadness and withdrawal. Although each of these behaviors is normal, tension may arise when one or more family members perceive that others are less caring, too emotional, or too detached.

The nurse should assess the characteristics of the family system and intervene in a manner that supports and enhances the cohesion of the family unit. Parameters for assessing the family facing life-threatening illness are identified in Chart 17-11. The nurse can patiently suggest that family members talk about their feelings and understand them in the broader context of anticipatory grief and mourning. Acknowledging and expressing feelings, continuing to interact with the patient in meaningful ways, and planning for the time of death and bereavement are adaptive family behaviors. Professional support provided by grief counselors, whether in the community, at a local hospital, in the long-term care facility, or associated with a hospice program, can help both the patient and the family sort out and acknowledge feelings and make the end of life as meaningful as possible.

Grief and Mourning After Death

When a loved one dies, the family members enter a new phase of grief and mourning as they begin to accept the loss, feel the pain of permanent separation, and prepare to live a life without the deceased. Even if the loved one died after a long illness, preparatory grief experienced during the terminal illness does not preclude the grief and mourning that follow the death. With a death after a long or difficult illness, family members may experience conflicting feelings of relief that the loved one's suffering has ended, compounded by guilt and grief related to unresolved issues or the circumstances of death. Grief work may be especially difficult if a patient's death was painful, prolonged, accompanied by unwanted interventions, or unattended. Families who had no preparation or support during the period of imminence and death may have a more difficult time finding a place for the painful memories.

Although some family members may experience prolonged or complicated mourning, most grief reactions fall within a "normal" range. The feelings are often profound, but bereaved people eventually reconcile the loss and find a way to reengage with their lives. Grief and mourning are affected by several factors, including individual characteristics, coping skills, and experiences with illness and death; the nature of the relationship to the deceased; factors surrounding the illness and the death; family dynamics; social support;

TABLE 17-4 Kübler-Ross's Five Stages of Dying

Stage	Nursing Implications
Denial: "This cannot be true." Feelings of isolation. May search for another health care professional who will give a more favorable opinion. May seek unproven therapies.	Denial can be an adaptive response, providing a buffer after bad news. It allows time to mobilize defenses but can be maladaptive when it prevents the patient or family from seeking help or when denial behaviors cause more pain or distress than the illness or interfere with everyday functions. Nurses should assess the patient's and family's coping style, information needs, and understanding of the illness and treatment to establish a basis for empathetic listening, education, and emotional support. Rather than confronting the patient with information he or she is not ready to hear, the nurse can encourage him or her to share fears and concerns. Open-ended questions or statements such as "Tell me more about how you are coping with this new information about your illness" can provide a springboard for expression of concerns.
Anger: "Why me?" Feelings of rage, resentment or envy directed at God, health care professionals, family, others.	Anger can be very isolating, and loved ones or clinicians may withdraw. Nurses should allow the patient and family to express anger, treating them with understanding, respect, and knowledge that the root of the anger is grief over impending loss.
Bargaining: "I just want to see my grandchild's birth, then I'll be ready. . . ." Patient and/or family plead for more time to reach an important goal. Promises are sometimes made with God.	Terminally ill patients are sometimes able to outlive prognoses and achieve some future goal. Nurses should be patient, allow expression of feelings, and support realistic and positive hope.
Depression: "I just don't know how my kids are going to get along after I'm gone." Sadness, grief, mourning for impending losses.	Normal and adaptive response. Clinical depression should be assessed and treated when present. Nurses should encourage the patient and family to fully express their sadness. Insincere reassurance or encouragement of unrealistic hopes should be avoided.
Acceptance: "I've lived a good life, and I have no regrets." Patient and/or family are neither angry nor depressed.	The patient may withdraw as his or her circle of interest diminishes. The family may feel rejected by the patient. Nurses need to support the family's expression of emotions and encourage them to continue to be present for the patient.

and cultural expectations and norms. Uncomplicated grief and mourning are characterized by emotional feelings of sadness, anger, guilt, and numbness; physical sensations such as hollowness in the stomach and tightness in the chest, weakness, and lack of energy; cognitions that include preoccupation with the loss and a sense of the deceased as still present; and behaviors such as crying, visiting places that are reminders of the deceased, social withdrawal, and restless overactivity (Worden, 1991).

After-death rituals, including preparation of the body, funeral practices, and burial rituals, are socially and culturally significant ways in which family members begin to accept the reality and finality of death. Preplanning of funerals is becoming increasingly common, and hospice professionals in particular help the family make plans for death, often involving the patient, who may wish to play an active role. Preplanning of the funeral relieves the family of the burden of making decisions in the intensely emotional period after a death.

In general, the period of mourning is an adaptive response to loss during which mourners come to accept the loss as real and permanent, acknowledge and experience the painful emotions that accompany the loss, experience life without the deceased, overcome impediments to adjustment, and find a new way of living in a world without the loved one. Particularly immediately after the death, mourners begin to recognize the reality and permanence of the loss by talking about the deceased and telling and retelling the story of the illness and death. Societal norms in the United States are frequently at odds with the normal grieving processes of people; time excused from work obligations is typically measured in days and mourners are often expected to get over the loss quickly and get on with life.

In reality, the work of grief and mourning takes time, and avoiding grief work after the death often leads to long-term adjustment difficulties. According to Rando (2000), mourning for a loss involves the "undoing" of psychosocial ties that bind mourners to the deceased, personal adaptation to the loss, and learning to live in the world without the deceased. Six key processes of mourning allow people to accommodate to the loss in a healthy way (Rando, 2000):

1. Recognition of the loss
2. Reaction to the separation, and experiencing and expressing the pain of the loss
3. Recollection and reexperiencing the deceased, the relationship, and the associated feelings
4. Relinquishing old attachments to the deceased
5. Readjustment to adapt to the new world without forgetting the old
6. Reinvestment

Similarly, Worden (1991) described four tasks of mourning:

1. Acceptance of the reality of the loss
2. Working through the pain of grief
3. Adjusting to the environment in which the deceased is gone

CHART 17-11

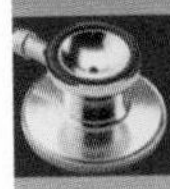

Assessing for Anticipatory Mourning in the Family Facing Life-Threatening Illness

FAMILY CONSTELLATION

- Identify the members who constitute the patient's family. Who is important to the patient?
- Identify roles and relationships among the family members.
  - Who is the primary caregiver?
  - By what authority is this person the primary caregiver?

COHESION AND BOUNDARIES

- How autonomous/interdependent are family members?
  - Degree of involvement with each other as individuals and as a family
  - Degree of bonding between family members
  - Degree of "teamwork" in the family
  - Degree of reliance on individual family members for specific tasks/roles
- How do family members differ in
  - Personality?
  - World view?
  - Priorities?
- What are the implicit and explicit expectations or "rules" for behavior within the family?

FLEXIBILITY AND ADAPTABILITY

- What is the family's ability to integrate new information?
- How does the family manage change?
- How able are the family members to assume new roles and responsibilities?

COMMUNICATION

- What is the style of communication in the family, in terms of
  - Openness?
  - Directness?
  - Clarity?
- What are the constraints on communication?
- What topics are avoided?

4. Emotional "relocation" of the deceased to move on with life

Although many people complete the work of mourning with the informal support of families and friends, many find that talking with others who have had a similar experience, such as in formal support groups, normalizes the feelings and experiences and provides a framework for learning new skills to cope with the loss and create a new life. Hospitals, hospices, religious organizations, and other community organizations often sponsor bereavement support groups. Groups for parents who have lost a child, children who have lost a parent, widows, widowers, and gay men and lesbians who have lost a life partner are some examples of specialized support groups available in many communities. Nursing interventions for those experiencing grief and mourning are identified in Chart 17-12.

Complicated Grief and Mourning

Complicated grief and mourning are characterized by prolonged feelings of sadness and feelings of general worthlessness or hopelessness that persist long after the death, prolonged symptoms that interfere with activities of daily living (anorexia, insomnia, fatigue, panic), or self-destructive behaviors such as alcohol or substance abuse and suicidal ideation or attempts. Complicated grief and mourning require professional assessment and can be treated with pharmacologic and psychological interventions.

Coping With Death and Dying: Professional Caregiver Issues

Whether practicing in the trauma center, intensive care unit or other acute care setting, home care, hospice, long-term care, or the many locations where patients and their families

CHART 17-12

Nursing Interventions for Grief and Mourning

SUPPORT THE EXPRESSION OF FEELINGS.

- Encourage the telling of the story using open-ended statements or questions (eg, "Tell me about your husband").
- Assist the mourner to find an outlet for his or her feelings: talking, attending a support group, keeping a journal, finding a safe outlet for angry feelings (writing letters that will not be mailed, physical activity)
- Assess emotional affect and reinforce the normalcy of feelings.
- Assess for guilt and regrets.
  - Are you especially troubled by a certain memory or thought?
  - How do you manage those memories?

ASSESS FOR THE PRESENCE OF SOCIAL SUPPORT.

- Do you have someone to whom you can talk about your husband?
- May I help you to find someone you can talk to?

ASSESS COPING SKILLS.

- How are you managing day to day?
- Have you experienced other losses? How did you manage those?
- Are there things you are having trouble doing?
- Do you have/need help with specific tasks?

ASSESS FOR SIGNS OF COMPLICATED GRIEF AND MOURNING AND OFFER PROFESSIONAL REFERRAL.

receive ambulatory services, the nurse is closely involved with complex and emotionally laden issues surrounding loss of life. To be most effective and satisfied with the care he or she provides, the nurse should attend to his or her own emotional responses to the losses he or she witnesses every day. Well before the nurse exhibits symptoms of stress or burnout, he or she should acknowledge the difficulty of coping with others' pain on a daily basis and put healthy practices in place that guard against emotional exhaustion. In hospice settings, where death, grief, and loss are expected outcomes of patient care, interdisciplinary colleagues rely on each other for support, using meeting time to express frustration, sadness, anger, and other emotions; to learn coping skills from each other; and to speak about how they were affected by the lives of those patients who have died since the last meeting. In many settings, staff members organize or attend memorial services to support families and other caregivers, who find comfort in joining each other to remember and celebrate the lives of patients. Finally, healthy personal habits, including diet, exercise, stress reduction activities (eg, dance, yoga, tai chi, meditation), and sleep, help guard against the detrimental effects of stress.

Critical Thinking Exercises

1 You are conducting your first home care visit to an 88-year-old man who has been hospitalized three times in the last 4 months with acute shortness of breath related to chronic obstructive pulmonary disease. Your assessment reveals that his respiratory rate is 24 breaths per minute, his nail beds and oropharynx are dusky, and he is using accessory muscles to breathe. He is very weak, has a poor appetite, and is able to move from bed to chair only with assistance. He tells you that when he has extreme difficulty breathing, his wife becomes very frightened, causing him to become very anxious as well. His wife, who is also 88 years of age, has heart failure and diabetes. She walks with a walker, and although she tries to take care of her husband, it is becoming increasingly difficult for her to do so. The couple have been married for almost 70 years and are very devoted to each other. What additional assessments would you conduct? What strategies would you implement to (1) relieve the patient's symptoms and discomfort, (2) assist his wife in management of his care, and (3) prepare both of them for his inevitable death?

2 A 55-year-old married mother of three adult children has been referred for hospice care. During your initial visit to the patient's home, you assess that she is experiencing severe pain in her ribs and pelvis (she reports a score of 8 on a 0-to-10 pain intensity scale). In addition, she reports that she is unable to sleep. Her physician has prescribed morphine for her pain, but you assess that she has used very few doses of the morphine. Her husband tells you privately that he has discouraged her use of the medicine because it has made her very sleepy and nauseated in the past. The interdisciplinary team is meeting to discuss the patient's treatment plan. What additional assessment data are needed to determine the wishes and expectations of the patient as well as the husband? What are the team's options for intervention? What are the pros and cons of each option?

3 You have been assigned to care for a 44-year-old married man who is in the end stages of AIDS. He was discharged home from the hospital yesterday and is being admitted to the local visiting nurse association's home palliative care program. When you ask him about his religion and beliefs as part of the spiritual assessment that is performed at the time of admission, he says to you, "I know that God is punishing me." How should you respond to his comment? Explain your rationale. What additional questions would you include in your spiritual assessment? Why? Discuss your plan for follow-up.

4 ebp Transcutaneous electrical stimulation (TENS) is prescribed for one of your patients in an effort to relieve his severe bone pain. You are responsible for teaching the patient and his wife how to use the TENS unit. What is the evidence for the effectiveness of TENS in relieving pain? How would you evaluate the strength of the evidence? What are the implications for practice based on the evidence for its effectiveness?

REFERENCES AND SELECTED READINGS

BOOKS

Abrahm, J. L. (2000). *A physician's guide to pain and symptom management in cancer patients*. Baltimore, MD: Johns Hopkins University Press.

Addington, T. G. (1991). *Communication and cancer*. Hershey, PA: Central Pennsylvania Oncology Group.

Amenta, M. O. & Bohnet, N. L. (1986). *Nursing care of the terminally ill*. New York: Little Brown.

American Nurses Association. (1994). Position statement on assisted suicide [online]. Available at: www.nursingworld.org/readroom/position/ethics/etsuic.htm (accessed March 31, 2006).

American Nurses Association. (2003). *Nursing's social policy statement*. Washington, DC: Author.

American Pain Society. (2003). *Principles of analgesic use in the treatment of acute pain and cancer pain* (5th ed.). Glenview, IL: Author.

Bailey, F. A. (2003). *The palliative response*. Birmingham, AL: Menasha Ridge.

Barnard, D., Towers, A., Boston, P. & Lambrinidou, Y. (2000). *Crossing over: Narratives of palliative care*. New York: Oxford.

Bennahum, D. A. (1996). The historical development of hospice and palliative care. In Sheehan, D. C. & Forman, W. B. (Eds.), *Hospice and palliative care: Concepts and practice*. Boston: Jones & Bartlett.

Byock, I. (1997). *Dying well: The prospect for growth at the end of life*. New York: Riverhead.

Callahan, D. (1993b). *The troubled dream of life*. New York: Simon & Schuster.

Doyle, D., Hanks, G. W. C., & MacDonald, N. (Eds.). (1998). *Oxford textbook of palliative medicine* (2nd ed.). New York: Oxford.

ExcelleRx, Inc. (2003). *Hospice pharmacia pharmaceutical care tool kit* (5th ed.). Philadelphia: Author.

Family Home Hospice of the Visiting Nurse Association of Greater Philadelphia. (1999). *Signs of approaching death*. Philadelphia: Author.

Federal Interagency Forum on Aging-Related Statistics. (2004). *Older Americans 2004: Key indicators of well-being.* Washington, DC: United States Government Printing Office.

Ferrell, B. R. & Coyle, N. (Eds.). (2001). *Textbook of palliative nursing.* New York: Oxford.

Field, M. J. & Cassel, C. K. (Eds.). (1997). *Approaching death: Improving care at the end of life.* Washington, DC: National Academy Press.

Frankl, V. E. (1984). *Man's search for meaning.* New York: Washington Square.

George H. Gallup International Institute. (1997). *Spiritual beliefs and the dying process.* Princeton, NJ: Author.

Glaser, B. G. & Strauss, A. (1965). *Awareness of dying.* Chicago: Aldine.

Hallenbeck, J. L. (2003). *Palliative care perspectives.* New York: Oxford.

Hogan, C., Lynn, J., Gabel, J., et al. (2000). *Medicare beneficiaries' costs and use of care in the last year of life.* Washington, DC: MedPAC.

Hospice Association of America. (2002). *Hospice facts and statistics.* Washington, DC: Author.

Jacox, A., Carr, D. B. & Payne, R. (1994). *Management of cancer pain.* Clinical practice guideline No. 9 (AHCPR Publication No. 94-0592). Washington, DC: Agency for Health Care Policy and Research, United States Department of Health and Human Services, Public Health Service.

Jennings, B., Ryndes, T., D'Onofrio, C. & Baily, M. A. (2003). *Access to hospice care: Expanding boundaries; overcoming barriers.* Hastings Center Report Supplement: S3.

Kübler-Ross, E. (1969). *On death and dying.* New York: MacMillan.

Lesparre, M. & Matherlee, K. (1998). *Delivering and financing care at the end of life.* Issue Brief (No. 711). Washington, DC: The George Washington University.

Lynn, J., Schuster, J. L. & Kabcenell, A. (2000). *Improving care for the end of life: A sourcebook for health care managers and clinicians.* New York: Oxford.

Matzo, M. L. & Sherman, D. W. (Eds.). (2001). *Palliative care nursing: Quality care to the end of life.* New York: Springer.

McSkimming, S. A., Super, A., Driever, M. J., et al. (1997). *Living and healing during life-threatening illness.* Portland, OR: Supportive Care of the Dying.

National Hospice and Palliative Care Organization. (2003). *Hospice facts and figures.* Alexandria, VA: Author.

Occupational Home Economics Education Series. (1977). Attitudes toward death. In *Care and independent living services for the aging* (Section III-A22). Washington, DC: U.S. Government Printing Office.

Office of the Inspector General, Department of Health and Human Services. (1997). *Hospice patients in nursing homes.* DHHS Publication No. OEI-05-95-00250. Washington, DC: U.S. Government Printing Office.

Plata-Salaman, C. (1997). Symptoms in terminal illness: A research workshop. Cachexia or wasting: Basic perspective [online]. Available at: ninr.nih.gov/ninr/wnew/symptoms_in_terminal_illness.html (accessed March 31, 2006).

Rando, T. A. (2000). Promoting healthy anticipatory mourning in intimates of the life-threatened or dying person. In Rando, T. A. (Ed.). *Clinical dimensions of anticipatory mourning.* Champaign, IL: Research Press.

Saunders, C. & Kastenbaum, R. (Eds.). (1997). *Hospice care on the international scene.* New York: Springer.

Smith, S. A. (2000). *Hospice concepts: A guide to palliative care in terminal illness.* Champaign, IL: Research Press.

Tilly, J. & Wiener, J. (2001). *Medicaid and end-of-life care.* Washington, DC: Last Acts.

Waller, A., & Caroline, N. A. (2000). *Handbook of palliative care in cancer* (2nd ed.). Boston: Butterworth-Heinemann.

Wentzel, K. B. (1981). *To those who need it most, hospice means hope.* Boston: Charles River.

World Health Organization. (1990). *Cancer pain relief and palliative care: Report of a WHO expert committee.* Technical Report Series, 804, 1–75. Geneva: World Health Organization.

Worden, J. W. (1991). *Grief counseling and grief therapy.* New York: Springer.

Wrede-Seaman, L. (1999). *Symptom management algorithms: A handbook for palliative care.* Yakima, WA: Intellicard.

JOURNALS

**An asterisk indicates a nursing research article.*

Ameling, A., & Povilonis, M. (2002). Spirituality, meaning, mental health, and nursing. *Journal of Psychosocial Nursing and Mental Health Services, 39*(4), 14–20.

Balaban, R. B. (2000). A physician's guide to talking about end-of-life care. *Journal of General Internal Medicine, 15*(3), 195–200.

Benoliel, J. Q. (1993). The moral context of oncology nursing. *Oncology Nursing Forum Supplement, 20*(10), 5–12.

Blackhall, L. J., Murphy, S. T., Frank, G., et al. (1995). Ethnicity and attitudes toward patient autonomy. *Journal of the American Medical Association, 274*(10), 820–825.

Block, S. D. (2000). Assessing and managing depression in the terminally ill patient. *Annals of Internal Medicine, 132*(3), 209–218.

Bolling, A. & Lynn, J. (1998). Hospice: Current practice, future possibilities. *Hospice Journal, 13*(1–2), 29–32.

Brant, J. M. (1998). The art of palliative care: Living with hope, dying with dignity. *Oncology Nursing Forum, 25*(96), 995–1004.

Brinson, S. V. & Brunk, Q. (2000). Hospice family caregivers: An experience in coping. *The Hospice Journal, 15*(3), 1–12.

Buchanan, J., Borland, R., Cosolo, W., et al. (1996). Patients' beliefs about cancer management. *Supportive Care in Cancer, 4*(2), 110–117.

Callahan, D. (1993a). Pursuing a peaceful death. *Hastings Center Report, 23*(4), 33–38.

Campbell, M. L. & Field, B. E. (1991). Management of the patient with do not resuscitate status: Compassion and cost containment. *Heart and Lung, 20*(4), 345–348.

Caralis, P. V., Davis, B., Wright, K., et al (1993). The influence of ethnicity and race on attitudes toward advance directives, life-prolonging treatments and euthanasia. *Journal of Clinical Ethics, 4*(2), 155–165.

Cassel, C. K., Ludden, J. M., & Moon, G. M. (2000). Perceptions of barriers to high-quality palliative care in hospitals. *Health Affairs, 19*(5), 166–172.

Chochinov, H. M., Tataryn, D. J., Wilson, K. G., et al. (2000). Prognostic awareness and the terminally ill. *Psychosomatics, 41*(6), 500–504.

Chow, E., Anderson, L., Wong, R., et al. (2001). Patients with advanced cancer: A survey of the understanding of their illness and expectations from palliative radiotherapy for symptomatic metastases. *Clinical Oncology, 13*(3), 204–208.

Christakis, N. A. & Lamont, E. B. (2000). Extent and determinants of error in doctors' prognoses in terminally ill patients: Prospective cohort study. *British Medical Journal, 320*(7233), 469–473.

Connor, S. R. (1992). Denial in terminal illness: To intervene or not to intervene. *Hospice Journal, 8*(4), 1–15.

Cook, D., Rocker, G., Marshall, J., et al. (2003). Withdrawal of mechanical ventilation in anticipation of death in the intensive care unit. *New England Journal of Medicine, 349*(12), 1123–1132.

Crawley, L. M., Marshall, P. A., Lo, B. & Koenig, B. A. (2002). Strategies for culturally effective end-of-life care. *Annals of Internal Medicine, 136*(9), 673–679.

Crawley, L., Payne, R., Bolden, J., et al. (2000). Palliative and end-of-life care in the African American community. *Journal of the American Medical Association, 284*(19), 2518–2521.

Dahlin, C. (2004). Oral complications at the end of life. *American Journal of Nursing, 104*(7), 40–47.

Department of Human Services, Office of Disease Prevention and Epidemiology. (March 6, 2006). Eighth annual report on Oregon's Death with Dignity Act. Available at: http://egov.oregon.gov/DHS/ph/pas/docs/year8.pdf (accessed May 24, 2006).

Egan, K. A. & Arnold, R. L. (2003). Grief and bereavement care. *American Journal of Nursing, 103*(9), 42–52.

Ersek, M., Kagawa-Singer, M., Barnes, D., et al. (1998). Multicultural considerations in the use of advance directives. *Oncology Nursing Forum, 25*(10), 1683–1690.

Ferrell, B. R. & Coyle, N. (2002). An overview of palliative nursing care. *American Journal of Nursing, 102*(5), 26–31.

Ferrell, B., Virani, R., Grant, M., et al. (2000). Beyond the Supreme Court decision: Nursing perspectives on end-of-life care. *Oncology Nursing Forum, 27*(3), 445–455.

Fetters, M. D., Churchill, L. & Danis, M. (2001). Conflict resolution at the end of life. *Critical Care Medicine, 29*(5), 921–925.

Finucane, T. (2002). Care of patients nearing death: Another view. *Journal of the American Geriatrics Society, 50*(3), 551–553.

Ganzini, L., Goy, E. R., Miller, L., et al. (2003). Nurses' experiences with hospice patients who refuse foods and fluids to hasten death. *New England Journal of Medicine, 349*(4), 359–365.

Gbrich, C. (2001). The emotions and coping strategies of caregivers of family members with a terminal cancer. *Journal of Palliative Care, 17*(1), 30–36.

Grady, P. A. (1999). Improving care at the end of life: Research issues. *Journal of Hospice and Palliative Nursing, 1*(94), 151–155.

Griffie, J., Nelson-Marten, P. & Muchka, S. (2004). Acknowledging the "Elephant": Communication in palliative care. *American Journal of Nursing, 104* (1), 48–57.

Helm, A. (1984). Debating euthanasia: An international perspective. *Journal of Gerontological Nursing, 10*(11), 20–24.

Hermann, C. P. (2001). Spiritual needs of dying patients: A qualitative study. *Oncology Nursing Forum, 28*(91), 67.

Hermann, C. & Looney, S. (2001). The effectiveness of symptom management in hospice patients during the last seven days of life. *Journal of Hospice and Palliative Nursing, 3*(3), 88–96.

Highfield, M. E. F. (2000). Providing spiritual care to patients with cancer. *Clinical Journal of Oncology Nursing, 4*(3), 115–120.

Inui, A. (2002). Cancer anorexia-cachexia syndrome: Current issues in research and management. *CA: A Cancer Journal for Clinicians, 52*(2), 72–91.

*Jezuit, D. L. (2000). Suffering of critical care nurses with end-of-life decisions. *MedSurg Nursing, 9*(3), 145–152.

Kagawa-Singer, M., & Blackhall, L. J. (2001). Negotiating cross-cultural issues at the end of life. *Journal of the American Medical Association, 286*(23), 2993–3001.

*Kirchhoff, K. T., Spuhler, V., Walker, L., et al. (2000). Intensive care nurses' experiences with end-of-life care. *American Journal of Critical Care 9*(1), 36–42.

Krisman-Scott, M. A. (2000). An historical analysis of disclosure of terminal status. *Journal of Nursing Scholarship, 32*(1), 47–52.

LaDuke, S. (2001). Terminal dyspnea and palliative care. *American Journal of Nursing 101*(11), 26–31.

Lawlor, P. G., Gagnon, B., Mancini, I. L., et al. (2000). Occurrence, causes, and outcome of delirium in patients with advanced cancer. *Archives of Internal Medicine, 160*(6), 786–794.

Mazanec, P. & Tyler, M. K. (2003). Cultural considerations in end-of-life care. *American Journal of Nursing, 103*(3), 50–58.

Maugans, T. A. (1996). The SPIRITual history. *Archives of Family Medicine, 5*(1), 11–16.

Means to a Better End: A Report on Dying in America Today. (2002). Available at: http://www.rwjf.org/files/publications/other/meansbetterend.pdf (accessed May 24, 2006).

Meier, D. E., Ahronheim, J. C., Morris, J., et al. (2001). High short-term mortality in hospitalized patients with advanced dementia: lack of benefit of tube feeding. *Archives of Internal Medicine, 161*(4), 594–599.

Morrison, R. S. & Meier, D. E. (2004). Palliative care. *New England Journal of Medicine, 350*(25), 2582–2590.

Morrison, R. S., Siu, A. L., Leipzig, R. M., et al. (2000). The hard task of improving care at the end of life. *Archives of Internal Medicine, 160*(6), 743–747.

Morse, J. M. (2000). On comfort and comforting. *American Journal of Nursing, 100*(9), 34–37.

Morse, J. M. & Doberneck, B. (1995). Delineating the concept of hope. *Image: Journal of Nursing Scholarship, 27,* 283–291.

National Institute of Nursing Research (NINR). Mission statement. Available at: ninr.nih.gov/ninr/research/diversity/mission.html (accessed March 31, 2006).

O'Gorman, M. L. (2002). Spiritual care at the end of life. *Critical Care Nursing Clinics of North America, 14*(2), 171–176.

Oregon Department of Human Services. (2004). Physician assisted suicide: Oregon's death with dignity act [online]. Available at: www.ohd.hr.state.or.us/chs/pas/pas.cfm (accessed March 31, 2006).

Paice, J. (2002). Managing psychological conditions in palliative care. *American Journal of Nursing, 102*(11), 36–42.

Patrick, D. L., Engelberg, R. A., & Curtis, J. R. (2001). Evaluating the quality of dying and death. *Journal of Pain and Symptom Management, 22*(3), 717–726.

Pitorak, E. F. (2003a). Care at the time of death. *American Journal of Nursing, 103*(7), 42–51.

Pitorak, E. F. (2003b). Respecting the dying patient's rights. *Home Healthcare Nurse, 21*(12), 833–836.

Post-White, J., Ceronsky, C., Kreitzer, M. J., et al. (1996). Hope, spirituality, sense of coherence, and quality of life in patients with cancer. *Oncology Nursing Forum, 23*(10), 1571–1579.

Quill, T. E., & Byock, I. R. (2000). Responding to intractable terminal suffering: The role of terminal sedation and voluntary refusal of foods and fluids. *Annals of Internal Medicine, 132*(5), 408–414.

Raudonis, B. M. (1992). Ethical considerations in qualitative research with hospice patients. *Qualitative Health Research, 2*(2), 238–249.

Ripamonti, C., Filiberti, A., Totis, A., et al. (1999). Suicide among patients with cancer cared for at home by palliative care teams. *Lancet, 354*(9193), 1877–1878.

Ross, H. M. (2001). Islamic tradition at the end of life. *MedSurg Nursing, 10*(2), 83–87.

Roth, A. J., & Breitbart, W. (1996). Psychiatric emergencies in terminally ill cancer patients. *Hematology/Oncology Clinics of North America, 10*(1), 235–258.

Rushton, C. H. (2004). Ethics and palliative care in pediatrics. *American Journal of Nursing, 104*(4), 54–63.

Sheehan, D. K. & Schirm, V. (2003) End-of-life care of older adults. *American Journal of Nursing, 103*(11), 48–58.

Silverman, P. R. (2002). Living with grief, rebuilding a world. *Journal of Palliative Medicine, 5*(3), 449–454.

Song, M. K. (2004). Effects of end-of-life discussions on patients' affective outcomes. *Nursing Outlook, 52*(3), 118–125.

Sorenson, B. F. (1991). Euthanasia: The "good death"? *Surgical Neurology, 35,* 827–830.

Spross, J. A. (1992). Cancer pain relief: An international perspective. *Oncology Nursing Forum, 19*(7), 5–19.

Stanley, K. J. (2000). Silence is not golden: Conversations with the dying. *Clinical Journal of Oncology Nursing, 4*(1), 34–40.

Steinhauser, K. E., Christakis, N. A., Clipp, E. C., et al. (2004). Family perspectives on end-of-life care at the last place of care. *Journal of the American Medical Association, 291*(1), 88–93.

SUPPORT Principal Investigators. (1995). A controlled trial to improve care for seriously ill hospitalized patients. *Journal of the American Medical Association, 274*(20), 1591–1598.

Teno, J. M., Fisher, E. S., Hamel, M. B., et al. (2002). Medical care inconsistent with patients' treatment goals: Association with 1-year Medicare resource use and survival. *Journal of American Geriatrics Society, 50*(3), 496–500.

Tilden, V. P. (2000). Policy perspectives: Advance directives. *American Journal of Nursing, 100*(12), 49–51.

Tolle, S. W., Tilden, V. P., Rosenfeld, A. G., et al. (2000). Family reports of barriers to optimal care of the dying. *Nursing Research, 49*(6), 310–317.

Tulsky, J. A. (2001). Preparing for the end of life: Preferences of patients, families, physicians and other care providers. *Journal of Pain and Symptom Management, 22*(3), 727–737.

Virani, R. & Sofer, D. (2003). Improving the quality of end-of-life care. *American Journal of Nursing, 103*(5), 52–60.

Virmani, J., Schneiderman, L. J. & Kaplan, R. M. (1994). Relationship of advance directives to physician-patient communication. *Archives of Internal Medicine, 154*(8), 909–913.

Waller, A., Hershkowitz, M. & Adunsky, A. (1994). The effects of intravenous fluid infusion on blood and urine parameters of hydration and on state of consciousness in terminally ill patients. *American Journal of Hospice and Palliative Care, 11*(6), 26–29.

Weissman, D. E. (2004). Decision making at a time of crisis near the end of life. *Journal of the American Medical Association, 292*(14), 1738–1743.

Wenger, N. S. & Rosenfeld, K. (2001). Quality indicators for end-of-life care in vulnerable elders. *Annals of Internal Medicine, 135*(8), 677–685.

Wenrich, M. D., Curtis, J. R., Shannon, S. E., et al. (2001). Communicating with dying patients within the spectrum of medical care from terminal diagnosis to death. *Archives of Internal Medicine, 161*(6), 868–874.

West, S. K. & Levi, L. (2004). Culturally appropriate end-of-life care for the Black American. *Home Healthcare Nurse, 22*(3), 164–168.

Yedidia, M. J. & MacGregor, B. (2001). Confronting the prospect of dying: Reports of terminally ill patients. *Journal of Pain and Symptom Management, 22*(4), 807–819.

Zerwekh, J. V. (1987). Should fluid and nutrition support be withheld from terminally ill patients? *American Journal of Hospice and Palliative Care, 4*(4), 37–38.

Zerwekh, J. (1994). The truth tellers: How hospice nurses help patients confront death. *American Journal of Nursing, 94*(2), 31–34.

Zerwekh, J. V. (1997). Do dying patients really need IV fluids? *American Journal of Nursing, 97*(3), 26–30.

Zerzan, J., Stearns, S. & Hanson, L. (2000). Access to palliative care and hospice in nursing homes. *Journal of the American Medical Association, 284*(19), 2489–2493.

RESOURCES

American Academy of Hospice and Palliative Medicine, 4700 West Lake Avenue, Glenview, IL 60025; 847-375-4712; http://www.aahpm.org/. Accessed March 31, 2006.

Americans for Better Care of the Dying (ABCD), 4125 Albemarle Street NW, Suite 210, Washington, DC 20016; (202) 895-9485, http://www.abcdcaring.org/. Accessed March 31, 2006.

Association for Death Education and Counseling (ADEC), 342 North Main Street West Hartford, CT 06117; 860-586-7503; fax 860-586-7550; http://www.adec.org/. Accessed March 31, 2006.

American Hospice Foundation, 2120 L Street NW, Suite 200, Washington, DC 20037; 202-223-0204; fax 202-223-0208; e-mail: ahf@msn.com; http://www.americanhospice.org/. Accessed March 31, 2006.

Caring Connections, a program of the National Hospice and Palliative Care Organization, 1700 Diagonal Road, Suite 625, Alexandria, VA 22314; http://www.caringinfo.org. Accessed May 24, 2006.

Center to Improve Care of the Dying (at George Washington University); offices located at the RAND Corporation, 1200 South Hayes Street, Arlington, VA 22202; 703-413-1100; http://www.gwu.edu/~cicd/. Accessed March 31, 2006.

Children's Hospice International, 2202 Mount Vernon Avenue, Suite 3C, Alexandria, VA 22301; 800-24-CHILD; http://www.chionline.org. Accessed March 31, 2006.

Compassion in Dying, 6312 SW Capital Highway, Suite 415, Portland, OR 97201; 503-221-9556; http://www.compassionindying.org/. Accessed March 31, 2006.

Department of Pain Medicine and Palliative Care at Beth Israel Medical Center, 1st Avenue at 16th Street, 12 Baird Hall, New York, NY 10003; 212-844-1472; http://www.stoppain.org. Accessed March 31, 2006.

End-of-Life Nursing Education Consortium; http://www.aacn.nche.edu/elnec/. Accessed March 31, 2006.

Growthhouse, Inc. (provides information and referral services for agencies working with death and dying issues), San Francisco, CA; 415-863-3045; http://www.growthhouse.org. Accessed March 31, 2006.

HMS Center for Palliative Care (Harvard Medical School), Massachusetts General Hospital, Founders House 606, 55 Fruit Street, Boston, MA 02114; 617-724-9509; http://www.hms.harvard.edu/cdi/pallcare/. Accessed March 31, 2006.

Hospice and Palliative Nurses Association (HPNA), Penn Center West One, Suite 229, Pittsburgh, PA 15276; 412-787-9301; http://www.hpna.org. Accessed March 31, 2006.

Hospice Association of America, National Association for Home Care, 228 Seventh Street SE, Washington, DC 20003; 202-547-7424; http://www.hospiceamerica.org/. Accessed March 31, 2006.

Hospice Education Institute, 190 Westbrook Road, Essex, CT 06426; 800-331-1620; http://www.hospiceworld.org/. Accessed March 31, 2006.

Hospice Foundation of America, 2001 S St. NW #300, Washington, DC 20009; 800-854-3402; http://www.hospicefoundation.org. Accessed March 31, 2006.

Hospice Net; http://www.hospicenet.org/index.html. Accessed March 31, 2006.

Hospice Web (links to other resources); http://www.hospiceweb.com/links.htm. Accessed March 31, 2006.

Last Acts Partnership, 1620 Eye Street NW, Suite 202, Washington, DC 20006; 800-989-WILL; http://www.caringinfo.org. Accessed March 31, 2006.

National Consensus Project for Quality Palliative Care (National Guidelines); http://www.nationalconsensusproject.org. Accessed March 31, 2006.

National Hospice and Palliative Care Organization, National Hospice Foundation, 1700 Diagonal Rd, Suite 625, Alexandria, VA 22314; 703-837-1500; http://www.nhpco.org. Accessed March 31, 2006.

National Prison Hospice Association, P.O. Box 4623, Boulder, CO 80306-4623; 303-447-8051; fax 303-447-8055; http://www.npha.org. Accessed March 31, 2006.

Palliative Care Nursing; http://www.palliativecarenursing.net/index.html. Accessed March 31, 2006.

Partnership for Caring: America's Voices for the Dying, National Office, 1620 Eye Street NW, Suite 202, Washington, DC 20006; 202-296-8071; http://www.partnershipforcaring.org. Accessed March 31, 2006.

Population-based Palliative Care Research Network, University of Colorado Health Sciences Center, 4200 East 9th Avenue, Denver, CO 80262; 866-372-9417; http://www.uchsc.edu/popcrn/. Accessed March 31, 2006.

Project on Death in America, Open Society Institute, 400 West 59th Street, New York, NY 10019; 212-548-0150; http://www.soros.org/initiatives/pdia. Accessed March 31, 2006.

Promoting Excellence in End-of-Life Care, The Practical Ethics Center, The University of Montana, 1000 East Beckwith Avenue, Missoula, MT 59812; 406-243-6601; fax 406-243-6633; http://www.promotingexcellence.org. Accessed March 31, 2006.

Supportive Care of the Dying: A Coalition for Compassionate Care; for more information, contact Sylvia McSkimming, PhD, RN, Executive Director, c/o Providence Health System, 4805 NE Glisan Street, 2E07, Portland, OR 97213; 503-215-5053; http://www.careofdying.org. Accessed March 31, 2006.

The Center to Advance Palliative Care at The Mount Sinai School of Medicine, 1255 5th Avenue, Suite C-2, New York, NY, 10029; main line: 212-201-2670; http://www.capcmssm.org. Accessed March 31, 2006.

Toolkit of Instruments to Measure End-of-life Care (TIME; Dr. Joan Teno at Brown University); http://www.chcr.brown.edu/pcoc/toolkit.htm. Accessed March 31, 2006.

Veterans Administration Hospice and Palliative Care Initiative, Office on Academic Affiliations, Department of Veterans Affairs; http://www.va.gov/oaa/flp/. Accessed March 31, 2006.

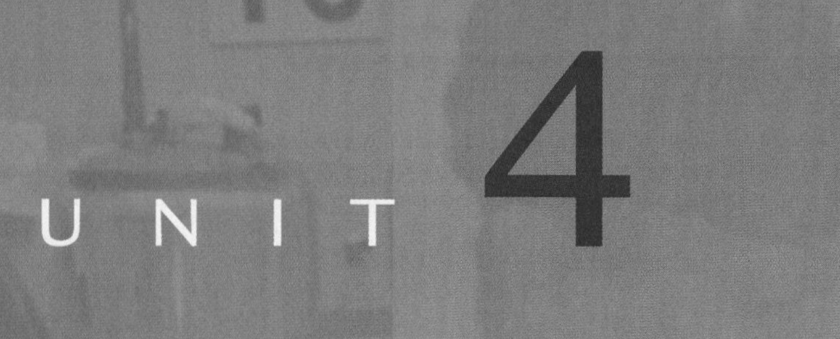

UNIT 4

Perioperative Concepts and Nursing Management

Case Study

Applying Concepts from NANDA, NIC, and NOC

A Patient Recovering From Abdominal Surgery

Mr. Dickson, a 60-year-old smoker, was admitted to the surgical unit 5 hours ago after colon resection for cancer. He is groggy but easily arousable. He can move all extremities with equal strength, but feels better lying still. In the last 4 hours, 125 mL of greenish material has drained from his nasogastric tube, which is connected to low intermittent suction. His abdomen is mildly distended; bowel sounds are absent. The large abdominal dressing has a reconstitutable bulb drain with 30 mL of serosanguineous drainage; the dressing's minimal visible drainage has not increased in several hours. A peripheral IV of D5W ½NS with 20 mEq of KCl is infusing at 125 mL/h. Mr. Dickson has voided 600 mL of clear urine. Vital signs are: Temp 97°F; HR 82, B/P 112/70; Resp 12 and shallow. Lung auscultation reveals scattered crackles throughout and a weak cough. After a 50-mg morphine injection, Mr. Dickson rates his pain at 3 (down from 7). He is reluctant to use his incentive spirometer for fear of more pain.

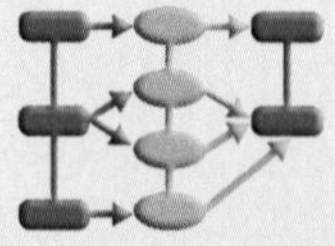

Turn to Appendix C to see a concept map that illustrates the relationships that exist between the nursing diagnoses, interventions, and outcomes for the patient's clinical problems.

Nursing Classifications and Languages

NANDA Nursing Diagnoses	NIC Nursing Interventions	NOC Nursing Outcomes Return to functional baseline status, stabilization of, or improvement in:
Risk for Impaired Gas Exchange—At risk for excess or deficit in oxygenation and/or carbon dioxide elimination at the alveolar-capillary membrane	**Respiratory Monitoring**—Collection and analysis of patient data to ensure airway patency and adequate gas exchange	**Anxiety Control**—Personal actions to eliminate or reduce feelings of apprehension and tension from an unidentifiable source
Risk for Ineffective Airway Clearance—At risk for inability to clear secretions or obstructions from the respiratory tract to maintain a clear airway	**Cough Enhancement**—Promotion of deep inhalation by the patient with subsequent generation of high intrathoracic pressures and compression of underlying lung parenchyma for the forceful expulsion of air	**Respiratory Status: Gas Exchange**—The alveolar exchange of O_2 and CO_2 to maintain arterial blood gas concentrations
Acute Pain—Unpleasant sensory and emotional experience arising from actual or potential tissue damage or described in terms of such damage	**Pain Management**—Alleviation of pain or reduction in pain to a level of comfort that is acceptable to the patient	**Pain Level**—Severity of observed or reported pain
Impaired Physical Mobility—Limitation in independent, purposeful physical movement of the body or of one or more extremities	**Teaching: Prescribed Activity/Exercise**—Preparing a patient to achieve and/or maintain a prescribed level of activity	**Mobility**—Ability to move purposefully in own environment independently with or without assistive device

NANDA International (2005). *Nursing diagnoses: Definitions & classification 2005–2006*. Philadelphia: North American Nursing Diagnosis Association.

Dochterman, J. M. & Bulechek, G. M. (2004). *Nursing interventions classification (NIC)* (4th ed.). St. Louis: Mosby.

Iowa Outcomes Project (2004). In Moorhead, S., Johnson, M. & Maas, M. (2004). *Nursing outcomes classification (NOC)* (3rd ed.). St. Louis: Mosby.

Dochterman, J. M. & Jones, D. A. (2003). *Unifying nursing languages: The harmonization of NANDA, NIC, and NOC*. Washington, D.C.: American Nurses Association.

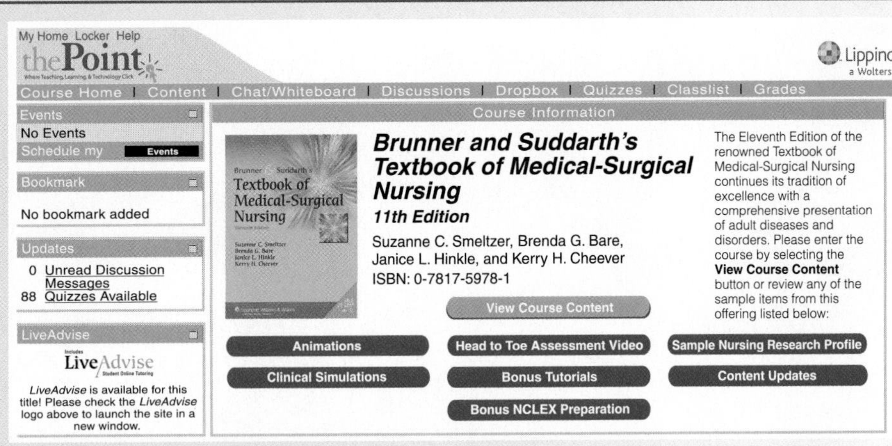

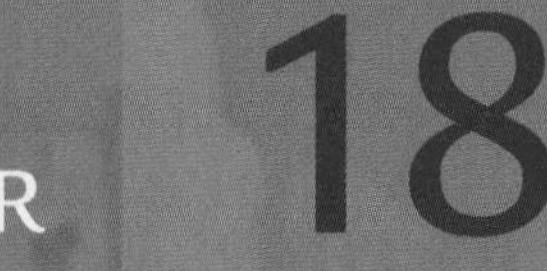

CHAPTER 18

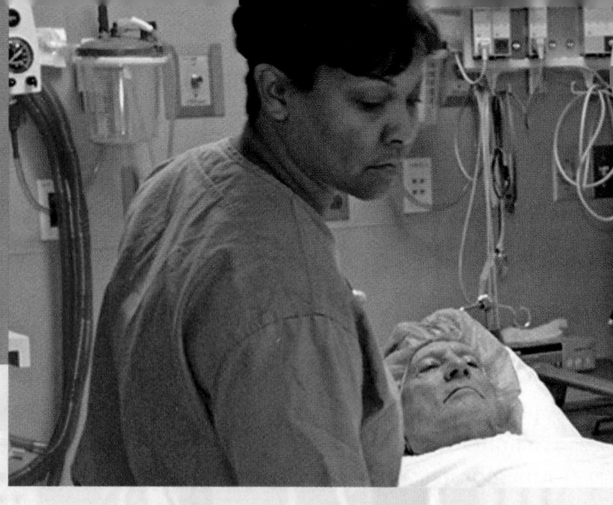

Preoperative Nursing Management

Learning Objectives

On completion of this chapter, the learner will be able to:

1. Define the three phases of perioperative nursing.
2. Describe a comprehensive preoperative assessment to identify surgical risk factors.
3. Identify health factors that affect patients preoperatively.
4. Identify legal and ethical considerations related to informed consent.
5. Describe preoperative nursing measures that decrease the risk for infection and other postoperative complications.
6. Describe the immediate preoperative preparation of the patient.
7. Develop a preoperative teaching plan designed to promote the patient's recovery from anesthesia and surgery, thus preventing postoperative complications.

Surgery, whether elective or emergent, is a stressful, complex event. Today, as a result of advances in surgical techniques and instrumentation as well as in anesthesia, many surgical procedures that were once performed in an inpatient setting now take place in ambulatory or outpatient settings. Approximately 60% of elective surgeries are now performed in an ambulatory or outpatient setting; this number is expected to continue to increase over the next decade (Conner, 2004). In the past, the patient scheduled for elective surgery was admitted to the hospital at least one day before surgery for evaluation and preparation; these activities are now completed before the patient is admitted to the hospital. Today, many patients arrive at the hospital on the morning of surgery and go home after recovering from the anesthesia in the postanesthesia care unit (PACU). Often, surgical patients who require hospital stays are trauma patients, acutely ill patients, patients undergoing major surgery, patients who require emergency surgery, and patients with a concurrent medical disorder. As a result, the acuity and complexity of surgical patients and procedures have increased in the inpatient setting. Although each setting (ambulatory, outpatient, or inpatient) offers its own unique advantages for the delivery of patient care, they all require a comprehensive preoperative nursing assessment and nursing interventions to prepare the patient and family before surgery.

Today's technology has led to more complex procedures, more complicated microsurgical and laser technology, more sophisticated bypass equipment, increased use of laparoscopic surgery, and more sensitive monitoring devices. Surgery today can involve the transplantation of multiple human organs, the implantation of mechanical devices, the reattachment of body parts, and the use of robots and minimally invasive procedures in the operating room (OR) (Lotan, Cadeddu & Gettman, 2004; Robinson & Stiegmann, 2004). Advances in anesthesia have kept pace with these surgical technologies. More sophisticated monitoring and new pharmacologic agents, such as short-acting anesthetics and more effective antiemetics, have improved postoperative pain management, reduced postoperative nausea and vomiting, and shortened procedure and recovery times.

Concurrent with technologic advances have been changes in the delivery of and payment for health care. Pressure to reduce hospital stays and contain costs has resulted in diagnostic **preadmission testing** (**PAT**) and preoperative preparation before admission to the hospital. Many facilities have a presurgical services department to facilitate PAT and to initiate the nursing assessment process, which focuses on patient demographics, health history, and other information pertinent to the surgical procedure (Halaszynski, Juda & Silverman, 2004). The increasing use of **ambulatory**, same-day, or short-stay surgery, means that patients leave the hospital sooner, which increases the need for teaching, discharge planning, preparation for self-care, and referral for home care and rehabilitation services. Competent care of ambulatory, same-day, or short-stay surgical patients requires a sound knowledge of all aspects of perioperative and perianesthesia nursing.

Perioperative and Perianesthesia Nursing

The special field known as perioperative and perianesthesia nursing includes a wide variety of nursing functions associated with the patient's surgical experience during the perioperative period. **Perioperative** and perianesthesia nursing addresses the nursing roles relevant to the three phases of the surgical experience: preoperative, intraoperative, and postoperative. Each phase begins and ends at a particular point in the sequence of events that constitutes the surgical experience, and each includes a wide range of activities the nurse performs using the nursing process and based on the standards of practice (American Society of PeriAnesthesia Nurses, 2002). Chart 18-1 presents nursing activities characteristic of the three perioperative phases of care.

Preoperative Phase

The **preoperative phase** begins when the decision to proceed with surgical intervention is made and ends with the transfer of the patient onto the OR table. The scope of nursing activities during this time involves establishing a baseline evaluation of the patient before surgery by carrying out a preoperative interview (which includes a physical

Glossary

ambulatory surgery: includes outpatient (same-day) surgery that does not require an overnight hospital stay or short stay, with admission to an inpatient hospital setting for less than 24 hours

informed consent: the patient's autonomous decision about whether to undergo a surgical procedure; based on the nature of the condition, the treatment options, and the risks and benefits involved

intraoperative phase: period of time from when the patient is transferred to the operating room table to when he or she is admitted to the postanesthesia care unit (PACU)

perioperative phase: period of time that constitutes the surgical experience; includes the preoperative, intraoperative, and postoperative phases of nursing care

postoperative phase: period of time that begins with the admission of the patient to the PACU and ends after a follow-up evaluation in the clinical setting or home

preadmission testing (PAT): diagnostic testing performed before admission to the hospital

preoperative phase: period of time from when the decision for surgical intervention is made to when the patient is transferred to the operating room table

CHART 18-1

Examples of Nursing Activities in the Perioperative Phases of Care

PREOPERATIVE PHASE

Preadmission Testing

1. Initiates initial preoperative assessment
2. Initiates teaching appropriate to patient's needs
3. Involves family in interview
4. Verifies completion of preoperative testing
5. Verifies understanding of surgeon-specific preoperative orders (eg, bowel preparation, preoperative shower)
6. Assesses patient's need for postoperative transportation and care

Admission to Surgical Center or Unit

1. Completes preoperative assessment
2. Assesses for risks for postoperative complications
3. Reports unexpected findings or any deviations from normal
4. Verifies that operative consent has been signed
5. Coordinates patient teaching with other nursing staff
6. Reinforces previous teaching
7. Explains phases in perioperative period and expectations
8. Answers patient's and family's questions
9. Develops a plan of care

In the Holding Area

1. Assesses patient's status, baseline pain and nutritional status
2. Reviews chart
3. Identifies patient
4. Verifies surgical site and marks site per institutional policy
5. Establishes intravenous line
6. Administers medications if prescribed
7. Takes measures to ensure patient's comfort
8. Provides psychological support
9. Communicates patient's emotional status to other appropriate members of the health care team

INTRAOPERATIVE PHASE

Maintenance of Safety

1. Maintains aseptic, controlled environment
2. Effectively manages human resources, equipment, and supplies for individualized patient care
3. Transfers patient to operating room bed or table
4. Positions the patient
   a. Functional alignment
   b. Exposure of surgical site
5. Applies grounding device to patient
6. Ensures that the sponge, needle, and instrument counts are correct
7. Completes intraoperative documentation

Physiologic Monitoring

1. Calculates effects on patient of excessive fluid loss or gain
2. Distinguishes normal from abnormal cardiopulmonary data
3. Reports changes in patient's vital signs
4. Institutes measures to promote normothermia

Psychological Support (Before Induction and When Patient Is Conscious)

1. Provides emotional support to patient
2. Stands near or touches patient during procedures and induction
3. Continues to assess patient's emotional status

POSTOPERATIVE PHASE

Transfer of Patient to Postanesthesia Care Unit

1. Communicates intraoperative information
   a. Identifies patient by name
   b. States type of surgery performed
   c. Identifies type of anesthetic used
   d. Reports patient's response to surgical procedure and anesthesia
   e. Describes intraoperative factors (eg, insertion of drains or catheters; administration of blood, analgesic agents, or other medications during surgery; occurrence of unexpected events)
   f. Describes physical limitations
   g. Reports patient's preoperative level of consciousness
   h. Communicates necessary equipment needs
   i. Communicates presence of family and/or significant others

Postoperative Assessment Recovery Area

1. Determines patient's immediate response to surgical intervention
2. Monitors patient's physiologic status
3. Assesses patient's pain level and administers appropriate pain relief measures
4. Maintains patient's safety (airway, circulation, prevention of injury)
5. Administers medications, fluid, and blood component therapy, if prescribed
6. Provides oral fluids if prescribed for ambulatory surgery patient
7. Assesses patient's readiness for transfer to in-hospital unit or for discharge home based on institutional policy (eg, Alderete score, see Chapter 20)

CHART 18-1 Examples of Nursing Activities in the Perioperative Phases of Care, continued

Surgical Unit

1. Continues close monitoring of patient's physical and psychological response to surgical intervention
2. Assesses patient's pain level and administers appropriate pain relief measures
3. Provides teaching to patient during immediate recovery period
4. Assists patient in recovery and preparation for discharge home
5. Determines patient's psychological status
6. Assists with discharge planning

Home or Clinic

1. Provides follow-up care during office or clinic visit or by telephone contact
2. Reinforces previous teaching and answers patient's and family's questions about surgery and follow-up care
3. Assesses patient's response to surgery and anesthesia and their effects on body image and function
4. Determines family's perception of surgery and its outcome

and emotional assessment, previous anesthetic and medical history, and identification of known allergies or genetics issues that may affect the surgical outcome), ensuring that necessary tests have been or will be performed in PAT, arranging appropriate consultations, and providing education about recovery from anesthesia and postoperative care (Garcia-Miguel, Serrano-Aguilar & Lopez-Bastida, 2003).

On the day of surgery, patient teaching is reviewed, the patient's identity and the surgical site are verified, informed consent is confirmed, and an intravenous (IV) infusion is started. If the patient is going home the same day, the availability of safe transport and the presence of an accompanying responsible adult are verified. Depending on when the preadmission evaluation and testing were done, nursing activities on the day of surgery include preoperative patient assessment and addressing questions the patient or family may have.

Intraoperative Phase

The **intraoperative phase** begins when the patient is transferred onto the OR table and ends with admission to the

NURSING RESEARCH PROFILE

The Effect of Preoperative Teaching on Outcomes

Oetker-Black, S. L., Jones, S., Estok, P., et al. (2003). Preoperative teaching and hysterectomy outcomes. *AORN Journal, 77*(6), 1215–1231.

Purpose

This study used a theoretical model of self-efficacy to determine whether an efficacy-enhancing teaching protocol was effective in improving immediate postoperative behaviors and selected short- and long-term health outcomes in women who underwent abdominal hysterectomy.

Design

A sample of 108 women admitted to a 486-bed teaching hospital in the Midwest for total abdominal hysterectomy was obtained by convenience sampling. Data collectors used the operating room schedule to identify potential participants based on predetermined criteria (eg, age, able to read English, alert and oriented). Those willing to participate in the 6-month study were randomly assigned to one of the study groups and received either the usual care protocol or the efficacy-enhancing teaching protocol. The efficacy-enhancing group received enhanced preoperative teaching. Sessions stressed the importance of early ambulation, included a detailed demonstration of the effective way to get out of bed, and required that participants demonstrate how to get out of bed.

Findings

There were no significant differences found between groups except in ambulation. Patients who received the efficacy-enhancing teaching ambulated significantly longer than those in the usual care group (330 seconds compared to a mean of 56 seconds).

Nursing Implications

The most common postoperative complications of hysterectomy or any major abdominal surgery are atelectasis, pneumonia, paralytic ileus, and deep vein thrombosis. Studies have previously shown that postoperative ambulation decreases or prevents all these complications. By incorporating enhanced preoperative patient instruction with return demonstrations, perioperative nurses can improve patients' postoperative ambulation.

PACU. In this phase, the scope of nursing activities includes providing for the patient's safety, maintaining an aseptic environment, ensuring proper function of equipment, providing the surgeon with specific instruments and supplies for the surgical field, and completing appropriate documentation. Nursing activities may include providing emotional support by holding the patient's hand during induction of general anesthesia; assisting in positioning the patient on the OR table using appropriate principles of body alignment; or acting as scrub nurse, circulating nurse, or registered nurse first assistant (RNFA).

Postoperative Phase

The **postoperative phase** begins with the admission of the patient to the PACU and ends with a follow-up evaluation in the clinical setting or home. The scope of nursing care covers a wide range of activities including maintaining the patient's airway, monitoring vital signs, assessing the effects of the anesthetic agents, assessing the patient for complications, and providing comfort and pain relief. Nursing activities also focus on promoting the patient's recovery and initiating the teaching, follow-up care, and referrals essential for recovery and rehabilitation after discharge. Each phase is reviewed in more detail in this chapter and in the other chapters in this unit.

A conceptual model of patient care, published by the Association of PeriOperative Registered Nurses, formerly known as the Association of Operating Room Nurses (still abbreviated AORN), helps delineate the relationships between various components of nursing practice and patient outcomes. The Perioperative Nursing Data Set (PNDS) categorizes the practice of perioperative nursing practice into four domains: safety, physiologic responses, behavioral responses, and health care systems (Fig. 18-1). The first three domains reflect phenomena of concern to perioperative nurses and are composed of nursing diagnoses, interventions, and outcomes. The fourth domain, the health care system, consists of structural data elements and focuses on clinical processes and outcomes. The model is used to depict the relationship of nursing process components to the achievement of optimal patient outcomes (Kleinbeck, 2004).

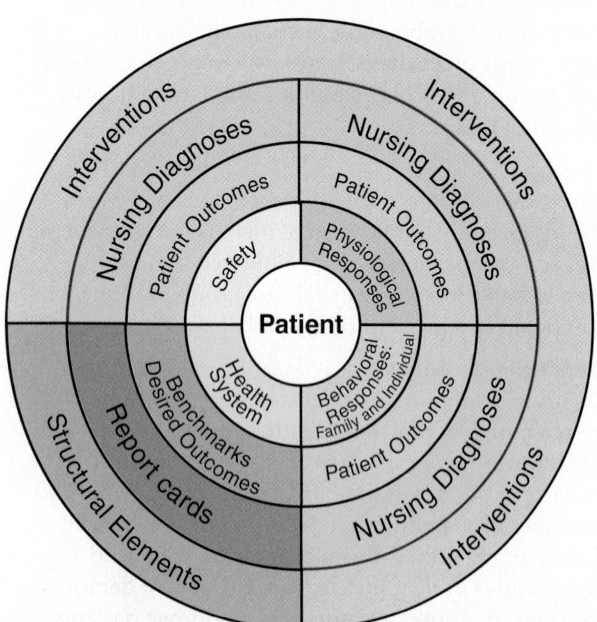

FIGURE 18-1. Perioperative patient-focused model. © With permission from Association of PeriOperative Registered Nurses, Inc., Denver, CO.

Surgical Classifications

Surgery may be performed for various reasons. A surgical procedure may be diagnostic (eg, biopsy, exploratory laparotomy), curative (eg, excision of a tumor or an inflamed appendix), or reparative (eg, multiple wound repair). It may be reconstructive or cosmetic (eg, mammoplasty or a facelift) or palliative (eg, to relieve pain or correct a problem—for instance, a gastrostomy tube may be inserted to compensate for the inability to swallow food). Surgery may also be classified according to the degree of urgency involved: emergent, urgent, required, elective, and optional (Table 18-1).

Preparation for Surgery

Informed Consent

Voluntary and written **informed consent** from the patient is necessary before nonemergent surgery can be performed. A written consent protects the patient from unsanctioned surgery and protects the surgeon from claims of an unauthorized operation. In the best interests of all parties concerned, sound medical, ethical, and legal principles are followed (Aiken, 2004). The nurse may ask the patient to sign the form and may witness the patient's signature. It is the physician's responsibility to provide appropriate information. Chart 18-2 lists the criteria for a valid informed consent (Bernat, 2004; Schroeter, 2003).

Many ethical principles are integral to informed consent (see Chapter 3). Before the patient signs the consent form, the surgeon must provide a clear and simple explanation of what the surgery will entail. The surgeon must also inform the patient of the benefits, alternatives, possible risks, complications, disfigurement, disability, and removal of body parts as well as what to expect in the early and late postoperative periods. If the patient requests additional information, the nurse notifies the physician. The nurse ascertains that the consent form has been signed before administering psychoactive premedication, because a consent may not be valid if it is obtained while the patient is under the influence of medications that can affect judgment and decision-making capacity. Informed consent is necessary in the following circumstances:

- Invasive procedures, such as a surgical incision, a biopsy, a cystoscopy, or paracentesis
- Procedures requiring sedation and/or anesthesia (see Chapter 19 for a discussion of anesthesia)
- A nonsurgical procedure, such as an arteriography, that carries more than slight risk to the patient
- Procedures involving radiation

TABLE 18-1 Categories of Surgery Based on Urgency

Classification	Indications for Surgery	Examples
I. Emergent—Patient requires immediate attention; disorder may be life-threatening	Without delay	Severe bleeding Bladder or intestinal obstruction Fractured skull Gunshot or stab wounds Extensive burns
II. Urgent—Patient requires prompt attention	Within 24–30 h	Acute gallbladder infection Kidney or ureteral stones
III. Required—Patient needs to have surgery	Plan within a few weeks or months	Prostatic hyperplasia without bladder obstruction Thyroid disorders Cataracts
IV. Elective—Patient should have surgery	Failure to have surgery not catastrophic	Repair of scars Simple hernia Vaginal repair
V. Optional—Decision rests with patient	Personal preference	Cosmetic surgery

The patient personally signs the consent if he or she is of legal age and is mentally capable. If the patient is a minor, is neurologically incapacitated, or is incompetent, permission must be obtained from a surrogate, who most often is a responsible family member (preferably next of kin) or legal guardian (Bernat, 2004). An emancipated minor (married or independently earning his or her own living) may sign his or her own consent form. State regulations and agency policy must be followed. In an emergency, it may be necessary for the surgeon to operate as a lifesaving measure without the patient's informed consent. However, every effort must be made to contact the patient's family. In such a situation, contact can be made by telephone, fax, or other electronic means.

If the patient has doubts and has not had the opportunity to investigate alternative treatments, a second opinion may be requested. No patient should be urged or coerced to give informed consent. Refusing to undergo a surgical procedure is a person's legal right and privilege. However, such information must be documented and relayed to the surgeon so that other arrangements can be made. For example, additional explanations may be provided to the patient and family, or the surgery may be rescheduled.

The consent process can be improved by providing audiovisual materials to supplement discussion, by ensuring that the wording of the consent form is understandable, and by using other strategies and resources as needed to help the patient understand its content. It may be necessary to have the consent available in multiple languages or have a trained medical interpreter available. Alternative formats of communication (eg, Braille, large print, sign interpreter) may be needed if the patient is elderly or has a disability (Saufl, 2004).

CHART 18-2

Criteria for Valid Informed Consent

VOLUNTARY CONSENT

Valid consent must be freely given, without coercion.

INCOMPETENT PATIENT

Legal definition: individual who is *not* autonomous and cannot give or withhold consent (eg, individuals who are cognitively impaired, mentally ill, or neurologically incapacitated)

INFORMED SUBJECT

Informed consent should be in writing. It should contain the following:

- Explanation of procedure and its risks
- Description of benefits and alternatives
- An offer to answer questions about procedure
- Instructions that the patient may withdraw consent
- A statement informing the patient if the protocol differs from customary procedure

PATIENT ABLE TO COMPREHEND

Information must be written and delivered in language understandable to the patient. Questions must be answered to facilitate comprehension if material is confusing.

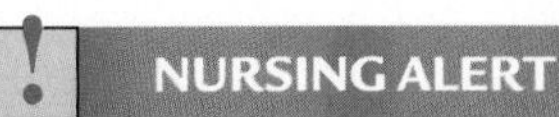

The signed consent form is placed in a prominent place on the patient's chart and accompanies the patient to the OR.

Assessment of Health Factors That Affect Patients Preoperatively

The goal in the preoperative period is for the patient to have as many positive health factors as possible. Many risk factors may lead to complications (Chart 18-3). Every attempt is made to stabilize those conditions that otherwise

CHART 18-3

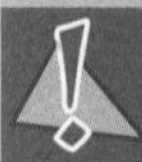

Risk Factors for Surgical Complications

- Hypovolemia
- Dehydration or electrolyte imbalance
- Nutritional deficits
- Extremes of age (very young, very old)
- Extremes of weight (emaciation, obesity)
- Infection and sepsis
- Toxic conditions
- Immunologic abnormalities
- Pulmonary disease
  - Obstructive disease
  - Restrictive disorder
  - Respiratory infection
- Renal or urinary tract disease
  - Decreased renal function
  - Urinary tract infection
  - Obstruction
- Pregnancy
  - Diminished maternal physiologic reserve
- Cardiovascular disease
  - Coronary artery disease or previous myocardial infarction
  - Cardiac failure
  - Dysrhythmias
  - Hypertension
  - Prosthetic heart valve
  - Thromboembolism
  - Hemorrhagic disorders
  - Cerebrovascular disease
- Endocrine dysfunction
  - Diabetes mellitus
  - Adrenal disorders
  - Thyroid malfunction
- Hepatic disease
  - Cirrhosis
  - Hepatitis
- Preexisting mental or physical disability

hinder recovery. When negative factors dominate, the risks of surgery and postoperative complications increase.

Before any surgical treatment is initiated, a health history is obtained, a physical examination is performed during which vital signs are noted, and a database is established for future comparisons. During the physical examination, many factors that have the potential to affect the patient undergoing surgery are considered (Bickley & Szilagyi, 2003). Health care providers should be alert for signs of abuse, which can occur at all ages and to men and women from all socioeconomic, ethnic, and cultural groups (Fuller, 2003). Findings need to be reported accordingly (see Chapter 5 for further discussion of signs of abuse). Blood tests, x-rays, and other diagnostic tests are prescribed when indicated by information obtained from the history and physical examination.

Nutritional and Fluid Status

Optimal nutrition is an essential factor in promoting healing and resisting infection and other surgical complications. Assessment of a patient's nutritional status identifies factors that can affect the patient's surgical course, such as obesity, undernutrition, weight loss, malnutrition, deficiencies in specific nutrients, metabolic abnormalities, and the effects of medications on nutrition. Nutritional needs may be determined by measurement of body mass index and waist circumference (U.S. Department of Health and Human Services, 2005). See Chapter 5 for further discussion of nutritional assessment.

Any nutritional deficiency, such as malnutrition, should be corrected before surgery to provide adequate protein for tissue repair. The nutrients needed for wound healing are summarized in Table 18-2.

Dehydration, hypovolemia, and electrolyte imbalances can lead to significant problems in patients with comorbid medical conditions or in patients who are elderly. The severity of fluid and electrolyte imbalances is often difficult to determine. Mild volume deficits may be treated during surgery; however, additional time may be needed to correct pronounced fluid and electrolyte deficits to promote the best possible preoperative condition.

Drug or Alcohol Use

People who abuse drugs or alcohol frequently deny or attempt to hide it. In such situations, the nurse who is obtaining the patient's health history needs to ask frank questions with patience, care, and a nonjudgmental attitude. See Chapter 5 for an assessment of alcohol and drug use.

Because acutely intoxicated people are susceptible to injury, surgery is postponed if possible. If emergency surgery is required, local, spinal, or regional block anesthesia is used for minor surgery. Otherwise, to prevent vomiting and potential aspiration, a nasogastric tube is inserted before general anesthesia is administered.

The person with a history of chronic alcoholism often suffers from malnutrition and other systemic problems that increase surgical risk. Alcohol withdrawal syndrome or delirium tremens may be anticipated between 48 and 72 hours after alcohol withdrawal (Schofield, 2004) and is associated with a significant mortality rate when it occurs postoperatively.

Respiratory Status

The goal for surgical patients is optimal respiratory function. The patient is taught breathing exercises and the use of an incentive spirometer if indicated. Because adequate ventilation is potentially compromised during all phases of surgical treatment, surgery is usually postponed if the patient has a respiratory infection. Patients with underlying respiratory disease (eg, asthma, chronic obstructive pulmonary disease) are assessed carefully for current threats to their pulmonary status. Patients also need to be assessed for comorbid conditions such as human immunodeficiency virus (HIV) in-

TABLE 18-2 Nutrients Important for Wound Healing

Nutrient	Rationale for Increased Need	Possible Deficiency Outcome
Protein	To allow collagen deposition and wound healing to occur	Collagen deposition leading to impaired/delayed wound healing Decreased skin and wound strength Increased wound infection rates
Arginine (amino acid)	To provide necessary substrate for collagen synthesis and nitric oxide (crucial for wound healing) at wound site To increase wound strength and collagen deposition To stimulate T-cell response Associated with a variety of essential reactions of intermediary metabolism	Impaired wound healing
Carbohydrates and fats	Primary source of energy in the body and consequently in the wound healing process To meet the demand for increased essential fatty acids needed for cellular function after an injury To spare protein To restore normal weight	Signs and symptoms of protein deficiency due to use of protein to meet energy requirements Extensive weight loss
Water	To replace fluid lost through vomiting, hemorrhage, exudates, fever, drainage, diuresis To maintain homeostasis	Signs, symptoms, and complications of dehydration, such as poor skin turgor, dry mucous membranes, oliguria, anuria, weight loss, increased pulse rate, decreased central venous pressure
Vitamin C	Important for capillary formation, tissue synthesis, and wound healing through collagen formation Needed for antibody formation	Impaired/delayed wound healing related to impaired collagen formation and increased capillary fragility and permeability Increased risk of infection related to decreased antibodies
Vitamin B complex	Indirect role in wound healing through their influence on host resistance	Decreased enzymes available for energy metabolism
Vitamin A	Increases inflammatory response in wounds, reduces anti-inflammatory effects of corticosteroids on wound healing	Impaired/delayed wound healing related to decreased collagen synthesis; impaired immune function Increased risk of infection
Vitamin K	Important for normal blood clotting Impaired intestinal synthesis associated with the use of antibiotics	Prolonged prothrombin time Hematomas contributing to impaired healing and predisposition to wound infections
Magnesium	Essential cofactor for many enzymes that are involved in the process of protein synthesis and wound repair	Impaired/delayed wound healing (impaired collagen production)
Copper	Required cofactor in the development of connective tissue	Impaired wound healing
Zinc	Involved DNA synthesis, protein synthesis, cellular proliferation needed for wound healing Essential to immune function	Impaired immune response

Table prepared and updated using information from Williams, J. & Barbul, A. (2003). Nutrition and wound healing. *Surgical Clinics of North America 83*(3), 571–596.

fection and Parkinson's disease, which may affect respiratory function (Galvez-Jimenez & Lang, 2004; Gotta, 2004).

Patients who smoke are urged to stop 4 to 8 weeks before surgery to significantly reduce pulmonary and wound healing complications, although many patients do not do so. These patients should be counseled to stop smoking at least 24 hours before surgery (Coleman, Cheater & Murphy, 2004).

Cardiovascular Status

The goal in preparing any patient for surgery is to ensure a well-functioning cardiovascular system to meet the oxygen, fluid, and nutritional needs of the perioperative period. If the patient has uncontrolled hypertension, surgery may be postponed until the blood pressure is under control. At times, surgical treatment can be modified to meet the cardiac tolerance of the patient. For example, in a patient with obstruction of the descending colon and coronary artery disease, a temporary simple colostomy may be performed rather than a more extensive colon resection that would require a prolonged period of anesthesia.

Hepatic and Renal Function

The presurgical goal is optimal function of the liver and urinary systems so that medications, anesthetic agents, body wastes, and toxins are adequately processed and removed from the body.

The liver is important in the biotransformation of anesthetic compounds. Therefore, any disorder of the liver has an effect on how anesthetic agents are metabolized. Because acute liver disease is associated with high surgical mortality (Wiklund, 2004), preoperative improvement in liver function is a goal. Careful assessment may include various liver function tests (see Chapter 39).

Because the kidneys are involved in excreting anesthetic medications and their metabolites and because acid–base status and metabolism are also important considerations in anesthesia administration, surgery is contraindicated if a patient has acute nephritis, acute renal insufficiency with oliguria or anuria, or other acute renal problems. The exception is surgery that is performed as a lifesaving measure or that is necessary to improve urinary function, as in the case of an obstructive uropathy.

Endocrine Function

The patient with diabetes who is undergoing surgery is at risk for hypoglycemia and hyperglycemia. Hypoglycemia may develop during anesthesia or postoperatively from inadequate carbohydrates or excessive administration of insulin. Hyperglycemia, which can increase the risk for surgical wound infection, may result from the stress of surgery, which can trigger increased levels of catecholamine (Lorenz, Lorenz & Cody, 2005). Other risks are acidosis and glucosuria. Although the surgical risk in the patient with controlled diabetes is no greater than in the patient without diabetes, the goal is to maintain the blood glucose level at or below 200 mg/dL (Lorenz et al., 2005). Frequent monitoring of blood glucose levels is important before, during, and after surgery (see Chapter 41 for discussion of the patient with diabetes undergoing surgery).

Patients who have received corticosteroids are at risk of adrenal insufficiency. Therefore, the use of corticosteroids for any purpose during the preceding year must be reported to the anesthesiologist, anesthetist (usually a nurse anesthetist), and surgeon. The patient is monitored for signs of adrenal insufficiency.

Patients with uncontrolled thyroid disorders are at risk for thyrotoxicosis (with hyperthyroid disorders) or respiratory failure (with hypothyroid disorders). Therefore, the patient is assessed for a history of these disorders.

Immune Function

An important function of the preoperative assessment is to determine the presence of allergies. It is especially important to identify and document any sensitivity to medications and past adverse reactions to these agents. The patient is asked to identify any substances that precipitated previous allergic reactions, including medications, blood transfusions, contrast agents, latex, and food products, and to describe the signs and symptoms produced by these substances. A sample latex allergy screening questionnaire is shown in Figure 18-2.

Immunosuppression is common with corticosteroid therapy, renal transplantation, radiation therapy, chemotherapy, and disorders affecting the immune system, such as AIDS and leukemia. The mildest symptoms or slightest temperature elevation must be investigated. Because patients who are immunosuppressed are highly susceptible to infection, great care is taken to ensure strict asepsis.

Previous Medication Use

A medication history is obtained from each patient because of the possible effects of medications on the patient's perioperative course, including the possibility of drug interactions. Any medication the patient is using or has used in the past is documented, including over-the-counter (OTC) preparations and herbal agents and the frequency with which they are used. Potent medications have an effect on physiologic functions; interactions of such medications with anesthetic agents can cause serious problems, such as arterial hypotension and circulatory collapse.

The potential effects of prior medication therapy are evaluated by the anesthesiologist or anesthetist, who considers the length of time the patient has used the medication, the physical condition of the patient, and the nature of the proposed surgery. Medications that cause particular concern are listed in Table 18-3.

In addition, many patients take self-prescribed or OTC medications. Aspirin is a common OTC medication that inhibits platelet aggregation; therefore, it is prudent to stop aspirin at least 7 to 10 days before surgery if possible, especially for surgeries in which excess bleeding would cause significant complications, such as brain or spinal cord surgeries (Bohan & Glass-Macenka, 2004; Mercado & Petty, 2003). Because of the effects of aspirin or other OTC medications and possible interactions with prescribed medications and anesthetic agents, it is important to ask a patient about their use. The information is noted in the patient's chart and conveyed to the anesthesiologist, anesthetist and surgeon.

The use of herbal medications is widespread among patients; approximately 15 million Americans report using these substances (Heyneman, 2003; MacKichan & Ruthman, 2004). The most commonly used herbal medications are echinacea, ephedra, garlic (*Allium sativum*), ginkgo biloba, ginseng, kava kava (*Piper methysticum*), St. John's wort (*Hypericum perforatum*), licorice (*Glycyrriza glabra*), and valerian (*Valeriana officinalis*). However, many patients fail to report using herbal medicines to their health care providers. Because of the potential effects of herbal medications on coagulation and potentially lethal interactions with other medications, the nurse must ask surgical patients specifically about the use of these agents, document their use, and inform the surgical team and anesthesiologist or anesthetist. Currently, it is recommended that the use of herbal

Ask the patient the following questions. Check "Yes" or "No" in the box.	YES	NO
1. Has a doctor ever told you that you are allergic to latex?		
2. Do you have on-the-job exposure to latex?		
3. Were you born with problems involving your spinal cord?		
4. Have you ever had allergies, asthma, hay fever, eczema or problems with rashes?		
5. Have you ever had respiratory distress, rapid heart rate or swelling?		
6. Have you ever had swelling, itching, hives or other symptoms after contact with a balloon?		
7. Have you ever had swelling, itching, hives or other symptoms after a dental examination or procedure?		
8. Have you ever had swelling, itching, hives or other symptoms following a vaginal or rectal examination or after contact with a diaphragm or condom?		
9. Have you ever had swelling, itching, hives or other symptoms during or within one hour after wearing rubber gloves?		
10. Have you ever had a rash on your hands that lasted longer than one week?		
11. Have you ever had swelling, itching, hives, runny nose, eye irritation, wheezing, or asthma after contact with any latex or rubber product?		
12. Have you ever had swelling, itching, hives or other symptoms after being examined by someone wearing rubber or latex gloves?		
13. Are you allergic to bananas, avocados, kiwi or chestnuts?		
14. Have you ever had an unexplained anaphylactic episode?		

Pre-op RN Signature: ______________________

Patient Name: ______________________

Procedure: ______________________

Scheduled Date / Time: ______________________

Surgeon: ______________________

FIGURE 18-2. Example of a latex allergy assessment form. Courtesy of Inova Fairfax Hospital, Falls Church, VA.

products be discontinued 2 to 3 weeks before surgery (MacKichan & Ruthman, 2004).

NURSING ALERT

Because of possible adverse interactions, the nurse must assess and document the patient's use of prescription medications, OTC medications (especially aspirin), and herbal agents. The nurse must clearly communicate this information to the anesthesiologist or anesthetist.

Psychosocial Factors

All patients have some type of emotional reaction before any surgical procedure, be it obvious or hidden, normal or abnormal. For example, preoperative anxiety may be an anticipatory response to an experience the patient views as a threat to his or her customary role in life, body integrity, or life itself. Psychological distress directly influences body functioning. Therefore, it is imperative to identify any anxiety the patient is experiencing (Defazio-Quinn & Schick, 2004).

Most patients who are about to undergo surgery have fears, including fear of the unknown, of death, of anesthesia, of pain, or of cancer. Concerns about loss of work time, loss of job, increased responsibilities or burden on family

TABLE 18-3 Examples of Medications With the Potential to Affect the Surgical Experience

Agent (Generic and Trade Example)	Effect of Interaction With Anesthetics
Corticosteroids Prednisone (Deltasone)	Cardiovascular collapse can occur if discontinued suddenly. Therefore, a bolus of corticosteroid may be administered intravenously immediately before and after surgery.
Diuretics Hydrochlorothiazide (HydroDIURIL)	During anesthesia, may cause excessive respiratory depression resulting from an associated electrolyte imbalance
Phenothiazines Chlorpromazine (Thorazine)	May increase the hypotensive action of anesthetics
Tranquilizers Diazepam (Valium)	May cause anxiety, tension, and even seizures if withdrawn suddenly
Insulin	Interaction between anesthetics and insulin must be considered when a patient with diabetes is undergoing surgery. Intravenous insulin may need to be administered to keep the blood glucose within the normal range.
Antibiotics Erythromycin (Ery-Tab)	When combined with a curariform muscle relaxant, nerve transmission is interrupted and apnea from respiratory paralysis may result.
Anticoagulants Warfarin (Coumadin)	Can increase the risk of bleeding during the intraoperative and postoperative periods; should be discontinued in anticipation of elective surgery. The surgeon will determine how long before the elective surgery the patient should stop taking an anticoagulant, depending on the type of planned procedure and the medical condition of the patient.
Antiseizure Medications	Intravenous administration of medication may be needed to keep the patient seizure-free in the intraoperative and postoperative periods.
Monoamine Oxidase (MAO) Inhibitors Phenelzine sulfate (Nardil)	May increase the hypotensive action of anesthetics
Thyroid Hormone Levothyroxine sodium (Levothyroid)	Intravenous administration may be needed during the postoperative period to maintain thyroid levels.

members, and the threat of permanent incapacity further contribute to the emotional strain created by the prospect of surgery. Less obvious concerns may occur because of previous experiences with the health care system and people the patient has known with the same condition.

People express fear in different ways. For example, some patients may repeatedly ask many questions, even though answers were given previously. Others may withdraw, deliberately avoiding communication, perhaps by reading, watching television, or talking about trivialities. Consequently, the nurse must be empathetic, listen well, and provide information that helps alleviate concerns.

An important outcome of the psychosocial assessment is the determination of the extent and role of the patient's support network. The value and reliability of all available support systems are assessed. Other information, such as usual level of functioning and typical daily activities, may assist in the patient's care and rehabilitation plans. Assessing the patient's readiness to learn and determining the best approach to maximize comprehension provides the basis for preoperative patient education.

Spiritual and Cultural Beliefs

Spiritual beliefs play an important role in how people cope with fear and anxiety. Regardless of the patient's religious affiliation, spiritual beliefs can be as therapeutic as medication. Every attempt must be made to help the patient obtain the spiritual support that he or she requests. Faith has great sustaining power. Therefore, the beliefs of each patient should be respected and supported. Some nurses avoid the subject of a clergy visit lest the suggestion alarm the patient. Asking whether the patient's spiritual advisor knows about the impending surgery is a caring, nonthreatening approach.

Showing respect for a patient's cultural values and beliefs facilitates rapport and trust. Some areas of assessment include identifying the ethnic group to which the patient relates and the customs and beliefs the patient holds about illness and health care providers. For example, patients from some cultural groups are unaccustomed to expressing feelings openly. Nurses need to consider this pattern of communication when assessing pain. As a sign of respect, people from some cultural groups may not make direct eye contact with others (Flowers, 2004). The nurse should know that this lack of eye contact is not avoidance or a lack of interest.

Perhaps the most valuable skill at the nurse's disposal is listening carefully to the patient, especially when obtaining the history. Invaluable information and insights may be gained through effective communication and interviewing skills. An unhurried, understanding, and caring nurse promotes confidence on the part of the patient.

Special Situations

In the preoperative period, attention needs to be paid to patients with special situations.

Patients Undergoing Ambulatory Surgery

The brief time the patient and family spend in the ambulatory setting is an important factor in the preoperative period. The nurse must quickly and comprehensively assess and anticipate the patient's needs and at the same time begin planning for discharge and follow-up home care.

The nurse needs to be sure that the patient and family understand that the patient will first go to the preoperative holding area before going to the OR for the surgical procedure and then will spend some time in the PACU before being discharged home with the family later that day. Other preoperative teaching content should also be verified and reinforced as needed (see later discussion). The nurse should ensure that any plans for follow-up home care are in place if needed.

Gerontologic Considerations

Preoperative pain assessment and teaching are important in the elderly patient. The older person undergoing surgery may have a combination of chronic illnesses and health issues in addition to the specific one for which surgery is indicated. Elderly people frequently do not report symptoms, perhaps because they fear a serious illness may be diagnosed or because they accept such symptoms as part of the aging process. Subtle clues alert the nurse to underlying problems. Research indicates that key predictors of perioperative complications in the elderly are the patient's preoperative condition and level of functioning (John & Sieber, 2004).

Health care staff must remember that the hazards of surgery for the aged are proportional to the number and severity of coexisting health problems and the nature and duration of the operative procedure. The underlying principle that guides the preoperative assessment, surgical care, and postoperative care is that the aged patient has less physiologic reserve (the ability of an organ to return to normal after a disturbance in its equilibrium) than a younger patient does. Cardiac reserves are lower, renal and hepatic functions are depressed, and gastrointestinal activity is likely to be reduced. Dehydration, constipation, and malnutrition may be evident. Sensory limitations, such as impaired vision or hearing and reduced tactile sensitivity, are often the reasons for falls and burns (Defazio-Quinn & Schick, 2004). Therefore, the nurse must be alert to maintaining a safe environment. Arthritis is common in older people and may affect mobility, making it difficult for the patient to turn from one side to the other or ambulate without discomfort. Protective measures include adequate padding for tender areas, moving the patient slowly, protecting bony prominences from prolonged pressure, and providing gentle massage to promote circulation.

The condition of the mouth is important to assess. Dental caries, dentures, and partial plates are particularly significant to the anesthesiologist or anesthetist, because decayed teeth or dental prostheses may become dislodged during intubation and occlude the airway.

As the body ages, its ability to perspire decreases. Because decreased perspiration leads to dry, itchy skin that becomes fragile and is easily abraded, precautions are taken when moving an elderly person. Decreased subcutaneous fat makes older people more susceptible to temperature changes. A lightweight cotton blanket is an appropriate cover when an elderly patient is moved to and from the OR.

Most elderly people have experienced personal illnesses and possibly life-threatening illnesses of friends and family. Such experiences may result in fears about the surgery and about the future. Providing an opportunity to express these fears enables the patient to gain some peace of mind.

Because the elderly patient may have greater risks during the perioperative period, the following factors are critical: (1) skillful preoperative assessment and treatment, (2) skillful anesthesia and surgery, and (3) meticulous and competent postoperative and postanesthesia management. In addition, the nurse should incorporate pain management information and pain communication skills when teaching the elderly patient how to obtain greater postoperative pain relief.

Patients Who Are Obese

Like age, obesity increases the risk and severity of complications associated with surgery. During surgery, fatty tissues are especially susceptible to infection. In addition, obesity increases technical and mechanical problems related to surgery. Therefore, dehiscence (wound separation) and wound infections are more common. Moreover, the obese patient may be more difficult to care for because of the added weight. The patient tends to have shallow respirations when supine, which increases the risk of hypoventilation and postoperative pulmonary complications. It has been estimated that for each 30 pounds of excess weight, about 25 additional miles of blood vessels are needed, and this places increased demands on the heart. As the incidence of obesity continues to grow, nurses will be called on to be part of multidisciplinary teams that will develop and implement clinical plans for patients who are obese (Charlebois & Wilmothe, 2004).

Patients With Disabilities

Special considerations for patients with mental or physical disabilities include the need for appropriate assistive devices, modifications in preoperative teaching, and additional assistance with and attention to positioning or transferring. Assistive devices include hearing aids, eyeglasses, braces, prostheses, and other devices. People who are hearing-impaired may need a sign interpreter or some alternative communication system perioperatively. If the patient relies on signing or speech (lip) reading and his or her eyeglasses or contact lenses are removed or the health care staff wear surgical masks, an alternative method of communication will be needed. These needs must be identified in the preoperative evaluation and clearly communicated to personnel. Specific strategies for accommodating the patient's needs must be identified in advance. Ensuring the security of assistive devices is important, because these devices are expensive and are likely to be lost.

Most patients are directed to move from the stretcher to the OR table and back again. In addition to being unable to see or hear instructions, the patient with a disability may be unable to move without special devices or a great deal of assistance. The patient with a disability that affects body position (eg, cerebral palsy, postpolio syndrome, other neuromuscular disorders) may need special positioning during surgery to prevent pain and injury. Moreover, these patients may be unable to sense whether their extremities are positioned incorrectly.

Patients with respiratory problems related to a disability (eg, multiple sclerosis, muscular dystrophy) may experience difficulties unless the problems are made known to the anesthesiologist or anesthetist and adjustments are made. These factors need to be clearly identified in the preoperative period and communicated to the appropriate personnel.

Patients Undergoing Emergency Surgery

Emergency surgeries are unplanned and occur with little time for preparation for the patient or the perioperative team. The unpredictable nature of trauma and emergency surgery poses unique challenges to the nurse throughout the perioperative period. In addition, research suggests that older patients undergoing urgent or emergent coronary artery bypass grafting surgery are at higher risk for prolonged mechanical ventilation compared with those undergoing a planned surgery (Bezanson, Weaver, Kinney, et al., 2004).

All of the previously discussed factors that affect patients preparing to undergo surgery apply to these patients, usually in a very condensed time frame. The only preoperative assessment may take place at the same time as resuscitation in the emergency department. For the unconscious patient, informed consent and essential information, such as pertinent past medical history and allergies, need to be obtained from a family member, if one is available. A quick visual survey of the patient is essential to identify all sites of injury if the emergency surgery is due to trauma (see Chapter 71 for more information). The patient, who may have undergone a very frightening experience, may need extra support and explanation of the surgery.

Preoperative Nursing Interventions

Preoperative Teaching

Nurses have long recognized the value of preoperative instruction (Rothrock, 2003). Each patient is taught as an individual, with consideration for any unique concerns or learning needs. Multiple teaching strategies should be used (eg, verbal, written, return demonstration), depending on the patient's needs and abilities (Saufl, 2004). Preoperative teaching is initiated as soon as possible. It should start in the physician's office or at the time of PAT and continue until the patient arrives in the OR.

When and What to Teach

Ideally, instruction is spaced over a period of time to allow the patient to assimilate information and ask questions as they arise. Frequently, teaching sessions are combined with various preparation procedures to allow for an easy and timely flow of information. The nurse should guide the patient through the experience and allow ample time for questions. For some patients, overly detailed descriptions increase anxiety; the nurse should be sensitive to this and provide less detail.

Teaching should go beyond descriptions of the procedure and should include explanations of the sensations the patient will experience. For example, telling the patient only that preoperative medication will cause relaxation before the operation is not as effective as also noting that the medication may result in lightheadedness and drowsiness. Knowing what to expect will help the patient anticipate these reactions and thus attain a higher degree of relaxation than might otherwise be expected. In addition, preoperative teaching includes instruction in breathing and leg exercises used to prevent postoperative complications such as pneumonia and deep vein thrombosis. These exercises may be performed in the hospital or at home (Chart 18-4).

The ideal timing for preoperative teaching is not on the day of surgery but during the preadmission visit, when diagnostic tests are performed. At this time, the nurse or resource person answers questions and provides important patient teaching. During this visit, the patient can meet and ask questions of the perioperative nurse, view audiovisual resources, receive written materials, and be given the telephone number to call as questions arise closer to the date of surgery. Most institutions provide written instructions (designed to be copied and given to patients) about many types of surgery. Patients who are elderly or have impaired vision may need a large-print version of written instructions (Saufl, 2004).

Deep-Breathing, Coughing, and Incentive Spirometry

One goal of preoperative nursing care is to teach the patient how to promote optimal lung expansion and consequent blood oxygenation after anesthesia. The patient assumes a sitting position to enhance lung expansion. The nurse then demonstrates how to take a deep, slow breath and how to

GENETICS IN NURSING PRACTICE

Perioperative Nursing

Nurses who are caring for patients undergoing surgery need to take various genetic considerations into account when assessing patients throughout the perioperative experience. For example, surgical outcomes may be altered by genetic conditions that may cause complications with anesthesia, including the following:

- Malignant hyperthermia
- Central core disease (CCD)
- Duchenne muscular dystrophy
- Hyperkalemic periodic paralysis
- King-Denborough Syndrome

NURSING ASSESSMENTS

Preoperative Family History Assessment

- Obtain a thorough assessment of personal and family history, inquiring about prior problems with surgery or anesthesia with specific attention to complications such as fever, rigidity, dark urine, and unexpected reactions.
- Inquire about any history of musculoskeletal complaints, history of heat intolerance, fevers of unknown origin, or unusual drug reaction.
- Assess for family history of any sudden or unexplained death, especially during participation in athletic events.

Patient Assessment

- Assess for subclinical muscle weakness.
- Assess for other physical features suggestive of an underlying genetic condition, such as contractures, kyphoscoliosis, and pterygium with progressive weakness.

Management Issues Specific to Genetics

- Inquire whether DNA mutation or other genetic testing has been performed on an affected family member.
- If indicated, refer for further genetic counseling and evaluation so that family members can discuss inheritance, risk to other family members, availability of diagnostic/genetic testing.
- Offer appropriate genetics information and resources.
- Assess patient's understanding of genetics information.
- Provide support to families with newly diagnosed malignant hyperthermia.
- Participate in management and coordination of care of patients with genetic conditions and individuals predisposed to develop or pass on a genetic condition.

GENETICS RESOURCES FOR NURSES AND THEIR PATIENTS ON THE WEB

Genetic Alliance, www.geneticalliance.org—a directory of support groups for patients and families with genetic conditions

Gene Clinics, www.geneclinics.org—a listing of common genetic disorders with up-to-date clinical summaries, genetic counseling and testing information

International Council of Nurses, www.icn.ch/matters_genetics.htm—ICN's statement re: genetics and nursing.

National Organization of Rare Disorders, www.rarediseases.org—a directory of support groups and information for patients and families with rare genetic disorders

OMIM: Online Mendelian Inheritance in Man, www.ncbi.nlm.nih.gov/entrez/query.fcgi?db-OMIM—a complete listing of inherited genetic conditions

exhale slowly. After practicing deep breathing several times, the patient is instructed to breathe deeply, exhale through the mouth, take a short breath, and cough from deep in the lungs (see Chart 18-4). The nurse also demonstrates how to use an incentive spirometer, a device that provides measurement and feedback related to breathing effectiveness (see Chapter 25). In addition to enhancing respiration, these exercises may help the patient relax.

If a thoracic or abdominal incision is anticipated, the nurse demonstrates how to splint the incision to minimize pressure and control pain. The patient should put the palms of both hands together, interlacing the fingers snugly. Placing the hands across the incisional site acts as an effective splint when coughing. In addition, the patient is informed that medications are available to relieve pain and should be taken regularly for pain relief so that effective deep-breathing and coughing exercises can be performed. The goal in promoting coughing is to mobilize secretions so that they can be removed. Deep breathing before coughing stimulates the cough reflex. If the patient does not cough effectively, atelectasis (collapse of the alveoli), pneumonia, or other lung complications may occur.

Mobility and Active Body Movement

The goals of promoting mobility postoperatively are to improve circulation, prevent venous stasis, and promote optimal respiratory function.

The nurse explains the rationale for frequent position changes after surgery and then shows the patient how to

CHART 18-4

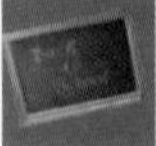

Patient Education

Preoperative Instructions to Prevent Postoperative Complications

DIAPHRAGMATIC BREATHING

Diaphragmatic breathing refers to a flattening of the dome of the diaphragm during inspiration, with resultant enlargement of the upper abdomen as air rushes in. During expiration, the abdominal muscles contract.

1. Practice in the same position you would assume in bed after surgery: a semi-Fowler's position, propped in bed with the back and shoulders well supported with pillows.
2. With your hands in a loose-fist position, allow the hands to rest lightly on the front of the lower ribs, with your fingertips against lower chest to feel the movement.

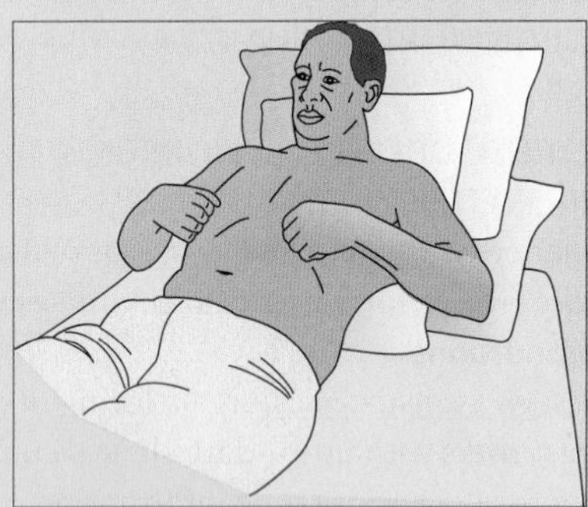

Diaphragmatic breathing

3. Breathe out gently and fully as the ribs sink down and inward toward midline.
4. Then take a deep breath through your nose and mouth, letting the abdomen rise as the lungs fill with air.
5. Hold this breath for a count of five.
6. Exhale and let out *all* the air through your nose and mouth.
7. Repeat this exercise 15 times with a short rest after each group of five.
8. Practice this twice a day preoperatively.

COUGHING

1. Lean forward slightly from a sitting position in bed, interlace your fingers together, and place your hands across the incisional site to act as a splintlike support when coughing.

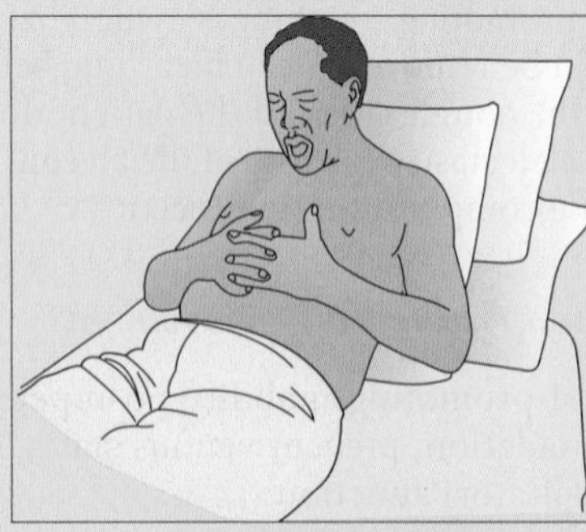

Splinting when coughing

2. Breathe with the diaphragm as described under "Diaphragmatic Breathing."
3. With your mouth slightly open, breathe in fully.
4. "Hack" out sharply for three short breaths.
5. Then, keeping your mouth open, take in a quick deep breath and immediately give a strong cough once or twice. This helps clear secretions from your chest. It may cause some discomfort but will not harm your incision.

LEG EXERCISES

1. Lie in a semi-Fowler's position and perform the following simple exercises to improve circulation.
2. Bend your knee and raise your foot—hold it a few seconds, then extend the leg and lower it to the bed.

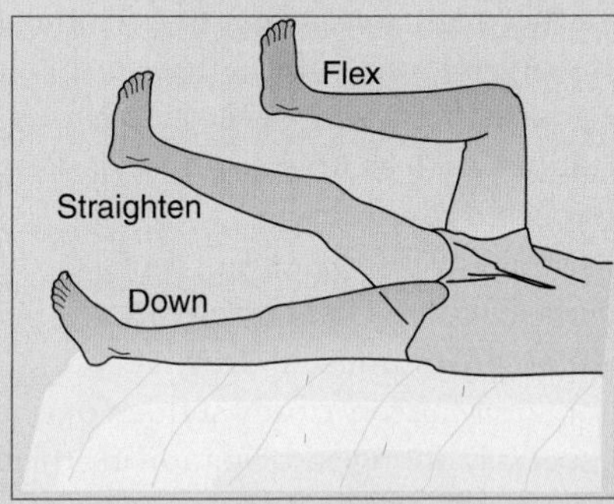

Leg exercises

3. Do this five times with one leg, then repeat with the other leg.
4. Then trace circles with the feet by bending them down, in toward each other, up, and then out.
5. Repeat these movements five times.

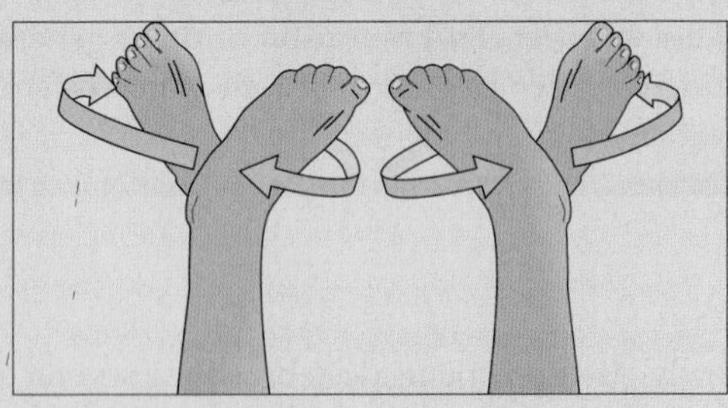

Foot exercises

TURNING TO THE SIDE

1. Turn on your side with the uppermost leg flexed most and supported on a pillow.
2. Grasp the side rail as an aid to maneuver to the side.
3. Practice diaphragmatic breathing and coughing while on your side.

GETTING OUT OF BED

1. Turn on your side.
2. Push yourself up with one hand as you swing your legs out of bed.

turn from side to side and how to assume the lateral position without causing pain or disrupting IV lines, drainage tubes, or other equipment. Any special position the patient needs to maintain after surgery (eg, adduction or elevation of an extremity) is discussed, as is the importance of maintaining as much mobility as possible despite restrictions. Reviewing the process before surgery is helpful, because the patient may be too uncomfortable or drowsy after surgery to absorb new information.

Exercise of the extremities includes extension and flexion of the knee and hip joints (similar to bicycle riding while lying on the side). The foot is rotated as though tracing the largest possible circle with the great toe (see Chart 18-4). The elbow and shoulder are also put through their range of motion. At first, the patient is assisted and reminded to perform these exercises. Later, the patient is encouraged to do them independently. Muscle tone is maintained so that ambulation will be easier.

The nurse should remember to use proper body mechanics and to instruct the patient to do the same. Whenever the patient is positioned, his or her body needs to be properly aligned.

Pain Management

A pain assessment should include differentiation between acute and chronic pain. Research suggests that, in older adults, teaching pain communication skills and pain management before surgery may result in greater pain relief during the early postoperative period (McDonald & Molony, 2004). A pain intensity scale should be introduced and explained to the patient to promote more effective postoperative pain management. Chapter 13 contains several examples of pain scales. Preoperative patient teaching also needs to include the difference between acute and chronic pain, so that the patient is prepared to differentiate acute postoperative pain from a chronic condition such as back pain (Nair & Podichetty, 2004).

Postoperatively, medications are administered to relieve pain and maintain comfort without increasing the risk of inadequate air exchange. The patient is instructed to take the medication as frequently as prescribed during the initial postoperative period for pain relief. Anticipated methods of administration of analgesic agents for inpatients include patient-controlled analgesia (PCA), epidural catheter bolus or infusion, or patient-controlled epidural analgesia (PCEA). A patient who is expected to go home will likely receive oral analgesic agents. These methods are discussed with the patient before surgery, and the patient's interest and willingness to use them are assessed.

Cognitive Coping Strategies

Cognitive strategies may be useful for relieving tension, overcoming anxiety, decreasing fear, and achieving relaxation. Examples of such strategies include the following:

- *Imagery:* The patient concentrates on a pleasant experience or restful scene.
- *Distraction:* The patient thinks of an enjoyable story or recites a favorite poem or song.
- *Optimistic self-recitation:* The patient recites optimistic thoughts ("I know all will go well").

Instruction for Patients Undergoing Ambulatory Surgery

Preoperative education for the same-day or ambulatory surgical patient comprises all the material presented earlier in this chapter as well as collaborative planning with the patient and family for discharge and follow-up home care. The major difference in outpatient preoperative education is the teaching environment.

Preoperative teaching content may be presented in a group class, on a videotape, at PAT, or by telephone in conjunction with the preoperative interview. In addition to answering questions and describing what to expect, the nurse tells the patient when and where to report, what to bring (insurance card, list of medications and allergies), what to leave at home (jewelry, watch, medications, contact lenses), and what to wear (loose-fitting, comfortable clothes; flat shoes). The nurse in the surgeon's office may initiate teaching before the perioperative telephone contact.

During the final preoperative telephone call, teaching is completed or reinforced as needed, and last-minute instructions are given. The patient is reminded not to eat or drink as directed.

Preoperative Psychosocial Interventions

Reducing Preoperative Anxiety

Cognitive strategies useful for reducing anxiety were addressed previously in this chapter. In addition to these strategies, music therapy is an easy-to-administer, inexpensive, noninvasive intervention that can reduce anxiety in the perioperative patient.

The general preoperative teaching addressed earlier in this section also helps decrease anxiety in many patients. Knowing ahead of time about the possible need for a ventilator, drainage tubes, or other types of equipment helps decrease anxiety in the postoperative period.

Decreasing Fear

During the preoperative assessment, the nurse should assist the patient to identify coping strategies that he or she has previously used to decrease fear. The patient benefits from knowing when family and friends will be able to visit after surgery and that a spiritual advisor will be available if desired.

Respecting Cultural, Spiritual, and Religious Beliefs

Psychosocial interventions include identifying and showing respect for cultural, spiritual, and religious beliefs. In some cultures, for example, people are stoic in regard to pain, whereas in others they are more expressive. These responses should be recognized as normal for those patients and families and should be respected by perioperative personnel (Flowers, 2004). If patients decline blood transfusions for religious reasons (Jehovah's Witnesses), this information needs to be clearly identified in the preoperative period, documented, and communicated to the appropriate personnel.

General Preoperative Nursing Interventions

Maintaining Patient Safety

Protecting patients from injury is one of the major roles of the perioperative nurse. Adherence to AORN recommended practices, the Joint Commission on Accreditation of Healthcare Organizations (JCAHO) recommendations, and national safety goals is crucial (Murphy, 2004). Seven main JCAHO patient safety goals apply throughout the perioperative period (Chart 18-5). These apply to hospitals as well as to ambulatory surgery centers and office-based surgery facilities (JCAHO, 2004).

Managing Nutrition and Fluids

The major purpose of withholding food and fluid before surgery is to prevent aspiration. Until recently, fluid and food were restricted preoperatively overnight and often longer. However, the American Society of Anesthesiologists reviewed this practice and has made new recommendations for people undergoing elective surgery who are otherwise healthy. Studies show that lengthy restriction of fluid and food is unnecessary in patients who do not have a compromised airway, coexisting disease, or disorders that affect gastric emptying or fluid volume (eg, pregnancy, obesity, diabetes, gastroesophageal reflux, enteral tube feeding, ileus, bowel obstruction) (Brady, Kinn & Stewart, 2004). Specific recommendations depend on the age of the patient and the type of food eaten. For example, adults may be advised to fast for 8 hours after eating fatty food and 4 hours after ingesting milk products. Most patients are currently allowed clear liquids up to 2 hours before an elective procedure (Brady et al., 2004).

Preparing the Bowel

Enemas are not commonly prescribed preoperatively unless the patient is undergoing abdominal or pelvic surgery. In this case, a cleansing enema or laxative may be prescribed the evening before surgery and may be repeated the morning of surgery. The goals of this preparation are to allow satisfactory visualization of the surgical site and to prevent trauma to the intestine or contamination of the peritoneum by feces. Unless the condition of the patient presents some contraindication, the toilet or bedside commode, rather than the bedpan, is used for evacuating the enema if the patient is hospitalized during this time. In addition, antibiotics may be prescribed to reduce intestinal flora.

CHART 18-5

Seven Primary National Patient Safety Goals for 2005

- Improve the accuracy of patient identification
- Improve effectiveness of communication among caregivers
- Improve safety of using medications
- Improve safety of using infusion pumps
- Reduce the risk of health care–associated infections
- Accurately and completely reconcile medications across continuum of care
- Reduce the risk of surgical fires

From Joint Commission on Accreditation of Healthcare Organizations (JCAHO). (2004). JCAHO issues 2005 Patient Safety Goals. *OR Manager, 20*(9), 5–8.

Preparing the Skin

The goal of preoperative skin preparation is to decrease bacteria without injuring the skin. If the surgery is not performed as an emergency, the patient may be instructed to use a soap containing a detergent-germicide to cleanse the skin area for several days before surgery to reduce the number of skin organisms; this preparation may be carried out at home.

Generally, hair is not removed preoperatively unless the hair at or around the incision site is likely to interfere with the operation. If hair must be removed, electric clippers are used for safe hair removal immediately before the operation.

Immediate Preoperative Nursing Interventions

The patient changes into a hospital gown that is left untied and open in the back. The patient with long hair may braid it, remove hairpins, and cover the head completely with a disposable paper cap.

The mouth is inspected, and dentures or plates are removed. If left in the mouth, these items could easily fall to the back of the throat during induction of anesthesia and cause respiratory obstruction.

Jewelry is not worn to the OR; wedding rings and jewelry of body piercings should be removed to prevent injury (Armstrong, 2004; Larkin, 2004). If a patient objects to removing a ring, some institutions allow the ring to be securely fastened to the finger with tape. All articles of value, including assistive devices, dentures, glasses, and prosthetic devices, are given to family members or are labeled clearly with the patient's name and stored in a safe and secure place according to the institution's policy.

All patients (except those with urologic disorders) should void immediately before going to the OR to promote continence during low abdominal surgery and to make abdominal organs more accessible. Urinary catheterization is performed in the OR as necessary.

Administering Preanesthetic Medication

The use of preanesthetic medication is minimal with ambulatory or outpatient surgery. If prescribed, it is usually administered in the preoperative holding area. If a preanesthetic medication is administered, the patient is kept in bed with the side rails raised, because the medication can cause lightheadedness or drowsiness. During this time, the nurse observes the patient for any untoward reaction to the medications. The immediate surroundings are kept quiet to promote relaxation.

Often, surgery is delayed or OR schedules are changed, and it becomes impossible to request that a medication be given at a specific time. In these situations, the preoperative medication is prescribed "on call to OR." The nurse can have the medication ready to administer as soon as a call is received from the OR staff. It usually takes 15 to 20 minutes to prepare the patient for the OR. If the nurse gives the medication before attending to the other details of preoperative preparation, the patient will have at least partial benefit from the preoperative medication and will have a smoother anesthetic and operative course.

Maintaining the Preoperative Record

Preoperative checklists contain critical elements that must be checked and verified preoperatively (Rothrock, 2003). The nurse completes the preoperative checklist (Fig. 18-3). The nurse also completes the verification form preoperatively, and others provide verification (Fig. 18-4). The completed chart (with the preoperative checklist and verification form) accompanies the patient to the OR with the surgical consent form attached, along with all laboratory reports and nurses' records. Any unusual last-minute observations that may have a bearing on anesthesia or surgery are noted prominently at the front of the chart.

Transporting the Patient to the Presurgical Area

The patient is transferred to the holding area or presurgical suite in a bed or on a stretcher about 30 to 60 minutes before the anesthetic is to be given. The stretcher should be as comfortable as possible, with a sufficient number of blankets to prevent chilling in an air-conditioned room. A small head pillow is usually provided.

The patient is taken to the preoperative holding area, greeted by name, and positioned comfortably on the

1. Patient's name: ______ Date: ______ Height: ______ Weight: ______
   Identification band present: ______
2. Informed consent signed: ______ Special permits signed: ______
3. Surgical site: ______ (Ex: Sterilization)
4. History & physical examination report present: ______ Date: ______
5. Laboratory records present: ______
   CBC: ______ Hgb: ______ Urinalysis: ______ Hct: ______

6. Item	Present	Removed
a. Natural teeth	______	______
Dentures; upper, lower, partial	______	______
Bridge, fixed; crown	______	______
b. Contact lenses	______	______
c. Other prostheses—type: ______	______	______
d. Jewelry:		
Wedding band (taped/tied)	______	______
Rings	______	______
Earrings: pierced, clip-on	______	______
Neck chains	______	______
Any other body piercings	______	______
e. Make-up	______	______
Nail polish	______	______
7. Clothing		
a. Clean patient gown	______	______
b. Cap	______	______
c. Sanitary pad, etc.	______	______

8. Family instructed where to wait? ______
9. Valuables secured? ______
10. Blood available? ______ Ordered? ______ Where? ______
11. Preanesthetic medication given: ______
    Type: ______ Time: ______
12. Voided: ______ Amount: ______ Time: ______ Catheter: ______
    Mouth care given: ______
13. Vital signs: Temperature: ______ Pulse: ______ Resp: ______ Blood Pressure: ______
14. Special problems/precautions: (Allergies, deafness, *etc.*): ______
15. Area of skin preparation: ______
16. ______ Date: ______ Time: ______
    Signature: Nurse releasing patient

FIGURE 18-3. Example of a preoperative checklist.

Operative/Invasive Procedure Checklist

Procedure Date
/ /

VERIFICATION #1

Location ☐ SDA/SPU ☐ Inpatient Room ☐ Other

Operative/Invasive Procedure ☐ Stated By Patient

☐ N/A ____ ☐ Other ____ Relationship to Patient ____

Procedure on Left Side of Body (complete form on Left Side)	**All Other Procedures** (complete form in center) (including non-lateral and bilateral)	**Procedure on Right Side of Body** (complete form on Right Side)
Consent Completed and In Chart ☐ Yes ☐ No Comments	Consent Completed and In Chart ☐ Yes ☐ No Comments	Consent Completed and In Chart ☐ Yes ☐ No Comments
Correct Patient Verification ☐ Name ☐ DOB	Correct Patient Verification ☐ Name ☐ DOB	Correct Patient Verification ☐ Name ☐ DOB
Staff Signature/Title	Staff Signature/Title	Staff Signature/Title

VERIFICATION #2 (Day of Procedure)

Location ☐ Holding ☐ ED ☐ Radiology ☐ Critical Care Bedside ☐ CVIR ☐ Procedure Room
☐ Endoscopy ☐ Invasive Cardiology ☐ Labor/Delivery ☐ Bronchoscopy ☐ Other

Operative/Invasive Procedure (as stated by patient)

☐ N/A ____

Procedure on Left Side of Body (complete form on Left Side)	**All Other Procedures** (complete form in center) (including non-lateral and bilateral)	**Procedure on Right Side of Body** (complete form on Right Side)
Consent Completed and In Chart ☐ Yes ☐ No Comments	Consent Completed and In Chart ☐ Yes ☐ No Comments	Consent Completed and In Chart ☐ Yes ☐ No Comments
Correct Patient Verification ☐ Name ☐ DOB	Correct Patient Verification ☐ Name ☐ DOB	Correct Patient Verification ☐ Name ☐ DOB
Physician Marking Site	Physician Marking Site	Physician Marking Site
Site Marked ☐ Yes ☐ No ☐ N/A	Site Marked ☐ Yes ☐ No ☐ N/A	Site Marked ☐ Yes ☐ No ☐ N/A
Site Verified By Patient ☐ Yes ☐ No ☐ N/A	Site Verified By Patient ☐ Yes ☐ No ☐ N/A	Site Verified By Patient ☐ Yes ☐ No ☐ N/A
Staff Signature/Title	Staff Signature/Title	Staff Signature/Title

VERIFICATION #3 (Immediately Prior to Procedure)

Operative/Invasive Procedure (as stated by patient)

☐ N/A ____

Procedure on Left Side of Body (complete form on Left Side)	**All Other Procedures** (complete form in center) (including non-lateral and bilateral)	**Procedure on Right Side of Body** (complete form on Right Side)
Verification Correct Patient/ Procedure/Site/Mark visible/ Consent read aloud ☐ Yes ☐ No Comments	**Verification Correct Patient/ Procedure/Site/Mark visible/ Consent read aloud** ☐ Yes ☐ No Comments	**Verification Correct Patient/ Procedure/Site/Mark visible/ Consent read aloud** ☐ Yes ☐ No Comments
Available in room: Special Equipment ☐ Yes ☐ No Comments Implants ☐ Yes ☐ No	Available in room: Special Equipment ☐ Yes ☐ No Comments Implants ☐ Yes ☐ No	Available in room: Special Equipment ☐ Yes ☐ No Comments Implants ☐ Yes ☐ No
Date/ Time	Date/ Time	Date/ Time
Physician Name	Physician Name	Physician Name
Anesthesia Name	Anesthesia Name	Anesthesia Name
Nurse/Tech Name	Nurse/Tech Name	Nurse/Tech Name
Nurse/Tech Name	Nurse/Tech Name	Nurse/Tech Name

FIGURE 18-4. Example of a verification form.

stretcher or bed. The surrounding area should be kept quiet if the preoperative medication is to have maximal effect. Unpleasant sounds or conversation should be avoided, because a sedated patient who overhears them might misinterpret them.

Patient safety in the preoperative area is a priority. Use of a process to verify patient identification, the surgical procedure, and the surgical site is imperative to maximize patient safety (see Fig. 18-4). This allows for prompt intervention if any discrepancies are identified.

NURSING ALERT

It is imperative that the entire perioperative team participate in verifying the correct patient identity, surgical procedure, and surgical site before proceeding to the OR.

Attending to Family Needs

Most hospitals and ambulatory surgery centers have a waiting room where family members and significant others can wait while the patient is undergoing surgery. This room may be equipped with comfortable chairs, television, telephones, and facilities for light refreshment. Volunteers may remain with the family, offer them coffee, and keep them informed of the patient's progress. After surgery, the surgeon may meet the family in the waiting room and discuss the outcome.

The family and significant others should never judge the seriousness of an operation by the length of time the patient is in the OR. A patient may be in surgery much longer than the actual operating time for several reasons:

- Patients are routinely transported well in advance of the actual operating time.
- The anesthesiologist or anesthetist often makes additional preparations that may take 30 to 60 minutes.
- The surgeon may take longer than expected with the preceding case, which delays the start of the next surgical procedure.

After surgery, the patient is taken to the PACU to ensure safe emergence from anesthesia. Family members and significant others waiting to see the patient after surgery should be informed that the patient may have certain equipment or devices (eg, IV lines, indwelling urinary catheter, nasogastric tube, oxygen lines, monitoring equipment, blood transfusion lines) in place when he or she returns from surgery. When the patient returns to the room, the nurse provides explanations regarding the frequent postoperative observations that will be made. However, it is the responsibility of the surgeon, not the nurse, to relay the surgical findings and the prognosis, even when the findings are favorable.

Expected Patient Outcomes

Expected patient outcomes in the preoperative phase of care are summarized in Chart 18-6.

CHART 18-6

Expected Patient Outcomes in the Preoperative Phase of Care

Relief of anxiety, evidenced when the patient
- Discusses with the anesthesiologist, anesthetist, or nurse anesthetist concerns related to types of anesthesia and induction
- Verbalizes an understanding of the preanesthetic medication and general anesthesia
- Discusses last-minute concerns with the nurse or physician
- Discusses financial concerns with the social worker, when appropriate
- Requests visit with spiritual advisor when appropriate
- Relaxes quietly after being visited by health care team members

Decreased fear, evidenced when the patient
- Discusses fears with health care professionals or a spiritual advisor, or both
- Verbalizes an understanding of any expected bodily changes, including expected duration of bodily changes

Understanding of the surgical intervention, evidenced when the patient
- Participates in preoperative preparation
- Demonstrates and describes exercises he or she is expected to perform postoperatively
- Reviews information about postoperative care
- Accepts preanesthetic medication, if prescribed
- Remains in bed once premedicated
- Relaxes during transportation to the OR or unit
- States rationale for use of side rails
- Discusses postoperative expectations

No evidence of preoperative complications

Critical Thinking Exercises

1 A morbidly obese man is scheduled for surgery on his right foot. The patient is noticeably favoring his left foot. What preoperative assessments are indicated? What nursing interventions are warranted?

2 ebp A male patient is scheduled for major surgery and asks how long before the surgery he will be without food and fluids. What resources would you use to identify the current fasting guidelines? What is the evidence base for the patient's being NPO after midnight as opposed to a 2-hour fast before surgery? Identify the criteria used to evaluate the strength of the evidence for this practice.

3 ebp Two patients are admitted to the same-day surgery unit for knee replacement surgery. What resources would you use to identify current safety practices during the perioperative period? Identify the evidence for and the criteria used to evaluate the strength of the evidence for the safety practices identified for these patients.

REFERENCES AND SELECTED READINGS

BOOKS

Aiken, T. D. (2004). *Legal, ethical, and political issues in nursing* (2nd ed.). Philadelphia: F. A. Davis.

American Society of PeriAnesthesia Nurses. (2002). *Standards of perianesthesia nursing practice.* Thorofare, NJ: ASPAN.

Bickley, L. S. & Szilagyi, P. G. (2003). *Bates' guide to physical examination and history taking* (8th ed.). Philadelphia: Lippincott Williams & Wilkins.

Clancy, J., McVicar, A. J. & Baird, N. (2002). *Perioperative practice: Fundamentals of homeostasis.* New York: Routledge.

Conner, R. (2004). *Ambulatory surgery principles and practices* (3rd ed.). Denver: AORN, Inc.

Defazio-Quinn, D. & Schick, L. (Eds). (2004). *Nursing core curriculum: Preoperative, phase I and phase II PACU nursing.* Philadelphia: W. B. Saunders.

Dudek, S. G. (2006). *Nutrition essentials for nursing practice* (5th ed.). Philadelphia: Lippincott Williams & Wilkins.

Kleinbeck, S. V. M. (2004). *Perioperative Nursing Data Set at work: Policies, procedures and pathways.* Denver: AORN, Inc.

Melnyk, B. M. & Fineout-Overholt, E. (2005). *Evidence-based practice in nursing and healthcare: A guide to best practices.* Philadelphia: Lippincott Williams & Wilkins.

Miller, R. D. (2005) *Miller's anesthesia* (6th ed.). New York: Elsevier/Churchill Livingstone.

Murray, M. J., Coursin, D. B., Pearl, R. G., et al. (2002). *Critical care medicine: Perioperative management* (2nd ed.). Philadelphia: Lippincott Williams & Wilkins.

National Institutes of Health, National Heart, Lung and Blood Institute, North American Association for the Study of Obesity. (2000). *The practical guide: Identification, evaluation, and treatment of overweight and obesity in adults.* NIH Publication Number 00-4084. Bethesda, MD: National Institutes of Health.

Phillips, N. (2004). *Berry and Kohn's operating room technique* (10th ed.). St. Louis: Mosby.

Rothrock, J. C. (Ed.). (2003). *Alexander's care of the patient in surgery* (12th ed.). St. Louis: Mosby.

U.S. Department of Health and Human Services, U. S. Department of Agriculture. (2005). *Dietary guidelines for Americans 2005.* Available at: www.healthierus.gov/dietaryguidelines (accessed May 7, 2006).

Weber, J. & Kelley, J. (2006). *Health assessment in nursing* (3rd ed.). Philadelphia: Lippincott Williams & Wilkins.

Worthington, P. H. (2004). *Practical aspects of nutritional support.* Philadelphia: W. B. Saunders.

JOURNALS

**An asterisk indicates a nursing research article.*

Perioperative

Armstrong, M. L. (2004). Caring for the patient with piercings. *RN, 67*(6), 46–53.

Bernat, J. L. (2004). Ethical issues in the perioperative management of neurologic patients. *Neurologic Clinics of North America, 22*(1), 457–471.

*Bezanson, J. L., Weaver, M., Kinney, M. R., et al. (2004). Presurgical risk factors for late extubation in Medicare recipients after cardiac surgery. *Nursing Research, 53*(1), 46–52.

Bohan, E. & Glass-Macenka, D. (2004). Surgical management of patients with primary brain tumors. *Seminars in Oncology Nursing, 29*(4), 240–252.

Coleman, T., Cheater, R. & Murphy, E. (2004). Qualitative study investigation the process of giving anti-smoking advice in general practice. *Patient Education and Counseling, 52*(2), 159–163.

Flowers, D. L. (2004). Culturally competent nursing care: A challenge for the 21st century. *Critical Care Nurse, 24*(4), 48–52.

Fuller, T. (2003). Elder abuse and neglect assessment. *Journal of Gerontological Nursing, 29*(1), 8–9.

Galvez-Jimenez, N. & Lang, A. E. (2004). The perioperative management of Parkinson's disease revisited. *Neurologic Clinics of North America, 22*(2), 367–377.

Gotta, A. W. (2004). Anesthetic management of the patient with HIV infection. *Current Reviews for Nurse Anesthetists, 27*(11), 117–128.

John, A. D. & Sieber, F. E. (2004). Age associated issues: Geriatrics. *Anesthesiology Clinic of North America, 22*(1), 45–58.

Joint Commission on Accreditation of Healthcare Organizations (JCAHO). (2004). JCAHO issues 2005 patient safety goals. *OR Manager, 20*(9), 5–8.

Lorenz, R. A., Lorenz, R. M. & Cody, J. E. (2005). Home study program: Perioperative blood glucose control during adult coronary artery bypass surgery. *AORN Journal, 81*(1), 126–150.

Lotan, Y., Cadeddu, J. A. & Gettman, M. T. (2004). The new economics of radical prostatectomy: Cost comparison of open, laparoscopic and robot assisted techniques. *Journal of Urology, 172*(4 Pt. 1), 1431–1435.

Matin, S. F., Abreu, S., Ramani, A., et al. (2003). Evaluation of age and comorbidity as risk factors after laparoscopic urological surgery. *Journal of Urology, 170*(4 Pt. 1), 1115–1120.

*McDonald, D. D. & Molony, S. L. (2004). Postoperative pain communication skills for older adults. *Western Journal of Nursing Research, 26*(8), 836–852.

Mercado, D. L. & Petty, B. G. (2003). Perioperative medication management. *Medical Clinics of North America, 87*(1), 41–57.

Pass, S. & Simpson, R. (2004). Discontinuation and reinstitution of medications during the perioperative period. *American Journal of Health-System Pharmacists, 61*(6), 899–912.

Robinson, T. N. & Stiegmann, G. V. (2004). Minimally invasive surgery. *Endoscopy, 36*(1), 48–51.

Saufl, N. M. (2004). Preparing the older adult for surgery and anesthesia. *Journal of Perianesthesia Nursing, 19*(6), 372–377.

Schofield, C. (2004). How do I care for a patient with alcohol withdrawal syndrome? *Nursing, 34*(8), 25.

Ziegeler, S., Tsusaki, B. & Charles, C. (2003). Influence of genotype on perioperative risk and outcome. *Anesthesiology, 99*(1), 212–219.

Preoperative Assessment

Barkhordarian, S. & Dardik, A. (2004). Preoperative assessment and management to prevent complications during high-risk vascular surgery. *Critical Care Medicine, 32*(4 Suppl.), S174–S185.

Brady, M., Kinn, S. & Stuart, P. (2004). Preoperative fasting for adults to prevent perioperative complications. *Cochrane Library (Oxford) (4)*, CD004423.

Bray, A. (2006). Preoperative nursing assessment of the surgical patient. *Nursing Clinics of North America, 41*(2), 135–150.

Charlebois, D. & Wilmothe, D. (2004). Critical care of patients with obesity. *Critical Care Nurse, 24*(4), 19–29.

DeFazio-Quinn, D. M. (2006). How religion, language and ethnicity impact perioperative nursing care. *Nursing Clinics of North America, 41*(2), 231–248.

Garcia-Miguel, F. J., Serrano-Aguilar, P. G. & Lopez-Bastida, J. (2003). Preoperative assessment. *Lancet, 362*(9397), 1749–1757.

Halaszynski, T. M., Juda, R. & Silverman, D. G. (2004). Optimizing postoperative outcomes with efficient preoperative assessment and management. *Critical Care Medicine, 32*(4), S76–S86.

Heyneman, C. (2003). Pharmacology. Preoperative considerations: Which herbal products should be discontinued before surgery? *Critical Care Nurse, 23*(2), 116–123.

Larkin, B. G. (2004). Home Study Program: The ins and outs of body piercing. *AORN Journal, 79*(2), 333–341.

MacKichan, C. & Ruthman, J. (2004). Herbal product use and perioperative patients. *AORN Journal, 79*(5), 947–959.

Mamaril, M. E. (2006). Nursing considerations in the geriatric surgical patient: The perioperative continuum of care. *Nursing Clinics of North America, 41*(2), 313–328.

Murphy, E. K. (2004). OR nursing law. Protecting patients from potential injuries. *AORN Journal, 79*(5), 1013–1016.

Nair, S. & Podichetty, V. K. (2004). The preoperative and postoperative assessment and care of patients with back pain. *Neurologic Clinics of North America, 22*(2), 441–456.

*Oetker-Black, S. L., Jones, S., Estok, P., et al. (2003). Preoperative teaching and hysterectomy outcomes. *AORN Journal, 77*(6), 1215–1231.

Pofahl, W. E. & Pories, W. J. (2003). Current status and future directions of geriatric general surgery. *Journal of American Geriatric Society, 51*(7 Suppl.), S351–S354.

Romanoski, S. (2006). Management of the special needs of the pregnant surgical patient. *Nursing Clinics of North America, 41*(2), 299–311.

Schroeter, K. (2003). Q & A: Informed consent. *Surgical Services Management, 9*(6), 52–54.

Wiklund, R. A. (2004). Preoperative preparation of patients with advanced liver disease. *Critical Care Medicine, 32*(4), S106–S115.

Williams, J. Z. & Barbul, A. (2003) Nutrition and wound healing. *Surgical Clinics of North America, 83*(3), 571–596.

RESOURCES

American Academy of Ambulatory Care Nursing, East Holly Ave., Box 56, Pitman, NJ, 08071; 856-256-2350, 800-AMB-NURS; http://www.aaacn.org. Accessed March 31, 2006.

American Society of PeriAnesthesia Nurses, 10 Melrose Ave., Suite 110, Cherry Hill, NJ 08003; toll-free 877-9696; fax 856-616-9621; http://www.aspan.org. Accessed March 31, 2006.

Association of Perioperative Registered Nurses, Inc., 2170 S. Parker Rd., Suite 300, Denver, CO 80231; 856-616-9600 or -9601; toll-free 1-877-737-9696; http://www.aorn.org. Accessed March 31, 2006.

Joint Commission on Accreditation of Healthcare Organizations, One Renaissance Blvd., Oakbrook Terrace, IL 60181; 630-792-5000; fax 630-792-5005; http://www.jcaho.org. Accessed March 31, 2006.

CHAPTER 19

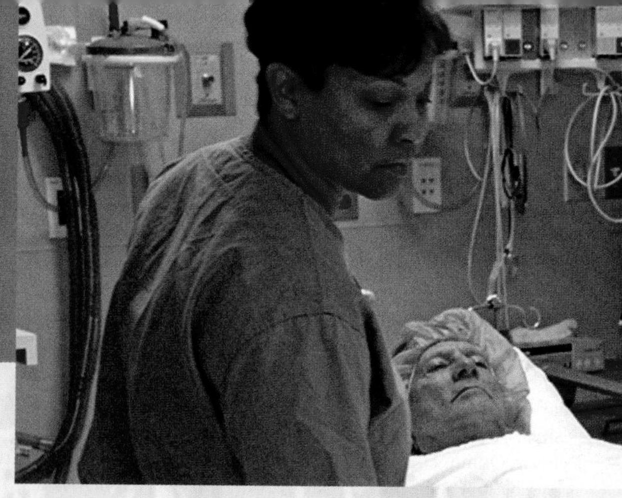

Intraoperative Nursing Management

Learning Objectives

On completion of this chapter, the learner will be able to:

1. Describe the interdisciplinary approach to the care of the patient during surgery.
2. Describe the principles of surgical asepsis.
3. Describe the roles of the surgical team members during the intraoperative phase of care.
4. Identify adverse effects of surgery and anesthesia.
5. Identify the surgical risk factors related to age-specific populations and nursing interventions to reduce those risks.
6. Compare various types of anesthesia with regard to uses, advantages, disadvantages, and nursing responsibilities.
7. Identify the use of the nursing process for optimizing patient outcomes during the intraoperative period.
8. Describe the role of the nurse in ensuring patient safety during the intraoperative period.

The intraoperative experience has undergone many changes that make it safer and less disturbing to patients. However, even with these advances, anesthesia and surgery place the patient at risk for several complications or adverse events. Consciousness or full awareness, mobility, protective biologic functions, and personal control are totally or partially relinquished by the patient when entering the operating room (OR). Staff from the departments of anesthesia, nursing, and surgery work collaboratively to implement professional standards of care, to control iatrogenic and individual risks, to prevent complications, and to promote high-quality patient outcomes.

The Surgical Team

The surgical team consists of the patient, the **anesthesiologist** or **anesthetist**, the surgeon, nurses, and the surgical technologists. The anesthesiologist or anesthetist (usually a nurse anesthetist) administers the **anesthetic** agent and monitors the patient's physical status throughout the surgery. The surgeon and assistants scrub and perform the surgery. The person in the scrub role, either a nurse or a surgical technologist, provides sterile instruments and supplies to the surgeon during the procedure. The circulating nurse coordinates the care of the patient in the OR. Care provided by the circulating nurse includes assisting with patient positioning, preparing the patient's skin for surgery, managing surgical specimens, and documenting intraoperative events.

The Patient

As the patient enters the OR, he or she may feel either relaxed and prepared or fearful and highly stressed. These feelings depend to a large extent on the amount and timing of preoperative sedation and the patient's level of fear and anxiety. Fears about loss of control, the unknown, pain, death, changes in body structure or function, and disruption of lifestyle all may contribute to generalized anxiety. These fears can increase the amount of anesthetic needed, the level of postoperative pain, and overall recovery time.

The patient is also subject to several risks. Infection, failure of the surgery to relieve symptoms, temporary or permanent complications related to the procedure or the anesthetic, and death are uncommon but potential outcomes of the surgical experience (Chart 19-1). In addition to fears and risks, the patient undergoing sedation and anesthesia temporarily loses both cognitive function and biologic self-protective mechanisms. Loss of pain sense, reflexes, and ability to communicate subjects the intraoperative patient to possible injury.

Gerontologic Considerations

Elderly patients face higher risks from anesthesia and surgery than younger adult patients do (Rothrock, 2003). Statistically, perioperative risk increases with each decade after 60 years of age, often because of the increased incidence of coexisting disease. Key predictors of perioperative complications in the elderly are the patient's preoperative condition and level of function (John & Sieber, 2004). Modifications tailored to the biologic changes of later life and the application of research findings can reduce the risks (Pofahl & Pories, 2003).

Biologic variations of particular importance include age-related cardiovascular and pulmonary changes. The aging heart and blood vessels have decreased ability to respond to stress. Reduced cardiac output and limited cardiac reserve make the elderly patient vulnerable to changes in circulating volume and blood oxygen levels. Excessive or rapid administration of intravenous (IV) solutions can cause pulmonary edema. A sudden or prolonged decline in blood

Glossary

anesthesia: a state of narcosis, analgesia, relaxation, and loss of reflexes

anesthesiologist: physician trained to deliver anesthesia and to monitor the patient's condition during surgery

anesthetic: the substance, such as a chemical or gas, used to induce anesthesia

anesthetist: health care professional, such as a nurse anesthetist, who is trained to deliver anesthesia and to monitor the patient's condition during surgery

circulating nurse (or circulator): registered nurse who coordinates and documents patient care in the operating room

moderate sedation: use of sedation to depress the level of consciousness without altering the patient's ability to maintain a patent airway and to respond to physical stimuli and verbal commands, previously referred to as conscious sedation

monitored anesthesia care (MAC): moderate sedation administered by an anesthesiologist or anesthetist

restricted zone: area in the operating room where scrub attire and surgical masks are required; includes operating room and sterile core areas

scrub role: registered nurse, licensed practical nurse, or surgical technologist who scrubs and dons sterile surgical attire, prepares instruments and supplies, and hands instruments to the surgeon during the procedure

semirestricted zone: area in the operating room where scrub attire is required; may include areas where surgical instruments are processed

surgical asepsis: absence of microorganisms in the surgical environment to reduce the risk for infection

unrestricted zone: area in the operating room that interfaces with other departments; includes patient reception area and holding area

CHART 19-1

Potential Adverse Effects of Surgery and Anesthesia

Anesthesia and surgery disrupt all major body systems. Although most patients can compensate for surgical trauma and the effects of anesthesia, all patients are at risk during the operative procedure. These risks include the following:

- Allergic reactions
- Cardiac dysrhythmia from electrolyte imbalance or adverse effect of anesthetic agents
- Myocardial depression, bradycardia, and circulatory collapse
- Central nervous system agitation, seizures, and respiratory arrest
- Oversedation or undersedation
- Agitation or disorientation, especially in elderly patients
- Hypoxemia or hypercarbia from hypoventilation and inadequate respiratory support during anesthesia
- Laryngeal trauma, oral trauma, and broken teeth from difficult intubation
- Hypothermia from cool operating room temperatures, exposure of body cavities, and impaired thermoregulation secondary to anesthetic agents
- Hypotension from blood loss or adverse effect of anesthesia
- Infection
- Thrombosis from compression of blood vessels or stasis
- Malignant hyperthermia secondary to adverse effect of anesthesia
- Nerve damage, skin breakdown from prolonged or inappropriate positioning
- Electrical shock or burns
- Laser burns
- Drug toxicity, faulty equipment, and human error

pressure may lead to cerebral ischemia, thrombosis, embolism, infarction, and anoxia. Reduced gas exchange can result in cerebral hypoxia.

The elderly patient needs fewer and smaller amounts of anesthetic agents to produce anesthesia and eliminates the anesthetic agent over a longer period of time, compared with a younger patient (Yellen, 2003). With increasing age, there is a decrease in the percentage of lean body tissue and a steady increase in fatty tissue (from 20 to 90 years of age). Anesthetic agents that have an affinity for fatty tissue concentrate in body fat and the brain. Lower doses of anesthetic agents are appropriate in an elderly patient if the patient is malnourished and has low plasma protein levels (Williams & Barbul, 2003). With decreased plasma proteins, more of the anesthetic agent remains free or unbound, and the result is more potent action.

In addition, body tissues of the older adult are made up predominantly of water, and those tissues with a rich blood supply, such as skeletal muscle, liver, and kidneys, shrink. Reduced liver size decreases the rate at which the liver can inactivate many anesthetic agents, and decreased kidney function slows the elimination of waste products and anesthetics. Other factors that affect the elderly surgical patient in the intraoperative period include the following:

- Impaired ability to increase metabolic rate and impaired thermoregulatory mechanisms increase susceptibility to hypothermia.
- Bone loss (25% in women, 12% in men) necessitates careful manipulation and positioning during surgery.
- Reduced ability to adjust rapidly to emotional and physical stress influences surgical outcomes and requires meticulous observation of vital functions.

As expected, mortality is higher with emergency surgery (commonly required for traumatic injuries) than with elective surgery, making continuous and careful monitoring and prompt intervention especially important for older surgical patients (Pofahl & Pories, 2003).

Nursing Care

Throughout surgery, nursing responsibilities include providing for the safety and well-being of the patient, coordinating the OR personnel, and performing scrub and circulating activities. Because the patient's emotional state remains a concern, the care begun by preoperative nurses is continued by the intraoperative nursing staff, who provide the patient with information and reassurance. The nurse supports coping strategies and reinforces the patient's ability to influence outcomes by encouraging his or her active participation in the plan of care.

As patient advocates, intraoperative nurses monitor factors that can cause injury, such as patient position, equipment malfunction, and environmental hazards, and they protect the patient's dignity and interests while the patient is anesthetized. Additional responsibilities include maintaining surgical standards of care and identifying and minimizing risks and complications.

The Circulating Nurse

The **circulating nurse** (also known as the **circulator**) is preferably a registered nurse (RN). In 20 states in the United States, the circulator is required by law to be an RN (Phillips, 2004). He or she manages the OR and protects the patient's safety and health by monitoring the activities of the surgical team, checking the OR conditions, and continually assessing the patient for signs of injury and implementing appropriate interventions. Main responsibilities include verifying consent; coordinating the team; and ensuring cleanliness, proper temperature, humidity, lighting, safe function of equipment, and the availability of supplies and materials. The circulating nurse monitors aseptic practices to avoid breaks in technique while coordinating the movement of related personnel (medical, x-ray, and laboratory), as well as implementing fire safety precautions. The circulating nurse also monitors the patient and documents specific activities throughout the operation to ensure the patient's safety and well-being.

In addition, the circulating nurse is responsible for ensuring that the second verification of the surgical procedure and site takes place and is documented (see Fig. 18-4 in Chapter 18). In some institutions, this is referred to as a "surgical or preprocedure pause" or "time-out" that takes place among the surgical team prior to incision. Every member of the surgical team verifies the patient's name, procedure, and surgical site using objective documentation and data before beginning the surgery, as mandated by the Joint Commission on Accreditation of Healthcare Organizations (JCAHO). Proper patient identification is one of the seven 2005 National Patient Safety Goals identified by JCAHO (2005) (see Chart 18-5 in Chapter 18).

The Scrub Role

Activities of the **scrub role** include performing a surgical hand scrub; setting up the sterile tables; preparing sutures, ligatures, and special equipment (eg, laparoscope); and assisting the surgeon and the surgical assistants during the procedure by anticipating the instruments and supplies that will be required, such as sponges, drains, and other equipment. As the surgical incision is closed, the scrub person and the circulator count all needles, sponges, and instruments to be sure they are accounted for and not retained as a foreign body in the patient (Gawande, Studdert, Orav, et al., 2003). Standards call for all sponges to be visible on x-ray and for sponge counts to take place at the beginning of surgery and twice at the end. Tissue specimens obtained during surgery are labeled by the scrub person and sent to the laboratory by the circulator.

The Surgeon

The surgeon performs the surgical procedure and heads the surgical team. He or she is a licensed physician (MD), osteopath (DO), oral surgeon (DDS or DMD), or podiatrist (DPM) who is specially trained and qualified. Qualifications may include certification by a specialty board, adherence to JCAHO standards, and adherence to hospital standards and admitting practices and procedures (Phillips, 2004).

The Registered Nurse First Assistant

The registered nurse first assistant (RNFA) is another member of the OR team. Although the scope of practice of the RNFA depends on each state's nurse practice act, the RNFA practices under the direct supervision of the surgeon. RNFA responsibilities may include handling tissue, providing exposure at the operative field, suturing, and maintaining hemostasis (Rothrock, 2003). The role requires a thorough understanding of anatomy and physiology, tissue handling, and the principles of **surgical asepsis**. The RNFA must be aware of the objectives of the surgery, must have the knowledge and ability to anticipate needs and to work as a skilled member of a team, and must be able to handle any emergency situation in the OR.

The Anesthesiologist and Anesthetist

An **anesthesiologist** is a physician specifically trained in the art and science of anesthesiology. An **anesthetist** is a qualified health care professional who administers anesthetics. Most anesthetists are nurses who have graduated from an accredited nurse anesthesia program and have passed examinations sponsored by the American Association of Nurse Anesthetists to become a certified registered nurse anesthetist (CRNA). The anesthesiologist or anesthetist assesses the patient before surgery, selects the anesthesia, administers it, intubates the patient if necessary, manages any technical problems related to the administration of the anesthetic agent, and supervises the patient's condition throughout the surgical procedure. Before the patient enters the OR, often at preadmission testing, the anesthesiologist or anesthetist visits the patient to supply information and answer questions. The type of anesthetic to be administered, previous reactions to anesthetics, and known anatomic abnormalities that would make airway management difficult are among the topics discussed.

The anesthesiologist or anesthetist uses the American Society of Anesthesiologists (ASA) Physical Status Classification System to determine the patient's status (Chart 19-2). If a patient has a classification of P2, P3, or P4, he or she has a systemic disease that may or may not be related to the cause of surgery. If a patient with a classification of P1, P2, P3, P4, or P5 requires emergency surgery, an E is added to the physical status designation (eg, P1E, P2E). Pb refers to a patient who is brain dead and is undergoing surgery as an organ donor. The abbreviations ASA1 through ASA6 are often used interchangeably with P1 to P6 to designate physical status (Phillips, 2004).

When the patient arrives in the OR, the anesthesiologist or anesthetist reassesses the patient's physical condition immediately prior to initiating anesthesia. The anesthetic is administered, and the patient's airway is maintained through either an endotracheal tube or a laryngeal mask airway (LMA). During surgery, the anesthesiologist or anesthetist monitors the patient's blood pressure, pulse, and respirations as well as the electrocardiogram (ECG), blood oxygen saturation level, tidal volume, blood gas levels, blood pH, alveolar gas concentrations, and body temperature. Monitoring by electroencephalography is sometimes required. Levels of anesthetics in the body can also be determined; a mass spectrometer can provide instant readouts of critical concentration levels on display terminals. This information helps personnel assess the patient's ability to breathe unassisted or the need for mechanical assistance if ventilation is poor and the patient is not breathing well independently.

The Surgical Environment

The surgical environment is known for its stark appearance and cool temperature. The surgical suite is behind double doors, and access is limited to authorized personnel. External precautions include adhering to principles of surgical asepsis; strict control of the OR environment is required, including traffic pattern restrictions. Policies governing this environment address such issues as the health of the staff; the cleanliness of the

CHART 19-2

American Society of Anesthesiologists Physical Status Classification System

Anesthetists and anesthesiologists use the American Society of Anesthesiologists Physical (P) Status Classification System to describe the patient's general status and identify potential risks during surgery. There are six classes of physical status.

- **P1.** A normal healthy patient
  Example: No systemic abnormality, localized infection without fever, benign tumor, hernia
- **P2.** A patient with mild systemic disease, without functional limitations
  Example: Well-controlled hypertension, well-controlled diabetes mellitus, chronic bronchitis, obesity, age over 80 years
- **P3.** A patient with severe systemic disease associated with functional limitations
  Example: Severe disease, compensated heart failure, myocardial infarction more than 6 months ago, angina pectoris, severe dysrhythmia, cirrhosis, poorly controlled diabetes or hypertension, ileus
- **P4.** A patient with an incapacitating systemic disease that is a constant threat to life
  Example: Severe heart failure, myocardial infarction less than 6 months ago, severe respiratory failure, advanced liver or renal failure
- **P5.** A moribund patient who is not expected to survive for 24 hours with or without operation
  Example: Unconscious patient with traumatic head injury and agonal respirations
- **P6.** Patient is brain dead and is being prepared as an organ donor

Adapted from American Society of Anesthesiologists. (1997). *Manual for anesthesia departments.* Park Ridge, IL: Author.

rooms; the sterility of equipment and surfaces; processes for scrubbing, gowning, and gloving; and OR attire.

To provide the best possible conditions for surgery, the OR is situated in a location that is central to all supporting services (eg, pathology, x-ray, laboratory). The OR has special air filtration devices to screen out contaminating particles, dust, and pollutants.

All seven of the JCAHO's 2005 National Patient Safety Goals pertain to the perioperative areas (see Chart 18-5 in Chapter 18), but the one that has the most direct relevance to the OR is the reduction of the risk of surgical fires. The surgical team must be educated about how to control heat sources, manage fuels, and minimize oxygen concentration under drapes (Salmon, 2004). Surgical drapes provide an opportunity for oxygen to concentrate; a stray spark could more easily ignite a fire. This occurs most commonly in ambulatory surgery settings (JCAHO, 2005). To further improve safety, electrical hazards, emergency exit clearances, and storage of equipment and anesthetic gases are monitored periodically by official agencies, such as the state department of health and JCAHO.

To help decrease microbes, the surgical area is divided into three zones: the **unrestricted zone**, where street clothes are allowed; the **semirestricted zone**, where attire consists of scrub clothes and caps; and the **restricted zone**, where scrub clothes, shoe covers, caps, and masks are worn. The surgeons and other surgical team members wear additional sterile clothing and protective devices during the operation.

The Association of PeriOperative Registered Nurses, formerly known as the Association of Operating Room Nurses (still abbreviated as AORN), recommends specific practices for personnel wearing surgical attire to promote a high level of cleanliness in a particular practice setting (AORN, 2004b). OR attire includes close-fitting cotton dresses, pantsuits, jumpsuits, and gowns. Knitted cuffs on sleeves and pant legs prevent organisms shed from the perineum, legs, and arms from being released into the immediate surroundings. Shirts and waist drawstrings should be tucked inside the pants to prevent accidental contact with sterile areas and to contain skin shedding. Wet or soiled garments should be changed.

Masks are worn at all times in the restricted zone of the OR. High-filtration masks decrease the risk of postoperative wound infection by containing and filtering microorganisms from the oropharynx and nasopharynx. Masks should fit tightly; should cover the nose and mouth completely; and should not interfere with breathing, speech, or vision. Masks must be adjusted to prevent venting from the sides. Disposable masks have a filtration efficiency exceeding 95%. Masks are changed between patients and should not be worn outside the surgical department. The mask must be either on or off; it must not be allowed to hang around the neck.

Headgear should completely cover the hair (head and neckline, including beard) so that single strands of hair, bobby pins, clips, and particles of dandruff or dust do not fall on the sterile field.

Shoes should be comfortable and supportive. Shoe covers are worn when it is reasonably anticipated that spills or splashes will occur. If worn, the covers should be changed whenever they become wet, torn, or soiled (Rothrock, 2003).

Barriers such as scrub attire and masks do not entirely protect the patient from microorganisms. Upper respiratory tract infections, sore throats, and skin infections in staff and patients are sources of pathogens and must be reported.

Because artificial fingernails harbor microorganisms and can cause nosocomial infections, a ban on artificial nails by OR personnel is supported by the Centers for Disease Control and Prevention (CDC), AORN, and the Association of Professionals in Infection Control. Short, natural fingernails are encouraged (Gupta, Della-Latta, Todd, et al., 2004).

Principles of Surgical Asepsis

Surgical asepsis prevents the contamination of surgical wounds. The patient's natural skin flora or a previously existing infection may cause postoperative wound infection. Rigorous adherence to the principles of surgical asepsis by OR personnel is basic to preventing surgical site infections.

All surgical supplies, instruments, needles, sutures, dressings, gloves, covers, and solutions that may come in contact with the surgical wound or exposed tissues must be sterilized before use (Rothrock, 2003). Traditionally, the surgeon, surgical assistants, and nurses prepared themselves by scrubbing their hands and arms with antiseptic soap and water, but this traditional practice is being challenged by research investigating the optimal length of time to scrub and the best preparation to use. In some institutions, an alcohol-based product or scrubless soap is used to prepare for surgery (Paulson, 2004; Rothrock, 2003).

Surgical team members wear long-sleeved, sterile gowns and gloves. Head and hair are covered with a cap, and a mask is worn over the nose and mouth to minimize the possibility that bacteria from the upper respiratory tract will enter the wound. During surgery, only personnel who have scrubbed, gloved, and gowned touch sterilized objects. Nonscrubbed personnel refrain from touching or contaminating anything sterile.

An area of the patient's skin considerably larger than that requiring exposure during the surgery is meticulously cleansed, and an antiseptic solution is applied (Phillips, 2004). If hair needs to be removed, this is done immediately before the procedure to minimize the risk of wound infection (Beyea, 2003). The remainder of the patient's body is covered with sterile drapes.

Environmental Controls

In addition to the protocols described previously, surgical asepsis requires meticulous cleaning and maintenance of the OR environment. Floors and horizontal surfaces are cleaned frequently with detergent, soap, and water or a detergent germicide. Sterilizing equipment is inspected regularly to ensure optimal operation and performance.

All equipment that comes into direct contact with the patient must be sterile. Sterilized linens, drapes, and solutions are used. Instruments are cleaned and sterilized in a unit near the OR. Individually wrapped sterile items are used when additional individual items are needed.

Airborne bacteria are a concern. To decrease the amount of bacteria in the air, standard OR ventilation provides 15 air exchanges per hour, at least 3 of which are fresh air (Phillips, 2004). A temperature of 20° to 24°C (68° to 73°F), humidity between 30% to 60%, and positive pressure relative to adjacent areas are maintained. Staff members shed skin scales, resulting in about 1000 bacteria-carrying particles (or colony-forming units [CFUs]) per cubic foot per minute. With the standard air exchanges, air counts of bacteria are reduced to 50 to 150 CFUs per cubic foot per minute. Systems with high-efficiency particulate air (HEPA) filters are needed to remove particles larger than 0.3 μm (Rothrock, 2003). Unnecessary personnel and physical movement may be restricted to minimize bacteria in the air and achieve an OR infection rate no greater than 3% to 5% in clean, infection-prone surgery.

Some ORs have laminar airflow units. These units provide 400 to 500 air exchanges per hour (Phillips, 2004). When used appropriately, laminar airflow units result in fewer than 10 CFUs per cubic foot per minute during surgery. The goal for a laminar airflow–equipped OR is an infection rate of less than 1%. An OR equipped with this unit is frequently used for total joint replacement or organ transplant surgery.

Despite these precautions, wound contamination may occur during surgery but may only become apparent days or weeks later in the form of a surgical site infection that results in a longer hospital stay (Pryor, Fahey, Lien, et al., 2004). Constant surveillance and conscientious technique in carrying out aseptic practices are necessary to reduce the risk of contamination and infection.

Basic Guidelines for Maintaining Surgical Asepsis

All practitioners involved in the intraoperative phase have a responsibility to provide and maintain a safe environment. Adherence to aseptic practice is part of this responsibility. The basic principles of aseptic technique follow:

- All materials in contact with the surgical wound or used within the sterile field must be sterile. Sterile surfaces or articles may touch other sterile surfaces or articles and remain sterile; contact with unsterile objects at any point renders a sterile area contaminated.
- Gowns of the surgical team are considered sterile in front from the chest to the level of the sterile field. The sleeves are also considered sterile from 2 inches above the elbow to the stockinette cuff.
- Sterile drapes are used to create a sterile field. Only the top surface of a draped table is considered sterile. During draping of a table or patient, the sterile drape is held well above the surface to be covered and is positioned from front to back.
- Items are dispensed to a sterile field by methods that preserve the sterility of the items and the integrity of the sterile field. After a sterile package is opened, the edges are considered unsterile. Sterile supplies, including solutions, are delivered to a sterile field or handed to a scrubbed person in such a way that the sterility of the object or fluid remains intact.
- The movements of the surgical team are from sterile to sterile areas and from unsterile to unsterile areas. Scrubbed persons and sterile items contact only sterile areas; circulating nurses and unsterile items contact only unsterile areas.
- Movement around a sterile field must not cause contamination of the field. Sterile areas must be kept in view during movement around the area. At least a 1-foot distance from the sterile field must be maintained to prevent inadvertent contamination.
- Whenever a sterile barrier is breached, the area must be considered contaminated. A tear or puncture of the drape permitting access to an unsterile surface underneath renders the area unsterile. Such a drape must be replaced.
- Every sterile field is constantly monitored and maintained. Items of doubtful sterility are considered unsterile. Sterile fields are prepared as close as possible to the time of use.
- The routine administration of hyperoxia (high levels of oxygen) is *not* recommended to reduce surgical site infections. In a study of 165 patients undergoing general surgery, the rate of surgical site infection was higher in patients who received 80% oxygen during surgery than in those who received 35% oxygen (Pryor et al., 2004).

Health Hazards Associated With the Surgical Environment

Safety issues in the OR include exposure to blood and body fluids; hazards associated with laser beams; and exposure to latex and adhesive substances, radiation, and toxic agents (Hammarsten, Hammarsten & Jemsby, 2003). Internal monitoring of the OR includes the analysis of surface swipe samples and air samples for infectious and toxic agents. In addition, policies and procedures for minimizing exposure to body fluids and reducing the dangers associated with lasers and radiation have been established.

An additional hazard is the unintentional leaving of an object in a person during a surgical procedure. The risk that foreign objects may be left in a person increases in the following situations: when the procedure is performed on an emergency basis, when there is an unplanned change in the procedure, and when the patient has a high body mass index. Complications from foreign bodies left after a surgical procedure include small bowel fistulas, obstruction, visceral perforation, and death (Gawande et al., 2003).

Laser Risks

The AORN has recommended practices for laser safety (Phillips, 2004). While lasers are in use, warning signs must be clearly posted to alert personnel. Safety precautions are implemented to reduce the possibility of exposing the eyes and skin to laser beams, to prevent inhalation of the laser plume (smoke and particulate matter), and to protect the patient and personnel from fire and electrical hazards. Several types of lasers are available for clinical use; perioperative personnel should be familiar with the unique features, specific operation, and safety measures for each type of laser used in the practice setting.

Nurses and other intraoperative personnel working with lasers must have a thorough eye examination before participating in procedures involving lasers. All personnel wear special protective goggles, specific to the type of laser used in the procedure (Andersen, 2004).

Whether protection is needed to avoid the laser plume and the effects of its inhalation is controversial. Smoke evacuators are used in some procedures to remove the laser plume from the operative field. In recent years, this technology has been used to protect the surgical team from the potential hazards associated with the generalized smoke plume generated by standard electrocautery units.

Exposure to Blood and Body Fluids

OR attire has changed dramatically since the advent of acquired immunodeficiency syndrome (AIDS). Double-gloving is routine in trauma and other types of surgery where sharp bone fragments are present. In addition to the routine scrub suit and double gloves, some surgical personnel wear rubber boots, a waterproof apron, and sleeve protectors. Goggles, or a wrap-around face shield, are worn to protect against splashing when the surgical wound is irrigated or when bone drilling is performed. In hospitals where numerous total joint procedures are performed, a complete bubble mask may be used. This mask provides full-barrier protection from bone fragments and splashes. Ventilation is accomplished through an accompanying hood with a separate air-filtration system.

Latex Allergy

The AORN has recommended standards of care for the patient with latex allergy (AORN, 2004a). These recommendations include early identification of patients with latex allergies, preparation of a latex allergy supply cart, and maintenance of latex allergy precautions throughout the perioperative period. Because of the increased number of patients with latex allergies, many latex-free products are now available. For safety, manufacturers and hospital material managers need to take responsibility for identifying the latex content in items used by patients and health care personnel. (See Chapters 18 and 53 for assessment for latex allergy.)

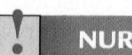

NURSING ALERT

It is the responsibility of all nurses, and particularly perianesthesia and perioperative nurses, to be aware of latex allergies, necessary precautions, and products that are latex-free. Hospital staff are also at risk for development of a latex allergy secondary to repeated exposure to latex products.

The Surgical Experience

During the surgical procedure, the patient will need sedation, anesthesia, or some combination of these.

Types of Anesthesia and Sedation

Anesthesia today is very safe; it is estimated that the number of anesthesia-related deaths is as low as 1 in 200,000 to 300,000 cases (Pine, Holt, & Lou, 2003). For the patient, the anesthesia experience consists of having an IV line inserted, if it was not inserted earlier; receiving a sedating agent prior to induction with an anesthetic agent; losing consciousness; being intubated, if indicated; and then receiving a combination of anesthetic agents. Typically the experience is a smooth one, and the patient has no recall of the events. The main types of anesthesia are general anesthesia, regional anesthesia, moderate sedation, monitored anesthesia care, and local anesthesia.

General Anesthesia

Anesthesia is a state of narcosis (severe central nervous system depression produced by pharmacologic agents), analgesia, relaxation, and reflex loss. Patients under general anesthesia are not arousable, not even to painful stimuli. They lose the ability to maintain ventilatory function and require assistance in maintaining a patent airway. Cardiovascular function may be impaired as well.

In 2004, JCAHO issued an alert regarding the phenomenon of patients being partially awake while under general

NURSING RESEARCH PROFILE

Preoperative Skin Testing of Materials Used in Surgical Procedures

Hammarsten, R., Hammarsten, J. & Jemsby, P. (2003). Preoperative skin testing of materials used in surgical procedures. *AORN Journal, 77*(4), 762–771.

Purpose

Postoperative skin complications due to allergic or toxic effects of adhesive substances increase health care costs and cause patient discomfort. The purpose of the study was to investigate the incidence of skin reactions with the application of different materials.

Design

Study participants included 101 consecutive patients with a history of atopic or contact eczema, allergy, or asthma as indicated by their medical history. The day before surgery, 10 patches containing different adhesive materials that the patient could potentially be exposed to in the operating room were placed on the right forearm or ring finger for 6 hours. The patches were removed and then evaluated for no reaction, redness, itching, rash, and blisters 30 minutes later. The statistical analysis of differences in skin reactions among the various tested patches was performed via chi-square analysis.

Findings

From 3% to 50% of the participants showed skin reactions after the preoperative skin test. Surgical drapes with tape caused a skin reaction 50% of the time. Skin reactions included redness, itching, rash, or blisters.

Nursing Implications

It is the nurse's responsibility to be the patient advocate during surgery; therefore, it is important to reduce the potential for harm or patient suffering, or even disruption in wound healing. For some time, adhesives have been known to be a source of allergy. Nurses need to be alert to adhesive materials that cause reactions and be instrumental in removing these materials from the OR.

anesthesia (referred to as anesthesia awareness). Patients at greatest risk of anesthesia awareness are cardiac, obstetric, and major trauma patients. The entire surgical team must be aware of this phenomenon and help prevent or manage it (JCAHO, 2004).

General anesthesia consists of four stages, each associated with specific clinical manifestations (Rothrock, 2003):

- *Stage I: beginning anesthesia.* As the patient breathes in the anesthetic mixture, warmth, dizziness, and a feeling of detachment may be experienced. The patient may have a ringing, roaring, or buzzing in the ears and, although still conscious, may sense an inability to move the extremities easily. During this stage, noises are exaggerated; even low voices or minor sounds seem loud and unreal. For this reason, unnecessary noises and motions are avoided when anesthesia begins.
- *Stage II: excitement.* The excitement stage, characterized variously by struggling, shouting, talking, singing, laughing, or crying, is often avoided if the anesthetic is administered smoothly and quickly. The pupils dilate, but they contract if exposed to light; the pulse rate is rapid, and respirations may be irregular. Because of the possibility of uncontrolled movements of the patient during this stage, the anesthesiologist or anesthetist must always be assisted by someone ready to help restrain the patient. A strap may be in place across the patient's thighs, and the hands may be secured to an armboard. The patient should not be touched except for purposes of restraint, but restraints should not be applied over the operative site. Manipulation increases circulation to the operative site and thereby increases the potential for bleeding.
- *Stage III: surgical anesthesia.* Surgical anesthesia is reached by continued administration of the anesthetic vapor or gas. The patient is unconscious and lies quietly on the table. The pupils are small but contract when exposed to light. Respirations are regular, the pulse rate and volume are normal, and the skin is pink or slightly flushed. With proper administration of the anesthetic, this stage may be maintained for hours in one of several planes, ranging from light (1) to deep (4), depending on the depth of anesthesia needed.
- *Stage IV: medullary depression.* This stage is reached when too much anesthesia has been administered. Respirations become shallow, the pulse is weak and thready, and the pupils become widely dilated and no longer contract when exposed to light. Cyanosis develops and, without prompt intervention, death rapidly follows. If this stage develops, the anesthetic is discontinued immediately and respiratory and circulatory support is initiated to prevent death. Stimulants, although rarely used, may be administered; narcotic antagonists can be used if the overdosage is due to opioids.

When opioid agents (narcotics) and neuromuscular blockers (relaxants) are administered, several of the stages are absent. During smooth administration of an anesthetic, there is no sharp division between stages I, II, and III, and there is no stage IV. The patient passes gradually from one stage to another, and it is through close observation of the signs exhibited by the patient that an anesthesiologist or anesthetist controls the situation. The responses of the pupils, the blood pressure, and the respiratory and cardiac rates are among the most reliable guides to the patient's condition.

Anesthetic agents used in general anesthesia are inhaled or administered by IV. Anesthetics produce anesthesia because they are delivered to the brain at a high partial pressure that enables them to cross the blood–brain barrier.

Relatively large amounts of anesthetic must be administered during induction and the early maintenance phases because the anesthetic is recirculated and deposited in body tissues. As these sites become saturated, smaller amounts of the anesthetic agent are required to maintain anesthesia because equilibrium or near equilibrium has been achieved between brain, blood, and other tissues.

Any condition that diminishes peripheral blood flow, such as vasoconstriction or shock, may reduce the amount of anesthetic required. Conversely, when peripheral blood flow is unusually high, as in a muscularly active or apprehensive patient, induction is slower, and greater quantities of anesthetic are required because the brain receives a smaller quantity of anesthetic.

INHALATION

Inhaled anesthetic agents include volatile liquid agents and gases. Volatile liquid anesthetics produce anesthesia when their vapors are inhaled. Commonly used inhalation agents are included in Table 19-1. All are administered with oxygen and usually with nitrous oxide as well.

Gas anesthetics are administered by inhalation and are always combined with oxygen. Nitrous oxide is the most commonly used gas anesthetic agent. When inhaled, the anesthetics enter the blood through the pulmonary capillaries and act on cerebral centers to produce loss of consciousness and sensation. When anesthetic administration is discontinued, the vapor or gas is eliminated through the lungs.

The vapor from inhalation anesthetics can be administered to the patient by several methods. The inhalation anesthetic may be administered through an LMA (Fig. 19-1A), a flexible tube with an inflatable silicone ring and cuff that can be inserted into the larynx. The endotracheal technique for administering anesthetics consists of introducing a soft rubber or plastic endotracheal tube into the trachea, usually by means of a laryngoscope. The endotracheal tube may be inserted through either the nose (see Fig. 19-1B) or mouth

℞ TABLE 19-1 Inhalation Anesthetic Agents

Agent	Administration	Advantages	Disadvantages	Implications/ Considerations
Volatile Liquids				
Halothane (Fluothane)	Inhalation; special vaporizer	Not explosive or flammable Induction rapid and smooth Useful in almost every type of surgery Low incidence of postoperative nausea and vomiting	Requires skillful administration to prevent overdosage May cause liver damage May produce hypotension Requires special vaporizer for administration	In addition to observation of pulse and respiration postoperatively, blood pressure must be monitored frequently.
Enflurane (Ethrane)	Inhalation	Rapid induction and recovery Potent analgesic Not explosive or flammable	Respiratory depression may develop rapidly, along with ECG abnormalities. Not compatible with epinephrine	Observe for possible respiratory depression. Administration with epinephrine may cause ventricular fibrillation.
Isoflurane (Forane)	Inhalation	Rapid induction and recovery Muscle relaxants are markedly potentiated.	A profound respiratory depressant	Respirations must be monitored closely and supported when necessary.
Sevoflurane (Ultrane)	Inhalation	Rapid induction and excretion; minimal side effects	Coughing and laryngospasm; trigger for malignant hyperthermia	Monitor for malignant hyperthermia.
Desflurane (Suprane)	Inhalation	Rapid induction and emergence; rare organ toxicity	Respiratory irritation; trigger for malignant hyperthermia	Monitor for malignant hyperthermia, dysrhythmias.
Gases				
Nitrous oxide (N_2O)	Inhalation (semi-closed method)	Induction and recovery rapid Nonflammable Useful with oxygen for short procedures Useful with other agents for all types of surgery	Poor relaxant Weak anesthetic May produce hypoxia	Most useful in conjunction with other agents with longer action Monitor for chest pain, hypertension, and stroke.
Oxygen (O_2)	Inhalation	Can increase O_2 available to tissues	High concentrations are hazardous	Increased fire risk when used with lasers

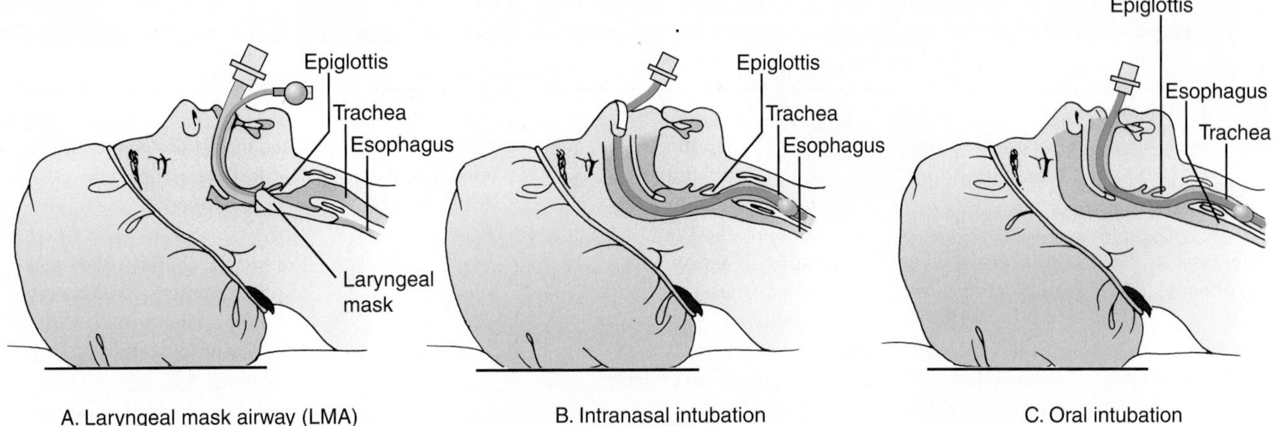

FIGURE 19-1. Anesthetic delivery methods: (**A**) laryngeal mask airway (LMA), (**B**) nasal endotracheal catheter (in position with cuff inflated), and (**C**) oral endotracheal intubation (tube is in position with cuff inflated).

(see Fig. 19-1C). When in place, the tube seals off the lungs from the esophagus so that, if the patient vomits, stomach contents do not enter the lungs.

INTRAVENOUS ADMINISTRATION

General anesthesia can also be produced by the IV administration of various substances, such as barbiturates, benzodiazepines, nonbarbiturate hypnotics, dissociative agents, and opioid agents. Table 19-2 lists commonly used IV anesthetic and analgesic agents, including IV medications used as muscle relaxants in the intraoperative period. These medications may be administered to induce (initiate) or maintain anesthesia. Although they are often used in combination with inhalation anesthetics, they may be used alone. They may also be used to produce moderate sedation, as discussed later in this chapter.

An advantage of IV anesthesia is that the onset of anesthesia is pleasant; there is none of the buzzing, roaring, or dizziness known to follow administration of an inhalation anesthetic. For this reason, induction of anesthesia usually begins with an IV agent and is often preferred by patients who have experienced various methods. The duration of action is brief, and the patient awakens with little nausea or vomiting.

The IV anesthetic agents are nonexplosive, require little equipment, and are easy to administer. The low incidence of postoperative nausea and vomiting makes the method useful in eye surgery, because in this setting vomiting would increase intraocular pressure and endanger vision in the operated eye. IV anesthesia is useful for short procedures but is used less often for the longer procedures of abdominal surgery. It is not indicated for children who have small veins or for those who require intubation because of their susceptibility to respiratory obstruction.

A disadvantage of an IV anesthetic such as thiopental (Pentothal) is its powerful respiratory depressant effect. It must be administered by a skilled anesthesiologist or anesthetist and only when some method of oxygen administration is available immediately in case of difficulty. Sneezing, coughing, and laryngospasm are sometimes noted with its use.

IV neuromuscular blockers (muscle relaxants) block the transmission of nerve impulses at the neuromuscular junction of skeletal muscles. Muscle relaxants are used to relax muscles in abdominal and thoracic surgery, relax eye muscles in certain types of eye surgery, facilitate endotracheal intubation, treat laryngospasm, and assist in mechanical ventilation.

Regional Anesthesia

Regional anesthesia is a form of local anesthesia in which an anesthetic agent is injected around nerves so that the area supplied by these nerves is anesthetized. The effect depends on the type of nerve involved. Motor fibers are the largest fibers and have the thickest myelin sheath. Sympathetic fibers are the smallest and have a minimal covering. Sensory fibers are intermediate. A local anesthetic blocks motor nerves least readily and sympathetic nerves most readily. An anesthetic cannot be regarded as having worn off until all three systems (motor, sensory, and autonomic) are no longer affected.

The patient receiving regional anesthesia is awake and aware of his or her surroundings unless medications are given to produce mild sedation or to relieve anxiety. The nurse must avoid careless conversation, unnecessary noise, and unpleasant odors; these may be noticed by the patient in the OR and may contribute to a negative response to the surgical experience. A quiet environment is therapeutic. The diagnosis must not be stated aloud if the patient is not to know it at this time.

EPIDURAL ANESTHESIA

Epidural anesthesia, a commonly used conduction block, is achieved by injecting a local anesthetic into the epidural space that surrounds the dura mater of the spinal cord (Fig. 19-2). (In contrast, spinal anesthesia involves injection through the dura mater into the subarachnoid space surrounding the spinal cord.) Epidural anesthesia blocks sensory, motor, and autonomic functions; it differs from spinal anesthesia by the site of the injection and the amount of anesthetic agent used. Epidural doses are much higher

TABLE 19-2 Commonly Used Intravenous Medications

Medication	Common Usage	Advantages	Disadvantages	Comments
Opioid Analgesics				
Morphine sulfate (MS)	Perioperative pain; premedication	Inexpensive; duration of action 4 to 5 hours; euphoria; good cardiovascular stability	Nausea and vomiting; histamine release; postural ↓ BP and ↓ SVR	Used intrathecally and epidurally for postoperative pain; elimination half-life 3 hours
Alfentanil (Alfenta)	Surgical analgesia in ambulatory patients	Duration of action 0.5 hour; used as bolus or infusion		Potency: 750 μg = 10 mg morphine sulfate; elimination half-life 1.6 hours
Fentanyl (Sublimaze)	Surgical analgesia: epidural infusion for postoperative analgesia; add to SAB	Good cardiovascular stability; duration of action 0.5 hour		Most commonly used opioid; potency: 100 μg = 10 mg morphine sulfate; elimination half-life 3.6 hours
Remifentanil (Ultiva)	IV infusion for surgical analgesia; small boluses for brief, intense pain	Easily titratable; metabolized by blood and tissue esterases; very short duration; good cardiovascular stability	New; expensive; requires mixing; may cause muscle rigidity	Potency: 25 μg = 10 mg morphine sulfate; 20 to 30 times potency of alfentanil; elimination half-life 3 to 10 min
Sufentanil (Sufenta)	Surgical analgesia	Good cardiovascular stability; duration of action 0.5 hour; prolonged analgesia	Prolonged respiratory depression	Potency: 15 μg = 10 mg morphine sulfate; elimination half-life 2.7 hours
Depolarizing Muscle Relaxants				
Succinylcholine (Anectine, Quelicin)	Intubation; short cases	Rapid onset; short duration	Requires refrigeration; may cause fasciculations, postoperative myalgias, and dysrhythmias; ↑ serum K^+ with burns, tissue trauma, paralysis, and muscle diseases; slight histamine release	Prolonged muscle relaxation with serum cholinesterase deficiency and certain antibiotics; trigger agent for malignant hyperthermia
Nondepolarizing Muscle Relaxants—Intermediate Onset and Duration				
Atracurium (Tracrium)	Intubation; maintenance of relaxation	No significant cardiovascular or cumulative effects; good with renal failure	Requires refrigeration; slight histamine release	Breakdown by Hofman elimination (non-enzymatic degradation) and ester hydrolysis
Cisatracurium (Nimbex)	Intubation; maintenance of relaxation	Similar to atracurium	No histamine release	Similar to atracurium
Mivacurium (Mivacron)	Intubation; maintenance of relaxation	Short acting; rapid metabolism by plasma cholinesterase; used as bolus or infusion	Expensive in longer cases	New; rarely need to reverse; prolonged effect with plasma cholinesterase deficiency
Rocuronium (Zemuron)	Intubation; maintenance of relaxation	Rapid onset (dose-dependent); elimination via kidney and liver	Vagolytic; may ↑ HR	Duration similar to atracurium and vecuronium
Vecuronium (Norcuron)	Intubation; maintenance of relaxation	No significant cardiovascular or cumulative effects; no histamine release	Requires mixing	Mostly eliminated in bile, some in urine

℞ TABLE 19-2 Commonly Used Intravenous Medications (Continued)

Medication	Common Usage	Advantages	Disadvantages	Comments
Nondepolarizing Muscle Relaxants—Longer Onset and Duration				
d-Tubocurarine	Maintenance of relaxation		May cause histamine release and transient ganglionic blockade	Mostly used for pretreatment with succinylcholine
Metocurine (Metubine)	Maintenance of relaxation	Good cardiovascular stability	Slight histamine release	Large bolus may cause ↓ BP
Pancuronium (Pavulon)	Maintenance of relaxation		May cause ↑ HR and ↑ BP	Mostly renal elimination
Intravenous Anesthetics				
Etomidate (Amidate)	Induction	Good cardiovascular stability; fast, smooth induction and recovery	May cause pain with injection and myotonic movements	
Diazepam (Valium, Dizac)	Amnesia; hypnotic; preoperative medication	Good sedation	Prolonged duration	Residual effects for 20 to 90 hr; increased effect with alcohol
Ketamine (Ketalar)	Induction, occasional maintenance (IV or IM)	Short acting; patient maintains airway; good in small children and burn patients	Large doses may cause hallucinations and respiratory depression	Need darkened, quiet room for recovery; often used in trauma cases
Midazolam (Versed)	Hypnotic; anxiolytic; sedation; often used as adjunct to induction	Excellent amnesia; water-soluble (no pain with IV injection); short-acting	Slower induction than thiopental	Often used for amnesia with insertion of invasive monitors or regional anesthesia
Propofol (Diprivan)	Induction and maintenance; sedation with regional anesthesia or MAC	Rapid onset; awakening in 4 to 8 min	May cause pain when injected	Short elimination half-life (34–64 min)
Sodium methohexital (Brevital)	Induction	Ultrashort-acting barbiturate	May cause hiccups	Can be given rectally
Thiopental sodium (Pentothal)	Induction	Induction	May cause laryngospasm; can be given rectally	Large doses may cause apnea and cardiovascular depression

BP, blood pressure; HR, heart rate; IM, intramuscular; IV, intravenous; MAC, monitored anesthesia care; PO, oral; SAB, subarachnoid block; SVR, stroke volume ratio.

Adapted with permission from Table 7-2, "Commonly Used Anesthetic Drugs," pp. 232–234 in Rothrock, J. C. (2003). *Alexander's care of the patient in surgery* (12th ed.). St. Louis: Mosby.

because the epidural anesthetic does not make direct contact with the spinal cord or nerve roots.

An advantage of epidural anesthesia is the absence of headache that occasionally results from spinal anesthesia. A disadvantage is the greater technical challenge of introducing the anesthetic into the epidural rather than the subarachnoid space. If inadvertent puncture of the dura occurs during epidural anesthesia and the anesthetic travels toward the head, high spinal anesthesia can result; this can produce severe hypotension and respiratory depression and arrest. Treatment of these complications includes airway support, IV fluids, and use of vasopressors.

SPINAL ANESTHESIA

Spinal anesthesia is an extensive conduction nerve block that is produced when a local anesthetic is introduced into the subarachnoid space at the lumbar level, usually between L4 and L5 (see Fig. 19-2). It produces anesthesia of the lower extremities, perineum, and lower abdomen. For the lumbar puncture procedure, the patient usually lies on the side in a knee–chest position. Sterile technique is used as a spinal puncture is made and the medication is injected through the needle. As soon as the injection has been made, the patient is positioned on his or her back. If a relatively high level of block is sought, the head and shoulders are lowered.

The spread of the anesthetic agent and the level of anesthesia depend on the amount of fluid injected, the speed with which it is injected, the positioning of the patient after the injection, and the specific gravity of the agent. If the specific gravity is greater than that of cerebrospinal fluid (CSF), the agent moves to the dependent position of the

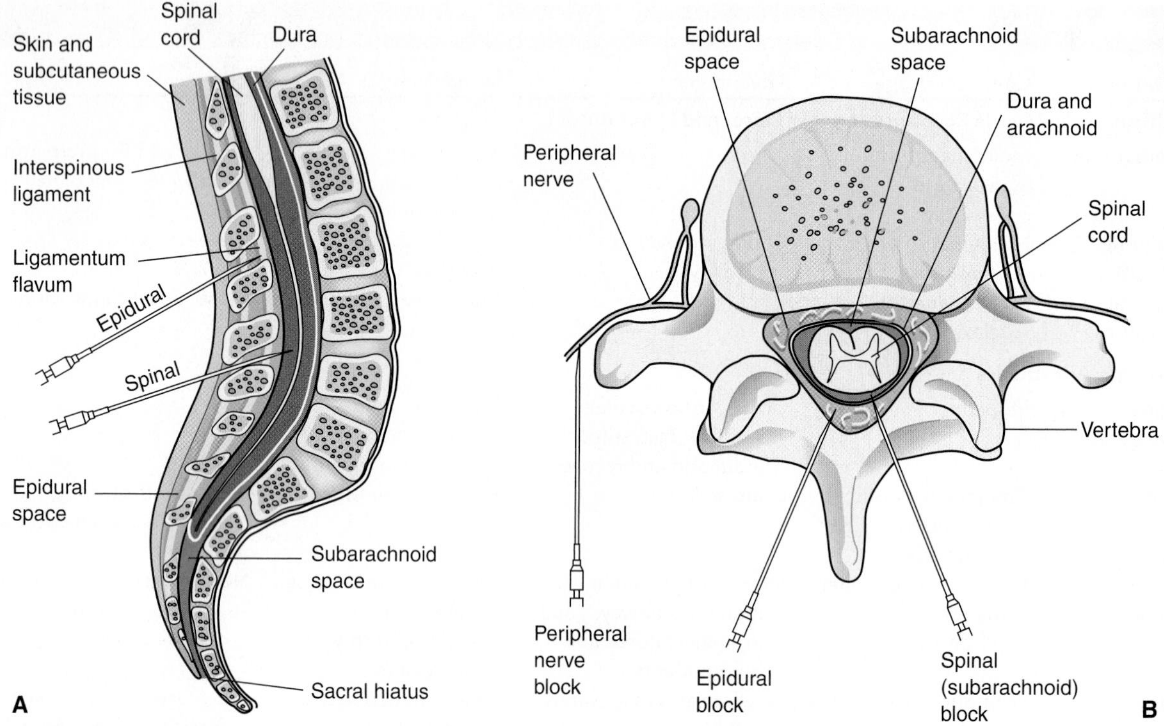

FIGURE 19-2. (**A**) Injection sites for spinal and epidural anesthesia. (**B**) Cross-section of injection sites for peripheral nerve, epidural, and spinal blocks.

subarachnoid space. If the specific gravity is less than that of CSF, the anesthetic moves away from the dependent position. The anesthesiologist or anesthetist controls the spread of the agent. Table 19-3 contains types of regional anesthesia agents.

A few minutes after induction of a spinal anesthetic, anesthesia and paralysis affect the toes and perineum and then gradually the legs and abdomen. If the anesthetic reaches the upper thoracic and cervical spinal cord in high concentrations, a temporary partial or complete respiratory paralysis results. Paralysis of the respiratory muscles is managed by mechanical ventilation until the effects of the anesthetic on the cranial and thoracic nerves have worn off.

Nausea, vomiting, and pain may occur during surgery when spinal anesthesia is used. As a rule, these reactions result from manipulation of various structures, particularly

℞ TABLE 19-3 Selected Regional and Local Anesthetic Agents

Agent	Administration	Advantages	Disadvantages	Implications/ Considerations
Lidocaine (Xylocaine)	Epidural, spinal, peripheral intravenous anesthesia, and local infiltration	Rapid Longer duration of action (compared with procaine) Free from local irritative effect	Occasional idiosyncrasy	Useful topically for cystoscopy Observe for untoward reactions—drowsiness, depressed respiration, seizures
Bupivacaine (Marcaine, Sensoricaine)	Epidural, spinal, peripheral intravenous anesthesia, and local infiltration	Duration is 2–3 times longer than lidocaine	Use cautiously in patients with known drug allergies or sensitivities.	A period of analgesia persists after return of sensation; therefore, need for strong analgesics is reduced. Greater potency and longer action than lidocaine
Tetracaine (Pontocaine)	Topical, infiltration, and nerve block	Long acting, produces good relaxation	Occasional allergic reaction	More than 10 times as potent as procaine (Novocaine)
Procaine (Novocaine)	Local infiltration		Occasional allergic reaction	Commonly used in oral or dental surgery

those within the abdominal cavity. The simultaneous IV administration of a weak solution of thiopental and inhalation of nitrous oxide may prevent such reactions.

Headache may be an after-effect of spinal anesthesia. Several factors are related to the incidence of headache: the size of the spinal needle used, the leakage of fluid from the subarachnoid space through the puncture site, and the patient's hydration status. Measures that increase cerebrospinal pressure are helpful in relieving headache. These include maintaining a quiet environment, keeping the patient lying flat, and keeping the patient well hydrated.

In continuous spinal anesthesia, the tip of a plastic catheter remains in the subarachnoid space during the surgical procedure so that more anesthetic may be injected as needed. This technique allows greater control of the dosage, but there is greater potential for postanesthetic headache because of the large-gauge needle used.

LOCAL CONDUCTION BLOCKS

Examples of common local conduction blocks are:

- Brachial plexus block, which produces anesthesia of the arm
- Paravertebral anesthesia, which produces anesthesia of the nerves supplying the chest, abdominal wall, and extremities
- Transsacral (caudal) block, which produces anesthesia of the perineum and, occasionally, the lower abdomen

Moderate Sedation/Analgesia

Moderate sedation (or moderate analgesia), previously referred to as conscious sedation, is a form of anesthesia that involves the IV administration of sedatives and/or analgesic medications to reduce patient anxiety and control pain during diagnostic or therapeutic procedures. It is being used increasingly for specific short-term surgical procedures in hospitals and ambulatory care centers (Rothrock, 2003). The goal is to depress a patient's level of consciousness to a moderate level to enable surgical, diagnostic, or therapeutic procedures to be performed while ensuring the patient's comfort during and cooperation with the procedures. With moderate sedation, the patient is able to maintain a patent airway, retain protective airway reflexes, and respond to verbal and physical stimuli (Morton, Fontaine, Hudak et al., 2005).

Moderate sedation can be administered by an anesthesiologist, anesthetist, or other specially trained and credentialed physician or nurse. The patient receiving moderate sedation is never left alone and is closely monitored by a physician or nurse who is knowledgeable and skilled in detecting dysrhythmias, administering oxygen, and performing resuscitation. The continual assessment of the patient's vital signs, level of consciousness, and cardiac and respiratory function is an essential component of moderate sedation. Pulse oximetry, ECG monitor, and frequent measurement of vital signs are used to monitor the patient. The regulations for use and administration of moderate sedation differ from state to state, and its administration is addressed by standards issued by JCAHO and by institutional policies and nursing specialty organizations, including the Association of PeriAnesthesia Nurses (2004).

Monitored Anesthesia Care

Monitored anesthesia care (MAC), also referred to as monitored sedation, is administered by an anesthesiologist or anesthetist. Although similar to moderate sedation, the health care provider who administers MAC, usually an anesthesiologist or anesthetist, must be prepared and qualified to convert to general anesthesia if necessary. The skills of an anesthesiologist or anesthetist may be necessary to manage the effects of a level of deeper sedation to return the patient to the appropriate level of sedation (Morton et al., 2005; American Society of Anesthesiologists, 2004). MAC may be used for healthy patients undergoing relatively minor surgical procedures and for some critically ill patients who may be unable to tolerate anesthesia without extensive invasive monitoring and pharmacologic support (Rothrock, 2003). Moderate sedation and monitored anesthesia care are compared in Table 19-4.

Local Anesthesia

Infiltration anesthesia is the injection of a solution containing the local anesthetic into the tissues at the planned incision site. Often it is combined with a local regional block by injecting the nerves immediately supplying the area. Advantages of local anesthesia are as follows:

- It is simple, economical, and nonexplosive.
- Equipment needed is minimal.
- Postoperative recovery is brief.
- Undesirable effects of general anesthesia are avoided.
- It is ideal for short and superficial surgical procedures.

Local anesthesia is often administered in combination with epinephrine. Epinephrine constricts blood vessels, which prevents rapid absorption of the anesthetic agent

℞ TABLE 19-4 Comparison of Moderate Sedation and Monitored Anesthesia Care

	Moderate Sedation	Monitored Anesthesia Care (MAC)
Responsiveness	Purposeful response to repeated or painful verbal or tactile stimulation	Purposeful response after stimulation
Airway	No intervention required	Intervention may be required
Spontaneous ventilation	Adequate	May be inadequate
Cardiovascular function	Usually maintained	Usually maintained

From Morton, P. G., Fontaine, D. K., Hudak, C. M. & Gallo, B. M. (2005). *Critical care nursing: A holistic approach* (8th ed.). Philadelphia: Lippincott Williams & Wilkins, p. 179.

and thus prolongs its local action. Rapid absorption of the anesthetic agent into the bloodstream, which could cause seizures, is also prevented. Agents that can be used as local anesthetic agents are listed in Table 19-3; some of the same agents used in regional anesthesia are used as local anesthetics.

Local anesthesia is the preferred method of choice in any surgical procedure in which it can be used. However, contraindications include high preoperative levels of anxiety, because surgery with local anesthesia may increase anxiety. A patient who requests general anesthesia rarely does well under local anesthesia. For some surgical procedures, local anesthesia is impractical because of the number of injections and the amount of anesthetic that would be required (eg, breast reconstruction).

The skin is prepared as for any surgical procedure, and a small-gauge needle is used to inject a modest amount of the anesthetic into the skin layers. This produces blanching or a wheal. Additional anesthetic is then injected into the skin until an area the length of the proposed incision is anesthetized. A larger, longer needle then is used to infiltrate deeper tissues with the anesthetic. The action of the agent is almost immediate, so surgery may begin as soon as the injection is complete. Anesthesia lasts 45 minutes to 3 hours, depending on the anesthetic and the use of epinephrine.

Potential Intraoperative Complications

The surgical patient is subject to several risks. Potential intraoperative complications include nausea and vomiting, anaphylaxis, hypoxia, hypothermia, malignant hyperthermia, and disseminated intravascular coagulopathy (DIC). The National Surgical Care Improvement Project (SCIP) set a national goal of a 25% reduction in surgical complications by 2010. Targeted areas include surgical site infections, as well as cardiac, respiratory, and venous thromboembolic complications. A SCIP committee has been formed to develop a quality improvement framework to improve both patient safety and the quality of surgical services nationwide (SCIP, 2005).

Nausea and Vomiting

Nausea and vomiting, or regurgitation, may affect patients during the intraoperative period. If gagging occurs, the patient is turned to the side, the head of the table is lowered, and a basin is provided to collect the vomitus. Suction is used to remove saliva and vomited gastric contents. The advent of new anesthetics has reduced the incidence; however, there is no single way to prevent nausea and vomiting. An interdisciplinary approach involving the surgeon, anesthesiologist or anesthetist, and nurse is best.

In some cases, the anesthesiologist or anesthetist administers antiemetics preoperatively or intraoperatively to counteract possible aspiration. If the patient aspirates vomitus, an asthma-like attack with severe bronchial spasms and wheezing is triggered. Pneumonitis and pulmonary edema can subsequently develop, leading to extreme hypoxia. Increasing medical attention is being paid to silent regurgitation of gastric contents (not related to preoperative fasting times), which occurs more frequently than previously realized. The volume and acidity of the aspirate determine the extent of damage to the lungs. Patients may be given Bicitra, a clear, nonparticulate antacid to increase gastric fluid pH or a histamine-2 (H_2) receptor antagonist such as cimetidine (Tagamet), ranitidine (Zantac), or famotidine (Pepcid) to decrease gastric acid production (Rothrock, 2003).

Anaphylaxis

Any time the patient comes into contact with a foreign substance, there is the potential for an anaphylactic reaction. Because medications are the most common cause of anaphylaxis, intraoperative nurses must be aware of the type and method of anesthesia used as well as the specific agents. An anaphylactic reaction can occur in response to many medications, latex, or other substances. The reaction may be immediate or delayed. Anaphylaxis is a life-threatening acute allergic reaction. See Chapters 15 and 53 for more details about the signs, symptoms, and treatment of anaphylaxis.

Fibrin sealants are used in a variety of surgical procedures, and cyanoacrylate tissue adhesives are used to close wounds without the use of sutures. These sealants have been implicated in allergic reactions and anaphylaxis (Phillips, 2004). Although these reactions are rare, the nurse must be alert to the possibility and observe the patient for changes in vital signs and symptoms of anaphylaxis when these products are used.

Hypoxia and Other Respiratory Complications

Inadequate ventilation, occlusion of the airway, inadvertent intubation of the esophagus, and hypoxia are significant potential complications associated with general anesthesia. Many factors can contribute to inadequate ventilation. Respiratory depression caused by anesthetic agents, aspiration of respiratory tract secretions or vomitus, and the patient's position on the operating table can compromise the exchange of gases. Anatomic variation can make the trachea difficult to visualize and result in the artificial airway's being inserted into the esophagus rather than into the trachea. In addition to these dangers, asphyxia caused by foreign bodies in the mouth, spasm of the vocal cords, relaxation of the tongue, or aspiration of vomitus, saliva, or blood can occur. Brain damage from hypoxia occurs within minutes; therefore, vigilant monitoring of the patient's oxygenation status is a primary function of the anesthesiologist or anesthetist and the circulating nurse. Peripheral perfusion is checked frequently, and pulse oximetry values are monitored continuously.

Hypothermia

During anesthesia, the patient's temperature may fall. Glucose metabolism is reduced, and, as a result, metabolic acidosis may develop. This condition is called hypothermia and is indicated by a core body temperature that is lower than normal (36.6°C [98.0°F] or less). Inadvertent hypothermia may occur as a result of a low temperature in the OR, infusion of cold fluids, inhalation of cold gases, open body wounds or cavities, decreased muscle activity, advanced age, or the pharmaceutical agents used (eg, vasodilators, phenothiazines, general anesthetics). Hypothermia may also be intentionally induced in selected surgical procedures (eg, cardiac surgeries requiring cardiopulmonary bypass) to reduce the patient's metabolic rate and energy demands (Seifert, 2002).

Preventing unintentional hypothermia is a major objective. If hypothermia occurs, the goal of intervention is to minimize or reverse the physiologic process. If hypothermia is intentional, the goal is safe return to normal body temperature. Environmental temperature in the OR can temporarily be set at 25° to 26.6°C (78° to 80°F). IV and irrigating fluids are warmed to 37°C (98.6°F). Wet gowns and drapes are removed promptly and replaced with dry materials, because wet linens promote heat loss. Whatever methods are used to rewarm the patient, warming must be accomplished gradually, not rapidly. Conscientious monitoring of core temperature, urinary output, ECG, blood pressure, arterial blood gas levels, and serum electrolyte levels is required.

Malignant Hyperthermia

Malignant hyperthermia is a rare inherited muscle disorder that is chemically induced by anesthetic agents (Rothrock, 2003). At one time, mortality rates exceeded 80%. Since the introduction of dantrolene sodium in 1979, the development of genetics testing, and early detection and treatment with specific protocols, fatalities have been reduced to approximately 10% (McCarthy, 2004). However, identification of patients at risk for malignant hyperthermia is imperative. Susceptible people include those with strong and bulky muscles, a history of muscle cramps or muscle weakness and unexplained temperature elevation, and an unexplained death of a family member during surgery that was accompanied by a febrile response (Litman & Rosenberg, 2005).

Pathophysiology

During anesthesia, potent agents such as inhalation anesthetics (halothane, enflurane) and muscle relaxants (succinylcholine) may trigger the symptoms of malignant hyperthermia (Rothrock, 2003). Stress and some medications, such as sympathomimetics (epinephrine), theophylline, aminophylline, anticholinergics (atropine), and cardiac glycosides (digitalis), can induce or intensify such a reaction.

The pathophysiology is related to a hypermetabolic condition in skeletal muscle cells that involves altered mechanisms of calcium function at the cellular level. This disruption of calcium causes clinical symptoms of hypermetabolism, which in turn increases muscle contraction (rigidity) and causes hyperthermia and subsequent damage to the central nervous system.

Clinical Manifestations

The initial symptoms of malignant hyperthermia are related to cardiovascular and musculoskeletal activity. Tachycardia (heart rate greater than 150 bpm) is often the earliest sign. In addition to the tachycardia, sympathetic nervous stimulation leads to ventricular dysrhythmia, hypotension, decreased cardiac output, oliguria, and, later, cardiac arrest. With the abnormal transport of calcium, rigidity or tetanus-like movements occur, often in the jaw. The rise in temperature is actually a late sign that develops rapidly; body temperature can increase 1° to 2°C (2° to 4°F) every 5 minutes (Rothrock, 2003). The core body temperature can reach or exceed 42°C (104°F) in a very short time and must be properly monitored and recorded during surgery (McCarthy, 2004).

Medical Management

Recognizing symptoms early and discontinuing anesthesia promptly are imperative. Goals of treatment are to decrease metabolism, reverse metabolic and respiratory acidosis, correct dysrhythmias, decrease body temperature, provide oxygen and nutrition to tissues, and correct electrolyte imbalance. The Malignant Hyperthermia Association of the United States (MHAUS) publishes a treatment protocol that should be posted in the OR and be readily available on a malignant hyperthermia cart.

As soon as the diagnosis is made, anesthesia and surgery are halted and the patient is hyperventilated with 100% oxygen. Dantrolene sodium (Dantrium), a skeletal muscle relaxant, and sodium bicarbonate are administered immediately (McCarthy, 2004). Continued monitoring of all parameters is necessary to evaluate the patient's status. Although malignant hyperthermia usually manifests about 10 to 20 minutes after induction of anesthesia, it can also occur during the first 24 hours after surgery.

Nursing Management

Although malignant hyperthermia is uncommon, the nurse must identify patients at risk, recognize the signs and symptoms, have the appropriate medication and equipment available, and be knowledgeable about the protocol to follow. This preparation may be lifesaving for the patient.

Disseminated Intravascular Coagulation

Disseminated intravascular coagulation (also referred to as coagulopathy [DIC]) is a life-threatening condition that is characterized by thrombus formation in the microcirculation and depletion of select coagulation proteins, causing hemorrhaging. The exact cause is unknown, but predisposing factors include many conditions that may occur with emergency surgery, such as massive trauma, head injury, massive transfusion, liver or kidney involvement, embolic events, and shock. The signs and symptoms, nursing assessment, and treatment of DIC are discussed in Chapter 33.

CHART 19-3

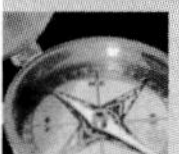

Ethics and Related Issues

To Resuscitate or Not?

SITUATION

Your ambulatory care center has developed a policy, authorized through the medical staff, that allows for patients to have a do-not-resuscitate order (DNR) in place during a surgical procedure. This policy follows the American Society of Anesthesiologists guidelines for DNR in the OR. You are preparing a patient for surgery, and the anesthesiologist who will be administering the anesthetic writes an order for the DNR to be rescinded during surgery. The physician is refusing to talk to the patient concerning the DNR.

PROBLEM

The patient believes his/her wishes will be followed with regard to resuscitation in the event of a cardiac arrest and the physician does not believe he can administer anesthesia if the DNR is in place.

DISCUSSION

- What are the rights of the patient with regard to advance directives?
- What can you do to advocate for the patient?
- Should you contact the ethics committee of the hospital?
- How do you contact the ethics committee?

Nursing Process

The Patient During Surgery

The Perioperative Nursing Data Set (PNDS) is a helpful model used by nurses in the intraoperative phase of care (see Fig. 18-1 in Chapter 18). Phenomena of concern to intraoperative nurses are nursing diagnoses, interventions, and outcomes that surgical patients and their families experience. Additional areas of concern include collaborative problems and expected goals.

Assessment

Nursing assessment of the intraoperative patient involves obtaining data from the patient and the patient's record to identify variables that can affect care and serve as guidelines for developing an individualized plan of patient care. The intraoperative nurse uses the focused preoperative nursing assessment documented on the patient record. This includes assessment of physiologic status (eg, health–illness level, level of consciousness), psychosocial status (eg, anxiety level, verbal communication problems, coping mechanisms), physical status (eg, surgical site, skin condition, and effectiveness of preparation; immobile joints), and ethical concerns (Chart 19-3).

Diagnosis

Nursing Diagnoses

Based on the assessment data, some major nursing diagnoses may include the following:

- Anxiety related to expressed concerns due to surgery or OR environment
- Risk for perioperative positioning injury related to positioning in the OR
- Risk for injury related to anesthesia and surgery
- Disturbed sensory perception (global) related to general anesthesia or sedation

Collaborative Problems/ Potential Complications

Based on the assessment data, potential complications may include the following:

- Nausea and vomiting
- Anaphylaxis
- Hypoxia
- Unintentional hypothermia
- Malignant hyperthermia
- DIC
- Infection

Planning and Goals

Goals for care of the patient during surgery include reducing anxiety, preventing positioning injuries, maintaining safety, maintaining the patient's dignity, and avoiding complications.

Nursing Interventions

Reducing Anxiety

The OR environment can seem cold, stark, and frightening to the patient, who may be feeling isolated and apprehensive. Introducing yourself, addressing the patient by name warmly and frequently, verifying details, providing explanations, and encouraging and answering questions provide a sense of professionalism and friendliness that can help the patient feel secure. When discussing what the patient can expect in surgery, the nurse uses basic communication skills, such as touch and eye contact, to reduce anxiety.

Attention to physical comfort (warm blankets, position changes) helps the patient feel more comfortable. Telling the patient who else will be present in the OR, how long the procedure is expected to take, and other details helps the patient prepare for the experience and gain a sense of control.

Preventing Intraoperative Positioning Injury

The patient's position on the operating table depends on the surgical procedure to be performed as well as on the patient's physical condition (Fig. 19-3). The potential for transient discomfort or permanent injury is present, because many positions are awkward. Hyperextending joints, compressing arteries, or pressing on nerves and bony prominences usually results in discomfort simply because the position must be sustained for a long period of time (Rothrock, 2003). Factors to consider include the following:

- The patient should be in as comfortable a position as possible, whether conscious or unconscious.
- The operative field must be adequately exposed.
- An awkward position, undue pressure on a body part, or use of stirrups or traction should not obstruct the vascular supply.
- Respiration should not be impeded by pressure of arms on the chest or by a gown that constricts the neck or chest.
- Nerves must be protected from undue pressure. Improper positioning of the arms, hands, legs, or feet can cause serious injury or paralysis. Shoulder braces must be well padded to prevent irreparable nerve injury, especially when the Trendelenburg position is necessary.
- Precautions for patient safety must be observed, particularly with thin, elderly, or obese patients and those with a physical deformity.
- The patient may need light restraint before induction in case of excitement.

The usual position for surgery, called the dorsal recumbent position, is flat on the back. One arm is positioned at the side of the table, with the hand placed palm down; the other is carefully positioned on an

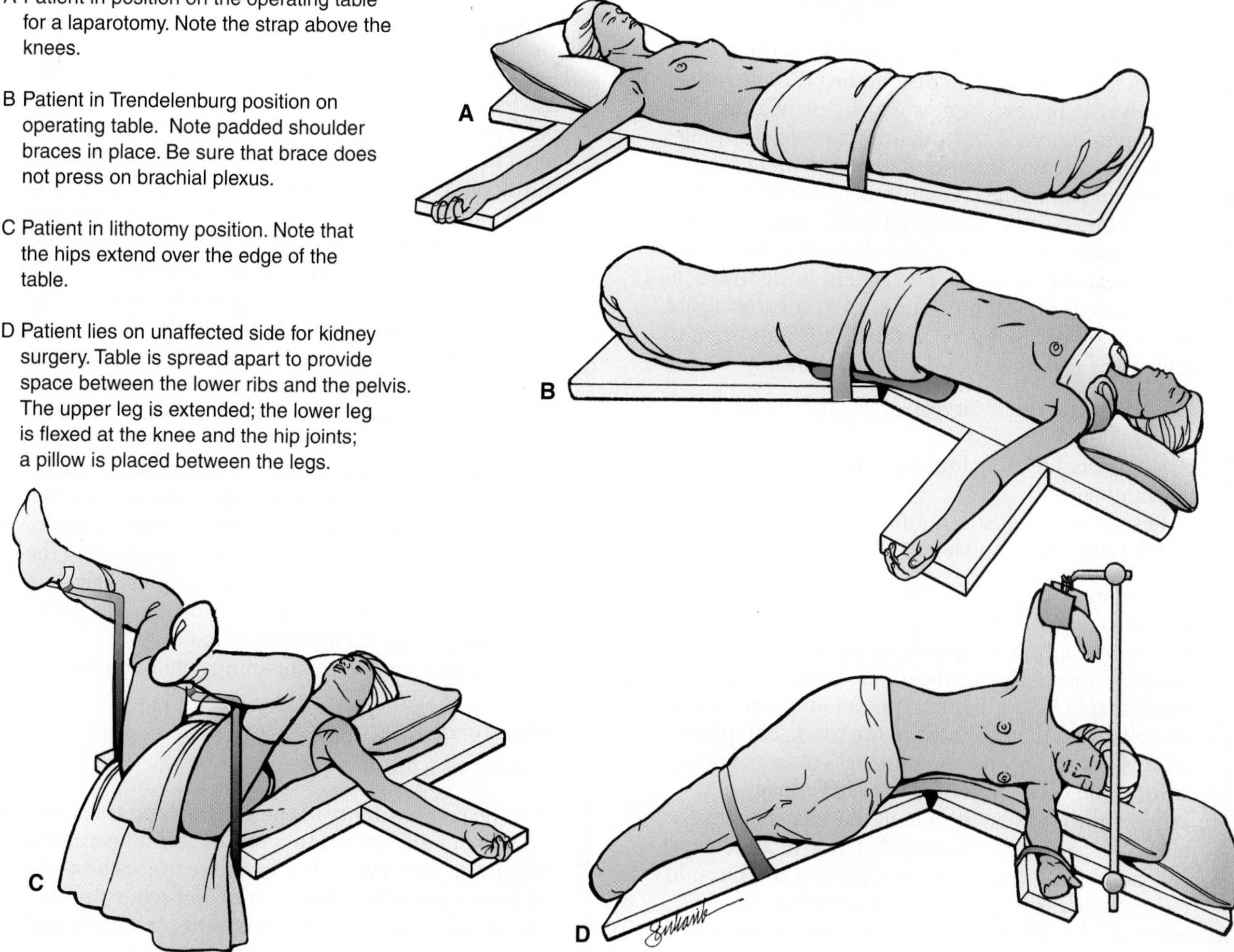

A Patient in position on the operating table for a laparotomy. Note the strap above the knees.
B Patient in Trendelenburg position on operating table. Note padded shoulder braces in place. Be sure that brace does not press on brachial plexus.
C Patient in lithotomy position. Note that the hips extend over the edge of the table.
D Patient lies on unaffected side for kidney surgery. Table is spread apart to provide space between the lower ribs and the pelvis. The upper leg is extended; the lower leg is flexed at the knee and the hip joints; a pillow is placed between the legs.
A
B
C
D

FIGURE 19-3. Positions on the operating table. Captions call attention to safety and comfort features. All surgical patients wear caps to cover the hair completely.

armboard to facilitate IV infusion of fluids, blood, or medications. This position is used for most abdominal surgeries except for surgery of the gallbladder or pelvis (see Fig. 19-3A).

The Trendelenburg position usually is used for surgery on the lower abdomen and pelvis to obtain good exposure by displacing the intestines into the upper abdomen. In this position, the head and body are lowered. The patient is held in position by padded shoulder braces (see Fig. 19-3B).

The lithotomy position is used for nearly all perineal, rectal, and vaginal surgical procedures (see Fig. 19-3C). The patient is positioned on the back with the legs and thighs flexed. The position is maintained by placing the feet in stirrups.

The Sims' or lateral position is used for renal surgery. The patient is placed on the nonoperative side with an air pillow 12.5 to 15 cm (5 to 6 inches) thick under the loin, or on a table with a kidney or back lift (see Fig. 19-3D).

Other procedures, such as neurosurgery or abdominothoracic surgery, may require unique positioning and supplemental apparatus, depending on the operative approach (Bohan & Glass-Macenka, 2004).

Protecting the Patient From Injury

A variety of activities are used to address the diverse patient safety issues that arise in the OR. The nurse protects the patient from injury by providing a safe environment. Verifying information, checking the chart for completeness, and maintaining surgical asepsis and an optimal environment are critical nursing responsibilities. Verifying that all required documentation is completed is one of the first functions of the intraoperative nurse. The patient is identified, and the planned surgical procedure, correct surgical site, and type of anesthesia are verified. It is important to review the patient's record for the following:

- Correct informed surgical consent, with patient's signature
- Completed records for health history and physical examination
- Results of diagnostic studies
- Allergies (including latex)

In addition to checking that all necessary patient data are complete, the perioperative nurse obtains the necessary equipment specific to the procedure. The need for nonroutine medications, blood components, instruments, and other equipment and supplies is assessed, and the readiness of the room, completeness of physical setup, and completeness of instrument, suture, and dressing setups are determined. Any aspects of the OR environment that may negatively affect the patient are identified. These include physical features, such as room temperature and humidity; electrical hazards; potential contaminants (dust, blood, and discharge on floor or surfaces, uncovered hair, faulty attire of personnel, jewelry worn by personnel); and unnecessary traffic. The circulating nurse also sets up and maintains suction equipment in working order, sets up invasive monitoring equipment, assists with insertion of vascular access and monitoring devices (arterial, Swan-Ganz, central venous pressure, IV lines), and initiates appropriate physical comfort measures for the patient.

Preventing physical injury includes using safety straps and side rails and not leaving the sedated patient unattended. Transferring the patient from the stretcher to the OR table requires safe transferring practices. Other safety measures include properly positioning the grounding pad under the patient to prevent electrical burns and shock, removing excess antiseptic solution from the patient's skin, and promptly and completely draping exposed areas after the sterile field has been created to decrease the risk for hypothermia.

Nursing measures to prevent injury from excessive blood loss include blood conservation using equipment such as a cell-saver (a device for recirculating the patient's own blood cells) and administration of blood products (Phillips, 2004). Few patients undergoing an elective procedure require blood transfusion, but those undergoing higher-risk procedures (such as orthopedic or cardiac surgeries) may require an intraoperative transfusion. The circulating nurse anticipates this need, checks that blood has been cross-matched and held in reserve, and is prepared to administer blood.

Serving as Patient Advocate

Because the patient undergoing general anesthesia or moderate sedation experiences temporary sensory/perceptual alteration or loss, he or she has an increased need for protection and advocacy. Patient advocacy in the OR entails maintaining the patient's physical and emotional comfort, privacy, rights, and dignity. Patients, whether conscious or unconscious, should not be subjected to excess noise, inappropriate conversation, or, most of all, derogatory comments. As surprising as this sounds, banter in the OR occasionally includes jokes about the patient's physical appearance, job, personal history, and so forth. Cases have been reported in which seemingly deeply anesthetized patients recalled the entire surgical experience, including disparaging personal remarks made by OR personnel. As an advocate, the nurse never engages in this conversation and discourages others from doing so. Other advocacy activities include minimizing the clinical, dehumanizing aspects of being a surgical patient by making sure the patient is treated as a person, respecting cultural and spiritual values, providing physical privacy, and maintaining confidentiality.

Monitoring and Managing Potential Complications

It is the responsibility of the surgeon and the anesthesiologist or anesthetist to monitor and manage complications. However, intraoperative nurses also play an important role. Being alert to and reporting changes in vital signs and symptoms of nausea and vomiting, anaphylaxis, hypoxia, hypothermia, malignant hyperthermia, or DIC and assisting with their management are important nursing functions. Each of these complications was discussed earlier. Maintaining asepsis and preventing infection are responsibilities of all members of the surgical team (Phillips, 2004; Rothrock, 2003).

Evaluation

Expected Patient Outcomes

Expected patient outcomes may include the following:

1. Exhibits low level of anxiety while awake during the intraoperative phase of care
2. Remains free of perioperative positioning injury
3. Experiences no unexpected threats to safety
4. Has dignity preserved throughout OR experience
5. Is free of complications (nausea and vomiting, anaphylaxis, hypoxia, hypothermia, malignant hyperthermia, or DIC) or experiences successful management of adverse effects of surgery and anesthesia should they occur.

Critical Thinking Exercises

1 An 80-year-old patient with Parkinson's disease is scheduled for surgery to replace a fractured hip. Identify the considerations and associated responsibilities of the OR nurse for safe intraoperative care of this patient.

2 ebp A patient has a large open lower-extremity wound caused by a motorcycle accident and is undergoing emergency surgery. What resources would you use to identify the current guidelines for surgical asepsis? What is the evidence base for current patient and environmental surgical asepsis practices? Identify the criteria used to evaluate the strength of the evidence for these practices.

3 A patient develops a temperature of 38°C (100°F) and becomes tachycardic halfway through an abdominal surgery. Five minutes later, the patient's temperature is 42°C (104°F). Describe the protocol you would follow and the medication you would administer for this condition.

4 ebp A patient with an infected wound is undergoing an incision and drainage in the OR. Develop an evidence-based plan of care that will reduce the risk of contamination and infection.

REFERENCES AND SELECTED READINGS

BOOKS

American Society of Anesthesiologists. (2004). *Distinguishing monitored anesthesia care ("MAC") from moderate sedation/analgesia (conscious sedation.)* http://www.asahq.org/publicationsAndServices/standards/35.pdf (accessed May 30, 2006).

American Society of PeriAnesthesia Nurses. (2002). *Standards of perianesthesia nursing practice.* Thorofare, NJ: ASPAN.

AORN standards, recommended practice, and guidelines (2004b). Denver: AORN, Inc.

Clancy, J., McVicar, A. J. & Baird, N. (2002). *Perioperative practice: Fundamentals of homeostasis.* New York: Routledge.

Conner, R. (2004). *Ambulatory surgery principles and practices* (3rd ed.). Denver: AORN, Inc.

Defazio-Quinn, D. & Schick, L. (Eds). (2004). *Nursing core curriculum-preoperative, phase I and phase II PACU nursing.* Philadelphia: W. B. Saunders.

Joint Commission on Accreditation of Healthcare Organizations (JCAHO). (2004). Sentinel alert: Patient alert under anesthesia. http://www.jcaho.org (accessed March 31, 2006).

Kleinbeck, S. V. M. (2004). *Perioperative nursing data set at work: Policies, procedures and pathways.* Denver: AORN, Inc.

Miller, R. D. (2005). *Miller's anesthesia* (6th ed.). Philadelphia: Elsevier.

Morton, P. G., Fontaine, D. K., Hudak, C. M., et al. (2005). *Critical care nursing: A holistic approach* (8th ed.). Philadelphia: Lippincott Williams & Wilkins.

Murray, M. J., Coursin, D. B., Pearl, R. G., et al. (2002). *Critical care medicine: Perioperative management* (2nd ed.). Philadelphia: Lippincott Williams & Wilkins.

NANDA International. (2005). NANDA: Nursing diagnoses: Definitions and classification. Philadelphia: NANDA International.

Phillips, N. (2004). *Berry and Kohn's operating room technique* (10th ed.). St. Louis: Mosby.

Rothrock, J. C. (Ed.). (2003). *Alexander's care of the patient in surgery* (12th ed.). St. Louis: Mosby.

Seifert, P. C. (2002). *Cardiac surgery: Perioperative patient care.* St Louis: Mosby.

Surgical Care Improvement Project (SCIP). (2005). Available at: http://www.medqic.org/scip/scip–contact.html. Accessed May 7, 2006.

Tighe, S. M. (2003). *Instrumentation for the operating room: A photographic manual.* St. Louis: Mosby.

JOURNALS

**Asterisks indicate nursing research articles.*

Andersen, K. (2004). Safe use of lasers in the operating room, *AORN Journal, 79*(1), 171–188.

AORN. (2004a). AORN latex guideline. *AORN Journal, 79*(3), 653–672.

Beyea, S. (2003). Keeping patients safe from infection. *AORN Journal, 78*(1), 133–140.

Bohan, E. & Glass-Macenka, D. (2004). Surgical management of patients with primary brain tumors. *Seminars in Oncology Nursing, 29*(4), 240–252.

DeFazio-Quinn, D. M. (2006). How religion, language and ethnicity impact perioperative nursing care. *Nursing Clinics of North America, 41*(2), 231–248.

Gawande, A. A., Studdert, D. M., Orav, E. J., et al. (2003). Risk for retained instruments and sponges after surgery. *New England Journal of Medicine, 348*(3), 229–235.

Gotta, A. W. (2004). Anesthetic management of the patient with HIV infection. *Current Reviews for Nurse Anesthetists, 27*(11), 117–128.

Gupta, A., Della-Latta, P., Todd, B., et al. (2004) Outbreak of extended-spectrum beta-lactamase-producing *Klebsiella pneumoniae* in a neonatal intensive care unit linked to artificial nails. *Infection Control and Hospital Epidemiology, 25*(3), 210–215.

*Hammarsten, R., Hammarsten, J. & Jemsby, P. (2003). Preoperative skin testing of materials used in surgical procedures. *AORN Journal, 77*(4), 762–771.

Houck, P. M. (2006). Comparison of operating room lasers: Uses, hazards, guidelines. *Nursing Clinics of North America, 41*(2), 193–218.

John, A. D. & Sieber, F. E. (2004). Age associated issues: Geriatrics. *Anesthesiology Clinic of North America, 22*(1), 45–58.

Joint Commission on Accreditation of Healthcare Organizations (JCAHO). (2005). JCAHO issues 2005 patient safety goals. *OR Manager, 20*(9), 5–8.

Litman, R. S. & Rosenberg H. (2005). Malignant hyperthermia: Update on susceptibility testing. *Journal of American Medical Association, 293*(23), 2918–2924.

McCarthy, E. (2004). Malignant hyperthermia. *AACN Clinical Issues, 15*(2), 231–237.

O'Connell, M. P. (2006). Positioning impact on the surgical patient. *Nursing Clinics of North America, 41*(2), 173–192.

Owens, T. M (2006). Bariatric surgery risks, benefits, and care of the morbidly obese. *Nursing Clinics of North America, 41*(2), 249–263.

Paulson, D. (2004). Hand scrub products-performance requirements. *AORN Journal, 80*(2), 225–234.

Pine, M., Holt, K. D. & Lou, Y. (2003). Surgical mortality and type of anesthesia provider. *AANA Journal, 71*(2), 109–116.

Pofahl, W. & Pories, W. (2003). Current status and future directions of geriatric general surgery. *Journal of American Geriatric Society, 51*(7), S351–S354.

Pryor, K. O., Fahey, T. J., Lien, C. A., et al. (2004). Surgical site infection and the routine use of perioperative hyperoxia in a general surgical population: A randomized controlled trial. *Journal of American Medical Association, 291*(1), 79–87.

Salmon, L. (2004). Fire in the OR: Prevention and preparedness. *AORN Journal, 80*(1), 41–54.

Saufl, N. M. (2004). Preparing the older adult for surgery and anesthesia. *Journal of PeriAnesthesia Nursing, 19*(6), 372–377.

Wadlund, D. L. (2006). Prevention, recognition, and management of nursing complications in the intraoperative and postoperative surgical patient. *Nursing Clinics of North America, 41*(2), 151–171.

Wadlund, D. L. (2006). Laparoscopy: Risks, benefits and complications. *Nursing Clinics of North America, 41*(2), 219–229.

Williams, J. & Barbul, A. (2003). Nutrition and wound healing. *Surgical Clinics of America, 83*(3), 571–596.

*Yellen, E. (2003). The influence of nurse-sensitive variables. *AORN Journal, 78*(5), 783–793.

RESOURCES

American Latex Allergy Association; toll-free 888-972-5378; fax 262-677-2808; http://www.latexallergyresources.org. Accessed March 31, 2006.

American Society of Anesthesiologists, 520 N. Northwest Highway, Park Ridge, IL, 60068; 847-825-2286; http://www.asahq.org. Accessed March 31, 2006.

American Society of PeriAnesthesia Nurses, 10 Melrose Ave., Suite 110, Cherry Hill, NJ 08003; toll-free 877-9696; fax 856-616-9621; http://www.aspan.org. Accessed March 31, 2006.

Association of PeriOperative Registered Nurses, Inc., 2170 S. Parker Rd., Suite 300, Denver, CO 80231; 800-755-2676; http://www.aorn.org. Accessed March 31, 2006.

Centers for Disease Control and Prevention, National Center for Injury Prevention and Control, Mailstop K65, 4770 Buford Highway NE, Atlanta, GA 30341; 770-488-1506; http://www.cdc.gov/nipc/. Accessed March 31, 2006.

Joint Commission on Accreditation Healthcare Organizations (JCAHO), 1 Renaissance Blvd., Oakbrook Terrace, IL; 877-223-6866; http://www.jcaho.org. Accessed March 31, 2006.

Malignant Hyperthermia Association of the United States (MHAUS), 39 East State Street, P.O. Box 1069, Sherburne, NY 13460; 607-674-7901; http://www.mhaus.org. Accessed March 31, 2006.

National SCIP Partnership, Oklahoma Foundation for Medical Quality, 14000 Quail Springs Parkway, Suite 400, Oklahoma City, OK 73134; 405-840-2891 ext. 278; http://www.medqic.org/scip. Accessed May 7, 2006.

CHAPTER 20

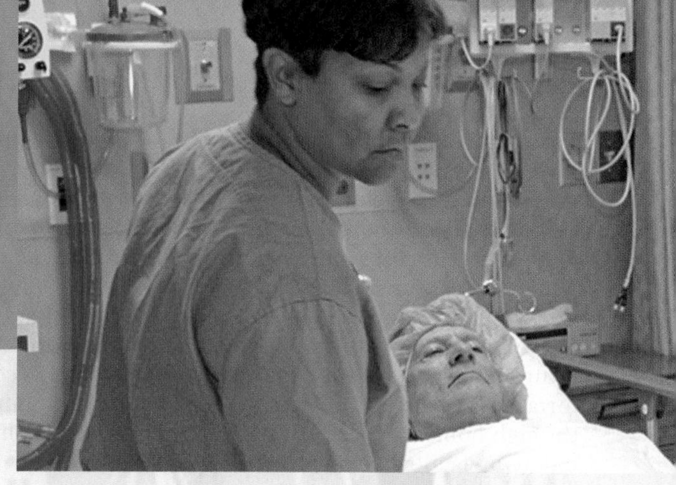

Postoperative Nursing Management

Learning Objectives

On completion of this chapter, the learner will be able to:

1. Describe the responsibilities of the postanesthesia care unit nurse in the prevention of immediate postoperative complications.
2. Compare postoperative care of the ambulatory surgery patient with that of the hospitalized surgery patient.
3. Identify common postoperative problems and their management.
4. Describe the gerontologic considerations related to postoperative management.
5. Describe variables that affect wound healing.
6. Demonstrate postoperative dressing techniques.
7. Identify assessment parameters appropriate for the early detection of postoperative complications.

The postoperative period extends from the time the patient leaves the operating room (OR) until the last follow-up visit with the surgeon. This may be as short as 1 week or as long as several months. During the postoperative period, nursing care focuses on reestablishing the patient's physiologic equilibrium, alleviating pain, preventing complications, and teaching the patient self-care. Careful assessment and immediate intervention assist the patient in returning to optimal function quickly, safely, and as comfortably as possible. Ongoing care in the community through home care, clinic visits, office visits, or telephone follow-up facilitates an uncomplicated recovery.

The Postanesthesia Care Unit

The **postanesthesia care unit (PACU)**, also called the recovery room or postanesthesia recovery room, is located adjacent to the operating rooms suite (Phillips, 2004). Patients still under anesthesia or recovering from anesthesia are placed in this unit for easy access to experienced, highly skilled nurses, anesthesiologists or anesthetists, surgeons, advanced hemodynamic and pulmonary monitoring and support, special equipment, and medications.

The PACU is kept quiet, clean, and free of unnecessary equipment. This area is painted in soft, pleasing colors and has indirect lighting. The PACU should also be well ventilated. These features benefit the patient by helping to decrease anxiety and promote comfort. The PACU bed provides easy access to the patient, is safe and easily movable, can readily be positioned to facilitate use of measures to counteract shock and other complications, and has features that facilitate care, such as intravenous (IV) poles, side rails and wheel brakes.

Phases of Postanesthesia Care

Postanesthesia care in some hospitals and ambulatory surgical centers is divided into three phases (Phillips, 2004). In the **phase I PACU**, used during the immediate recovery phase, intensive nursing care is provided. In the **phase II PACU**, the patient is prepared for self-care or care in the hospital or an extended care setting. In **phase III PACU**, the patient is prepared for discharge. Recliners rather than stretchers or beds are standard in many phase III units, which may also be referred to as step-down, sit-up, or progressive care units. Patients may remain in a PACU unit for as long as 4 to 6 hours, depending on the type of surgery and any preexisting conditions. In facilities without separate phase I, II, and III units, the patient remains in the PACU and may be discharged home directly from this unit.

All PACU nurses have special skills, including strong assessment skills. The PACU nurse provides frequent (every 15 minutes) monitoring of the patient's pulse, electrocardiogram, respiratory rate, blood pressure, and pulse oximeter value (blood oxygen level). In some cases, the end-tidal carbon dioxide ($ETCO_2$) level is monitored as well. The patient's airway may become obstructed because of the latent effects of recent anesthesia, and the PACU nurse must be prepared to assist in reintubation and in handling other emergencies that may occur. Nurses in the phase II and III PACUs must also possess excellent patient teaching skills.

Admitting the Patient to the PACU

Transferring the postoperative patient from the OR to the PACU is the responsibility of the anesthesiologist or anesthetist. During transport from the OR to the PACU, the anesthesia provider remains at the head of the stretcher (to maintain the airway), and a surgical team member remains at the opposite end. Transporting the patient involves special consideration of the incision site, potential vascular changes, and exposure. The surgical incision is considered every time the postoperative patient is moved; many wounds are closed under considerable tension, and every effort is made to prevent further strain on the incision. The patient is positioned so that he or she is not lying on and obstructing drains or drainage tubes. Serious orthostatic hypotension may occur when a patient is moved too quickly from one position to another (eg, from a lithotomy position to a horizontal position or from a lateral to a supine position), so the patient must be moved slowly and carefully. As soon as the patient is placed on the stretcher or bed, the soiled gown is removed and replaced with a dry gown. The patient

Glossary

dehiscence: partial or complete separation of wound edges

evisceration: protrusion of organs through the surgical incision

first-intention healing: method of healing in which wound edges are surgically approximated and integumentary continuity is restored without granulation

Phase I PACU: area designated for care of surgical patients immediately after surgery and for patients whose condition warrants close monitoring

Phase II PACU: area designated for care of surgical patients who have been transferred from a phase I PACU because their condition no longer requires the close monitoring provided in a phase I PACU

Phase III PACU: setting in which the patient is cared for in the immediate postoperative period and then prepared for discharge from the facility

postanesthesia care unit (PACU): area where postoperative patients are monitored as they recover from anesthesia; formerly referred to as the recovery room or postanesthesia recovery room

second-intention healing: method of healing in which wound edges are not surgically approximated and integumentary continuity is restored by the process known as granulation

third-intention healing: method of healing in which surgical approximation of wound edges is delayed and integumentary continuity is restored by apposing areas of granulation

is covered with lightweight blankets and warmed. Three side rails may be raised to prevent falls.

The nurse who admits the patient to the PACU reviews essential information with the anesthesiologist or anesthetist (Chart 20-1) (Defazio-Quinn & Schick, 2004; Morton, Fontaine, Hudak, et al., 2005).

Nursing Management in the PACU

The nursing management objectives for the patient in the PACU are to provide care until the patient has recovered from the effects of anesthesia (eg, until resumption of motor and sensory functions), is oriented, has stable vital signs, and shows no evidence of hemorrhage or other complications.

Assessing the Patient

Frequent, skilled assessments of the blood oxygen saturation level, pulse rate and regularity, depth and nature of respirations, skin color, level of consciousness, and ability to respond to commands are the cornerstones of nursing care in the PACU. The nurse performs a baseline assessment, then checks the surgical site for drainage or hemorrhage and makes sure that all drainage tubes and monitoring lines are connected and functioning. The nurse checks any IV fluids or medications currently infusing and verifies dosage and rate.

After the initial assessment, the patient's vital signs and general physical status are assessed at least every 15 minutes (Defazio-Quinn & Schick, 2004). Patency of the airway and respiratory function are always evaluated first, followed by assessment of cardiovascular function, the condition of the surgical site, and function of the central nervous system. The nurse must be aware of any pertinent information from the patient's history that may be significant (eg, patient is deaf or hard of hearing, has a history of seizures, has diabetes, is allergic to certain medications or to latex).

CHART 20-1

Anesthesia Provider-to-Nurse Report: Information to Convey

- Name of patient
- Surgical procedure
- Anesthetic options (agents and reversal agents used)
- Estimated blood loss/fluid loss
- Fluid/blood replacement
- Vital signs—significant problems
- Complications encountered (anesthetic or surgical)
- Preoperative condition (eg, diabetes, hypertension, allergies)
- Considerations for immediate postoperative period (pain management, reversals, ventilator settings)
- Language barrier

Ideally, the anesthesia provider should not leave the patient until the nurse is satisfied with the patient's airway and immediate condition.

From Morton, P. G., Fontaine D. K., Hudak, C. M., et al. (2005). *Critical care nursing: A holistic approach* (8th ed.). Philadelphia: Lippincott Williams & Wilkins.

Maintaining a Patent Airway

The primary objective in the immediate postoperative period is to maintain pulmonary ventilation and thus prevent hypoxemia (reduced oxygen in the blood) and hypercapnia (excess carbon dioxide in the blood). Both can occur if the airway is obstructed and ventilation is reduced (hypoventilation). Besides checking the physician's orders for and administering supplemental oxygen, the nurse assesses respiratory rate and depth, ease of respirations, oxygen saturation, and breath sounds.

Patients who have experienced prolonged anesthesia usually are unconscious, with all muscles relaxed. This relaxation extends to the muscles of the pharynx. When the patient lies on his or her back, the lower jaw and the tongue fall backward and the air passages become obstructed (Fig. 20-1A). This is called hypopharyngeal obstruction. Signs of occlusion include choking; noisy and irregular respirations; decreased oxygen saturation scores; and within minutes, a blue, dusky color (cyanosis) of the skin. Because movement of the thorax and the diaphragm does not necessarily indicate that the patient is breathing, the nurse needs to place the palm of the hand at the patient's nose and mouth to feel the exhaled breath.

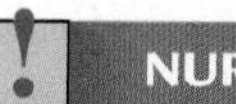

NURSING ALERT

The treatment of hypopharyngeal obstruction involves tilting the head back and pushing forward on the angle of the lower jaw, as if to push the lower teeth in front of the upper teeth (see Fig. 20-1B,C). This maneuver pulls the tongue forward and opens the air passages.

The anesthesiologist or anesthetist may leave a hard rubber or plastic airway in the patient's mouth (Fig. 20-2) to maintain a patent airway. Such a device should not be removed until signs such as gagging indicate that reflex action is returning. Alternatively, the patient may enter the PACU with an endotracheal tube still in place and may require continued mechanical ventilation. The nurse assists in initiating the use of the ventilator and in the weaning and extubation processes. Some patients, particularly those who have had extensive or lengthy surgical procedures, may be transferred from the OR directly to the intensive care unit (ICU) or from the PACU to the ICU while still intubated and receiving mechanical ventilation.

Respiratory difficulty can also result from excessive secretion of mucus or aspiration of vomitus. Turning the patient to one side allows the collected fluid to escape from the side of the mouth (Defazio-Quinn & Schick, 2004). If the teeth are clenched, the mouth may be opened manually but cautiously with a padded tongue depressor. The head of the bed is elevated 15 to 30 degrees unless contraindicated, and

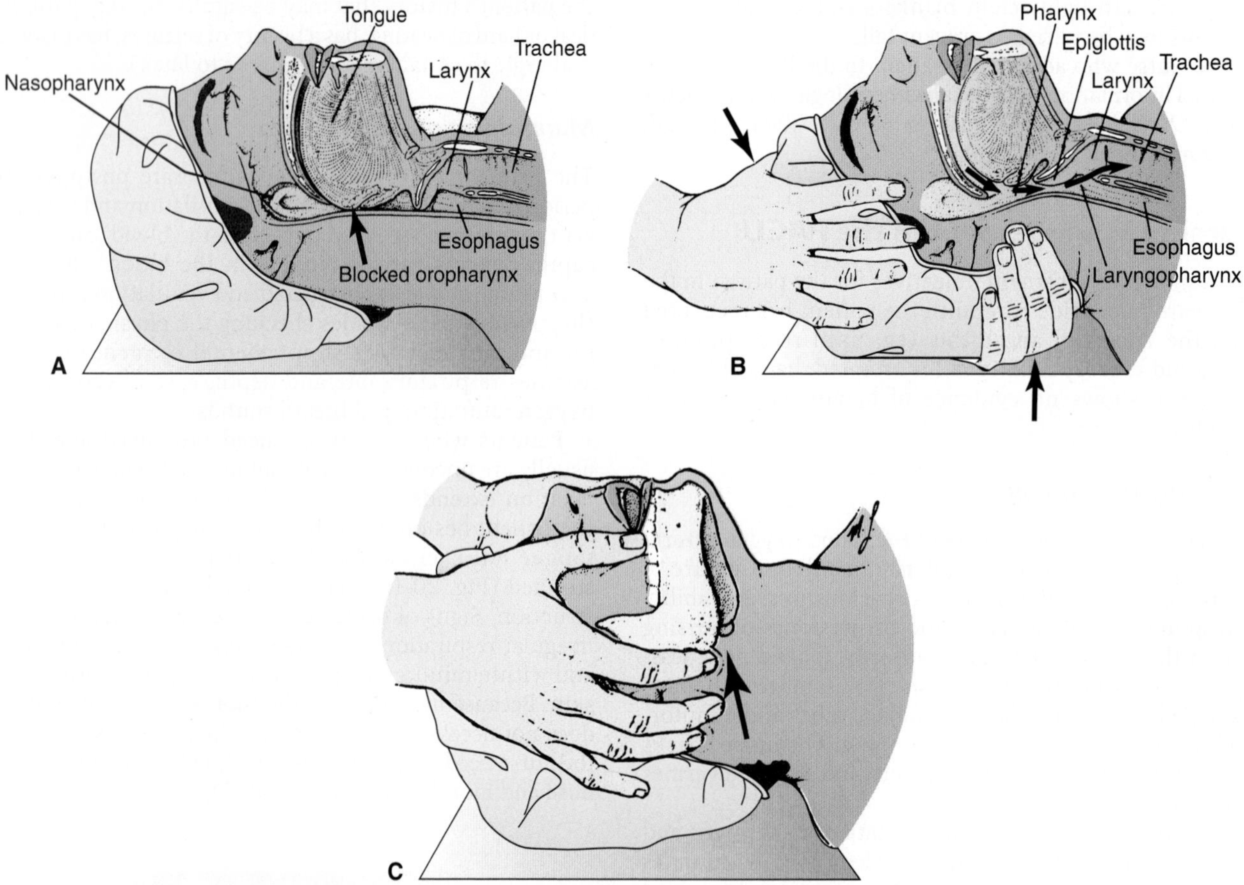

FIGURE 20-1. (**A**) A hypopharyngeal obstruction occurs when neck flexion permits the chin to drop toward the chest; obstruction almost always occurs when the head is in the midposition. (**B**) Tilting the head back to stretch the anterior neck structure lifts the base of the tongue off the posterior pharyngeal wall. The direction of the *arrows* indicates the pressure of the hands. (**C**) Opening the mouth is necessary to correct valvelike obstruction of the nasal passage during expiration, which occurs in about 30% of unconscious patients. Open the patient's mouth (separate lips and teeth) and move the lower jaw forward so that the lower teeth are in front of the upper teeth. To regain backward tilt of the neck, lift with both hands at the ascending rami of the mandible.

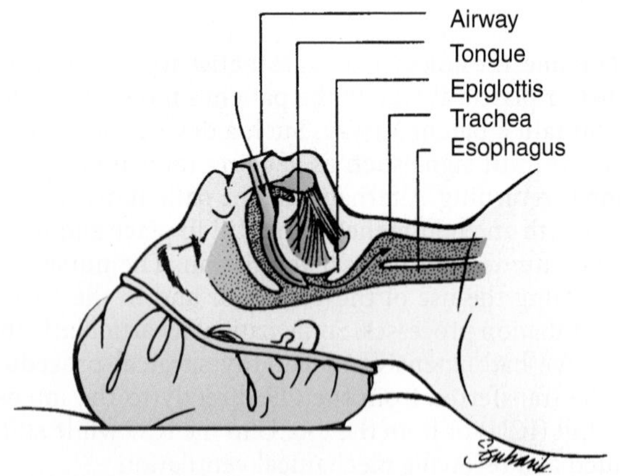

FIGURE 20-2. Use of an airway to maintain a patent airway after anesthesia. The airway passes over the base of the tongue and permits air to pass into the pharynx in the region of the epiglottis. Patients often leave the operating room with an airway in place. The airway should remain in place until the patient recovers sufficiently to breathe normally. As the patient regains consciousness, the airway usually causes irritation and should be removed.

the patient is closely monitored to maintain the airway as well as to minimize the risk of aspiration. If vomiting occurs, the patient is turned to the side to prevent aspiration and the vomitus is collected in the emesis basin. Mucus or vomitus obstructing the pharynx or the trachea is suctioned with a pharyngeal suction tip or a nasal catheter introduced into the nasopharynx or oropharynx. The catheter can be passed into the nasopharynx or oropharynx safely to a distance of 15 to 20 cm (6 to 8 inches). Caution is necessary in suctioning the throat of a patient who has had a tonsillectomy or other oral or laryngeal surgery because of risk of bleeding and discomfort.

Maintaining Cardiovascular Stability

To monitor cardiovascular stability, the nurse assesses the patient's mental status; vital signs; cardiac rhythm; skin temperature, color, and moisture; and urine output. Central venous pressure, pulmonary artery pressure, and arterial lines are monitored if the patient's condition requires such assessment. The nurse also assesses the patency of all IV

NURSING RESEARCH PROFILE

Risk Factors for Extended Mechanical Ventilation Following Surgery

Bezanson, J. L., Weaver, M., Kinney, M., et al. (2004). Presurgical risk factors for late extubation in Medicare recipients after cardiac surgery. *Nursing Research, 53*(1), 46–52.

Purpose

The number of Medicare recipients undergoing coronary artery bypass grafting surgery (CABG) is increasing. This study developed and validated a model using selected presurgical patient characteristics to assess the probability of prolonged mechanical ventilation after CABG in Medicare recipients.

Design

A retrospective nonexperimental design was used to study 548 Medicare recipients (all 65 years of age or older) who had undergone a CABG. An existing database for the year 1998 was used to assess risks for prolonged mechanical ventilation. 74% of the sample were male, 92% were Caucasian, and the mean age was 72.8 years (SD = 4.99). Logistic regression modeling was used to identify predictors of late extubation.

Findings

Based on the time of extubation, the sample was divided into two groups. Group 1, early extubation ($n = 205$), had a mechanical ventilation time of 5 hours or less. Group 2, late extubation ($n = 343$), had a mechanical ventilation time of more than 5 hours. Predictors of late extubation were found to include (1) age 80 years or older, (2) female gender (OR = 1.76, $P = .011$), (3) hypertension (OR = 1.60, $P = .18$), and (4) urgent or emergent preoperative clinical status (OR = 3.04, $P = .002$).

Nursing Implications

A better understanding of predictors of prolonged mechanical ventilation may provide information for nurses to optimize the preoperative health status of elderly patients. During preoperative assessments, nurses should note the presence of predictors of prolonged mechanical ventilation and communicate these to the intraoperative and postoperative health care providers.

lines. The primary cardiovascular complications seen in the PACU include hypotension and shock, hemorrhage, hypertension, and dysrhythmias.

HYPOTENSION AND SHOCK

Hypotension can result from blood loss, hypoventilation, position changes, pooling of blood in the extremities, or side effects of medications and anesthetics. The most common cause is loss of circulating volume through blood and plasma loss. If the amount of blood loss exceeds 500 mL (especially if the loss is rapid), replacement is usually indicated.

Shock, one of the most serious postoperative complications, can result from hypovolemia and decreased intravascular volume. The types of shock are classified as hypovolemic, cardiogenic, neurogenic, anaphylactic, and septic shock. The classic signs of hypovolemic shock (the most common type of shock) are

- Pallor
- Cool, moist skin
- Rapid breathing
- Cyanosis of the lips, gums, and tongue
- Rapid, weak, thready pulse
- Narrowing pulse pressure
- Low blood pressure
- Concentrated urine

See Chapter 15 for a detailed discussion of shock.

Hypovolemic shock can be avoided largely by the timely administration of IV fluids, blood, blood products, and medications that elevate blood pressure. Volume replacement is the primary intervention for shock (Defazio-Quinn & Schick, 2004). An infusion of lactated Ringer's solution, 0.9% sodium chloride solution, colloids, or blood component therapy is initiated (see Table 15-2 in Chapter 15). Oxygen is administered by nasal cannula, face mask, or mechanical ventilation. If fluid administration fails to reverse hypovolemic shock, then various cardiac, vasodilator, and corticosteroid medications may be prescribed to improve cardiac function and reduce peripheral vascular resistance. The patient is placed flat in bed with the legs elevated. Respiratory rate, pulse rate, blood pressure, blood oxygen concentration, urinary output, level of consciousness, central venous pressure, pulmonary artery pressure, pulmonary capillary wedge pressure, and cardiac output are monitored to provide information on the patient's respiratory and cardiovascular status. Vital signs are monitored continuously until the patient's condition has stabilized.

Other factors can contribute to hemodynamic instability, and the PACU nurse implements multiple measures to manage these factors. Pain is controlled by making the patient as comfortable as possible and by using opioids judiciously. The patient is kept warm while avoiding overheating to prevent cutaneous vessels from dilating and depriving vital organs of blood. Exposure is avoided, and normothermia is maintained to prevent vasodilation.

HEMORRHAGE

Hemorrhage is an uncommon yet serious complication of surgery that can result in death. It can present insidiously or emergently at any time in the immediate postoperative period or up to several days after surgery (Table 20-1). When blood loss is extreme, the patient is apprehensive, restless,

TABLE 20-1 Classifications of Hemorrhage

Classification	Defining Characteristic
Time Frame	
Primary	Hemorrhage occurs at the time of surgery.
Intermediary	Hemorrhage occurs during the first few hours after surgery when the rise of blood pressure to its normal level dislodges insecure clots from untied vessels.
Secondary	Hemorrhage may occur some time after surgery if a suture slips because a blood vessel was not securely tied, became infected, or was eroded by a drainage tube.
Type of Vessel	
Capillary	Hemorrhage is characterized by a slow, general ooze.
Venous	Darkly colored blood bubbles out quickly.
Arterial	Blood is bright red and appears in spurts with each heartbeat.
Visibility	
Evident	Hemorrhage is on the surface and can be seen.
Concealed	Hemorrhage is in a body cavity and cannot be seen.

and thirsty; the skin is cold, moist, and pale. The pulse rate increases, the temperature falls, and respirations are rapid and deep, often of the gasping type spoken of as "air hunger." If hemorrhage progresses untreated, cardiac output decreases, arterial and venous blood pressure and hemoglobin level fall rapidly, the lips and the conjunctivae become pale, spots appear before the eyes, a ringing is heard in the ears, and the patient grows weaker but remains conscious until near death (Defazio-Quinn & Schick, 2004).

Transfusing blood or blood products and determining the cause of hemorrhage are the initial therapeutic measures. The surgical site and incision should always be inspected for bleeding. If bleeding is evident, a sterile gauze pad and a pressure dressing are applied, and the site of the bleeding is elevated to heart level if possible. The patient is placed in the shock position (flat on back; legs elevated at a 20-degree angle; knees kept straight). If hemorrhage is suspected but cannot be visualized, the patient may be taken back to the OR for emergency exploration of the surgical site.

If hemorrhage is suspected, the nurse should be aware of any special considerations related to blood loss replacement. Certain patients may decline blood transfusions for religious or cultural reasons and may identify this request on their advance directives or living will.

HYPERTENSION AND DYSRHYTHMIAS

Hypertension is common in the immediate postoperative period secondary to sympathetic nervous system stimulation from pain, hypoxia, or bladder distention. Dysrhythmias are associated with electrolyte imbalance, altered respiratory function, pain, hypothermia, stress, and anesthetic agents. Both hypertension and dysrhythmias are managed by treating the underlying causes.

Relieving Pain and Anxiety

Opioid analgesics are administered judiciously and often by IV in the PACU (Rothrock, 2003). IV opioids provide immediate pain relief and are short-acting, thus minimizing the potential for drug interactions or prolonged respiratory depression while anesthetics are still active in the patient's system. The PACU nurse monitors the patient's physiologic status, manages pain, and provides psychological support in an effort to relive the patient's fears and concerns. The nurse checks the medical record for special needs and concerns of the patient. When the patient's condition permits, a close member of the family may visit in the PACU for a few moments. This often decreases the family's anxiety and makes the patient feel more secure.

Controlling Nausea and Vomiting

Nausea and vomiting are common issues in the PACU. The nurse should intervene at the patient's first report of nausea to control the problem rather than wait for it to progress to vomiting.

Many medications are available to control nausea and vomiting without oversedating the patient; they are commonly administered during surgery as well as in the PACU. Medications such as metoclopramide (Reglan), prochlorperazine (Compazine), promethazine (Phenergan), dimenhydrinate (Dramamine), hydroxyzine (Vistaril, Atarax) and scopolamine (Transderm-Scop) are commonly prescribed (Rothrock, 2003). Although it is costly, ondansetron (Zofran) is frequently used as an effective antiemetic with few side effects.

A panel of anesthesiologists has reviewed the literature and developed guidelines for the treatment of postoperative nausea and vomiting (PONV). The panel concluded that it was important to evaluate the patient's level of risk for PONV. Based on the risk level, the panel recommended a range of treatments, from no prophylactic antiemetics (for low-risk patients) to double and triple antiemetic combinations for patients at high risk for PONV. The panel identified high-risk patients as females, nonsmokers, those with a history of PONV or motion sickness, and patients undergoing surgical procedures lasting longer than 2 hours (Gan, Meyer, Apfel, et al., 2003).

NURSING ALERT

At the slightest indication of nausea, the patient is turned completely to one side to promote mouth drainage and prevent aspiration of vomitus, which can cause asphyxiation and death.

Gerontologic Considerations

The elderly patient, like all other patients, is transferred from the OR table to the bed or stretcher slowly and gently. The effects of this action on blood pressure and ventilation are monitored. Special attention is given to keeping the patient warm, because elderly patients are more susceptible to hypothermia. The patient's position is changed frequently to stimulate respirations and to promote circulation and comfort.

Immediate postoperative care for the elderly patient is the same as for any surgical patient, but additional support is given if cardiovascular, pulmonary, or renal function is impaired. With careful monitoring, it is possible to detect cardiopulmonary deficits before signs and symptoms are apparent. The elderly patient has less physiologic reserve, and physiologic responses to stress are diminished or slowed. These changes reinforce the need for close monitoring and prompt treatment of hypotension, shock, and hemorrhage. Because of monitoring and improved individualized preoperative preparation, many older adults tolerate surgery well and have an uneventful recovery. Treating postoperative pain in the elderly patient requires an understanding of the normal changes associated with aging and the impact of aging on metabolism of medications (Barnett, 2003).

Postoperative confusion and delirium affect as many as 51% of older patients (Cofer, 2005; Saufl, 2004). Acute confusion may be caused by pain, analgesic agents, hypotension, fever, hypoglycemia, fluid loss, fecal impaction, urinary retention, or anemia (Cofer, 2005). Providing adequate hydration; reorienting the patient to the environment; and reassessing the doses of sedatives, anesthetics, and analgesics may reduce the risk for confusion. Hypoxia can present as confusion and restlessness, as can blood loss and electrolyte imbalances. Exclusion of all other causes of confusion must precede the assumption that confusion is related to age, circumstances, and medications.

Determining Readiness for Discharge from the PACU

A patient remains in the PACU until fully recovered from the anesthetic agent. Indicators of recovery include stable blood pressure, adequate respiratory function, adequate oxygen saturation level compared with baseline, and spontaneous movement or movement on command. Ordinarily, the following measures are used to determine the patient's readiness for discharge from the PACU (Defazio-Quinn & Schick, 2004):

- Stable vital signs
- Orientation to person, place, events, and time
- Uncompromised pulmonary function
- Pulse oximetry readings indicating adequate blood oxygen saturation
- Urine output at least 30 mL/hour
- Nausea and vomiting absent or under control
- Minimal pain

Many hospitals use a scoring system (eg, Aldrete score) to determine the patient's general condition and readiness for transfer from the PACU. Throughout the recovery period, the patient's physical signs are observed and evaluated by means of a scoring system based on a set of objective criteria (Aldrete & Wright, 1992). This evaluation guide allows an objective assessment of the patient's condition in the PACU (Fig. 20-3). The patient is assessed at regular intervals (eg, every 15 minutes), and a total score is calculated and recorded on the assessment record. Patients with a score of less than 7 must remain in the PACU until their condition improves or be transferred to an intensive care area, depending on their preoperative baseline score.

The patient is discharged from the phase I PACU by the anesthesiologist or anesthetist to the critical care unit, the medical-surgical unit, the phase II PACU, or home with a responsible family member. In some hospitals and ambulatory care centers, patients are discharged to a phase III PACU, where they are prepared for discharge.

Preparing the Postoperative Patient for Direct Discharge

Because approximately 60% of elective surgeries are now performed in ambulatory or outpatient settings, the majority of patients are discharged directly home from the PACU (Conner, 2004). Patients being discharged directly to home require verbal and written instructions and information about follow-up care.

Promoting Home and Community-Based Care

To ensure patient safety and recovery, expert patient teaching and discharge planning are necessary when a patient undergoes same-day or ambulatory surgery. Because anesthetics cloud memory for concurrent events, verbal and written instructions should be given to both the patient and the adult who will be accompanying the patient home. Alternative formats (eg, large print, Braille) of instructions or use of a sign interpreter may be required to ensure patient and family understanding. A translator may be required if the patient and family members do not understand English.

TEACHING PATIENTS SELF-CARE

The patient and caregiver (eg, family member or friend) are informed about expected outcomes and immediate postoperative changes anticipated. Written instructions about wound care, activity and dietary recommendations, medications, and follow-up visits to the same-day surgery unit or the surgeon are provided. Written instructions (designed to be copied and given to patients) about postoperative care after many types of surgery are usually provided. The patient's caregiver at home is provided with verbal and written instructions about what to look for and about the actions to take if complications occur. Prescriptions are given to the patient. The nurse's or surgeon's telephone number is provided, and the patient and caregiver are encouraged to call with questions and to schedule follow-up appointments (Chart 20-2).

Although recovery time varies depending on the type and extent of surgery and the patient's overall condition, instructions usually advise limited activity for 24 to 48 hours. During this time, the patient should not drive a vehicle, drink alcoholic beverages, or perform tasks that require energy or skill. Fluids may be consumed as desired, and smaller-than-normal amounts may be eaten at mealtime. Patients are cautioned not to make important decisions at this time, because the medications, anesthesia, and surgery may affect their decision-making ability.

Post Anesthesia Care Unit

MODIFIED ALDRETE SCORE

Patient: ______________________ Final score: ______________________

Room: ______________________ Surgeon: ______________________

Date: ______________________ PACU nurse: ______________________

Area of Assessment	Point Score	Upon Admission	After 15 min	After 30 min	After 45 min	After 60 min
Activity						
(Able to move spontaneously or on command)						
• Ability to move all extremities	2					
• Ability to move 2 extremities	1					
• Unable to control any extremity	0					
Respiration						
• Ability to breathe deeply and cough	2					
• Limited respiratory effort (dyspnea or splinting)	1					
• No spontaneous effort	0					
Circulation						
• BP ± 20% of preanesthetic level	2					
• BP ± 20% –49% of preanesthetic level	1					
• BP ± 50% of preanesthetic level	0					
Consciousness						
• Fully awake	2					
• Arousable on calling	1					
• Not responding	0					
O_2 Saturation						
• Able to maintain O_2 sat >92% on room air	2					
• Needs O_2 inhalation to maintain O_2 sat >90%	1					
• O_2 sat <90% even with O_2 supplement	0					
Totals:						

Required for discharge from Post Anesthesia Care Unit: 7–8 points

______________________ ______________________

Time of release Signature of nurse

FIGURE 20-3. Post anesthesia care unit record; Modified Aldrete Score. (O_2 sat = oxygen saturation; BP = blood pressure.) Modified from Aldrete, A., & Wright, A. (1992). Revised Aldrete score for discharge. *Anesthesiology News, 18*(1), 17.

CONTINUING CARE

Although most patients who undergo ambulatory surgery recover quickly and without complications, some patients require referral for home care. These may be elderly or frail patients, those who live alone, and patients with other health care problems or disabilities that might interfere with self-care or resumption of usual activities. The home care nurse assesses the patient's physical status (eg, respiratory and cardiovascular status, adequacy of pain management, the surgical incision) and the patient's and family's ability to adhere to the recommendations given at the time of discharge. Previous teaching is reinforced as needed. The home care nurse may change surgical dressings, monitor the patency of a drainage system, or administer medications. The patient is assessed for any surgical complications. The patient and family are reminded about the importance of keeping follow-

CHART 20-2

HOME CARE CHECKLIST • Discharge After Surgery

At the completion of the home care instruction, the patient or caregiver will be able to:	Patient	Caregiver
• Name the procedure that was performed and identify any permanent changes in anatomic structure or function.	✔	✔
• Describe ongoing postoperative therapeutic regimen, including medications, diet, activities to perform, (eg, walking and breathing exercises) and to avoid (eg, driving a car; contact sports), adjuvant therapies, dressing changes and wound care, and any other treatments.	✔	✔
• Describe signs and symptoms of complications.	✔	✔
• State time and date of follow-up appointments.	✔	✔
• Identify interventions and strategies to use in adapting to any permanent changes in structure or function.	✔	✔
• Relate how to reach health care provider with questions or complications.	✔	✔
• State understanding of community resources and referrals (if any).	✔	✔
• Describe pertinent health promotion activities (eg, weight reduction, smoking cessation, stress management).	✔	✔

up appointments with the surgeon. Follow-up phone calls from the nurse or surgeon may also be used to assess the patient's progress and to answer any questions.

The Hospitalized Postoperative Patient

The majority of surgeries are now performed in ambulatory care centers, and surgical patients who require hospital stays are trauma patients, acutely ill patients, patients undergoing major surgery, patients who require emergency surgery, and patients with a concurrent medical disorder. Seriously ill patients and those who have undergone major cardiovascular, pulmonary, or neurologic surgery may be admitted to specialized ICUs for close monitoring and advanced interventions and support. The care required by these patients in the immediate postoperative period is discussed in specific chapters. Patients admitted to the clinical unit for postoperative care have multiple needs and stay for a short period of time. Postoperative care for those surgical patients returning to the general medical-surgical unit is discussed later.

Receiving the Patient in the Clinical Unit

The patient's room is readied by assembling the necessary equipment and supplies: IV pole, drainage receptacle holder, suction equipment, oxygen, emesis basin, tissues, disposable pads, blankets, and postoperative documentation forms. When the call comes to the unit about the patient's transfer from the PACU, the need for any additional items is communicated. The PACU nurse reports data about the patient to the receiving nurse. The report includes relevant demographic data, medical diagnosis, procedure performed, comorbid conditions, allergies, unexpected intraoperative events, estimated blood loss, types and amounts of fluids received, medications administered for pain, types of IV fluids or medications infused, whether the patient has voided, and information that the patient and family have received about the patient's condition. Usually the surgeon speaks to the family after surgery and relates the general condition of the patient. The receiving nurse reviews the postoperative orders, admits the patient to the unit, performs an initial assessment, and attends to the patient's immediate needs (Chart 20-3).

Nursing Management After Surgery

During the first 24 hours after surgery, nursing care of the hospitalized patient on the general medical-surgical unit involves continuing to help the patient recover from the effects of anesthesia, frequently assessing the patient's physiologic status, monitoring for complications, managing pain, and implementing measures designed to achieve the long-range goals of independence with self-care, successful management of the therapeutic regimen, discharge to home, and full recovery. In the initial hours after admission to the clinical unit, adequate ventilation, hemodynamic stability, incisional pain, surgical site integrity, nausea and vomiting, neurologic status, and spontaneous voiding are primary concerns. The pulse rate, blood pressure, and respiration rate are recorded at least every 15 minutes for the first hour and every 30 minutes for the next 2 hours (Defazio-Quinn & Schick, 2004). Thereafter, they are measured less frequently if they remain stable. The temperature is monitored every 4 hours for the first 24 hours.

Patients usually begin to return to their usual state of health several hours after surgery or after waking up the next morning. Although pain may still be intense, many patients

CHART 20-3

Guidelines for Immediate Postoperative Nursing Interventions

NURSING INTERVENTIONS	RATIONALE
1. Assess breathing and administer supplemental oxygen, if prescribed.	1. Assessment provides a baseline and helps identify signs and symptoms of respiratory distress early.
2. Monitor vital signs and note skin warmth, moisture, and color.	2. A careful baseline assessment helps identify signs and symptoms of shock early.
3. Assess the surgical site and wound drainage systems. Connect all drainage tubes to gravity or suction as indicated and monitor closed drainage systems.	3. Assessment provides a baseline and helps identify signs and symptoms of hemorrhage early.
4. Assess level of consciousness, orientation, and ability to move extremities.	4. These parameters provide a baseline and help identify signs and symptoms of neurologic complications.
5. Assess pain level, pain characteristics (location, quality) and timing, type, and route of administration of last dose of analgesic.	5. Assessment provides a baseline of current pain level and for assessment of effectiveness of pain management strategies.
6. Administer analgesics as prescribed and assess their effectiveness in relieving pain.	6. Administration of analgesics helps decrease pain.
7. Place the call light, emesis basin, ice chips (if allowed), and bedpan or urinal within reach.	7. Attending to these needs provides for comfort and safety.
8. Position the patient to enhance comfort, safety, and lung expansion.	8. This promotes safety and reduces risk of postoperative complications.
9. Assess IV sites for patency and infusions for correct rate and solution.	9. Assessing IV sites and infusions helps detect phlebitis and prevents errors in rate and solution type.
10. Assess urine output in closed drainage system or the patient's urge to void and bladder distention.	10. Assessment provides a baseline and helps identify signs of urinary retention.
11. Reinforce the need to begin deep-breathing and leg exercises.	11. These activities help to prevent complications.
12. Provide information to the patient and family.	12. Patient teaching helps to decrease the patient's and family's anxiety.

feel more alert, less nauseous, and less anxious. They have begun their breathing and leg exercises, and many will have dangled their legs over the edge of the bed, stood, and ambulated a few feet or been assisted out of bed to the chair at least once. Many will have tolerated a light meal and had IV fluids discontinued. The focus of care shifts from intense physiologic management and symptomatic relief of the adverse effects of anesthesia to regaining independence with self-care and preparing for discharge. Despite these gains, the postoperative patient is still at risk for complications. Atelectasis, pneumonia, deep vein thrombosis, pulmonary embolism, bleeding, constipation, paralytic ileus, and wound infection are ongoing threats for the postoperative patient (Fig. 20-4).

Nursing Process

The Hospitalized Patient Recovering From Surgery

Nursing care of the hospitalized patient recovering from surgery takes place in a compressed time frame, with much of the healing and recovery occurring after the patient is discharged to home or to a rehabilitation center. The Perioperative Nursing Data Set (PNDS) is a helpful model used by nurses in the postoperative phase of care (see Figure 18-1 in Chapter 18). Phenomena of concern to nurses on the clinical unit in the postoperative phase of care include nursing diagnoses, interventions, and outcomes for patients and their families. Additional areas of concern include collaborative problems and expected goals.

Assessment

Assessment of the hospitalized postoperative patient includes monitoring vital signs and completing a review of the systems on arrival of the patient to the clinical unit (see Chart 20-3) and at regular intervals thereafter.

Respiratory status is important, because pulmonary complications are among the most frequent and serious problems encountered by the surgical patient. The nurse observes for airway patency, watching for laryngeal edema (Letizia, O'Leary & Vodvarka, 2003). The quality of respirations, including depth, rate, and sound, are assessed regularly. Chest auscultation verifies that breath sounds are normal (or abnormal) bilaterally, and the findings are documented as a

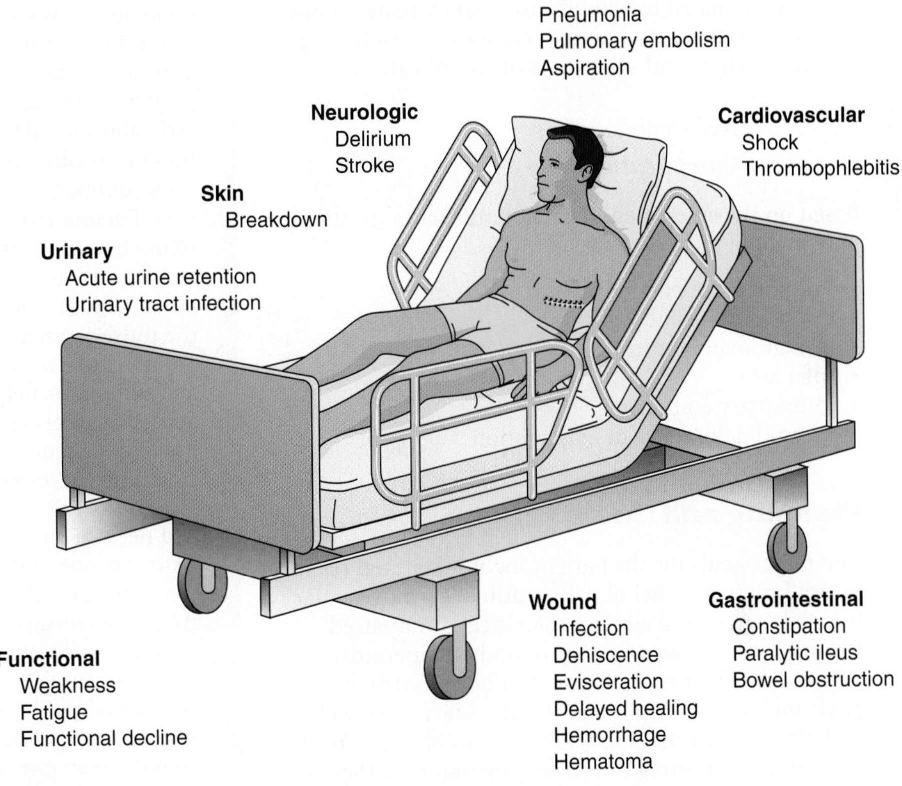

FIGURE 20-4. The postoperative patient is subject to a number of potential complications.

baseline for later comparisons. Often, because of the effects of analgesic and anesthetic medications, respirations are slow. Shallow and rapid respirations may be caused by pain, constricting dressings, gastric dilation, abdominal distention, or obesity. Noisy breathing may be due to obstruction by secretions or the tongue.

The nurse assesses the patient's pain level using a verbal or visual analogue scale and assesses the characteristics of the pain. The patient's appearance, pulse, respirations, blood pressure, skin color (adequate or cyanotic), and skin temperature (cold and clammy, warm and moist, or warm and dry) are clues to cardiovascular function. When the patient arrives in the clinical unit, the surgical site is observed for bleeding, type and integrity of dressings, and drains.

The nurse also assesses the patient's mental status and level of consciousness, speech, and orientation and compares them with the preoperative baseline. Although a change in mental status or postoperative restlessness may be related to anxiety, pain, or medications, it may also be a symptom of oxygen deficit or hemorrhage. These serious causes must be investigated and excluded before other causes are pursued.

General discomfort resulting from lying in one position on the operating table, the surgeon's handling of tissues, the body's reaction to anesthesia, and anxiety are also common causes of restlessness. These discomforts may be relieved by administering the prescribed analgesics, changing the patient's position frequently, and assessing and alleviating the cause of anxiety. If tight, drainage-soaked bandages are causing discomfort, reinforcing or changing the dressing completely as prescribed by the physician may make the patient more comfortable. The bladder is assessed for distention, because urinary retention can also cause restlessness.

Diagnosis

Nursing Diagnoses

Based on the assessment data, major nursing diagnoses may include the following:

- Risk for ineffective airway clearance related to depressed respiratory function, pain, and bed rest
- Acute pain related to surgical incision
- Decreased cardiac output related to shock or hemorrhage
- Risk for activity intolerance related to generalized weakness secondary to surgery
- Impaired skin integrity related to surgical incision and drains
- Ineffective thermoregulation related to surgical environment and anesthetic agents
- Risk for imbalanced nutrition, less than body requirements related to decreased intake and increased need for nutrients secondary to surgery
- Risk for constipation related to effects of medications, surgery, dietary change, and immobility
- Risk for urinary retention related to anesthetic agents
- Risk for injury related to surgical procedure/positioning or anesthetic agents

- Anxiety related to surgical procedure
- Risk for ineffective management of therapeutic regimen related to wound care, dietary restrictions, activity recommendations, medications, follow-up care, or signs and symptoms of complications

Collaborative Problems/ Potential Complications

Based on the assessment data, potential complications may include the following:

- Pulmonary infection/hypoxia
- Deep vein thrombosis
- Hematoma/hemorrhage
- Infection
- Pulmonary embolism
- Wound dehiscence or evisceration

Planning and Goals

The major goals for the patient include optimal respiratory function, relief of pain, optimal cardiovascular function, increased activity tolerance, unimpaired wound healing, maintenance of body temperature, and maintenance of nutritional balance. Further goals include resumption of usual pattern of bowel and bladder elimination, identification of any perioperative positioning injury, acquisition of sufficient knowledge to manage self-care after discharge, and absence of complications.

Nursing Interventions

Preventing Respiratory Complications

Respiratory depressive effects of opioid medications, decreased lung expansion secondary to pain, and decreased mobility combine to put the patient at risk for common respiratory complications, particularly atelectasis (alveolar collapse; incomplete expansion of the lung), pneumonia, and hypoxemia (Rothrock, 2003). Atelectasis remains a risk for the patient who is not moving well or ambulating or who is not performing deep-breathing and coughing exercises or using an incentive spirometer. Signs and symptoms include decreased breath sounds over the affected area, crackles, and cough. Pneumonia is characterized by chills and fever, tachycardia, and tachypnea. Cough may or may not be present and may or may not be productive. Hypostatic pulmonary congestion, caused by a weakened cardiovascular system that permits stagnation of secretions at lung bases, may develop; this condition occurs most frequently in elderly patients who are not mobilized effectively. The symptoms are often vague, with perhaps a slight elevation of temperature, pulse, and respiratory rate, as well as a cough. Physical examination reveals dullness and crackles at the base of the lungs. If the condition progresses, the outcome may be fatal.

The types of hypoxemia that can affect postoperative patients are subacute and episodic. Subacute hypoxemia is a constant low level of oxygen saturation, although breathing appears normal. Episodic hypoxemia develops suddenly, and the patient may be at risk for cerebral dysfunction, myocardial ischemia, and cardiac arrest. Risk for hypoxemia is present in patients who have undergone major surgery (particularly abdominal), are obese, or have preexisting pulmonary problems. Hypoxemia can be detected by pulse oximetry, which measures blood oxygen saturation. Factors that may affect the accuracy of pulse oximetry readings include cold extremities, tremors, atrial fibrillation, acrylic nails, and black or blue nail polish (these colors interfere with the functioning of the pulse oximeter; other colors do not).

Preventive measures and timely recognition of signs and symptoms help avert pulmonary complications. Strategies to prevent respiratory complications include use of an incentive spirometer and deep-breathing and coughing exercises. Crackles indicate static pulmonary secretions that need to be mobilized by coughing and deep-breathing exercises. When a mucus plug obstructs one of the bronchi entirely, the pulmonary tissue beyond the plug collapses, and massive atelectasis results.

To clear secretions and prevent pneumonia, the nurse encourages the patient to turn frequently and take deep breaths at least every 2 hours. Coughing is also encouraged to dislodge mucus plugs. These pulmonary exercises should begin as soon as the patient arrives on the clinical unit and continue until the patient is discharged. Even if he or she is not fully awake from anesthesia, the patient can be asked to take several deep breaths. This helps expel residual anesthetic agents, mobilize secretions, and prevent alveolar collapse (atelectasis). Careful splinting of abdominal or thoracic incision sites helps the patient overcome the fear that the exertion of coughing might open the incision. Analgesic agents are administered to permit more effective coughing, and oxygen is administered as prescribed to prevent or relieve hypoxia. To encourage lung expansion, the patient is encouraged to yawn or take sustained maximal inspirations to create a negative intrathoracic pressure of −40 mm Hg and expand lung volume to total capacity. Chest physical therapy may be prescribed if indicated.

Coughing is contraindicated in patients who have head injuries or who have undergone intracranial surgery (because of the risk for increasing intracranial pressure), as well as in patients who have undergone eye surgery (because of the risk for increasing intraocular pressure) or plastic surgery (because of the risk for increasing tension on delicate tissues). In patients with an abdominal or thoracic incision, the nurse teaches the patient how to splint the incision while coughing.

Most postoperative patients, especially the elderly and those with an abdominal or thoracic incision, are given an incentive spirometer and instructed in its use. A common recommendation for use of the incentive spirometer is 10 deep breaths every hour while awake. Refer to Chapter 25 for additional discussion of incentive spirometry and other respiratory modalities.

Early ambulation increases metabolism and pulmonary aeration and, in general, improves all body functions. The patient is encouraged to be out of bed as soon as possible (ie, on the day of surgery, or no later than the first postoperative day). This practice is especially valuable in preventing pulmonary complications in older patients.

Relieving Pain

Most patients experience some pain after a surgical procedure. Many factors (motivational, affective, cognitive, and emotional) influence the pain experience. The degree and severity of postoperative pain and the patient's tolerance for pain depend on the incision site, the nature of the surgical procedure, the extent of surgical trauma, the type of anesthetic agent, and how the agent was administered. The preoperative preparation received by the patient (including information about what to expect, reassurance, psychological support, and teaching specific communication techniques related to pain) is a significant factor in decreasing anxiety, apprehension, and even the amount of postoperative pain (McDonald & Molony, 2004; Nair & Podichetty, 2004).

The reasons for controlling pain are compelling. There is a well-known correlation between frequency of complications and intensity of pain (Barnett, 2003; Milgrom, Brooks, Qi, et al. 2004). Intense pain stimulates the stress response, which adversely affects the cardiac and immune systems. When pain impulses are transmitted, both muscle tension and local vasoconstriction increase. The ischemia in the affected area causes further stimulation of pain receptors. When these impulses travel centrally, sympathetic activity is compounded, which increases myocardial demand and oxygen consumption. Research suggests that outcomes are improved and complications prevented with good pain control in the postoperative period (Barnett & Ochroch, 2004). Cardiovascular insufficiency occurs three times more frequently, and the incidence of infection is five times greater, in people with poor postoperative pain control (Moline, 2001). The hypothalamic stress response is also responsible for an increase in blood viscosity and platelet aggregation; this can lead to phlebothrombosis and pulmonary embolism.

Often the physician has prescribed different medications or dosages to cover various levels of pain. The nurse discusses these options with the patient to determine the best medication. Then the nurse assesses the effectiveness of the medication periodically, beginning 30 minutes after administration, or sooner if the medication is being delivered by patient-controlled analgesia (PCA).

OPIOID ANALGESICS

About one third of patients report severe pain, one third moderate pain, and one third little or no pain. This does not mean that the patients in the last group have no pain; rather, they appear to activate psychodynamic mechanisms that impair the registering of pain ("gate closing" theory and nociceptive transmission). See Chapter 13 for a more detailed discussion of pain, the factors influencing the pain experience, and use of pain relief strategies.

Opioid analgesics are commonly prescribed for pain and immediate postoperative restlessness. A preventive approach, rather than an "as needed" (PRN) approach, is more effective in relieving pain. With a preventive approach, the medication is administered at prescribed intervals rather than when the pain becomes severe or unbearable. Many patients (and some health care providers) are overly concerned about the risk of drug addiction in the postoperative patient. However, this risk is negligible with the use of opioid medications for short-term pain control.

The postoperative level of opiate analgesia required also depends on whether the patient is a smoker or nonsmoker. Patients who smoke require greater amounts of opioids in the first 48 hours after cardiac surgery (Creekmore, Lugo & Weiland, 2004).

PATIENT-CONTROLLED ANALGESIA

Given the negative impact of pain on recovery, nurses need to think "pain prevention" rather than sporadic pain control and should encourage the use of PCA. Patients recover more quickly when adequate pain relief measures are used, and PCA permits patients to administer their own pain medication when needed (Defazio-Quinn & Schick, 2004). The amount of medication delivered by the IV or epidural route and the time span during which the opioid medication is released are controlled by the PCA device. Self-administration promotes patient participation in care, eliminates delayed administration of analgesics, and maintains a therapeutic drug level.

Most patients are candidates for PCA. The two requirements for PCA are an understanding of the need to self-dose and the physical ability to self-dose. On sensing pain, the patient activates the medication-delivering pump with a handheld button. PCA enables the patient to move, turn, cough, and take deep breaths with less pain, thus reducing postoperative pulmonary complications.

EPIDURAL INFUSIONS AND INTRAPLEURAL ANESTHESIA

For thoracic, orthopedic, obstetric, and major abdominal surgery, certain opioid analgesics may be administered by epidural or intrathecal infusion (Defazio-Quinn & Schick, 2004). Epidural infusions provide better postoperative analgesia compared with parenteral opioids (Block, Liu, Rowlingson, et al., 2003; Pasero, 2003). Epidural infusions are used with caution in chest procedures because the analgesic may ascend along the spinal cord and affect respiration. Intrapleural anesthesia involves the administration of local anesthetic by a catheter between the parietal and visceral pleura. It provides sensory anesthesia without affecting motor function to the intercostal muscles. This anesthesia allows more effective coughing and deep breathing in conditions such as cholecystectomy, renal surgery, and rib fractures in which pain in the thoracic region would interfere with these exercises.

A local opioid or a combination anesthetic (opioid plus local anesthetic agent) is used in the epidural infusion. Other local anesthetic methods may be used to provide analgesia and anesthesia. Intrapleural anesthesia has fewer adverse effects than systemic or spinal opioids and is associated with a lowered incidence of urinary retention, vomiting, and pruritus when compared with thoracic epidural opioids (Moline, 2001).

OTHER PAIN RELIEF MEASURES

For pain that is difficult to control, a subcutaneous pain management system may be used. This is a silicone catheter that is inserted at the site of the affected area. The catheter is attached to a pump that delivers a continuous amount of local anesthetic at a specific amount determined and prescribed by the physician (Fig. 20-5).

Complete absence of pain in the area of the surgical incision may not occur for a few weeks, depending on the site and nature of the surgery, but the intensity of postoperative pain gradually subsides on subsequent days. However, pain control continues to be an important concern for the patient and the nurse. Effective pain management allows the patient to participate in care, perform deep-breathing and leg exercises, and tolerate activity. As stated previously, poor pain control contributes to postoperative complications and increased length of stay. The nurse continues to assess the pain level, the effectiveness of analgesic agents, and factors that influence pain tolerance (eg, energy level, stress level, cultural background, meaning of pain to the patient). The nurse explains that taking an analgesic agent before the pain becomes intense is more effective and offers medication to the patient at intervals rather than waiting for the patient to request it.

Nonpharmacologic pain relief measures, such as imagery, music, relaxation, massage, application of heat or cold (if prescribed), and distraction, can be used to supplement medications (Ikonomidou, Rehnstrom, Naesh, et al., 2004; McRee, Noble & Pasvogel, 2003; Taylor, Galper, Taylor, et al., 2003). Changing the patient's position, using distraction, applying cool washcloths to the face, and rubbing the back with a soothing lotion may be useful in relieving general discomfort temporarily, promoting relaxation, and rendering medication more effective when it is administered.

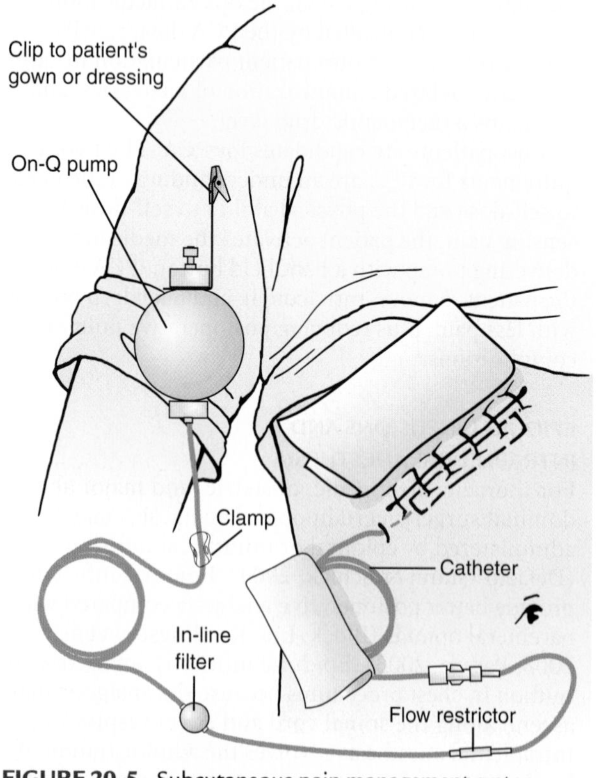

FIGURE 20-5. Subcutaneous pain management system consists of a pump, filter, and catheter that delivers a specific amount of prescribed local anesthetic at the rate determined by the physician. Used with permission from I-Flow Corporation, Lake Forest, CA.

Promoting Cardiac Output

If signs and symptoms of shock or hemorrhage occur, treatment and nursing care are implemented as described in the discussion of care in the PACU.

> **NURSING ALERT**
>
> **A systolic blood pressure of less than 90 mm Hg is usually considered reportable at once. However, the patient's preoperative or baseline blood pressure is used to make informed postoperative comparisons. A previously stable blood pressure that shows a downward trend of 5 mm Hg at each 15-minute reading should also be reported.**

Although most patients do not hemorrhage or go into shock, changes in circulating volume, the stress of surgery, and the effects of medications and preoperative preparations all affect cardiovascular function. IV fluid replacement is standard for up to 24 hours after surgery or until the patient is stable and tolerating oral fluids. Close monitoring is indicated to detect and correct conditions such as fluid volume deficit, altered tissue perfusion, and decreased cardiac output, all of which can increase the patient's discomfort, place him or her at risk of complications, and prolong the hospital stay. Some patients are at risk of fluid volume excess secondary to existing cardiovascular or renal disease, advanced age, or the release of adrenocorticotropic hormone and antidiuretic hormone as a result of the stress of surgery (Defazio-Quinn & Schick, 2004). Consequently, fluid replacement must be carefully managed, and intake and output records must be accurate.

Nursing management includes assessing the patency of the IV lines and ensuring that the correct fluids are administered at the prescribed rate. Intake and output, including emesis and output from wound drainage systems, are recorded separately and totaled to determine fluid balance. If the patient has an indwelling urinary catheter, hourly outputs are monitored and rates of less than 30 mL/hour are reported; if the patient is voiding, an output of less than 240 mL per 8-hour shift is reported. Electrolyte levels and hemoglobin and hematocrit levels are monitored. Decreased hemoglobin and hematocrit levels can indicate blood loss or dilution of circulating volume by IV fluids. If dilution is contributing to the decreased levels, the hemoglobin and hematocrit will rise as the stress response abates and fluids are mobilized and excreted.

Venous stasis from dehydration, immobility, and pressure on leg veins during surgery put the patient at risk for deep vein thrombosis. Leg exercises and frequent position changes are initiated early in the postoperative period to stimulate circulation. Patients should avoid positions that compromise venous return, such as raising the bed's knee gatch, placing a pillow under the knees, sitting for long periods, and dangling the legs with pressure at the back of the knees. Venous return is promoted by elastic compression stockings and early ambulation. Early ambulation has a significant effect on recovery and the prevention of complications and can begin, in many instances, on the evening of surgery. Postoperative activity orders are checked before the patient is assisted to get out of bed. Sitting up at the edge of the bed for a few minutes may be all that the patient who has undergone a major surgical procedure can tolerate at first.

Encouraging Activity

Most surgical patients are encouraged to be out of bed as soon as possible. Early ambulation reduces the incidence of postoperative complications, such as atelectasis, hypostatic pneumonia, gastrointestinal discomfort, and circulatory problems (Oetker-Black, Jones, Estok, et al., 2003; Rothrock, 2003). Ambulation increases ventilation and reduces the stasis of bronchial secretions in the lungs. It also reduces postoperative abdominal distention by increasing gastrointestinal tract and abdominal wall tone and stimulating peristalsis. Early ambulation prevents stasis of blood by increasing the rate of circulation in the extremities; as a result, thrombophlebitis or phlebothrombosis occurs less frequently. Pain is often decreased when early ambulation is possible, and the hospital stay is shorter and less costly, a further advantage to the patient and the hospital.

Despite the advantages of early ambulation, patients may be reluctant to get out of bed on the evening of surgery. Reminding them of the importance of early mobility in preventing complications may help patients overcome their fears. When a patient gets out of bed for the first time, orthostatic hypotension, also called postural hypotension, is a concern. Orthostatic hypotension is an abnormal drop in blood pressure that occurs as the patient changes from a supine to a standing position. It is common after surgery because of changes in circulating blood volume and bed rest. Signs and symptoms include a decrease of 20 mm Hg in systolic blood pressure or 10 mm Hg in diastolic blood pressure, weakness, dizziness, and fainting. Older adults are at increased risk for orthostatic hypotension secondary to age-related changes in vascular tone. To detect orthostatic hypotension, the nurse assesses the patient's blood pressure first in the supine position, after the patient sits up, again after the patient stands, and 2 to 3 minutes later. Gradual position change gives the circulatory system time to adjust. If the patient becomes dizzy, he or she should be returned to the supine position, and getting out of bed should be delayed for several hours.

To assist the postoperative patient in getting out of bed for the first time after surgery, the nurse

1. Helps the patient move gradually from the lying position to the sitting position by raising the head of the bed and encourages the patient to splint the incision when applicable.
2. Positions the patient completely upright (sitting) and turned so that both legs are hanging over the edge of the bed.
3. Helps the patient stand beside the bed.

After becoming accustomed to the upright position, the patient may start to walk. The nurse should be at the patient's side to give physical support and encouragement. Care must be taken not to tire the patient; the extent of the first few periods of ambulation varies with the type of surgical procedure and the patient's physical condition and age.

Whether or not the patient can ambulate early in the postoperative period, bed exercises are encouraged to improve circulation. Bed exercises consist of the following:

- Arm exercises (full range of motion, with specific attention to abduction and external rotation of the shoulder)
- Hand and finger exercises
- Foot exercises to prevent deep vein thrombosis, foot drop, and toe deformities and to aid in maintaining good circulation
- Leg flexion and leg-lifting exercises to prepare the patient for ambulation
- Abdominal and gluteal contraction exercises

Hampered by pain, dressings, IV lines, or drains, many patients cannot engage in activity without assistance. Prolonged inactivity may lead to pressure ulcers, deep vein thrombosis, atelectasis, or hypostatic pneumonia. Helping the patient increase his or her activity level on the first postoperative day is an important nursing function. One way to increase the patient's activity is to have the patient perform as much routine hygiene care as possible. Setting up the patient to bathe with a bedside wash basin or, if possible, assisting the patient to the bathroom to sit in a chair at the sink not only gets the patient moving but helps restore a sense of self-control and prepares the patient for discharge.

To be safely discharged to home, patients need to be able to ambulate a functional distance (eg, length of the house or apartment), get in and out of bed unassisted, and be independent with toileting. Patients can be asked to perform as much as they can and then to call for assistance. The patient and the nurse can collaborate on a schedule for progressive activity that includes ambulating in the room and hallway and sitting out of bed in the chair. Assessing the patient's vital signs before, during, and after a scheduled activity helps the nurse and patient determine the rate of progression. By providing physical support, the nurse maintains the patient's safety; by communicating a positive attitude about the patient's ability to perform the activity, the nurse promotes the patient's confidence. The nurse should make sure the patient continues to perform bed exercises, wears pneumatic compression or thigh-high elastic compression stockings when in bed, and rests as needed. If the patient has had orthopedic surgery of the lower extremities or will require a mobility aid (ie, walker, crutches) at home, a physical therapist may be involved the first time the patient gets out of bed to teach him or her to ambulate safely or to use the mobility aid correctly.

Promoting Wound Healing

CONCEPTS in action ANIMATION

Ongoing assessment of the surgical site involves inspection for approximation of wound edges, integrity of sutures or staples, redness, discoloration, warmth, swelling, unusual tenderness, or drainage. The area around the wound should also be inspected for a reaction to tape or trauma from tight bandages.

Nursing interventions to promote wound healing also include management of surgical drains and dressings. Wound drains are tubes that exit the peri-incisional area, either into a portable wound suction device (closed) or into the dressings (open). The principle involved is to allow the escape of blood and serous fluids that could otherwise serve as a culture medium for bacteria. In portable wound suction, the use of gentle, constant suction enhances drainage of these fluids and collapses the skin flaps against the underlying tissue, thus removing "dead space." Types of wound drains include the Penrose, Hemovac, and Jackson-Pratt drains (Fig. 20-6). Output from wound drainage systems and all new drainage is recorded. The amount of bloody drainage on the surgical dressing is assessed frequently. Spots of drainage on the dressings are outlined with a pen, and the date and time of the outline are recorded on the dressing so that increased drainage can be easily seen. A certain amount of bloody drainage in a wound drainage system or on the dressing is expected, but excessive amounts should be reported to the surgeon. Increasing amounts of fresh blood on the dressing should be reported immediately. Some wounds are irrigated heavily before closure in the OR, and open drains exiting the wound may be embedded in the dressings. These wounds may drain large amounts of blood-tinged fluid that saturate the dressing. The dressing can be reinforced with sterile gauze bandages; the time at which they were reinforced should be documented. If drainage continues, the surgeon should be notified so that the dressing can be changed. Multiple similar drains are numbered or otherwise labeled (eg, left lower quadrant, left upper quadrant) so that output measurements can be reliably and consistently recorded.

Surgical wound healing occurs in three phases: the inflammatory, proliferative, and maturation phases (Table 20-2) (Hogan, 2004). Wounds also heal by different mechanisms, depending on the condition of the wound. These mechanisms are first-, second-, and third-intention wound healing (Fig. 20-7) (Rothrock, 2003). With shorter hospital stays, much of the healing takes place at home, and both the hospital and home care nurse should be informed about the principles of wound healing.

FIRST-INTENTION HEALING

Wounds made aseptically with a minimum of tissue destruction that are properly closed heal with little tissue reaction by first intention (primary union). When wounds heal by **first-intention healing**, gran-

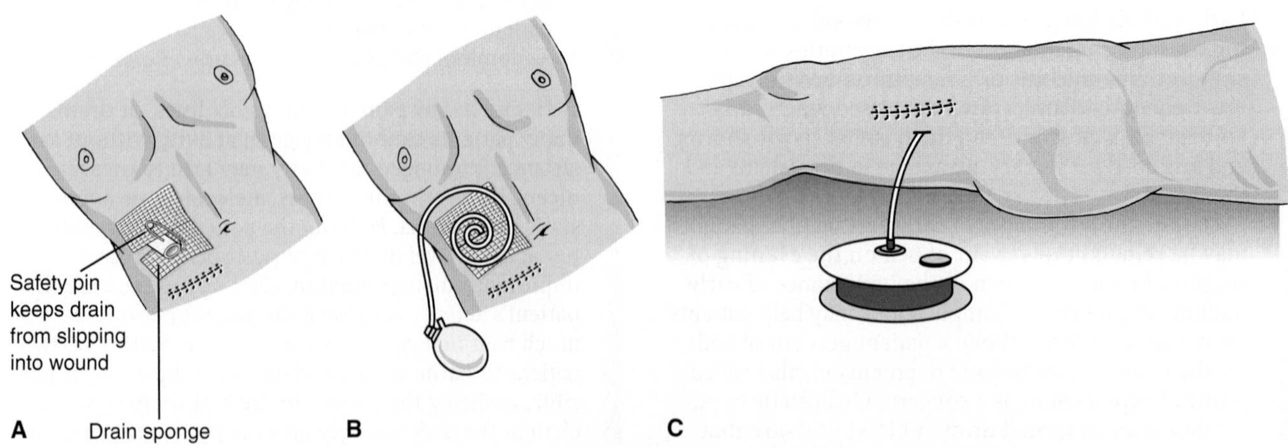

FIGURE 20-6. Types of surgical drains: (A) Penrose, (B) Jackson-Pratt, (C) Hemovac.

TABLE 20-2 Phases of Wound Healing

Phase	Duration	Events
Inflammatory (also called lag or exudative phase)	1–4 days	Blood clot forms Wound becomes edematous Debris of damaged tissue and blood clot are phagocytosed
Proliferative (also called fibroblastic or connective tissue phase)	5–20 days	Collagen produced Granulation tissue forms Wound tensile strength increases
Maturation (also called differentiation, resorptive, remodeling, or plateau phase)	21 days to months or even years	Fibroblasts leave wound Tensile strength increases Collagen fibers reorganize and tighten to reduce scar size

ulation tissue is not visible and scar formation is minimal. Postoperatively, many of these wounds are covered with a dry sterile dressing. If a cyanoacrylate tissue adhesive (Liquiband) was used to close the incision without sutures, a dressing is contraindicated.

SECOND-INTENTION HEALING

Second-intention healing (granulation) occurs in infected wounds (abscess) or in wounds in which the edges have not been approximated. When an abscess is incised, it collapses partly, but the dead and the dying cells forming its walls are still being released

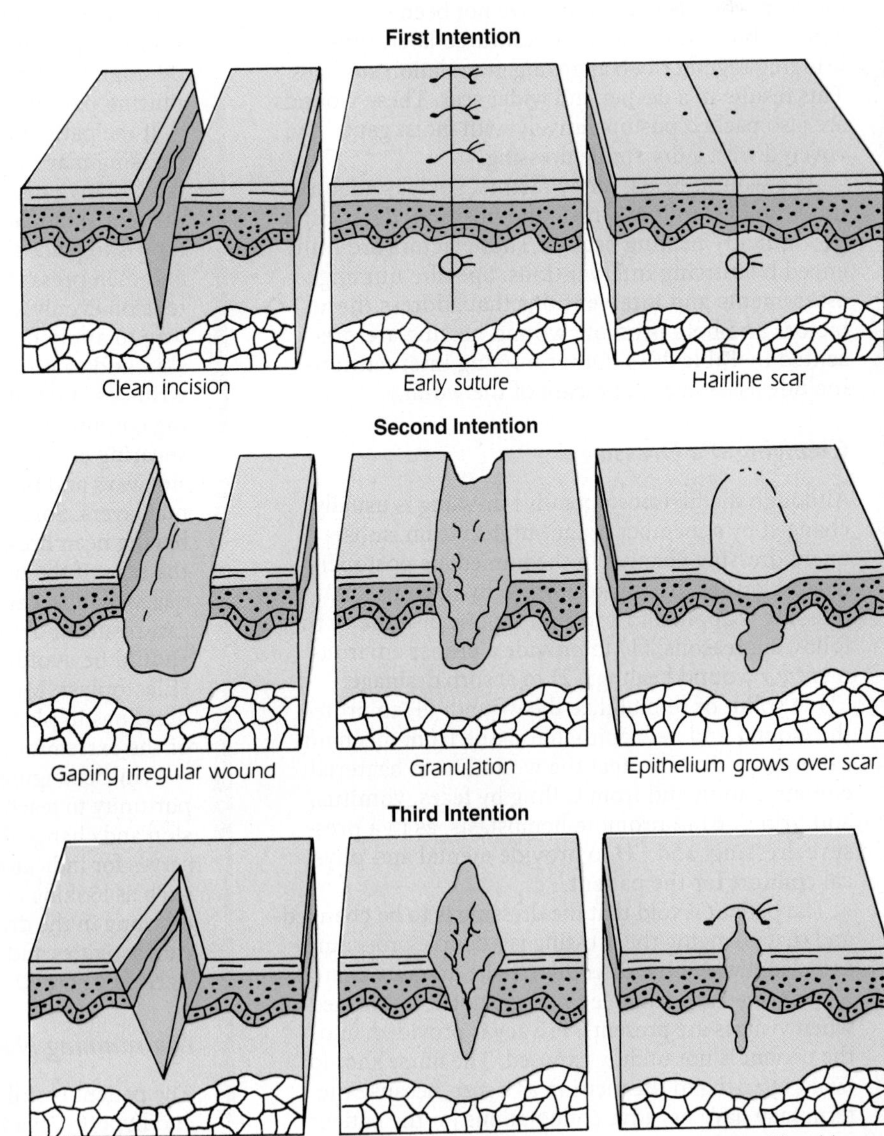

FIGURE 20-7. Types of wound healing: first-intention healing, second-intention healing, and third-intention healing.

into the cavity. For this reason, drainage tubes or gauze packing is inserted into the abscess pocket to allow drainage to escape easily. Gradually, the necrotic material disintegrates and escapes, and the abscess cavity fills with a red, soft, sensitive tissue that bleeds easily. This tissue is composed of minute, thin-walled capillaries and buds that later form connective tissue. These buds, called granulations, enlarge until they fill the area left by the destroyed tissue (see Fig. 20-7). The cells surrounding the capillaries change their round shape to become long, thin, and intertwined to form a scar (cicatrix). Healing is complete when skin cells (epithelium) grow over these granulations. This method of repair is called healing by granulation, and it takes place whenever pus is formed or when loss of tissue has occurred for any reason. When the postoperative wound is to be allowed to heal by secondary intention, it is usually packed with saline-moistened sterile dressings and covered with a dry sterile dressing.

THIRD-INTENTION HEALING

Third-intention healing (secondary suture) is used for deep wounds that either have not been sutured early or break down and are resutured later, thus bringing together two apposing granulation surfaces. This results in a deeper and wider scar. These wounds are also packed postoperatively with moist gauze and covered with a dry sterile dressing.

As a wound heals, many factors, such as adequate nutrition, cleanliness, rest, and position, determine how quickly healing occurs. These factors are influenced by nursing interventions. Specific nursing assessments and interventions that address these factors and help promote wound healing are presented in Table 20-3. Other nursing interventions include assessment and care of the wound.

Changing the Dressing

Although the first postoperative dressing is usually changed by a member of the surgical team, subsequent dressing changes in the immediate postoperative period are usually performed by the nurse. A dressing is applied to a wound for one or more of the following reasons: (1) to provide a proper environment for wound healing; (2) to absorb drainage; (3) to splint or immobilize the wound; (4) to protect the wound and new epithelial tissue from mechanical injury; (5) to protect the wound from bacterial contamination and from soiling by feces, vomitus, and urine; (6) to promote hemostasis, as in a pressure dressing; and (7) to provide mental and physical comfort for the patient.

The patient is told that the dressing is to be changed and that changing the dressing is a simple procedure associated with little discomfort. The dressing change is performed at a suitable time (eg, not at mealtimes or when visitors are present). Privacy is provided, and the patient is not unduly exposed. The nurse should avoid referring to the incision as a scar, because the term may have negative connotations for the patient.

NURSING ALERT

If disruption of a wound occurs, the patient is placed in low Fowler's position and instructed to lie quietly. These actions minimize protrusion of body tissues. The protruding coils of intestine are covered with sterile dressings moistened with sterile saline solution, and the surgeon is notified at once.

Assurance is given that the incision will shrink as it heals and that the redness will fade.

The nurse carries out hand hygiene before and after the dressing change and wears disposable gloves for the dressing change itself. The tape or adhesive portion of the dressing is removed by pulling it parallel with the skin surface and in the direction of hair growth, rather than at right angles. Alcohol wipes or nonirritating solvents aid in removing adhesive painlessly and quickly. The old dressing is removed and then deposited in a container designated for disposal of biomedical waste. In accordance with standard precautions, dressings are never touched by ungloved hands because of the danger of transmitting pathogenic organisms.

If the patient is sensitive to adhesive tape, the dressing may be held in place with hypoallergenic tape. Many tapes are porous to permit ventilation and prevent skin maceration. The correct way to apply tape is to place the tape at the center of the dressing and then press the tape down on both sides, applying tension evenly away from the midline. The incorrect way to apply tape—to fix one end of the tape to the skin and to pull it tight over the dressing—often wrinkles and pulls the skin in the process. The resulting continuous and forceful traction produces a shearing effect, causing the epidermal layer to slip sideways and become separated from the deeper dermal layers. Some wounds become edematous after having been dressed, causing considerable tension on the tape. If the tape is not flexible, the stretching bandage will also cause a shear injury to the skin. This can result in denuded areas or large blisters and should be avoided. An elastic adhesive bandage (Elastoplast, Microfoam-3M) may be used to hold dressings in place over mobile areas, such as the neck or the extremities, or where pressure is required.

While changing the dressing, the nurse has an opportunity to teach the patient how to care for the incision and change the dressings at home. The nurse observes for indicators of the patient's readiness to learn, such as looking at the incision, expressing interest, or assisting in the dressing change. Information on self-care activities and possible signs of infection is summarized in Chart 20-4.

Maintaining Normal Body Temperature

The patient is still at risk for malignant hyperthermia and hypothermia in the postoperative period. Efforts

TABLE 20-3 Factors Affecting Wound Healing

Factors	Rationale	Nursing Interventions
Age of patient	The older the patient, the less resilient the tissues.	Handle all tissues gently.
Handling of tissues	Rough handling causes injury and delayed healing.	Handle tissues carefully and evenly.
Hemorrhage	Accumulation of blood creates dead spaces as well as dead cells that must be removed. The area becomes a growth medium for organisms.	Monitor vital signs. Observe incision site for evidence of bleeding and infection.
Hypovolemia	Insufficient blood volume leads to vasoconstriction and reduced oxygen and nutrients available for wound healing.	Monitor for volume deficit (circulatory impairment). Correct by fluid replacement as prescribed.
Local factors		
Edema	Reduces blood supply by exerting increased interstitial pressure on vessels	Elevate part; apply cool compresses.
Inadequate dressing technique		
Too small	Permits bacterial invasion and contamination	Follow guidelines for proper dressing technique.
Too tight	Reduces blood supply carrying nutrients and oxygen	
Nutritional deficits	Protein–calorie depletion may occur. Insulin secretion may be inhibited, causing blood glucose to rise.	Correct deficits; this may require parenteral nutritional therapy. Monitor blood glucose levels. Administer vitamin supplements as prescribed.
Foreign bodies	Foreign bodies retard healing.	Keep wounds free of dressing threads and talcum powder from gloves.
Oxygen deficit (tissue oxygenation insufficient)	Insufficient oxygen may be due to inadequate lung and cardiovascular function as well as localized vasoconstriction.	Encourage deep breathing, turning, controlled coughing.
Drainage accumulation	Accumulated secretions hamper healing process.	Monitor closed drainage systems for proper functioning. Institute measures to remove accumulated secretions.
Medications		
Corticosteroids	May mask presence of infection by impairing normal inflammatory response	Be aware of action and effect of medications patient is receiving.
Anticoagulants	May cause hemorrhage	
Broad-spectrum and specific antibiotics	Effective if administered immediately before surgery for specific pathology or bacterial contamination. If administered after wound is closed, ineffective because of intravascular coagulation.	
Patient overactivity	Prevents approximation of wound edges. Resting favors healing.	Use measures to keep wound edges approximated: taping, bandaging, splints. Encourage rest.
Systemic disorders Hemorrhagic shock Acidosis Hypoxia Renal failure Hepatic disease Sepsis	These depress cell functions that directly affect wound healing.	Be familiar with the nature of the specific disorder. Administer prescribed treatment. Cultures may be indicated to determine appropriate antibiotic.
Immunosuppressed state	Patient is more vulnerable to bacterial and viral invasion; defense mechanisms are impaired.	Provide maximum protection to prevent infection. Restrict visitors with colds; institute mandatory hand hygiene by all staff.
Wound stressors Vomiting Valsalva maneuver Heavy coughing Straining	Produce tension on wounds, particularly of the torso.	Encourage frequent turning and ambulation and administer antiemetic medications as prescribed. Assist patient in splinting incision.

CHART 20-4

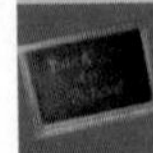

Patient Education

Wound Care Instructions

UNTIL SUTURES ARE REMOVED

1. Keep the wound dry and clean.
   - If there is no dressing, ask your nurse or physician if you can bathe or shower.
   - If a dressing or splint is in place, do not remove it unless it is wet or soiled.
   - If wet or soiled, change dressing yourself if you have been taught to do so; otherwise, call your nurse or physician for guidance.
   - If you have been taught, instruction might be as follows:
     - Cleanse area *gently* with sterile normal saline once or twice daily.
     - Cover with a sterile Telfa pad or gauze square large enough to cover wound.
     - Apply hypoallergenic tape (Dermacel or paper). Adhesive is not recommended because it is difficult to remove without possible injury to the incisional site.
2. Immediately report any of these signs of infection:
   - Redness, marked swelling exceeding ½ inch (2.5 cm) from incision site; tenderness; or increased warmth around wound
   - Red streaks in skin near wound
   - Pus or discharge, foul odor
   - Chills or temperature higher than 37.7°C (100°F)
3. If soreness or pain causes discomfort, apply a dry cool pack (containing ice or cold water) or take prescribed acetaminophen tablets (2) every 4–6 hours. Avoid using aspirin without direction or instruction because bleeding can occur with its use.
4. Swelling after surgery is common. To help reduce swelling, elevate the affected part to the level of the heart.
   - Hand or arm
     - Sleep—elevate arm on pillow at side
     - Sitting—place arm on pillow on adjacent table
     - Standing—rest affected hand on opposite shoulder; support elbow with unaffected hand
   - Leg or foot
     - Sitting—place a pillow on a facing chair; provide support underneath the knee
     - Lying—place a pillow under affected leg

AFTER SUTURES ARE REMOVED

Although the wound appears to be healed when sutures are removed, it is still tender and will continue to heal and strengthen for several weeks.

1. Follow recommendations of physician or nurse regarding extent of activity.
2. Keep suture line clean; do not rub vigorously; pat dry. Wound edges may look red and may be slightly raised. This is normal.
3. If the site continues to be red, thick, and painful to pressure after 8 weeks, consult the health care provider. (This may be due to excessive collagen formation and should be checked.)

are made to identify malignant hyperthermia and to treat it early and promptly (McCarthy, 2004; Rothrock, 2003). (See the discussion of malignant hyperthermia in Chapter 19.)

Patients who have been anesthetized are susceptible to chills and drafts. Attention to hypothermia management, begun in the intraoperative period, extends into the postoperative period to prevent significant nitrogen loss and catabolism. Signs of hypothermia are reported to the physician. The room is maintained at a comfortable temperature, and blankets are provided to prevent chilling. Treatment includes oxygen administration, adequate hydration, and proper nutrition. The patient is also monitored for cardiac dysrhythmias. The risk of hypothermia is greater in the elderly and in patients who were in the cool OR environment for a prolonged period.

Managing Gastrointestinal Function and Resuming Nutrition

Gastrointestinal discomfort (nausea, vomiting, hiccups) and resumption of oral intake are issues for both the patient and the nurse. Nausea and vomiting are common after anesthesia (Rothrock, 2003). They are more common in women, in obese people (fat cells act as reservoirs for the anesthetic), in patients prone to motion sickness, and in patients who have undergone lengthy surgical procedures. Other causes of postoperative vomiting include an accumulation of fluid in the stomach, inflation of the stomach, and the ingestion of food and fluid before peristalsis resumes.

If vomiting is likely because of the nature of surgery, a nasogastric tube is inserted preoperatively and remains in place throughout the surgery and the immediate postoperative period. A nasogastric tube also may be inserted before surgery if postoperative distention is anticipated. In addition, a nasogastric tube may be inserted if a patient who has food in the stomach requires emergency surgery.

Hiccups, produced by intermittent spasms of the diaphragm secondary to irritation of the phrenic nerve, can occur after surgery. The irritation may be direct, such as from stimulation of the nerve by a distended stomach, subdiaphragmatic abscess, or abdominal distention; indirect, such as from toxemia or uremia that stimulates the nerve; or reflexive, such as irritation from a drainage tube or obstruction of the intestines. Usually these occurrences are mild, transitory attacks that cease spontaneously. If hiccups persist, they may produce considerable distress and serious effects such as vomiting, exhaustion, and wound dehiscence. The physician may prescribe phenothiazine medications (e.g., Thorazine) for intractable hiccups (Zunderman & Doyle, 2006).

Once nausea and vomiting have subsided and the patient is fully awake and alert, the sooner he or she can tolerate a usual diet, the more quickly normal gastrointestinal function will resume. Taking food by mouth stimulates digestive juices and promotes gastric function and intestinal peristalsis. The return to normal dietary intake should proceed at a pace set by the patient. Of course, the nature of the surgery and the type of anesthesia directly affect the rate at which normal gastric activity resumes. Liquids are typically the first substances desired and tolerated by the patient after surgery. Water, juice, and tea may be given in increasing amounts. Cool fluids are tolerated more easily than those that are ice cold or hot. Soft foods (gelatin, custard, milk, and creamed soups) are added gradually after clear fluids have been tolerated. As soon as the patient tolerates soft foods well, solid food may be given.

Assessment and management of gastrointestinal function are important after surgery because the gastrointestinal tract is subject to uncomfortable or potentially life-threatening complications. Any postoperative patient may suffer from distention. Postoperative distention of the abdomen results from the accumulation of gas in the intestinal tract. Manipulation of the abdominal organs during surgery may produce a loss of normal peristalsis for 24 to 48 hours, depending on the type and extent of surgery. Even though nothing is given by mouth, swallowed air and gastrointestinal secretions enter the stomach and intestines; if not propelled by peristalsis, they collect in the intestines, producing distention and causing the patient to complain of fullness or pain in the abdomen. Most often, the gas collects in the colon. Abdominal distention is further increased by immobility, anesthetic agents, and the use of opioid medications.

After major abdominal surgery, distention may be avoided by having the patient turn frequently, exercise, and ambulate as early as possible. This also alleviates distention produced by swallowing air, which is common in anxious patients. A nasogastric tube inserted before surgery may remain in place until full peristaltic activity (indicated by the passage of flatus) has resumed. The nurse can determine when peristaltic bowel sounds return by listening to the abdomen with a stethoscope. Bowel sounds are documented so that diet progression can occur.

Paralytic ileus and intestinal obstruction are potential postoperative complications that occur more frequently in patients undergoing intestinal or abdominal surgery. Refer to Chapter 37 for discussion of treatment.

Promoting Bowel Function

Constipation is common after surgery and can range from a minor to a serious complication. Decreased mobility, decreased oral intake, and opioid analgesics contribute to difficulty having a bowel movement. In addition, irritation and trauma to the bowel during surgery may inhibit intestinal movement for several days. The combined effect of early ambulation, improved dietary intake, and a stool softener (if prescribed) promotes bowel elimination. Until the patient reports return of normal bowel function, the nurse should assess the abdomen for distention and the presence and frequency of bowel sounds. If the abdomen is not distended and bowel sounds are normal, and if the patient does not have a bowel movement by the second or third postoperative day, the physician should be notified so that a laxative can be given that evening.

Managing Voiding

Urinary retention after surgery can occur for various reasons. Anesthetics, anticholinergic agents, and opioids interfere with the perception of bladder fullness and the urge to void and inhibit the ability to initiate voiding and completely empty the bladder. Abdominal, pelvic, and hip surgery may increase the likelihood of retention secondary to pain. In addition, some patients find it difficult to use the bedpan or urinal in the recumbent position.

Bladder distention and the urge to void should be assessed at the time of the patient's arrival on the unit and frequently thereafter. The patient is expected to void within 8 hours after surgery (this includes time spent in the PACU). If the patient has an urge to void and cannot, or if the bladder is distended and no urge is felt or the patient cannot void, catheterization is not delayed solely on the basis of the 8-hour time frame. All methods to encourage the patient to void should be tried (eg, letting water run, applying heat to the perineum). The bedpan should be warm; a cold bedpan causes discomfort and automatic tightening of muscles (including the urethral sphincter). If the patient cannot void on a bedpan, it may be possible to use a commode rather than resorting to catheterization. Male patients are often permitted to sit up or stand beside the bed to use the urinal, but safeguards should be taken to prevent the patient from falling or fainting due to loss of coordination from medications or orthostatic hypotension. If the patient cannot void in the specified time frame, the patient is catheterized and the catheter is removed after the bladder has emptied. Straight intermittent catheterization is preferred over indwelling catheterization, because the risk of infection is increased with an indwelling catheter.

Even if the patient voids, the bladder may not necessarily be empty. The nurse notes the amount of urine voided and palpates the suprapubic area for distention or tenderness. A portable ultrasound device may also be used to assess residual volume. Intermittent catheterization may be prescribed every 4 to 6 hours until the patient can void spontaneously and the postvoid residual is less than 100 mL.

Maintaining a Safe Environment

During the immediate postoperative period, the patient recovering from anesthesia should have three side rails up, and the bed should be in the low position. The nurse assesses the patient's level of consciousness and orientation and determines whether the patient needs his or her eyeglasses or hearing aid, because impaired vision, inability to hear postoperative instructions, or inability to communicate verbally places the patient at risk for injury. All objects the patient may need should be within reach, especially the call light. Any immediate postoperative orders concerning special positioning, equipment, or interventions should be implemented as soon as possible. The patient is instructed to ask for assistance with any activity. Although restraints are occasionally necessary for the disoriented patient, they should be avoided if at all possible. Agency policy on the use of restraints must be consulted and followed.

Any surgical procedure has the potential for injury due to disrupted neurovascular integrity resulting from prolonged awkward positioning in the OR, manipulation of tissues, inadvertent severing of nerves, or tight bandages. Any orthopedic surgery or surgery involving the extremities carries a risk of peripheral nerve damage. Vascular surgeries, such as replacing sections of diseased peripheral arteries or inserting an arteriovenous graft, put the patient at risk for thrombus formation at the surgical site and subsequent ischemia of tissues distal to the thrombus. Assessment includes having the patient move the hand or foot distal to the surgical site through a full range of motion, assessing all surfaces for intact sensation, and assessing peripheral pulses (Rothrock, 2003).

Providing Emotional Support to the Patient and Family

Although patients and families are undoubtedly relieved that surgery is over, anxiety levels may remain high in the immediate postoperative period. Many factors contribute to this anxiety: pain, being in an unfamiliar environment, inability to control one's circumstances or care for oneself, fear of the long-term effects of surgery, fear of complications, fatigue, spiritual distress, altered role responsibilities, ineffective coping, and altered body image are all potential reactions to the surgical experience. The nurse helps the patient and family work through their anxieties by providing reassurance and information and by spending time listening to and addressing their concerns. The nurse describes hospital routines and what to expect in the ensuing hours and days until discharge and explains the purpose of nursing assessments and interventions. Informing patients when they will be able to drink fluids or eat, when they will be getting out of bed, and when tubes and drains will be removed helps them gain a sense of control and participation in recovery and engages them in the plan of care. Acknowledging family members' concerns and accepting and encouraging their participation in the patient's care assists them in feeling that they are helping their loved one. The nurse can modify the environment to enhance rest and relaxation by providing privacy, reducing noise, adjusting lighting, providing enough seating for family members, and encouraging a supportive atmosphere.

Managing Potential Complications

DEEP VEIN THROMBOSIS

Deep vein thrombosis and other complications, such as pulmonary embolism, are serious potential complications of surgery (Chart 20-5) (Defazio-Quinn & Schick, 2004). The stress response that is initiated by

CHART 20-5

Risk Factors for Postoperative Complications

DEEP VEIN THROMBOSIS

- Orthopedic patients having hip surgery, knee reconstruction, and other lower extremity surgery
- Urologic patients having transurethral prostatectomy and older patients having urologic surgery
- General surgical patients older than 40 years of age, those who are obese, those with a malignancy, those who have had prior deep vein thrombosis or pulmonary embolism, and those undergoing extensive, complicated surgical procedures
- Gynecologic (and obstetric) patients older than 40 years of age with added risk factors (varicose veins, previous venous thrombosis, infection, malignancy, obesity)
- Neurosurgical patients, similar to other surgical high-risk groups (in patients with stroke, for instance, the risk of deep vein thrombosis in the paralyzed leg is as high as 75%)

PULMONARY COMPLICATIONS

- Type of surgery—greater incidence after all forms of abdominal surgery when compared with peripheral surgery
- Location of incision—the closer the incision to the diaphragm, the higher the incidence of pulmonary complications
- Preoperative respiratory problems
- Age—greater risk after age 40 than before age 40
- Sepsis
- Obesity—weight greater than 110% of ideal body weight
- Prolonged bed rest
- Duration of surgical procedure—more than 3 hours
- Aspiration
- Dehydration
- Malnutrition
- Hypotension and shock
- Immunosuppression

surgery inhibits the fibrinolytic system, resulting in blood hypercoagulability. Dehydration, low cardiac output, blood pooling in the extremities, and bed rest add to the risk of thrombosis formation. Although all postoperative patients are at some risk, factors such as a history of thrombosis, malignancy, trauma, obesity, indwelling venous catheters, and hormone (eg, estrogen) use increase the risk (Farray, Carman & Fernandez, 2004). The first symptom of deep vein thrombosis may be a pain or cramp in the calf. Initial pain and tenderness may be followed by a painful swelling of the entire leg, often accompanied by a fever, chills, and diaphoresis.

Prophylactic treatment for postoperative patients at risk is common practice. Low-dose heparin may be prescribed and administered subcutaneously until the patient is ambulatory (Roper, Gress, Diringer, et al., 2004). Low-molecular-weight heparin and low-dose warfarin are other anticoagulants that may be used. External pneumatic compression and thigh-high elastic compression stockings can be used alone or in combination with low-dose heparin.

The benefits of early ambulation and hourly leg exercises in preventing deep vein thrombosis cannot be overemphasized, and these activities are recommended for all patients, regardless of their risk. It is important to avoid the use of blanket rolls, pillow rolls, or any form of elevation that can constrict vessels under the knees. Even prolonged "dangling" (having the patient sit on the edge of the bed with legs hanging over the side) can be dangerous and is not recommended in susceptible patients because pressure under the knees can impede circulation. Adequate hydration is also encouraged; the patient can be offered juices and water throughout the day to avoid dehydration. Refer to Chapter 30 for a complete discussion of deep vein thrombosis and to Chapter 23 for discussion of pulmonary embolus.

HEMATOMA

At times, concealed bleeding occurs beneath the skin at the surgical site. This hemorrhage usually stops spontaneously but results in clot (hematoma) formation within the wound. If the clot is small, it will be absorbed and need not be treated. If the clot is large, the wound usually bulges somewhat, and healing will be delayed unless the clot is removed. After several sutures are removed by the physician, the clot is evacuated and the wound is packed lightly with gauze. Healing occurs usually by granulation, or a secondary closure may be performed.

INFECTION (WOUND SEPSIS)

The creation of a surgical wound disrupts the integrity of the skin and its protective function. Exposure of deep body tissues to pathogens in the environment places the patient at risk for infection of the surgical site, a potentially life-threatening complication. Surgical site infection increases hospital length of stay, costs of care, and risk of further complications. In postoperative patients, surgical site infection is the most common nosocomial infection, with 67% of these infections occurring within the incision and 33% occurring in an organ or space around the surgical site. The administration of supplemental oxygen during colorectal resection and for 2 hours postoperatively has been shown to reduce the incidence of postoperative infection (Hopf, Hunt & Rosen, 2004).

Multiple factors place the patient at risk of wound infection. One risk factor relates to the type of wound. Surgical wounds are classified according to the degree of contamination. Table 20-4 defines the

TABLE 20-4 Wound Classification and Associated Surgical Site Infection Risk

Surgical Category	Determinants of Category	Expected Risk of Postsurgical Infection (%)
Clean	Nontraumatic site Uninfected site No inflammation No break in aseptic technique No entry into respiratory, alimentary, genitourinary, or oropharyngeal tracts	1–3
Clean-contaminated	Entry into respiratory, alimentary, genitourinary or oropharyngeal tracts without unusual contamination Appendectomy Minor break in aseptic technique Mechanical drainage	3–7
Contaminated	Open, newly experienced traumatic wounds Gross spillage from gastrointestinal tract Major break in aseptic technique Entry into genitourinary or biliary tract when urine or bile is infected	7–16
Dirty	Traumatic wound with delayed repair, devitalized tissue, foreign bodies, or fecal contamination Acute inflammation and purulent drainage encountered during procedure	16–29

terms used to describe surgical wounds and gives the expected rate of wound infection per category. Other risk factors include both patient-related factors and those associated with the surgical procedure. Patient-related factors include age, nutritional status, diabetes, smoking, obesity, remote infections, endogenous mucosal microorganisms, altered immune response, length of preoperative stay, and severity of illness (Defazio-Quinn & Schick, 2004; Worley, 2004). Factors related to the surgical procedure include the method of preoperative skin preparation, surgical attire of the team, method of sterile draping, duration of surgery, antimicrobial prophylaxis, aseptic technique, factors related to surgical technique, drains or foreign material, OR ventilation, length of procedure, and exogenous microorganisms. Efforts to prevent wound infection are directed at reducing these risks. Preoperative and intraoperative risks and interventions are discussed in Chapters 18 and 19. Although the conditions for surgical site infection and serious contamination of the wound occur in the preoperative and intraoperative time frames, postoperative care of the wound centers on assessing the wound, preventing contamination and infection before wound edges have sealed, and enhancing healing.

Wound infection may not be evident until at least postoperative day 5. Most patients are discharged before that time, and more than half of wound infections are diagnosed after discharge, highlighting the importance of patient education regarding wound care. Risk factors for wound sepsis include wound contamination, foreign body, faulty suturing technique, devitalized tissue, hematoma, debilitation, dehydration, malnutrition, anemia, advanced age, extreme obesity, shock, length of preoperative hospitalization, duration of surgical procedure, and associated disorders (eg, diabetes mellitus, immunosuppression). Signs and symptoms of wound infection include increased pulse rate and temperature; an elevated white blood cell count; wound swelling, warmth, tenderness, or discharge; and incisional pain. Local signs may be absent if the infection is deep. *Staphylococcus aureus* accounts for many postoperative wound infections. Other infections may result from *Escherichia coli, Proteus vulgaris, Aerobacter aerogenes, Pseudomonas aeruginosa,* and other organisms. Although they are rare, beta-hemolytic streptococcal or clostridial infections can be rapid and deadly. If wound infection due to beta-hemolytic streptococcus or clostridium occurs, strict infection control practices are needed to prevent the spread of infection to others. Intensive medical and nursing care is essential if the patient is to survive.

When a wound infection is diagnosed in a surgical incision, the surgeon may remove one or more sutures or staples and, using aseptic precautions, separate the wound edges with a pair of blunt scissors or a hemostat. Once the incision is opened, a drain is inserted. If the infection is deep, an incision and drainage procedure may be necessary. Antimicrobial therapy and a wound care regimen are also initiated.

WOUND DEHISCENCE AND EVISCERATION

Wound **dehiscence** (disruption of surgical incision or wound) and **evisceration** (protrusion of wound contents) are serious surgical complications (Fig. 20-8). Dehiscence and evisceration are especially serious when they involve abdominal incisions or wounds. These complications result from sutures giving way, from infection, or, more frequently, from marked distention or strenuous cough. They may also occur because of increasing age, poor nutritional status, or pulmonary or cardiovascular disease in patients undergoing abdominal surgery.

When the wound edges separate slowly, the intestines may protrude gradually or not at all, and the earliest sign may be a gush of bloody (serosanguineous) peritoneal fluid from the wound. When a wound ruptures suddenly, coils of intestine may push out of the abdomen. The patient may report that "something gave way." The evisceration causes pain and may be associated with vomiting.

An abdominal binder, properly applied, is an excellent prophylactic measure against an evisceration and often is used along with the primary dressing, especially in patients with weak or pendulous abdominal walls or when rupture of a wound has occurred.

Gerontologic Considerations

Elderly patients recover more slowly, have longer hospital stays, and are at greater risk for development of postoperative complications. Delirium, pneumonia, decline in functional ability, exacerbation

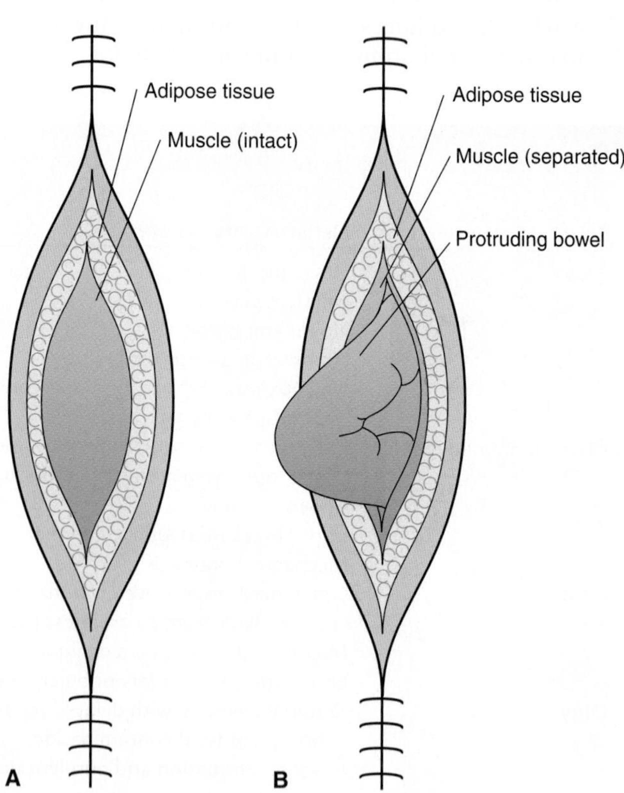

FIGURE 20-8. (**A**) Wound dehiscence; (**B**) wound evisceration.

of comorbid conditions, pressure ulcers, decreased oral intake, gastrointestinal disturbance, and falls are all threats to recovery in the older adult (Saufl, 2004). Expert nursing care can help the older adult avoid these complications or minimize their effects.

Postoperative delirium, characterized by confusion, perceptual and cognitive deficits, altered attention levels, disturbed sleep patterns, and impaired psychomotor skills, is a significant problem for older adults. Causes of delirium are multifactorial (Chart 20-6). Skilled and frequent assessment of mental status and of all physiologic factors influencing mental status helps the nurse plan care, because delirium may be the initial or only early indicator of infection, fluid and electrolyte imbalance, or deterioration of respiratory or hemodynamic status in the elderly patient. Factors that determine whether a patient is at risk for delirium include age, history of alcohol abuse, preoperative cognitive function, physical function, serum chemistries, and type of surgery.

Recognizing postoperative delirium and identifying and treating its underlying cause are the goals of care. Postoperative delirium is sometimes mistaken for preexisting dementia or is attributed to age. In addition to monitoring and managing identifiable causes, the nurse implements supportive interventions. Keeping the patient in a well-lit room and close to the nurses' station can help with sensory deprivation. At the same time, distracting and unfamiliar noises should be minimized. Because pain can contribute to postoperative delirium, adequate pain control is essential. The nurse collaborates with the physician or geriatric nurse specialist and the patient to achieve pain relief without oversedation (Barnett, 2003).

The patient is reoriented as often as necessary, and staff should introduce themselves each time they come in contact with the patient. Engaging the patient in conversation and care activities and placing a clock and calendar nearby may improve cognitive function. Physical activity should not be neglected while the patient is confused, because physical deterioration can worsen delirium and place the patient at increased risk for other complications. Restraints should be avoided, because they can also worsen confusion. If possible, a family member or staff member is asked to stay with the patient instead. Haloperidol (Haldol) or lorazepam (Ativan) may be administered during episodes of acute confusion, but these medications should be discontinued as soon as possible to avoid side effects.

Other problems confronting the elderly postoperative patient, such as pneumonia, altered bowel function, deep vein thrombosis, weakness, and functional decline, often can be prevented by early and progressive ambulation. Ambulation means walking, not just getting out of bed and sitting in a chair. Prolonged sitting positions that promote venous stasis in the lower extremities should be avoided. Assistance with ambulation may be required to keep the patient from bumping into objects and falling. A physical therapy referral may be indicated to promote safe, regular exercise for the older adult.

Urinary incontinence can be prevented by providing easy access to the call bell and the commode and by prompting voiding. Early ambulation and familiarity with the room help the patient to become self-sufficient sooner.

Optimal nutritional status is important for wound healing, return of normal bowel function, and fluid and electrolyte balance. The nurse and patient can consult with the dietitian to plan appealing, high-protein meals that provide sufficient fiber, calories, and vitamins. Nutritional supplements, such as Ensure or Sustacal, may be recommended. Multivitamins, iron, and vitamin C supplements aid in tissue healing, formation of new red blood cells, and overall nutritional status and are commonly prescribed postoperatively.

In addition to monitoring and managing physiologic recovery of the older adult, the nurse identifies and addresses psychosocial needs. The older adult may require much encouragement and support to resume activities, and the pace may be slow. Sensory deficits may require frequent repetition of instructions, and decreased physiologic reserve may necessitate frequent rest periods. The older adult may require extensive discharge planning to coordinate both professional and family care providers, and the nurse, social

CHART 20-6

Causes of Postoperative Delirium

- Acid–base disturbances
- Age greater than 80 years
- Fluid and electrolyte imbalance
- Dehydration
- History of dementia-like symptoms
- Hypoxia
- Hypercarbia
- Infection (urinary tract, wound, respiratory)
- Medications (anticholinergics, benzodiazepines, central nervous system depressants)
- Unrelieved pain
- Blood loss
- Decreased cardiac output
- Cerebral hypoxia
- Heart failure
- Acute myocardial infarction
- Hypothermia or hyperthermia
- Unfamiliar surroundings and sensory deprivation
- Emergent surgery
- Alcohol withdrawal
- Urinary retention
- Fecal impaction
- Polypharmacy
- Presence of multiple diseases
- Sensory impairments
- High stress or anxiety levels

worker, or nurse case manager may institute the plan for continuing care.

Promoting Home and Community-Based Care

TEACHING PATIENTS SELF-CARE

Patients have always required detailed discharge instructions to become proficient in special self-care needs after surgery; however, dramatically reduced hospital lengths of stay during the past decade have greatly increased the amount of information needed while reducing the amount of time in which to provide it. Although needs are specific to individual patients and the procedures they have undergone, general patient education needs for postoperative care have been identified (see Chart 20-2).

CONTINUING CARE

Continuing care provided by community-based services is frequently necessary after surgery. Older patients, patients who live alone, patients without family support, and patients with preexisting chronic illness or disabilities are often in greatest need. Planning for discharge involves arranging for necessary services early in the acute care hospitalization. Wound care, drain management, catheter care, infusion therapy, and physical or occupational therapy are some of the needs addressed by community-based health care providers. The home care nurse coordinates these activities and services.

During home care visits, the nurse assesses the patient for postoperative complications; the nurse also assesses the surgical incision, respiratory and cardiovascular status, adequacy of pain management, fluid and nutritional status, and the patient's progress in returning to preoperative status. The nurse assesses the patient's and family's ability to manage dressing changes and drainage systems and other devices and to administer prescribed medications. The nurse may change dressings or catheters if needed. The nurse determines whether any additional services are needed and assists the patient and family to arrange for them. Previous teaching is reinforced, and the patient is reminded to keep follow-up appointments. The patient and family are instructed about signs and symptoms to be reported to the surgeon. In addition, the nurse provides information about how to obtain needed supplies and suggests resources or support groups the patient may want to contact. In many settings, postoperative telephone calls are made to answer questions, assess recovery, and reassure patients and families.

Evaluation

Expected Patient Outcomes

Expected patient outcomes may include the following:

1. Maintains optimal respiratory function
   a. Performs deep-breathing exercises
   b. Displays clear breath sounds
   c. Uses incentive spirometer as prescribed
   d. Splints incisional site when coughing to reduce pain
2. Indicates that pain is decreased in intensity
3. Increases activity as prescribed
   a. Alternates periods of rest and activity
   b. Progressively increases ambulation
   c. Resumes normal activities within prescribed time frame
   d. Performs activities related to self-care
4. Wound heals without complication
5. Maintains body temperature within normal limits
6. Resumes oral intake
   a. Reports absence of nausea and vomiting
   b. Eats at least 75% of usual diet
   c. Is free of abdominal distress and gas pains
   d. Exhibits normal bowel sounds
7. Reports resumption of usual bowel elimination pattern
8. Resumes usual voiding pattern
9. Is free of injury
10. Exhibits decreased anxiety
11. Acquires knowledge and skills necessary to manage therapeutic regimen
12. Experiences no complications

Critical Thinking Exercises

1 A 35-year-old woman who has had a right-sided mastectomy for cancer is admitted to the phase II PACU. Identify what information is essential to obtain during report from the OR, describe the Aldrete scoring system, and explain how you will know when the patient is ready to be discharged from the PACU.

2 A frail 75-year-old man, who was brought in to the emergency department last night, has undergone an appendectomy. How would you direct your assessment to identify the factors that might affect his recovery? How would you prioritize his care needs, and what complications would you anticipate? Create a nursing care plan for this patient that addresses discharge to home in the next 24 hours.

3 ebp An obese woman is admitted to the PACU after knee surgery, and she is complaining of nausea. What resources would you use to identify the current guidelines for treatment of PONV? What is the evidence base for PONV management practices? Identify the criteria used to evaluate the strength of the evidence for these practices.

4 ebp A 45-year-old patient who is a smoker is admitted to the postoperative nursing unit after abdominal surgery and is complaining of severe pain. Develop an evidence-based plan of care for this patient, addressing priorities from admission to the unit until discharge to home.

REFERENCES AND SELECTED READINGS

BOOKS

American Society of PeriAnesthesia Nurses. (2002). *Standards of perianesthesia nursing practice.* Thorofare, NJ: ASPAN.

Clancy, J., McVicar, A. J. & Baird, N. (2002). *Perioperative practice: Fundamentals of homeostasis.* New York: Routledge.

Conner, R. (2004). *Ambulatory surgery principles and practices* (3rd ed.). Denver: AORN.

Defazio-Quinn, D. & Schick, L. (Eds.). (2004). *Nursing core curriculum: Preoperative, phase I and phase II PACU nursing.* Philadelphia: W. B. Saunders.

Dudek, S. G. (2006). *Nutrition essentials for nursing practice* (5th ed.). Philadelphia: Lippincott Williams & Wilkins.

Kost, M. (2004). *Moderate sedations/analgesia: Core competencies for practice.* Philadelphia: W. B. Saunders.

Miller, R. D. (2005) *Miller's anesthesia* (6th ed.). Philadelphia: Elsevier.

Morton, P. G., Fontaine, D. K., Hudak, C. M., et al. (2005). *Critical care nursing: A holistic approach* (8th ed.). Philadelphia: Lippincott Williams & Wilkins.

Murray, M. J., Coursin, D. B., Pearl, R. G., et al. (2002). *Critical care medicine: Perioperative management* (2nd ed.). Philadelphia: Lippincott Williams & Wilkins.

Phillips, N. (2004). *Berry and Kohn's operating room technique* (10th ed.). St. Louis: Mosby.

Roper, A. H., Gress, D., Diringer, M. N., et al. (2004). *Neurological and neurosurgical intensive care* (4th ed.). Philadelphia: Lippincott Williams & Wilkins.

Rothrock, J. C. (Ed.). (2003). *Alexander's care of the patient in surgery* (12th ed.). St. Louis: Mosby.

Seifert, P. C. (2002). *Cardiac surgery: Perioperative patient care.* St Louis: Mosby.

Zonderman, J. & Doyle, R. (2006). *Springhouse nurse's drug guide 2006.* Philadelphia: Lippincott Williams & Wilkins.

JOURNALS

**Asterisks indicate nursing research articles.*

Aldrete, A. & Wright, A. (1992). Revised Aldrete score for discharge. *Anesthesiology News, 18*(1), 17.

Barnett, R. & Ochroch, E. (2004). Epidural analgesia: Management and outcomes. *Annals of Long-Term Care, 11*(11), 33–38.

Barnett, S. (2003). Acute pain in the elderly surgical patient. *Clinical Geriatrics, 11*(9), 30–35.

*Bezanson, J. L., Weaver, M., Kinney, M., et al. (2004). Presurgical risk factors for late extubation in Medicare recipients after cardiac surgery. *Nursing Research, 53*(1), 46–52.

Block, B. M., Liu, S. S., Rowlingson, A. J., et al. (2003). Efficacy of postoperative epidural analgesia. *Journal of the American Medical Association, 290*(18), 2455–2463.

Cofer, M. J. (2005). Unwelcome companion to older patients: Postoperative delirium. *Nursing, 35*(1), 32hn1–32hn3.

Creekmore, F., Lugo, R. A., & Weiland, K. J. (2004). Postoperative opiate analgesic requirements of smokers and nonsmokers. *Annals of Pharmacotherapy, 38*(4), 949–953.

DeFazio-Quinn, D. M. (2006). How religion, language and ethnicity impact perioperative nursing care. *Nursing Clinics of North America, 41*(2), 231–248.

Farray, D., Carman, T. L. & Fernandez, B. B. (2004). The treatment and prevention of deep vein thrombosis in the preoperative management of patients who have neurologic diseases. *Neurologic Clinics of North America, 22*(2), 423–439.

Gan, T., Meyer, T., Apfel, C., et al. (2003). Consensus guidelines for managing postoperative nausea and vomiting. *Anesthesia and Analgesia, 97*(1), 62–71.

Happ, M. B., Roesch, T. & Kagan, S. (2004). Communication needs, methods and perceived voice quality following head and neck surgery: A literature review. *Cancer Nursing, 27*(1), 1–9.

Hogan, S. L. (2004). How to help wounds heal. *RN, 67*(8), 26–31.

Holmes, C. L. & Walley, K. R. (2003). The evaluation and management of shock. *Clinics in Chest Medicine, 24*(4), 775–789.

Hopf, H., Hunt, T. & Rosen, N. (2004). Supplemental oxygen and risk of surgical site infection. *Journal of the American Medical Association, 291*(1), 79–87.

*Ikonomidou, E., Rehnstrom, A., Naesh, O., et al. (2004). Effect of music on vital signs and postoperative pain. *AORN Journal, 80*(2), 269–278.

Letizia, M., O'Leary, J. & Vodvarka, J. (2003). Laryngeal edema: Perioperative nursing considerations. *MedSurg Nursing, 12*(2), 111–115.

McCarthy, E. (2004). Malignant hyperthermia. *AACN Clinical Issues, 15*(2), 231–237.

*McDonald, D. D. & Molony, S. L. (2004). Postoperative pain communication skills for older adults. *Western Journal of Nursing Research, 25*(8), 836–852.

*McRee, L., Noble, S. & Pasvogel, A. (2003). Using massage and music therapy to improve postoperative outcomes. *AORN Journal, 78*(3), 433–447.

Milgrom, L. B., Brooks, J. A., Qi, R., et al. (2004). Pain levels experienced with activities after cardiac surgery. *American Journal of Critical Care, 13*(2), 116–125.

Moline, B. M. (2001). Pain management in the ambulatory surgical population. *Journal of Perianesthesia Nursing, 16*(6), 388–398.

Nair, S. & Podichetty, V. K. (2004). The preoperative and postoperative assessment and care of patients with back pain. *Neurologic Clinics of North America, 22*(2), 441–456.

*Oetker-Black, S. L., Jones, S., Estok, P., et al. (2003). Preoperative teaching and hysterectomy outcomes. *AORN Journal, 77*(6), 1215–1231.

Pasero, C. (2003). Epidural analgesia for postoperative pain. *American Journal of Nursing, 103*(10), 62–65.

Saufl, N. M. (2004). Preparing the older adult for surgery and anesthesia. *Journal of Perianesthesia Nursing, 19*(6), 372–377.

Taylor, A., Galper, D., Taylor, P., et al. (2003). Effects of adjunctive Swedish massage and vibration therapy on short-term postoperative outcomes: A randomized, controlled trial. *Journal of Alternative and Complementary Medicine, 9*(1), 77–89.

Wadlund, D. L. (2006). Prevention, recognition, and management of nursing complications in the intraoperative and postoperative surgical patient. *Nursing Clinics of North America, 41*(2), 151–171.

Worley, C. (2004). "Why won't this wound heal?" Factors affecting wound healing. *Dermatology Nursing, 16*(4), 360–362.

*Yellen, E. (2003). The influence of nurse-sensitive variables on patient satisfaction. *AORN Journal, 78*(5), 783–793.

*Zalon, M. L. (2004). Correlates of recovery among older adults after major abdominal surgery. *Nursing Research, 53*(2), 99–106.

RESOURCES

American Academy of Ambulatory Care Nursing, East Holly Ave., Box 56, Pitman, NJ, 08071; 856-256-2350 or 800-AMB-NURS; http://www.aacn.org. Accessed March 31, 2006.

American Society of PeriAnesthesia Nurses, 10 Melrose Ave., Suite 110, Cherry Hill, NJ 08003; 856-616-9600 or -9601; toll-free 877-737-9696; fax 856-616-9621; http://www.aspan.org. Accessed March 31, 2006.

Association of PeriOperative Registered Nurses, Inc., 2170 S. Parker Road, Suite 300, Denver, CO 80231; 800-755-2676 or 303-755-6304; http://www.aorn.org. Accessed March 31, 2006.

Centers for Disease Control and Prevention, Surgical Site Infection Guideline, Division of Healthcare Quality Promotion, National Center for Infectious Diseases, Atlanta, GA 30333; 404-639-3534 or 800-311-3435; http://www.cdc.gov/ncidod/dhqp/gl_surgicalsite.html. Accessed March 31, 2006.

Malignant Hyperthermia Association of the United States (MHAUS), 39 East State Street, P.O. Box 1069, Sherburne, NY 13460; 607-674-7901; http://www.mhaus.org. Accessed March 31, 2006.

UNIT 5

Gas Exchange and Respiratory Function

Case Study

Applying Concepts from NANDA, NIC, and NOC

A Patient With Impaired Cough Reflex

Mrs. Lewis, age 77 years, is admitted to the hospital for left lower lobe pneumonia. Her vital signs are: Temp 100.6°F; HR 90 and regular; B/P: 142/74; Resp 28. She has a weak cough, diminished breath sounds over the lower left lung field, and coarse rhonchi over the midtracheal area. She can expectorate some sputum, which is thick and grayish-green. She has a history of stroke. Secondary to the stroke she has impaired gag and cough reflexes and mild weakness of her left side. She is allowed food and fluids because she can swallow safely if she uses the chin-tuck maneuver.

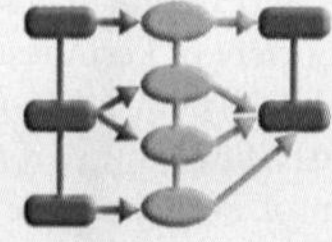

Turn to Appendix C to see a concept map that illustrates the relationships that exist between the nursing diagnoses, interventions, and outcomes for the patient's clinical problems.

Nursing Classifications and Languages

NANDA Nursing Diagnoses	NIC Nursing Interventions	NOC Nursing Outcomes Return to functional baseline status, stabilization of, or improvement in:
Ineffective Airway Clearance—Inability to clear secretions or obstructions from the respiratory tract to maintain a clear airway	**Respiratory Monitoring**—Collection and analysis of patient data to ensure airway patency and adequate gas exchange	**Respiratory Status: Airway Patency**—Extent to which the tracheobronchial passages remain open
Impaired Gas Exchange—Excess or deficit in oxygenation and/or carbon dioxide elimination at the alveolar-capillary membrane	**Airway Management**—Facilitation of patency of air passages	**Respiratory Status: Gas Exchange**—The alveolar exchange of O_2 and CO_2 to maintain arterial blood gas concentrations
Ineffective Breathing Pattern—Inspiration and/or expiration that does not provide adequate ventilation	**Cough Enhancement**—Promotion of deep inhalation by the patient with subsequent generation of high intrathoracic pressures and compression of underlying lung parenchyma for the forceful expulsion of air	**Respiratory Status: Ventilation**—Movement of air in and out of the lungs
Risk for Aspiration—At risk for entry of gastrointestinal secretions, oropharyngeal secretions, solids, or fluids into tracheobronchial passages	**Airway Suctioning**—Removal of airway secretions by inserting a suction catheter into the patient's oral airway and/or trachea	
	Aspiration Precautions—Prevention or minimization of risk factors in the patient at risk for aspiration	

NANDA International (2005). *Nursing diagnoses: Definitions & classification 2005–2006.* Philadelphia: North American Nursing Diagnosis Association.
Dochterman, J. M. & Bulechek, G. M. (2004). *Nursing interventions classification (NIC)* (4th ed.). St. Louis: Mosby.
Iowa Outcomes Project (2004). In Moorhead, S., Johnson, M. & Maas, M. (2004). *Nursing outcomes classification (NOC)* (3rd ed.). St. Louis: Mosby.
Dochterman, J. M. & Jones, D. A. (2003). *Unifying nursing languages: The harmonization of NANDA, NIC, and NOC.* Washington, D.C.: American Nurses Association.

CHAPTER 21

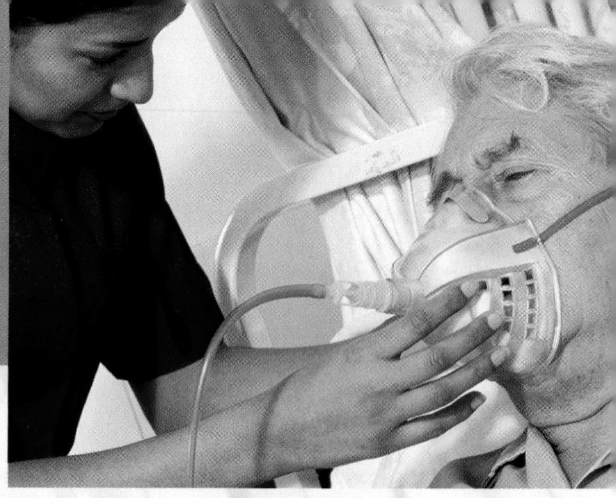

Assessment of Respiratory Function

Learning Objectives

On completion of this chapter, the learner will be able to:

1. Describe the structures and functions of the upper and lower respiratory tracts.
2. Describe ventilation, perfusion, diffusion, shunting, and the relationship of pulmonary circulation to these processes.
3. Discriminate between normal and abnormal breath sounds.
4. Use assessment parameters appropriate for determining the characteristics and severity of the major symptoms of respiratory dysfunction.
5. Identify the nursing implications of the various procedures used for diagnostic evaluation of respiratory function.

Disorders of the respiratory system are common and are encountered by nurses in every setting from the community to the intensive care unit. To assess the respiratory system, the nurse must be skilled at differentiating between normal and abnormal assessment findings. Expert assessment skills must be developed and used when caring for patients with acute and chronic respiratory problems. In addition, an understanding of respiratory function and the significance of abnormal diagnostic test results is essential.

Anatomic and Physiologic Overview

The respiratory system is composed of the upper and lower respiratory tracts. Together, the two tracts are responsible for **ventilation** (movement of air in and out of the airways). The upper tract, known as the upper airway, warms and filters inspired air so that the lower respiratory tract (the lungs) can accomplish gas exchange. Gas exchange involves delivering oxygen to the tissues through the bloodstream and expelling waste gases, such as carbon dioxide, during expiration. The respiratory system works in concert with the cardiovascular system; the respiratory system is responsible for ventilation and diffusion, and the cardiovascular system is responsible for perfusion (Farquhar & Fantasia, 2005).

Anatomy of the Upper Respiratory Tract

Upper airway structures consist of the nose, sinuses and nasal passages, pharynx, tonsils and adenoids, larynx, and trachea.

Nose

The nose is composed of an external and an internal portion. The external portion protrudes from the face and is supported by the nasal bones and cartilage. The anterior nares (nostrils) are the external openings of the nasal cavities.

The internal portion of the nose is a hollow cavity separated into the right and left nasal cavities by a narrow vertical divider, the septum. Each nasal cavity is divided into three passageways by the projection of the turbinates (also called conchae) from the lateral walls. The nasal cavities are lined with highly vascular ciliated mucous membranes called the nasal mucosa. Mucus, secreted continuously by goblet cells, covers the surface of the nasal mucosa and is moved back to the nasopharynx by the action of the **cilia** (fine hairs).

The nose serves as a passageway for air to pass to and from the lungs. It filters impurities and humidifies and warms the air as it is inhaled. It is responsible for olfaction (smell) because the olfactory receptors are located in the nasal mucosa. This function diminishes with age.

Paranasal Sinuses

The paranasal sinuses include four pairs of bony cavities that are lined with nasal mucosa and ciliated pseudostratified columnar epithelium. These air spaces are connected by a series of ducts that drain into the nasal cavity. The sinuses are named by their location: frontal, ethmoidal, sphenoidal, and maxillary (Fig. 21-1). A prominent function of the sinuses is to serve as a resonating chamber in speech. The sinuses are a common site of infection.

Turbinate Bones (Conchae)

The turbinate bones are also called conchae (the name suggested by their shell-like appearance). Because of their curves, these bones increase the mucous membrane surface of the nasal passages and slightly obstruct the air flowing through them (Fig. 21-2).

Air entering the nostrils is deflected upward to the roof of the nose, and it follows a circuitous route before it reaches the nasopharynx. It comes into contact with a large surface of moist, warm mucous membrane that traps practically all the dust and organisms in the inhaled air. The air is moistened, warmed to body temperature, and brought into contact with sensitive nerves. Some of these nerves detect odors; others provoke sneezing to expel irritating dust.

Glossary

bronchoscopy: direct examination of larynx, trachea, and bronchi using an endoscope

cilia: short hairs that provide a constant whipping motion that serves to propel mucus and foreign substances away from the lung toward the larynx

crackles: soft, high-pitched, discontinuous popping sounds during inspiration caused by delayed reopening of the airways

diffusion: exchange of gas molecules from areas of high concentration to areas of low concentration

dyspnea: labored breathing or shortness of breath

hemoptysis: expectoration of blood from the respiratory tract

hypoxemia: decrease in arterial oxygen tension in the blood

hypoxia: decrease in oxygen supply to the tissues and cells

orthopnea: inability to breathe easily except in an upright position

physiologic dead space: portion of the tracheobronchial tree that does not participate in gas exchange

pulmonary perfusion: blood flow through the pulmonary vasculature

respiration: gas exchange between atmospheric air and the blood and between the blood and cells of the body

ventilation: movement of air in and out of airways

wheezes: continuous musical sounds associated with airway narrowing or partial obstruction

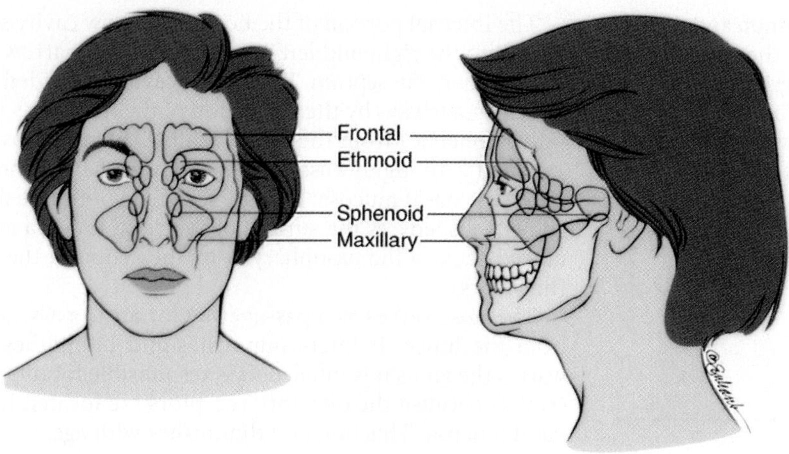

FIGURE 21-1. The paranasal sinuses.

Pharynx, Tonsils, and Adenoids

The pharynx, or throat, is a tubelike structure that connects the nasal and oral cavities to the larynx. It is divided into three regions: nasal, oral, and laryngeal. The nasopharynx is located posterior to the nose and above the soft palate. The oropharynx houses the faucial, or palatine, tonsils. The laryngopharynx extends from the hyoid bone to the cricoid cartilage. The epiglottis forms the entrance to the larynx.

The adenoids, or pharyngeal tonsils, are located in the roof of the nasopharynx. The tonsils, the adenoids, and other lymphoid tissue encircle the throat. These structures are important links in the chain of lymph nodes guarding the body from invasion by organisms entering the nose and the throat. The pharynx functions as a passageway for the respiratory and digestive tracts.

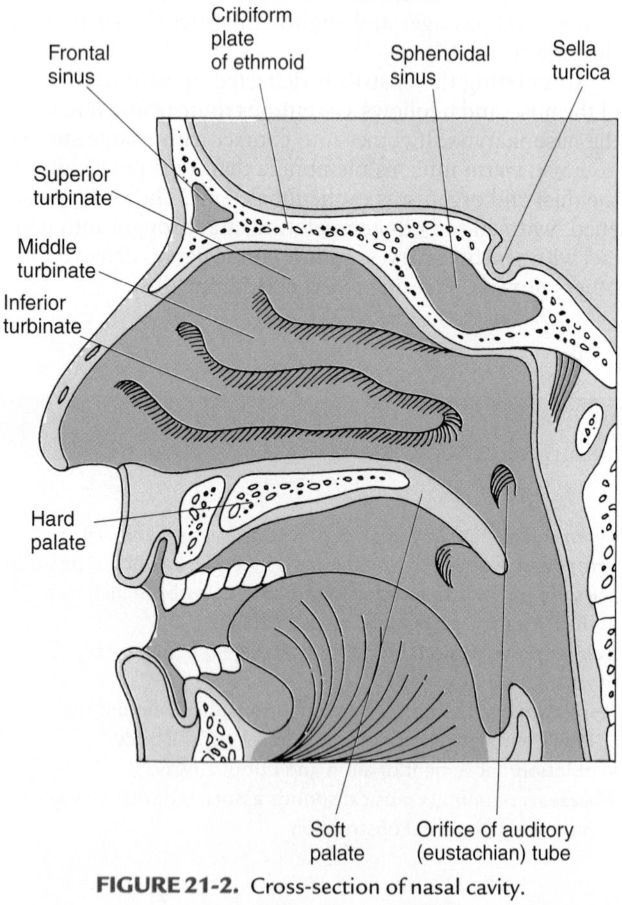

Cribiform plate of ethmoid
Frontal sinus
Sphenoidal sinus
Sella turcica
Superior turbinate
Middle turbinate
Inferior turbinate
Hard palate
Soft palate
Orifice of auditory (eustachian) tube

FIGURE 21-2. Cross-section of nasal cavity.

Larynx

The larynx, or voice organ, is a cartilaginous epithelium-lined structure that connects the pharynx and the trachea. The major function of the larynx is vocalization. It also protects the lower airway from foreign substances and facilitates coughing. It is frequently referred to as the voice box and consists of the following:

- Epiglottis—a valve flap of cartilage that covers the opening to the larynx during swallowing
- Glottis—the opening between the vocal cords in the larynx
- Thyroid cartilage—the largest of the cartilage structures; part of it forms the Adam's apple
- Cricoid cartilage—the only complete cartilaginous ring in the larynx (located below the thyroid cartilage)
- Arytenoid cartilages—used in vocal cord movement with the thyroid cartilage
- Vocal cords—ligaments controlled by muscular movements that produce sounds; located in the lumen of the larynx

Trachea

The trachea, or windpipe, is composed of smooth muscle with C-shaped rings of cartilage at regular intervals. The cartilaginous rings are incomplete on the posterior surface and give firmness to the wall of the trachea, preventing it from collapsing. The trachea serves as the passage between the larynx and the bronchi.

Anatomy of the Lower Respiratory Tract

The lower respiratory tract consists of the lungs, which contain the bronchial and alveolar structures needed for gas exchange.

Lungs

The lungs are paired elastic structures enclosed in the thoracic cage, which is an airtight chamber with distensible walls (Fig. 21-3). Ventilation requires movement of the walls of the thoracic cage and of its floor, the diaphragm. The effect of these movements is alternately to increase and decrease the capacity of the chest. When the capacity of the chest is increased, air enters through the trachea (inspiration) because of the lowered pressure within and inflates the lungs. When the chest wall and diaphragm return to their previous positions (expiration), the lungs recoil and force the air out through the bronchi and trachea. Inspiration occurs during the first third of the respiratory cycle, expiration during the latter two thirds. The inspiratory phase of respiration normally requires energy; the expiratory phase is normally passive requiring very little energy. In respiratory diseases, such as chronic obstructive pulmonary disease (COPD), expiration requires energy.

PLEURA

The lungs and wall of the thorax are lined with a serous membrane called the pleura. The visceral pleura covers the lungs; the parietal pleura lines the thorax. The visceral and parietal pleura and the small amount of pleural fluid between these two membranes serve to lubricate the thorax and lungs and permit smooth motion of the lungs within the thoracic cavity with each breath.

MEDIASTINUM

The mediastinum is in the middle of the thorax, between the pleural sacs that contain the two lungs. It extends from the sternum to the vertebral column and contains all the thoracic tissue outside the lungs.

LOBES

Each lung is divided into lobes. The left lung consists of an upper and lower lobe, whereas the right lung has an upper, middle, and lower lobe (Fig. 21-4). Each lobe is further

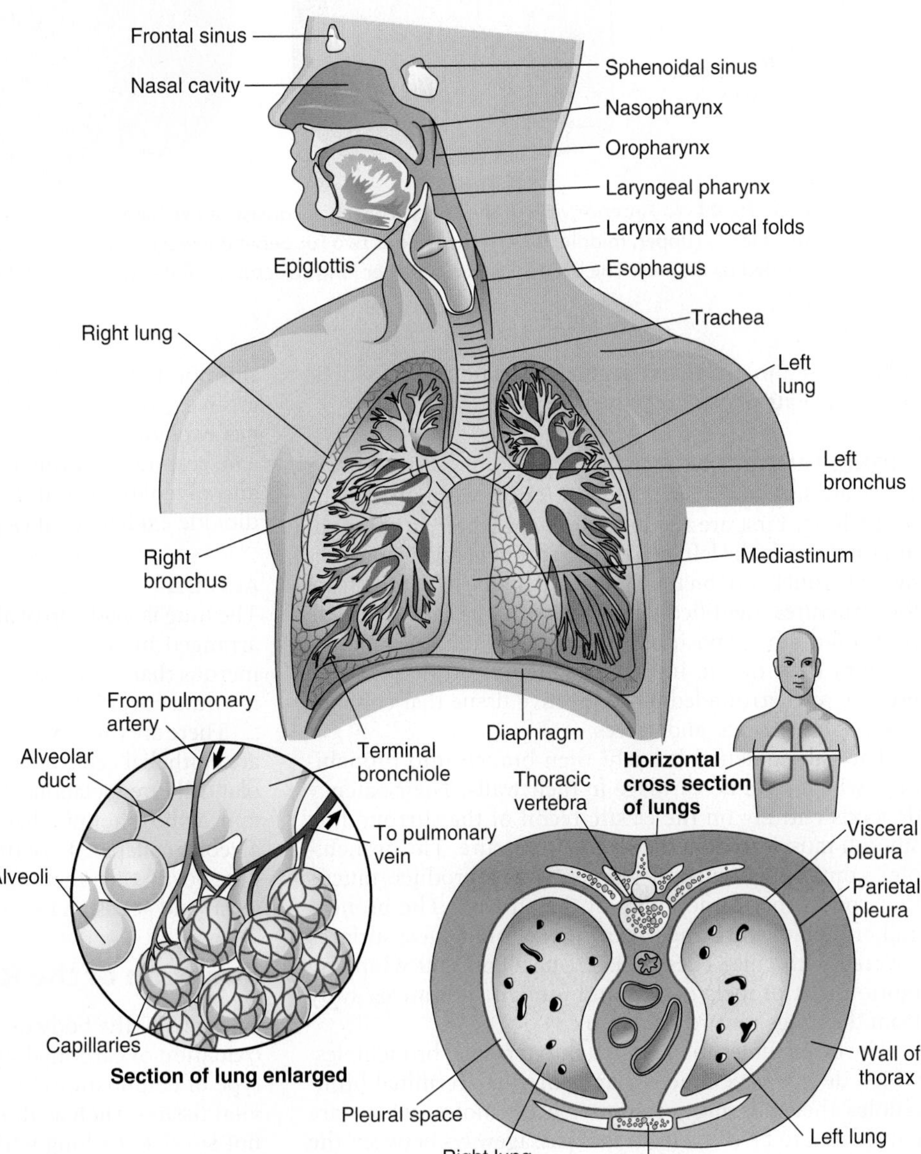

FIGURE 21-3. The respiratory system; upper respiratory structures and the structures of the thorax (*top*); alveoli and a horizontal cross section of the lungs (*bottom*).

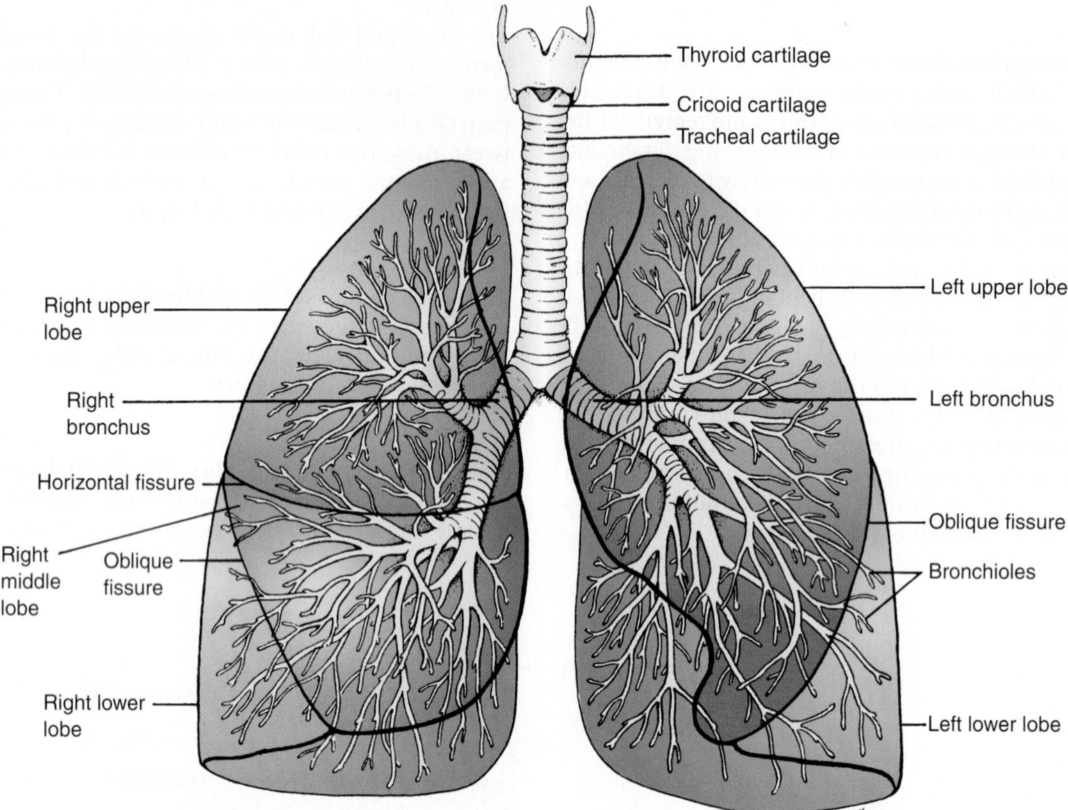

FIGURE 21-4. Anterior view of the lungs. The lungs consist of five lobes. The right lung has three lobes (upper, middle, lower); the left has two (upper and lower). The lobes are further subdivided by fissures. The bronchial tree, another lung structure, inflates with air to fill the lobes.

subdivided into two to five segments separated by fissures, which are extensions of the pleura.

BRONCHI AND BRONCHIOLES

There are several divisions of the bronchi within each lobe of the lung. First are the lobar bronchi (three in the right lung and two in the left lung). Lobar bronchi divide into segmental bronchi (10 on the right and 8 on the left), which are the structures identified when choosing the most effective postural drainage position for a given patient. Segmental bronchi then divide into subsegmental bronchi. These bronchi are surrounded by connective tissue that contains arteries, lymphatics, and nerves.

The subsegmental bronchi then branch into bronchioles, which have no cartilage in their walls. Their patency depends entirely on the elastic recoil of the surrounding smooth muscle and on the alveolar pressure. The bronchioles contain submucosal glands, which produce mucus that covers the inside lining of the airways. The bronchi and bronchioles are lined also with cells that have surfaces covered with cilia. These cilia create a constant whipping motion that propels mucus and foreign substances away from the lungs toward the larynx.

The bronchioles then branch into terminal bronchioles, which do not have mucus glands or cilia. Terminal bronchioles then become respiratory bronchioles, which are considered to be the transitional passageways between the conducting airways and the gas exchange airways. Up to this point, the conducting airways contain about 150 mL of air in the tracheobronchial tree that does not participate in gas exchange. This is known as **physiologic dead space.** The respiratory bronchioles then lead into alveolar ducts and alveolar sacs and then alveoli. Oxygen and carbon dioxide exchange takes place in the alveoli.

ALVEOLI

The lung is made up of about 300 million alveoli, which are arranged in clusters of 15 to 20. These alveoli are so numerous that if their surfaces were united to form one sheet, it would cover 70 square meters—the size of a tennis court.

There are three types of alveolar cells. Type I alveolar cells are epithelial cells that form the alveolar walls. Type II alveolar cells are metabolically active. These cells secrete surfactant, a phospholipid that lines the inner surface and prevents alveolar collapse. Type III alveolar cell macrophages are large phagocytic cells that ingest foreign matter (eg, mucus, bacteria) and act as an important defense mechanism.

Function of the Respiratory System

The cells of the body derive the energy they need from the oxidation of carbohydrates, fats, and proteins. As with any type of combustion, this process requires oxygen. Certain vital tissues, such as those of the brain and the heart, cannot survive for long without a continuous supply of oxygen. However, as a result of oxidation in the body tissues, carbon dioxide is produced and must be removed from the cells to prevent the buildup of acid waste products. The respiratory system performs this function by facilitating life-sustaining processes such as oxygen transport, respiration and ventilation, and gas exchange.

Oxygen Transport

Oxygen is supplied to, and carbon dioxide is removed from, cells by way of the circulating blood. Cells are in close contact with capillaries, the thin walls of which permit easy passage or exchange of oxygen and carbon dioxide. Oxygen diffuses from the capillary through the capillary wall to the interstitial fluid. At this point, it diffuses through the membrane of tissue cells, where it is used by mitochondria for cellular respiration. The movement of carbon dioxide occurs by diffusion in the opposite direction—from cell to blood.

Respiration

After these tissue capillary exchanges, blood enters the systemic veins (where it is called venous blood) and travels to the pulmonary circulation. The oxygen concentration in blood within the capillaries of the lungs is lower than in the lungs' air sacs (alveoli). Because of this concentration gradient, oxygen diffuses from the alveoli to the blood. Carbon dioxide, which has a higher concentration in the blood than in the alveoli, diffuses from the blood into the alveoli. Movement of air in and out of the airways (ventilation) continually replenishes the oxygen and removes the carbon dioxide from the airways and lungs. This whole process of gas exchange between the atmospheric air and the blood and between the blood and cells of the body is called **respiration.**

Ventilation

During inspiration, air flows from the environment into the trachea, bronchi, bronchioles, and alveoli. During expiration, alveolar gas travels the same route in reverse.

Physical factors that govern air flow in and out of the lungs are collectively referred to as the mechanics of ventilation and include air pressure variances, resistance to air flow, and lung compliance.

AIR PRESSURE VARIANCES

Air flows from a region of higher pressure to a region of lower pressure. During inspiration, movement of the diaphragm and other muscles of respiration enlarges the thoracic cavity and thereby lowers the pressure inside the thorax to a level below that of atmospheric pressure. As a result, air is drawn through the trachea and bronchi into the alveoli. During expiration, the diaphragm relaxes and the lungs recoil, resulting in a decrease in the size of the thoracic cavity. The alveolar pressure then exceeds atmospheric pressure, and air flows from the lungs into the atmosphere.

AIRWAY RESISTANCE

Resistance is determined chiefly by the radius or size of the airway through which the air is flowing. Any process that changes the bronchial diameter or width affects airway resistance and alters the rate of air flow for a given pressure gradient during respiration (Chart 21-1). With increased resistance, greater-than-normal respiratory effort is required to achieve normal levels of ventilation.

CHART 21-1

Causes of Increased Airway Resistance

Common phenomena that may alter bronchial diameter, which affects airway resistance, include the following:

- Contraction of bronchial smooth muscle—as in asthma
- Thickening of bronchial mucosa—as in chronic bronchitis
- Obstruction of the airway—by mucus, a tumor, or a foreign body
- Loss of lung elasticity—as in emphysema, which is characterized by connective tissue encircling the airways, thereby keeping them open during both inspiration and expiration

COMPLIANCE

The pressure gradient between the thoracic cavity and the atmosphere causes air to flow in and out of the lungs. When pressure changes occur in the normal lung, there is a proportional change in the lung volume. A measure of the elasticity, expandability, and distensibility of the lungs and thoracic structures is called compliance. Factors that determine lung compliance are the surface tension of the alveoli (normally low with the presence of surfactant) and the connective tissue (ie, collagen and elastin) of the lungs.

Compliance is determined by examining the volume–pressure relationship in the lungs and the thorax. Compliance is normal (1.0 L/cm H_2O) if the lungs and thorax easily stretch and distend when pressure is applied. High or increased compliance occurs if the lungs have lost their elasticity and the thorax is overdistended (ie, in emphysema). Low or decreased compliance occurs if the lungs and thorax are "stiff." Conditions associated with decreased compliance include pneumothorax, hemothorax, pleural effusion, pulmonary edema, atelectasis, pulmonary fibrosis, and acute respiratory distress syndrome (ARDS), all of which are discussed in later chapters in this unit. Measurement of compliance is one method used to assess the progression and improvement in patients with ARDS. Lungs with decreased compliance require greater-than-normal energy expenditure by the patient to achieve normal levels of ventilation. Compliance is usually measured under static conditions.

Lung Volumes and Capacities

Lung function, which reflects the mechanics of ventilation, is viewed in terms of lung volumes and lung capacities. Lung volumes are categorized as tidal volume, inspiratory reserve volume, expiratory reserve volume, and residual volume. Lung capacity is evaluated in terms of vital capacity, inspiratory capacity, functional residual capacity, and total lung capacity. These terms are described in Table 21-1.

Diffusion and Perfusion

Diffusion is the process by which oxygen and carbon dioxide are exchanged at the air–blood interface. The alveolar–

TABLE 21-1 Lung Volumes and Lung Capacities

Term	Symbol	Description	Normal Value*	Significance
Lung Volumes				
Tidal volume	VT or TV	The volume of air inhaled and exhaled with each breath	500 mL or 5–10 mL/kg	The tidal volume may not vary, even with severe disease.
Inspiratory reserve volume	IRV	The maximum volume of air that can be inhaled after a normal inhalation	3000 mL	
Expiratory reserve volume	ERV	The maximum volume of air that can be exhaled forcibly after a normal exhalation	1100 mL	Expiratory reserve volume is decreased with restrictive conditions, such as obesity, ascites, pregnancy.
Residual volume	RV	The volume of air remaining in the lungs after a maximum exhalation	1200 mL	Residual volume may be increased with obstructive disease.
Lung Capacities				
Vital capacity	VC	The maximum volume of air exhaled from the point of maximum inspiration VC = TV + IRV + ERV	4600 mL	A decrease in vital capacity may be found in neuromuscular disease, generalized fatigue, atelectasis, pulmonary edema, and COPD.
Inspiratory capacity	IC	The maximum volume of air inhaled after normal expiration IC = TV + IRV	3500 mL	A decrease in inspiratory capacity may indicate restrictive disease.
Functional residual capacity	FRC	The volume of air remaining in the lungs after a normal expiration FRV = ERV + RV	2300 mL	Functional residual capacity may be increased with COPD and decreased in ARDS.
Total lung capacity	TLC	The volume of air in the lungs after a maximum inspiration TLC = TV + IRV + ERV + RV	5800 mL	Total lung capacity may be decreased with restrictive disease (atelectasis, pneumonia) and increased in COPD.

* Values for healthy men; women are 20–25% less.
ARDS, acute respiratory distress syndrome; COPD, chronic obstructed pulmonary disease.

capillary membrane is ideal for diffusion because of its thinness and large surface area. In the normal healthy adult, oxygen and carbon dioxide travel across the alveolar–capillary membrane without difficulty as a result of differences in gas concentrations in the alveoli and capillaries.

Pulmonary perfusion is the actual blood flow through the pulmonary circulation. The blood is pumped into the lungs by the right ventricle through the pulmonary artery. The pulmonary artery divides into the right and left branches to supply both lungs. These two branches divide further to supply all parts of each lung. Normally about 2% of the blood pumped by the right ventricle does not perfuse the alveolar capillaries. This shunted blood drains into the left side of the heart without participating in alveolar gas exchange.

The pulmonary circulation is considered a low-pressure system because the systolic blood pressure in the pulmonary artery is 20 to 30 mm Hg and the diastolic pressure is 5 to 15 mm Hg. Because of these low pressures, the pulmonary vasculature normally can vary its capacity to accommodate the blood flow it receives. However, when a person is in an upright position, the pulmonary artery pressure is not great enough to supply blood to the apex of the lung against the force of gravity. Thus, when a person is upright, the lung may be considered to be divided into three sections: an upper part with poor blood supply, a lower part with maximal blood supply, and a section between the two with an intermediate supply of blood. When a person lying down turns to one side, more blood passes to the dependent lung.

Perfusion also is influenced by alveolar pressure. The pulmonary capillaries are sandwiched between adjacent alveoli. If the alveolar pressure is sufficiently high, the capillaries are squeezed. Depending on the pressure, some capillaries completely collapse, whereas others narrow.

Pulmonary artery pressure, gravity, and alveolar pressure determine the patterns of perfusion. In lung disease these factors vary, and the perfusion of the lung may become very abnormal.

Ventilation and Perfusion Balance and Imbalance

Ventilation is the flow of gas in and out of the lungs, and perfusion is the filling of the pulmonary capillaries with blood. Adequate gas exchange depends on an adequate ventilation–perfusion ($\dot{V}/\dot{Q}$) ratio. In different areas of the lung, the $\dot{V}/\dot{Q}$ ratio varies. Alterations in perfusion may occur with a change in the pulmonary artery pressure, alveolar pressure, or gravity. Airway blockages, local changes in compliance, and gravity may alter ventilation.

$\dot{V}/\dot{Q}$ imbalance occurs as a result of inadequate ventilation, inadequate perfusion, or both. There are four possible $\dot{V}/\dot{Q}$ states in the lung: normal $\dot{V}/\dot{Q}$ ratio, low $\dot{V}/\dot{Q}$ ratio (shunt), high $\dot{V}/\dot{Q}$ ratio (dead space), and absence of ventilation and perfusion (silent unit) (Chart 21-2). $\dot{V}/\dot{Q}$ imbalance causes shunting of blood, resulting in **hypoxia** (low level of cellular oxygen). Shunting appears to be the main cause of hypoxia after thoracic or abdominal surgery and most types of respiratory failure. Severe hypoxia results when the amount of shunting exceeds 20%. Supplemental oxygen may eliminate hypoxia, depending on the type of $\dot{V}/\dot{Q}$ imbalance.

Gas Exchange

CONCEPTS in action **ANIMATION**

The air we breathe is a gaseous mixture consisting mainly of nitrogen (78.62%) and oxygen (20.84%), with traces of carbon dioxide (0.04%), water vapor (0.05%), helium, and argon. The atmospheric pressure at sea level is about 760 mm Hg. Partial pressure is the pressure exerted by

CHART 21-2

Ventilation-Perfusion Ratios

NORMAL RATIO (A)
In the healthy lung, a given amount of blood passes an alveolus and is matched with an equal amount of gas (**A**). The ratio is 1:1 (ventilation matches perfusion).

LOW VENTILATION–PERFUSION RATIO: SHUNTS (B)
Low ventilation–perfusion states may be called shunt-producing disorders. When perfusion exceeds ventilation, a shunt exists (**B**). Blood bypasses the alveoli without gas exchange occurring. This is seen with obstruction of the distal airways, such as with pneumonia, atelectasis, tumor, or a mucus plug.

HIGH VENTILATION–PERFUSION RATIO: DEAD SPACE (C)
When ventilation exceeds perfusion, dead space results (**C**). The alveoli do not have an adequate blood supply for gas exchange to occur. This is characteristic of a variety of disorders, including pulmonary emboli, pulmonary infarction, and cardiogenic shock.

SILENT UNIT (D)
In the absence of ventilation and perfusion or with limited ventilation and perfusion, a condition known as a silent unit occurs (**D**). This is seen with pneumothorax and severe acute respiratory distress syndrome.

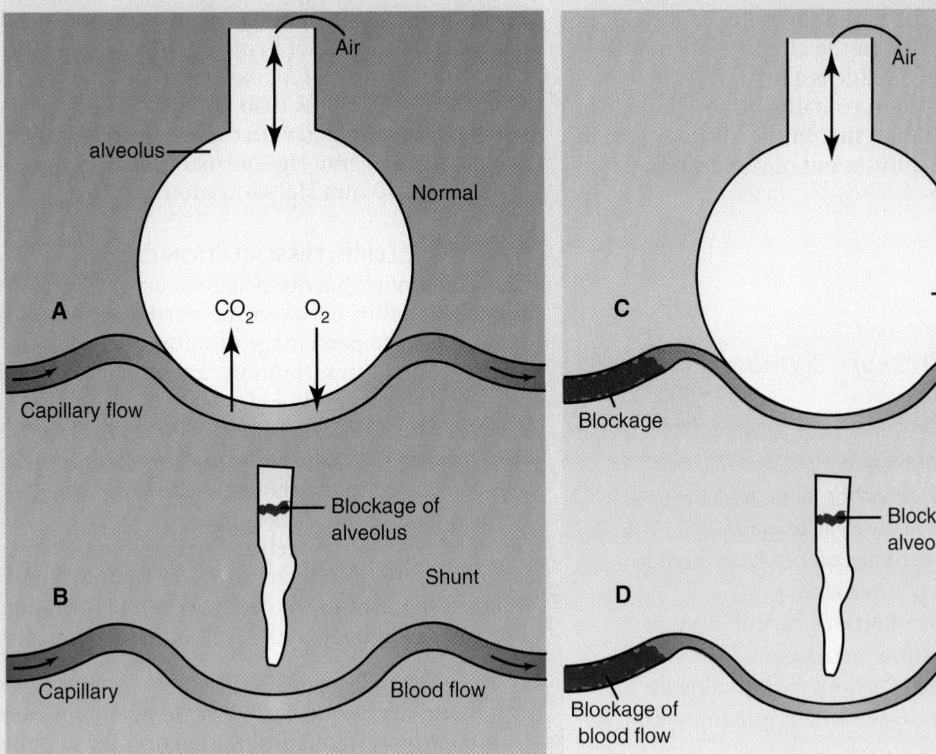

each type of gas in a mixture of gases. The partial pressure of a gas is proportional to the concentration of that gas in the mixture. The total pressure exerted by the gaseous mixture is equal to the sum of the partial pressures.

PARTIAL PRESSURE OF GASES

Based on these facts, the partial pressures of nitrogen and oxygen can be calculated. The partial pressure of nitrogen is 79% of 760 (0.79×760), or 600 mm Hg; that of oxygen is 21% of 760 (0.21×760), or 160 mm Hg. Chart 21-3 identifies and defines terms and abbreviations related to partial pressure of gases.

Once the air enters the trachea, it becomes fully saturated with water vapor, which displaces some of the gases so that the air pressure within the lung remains equal to the air pressure outside (760 mm Hg). Water vapor exerts a pressure of 47 mm Hg when it fully saturates a mixture of gases at the body temperature of 37°C (98.6°F). Nitrogen and oxygen are responsible for the remaining 713 mm Hg (760–47) pressure. Once this mixture enters the alveoli, it is further diluted by carbon dioxide. In the alveoli, the water vapor continues to exert a pressure of 47 mm Hg. The remaining 713 mm Hg pressure is now exerted as follows: nitrogen, 569 mm Hg (74.9%); oxygen, 104 mm Hg (13.6%); and carbon dioxide, 40 mm Hg (5.3%).

PARTIAL PRESSURE IN GAS EXCHANGE

When a gas is exposed to a liquid, the gas dissolves in the liquid until an equilibrium is reached. The dissolved gas also exerts a partial pressure. At equilibrium, the partial pressure of the gas in the liquid is the same as the partial pressure of the gas in the gaseous mixture. Oxygenation of venous blood in the lung illustrates this point. In the lung, venous blood and alveolar oxygen are separated by a very thin alveolar membrane. Oxygen diffuses across this membrane to dissolve in the blood until the partial pressure of oxygen in the blood is the same as that in the alveoli (104 mm Hg). However, because carbon dioxide is a byproduct of oxidation in the cells, venous blood contains carbon dioxide at a higher partial pressure than that in the alveolar gas. In the lung, carbon dioxide diffuses out of venous blood into the alveolar gas. At equilibrium, the partial pressure of carbon dioxide in the blood and in alveolar gas is the same (40 mm Hg). The changes in partial pressure are shown in Figure 21-5.

CHART 21-3

Partial Pressure Symbols

P = pressure
PO_2 = partial pressure of oxygen
PCO_2 = partial pressure of carbon dioxide
PAO_2 = partial pressure of alveolar oxygen
$PACO_2$ = partial pressure of alveolar carbon dioxide
PaO_2 = partial pressure of arterial oxygen
$PaCO_2$ = partial pressure of arterial carbon dioxide
$P\bar{v}O_2$ = partial pressure of venous oxygen
$P\bar{v}CO_2$ = partial pressure of venous carbon dioxide
P_{50} = partial pressure of oxygen when the hemoglobin is 50% saturated

EFFECTS OF PRESSURE ON OXYGEN TRANSPORT

CONCEPTS in action ANIMATION

Oxygen and carbon dioxide are transported simultaneously dissolved in blood or combined with some of the elements of blood. Oxygen is carried in the blood in two forms: first as physically dissolved oxygen in the plasma, and second in combination with the hemoglobin of the red blood cells. Each 100 mL of normal arterial blood carries 0.3 mL of oxygen physically dissolved in the plasma and 20 mL of oxygen in combination with hemoglobin. Large amounts of oxygen can be transported in the blood because oxygen combines easily with hemoglobin to form oxyhemoglobin:

$$O_2 + Hgb \leftrightarrow HgbO_2$$

The volume of oxygen physically dissolved in the plasma varies directly with the partial pressure of oxygen in the arteries (PaO_2). The higher the PaO_2, the greater the amount of oxygen dissolved. For example, at a PaO_2 of 10 mm Hg, 0.03 mL of oxygen is dissolved in 100 mL of plasma. At 20 mm Hg, twice this amount is dissolved in plasma, and at 100 mm Hg, 10 times this amount is dissolved. Therefore, the amount of dissolved oxygen is directly proportional to the partial pressure, regardless of how high the oxygen pressure becomes.

The amount of oxygen that combines with hemoglobin also depends on PaO_2, but only up to a PaO_2 of about 150 mm Hg. When the PaO_2 is 150 mm Hg, hemoglobin is 100% saturated and does not combine with any additional oxygen. When hemoglobin is 100% saturated, 1 g of hemoglobin combines with 1.34 mL of oxygen. Therefore, in a person with 14 g/dL of hemoglobin, each 100 mL of blood contains about 19 mL of oxygen associated with hemoglobin. If the PaO_2 is less than 150 mm Hg, the percentage of hemoglobin saturated with oxygen decreases. For example, at a PaO_2 of 100 mm Hg (normal value), saturation is 97%; at a PaO_2 of 40 mm Hg, saturation is 70%.

OXYHEMOGLOBIN DISSOCIATION CURVE

The oxyhemoglobin dissociation curve (Chart 21-4) shows the relationship between the partial pressure of oxygen (PaO_2) and the percentage of saturation of oxygen (SaO_2). The percentage of saturation can be affected by the following factors: carbon dioxide, hydrogen ion concentration, temperature, and 2,3-diphosphoglycerate. An increase in these factors shifts the curve to the right, so that more oxygen is released to the tissues at the same PaO_2. A decrease in these factors causes the curve to shift to the left, making the bond between oxygen and hemoglobin stronger, so that less oxygen is given up to the tissues at the same PaO_2. The unusual shape of the oxyhemoglobin dissociation curve is a distinct advantage to the patient for two reasons:

1. If the PaO_2 decreases from 100 to 80 mm Hg as a result of lung disease or heart disease, the hemoglobin of the arterial blood remains almost maximally saturated (94%), and the tissues do not suffer from hypoxia.

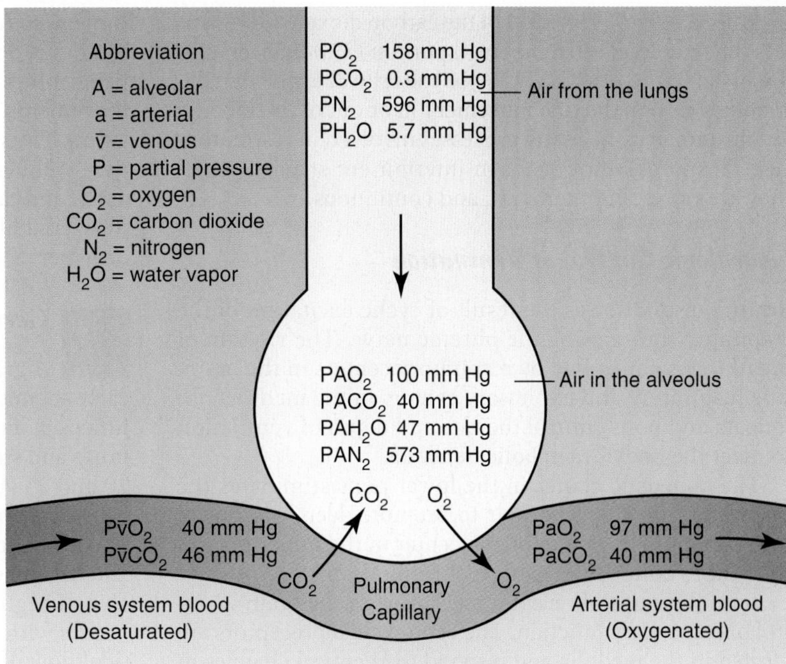

FIGURE 21-5. Changes occur in the partial pressure of gases during respiration. These values vary as a result of the exchange of oxygen and carbon dioxide and the changes that occur in their partial pressures as venous blood flows through the lungs.

CHART 21-4

Oxyhemoglobin Dissociation Curve

The oxyhemoglobin dissociation curve is marked to show three oxygen levels:

1. Normal levels—PaO_2 above 70 mm Hg
2. Relatively safe levels—PaO_2 45 to 70 mm Hg
3. Dangerous levels—PaO_2 below 40 mm Hg

The normal (middle) curve (N) shows that 75% saturation occurs at a PaO_2 of 40 mm Hg. If the curve shifts to the right (R), the same saturation (75%) occurs at the higher PaO_2 of 57 mm Hg. If the curve shifts to the left (L), 75% saturation occurs at a PaO_2 of 25 mm Hg.

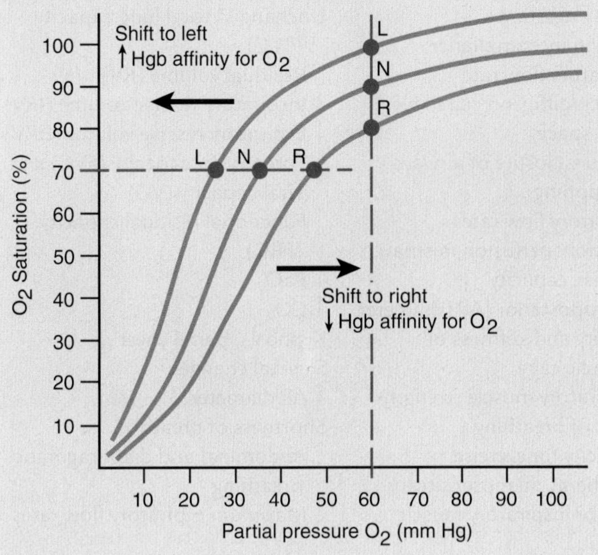

2. When the arterial blood passes into tissue capillaries and is exposed to the tissue tension of oxygen (about 40 mm Hg), hemoglobin gives up large quantities of oxygen for use by the tissues.

With a normal value for PaO_2 of 80 to 100 mm Hg (95% to 98% saturation), there is a 15% margin of excess oxygen available to the tissues. With a normal hemoglobin level of 15 mg/dL and a PaO_2 level of 40 mm Hg (oxygen saturation 75%), there is adequate oxygen available for the tissues but no reserve for physiologic stresses that increase tissue oxygen demand. When a serious incident occurs (eg, bronchospasm, aspiration, hypotension, or cardiac dysrhythmias) that reduces the intake of oxygen from the lungs, tissue hypoxia results.

An important consideration in the transport of oxygen is cardiac output, which determines the amount of oxygen delivered to the body and which affects lung and tissue perfusion. If the cardiac output is normal (5 L/min), the amount of oxygen delivered to the body per minute is normal. If cardiac output falls, the amount of oxygen delivered to the tissues also falls. Under normal conditions, most of the oxygen delivered to the body is not used. In fact, only 250 mL of oxygen is used per minute. Under normal conditions, this is approximately 25% of available oxygen. The rest of the oxygen returns to the right side of the heart, and the PaO_2 of venous blood drops from 80 to 100 mm Hg to about 40 mm Hg.

Carbon Dioxide Transport

At the same time that oxygen diffuses from the blood into the tissues, carbon dioxide diffuses in the opposite direction (ie, from tissue cells to blood) and is transported to the lungs for excretion. The amount of carbon dioxide in transit is one of the major determinants of the acid–base balance of the body. Normally, only 6% of the venous carbon dioxide is removed, and enough remains in the arterial blood to exert a pressure of 40 mm Hg. Most of the carbon dioxide (90%) enters the red blood cells; the small portion (5%) that remains dissolved in the plasma (PCO_2) is the critical factor that determines carbon dioxide movement in or out of the blood.

In summary, the many processes involved in respiratory gas transport do not occur in intermittent stages; rather, they are rapid, simultaneous, and continuous.

Neurologic Control of Ventilation

Resting respiration is the result of cyclic excitation of the respiratory muscles by the phrenic nerve. The rhythm of breathing is controlled by respiratory centers in the brain. The inspiratory and expiratory centers in the medulla oblongata and pons control the rate and depth of ventilation to meet the body's metabolic demands.

The apneustic center in the lower pons stimulates the inspiratory medullary center to promote deep, prolonged inspirations. The pneumotaxic center in the upper pons is thought to control the pattern of respirations.

Several groups of receptor sites assist in the brain's control of respiratory function. The central chemoreceptors are located in the medulla and respond to chemical changes in the cerebrospinal fluid, which result from chemical changes in the blood. These receptors respond to an increase or decrease in the pH and convey a message to the lungs to change the depth and then the rate of ventilation to correct the imbalance. The peripheral chemoreceptors are located in the aortic arch and the carotid arteries and respond first to changes in PaO_2, then to $PaCO_2$ and pH. The Hering–Breuer reflex is activated by stretch receptors in the alveoli. When the lungs are distended, inspiration is inhibited; as a result, the lungs do not become overdistended. In addition, proprioceptors in the muscles and joints respond to body movements, such as exercise, causing an increase in ventilation. Thus, range-of-motion exercises in an immobile patient stimulate breathing. Baroreceptors, also located in the aortic and carotid bodies, respond to an increase or decrease in arterial blood pressure and cause reflex hypoventilation or hyperventilation.

Gerontologic Considerations

A gradual decline in respiratory function begins in early to middle adulthood and affects the structure and function of the respiratory system. The vital capacity of the lungs and strength of the respiratory muscles peak between 20 and 25 years of age and decrease thereafter. With aging (40 years and older), changes occur in the alveoli that reduce the surface area available for the exchange of oxygen and carbon dioxide. At approximately 50 years of age, the alveoli begin to lose elasticity. A decrease in vital capacity occurs with loss of chest wall mobility, which restricts the tidal flow of air. The amount of respiratory dead space increases with age. These changes result in a decreased diffusion capacity for oxygen with increasing age, producing lower oxygen levels in the arterial circulation. Elderly people have a decreased ability to rapidly move air in and out of the lungs.

Gerontologic changes in the respiratory system are summarized in Table 21-2. Despite these changes, in the absence of chronic pulmonary disease, elderly people are

TABLE 21-2 Age-Related Changes in the Respiratory System

	Structural Changes	Functional Changes	History and Physical Findings
Defense mechanisms (respiratory and nonrespiratory)	↓ Number of cilia and ↓ mucus ↓ Cough and gag reflex Loss of surface area of the capillary membrane Lack of a uniform or consistent ventilation and/or blood flow	↓ Protection against foreign particles ↓ Protection against aspiration ↓ Antibody response to antigens ↓ Response to hypoxia and hypercapnia (chemoreceptors)	↓ Cough reflex and mucus ↑ Infection rate History of respiratory infections, COPD, pneumonia. Risk factors: smoking, environmental exposure, TB exposure
Lung	↓ Size of airway ↑ Diameter of alveolar ducts ↑ Collagen of alveolar walls ↑ Thickness of alveolar membranes ↓ Elasticity of alveolar sacs	↑ Airway resistance ↑ Pulmonary compliance ↓ Expiratory flow rate ↓ Oxygen diffusion capacity ↑ Dead space Premature closure of airways ↑ Air trapping ↓ Expiratory flow rates Ventilation–perfusion mismatch ↓ Exercise capacity ↑ Anteroposterior (AP) diameter	Unchanged total lung capacity (TLC) ↑ Residual volume (RV) ↓ Inspiratory reserve volume (IRV) ↓ Expiratory reserve volume (ERV) ↓ Forced vital capacity (FVC) and vital capacity (VC) ↑ Functional residual capacity (FRC) ↓ PaO_2 ↑ CO_2
Chest wall and muscles	Calcification of intercostal cartilages Arthritis of costovertebral joints ↓ Continuity of diaphragm Osteoporotic changes ↓ Muscle mass Muscle atrophy	↑ Rigidity and stiffness of thoracic cage ↓ Respiratory muscle strength ↑ Work of breathing ↓ Capacity for exercise ↓ Peripheral chemosensitivity ↑ Risk for inspiratory muscle fatigue	Kyphosis, barrel chest Skeletal changes ↑ AP diameter Shortness of breath ↑ Abdominal and diaphragmatic breathing ↓ Maximum expiratory flow rates

able to carry out activities of daily living, but they may have decreased tolerance for and require additional rest after prolonged or vigorous activity.

Assessment

Health History

The health history focuses on the physical and functional problems of the patient and the effects of these problems on the patient, including his or her ability to carry out activities of daily living. The reason the patient is seeking health care often is related to one of the following: **dyspnea** (shortness of breath), pain, accumulation of mucus, wheezing, **hemoptysis** (blood spit up from the respiratory tract), edema of the ankles and feet, cough, and general fatigue and weakness. If the patient is experiencing severe dyspnea, the nurse may need to modify or abbreviate the questions asked and the timing of the health history to avoid increasing the patient's breathlessness and anxiety.

In addition to identifying the chief reason why the patient is seeking health care, the nurse tries to determine when the health problem or symptom started, how long it lasted, if it was relieved at any time, and how relief was obtained. The nurse obtains information about precipitating factors, duration, severity, and associated factors or symptoms and also assesses for risk factors and genetics factors that may contribute to the patient's lung condition (Chart 21-5).

The nurse assesses the impact of signs and symptoms on the patient's ability to perform activities of daily living and to participate in usual work and family activities. In addition, psychosocial factors that may affect the patient are explored (Chart 21-6). These factors include anxiety, role changes, family relationships, financial problems, employment status, and the strategies the patient uses to cope with them.

Many respiratory diseases are chronic and progressively debilitating and disabling. Therefore, ongoing assessment of the patient's physical abilities, psychosocial supports, and quality of life is needed to plan appropriate interventions. It is important that the patient with a respiratory disorder understand the condition and be familiar with necessary self-care interventions. The nurse evaluates these factors over time and provides education as needed.

The major signs and symptoms of respiratory disease are dyspnea, cough, sputum production, chest pain, wheezing, clubbing of the fingers, hemoptysis, and cyanosis. These clinical manifestations are related to the duration and severity of the disease.

CHART 21-5

Risk Factors for Respiratory Disease

- Smoking (the single most important contributor to lung disease)
- Exposure to secondhand smoke
- Personal or family history of lung disease
- Genetic make-up
- Allergens and environmental pollutants
- Recreational and occupational exposure

Dyspnea

Dyspnea (difficult or labored breathing, breathlessness, shortness of breath) is a symptom common to many pulmonary and cardiac disorders, particularly when there is decreased lung compliance or increased airway resistance. The right ventricle of the heart is affected ultimately by lung disease because it must pump blood through the lungs against greater resistance. It may also be associated with neurologic or neuromuscular disorders (ie, myasthenia gravis, Guillain-Barré syndrome, muscular dystrophy) that affect respiratory function. Dyspnea can also occur after physical exercise in people without disease (Porth, 2005). It is also common at the end of life in patients with a variety of disorders.

CLINICAL SIGNIFICANCE

In general, acute diseases of the lungs produce a more severe grade of dyspnea than do chronic diseases. Sudden dyspnea in a healthy person may indicate pneumothorax (air in the pleural cavity), acute respiratory obstruction, or ARDS. In immobilized patients, sudden dyspnea may denote pulmonary embolism. **Orthopnea** (inability to breathe easily except in an upright position) may be found in patients with heart disease and occasionally in patients with COPD; dyspnea with an expiratory wheeze occurs with COPD. Noisy breathing may result from a narrowing of the airway or localized obstruction of a major bronchus by a tumor or foreign body. The presence of both inspiratory and expiratory wheezing usually signifies asthma if the patient does not have heart failure. Because dyspnea can occur with other disorders (eg, cardiac disease, anaphylactic reactions, severe anemia), these disorders also need to be considered when obtaining the patient's health history (Zoorob & Campbell, 2003).

The circumstance that produces the dyspnea must be determined. Therefore, it is important to ask the patient the following questions:

1. How much exertion triggers shortness of breath?
2. Is there an associated cough?
3. Is the shortness of breath related to other symptoms?
4. Was the onset of shortness of breath sudden or gradual?
5. At what time of day or night does the shortness of breath occur?
6. Is the shortness of breath worse when the patient is flat in bed?
7. Does the shortness of breath occur at rest? With exercise? Running? Climbing stairs?
8. Is the shortness of breath worse while walking? If so, when walking how far? How fast?

Other issues that are important in assessment of dyspnea include the following: the patient's rating of the intensity of breathlessness, the effort required to breathe, and the severity of the breathlessness or dyspnea. Patients use a variety of terms and phrases to describe breathlessness, and the nurse needs to clarify what terms are most familiar to the patient and what these terms mean (Bailey, 2004; de Souza Caroci & Lareau, 2004; Michaels & Meek, 2004). Several scales are available to assess the severity of dyspnea,

GENETICS IN NURSING PRACTICE

Genetic Influences

Various conditions that affect gas exchange and respiratory function are influenced by genetics factors, including:

- Asthma
- Chronic obstructive pulmonary disease
- Cystic fibrosis
- Alpha-1 antitrypsin deficiency

NURSING ASSESSMENTS

Family History Assessment

- Assess family history for other family members with histories of respiratory impairment.
- Assess family history for individuals with early-onset chronic pulmonary disease, family history of hepatic disease in infants (clinical symptoms of alpha-1 antitrypsin deficiency).
- Inquire about family history of genetic cystic fibrosis.

PATIENT ASSESSMENT

- Assess for symptoms such as changes in respiratory status associated with asthma (eg, wheezing, hyperresponsiveness, mucosal edema, and mucus production).
- Assess for multisystem effects characteristic of cystic fibrosis (eg, productive cough, wheezing, obstructive airways disease, gastrointestinal problems including pancreatic insufficiency, clubbing of the fingers).

MANAGEMENT ISSUES SPECIFIC TO GENETICS

- Inquire whether DNA mutation or other genetic testing has been performed on affected family members.
- Refer for further genetics counseling and evaluation so that family members can discuss inheritance, risk to other family members, availability of genetics testing and gene-based interventions.
- Offer appropriate genetics information and resources.
- Assess patient's understanding of genetics information.
- Provide support to families with newly diagnosed genetic-related respiratory disorders.
- Participate in management and coordination of care of patients with genetic conditions, individuals predisposed to develop or pass on a genetic condition.

GENETIC RESOURCES

American Lung Association, www.lungusa.org

Cystic Fibrosis Foundation, www.cff.org

Genetic Alliance, www.geneticalliance.org—a directory of support groups for patients and families with genetic conditions

Gene Clinics, www.geneclinics.org—a listing of common genetic disorders with clinical summaries, genetics counseling and testing information

National Organization of Rare Disorders, www.rarediseases.org—a directory of support groups and information for patients and families with rare genetic disorders

OMIM: Online Mendelian Inheritance in Man, www.ncbi.nlm.nih.gov/cntrez/query.fcgi?db=OMIM—a complete listing of inherited genetic conditions

including visual analog scales that can be used to assess changes in its severity over time (Leidy, Rennard, Schmier, et al., 2003; Porth, 2005).

RELIEF MEASURES

The management of dyspnea is aimed at identifying and correcting its cause. Relief of the symptom sometimes is achieved by placing the patient at rest with the head elevated (high Fowler's position) and, in severe cases, by administering oxygen. Strategies that enable patients with chronic or persistent dyspnea to decrease or prevent breathlessness and to cope with it can lead to improved quality of life (Hately, Laurence, Scott, et al. 2003).

Cough

Although cough is a reflex that protects the lungs from the accumulation of secretions or the inhalation of foreign bodies, it can also be a symptom of a number of disorders of the pulmonary system or it can be suppressed in other disorders. The cough reflex may be impaired by weakness or paralysis of the respiratory muscles, prolonged inactivity, the presence of a nasogastric tube, or depressed function of the medullary centers in the brain (eg, anesthesia, brain disorders) (Ebihara, Saito, Kanda, et al., 2003; Porth, 2005).

Cough results from irritation of the mucous membranes anywhere in the respiratory tract. The stimulus that produces a cough may arise from an infectious process or from an airborne irritant, such as smoke, smog, dust, or a gas. A persistent and frequent cough can be exhausting and cause pain. Cough may indicate serious pulmonary disease, but it may be caused by a variety of other problems as well, including cardiac disease, medications (eg, amiodarone, angiotensin-converting enzyme [ACE] inhibitors), smoking, and gastroesophageal reflux disease (Ott, Khoor, Leventhal, et al. 2003; Poe & Kallay, 2003).

CLINICAL SIGNIFICANCE

To help determine the cause of the cough, the nurse describes the cough: dry, hacking, brassy, wheezing, loose, or severe. A dry, irritative cough is characteristic of an upper respiratory tract infection of viral origin, or it may

CHART 21-6

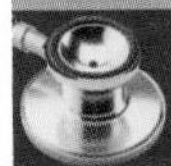

Assessing for Psychosocial Factors Related to Pulmonary Disease and Respiratory Function

- What strategies does the patient use to cope with the signs and symptoms and challenges associated with pulmonary disease?
- What effect has the pulmonary disease had on the patient's quality of life, goals, role within the family, and occupation?
- What changes has the pulmonary disease had on the patient's family and relationships with family members?
- Does the patient exhibit depression, anxiety, anger, hostility, dependency, withdrawal, isolation, avoidance, noncompliance, acceptance, or denial?
- What support systems does the patient use to cope with the illness?
- Are resources (relatives, friends, or community groups) available? Do the patient and family use them effectively?

be a side effect of ACE inhibitor therapy. Laryngotracheitis causes an irritative, high-pitched cough. Tracheal lesions produce a brassy cough. A severe or changing cough may indicate bronchogenic carcinoma. Pleuritic chest pain that accompanies coughing may indicate pleural or chest wall (musculoskeletal) involvement.

The time of coughing is also noted. Coughing at night may herald the onset of left-sided heart failure or bronchial asthma. A cough in the morning with sputum production may indicate bronchitis. A cough that worsens when the patient is supine suggests postnasal drip (sinusitis). Coughing after food intake may indicate aspiration of material into the tracheobronchial tree. A cough of recent onset is usually from an acute infection.

A persistent cough may affect a patient's quality of life and may produce embarrassment, exhaustion, inability to sleep, and pain. Therefore, the effect of a chronic cough on the patient and the patient's view about the significance of the cough and its effect on his or her life should also be obtained during the health history (French, Fletcher & Irwin, 2004).

RELIEF MEASURES

Cough suppressants must be used with caution, because they may relieve the cough but do not address the cause of the cough. If used inappropriately, they may prevent the patient from clearing mucus from the airways and result in a delay in seeking indicated health care. If the cause of the cough has been investigated and addressed but the cough persists, cough suppressants may be prescribed. If the cough is a result of irritation, smoking cessation strategies are indicated. Drinking warm beverages may relieve cough caused by throat irritation.

The American College of Chest Physicians (ACCP) issued guidelines for the assessment and management of acute cough (a cough that lasts for less than 3 weeks), subacute cough (a cough that lasts 3 to 8 weeks), and chronic cough (a cough that lasts for more than 8 weeks) (Irwin, Baumann, Bolser, et al., 2006). The guidelines recommend use of first-generation antihistamines with a decongestant for treatment of acute cough or upper airway cough syndrome secondary to rhinosinus disease (previously referred to as postnasal drip syndrome) instead of over-the-counter cough expectorants or suppressants (ie, cough syrups and cough drops). The guidelines contain a number of algorithms for use in evaluating different patterns of cough and identifying appropriate treatment strategies (Irwin et al., 2006).

Sputum Production

A patient who coughs long enough almost invariably produces sputum. Violent coughing causes bronchial spasm, obstruction, and further irritation of the bronchi and may result in syncope (fainting). A severe, repeated, or uncontrolled cough that is nonproductive is exhausting and potentially harmful. Sputum production is the reaction of the lungs to any constantly recurring irritant. It also may be associated with a nasal discharge.

CLINICAL SIGNIFICANCE

The nature of the sputum is indicative of the causal condition. A profuse amount of purulent sputum (thick and yellow, green, or rust-colored) or a change in color of the sputum is a common sign of a bacterial infection. Thin, mucoid sputum frequently results from viral bronchitis. A gradual increase of sputum over time may indicate the presence of chronic bronchitis or bronchiectasis. Pink-tinged mucoid sputum suggests a lung tumor. Profuse, frothy, pink material, often welling up into the throat, may indicate pulmonary edema. Foul-smelling sputum and bad breath point to the presence of a lung abscess, bronchiectasis, or an infection caused by fusospirochetal or other anaerobic organisms.

RELIEF MEASURES

If the sputum is too thick for the patient to expectorate, it is necessary to decrease its viscosity by increasing its water content through adequate hydration (drinking water) and inhalation of aerosolized solutions, which may be delivered by any type of nebulizer. Strategies to help the patient cough productively are discussed later in this chapter.

Smoking is contraindicated with excessive sputum production because it interferes with ciliary action, increases bronchial secretions, causes inflammation and hyperplasia of the mucous membranes, and reduces production of surfactant. Thus, smoking impairs bronchial drainage. When a person stops smoking, sputum volume decreases and resistance to bronchial infections increases.

The patient's appetite may decrease because of the odor of the sputum or the taste it leaves in the mouth. The nurse encourages adequate oral hygiene and wise selection of food, measures that stimulate the appetite. In addition, the nurse encourages the patient and family to remove sputum cups, emesis basins, and soiled tissues before mealtime. Encouraging the patient to drink citrus juices at the beginning of the meal may increase the palatability of the rest of

NURSING RESEARCH PROFILE

Patients' Descriptions of Respiratory Symptoms

Michaels, C. & Meek, P. M. (2004). The language of breathing among individuals with chronic obstructive pulmonary disease. *Heart and Lung, 33*(6), 390–400.

Purpose

The words patients use to describe pulmonary symptoms and changes in their symptoms to their health care providers may determine whether further assessment and treatment are performed. Difficulty with breathing can include effort required to breathe and the distress associated with impaired breathing. The purpose of this study was to examine the everyday language used by people with moderate to severe chronic obstructive pulmonary disease (COPD) to describe the effort of breathing and the distress associated with breathlessness.

Design

A longitudinal study was conducted using descriptive naturalistic research methods. The convenience sample included 15 people with a clinical diagnosis of COPD, moderate to severe pulmonary impairment based on results of pulmonary function tests, and no history of an exacerbation of COPD in the 3 months before enrollment in the study. Study participants were asked to perform each of the following tasks:

- From a list of 20 terms used in other studies, select the word or phrase that most accurately describes their breathing each day for 28 consecutive days.
- Complete a daily description and rating of breathing intensity for 28 days using a visual analogue scale (VAS) for breathing distress and another VAS for breathing effort.
- Describe the experience of breathing intensity during the previous 24 hours and record their breathing at the same time each day.
- Record physical sensations, associated emotions, or details they believed pertinent to the study.

Participants were visited at home weekly for 4 weeks. At each home visit, the daily logs and VAS scores for the previous week were reviewed. Terminology used was analyzed using qualitative data analysis techniques, and mean VAS scores on breathing effort and breathing distress were calculated.

Findings

Data were available from 11 of 15 participants who were originally recruited into the study. The mean VAS score (on a scale ranging from 0 = no distress or no effort to 100 = greatest distress or greatest effort possible) was 28.4 (SD ± 18.5) for breathing distress and 31.3 (SD ± 18.2) for breathing effort. Ten participants reported at least one episode of breathing distress or effort greater than 20 mm above their baseline VAS scores. In 30 instances, breathing distress and/or effort exceeded individual means by greater than 20 mm, representing 1% of the total days reviewed. Distress and effort both increased 50% of the time. In the remaining instances, distress was increased above effort 8 times, and effort was increased above distress 7 times. Descriptors that were frequently identified included "hard to breathe," "difficulty breathing," and "out of breath." Other terms that were often reported were "short of breath," "tightness," and "breathless." Occasionally, participants used more than one term or phrase to describe their breathing each day. The use of more intense wording or phrases to describe breathing difficulty tended to be associated with VAS scores indicating more breathing effort and greater breathing distress.

Typically, the highest VAS scores reported for distress and effort occurred on the same day, although there were inconsistencies. For example, "no problem" was used to describe breathing on days with high breathing distress and effort scores when participants had ceased all physical activity to minimize respiratory distress.

Nursing Implications

This study provides some insight into the everyday language used by people with moderate to severe COPD to describe their breathing effort and breathing distress. In a natural setting (ie, patients' homes), factors other than altered breathing may contribute to wording used by patients to describe their breathing. Participants used some of the words or phrases identified in previous research conducted in laboratory settings, added other words or phrases, and described the range of intensity of breathing difficulty. It is important that health care professionals understand the nuances of a patient's descriptions of changes in breathing, because the patient's language is essential for communication about problems that necessitate self-care and those that require professional treatment. To detect significant breathing changes, it is essential that nurses and other clinicians be sensitive to the various words and phrases patients use in describing their breathing difficulties and clarify terms used by patients.

NURSING RESEARCH PROFILE

Dyspnea-Anxiety-Dyspnea Cycle in Patients With Chronic Obstructive Pulmonary Disease

Bailey, P. H. (2004). The dyspnea-anxiety-dyspnea cycle—COPD patients' stories of breathlessness: "It's scary when you can't breathe." *Qualitative Health Research, 14*(6), 760–778.

Purpose

Dyspnea, or the sensation of breathlessness, is a major subjective symptom of chronic obstructive pulmonary disease (COPD) that is invisible to others because it is subjective. The purpose of this study was to explore the affective component of dyspnea, specifically anxiety, as described by patients and family caregivers, associated with acute exacerbations of COPD characterized by severe dyspnea.

Design

The researcher used qualitative research methods to gain insight into the meaning and experience of severe dyspnea associated with acute exacerbations of COPD. Ten patients with advanced COPD and at least two previous hospital admissions for acute exacerbations of COPD and 15 of their family caregivers participated in in-depth interviews about their experiences. Narrative analysis of the transcriptions of the interviews was used to examine the data.

Findings

Patients with COPD and their caregivers identified and described a close relationship between acute dyspnea and patients' physical and emotional functioning. Stories about the experiences of acute dyspnea and the relationship between dyspnea and patients' emotional function, labeled Emotional Vulnerability Stories by the researcher, revealed that patients were often unable to cope emotionally with everyday experiences (eg, having a heated discussion with others, becoming excited about an event) because of intractable breathlessness. Normal emotional responses to everyday events often produced an increase in patients' feelings of breathlessness. Patients who were emotionally disabled because of increased breathlessness were unable to participate in normal physical or emotional activities because doing so increased the likelihood of even greater breathlessness.

Nursing Implications

The findings of this study demonstrate the complex and often circular relationship between dyspnea and emotional functioning in patients with severe COPD. Other researchers have described a cycle of anxiety-breathlessness-anxiety, in which patients' emotional reactions to being dyspneic have further increased their sense of breathlessness and have led to greater anxiety. However, the findings of this study suggest a cycle of dyspnea–anxiety–dyspnea in which anxiety is not the underlying cause of acute episodes of dyspnea. Patients who can control or suppress their emotional reactions can decrease the severity of their dyspnea. Thus, when they feel anxious, their anxiety is not a cause of dyspnea; rather, their acute episodes of anxiety may be indicators of increasing breathlessness. This study suggests that nurses and other health care providers should consider anxiety as a sign of increasing dyspnea rather than as a cause of the breathlessness in patients with COPD who are in acute respiratory distress.

the meal, because these juices cleanse the palate of the sputum taste.

Chest Pain

Chest pain or discomfort may be associated with pulmonary or cardiac disease. Chest pain associated with pulmonary conditions may be sharp, stabbing, and intermittent, or it may be dull, aching, and persistent. The pain usually is felt on the side where the pathologic process is located, but it may be referred elsewhere—for example, to the neck, back, or abdomen.

CLINICAL SIGNIFICANCE

Chest pain may occur with pneumonia, pulmonary embolism with lung infarction, and pleurisy. It also may be a late symptom of bronchogenic carcinoma. In carcinoma, the pain may be dull and persistent because the cancer has invaded the chest wall, mediastinum, or spine.

Lung disease does not always cause thoracic pain, because the lungs and the visceral pleura lack sensory nerves and are insensitive to pain stimuli. However, the parietal pleura has a rich supply of sensory nerves that are stimulated by inflammation and stretching of the membrane. Pleuritic pain from irritation of the parietal pleura is sharp and seems to "catch" on inspiration; patients often describe it as "like the stabbing of a knife." Patients are more comfortable when they lie on the affected side, because this splints the chest wall, limits expansion and contraction of the lung, and reduces the friction between the injured or diseased pleurae on that side. Pain associated with cough may be reduced manually by splinting the rib cage.

The nurse assesses the quality, intensity, and radiation of pain and identifies and explores precipitating factors and their relationship to the patient's position. In addition, it is important to assess the relationship of pain to the inspiratory and expiratory phases of respiration.

RELIEF MEASURES

Analgesic medications may be effective in relieving chest pain, but care must be taken not to depress the respiratory center or a productive cough, if present. Nonsteroidal anti-inflammatory drugs (NSAIDs) achieve this goal and therefore are used for pleuritic pain. A regional anesthetic block may be performed to relieve extreme pain.

Wheezing

Wheezing is often the major finding in a patient with bronchoconstriction or airway narrowing. It is heard with or without a stethoscope, depending on its location. Wheezing is a high-pitched, musical sound heard mainly on expiration.

Oral or inhalant bronchodilator medications reverse wheezing in most instances.

Clubbing of the Fingers

Clubbing of the fingers is a sign of lung disease that is found in patients with chronic hypoxic conditions, chronic lung infections, or malignancies of the lung (Bickley & Szilagyi, 2003). This finding may be manifested initially as sponginess of the nail bed and loss of the nail bed angle (Fig. 21-6).

Hemoptysis

Hemoptysis (expectoration of blood from the respiratory tract) is a symptom of both pulmonary and cardiac disorders. The onset of hemoptysis is usually sudden, and it may be intermittent or continuous. Signs, which vary from blood-stained sputum to a large, sudden hemorrhage, always merit investigation. The most common causes are

- Pulmonary infection
- Carcinoma of the lung
- Abnormalities of the heart or blood vessels
- Pulmonary artery or vein abnormalities
- Pulmonary embolus and infarction

Diagnostic evaluation to determine the cause includes several studies: chest x-ray, chest angiography, and bronchoscopy. A careful history and physical examination are necessary to diagnose the underlying disease, irrespective of whether the bleeding involved a very small amount of blood in the sputum or a massive hemorrhage. The amount of blood produced is not always proportional to the seriousness of the cause.

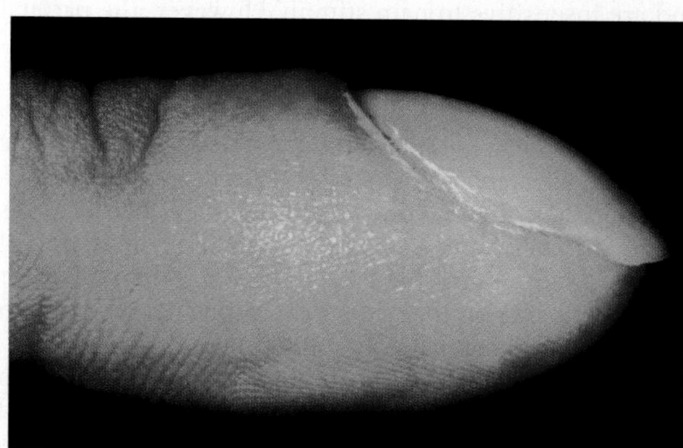

FIGURE 21-6. Clubbed finger. In clubbing, the distal phalanx of each finger is rounded and bulbous. The nail plate is more convex, and the angle between the plate and the proximal nail fold increases to 180 degrees or more. The proximal nail fold, when palpated, feels spongy or floating. Among the many causes are chronic hypoxia and lung cancer.

First, it is important to determine the source of the bleeding—the gums, nasopharynx, lungs, or stomach. The nurse may be the only witness to the episode. When documenting the bleeding episode, the nurse considers the following points:

- Bloody sputum from the nose or the nasopharynx is usually preceded by considerable sniffing, with blood possibly appearing in the nose.
- Blood from the lung is usually bright red, frothy, and mixed with sputum. Initial symptoms include a tickling sensation in the throat, a salty taste, a burning or bubbling sensation in the chest, and perhaps chest pain, in which case the patient tends to splint the bleeding side. The term "hemoptysis" is reserved for the coughing up of blood arising from a pulmonary hemorrhage. This blood has an alkaline pH (greater than 7.0).
- If the hemorrhage is in the stomach, the blood is vomited (hematemesis) rather than coughed up. Blood that has been in contact with gastric juice is sometimes so dark that it is referred to as "coffee grounds." This blood has an acid pH (less than 7.0).

Cyanosis

Cyanosis, a bluish coloring of the skin, is a very late indicator of hypoxia. The presence or absence of cyanosis is determined by the amount of unoxygenated hemoglobin in the blood. Cyanosis appears when there is at least 5 g/dL of unoxygenated hemoglobin. A patient with a hemoglobin level of 15 g/dL does not demonstrate cyanosis until 5 g/dL of that hemoglobin becomes unoxygenated, reducing the effective circulating hemoglobin to two thirds of the normal level.

A patient with anemia rarely manifests cyanosis, and a patient with polycythemia may appear cyanotic even if adequately oxygenated. Therefore, cyanosis is *not* a reliable sign of hypoxia.

Assessment of cyanosis is affected by room lighting, the patient's skin color, and the distance of the blood vessels from the surface of the skin. In the presence of a pulmonary condition, central cyanosis is assessed by observing the color of the tongue and lips. This indicates a decrease in oxygen tension in the blood. Peripheral cyanosis results from decreased blood flow to a certain area of the body, as in vasoconstriction of the nail beds or earlobes from exposure to cold, and does not necessarily indicate a central systemic problem.

Physical Assessment of the Upper Respiratory Structures

For a routine examination of the upper airway, only a simple light source, such as a penlight, is necessary. A more thorough examination requires the use of a nasal speculum.

Nose and Sinuses

The nurse inspects the external nose for lesions, asymmetry, or inflammation and then asks the patient to tilt the head backward. Gently pushing the tip of the nose upward, the nurse examines the internal structures of the nose, inspecting the mucosa for color, swelling, exudate, or bleeding. The nasal mucosa is normally redder than the oral mucosa. It may appear swollen and hyperemic if the patient has a common cold, but in allergic rhinitis the mucosa appears pale and swollen.

Next the nurse inspects the septum for deviation, perforation, or bleeding. Most people have a slight degree of septal deviation, but actual displacement of the cartilage into either the right or left side of the nose may produce nasal obstruction. Such deviation usually causes no symptoms.

While the head is still tilted back, the nurse inspects the inferior and middle turbinates. In chronic rhinitis, nasal polyps may develop between the inferior and middle turbinates; they are distinguished by their gray appearance. Unlike the turbinates, they are gelatinous and freely movable.

Next the nurse may palpate the frontal and maxillary sinuses for tenderness (Fig. 21-7). Using the thumbs, the nurse applies gentle pressure in an upward fashion at the supraorbital ridges (frontal sinuses) and in the cheek area adjacent to the nose (maxillary sinuses). Tenderness in either area suggests inflammation. The frontal and maxillary sinuses can be inspected by transillumination (passing a strong light through a bony area, such as the sinuses, to inspect the cavity; Fig. 21-8). If the light fails to penetrate, the cavity likely contains fluid or pus.

Pharynx and Mouth

After the nasal inspection, the nurse assesses the mouth and pharynx, instructing the patient to open the mouth wide and take a deep breath. Usually this flattens the posterior tongue and briefly allows a full view of the anterior and posterior pillars, tonsils, uvula, and posterior pharynx (Fig. 21-9). The nurse inspects these structures for color, symmetry, and evidence of exudate, ulceration, or enlargement. If a tongue blade is needed to depress the tongue to visualize the pharynx, it is pressed firmly beyond the midpoint of the tongue to avoid a gagging response.

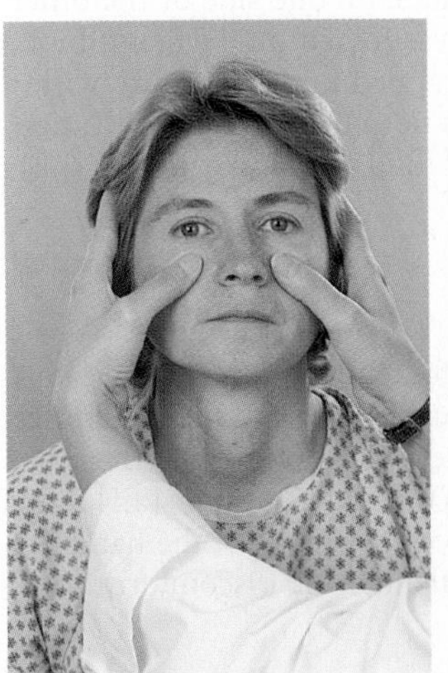
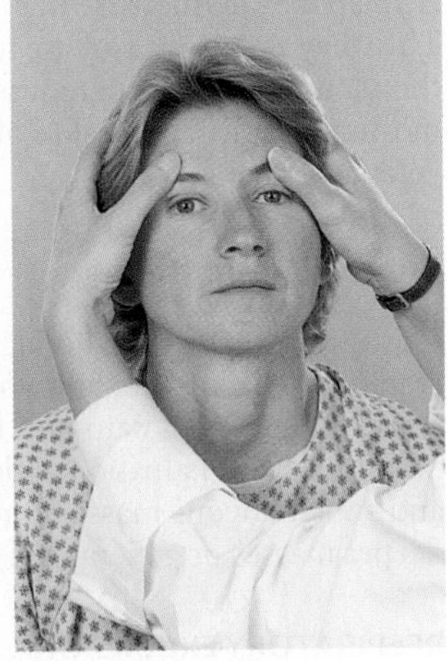

FIGURE 21-7. Technique for palpating the frontal sinuses at left and the maxillary sinuses at right. From Weber, J. & Kelley, J. (2003). *Health assessment in nursing* (2nd ed.). Philadelphia: Lippincott Williams & Wilkins.

Trachea

Next the position and mobility of the trachea are noted by direct palpation. This is performed by placing the thumb and index finger of one hand on either side of the trachea just above the sternal notch. The trachea is highly sensitive, and palpating too firmly may trigger a coughing or gagging response. The trachea is normally in the midline as it enters the thoracic inlet behind the sternum, but it may be deviated by masses in the neck or mediastinum. Pleural or pulmonary disorders, such as a pneumothorax, may also displace the trachea.

Physical Assessment of the Lower Respiratory Structures and Breathing

Thorax

Inspection of the thorax provides information about the musculoskeletal structure, the patient's nutritional status, and the respiratory system. The nurse observes the skin over the thorax for color and turgor and for evidence of loss of subcutaneous tissue. It is important to note asymmetry, if present. In recording or reporting the findings, anatomic landmarks are used as points of reference (Chart 21-7).

CHEST CONFIGURATION

Normally, the ratio of the anteroposterior diameter to the lateral diameter is 1:2. However, there are four main deformities of the chest associated with respiratory disease that alter this relationship: barrel chest, funnel chest (pectus excavatum), pigeon chest (pectus carinatum), and kyphoscoliosis.

Barrel Chest. Barrel chest occurs as a result of overinflation of the lungs. There is an increase in the anteroposterior diameter of the thorax. In a patient with emphysema, the ribs are more widely spaced and the intercostal spaces tend

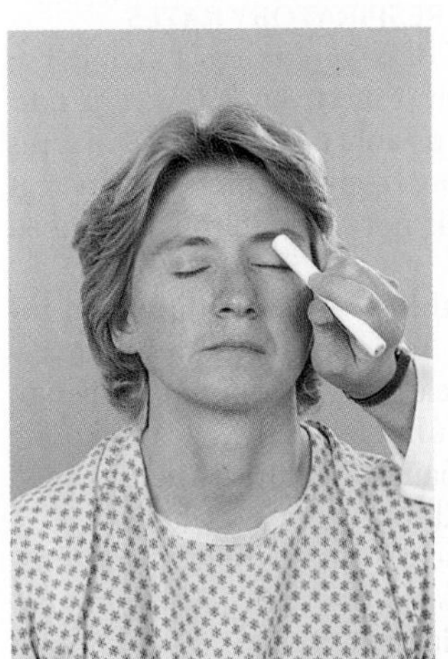
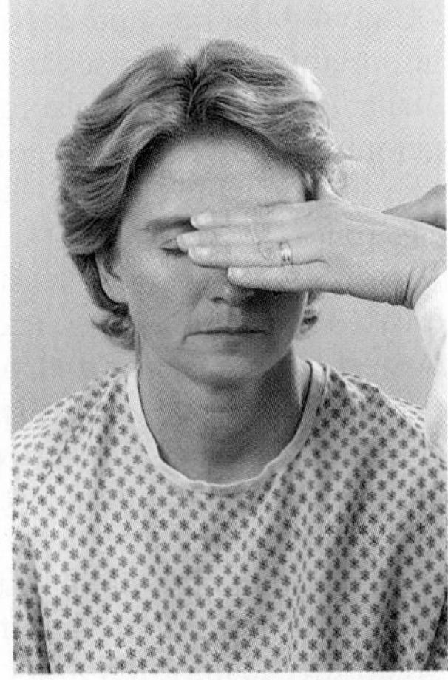

FIGURE 21-8. At left, the nurse positions the light source for transillumination of the frontal sinus. At right, the nurse shields the patient's brow and shines the light. In normal conditions (a darkened room), the light should shine through the tissues and appear as a reddish glow (above the nurse's hand) over the sinus. From Weber, J. & Kelley, J. (2003). *Health assessment in nursing* (2nd ed.). Philadelphia: Lippincott Williams & Wilkins.

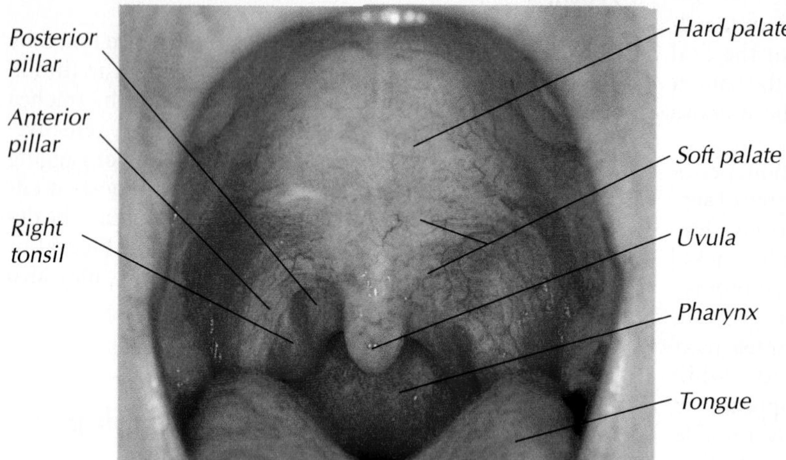

FIGURE 21-9. The pharynx and other oral structures—pillars, tonsils, uvula, hard and soft palates, posterior pharynx, and tongue—are easily seen when the mouth is open.

to bulge on expiration. The appearance of the patient with advanced emphysema is thus quite characteristic and often allows the observer to detect its presence easily, even from a distance.

Funnel Chest (Pectus Excavatum). Funnel chest occurs when there is a depression in the lower portion of the sternum. This may compress the heart and great vessels, resulting in murmurs. Funnel chest may occur with rickets or Marfan's syndrome.

Pigeon Chest (Pectus Carinatum). A pigeon chest occurs as a result of displacement of the sternum. There is an increase in the anteroposterior diameter. This may occur with rickets, Marfan's syndrome, or severe kyphoscoliosis.

Kyphoscoliosis. A kyphoscoliosis is characterized by elevation of the scapula and a corresponding S-shaped spine. This deformity limits lung expansion within the thorax. It may occur with osteoporosis and other skeletal disorders that affect the thorax.

BREATHING PATTERNS AND RESPIRATORY RATES

Observing the rate and depth of respiration is a simple but important aspect of assessment (Finesilver, 2003). The normal adult who is resting comfortably takes 12 to 18 breaths per minute. Except for occasional sighs, respirations are regular in depth and rhythm. This normal pattern is described as eupnea.

Bradypnea, or slow breathing, is associated with increased intracranial pressure, brain injury, and drug overdose. Tachypnea, or rapid breathing, is commonly seen in patients with pneumonia, pulmonary edema, metabolic acidosis, septicemia, severe pain, or rib fracture. Shallow, irregular breathing is referred to as hypoventilation.

Hyperpnea is an increase in depth of respirations. Hyperventilation is an increase in both rate and depth that results in a decreased arterial $PaCO_2$ level. With rapid breathing, inspiration and expiration are nearly equal in duration. Hyperventilation that is marked by an increase in rate and depth, associated with severe acidosis of diabetic or renal origin, is called Kussmaul's respiration.

Apnea describes varying periods of cessation of breathing. If sustained, apnea is life-threatening.

Cheyne-Stokes respiration is characterized by alternating episodes of apnea (cessation of breathing) and periods of deep breathing. Deep respirations become increasingly shallow, followed by apnea that may last approximately 20 seconds. The cycle repeats after each apneic period. The duration of the period of apnea may vary and may progressively lengthen; therefore, it is timed and reported. Cheyne-Stokes respiration is usually associated with heart failure and damage to the respiratory center (drug-induced, tumor, trauma).

Biot's respirations, or cluster breathing, are cycles of breaths that vary in depth and have varying periods of apnea. Biot's respirations are seen with some central nervous system disorders.

Certain patterns of respiration are characteristic of specific disease states. Respiratory rhythms and their deviation from normal are important observations that the nurse reports and documents. The rate and depth of various patterns of respiration are presented in Table 21-3.

In thin people, it is quite normal to note a slight retraction of the intercostal spaces during quiet breathing. Bulging of the intercostal spaces during expiration implies obstruction of expiratory airflow, as in emphysema. Marked retraction on inspiration, particularly if asymmetric, implies blockage of a branch of the respiratory tree. Asymmetric bulging of the intercostal spaces, on one side or the other, is created by an increase in pressure within the hemithorax. This may be a result of air trapped under pressure within the pleural cavity, where it is not normally present (pneumothorax), or the pressure of fluid within the pleural space (pleural effusion).

Thoracic Palpation

The nurse palpates the thorax for tenderness, masses, lesions, respiratory excursion, and vocal fremitus. If the patient has reported an area of pain or if lesions are apparent, the nurse performs direct palpation with the fingertips (for skin lesions and subcutaneous masses) or with the ball of the hand (for deeper masses or generalized flank or rib discomfort).

RESPIRATORY EXCURSION

Respiratory excursion is an estimation of thoracic expansion and may disclose significant information about thoracic movement during breathing. The nurse assesses the patient for range and symmetry of excursion. The

CHART 21-7

Locating Thoracic Landmarks

With respect to the thorax, location is defined both horizontally and vertically. With respect to the lungs, location is defined by lobe.

HORIZONTAL REFERENCE POINTS

Horizontally, thoracic locations are identified according to their proximity to the rib or the intercostal space under the examiner's fingers. On the anterior surface, identification of a specific rib is facilitated by first locating the angle of Louis. This is where the manubrium joins the body of the sternum in the midline. The second rib joins the sternum at this prominent landmark.

Other ribs may be identified by counting down from the second rib. The intercostal spaces are referred to in terms of the rib immediately above the intercostal space; for example, the fifth intercostal space is directly below the fifth rib.

Locating ribs on the posterior surface of the thorax is more difficult. The first step is to identify the spinous process. This is accomplished by finding the seventh cervical vertebra (*vertebra prominens*), which is the most prominent spinous process. When the neck is slightly flexed, the seventh cervical spinous process stands out. Other vertebrae are then identified by counting downward.

VERTICAL REFERENCE POINTS

Several imaginary lines are used as vertical referents or landmarks to identify the location of thoracic findings. The *midsternal line* passes through the center of the sternum. The *midclavicular line* is an imaginary line that descends from the middle of the clavicle. The *point of maximal impulse* of the heart normally lies along this line on the left thorax.

When the arm is abducted from the body at 90°, imaginary vertical lines may be drawn from the anterior axillary fold, from the middle of the axilla, and from the posterior axillary fold. These lines are called, respectively, the *anterior axillary line*, the *midaxillary line*, and the *posterior axillary line*. A line drawn vertically through the superior and inferior poles of the scapula is called the *scapular line*, and a line drawn down the center of the vertebral column is called the *vertebral line*. Using these landmarks, for example, the examiner communicates findings by referring to an area of dullness extending from the vertebral to the scapular line between the seventh and tenth ribs on the right.

LOBES OF THE LUNGS

The lobes of the lung may be mapped on the surface of the chest wall in the following manner. The line between the upper and lower lobes on the left begins at the fourth thoracic spinous process posteriorly, proceeds around to cross the fifth rib in the midaxillary line, and meets the sixth rib at the sternum. This line on the right divides the right middle lobe from the right lower lobe. The line dividing the right upper lobe from the middle lobe is an incomplete one that begins at the fifth rib in the midaxillary line, where it intersects the line between the upper and lower lobes and traverses horizontally to the sternum. Thus, the upper lobes are dominant on the anterior surface of the thorax and the lower lobes are dominant on the posterior surface. There is no presentation of the right middle lobe on the posterior surface of the chest.

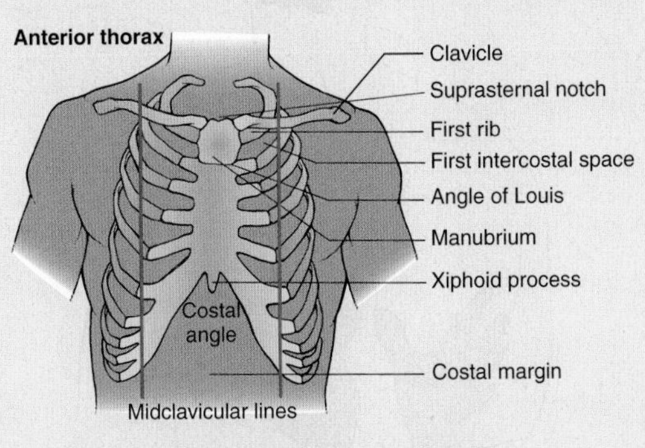

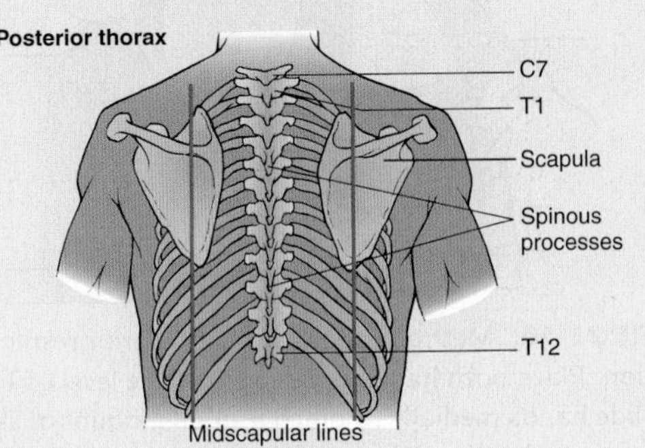

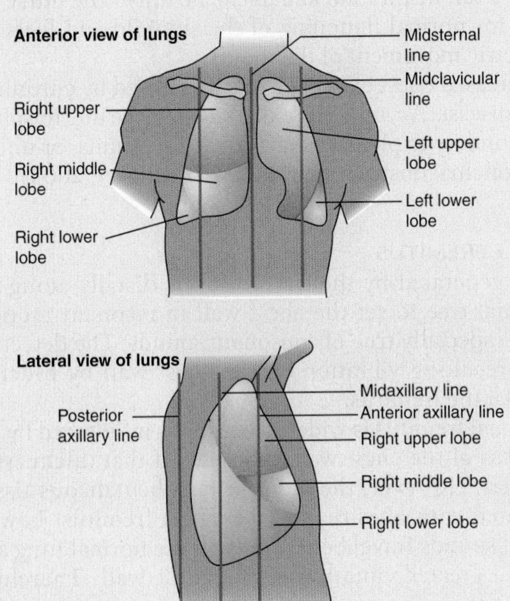

TABLE 21-3 Rates and Depths of Respiration

	Definition	Graphic Representation
Eupnea	Normal, breathing at 12–18 breaths/minute	
Bradypnea	Slower than normal rate (<10 breaths/minute), with normal depth and regular rhythm	
Tachypnea	Rapid, shallow breathing >24 breaths/minute	
Hypoventilation	Shallow, irregular breathing	
Hyperventilation	Increased rate and depth of breathing (called Kussmaul's respiration if caused by diabetic ketoacidosis)	
Apnea	Period of cessation of breathing. Time duration varies; apnea may occur briefly during other breathing disorders, such as with sleep apnea. Life threatening if sustained.	
Cheyne-Stokes	Regular cycle where the rate and depth of breathing increase, then decrease until apnea (usually about 20 seconds) occurs.	
Biot's respiration	Periods of normal breathing (3–4 breaths) followed by a varying period of apnea (usually 10–60 seconds).	

patient is instructed to inhale deeply while the movement of the nurse's thumbs (placed along the costal margin on the anterior chest wall) during inspiration and expiration is observed. This movement is normally symmetric (Bickley & Szilagyi, 2003).

Posterior assessment is performed by placing the thumbs adjacent to the spinal column at the level of the tenth rib (Fig. 21-10). The hands lightly grasp the lateral rib cage. Sliding the thumbs medially about 2.5 cm (1 inch) raises a small skinfold between the thumbs. The patient is instructed to take a full inspiration and to exhale fully. The nurse observes for normal flattening of the skinfold and feels the symmetric movement of the thorax.

Decreased chest excursion may be caused by chronic fibrotic disease. Asymmetric excursion may be due to splinting secondary to pleurisy, fractured ribs, trauma, or unilateral bronchial obstruction (Bickley & Szilagyi, 2003).

TACTILE FREMITUS

Sound generated by the larynx travels distally along the bronchial tree to set the chest wall in resonant motion. This is especially true of consonant sounds. The detection of the resulting vibration on the chest wall by touch is called tactile fremitus.

Normal fremitus is widely varied. It is influenced by the thickness of the chest wall, especially if that thickness is muscular. However, the increase in subcutaneous tissue associated with obesity may also affect fremitus. Lower-pitched sounds travel better through the normal lung and produce greater vibration of the chest wall. Therefore, fremitus is more pronounced in men than in women because of the deeper male voice. Normally, fremitus is most pronounced where the large bronchi are closest to the chest wall and least palpable over the distant lung fields. Therefore, it is most palpable in the upper thorax, anteriorly and posteriorly.

The patient is asked to repeat "ninety-nine" or "one, two, three," or "eee, eee, eee" as the nurse's hands move down

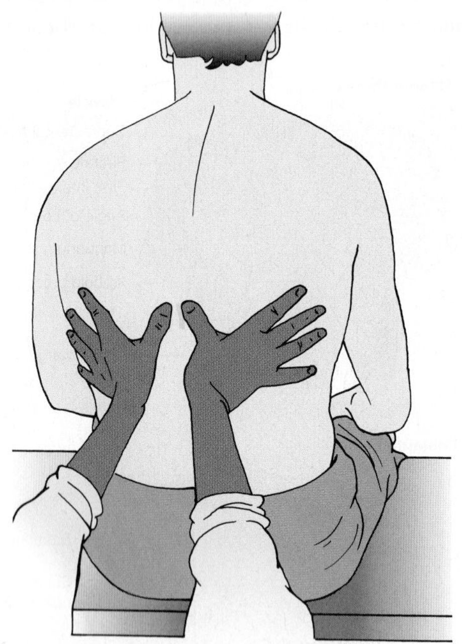

FIGURE 21-10. Method for assessing posterior respiratory excursion. Place both hands posteriorly at the level of T9 or T10. Slide hands medially to pinch a small amount of skin between your thumbs. Observe for symmetry as the patient exhales fully following a deep inspiration.

the patient's thorax. The vibrations are detected with the palmar surfaces of the fingers and hands, or the ulnar aspect of the extended hands, on the thorax. The hand or hands are moved in sequence down the thorax. Corresponding areas of the thorax are compared (Fig. 21-11). Bony areas are not tested.

Air does not conduct sound well, but a solid substance such as tissue does, provided that it has elasticity and is not compressed. Therefore, an increase in solid tissue per unit volume of lung enhances fremitus, and an increase in air per unit volume of lung impedes sound. Patients with emphysema, which results in the rupture of alveoli and trapping of air, exhibit almost no tactile fremitus. A patient with consolidation of a lobe of the lung from pneumonia has increased tactile fremitus over that lobe. Air in the pleural space does not conduct sound (Bickley & Szilagyi, 2003).

Thoracic Percussion

Percussion sets the chest wall and underlying structures in motion, producing audible and tactile vibrations. The nurse uses percussion to determine whether underlying tissues are filled with air, fluid, or solid material (Finesilver, 2003). Percussion also is used to estimate the size and location of certain structures within the thorax (eg, diaphragm, heart, liver).

Percussion usually begins with the posterior thorax. Ideally, the patient is in a sitting position with the head flexed forward and the arms crossed on the lap. This position separates the scapulae widely and exposes more lung area for assessment. The nurse percusses across each shoulder top, locating the 5-cm width of resonance overlying the lung apices (Fig. 21-12). Then the nurse proceeds down the posterior thorax, percussing symmetric areas at intervals of 5 to 6 cm (2 to 2.5 inches). The middle finger is positioned parallel to the ribs in the intercostal space; the finger is placed firmly against the chest wall before it is struck with the middle finger of the opposite hand. Bony structures (scapulae or ribs) are not percussed.

Percussion over the anterior chest is performed with the patient in an upright position with shoulders arched backward and arms at the side. The nurse begins in the supraclavicular area and proceeds downward, from one intercostal space to the next. In the female patient, it may be necessary to displace the breasts for an adequate examination. Dullness noted to the left of the sternum between the third and fifth intercostal spaces is a normal finding, because that is the location of the heart. Similarly, there is a normal span of liver dullness in the right thorax, from the fifth intercostal space to the right costal margin at the midclavicular line (Bickley & Szilagyi, 2003).

The anterior and lateral thorax is examined with the patient in a supine position. If the patient cannot sit up, percussion of the posterior thorax is performed with the patient positioned on the side.

Dullness over the lung occurs when air-filled lung tissue is replaced by fluid or solid tissue. Table 21-4 reviews percussion sounds and their characteristics.

DIAPHRAGMATIC EXCURSION

The normal resonance of the lung stops at the diaphragm. The position of the diaphragm is different during inspiration and expiration.

To assess the position and motion of the diaphragm, the nurse instructs the patient to take a deep breath and hold it while the maximal descent of the diaphragm is percussed. The point at which the percussion note at the midscapular line changes from resonance to dullness is marked with a pen. The patient is then instructed to exhale fully and hold it while the nurse again percusses downward to the dullness

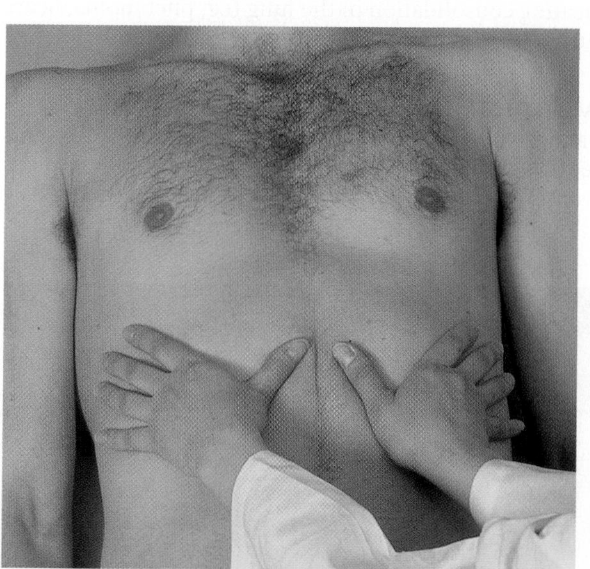

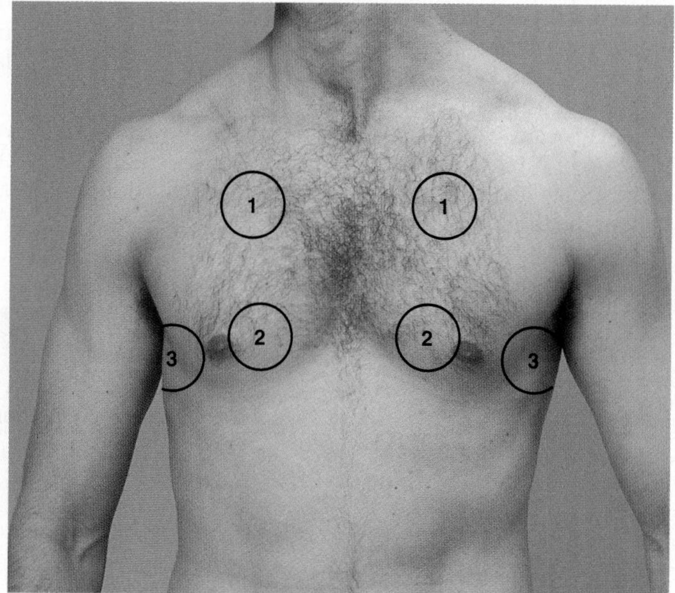

FIGURE 21-11. When palpating for tactile fremitus (*left*), the nurse places the ball or ulnar surface of the hands on the chest area being assessed. The palpation sequence is at *right*. From Bickley, L. S. & Szilagyi, P. G. (2003). *Bates' guide to physical examination and history taking* (8th ed.). Philadelphia: Lippincott Williams & Wilkins.

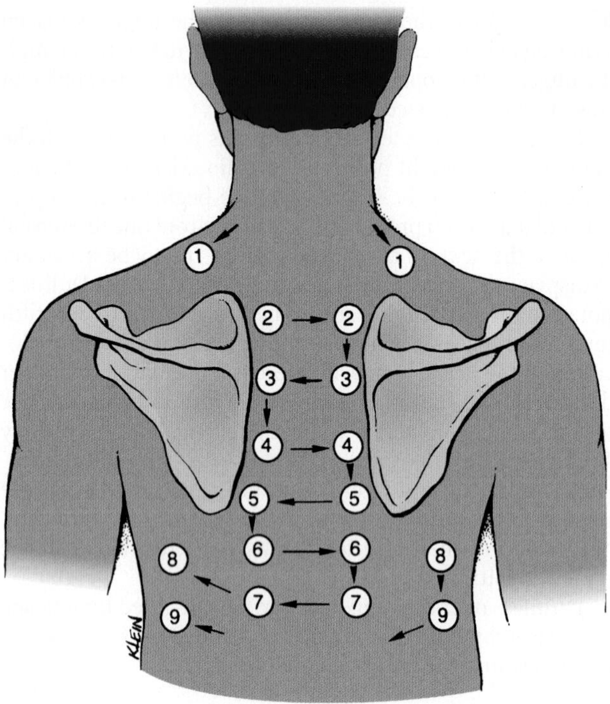

FIGURE 21-12. Percussion of the posterior thorax. With the patient in a sitting position, symmetric areas of the lungs are percussed at 5-cm intervals. This progression starts at the apex of each lung and concludes with percussion of each lateral chest wall.

of the diaphragm. This point is also marked. The distance between the two markings indicates the range of motion of the diaphragm.

Maximal excursion of the diaphragm may be as much as 8 to 10 cm (3 to 4 inches) in healthy, tall young men, but for most people it is usually 5 to 7 cm (2 to 2.75 inches). Normally, the diaphragm is about 2 cm (0.75 inches) higher on the right because of the position of the heart and the liver above and below the left and right segments of the diaphragm, respectively. Decreased diaphragmatic excursion may occur with pleural effusion and emphysema. An increase in intra-abdominal pressure, as in pregnancy or ascites, may account for a diaphragm that is positioned high in the thorax (Bickley & Szilagyi, 2003).

Thoracic Auscultation

Auscultation is useful in assessing the flow of air through the bronchial tree and in evaluating the presence of fluid or solid obstruction in the lung. The nurse auscultates for normal breath sounds, adventitious sounds, and voice sounds (Finesilver, 2003).

Examination includes auscultation of the anterior, posterior, and lateral thorax and is performed as follows. The nurse places the diaphragm of the stethoscope firmly against the chest wall as the patient breathes slowly and deeply through the mouth. Corresponding areas of the chest are auscultated in a systematic fashion from the apices to the bases and along midaxillary lines. The sequence of auscultation and the positioning of the patient are similar to those used for percussion. It often is necessary to listen to two full inspirations and expirations at each anatomic location for valid interpretation of the sound heard. Repeated deep breaths may result in symptoms of hyperventilation (eg, lightheadedness); this is avoided by having the patient rest and breathe normally periodically during the examination.

BREATH SOUNDS

Normal breath sounds are distinguished by their location over a specific area of the lung and are identified as vesicular, bronchovesicular, and bronchial (tubular) breath sounds (Table 21-5).

The location, quality, and intensity of breath sounds are determined during auscultation. When airflow is decreased by bronchial obstruction (atelectasis) or when fluid (pleural effusion) or tissue (obesity) separates the air passages from the stethoscope, breath sounds are diminished or absent. For example, the breath sounds of the patient with emphysema are faint or often completely inaudible. When they are heard, the expiratory phase is prolonged. Bronchial and bronchovesicular sounds that are audible anywhere except over the main bronchus in the lungs signify pathology, usually indicating consolidation in the lung (eg, pneumonia, heart failure). This finding requires further evaluation.

ADVENTITIOUS SOUNDS

An abnormal condition that affects the bronchial tree and alveoli may produce adventitious (additional) sounds. Adventitious sounds are divided into two categories: dis-

TABLE 21-4 Characteristics of Percussion Sounds

Sound	Relative Intensity	Relative Pitch	Relative Duration	Location Example	Examples
Flatness	Soft	High	Short	Thigh	Large pleural effusion
Dullness	Medium	Medium	Medium	Liver	Lobar pneumonia
Resonance	Loud	Low	Long	Normal lung	Simple chronic bronchitis
Hyperresonance	Very loud	Lower	Longer	None normally	Emphysema, pneumothorax
Tympany	Loud	High*	—*	Gastric air bubble or puffed-out cheek	Large pneumothorax

*Distinguished mainly by its musical timbre.

TABLE 21-5 Breath Sounds

	Duration of Sounds	Intensity of Expiratory Sound	Pitch of Expiratory Sound	Locations Where Heard Normally
Vesicular*	Inspiratory sounds last longer than expiratory ones	Soft	Relatively low	Entire lung field except over the upper sternum and between the scapulae
Broncho-vesicular	Inspiratory and expiratory sounds are about equal	Intermediate	Intermediate	Often in the 1st and 2nd interspaces anteriorly and between the scapulae (over the main bronchus)
Bronchial	Expiratory sounds last longer than inspiratory ones	Loud	Relatively high	Over the manubrium, if heard at all
Tracheal	Inspiratory and expiratory sounds are about equal	Very loud	Relatively high	Over the trachea in the neck

*The thickness of the bars indicates intensity of breath sounds; the steeper their incline, the higher the pitch of the sounds.

crete, noncontinuous sounds (crackles) and continuous musical sounds (wheezes). The duration of the sound is the important distinction to make in identifying the sound as noncontinuous or continuous.

Crackles (formerly referred to as rales) are discrete, noncontinuous sounds that result from delayed reopening of deflated airways. Crackles may or may not be cleared by coughing. They reflect underlying inflammation or congestion and are often present in such conditions as pneumonia, bronchitis, heart failure, bronchiectasis, and pulmonary fibrosis. Crackles are usually heard on inspiration, but they may also be heard on expiration.

Pleural friction rubs are specific examples of crackles (Table 21-6). Friction rubs result from inflammation of the

TABLE 21-6 Abnormal (Adventitious) Breath Sounds

Breath Sound	Description	Etiology
Crackles		
Crackles in general	Soft, high-pitched, discontinuous popping sounds that occur during inspiration	Secondary to fluid in the airways or alveoli or to opening of collapsed alveoli
Coarse crackles	Discontinuous popping sounds heard in early inspiration; harsh, moist sound originating in the large bronchi	Associated with obstructive pulmonary disease
Fine crackles	Discontinuous popping sounds heard in late inspiration; sounds like hair rubbing together; originates in the alveoli	Associated with interstitial pneumonia, restrictive pulmonary disease (eg, fibrosis). Fine crackles in early inspiration are associated with bronchitis or pneumonia.
Wheezes		
Sonorous wheezes (rhonchi)	Deep, low-pitched rumbling sounds heard primarily during expiration; caused by air moving through narrowed tracheobronchial passages	Secretions or tumor
Sibilant wheezes	Continuous, musical, high-pitched, whistle-like sounds heard during inspiration and expiration caused by air passing through narrowed or partially obstructed airways; may clear with coughing	Bronchospasm, asthma, and buildup of secretions
Friction rubs		
Pleural friction rub	Harsh, crackling sound, like two pieces of leather being rubbed together. Heard during inspiration alone or during both inspiration and expiration. May subside when patient holds breath. Coughing will not clear sound.	Secondary to inflammation and loss of lubricating pleural fluid

pleural surfaces that induces a crackling, grating sound usually heard in inspiration and expiration. The sound can be enhanced by applying pressure to the chest wall with the diaphragm of the stethoscope. The sound is imitated by rubbing the thumb and index finger together near the ear. A friction rub is best heard over the lower lateral anterior surface of the thorax.

Wheezes are associated with bronchial wall oscillation and changes in airway diameter. Like crackles, wheezes are usually heard on expiration but may be heard on inspiration. They are commonly heard in patients with asthma, chronic bronchitis, or bronchiectasis.

VOICE SOUNDS

The sound heard through the stethoscope as the patient speaks is known as vocal resonance. The vibrations produced in the larynx are transmitted to the chest wall as they pass through the bronchi and alveolar tissue. During the process, the sounds are diminished in intensity and altered so that syllables are not distinguishable. Voice sounds are usually assessed by having the patient repeat "ninety-nine" or "eee" while the nurse listens with the stethoscope in corresponding areas of the chest from the apices to the bases.

Bronchophony describes vocal resonance that is more intense and clearer than normal. Egophony describes voice sounds that are distorted. It is best appreciated by having the patient repeat the letter E. The distortion produced by consolidation transforms the sound into a clearly heard A rather than E. Bronchophony and egophony have precisely the same significance as bronchial breathing with an increase in tactile fremitus. When an abnormality is detected, it should be evident using more than one assessment method. A change in tactile fremitus is more subtle and can be missed, but bronchial breathing and bronchophony can be noted loudly and clearly.

Whispered pectoriloquy is a very subtle finding, which is heard only in the presence of rather dense consolidation of the lungs. Transmission of high-frequency components of sound is so enhanced by the consolidated tissue that even whispered words are heard, a circumstance not noted in normal physiology. The significance is the same as that of bronchophony (Bickley & Szilagyi, 2003). The physical findings for the most common respiratory diseases are summarized in Table 21-7.

Assessment of Respiratory Function in the Acutely or Critically Ill Patient

Assessment of respiratory status is essential for the well-being of the patient who is acutely or critically ill. Often, such a patient is intubated and receiving mechanical ventilation. This requires that the nurse have expertise in physical assessment, be skilled in monitoring techniques, and be knowledgeable about possible ventilator-induced lung injury (Winters & Munro, 2004). The nurse reviews the patient's health history, including the history of disorders affecting lung function, signs and symptoms, and exposure to medications and other agents that can affect respiratory status. The nurse also observes the patient's respiratory status to analyze and interpret a variety of clinical findings and laboratory test results. Checking the ventilator settings to make sure that they are set as prescribed and that alarms are always in the "on" position, the nurse must assess for patient–ventilator synchrony as well as for agitation, restlessness, and other signs of respiratory distress (nasal flaring, excessive use of intercostals and accessory muscles, uncoordinated movement of the chest and abdomen, and a report by the patient of shortness of breath). The nurse must note changes in the patient's vital signs and evidence of hemodynamic instability and report them to the physician, because they may indicate that the mechanical ventilation is ineffective or that the patient's status has deteriorated. It is necessary to assess the position of the patient to be certain that the head of the bed is elevated to prevent aspiration, especially if the patient is receiving enteral feedings. In addition, the patient's mental status should be assessed and compared to previous status. Lethargy and somnolence may be signs of increasing carbon dioxide levels and should not be considered insignificant, even if the patient is receiving sedation or analgesic agents (Johnson, 2004).

TABLE 21-7 Assessment Findings in Common Respiratory Disorders

Disorder	Tactile Fremitus	Percussion	Auscultation
Consolidation (eg, pneumonia)	Increased	Dull	Bronchial breath sounds, crackles, bronchophony, egophony, whispered pectoriloquy
Bronchitis	Normal	Resonant	Normal to decreased breath sounds, wheezes
Emphysema	Decreased	Hyperresonant	Decreased intensity of breath sounds, usually with prolonged expiration
Asthma (severe attack)	Normal to decreased	Resonant to hyperresonant	Wheezes
Pulmonary edema	Normal	Resonant	Crackles at lung bases, possibly wheezes
Pleural effusion	Absent	Dull to flat	Decreased to absent breath sounds, bronchial breath sounds and bronchophony, egophony, and whispered pectoriloquy above the effusion over the area of compressed lung
Pneumothorax	Decreased	Hyperresonant	Absent breath sounds
Atelectasis	Absent	Flat	Decreased to absent breath sounds

Chest auscultation, percussion, and palpation are essential parts of the evaluation of the critically ill patient with or without mechanical ventilation. Assessment of the anterior and posterior lung fields is part of the nurse's routine evaluation. If the patient is recumbent, it is essential to turn the patient to assess all lung fields so that dependent areas can be assessed for breath sounds, including the presence of normal breath sounds and adventitious sounds. Failure to examine the dependent areas of the lungs can result in missing the findings associated with disorders such as atelectasis or pleural effusion. Percussion is performed to assess for pleural effusion; if pleural effusion is present, the affected lung fields are dull to percussion and breath sounds are absent. A pleural friction rub may also be present (Winters & Munro, 2004).

Tests of the patient's respiratory status are easily performed at the bedside by measuring the respiratory rate (see earlier discussion), tidal volume, minute ventilation, vital capacity, inspiratory force, and compliance. These tests are particularly important for patients who are at risk for pulmonary complications, including those who have undergone chest or abdominal surgery, have had prolonged anesthesia, have preexisting pulmonary disease, or are elderly. These tests are also used routinely for mechanically ventilated patients.

The patient whose chest expansion is limited by external restrictions such as obesity or abdominal distention and who cannot breathe deeply because of postoperative pain or sedation will inhale and exhale a low volume of air (referred to as low tidal volumes). Prolonged hypoventilation at low tidal volumes can produce alveolar collapse (atelectasis). The amount of air remaining in the lungs after a normal expiration (functional residual capacity) decreases, the ability of the lungs to expand (compliance) is reduced, and the patient must breathe faster to maintain the same degree of tissue oxygenation. These events can be exaggerated in patients who have preexisting pulmonary diseases and in elderly patients whose airways are less compliant, because the small airways may collapse during expiration. More details of the assessment of the patient with lung disease, including arterial blood gas (ABG) analysis, are described in subsequent chapters in this unit and in Chapter 14.

NURSING ALERT

One should not rely only on visual inspection of the rate and depth of a patient's respiratory excursions to determine the adequacy of ventilation. Respiratory excursions may appear normal or exaggerated due to an increased work of breathing, but the patient may actually be moving only enough air to ventilate the dead space. If there is any question regarding adequacy of ventilation, auscultation or pulse oximetry (or both) should be used for additional assessment of respiratory status.

Tidal Volume

The volume of each breath is referred to as the tidal volume (see Table 21-1 to review lung capacities and volumes). A spirometer is an instrument that can be used at the bedside to measure volumes. If the patient is breathing through an endotracheal tube or tracheostomy, the spirometer is directly attached to it and the exhaled volume is obtained from the reading on the gauge. In other patients, the spirometer is attached to a face mask or a mouthpiece positioned so that it is airtight, and the exhaled volume is measured.

The tidal volume may vary from breath to breath. To ensure that the measurement is reliable, it is important to measure the volumes of several breaths and to note the range of tidal volumes, together with the average tidal volume.

Minute Ventilation

Respiratory rates and tidal volume alone are unreliable indicators of adequate ventilation, because both can vary widely from breath to breath. However, together the tidal volume and respiratory rate are important because the minute ventilation, which is useful in detecting respiratory failure, can be determined from them. Minute ventilation is the volume of air expired per minute. It is equal to the product of the tidal volume in liters multiplied by the respiratory rate or frequency. In practice, the minute ventilation is not calculated but is measured directly using a spirometer.

Minute ventilation may be decreased by a variety of conditions that result in hypoventilation. When the minute ventilation falls, alveolar ventilation in the lungs also decreases, and the $PaCO_2$ increases. Risk factors for hypoventilation are listed in Chart 21-8.

Vital Capacity

Vital capacity is measured by having the patient take in a maximal breath and exhale fully through a spirometer. The normal value depends on the patient's age, gender, body build, and weight.

CHART 21-8

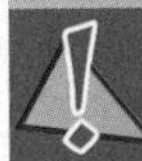

Risk Factors for Hypoventilation

- Limited neurologic impulses transmitted from the brain to the respiratory muscles, as in spinal cord trauma, cerebrovascular accidents, tumors, myasthenia gravis, Guillain-Barré syndrome, polio, and drug overdose
- Depressed respiratory centers in the medulla, as with anesthesia, sedation, and drug overdose
- Limited thoracic movement (kyphoscoliosis), limited lung movement (pleural effusion, pneumothorax), or reduced functional lung tissue (chronic pulmonary diseases, severe pulmonary edema)

NURSING ALERT

Most patients can generate a vital capacity twice the volume they normally breathe in and out (tidal volume). If the vital capacity is less than 10 mL/kg, the patient will be unable to sustain spontaneous ventilation and will require respiratory assistance.

When the vital capacity is exhaled at a maximal flow rate, the forced vital capacity is measured. Most patients can exhale at least 80% of their vital capacity in 1 second (forced expiratory volume in 1 second, or FEV_1) and almost all of it in 3 seconds (FEV_3). A reduction in FEV_1 suggests abnormal pulmonary air flow. If the patient's FEV_1 and forced vital capacity are proportionately reduced, maximal lung expansion is restricted in some way. If the reduction in FEV_1 greatly exceeds the reduction in forced vital capacity, the patient may have some degree of airway obstruction.

Inspiratory Force

Inspiratory force evaluates the effort the patient is making during inspiration. It does not require patient cooperation and therefore is a useful measurement in the unconscious patient. The equipment needed for this measurement includes a manometer that measures negative pressure and adapters that are connected to an anesthesia mask or a cuffed endotracheal tube. The manometer is attached and the airway is completely occluded for 10 to 20 seconds while the inspiratory efforts of the patient are registered on the manometer. The normal inspiratory pressure is about 100 cm H_2O. If the negative pressure registered after 15 seconds of occluding the airway is less than about 25 cm H_2O, mechanical ventilation is usually required because the patient lacks sufficient muscle strength for deep breathing or effective coughing.

Diagnostic Evaluation

A wide range of diagnostic studies, described on the following pages, may be performed in patients with respiratory conditions.

Pulmonary Function Tests

Pulmonary function tests (PFTs) are routinely used in patients with chronic respiratory disorders. They are performed to assess respiratory function and to determine the extent of dysfunction. Such tests include measurements of lung volumes, ventilatory function, and the mechanics of breathing, diffusion, and gas exchange (Table 21-8).

PFTs are useful in monitoring the course of a patient with an established respiratory disease and assessing the response to therapy (Conner & Meng, 2003). They are useful as screening tests in potentially hazardous industries, such as coal mining and those that involve exposure to asbestos and other noxious fumes, dusts, or gases. They are used to screen patients who are scheduled for thoracic and upper abdominal surgery (Beckles, Spiro, Colice, et al., 2003; Wang, 2004) and symptomatic patients with a history suggesting high risk. In addition, PFTs may be used for evaluation of respiratory symptoms and disability for insurance or legal purposes (Porth, 2005) and to diagnose occupational respiratory disease (Anees, 2003).

PFTs generally are performed by a technician using a spirometer that has a volume-collecting device attached to a recorder that demonstrates volume and time simultaneously. A number of tests are carried out, because no single measurement provides a complete picture of pulmonary function. The most frequently used PFTs are described in Table 21-8. Technology is available that allows for more complex assessment of pulmonary function. Methods include exercise tidal flow–volume loops, negative expiratory pressure, nitric oxide, and forced oscillation. These assessment methods

TABLE 21-8 Pulmonary Function Tests

Term Used	Symbol	Description	Remarks
Forced vital capacity	FVC	Vital capacity performed with a maximally forced expiratory effort	Forced vital capacity is often reduced in COPD because of air trapping.
Forced expiratory volume (qualified by subscript indicating the time interval in seconds)	FEV_t (usually FEV_1)	Volume of air exhaled in the specified time during the performance of forced vital capacity; FEV_1 is volume exhaled in 1 second	A valuable clue to the severity of the expiratory airway obstruction
Ratio of timed forced expiratory volume to forced vital capacity	FEV_t/FVC%, usually FEV_1/FVC%	FEV_t expressed as a percentage of the forced vital capacity	Another way of expressing the presence or absence of airway obstruction
Forced expiratory flow	$FEF_{200-1200}$	Mean forced expiratory flow between 200 and 1200 mL of the FVC	An indicator of large airway obstruction
Forced midexpiratory flow	$FEF_{25-75\%}$	Mean forced expiratory flow during the middle half of the FVC	Slowed in small airway obstruction
Forced end expiratory flow	$FEF_{75-85\%}$	Mean forced expiratory flow during the terminal portion of the FVC	Slowed in obstruction of smallest airways
Maximal voluntary ventilation	MVV	Volume of air expired in a specified period (12 seconds) during repetitive maximal effort	An important factor in exercise tolerance

allow for detailed evaluation of expiratory flow limitations and airway inflammation (Conner & Meng, 2003).

PFT results are interpreted on the basis of the degree of deviation from normal, taking into consideration the patient's height, weight, age, and gender. Because there is a wide range of normal values, PFTs may not detect early localized changes. The patient with respiratory symptoms (dyspnea, wheezing, cough, sputum production) usually undergoes a complete diagnostic evaluation, even if the results of PFTs are "normal." Trends of results provide information about disease progression as well as the patient's response to therapy (Conner & Meng, 2003).

Patients with respiratory disorders may be taught how to measure their peak flow rate (which reflects maximal expiratory flow) at home using a spirometer (Ramirez, 2003). This allows them to monitor the progress of therapy, to alter medications and other interventions as needed based on caregiver guidelines, and to notify the health care provider if there is inadequate response to their own interventions. Home care teaching instructions are described in Chapter 24, which discusses asthma.

Arterial Blood Gas Studies

Measurements of blood pH and of arterial oxygen and carbon dioxide tensions are obtained when managing patients with respiratory problems and adjusting oxygen therapy as needed. The arterial oxygen tension (PaO_2) indicates the degree of oxygenation of the blood, and the arterial carbon dioxide tension ($PaCO_2$) indicates the adequacy of alveolar ventilation. ABG studies aid in assessing the ability of the lungs to provide adequate oxygen and remove carbon dioxide and the ability of the kidneys to reabsorb or excrete bicarbonate ions to maintain normal body pH. Serial ABG analysis also is a sensitive indicator of whether the lung has been damaged after chest trauma. ABG levels are obtained through an arterial puncture at the radial, brachial, or femoral artery or through an indwelling arterial catheter. ABG levels are discussed in detail in Chapter 14.

Patients whose ABG levels are monitored repeatedly with blood obtained from arterial punctures should receive an explanation of the purpose of the procedure. It has been reported that patients often experience considerable pain with repeated ABG levels yet are often unaware of the purpose of the puncture and the fact that the ABG results could make a major difference in their treatment (Crawford, 2004).

Pulse Oximetry

Pulse oximetry is a noninvasive method of continuously monitoring the oxygen saturation of hemoglobin (SaO_2). When oxygen saturation is measured with pulse oximetry, it is referred to as SpO_2 (Johnson, 2004; Woodrow, 2004). Although pulse oximetry does not replace ABG measurement, it is an effective tool to monitor for subtle or sudden changes in oxygen saturation. It is used in all settings where oxygen saturation monitoring is needed, such as the home, clinics, ambulatory surgical settings, and hospitals.

A probe or sensor is attached to the fingertip (Fig. 21-13), forehead, earlobe, or bridge of the nose. The sensor detects changes in oxygen saturation levels by monitoring light

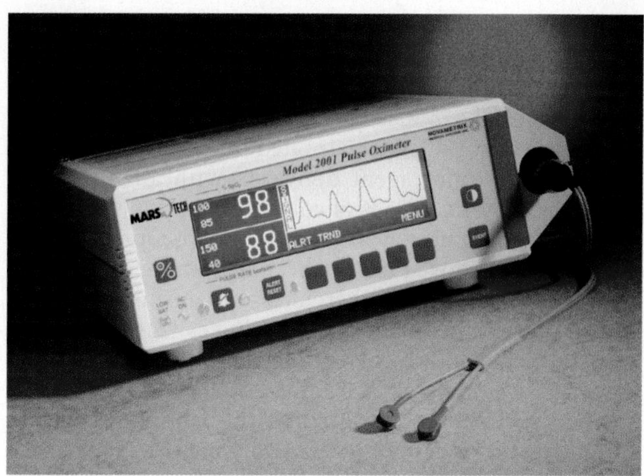

FIGURE 21-13. Measuring blood oxygenation with pulse oximetry reduces the need for invasive procedures, such as drawing blood for analysis of oxygen levels. After the pulse oximeter sensor slips easily over a patient's finger, the oxygen saturation level appears on the monitor. The oximeter is portable and ideal for home use. Courtesy of Novametrix Medical Systems, Inc.

signals generated by the oximeter and reflected by blood pulsing through the tissue at the probe. Normal SpO_2 values are 95% to 100%. Values less than 85% indicate that the tissues are not receiving enough oxygen, and further evaluation is needed. SpO_2 values obtained by pulse oximetry are unreliable in cardiac arrest and shock, if dyes (ie, methylene blue) or vasoconstrictor medications have been used, or if the patient has severe anemia or a high carbon monoxide level. Furthermore, they are not reliable detectors of hypoventilation if the patient is receiving supplemental oxygen (Fu, Downs, Schweiger, et al., 2004).

Cultures

Throat cultures may be performed to identify organisms responsible for pharyngitis. Throat culture may also assist in identifying organisms responsible for infection of the lower respiratory tract. Nasal swabs also may be performed for the same purpose.

Sputum Studies

Sputum is obtained for analysis to identify pathogenic organisms and to determine whether malignant cells are present. It also may be used to assess for hypersensitivity states (in which there is an increase in eosinophils). Periodic sputum examinations may be necessary for patients receiving antibiotics, corticosteroids, and immunosuppressive medications for prolonged periods, because these agents are associated with opportunistic infections. In general, sputum cultures are used in diagnosis, for drug sensitivity testing, and to guide treatment.

Expectoration is the usual method for collecting a sputum specimen. The patient is instructed to clear the nose and throat and rinse the mouth to decrease contamination of the sputum. After taking a few deep breaths, the patient coughs (rather than spits), using the diaphragm, and expectorates into a sterile container.

If the sputum cannot be raised spontaneously, the patient often can be induced to cough deeply by breathing an irritating aerosol of supersaturated saline, propylene glycol, or some other agent delivered with an ultrasonic nebulizer. Other methods of collecting sputum specimens include endotracheal aspiration, bronchoscopic removal, bronchial brushing, transtracheal aspiration, and gastric aspiration—usually for tuberculosis organisms (see Chapter 23). Generally, the deepest specimens (those from the base of the lungs) are obtained in the early morning after they have accumulated overnight.

The specimen is delivered to the laboratory within 2 hours by the patient or nurse. Allowing the specimen to stand for several hours in a warm room results in the overgrowth of contaminant organisms and may make it difficult to identify the pathogenic organisms (especially *Mycobacterium tuberculosis*). The home care nurse may assist patients who need help obtaining the sample or who cannot deliver the specimen to the laboratory in a timely fashion.

Imaging Studies

Imaging studies, including x-rays, computed tomography (CT), magnetic resonance imaging (MRI), contrast studies, and radioisotope diagnostic scans may be part of any diagnostic workup, ranging from a determination of the extent of infection in sinusitis to tumor growth in cancer.

Chest X-Ray

Normal pulmonary tissue is radiolucent; therefore, densities produced by fluid, tumors, foreign bodies, and other pathologic conditions can be detected by x-ray examination. A chest x-ray may reveal an extensive pathologic process in the lungs in the absence of symptoms. The routine chest x-ray consists of two views—the posteroanterior projection and the lateral projection. Chest x-rays are usually taken after full inspiration (a deep breath), because the lungs are best visualized when they are well aerated. Also, the diaphragm is at its lowest level and the largest expanse of lung is visible. If taken on expiration, x-ray films may accentuate an otherwise unnoticed pneumothorax or obstruction of a major artery.

Computed Tomography

CT is an imaging method in which the lungs are scanned in successive layers by a narrow-beam x-ray. The images produced provide a cross-sectional view of the chest. Whereas a chest x-ray shows major contrasts between body densities such as bone, soft tissue, and air, CT can distinguish fine tissue density. CT may be used to define pulmonary nodules and small tumors adjacent to pleural surfaces that are not visible on routine chest x-rays and to demonstrate mediastinal abnormalities and hilar adenopathy, which are difficult to visualize with other techniques. Contrast agents are useful when evaluating the mediastinum and its contents.

Magnetic Resonance Imaging

MRI is similar to CT except that magnetic fields and radiofrequency signals are used instead of a narrow-beam x-ray. MRI yields a much more detailed diagnostic image than CT. MRI is used to characterize pulmonary nodules, to help stage bronchogenic carcinoma (assessment of chest wall invasion), and to evaluate inflammatory activity in interstitial lung disease, acute pulmonary embolism, and chronic thrombolytic pulmonary hypertension.

Fluoroscopic Studies

Fluoroscopy is used to assist with invasive procedures, such as a chest needle biopsy or transbronchial biopsy, that are performed to identify lesions. It also may be used to study the movement of the chest wall, mediastinum, heart, and diaphragm; to detect diaphragm paralysis; and to locate lung masses.

Pulmonary Angiography

Pulmonary angiography is most commonly used to investigate thromboembolic disease of the lungs, such as pulmonary emboli, and congenital abnormalities of the pulmonary vascular tree. It involves the rapid injection of a radiopaque agent into the vasculature of the lungs for radiographic study of the pulmonary vessels. It can be performed by injecting the radiopaque agent into a vein in one or both arms (simultaneously) or into the femoral vein, with a needle or catheter. The agent also can be injected into a catheter that has been inserted in the main pulmonary artery or its branches or into the great veins proximal to the pulmonary artery.

Radioisotope Diagnostic Procedures (Lung Scans)

Several types of lung scans—V/Q scan, gallium scan, and positron emission tomography (PET)—are used to assess normal lung functioning, pulmonary vascular supply, and gas exchange.

A V/Q lung scan is performed by injecting a radioactive agent into a peripheral vein and then obtaining a scan of the chest to detect radiation. The isotope particles pass through the right side of the heart and are distributed into the lungs in proportion to the regional blood flow, making it possible to trace and measure blood perfusion through the lung. This procedure is used clinically to measure the integrity of the pulmonary vessels relative to blood flow and to evaluate blood flow abnormalities, as seen in pulmonary emboli. The imaging time is 20 to 40 minutes, during which the patient lies under the camera with a mask fitted over the nose and mouth. This is followed by the ventilation component of the scan. The patient takes a deep breath of a mixture of oxygen and radioactive gas, which diffuses throughout the lungs. A scan is performed to detect ventilation abnormalities in patients who have regional differences in ventilation. It may be helpful in the diagnosis of bronchitis, asthma, inflammatory fibrosis, pneumonia, emphysema, and lung cancer. Ventilation without perfusion is seen with pulmonary emboli.

A gallium scan is a radioisotope lung scan used to detect inflammatory conditions, abscesses, adhesions, and the presence, location, and size of tumors. It is used to stage bronchogenic cancer and document tumor regression after chemotherapy or radiation. Gallium is injected intravenously, and scans are taken at intervals (eg, 6, 24, and 48 hours) to evaluate gallium uptake by the pulmonary tissues.

PET is a radioisotope study with advanced diagnostic capabilities that is used to evaluate lung nodules for malignancy. PET can detect and display metabolic changes in tissue, distinguish normal tissue from diseased tissue (such as in cancer), differentiate viable from dead or dying tissue, show regional blood flow, and determine the distribution and fate of medications in the body. PET is more accurate in detecting malignancies than CT and has equivalent accuracy in detecting malignant nodules when compared with invasive procedures such as thoracoscopy.

Endoscopic Procedures

Bronchoscopy

Bronchoscopy is the direct inspection and examination of the larynx, trachea, and bronchi through either a flexible fiberoptic bronchoscope or a rigid bronchoscope (Fig. 21-14). The fiberoptic scope is used more frequently in current practice.

The purposes of diagnostic bronchoscopy are: (1) to examine tissues or collect secretions, (2) to determine the location and extent of the pathologic process and to obtain a tissue sample for diagnosis (by biting or cutting forceps, curettage, or brush biopsy), (3) to determine whether a tumor can be resected surgically, and (4) to diagnose bleeding sites (source of hemoptysis).

Therapeutic bronchoscopy is used to (1) remove foreign bodies from the tracheobronchial tree, (2) remove secretions obstructing the tracheobronchial tree when the patient cannot clear them, (3) treat postoperative atelectasis, and (4) destroy and excise lesions. It has also been used to insert stents to relieve airway obstruction that is caused by tumors or miscellaneous benign conditions or that occurs as a complication of lung transplantation (Saad, Murthy, Krizmanich, et al., 2003).

The fiberoptic bronchoscope is a thin, flexible bronchoscope that can be directed into the segmental bronchi. Because of its small size, its flexibility, and its excellent optical system, it allows increased visualization of the peripheral airways and is ideal for diagnosing pulmonary lesions. Fiberoptic bronchoscopy allows biopsy of previously inaccessible tumors and can be performed at the bedside. It also can be performed through endotracheal or tracheostomy tubes of patients on ventilators. Cytologic examinations can be performed without surgical intervention.

The rigid bronchoscope is a hollow metal tube with a light at its end. It is used mainly for removing foreign substances, investigating the source of massive hemoptysis, or performing endobronchial surgical procedures. Rigid bronchoscopy is performed in the operating room, not at the bedside.

Possible complications of bronchoscopy include a reaction to the local anesthetic, infection, aspiration, bronchospasm, **hypoxemia** (low blood oxygen level), pneumothorax, bleeding, and perforation.

NURSING INTERVENTIONS

Before the procedure, a signed consent form is obtained from the patient. Food and fluids are withheld for 6 hours before the test to reduce the risk of aspiration when the cough reflex is blocked by anesthesia. The nurse explains the procedure to the patient to reduce fear and decrease anxiety and administers preoperative medications (usually atropine and a sedative or opioid) as prescribed to inhibit vagal stimulation (thereby guarding against bradycardia, dysrhythmias, and hypotension), suppress the cough reflex, sedate the patient, and relieve anxiety.

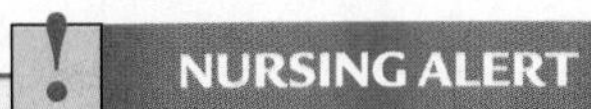

Sedation given to patients with respiratory insufficiency may precipitate respiratory arrest.

The patient must remove dentures and other oral prostheses. The examination is usually performed under local anesthesia or moderate sedation, but general anesthesia may be used for rigid bronchoscopy. A topical anesthetic such as lidocaine (Xylocaine) may be sprayed on the pharynx or

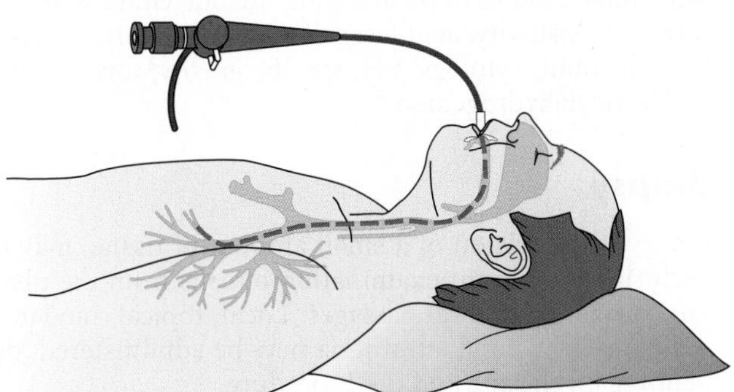

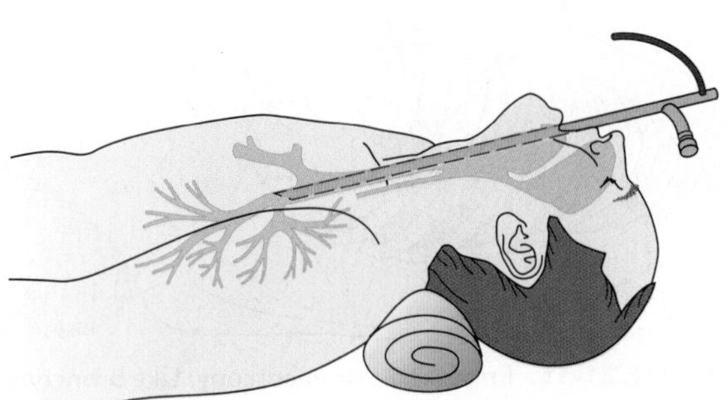

FIGURE 21-14. Endoscopic bronchoscopy permits visualization of bronchial structures. The bronchoscope is advanced into bronchial structures orally. Bronchoscopy permits the clinician not only to diagnose but also to treat various lung problems.

dropped on the epiglottis and vocal cords and into the trachea to suppress the cough reflex and minimize discomfort. Sedatives or opioids are administered intravenously as prescribed to provide moderate sedation.

After the procedure, it is important that the patient takes nothing by mouth until the cough reflex returns, because the preoperative sedation and local anesthesia impair the protective laryngeal reflex and swallowing for several hours. Once the patient demonstrates a cough reflex, the nurse may offer ice chips and eventually fluids. In the elderly patient, the nurse assesses for confusion and lethargy, which may be due to the large doses of lidocaine administered during the procedure. The nurse also monitors the patient's respiratory status and observes for hypoxia, hypotension, tachycardia, dysrhythmias, hemoptysis, and dyspnea. Any abnormality is reported promptly. The patient is not discharged from the recovery area until adequate cough reflex and respiratory status are present. The nurse instructs the patient and family caregivers to report any shortness of breath or bleeding immediately.

Thoracoscopy

Thoracoscopy is a diagnostic procedure in which the pleural cavity is examined with an endoscope (Fig. 21-15). Small incisions are made into the pleural cavity in an intercostal space; the location of the incision depends on the clinical and diagnostic findings. After any fluid present in the pleural cavity is aspirated, the fiberoptic mediastinoscope is inserted into the pleural cavity, and its surface is inspected through the instrument. After the procedure, a chest tube may be inserted, and the pleural cavity is drained by negative-pressure water-seal drainage.

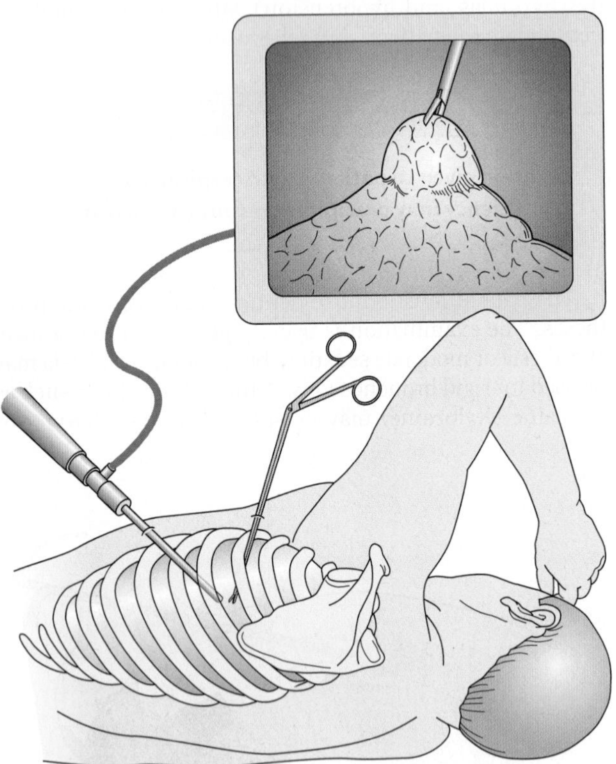

FIGURE 21-15. Endoscopic thoracoscopy. Like bronchoscopy, thoracoscopy uses fiberoptic instruments and video cameras for visualizing thoracic structures. Unlike bronchoscopy, thoracoscopy usually requires the surgeon to make a small incision before inserting the endoscope. A combined diagnostic–treatment procedure, thoracoscopy includes excising tissue for biopsy.

Thoracoscopy is primarily indicated in the diagnostic evaluation of pleural effusions, pleural disease, and tumor staging. Biopsies of the lesions can be performed under visualization for diagnosis.

Thoracoscopic procedures have expanded with the availability of video monitoring, which permits improved visualization of the lung. Video-assisted thoracoscopy may be used in the diagnosis and treatment of empyema, pleural effusion, and other respiratory disorders (Luh, Chou, Wang, et al., 2005). Such procedures also have been used with the carbon dioxide laser in the removal of pulmonary blebs and bullae and in the treatment of spontaneous pneumothorax. Lasers have also been used in the excision of peripheral pulmonary nodules. Although the laser does not replace the need for thoracotomy in the treatment of some lung cancers, its use continues to expand, because it is less invasive than open surgical procedures and hospitalization and recovery are shorter.

NURSING INTERVENTIONS

Follow-up care in the health care facility and at home involves monitoring the patient for shortness of breath (which might indicate a pneumothorax) and minor activity restrictions, which vary depending on the intensity of the procedure. If a chest tube was inserted during the procedure, monitoring of the chest drainage system and chest tube insertion site is essential (see Chapter 25).

Thoracentesis

A thin layer of pleural fluid normally remains in the pleural space. An accumulation of pleural fluid may occur with some disorders. A sample of this fluid can be obtained by thoracentesis (aspiration of pleural fluid for diagnostic or therapeutic purposes). It is important to position the patient as shown in Chart 21-9. When thoracentesis is performed under ultrasound guidance, it has a lower rate of complications than when it is performed without ultrasound guidance (Jones, Moyers, Rogers, et al., 2003; Mayo, Goltz, Tafreshi, et al., 2004).

A needle biopsy of the pleura may be performed at the same time. Studies of pleural fluid include Gram stain culture and sensitivity, acid-fast staining and culture, differential cell count, cytology, pH, specific gravity, total protein, and lactic dehydrogenase.

Biopsy

Biopsy, the excision of a small amount of tissue, may be performed to permit examination of cells from the pharynx, larynx, and nasal passages. Local, topical, moderate sedation, or general anesthesia may be administered, depending on the site and the procedure.

Pleural Biopsy

Pleural biopsy is accomplished by needle biopsy of the pleura or by pleuroscopy, a visual exploration through a fiberoptic

CHART 21-9 Guidelines for Assisting the Patient Undergoing Thoracentesis

A thoracentesis (aspiration of fluid or air from the pleural space) is performed on patients with various clinical problems. A diagnostic or therapeutic procedure, thoracentesis may be used for

- Removal of fluid and air from the pleural cavity
- Aspiration of pleural fluid for analysis
- Pleural biopsy
- Instillation of medication into the pleural space

The responsibilities of the nurse and rationale for the nursing actions are summarized below.

NURSING ACTIVITIES	RATIONALE
1. Ascertain in advance that a chest x-ray has been ordered and completed and the consent form has been signed.	1. Posteroanterior and lateral chest x-ray films are used to localize fluid and air in the pleural cavity and to aid in determining the puncture site. When fluid is loculated (isolated in a pocket of pleural fluid), ultrasound scans are performed to help select the best site for needle aspiration.
2. Assess the patient for allergy to the local anesthetic to be used.	2. If the patient is allergic to the initially prescribed anesthetic, assessment findings provide an opportunity to use a safer anesthetic.
3. Administer sedation if prescribed	3. Sedation enables the patient to cooperate with the procedure and promotes relaxation
4. Inform the patient about the nature of the procedure and a. The importance of remaining immobile b. Pressure sensations to be experienced c. That minimal discomfort is anticipated after the procedure	4. An explanation helps to orient the patient to the procedure, assists the patient to mobilize resources, and provides an opportunity to ask questions and verbalize anxiety.
5. Position the patient comfortably with adequate supports. If possible, place the patient upright or in one of the following positions: a. Sitting on the edge of the bed with the feet supported and arms and head on a padded over-the-bed table	5. The upright position facilitates the removal of fluid that usually localizes at the base of the thorax. A position of comfort helps the patient to relax.

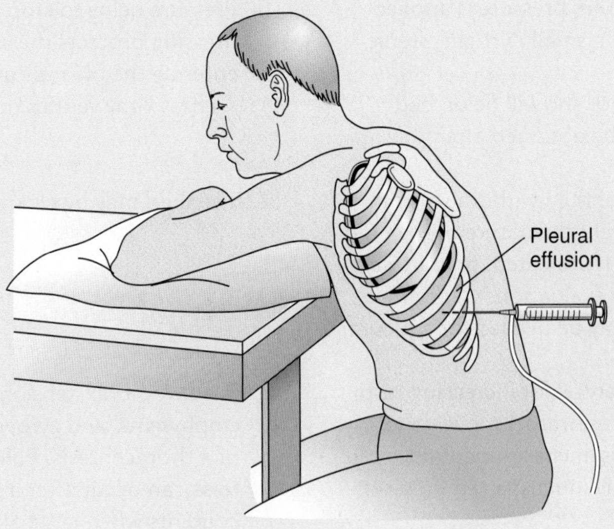

continued >

CHART 21-9 Guidelines for Assisting the Patient Undergoing Thoracentesis, continued

NURSING ACTIVITIES	RATIONALE
b. Straddling a chair with arms and head resting on the back of the chair	
c. Lying on the unaffected side with the head of the bed elevated 30 to 45 degrees if unable to assume a sitting position	
6. Support and reassure the patient during the procedure.	6. Sudden and unexpected movement, such as coughing, by the patient can traumatize the visceral pleura and lung.
a. Prepare the patient for the cold sensation of skin germicide solution and for a pressure sensation from infiltration of local anesthetic agent.	
b. Encourage the patient to refrain from coughing.	
7. Expose the entire chest. The site for aspiration is visualized by chest x-ray and percussion. If fluid is in the pleural cavity, the thoracentesis site is determined by the chest x-ray, ultrasound scanning, and physical findings, with attention to the site of maximal dullness on percussion.	7. If air is in the pleural cavity, the thoracentesis site is usually in the second or third intercostal space in the midclavicular line because air rises in the thorax.
8. The procedure is performed under aseptic conditions. After the skin is cleansed, the physician uses a small-caliber needle to inject a local anesthetic slowly into the intercostal space.	8. An intradermal wheal is raised slowly; rapid injection causes pain. The parietal pleura is very sensitive and should be well infiltrated with anesthetic before the physician passes the thoracentesis needle through it.
9. The physician advances the thoracentesis needle with the syringe attached. When the pleural space is reached, suction may be applied with the syringe.	9. Use of thoracentesis needle allows proper insertion.
a. A 20-mL syringe with a three-way stopcock is attached to the needle (one end of the adapter is attached to the needle and the other to the tubing leading to a receptacle that receives the fluid being aspirated).	a. When a large quantity of fluid is withdrawn, a three-way stopcock serves to keep air from entering the pleural cavity.
b. If a considerable quantity of fluid is removed, the needle is held in place on the chest wall with a small hemostat.	b. The hemostat steadies the needle on the chest wall. Sudden pleuritic chest pain or shoulder pain may indicate that the needle point is irritating the visceral or the diaphragmatic pleura.
10. After the needle is withdrawn, pressure is applied over the puncture site and a small, airtight, sterile dressing is fixed in place.	10. Pressure helps to stop bleeding, and the airtight dressing protects the site and prevents air from entering the pleural cavity.
11. Advise the patient that he or she will be on bed rest and a chest x-ray will be obtained after thoracentesis.	11. A chest x-ray verifies that there is no pneumothorax.
12. Record the total amount of fluid withdrawn from the procedure and document the nature of the fluid, its color, and its viscosity. If indicated, prepare samples of fluid for laboratory evaluation. A specimen container with formalin may be needed for a pleural biopsy.	12. The fluid may be clear, serous, bloody, purulent, etc.
13. Monitor the patient at intervals for increasing respiratory rate; asymmetry in respiratory movement; faintness; vertigo; tightness in chest; uncontrollable cough; blood-tinged, frothy mucus; a rapid pulse; and signs of hypoxemia.	13. Pneumothorax, tension pneumothorax, subcutaneous emphysema, and pyrogenic infection are complications of a thoracentesis. Pulmonary edema or cardiac distress can occur after a sudden shift in mediastinal contents when large amounts of fluid are aspirated.

bronchoscope inserted into the pleural space. Pleural biopsy is performed when there is pleural exudate of undetermined origin or when there is a need to culture or stain the tissue to identify tuberculosis or fungi.

Lung Biopsy Procedures

If the chest x-ray findings are inconclusive or show pulmonary density (indicating an infiltrate or lesion), biopsy may be performed to obtain lung tissue for examination to identify the nature of the lesion. Several nonsurgical lung biopsy techniques are used because they yield accurate information with low morbidity: (1) transcatheter bronchial brushing, (2) transbronchial lung biopsy, and (3) percutaneous (through-the-skin) needle biopsy.

In transcatheter bronchial brushing, a fiberoptic bronchoscope is introduced into the bronchus under fluoroscopy. A small brush attached to the end of a flexible wire is inserted through the bronchoscope. Under direct visualization, the area under suspicion is brushed back and forth, causing cells to slough off and adhere to the brush. The catheter port of the bronchoscope may be used to irrigate the lung tissue with saline solution to secure material for additional studies. The brush is removed from the bronchoscope and a slide is made for examination under the microscope. The brush may be cut off and sent to the pathology laboratory for analysis.

This procedure is useful for cytologic evaluations of lung lesions and for the identification of pathogenic organisms (eg, *Nocardia, Aspergillus, Pneumocystis carinii*). It is especially useful in the immunologically compromised patient.

Another method of bronchial brushing involves the introduction of the catheter through the transcricothyroid membrane by needle puncture. After this procedure, the patient is instructed to hold a finger or thumb over the puncture site while coughing to prevent air from leaking into the surrounding tissues.

In transbronchial lung biopsy, biting or cutting forceps are introduced by a fiberoptic bronchoscope. A biopsy is indicated when a lung lesion is suspected and the results of routine sputum samples and bronchoscopic washings are negative.

In percutaneous needle biopsy, a cutting needle or a spinal-type needle is used to obtain a tissue specimen for histologic study. Analgesia may be administered before the procedure. The skin over the biopsy site is cleansed and anesthetized, and a small incision is made. The biopsy needle is inserted through the incision into the pleura with the patient holding the breath in midexpiration. Using fluoroscopic monitoring, the surgeon guides the needle into the periphery of the lesion and obtains a tissue sample from the mass. Possible complications include pneumothorax, pulmonary hemorrhage, and empyema.

NURSING INTERVENTIONS

After the procedure, recovery and home care are similar to those for bronchoscopy and thoracoscopy. Nursing care involves monitoring the patient for shortness of breath, bleeding, and infection. In preparation for discharge, the patient and family are instructed to report pain, shortness of breath, visible bleeding, redness of the biopsy site, or purulent drainage (pus) to the health care provider immediately. Patients who have undergone biopsy are often anxious because of the need for the biopsy and the potential findings; the nurse must consider this in providing postbiopsy care and teaching.

Lymph Node Biopsy

The scalene lymph nodes are enmeshed in the deep cervical pad of fat overlying the scalenus anterior muscle. They drain the lungs and mediastinum and may show histologic changes from intrathoracic disease. If these nodes are palpable on physical examination, a scalene node biopsy may be performed. A biopsy of these nodes may be performed to detect spread of pulmonary disease to the lymph nodes and to establish a diagnosis or prognosis in such diseases as Hodgkin disease, sarcoidosis, fungal disease, tuberculosis, and carcinoma.

Mediastinoscopy is the endoscopic examination of the mediastinum for exploration and biopsy of mediastinal lymph nodes that drain the lungs; this examination does not require a thoracotomy. Biopsy is usually performed through a suprasternal incision. Mediastinoscopy is carried out to detect mediastinal involvement of pulmonary malignancy and to obtain tissue for diagnostic studies of other conditions (eg, sarcoidosis).

An anterior mediastinotomy is thought to provide better exposure and diagnostic possibilities than a mediastinoscopy. An incision is made in the area of the second or third costal cartilage. The mediastinum is explored, and biopsies are performed on any lymph nodes found. Chest tube drainage is required after the procedure. Mediastinotomy is particularly valuable to determine whether a pulmonary lesion is resectable.

NURSING INTERVENTIONS

Postprocedure care focuses on providing adequate oxygenation, monitoring for bleeding, and providing pain relief. The patient may be discharged a few hours after the chest drainage system is removed. The nurse should instruct the patient and family about monitoring for changes in respiratory status, taking into consideration the impact of anxiety about the potential findings of the biopsy on their ability to remember those instructions.

Critical Thinking Exercises

1 A man with a long history of smoking (60 pack-years) is scheduled for surgery to remove a nonfunctioning kidney. In preparation for surgery, he is scheduled for PFTs, which he refuses to have because he says his breathing has nothing to do with his kidney problem or his scheduled kidney surgery. How would you respond to his statement? What impact does his 60-pack-year history of cigarette smoking have on your preoperative, intraoperative, and postoperative assessment?

2 When obtaining a health history from a 55-year-old patient who is seeking health care because of a persistent cough and extreme fatigue, you note that she is able to speak only in short sentences before having to stop to catch her breath. What specific information about signs and symptoms would you obtain during the health history? How would you modify your physical examination based on your observations? What initial laboratory tests would you anticipate will be ordered for this patient?

3 A patient who has cancer of the lung has undergone a thoracentesis for removal of pleural fluid in an effort to relieve his shortness of breath. Soon after the procedure is completed, the patient reports that his shortness of breath has increased rather than decreased. Based on your knowledge of risks associated with thoracentesis, what assessment data would you obtain from this patient and report to the physician? What additional nursing measures are warranted for the patient at this time? How would you respond if the patient had been discharged an hour after the thoracentesis and provided this information to you by telephone from home?

4 ebp A woman reports that she has had a cough with sputum production in the morning for the past 2 weeks. She says that she is a smoker and has a 20-pack-year history of smoking. Her primary health care provider explains to her why smoking is contraindicated with cough and sputum production and explains the importance of smoking cessation. As the nurse in the clinic, your role is to discuss smoking cessation techniques with her and to identify a plan that is likely to be successful for her. Describe the specific smoking cessation strategies that you will discuss with this patient. Identify the evidence base that supports the use of the smoking cessation strategies selected. What is the strength of the evidence, and what criteria will you use to evaluate the effectiveness of various smoking cessation strategies?

REFERENCES AND SELECTED READINGS

BOOKS

Bickley, L. S. & Szilagyi, P. G. (2003). *Bates' guide to physical examination and history taking* (8th ed.). Philadelphia: Lippincott Williams & Wilkins.

Levitzky, M. G. (2003). *Pulmonary physiology* (6th ed.). New York: McGraw-Hill Medical.

Morton, P. G., Fontaine, D. K., Hudak, C. M., et al. (2005). *Critical care nursing: A holistic approach* (8th ed.). Philadelphia: Lippincott Williams & Wilkins.

Porth, C. M. (2005). *Pathophysiology: Concepts of altered health states* (7th ed.). Philadelphia: Lippincott Williams & Wilkins.

Sole, M. L., Klein, D. G., & Moseley, M. J. (2005). *Introduction to critical care nursing* (4th ed.). St. Louis: Elsevier Saunders.

Stanley, M., Blair, K. A. & Beare, P. G. (2005). *Gerontological nursing: Promoting successful aging with older adults* (3rd ed.). Philadelphia: F. A. Davis.

Urden, L. D., Stacy, K. M. & Lough, M. E. (2002). *Thelan's critical care nursing: Diagnosis and management* (4th ed.). St. Louis: Mosby.

Weber, J. & Kelley, J. (2003). *Health assessment in nursing* (2nd ed.). Philadelphia: Lippincott Williams & Wilkins.

West, J. B. (2004). *Respiratory physiology* (7th ed.). Philadelphia: Lippincott Williams & Wilkins.

Wilkins, R. L., Sheldon, R. L. & Krider, S. J. (2005). *Clinical assessment in respiratory care* (5th ed.). St. Louis: Elsevier Mosby.

JOURNALS

**Asterisks indicate nursing research articles.*

Anees, W. (2003). Use of pulmonary function tests in the diagnosis of occupational asthma. *Annals of Allergy, Asthma, and Immunology, 90*(5 Suppl. 2), 47–51.

Ayers, D. M. M. & Lappin, J. S. (2004). Act fast when your patient has dyspnea. *Nursing, 34*(7), 36–42.

Bahhady, I. J. & Unterborn, J. (2003a). Pulmonary function tests: An update. *Consultant, 43*(7), 813–818,820.

Bahhady, I. J. & Unterborn, J. (2003b). What pulmonary function tests can and cannot tell you: Results help assess disease severity in ILD and COPD. *Journal of Respiratory Diseases, 24*(4), 170–176.

*Bailey, P. H. (2004). The dyspnea-anxiety-dyspnea cycle—COPD patients' stories of breathlessness: "It's scary when you can't breathe." *Qualitative Health Research, 14*(6), 760–778.

Beckles, M. A., Spiro, S. G., Colice, G. L., et al. (2003). The physiologic evaluation of patients with lung cancer being considered for resectional surgery. *Chest, 123*(1 Suppl.), 105S–114S.

Bledsoe, B. E., Porter, R. S., & Cherry, R. A. (2005). 25 Physical examination pearls: Important tips to help you polish your hands-on patient assessment skills. *JEMS: Journal of Emergency Medical Services, 30*(3), 58–60, 62–63, 64–74.

Boyle, A. H. & Waters, H. F. (2000). Issues in respiratory nursing. Focus on prevention: Recommendations of the National Lung Health Education Program. *Heart and Lung, 29*(6), 446–449.

Burki, N. (2003). Evaluating dyspnea: A practical guide. *Journal of Respiratory Diseases, 24*(1), 10–15.

*Chernecky, C., Sarna, L., Waller, J. L., et al. (2004). Assessing coughing and wheezing in lung cancer: A pilot study. *Oncology Nursing Forum, 31*(6), 1095–1101.

Conklin B. (2005). B-type natriuretic peptide: A new measurement to distinguish cardiac from pulmonary causes of acute dyspnea. *Journal of Emergency Nursing, 31*(1), 73–75,117–123.

Conner, B. & Meng, A. (2003). Pulmonary function testing in asthma: Nursing applications. *Nursing Clinics of North America, 38*(4), 571–583.

Considine, J. (2005). The role of nurses in preventing adverse events related to respiratory dysfunction: Literature review. *Journal of Advanced Nursing, 49*(6), 624–633.

Crawford, A. (2004). Respiratory nursing. An audit of the patient's experience of arterial blood gas testing. *British Journal of Nursing, 13*(9), 529–532.

Davis, M. & Holliday, J. Jr. (2005). Differentiating causes of respiratory distress. *Emergency Medical Services, 34*(1), 72–73.

*de Souza Caroci, A. D. S. & Lareau, S. C. (2004). Descriptors of dyspnea by patients with chronic obstructive pulmonary disease versus congestive heart failure. *Heart and Lung, 33*(2), 102–110.

Ebihara, S., Saito, H., Kanda, A., et al. (2003). Impaired efficacy of cough in patients with Parkinson disease. *Chest, 124*(3), 1009–1015.

Farquhar, S. L. & Fantasia, L. (2005). Pulmonary anatomy and physiology and the effects of COPD. *Home Healthcare Nurse, 23*(3), 167–176.

Finesilver, C. (2003). Pulmonary assessment: What you need to know. *Progress in Cardiovascular Nursing, 18*(2), 83–92.

French, C. T., Fletcher, K. E. & Irwin, R. S. (2004). Gender differences in health-related quality of life in patients complaining of chronic cough. *Chest, 125*(2), 482–488.

Fu, E. S., Downs, J. B., Schweiger, J. W., et al. (2004). Supplemental oxygen impairs detection of hypoventilation by pulse oximetry. *Chest, 126*(5), 1552–1558.

Garrett, K., Laurer, K., & Christopher, B. (2004). The effects of obesity on the cardiopulmonary system: Implications for critical care nursing. *Progress in Cardiovascular Nursing, 19*(4), 155–161.

Hardie, J. A., Vollmer, W. M., Buist, A. S., et al. (2004). Reference values for arterial blood gases in the elderly. *Chest, 125*(6), 2053–2060.

Hately, J., Laurence, V., Scott, A., et al. (2003). Breathlessness clinics within specialist palliative care settings can improve the quality of life and functional capacity of patients with lung cancer. *Palliative Medicine, 17*(5), 410–417.

Irwin, R. S., Baumann, M. H., Bolser, D. C., et al. (2006). Diagnosis and management of cough: Executive summary. ACCP evidence-based clinical practice guidelines. *Chest, 129*(1 Suppl.), 1S–23S.

Johnson, K. L. (2004). Diagnostic measures to evaluate oxygenation in critically ill adults: Implications and limitations. *AACN Clinical Issues: Advanced Practice in Acute and Critical Care, 15*(4), 506–524, 640–642.

Jones, P. W., Moyers, J. P., Rogers, J. T., et al. (2003). Ultrasound-guided thoracentesis: Is it a safer method? *Chest, 123*(2), 418–423.

Karnani, N. G., Reisfield, G. M. & Wilson, G. R. (2005). Evaluation of chronic dyspnea. *American Family Physician, 71*(8), 1529–1538, 1473–1475, 1612.

Leidy, N. K., Rennard, S. I., Schmier, J., et al. (2003). The Breathlessness, Cough, and Sputum Scale: The development of empirically based guidelines for interpretation. *Chest, 124*(6), 2182–2191.

Lim, K. G. & Morgenthaler, T. I. (2005). Defining obstruction or restriction remains the goal: Pulmonary function tests. Part 1: Applying the basics. *Journal of Respiratory Diseases, 26*(1), 26–30,32.

Luh, S. P., Chou, M. C., Wang, L. S., et al. (2005). Video-assisted thoracoscopic surgery in the treatment of complicated parapneumonic effusions or empyemas: Outcome of 234 patients. *Chest, 127*(4), 1427–1432.

Lung, C. L. & Lung, M. L. (2003). General principles of asthma management: Symptom monitoring. *Nursing Clinics of North America, 38*(4), 585–596.

Mahler, D. A., Fierro-Carrion, G., & Baird, J. C. (2003). Evaluation of dyspnea in the elderly. *Clinics in Geriatric Medicine, 19*(1), 19–33.

Mayo, P. H., Goltz, H. R., Tafreshi, M., et al. (2004). Safety of ultrasound-guided thoracentesis in patients receiving mechanical ventilation. *Chest, 125*(3), 1059–1067.

*Meek, P. M., Lareau, S. C., & Hu, J. (2003). Are self-reports of breathing effort and breathing distress stable and valid measures among persons with asthma, persons with COPD, and healthy persons? *Heart and Lung, 32*(5), 335–346.

Mehta, M. (2003). Assessing respiratory status: Learn how to evaluate your patient's lungs through sight, sound, and touch. *Nursing, 33*(2), 54–56.

Meng, A. & McConnell, S. (2003). Symptom perception and respiratory sensation: Clinical applications. *Nursing Clinics of North America, 38*(4), 737–748.

*Michaels, C. & Meek, P. M. (2004). The language of breathing among individuals with chronic obstructive pulmonary disease. *Heart and Lung, 33*(6), 390–400.

*Moody, L. E., Webb, M., Cheung, R., et al. (2004). A focus group for caregivers of hospice patients with severe dyspnea. *American Journal of Hospice and Palliative Care, 21*(2), 121–130, 160.

Noppen, M., Poppe, K., D'Haese, J., et al. (2004). Interventional bronchoscopy for treatment of tracheal obstruction secondary to benign or malignant thyroid disease. *Chest, 125*(2), 723–730.

*Nguyen, H. Q., Carrieri-Kuhlman, V., Rankin, S. H., et al. (2005). Is Internet-based support for dyspnea self-management in patients with chronic obstructive pulmonary disease possible? Results of a pilot study. *Heart and Lung, 34*(1), 51–62.

Ott, M. C., Khoor, A., Leventhal, J. P., et al. (2003). Pulmonary toxicity in patients receiving low-dose amiodarone. *Chest, 123*(2), 646–651.

Pezzoli, L., Giardini, G., Consonni, S., et al. (2003). Quality of spirometric performance in older people. *Age and Ageing, 21*(1), 43–46.

Poe, R. H. & Kallay, M. C. (2003). Chronic cough and gastroesophageal reflux disease: Experience with specific therapy for diagnosis and treatment. *Chest, 123*(3), 679–684.

Prigmore, S. (2005). Respiratory care: Assessment and nursing care of the patient with dyspnoea. *Nursing Times, 101*(4), 50–53.

Ramirez, E. G. (2003). Management of asthma emergencies. *Nursing Clinics of North America, 38*(4), 713–724.

Saad, C. P., Murthy, S., Krizmanich, G., et al. (2003). Bronchoscopy. Self-expandable metallic airway stents and flexible bronchoscopy: Long-term outcomes analysis. *Chest, 124*(5), 1993–1999.

Simpson, H. (2004). Respiratory nursing. Interpretation of arterial blood gases: A clinical guide for nurses. *British Journal of Nursing, 13*(9), 522–528.

Smetana, G. W. (2003). Preoperative pulmonary assessment of the older adult. *Clinics in Geriatric Medicine, 19*(1), 35–55.

Vrijhoef, H. J. M., Diederiks, J. P. M., Wesseling, G. J., et al. (2003). Undiagnosed patients and patients at risk for COPD in primary health care: Early detection with the support of non-physicians. *Journal of Clinical Nursing, 12*(3), 366–373.

Wang, J. S. (2004). Pulmonary function tests in preoperative pulmonary evaluation. *Respiratory Medicine, 98*(7), 598–605.

Winters, A. C. & Munro, N. (2004). Assessment of the mechanically ventilated patient: An advanced practice approach. *AACN Clinical Issues: Advanced Practice in Acute and Critical Care, 15*(4), 525–533.

Woodrow, P. (2004). Arterial blood gas analysis. *Nursing Standard, 18*(21), 45–52.

*Wu, H., Wu, S., Lin, J., et al. (2004). Effectiveness of acupressure in improving dyspnoea in chronic obstructive pulmonary disease. *Journal of Advanced Nursing, 45*(3), 252–259.

Zeleznik, J. (2003). Normative aging of the respiratory system. *Clinics in Geriatric Medicine, 19*(1), 1–18.

Zoorob, R. J. & Campbell, J. S. (2003). Acute dyspnea in the office. *American Family Physician, 68*(9), 1803–1810.

RESOURCES

American Association for Respiratory Care, 11030 Ables Lane, Dallas, TX 75229; 972-243-2272; http://www.aarc.org. Accessed March 31, 2006.

American Lung Association, 1740 Broadway, New York, NY 10019; 212-315-8700 or 800-LUNG USA; http://www.lungusa.org. Accessed March 31, 2006.

National Heart, Lung, and Blood Institute/National Institutes of Health, Rockville Pike, Bldg. 31, Bethesda, MD 20892; 301-496-5166; http://www.nhlbi.nih.gov/index.htm. Accessed March 31, 2006.

National Lung Health Education Program; http://www.nlhep.org. Accessed March 31, 2006. Has easy-to-read teaching resources for patients.

CHAPTER 22

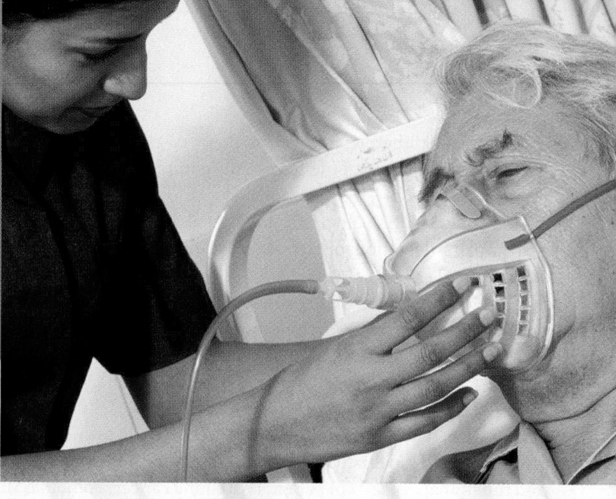

Management of Patients With Upper Respiratory Tract Disorders

Learning Objectives

On completion of this chapter, the learner will be able to:

1. Describe nursing management of patients with upper airway disorders.
2. Compare and contrast the upper respiratory tract infections with regard to cause, incidence, clinical manifestations, management, and the significance of preventive health care.
3. Use the nursing process as a framework for care of patients with upper airway infection.
4. Describe nursing management of the patient with epistaxis.
5. Use the nursing process as a framework for care of patients undergoing laryngectomy.

Many upper airway disorders are relatively minor, and their effects are limited to mild and temporary discomfort and inconvenience for the patient. Others, however, are acute, severe, and life-threatening and may require permanent alterations in breathing and speaking. Therefore, the nurse must have expert assessment skills, an understanding of the wide variety of disorders that may affect the upper airway, and an awareness of the impact of these alterations on patients. Because many of the disorders are treated outside the hospital or at home by patients themselves, patient teaching is an important aspect of nursing care. When caring for patients with acute, life-threatening disorders, the nurse needs highly developed assessment and clinical management skills, along with a focus on rehabilitation needs.

Upper Airway Infections

Upper airway infections are the most common cause of illness and affect most people on occasion. Some infections are acute, with symptoms that last several days; others are chronic, with symptoms that last a long time or recur. Patients with these conditions seldom require hospitalization. However, nurses working in community settings or long-term care facilities may encounter patients who have these infections. Therefore, it is important for the nurse to recognize the signs and symptoms and to provide appropriate care.

Infections of the upper airway are also known as upper respiratory tract infections (URIs). They occur when microorganisms such as viruses and bacteria are inhaled. URIs are the most common reason for seeking health care and for absences from school and work throughout the year. There are many causative organisms, and people are susceptible throughout life.

URIs affect the nasal cavity; ethmoidal air cells; and frontal, maxillary, and sphenoid sinuses, as well as the larynx and trachea. About 90% of upper respiratory disorders stem from a viral infection of the upper respiratory passages and subsequent mucous membrane inflammation. Although patients with these conditions rarely require hospitalization, the nurse can influence patient outcomes in community settings and in long-term facilities through patient teaching and use of resources when warranted.

Special considerations with regard to URIs in the elderly are summarized in Chart 22-1.

Rhinitis

Rhinitis is a group of disorders characterized by inflammation and irritation of the mucous membranes of the nose. It may be acute or chronic, nonallergic or allergic. It is estimated that 20% of the population of the United States has allergic rhinitis (Bush, 2004). Allergic rhinitis is further classified as seasonal or perennial rhinitis. Seasonal rhinitis occurs during pollen seasons, and perennial rhinitis occurs throughout the year. Allergies, including allergic rhinitis, affect more than 40 million people in the United States yearly (National Institute of Allergy and Infectious Diseases, 2005). Allergic disorders are described in detail in Chapter 53.

Pathophysiology

Nonallergic rhinitis may be caused by a variety of factors, including environmental factors such as changes in temperature or humidity, odors, or foods; infection; age; systemic disease; drugs (eg, cocaine), over-the-counter (OTC) and prescribed nasal decongestants, and other medications; and the presence of a foreign body. The most common cause of nonallergic rhinitis is the common cold. Drug-induced rhinitis is associated with use of antihypertensive agents and oral contraceptives and chronic use of nasal decongestants. Other causes of rhinitis are identified in Table 22-1. Figure 22-1 shows the pathologic processes involved in rhinitis and sinusitis.

Glossary

alaryngeal communication: alternative modes of speaking that do not involve the normal larynx; used by patients whose larynx has been surgically removed

aphonia: impaired ability to use one's voice due to disease or injury to the larynx

apnea: cessation of breathing

dysphagia: difficulties in swallowing

epistaxis: hemorrhage from the nose due to rupture of tiny, distended vessels in the mucous membrane of any area of the nose

herpes simplex: cold sore (cutaneous viral infection with painful vesicles and erosions on the tongue, palate, gingiva, buccal membranes, or lips)

laryngitis: inflammation of the larynx; may be caused by voice abuse, exposure to irritants, or infectious organisms

laryngectomy: removal of all or part of the larynx and surrounding structures

nuchal rigidity: stiffness of the neck or inability to bend the neck

pharyngitis: inflammation of the throat; usually viral or bacterial in origin

rhinitis: inflammation of the mucous membranes of the nose; may be infectious, allergic, or inflammatory in origin

rhinorrhea: drainage of a large amount of fluid from the nose

sinusitis: inflammation of the sinuses; may be acute or chronic; may be viral, bacterial, or fungal in origin

submucosal resection: surgical procedure to correct nasal obstruction due to deviated septum; also called septoplasty

tonsillitis: inflammation of the tonsils, usually due to an acute infection

xerostomia: dryness of the mouth from a variety of causes

CHART 22-1

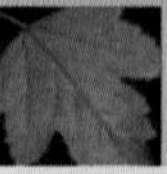

Upper Respiratory Tract Disorders in the Elderly

- Upper respiratory infections in the elderly may have more serious consequences if patients have concurrent medical problems that compromise their respiratory or immune status.
- Antihistamines to treat upper respiratory disorders must be used cautiously in the elderly because of their side effects and potential interactions with other medications.
- Sinusitis in the elderly is often preceded by nasal packing for treatment of epistaxis.
- Laryngitis in the elderly is common and most frequently occurs secondary to gastroesophageal reflux disease (GERD). The elderly are more likely to have impaired esophageal peristalsis and a weaker esophageal sphincter. Treatment measures include sleeping with the head of the bed elevated and the use of medications such as H_2-receptor blockers (eg, famotidine [Pepcid], ranitidine [Zantac]) or proton pump inhibitors (omeprazole [Prilosec]).

TABLE 22-1 Causes of Rhinitis

Category	Causes
Vasomotor	Idiopathic
	Abuse of nasal decongestants (rhinitis medicamentosa)
	Psychological stimulation (anger, sexual arousal)
	Irritants (smoke, air pollution, exhaust fumes, cocaine)
Mechanical	Tumor
	Deviated septum
	Crusting
	Hypertrophied turbinates
	Foreign body
	Cerebrospinal fluid leak
Chronic inflammatory	Polyps (in cystic fibrosis)
	Sarcoidosis
	Wegener's granulomatosis
	Midline granuloma
Infectious	Acute viral infection
	Acute or chronic sinusitis
	Rare nasal infections (syphilis, tuberculosis)
Hormonal	Pregnancy
	Use of oral contraceptives
	Hypothyroidism

Adapted from Carr, M. M. Differential diagnosis of rhinitis. Available at: icarus.med.utoronto.ca/carr/manual/ddxrhinitis.html (accessed March 31, 2006).

Physiology/Pathophysiology

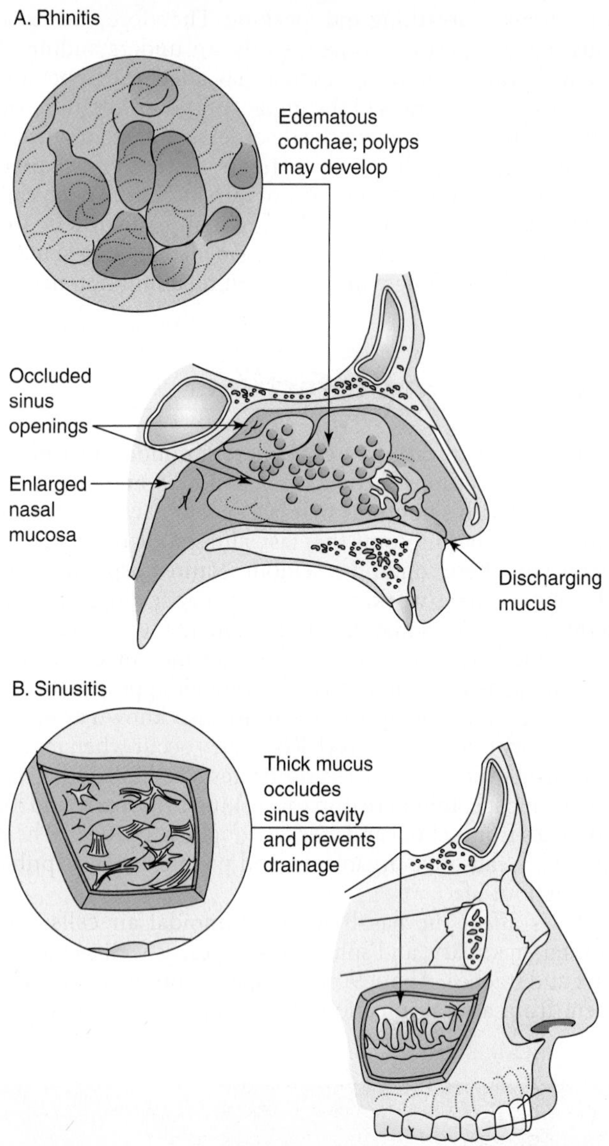

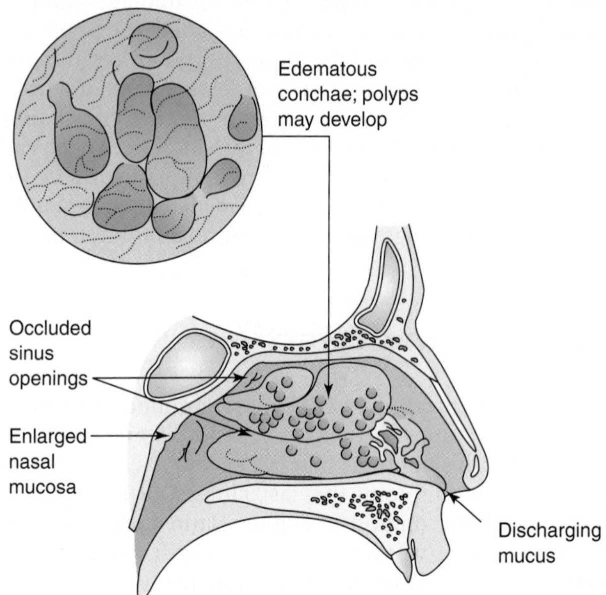

FIGURE 22-1. Pathophysiologic processes in rhinitis and sinusitis. Although pathophysiologic processes are similar in rhinitis and sinusitis, they affect different structures. In rhinitis **(A)**, the mucous membranes lining the nasal passages become inflamed, congested, and edematous. The swollen nasal conchae block the sinus openings, and mucus is discharged from the nostrils. Sinusitis **(B)** is also marked by inflammation and congestion, with thickened mucous secretions filling the sinus cavities and occluding the openings.

Clinical Manifestations

The signs and symptoms of nonallergic rhinitis include **rhinorrhea** (excessive nasal drainage, runny nose); nasal congestion; nasal discharge (purulent with bacterial rhinitis); sneezing; and pruritus of the nose, roof of the mouth, throat, eyes, and ears. Headache may occur, particularly if sinusitis is also present. Nonallergic rhinitis can occur throughout the year.

Medical Management

The management of rhinitis depends on the cause, which may be identified through the history and physical examination. The examiner asks the patient about recent symptoms as well as possible exposure to allergens in the home, environment, or workplace. If viral rhinitis is the cause, medications are given to relieve the symptoms. In allergic rhinitis, tests may be performed to identify possible allergens. Depending on the severity of the allergy, desensitizing immunizations and corticosteroids may be required (see Chapter 53 for more details). If symptoms suggest a bacterial infection, an antimicrobial agent will be used (see later discussion of sinusitis). Patients with nasal septal deformities or nasal polyps may be referred to an ear, nose, and throat specialist.

Pharmacologic Therapy

Medication therapy for allergic and nonallergic rhinitis focuses on symptom relief. Antihistamines are administered for sneezing, pruritus, and rhinorrhea. Examples of first-generation antihistamines include diphenhydramine (Benadryl), chlorpheniramine (Chlor-Trimeton), and brompheniramine. Newer, second-generation antihistamines used to treat rhinitis include loratadine (Alavert, Claritin), fexofenadine (Allegra), and cetirizine (Zyrtec). Dimetapp (brompheniramine/pseudoephedrine) is an example of a combination antihistamine. Oral decongestant agents are used for nasal obstruction. Another medication used in the treatment of rhinitis is cromolyn (Nasalcrom), which inhibits the release of histamine and other chemicals. Use of saline nasal spray can act as a mild decongestant and can liquefy mucus to prevent crusting. Two inhalations of intranasal ipratropium (Atrovent) can be administered in each nostril 2 to 3 times per day for symptomatic relief of rhinorrhea. In addition, intranasal corticosteroids may be used for severe congestion, and ophthalmic agents are used to relieve irritation, itching, and redness of the eyes. The choice of medications depends on the symptoms, adverse reactions, adherence factors, risk of drug interactions, and cost to the patient.

Nursing Management

Teaching Patients Self-Care

The nurse instructs the patient with allergic rhinitis to avoid or reduce exposure to allergens and irritants, such as dusts, molds, animals, fumes, odors, powders, sprays, and tobacco smoke. Patient education is essential when assisting the patient in the use of OTC medications. To prevent possible drug interactions, the nurse teaches the patient to read drug labels before taking any OTC medication.

The nurse instructs the patient about the importance of controlling the environment at home and at work. Saline nasal or aerosol sprays may be helpful in soothing mucous membranes, softening crusted secretions, and removing irritants. The nurse instructs the patient in the proper technique for administrating nasal medications. To achieve maximal relief, the patient is instructed to blow the nose before applying any medication into the nasal cavity. In addition, the patient is taught to keep the head upright; spray quickly and firmly into each nostril away from the nasal septum, and wait at least 1 minute before administering the second spray. The container should be cleaned after each use.

In the case of infectious rhinitis, the nurse reviews hand hygiene technique with the patient as a measure to prevent transmission of organisms. This is especially important for infected people who are in contact with vulnerable populations such as the very young, the elderly, or people who are immunosuppressed (eg, patients with HIV infection, those taking immunosuppressive medications). The nurse teaches methods to treat symptoms of viral rhinitis. In the elderly and other high-risk populations, the nurse reviews the value of receiving an influenza vaccination each year to achieve immunity before the beginning of the "flu season."

Viral Rhinitis (Common Cold)

Viral rhinitis is the most frequent viral infection in the general population. The term "common cold" often is used when referring to a URI that is self-limited and caused by a virus. The term "cold" refers to an afebrile, infectious, acute inflammation of the mucous membranes of the nasal cavity characterized by nasal congestion, rhinorrhea, sneezing, sore throat, and general malaise. More broadly, the term refers to an acute URI, whereas terms such as "rhinitis," "pharyngitis," and "laryngitis" distinguish the sites of the symptoms. It is also used when the causative virus is influenza ("the flu"). Colds are highly contagious, because virus is shed for about 2 days before the symptoms appear and during the first part of the symptomatic phase.

Adults in the United States average two to three colds each year (American Lung Association, 2005). Adult women are more susceptible than adult men. In the United States, colds are more frequent during the late fall and winter seasons. The incidence of viral rhinitis follows a specific pattern during the year, depending on the causative agent (Fig. 22-2). Even though viral rhinitis can occur at any time of the year, three time periods account for the epidemics in the United States:

- In September, just after the opening of school
- In late January
- Toward the end of April

Colds are believed to be caused by as many as 200 different viruses. Rhinoviruses are the most likely causative organisms and are believed to cause more than 40% of colds. Other viruses implicated in the common cold include coronaviruses, adenovirus, respiratory syncytial virus (RSV), influenza virus, and parainfluenza virus. Each virus may have multiple strains. Because of this diversity, development of a vaccine is almost impossible. Immunity after recovery is variable and depends on many factors, including a person's natural host resistance and the specific virus that caused the cold. Despite popular belief, cold temperatures and exposure to cold rainy weather do not increase the incidence or severity of the common cold.

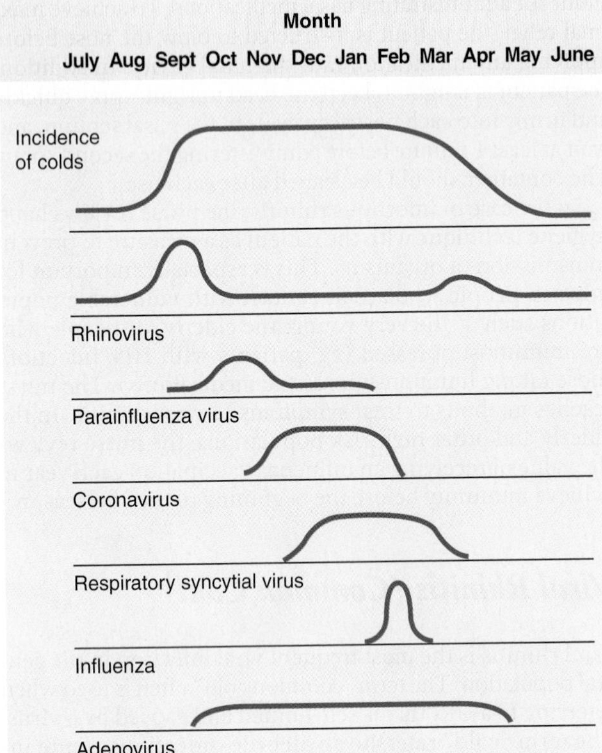

FIGURE 22-2. Schematic diagram incidence of viral rhinitis (common cold) in the United States and the frequency of the causative agents. Redrawn from Goldman, L. & Bennett, J. C. (Eds.) (2000). *Cecil textbook of medicine* (21st ed., Vol. 2). Philadelphia: W. B. Saunders, p. 1791.

Clinical Manifestations

Signs and symptoms of viral rhinitis are nasal congestion, rhinorrhea and nasal discharge, sneezing, tearing watery eyes, "scratchy" or sore throat, general malaise, low-grade fever, chills, and often headache and muscle aches. As the illness progresses, cough usually appears. In some people, the virus exacerbates **herpes simplex**, commonly called a "cold sore" (Chart 22-2).

The symptoms of viral rhinitis may last from 1 to 2 weeks. If there is significant fever or more severe systemic respiratory symptoms, it is no longer considered viral rhinitis but one of the other acute URIs. Allergic conditions can also affect the nose, mimicking the symptoms of a cold.

Medical Management

Management consists of symptomatic therapy. Some measures include providing adequate fluid intake, encouraging rest, preventing chilling, and using expectorants as needed. Warm salt-water gargles soothe the sore throat, and nonsteroidal anti-inflammatory agents (NSAIDs), such as aspirin or ibuprofen, relieve the aches, pains, and fever in adults. Antihistamines are used to relieve sneezing, rhinorrhea, and nasal congestion. Topical (nasal) decongestant agents may relieve nasal congestion; however, if they are overused they

CHART 22-2

Colds and Cold Sores (Herpes Simplex Virus HSV-1)

Herpes labialis is an infection that is caused by the herpes simplex virus. It is characterized by an eruption of small, painful blisters on the skin of the lips, mouth, gums, tongue, or the skin around the mouth. The blisters are commonly referred to as "cold sores" or "fever blisters." Once the person is infected with this virus, it can lie latent in the cells for a period of time. The incubation period is about 2 to 12 days. It is activated by overexposure to sunlight or wind, colds, influenza and similar infections, heavy alcohol use, and physical or emotional stress.

Herpes labialis is extremely common and is caused by the herpes simplex virus type 1. (Herpes type 2 virus causes genital herpes.) Most Americans are infected with the type 1 virus by 20 years of age. Herpes labialis is extremely contagious and can be spread through contaminated razors, towels, and dishes. Oral/genital contact can spread oral herpes to the genitals (and vice versa). People with active herpetic lesions should avoid oral sex. It is extremely important for patients to understand that the virus can be transmitted by asymptomatic people.

Early symptoms of herpes labialis include burning, itching and increased sensitivity or tingling sensation. These symptoms occur about 2 days before the appearance of lesions. The lesions appear as small blisters (vesicles) that are filled with clear, yellowish fluid. They are raised, red, and painful and can break and ooze. Eventually yellow crusts slough to reveal pink, healing skin.

The lesions will eventually subside (10 to 14 days). Medications used in the management of herpes labialis include acyclovir (Zovirax) and valacyclovir (Valtrex), which help to minimize the symptoms and the duration or length of flare-up. Other medications used for analgesia include acetaminophen with codeine and other milder forms of opioids. Topical anesthetics such as xylocaine or over-the-counter medications such as Herpecin-L or docosanol [Abreva] can help in the control of discomfort.

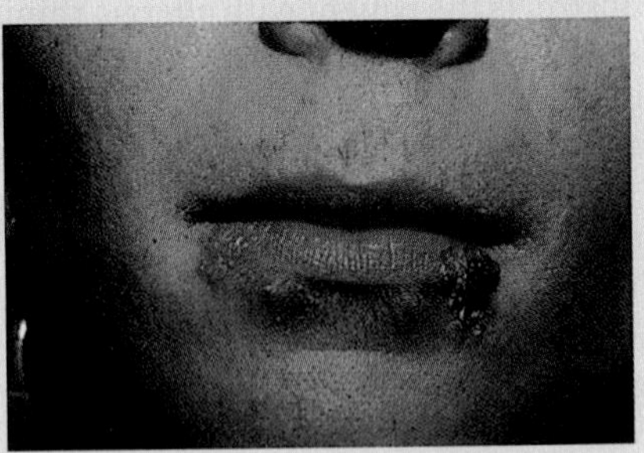

may create a rebound congestion that can be worse than the original symptoms. Some research suggests that zinc lozenges may reduce the duration of cold symptoms if taken within the first 24 hours of onset (Marshall, 2006). Amantadine (Symmetrel) or rimantadine (Flumadine) may be prescribed prophylactically to decrease the signs and symptoms as well. Antimicrobial agents (antibiotics) should not be used, because they do not affect the virus or reduce the incidence of bacterial complications.

Most patients treat the common cold with OTC medications that produce moderate clinical benefits. OTC medications provide symptomatic relief along with other measures to improve well-being through the course of the illness. Other treatment measures include adequate fluid intake, adequate rest, and warm salt-water gargles to soothe the sore throat. Acetaminophen or NSAIDs such as ibuprofen can relieve generalized aches, pains, and fevers. Antihistamines and decongestants can be used to treat sneezing and congestion. Topical nasal decongestants can be used with caution. Topical therapy delivers medication directly to the nasal mucosa, but its overuse can produce rhinitis medicamentosa or rebound rhinitis.

Nursing Management

Teaching Patients Self-Care

Most viruses can be transmitted in several ways: direct contact with infected secretions; inhalation of large particles from others' coughing or sneezing; or inhalation of small particles (aerosol) that may be suspended in the air for up to an hour. The nurse teaches the patient how to break the chain of infection. Handwashing remains the most effective measure to prevent transmission of organisms. The nurse teaches methods to treat symptoms of the common cold and preventive measures (Chart 22-3) and provides both verbal and written information to assist the patient in the prevention and management of URIs.

NURSING ALERT

Due to the risk of gastrointestinal bleeding, aspirin, ibuprofen, and naproxen should be avoided by persons who are not eating well, have a history of peptic ulcer or related disorder, have aspirin-sensitive asthma, or have renal dysfunction.

Patients who have high blood pressure, diabetes, or thyroid disease, and those who are pregnant should check with their physician before using a decongestant.

Patients should avoid use of zinc and dextromethorphan (Benylin) if pregnancy is possible.

Patients taking monoamine oxidase (MAO) inhibitors (eg, phenelzine sulfate [Nardil], tranylcypromine [Parnate]) should not use dextromethorphan [Robitussin].

Acute Sinusitis

The sinuses, mucus-lined cavities filled with air, normally drain into the nose and are involved in many URIs. If their openings into the nasal passages are clear, the infections resolve promptly. However, if their drainage is obstructed by a deviated septum or by hypertrophied turbinates, spurs, or nasal polyps or tumors, sinus infection may persist as a smoldering (persistent) secondary infection or progress to an acute suppurative process (causing purulent discharge). **Sinusitis** (inflammation of the sinuses) affects 14% to 16% of the population and accounts for billions of dollars in direct health care costs (Shashy, Moore & Weaver, 2004). Some people are more prone to sinusitis because of their occupations. For example, continuous exposure to environmental hazards such as paint, sawdust, and chemicals may result in chronic inflammation of the nasal passages.

Pathophysiology

Acute sinusitis is an infection of the mucous membranes that line the paranasal sinuses. Five subtypes of sinusitis have been identified: acute, subacute, chronic, allergic, and hyperplastic sinusitis. Acute sinusitis refers to rapid-onset infection in one or more of the paranasal sinuses that resolves with treatment, whereas subacute sinusitis is persistent purulent nasal discharge despite therapy with symptoms lasting less than 3 months. Chronic sinusitis occurs with episodes of prolonged inflammation and with repeated or inadequate treatment of acute infections. Irreversible damage to the mucosa may occur. Symptoms last for longer than 3 months. Sinusitis often follows a URI or cold, such as an unresolved viral or bacterial infection, or an exacerbation of allergic rhinitis. Nasal congestion, caused by inflammation, edema, and transudation of fluid secondary to URI, leads to obstruction of the sinus cavities (see Fig. 22-1). This provides an excellent medium for bacterial growth. Other conditions that can block the normal flow of sinus secretions include abnormal structures of the nose, enlarged adenoids, diving and swimming, tooth infection, trauma to the nose, tumors, and the pressure of foreign objects. Bacterial organisms account for more than 60% of the cases of acute sinusitis. *Streptococcus pneumonia, Haemophilus influenzae,* and *Moraxella catarrhalis* are the most common organisms associated with sinusitis. Less common organisms include *Chlamydia pneumoniae, Streptococcus pyogenes,* viruses, and fungi (*Aspergillus fumigatus*). Fungal infections occur most often in immunosuppressed patients. Pathogens in chronic or subacute sinusitis are likely to be polymicrobial, involving anaerobic bacteria (Uphold & Graham, 2003).

Clinical Manifestations

Symptoms of sinusitis vary among people and are dependent on the age of the person. Most infections in adults involve the maxillary and anterior ethmoidal sinuses. Symptoms may include facial pain or pressure over the affected sinus area, nasal obstruction, fatigue, purulent nasal discharge, fever, headache, ear pain and a sense of fullness, dental pain, decreased sense of smell, sore throat, early morning

CHART 22-3

HOME CARE CHECKLIST • Preventing and Managing Upper Respiratory Infections

At the completion of home care instructions, the patient and significant other will be able to:	Patient	Caregiver
Prevention		
• Identify strategies to prevent infection and, if infected, to prevent the spread of infection to others.		
• Perform hand hygiene often	✔	✔
• Use disposable tissues	✔	
• Cover mouth when coughing or sneezing	✔	
• Avoid crowds during the flu season	✔	
• Avoid people with infections	✔	
• Obtain annual influenza vaccination (especially if patient is elderly or has a chronic illness or disability)	✔	
• Practice good health habits		
• Eat a nutritious diet	✔	
• Get adequate sleep, rest, and exercise	✔	
• Avoid the use of tobacco in all forms	✔	
• Avoid secondhand smoke	✔	
• Increase the humidity in the home (especially in the winter)	✔	✔
• Avoid irritants (dust, chemicals) to include exposure to animals	✔	✔
• Use central air conditioning with microstatic air filters	✔	✔
Management		
• Describe strategies to relieve symptoms of upper respiratory infection		
• Increase fluid intake. Warm fluids (eg, chicken soup) are especially soothing for irritated throats.	✔	✔
• Elevate head of bed.	✔	✔
• Gargle with salt water frequently for sore throat (1/4 teaspoon of salt dissolved in eight ounces warm water)	✔	
• Use throat lozenge for sore throat or cough.	✔	
• Use saline nose drops/sprays (1/4 teaspoon salt dissolved in eight ounces warm water; use dropper, or purchase prepared saline drops)	✔	
• Recognize signs and symptoms of infection and state when to contact health care provider		
• If symptoms worsen after 3 to 5 days; new symptoms develop or symptoms do not improve after 14 days.	✔	✔
• If the following signs or symptoms occur, obtain immediate health care:		
• Upper respiratory distress (stridor, drooling, inability to swallow)	✔	✔
• Lower respiratory distress (moderate to severe dyspnea)	✔	✔
• Severe headache ("worst ever," rigid neck, altered mental state, focal neurologic symptoms)	✔	

periorbital edema, and cough that worsens when the patient is supine. Acute sinusitis can be difficult to differentiate from a URI or allergic rhinitis. The presence of fewer than two symptoms rules out acute bacterial sinusitis, and four or more symptoms suggest acute bacterial sinusitis (DeAlleaume, Parker & Reider, 2003).

Assessment and Diagnostic Findings

A careful history and physical examination are performed. The head and neck, particularly the nose, ears, teeth, sinuses, pharynx, and chest, are examined. There may be tenderness to palpation over the infected sinus area. The sinuses are percussed using the index finger, tapping lightly to determine whether the patient experiences pain. The affected area is also transilluminated; with sinusitis, there is a decrease in the transmission of light (see Chapter 21). Diagnostic tests are not indicated for sinusitis with a typical presentation or for the first episode of acute sinusitis. Sinus x-rays and computed tomography (CT) scans may be obtained for patients with frontal headaches, in refractory cases, if complications are suspected, or when the diagnosis is unclear (Reider, Nashelsky & Neher, 2003; Uphold & Graham, 2003). To confirm the diagnosis of maxillary and frontal sinusitis and identify the pathogen, sinus aspirates may be obtained. Flexible endoscopic culture techniques have been used for this purpose as well as swabbing of the sinuses.

Complications

If untreated, acute sinusitis may lead to severe and occasionally life-threatening complications such as meningitis, brain abscess, ischemic brain infarction, and osteomyelitis. Other complications of sinusitis, although uncommon, include severe orbital cellulitis, subperiosteal abscess, cavernous sinus thrombosis, and meningitis. Brain abscesses occur by direct spread and can be life-threatening. Frontal epidural abscesses are usually quiescent and can be detected by CT scan.

Medical Management

The goals of treatment of acute sinusitis are to treat the infection, shrink the nasal mucosa, and relieve pain. Because of growing concern about the inappropriate use of antibiotics for viral URIs and the resulting resistance that has occurred, careful consideration must be given to the potential pathogen before antimicrobial agents are prescribed.

Antibiotic therapy is used to eradicate the infecting organism. First-line antibiotics include amoxicillin, ampicillin, trimethoprim/sulfamethoxazole (Bactrin, Septra), and erythromycin. Second-line antibiotic therapy includes cephalosporins such as cefuroxime axetil (Ceftin) and cefprozil (Cefzil) and amoxicillin clavulanate (Augmentin). Newer and more expensive antibiotics such as macrolides (clarithromycin [Biaxin], azithromycin [Zithromax]) and quinolones such as levofloxacin (Levaquin) can be used if the patient has a severe allergy to penicillin. Studies suggest that most patients will improve spontaneously, and antibiotics should be reserved for those with prolonged symptoms (Lindbaek, 2004). However, deep-seated bacterial sinusitis can be a serious infection that requires antibiotic treatment for 2 to 3 weeks. A narrow-spectrum antibiotic such as amoxicillin is often a good initial choice (Jackson, 2003).

Treatment of acute sinusitis typically involves nasal decongestants (pseudoephedrine hydrochloride [Sudafed]). Decongestants or nasal saline spray can improve patency of the ostiomeatal unit and improve drainage of the sinuses. Topical decongestants are used only in adults and should not be used for longer than 3 or 4 days. Oral decongestants must be used cautiously in patients with hypertension. OTC antihistamines, including diphenhydramine (Benadryl) and antihistamines (cetirizine, fexofenadine) are used if an allergic component is suspected.

Heated mist and saline irrigation also may be effective for opening blocked passages. If the patient continues to have symptoms after 7 to 10 days, the sinuses may need to be irrigated and hospitalization may be required.

Nursing Management

Teaching Patients Self-Care

Patient teaching is an important aspect of nursing care for the patient with acute sinusitis. The nurse instructs the patient about symptoms of complications that require immediate follow-up. Referral to a physician is indicated if periorbital edema and severe pain on palpation occur. The nurse instructs the patient about methods to promote drainage of the sinuses, including humidification of the air in the home and use of steam inhalation and warm compresses to relieve pressure. The patient is advised to avoid swimming, diving, and air travel during the acute infection. Patients using tobacco are instructed to immediately stop smoking or using any form of tobacco. The nurse also teaches the patient about the side effects of nasal sprays and about rebound congestion. In the case of rebound congestion, the body's receptors have become dependent on the decongestant sprays to keep the nasal passages open. Once the decongestant is discontinued, the nasal passages close and congestion results. Patients with recurrent sinusitis should be instructed to begin decongestants at the first sign of sinusitis. This will promote drainage and decrease the risk of bacterial infection.

The nurse stresses the importance of following the recommended antibiotic regimen, because a consistent blood level of the medication is critical to treat the infection. The nurse teaches the patient the early signs of a sinus infection and recommends preventive measures such as following healthy practices and avoiding contact with people who have URIs (see Chart 22-3).

The nurse explains to the patient that fever, severe headache, and **nuchal rigidity** (stiffness of the neck/inability to bend the neck) are signs of potential complications. Patients with chronic symptoms of sinusitis who do not have marked improvement in 4 weeks with continuous medical treatment may be candidates for aspiration of the sinus or sinus surgery.

Chronic Sinusitis

Chronic sinusitis is one of the most common illnesses in the United States, reportedly affecting up to 16% of the population. It affects more than 32 million persons each year and ranks fifth in frequency of antibiotic use associated with treatment. It is considered a common disease worldwide. The data on the incidence, however, rely largely on patients' self report and can lead to inaccuracies and likely overestimation (Shashy et al., 2004). Chronic sinusitis is a result of prolonged inflammation or repeated or inadequately treated acute sinus infections. People with symptoms lasting longer than 3 months are usually classified as having chronic sinusitis.

Pathophysiology

Mechanical obstruction in the ostia of the frontal, maxillary, and anterior ethmoid sinuses (known collectively as the ostiomeatal complex) is the usual cause of chronic sinusitis. Obstruction prevents adequate drainage to the nasal passages. Blockage that persists longer than 3 weeks in an adult may occur because of infection, allergy, or structural abnormalities. This results in stagnant secretions, an ideal medium for growth of bacteria. The organisms that cause chronic sinusitis are the same as those implicated in acute sinusitis. Immunocompromised patients, however, are at increased risk for development of fungal sinusitis. Fungal sinusitis in immunocompromised patients can be divided into three categories: (1) fungus ball, (2) chronic erosive (noninvasive) sinusitis, and (3) allergic fungal sinusitis. *A. fumigatus* is the most common organism associated with fungal sinusitis.

Clinical Manifestations

Clinical manifestations of chronic sinusitis include impaired mucociliary clearance and ventilation, cough (because the thick discharge constantly drips backward into the nasopharynx), chronic hoarseness, chronic headaches in the periorbital area, and facial pain. As a result of chronic nasal congestion, the patient is usually required to breathe through the mouth. Snoring, sore throat, and, in some situations, adenoidal hypertrophy may also occur. Periorbital edema and facial pain are common. These symptoms are generally most pronounced on awakening in the morning. Fatigue and nasal congestion are also common. Many patients experience a decrease in smell and taste and a sense of fullness in the ears.

Assessment and Diagnostic Findings

The health assessment focuses on onset and duration of symptoms. It addresses the quantity and quality of nasal discharge and cough, the presence of pain, factors that relieve or aggravate the pain, and allergies. It is essential to obtain any history of comorbid conditions, including asthma, and history of tobacco use. A history of fever, fatigue, previous episodes and treatments, and previous response to therapies is also obtained. The physical assessment includes vital signs and examination of the eyes, nasal mucosa, ears, throat, mouth, and pharynx for signs of erythema and exudates. The nose is inspected for septal deviation and polyps and the eyes for periorbital edema. Pain on examination of the teeth and tapping them with a tongue blade suggests tooth infection. The frontal and maxillary sinuses are palpated, and the patient is asked whether this produces tenderness.

Diagnostic tests may include CT scan or magnetic resonance imaging (if fungal sinusitis is suspected) of the sinuses to rule out other local or systemic disorders, such as tumor, fistula, and allergy. Nasal endoscopy may be indicated to rule out underlying diseases such as tumors and sinus mycetomas (fungus balls). The fungus ball is usually a brown or greenish-black material with the consistency of peanut butter or cottage cheese.

Complications

Complications of chronic sinusitis, although uncommon, include severe orbital cellulitis, subperiosteal abscess, cavernous sinus thrombosis, meningitis, encephalitis, and ischemic infarction.

Medical Management

Medical management of chronic sinusitis is almost the same as for acute sinusitis. The antimicrobial agents of choice include amoxicillin clavulanate (Augmentin) or ampicillin (Ampicin). Clarithromycin (Biaxin) and third-generation cephalosporins such as cefuroxime axetil (Ceftin), cefpodoxime (Vantin), and cefprozil (Cefzil) have also been effective. Macrolides (eg, clarithromycin [Biaxin]) increase mucociliary clearance and improve sinusitis symptoms and are known to decrease nasal secretions and polyp size associated with chronic sinusitis. In addition to their antimicrobial activity, the macrolides' immunomodulatory properties may be effective in chronic inflammation (Gotfried, 2004). Levofloxacin (Levaquin), a quinolone, may also be used. The course of treatment may be 3 to 4 weeks. As with acute sinusitis, decongestant agents, antihistamines, saline sprays, and heated mist may also provide some symptom relief.

The use of intranasal nebulized medications is emerging as a treatment of chronic sinusitis. Specially formulated medication compounds delivered by nebulizer are an innovative and advanced approach to treating acute and chronic sinusitis. The role of leukotriene inhibitors in patients with paranasal sinus disease is also under study. This class of medications blocks the binding of leukotrienes (inflammatory mediators) to receptors and in a number of studies has demonstrated a role in inhibiting nasal symptoms in asthmatic patients (Chung & Adcock, 2004; Singh, 2004). As a result, studies are ongoing to determine the role of these agents in patients with chronic sinusitis and their role in endoscopic surgical treatment. Endoscopic sinus surgery has evolved over the past 20 years as an accepted treatment for people with chronic sinusitis refractory to medical management (Colclasure, Gross & Kountakis, 2004).

Surgical Management

If standard medical therapy fails and symptoms persist, surgery, usually endoscopic, may be indicated to correct structural deformities that obstruct the ostia (openings) of the sinuses. Minimally invasive surgical procedures are used, reducing postoperative discomfort and producing significant improvement in the patient's quality of life. Excising and cauterizing nasal polyps, correcting a deviated septum, incising and draining the sinuses, aerating the sinuses, and removing tumors are some of the specific procedures performed. If sinusitis is caused by a fungal infection, surgery is required to excise the fungus ball and necrotic tissue and drain the sinuses. Antimicrobial agents are administered before and after surgery. Some patients with severe chronic sinusitis obtain relief only by moving to a dry climate.

Nursing Management

Because the patient usually performs care measures for sinusitis at home, nursing management consists mainly of patient teaching.

Teaching Patients Self-Care

Many people with sinus infections tend to blow their nose frequently and with force to clear their nasal passages. Doing so, however, often increases the symptoms. Therefore, the patient is instructed to blow the nose gently and to use tissue to remove the nasal drainage. Increasing the environmental humidity (eg, steam bath, hot shower, vaporizer), increasing fluid intake, applying local heat (hot wet packs), and elevating the head of the bed promote drainage of the sinuses. The nurse also instructs the patient about the importance of following the medication regimen. Instructions on the early signs of a sinus infection are provided, and preventive measures are reviewed. The nurse instructs the patient about signs and symptoms that require follow-up and provides these instructions in writing.

Acute Pharyngitis

Acute **pharyngitis** is a sudden inflammation of the pharynx that is more common in patients younger than 25 years of age (particularly between 5 and 15 years). It is most common in adolescents and young adults. It occurs less frequently in the elderly. The primary symptom is a sore throat.

Pathophysiology

Most cases of acute pharyngitis are caused by viral infection. Responsible viruses include the adenovirus, influenza virus, Epstein-Barr virus and herpes simplex virus. Bacterial organisms known to cause pharyngitis include group A beta-hemolytic streptococci, *Neisseria gonorrhoeae, H. influenzae* type B, and *Mycoplasma.* When group A beta-hemolytic streptococcus, the most common bacterial organism, causes acute pharyngitis, the condition is known as strep throat (Wald & Fischer, 2004). The body responds by triggering an inflammatory response in the pharynx. This results in pain, fever, vasodilation, edema, and tissue damage, manifested by redness and swelling in the tonsillar pillars, uvula, and soft palate. A creamy exudate may be present in the tonsillar pillars (Fig. 22-3).

Uncomplicated viral infections usually subside promptly, within 3 to 10 days after the onset. However, pharyngitis caused by more virulent bacteria, such as group A beta-hemolytic streptococci, is a more severe illness. If left untreated, the complications can be severe and life-threatening. Complications include sinusitis, otitis media, peritonsillar abscess, mastoiditis, and cervical adenitis. In rare cases, the infection may lead to bacteremia, pneumonia, meningitis, rheumatic fever, or nephritis.

Clinical Manifestations

The signs and symptoms of acute pharyngitis include a fiery-red pharyngeal membrane and tonsils, lymphoid follicles that are swollen and flecked with white-purple exudate, enlarged and tender cervical lymph nodes, and no cough. Fever, malaise, and sore throat also may be present. Occasionally patients with group A beta-hemolytic streptococcal pharyngitis exhibit vomiting, anorexia, and a scarlatina-form rash with urticaria.

Assessment and Diagnostic Findings

Diagnosis of group A streptococcal pharyngitis must be made by laboratory testing rather than by clinical findings alone. Rapid strep test (RST) and strep culture (sometimes referred to as STCX) require proper collection technique, because improper collection reduces the accuracy of the test. RST must be performed according to the manufacturer's guidelines. When the test is performed correctly, the swabs touch both the tonsillar pillars and the posterior pharyngeal wall; the tongue should not be included. If the RST result is negative, a second culture should be performed. Treatment is usually delayed until the culture results are available (Armengol, Schlager & Hendley, 2004; Neuner,

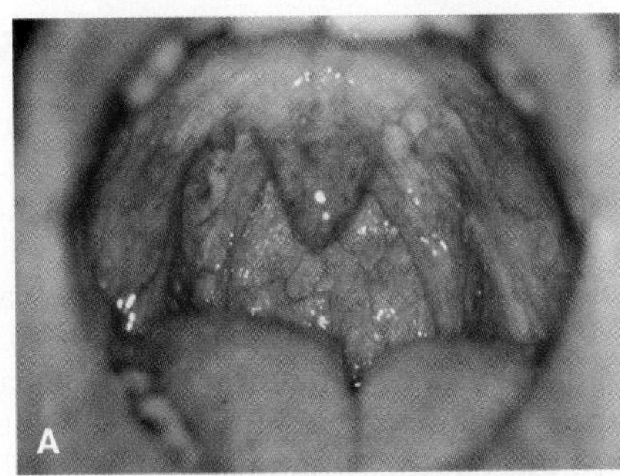

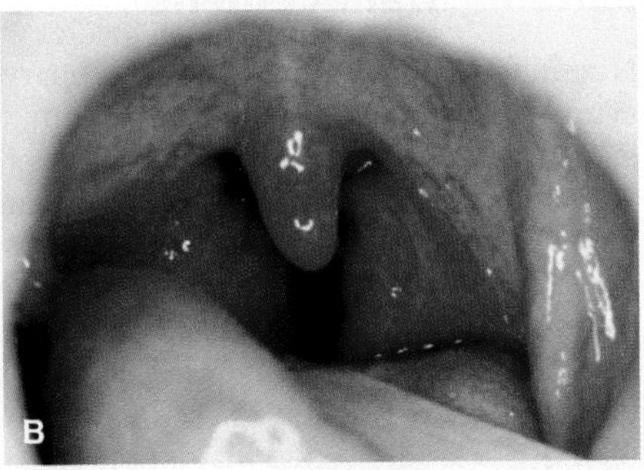

FIGURE 22-3. Pharyngitis—inflammation without exudate. (**A**) Redness and vascularity of the pillars and uvula are mild to moderate. (**B**) Redness is diffuse and intense. Each patient would probably complain of a sore throat. From Bickley, L. S. & Szilagyi, P. G. (2003). *Bates' guide to physical examination and history taking* (8th ed.). Philadelphia: Lippincott Williams & Wilkins.

Hamel, Phillips et al., 2003). In most communities, preliminary culture reports are available in 24 hours. Rapid screenings include the latex agglutination (LA) antigen test and solid-phase enzyme immunoassays (ELISA), optical immunoassay (OIA), and streptolysin titers. Nasal swabs and blood cultures may also be necessary to identify the organism.

Medical Management

Viral pharyngitis is treated with supportive measures, because antibiotics will have no effect on the organism. Bacterial pharyngitis is treated with a variety of antimicrobial agents.

Pharmacologic Therapy

If a bacterial cause is suggested or demonstrated, penicillin is usually the treatment of choice. For patients who are allergic to penicillin or have organisms that are resistant to erythromycin (one fifth of group A beta-hemolytic streptococci and most *Staphylococcus aureus* organisms are resistant to penicillin and erythromycin), cephalosporins and macrolides (clarithromycin and azithromycin) may be used. Antibiotics are administered for at least 10 days to eradicate the infection from the oropharynx.

Severe sore throats can also be relieved by analgesic medications, as prescribed. For example, aspirin or acetaminophen (Tylenol) can be taken at 3- to 6-hour intervals; if required, acetaminophen with codeine can be taken three or four times daily. Antitussive medication, in the form of codeine, dextromethorphan (Robitussin DM), or hydrocodone bitartrate (Hycodan), may be required to control the persistent and painful cough that often accompanies acute pharyngitis.

Nutritional Therapy

A liquid or soft diet is provided during the acute stage of the disease, depending on the patient's appetite and the degree of discomfort that occurs with swallowing. Cool beverages, warm liquids, and flavored frozen desserts such as popsicles are often soothing. Occasionally, the throat is so sore that liquids cannot be taken in adequate amounts by mouth. In severe situations, IV fluids may be needed. Otherwise, the patient is encouraged to drink as much fluid as possible (at least 2 to 3 L per day).

Nursing Management

Nursing care for patients with viral pharyngitis focuses on symptomatic management. For patients who demonstrate signs of strep throat and have a history of rheumatic fever, who appear toxic, who have clinical scarlet fever, or who have symptoms suggesting peritonsillar abscess, nursing care focuses on prompt initiation and correct administration of prescribed antibiotic therapy. The nurse instructs the patient about signs and symptoms that warrant prompt contact with the physician. These include dyspnea, drooling, inability to swallow, and inability to fully open the mouth.

The nurse instructs the patient to stay in bed during the febrile stage of illness and to rest frequently once up and about. Used tissues should be disposed of properly to prevent the spread of infection. The nurse (or the patient or family member, if the patient is not hospitalized) should examine the skin once or twice daily for possible rash, because acute pharyngitis may precede some other communicable diseases (eg, rubella).

Depending on the severity of the lesion and the degree of pain, warm saline gargles or throat irrigations are used. The benefits of this treatment depend on the degree of heat that is applied. The nurse teaches the patient about these procedures and about the recommended temperature of the solution: high enough to be effective and as warm as the patient can tolerate, usually 105°F to 110°F (40.6°C to 43.3°C). Irrigating the throat properly is an effective means of reducing spasm in the pharyngeal muscles and relieving soreness of the throat.

An ice collar also can relieve severe sore throats. Mouth care may add greatly to the patient's comfort and prevent the development of fissures (cracking) of the lips and oral inflammation when bacterial infection is present. The nurse instructs the patient to resume activity gradually and to delay returning to work or school until after 24 hours of antibiotic therapy. A full course of antibiotic therapy is indicated in patients with group A beta-hemolytic streptococcal infection because of the potential complications such as nephritis and rheumatic fever, which may have their onset 2 or 3 weeks after the pharyngitis has subsided. The nurse instructs the patient and family about the importance of taking the full course of therapy and informs them about the symptoms to watch for that may indicate complications.

Chronic Pharyngitis

Chronic pharyngitis is a persistent inflammation of the pharynx. It is common in adults who work or live in dusty surroundings, use their voice to excess, suffer from chronic cough, or habitually use alcohol and tobacco.

There are three types of chronic pharyngitis:

- Hypertrophic: characterized by general thickening and congestion of the pharyngeal mucous membrane
- Atrophic: probably a late stage of the first type (the membrane is thin, whitish, glistening, and at times wrinkled)
- Chronic granular ("clergyman's sore throat"), characterized by numerous swollen lymph follicles on the pharyngeal wall.

Clinical Manifestations

Patients with chronic pharyngitis complain of a constant sense of irritation or fullness in the throat, mucus that collects in the throat and can be expelled by coughing, and difficulty swallowing. This is often associated with intermittent postnasal drip that causes minor irritation and inflammation of the pharynx. A sore throat that is worse with swallowing in the absence of pharyngitis suggests the possibility of thyroiditis, and patients with this symptom are referred for evaluation for possible thyroiditis.

Medical Management

Treatment of chronic pharyngitis is based on relieving symptoms, avoiding exposure to irritants, and correcting any upper respiratory, pulmonary, or cardiac condition that might be responsible for a chronic cough.

Nasal congestion may be relieved by short-term use of nasal sprays or medications containing ephedrine sulfate (Kondon's Nasal) or phenylephrine hydrochloride (Neo-Synephrine). For a patient with a history of allergy, one of the antihistamine decongestant medications, such as Drixoral or Dimetapp, is prescribed orally every 4 to 6 hours. Aspirin or acetaminophen is recommended for its anti-inflammatory and analgesic properties.

Nursing Management

Teaching Patients Self-Care

To prevent the infection from spreading, the nurse instructs the patient to avoid contact with others until the fever subsides. The nurse recommends avoidance of alcohol, tobacco, secondhand smoke, and exposure to cold or to environmental or occupational pollutants. The patient may minimize exposure to pollutants by wearing a disposable facemask. The nurse encourages the patient to drink plenty of fluids. Gargling with warm saline solution may relieve throat discomfort. Lozenges will keep the throat moistened.

Tonsillitis and Adenoiditis

The tonsils are composed of lymphatic tissue and are situated on each side of the oropharynx. The faucial or palatine tonsils and lingual tonsils are located behind the pillars of fauces and tongue, respectively. They frequently serve as the site of acute infection (**tonsillitis**). Acute tonsillitis can be confused with pharyngitis. Chronic tonsillitis is less common and may be mistaken for other disorders such as allergy, asthma, and sinusitis.

The adenoids or pharyngeal tonsils consist of lymphatic tissue near the center of the posterior wall of the nasopharynx. Infection of the adenoids frequently accompanies acute tonsillitis. Group A beta-hemolytic streptococcus is the most common organism associated with tonsillitis and adenoiditis. Often thought of as a childhood disorder, tonsillitis can also occur in adults.

Clinical Manifestations

The symptoms of tonsillitis include sore throat, fever, snoring, and difficulty swallowing. Enlarged adenoids may cause mouth-breathing, earache, draining ears, frequent head colds, bronchitis, foul-smelling breath, voice impairment, and noisy respiration. Unusually enlarged adenoids fill the space behind the posterior nares, making it difficult for the air to travel from the nose to the throat and resulting in nasal obstruction. Infection can extend to the middle ears by way of the auditory (eustachian) tubes and may result in acute otitis media, which can lead to spontaneous rupture of the tympanic membranes (eardrums) and further extension of the infection into the mastoid cells, causing acute mastoiditis. The infection also may reside in the middle ear as a chronic, low-grade, smoldering process that eventually may cause permanent deafness.

Assessment and Diagnostic Findings

A thorough physical examination is performed, and a careful history is obtained to rule out related or systemic conditions. The tonsillar site is cultured to determine the presence of bacterial infection. In adenoiditis, if recurrent episodes of suppurative otitis media result in hearing loss, the patient should be given a comprehensive audiometric examination (see Chapter 59).

Medical Management

Tonsillitis is treated through the use of supportive measures that include increased fluid intake, analgesics, salt-water gargles, and rest. Bacterial infections are treated with penicillin as first-line therapy. Viral tonsillitis is not effectively treated by antibiotic therapy.

Tonsillectomy or adenoidectomy is indicated if the patient has had repeated episodes of tonsillitis despite antibiotic therapy; hypertrophy of the tonsils and adenoids that could cause obstruction and obstructive sleep apnea; repeated attacks of purulent otitis media; suspected hearing loss due to serous otitis media that has occurred in association with enlarged tonsils and adenoids; and in some other conditions, such as an exacerbation of asthma or rheumatic fever. Surgery is also indicated if the patient has developed a peritonsillar abscess that occludes the pharynx, making swallowing difficult and endangering the patency of the airway (particularly during sleep). Enlargement of the tonsils is rarely an indication for their removal; most children normally have large tonsils, which decrease in size with age. Despite the continuing debate over the effectiveness of tonsillectomy, it is a common surgical procedure in the United States (Discolo, Darrow & Koltai, 2003). Appropriate antibiotic therapy is initiated for patients undergoing tonsillectomy or adenoidectomy. The most common antimicrobial agent is oral penicillin, which is prescribed for 7 to 10 days. Amoxicillin and erythromycin are alternatives. Indications for adenoidectomy include chronic nasal airway obstruction, chronic rhinorrhea, obstruction of the eustachian tube with related ear infections, and abnormal speech.

Nursing Management

Providing Postoperative Care

Continuous nursing observation is required in the immediate postoperative and recovery periods because of the significant risk of hemorrhage. In the immediate postoperative period, the most comfortable position is prone with the head turned to the side to allow drainage from the mouth and pharynx. The nurse must not remove the oral airway until the patient's gag and swallowing reflexes have returned. The nurse applies an ice collar to the neck, and a basin and tissues are provided for the expectoration of blood and mucus.

Symptoms of postoperative complications include fever, throat pain, ear pain, and bleeding. Pain is effectively controlled with analgesic medications. Bleeding may be bright red if the patient expectorates blood before swallowing it. If the patient swallows the blood, it becomes brown because of the action of the acidic gastric juice. Hemorrhage is a potential complication after tonsillectomy and adenoidectomy. Risk factors associated with post-tonsillectomy hemorrhage include male gender, age older than 70 years, infectious mononucleosis, and history of recurrent tonsillitis (Windfuhr & Chen, 2003). Postoperative hemorrhage rates are not significantly different with tonsillectomy by electrodissection versus sharp dissection (Leinbach, Markwell, Colliver, et al., 2003).

If the patient vomits large amounts of dark blood or bright-red blood at frequent intervals, or if the pulse rate and temperature rise and the patient is restless, the nurse notifies the surgeon immediately. The nurse should have the following items ready for examination of the surgical site for bleeding: a light, a mirror, gauze, curved hemostats, and a waste basin.

Occasionally, suture or ligation of the bleeding vessel is required. In such cases, the patient is taken to the operating room and given general anesthesia. After ligation, continuous nursing observation and postoperative care are required, as in the initial postoperative period. If there is no bleeding, water and ice chips may be given to the patient as soon as desired. The patient is instructed to refrain from too much talking and coughing, because these activities can produce throat pain.

Teaching Patients Self-Care

Tonsillectomy and adenoidectomy are usually performed as outpatient surgery with a short length of stay. Because the patient will be sent home soon after surgery, the patient and family must understand the signs and symptoms of hemorrhage. Hemorrhage usually occurs in the first 12 to 24 hours; however, the risk is present for up to 18 days after the procedure (Windfuhr & Chen, 2003). The patient is instructed to report frank red bleeding to the physician.

Alkaline mouthwashes and warm saline solutions are useful in coping with the thick mucus and halitosis that may be present after surgery. The nurse should explain to the patient that a sore throat, stiff neck, and vomiting may occur in the first 24 hours. A liquid or semiliquid diet is given for several days. Sherbet and gelatin are acceptable foods. The patient should avoid spicy, hot, acidic, or rough foods. Milk and milk products (ice cream and yogurt) may be restricted because they make removal of mucus more difficult for some patients. The patient is informed that halitosis and some minor ear pain may occur for the first few days. The nurse instructs the patient to avoid vigorous tooth brushing or gargling, because these activities can cause bleeding.

Peritonsillar Abscess

Peritonsillar abscess is a collection of purulent exudate between the tonsillar capsule and the surrounding tissues, including the soft palate. It may develop after an acute tonsillar infection that progresses to a local cellulitis and abscess. Beta-hemolytic streptococcus is the usual organism responsible for peritonsillar abscesses (Brook, 2004). In more severe cases, the infection can spread over the palate and to the neck and chest. Edema can cause airway obstruction, which can become life-threatening and is a medical emergency. Peritonsillar abscess is an uncommon infection in older adults. However, the possibility of a peritonsillar abscess as well as pharyngeal space abscess should be considered in afebrile, nontoxic patients older than 50 years of age who have complaints of new-onset sore throat and **dysphagia** (difficulty swallowing) lasting several days (Franzese & Isaacson, 2003).

Clinical Manifestations

The person with a peritonsillar abscess appears acutely ill. The patient often has fever, trismus (inability to open the mouth), and drooling. Local symptoms include a raspy voice, odynophagia (a severe sensation of burning, squeezing pain while swallowing), dysphagia, and otalgia (pain in the ear). The patient may also demonstrate tender and enlarged cervical lymph nodes. On physical examination, the patient shows signs of marked swelling of the soft palate, often occluding almost half of the opening from the mouth into the pharynx; unilateral tonsillar hypertrophy; and dehydration. The patient may also present with erythema of the skin of the chest.

Assessment and Diagnostic Findings

Emergency room physicians are often required to make the diagnosis of peritonsillar abscess and to decide whether aspiration, an invasive procedure, should be carried out based on the patient's clinical picture. Intraoral ultrasound is used in the management of peritonsillar abscess to assist in distinguishing between peritonsillar cellulitis (inflammation) and abscess. This diagnostic tool also helps to provide ultrasound needle guidance during peritonsillar abscess drainage, avoiding the multiple attempts to aspirate the abscess that often occur with a blind approach (Blaivas, Theodoro & Duggal, 2003). The aspirated material is sent for culture and Gram stain. A CT scan may be performed if it is not possible to aspirate the abscess or to confirm the diagnosis before surgical intervention.

Medical Management

Studies have evaluated the best treatment for peritonsillar abscess, including use of corticosteroids, permucosal aspiration with a fine needle versus incision and drainage, and tonsillectomy (Johnson, Stewart & Wright, 2003). Rarely, the patient with a peritonsillar abscess may present with acute airway obstruction and require immediate airway management. Procedures may include intubation, cricothyroidotomy, or tracheotomy. Antibiotics (usually penicillin) are extremely effective in controlling the infection in peritonsillar abscess. If antibiotics are prescribed early in the course of the disease, the abscess may resolve without needing to be incised. Patients with signs of toxicity or complications require hospitalization for IV antibiotics, imaging studies, observation, and proper airway management.

Surgical Management

If pharmacologic treatment is delayed or ineffective, the abscess must be evacuated as soon as possible. Untreated abscesses can rupture spontaneously into the pharynx and cause catastrophic aspiration and death (Brook, 2004). Fine needle aspiration of purulent material (pus) has traditionally been the treatment of choice once the diagnosis has been made. Evidence suggests that these treatment methods (ie, aspiration, incision and drainage) are equally effective, with low rates of recurrence of peritonsillar abscess (Johnson et al., 2003). The mucous membrane over the swelling is first sprayed with a topical anesthetic and then injected with a local anesthetic. Single or repeated needle aspirations are performed to decompress the abscess. Alternatively, the abscess may be incised and drained. These procedures are performed best with the patient in the sitting position to make it easier to expectorate the pus and blood that accumulate in the pharynx. Almost immediate relief is experienced. In a small number of cases, needle aspiration is unsuccessful, so incision and drainage therapy will be used with later tonsillectomy. Approximately 30% of patients with peritonsillar abscess have indications for tonsillectomy (Tierney, McPhee & Papadakis, 2005).

If the patient requires intubation, cricothyroidotomy, or tracheotomy to treat airway obstruction, the nurse assists with the procedure and provides support to the patient before, during, and after the procedure. The nurse also assists with the needle aspiration when indicated.

Considerable relief may be obtained by the use of topical anesthetic agents and throat irrigations or the frequent use of mouthwashes or gargles, using saline or alkaline solutions at a temperature of 105°F to 110°F (40.6°C to 43.3°C). Gentle gargling after the procedure with a cool normal saline gargle may relieve discomfort. The patient must be upright and clearly expectorate forward. The nurse instructs the patient to gargle *gently* at intervals of 1 or 2 hours for 24 to 36 hours. Liquids that are cool or at room temperature are usually well tolerated. Adequate fluids must be provided to treat dehydration and prevent its recurrence.

Laryngitis

Laryngitis, an inflammation of the larynx, often occurs as a result of voice abuse or exposure to dust, chemicals, smoke, and other pollutants, or as part of a URI. It also may be caused by isolated infection involving only the vocal cords.

Laryngitis is very often caused by the same pathogens that cause the common cold and pharyngitis; the most common cause is a virus and laryngitis is often associated with allergic rhinitis or pharyngitis. Bacterial invasion may be secondary. The onset of infection may be associated with exposure to sudden temperature changes, dietary deficiencies, malnutrition, or an immunosuppressed state. Viral laryngitis is common in the winter and is easily transmitted to others.

Clinical Manifestations

Signs of acute laryngitis include hoarseness or **aphonia** (complete loss of voice) and severe cough. Chronic laryngitis is marked by persistent hoarseness. Laryngitis may be a complication of URIs. Other signs of acute laryngitis include sudden onset made worse by cold dry wind. The throat feels worse in the morning and improves when the patient is indoors in a warmer climate. At times the patient presents with a dry cough and a dry, sore throat that worsens in the evening hours. If allergies are present, the uvula will be visibly edematous. Many patients also complain of a "tickle" in the throat that is made worse by cold air or cold liquids. Chronic laryngitis is marked by persistent hoarseness. Laryngitis may be a complication of a URI.

Medical Management

Management of acute laryngitis includes resting the voice, avoiding irritants (including smoking), resting, and inhaling cool steam or an aerosol. If the laryngitis is part of a more extensive respiratory infection caused by a bacterial organism or if it is severe, appropriate antibacterial therapy is instituted. The majority of patients recover with conservative treatment; however, laryngitis tends to be more severe in elderly patients and may be complicated by pneumonia.

For chronic laryngitis, the treatment includes resting the voice, eliminating any primary respiratory tract infection, eliminating smoking, and avoiding secondhand smoke. Topical corticosteroids, such as beclomethasone dipropionate (Vanceril), may also be given by inhalation. These preparations have few systemic or long-lasting effects and may reduce local inflammatory reactions.

Nursing Management

The nurse instructs the patient to rest the voice and to maintain a well-humidified environment. If laryngeal secretions are present during acute episodes, expectorant agents are suggested, along with a daily fluid intake of 2 to 3 L to thin secretions. In cases involving infection, the nurse informs the patient that the symptoms of laryngitis often extend a week to 10 days after completion of antibiotic therapy. The nurse also informs the patient of signs and symptoms that require contacting the health care provider. These signs and symptoms include loss of voice with sore throat that makes swallowing saliva difficult, hemoptysis, and noisy respirations. Continued hoarseness after voice rest or laryngitis that persists for longer than 5 days should be reported because of the possibility of malignancy.

Nursing Process

The Patient With Upper Airway Infection

Assessment

A health history may reveal signs and symptoms of headache, sore throat, pain around the eyes and on either side of the nose, difficulty in swallowing, cough, hoarseness, fever, stuffiness, and generalized discomfort and fatigue. Determining when the symptoms began, what precipitated them, what if anything relieves them, and what aggravates them is part of the assessment. The nurse should also determine any history of allergy or the existence of a concomitant illness. Inspection may reveal swelling, lesions, or asymmetry of the nose as well as bleeding or discharge. The nurse inspects the nasal mucosa for abnormal findings such as increased redness, swelling, exudate, and nasal polyps, which may develop in chronic rhinitis. The nurse palpates the frontal and maxillary sinuses for tenderness, which suggests inflammation, and then inspects the throat by having the patient open the mouth wide and take a deep breath. The tonsils and pharynx are inspected for abnormal findings such as redness, asymmetry, or evidence of drainage, ulceration, or enlargement. The nurse also palpates the trachea to determine the midline position in the neck and to detect any masses or deformities. The neck lymph nodes are palpated for enlargement and tenderness.

Diagnosis

Nursing Diagnoses

Based on the assessment data, the patient's major nursing diagnoses may include the following:

- Ineffective airway clearance related to excessive mucus production secondary to retained secretions and inflammation
- Acute pain related to upper airway irritation secondary to an infection
- Impaired verbal communication related to physiologic changes and upper airway irritation secondary to infection or swelling
- Deficient fluid volume related to decreased fluid intake and increased fluid loss secondary to diaphoresis associated with a fever
- Deficient knowledge regarding prevention of URIs, treatment regimen, surgical procedure, or postoperative care

Collaborative Problems/ Potential Complications

Based on assessment data, potential complications include

- Sepsis
- Meningitis
- Peritonsillar abscess
- Otitis media
- Sinusitis

Planning and Goals

The major goals for the patient may include maintenance of a patent airway, relief of pain, maintenance of effective means of communication, normal hydration, knowledge of how to prevent upper airway infections, and absence of complications.

Nursing Interventions

Maintaining a Patent Airway

An accumulation of secretions can block the airway in patients with an upper airway infection. As a result, changes in the respiratory pattern occur, and the work of breathing increases to compensate for the blockage. The nurse can implement several measures to loosen thick secretions or to keep the secretions moist so that they can be easily expectorated. Increasing fluid intake helps thin the mucus. Use of room vaporizers or steam inhalation also loosens secretions and reduces inflammation of the mucous membranes. To enhance drainage from the sinuses, the nurse instructs the patient about the best position to assume; this depends on the location of the infection or inflammation. For example, drainage for sinusitis or rhinitis is achieved in the upright position. In some conditions, topical or systemic medications, when prescribed, help to relieve nasal or throat congestion.

Promoting Comfort

URIs usually produce localized discomfort. In sinusitis, pain may occur in the area of the sinuses, or a general headache may be produced. In pharyngitis, laryngitis, or tonsillitis, a sore throat occurs. The nurse encourages the patient to take analgesics, such as acetaminophen with codeine, as prescribed, to relieve this discomfort. A pain intensity rating scale (see Chapter 13) may be used to assess effectiveness of pain relief measures. Other helpful measures include topical anesthetic agents for symptomatic relief of herpes simplex blisters (see Chart 22-2) and sore throats, hot packs to relieve the congestion of sinusitis and promote drainage, and warm-water gargles or irrigations to relieve the pain of a sore throat. The nurse encourages rest to relieve the generalized discomfort and fever that accompany many upper airway conditions (especially rhinitis, pharyngitis, and laryngitis). The nurse instructs the patient in general hygiene techniques to prevent the spread of infection. For postoperative care after tonsillectomy and adenoidectomy, an ice collar may reduce swelling and decrease bleeding.

Promoting Communication

Upper airway infections may result in hoarseness or loss of speech. The nurse instructs the patient to refrain from speaking as much as possible and, if possible, to communicate in writing instead. Additional strain on the vocal cords may delay full return of the voice. The nurse encourages the patient and family to use alternative forms of communication, such as a memo pad and a bell to signal for assistance when needed.

Encouraging Fluid Intake

In upper airway infections, the work of breathing and the respiratory rate increase as inflammation and secretions develop. This, in turn, may increase insensible fluid loss. Fever further increases the metabolic rate, diaphoresis, and fluid loss.

Sore throat, malaise, and fever may interfere with a patient's willingness to eat and drink. The nurse provides a list of easily ingested foods to increase caloric intake during the acute phase of illness. These include soups, pudding, yogurt, cottage cheese, high protein drinks, and popsicles. The nurse encourages the patient to drink 2 to 3 L of fluid per day during the acute stage of airway infection, unless contraindicated, to thin the secretions and promote drainage. Liquids (hot or cold) may be soothing, depending on the disorder.

Promoting Home and Community-Based Care

TEACHING PATIENTS SELF-CARE

Prevention of most upper airway infections is difficult because of the many potential causes. But because most URIs are transmitted by hand-to-hand contact, the nurse teaches the patient and family techniques to minimize the spread of infection to others, including frequent handwashing. Other preventive strategies are identified in Chart 22-3. The nurse advises the patient to avoid exposure to people who are at risk for serious illness if respiratory infection is transmitted. Those at risk include elderly adults, immunosuppressed people, and those with chronic health problems.

The nurse teaches patients and their families strategies to relieve symptoms of URIs. These include increasing the humidity level, encouraging adequate fluid intake, getting adequate rest, using warm-water gargles or irrigations and topical anesthetic agents to relieve sore throat, and applying hot packs to relieve congestion. The nurse reinforces the need to complete the treatment regimen, particularly when antibiotics are prescribed.

CONTINUING CARE

Referral for home care is rare. However, it may be indicated for people whose health status was compromised before the onset of the respiratory infection and for those who cannot manage self-care without assistance. In such circumstances, the home care nurse assesses the patient's respiratory status and progress in recovery. The nurse may advise elderly patients and those who would be at increased risk from a respiratory infection to consider an annual influenza vaccine. A follow-up appointment with the primary care provider may be indicated for patients with compromised health status to ensure that the respiratory infection has resolved.

Monitoring and Managing Potential Complications

Although major complications of URIs are rare, the nurse must be aware of them and assess the patient for them. Because most patients with URIs are managed at home, patients and their families must be instructed to monitor for signs and symptoms and to seek immediate medical care if the patient's condition does not improve or if the patient's physical status appears to be worsening.

Sepsis and meningitis may occur in patients with compromised immune status or in those with an overwhelming bacterial infection. The patient with a URI and family members are instructed to seek medical care if the patient's condition fails to improve within several days after the onset of symptoms, if unusual symptoms develop, or if the patient's condition deteriorates. They are instructed about signs and symptoms that require further attention: persistent or high fever, increasing shortness of breath, confusion, and increasing weakness and malaise. The patient with sepsis requires expert care to treat the infection, stabilize vital signs, and prevent or treat septicemia and shock. Deterioration of the patient's condition necessitates intensive care measures (eg, hemodynamic monitoring and administration of vasoactive medications, IV fluids, nutritional support, corticosteroids) to monitor the patient's status and to support the patient's vital signs. High doses of antibiotics may be administered to treat the causative organism. The nurse's role is to monitor the patient's vital signs, hemodynamic status, and laboratory values, administer needed treatment, alleviate the patient's physical discomfort, and provide explanations, teaching, and emotional support to the patient and family.

Peritonsillar abscess may develop after an acute infection of the tonsils. The patient requires treatment to drain the abscess and receives antibiotics for infection and topical anesthetic agents and throat irrigations to relieve pain and sore throat. Follow-up is necessary to ensure that the abscess resolves; tonsillectomy may be required. The nurse assists the patient in administering throat irrigations and instructs the patient and family about the importance of adhering to the prescribed treatment regimen and recommended follow-up appointments.

Otitis media and sinusitis may develop with URI. The patient and family are instructed about the signs and symptoms of otitis media and sinusitis and about the importance of follow-up with the primary health care practitioner to ensure adequate evaluation and treatment of these conditions.

Evaluation

Expected Patient Outcomes

Expected patient outcomes may include the following:

1. Maintains a patent airway by managing secretions
   a. Reports decreased congestion
   b. Assumes best position to facilitate drainage of secretions
   c. Uses self-care measures appropriately and consistently to manage secretions during the acute phase of illness

2. Reports relief of pain and discomfort using pain intensity scale
   a. Uses comfort measures: analgesics, hot packs, gargles, rest
   b. Demonstrates adequate oral hygiene
3. Demonstrates ability to communicate needs, wants, level of comfort
4. Maintains adequate fluid and nutrition intake
5. Utilizes strategies to prevent upper airway infections and allergic reactions
   a. Demonstrates hand hygiene technique
   b. Identifies the value of the influenza vaccine
6. Demonstrates an adequate level of knowledge and performs self-care adequately
7. Becomes free of signs and symptoms of infection
   a. Exhibits normal vital signs (temperature, pulse, respiratory rate)
   b. Absence of purulent drainage
   c. Free of pain in ears, sinuses, and throat
   d. Absence of signs of inflammation
8. Absence of complications
   a. No signs of sepsis: fever, hypotension, deterioration of cognitive status
   b. Vital signs and hemodynamic status normal
   c. No evidence of neurologic involvement
   d. No signs of development of peritonsillar abscess
   e. Resolution of URI without development of otitis media or sinusitis

Obstruction and Trauma of the Upper Respiratory Airway

Obstruction During Sleep

A variety of respiratory disorders are associated with sleep, the most common being sleep apnea syndrome. Chronic loss of sleep, along with untreated sleep disorders, affects the health and quality of life of 70 million people in the United States. Health care costs for sleep disorders average $15 billion annually plus $50 billion in lost productivity (Lamberg, 2004). Sleep apnea syndrome is defined as cessation of breathing (**apnea**) during sleep usually caused by repetitive upper airway obstruction. It interferes with the person's ability to obtain adequate rest and ultimately can affect memory, learning, and decision making.

Various definitions of obstructive sleep apnea (OSA)—also referred to as obstructive sleep apnea/hypopnea syndrome (OSAHS)—exist, leading to overestimation of the prevalence of this syndrome. More research is needed to accurately estimate the number of people with sleep apnea syndrome (Stradling & Davis, 2004). It is currently estimated that 12 million Americans each year suffer from chronic sleep disorders, including sleep apnea. Sleep apnea is more prevalent in men, especially those who are older and overweight. However, patients who are not obese should also be evaluated for OSA, because it is not always associated with obesity. Cigarette smoking has also been identified as another possible risk factor, although more studies on this topic are needed (Young, Skatrud & Peppard, 2004).

Pathophysiology

Sleep apnea is classified into three types:

- Obstructive—lack of air flow due to pharyngeal occlusion
- Central—simultaneous cessation of both air flow and respiratory movements
- Mixed—a combination of central and obstructive apnea within one apneic episode

The most common type of sleep apnea syndrome, OSA, will be presented here. The obstruction may be caused by mechanical factors such as a reduced diameter of the upper airway or dynamic changes in the upper airway during sleep. The tone of the muscles of the upper air-way is reduced during sleep. These sleep-related changes may predispose the patient to upper airway collapse when small amounts of negative pressure are generated during inspiration.

Clinical Manifestations

OSA is characterized by frequent and loud snoring with breathing cessation for 10 seconds or longer, for at least five episodes per hour, followed by awakening abruptly with a loud snort as the blood oxygen level drops. Patients with sleep apnea may experience anywhere from five apneic episodes per hour to several hundred per night. Signs and symptoms of OSA are given in (Chart 22-4).

OSA may be associated with obesity and with other conditions that reduce pharyngeal muscle tone (eg, neuromuscular disease, sedative/hypnotic medications, acute ingestion of alcohol). The diagnosis of sleep apnea is based on clinical features plus polysomnographic findings (sleep study), in which the patient's cardiopulmonary status, eye

CHART 22-4

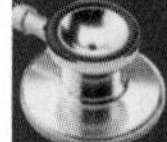

Assessing for Obstructive Sleep Apnea (OSA)

Be alert for the following signs and symptoms:

- Excessive daytime sleepiness
- Frequent nocturnal awakening
- Insomnia
- Loud snoring
- Morning headaches
- Intellectual deterioration
- Personality changes, irritability
- Impotence
- Systemic hypertension
- Dysrhythmias
- Pulmonary hypertension, cor pulmonale
- Polycythemia
- Enuresis

movements, and muscle activity are monitored during an episode of sleep (Merritt & Berger, 2004).

The patient with OSA is at high risk for coronary artery disease, cerebrovascular disease, and premature death (von Känel & Dimsdale, 2003). Repetitive apneic events result in hypoxia and hypercapnia, which triggers a sympathetic response. As a consequence, patients have a high prevalence of hypertension and an increased risk of myocardial infarction and stroke. In patients with underlying cardiovascular disease, the nocturnal hypoxemia may predispose to dysrhythmias.

Medical Management

Patients usually seek medical treatment because their sleeping partners express concern or because they experience excessive sleepiness at inappropriate times or settings (eg, while driving a car). A variety of treatments are used. In mild cases, the patient is advised to avoid sleeping on the back, avoid alcohol and medications that depress the upper airway, and lose weight. In more severe cases involving hypoxemia with severe carbon dioxide retention (hypercapnia), the treatment includes continuous positive airway pressure (CPAP) or bilevel positive airway pressure (BiPAP) therapy with supplemental oxygen via nasal cannula. These treatment methods are described in Chapter 25. CPAP is used to prevent airway collapse, whereas BiPAP makes breathing easier and results in a lower average airway pressure.

Surgical procedures (eg, uvulopalatopharyngoplasty) may be performed to correct the obstruction. As a last resort, a tracheostomy is performed to bypass the obstruction if the potential for respiratory failure or life-threatening dysrhythmias exists. The tracheostomy is unplugged only during sleep. Although this is an effective treatment, it is used in a limited number of patients because of its associated physical disfigurement (Thatcher & Maisel, 2003).

Pharmacologic Therapy

Although medications are not generally recommended for OSA, some preliminary data suggest that modafinil (Provigil) may help reduce daytime sleepiness (Boutrel & Koob, 2004). Protriptyline (Triptil) given at bedtime may increase the respiratory drive and improve upper airway muscle tone. Medroxyprogesterone acetate (Provera) and acetazolamide (Diamox) have been recommended for sleep apnea associated with chronic alveolar hypoventilation, but their benefits have not been well established. The patient must understand that these medications are not a substitute for CPAP or BiPAP. Administration of low-flow nasal oxygen at night can help relieve hypoxemia in some patients but has little effect on the frequency or severity of apnea. Clinical trials are needed to assess the effectiveness of these treatment approaches.

Nursing Management

The patient with OSA may not recognize the potential consequences of the disorder. Therefore, the nurse explains the disorder in terms that are understandable to the patient and relates symptoms (daytime sleepiness) to the underlying disorder. The nurse also instructs the patient and family about treatments, including the correct and safe use of CPAP, BiPAP, and oxygen therapy, if prescribed.

Epistaxis (Nosebleed)

Epistaxis, a hemorrhage from the nose, is caused by the rupture of tiny, distended vessels in the mucous membrane of any area of the nose. Rarely does epistaxis originate in the densely vascular tissue over the turbinates. Most commonly, the site is the anterior septum, where three major blood vessels enter the nasal cavity: (1) the anterior ethmoidal artery on the forward part of the roof (Kiesselbach's plexus), (2) the sphenopalatine artery in the posterosuperior region, and (3) the internal maxillary branches (the plexus of veins located at the back of the lateral wall under the inferior turbinate).

A variety of causes are associated with epistaxis (Chart 22-5).

Medical Management

Management of epistaxis depends on its cause and the location of the bleeding site. A nasal speculum, penlight, or headlight may be used to determine the site of bleeding in the nasal cavity. Most nosebleeds originate from the anterior portion of the nose. Initial treatment may include applying direct pressure. The patient sits upright with the head tilted forward to prevent swallowing and aspiration of blood and is directed to pinch the soft outer portion of the nose against the midline septum for 5 or 10 minutes continuously. If this measure is unsuccessful, additional treatment is indicated. In anterior nosebleeds, the area may be treated with a silver nitrate applicator and Gelfoam, or by electrocautery.

Topical vasoconstrictors, such as adrenaline (1:1,000), cocaine (0.5%), and phenylephrine may be prescribed.

CHART 22-5

Risk Factors for Epistaxis

- Local infections (vestibulitis, rhinitis, sinusitis)
- Systemic infections (scarlet fever, malaria)
- Drying of nasal mucous membranes
- Nasal inhalation of illicit drugs (eg, cocaine)
- Trauma (digital trauma as in picking the nose; blunt trauma; fracture; forceful nose blowing)
- Arteriosclerosis
- Hypertension
- Tumor (sinus or nasopharynx)
- Thrombocytopenia
- Use of aspirin
- Liver disease
- Redu-Osler-Weber syndrome (hereditary hemorrhagic telangiectasia)

Cotton pledgets soaked in a vasoconstricting solution (ie, epinephrine, ephedrine, cocaine) may be inserted into the nose to reduce the blood flow and improve the examiner's view of the bleeding site. Alternatively, a cotton tampon may be used to try to stop the bleeding. Suction may be used to remove excess blood and clots from the field of inspection. The search for the bleeding site should shift from the anteroinferior quadrant to the anterosuperior, then to the posterosuperior, and finally to the posteroinferior area. The field is kept clear by using suction and by shifting the cotton tampon. Only about 60% of the total nasal cavity can actually be seen, however.

If the origin of the bleeding cannot be identified, the nose may be packed with gauze impregnated with petrolatum jelly or antibiotic ointment; a topical anesthetic spray and decongestant agent may be used before the gauze packing is inserted, or a balloon-inflated catheter may be used (Fig. 22-4). Alternatively, a compressed nasal sponge may be used. Once the sponge becomes saturated with blood or is moistened with a small amount of saline, it will expand and produce tamponade to halt the bleeding. The packing may remain in place for 48 hours or up to 5 or 6 days if necessary to control bleeding. Antibiotics may be prescribed because of the risk of iatrogenic sinusitis and toxic shock syndrome.

Nursing Management

The nurse monitors the patient's vital signs, assists in the control of bleeding, and provides tissues and an emesis basin to allow the patient to expectorate any excess blood. It is common for patients to be anxious in response to a nosebleed. Blood loss on clothing and handkerchiefs can be frightening, and the nasal examination and treatment are uncomfortable. Assuring the patient in a calm, efficient manner that bleeding can be controlled can help reduce anxiety. The nurse continuously assesses the patient's airway and breathing as well as vital signs. On rare occasions, a patient with significant hemorrhage requires IV infusions of crystalloid solutions (normal saline) as well as cardiac and pulse oximetry monitoring.

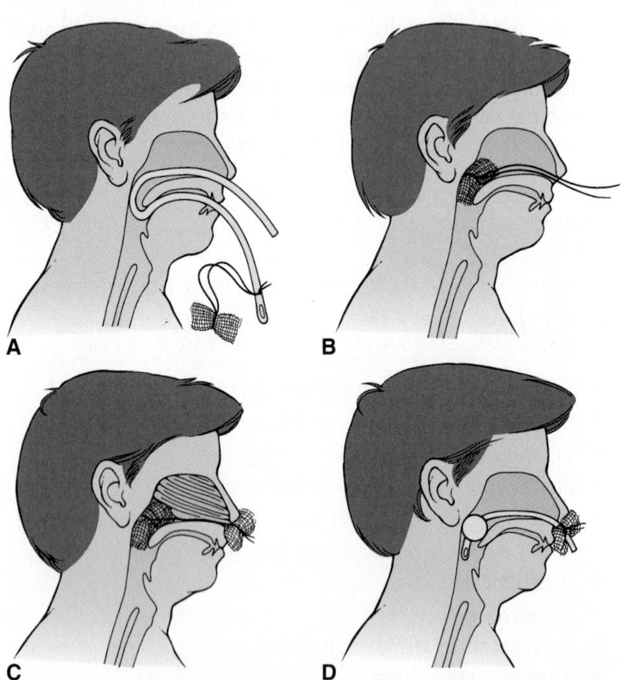

FIGURE 22-4. Packing to control bleeding from the posterior nose. (**A**) Catheter is inserted and packing is attached. (**B**) Packing is drawn into position as the catheter is removed. (**C**) Strip is tied over a bolster to hold the packing in place with an anterior pack installed "accordion pleat" style. (**D**) Alternative method, using a balloon catheter instead of gauze packing.

Teaching Patients Self-Care

Discharge teaching includes reviewing ways to prevent epistaxis: avoiding forceful nose blowing, straining, high altitudes, and nasal trauma (including nose picking). Adequate humidification may prevent drying of the nasal passages. The nurse instructs the patient how to apply direct pressure to the nose with the thumb and the index finger for 15 minutes in the case of a recurrent nosebleed. If recurrent bleeding cannot be stopped, the patient is instructed to seek additional medical attention.

Nasal Obstruction

The passage of air through the nostrils is frequently obstructed by a deviation of the nasal septum, hypertrophy of the turbinate bones, or the pressure of nasal polyps, which are grapelike swellings that arise from the mucous membrane of the sinuses, especially the ethmoids. Chronic nasal congestion seriously affects the patient throughout the day as well as during sleep. It forces the patient to breath through the mouth, thus producing dryness of the oral mucosa and associated problems including persistent dry, cracked lips. Patients with chronic nasal congestion often suffer from sleep deprivation due to difficulty maintaining an adequate airway while lying flat and during sleep.

Persistent nasal obstruction also may lead to chronic infection of the nose and result in frequent episodes of nasopharyngitis. Frequently, the infection extends to the nasal sinuses. When sinusitis develops and the drainage from these cavities is obstructed by deformity or swelling within the nose, pain is experienced in the region of the affected sinus.

Medical Management

The treatment of nasal obstruction requires the removal of the obstruction, followed by measures to treat whatever chronic infection exists. In many patients an underlying allergy also requires treatment. Measures to reduce or alleviate nasal obstruction include nonsurgical as well as surgical techniques. Commonly used medications include fluticasone propionate aqueous nasal spray (Flonase) and montelukast (Singulair). Additional medications may include antibiotics for the treatment of underlying infection or antihistamines for management of allergies. Hypertrophied turbinates may be treated by applying an astringent agent to shrink them.

A more aggressive approach in treating nasal obstruction caused by turbinate hypertrophy involves surgical reduction of the hypertrophy. Available surgical procedures include turbinectomy, laser cautery, electrocautery, cryotherapy, submucosal resection, and submucosal resection with lateral displacement (Passali, Passali, Damiani, et al., 2003). During **submucosal resection** to treat a deviated septum, the surgeon makes an incision into the mucous membrane and, after raising it from the bone, removes the deviated bone and cartilage with bone forceps. The mucosa then is allowed to fall back in place and is held there by tight packing. Generally, the packing is soaked in liquid petrolatum so that it can be removed easily after 24 to 36 hours. At times endoscopic surgery is also indicated to drain the nasal sinuses. The specific procedure performed depends on the type of nasal obstruction found. Nasal polyps are removed by clipping them at their base with a wire snare. Usually, these surgical procedures are performed under local anesthesia.

Nursing Management

Most of these procedures are performed on an outpatient basis. The nurse explains the procedure after the physician provides the initial instruction. Postoperatively, the nurse elevates the head of the bed to promote drainage and to alleviate discomfort from edema. Frequent oral hygiene is encouraged to overcome dryness caused by breathing through the mouth. Before discharge from the outpatient or same-day surgical unit, the patient is instructed to avoid blowing the nose with force during the postoperative recovery period. The patient is also instructed about the signs and symptoms of bleeding and infection and when to contact the physician. The patient is provided with written postoperative instructions including emergency phone numbers.

Fractures of the Nose

The location of the nose makes it susceptible to injury. Nasal fracture is the most common facial fracture and the most common fracture in the body. Fractures of the nose usually result from a direct assault. Nasal fractures may affect the ascending process of the maxilla and the septum. The torn mucous membrane results in a nosebleed. In a series of complications, the patient could ultimately experience a hematoma, infection, abscess, and avascular/septic necrosis. However, as a rule, serious consequences usually do not occur.

Clinical Manifestations

The signs and symptoms of a nasal fracture are pain, bleeding from the nose externally and internally into the pharynx, swelling of the soft tissues adjacent to the nose, periorbital ecchymosis, nasal obstruction, and deformity. The patient's nose may have an asymmetric appearance that may not be obvious until the edema subsides.

Assessment and Diagnostic Findings

The nose is examined internally to rule out the possibility that the injury may be complicated by a fracture of the nasal septum and a submucosal septal hematoma. Because of the swelling and bleeding that occur with a nasal fracture, an accurate diagnosis can be made only after the swelling subsides.

Clear fluid draining from either nostril suggests a fracture of the cribriform plate with leakage of cerebrospinal fluid. Because cerebrospinal fluid contains glucose, it can readily be differentiated from nasal mucus by means of a dipstick (Dextrostix). Usually, careful inspection or palpation discloses any deviations of the bone or disruptions of the nasal cartilages. An x-ray may reveal displacement of the fractured bones and may help rule out extension of the fracture into the skull.

Medical Management

The nose is assessed for symmetry either before swelling has occurred or after it has subsided. A nasal fracture very often produces bleeding from the nasal passage. As a rule, bleeding is controlled with the use of packing. Cold compresses are used to prevent or reduce edema. For the patient who has sustained enough trauma to break the nose or any facial bone, the emergency medical team must consider the possibility of a cervical spine fracture. Therefore, it is essential to ensure a patent airway and to rule out a cervical spine fracture. Uncomplicated nasal fractures may be treated initially with antibiotics, analgesic agents, and a decongestant nasal spray.

Treatment of nasal fractures is aimed at restoring nasal function and returning the aesthetic appearance of the nose to baseline. The patient is referred to a specialist, usually 3 to 5 days after the injury, to evaluate the need to realign the bones. Although improved outcomes are obtained when reduction of the fracture is performed during the first 3 hours after the injury, this is often not possible because of the edema. If immediate reduction of the fracture is not possible, it is performed within 3 to 7 days. Timing is important when treating nasal fractures because a delay in treatment longer than 7 to 10 days may result in significant bone healing, which ultimately may require surgical intervention that includes rhinoplasty to reshape the external appearance of the nose. A septorhinoplasty is performed when the nasal septum needs to be repaired. In patients who develop a septal hematoma, the physician will drain the hematoma through a small incision. A septal hematoma that is not drained can lead to permanent deformity of the nose.

Nursing Management

Immediately after the fracture, the nurse applies ice and encourages the patient to keep the head elevated. The nurse instructs the patient to apply ice packs to the nose for 20 minutes four times each day to decrease swelling. The patient who experiences bleeding from the nose (epistaxis) is usually frightened and anxious and needs reassurance. The packing inserted to stop the bleeding may be uncomfortable and unpleasant, and obstruction of the nasal passages by the packing forces the patient to breathe through the mouth. This in turn causes the oral mucous membranes to become dry. Mouth rinses help to moisten the mucous membranes and to reduce the odor and taste of dried blood in the oropharynx and nasopharynx. Use of analgesic agents such as acetaminophen or NSAIDs such as ibuprofen or naproxen is encouraged. For people younger than 20 years of age, aspirin is avoided because of the risk of Reye's syndrome. When removing the cotton pledgets, the nurse carefully inspects the mucosa for lacerations or a septal hematoma. The nurse reminds the patient to avoid sports activities for 6 weeks.

Laryngeal Obstruction

Obstruction of the larynx because of edema is a serious, often fatal, condition. The larynx is a stiff box that will not stretch. It contains a narrow space between the vocal cords (glottis), through which air must pass. Swelling of the laryngeal mucous membranes may close off the opening tightly, leading to life-threatening hypoxia or suffocation. Edema of the glottis occurs rarely in patients with acute laryngitis, occasionally in patients with urticaria, and more frequently in patients with severe inflammation of the throat, as in scarlet fever. It is an occasional but usually preventable cause of death in severe anaphylaxis (angioneurotic edema).

Hereditary angioedema (HAE) is also characterized by episodes of life-threatening laryngeal edema. Laryngeal edema in people with HAE can occur at any age, although young adults are at greatest risk. Risk factors for laryngeal obstruction are given in Table 22-2.

Foreign bodies frequently are aspirated into the pharynx, the larynx, or the trachea and cause a twofold problem. First, they obstruct the air passages and cause difficulty in breathing, which may lead to asphyxia; later, they may be drawn farther down, entering the bronchi or a bronchial branch and causing symptoms of irritation, such as a croupy cough, expectoration of blood or mucus, or labored breathing. The physical signs and x-ray findings confirm the diagnosis.

TABLE 22-2 Risk Factors for Laryngeal Obstruction

Precipitating Event	Mechanism of Obstruction
History of allergies; exposure to medications, latex, foods (tree nuts [eg, walnuts, pecans]), bee stings	Anaphylaxis
Foreign body	Inhalation/ingestion of meat or other food items, coin, chewing gum, balloon fragments, drug packets (ingested to avoid arrest)
Heavy alcohol consumption; heavy tobacco use	Obstruction from tumor
Family history of airway problems	Suggests angioedema (type I hypersensitivity reaction)
Use of angiotensin-converting enzyme (ACE) inhibitors	Increased risk for angioedema of the mucous membranes
Recent throat pain or recent fever	Infectious process
History of surgery or previous tracheostomy	Possible subglottic stenosis

Clinical Manifestations

The patient's clinical presentation and x-ray findings confirm the diagnosis of laryngeal obstruction. The patient may demonstrate lowered oxygen saturation; however, a normal oxygen saturation should not be interpreted as a sign that the obstruction is not significant. Use of accessory muscles to maximize airflow may occur and is often manifested by retractions in the neck or abdomen during inspirations. Patients who demonstrate these symptoms are at an immediate risk of collapse, and respiratory support (ie, mechanical ventilation or positive-pressure ventilation) is considered.

Assessment and Diagnostic Findings

A thorough history can be very useful to the health care team in diagnosing and treating the patient with a laryngeal obstruction. However, emergency measures to secure the patient's airway should not be delayed to obtain a history or perform tests. If possible, the nurse obtains a history from the patient or family about heavy alcohol or tobacco consumption, current medications, family history of airway problems, recent infections, pain or fever, dental pain or poor dentition, and any previous surgeries or trauma.

Medical Management

Medical management is based on the initial evaluation of the patient and the need to ensure a patent airway. If the airway is obstructed by a foreign body and signs of asphyxia are apparent, immediate treatment is necessary. Frequently, if the foreign body has lodged in the pharynx and can be visualized, the finger can dislodge it. If the obstruction is in the larynx or the trachea, the clinician or other rescuer tries the subdiaphragmatic abdominal thrust maneuver (Chart 22-6). If all efforts are unsuccessful, an immediate tracheotomy is necessary (see Chapter 25 for further discussion). If the obstruction is caused by edema resulting from an allergic reaction, treatment may include administration of subcutaneous epinephrine and a corticosteroid (see Chapter 53). Ice may be applied to the neck in an effort to reduce edema. Continuous pulse oximetry is essential in the patient who has experienced acute upper airway obstruction.

Cancer of the Larynx

Cancer of the larynx is a malignant tumor in and around the larynx (voice box). Squamous cell carcinoma is the most common form of cancer of the larynx (95%). Adenocarcinoma or sarcoma of the larynx is diagnosed less often. More than 10,000 new cases of cancer of the larynx occur annually. Cancer of the larynx occurs more frequently in men than in women, and it is most common in people between the ages of 50 and 70 years. The incidence of laryngeal cancer continues to decline, but the incidence in women versus men continues to increase. The disease is also about 50% more common among African Americans than among Caucasian Americans.

Carcinogens that have been associated with laryngeal cancer include tobacco (smoke, smokeless) and alcohol

CHART 22-6

Performing the Abdominal Thrust Maneuver

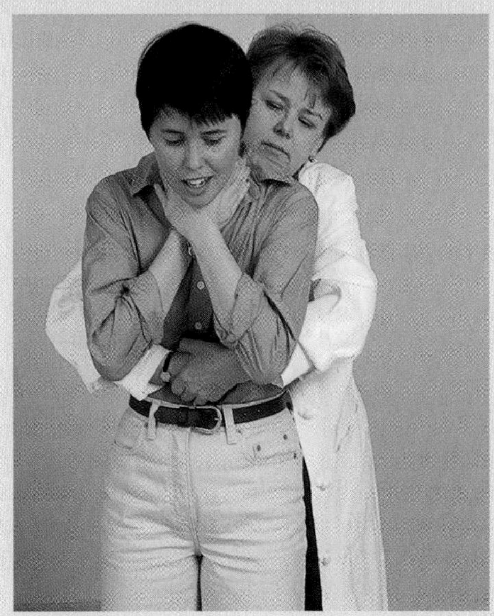

To assist a patient or other person who is choking on a foreign object, the nurse performs the abdominal thrust maneuver (sometimes called the Heimlich maneuver) according to guidelines set forth by the American Heart Association. (*Note:* Hands crossed at the neck is the universal sign for choking.)

1. Stand behind the person who is choking.
2. Place both arms around the person's waist.
3. Make a fist with one hand with the thumb outside the fist.
4. Place thumb side of fist against the person's abdomen above the navel and below the xiphoid process.
5. Grasp fist with other hand.
6. Quickly and forcefully exert pressure against the person's diaphragm, pressing upward with quick, firm thrusts.
7. Apply thrusts 6 to 10 times until the obstruction is cleared.
8. The pressure from the thrusts should lift the diaphragm, force air into the lungs, and create an artificial cough powerful enough to expel the aspirated object.

and their combined effects, as well as exposure to asbestos, mustard gas, wood dust, cement dust, tar products, leather, and metals (Dietz, Ramroth, Urban, et al., 2004). Other contributing factors include straining the voice, chronic laryngitis, nutritional deficiencies (riboflavin), and family predisposition (Chart 22-7).

Laryngeal cancer can be classified into three categories: supraglottic (false vocal cords), glottic (true vocal cords), and subglottic (downward extension of disease from the vocal cords) (National Cancer Institute, 2003). Two thirds of laryngeal cancers are in the glottic area. Supraglottic cancers account for approximately one third of the cases, subglottic tumors for fewer than 1%. Glottic tumors seldom spread if found early, because of the limited lymph vessels found in the vocal cords.

Approximately 25% to 50% of patients with laryngeal cancer present with involved lymph nodes. Metastatic disease from the true vocal cords is very rare, because they are devoid of lymph nodes. The prognosis for patients who have small laryngeal cancers without evidence of spread to the lymph nodes is about 75% to 95%. Recurrence occurs usually within the first 2 to 3 years after diagnosis. The presence of disease after 5 years is very often secondary to a new primary malignancy (National Cancer Institute, 2003).

Clinical Manifestations

Hoarseness of more than 2 weeks' duration occurs in the patient with cancer in the glottic area, because the tumor impedes the action of the vocal cords during speech. The

CHART 22-7

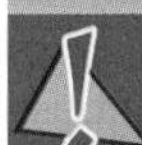

Risk Factors for Laryngeal Cancer

CARCINOGENS

- Tobacco (smoke, smokeless)
- Combined effects of alcohol and tobacco
- Asbestos
- Secondhand smoke
- Paint fumes
- Wood dust
- Cement dust
- Chemicals
- Tar products
- Mustard gas
- Leather and metals

OTHER FACTORS

- Straining the voice
- Chronic laryngitis
- Nutritional deficiencies (riboflavin)
- History of alcohol abuse
- Familial predisposition
- Age (higher incidence after 60 years of age)
- Gender (more common in men)
- Race (more prevalent in African Americans)
- Weakened immune system

voice may sound harsh, raspy, and lower in pitch. Affected voice sounds are not early signs of subglottic or supraglottic cancer. The patient may complain of a persistent cough or sore throat and pain and burning in the throat, especially when consuming hot liquids or citrus juices. A lump may be felt in the neck. Later symptoms include dysphagia, dyspnea (difficulty breathing), unilateral nasal obstruction or discharge, persistent hoarseness, persistent ulceration, and foul breath. Cervical lymph adenopathy, unintentional weight loss, a general debilitated state, and pain radiating to the ear may occur with metastasis.

Assessment and Diagnostic Findings

An initial assessment includes a complete history and physical examination of the head and neck. This includes identification of risk factors, family history, and any underlying medical conditions. An indirect laryngoscopy, using a flexible endoscope, is initially performed in the otolaryngologist's office to visually evaluate the pharynx, larynx, and possible tumor. Mobility of the vocal cords is assessed; if normal movement is limited, the growth may affect muscle, other tissue, and even the airway. The neck and the thyroid gland are palpated for enlarged lymph nodes (Timon, Toner & Conlon, 2003).

If a tumor of the larynx is suspected on an initial examination, a direct laryngoscopic examination is performed under local or general anesthesia to evaluate all areas of the larynx. In some cases, intraoperative examination obtained by direct microscopic visualization and palpation of the vocal folds may yield a more accurate diagnosis. Samples of the suspicious tissue are obtained for histologic evaluation. The tumor may involve any of the three areas of the larynx and may vary in appearance. Additionally, tumor markers (p53 and cyclin D1) obtained through analysis of biopsy tissue provide information about the prognosis of patients with laryngeal epidermoid carcinomas (Vielba, Bilbao, Ispizua, et al., 2003).

The stage of the tumor serves as a basis for the therapeutic regimen. The TNM classification system, developed by the American Joint Committee on Cancer (AJCC), is used to classify head and neck tumors. The classification of the tumor is used to determine treatment modalities. The presence of metastatic disease in lymph nodes is the foremost prognostic indicator (Timon et al., 2003). Because many of these lesions are submucosal, obtaining tissue for biopsy may require an incision made with microlaryngeal techniques or with the use of a CO_2 laser to transect the mucosa and reach the tumor.

CT and magnetic resonance imaging (MRI) are used to assess regional adenopathy and soft tissue and to help stage and determine the extent of a tumor. MRI is also helpful in post-treatment follow-up to detect a recurrence. Positron emission tomography (PET) scanning may also be used to detect recurrence of a laryngeal tumor after treatment.

Medical Management

Treatment of laryngeal cancer depends on the staging of the tumor, which includes the location, size, and histology of the tumor and the presence and extent of cervical lymph node involvement. Treatment options include surgery, radiation therapy, and chemotherapy. The prognosis depends on a variety of factors: tumor stage, the patient's gender and age, and pathologic features of the tumor, including the grade and depth of infiltration. The treatment plan also depends on whether this is an initial diagnosis or a recurrence.

Patients with early-stage disease (stage I or II) can be treated with either radiation therapy or surgery. Survival with radiation alone is 80% to 90% for patients with stage I disease and 70% to 80% for patients with stage II disease. Surgery alone can be used; however, voice preservation is better with radiation alone than with partial laryngectomy (American Cancer Society, 2005). Patients with stage III or IV or advanced tumors require a combined treatment modality approach consisting of either surgery and irradiation, radiation therapy and chemotherapy, or all three treatment regimens. Because of the advanced nature of the disease, surgery often requires the complete removal of the larynx. Patients with advanced laryngeal cancer have longer disease-free survival when treated with chemotherapy along with radiotherapy rather than with radiotherapy alone (Forastiere, Goepfert, Maor, et al., 2003).

Treatment with hyperfractionated accelerated irradiation and concomitant cisplatin has also been effective against locally advanced laryngeal carcinomas. In hyperfractionated radiotherapy, the patient receives a radiation treatment twice daily for a prescribed period of time (DeVita, Hellman & Rosenberg, 2005).

Surgery and radiation therapy are both effective methods in the early stages of cancer of the larynx. Chemotherapy traditionally has been used for recurrence or metastatic disease. It has also been used more recently in conjunction with radiation therapy, to avoid a total laryngectomy, or preoperatively, to shrink a tumor before surgery.

The highest risk of laryngeal cancer recurrence is in the first 2 to 3 years. Combined treatment for patients with stage III cancers yields a survival rate of 30% to 50% at 3 years. The survival rate decreases to 20% to 30% at 5 years. Patients with resectable stage IV disease treated with combined therapy have a 5-year survival rate of 15% to 25% (American Cancer Society, 2005).

Before treatment, a complete dental examination is performed to rule out any oral disease. Any dental problems are resolved, if possible, before surgery and radiotherapy. If surgery is to be performed, a multidisciplinary team evaluates the needs of the patient and family to develop a successful plan of care (Harrison, Dale, Haverman, et al., 2003; Marques & Dib, 2004).

Surgical Management

Surgical management depends largely on the stage of the disease. The overall goals for the patient include minimizing the effects of surgery on speech, swallowing, and breathing while maximizing the cure of the cancer. Complete removal of the larynx (total **laryngectomy**) can provide the desired cure, but it also leaves the patient with significant loss of the natural voice and the need to breathe through an opening (stoma) created in the lower neck. Advances in surgical techniques for treating laryngeal cancer may minimize the cosmetic and functional deficits previously seen with total laryngectomy. Partial laryngectomy is often used for smaller cancers of the larynx. Several different curative procedures are available that can offer voice-sparing results for the patient who has an early laryngeal carcinoma while achieving a positive cure rate. Some microlaryngeal surgery can be performed endoscopically. The CO_2 laser can be used for the treatment of many laryngeal tumors, with the exception of large vascular tumors.

Some less extensive procedures are used to treat dysplasia, hyperkeratosis, and leukoplakia. Complete stripping of the cord is often the curative treatment for this classification of lesions. Stripping of the cord involves removal of the mucosa of the edge of the cord. It is performed with use of an operating microscope. Early vocal cord lesions are initially treated with radiation therapy. An excision of the vocal cord (cordectomy) is usually performed via transoral laser. This procedure is used for confined lesions involving the middle third of the vocal cord. The probability of poor voice quality is related to the extent of tissue removed. High-volume, bilateral, advanced lesions in patients who either refuse laryngectomy or are unable to tolerate surgery may be treated with radiation therapy, with a cure rate of 10% to 20%. Patients with a fixed cord but minimal total tumor bulk may be treated with radiation therapy. Chemotherapy is often considered, and the patients are informed that the need for a subsequent total laryngectomy will be based on clinical suspicion of disease recurrence (ie, in the absence of a biopsy).

Several different types of laryngectomy (surgical removal of part or all of the larynx and surrounding structures) are considered for patients with more extensive involvement:

- Partial laryngectomy
- Supraglottic laryngectomy
- Hemilaryngectomy
- Total laryngectomy
- Other surgical procedures

PARTIAL LARYNGECTOMY. A partial laryngectomy (laryngofissure–thyrotomy) is recommended in the early stages of cancer in the glottic area when only one vocal cord is involved. The surgery is associated with a very high cure rate. It may also be performed for recurrence when high-dose radiation has failed. A portion of the larynx is removed, along with one vocal cord and the tumor; all other structures remain. The airway remains intact, and the patient is expected to have no difficulty swallowing. The voice quality may change, or the patient may sound hoarse.

SUPRAGLOTTIC LARYNGECTOMY. This is a voice-sparing operation that can be tailored to the supraglottic lesion. It is used for lesions that involve the epiglottis, a single arytenoid cartilage, the aryepiglottic fold, and false vocal cords. A neck dissection of one or both sides may also be performed. Postoperative irradiation is indicated based on the pathologic findings from the surgery. A supraglottic laryngectomy is indicated in the management of early (stage I) supraglottic and stage II lesions. The hyoid bone, glottis, and false cords are removed. The true vocal cords, cricoid cartilage, and trachea remain intact. A tracheostomy tube (see Chapter 25) is left in the trachea until the glottic airway is established. It is usually removed after a few days, and the stoma is allowed to close. Nutrition is provided through enteral feedings until there is healing, followed by a semisolid diet. Postoperatively, the patient may experience some difficulty swallowing for the first 2 weeks. Aspiration is a potential complication, because the patient must learn a new method of swallowing (supraglottic swallowing). The chief advantage of this surgical procedure is that it preserves the voice, even though the quality of the voice may change. Speech therapy is required before and after surgery. The major problem is the high risk for recurrence of the cancer; therefore, patients are selected carefully. For patients with early disease, the surgeon may consider an endoscopic supraglottic laryngectomy with postoperative radiation therapy (Davis, Kriskovich, Galloway, et al., 2004).

HEMILARYNGECTOMY. A hemilaryngectomy is performed when the tumor extends beyond the vocal cord but is less than 1 cm in size and is limited to the subglottic area. It may be used in stage I glottic lesions. In this procedure, the thyroid cartilage of the larynx is split in the midline of the neck, and the portion of the vocal cord (one true cord and one false cord) is removed with the tumor. The arytenoid cartilage and half of the thyroid are removed. The patient will have a tracheostomy tube and nasogastric tube in place for a number of days after the surgery. The patient is at risk for aspiration postoperatively. Some change may occur in the voice quality. The voice may be rough, raspy, and hoarse and have limited projection. The airway and swallowing remain intact. Usually, this procedure is reserved for patients with lesions that involve only one cord. Extension of the lesion to the epiglottis, false cord, or intra-arytenoid areas is a contraindication to a hemilaryngectomy.

TOTAL LARYNGECTOMY. A total laryngectomy is performed in most advanced stage IV laryngeal cancers, when the tumor extends beyond the vocal cords, or for cancer that recurs or persists after radiation therapy. In a total laryngectomy, the laryngeal structures are removed, including the hyoid bone, epiglottis, cricoid cartilage, and two or three rings of the trachea. The tongue, pharyngeal walls, and trachea are preserved. A total laryngectomy results in permanent loss of the voice and a change in the airway, requiring a permanent tracheostomy (Fig. 22-5). Patients who have this procedure require alternatives to normal speech; these may include a prosthetic device such as the Singer-Blom valve to speak without aspirating.

Although this procedure can be performed with or without neck dissection, many surgeons recommend that a radical neck dissection be performed on the same side as the lesion even if no lymph nodes are palpable, because metastasis to the cervical lymph nodes is common. Surgery is more difficult when the lesion involves the midline structures or both vocal cords. With or without neck dissection, a total laryngectomy requires a permanent tracheal stoma, because the larynx that provides the protective sphincter is no longer present. The tracheal stoma prevents the aspiration of food and fluid into the lower respiratory tract. The patient will have no voice but will have normal swallowing. A total laryngectomy changes the manner in which airflow is used for breathing and speaking, as depicted in Figure 22-5. Complications that may occur include a salivary leak, wound infection from the development of a pharyngocutaneous fistula, stomal stenosis, and dysphagia secondary to pharyngeal and cervical esophageal stricture.

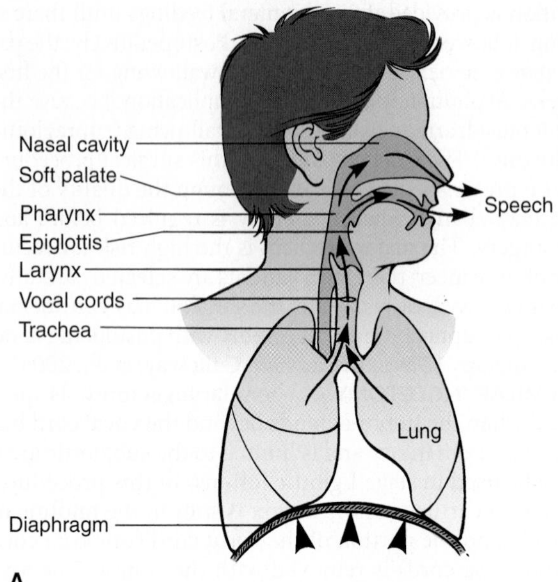

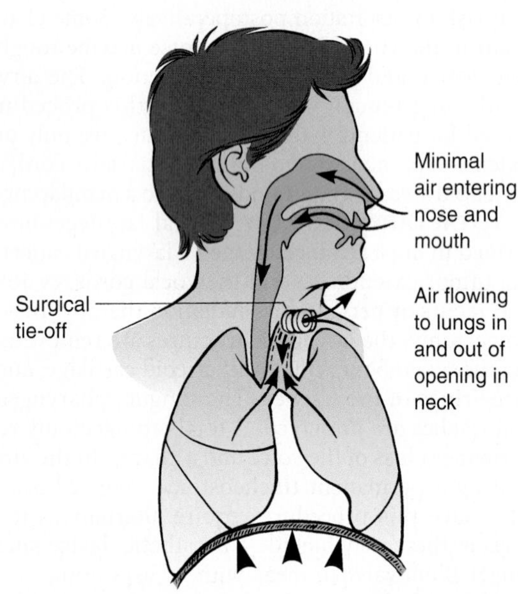

FIGURE 22-5. Total laryngectomy produces a change in airflow for breathing and speaking. **(A)** Normal airflow. **(B)** Airflow after total laryngectomy.

In some cases, the patient may be a candidate for a near-total laryngectomy (NTL). In this situation, the patient would be a candidate for chemotherapy and radiotherapy regimens postoperatively. Voice preservation can be achieved in most cases. NTL enhances speech rehabilitation options for the patient by adding a physiologic, nonprosthetic tissue technique (ie, the myomucosal shunt) that provides a prosthesis-free method for rehabilitating the voice (Kasperbauer & Thomas, 2004).

OTHER SURGICAL APPROACHES. Other surgical procedures include the supracricoid laryngectomy, which was initially developed in the late 1950s as an alternative to total laryngectomy but was not widely adopted in the United States until 30 years later. Two types of this procedure exist; they differ in the extent of resection and reconstruction. Both procedures are alternatives to the total laryngectomy and have been used to preserve or restore speech in patients with more advanced larynx cancers (Shiotani, Araki, Moro, et al., 2004).

In the supracricoid partial laryngectomy (SCPL), the true and false cords, both paraglottic spaces, and the thyroid cartilage are resected. The reconstruction requires suturing of the cricoid to the hyoid and the epiglottis. The procedure is thus termed cricohyoidoepiglottopexy (CHEP).

The second procedure involves the resection of both true and false cords, both paraglottic spaces, the entire preepiglottic space, the epiglottis, and the entire thyroid cartilage. The reconstruction is extensive and requires suturing of the cricoid to the hyoid. The procedure is therefore termed cricohyoidopexy (CHP).

Radiation Therapy

The goal of radiation therapy is to eradicate the cancer and preserve the function of the larynx. The decision to use radiation therapy is based on several factors, including the staging of the tumor (usually used for stage I and stage II tumors as a standard treatment option) and the patient's overall health status, lifestyle (including occupation), and personal preference. Excellent results have been achieved with radiation therapy in patients with early-stage (stage I or II) glottic tumors when only one vocal cord is involved and there is normal mobility (ie, with phonation), as well as in small supraglottic lesions. One of the benefits of radiation therapy is that patients retain a near-normal voice. A few may develop chondritis (inflammation of the cartilage) or stenosis; a small number may later require laryngectomy.

Radiation therapy may also be used preoperatively to reduce the tumor size. Radiation therapy is combined with surgery in advanced laryngeal cancer (stages III and IV) as adjunctive therapy to surgery or chemotherapy and as a palliative measure. A variety of clinical trials have combined chemotherapy and radiation therapy in the treatment of advanced laryngeal tumors.

Advances in research and treatment of these tumors with surgery, chemotherapy, and radiation therapy have improved outcomes and decreased the incidence of post-treatment morbidities (DeVita et al., 2005). Radiation therapy combined with chemotherapy may be an alternative to a total laryngectomy.

Complications from radiation therapy are a result of external radiation to the head and neck area, which may also include the parotid gland, which is responsible for mucus production. Symptoms may include acute mucositis, ulceration of the mucous membranes, pain, **xerostomia** (dry mouth), loss of taste, dysphasia, fatigue, and skin reactions. Later complications may include laryngeal necrosis, edema, and fibrosis.

Speech Therapy

The patient who undergoes a laryngectomy faces potentially complex and frustrating communication problems. These are related to alterations in communication methods, perceived voice quality, and perceptions of quality of life related to communication, disfigurement, and socialization (Happ, Roesch & Kagan, 2004). Often, communication needs and voice quality of patients are ignored during the hospital stay. To minimize anxiety and frustration on the part of the patient and family, the loss or alteration of speech is discussed with the patient and family before surgery, and the speech therapist conducts a preoperative evaluation. During this time, the nurse discusses with the patient and family methods of communication that will be available in the immediate postoperative period. These include writing, lip speaking, and communication or word boards. A system of communication is established with the patient, family, nurse, and physician and is implemented consistently after surgery.

In addition, a long-term postoperative communication plan for **alaryngeal communication** is developed. The three most common techniques of alaryngeal communication are esophageal speech, artificial larynx (electrolarynx), and tracheoesophageal puncture. Training in these techniques begins once medical clearance is obtained from the physician.

ESOPHAGEAL SPEECH. Esophageal speech was the primary method of alaryngeal speech taught to patients until the 1980s. The patient needs the ability to compress air into the esophagus and expel it, setting off a vibration of the pharyngeal esophageal segment. The technique can be taught once the patient begins oral feedings, approximately 1 week after surgery. First, the patient learns to belch and is reminded to do so an hour after eating. Then the technique is practiced repeatedly. Later, this conscious belching action is transformed into simple explosions of air

NURSING RESEARCH PROFILE

Communication Needs after Head and Neck Surgery

Happ, M. B., Roesch, T. & Kagan, S. H. (2004). Communication needs, methods, and perceived voice quality following head and neck surgery: A literature review. *Cancer Nursing, 27*(1), 1–9.

Purpose

Limited data on the topic of communication immediately after surgery for treatment of head and neck cancer stimulated this review. The authors conducted a review and critique of research and related medical, nursing, and psychological literature on in-hospital postoperative communication with adult patients with head and neck cancer.

Design

The authors conducted a comprehensive literature review of available research to address the communication needs, methods, or perceived voice quality of patients with head and neck cancer during the postoperative period. A combined computerized and hand search of the medical, psychological and nursing literature was evaluated through MEDLINE, Cancerlit, and CINHL, as well as a review of health and psychosocial instruments. The search included the following terms: head and neck cancer, head and neck surgery, head and neck surgery complications, and nonverbal communication. Due to the significant lack of in-hospital research, the authors expanded their search to include the first 12 months after surgery. Ten published research articles and one clinical case report were used in the analysis.

Findings

The review and synthesis of the articles included in this review addressed the communication needs, communication methods, and perceptions of voice quality of patients with head and neck cancer in the postoperative period. Three major themes emerged from the small body of research; these themes included (1) information needs, (2) communication methods and perceived voice quality, and (3) quality-of-life perceptions related to communication, disfigurement and socialization.

The patients and family members addressed in the studies reported the need for more information about the consequences of head and neck surgery, specifically the loss of speech and the alternative communication methods available to them. The patients' experiences of being voiceless immediately after surgery were largely ignored during their hospital stays. The emotional and social changes associated with loss of voice and the lack of congruence between actual voice quality and expected voice quality were significant issues for patients in the studies. The effect of surgery, disfigurement, and loss of socialization on perceived quality of life was addressed in several studies. The authors reported that disfigurement and perceptions of disfigurement are factors that influence social interaction and quality of life after head and neck cancer surgery.

Nursing Implications

The results of this critical review and synthesis of articles revealed that health care personnel, including nurses, need to address the physical, emotional and social changes resulting from surgery to treat head and neck cancer. Educational needs and preparation for postoperative communication impairment remain largely unaddressed in caring for the patient with head and neck cancer. Strategies to address patients' and families' educational, emotional, and communication needs are needed and should be subjected to research studies to determine best practices.

from the esophagus for speech purposes. The speech therapist continues to work with the patient to make speech intelligible and as close to normal as possible. Because it takes a long time to become proficient, the success rate is low.

ELECTRIC LARYNX. If esophageal speech is not successful, or until the patient masters the technique, an electric larynx may be used for communication. This battery-powered apparatus projects sound into the oral cavity. When the mouth forms words (articulated), the sounds from the electric larynx become audible words. The voice that is produced sounds mechanical, and some words may be difficult to understand. The advantage is that the patient is able to communicate with relative ease while working to become proficient at either esophageal or tracheoesophageal puncture speech.

TRACHEOESOPHAGEAL PUNCTURE. The third technique of alaryngeal speech is tracheoesophageal puncture (Fig. 22-6). This technique has become the most widely used because the speech associated with it most resembles normal speech (the sound produced is a combination of esophageal speech and voice), and it is easily learned. A valve is placed in the tracheal stoma to divert air into the esophagus and out the mouth. Once the puncture is surgically created and has healed, a voice prosthesis (Singer–Blom) is fitted over the puncture site. A speech therapist teaches the patient how to produce sounds. Moving the tongue and lips to form the sound into words produces speech as before. To prevent airway obstruction, the prosthesis is removed and cleaned when mucus builds up.

The success of these various approaches to preserve or restore speech varies. In one study that evaluated the effectiveness of these methods, the electric larynx was used more often than the other methods of speaking, and tracheoesophageal speech was preferred over esophageal speech. (DeVita et al., 2005).

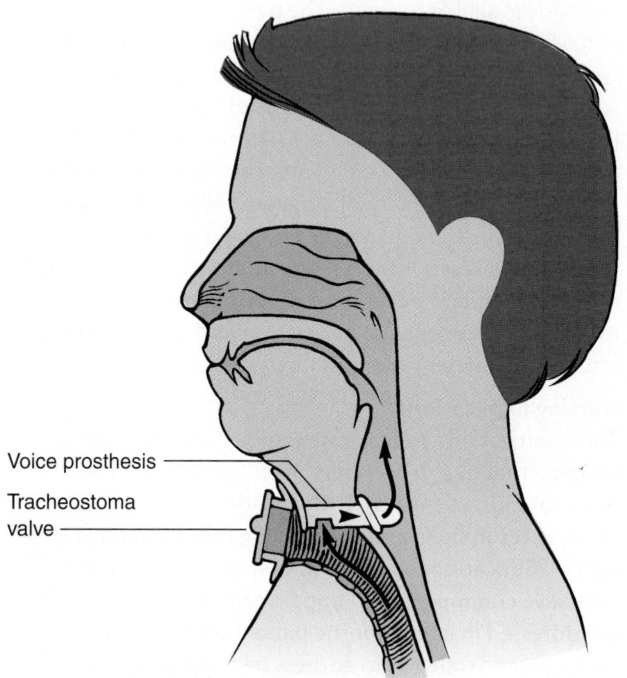

FIGURE 22-6. Schematic representation of tracheoesophageal puncture speech (TEP). Air travels from the lung through a puncture in the posterior wall of the trachea into the esophagus and out the mouth. A voice prosthesis is fitted over the puncture site.

Nursing Process

The Patient Undergoing Laryngectomy

Assessment

The nurse obtains a health history and assesses the patient's physical, psychosocial, and spiritual domains. The health history addresses the following symptoms: hoarseness, sore throat, dyspnea, dysphagia, and pain or burning in the throat. The physical assessment includes a thorough head and neck examination with an emphasis on the patient's airway. In addition, the neck is palpated for swelling or adenopathy.

The nurse also assesses the patient's general state of nutrition, including height and weight and body mass index and reviews laboratory values that assist in determining the patient's nutritional status (albumin, protein, glucose, and electrolyte levels). If treatment includes surgery, the nurse must know the nature of the surgery to plan appropriate care. If the patient is expected to have no voice as a result of the surgical procedure, a preoperative evaluation by the speech therapist is essential. The patient's ability to hear, see, read, and write is assessed. Visual impairment and functional illiteracy may create additional problems with communication and may require creative approaches to ensure that the patient is able to communicate any needs. Because alcohol abuse is a risk factor for cancer of the larynx, it is essential to assess the patient's pattern of alcohol intake. Patients who are accustomed to daily consumption of alcohol are at risk for alcohol withdrawal syndrome (delirium tremens) when alcohol intake is stopped suddenly.

In addition, the nurse determines the psychological readiness of the patient and family. The thought of having cancer is frightening to most people. Fear is compounded by the possibility of permanent voice loss and, in some cases, some degree of disfigurement (Chart 22-8). The nurse evaluates the patient's and family's knowledge of the planned surgical procedure and expected postoperative course, and assesses the patient's and family's coping methods and support systems. The nurse assesses the patient's spirituality needs based on the patient's individual preferences, beliefs, and culture.

Diagnosis

Nursing Diagnoses

Based on all the assessment data, major nursing diagnoses may include the following:

CHART 22-8

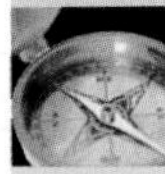

Ethics and Related Issues

SITUATION

A 60-year-old singer was diagnosed with cancer of the larynx 6 years ago. He was treated successfully with radiation therapy, resulting in an altered voice quality. Recently, he has complained of shortness of breath and difficulty swallowing. In the past few months, he also has noticed a marked change in his voice and physical condition, yet has not sought health care.

After a complete physical examination and an extensive diagnostic workup and biopsy, it is determined that the cancer has recurred. His health care provider recommends surgery (a total laryngectomy) and chemotherapy as the best options. The patient states that he is not willing to "lose my voice and my livelihood" but instead will "take my chances." He has also expressed concern about his quality of life after surgery. His family has approached you about trying to convince him to have surgery.

DILEMMA

The patient's right to refuse treatment conflicts with the family's wishes and recommendation from his health care provider.

DISCUSSION

1. Is the patient making a decision based upon all pertinent information concerning his health status, treatment, options, risk/benefits, and long-term prognosis?
2. What arguments can be made to support the patient's decision to forego treatment?
3. What arguments can be made to question the patient's decision to forego treatment?

- Deficient knowledge about the surgical procedure and postoperative course
- Anxiety and depression related to the diagnosis of cancer and impending surgery
- Ineffective airway clearance related to excess mucus production secondary to surgical alterations in the airway
- Impaired verbal communication related to anatomic deficit secondary to removal of the larynx and to edema
- Imbalanced nutrition: less than body requirements, related to inability to ingest food secondary to swallowing difficulties
- Disturbed body image and low self-esteem secondary to major neck surgery, change in appearance, and altered structure and function
- Self-care deficit related to pain, weakness, fatigue, musculoskeletal impairment related to surgical procedure and postoperative course

Collaborative Problems/ Potential Complications

Based on assessment data, potential complications that may develop include the following:

- Respiratory distress (hypoxia, airway obstruction, tracheal edema)
- Hemorrhage
- Infection
- Wound breakdown
- Aspiration

Planning and Goals

The major goals for the patient may include attainment of an adequate level of knowledge, reduction in anxiety, maintenance of a patent airway (patient is able to handle own secretions), effective use of alternative means of communication, attainment of optimal levels of nutrition and hydration, improvement in body image and self-esteem, improved self-care management, and absence of complications.

Nursing Interventions

Teaching the Patient Preoperatively

The diagnosis of laryngeal cancer often produces misconceptions and fears. Many people assume that loss of speech and disfigurement are inevitable with this condition. Once the physician explains the diagnosis and discusses treatment options with the patient and family, the nurse clarifies any misconceptions by identifying the location of the larynx, its function, the nature of the planned surgical procedure, and its effect on speech. Informational materials (written and audiovisual) about the surgery are given to the patient and family for review and reinforcement. If a complete laryngectomy is planned, the patient must understand that the natural voice will be lost, but that special training can provide a means for communicating. The patient needs to know that until this training is started, communication will be possible by using the call light, by writing, or by using a special communication board. The nurse answers questions about the nature of the surgery and reinforces the physician's explanation that the patient will lose the ability to vocalize, but that a rehabilitation program is available. The patient's ability to sing, laugh, and whistle will be lost. The interdisciplinary team conducts an initial assessment of the patient and family. The team might include the nurse, physician, speech therapist, respiratory therapist, clinical nurse specialist, social worker, dietitian, and home care nurse. The services of a spiritual advisor are made available to the patient and family, as appropriate.

The nurse also reviews equipment and treatments for postoperative care with the patient and family, teaches important coughing and deep-breathing exercises, and assists the patient to perform return demonstrations. The nurse clarifies the patient's role in the postoperative and rehabilitation periods.

Reducing Anxiety and Depression

Because surgery of the larynx is performed most commonly for a malignant tumor, the patient may have many questions: Will the surgeon be able to remove all of the tumor? Is it cancer? Will I die? Will I choke? Will I suffocate? Will I ever speak again? What will I look like? Because of these and other questions, the psychological preparation of the patient is as important as the physical preparation.

Any patient undergoing surgery may have many fears. In laryngeal surgery, these fears may relate to the diagnosis of cancer and the possibility of permanent loss of the voice and disfigurement. The nurse provides the patient and family with opportunities to ask questions, verbalize feelings, and discuss perceptions. The nurse should address any questions and misconceptions the patient and family have. During the preoperative or postoperative period, a visit from someone who has had a laryngectomy may reassure the patient that people are available to assist and that rehabilitation is possible.

In the immediate postoperative period, the nurse attempts to spend time with the patient that is uninterrupted and focused on building trust and reducing the patient's anxiety. Active listening provides an environment that promotes open communication and allows the patient to verbalize feelings. Clear instructions and explanations are given to the patient and family in a calm, reassuring manner before and during each contact with the patient. The nurse listens attentively, encourages the patient, and identifies and reduces environmental stressors. The nurse seeks to learn from the patient what activities promote feelings of comfort and assists the patient in such activities (eg, listening to music, reading). The nurse remains with the patient during episodes of severe anxiety and includes the patient in decision making. The nurse also supports the family by allowing extra visiting periods if indicated. Relaxation techniques such as guided imagery and meditation are often helpful to the patient.

Maintaining a Patent Airway

The nurse promotes a patent airway by positioning the patient in the semi-Fowler's or Fowler's position after recovery from anesthesia. This position decreases surgical edema and promotes lung expansion. Observing the patient for restlessness, labored breathing, apprehension, and increased pulse rate helps to identify possible respiratory or circulatory problems. The nurse assesses the patient's lung sounds and reports changes that may indicate impending complications. Medications that depress respiration, particularly opioids, should be used cautiously. However, adequate use of analgesic medications is essential for pain relief, because postoperative pain can result in shallow breathing and an ineffective cough. As with other surgical patients, the nurse encourages the patient to turn, cough, and take deep breaths. If necessary, suctioning may be performed to remove secretions, but the nurse must avoid disruption of suture lines. The nurse also encourages and assists the patient with early ambulation to prevent atelectasis, pneumonia, and deep vein thrombosis. Pulse oximetry is used to monitor the patient's oxygen saturation level.

If a total laryngectomy was performed, a laryngectomy tube will most likely be in place. In some instances a laryngectomy tube is not used; in others it is used temporarily; and in many it is used permanently. The laryngectomy tube, which is shorter than a tracheostomy tube but has a larger diameter, is the patient's only airway. The care of this tube is the same as for a tracheostomy tube (see Chapter 25). The nurse changes the inner cannula of the tube every 8 hours if it is disposable. Although nondisposable tubes are used infrequently, if one is used, the nurse cleans the inner cannula every 8 hours. If a tracheostomy tube without an inner cannula is used, humidification and suctioning of this tube is essential to prevent formation of mucous plugs. The nurse must suction both sides of the T-tube to relieve the obstruction (Shores, Hacking & Triana, 2004). This prevents obstruction of the airway due to copious secretions. The nurse should also maintain secure tracheostomy ties to prevent tube dislodgement.

The nurse cleans the stoma daily with saline solution or another prescribed solution. If a non–oil-based antibiotic ointment is prescribed, the nurse applies it around the stoma and suture line. If crusting appears around the stoma, the nurse removes the crusts with sterile tweezers and applies additional ointment.

Wound drains, inserted during surgery, may be in place to assist in removal of fluid and air from the surgical site. Suction also may be used, but cautiously, to avoid trauma to the surgical site and incision. The nurse observes, measures, and records drainage. When drainage is less than 50 to 60 mL/day, the physician usually removes the drains.

Frequently, the patient coughs up large amounts of mucus through this opening. Because air passes directly into the trachea without being warmed and moistened by the upper respiratory mucosa, the tracheobronchial tree compensates by secreting excessive amounts of mucus. Therefore, the patient will have frequent coughing episodes and may develop a brassy-sounding, mucus-producing cough. The nurse reassures the patient that these problems will diminish in time, as the tracheobronchial mucosa adapts to the altered physiology.

After the patient coughs, the tracheostomy opening must be wiped clean and clear of mucus. A simple gauze dressing, washcloth, or even paper towel (because of its size and absorbency) worn below the tracheostomy may serve as a barrier to protect the clothing from the copious mucus that the patient may initially expel.

One of the most important factors in decreasing cough, mucus production, and crusting around the stoma is adequate humidification of the environment. Mechanical humidifiers and aerosol generators (nebulizers) increase the humidity and are important for the patient's comfort. The laryngectomy tube may be removed when the stoma is well healed, within 3 to 6 weeks after surgery. The nurse teaches the patient how to clean and change the tube (see Chapter 25) and remove secretions.

Promoting Alternative Communication Methods

Understanding and anticipating the patient's postoperative needs are critical. Alternative means of communication are established preoperatively and must be used consistently by all personnel who come in contact with the patient postoperatively. For example, a call bell or hand bell must be placed within easy reach of the patient. Because a Magic Slate often is used for communication, the nurse documents which hand the patient uses for writing so that the opposite arm can be used for IV infusions. (To ensure the patient's privacy, the nurse discards any old notes used for communication.) If the patient cannot write, a picture-word-phrase board or hand signals can be used.

Writing everything or communicating through gestures can be very time-consuming and frustrating. The patient must be given adequate time to communicate his or her needs. The patient may become impatient and angry when not understood. In addition, other staff members need to be alerted to the problem and also be aware that the patient will be unable to use the intercom system.

Establishing an effective means of communication is usually the ultimate goal in the rehabilitation of the laryngectomy patient. The nurse works with the patient, speech therapist, and family to encourage use of alternative communication methods.

Promoting Adequate Nutrition and Hydration

Postoperatively, the patient may not be permitted to eat or drink for several days. Alternative sources of nutrition and hydration include IV fluids, enteral feedings through a nasogastric or gastrostomy tube, and parenteral nutrition.

When the patient is ready to start oral feedings, a speech therapist or radiologist may conduct a swallow study (a video fluoroscopy radiology procedure) to evaluate the patient's risk for aspiration. Once the patient is cleared for oral feedings, the nurse explains that thick liquids will be used first, because they are easy to swallow. Different swallowing maneuvers are attempted with various food consistencies. Once the patient is cleared for food intake, the nurse stays with the patient during initial oral feedings and keeps a suction setup at the bedside for needed suctioning. The nurse instructs the patient to avoid sweet foods, which increase salivation and suppress the appetite. Solid foods are introduced as tolerated. The patient is instructed to rinse the mouth with warm water or mouthwash after oral feedings and to brush the teeth frequently.

Because taste and smell are so closely related, taste sensations are altered for a while after surgery because inhaled air passes directly into the trachea, bypassing the nose and the olfactory end organs. In time, however, the patient usually accommodates to this change and olfactory sensation adapts, often with return of interest in eating. The nurse observes the patient for any difficulty swallowing, particularly when eating resumes, and reports its occurrence to the physician.

The patient's weight and laboratory data are monitored to ensure that nutritional and fluid intake are adequate. In addition, skin turgor and vital signs are assessed for signs of decreased fluid volume.

Promoting Positive Body Image and Self-Esteem

Disfiguring surgery and an altered communication pattern are a threat to a patient's body image and self-esteem. The reaction of family members and friends is a major concern for the patient. The nurse encourages the patient to express feelings about the changes brought about by surgery, particularly feelings related to fear, anger, depression, and isolation. Encouraging use of previous effective coping strategies may be helpful. Referral to a support group, such as Lost Chord or New Voice clubs (through the International Association of Laryngectomees [IAL]) and I Can Cope (through the American Cancer Society), may help the patient and family deal with the changes in their lives.

Promoting Self-Care Management

A positive approach is important when caring for the patient and includes promotion of self-care activities. The patient and family should begin participating in self-care activities as soon as possible. The nurse assesses the patient's readiness for decision making and encourages the patient to participate actively in performing care. The nurse provides positive reinforcement when the patient makes an effort in self-care. The nurse needs to be a good listener and a support to the family, especially when explaining the tubes, dressings, and drains that are in place postoperatively. Groups such as Lost Chord and New Voice promote and support the rehabilitation of people who have had a laryngectomy by providing an opportunity for exchanging ideas and sharing information.

In addition to its work through support groups, the International Association of Laryngectomees encourages an exchange of ideas and methods for learning and teaching alaryngeal methods of communication. It also works to promote employers' understanding about cancer of the larynx, to enable patients to retain or obtain employment after surgery.

Monitoring and Managing Potential Complications

The potential complications after laryngectomy include respiratory distress and hypoxia, hemorrhage, infection, wound breakdown, and aspiration.

RESPIRATORY DISTRESS AND HYPOXIA

The nurse monitors the patient for signs and symptoms of respiratory distress and hypoxia, particularly restlessness, irritation, agitation, confusion, tachypnea, use of accessory muscles, and decreased oxygen saturation on pulse oximetry (SpO_2). Any change in respiratory status requires immediate intervention. Hypoxia may cause restlessness and an initial rise in blood pressure; this is followed by hypotension and somnolence. Cyanosis is a late sign of hypoxia. Obstruction needs to be ruled out immediately by suctioning and by having the patient cough and breathe deeply. Hypoxia and airway obstruction, if not immediately treated, are life-threatening.

Other nursing measures include repositioning of the patient to ensure an open airway and administering oxygen as prescribed and used with caution in patients with chronic obstructive pulmonary disease. The nurse should always be prepared for possible intubation and mechanical ventilation. The nurse must be knowledgeable about the hospital's emergency code protocols and skilled in use of emergency equipment. The nurse must remain with the patient at all times during respiratory distress. The emergency call bell and telephone should be used to initiate a code, call for further assistance, and summon the physician immediately if nursing measures do not improve the patient's respiratory status.

HEMORRHAGE

Bleeding from the drains at the surgical site or with tracheal suctioning may signal the occurrence of hemorrhage. The nurse promptly notifies the surgeon of any active bleeding, which can occur at a variety of sites, including the surgical site, drains, and trachea. Rupture of the carotid artery is especially dangerous. Should this occur, the nurse must apply direct pressure over the artery, summon assistance, and provide emotional support to the patient until the vessel is ligated. The nurse monitors vital signs for changes, particularly increased pulse rate, decreased blood pressure, and rapid deep respirations. Cold, clammy, pale skin may indicate active bleeding. IV fluids and blood components may be administered and other measures implemented to prevent or treat hemorrhagic shock. Management of the patient with shock is discussed in detail in Chapter 15.

INFECTION

The nurse monitors the patient for signs of postoperative infection. These include an increase in temperature and pulse, a change in the type of wound drainage, and increased areas of redness or tenderness at the surgical site. Other signs include purulent drainage, odor, and increased wound drainage. The nurse monitors the patient's white blood cell (WBC) count; a rise in WBCs may indicate the body's effort to combat infection. In elderly patients, infection can be present without an increase in the patient's WBC count; therefore, the nurse must monitor the patient for more subtle signs. WBCs will be suppressed in the patient with decreased immune function (eg, patients with HIV infection, those receiving chemotherapy or radiation therapy); this predisposes the patient to a severe infection and sepsis. Antimicrobial (antibiotic) medications must be administered as scheduled. All suspicious drainage is cultured, and the patient may be placed in isolation as indicated. Strategies are implemented to minimize the exposure of the patient to microorganisms and their spread to others. The nurse reports any significant change in the patient's status to the surgeon.

WOUND BREAKDOWN

Wound breakdown caused by infection, poor wound healing, development of a fistula, radiation therapy, or tumor growth can create a life-threatening emergency. The carotid artery, which is close to the stoma, may rupture from erosion if the wound does not heal properly. The nurse observes the stoma area for wound breakdown, hematoma, and bleeding and reports their occurrence to the surgeon. If wound breakdown occurs, the patient must be monitored carefully and identified as being at high risk for carotid hemorrhage.

ASPIRATION

The patient who has undergone a laryngectomy is at risk for aspiration and aspiration pneumonia due to depressed cough, the sedating effects of anesthetic and analgesic medications, alteration in the airway, impaired swallowing, and the administration of tube feedings. The nurse assesses for the presence of nausea and administers antiemetic medications, as prescribed. The nurse keeps a suction set-up available in the hospital and instructs the family to do so at home for use if needed. Patients receiving tube feedings are positioned with the head of the bed at 30 degrees or higher during feedings and for 30 to 45 minutes after tube feedings. Adding a small amount of food coloring to the tube feedings assists in distinguishing tube feeding aspirate from other secretions from the pulmonary system. When the patient begins oral feeding, the nurse maintains the head of the bed in an upright position for 30 to 45 minutes after each feeding. For patients with a nasogastric or gastrostomy tube, the placement of the tube and residual gastric volume must be checked before each feeding. High amounts of residual volume (greater than 50% of previous intake) indicate delayed gastric emptying; this can lead to reflux and aspiration. Signs or symptoms of aspiration are reported to the physician immediately.

Promoting Home and Community-Based Care

TEACHING PATIENTS SELF-CARE

The nurse has an important role in the recovery and rehabilitation of the patient who has had a laryngectomy. In an effort to facilitate the patient's ability to manage self-care, discharge instruction begins as soon as the patient is able to participate. Nursing care and patient teaching in the hospital, outpatient setting, and rehabilitation or long-term care facility must take into consideration the many emotions, physical changes, and lifestyle changes experienced by the patient. In preparing the patient to go home, the nurse assesses the patient's readiness to learn and the level of knowledge about self-care management. The nurse also reassures the patient and family that most self-care management strategies can be mastered. The patient will need to learn a variety of self-care behaviors, including tracheostomy and stoma care, wound care, and oral hygiene. The nurse also instructs the patient about the need for adequate dietary intake, safe hygiene, and recreational activities.

Tracheostomy and Stoma Care. The nurse provides specific instructions to the patient and family about what to expect with a tracheostomy and its management. The nurse teaches the patient and caregiver to perform suctioning and emergency measures and tracheostomy and stoma care. The nurse stresses the importance of humidification at home and instructs the family to obtain and set up a humidification system before the patient returns home. In addition, the nurse cautions the patient and family that air-conditioned air may be too cool or too dry, and therefore irritating for the patient with a new laryngectomy. (See Chapter 25 for details about tracheostomy care.)

Hygiene and Safety Measures. The nurse instructs the patient and family about safety precautions that are needed because of the changes in structure and function resulting from the surgery. Special precautions are needed in the shower to prevent water from entering the stoma. Wearing a loose-fitting plastic bib over the tracheostomy or simply holding a hand over the opening is effective. Swimming is not recommended, because a person with a laryngectomy can drown without submerging his or her face. Barbers and beauticians need to be alerted so that hair sprays, loose hair, and powder do not get near the stoma, because they can block or irritate the trachea and possibly cause infection. These self-care points are summarized in Chart 22-9.

The nurse teaches the patient and caregiver the signs and symptoms of infection and identifies indications that require contacting the physician after discharge. A discussion regarding cleanliness and infection control behaviors is essential in the education of the patient. The nurse teaches the patient and family to wash their hands before and after caring for the tracheostomy, to use tissue to remove mucus, and to dispose of soiled dressings and equipment properly. If the patient's surgery included cervical lymph node dissection, the nurse teaches the patient exercises for strengthening the shoulder and neck muscles.

CHART 22-9

HOME CARE CHECKLIST • The Patient With a Laryngectomy

At the completion of the home care instruction, the patient or caregiver will be able to:	Patient	Caregiver
• Demonstrate methods to clear the airway and handle secretions	✔	✔
• Explain the rationale for maintaining adequate humidification with a humidifier or nebulizer	✔	✔
• Demonstrate how to clean the skin around the stoma and how to use ointments and tweezers to remove encrustations	✔	✔
• State the rationale for wearing a loose-fitting protective cloth at the stoma	✔	✔
• Discuss the need to avoid cold air from air conditioning and the environment to prevent irritation of the airway	✔	✔
• Demonstrate safe technique in changing the laryngectomy/tracheostomy tube	✔	✔
• Identify the signs and symptoms of wound infection and state what to do about them	✔	✔
• Describe safety or emergency measures to implement in case of breathing difficulty or bleeding	✔	✔
• State the rationale for wearing or carrying special medical identification and ways to obtain help in an emergency	✔	✔
• Explain the importance of covering the stoma when showering or bathing	✔	✔
• Identify fluid and caloric needs	✔	✔
• Describe mouth care and discuss its importance	✔	✔
• Demonstrate alternative communication methods	✔	
• Identify support groups and agency resources	✔	✔
• State the need for regular checkups and reporting of any problems immediately	✔	✔

Recreation and exercise are important for the patient's well-being and quality of life, and all but very strenuous exercise can be enjoyed safely. Avoidance of strenuous exercise and fatigue is important because the patient will have more difficulty speaking when tired, which can be discouraging. Additional safety points to address include the need for the patient to wear or carry medical identification, such as a bracelet or card, to alert medical personnel to the special requirements for resuscitation should this need arise. If resuscitation is needed, direct mouth-to-stoma ventilation should be performed. For home emergency situations, prerecorded emergency messages for police, the fire department, or other rescue services can be kept near the phone to be used quickly.

The nurse instructs and encourages the patient to perform oral care on a regular basis to prevent halitosis and infection. If the patient is receiving radiation therapy, synthetic saliva may be required because of decreased saliva production. The nurse instructs the patient to drink water or sugar-free liquids throughout the day and to use a humidifier at home. Brushing the teeth or dentures and rinsing the mouth several times a day will assist in maintaining proper oral hygiene.

CONTINUING CARE

Referral for home care is an important aspect of postoperative care for the patient who has had a laryngectomy and will assist the patient and family in the transition to the home. The home care nurse assesses the patient's general health status and the ability of the patient and family to care for the stoma and tracheostomy. The nurse assesses the surgical incisions, nutritional and respiratory status, and adequacy of pain management. The nurse assesses for signs and symptoms of complications and the patient's and family's knowledge of signs and symptoms to be reported to the physician. During the home visit, the nurse identifies and addresses other learning needs and concerns of the patient and family, such as adaptation to physical, lifestyle, and functional changes, as well as the patient's progress with learning and using new communication strategies. The nurse assesses the patient's psychological status as well. The home care nurse reinforces previous teaching and provides reassurance and support to the patient and family as needed.

The nurse encourages the person who has had a laryngectomy to have regular physical examinations and to seek advice concerning any problems related to recovery and rehabilitation. The patient is also reminded to participate in health promotion activities and health screening and about the importance of keeping scheduled appointments with the physician, speech therapist, and other health care providers.

Evaluation

Expected Patient Outcomes

Expected patient outcomes may include the following:

1. Demonstrates an adequate level of knowledge, verbalizing an understanding of the surgical procedure and performing self-care adequately
2. Demonstrates less anxiety and depression
   a. Expresses a sense of hope
   b. Is aware of available community organizations and agencies such as the Lost Chord and New Voice groups
   c. Participates in support group, such as I Can Cope.
3. Maintains a clear airway and handles own secretions; also demonstrates practical, safe, and correct technique for cleaning and changing the laryngectomy tube
4. Acquires effective communication techniques
   a. Uses assistive devices and strategies for communication (Magic Slate, call bell, picture board, sign language, lip reading, computer aids)
   b. Follows the recommendations of the speech therapist
   c. Demonstrates ability to communicate with new communication strategy
   d. Reports availability of prerecorded messages to summon emergency assistance by telephone
5. Maintains adequate nutrition and adequate fluid intake
6. Exhibits improved body image, self-esteem, and self-concept
   a. Expresses feelings and concerns
   b. Participates in self-care and decision making
   c. Accepts information about support group
7. Adheres to rehabilitation and home care program
   a. Practices recommended speech therapy
   b. Demonstrates proper methods for caring for stoma and laryngectomy or tracheostomy tube (if present)
   c. Verbalizes understanding of symptoms that require medical attention
   d. States safety measures to take in emergencies
   e. Performs oral hygiene as prescribed
8. Absence of complications
   a. Demonstrates a patent airway
   b. No bleeding from surgical site and minimal bleeding from drains; vital signs (blood pressure, temperature, pulse, respiratory rate) normal
   c. No redness, tenderness, or purulent drainage at surgical site
   d. No wound breakdown
   e. Clear breath sounds; oxygen saturation level within acceptable range; chest x-ray clear

Critical Thinking Exercises

1 A 49-year-old man presents to the employee health clinic with generalized fatigue and low-grade fever. He reports a history of recently "having a cold" that "lasted 3 weeks." He also states that he is "stuffy all the time." What further information would you request from the patient to obtain a more accurate health history? Is the patient at risk for sinusitis? What are the symptoms of acute and chronic sinusitis? What teaching is warranted for a patient with acute sinusitis? How does teaching for a patient with chronic sinusitis differ?

2 A 75-year-old woman comes to the clinic today with complaints of a persistent runny nose that is producing yellow to greenish drainage. She lives in an assisted-living environment and is accompanied to the clinic by an aide from the facility. The aide reports that the patient has complained of a sore throat and that she "sleeps all the time" and had a fever of 100.6°F early this morning. Discuss your assessment of this patient. You suspect that the patient is at risk for which upper respiratory illnesses? As a community health nurse, what actions would you take to ensure control of the infection at the assisted-living facility?

3 ebp A 55-year-old woman is brought to the emergency department by her husband, who tells you that her nose has been bleeding for more than 3 hours. The patient reports that she takes one aspirin a day (325 mg), has a history of atrial fibrillation, and takes medication for hypertension. What immediate action would you take to care for this patient? What are the risk factors for epistaxis in this patient? What medical treatment would you anticipate for her? What nursing measures would you provide for this patient? How would you modify your discharge instructions if the patient lived alone? What strategies would you recommend to the patient and her husband to stop a nosebleed if it occurs again at home? What is the evidence for your recommendations? How will you determine the strength of the evidence on which your recommendations are based?

4 You are caring for a 78-year-old patient on a medical-surgical nursing unit. He has recently been diagnosed with cancer of the larynx and is scheduled for a total laryngectomy in the morning. What patient education is needed before this patient's surgery? Discuss nursing management of the patient's airway in the immediate postoperative period. What critical elements would you include in teaching the patient how to care for his tracheostomy? What community resources would you provide or arrange for this patient once he is discharged? What modifications in teaching and care would be necessary if this man had one-sided weakness secondary to an earlier stroke?

5 A 65-year-old man is referred for home care after a total laryngectomy performed to treat cancer of the larynx. As the home health nurse, you are responsible to provide continued patient education regarding tracheostomy care and gastric tube feedings. The overall plan is for the patient to begin oral feedings; however, both the patient and his wife believe that he is not ready to begin to eat. What are your priorities in terms of assessment of this patient? What are your recommendations to the patient regarding fear, anxiety, communication, and nutrition? What additional medical and support services will the patient need to assist him in his recovery? How would your care differ if this patient lived alone?

REFERENCES AND SELECTED READINGS

BOOKS

Abeloff, M., Armitage, J., Niederhuber, J., et al. (2004). *Clinical oncology*. Philadelphia: Churchill Livingstone.

American Cancer Society. (2005). *Cancer facts and figures*. Atlanta: American Cancer Society Inc.

American Lung Association. (2005). *Guidelines for the prevention and treatment of influenza and the common cold*. www.lungusa.org/site/pp.asp?c=dvLUK9O0E&b=23161 (accessed May 30, 2006).

Bickley, L. S. & Szilagyi, P. G. (2003). *Bates' guide to physical examination and history taking* (8th ed.). Philadelphia: Lippincott Williams & Wilkins.

Cameron, J. L. (2004). *Current surgical therapy*. St. Louis: Mosby.

Casciato, D. A. (2004). *Manual of clinical oncology* (5th ed.). Philadelphia: Lippincott Williams & Wilkins.

De Vita, V. T., Hellman, S. & Rosenberg, S. A. (Eds.)(2004). *Cancer: Principles and practice of oncology* (7th ed.). Philadelphia: Lippincott Williams & Wilkins.

Evans, P. R., Montgomery, P. Q. & Gullane, P. J. (2003). *Principles and practice of head and neck oncology*. London: Taylor & Francis Group.

Goldman, L. & Ausiello, D. A. (Eds.)(2003). *Cecil textbook of medicine* (22nd ed.). Philadelphia: Saunders.

Green, F., Balch, C., Flemming, I., et al. (Eds.)(2002). *AJCC cancer staging manual* (6th ed), New York: Springer.

Gulanick, M. & Myers, J. (2003). *Nursing care plans: Nursing diagnosis and intervention* (5th ed.). St. Louis: Mosby.

Kufe, D., Pollock, R., Weichselbaum, R., et al. (2003). *Holland-Frei cancer medicine* (6th ed.). Hamilton, Ontario: B. C. Decker.

Mandell, G. L., Bennett, J. E. & Dolin, R. (Eds.). (2004). *Principles and practice of infectious diseases* (6th ed.). Philadelphia: Churchill Livingstone.

Murray, J. F. & Nadel, J. A. (2005). *Textbook of respiratory medicine* (4th ed.). Philadelphia: Saunders.

National Cancer Institute. (2003). *What you need to know about cancer of the larynx*. NIH Publication No. 02-1568. Washington, DC: U.S. Department of Health and Human Services. http://www.cancer.gov/cancertopics/wyntk/larynx (accessed May 30, 2006).

National Institute of Allergy and Infectious Diseases. (2005). *Allergy statistics*. http://www.niaid.nih.gov/factsheets/allergystat.htm (accessed May 30, 2006).

National Institute of Allergy and Infectious Diseases. (2004). *The common cold*. http://www.niaid.nih.gov/factsheets/cold.htm (accessed May 30, 2006).

Shores, C., Hacking, T. & Triana, R. (2004). Complications of airway management. In Tintinalli, J., Kelan, G. & Stapczynski, S. (Eds.). *Emergency medicine: A comprehensive study guide* (6th ed.). New York: McGraw-Hill.

Tierney, L. M., McPhee, S. J. & Papadakis, M. A. (Eds.). (2005). *Current medical diagnosis and treatment* (44th ed.). New York: McGraw-Hill.

Townsend, C. M., Beauchamp, R. D., Evans, B. M., et al. (Ed.)(2004). *Sabiston textbook of surgery* (17th ed.). Philadelphia: Saunders.

Uphold, C. & Graham, M. (2003). *Clinical guidelines in family practice* (4th ed.). Gainesville: Barmarrae Books.

Yunglinger, J., Busse, W., Bochner, B., et al. (2003). *Allergy: Principles and practice* (6th ed.). St. Louis: Mosby.

JOURNALS

**Asterisks indicate nursing research articles.*

General

Banerjee, D., Vitiello, M. V. & Grunstein, R. R. (2004). Pharmacology for excessive daytime sleepiness. *Sleep Medicine Reviews, 8*(5), 319–354.

Boutrel, B. & Koob, G. G. (2004). What keeps us awake: The neuropharmacology of stimulants and wakefulness-promoting medications. *Sleep, 27*(6), 1181–1194.

Bush, R. K. (2004). Etiopathogenesis and management of perennial allergic rhinitis: A state-of-the-art review. *Treatments in Respiratory Medicine, 3*(1), 45–57.

Colclasure, J. C., Gross, C. W. & Kountakis, S. E. (2004). Endoscopic sinus surgery in patients older than sixty. *Otolaryngology Head & Neck Surgery, 131*(6), 946–949.

Lamberg, L. (2004). Promoting adequate sleep finds a place on the public health agenda. *Journal of the American Medical Association, 291*(20), 2415–2417.

Leinbach, R. F., Markwell, S. J., Colliver, J. A., et al. (2003). Hot versus cold tonsillectomy: A systematic review of the literature. *Otolaryngology Head & Neck Surgery, 129*(4), 360–364.

Marshall, I. (2006). Zinc for the common cold. *Cochrane Database of Systematic Reviews (2),* CD001364.

Parmet, S. (2004). Sore throat. *Journal of the American Medical Association, 291*(13), 1664.

Reider, J. M., Nashelsky, J. & Neher, J. (2003). Do imaging studies aid diagnosis of acute sinusitis? *Journal of Family Practice, 52*(7), 565–567.

Windfuhr, J. P. & Chen, Y. S. (2003). Post-tonsillectomy and adenoidectomy hemorrhage in nonselected patients. *Annals of Otology, Rhinology and Laryngology, 112*(1), 63–70.

Upper Respiratory Infections

Armengol, C. E., Schlager, T. A. & Hendley, J. O. (2004). Sensitivity of a rapid antigen detection test for group A streptococci in a private pediatric office setting: Answering the Red book's request for validation. *Pediatrics, 113*(4), 924–926.

Blaivas, M., Theodoro, D. & Duggal, S. (2003). Ultrasound-guided drainage of peritonsillar abscess by the emergency physician. *American Journal of Emergency Medicine, 21*(2), 155–158.

Brook, I. (2004). Microbiology and management of peritonsillar, retropharyngeal, and parapharyngeal abscesses. *Journal of Oral and Maxillofacial Surgery, 62*(12), 1545–1550.

DeAlleaume, L., Parker, S. & Reider, J. M. (2003). What findings distinguish acute bacterial sinusitis? *Journal of Family Practice, 52*(7), 563–565.

Del Mar, C. B., Glasziou, P. P. & Spinks, A. B. (2004). Antibiotics for sore throat. *Cochrane Database of Systematic Reviews (2),* CD000023.

Discolo, C. M., Darrow, D. H. & Koltai, P. J. (2003). Infectious indications for tonsillectomy. *Pediatric Clinics of North America, 50*(2), 445–458.

Eiles, W. & Huber, K. (2004). Short-course therapy for acute sinusitis: How long is enough? *Treatments in Respiratory Medicine, 3*(5), 269–277.

Franzese, C. B. & Isaacson, J. E. (2003). Peritonsillar and parapharyngeal space abscess in the older adult. *American Journal of Otolaryngology, 24*(3), 169–173.

Gotfried, M. H. (2004). Macrolides for the treatment of chronic sinusitis, asthma, and COPD. *Chest, 125*(2), 52S–61S.

Jackson, E. A. (2003). Amoxicillin-clavulanate ineffective for suspected acute sinusitis. *Journal of Family Practice, 529*(12), 930, 932.

Johnson, R. F., Stewart, M. G. & Wright, C. C. (2003). An evidence-based review of the treatment of peritonsillar abscess. *Otolaryngology Head & Neck Surgery, 128*(3), 332–343.

Jull, A. (2003). Review: Specific signs and symptoms can help practitioners to diagnose acute purulent sinusitis in general practice. *Evidence-Based Nursing, 6*(1), 24.

Lindbaek, M. (2004). Acute sinusitis: Guide to selection of antibacterial therapy. *Drugs, 64*(8), 805–819.

Neuner, J. M., Hamel, M. B., Phillips, R. S., et al. (2003). Diagnosis and management of adults with pharyngitis a cost effective analysis. *Annals of Internal Medicine, 139*(2), 113–122.

Scheid, D. C. & Hamm, R. M. (2004). Acute bacterial rhinosinusitis in adults: Part I. Evaluation. *American Family Physician, 70*(9), 1685–1692.

Shashy, R. G., Moore, E. J. & Weaver, A. (2004). Prevalence of the chronic sinusitis in Olmsted County, Minnesota. *Archives of Otolaryngology Head & Neck Surgery, 130*(3), 320–323.

Singh, M. (2004). Newer drugs for asthma. *Indian Journal of Pediatrics, 71*(8), 721–727

Wald, E. R. & Fischer, D. R. (2004). Diagnosing and treating strep throat. *Family Practice Management, 11*(2), 20.

Williams, J. W., Jr., Aguilar, C., Cornell, J., et al. (2004). Antibiotics for acute maxillary sinusitis. *Cochrane Database of Systematic Reviews (2),* CD000243.

Obstruction and Trauma of the Airway

Chung, K. F. & Adcock, I. M. (2004). Combination therapy of long-acting beta2-adrenoceptor agonists and corticosteroids for asthma. *Treatments in Respiratory Medicine, 3*(5), 279–289.

Letizia, M., O'Leary, J. & Vodvarka, J. (2003). Laryngeal edema: Perioperative nursing considerations. *MedSurg Nursing, 12*(2), 111–115.

Merritt, S. L. (2004). Sleep-disordered breathing and the association with cardiovascular risk. *Progress in Cardiovascular Nursing, 19*(1), 19–27.

Merritt, S. L. & Berger, B. E. (2004). Obstructive sleep apnea-hypopnea syndrome. *American Journal of Nursing, 104*(7), 49–52.

Passali, D., Passali, F. M., Damiani, V., et al. (2003). Treatment of inferior turbinate hypertrophy: A randomized clinical trial. *Annals of Otology, Rhinology & Laryngology, 112*(8), 683–688.

Stradling, J. R. & Davies, R. J. O. (2004). Sleep. 1: Obstructive sleep apnoea/hypopnea syndrome: Definitions, epidemiology, and natural history. *Thorax, 59*(1), 73–78.

Thatcher, G. W. & Maisel, R. H. (2003). The long-term evaluation of tracheostomy in the management of severe obstructive sleep apnea. *Laryngoscope, 113*(2), 201–204.

Von Känel, R. & Dimsdale, J. E. (2003). Hemostatic alterations in patients with obstructive sleep apnea and the implications for cardiovascular disease. *Chest, 124*(5), 1956–1967.

Yantis, M. A. & Neatherlin, J. (2005). Obstructive sleep apnea in neurological patients. *Journal of Neuroscience Nursing, 37*(3), 150–155.

Young, T., Skatrud, J. & Peppard, P. E. (2004). Risk factors for obstructive sleep apnea in adults. *Journal of the American Medical Association, 291*(16), 2013–2016.

Cancer of the Larynx

Davis, R. K., Kriskovich, M. D., Galloway, E. B., III, et al. (2004). Endoscopic supraglottic laryngectomy with postoperative irradiation. *Annals of Otology, Rhinology, and Laryngology, 113*(2), 132–138.

Dietz, A., Ramroth, H., Urban, T., et al. (2004). Exposure to cement dust, related occupational groups and laryngeal cancer risk: Results of a population based case control study. *International Journal of Cancer, 108*(6), 907–911.

Forastiere, A. A., Goepfert, H., Maor, M., et al. (2003). Concurrent chemotherapy and radiotherapy for organ preservation in advanced laryngeal cancer. *New England Journal of Medicine, 249*(22), 2091.

*Happ, M. B., Roesch, T. & Kagan, S. H. (2004). Communication needs, methods, and perceived voice quality following head and neck surgery: A literature review. *Cancer Nursing, 27*(1), 1–9.

Harrison, J. S., Dale, R. A., Haverman, C. W., et al. (2003). Oral complications in radiation therapy. *General Dentistry, 51*(6), 552–560.

International Association of Laryngectomees, 2004

Kasperbauer, J. L. & Thomas, J. E. (2004). Voice rehabilitation after near-total laryngectomy. *Otolaryngologic Clinics of North America, 37*(3), 655–657.

*Krouse, H. J., Rudy, S. F., Vallerand, A. H., et al. (2004). Impact of tracheostomy or laryngectomy on spousal and caregiver relationships. *ORL Head & Neck Nursing, 22*(1), 10–25.

Marques, M. A. & Dib, L. L. (2004). Peridontal changes in patients undergoing radiotherapy. *Journal of Periodontology, 75*(9), 1178–1187.

*Rodriguez, C. S. & VanCott, M. L. (2005). Speech impairment in the postoperative head and neck and neck cancer patient: Nurses' and patients' perceptions. *Qualitative Health Research, 15*(7), 897–911.

Shiotani, A., Araki, K., Moro, K., et al. (2003). CHEP with the total removal of the arytenoids on the tumor-bearing side. *Journal of the Oto-Rhino-Laryngological Society of Japan, 106*(11), 1100–1103.

Timon, C. V., Toner, M. & Conlon, B. J. (2003). Paratracheal lymph node involvement in advanced cancer of the larynx, hypopharynx, and cervical esophagus. *Laryngoscope, 113*(9), 595–1599.

Vielba, R., Bilbao, J., Ispizua, A. et al. (2003). P53 and cyclin D1 as prognostic factors in squamous cell carcinoma of the larynx. *Laryngoscope, 113*(1), 167–172.

RESOURCES

American Cancer Society, 1599 Clifton Rd. NE, Atlanta, GA 30329; 404-320-3333 or 800-ACS-2345; http://www.cancer.org. Accessed March 31, 2006.

American Lung Association, 1740 Broadway, New York, NY 10019; 212-315-8700; http://www.lungusa.org. Accessed March 31, 2006.

American Sleep Apnea Association, 1424 K Street NW, Suite 302, Washington, DC 20005; 202-293-3650; http://www.sleepapnea.org. Accessed March 31, 2006.

Differential Diagnosis of Rhinitis; http://icarus.med.utoronto.ca/carr/manual/ddxrhinitis.html. Accessed March 31, 2006; by M. M. Carr, Otolaryngologist, Department of Otolaryngology, Toronto General Hospital, 200 Elizabeth Street, Toronto, Ontario, Canada M5G 2C4, 416-340-3490; fax 416-340-5116.

E-Medicine: Instant Access to the Minds of Medicine. http://www.emedicine.com. Accessed March 31, 2006.

International Association of Laryngectomees, 7400 N. Shadeland Ave., Suite 100, Indianapolis, IN 46250; 317-570-4568; http://www.larynxlink.com. Accessed March 31, 2006.

National Cancer Institute (NCI), Bldg. 31, 31 Center Drive, MSC 2580, Bethesda, MD 20892; http://cancernet.nci.nih.gov. Accessed March 31, 2006.

National Cancer Institute: US National Institutes of Health. http://www.cancer.gov. Accessed March 31, 2006); NCI Public Inquiries, Office 6116, Executive Boulevard Room 3036A, Bethesda, MD 20892, 1-800-422-6237.

National Heart, Lung, and Blood Institute (NHBLI), National Institutes of Health, Bldg. 31, Rm. 4A21, Bethesda, MD 20892; 301-592-8573 or 800-575-9355; http://www.nhlbi.nih.gov. Accessed March 31, 2006.

National Institute of Allergy and Infectious Disease, Building 31, 31 Center Drive MSC 2520, Bethesda, MD 20892; http://www.niaid.nih.gov. Accessed March 31, 2006.

National Sleep Foundation, 1522 K Street NW, Suite 500, Washington, DC 20005; 202-437-3471; fax 202-347-3472; http://www.sleepfoundation.org. Accessed March 31, 2006.

Voice Center at Eastern Virginia Medical School, Department of Otolaryngology, P.O. Box 1980, Norfolk, VA 23507; 757-446-5934, http://www.evms.edu/about/centers.html. Accessed March 31, 2006.

University of Kansas Medical Center—Head and Neck Surgery, 3001 Eaton, Kansas City, KS 66160; 913-588-6719; http://www2.kumc.edu/otolaryngology/. Accessed March 31, 2006.

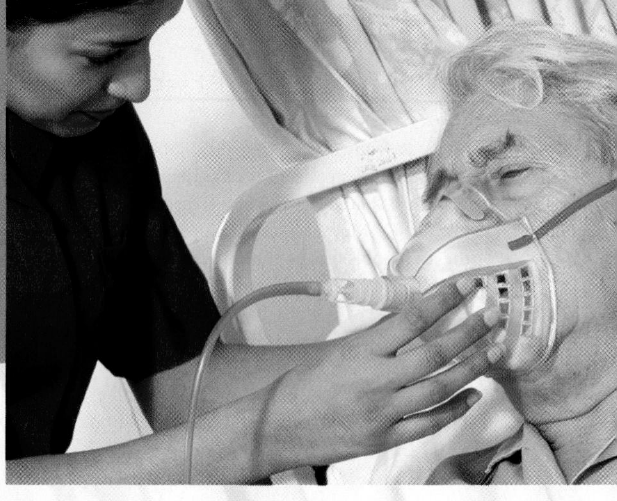

CHAPTER 23

Management of Patients With Chest and Lower Respiratory Tract Disorders

Learning Objectives

On completion of this chapter, the learner will be able to:

1. Identify patients at risk for atelectasis and nursing interventions related to its prevention and management.
2. Compare the various pulmonary infections with regard to causes, clinical manifestations, nursing management, complications, and prevention.
3. Use the nursing process as a framework for care of the patient with pneumonia.
4. Relate pleurisy, pleural effusion, and empyema to pulmonary infection.
5. Describe smoking and air pollution as causes of pulmonary disease.
6. Relate the therapeutic management techniques of acute respiratory distress syndrome to the underlying pathophysiology of the syndrome.
7. Describe risk factors and measures appropriate for prevention and management of pulmonary embolism.
8. Describe preventive measures appropriate for controlling and eliminating occupational lung disease.
9. Discuss the modes of therapy and related nursing management for patients with lung cancer.
10. Describe the complications of chest trauma and their clinical manifestations and nursing management.
11. Describe nursing measures to prevent aspiration.

Conditions affecting the lower respiratory tract range from acute problems to chronic disorders. Many of these disorders are serious and often life-threatening. Patients with lower respiratory tract disorders require care from nurses with astute assessment and clinical management skills who also understand the impact of the particular disorder on the patient's quality of life and ability to carry out usual activities of daily living. Patient and family teaching is an important nursing intervention in the management of all lower respiratory tract disorders.

Atelectasis

Atelectasis refers to closure or collapse of alveoli and often is described in relation to x-ray findings and clinical signs and symptoms. Atelectasis may be acute or chronic and may cover a broad range of pathophysiologic changes, from microatelectasis (which is not detectable on chest x-ray) to macroatelectasis with loss of segmental, lobar, or overall lung volume. The most commonly described atelectasis is acute atelectasis, which occurs frequently in the postoperative setting or in people who are immobilized and have a shallow, monotonous breathing pattern. Excess secretions or mucus plugs may also cause obstruction of airflow and result in atelectasis in an area of the lung. Atelectasis also is observed in patients with a chronic airway obstruction that impedes or blocks air flow to an area of the lung (eg, obstructive atelectasis in the patient with lung cancer that is invading or compressing the airways). This type of atelectasis is more insidious and slower in onset.

Pathophysiology

Atelectasis may occur in adults as a result of reduced alveolar ventilation or any type of blockage that impedes passage of air to and from the alveoli that normally receive air through the bronchi and network of airways. The trapped alveolar air becomes absorbed into the bloodstream, and no additional air can enter into the alveoli because of the blockage. As a result, the affected portion of the lung becomes airless and the alveoli collapse. This may result from altered

Glossary

acute lung injury (ALI): an umbrella term for hypoxemic, respiratory failure; ARDS is a severe form of ALI

acute respiratory distress syndrome (ARDS): nonspecific pulmonary response to a variety of pulmonary and nonpulmonary insults to the lung; characterized by interstitial infiltrates, alveolar hemorrhage, atelectasis, decreased compliance, and refractory hypoxemia

asbestosis: diffuse lung fibrosis resulting from exposure to asbestos fibers

atelectasis: collapse or airless condition of the alveoli caused by hypoventilation, obstruction to the airways, or compression

central cyanosis: bluish discoloration of the skin or mucous membranes due to hemoglobin carrying reduced amounts of oxygen

consolidation: lung tissue that has become more solid in nature due to collapse of alveoli or infectious process (pneumonia)

cor pulmonale: "heart of the lungs"; enlargement of the right ventricle from hypertrophy or dilation or as a secondary response to disorders that affect the lungs

empyema: accumulation of purulent material in the pleural space

fine-needle aspiration: insertion of a needle through the chest wall to obtain cells of a mass or tumor; usually performed under fluoroscopy or chest CT guidance

hemoptysis: the coughing up of blood from the lower respiratory tract

hemothorax: partial or complete collapse of the lung due to blood accumulating in the pleural space; may occur after surgery or trauma

induration: an abnormally hard lesion or reaction, as in a positive tuberculin skin test

nosocomial: pertaining to or originating from a hospitalization; not present at the time of hospital admission

open lung biopsy: biopsy of lung tissue performed through a limited thoracotomy incision

orthopnea: shortness of breath when reclining or in the supine position

pleural effusion: abnormal accumulation of fluid in the pleural space

pleural friction rub: localized grating or creaking sound caused by the rubbing together of inflamed parietal and visceral pleurae

pleural space: the area between the parietal and visceral pleurae; a potential space

pneumothorax: partial or complete collapse of the lung due to positive pressure in the pleural space

pulmonary edema: increase in the amount of extravascular fluid in the lung

pulmonary embolism: obstruction of the pulmonary vasculature with an embolus; embolus may be due to blood clot, air bubbles, or fat droplets

purulent: consisting of, containing, or discharging pus

restrictive lung disease: disease of the lung that causes a decrease in lung volumes

tension pneumothorax: pneumothorax characterized by increasing positive pressure in the pleural space with each breath; this is an emergency situation and the positive pressure needs to be decompressed or released immediately

thoracentesis: insertion of a needle into the pleural space to remove fluid that has accumulated and decrease pressure on the lung tissue; may also be used diagnostically to identify potential causes of a pleural effusion

transbronchial: through the bronchial wall, as in a transbronchial lung biopsy

ventilation–perfusion ratio: the ratio between ventilation and perfusion in the lung; matching of ventilation to perfusion optimizes gas exchange

breathing patterns, retained secretions, pain, alterations in small airway function, prolonged supine positioning, increased abdominal pressure, reduced lung volumes due to musculoskeletal or neurologic disorders, restrictive defects, and specific surgical procedures (eg, upper abdominal, thoracic, or open heart surgery). Persistent low lung volumes, secretions or a mass obstructing or impeding airflow, and compression of lung tissue may all cause collapse or obstruction of the airways, which leads to atelectasis.

Patients are at high risk for atelectasis postoperatively because of the numerous respiratory changes that may occur. A monotonous, low tidal breathing pattern may cause small airway closure and alveolar collapse. This can result from the effects of anesthesia or analgesic agents, supine positioning, splinting of the chest wall because of pain, or abdominal distention. Postoperative patients may also have secretion retention, airway obstruction, and an impaired cough reflex, or they may be reluctant to cough because of pain. Figure 23-1 shows the pathogenic mechanisms and consequences of acute atelectasis in postoperative patients.

Atelectasis resulting from bronchial obstruction by secretions may occur in postoperative patients, in those with impaired cough mechanisms (eg, musculoskeletal or neurologic disorders), and in debilitated, bedridden patients. Atelectasis may also result from excessive pressure on the lung tissue, which restricts normal lung expansion on inspiration. Such pressure may be produced by fluid accumulating within the pleural space (**pleural effusion**), air in the pleural space (**pneumothorax**), or blood in the pleural space (**hemothorax**). The **pleural space** is the area between the parietal and the visceral pleurae. Pressure may also be produced by a pericardium distended with fluid (pericardial effusion), tumor growth within the thorax, or an elevated diaphragm.

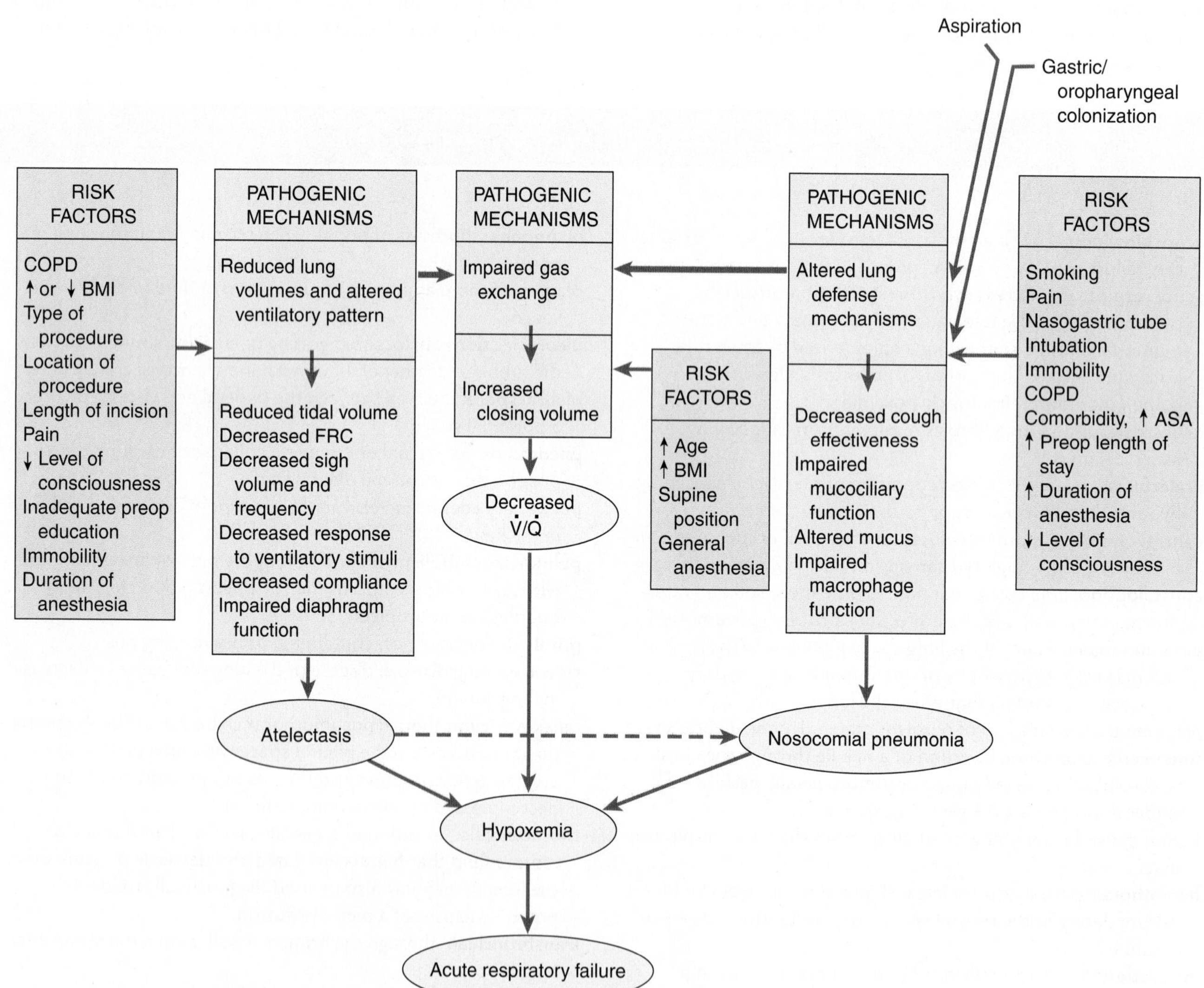

FIGURE 23-1. Relationship of risk factors, pathogenic mechanisms, and consequences of acute atelectasis in the postoperative patient. COPD, chronic obstructive pulmonary disease; BMI, body mass index; FRC, functional residual capacity; diaphragm fx, diaphragm function; ASA, American Society of Anesthesiology physical status; $\dot{V}/\dot{Q}$, ventilation-perfusion ratio. From the work of Jo Ann Brooks-Brunn, DNS, RN, FAAN, FCCP, Indiana University Medical Center, Indianapolis.

Clinical Manifestations

The development of atelectasis usually is insidious. Signs and symptoms include cough, sputum production, and low-grade fever. Fever is universally cited as a clinical sign of atelectasis, but there are few data to support this. Most likely, the fever that accompanies atelectasis is due to infection or inflammation distal to the obstructed airway.

In acute atelectasis involving a large amount of lung tissue (lobar atelectasis), marked respiratory distress may be observed. In addition to the previously mentioned signs and symptoms, dyspnea, tachycardia, tachypnea, pleural pain, and **central cyanosis** (a bluish skin hue that is a late sign of hypoxemia) may be anticipated. Patients characteristically have difficulty breathing in the supine position and are anxious.

In chronic atelectasis, signs and symptoms are similar to those of acute atelectasis. The chronic nature of the alveolar collapse predisposes patients to infection distal to the obstruction. Therefore, the signs and symptoms of a pulmonary infection also may be present.

Assessment and Diagnostic Findings

When clinically significant atelectasis develops, it is generally characterized by increased work of breathing and hypoxemia. The patient may demonstrate an increased respiratory rate and appear to labor with breathing. Decreased breath sounds and crackles are heard over the affected area. In addition, chest x-ray findings may reveal patchy infiltrates or consolidated areas. In patients who are confined to bed, atelectasis is usually diagnosed by chest x-ray or identified by physical assessment in the dependent, posterior, basilar areas of the lungs. Depending on the degree of hypoxemia, pulse oximetry (SpO_2) may demonstrate a low saturation of hemoglobin with oxygen (less than 90%) or a lower-than-normal partial pressure of arterial oxygen (PaO_2).

Prevention

Nursing measures to prevent atelectasis include frequent turning, early mobilization, and strategies to expand the lungs and to manage secretions. Voluntary deep-breathing maneuvers (at least every 2 hours) assist in preventing and treating atelectasis. The performance of these maneuvers requires the patient to be alert and cooperative. Patient education and reinforcement are key to the success of these interventions. The use of incentive spirometry or voluntary deep breathing enhances lung expansion, decreases the potential for airway closure, and may generate a cough. Secretion management techniques include directed cough, suctioning, aerosol nebulizer treatments followed by chest physical therapy (postural drainage and chest percussion), and bronchoscopy. In some settings, a metered-dose inhaler is used to dispense a bronchodilator rather than an aerosol nebulizer. Chart 23-1 summarizes measures used to prevent atelectasis.

CHART 23-1

Preventing Atelectasis

- Change patient's position frequently, especially from supine to upright position, to promote ventilation and prevent secretions from accumulating.
- Encourage early mobilization from bed to chair followed by early ambulation.
- Encourage appropriate deep breathing and coughing to mobilize secretions and prevent them from accumulating.
- Teach/reinforce appropriate technique for incentive spirometry.
- Administer prescribed opioids and sedatives judiciously to prevent respiratory depression.
- Perform postural drainage and chest percussion, if indicated.
- Institute suctioning to remove tracheobronchial secretions, if indicated.

Management

The goal of treatment is to improve ventilation and remove secretions. Strategies to prevent atelectasis, which include frequent turning, early ambulation, lung volume expansion maneuvers (eg, deep-breathing exercises, incentive spirometry), and coughing, also serve as the first-line measures to minimize or treat atelectasis by improving ventilation. In patients who do not respond to first-line measures or who cannot perform deep-breathing exercises, other treatments such as positive end-expiratory pressure (PEEP; a simple mask and one-way valve system that provides varying amounts of expiratory resistance, usually 5 to 15 cm H_2O), continuous or intermittent positive pressure-breathing (IPPB), or bronchoscopy may be used. An older therapy, IPPB continues to be used in some settings to improve lung volume expansion; however, other types of lung volume expansion maneuvers should be tried first in the postoperative setting (Sorenson & Shelledy, 2003). Before initiating more complex, costly, and labor-intensive therapies, nurses should ask several questions:

- Has the patient been given an adequate trial of deep-breathing exercises?
- Has the patient received adequate education, supervision, and coaching to carry out the deep-breathing exercises?
- Have other factors been evaluated that may impair ventilation or prevent a good patient effort (eg, lack of turning, mobilization; excessive pain; excessive sedation)?

If the cause of atelectasis is bronchial obstruction from secretions, the secretions must be removed by coughing or suctioning to allow air to re-enter that portion of the lung. Chest physical therapy (chest percussion and postural drainage) may also be used to mobilize secretions. Nebulizer treatments with a bronchodilator or sodium bicarbonate may be used to assist patients in the expectoration of secretions. If respiratory care measures fail to remove the obstruction, a bronchoscopy is performed. Although bronchoscopy is an excellent measure to acutely remove secretions and increase ventilation, it is imperative for the nurse to assist the patient with maintaining the patency of the airways after bronchoscopy, using the traditional techniques of deep breathing, coughing, and suctioning. Severe or massive atelectasis may lead to acute respiratory failure, especially in patients with underlying lung disease. Endotracheal intubation and mechanical ventilation may be necessary. Prompt treatment reduces the risk for development of acute respiratory failure, pneumonia, or both.

If the cause of atelectasis is compression of lung tissue, the goal is to decrease the compression. With a large pleural effusion that is compressing lung tissue and causing alveolar collapse, treatment may include **thoracentesis** (removal of the fluid by needle aspiration) or insertion of a chest tube. The measures to increase lung expansion described previously also are used.

Management of chronic atelectasis focuses on removing the cause of the obstruction of the airways or the compression of the lung tissue. For example, bronchoscopy may be used to open an airway obstructed by lung cancer or a nonmalignant lesion, and the procedure may involve cryotherapy or laser therapy. If the atelectasis is a result of obstruction caused by lung cancer, an airway stent or radiation therapy to shrink a tumor may be used to open the airways and provide ventilation to the collapsed area. However, in patients who have experienced chronic, long-term collapse, it may not be possible to reopen the airways and reaerate the area of the lung. In some cases, surgical management may be indicated.

Respiratory Infections

Acute Tracheobronchitis

Acute tracheobronchitis, an acute inflammation of the mucous membranes of the trachea and the bronchial tree, often follows infection of the upper respiratory tract. Patients with viral infections have decreased resistance and can readily develop a secondary bacterial infection. Adequate treatment of upper respiratory tract infection is one of the major factors in the prevention of acute bronchitis.

Pathophysiology

In acute tracheobronchitis, the inflamed mucosa of the bronchi produces mucopurulent sputum, often in response to infection by *Streptococcus pneumoniae, Haemophilus influenzae,* or *Mycoplasma pneumoniae.* In addition, a fungal infection (eg, *Aspergillus*) may also cause tracheobronchitis. A sputum culture is essential to identify the specific causative organism. In addition to infection, inhalation of physical and chemical irritants, gases, or other air contaminants can also cause acute bronchial irritation.

Clinical Manifestations

Initially, the patient has a dry, irritating cough and expectorates a scanty amount of mucoid sputum. The patient may report sternal soreness from coughing and have fever or chills, night sweats, headache, and general malaise. As the infection progresses, the patient may be short of breath, have noisy inspiration and expiration (inspiratory stridor and expiratory wheeze), and produce **purulent** (pus-filled) sputum. In severe tracheobronchitis, blood-streaked secretions may be expectorated as a result of the irritation of the mucosa of the airways.

Medical Management

Antibiotic treatment may be indicated depending on the symptoms, sputum purulence, and results of the sputum culture. Antihistamines usually are not prescribed, because they can cause excessive drying and make secretions more difficult to expectorate. Expectorants may be prescribed, although their efficacy is questionable. Fluid intake is increased to thin the viscous and tenacious secretions. Copious, purulent secretions that cannot be cleared by coughing place patients at risk for increasing airway obstruction and the development of more severe lower respiratory tract infections, such as pneumonia. Suctioning and bronchoscopy may be needed to remove secretions. Rarely, endotracheal intubation may be necessary in cases of acute tracheobronchitis leading to acute respiratory failure, such as in patients who are severely debilitated or who have coexisting diseases that also impair the respiratory system.

In most cases, treatment of tracheobronchitis is largely symptomatic. Increasing the vapor pressure (moisture content) in the air reduces airway irritation. Cool vapor therapy or steam inhalations may help relieve laryngeal and tracheal irritation. Moist heat to the chest may relieve the soreness and pain. Mild analgesics or antipyretics may be indicated.

Nursing Management

Acute tracheobronchitis is usually treated in the home setting. A primary nursing function is to encourage bronchial hygiene, such as increased fluid intake and directed coughing to remove secretions. The nurse encourages and assists the patient to sit up frequently to cough effectively and to prevent retention of mucopurulent sputum. If the patient is taking antibiotics for an underlying infection, it is important to emphasize the need to complete the full course of antibiotics prescribed. Fatigue is a consequence of tracheobronchitis; therefore, the nurse cautions the patient against overexertion, which can induce a relapse or exacerbation of the infection. The patient is advised to rest.

Pneumonia

Pneumonia is an inflammation of the lung parenchyma caused by various microorganisms, including bacteria, mycobacteria, chlamydiae, mycoplasma, fungi, parasites, and viruses. “Pneumonitis” is a more general term that describes an inflammatory process in the lung tissue that may predispose or place the patient at risk for microbial invasion. Pneumonia is the most common cause of death from infectious diseases in the United States. It accounts for almost 66,000 deaths per year and ranks as the seventh leading cause of death in the United States (Kochanek & Smith, 2004). A costly disorder, pneumonia occurs in both inpatients and outpatients.

Classification

Several systems are used to classify pneumonias. Classically, pneumonia has been categorized into one of four categories: bacterial or typical, atypical, anaerobic/cavitary, and opportunistic. However, there is overlap in the microorganisms thought to be responsible for typical and atypical pneumonias. A more widely used classification scheme categorizes the major pneumonias as community-acquired pneumonia (CAP), hospital-acquired (nosocomial) pneumonia (HAP), pneumonia in the immunocompromised host, and aspiration pneumonia (Table 23-1). There is overlap in how specific pneumonias are classified, because they may occur in differing settings.

Community-Acquired Pneumonia

CAP occurs either in the community setting or within the first 48 hours after hospitalization or institutionalization. The need for hospitalization for CAP depends on the severity of the pneumonia. The causative agents for CAP that requires hospitalization are most frequently *S. pneumoniae, H. influenzae, Legionella, Pseudomonas aeruginosa,* and other gram-negative rods. The specific etiologic agent is identified in about 50% of cases. More than 5.5 million people develop CAP and as many as 1.1 million of these require hospitalization each year. (The absence of a responsible caregiver in the home may be another indication for hospitalization.) In the United States, CAP is the major cause of death from infectious disease (Andrews, Nadjm, Gant, et al., 2003).

Pneumonia caused by *S. pneumoniae* (pneumococcus) is the most common CAP in people younger than 60 years of age without comorbidity and in those 60 years and older with comorbidity. It is most prevalent during the winter and spring, when upper respiratory tract infections are most frequent. *S. pneumoniae* is a gram-positive, capsulated, nonmotile coccus that resides naturally in the upper respiratory tract. The organism colonizes the upper respiratory tract and can cause the following types of illnesses: disseminated invasive infections, pneumonia and other lower respiratory tract infections, and upper respiratory tract infections, including otitis media and sinusitis. It may occur as a lobar or bronchopneumonic form in patients of any age and may follow a recent respiratory illness.

Mycoplasma pneumonia, another type of CAP, is caused by *M. pneumoniae.* Mycoplasma pneumonia occurs most often in older children and young adults and is spread by infected respiratory droplets through person-to-person contact. Patients can be tested for mycoplasma antibodies. The inflammatory infiltrate is primarily interstitial rather than alveolar. It spreads throughout the entire respiratory tract, including the bronchioles, and has the characteristics of a bronchopneumonia. Earache and bullous myringitis are common. Impaired ventilation and diffusion may occur.

H. influenzae is another cause of CAP. This type of pneumonia frequently affects elderly people and those with comorbid illnesses (eg, chronic obstructive pulmonary disease [COPD], alcoholism, diabetes mellitus). The presentation is indistinguishable from that of other forms of bacterial CAP and may be subacute, with cough or low-grade fever for weeks before diagnosis. Chest x-rays may reveal multilobar, patchy bronchopneumonia or areas of **consolidation** (tissue that solidifies as a result of collapsed alveoli or pneumonia).

Viruses are the most common cause of pneumonia in infants and children but are relatively uncommon causes of CAP in adults. In immunocompetent adults, the chief causes of viral pneumonia are influenza viruses types A and B, adenovirus, parainfluenza virus, coronavirus, and varicella-zoster virus. In immunocompromised adults, cytomegalovirus is the most common viral pathogen, followed by herpes simplex virus, adenovirus, and respiratory syncytial virus. The acute stage of a viral respiratory infection occurs within the ciliated cells of the airways. This is followed by infiltration of the tracheobronchial tree. With pneumonia, the inflammatory process extends into the alveolar area, resulting in edema and exudation. The clinical signs and symptoms of a viral pneumonia are often difficult to distinguish from those of a bacterial pneumonia.

Hospital-Acquired Pneumonia

HAP, also known as **nosocomial** pneumonia, is defined as the onset of pneumonia symptoms more than 48 hours after admission in patients with no evidence of infection at the time of admission. HAP accounts for approximately 15% of hospital-acquired infections but is the most lethal nosocomial infection. It is estimated to occur in 0.5% to 1% of all hospitalized patients and in 15% to 20% of intensive care patients (Centers for Disease Control and Prevention [CDC], 2004d). Ventilator-associated pneumonia can be considered a type of nosocomial pneumonia that is associated with endotracheal intubation and mechanical ventilation. Ventilator-associated pneumonia is defined as bacterial pneumonia that develops in patients with acute respiratory failure who have been receiving mechanical ventilation for at least 48 hours.

HAP occurs when at least one of three conditions exists: host defenses are impaired, an inoculum of organisms reaches the lower respiratory tract and overwhelms the host's defenses, or a highly virulent organism is present. Certain factors may predispose patients to HAP because of impaired host defenses (eg, severe acute or chronic illness), a variety of comorbid conditions, supine positioning and aspiration, coma, malnutrition, prolonged hospitalization, hypotension, and metabolic disorders. Hospitalized patients are also exposed to potential bacteria from other sources (eg, respiratory therapy devices and equipment, transmission of pathogens by the hands of health care personnel). Numerous intervention-related factors also may play a role in the development of HAP (eg, therapeutic agents leading to central nervous system depression with decreased ventilation, impaired removal of secretions, or potential aspiration; prolonged or complicated thoracoabdominal procedures, which may impair mucociliary function and cellular host defenses; endotracheal intubation; prolonged or inappropriate use of antibiotics; use of nasogastric tubes). In addition, immunocompromised patients are at particular risk. HAP is associated with a high mortality rate, in part because of the virulence of the organisms, their resistance to antibiotics, and the patient's underlying disorder.

The common organisms responsible for HAP include the pathogens *Enterobacter* species, *Escherichia coli, H. influenzae,*

(text continues on page 633)

TABLE 23-1 Commonly Encountered Pneumonias

Type	Organism Responsible	Epidemiology	Clinical Features	Treatment	Comments
Community-Acquired Pneumonia					
Streptococcal pneumonia (pneumococcal)	*Streptococcus pneumoniae*	Highest occurrence in winter months. Incidence greatest in the elderly and in patients with COPD, heart failure, alcoholism, asplenia, and after influenza. Leading infectious cause of illness worldwide among young children, persons with underlying chronic health conditions, and the elderly. Death occurs in 14% of hospitalized adults with invasive disease.	Abrupt onset, toxic appearance, pleuritic chest pain. Usually involves one or more lobes. Lobar infiltrate common on chest x-ray or bronchopneumonia pattern. Bacteremia in 15% to 25% of all patients.	Penicillins Alternative antibiotic therapy, such as cefotaxime or ceftriaxone; antipseudomonal fluoroquinolones (levofloxacin, gatifloxacin, moxifloxacin).	Complications include shock, pleural effusion, superinfections, pericarditis, and otitis media.
Haemophilus influenzae	*Haemophilus influenzae*	Incidence greatest in alcoholics, the elderly, patients in long-term care facilities and nursing homes, patients with diabetes or COPD, and children <5 years of age. Accounts for 5–20% of community-acquired pneumonias. Mortality rate: 30%.	Frequently insidious onset associated with upper respiratory tract infection 2 to 6 weeks before onset of illness. Fever, chills, productive cough. Usually involves one or more lobes. Bacteremia is common. Infiltrate, occasional bronchopneumonia pattern on chest x-ray.	Ampicillin, third- or fourth-generation cephalosporin, macrolides (azithromycin, clarithromycin), fluoroquinolones	Complications include lung abscess, pleural effusion, meningitis, arthritis, pericarditis, epiglottitis.
Legionnaires' disease	*Legionella pneumophila*	Highest occurrence in summer and fall. May cause disease sporadically or as part of an epidemic. Incidence greatest in middle-aged and older men, smokers, patients with chronic diseases, those receiving immunosuppressive therapy, and those in close proximity to excavation sites. Accounts for 15% of community-acquired pneumonias. Mortality rate: 15–50%.	Flulike symptoms. High fevers, mental confusion, headache, pleuritic pain, myalgias, dyspnea, productive cough, hemoptysis, leukocytosis. Bronchopneumonia, unilateral or bilateral disease, lobar consolidation.	Erythromycin +/− rifampin (in severely compromised patient) or clarithromycin, or a macrolide (azithromycin), or a fluoroquinolone (ofloxacin, levofloxacin, sparfloxacin).	Complications include hypotension, shock, and acute renal failure.

TABLE 23-1 Commonly Encountered Pneumonias (Continued)

Type	Organism Responsible	Epidemiology	Clinical Features	Treatment	Comments
Mycoplasma pneumoniae	*Mycoplasma pneumoniae*	Increase in fall and winter. Responsible for epidemics of respiratory illness. Most common type of atypical pneumonia. Accounts for 20% of community-acquired pneumonias. More common in children and young adults. Mortality rate: <0.1%.	Onset is usually insidious. Patients not usually as ill as in other pneumonias. Sore throat, nasal congestion, ear pain, headache, low-grade fever, pleuritic pain, myalgias, diarrhea, erythematous rash, pharyngitis. Interstitial infiltrates on chest x-ray.	Doxycycline, macrolide or fluoroquinolone.	Complications include aseptic meningitis, meningoencephalitis, transverse myelitis, cranial nerve palsies, pericarditis, myocarditis.
Viral pneumonia	Influenza viruses types A, B adenovirus, parainfluenza, cytomegalovirus, coronavirus	Incidence greatest in winter months. Epidemics occur every 2 to 3 years. Most common causative organisms in adults. Other organisms in children (eg, cytomegalovirus, respiratory syncytial virus). Accounts for 20% of community-acquired pneumonias.	Patchy infiltrate, small pleural effusion on chest x-ray. In most patients, influenza begins as an acute upper respiratory infection; others have bronchitis, pleurisy, and so on, and still others develop gastrointestinal symptoms.	Type A: amantadine and rimantadine Type A/B: zanamivir, oseltamivir phosphate. Treated symptomatically. Does not respond to treatment with currently available antimicrobials.	Complications include a superimposed bacterial infection, bronchopneumonia.
Chlamydial pneumonia (TWAR agent)	*Chlamydia pneumoniae*	Reported mainly in college students, military recruits, and the elderly. May be a common cause of community-acquired pneumonia or observed in combination with other pathogens. Mortality rate is low because the majority of cases are relatively mild. The elderly with coexistent infections, comorbidities, and reinfections may require hospitalization.	Hoarseness, fever, chills, pharyngitis, rhinitis, nonproductive cough, myalgias, arthralgias. Single infiltrate on chest x-ray; pleural effusion possible.	Tetracycline, erythromycin, macrolide, quinolone.	Complications include reinfection and acute respiratory failure.

continued >

TABLE 23-1 Commonly Encountered Pneumonias (Continued)

Type	Organism Responsible	Epidemiology	Clinical Features	Treatment	Comments
Hospital-Acquired Pneumonia					
Pseudomonas pneumonia	*Pseudomonas aeruginosa*	Incidence greatest in those with pre-existing lung disease, cancer (particularly leukemia); those with homograft transplants, burns; debilitated persons; and patients receiving antimicrobial therapy and treatments such as tracheostomy, suctioning, and in post-operative settings. Almost always of nosocomial origin. Accounts for 15% of hospital-acquired pneumonias. Mortality rate: 40–60%.	Diffuse consolidation on chest x-ray. Toxic appearance: fever, chills, productive cough, relative bradycardia, leukocytosis.	Aminoglycoside and anti-pseudomonal agents (ticarcillin, piperacillin, mezlocillin, ceftazidine).	Complications include lung cavitation. Has capacity to invade blood vessels, causing hemorrhage and lung infarction. Usually requires hospitalization.
Staphylococcal pneumonia	*Staphylococcus aureus*	Incidence greatest in immunocompromised patients, IV drug users, and as a complication of epidemic influenza. Commonly nosocomial in origin. Accounts for 10–30% of hospital-acquired pneumonias. Mortality rate: 25–60%.	Severe hypoxemia, cyanosis, necrotizing infection. Bacteremia is common.	Nafcillin/oxacillin; clindamycin or linezolid; methicillin-resistant: vancomycin or linezolid	Complications include pleural effusion/pneumothorax, lung abscess, empyema, meningitis, endocarditis. Frequently requires hospitalization. Treatment must be vigorous and prolonged because disease tends to destroy lung tissue.
Klebsiella pneumonia	*Klebsiella pneumoniae* (Friedlander's bacillus-encapsulated gram-negative aerobic bacillus)	Incidence greatest in the elderly; alcoholics; patients with chronic disease, such as diabetes, heart failure, COPD; patients in chronic care facilities and nursing homes. Accounts for 2–5% of community-acquired and 10–30% of hospital-acquired pneumonias. Mortality rate: 40–50%.	Tissue necrosis occurs rapidly. Toxic appearance: fever, cough, sputum production, bronchopneumonia, lung abscess. Lobar consolidation, bronchopneumonia pattern on chest x-ray.	Third- and/or fourth-generation cephalosporins (cefotaxime, ceftriaxone) plus aminoglycoside, antipseudomonal penicillin, monobactam (aztreonam), or quinolone.	Complications include multiple lung abscesses with cyst formation, empyema, pericarditis, pleural effusion. May be fulminating, progressing to fatal outcome.

TABLE 23-1 Commonly Encountered Pneumonias (Continued)

Type	Organism Responsible	Epidemiology	Clinical Features	Treatment	Comments
Pneumonia in Immunocompromised Host					
Pneumocystis pneumonia (PCP)	*Pneumocystis jiroveci*	Incidence greatest in patients with AIDS and patients receiving immunosuppressive therapy for cancer, organ transplantation, and other disorders. Frequently seen with cytomegalovirus infection. Mortality rate 15–20% in hospitalized patients and fatal if not treated.	Pulmonary infiltrates on chest x-ray. Nonproductive cough, fever, dyspnea.	Trimethoprim/sulfamethoxazole (TMP-SMZ), dapsone-trimethoprim, pentamidine, primequine plus clindamycin.	Complications include respiratory failure.
Fungal pneumonia	*Aspergillus fumigatus*	Incidence greatest in immunocompromised and neutropenic patients. Mortality rate: 15–20%.	Cough, hemoptysis, infiltrates, fungus ball on chest x-ray.	Flucytosine with amphotericin B in non-neutropenic patients, amphotericin B, itraconazole, ketoconazole. Lobectomy for fungus ball.	Complications include dissemination to brain, myocardium, and/or thyroid gland.
Tuberculosis	*Mycobacterium tuberculosis*	Incidence increased in indigent, immigrant, and prison populations, people with AIDS, and the homeless. Mortality rate <1% (depending on comorbidity)	Weight loss, fever, night sweats, cough, sputum production, hemoptysis, nonspecific infiltrate (lower lobe), hilar node enlargement, pleural effusion on chest x-ray.	Rifampin, ethambutol, INH (isoniazid), pyrazinamide	Complications include reinfection and acute respiratory infection.

+/– may add depending upon situation; COPD, chronic obstructive pulmonary disease.

Klebsiella species, *Proteus*, *Serratia marcescens*, *P. aeruginosa*, methicillin-sensitive or methicillin-resistant *Staphylococcus aureus* (MRSA), and *S. pneumoniae*. Some risk factors for infection are shared, and others are unique to the specific organisms; however, most patients with HAP are colonized with multiple organisms. Pseudomonal pneumonia, which accounts for 15% of cases of HAP, occurs in patients who are debilitated, those with altered mental status, and those with prolonged intubation or with tracheostomy. Staphylococcal pneumonia, which accounts for more than 30% of cases of HAP but less than 10% of cases of CAP, can occur through inhalation of the organism or spread through the hematogenous route. It is often accompanied by bacteremia and positive blood cultures. Its mortality rate is high. Specific strains of staphylococci are resistant to all available antimicrobial agents except vancomycin. Overuse and misuse of antimicrobial agents are major risk factors for the emergence of these resistant pathogens. Because MRSA is highly virulent, steps must be taken to prevent its spread. Patients with MRSA are isolated in a private room, and contact precautions (gown, mask, glove, and antibacterial soap) are used. The number of people in contact with affected patients is minimized, and appropriate precautions must be taken when transporting these patients within or between facilities.

The usual presentation of HAP is a new pulmonary infiltrate on chest x-ray combined with evidence of infection such as fever, respiratory symptoms, purulent sputum, or leukocytosis. Pneumonias from *Klebsiella* or other gram-negative organisms (*E. coli*, *Proteus*, *Serratia*) are characterized by destruction of lung structure and alveolar walls, consolidation, and bacteremia. Elderly patients and those with alcoholism, chronic lung disease, or diabetes are at particular risk. Development of a cough or increased cough and sputum production are common presentations, along with low-grade fever and general malaise. In debilitated or dehydrated patients, sputum production may be minimal or absent. Pleural effusion, high fever, and tachycardia are common. Even with treatment, the mortality rate remains high.

Pneumonia in the Immunocompromised Host

Pneumonia in immunocompromised hosts includes *Pneumocystis* pneumonia (PCP), fungal pneumonias, and *Mycobacterium tuberculosis.* The organism that causes PCP is now known as *Pneumocystis jiroveci* instead of *Pneumocystis carinii.* The acronym PCP still applies because it can be read "*Pneumocystis* pneumonia."

Pneumonia in the immunocompromised host occurs with use of corticosteroids or other immunosuppressive agents, chemotherapy, nutritional depletion, use of broad-spectrum antimicrobial agents, acquired immunodeficiency syndrome (AIDS), genetic immune disorders, and long-term advanced life-support technology (mechanical ventilation). It is seen with increasing frequency because affected patients constitute a growing portion of the population; however, pneumonias that typically occur in immunocompromised people may also occur in immunocompetent people. Patients with compromised immune systems commonly develop pneumonia from organisms of low virulence. In addition, increasing numbers of patients with impaired defenses develop HAP from gram-negative bacilli (*Klebsiella, Pseudomonas, E. coli,* Enterobacteriaceae, *Proteus, Serratia*).

Pneumonia in immunocompromised hosts may be caused by the organisms also observed in CAP or HAP (*S. pneumoniae, S. aureus, H. influenzae, P. aeruginosa, M. tuberculosis*). PCP is rarely observed in immunocompetent hosts and is often an initial AIDS-defining complication. Whether patients are immunocompromised or immunocompetent, the clinical presentation of pneumonia is similar. PCP has a subtle onset, with progressive dyspnea, fever, and a nonproductive cough.

Aspiration Pneumonia

Aspiration pneumonia refers to the pulmonary consequences resulting from entry of endogenous or exogenous substances into the lower airway. The most common form of aspiration pneumonia is bacterial infection from aspiration of bacteria that normally reside in the upper airways. Aspiration pneumonia may occur in the community or hospital setting. Common pathogens are *S. pneumoniae, H. influenzae,* and *S. aureus.* Substances other than bacteria may be aspirated into the lung, such as gastric contents, exogenous chemical contents, or irritating gases. This type of aspiration or ingestion may impair the lung defenses, cause inflammatory changes, and lead to bacterial growth and a resulting pneumonia. (See later discussion of aspiration.)

Pathophysiology

Upper airway characteristics normally prevent potentially infectious particles from reaching the sterile lower respiratory tract. Pneumonia arises from normal flora present in patients whose resistance has been altered or from aspiration of flora present in the oropharynx; patients often have an acute or chronic underlying disease that impairs host defenses. Pneumonia may also result from bloodborne organisms that enter the pulmonary circulation and are trapped in the pulmonary capillary bed.

Pneumonia affects both ventilation and diffusion. An inflammatory reaction can occur in the alveoli, producing an exudate that interferes with the diffusion of oxygen and carbon dioxide. White blood cells, mostly neutrophils, also migrate into the alveoli and fill the normally air-containing spaces. Areas of the lung are not adequately ventilated because of secretions and mucosal edema that cause partial occlusion of the bronchi or alveoli, with a resultant decrease in alveolar oxygen tension. Bronchospasm may also occur in patients with reactive airway disease. Because of hypoventilation, a ventilation–perfusion mismatch occurs in the affected area of the lung. Venous blood entering the pulmonary circulation passes through the underventilated area and travels to the left side of the heart poorly oxygenated. The mixing of oxygenated and unoxygenated or poorly oxygenated blood eventually results in arterial hypoxemia.

If a substantial portion of one or more lobes is involved, the disease is referred to as "lobar pneumonia." The term "bronchopneumonia" is used to describe pneumonia that is distributed in a patchy fashion, having originated in one or more localized areas within the bronchi and extending to the adjacent surrounding lung parenchyma. Bronchopneumonia is more common than lobar pneumonia (Fig. 23-2).

Risk Factors

Being knowledgeable about the factors and circumstances that commonly predispose people to pneumonia helps identify patients at high risk for the disease (Table 23-2).

Increasing numbers of patients who have compromised defenses against infections are susceptible to pneumonia. Some types of pneumonia, such as those caused by viral infections, occur in previously healthy people, often after a viral illness.

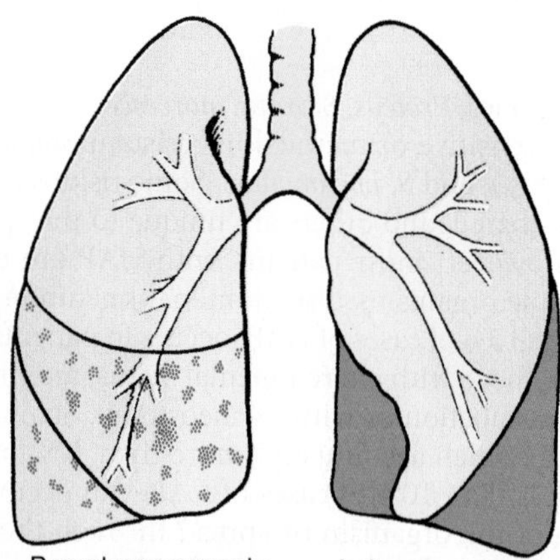

FIGURE 23-2. Distribution of lung involvement in bronchial and lobar pneumonia. In bronchopneumonia (*left*), patchy areas of consolidation occur. In lobar pneumonia (*right*), an entire lobe is consolidated.

TABLE 23-2 Risk Factors and Preventive Measures for Pneumonia

Risk Factor	Preventive Measure
Conditions that produce mucus or bronchial obstruction and interfere with normal lung drainage (eg, cancer, cigarette smoking, COPD)	Promote coughing and expectoration of secretions. Encourage smoking cessation.
Immunosuppressed patients and those with a low neutrophil count (neutropenic)	Initiate special precautions against infection.
Smoking; cigarette smoke disrupts both mucociliary and macrophage activity	Encourage smoking cessation.
Prolonged immobility and shallow breathing pattern	Reposition frequently and promote lung expansion exercises and coughing. Initiate suctioning and chest physical therapy if indicated.
Depressed cough reflex (due to medications, a debilitated state, or weak respiratory muscles); aspiration of foreign material into the lungs during a period of unconsciousness (head injury, anesthesia, depressed level of consciousness), or abnormal swallowing mechanism	Reposition frequently to prevent aspiration and administer medications judiciously, particularly those that increase risk for aspiration. Perform suctioning and chest physical therapy if indicated.
Nothing-by-mouth (NPO) status; placement of nasogastric, orogastric, or endotracheal tube	Promote frequent oral hygiene. Minimize risk for aspiration by checking placement of tube and proper positioning of patient.
Supine positioning in patients unable to protect their airway	Elevate head of bed at least 30 degrees.
Antibiotic therapy (in very ill people, the oropharynx is likely to be colonized by gram-negative bacteria)	Monitor patients receiving antibiotic therapy for signs and symptoms of pneumonia.
Alcohol intoxication (because alcohol suppresses the body's reflexes, may be associated with aspiration, and decreases white cell mobilization and tracheobronchial ciliary motion)	Encourage reduced or moderate alcohol intake (in case of alcohol stupor, position patient to prevent aspiration).
General anesthetic, sedative, or opioid preparations that promote respiratory depression, which causes a shallow breathing pattern and predisposes to the pooling of bronchial secretions and potential development of pneumonia	Observe the respiratory rate and depth during recovery from general anesthesia and before giving medications. If respiratory depression is apparent, withhold the medication and contact the physician.
Advanced age, because of possible depressed cough and glottic reflexes and nutritional depletion	Promote frequent turning, early ambulation and mobilization, effective coughing, breathing exercises, and nutritious diet.
Respiratory therapy with improperly cleaned equipment	Make sure that respiratory equipment is cleaned properly; participate in continuous quality improvement monitoring with the respiratory care department.
Transmission of organisms from health care providers	Use strict hand hygiene and gloves. Implement health care provider education.

Pneumonia occurs in patients with certain underlying disorders such as heart failure, diabetes, alcoholism, COPD, and AIDS. Certain diseases also have been associated with specific pathogens. For example, staphylococcal pneumonia has been noted after epidemics of influenza, and patients with COPD are at increased risk for development of pneumonia caused by pneumococci or *H. influenzae*. In addition, cystic fibrosis is associated with respiratory infection caused by pseudomonal and staphylococcal organisms, and PCP has been associated with AIDS. Pneumonias occurring in hospitalized patients often involve organisms not usually found in CAP, including enteric gram-negative bacilli and *S. aureus*.

The CDC (2004d) has identified four specific strategies for preventing HAP: (1) staff education and involvement in infection prevention, (2) infection and microbiologic surveillance, (3) prevention of transmission of microorganisms, and (4) modifying host risk for infection. The CDC (2003a) has also established guidelines for environmental infection control in health care facilities. Providing anticipatory interventions and preventive care are important nursing measures.

Pneumococcal disease is more prevalent (threefold to fivefold higher) in African American adults as compared with Caucasians. Pneumococcal vaccination has been demonstrated to prevent pneumonia in otherwise healthy populations with an efficiency of 65% to 85% (Niederman & Ahmed, 2003). To reduce or prevent serious complications of CAP in high-risk groups, vaccination against pneumococcal infection is advised for the following:

- People 65 years of age or older
- Immunocompetent people who are at increased risk for illness and death associated with pneumococcal disease because of chronic illness (eg, cardiovascular disease, pulmonary disease, diabetes mellitus, chronic liver disease) or disability
- People with functional or anatomic asplenia
- People living in environments or social settings in which the risk of disease is high
- Immunocompromised people at high risk for infection

The vaccine provides specific prevention against pneumococcal pneumonia and other infections caused by *S. pneumoniae* (otitis media, other upper respiratory tract infections). Vaccines should be avoided during the first trimester of pregnancy.

Clinical Manifestations

Pneumonia varies in its signs and symptoms depending on the causal organism and the presence of underlying disease. However, it is not possible to diagnose a specific type of pneumonia (CAP, HAP, immunocompromised host, or aspiration) by clinical manifestations alone. The patient with streptococcal (pneumococcal) pneumonia usually has a sudden onset of chills, rapidly rising fever (38.5° to 40.5°C [101° to 105°F]), and pleuritic chest pain that is aggravated by deep breathing and coughing. The patient is severely ill, with marked tachypnea (25 to 45 breaths/min), accompanied by other signs of respiratory distress (eg, shortness of breath, use of accessory muscles in respiration). The pulse is rapid and bounding, and it usually increases about 10 bpm for every degree (Celsius) of temperature elevation. A relative bradycardia for the amount of fever may suggest viral infection, mycoplasma infection, or infection with a *Legionella* organism.

Some patients exhibit an upper respiratory tract infection (nasal congestion, sore throat), and the onset of symptoms of pneumonia is gradual and nonspecific. The predominant symptoms may be headache, low-grade fever, pleuritic pain, myalgia, rash, and pharyngitis. After a few days, mucoid or mucopurulent sputum is expectorated. In severe pneumonia, the cheeks are flushed and the lips and nail beds demonstrate central cyanosis (a late sign of poor oxygenation [hypoxemia]).

The patient may exhibit **orthopnea** (shortness of breath when reclining), preferring to be propped up or sitting in bed leaning forward (orthopneic position) in an effort to achieve adequate gas exchange without coughing or breathing deeply. Appetite is poor, and the patient is diaphoretic and tires easily. Sputum is often purulent; however, this is not a reliable indicator of the etiologic agent. Rusty, blood-tinged sputum may be expectorated with streptococcal (pneumococcal), staphylococcal, and *Klebsiella* pneumonia.

Signs and symptoms of pneumonia may also depend on a patient's underlying condition. Different signs occur in patients with conditions such as cancer, and in those who are undergoing treatment with immunosuppressants, which decrease the resistance to infection. Such patients have fever, crackles, and physical findings that indicate consolidation of lung tissue, including increased tactile fremitus (vocal vibration detected on palpation), percussion dullness, bronchial breath sounds, egophony (when auscultated, the spoken "E" becomes a loud, nasal-sounding "A"), and whispered pectoriloquy (whispered sounds are easily auscultated through the chest wall). These changes occur because sound is transmitted better through solid or dense tissue (consolidation) than through normal air-filled tissue; these sounds are described in Chapter 21.

Purulent sputum or slight changes in respiratory symptoms may be the only sign of pneumonia in patients with COPD. It may be difficult to determine whether an increase in symptoms is an exacerbation of the underlying disease process or an additional infectious process.

Assessment and Diagnostic Findings

The diagnosis of pneumonia is made by history (particularly of a recent respiratory tract infection), physical examination, chest x-ray, blood culture (bloodstream invasion, called bacteremia, occurs frequently), and sputum examination. The sputum sample is obtained by having patients do the following: (1) rinse the mouth with water to minimize contamination by normal oral flora, (2) breathe deeply several times, (3) cough deeply, and (4) expectorate the raised sputum into a sterile container.

More invasive procedures may be used to collect specimens. Sputum may be obtained by nasotracheal or orotracheal suctioning with a sputum trap or by fiberoptic bronchoscopy (see Chapter 21). Bronchoscopy is often used in patients with acute severe infection, in patients with chronic or refractory infection, in immunocompromised patients when a diagnosis cannot be made from an expectorated or induced specimen, and in mechanically ventilated patients.

Medical Management

Pharmacologic Therapy

The treatment of pneumonia includes administration of the appropriate antibiotic as determined by the results of a Gram stain. However, an etiologic agent is not identified in half of CAP cases, and empiric therapy must be initiated. Therapy for CAP is continuing to evolve. Guidelines exist to guide antibiotic choice; however, the resistance patterns, prevalence of etiologic agents, patient risk factors, and costs and availability of newer antibiotic agents must all be considered.

Several organizations have published guidelines and comprehensive reviews of the medical management of CAP (File, Garau, Blasi, et al., 2004; Institute for Clinical Systems Improvement [ICSI], 2003; Mandell, Bartlett, Dowell, et al., 2003). However, guidelines take time to develop, and by the time they are published, they are often out-of-date. In addition, different organizations may publish slightly different recommendations, making treatment decisions even more difficult (File et al., 2004). Guidelines may be classified in terms of risk factors, treatment setting (inpatient versus outpatient), or specific pathogens. Examples of risk factors that may increase the risk of infection with certain types of pathogens appear in Chart 23-2.

Prompt administration (within 4 to 8 hours) of antibiotics in patients in whom CAP is strongly suspected or confirmed is a key treatment measure. For outpatients with CAP who have no cardiopulmonary disease or other modifying factors, treatment should include an oral macrolide (azithromycin [Zithromax] or clarithromycin [Biaxin]), doxycycline (Vibramycin), or a fluoroquinolone (eg, gatifloxacin [Tequin], levofloxacin [Levaquin]) with enhanced activity against *S. pneumoniae* (File et al. 2004; ICSI, 2003). For outpatients with CAP who have cardiopulmonary disease or other modifying factors, treatment should include a beta-lactam agent (oral cefpodoxime [Vantin], cefurox-

CHART 23-2

Risk Factors for Pathogenic Lung Infections

RISK FACTORS FOR INFECTION WITH PENICILLIN-RESISTANT AND DRUG-RESISTANT PNEUMOCOCCI

- Age over 65 years
- Alcoholism
- Beta-lactam therapy (eg, cephalosporins) in past 3 months
- Immunosuppressive disorders
- Multiple medical comorbidities
- Exposure to a child in a day care facility

RISK FACTORS FOR INFECTION WITH ENTERIC GRAM-NEGATIVE BACTERIA

- Residency in a long-term care facility
- Underlying cardiopulmonary disease
- Multiple medical comorbidities
- Recent antibiotic therapy

RISK FACTORS FOR INFECTION WITH *PSEUDOMONAS AERUGINOSA*

- Structural lung disease (eg, bronchiectasis)
- Corticosteroid therapy
- Broad-spectrum antibiotic therapy (more than 7 days in the past month)
- Malnutrition

ime [Zinacef, Ceftin], high-dose amoxicillin or amoxicillin/clavulanate [Augmentin, Clavulin]) plus a macrolide or doxycycline. Also, a beta-lactam agent plus an antipneumococcal fluoroquinolone can be used (File et al., 2004; ICSI, 2003). For older patients with multiple comorbidities, a fluoroquinolone may be preferred. Fluoroquinolones are sometimes reserved for use in higher-risk or drug-intolerant patients to slow the emergence of resistance to this class of antibiotics (File et al., 2004; ICSI, 2003). These are guidelines only; treatment regimens may be modified for individual patients.

For patients with CAP who are hospitalized and do not have cardiopulmonary disease or other significant risk factors, management consists of intravenous (IV) azithromycin or doxycycline plus a beta-lactam agent or monotherapy with an antipneumococcal fluoroquinolone. For inpatients with cardiopulmonary disease or other significant risk factors who are not in the intensive care unit, treatment involves IV ceftriaxone plus azithromycin. For acutely ill patients admitted to the intensive care unit, management includes an IV beta-lactam agent plus either an IV macrolide or fluoroquinolone. In a setting in which MRSA is a potential organism, an IV fluoroquinolone plus vancomycin or linezolid may be administered. For patients at high risk for *P. aeruginosa,* more select antipseudomonal antibiotics are administered by IV.

If specific pathogens responsible for the CAP are identified, more specific agents may be used. Mycoplasma pneumonia is treated with doxycycline or a macrolide. PCP responds best to pentamidine (Pentacarinat, NebuPent) or trimethoprim–sulfamethoxazole (TMP-SMZ [Bactrim, Septra]). Amantadine (Symmetrel) and rimantadine (Flumadine) are effective with influenza type A, and zanamivir and oseltamivir are effective with influenza type A/B. These medications have been shown to reduce the duration of fever and other systemic complications when administered within 24 to 48 hours of the onset of an uncomplicated influenza infection (CDC, 2004e). These medications also reduce the duration and quantity of virus shed in the respiratory secretions. They are most effective when used in combination with influenza vaccine. Ganciclovir (Cytovene, Vitrasert) is used to treat cytomegalovirus in patients who do not have AIDS; cytomegalovirus immunoglobulin may also be used.

HAP has a different etiology from CAP. In suspected HAP or nosocomial pneumonia, empiric treatment is usually initiated with a broad-spectrum IV antibiotic and may be monotherapy or combination therapy. In patients who are mildly to moderately ill with a low risk of *Pseudomonas* infection, the following antibiotics may be used: second-generation cephalosporins (eg, cefuroxime [Ceftin, Zinacef], cefamandole [Mandol]), nonpseudomonal third-generation cephalosporins (ceftriaxone [Rocephin], cefotaxime [Claforan], ampicillin-sulbactam [Unasyn]), fluoroquinolones (eg, ciprofloxacin [Cipro], levofloxacin [Levaquin]), or a carbapenem (meropenem [Merrem]). For combination therapy, any of these may be used with an aminoglycoside.

For patients who are at high risk for *Pseudomonas* infection, an antipseudomonal penicillin plus an aminoglycoside (amikacin [Amikin], gentamicin) or a beta-lactamase inhibitor (ampicillin/sulbactam [Unasyn], ticarcillin/clavulanate [Timentin]) may be used. Other types of combination therapy may also be used, depending on patient characteristics.

For patients with MRSA infection, vancomycin (Vancocin) or linezolid (Zyvox) is used. For patients with methicillin-sensitive *S. aureus,* nafcillin (Unipen), clindamycin (Cleocin), or linezolid (Zyvox) may be used.

Of concern is the rampant rise in respiratory pathogens that are resistant to available antibiotics. Examples include vancomycin-resistant enterococcus (VRE), MRSA, and drug-resistant *S. pneumoniae.* There is a tendency for clinicians to use antibiotics aggressively and inappropriately; they may use broad-spectrum agents when narrow-spectrum agents are more appropriate. Mechanisms to monitor and minimize the inappropriate use of antibiotics are in place. Education of clinicians about the use of evidence-based guidelines in the treatment of respiratory infection is important, and some institutions have implemented algorithms to assist clinicians in making the appropriate choice of antibiotics. Monitoring and surveillance of susceptibility patterns for pathogens are also important.

Usually, therapy with parenteral agents is changed to oral antimicrobial agents when there is evidence of a clinical response and patients are stable and able to tolerate oral medications. The recommended duration of treatment for pneumococcal pneumonia is 72 hours after the patient become afebrile. Patients with most other forms of pneumonia caused by bacterial pathogens are treated for 1 to 2 weeks after they become afebrile. Those with atypical pneumonia (eg, *Legionella*, *M. pneumoniae*) are usually treated for 10 to 21 days.

Other Therapeutic Regimens

Antibiotics are ineffective in viral upper respiratory tract infections and pneumonia, and their use may be associated with adverse effects. Treatment of viral infections with antibiotics is a major reason for the overuse of these medications in the United States. Antibiotics are indicated with a viral respiratory infection *only* if a secondary bacterial pneumonia, bronchitis, or sinusitis is present. With the exception of the use of antimicrobial therapy, treatment of viral pneumonia is the same as that for bacterial pneumonia.

Treatment of viral pneumonia is primarily supportive. Hydration is a necessary part of therapy, because fever and tachypnea may result in insensible fluid losses. Antipyretics may be used to treat headache and fever; antitussive medications may be used for the associated cough. Warm, moist inhalations are helpful in relieving bronchial irritation. Antihistamines may provide benefit with reduced sneezing and rhinorrhea. Nasal decongestants may also be used to treat symptoms and improve sleep; however, excessive use can cause rebound nasal congestion. Bed rest is prescribed until the infection shows signs of clearing. If the patient is hospitalized, he or she is observed carefully until the clinical condition improves.

If hypoxemia develops, oxygen is administered. Pulse oximetry or arterial blood gas analysis is performed to determine the need for oxygen and to evaluate the effectiveness of the therapy. Arterial blood gases may be used to obtain a baseline measure of the patient's oxygenation and acid–base status; however, pulse oximetry is used to continuously monitor the patient's oxygen saturation and response to therapy. A high concentration of oxygen is contraindicated in the patient with COPD because it may worsen alveolar ventilation by decreasing the patient's ventilatory drive, leading to further respiratory decompensation. More aggressive respiratory support measures include administration of high concentrations of oxygen (fraction of inspired oxygen [FIO_2]), endotracheal intubation, and mechanical ventilation. Different modes of mechanical ventilation may be required; see Chapter 25. Figure 23-3 provides an example of a treatment algorithm for patients with suspected CAP.

Gerontologic Considerations

Pneumonia in elderly patients may occur as a primary diagnosis or as a complication of a chronic disease process. Pulmonary infections in older people frequently are difficult to treat and result in a higher mortality rate than in younger people. General deterioration, weakness, abdominal symptoms, anorexia, confusion, tachycardia, and tachypnea may signal the onset of pneumonia. The diagnosis of pneumonia may be missed because the classic symptoms of cough, chest pain, sputum production, and fever may be absent or masked in elderly patients. Also, the presence of some signs may be misleading. Abnormal breath sounds, for example, may be caused by microatelectasis that occurs as a result of decreased mobility, decreased lung volumes, or other respiratory function changes. It may be necessary to obtain chest x-rays to differentiate chronic heart failure, which is often seen in the elderly, from pneumonia as the cause of clinical signs and symptoms.

Supportive treatment includes hydration (with caution and with frequent assessment because of the risk of fluid overload in the elderly), supplemental oxygen therapy, and assistance with deep breathing, coughing, frequent position changes, and early ambulation. All of these are particularly important in the care of elderly patients with pneumonia. To reduce or prevent serious complications of pneumonia in the elderly, vaccination against pneumococcal and influenza infections is recommended.

Complications

Shock and Respiratory Failure

Severe complications of pneumonia include hypotension and shock and respiratory failure (especially with gram-negative bacterial disease in elderly patients). These complications are encountered chiefly in patients who have received no specific treatment or inadequate or delayed treatment. These complications are also encountered when the infecting organism is resistant to therapy, when a comorbid disease complicates the pneumonia, or when the patient is immunocompromised.

If the patient is seriously ill, aggressive therapy may include hemodynamic and ventilatory support to combat peripheral collapse, maintain arterial blood pressure, and provide adequate oxygenation. A vasopressor agent may be administered by continuous IV infusion and at a rate adjusted in accordance with the pressure response. Corticosteroids may be administered parenterally to combat shock and toxicity in patients who are extremely ill with pneumonia and at apparent risk for death from the infection. Patients may require endotracheal intubation and mechanical ventilation. Heart failure, cardiac dysrhythmias, pericarditis, and myocarditis also are complications of pneumonia that may lead to shock.

Atelectasis and Pleural Effusion

Atelectasis (from obstruction of a bronchus or small airways by accumulated secretions) may occur at any stage of acute pneumonia. Parapneumonic pleural effusions occur in at least 40% of bacterial pneumonias. A parapneumonic effusion is any pleural effusion associated with bacterial pneumonia, lung abscess, or bronchiectasis. After the pleural effusion is detected on a chest x-ray, a thoracentesis may be performed to remove the fluid. The fluid is sent to the laboratory for analysis. There are three stages of parapneumonic pleural effusions based on pathogenesis: uncomplicated, complicated, and thoracic empyema. An **empyema** occurs when thick, purulent fluid accumulates within the pleural space, often with fibrin development and a loculated (walled-off) area where the infection is located (see later discussion). A chest tube may be inserted to treat pleural infection by establishing proper drainage of the empyema. Sterilization of the empyema cavity requires 4 to 6 weeks of antibiotics. Frequently used antibiotics include clindamycin (Cleocin), meropenem (Merrem), or piperacillin/tazobactam (Zosyn). Sometimes surgical management is required.

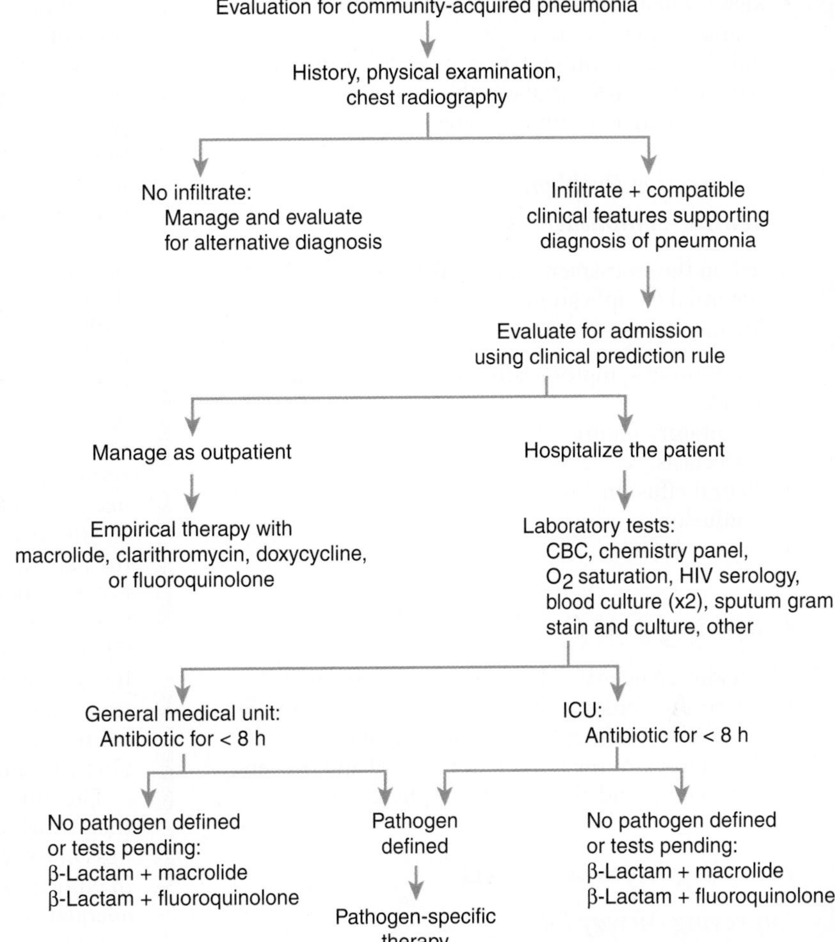
Evaluation for community-acquired pneumonia
History, physical examination, chest radiography
No infiltrate: Manage and evaluate for alternative diagnosis
Infiltrate + compatible clinical features supporting diagnosis of pneumonia
Evaluate for admission using clinical prediction rule
Manage as outpatient
Hospitalize the patient
Empirical therapy with macrolide, clarithromycin, doxycycline, or fluoroquinolone
Laboratory tests: CBC, chemistry panel, O2 saturation, HIV serology, blood culture (x2), sputum gram stain and culture, other
General medical unit: Antibiotic for < 8 h
ICU: Antibiotic for < 8 h
No pathogen defined or tests pending: β-Lactam + macrolide β-Lactam + fluoroquinolone
Pathogen defined
Pathogen-specific therapy
No pathogen defined or tests pending: β-Lactam + macrolide β-Lactam + fluoroquinolone

FIGURE 23-3. Example of a treatment algorithm for patient with suspected community-acquired pneumonia (CAP). From Bartlett, J. G., Dowell, S. F., Mandell, F. A., et al. (2000). Practice guidelines for the management of community-acquired pneumonia in adults. *Clinical Infectious Diseases, 31*(2), 347–382.

Superinfection

Superinfection may occur with the administration of very large doses of antibiotics, such as penicillin, or with combinations of antibiotics. Superinfection may also occur in patients who have been receiving numerous courses and types of antibiotics. In such cases, bacteria may become resistant to the antibiotic therapy. If the patient improves and fever decreases after initial antibiotic therapy, but subsequently a rise in temperature occurs with increasing cough and evidence that the pneumonia has spread, a superinfection is likely. Antibiotics are changed appropriately or discontinued entirely in some cases to reevaluate the causative organisms, antibiotic resistance, and sensitivity.

Nursing Process

The Patient With Pneumonia

Assessment

Nursing assessment is critical in detecting pneumonia. Fever, chills, or night sweats in a patient who also has respiratory symptoms should alert the nurse to the possibility of bacterial pneumonia. Respiratory assessment further identifies the clinical manifestations of pneumonia: pleuritic-type pain, fatigue, tachypnea, use of accessory muscles for breathing, bradycardia or relative bradycardia, coughing, and purulent sputum. The nurse monitors the patient for the following:

- Changes in temperature and pulse
- Amount, odor, and color of secretions
- Frequency and severity of cough
- Degree of tachypnea or shortness of breath
- Changes in physical assessment findings (primarily assessed by inspecting and auscultating the chest)
- Changes in the chest x-ray findings

In addition, it is important to assess elderly patients for unusual behavior, altered mental status, dehydration, excessive fatigue, and concomitant heart failure.

Diagnosis

Nursing Diagnoses

Based on the assessment data, the major nursing diagnoses may include the following:

- Ineffective airway clearance related to copious tracheobronchial secretions
- Activity intolerance related to impaired respiratory function

- Risk for deficient fluid volume related to fever and a rapid respiratory rate
- Imbalanced nutrition: less than body requirements
- Deficient knowledge about the treatment regimen and preventive health measures

Collaborative Problems/ Potential Complications

Based on the assessment data, collaborative problems or potential complications that may occur include the following:

- Continuing symptoms after initiation of therapy
- Shock
- Respiratory failure
- Atelectasis
- Pleural effusion
- Confusion
- Superinfection

Planning and Goals

The major goals may include improved airway patency, rest to conserve energy, maintenance of proper fluid volume, maintenance of adequate nutrition, an understanding of the treatment protocol and preventive measures, and absence of complications.

Nursing Interventions

Improving Airway Patency

Removing secretions is important, because retained secretions interfere with gas exchange and may slow recovery. The nurse encourages hydration (2 to 3 L/day), because adequate hydration thins and loosens pulmonary secretions. Hydration must be achieved more slowly and with careful monitoring in patients with preexisting conditions, such as heart failure. Humidification may be used to loosen secretions and improve ventilation. A high-humidity face mask (using either compressed air or oxygen) delivers warm, humidified air to the tracheobronchial tree, helps to liquefy secretions, and relieves tracheobronchial irritation. Coughing can be initiated either voluntarily or by reflex. Lung expansion maneuvers, such as deep breathing with an incentive spirometer, may induce a cough. A directed cough may be necessary to improve airway patency. The nurse encourages the patient to perform an effective, directed cough, which includes correct positioning, a deep inspiratory maneuver, glottic closure, contraction of the expiratory muscles against the closed glottis, sudden glottic opening, and an explosive expiration. In some cases, the nurse may assist the patient by placing both hands on the lower rib cage (either anteriorly or posteriorly) to focus the patient on a slow deep breath, and then manually assisting the patient by applying constant, external pressure during the expiratory phase.

Chest physiotherapy (percussion and postural drainage) is important in loosening and mobilizing secretions (see Chapter 25). Indications for chest physiotherapy include sputum retention not responsive to spontaneous or directed cough, a history of pulmonary problems previously treated with chest physiotherapy, continued evidence of retained secretions (decreased or abnormal breath sounds, change in vital signs), abnormal chest x-ray findings consistent with atelectasis or infiltrates, and deterioration in oxygenation. The patient is placed in the proper position to drain the involved lung segments, and then the chest is percussed and vibrated either manually or with a mechanical percussor. Other devices, such as the Flutter device (Axcan Pharma), assist in secretion removal. The nurse may consult the respiratory therapy department for volume-expansion protocols and secretion-management protocols that help direct the respiratory care of the patient and match the patient's needs with appropriate treatment schedules.

After each position change, the nurse encourages the patient to breathe deeply and cough. If the patient is too weak to cough effectively, the nurse may need to remove the mucus by nasotracheal suctioning (see Chapter 25). It may take time for secretions to mobilize and move into the central airways for expectoration. Therefore, it is important for the nurse to monitor the patient for cough and sputum production after the completion of chest physiotherapy.

The nurse also administers and titrates oxygen therapy as prescribed or via protocols. The effectiveness of oxygen therapy is monitored by improvement in clinical signs and symptoms, patient comfort, and adequate oxygenation values as measured by pulse oximetry or arterial blood gas analysis.

Promoting Rest and Conserving Energy

The nurse encourages the debilitated patient to rest and avoid overexertion and possible exacerbation of symptoms. The patient should assume a comfortable position to promote rest and breathing (eg, semi-Fowler's position) and should change positions frequently to enhance secretion clearance and ventilation and perfusion in the lungs. It is important to instruct outpatients not to overexert themselves and to engage in only moderate activity during the initial phases of treatment.

Promoting Fluid Intake

The respiratory rate of patients with pneumonia increases because of the increased workload imposed by labored breathing and fever. An increased respiratory rate leads to an increase in insensible fluid loss during exhalation and can lead to dehydration. Therefore, it is important to encourage increased fluid intake (at least 2 L/day), unless contraindicated.

Maintaining Nutrition

Many patients with shortness of breath and fatigue have a decreased appetite and consume only fluids. Fluids with electrolytes (commercially available drinks, such as Gatorade) may help provide fluid, calories, and electrolytes. Other nutritionally enriched drinks or shakes may be helpful. In addition, IV fluids and nutrients may be administered if necessary.

Promoting Patients' Knowledge

The patient and family are instructed about the cause of pneumonia, management of symptoms of pneumonia, signs and symptoms that should be reported to the physician or nurse, and the need for follow-up. The patient also needs information about factors (both patient risk factors and external factors) that may have contributed to development of pneumonia and strategies to promote recovery and prevent recurrence. If the patient is hospitalized, he or she is instructed about the purpose and importance of management strategies that have been implemented and about the importance of adhering to them during and after the hospital stay. Explanations should be given simply and in language that the patient can understand. If possible, written instructions and information should be provided, and alternative formats should be provided for patients with hearing or vision loss, if necessary. Because of the severity of symptoms, the patient may require that instructions and explanations be repeated several times.

Monitoring and Managing Potential Complications

CONTINUING SYMPTOMS AFTER INITIATION OF THERAPY

The patient is observed for response to antibiotic therapy; patients usually begin to respond to treatment within 24 to 48 hours after antibiotic therapy is initiated. If the patient started taking antibiotics before evaluation by culture and sensitivity of the causative organisms, antibiotics may need to be changed once the results are available. The patient is monitored for changes in physical status (deterioration of condition or resolution of symptoms) and for persistent recurrent fever, which may be a result of medication allergy (signaled possibly by a rash); medication resistance or slow response (greater than 48 hours) of the susceptible organism to therapy; superinfection; pleural effusion; or pneumonia caused by an unusual organism, such as *P. jiroveci* or *Aspergillus fumigatus*. Failure of the pneumonia to resolve or persistence of symptoms despite changes on the chest x-ray raises the suspicion of other underlying disorders, such as lung cancer. As previously described, lung cancers may invade or compress airways, causing an obstructive atelectasis that may lead to pneumonia.

In addition to monitoring for continuing symptoms of pneumonia, the nurse also monitors for other complications, such as shock and multisystem failure and atelectasis, which may develop during the first few days of antibiotic treatment.

SHOCK AND RESPIRATORY FAILURE

The nurse assesses for signs and symptoms of shock and respiratory failure by evaluating the patient's vital signs, pulse oximetry values, and hemodynamic monitoring parameters. The nurse reports signs of deteriorating patient status and assists in administering IV fluids and medications prescribed to combat shock. Intubation and mechanical ventilation may be required if respiratory failure occurs. Shock is described in detail in Chapter 15, and care of the patient receiving mechanical ventilation is described in Chapter 25.

ATELECTASIS AND PLEURAL EFFUSION

The patient is assessed for atelectasis, and preventive measures are initiated to prevent its development. If pleural effusion develops and thoracentesis is performed to remove fluid, the nurse assists in the procedure and explains it to the patient. After thoracentesis, the nurse monitors the patient for pneumothorax or recurrence of pleural effusion. If a chest tube needs to be inserted, the nurse monitors the patient's respiratory status (see Chapter 25 for more information on care of patients with chest tubes).

SUPERINFECTION

The patient is monitored for manifestations of superinfection (ie, minimal improvement in signs and symptoms, increase in temperature with increasing cough, increasing fremitus and adventitious breath sounds on auscultation of the lungs). These signs are reported, and the nurse assists in implementing therapy to treat superinfection.

CONFUSION

A patient with pneumonia is assessed for confusion and other more subtle changes in cognitive status. Confusion and changes in cognitive status resulting from pneumonia are poor prognostic signs. Confusion may be related to hypoxemia, fever, dehydration, sleep deprivation, or developing sepsis. The patient's underlying comorbid conditions may also play a part in the development of confusion. Addressing the underlying factors and ensuring patient safety are important nursing interventions.

Promoting Home and Community-Based Care

TEACHING PATIENTS SELF-CARE

Depending on the severity of the pneumonia, treatment may occur in the hospital or in the outpatient setting. Patient education is crucial regardless of the setting, and the proper administration of antibiotics is important. In some instances, the patient may be initially treated with IV antibiotics as an inpatient and then discharged to continue the IV antibiotics at home. It is important that a seamless system of care be maintained for the patient from hospital to home; this includes communication between the nurses caring for the patient in both settings.

If oral antibiotics are prescribed, it is important to teach the patient about their proper administration and potential side effects. The patient should be instructed about symptoms that require contacting the health care provider: difficulty breathing, worsening cough, recurrent/increasing fever, and medication intolerance.

After the fever subsides, the patient may gradually increase activities. Fatigue and weakness may be prolonged after pneumonia, especially in the elderly. The nurse encourages breathing exercises to promote secretion clearance and volume expansion. A patient who is being treated as an outpatient should be contacted by the health care team or instructed to contact the health care provider 24 to 48 hours after starting therapy. The patient is also instructed to return to the clinic or physician's office for a follow-up chest x-ray and physical examination. Often improvement in chest x-ray findings lags behind improvement in clinical signs and symptoms.

The nurse encourages the patient to stop smoking. Smoking inhibits tracheobronchial ciliary action, which is the first line of defense of the lower respiratory tract. Smoking also irritates the mucous cells of the bronchi and inhibits the function of alveolar macrophage (scavenger) cells. The patient is instructed to avoid stress, fatigue, sudden changes in temperature, and excessive alcohol intake, all of which lower resistance to pneumonia. The nurse reviews with the patient the principles of adequate nutrition and rest, because one episode of pneumonia may make a patient susceptible to recurring respiratory tract infections.

CONTINUING CARE

A patient who is severely debilitated or who cannot care for himself or herself may require referral for home care. During home visits, the nurse assesses the patient's physical status, monitors for complications, assesses the home environment, and reinforces previ-

NURSING RESEARCH PROFILE

Tobacco-Related Nursing Interventions

Ratner, P. A., Johnson, J. L., Richardson, C. G., et al. (2004). Efficacy of a smoking-cessation intervention for elective-surgical patients. *Research in Nursing & Health, 27*(3), 148–161.

Purpose

Smoking remains a major cause of morbidity and mortality in the United States. The purpose of this study was to evaluate a smoking-cessation intervention for elective surgical patients to determine whether patients could (1) abstain from cigarette use just prior to surgery, (2) sustain abstinence from tobacco in the postoperative period, and (3) maintain long-term 12-month post-surgery abstinence.

Design

This randomized, pretest-posttest study targeted patients admitted for presurgical assessment who smoked tobacco. Variables assessed were smoking status, smoking-cessation self-efficacy, smoking stage of change, demographic and personal information, smoking history/nicotine dependence, and psychological state. There were 120 subjects in the control group and 117 in the intervention group. Subjects in the intervention group received the following:

- A 15-minute counseling session in the preoperative assessment clinic, including one-on-one counseling, written information, nicotine replacement therapy, and phone numbers for assistance/information
- Nurse visitation within 24 hours after surgery (or when stable) for provision of reinforcement information regarding smoking cessation
- Telephone contact approximately 1 week later and weekly thereafter
- Final telephone contact to provide educational information at 16 weeks after discharge
- Telephone contact at 6 and 12 months regarding smoking habits

Subjects assigned to the control group received routine care and were seen by the study nurse immediately after surgery and contacted by telephone at 6 and 12 months.

Findings

Subjects in the intervention group were more likely to abstain from smoking prior to surgery ($P = .003$) than subjects in the control group and were more likely to abstain from smoking at 6 months after surgery (31.2% versus 20.2%; however, the unadjusted effect of treatment was not statistically significant). There was no significant difference in the abstinence rates at 12 months in subjects in the two groups (18.8% versus 19.2%).

Nursing Implications

Nurses have frequent contacts with active smokers in inpatient and outpatient settings. Therefore, nurses could have a tremendous impact on smoking prevention and cessation. This study demonstrates that educating patients prior to surgery may be an excellent strategy to begin the process of smoking cessation. In addition, these results show that continued contact and support with patients may increase the probability of cessation. Nurses need advanced education regarding evidence-based guidelines for smoking cessation techniques. Nurses need to raise the issue of tobacco use with patients, discuss smoking cessation, and provide potential resources that are accessible to patients.

ous teaching. The nurse evaluates the patient's adherence to the therapeutic regimen (ie, taking medications as prescribed, performing breathing exercises, consuming adequate fluid and dietary intake, and avoiding smoking, alcohol, and excessive activity). The nurse stresses to the patient and family the importance of monitoring for complications or exacerbation of the pneumonia. The nurse encourages the patient to obtain an influenza vaccination at the prescribed times, because influenza increases susceptibility to secondary bacterial pneumonia, especially that caused by staphylococci, *H. influenzae*, and *S. pneumoniae* (CDC, 2004e). The nurse also urges the patient to seek medical advice about receiving the vaccine (Pneumovax) against *S. pneumoniae*.

Evaluation

Expected Patient Outcomes

Expected patient outcomes may include the following:

1. Demonstrates improved airway patency, as evidenced by adequate oxygenation by pulse oximetry or arterial blood gas analysis, normal temperature, normal breath sounds, and effective coughing
2. Rests and conserves energy by limiting activities and remaining in bed while symptomatic and then slowly increasing activities
3. Maintains adequate hydration, as evidenced by an adequate fluid intake and urine output and normal skin turgor
4. Consumes adequate dietary intake, as evidenced by maintenance or increase in body weight without excess fluid gain
5. States explanation for management strategies
6. Complies with management strategies
7. Exhibits no complications
    a. Exhibits acceptable vital signs, pulse oximetry, and arterial blood gas measurements
    b. Reports productive cough that diminishes over time
    c. Has absence of signs or symptoms of shock, respiratory failure, or pleural effusion
    d. Remains oriented and aware of surroundings
    e. Maintains or increases weight
8. Complies with treatment protocol and prevention strategies

Severe Acute Respiratory Syndrome

Severe acute respiratory syndrome (SARS) is a viral respiratory illness caused by a coronavirus, called SARS-associated coronavirus (Denison, 2004). SARS was first reported in Asia in February 2003. The illness quickly spread to countries in North America, South America, Europe, and Asia. The World Health Organization (WHO) reported that 8098 people worldwide became sick with SARS during the 2003 outbreak, and 774 died (CDC, 2004c).

The SARS-associated coronavirus is transmitted via respiratory droplets when an infected person coughs or sneezes; the droplets may be deposited on the mucous membranes (mouth, nose, eyes) of a nearby person. The virus may also be spread when a person touches a surface or object contaminated by the droplets and then touches his or her mucous membranes. The SARS virus may be transmitted in other ways, but those methods of transmission are unknown at this time.

The constellation of symptoms characteristic of SARS are a high fever in association with headache, overall discomfort, and body aches. Mild respiratory symptoms may also be present. Approximately 10% to 20% of patients develop diarrhea. After 2 to 7 days, a dry cough may develop, which often includes progressive hypoxemia and subsequent pneumonia. Based on available information, SARS is most likely to be contagious only when symptoms are present; patients are most contagious during the second week of illness. It is recommended that people with SARS limit interactions outside the home until 10 days after the fever is no longer present and respiratory symptoms have improved. At this time, treatment of SARS is the same for a severe community-acquired atypical pneumonia (CDC, 2004c).

Infection control measures designed to limit transmission of SARS are a priority. In health care settings, the general CDC guidelines for infection control in health care facilities should be followed; in addition, specific strategies for SARS should be in place regarding use of negative pressure isolation rooms, personal protective equipment, hand hygiene, environmental cleaning and disinfection techniques, and source control measures to contain patients' secretions (CDC, 2003a; Levy, Baylor, Bernard, et al., 2005).

Pulmonary Tuberculosis

Tuberculosis (TB) is an infectious disease that primarily affects the lung parenchyma. It also may be transmitted to other parts of the body, including the meninges, kidneys, bones, and lymph nodes. The primary infectious agent, *M. tuberculosis,* is an acid-fast aerobic rod that grows slowly and is sensitive to heat and ultraviolet light. *Mycobacterium bovis* and *Mycobacterium avium* have rarely been associated with the development of a TB infection.

TB is a worldwide public health problem, and mortality and morbidity rates continue to rise. *M. tuberculosis* infects an estimated one third of the world's population and remains the leading cause of death from infectious disease in the world. The World Health Organization estimates that TB is the cause of death for 11% of all patients with AIDS (Corbett, Walt, Walker, et al., 2003). TB is closely associated with poverty, malnutrition, overcrowding, substandard housing, and inadequate health care.

In 1952, anti-TB medications were introduced, and the rate of reported cases of TB in the United States declined an average of 6% each year between 1953 and 1985. It was thought that, by the early part of the 21st century, TB might be eliminated in the United States. However, since 1985 the trend has reversed, and the number of cases has increased. This change has been attributed to several factors, including increased immigration, the human immunodeficiency virus (HIV) epidemic, the emergence of multidrug-resistant strains of TB, increased homelessness, decreased interest and detection by health care providers, and inadequate funding of the United States public health system. Almost 15,000 cases of TB are reported annually to the CDC (2005). Progress toward TB elimination in the United States focuses on programs that provide services to foreign-born persons with latent TB infection, collaborative efforts that reduce the burden of TB globally, and intensified TB control efforts that address higher rates in the population of non-Hispanic blacks born in the United States (CDC, 2003c).

Transmission and Risk Factors

TB spreads from person to person by airborne transmission. An infected person releases droplet nuclei (usually particles 1 to 5 μm in diameter) through talking, coughing, sneezing, laughing, or singing. Larger droplets settle; smaller droplets remain suspended in the air and are inhaled by a susceptible person. Risk factors for TB are listed in Chart 23-3.

CHART 23-3

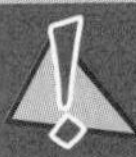

Risk Factors for Tuberculosis

- Close contact with someone who has active TB. Inhalation of airborne nuclei from an infected person is proportional to the amount of time spent in the same air space, the proximity of the person, and the degree of ventilation.
- Immunocompromised status (eg, those with HIV infection, cancer, transplanted organs, and prolonged high-dose corticosteroid therapy)
- Substance abuse (IV/injection drug users and alcoholics)
- Any person without adequate health care (the homeless; impoverished; minorities, particularly children under age 15 y and young adults between ages 15 and 44 y)
- Preexisting medical conditions or special treatment (eg, diabetes, chronic renal failure, malnourishment, selected malignancies, hemodialysis, transplanted organ, gastrectomy, jejunoileal bypass)
- Immigration from countries with a high prevalence of TB (southeastern Asia, Africa, Latin America, Caribbean)
- Institutionalization (eg, long-term care facilities, psychiatric institutions, prisons)
- Living in overcrowded, substandard housing
- Being a health care worker performing high-risk activities: administration of aerosolized pentamidine and other medications, sputum induction procedures, bronchoscopy, suctioning, coughing procedures, caring for the immunosuppressed patient, home care with the high-risk population, and administering anesthesia, and related procedures (eg, intubation, suctioning)

Chart 23-4 summarizes the CDC's recommendations for prevention of TB transmission in health care settings.

Pathophysiology

TB begins when a susceptible person inhales mycobacteria and becomes infected. The bacteria are transmitted through the airways to the alveoli, where they are deposited and begin to multiply. The bacilli also are transported via the lymph system and bloodstream to other parts of the body (kidneys, bones, cerebral cortex) and other areas of the lungs (upper lobes). The body's immune system responds by initiating an inflammatory reaction. Phagocytes (neutrophils and macrophages) engulf many of the bacteria, and TB-specific lymphocytes lyse (destroy) the bacilli and normal tissue. This tissue reaction results in the accumulation of exudate in the alveoli, causing bronchopneumonia. The initial infection usually occurs 2 to 10 weeks after exposure.

Granulomas, new tissue masses of live and dead bacilli, are surrounded by macrophages, which form a protective wall. They are then transformed to a fibrous tissue mass, the central portion of which is called a Ghon tubercle. The material (bacteria and macrophages) becomes necrotic, forming a cheesy mass. This mass may become calcified and form a collagenous scar. At this point, the bacteria become dormant, and there is no further progression of active disease.

After initial exposure and infection, active disease may develop because of a compromised or inadequate immune system response. Active disease also may occur with reinfection and activation of dormant bacteria. In this case, the Ghon tubercle ulcerates, releasing the cheesy material into the bronchi. The bacteria then become airborne, resulting in further spread of the disease. Then the ulcerated tubercle heals and forms scar tissue. This causes the infected lung to become more inflamed, resulting in further development of bronchopneumonia and tubercle formation.

Unless the process is arrested, it spreads slowly downward to the hilum of the lungs and later extends to adjacent lobes. The process may be prolonged and is characterized by long remissions when the disease is arrested, followed by periods of renewed activity. Approximately 10% of people who are initially infected develop active disease. Some people develop reactivation TB (also called adult-type TB). This type of TB results from a breakdown of the host defenses. It most commonly occurs in the lungs, usually in the apical or posterior segments of the upper lobes or the superior segments of the lower lobes.

Clinical Manifestations

The signs and symptoms of pulmonary TB are insidious. Most patients have a low-grade fever, cough, night sweats, fatigue, and weight loss. The cough may be nonproductive, or mucopurulent sputum may be expectorated. Hemoptysis also may occur. Both the systemic and the pulmonary symptoms are chronic and may have been present for weeks to months. Elderly patients usually present with less pronounced symptoms than younger patients do. Extrapulmonary disease occurs in up to 16% of cases in the United States. In patients with AIDS, extrapulmonary disease is more prevalent.

CHART 23-4

CDC Recommendations for Preventing Transmission of Tuberculosis in Health Care Settings

1. Early identification and treatment of persons with active TB
   a. Maintain a high index of suspicion for TB to identify cases rapidly.
   b. Promptly initiate effective multidrug anti-TB therapy based on clinical and drug-resistance surveillance data.
2. Prevention of spread of infectious droplet nuclei by source control methods and by reduction of microbial contamination of indoor air
   a. Initiate acid-fast bacilli (AFB) isolation precautions immediately for all patients who are suspected or confirmed to have active TB and who may be infectious. AFB isolation precautions include use of a private room with negative pressure in relation to surrounding areas and a minimum of six air exchanges per hour. Air from the room should be exhausted directly to the outside. Use of ultraviolet lamps and/or high-efficiency particulate air filters to supplement ventilation may be considered.
   b. Persons entering the AFB isolation room should use disposable particulate respirators that fit snugly around the face.
   c. Continue AFB isolation precautions until there is clinical evidence of reduced infectiousness (ie, cough has substantially decreased, and the number of organisms on sequential sputum smears is decreasing). If drug resistance is suspected or confirmed, continue AFB precautions until the sputum smear is negative for AFB.
   d. Use special precautions during cough-inducing procedures.
3. Surveillance for TB transmission
   a. Maintain surveillance for TB infection among health care workers (HCWs) by routine, periodic tuberculin skin testing. Recommend appropriate preventive therapy for HCWs when indicated.
   b. Maintain surveillance for TB cases among patients and HCWs.
   c. Promptly initiate contact investigation procedures among HCWs, patients, and visitors exposed to an untreated, or ineffectively treated, patient with infectious TB for whom appropriate AFB procedures are not in place. Recommend appropriate therapy or preventive therapy for contacts with disease or TB infection without current disease. Therapeutic regimens should be chosen based on the clinical history and local drug-resistance surveillance data.

Assessment and Diagnostic Findings

A complete history, physical examination, tuberculin skin test, chest x-ray, acid-fast bacillus smear, and sputum culture are used to diagnose TB. If the patient is infected with TB, the chest x-ray usually reveals lesions in the upper lobes, and the acid-fast bacillus smear contains mycobacteria.

Tuberculin Skin Test

The Mantoux test is used to determine whether a person has been infected with the TB bacillus. The Mantoux test is a standardized procedure and should be performed only by those trained in its administration and reading. Tubercle bacillus extract (tuberculin), purified protein derivative (PPD), is injected into the intradermal layer of the inner aspect of the forearm, approximately 4 inches below the elbow (Fig. 23-4). Intermediate-strength PPD, in a tuberculin syringe with a half-inch 26- or 27-gauge needle, is used. The needle, with the bevel facing up, is inserted beneath the skin. Then 0.1 mL of PPD is injected, creating an elevation in the skin, a wheal or bleb. The site, antigen name, strength, lot number, date, and time of the test are recorded. The test result is read 48 to 72 hours after injection. Tests read after 72 hours tend to underestimate the true size of **induration** (hardening). A delayed localized reaction indicates that the person is sensitive to tuberculin.

A reaction occurs when both induration and erythema (redness) are present. After the area is inspected for induration, it is lightly palpated across the injection site, from the area of normal skin to the margins of the induration. The diameter of the induration (not erythema) is measured in millimeters at its widest part (see Fig. 23-4), and the size of the induration is documented. Erythema without induration is not considered significant.

Interpretation of Results

The size of the induration determines the significance of the reaction. A reaction of 0 to 4 mm is considered not significant; a reaction of 5 mm or greater may be significant in people who are considered to be at risk. An induration of 10 mm or greater is usually considered significant in people who have normal or mildly impaired immunity. A significant reaction indicates past exposure to *M. tuberculosis* or vaccination with bacille Calmette-Guérin (BCG) vaccine. The BCG vaccine is given to produce a greater resistance to development of TB. It is effective in up to 76% of people who receive it. The BCG vaccine is used in Europe and Latin America but not routinely in the United States.

A reaction of 5 mm or greater is defined as positive in patients who are HIV-positive or have HIV risk factors and are of unknown HIV status; in those who are close contacts

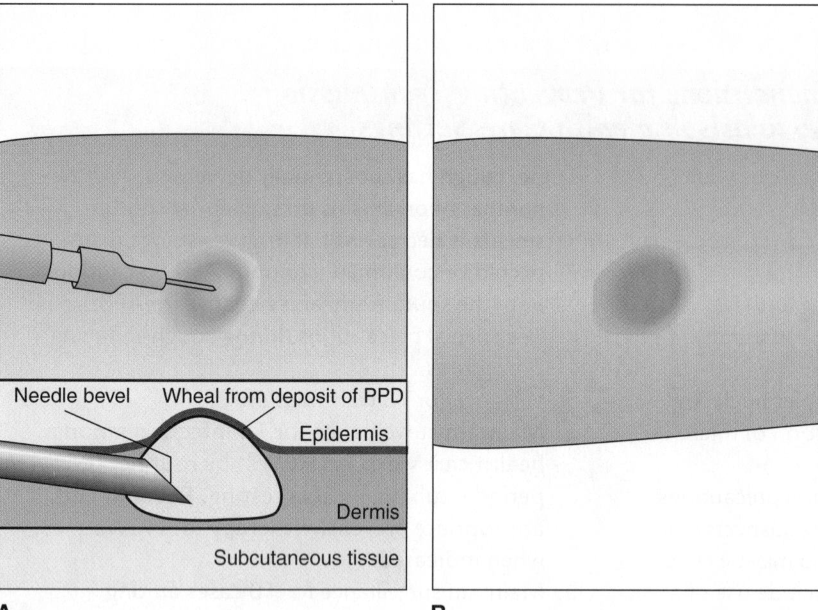

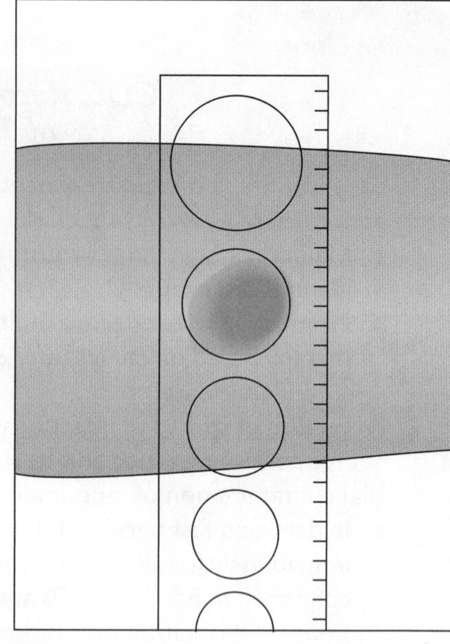

FIGURE 23-4. The Mantoux test for tuberculosis. (**A**) Correct technique for inserting the needle involves depositing the PPD subcutaneously with the needle bevel facing upward. (**B**) The reaction to the Mantoux test usually consists of a wheal, a hivelike, firm welt. (**C**) To determine the extent of the reaction, the wheal is measured using a commercially prepared gauge. Interpretation of the Mantoux test is discussed in the text.

of someone with active TB; and in those who have chest x-ray results consistent with TB.

A significant (positive) reaction does not necessarily mean that active disease is present in the body. More than 90% of people who are tuberculin-significant reactors do not develop clinical TB. However, all significant reactors are candidates for active TB. In general, the more intense the reaction, the greater the likelihood of an active infection.

A nonsignificant (negative) skin test does not exclude TB infection or disease, because patients who are immunosuppressed cannot develop an immune response that is adequate to produce a positive skin test. This is referred to as anergy.

QuantiFERON-TB Gold (QFT-G) Test

In 2005, the U.S. Food and Drug Administration approved a new test for the detection of TB. The QuantiFERON-TB Gold (QFT-G) test is an enzyme-linked immunosorbent assay (ELISA) that detects the release of interferon-gamma by white blood cells when the blood of a patient with TB is incubated with peptides similar to those in *M. tuberculosis*. The results of the QFT-G test are available in less than 24 hours and are not affected by prior vaccination with BCG. The test results are also less influenced than those of TST by previous infection with nontuberculous mycobacteria. The CDC has recommended that the QFT-G be used in place of, rather than in addition to, the TST, although the new test is not yet widely used. Additional studies of the QFT-G test are under way to evaluate the use of this new diagnostic test (CDC, 2005).

Classification

Data from the history, physical examination, TB test, chest x-ray, and microbiologic studies are used to classify TB into one of five classes. A classification scheme provides public health officials with a systematic way to monitor epidemiology and treatment of the disease (American Thoracic Society, 2000).

- Class 0: no exposure; no infection
- Class 1: exposure; no evidence of infection
- Class 2: latent infection; no disease (eg, positive PPD reaction but no clinical evidence of active TB)
- Class 3: disease; clinically active
- Class 4: disease; not clinically active
- Class 5: suspected disease; diagnosis pending

Gerontologic Considerations

TB may have atypical manifestations in elderly patients, whose symptoms may include unusual behavior and altered mental status, fever, anorexia, and weight loss. In many elderly patients, the tuberculin skin test produces no reaction (loss of immunologic memory) or delayed reactivity for up to 1 week (recall phenomenon). A second skin test is performed in 1 to 2 weeks.

Medical Management

Pulmonary TB is treated primarily with chemotherapeutic agents (antituberculosis agents) for 6 to 12 months. A prolonged treatment duration is necessary to ensure eradication of the organisms and to prevent relapse. The continuing (since the 1950s) and increasing resistance of *M. tuberculosis* to TB medications is a worldwide concern and challenge in TB therapy. Several types of drug resistance must be considered when planning effective therapy:

- Primary drug resistance: resistance to one of the first-line antituberculosis agents in people who have not had previous treatment
- Secondary or acquired drug resistance: resistance to one or more antituberculosis agents in patients undergoing therapy
- Multidrug resistance: resistance to two agents, isoniazid (INH) and rifampin. The populations at greatest risk for multidrug resistance are those who are HIV-positive, institutionalized, or homeless.

The increasing prevalence of drug resistance points out the need to begin TB treatment with four or more medications, to ensure completion of therapy, and to develop and evaluate new anti-TB medications.

Pharmacologic Therapy

In current TB therapy, four first-line medications are used (Table 23-3), INH, rifampin, pyrazinamide, and ethambutol. Combination medications, such as INH and rifampin (Rifamate) or INH, pyrazinamide, and rifampin (Rifater) and medications administered twice a week (eg, rifapentine) are available to help improve patient adherence. Capreomycin, ethionamide, para-aminosalicylate sodium, and cycloserine are second-line medications. Additional potentially effective medications include other aminoglycosides, quinolones, rifabutin, clofazimine, and combinations of medications.

℞ TABLE 23-3 First-Line Antituberculosis Medications

Commonly Used Agents	Adult Daily Dosage*	Most Common Side Effects	Drug Interactions†	Remarks*
Isoniazid (INH)	5 mg/kg (300 mg maximum daily)	Peripheral neuritis, hepatic enzyme elevation, hepatitis, hypersensitivity	Phenytoin—synergistic Antabuse Alcohol	Bactericidal. Pyridoxine is used as prophylaxis for neuritis. Monitor AST and ALT.
Rifampin (Rifadin)	10 mg/kg (600 mg maximum daily)	Hepatitis, febrile reaction, purpura (rare), nausea, vomiting	Rifampin increases metabolism of oral contraceptives, quinidine, corticosteroids, coumarin derivatives and methadone, digoxin, oral hypoglycemics; PAS may interfere with absorption of rifampin.	Bactericidal. Orange urine and other body secretions. Discoloring of contact lenses. Monitor AST and ALT.
Rifabutin (Mycobutin)	5 mg/kg (300 mg maximum daily)			
Rifapentine (Priftin)	10 mg/kg (600 mg twice weekly)	Hepatotoxicity, thrombocytopenia	Avoid protease inhibitors	Orange-red coloration of body secretions, contact lenses, dentures. Use with caution in elderly or in those with renal disease.
Pyrazinamide	15 to 30 mg/kg (2.0 g maximum daily)*	Hyperuricemia, hepatotoxicity, skin rash, arthralgias, GI distress		Bactericidal. Monitor uric acid, AST, ALT.
Ethambutol (Myambutol)	15 to 25 mg/kg (no maximum daily dose, but base on lean body wt)*	Optic neuritis (may lead to blindness; very rare at 15 mg/kg), skin rash		Bacteriostatic. Use with caution with renal disease or when eye testing is not feasible. Monitor visual acuity, color discrimination.‡
Combinations: INH + rifampin (eg, Rifamate)	150-mg & 300-mg caps (2 caps daily)			

*Check product labeling for detailed information on dose, contraindications, drug interaction, adverse reactions, and monitoring.
† Refer to current literature, particularly on rifampin, because it increases hepatic microenzymes and therefore interacts with many drugs.
‡ Initial examination should be performed at start of treatment.

Recommended treatment guidelines for newly diagnosed cases of pulmonary TB (CDC, 2003b) have two parts: an initial treatment phase and a continuation phase. The initial phase consists of a multiple-medication regimen of INH, rifampin, pyrazinamide, and ethambutol. This initial intensive-treatment regimen is administered daily for 8 weeks, after which options for the continuation phase of treatment include INH and rifampin or INH and rifapentine. The continuation course of treatment lasts for an additional 4 or 7 months. The 4-month period is used for the large majority of patients (CDC, 2003b). The 7-month period is recommended for patients with cavitary pulmonary TB whose sputum culture after the initial 2 months of treatment is positive, for those whose initial phase of treatment did not include pyrazinamide (PZA), and for those being treated once weekly with INH and rifapentine whose sputum culture is positive at the end of the initial phase of treatment. People are considered noninfectious after 2 to 3 weeks of continuous medication therapy. Vitamin B (pyridoxine) is usually administered with INH to prevent INH-associated peripheral neuropathy (see Table 23-3). The total number of doses taken, not simply the duration of treatment, more accurately determines whether a course of therapy has been completed.

INH also may be used as a prophylactic (preventive) measure for people who are at risk for significant disease, including

- Household family members of patients with active disease
- Patients with HIV infection who have a PPD test reaction with 5 mm of induration or more
- Patients with fibrotic lesions suggestive of old TB detected on a chest x-ray and a PPD reaction with 5 mm of induration or more
- Patients whose current PPD test results show a change from former test results, suggesting recent exposure to TB and possible infection (skin test converters)
- Users of IV/injection drugs who have PPD test results with 10 mm of induration or more
- Patients with high-risk comorbid conditions and a PPD result with 10 mm of induration or more

Other candidates for preventive INH therapy are those 35 years or younger who have PPD test results with 10 mm of induration or more and one of the following criteria:

- Foreign-born individuals from countries with a high prevalence of TB
- High-risk, medically underserved populations
- Institutionalized patients

Prophylactic INH treatment involves taking daily doses for 6 to 12 months. Liver enzymes, blood urea nitrogen (BUN), and creatinine levels are monitored monthly. Sputum culture results are monitored for acid-fast bacillus to evaluate the effectiveness of treatment and the patient's adherence to the treatment regimen.

In 1998, the federal Advisory Council for the Elimination of Tuberculosis published recommendations for the development of TB vaccines. The recommendations include a focus on a "postinfection vaccine" to prevent people who are infected with TB from developing active disease. To date, this vaccine has not become clinically available. Recommendations regarding the treatment of latent TB infection were released in 2000 and updated in 2003 and 2005 (CDC, 2003b, 2005a). The 2000 recommendations focused on treating latent infections for a shorter period of time. The CDC released case reports of liver injury associated with the 2-month rifampin-pyrazinamide (RIF-PZA) dosing regimen in August 2001. RIF plus PZA is no longer recommended for treatment of latent tuberculosis infection (CDC, 2003b). Nine months of daily INH remains the preferred treatment, and 4 months of daily RIF is an acceptable alternative.

Nursing Process

The Patient With Tuberculosis

Assessment

The nurse performs a complete history and physical examination. Clinical manifestations of fever, anorexia, weight loss, night sweats, fatigue, cough, and sputum production prompt a more thorough assessment of respiratory function—for example, assessing the lungs for consolidation by evaluating breath sounds (diminished, bronchial sounds, crackles), fremitus, egophony, and dullness on percussion. Enlarged, painful lymph nodes may be palpated as well. The nurse also assesses the patient's living arrangements, perceptions and understanding of TB and its treatment, and readiness to learn.

Diagnosis

Nursing Diagnoses

Based on the assessment data, nursing diagnoses may include the following:

- Ineffective airway clearance related to copious tracheobronchial secretions
- Deficient knowledge about treatment regimen and preventive health measures and related ineffective individual management of the therapeutic regimen (noncompliance)
- Activity intolerance related to fatigue, altered nutritional status, and fever

Collaborative Problems/ Potential Complications

Based on the assessment data, collaborative problems or potential complications that may occur include the following:

- Malnutrition
- Adverse side effects of medication therapy: hepatitis, neurologic changes (deafness or neuritis), skin rash, gastrointestinal upset
- Multidrug resistance
- Spread of TB infection (miliary TB)

Planning and Goals

The major goals include maintenance of a patent airway, increased knowledge about the disease and treatment regimen and adherence to the medication regimen, increased activity tolerance, and absence of complications.

Nursing Interventions

Promoting Airway Clearance

Copious secretions obstruct the airways in many patients with TB and interfere with adequate gas exchange. Increasing the fluid intake promotes systemic hydration and serves as an effective expectorant. The nurse instructs the patient about correct positioning to facilitate airway drainage (postural drainage); this is described in Chapter 25.

Advocating Adherence to Treatment Regimen

The multiple-medication regimen that the patient must follow can be quite complex. Understanding of the medications, schedule, and side effects is important. The patient must understand that TB is a communicable disease and that taking medications is the most effective means of preventing transmission. The major reason treatment fails is that patients do not take their medications regularly and for the prescribed duration. The nurse carefully instructs the patient about important hygiene measures, including mouth care, covering the mouth and nose when coughing and sneezing, proper disposal of tissues, and handwashing. The nurse's positive reinforcement and monitoring of the patient's adherence are important follow-up measures.

Promoting Activity and Adequate Nutrition

Patients with TB are often debilitated from prolonged chronic illness and impaired nutritional status. The nurse plans a progressive activity schedule that focuses on increasing activity tolerance and muscle strength. Anorexia, weight loss, and malnutrition are common in patients with TB. The patient's willingness to eat may be altered by fatigue from excessive coughing, sputum production, chest pain, generalized debilitated state, or cost, if the patient has few resources. A nutritional plan that allows for small, frequent meals may be required. Liquid nutritional supplements may assist in meeting basic caloric requirements.

Monitoring and Managing Potential Complications

MALNUTRITION

Malnutrition may be a consequence of the patient's lifestyle, lack of knowledge about adequate nutrition and its role in health maintenance, lack of resources, fatigue, or lack of appetite because of coughing and mucus production. To counter the effects of these factors, the nurse collaborates with the dietitian, physician, social worker, family, and patient to identify strategies to ensure an adequate nutritional intake and availability of nutritious food. Identifying facilities (eg, shelters, soup kitchens, Meals on Wheels) that provide meals in the patient's neighborhood may increase the likelihood that the patient with limited resources and energy will have access to a more nutritious intake. High-calorie nutritional supplements may be suggested as a strategy for increasing dietary intake using food products normally found in the home. Purchasing food supplements may be beyond the patient's budget, but dietitians can help develop recipes to increase caloric intake despite minimal resources.

SIDE EFFECTS OF MEDICATION THERAPY

It is important to assess medication side effects, because they are often a reason why patients fail to adhere to the prescribed medication regimen. Efforts are made to reduce the side effects and to motivate the patient to take the medications as prescribed.

The nurse instructs the patient to take the medication either on an empty stomach or at least 1 hour before meals, because food interferes with medication absorption (although taking medications on an empty stomach frequently results in gastrointestinal upset). Patients taking INH should avoid foods that contain tyramine and histamine (tuna, aged cheese, red wine, soy sauce, yeast extracts), because eating them while taking INH may result in headache, flushing, hypotension, lightheadedness, palpitations, and diaphoresis.

In addition, rifampin can increase the metabolism of certain other medications, making them less effective. These medications include beta-blockers, oral anticoagulants such as warfarin (Coumadin), digoxin, quinidine, corticosteroids, oral hypoglycemic agents, oral contraceptives, theophylline, and verapamil (Calan, Isoptin). This issue should be discussed with the physician and pharmacist so that medication dosages can be adjusted accordingly. The nurse informs the patient that rifampin may discolor contact lenses and that the patient may want to wear eyeglasses during treatment. The nurse monitors for other side effects of anti-TB medications, including hepatitis, neurologic changes (hearing loss, neuritis), and rash. Liver enzymes, BUN, and serum creatinine levels are monitored to detect changes in liver and kidney function. Sputum culture results are monitored for acid-fast bacilli to evaluate the effectiveness of the treatment regimen and adherence to therapy.

MULTIDRUG RESISTANCE

The nurse carefully monitors vital signs and observes for spikes in temperature or changes in the patient's clinical status. Changes in the patient's respiratory status are reported to the primary health care provider. The nurse instructs the patient about the risk of drug resistance if the medication regimen is not strictly and continuously followed.

SPREAD OF TUBERCULOSIS INFECTION

Spread or dissemination of TB infection to nonpulmonary sites of the body is known as miliary TB. It is the result of invasion of the bloodstream by the tubercle bacillus (Ghon tubercle). Usually it results from late reactivation of a dormant infection in the lung or elsewhere. The origin of the bacilli that enter the bloodstream is either a chronic focus that has ulcerated into a blood vessel or multitudes of miliary tubercles lining the inner surface of the thoracic duct. The organisms migrate from these foci into the bloodstream, are carried throughout the body, and disseminate throughout all tissues, with tiny miliary tubercles developing in the lungs, spleen, liver, kidneys, meninges, and other organs.

The clinical course of miliary TB may vary from an acute, rapidly progressive infection with high fever to a slowly developing process with low-grade fever, anemia, and debilitation. At first, there may be no localizing signs except an enlarged spleen and a reduced number of leukocytes. However, within a few weeks, the chest x-ray reveals small densities scattered diffusely throughout both lung fields; these are the miliary tubercles, which gradually grow.

The possibility of spread to nonpulmonary sites in the body requires careful monitoring for this very serious form of TB. The nurse monitors vital signs and observes for spikes in temperature as well as changes in renal and cognitive function. Few physical signs may be elicited on physical examination of the chest, but at this stage the patient has a severe cough and dyspnea. Treatment of miliary TB is the same as for pulmonary TB.

Promoting Home and Community-Based Care

TEACHING PATIENTS SELF-CARE

The nurse plays a vital role in caring for the patient with TB and the family, which includes assessing the patient's ability to continue therapy at home. The nurse instructs the patient and family about infection control procedures, such as proper disposal of tissues, covering the mouth during coughing, and frequent handwashing. Assessment of the patient's adherence to the medication regimen is essential because of the risk of emergence of resistance if the regimen is not followed faithfully. In some cases, when the patient's ability to comply with the medication regimen is in question, referral to an outpatient clinic for daily medication administration may be required. This is referred to as directly observed therapy (DOT).

CONTINUING CARE

The nurse evaluates the patient's environment, including the home or workplace and social setting, to identify other people who may have been in contact with the patient during the infectious stage. It is important to arrange follow-up screening for any such contacts. The nurse who has contact with a patient in the home, shelter, hospital, clinic, or work setting continues to assess the patient's physical and psychological status and ability to adhere to the prescribed treatment. The nurse also assesses the patient for adverse effects of medications and adherence to the therapeutic regimen (eg, taking medications as prescribed, practicing safe hygiene, consuming a nutritious and adequate diet, and participating in an appropriate level of activity). In addition, the nurse reinforces previous teaching, emphasizes the importance of keeping scheduled appointments with the primary health care provider, and reminds the patient about the importance of other health promotion activities and recommended health screening.

Evaluation

Expected Patient Outcomes

Expected patient outcomes may include the following:

1. Maintains a patent airway by managing secretions with hydration, humidification, coughing, and postural drainage
2. Demonstrates an adequate level of knowledge
   a. Lists medications by name and the correct schedule for taking them
   b. Identifies expected side effects of medications
   c. Identifies how and when to contact health care provider
3. Adheres to treatment regimen by taking medications as prescribed and reporting for follow-up screening
4. Participates in preventive measures
   a. Disposes of used tissues properly
   b. Encourages people who are close contacts to undergo testing
   c. Adheres to handwashing or hand hygiene recommendations
5. Maintains activity schedule
6. Exhibits no complications
   a. Maintains adequate weight or gains weight if indicated
   b. Exhibits normal results of tests of liver and kidney function
7. Takes steps to minimize side effects of medications
   a. Takes supplemental vitamins (vitamin B), as prescribed, to minimize peripheral neuropathy
   b. Avoids use of alcohol
   c. Avoids foods containing tyramine and histamine
   d. Has regular physical examinations and blood tests to evaluate liver and kidney function, neuropathy, hearing and visual acuity

Lung Abscess

A lung abscess is a localized necrotic lesion of the lung parenchyma containing purulent material that collapses and forms a cavity. It is generally caused by aspiration of anaerobic bacteria. In a lung abscess, by definition, the chest x-ray demonstrates a cavity of at least 2 cm. Patients who have impaired cough reflexes and cannot close the glottis, and those with swallowing difficulties, are at risk for aspiration of foreign material and development of a lung abscess. Other at-risk patients include those with central nervous system disorders (eg, seizure, stroke), drug addiction, alcoholism, esophageal disease, or compromised immune function; patients without teeth and those receiving nasogastric tube feedings; and patients with an altered state of consciousness due to anesthesia.

Pathophysiology

Most lung abscesses are a complication of bacterial pneumonia or are caused by aspiration of oral anaerobes into the lung. Abscesses also may occur secondary to mechanical or functional obstruction of the bronchi by a tumor, foreign body, or bronchial stenosis, or from necrotizing pneumonias, TB, pulmonary embolism (PE), or chest trauma.

Most lung abscesses are found in areas of the lung that may be affected by aspiration. The site of the lung abscess is related to gravity and is determined by position. For patients who are confined to bed, the posterior segment of an upper lobe and the superior segment of the lower lobe are the most common areas in which lung abscess occurs. However, atypical presentations may occur, depending on the position of the patient when the aspiration occurred.

Initially, the cavity in the lung may or may not extend directly into a bronchus. Eventually, the abscess becomes surrounded, or encapsulated, by a wall of fibrous tissue. The necrotic process may extend until it reaches the lumen of a bronchus or the pleural space and establishes communication with the respiratory tract, the pleural cavity, or both. If the bronchus is involved, the purulent contents are expectorated continuously in the form of sputum. If the pleura is involved, an empyema results. A communication or connection between the bronchus and pleura is known as a bronchopleural fistula.

The organisms frequently associated with lung abscesses are *S. aureus*, *Klebsiella*, and other gram-negative species. However, anaerobic organisms may also be present. The organisms vary depending on the underlying predisposing factors.

Clinical Manifestations

The clinical manifestations of a lung abscess may vary from a mild productive cough to acute illness. Most patients have a fever and a productive cough with moderate to copious amounts of foul-smelling, sometimes bloody, sputum. The fever and cough may develop insidiously and may have been present for several weeks before diagnosis. Leukocytosis may be present. Pleurisy or dull chest pain, dyspnea, weakness, anorexia, and weight loss are common.

Assessment and Diagnostic Findings

Physical examination of the chest may reveal dullness on percussion and decreased or absent breath sounds with an intermittent **pleural friction rub** (grating or rubbing sound) on auscultation. Crackles may be present. Confirmation of the diagnosis is made by chest x-ray, sputum culture, and, in some cases, fiberoptic bronchoscopy. The chest x-ray reveals an infiltrate with an air–fluid level. A computed tomography (CT) scan of the chest may be required to provide more detailed pictures of different cross-sectional areas of the lung.

Prevention

The following measures reduce the risk of lung abscess:

- Appropriate antibiotic therapy before any dental procedures in patients who must have teeth extracted while their gums and teeth are infected
- Adequate dental and oral hygiene, because anaerobic bacteria play a role in the pathogenesis of lung abscess
- Appropriate antimicrobial therapy for patients with pneumonia

Medical Management

The findings of the history, physical examination, chest x-ray, and sputum culture indicate the type of organism and the treatment required. Adequate drainage of the lung abscess may be achieved through postural drainage and chest physiotherapy. Patients should be assessed for an adequate cough. Some patients require insertion of a percutaneous chest catheter for long-term drainage of the abscess. Therapeutic use of bronchoscopy to drain an abscess is uncommon. A diet high in protein and calories is necessary, because chronic infection is associated with a catabolic state, necessitating increased intake of calories and protein to facilitate healing. Surgical intervention is rare, but pulmonary resection (lobectomy) is performed if massive **hemoptysis** (coughing up of blood) occurs or if there is little or no response to medical management.

Pharmacologic Therapy

IV antimicrobial therapy depends on the results of the sputum culture and sensitivity and is administered for an extended period. Antibiotics used include clindamycin (Cleocin), meropenem (Merrem), or piperacillin/tazobactam (Zosyn). Large IV doses are usually required, because the antibiotic must penetrate the necrotic tissue and the fluid in the abscess. The IV dose is continued until there is evidence of symptom improvement.

Long-term therapy with oral antibiotics replaces IV therapy after the patient shows signs of improvement (usually 3 to 5 days). Improvement is demonstrated by normal temperature, decreased white blood cell count, and improvement on chest x-ray (resolution of surrounding infiltrate, reduction in cavity size, absence of fluid). Oral administration of antibiotic therapy is continued for an additional 4 to 8 weeks. If treatment is stopped too soon, a relapse may occur.

Nursing Management

The nurse administers antibiotics and IV treatments as prescribed and monitors for adverse effects. Chest physiotherapy is initiated as prescribed to facilitate drainage of the abscess. The nurse teaches the patient to perform deep-breathing and coughing exercises to help expand the lungs.

To ensure proper nutritional intake, the nurse encourages a diet that is high in protein and calories. The nurse also offers emotional support, because the abscess may take a long time to resolve.

Promoting Home and Community-Based Care

TEACHING PATIENTS SELF-CARE. A patient who has had surgery may return home before the wound closes entirely or with a drain or tube in place. In these cases, the patient or caregivers require instruction about how to change the dressings to prevent skin excoriation and odor, how to monitor for signs and symptoms of infection, and how to care for and maintain the drain or tube. The nurse instructs the patient to perform deep-breathing and coughing exercises every 2 hours during the day and shows caregivers how to perform chest percussion and postural drainage to facilitate expectoration of lung secretions.

CONTINUING CARE. A patient whose condition requires therapy at home may need referral for home care. During home visits, the nurse assesses the physical condition, nutritional status, and home environment of the patient, as well as the ability of the patient and family to carry out the therapeutic regimen. Patient teaching is reinforced, and nutritional counseling is provided with the goal of attaining and maintaining an optimal state of nutrition. To prevent relapses, the nurse emphasizes the importance of completing the antibiotic regimen and of following suggestions for rest and appropriate activity. If IV antibiotic therapy is to continue at home, the services of home care nurses may be arranged to initiate IV therapy and to evaluate its administration by the patient or family.

Although most outpatient IV therapy is administered in the home setting, the patient may visit a nearby clinic or physician's office for this treatment. In some cases, patients with lung abscess may have ignored their health. Therefore, it is important to use this opportunity to address health promotion strategies and health screening with the patient.

Pleural Conditions

Pleural conditions are disorders that involve the membranes covering the lungs (visceral pleura) and the surface of the chest wall (parietal pleura) or disorders affecting the pleural space.

Pleurisy

Pathophysiology

Pleurisy (pleuritis) refers to inflammation of both layers of the pleurae (parietal and visceral). Pleurisy may develop in conjunction with pneumonia or an upper respiratory tract infection, TB, or collagen disease; after trauma to the chest, pulmonary infarction, or PE; in patients with primary or metastatic cancer; and after thoracotomy. The parietal pleura has nerve endings; the visceral pleura does not. When the inflamed pleural membranes rub together during respiration (intensified on inspiration), the result is severe, sharp, knifelike pain.

Clinical Manifestations

The key characteristic of pleuritic pain is its relationship to respiratory movement. Taking a deep breath, coughing, or sneezing worsens the pain. Pleuritic pain is limited in distribution rather than diffuse; it usually occurs only on one side. The pain may become minimal or absent when the breath is held. It may be localized or radiate to the shoulder or abdomen. Later, as pleural fluid develops, the pain decreases.

Assessment and Diagnostic Findings

In the early period, when little fluid has accumulated, a pleural friction rub can be heard with the stethoscope, only to disappear later as more fluid accumulates and separates the inflamed pleural surfaces. Diagnostic tests may include chest x-rays, sputum examinations, thoracentesis to obtain a specimen of pleural fluid for examination, and, less commonly, a pleural biopsy.

Medical Management

The objectives of treatment are to discover the underlying condition causing the pleurisy and to relieve the pain. As the underlying disease (pneumonia, infection) is treated, the pleuritic inflammation usually resolves. At the same time, it is necessary to monitor for signs and symptoms of pleural effusion, such as shortness of breath, pain, assumption of a position that decreases pain, and decreased chest wall excursion.

Prescribed analgesics and topical applications of heat or cold provide symptomatic relief. Indomethacin (Indocin), a nonsteroidal anti-inflammatory agent, may provide pain relief while allowing the patient to take deep breaths and cough more effectively. If the pain is severe, an intercostal nerve block may be required.

Nursing Management

Because the patient has considerable pain on inspiration, the nurse offers suggestions to enhance comfort, such as turning frequently onto the affected side to splint the chest wall and reduce the stretching of the pleurae. The nurse also teaches the patient to use the hands or a pillow to splint the rib cage while coughing.

Pleural Effusion

Pleural effusion, a collection of fluid in the pleural space, is rarely a primary disease process but is usually occurs secondary to other diseases. Normally, the pleural space contains a small amount of fluid (5 to 15 mL), which acts as a lubricant that allows the pleural surfaces to move without friction (Fig. 23-5). Pleural effusion may be a complication of heart failure, TB, pneumonia, pulmonary infections (par-

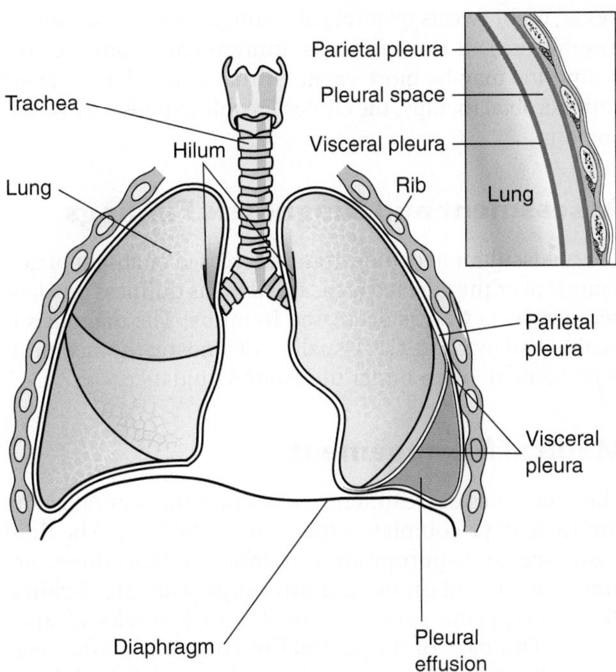

FIGURE 23-5. In pleural effusion, an abnormal volume of fluid collects in the pleural space, causing pain and shortness of breath. Pleural effusion is usually secondary to other disease processes.

ticularly viral infections), nephrotic syndrome, connective tissue disease, pulmonary embolus, and neoplastic tumors. The most common malignancy associated with a pleural effusion is bronchogenic carcinoma.

Pathophysiology

In certain disorders, fluid may accumulate in the pleural space to a point at which it becomes clinically evident. This almost always has pathologic significance. The effusion can be composed of a relatively clear fluid, or it can be bloody or purulent. An effusion of clear fluid may be a transudate or an exudate. A transudate (filtrate of plasma that moves across intact capillary walls) occurs when factors influencing the formation and reabsorption of pleural fluid are altered, usually by imbalances in hydrostatic or oncotic pressures. The finding of a transudative effusion generally implies that the pleural membranes are not diseased. A transudative effusion most commonly results from heart failure. An exudate (extravasation of fluid into tissues or a cavity) usually results from inflammation by bacterial products or tumors involving the pleural surfaces.

Clinical Manifestations

Usually, the clinical manifestations are caused by the underlying disease. Pneumonia causes fever, chills, and pleuritic chest pain, whereas a malignant effusion may result in dyspnea, difficulty lying flat, and coughing. The severity of symptoms is determined by the size of the effusion, the speed of its formation, and the underlying lung disease. A large pleural effusion causes dyspnea (shortness of breath). A small to moderate pleural effusion causes minimal or no dyspnea.

Assessment and Diagnostic Findings

Assessment of the area of the pleural effusion reveals decreased or absent breath sounds, decreased fremitus, and a dull, flat sound on percussion. In the case of an extremely large pleural effusion, the assessment reveals a patient in acute respiratory distress. Tracheal deviation away from the affected side may also be apparent.

Physical examination, chest x-ray, chest CT, and thoracentesis confirm the presence of fluid. In some instances, a lateral decubitus x-ray is obtained. For this x-ray, the patient lies on the affected side in a side-lying position. A pleural effusion can be diagnosed because this position allows for the "layering out" of the fluid, and an air–fluid line is visible.

Pleural fluid is analyzed by bacterial culture, Gram stain, acid-fast bacillus stain (for TB), red and white blood cell counts, chemistry studies (glucose, amylase, lactic dehydrogenase, protein), cytologic analysis for malignant cells, and pH. A pleural biopsy also may be performed as a diagnostic tool.

Medical Management

The objectives of treatment are to discover the underlying cause of the pleural effusion; to prevent reaccumulation of fluid; and to relieve discomfort, dyspnea, and respiratory compromise. Specific treatment is directed at the underlying cause (eg, heart failure, pneumonia, cirrhosis). If the pleural fluid is an exudate, more extensive diagnostic procedures are performed to determine the cause. Treatment for the primary cause is then instituted.

Thoracentesis is performed to remove fluid, to obtain a specimen for analysis, and to relieve dyspnea and respiratory compromise (see Chapter 21). Thoracentesis may be performed under ultrasound guidance. Depending on the size of the pleural effusion, the patient may be treated by removing the fluid during the thoracentesis procedure or by inserting a chest tube connected to a water-seal drainage system or suction to evacuate the pleural space and reexpand the lung.

However, if the underlying cause is a malignancy, the effusion tends to recur within a few days or weeks. Repeated thoracenteses result in pain, depletion of protein and electrolytes, and sometimes pneumothorax. Once the pleural space is adequately drained, a chemical pleurodesis may be performed to obliterate the pleural space and prevent reaccumulation of fluid. Pleurodesis may be performed using either a thoracoscopic approach or a chest tube. A chemically irritating agent (eg., talc) is instilled or aerosolized into the pleural space. With the chest tube approach, after the agent is instilled, the chest tube is clamped for 60 to 90 minutes and the patient is assisted to assume various positions to promote uniform distribution of the agent and to maximize its contact with the pleural surfaces. The tube is unclamped as prescribed, and chest drainage may be continued several days longer to prevent reaccumulation of fluid and to promote the formation of adhesions between the visceral and parietal pleurae.

Other treatments for malignant pleural effusions include surgical pleurectomy, insertion of a small catheter attached to a drainage bottle for outpatient management (Pleurx catheter [Denver Biomedical]), or implantation of a pleuroperitoneal shunt. A pleuroperitoneal shunt consists of two catheters connected by a pump chamber containing two one-way valves. Fluid moves from the pleural space to the pump chamber and then to the peritoneal cavity. The patient manually pumps on the reservoir daily to move fluid from the pleural space to the peritoneal space.

Nursing Management

The nurse's role in the care of patients with a pleural effusion includes implementing the medical regimen. The nurse prepares and positions the patient for thoracentesis and offers support throughout the procedure. The nurse is responsible for making sure the thoracentesis fluid amount is recorded and sent for appropriate laboratory testing. If a chest tube drainage and water-seal system is used, the nurse is responsible for monitoring the system's function and recording the amount of drainage at prescribed intervals. Nursing care related to the underlying cause of the pleural effusion is specific to the underlying condition. Care of the patient with a chest tube is discussed in Chapter 25.

If a chest tube is inserted for talc instillation, pain management is a priority and the nurse helps the patient assume positions that are the least painful. However, frequent turning and movement are important to facilitate adequate spreading of the talc over the pleural surface. The nurse evaluates the patient's pain level and administers analgesics as prescribed and as needed.

If the patient is to be managed as an outpatient with a pleural catheter for drainage, the nurse is responsible for educating the patient and family regarding management and care of the catheter and drainage system.

Empyema

An empyema is an accumulation of thick, purulent fluid within the pleural space, often with fibrin development and a loculated (walled-off) area where infection is located.

Pathophysiology

Most empyemas occur as complications of bacterial pneumonia or lung abscess. They also result from penetrating chest trauma, hematogenous infection of the pleural space, nonbacterial infections, and iatrogenic causes (after thoracic surgery or thoracentesis). At first the pleural fluid is thin, with a low leukocyte count, but it frequently progresses to a fibropurulent stage and, finally, to a stage where it encloses the lung within a thick exudative membrane (loculated empyema).

Clinical Manifestations

The patient is acutely ill and has signs and symptoms similar to those of an acute respiratory infection or pneumonia (fever, night sweats, pleural pain, cough, dyspnea, anorexia, weight loss). If the patient is immunocompromised, the symptoms may be more vague. If the patient has received antimicrobial therapy, the clinical manifestations may be less obvious.

Assessment and Diagnostic Findings

Chest auscultation demonstrates decreased or absent breath sounds over the affected area, and there is dullness on chest percussion as well as decreased fremitus. The diagnosis is established by chest CT. Usually a diagnostic thoracentesis is performed, often under ultrasound guidance.

Medical Management

The objectives of treatment are to drain the pleural cavity and to achieve complete expansion of the lung. The fluid is drained, and appropriate antibiotics, in large doses, are prescribed based on the causative organism. Sterilization of the empyema cavity requires 4 to 6 weeks of antibiotics. Drainage of the pleural fluid depends on the stage of the disease and is accomplished by one of the following methods:

- Needle aspiration (thoracentesis) with a thin percutaneous catheter, if the volume is small and the fluid is not too purulent or too thick
- Tube thoracostomy (chest drainage using a large-diameter intercostal tube attached to water-seal drainage [see Chapter 25]) with fibrinolytic agents instilled through the chest tube in patients with loculated or complicated pleural effusions
- Open chest drainage via thoracotomy, including potential rib resection, to remove the thickened pleura, pus, and debris and to remove the underlying diseased pulmonary tissue

With long-standing inflammation, an exudate can form over the lung, trapping it and interfering with its normal expansion. This exudate must be removed surgically (decortication). The drainage tube is left in place until the pus-filled space is obliterated completely. The complete obliteration of the pleural space is monitored by serial chest x-rays, and the patient should be informed that treatment may be long term. Patients are frequently discharged from the hospital with a chest tube in place, with instructions to monitor fluid drainage at home.

Nursing Management

Resolution of empyema is a prolonged process. The nurse helps the patient cope with the condition and instructs the patient in lung-expanding breathing exercises to restore normal respiratory function. The nurse also provides care specific to the method of drainage of the pleural fluid (eg, needle aspiration, closed chest drainage, rib resection and drainage). When the patient is discharged home with a drainage tube or system in place, the nurse instructs the patient and family on care of the drainage system and drain site, measurement and observation of drainage, signs and symptoms of infection, and how and when to contact the health care provider. (See Nursing Process: The Patient Undergoing Thoracic Surgery in Chapter 25.)

Pulmonary Edema

Pulmonary edema is defined as abnormal accumulation of fluid in the lung tissue, the alveolar space, or both. It is a severe, life-threatening condition.

Pathophysiology

Pulmonary edema most commonly occurs as a result of increased microvascular pressure from abnormal cardiac function. The backup of blood into the pulmonary vasculature resulting from inadequate left ventricular function causes an increased microvascular pressure, and fluid begins to leak into the interstitial space and the alveoli. Other causes of pulmonary edema are hypervolemia or a sudden increase in the intravascular pressure in the lung. One example occurs in the patient who has undergone pneumonectomy. When one lung has been removed, all the cardiac output goes to the remaining lung. If the patient's fluid status is not monitored closely, pulmonary edema can quickly develop in the postoperative period as the patient's pulmonary vasculature attempts to adapt. This type of pulmonary edema is sometimes termed "flash" pulmonary edema. A second example is called re-expansion pulmonary edema. This may result from a rapid reinflation of the lung after removal of air from a pneumothorax or evacuation of fluid from a large pleural effusion.

Clinical Manifestations

Increasing respiratory distress, characterized by dyspnea, air hunger, and central cyanosis, is present. Patients are usually very anxious and often agitated. As the fluid leaks into the alveoli and mixes with air, a foam or froth is formed. The patient coughs up (or the nurse suctions out) these foamy, frothy, and often blood-tinged secretions. The patient experiences acute respiratory distress and may become confused or stuporous.

Assessment and Diagnostic Findings

Auscultation reveals crackles in the lung bases (especially in the posterior bases) that rapidly progress toward the apices of the lungs. These crackles are caused by the movement of air through the alveolar fluid. The chest x-ray reveals increased interstitial markings. The patient may have tachycardia. Pulse oximetry values begin to fall, and arterial blood gas analysis demonstrates worsening hypoxemia.

Medical Management

Management focuses on correcting the underlying disorder. If the pulmonary edema is cardiac in origin, then improvement in left ventricular function is the goal. Vasodilators, inotropic medications, afterload or preload agents, or contractility medications may be administered. Additional cardiac measures (eg, intra-aortic balloon pump) may be indicated if there is no response. If the problem is fluid overload, diuretics are administered and fluids are restricted. Oxygen is administered to correct the hypoxemia; in some circumstances, intubation and mechanical ventilation are necessary. The patient is extremely anxious, and morphine is prescribed to reduce anxiety and control pain.

Nursing Management

Nursing management includes assisting with administration of oxygen and intubation and mechanical ventilation if respiratory failure occurs. The nurse also administers medications (eg, morphine, vasodilators, inotropic medications, preload and afterload agents) as prescribed and monitors the patient's responses. Nursing management in pulmonary edema is described in more detail in Chapter 30.

Acute Respiratory Failure

Respiratory failure is a sudden and life-threatening deterioration of the gas exchange function of the lung. It exists when the exchange of oxygen for carbon dioxide in the lungs cannot keep up with the rate of oxygen consumption and carbon dioxide production by the cells of the body. Acute respiratory failure (ARF) is defined as a decrease in arterial oxygen tension (PaO_2) to less than 50 mm Hg (hypoxemia) and an increase in arterial carbon dioxide tension ($PaCO_2$) to greater than 50 mm Hg (hypercapnia), with an arterial pH of less than 7.35.

It is important to distinguish between ARF and chronic respiratory failure. Chronic respiratory failure is defined as a deterioration in the gas exchange function of the lung that has developed insidiously or has persisted for a long period after an episode of ARF. The absence of acute symptoms and the presence of a chronic respiratory acidosis suggest the chronicity of the respiratory failure. Two causes of chronic respiratory failure are COPD (discussed in Chapter 24) and neuromuscular diseases (discussed in Chapter 65). Patients with these disorders develop a tolerance to the gradually worsening hypoxemia and hypercapnia. However, patients with chronic respiratory failure can develop ARF. For example, a patient with COPD may develop an exacerbation or infection that causes additional deterioration of gas exchange. The principles of management of acute versus chronic respiratory failure are different; the following discussion is limited to ARF.

Pathophysiology

In ARF, the ventilation or perfusion mechanisms in the lung are impaired. Impaired respiratory system mechanisms leading to ARF include

- Alveolar hypoventilation
- Diffusion abnormalities
- Ventilation–perfusion mismatching
- Shunting

Common causes of ARF can be classified into four categories: decreased respiratory drive, dysfunction of the chest wall, dysfunction of the lung parenchyma, and other causes.

Decreased Respiratory Drive

Decreased respiratory drive may occur with severe brain injury, large lesions of the brainstem (multiple sclerosis), use of sedative medications, and metabolic disorders such as severe hypothyroidism. These disorders impair the response of chemoreceptors in the brain to normal respiratory stimulation.

Dysfunction of the Chest Wall

The impulses arising in the respiratory center travel through nerves that extend from the brainstem down the spinal cord to receptors in the muscles of respiration. Any disease or disorder of the nerves, spinal cord, muscles, or neuromuscular junction involved in respiration seriously affects ventilation and may ultimately lead to ARF. These include musculoskeletal disorders (muscular dystrophy, polymyositis), neuromuscular junction disorders (myasthenia gravis, poliomyelitis), some peripheral nerve disorders, and spinal cord disorders (amyotrophic lateral sclerosis, Guillain-Barré syndrome, and cervical spinal cord injuries).

Dysfunction of Lung Parenchyma

Pleural effusion, hemothorax, pneumothorax, and upper airway obstruction are conditions that interfere with ventilation by preventing expansion of the lung. These conditions, which may cause respiratory failure, usually are produced by an underlying lung disease, pleural disease, or trauma and injury. Other diseases and conditions of lung parenchyma that lead to ARF include pneumonia, status asthmaticus, lobar atelectasis, PE, and pulmonary edema.

Other Causes

In the postoperative period, especially after major thoracic or abdominal surgery, inadequate ventilation and respiratory failure may occur because of several factors. During this period, for example, ARF may be caused by the effects of anesthetic agents, analgesics, and sedatives, which may depress respiration (as described earlier) or enhance the effects of opioids and lead to hypoventilation. Pain may interfere with deep breathing and coughing. A ventilation–perfusion mismatch is the usual cause of respiratory failure after major abdominal, cardiac, or thoracic surgery.

Clinical Manifestations

Early signs are those associated with impaired oxygenation and may include restlessness, fatigue, headache, dyspnea, air hunger, tachycardia, and increased blood pressure. As the hypoxemia progresses, more obvious signs may be present, including confusion, lethargy, tachycardia, tachypnea, central cyanosis, diaphoresis, and finally respiratory arrest. Physical findings are those of acute respiratory distress, including use of accessory muscles, decreased breath sounds if the patient cannot adequately ventilate, and other findings related specifically to the underlying disease process and cause of ARF.

Medical Management

The objectives of treatment are to correct the underlying cause and to restore adequate gas exchange in the lung. Intubation and mechanical ventilation may be required to maintain adequate ventilation and oxygenation while the underlying cause is corrected.

Nursing Management

Nursing management of patients with ARF includes assisting with intubation and maintaining mechanical ventilation (described in Chapter 25). Patients are usually managed in the intensive care unit. The nurse assesses the patient's respiratory status by monitoring the level of responsiveness, arterial blood gases, pulse oximetry, and vital signs. In addition, the nurse assesses the entire respiratory system and implements strategies (eg, turning schedule, mouth care, skin care, range of motion of extremities) to prevent complications. The nurse also assesses the patient's understanding of the management strategies that are used and initiates some form of communication to enable the patient to express concerns and needs to the health care team.

Finally, the nurse addresses the problems that led to the ARF. As the patient's status improves, the nurse assesses the patient's knowledge of the underlying disorder and provides teaching as appropriate to address the disorder.

Acute Respiratory Distress Syndrome

Acute respiratory distress syndrome (ARDS; previously called adult respiratory distress syndrome) is a severe form of **acute lung injury**. This clinical syndrome is characterized by a sudden and progressive pulmonary edema, increasing bilateral infiltrates on chest x-ray, hypoxemia refractory to oxygen supplementation, and reduced lung compliance. These signs occur in the absence of left-sided heart failure. Patients with ARDS usually require mechanical ventilation with a higher-than-normal airway pressure. A wide range of factors are associated with the development of ARDS (Chart 23-5), including direct injury to the lungs (eg, smoke inhalation) or indirect insult to the lungs (eg, shock). ARDS has been associated with a mortality rate as high as 50% to 60%. The major cause of death in ARDS is nonpulmonary multiple-system organ failure, often with sepsis.

Pathophysiology

ARDS occurs as a result of an inflammatory trigger that initiates the release of cellular and chemical mediators, causing injury to the alveolar capillary membrane. This leads to leakage of fluid into the alveolar interstitial spaces and alterations in the capillary bed.

Severe ventilation–perfusion mismatching occurs in ARDS. Alveoli collapse because of the inflammatory infiltrate, blood, fluid, and surfactant dysfunction. Small air-

CHART 23-5

Etiologic Factors Related to Acute Respiratory Distress Syndrome (ARDS)

- Aspiration (gastric secretions, drowning, hydrocarbons)
- Drug ingestion and overdose
- Hematologic disorders (disseminated intravascular coagulopathy [DIC], massive transfusions, cardiopulmonary bypass)
- Prolonged inhalation of high concentrations of oxygen, smoke, or corrosive substances
- Localized infection (bacterial, fungal, viral pneumonia)
- Metabolic disorders (pancreatitis, uremia)
- Shock (any cause)
- Trauma (pulmonary contusion, multiple fractures, head injury)
- Major surgery
- Fat or air embolism
- Systemic sepsis

ways are narrowed because of interstitial fluid and bronchial obstruction. Lung compliance becomes markedly decreased (stiff lungs), and the result is a characteristic decrease in functional residual capacity and severe hypoxemia. The blood returning to the lung for gas exchange is pumped through the nonventilated, nonfunctioning areas of the lung, causing shunting. This means that blood is interfacing with nonfunctioning alveoli and gas exchange is markedly impaired, resulting in severe, refractory hypoxemia. Figure 23-6 shows the sequence of pathophysiologic events leading to ARDS.

Clinical Manifestations

Clinically, the acute phase of ARDS is marked by a rapid onset of severe dyspnea that usually occurs 12 to 48 hours after the initiating event. A characteristic feature is arterial hypoxemia that does not respond to supplemental oxygen. On chest x-ray, the findings are similar to those seen with cardiogenic pulmonary edema and appear as bilateral infiltrates that quickly worsen. The acute lung injury then progresses to fibrosing alveolitis with persistent, severe hypoxemia. The patient also has increased alveolar dead space (ventilation to alveoli, but poor perfusion) and decreased pulmonary compliance ("stiff lungs," which are difficult to ventilate). Clinically, the patient is thought to be in the recovery phase if the hypoxemia gradually resolves, the chest x-ray improves, and the lungs become more compliant.

Assessment and Diagnostic Findings

Intercostal retractions and crackles, as the fluid begins to leak into the alveolar interstitial space, are evident on physical examination. A diagnosis of ARDS may be made based on the following criteria: a history of systemic or pulmonary risk factors, acute onset of respiratory distress, bilateral pulmonary infiltrates, clinical absence of left-sided heart failure, and a ratio of PaO_2 to fraction of inspired oxygen (FiO_2) less than 200 mm Hg (severe refractory hypoxemia).

Medical Management

The primary focus in the management of ARDS includes identification and treatment of the underlying condition. Aggressive, supportive care must be provided to compensate for the severe respiratory dysfunction. This supportive therapy almost always includes intubation and mechanical

Physiology/Pathophysiology

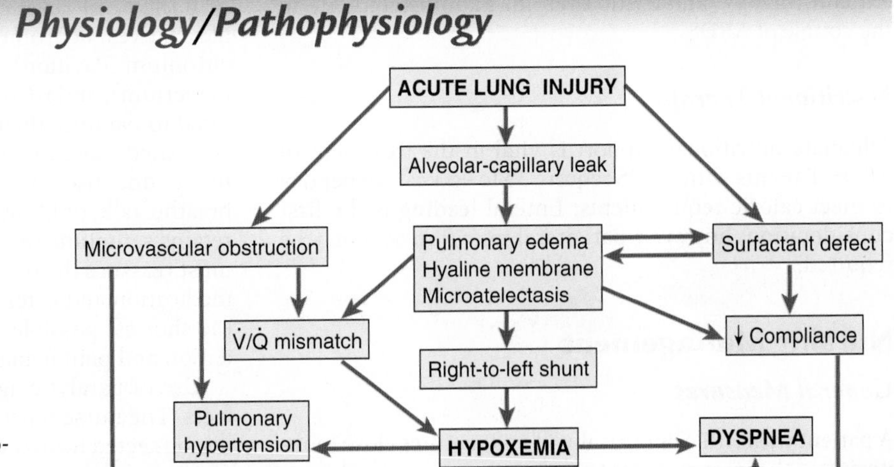

FIGURE 23-6. Pathogenesis and pathophysiology of acute respiratory distress syndrome. Adapted from Farzan, S. (1997). *A concise handbook of respiratory diseases* (4th ed.). Stamford, CT: Appleton & Lange.

ventilation. In addition, circulatory support, adequate fluid volume, and nutritional support are important. Supplemental oxygen is used as the patient begins the initial spiral of hypoxemia. As the hypoxemia progresses, intubation and mechanical ventilation are instituted. The concentration of oxygen and ventilator settings and modes are determined by the patient's status. This is monitored by arterial blood gas analysis, pulse oximetry, and bedside pulmonary function testing.

PEEP is a critical part of the treatment of ARDS. PEEP usually improves oxygenation, but it does not influence the natural history of the syndrome. Use of PEEP helps increase functional residual capacity and reverse alveolar collapse by keeping the alveoli open, resulting in improved arterial oxygenation and a reduction in the severity of the ventilation–perfusion imbalance. By using PEEP, a lower FiO_2 may be required. The goal is a PaO_2 greater than 60 mm Hg or an oxygen saturation level of greater than 90% at the lowest possible FiO_2. Evidence suggests that ARDS should be managed with a low tidal volume, pressure-limited approach with low or moderately high PEEP (Kallet, 2004; Young, Manning, Wilson, et al., 2004). PEEP and modes of mechanical ventilation are discussed in Chapter 25.

Systemic hypotension may occur in ARDS as a result of hypovolemia secondary to leakage of fluid into the interstitial spaces and depressed cardiac output from high levels of PEEP therapy. Hypovolemia must be carefully treated without causing further overload. IV crystalloid solutions are administered, with careful monitoring of pulmonary status. Inotropic or vasopressor agents may be required. Pulmonary artery pressure catheters are used to monitor the patient's fluid status and the severe and progressive pulmonary hypertension sometimes observed in ARDS.

Pharmacologic Therapy

Numerous pharmacologic treatments are under investigation to stop the cascade of events leading to ARDS. These include human recombinant interleukin-1 receptor antagonist, neutrophil inhibitors, pulmonary-specific vasodilators, surfactant replacement therapy, antisepsis agents, antioxidant therapy, and corticosteroids administered late in the course of ARDS.

Nutritional Therapy

Adequate nutritional support is vital in the treatment of ARDS. Patients with ARDS require 35 to 45 kcal/kg per day to meet caloric requirements. Enteral feeding is the first consideration; however, parenteral nutrition also may be required.

Nursing Management

General Measures

A patient with ARDS is critically ill and requires close monitoring in the intensive care unit, because the patient's condition could quickly become life-threatening. Most of the respiratory modalities discussed in Chapter 25 are used in this situation (oxygen administration, nebulizer therapy, chest physiotherapy, endotracheal intubation or tracheostomy, mechanical ventilation, suctioning, bronchoscopy). Frequent assessment of the patient's status is necessary to evaluate the effectiveness of treatment.

In addition to implementing the medical plan of care, the nurse considers other needs of the patient. Positioning is important. The nurse turns the patient frequently to improve ventilation and perfusion in the lungs and enhance secretion drainage. However, the nurse must closely monitor the patient for deterioration in oxygenation with changes in position. Oxygenation in patients with ARDS is sometimes improved in the prone position. This position may be evaluated for improvement in oxygenation and used in special circumstances. Devices and specialty beds are available to assist the nurse in placing the patient in a prone position ("proning") (Powers & Daniels, 2004).

The patient is extremely anxious and agitated because of the increasing hypoxemia and dyspnea. The nurse explains all procedures and provides care in a calm, reassuring manner. It is important to reduce the patient's anxiety, because anxiety increases oxygen expenditure by preventing rest. Rest is essential to limit oxygen consumption and reduce oxygen needs.

Ventilator Considerations

If the patient is intubated and receiving mechanical ventilation with PEEP, several considerations must be addressed. PEEP, which causes increased end-expiratory pressure, is an unnatural pattern of breathing and feels strange to patients. The patients may be anxious and "fight" the ventilator. Nursing assessment is important to assess for problems with ventilation that may be causing the anxiety reaction: tube blockage by kinking or retained secretions; other acute respiratory problems (eg, pneumothorax, pain); a sudden decrease in the oxygen level; the level of dyspnea; or ventilator malfunction. In some cases, sedation may be required to decrease the patient's oxygen consumption, allow the ventilator to provide full support of ventilation, and decrease the patient's anxiety. Sedatives that may be used are lorazepam (Ativan), midazolam (Versed), dexmedetomidine (Precedex), propofol (Diprivan), and short-acting barbiturates.

If the PEEP level cannot be maintained despite the use of sedatives, neuromuscular blocking agents, such as pancuronium (Pavulon), vecuronium (Norcuron), atracurium (Tracrium), and rocuronium (Zemuron), may be administered to paralyze the patient. This allows the patient to be ventilated more easily. With paralysis, the patient appears to be unconscious; loses motor function; and cannot breathe, talk, or blink independently. However, the patient retains sensation and is awake and able to hear. The nurse must reassure the patient that the paralysis is a result of the medication and is temporary. Paralysis should be used for the shortest possible time and never without adequate sedation and pain management.

Use of paralytic agents has many dangers and side effects. The nurse must be sure the patient does not become disconnected from the ventilator, because respiratory muscles are paralyzed and the patient will be apneic. Consequently, the nurse ensures that the patient is closely monitored, and all ventilator and patient alarms must be on at all times. Eye care is important as well, because the patient cannot blink, increasing the risk of corneal abrasions.

Neuromuscular blockers predispose the patient to deep venous thrombi, muscle atrophy, and skin breakdown. Nursing assessment is essential to minimize the complications related to neuromuscular blockade. The patient may have discomfort or pain but cannot communicate these sensations. Analgesia is usually administered concurrently with neuromuscular blocking agents. The nurse must anticipate the patient's needs regarding pain and comfort. The nurse checks the patient's position to ensure it is comfortable and in normal alignment and talks to, and not about, the patient while in the patient's presence.

In addition, it is important for the nurse to describe the purpose and effects of the paralytic agents to the patient's family. If family members are unaware that these agents have been administered, they may become distressed by the change in the patient's status.

Pulmonary Arterial Hypertension

Pulmonary arterial hypertension exists when the systolic pulmonary artery pressure exceeds 30 mm Hg or the mean pulmonary artery pressure exceeds 25 mm Hg at rest or 30 mm Hg with activities. These pressures cannot be measured indirectly as can systemic blood pressure; instead, they must be measured during right-sided heart catheterization. In the absence of these measurements, clinical recognition becomes the only indicator for the presence of pulmonary hypertension. However, pulmonary arterial hypertension is a condition that is not clinically evident until late in its progression.

There are two types of pulmonary arterial hypertension: idiopathic (or primary) pulmonary arterial hypertension and pulmonary arterial hypertension due to a known cause (American College of Chest Physicians, 2004). Idiopathic hypertension is an uncommon disease; the incidence is 1 to 2 cases per million persons per year (Eells, 2004). It occurs most often in women 20 to 40 years of age, either sporadically or in patients with a family history, and is usually fatal within 5 years of diagnosis. There are several possible causes, but the exact cause is unknown (Chart 23-6). The clinical presentation may occur with no evidence of pulmonary or cardiac disease or PE.

In contrast, pulmonary arterial hypertension due to a known cause is more common and results from existing cardiac or pulmonary disease. The prognosis depends on the severity of the underlying disorder and the changes in the pulmonary vascular bed. A common cause of pulmonary arterial hypertension is pulmonary artery constriction due to hypoxemia from COPD (cor pulmonale).

Pathophysiology

Conditions such as collagen vascular disease, congenital heart disease, portal hypertension, and HIV infection increase the risk for pulmonary arterial hypertension in susceptible patients. Vascular injury occurs with endothelial dysfunction and vascular smooth muscle dysfunction, which leads to disease progression (vascular smooth muscle hypertrophy, adventitial and intimal proliferation [thickening of the wall], and advanced vascular lesion formation). Normally, the pulmonary vascular bed can handle the blood volume delivered by the right ventricle. It has a low resistance to blood flow and compensates for increased blood volume by dilation of the vessels in the pulmonary circulation. However, if the pulmonary vascular bed is destroyed or obstructed, as in pulmonary hypertension, the ability to handle whatever flow or volume of blood it receives is impaired, and the increased blood flow then increases the pulmonary artery pressure. As the pulmonary arterial pressure increases, the pulmonary vascular resistance also increases. Both pulmonary artery constriction (as in hypoxemia or hypercapnia) and a reduction of the pulmonary vascular bed (which occurs with pulmonary emboli) result in increased pulmonary vascular resistance and pressure. This increased workload affects right ventricular function. The myocardium ultimately cannot meet the increasing demands imposed on it, leading to right ventricular hypertrophy (enlargement and dilation) and failure.

CHART 23-6

Causes of Pulmonary Arterial Hypertension

IDIOPATHIC (PRIMARY) ARTERIAL HYPERTENSION AND PULMONARY ARTERIAL HYPERTENSION DUE TO A KNOWN CAUSE

- Collagen vascular diseases
- Congenital systemic-to-pulmonary shunts
- Portal hypertension
- Altered immune mechanisms (HIV infection)
- Diseases associated with significant venous or capillary involvement
- Chronic thrombotic or embolic disease
- Pulmonary venous hypertension
- Pulmonary vasoconstriction due to hypoxemia
- Chronic obstructive pulmonary disease (COPD), interstitial lung disease, sleep-disordered breathing
- Miscellaneous causes: sarcoidosis, histiocytosis, compression of pulmonary vessels

Clinical Manifestations

Dyspnea, the main symptom of pulmonary hypertension, occurs at first with exertion and eventually at rest. Substernal chest pain also is common, affecting 25% to 50% of patients. Other signs and symptoms include weakness, fatigue, syncope, occasional hemoptysis, and signs of right-sided heart failure (peripheral edema, ascites, distended neck veins, liver engorgement, crackles, heart murmur).

Assessment and Diagnostic Findings

Several tests are used to determine whether there is a known cause for the pulmonary hypertension. If the diagnostic tests and thorough evaluation of the patient reveal no known cause, a diagnosis of primary pulmonary hypertension is made. Complete diagnostic evaluation includes a history, physical examination, chest x-ray, pulmonary function studies, electrocardiogram (ECG), echocardiogram, ventilation–perfusion scan, sleep studies, autoantibody tests (to identify diseases of collagen vascular origin), HIV tests, liver function testing, and cardiac catheterization. Pulmonary function studies may be normal or show a slight decrease in vital capacity and lung compliance, with a mild decrease in the diffusing capacity. The PaO_2 also is decreased (hypoxemia). The ECG reveals right ventricular hypertrophy, right axis deviation, and tall peaked P waves in inferior leads; tall anterior R waves; and ST-segment depression, T-wave inversion, or both anteriorly. An echocardiogram can assess the progression of the disease and rule out other conditions with similar signs and symptoms. A ventilation–perfusion scan or pulmonary angiography detects defects in pulmonary vasculature, such as pulmonary emboli. Cardiac catheterization of the right side of the heart reveals elevated pulmonary arterial pressure and determines whether there is a vasoactive component to the pulmonary hypertension.

Medical Management

The goal of treatment is to manage the underlying condition related to pulmonary hypertension of known cause. Most patients with pulmonary hypertension do not have hypoxemia at rest but require supplemental oxygen with exercise. However, patients with severe right ventricular failure, decreased cardiac output, and progressive disease may have resting hypoxemia and require continuous oxygen supplementation. Appropriate oxygen therapy (see Chapter 25) reverses the vasoconstrictive effect and reduces the pulmonary hypertension in a relatively short time.

Bosentan, an endothelin receptor antagonist, causes vasodilation and is prescribed for its antihypertensive effects in patients with pulmonary hypertension (Eells, 2004). Other medications, including diuretics, digoxin, anticoagulant therapy, and calcium-channel blockers (nifedipine [Procardia], diltiazem [Cardizem]) may be prescribed. Because calcium-channel blockers are effective in only a small percentage of patients, other treatment options, including prostacyclin, are often necessary (Humbert, Sitbon & Simonneau, 2004).

Prostaglandin (prostacyclin) relaxes vascular smooth muscle by stimulating the production of cyclic adenosine monophosphate (AMP) and inhibiting the growth of smooth muscle cells. Additionally, it inhibits platelet aggregation. Because of its short-half life in the circulation (ie, 3 minutes), IV prostacyclin (epoprostenol [Flolan]) can be administered only by continuous IV infusion (Humbert et al., 2004). It helps to decrease pulmonary hypertension by reducing pulmonary vascular resistance and pressures and increasing cardiac output. For long-term administration, epoprostenol can be infused with the use of a portable infusion pump connected to a permanent catheter inserted in the subclavian vein. The use of epoprostenol has led to improvement in some patients without lung transplantation, which had previously been the only treatment.

Despite its role in improving function in some patients, epoprostenol is not an ideal treatment because it has significant side effects, is uncomfortable for patients, and is very costly. Continuous subcutaneous infusion of treprostinil (Remodulin), a prostacyclin analogue, was approved for treatment of pulmonary hypertension in 2002 and is an alternative for some patients. Iloprost (Ventavis) is an inhaled, synthetic form of prostacyclin and a powerful vasodilator of the pulmonary arteries. It has been shown to improve patients' overall symptoms and their ability to exercise (walk). Bosentan is an oral endothelin-receptor antagonist; other agents with similar action are under investigation.

Nitric oxide, sildenafil, vasoactive intestinal peptide, and selective serotonin-reuptake inhibitors (SSRIs), and various combinations of these agents are undergoing studies to determine if they have a role in the treatment of patients with pulmonary hypertension (Humbert et al., 2004). Although several treatments for pulmonary arterial hypertension (epoprostenol, treprostinil, and bosentan) are now approved for use in the United States, the long-term effects of many of these therapies are unknown. Lung transplantation remains an option for all eligible patients who have severe disease and symptoms after 3 months of receiving epoprostenol. Atrial septostomy may be considered for selected patients with severe disease (Humbert et al., 2004).

Nursing Management

The major nursing goal is to identify patients at high risk for pulmonary arterial hypertension, such as those with COPD, pulmonary emboli, congenital heart disease, and mitral valve disease. The nurse also must be alert for signs and symptoms, administer oxygen therapy appropriately, and instruct the patient and family about the use of home oxygen supplementation. In patients treated with prostacyclin (ie, epoprostenol or treprostinil), education about the need for central venous access (epoprostenol), subcutaneous infusion (treprostinil), proper administration and dosing of the medication, pain at the injection site, and potential severe side effects is extremely important. Emotional and psychosocial aspects of this disease must be addressed. Formal and informal support groups for patients and families are extremely valuable (Eells, 2004).

Pulmonary Heart Disease (Cor Pulmonale)

Cor pulmonale is a condition in which the right ventricle of the heart enlarges (with or without right-sided heart failure) as a result of diseases that affect the structure or function of the lung or its vasculature. It is a type of pulmonary arterial hypertension due to a known cause. Any disease affecting the lungs and accompanied by hypoxemia may result in cor pulmonale. The most frequent cause is severe COPD (see Chapter 24), in which changes in the airway and retained secretions reduce alveolar ventilation. Other causes are conditions that restrict or compromise ventilatory function, leading to hypoxemia or acidosis (eg, deformities of the thoracic cage, massive obesity) and conditions that reduce the pulmonary vascular bed (eg, primary idiopathic pulmonary arterial hypertension, pulmonary embolus). Certain disorders of the nervous system, respiratory muscles, chest wall, and pulmonary arterial tree also may be responsible for cor pulmonale.

Pathophysiology

Pulmonary disease can produce physiologic changes that in time affect the heart and cause the right ventricle to enlarge and eventually fail. Any condition that deprives the lungs of oxygen can cause hypoxemia and hypercapnia, resulting in ventilatory insufficiency. Hypoxemia and hypercapnia cause pulmonary arterial vasoconstriction and possibly reduction of the pulmonary vascular bed, as in emphysema or pulmonary emboli. The result is increased resistance in the pulmonary circulatory system, with a subsequent rise in pulmonary blood pressure (pulmonary hypertension). A mean pulmonary arterial pressure of 45 mm Hg or more may occur in cor pulmonale. Right ventricular hypertrophy may result, followed by right ventricular failure. In short, cor pulmonale results from pulmonary hypertension, which causes the right side of the heart to enlarge because of the increased work required to pump blood against high resistance through the pulmonary vascular system.

Clinical Manifestations

Symptoms of cor pulmonale are usually related to the underlying lung disease, such as COPD. With right ventricular failure, the patient may develop increasing edema of the feet and legs, distended neck veins, an enlarged palpable liver, pleural effusion, ascites, and heart murmurs. Headache, confusion, and somnolence may occur as a result of increased levels of carbon dioxide (hypercapnia). Patients often complain of increasing shortness of breath, wheezing, cough, and fatigue.

Medical Management

The objectives of treatment are to improve ventilation and to treat both the underlying lung disease and the manifestations of heart disease. Supplemental oxygen is administered to improve gas exchange and to reduce pulmonary arterial pressure and pulmonary vascular resistance. Improved oxygen transport relieves the pulmonary hypertension that is causing the cor pulmonale.

Continuous, 24-hour oxygen therapy in patients with severe hypoxemia reportedly leads to better survival rates and greater reduction in pulmonary vascular resistance. Substantial improvement may require 4 to 6 weeks of oxygen therapy, usually in the home. Periodic assessment of pulse oximetry and arterial blood gases is necessary to determine the adequacy of alveolar ventilation and to monitor the effectiveness of oxygen therapy.

Chest physical therapy and bronchial hygiene maneuvers as indicated to remove accumulated secretions and the administration of bronchodilators further improve ventilation. Additional measures depend on the patient's condition. If the patient is in respiratory failure, endotracheal intubation and mechanical ventilation may be necessary. If the patient is in heart failure, hypoxemia and hypercapnia must be relieved to improve cardiac function and output. Bed rest, sodium restriction, and diuretic therapy also are instituted judiciously to reduce peripheral edema (ie, to lower pulmonary arterial pressure through a decrease in total blood volume) and the circulatory load on the right side of the heart. Digitalis may be prescribed to relieve pulmonary hypertension if the patient also has left ventricular failure, a supraventricular dysrhythmia, or right ventricular failure that does not respond to other therapy.

ECG monitoring may be indicated because of the high incidence of dysrhythmias in patients with cor pulmonale. Any respiratory infection must be treated promptly to avoid further impaired gas exchange and exacerbations of hypoxemia and pulmonary heart disease. The prognosis depends on whether the pulmonary hypertension is reversible. (See earlier discussion of the management of acute respiratory failure.)

Nursing Management

Nursing care addresses the underlying disorder leading to cor pulmonale as well as the problems related to pulmonary hyperventilation and right-sided cardiac failure. If intubation and mechanical ventilation are required to manage ARF, the nurse assists with the intubation procedure and maintains mechanical ventilation. The nurse assesses the patient's respiratory and cardiac status and administers medications as prescribed.

During the patient's hospital stay, the nurse instructs the patient about the importance of close self-monitoring (fluid retention, weight gain, edema) and adherence to the therapeutic regimen, especially the 24-hour use of oxygen. It is important to address factors that affect the patient's adherence to the treatment regimen.

Promoting Home and Community-Based Care

TEACHING PATIENTS SELF-CARE

Because cor pulmonale is a chronic disorder, most of the care and monitoring of patients with cor pulmonale is performed by patients and families in the home. If supplemental oxygen is administered, the nurse instructs the patient and family in its safe and correct use. Nutrition counseling is warranted if the patient is on a sodium-restricted diet or is taking diuretics. The nurse teaches the family to monitor for signs and symptoms of right ventricular failure and about emergency interventions and when to call for assistance. Most importantly, the nurse works with the patient to stop smoking.

CONTINUING CARE

Referral for home care may be warranted for patients who cannot manage self-care and for those whose physical condition warrants close assessment. During home visits, the home care nurse evaluates the patient's status and the patient's and family members' understanding of the therapeutic regimen and their adherence to it. If oxygen is used in the home, the nurse determines whether it is being administered safely and as prescribed. It is important to assess the patient's progress in stopping smoking and to reinforce the importance of smoking cessation with the patient and family. The nurse identifies strategies to assist with smoking cessation and refers the patient and family to community support groups. In addition, the nurse reminds the patient about the importance of other health promotion and screening practices.

Pulmonary Embolism

Pulmonary embolism (PE) refers to the obstruction of the pulmonary artery or one of its branches by a thrombus (or thrombi) that originates somewhere in the venous system or in the right side of the heart. It is estimated that more than half a million people develop PE yearly, resulting in more than 50,000 deaths (Goldhaber, 2004). PE is a common disorder and often is associated with trauma, surgery (orthopedic, major abdominal, pelvic, gynecologic), pregnancy, heart failure, age older than 50 years, hypercoagulable states, and prolonged immobility. It also may occur in apparently healthy people. Risk factors for PE are identified in Chart 23-7.

CHART 23-7

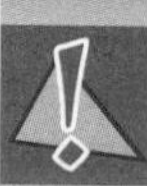

Risk Factors for Pulmonary Embolus

VENOUS STASIS (SLOWING OF BLOOD FLOW IN VEINS)

- Prolonged immobilization (especially postoperative)
- Prolonged periods of sitting/traveling
- Varicose veins
- Spinal cord injury

HYPERCOAGULABILITY (DUE TO RELEASE OF TISSUE THROMBOPLASTIN AFTER INJURY/SURGERY)

- Injury
- Tumor (pancreatic, gastrointestinal, genitourinary, breast, lung)
- Increased platelet count (polycythemia, splenectomy)

VENOUS ENDOTHELIAL DISEASE

- Thrombophlebitis
- Vascular disease
- Foreign bodies (IV/central venous catheters)

CERTAIN DISEASE STATES (COMBINATION OF STASIS, COAGULATION ALTERATIONS, AND VENOUS INJURY)

- Heart disease (especially heart failure)
- Trauma (especially fracture of hip, pelvis, vertebra, lower extremities)
- Postoperative state/postpartum period
- Diabetes mellitus
- Chronic obstructive pulmonary disease (COPD)

OTHER PREDISPOSING CONDITIONS

- Advanced age
- Obesity
- Pregnancy
- Oral contraceptive use
- History of previous thrombophlebitis, pulmonary embolism
- Constrictive clothing

Pathophysiology

Most commonly, PE is due to a blood clot or thrombus. However, there are other types of emboli: air, fat, amniotic fluid, and septic (from bacterial invasion of the thrombus). Although most thrombi originate in the deep veins of the legs, other sites include the pelvic veins and the right atrium of the heart. Venous thrombosis can result from slowing of blood flow (stasis) secondary to damage to the blood vessel wall (particularly the endothelial lining) or changes in the blood coagulation mechanism. Atrial fibrillation also causes PE. An enlarged right atrium in fibrillation causes blood to stagnate and form clots in this area. These clots are prone to travel into the pulmonary circulation.

When a thrombus completely or partially obstructs a pulmonary artery or its branches, the alveolar dead space is increased. The area, although continuing to be ventilated, receives little or no blood flow. Therefore, gas exchange is impaired or absent in this area. In addition, various substances are released from the clot and surrounding area that cause regional blood vessels and bronchioles to constrict. This results in an increase in pulmonary vascular resistance. This reaction compounds the ventilation–perfusion imbalance.

The hemodynamic consequences are increased pulmonary vascular resistance due to the regional vasoconstriction and reduced size of the pulmonary vascular bed. This results in an increase in pulmonary arterial pressure and, in turn, an increase in right ventricular work to maintain pulmonary blood flow. When the work requirements of the right ventricle exceed its capacity, right ventricular failure occurs, leading to a decrease in cardiac output followed by a decrease in systemic blood pressure and the development of shock.

Clinical Manifestations

Symptoms depend on the size of the thrombus and the area of the pulmonary artery occluded by the thrombus; they may be nonspecific. Dyspnea is the most frequent symptom; tachypnea (very rapid respiratory rate) is the most frequent sign (Goldhaber, 2004). The duration and intensity of the dyspnea depend on the extent of embolization. Chest pain is common and is usually sudden and pleuritic in origin. It may be substernal and may mimic angina pectoris or a myocardial infarction. Other symptoms include anxiety, fever, tachycardia, apprehension, cough, diaphoresis, hemoptysis, and syncope.

Deep venous thrombosis is closely associated with development of PE. Typically, patients report sudden onset of pain and/or swelling and warmth of the proximal or distal extremity, skin discoloration, and superficial vein distention. The pain is usually relieved with elevation.

A massive PE is best defined by the degree of hemodynamic instability rather than the percentage of pulmonary vasculature occlusion. It is described as an occlusion of the outflow tract of the main pulmonary artery or of the bifurcation of the pulmonary arteries that produces pronounced dyspnea, sudden substernal pain, rapid and weak pulse, shock, syncope, and sudden death. Multiple small emboli can lodge in the terminal pulmonary arterioles, producing multiple small infarctions of the lungs. A pulmonary infarction causes ischemic necrosis of an area of the lung. The clinical picture may mimic that of bronchopneumonia or heart failure. In atypical instances, PE causes few signs and symptoms, whereas in other instances it mimics various other cardiopulmonary disorders.

Assessment and Diagnostic Findings

Death from PE commonly occurs within 1 hour after the onset of symptoms; therefore, early recognition and diagnosis are priorities. Because the symptoms of PE can vary from few to severe, a diagnostic workup is performed to rule out other diseases. The initial diagnostic workup includes chest x-ray, ECG, peripheral vascular studies, arterial blood gas analysis, and ventilation–perfusion ($\dot{V}/\dot{Q}$) scan.

The chest x-ray is usually normal but may show infiltrates, atelectasis, elevation of the diaphragm on the affected side, or a pleural effusion. The chest x-ray is most helpful in excluding other possible causes. The ECG usually shows sinus tachycardia, PR-interval depression, and nonspecific T-wave changes. Peripheral vascular studies may include impedance plethysmography, Doppler ultrasonography, or venography (see Chapter 31). Test results confirm or exclude the diagnosis of PE. Arterial blood gas analysis may show hypoxemia and hypocapnia (from tachypnea); however, arterial blood gas measurements may be normal even in the presence of PE.

The $\dot{V}/\dot{Q}$ scan was once the second choice for diagnosis of a PE (with pulmonary angiogram [discussed below] considered the best diagnostic procedure). It is still used, especially in facilities that do not have access to a spiral CT scanner. The $\dot{V}/\dot{Q}$ scan is minimally invasive, involving the IV administration of a contrast agent. This scan evaluates different regions of the lung (upper, middle, lower) and allows comparisons of the percentage of ventilation and perfusion in each area. This test has a high sensitivity but can be more cumbersome then a CT scan and is not as accurate as a pulmonary angiogram.

A high suspicion of PE may warrant a spiral computed CT scan of the lung, D-dimer assay (blood test for evidence of blood clots), and pulmonary arteriogram. Spiral CT of the chest may also assist in the diagnosis. Spiral CT scan has recently gained popularity for use in the diagnosis of PE; it is more advanced and quicker than routine tomography. The term "spiral" comes from the shape of the path taken by the x-ray beam during scanning. The examination table advances at a constant rate through the scanner while the x-ray tube rotates continuously around the patient, following a spiral path, thus allowing the gathering of continuous data with no gaps between images. Unlike the traditional CT scan, the spiral CT scan evaluates slices as narrow as 1.0 mm, as compared with 5.0 mm slices obtained by traditional CT scan. This allows for a more accurate visualization of a PE. However, spiral CT has limitations. It cannot be performed at the bedside, so unstable patients must be transported to a CT scanner. In addition, IV infusion of contrast agent is necessary for visualization.

The D-dimer assay is becoming a more commonly used method for evaluating patients with possible PE. Because it is a simple test to perform, involving only a venipuncture, it has been studied as a possible method for ruling out PE; it is not used to make the diagnosis of PE. Emergency departments in particular have used this as a rapid, cost-effective test. D-dimer is a product of fibrin degradation and occurs as a result of fibrin lysis. An increased D-dimer value is usually indicative of a clotting abnormality. When a clot is dislodged, similar elevations of clotting factors should be present in the blood, especially in the case of a large embolus.

Pulmonary angiography is considered the best method to diagnose PE; however, it may not be feasible, cost-effective, or easily performed, especially with critically ill patients. The pulmonary angiogram allows for direct visualization under fluoroscopy of the arterial obstruction and accurate assessment of the perfusion deficit. A catheter is threaded through the vena cava to the right side of the heart to inject dye, similar to a cardiac catheterization, and a specially trained team must be available to perform the procedure.

Prevention

For patients at risk for PE, the most effective approach for prevention is to prevent deep venous thrombosis. Active leg exercises to avoid venous stasis, early ambulation, and use of elastic compression stockings are general preventive measures. Additional strategies for prevention are listed in Chart 23-8.

Anticoagulant therapy may be prescribed for patients who are older than 40 years of age, whose hemostasis is adequate, and who are undergoing major elective abdominal or thoracic surgery. Low doses of heparin may be administered before surgery to reduce the risk of postoperative deep venous thrombus and PE. Heparin should be administered subcutaneously 2 hours before surgery and continued every 8 to 12 hours until the patient is discharged. Low-dose heparin is thought to enhance the activity of antithrombin III, a major plasma inhibitor of clotting factor X. This regimen is not recommended for patients with an active thrombotic process or for those undergoing major orthopedic surgery, open prostatectomy, or surgery on the eye or brain. Low-molecular-weight heparin (eg, enoxaparin [Lovenox]) is an alternative therapy. It has a longer half-life, enhanced subcutaneous absorption, a reduced incidence of thrombocytopenia, and reduced interaction with platelets, compared with unfractionated heparin (Goldhaber, 2004).

Sequential compression devices (SCDs) are often used to prevent venous stasis through compression and relaxation of the calf muscles, similar to the effect of muscle contraction. SCDs have been proven to effectively reduce the risk of deep venous thrombosis and have been shown to be an effective primary therapy for patients who are unable to receive anticoagulation therapy (Nagahiro, Andou, Aoe, et al., 2004; Ramirez, Pantelis, Gonzalez-Ruiz, et al., 2003). Several types of SCDs, using foot, calf, and thigh-high compression as well as graduated, asymmetric, and circumferential compression, are available. There is little evidence favoring any particular type of compression. Graduated compression involves the sequential movement of air in the sleeve up the leg, followed by relaxation of the sleeve. The advantage of this therapy is the extended duration of compression compared with standard inflation. Asymmetric compression involves inflating only the area on the back of the leg or foot. Circumferential compression involves even compression of the entire leg.

CHART 23-8

HOME CARE CHECKLIST • Prevention of Recurrent Pulmonary Embolism

At the completion of the home care instruction, the patient or caregiver will be able to:	Patient	Caregiver
• Describe the underlying process leading to pulmonary embolism.	✔	✔
• Describe the need for continued anticoagulant therapy after the initial embolism.	✔	✔
• Name the anticoagulant prescribed and identify dosage and schedule of administration.	✔	✔
• Describe potential side effects of coagulation such as bruising and bleeding and identify ways to prevent bleeding.	✔	✔
• Avoid the use of sharps (razors, knives, etc.) to prevent cuts; shave with an electric shaver.		
• Use a toothbrush with soft bristles to prevent gum injury.		
• Do not take aspirin or antihistamines while taking warfarin sodium (Coumadin).		
• Always check with health care provider before taking any medicine, including over-the-counter medications.		
• Avoid laxatives, because they may affect vitamin K absorption.		
• Report the occurrence of dark, tarry stools to the health care provider immediately.		
• Wear an identification bracelet or carry a medicine card stating that you are taking anticoagulants.		
• Describe strategies to prevent recurrent deep venous thrombosis and pulmonary emboli:	✔	✔
• Continue to wear elastic pressure stockings (compression hose) as long as directed.		
• Avoid sitting with legs crossed or sitting for prolonged periods of time.		
• When traveling, change position regularly, walk occasionally, and do active exercises of moving the legs and ankles while sitting.		
• Drink fluids, especially while traveling and in warm weather, to avoid hemoconcentration due to fluid deficit.		
• Describe the signs and symptoms of lower extremity circulatory compromise and potential deep venous thrombosis: calf or leg pain, swelling, pedal edema.	✔	✔
• Describe the signs and symptoms of pulmonary compromise related to recurrent pulmonary embolism.	✔	✔
• Describe how and when to contact the health care provider if symptoms of circulatory compromise or pulmonary compromise are identified.	✔	✔

Medical Management

Because PE is often a medical emergency, emergency management is of primary concern. After emergency measures have been initiated and the patient is stabilized, the treatment goal is to dissolve (lyse) the existing emboli and prevent new ones from forming. Treatment may include a variety of modalities:

- General measures to improve respiratory and vascular status
- Anticoagulation therapy
- Thrombolytic therapy
- Surgical intervention

Emergency Management

Massive PE is a life-threatening emergency. The immediate objective is to stabilize the cardiopulmonary system. A sudden increase in pulmonary resistance increases the work of the right ventricle, which can cause acute right-sided heart failure with cardiogenic shock. Emergency management consists of the following actions:

- Nasal oxygen is administered immediately to relieve hypoxemia, respiratory distress, and central cyanosis.
- Intravenous infusion lines are inserted to establish routes for medications or fluids that will be needed.
- A perfusion scan, hemodynamic measurements, and arterial blood gas determinations are performed. spiral (helical) CT or pulmonary angiography may be performed.
- Hypotension is treated by a slow infusion of dobutamine (Dobutrex), which has a dilating effect on the pulmonary vessels and bronchi, or dopamine (Intropin).
- The ECG is monitored continuously for dysrhythmias and right ventricular failure, which may occur suddenly.
- Digitalis glycosides, IV diuretics, and antiarrhythmic agents are administered when appropriate.

- Blood is drawn for serum electrolytes, complete blood count, and hematocrit.
- If clinical assessment and arterial blood gas analysis indicate the need, the patient is intubated and placed on a mechanical ventilator.
- If the patient has suffered massive embolism and is hypotensive, an indwelling urinary catheter is inserted to monitor urinary output.
- Small doses of IV morphine or sedatives are administered to relieve patient anxiety, to alleviate chest discomfort, to improve tolerance of the endotracheal tube, and to ease adaptation to the mechanical ventilator.

General Management

Measures are initiated to improve respiratory and vascular status. Oxygen therapy is administered to correct the hypoxemia, relieve the pulmonary vascular vasoconstriction, and reduce the pulmonary hypertension. Use of elastic compression stockings or intermittent pneumatic leg compression devices reduces venous stasis. These measures compress the superficial veins and increase the velocity of blood in the deep veins by redirecting the blood through the deep veins. Elevating the leg (above the level of the heart) also increases venous flow.

Pharmacologic Therapy

ANTICOAGULATION THERAPY

Anticoagulant therapy (heparin, warfarin sodium) has traditionally been the primary method for managing acute deep vein thrombosis and PE (Goldhaber, 2004; Karin, 2003). Heparin is used to prevent recurrence of emboli but has no effect on emboli that are already present. Heparin is generally recommended for all patients who have been diagnosed with PE. Generally, a therapeutic heparin dose is administered as a one-time 5000-unit bolus and a continuous IV infusion is then started to maintain the partial thromboplastin time (PTT) at 1.5 to 2.0 times the normal level.

Heparin administration is associated with several concerns. Because the half-life of heparin is dose dependent, it is difficult and time-consuming to adjust and maintain the IV drip infusion at a therapeutic level; frequent laboratory testing is necessary. With long-term heparin use, there is also the risk of antibody formation and bleeding. Despite the risks, anticoagulation after initial clot formation and dislodgement is necessary because of the high risk for a recurrent thrombus. Therapy may be changed to an oral regimen, such as warfarin (Coumadin), as soon as the patient is able to take oral medications. Heparin must be continued until the international normalized ratio (INR) is within a therapeutic range, typically 2.0 to 2.5. Once the patient starts an oral regimen, it is important that he or she continue to take the same brand of warfarin, because the bioavailability may vary greatly among brands.

High doses of subcutaneous low-molecular-weight heparin or heparinoids may also be used to maintain a therapeutic PTT while oral anticoagulation therapy is being adjusted. Lepirudin (Refludan) and argatroban are alternatives for patients in whom heparin or heparinoids are contraindicated. These agents are direct thrombin inhibitors; therefore, they require less frequent monitoring and dose adjustment. Both medications have contraindications and side effects that the nurse must be aware of before administration. Lepirudin and argatroban are both contraindicated in patients with overt major bleeding and in patients who are hypersensitive to these agents or at high risk for bleeding (eg, recent cerebrovascular accident [CVA, brain attack], anomaly of vessels or organs, recent major surgery, recent puncture of large vessels or organ biopsy). Major side effects are bleeding anywhere in the body and anaphylactic reaction resulting in shock or death. Other side effects include fever, abnormal liver function, and allergic skin reaction. All patients must continue to take some form of anticoagulation for at least 3 to 6 months after the embolic event.

THROMBOLYTIC THERAPY

Thrombolytic therapy (urokinase, streptokinase, alteplase, anistreplase, reteplase) also may be used in treating PE, particularly for patients who are severely compromised (eg, those who are hypotensive and have significant hypoxemia despite oxygen supplementation). Thrombolytic therapy resolves the thrombi or emboli more quickly and restores more normal hemodynamic functioning of the pulmonary circulation, thereby reducing pulmonary hypertension and improving perfusion, oxygenation, and cardiac output. However, bleeding is a significant side effect. Contraindications to thrombolytic therapy include a CVA within the past 2 months, other active intracranial processes, active bleeding, surgery within 10 days of the thrombotic event, recent labor and delivery, trauma, or severe hypertension. Consequently, thrombolytic agents are advocated only for PE affecting a significant area of blood flow to the lung and causing hemodynamic instability.

Before thrombolytic therapy is started, INR, PTT, hematocrit, and platelet counts are obtained. Heparin is stopped prior to administration of a thrombolytic agent. During therapy, all but essential invasive procedures are avoided because of potential bleeding. If necessary, fresh whole blood, packed red cells, cryoprecipitate, or frozen plasma is administered to replace blood loss and reverse the bleeding tendency. After the thrombolytic infusion is completed (which varies in duration according to the agent used and the condition being treated), anticoagulant therapy is initiated.

Surgical Management

A surgical embolectomy is rarely performed but may be indicated if the patient has a massive PE or hemodynamic instability or if there are contraindications to thrombolytic therapy. This invasive procedure involves removal of the actual clot and must be performed by a cardiovascular surgical team with the patient on cardiopulmonary bypass. It may be used for patients who fail to improve with thrombolytic therapy, have contraindications to thrombolytic therapy and have had a massive PE, or must have the clot removed to help reduce right-sided heart failure. Although surgical embolectomy ensures removal of the clot, it is not without risk. The procedure has a high intraoperative mortality rate and has typical postoperative complications.

Transvenous catheter embolectomy is a technique in which a vacuum-cupped catheter is introduced transvenously into the affected pulmonary artery. Suction is applied to the end of the embolus, and the embolus is aspirated into the cup. The surgeon maintains suction to hold the embolus within the cup, and the entire catheter is withdrawn through the right side of the heart and out the femoral vein. Catheters are available that pulverize the clot with high-velocity jets of normal saline solution. An inferior vena cava filter is usually inserted at the time of surgery to protect against a recurrence.

Interrupting the inferior vena cava is another surgical technique used when PE recurs or when the patient does not tolerate anticoagulant therapy. This approach prevents dislodged thrombi from being swept into the lungs while allowing adequate blood flow. The preferred approach is the application of Teflon clips to the inferior vena cava to divide the lumen into small channels without occluding caval blood flow. Also, the use of transvenous devices that occlude or filter the blood through the inferior vena cava is a fairly safe way to prevent recurrent PE. One such technique involves insertion of a filter (eg, Greenfield filter) through the internal jugular vein or common femoral vein (Fig. 23-7). This filter is advanced into the inferior vena cava, where it is opened. The perforated umbrella permits the passage of blood but prevents the passage of large thrombi. It is recommended that anticoagulation be continued in patients with a vena cava filter, if there are no contraindications to its use.

Nursing Management

Minimizing the Risk of Pulmonary Embolism

A key role of the nurse is to identify the patient at high risk for PE and to minimize the risk of PE in all patients. The nurse must have a high degree of suspicion for PE in all patients, but particularly in those with conditions predisposing to a slowing of venous return (see Chart 23-7).

Preventing Thrombus Formation

Preventing thrombus formation is a major nursing responsibility. The nurse encourages ambulation and active and passive leg exercises to prevent venous stasis in patients prescribed bed rest. The nurse instructs the patient to move the legs in a "pumping" exercise so that the leg muscles can help increase venous flow. The nurse also advises the patient not to sit or lie in bed for prolonged periods, not to cross the legs, and not to wear constrictive clothing. Legs should not be dangled or feet placed in a dependent position while the patient sits on the edge of the bed; instead, feet should rest on the floor or on a chair. In addition, IV catheters (for parenteral therapy or measurements of central venous pressure) should not be left in place for prolonged periods.

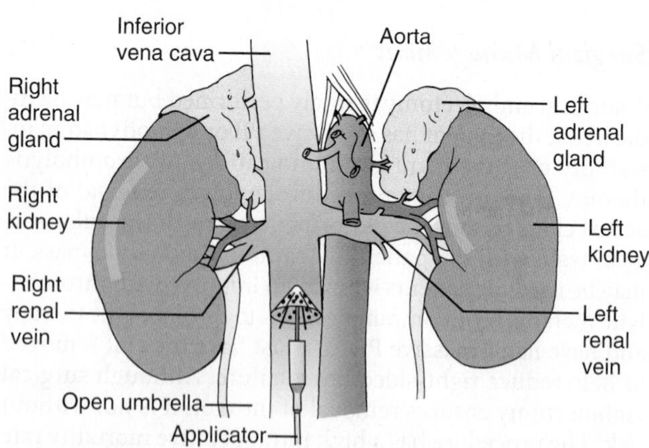

FIGURE 23-7. An umbrella filter is in place in the inferior vena cava to prevent pulmonary embolism. The filter (compressed within an applicator catheter) is inserted through an incision in the right internal jugular vein. The applicator is withdrawn when the filter fixes itself to the wall of the inferior vena cava after ejection from the applicator.

Assessing Potential for Pulmonary Embolism

All patients are evaluated for risk factors for thrombus formation and pulmonary embolus. The nurse does a careful assessment of the patient's health history, family history, and medication record. On a daily basis, the patient is asked about pain or discomfort in the extremities. In addition, the extremities are evaluated for warmth, redness, and inflammation.

Monitoring Thrombolytic Therapy

The nurse is responsible for monitoring thrombolytic and anticoagulant therapy. Thrombolytic therapy (streptokinase, urokinase, tissue plasminogen activator) causes lysis of deep vein thrombi and pulmonary emboli, which helps dissolve the clots. During thrombolytic infusion, while the patient remains on bed rest, vital signs are assessed every 2 hours and invasive procedures are avoided. Tests to determine INR or PTT are performed 3 to 4 hours after the thrombolytic infusion is started to confirm that the fibrinolytic systems have been activated. See Chapter 31 for nursing management for the patient receiving anticoagulant or thrombolytic therapy.

NURSING ALERT

Because of the prolonged clotting time, only essential arterial punctures or venipunctures are performed, and manual pressure is applied to any puncture site for at least 30 minutes. Pulse oximetry is used to monitor changes in oxygenation. The thrombolytic infusion is discontinued immediately if uncontrolled bleeding occurs.

Managing Pain

Chest pain, if present, is usually pleuritic rather than cardiac in origin. A semi-Fowler's position provides a more comfortable position for breathing. However, it is important to continue to turn patients frequently and reposition them to improve the **ventilation–perfusion ratio** in the lung. The nurse administers opioid analgesics as prescribed for severe pain.

Managing Oxygen Therapy

Careful attention is given to the proper use of oxygen. It is important to ensure that the patient understands the need for continuous oxygen therapy. The nurse assesses the patient frequently for signs of hypoxemia and monitors the pulse oximetry values to evaluate the effectiveness of the oxygen therapy. Deep breathing and incentive spirometry are indicated for all patients to minimize or prevent atelectasis and improve ventilation. Nebulizer therapy or percussion and postural drainage may be used for management of secretions.

Relieving Anxiety

The nurse encourages the stabilized patient to talk about any fears or concerns related to this frightening episode, answers the patient's and family's questions concisely and accurately, explains the therapy, and describes how to recognize untoward effects early.

Monitoring for Complications

When caring for a patient who has had PE, the nurse must be alert for the potential complication of cardiogenic shock or right ventricular failure subsequent to the effect of PE on the cardiovascular system. Nursing activities for managing shock are found in Chapter 15.

Providing Postoperative Nursing Care

The nurse measures the patient's pulmonary arterial pressure and urinary output. The nurse also assesses the insertion site of the arterial catheter for hematoma formation and infection. It is important to maintain the blood pressure at a level that supports perfusion of vital organs. To prevent peripheral venous stasis and edema of the lower extremities, the nurse elevates the foot of the bed and encourages isometric exercises, use of elastic compression stockings, and walking when the patient is permitted out of bed. Sitting is discouraged, because hip flexion compresses the large veins in the legs.

Promoting Home and Community-Based Care

TEACHING PATIENTS SELF-CARE

Before hospital discharge and at follow-up visits to the clinic, the nurse instructs the patient about preventing recurrence and reporting signs and symptoms. Patient instructions, as presented in Chart 23-8, are intended to help prevent recurrences and side effects of treatment.

CONTINUING CARE

During follow-up or home care visits, the nurse monitors the patient's adherence to the prescribed management plan and reinforces previous instructions. The nurse also monitors the patient for residual effects of the PE and recovery. The patient is reminded about the importance of keeping follow-up appointments for coagulation tests and appointments with the primary care provider. The nurse also reminds the patient about the importance of participation in health promotion activities (eg, immunizations) and health screening.

Sarcoidosis

Sarcoidosis is a multisystem, granulomatous disease of unknown etiology. It may involve almost any organ or tissue but most commonly involves the lungs, lymph nodes, liver, spleen, central nervous system, skin, eyes, fingers, and parotid glands. The disease is not gender-specific, but some manifestations are more common in women. Prevalence rates are 10 to 40 cases per 100,000 population. In the United States, the disease is more common in African Americans (36 cases per 100,000) than in Caucasians (11 cases per 100,000), and the disease usually begins in the third or fourth decade of life (Doty & Judson, 2004).

Pathophysiology

Sarcoidosis is thought to be a hypersensitivity response to one or more agents (bacteria, fungi, virus, chemicals) in people with an inherited or acquired predisposition to the disorder. The hypersensitivity response results in noncaseating granuloma formation due to the release of cytokines and other substances that promote replication of fibroblasts. In the lung, granuloma infiltration and fibrosis may occur, resulting in low lung compliance, impaired diffusing capacity, and reduced lung volumes.

Clinical Manifestations

Hallmarks of sarcoidosis are its insidious onset and lack of prominent clinical signs or symptoms. The clinical picture depends on the systems affected. The lung is most commonly involved; signs and symptoms may include dyspnea, cough, hemoptysis, and congestion. Generalized symptoms include anorexia, fatigue, and weight loss. Other signs include uveitis, joint pain, fever, and granulomatous lesions of the skin, liver, spleen, kidney, and central nervous system. The granulomas may disappear or gradually convert to fibrous tissue. With multisystem involvement, patients may also have fatigue, fever, anorexia, and weight loss.

Assessment and Diagnostic Findings

Chest x-rays and CT are used to assess pulmonary adenopathy. These may show hilar adenopathy and disseminated miliary and nodular lesions in the lungs. A mediastinoscopy or **transbronchial** biopsy (in which a tissue specimen is obtained through the bronchial wall) may be used to confirm the diagnosis. In rare cases, an **open lung biopsy** is performed. Diagnosis is confirmed by a biopsy that shows noncaseating granulomas. Pulmonary function test results are abnormal if there is restriction of lung function (reduction in total lung capacity). Arterial blood gas measurements may be normal or may show reduced oxygen levels (hypoxemia) and increased carbon dioxide levels (hypercapnia).

Medical Management

Many patients undergo remission without specific treatment. Corticosteroids may be beneficial because of their anti-inflammatory effects, which relieve symptoms and improve organ function. They are useful in patients with ocular and myocardial involvement, skin involvement, extensive pulmonary disease that compromises pulmonary function, hepatic involvement, and hypercalcemia. Other cytotoxic and immunosuppressive agents have been used, but without the benefit of controlled clinical trials. There is no single test that monitors the progression or recurrence of sarcoidosis. Multiple tests are used to monitor involved systems.

Occupational Lung Diseases: Pneumoconioses

Pneumoconiosis refers to a nonneoplastic alteration of the lung resulting from inhalation of mineral or inorganic dust (eg, "dusty lung"). Pneumoconioses are caused by inhalation and deposition of mineral dusts in the lungs, resulting in pulmonary fibrosis and parenchymal changes. Many people with early pneumoconiosis are asymptomatic, but advanced disease often is accompanied by disability and premature death (CDC, 2004b). Between 1968 and 2000, pneumoconiosis was cited as the cause of death of 124,846 people in the United States (CDC, 2004b).

Diseases of the lungs occur in numerous occupations as a result of exposure to several different types of agents. Examples include mineral dusts (asbestos, silica, coal), metal dusts, biological dusts (spores, mycelia, bird droppings), manufactured fibers (glass or ceramic fibers), and toxic fumes (nitrogen dioxide, sulfur dioxide, chlorine, ammonia). The effects of inhaling these materials depend on the composition of the substance, its concentration, its ability to initiate an immune response, its irritating properties, the duration of exposure, and the individual's response or susceptibility to the irritant. Smoking may compound the problem and may increase the risk of lung cancers in people exposed to the mineral asbestos and other potential carcinogens.

Key aspects of any assessment of patients with a potential occupational respiratory history include job and job activities, exposure levels, general hygiene, time frame of exposure, amount of respiratory protection used, and direct versus indirect exposures. Specific information that should be obtained includes the following:

- Exposure to an agent known to cause an occupational disorder
- Length of time from exposure of agent to onset of symptoms
- Congruence of symptoms with those of known exposure-related disorder
- Lack of other more likely explanations of the signs and symptoms

Occupational health nurses serve as employee advocates, making every effort to promote measures to reduce the exposure of workers to industrial products. Resources for occupational health nurses include the United States Department of Labor Occupational Safety and Health Administration (OSHA) as well as state-specific resources. The mission of OSHA is to ensure the safety and health of America's workers by setting and enforcing standards; providing training, outreach, and education; establishing partnerships; and encouraging continual improvement in workplace safety and health. Laws require that the work environment be ventilated properly to remove any noxious agent.

Dust control can prevent many of the pneumoconioses. Dust control includes ventilation, spraying an area with water to control dust, and effective and frequent floor cleaning. Air samples need to be monitored. Toxic substances should be enclosed and placed in restricted areas. Workers must wear or use protective devices (face masks, hoods, industrial respirators) to provide a safe air supply when a toxic element is present. Employees who are at risk should be carefully screened and monitored. There is a risk of developing serious smoking-related illness (cancer) in industries in which there are unsafe levels of certain gases, dusts, fumes, fluids, and other toxic substances. In addition, there is the potential for second-hand exposure. Asbestos and toxic dusts and substances may be transferred to others through the handling of clothing or shoes that have been exposed. Ongoing educational programs should be designed to teach workers to take responsibility for their own health and to stop smoking and receive an influenza vaccination.

Federal "right to know" laws stipulate that employees must be informed about all hazardous and toxic substances in the workplace. Specifically, they must be informed about any hazardous or toxic substances they work with, what effects these substances can have on their health, and the measures they can take to protect themselves. The responsibility for implementing these controls inevitably falls on the federal or state government.

In addition to teaching preventive measures to patients and their families, the nurse assesses patients for a history of exposure to environmental agents (eg, dusts, fibers, fumes) and makes referrals so that pulmonary function can be evaluated and the patient can be treated early in the course of the disease. Patients with occupational lung disease often experience increasing chronic dyspnea, cough, and a prolonged illness culminating in respiratory failure. Strategies to prevent superimposed infection are implemented, and the patient and family are assisted in coping with the increasing disability that accompanies occupational lung disease. Home care referrals are often helpful in identifying measures to decrease the patient's dyspnea, ensure appropriate and safe use of oxygen, and make the patient as comfortable as possible. In addition, referral to a pulmonary rehabilitation program may be considered in some patients.

The most common pneumoconioses are silicosis, asbestosis, and coal worker's pneumoconiosis.

Silicosis

Silicosis is a chronic fibrotic pulmonary disease caused by inhalation of silica dust (crystalline silicon dioxide particles). Exposure to silica and silicates occurs in almost all mining, quarrying, and tunneling operations. Glass manufacturing, stone-cutting, manufacturing of abrasives and pottery, and foundry work are other occupations with exposure hazards. Finely ground silica, such as that found in soaps, polishes and filters, is extremely dangerous.

Pathophysiology

When the silica particles, which have fibrogenic properties, are inhaled, nodular lesions are produced throughout the lungs. With the passage of time and further exposure, the nodules enlarge and coalesce. Dense masses form in the upper portion of the lungs, resulting in the loss of pulmonary volume. **Restrictive lung disease** (disease of the lungs that limits their ability to expand fully) and obstructive lung disease from secondary emphysema result. Cavities can form as a result of superimposed TB. Exposure of 15 to 20 years is usually required before the onset of the disease and shortness of breath occurs. Fibrotic destruction of pulmonary tissue can lead to emphysema, pulmonary hypertension, and cor pulmonale.

Clinical Manifestations

Patients with acute silicosis present with dyspnea, fever, cough, and weight loss, and progression of the disease is rapid. Symptoms are more severe in patients whose disease is complicated by progressive massive fibrosis. More commonly, this disease is a chronic problem with a long latency period. Patients may have slowly progressive symptoms indicative of hypoxemia, severe air-flow obstruction, and right-sided heart failure. Edema may occur because of the cardiac failure.

Medical Management

There is no specific treatment for silicosis, because the fibrotic process in the lung is irreversible. Supportive therapy is directed at managing complications and preventing infection. Testing is performed to rule out other lung diseases, such as TB, lung cancer, and sarcoidosis. If TB is present, it is aggressively treated. Additional therapy may include oxygen, diuretics, inhaled beta-adrenergic agonists, anticholinergics, and bronchodilator therapy.

Asbestosis

Asbestosis is a disease characterized by diffuse pulmonary fibrosis from the inhalation of asbestos dust. Current laws restrict the use of asbestos, but many industries used it in the past. Therefore, exposure occurred, and may still occur, in people in numerous occupations, including asbestos mining and manufacturing, shipbuilding, demolition of structures containing asbestos, and roofing. Materials such as shingles, cement, vinyl asbestos tile, fireproof paint and clothing, brake linings, and filters all contained asbestos at one time, and many of these materials are still in existence. Chronic exposure may also occur by washing clothes that have been in contact with asbestos. Additional diseases related to asbestos exposure include lung cancer, mesothelioma, and asbestos-related pleural effusion.

Pathophysiology

Inhaled asbestos fibers enter the alveoli, where they are surrounded by fibrous tissue. The fibrous tissue eventually obliterates the alveoli. Fibrous changes also affect the pleura, which thickens and develops plaque. The result of these physiologic changes is a restrictive lung disease, with a decrease in lung volume, diminished exchange of oxygen and carbon dioxide, and hypoxemia.

Clinical Manifestations

The onset of the disease is insidious, and patients have progressive dyspnea, persistent, dry cough, mild to moderate chest pain, anorexia, weight loss, and malaise. Early physical findings include bibasilar fine, end-inspiratory crackles and, in more advanced cases, clubbing of the fingers. As the disease progresses, cor pulmonale and respiratory failure occur. A high proportion of workers who have been exposed to asbestos dust, especially those who smoke or have a history of smoking, die of lung cancer. Malignant mesothelioma, a rare cancer of the pleura or peritoneum that is strongly associated with asbestos exposure, may also occur.

Medical Management

There is no effective treatment for asbestosis, because the lung damage is permanent and often progressive. Management is directed at controlling infection and treating the lung disease. When oxygen–carbon dioxide exchange becomes severely impaired, continuous oxygen therapy may help improve activity tolerance. The patient must be instructed to avoid additional exposure to asbestos and to stop smoking. A significant contributing cause to mortality in this population is the high incidence of lung carcinoma.

Coal Worker's Pneumoconiosis

Coal worker's pneumoconiosis ("black lung disease") includes a variety of respiratory diseases found in coal workers who have inhaled coal dust over the years. Coal miners are exposed to dusts that are mixtures of coal, kaolin, mica, and silica.

Pathophysiology

When coal dust is deposited in the alveoli and respiratory bronchioles, macrophages engulf the particles (by phagocytosis) and transport them to the terminal bronchioles, where they are removed by mucociliary action. In time, the clearance mechanisms cannot handle the excessive dust load, and the macrophages aggregate in the respiratory bronchioles and alveoli. Fibroblasts appear and a network of reticulin is laid down surrounding the dust-laden macrophages. The bronchioles and the alveoli become clogged with coal dust, dying macrophages, and fibroblasts. This leads to the formation of the coal macule, the primary lesion of the disorder. Macules appear as blackish dots on the lungs. Fibrotic lesions develop and, as the macules enlarge, the weakening bronchioles dilate, with subsequent development of localized emphysema. The disease begins in the upper lobes of the lungs but may progress to the lower lobes.

Clinical Manifestations

The first signs are a chronic cough and sputum production, similar to the signs encountered in chronic bronchitis. As the disease progresses, patients develop dyspnea and cough up large amounts of sputum with varying amounts of black fluid (melanoptysis), particularly if they are smokers. Eventually, cor pulmonale and respiratory failure result. The diagnosis may first be made based on chest x-ray findings and history of exposure.

Medical Management

Preventing this disease is key, because there is no effective treatment. Instead, treatment focuses on early diagnosis and management of complications. (See Chapter 24 for discussion of emphysema.)

Chest Tumors

Tumors of the lung may be benign or malignant. A malignant chest tumor can be primary, arising within the lung, chest wall, or mediastinum, or it can be a metastasis from a primary tumor site elsewhere in the body. Metastatic lung tumors occur frequently because the bloodstream transports cancer cells from primary cancers elsewhere in the body to the lungs.

Lung Cancer (Bronchogenic Carcinoma)

Lung cancer is the leading cancer killer among men and women in the United States. In 2005, there were an estimated 172,500 new cases of cancer of the lung and bronchus (93,000 men and 79,500 women). In the same year, it was estimated that 163,500 would die from this disease (American Cancer Society, 2005). For men, the incidence of lung cancer has remained relatively constant and in women it has begun to plateau after a continuous rise over the past 30 years (American Cancer Society, 2005). Two thirds of the United States population with lung cancer is 65 years of age or older (Hurria & Kris, 2003).

In approximately 70% of patients with lung cancer, the disease has spread to regional lymphatics and other sites by the time of diagnosis. As a result, the long-term survival rate is low.

Pathophysiology

Between 80% and 90% of lung cancers are caused by inhaled carcinogens, most commonly cigarette smoke (Baldwin, 2003); other carcinogens include radon gas and occupational and environmental agents. Lung cancers arise from a single transformed epithelial cell in the tracheobronchial airways, in which the carcinogen binds to and damages the cell's DNA. This damage results in cellular changes, abnormal cell growth, and eventually a malignant cell. As the damaged DNA is passed on to daughter cells, the DNA undergoes further changes and becomes unstable. With the accumulation of genetic changes, the pulmonary epithelium undergoes malignant transformation from normal epithelium eventually to invasive carcinoma. Evidence indicates that carcinoma tends to arise at sites of previous scarring (TB, fibrosis) in the lung.

Classification and Staging

For purposes of staging and treatment, most lung cancers are classified into one of two major categories: small cell lung cancer and non–small cell lung cancer. Non–small cell lung cancer is further classified with cell types. Squamous cell cancer is usually more centrally located and arises more commonly in the segmental and subsegmental bronchi. Adenocarcinoma is the most prevalent carcinoma of the lung in both men and women; it occurs peripherally as peripheral masses or nodules and often metastasizes. Large cell carcinoma (also called undifferentiated carcinoma) is a fast-growing tumor that tends to arise peripherally. Bronchoalveolar cell cancer is found in the terminal bronchi and alveoli and is usually slower growing compared with other bronchogenic carcinomas.

Non–small cell lung carcinoma (NSCLC) represents 75% to 80% of tumors; small cell carcinoma represents 15% to 20% of tumors. In NSCLC, the cell types include squamous cell carcinoma (20% to 30%), large cell carcinoma (10%), and adenocarcinoma (30% to 40%), including bronchoalveolar carcinoma. Most small cell carcinomas arise in the major bronchi and spread by infiltration along the bronchial wall. Small cell lung cancer accounts for 20% to 25% of all bronchogenic cancers (Baldwin, 2003).

In addition to classification according to cell type, lung cancers are staged. The stage of the tumor refers to the size of the tumor, its location, whether lymph nodes are involved, and whether the cancer has spread (American Joint Committee on Cancer, 2002). NSCLC is staged as I to IV. Stage I is the earliest stage and has the highest cure rates, whereas stage IV designates metastatic spread. Estimated 5-year survival rates for the stages of NSCLC are as follows: stages IA and IB, 50% to 80%; stage IIA and IIB, 30% to 50%; stage IIIA, 10% to 40%; stage IIIB, 5% to 20%; and stage IV, less than 5% (Baldwin, 2003). Small cell lung cancers are classified as limited or extensive. Diagnostic tools and further information on staging are described in Chapter 16.

Risk Factors

Various factors have been associated with the development of lung cancer, including tobacco smoke, secondhand (passive) smoke, environmental and occupational exposures, gender, genetics, and dietary deficits. Other factors that have been associated with lung cancer include genetic predisposition and underlying respiratory diseases, such as COPD and TB.

Tobacco Smoke

Tobacco use is responsible for more than one of every six deaths in the United States from pulmonary and cardiovascular diseases. Smoking is the most important single preventable cause of death and disease in this country. Lung cancer is 10 times more common in cigarette smokers than nonsmokers. Risk is determined by the pack-year history (number of packs of cigarettes used each day, multiplied by the number of years smoked), the age of initiation of smoking, the depth of inhalation, and the tar and nicotine levels in the cigarettes smoked. The younger a person is when he or she starts smoking, the greater the risk of developing lung cancer. The risk of cancer is always higher for former smokers than for people who have never smoked. However, the risk decreases beginning at approximately 5 years after smoking cessation occurs and continues to decrease over time.

Secondhand Smoke

Passive smoking has been identified as a possible cause of lung cancer in nonsmokers. It is estimated that secondhand smoke causes about 3000 deaths per year (Baldwin, 2003). When compared with unexposed nonsmokers, people who are involuntarily exposed to tobacco smoke in a closed environment (house, automobile, building) have an increased risk of lung cancer.

Environmental and Occupational Exposure

Various carcinogens have been identified in the atmosphere, including motor vehicle emissions and pollutants from refineries and manufacturing plants. Evidence suggests that the incidence of lung cancer is greater in urban areas as a result of the buildup of pollutants and motor vehicle emissions.

Radon is a colorless, odorless gas found in soil and rocks. For many years it has been associated with uranium mines, but it is now known to seep into homes through ground rock. High levels of radon have been associated with the development of lung cancer, especially when combined with cigarette smoking. Homeowners are advised to have radon levels checked in their houses and to arrange for special venting if the levels are high.

Chronic exposure to industrial carcinogens, such as arsenic, asbestos, mustard gas, chromates, coke oven fumes, nickel, oil, and radiation, has been associated with the development of lung cancer. Laws have been passed to control exposure to these carcinogens in the workplace.

Genetics

Some familial predisposition to lung cancer seems apparent, because the incidence of lung cancer in close relatives of patients with lung cancer appears to be two to three times that in the general population regardless of smoking status.

Dietary Factors

Smokers who eat a diet low in fruits and vegetables have an increased risk of developing lung cancer. The actual active agents in a diet rich in fruits and vegetables have yet to be determined. It has been hypothesized that carotenoids, particularly carotene or vitamin A, may be important. Several ongoing trials may help determine whether carotene supplementation has anticancer properties. Other nutrients, including vitamin E, selenium, vitamin C, fat, and retinoids, are also being evaluated regarding their protective role against lung cancer.

Clinical Manifestations

Often, lung cancer develops insidiously and is asymptomatic until late in its course. The signs and symptoms depend on the location and size of the tumor, the degree of obstruction, and the existence of metastases to regional or distant sites.

The most frequent symptom of lung cancer is cough or change in a chronic cough. People frequently ignore this symptom and attribute it to smoking or a respiratory infection. The cough starts as a dry, persistent cough, without sputum production. When obstruction of airways occurs, the cough may become productive due to infection.

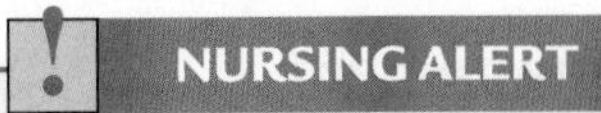

A cough that changes in character should arouse suspicion of lung cancer.

Dyspnea occurs in 35% to 50% of patients (Baldwin, 2003). Hemoptysis or blood-tinged sputum may be expectorated. Chest or shoulder pain may indicate chest wall or pleural involvement by a tumor. Pain also is a late manifestation and may be related to metastasis to the bone.

In some patients, a recurring fever is an early symptom in response to a persistent infection in an area of pneumonitis distal to the tumor. In fact, cancer of the lung should be suspected in people with repeated unresolved upper respiratory tract infections. If the tumor spreads to adjacent structures and regional lymph nodes, the patient may present with chest pain and tightness, hoarseness (involving the recurrent laryngeal nerve), dysphagia, head and neck edema, and symptoms of pleural or pericardial effusion. The most common sites of metastases are lymph nodes, bone, brain, contralateral lung, adrenal glands, and liver. Nonspecific symptoms of weakness, anorexia, and weight loss also may be present.

Assessment and Diagnostic Findings

If pulmonary symptoms occur in heavy smokers, cancer of the lung should always be considered. A chest x-ray is performed to search for pulmonary density, a solitary pulmonary nodule (coin lesion), atelectasis, and infection. CT scans of the chest are used to identify small nodules not easily visualized on the chest x-ray and also to serially examine areas for lymphadenopathy.

Sputum cytology is rarely used to make a diagnosis of lung cancer. Fiberoptic bronchoscopy is more commonly used; it provides a detailed study of the tracheobronchial tree and allows for brushings, washings, and biopsies of suspicious areas. For peripheral lesions not amenable to bronchoscopic biopsy, a transthoracic **fine-needle aspiration** may be performed under CT guidance to aspirate cells from a suspicious area. In some circumstances, an endoscopy with esophageal ultrasound may be used to obtain a transesophageal biopsy of enlarged subcarinal lymph nodes that are not easily accessible by other means.

A variety of scans may be used to assess for metastasis of the cancer. These may include bone scans, abdominal scans, positron emission tomography (PET) scans, and liver ultrasound. CT of the brain, magnetic resonance imaging (MRI), and other neurologic diagnostic procedures are used to detect central nervous system metastases. Mediastinoscopy or mediastinotomy may be used to obtain biopsy samples from lymph nodes in the mediastinum.

If surgery is a potential treatment, the patient is evaluated to determine whether the tumor is resectable and whether the patient can tolerate the physiologic impairment resulting from such surgery. Pulmonary function tests, arterial blood gas analysis, V̇/Q scans, and exercise testing may all be used as part of the preoperative assessment.

CHART 23-9

Types of Lung Resection

- Lobectomy: a single lobe of lung is removed
- Bilobectomy: two lobes of the lung are removed
- Sleeve resection: cancerous lobe(s) is removed and a segment of the main bronchus is resected
- Pneumonectomy: removal of entire lung
- Segmentectomy: a segment of the lung is removed*
- Wedge resection: removal of a small, pie-shaped area of the segment*
- Chest wall resection with removal of cancerous lung tissue: for cancers that have invaded the chest wall

*Not recommended as curative resection for lung cancer.

Medical Management

The objective of management is to provide a cure, if possible. Treatment depends on the cell type, the stage of the disease, and the patient's physiologic status (particularly cardiac and pulmonary status). In general, treatment may involve surgery, radiation therapy, or chemotherapy—or a combination of these. Newer and more specific therapies to modulate the immune system (gene therapy, therapy with defined tumor antigens) are under study and show promise.

Surgical Management

Surgical resection is the preferred method of treating patients with localized non–small cell tumors, no evidence of metastatic spread, and adequate cardiopulmonary function. If the patient's cardiovascular status, pulmonary function, and functional status are satisfactory, surgery is generally well tolerated. However, coronary artery disease, pulmonary insufficiency, and other comorbidities may contraindicate surgical intervention. The cure rate of surgical resection depends on the type and stage of the cancer. Surgery is primarily used for NSCLCs, because small cell cancer of the lung grows rapidly and metastasizes early and extensively. Lesions of many patients with bronchogenic cancer are inoperable at the time of diagnosis.

Several different types of lung resection may be performed (Chart 23-9). The most common surgical procedure for a small, apparently curable tumor of the lung is lobectomy (removal of a lobe of the lung). In some cases, an entire lung may be removed (pneumonectomy) (see Chapter 25 for further details).

Radiation Therapy

Radiation therapy may offer cure in a small percentage of patients. It is useful in controlling neoplasms that cannot be surgically resected but are responsive to radiation. Irradiation also may be used to reduce the size of a tumor, to make an inoperable tumor operable, or to relieve the pressure of the tumor on vital structures. It can reduce symptoms of spinal cord metastasis and superior vena caval compression. Also, prophylactic brain irradiation is used in certain patients to treat microscopic metastases to the brain. Radiation therapy may help relieve cough, chest pain, dyspnea, hemoptysis, and bone and liver pain. Relief of symptoms may last from a few weeks to many months and is important in improving the quality of the remaining period of life.

Radiation therapy usually is toxic to normal tissue within the radiation field, and this may lead to complications such as esophagitis, pneumonitis, and radiation lung fibrosis. These may impair ventilatory and diffusion capacity and significantly reduce pulmonary reserve. The patient's nutritional status, psychological outlook, fatigue level, and signs of anemia and infection are monitored throughout the treatment. See Chapter 16 for management of the patient receiving radiation therapy.

Chemotherapy

Chemotherapy is used to alter tumor growth patterns, to treat distant metastases or small cell cancer of the lung, and as an adjunct to surgery or radiation therapy. Chemotherapy may provide relief, especially of pain, but it does not usually cure the disease or prolong life to any great degree. Chemotherapy is also accompanied by side effects. It is valuable in reducing pressure symptoms of lung cancer and in treating brain, spinal cord, and pericardial metastasis. See Chapter 16 for a discussion of chemotherapy for the patient with cancer.

The choice of agent depends on the growth of the tumor cell and the specific phase of the cell cycle that the medication affects. In combination with surgery, chemotherapy may be administered before surgery (neoadjuvant therapy) or after surgery (adjuvant therapy). Combinations of two or more medications may be more beneficial than single-dose regimens. A variety of agents are used, including platinum analogues (cisplatin and carboplatin) and non–platinum-containing agents—taxanes (paclitaxel, docetaxel), vinca alkaloids (vinblastine and vindesine), doxorubicin, gemcitabine, vinorelbine, irinotecan (CPT-11), etoposide (VP-16), and pemetrexed (Alimta). Recently approved chemotherapeutic agents in oral form are gefitinib (Iressa) and erlotinib (Tarceva), which are epidermal growth factor tyrosine kinase inhibitors. Numerous new agents with cellular targets, including protein kinase C, vascular endothelial growth factor, cyclooxygenase-2, and farnesyl transferase, are being tested for various types of lung cancer.

Palliative Therapy

Palliative therapy may include radiation therapy to shrink the tumor to provide pain relief, a variety of bronchoscopic interventions to open a narrowed bronchus or airway, and pain management and other comfort measures. Evaluation and referral for hospice care are important in planning for comfortable and dignified end-of-life care for the patient and family.

Treatment-Related Complications

A variety of complications may occur as a result of treatment for lung cancer. Surgical resection may result in respiratory failure, particularly if the cardiopulmonary system is compromised before surgery. Surgical complications and prolonged mechanical ventilation are potential outcomes. Radiation therapy may result in diminished cardiopulmonary function and other complications, such as pulmonary fibrosis, pericarditis, myelitis, and cor pulmonale. Chemotherapy, particularly in combination with radiation therapy, can cause pneumonitis. Pulmonary toxicity is a potential side effect of chemotherapy.

Nursing Management

Nursing care of patients with lung cancer is similar to that for other patients with cancer (see Chapter 16) and addresses the physiologic and psychological needs of the patient. The physiologic problems are primarily due to the respiratory manifestations of the disease. Nursing care includes strategies to ensure relief of pain and discomfort and to prevent complications.

Managing Symptoms

The nurse instructs the patient and family about the potential side effects of the specific treatment and strategies to manage them. Strategies for managing such symptoms as dyspnea, fatigue, nausea and vomiting, and anorexia help the patient and family cope with therapeutic measures.

Relieving Breathing Problems

Airway clearance techniques are key to maintaining airway patency through the removal of excess secretions. This may be accomplished through deep-breathing exercises, chest physiotherapy, directed cough, suctioning, and in some instances bronchoscopy. Bronchodilator medications may be prescribed to promote bronchial dilation. As the tumor enlarges or spreads, it may compress a bronchus or involve a large area of lung tissue, resulting in an impaired breathing pattern and poor gas exchange. At some stage of the disease, supplemental oxygen will probably be necessary.

Nursing measures focus on decreasing dyspnea by encouraging the patient to assume positions that promote lung expansion and to perform breathing exercises for lung expansion and relaxation. Patient education about energy conservation and airway clearance techniques is also necessary. Many of the techniques used in pulmonary rehabilitation can be applied to patients with lung cancer. Depending on the severity of disease and the patient's wishes, a referral to a pulmonary rehabilitation program may be helpful in managing respiratory symptoms.

Reducing Fatigue

Fatigue is a devastating symptom that affects quality of life in patients with cancer. It is commonly experienced by patients with lung cancer and may be related to the disease itself, the cancer treatment and complications (eg, anemia), sleep disturbances, pain and discomfort, hypoxemia, poor nutrition, or the psychological ramifications of the disease (eg, anxiety, depression). The nurse is pivotal in thoroughly assessing the patient's level of fatigue, identifying potentially treatable causes, and validating with the patient that fatigue is indeed an important symptom. Educating the patient about energy conservation techniques or referral to physical therapy, occupational therapy, or pulmonary rehabilitation programs may be helpful. In addition, guided exercise has been recently identified as a potential intervention for treating fatigue in cancer patients. This is an important area for research, because few studies have been conducted, and only in select populations of patients with cancer.

Providing Psychological Support

Another important part of the nursing care of patients with lung cancer is provision of psychological support and identification of potential resources for the patient and family. Often, the nurse must help the patient and family deal with the following:

- The poor prognosis and relatively rapid progression of this disease
- Informed decision making regarding the possible treatment options
- Methods to maintain the patient's quality of life during the course of this disease
- End-of-life treatment options

Gerontologic Considerations

At the time of diagnosis of lung cancer, most patients are older than 65 years of age and have stage III or IV disease (Hurria & Kris, 2003). Although age is not a significant prognostic factor for overall survival and response to treatment for either NSCLC or small cell lung cancer, older patients have specific needs (Hurria & Kris, 2003). Depending on the comorbidities and functional status of elderly patients, chemotherapy agents, doses, and cycles may need to be adjusted to maintain quality of life. Issues that must be considered in care of elderly patients with lung cancer include functional status, comorbid conditions, nutritional status, cognition, concomitant medications, and psychological

NURSING RESEARCH PROFILE

Lung Cancer

Gift, A. G., Stommel, M., Jablonski, A., et al. (2003). A cluster of symptoms over time in patients with lung cancer. *Nursing Research, 52*(6), 393–400.

Purpose

Lung cancer is a leading type of cancer diagnosed in both men and women. The purpose of this study was to determine whether the symptom cluster identified at the time of diagnosis remained constant at 3 and 6 months after diagnosis and whether there was a difference in the number or severity of symptoms. Lastly, the ability of number of symptoms and cluster of symptoms to predict survival was explored.

Design

An existing data set of 112 patients (58 men and 54 women) with newly diagnosed lung cancer was evaluated. Only patients who survived at least 6 months after diagnosis were included in the analysis. Symptoms were assessed using the Physical Symptom Experience technique, a self-report measure used to assess the occurrence and severity of 37 common symptoms. Symptom clusters were evaluated at the time of diagnosis and 3 and 6 months later. Survival was evaluated at 19 months after diagnosis.

Findings

A cluster of seven symptoms (fatigue, weakness, weight loss, appetite loss, nausea, vomiting, altered taste) was identified at diagnosis. Both the mean number and severity of symptoms declined over time. Correlations between severity of vomiting and weight loss at diagnosis, at 3 months, and at 6 months were low; however, fatigue, weakness, poor appetite, altered taste, and nausea were reported more consistently over time. Stage of cancer at diagnosis was the most predictive of the number of cluster symptoms reported, and death occurring 6 to 19 months after diagnosis was predicted by age, stage at diagnosis, and symptom severity at 6 months.

Nursing Implications

Symptom management is a major nursing priority in patients with cancer. Many nurses focus on only one symptom; however, multiple symptoms are frequently experienced. These clusters of symptoms most likely have a multiplicative effect on patients and their cancers. These symptoms relate not only to the cancer diagnosis but also to the patient's comorbidities, treatment regimen, or palliative care plan. It is important to identify symptom clusters and symptom distress in patients with cancer and to further develop and evaluate nursing interventions to help patients deal with different symptom clusters.

and social support (Barrocas, Purdy, Brady, et al., 2002; Hurria & Kris, 2003).

Tumors of the Mediastinum

Tumors of the mediastinum include neurogenic tumors, tumors of the thymus, lymphomas, germ cell tumors, cysts, and mesenchymal tumors. These tumors may be malignant or benign. They are usually described in relation to location: anterior, middle, or posterior masses or tumors.

Clinical Manifestations

Nearly all symptoms of mediastinal tumors result from the pressure of the mass against important intrathoracic organs. Symptoms may include cough, wheezing, dyspnea, anterior chest or neck pain, bulging of the chest wall, heart palpitations, angina, other circulatory disturbances, central cyanosis, superior vena cava syndrome (ie, swelling of the face, neck, and upper extremities), marked distention of the veins of the neck and the chest wall (evidence of the obstruction of large veins of the mediastinum by extravascular compression or intravascular invasion), and dysphagia and weight loss from pressure or invasion into the esophagus.

Assessment and Diagnostic Findings

Chest x-rays are the major method used initially to diagnose mediastinal tumors and cysts. CT is the standard diagnostic test for assessment of the mediastinum and surrounding structures. MRI, as well as PET, may be used in some circumstances.

Medical Management

If the tumor is malignant and has infiltrated the surrounding tissue and complete surgical removal is not feasible, radiation therapy, chemotherapy, or both are used.

Surgical Management

Many mediastinal tumors are benign and operable. The location of the tumor (anterior, middle, or posterior compartment) in the mediastinum dictates the type of incision. The common incision used is a median sternotomy; however, a thoracotomy may be used, depending on the location of the tumor. Additional approaches include a bilateral anterior thoracotomy (clamshell incision) and video-assisted thoracoscopic surgery (see Chapter 25). The care is the same as for any patient undergoing thoracic surgery. Major complications include hemorrhage, injury to the phrenic or recurrent laryngeal nerve, and infection.

Chest Trauma

Major chest trauma may occur alone or in combination with multiple other injuries. Chest trauma is classified as either blunt or penetrating. Blunt chest trauma results from sudden compression or positive pressure inflicted to the chest wall. Penetrating trauma occurs when a foreign object penetrates the chest wall.

Blunt Trauma

Blunt thoracic injures are responsible for approximately 8% of all trauma admissions (Karmy-Jones & Jurkovich, 2004). Although blunt chest trauma is more common than penetrating trauma, it is often difficult to identify the extent of the damage because the symptoms may be generalized and vague. In addition, patients may not seek immediate medical attention, which may complicate the problem.

Overview

Pathophysiology

The most common causes of blunt chest trauma are motor vehicle crashes (trauma from steering wheel, seat belt), falls, and bicycle crashes (trauma from handlebars). Mechanisms of blunt chest trauma include acceleration (moving object hitting the chest or patient being thrown into an object), deceleration (sudden decrease in rate of speed or velocity, such as a motor vehicle crash), shearing (stretching forces to areas of the chest causing tears, ruptures, or dissections), and compression (direct blow to the chest, such as a crush injury). Injuries to the chest are often life-threatening and result in one or more of the following pathologic states:

- Hypoxemia from disruption of the airway; injury to the lung parenchyma, rib cage, and respiratory musculature; massive hemorrhage; collapsed lung; and pneumothorax
- Hypovolemia from massive fluid loss from the great vessels, cardiac rupture, or hemothorax
- Cardiac failure from cardiac tamponade, cardiac contusion, or increased intrathoracic pressure

These pathologic states frequently result in impaired ventilation and perfusion leading to ARF, hypovolemic shock, and death.

Assessment and Diagnostic Findings

Time is critical in treating chest trauma. Therefore, it is essential to assess the patient immediately to determine the following:

- Time elapsed since injury occurred
- Mechanism of injury
- Level of responsiveness
- Specific injuries
- Estimated blood loss
- Recent drug or alcohol use
- Prehospital treatment

Initial assessment of thoracic injuries includes assessment for airway obstruction, tension pneumothorax, open pneumothorax, massive hemothorax, flail chest, and cardiac tamponade. These injuries are life-threatening and require immediate treatment. Secondary assessment includes assessment for simple pneumothorax, hemothorax, pulmonary contusion, traumatic aortic rupture, tracheobronchial disruption, esophageal perforation, traumatic diaphragmatic injury, and penetrating wounds to the mediastinum. Although listed as secondary, these injuries may be life-threatening as well.

The physical examination includes inspection of the airway, thorax, neck veins, and breathing difficulty. Specifics include assessing the rate and depth of breathing for abnormalities such as stridor, cyanosis, nasal flaring, use of accessory muscles, drooling, and overt trauma to the face, mouth, or neck. The chest is assessed for symmetric movement, symmetry of breath sounds, open chest wounds, entrance or exit wounds, impaled objects, tracheal shift, distended neck veins, subcutaneous emphysema, and paradoxical chest wall motion. In addition, the chest wall is assessed for bruising, petechiae, lacerations, and burns. The vital signs and skin color are assessed for signs of shock. The thorax is palpated for tenderness and crepitus, and the position of the trachea is also assessed.

The initial diagnostic workup includes a chest x-ray, CT scan, complete blood count, clotting studies, type and cross-match, electrolytes, oxygen saturation, arterial blood gas analysis, and ECG. The patient is completely undressed to avoid missing additional injuries that may complicate care. Many patients with injuries involving the chest have associated head and abdominal injuries that require attention. Ongoing assessment is essential to monitor the patient's response to treatment and to detect early signs of clinical deterioration.

Medical Management

The goals of treatment are to evaluate the patient's condition and to initiate aggressive resuscitation. An airway is immediately established with oxygen support and, in some cases, intubation and ventilatory support. Reestablishing fluid volume and negative intrapleural pressure and draining intrapleural fluid and blood are essential.

The potential for massive blood loss and exsanguination with blunt or penetrating chest injuries is high because of injury to the great blood vessels. Many patients die at the scene of the injury or are in shock by the time help arrives. Agitation and irrational and combative behavior are signs of decreased oxygen delivery to the cerebral cortex. Strategies to restore and maintain cardiopulmonary function include ensuring an adequate airway and ventilation; stabilizing and reestablishing chest wall integrity; occluding any opening into the chest (open pneumothorax); and draining or removing any air or fluid from the thorax to relieve pneumothorax, hemothorax, or cardiac tamponade. Hypovolemia and low cardiac output must be corrected. Many of these treatment efforts, along with the control of hemorrhage, are carried out simultaneously at the scene of the injury or in the emergency department. Depending on the success of efforts to control the hemorrhage in the emergency department, the patient may be taken immediately to the operating room. Principles of management are essentially those pertaining to care of the postoperative thoracic patient (see Chapter 25).

Sternal and Rib Fractures

Sternal fractures are most common in motor vehicle crashes with a direct blow to the sternum via the steering wheel. Rib fractures are the most common type of chest trauma, occurring in more than 60% of patients admitted with blunt chest injury (Karmy-Jones & Jurkovich, 2004). Most rib fractures are benign and are treated conservatively. Fractures of the first three ribs are rare but can result in a high mortality rate because they are associated with laceration of the subclavian artery or vein. The fifth through ninth ribs are the most common sites of fractures. Fractures of the lower ribs are associated with injury to the spleen and liver, which may be lacerated by fragmented sections of the rib.

Clinical Manifestations

Patients with sternal fractures have anterior chest pain, overlying tenderness, ecchymosis, crepitus, swelling, and possible chest wall deformity. For patients with rib fractures, clinical manifestations are similar: severe pain, point tenderness, and muscle spasm over the area of the fracture that are aggravated by coughing, deep breathing, and movement. The area around the fracture may be bruised. To reduce the pain, the patient splints the chest by breathing in a shallow manner and avoids sighs, deep breaths, coughing, and movement. This reluctance to move or breathe deeply results in diminished ventilation, atelectasis (collapse of unaerated alveoli), pneumonitis, and hypoxemia. Respiratory insufficiency and failure can be the outcomes of such a cycle.

Assessment and Diagnostic Findings

The patient must be closely evaluated for underlying cardiac injuries. A crackling, grating sound in the thorax (subcutaneous crepitus) may be detected with auscultation. The diagnostic workup may include a chest x-ray, rib films of a specific area, ECG, continuous pulse oximetry, and arterial blood gas analysis.

Medical Management

Medical management is directed toward relieving pain, avoiding excessive activity, and treating any associated injuries. Surgical fixation is rarely necessary unless fragments are grossly displaced and pose a potential for further injury.

The goals of treatment for rib fractures are to control pain and to detect and treat the injury. Sedation is used to relieve pain and to allow deep breathing and coughing. Care must be taken to avoid oversedation and suppression of respiratory drive. Alternative strategies to relieve pain include an intercostal nerve block and ice over the fracture site. A chest binder may be used as supportive treatment to provide stability to the chest wall and may decrease pain. The patient is instructed to apply the binder snugly enough to provide support, but not to impair respiratory excursion. Usually the pain abates in 5 to 7 days, and discomfort can be relieved with epidural analgesia, patient-controlled analgesia, or nonopioid analgesia. Most rib fractures heal in 3 to 6 weeks. The patient is monitored closely for signs and symptoms of associated injuries.

Flail Chest

Flail chest is frequently a complication of blunt chest trauma from a steering wheel injury. It usually occurs when three or more adjacent ribs (multiple contiguous ribs) are fractured at two or more sites, resulting in free-floating rib segments. It may also result as a combination fracture of ribs and costal cartilages or sternum. As a result, the chest wall loses stability, causing respiratory impairment and usually severe respiratory distress.

Pathophysiology

During inspiration, as the chest expands, the detached part of the rib segment (flail segment) moves in a paradoxical manner (pendelluft movement) in that it is pulled inward during inspiration, reducing the amount of air that can be drawn into the lungs. On expiration, because the intrathoracic pressure exceeds atmospheric pressure, the flail segment bulges outward, impairing the patient's ability to exhale. The mediastinum then shifts back to the affected side (Fig. 23-8). This paradoxical action results in increased dead space, a reduction in alveolar ventilation, and decreased compliance. Retained airway secretions and atelectasis frequently accompany flail chest. The patient has hypoxemia, and if gas exchange is greatly compromised, respiratory acidosis develops as a result of carbon dioxide retention. Hypotension, inadequate tissue perfusion, and metabolic acidosis often follow as the paradoxical motion of the mediastinum decreases cardiac output.

Medical Management

As with rib fracture, treatment of flail chest is usually supportive. Management includes providing ventilatory support, clearing secretions from the lungs, and controlling pain. Specific management depends on the degree of respiratory dysfunction. If only a small segment of the chest is involved, the objectives are to clear the airway through positioning, coughing, deep breathing, and suctioning to aid in the expansion of the lung, and to relieve pain by intercostal nerve blocks, high thoracic epidural blocks, or cautious use of IV opioids.

For mild to moderate flail chest injuries, the underlying pulmonary contusion is treated by monitoring fluid intake and appropriate fluid replacement while relieving chest pain. Pulmonary physiotherapy focusing on lung volume expansion, and secretion management techniques are performed. The patient is closely monitored for further respiratory compromise.

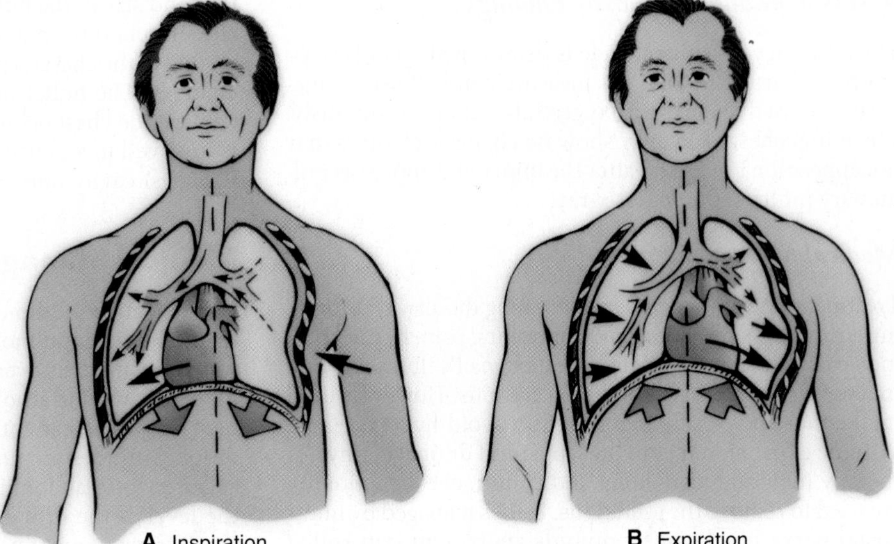

FIGURE 23-8. Flail chest is caused by a free-floating segment of rib cage resulting from multiple rib fractures. (**A**) Paradoxical movement on inspiration occurs when the flail rib segment is sucked inward and the mediastinal structures shift to the unaffected side. The amount of air drawn into the affected lung is reduced. (**B**) On expiration, the flail segment bulges outward and the mediastinal structures shift back to the affected side.

For severe flail chest injuries, endotracheal intubation and mechanical ventilation are required to provide internal pneumatic stabilization of the flail chest and to correct abnormalities in gas exchange. This helps treat the underlying pulmonary contusion, serves to stabilize the thoracic cage to allow the fractures to heal, and improves alveolar ventilation and intrathoracic volume by decreasing the work of breathing. This treatment modality requires endotracheal intubation and ventilator support. Differing modes of ventilation are used depending on the patient's underlying disease and specific needs.

In rare circumstances, surgery may be required to more quickly stabilize the flail segment. This may be used for patients who are difficult to ventilate or for high-risk patients with underlying lung disease who may be difficult to wean from mechanical ventilation.

Regardless of the type of treatment, the patient is carefully monitored by serial chest x-rays, arterial blood gas analysis, pulse oximetry, and bedside pulmonary function monitoring. Pain management is key to successful treatment. Patient-controlled analgesia, intercostal nerve blocks, epidural analgesia, and intrapleural administration of opioids may be used to relieve or manage thoracic pain.

Pulmonary Contusion

Pulmonary contusion is a common thoracic injury and is frequently associated with flail chest. It is defined as damage to the lung tissues resulting in hemorrhage and localized edema. It is associated with chest trauma when there is rapid compression and decompression to the chest wall (ie, blunt trauma). Pulmonary contusion represents a spectrum of lung injury characterized by the development of infiltrates and various degrees of respiratory dysfunction and sometimes respiratory failure. It is often cited as the most common potentially life-threatening chest injury; however, mortality is often attributed to other associated injuries (Karmy-Jones & Jurkovich, 2004). A contusion is sustained in 30% to 70% of patients who experience blunt force trauma. Pulmonary contusion may not be evident initially on examination but develops in the posttraumatic period; it may involve a small portion of one lung, a massive section of a lung, one entire lung, or both lungs.

Pathophysiology

The primary pathologic defect is an abnormal accumulation of fluid in the interstitial and intra-alveolar spaces. It is thought that injury to the lung parenchyma and its capillary network results in a leakage of serum protein and plasma. The leaking serum protein exerts an osmotic pressure that enhances loss of fluid from the capillaries. Blood, edema, and cellular debris (from cellular response to injury) enter the lung and accumulate in the bronchioles and alveoli, where they interfere with gas exchange. An increase in pulmonary vascular resistance and pulmonary artery pressure occurs. The patient has hypoxemia and carbon dioxide retention. Occasionally, a contused lung occurs on the other side of the point of body impact; this is called a contrecoup contusion.

Clinical Manifestations

Pulmonary contusion may be mild, moderate, or severe. The clinical manifestations vary from decreased breath sounds, tachypnea, tachycardia, chest pain, hypoxemia, and blood-tinged secretions to more severe tachypnea, tachycardia, crackles, frank bleeding, severe hypoxemia (cyanosis), and respiratory acidosis. Changes in sensorium, including increased agitation or combative irrational behavior, may be signs of hypoxemia.

In addition, patients with moderate pulmonary contusion have a large amount of mucus, serum, and frank blood in the tracheobronchial tree; patients often have a constant cough but cannot clear the secretions. Patients with severe pulmonary contusion have the signs and symptoms of ARDS; these may include central cyanosis, agitation, combativeness, and productive cough with frothy, bloody secretions.

Assessment and Diagnostic Findings

The efficiency of gas exchange is determined by pulse oximetry and arterial blood gas measurements. Pulse oximetry is also used to measure oxygen saturation continuously. The initial chest x-ray may show no changes; changes may not appear for 1 or 2 days after the injury and appear as pulmonary infiltrates on chest x-ray.

Medical Management

Treatment priorities include maintaining the airway, providing adequate oxygenation, and controlling pain. In mild pulmonary contusion, adequate hydration via IV fluids and oral intake is important to mobilize secretions. However, fluid intake must be closely monitored to avoid hypervolemia. Volume expansion techniques, postural drainage, physiotherapy including coughing, and endotracheal suctioning are used to remove the secretions. Pain is managed by intercostal nerve blocks or by opioids via patient-controlled analgesia or other methods. Usually, antimicrobial therapy is administered because the damaged lung is susceptible to infection. Supplemental oxygen is usually given by mask or cannula for 24 to 36 hours.

In patients with moderate pulmonary contusions, bronchoscopy may be required to remove secretions. Intubation and mechanical ventilation with PEEP (see Chapter 25) may also be necessary to maintain the pressure and keep the lungs inflated. Diuretics may be administered to reduce edema. A nasogastric tube is inserted to relieve gastrointestinal distention.

In patients with severe contusion, who may develop respiratory failure, aggressive treatment with endotracheal intubation and ventilatory support, diuretics, and fluid restriction may be necessary. Colloids and crystalloid solutions may be used to treat hypovolemia.

Antimicrobial medications may be prescribed for the treatment of pulmonary infection. This is a common complication of pulmonary contusion (especially pneumonia in the contused segment), because the fluid and blood that extravasates into the alveolar and interstitial spaces serve as an excellent culture medium.

Penetrating Trauma: Gunshot and Stab Wounds

Gunshot and stab wounds are the most common causes of penetrating chest trauma. These wounds are classified according to their velocity. Stab wounds are generally considered low-velocity trauma because the weapon destroys a small area around the wound. Knives and switchblades cause most stab wounds. The appearance of the external wound may be very deceptive, because pneumothorax, hemothorax, lung contusion, and cardiac tamponade, along with severe and continuing hemorrhage, can occur from any small wound, even one caused by a small-diameter instrument such as an ice pick.

Gunshot wounds may be classified as low, medium, or high velocity. The factors that determine the velocity and resulting extent of damage include the distance from which the gun was fired, the caliber of the gun, and the construction and size of the bullet. A bullet can cause damage at the site of penetration and along its pathway, and a gunshot wound to the chest can produce a variety of pathophysiologic changes. The bullet may ricochet off bony structures and damage the chest organs and great vessels. If the diaphragm is involved in a gunshot wound or a stab wound, injury to the chest cavity must be considered.

Medical Management

The objective of immediate management is to restore and maintain cardiopulmonary function. After an adequate airway is ensured and ventilation is established, examination for shock and intrathoracic and intra-abdominal injuries is necessary. The patient is undressed completely so that additional injuries are not missed. There is a high risk for associated intra-abdominal injuries with stab wounds below the level of the fifth anterior intercostal space. Death can result from exsanguinating hemorrhage or intra-abdominal sepsis.

The diagnostic workup includes a chest x-ray, chemistry profile, arterial blood gas analysis, pulse oximetry, and ECG. The patient's blood is typed and cross-matched in case blood transfusion is required. After the status of the peripheral pulses is assessed, a large-bore IV line is inserted. An indwelling catheter is inserted to monitor urinary output. A nasogastric tube is inserted and connected to low suction to prevent aspiration, minimize leakage of abdominal contents, and decompress the gastrointestinal tract.

Shock is treated simultaneously with colloid solutions, crystalloids, or blood, as indicated by the patient's condition. Diagnostic procedures are carried out as dictated by the needs of the patient (eg, CT scans of chest or abdomen, flat plate x-ray of the abdomen, abdominal tap to check for bleeding).

A chest tube is inserted into the pleural space in most patients with penetrating wounds of the chest to achieve rapid and continuing reexpansion of the lungs. The insertion of the chest tube frequently results in a complete evacuation of the blood and air. The chest tube also allows early recognition of continuing intrathoracic bleeding, which would make surgical exploration necessary. If the patient has a penetrating wound of the heart or great vessels, the esophagus, or the tracheobronchial tree, surgical intervention is required.

Pneumothorax

Pneumothorax occurs when the parietal or visceral pleura is breached and the pleural space is exposed to positive atmospheric pressure. Normally the pressure in the pleural space is negative or subatmospheric; this negative pressure is required to maintain lung inflation. When either pleura is breached, air enters the pleural space, and the lung or a portion of it collapses.

Types of Pneumothorax

Types of pneumothorax include simple, traumatic, and tension pneumothorax.

Simple Pneumothorax

A simple, or spontaneous, pneumothorax occurs when air enters the pleural space through a breach of either the parietal or visceral pleura. Most commonly this occurs as air enters the pleural space through the rupture of a bleb or a bronchopleural fistula. A spontaneous pneumothorax may occur in an apparently healthy person in the absence of trauma due to rupture of an air-filled bleb, or blister, on the surface of the lung, allowing air from the airways to enter the pleural cavity. It may be associated with diffuse interstitial lung disease and severe emphysema.

Traumatic Pneumothorax

A traumatic pneumothorax occurs when air escapes from a laceration in the lung itself and enters the pleural space or enters the pleural space through a wound in the chest wall. It may result from blunt trauma (eg, rib fractures), penetrating chest or abdominal trauma (eg, stab wounds or gunshot wounds), or diaphragmatic tears. Traumatic pneumothorax may occur during invasive thoracic procedures (ie, thoracentesis, transbronchial lung biopsy, insertion of a subclavian line) in which the pleura is inadvertently punctured, or with barotrauma from mechanical ventilation.

A traumatic pneumothorax resulting from major injury to the chest is often accompanied by hemothorax (collection of blood in the pleural space resulting from torn intercostal vessels, lacerations of the great vessels, or lacerations of the lungs). Often both blood and air are found in the chest cavity (hemopneumothorax) after major trauma. Chest surgery can be classified as a traumatic pneumothorax as a result of the entry into the pleural space and the accumulation of air and fluid in the pleural space.

Open pneumothorax is one form of traumatic pneumothorax. It occurs when a wound in the chest wall is large enough to allow air to pass freely in and out of the thoracic cavity with each attempted respiration. Because the rush of air through the wound in the chest wall produces a sucking sound, such injuries are termed sucking chest wounds. In such patients, not only does the lung collapse, but the structures of the mediastinum (heart and great vessels) also shift toward the uninjured side with each inspiration and in the opposite direction with expiration. This is termed mediastinal flutter or swing, and it produces serious circulatory problems.

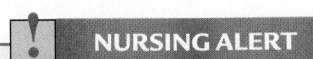

Traumatic open pneumothorax calls for emergency interventions. Stopping the flow of air through the opening in the chest wall is a life-saving measure.

Tension Pneumothorax

A **tension pneumothorax** occurs when air is drawn into the pleural space from a lacerated lung or through a small opening or wound in the chest wall. It may be a complication of other types of pneumothorax. In contrast to open pneumothorax, the air that enters the chest cavity with each inspiration is trapped; it cannot be expelled during expiration through the air passages or the opening in the chest wall. In effect, a one-way valve or ball valve mechanism occurs where air enters the pleural space but cannot escape. With each breath, tension (positive pressure) is increased within the affected pleural space. This causes the lung to collapse and the heart, the great vessels, and the trachea to shift toward the unaffected side of the chest (mediastinal shift). Both respiration and circulatory function are compromised because of the increased intrathoracic pressure, which decreases venous return to the heart, causing decreased cardiac output and impairment of peripheral circulation. In extreme cases, the pulse may be undetectable—this is known as pulseless electrical activity.

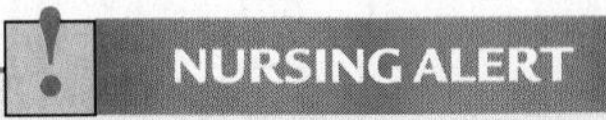

Relief of tension pneumothorax is considered an emergency measure.

Clinical Manifestations

The signs and symptoms associated with pneumothorax depend on its size and cause. Pain is usually sudden and may be pleuritic. The patient may have only minimal respiratory distress with slight chest discomfort and tachypnea with a small simple or uncomplicated pneumothorax. If the pneumothorax is large and the lung collapses totally, acute respiratory distress occurs. The patient is anxious, has dyspnea and air hunger, has increased use of the accessory muscles, and may develop central cyanosis from severe hypoxemia. In assessing the chest for any type of pneumothorax, the nurse assesses tracheal alignment, expansion of the chest, breath sounds and percussion of the chest. In a simple pneumothorax the trachea is midline, expansion of the chest is decreased, breath sounds may be diminished, and percussion of the chest may reveal normal sounds or hyperresonance depending on the size of the pneumothorax.

In a tension pneumothorax, the trachea is shifted away from the affected side, chest expansion may be decreased or fixed in a hyperexpansion state, breath sounds are diminished or absent, and percussion to the affected side is hyperresonant. The clinical picture is one of air hunger, agitation, increasing hypoxemia, central cyanosis, hypotension, tachycardia, and profuse diaphoresis. Figure 23-9 compares open and tension pneumothorax.

Medical Management

Medical management of pneumothorax depends on its cause and severity. The goal of treatment is to evacuate the air or blood from the pleural space. A small chest tube (28 French) is inserted near the second intercostal space; this space is used because it is the thinnest part of the chest wall, minimizes the danger of contacting the thoracic nerve, and leaves

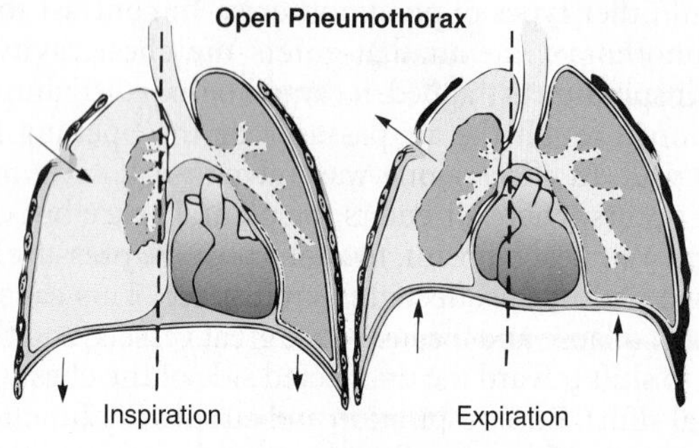

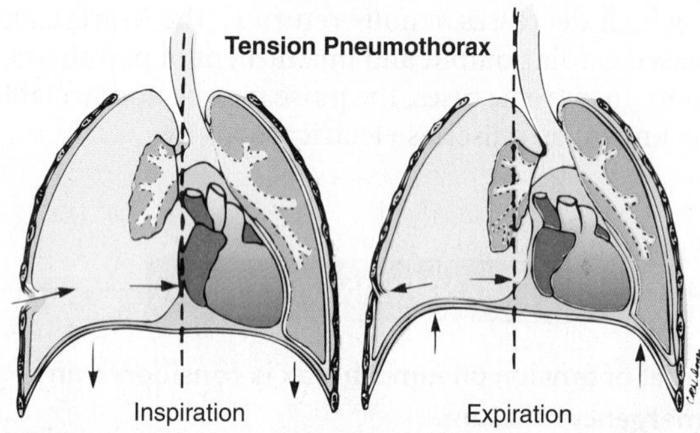

FIGURE 23-9. Open pneumothorax (*top*) and tension pneumothorax (*bottom*). In open pneumothorax, air enters the chest during inspiration and exits during expiration. A slight shift of the affected lung may occur because of a decrease in pressure as air moves out of the chest. In tension pneumothorax, air enters but cannot leave the chest. As the pressure increases, the heart and great vessels are compressed and the mediastinal structures are shifted toward the opposite side of the chest. The trachea is pushed from its normal midline position toward the opposite side of the chest, and the unaffected lung is compressed.

a less visible scar. If a patient also has a hemothorax, a large-diameter chest tube (32 French or greater) is inserted, usually in the fourth or fifth intercostal space at the midaxillary line. The tube is directed posteriorly to drain the fluid and air. Once the chest tube or tubes are inserted and suction is applied (usually to 20 mm Hg suction), effective decompression of the pleural cavity (drainage of blood or air) occurs.

If an excessive amount of blood enters the chest tube in a relatively short period, an autotransfusion may be needed. This technique involves taking the patient's own blood that has been drained from the chest, filtering it, and then transfusing it back into the vascular system.

In such an emergency, anything may be used that is large enough to fill the chest wound—a towel, a handkerchief, or the heel of the hand. If conscious, the patient is instructed to inhale and strain against a closed glottis. This action assists in reexpanding the lung and ejecting the air from the thorax. In the hospital, the opening is plugged by sealing it with gauze impregnated with petrolatum. A pressure dressing is applied. Usually, a chest tube connected to water-seal drainage is inserted to permit air and fluid to drain. Antibiotics usually are prescribed to combat infection from contamination.

The severity of open pneumothorax depends on the amount and rate of thoracic bleeding and the amount of air in the pleural space. The pleural cavity can be decompressed by needle aspiration (thoracentesis) or by chest tube drainage of the blood or air. The lung is then able to re-expand and resume the function of gas exchange. As a rule of thumb, the chest wall is opened surgically (thoracotomy) if more than 1500 mL of blood is aspirated initially by thoracentesis (or is the initial chest tube output) or if chest tube output continues at greater than 200 mL/hour. The urgency with which the blood must be removed is determined by the degree of respiratory compromise. An emergency thoracotomy may also be performed in the emergency department if a cardiovascular injury secondary to chest or penetrating trauma is suspected. The patient with a possible tension pneumothorax should immediately be given a high concentration of supplemental oxygen to treat the hypoxemia, and pulse oximetry should be used to monitor oxygen saturation. In an emergency situation, a tension pneumothorax can be decompressed or quickly converted to a simple pneumothorax by inserting a large-bore needle (14-gauge) at the second intercostal space, midclavicular line on the affected side. This relieves the pressure and vents the positive pressure to the external environment. A chest tube is then inserted and connected to suction to remove the remaining air and fluid, reestablish the negative pressure, and reexpand the lung. If the lung reexpands and air leakage from the lung parenchyma stops, further drainage may be unnecessary. If a prolonged air leak continues despite chest tube drainage to underwater seal, surgery may be necessary to close the leak.

Cardiac Tamponade

Cardiac tamponade is compression of the heart resulting from fluid or blood within the pericardial sac. It usually is caused by blunt or penetrating trauma to the chest. A penetrating wound of the heart is associated with a high mortality rate. Cardiac tamponade also may follow diagnostic cardiac catheterization, angiographic procedures, and pacemaker insertion, which can produce perforations of the heart and great vessels. Pericardial effusion with fluid compressing the heart also may develop from metastases to the pericardium from malignant tumors of the breast, lung, or mediastinum and may occur with lymphomas and leukemias, renal failure, TB, and high-dose radiation to the chest. Cardiac tamponade is discussed in detail in Chapter 30.

Subcutaneous Emphysema

No matter what kind of chest trauma a patient has, when the lung or the air passages are injured, air may enter the tissue planes and pass for some distance under the skin (eg, neck, chest). The tissues give a crackling sensation when palpated, and the subcutaneous air produces an alarming appearance as the face, neck, body, and scrotum become misshapen by subcutaneous air. Fortunately, subcutaneous emphysema is of itself usually not a serious complication. The subcutaneous air is spontaneously absorbed if the underlying air leak is treated or stops spontaneously. In severe cases in which there is widespread subcutaneous emphysema, a tracheostomy is indicated if airway patency is threatened.

Aspiration

Aspiration of stomach contents into the lungs is a serious complication that can cause pneumonia and result in the following clinical picture: tachycardia, dyspnea, central cyanosis, hypertension, hypotension, and finally death. It can occur when the protective airway reflexes are decreased or absent due to a variety of factors (Chart 23-10).

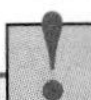

NURSING ALERT

When a nonfunctioning nasogastric tube allows the gastric contents to accumulate in the stomach, a condition known as silent aspiration may result. Silent aspiration often occurs unobserved and may be more common than suspected. If untreated, massive inhalation of gastric contents develops in a period of several hours.

Pathophysiology

The primary factors responsible for death and complications after aspiration of gastric contents are the volume and character of the aspirated gastric contents. For example, a small, localized aspiration from regurgitation can cause pneumonia and acute respiratory distress; a massive aspiration is usually fatal.

A full stomach contains solid particles of food. If these are aspirated, the problem then becomes one of mechanical blockage of the airways and secondary infection. During periods of fasting, the stomach contains acidic gastric juice, which, if aspirated, can be very destructive to the alveoli and capillaries. Fecal contamination (more likely seen in intestinal obstruction) increases the likelihood of death, because the endotoxins produced by intestinal organisms may be absorbed systemically, or the thick proteinaceous material found in the intestinal contents may obstruct the airway, leading to atelectasis and secondary bacterial invasion.

Aspiration pneumonitis may develop from aspiration of substances with a pH of less than 2.5 and a volume of gastric aspirate greater than 0.3 mL per kilogram of body weight (approximately 20 to 25 mL in adults) (Marik, 2001). Aspiration of gastric contents causes a chemical burn of the tracheobronchial tree and pulmonary parenchyma (Marik, 2001). An inflammatory response occurs. This results in the destruction of alveolar–capillary endothelial cells, with a consequent outpouring of protein-rich fluids into the interstitial and intra-alveolar spaces. As a result, surfactant is lost, which in turn causes the airways to close and the alveoli to collapse. Finally, the impaired exchange of oxygen and carbon dioxide causes respiratory failure.

Aspiration pneumonia develops after inhalation of colonized oropharyngeal material. The pathologic process involves an acute inflammatory response to bacteria and bacterial products. Most commonly, the bacteriologic findings include gram-positive cocci, gram-negative rods, and occasionally anaerobic bacteria (Marik, 2001).

CHART 23-10

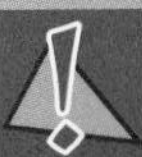

Risk Factors for Aspiration

- Seizure activity
- Decreased level of consciousness from trauma, drug or alcohol intoxication, excessive sedation, or general anesthesia
- Nausea and vomiting in the patient with a decreased level of consciousness
- Stroke
- Swallowing disorders
- Cardiac arrest
- Silent aspiration

Prevention

Prevention is the primary goal when caring for patients at risk for aspiration. Examples of risk factors for aspiration include decreased level of consciousness, supine positioning, presence of a nasogastric tube, tracheal intubation and mechanical ventilation, bolus or intermittent feeding delivery methods, and advanced age (Metheny, 2002). Evidence confirms that one of the main preventive measures for aspiration is placing at-risk patients in a semirecumbent position (elevation of the head of the bed to a 30- to 45-degree angle) (CDC, 2004d; Keithley & Swanson, 2004).

Compensating for Absent Reflexes

Aspiration may occur if the patient cannot adequately coordinate protective glottic, laryngeal, and cough reflexes. This hazard is increased if the patient has a distended abdomen, is supine, has the upper extremities immobilized by IV infusions or hand restraints, receives local anesthetics to the oropharyngeal or laryngeal area for diagnostic procedures, has been sedated, or has had long-term intubation.

When vomiting, people can normally protect their airway by sitting up or turning on the side and coordinating breathing, coughing, gag, and glottic reflexes. If these reflexes are active, an oral airway should not be inserted. If an airway is in place, it should be pulled out the moment the patient gags so as not to stimulate the pharyngeal gag reflex and promote vomiting and aspiration. Suctioning of oral secretions with a catheter should be performed with minimal pharyngeal stimulation.

Assessing Feeding Tube Placement

When a patient is intubated, aspiration may occur even with a nasogastric tube in place and may result in nosocomial pneumonia. Assessment of nasogastric tube placement is key to prevention of aspiration. The best method for determining tube placement is via an x-ray. Other methods have been studied; observation of the aspirate and testing of its pH are the most reliable. Gastric fluid may be grassy green, brown, clear, or colorless. An aspirate from the lungs may be off-white or tan mucus. Pleural fluid is watery and usually straw-colored. Gastric pH values are typically lower (more acidic) than those of the intestinal or respiratory tract. Gastric pH is usually between 1 and 5, whereas intestinal or respiratory pH is 7 or higher. There are differences in assessing tube placement with continuous versus intermittent feedings. For intermittent feedings with small-bore tubes, observation of aspirated contents and pH evaluation should be performed. For continuous feedings, the pH method is not clinically useful because of the infused formula (Metheny, 2002; Metheny & Titler, 2001).

Patients who receive continuous or timed-interval tube feedings must be positioned properly. Patients receiving continuous infusions are given small volumes under low pressure in an upright position, which helps prevent aspiration. Patients receiving tube feedings at timed intervals are maintained in an upright or semirecumbent position (elevation of the head of the bed to a 30- to 45-degree angle) during the feeding and for a minimum of 30 minutes afterward to allow the stomach to empty partially (Keithley & Swanson, 2004). Tube feedings must be given only when it is certain that the feeding tube is positioned correctly in the stomach. Many patients today receive enteral feeding directly into the duodenum through a small-bore flexible feeding tube or surgically implanted tube. Feedings are given slowly and are regulated by a feeding pump. Correct placement is confirmed by chest x-ray.

Identifying Delayed Stomach Emptying

A full stomach can cause aspiration because of increased intragastric or extragastric pressure. The following clinical situations delay emptying of the stomach and may contribute to aspiration: intestinal obstruction; increased gastric secretions in gastroesophageal reflex disease; increased gastric secretions during anxiety, stress, or pain; and abdominal distention because of ileus, ascites, peritonitis, use of opioids or sedatives, severe illness, or vaginal delivery.

When a feeding tube is present, contents are aspirated, usually every 4 hours, to determine the amount of the last feeding left in the stomach (residual volume). Preliminary evidence in this area suggests that gastric residuals are insensitive and unreliable markers of tolerance to tube feedings. Except in high-risk, selected patients, few data support withholding tube feedings in patients with gastric residuals less than 500 mL (Keithley & Swanson, 2004).

Managing Effects of Prolonged Intubation

Prolonged endotracheal intubation or tracheostomy can depress the laryngeal and glottic reflexes because of disuse. Patients with prolonged tracheostomies are encouraged to phonate and exercise their laryngeal muscles. For patients who have had long-term intubation or tracheostomies, it may be helpful to have a rehabilitation therapist experienced in speech and swallowing disorders (ie, speech therapist) work with the patient to assess the swallowing reflex.

Critical Thinking Exercises

1 ebp You are caring for an 82-year-old woman who was recently transferred to the hospital from a nursing home with the diagnosis of presumed nursing home–acquired pneumonia. She has a nasogastric feeding tube in place and is lethargic, dehydrated, and confused. What strategies would you initiate to prevent aspiration? What nursing care interventions would you use to assess for aspiration? What is the evidence base for the interventions that you consider? How will you evaluate the strength of the evidence? What suggestions might you have regarding appropriate devices for long-term enteral feeding in this patient once she is discharged back to the nursing home?

2 On a surgical unit, you are caring for a 42-year-old woman who underwent a total abdominal hysterectomy and bilateral salpingo-oophorectomy and has developed severe postoperative deep venous thrombosis that resulted in a pulmonary embolism. She is a smoker and is taking multiple medications. She was stable when you started your shift, but she has become increasingly anxious with some shortness of breath in the past hour. What are potential risk factors you might observe or identify in this patient? What assessment strategies would you use to evaluate changes in her respiratory status? What decision process would you use to determine when the physician should be contacted?

3 You are caring for a patient who experienced blunt chest trauma in a motor vehicle crash. A chest tube has been inserted to treat a simple pneumothorax and hemothorax. The chest drainage system has drained 400 mL of light red fluid during the first 6 hours after insertion. The patient has become increasingly short of breath during the past hour. What physical assessment skills and strategies would you use to determine potential changes in the patient's respiratory condition? What are potential causes of this increasing shortness of breath? What would you do to prepare for an emergency situation in this patient?

4 ebp On a surgical unit, you are caring for a 62-year-old man who has undergone right upper lobectomy for lung cancer. The patient has chronic obstructive pulmonary disease (COPD) and has continued to smoke despite the diagnoses of COPD and lung cancer. What strategies would you use to prevent or minimize pulmonary complications in this patient? What are methods you might use to assess the patient's progress from a respiratory standpoint? What strategies would you consider to encourage the patient to stop smoking? What is the evidence base for the strategies that you consider? How will you evaluate the strength of the evidence?

REFERENCES AND SELECTED READINGS

BOOKS

Agency for Healthcare Research and Quality. (2003). *Diagnosis and treatment of deep venous thrombosis and pulmonary embolism.* Rockville, MD: Agency for Healthcare Research and Quality.

Albert, R., Spiro, S. & Jett, J. (2004). *Clinical respiratory medicine* (2nd ed.). St. Louis: Mosby.

American Cancer Society. (2005). *Cancer facts and figures.* Atlanta: American Cancer Society.

American Joint Committee on Cancer (AJCC). (2002). *Cancer staging manual* (6th ed.). New York: Springer-Verlag.

Fossella, F. V., Putnam, J. B. & Komaki, K. (2003). *Lung cancer.* New York: Springer-Verlag.

Haas, M. (2003). *Contemporary issues in lung cancer: A nursing perspective.* Sudbury, MA: Jones and Bartlett.

Pazdur, R., Coia, L. R., Hoskins, W. J., et al. (2003). *Cancer management: A multidisciplinary approach* (7th ed.). New York: The Oncology Group.

Schwartz, A. L. (2004). *Pocket guide to managing cancer fatigue.* Sudbury, MA: Jones and Bartlett.

Tapson, V. F. (2003). *Venous thromboembolism.* Philadelphia: Saunders.

Williams, N. R. & Harrison, J. (2004). *Atlas of occupational health and disease.* Oxford, UK: Oxford University Press.

JOURNALS

**Asterisks indicate nursing research articles.*

General

American College of Chest Physicians. (2004). Diagnosis and management of pulmonary arterial hypertension: ACCP evidence-based clinical practice guidelines. *Chest, 126*(1 Suppl.), 4S–92S.

American Thoracic Society and European Respiratory Society. (2000). Idiopathic pulmonary fibrosis: Diagnosis and treatment. International consensus statement. *American Journal of Respiratory and Critical Care Medicine, 161*(2), 646–664.

Azoulay, E. (2003). Pleural effusions in the intensive care unit. *Current Opinions in Pulmonary Medicine, 9*(4), 291–297.

Barrocas, A., Purdy, D., Brady, P., et al. (2002). Cancer: Nutritional management for older adults. From *A physician's guide to nutrition in chronic disease management in older adults.* Washington, DC: Nutrition Screening Initiative.

Centers for Disease Control and Prevention. (2004b). Changing patterns of pneumoconiosis mortality United States, 1968–2000. *MMWR Morbidity and Mortality Weekly Report, 53*(28), 627–632.

Davies, R. J. O. & Gleeson, F. V. (2003). Introduction to methods used in the generation of the British Thoracic Society guidelines for the management of pleural diseases. *Thorax, 58*(Suppl. II), ii1–ii7.

Doty, J. D. & Judson, M. A. (2004). Sarcoidosis, part 1: A thorough look at the clinical aspects. *Journal of Respiratory Diseases, 25*(1), 31–36.

Eells, P. L. (2004). Advances in prostacyclin therapy for pulmonary arterial hypertension. *Critical Care Nursing, 24*(2), 42–54.

Goldhaber, S. Z. (2004). Pulmonary embolism. *Lancet, 363*(9417), 1295–1305.

Humbert, M., Sitbon, O. & Simonneau, G. (2004). Drug therapy: Treatment of pulmonary arterial hypertension. *New England Journal of Medicine, 351*(14), 1425–1436.

Kaboli, P., Henderson, M. C., & White, R. H. (2003). DVT prophylaxis and anticoagulation in the surgical patient. *Medical Clinics of North America, 87*(1), 77–110.

Karin, J. (2003). Managing pulmonary embolism. *British Medical Journal, 326*(7403), 1341–1342.

Keithley, J. K., & Swanson, B. (2004). Enteral nutrition: An update on practice recommendations. *MedSurg Nursing, 13*(2), 131–134.

Marik, P. E. (2001). Aspiration pneumonitis and aspiration pneumonia. *New England Journal of Medicine, 344*(9), 665–671.

McClave, S. A., DeMeo, M. T., DeLegge, M. H., et al. (2002). North American summit on aspiration in the critically ill patient: Consensus statement. *Journal of Parenteral and Enteral Nutrition, 26*(6 Suppl), S80–S85.

Metheny, N. A. (2002). Risk factors for aspiration. *Journal of Parenteral and Enteral Nutrition, 26*(Suppl 6), S26–S33.

Metheny, N. A. & Titler, M. G. (2001). Assessing placement of feeding tubes. *American Journal of Nursing, 101*(5), 36–45.

Morris, R. J. & Woodcock, J. P. (2004). Evidence-based compression: prevention of stasis and deep vein thrombosis. *Annals of Surgery, 239*(2), 162–171.

Nagahiro, I., Andou, A., Aoe, M., et al. (2004). Intermittent pneumatic compression is effective in preventing symptomatic pulmonary embolism after thoracic surgery. *Surgery Today, 34*(1), 6–10.

Ramirez, J., Pantelis, V., Gonzalez-Ruiz, C., et al. (2003). Sequential compression devices as prophylaxis for venous thromboembolism in high-risk colorectal surgery patients: Reconsidering American Society of Colorectal Surgeons parameters. *American Surgeon, 69*(11), 941–945.

*Ratner, P. A., Johnson, J. L., Richardson, C. G., et al. (2004). Efficacy of a smoking-cessation intervention for elective-surgical patients. *Research in Nursing and Health, 27*(3), 148–161.

Sorenson, H. M. & Shelledy, D. C. (2003). AARC clinical practice guideline. Intermittent positive pressure breathing—2003 revision and update. *Respiratory Care, 48*(5), 540–546.

Wood, K., & Joffe, A. (2003). Major pulmonary embolism part 3: A practical treatment strategy. *The Journal of Respiratory Diseases, 24*(10), 446–451.

Acute Respiratory Failure and ARDS

Bernard, G. R., Artigas, A., Brigham, K. L., et al. (1994). Report of the American-European consensus conference on acute respiratory distress syndrome: Definitions, mechanisms, relevant outcomes, and clinical trial coordination. *American Journal of Critical Care Medicine, 9*(1), 72–81.

Kallet, R. H. (2004). Evidence-based management of acute lung injury and acute respiratory distress syndrome. *Respiratory Care, 49*(7), 793–809.

Marini, J. (2004). Advances in the understanding of acute respiratory distress syndrome: Summarizing a decade of progress. *Current Opinion in Critical Care, 10*(4), 265–271.

Powers, J., & Daniels, D. (2004). Turning points: Implementing kinetic therapy in the ICU. *Nursing Management, 35*(Suppl. 3), 2–7.

Young, M. P., Manning, H. L., Wilson, D. L., et al. (2004). Ventilation of patients with acute lung injury and acute respiratory distress syndrome: Has new evidence changed clinical practice? *Critical Care Medicine, 32*(6), 1260–1265.

Lung Cancer

Baldwin, P. D. (2003). Lung cancer. *Clinical Journal of Oncology Nursing, 7*(6), 699–702.

Centers for Disease Control and Prevention. (2004a). Cancer mortality surveillance—United States, 1990–2000. *MMWR Morbidity and Mortality Weekly Report, 53*(SS03), 1–108.

*Gift, A. G., Stommel, M., Jablonski, A., et al. (2003). A cluster of symptoms over time in patients with lung cancer. *Nursing Research, 52*(6), 393–400.

Gohagan, J., Marcus, P., Fagerstsrom, R., et al. (2004). Baseline findings of a randomized feasibility trial of lung cancer screening with spiral CT scan vs. chest radiograph. *Chest, 126*(1), 114–121.

Hurria, A. & Kris, M. G. (2003). Management of lung cancer in older adults. *CA: A Cancer Journal for Clinicians, 53*(6), 325–341.

Jemal, A., Tiwari, R. C., Murray, T., et al. (2004). Cancer statistics 2004. *CA: A Cancer Journal for Clinicians, 54*(1), 8–29.

Mulshine, J. L. & Sullivan, D. C. (2005). Lung cancer screening. *New England Journal of Medicine, 352*(26), 2714–2719.

Spira, A. & Ettinger, D. S. (2004). Drug therapy: Multidisciplinary management of lung cancer. *New England Journal of Medicine, 350*(4), 379–392.

Pulmonary Infections

Andrews, J., Nadjm, B., Gant, V., et al. (2003). Community acquired pneumonia. *Current Opinion in Pulmonary Medicine, 9*(3), 175–180.

Centers for Disease Control and Prevention. (2003a). Guidelines for environmental infection control in health-care facilities: Recommendations of CDC and the Healthcare Infection Control Practice Advisory Committee (HICPAC). *MMWR Morbidity and Mortality Weekly Report,* 52(RR10).

Centers for Disease Control and Prevention. (2004c). Clinical guidance on the identification and evaluation of possible SARS-CoV disease among persons presenting with community-acquired illness, version 2. January, 2004.

Centers for Disease Control and Prevention. (2004d). Guidelines for preventing health-care–associated pneumonia, 2004. *MMWR Morbidity and Mortality Weekly Report,* 53(RR03), 1–36.

Centers for Disease Control and Prevention. (2004e). Prevention and control of influenza: recommendations of the Advisory Committee on Immunization Practices (ACIP). *MMWR Morbidity and Mortality Weekly Report, 53*(RR-6), 1–40.

Collard, H. R., Saint, S., & Matthay, M. A. (2003). Prevention of ventilator-associated pneumonia: An evidence-based systematic review. *Annals of Internal Medicine, 138*(6), 494–501.

Denison, M. R. (2004). Severe acute respiratory syndrome coronavirus pathogenesis, disease and vaccines: An update. *Pediatric Infectious Disease Journal, 23*(11), S207–S214.

File, T. M., Garau, J., Blasi, F., et al. (2004). Guidelines for empiric antimicrobial prescribing in community-acquired pneumonia. *Chest, 125*(5), 1888–1901.

Frazee, B. W. (2004). Community-acquired pneumonia: Getting down to the basics. *Journal of Respiratory Diseases, 25*(1), 37–44.

Institute for Clinical Systems Improvement (ISCI). (2003). Community acquired pneumonia in adults. Bloomington, MN: Institute for Clinical Systems Improvement.

Kochanek, K. D., & Smith, B. L. (2004). Deaths: Preliminary data for 2002. *National Vital Statistics Reports, 52*(13). Hyattsville, MD: National Center for Heath Statistics.

Levy, M. M., Baylor, M. S., Bernard, G. R., et al. (2005). Clinical issues and research in respiratory failure from severe acute respiratory syndrome. *American Journal of Respiratory and Critical Care Medicine, 171*(5), 518–526.

Mandell, L. A., Bartlett, J. G., Dowell, S. F., et al. (2003). Update of practice guidelines for the management of community-acquired pneumonia in immunocompetent adults. *Clinical Infectious Diseases, 37*(11), 1405–1433.

Niederman, M. S. & Ahmed, Q. A. (2003). Community-acquired pneumonia in elderly patients. *Clinical Geriatric Medicine, 21*(1), 101–120.

Stringer, J. R., Beard, C. B., Miller, R. F., et al. (2002). A new name (*Pneumocystis jiroveci*) for pneumocystis from humans. *Emerging Infectious Diseases, 8*(9), 891–896.

Wilkinson, M. & Woodhead, M. A. (2004). Guidelines for community-acquired pneumonia in the ICU. *Current Opinions in Critical Care, 10*(1), 59–64.

Trauma

Karmy-Jones, R. & Jurkovich, G. J. (2004). Blunt chest trauma. *Current Problems in Surgery, 41*(3), 223–380.

Kulshrestha, P., Munshi, I., & Wait, R. (2004). Profile of chest trauma in a level 1 trauma center. *Journal of Trauma Injury, Infection and Critical Care, 57*(3), 576–581.

Sirmali, M., Turut, H., Topcu, S. et al. (2003). A comprehensive analysis of traumatic rib fractures: Morbidity, mortality and management. *European Journal of Cardio-thoracic Surgery, 24*(2003), 133–138.

Wanek, S. & Mayberry, J. C. (2004). Blunt thoracic trauma: Flail chest, pulmonary contusion and blast injury. *Critical Care Clinics, 20*(1), 71–81.

Tuberculosis

American Thoracic Society. (2000). Diagnostic standards and classification of tuberculosis in adults and children. *American Journal of Respiratory and Critical Care Medicine, 161*(4), 1376–1395.

Centers for Disease Control and Prevention. (2003b). Treatment of tuberculosis. American Thoracic Society, CDC, and Infectious Diseases Society of America. *MMWR Morbidity and Mortality Weekly Report,* 52(RR-11), 1–74.

Centers for Disease Control and Prevention. (2003c). Trends in tuberculosis morbidity—United States, 1992–2002. *MMWR Morbidity and Mortality Weekly Report, 52*(11), 217–222.

Centers for Disease Control and Prevention. (2004f). Trends in tuberculosis—United States, 1998–2003. *MMWR Morbidity and Mortality Weekly Report, 53*(10), 209–214.

Centers for Disease Control and Prevention. (2005a). Treatment options for latent tuberculosis infection. Document 250004. CDC, Atlanta, GA.

Centers for Disease Control and Prevention. (2005b). Guidelines for using the QuantiFERON®-TB Gold Test for detecting *Mycobacterium tuberculosis* infection, United States. *MMWR Morbidity and Mortality Weekly Report, 54*(RR 15), 49–55.

Corbett, E. L., Watt, C. J., Walker, N., et al. (2003). The growing burden of tuberculosis: Global trends and interactions with the HIV epidemic. *Archives of Internal Medicine, 163*(9), 1009–1021.

RESOURCES

Agency for Healthcare Quality and Research, John M. Eisenberg Bldg, 540 Gaither Road, Rockville, MD 20850; 301-427-1364; http://www.ahrq.gov. Accessed March 31, 2006.

American Association for Respiratory Care, 9425 N. MacArthur Blvd., Suite 100, Irving, TX 75063; 972-243-2272; http://www.aarc.org. Accessed March 31, 2006.

American Cancer Society, 1599 Clifton Road NE, Atlanta, GA 30329; 888-ACS-2345; http://www.cancer.org. Accessed March 31, 2006.

American College of Chest Physicians, 3300 Dundee Road, Northbrook, IL 60062; 847-498-1400; http://www.chestnet.org. Accessed March 31, 2006.

American Lung Association, 61 Broadway 6th Floor, New York, NY 10006; 800-LUNGUSA; http://www.lungusa.org. Accessed March 31, 2006.

American Thoracic Society, 61 Broadway, New York, NY 10006; 212-315-8600; http://www.thoracic.org. Accessed March 31, 2006.

Centers for Disease Control and Prevention, 1600 Clifton Road NE, Atlanta, GA 30333; 800-311-3435; http://www.cdc.gov. Accessed March 31, 2006.

National Cancer Institute, National Institutes of Health, 6116 Executive Blvd, Room 3036A, Bethesda, MD 20892; 800-4-CANCER (Cancer Information Services); http://www.cancer.gov. Accessed March 31, 2006.

National Heart, Lung and Blood Institute, National Institutes of Health, Bldg. 31, 31 Center Drive MSC, Bethesda, MD 20892; 301-592-8573; http://www.nhlbi.nih.gov. Accessed March 31, 2006.

Occupational Safety and Health Administration (OSHA), United States Department of Labor, 200 Constitution Avenue NW., Washington, DC 20210; 800-321-6742; http://www.osha.gov. Accessed March 31, 2006.

Respiratory Nursing Society, c/o NYSNA, 11 Cornell Road, Latham, NY 12110; 518-782-9400 ×286; http://www.respiratorynursingsociety.org. Accessed March 31, 2006.

CHAPTER 24

Management of Patients With Chronic Obstructive Pulmonary Disorders

Learning Objectives

On completion of this chapter, the learner will be able to:

1. Describe the pathophysiology of chronic obstructive pulmonary disease (COPD).
2. Discuss the major risk factors for developing COPD and nursing interventions to minimize or prevent these risk factors.
3. Use the nursing process as a framework for care of patients with COPD.
4. Develop a teaching plan for patients with COPD.
5. Describe the pathophysiology of asthma.
6. Discuss the medications used in asthma management.
7. Describe asthma self-management strategies.
8. Describe the pathophysiology of cystic fibrosis.

Chronic pulmonary disorders are a leading cause of morbidity and mortality in the United States. Nurses are involved with patients with chronic pulmonary disease across the spectrum of care, from outpatient and home care to critical care and the hospice setting. Patients with chronic pulmonary disorders need care from nurses who not only have astute assessment and clinical management skills but who also understand how these disorders can affect quality of life. In addition, the nurse's knowledge of palliative and end-of-life care is important for affected patients. Patient and family teaching is an important nursing intervention to enhance self-management in patients with any chronic pulmonary disorder.

Chronic Obstructive Pulmonary Disease

Chronic obstructive pulmonary disease (COPD) is a disease state characterized by airflow limitation that is not fully reversible. This newest definition of COPD, provided by the Global Initiative for Chronic Obstructive Lung Disease (GOLD), is a broad description that better explains this disorder and its signs and symptoms (GOLD, World Health Organization [WHO] & National Heart, Lung and Blood Institute [NHLBI], 2004). Although previous definitions have included emphysema and chronic bronchitis under the umbrella classification of COPD, this was often confusing because most patients with COPD present with overlapping signs and symptoms of these two distinct disease processes.

COPD may include diseases that cause airflow obstruction (eg, emphysema, chronic bronchitis) or any combination of these disorders. Other diseases such as cystic fibrosis, bronchiectasis, and asthma that were previously classified as types of chronic obstructive lung disease are now classified as chronic pulmonary disorders. However, asthma is now considered a separate disorder and is classified as an abnormal airway condition characterized primarily by reversible inflammation. COPD can coexist with asthma. Both of these diseases have the same major symptoms; however, symptoms are generally more variable in asthma than in COPD. This chapter discusses COPD as a disease and describes chronic bronchitis and emphysema as distinct disease states, providing a foundation for understanding the pathophysiology of COPD. Bronchiectasis, asthma, and cystic fibrosis are discussed separately.

Currently, COPD is the fourth leading cause of mortality and the 12th leading cause of disability in the United States; however, by the year 2020 it is estimated that COPD will be the third leading cause of death and the fifth leading cause of disability (Sin, McAlister, Man, et al., 2003). In 2001, chronic pulmonary disorders caused 123,013 deaths in people of all ages, regardless of gender, and the male/female age-adjusted ratio was 1:4 (Arias, Anderson, Hsiang-Ching, et al., 2003). At present, approximately 16 million people in the United States have some form of COPD. The annual cost of COPD is approximately $32.1 billion, including health care expenditures of $18.0 billion and indirect costs of $14.1 billion (American Lung Association, 2004).

People with COPD commonly become symptomatic during the middle adult years, and the incidence of the disease increases with age. Although certain aspects of lung function normally decrease with age—for example, vital capacity and forced expiratory volume in 1 second (FEV_1), COPD accentuates and accelerates these physiologic changes.

Pathophysiology

In COPD, the airflow limitation is both progressive and associated with an abnormal inflammatory response of the lungs to noxious particles or gases. The inflammatory response occurs throughout the airways, parenchyma, and pulmonary vasculature (GOLD, WHO & NHLBI, 2004). Because of the chronic inflammation and the body's attempts to repair it, narrowing occurs in the small peripheral airways. Over time, this injury-and-repair process causes

Glossary

air trapping: incomplete emptying of alveoli during expiration due to loss of lung tissue elasticity (emphysema), bronchospasm (asthma), or airway obstruction

alpha$_1$-antitrypsin deficiency: genetic disorder resulting from deficiency of alpha$_1$ antitrypsin, a protective agent for the lung; increases patient's risk for developing panacinar emphysema even in the absence of smoking

asthma: a disease with multiple precipitating mechanisms resulting in a common clinical outcome of reversible airflow obstruction; no longer considered a category of COPD

bronchiectasis: chronic dilation of a bronchus or bronchi; the dilated airways become saccular and are a medium for chronic infection. No longer considered a category of COPD.

bronchitis: a disease of the airways defined as the presence of cough and sputum production for at least a combined total of 3 months in each of 2 consecutive years; a category of COPD

chronic obstructive pulmonary disease: disease state characterized by airflow limitation that is not fully reversible; sometimes referred to as chronic airway obstruction or chronic obstructive lung disease

emphysema: a disease of the airways characterized by destruction of the walls of overdistended alveoli; a category of COPD

metered-dose inhaler (MDI): patient-activated medication canister that provides aerosolized medication that the patient inhales into the lungs

polycythemia: increase in the red blood cell concentration in the blood; in COPD, the body attempts to improve oxygen carrying capacity by producing increasing amounts of red blood cells

spirometry: pulmonary function tests that measure specific lung volumes (eg, FEV_1, FVC) and rates ($FEF_{25-75\%}$); may be measured before and after bronchodilator administration

scar tissue formation and narrowing of the airway lumen. Airflow obstruction may also be caused by parenchymal destruction, as is seen with emphysema, a disease of the alveoli or gas exchange units.

In addition to inflammation, processes related to imbalances of proteinases and antiproteinases in the lung may be responsible for airflow limitation. When activated by chronic inflammation, proteinases and other substances may be released, damaging the parenchyma of the lung. The parenchymal changes may occur as a consequence of inflammation or environmental or genetic factors (eg, alpha$_1$-antitrypsin deficiency).

Early in the course of COPD, the inflammatory response causes pulmonary vasculature changes that are characterized by thickening of the vessel wall. These changes may result from (1) exposure to cigarette smoke, (2) use of tobacco products, or (3) the release of inflammatory mediators (GOLD, WHO & NHLBI, 2004).

Chronic Bronchitis

Chronic **bronchitis**, a disease of the airways, is defined as the presence of cough and sputum production for at least 3 months in each of two consecutive years. In many cases, smoke or other environmental pollutants irritate the airways, resulting in hypersecretion of mucus and inflammation. This constant irritation causes the mucus-secreting glands and goblet cells to increase in number. Ciliary function is reduced, and more mucus is produced. The bronchial walls become thickened, the bronchial lumen narrows, and mucus may plug the airway (Fig. 24-1). Alveoli adjacent to the bronchioles may become damaged and fibrosed, resulting in altered function of the alveolar macrophages. This is significant because the macrophages play an important role in destroying foreign particles, including bacteria. As a result, the patient becomes more susceptible to respiratory infection. A wide range of viral, bacterial, and mycoplasmal infections can produce acute episodes of bronchitis. Exacerbations of chronic bronchitis are most likely to occur during the winter.

Emphysema

In **emphysema**, impaired gas oxygen and carbon dioxide exchange results from destruction of the walls of overdistended alveoli. "Emphysema" is a pathologic term that describes an abnormal distention of the air spaces beyond the terminal bronchioles, with destruction of the walls of the alveoli. It is the end stage of a process that has progressed slowly for many years. As the walls of the alveoli are destroyed (a process accelerated by recurrent infections), the alveolar surface area in direct contact with the pulmonary capillaries continually decreases, causing an increase in dead space (lung area where no gas exchange can occur) and impaired oxygen diffusion, which leads to hypoxemia. In the later stages of disease, carbon dioxide elimination is impaired, resulting in increased carbon dioxide tension in arterial blood (hypercapnia) and causing respiratory acidosis. As the alveolar walls continue to break down, the pulmonary capillary bed is reduced in size. Consequently, resistance to pulmonary blood flow is increased, forcing the right ventricle to maintain a higher blood pressure in the pulmonary artery. Hypoxemia may further increase pulmonary artery pressures. For this reason, right-sided heart failure (cor pulmonale) is one of the complications of emphysema. Congestion, dependent edema, distended neck veins, or pain in the region of the liver suggests the development of cardiac failure.

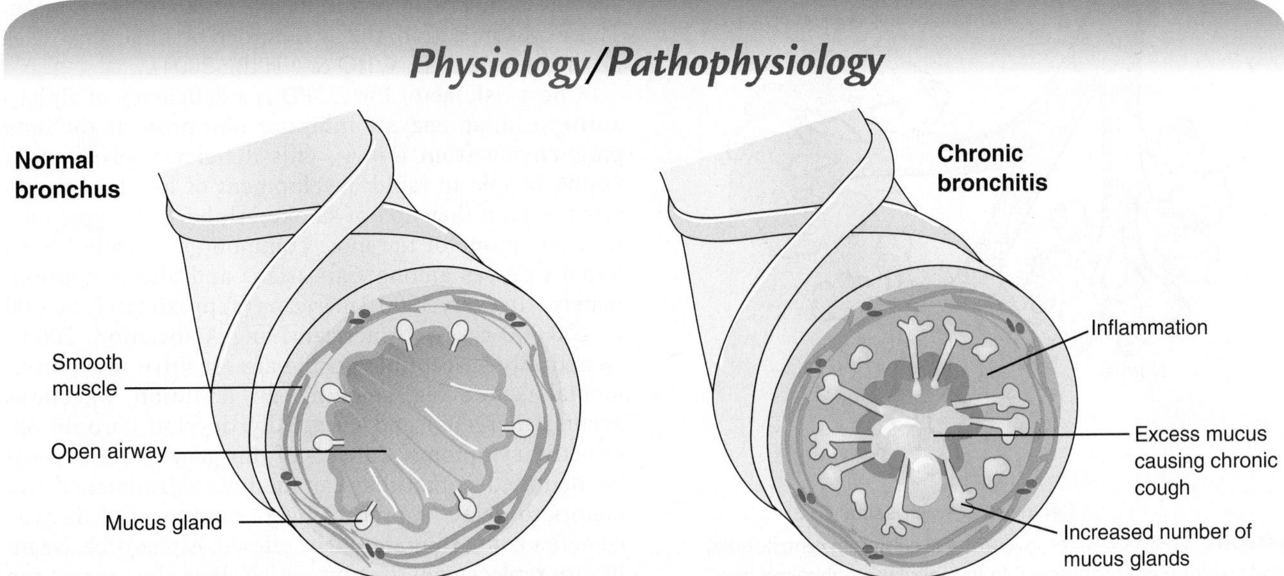

FIGURE 24-1. Pathophysiology of chronic bronchitis as compared to a normal bronchus. The bronchus in chronic bronchitis is narrowed and has impaired air flow due to multiple mechanisms: inflammation, excess mucus production, and potential smooth muscle constriction (bronchospasm).

There are two main types of emphysema, based on the changes taking place in the lung (Fig. 24-2). Both types may occur in the same patient.

In the panlobular (panacinar) type of emphysema, there is destruction of the respiratory bronchiole, alveolar duct, and alveolus. All air spaces within the lobule are essentially enlarged, but there is little inflammatory disease. A hyperinflated (hyperexpanded) chest (barrel chest on physical examination), marked dyspnea on exertion, and weight loss typically occur. To move air into and out of the lungs, negative pressure is required during inspiration, and an adequate level of positive pressure must be attained and maintained during expiration. The resting position is one of inflation. Instead of being an involuntary passive act, expiration becomes active and requires muscular effort. Patients become increasingly short of breath; the chest becomes rigid, and the ribs are fixed at their joints.

In the centrilobular (centroacinar) form, pathologic changes take place mainly in the center of the secondary lobule, preserving the peripheral portions of the acinus. Frequently, there is a derangement of ventilation–perfusion ratios, producing chronic hypoxemia, hypercapnia, **polycythemia**, and episodes of right-sided heart failure. This leads to central cyanosis and respiratory failure. The patient also develops peripheral edema, which is treated with diuretic therapy.

Risk Factors

Risk factors for COPD include environmental exposures and host factors (Chart 24-1). The most important risk factor for COPD is cigarette smoking. Other risk factors are pipe, cigar, and other types of tobacco smoking. In addition, passive smoking contributes to respiratory symptoms and COPD (NIH, 2001). Smoking depresses the activity of scavenger cells and affects the respiratory tract's ciliary cleansing mechanism, which keeps breathing passages free of inhaled irritants, bacteria, and other foreign matter. When smoking damages this cleansing mechanism, airflow is obstructed and air becomes trapped behind the obstruction. The alveoli greatly distend, diminishing lung capacity. Smoking also irritates the goblet cells and mucus glands, causing an increased accumulation of mucus, which in turn produces more irritation, infection, and damage to the lung. In addition, carbon monoxide (a byproduct of smoking) combines with hemoglobin to form carboxyhemoglobin. Hemoglobin that is bound by carboxyhemoglobin cannot carry oxygen efficiently.

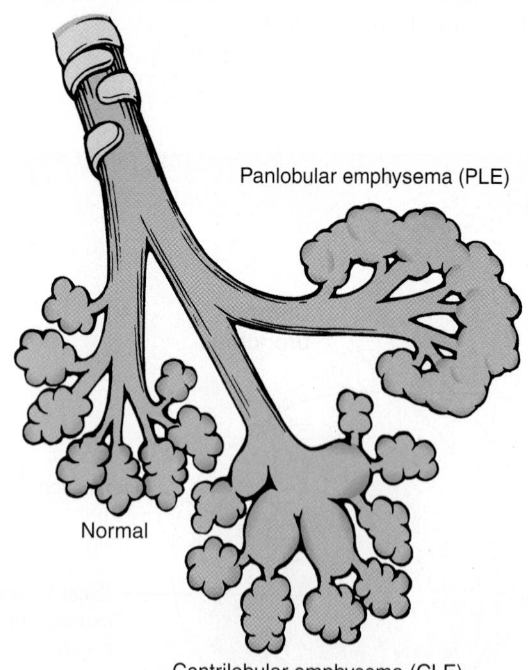

FIGURE 24-2. Changes in alveolar structure in centrilobular and panlobular emphysema. In panlobular emphysema, the bronchioles, alveolar ducts, and alveoli are destroyed, and the air spaces within the lobule are enlarged. In centrilobular emphysema, the pathologic changes occur in the lobule, whereas the peripheral portions of the acinus are preserved.

CHART 24-1

Risk Factors for Chronic Obstructive Pulmonary Disease (COPD)

- Exposure to tobacco smoke accounts for an estimated 80% to 90% of COPD cases
- Passive smoking
- Occupational exposure
- Ambient air pollution
- Genetic abnormalities, including a deficiency of alpha$_1$-antitrypsin, an enzyme inhibitor that normally counteracts the destruction of lung tissue by certain other enzymes

Other factors that put people at risk for COPD include prolonged and intense exposure to occupational dusts and chemicals, indoor air pollution, and outdoor air pollution. This exposure adds to the total burden of inhaled particles on the lung (GOLD, WHO & NHLBI, 2004).

A host risk factor for COPD is a deficiency of alpha$_1$-antitrypsin, an enzyme inhibitor that protects the lung parenchyma from injury. This deficiency predisposes young people to rapid development of lobular emphysema, even if they do not smoke. **Alpha$_1$-antitrypsin deficiency** is one of the most common genetically linked lethal diseases among Caucasians and affects approximately 1 in every 3000 Americans (approximately 80,000 to 100,000 cases) (American Lung Association, 2005). Genetically susceptible people are sensitive to environmental factors (eg, smoking, air pollution, infectious agents, allergens) and eventually develop chronic obstructive symptoms. Carriers of this genetic defect must be identified so that they can modify environmental risk factors to delay or prevent overt symptoms of disease. Genetics counseling should be offered. Alpha-protease inhibitor replacement therapy, which slows the progression of the disease, is available for patients with this genetic defect and for those with severe disease. However, this intermittent infusion therapy is costly and is required on an ongoing basis.

Clinical Manifestations

COPD is characterized by three primary symptoms: chronic cough, sputum production, and dyspnea on exertion (GOLD, WHO & NHLBI, 2004). These symptoms often worsen over time. Chronic cough and sputum production often precede the development of airflow limitation by many years. However, not all people with cough and sputum production develop COPD. Dyspnea may be severe and often interferes with the patient's activities. Weight loss is common, because dyspnea interferes with eating and the work of breathing is energy-depleting. Often patients cannot participate in even mild exercise because of dyspnea; as COPD progresses, dyspnea occurs even at rest. As the work of breathing increases over time, the accessory muscles are recruited in an effort to breathe. Patients with COPD are at risk for respiratory insufficiency and respiratory infections, which in turn increase the risk of acute and chronic respiratory failure.

In patients with COPD that has a primary emphysematous component, chronic hyperinflation leads to the "barrel chest" thorax configuration. This results from fixation of the ribs in the inspiratory position (due to hyperinflation) and from loss of lung elasticity (Fig. 24-3). Retraction of the supraclavicular fossae occurs on inspiration, causing the shoulders to heave upward (Fig. 24-4). In advanced emphysema, the abdominal muscles also contract on inspiration.

Assessment and Diagnostic Findings

The nurse should obtain a thorough health history for patients with known or potential COPD. Chart 24-2 lists the key factors to assess. Pulmonary function studies are used to help confirm the diagnosis of COPD, determine disease severity, and monitor disease progression. **Spirometry** is used to evaluate airflow obstruction, which is determined by the ratio of FEV_1 to forced vital capacity (FVC). Spirometric results are expressed as an absolute volume and as a percentage of the predicted value using appropriate normal values for gender, age, and height. With obstruction, the patient either has difficulty exhaling or cannot forcibly exhale air from the lungs, reducing the FEV_1. Obstructive lung disease is defined as a FEV_1/FVC ratio of less than 70%.

In addition, bronchodilator reversibility testing may be performed to rule out the diagnosis of asthma and to guide initial treatment. With this type of testing, spirometry is first obtained, then the patient is given an inhaled bronchodilator treatment according to a protocol, and finally spirometry is repeated. The patient demonstrates a degree of reversibility if the pulmonary function values improve after administration of the bronchodilator. Even patients who do not show a significant response to a short-acting bronchodilator test may benefit symptomatically from long-term bronchodilator treatment.

Arterial blood gas measurements may also be obtained to assess baseline oxygenation and gas exchange and are especially important in advanced COPD. In addition, a chest x-ray may be obtained to exclude alternative diagnoses. A chest x-ray is seldom diagnostic in COPD unless obvious bullous disease is present. A computed tomography (CT) scan is not routinely obtained in the diagnosis of COPD, but a high-resolution CT scan may help in the differential diagnosis. Lastly, screening for alpha$_1$-antitrypsin deficiency

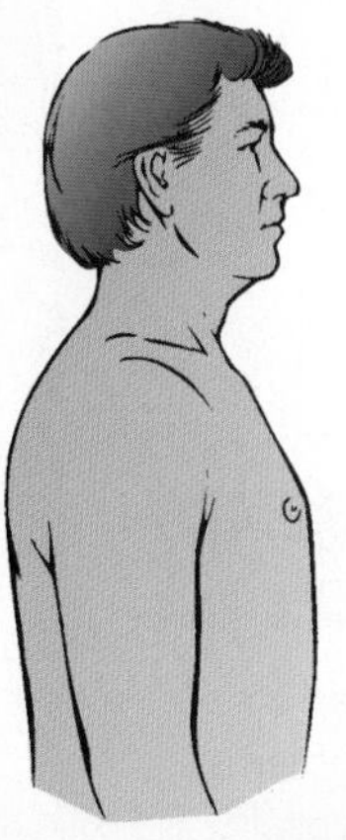

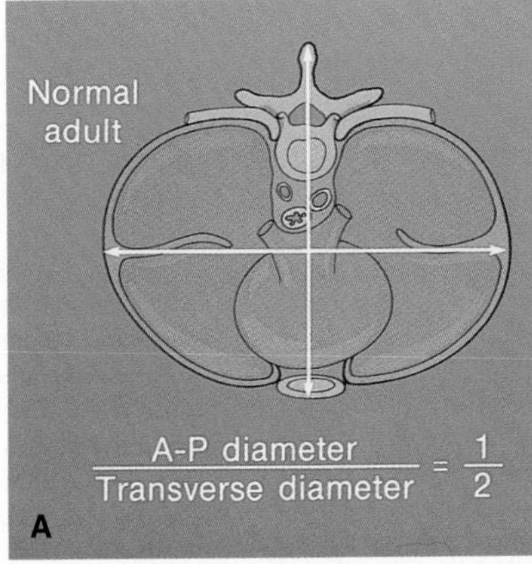

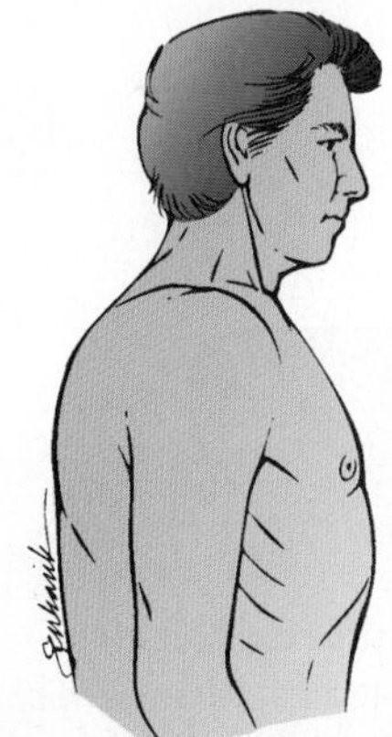

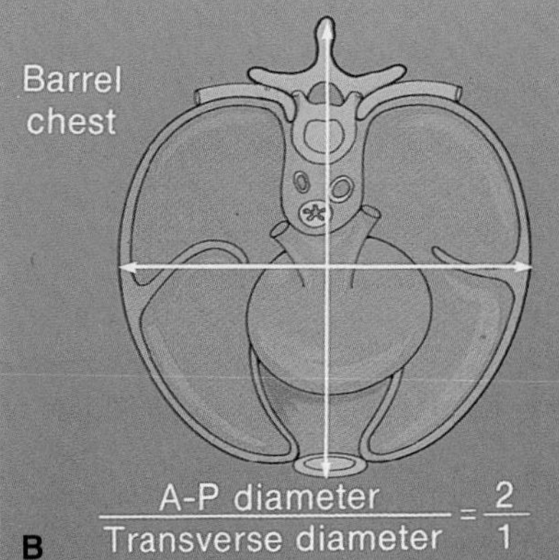

FIGURE 24-3. Characteristics of normal chest wall and chest wall in emphysema. (**A**) The normal chest wall and its cross-section. (**B**) The barrel-shaped chest of emphysema and its cross-section.

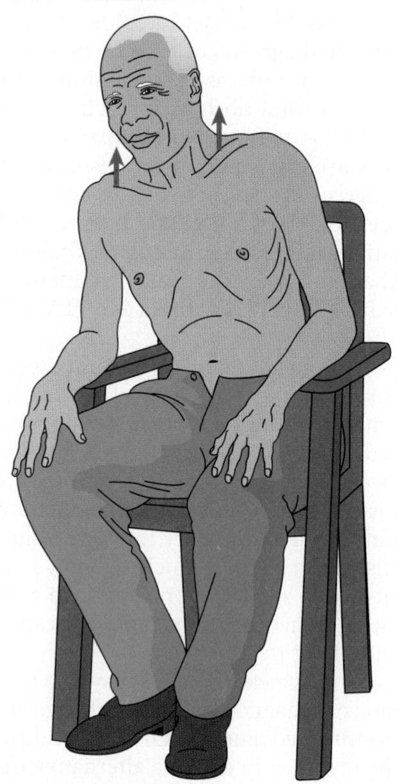

FIGURE 24-4. Typical posture of a person with chronic obstructive pulmonary disease (COPD)—primarily emphysema. The person tends to lean forward and uses the accessory muscles of respiration to breathe, forcing the shoulder girdle upward and causing the supraclavicular fossae to retract on inspiration.

may be performed for patients younger than 45 years and for those with a strong family history of COPD.

COPD is classified into five stages depending on severity (Table 24-1) (GOLD, WHO & NHLBI, 2004). Factors that determine the clinical course and survival of patients with COPD include history of cigarette smoking, passive smoking exposure, age, rate of decline of FEV_1, hypoxemia, pulmonary artery pressure, resting heart rate, weight loss, and reversibility of airflow obstruction.

In diagnosing COPD, several differential diagnoses must be ruled out. The primary differential diagnosis is asthma. Key characteristics of asthma often include onset early in life; variation in daily symptoms and day-to-day occurrence or timing of symptoms; symptoms at night or in the early morning; family history of asthma; potential presence of allergy, rhinitis, or eczema; and a largely reversible airflow obstruction. It may be difficult to differentiate between a patient with COPD and one with chronic asthma. Key parts of differentiation are the patient history and the patient's responsiveness to bronchodilators. Other diseases that must be considered in the differential diagnosis include heart failure, bronchiectasis, tuberculosis, obliterative bronchiolitis, and diffuse panbronchiolitis (GOLD, WHO & NHLBI, 2004).

Complications

Respiratory insufficiency and failure are major life-threatening complications of COPD. The acuity of the onset

CHART 24-2

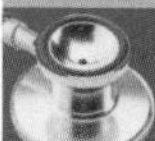

Assessing Key Factors in the Health History of Patients with COPD

- Exposure to risk factors—types, intensity, duration
- Past medical history—respiratory diseases/problems, including asthma, allergy, sinusitis, nasal polyps, history of respiratory infections
- Family history of COPD or other chronic respiratory diseases
- Pattern of symptom development
- History of exacerbations or previous hospitalizations for respiratory problems
- Presence of comorbidities
- Appropriateness of current medical treatments
- Impact of the disease on quality of life
- Available social and family support for patient
- Potential for reducing risk factors (eg, smoking cessation)

TABLE 24-1 Classifications of Chronic Obstructive Pulmonary Disease (COPD) by Severity

Stage	Characteristics
0 (at risk)	Normal spirometry Chronic symptoms of cough, sputum production
I (mild COPD)	$FEV_1/FVC < 70\%$ $FEV_1 \geq 80\%$ predicted With or without chronic symptoms of cough, sputum production
II (moderate COPD)	$FEV_1/FVC < 70\%$ FEV_1 50–80% predicted With or without chronic symptoms of cough, sputum production
III (severe COPD)	$FEV_1/FVC < 70\%$ $FEV_1 <$ 30–50% predicted With or without chronic symptoms
IV (very severe COPD)	$FEV_1/FVC < 70\%$ $FEV_1 <$ 30–50% predicted Chronic respiratory failure

COPD, chronic obstructive pulmonary disease; FEV_1, forced expiratory volume in 1 second; FVC, forced vital capacity.

From Global Initiative for Chronic Obstructive Lung Disease (GOLD), World Health Organization (WHO), & National Heart, Lung and Blood Institute (NHLBI). (2004). *Global strategy for the diagnosis, management, and prevention of chronic obstructive pulmonary disease.* Bethesda, MD: National Heart, Lung and Blood Institute.

NURSING RESEARCH PROFILE

Fatigue in Patients With COPD

Theander, K. & Unosson, M. (2004). Fatigue in patients with chronic obstructive pulmonary disease. *Journal of Advanced Nursing, 45*(2), 172–177.

Purpose

This study described the frequency, duration, and severity of fatigue in patients with COPD. In addition, it compared the impact of perceived fatigue on cognitive, physical, and psychosocial functioning between patients with COPD and control subjects.

Design

The convenience sample in this study was made up of 36 patients with COPD (19 women and 17 men) with mean ages of 63 ± 4.6 years and 68 ± 5.3 years, respectively. Using a control group comparison design, two gender- and age-matched controls were randomly assigned for each patient with COPD (control group, $n = 88$). A total of 36 patients with COPD and 37 controls completed questionnaires that included a demographic form and the Fatigue Impact Scale, which was used to assess perceptions of the impact of functional limitations due to fatigue on cognitive, physical, and psychosocial functioning during the past 4 weeks.

Findings

Forty-seven percent of patients with COPD reported fatigue every day during the preceding month compared to 13.5% of the control group ($p < .001$). In evaluation of the duration of fatigue, 52.7% of the patients with COPD reported fatigue more than 6 hours per day versus 18.9% of the controls ($p < .001$). In rating the impact of fatigue, 44.4% of patients with COPD reported fatigue as either the worst or one of the worst symptoms experienced, while 10.8% of the control group did so ($p < .01$). Patients with COPD reported a significantly greater ($p < .001$) impact of fatigue on cognitive, physical, and psychosocial functioning than did members of the control group.

Nursing Implications

Fatigue is a common symptom experienced by patients with COPD on a daily basis. Nursing interventions must include assessment of this symptom and the impact of all dimensions of fatigue (cognitive, physical, and psychosocial) on activities of daily living and quality of life. Future studies must focus on specific interventions related to fatigue for the COPD population.

and the severity of respiratory failure depend on baseline pulmonary function, pulse oximetry or arterial blood gas values, comorbid conditions, and the severity of other complications of COPD. Respiratory insufficiency and failure may be chronic (with severe COPD) or acute (with severe bronchospasm or pneumonia in a patient with severe COPD). Acute respiratory insufficiency and failure may necessitate ventilatory support until other acute complications, such as infection, can be treated. Management of the patient requiring ventilatory support is discussed in Chapter 25. Other complications of COPD include pneumonia, atelectasis, pneumothorax, and pulmonary arterial hypertension (cor pulmonale).

Medical Management

Risk Reduction

Smoking cessation is the only intervention proven to slow the accelerated decline in lung function and the progression of COPD (GOLD, WHO & NHLBI, 2004; Sin et al., 2003). Recent surveys indicate that 22.5% (46.2 million) of all American adults smoke. According to the Centers for Disease Control and Prevention (CDC), 28.5% of all high school students report that they smoke (CDC, 2004). Smoking cessation is difficult to achieve and even more difficult to sustain in the long term. Nurses play a key role in promoting smoking cessation and educating patients about ways to do so. Patients diagnosed with COPD who continue to smoke must be encouraged and assisted to quit. Factors associated with continued smoking vary among patients and may include the strength of the nicotine addiction, continued exposure to smoking-associated stimuli (at work or in social settings), stress, depression, and habit. Continued smoking is also more prevalent among those with low incomes, low levels of education, or psychosocial problems (CDC, 2004).

Because multiple factors are associated with continued smoking, successful cessation often requires multiple strategies. Health care providers should promote cessation by explaining the risks of smoking and personalizing the "at-risk" message to the patient. After giving a strong warning about smoking, health care providers should work with the patient to set a definite "quit date." Referral to a smoking cessation program may be helpful. Follow-up within 3 to 5 days after the "quit date" to review progress and to address any problems is associated with an increased rate of success; this should be repeated as needed. Continued reinforcement with telephone calls or clinic visits is extremely beneficial. Relapses should be analyzed, and the patient and health care provider should jointly identify possible solutions to prevent future backsliding. It is important to emphasize successes rather than failures. First-line pharmacotherapy that reliably increases long-term smoking abstinence rates is nicotine replacement (gum, inhaler, nasal spray, transdermal patch, sublingual tablet, or lozenges). Bupropion SR (Zyban,

Wellbutrin) and nortriptyline (Aventyl) may also increase long-term quit rates. Second-line pharmacotherapy includes the antihypertensive agent clonidine (Catapres); however, its use is limited by its side effects (GOLD, WHO & NHLBI, 2004). Patients with medical contraindications, light smokers (less than 10 cigarettes per day), and pregnant and adolescent smokers are not appropriate candidates for the use of pharmacotherapy.

Smoking cessation can begin in a variety of health care settings—outpatient clinic, pulmonary rehabilitation, community, hospital, and the home. Regardless of the setting, nurses have the opportunity to teach patients about the risks of smoking and the benefits of smoking cessation. Various materials, resources, and programs developed by several organizations (eg, Agency for Healthcare Research and Quality, U.S. Public Health Service, CDC, National Cancer Institute, American Lung Association, American Cancer Society) are available to assist with this effort.

Pharmacologic Therapy

BRONCHODILATORS. Bronchodilators relieve bronchospasm and reduce airway obstruction by allowing increased oxygen distribution throughout the lungs and improving alveolar ventilation. These medications, which are central in the management of COPD (GOLD, WHO & NHLBI, 2004), are delivered through a metered-dose inhaler or other type of inhaler, by nebulization, or via the oral route in pill or liquid form. Bronchodilators are often administered regularly throughout the day as well as on an as-needed basis. They may also be used prophylactically to prevent breathlessness by having the patient use them before participating in or completing an activity, such as eating or walking.

A **metered-dose inhaler** (MDI) is a pressurized device that contains an aerosolized powder of medication. A precise amount of medication is released with each activation of the canister. Patients must be instructed on the correct use of the device. A spacer (holding chamber) may also be used to enhance deposition of the medication in the lung and help the patient coordinate activation of the MDI with inspiration. Spacers come in several designs, but all are attached to the MDI and have a mouthpiece on the opposite end (Fig. 24-5). Once the canister is activated, the spacer holds the aerosol in the chamber until the patient inhales. The patient should take a slow, 3- to 5-second inhalation immediately after activation of the MDI (Expert Panel Report, 1997; NHLBI/WHO, 2001). Other types of inhalers include the discus inhaler (Serevent) and the Aerolizer inhaler (Foradil). Specific package insert information is available on the use of these inhalers.

Several classes of bronchodilators are used, including beta-adrenergic agonists, anticholinergic agents, methylxanthines, and combination agents. These medications may be used in combination to optimize bronchodilation. Some of these medications are short-acting, and others are long-acting. Long-acting bronchodilators are more convenient for patient use. Examples of medications are shown in Table 24-2. Nebulized medications (nebulization of medication via an air compressor) may also be effective in patients who cannot use an MDI properly or who prefer this method of administration.

CORTICOSTEROIDS. Inhaled and systemic corticosteroids (oral or intravenous) may also be used in COPD but are used more frequently in asthma. They may improve symptoms, but it has been shown that they do not slow the decline in lung function. A short trial course of oral corticosteroids may be prescribed for patients to determine

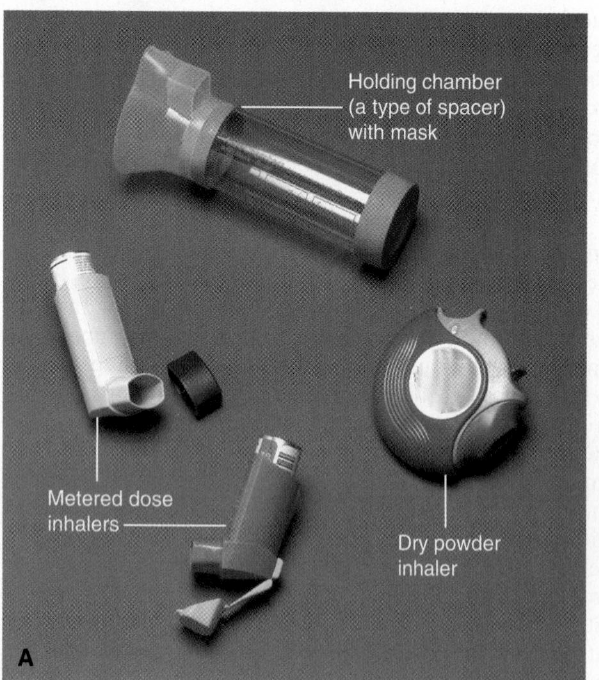

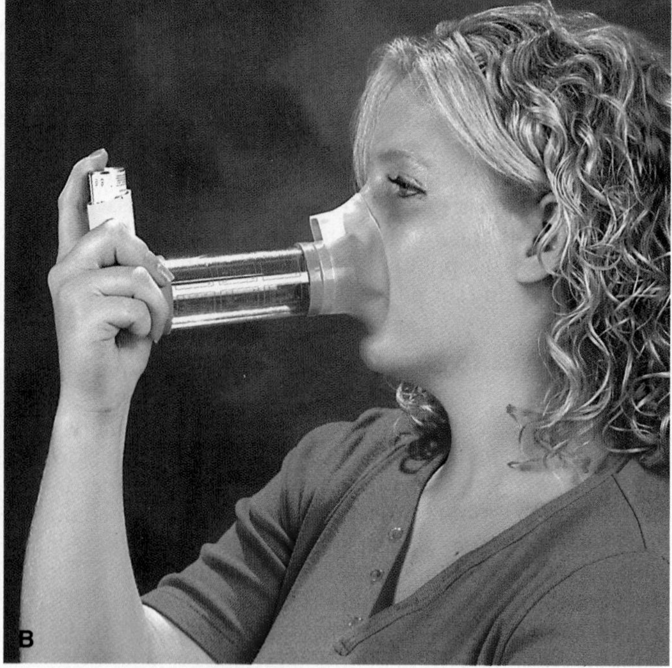

FIGURE 24-5. (**A**) Examples of metered-dose inhalers and spacers. (**B**) A metered-dose inhaler and spacer in use.

TABLE 24-2 Common Types of Bronchodilator Medications

	Method of Administration			
Class/Drug	***Inhaler****	***Nebulizer***	***Oral***	***Duration of Action***
Beta$_2$-Adrenergic Agonist Agents				
Albuterol (Proventil, Ventolin, Volmax)	X	X	X	Short
Bitolterol (Tornalate)		X		Long
Formoterol (Foradil)	X			Long
Levalbuterol (Xopenax)		X		Medium
Metaproterenol (Alupent)	X	X	X	Short
Pirbuterol (Maxair)	X			Short
Salmeterol (Serevent Diskus)	X			Long
Anticholinergic Agents				
Ipratropium bromide (Atrovent)	X			Short
Oxitropium bromide (Oxivent)	X	X		Medium
Methylxanthines				
Aminophylline (Phyllocontin)			X	Variable
Theophylline (Slo-bid, Theo-Dur)			X	Variable

Short-acting, 4–6 hours; medium-acting, 6–9 hours; long-acting, 12+ hours.
*Inhaler may include metered-dose inhaler, powdered inhalation with inhaler, or discus.

whether pulmonary function improves and symptoms decrease. Regular treatment with inhaled glucocorticosteroids is appropriate for symptomatic stage III and IV patients and for those with repeated exacerbations of the disease (eg, three episodes in the past 3 years). Long-term treatment with oral corticosteroids is not recommended in COPD and can cause steroid myopathy, leading to muscle weakness, decreased ability to function, and, in advanced disease, respiratory failure (GOLD, WHO & NHLBI, 2004). Examples of corticosteroids in the inhaled form are beclomethasone (Beclo-vent, Vanceril, Qvar), budesonide (Pulmicort Turbuhaler, Pulmicort Respules), flunisolide (AeroBid), fluticasone (Flovent), and triamcinolone (Azmacort).

Medication regimens used to manage COPD are based on disease severity. For stage I (mild) COPD, a short-acting bronchodilator may be prescribed. For stage II or III COPD, a short-acting bronchodilator along with regular treatment of one or more long-acting bronchodilators may be used. For stage III or IV (severe or very severe) COPD, medication therapy includes regular treatment with one or more bronchodilators and inhaled corticosteroids for repeated exacerbations (GOLD, WHO & NHLBI, 2004).

OTHER MEDICATIONS. There is little evidence regarding the usefulness of influenza and pneumococcal vaccinations specifically for patients with COPD. However, it has been demonstrated that influenza and pneumococcal vaccinations reduce the incidence of pneumonia, hospitalizations for cardiac conditions, and deaths in the general elderly population (Sin et al., 2003). As a preventive measure, patients should receive a yearly influenza vaccine and the pneumococcal vaccine every 5 to 7 years. In most healthy adults, pneumococcal vaccine titers persist for 5 or more years. Other pharmacologic treatments that may be used in COPD include alpha1-antitrypsin augmentation therapy, antibiotic agents, mucolytic agents, and antitussive agents.

Management of Exacerbations

An exacerbation of respiratory symptoms requiring medical intervention is an important clinical event in COPD. An exacerbation of COPD is difficult to diagnose, but signs and symptoms may include increased dyspnea, increased sputum production and purulence, respiratory failure, changes in mental status, or worsening blood gas abnormalities. Primary causes of an acute exacerbation include tracheobronchial infection and air pollution. However, the cause of approximately one third of severe exacerbations cannot be identified (GOLD, WHO & NHLBI, 2004). First the primary cause of the exacerbation is identified, if possible, and then specific treatment is administered. Optimization of bronchodilator medications is the first-line therapy and involves identifying the best medication or combinations of medications taken on a regular schedule for a specific patient. Depending on the signs and symptoms, corticosteroids, antibiotic agents, oxygen therapy, and intensive respiratory interventions may also be used. Indications for hospitalization for acute exacerbation of COPD include severe dyspnea that does not respond adequately to initial therapy, confusion or lethargy, respiratory muscle fatigue, paradoxical chest wall movement, peripheral edema, worsening or new onset of central cyanosis, persistent or worsening hypoxemia, and need for noninvasive or invasive assisted mechanical ventilation (GOLD, WHO & NHLBI, 2004). The risk of death from an exacerbation of COPD is closely related to the development of respiratory acidosis, the presence of significant comorbidities, and the need for noninvasive or invasive positive-pressure ventilatory support.

The GOLD, WHO & NHLBI guidelines (2004) provide indications for assessment, hospital admission, and intensive care admission for patients with exacerbation of COPD.

Oxygen Therapy

Oxygen therapy can be administered as long-term continuous therapy, during exercise, or to prevent acute dyspnea. Supplemental oxygen is effective in prolonging survival of patients with COPD who have a resting partial arterial pressure of oxygen (PaO_2) of less than 60 mm Hg at sea level (Sin et al., 2003). Long-term oxygen therapy (more than 15 hours per day) has also been shown to improve quality of life, has a mild beneficial effect on pulmonary arterial pressure, and decreases dyspnea (Sin et al., 2003). Long-term oxygen therapy is usually introduced in stage IV (very severe) COPD, and indications generally include a PaO_2 of 55 mm Hg or less or evidence of tissue hypoxia and organ damage such as cor pulmonale, secondary polycythemia, edema from right-sided heart failure, or impaired mental status (GOLD, WHO & NHLBI, 2004). For patients with exercise-induced hypoxemia, oxygen supplementation during exercise may improve performance. However, there is no evidence to support the idea that short bursts of oxygen before or after exercise provide any symptomatic relief (GOLD, WHO & NHLBI, 2004). Patients who are hypoxemic while awake are likely to be so during sleep. Therefore, nighttime oxygen therapy is recommended as well, and the prescription for oxygen therapy is for continuous, 24-hour use. Intermittent oxygen therapy is indicated for patients who desaturate only during exercise or sleep.

For years, the hypoxic drive theory has influenced clinicians. This theory proposed that administering oxygen to patients with COPD could result in apnea, cardiopulmonary arrest, or death as a result of blunting of the hypoxic drive to breathe (Simmons & Simmons, 2004). This theory is now considered obsolete. A small subset of COPD patients with chronic hypercapnia (elevated $PaCO_2$ levels) may be oxygen sensitive; however, the theories of ventilation–perfusion mismatch in the lungs and the Haldane effect are probably more important. The Haldane effect relates to the ability of hemoglobin to carry oxygen and carbon dioxide. When supplemental oxygen is administered, increased oxygen saturation results, and carbon dioxide is unable to be carried by the hemoglobin or is cast off by the hemoglobin. It must be transported in the dissolved form or as bicarbonate. This results in an overall increased load of carbon dioxide in the body. When patients with COPD cannot increase ventilation to adjust for this increased load, increasing hypercapnia occurs (Simmons & Simmons, 2004). Key in the care of patients with COPD on supplemental oxygen is monitoring and assessment. Pulse oximetry is helpful in assessing response to therapy but does not assess $PaCO_2$ levels. Optimal oxygenation of patients is important while monitoring for any possible complications of oxygen supplementation (Simmons & Simmons, 2004).

Surgical Management

BULLECTOMY. A bullectomy is a surgical option for select patients with bullous emphysema. Bullae are enlarged airspaces that do not contribute to ventilation but occupy space in the thorax; these areas may be surgically excised. Many times these bullae compress areas of the lung that do have adequate gas exchange. Bullectomy may help reduce dyspnea and improve lung function. It can be performed thoracoscopically (with a video-assisted thoracoscope) or via a limited thoracotomy incision (see Chapter 25).

LUNG VOLUME REDUCTION SURGERY. Treatment options for patients with end-stage COPD (stage IV) with a primary emphysematous component are limited, although lung volume reduction surgery is an option for a selected subset of patients. This subset includes patients with homogenous disease or disease that is focused in one area and not widespread throughout the lungs. Lung volume reduction surgery involves the removal of a portion of the diseased lung parenchyma. This reduces hyperinflation and allows the functional tissue to expand, resulting in improved elastic recoil of the lung and improved chest wall and diaphragmatic mechanics. This type of surgery does not cure the disease or improve life expectancy, but it may decrease dyspnea, improve lung function, and improve the patient's overall quality of life (GOLD, WHO & NHLBI, 2004).

Careful selection of patients for lung volume reduction surgery is essential to decrease morbidity and mortality. The National Emphysema Treatment Trial found that the addition of lung volume reduction surgery to optimal medical management and rehabilitation led to overall improvement in exercise tolerance and survival in a subgroup of patients with predominantly upper lobe disease (National Emphysema Treatment Trial Research Group, 2003).

LUNG TRANSPLANTATION. Lung transplantation is a viable alternative for definitive surgical treatment of end-stage emphysema. It has been shown to improve quality of life and functional capacity in a selected group of patients with COPD (GOLD, WHO & NHLBI, 2004). Single-lung transplantation may be considered for patients with end-stage emphysema who have an FEV_1 less than 25% of the predicted normal and who have complications such as pulmonary hypertension, marked hypoxemia, and hypercapnia. However, surgery does not appear to significantly improve survival (Sutherland & Cherniack, 2004). Specific criteria exist for referral for lung transplantation. Organs are in short supply, and many patients die while waiting for a transplant.

Pulmonary Rehabilitation

Pulmonary rehabilitation for patients with COPD is well established and widely accepted as a means to alleviate symptoms and optimize functional status. The primary goals of rehabilitation are to reduce symptoms, improve quality of life, and increase physical and emotional participation in everyday activities (GOLD, WHO & NHLBI, 2004). Pulmonary rehabilitation services are multidisciplinary and include assessment, education, physical reconditioning, skills training, and psychological support. Patients are taught methods to alleviate symptoms. Breathing exercises as well as retraining and exercise programs are used to improve functional status.

Pulmonary rehabilitation may be used therapeutically in other disorders besides COPD, including asthma, cystic fibrosis, lung cancer, interstitial lung disease, thoracic surgery, and lung transplantation. It may be conducted in inpatient, outpatient, or home settings, and the lengths of programs vary. Patients at all stages of COPD may benefit from pulmonary rehabilitation. The minimum length of an effective program is 2 months, and the longer the program continues, the more effective the results (GOLD, WHO &

NHLBI, 2004). Selection of a program depends on the patient's physical, functional, and psychosocial status; insurance coverage; availability of programs; and preference.

Nursing Management

Nurses play a key role in identifying potential candidates for pulmonary rehabilitation and in facilitating and reinforcing the material learned in the rehabilitation program. Not all patients have access to a formal rehabilitation program. However, nurses can be instrumental in teaching patients and families as well as facilitating specific services, such as respiratory therapy education, physical therapy for exercise and breathing retraining, occupational therapy for conserving energy during activities of daily living, and nutritional counseling.

Numerous educational materials are available to assist nurses in teaching patients with COPD. Potential resources include those of organizations such as the American Lung Association, the American Association of Cardiovascular and Pulmonary Rehabilitation, the American Thoracic Society, the American College of Chest Physicians, and the American Association for Respiratory Therapy.

Patient Education

Patient education is a major component of pulmonary rehabilitation and includes a broad variety of topics. Depending on the length and setting of the educational program, topics may include normal anatomy and physiology of the lung, pathophysiology and changes with COPD, medications and home oxygen therapy, nutrition, respiratory therapy treatments, symptom alleviation, smoking cessation, sexuality and COPD, coping with chronic disease, communicating with the health care team, and planning for the future (advance directives, living wills, informed decision making about health care alternatives).

BREATHING EXERCISES. The breathing pattern of most people with COPD is shallow, rapid, and inefficient; the more severe the disease, the more inefficient the breathing pattern. With practice, this type of upper chest breathing can be changed to diaphragmatic breathing, which reduces the respiratory rate, increases alveolar ventilation, and sometimes helps expel as much air as possible during expiration (see Chapter 25 for technique). Pursed-lip breathing helps slow expiration, prevents collapse of small airways, and helps the patient control the rate and depth of respiration. It also promotes relaxation, enabling the patient to gain control of dyspnea and reduce feelings of panic.

INSPIRATORY MUSCLE TRAINING. Once the patient masters diaphragmatic breathing, a program of inspiratory muscle training may be prescribed to help strengthen the muscles used in breathing. This program involves use of a respiratory training device, which is placed in the mouth. The patient is instructed to inhale against a set resistance for a prescribed amount of time every day. As the resistance is gradually increased, the muscles become better conditioned. To be effective, inspiratory muscle training must be intense, and it is not recommended for all patients with COPD.

ACTIVITY PACING. People with COPD have decreased exercise tolerance during specific periods of the day, especially in the morning on arising, because bronchial secretions have collected in the lungs during the night while the person was lying down. The patient may have difficulty bathing or dressing and may become fatigued. Activities that require the arms to be supported above the level of the thorax may produce fatigue or respiratory distress but may be tolerated better after the patient has been up and moving around for an hour or more. The nurse can help the patient reduce these limitations by planning self-care activities and determining the best times for bathing, dressing, and other daily activities.

SELF-CARE ACTIVITIES. As gas exchange, airway clearance, and the breathing pattern improve, the patient is encouraged to assume increasing participation in self-care activities. The patient is taught to coordinate diaphragmatic breathing with activities such as walking, bathing, bending, or climbing stairs. The patient should bathe, dress, and take short walks, resting as needed to avoid fatigue and excessive dyspnea. Fluids should always be readily available, and the patient should begin to drink fluids without having to be reminded. If secretion management is a problem and some type of postural drainage or airway clearance maneuver is to be performed at home, the nurse or respiratory therapist instructs and supervises the patient before discharge or in an outpatient setting.

PHYSICAL CONDITIONING. People with COPD of all stages benefit from exercise training programs, which result in increased exercise tolerance and decreased dyspnea and fatigue (GOLD, WHO & NHLBI, 2004). Physical conditioning techniques include breathing exercises and general exercises intended to conserve energy and increase pulmonary ventilation. There is a close relationship between physical fitness and respiratory fitness (Covey & Larson, 2004). Graded exercises and physical conditioning programs using treadmills, stationary bicycles, and measured level walks can improve symptoms and increase work capacity and exercise tolerance. Any physical activity that can be performed regularly is helpful. Walking aids may be beneficial (GOLD, WHO & NHLBI, 2004). Lightweight portable oxygen systems are available for ambulatory patients who require oxygen therapy during physical activity.

OXYGEN THERAPY. Oxygen supplied to the home comes in compressed gas, liquid, or concentrator systems. Portable oxygen systems allow the patient to exercise, work, and travel. To help the patient adhere to the oxygen prescription, the nurse explains the proper flow rate and required number of hours for oxygen use as well as the dangers of arbitrary changes in flow rate or duration of therapy (Simmons & Simmons, 2004). The nurse should caution the patient that smoking with or near oxygen is extremely dangerous. The nurse also reassures the patient that oxygen is not "addictive" and explains the need for regular evaluations of blood oxygenation by pulse oximetry or arterial blood gas analysis.

NUTRITIONAL THERAPY. Nutritional assessment and counseling are important aspects in the rehabilitation process for patients with COPD. Weight loss as well as a depletion of muscle mass may be observed in stable patients with COPD, irrespective of the degree of airflow limitation. Weight loss and loss of fat mass are primarily the result of a negative balance between dietary intake and energy expenditure, whereas muscle wasting is a consequence of an impaired balance between protein synthesis and protein breakdown (American Thoracic Society & European Respiratory

Society, 2004). A thorough assessment of caloric needs and counseling about meal planning and supplementation is part of the rehabilitation process. Continual monitoring of weight and interventions as necessary are important parts of the care of patients with COPD.

COPING MEASURES. Any factor that interferes with normal breathing quite naturally induces anxiety, depression, and changes in behavior. Many patients find the slightest exertion exhausting, and fatigue is a major symptom of patients with COPD (Theander & Unosson, 2004). Constant shortness of breath and fatigue may make the patient irritable and apprehensive to the point of panic. Restricted activity (and reversal of family roles due to loss of employment), the frustration of having to work to breathe, and the realization that the disease is prolonged and unrelenting may cause the patient to become angry, depressed, and demanding (Andenaes, Kalfoss & Wahl, 2004). Sexual function may be compromised, which also diminishes self-esteem. The nurse should provide education and support to spouses or significant others and families, because the caregiver role in end-stage COPD can be difficult.

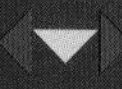

Nursing Process

The Patient With COPD

Assessment

Assessment involves obtaining information about current symptoms as well as previous disease manifestations. Chart 24-3 lists sample questions that may be used to obtain a clear history of the disease process. In addition to the history, nurses review the results of available diagnostic tests.

Diagnosis

Nursing Diagnoses

Based on the assessment data, major nursing diagnoses may include the following:

- Impaired gas exchange and airway clearance due to chronic inhalation of toxins
- Impaired gas exchange related to ventilation–perfusion inequality
- Ineffective airway clearance related to bronchoconstriction, increased mucus production, ineffective cough, bronchopulmonary infection, and other complications
- Ineffective breathing pattern related to shortness of breath, mucus, bronchoconstriction, and airway irritants
- Activity intolerance due to fatigue, ineffective breathing patterns, and hypoxemia
- Deficient knowledge of self-care strategies to be performed at home
- Ineffective coping related to reduced socialization, anxiety, depression, lower activity level, and the inability to work

CHART 24-3

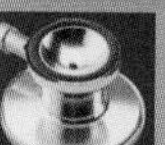

Assessing Patients With Chronic Obstructive Pulmonary Disease

HEALTH HISTORY

- How long has the patient had respiratory difficulty?
- Does exertion increase the dyspnea? What type of exertion?
- What are the limits of the patient's tolerance for exercise?
- At what times during the day does the patient complain most of fatigue and shortness of breath?
- Which eating and sleeping habits have been affected?
- What does the patient know about the disease and his or her condition?
- What is the patient's smoking history (primary and secondary)?
- Is there occupational exposure to smoke or other pollutants?
- What are the triggering events (eg, exertion, strong odors, dust, exposure to animals)?

PHYSICAL ASSESSMENT

- What position does the patient assume during the interview?
- What are the pulse and the respiratory rates?
- What is the character of respirations? Even and without effort? Other?
- Can the patient complete a sentence without having to take a breath?
- Does the patient contract the abdominal muscles during inspiration?
- Does the patient use accessory muscles of the shoulders and neck when breathing?
- Does the patient take a long time to exhale (prolonged expiration)?
- Is central cyanosis evident?
- Are the patient's neck veins engorged?
- Does the patient have peripheral edema?
- Is the patient coughing?
- What is the color, amount, and consistency of the sputum?
- Is clubbing of the fingers present?
- What types of breath sounds (ie, clear, diminished or distant, crackles, wheezes) are heard? Describe and document findings and locations.
- What is the status of the patient's sensorium?
- Is there short-term or long-term memory impairment?
- Is there increasing stupor?
- Is the patient apprehensive?

Collaborative Problems/ Potential Complications

Based on the assessment data, potential complications may include the following:

- Respiratory insufficiency or failure
- Atelectasis
- Pulmonary infection
- Pneumonia
- Pneumothorax
- Pulmonary hypertension

Planning and Goals

Major patient goals may include smoking cessation, improved gas exchange, airway clearance, improved breathing pattern, improved activity tolerance, maximal self-management, improved coping ability, adherence to the therapeutic program and home care, and absence of complications.

Nursing Interventions

Promoting Smoking Cessation

Because smoking has such a detrimental effect on the lungs, the nurse must discuss smoking cessation strategies with the patient. Although the patient may believe that smoking cessation is futile, because it is too late to reverse the damage caused by years of smoking, the nurse should inform the patient that continuing to smoke impairs the mechanisms used to clear the airways and keep them free of irritants. The nurse should educate the patient regarding the hazards of smoking and cessation strategies and provide resources regarding smoking cessation, counseling, and formalized programs available in the community.

Improving Gas Exchange

Bronchospasm, which occurs in many pulmonary diseases, reduces the caliber of the small bronchi and may cause dyspnea, static secretions, and infection. Bronchospasm can sometimes be detected on auscultation with a stethoscope when wheezing or diminished breath sounds are heard. Increased mucus production, along with decreased mucociliary action, contributes to further reduction in the caliber of the bronchi and results in decreased airflow and decreased gas exchange. This is further aggravated by the loss of lung elasticity that occurs with COPD (GOLD, WHO & NHLBI, 2004). These changes in the airway require that the nurse monitor the patient for dyspnea and hypoxemia. If bronchodilators or corticosteroids are prescribed, the nurse must administer the medications properly and be alert for potential side effects. The relief of bronchospasm is confirmed by measuring improvement in expiratory flow rates and volumes (the force of expiration, how long it takes to exhale, and the amount of air exhaled) as well as by assessing the dyspnea and making sure that it has lessened.

Achieving Airway Clearance

Diminishing the quantity and viscosity of sputum can clear the airway and improve pulmonary ventilation and gas exchange. All pulmonary irritants should be eliminated or reduced, particularly cigarette smoking, which is the most persistent source of pulmonary irritation. The nurse instructs the patient in directed or controlled coughing, which is more effective and reduces the fatigue associated with undirected forceful coughing. Directed coughing consists of a slow, maximal inspiration followed by breath-holding for several seconds and then two or three coughs. "Huff" coughing may also be effective. The technique consists of one or two forced exhalations ("huffs") from low to medium lung volumes with the glottis open.

Chest physiotherapy with postural drainage, intermittent positive-pressure breathing, increased fluid intake, and bland aerosol mists (with normal saline solution or water) may be useful for some patients with COPD. The use of these measures must be based on the response and tolerance of the particular patient.

Improving Breathing Patterns

Ineffective breathing patterns and shortness of breath are due to the ineffective respiratory mechanics of the chest wall and lung resulting from **air trapping**, ineffective diaphragmatic movement, airway obstruction, the metabolic cost of breathing, and stress. Inspiratory muscle training and breathing retraining may help improve breathing patterns. Training in diaphragmatic breathing reduces the respiratory rate, increases alveolar ventilation, and sometimes helps expel as much air as possible during expiration. Pursed-lip breathing helps slow expiration, prevent collapse of small airways, and control the rate and depth of respiration. It also promotes relaxation, which allows patients to gain control of dyspnea and reduce feelings of panic.

Improving Activity Tolerance

Patients with COPD experience progressive activity and exercise intolerance and disability. Education is focused on rehabilitative therapies to promote independence in executing activities of daily living. These may include pacing activities throughout the day or using supportive devices to decrease energy expenditure. The nurse evaluates the patient's activity tolerance and limitations and uses teaching strategies to promote independent activities of daily living. The patient may be a candidate for exercise training to strengthen the muscles of the upper and lower extremities and to improve exercise tolerance and endurance. Use of walking aids may be recommended to improve activity levels and ambulation (GOLD, WHO & NHLBI, 2004). Other health care professionals (rehabilitation therapist, occupational therapist, physical therapist) may be consulted as additional resources.

Enhancing Self-Care Strategies

In addition to a pulmonary rehabilitation program, the nurse helps the patient manage self-care by emphasizing the importance of setting realistic goals, avoiding temperature extremes, and modifying lifestyle (particularly stopping smoking) as applicable.

SETTING REALISTIC GOALS

A major area of teaching is the importance of setting and accepting realistic short-term and long-range goals. If the patient is severely disabled, the objectives of treatment are to preserve current pulmonary function and relieve symptoms as much as possible. If the COPD is mild, the objectives are to increase exercise tolerance and prevent further loss of pulmonary function. It is important to plan and share the goals and expectations of treatment with the patient. Both the patient and the care provider need patience to achieve these goals.

AVOIDING TEMPERATURE EXTREMES

The nurse instructs the patient to avoid extremes of heat and cold. Heat increases the body temperature, thereby raising oxygen requirements, and cold tends to promote bronchospasm. Air pollutants such as fumes, smoke, dust, and even talcum, lint, and aerosol sprays may initiate bronchospasm. High altitudes aggravate hypoxemia.

MODIFYING LIFESTYLES

A patient with COPD should adopt a lifestyle of moderate activity, ideally in a climate with minimal shifts in temperature and humidity. The patient should avoid emotional disturbances and stressful situations that might trigger a coughing episode as much as possible. The medication regimen can be quite complex; patients receiving aerosol medications by an MDI or other type of inhaler may be particularly challenged. It is crucial to review educational information and to have the patient demonstrate correct MDI use before discharge, during follow-up visits to a caregiver's office or clinic, and during home visits (Chart 24-4).

Smoking cessation goes hand in hand with lifestyle changes, and reinforcement of the patient's efforts is a key nursing activity. Smoking cessation is the single most important therapeutic intervention for patients with COPD. There are many strategies, including prevention, cessation with or without oral or topical patch medications, and behavior modification techniques.

Enhancing Individual Coping Strategies

COPD and its progression promote a cycle of physical, social, and psychological consequences, all of which are interrelated. The patient experiences depression, altered mood states, social isolation, and altered functional status. The nurse is crucial to identifying this cycle and promoting interventions for improved physical functioning, psychological and emotional stability, and social support. After the initial assessment of the patient, the nurse may provide referrals to health care professionals in these specific areas.

Monitoring and Managing Potential Complications

The nurse must assess for various complications of COPD, such as life-threatening respiratory insufficiency and failure, as well as respiratory infection and atelectasis, which may increase the risk of respiratory failure. The nurse monitors for cognitive changes (personality and behavioral changes, memory impairment), increasing dyspnea, tachypnea, and tachycardia, which may indicate increasing hypoxemia and impending respiratory failure.

The nurse monitors pulse oximetry values to assess the patient's need for oxygen and administers supplemental oxygen as prescribed. The nurse also instructs the patient about signs and symptoms of respiratory infection that may worsen hypoxemia and reports changes in the patient's physical and cognitive status to the physician. The nurse also assists with the management of developing complications, with possible noninvasive positive-pressure ventilation or intubation, and with mechanical ventilation (see Chapter 25).

Bronchopulmonary infections must be controlled to diminish inflammatory edema and to permit recovery of normal ciliary action. Minor respiratory infections that are of no consequence to people with normal lungs can be life-threatening to people with COPD. The cough associated with bronchial infection introduces a vicious cycle with further trauma and damage to the lungs, progression of symptoms, increased bronchospasm, and increased susceptibility to bronchial infection. Infection compromises lung function and is a common cause of respiratory failure in people with COPD.

In COPD, infection may be accompanied by subtle changes. The nurse instructs the patient to report any signs of infection, such as a fever or change in sputum color, character, consistency, or amount. Any worsening of symptoms (increased tightness of the chest, increased dyspnea and fatigue) also suggests infection and must be reported. Viral infections are hazardous to the patient because they are often followed by infections caused by bacterial organisms, such as *Streptococcus pneumoniae* and *Haemophilus influenzae*.

To prevent infection, the nurse should encourage the patient with COPD to be immunized against influenza and *S. pneumoniae,* because the patient is prone to respiratory infection. It is important to caution the patient to avoid going outdoors if the pollen count is high or if there is significant air pollution, because of the risk of bronchospasm. The patient also should avoid exposure to high outdoor temperatures with high humidity.

Pneumothorax is a potential complication of COPD and can be life-threatening in patients with COPD who have minimal pulmonary reserve. Patients with severe emphysematous changes can develop large bullae, which may rupture and cause a pneumo-

CHART 24-4

HOME CARE CHECKLIST • Use of Metered-Dose Inhaler (MDI)

At the completion of the home care instruction, the patient or caregiver will be able to:	Patient	Caregiver
• Describe the rationale for using the MDI to administer inhaled medicine.	✔	✔
• Describe how the medication enters the lungs.	✔	✔
• Demonstrate the correct steps in administering medication with an MDI:		
• Remove the cap and hold the inhaler upright.	✔	
• Shake the inhaler.	✔	
• Tilt your head back slightly and breathe out slowly.	✔	
• Position the inhaler approximately 1–2 inches away from the open mouth, or use a spacer/holding chamber. When using a medicine chamber, place the lips around the mouthpiece.	✔	
• Press down on the inhaler to release the medication as you start to breathe in slowly through the mouth. Continue breathing in as the medication is released (press the cartridge down).	✔	

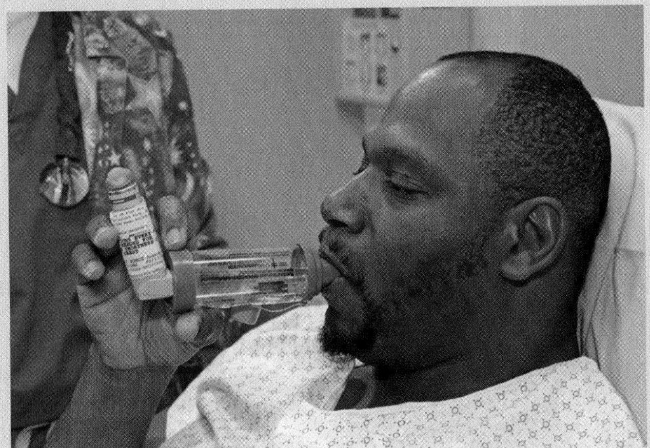

	Patient	Caregiver
• Breathe in slowly and deeply for 3–5 seconds.	✔	
• Hold your breath for 8–10 seconds to allow the medication to reach down into your airways.	✔	
• Repeat puffs as directed, allowing 1–2 minutes between puffs.	✔	
• Apply the cap to the MDI for storage.	✔	
• After inhalation, rinse mouth with water when using a corticosteroid-containing MDI.	✔	
• Describe how to clean the MDI.	✔	✔
• Describe how to assess the amount of medication remaining in the MDI.	✔	✔
• Describe how and when to contact the health care provider for assessment, and how to obtain a refill of the MDI prescription.	✔	✔

Expert Panel Report II. (1997). *Guidelines for the diagnosis and management of asthma*. Bethesda, MD: National Asthma Education and Prevention Program, National Institutes of Health.

thorax. Development of a pneumothorax may be spontaneous or related to an activity such as severe coughing or large intrathoracic pressure changes. If a rapid onset of shortness of breath occurs, the nurse should quickly evaluate the patient for potential pneumothorax by assessing the symmetry of chest movement, differences in breath sounds, and pulse oximetry.

Over time, pulmonary hypertension may occur as a result of chronic hypoxemia. The pulmonary arteries respond to hypoxemia by constricting, which results in pulmonary hypertension. The complication may be prevented by maintaining adequate oxygenation through an adequate hemoglobin level, improved ventilation–perfusion of the lungs, or continuous administration of supplemental oxygen (if needed).

Promoting Home and Community-Based Care

TEACHING PATIENTS SELF-CARE

Teaching is essential throughout the course of COPD and should be part of the nursing care given to all patients with COPD. The knowledge of patients and family members and their comfort level with this knowledge should be assessed and considered when providing instructions about self-management strategies. In addition to the previously described aspects of patient education, patients and family members must become familiar with the medications prescribed and knowledgeable about potential side effects. Patients and family members need to learn the early signs and symptoms of infection and other complications so that they seek appropriate health care promptly.

CONTINUING CARE

Referral for home care is important to enable the nurse to assess the patient's home environment and physical and psychological status, to evaluate the patient's adherence to a prescribed regimen, and to assess the patient's ability to cope with changes in lifestyle and physical status. The nurse assesses the patient's and family's understanding of the complications and side effects of medications. Home care visits provide an opportunity to reinforce the information and activities learned in the inpatient or outpatient pulmonary rehabilitation program and to have the patient and family demonstrate correct administration of medications and oxygen, if indicated, and performance of exercises. If the patient does not have access to a formal pulmonary rehabilitation program, it is important to provide the education and breathing retraining necessary to optimize the patient's functional status.

The nurse may direct the patient to community resources such as pulmonary rehabilitation programs and smoking cessation programs to help improve the patient's ability to cope with his or her chronic condition and the therapeutic regimen and to give the patient a sense of worth, hope, and well-being. In addition, the nurse reminds the patient and family about the importance of participating in general health promotion activities and health screening.

It is important to address quality of life and issues surrounding the end of life in patients with end-stage COPD. Patients with COPD have identified lack of information about diagnosis and the disease process, treatment, prognosis, advance care planning, and the dying process as areas of major concern (Curtis, Wenrich, Carline et al., 2002). Areas identified as being of major importance in palliative care for patients with end-stage COPD include symptom management, psychological and emotional needs, spiritual needs, privacy and dignity, equitable care at the end of life, and safety (Blackler, Mooney & Jones, 2004). It is crucial that patients know what to expect as the disease progresses. In addition, they should have information about their role in decisions regarding aggressiveness of care near the end of life and access to specialists who may help them and their families. As the disease course progresses, a holistic assessment of physical and psychological needs should be undertaken at each hospitalization, clinic visit, or home visit. This helps to gauge the patient's assessment of the progression of the disease and its impact on quality of life and guides planning for future interventions and management.

Evaluation

Expected Patient Outcomes

Expected patient outcomes may include the following:

1. Demonstrates knowledge of hazards of smoking
   a. Verbalizes willingness/interest to quit smoking
   b. Verbalizes information about smoking, risks of continuing, benefits of quitting, and techniques to optimize cessation efforts
2. Demonstrates improved gas exchange
   a. Shows no signs of restlessness, confusion, or agitation
   b. Has stable pulse oximetry or arterial blood gas values (but not necessarily normal values due to chronic changes in the gas exchange ability of the lungs)
3. Achieves maximal airway clearance
   a. Stops smoking
   b. Avoids noxious substances and extremes of temperature
   c. Maintains adequate hydration
   d. If indicated, performs postural drainage correctly
   e. Knows signs of early infection and is aware of how and when to report them if they occur
   f. Performs controlled coughing without experiencing excessive fatigue
4. Improves breathing pattern
   a. Practices and uses pursed-lip and diaphragmatic breathing
   b. Shows signs of decreased respiratory effort (decreased respiratory rate, less dyspnea)
5. Demonstrates knowledge of strategies to improve activity tolerance and maintain maximum level of self-care
   a. Performs self-care activities within tolerance range
   b. Paces self to avoid fatigue and dyspnea
   c. Uses controlled breathing while performing activities
   d. Uses assistive devices to increase activity tolerance and decrease energy expenditure
6. Demonstrates knowledge of self-care strategies
   a. Participates in determining the therapeutic program
   b. Understands the rationale for activities and medications
   c. Follows the medication plan
   d. Uses bronchodilators and oxygen therapy as prescribed
   e. Stops smoking
   f. Maintains acceptable activity level

NURSING RESEARCH PROFILE

Psychological Distress and Quality of Life in Hospitalized Patients With COPD

Andenaes, R., Kalfoss, M. H. & Wahl, A. (2004). Psychological distress and quality of life in hospitalized patients with chronic obstructive pulmonary disease. *Journal of Advanced Nursing, 46*(5), 522–530.

Purpose

The purpose of this study was to describe the influence of psychological distress on health status and self-reported quality of life in hospitalized patients with COPD.

Design

This longitudinal study evaluated a convenience sample of 92 acutely ill hospitalized patients with COPD. Inclusion criteria included diagnosis of COPD, 45 years of age and older with no other chronic disabling diseases, and ability to communicate in the native language (Norwegian). Participants were evaluated after hospitalization and up to 9 months after discharge. Background and demographic information was collected for each participant. Questionnaires were used to assess health status (St. George's Respiratory Questionnaire), psychological distress (Hopkins Symptom Checklist-25), and quality of life (World Health Organization Quality of Life Abbreviated Questionnaire). Correlational coefficient analysis and multiple linear regression were used to assess relationships between disease factors, psychological distress, and quality-of-life variables.

Findings

The majority of the subjects were older (mean age, 69.1 years), lived alone, and had a low educational level. Their physiologic status was poor, with a mean FEV_1% of 38.9%, indicating severe COPD according to the GOLD classification system. There were significant relationships demonstrated between the St. George's Respiratory Questionnaire Total Impact subscores (measure of social functioning and the psychological disturbances resulting from airways disease) with psychological distress (Hopkins Symptom Checklist-25). Physiologic status as measured by pulmonary function tests was moderately associated with perceived quality of life. Psychological distress was significantly associated with quality of life and accounted for 34% of the total 39% variance explained in the regression model.

Nursing Implications

There is a relationship between psychological distress and perceived quality of life, and care of patients with COPD includes planning for interventions related not only to patients' physiologic needs but also their psychological needs. Nursing interventions must focus on helping patients decrease psychological distress to improve perceived quality of life.

7. Uses effective coping mechanisms to deal with consequences of disease
   a. Uses self-care strategies to lessen stress associated with disease
   b. Verbalizes resources available to deal with psychological burden of disease
   c. Participates in pulmonary rehabilitation, if appropriate
8. Uses community resources and home-based care
   a. Verbalizes knowledge of community resources (eg, smoking cessation, hospital/community-based support groups)
   b. Participates in pulmonary rehabilitation, if appropriate
   c. Identifies preferences for care as the disease progresses
9. Avoids or reduces complications
   a. Has no evidence of respiratory failure or insufficiency
   b. Maintains adequate pulse oximetry and arterial blood gas values
   c. Shows no signs or symptoms of infection, pneumothorax, or pulmonary hypertension

For more information, see the plan of nursing care for the patient with COPD given in Chart 24-5.

Bronchiectasis

Bronchiectasis is a chronic, irreversible dilation of the bronchi and bronchioles. Under the new definition of COPD, it is considered a separate disease process from COPD (GOLD, WHO & NHLBI, 2004). Bronchiectasis may be caused by a variety of conditions, including

- Airway obstruction
- Diffuse airway injury
- Pulmonary infections and obstruction of the bronchus or complications of long-term pulmonary infections
- Genetic disorders such as cystic fibrosis
- Abnormal host defense (eg, ciliary dyskinesia or humoral immunodeficiency)
- Idiopathic causes

People may be predisposed to bronchiectasis as a result of recurrent respiratory infections in early childhood, measles, influenza, tuberculosis, or immunodeficiency disorders.

(text continues on page 708)

CHART 24-5

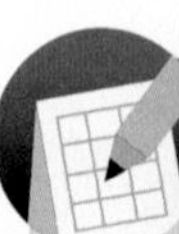

Plan of Nursing Care — Care of the Patient With COPD

Nursing Diagnosis: Impaired gas exchange and airway clearance due to chronic inhalation of toxins
Goal: Improvement in gas exchange

NURSING INTERVENTIONS	RATIONALE	EXPECTED OUTCOMES
1. Evaluate current smoking status, educate regarding smoking cessation, and facilitate efforts to quit. a. Evaluate current smoking habits of patient and family. b. Educate regarding hazards of smoking and relationship to COPD. c. Evaluate previous smoking cessation attempts. d. Provide educational materials. e. Refer to a smoking cessation program or resource.	1. Smoking causes permanent damage to the lung and diminishes the lungs' protective mechanisms. Airflow is obstructed, secretions are increased, and lung capacity is reduced. Continued smoking increases morbidity and mortality in COPD and is also a risk factor for lung cancer.	• Identifies the hazards of cigarette smoking • Identifies resources for smoking cessation • Enrolls in smoking cessation program • Reports success in stopping smoking • Verbalizes types of inhaled toxins • Minimizes or eliminates exposures • Monitors public announcements regarding air quality and minimizes or eliminates exposures during episodes of severe pollution
2. Evaluate current exposure to occupational toxins or pollutants and indoor/outdoor pollution. a. Evaluate current exposures to occupational toxins, indoor and outdoor air pollution (eg, smog, toxic fumes, chemicals). b. Emphasize primary prevention to occupational exposures. This is best achieved by elimination or reduction of exposures in the workplace. c. Educate regarding types of indoor and outdoor air pollution (eg, biomass fuel burned for cooking and heating in poorly ventilated buildings, outdoor air pollution). d. Advise patient to monitor public announcements regarding air quality.	2. Chronic inhalation of both indoor and outdoor toxins causes damage to the airways and impairs gas exchange.	

Nursing Diagnosis: Impaired gas exchange related to ventilation–perfusion inequality
Goal: Improvement in gas exchange

NURSING INTERVENTIONS	RATIONALE	EXPECTED OUTCOMES
1. Administer bronchodilators as prescribed: a. Inhalation is the preferred route.	1. Bronchodilators dilate the airways. The medication dosage is carefully adjusted for each patient, in accordance with clinical response.	• Verbalizes need for bronchodilators and for taking them as prescribed • Evidences minimal side effects; heart rate near normal, absence of dysrhythmias, normal mentation

CHART 24-5

Plan of Nursing Care — Care of the Patient With COPD (Continued)

NURSING INTERVENTIONS	RATIONALE	EXPECTED OUTCOMES
b. Observe for side effects: tachycardia, dysrhythmias, central nervous system excitation, nausea, and vomiting. c. Assess for correct technique of metered-dose inhaler (MDI) or other type of administration.		• Reports a decrease in dyspnea • Shows an improved expiratory flow rate • Uses and cleans respiratory therapy equipment as applicable • Demonstrates diaphragmatic breathing and coughing • Uses oxygen equipment appropriately when indicated • Evidences improved arterial blood gases or pulse oximetry • Demonstrates correct technique for use of MDI
2. Evaluate effectiveness of nebulizer or MDI treatments. a. Assess for decreased shortness of breath, decreased wheezing or crackles, loosened secretions, decreased anxiety. b. Ensure that treatment is given before meals to avoid nausea and to reduce fatigue that accompanies eating.	2. Combining medication with aerosolized bronchodilators is typically used to control bronchoconstriction in an acute exacerbation. Generally, however, the MDI with spacer is the preferred route (less cost and time to treatment).	
3. Instruct and encourage patient in diaphragmatic breathing and effective coughing.	3. These techniques improve ventilation by opening airways to facilitate clearing the airways of sputum. Gas exchange is improved and fatigue is minimized.	
4. Administer oxygen by the method prescribed. a. Explain rationale and importance to patient. b. Evaluate effectiveness; observe for signs of hypoxemia. Notify physician if restlessness, anxiety, somnolence, cyanosis, or tachycardia is present. c. Analyze arterial blood gases and compare with baseline values. When arterial puncture is performed and a blood sample is obtained, hold puncture site for 5 minutes to prevent arterial bleeding and development of ecchymoses. d. Initiate pulse oximetry to monitor oxygen saturation. e. Explain that no smoking is permitted by patient or visitors while oxygen is in use.	4. Oxygen will correct the hypoxemia. Careful observation of the liter flow or the percentage administered and its effect on the patient is important. These patients generally require low-flow oxygen rates of 1 to 2 L/min. Monitor and titrate to achieve desired PaO_2. Periodic arterial blood gases and pulse oximetry help evaluate adequacy of oxygenation. Smoking may render pulse oximetry inaccurate because the carbon monoxide from cigarette smoke also saturates hemoglobin.	

continued >

CHART 24-5

Plan of Nursing Care — Care of the Patient With COPD (Continued)

Nursing Diagnosis: Ineffective airway clearance related to bronchoconstriction, increased mucus production, ineffective cough, bronchopulmonary infection, and other complications
Goal: Achievement of airway clearance

NURSING INTERVENTIONS	RATIONALE	EXPECTED OUTCOMES
1. Adequately hydrate the patient.	1. Systemic hydration keeps secretions moist and easier to expectorate. Fluids must be given with caution if right- or left-sided heart failure is present.	• Verbalizes need to drink fluids • Demonstrates diaphragmatic breathing and coughing • Performs postural drainage correctly • Coughing is minimized • Does not smoke • Verbalizes that pollens, fumes, gases, dusts, and extremes of temperature and humidity are irritants to be avoided • Identifies signs of early infection • Is free of infection (no fever, no change in sputum, lessening of dyspnea) • Verbalizes need to notify health care provider at the earliest sign of infection • Verbalizes need to stay away from crowds or people with colds in flu season • Discusses flu and pneumonia vaccines with clinician to help prevent infection
2. Teach and encourage the use of diaphragmatic breathing and coughing techniques.	2. These techniques help to improve ventilation and mobilize secretions without causing breathlessness and fatigue.	
3. Assist in administering nebulizer or MDI.	3. This ensures adequate delivery of medication to the airways.	
4. If indicated, perform postural drainage with percussion and vibration in the morning and at night as prescribed.	4. Uses gravity to help raise secretions so they can be more easily expectorated or suctioned.	
5. Instruct patient to avoid bronchial irritants such as cigarette smoke, aerosols, extremes of temperature, and fumes.	5. Bronchial irritants cause bronchoconstriction and increased mucus production, which then interfere with airway clearance.	
6. Teach early signs of infection that are to be reported to the clinician immediately: a. Increased sputum production b. Change in color of sputum c. Increased thickness of sputum d. Increased shortness of breath, tightness in chest, or fatigue e. Increased coughing f. Fever or chills	6. Minor respiratory infections that are of no consequence to the person with normal lungs can produce fatal disturbances in the lungs of the person with emphysema. Early recognition is crucial.	
7. Administer antibiotics as prescribed.	7. Antibiotics may be prescribed to prevent or treat infection.	
8. Encourage patient to be immunized against influenza and *Streptococcus pneumoniae*.	8. People with respiratory conditions are prone to respiratory infections and are encouraged to be immunized.	

Nursing Diagnosis: Ineffective breathing pattern related to shortness of breath, mucus, bronchoconstriction, and airway irritants
Goal: Improvement in breathing pattern

NURSING INTERVENTIONS	RATIONALE	EXPECTED OUTCOMES
1. Teach patient diaphragmatic and pursed-lip breathing.	1. Helps patient prolong expiration time and decreases air trapping. With these techniques, patient will breathe more efficiently and effectively.	• Practices pursed-lip and diaphragmatic breathing and uses them when short of breath and with activity

CHART 24-5

Plan of Nursing Care — Care of the Patient With COPD (Continued)

NURSING INTERVENTIONS	RATIONALE	EXPECTED OUTCOMES
2. Encourage alternating activity with rest periods. Allow patient to make some decisions (bath, shaving) about care based on tolerance level.	2. Pacing activities permits patient to perform activities without excessive distress.	• Shows signs of decreased respiratory effort and paces activities • Uses inspiratory muscle trainer as prescribed
3. Encourage use of an inspiratory muscle trainer if prescribed.	3. Strengthens and conditions the respiratory muscles.	

Nursing Diagnosis: Self-care deficits related to fatigue secondary to increased work of breathing and insufficient ventilation and oxygenation
Goal: Independence in self-care activities

NURSING INTERVENTIONS	RATIONALE	EXPECTED OUTCOMES
1. Teach patient to coordinate diaphragmatic breathing with activity (eg, walking, bending).	1. This will allow the patient to be more active and to avoid excessive fatigue or dyspnea during activity.	• Uses controlled breathing while bathing, bending, and walking • Paces activities of daily living to alternate with rest periods to reduce fatigue and dyspnea • Describes energy conservation strategies • Performs same self-care activities as before • Performs postural drainage correctly
2. Encourage patient to begin to bathe self, dress self, walk, and drink fluids. Discuss energy conservation measures.	2. As condition resolves, patient will be able to do more but needs to be encouraged to avoid increasing dependence.	
3. Teach postural drainage if appropriate.	3. Encourages patient to become involved in own care. Prepares patient to manage at home.	

Nursing Diagnosis: Activity intolerance due to fatigue, hypoxemia, and ineffective breathing patterns
Goal: Improvement in activity tolerance

NURSING INTERVENTIONS	RATIONALE	EXPECTED OUTCOMES
1. Support patient in establishing a regular regimen of exercise using treadmill and exercise bicycle, walking, or other appropriate exercises, such as mall walking. a. Assess the patient's current level of functioning and develop exercise plan based on baseline functional status. b. Suggest consultation with a physical therapist or pulmonary rehabilitation program to determine an exercise program specific to the patient's capability. Have portable oxygen unit available if oxygen is prescribed for exercise.	1. Muscles that are deconditioned consume more oxygen and place an additional burden on the lungs. Through regular, graded exercise, these muscle groups become more conditioned, and the patient can do more without getting as short of breath. Graded exercise breaks the cycle of debilitation.	• Performs activities with less shortness of breath • Verbalizes need to exercise daily and demonstrates an exercise plan to be carried out at home • Walks and gradually increases walking time and distance to improve physical condition • Exercises both upper and lower body muscle groups

continued >

CHART 24-5

Plan of Nursing Care — Care of the Patient With COPD (Continued)

Nursing Diagnosis: Ineffective coping related to reduced socialization, anxiety, depression, lower activity level, and the inability to work
Goal: Attainment of an optimal level of coping

NURSING INTERVENTIONS	RATIONALE	EXPECTED OUTCOMES
1. Help the patient develop realistic goals.	1. Developing realistic goals will promote a sense of hope and accomplishment rather than defeat and hopelessness.	• Expresses interest in the future • Participates in the discharge plan • Discusses activities or methods that can be performed to ease shortness of breath • Uses relaxation techniques appropriately • Expresses interest in a pulmonary rehabilitation program
2. Encourage activity to level of symptom tolerance.	2. Activity reduces tension and decreases degree of dyspnea as patient becomes conditioned.	
3. Teach relaxation technique or provide a relaxation tape for patient.	3. Relaxation reduces stress, anxiety, and dyspnea and helps patient to cope with disability.	
4. Enroll patient in pulmonary rehabilitation program where available.	4. Pulmonary rehabilitation programs have been shown to promote a subjective improvement in a patient's status and self-esteem as well as increased exercise tolerance and decreased hospitalizations.	

Nursing Diagnosis: Deficient knowledge about self-management to be performed at home.
Goal: Adherence to therapeutic program and home care

NURSING INTERVENTIONS	RATIONALE	EXPECTED OUTCOMES
1. Help patient identify/develop short- and long-term goals. a. Teach the patient about disease, medications, procedures, and how and when to seek help. b. Refer patient to pulmonary rehabilitation.	1. Patient needs to be a partner in developing the plan of care and needs to know what to expect. Teaching about the condition is one of the most important aspects of care; it will prepare the patient to live and cope with the condition and improve quality of life.	• Understands disease and what affects it • Verbalizes the need to preserve existing lung function by adhering to the prescribed program • Understands purposes and proper administration of medications • Stops smoking or enrolls in a smoking cessation program • Identifies when and whom to call for assistance
2. Give strong message to stop smoking. Discuss smoking cessation strategies. Provide information about resource groups (eg, SmokEnders, American Cancer Society, American Lung Association).	2. Smoking causes permanent damage to the lung and diminishes the lungs' protective mechanisms. Air flow is obstructed and lung capacity is reduced. Smoking increases morbidity and mortality and is also a risk factor for lung cancer.	

CHART 24-5

Plan of Nursing Care — Care of the Patient With COPD (Continued)

Collaborative Problem: Atelectasis
Goal: Absence of atelectasis on x-ray and physical examination

NURSING INTERVENTIONS	RATIONALE	EXPECTED OUTCOMES
1. Monitor respiratory status, including rate and pattern of respirations, breath sounds, signs and symptoms of respiratory distress, and pulse oximetry.	1. A change in respiratory status, including tachypnea, dyspnea, and diminished or absent breath sounds, may indicate atelectasis.	• Normal (baseline for patient) respiratory rate and pattern • Normal breath sounds for patient • Demonstrates diaphragmatic breathing and effective coughing • Performs deep-breathing exercises, incentive spirometry as prescribed • Pulse oximetry is ≥ 90%
2. Instruct in and encourage diaphragmatic breathing and effective coughing techniques.	2. These techniques improve ventilation and lung expansion and ideally improve gas exchange.	
3. Promote use of lung expansion techniques (eg, deep-breathing exercises, incentive spirometry) as prescribed.	3. Deep-breathing exercises and incentive spirometry promote maximal lung expansion.	

Collaborative Problem: Pneumothorax
Goal: Absence of signs and symptoms of pneumothorax

NURSING INTERVENTIONS	RATIONALE	EXPECTED OUTCOMES
1. Monitor respiratory status, including rate and pattern of respirations, symmetry of chest wall movement, breath sounds, signs and symptoms of respiratory distress, and pulse oximetry.	1. Dyspnea, tachypnea, tachycardia, acute pleuritic chest pain, tracheal deviation away from the affected side, absence of breath sounds on the affected side, and decreased tactile fremitus may indicate pneumothorax.	• Normal respiratory rate and pattern for patient • Normal breath sounds bilaterally • Normal pulse for patient • Normal tactile fremitus • Absence of pain • Tracheal position is midline • Pulse oximetry ≥ 90% • Maintains normal oxygen saturation and arterial blood gas measurements for patient • Exhibits no hypoxemia and hypercapnia (or returns to baseline values) • Absence of pain • Symmetric chest wall movement • Lung is reexpanded on chest x-ray • Breath sounds are heard on the affected side
2. Assess pulse.	2. Tachycardia is associated with pneumothorax and anxiety.	
3. Assess for chest pain and precipitating factors.	3. Pain may accompany pneumothorax.	
4. Palpate for tracheal deviation/shift away from the affected side.	4. Early detection of pneumothorax and prompt intervention will prevent other serious complications.	
5. Monitor pulse oximetry and if indicated arterial blood gases.	5. Recognition of a deterioration in respiratory function will prevent serious complications.	
6. Administer supplemental oxygen therapy, as indicated.	6. Oxygen will correct hypoxemia; administer it with caution.	
7. Administer analgesics, as indicated, for chest pain.	7. Pain interferes with deep breathing, resulting in a decrease in lung expansion.	
8. Assist with chest tube insertion and use pleural drainage system, as prescribed.	8. Removal of air from the pleural space will reexpand the lung.	

continued >

CHART 24-5

Plan of Nursing Care — Care of the Patient With COPD (Continued)

Collaborative Problem: Respiratory failure
Goal: Absence of signs and symptoms of respiratory failure; no evidence of respiratory failure on laboratory tests

NURSING INTERVENTIONS	RATIONALE	EXPECTED OUTCOMES
1. Monitor respiratory status, including rate and pattern of respirations, breath sounds, and signs and symptoms of acute respiratory distress.	1. Early recognition of a deterioration in respiratory function will avert further complications, such as respiratory failure, severe hypoxemia, and hypercapnia.	• Normal respiratory rate and pattern for patient with no acute distress • Recognizes symptoms of hypoxemia and hypercapnia • Maintains normal arterial blood gases/pulse oximetry or returns to baseline values
2. Monitor pulse oximetry and arterial blood gases.	2. Recognition of changes in oxygenation and acid–base balance will guide in correcting and preventing complications.	
3. Administer supplemental oxygen and initiate mechanisms for mechanical ventilation, as prescribed.	3. Acute respiratory failure is a medical emergency. Hypoxemia is a hallmark sign. Administration of oxygen therapy and mechanical ventilation (if indicated) are critical to survival.	

Collaborative Problem: Pulmonary arterial hypertension
Goal: Absence of evidence of pulmonary arterial hypertension on physical examination or laboratory tests

NURSING INTERVENTIONS	RATIONALE	EXPECTED OUTCOMES
1. Monitor respiratory status, including rate and pattern of respirations, breath sounds, pulse oximetry, and signs and symptoms of acute respiratory distress.	1. Dyspnea is the primary symptom of pulmonary arterial hypertension. Other symptoms include fatigue, angina, near syncope, edema, and palpitations.	• Normal respiratory rate and pattern for patient • Exhibits no signs and symptoms of right-sided failure • Maintains baseline pulse oximetry values and arterial blood gases
2. Assess for signs and symptoms of right-sided heart failure, including peripheral edema, ascites, distended neck veins, crackles, and heart murmur.	2. Right-sided heart failure is a common clinical manifestation of pulmonary arterial hypertension due to increased right ventricular workload.	
3. Administer oxygen therapy, as prescribed.	3. Continuous oxygen therapy is a major component of management of pulmonary arterial hypertension by preventing hypoxemia and thereby reducing pulmonary vascular constriction (resistance) secondary to hypoxemia.	

Pathophysiology

The inflammatory process associated with pulmonary infections damages the bronchial wall, causing a loss of its supporting structure and resulting in thick sputum that ultimately obstructs the bronchi. The walls become permanently distended and distorted, impairing mucociliary clearance. The inflammation and infection extend to the peribronchial tissues; in the case of saccular bronchiectasis, each dilated tube virtually amounts to a lung abscess, the exudate of which drains freely through the bronchus. Bronchiectasis is usually localized, affecting a segment or lobe of a lung, most frequently the lower lobes.

The retention of secretions and subsequent obstruction ultimately cause the alveoli distal to the obstruction to collapse (atelectasis). Inflammatory scarring or fibrosis replaces functioning lung tissue. In time, the patient develops respiratory insufficiency with reduced vital capacity, decreased ventilation, and an increased ratio of residual volume to total lung capacity. There is impairment in the matching of ventilation to perfusion (ventilation–perfusion imbalance) and hypoxemia.

Clinical Manifestations

Characteristic symptoms of bronchiectasis include chronic cough and the production of purulent sputum in copious amounts. Many patients with this disease have hemoptysis. Clubbing of the fingers also is common because of respiratory insufficiency. Patients usually have repeated episodes of pulmonary infection. Even with modern treatment approaches, the average age at death is approximately 55 years.

Assessment and Diagnostic Findings

Bronchiectasis is not readily diagnosed because the symptoms can be mistaken for those of simple chronic bronchitis. A definite sign is offered by the prolonged history of productive cough, with sputum consistently negative for tubercle bacilli. The diagnosis is established by a CT scan, which demonstrates either the presence or absence of bronchial dilation.

Medical Management

Treatment objectives are to promote bronchial drainage to clear excessive secretions from the affected portion of the lungs and to prevent or control infection. Postural drainage is part of all treatment plans, because draining of the bronchiectatic areas by gravity reduces the amount of secretions and the degree of infection. Sometimes mucopurulent sputum must be removed by bronchoscopy. Chest physiotherapy, including percussion and postural drainage, is important in the management of secretions.

Smoking cessation is important, because smoking impairs bronchial drainage by paralyzing ciliary action, increasing bronchial secretions, and causing inflammation of the mucous membranes, resulting in hyperplasia of the mucous glands. Infection is controlled with antimicrobial therapy based on the results of sensitivity studies on organisms cultured from sputum. A year-round regimen of antibiotic agents may be prescribed, with different types of antibiotics at intervals. Some clinicians prescribe antibiotic agents throughout the winter or when acute upper respiratory tract infections occur. Patients should be vaccinated against influenza and pneumococcal pneumonia. Bronchodilators, which may be prescribed for patients who also have reactive airway disease, may also assist with secretion management.

Surgical intervention, although used infrequently, may be indicated for patients who continue to expectorate large amounts of sputum and have repeated bouts of pneumonia and hemoptysis despite adherence to treatment regimens. The disease must involve only one or two areas of the lung that can be removed without producing respiratory insufficiency. The goals of surgical treatment are to conserve normal pulmonary tissue and to avoid infectious complications. Diseased tissue is removed, provided that postoperative lung function will be adequate. It may be necessary to remove a segment of a lobe (segmental resection), a lobe (lobectomy), or rarely an entire lung (pneumonectomy). (See Chart 25-16 in Chapter 25 for further information.) Segmental resection is the removal of an anatomic subdivision of a pulmonary lobe. The chief advantage is that only diseased tissue is removed, and healthy lung tissue is conserved.

The surgery is preceded by a period of careful preparation. The objective is to obtain a dry (free of infection) tracheobronchial tree to prevent complications (atelectasis, pneumonia, bronchopleural fistula, and empyema). This is accomplished by postural drainage or, depending on the location, by direct suction through a bronchoscope. A course of antibacterial therapy may be prescribed. After surgery, care is the same as for any patient who has undergone chest surgery (see Chapter 25).

Nursing Management

Nursing management of patients with bronchiectasis focuses on alleviating symptoms and helping patients clear pulmonary secretions. Patient teaching targets smoking and other factors that increase the production of mucus and hamper its removal. Patients and families are taught to perform postural drainage and to avoid exposure to people with upper respiratory or other infections. If the patient experiences fatigue and dyspnea, he or she is informed about strategies to conserve energy while maintaining as active a lifestyle as possible. The patient is taught about the early signs of respiratory infection and the progression of the disorder, so that appropriate treatment can be implemented promptly. The presence of a large amount of mucus may decrease the patient's appetite and result in an inadequate dietary intake; therefore, the patient's nutritional status is assessed and strategies are implemented to ensure an adequate diet.

Asthma

Asthma is a chronic inflammatory disease of the airways that causes airway hyperresponsiveness, mucosal edema, and mucus production. This inflammation ultimately leads to recurrent episodes of asthma symptoms: cough, chest tightness, wheezing, and dyspnea (Fig. 24-6). In 2001, there were 11.3 million visits to physicians' offices for treatment of asthma and approximately 4300 deaths attributable to asthma. In 2002, 1.9 million hospital emergency department visits were due to asthma. In that same year, 14 million noninstitutionalized adults and 6.4 million children were diagnosed with asthma in the United States (CDC, 2004).

Asthma differs from other obstructive lung diseases in that it is largely reversible, either spontaneously or with treatment. Patients with asthma may experience symptom-free periods alternating with acute exacerbations that last from minutes to hours or days. Asthma is the most common

Physiology/Pathophysiology

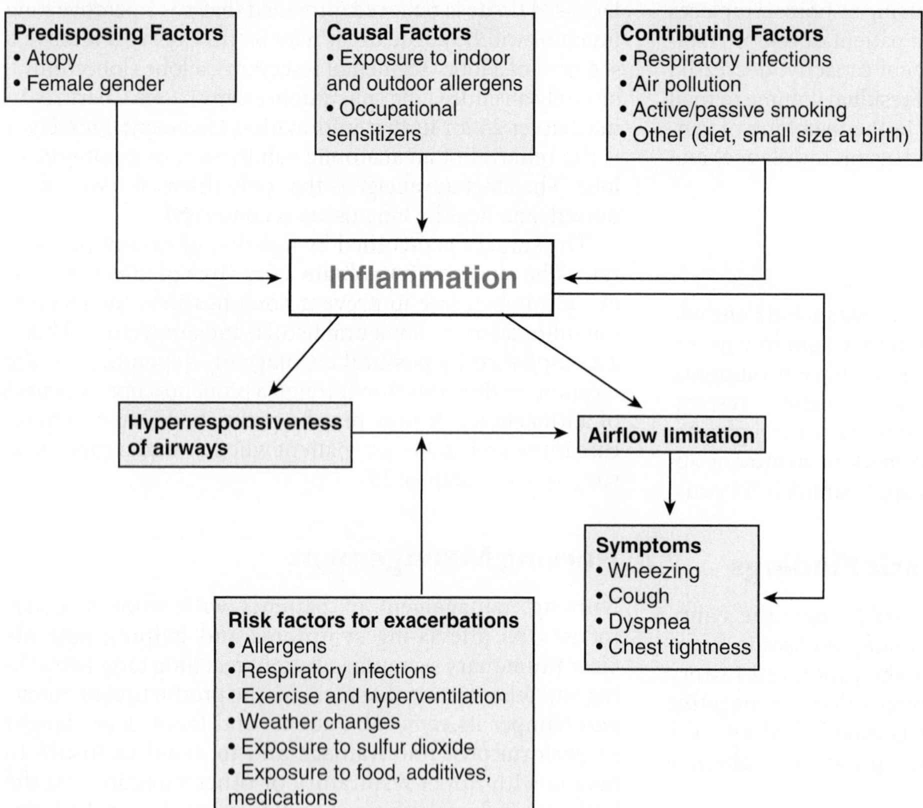

FIGURE 24-6. Pathophysiology of asthma. Adapted from materials developed for the Global Initiative for Asthma (GINA): Global Strategy for Asthma Management and Prevention, National Institutes of Health, National Heart, Lung, and Blood Institute (revised 2003).

chronic disease of childhood and can occur at any age. Despite increased knowledge regarding the pathology of asthma and the development of better medications and management plans, the death rate from this disease continues to increase. For most patients, asthma is a disruptive disease, affecting school and work attendance, occupational choices, physical activity, and general quality of life.

Allergy is the strongest predisposing factor for asthma. Chronic exposure to airway irritants or allergens also increases the risk of asthma. Common allergens can be seasonal (grass, tree, and weed pollens) or perennial (eg, mold, dust, roaches, animal dander). Common triggers for asthma symptoms and exacerbations include airway irritants (eg, air pollutants, cold, heat, weather changes, strong odors or perfumes, smoke), exercise, stress or emotional upset, sinusitis with postnasal drip, medications, viral respiratory tract infections, and gastroesophageal reflux. Most people who have asthma are sensitive to a variety of triggers. A person's asthma changes depending on the environment, activities, management practices, and other factors (American Thoracic Society, 2004).

Pathophysiology

CONCEPTS in action ANIMATION

The underlying pathology in asthma is reversible and diffuse airway inflammation. The inflammation leads to obstruction due to the following factors: (1) swelling of the membranes that line the airways (mucosal edema), which reduces the airway diameter; (2) contraction of the bronchial smooth muscle that encircles the airways (bronchospasm), which causes further narrowing; and (3) increased mucus production, which diminishes airway size and may entirely plug the bronchi.

The bronchial muscles and mucous glands enlarge; thick, tenacious sputum is produced; and the alveoli hyperinflate. Some patients have airway subbasement membrane fibrosis. This is called airway "remodeling" and occurs in response to chronic inflammation. The fibrotic changes in the airway lead to airway narrowing and potentially irreversible airflow limitation (Expert Panel Report, 2003). Cells that play a key role in the inflammation of asthma are mast cells, neutrophils, eosinophils, and lymphocytes. Mast cells, when activated, release several chemicals called mediators. These chemicals, which include histamine, bradykinin, prostaglandins, and leukotrienes, perpetuate the inflammatory response, causing increased blood flow, vasoconstriction, fluid leak from the vasculature, attraction of white blood cells to the area, and bronchoconstriction (Expert Panel Report, 2003). Regulation of these chemicals is the aim of much of the current research regarding pharmacologic therapy for asthma.

In addition, alpha- and beta$_2$-adrenergic receptors of the sympathetic nervous system located in the bronchi play a role. When the alpha-adrenergic receptors are stimulated, bronchoconstriction occurs. When the beta$_2$-adrenergic receptors are stimulated, bronchodilation occurs. The balance between alpha and beta$_2$-adrenergic receptors is controlled primarily by cyclic adenosine monophosphate (cAMP). Alpha-adrenergic receptor stimulation results in a decrease in cAMP, which leads to an increase of chemical mediators released by the mast cells and bronchoconstriction. Beta$_2$-adrenergic stimulation results in increased levels of cAMP, which inhibits the release of chemical mediators and causes bronchodilation.

Clinical Manifestations

The three most common symptoms of asthma are cough, dyspnea, and wheezing. In some instances, cough may be the only symptom. An asthma attack often occurs at night or early in the morning, possibly because of circadian variations that influence airway receptor thresholds.

An asthma exacerbation may begin abruptly but most frequently is preceded by increasing symptoms over the previous few days. There is cough, with or without mucus production. At times the mucus is so tightly wedged in the narrowed airway that the patient cannot cough it up. There may be generalized wheezing (the sound of airflow through narrowed airways), first on expiration and then possibly during inspiration as well. Generalized chest tightness and dyspnea occur. Expiration requires effort and becomes prolonged. As the exacerbation progresses, diaphoresis, tachycardia, and a widened pulse pressure may occur along with hypoxemia and central cyanosis (a late sign of poor oxygenation). Although life-threatening and severe hypoxemia can occur in asthma, it is relatively uncommon. The hypoxemia is secondary to a ventilation–perfusion mismatch and readily responds to supplemental oxygenation.

Symptoms of exercise-induced asthma include maximal symptoms during exercise, absence of nocturnal symptoms, and sometimes only a description of a "choking" sensation during exercise.

Asthma is categorized according to symptoms and objective measures of airflow obstruction (Table 24-3) (Expert Panel Report, 2003).

Assessment and Diagnostic Findings

A complete family, environmental, and occupational history is essential. To establish the diagnosis, the clinician must determine that periodic symptoms of airflow obstruction are present, airflow is at least partially reversible, and other causes have been excluded. A positive family history and environmental factors, including seasonal changes, high pollen counts, mold, pet dander, climate changes (particularly cold air), and air pollution, are primarily associated with asthma. In addition, asthma is associated with a variety of occupation-related chemicals and compounds, including metal salts, wood and vegetable dust, medications (eg, aspirin, antibiotics, piperazine, cimetidine), industrial chemicals and plastics, biologic enzymes (eg, laundry detergents), animal and insect dusts, sera, and secretions. Comorbid conditions that may accompany asthma include gastroesophageal reflux, drug-induced asthma, and allergic bronchopulmonary aspergillosis. Other possible allergic reactions that may accompany asthma include eczema, rashes, and temporary edema.

During acute episodes, sputum and blood tests may disclose eosinophilia (elevated levels of eosinophils). Serum levels of immunoglobulin E may be elevated if allergy is present. Arterial blood gas analysis and pulse oximetry reveal hypoxemia during acute attacks. Initially, hypocapnia and respiratory alkalosis are present. As the patient's condition worsens and he or she becomes more fatigued, the $PaCO_2$ may increase. A normal $PaCO_2$ value may be a signal of impending respiratory failure. Because carbon dioxide is 20 times more diffusible than oxygen, it is rare for $PaCO_2$ to be normal or elevated in a person who is breathing very rapidly. During an exacerbation, the FEV_1 and FVC are markedly decreased but improve with bronchodilator administration (demonstrating reversibility). Pulmonary function is usually normal between exacerbations.

The occurrence of a severe, continuous reaction is referred to as status asthmaticus and is considered life-threatening (see later discussion).

Prevention

Patients with recurrent asthma should undergo tests to identify the substances that precipitate the symptoms. Possible causes are dust, dust mites, roaches, certain types of cloth, pets, horses, detergents, soaps, certain foods, molds, and pollens. If the attacks are seasonal, pollens can be strongly suspected. Patients are instructed to avoid the causative agents whenever possible. Knowledge is the key to quality asthma care. National guidelines are available for the care of patients with asthma. Unfortunately, not all health care providers follow them.

Complications

Complications of asthma may include status asthmaticus, respiratory failure, pneumonia, and atelectasis. Airway obstruction, particularly during acute asthmatic episodes, often results in hypoxemia, requiring the administration of oxygen and the monitoring of pulse oximetry and arterial blood gases. Fluids are administered, because people with asthma are frequently dehydrated from diaphoresis and insensible fluid loss with hyperventilation.

Medical Management

Immediate intervention is necessary, because the continuing and progressive dyspnea leads to increased anxiety, aggravating the situation.

Pharmacologic Therapy

There are two general classes of asthma medications: quick-relief medications for immediate treatment of asthma symptoms and exacerbations (see Table 24-2) and long-acting medications to achieve and maintain control of persistent asthma (Table 24-4). Because the underlying pathology of asthma is inflammation, control of persistent asthma is accomplished primarily with regular use of anti-inflammatory medications. These medications have systemic side effects

TABLE 24-3 Stepwise Approach for Managing Asthma in Adults and Children Older Than 5 Years of Age: Treatment

Classify Severity: Clinical Features Before Treatment or Adequate Control	Symptoms/Day / Symptoms/Night	PEF or FEV_1 / PEF Variability	Medications Required To Maintain Long-Term Control: Daily Medications
Step 4 *Severe Persistent*	Continual / Frequent	≤60% / >30%	• Preferred treatment: – High-dose inhaled corticosteroids AND – Long-acting inhaled $beta_2$-agonists AND, if needed, – Corticosteroid tablets or syrup long term (2 mg/kg/day, generally do not exceed 60 mg per day). (Make repeat attempts to reduce systemic corticosteroids and maintain control with high-dose inhaled corticosteroids.)
Step 3 *Moderate Persistent*	Daily / >1 night/week	>60% – <80% / >30%	• Preferred treatment: – Low-to-medium dose inhaled corticosteroids and long-acting inhaled $beta_2$-agonists. • Alternative treatment (listed alphabetically): – Increase inhaled corticosteroids within medium-dose range OR – Low-to-medium dose inhaled corticosteroids and either leukotriene modifier or theophylline. If needed (particularly in patients with recurring severe exacerbations): • Preferred treatment: – Increase inhaled corticosteroids within medium-dose range and add long-acting inhaled $beta_2$-agonists. • Alternative treatment (listed alphabetically): – Increase inhaled corticosteroids within medium-dose range and add either leukotriene modifier or theophylline.
Step 2 *Mild Persistent*	>2 weeks but < 1x/day / >2 nights/month	≥80% / 20–30%	• Preferred treatment: – Low-dose inhaled corticosteroids. • Alternative treatment: (listed alphabetically): cromolyn, leukotriene modifier, nedocromil, OR sustained-release theophylline to serum concentration of 5–15 mcg/mL.
Step 1 *Mild Intermittent*	≤2 days/week / ≤2 nights/month	≥80% / < 20%	• No daily medication needed • Severe exacerbations may occur, separated by long periods of normal lung function and no symptoms. A course of systemic corticosteroids is recommended.
Quick Relief *All Patients*	• Short-acting bronchodilator: 2–4 puffs short-acting inhaled $beta_2$-agonists as needed for symptoms. • Intensity of treatment will depend on severity of exacerbation; up to 3 treatments at 20-minute intervals or a single nebulizer treatment as needed. Course of systemic corticosteroids may be needed. • Use of short-acting $beta_2$-agonists >2 times a week in intermittent asthma (daily, or increasing use in persistent asthma) may indicate the need to initiate (increase) long-term-control therapy.		

↓ Step down

Review treatment every 1 to 6 months: a gradual stepwise reduction in treatment may be possible.

↑ Step up

If control is not maintained, consider step up. First, review patient medication technique, adherence, and environmental control.

Goals of Therapy: Asthma Control

- Minimal or no chronic symptoms day or night
- Minimal or no exacerbations
- No limitations on activities; no school/work missed
- Maintain (near) normal pulmonary function
- Minimal use of short-acting inhaled $beta_2$-agonist
- Minimal or no adverse effects from medications

Note

- The stepwise approach is meant to assist, not replace, the clinical decision-making required to meet individual patient needs.
- Classify severity: assign patient to most severe step in which any feature occurs (PEF is % of personal best; FEV_1 is % predicted).
- Gain control as quickly as possible (consider a short course of systemic corticosteroids); then step down to the least medication necessary to maintain control.
- Minimize use of short-acting inhaled $beta_2$-agonists. Overreliance on short-acting inhaled $beta_2$-agonists (e.g., use of approximately one canister a month even if not using it every day) indicates inadequate control of asthma and the need to initiate or intensify long-term-control therapy.
- Provide education on self-management and controlling environmental factors that make asthma worse (e.g., allergens and irritants).
- Refer to an asthma specialist if there are difficulties controlling asthma or if step 4 care is required. Referral may be considered if step 3 care is required.

From Expert Panel Report (2003). *Guidelines for the diagnosis and management of asthma: Update on selected topics 2002.* NIH Publication No 02-5074. Bethesda, MD: National Institutes of Health, National Heart, Lung and Blood Institute.

TABLE 24-4 Usual Dosages for Long-Term Asthma Control Medications

Medication	Dosage Form	Adult Dose
Inhaled Corticosteroids *(See Guidelines for the diagnosis and management of asthma: update on selected topics, 2002, for comparative daily dosages for inhaled corticosteroids.)*		
Systemic Corticosteroids *(Applies to all three corticosteroids.)*		
Methylprednisolone	2, 4, 8, 16, 32 mg tablets	• 7.5–60 mg daily in a single dose in a.m. or qod as needed for control • Short-course "burst" to achieve control: 40–60 mg per day as single or 2 divided doses for 3–10 days
Prednisolone	5 mg tablets, 5 mg/5 mL, 15 mg/5 mL	
Prednisone	1, 2.5, 5, 10, 20, 50 mg tablets; 5 mg/mL, 5 mg/5 mL	
Long-Acting Inhaled Beta$_2$-Agonists *(Should not be used for symptom relief or for exacerbations. Use with inhaled corticosteroids.)*		
Salmeterol	MDI 21 mcg/puff DPI 50 mcg/blister	2 puffs q12h 1 blister q12h
Formoterol	DPI 12 mcg/single-use capsule	1 capsule q12h
Combined Medication		
Fluticasone/Salmeterol	DPI 100, 250, or 500 mcg/50 mcg	1 inhalation bid; dose depends on severity of asthma
Cromolyn and Nedocromil		
Cromolyn	MDI 1 mg/puff Nebulizer 20 mg/ampule	2–4 puffs tid–qid 1 ampule tid–qid
Nedocromil	MDI 1.75 mg/puff	2–4 puffs tid–qid
Leukotriene Modifiers		
Montelukast	5 mg chewable tablet 10 mg tablet	10 mg qhs
Zafirlukast	10 or 20 mg tablet	40 mg daily (20 mg tablet bid)
Zileuton	300 or 600 mg tablet	2,400 mg daily (give tablets qid)
Methylxanthines *(Serum monitoring is important, serum concentration of 5–15 mcg/mL at steady state)*		
Theophylline	Liquids, sustained-release tablets, and capsules	Starting dose 10 mg/kg/day up to 300 mg max; usual max 800 mg/day

DPI, dry powder inhaler; MDI, metered-dose inhaler.

Expert Panel Report (2003). *Guidelines for the diagnosis and management of asthma: Update on selected topics 2002.* NIH Publication No 02-5074. Bethesda, MD: National Institutes of Health, National Heart, Lung and Blood Institute.

when used over the long term. The route of choice for administration of these medications is an MDI or other type of inhaler, because it allows for topical administration. Critical to the success of inhaled therapy is the proper use of the MDI (see Chart 24-4). If patients have difficulty with this procedure, a spacer device may be used. Management of asthma involves a stepwise approach (see Table 24-3) (Expert Panel Report, 2003).

LONG-ACTING CONTROL MEDICATIONS. Corticosteroids are the most potent and effective anti-inflammatory medications currently available. They are broadly effective in alleviating symptoms, improving airway function, and decreasing peak flow variability. Initially, an inhaled form is used. A spacer should be used with inhaled corticosteroids, and the patient should rinse his or her mouth after administration to prevent thrush, a common complication associated with use of inhaled corticosteroids. A systemic preparation may be used to gain rapid control of the disease; to manage severe, persistent asthma; to treat moderate to severe exacerbations; to accelerate recovery; and to prevent recurrence. Cromolyn sodium (Intal) and nedocromil (Tilade) are mild to moderate anti-inflammatory agents that are used more commonly in children. They also are effective on a prophylactic basis to prevent exercise-induced asthma or in unavoidable exposure to known triggers. These medications are contraindicated in acute asthma exacerbations.

Long-acting beta$_2$-adrenergic agonists are used with anti-inflammatory medications to control asthma symptoms, particularly those that occur during the night. These agents are also effective in the prevention of exercise-induced asthma. Long-acting beta$_2$-adrenergic agonists are not indicated for immediate relief of symptoms. Theophylline (Slo-bid, Theo-24, Theo-Dur) is a mild to moderate bronchodilator that is usually used in addition to inhaled corticosteroids, mainly for relief of nighttime asthma symptoms.

Leukotriene modifiers (inhibitors), or antileukotrienes, are a new class of medications that include montelukast (Singulair), zafirlukast (Accolate), and zileuton (Zyflo). Leukotrienes, which are synthesized from membrane phospholipids through a cascade of enzymes, are potent bronchoconstrictors that also dilate blood vessels and alter permeability. Leukotriene inhibitors act either by interfering with leukotriene synthesis or by blocking the receptors where leukotrienes exert their action. They may provide an alternative to inhaled corticosteroids for mild persistent asthma, or they may be added to a regimen of inhaled corticosteroids in more severe asthma to attain further control.

QUICK-RELIEF MEDICATIONS. Short-acting beta$_2$-adrenergic agonists are the medications of choice for relief of acute symptoms and prevention of exercise-induced asthma (see Table 24-2). They have a rapid onset of action. Anticholinergics (eg, ipratropium bromide [Atrovent]) may have an added benefit in severe exacerbations of asthma, but they are used more frequently in COPD.

Management of Exacerbations

Asthma exacerbations are best managed by early treatment and education, including the use of written action plans as part of any overall effort to educate patients about self-management techniques, especially those with moderate or severe persistent asthma and those with a history of severe exacerbations (Expert Panel Report, 2003). Quick-acting beta$_2$-adrenergic agonist medications are first used for prompt relief of airflow obstruction. Systemic corticosteroids may be necessary to decrease airway inflammation in patients who fail to respond to inhaled beta-adrenergic medications. In some patients, oxygen supplementation may be required to relieve hypoxemia associated with moderate to severe exacerbations (Expert Panel Report, 2003). In addition, response to treatment may be monitored by serial measurements of lung function.

Evidence from clinical trials suggests that antibiotic therapy, whether administered routinely or when suspicion of bacterial infection is low, is not beneficial for asthma exacerbations (Expert Panel Report, 2003). Antibiotics may be appropriate in the treatment of acute asthma exacerbations in patients with comorbid conditions (eg, fever and purulent sputum, evidence of pneumonia, suspected bacterial sinusitis).

Despite insufficient data supporting or refuting the benefits of using a written asthma action plan as compared to medical management alone, the 2003 Expert Panel Report continues to recommend the use of a written plan to educate patients about self-management (Fig. 24-7). Such a plan gives patients self-management strategies to combat exacerbations and provides instructions about early warning signs of worsening asthma. Patient self-management and early recognition of problems lead to more efficient communication with health care providers about asthma exacerbations (Expert Panel Report, 2003).

Peak Flow Monitoring

Peak flow meters measure the highest airflow during a forced expiration (Fig. 24-8). Daily peak flow monitoring is recommended for all patients with moderate or severe asthma, because it helps measure asthma severity and, when added to symptom monitoring, indicates the current degree of asthma control. The patient is instructed in the proper technique (Chart 24-6), particularly about giving maximal effort, and peak flows are monitored for 2 or 3 weeks after receipt of optimal asthma therapy. Then the patient's "personal best" value is measured. The green (80% to 100% of personal best), yellow (60% to 80%), and red (less than 60%) zones are determined, and specific actions are delineated for each zone, enabling the patient to monitor and manipulate his or her own therapy after careful instruction (Expert Panel Report, 1997).

The 2003 Expert Panel Report recommends that peak flow monitoring should be considered as an adjunct to asthma management for patients with moderate to severe persistent asthma. Peak flow monitoring plans may enhance communication between the patient and health care providers and may increase the patient's awareness of disease status and control (Expert Panel Report, 2003).

Nursing Management

The immediate nursing care of patients with asthma depends on the severity of symptoms. The patient may be treated successfully as an outpatient if asthma symptoms are relatively mild or may require hospitalization and intensive care if symptoms are acute and severe. The patient and family are often frightened and anxious because of the patient's dyspnea. Therefore, a calm approach is an important aspect of care. The nurse assesses the patient's respiratory status by monitoring the severity of symptoms, breath sounds, peak flow, pulse oximetry, and vital signs.

The nurse generally performs the following tasks:

- Obtains a history of allergic reactions to medications before administering medications.
- Identifies medications the patient is currently taking.
- Administers medications as prescribed and monitors the patient's responses to those medications. An antibiotic may be prescribed if the patient has an underlying respiratory infection.
- Administers fluids if the patient is dehydrated.

If the patient requires intubation because of acute respiratory failure, the nurse assists with the intubation procedure, continues close monitoring of the patient, and keeps the patient and family informed about procedures.

Promoting Home and Community-Based Care

TEACHING PATIENTS SELF-CARE. A major challenge is to implement basic asthma management principles at the community level. Key issues include education of health care providers, establishment of programs for asthma education (for patients and providers), use of outpatient follow-up care for patients, and a focus on chronic management versus acute episodic care. Nurses are pivotal to achievement of these objectives.

Patient teaching is a critical component of care for patients with asthma. Multiple inhalers, different types of inhalers, antiallergy therapy, antireflux medications, and avoidance measures are essential for long-term control. This complex therapy requires a partnership between the patient and the health care providers to determine the desired outcomes and to formulate a plan to achieve those outcomes. The patient then carries out daily therapy as part of self-care management, with input and guidance by his or her health care providers. Before a partnership can be established, the patient must understand the following:

- The nature of asthma as a chronic inflammatory disease
- The definition of inflammation and bronchoconstriction
- The purpose and action of each medication
- Triggers to avoid, and how to do so
- Proper inhalation technique
- How to perform peak flow monitoring (see Chart 24-6)

ASTHMA ACTION PLAN FOR ____________________ Doctor's Name ____________________ Date __________

Doctor's Phone Number ____________________ Hospital/Emergency Room Phone Number ____________________

GREEN ZONE: Doing Well

- No cough, wheeze, chest tightness, or shortness of breath during the day or night
- Can do usual activities

And, if a peak flow meter is used,
Peak flow: more than __________
(80% or more of my best peak flow)

My best peak flow is: __________

Take These Long-Term-Control Medicines Each Day (include an anti-inflammatory)

Medicine	How much to take	When to take it

Before exercise ❑ __________ ❑ 2 or ❑ 4 puffs 5 to 60 minutes before exercise

YELLOW ZONE: Asthma Is Getting Worse

- Cough, wheeze, chest tightness, or shortness of breath, or
- Waking at night due to asthma, or
- Can do some, but not all, usual activities

-Or-

Peak flow: ______ to ______
(50% - 80% of my best peak flow)

FIRST → **Add: Quick-Relief Medicine - and keep taking your GREEN ZONE medicine**

__________ (short-acting beta$_2$-agonist) ❑ 2 or ❑ 4 puffs, every 20 minutes for up to 1 hour
❑ Nebulizer, once

SECOND → **If your symptoms (and peak flow, if used) *return to GREEN ZONE* after 1 hour of above treatment:**

❑ Take the quick-relief medicine every 4 hours for 1 to 2 days.
❑ Double the dose of your inhaled steroid for __________ (7-10) days.

-Or-

If your symptoms (and peak flow, if used) *do not return to GREEN ZONE* after 1 hour of above treatment:

❑ Take: __________ (short-acting beta$_2$-agonist) ❑ 2 or ❑ 4 puffs or ❑ Nebulizer
❑ Add: __________ (oral steroid) mg. per day For ______ (3-10) days
❑ Call the doctor ❑ before/ ❑ within __________ hours after taking the oral steroid.

RED ZONE: Medical Alert!

- Very short of breath, or
- Quick-relief medicines have not helped, or
- Cannot do usual activities, or
- Symptoms are same or get worse after 24 hours in Yellow Zone

-Or-

Peak flow: less than ______
(50% of my best peak flow)

Take this medicine:

❑ __________ (short-acting beta$_2$-agonist) ❑ 4 or ❑ 6 puffs or ❑ Nebulizer
❑ __________ (oral steroid) __________ mg.

Then call your doctor *NOW*. Go to the hospital or call for an ambulance if:

- You are still in the red zone after 15 minutes AND
- You have not reached your doctor.

DANGER SIGNS

- **Trouble walking and talking due to shortness of breath**
- **Lips or fingernails are blue**

→

- **Take ❑ 4 or ❑ 6 puffs of your quick-relief medicine *AND***
- **Go to the hospital or call for an ambulance (__________) *NOW!***

FIGURE 24-7. Asthma action plan. From *Facts about controlling asthma,* National Asthma Education and Prevention Program, National Heart, Lung, and Blood Institute. NIH Publication No. 97-2339. Bethesda, MD: National Institutes of Health.

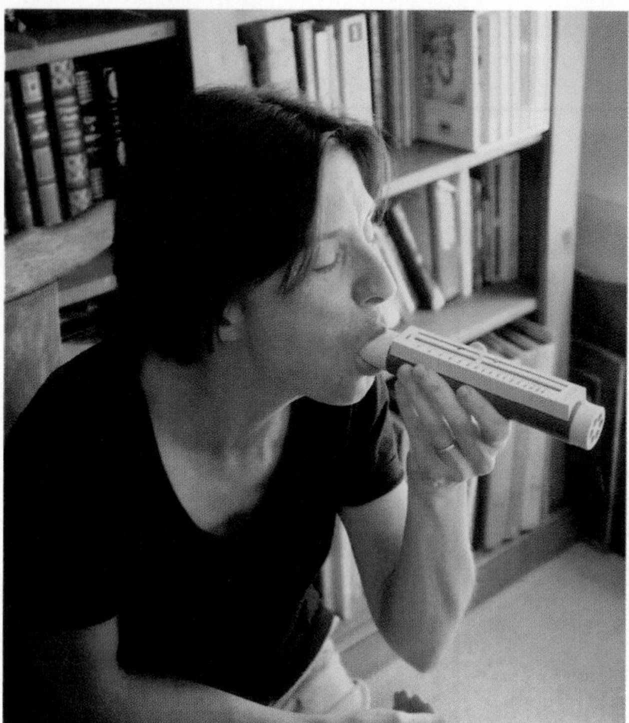

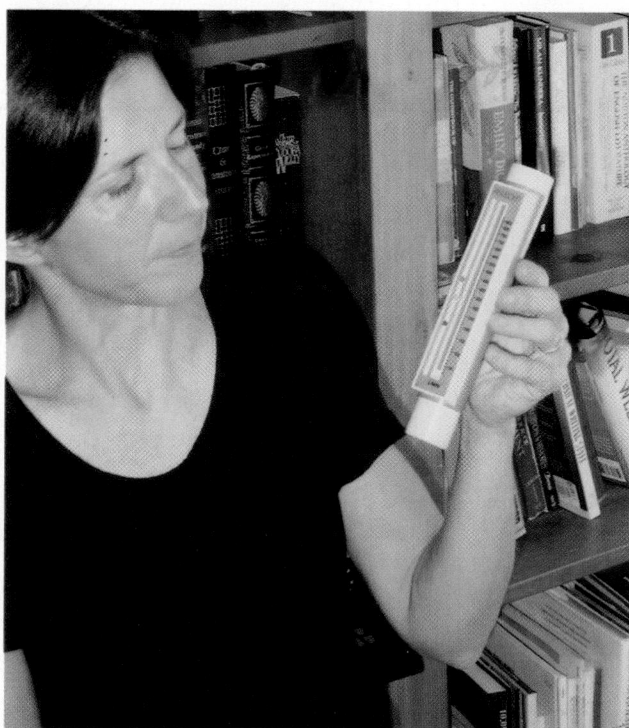

FIGURE 24-8. Peak flow meters measure the highest volume of air flow during a forced expiration (*left*). Volume is measured in color-coded zones (*right*): the green zone signifies 80% to 100% of personal best; yellow, 60% to 80%; and red, less than 60%. If peak flow falls below the red zone, the patient should take the appropriate actions prescribed by his or her health care provider.

CHART 24-6

HOME CARE CHECKLIST • Use of Peak Flow Meter

At the completion of the home care instruction, the patient or caregiver will be able to:	Patient	Caregiver
• Describe the rationale for using a peak flow meter in asthma management.	✔	✔
• Explain how peak flow monitoring is used along with symptoms to determine severity of asthma.	✔	✔
• Demonstrate steps for using the peak flow meter correctly:	✔	
• Move the indicator to the bottom of the numbered scale.	✔	
• Stand up.	✔	
• Take a deep breath and fill the lungs completely.	✔	
• Place mouthpiece in mouth and close lips around mouthpiece (do not put tongue inside opening).	✔	
• Blow out hard and fast with a single blow.	✔	
• Record the number achieved on the indicator.	✔	
• Repeat steps 1–5 two more times and write the highest number in the asthma diary.	✔	
• Explain how to determine the “personal best” peak flow reading.	✔	✔
• Describe the significance of the color zones for peak flow monitoring.	✔	✔
• Demonstrate how to clean the peak flow meter.	✔	✔
• Discuss how and when to contact the health care provider about changes or decreases in peak flow values.	✔	✔

- How to implement an action plan
- When to seek assistance, and how to do so

An assortment of excellent educational materials is available from the NHLBI and other sources. The nurse should obtain current educational materials for the patient based on the patient's diagnosis, causative factors, educational level, and cultural background. If a patient has a coexisting sensory impairment (ie, vision loss or hearing impairment), materials should be provided in an alternative format.

CONTINUING CARE. Nurses who have contact with patients in the hospital, clinic, school, or office use the opportunity to assess the patient's respiratory status and ability to manage self-care to prevent serious exacerbations. Nurses emphasize adherence to the prescribed therapy, preventive measures, and the need to keep follow-up appointments with health care providers. Home visits to assess the home environment for allergens may be indicated for patients with recurrent exacerbations. Nurses refer patients to community support groups. In addition, nurses remind patients and families about the importance of health promotion strategies and recommended health screening.

Status Asthmaticus

Status asthmaticus is severe and persistent asthma that does not respond to conventional therapy. The attacks can occur with little or no warning and can progress rapidly to asphyxiation. Infection, anxiety, nebulizer abuse, dehydration, increased adrenergic blockage, and nonspecific irritants may contribute to these episodes. An acute episode may be precipitated by hypersensitivity to aspirin.

Pathophysiology

The basic characteristics of asthma (inflammation of bronchial mucosa, constriction of the bronchiolar smooth muscle, and thickened secretions) decrease the diameter of the bronchi and occur in status asthmaticus. The most common scenario is severe bronchospasm, with mucus plugging leading to asphyxia. A ventilation–perfusion abnormality results in hypoxemia and respiratory alkalosis initially, followed by respiratory acidosis. There is a reduced PaO_2 and initial respiratory alkalosis, with a decreased $PaCO_2$ and an increased pH. As status asthmaticus worsens, the $PaCO_2$ increases and the pH decreases, reflecting respiratory acidosis.

Clinical Manifestations

The clinical manifestations are the same as those seen in severe asthma; signs and symptoms include labored breathing, prolonged exhalation, engorged neck veins, and wheezing. However, the extent of wheezing does not indicate the severity of the attack. As the obstruction worsens, the wheezing may disappear; this is frequently a sign of impending respiratory failure.

Assessment and Diagnostic Findings

Pulmonary function studies are the most accurate means of assessing acute airway obstruction. Arterial blood gas measurements are obtained if the patient cannot perform pulmonary function maneuvers because of severe obstruction or fatigue, or if the patient does not respond to treatment. Respiratory alkalosis (low $PaCO_2$) is the most common finding in patients with asthma. An increasing $PaCO_2$ (to normal levels or levels indicating respiratory acidosis) frequently is a danger sign indicating impending respiratory failure.

Medical Management

Close monitoring of the patient and objective reevaluation for response to therapy are key in status asthmaticus. In the emergency setting, the patient is treated initially with a short-acting beta$_2$-adrenergic agonist and subsequently a short course of systemic corticosteroids, especially if the patient does not respond to the short-acting beta$_2$-adrenergic agonist. Corticosteroids are critical in the therapy of status asthmaticus and are used to decrease the intense airway inflammation and swelling. Short-acting inhaled beta$_2$-adrenergic agonists provide the most rapid relief from bronchospasm. An MDI with or without a spacer may be used for nebulization of the drugs. The patient usually requires supplemental oxygen and IV fluids for hydration. Oxygen therapy is initiated to treat dyspnea, central cyanosis, and hypoxemia. High-flow supplemental oxygen is best delivered using a partial or complete non-rebreather mask with the objective of maintaining the PaO_2 at a minimum of 92 mm Hg or O_2 saturation greater than 95% (Higgins, 2003). Sedative medications are contraindicated. Magnesium sulfate, a calcium antagonist, may be administered to induce smooth muscle relaxation. In trials, magnesium sulfate has improved symptoms of patients with severe asthma who did not respond to other treatments. Magnesium may be beneficial in patients who are prone to hypomagnesemia because of prolonged use of inhaled beta$_2$-adrenergic agonists (Higgins, 2003). In addition, magnesium can relax smooth muscle and hence cause bronchodilation by competing with calcium at calcium-mediated smooth muscle binding sites. Adverse effects of magnesium sulfate may include facial warmth, flushing, tingling, nausea, central nervous system depression, respiratory depression, and hypotension.

If there is no response to repeated treatments, hospitalization is required. Other criteria for hospitalization include poor pulmonary function test results and deteriorating blood gas levels (respiratory acidosis), which may indicate that the patient is tiring and will require mechanical ventilation. Most patients do not need mechanical ventilation, but it is used for patients in respiratory failure, for those who tire and are too fatigued by the attempt to breathe, and for those whose conditions do not respond to initial treatment.

Death from asthma is associated with several risk factors, including the following (Expert Panel Report, 1997):

- Past history of sudden and severe exacerbations
- Prior endotracheal intubation for asthma
- Prior admission to the intensive care unit for an asthma exacerbation
- Two or more hospitalizations for asthma within the past year
- Three or more emergency care visits for asthma in the past year
- Excessive use of short-acting beta-adrenergic inhalers (more than two canisters per month)

- Recent withdrawal from systemic corticosteroids
- Comorbidity of cardiovascular disease or COPD
- Psychiatric disease
- Low socioeconomic status
- Urban residence

Nursing Management

The main focus of nursing management is to actively assess the airway and the patient's response to treatment. The nurse should be prepared for the next intervention if the patient does not respond to treatment.

The nurse constantly monitors the patient for the first 12 to 24 hours, or until status asthmaticus is under control. The nurse also assesses the patient's skin turgor for signs of dehydration. Fluid intake is essential to combat dehydration, to loosen secretions, and to facilitate expectoration. Nurses administer IV fluids as prescribed, up to 3 to 4 L/day, unless contraindicated. Blood pressure and cardiac rhythm should be monitored continuously during the acute phase and until the patient stabilizes and responds to therapy. The patient's energy needs to be conserved, and his or her room should be quiet and free of respiratory irritants, including flowers, tobacco smoke, perfumes, or odors of cleaning agents. Nonallergenic pillows should be used.

Cystic Fibrosis

Cystic fibrosis (CF) is the most common fatal autosomal recessive disease among the Caucasian population. A person must inherit a defective copy of the CF gene (one from each parent) to have CF. One in 31 Americans are unknowing carriers of this gene, and approximately 30,000 children and adults in the United States have CF (Cystic Fibrosis Foundation, 2004).

The frequency of CF is 1 in 1900 to 1 in 3700 live births among Caucasian Americans (Aronson & Marquis, 2004). CF is less frequently found among Hispanic, Asian, and African Americans. Although CF was once considered a fatal childhood disease, approximately 37% of people living with the disease are 18 years of age or older. Researchers have documented survival past age 76 years (Aronson & Marquis, 2004).

This multisystem genetic disease is usually diagnosed in infancy or early childhood but may be diagnosed later in life. Respiratory symptoms are frequently the major manifestation of CF when it is diagnosed later in life.

Pathophysiology

CF is caused by mutations in the CF transmembrane conductance regulator protein, which is a chloride channel found in all exocrine tissues. Chloride transport problems lead to thick, viscous secretions in the lungs, pancreas, liver, intestine, and reproductive tract as well as increased salt content in sweat gland secretions. The CF gene was discovered in 1989 and mapped to a single locus on the long arm of chromosome 7. More than 1000 mutations have been identified on the CF transmembrane conductance regulator gene, thus creating multiple variations in presentation and progression of the disease (Aronson & Marquis, 2004).

The ability to detect the common mutations of this gene allows for routine screening for CF and the detection of carriers of the disease. Genetics counseling is an important part of health care for couples at risk. People who are heterozygous for CF (ie, having one defective gene and one normal gene) do not have the disease but can be carriers and pass the defective gene on to their children. If both parents are carriers, their risk of having a child with CF is 1 in 4 (25%) with each pregnancy. Genetics testing should be offered to adults with a positive family history of CF and to partners of people with CF who are planning a pregnancy or seeking prenatal counseling. Currently, genetics testing for CF is not recommended for the general population.

Clinical Manifestations

The pulmonary manifestations of CF include a productive cough, wheezing, hyperinflation of the lung fields on chest x-ray, and pulmonary function test results consistent with obstructive disease of the airways. Chronic respiratory inflammation and infection are caused by impaired mucus clearance. Colonization of the airways with pathogenic bacteria usually occurs early in life. *Staphylococcus aureus* and *H. influenzae* are common organisms during early childhood. As the disease progresses, *Pseudomonas aeruginosa* is ultimately isolated from the sputum of most patients. Upper respiratory manifestations of the disease include sinusitis and nasal polyps.

Nonpulmonary clinical manifestations include gastrointestinal problems (eg, pancreatic insufficiency, recurrent abdominal pain, biliary cirrhosis, vitamin deficiencies, recurrent pancreatitis, weight loss), CF-related diabetes, genitourinary problems (male and female infertility), and clubbing of the digits (fingers and toes). (See Chapter 40 for a discussion of pancreatitis.)

Assessment and Diagnostic Findings

The diagnosis of CF is suspected in patients with typical clinical features of CF, once other diseases have been excluded. Diagnosis is based on an elevated sweat chloride concentration, together with clinical signs and symptoms consistent with the disease. Repeated sweat chloride values of greater than 60 mEq/L distinguish most people with CF from those with other obstructive diseases. The only acceptable procedure for sweat testing is the quantitative pilocarpine iontophoresis sweat test. It should be performed in a laboratory that frequently does this test. A molecular diagnosis or genetics evaluation may also be used in evaluating common genetic mutations of the CF gene.

Medical Management

Pulmonary problems remain the leading cause of morbidity and mortality in CF and account for death in more than 95% of patients (Aronson & Marquis, 2004). A variety of management techniques are necessary.

Because chronic bacterial infection of the airways occurs in CF, control of infections is essential to treatment. Antibiotic medications are routinely prescribed for acute pulmonary exacerbations of the disease. Depending on the severity of the exacerbation, aerosolized, oral, or IV antibiotic therapy may be used. Antibiotic agents are selected based on the results of a sputum culture and sensitivity. Patients with CF may be infected with bacteria that are resistant to multiple antibiotics and require multiple courses of antibiotic agents over long periods.

Bronchodilators, including beta$_2$-adrenergic agonists and anticholinergics, are frequently administered to treat airway hyperactivity and to reverse bronchospasm.

Airway clearance is a key intervention in the care of patients with CF, and various pulmonary techniques are used to enhance secretion clearance. Examples include manual postural drainage and chest physical therapy, high-frequency chest wall oscillation, autogenic drainage (a combination of breathing techniques at different lung volume levels to move the secretions to where they can be "huff"-coughed out), and other devices that assist in airway clearance, such as masks that generate positive expiratory pressure (PEP masks) and "flutter devices" (devices that provide an oscillatory expiratory pressure pattern with positive expiratory pressure and assist with expectoration of secretions). Inhaled mucolytic agents such as dornase alfa (Pulmozyme) or *N*-acetylcysteine (Mucomyst) may also be used. These agents help decrease the viscosity of the sputum and promote expectoration of secretions.

To decrease the inflammation and ongoing destruction of the airways, anti-inflammatory agents, including inhaled corticosteroids or systemic therapy, may also be used. Corticosteroids are used in late-stage disease and during severe respiratory exacerbations. Their routine use is not recommended because of unacceptable short-term and long-term side effects (Aronson & Marquis, 2004). Other anti-inflammatory medications have also been studied in CF. Ibuprofen has been studied in younger patients, and some benefit has been demonstrated in reducing the rate of deterioration of pulmonary function in specific groups of patients; however, it is not routinely used to treat CF.

Supplemental oxygen is used to treat the progressive hypoxemia that occurs with CF. It helps correct the hypoxemia and may minimize the complications seen with chronic hypoxemia (pulmonary hypertension).

Lung transplantation is an option for a small, selected population of patients with CF. A double-lung transplantation technique is used because of chronic infection of both lungs in end-stage CF. Because there is a long waiting list for lung transplants, many patients die while waiting for suitable lungs for transplantation.

Gene therapy is a promising approach to management, and clinical trials are underway. It is hoped that techniques will be developed to carry healthy genes to the damaged cells and correct defective CF cells. Efforts are underway to develop innovative methods of delivering therapy to the CF cells of the airways. In addition, clinical trials are focusing on chloride channel therapies and anti-inflammatory therapies for CF (Cystic Fibrosis Foundation, 2004).

Nursing Management

Nursing is crucial to the interdisciplinary approach required for care of adults with CF. Nursing care includes helping patients manage pulmonary symptoms and prevent complications of CF. Specific nursing measures include strategies that promote removal of pulmonary secretions; chest physiotherapy (including postural drainage, chest percussion, and vibration); and breathing exercises, which are implemented and are taught to the patient and family when the patient is very young. The patient is reminded of the need to reduce risk factors associated with respiratory infections (eg, exposure to crowds or to persons with known infections). In addition, the patient is taught the early signs and symptoms of respiratory infection and disease progression that indicate the need to notify a primary health care provider.

Nurses emphasize the importance of an adequate fluid and dietary intake to promote removal of secretions and to ensure an adequate nutritional status. Because CF is a lifelong disorder, patients often have learned to modify their daily activities to accommodate their symptoms and treatment modalities. However, as the disease progresses, assessment of the home environment may be warranted to identify modifications required to address changes in the patient's needs, increasing dyspnea and fatigue, and nonpulmonary symptoms.

Although gene therapy and double-lung transplantation are promising therapies for CF, they are limited in availability and are largely experimental. As a result, the overall life expectancy of adults with CF is shortened. Despite this, pregnancy is possible in patients with CF. Preconception counseling and evaluation are needed because of high risks associated with pregnancy. Very frequent monitoring is needed throughout pregnancy and delivery in women with CF. End-of-life issues and concerns need to be addressed with the patient when warranted. For the patient whose disease is progressing and who is developing increasing hypoxemia, preferences for end-of-life care should be discussed, documented, and honored (see Chapter 17). Patients and family members require support as they face a shortened life span and an uncertain future.

Critical Thinking Exercises

1 A 74-year-old man with end-stage COPD has been admitted with impending respiratory failure. He is extremely anxious and short of breath and shows signs of central cyanosis. He is unable to lie flat in bed and is on supplemental oxygen at 2 L/min. What tests or examinations might be appropriate to assess the severity of the patient's respiratory failure and his oxygenation status? What comfort measures would you institute for this patient?

2 ebp A 69-year-old farmer with COPD reports that he has been using continuous oxygen for the past 5 years. He reports increasing shortness of breath and asks you to increase his oxygen flow. How do you respond to his request? What is the evidence base for your response? How do you evaluate the strength of the evidence?

3 As a nurse in an outpatient asthma clinic in a tertiary care medical center, you see a 35-year-old Mexican-American mother with asthma. When you inquire about symptom

management and medication history, she provides minimal information and reports that she does not take any medication on a regular basis but has an MDI. In her medical record, you note that use of an MDI on a regular daily schedule has been repeatedly prescribed for her, but she reports that she does not use it except as needed when she is extremely short of breath. Describe the assessment method you would use to evaluate her asthma symptoms and severity. Describe teaching techniques you might use to assess the patient's knowledge of her medications and provide education about the action of the MDI, frequency of use, and correct administration of medication. What methods would you use to monitor use of the MDI and reinforce education about its use?

4 As a nurse in your hospital's community outreach clinic, you are responsible for providing group education and counseling to patients with newly diagnosed asthma. What areas would you address regarding triggers for asthma? How might you have patients assess or change their home and work environments? What resources might you suggest?

5 A 35-year-old woman with CF is admitted to your unit from the emergency room. Her husband accompanies her and states that this is the first time she has been admitted to the hospital for her disease. She cannot lie flat in bed, is extremely short of breath, and is having paroxysms of coughing. The cough is productive of thick, yellow sputum. What is the pathophysiology associated with these findings? What medical and nursing interventions might be used to decrease or alleviate these signs and symptoms? What members of the health care team would you consult to be involved in her care and why?

REFERENCES AND SELECTED READINGS

BOOKS

American Lung Association. (2004). *Chronic obstructive pulmonary disease fact sheet.* New York: Author.

Brown, E. S. (Ed.). (2003). *Asthma: Social and psychological factors and psychosomatic syndromes.* New York: Karger.

Cazzola, M. (2004). *Therapeutic strategies in COPD.* London: Taylor & Francis.

Expert Panel Report. (1997). *Guidelines for the diagnosis and management of asthma.* Bethesda, MD: National Asthma Education and Prevention Program, National Institutes of Health.

Expert Panel Report. (2003). *Guidelines for the diagnosis and management of asthma-update on selected topics 2002.* NIH Publication No. 02-5074. Bethesda, MD: National Institutes of Health, National Heart, Lung and Blood Institute.

Global Initiative for Asthma Management and Prevention. (2004). *National Heart, Lung and Blood Institute NHLBI/World Health Organization WHO workshop report, 2004.* NIH Publication No. 02-3659. Bethesda, MD: National Institutes of Health.

Global Initiative for Asthma Management and Prevention. (2001). *Inhaler Charts for Use with GINA Documents.* National Heart, Lung and Blood Institute NHLBI/World Health Organization. Geneva: WHO.

Global Initiative for Chronic Obstructive Lung Disease (GOLD), World Health Organization (WHO) & National Heart, Lung and Blood Institute (NHLBI). (2004). *Global strategy for the diagnosis, management, and prevention of chronic obstructive pulmonary disease.* Bethesda, MD: National Heart, Lung and Blood Institute.

Hansel, T. T. & Barnes, P. (2004). *An atlas of chronic obstructive pulmonary disease: COPD. A resource for reference, teaching and lecturing.* London: Taylor & Francis.

Institute for Clinical Systems Improvement (ICSI). (2003). *Chronic obstructive pulmonary disease.* Bloomington, MN: Author.

National Heart, Lung and Blood Institute & World Health Organization. (2004). *NHLBI/WHO Workshop Report: Global initiative for asthma management and prevention.* NIH Publication No. 02-3659. Bethesda, MD: National Heart, Lung and Blood Institute.

National Institutes of Health. (2001). *Global initiative for chronic obstructive lung disease: Global strategy for the diagnosis, management, and prevention of chronic obstructive pulmonary disease.* NIH Publication No. 2701B. Washington, DC: U.S. Department of Health and Human Services.

Petty, T. L. (2003). *Coping with COPD: Understanding, treating, and living with chronic obstructive pulmonary disease.* New York: St. Martin's Press.

Reid, W. D. (2004). *Clinical management notes and case histories in cardiopulmonary physical therapy.* Thorofare, NJ: Slack.

Ruppel, G. (2003). *Manual of pulmonary function testing.* St. Louis: Mosby.

JOURNALS

**Asterisks indicate nursing research articles.*

General

ACCP/AACVPR Pulmonary Rehabilitation Guidelines Panel. (1997). Pulmonary rehabilitation: Joint ACCP/AACVPR evidence-based guidelines. *Chest, 112*(5), 1363–1396.

American Thoracic Society. (1999). Statement on pulmonary rehabilitation. *American Journal of Respiratory and Critical Care Medicine, 159*(5), 1666–1682.

Asthma

Adams, R. J., Wilson, D. H., Taylor, A. W., et al. (2004). Psychological factors and asthma quality of life: A population based study. *Thorax, 59*(11), 930–935.

American Thoracic Society. (2004). Guidelines for assessing and managing asthma risk at work, school, and recreation. *American Journal of Respiratory and Critical Care Medicine, 169*(7), 873–881.

Bender, B. G. & Bender S. E. (2005). Patient-identified barriers to asthma treatment adherence: Responses to interviews, focus groups, and questionnaires. *Immunology and Allergy Clinics of North America, 25*(1), 107–130.

Centers for Disease Control and Prevention. (2004). *Fast stats sheet: Asthma.* Atlanta: National Center for Health Statistics.

Gelb, A. F., Schein, A., Nussbaum, E., et al. (2004). Risk factors for near-fatal asthma. *Chest, 126*(4), 1138–1146.

Higgins, J. C. (2003). The "crashing asthmatic." *American Family Physician, 67*(5), 997–1004.

Sin, D. D., Man, J., Sharpe, H., et al. (2004). Pharmacological management to reduce exacerbations in adults with asthma: A systematic review and meta-analysis. *Journal of the American Medical Association, 293*(2), 367–376.

Chronic Obstructive Pulmonary Disease

American Lung Association. (2005). Alpha-1 related emphysema. Available at: http://www.lungusa.org. Accessed June 17, 2006.

American Thoracic Society & European Respiratory Society. (2004). *ATS and ERS standards for the diagnosis and management of patients with COPD.* Available at: www.thoracic.org. Accessed April 20, 2006.

Andenaes, R., Kalfoss, M. H. & Wahl, A. (2004). Psychological distress and quality of life in hospitalized patients with chronic obstructive pulmonary disease. *Journal of Advance Nursing, 46*(5), 522–530.

Arias, E., Anderson, R. N., Hsiang-Ching, K., et al. (2003). Deaths: Final data for 2001. *National Vital Statistics Reports, 52*(3), 1–116.

Blackler, L., Mooney, C. & Jones, C. (2004). Palliative care in the management of chronic obstructive pulmonary disease. *British Journal of Nursing, 13*(9), 518–521.

Brenner, M., Hanna, N. M., Mina-Araghi, R., et al. (2004). Innovative approaches to lung volume reduction for emphysema. *Chest, 126*(1), 238–248.

Centers for Disease Control and Prevention. (2004). *Smoking fact sheets.* Atlanta: Office on Smoking and Heath.

Covey, M. K. & Larson, J. L. (2004). Exercise and COPD. *American Journal of Nursing, 104*(5), 40–43.

Curtis, J., Wenrich, M., Carline, J., et al. (2002). Patients' perspectives on physician skill in end-of-life care. Differences between patients with COPD, cancer and AIDS. *Chest, 122*(1), 356–362.

*Meek, P. M. & Lareau, S. C. (2003). Critical outcomes in pulmonary rehabilitation: Assessment and evaluation of dyspnea and fatigue. *Journal of Rehabilitation Research and Development, 50*(5), 13–24.

National Emphysema Treatment Trial Research Group. (2003). A randomized trial comparing lung-volume reduction surgery with medical therapy for severe emphysema. *New England Journal of Medicine, 348*(21), 2059–2073.

Simmons, P. & Simmons, M. (2004). Informed nursing practice: The administration of oxygen to patients with COPD. *MedSurg Nursing, 13*(2), 82–85.

Sin, D., McAlister, F., Man, S. F. P., et al. (2003). Contemporary management of chronic obstructive pulmonary disease: Scientific review. *Journal of the American Medical Association, 290*(7), 2301–2312.

Sutherland, R. E. & Cherniack, R. M. (2004). Management of chronic obstructive pulmonary disease. *New England Journal of Medicine, 350*(26), 2689–2697.

Theander, K. & Unosson, M. (2004). Fatigue in patients with chronic obstructive pulmonary disease. *Journal of Advanced Nursing, 45*(2), 172–177.

Cystic Fibrosis

Aronson, B. S. & Marquis, M. (2004). Care of the adult with cystic fibrosis. *MedSurg Nursing, 13*(3), 143–154

Cystic Fibrosis Adult Care: Consensus Committee Report. (2004). *Chest, 125*(1 Suppl.), 1S–39S.

Cystic Fibrosis Foundation. (2004). What is cystic fibrosis? Available at: http://www.cff.org/about_cystic_fibrosis. Accessed June 16, 2006.

RESOURCES

Agency for Healthcare Research and Quality, John M. Eisenberg Bldg, 540 Gaither Road, Rockville, MD 20850; 1-301-427-1364; http://www.ahrq.gov or www.ahcpr.gov. Accessed April 20, 2006.

Alpha-1 Association, 275 West Street, Suite 210, Annapolis, MD 21401; 1-800-521-3025; http://www.alpha1.org. Accessed April 20, 2006.

American Academy of Allergy, Asthma, and Immunology, 611 E. Wells St. Suite 1100, Milwaukee, WI 53202; 414-272-6071; http://www.aaaai.org. Accessed April 20, 2006.

American Association of Cardiovascular and Pulmonary Rehabilitation, 401 North Michigan Ave, Suite 2200, Chicago, IL 60611; 312-321-5146; http://www.aacvpr.org. Accessed April 20, 2006.

American Association for Respiratory Care, 9425 N. MacArthur Blvd., Suite 100, Irving, TX 75063; 1-972-243-2272; http://www.aarc.org. Accessed April 20, 2006.

American College of Chest Physicians, 3300 Dundee Road, Northbrook, IL 60062; 1-847-498-1400; http://www.chestnet.org. Accessed April 20, 2006.

American Lung Association, 61 Broadway 6th Floor, New York, NY 10006; 1-800-LUNGUSA; http://www.lungusa.org. Accessed April 20, 2006.

American Thoracic Society, 61 Broadway, New York, NY 10006; 1-212-315-8600; http://www.thoracic.org. Accessed June 17, 2006.

Centers for Disease Control and Prevention, 1600 Clifton Road, NE, Atlanta, GA 30333; 1-800-311-3435; http://www.cdc.gov. Accessed June 17, 2006.

Cystic Fibrosis Foundation, 6931 Arlington Road, Bethesda, MD 20814; 310-951-4422 or 800-FIGHT-CF; http://www.cff.org. Accessed April 20, 2006.

National Heart, Lung and Blood Institute, National Institutes of Health, Bldg. 31, 31 Center Drive MSC, Bethesda, MD 20892; 1-301-592-8573; http://www.nhlbi.nih.gov. Accessed April 20, 2006.

Respiratory Nursing Society, c/o NYSNA, 11 Cornell Road, Latham, NY 12110; 1-518-782-9400 × 286; http://www.respiratorynursingsociety.org. Accessed April 20, 2006.

U.S. Department of Health and Human Services, Department of Health and Human Services, 200 Independence Avenue, S.W., Washington DC 20201; 202-619-0257; http://www.hhs.gov or http://www.healthfinder.gov. Accessed April 20, 2006.

CHAPTER 25

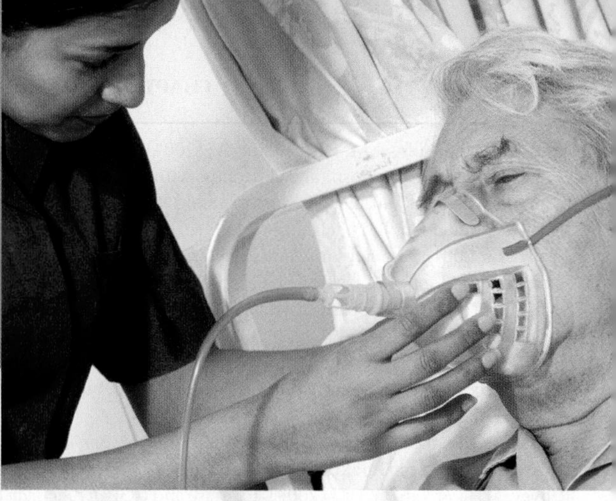

Respiratory Care Modalities

Learning Objectives

On completion of this chapter, the learner will be able to:

1. Describe the nursing management for patients receiving oxygen therapy, intermittent positive-pressure breathing, mini-nebulizer therapy, incentive spirometry, chest physiotherapy, and breathing retraining.
2. Describe the patient education and home care considerations for patients receiving oxygen therapy.
3. Describe the nursing care for a patient with an endotracheal tube and for a patient with a tracheostomy.
4. Demonstrate the procedure of tracheal suctioning.
5. Use the nursing process as a framework for care of patients who are mechanically ventilated.
6. Describe the process of weaning the patient from mechanical ventilation.
7. Describe the significance of preoperative nursing assessment and patient teaching for the patient who is to have thoracic surgery.
8. Explain the principles of chest drainage and the nursing responsibilities related to the care of the patient with a chest drainage system.
9. Describe the patient education and home care considerations for patients who have had thoracic surgery.

Numerous treatment modalities are used when caring for patients with various respiratory conditions. The choice of modality is based on the oxygenation disorder and whether there is a problem with gas ventilation, diffusion, or both. Therapies range from simple and noninvasive (oxygen and nebulizer therapy, chest physiotherapy, breathing retraining) to complex and highly invasive treatments (intubation, mechanical ventilation, surgery). Assessment and management of the patient with respiratory disorders are best accomplished when the approach is multidisciplinary and collaborative.

Noninvasive Respiratory Therapies

Noninvasive respiratory therapies include oxygen therapy, incentive spirometry, mini-nebulizer therapy, intermittent positive-pressure breathing, and chest physiotherapy.

Oxygen Therapy

Oxygen therapy is the administration of oxygen at a concentration greater than that found in the environmental atmosphere. At sea level, the concentration of oxygen in room air is 21%. The goal of oxygen therapy is to provide adequate transport of oxygen in the blood while decreasing the work of breathing and reducing stress on the myocardium.

Oxygen transport to the tissues depends on factors such as cardiac output, arterial oxygen content, concentration of hemoglobin, and metabolic requirements. These factors must be kept in mind when oxygen therapy is considered. (Respiratory physiology and oxygen transport are discussed in Chapter 21.)

Glossary

airway pressure release ventilation (APRV): mode of mechanical ventilation that allows unrestricted, spontaneous breaths throughout the ventilatory cycle; produces tidal ventilation by release of airway pressure from an elevated baseline airway pressure to simulate expiration

assist–control ventilation: mode of mechanical ventilation in which the patient's breathing pattern may trigger the ventilator to deliver a preset tidal volume; in the absence of spontaneous breathing, the machine delivers a controlled breath at a preset minimum rate and tidal volume

chest drainage system: use of a chest tube and closed drainage system to reexpand the lung and to remove excess air, fluid, and blood

chest percussion: manually cupping over the chest wall to mobilize secretions by mechanically dislodging viscous or adherent secretions in the lungs

chest physiotherapy (CPT): therapy used to remove bronchial secretions, improve ventilation, and increase the efficiency of the respiratory muscles. Types include postural drainage, chest percussion, and vibration.

continuous positive airway pressure (CPAP): positive pressure applied throughout the respiratory cycle to a spontaneously breathing patient to promote alveolar and airway stability; may be administered with endotracheal or tracheostomy tube, or by mask

controlled ventilation: mode of mechanical ventilation in which the ventilator completely controls the patient's ventilation according to preset tidal volumes and respiratory rate. Because of problems with synchrony, it is rarely used except in paralyzed or anesthetized patients.

endotracheal intubation: insertion of a breathing tube through the nose or mouth into the trachea

fraction of inspired oxygen (FiO_2): concentration of oxygen delivered (1.0 = 100% oxygen)

hypoxemia: decrease in arterial oxygen tension in the blood

hypoxia: decrease in oxygen supply to the tissues and cells

incentive spirometry: method of deep breathing that provides visual feedback to help the patient inhale deeply and slowly and achieve maximum lung inflation

intermittent mandatory ventilation (IMV): mode of mechanical ventilation that provides a combination of mechanically assisted breaths and spontaneous breaths

mechanical ventilator: a positive- or negative-pressure breathing device that supports ventilation and oxygenation

pneumothorax: partial or complete collapse of the lung due to positive pressure in the pleural space

positive end-expiratory pressure (PEEP): positive pressure maintained by the ventilator at the end of exhalation (instead of a normal zero pressure) to increase functional residual capacity and open collapsed alveoli; improves oxygenation with lower FiO_2

postural drainage: positioning the patient to allow drainage from all the lobes of the lungs and airways

pressure support ventilation (PSV): mode of mechanical ventilation in which preset positive pressure is delivered with spontaneous breaths to decrease work of breathing

proportional assist ventilation (PAV): mode of mechanical ventilation that provides partial ventilatory support in proportion to the patient's inspiratory efforts; decreases the work of breathing

respiratory weaning: process of gradual, systematic withdrawal and/or removal of ventilator, breathing tube, and oxygen

synchronized intermittent mandatory ventilation (SIMV): mode of mechanical ventilation in which the ventilator allows the patient to breathe spontaneously while providing a preset number of breaths to ensure adequate ventilation; ventilated breaths are synchronized with spontaneous breathing

thoracotomy: surgical opening into the chest cavity

tracheotomy: surgical opening into the trachea

tracheostomy tube: indwelling tube inserted directly into the trachea to assist with ventilation

vibration: a type of massage administered by quickly tapping the chest with the fingertips or alternating the fingers in a rhythmic manner, or by using a mechanical device to assist in mobilizing lung secretions

Indications

A change in the patient's respiratory rate or pattern may be one of the earliest indicators of the need for oxygen therapy. The change in respiratory rate or pattern may result from hypoxemia or hypoxia. **Hypoxemia** (a decrease in the arterial oxygen tension in the blood) is manifested by changes in mental status (progressing through impaired judgment, agitation, disorientation, confusion, lethargy, and coma), dyspnea, increase in blood pressure, changes in heart rate, dysrhythmias, central cyanosis (late sign), diaphoresis, and cool extremities. Hypoxemia usually leads to **hypoxia,** which is a decrease in oxygen supply to the tissues. Hypoxia, if severe enough, can be life-threatening.

The signs and symptoms signaling the need for oxygen may depend on how suddenly this need develops. With rapidly developing hypoxia, changes occur in the central nervous system because the higher neurologic centers are very sensitive to oxygen deprivation. The clinical picture may resemble that of alcohol intoxication, with the patient exhibiting lack of coordination and impaired judgment. Longstanding hypoxia (as seen in chronic obstructive pulmonary disease [COPD] and chronic heart failure) may produce fatigue, drowsiness, apathy, inattentiveness, and delayed reaction time. The need for oxygen is assessed by arterial blood gas analysis and pulse oximetry as well as by clinical evaluation. More information about hypoxia is presented in Chart 25-1.

CHART 25-1

Types of Hypoxia

Hypoxia can occur from either severe pulmonary disease (inadequate oxygen supply) or from extrapulmonary disease (inadequate oxygen delivery) affecting gas exchange at the cellular level. The four general types of hypoxia are hypoxemic hypoxia, circulatory hypoxia, anemic hypoxia, and histotoxic hypoxia.

HYPOXEMIC HYPOXIA

Hypoxemic hypoxia is a decreased oxygen level in the blood resulting in decreased oxygen diffusion into the tissues. It may be caused by hypoventilation, high altitudes, ventilation–perfusion mismatch (as in pulmonary embolism), shunts in which the alveoli are collapsed and cannot provide oxygen to the blood (commonly caused by atelectasis), and pulmonary diffusion defects. It is corrected by increasing alveolar ventilation or providing supplemental oxygen.

CIRCULATORY HYPOXIA

Circulatory hypoxia is hypoxia resulting from inadequate capillary circulation. It may be caused by decreased cardiac output, local vascular obstruction, low-flow states such as shock, or cardiac arrest. Although tissue partial pressure of oxygen (PO_2) is reduced, arterial oxygen (PaO_2) remains normal. Circulatory hypoxia is corrected by identifying and treating the underlying cause.

ANEMIC HYPOXIA

Anemic hypoxia is a result of decreased effective hemoglobin concentration, which causes a decrease in the oxygen-carrying capacity of the blood. It is rarely accompanied by hypoxemia. Carbon monoxide poisoning, because it reduces the oxygen-carrying capacity of hemoglobin, produces similar effects but is not strictly anemic hypoxia because hemoglobin levels may be normal.

HISTOTOXIC HYPOXIA

Histotoxic hypoxia occurs when a toxic substance, such as cyanide, interferes with the ability of tissues to use available oxygen.

Complications

As with other medications, the nurse administers oxygen with caution and carefully assesses its effects on each patient. Oxygen is a medication, and except in emergency situations it is administered only when prescribed by a physician.

In general, patients with respiratory conditions are given oxygen therapy only to increase the arterial oxygen pressure (PaO_2) back to the patient's normal baseline, which may vary from 60 to 95 mm Hg. In terms of the oxyhemoglobin dissociation curve (see Chapter 21), the blood at these levels is 80% to 98% saturated with oxygen; higher **fraction of inspired oxygen (FiO_2)** flow values add no further significant amounts of oxygen to the red blood cells or plasma. Instead of helping, increased amounts of oxygen may produce toxic effects on the lungs and central nervous system or may depress ventilation (see later discussion).

It is important to observe for subtle indicators of inadequate oxygenation when oxygen is administered by any method. Therefore, the nurse assesses the patient frequently for confusion, restlessness progressing to lethargy, diaphoresis, pallor, tachycardia, tachypnea, and hypertension. Intermittent or continuous pulse oximetry is used to monitor oxygen levels.

Oxygen Toxicity

Oxygen toxicity may occur when too high a concentration of oxygen (greater than 50%) is administered for an extended period (longer than 48 hours). It is caused by overproduction of oxygen free radicals, which are byproducts of cell metabolism. If oxygen toxicity is untreated, these radicals can severely damage or kill cells. Antioxidants such as vitamin E, vitamin C, and beta-carotene may help defend against oxygen free radicals. The dietitian can adjust the patient's diet so that it is rich in antioxidants; supplements are also available for patients who have a decreased appetite or who are unable to eat.

Signs and symptoms of oxygen toxicity include substernal discomfort, paresthesias, dyspnea, restlessness, fatigue, malaise, progressive respiratory difficulty, refractory hypoxemia, alveolar atelectasis, and alveolar infiltrates evident on chest x-rays.

Prevention of oxygen toxicity is achieved by using oxygen only as prescribed. If high concentrations of oxygen are necessary, it is important to minimize the duration of administration and reduce its concentration as soon as possible. Often, **positive end-expiratory pressure (PEEP)** or **continuous positive airway pressure (CPAP)** is used with oxygen therapy to reverse or prevent microatelectasis, thus allowing a lower percentage of oxygen to be used. The level of PEEP that allows the best oxygenation without hemodynamic compromise is known as "best PEEP."

Suppression of Ventilation

In many patients with COPD, the stimulus for respiration is a decrease in blood oxygen rather than an elevation in carbon dioxide levels. The administration of a high concentration of oxygen removes the respiratory drive that has been created largely by the patient's chronic low oxygen tension. The resulting decrease in alveolar ventilation can cause a progressive increase in arterial carbon dioxide pressure ($PaCO_2$). This hypoventilation can, in rare cases, lead to acute respiratory failure secondary to carbon dioxide narcosis, acidosis, and death. Oxygen-induced hypoventilation is prevented by administering oxygen at low flow rates (1 to 2 L/min) and by closely monitoring the respiratory rate and the oxygen saturation as measured by pulse oximetry (SpO_2).

Other Complications

Because oxygen supports combustion, there is always a danger of fire when it is used. It is important to post "No Smoking" signs when oxygen is in use. Oxygen therapy equipment is also a potential source of bacterial cross-infection; therefore, the nurse (or respiratory therapist) changes the tubing according to infection control policy and the type of oxygen delivery equipment.

Methods of Oxygen Administration

Oxygen is dispensed from a cylinder or a piped-in system. A reduction gauge is necessary to reduce the pressure to a working level, and a flow meter regulates the flow of oxygen in liters per minute. When oxygen is used at high flow rates, it should be moistened by passing it through a humidification system to prevent it from drying the mucous membranes of the respiratory tract.

The use of oxygen concentrators is another means of providing varying amounts of oxygen, especially in the home setting. These devices are relatively portable, easy to operate, and cost-effective. However, they require more maintenance than tank or liquid systems and probably cannot deliver oxygen flows in excess of 4 L/min, which provides an FiO_2 of about 36%.

Many different oxygen devices are used, and all deliver oxygen if they are used as prescribed and maintained correctly (Table 25-1). The amount of oxygen delivered is expressed as a percentage concentration (eg, 70%). The

TABLE 25-1 Oxygen Administration Devices

Device	Suggested Flow Rate (L/min)	O_2 Percentage Setting	Advantages	Disadvantages
Low-Flow Systems				
Cannula	1–2 3–5 6	23–30 30–40 42	Lightweight, comfortable, inexpensive, continuous use with meals and activity	Nasal mucosal drying, variable FiO_2
Oropharyngeal catheter	1–6	23–42	Inexpensive, does not require a tracheostomy	Nasal mucosa irritation; catheter should be changed frequently to alternate nostril
Mask, simple	6–8	40–60	Simple to use, inexpensive	Poor fitting, variable FiO_2, must remove to eat
Mask, partial rebreather	8–11	50–75	Moderate O_2 concentration	Warm, poorly fitting, must remove to eat
Mask, non-rebreather	12	80–100	High O_2 concentration	Poorly fitting
High-Flow Systems				
Transtracheal catheter	¼–4	60–100	More comfortable, concealed by clothing, less oxygen liters per minute needed than nasal cannula	Requires frequent and regular cleaning, requires surgical intervention
Mask, Venturi	4–6 6–8	24, 26, 28 30, 35, 40	Provides low levels of supplemental O_2 Precise FiO_2, additional humidity available	Must remove to eat
Mask, aerosol	8–10	30–100	Good humidity, accurate FiO_2	Uncomfortable for some
Tracheostomy collar	8–10	30–100	Good humidity, comfortable, fairly accurate FiO_2	
T-piece	8–10	30–100	Same as tracheostomy collar	Heavy with tubing
Face tent	8–10	30–100	Good humidity, fairly accurate FiO_2	Bulky and cumbersome
Oxygen Conserving Devices				
Pulse dose (or demand)	10–40 mL/breath		Deliver O_2 only on inspiration, conserve 50% to 75% of O_2 used	Must carefully evaluate function individually

appropriate form of oxygen therapy is best determined by arterial blood gas levels, which indicate the patient's oxygenation status.

Oxygen delivery systems are classified as low-flow or high-flow delivery systems. Low-flow systems contribute partially to the inspired gas the patient breathes, which means that the patient breathes some room air along with the oxygen. These systems do not provide a constant or known concentration of inspired oxygen. The amount of inspired oxygen changes as the patient's breathing changes. Examples of low-flow systems include nasal cannula, oropharyngeal catheter, simple mask, partial-rebreather, and non-rebreather masks. In contrast, high-flow systems provide the total amount of inspired air. A specific percentage of oxygen is delivered independent of the patient's breathing. High-flow systems are indicated for patients who require a constant and precise amount of oxygen. Examples of such systems include transtracheal catheters, Venturi masks, aerosol masks, tracheostomy collars, T-pieces, and face tents.

A nasal cannula is used when the patient requires a low to medium concentration of oxygen for which precise accuracy is not essential. This method is relatively simple and allows the patient to move about in bed, talk, cough, and eat without interrupting oxygen flow. Flow rates in excess of 6 to 8 L/min may lead to swallowing of air or may cause irritation and drying of the nasal and pharyngeal mucosa.

The oropharyngeal catheter is rarely used but may be prescribed for short-term therapy to administer low to moderate concentrations of oxygen. The catheter should be changed every 8 hours, alternating nostrils to prevent nasal irritation and infection.

When oxygen is administered via cannula or catheter, the percentage of oxygen reaching the lungs varies with the depth and rate of respirations, particularly if the nasal mucosa is swollen or if the patient is a mouth breather.

Oxygen masks come in several forms. Each is used for different purposes (Fig. 25-1). *Simple masks* are used to administer low to moderate concentrations of oxygen. The body of the mask itself gathers and stores oxygen between breaths. The patient exhales directly through openings or ports in the body of the mask. If oxygen flow ceases, the patient can draw air in through these openings around the mask edges. Although widely used, these masks cannot be used for controlled oxygen concentrations and must be adjusted for proper fit. They should not press too tightly against the skin, because this can cause a sense of claustrophobia as well as skin breakdown; adjustable elastic bands are provided to ensure comfort and security.

Partial-rebreathing masks have a reservoir bag that must remain inflated during both inspiration and expiration. The nurse adjusts the oxygen flow to ensure that the bag does not collapse during inhalation. A high concentration of oxygen can be delivered, because both the mask and the bag serve as reservoirs for oxygen. Oxygen enters the mask through small-bore tubing that connects at the junction of the mask and bag. As the patient inhales, gas is drawn from the mask, from the bag, and potentially from room air through the exhalation ports. As the patient exhales, the first third of the exhalation fills the reservoir bag. This is mainly dead space and does not participate in gas exchange in the lungs. Therefore, it has a high oxygen concentration. The remainder of the exhaled gas is vented through the exhalation ports. The actual percentage of oxygen delivered is influenced by the patient's ventilatory pattern (Kacmarek, Dimas, & Mack, 2005).

Non-rebreathing masks are similar in design to partial-rebreathing masks except that they have additional valves. A one-way valve located between the reservoir bag and the base of the mask allows gas from the reservoir bag to enter the mask on inhalation but prevents gas in the mask from flowing back into the reservoir bag during exhalation. One-way valves located at the exhalation ports prevent room air from entering the mask during inhalation. They also allow the patient's exhaled gases to exit the mask on exhalation.

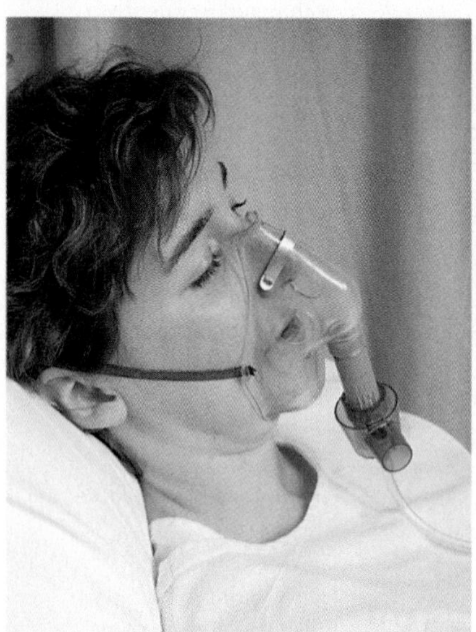

Venturi mask

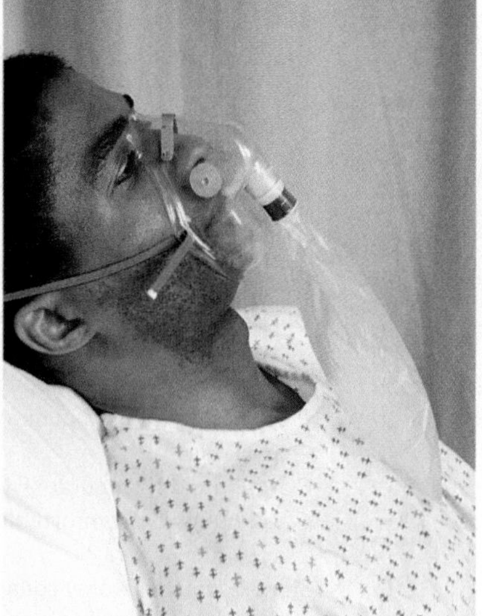

Nonrebreathing mask

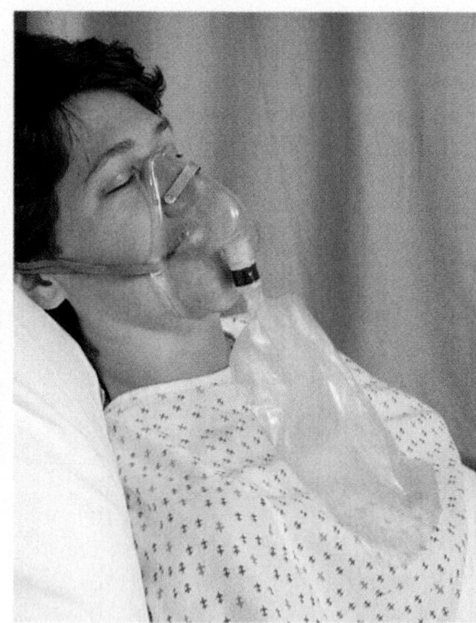

Partial rebreathing mask

FIGURE 25-1. Types of oxygen masks used to deliver varying concentrations of oxygen. Photos © Ken Kaspar.

As with the partial-rebreathing mask, it is important to adjust the oxygen flow so that the reservoir bag does not completely collapse on inspiration. In theory, if the non-rebreathing mask fits the patient snugly and both side exhalation ports have one-way valves, it is possible for the patient to receive 100% oxygen, making the non-rebreathing mask a high-flow oxygen system. However, because it is difficult to get an exact fit from the mask on every patient, and some non-rebreathing masks have only one one-way exhalation valve, it is almost impossible to ensure 100% oxygen delivery, making it a low-flow oxygen system.

The *Venturi mask* is the most reliable and accurate method for delivering precise concentrations of oxygen through noninvasive means. The mask is constructed in a way that allows a constant flow of room air blended with a fixed flow of oxygen. It is used primarily for patients with COPD because it can accurately provide appropriate levels of supplemental oxygen, thus avoiding the risk of suppressing the hypoxic drive.

The Venturi mask uses the Bernoulli principle of air entrainment (trapping the air like a vacuum), which provides a high air flow with controlled oxygen enrichment. For each liter of oxygen that passes through a jet orifice, a fixed proportion of room air is entrained. A precise volume of oxygen can be delivered by varying the size of the jet orifice and adjusting the flow of oxygen. Excess gas leaves the mask through the two exhalation ports, carrying with it the exhaled carbon dioxide. This method allows a constant oxygen concentration to be inhaled regardless of the depth or rate of respiration.

The mask should fit snugly enough to prevent oxygen from flowing into the patient's eyes. The nurse checks the patient's skin for irritation. It is necessary to remove the mask so that the patient can eat, drink, and take medications, at which time supplemental oxygen is provided through a nasal cannula.

The *transtracheal oxygen catheter* is inserted directly into the trachea and is indicated for patients with chronic oxygen therapy needs. These catheters are more comfortable, less dependent on breathing patterns, and less obvious than other oxygen delivery methods. Because no oxygen is lost into the surrounding environment, the patient achieves adequate oxygenation at lower rates, making this method less expensive and more efficient.

The *T-piece* connects to the endotracheal tube and is useful in weaning patients from mechanical ventilation (Fig. 25-2).

Other oxygen devices include *aerosol masks, tracheostomy collars,* and *face tents,* all of which are used with aerosol devices (nebulizers) that can be adjusted for oxygen concentrations from 27% to 100% (0.27 to 1.00). If the gas mixture flow falls below patient demand, room air is pulled in, diluting the concentration. The aerosol mist must be available for the patient during the entire inspiratory phase.

Although most oxygen therapy is administered as continuous flow oxygen, new methods of oxygen conservation are coming into use. The *demand oxygen delivery system* (DODS) interrupts the flow of oxygen during exhalation, when it is otherwise mostly wasted. Several versions of the DODS are being evaluated for their effectiveness. Studies show that DODS models conserve oxygen and maintain oxygen saturations better than continuous-flow oxygen systems when the respiratory rate increases (Langenhof & Fichter, 2005).

Hyperbaric oxygen therapy is the administration of oxygen at pressures greater than 1 atmosphere. As a result, the amount of oxygen dissolved in plasma is increased, which increases oxygen levels in the tissues.

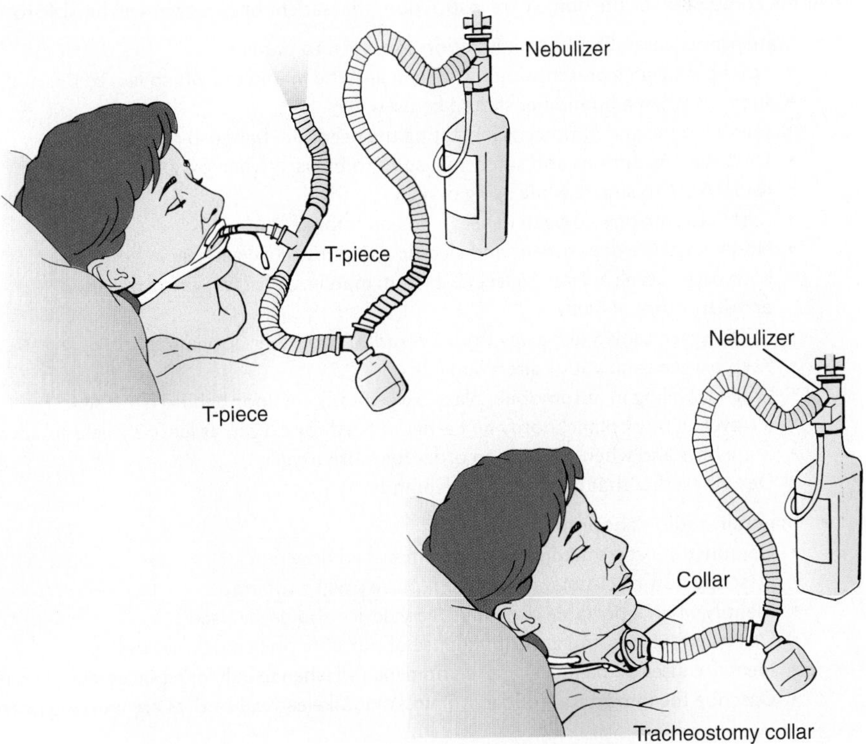

FIGURE 25-2. T-pieces and tracheostomy collars are devices used when weaning patients from mechanical ventilation.

During therapy, the patient is placed in a small (single patient use) or large (multiple patient use) cylinder chamber. Hyperbaric oxygen therapy is used to treat conditions such as air embolism, carbon monoxide poisoning, gangrene, tissue necrosis, and hemorrhage.

Other, more controversial, uses for this therapy include treatment for multiple sclerosis (Bennett & Heard, 2004; Moon, 2002), diabetic foot ulcers (Broussard, 2003;. Roeckl-Wiedmann, Bennett & Kranke, 2005), closed head trauma (Bennett, Trytko, & Jonker, 2004; McDonagh, Helfand, Carson et al., 2004), and acute myocardial infarction (Dekleva, Neskovic, Vlahovic, et al., 2004; Sharifi, Fares, Abdel-Karim, et al., 2004). Potential side effects include ear trauma, central nervous system disorders, and oxygen toxicity.

Gerontologic Considerations

The respiratory system changes throughout the aging process, and it is important for nurses to be aware of these changes when assessing patients who are receiving oxygen therapy. As the respiratory muscles weaken and the large bronchi and alveoli become enlarged, the available surface area of the lungs decreases, resulting in reduced ventilation and respiratory gas exchange. The number of functional cilia is also reduced, decreasing ciliary action and the cough reflex. As a result of osteoporosis and calcification of the costal cartilages, chest wall compliance is decreased. Patients may display increased chest rigidity and respiratory rate and decreased PaO_2 and lung expansion. Nurses should be aware that the older adult is at risk for aspiration and infection related to these changes. In addition, patient education regarding adequate nutrition is essential, because appropriate dietary intake can help diminish the excess buildup of carbon dioxide and maintain optimal respiratory functioning.

Nursing Management

Promoting Home and Community-Based Care

TEACHING PATIENTS SELF-CARE

At times oxygen must be administered to the patient at home. The nurse instructs the patient or family in the methods for administering oxygen safely and informs the patient and family that oxygen is available in gas, liquid, and concentrated forms. The gas and liquid forms come in portable devices so that the patient can leave home while receiving oxygen therapy. Humidity must be provided while oxygen is used (except with portable devices) to counteract the dry, irritating effects of compressed oxygen on the airway (Chart 25-2).

CONTINUING CARE

Home visits by a home health nurse or respiratory therapist may be arranged based on the patient's status and needs. It is important to assess the patient's home envi-

CHART 25-2

HOME CARE CHECKLIST • Oxygen Therapy

At the completion of the home care instruction, the patient or caregiver will be able to:	Patient	Caregiver
• State proper care of and administration of oxygen to patient		
• State physician's prescription for oxygen and the manner in which it is to be used	✔	✔
• Indicate when a humidifier should be used	✔	✔
• Identify signs and symptoms indicating the need for change in oxygen therapy	✔	✔
• Describe precautions and safety measures to be used when oxygen is in use	✔	✔
• Know ***NOT*** to smoke while using oxygen	✔	✔
• Post "No smoking—oxygen in use" signs on doors	✔	✔
• Notify local fire department and electric company of oxygen use in home	✔	✔
• Keep oxygen tank at least 15 feet away from matches, candles, gas stove, or other source of flame	✔	✔
• Keep oxygen tank 5 feet away from TV, radio, and other appliances	✔	✔
• Keep oxygen tank out of direct sunlight	✔	✔
• When traveling in automobile, place oxygen tank on floor behind front seat	✔	✔
• If traveling by airplane, notify air carrier of need for oxygen at least 2 weeks in advance	✔	✔
• State how and when to place an order for more oxygen	✔	✔
• Describe a diet that meets energy demands	✔	✔
• Maintain equipment properly		
• Demonstrate correct adjustment of prescribed flow rate	✔	✔
• Describe how to clean and when to replace oxygen tubing	✔	✔
• Identify when a portable oxygen delivery device should be used	✔	✔
• Demonstrate safe and appropriate use of portable oxygen delivery device	✔	✔
• Identify causes of malfunction of equipment and when to call for replacement of equipment	✔	✔
• Describe the importance of determining that all electrical outlets are working properly	✔	✔

ronment, the patient's physical and psychological status, and the need for further teaching. The nurse reinforces the teaching points on how to use oxygen safely and effectively, including fire safety tips. To maintain a consistent quality of care and to maximize the patient's financial reimbursement for home oxygen therapy, the nurse ensures that the physician's prescription includes the diagnosis, the prescribed oxygen flow, and conditions for use (eg, continuous use, nighttime use only). Because oxygen is a medication, the nurse reminds the patient receiving long-term oxygen therapy and the family about the importance of keeping follow-up appointments with the physician. The patient is instructed to see the physician every 6 months or more often, if indicated. Arterial blood gas measurements and laboratory tests are repeated annually, or more often if the patient's condition changes.

Incentive Spirometry (Sustained Maximal Inspiration)

Incentive spirometry is a method of deep breathing that provides visual feedback to encourage the patient to inhale slowly and deeply to maximize lung inflation and prevent or reduce atelectasis. Ideally, the patient assumes a sitting or semi-Fowler's position to enhance diaphragmatic excursion (Chart 25-3). However, this procedure may be performed with the patient in any position.

Incentive spirometers are available in two types: volume or flow. In the volume type, the tidal volume of the spirometer is set according to the manufacturer's instructions. The purpose of the device is to ensure that the volume of air inhaled is increased gradually as the patient takes deeper and deeper breaths. The patient takes a deep breath through the mouthpiece, pauses at peak lung inflation, and then relaxes and exhales. Taking several normal breaths before attempting another with the incentive spirometer helps avoid fatigue. The volume is periodically increased as tolerated.

A flow spirometer has the same purpose as a volume spirometer, but the volume is not preset. The spirometer contains a number of movable balls that are pushed up by the force of the breath and held suspended in the air while the patient inhales. The amount of air inhaled and the flow of the air are estimated by how long and how high the balls are suspended.

Indications

Incentive spirometry is used after surgery, especially thoracic and abdominal surgery, to promote the expansion of the alveoli and to prevent or treat atelectasis.

CHART 25-3

Assisting the Patient to Perform Incentive Spirometry

- Explain the reason and objective for the therapy: the inspired air helps to inflate the lungs. The ball or weight in the spirometer will rise in response to the intensity of the intake of air. The higher the ball rises, the deeper the breath.
- Assess the patient's level of pain and administer pain medication if prescribed.
- Position the patient in semi-Fowler's position or in an upright position (although any position is acceptable).
- Demonstrate how to use diaphragmatic breathing.
- Instruct the patient to place the mouthpiece of the spirometer firmly in the mouth, to breathe air in (inspire), and to hold the breath at the end of inspiration for about 3 seconds. The patient then exhales slowly.
- Encourage the patient to perform the procedure approximately 10 times in succession, repeating the 10 breaths with the spirometer each hour during waking hours.
- Set a reasonable volume and repetition goal (to provide encouragement and give the patient a sense of accomplishment).
- Encourage coughing during and after each session.

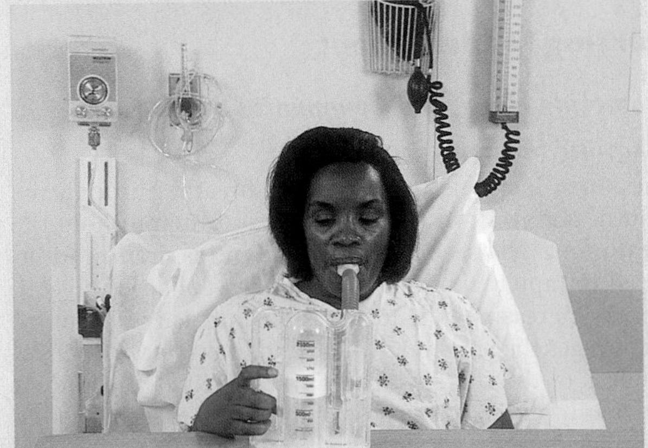

© B. Proud

- Assist the patient to splint the incision when coughing postoperatively.
- Place the spirometer within easy reach of the patient.
- For the postoperative patient, begin the therapy immediately. (If the patient begins to hypoventilate, atelectasis can start to develop within an hour.)
- Record how effectively the patient performs the therapy and the number of breaths achieved with the spirometer every 2 hours.

Nursing Management

Nursing management of the patient using incentive spirometry includes placing the patient in the proper position, teaching the technique for using the incentive spirometer, setting realistic goals for the patient, and recording the results of the therapy.

Mini-Nebulizer Therapy

The mini-nebulizer is a handheld apparatus that disperses a moisturizing agent or medication, such as a bronchodilator or mucolytic agent, into microscopic particles and delivers it to the lungs as the patient inhales. The mini-nebulizer is usually air-driven by means of a compressor through connecting tubing. In some instances, the nebulizer is oxygen-driven rather than air-driven. To be effective, a visible mist must be available for the patient to inhale.

Indications

The indications for use of a mini-nebulizer include difficulty in clearing respiratory secretions, reduced vital capacity with ineffective deep breathing and coughing, and unsuccessful trials of simpler and less costly methods for clearing secretions, delivering aerosol, or expanding the lungs. The patient must be able to generate a deep breath. Diaphragmatic breathing (Chart 25-4) is a helpful technique to prepare for proper use of the mini-nebulizer. Mini-nebulizers are frequently used for patients with COPD to dispense inhaled medications, and they are commonly used at home on a long-term basis.

Nursing Management

Promoting Home and Community-Based Care

TEACHING PATIENTS SELF-CARE

The nurse instructs the patient to breathe through the mouth, taking slow, deep breaths, and then to hold the breath for a few seconds at the end of inspiration to increase intrapleural pressure and reopen collapsed alveoli, thereby increasing functional residual capacity. The nurse encourages the patient to cough and to monitor the effectiveness of the therapy. The nurse instructs the patient and family about the purpose of the treatment, equipment setup, medication additive, and proper cleaning and storage of the equipment.

Intermittent Positive-Pressure Breathing

Intermittent positive-pressure breathing (IPPB) is an older form of assisted or controlled respiration in which compressed gas is delivered under positive pressure into a person's airways until a preset pressure is reached. Passive exhalation is allowed through a valve.

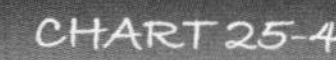

CHART 25-4

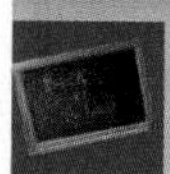

Patient Education

Breathing Exercises

GENERAL INSTRUCTIONS

- Breathe slowly and rhythmically to exhale completely and empty the lungs completely.
- Inhale through the nose to filter, humidify, and warm the air before it enters the lungs.
- If you feel out of breath, breathe more slowly by prolonging the exhalation time.
- Keep the air moist with a humidifier.

DIAPHRAGMATIC BREATHING

Goal: To use and strengthen the diaphragm during breathing

- Place one hand on the abdomen (just below the ribs) and the other hand on the middle of the chest to increase the awareness of the position of the diaphragm and its function in breathing.
- Breathe in slowly and deeply through the nose, letting the abdomen protrude as far as possible.
- Breathe out through pursed lips while tightening (contracting) the abdominal muscles.
- Press firmly inward and upward on the abdomen while breathing out.
- Repeat for 1 minute; follow with a rest period of 2 minutes.
- Gradually increase duration up to 5 minutes, several times a day (before meals and at bedtime).

PURSED-LIP BREATHING

Goal: To prolong exhalation and increase airway pressure during expiration, thus reducing the amount of trapped air and the amount of airway resistance.

- Inhale through the nose while slowly counting to 3—the amount of time needed to say "Smell a rose."
- Exhale slowly and evenly against pursed lips while tightening the abdominal muscles. (Pursing the lips increases intratracheal pressure; exhaling through the mouth offers less resistance to expired air.)
- Count to 7 slowly while prolonging expiration through pursed lips—the length of time to say "Blow out the candle."
- While sitting in a chair:
  Fold arms over the abdomen.
  Inhale through the nose while counting to 3 slowly.
  Bend forward and exhale slowly through pursed lips while counting to 7 slowly.
- While walking:
  Inhale while walking two steps.
  Exhale through pursed lips while walking four or five steps.

Indications

IPPB is indicated for patients who need to increase lung expansion. Although it has been used to administer aerosolized medications, spontaneous inhalation of medications using a metered-dose inhaler or a nebulizer is equally effective (Kacmarek et al., 2005).

Complications

IPPB therapy is used rarely today because of its inherent hazards, which include pneumothorax, mucosal drying, increased intracranial pressure (ICP), hemoptysis, gastric distention, vomiting with possible aspiration, psychological dependency (especially with long-term use, as in patients with COPD), hyperventilation, excessive oxygen administration, and cardiovascular problems.

Chest Physiotherapy

Chest physiotherapy (CPT) includes **postural drainage**, **chest percussion** and **vibration**, and breathing retraining. In addition, teaching the patient effective coughing technique is an important part of CPT. The goals of CPT are to remove bronchial secretions, improve ventilation, and increase the efficiency of the respiratory muscles.

Postural Drainage (Segmented Bronchial Drainage)

Postural drainage uses specific positions that allow the force of gravity to assist in the removal of bronchial secretions. The secretions drain from the affected bronchioles into the bronchi and trachea and are removed by coughing or suctioning. Postural drainage is used to prevent or relieve bronchial obstruction caused by accumulation of secretions.

Because the patient usually sits in an upright position, secretions are likely to accumulate in the lower parts of the lungs. With postural drainage, different positions (Fig. 25-3) are used so that the force of gravity helps move secretions from the smaller bronchial airways to the main bronchi and trachea. The secretions then are removed by coughing. The nurse instructs the patient to inhale bronchodilators and mucolytic agents, if prescribed, before postural drainage, because these medications improve drainage of the bronchial tree.

Postural drainage exercises can be directed at any of the segments of the lungs. The lower and middle lobe bronchi drain more effectively when the head is down; the upper lobe bronchi drain more effectively when the head is up. Frequently, five positions are used, one for drainage of each lobe: head down, prone, right and left lateral, and sitting upright.

Nursing Management

The nurse should be aware of the patient's diagnosis as well as the lung lobes or segments involved, the cardiac status, and any structural deformities of the chest wall and spine. Auscultating the chest before and after the procedure helps identify the areas needing drainage and assess the effectiveness of treatment. The nurse teaches family members who will be assisting the patient at home to evaluate breath sounds before and after treatment. The nurse explores strategies that will enable the patient to assume the indicated positions at home. This may require the creative use of objects readily available at home, such as pillows, cushions, or cardboard boxes.

Postural drainage is usually performed two to four times daily, before meals (to prevent nausea, vomiting, and aspiration) and at bedtime. Prescribed bronchodilators, water, or saline may be nebulized and inhaled before postural drainage to dilate the bronchioles, reduce bronchospasm, decrease the thickness of mucus and sputum, and combat edema of the bronchial walls. The recommended sequence starts with positions to drain the lower lobes, followed by positions to drain the upper lobes.

The nurse makes the patient as comfortable as possible in each position and provides an emesis basin, sputum cup, and paper tissues. The nurse instructs the patient to remain in each position for 10 to 15 minutes and to breathe in slowly through the nose and out slowly through pursed lips to help keep the airways open so that secretions can drain while in each position. If a position cannot be tolerated, the nurse helps the patient assume a modified position. When the patient changes position, the nurse explains how to cough and remove secretions (Chart 25-5).

If the patient cannot cough, the nurse may need to suction the secretions mechanically. It also may be necessary to use chest percussion and vibration or a high-frequency chest wall oscillation (HFCWO) vest to loosen bronchial secretions and mucus plugs that adhere to the bronchioles and bronchi and to propel sputum in the direction of gravity drainage (see later discussion). If suctioning is required at home, the nurse instructs caregivers in safe suctioning technique and care of the suctioning equipment.

After the procedure, the nurse notes the amount, color, viscosity, and character of the expelled sputum. It is important to evaluate the patient's skin color and pulse the first few times the procedure is performed. It may be necessary to administer oxygen during postural drainage.

If the sputum is foul-smelling, it is important to perform postural drainage in a room away from other patients or family members. (Deodorizers may be used to counteract the odor, but aerosol sprays can cause bronchospasm and irritation; therefore, they should be used sparingly and with caution.) After the procedure, the patient may find it refreshing to brush the teeth and use a mouthwash before resting.

Chest Percussion and Vibration

Thick secretions that are difficult to cough up may be loosened by tapping (percussing) and vibrating the chest or through use of an HFCWO vest. Chest percussion and vibration help dislodge mucus adhering to the bronchioles and bronchi.

Percussion is carried out by cupping the hands and lightly striking the chest wall in a rhythmic fashion over the lung segment to be drained. The wrists are alternately flexed and extended so that the chest is cupped or clapped in a painless manner (Fig. 25-4). A soft cloth or towel may be placed over the segment of the chest that is being cupped to prevent skin irritation and redness from direct contact.

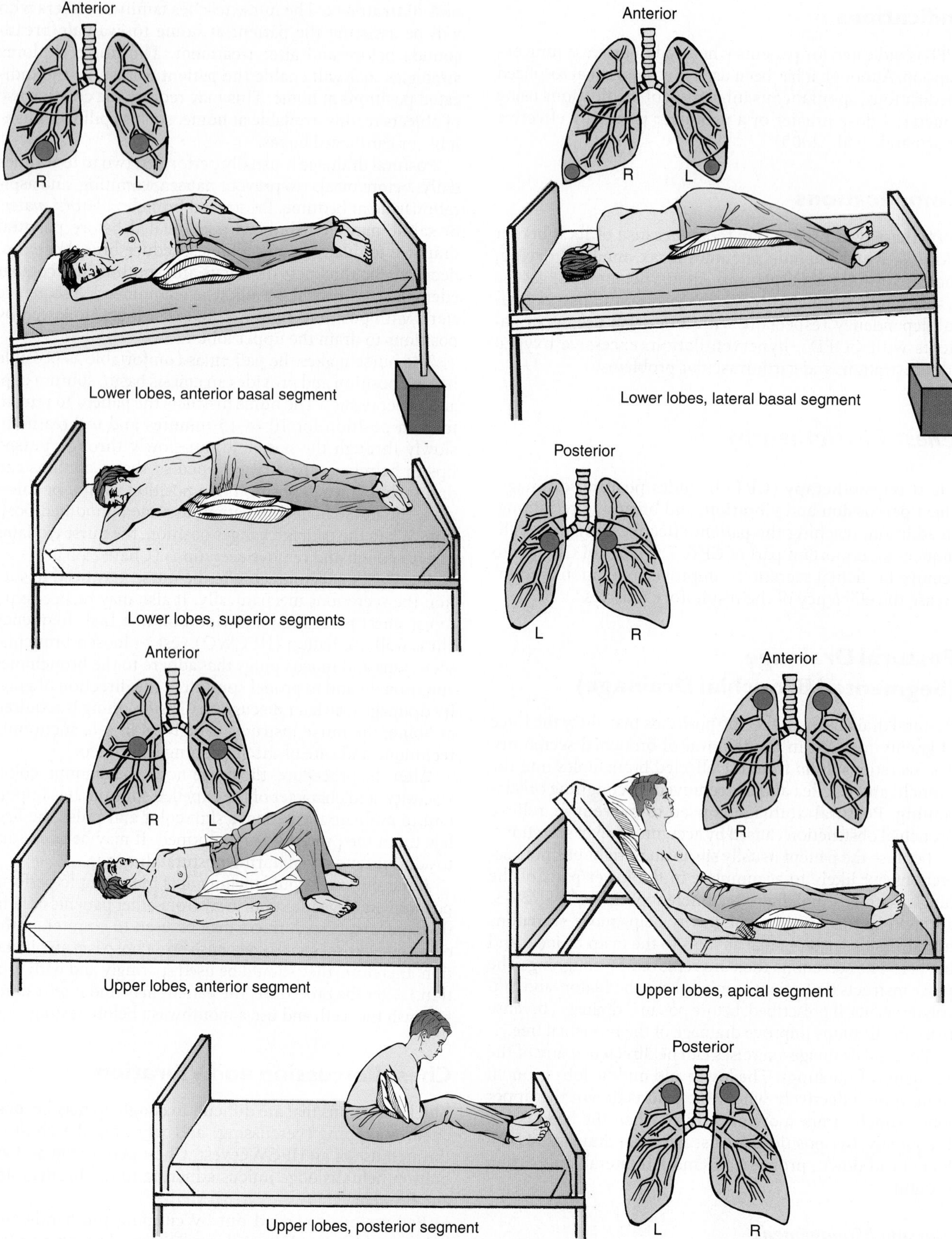

FIGURE 25-3. Postural drainage positions and the areas of lung drained by each position.

CHART 25-5

Effective Coughing Technique

1. The patient assumes a sitting position and bends slightly forward. This upright position permits a stronger cough.
2. The patient's knees and hips are flexed to promote relaxation and reduce the strain on the abdominal muscles while coughing.
3. The patient inhales slowly through the nose and exhales through pursed lips several times.
4. The patient should cough twice during each exhalation while contracting (pulling in) the abdomen sharply with each cough.
5. The patient splints the incisional area, if any, with firm hand pressure or supports it with a pillow or rolled blanket while coughing (see Fig. 25-12). (The nurse can initially demonstrate this by using the patient's hands.)

Percussion, alternating with vibration, is performed for 3 to 5 minutes for each position. The patient uses diaphragmatic breathing during this procedure to promote relaxation (see later discussion). As a precaution, percussion over chest drainage tubes, the sternum, spine, liver, kidneys, spleen, or breasts (in women) is avoided. Percussion is performed cautiously in the elderly because of their increased incidence of osteoporosis and risk of rib fracture.

Vibration is the technique of applying manual compression and tremor to the chest wall during the exhalation phase of respiration (see Fig. 25-4). This helps increase the velocity of the air expired from the small airways, thus freeing the mucus. After three or four vibrations, the patient is encouraged to cough, using the abdominal muscles. (Contracting the abdominal muscles increases the effectiveness of the cough.)

An inflatable HFCWO vest (Fig. 25-5) may be used to provide chest therapy. The vest uses air pulses to compress the chest wall 8 to 18 times/second, causing secretions to detach from the airway wall, enabling the patient to expel them by coughing. Vest therapy is considered more effective than manual percussion because it is more gentle and acts on all lobes of the lung simultaneously (Oermann, Sockrider, Giles, et al., 2001).

A scheduled program of coughing and clearing sputum, together with hydration, reduces the amount of sputum in most patients. The number of times the percussion and coughing cycle is repeated depends on the patient's tolerance and clinical response. It is important to evaluate breath sounds before and after the procedures.

To increase the effectiveness of coughing, a flutter valve is sometimes used, especially by people who have cystic fibrosis. The flutter valve looks like a pipe but has a cap covering the bowl, which contains a steel ball. When the patient exhales actively into the valve, movement of the ball causes pressure oscillations, thereby decreasing mucus viscosity, allowing it to move within the airways and be coughed out.

Nursing Management

When performing CPT, the nurse ensures that the patient is comfortable, is not wearing restrictive clothing, and has not just eaten. The uppermost areas of the lung are treated first. The nurse gives medication for pain, as prescribed, before percussion and vibration and splints any incision and provides pillows for support as needed. The positions are varied, but focus is placed on the affected areas. On completion of the treatment, the nurse assists the patient to assume a comfortable position.

If an HFCWO vest is being used, the patient may assume whatever position is most comfortable and may even continue to perform light activity during therapy within the length of the compressed air hose. It is not necessary for the patient to assume specific positions for the vest to be effective.

The nurse must stop treatment if any of the following occur: increased pain, increased shortness of breath, weakness, lightheadedness, or hemoptysis. Therapy is indicated

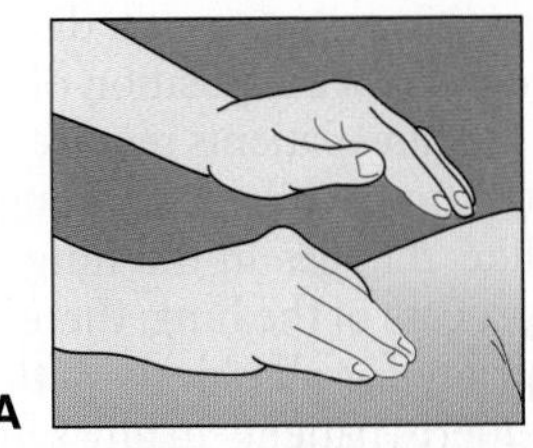

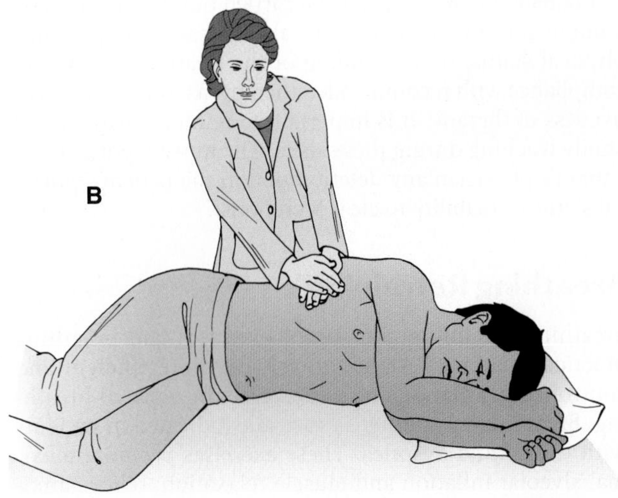

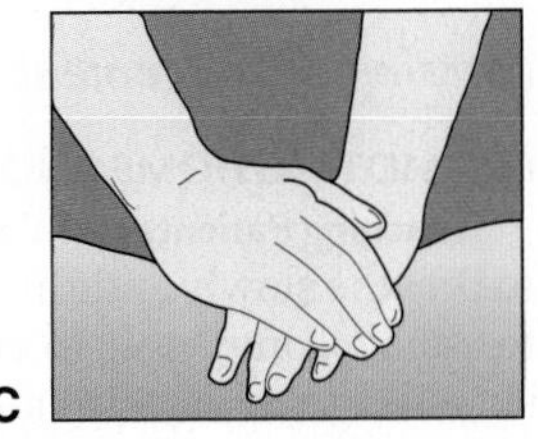

FIGURE 25-4. Percussion and vibration. (**A**) Proper hand position for percussion. (**B**) Proper technique for vibration. The wrists and elbows remain stiff; the vibrating motion is produced by the shoulder muscles. (**C**) Proper hand position for vibration.

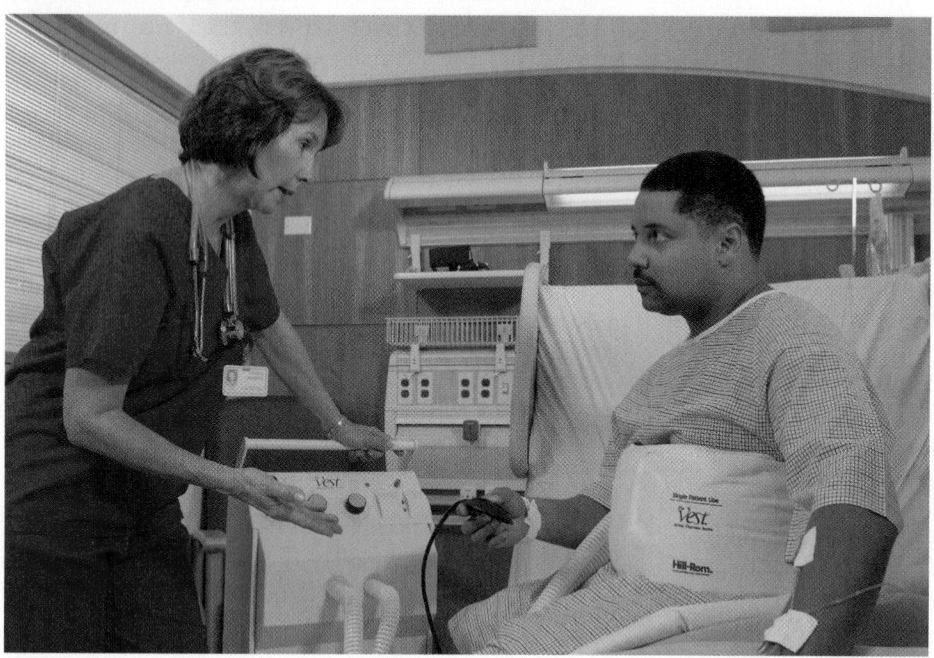

FIGURE 25-5. High-frequency chest wall oscillation vest. © 2005 Hill-Rom Services, Inc. Reprinted with permission—all rights reserved.

until the patient has normal respirations, can mobilize secretions, and has normal breath sounds, and until the chest x-ray findings are normal.

PROMOTING HOME AND COMMUNITY-BASED CARE

Teaching Patients Self-Care. CPT is frequently indicated at home for patients with COPD, bronchiectasis, or cystic fibrosis. The techniques are the same as described previously, but gravity drainage is achieved by placing the hips over a box, a stack of magazines, or pillows (unless a hospital bed is available). The nurse instructs the patient and family in the positions and techniques of percussion and vibration so that therapy can be continued in the home. In addition, the nurse instructs the patient to maintain an adequate fluid intake and air humidity to prevent secretions from becoming thick and tenacious. It also is important to teach the patient to recognize early signs of infection, such as fever and a change in the color or character of sputum. Resting 5 to 10 minutes in each postural drainage position before CPT maximizes the amount of secretions obtained.

Continuing Care. CPT may be carried out during visits by a home care nurse. The nurse also assesses the patient's physical status, understanding of the treatment plan, and compliance with recommended therapy, as well as the effectiveness of therapy. It is important to reinforce patient and family teaching during these visits. The nurse reports to the patient's physician any deterioration in the patient's physical status or inability to clear secretions.

Breathing Retraining

Breathing retraining consists of exercises and breathing practices that are designed to achieve more efficient and controlled ventilation and to decrease the work of breathing. Breathing retraining is especially indicated in patients with COPD and dyspnea. These exercises promote maximal alveolar inflation and muscle relaxation; relieve anxiety; eliminate ineffective, uncoordinated patterns of respiratory muscle activity; slow the respiratory rate; and decrease the work of breathing. Slow, relaxed, and rhythmic breathing also helps to control the anxiety that occurs with dyspnea. Specific breathing exercises include diaphragmatic and pursed-lip breathing (see Chart 25-4).

The goal of diaphragmatic breathing is to use and strengthen the diaphragm during breathing. Diaphragmatic breathing can become automatic with sufficient practice and concentration. Pursed-lip breathing, which improves oxygen transport, helps induce a slow, deep breathing pattern and assists the patient to control breathing, even during periods of stress. This type of breathing helps prevent airway collapse secondary to loss of lung elasticity in emphysema. The goal of pursed-lip breathing is to train the expiratory muscles to prolong exhalation and increase airway pressure during expiration, thus lessening the amount of airway trapping and resistance. The nurse instructs the patient in diaphragmatic breathing and pursed-lip breathing, as described earlier in Chart 25-4. Breathing exercises may be practiced in several positions, because air distribution and pulmonary circulation vary with the position of the chest.

Many patients require additional oxygen, using a low-flow method, while performing breathing exercises. Emphysema-like changes in the lung occur as part of the natural aging process of the lung; therefore, breathing exercises are appropriate for all elderly patients who are hospitalized and for elderly patients in any setting who are sedentary, even without primary lung disease.

Nursing Management

PROMOTING HOME AND COMMUNITY-BASED CARE

Teaching Patients Self-Care. The nurse instructs the patient to breathe slowly and rhythmically in a relaxed manner and to exhale completely to empty the lungs. The patient is instructed to always inhale through the nose because this filters, humidifies, and warms the air. If short of breath, the patient should concentrate on breathing slowly and rhythmically. To avoid initiating a cycle of increasing shortness of breath and panic, it is often helpful to instruct the patient to concentrate on prolonging the length of exhalation rather than merely slowing the rate of breathing. Minimizing the amount of dust or particles in the air and providing adequate humidification may also make it easier for the patient to breathe. Strategies to decrease dust or particles in the air include removing drapes and upholstered furniture, using air filters, and washing floors, dusting, and vacuuming frequently.

The nurse instructs the patient that an adequate dietary intake promotes gas exchange and increases energy levels. It is important to provide adequate nutrition without overfeeding the patient. The nurse teaches the patient to consume small, frequent meals and snacks. Having ready-prepared meals and favorite foods available helps encourage nutrient consumption. Gas-producing foods such as beans, legumes, broccoli, cabbage, and Brussels sprouts should be avoided to prevent gastric distress. Because many of these patients lack the energy to eat, they should be taught to rest before and after meals to conserve energy.

Airway Management

Adequate ventilation is dependent on free movement of air through the upper and lower airways. In many disorders, the airway becomes narrowed or blocked as a result of disease, bronchoconstriction (narrowing of airway by contraction of muscle fibers), a foreign body, or secretions. Maintaining a patent (open) airway is achieved through meticulous airway management, whether in an emergency situation such as airway obstruction or in long-term management, as in caring for a patient with an endotracheal or a tracheostomy tube.

Emergency Management of Upper Airway Obstruction

Upper airway obstruction has a variety of causes. Acute upper airway obstruction may be caused by food particles, vomitus, blood clots, or any other particle that enters and obstructs the larynx or trachea. It also may occur from enlargement of tissue in the wall of the airway, as in epiglottitis, obstructive sleep apnea, laryngeal edema, laryngeal carcinoma, or peritonsillar abscess, or from thick secretions. Pressure on the walls of the airway, as occurs in retrosternal goiter, enlarged mediastinal lymph nodes, hematoma around the upper airway, and thoracic aneurysm, also may result in upper airway obstruction.

The patient with an altered level of consciousness from any cause is at risk for upper airway obstruction because of loss of the protective reflexes (cough and swallowing) and loss of the tone of the pharyngeal muscles, which causes the tongue to fall back and block the airway.

The nurse makes the following rapid observations to assess for signs and symptoms of upper airway obstruction:

- Inspection: Is the patient conscious? Is there any inspiratory effort? Does the chest rise symmetrically? Is there use or retraction of accessory muscles? What is the skin color? Are there any obvious signs of deformity or obstruction (trauma, food, teeth, vomitus)? Is the trachea midline?
- Palpation: Do both sides of the chest rise equally with inspiration? Are there any specific areas of tenderness, fracture, or subcutaneous emphysema (crepitus)?
- Auscultation: Is there any audible air movement, stridor (inspiratory sound), or wheezing (expiratory sound)? Are breath sounds present over the lower trachea and bilaterally in all lobes?

As soon as an upper airway obstruction is identified, the nurse takes emergency measures (Chart 25-6). (See Chapter 71 for more details on managing a foreign body airway obstruction, or see Chapter 22.)

Endotracheal Intubation

Endotracheal intubation involves passing an endotracheal tube through the mouth or nose into the trachea (Fig. 25-6). Intubation provides a patent airway when the patient is having respiratory distress that cannot be treated with simpler methods. It is the method of choice in emergency care. Endotracheal intubation is a means of providing an airway for patients who cannot maintain an adequate airway on their own (eg, comatose patients, patients with upper airway obstruction), for patients needing mechanical ventilation, and for suctioning secretions from the pulmonary tree.

An endotracheal tube usually is passed with the aid of a laryngoscope by specifically trained medical, nursing, or respiratory therapy personnel (see Chapter 71). Once the tube is inserted, a cuff is inflated to prevent air from leaking around the outer part of the tube, to minimize the possibility of subsequent aspiration, and to prevent movement of the tube.

The nurse should be aware that complications could occur from pressure exerted by the cuff on the tracheal wall. Cuff pressures should be checked with a calibrated aneroid manometer device every 6 to 8 hours to maintain cuff pressure between 15 and 20 mm Hg (Morton, Fontaine, Hudak, et al., 2005). High cuff pressure can cause tracheal bleeding, ischemia, and pressure necrosis, whereas low cuff pressure can increase the risk for aspiration pneumonia. Routine deflation of the cuff is not recommended because of the increased risk for aspiration and hypoxia. The cuff is deflated before the endotracheal tube is removed. Tracheobronchial secretions are suctioned through the tube. Warmed, humidified oxygen should always be introduced through the tube, whether the patient is breathing spontaneously or is receiving ventilatory support. Endotracheal intubation may be used for no longer than 3 weeks, by which time a tracheostomy must be considered to decrease irritation of and trauma to the tracheal lining, to reduce the incidence of vocal cord paralysis (secondary to laryngeal nerve damage), and to decrease the work of breathing. Chart 25-7 discusses the nursing care of the patient with an endotracheal tube.

Endotracheal and tracheostomy tubes have several disadvantages. The tubes cause discomfort. The cough reflex is depressed because closure of the glottis is hindered.

CHART 25-6

Clearing an Upper Airway Obstruction

CLEARING THE AIRWAY

- Hyperextend the patient's neck by placing one hand on the forehead and placing the fingers of the other hand underneath the jaw and lifting upward and forward. This action pulls the tongue away from the back of the pharynx.

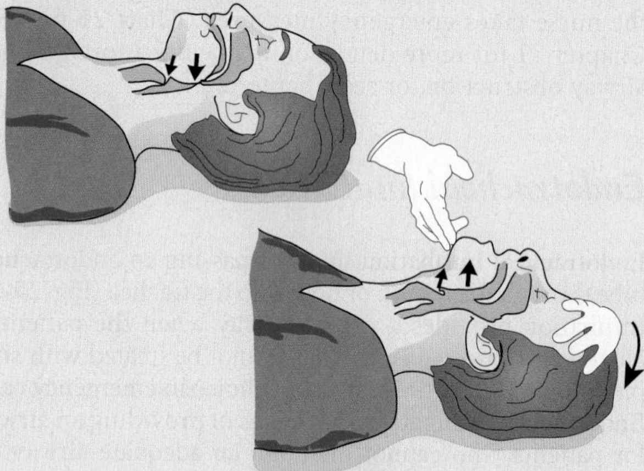

Opening the airway.

- Assess the patient by observing the chest and listening and feeling for the movement of air.
- Use a cross-finger technique to open the mouth and observe for obvious obstructions such as secretions, blood clots, or food particles.
- If no passage of air is detected, apply five quick sharp abdominal thrusts just below the xiphoid process to expel the obstruction. Repeat this procedure until the obstruction is expelled.
- After the obstruction is expelled, roll the patient as a unit onto the side for recovery.
- When the obstruction is relieved, if the patient can breathe spontaneously but not cough, swallow, or gag, insert an oral or nasopharyngeal airway.

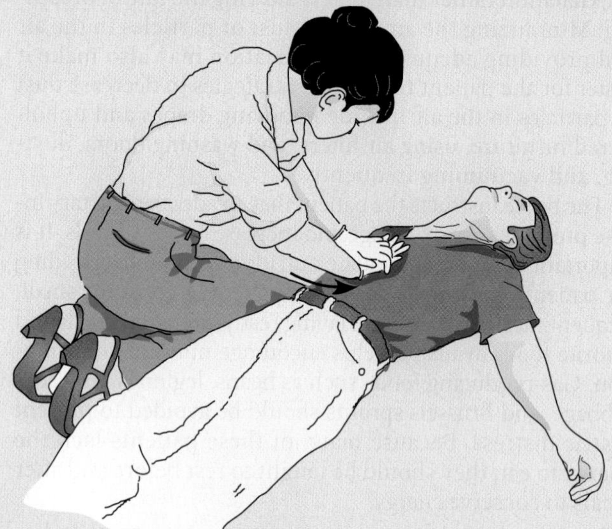

Abdominal thrust (Heimlich) maneuver administered to unconscious patient.

BAG AND MASK RESUSCITATION

- Use a resuscitation bag and mask if assisted ventilation is required.
- Apply the mask to the patient's face and create a seal by pressing the thumb of the nondominant hand on the bridge of the nose and the index finger on the chin. Using the rest of the fingers on that hand, pull on the chin and the angle of the mandible to maintain the head in extension. Use the dominant hand to inflate the lungs by squeezing the bag to its full volume.

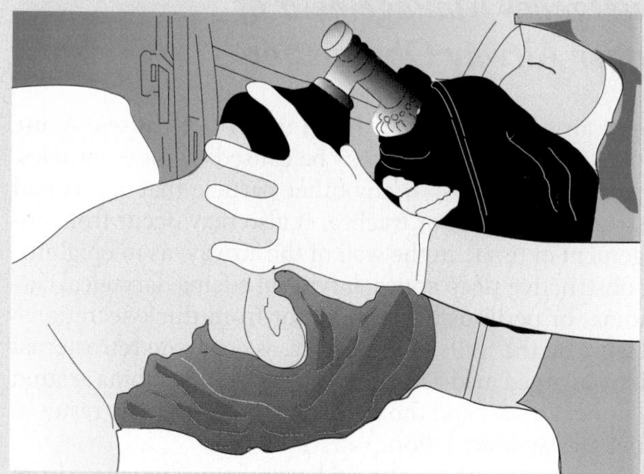

Resuscitation via bag and mask apparatus.

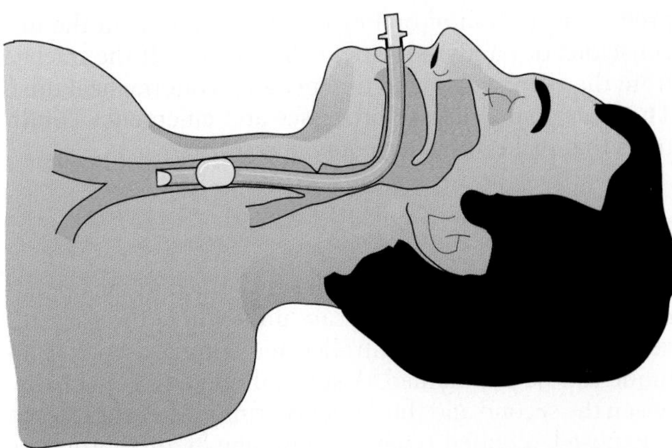

FIGURE 25-6. Endotracheal tube in place. The tube has been inserted using the oral route. The cuff has been inflated to maintain the tube's position and to minimize the risk of aspiration.

Secretions tend to become thicker because the warming and humidifying effect of the upper respiratory tract has been bypassed. The swallowing reflexes, composed of the glottic, pharyngeal, and laryngeal reflexes, are depressed because of prolonged disuse and the mechanical trauma produced by the endotracheal or tracheostomy tube, increasing the risk of aspiration. In addition, ulceration and stricture of the larynx or trachea may develop. Of great concern to the patient is the inability to talk and to communicate needs.

Unintentional or premature removal of the tube is a potentially life-threatening complication of endotracheal intubation. Removal of the tube is a frequent problem in intensive care units and occurs mainly during nursing care or by the patient. It is important that nurses instruct patients and family members about the purpose of the tube and the dangers of removing it. Baseline and ongoing assessment of the patient and of the equipment ensures effective care. Providing comfort measures, including opioid analgesia and sedation, can improve the patient's tolerance of the endotracheal tube.

CHART 25-7

Care of the Patient With an Endotracheal Tube

IMMEDIATELY AFTER INTUBATION

1. Check symmetry of chest expansion.
   a. Auscultate breath sounds of anterior and lateral chest bilaterally.
   b. Obtain order for chest x-ray to verify proper tube placement.
   c. Check cuff pressure every 8–12 hours.
   d. Monitor for signs and symptoms of aspiration.
2. Ensure high humidity; a visible mist should appear in the T-piece or ventilator tubing.
3. Administer oxygen concentration as prescribed by physician.
4. Secure the tube to the patient's face with tape, and mark the proximal end for position maintenance.
   a. Cut proximal end of tube if it is longer than 7.5 cm (3 inches) to prevent kinking.
   b. Insert an oral airway or mouth device to prevent the patient from biting and obstructing the tube.
5. Use sterile suction technique and airway care to prevent iatrogenic contamination and infection.
6. Continue to reposition patient every 2 hours and as needed to prevent atelectasis and to optimize lung expansion.
7. Provide oral hygiene and suction the oropharynx whenever necessary.

EXTUBATION (REMOVAL OF ENDOTRACHEAL TUBE)

1. Explain procedure.
2. Have self-inflating bag and mask ready in case ventilatory assistance is required immediately after extubation.
3. Suction the tracheobronchial tree and oropharynx, remove tape, and then deflate the cuff.
4. Give 100% oxygen for a few breaths, then insert a new, sterile suction catheter inside tube.
5. Have the patient inhale. At peak inspiration remove the tube, suctioning the airway through the tube as it is pulled out.

Note: In some hospitals this procedure can be performed by respiratory therapists; in others, by nurses. Check hospital policy.

CARE OF PATIENT FOLLOWING EXTUBATION

1. Give heated humidity and oxygen by face mask and maintain the patient in a sitting or high Fowler's position.
2. Monitor respiratory rate and quality of chest excursions. Note stridor, color change, and change in mental alertness or behavior.
3. Monitor the patient's oxygen level using a pulse oximeter.
4. Keep NPO or give only ice chips for next few hours.
5. Provide mouth care.
6. Teach patient how to perform coughing and deep-breathing exercises.

NURSING ALERT

Inadvertent removal of an endotracheal tube can cause laryngeal swelling, hypoxemia, bradycardia, hypotension, and even death. Measures must be taken to prevent premature or inadvertent removal.

To prevent tube removal by the patient, the nurse can use the following strategies: explain to the patient and family the purpose of the tube, distract the patient through one-to-one interaction with the nurse and family or with television, and maintain comfort measures. As a last resort, soft wrist restraints may be used. Discretion and caution must always be used before applying any restraint. If the patient cannot move the arms and hands to the endotracheal tube, restraints are not needed. If the patient is alert, oriented, able to follow directions, and cooperative to the point that it is highly unlikely that he or she will remove the endotracheal tube, restraints are not needed. However, if the nurse determines there is a risk that the patient may try to remove the tube, soft wrist restraints are appropriate with a physician's order (check agency policy). Close monitoring of the patient is essential to ensure safety and prevent harm.

Tracheostomy

A **tracheotomy** is a surgical procedure in which an opening is made into the trachea. The indwelling tube inserted into the trachea is called a **tracheostomy tube.** A tracheostomy may be either temporary or permanent (Fig. 25-7).

A tracheostomy is used to bypass an upper airway obstruction, to allow removal of tracheobronchial secretions, to permit the long-term use of mechanical ventilation, to prevent aspiration of oral or gastric secretions in the unconscious or paralyzed patient (by closing off the trachea from the esophagus), and to replace an endotracheal tube. There are many disease processes and emergency conditions that make a tracheostomy necessary.

Procedure

The surgical procedure is usually performed in the operating room or in an intensive care unit, where the patient's ventilation can be well controlled and optimal aseptic technique can be maintained. A surgical opening is made between the second and third tracheal rings. After the trachea is exposed, a cuffed tracheostomy tube of an appropriate size is inserted. The cuff is an inflatable attachment to the tracheostomy tube that is designed to occlude the space between the tracheal walls and the tube, to permit effective mechanical ventilation and to minimize the risk of aspiration. See Figure 25-7 for types of tracheostomy tubes.

The tracheostomy tube is held in place by tapes fastened around the patient's neck. Usually a square of sterile gauze is placed between the tube and the skin to absorb drainage and reduce the risk for infection.

Complications

Complications may occur early or late in the course of tracheostomy tube management. They may even occur years after the tube has been removed. Early complications include bleeding, pneumothorax, air embolism, aspiration, subcutaneous or mediastinal emphysema, recurrent laryngeal nerve damage, and posterior tracheal wall penetration. Long-term complications include airway obstruction from accumulation of secretions or protrusion of the cuff over the opening of the tube, infection, rupture of the innominate artery, dysphagia, tracheoesophageal fistula, tracheal dilation, and tracheal ischemia and necrosis. Tracheal

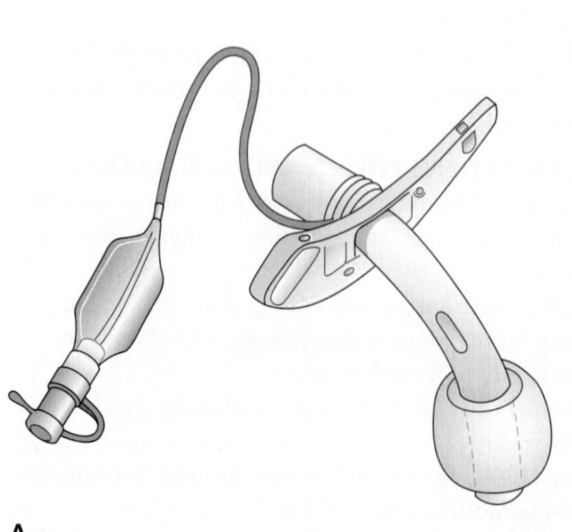

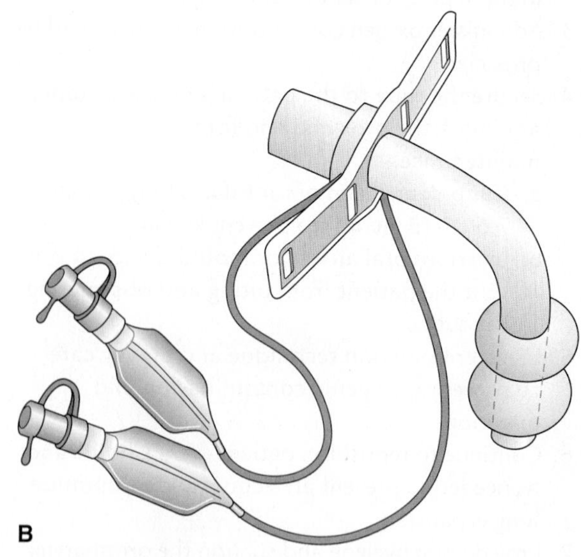

FIGURE 25-7. Tracheostomy tubes. (**A**) Fenestrated tube, which allows patient to talk. (**B**) Double-cuffed tube. Inflating the two cuffs alternately can help prevent tracheal damage. Courtesy of Smiths Medical, Keene, NH.

stenosis may develop after the tube is removed. Chart 25-8 outlines measures nurses can take to prevent complications.

Nursing Management

The patient requires continuous monitoring and assessment. The newly made opening must be kept patent by proper suctioning of secretions. After the vital signs are stable, the patient is placed in a semi-Fowler's position to facilitate ventilation, promote drainage, minimize edema, and prevent strain on the suture lines. Analgesia and sedative agents must be administered with caution because of the risk of suppressing the cough reflex.

Major objectives of nursing care are to alleviate the patient's apprehension and to provide an effective means of communication. The nurse keeps paper and pencil or a Magic Slate and the call light within the patient's reach at all times to ensure a means of communication. The care of the patient with a tracheostomy tube is summarized in Chart 25-9.

Suctioning the Tracheal Tube (Tracheostomy or Endotracheal Tube)

When a tracheostomy or endotracheal tube is in place, it is usually necessary to suction the patient's secretions because of the decreased effectiveness of the cough mechanism. Tracheal suctioning is performed when adventitious breath sounds are detected or whenever secretions are obviously present. Unnecessary suctioning can initiate bronchospasm and cause mechanical trauma to the tracheal mucosa.

All equipment that comes into direct contact with the patient's lower airway must be sterile to prevent overwhelming pulmonary and systemic infections. The procedure for suctioning a tracheostomy is presented in Chart 25-10. In mechanically ventilated patients, an in-line suction catheter may be used to allow rapid suction when needed and to minimize cross-contamination by airborne pathogens. An in-line suction device allows the patient to be suctioned without being disconnected from the ventilator circuit.

Managing the Cuff

As a general rule, the cuff on an endotracheal or tracheostomy tube should be inflated. The pressure within the cuff should be the lowest possible pressure that allows delivery of adequate tidal volumes and prevents pulmonary aspiration. Usually the pressure is maintained at less than 25 mm Hg to prevent injury and at more than 15 mm Hg to prevent aspiration. Cuff pressure must be monitored at least every 8 hours by attaching a handheld pressure gauge to the pilot balloon of the tube or by using the minimal leak volume or minimal occlusion volume technique. With long-term intubation, higher pressures may be needed to maintain an adequate seal.

Promoting Home and Community-Based Care

TEACHING PATIENTS SELF-CARE

If the patient is at home with a tracheostomy, the nurse instructs the patient and family about daily care, including techniques to prevent infection, as well as measures to take in an emergency. The nurse provides the patient and family with a list of community contacts for education and support needs.

CONTINUING CARE

A referral for home care is indicated for ongoing assessment of the patient and of the ability of the patient and family to provide appropriate and safe care. The home care nurse assesses the patient's and family's ability to cope with the physical changes and psychological issues associated with having a tracheostomy. The nurse also identifies resources and makes referrals for appropriate services to assist the patient and family to manage the tracheostomy at home.

CHART 25-8

Preventing Complications Associated With Endotracheal and Tracheostomy Tubes

- Administer adequate warmed humidity.
- Maintain cuff pressure at appropriate level.
- Suction as needed per assessment findings.
- Maintain skin integrity. Change tape and dressing as needed or per protocol.
- Auscultate lung sounds.
- Monitor for signs and symptoms of infection, including temperature and white blood cell count.
- Administer prescribed oxygen and monitor oxygen saturation.
- Monitor for cyanosis.
- Maintain adequate hydration of the patient.
- Use sterile technique when suctioning and performing tracheostomy care.

Mechanical Ventilation

Mechanical ventilation may be required for a variety of reasons: to control the patient's respirations during surgery or during treatment of severe head injury, to oxygenate the blood when the patient's ventilatory efforts are inadequate, and to rest the respiratory muscles, among others. Many patients placed on a ventilator can breathe spontaneously, but the effort needed to do so may be exhausting.

A mechanical ventilator is a positive- or negative-pressure breathing device that can maintain ventilation and oxygen delivery for a prolonged period. Caring for a patient on mechanical ventilation has become an integral part of nursing care in critical care or general medical-surgical units, extended care facilities, and the home. Nurses, physicians, and respiratory therapists must understand each patient's specific pulmonary needs and work together to set realistic goals. Positive patient outcomes depend on an understanding of the principles of mechanical ventilation and the patient's care needs as well as open communication among members of the health care team about the goals of therapy, weaning plans, and the patient's tolerance of changes in ventilator settings.

CHART 25-9 Guidelines for Care of the Patient With a Tracheostomy Tube

ACTIONS	RATIONALE
1. Gather the needed equipment, including sterile gloves, hydrogen peroxide, normal saline solution or sterile water, cotton-tipped applicators, dressing and twill tape (and the type of tube prescribed, if the tube is to be changed).	Everything needed to care for a tracheostomy should be readily on hand for the most effective care.
A cuffed tube (air injected into cuff) is required during mechanical ventilation. A low-pressure cuff is most commonly used.	A cuffed tube prevents air from leaking during positive-pressure ventilation and also prevents tracheal aspiration of gastric contents. An adequate seal is indicated by the disappearance of any air leakage from the mouth or tracheostomy or by the disappearance of the harsh, gurgling sound of air coming from the throat.
Patients requiring long-term use of a tracheostomy tube and who can breathe spontaneously commonly use an uncuffed, metal tube.	Low-pressure cuffs exert minimal pressure on the tracheal mucosa and thus reduce the danger of tracheal ulceration and stricture.
2. Provide patient and family instruction on the key points for tracheostomy care, beginning with how to inspect the tracheostomy dressing for moisture or drainage.	The tracheostomy dressing is changed as needed to keep the skin clean and dry. To prevent potential breakdown, moist or soiled dressings should not remain on the skin.
3. Perform hand hygiene.	Hand hygiene reduces bacteria on hands.
4. Explain procedure to patient and family as appropriate.	A patient with a tracheostomy is apprehensive and requires ongoing assurance and support.
5. Put on clean gloves; remove and discard the soiled dressing in a biohazard container.	Observing body substance isolation reduces cross-contamination from soiled dressings.
6. Prepare sterile supplies, including hydrogen peroxide, normal saline solution or sterile water, cotton-tipped applicators, dressing, and tape.	Having necessary supplies and equipment readily available allows the procedure to be completed efficiently.
7. Put on sterile gloves. (Some physicians approve clean technique for long-term tracheostomy patients in the home.)	Sterile equipment minimizes transmission of surface flora to the sterile respiratory tract. Clean technique may be used in the home because of decreased exposure to potential pathogens.
8. Cleanse the wound and the plate of the tracheostomy tube with sterile cotton-tipped applicators moistened with hydrogen peroxide. Rinse with sterile saline solution.	Hydrogen peroxide is effective in loosening crusted secretions. Rinsing prevents skin residue.
9. Soak inner cannula in peroxide or sterile saline, per manufacturer's instructions; rinse with saline solution; and inspect to be sure all dried secretions have been removed. Dry and reinsert inner cannula or replace with a new disposable inner cannula.	Soaking loosens and removes secretions from the inner lumen of the tracheostomy tube. Retained secretions could harbor bacteria, leading to infection. Some plastic tracheostomy tubes may be damaged by using peroxide.
10. Place clean twill tape in position to secure the tracheostomy tube by inserting one end of the tape through the side opening of the outer cannula. Take the tape around the back of the patient's neck and thread it through the opposite opening of the outer cannula. Bring both ends around so that they meet on one side of the neck. Tighten the tape until only two fingers can be comfortably inserted under it. Secure with a knot. For a new tracheostomy, two people should assist with tape changes. Remove soiled twill tape after the new tape is in place.	This taping technique provides a double thickness of tape around the neck, which is needed because the tracheostomy tube can be dislodged by movement or by a forceful cough if left unsecured. A dislodged tracheostomy tube is difficult to reinsert, and respiratory distress may occur. Dislodgement of a new tracheostomy is a medical emergency.

CHART 25-9 Guidelines for Care of the Patient With a Tracheostomy Tube, continued

ACTIONS	RATIONALE
11. Remove old tapes and discard in a biohazard container after the new tape is in place.	Tapes with old secretions may harbor bacteria.
12. Although some long-term tracheostomies with healed stomas may not require a dressing, other tracheostomies do. In such cases, use a sterile tracheostomy dressing, fitting it securely under the twill tapes and flange of tracheostomy tube so that the incision is covered, as shown below.	Healed tracheostomies with minimal secretions do not need a dressing. Dressings that will shred are not used around a tracheostomy because of the risk that pieces of material, lint, or thread may get into the tube, and eventually into the trachea, causing obstruction or abscess formation. Special dressings that do not have a tendency to shred are used.

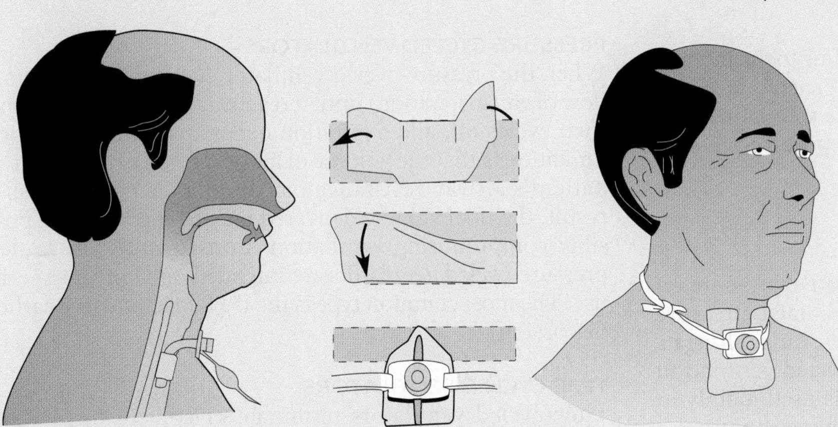

(**A**) The cuff of the tracheostomy tube fits smoothly and snugly in the trachea in a way that promotes circulation but seals off the escape of secretions and air surrounding the tube. (**B**) For a dressing change, a 4 × 4-inch gauze pad may be folded (cutting would promote shredding, placing the patient at risk for aspiration) around the tracheostomy tube and (**C**) stabilized by slipping the neck tape ties through the neck plate slots of the tracheostomy tube. The ties may be fastened to the side of the neck to eliminate the discomfort of lying on the knot.

CHART 25-10 *Performing Tracheal Suction*

EQUIPMENT

- Suction catheters
- Gloves (sterile and nonsterile), gown, mask, and goggles
- Goggles for eye protection
- Basin for sterile normal saline solution for irrigation
- Manual resuscitation bag with supplemental oxygen
- Suction source

PROCEDURE

1. Explain the procedure to the patient before beginning and offer reassurance during suctioning; the patient may be apprehensive about choking and about an inability to communicate.
2. Begin by performing hand hygiene. Put on nonsterile gloves, goggles, gown, and mask.
3. Turn on suction source (pressure should not exceed 120 mm Hg).
4. Open suction catheter kit.
5. Fill basin with sterile normal saline solution.
6. Ventilate the patient with manual resuscitation bag and high-flow oxygen.
7. Put sterile glove on dominant hand.
8. Pick up suction catheter in sterile gloved hand and connect to suction.
9. Hyperoxygenate the patient's lungs for several deep breaths. Instill normal saline solution into airway only if there are thick, tenacious secretions.
10. Insert suction catheter at least as far as the end of the tube without applying suction, just far enough to stimulate the cough reflex.
11. Apply suction while withdrawing and gently rotating the catheter 360° (no longer than 10 to 15 seconds, because hypoxia and dysrhythmias may develop, leading to cardiac arrest).
12. Reoxygenate and inflate the patient's lungs for several breaths.
13. Repeat previous three steps until the airway is clear.
14. Rinse catheter by suctioning a few milliliters of sterile saline solution from the basin between suction attempts.
15. Suction oropharyngeal cavity after completing tracheal suctioning.
16. Rinse suction tubing.
17. Discard catheter, gloves, and basin appropriately.

Indications

If a patient has a continuous decrease in oxygenation (PaO_2), an increase in arterial carbon dioxide levels ($PaCO_2$), and a persistent acidosis (decreased pH), mechanical ventilation may be necessary. Conditions such as thoracic or abdominal surgery, drug overdose, neuromuscular disorders, inhalation injury, COPD, multiple trauma, shock, multisystem failure, and coma all may lead to respiratory failure and the need for mechanical ventilation. The criteria for mechanical ventilation (Chart 25-11) guide the decision to place a patient on a ventilator. A patient with apnea that is not readily reversible also is a candidate for mechanical ventilation.

Classification of Ventilators

Mechanical ventilators are classified according to the method by which they support ventilation. The two general categories are negative-pressure and positive-pressure ventilators. The most common category in use today is the positive-pressure ventilator.

Negative-Pressure Ventilators

Negative-pressure ventilators exert a negative pressure on the external chest. Decreasing the intrathoracic pressure during inspiration allows air to flow into the lung, filling its volume. Physiologically, this type of assisted ventilation is similar to spontaneous ventilation. It is used mainly in chronic respiratory failure associated with neuromuscular conditions, such as poliomyelitis, muscular dystrophy, amyotrophic lateral sclerosis, and myasthenia gravis. It is inappropriate for the patient whose condition is unstable or complex or who requires frequent ventilatory changes. Negative-pressure ventilators are simple to use and do not require intubation of the airway; consequently, they are especially adaptable for home use.

There are several types of negative-pressure ventilators: iron lung, body wrap, and chest cuirass.

IRON LUNG (DRINKER RESPIRATOR TANK). The iron lung is a negative-pressure chamber used for ventilation. It was used extensively during polio epidemics in the past and currently is used by a few polio survivors and patients with other neuromuscular disorders (eg, amyotrophic lateral sclerosis, muscular dystrophy).

BODY WRAP (PNEUMO-WRAP) AND CHEST CUIRASS (TORTOISE SHELL). Both of these portable devices require a rigid cage or shell to create a negative-pressure chamber around the thorax and abdomen. Because of problems with proper fit and system leaks, these types of ventilators are used only with carefully selected patients.

CHART 25-11

Indications for Mechanical Ventilation

$PaO_2 < 50$ mm Hg with $FiO_2 > 0.60$
$PaO_2 > 50$ mm Hg with pH < 7.25
Vital capacity < 2 times tidal volume
Negative inspiratory force < 25 cm H_2O
Respiratory rate > 35/min

Positive-Pressure Ventilators

Positive-pressure ventilators inflate the lungs by exerting positive pressure on the airway, similar to a bellows mechanism, forcing the alveoli to expand during inspiration. Expiration occurs passively. Endotracheal intubation or tracheostomy is necessary in most cases. These ventilators are widely used in the hospital setting and are increasingly used in the home for patients with primary lung disease. There are three types of positive-pressure ventilators, which are classified by the method of ending the inspiratory phase of respiration: pressure-cycled, time-cycled, and volume-cycled. Another type of positive-pressure ventilator used for selected patients is noninvasive positive-pressure ventilation (NIPPV), which does not require intubation.

PRESSURE-CYCLED VENTILATORS

When the pressure-cycled ventilator cycles on, it delivers a flow of air (inspiration) until it reaches a preset pressure, and then cycles off, and expiration occurs passively. Its major limitation is that the volume of air or oxygen can vary as the patient's airway resistance or compliance changes. As a result, the tidal volume delivered may be inconsistent, possibly compromising ventilation. Consequently, in adults, pressure-cycled ventilators are intended only for short-term use. The most common type is the IPPB machine (see earlier discussion).

TIME-CYCLED VENTILATORS

Time-cycled ventilators terminate or control inspiration after a preset time. The volume of air the patient receives is regulated by the length of inspiration and the flow rate of the air. Most ventilators have a rate control that determines the respiratory rate, but pure time-cycling is rarely used for adults. These ventilators are used in newborns and infants.

VOLUME-CYCLED VENTILATORS

Volume-cycled ventilators are by far the most commonly used positive-pressure ventilators today (Fig. 25-8). With this type of ventilator, the volume of air to be delivered with each inspiration is preset. Once this preset volume is delivered to the patient, the ventilator cycles off and exhalation occurs passively. From breath to breath, the volume of air delivered by the ventilator is relatively constant, ensuring consistent, adequate breaths despite varying airway pressures.

NONINVASIVE POSITIVE-PRESSURE VENTILATION

Positive-pressure ventilation can be given via face masks that cover the nose and mouth, nasal masks, or other oral or nasal devices such as the nasal pillow (a small nasal cannula that seals around the nares to maintain the prescribed pressure). NIPPV eliminates the need for endotracheal intubation or tracheostomy and decreases the risk for nosocomial infections such as pneumonia. The most comfortable mode for the patient is pressure-controlled ventilation with pressure support. This eases the work of breathing and enhances gas exchange. The ventilator can be set with a minimum backup rate for patients with periods of apnea.

Patients are considered candidates for noninvasive ventilation if they have acute or chronic respiratory failure, acute pulmonary edema, COPD, chronic heart failure, or a sleep-related breathing disorder. The device also may be used at home to improve tissue oxygenation and to rest the respiratory muscles while the patient sleeps at night. NIPPV is contraindicated for those who have experienced respiratory ar-

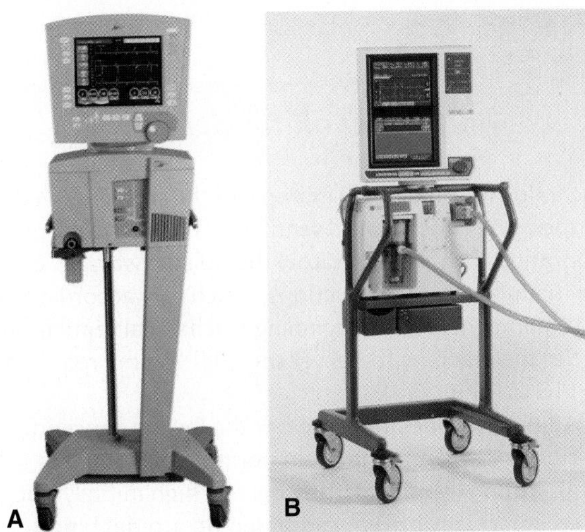

FIGURE 25-8. Positive-pressure ventilators. **(A)** The AVEA can be used to both ventilate and monitor neonatal, pediatric, and adult patients. It can also deliver noninvasive ventilation with Heliox to adult and pediatric patients. Courtesy of VIASYS Healthcare, Inc., Yorba Linda, CA. **(B)** The Puritan-Bennett 840 Ventilator System has volume, pressure, and mixed modes designed for adult, pediatric, and infant ventilation. Courtesy of Tyco Healthcare/Nelicor Puritan Bennett, Pleasanton, CA.

rest, serious dysrhythmias, cognitive impairment, or head or facial trauma. Noninvasive ventilation may also be used for obstructive sleep apnea, for patients at the end of life, and for those who do not want endotracheal intubation but may need short- or long-term ventilatory support.

Continuous positive airway pressure (CPAP) provides positive pressure to the airways throughout the respiratory cycle. Although it can be used as an adjunct to mechanical ventilation with a cuffed endotracheal tube or tracheostomy tube to open the alveoli, it is also used with a leakproof mask to keep alveoli open, thereby preventing respiratory failure. CPAP is the most effective treatment for obstructive sleep apnea, because the positive pressure acts as a splint, keeping the upper airway and trachea open during sleep. To use CPAP, the patient must be breathing independently.

Bilevel positive airway pressure (bi-PAP) ventilation offers independent control of inspiratory and expiratory pressures while providing pressure support ventilation. It delivers two levels of positive airway pressure provided via a nasal or oral mask, nasal pillow, or mouthpiece with a tight seal and a portable ventilator. Each inspiration can be initiated either by the patient or by the machine if it is programmed with a backup rate. The backup rate ensures that the patient will receive a set number of breaths per minute. Bi-PAP is most often used for patients who require ventilatory assistance at night, such as those with severe COPD or sleep apnea. Tolerance is variable; bi-PAP usually is most successful with highly motivated patients.

Ventilator Modes

Ventilator mode refers to how breaths are delivered to the patient. The most commonly used modes are assist–control, intermittent mandatory ventilation, synchronized intermittent mandatory ventilation, pressure support ventilation, and airway pressure release ventilation (Fig. 25-9).

Assist–control ventilation provides full ventilatory support by delivering a preset tidal volume and respiratory rate. If the patient initiates a breath between the machine's breaths, the ventilator delivers at the preset volume (assisted breath). The cycle does not adapt to the patient's spontaneous efforts; every breath is the preset volume.

Intermittent mandatory ventilation (IMV) provides a combination of mechanically assisted breaths and spontaneous breaths. Therefore, the patient can increase the respi-

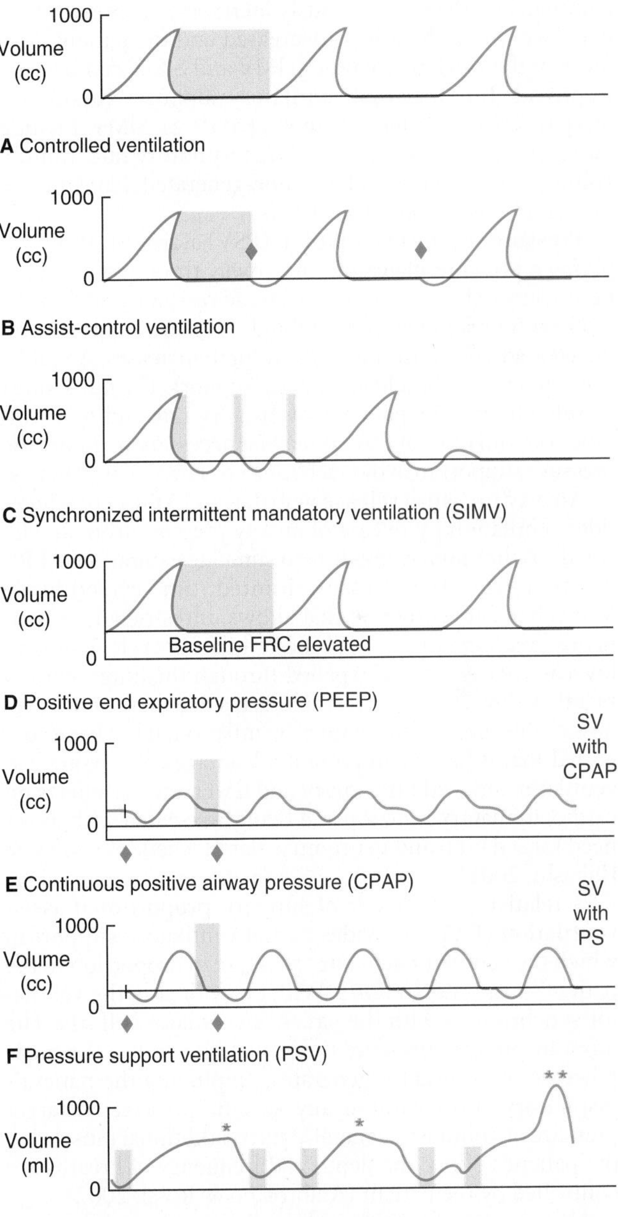

— Inspiration/airflow
Exhalation
♦ Patient-triggered breath
* Spontaneous inspiration on low pressure level
** Spontaneous inspiration on high pressure level

FIGURE 25-9. Modes of mechanical ventilation with airflow waveforms.

ratory rate, but each spontaneous breath is limited to the tidal volume the patient generates. Mechanical breaths are delivered at preset intervals and a preselected tidal volume, regardless of the patient's efforts. IMV allows patients to use their own muscles of ventilation to help prevent muscle atrophy. It lowers mean airway pressure, which can assist in preventing barotrauma. However, bucking the ventilator may be increased.

Synchronized intermittent mandatory ventilation (SIMV) also delivers a preset tidal volume and number of breaths per minute. Between ventilator-delivered breaths, the patient can breathe spontaneously with no assistance from the ventilator on those extra breaths. As the patient's ability to breathe spontaneously increases, the preset number of ventilator breaths is decreased and the patient does more of the work of breathing. IMV and SIMV can be used to provide full or partial ventilatory support. Nursing interventions for patients receiving IMV or SIMV include monitoring progress by recording respiratory rate, minute volume, spontaneous and machine-generated tidal volume, FiO_2, and arterial blood gas levels.

Pressure support ventilation (PSV) assists SIMV by applying a pressure plateau to the airway throughout the patient-triggered inspiration to decrease resistance within the tracheal tube and ventilator tubing. Pressure support is reduced gradually as the patient's strength increases. An SIMV backup rate may be added for extra support. The nurse must closely observe the patient's respiratory rate and tidal volumes on initiation of PSV. It may be necessary to adjust the pressure support to avoid tachypnea or large tidal volumes.

Airway pressure release ventilation (APRV) produces tidal ventilation by release of airway pressure from an elevated baseline airway pressure to simulate expiration. APRV is a time-triggered, pressure-limited, time-cycled mode of mechanical ventilation that allows unrestricted, spontaneous breathing throughout the ventilatory cycle. It also allows alveolar gas to be expelled through the lungs' natural recoil. Although further research is needed on the effectiveness of this mode of mechanical ventilation, it has been suggested that it has the important advantages of causing less ventilator-induced lung injury and fewer adverse effects on cardiocirculatory function and being associated with lower need for sedation and neuromuscular blockade (Frawley & Habashi, 2001).

A relatively new mode of support, **proportional assist ventilation (PAV)**, provides partial ventilatory support in which the ventilator generates pressure in proportion to the patient's inspiratory efforts. With every breath, the ventilator synchronizes with the patient's ventilatory efforts. The more inspiratory pressure the patient generates, the more pressure the ventilator generates, amplifying the patient's inspiratory effort without any specific preselected target pressure or volume. It generally adds "additional muscle" to the patient's effort; the depth and frequency of breaths are controlled by the patient (Ambrosino & Rossi, 2002).

New modes of mechanical ventilation that incorporate computerized control of ventilation are being developed. In some of these modes, the ventilator constantly monitors many variables and adjusts gas delivery during individual breaths; these within-breath adjustment systems include automatic tube compensation, volume-assured pressure support, and proportional support ventilation. In other modes, the ventilator evaluates gas delivery during one breath and uses that information to adjust the next breath; these between-breath adjustment systems can be made to ensure a preset tidal volume by adjusting pressure, up to a preset maximum, and include pressure volume support, pressure-regulated volume control, and adaptive support ventilation.

CHART 25-12

Initial Ventilator Settings

The following guide is an example of the steps involved in operating a mechanical ventilator. The nurse, in collaboration with the respiratory therapist, always reviews the manufacturer's instructions, which vary according to the equipment, before beginning mechanical ventilation.

1. Set the machine to deliver the tidal volume required (10 to 15 mL/kg).
2. Adjust the machine to deliver the lowest concentration of oxygen to maintain normal PaO_2 (80 to 100 mm Hg). This setting may be high initially but will gradually be reduced based on arterial blood gas results.
3. Record peak inspiratory pressure.
4. Set mode (assist–control or synchronized intermittent mandatory ventilation) and rate according to physician order. (See the glossary for definitions of modes of mechanical ventilation.) Set PEEP and pressure support if ordered.
5. Adjust sensitivity so that the patient can trigger the ventilator with a minimal effort (usually 2 mm Hg negative inspiratory force).
6. Record minute volume and obtain ABGs to measure carbon dioxide partial pressure ($PaCO_2$), pH, and PaO_2 after 20 minutes of continuous mechanical ventilation.
7. Adjust setting (FiO_2 and rate) according to results of arterial blood gas analysis to provide normal values or those set by the physician.
8. If the patient suddenly becomes confused or agitated or begins bucking the ventilator for some unexplained reason, assess for hypoxia and manually ventilate on 100% oxygen with a resuscitation bag.

Adjusting the Ventilator

The ventilator is adjusted so that the patient is comfortable and breathes "in sync" with the machine. Minimal alteration of the normal cardiovascular and pulmonary dynamics is desired. Modes of mechanical ventilation are described in Figure 25-9. If the volume ventilator is adjusted appropriately, the patient's arterial blood gas values will be satisfactory and there will be little or no cardiovascular compromise. Chart 25-12 discusses how to achieve adequate mechanical ventilation for each patient.

Assessing the Equipment

The ventilator needs to be assessed to make sure that it is functioning properly and that the settings are appropriate.

Even though the nurse may not be primarily responsible for adjusting the settings on the ventilator or measuring ventilator parameters (these are usually responsibilities of the respiratory therapist), the nurse is responsible for the patient and therefore needs to evaluate how the ventilator affects the patient's overall status.

When monitoring the ventilator, the nurse notes the following:

- Type of ventilator (eg, volume-cycled, pressure-cycled, negative-pressure)
- Controlling mode (eg, **controlled ventilation**, assist–control ventilation, synchronized intermittent mandatory ventilation)
- Tidal volume and rate settings (tidal volume is usually set at 6 to 12 mL/kg [ideal body weight]; rate is usually set at 12 to 16 breaths/min)
- FiO_2 setting
- Inspiratory pressure reached and pressure limit (normal is 15 to 20 cm H_2O; this increases if there is increased airway resistance or decreased compliance)
- Sensitivity (a 2-cm H_2O inspiratory force should trigger the ventilator)
- Inspiratory-to-expiratory ratio (usually 1:3 [1 second of inspiration to 3 seconds of expiration] or 1:2)
- Minute volume (tidal volume × respiratory rate, usually 6 to 8 L/min)
- Sigh settings (usually set at 1.5 times the tidal volume and ranging from 1 to 3 per hour), if applicable
- Water in the tubing, disconnection or kinking of the tubing
- Humidification (humidifier filled with water) and temperature
- Alarms (turned on and functioning properly)
- PEEP and/or pressure support level, if applicable (PEEP is usually set at 5 to 15 cm H_2O)

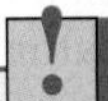

NURSING ALERT

If the ventilator system malfunctions and the problem cannot be identified and corrected immediately, the nurse must ventilate the patient with a manual resuscitation bag until the problem is resolved.

Problems With Mechanical Ventilation

Because of the seriousness of the patient's condition and the highly complex and technical nature of mechanical ventilation, a number of problems or complications can occur. Such situations fall into two categories: ventilator problems and patient problems (Table 25-2). In either case,

TABLE 25-2 Troubleshooting Problems with Mechanical Ventilation

Problem	Cause	Solution
Ventilator Problems		
Increase in peak airway pressure	Coughing or plugged airway tube	Suction airway for secretions, empty condensation fluid from circuit.
	Patient "bucking" ventilator	Adjust sensitivity.
	Decreasing lung compliance	Manually ventilate patient. Assess for hypoxia or bronchospasm. Check arterial blood gas values. Sedate only if necessary.
	Tubing kinked	Check tubing; reposition patient; insert oral airway if necessary.
	Pneumothorax	Manually ventilate patient; notify physician.
	Atelectasis or bronchospasm	Clear secretions.
Decrease in pressure or loss of volume	Increase in compliance	None
	Leak in ventilator or tubing; cuff on tube/humidifier not tight	Check entire ventilator circuit for patency. Correct leak.
Patient Problems		
Cardiovascular compromise	Decrease in venous return due to application of positive pressure to lungs	Assess for adequate volume status by measuring heart rate, blood pressure, central venous pressure, pulmonary capillary wedge pressure, and urine output. Notify physician if values are abnormal.
Barotrauma/pneumothorax	Application of positive pressure to lungs; high mean airway pressures lead to alveolar rupture	Notify physician. Prepare patient for chest tube insertion. Avoid high pressure settings for patients with COPD, ARDS, or history of pneumothorax.
Pulmonary infection	Bypass of normal defense mechanisms; frequent breaks in ventilator circuit; decreased mobility; impaired cough reflex	Use meticulous aseptic technique. Provide frequent mouth care. Optimize nutritional status.

the patient must be supported while the problem is identified and corrected.

Bucking the Ventilator

The patient is "in sync" with the ventilator when thoracic expansion coincides with the inspiratory phase of the machine and exhalation occurs passively. The patient is said to fight or buck the ventilator when he or she is out of phase with the machine. This is manifested when the patient attempts to breathe out during the ventilator's mechanical inspiratory phase or when there is jerky and increased abdominal muscle effort. The following factors contribute to this problem: anxiety, hypoxia, increased secretions, hypercapnia, inadequate minute volume, and pulmonary edema. These problems must be corrected before resorting to the use of paralyzing agents to reduce bucking; otherwise, the underlying problem is simply masked and the patient's condition will continue to deteriorate.

Muscle relaxants, tranquilizers, analgesic agents, and paralyzing agents are sometimes administered to patients receiving mechanical ventilation. Their purpose is ultimately to increase the patient–machine synchrony by decreasing the patient's anxiety, hyperventilation, or excessive muscle activity. The selection and dose of the appropriate medication are determined carefully and are based on the patient's requirements and the cause of his or her restlessness. Paralyzing agents are always used as a last resort, and always in conjunction with a sedative medication and often an analgesic medication.

Nursing Management

Promoting Home and Community-Based Care

Increasingly, patients are being cared for in extended care facilities or at home while receiving mechanical ventilation, with a tracheostomy tube, or receiving oxygen therapy.

NURSING RESEARCH PROFILE

Oral Care in the Prevention of Ventilator-Associated Pneumonia

Grap, M. J., Munro, C. L., Elswick, R. K., et al. (2004). Duration of action of a single, early oral application of chlorhexidine on oral microbial flora in mechanically ventilated patients: A pilot study. *Heart & Lung, 33*(2), 83–91.

Purpose

Although good oral care has been shown to reduce the incidence of ventilator-associated pneumonia (VAP), oral care is not a high-priority intervention for patients who are intubated on an emergent basis. Therefore, they remain at high risk of VAP. This study was conducted to examine the effect of a single application of chlorhexidine gluconate (CHG) by spray or swab and oral care on subsequent oral microbial flora and on the occurrence of VAP in intubated patients.

Design

Thirty-four intubated adults receiving mechanical ventilation were randomly assigned to one of three groups. Adults in two groups received 2 mL of CHG by either oral spray or swab shortly after intubation, and adults in the third group received routine oral care. CHG is a broad-spectrum antibacterial agent used in healthy populations as a daily oral rinse to control plaque and to prevent and treat gingivitis. Oral cultures for specific respiratory pathogens were obtained at baseline, 12 hours, and every 24 hours up to and including 72 hours after intubation. The presence of VAP was assessed using the Clinical Pulmonary Infection Score (CPIS), which is based on six clinical and laboratory variables. Possible scores range from 0 to 12, with a score of 6 or greater considered indicative of pneumonia.

Findings

As predicted, there were fewer positive oral cultures and decreased growth of oral respiratory bacteria from baseline to 48 hours (duration of intubation required for a definition of VAP) in the group that received CHG. In contrast, the usual oral care group experienced an increase in positive culture results. Although complete data were available on only 12 patients at 48 hours because of extubation or patient death, important trends were detected. In the two groups treated with CHG, the mean CPIS increased only slightly, from 5.17 to 5.57, whereas the mean CPIS in the usual care group increased from 4.7 to 6.6, a level indicating pneumonia.

Nursing Implications

Although statistically significant differences in oral bacterial culture results were not detected, trends in the data suggest that swabbing or spraying the mouth with CHG shortly after intubation may decrease bacterial colonization of the mouth and the risk of VAP. The results of this study suggest the need for early oral care after intubation; however, the study needs to be repeated in a larger group to determine whether oral CHG (or other antibacterial intervention) significantly affects the incidence of VAP.

Patients receiving home ventilator care usually have a chronic neuromuscular condition or COPD. Providing the opportunity for ventilator-dependent patients to return home to live with their families in familiar surroundings can be a positive experience. The ultimate goal of home ventilator therapy is to enhance the patient's quality of life, not simply to support or prolong life.

TEACHING PATIENTS SELF-CARE

Caring for the patient with mechanical ventilator support at home can be accomplished successfully, but the family must be emotionally, educationally, and physically able to assume the role of primary caregiver. A home care team consisting of the nurse, physician, respiratory therapist, social service or home care agency, and equipment supplier is needed. The home is evaluated to determine whether the electrical equipment needed can be operated safely. A summary of the basic assessment criteria needed for successful home care is presented in Chart 25-13.

Once the decision to initiate mechanical ventilation at home is made, the nurse prepares the patient and family for home care. The nurse teaches the patient and family about the ventilator, suctioning, tracheostomy care, signs of pulmonary infection, cuff inflation and deflation, and assessment of vital signs. Teaching begins in the hospital and continues at home. Nursing responsibilities include evaluating the patient's and family's understanding of the information presented.

The nurse teaches the family cardiopulmonary resuscitation, including mouth-to-tracheostomy tube (instead of mouth-to-mouth) breathing. The nurse also explains how to handle a power failure, which usually involves converting the ventilator from an electrical power source to a battery power source. Conversion is automatic in most types of home ventilators and lasts approximately 1 hour. The nurse instructs the family on the use of a manual self-inflation bag should it be necessary. Some of the patient's and family's responsibilities are listed in Chart 25-14.

CONTINUING CARE

A home care nurse monitors and evaluates how well the patient and family are adapting to providing care in the home. The nurse assesses the adequacy of the patient's ventilation and oxygenation as well as airway patency. The nurse addresses any unique adaptation problems the patient may have and listens to the patient's and family's anxieties and frustrations, offering support and encouragement where possible. The home care nurse helps identify and contact community resources that may assist in home management of the patient with mechanical ventilation.

The technical aspects of the ventilator are managed by vendor follow-up. A respiratory therapist usually is assigned to the patient and makes frequent home visits to evaluate the patient and perform a maintenance check of the ventilator.

Transportation services are identified in case the patient requires transportation in an emergency. These arrangements must be made before an emergency arises.

CHART 25-13

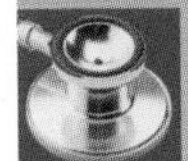

Assessment

Criteria for Successful Home Ventilator Care

The decision to proceed with home ventilation therapy is usually based on the following parameters.

PATIENT CRITERIA

- The patient has a chronic underlying pulmonary or neuromuscular disorder.
- The patient's clinical pulmonary status is stable.
- The patient is willing to go home on mechanical ventilation.

HOME CRITERIA

- The home environment is conducive to care of the patient.
- The electrical facilities are adequate to operate all equipment safely.
- The home environment is controlled, without drafts in cold weather and with proper ventilation in warm weather.
- Space is available for cleaning and storing ventilator equipment.

FAMILY CRITERIA

- Family members are competent, dependable, and willing to spend the time required for proper training with available professional support.
- Family members understand the diagnosis and prognosis.
- Family has sufficient financial and supportive resources.

Nursing Process

The Patient Receiving Mechanical Ventilation

Assessment

The nurse plays a vital role in assessing the patient's status and the functioning of the ventilator.

In assessing the patient, the nurse evaluates the patient's physiologic status and how he or she is coping with mechanical ventilation. Physical assessment includes systematic assessment of all body systems, with an in-depth focus on the respiratory system. Respiratory assessment includes vital signs, respiratory rate and pattern, breath sounds, evalua-

CHART 25-14

HOME CARE CHECKLIST • Ventilator Care

At the completion of the home care instruction, the patient or caregiver will be able to:	Patient	Caregiver
• State proper care of patient on ventilator		
• Observe physical signs such as color, secretions, breathing pattern, and state of consciousness.		✔
• Perform physical care such as suctioning, postural drainage, and ambulation.		✔
• Observe the tidal volume and pressure manometer regularly. Intervene when they are abnormal (ie, suction if airway pressure increases).		✔
• Provide a communication method for the patient (eg, pad and pencil, electric larynx, talking tracheostomy, sign language).		✔
• Monitor vital signs as directed.		✔
• Use a predetermined signal to indicate when feeling short of breath or in distress.	✔	
• Care for and maintain equipment properly		
• Check the ventilator settings twice each day and whenever the patient is removed from the ventilator.		✔
• Adjust the volume and pressure alarms if needed.		✔
• Fill humidifier as needed and check its level three times a day.		✔
• Empty water in tubing as needed.	✔	✔
• Use a clean humidifier when circuitry is changed.		✔
• Keep exterior of ventilator clean and free of any objects.		✔
• Change external circuitry once a week or more often as indicated.		✔
• Report malfunction or strange noises immediately	✔	✔

tion of spontaneous ventilatory effort, and potential evidence of hypoxia (eg, skin color). Increased adventitious breath sounds may indicate a need for suctioning. The nurse also evaluates the settings and functioning of the mechanical ventilator, as described previously.

Assessment also addresses the patient's neurologic status and effectiveness of coping with the need for assisted ventilation and the changes that accompany it. The nurse assesses the patient's comfort level and ability to communicate as well. Because weaning from mechanical ventilation requires adequate nutrition, it is important to assess the patient's gastrointestinal system and nutritional status.

Diagnosis

Nursing Diagnoses

Based on the assessment data, the patient's major nursing diagnoses may include:

- Impaired gas exchange related to underlying illness, ventilator setting adjustment during stabilization, or weaning.
- Ineffective airway clearance related to increased mucus production associated with presence of the tube in trachea or continuous positive-pressure mechanical ventilation
- Risk for trauma and infection related to endotracheal intubation or tracheostomy
- Impaired physical mobility related to ventilator dependency
- Impaired verbal communication related to endotracheal tube and attachment to ventilator
- Defensive coping and powerlessness related to ventilator dependency

Collaborative Problems/ Potential Complications

Based on the assessment data, potential complications may include the following:

- Alterations in cardiac function
- Barotrauma (trauma to the alveoli) and pneumothorax
- Pulmonary infection
- Sepsis

Planning and Goals

The major goals for the patient may include achievement of optimal gas exchange, maintenance of a patent airway, absence of trauma or infection, attainment of optimal mobility, adjustment to nonverbal methods of communication, acquisition of successful coping measures, and absence of complications.

Nursing Interventions

Nursing care of the mechanically ventilated patient requires expert technical and interpersonal skills. Nursing interventions are similar regardless of the setting; however, the frequency of interventions and the stability of the patient vary from setting to setting. Nursing interventions for the mechanically ventilated patient are not uniquely different from those for patients with other pulmonary disorders, but astute nursing assessment and a therapeutic nurse–patient relationship are critical. The specific interventions used by the nurse are determined by the underlying disease process and the patient's response.

Two general nursing interventions that are important in the care of the mechanically ventilated patient are pulmonary auscultation and interpretation of arterial blood gas measurements. The nurse is often the first to note changes in physical assessment findings or significant trends in blood gases that signal the development of a serious problem (eg, pneumothorax, tube displacement, pulmonary embolus).

Enhancing Gas Exchange

The purpose of mechanical ventilation is to optimize gas exchange by maintaining alveolar ventilation and oxygen delivery. The alteration in gas exchange may be caused by the underlying illness or by mechanical factors related to adjustment of the machine to the patient. The health care team, including nurse, physician, and respiratory therapist, continually assesses the patient for adequate gas exchange, signs and symptoms of hypoxia, and response to treatment. Therefore, the nursing diagnosis of impaired gas exchange is, by its complex nature, multidisciplinary and collaborative. The team members must share goals and information freely. All other goals directly or indirectly relate to this primary goal.

Nursing interventions to promote optimal gas exchange include judicious administration of analgesic agents to relieve pain without suppressing the respiratory drive and frequent repositioning to diminish the pulmonary effects of immobility. The nurse also monitors for adequate fluid balance by assessing for the presence of peripheral edema, calculating daily intake and output, and monitoring daily weights. The nurse administers medications prescribed to control the primary disease and monitors for their side effects.

Promoting Effective Airway Clearance

Continuous positive-pressure ventilation increases the production of secretions regardless of the patient's underlying condition. The nurse assesses for the presence of secretions by lung auscultation at least every 2 to 4 hours. Measures to clear the airway of secretions include suctioning, CPT, frequent position changes, and increased mobility as soon as possible. Frequency of suctioning should be determined by patient assessment. If excessive secretions are identified by inspection or auscultation techniques, suctioning should be performed. Sputum is not produced continuously or every 1 to 2 hours but as a response to a pathologic condition. Therefore, there is no rationale for routine suctioning of all patients every 1 to 2 hours. Although suctioning is used to aid in the clearance of secretions, it can damage the airway mucosa and impair cilia action.

The sigh mechanism on the ventilator may be adjusted to deliver at least 1 to 3 sighs per hour at 1.5 times the tidal volume if the patient is receiving assist–control ventilation. Periodic sighs prevent atelectasis and the further retention of secretions. Because of the risk for hyperventilation and trauma to pulmonary tissue from excess ventilator pressure (barotrauma, pneumothorax), the sigh feature is not used frequently. If the SIMV mode is being used, the mandatory ventilations act as sighs because they are of greater volume than the patient's spontaneous breaths.

Humidification of the airway via the ventilator is maintained to help liquefy secretions so that they are more easily removed. Bronchodilators are administered to dilate the bronchioles and are classified as adrenergic or anticholinergic. Adrenergic bronchodilators are mostly inhaled and work by stimulating the beta-receptor sites, mimicking the effects of epinephrine in the body. The desired effect is smooth muscle relaxation, which dilates the constricted bronchial tubes. Medications include albuterol (Proventil, Ventolin), isoetharine (Bronkosol), isoproterenol (Isuprel), metaproterenol (Alupent, Metaprel), pirbuterol acetate (Maxair), salmeterol (Serevent), and terbutaline (Brethine, Brethaire, Bricanyl). Tachycardia, heart palpitations, and tremors have been reported with use of these medications. Anticholinergic bronchodilators such as ipratropium (Atrovent), tiotropium (Spiriva), and ipratropium with albuterol (Combivent) produce airway relaxation by blocking cholinergic-induced bronchoconstriction. Patients receiving bronchodilator therapy of either type should be monitored for adverse effects, including dizziness, nausea, decreased oxygen saturation, hypokalemia, increased heart rate, and urine retention. Mucolytic agents such as acetylcysteine (Mucomyst) are administered to liquefy secretions so that they are more easily mobilized. Nursing management of patients receiving mucolytic therapy includes assessment for an adequate cough reflex, sputum characteristics, and (in patients not receiving mechanical ventilation) improvement in incentive spirometry. Side effects include nausea, vomiting, bronchospasm, stomatitis (oral ulcers), urticaria, and rhinorrhea (runny nose).

Preventing Trauma and Infection

Maintaining the endotracheal or tracheostomy tube is an essential part of airway management. The nurse positions the ventilator tubing so that there is minimal pulling or distortion of the tube in the trachea, reducing the risk of trauma to the trachea. Cuff pressure is monitored every 6 to 8 hours to maintain the pressure at less than 25 mm Hg (optimal cuff pressure is 15 to 20 mm Hg). The nurse assesses for the presence of a cuff leak at the same time.

Patients with endotracheal intubation or a tracheostomy tube do not have the normal defenses of the upper airway. In addition, these patients frequently have multiple additional body system disturbances that lead to immunocompromise. Tracheostomy care is performed at least every 8 hours, and more frequently if needed, because of the increased risk for infection. The ventilator circuit tubing and in-line suction tubing are replaced periodically, according to infection control guidelines, to decrease the risk for infection.

The nurse administers oral hygiene frequently, because the oral cavity is a primary source of contamination of the lungs in the intubated and compromised patient. The presence of a nasogastric tube in the intubated patient can increase the risk for aspiration, leading to nosocomial pneumonia. The nurse positions the patient with the head elevated above the stomach as much as possible. Although antiulcer medications such as cimetidine (Tagamet) or ranitidine (Zantac) are sometimes administered, an oral antiulcer medication such as sucralfate (Carafate) is preferable because it maintains normal gastric pH, decreasing the incidence of aspiration pneumonia.

Promoting Optimal Level of Mobility

Being connected to a ventilator limits the patient's mobility. The nurse helps the patient whose condition has become stable to get out of bed and move to a chair as soon as possible. Mobility and muscle activity are beneficial because they stimulate respirations and improve morale. If the patient is unable to get out of bed, the nurse encourages performance of active range-of-motion exercises every 6 to 8 hours. If the patient cannot perform these exercises, the nurse performs passive range-of-motion exercises every 8 hours to prevent contractures and venous stasis.

Promoting Optimal Communication

It is important to develop alternative methods of communication for the patient who is receiving mechanical ventilation. The nurse assesses the patient's communication abilities to evaluate for limitations. Questions to consider when assessing the ventilator-dependent patient's ability to communicate include the following:

- Is the patient conscious and able to communicate? Can the patient nod or shake his or her head?
- Is the patient's mouth unobstructed by the tube so that words can be mouthed?
- Is the patient's dominant hand strong and available for writing? For example, if the patient is right-handed, the intravenous (IV) line should be placed in the left arm if possible so that the right hand is free.
- Is the patient a candidate for a Passy-Muir valve, which permits talking?

Once the patient's limitations are known, the nurse offers several appropriate communication approaches: lip reading (use single key words), pad and pencil or Magic Slate, communication board, gesturing, sign language, or electric larynx. Use of a "talking" or fenestrated tracheostomy tube may be suggested to the physician; this allows the patient to talk while on the ventilator. The nurse makes sure that the patient's eyeglasses, hearing aid, sign interpreter, and language translator are available if needed to enhance the patient's ability to communicate.

The patient must be assisted to find the most suitable communication method. Some methods may be frustrating to the patient, family, and nurse; these need to be identified and minimized. A speech therapist can assist in determining the most appropriate method.

Promoting Coping Ability

Dependence on a ventilator is frightening to both the patient and the family and disrupts even the most stable families. Encouraging the family to verbalize their feelings about the ventilator, the patient's condition, and the environment in general is beneficial. Explaining procedures every time they are performed helps reduce anxiety and familiarizes the patient with ventilator procedures. To restore a sense of control, the nurse encourages the patient to participate in decisions about care, schedules, and treatment when possible. The patient may become withdrawn or depressed while receiving mechanical ventilation, especially if its use is prolonged. To promote effective coping, the nurse informs the patient about progress when appropriate. It is important to provide diversions such as watching television, playing music, or taking a walk (if appropriate and possible). Stress reduction techniques (eg, a back rub, relaxation measures) help relieve tension and help the patient deal with anxieties and fears about both the condition and the dependence on the ventilator.

Monitoring and Managing Potential Complications

ALTERATIONS IN CARDIAC FUNCTION

Alterations in cardiac output may occur as a result of positive-pressure ventilation. The positive intrathoracic pressure during inspiration compresses the heart and great vessels, thereby reducing venous return and cardiac output. This is usually corrected during exhalation when the positive pressure is off. The patient may have decreased cardiac output and resultant decreased tissue perfusion and oxygenation.

To evaluate cardiac function, the nurse first observes for signs and symptoms of hypoxia (restlessness, apprehension, confusion, tachycardia, tachypnea, labored breathing, pallor progressing to cyanosis, diaphoresis, transient hypertension, and decreased urine output). If a pulmonary artery catheter is in place, cardiac output, cardiac index, and other hemodynamic values can be used to assess the patient's status.

BAROTRAUMA AND PNEUMOTHORAX

Excessive positive pressure can cause barotrauma, which results in a spontaneous **pneumothorax.** This may quickly develop into a tension pneumothorax, further compromising venous return, cardiac output, and blood pressure. The nurse considers any sudden changes in oxygen saturation or the onset of respiratory distress to be a life-threatening emergency requiring immediate action.

PULMONARY INFECTION

The patient is at high risk for infection, as described earlier. The nurse reports fever or a change in the color or odor of sputum to the physician for follow-up.

Evaluation

Expected Patient Outcomes

Expected patient outcomes may include the following:

1. Exhibits adequate gas exchange, as evidenced by normal breath sounds, acceptable arterial blood gas levels, and vital signs
2. Demonstrates adequate ventilation with minimal mucus accumulation
3. Is free of injury or infection, as evidenced by normal temperature, white blood cell count, and clear sputum
4. Is mobile within limits of ability
   a. Gets out of bed to chair, bears weight, or ambulates as soon as possible
   b. Performs range-of-motion exercises every 6 to 8 hours
5. Communicates effectively through written messages, gestures, or other communication strategies
6. Copes effectively
   a. Verbalizes fears and concerns about condition and equipment
   b. Participates in decision making when possible
   c. Uses stress reduction techniques when necessary
7. Absence of complications
   a. Absence of cardiac compromise, as evidenced by stable vital signs and adequate urine output
   b. Absence of pneumothorax, as evidenced by bilateral chest excursion, normal chest x-ray, and adequate oxygenation
   c. Absence of pulmonary infection, as evidenced by normal temperature, clear pulmonary secretions, and negative sputum cultures

Weaning the Patient From the Ventilator

Respiratory weaning, the process of withdrawing the patient from dependence on the ventilator, takes place in three stages: the patient is gradually removed from the ventilator, then from the tube, and finally from oxygen. Weaning from mechanical ventilation is performed at the earliest possible time consistent with patient safety. The decision must be made from a physiologic rather than a mechanical viewpoint. A thorough understanding of the patient's clinical status is required in making this decision. Weaning is started when the patient is recovering from the acute stage of medical and surgical problems and when the cause of respiratory failure is sufficiently reversed.

Successful weaning involves collaboration among the physician, respiratory therapist, and nurse. Each health care provider must understand the scope and function of other team members in relation to patient weaning to conserve the patient's strength, use resources efficiently, and maximize successful outcomes.

Criteria for Weaning

Careful assessment is required to determine whether the patient is ready to be removed from mechanical ventilation. If the patient is stable and showing signs of improvement or reversal of the disease or condition that caused the need for mechanical ventilation, weaning indices should be assessed. These indices include the following:

- Vital capacity—the amount of air expired after maximum inspiration. It is used to assess the patient's ability to take deep breaths and should be 10 to 15 mL/kg to meet the criteria for weaning.
- Maximum inspiratory pressure—used to assess the patient's respiratory muscle strength. It is also known as negative inspiratory pressure and should be at least –20 cm H_2O.
- Tidal volume—the volume of air that is inhaled or exhaled from the lungs during an effortless breath. It should be more than 3.5 mL/kg for weaning (Kacmarek et al., 2005).
- Minute ventilation—equal to the respiratory rate multiplied by tidal volume. Normal is about 6 L/min.
- Rapid/shallow breathing index—calculated by dividing the respiratory rate by the tidal volume. It is used to as-

sess the breathing pattern, and patients with indices lower than 105 breaths/min/L are more likely to be successful at weaning.

Other measurements used to assess readiness for weaning include a PaO_2 of greater than 60 mm Hg with an FiO_2 of less than 50% (Kacmarek et al., 2005). Stable vital signs and arterial blood gases are also important predictors of successful weaning. Once readiness has been determined, the nurse records baseline measurements of weaning indices to monitor progress.

Patient Preparation

To maximize the chances of success of weaning, the nurse must consider the patient as a whole, taking into account factors that impair the delivery of oxygen and elimination of carbon dioxide as well as those that increase oxygen demand (eg, sepsis, seizures, thyroid imbalances) or decrease the patient's overall strength (eg, inadequate nutrition, neuromuscular disease). Adequate psychological preparation is necessary before and during the weaning process. Patients need to know what is expected of them during the procedure. They are often frightened by having to breathe on their own again and need reassurance that they are improving and are well enough to handle spontaneous breathing. The nurse explains what will happen during weaning and what role the patient will play in the procedure. The nurse emphasizes that someone will be with or near the patient at all times and answers any questions simply and concisely. Proper preparation of the patient can shorten the time required for successful weaning.

Methods of Weaning

Successful weaning depends on the combination of adequate patient preparation, available equipment, and an interdisciplinary approach to solving patient problems (Chart 25-15). All usual modes of ventilation can be used for weaning.

When assist–control ventilation is used, the control rate is decreased, so that the patient strengthens the respiratory muscles by triggering progressively more breaths. The nurse assesses the patient for the following signs of distress: rapid/shallow breathing, use of accessory muscles, reduced level of consciousness, increase in carbon dioxide levels, decrease in oxygen saturation, and tachycardia.

SIMV is indicated if the patient satisfies all the criteria for weaning but cannot sustain adequate spontaneous ventilation for long periods. As the patient's respiratory muscles become stronger, the rate is decreased until the patient is breathing spontaneously.

The PAV mode of partial ventilatory support allows the ventilator to generate pressure in proportion to the patient's efforts. With every breath, the ventilator synchronizes with the patient's ventilatory efforts. Nursing assessment includes careful monitoring of the patient's respiratory rate, arterial blood gases, tidal volume, minute ventilation, and breathing pattern.

CPAP allows the patient to breathe spontaneously while applying positive pressure throughout the respiratory cycle to keep the alveoli open and promote oxygenation. Providing CPAP during spontaneous breathing also offers the advantage of an alarm system and may reduce patient anxiety if the patient has been taught that the machine is keeping track of breathing. It also maintains lung volumes and improves the patient's oxygenation status. CPAP is often used in conjunction with PSV. Nurses should carefully assess for tachypnea, tachycardia, reduced tidal volumes, decreasing oxygen saturations, and increasing carbon dioxide levels.

When the patient can breathe spontaneously, weaning trials using a T-piece or tracheostomy mask (see Fig. 25-2) are normally conducted with the patient disconnected from the ventilator, receiving humidified oxygen only, and performing all work of breathing. Because patients do not have to overcome the resistance of the ventilator, they may find this mode more comfortable, or they may become anxious as they breathe with no support from the ventilator. During T-piece trials, the nurse monitors the patient closely and provides encouragement. This method of weaning is usually used when the patient is awake and alert, is breathing without difficulty, has good gag and cough reflexes, and is hemodynamically stable. During the weaning process, the patient is maintained on the same or a higher oxygen concentration than when receiving mechanical ventilation. While the patient is using the T-piece, he or she is observed for signs and symptoms of hypoxia, increasing respiratory muscle fatigue, or systemic fatigue. These include restlessness, increased respiratory rate (greater than 35 breaths/min), use of accessory muscles, tachycardia with premature ventricular contractions, and paradoxical chest movement (asynchronous breathing, chest contraction during inspiration and expansion during expiration). Fatigue or exhaustion is initially manifested by an increased respiratory rate associated with a gradual reduction in tidal volume; later there is a slowing of the respiratory rate.

If the patient appears to be tolerating the T-piece trial, a second set of arterial blood gas measurements is drawn 20 minutes after the patient has been on spontaneous ventilation at a constant FiO_2 pressure support ventilation. (Alveolar–arterial equilibration takes 15 to 20 minutes to occur.)

Signs of exhaustion and hypoxia correlated with deterioration in the blood gas measurements indicate the need for ventilatory support. The patient is placed back on the ventilator each time signs of fatigue or deterioration develop.

If clinically stable, the patient usually can be extubated within 2 or 3 hours after weaning and allowed spontaneous ventilation by means of a mask with humidified oxygen. Patients who have had prolonged ventilatory assistance usually require more gradual weaning; it may take days or even weeks. They are weaned primarily during the day and placed back on the ventilator at night to rest.

Because patients respond in different manners to the various weaning methods, there is no definitive way to assess

CHART 25-15

Guidelines for Care of the Patient Being Weaned From Mechanical Ventilation

ACTIONS	RATIONALE
1. Assess patient for weaning criteria: Vital capacity—10 to 15 mL/kg Maximum inspiratory pressure (MIP) at least −20 cm H_2O Tidal volume—7 to 9 mL/kg Minute ventilation—6 L/min Rapid/shallow breathing index—below 100 breaths/minute/L PaO_2 greater than 60 mm Hg with FiO_2 less than 40%	1. Careful assessment of multiple weaning indices helps to determine readiness for weaning. When the criteria have been met, the patient's likelihood of successful weaning increases.
2. Monitor activity level, assess dietary intake, and monitor results of laboratory tests of nutritional status.	2. Reestablishing independent spontaneous ventilation can be physically exhausting. It is crucial that the patient have enough energy reserves to succeed. Providing periods of rest and recommended nutritional intake can increase the likelihood of successful weaning.
3. Assess the patient's and family's understanding of the weaning process and address any concerns about the process. Explain that the patient may feel short of breath initially and provide encouragement as needed. Reassure the patient that he or she will be attended closely and that if the weaning attempt is not successful, it can be tried again later.	3. The weaning process can be psychologically tiring; emotional support can help promote a sense of security. Explaining that weaning will be attempted again later helps reduce the sense of failure if the first attempts are unsuccessful.
4. Implement the weaning method prescribed: A/C, IMV, SIMV, PSV, PAV, CPAP, or T-piece.	4. The prescribed weaning method should reflect the patient's individualized criteria for weaning and weaning history. By having different methods to choose from, the physician can select the one that best fits the patient.
5. Monitor vital signs, pulse oximetry, ECG, and respiratory pattern constantly for the first 20 to 30 minutes and every 5 minutes after that until weaning is complete.	5. Monitoring the patient closely provides ongoing indications of success or failure.
6. Maintain a patent airway; monitor arterial blood gas levels and pulmonary function tests. Suction the airway as needed.	6. These values can be compared to baseline measurements to evaluate weaning. Suctioning helps to reduce the risk of aspiration and maintain the airway.
7. In collaboration with the physician, terminate the weaning process if adverse reactions occur. These include a heart rate increase of 20 beats/min, systolic blood pressure increase of 20 mm Hg, a decrease in oxygen saturation to less than 90%, respiratory rate less than 8 or greater than 20 breaths/minute, ventricular dysrhythmias, fatigue, panic, cyanosis, erratic or labored breathing, paradoxical chest movement.	7. These signs and symptoms indicate an unstable patient at risk for hypoxia and ventricular dysrhythmias. Continuing the weaning process can lead to cardiopulmonary arrest.
8. If the weaning process continues, measure tidal volume and minute ventilation every 20 to 30 minutes; compare with the patient's desired values, which have been determined in collaboration with the physician.	8. These values help to determine if weaning is successful and should be continued.
9. Assess for psychological dependence if the physiologic parameters indicate weaning is feasible and the patient still resists.	9. Psychological dependence is a common problem after mechanical ventilation. Possible causes include fear of dying and depression from chronic illness. It is important to address this issue before the next weaning attempt.

which method is best. Regardless of the weaning method being used, ongoing assessment of respiratory status is essential to monitor patient progress.

Successful weaning from the ventilator is supplemented by intensive pulmonary care. The following methods are used:

- Oxygen therapy
- Arterial blood gas evaluation
- Pulse oximetry
- Bronchodilator therapy
- CPT
- Adequate nutrition, hydration, and humidification
- Incentive spirometry

These patients still have borderline pulmonary function and need vigorous supportive therapy before their respiratory status returns to a level that supports activities of daily living.

Weaning From the Tube

Weaning from the tube is considered when the patient can breathe spontaneously, maintain an adequate airway by effectively coughing up secretions, swallow, and move the jaw. If frequent suctioning is needed to clear secretions, tube weaning may be unsuccessful. Secretion clearance and aspiration risks are assessed to determine whether active pharyngeal and laryngeal reflexes are intact.

Once the patient can clear secretions adequately, a trial period of mouth breathing or nose breathing is conducted. This can be accomplished by several methods. The first method requires changing to a smaller size tube to increase the resistance to airflow or plugging the tracheostomy tube (deflating the cuff first). The smaller tube is sometimes replaced by a cuffless tracheostomy tube, which allows the tube to be plugged at lengthening intervals to monitor patient progress. A second method involves changing to a fenestrated tube (a tube with an opening or window in its bend). This permits air to flow around and through the tube to the upper airway and enables talking. A third method involves switching to a smaller tracheostomy button (stoma button). A tracheostomy button is a plastic tube approximately 1 inch long that helps keep the windpipe open after the larger tracheostomy tube has been removed. Finally, when the patient demonstrates the ability to maintain a patent airway, the tube can be removed. An occlusive dressing is placed over the stoma, which heals in several days to weeks.

Weaning From Oxygen

The patient who has been successfully weaned from the ventilator, cuff, and tube and has adequate respiratory function is then weaned from oxygen. The FiO_2 is gradually reduced until the PaO_2 is in the range of 70 to 100 mm Hg while the patient is breathing room air. If the PaO_2 is less than 70 mm Hg on room air, supplemental oxygen is recommended. To be eligible for financial reimbursement from the Centers for Medicare and Medicaid Services for in-home oxygen, the patient must have a PaO_2 of less than 55 mm Hg while awake and at rest.

Nutrition

Success in weaning the long-term ventilator-dependent patient requires early and aggressive but judicious nutritional support. The respiratory muscles (diaphragm and especially intercostals) become weak or atrophied after just a few days of mechanical ventilation and may be catabolized for energy, especially if nutrition is inadequate. Because the metabolism of fat produces less carbon dioxide than the metabolism of carbohydrate, a high-fat diet may assist patients with respiratory failure, both during mechanical ventilation and while being weaned (Baudouin & Evans, 2003). The evidence on the value of a limited carbohydrate intake versus a carbohydrate-enriched diet is contradictory (Goris, Vermeeren, Wouters, et al., 2003). A high-fat diet may provide as much as 50% of the total daily kilocalories. Adequate protein intake is important in increasing respiratory muscle strength. Protein intake should be approximately 25% of total daily kilocalories, or 1.2 to 1.5 g/kg/day. Care must be taken not to overfeed the patient, because excessive intake can increase the demand for oxygen and the production of carbon dioxide. Daily nutrition should be closely monitored.

Soon after the patient is admitted, a consultation with a dietitian or nutrition support team should be arranged to plan the best form of nutritional replacement. Adequate nutrition may decrease the duration of mechanical ventilation and prevent other complications, especially sepsis. Sepsis can occur if bacteria enter the bloodstream and release toxins that, in turn, cause vasodilation and hypotension, fever, tachycardia, increased respiratory rate, and coma. Aggressive treatment of sepsis is essential to reverse this threat to survival and to promote weaning from the ventilator when the patient's condition improves. Optimal nutritional intake is an essential part of the treatment of sepsis.

The Patient Undergoing Thoracic Surgery

Assessment and management are particularly important for the patient undergoing thoracic surgery. Frequently, patients undergoing such surgery also have obstructive pulmonary disease with compromised breathing. Preoperative preparation and careful postoperative management are crucial for successful patient outcomes, because these patients may have a narrow range between their physical tolerance for certain activities and their limitations, which, if exceeded, can lead to distress. Various types of thoracic surgical procedures are performed to relieve disease conditions such as lung abscesses, lung cancer, cysts, benign tumors, and emphysema (Chart 25-16). An exploratory **thoracotomy** (creation of a surgical opening into the thoracic cavity) may be performed to diagnose lung or chest disease. A biopsy may be performed in this procedure with a small amount of lung tissue removed for analysis; the chest incision is then closed.

The objectives of preoperative care for the patient undergoing thoracic surgery are to ascertain the patient's

CHART 25-16

Thoracic Surgeries and Procedures

PNEUMONECTOMY

The removal of an entire lung (pneumonectomy) is performed chiefly for cancer when the lesion cannot be removed by a less extensive procedure. It also may be performed for lung abscesses, bronchiectasis, or extensive unilateral tuberculosis. The removal of the right lung is more dangerous than the removal of the left, because the right lung has a larger vascular bed and its removal imposes a greater physiologic burden.

A posterolateral or anterolateral thoracotomy incision is made, sometimes with resection of a rib. The pulmonary artery and the pulmonary veins are ligated and severed. The main bronchus is divided and the lung removed. The bronchial stump is stapled, and usually no drains are used because the accumulation of fluid in the empty hemithorax prevents mediastinal shift.

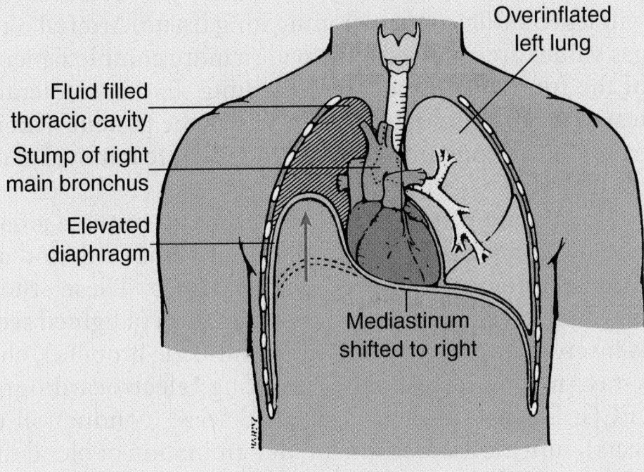

Pneumonectomy

LOBECTOMY

When the pathology is limited to one area of a lung, a lobectomy (removal of a lobe of a lung) is performed. Lobectomy, which is more common than pneumonectomy, may be carried out for bronchogenic carcinoma, giant emphysematous blebs or bullae, benign tumors, metastatic malignant tumors, bronchiectasis, and fungus infections.

The surgeon makes a thoracotomy incision: its exact location depends on the lobe to be resected. When the pleural space is entered, the involved lung collapses and the lobar vessels and the bronchus are ligated and divided. After the lobe is removed, the remaining lobes of the lung are reexpanded. Usually, two chest catheters are inserted for drainage. The upper tube is for air removal; the lower one is for fluid drainage. Sometimes, only one catheter is needed. The chest tube is connected to a chest drainage apparatus for several days.

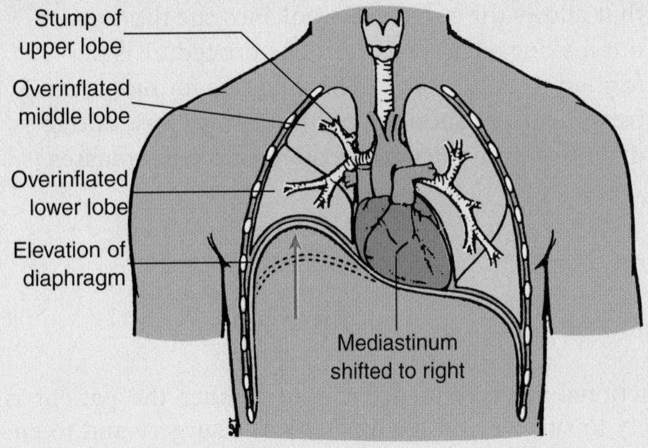

Lobectomy

SEGMENTECTOMY (SEGMENTAL RESECTION)

Some lesions are located in only one segment of the lung. Bronchopulmonary segments are subdivisions of the lung that function as individual units. They are held together by delicate connective tissue. Disease processes may be limited to a single segment. Care is used to preserve as much healthy and functional lung tissue as possible, especially in patients who already have limited cardiopulmonary reserve. Single segments can be removed from any lobe; the right middle lobe, which has only two small segments, invariably is removed entirely. On the left side, corresponding to a middle lobe, is a “lingular” segment of the upper lobe. This can be removed as a single segment or by lingulectomy. This segment frequently is involved in bronchiectasis.

WEDGE RESECTION

A wedge resection of a small, well-circumscribed lesion may be performed without regard for the location of the intersegmental planes. The pleural cavity usually is drained because of the possibility of an air or blood leak. This procedure is performed for diagnostic lung biopsy and for the excision of small peripheral nodules.

BRONCHOPLASTIC OR SLEEVE RESECTION

Bronchoplastic resection is a procedure in which only one lobar bronchus, together with a part of the right or left bronchus, is excised. The distal bronchus is reanastomosed to the proximal bronchus or trachea.

LUNG VOLUME REDUCTION

Lung volume reduction is a surgical procedure involving the removal of 20% to 30% of a patient’s lung through a midsternal incision or video thoracoscopy. The diseased lung tissue is identified on a lung perfusion scan. This surgery leads to significant improvements in dyspnea, exercise capacity, quality of life, and survival of a subgroup of people with end-stage emphysema (Naunheim, 2004).

continued >

CHART 25-16 Thoracic Surgeries and Procedures, continued

VIDEO THORACOSCOPY

A video thoracoscopy is an endoscopic procedure that allows the surgeon to look into the thorax without making a large incision. The procedure is performed to obtain specimens of tissue for biopsy, to treat recurrent spontaneous pneumothorax, and to diagnose either pleural effusions or pleural masses.

Thoracoscopy has also been found to be an effective diagnostic and therapeutic alternative for the treatment of mediastinal disorders (Cirino, Campos, Jatene, et al., 2000). Some advantages of video thoracoscopy are rapid diagnosis and treatment of some conditions, a decrease in postoperative complications, and a shortened hospital stay (see Chapter 21).

functional reserve, to determine whether the patient is likely to survive and recover from the surgery and to ensure that the patient is in optimal condition for surgery.

Preoperative Management

Assessment and Diagnostic Findings

The nurse performs chest auscultation to assess breath sounds in all regions of the lungs (see Chapter 21). It is important to note whether breath sounds are normal, indicating a free flow of air in and out of the lungs. (In the patient with emphysema, the breath sounds may be markedly decreased or even absent on auscultation.) The nurse notes crackles and wheezes and assesses for hyperresonance and decreased diaphragmatic motion. Unilateral diminished breath sounds and rhonchi can be the result of occlusion of the bronchi by mucus plugs. The nurse assesses for retained secretions during auscultation by asking the patient to cough. It is important to note any signs of rhonchi or wheezing. The patient history and assessment should include the following questions:

- What signs and symptoms (cough, sputum expectorated [amount and color], hemoptysis, chest pain, dyspnea) are present?
- If there is a smoking history, how long has the patient smoked? Does the patient smoke currently? How many packs a day?
- What is the patient's cardiopulmonary tolerance while resting, eating, bathing, and walking?
- What is the patient's breathing pattern? How much exertion is required to produce dyspnea?
- Does the patient need to sleep in an upright position or with more than two pillows?
- What is the patient's general physiologic status (eg, general appearance, mental alertness, behavior, nutritional status)?
- What other medical conditions exist (eg, allergies, cardiac disorders, diabetes)?

A number of tests are performed to determine the patient's preoperative status and to assess the patient's physical assets and limitations. Many patients are seen by their surgeons in the office, and many tests and examinations are performed on an outpatient basis. The decision to perform any pulmonary resection is based on the patient's cardiovascular status and pulmonary reserve. Pulmonary function studies (especially lung volume and vital capacity) are performed to determine whether the planned resection will leave sufficient functioning lung tissue. Arterial blood gas values are assessed to provide a more complete picture of the functional capacity of the lung. Exercise tolerance tests are useful to determine whether the patient who is a candidate for pneumonectomy can tolerate removal of one of the lungs.

Preoperative studies are performed to provide a baseline for comparison during the postoperative period and to detect any unsuspected abnormalities. These studies may include a bronchoscopic examination (a lighted scope is inserted into the airways to examine the bronchi), chest x-ray, magnetic resonance imaging, electrocardiogram (ECG; for arteriosclerotic heart disease, conduction defects), nutritional assessment, determination of blood urea nitrogen and serum creatinine levels (to assess renal function), determination of glucose tolerance or blood glucose level (to check for diabetes), assessment of serum electrolytes and protein levels, blood volume determinations, and complete blood cell count.

Preoperative Nursing Management

IMPROVING AIRWAY CLEARANCE

The underlying lung condition often is associated with increased respiratory secretions. Before surgery, the airway is cleared of secretions to reduce the possibility of postoperative atelectasis or infection. Risk factors for postoperative atelectasis and pneumonia are listed in Chart 25-17. Strategies to reduce the risk for atelectasis and infection include humidification, postural drainage, and chest percussion after bronchodilators are administered, if prescribed. The nurse estimates the volume of sputum if the patient expectorates large amounts of secretions. Such measurements are carried out to determine whether and when the amount decreases. Antibiotics are

CHART 25-17

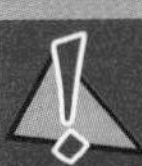

Risk Factors for Surgery-Related Atelectasis and Pneumonia

PREOPERATIVE RISK FACTORS

- Increased age
- Obesity
- Poor nutritional status
- Smoking history
- Abnormal pulmonary function tests
- Preexisting lung disease
- Emergency surgery
- History of aspiration
- Comorbid states
- Preexisting disability

INTRAOPERATIVE RISK FACTORS

- Thoracic incision
- Prolonged anesthesia

POSTOPERATIVE RISK FACTORS

- Immobilization
- Supine position
- Decreased level of consciousness
- Inadequate pain management
- Prolonged intubation/mechanical ventilation
- Presence of nasogastric tube
- Inadequate preoperative education

administered as prescribed for infection, which may be causing the excessive secretions.

TEACHING THE PATIENT

Increasingly, patients are admitted on the day of surgery, which does not provide much time for the acute care nurse to talk with the patient. Nurses in all settings must take an active role in educating the patient and relieving anxiety. The nurse informs the patient what to expect, from administration of anesthesia to thoracotomy and the likely use of chest tubes and a drainage system in the postoperative period. The patient is also informed about the usual postoperative administration of oxygen to facilitate breathing and the possible use of a ventilator. It is essential to explain the importance of frequent turning to promote drainage of lung secretions. Instruction in the use of incentive spirometry begins before surgery to familiarize the patient with its correct use. The nurse teaches diaphragmatic and pursed-lip breathing, and the patient should begin practicing these techniques (see Charts 25-3 and 25-4).

Because a coughing schedule is necessary in the postoperative period to promote the clearance or removal of secretions, the nurse instructs the patient in the technique of coughing and warns the patient that the coughing routine may be uncomfortable. The nurse teaches the patient to splint the incision with the hands, a pillow, or a folded towel (see Chart 25-5).

Another technique, "huffing," may be helpful for the patient with diminished expiratory flow rates or for the patient who refuses to cough because of severe pain. Huffing is the expulsion of air through an open glottis. This type of forced expiration technique (FET) stimulates pulmonary expansion and assists in alveolar inflation. The nurse instructs the patient as follows:

- Take a deep diaphragmatic breath and exhale forcefully against your hand in a quick, distinct pant, or huff.
- Practice doing small huffs and progress to one strong huff during exhalation.

Patients should be informed preoperatively that blood and other fluids may be administered, oxygen will be administered, and vital signs will be checked often for several hours after surgery. If a chest tube is needed, the patient should be informed that it will drain the fluid and air that normally accumulate after chest surgery. The patient and family are informed that the patient may be admitted to the intensive care unit for 1 to 2 days after surgery, that the patient may experience pain at the incision site, and that medication is available to relieve pain and discomfort.

RELIEVING ANXIETY

The nurse listens to the patient to evaluate his or her feelings about the illness and proposed treatment. The nurse also determines the patient's motivation to return to normal or baseline function. The patient may reveal significant concerns: fear of hemorrhage because of bloody sputum, fear of discomfort from a chronic cough and chest pain, fear of ventilator dependence, or fear of death because of dyspnea and the underlying disease (eg, tumor).

The nurse helps the patient to overcome these fears and to cope with the stress of surgery by correcting any misconceptions, supporting the patient's decision to undergo surgery, reassuring the patient that the incision will "hold," and dealing honestly with questions about pain and discomfort and their treatment. The management and control of pain begin before surgery, when the nurse informs the patient that many postoperative problems can be overcome by following certain routines related to deep breathing, coughing, turning, and moving. If patient-controlled analgesia (PCA) or epidural analgesia is to be used after surgery, the nurse instructs the patient in its use.

Postoperative Management

After surgery, the vital signs are checked frequently. Oxygen is administered by a mechanical ventilator, nasal cannula, or mask for as long as necessary. A reduction in lung capacity requires a period of physiologic adjustment, and fluids may be given at a low hourly rate to prevent fluid overload and pulmonary edema. After the patient is conscious and the vital signs have stabilized, the head of the bed may be elevated 30 to 45 degrees. Careful positioning of the patient is important. After pneumonectomy, a patient is usually turned every hour from the back to the operative side and should not be completely turned to the unoperated side. This allows the fluid left in the space to consolidate and prevents the remaining lung and the heart from shifting (mediastinal shift) toward the operative side. The patient with a lobectomy may be turned to either side, and a patient with a segmental resection usually is not turned onto the operative side unless the surgeon prescribes this position.

Medication for pain is needed for several days after surgery. Because coughing can be painful, the patient should be taught to splint the chest. Exercises are resumed early in the postoperative period to facilitate lung ventilation. The nurse assesses for signs of complications, including cyanosis, dyspnea, and acute chest pain. These may indicate atelectasis and should be reported immediately. Increased temperature or white blood cell count may indicate an infection, and pallor and increased pulse may indicate internal hemorrhage. Dressings are assessed for fresh bleeding.

Mechanical Ventilation

Depending on the nature of the surgery, the patient's underlying condition, the intraoperative course, and the depth of anesthesia, the patient may require mechanical ventilation after surgery. The physician is responsible for determining the ventilator settings and modes, as well as determining the overall method and pace of weaning. However, the physician, nurse, and respiratory therapist work together closely to assess the patient's tolerance and weaning progress. Early extubation from mechanical ventilation can also lead to earlier removal of arterial lines.

Chest Drainage

A crucial intervention for improving gas exchange and breathing in the postoperative period is the proper management of chest drainage and the **chest drainage system**. After thoracic surgery, chest tubes and a closed drainage system are used to re-expand the involved lung and to remove excess air, fluid, and blood. Chest drainage systems also are used in treatment of spontaneous pneumothorax and trauma resulting in pneumothorax. Table 25-3 describes and compares the main features of these systems. Management of chest drainage systems is explained in Chart 25-18. Prevention of cardiopulmonary complications after thoracic surgery is discussed in Chart 25-19.

The normal breathing mechanism operates on the principle of negative pressure; that is, the pressure in the chest

TABLE 25-3 Comparison of Chest Drainage Systems*

Types of Chest Drainage Systems	Description	Comments
Traditional Water Seal		
Also referred to as wet suction	Has three chambers: a collection chamber, water seal chamber (middle chamber), and wet suction control chamber	Requires that sterile fluid be instilled into water seal and suction chambers Has positive- and negative-pressure release valves Intermittent bubbling indicates that the system is functioning properly Additional suction can be added by connecting system to a suction source
Dry Suction Water Seal		
Also referred to as dry suction	Has three chambers: a collection chamber, water seal chamber (middle chamber), and wet suction control chamber	Requires that sterile fluid be instilled in water seal chamber at 2-cm level No need to fill suction chamber with fluid Suction pressure is set with a regulator Has positive- and negative-pressure release valves Has an indicator to signify that the suction pressure is adequate Quieter than traditional water seal systems
Dry Suction		
Also referred to as one-way valve system	Has a one-way mechanical value that allows air to leave the chest and prevents air from moving back into the chest	No need to fill suction chamber with fluid; thus, can be set up quickly in an emergency Works even if knocked over, making it ideal for patients who are ambulatory

*If no fluid drainage is expected, a drainage collection device may not be needed.

CHART 25-18

Guidelines for Managing Chest Drainage Systems

ACTIONS	RATIONALE
1. If using a chest drainage system with a water seal, fill the water seal chamber with sterile water to the level specified by the manufacturer.	Water seal drainage allows air and fluid to escape into a drainage chamber. The water acts as a seal and keeps the air from being drawn back into the pleural space.
2. When using suction in chest drainage systems with a water seal, fill the suction control chamber with sterile water to the 20-cm level or as prescribed. In systems without a water seal, set the regulator dial at the appropriate suction level.	The water level regulator dial setting determines the degree of suction applied.
3. Attach the drainage catheter exiting the thoracic cavity to the tubing coming from the collection chamber. Tape securely with adhesive tape.	In chest drainage units, the system is closed. The only connection is the one to the patient's catheter.
4. If suction is used, connect the suction control chamber tubing to the suction unit. If using a wet suction system, turn on the suction unit and increase pressure until slow but steady bubbling appears in the suction control chamber. If using a chest drainage system with a dry suction control chamber, turn the regulator dial to 20 cm H_2O.	With a wet suction system, the degree of suction is determined by the amount of water in the suction control chamber and is not dependent on the rate of bubbling or the pressure gauge setting on the suction unit. With a dry suction control chamber, the regulator dial replaces the water.

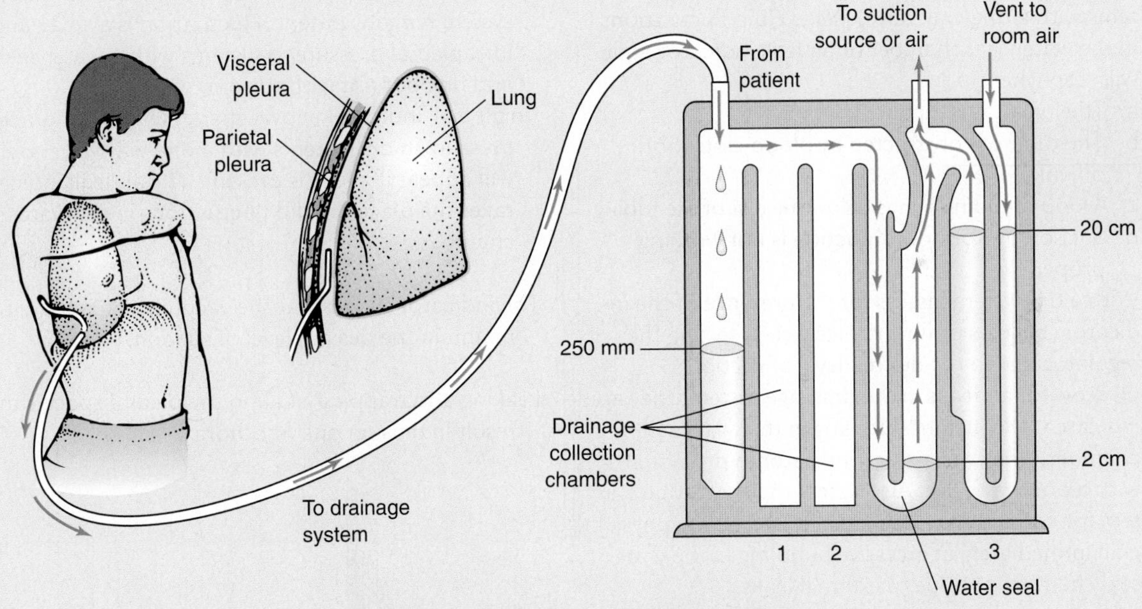

Example of a disposable chest drainage system.

ACTIONS	RATIONALE
5. Mark the drainage from the collection chamber with tape on the outside of the drainage unit. Mark hourly/daily increments (date and time) at the drainage level.	This marking shows the amount of fluid loss and how fast fluid is collecting in the drainage chamber. It serves as a basis for determining the need for blood replacement, if the fluid is blood. Visibly bloody drainage will appear in the chamber in the immediate postoperative period but should gradually becomes serous. If the patient is bleeding as heavily as 100 mL every 15 minutes, check the drainage every few minutes. A reoperation or autotransfusion may be needed. The transfusion of blood collected in the drainage chamber must be reinfused within 4 to 6 hours. Usually, however, drainage decreases progressively in the first 24 hours.

continued >

CHART 25-18 Guidelines for Managing Chest Drainage Systems, continued

ACTIONS	RATIONALE
6. Ensure that the drainage tubing does not kink, loop, or interfere with the patient's movements.	Kinking, looping, or pressure on the drainage tubing can produce back-pressure, which may force fluid back into the pleural space or impede its drainage.
7. Encourage the patient to assume a comfortable position with good body alignment. With the lateral position, make sure that the patient's body does not compress the tubing. The patient should be turned and repositioned every 1.5 to 2 hours. Provide adequate analgesia.	Frequent position changes promote drainage, and good body alignment helps prevent postural deformities and contractures. Proper positioning also helps breathing and promotes better air exchange. Analgesics may be needed to promote comfort.
8. Assist the patient with range-of-motion exercises for the affected arm and shoulder several times daily. Provide adequate analgesia.	Exercise helps to prevent ankylosis of the shoulder and to reduce postoperative pain and discomfort. Analgesics may be needed to relieve pain.
9. Gently "milk" the tubing in the direction of the drainage chamber as needed.	"Milking" prevents the tubing from becoming obstructed by clots and fibrin. Constant attention to maintaining the patency of the tube facilitates prompt expansion of the lung and minimizes complications.
10. Make sure there is fluctuation ("tidaling") of the fluid level in the water seal chamber (in wet systems), or check the air leak indicator for leaks (in dry systems with a one-way valve). *Note:* Fluid fluctuations in the water seal chamber or air leak indicator area will stop when: a. The lung has reexpanded b. The tubing is obstructed by blood clots, fibrin, or kinks c. A loop of tubing hangs below the rest of the tubing d. Suction motor or wall suction is not working properly	Fluctuation of the water level in the water seal shows effective connection between the pleural cavity and the drainage chamber and indicates that the drainage system remains patent. Fluctuation is also a gauge of intrapleural pressure in systems with a water seal (wet and dry, but not with the one-way valve). An air leak indicator shows changes in intrathoracic pressure in dry systems with a one-way valve. Bubbles will appear if a leak is present. The air leak indicator takes the place of fluid fluctuations in the water seal chamber.
11. With a dry system, assess for the presence of the indicator (bellows or float device) when setting the regulator dial to the desired level of suction.	The indicator shows that the vacuum is adequate to maintain the desired level of suction.
12. Observe for air leaks in the drainage system; they are indicated by constant bubbling in the water seal chamber, or by the air leak indicator in dry systems with a one-way valve. Also assess the chest tube system for correctable external leaks. Notify the physician immediately of excessive bubbling in the water seal chamber not due to external leaks.	Leaking and trapping of air in the pleural space can result in tension pneumothorax.
13. When turning down the dry suction, depress the manual high-negativity vent, and assess for a rise in the water level of the water seal chamber.	A rise in the water level of the water seal chamber indicates high negative pressure in the system that could lead to increased intrathoracic pressure.
14. Observe and immediately report rapid and shallow breathing, cyanosis, pressure in the chest, subcutaneous emphysema, symptoms of hemorrhage, or significant changes in vital signs.	Many clinical conditions can cause these signs and symptoms, including tension pneumothorax, mediastinal shift, hemorrhage, severe incisional pain, pulmonary embolus, and cardiac tamponade. Surgical intervention may be necessary.
15. Encourage the patient to breathe deeply and cough at frequent intervals. Provide adequate analgesia. If needed, request an order for patient-controlled analgesia. Also teach the patient how to perform incentive spirometry.	Deep breathing and coughing help to raise the intrapleural pressure, which promotes drainage of accumulated fluid in the pleural space. Deep breathing and coughing also promote removal of secretions from the tracheobronchial tree, which in turn promotes lung expansion and prevents atelectasis (alveolar collapse).

CHART 25-18

Guidelines for Managing Chest Drainage Systems, continued

ACTIONS	RATIONALE
16. If the patient is lying on a stretcher and must be transported to another area, place the drainage system below the chest level. If the tubing disconnects, cut off the contaminated tips of the chest tube and tubing, insert a sterile connector in the cut ends, and reattach to the drainage system. Do *not* clamp the chest tube during transport.	The drainage apparatus must be kept at a level lower than the patient's chest to prevent fluid from flowing backward into the pleural space. Clamping can result in a tension pneumothorax.
17. When assisting in the chest tube's removal, instruct the patient to perform a gentle Valsalva maneuver or to breathe quietly. The chest tube is then clamped and quickly removed. Simultaneously, a small bandage is applied and made airtight with petrolatum gauze covered by a 4 × 4-inch gauze pad and thoroughly covered and sealed with nonporous tape.	The chest tube is removed as directed when the lung is reexpanded (usually 24 hours to several days), depending on the cause of the pneumothorax. During tube removal, the chief priorities are preventing air from entering the pleural cavity as the tube is withdrawn and preventing infection.

CHART 25-19

Preventing Postoperative Cardiopulmonary Complications After Thoracic Surgery

PATIENT MANAGEMENT

- Auscultate lung sounds and assess for rate, rhythm, and depth.
- Monitor oxygenation with pulse oximetry.
- Monitor electrocardiogram for rate and rhythm changes.
- Assess capillary refill, skin color, and status of the surgical dressing.
- Encourage and assist the patient to turn, cough, and take deep breaths.

CHEST DRAINAGE MANAGEMENT

- Verify that all connection tubes are patent and connected securely.
- Assess that the water seal is intact when using a wet suction system and assess the regulator dial in dry suction systems.
- Monitor characteristics of drainage including color, amount, and consistency. Assess for significant increases or decreases in drainage output.
- Note fluctuations in the water seal chamber for wet suction systems and the air leak indicator for dry suction systems.
- Keep system below the patient's chest level.
- Assess suction control chamber for bubbling in wet suction systems.
- Keep suction at prescribed level.
- Maintain appropriate fluid in water seal for wet suction systems.
- Keep air vent open when suction is off.

cavity normally is lower than the pressure of the atmosphere, causing air to move into the lungs during inspiration. Whenever the chest is opened, there is a loss of negative pressure, which can result in collapse of the lung. The collection of air, fluid, or other substances in the chest can compromise cardiopulmonary function and can also cause the lung to collapse. Pathologic substances that collect in the pleural space include fibrin or clotted blood, liquids (serous fluids, blood, pus, chyle), and gases (air from the lung, tracheobronchial tree, or esophagus).

Chest tubes may be inserted to drain fluid or air from any of the three compartments of the thorax (the right and left pleural spaces and the mediastinum). The pleural space, located between the visceral and parietal pleura, normally contains 20 mL or less of fluid, which helps lubricate the visceral and parietal pleura. Surgical incision of the chest wall almost always causes some degree of pneumothorax (air accumulating in the pleural space) or hemo-thorax (buildup of serous fluid or blood in the pleural space). Air and fluid collect in the pleural space, restricting lung expansion and reducing gas exchange. Placement of a chest tube in the pleural space restores the negative intrathoracic pressure needed for lung re-expansion after surgery or trauma.

The mediastinal space is an extrapleural space that lies between the right and left thoracic cavities and contains the large blood vessels, heart, mainstem bronchus, and thymus gland. If fluid accumulates here, the heart can become compressed and stop beating, causing death. Mediastinal chest tubes can be inserted either anteriorly or posteriorly to the heart to drain blood after surgery.

There are two types of chest tubes: small-bore and large-bore catheters. Small-bore catheters (7F to 12F) have a one-way valve apparatus to prevent air from moving back into the patient. They can be inserted through a small skin incision. Large-bore catheters, which range in size up to 40F, are usually connected to a chest drainage system to collect any pleural fluid and monitor for air leaks. After the chest tube is positioned, it is sutured to the skin and connected to a drainage apparatus (Fig. 25-10) to remove the residual air and fluid from the pleural or mediastinal space. This results in the re-expansion of remaining lung tissue.

CHEST DRAINAGE SYSTEMS

Chest drainage systems have a suction source, a collection chamber for pleural drainage, and a mechanism to prevent air from reentering the chest with inhalation. Various types of chest drainage systems are available for use in removal of air and fluid from the pleural space and re-expansion of the lungs. Chest drainage systems come with either wet (water seal) or dry suction control. In wet suction systems, the amount of suction is determined by the amount of water instilled in the suction chamber. The amount of bubbling in the suction chamber indicates how strong the suction is. Wet systems use

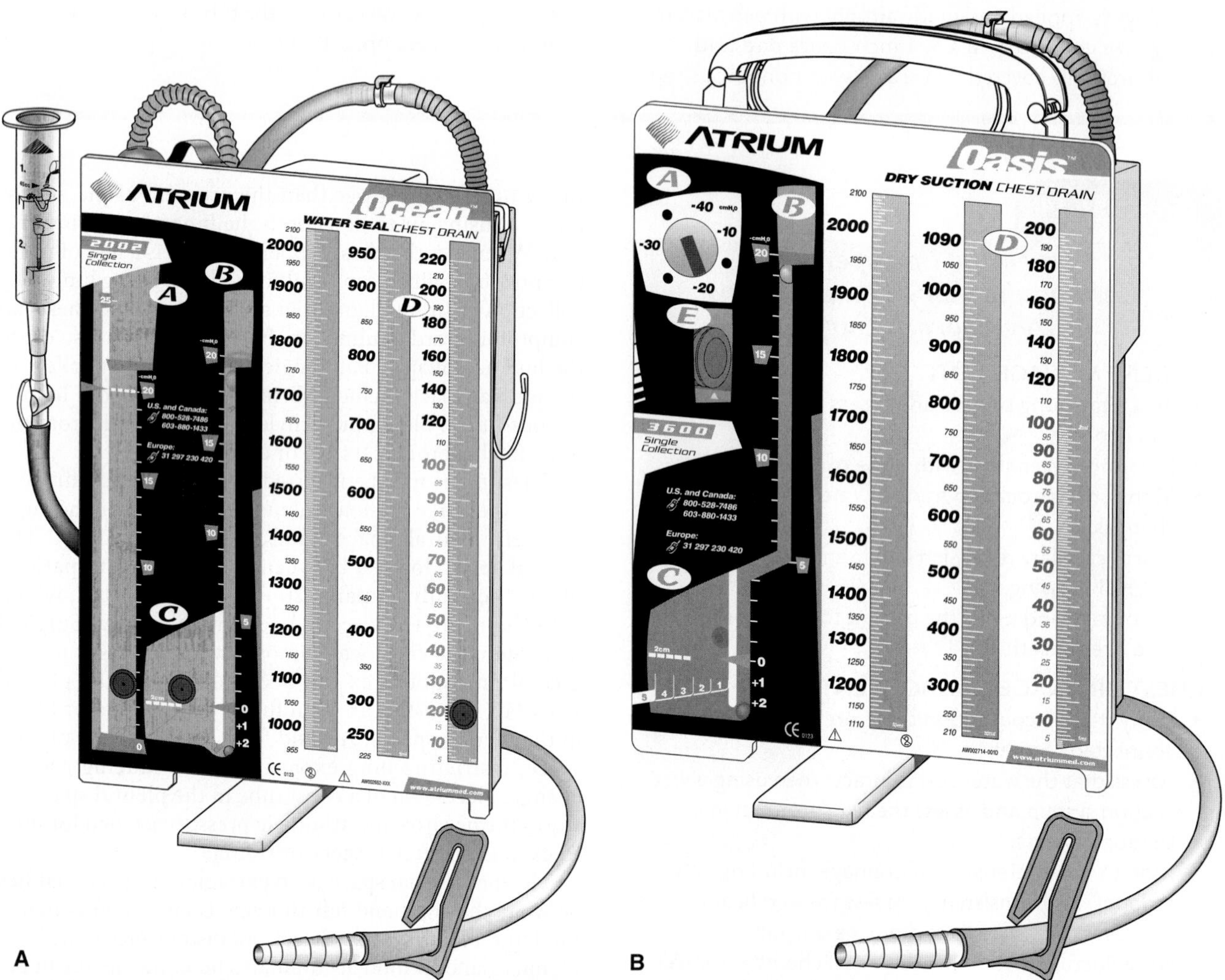

FIGURE 25-10. Chest drainage systems. (**A**) The Atrium Ocean is an example of a water seal chest drain system composed of a drainage chamber and water seal chamber. The suction control is determined by the height of the water column in that chamber (usually 20 cm). *A,* suction control chamber; *B,* water seal chamber; *C,* air leak zone; *D,* collection chamber. (**B**) The Atrium Oasis is an example of a dry suction water seal system that uses a mechanical regulator for vacuum control, a water seal chamber, and a drainage chamber. *A,* dry suction regulator; *B,* water seal chamber; *C,* air leak monitor; *D,* collection chamber; *E,* suction monitor bellows. Art redrawn with permission from Atrium Medical Corporation, Hudson, NH. Reprinted from Morton P. G., Fontaine, D. K., Hudak, C. M., et al. (2005). *Critical care nursing: A holistic approach* (8th ed.). Philadelphia: Lippincott Williams & Wilkins.

a water seal to prevent air from moving back into the chest on inspiration. Dry systems use a one-way valve and may have a suction control dial in place of the water. Both systems can operate by gravity drainage, without a suction source.

Water Seal Systems. The traditional water seal system (or wet suction) for chest drainage has three chambers: a collection chamber, a water seal chamber, and a wet suction control chamber. The collection chamber acts as a reservoir for fluid draining from the chest tube. It is graduated to permit easy measurement of drainage. Suction may be added to create negative pressure and promote drainage of fluid and removal of air. The suction control chamber regulates the amount of negative pressure applied to the chest. The amount of suction is determined by the water level. It is usually set at 20-cm H_2O; adding more fluid results in more suction. After the suction is turned on, bubbling appears in the suction chamber. A positive-pressure valve is located at the top of the suction chamber that automatically opens with increases in positive pressure within the system. Air is automatically released through a positive-pressure relief valve if the suction tubing is inadvertently clamped or kinked.

The water seal chamber has a one-way valve or water seal that prevents air from moving back into the chest when the patient inhales. There is an increase in the water level with inspiration and a return to the baseline level during exhalation; this is referred to as tidaling. Intermittent bubbling in the water seal chamber is normal, but continuous bubbling can indicate an air leak. Bubbling and tidaling do not occur when the tube is placed in the mediastinal space; however, fluid may pulsate with the patient's heartbeat. If the chest tube is connected to gravity drainage only, suction is not used. The pressure is equal to the water seal only. Two-chamber chest drainage systems (water seal chamber and collection chamber) are available for use with patients who need only gravity drainage.

The water level in the water seal chamber reflects the negative pressure present in the intrathoracic cavity. A rise in the water level indicates negative pressure in the pleural or mediastinal space. Excessive negative pressure can cause trauma to tissue. Most chest drainage systems have an automatic means to prevent excessive negative pressure. By pressing and holding a manual high-negativity vent (usually located on the top of the chest drainage system) until the water level in the water seal chamber returns to the 2-cm mark, excessive negative pressure is avoided, preventing damage to tissue.

NURSING ALERT

When the wall vacuum is turned off, the drainage system must be open to the atmosphere so that intrapleural air can escape from the system. This can be done by detaching the tubing from the suction port to provide a vent.

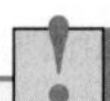

NURSING ALERT

If the chest tube and drainage system become disconnected, air can enter the pleural space, producing a pneumothorax. To prevent pneumothorax if the chest tube is inadvertently disconnected from the drainage system, a temporary water seal can be established by immersing the chest tube's open end in a bottle of sterile water.

Dry Suction Water Seal Systems. Dry suction water seal systems, also referred to as dry suction, have a collection chamber for drainage, a water seal chamber, and a dry suction control chamber. The water seal chamber is filled with water to the 2-cm level. Bubbling in this area can indicate an air leak. The dry suction control chamber contains a regulator dial that conveniently regulates vacuum to the chest drain. Water is not needed for suction in these systems. Without the bubbling in the suction chamber, the machine is quieter. However, if the container is knocked over, the water seal may be lost.

Once the tube is connected to the suction source, the regulator dial allows the desired level of suction to be dialed in; the suction is increased until an indicator appears. The indicator has the same function as the bubbling in the traditional water seal system; that is, it indicates that the vacuum is adequate to maintain the desired level of suction. Some drainage systems use a bellows (a chamber that can be expanded or contracted) or an orange-colored float device as an indicator of when the suction control regulator is set.

When the water in the water seal rises above the 2-cm level, intrathoracic pressure increases. Dry suction water seal systems have a manual high-negativity vent located on top of the drain. The manual high-negativity vent is pressed until the indicator appears (either a float device or bellows) and the water level in the water seal returns to the desired level, indicating that the intrathoracic pressure is decreased.

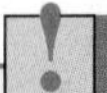

NURSING ALERT

The manual vent should not be used to lower the water level in the water seal when the patient is on gravity drainage (no suction) because intrathoracic pressure is equal to the pressure in the water seal.

Dry Suction Systems with a One-Way Valve. A third type of chest drainage system is dry suction with a one-way mechanical valve. This system has a collection chamber, a one-way mechanical valve, and a dry suction control chamber. The valve permits air and fluid to leave the chest but prevents their movement back into the pleural space. This model lacks a water seal chamber and therefore can be set up quickly in emergency situations, and the dry control drain still works even if it is knocked over. This makes the dry suction systems useful for the patient who is ambulating or being transported. However, without the water seal chamber, there is no way to tell by inspection whether the pressure in the chest has changed, even though an air leak indicator is present so that the system can be checked. If an air leak is suspected, 30 mL of water is injected into the air leak indicator or the container is tipped so that fluid enters the air leak detection chamber. Bubbles will appear if a leak is present.

If the chest tube has been inserted to re-expand a lung after pneumothorax, or if very little fluid drainage is expected, a one-way valve (Heimlich valve) may be connected to the chest tube. This valve may be attached to a collection bag (Fig. 25-11) or covered with a sterile dressing if no drainage is expected.

Nursing Process

The Patient Undergoing Thoracic Surgery

Postoperative Assessment

The nurse monitors the heart rate and rhythm by auscultation and ECG, because episodes of major dysrhythmias are common after thoracic and cardiac surgery. In the immediate postoperative period, an arterial line may be maintained to allow frequent monitoring of arterial blood gases, serum electrolytes, hemoglobin and hematocrit values, and arterial pressure. Central venous pressure may be monitored to detect early signs of fluid volume disturbances; however, central venous pressure monitoring devices are being used less than in the past. Early extubation from mechanical ventilation can also lead to earlier removal of arterial lines. Another important component of postoperative assessment is to note the results of the preoperative evaluation of the patient's lung reserve by pulmonary function testing. A preoperative FEV_1 (the volume of air that the patient can forcibly exhale in 1 second) of more than 2 L or more than 70% of predicted value indicates a good lung reserve. Patients who have a postoperative FEV_1 of less than 40% of predicted value have decreased tidal volume, which places them at risk for respiratory failure, other morbidity, and death.

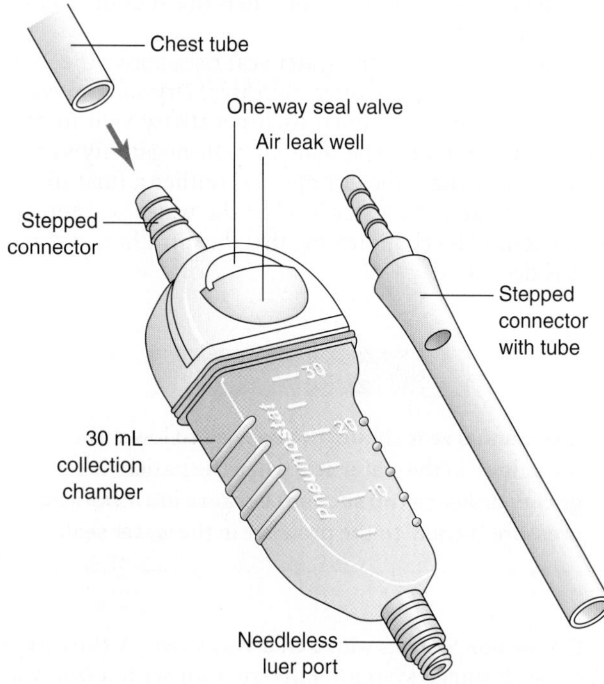

FIGURE 25-11. One-way (Heimlich) valve, a disposable, single-use chest drainage system with 30 mL collection volume. Used when minimal volume of chest drainage is expected.

Diagnosis

Nursing Diagnoses

Based on the assessment data, the patient's major postoperative nursing diagnoses may include:

- Impaired gas exchange related to lung impairment and surgery
- Ineffective airway clearance related to lung impairment, anesthesia, and pain
- Acute pain related to incision, drainage tubes, and the surgical procedure
- Impaired physical mobility of the upper extremities related to thoracic surgery
- Risk for imbalanced fluid volume related to the surgical procedure
- Imbalanced nutrition, less than body requirements related to dyspnea and anorexia
- Deficient knowledge about self-care procedures at home

Collaborative Problems/ Potential Complications

Based on assessment data, potential complications may include the following:

- Respiratory distress
- Dysrhythmias
- Atelectasis, pneumothorax, and bronchopleural fistula
- Blood loss and hemorrhage
- Pulmonary edema

Planning and Goals

The major goals for the patient may include improvement of gas exchange and breathing, improvement of airway clearance, relief of pain and discomfort, increased arm and shoulder mobility, maintenance of adequate fluid volume and nutritional status, understanding of self-care procedures, and absence of complications.

Nursing Interventions

Improving Gas Exchange and Breathing

Gas exchange is determined by evaluating oxygenation and ventilation. In the immediate postoperative period, this is achieved by measuring vital signs (blood pressure, pulse, and respirations) at least every 15 minutes for the first 1 to 2 hours, then less frequently as the patient's condition stabilizes.

Pulse oximetry is used for continuous monitoring of the adequacy of oxygenation. It is important to draw blood for arterial blood gas measurements early in the postoperative period, to establish a baseline to assess the adequacy of oxygenation and ventilation and the possible retention of carbon dioxide. The frequency with which postoperative arterial blood gases are measured depends on whether the patient is mechanically ventilated and whether he or she exhibits signs of respiratory distress; these measurements can help determine appropriate therapy. It also is common practice for patients to have an arterial line in place to obtain blood for blood gas measurements and to monitor blood pressure closely. Hemodynamic monitoring may be used to assess hemodynamic stability.

Breathing techniques, such as diaphragmatic and pursed-lip breathing, that were taught before surgery should be performed by the patient every 2 hours to expand the alveoli and prevent atelectasis. Another technique to improve ventilation is sustained maximal inspiration therapy or incentive spirometry. This technique promotes lung inflation, improves the cough mechanism, and allows early assessment of acute pulmonary changes. (See Charts 25-3 and 25-4 for more information.)

Positioning also improves breathing. If the patient is oriented and blood pressure is stabilized, the head of the bed is elevated 30 to 40 degrees during the immediate postoperative period. This facilitates ventilation, promotes chest drainage from the lower chest tube, and helps residual air to rise in the upper portion of the pleural space, where it can be removed through the upper chest tube.

The nurse consults with the surgeon about patient positioning. There is controversy regarding the best side-lying position. In general, the patient should be positioned from back to side frequently and moved from a flat to a semiupright position as soon as tolerated. Most commonly, the patient is instructed to lie on the operative side. However, the patient with unilateral lung pathology may not be able to turn well onto that side because of pain. In addition, positioning the patient with the "good lung" (the nonoperated lung) down allows a better match of ventilation and perfusion and therefore may actually improve oxygenation. The patient's position is changed from flat to semiupright as soon as possible, because remaining in one position tends to promote the retention of secretions in the dependent portion of the lungs, and the upright position increases diaphragmatic excursion, enhancing lung expansion. After a pneumonectomy, the operated side should be dependent so that fluid in the pleural space remains below the level of the bronchial stump and the other lung can fully expand.

The procedure for turning the patient is as follows:

- Instruct the patient to bend the knees and use the feet to push.
- Have the patient shift hips and shoulders to the opposite side of the bed while pushing with the feet.
- Bring the patient's arm over the chest, pointing it in the direction toward which the patient is being turned. Have the patient grasp the side rail with the hand.
- Turn the patient in log-roll fashion to prevent twisting at the waist and pain from possible pulling on the incision.

Improving Airway Clearance

Retained secretions are a threat to the patient after thoracotomy surgery. Trauma to the tracheobronchial tree during surgery, diminished lung ventilation, and diminished cough reflex all result in the accumulation of excessive secretions. If the secretions are retained, airway obstruction occurs. This, in turn, causes the air in the alveoli distal to the obstruction to become absorbed and the affected portion of the lung to collapse. Atelectasis, pneumonia, and respiratory failure may result.

Several techniques are used to maintain a patent airway. First, secretions are suctioned from the tracheobronchial tree before the endotracheal tube is discontinued. Secretions continue to be removed by suctioning until the patient can cough up secretions effectively. Nasotracheal suctioning may be needed to stimulate a deep cough and aspirate secretions that the patient cannot clear by coughing. However, it should be used only after other methods to raise secretions have been unsuccessful (Chart 25-20).

Coughing technique is another measure used to maintain a patent airway. The patient is encouraged to cough effectively; ineffective coughing results in exhaustion and retention of secretions (see Chart 25-5). To be effective, the cough must be low-pitched, deep, and controlled. Because it is difficult to cough in a supine position, the patient is helped to a sitting position on the edge of the bed, with the feet resting

CHART 25-20

Performing Nasotracheal Suction

STERILE TECHNIQUE TO BE USED

1. Explain procedure to the patient.
2. Medicate patient for pain if necessary.
3. Place the patient in a sitting or semi-Fowler's position. Make sure the patient's head is not flexed forward. Remove excess pillows if necessary.
4. Oxygenate the patient several minutes before initiating the suctioning procedure. Have oxygen source ready nearby during procedure.
5. Put on sterile gloves.
6. Lubricate catheter with water-soluble gel.
7. Gently pass catheter through the patient's nose to the pharynx. If it is difficult to pass the catheter, and repeated suctioning is expected, a soft rubber nasal trumpet may be placed nasopharyngeally to provide easier catheter passage. Check the position of the tip of the catheter by asking the patient to open the mouth and inspecting it; the tip of the catheter should be in the lower pharynx.
8. Instruct the patient to take a deep breath or stick out the tongue. This action opens the epiglottis and promotes downward movement of the catheter.
9. Advance the catheter into the trachea only during inspiration. Listen for cough or for passage of air through the catheter.
10. Attach the catheter to suction apparatus. Apply intermittent suction while slowly withdrawing the catheter. Do not let suction exceed 120 mm Hg.
11. Do not suction for longer than 10 to 15 seconds, as dysrhythmias, bradycardia, or cardiac arrest may occur in patients with borderline oxygenation.
12. If additional suctioning is needed, withdraw the catheter to the back of the pharynx. Reassure patient and oxygenate for several minutes before resuming suctioning.

on a chair. The patient should cough at least every hour during the first 24 hours and when necessary thereafter. If audible crackles are present, it may be necessary to use chest percussion with the cough routine until the lungs are clear. Aerosol therapy is helpful in humidifying and mobilizing secretions so that they can easily be cleared with coughing. To minimize incisional pain during coughing, the nurse supports the incision or encourages the patient to do so (Fig. 25-12).

After helping the patient to cough, the nurse listens to both lungs, anteriorly and posteriorly, to determine whether there are any changes in breath sounds. Diminished breath sounds may indicate collapsed or hypoventilated alveoli.

CPT is the final technique for maintaining a patent airway. If a patient is identified as being at high risk for postoperative pulmonary complications, then CPT is started immediately (perhaps even before surgery). The techniques of postural drainage, vibration, and percussion help loosen and mobilize the secretions so that they can be coughed up or suctioned.

Relieving Pain and Discomfort

Pain after a thoracotomy may be severe, depending on the type of incision and the patient's reaction to and ability to cope with pain. Deep inspiration is very painful after thoracotomy. Pain can lead to postoperative complications if it reduces the patient's ability to breathe deeply and cough and if it further limits chest excursions so that ventilation becomes ineffective.

Immediately after the surgical procedure and before the incision is closed, the surgeon may perform a nerve block with a long-acting local anesthetic such as bupivacaine (Marcaine, Sensorcaine). Bupivacaine is titrated to relieve postoperative pain while allowing the patient to cooperate in deep breathing, coughing, and mobilization. However, it is important to avoid depressing the respiratory system with excessive analgesia: the patient should not be so sedated as to be unable to cough. There is controversy about the effectiveness of injections of local anesthetic for pain relief after thoracotomy. Research has shown that local injections of bupivacaine combined with PCA with IV morphine are as effective in relieving pain as epidural analgesia (Concha, Dagnino, Cariaga, et al., 2004).

Lidocaine and prilocaine are local anesthetic agents used to treat pain at the site of the chest tube insertion. These medications are administered as topical transdermal analgesics that penetrate the skin. Lidocaine and prilocaine have also been found to be effective when used together. EMLA cream, which is a mixture of the two medications, has been found to be effective in treating pain from chest tube removal, and one study showed it to be more effective than IV morphine (Valenzuela & Rosen, 1999). However, many physicians prefer not to use analgesia when removing chest tubes because the pain, although severe, is of short duration (usually less than a few minutes) and the analgesia might interfere with respiratory effort.

PCA is often used postoperatively because of the need to maximize patient comfort without depressing the respiratory drive. Opioid analgesic agents such as morphine are commonly used. PCA, administered through an IV pump or an epidural catheter, allows the patient to control the frequency and total dosage. Preset limits on the pump avoid overdosage. With proper instruction, PCA is well

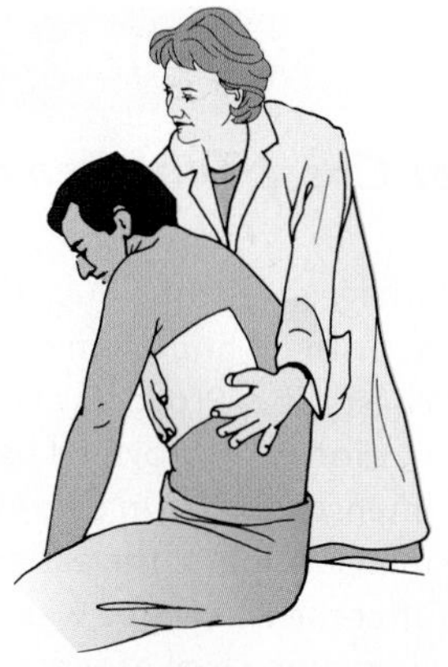

A The nurse's hands should support the chest incision anteriorly and posteriorly. The patient is instructed to take several deep breaths, inhale, and then cough forcibly.

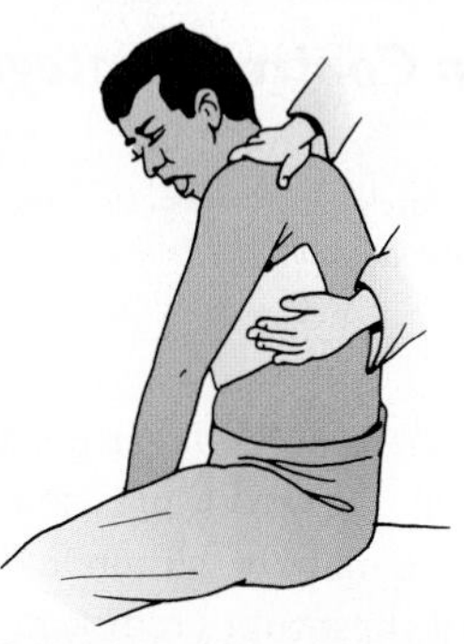

B With one hand, the nurse exerts downward pressure on the shoulder of the affected side while firmly supporting the area beneath the wound with the other hand. The patient is instructed to take several deep breaths, inhale, and then cough forcibly.

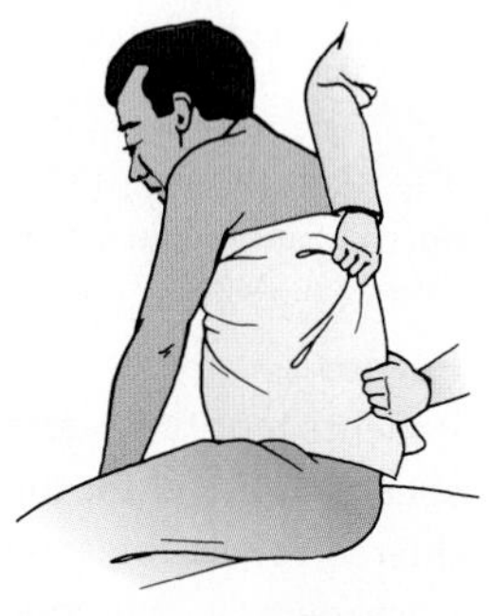

C The nurse can wrap a towel or sheet around the patient's chest and hold the ends together, pulling slightly as the patient coughs, and releasing during deep breaths.

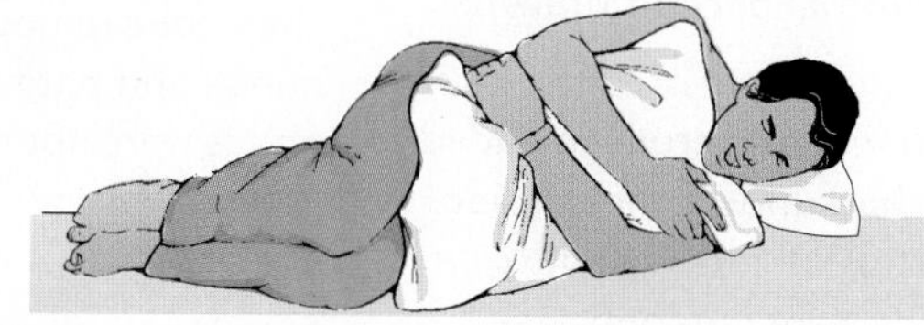

D The patient can be taught to hold a pillow firmly against the incision while coughing. This can be done while lying down or sitting in an upright position.

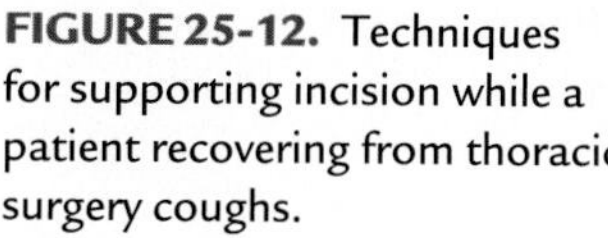

FIGURE 25-12. Techniques for supporting incision while a patient recovering from thoracic surgery coughs.

tolerated and allows earlier mobilization and cooperation with the treatment regimen. (See Chapter 13 for a more extensive discussion of PCA and pain management.)

NURSING ALERT

It is important not to confuse the restlessness of hypoxia with the restlessness caused by pain. Dyspnea, restlessness, increasing respiratory rate, increasing blood pressure, and tachycardia are warning signs of impending respiratory insufficiency. Pulse oximetry is used to monitor oxygenation and to differentiate causes of restlessness.

Promoting Mobility and Shoulder Exercises

Because large shoulder girdle muscles are transected during a thoracotomy, the arm and shoulder must be mobilized by full range of motion of the shoulder. As soon as physiologically possible, usually within 8 to 12 hours, the patient is helped to get out of bed. Although this may be painful initially, the earlier the patient moves, the sooner the pain will subside. In addition to getting out of bed, the patient begins arm and shoulder exercises to restore movement and prevent painful stiffening of the affected arm and shoulder (Chart 25-21).

Maintaining Fluid Volume and Nutrition

INTRAVENOUS THERAPY

During the surgical procedure or immediately after, the patient may receive a transfusion of blood products, followed by a continuous IV infusion. Because a reduction in lung capacity often occurs after thoracic surgery, a period of physiologic adjustment is needed. Fluids should be administered at a low hourly rate and titrated (as prescribed) to prevent overloading the vascular system and precipitating pulmonary edema. The nurse performs careful respiratory and cardiovascular assessments, as well as intake and output, vital signs, and assessment of jugular vein distention. The nurse also monitors the infusion site for signs of infiltration, including swelling, tenderness, and redness.

NUTRITION

It is not unusual for patients undergoing thoracotomy to have poor nutritional status before surgery because of dyspnea, sputum production, and poor appetite. Therefore, it is especially important that adequate nutrition be provided. A liquid diet is provided as soon as bowel sounds return, and the patient is progressed to a full diet as soon as possible. Small, frequent meals are better tolerated and are crucial to the recovery and maintenance of lung function.

Monitoring and Managing Potential Complications

Complications after thoracic surgery are always a possibility and must be identified and managed early.

NURSING RESEARCH PROFILE

Pain Control Strategies for Chest Tube Removal

Puntillo, K. & Ley, S. J. (2004). Appropriately timed analgesics control pain due to chest tube removal. *American Journal of Critical Care, 13*(4), 292–301.

Purpose

Patients report moderate to severe pain and distress associated with chest tube removal. This study was conducted to test four approaches to managing pain in postoperative patients who had chest tubes removed. It examined the effects of two analgesic agents (morphine versus ketorolac, a nonsteroidal noninflammatory agent) and two educational approaches (information about the procedure versus the same information about the procedure *plus* information about sensations that could be expected with removal of chest tubes).

Design

This double-blind, quasi-experimental study included a sample of 74 patients who had undergone cardiac surgery about 1 day previously. Patients who gave informed consent for the study were randomly assigned to one of four pain relief strategies: (1) intravenous (IV) morphine and procedural information; (2) IV ketorolac and procedural information; (3) IV morphine and procedural plus sensory information; and (4) IV ketorolac and procedural plus sensory information. Patients were instructed on the use of rating scales to assess pain intensity and pain distress. Morphine or ketorolac was administered before removal of the tube at a time that corresponded with the peak effect of each medication (60 minutes before removal for ketorolac, 20 minutes for morphine). To blind the patient and data collector to the analgesic agent used, an injection of normal saline was administered to all patients in addition to the assigned analgesic agent; thus, all patients received injections at both 60 and 20 minutes before removal of the chest tube. Procedural information and sensory information were provided using prepared scripts. Pain intensity and pain distress were measured before administration of the assigned analgesic, immediately after the chest tube was removed, and again 20 minutes later. Level of sedation was also measured before and 20 minutes after chest tube removal. Differences in effectiveness of pain relief strategies and level of sedation were analyzed over time.

Findings

Patients reported mild levels of pain and distress during chest tube removal. Sedation levels as assessed by nurses and patients' pain intensity and pain distress scores were not significantly different across the four groups. Patients remained alert, regardless of which analgesic agent was received.

Nursing Implications

Many clinicians elect not to medicate patients before removal of chest tubes because the severe pain associated with removal is of short duration and because of the risk of prolonged sedation associated with analgesic agents. The findings of this study indicate that timing the administration of analgesics so that their effect peaks at the time of chest tube removal reduces pain associated with the procedure and does not increase sedation. These findings suggest that nurses should time administration of analgesics so that their effects are beneficial to patients. Furthermore, they suggest that several safe and effective interventions are available to reduce pain and distress associated with chest tube removal.

In addition, the nurse monitors the patient at regular intervals for signs of respiratory distress or developing respiratory failure, dysrhythmias, bronchopleural fistula, hemorrhage and shock, atelectasis, and pulmonary infection.

Respiratory distress is treated by identifying and eliminating its cause while providing supplemental oxygen. If the patient progresses to respiratory failure, intubation and mechanical ventilation are necessary.

Dysrhythmias are often related to the effects of hypoxia or the surgical procedure. They are treated with antiarrhythmic medication and supportive therapy (see Chapter 27). Pulmonary infections or effusion, often preceded by atelectasis, may occur a few days into the postoperative course.

Pneumothorax may occur after thoracic surgery if there is an air leak from the surgical site to the pleural cavity or from the pleural cavity to the environment. Failure of the chest drainage system prevents return of negative pressure in the pleural cavity and results in pneumothorax. In the postoperative patient, pneumothorax is often accompanied by hemothorax. The nurse maintains the chest drainage system and monitors the patient for signs and symptoms of pneumothorax: increasing shortness of breath, tachycardia, increased respiratory rate, and increasing respiratory distress.

Bronchopleural fistula is a serious but rare complication that prevents the return of negative intrathoracic pressure and lung re-expansion. Depending on its severity, it is treated with closed chest drainage, me-

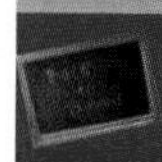

CHART 25-21

Patient Education

Performing Arm and Shoulder Exercises

Arm and shoulder exercises are performed after thoracic surgery to restore movement, prevent painful stiffening of the shoulder, and improve muscle power.

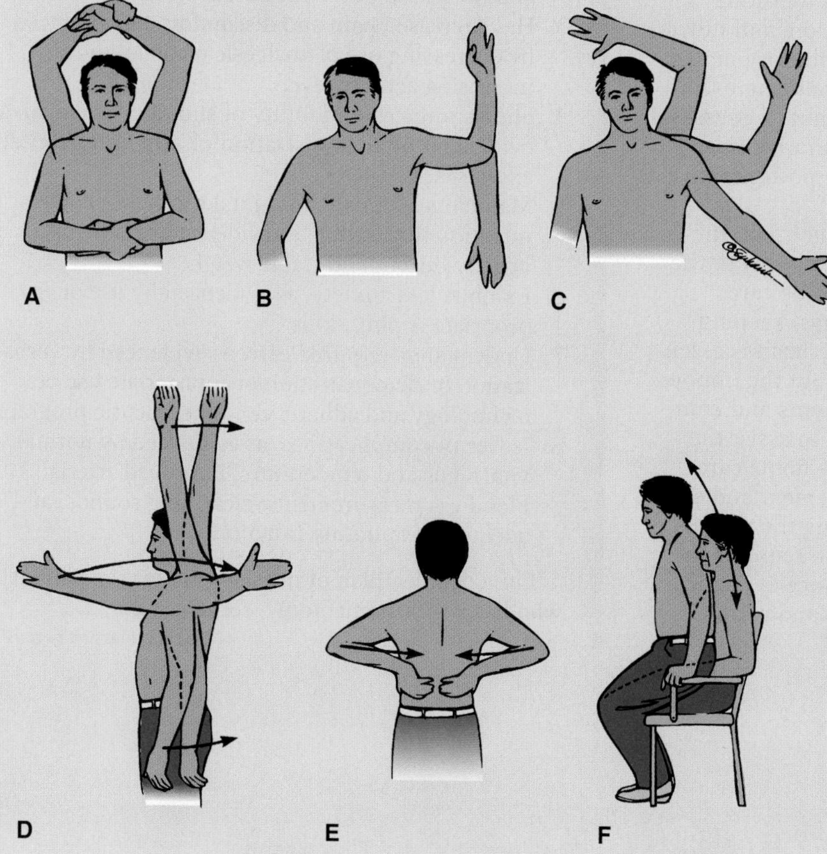

(**A**) Hold hand of the affected side with the other hand, palms facing in. Raise the arms forward, upward, and then overhead, while taking a deep breath. Exhale while lowering the arms. Repeat five times. (**B**) Raise arm sideward, upward, and downward in a waving motion. (**C**) Place arm at side. Raise arm sideward, upward, and over the head. Repeat five times. These exercises can also be performed while lying in bed. (**D**) Extend the arm up and back, out to the side and back, down at the side and back. (**E**) Place hands in small of back. Push elbows as far back as possible. (**F**) Sit erect in an armchair; place the hands on the arms of the chair directly opposite the sides of the body. Press down on hands, consciously pulling the abdomen in and stretching up from the waist. Inhale while raising the body until the elbows are extended completely. Hold this position a moment, and begin exhaling while lowering the body slowly to the original position.

chanical ventilation, and possibly talc pleurodesis (described in Chapter 23).

Hemorrhage and shock are managed by treating the underlying cause, whether by reoperation or by administration of blood products or fluids. Pulmonary edema from overinfusion of IV fluids is a significant danger. Early symptoms are dyspnea, crackles, bubbling sounds in the chest, tachycardia, and pink, frothy sputum. This constitutes an emergency and must be reported and treated immediately.

Promoting Home and Community-Based Care

TEACHING PATIENTS SELF-CARE

The nurse instructs the patient and family about postoperative care that will be continued at home. The nurse explains signs and symptoms that should be reported to the physician. These include the following:

- Change in respiratory status: increasing shortness of breath, fever, increased restlessness or other changes in mental or cognitive status, increased respiratory rate, change in respiratory pattern, change in amount or color of sputum
- Bleeding or other drainage from the surgical incision or chest tube exit sites
- Increased chest pain

In addition, respiratory care and other treatment modalities (oxygen, incentive spirometry, CPT, and oral, inhaled, or IV medications) may be continued at home. Therefore, the nurse needs to instruct the patient and family in their correct and safe use.

The nurse emphasizes the importance of progressively increased activity. The nurse instructs the patient to ambulate within limits and explains that return of strength is likely to be very gradual. Another important aspect of patient teaching addresses shoulder exercises. The patient is instructed to do these exercises five times daily. Additional patient teaching is described in Chart 25-22.

CONTINUING CARE

Depending on the patient's physical status and the availability of family assistance, a home care referral may be indicated. The home care nurse assesses the patient's recovery from surgery, with special attention to respiratory status, the surgical incision, chest drainage, pain control, ambulation, and nutritional status. The patient's use of respiratory modalities is assessed to ensure that they are being used correctly and safely. In addition, the nurse assesses the patient's adherence to the postoperative treatment plan and identifies acute or late postoperative complications.

The recovery process may take longer than the patient had expected, and providing support to the patient is an important task for the home care nurse. Because of shorter hospital stays, keeping follow-up appointments with the physician is essential. The nurse teaches the patient about the importance of keeping follow-up appointments and completing laboratory tests as prescribed to assist the physician in evaluating recovery. The home care nurse provides continuous encouragement and education to the patient and family during the process. As recovery progresses, the nurse also reminds the patient and family about the importance of participating in health promotion activities and recommended health screening.

Evaluation

Expected Patient Outcomes

Expected patient outcomes may include the following:

1. Demonstrates improved gas exchange, as evidenced by improved arterial blood gas measurements.
2. Shows improved airway clearance, as evidenced by deep, controlled coughing and clear breath sounds and decreased or absent adventitious sounds
3. Has decreased pain and discomfort, as evidenced by decreasing use of analgesic medications and increasing activity level
4. Shows improved mobility of shoulder and arm, as evidenced by demonstration of arm and shoulder exercises.
5. Maintains adequate fluid intake and maintains nutrition for healing, as evidenced by adequate urinary output and stable weight.
6. Exhibits less anxiety, as evidenced by use of appropriate coping skills
7. Understands required care, as evidenced by verbalization or demonstration of appropriate use of technology and adherence to therapeutic program
8. Is free of complications, as evidenced by normal vital signs and temperature, improved arterial blood gas measurements, clear lung sounds, and adequate respiratory function

For a detailed plan of nursing care for the patient who has had a thoracotomy, see Chart 25-23.

(text continues on page 775)

CHART 25-22

HOME CARE CHECKLIST • The Patient With a Thoracotomy

At the completion of the home care instruction, the patient or caregiver will be able to:	Patient	Caregiver
• Use local heat and oral analgesia to relieve intercostal pain.	✔	✔
• Alternate walking and other activities with frequent rest periods, expecting weakness and fatigue for the first 3 weeks.	✔	✔
• Perform breathing exercises several times daily for the first few weeks at home.	✔	
• Avoid lifting more than 20 pounds until complete healing has taken place; the chest muscles and incision may be weaker than normal for 3 to 6 months after surgery.	✔	
• Walk at a moderate pace, gradually and persistently extending walking time and distance.	✔	
• Immediately stop any activity that causes undue fatigue, increased shortness of breath, or chest pain.	✔	
• Avoid bronchial irritants (smoke, fumes, air pollution, aerosol sprays).	✔	✔
• Avoid others with known colds or lung infections.	✔	✔
• Obtain an annual influenza vaccine and discuss vaccination against pneumonia with the physician.	✔	
• Report for follow-up care by the surgeon or clinic as necessary.	✔	✔
• Stop smoking, if applicable, and avoid exposure to secondhand smoke.	✔	✔

CHART 25-23

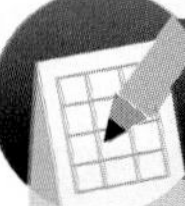

Plan of Nursing Care: Care of the Patient After Thoracotomy

Nursing Diagnosis: Impaired gas exchange related to lung impairment and surgery
Goal: Improvement of gas exchange and breathing

NURSING INTERVENTIONS	RATIONALE	EXPECTED OUTCOMES
1. Monitor pulmonary status as directed and as needed: a. Auscultate breath sounds. b. Check rate, depth, and pattern of respirations. c. Assess blood gases for signs of hypoxemia or CO_2 retention. d. Evaluate patient's color for cyanosis.	1. Changes in pulmonary status indicate improvement or onset of complications.	• Lungs are clear on auscultation • Respiratory rate is within acceptable range with no episodes of dyspnea • Vital signs are stable • Dysrhythmias are not present or are under control • Demonstrates deep, controlled, effective breathing to allow maximal lung expansion • Uses incentive spirometer every 2 hours while awake • Demonstrates deep, effective coughing technique • Lungs are expanded to capacity (evidenced by chest x-ray)
2. Monitor and record blood pressure, apical pulse, and temperature every 2–4 hours, central venous pressure (if indicated) every 2 hours.	2. Aid in evaluating effect of surgery on cardiac status.	
3. Monitor continuous electrocardiogram for pattern and dysrhythmias.	3. Dysrhythmias (especially atrial fibrillation and atrial flutter) are more frequently seen after thoracic surgery. A patient with total pneumonectomy is especially prone to cardiac irregularity.	
4. Elevate head of bed 30–40 degrees when patient is oriented and hemodynamic status is stable.	4. Maximum lung excursion is achieved when patient is as close to upright as possible.	
5. Encourage deep-breathing exercises (see section on Breathing Retraining) and effective use of incentive spirometer (sustained maximal inspiration).	5. Helps to achieve maximal lung inflation and to open closed airways.	
6. Encourage and promote an effective cough routine to be performed every 1–2 hours during first 24 hours.	6. Coughing is necessary to remove retained secretions.	
7. Assess and monitor the chest drainage system:* a. Assess for leaks and patency as needed. b. Monitor amount and character of drainage and document every 2 hours. Notify physician if drainage is 150 mL/h or greater. c. See Chart 25-18 for summary of nurse's role in management of chest drainage systems.	7. System is used to eliminate any residual air or fluid after thoracotomy.	

*A patient with a pneumonectomy usually does not have water seal chest drainage because it is desirable that the pleural space fill with an effusion, which eventually obliterates this space. Some surgeons do use a modified water seal system.

continued >

CHART 25-23

Plan of Nursing Care — Care of the Patient After Thoracotomy (Continued)

Nursing Diagnosis: Ineffective airway clearance related to lung impairment, anesthesia, and pain
Goal: Improvement of airway clearance and achievement of a patent airway

NURSING INTERVENTIONS	RATIONALE	EXPECTED OUTCOMES
1. Maintain an open airway.	1. Provides for adequate ventilation and gas exchange	• Airway is patent • Coughs effectively • Splints incision while coughing • Sputum is clear or colorless • Lungs are clear on auscultation
2. Perform endotracheal suctioning until patient can raise secretions effectively.	2. Endotracheal secretions are present in excessive amounts in post-thoracotomy patients due to trauma to the tracheobronchial tree during surgery, diminished lung ventilation, and cough reflex.	
3. Assess and medicate for pain. Encourage deep-breathing and coughing exercises. Help splint incision during coughing.	3. Helps to achieve maximal lung inflation and to open closed airways. Coughing is painful; incision needs to be supported.	
4. Monitor amount, viscosity, color, and odor of sputum. Notify physician if sputum is excessive or contains bright-red blood.	4. Changes in sputum suggest presence of infection or change in pulmonary status. Colorless sputum is not unusual; opacification or coloring of sputum may indicate dehydration or infection.	
5. Administer humidification and mini-nebulizer therapy as prescribed.	5. Secretions must be moistened and thinned if they are to be raised from the chest with the least amount of effort.	
6. Perform postural drainage, percussion, and vibration as prescribed. Do not percuss or vibrate directly over operative site.	6. Chest physiotherapy uses gravity to help remove secretions from the lung.	
7. Auscultate both sides of chest to determine changes in breath sounds.	7. Indications for tracheal suctioning are determined by chest auscultation.	

Nursing Diagnosis: Acute pain related to incision, drainage tubes, and the surgical procedure
Goal: Relief of pain and discomfort

NURSING INTERVENTIONS	RATIONALE	EXPECTED OUTCOMES
1. Evaluate location, character, quality, and severity of pain. Administer analgesic medication as prescribed and as needed. Observe for respiratory effect of opioid. Is patient too somnolent to cough? Are respirations depressed?	1. Pain limits chest excursions and thereby decreases ventilation.	• Asks for pain medication, but verbalizes that he or she expects some discomfort while deep breathing and coughing • Verbalizes that he or she is comfortable and not in acute distress • No signs of incisional infection evident

CHART 25-23

Plan of Nursing Care Care of the Patient After Thoracotomy (Continued)

NURSING INTERVENTIONS	RATIONALE	EXPECTED OUTCOMES
2. Maintain care postoperatively in positioning the patient: a. Place patient in semi-Fowler's position. b. Patients with limited respiratory reserve may not be able to turn on unoperated side. c. Assist or turn patient every 2 hours.	2. The patient who is comfortable and free of pain will be less likely to splint the chest while breathing. A semi-Fowler's position permits residual air in the pleural space to rise to upper portion of pleural space and be removed via the upper chest catheter.	
3. Assess incision area every 8 hours for redness, heat, induration, swelling, separation, and drainage.	3. These signs indicate possible infection.	
4. Request order for patient-controlled analgesia pump if appropriate for patient.	4. Allowing patient control over frequency and dose improves comfort and compliance with treatment regimen.	

Nursing Diagnosis: Anxiety related to outcomes of surgery, pain, technology
Goal: Reduction of anxiety to a manageable level

NURSING INTERVENTIONS	RATIONALE	EXPECTED OUTCOMES
1. Explain all procedures in understandable language.	1. Explaining what can be expected in understandable terms decreases anxiety and increases cooperation.	• States that anxiety is at a manageable level • Participates with health care team in treatment regimen • Uses appropriate coping skills (verbalization, pain relief strategies, use of support systems such as family, clergy) • Demonstrates basic understanding of technology used in care
2. Assess for pain and medicate, especially before potentially painful procedures.	2. Premedication before painful procedures or activities improves comfort and minimizes undue anxiety.	
3. Silence all *unnecessary* alarms on technology (monitors, ventilators).	3. *Unnecessary* alarms increase the risk of sensory overload and may increase anxiety. *Essential* alarms must be turned on at all times.	
4. Encourage and support patient while increasing activity level.	4. Positive reinforcement improves patient motivation and independence.	
5. Mobilize resources (family, clergy, social worker) to help patient cope with outcomes of surgery (diagnosis, change in functional abilities).	5. A multidisciplinary approach promotes the patient's strengths and coping mechanisms.	

continued >

CHART 25-23

Plan of Nursing Care — Care of the Patient After Thoracotomy (Continued)

Nursing Diagnosis: Impaired physical mobility of the upper extremities related to thoracic surgery
Goal: Increased mobility of the affected shoulder and arm

NURSING INTERVENTIONS	RATIONALE	EXPECTED OUTCOMES
1. Assist patient with normal range of motion and function of shoulder and trunk: a. Teach breathing exercises to mobilize thorax. b. Encourage skeletal exercises to promote abduction and mobilization of shoulder (see Chart 25-21). c. Assist out of bed to chair as soon as pulmonary and circulatory systems are stable (usually by evening of surgery).	1. Necessary to regain normal mobility of arm and shoulder and to speed recovery and minimize discomfort	• Demonstrates arm and shoulder exercises and verbalizes intent to perform them on discharge • Regains previous range of motion in shoulder and arm
2. Encourage progressive activities according to level of fatigue.	2. Increases patient's use of affected shoulder and arm	

Nursing Diagnosis: Risk for imbalanced fluid volume related to the surgical procedure
Goal: Maintenance of adequate fluid volume

NURSING INTERVENTIONS	RATIONALE	EXPECTED OUTCOMES
1. Monitor and record hourly intake and output. Urine output should be at least 30 mL/h after surgery.	1. Fluid management may be altered before, during, and after surgery, and patient's response to and need for fluid management must be assessed.	• Patient is adequately hydrated, as evidenced by: • Urine output greater than 30 mL/h • Vital signs stable, heart rate, and central venous pressure approaching normal • No excessive peripheral edema
2. Administer blood component therapy and parenteral fluids and/or diuretics as prescribed to restore and maintain fluid volume.	2. Pulmonary edema due to transfusion or fluid overload is an ever-present threat; after pneumonectomy, the pulmonary vascular system has been greatly reduced.	

Nursing Diagnosis: Deficient knowledge of home care procedures
Goal: Increased ability to carry out care procedures at home

NURSING INTERVENTIONS	RATIONALE	EXPECTED OUTCOMES
1. Encourage patient to practice arm and shoulder exercises five times daily at home.	1. Exercise accelerates recovery of muscle function and reduces long-term pain and discomfort.	• Demonstrates arm and shoulder exercises • Verbalizes need to try to assume an erect posture
2. Instruct patient to practice assuming a functionally erect position in front of a full-length mirror.	2. Practice will help restore normal posture.	

CHART 25-23

Plan of Nursing Care — Care of the Patient After Thoracotomy (Continued)

NURSING INTERVENTIONS	RATIONALE	EXPECTED OUTCOMES
3. Instruct patient in following aspects of home care:	3. Knowing what to expect facilitates recovery.	• Verbalizes the importance of relieving discomfort, alternating walking and rest, performing breathing exercises, avoiding heavy lifting, avoiding undue fatigue, avoiding bronchial irritants, preventing colds or lung infections, getting influenza vaccine, keeping follow-up visits, and stopping smoking
a. Relieve intercostal pain by local heat or oral analgesia.	a. Some soreness may persist for several weeks.	
b. Alternate activities with frequent rest periods.	b. Weakness and fatigue are common for the first 3 weeks or longer.	
c. Practice breathing exercises at home.	c. Effective breathing is necessary to prevent splinting of affected side, which may lead to atelectasis.	
d. Avoid heavy lifting until complete healing has occurred.	d. Chest muscles and incision may be weaker than normal for 3–6 months.	
e. Avoid undue fatigue, increased shortness of breath, or chest pain.	e. Undue stress may prolong the healing process.	
f. Avoid bronchial irritants.	f. The lung is more susceptible to irritants.	
g. Prevent colds or lung infection.	g. The lung is more susceptible to infection during the recovery phase.	
h. Get annual influenza vaccine.	h. Vaccination helps prevent flu.	
i. Keep follow-up appointment with physician.	i. This allows timely follow-up assessment.	
j. Stop smoking.	j. Smoking will slow healing process by decreasing oxygen delivery to tissues and make lung susceptible to infection and other complications.	

Critical Thinking Exercises

1 The morning after a man has undergone thoracic surgery, he gets out of bed unassisted and disconnects the chest tube from the drainage system. What immediate complications are of greatest concern, and what actions should the nurse take to prevent these complications? What nursing assessments and nursing interventions are needed to (1) prevent recurrence of this situation and (2) identify and treat other complications?

2 ebp A patient with long-standing pulmonary disease is instructed to perform postural drainage three times a day. What is the evidence base for use of postural drainage? What is the strength of that evidence, and what criteria did you use to assess the strength of that evidence? What patient teaching is important for the patient and family member if the patient is to continue postural drainage at home?

3 Oxygen therapy is required for the following patients: a 44-year-old patient who has undergone a right lower lobe lobectomy and requires short-term oxygen therapy; a 68-year-old patient with advanced COPD who has been admitted to the hospital repeatedly in the past 2 years; and a 78-year-old patient with dyspnea secondary to advanced lung cancer. Compare and contrast the similarities and differences in the oxygen therapy necessary for each patient, and discuss teaching and safety precautions indicated for each patient and his or her family. Describe the patient teaching that will be required if each of these patients is discharged from the hospital with a prescription for oxygen therapy.

4 ebp A woman is scheduled to have a tracheostomy performed in the operating room to allow her to continue to receive mechanical ventilation to treat temporary paralysis of her respiratory muscles secondary to a neuromuscular disorder. For the past week, she has been intubated with an endotracheal tube and has been receiving mechanical ventilation. What preprocedure preparation and teaching and what safety precautions are warranted for this patient? Develop an evidence-based protocol for addressing her needs related to tracheostomy care and positive-pressure mechanical ventilation.

5 Your patient has just returned from the operating room after thoracic surgery. She has an endotracheal tube, two chest tubes, two IV lines, a cardiac monitor, and an indwelling urinary catheter in place. What are your immediate priorities for assessment for this patient? What observations need to be reported to the surgeon immediately? What other nursing interventions are warranted immediately? In 8 hours? At 24 hours and 48 hours postoperatively?

REFERENCES AND SELECTED READINGS

BOOKS

Doenges, M. E., Moorhouse, M. F. & Murr, A. C. (2004). *Nurse's pocket guide: Diagnoses, interventions, and rationales* (9th ed.). Philadelphia: F. A. Davis.

Ebersole, P., Hess, P. & Luggen, A. S. (2003). *Toward healthy aging: Human needs and nursing response* (6th ed.). St. Louis: C. V. Mosby.

Grodner, M., Long, S. & Deyoung, S. (2003). *Foundations and clinical application of nutrition: A nursing approach* (3rd ed.). St. Louis: C. V. Mosby.

Hess, D. R. & Kacmarek, R. M. (2002). *Essentials of mechanical ventilation* (2nd ed.): New York: McGraw-Hill Medical.

Kacmarek, R. M., Dimas, S. & Mack, C. W. (2005). *The essentials of respiratory care* (4th ed.). St. Louis: Elsevier Mosby.

Kee, J. L. & Hayes, E. R. (2002). *Pharmacology: A nursing process approach* (4th ed.). Philadelphia: W. B. Saunders.

MacIntyre, N. R., Mishoe, S. C., Galvin, W. F., et al. (2001). *Respiratory care: Principles and practice* (1st ed.). Philadelphia: W. B. Saunders.

Morton, P. G., Fontaine, D. K., Hudak, C. M., et al. (2005). *Critical care nursing: A holistic approach* (8th ed.). Philadelphia: Lippincott Williams & Wilkins.

NHS Quality Improvement Scotland (2003). *Caring for the patient with a tracheostomy: Best practice statement.* Edinburgh: Nursing & Midwifery Practice Development Unit.

Sole, M. L., Klein, D. & Moseley, M. (2004). *Introduction to critical care nursing* (4th ed.). Philadelphia: W. B. Saunders.

Wilkins, R. L., Stoller, J. K. & Scanlon, C. l. (2003). *Egan's fundamentals of respiratory care* (8th ed.). St. Louis: Mosby.

JOURNALS

**Asterisks indicate nursing research articles.*

Allibone, L. (2003). Nursing management of chest drains. *Nursing Standard, 17*(22), 45–54.

Ambrosino, N. & Rossi, A. (2002). Proportional assist ventilation (PAV): A significant advance or a futile struggle between logic and practice. *Thorax, 57*(3), 272–276.

Andrs, K. (2004). Chest drainage to go. *Nursing, 34*(5), 54–55.

Baudouin, S. V. & Evans, T. W. (2003). Nutritional support in critical care. *Clinics in Chest Medicine 24*(3), 633–644.

Benditt, J. O. (2004). Surgical therapies for chronic obstructive pulmonary disease. *Respiratory Care, 49*(1), 53–61.

Bennett, M. & Heard, R. (2004). Hyperbaric oxygen therapy for multiple sclerosis. *Cochrane Database of Systematic Reviews,* CD003057.

Bennett, M. H., Trytko, B. & Jonker, B. (2004). Hyperbaric oxygen therapy for the adjunctive treatment of traumatic brain injury. *Cochrane Database of Systematic Reviews,* CD004609.

Bliss, P. L., McCoy, R. W. & Adams, A. B. (2004). Characteristics of demand oxygen delivery systems: Maximum output and setting recommendations. *Respiratory Care, 49*(2), 160–165.

Bond, P., Grant, F., Coltart, L., et al. (2003). Best practice in the care of patients with a tracheostomy. *Nursing Times, 99*(30), 24–25.

Broussard, C. L. (2003). Hyperbaric oxygenation and wound healing. *Journal of WOCN, 30*(4), 210–216.

Burns, S. M. (2004). The science of weaning: When and how? *Critical Care Nursing Clinics of North America, 16*(3), 379–386.

Cirino, L. M., Campos, L., Jatene, F., et al. (2000). Diagnosis and treatment of mediastinal tumors by thoracoscopy. *Chest, 117*(6), 1787–1792.

Concha, M., Dagnino, J., Cariaga, M., et al. (2004). Analgesia after thoracotomy: Epidural fentanyl/bupivacaine compared with intercostal nerve block plus intravenous morphine. *Journal of Cardiothoracic and Vascular Anesthesia, 18*(3), 322–326.

Dekleva, M., Neskovic, A., Vlahovic, A., et al. (2004). Adjunctive effect of hyperbaric oxygen treatment after thrombolysis on left ventricular function in patients with acute myocardial infarction. *American Heart Journal, 148*(4), E14.

Doherty, D. E. & Briggs, D. D., Jr. (2004). Long-term nonpharmacologic management of patients with chronic obstructive pulmonary disease. *Clinical Cornerstone, 6*(Suppl. 2), S29–S34.

Frawley, P. M. & Habashi, N. M. (2001). Airway pressure release ventilation: Theory and practice. *AACN Clinical Issues, 12*(2), 234–246.

Fuhrman, C., Chouaid, C., Herigault, R., et al. (2004). Comparison of four demand oxygen delivery systems at rest and during exercise for chronic obstructive pulmonary disease. *Respiratory Medicine, 98*(10), 938–944.

*Gelsthorpe, T., & Crocker, C. (2004). A study exploring factors which influence the decision to commence nurse-led weaning. *Nursing in Critical Care, 9*(5), 213–221.

*Goris, A. H., Vermeeren, M. A., Wouters, E. F., et al. (2003). Energy balance in depleted ambulatory patients with chronic obstructive pulmonary disease: The effect of physical activity and oral nutritional supplementation. *British Journal of Nutrition, 89*(5), 725–729.

*Grap, M. J., Munro, C. L., Elswick, R. K., et al. (2004). Duration of action of a single, early oral application of chlorhexadine on oral microbial flora in mechanically ventilated patients: A pilot study. *Heart & Lung, 33*(2), 83–91.

Habashi, N. M. (2005). Other approaches to open-lung ventilation: Airway pressure release ventilation. *Critical Care Medicine, 33*(3 Suppl.), S228–S240.

Harper, A. & Croft-Baker, J. (2004). Carbon monoxide poisoning: Undetected by both patients and their doctors. *Age and Ageing, 33*(2), 105–109.

Hess, D. R. (2005). Facilitating speech in the patient with a tracheostomy. *Respiratory Care, 50*(4), 519–525.

Higgins, D. (2005a). Oxygen therapy. *Nursing Times, 101*(4), 30–31.

Higgins, D. (2005b). Tracheal suction. *Nursing Times, 101*(8), 36–37.

Langenhof, S. & Fichter, J. (2005). Comparison of two demand oxygen delivery devices for administration of oxygen in COPD. *Chest, 128*(4), 2082–2087.

Lindgren, V. A. & Ames, N. J. (2005). Caring for patients on mechanical ventilation. *American Journal of Nursing, 105*(5), 50–60.

*Lorente, L., Lecuona, M., Galvan, R., et al. (2004). Periodically changing ventilator circuits is not necessary to prevent ventilator-associated

pneumonia when a heat and moisture exchanger is used. *Infection Control and Hospital Epidemiology, 25*(12), 1077–1082.
*Lorente, L., Lecuona, M., Martin, M. M., et al. (2005). Ventilator-associated pneumonia using a closed versus an open tracheal suction system. *Critical Care Medicine, 33*(1), 115–119.
MacIntyre, N. R. (2004). Evidence-based ventilator weaning and discontinuation. *Respiratory Care, 49*(7), 830–836.
Mathews, P. J., Roark-Sample, B., Schmidt, J., et al. (2004). The latest in respiratory care. *Nursing Management, 20*(Suppl.), 22–24.
McDonagh, M., Helfand, M., Carson, S., et al. (2004). Hyperbaric oxygen therapy for traumatic brain injury: A systematic review of the evidence. *Archives of Physical Medicine and Rehabilitation, 85*(7), 1198–1204.
Moon, R. E. (2002). Mini-forum on multiple sclerosis (MS) and hyperbaric oxygen therapy. *Undersea and Hyperbaric Medicine, 29*(4), 235–236.
Naunheim, K. S. (2004). Update on lung volume reduction. *Journal of Surgical Research, 117*(1), 134–143.
Oermann, C., Sockrider, M. M. D., Giles, D. M. K., et al. (2001). Comparison of high-frequency chest wall oscillation and oscillating positive expiratory pressure in the home management of cystic fibrosis: A pilot study. *Pediatric Pulmonology, 32*(5), 372–377.
Pawson, S. R., & DePriest, J. L. (2004). Are blood gases necessary in mechanically ventilated patients who have successfully completed a spontaneous breathing trial? *Respiratory Care, 49*(11), 1316–1319.
*Puntillo, K., & Ley, S. J. (2004). Appropriately timed analgesics control pain due to chest tube removal. *American Journal of Critical Care, 13*(4), 292–303.
*Robinson, T. (2005). Living with severe hypoxic COPD: The patients' experience. *Nursing Times, 101*(7), 38–42.
Roeckl-Wiedmann, I., Bennett, M. & Kranke, P. (2005). Systematic review of hyperbaric oxygen in the management of chronic wounds. *British Journal of Surgery, 92*(1), 24–32.
Roman, M. (2005). Tracheostomy tubes. *MedSurg Nursing, 14*(2), 143–145.
*Salam, A., Smina, M., Gada, P., et al. (2003). The effect of arterial blood gas values on extubation decisions. *Respiratory Care, 48*(11), 1033–1037.
Schweickert, W. D., Gelbach, B. K., Pohlman, A. S., et al. (2004). Daily interruption of sedative infusions and complications of critical illness in mechanically ventilated patients. *Critical Care Medicine, 32*(6), 1272–1276.
Sharifi, M., Fares, W., Abdel-Karim, I., et al. (2004). Usefulness of hyperbaric oxygen therapy to inhibit restenosis after percutaneous coronary intervention for acute myocardial infarction or unstable angina pectoris. *American Journal of Cardiology, 93*(12), 1533–1535.
Smith, B. (2005). The nursing of a patient following lung volume reduction surgery. *Nursing Times, 101*(6), 61–63.
Spritzer, C. J. (2003). Unraveling the mysteries of mechanical ventilation: A helpful step-by-step guide. *Journal of Emergency Nursing, 29*(1), 29–36.
St. John, R. E. & Malen, J. F. (2004). Contemporary issues in adult tracheostomy management. *Critical Care Nursing Clinics of North America, 16*(3), 413–430.
Stoller, J. K. (2000). Oxygen and air travel. *Respiratory Care, 45*(2), 214–221.
Torres, L. Y. & Sirbegovic, D. J. (2004). Early intervention with a tracheostomy and ventilator speaking valve: Physiological benefits begin in the ICU. *AACN News, 21*(6), 10–13.
Valenzuela, R. & Rosen, D. (1999). Topical lidocaine-prilocaine cream (EMLA) for thoracostomy tube removal. *Anesthesia and Analgesia, 88*(1), 1107–1108.

RESOURCES

American Association for Respiratory Care, 11030 Ables Lane, Dallas, TX 75229; 972-243-2272; http://www.aarc.org. Accessed April 20, 2006.

American Lung Association, 1740 Broadway, New York, NY 10019; 212-315-8700, 800-LUNG-USA; http://www.lungusa.org. Accessed April 20, 2006.

American Thoracic Society, 1740 Broadway, New York, NY 10019; 212-315-8700; http://www.thoracic.org. Accessed April 20, 2006.

National Heart, Lung and Blood Institute, National Institutes of Health, 9000 Rockville Pike, Bldg 31, Rm 5A52, Bethesda, MD 20892; 301-496-5166 or 301-496-4236; http://www.nhlbi.nih.gov. Accessed April 20, 2006.

UNIT 6

Cardiovascular, Circulatory, and Hematologic Function

Case Study

Applying Concepts from NANDA, NIC, and NOC

A Patient Who Has Intermittent Claudication and Ulceration

Mr. Black, age 73 years, has a history of peripheral arterial occlusive disease (2 years), hypertension, hypercholesterolemia, type 2 diabetes, and smoking. He eats low-fat foods and cut back on smoking to half a pack a day. His home-monitored blood glucose levels range from 180 to 215 mg/dL. Because he has severe calf pain after walking, he now walks only two blocks a day: one block from home and one block back. He now receives medical treatment for a nonhealing ulcer on the plantar aspect of his left foot.

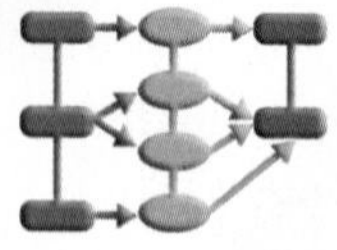

Turn to Appendix C to see a concept map that illustrates the relationships that exist between the nursing diagnoses, interventions, and outcomes for the patient's clinical problems.

Nursing Classifications and Languages

NANDA Nursing Diagnoses	NIC Nursing Interventions	NOC Nursing Outcomes Return to functional baseline status, stabilization of, or improvement in:
Ineffective Peripheral Tissue Perfusion—Decrease in oxygen resulting in the failure to nourish tissues at the capillary level	**Circulatory Care: Arterial Insufficiency**—Promotion of arterial circulation **Circulatory Precautions**—Protection of localized area with limited perfusion	**Circulation Status**—Unobstructed, unidirectional blood flow at an appropriate pressure through large vessels of the systemic and pulmonary circuits **Peripheral Tissue Perfusion**—Adequacy of blood flow through the small vessels of the extremities to maintain tissue function
Chronic Pain—Unpleasant sensory and emotional experience arising from actual or potential tissue damage or described in terms of such damage; sudden or slow onset of any intensity from mild to severe, constant or recurring without an anticipated or predictable end and a duration of greater than 6 months	**Pain Management**—Alleviation of pain or reduction in pain to a level of comfort that is acceptable to the patient	**Symptom Control**—Personal actions to minimize perceived adverse changes in physical and emotional functioning **Comfort Level**—Extent of positive perception of physical and psychological ease
Activity Intolerance—Insufficient physiological or psychological energy to endure or complete required or desired daily activities	**Exercise Therapy: Ambulation**—Promotion and assistance with walking to maintain or restore autonomic and voluntary body functions during treatment and recovery from illness or injury	**Activity Tolerance**—Physiologic response to energy-consuming movements with daily activities

NANDA International (2005). *Nursing diagnoses: Definitions & classification 2005–2006.* Philadelphia: North American Nursing Diagnosis Association.

Dochterman, J. M., & Bulechek, G. M. (2004). *Nursing Interventions Classification (NIC)* (4th ed.). St. Louis: Mosby.

Iowa Outcomes Project, 2004. In S. Moorhead, M. Johnson, & M. Maas, eds. (2004). *Nursing outcomes classification (NOC)* (3rd ed.). St. Louis: Mosby.

Dochterman, J. M., & Jones, D. A. (2003). *Unifying nursing languages: The harmonization of NANDA, NIC, and NOC.* Washington, D.C.: American Nurses Association.

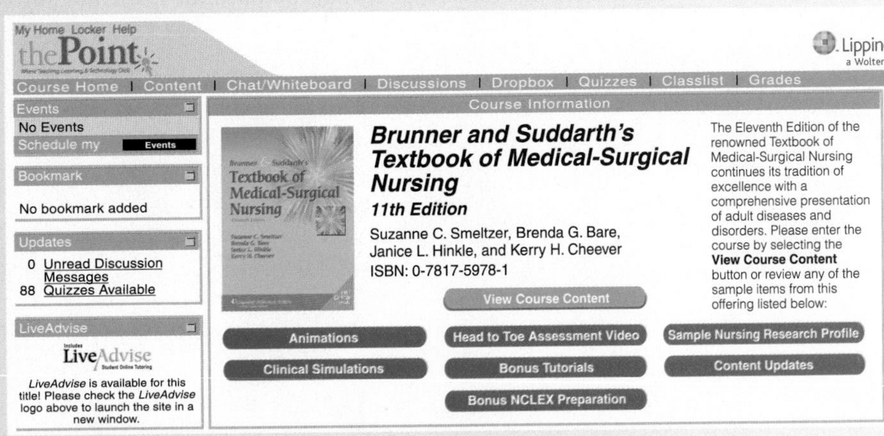

CHAPTER 26

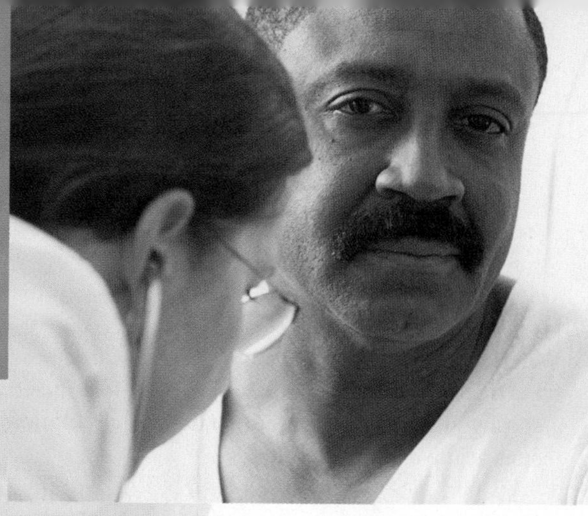

Assessment of Cardiovascular Function

Learning Objectives

On completion of this chapter, the learner will be able to:

1. Explain cardiac physiology in relation to cardiac anatomy and the conduction system of the heart.
2. Incorporate assessment of functional health patterns and cardiac risk factors into the health history and physical assessment of the patient with cardiovascular disease.
3. Discuss the clinical indications, patient preparation, and other related nursing implications for common tests and procedures used to assess cardiovascular function and diagnose cardiovascular diseases.
4. Compare the various methods of hemodynamic monitoring (eg, central venous pressure, pulmonary artery pressure, and arterial pressure monitoring) with regard to indications for use, potential complications, and nursing responsibilities.

More than 71 million Americans have one or more types of cardiovascular disease (CVD), including hypertension, coronary artery disease (CAD), heart failure (HF), stroke, and congenital cardiovascular defects (American Heart Association [AHA], 2006). Because of the prevalence of CVD, nurses practicing in any setting across the continuum of care, whether in the home, office, hospital, nursing home, or rehabilitation facility, must be capable of assessing the cardiovascular system. Key components of assessment include a health history, physical examination, and monitoring of a variety of laboratory and diagnostic test results. An accurate and timely assessment of cardiovascular function provides the data necessary to identify nursing diagnoses, formulate an individualized plan of care, evaluate the response of the patient to the care provided, and revise the plan as needed. An understanding of the structure and function of the heart in health and in disease is essential to develop cardiovascular assessment skills.

Anatomic and Physiologic Overview

The heart is a hollow, muscular organ located in the center of the thorax, where it occupies the space between the lungs (mediastinum) and rests on the diaphragm. It weighs approximately 300 g (10.6 oz); heart weight and size are influenced by age, gender, body weight, extent of physical exercise and conditioning, and heart disease. The heart pumps blood to the tissues, supplying them with oxygen and other nutrients.

The pumping action of the heart is accomplished by the rhythmic contraction and relaxation of its muscular wall. During **systole** (contraction of the muscle), the chambers of the heart become smaller as the blood is ejected. During **diastole** (relaxation of the muscle), the heart chambers fill with blood in preparation for subsequent ejection. A normal

Glossary

afterload: the amount of resistance to ejection of blood from the ventricle

apical impulse (also called point of maximum impulse [PMI]): impulse normally palpated at the fifth intercostal space, left midclavicular line; caused by contraction of the left ventricle

baroreceptors: nerve fibers located in the aortic arch and carotid arteries that are responsible for reflex control of the blood pressure

cardiac catheterization: an invasive procedure used to measure cardiac chamber pressures and assess patency of the coronary arteries

cardiac conduction system: specialized heart cells strategically located throughout the heart that are responsible for methodically generating and coordinating the transmission of electrical impulses to the myocardial cells

cardiac output: amount of blood pumped by each ventricle in liters per minute; normal cardiac output is 5 L per minute in the resting adult heart

cardiac stress test: a test used to evaluate the functioning of the heart during a period of increased oxygen demand

contractility: ability of the cardiac muscle to shorten in response to an electrical impulse

depolarization: electrical activation of a cell caused by the influx of sodium into the cell while potassium exits the cell

diastole: period of ventricular relaxation resulting in ventricular filling

ejection fraction: percentage of the end-diastolic blood volume ejected from the ventricle with each heartbeat

hemodynamic monitoring: use of monitoring devices to measure cardiovascular function

hypertension: blood pressure greater than 140/90 mm Hg

hypotension: a decrease in blood pressure to less than 100/60 mm Hg

international normalized ratio (INR): a standard method for reporting prothrombin levels, eliminating the variation in test results from laboratory to laboratory

murmurs: sounds created by abnormal, turbulent flow of blood in the heart

myocardial ischemia: condition in which heart muscle cells receive less oxygen than needed

myocardium: muscle layer of the heart responsible for the pumping action of the heart

normal heart sounds: sounds produced when the valves close; normal heart sounds are S1 (atrioventricular valves) and S2 (semilunar valves)

postural (orthostatic) hypotension: a significant drop in blood pressure (usually 10 mm Hg systolic or more) after an upright posture is assumed

preload: degree of stretch of the cardiac muscle fibers at the end of diastole

pulmonary vascular resistance: resistance to right ventricle ejection of blood

radioisotopes: unstable atoms that emit small amounts of energy in the form of gamma rays; used in cardiac nuclear medicine studies

repolarization: return of the cell to resting state, caused by reentry of potassium into the cell while sodium exits the cell

sinoatrial (SA) node: primary pacemaker of the heart, located in the right atrium

stroke volume: amount of blood ejected from the ventricle per heartbeat; normal stroke volume is 70 mL in the resting heart

systemic vascular resistance: resistance to left ventricle ejection

systole: period of ventricular contraction resulting in ejection of blood from the ventricles into the pulmonary artery and aorta

telemetry: the process of continuous electrocardiographic monitoring by the transmission of radiowaves from a battery-operated transmitter worn by the patient

venodilating agent: medication causing dilation of veins

resting adult heart beats approximately 60 to 80 times per minute. Each ventricle ejects approximately 70 mL of blood per beat and has an output of approximately 5 L per minute.

Anatomy of the Heart

The heart is composed of three layers (Fig. 26-1). The inner layer, or endocardium, consists of endothelial tissue and lines the inside of the heart and valves. The middle layer, or **myocardium**, is made up of muscle fibers and is responsible for the pumping action. The exterior layer of the heart is called the epicardium.

The heart is encased in a thin, fibrous sac called the pericardium, which is composed of two layers. Adhering to the epicardium is the visceral pericardium. Enveloping the visceral pericardium is the parietal pericardium, a tough fibrous tissue that attaches to the great vessels, diaphragm, sternum, and vertebral column and supports the heart in the mediastinum. The space between these two layers (pericardial space) is filled with about 30 mL of fluid, which lubricates the surface of the heart and reduces friction during systole.

Heart Chambers

The four chambers of the heart constitute the right- and left-sided pumping systems. The right side of the heart, made up of the right atrium and right ventricle, distributes venous blood (deoxygenated blood) to the lungs via the pulmonary artery (pulmonary circulation) for oxygenation. The right atrium receives blood returning from the superior vena cava (head, neck, and upper extremities), inferior vena cava (trunk and lower extremities), and coronary sinus (coronary circulation). The left side of the heart, composed of the left atrium and left ventricle, distributes oxygenated blood to the remainder of the body via the aorta (systemic circulation). The left atrium receives oxygenated blood from the pulmonary circulation via the pulmonary veins. The relationships of the four heart chambers are shown in Figure 26-1.

The varying thicknesses of the atrial and ventricular walls relate to the workload required by each chamber. The atria are thin-walled because blood returning to these chambers generates low pressures. In contrast, the ventricular walls are thicker because they generate greater pressures during systole. The right ventricle contracts against low pulmonary

Physiology/Pathophysiology

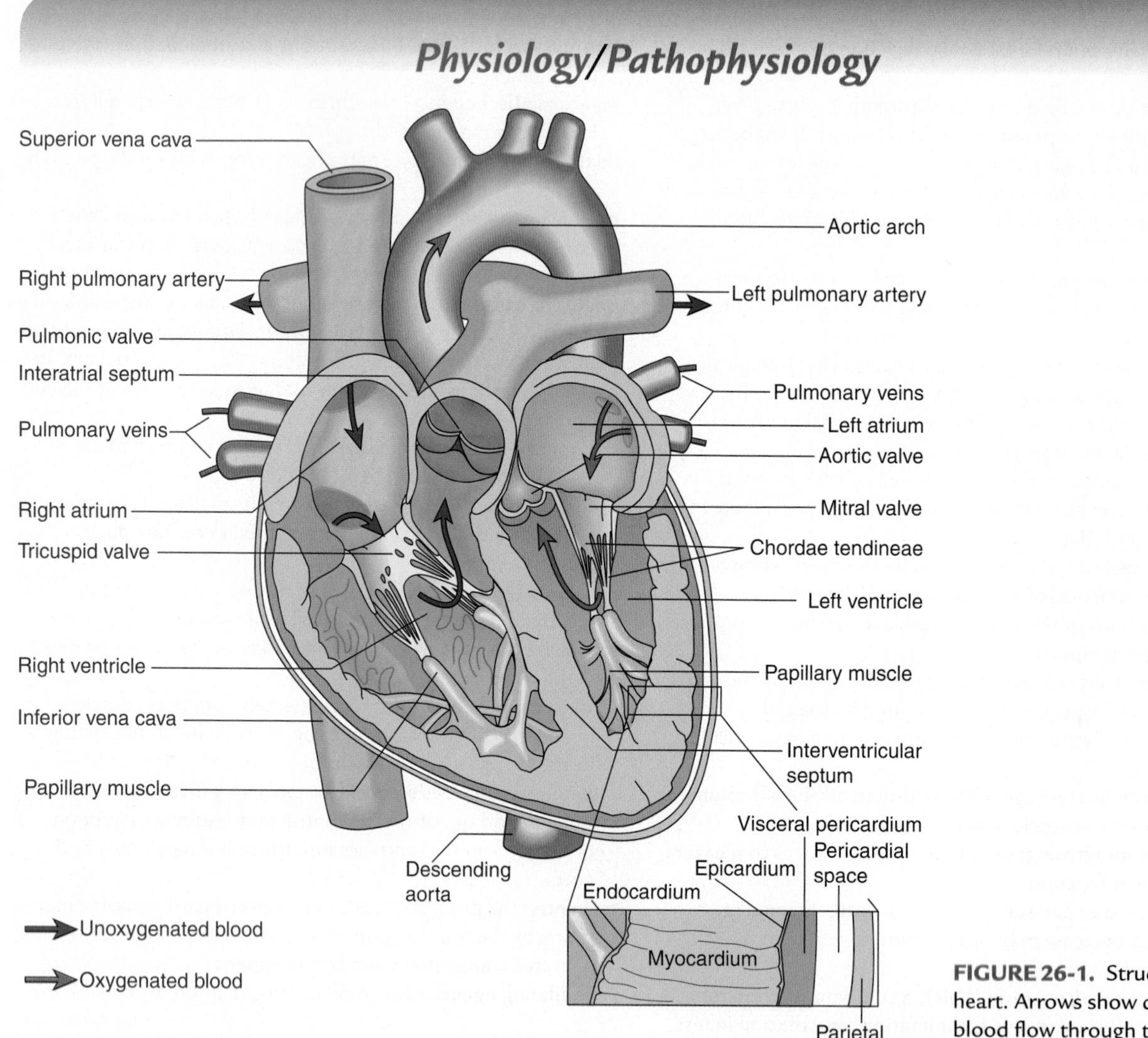

FIGURE 26-1. Structure of the heart. Arrows show course of blood flow through the heart chambers.

vascular pressure and has thinner walls than the left ventricle. The left ventricle, with walls two-and-a-half times more muscular than those of the right ventricle, contracts against high systemic pressure.

Because the heart lies in a rotated position within the chest cavity, the right ventricle lies anteriorly (just beneath the sternum) and the left ventricle is situated posteriorly. The left ventricle is responsible for the apical beat or the point of maximum impulse (PMI), which is normally palpable in the left midclavicular line of the chest wall at the fifth intercostal space.

Heart Valves

The four valves in the heart permit blood to flow in only one direction. The valves, which are composed of thin leaflets of fibrous tissue, open and close in response to the movement of blood and pressure changes within the chambers. There are two types of valves: atrioventricular and semilunar.

ATRIOVENTRICULAR VALVES

The valves that separate the atria from the ventricles are termed atrioventricular valves. The tricuspid valve, so named because it is composed of three cusps or leaflets, separates the right atrium from the right ventricle. The mitral or bicuspid (two cusps) valve lies between the left atrium and the left ventricle (see Fig. 26-1).

Normally, when the ventricles contract, ventricular pressure increases, closing the atrioventricular valve leaflets. Two additional structures, the papillary muscles and the chordae tendineae, maintain valve closure. The papillary muscles, located on the sides of the ventricular walls, are connected to the valve leaflets by thin fibrous bands called chordae tendineae. During systole, contraction of the papillary muscles causes the chordae tendineae to become taut, keeping the valve leaflets approximated and closed.

SEMILUNAR VALVES

The two semilunar valves are composed of three half-moon–like leaflets. The valve between the right ventricle and the pulmonary artery is called the pulmonic valve. The valve between the left ventricle and the aorta is called the aortic valve.

Coronary Arteries

CONCEPTS in action ANIMATION

The left and right coronary arteries and their branches supply arterial blood to the heart. These arteries originate from the aorta just above the aortic valve leaflets. The heart has large metabolic requirements, extracting approximately 70% to 80% of the oxygen delivered (other organs extract, on average, 25%). Unlike other arteries, the coronary arteries are perfused during diastole. An increase in heart rate shortens diastole and can decrease myocardial perfusion. Patients, particularly those with CAD, can develop **myocardial ischemia** (inadequate oxygen supply) when the heart rate accelerates.

The left coronary artery has three branches. The artery from the point of origin to the first major branch is called the left main coronary artery. Two branches arise off the left main coronary artery: the left anterior descending artery, which courses down the anterior wall of the heart, and the circumflex artery, which circles around to the lateral left wall of the heart.

The right side of the heart is supplied by the right coronary artery, which progresses around to the bottom or inferior wall of the heart. The posterior wall of the heart receives its blood supply by an additional branch from the right coronary artery called the posterior descending artery.

Superficial to the coronary arteries are the coronary veins. Venous blood from these veins returns to the heart primarily through the coronary sinus, which is located posteriorly in the right atrium.

Cardiac Muscle

The myocardium is the middle, muscular layer of the atrial and ventricular walls. It is composed of specialized cells called myocytes, which form an interconnected network of muscle fibers. These fibers encircle the heart in a figure-of-eight pattern, forming a spiral from the base of the heart to the apex. During contraction, this muscular configuration facilitates a twisting and compressive movement of the heart that begins in the atria and moves to the ventricles. The sequential and rhythmic pattern of contraction, followed by relaxation of the muscle fibers, maximizes the volume of blood ejected with each contraction. This cyclical pattern of myocardial contraction is controlled by the conduction system.

Physiology of the Heart

Cardiac Electrophysiology

The **cardiac conduction system** generates and transmits electrical impulses that stimulate contraction of the myocardium. Under normal circumstances, the conduction system first stimulates contraction of the atria and then the ventricles. The synchronization of the atrial and ventricular events allows the ventricles to fill completely before ventricular ejection, thereby maximizing cardiac output. Three physiologic characteristics of two specialized electrical cells, the **nodal cells** and the **Purkinje cells**, provide this synchronization:

Automaticity: ability to initiate an electrical impulse
Excitability: ability to respond to an electrical impulse
Conductivity: ability to transmit an electrical impulse from one cell to another

Both the **sinoatrial (SA) node** and the **atrioventricular (AV) node** are composed of nodal cells. The SA node, the primary pacemaker of the heart, is located at the junction of the superior vena cava and the right atrium (Fig. 26-2). The SA node in a normal resting adult heart has an inherent firing rate of 60 to 100 impulses per minute, but the rate can change in response to the metabolic demands of the body.

The electrical impulses initiated by the SA node are conducted along the myocardial cells of the atria via specialized tracts called internodal pathways. The impulses cause electrical stimulation and subsequent contraction of the atria. The impulses are then conducted to the AV node, which is located in the right atrial wall near the tricuspid valve (see Fig. 26-2). The AV node coordinates the incoming electrical

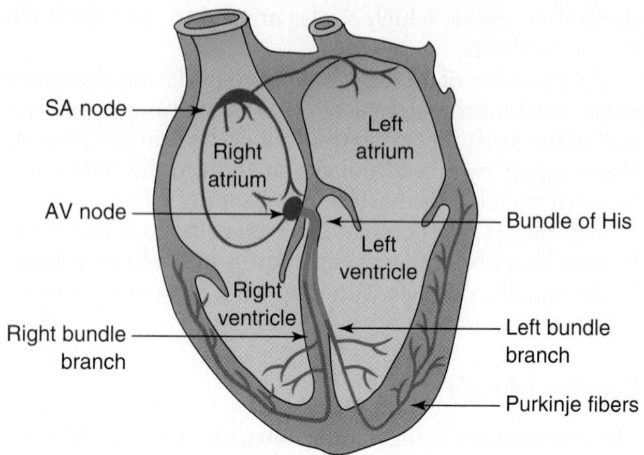

FIGURE 26-2. Cardiac conduction system. AV, atrioventricular; SA, sinoatrial.

impulses from the atria and after a slight delay (allowing the atria time to contract and complete ventricular filling) relays the impulse to the ventricles.

Initially, the impulse is conducted through a bundle of specialized conducting tissue, referred to as the bundle of His, which then divides into the right bundle branch (conducting impulses to the right ventricle) and the left bundle branch (conducting impulses to the left ventricle). To transmit impulses to the left ventricle, the largest chamber of the heart, the left bundle branch divides into the left anterior and left posterior bundle branches. Impulses travel through the bundle branches to reach the terminal point in the conduction system, called the Purkinje fibers. These fibers are composed of Purkinje cells, specialized to rapidly conduct the impulses through the thick walls of the ventricles. This is the point at which the myocardial cells are stimulated, causing ventricular contraction.

The heart rate is determined by the myocardial cells with the fastest inherent firing rate. Under normal circumstances, the SA node has the highest inherent rate (60 to 100 impulses per minute), the AV node has the second-highest inherent rate (40 to 60 impulses per minute), and the ventricular pacemaker sites have the lowest inherent rate (30 to 40 impulses per minute). If the SA node malfunctions, the AV node generally takes over the pacemaker function of the heart at its inherently lower rate. Should both the SA and the AV nodes fail in their pacemaker function, a pacemaker site in the ventricle will fire at its inherent bradycardic rate of 30 to 40 impulses per minute.

CARDIAC ACTION POTENTIAL

The nodal and Purkinje cells (electrical cells) generate and transmit impulses across the heart, stimulating the cardiac myocytes (working cells) to contract. Stimulation of the cardiac working cells occurs due to the exchange of electrically charged particles, called ions, across channels located in the cell membrane. The channels regulate the movement and speed of specific ions, namely sodium, potassium, and calcium, as they enter and exit the cell. Sodium rapidly enters into the cell through sodium fast channels, in contrast to calcium, which enters the cell through calcium slow channels. In the resting or polarized state, sodium is the primary extracellular ion, whereas potassium is the primary intracellular ion. This difference in ion concentration means that the inside of the cell has a negative charge compared to the positive charge on the outside. This relationship changes during cellular stimulation, when sodium or calcium crosses the cell membrane into the cell and potassium ions exit into the extracellular space. This exchange of ions creates a positively charged intracellular space and a negatively charged extracellular space that characterizes the period known as **depolarization.** Once depolarization is complete, the exchange of ions reverts back to its resting state; this period is known as **repolarization.** The repeated cycle of depolarization and repolarization is called the cardiac action potential.

As shown in Figure 26-3, the cardiac action potential has five phases:

- Phase 0: Cellular depolarization is initiated as positive ions influx into the cell. During this phase, the working cells (atrial and ventricular myocytes) rapidly depolarize as sodium moves into the cells through sodium fast channels. The myocytes have a fast response action potential. In contrast, the cells of the SA and AV node depolarize when calcium enters these cells through calcium slow channels. These cells have a slow response action potential.
- Phase 1: Early cellular repolarization begins during this phase as potassium exits the intracellular space.
- Phase 2: This phase is called the plateau phase because the rate of repolarization slows. Calcium ions enter the intracellular space.
- Phase 3: This phase marks the completion of repolarization and return of the cell to its resting state.
- Phase 4: This phase is considered the resting phase before the next depolarization.

Knowledge of the differences between fast- and slow-response action potentials enhances the nurse's understanding of the indications for and actions of antiarrhythmic medications. For example, class I antiarrhythmic medications such as lidocaine (Xylocaine), quinidine (Quinalan), and propafenone (Rythmol) are administered to suppress dysrhythmia formation. These medications act by blocking the influx of sodium into the cells that have a fast-response

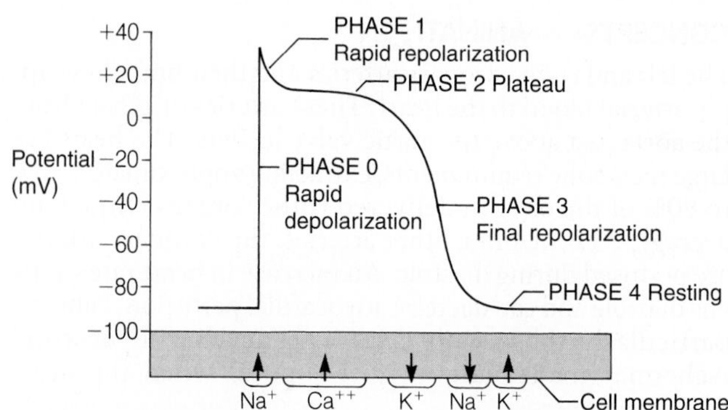

FIGURE 26-3. Cardiac action potential of a fast-response Purkinje fiber. The arrows indicate the approximate time and direction of movement of each ion influencing membrane potential. Ca^{++} movement out of the cell is not well defined but is thought to occur during phase 4.

action potential. This action prevents rapid depolarization or phase 0, thereby preventing the dysrhythmia. Class II agents or beta-blockers (eg, metoprolol [Lopressor], sotalol [Betapace]) decrease automaticity and help slow tachycardias. Class III agents such as amiodarone (Cordarone) prolong repolarization and are useful in suppressing atrial or ventricular dysrhythmias. Class IV agents or calcium channel blockers (eg, verapamil [Calan], diltiazem [Cardizem]) are used to treat tachycardias. These medications block the influx of calcium in phase 0 of the SA and AV nodes that have a slow-response action potential. This action slows AV node conduction of impulses into the ventricle, resulting in a slower ventricular rate of depolarization and subsequent contraction.

REFRACTORY PERIODS

Under normal circumstances, the myocardial cell must complete repolarization before it can enter a new phase of depolarization. During this phase, called the refractory period, the cells are incapable of being stimulated. There are two phases of the refractory period of the action potential, commonly referred to as the effective (or absolute) refractory period and the relative refractory period. During the effective refractory period, the cell is completely unresponsive to any electrical stimulus; it is incapable of initiating an early depolarization. The effective refractory period corresponds with the time in phase 0 to the middle of phase 3 of the action potential. The relative refractory period corresponds with the short time at the end of phase 3. During the relative refractory period, if an electrical stimulus is stronger than normal, the cell may depolarize prematurely. Early depolarizations of the atrium or ventricle cause premature contractions, placing the patient at risk for dysrhythmias. Premature ventricular contractions in certain situations, such as the setting of myocardial ischemia, are worrisome because these early ventricular depolarizations can trigger life-threatening dysrhythmias, including ventricular tachycardia or ventricular fibrillation. These dysrhythmias and others are discussed in detail in Chapter 27.

Several circumstances make the heart more susceptible to early depolarization during the relative refractory period, thus increasing the risk for serious dysrhythmias. These conditions include electrolyte disturbances (hypokalemia, hypomagnesemia), hypoxemia, acidosis, hypercarbia, hypothermia, an increase in catecholamines, myocardial injury (eg, acute myocardial infarction [MI]), and chamber enlargement (eg, HF, hypertension, ventricular aneurysm).

Cardiac Hemodynamics

An important determinant of blood flow in the cardiovascular system is the principle that fluid flows from a region of higher pressure to one of lower pressure. The pressures responsible for blood flow in the normal circulation are generated during systole and diastole. Figure 26-4 depicts the pressure differences in the great vessels and in the four chambers of the heart during systole and diastole.

Physiology/Pathophysiology

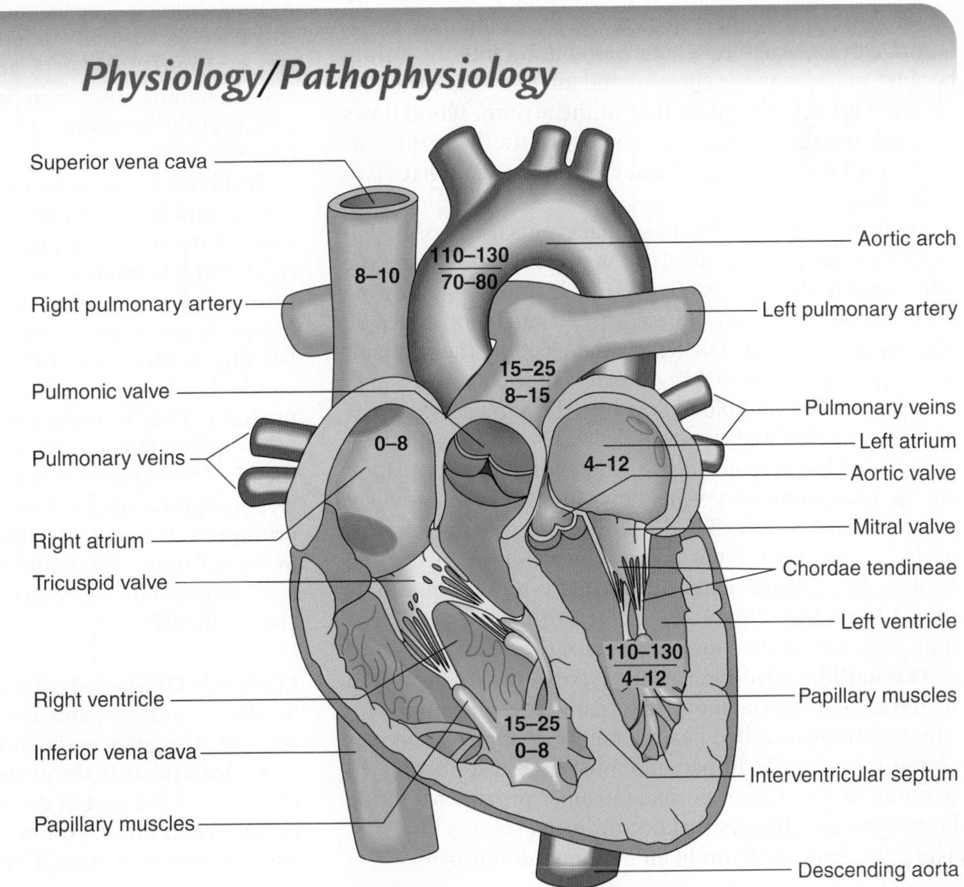

FIGURE 26-4. Great vessel and chamber pressures. Pressures are identified in mm Hg as mean pressure or systolic over diastolic pressure.

CARDIAC CYCLE

CONCEPTS in action ANIMATION

Beginning with systole, the pressure inside the ventricles rapidly increases, forcing the atrioventricular valves to close. As a result, blood ceases to flow from the atria into the ventricles, and regurgitation (backflow) of blood into the atria is prevented. The rapid increase of pressure inside the right and left ventricles forces the pulmonic and aortic valves to open, and blood is ejected into the pulmonary artery and aorta, respectively. The exit of blood is at first rapid; then, as the pressure in each ventricle and its corresponding artery equalizes, the flow of blood gradually decreases. At the end of systole, pressure within the right and left ventricles rapidly decreases. This decreases pulmonary artery and aortic pressure, causing closure of the semilunar valves. These events mark the onset of diastole.

During diastole, when the ventricles are relaxed and the atrioventricular valves are open, blood returning from the veins flows into the atria and then into the ventricles. Toward the end of this diastolic period, the atrial muscles contract in response to an electrical impulse initiated by the SA node (atrial systole). The resultant contraction increases the pressure inside the atria, ejecting blood into the ventricles. Atrial systole augments ventricular blood volume by 15% to 25% and is sometimes referred to as the "atrial kick." At this point, ventricular systole begins in response to propagation of the electrical impulse that began in the SA node some milliseconds previously.

Chamber Pressures. In the right side of the heart, the pressure generated during ventricular systole (15 to 25 mm Hg) exceeds the pulmonary artery diastolic pressure (8 to 15 mm Hg), and blood is ejected into the pulmonary circulation. During diastole, venous blood flows into the atrium because pressure in the superior and inferior vena cava (8 to 10 mm Hg) is higher than that in the atrium. Blood flows through the open tricuspid valve and into the right ventricle until the two right chamber pressures equalize (0 to 8 mm Hg).

In the left side of the heart, similar events occur, although higher pressures are generated. As pressure mounts in the left ventricle during systole (110 to 130 mm Hg), resting aortic pressure (80 mm Hg) is exceeded and blood is ejected into the aorta. During left ventricular ejection, the resultant aortic pressure (110 to 130 mm Hg) forces blood through the arteries. Forward blood flow into the aorta ceases as the ventricle relaxes and pressure decreases. During diastole, oxygenated blood returning from the pulmonary circulation via the four pulmonary veins flows into the atrium, where pressure remains low. Blood readily flows into the left ventricle because ventricular pressure is also low. At the end of diastole, pressures in the atrium and ventricle equilibrate (4 to 12 mm Hg). Figure 26-4 depicts the systolic and diastolic pressures in the four chambers of the heart.

Pressure Measurement. Chamber pressures are measured with the use of special monitoring catheters and equipment. This technique is called hemodynamic monitoring. Nurses caring for critically ill patients must have a sophisticated working knowledge of normal chamber pressures and the hemodynamic changes that occur during serious illnesses. The data obtained from hemodynamic monitoring assist with the diagnosis and management of pathophysiologic conditions affecting critically ill patients. Methods of hemodynamic monitoring are covered in more detail at the end of this chapter.

Cardiac Output

Cardiac output refers to the amount of blood pumped by each ventricle during a given period. The cardiac output in a resting adult is about 5 liters per minute but varies greatly depending on the metabolic needs of the body. Cardiac output is computed by multiplying the stroke volume by the heart rate. **Stroke volume** is the amount of blood ejected per heartbeat. The average resting stroke volume is about 70 mL, and the heart rate is 60 to 80 beats per minute (bpm). Cardiac output can be affected by changes in either stroke volume or heart rate.

CONTROL OF HEART RATE

Cardiac output must be responsive to changes in the metabolic demands of the tissues. For example, during exercise the total cardiac output may increase fourfold, to 20 liters per minute. This increase is normally accomplished by approximate doubling of both the heart rate and the stroke volume. Changes in heart rate are accomplished by reflex controls mediated by the autonomic nervous system, including its sympathetic and parasympathetic divisions. The parasympathetic impulses, which travel to the heart through the vagus nerve, can slow the cardiac rate, whereas sympathetic impulses increase it. These effects on heart rate result from action on the SA node, to either decrease or increase its inherent rate. The balance between these two reflex control systems normally determines the heart rate. The heart rate is stimulated also by an increased level of circulating catecholamines (secreted by the adrenal gland) and by excess thyroid hormone, which produces a catecholamine-like effect.

In addition, the heart rate is affected by central nervous system and baroreceptor activity. **Baroreceptors** are specialized nerve cells located in the aortic arch and in both right and left internal carotid arteries (at the point of bifurcation from the common carotid arteries). The baroreceptors are sensitive to changes in blood pressure (BP). During elevations in BP (**hypertension**), these cells increase their rate of discharge, transmitting impulses to the medulla. This initiates parasympathetic activity and inhibits sympathetic response, lowering the heart rate and the BP. The opposite is true during **hypotension** (low BP). Hypotension results in less baroreceptor stimulation, which prompts a decrease in parasympathetic inhibitory activity in the SA node, allowing for enhanced sympathetic activity. The resultant vasoconstriction and increased heart rate elevate the BP.

CONTROL OF STROKE VOLUME

Stroke volume is primarily determined by three factors: preload, afterload, and contractility.

Preload refers to the degree of stretch of the cardiac muscle fibers at the end of diastole. The end of diastole is the period when filling volume in the ventricles is the highest and the degree of stretch on the muscle fibers is the greatest. The volume of blood within the ventricle at the end of diastole determines preload, which directly affects stroke volume. As the volume of blood returning to the heart increases, muscle fiber stretch also increases (increased preload), resulting in stronger contraction and a greater stroke volume. This relationship, called the Frank-Starling (or Starling) law of the heart, is maintained until the physiologic limit of the muscle is reached.

The Frank-Starling law is based on the fact that, within limits, the greater the initial length or stretch of the cardiac muscle cells (sarcomeres), the greater the degree of shortening that occurs. This result is caused by increased interaction between the thick and thin filaments within the cardiac muscle cells. Preload is decreased by a reduction in the volume of blood returning to the ventricles. Diuresis, **venodilating agents** (eg, nitrates), and low fluid volume or excessive fluid loss reduce preload. Preload is increased by increasing the return of circulating blood volume to the ventricles. Controlling the loss of blood or body fluids and replacing fluids (ie, blood transfusions and intravenous [IV] fluid administration) are examples of ways to increase preload.

Afterload, the amount of resistance to ejection of blood from the ventricle, is the second determinant of stroke volume. The resistance of the systemic BP to left ventricular ejection is called **systemic vascular resistance.** The resistance of the pulmonary BP to right ventricular ejection is called **pulmonary vascular resistance.** There is an inverse relationship between afterload and stroke volume. For example, afterload is increased by arterial vasoconstriction, which leads to decreased stroke volume. The opposite is true with arterial vasodilation: afterload is reduced because there is less resistance to ejection, and stroke volume increases.

Contractility refers to the force generated by the contracting myocardium under any given condition. Contractility is enhanced by circulating catecholamines, sympathetic neuronal activity, and certain medications (eg, digoxin [Lanoxin], IV dopamine [Intropin], or dobutamine [Dobutrex]). Increased contractility results in increased stroke volume. Contractility is depressed by hypoxemia, acidosis, and certain medications (eg, beta-adrenergic blocking agents such as atenolol [Tenormin]).

The heart can achieve a greatly increased stroke volume (eg, during exercise) if preload is increased (through increased venous return), if contractility is increased (through sympathetic nervous system discharge), and if afterload is decreased (through peripheral vasodilation with decreased aortic pressure).

The percentage of the end-diastolic volume that is ejected with each stroke is called the **ejection fraction.** With each stroke, about 42% (right ventricle) to 50% (left ventricle) or more of the end-diastolic volume is ejected by the normal heart. The ejection fraction can be used as an index of myocardial contractility: the ejection fraction decreases if contractility is depressed.

Gerontologic Considerations

Changes in cardiac structure and function are clearly observable in the aging heart. To understand the changes specifically related to aging, it is helpful to distinguish the normal aging process from changes related to CVD. The anatomic and functional changes in the aging heart are summarized in Table 26-1.

The normal aging heart can maintain an adequate cardiac output under ordinary circumstances but may have a limited ability to respond to situations that cause physical or emotional stress. In an elderly person who is less active, the left ventricle may become smaller (atrophy) as a consequence of physical deconditioning. Aging also results in decreased elasticity and widening of the aorta, thickening and rigidity of the cardiac valves, and increased connective tissue in the SA and AV nodes and bundle branches.

These changes lead to decreased myocardial contractility, increased left ventricular ejection time (prolonged systole), and delayed conduction. Therefore, stressful physical and emotional conditions, especially those that occur suddenly, may have adverse effects on the aged person. The heart cannot respond to such conditions with an adequate rate increase and needs more time to return to a normal resting rate after even a minimal increase in heart rate. In some patients, the added stress may precipitate HF.

Gender Differences in Cardiac Structure and Function

Structural differences between the hearts of men and women have significant implications. Compared with a man's heart, a woman's heart tends to be smaller. It weighs less and has smaller coronary arteries. Because the coronary arteries of a woman are smaller, they occlude from atherosclerosis more easily, making procedures such as cardiac catheterization and angioplasty technically more difficult, with a higher incidence of postprocedural complications. In addition, the resting rate, stroke volume, and ejection fraction of a woman's heart are higher than those of a man's heart, and the conduction time of an electrical impulse coursing from the SA node through the AV node to the Purkinje fibers is briefer.

For many years, it was believed that the female hormone estrogen had cardioprotective effects. Hormone therapy was routinely prescribed for postmenopausal women in the belief that this pharmacologic therapy would deter the onset and progression of coronary atherosclerosis. This belief was supported by anecdotal evidence that the onset of heart disease in women tends to occur later than in men, at a time when most women had experienced menopause and were largely bereft of estrogen. However, data from the Women's Health Initiative refuted this belief (see Chapter 28 for additional information) (Mosca, Appel, Benjamin, et al., 2004).

Assessment

The frequency and extent of the nursing assessment of cardiovascular function are based on several factors, including the severity of the patient's symptoms, the presence of risk factors, the practice setting, and the purpose

TABLE 26-1 Age-Related Changes of the Cardiac System

Cardiovascular System	Structural Changes	Functional Changes	History and Physical Findings
Atria	↑ Size of left atrium Thickening of the endocardium	↑ Atrial irritability	Irregular heart rhythm from atrial dysrhythmias
Left ventricle	Endocardial fibrosis Myocardial thickening (hypertrophy) Infiltration of fat into myocardium	Left ventricle stiff and less compliant Progressive decline in cardiac output ↑ Risk for ventricular dysrhythmias Prolonged systole	Fatigue ↓ Exercise tolerance Signs and symptoms of HF or ventricular dysrhythmias Point of maximal impulse palpated lateral to the midclavicular line ↓ Intensity S_1, S_2; split S_2 S_4 may be present
Valves	Thickening and rigidity of AV valves Calcification of aortic valve	Abnormal blood flow across valves during cardiac cycle	Murmurs may be present Thrill may be palpated if significant murmur is present
Conduction system	Connective tissue collects in SA node, AV node, and bundle branches ↓ Number SA node cells ↓ Number AV, bundle of His, right and left bundle branch cells	Slower SA node rate of impulse discharge Slowed conduction across AV node and ventricular conduction system	Bradycardia Heart block ECG changes consistent with slowed conduction (↑ PR interval, widened QRS complex)
Sympathetic nervous system	↓ Response to beta-adrenergic stimulation	↓ Adaptive response to exercise: contractility and heart rate slower to respond to exercise demands Heart rate takes more time to return to baseline	Fatigue Diminished exercise tolerance ↓ Ability to respond to stress
Aorta and arteries	Stiffening of vasculature ↓ Elasticity and widening of aorta Elongation of aorta, displacing the brachiocephalic artery upward	Left ventricular hypertrophy	Progressive increase in systolic BP; slight ↑ in diastolic BP Widening pulse pressure Pulsation visible above right clavicle
Baroreceptor response	↓ Sensitivity of baroreceptors in the carotid artery and aorta to transient episodes of hypertension and hypotension	Baroreceptors unable to regulate heart rate and vascular tone, causing slow response to postural changes in body position	Postural blood pressure changes and reports feeling dizzy, fainting when moving from lying to sitting or standing position

AV, atrioventricular; BP, blood pressure; ECG, electrocardiographic; HF, heart failure; SA, sinoatrial.

of the assessment. An acutely ill patient with CVD who is admitted to the emergency department or coronary intensive care unit requires a very different assessment than a person who is being examined for a chronic stable condition. Although the key components of the cardiovascular assessment remain the same (health history, physical examination, and monitoring of laboratory and diagnostic test results), the assessment priorities vary according to the needs of the patient. For example, an emergency department nurse caring for a patient who is admitted with symptoms associated with acute coronary syndrome (ACS) performs a rapid and focused assessment because treatment of ACS is time-dependent. The nurse obtains the patient's history of current illness, including the signs and symptoms that prompted the patient to come to the emergency department, cardiac risk factors, and current medications. The physical assessment is ongoing and concentrates on evaluating the patient for ACS complications, such as dysrhythmias and HF, and determining the effectiveness of medical treatment.

Health History and Clinical Manifestations

The health history allows the nurse to obtain important information about the health status of the patient. In addition, it gives the patient the opportunity to share his or her impressions of relevant symptoms, current state of illness, and experiences associated with managing his or her health (see "Health Perception and Management" later in this chapter). Nurses, physicians, and other health care professionals often obtain health histories from the same patient for similar reasons. It is important for the nurse to be aware of the information obtained by other members of the health care team. This knowledge allows the nurse to validate the findings of others, such as a history of allergies or use of current medications, leaving more time to explore other important topics. Health histories taken by members of each discipline should complement one another and not be repetitive or burdensome to the patient. For example, a patient who is asked about his or her allergies or medications multiple times during the same hospitalization may believe that the nurses and other health care professionals do not communicate with each other.

It is the nurse's responsibility to ensure that the information obtained from the health history accurately reflects the patient's current health. Questions are formulated based on the setting. For example, in the emergency department, the goal of the triage nurse is to assess the patient's major complaint accurately and then rapidly decide what level of care the patient requires. Once the patient's condition stabilizes, a more extensive history can be obtained. In nonemergency situations and with stable patients, it is possible and advisable to obtain a complete health history during the initial contact.

During a health history, the primary source of information is the patient. If the patient does not speak English, a reliable professional interpreter who is cognizant of the importance of confidentiality should be used. It is often helpful to have spouses or partners available during the health history interview. For patients who cannot communicate, the family or the prior medical record are important sources of information. The source of information obtained during the health history is documented in the patient's medical record.

Initially, demographic information regarding age, gender, and ethnic origin is obtained. The family history and the physical examination include assessment for genetic abnormalities associated with cardiovascular disorders. Height and current weight are measured. (If there has been a recent weight loss or gain, the patient is asked about his or her usual weight.) During the interview, the nurse must be sensitive to the cultural background and religious practices of the patient. Having a heightened awareness of cultural diversity prevents barriers to communication that can result

GENETICS IN NURSING PRACTICE

Cardiovascular Disorders

Several cardiovascular disorders are associated with genetic abnormalities. Some examples are:

- Familial hypercholesterolemia
- Hypertrophic cardiomyopathy
- Long QT syndrome
- Hereditary hemochromatosis
- Elevated homocysteine levels

NURSING ASSESSMENTS

Family History Assessment

- Assess all patients with cardiovascular symptoms for coronary artery disease (CAD), regardless of age (early-onset CAD occurs).
- Assess family history of sudden death in persons who may or may not have been diagnosed with coronary disease (especially of early onset).
- Ask about sudden death in a previously asymptomatic child, adolescent, or adult.
- Ask about other family members with biochemical or neuromuscular conditions (eg, hemochromatosis or muscular dystrophy).
- Assess whether DNA mutation or other genetic testing has been performed on an affected family member.

Patient Assessment

- Assess for signs and symptoms of hyperlipidemias (xanthomas, corneal arcus, abdominal pain of unexplained origin).
- Assess for muscular weakness.

MANAGEMENT ISSUES SPECIFIC TO GENETICS

- If indicated, refer for further genetic counseling and evaluation so that the family can discuss inheritance, risk to other family members, availability of genetic testing, and gene-based interventions.
- Offer appropriate genetics information and resources (eg, Genetic Alliance website, American Heart Association, Muscular Dystrophy Association).
- Provide support to families newly diagnosed with genetics-related cardiovascular disease.

GENETICS RESOURCES

Genetic Alliance—a directory of support groups for patients and families with genetic conditions, http://www.geneticalliance.org

Gene Clinics—a listing of common genetic disorders with up-to-date clinical summaries, genetic counseling, and testing information, http://www.geneclinics.org

National Organization of Rare Disorders—a directory of support groups and information for patients and families with rare genetic disorders, http://www.rarediseases.org

OMIM: Online Mendelian Inheritance in Man—a complete listing of inherited genetic conditions, http://www.ncbi.nlm.nih.gov/omim/stats/html

when the interview is based on the nurse's personal frame of reference. For example, patients whose cultural or ethnic norms vary from those of the nurse may differ in their description of symptoms such as pain. In addition, they may engage in nontraditional health practices before seeking formal health care.

The information derived from the history assists in identifying pertinent issues related to the patient's condition and educational and self-care needs. Once these issues are clearly defined and possibly verified through the physical assessment, a plan of care is developed and implemented. During subsequent contacts or visits with the patient, a more focused health history is performed to:

- Determine whether the patient is progressing toward the established goals
- Reevaluate the existing plan of care and revise it as needed
- Evaluate the patient's health status so current issues can be resolved and new issues identified

Clinical Manifestations

The signs and symptoms experienced by people with CVD are related to dysrhythmias and conduction problems (see Chapter 27); CAD (see Chapter 28); structural, infectious, and inflammatory disorders of the heart (see Chapter 29); and complications of CVD such as HF and cardiogenic shock (see Chapter 30). These disorders have many signs and symptoms in common; therefore, the nurse must be skillful at recognizing these signs and symptoms so that patients are given appropriate and often life-saving care.

CAD, which may be characterized by a history of angina pectoris, MI, or both, is the most prevalent of all forms of CVD and deserves further discussion before common clinical manifestations of CVD are reviewed. More than 13 million Americans have CAD; it is responsible for more than 54% of all CVD-related deaths (AHA, 2006). ACS, a serious manifestation of CAD, develops when an atheromatous plaque in a diseased coronary artery ruptures and forms an obstructive thrombus. The spectrum of diagnoses associated with ACS include unstable angina, non-ST-elevation myocardial infarction (NSTEMI), and ST-elevation myocardial infarction (STEMI) (see Chapter 28). Approximately 50% of people with ACS experience similar symptoms that include chest pain or discomfort associated with myocardial ischemia; therefore, the specific diagnosis cannot be made based on presenting signs and symptoms alone. Further testing with a 12-lead electrocardiogram (ECG) and serum laboratory analysis of cardiac biomarkers is necessary to determine whether the patient has NSTEMI, STEMI, or unstable angina (see Chapter 28).

The following are the most common signs and symptoms of CVD, with related medical diagnoses in parentheses:

- Chest pain or discomfort (angina pectoris, ACS, dysrhythmias, valvular heart disease)
- Shortness of breath or dyspnea (ACS, cardiogenic shock, HF, valvular heart disease)
- Peripheral edema and weight gain (HF)
- Palpitations (tachycardia from a variety of causes, including ACS, caffeine or other stimulants, electrolyte imbalances, stress, valvular heart disease, ventricular aneurysms)
- Fatigue (early warning symptom of ACS, HF, valvular heart disease)
- Dizziness, syncope, or changes in level of consciousness (cardiogenic shock, cerebrovascular disorders, dysrhythmias, hypotension, postural hypotension, vasovagal episode)

Not all chest symptoms, including chest pain or discomfort, reflect myocardial ischemia. When a patient experiences chest pain, the nurse asks questions that aid in differentiating cardiac-related chest symptoms from other sources. Table 26-2 summarizes the characteristics and patterns of the more common cardiac and noncardiac causes of chest symptoms. During the assessment the patient is asked to describe the character or quality of the pain or discomfort and its location. The nurse needs to determine whether there is radiation to or discomfort in other areas and must assess for key signs and symptoms such as diaphoresis or nausea. It is important to identify the events that precipitate symptom onset, the duration of the symptom, and measures that aggravate or relieve the symptom. Chart 26-1 provides examples of questions used to assess common cardiac signs and symptoms. Some of the patient's responses may require clarification and follow-up.

Nurses and other health care professionals must take a patient's complaint of chest pain or discomfort seriously until the cause is determined. The following points should be remembered when assessing patients who may have cardiac symptoms:

- All patients reporting chest symptoms, particularly those at risk for CAD or who have a history of CAD, should be evaluated initially for ACS.
- The location of chest symptoms is not well correlated with the cause of the pain. For example, substernal chest pain can result from a number of causes (see Table 26-2).
- The severity or duration of chest pain or discomfort does not predict the seriousness of its cause. For example, a patient experiencing esophageal spasm may rate chest pain as a "10/10" (eg, the worst pain the patient has ever felt), whereas a patient experiencing an acute MI may report only mild to moderate chest pressure.
- Elderly people and patients with diabetes may not experience chest pain as a typical symptom associated with angina and ACS because of neuropathies. Atypical symptoms, such as fatigue or shortness of breath, are predominant symptoms in these patients.
- Women with ACS are more likely than men to present with atypical symptoms, including shoulder or upper back pain, shortness of breath, or extreme fatigue (Ryan, DeVon, & Zerwic, 2005).
- More than one clinical cardiac condition may occur simultaneously. During an acute MI, patients may report chest pain from myocardial ischemia, shortness of breath from HF, and palpitations from dysrhythmias. Both HF and dysrhythmias are complications of acute MI.

TABLE 26-2 Assessing Chest Pain

Location	Character	Duration	Precipitating Events and Aggravating Factors	Alleviating Factors
Angina pectoris—acute coronary syndrome (unstable angina, myocardial infarction [MI]) 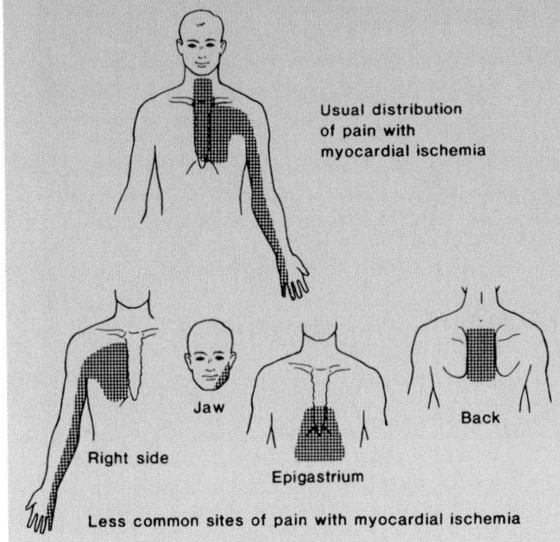 Usual distribution of pain with myocardial ischemia Right side, Jaw, Epigastrium, Back Less common sites of pain with myocardial ischemia	Angina: Uncomfortable pressure, squeezing, or fullness in substernum, Can radiate across chest or to the medial aspect of one or both arms and hands, or to the jaw, shoulders, back,or epigastrium. Radiation to arms and hands is described as numbness, tingling, or aching.	Angina: 5–15 min	Angina: Physical exertion, emotional upset, eating large meal, or exposure to extremes in temperature	Angina: Rest, nitroglycerin, oxygen
	MI: Similar symptom presentation as in angina pectoris. Often associated with shortness of breath, diaphoresis, palpitations, fatigue, and nausea or vomiting.	MI: >15 min	MI: Emotional upset or unusual physical exertion occurring within 24 hours of symptom onset. Can occur at rest or while asleep.	MI: Morphine sulfate, reperfusion of coronary artery with thrombolysis or percutaneous coronary intervention
Pericarditis 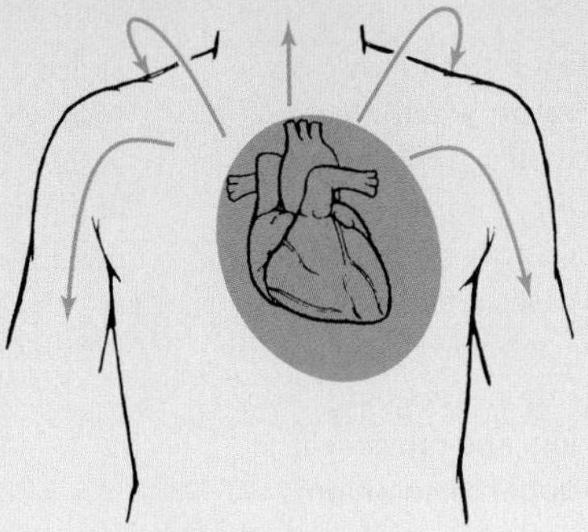	Sharp, severe substernal or epigastric pain. Can radiate to neck, arms, and back. Other associated symptoms are fever, malaise, dyspnea, cough, nausea, dizziness, and palpitations.	Intermittent	Sudden onset. Pain increases with inspiration, swallowing, coughing, and rotation of trunk.	Sitting upright, analgesia, anti-inflammatory medications
Pulmonary disorders (pneumonia, pulmonary embolism) 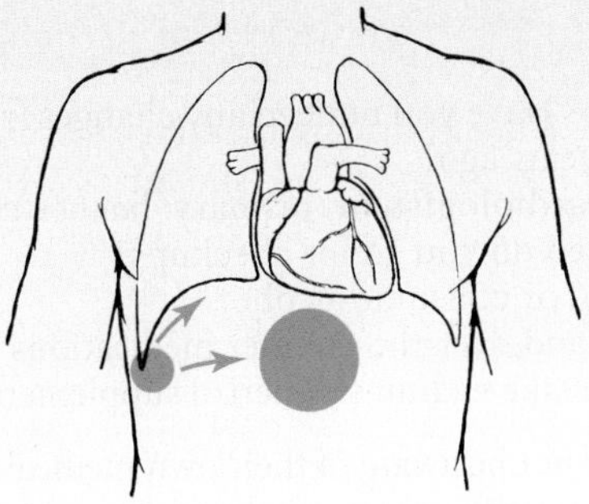	Sharp, severe substernal or epigastric pain arising from inferior portion of pleura. Patient may be able to localize the pain.	30+ min	Follows an infectious or noninfectious process (acute MI, cardiac surgery, cancer, immune disorders, uremia). Pleuritic pain increases with inspiration, coughing, movement and supine positioning. Occurs in conjunction with community-acquired or nosocomial lung infections (pneumonia) or deep vein thrombosis (pulmonary embolism).	Treatment of underlying cause

continued >

TABLE 26-2 Assessing Chest Pain (Continued)

Location	Character	Duration	Precipitating Events and Aggravating Factors	Alleviating Factors
Esophageal disorders (hiatal hernia, reflux esophagitis or spasm)	Substernal pain described as sharp, burning, or heavy; often mimics angina; can radiate to neck, arm, or shoulders.	5–60 min	Recumbency, cold liquids, exercise.	Food, antacid. Nitroglycerin relieves spasm.
Anxiety and panic disorders	Pain described as stabbing to dull ache. Associated with diaphoresis, palpitations, shortness of breath, tingling of hands or mouth, feeling of unreality, or fear of losing control.	Peaks in 10 min	No associated trigger (unexpected) or situation where symptoms are associated with anticipating or experiencing a specific trigger.	Removal of stimulus, relaxation, medications to treat anxiety or antidepressant medication
Musculoskeletal disorders (costochondritis)	Sharp or stabbing pain localized in anterior chest. Most often unilateral. Can radiate across chest to epigastrium or back. Patient able to localize pain.	Hours to days	Most often follows respiratory tract infection with significant coughing, vigorous exercise, or post trauma. Some cases are idiopathic. Exacerbated by deep inspiration, coughing, sneezing, and movement of upper torso or arms.	Rest, ice, or heat; analgesic or anti-inflammatory medications

Health Perception and Management

In an effort to determine how the patient perceives his or her current health status, the nurse might ask some of the following questions:

- What type of health concerns do you have? Are you able to identify any family history or behaviors (risk factors) that put you at risk for this health problem?
- What are your risk factors for heart disease? What do you do to stay healthy and take care of your heart?
- How is your health? Have you noticed any changes from last year? From 5 years ago?
- Do you have a cardiologist or primary health care provider? How often do you go for checkups?
- Do you use tobacco or consume alcohol?
- What prescription and over-the-counter medications are you taking? Do you take vitamins or herbal supplements?

Some patients may not be aware of their own medical diagnosis. For example, patients may not realize that their heart attack was caused by CAD. Patients who do not understand

CHART 26-1

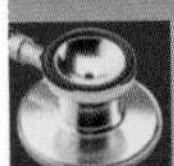

Assessing for Cardiac Signs and Symptoms

SYMPTOMS	ASSESSMENT QUESTIONS	ASSESSING PATIENT'S CAPACITY FOR SELF-MANAGEMENT
Chest pain, chest discomfort, angina pain	• Where is your pain? (ask patient to point to location on chest) • What does the pain feel like? (pressure, heaviness, burning) • How severe is it on a scale of 0 to 10? • What causes the pain? (exertion, stress) • Does anything relieve it? (rest, nitroglycerin) • Does it spread to your arms, neck, jaw, shoulders, or back? • How long does the pain last? • Do you have any additional symptoms? (shortness of breath, palpitations, dizziness, sweating)	*Symptom Recognition* • If you have angina, what does it usually feel like? • If you have angina, how do your angina symptoms differ from the discomfort caused by your other medical conditions? (indigestion, GI disorders) • How do you think you would tell the difference between the symptoms of angina and a heart attack? • What were you doing when the pain started? *Symptom Management* • What did you do when the pain started? • How long did you wait before seeking medical attention (calling the doctor, coming to the emergency department, or calling the ambulance)? *Use of Nitroglycerin* • Do you have a prescription for nitroglycerin (NTG) tablets or spray? • At the time of your chest pain, did you use your NTG? • How many tablets or sprays did you use and how frequently? • If you have NTG and did not take it with this angina episode, why do you think you did not take it? • When did you first open your NTG container? Where is it stored?
Shortness of breath, edema, weight gain	• When did you first notice feeling short of breath? • What makes you short of breath? Does anything make your breathing better or worse? • What activities are you no longer able to do because you are short of breath? • Do you ever wake up at night feeling short of breath? • Do you have a cough? If yes, what do you cough up? • What is your normal weight? • Have you had a recent weight gain? • Do you get up at night to urinate? Have you noticed an increase or decrease in the amount you usually urinate?	• Has anyone ever told you that you have heart failure? What does this mean to you? • Do you ever forget to take your diuretic medication (water pill) or other heart medicines or decide not to take them? If so, why do you think this happens? • What do you typically eat or drink? Who does the food shopping and meal preparation? • Are you on a sodium- or fluid-restricted diet? Have you been able to follow your special diet? • Do you have a scale to weigh yourself? How often do you weigh yourself? • What are important signs or symptoms to report to your doctor?

continued >

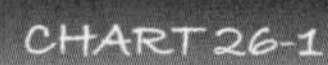

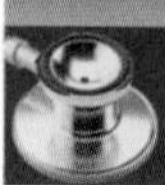

Assessing for Cardiac Signs and Symptoms, continued

SYMPTOMS	ASSESSMENT QUESTIONS	ASSESSING PATIENT'S CAPACITY FOR SELF-MANAGEMENT
	• Have you noticed any weight gain or swelling in your feet, ankles, legs, or abdomen? (sacrum if bedridden) Do your shoes feel tight or clothes feel tight around your waist? • On how many pillows do you sleep, and has this changed recently? • Do you sleep in your bed, or do you breathe easier sleeping in a chair?	
Palpitations	• Do you ever feel your heart racing, skipping beats, or pounding? • Do you ever feel lightheaded or dizzy? • Are there any other symptoms that occur at the same time? • How much caffeine do you consume? • Do you use tobacco? (cigarettes, cigars, chew) • Do you use any other stimulants, recreational drugs? • Do you use any nutritional supplements or herbs? • Have there been any changes in the amount of stress you experience?	• What did you do when your symptoms first occurred? • Is your primary health care provider aware of these symptoms? • Are you taking medication for this condition, and have you been taking it as directed?
Fatigue	• How would you describe your usual activity level? • What is your current activity level? • What were you able to do 1 month and 6 months ago? • What activities can you no longer do because of fatigue? • Do you feel rested when you wake up in the morning? • Can you rest during the day? • How often do you awaken at night, and for what reason?	• Have you spoken with your primary health care provider about decreases in your activity level? • Has anyone ever taught you energy conservation techniques? If so, are you able to use them?
Dizziness, syncope (loss of consciousness)	• Do you ever feel dizzy or lightheaded? • Do you ever pass out or have fainting spells? • Does this happen when you move from a lying to a sitting or standing position? • Do you strain while having a bowel movement or when urinating? • Have you been urinating more than usual? • Have you decreased the amount of fluids you normally drink? • Do you have headaches?	• Have you ever been told you have high or low blood pressure? Has it been checked recently? • Are you taking any medications that can lower your blood pressure? • Before standing from a lying position, do you sit for a few minutes? Does that relieve the dizziness? • What are you using to prevent constipation?

that their behaviors or diagnoses pose a threat to their health may be less motivated to make lifestyle changes or to manage their illness effectively. On the other hand, patients who perceive that their modifiable risk factors for heart disease affect their health and believe that they have the power to modify or change them may be more likely to change these behaviors (Chart 26-2).

The patient's ability to recognize cardiac symptoms and to know what to do when they occur is essential for effective self-care management. All too often, a patient's new symptoms or symptoms of progressing cardiac dysfunction go unrecognized. This results in prolonged delays in seeking life-saving treatment. Major barriers to seeking prompt medical care include lack of knowledge about the symp-

NURSING RESEARCH PROFILE

Women and Symptoms of Myocardial Infarction

McSweeney, J. C., Cody, M., O'Sullivan, P., et al. (2003). Women's early warning symptoms of acute myocardial infarction. *Circulation, 108*, 2619–2623.

Purpose

Chest pain is referred to as the typical acute symptom of coronary heart disease (CHD), and symptoms other than chest pain are referred to as atypical. However, this determination was based on the results of studies on middle-aged, white men. This study was conducted to determine how women present with acute symptoms of CHD, with a focus on early warning or prodromal symptoms of acute myocardial infarction (MI). The researchers sought to determine the most frequent prodromal symptoms of acute MI among women, how prodromal and acute symptoms relate to comorbidities and risk factors for CHD among women, and whether prodromal symptoms are predictive of acute MI symptomatology among women.

Design

Women who were discharged from the hospital after experiencing an acute MI were recruited from five sites in Arkansas, North Carolina, and Ohio. To be eligible for inclusion in the study, participants had to be cognitively intact, speak English, and have telephone access. Once consent was obtained from each participant, nurse research assistants conducted a 60-minute telephone interview using the McSweeney Acute and Prodromal Myocardial Infarction Symptom Survey (MAPMISS). The MAPMISS was developed by the researchers to survey 33 prodromal and 37 acute symptoms of CHD. Prodromal symptoms were defined as symptoms that are intermittent; new or changed in intensity or frequency; or disappear or return to previous levels after the acute MI. Acute symptoms were defined as those that begin at the time of acute MI and resolve after treatment.

Of the 515 women who completed the survey, 93% were white, 6% were black, and 2% were Native American. The mean age was 66.4 (± 12) years. A small percentage (13%) of the women had attended school through eighth grade or less, and about 33% had some college education. More than 44% of the subjects reported a yearly income of $20,000 or less.

Findings

Women had an average of 5.71 (± 4.36) prodromal and 7.3 (± 4.8) acute symptoms. Most women (95%) experienced prodromal symptoms such as unusual fatigue (71%), sleep disturbances (48%), and shortness of breath (42%), and they reported the first two symptoms as being severe. These symptoms occurred daily or less frequently at least 1 month before the acute MI. Acute symptoms most frequently reported were shortness of breath (58%), weakness (55%), and fatigue (43%), whereas only 30% described chest discomfort. Prodromal and acute symptom scores were found to be significantly associated with most cardiac risk factors. The prodromal scores were an important predictor of acute symptom scores, more so than cardiac risk factors such as diabetes, hypertension, and hyperlipidemia.

Nursing Implications

Although the results of this study are limited by the sample demographics, they provide important contributions to the knowledge of early symptoms of acute MI among women. Symptoms described by women in this study were not the typical symptom of chest pain most commonly associated with acute MI among men. It is important for nurses to be aware of the spectrum of symptoms that can be experienced by women for 1 month or longer before acute MI. A thorough health history should include questions about prodromal symptoms. Women with suspected CHD should be asked about the recent onset of new or changing symptoms, especially fatigue, sleep disturbances, or shortness of breath. Women with these symptoms benefit from further cardiac diagnostic testing. Education targeted at women concerning the symptoms of an acute MI should include information about prodromal symptoms as well as the importance of reporting these symptoms to a health care provider.

---

toms of heart disease, attributing symptoms to a benign source, denying symptom significance, and feeling embarrassed about having symptoms (Zerwic & Ryan, 2004).

An additional issue to consider is the patient's medication history, dosages, and schedules. Is the patient independent in taking medications? Are the medications taken as prescribed? Does the patient understand why the medication regimen is important? Are doses ever forgotten or skipped, or does the patient ever decide to stop taking a medication? An aspirin a day is a common nonprescription medication that improves patient outcomes after an MI. However, if patients are not aware of this benefit, they may be inclined to stop taking aspirin if they think it is a trivial medication. A careful medication history often uncovers common medication errors and causes for nonadherence to the medication regimen.

Nutrition and Metabolism

Dietary modifications, exercise, weight loss, and careful monitoring are important strategies for managing three major

CHART 26-2

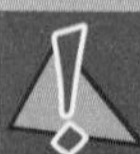

Risk Factors for Coronary Artery Disease (CAD)

Nonmodifiable Risk Factors

- Family history of CAD
- Increasing age
- Male gender (although postmenopausal women have 2 to 3 times the CAD rates of premenopausal women of the same age)
- Race (higher incidence in African Americans than Caucasians due to greater risk of hypertension)

Modifiable Risk Factors*

- Hyperlipidemia (LDL < 100 mg/dL and preferably < 70 mg/dL if CAD present; LDL <160 mg/dL if ≤1 risk factor or 130 mg/dL if ≤2 risk factors; HDL >40 mg/dL and triglycerides < 150 mg/dL)
- Hypertension (<140/90 mm Hg; <130/80 if diabetes or chronic renal disease present)
- Cigarette smoking, exposure to tobacco smoke (no tobacco use or secondhand exposure)
- Diabetes mellitus (fasting serum glucose < 110 mg/dL and hemoglobin A_{1c} < 7%)
- Obesity (BMI 18.5 to 24.9 kg/m^2; waist circumference: male ≤40 inches, female ≤35 inches)
- Physical inactivity (30 to 60 minutes moderate-intensity aerobic activity on all or most days)

*American Heart Association–recommended goals are given in parentheses.

cardiovascular risk factors: hyperlipidemia, hypertension, and diabetes mellitus. Diets that are restricted in sodium, fat, cholesterol, and/or calories are commonly prescribed. The nurse obtains the following information:

- The patient's current height and weight (to determine Body Mass Index), waist measurement (assessment for obesity), BP, and any laboratory test results such as blood glucose, glycosylated hemoglobin (diabetes), total blood cholesterol, high-density and low-density lipoprotein levels, and triglyceride levels (hyperlipidemia)
- How often the patient self-monitors BP, blood glucose, and weight as appropriate to the medical diagnoses
- The patient's level of awareness regarding his or her target goals for each of the risk factors, and any problems achieving or maintaining these goals
- What the patient normally eats and drinks in a typical day and any food preferences (including cultural or ethnic preferences)
- Eating habits (canned or commercially prepared foods versus fresh foods, restaurant cooking versus home cooking, assessing for high-sodium foods, dietary intake of fats)
- Who shops for groceries and prepares meals

Elimination

Typical bowel and bladder habits need to be identified. Nocturia (awakening at night to urinate) is common in patients with HF. Fluid collected in the dependent tissues (extremities) during the day redistributes into the circulatory system once the patient is recumbent at night. The increased circulatory volume is excreted by the kidneys (increased urine production).

When straining during defecation, the patient bears down (the Valsalva maneuver), which momentarily increases pressure on the baroreceptors. This triggers a vagal response, causing the heart rate to slow and resulting in syncope in some patients. Straining during urination can produce the same response.

Because many cardiac medications can cause gastrointestinal side effects or bleeding, the nurse asks about bloating, diarrhea, constipation, stomach upset, heartburn, loss of appetite, nausea, and vomiting. Patients taking platelet-inhibiting medications such as aspirin and clopidogrel (Plavix); platelet aggregation inhibitors such as abciximab (ReoPro), eptifibatide (Integrilin), and tirofiban (Aggrastat); and anticoagulants such as low-molecular-weight heparin (ie, dalteparin [Fragmin], enoxaparin [Lovenox]), heparin, or warfarin (Coumadin) are screened for bloody urine or stools.

Activity and Exercise

As the nurse assesses the patient's activity and exercise history, it is important to note that decreases in activity tolerance are typically gradual and may go unnoticed by the patient. Therefore, the nurse needs to determine whether there has been a change in the activity pattern during the past 6 to 12 months. The patient's subjective response to activity is an essential assessment parameter. New symptoms or a change in the usual anginal symptoms during activity is a significant finding. Fatigue, associated with a low left ventricular ejection fraction (less than 40%) and certain medications (eg, beta-adrenergic blocking agents), can result in activity intolerance. Patients with fatigue may benefit from having their medications adjusted and learning energy-conservation techniques.

Additional areas to ask about include possible architectural barriers and challenges in the home, and what the patient does for exercise. If the patient exercises, the nurse asks additional questions: What is the intensity, and how long and how often is exercise performed? Has the patient ever participated in a cardiac rehabilitation program? Functional levels are known to improve for almost all patients who participate in a cardiac rehabilitation program, and participation is highly recommended (Leon, Franklin, Costa, et al., 2005; Smith, Allen, Blair, et al., 2006). Patients with disabilities may require an individually tailored exercise program.

Sleep and Rest

Clues to worsening cardiac disease, especially HF, can be revealed by sleep-related events. Determining where the patient sleeps or rests is important. Recent changes, such as sleeping upright in a chair instead of in bed, increasing the number of pillows used, awakening short of breath at night (paroxysmal nocturnal dyspnea), or awakening with angina (nocturnal angina), are all indicative of worsening HF.

Cognition and Perception

Evaluating cognitive ability helps determine whether the patient has the mental capacity to manage safe and effective self-care. Is the patient's short-term memory intact? Is there any history of dementia? Is there evidence of depression or anxiety? Can the patient read? Can the patient read English? What is the patient's reading level? What is the patient's preferred learning style? What information does the patient perceive as important? Providing the patient with written information can be a valuable part of patient education, but only if the patient can read and comprehend the information.

Related assessments include possible hearing or visual impairments. If vision is impaired, patients with HF may not be able to weigh themselves independently or keep records of weight, BP, pulse, or other data requested by the health care team.

Self-Perception and Self-Concept

Personality factors may be associated with the development of and recovery from CAD. Most commonly cited is "type A behavior," which is characterized by competitive, hard-driving behaviors and a sense of time urgency. Although this behavior is not an independent risk factor for CAD, anger and hostility (personality traits common in people with "type A behavior") do affect the heart. People with these traits react to frustrating situations with an increase in BP, heart rate, and neuroendocrine responses. This physiologic activation, called cardiac reactivity, is thought to trigger acute cardiovascular events (Woods, Froelicher, & Motzer, 2004).

During the health history, the nurse discovers how patients feel about themselves by asking questions such as: How would you describe yourself? Do you find that you are easily angered or hostile? How do you feel right now? What helps you manage these feelings? Assistance from a psychiatric advanced practice nurse, psychologist, psychiatrist, or social worker may be necessary.

Roles and Relationships

Determining the patient's social support systems is important in today's health care environment. Hospital stays for cardiac disorders have shortened, with many invasive diagnostic cardiac procedures, such as cardiac catheterization and percutaneous coronary intervention (PCI), being performed as outpatient procedures.

To assess support systems, the nurse needs to ask: Who is the primary caregiver? With whom does the patient live? Are there adequate services in place to provide a safe home environment? The nurse also assesses for any significant effects the cardiac illness has had on the patient's role in the family. Are there adequate finances and health insurance? The answers to these questions help the nurse develop a plan to meet the patient's home care needs.

Sexuality and Reproduction

Although people recovering from cardiac illnesses or procedures are often concerned about sexual activity, they are less likely to ask their nurse or other health care provider for information to help them resume their normal sex life. Reduced frequency of and satisfaction with sexual activity are often caused by fear and lack of correct information. Therefore, the nurse needs to initiate a discussion about sexuality with the patient, as opposed to waiting for the patient to bring the subject up in conversation.

The most commonly cited reasons for changes in sexual activity are fear of another heart attack or sudden death; untoward symptoms such as angina, dyspnea, or palpitations; and problems with impotence or depression. In men, impotence may develop as a side effect of cardiac medications (eg, beta-blockers); some men will stop taking their medication as a result. Other medications may be substituted, so patients should be encouraged to discuss this problem with their health care providers. Often, patients and their partners do not have adequate information about the physical demands related to sexual activity and ways in which these demands can be modified. The physiologic demands are greatest during orgasm, reaching 5 or 6 metabolic equivalents (METs). This level of activity is equivalent to walking 3 to 4 miles per hour on a treadmill. The METs expended before and after orgasm are considerably less, at 3.7 METs (Steinke & Swan, 2004). Sharing this information may make the patient and his or her partner more comfortable about resuming sexual activity.

A reproductive history is necessary for women of childbearing age, particularly those with seriously compromised cardiac function. These women may be advised by their physicians not to become pregnant. The reproductive history includes information about previous pregnancies, plans for future pregnancies, oral contraceptive use (especially in women older than 35 years of age who smoke), menopausal status, and use of hormone therapy.

Coping and Stress Tolerance

It is important to determine the presence of psychosocial factors that adversely affect cardiac health. Anxiety, depression, and stress are known to influence both the development of and recovery from CAD. High levels of anxiety are associated with an increased incidence of CAD and increased in-hospital complication rates after MI. People with depression have an increased risk of MI- and heart disease–related death compared to people without depression. Although the association between depression and CAD is not completely understood, it is postulated that both biologic factors (eg, platelet abnormalities, inflammatory responses) and lifestyle factors contribute to the development of CAD. People who are depressed may be less motivated to adhere to the recommended lifestyle changes and medical regimens necessary to prevent future cardiac events (Glassman, Shapiro, Ford, et al., 2003).

Stress initiates a variety of physiologic responses, including increases in the circulation of catecholamines and cortisol, and has been strongly linked to cardiovascular events. Therefore, the patient needs to be assessed for the presence of labile emotions, as well as sources of stress. This is achieved by asking questions about recent or ongoing stressors, previous coping styles and effectiveness, and the patient's perception of his or her current mood and coping ability. Consultation with a psychiatric advanced practice nurse, psychologist, psychiatrist, or social worker may be indicated.

Prevention Strategies

Additional features of the health history include identification of risk factors for heart disease and measures taken by the patient to prevent disease. The nurse's questions need to focus on the patient's health promotion practices. Epidemiologic studies show that certain conditions or behaviors (ie, risk factors) are associated with a greater incidence of coronary artery, peripheral vascular, and cerebrovascular disease (AHA, 2006). Risk factors are classified by the extent to which they can be modified by changing one's lifestyle or modifying personal behaviors (see Chart 26-2).

Once a patient's risk factors are determined, the nurse assesses whether the patient has a plan for making necessary behavioral changes and whether assistance is needed to support these lifestyle changes. For example, tobacco use is one of the most commonly implicated and readily modifiable risk factors for CAD. The first step in treating this health risk is to identify patients who use tobacco products and those who have recently quit. Because 70% of people who smoke visit a health care facility each year, nurses have ample opportunities to assess patients for tobacco use and motivation to quit, and to provide referrals to smoking cessation programs as appropriate. For patients who are obese or who have hyperlipidemia, hypertension, or diabetes, the nurse determines any problems the patient may be having following the prescribed management plan (ie, diet, exercise, and medications). It may be necessary to clarify the patient's responsibilities, assist with finding additional resources, or make alternative plans for risk factor modification.

Physical Assessment

A physical examination is performed to confirm some of the data obtained in the health history. The nurse observes the patient's general appearance and performs a focused cardiac physical examination that includes evaluation of the following:

- Effectiveness of the heart as a pump
- Filling volumes and pressures
- Cardiac output
- Compensatory mechanisms

Indicators that the heart is not functioning effectively as a pump include reduced pulse pressure, cardiac enlargement, and abnormal heart sounds (eg, murmurs or gallop rhythms).

The amount of blood filling the atria and ventricles and the resulting pressures (called filling volumes and pressures) are estimated by the degree of jugular vein distention and the presence or absence of congestion in the lungs, peripheral edema, and postural changes in BP that occur when the patient sits up or stands.

Cardiac output is reflected by cognition, heart rate, pulse pressure, color and texture of the skin, and urine output. Examples of compensatory mechanisms that help maintain cardiac output are increased filling volumes and elevated heart rate. The findings on the physical examination are correlated with data obtained from diagnostic procedures, such as hemodynamic monitoring (discussed later in this chapter).

The examination, which proceeds logically (eg, from head to toe), can be performed in about 10 minutes with practice and covers the following areas: (1) general appearance, (2) cognition, (3) skin, (4) BP, (5) arterial pulses, (6) jugular venous pulsations and pressures, (7) heart, (8) extremities, (9) lungs, and (10) abdomen.

General Appearance and Cognition

The nurse observes the patient's level of distress, level of consciousness, and thought processes as an indication of the heart's ability to propel oxygen to the brain (cerebral perfusion). The nurse also observes for evidence of anxiety, along with any effects that emotional factors may have on cardiovascular status. The nurse attempts to put the anxious patient at ease throughout the examination.

Inspection of the Skin

Examination of the skin begins during the evaluation of the patient's general appearance and continues throughout the assessment. It includes all body surfaces, starting with the head and finishing with the lower extremities. Skin color, temperature, and texture are assessed. The more common findings associated with cardiovascular disease are as follows:

- Pallor—a decrease in the color of the skin—is caused by lack of oxyhemoglobin. It is a result of anemia or decreased arterial perfusion. Pallor is best observed around the fingernails, lips, and oral mucosa. In patients with dark skin, the nurse observes the palms of the hands and soles of the feet.
- Peripheral cyanosis—a bluish tinge, most often of the nails and skin of the nose, lips, earlobes, and extremities—suggests decreased blood flow to a particular area, which allows more time for the hemoglobin molecule to become desaturated. This may occur normally in peripheral vasoconstriction associated with a cold environment, in patients with anxiety, or in disease states such as HF.
- Central cyanosis—a bluish tinge observed in the tongue and buccal mucosa—denotes serious cardiac disorders (pulmonary edema and congenital heart disease) in which venous blood passes through the pulmonary circulation without being oxygenated.
- Xanthelasma—yellowish, slightly raised plaques in the skin—may be observed along the nasal portion of one or both eyelids and may indicate elevated cholesterol levels (hypercholesterolemia).
- Reduced skin turgor occurs with dehydration and aging.
- Temperature and moistness are controlled by the autonomic nervous system. Normally the skin is warm and dry. Under stress, the hands may become cool and moist. In cardiogenic shock, sympathetic nervous system stimulation causes vasoconstriction, and the skin becomes cold and clammy. During an acute MI, diaphoresis is common.
- Ecchymosis (bruise)—a purplish-blue color fading to green, yellow, or brown over time—is associated with blood outside of the blood vessels and is usually caused by trauma. Patients who are receiving anticoagulant therapy should be carefully observed for unexplained ecchymosis. In these patients, excessive bruising indicates prolonged clotting times (prothrombin or partial thromboplastin time) caused by an anticoagulant dosage that is too high.

- Wounds, scars, and tissue surrounding implanted devices should also be examined. Wounds are assessed for adequate healing, and any scars from previous surgeries are noted. The skin surrounding a pacemaker or implantable cardioverter–defibrillator generator is examined for thinning, which could indicate erosion of the device through the skin.

Blood Pressure

Systemic arterial BP is the pressure exerted on the walls of the arteries during ventricular systole and diastole. It is affected by factors such as cardiac output; distention of the arteries; and the volume, velocity, and viscosity of the blood. Normal adult BP values range from 100/60 to 135/85 mm Hg. The average normal BP usually cited is 120/80 mm Hg. An increase in BP above the upper normal range is called hypertension (see Chapter 32 for additional definitions, measurement, and management), whereas a decrease below the lower range is called hypotension.

PULSE PRESSURE

The difference between the systolic and the diastolic pressures is called the pulse pressure. It is a reflection of stroke volume, ejection velocity, and systemic vascular resistance. Pulse pressure, which normally is 30 to 40 mm Hg, indicates how well the patient maintains cardiac output. The pulse pressure increases in conditions that elevate the stroke volume (anxiety, exercise, bradycardia), reduce systemic vascular resistance (fever), or reduce distensibility of the arteries (atherosclerosis, aging, hypertension). Decreased pulse pressure reflects reduced stroke volume and ejection velocity (shock, HF, hypovolemia, mitral regurgitation) or obstruction to blood flow during systole (mitral or aortic stenosis). A pulse pressure of less than 30 mm Hg signifies a serious reduction in cardiac output and requires further cardiovascular assessment.

POSTURAL BLOOD PRESSURE CHANGES

Postural (orthostatic) hypotension occurs when the BP decreases significantly after the patient assumes an upright posture. It is usually accompanied by dizziness, lightheadedness, or syncope.

Although there are many causes of postural hypotension, the three most common causes in patients with cardiac problems are a reduced volume of fluid or blood in the circulatory system (intravascular volume depletion, dehydration), inadequate vasoconstrictor mechanisms, and insufficient autonomic effect on vascular constriction. Postural changes in BP and an appropriate history help health care providers differentiate among these causes. The following recommendations are important when assessing postural BP changes:

- The patient should be positioned supine and flat (as symptoms permit) for 10 minutes before taking the initial BP and heart rate measurements.
- Supine measurements should be checked before checking upright measurements.
- The BP cuff should not be removed between position changes, but the nurse should check to see that it is still correctly placed.
- Postural BP changes should be assessed with the patient sitting on the edge of the bed with feet dangling and, if appropriate, with the patient standing at the side of the bed.
- One to three minutes should elapse after each postural change before measuring BP and heart rate.
- If the patient exhibits any signs or symptoms of distress, he or she is returned to a supine position before completing the test.
- Both heart rate and BP are recorded. The patient's position (eg, supine, sitting, standing) and any signs or symptoms that accompany the postural change are also noted.

Normal postural responses that occur when a person stands up or changes from a lying to a sitting position include (1) a heart rate increase of 5 to 20 bpm above the resting rate (to offset reduced stroke volume and maintain cardiac output); (2) an unchanged systolic pressure, or a slight decrease of up to 10 mm Hg; and (3) a slight increase of 5 mm Hg in diastolic pressure.

A decrease in the amount of blood or fluid in the circulatory system should be suspected after diuretic therapy or bleeding, when a postural change results in an increased heart rate and either a decrease in systolic pressure by 15 mm Hg or a decrease in diastolic pressure by 10 mm Hg. Vital signs alone do not differentiate between a decrease in intravascular volume and inadequate constriction of the blood vessels as a cause of postural hypotension. With intravascular volume depletion, the reflexes that maintain cardiac output (increased heart rate and peripheral vasoconstriction) function correctly; the heart rate increases and the peripheral vessels constrict. However, because of lost volume, the BP falls. With inadequate vasoconstrictor mechanisms, the heart rate again responds appropriately, but because of diminished peripheral vasoconstriction the BP drops. The following is an example of a postural BP recording showing either intravascular volume depletion or inadequate vasoconstrictor mechanisms:

Supine: BP 120/70 mm Hg, heart rate 70 bpm
Sitting: BP 100/55 mm Hg, heart rate 90 bpm
Standing: BP 98/52 mm Hg, heart rate 94 bpm

In autonomic insufficiency, the heart rate cannot increase to completely compensate for the gravitational effects of an upright posture. Peripheral vasoconstriction may be absent or diminished. Autonomic insufficiency does not rule out a concurrent decrease in intravascular volume. The following is an example of autonomic insufficiency as demonstrated by postural BP changes:

Supine: BP 150/90 mm Hg, heart rate 60 bpm
Sitting: BP 100/60 mm Hg, heart rate 60 bpm

Arterial Pulses

Factors to be evaluated in examining the pulse are rate, rhythm, quality, configuration of the pulse wave, and quality of the arterial vessel.

PULSE RATE

The normal pulse rate varies from a low of 50 bpm in healthy, athletic young adults to rates well in excess of 100 bpm after exercise or during times of excitement. Anxiety frequently raises the pulse rate during the physical examination. If the rate is higher than expected, it is appropriate to reassess it near the end of the physical examination, when the patient may be more relaxed.

PULSE RHYTHM

The rhythm of the pulse is as important to assess as the rate. Minor variations in regularity of the pulse are normal. The pulse rate may increase during inhalation and slow during exhalation. This phenomenon, called sinus arrhythmia, occurs most commonly in children and young adults.

For the initial cardiac examination, or if the pulse rhythm is irregular, the heart rate should be counted by auscultating the apical pulse for a full minute while simultaneously palpating the radial pulse. Any discrepancy between contractions heard and pulses felt is noted. Disturbances of rhythm (dysrhythmias) often result in a pulse deficit, a difference between the apical rate (the heart rate heard at the apex of the heart) and the peripheral rate. Pulse deficits commonly occur with atrial fibrillation, atrial flutter, premature ventricular contractions, and varying degrees of heart block (see Chapter 27 for a detailed discussion of these dysrhythmias).

Understanding the complexity of dysrhythmias requires a sophisticated knowledge of cardiac electrophysiology, which is obtained through advanced education and training.

PULSE QUALITY

The quality, or amplitude, of the pulse can be described as absent, diminished, normal, or bounding. It should be assessed bilaterally. Scales can be used to rate the strength of the pulse. The following is an example of a 0-to-4 scale:

0: pulse not palpable or absent
+1: weak, thready pulse; difficult to palpate; obliterated with pressure
+2: diminished pulse; cannot be obliterated
+3: easy to palpate, full pulse; cannot be obliterated
+4: strong, bounding pulse; may be abnormal

The numerical classification is quite subjective; therefore, when documenting the pulse quality, it helps to specify a scale range (eg, "left radial +3/+4").

PULSE CONFIGURATION

The configuration (contour) of the pulse conveys important information. In patients with stenosis of the aortic valve, the valve opening is narrowed, reducing the amount of blood ejected into the aorta. The pulse pressure is narrow, and the pulse feels feeble. In aortic insufficiency, the aortic valve does not close completely, allowing blood to flow back from the aorta into the left ventricle. The rise of the pulse wave is abrupt and strong, and its fall is precipitous—a "collapsing" or "water hammer" pulse. The true configuration of the pulse is best appreciated by palpating over the carotid artery rather than the distal radial artery, because the dramatic characteristics of the pulse wave may be distorted when the pulse is transmitted to smaller vessels.

EFFECT OF VESSEL QUALITY ON PULSE

The condition of the vessel wall also influences the pulse and is of concern, especially in older patients. Once rate and rhythm have been determined, the nurse assesses the quality of the vessel by palpating along the radial artery and comparing it with normal vessels. Does the vessel wall feel thickened? Is it tortuous?

To assess peripheral circulation, the nurse locates and evaluates all arterial pulses. Arterial pulses are palpated at points where the arteries are near the skin surface and are easily compressed against bones or firm musculature. Pulses are detected over the temporal, carotid, brachial, radial, femoral, popliteal, dorsalis pedis, and posterior tibial arteries. A reliable assessment of the pulses of the lower extremities depends on accurate identification of the location of the artery and careful palpation of the area. Light palpation is essential; firm finger pressure can easily obliterate the dorsalis pedis and posterior tibial pulses and confuse the examiner. In approximately 10% of patients, the dorsalis pedis pulses are not palpable. In such circumstances, both are usually absent together, and the posterior tibial arteries alone provide adequate blood supply to the feet. Arteries in the extremities are often palpated simultaneously to facilitate comparison of quality.

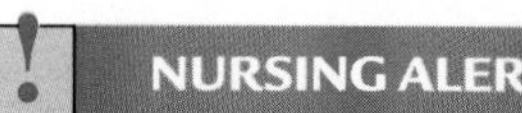

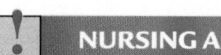

Do not simultaneously palpate the temporal or carotid arteries bilaterally, because it is possible to decrease the blood flow to the brain.

Jugular Venous Pulsations

Right-sided heart function can be estimated by observing the pulsations of the jugular veins of the neck and the central venous pressure (CVP), which reflects right atrial or right ventricular end-diastolic pressure (the pressure immediately preceding the contraction of the right ventricle).

Pulsations of the internal jugular veins are most commonly assessed. If they are difficult to see, pulsations of the external jugular veins may be noted. These veins are more superficial and are visible just above the clavicles, adjacent to the sternocleidomastoid muscles. The external jugular veins are frequently distended while the patient lies supine on the examining table or bed. As the patient's head is elevated, distention of the veins normally disappears. The veins normally are not apparent if the patient's head is elevated more than 30 degrees.

Obvious distention of the veins with the patient's head elevated 45 to 90 degrees indicates an abnormal increase in the volume of the venous system. This occurs with right-sided HF, less commonly with obstruction of blood flow in the superior vena cava, and rarely with acute massive pulmonary embolism.

Heart Inspection and Palpation

The heart is examined indirectly by inspection, palpation, percussion, and auscultation of the chest wall. A systematic approach is used to examine the chest wall in the following six areas (Fig. 26-5):

1. *Aortic area*—second intercostal space to the right of the sternum. To determine the correct intercostal space, start at the angle of Louis by locating the bony ridge near

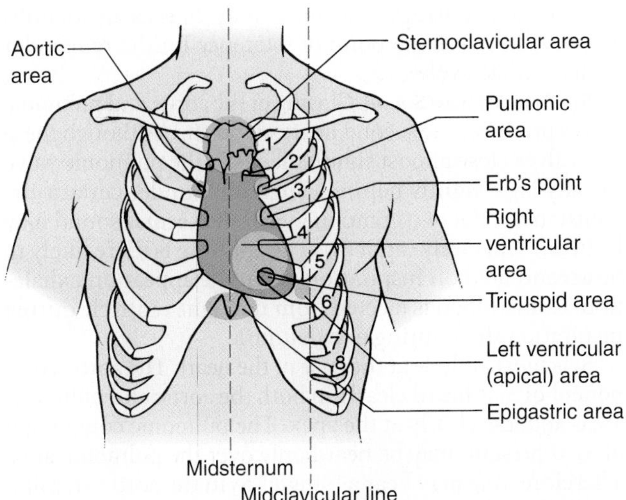

FIGURE 26-5. Areas of the precordium to be assessed when evaluating heart function. (Numerals identify ribs of adjacent intercostal spaces.)

the top of the sternum, at the junction of the body and the manubrium. From this angle, locate the second intercostal space by sliding one finger to the left or right of the sternum. Subsequent intercostal spaces are located from this reference point by palpating down the rib cage.

2. *Pulmonic area*—second intercostal space to the left of the sternum
3. *Erb's point*—third intercostal space to the left of the sternum
4. *Right ventricular or tricuspid area*—fourth and fifth intercostal spaces to the left of the sternum
5. *Left ventricular or apical area*—the point of maximal impulse (PMI), the location on the chest where heart contractions can be palpated
6. *Epigastric area*—below the xiphoid process

For most of the examination, the patient lies supine, with the head of the bed slightly elevated. A right-handed examiner stands at the right side of the patient, a left-handed examiner at the left side.

Each area of the precordium is inspected and then palpated. Oblique lighting is used to assist the examiner in identifying subtle pulsation. A normal impulse that is distinct and located over the apex of the heart is called the **apical impulse**, also referred to as the PMI. It may be observed in young people and in older people who are thin. The apical impulse is normally located and auscultated in the left fifth intercostal space at the midclavicular line (Fig. 26-6).

In many cases, the apical impulse is palpable and is normally felt as a light pulsation, 1 to 2 cm in diameter. It is felt at the onset of the first heart sound and lasts for only half of systole (see the next section for a discussion of heart sounds). The nurse uses the palm of the hand to locate the apical impulse initially and the fingerpads to assess its size and quality. A broad and forceful apical impulse is known as a left ventricular heave or lift because it appears to lift the hand from the chest wall during palpation.

An apical impulse below the fifth intercostal space or lateral to the midclavicular line usually denotes left ventricular enlargement from left ventricular failure. Normally,

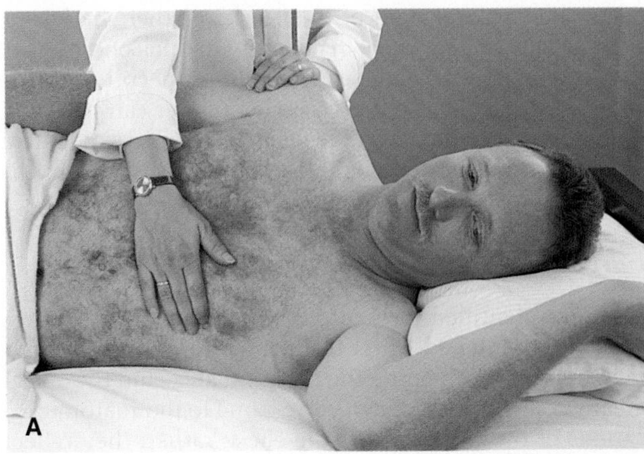

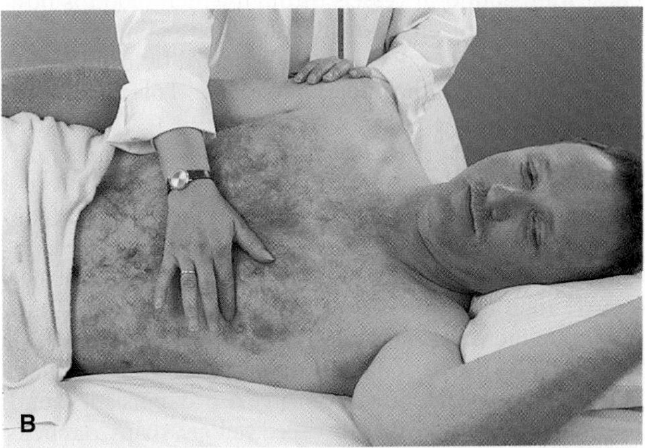

FIGURE 26-6. Locating (**A**) and palpating (**B**) the apical impulse (also called the point of maximal impulse [PMI]). The apical impulse normally is located at the fifth intercostal space to the left of the sternum at the midclavicular line. The nurse locates the impulse with the palm of the hand and palpates with the fingerpads. © B. Proud in Weber, J. W., & Kelley, J. (2003). *Health assessment in nursing* (2nd ed.). Philadelphia: Lippincott Williams & Wilkins.

the apical impulse is palpable in only one intercostal space; palpability in two or more adjacent intercostal spaces indicates left ventricular enlargement. If the apical impulse can be palpated in two distinctly separate areas and the pulsation movements are paradoxical (not simultaneous), a ventricular aneurysm may be suspected.

Abnormal, turbulent blood flow within the heart may be palpated with the palm of the hand as a purring sensation. This phenomenon is called a thrill and is associated with a loud murmur. A thrill is always indicative of significant pathology within the heart. Thrills also may be palpated over vessels when blood flow is significantly and substantially obstructed and over the carotid arteries if aortic stenosis is present or if the aortic valve is narrowed.

Chest Percussion

Normally, only the left border of the heart can be detected by percussion. It extends from the sternum to the midclavicular line in the third to fifth intercostal spaces. The right border lies under the right margin of the sternum and is not detectable. Enlargement of the heart to either the left or right usually can be noted. In people with thick chests, obesity, or emphysema, the heart may lie so deep under the thoracic surface that not even its left border can be noted unless the heart is enlarged. In such cases, unless the nurse detects a displaced apical impulse and suspects cardiac enlargement, percussion is omitted.

Cardiac Auscultation

All areas identified in Figure 26-5, except the epigastric area, are auscultated. These include the aortic area, the pulmonary area, Erb's point, the tricuspid area, and the apical area. These locations do not correspond to the anatomic locations of the valves within the chest; rather, they reflect the patterns by which heart sounds radiate toward the chest wall. Sound in vessels through which blood is flowing is always reflected downstream. For example, the actions of the mitral valve are usually heard best in the fifth intercostal space at the midclavicular line. This is called the mitral valve area.

HEART SOUNDS

The **normal heart sounds,** S_1 and S_2, are produced primarily by the closing of the heart valves. The time between S_1 and S_2 corresponds to systole (Fig. 26-7). This is normally shorter than the time between S_2 and S_1 (diastole). As the heart rate increases, diastole shortens.

Normally, the periods of systole and diastole are silent. However, ventricular disease can give rise to transient sounds in systole and diastole that are called gallops, snaps, or clicks. Significant narrowing of the valve orifices at times when they should be open, or residual gapping of valves at times when they should be closed, produces prolonged sounds called **murmurs.**

S_1—First Heart Sound. Closure of the mitral and tricuspid valves creates the first heart sound (S_1), although vibration of the myocardial wall also may contribute to this sound. Although S_1 is heard over the entire precordium, it is heard best at the apex of the heart (apical area). Its intensity increases when the valve leaflets are made rigid by calcium in rheumatic heart disease and in any circumstance in which ventricular contraction occurs at a time when the valve is caught wide open (eg, when a premature ventricular contraction interrupts the normal cardiac cycle). S_1 varies in intensity from beat to beat when atrial contraction is not synchronous with ventricular contraction because the valve may be fully or partially closed on one beat and open on the next one due to irregular atrial activity. S_1 is easily identifiable and serves as the point of reference for the remainder of the cardiac cycle.

S_2—Second Heart Sound. Closing of the aortic and pulmonic valves produces the second heart sound (S_2). Although these two valves close almost simultaneously, the pulmonic valve usually lags slightly behind. Therefore, under certain circumstances, the two components of the second sound may be heard separately (split S_2). The splitting is more likely to be accentuated on inspiration and to disappear on exhalation. (More blood is ejected from the right ventricle during inspiration than during exhalation.)

S_2 is most audible at the base of the heart. The aortic component of S_2 is heard clearly in both the aortic and pulmonic areas and less clearly at the apex. The pulmonic component of S_2, if present, may be heard only over the pulmonic area. Therefore, one may hear a "single" S_2 in the aortic area and a split S_2 in the pulmonic area.

Gallop Sounds. If the blood filling the ventricle is impeded during diastole, as occurs in certain disease states, then a temporary vibration may occur in diastole that is similar to, although usually softer than, S_1 and S_2. The heart sounds then come in triplets and have the acoustic effect of a galloping horse; they are called gallops. This may occur early in diastole, during the rapid-filling phase of the cardiac cycle, or later at the time of atrial contraction.

Gallop sounds are very low-frequency sounds and may be heard only with the bell of the stethoscope placed very lightly against the chest. They are heard best at the apex, although occasionally, when emanating from the right ventricle, they may be heard to the left of the sternum.

A gallop sound that occurs during rapid ventricular filling is called a third heart sound (S_3); it may represent a normal finding in children and young adults (Fig. 26-8A). Such a

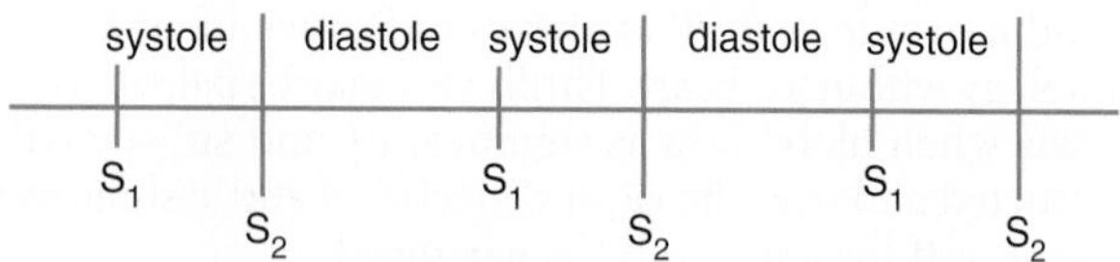

FIGURE 26-7. Normal heart sounds. The first heart sound (S_1) is produced by the closing of the mitral and tricuspid valves and is best heard at the apex of the heart (left ventricular or apical area). The second heart sound (S_2) is produced by the closing of the aortic and pulmonic valves and is loudest at the base of the heart. The time between S_1 and S_2 corresponds to systole. The time between S_2 and S_1 is diastole.

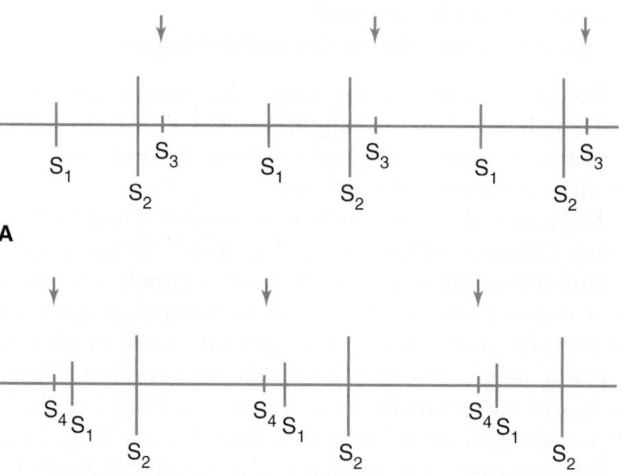

FIGURE 26-8. Gallops. (**A**) An S_3 gallop is heard immediately following the S_2 and occurs when the blood filling the ventricle is impeded during diastole, resulting in temporary vibrations. The heart sounds come in triplets and resemble the sound of a galloping horse. Myocardial disease and heart failure are associated with this sound. (**B**) An S_4 gallop is heard immediately preceding the S_1. The S_4 sound occurs during atrial contraction and is often heard when the ventricle is enlarged or hypertrophied. Associated conditions include coronary artery disease, hypertension, and aortic stenosis.

sound is heard in patients who have myocardial disease or in those who have HF and whose ventricles fail to eject all of their blood during systole. An S_3 gallop is heard best with the patient lying on the left side.

A gallop sound that occurs during atrial contraction is called a fourth heart sound (S_4) (see Fig. 26-8B). An S_4 is often heard when the ventricle is enlarged or hypertrophied and therefore resistant to filling. Such a circumstance may be associated with CAD, hypertension, or stenosis of the aortic valve. On rare occasions, all four heart sounds are heard within a single period of cardiac contraction, ejection, refilling, and resting, referred to as a cardiac cycle, giving rise to what is called a quadruple rhythm.

Snaps and Clicks. Stenosis of the mitral valve resulting from rheumatic heart disease gives rise to an unusual high-pitched sound very early in diastole that is best heard along the left sternal border. The sound is caused by high pressure in the left atrium with abrupt displacement of a rigid mitral valve. The sound is called an opening snap. It occurs too long after S_2 to be mistaken for a split S_2 and too early in diastole to be mistaken for a gallop. It almost always is associated with the murmur of mitral stenosis and is specific to this disorder.

In a similar manner, stenosis of the aortic valve gives rise to a short, high-pitched sound immediately after S_1 that is called an ejection click. This is caused by very high pressure within the ventricle, displacing a rigid and calcified aortic valve.

Murmurs. Murmurs are created by turbulent flow of blood. The causes of the turbulence may be a critically narrowed valve, a malfunctioning valve that allows regurgitant blood flow, a congenital defect of the ventricular wall, a defect between the aorta and the pulmonary artery, or an increased flow of blood through a normal structure (eg, with fever, pregnancy, hyperthyroidism). Murmurs are characterized and consequently described by several characteristics, including their timing in the cardiac cycle, location on the chest wall, intensity, pitch, quality, and pattern of radiation (Chart 26-3).

Friction Rub. In pericarditis, a harsh, grating sound that can be heard in both systole and diastole is called a friction rub. It is caused by abrasion of the pericardial surfaces during the cardiac cycle. Because a friction rub may be confused with a murmur, care should be taken to identify the sound and to distinguish it from murmurs that may be heard in both systole and diastole. A pericardial friction rub can be heard best using the diaphragm of the stethoscope, with the patient sitting up and leaning forward.

AUSCULTATION PROCEDURE

During auscultation, the patient remains supine and the examining room is as quiet as possible. A stethoscope with a diaphragm and a bell is necessary for accurate auscultation of the heart.

Using the diaphragm of the stethoscope, the examiner starts at the apical area and progresses upward along the left sternal border to the pulmonic and aortic areas. Alternatively, the examiner may begin the examination at the aortic and pulmonic areas and progress downward to the apex of the heart. Initially, S_1 is identified and evaluated with respect to its intensity and splitting. Next, S_2 is identified, and its intensity and any splitting are noted. After

CHART 26-3

Characteristics of Heart Murmurs

Heart murmurs are described in terms of location, timing, intensity, pitch, quality, and radiation. These characteristics provide data about the location and nature of the cardiac abnormality.

Location

The location of the murmur (where it is detected on the chest wall) is crucial. Depending on the type of valvular disorder, a murmur can be heard only at the apex or more widely over the chest wall, or along the left sternal border between the third and fourth interspaces.

Timing

Timing of the murmur in the cardiac cycle is vital. The examiner first determines whether the murmur is occurring in systole or in diastole. Then, does it begin simultaneously with a heart sound, or is there some delay between the sound and the beginning of the murmur? Does the murmur continue to (or through) the second heart sound, or is there a delay between the end of the murmur and the second heart sound? Are diastolic murmurs (between the second and first heart sounds) continuous, or do they subside in mid- or late diastole?

Intensity

The intensity of murmurs is conventionally graded from I through VI. Sometimes, grade I murmurs are difficult to hear. However, a grade II cardiac murmur can be easily perceived by the experienced examiner. Murmurs of grades IV or louder are usually associated with thrills that may be palpated on the surface of the chest wall. A grade VI murmur can be heard with the stethoscope off the chest. A murmur may vary in intensity from its beginning to its conclusion. This is very characteristic of certain valvular disorders.

Pitch

The next important characteristic of a murmur is its pitch, which may be low, often heard only with the bell of the stethoscope placed lightly on the chest wall, or a very high-pitched murmur, heard best with the stethoscope's diaphragm. Other murmurs contain the full spectrum of sound frequency.

Quality

In addition to the intensity and pitch, noting the character of the sound is vital. A murmur may be described as rumbling, blowing, whistling, harsh, or musical.

Radiation

The last feature of concern is radiation of the murmur. A murmur can radiate into the axilla, the carotid arteries in the neck, the left shoulder, or the back.

concentrating on S_1 and S_2, the examiner listens for extra sounds in systole and then in diastole.

Sometimes it helps to ask the following questions: Do I hear snapping or clicking sounds? Do I hear any high-pitched blowing sounds? Is this sound in systole, or diastole, or both? The examiner again proceeds to move the stethoscope to all of the designated areas of the precordium, listening carefully for these sounds. Finally, the patient is turned on the left side and the stethoscope is placed on the apical area, where an S_3, an S_4, and a mitral murmur are more readily detected.

Once an abnormality is heard, the entire chest surface is reexamined to determine the exact location of the sound and its radiation. The patient may be concerned about the prolonged examination and must be supported and reassured. The auscultatory findings, particularly murmurs, are documented by identifying the following characteristics:

- Location on chest wall
- Timing of sound as either during systole or during diastole; described as early, middle, or late (if heard throughout systole, the sound is often referred to as pansystolic or holosystolic)
- Intensity of the sound (I, very faint; II, quiet; III, moderately loud; IV, loud; V, very loud; or VI, heard with stethoscope removed from the chest)
- Pitch, described as high, medium, or low
- Quality of the sound, commonly described as blowing, harsh, or musical
- Location of radiation of the sound away from where it is heard the loudest

INTERPRETATION OF CARDIAC SOUNDS

Interpreting cardiac sounds requires detailed knowledge of cardiac physiology and the pathophysiology of cardiac diseases. When nurses evaluate cardiac sounds, they may be expected to perform at different levels. The first level involves simply recognizing that what one is hearing is not normal—such as a third heart sound, a murmur in systole or diastole, a pericardial friction rub over the midsternum, or a second heart sound that is widely split. These findings are reported to the physician and acted on accordingly. This level of function is useful in screening. It is the kind of activity involved in performing physical examinations in schools on normal children or in performing routine physical examinations or screening examinations.

The second level involves recognizing patterns. The nurse correctly observes the findings and recognizes the diagnostic significance of common heart sounds. Highly skilled nurses can differentiate among dysrhythmias and respond accordingly. They can determine the significance of the appearance and disappearance of gallops during the treatment of patients who have had MIs or who have HF. This is the role of coronary care and cardiovascular advanced practice nurses as they work collaboratively with other health care professionals.

Inspection of the Extremities

The hands, arms, legs, and feet are observed for skin and vascular changes. The most noteworthy changes include the following:

- Decreased capillary refill time indicates a slower peripheral flow rate from sluggish reperfusion and is often observed in patients with hypotension or HF. Capillary refill time provides the basis for estimating the rate of peripheral blood flow. To test capillary refill, the nurse briefly compresses the nailbed so that it blanches, and then releases the pressure. Normally, reperfusion occurs within 3 seconds, as evidenced by the return of color.
- Vascular changes from decreased arterial circulation include a decrease in quality or loss of pulse, discomfort or pain, paresthesia, numbness, decrease in temperature, pallor, and loss of movement. During the first few hours after invasive cardiac procedures (eg, cardiac catheterization), affected extremities should be assessed frequently for vascular changes.
- Hematoma, or a localized collection of clotted blood in the tissue, may be observed in patients who have undergone invasive cardiac procedures such as cardiac catheterization, PCI, or cardiac electrophysiology testing. Major blood vessels of the arms and legs are used for catheter insertion. During these procedures, systemic anticoagulation with heparin is necessary, and minor or small hematomas may occur at the catheter puncture site. However, large hematomas are a serious complication that can compromise circulating blood volume and cardiac output, requiring blood transfusions. Patients who have undergone these procedures must have their puncture sites frequently observed until hemostasis is adequately achieved.
- Peripheral edema is fluid accumulation in dependent areas of the body (feet and legs, sacrum in the bedridden patient). Pitting edema (a depression over an area of pressure) is assessed by pressing firmly for 5 seconds with the thumb over the dorsum of each foot, behind each medial malleolus, and over the shins. It is graded as absent or as present on a scale from slight (1+ = 0 to 2 mm) to very marked (4+ = more than 8 mm). Peripheral edema is observed in patients with HF and in those with peripheral vascular diseases such as deep vein thrombosis or chronic venous insufficiency.
- Clubbing of the fingers and toes implies chronic hemoglobin desaturation, as in congenital heart disease.
- Lower extremity ulcers are observed in patients with arterial or venous insufficiency (see Chapter 31 for a complete description of these conditions).

Other Systems

LUNGS

The details of respiratory assessment are described in Chapter 21. Findings frequently exhibited by patients with cardiac disorders include the following:

Tachypnea: Rapid, shallow breathing may be noted in patients who have HF, pain, or anxiety.

Cheyne-Stokes respirations: Patients with severe left ventricular failure may exhibit Cheyne-Stokes breathing, a pattern of rapid respirations alternating with apnea. It is important to note the duration of the apnea.

Hemoptysis: Pink, frothy sputum is indicative of acute pulmonary edema.

Cough: A dry, hacking cough from irritation of small airways is common in patients with pulmonary congestion from HF.

Crackles: HF or atelectasis associated with bed rest, splinting from ischemic pain, or the effects of analgesics, sedatives, or anesthetic agents often results in the development of crackles. Typically, crackles are first noted at the bases (because of gravity's effect on fluid accumulation and decreased ventilation of basilar tissue), but they may progress to all portions of the lung fields.

Wheezes: Compression of the small airways by interstitial pulmonary edema may cause wheezing. Beta-adrenergic blocking agents (beta-blockers), such as propranolol (Inderal), may cause airway narrowing, especially in patients with underlying pulmonary disease.

ABDOMEN

For the patient with a cardiovascular disorder, two components of the abdominal examination are relevant:

Hepatojugular reflux: Liver engorgement occurs because of decreased venous return secondary to right ventricular failure. The liver is enlarged, firm, nontender, and smooth. The hepatojugular reflux may be demonstrated by pressing firmly over the right upper quadrant of the abdomen for 30 to 60 seconds and noting an increase of 1 cm or more in jugular venous pressure. This increase indicates an inability of the right side of the heart to accommodate increased volume.

Bladder distention: Urine output is an important indicator of cardiac function. Reduced urine output may indicate inadequate renal perfusion or a less serious problem such as one caused by urinary retention. When the urine output is decreased, the patient must be assessed for a distended bladder or difficulty voiding. The bladder may be assessed with an ultrasound scanner or the suprapubic area palpated for an oval mass and percussed for dullness, indicative of a full bladder.

Gerontologic Considerations

When performing a cardiovascular examination on an elderly patient, the nurse may note such differences as more readily palpable peripheral pulses because of decreased elasticity of the arteries and a loss of adjacent connective tissue. Palpation of the precordium in the elderly is affected by the changes in the shape of the chest. For example, a cardiac impulse may not be palpable in patients with chronic obstructive pulmonary disease, because these patients usually have an increased anterior–posterior chest diameter. Kyphoscoliosis, a spinal deformity that occurs frequently in elderly patients, may dislocate the cardiac apex downward so that palpation of the apical impulse is obscured.

Systolic BP increases with age, but diastolic BP usually plateaus after 50 years. Isolated systolic hypertension occurs most commonly among the elderly and is associated with significant cardiovascular morbidity and mortality. Orthostatic hypotension may reflect decreased sensitivity of postural reflexes, which must be considered when medication therapy is prescribed.

An S_4 is heard in about 90% of elderly patients and is thought to be due to decreased compliance of the left ventricle. The S_2 is usually split. At least 60% of elderly patients have murmurs, the most common being a soft systolic ejection murmur resulting from sclerotic changes of the aortic leaflets (see Table 26-1).

Diagnostic Evaluation

Diagnostic tests and procedures are used to confirm the data obtained by the history and physical assessment. Some tests are easy to interpret, but others must be interpreted by expert clinicians. All tests should be explained to the patient. Some necessitate special preparation before they are performed and special monitoring by the nurse after the procedure.

Laboratory Tests

Laboratory tests may be performed for the following reasons:

- To assist in identifying the cause of cardiac-related signs and symptoms
- To identify abnormalities in the blood that affect the prognosis of a patient with CVD
- To assess the degree of inflammation
- To screen for risk factors associated with CAD
- To determine baseline values before initiating therapeutic interventions
- To ensure that therapeutic levels of medications (eg, antiarrhythmic agents and warfarin) are maintained
- To assess the effects of medications (eg, the effects of diuretics on serum potassium levels)
- To screen generally for abnormalities

Because different laboratories use different equipment and different methods of measurements, normal test values may vary depending on the laboratory and the health care institution.

Cardiac Biomarker Analysis

Plasma analysis of key cardiac isoenzymes and other biomarkers is part of a diagnostic profile for acute MI that also includes the health history, symptoms, and ECG. Enzymes are released from injured cells when the cell membranes rupture. Most enzymes are nonspecific in relation to the particular organ that has been damaged. However, certain isoenzymes come only from myocardial cells and are released when those cells are damaged by sustained hypoxia or trauma that results in infarction. The isoenzymes leak into the interstitial spaces of the myocardium and are carried into the general circulation by the lymphatic system and the coronary circulation, resulting in elevated serum enzyme concentrations.

Because different enzymes move into the blood at varying periods after MI, enzyme levels should be tested in relation to the time of onset of chest discomfort or other symptoms. Creatine kinase (CK) and its isoenzyme CK-MB are the most specific enzymes analyzed in acute MI, and they are the first enzyme levels to increase. Lactic dehydrogenase and its isoenzymes may also be analyzed but only in select patients who have delayed seeking medical attention, because the blood levels of these substances peak in 2 to 3 days, much later than CK levels.

Other important cardiac biomarkers that are assessed include the myoglobin and troponin T or I. Myoglobin, an early marker of MI, is a heme protein with a small molecular weight. This allows it to be rapidly released from damaged myocardial tissue and accounts for its early increase, within 1 to 3 hours after the onset of an acute MI. Myoglobin peaks in 4 to 12 hours and returns to normal in 24 hours. Myoglobin is not used alone to diagnose MI, because elevations can also occur in patients with renal or musculoskeletal disease. However, negative results are helpful in ruling out an early diagnosis of MI.

Troponin T and I are laboratory tests that have several advantages over traditional enzyme studies such as CK-MB. Troponin T and I are proteins found only in cardiac muscle. After myocardial injury, elevated serum troponin T and I concentrations can be detected within 3 to 4 hours; they peak in 4 to 24 hours and remain elevated for 1 to 3 weeks. These early and prolonged elevations make very early diagnosis of MI possible or allow for late diagnosis if the patient has delayed seeking treatment (see Table 28-3 in Chapter 28 for the time course of cardiac biomarkers).

Blood Chemistry, Hematology, and Coagulation Studies

Table 26-3 provides information about some common serum laboratory tests and the implications for patients with CVD. Lipid measurements are discussed below.

LIPID PROFILE

Cholesterol, triglycerides, and lipoproteins are measured to evaluate a person's risk of developing atherosclerotic disease, especially if there is a family history of premature heart disease, or to diagnose a specific lipoprotein abnormality. Cholesterol and triglycerides are transported in the blood by combining with protein molecules to form lipoproteins. The lipoproteins are referred to as low-density lipoproteins (LDL) and high-density lipoproteins (HDL). The risk of CAD increases as the ratio of LDL to HDL or the ratio of total cholesterol (LDL + HDL) to HDL increases. Although cholesterol levels remain relatively constant over 24 hours, the blood specimen for the lipid profile should be obtained after a 12-hour fast.

CHOLESTEROL LEVELS

Cholesterol (normal level is less than 200 mg/dL) is a lipid required for hormone synthesis and cell membrane formation. It is found in large quantities in brain and nerve tissue. Two major sources of cholesterol are diet (animal products) and the liver, where cholesterol is synthesized. Elevated cholesterol levels are known to increase the risk of CAD. Factors that contribute to variations in cholesterol levels include age, gender, diet, exercise patterns, genetics, menopause, tobacco use, and stress levels.

LDLs (normal level is less than 160 mg/dL) are the primary transporters of cholesterol and triglycerides into the cell. One harmful effect of LDL is the deposition of these substances in the walls of arterial vessels. Elevated LDL levels are associated with a greater incidence of CAD. In people with known CAD or diabetes, the primary goal for lipid management is reduction of LDL levels to less than 70 mg/dL.

HDLs (normal range in men is 35 to 70 mg/dL; in women, 35 to 85 mg/dL) have a protective action. They transport cholesterol away from the tissue and cells of the arterial wall to the liver for excretion. Therefore, there is an inverse relationship between HDL levels and risk of CAD. Factors that lower HDL levels include smoking, diabetes, obesity, and physical inactivity. In patients with CAD, a secondary goal of lipid management is the increase of HDL levels to more than 40 mg/dL.

TRIGLYCERIDES

Triglycerides (normal range is 100 to 200 mg/dL), composed of free fatty acids and glycerol, are stored in the adipose tissue and are a source of energy. Triglyceride levels increase after meals and are affected by stress. Diabetes, alcohol use, and obesity can elevate triglyceride levels. These levels have a direct correlation with LDL and an inverse one with HDL.

Brain (B-Type) Natriuretic Peptide

Brain (B-type) natriuretic peptide (BNP) is a neurohormone that helps regulate BP and fluid volume. It is primarily secreted from the ventricles in response to increased preload with resulting elevated ventricular pressure. The level of BNP in the blood increases as the ventricular walls expand from increased pressure, making it an excellent diagnostic, monitoring, and prognostic tool in the setting of HF. Because this serum laboratory test can be quickly obtained, BNP levels are useful for prompt diagnosis of HF in settings such as the emergency department. A BNP level of 51.2 pg/mL or greater is correlated with mild HF, and levels greater than 1000 pg/mL are associated with severe HF (Gordon & Rempher, 2003).

C-Reactive Protein

High-sensitivity assay for C-reactive protein (hs-CRP) is a venous blood test that measures levels of CRP, a protein produced by the liver in response to systemic inflammation. Inflammation is thought to play a role in the development and progression of atherosclerosis. Therefore, hs-CRP is used as an adjunct to other tests to predict CVD risk. People with high levels of hs-CRP (3.0 mg/dL) are at greatest risk for CVD compared to people with moderate (1.0 to 3.0 mg/dL) or low (less than 1.0 mg/dL) levels of hs-CRP. In addition, an elevated hs-CRP places patients with ACS at high risk for recurrent cardiac events, including unstable angina and acute MI, higher mortality, and increased risk of restenosis of coronary arteries after PCI (Koenig, 2005).

Homocysteine

Determining the homocysteine level enhances the clinician's ability to assess the patient's risk for CVD. An elevated blood level of homocysteine, an amino acid, is thought to indicate a high risk for CAD, stroke, and peripheral vascular disease, although it is not an independent predictor of CAD (AHA, 2005). Homocysteine is linked to the development of atherosclerosis, the underlying disorder in CAD, stroke, and peripheral vascular disease, because it can damage the endothelial lining of arteries and promote thrombus formation. Genetic factors and a diet low in folic acid, vitamin B_6, and vitamin B_{12} are associated with elevated homocysteine levels. A 12-hour fast is necessary before drawing a blood sample for an accurate serum measurement. Test results are interpreted as normal (5 to 15 μmol/L), mod-

TABLE 26-3 Common Serum Laboratory Tests and Implications for Patients with Cardiovascular Disease (CVD)

Laboratory Test	Implications
Blood Chemistries	
Sodium (Na^+)	Low or high serum sodium levels do not directly affect cardiac function. *Hyponatremia:* Decreased sodium levels indicate fluid excess and can be caused by heart failure or administration of thiazide diuretics. *Hypernatremia:* Increased sodium levels indicate fluid deficits and can result from decreased water intake or loss of water through excessive sweating or diarrhea.
Potassium (K^+)	Potassium has a major role in cardiac electrophysiologic function. *Hypokalemia:* Decreased potassium levels due to administration of potassium-excreting diuretics can cause many forms of dysrhythmias, including life-threatening ventricular tachycardia or ventricular fibrillation, and predispose patients taking digitalis preparations to digitalis toxicity. *Hyperkalemia:* Increased potassium levels can result from an increased intake of potassium (eg, foods high in potassium or potassium supplements), decreased renal excretion of potassium, use of potassium-sparing diuretics (eg, spironolactone), or use of angiotensin-converting enzyme inhibitors (ACE inhibitors) that inhibit aldosterone function. Serious consequences of hyperkalemia include heart block, asystole, and life-threatening ventricular dysrhythmias.
Calcium (Ca^{++})	Calcium is necessary for blood coagulability, neuromuscular activity, and automaticity of the nodal cells (sinus and atrioventricular nodes). *Hypocalcemia:* Decreased calcium levels slow nodal function and impair myocardial contractility. The latter effect increases the risk for heart failure. *Hypercalcemia:* Increased calcium levels can occur with the administration of thiazide diuretics because these medications reduce renal excretion of calcium. Hypercalcemia potentiates digitalis toxicity, causes increased myocardial contactility, and increases the risk for varying degrees of heart block and sudden death from ventricular fibrillation.
Magnesium (Mg^{++})	Magnesium is necessary for the absorption of calcium, maintenance of potassium stores, and metabolism of adenosine triphosphate. It plays a major role in protein and carbohydrate synthesis and muscular contraction. *Hypomagnesemia:* Decreased magnesium levels are due to enhanced renal excretion of magnesium from the use of diuretic or digitalis therapy. Low magnesium levels predispose patients to atrial or ventricular tachycardias. *Hypermagnesemia:* Increased magnesium levels are commonly caused by the use of cathartics or antacids containing magnesium. Increased magnesium levels depress contractility and excitability of the myocardium, causing heart block and, if severe, asystole.
Blood urea nitrogen (BUN) Creatinine	BUN and creatinine are end products of protein metabolism excreted by the kidneys. Elevated BUN reflects reduced renal perfusion from decreased cardiac output or intravascular fluid volume deficit as a result of diuretic therapy or dehydration. Both laboratory values are used to assess renal function, although creatinine is a more sensitive measure. Renal impairment is detected by an increase in both BUN and creatinine. A normal creatinine level and an elevated BUN detect an intravascular fluid volume deficit.
Glucose	Glucose levels are elevated in stressful situations, when mobilization of endogenous epinephrine results in conversion of liver glycogen to glucose. Serum glucose levels are drawn in a fasting state.
Glycosylated hemoglobin (hemoglobin A_{1c})	Glycosylated hemoglobin (hemoglobin A_{1C}) is monitored in people with diabetes. It reflects the blood glucose levels over 2 to 3 months. The glycemic goal is to maintain the hemoglobin A_{1C} below 7% (normal range 4%–6%), reflecting consistent near-normal blood glucose levels.
Coagulation Studies	Injury to a vessel wall or tissue initiates the formation of a thrombus. This injury activates the coagulation cascade, the complex interactions among phospholipids, calcium, and clotting factors that convert prothrombin to thrombin. The coagulation cascade has two pathways, the intrinsic and extrinsic pathways. Coagulation studies are routinely performed before invasive procedures, such as cardiac catheterization, electrophysiology testing, and coronary or cardiac surgery.

continued >

TABLE 26-3 Common Serum Laboratory Tests and Implications for Patients with Cardiovascular Disease (CVD) (Continued)

Laboratory Test	Implications
Partial thromboplastin time (PTT) Activated partial thromboplastin time (aPTT)	PTT or aPTT measures the activity of the intrinsic pathway and is used to assess the effects of unfractionated heparin. A therapeutic range is 1.5 to 2.5 times baseline values. Adjustment of heparin dose is required for aPTT < 50 seconds (↑ dose) or >100 seconds (↓ dose).
Prothrombin time (PT)	PT measures the extrinsic pathway activity and is used to monitor the level of anticoagulation with warfarin (Coumadin).
International Normalized Ratio (INR)	The INR, reported with the PT, provides a standard method for reporting PT levels and eliminates the variation of PT results from different laboratories. The INR, rather than the PT alone, is used to monitor the effectiveness of warfarin. The therapeutic range for INR is 2.0–3.5, although specific ranges vary based on diagnosis.
Hematologic Studies	
Complete blood count (CBC)	The CBC identifies the total number of white and red blood cells and platelets, and measures hemoglobin and hematocrit. The CBC is carefully monitored in patients with cardiovascular disease.
White blood cell (WBC) count	WBC counts are monitored in immunocompromised patients, including patients with heart transplants or in situations where there is concern for infection (eg, after invasive procedures or surgery).
Hemoglobin and hematocrit	The hematocrit represents the percentage of red blood cells found in 100 mL of whole blood. The red blood cells contain hemoglobin, which transports oxygen to the cells. Low hemoglobin and hematocrit levels have serious consequences for patients with cardiovascular disease, such as more frequent angina episodes or acute myocardial infarction.
Platelets	Platelets are the first line of protection against bleeding. Once activated by blood vessel wall injury or rupture of atherosclerotic plaque, platelets undergo chemical changes that form a thrombus. Several medications inhibit platelet function, including aspirin, clopidogrel (Plavix), and IV GP IIb/IIIa inhibitors (abciximab [ReoPro], eptifibatide [Integrilin], and tirofiban [Aggrastat]). When these medications are administered, it is essential to monitor for thrombocytopenia (low platelet counts).

erate (16 to 30 μmol/L), intermediate (31 to 100 μmol/L), and severe (more than 100 μmol/L).

Chest X-Ray and Fluoroscopy

A chest x-ray is obtained to determine the size, contour, and position of the heart. It reveals cardiac and pericardial calcifications and demonstrates physiologic alterations in the pulmonary circulation. Although it does not help diagnose acute MI, it can help diagnose some complications (eg, HF). Correct placement of cardiac catheters, such as pacemakers and pulmonary artery catheters, is also confirmed by chest x-ray.

Fluoroscopy allows visualization of the heart on an x-ray screen. It shows cardiac and vascular pulsations and unusual cardiac contours. Fluoroscopy is useful for positioning IV pacing electrodes and for guiding catheter insertion during cardiac catheterization.

Electrocardiography

The ECG is a diagnostic tool used in assessing the cardiovascular system. It is a graphic recording of the electrical activity of the heart. The ECG is obtained by placing disposable electrodes in standard positions on the skin of the chest wall and extremities. The heart's electrical impulses are recorded on special graph paper, with 12, 15, or 18 leads, showing the activity from those different reference points.

The standard 12-lead ECG is used to diagnose dysrhythmias, conduction abnormalities, enlarged heart chambers, and myocardial ischemia or infarction and to monitor high or low calcium and potassium levels and the effects of some medications. A 15-lead ECG adds 3 additional chest leads across the right precordium and is used for early diagnosis of right ventricular and posterior left ventricular infarction. The 18-lead ECG adds 3 posterior leads to the 15-lead ECG and is useful for early detection of myocardial ischemia and injury. To enhance interpretation of the ECG, the patient's age, gender, BP, height, weight, symptoms, and medications (especially digitalis and antiarrhythmic agents) are noted on the ECG requisition. The details of electrocardiography are presented in Chapter 27.

Continuous Electrocardiographic Monitoring

Continuous ECG monitoring to detect abnormalities in heart rate and rhythm is standard for patients who are at high risk for dysrhythmias. In addition, it is often possible to monitor the ST segment of the ECG to identify changes indicative of myocardial ischemia or infarction (see Chapter 28). Two continuous ECG monitoring techniques are hardwire monitoring, found in emergency departments, critical care units, and progressive care units (sometimes called specialty step-down units), and telemetry, found in general nursing care units. Patients monitored continuously need to be informed of the purpose of the monitoring and cautioned that it does not detect symptoms such as dyspnea or chest pain. Therefore, patients need to be advised to report symptoms to the nurse whenever they occur.

HARDWIRE CARDIAC MONITORING

The patient's ECG can be continuously observed for dysrhythmias and conduction disorders on an oscilloscope at the bedside or at a central monitoring station by a hardwire monitoring system. This system is composed of three to five electrodes positioned on the patient's chest, a lead cable, and a bedside monitor. Hardwire monitoring systems vary in sophistication but in general can do the following:

- Monitor more than one lead simultaneously
- Monitor ST segments (ST-segment depression is a marker of myocardial ischemia; ST-segment elevation provides evidence of an evolving MI)
- Provide graded visual and audible alarms (based on priority, asystole would be highest)
- Computerize rhythm monitoring (dysrhythmias are interpreted and stored in memory)
- Print a rhythm strip
- Record a 12-lead ECG

Two leads commonly used for continuous monitoring are leads II and V1 or a modification of V1 (MCL1) (Fig. 26-9). Lead II provides the best visualization of atrial depolarization (represented by the P wave). Leads V1 and MCL1 best record ventricular depolarization and are most helpful when monitoring for ventricular dysrhythmias (eg, premature ventricular contractions or ventricular tachycardia).

TELEMETRY

In addition to hardwire monitoring systems, the ECG can be continuously observed by **telemetry**, the transmission of radiowaves from a battery-operated transmitter worn by the patient to a central bank of monitors. Although telemetry systems have the same capabilities as hardwire systems, they are wireless, allowing the patient to ambulate while being monitored. To ensure good conduction and a clear picture of the patient's rhythm on the monitor, it is important to adhere to the following guidelines for electrode placement:

- Clean the skin surface with soap and water and dry well (or as recommended by the manufacturer) before applying the electrodes. If the patient has much hair where the electrodes need to be placed, shave or clip the hair.
- Apply a small amount of benzoin to the skin if the patient is diaphoretic (sweaty) and the electrodes do not adhere well.
- Change the electrodes every 24 to 48 hours and examine the skin for irritation. Apply the electrodes to different locations each time they are changed.
- If the patient is sensitive to the electrodes, use hypoallergenic electrodes.

SIGNAL-AVERAGED ELECTROCARDIOGRAM

For some patients who are considered to be at high risk for sudden cardiac death, a signal-averaged ECG is performed. This high-resolution ECG assists in identifying the risk for life-threatening dysrhythmias and helps determine the need for invasive diagnostic procedures. Signal averaging works by averaging about 150 to 300 QRS waveforms (QRS waveforms represent depolarization of the ventricle). The resulting averaged QRS complex is analyzed for certain characteristics that are likely to lead to lethal ventricular dysrhythmias. The recording is performed at the bedside and requires about 15 minutes.

CONTINUOUS AMBULATORY MONITORING

In ambulatory ECG monitoring, which may occur in the hospital but is more commonly used for outpatients, one lead of the patient's ECG is monitored by a Holter monitor. This monitor is a small tape recorder that continuously (for 10 to 24 hours) documents the heart's electrical activity on a magnetic tape. The tape recorder weighs approximately 2 pounds and can be carried over the shoulder or worn around the waist day and night to detect dysrhythmias or evidence of myocardial ischemia during activities of daily living. The patient keeps a diary of activity, noting the time of any symptoms, experiences, or performance of unusual activities. The tape recording is then examined with a special scanner,

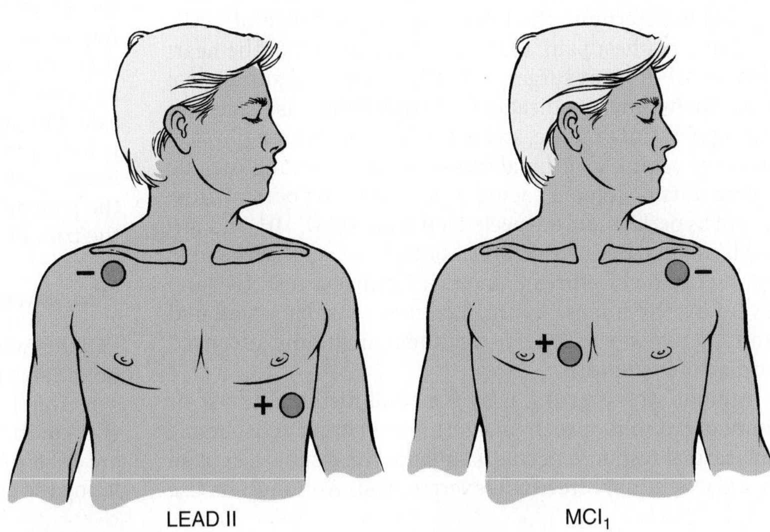

FIGURE 26-9. Two leads (views of the heart) commonly used for continuous monitoring. To monitor lead II, the negative electrode is placed on the right upper chest; the positive electrode is placed on the left lower chest. To monitor MCL_1, the negative electrode is placed on the left upper chest; the positive electrode is placed in the V1 position. If three electrodes are used, the third electrode, which is the ground electrode, can be placed anywhere on the chest.

analyzed, and interpreted. Evidence obtained in this way helps the physician diagnose dysrhythmias and myocardial ischemia and evaluate therapy, such as antiarrhythmic and antianginal medications or pacemaker function.

TRANSTELEPHONIC MONITORING

Another method of evaluating the ECG of a patient at home is by transtelephonic monitoring. The patient attaches a specific lead system for transmitting the signals and places a telephone mouthpiece over the transmitter box, and the ECG is recorded and evaluated at another location. This method is often used for diagnosing dysrhythmias and in follow-up evaluation of permanent cardiac pacemakers.

WIRELESS MOBILE CARDIAC MONITORING SYSTEMS

This emerging technology allows health care professionals to monitor and transmit the ECG of patients outside of the hospital or office setting continuously. The wireless method has a number of advantages compared to Holter and transtelephonic monitoring. It is lightweight, can monitor the patient 24 hours a day 7 days a week, and does not require patients to transmit their ECG by telephone. Patients wear a small sensing device that transmits each heartbeat to a small monitor. When a dysrhythmia is detected, the system automatically transmits the patient's ECG to a monitoring center through either the patient's telephone line when at home or through wireless communications systems when outside of the home. This system enhances detection and early treatment of dysrhythmias that might otherwise be diagnosed only after the patient develops serious symptoms (Frantz, 2003; Tachakra, Wang, Istepanian, et al., 2003).

Cardiac Stress Testing

Normally, the coronary arteries dilate to four times their usual diameter in response to increased metabolic demands for oxygen and nutrients. However, coronary arteries affected by atherosclerosis dilate much less, compromising blood flow to the myocardium and causing ischemia. Therefore, abnormalities in cardiovascular function are more likely to be detected during times of increased demand, or "stress." The **cardiac stress test** procedures—the exercise stress test, the pharmacologic stress test, and more recently the mental or emotional stress test—are noninvasive ways to evaluate the response of the cardiovascular system to stress. The stress test helps determine the following: (1) presence of CAD, (2) cause of chest pain, (3) functional capacity of the heart after an MI or heart surgery, (4) effectiveness of antianginal or antiarrhythmic medications, (5) dysrhythmias that occur during physical exercise, and (6) specific goals for a physical fitness program. Contraindications to stress testing include severe aortic stenosis, acute myocarditis or pericarditis, severe hypertension, suspected left main CAD, HF, and unstable angina. Because complications associated with stress testing can be life-threatening (MI, cardiac arrest, HF, and severe dysrhythmias), testing facilities must have staff and equipment ready to provide treatment, including advanced cardiac life support.

Mental stress testing uses a mental arithmetic test or simulated public speech to determine whether an ischemic myocardial response occurs, similar to the response evoked by a conventional treadmill exercise test. Although its use for diagnostic purposes in patients with CAD is currently investigational, preliminary results indicate that the ischemic and hemodynamic measures obtained from mental stress testing may be useful in assessing the prognosis of patients with CHD who have had a positive exercise test (Kim, Bartholomew, Mastin, et al., 2003).

Stress testing is often combined with echocardiography or radionuclide imaging (discussed later). These techniques are performed during the resting state and immediately after stress.

Exercise Stress Testing

In an exercise stress test, the patient walks on a treadmill (most common) or pedals a stationary bicycle or arm crank. Exercise intensity progresses according to established protocols. The Bruce protocol, for example, is a common treadmill protocol in which the speed and grade of the treadmill are increased every 3 minutes. The goal of the test is to increase the heart rate to the "target heart rate." This is 80% to 90% of the maximum predicted heart rate and is based on the patient's age and gender. During the test, the following are monitored: two or more ECG leads for heart rate, rhythm, and ischemic changes; BP; skin temperature; physical appearance; perceived exertion; and symptoms, including chest pain, dyspnea, dizziness, leg cramping, and fatigue. The test is terminated when the target heart rate is achieved or when the patient experiences chest pain, extreme fatigue, a decrease in BP or pulse rate, serious dysrhythmias or ST-segment changes on the ECG, or other complications. When significant ECG abnormalities occur during the stress test (ST-segment depressions or elevations), the test result is reported as positive and further diagnostic testing such as coronary angiography is required.

NURSING INTERVENTIONS

In preparation for the exercise stress test, the patient is instructed to fast for 4 hours before the test and to avoid stimulants such as tobacco and caffeine. Medications may be taken with sips of water. The physician may instruct the patient not to take certain cardiac medications, such as beta-adrenergic blocking agents, before the test. Clothes and sneakers or rubber-soled shoes suitable for exercising are to be worn. Women are advised to wear a bra that provides adequate support. The nurse describes the equipment used and the sensations and experiences that the patient may have during the test. The nurse explains the monitoring equipment used, the need to have an IV line placed, and the symptoms to report. The type of exercise is reviewed, and the patient is asked to put forth his or her best exercise effort. If the test is to be performed with echocardiography or radionuclide imaging, this information is reviewed as well. After the test, the patient is monitored for 10 to 15 minutes. Once stable, the patient may resume his or her usual activities.

Pharmacologic Stress Testing

Patients who are physically disabled or deconditioned will not be able to achieve their target heart rate by exercising on a treadmill or bicycle. Two vasodilating agents, dipyridamole (Persantine) and adenosine (Adenocard), administered IV, are used to mimic the effects of exercise by maximally dilating the coronary arteries. The effects of dipyridamole last about 15 to 30 minutes. The side effects are related to its vasodilating action and include chest discomfort, dizziness, headache, flushing, and nausea. Adenosine has similar side effects, although patients report these symptoms as more severe. Adenosine has an extremely short half-life (less than 10 seconds), so any severe effects rapidly subside. Dipyridamole and adenosine are the agents of choice used in conjunction with radionuclide imaging techniques. Theophylline and other xanthines, such as caffeine, block the effects of dipyridamole and adenosine and must be avoided before either of these pharmacologic stress tests.

Dobutamine (Dobutrex) is another medication that may be used if the patient cannot exercise. Dobutamine, a synthetic sympathomimetic, increases heart rate, myocardial contractility, and BP, thereby increasing the metabolic demands of the heart. It is the agent of choice when echocardiography is used because of its effects on altering myocardial wall motion (due to enhanced contractility). Dobutamine is also used for patients who have bronchospasm or pulmonary disease and cannot tolerate having doses of theophylline withheld.

NURSING INTERVENTIONS

In preparation for the pharmacologic stress test, the patient is instructed not to eat or drink anything for at least 4 hours before the test. This includes chocolate, caffeine, caffeine-free coffee, tea, carbonated beverages, or medications that contain caffeine (eg, Anacin, Darvon). If caffeine is ingested before a dipyridamole or adenosine stress test, the test will have to be rescheduled. Patients taking aminophylline or theophylline are instructed to stop taking these medications for 24 to 48 hours before the test (if tolerated). Oral doses of dipyridamole are withheld as well. The patient is informed about the transient sensations that may occur during infusion of the vasodilating agent, such as flushing or nausea, which will disappear quickly. The patient is instructed to report any other symptoms occurring during the test to the cardiologist or nurse. An explanation of echocardiography or radionuclide imaging is also provided as necessary. The stress test may take about 1 hour, or up to 3 hours if imaging is performed.

Echocardiography

Traditional Echocardiography

Echocardiography is a noninvasive ultrasound test that is used to examine the size, shape, and motion of cardiac structures. It is particularly useful for diagnosing pericardial effusions, determining chamber size and the etiology of heart murmurs, evaluating the function of prosthetic heart valves, and evaluating ventricular wall motion. It involves transmission of high-frequency sound waves into the heart through the chest wall and recording of the return signals. The ultrasound is generated by a hand-held transducer applied to the front of the chest. The transducer picks up the echoes, converts them to electrical impulses, and transmits them to the echocardiography machine for display on an oscilloscope and recording on a videotape. An ECG is recorded simultaneously to assist with interpreting the echocardiogram.

M-mode (motion), the unidimensional mode that was first introduced, provides information about the cardiac structures and their motion. Two-dimensional or cross-sectional echocardiography, an enhancement of the technique, creates a sophisticated, spatially correct image of the heart. Other techniques, such as Doppler and color flow imaging echocardiography, show the direction and velocity of the blood flow through the heart.

Echocardiography may be performed with an exercise or pharmacologic stress test; resting and stress images are obtained. Myocardial ischemia from decreased perfusion during stress causes abnormalities in ventricular wall motion and is easily detected by echocardiography. A stress test using echocardiography is considered positive if abnormalities in ventricular wall motion are detected during stress but not during rest. These findings are highly suggestive of CAD and require further evaluation, such as a cardiac catheterization.

NURSING INTERVENTIONS

Before echocardiography, the nurse informs the patient about the test, explaining that it is painless. Echocardiographic monitoring is performed while a transducer that emits the sound waves is moved on the surface of the chest wall. Gel applied to the skin helps transmit the sound waves. Periodically, the patient will have to turn onto the left side or hold a breath. The test takes about 30 to 45 minutes. If the patient is to undergo an exercise or pharmacologic stress test with echocardiography, information on stress testing is also reviewed with the patient.

Transesophageal Echocardiography (TEE)

A significant limitation of traditional echocardiography has been the poor quality of the images produced. Ultrasound loses its clarity as it passes through tissue, lung, and bone. Another echocardiographic technique involves threading a small transducer through the mouth and into the esophagus. This technique, called transesophageal echocardiography (TEE), provides clearer images because ultrasound waves are passing through less tissue. Pharmacologic stress testing using dobutamine and TEE can also be performed. The high-quality imaging obtained during TEE makes this technique an important first-line diagnostic tool for evaluating patients with many types of CVD, including those with HF, valvular heart disease, and intracardiac thrombi. It is frequently used during cardiac surgery to continuously monitor the response of the heart to the surgical procedure (eg, valve replacement or coronary artery bypass). Complications are uncommon during TEE, but if they do occur they are serious. These complications are caused by sedation and impaired swallowing resulting from the topical anesthesia (respiratory depression and aspiration) and by insertion and manipulation of the transducer into the esophagus and stomach (vasovagal response or esophageal perforation). The patient must be assessed before TEE for a history of dysphagia or radiation therapy to the chest, which increases the risk of complications.

NURSING INTERVENTIONS

The following protocol is usually implemented to prepare for a TEE study:

- The patient must fast for 6 hours before the study.
- An IV line is started for administering a sedative and any pharmacologic stress testing medications.

- The patient is maintained on moderate sedation, defined as a state of depressed consciousness during which time the patient responds appropriately to commands and can maintain a patent airway (see Chapter 19).
- The patient's throat is anesthetized before the probe is inserted. The patient is then asked to swallow the probe until it is correctly positioned in the esophagus.
- BP, ECG, respiration, and oxygen saturation (SpO_2) are monitored throughout the study.
- During recovery from moderate sedation, frequent assessments of the parameters previously identified are made as well as the patient's level of consciousness. The patient must continue to fast until fully alert and the effects of the topical anesthetic are reversed, usually 2 hours after the procedure. The patient may have a sore throat for the next 24 hours. If the procedure is performed in an outpatient setting, someone must be available to transport the patient home from the test site.

Radionuclide Imaging

Radionuclide imaging studies involve the use of radioisotopes to evaluate coronary artery perfusion noninvasively, to detect myocardial ischemia and infarction, and to assess left ventricular function. **Radioisotopes** are atoms in an unstable form. Thallium 201 (Tl^{201}) and technetium 99m (Tc^{99m}) are two radioisotopes used in cardiac nuclear medicine studies. As they decay, they give off small amounts of energy in the form of gamma rays. When they are injected into the bloodstream, the energy emitted can be detected by a gamma scintillation camera positioned over the body. Planar imaging, used with thallium, provides a one-dimensional view of the heart from three locations. Single photon emission computed tomography (SPECT) provides three-dimensional images. With SPECT, the patient is positioned supine with arms raised above the head, while the camera moves around the patient's chest in a 180- to 360-degree arc to identify the areas of decreased myocardial perfusion more precisely.

Myocardial Perfusion Imaging

The radioisotope Tl^{201} is used to assess myocardial perfusion. It resembles potassium and readily crosses into the cells of healthy myocardium. It is taken up more slowly and in smaller amounts by myocardial cells that are ischemic from decreased blood flow. However, thallium does not cross into the necrotic tissue that results from an MI.

Often, thallium is used with stress testing to assess changes in myocardial perfusion immediately after exercise (or after injection of one of the pharmacologic agents used in stress testing) and at rest. One or two minutes before the end of the stress test, a dose of Tl^{201} is injected into the IV line, allowing the radioisotope to be distributed into the myocardium. Images are taken immediately. Areas that do not show thallium uptake indicate areas of either MI or stress-induced myocardial ischemia. Resting images, taken 3 hours later, help differentiate infarction from ischemia. Infarcted tissue cannot take up thallium regardless of when the scan is taken; the defect remains the same size during exercise or rest. This is called a fixed defect, indicating that there is no perfusion in that area of the myocardium. Ischemic myocardium, on the other hand, recovers in a few hours. If perfusion is restored, thallium crosses into the myocardial cells, and the area of defect on the resting images is either smaller or completely reversed. These reversible defects constitute positive stress test findings. Usually, cardiac catheterization is recommended after a positive test result to determine whether PCI or coronary artery bypass graft surgery is needed.

Another radioisotope used for cardiac imaging is Tc^{99m}. Technetium can be combined with various chemical compounds, giving it an affinity for different types of cells. For example, Tc^{99m} sestamibi (Cardiolite) is distributed to myocardial cells in proportion to its perfusion, making this an excellent tracer for assessing perfusion to the myocardium. The procedure for cardiac imaging using Tc^{99m} sestamibi with stress testing is similar to the one using thallium, with two differences. Patients receiving Tc^{99m} sestamibi can have their resting images recorded before or after the exercise images. Timing of the images is not important because the half-life of Tc^{99m} is short, and Tc^{99m} needs to be injected before each scan. Also, SPECT imaging with Tc^{99m} sestamibi provides high-quality images.

NURSING INTERVENTIONS

The patient undergoing nuclear imaging techniques with stress testing should be prepared for the type of stressor to be used (exercise or drug) and the type of imaging technique (planar or SPECT). The patient may be concerned about receiving a radioactive substance and needs to be reassured that these tracers are safe—the radiation exposure is similar to that of other diagnostic x-ray studies. No post-procedure radiation precautions are necessary.

When providing teaching for a patient undergoing SPECT, the nurse instructs the patient that the arms will need to be positioned over the head for about 20 to 30 minutes. If the patient is physically unable to do this, thallium with planar imaging can be used.

Test of Ventricular Function and Wall Motion

Equilibrium radionuclide angiocardiography (ERNA), also known as multiple-gated acquisition (MUGA) scanning, is a common noninvasive technique that uses a conventional scintillation camera interfaced with a computer to record images of the heart during several hundred heartbeats. The computer processes the data and allows for sequential viewing of the functioning heart. The sequential images are analyzed to evaluate left ventricular function, wall motion, and ejection fraction. MUGA scanning can also be used to assess the differences in left ventricular function during rest and exercise.

The patient is reassured that there is no known radiation danger and is instructed to remain motionless during the scan.

Computed Tomography

Computed tomography (CT), also called computerized axial tomographic (CAT) scanning or electron-beam computed tomography (EBCT), uses x-rays to provide cross-sectional images of the chest, including the heart and great vessels. These techniques are used to evaluate cardiac masses and diseases of the aorta and pericardium.

EBCT, also known as the ultrafast CT, is an especially fast x-ray scanning technique that results in much faster image acquisition with a higher degree of resolution than traditional x-ray or CT scanning provides. It is used to evaluate bypass graft patency, congenital heart lesions, left and right ventricular muscle mass, chamber volumes, cardiac output, and ejection fraction. For people without previous MI, PCI, or coronary artery bypass surgery, the EBCT is used to determine the amount of calcium deposits in the coronary arteries and underlying atherosclerosis. From this scan, a calcium score is derived that predicts the incidence of cardiac events, such as MI or the need for a revascularization procedure within the next 1 to 2 years.

The EBCT is not widely used, but it does show great promise in the early detection of CAD that is not yet clinically significant and that would not be identified by traditional testing methods such as the exercise stress test.

NURSING INTERVENTIONS

Patient preparation for these tests is the primary role of the nurse. The nurse explains to the patient that he or she will be positioned on a table during the scan while the scanner rotates around him or her. The procedure is noninvasive and painless. However, to obtain adequate images, the patient must lie perfectly still during the scanning process. An IV access line is necessary if contrast enhancement is to be used.

Positron Emission Tomography

Positron emission tomography (PET) is a noninvasive scanning method that has been used primarily to study neurologic dysfunction. More recently, and with increasing frequency, PET has been used to diagnose cardiac dysfunction. PET provides more specific information about myocardial perfusion and viability than does TEE or thallium scanning. For cardiac patients, including those without symptoms, PET helps in planning treatment (eg, coronary artery bypass surgery, PCIs). PET also helps evaluate the patency of native and previously grafted vessels and the collateral circulation.

During a PET scan, radioisotopes are administered by injection; one compound is used to determine blood flow in the myocardium, and another shows the metabolic function. The PET camera provides detailed three-dimensional images of the distributed compounds. The viability of the myocardium is determined by comparing the extent of glucose metabolism in the myocardium to the degree of blood flow. For example, ischemic but viable tissue would show decreased blood flow and elevated metabolism. For a patient with this finding, revascularization through surgery or angioplasty would probably be indicated to improve heart function. Restrictions of food intake before the test vary among institutions, but because PET evaluates glucose metabolism, the patient's blood glucose level should be in the normal range before testing. Although PET equipment is costly, it is increasingly available.

NURSING INTERVENTIONS

Nurses involved in PET and other scanning procedures may instruct the patient to refrain from using tobacco and ingesting caffeine for 4 hours before the procedure. They should also reassure the patient that radiation exposure is at safe and acceptable levels, similar to those of other diagnostic x-ray studies.

Magnetic Resonance Imaging

Magnetic resonance imaging (MRI) is a noninvasive, painless technique that is used to examine both the physiologic and anatomic properties of the heart. MRI uses a powerful magnetic field and computer-generated pictures to image the heart and great vessels. It is valuable in diagnosing diseases of the aorta, heart muscle, and pericardium, as well as congenital heart lesions. The application of this technique to the evaluation of coronary artery anatomy, cardiac blood flow, and myocardial viability in conjunction with pharmacologic stress testing is being investigated.

NURSING INTERVENTIONS

Because of the strong magnetic field used during MRI, diagnostic centers where these procedures are performed carefully screen patients for contraindications. Standardized questionnaires are commonly used to determine whether the patient has a pacemaker, metal plates, prosthetic joints, or other metallic implants that can become dislodged if exposed to MRI. The patient is instructed to remove any jewelry, watches, or other metal items. Transdermal patches that contain a heat-conducting aluminized layer (eg, NicoDerm, Androderm, Transderm Nitro, Transderm Scop, Catapres-TTS) must be removed before MRI to prevent burning of the skin. During an MRI, the patient is positioned supine on a table that is placed into an enclosed imager or tube containing the magnetic field. People who are claustrophobic may need to receive a mild sedative before undergoing an MRI. As the MRI is performed, there is an intermittent clanking or thumping sound from the magnetic coils that can be annoying to the patient, so patients may be offered headsets to listen to music. The scanner is equipped with a microphone so that the patient can communicate with the staff. The patient is instructed to remain motionless during the scan.

Cardiac Catheterization

Cardiac catheterization is an invasive diagnostic procedure in which radiopaque arterial and venous catheters are introduced into selected blood vessels of the right and left sides of the heart. Catheter advancement is guided by fluoroscopy. Most commonly, the catheters are inserted percutaneously through the blood vessels, or via a cutdown procedure if the patient has poor vascular access. Pressures and oxygen saturation levels in the four heart chambers are measured.

Cardiac catheterization is most frequently used to diagnose CAD, assess coronary artery patency, and determine the extent of atherosclerosis based on the percentage of coronary artery obstruction. These results determine whether revascularization procedures, including PCI or coronary artery bypass surgery, may be of benefit to the patient (see Chapter 28). Cardiac catheterization is also used to diagnose pulmonary arterial hypertension or to treat stenotic heart valves via percutaneous balloon valvuloplasty.

During cardiac catheterization, the patient has an IV line in place for the administration of sedatives, fluids, heparin, and other medications. Noninvasive hemodynamic monitoring that includes BP and multiple ECG tracings is necessary to continuously observe for dysrhythmias or hemodynamic instability. The myocardium can become ischemic and trigger dysrhythmias as catheters are positioned in the coronary arteries or during injection of contrast agents. Resuscitation equipment must be readily available during the procedure. Staff must be prepared to provide advanced cardiac life support measures as necessary.

Radiopaque contrast agents are used to visualize the coronary arteries. Some contrast agents contain iodine, and the patient is assessed before the procedure for previous reactions to contrast agents or allergies to iodine-containing substances (eg, seafood). If the patient has a suspected or known allergy to the substance, antihistamines or methylprednisolone (Solu-Medrol) may be administered before the procedure. In addition, the following blood tests are performed to identify abnormalities that may complicate recovery: blood urea nitrogen (BUN) and creatinine levels, **International Normalized Ratio (INR)** or prothrombin time (PT), activated thromboplastin time (aPTT), hematocrit and hemoglobin values, platelet count, and electrolyte levels.

Patients who have comorbid conditions—including diabetes, renal insufficiency, HF, preexisting renal failure, nephrotic syndrome, hypotension, or dehydration—who undergo cardiac catheterization are at risk for contrast-induced acute renal failure. Preventive strategies under investigation for these patients may include preprocedure administration of IV fluids and the antioxidant acetylcysteine (Mucomyst) (Ferrone, 2004).

Diagnostic cardiac catheterizations are commonly performed on an outpatient basis and require 2 to 6 hours of bed rest after the procedure before the patient ambulates. Variations in time to ambulation are related to the size of the catheter used during the procedure, the site of catheter insertion (femoral or radial artery), the anticoagulation status of the patient, and other patient variables (eg, advanced age, obesity, bleeding disorder). The use of smaller (4 or 6 French) catheters, which are associated with shorter recovery times, is common in diagnostic cardiac catheterizations. Several options to achieve arterial hemostasis after catheter removal, including manual pressure, mechanical compression devices such as the FemoStop (placed over puncture site for 30 minutes), and percutaneously deployed devices, are used. The latter devices are positioned at the femoral arterial puncture site after completion of the procedure. They deploy a saline-soaked gelatin sponge (QuickSeal), collagen (VasoSeal), sutures (Perclose, Techstar), or a combination of both collagen and sutures (Angio-Seal). Other newer products that expedite arterial hemostasis include external patches (Syvek Patch, Clo-Sur PAD). These products are placed over the puncture site as the catheter is removed and manual pressure is applied for 4 to 10 minutes. Once hemostasis is achieved, the patch is covered with a dressing that remains in place for 24 hours (Hirsch, Reddy, Capasso, et al., 2003).

Major benefits of the vascular closure devices include reliable, immediate hemostasis and a shorter time on bed rest without a significant increase in bleeding or other complications (Hoffer & Block, 2003). A number of factors determine which closure devices are used, such as the physician's preference, the patient's condition, cost, and institutional availability of these devices.

Patients hospitalized for angina or acute MI who require cardiac catheterization usually return to their hospital rooms for recovery. In some cardiac catheterization laboratories, an angioplasty (discussed in Chapter 28) may be performed immediately during the catheterization if indicated.

Angiography

Cardiac catheterization is usually performed with angiography, a technique in which a contrast agent is injected into the vascular system to outline the heart and blood vessels. When a specific heart chamber or blood vessel is singled out for study, the procedure is known as selective angiography. Angiography makes use of cineangiograms, a series of rapidly changing films on an intensified fluoroscopic screen that record the passage of the contrast agent through the vascular site or sites. The recorded information allows for comparison of data over time.

Common Sites

Common sites for selective angiography are the aorta, the coronary arteries, and the right and left sides of the heart.

AORTOGRAPHY

An aortogram is a form of angiography that outlines the lumen of the aorta and the major arteries arising from it. In thoracic aortography, a contrast agent is used to study the aortic arch and its major branches. The catheter may be introduced into the aorta using the translumbar or retrograde brachial or femoral artery approach.

CORONARY ARTERIOGRAPHY

In coronary arteriography, the catheter is introduced into the right or left brachial or femoral artery, then passed into the ascending aorta and manipulated into the right and left coronary arteries. Coronary arteriography is used to evaluate the degree of atherosclerosis and to determine treatment. It is also used to study suspected congenital anomalies of the coronary arteries.

RIGHT HEART CATHETERIZATION

Right heart catheterization usually precedes left heart catheterization. It involves the passage of a catheter from an antecubital or femoral vein into the right atrium, right ventricle, pulmonary artery, and pulmonary arterioles. Pressures and oxygen saturation levels from each of these areas are obtained and recorded.

Although right heart catheterization is considered relatively safe, potential complications include cardiac dysrhythmias, venous spasm, infection of the insertion site, cardiac perforation, and, rarely, cardiac arrest.

LEFT HEART CATHETERIZATION

Left heart catheterization is performed to evaluate the patency of the coronary arteries and the function of the left ventricle and the mitral and aortic valves. Potential complications include dysrhythmias, MI, perforation of the heart or great vessels, and systemic embolization. Left heart catheterization is performed by retrograde catheterization of the left ventricle. In this approach, the physician usually inserts the catheter into the right brachial artery or a femoral artery and advances it into the aorta and left ventricle.

After the procedure, the catheter is carefully withdrawn and arterial hemostasis is achieved using manual pressure or other techniques previously described. If the physician performed an arterial or venous cutdown, the site is sutured and a sterile dressing is applied.

Nursing Interventions

Nursing responsibilities before cardiac catheterization include the following:

- The patient is instructed to fast, usually for 8 to 12 hours, before the procedure. If catheterization is to be performed as an outpatient procedure, a friend, family member, or other responsible person must transport the patient home.
- The patient is informed of the expected duration of the procedure and advised that it will involve lying on a hard table for less than 2 hours.
- The patient is reassured that mild sedatives or moderate sedation will be given IV.
- The patient is informed about certain sensations that will be experienced during the catheterization. Knowing what to expect can help the patient cope with the experience. The nurse explains that an occasional pounding sensation (palpitation) may be felt in the chest because of extrasystoles that almost always occur, particularly when the catheter tip touches the myocardium. The patient may be asked to cough and to breathe deeply, especially after the injection of contrast agent. Coughing may help disrupt a dysrhythmia and clear the contrast agent from the arteries. Breathing deeply and holding the breath help lower the diaphragm for better visualization of heart structures. The injection of a contrast agent into either side of the heart may produce a flushed feeling throughout the body and a sensation similar to the need to void, which subsides in 1 minute or less.
- The patient is encouraged to express fears and anxieties. The nurse provides teaching and reassurance to reduce apprehension.

Nursing responsibilities after cardiac catheterization may include the following:

- The catheter access site is observed for bleeding or hematoma formation. Peripheral pulses in the affected extremity (dorsalis pedis and posterior tibial pulses in the lower extremity, radial pulse in the upper extremity) are assessed every 15 minutes for 1 hour, and then every 1 to 2 hours until the pulses are stable.
- Temperature and color of the affected extremity are evaluated, as well as any patient complaints of pain, numbness, or tingling sensations, to detect arterial insufficiency. Any changes are reported promptly.
- Dysrhythmias are carefully assessed by observing the cardiac monitor or by assessing the apical and peripheral pulses for changes in rate and rhythm. A vasovagal reaction, consisting of bradycardia, hypotension, and nausea, can be precipitated by a distended bladder or by discomfort during removal of the arterial catheter, especially if a femoral site has been used. Prompt intervention is critical; this includes raising the feet and legs above the head, administering IV fluids, and administering IV atropine.
- Bed rest must be maintained for 2 to 6 hours after the procedure. If manual or mechanical pressure is used without vascular closure devices, the patient must remain on bed rest for up to 6 hours with the affected leg straight and the head elevated to 30 degrees. For comfort, the patient may be turned from side to side with the affected extremity straight. If the cardiologist used deployed closure devices or patches, the nurse checks local nursing care standards and anticipates that the patient will have fewer activity restrictions, such as elevation of the head of the bed, and that the patient will be allowed to ambulate in 2 hours or less. Analgesic medication is administered as prescribed for discomfort.
- The patient is instructed to report chest pain and bleeding or sudden discomfort from the catheter insertion sites immediately.
- The patient is monitored for contrast agent–induced renal failure that may be suspected if there is an increase in the BUN and creatinine levels. An accurate record of intake and output must be maintained, and both oral and IV fluids are encouraged to increase urinary output and flush the agent from the urinary tract.
- Safety is ensured by instructing the patient to ask for help when getting out of bed the first time after the procedure, because orthostatic hypotension may occur and the patient may feel dizzy and lightheaded.

For patients being discharged from the hospital on the same day as the procedure, additional instructions are provided (Chart 26-4).

CHART 26-4

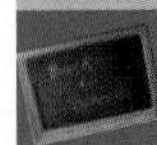

Patient Education

Self-Management After Cardiac Catheterization

After discharge from the hospital for cardiac catheterization, guidelines for self-care include the following:

- For the next 24 hours, do not bend at the waist (to lift anything), strain, or lift heavy objects.
- Avoid tub baths, but shower as desired.
- Talk with your physician about when you may return to work, drive, or resume strenuous activities.
- Call your physician if any of the following occur: bleeding, swelling, new bruising or pain from your procedure puncture site, temperature of 101.5°F (38.6°C) or more.
- If test results show that you have coronary artery disease, talk with your physician about options for treatment, including cardiac rehabilitation programs in your community.
- Talk with your physician and nurse about lifestyle changes to reduce your risk for further or future heart problems, such as quitting smoking, lowering your cholesterol level, initiating dietary changes, beginning an exercise program, or losing weight.

Electrophysiologic Testing

The electrophysiology study (EPS) is an invasive procedure that plays a major role in the diagnosis and management of serious dysrhythmias. EPS is indicated for patients with syncope, palpitations, or both, and for survivors of cardiac arrest from ventricular fibrillation (sudden cardiac death). EPS is used to:

- Distinguish atrial from ventricular tachycardias when the determination cannot be made from the 12-lead ECG
- Evaluate how readily a life-threatening dysrhythmia (eg, ventricular tachycardia, ventricular fibrillation) can be induced
- Evaluate AV node function
- Evaluate the effectiveness of antiarrhythmic medications in suppressing the dysrhythmia
- Determine the need for other therapeutic interventions, such as a pacemaker, implantable cardioverter–defibrillator, or radiofrequency ablation (discussed in Chapter 27)

The initial study can take up to 4 hours. The patient receives moderate sedation. Catheters with recording and electrical stimulating (pacing) capabilities are inserted into the heart through the femoral and right subclavian veins to record electrical activity in the right and left atrium, bundle of His, and right ventricle. Fluoroscopy guides the positioning of these catheters. Baseline intracardiac recordings are obtained; programmed electrical stimulations of the atrium or ventricle are then administered in an attempt to induce the patient's dysrhythmia. If the dysrhythmia is induced, various antiarrhythmic medications are administered IV. The study is repeated after each medication to evaluate which medication or combination of medications is most effective in controlling the dysrhythmia.

After the study, the patient receives an equivalent oral antiarrhythmic agent; subsequent studies may be necessary to evaluate the effectiveness of that medication. Results of the study may indicate the need for other therapeutic interventions, such as a pacemaker or implantable cardioverter–defibrillator.

During EPS, lethal dysrhythmias may be induced; therefore, the procedure must be performed in a controlled environment with resuscitation equipment (eg, defibrillator) readily available. Possible complications include bleeding and hematoma from the catheter insertion sites, pneumothorax (air in the pleural cavity that may collapse portions of the lung), deep vein thrombosis, stroke, and sudden death.

Nursing Interventions

Patients receive nothing to eat or drink for 8 hours before the procedure. Antiarrhythmic medications are withheld for at least 24 hours before the initial study, and the patient's cardiac rate and rhythm are carefully monitored for dysrhythmias. Other medications may be taken with sips of water.

Thorough preparation before EPS helps minimize patient anxiety. The nurse ensures that the patient understands the reason for the study and is aware of the common sensations and experiences expected during and after the study. Often the EPS laboratory has relaxation strategies available for patients, such as headsets with music. Also, the patient needs to be aware that the nurses in the EPS laboratory will be monitoring carefully for signs of discomfort and will offer IV medications to reduce discomfort or anxiety. The patient is reminded to request these medications if necessary. Postprocedure interventions include careful monitoring for complications. The nurse takes vital signs, reviews tracings of continuous ECG monitoring, assesses the apical pulse, auscultates for pericardial friction rub (which indicates bleeding into the pericardial sac), and inspects the catheter insertion sites for bleeding or hematoma formation.

In addition, the nurse assists the patient to maintain bed rest with the affected extremity kept straight and the head of the bed elevated to 30 degrees for 4 to 6 hours. The frequency of assessments and the duration of bed rest may vary based on institutional policy and physician preference.

Hemodynamic Monitoring

Critically ill patients require continuous assessment of their cardiovascular system to diagnose and manage their complex medical conditions. This is most commonly achieved by the use of direct pressure monitoring systems, often referred to as **hemodynamic monitoring.** CVP, pulmonary artery pressure, and intra-arterial BP monitoring are common forms of hemodynamic monitoring. Patients requiring hemodynamic monitoring are typically cared for in critical care units. Some progressive care units also admit stable patients with CVP or intra-arterial BP monitoring. Noninvasive hemodynamic monitoring is used in some facilities.

To perform invasive hemodynamic monitoring, specialized equipment is necessary, such as the following:

- A CVP, pulmonary artery, or arterial catheter, which is introduced into the appropriate blood vessel or heart chamber
- A flush system composed of IV solution (which may include heparin), tubing, stopcocks, and a flush device, which provides for continuous and manual flushing of the system
- A pressure bag placed around the flush solution that is maintained at 300 mm Hg of pressure; the pressurized flush system delivers 3 to 5 mL of solution per hour through the catheter to prevent clotting and backflow of blood into the pressure monitoring system
- A transducer to convert the pressure coming from the artery or heart chamber into an electrical signal
- An amplifier or monitor, which increases the size of the electrical signal for display on an oscilloscope

Only nurses who have demonstrated knowledge and skill in the use of hemodynamic monitoring should manage patients who require this highly sophisticated type of monitoring. To ensure accuracy of the measurements, an evidence-based approach is necessary. The most important nursing responsibilities when caring for a patient who is undergoing hemodynamic monitoring are the following:

- The nurse makes sure that the system is set up and maintained properly. For example, the connecting tubing used for the monitoring system, called pressure tubing, is specifically manufactured for this purpose. The pressure tubing typically used for adults has a large diameter (7 French) and is no more than 3 to 4 feet long. The pressure monitoring system must be kept patent and free of air bubbles.

- Before the pressure monitoring system is used, the nurse checks to make sure that the stopcock of the transducer is positioned at the level of the right atrium; this is referred to as the phlebostatic level. Figure 26-10 shows how to locate this landmark. The nurse uses a marker to identify this level on the chest wall, which provides a stable reference point for subsequent pressure readings.
- To ensure that the pressure system is properly functioning at atmospheric pressure, the nurse establishes the zero reference point. This process is accomplished by placing the stopcock of the transducer at the phlebostatic level, opening the transducer to air, and activating the zero function key on the bedside monitor. Measurements of CVP, BP, and pulmonary artery pressures can be made with the head of the patient's bed elevated up to 60 degrees, but the system must be repositioned to the phlebostatic level to ensure an accurate reading.

Central Venous Pressure Monitoring

The CVP, the pressure in the vena cava or right atrium, is used to assess right ventricular function and venous blood return to the right side of the heart. The CVP can be continuously measured by connecting either a catheter positioned in the vena cava or the proximal port of a pulmonary artery catheter to a pressure monitoring system. The pulmonary artery catheter, described in greater detail later, is used for monitoring critically ill patients. Patients in general medical-surgical units who require CVP monitoring may have a single-lumen or multilumen catheter placed into the superior vena cava. Intermittent measurement of the CVP can then be obtained with the use of a water manometer.

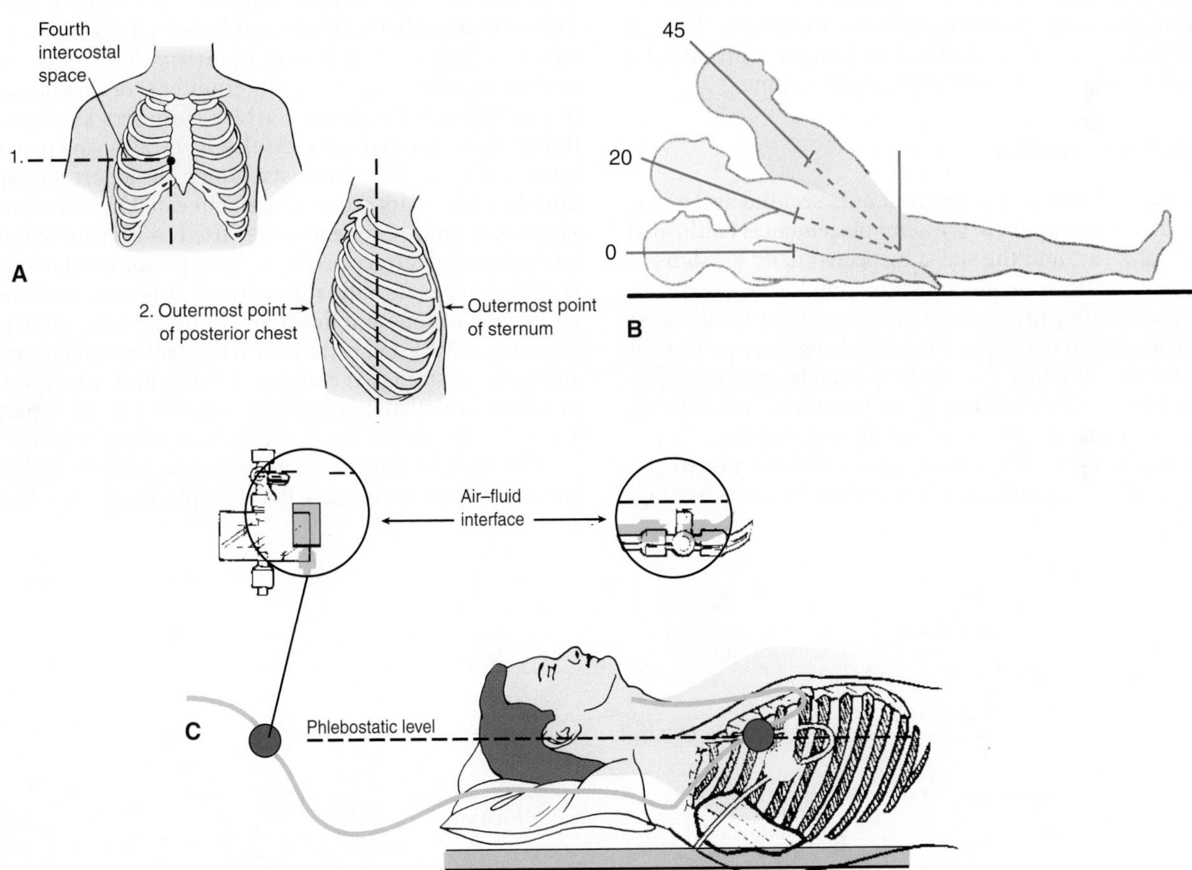

FIGURE 26-10. The phlebostatic axis and the phlebostatic level. (**A**) The phlebostatic axis is the crossing of two reference lines: (1) a line from the fourth intercostal space at the point where it joins the sternum, drawn out to the side of the body beneath the axilla; and (2) a line midway between the anterior and posterior surfaces of the chest. (**B**) The phlebostatic level is a horizontal line through the phlebostatic axis. The air–fluid interface of the stopcock of the transducer, or the zero mark on the manometer, must be level with this axis for accurate measurements. When moving from the flat to erect positions, the patient moves the chest and therefore the reference level; the phlebostatic level stays horizontal through the same reference point. (**C**) Two methods for referencing the pressure system to the phlebostatic axis. The system can be referenced by placing the air–fluid interface of either the in-line stopcock or the stopcock on top of the transducer at the phlebostatic level.

Because the pressures in the right atrium and right ventricle are equal at the end of diastole (0 to 8 mm Hg), the CVP is also an indirect method of determining right ventricular filling pressure (preload). This makes the CVP a useful hemodynamic parameter to observe when managing an unstable patient's fluid volume status. CVP monitoring is most valuable when pressures are monitored over time and are correlated with the patient's clinical status. An increasing pressure may be caused by hypervolemia or by a condition such as HF that results in a decrease in myocardial contractility. Pulmonary artery monitoring is preferred for the patient with HF. Decreased CVP indicates reduced right ventricular preload, most often caused by hypovolemia. This diagnosis can be substantiated when a rapid IV infusion causes the CVP to increase. (CVP monitoring is not clinically useful in a patient with HF in whom left ventricular failure precedes right ventricular failure, because in these patients an elevated CVP is a very late sign of HF.)

Before insertion of a CVP catheter, the site is prepared by shaving excessive hair, if necessary, and by cleansing with an antiseptic solution. A local anesthetic is used. The physician threads a single-lumen or multilumen catheter through the external jugular, antecubital, or femoral vein into the vena cava just above or within the right atrium.

Nursing Interventions

Once the CVP catheter is inserted, it is secured and a dry, sterile dressing is applied. Catheter placement is confirmed by a chest x-ray, and the site is inspected daily for signs of infection. The dressing and pressure monitoring system are changed according to hospital policy. In general, the dressing is kept dry and air occlusive. Dressing changes are performed using sterile technique. CVP catheters can be used for infusing IV fluids, administering IV medications, and drawing blood specimens in addition to monitoring pressure.

To measure the CVP, the transducer must be placed at a standard reference point, called the phlebostatic axis (see Fig. 26-10). When the phlebostatic axis is used, then the CVP can be measured correctly with the patient supine at any backrest position up to 45 degrees. The range for a normal CVP is 0 to 8 mm Hg. The most common complications of CVP monitoring are infection, pneumothorax, and air embolism.

Pulmonary Artery Pressure Monitoring

Pulmonary artery pressure monitoring is an important tool used in critical care for assessing left ventricular function (cardiac output), diagnosing the etiology of shock, and evaluating the patient's response to medical interventions (eg, fluid administration, vasoactive medications). Pulmonary artery pressure monitoring involves the use of a pulmonary artery catheter and pressure monitoring system. The pressure monitoring system acts as a fluid-filled conduit for detecting pressure changes within the chambers of the heart and the pulmonary arteries.

Pulmonary catheters are available in a variety of models. The type of catheter is selected based on its capabilities, which include cardiac pacing, oximetry, or cardiac output measurement (continuous or intermittent) or a combination of capabilities. Pulmonary artery catheters are balloon-tipped, flow-directed catheters that have distal and proximal lumens (Fig. 26-11). The distal lumen has a port that opens into the pulmonary artery. Once connected by its hub to the pressure monitoring system, it is used to measure continuous pulmonary artery pressures. The proximal lumen has a port that opens into the right atrium. It is used to administer IV medications and fluids or to monitor right atrial pressures (eg, CVP). Each catheter has a balloon inflation hub and valve. A syringe is connected to the hub, which is used to inflate or deflate the balloon with air (1.5-mL capacity). The valve opens and closes the balloon inflation lumen.

A pulmonary artery catheter with specialized capabilities has additional components. For example, the thermodilution

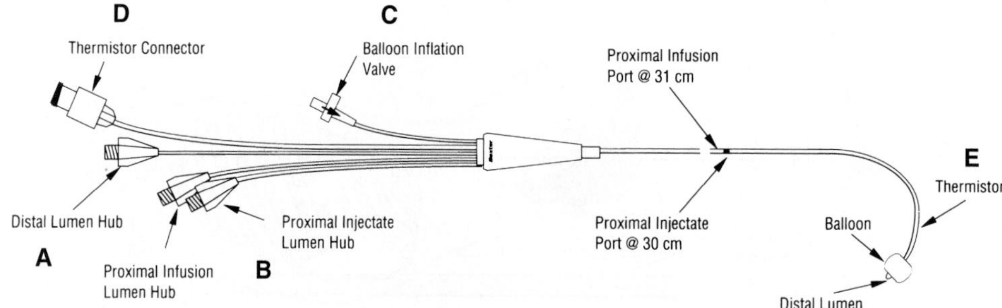

FIGURE 26-11. The pulmonary artery monitoring catheter used for obtaining pressure measurements and cardiac output. (**A**) The pressure monitoring system is connected to the distal lumen hub. (**B**) IV solutions are infused through the proximal infusion and injectate lumen hubs. (**C**) An air-filled syringe connected to the balloon inflation valve is used for balloon inflation during catheter insertion and pulmonary artery wedge pressure measurements. (**D**) To obtain cardiac output, the thermistor connector is inserted into the cardiac output component of the bedside cardiac monitor and 5 to 10 mL of normal saline is injected in 4 seconds into the proximal injectate port. (**E**) The thermistor located near the balloon is used to calculate the cardiac output. (Courtesy of Baxter Healthcare Corporation, Edwards Critical Care Division, Santa Ana, CA; used in Woods, S. L., Froelicher, E. S., & Motzer, S. A. [2004]. *Cardiac nursing* [5th ed.]. Philadelphia: Lippincott Williams & Wilkins.)

catheter has three additional features that enable it to measure cardiac output: a thermistor connector attached to the cardiac output computer of the bedside monitor, a proximal injectate port used for injecting fluids when obtaining the cardiac output, and a thermistor (positioned near the distal port) (see Fig. 26-11).

The pulmonary artery catheter, covered with a sterile sleeve, is inserted into a large vein (subclavian, jugular, or femoral) through a sheath. The sheath is equipped with a side port for infusing IV fluids and medications. The catheter is then passed into the vena cava and right atrium. In the right atrium, the balloon tip is inflated, and the catheter is carried rapidly by the flow of blood through the tricuspid valve into the right ventricle, through the pulmonic valve, and into a branch of the pulmonary artery. When the catheter reaches the pulmonary artery, the balloon is deflated and the catheter is secured with sutures (Fig. 26-12). Fluoroscopy may be used during insertion to visualize the progression of the catheter through the heart chambers to the pulmonary artery. This procedure can be performed in the operating room or cardiac catheterization laboratory or at the bedside in the critical care unit. During insertion of the pulmonary artery catheter, the bedside monitor is observed for waveform and ECG changes as the catheter progresses

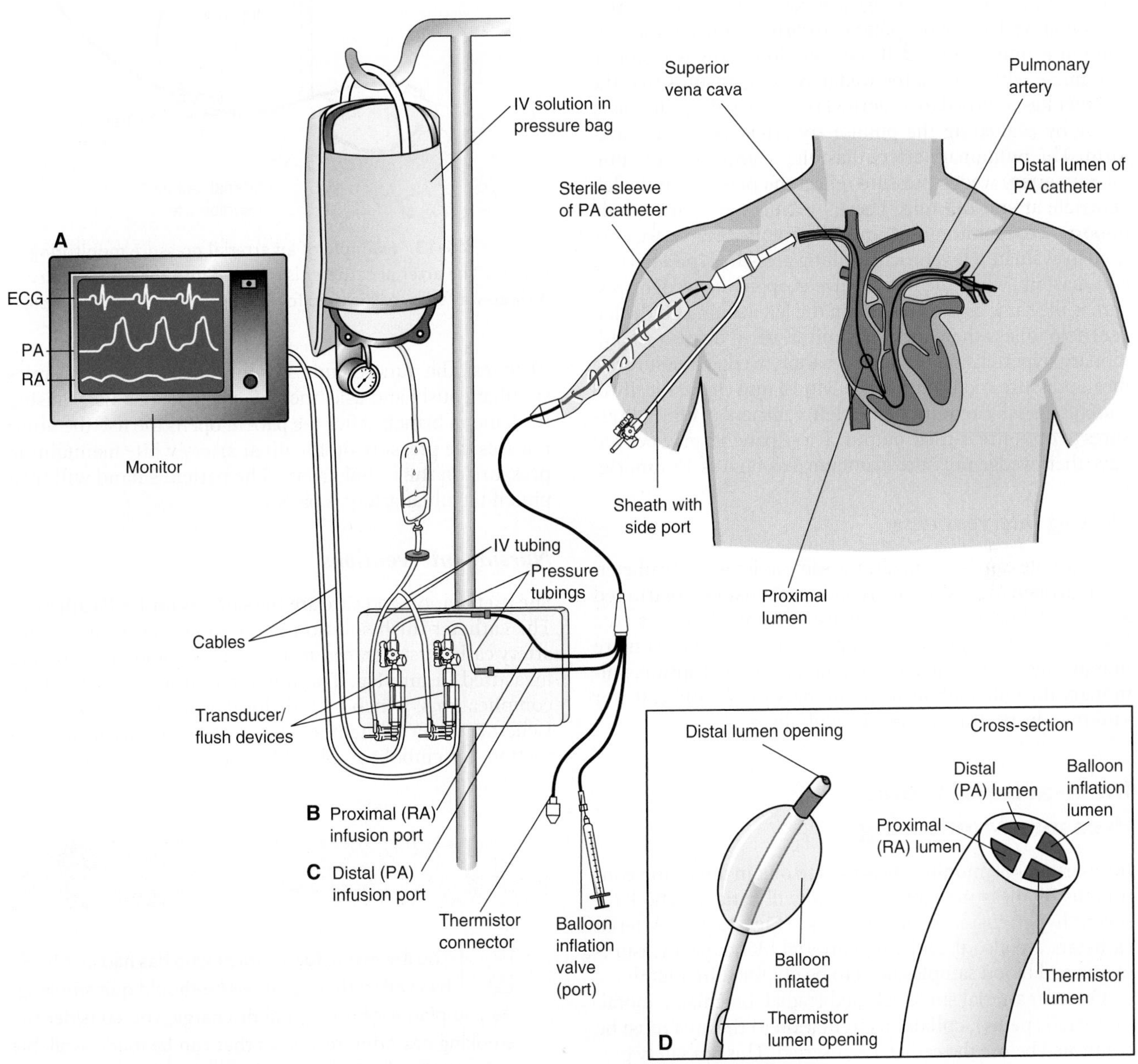

FIGURE 26-12. Pulmonary artery (PA) catheter and pressure monitoring systems. (**A**) Bedside cardiac monitoring. (**B**) Right atria (RA) or central venous pressure monitoring system connected to proximal infusion lumen hub. (**C**) PA monitoring system connected to distal infusion lumen hub. Each system is attached to pressurized IV fluid, a transducer with stopcock and flush device, and pressure tubing. A cable attaches each transducer to the bedside monitor. (**D**) Magnified view of distal end of PA catheter with cross-section of catheter lumen.

through the right-sided heart chambers and into the pulmonary artery.

After the catheter is correctly positioned, the following pressures can be measured: right atrial, pulmonary artery systolic, pulmonary artery diastolic, mean pulmonary artery, and pulmonary artery wedge. Systemic vascular resistance and pulmonary vascular resistance are examples of additional measures that can be calculated.

Normal pulmonary artery pressure is 25/9 mm Hg, with a mean pressure of 15 mm Hg (see Fig. 26-4 for normal ranges). When the balloon tip is inflated, the catheter floats into the pulmonary artery until it becomes wedged. This is an occlusive maneuver that impedes blood flow through that segment of the pulmonary artery. A pressure measurement, called pulmonary artery wedge pressure, is taken within seconds after wedging of the pulmonary artery catheter; then the balloon is immediately deflated and blood flow is restored. The nurse who obtains the wedge reading ensures that the catheter has returned to its normal position in the pulmonary artery by evaluating the pulmonary artery pressure waveform. The pulmonary artery diastolic reading and the pulmonary artery wedge pressure reflect the pressure in the left ventricle at end-diastole. These measures are particularly important to monitor in critically ill patients because they are used to evaluate left ventricular filling pressures (preload). At end-diastole, when the mitral valve is open, the wedge pressure is the same as the pressure in the left atrium and the left ventricle unless the patient has mitral valve disease or pulmonary hypertension. Pulmonary artery wedge pressure is a mean pressure and is normally 4.5 to 13 mm Hg. Critically ill patients usually require higher left ventricular filling pressures to optimize cardiac output. These patients may need to have their wedge pressure maintained as high as 18 mm Hg.

Nursing Interventions

Catheter site care is essentially the same as for a CVP catheter. As in measuring CVP, the transducer must be positioned at the phlebostatic axis to ensure accurate readings (see Fig. 26-10). Complications of pulmonary artery pressure monitoring include infection, pulmonary artery rupture, pulmonary thromboembolism, pulmonary infarction, catheter kinking, dysrhythmias, and air embolism.

Intra-arterial Blood Pressure Monitoring

Intra-arterial BP monitoring is used to obtain direct and continuous BP measurements in critically ill patients who have severe hypertension or hypotension (Fig. 26-13). Arterial catheters are also useful when arterial blood gas measurements and blood samples need to be obtained frequently.

Once an arterial site is selected (radial, brachial, femoral, or dorsalis pedis), collateral circulation to the area must be confirmed before the catheter is inserted. This is a safety precaution to prevent compromised arterial perfusion to the area distal to the arterial catheter insertion site. If no collateral circulation existed and the cannulated artery became occluded, ischemia and infarction of the area distal to that artery could occur. Collateral circulation to the hand can be checked by the Allen test to evaluate the radial and ulnar arteries or by an ultrasonic Doppler test for any of the arteries. To perform the Allen test, the nurse compresses the radial and ulnar arteries simultaneously and asks the patient to make a fist, causing the hand to blanch. After the patient opens the fist, the nurse releases the pressure on the ulnar artery while maintaining pressure on the radial artery. The patient's hand will turn pink if the ulnar artery is patent.

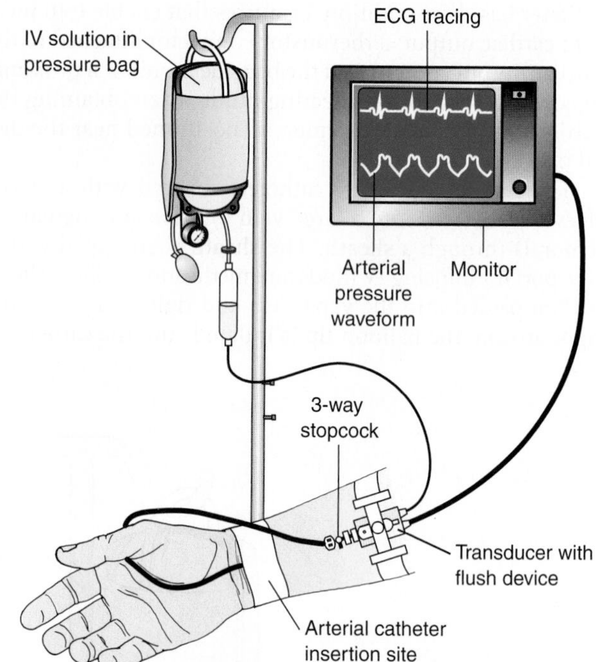

FIGURE 26-13. Example of an arterial pressure monitoring system. The arterial catheter is inserted into the radial artery. A three-way stopcock is used for drawing arterial blood samples.

Nursing Interventions

Site preparation and care are the same as for CVP catheters. The catheter flush solution is the same as for pulmonary artery catheters. A transducer is attached, and pressures are measured in mm Hg. The nurse monitors the patient for complications, which include local obstruction with distal ischemia, external hemorrhage, massive ecchymosis, dissection, air embolism, blood loss, pain, arteriospasm, and infection.

Critical Thinking Exercises

1 ebp You are caring for a patient who has had an MI. He has stated that he knows he should quit smoking. As you plan for his hospital discharge, you consider the smoking cessation resources that can be made available to him. What is the evidence base regarding smoking cessation strategies in discharge planning? Discuss the strength of the evidence and the effectiveness of smoking cessation strategies and techniques.

2 The president of a community organization you belong to has asked for your help in organizing a health fair for its

members. You are informed that the fair will focus on cardiovascular health. It will take place on a Saturday morning and approximately 200 people will attend. What cardiac risk factors will you screen for? Where will you obtain educational materials needed for distribution at the health fair? What supplies and equipment will you need? How many volunteers will you need to run the health fair? What advice will you give to people who are found to be at risk for heart disease?

3 To reduce the morbidity and mortality associated with acute MI, patients who experience symptoms of ACS must receive life-saving care as quickly as possible. Chest pain is a common symptom of ACS, but what are some of the other associated symptoms? If chest pain is the primary symptom, what key questions should you ask patients to help determine if the chest pain is cardiac in origin? What physical assessment parameters and tests are needed to reach a rapid and accurate diagnosis? During a home visit, if you suspect that your patient has ACS, what should you do?

REFERENCES AND SELECTED READINGS

BOOKS

American Heart Association. (2006). *Heart disease and stroke statistics—2006 update*. Accessed May 31, 2006. http://www.americanheart.org.

Bickley, L. S., & Szilagyi, P. G. (2005). *Bates' guide to physical examination* (9th ed.). Philadelphia: Lippincott Williams & Wilkins.

Chernecky, C. C., & Berger, B. J. (2004). *Laboratory tests and diagnostic procedures* (4th ed.). Philadelphia: W. B. Saunders.

Darovic, G. O. (2004). *Handbook of hemodynamic monitoring* (2nd ed.). Philadelphia: W. B. Saunders.

Kern, M. J. (2004). *The interventional cardiac catheterization handbook* (2nd ed.). St. Louis: C. V. Mosby.

Topol, E. J., Califf, R. M., Isner, J., et al. (2002). *The textbook of cardiovascular medicine* (2nd ed.). Philadelphia: Lippincott Williams & Wilkins.

Weber, J., & Kelley, J. (2003). *Health assessment in nursing* (2nd ed.). Philadelphia: Lippincott Williams & Wilkins.

Woods, S. L., Froelicher, E. S., Motzer, S. A., et al. (2004). *Cardiac nursing* (5th ed.). Philadelphia: Lippincott Williams & Wilkins.

JOURNALS

**Asterisks indicate nursing research articles.*

Anderson, J. E., Jorenby, D. E., Scott, W. J., et al. (2002). Treating tobacco use and dependence: An evidence-based clinical practice guideline for tobacco cessation. *Chest, 121*(3), 932–941.

Drew, B. J., Califf, R. M., Funk, M., et al. (2005). AHA scientific statement: Practice standards for electrocardiographic monitoring in hospital settings: An American Heart Association Scientific Statement from the Councils on Cardiovascular Nursing, Clinical Cardiology, and Cardiovascular Disease in the Young: Endorsed by the International Society of Computerized Electrocardiology and the American Association of Critical-Care Nurses. *Journal of Cardiovascular Nursing, 20*(2), 76–106.

Ferrone, M. (2004). Pharmocotherapeutic options to prevent radiocontrast-induced acute renal failure. *Formulary, 39*(11), 163–185.

Frantz, A. K. (2003). Current issues related to home monitoring. *AACN Clinical Issues, 14*(2), 232–239.

*Funk, M., Chrostowski, V. M., Richards, S., et al. (2005). Feasibility of using ambulatory electrocardiographic monitors following discharge after cardiac surgery. *Home Healthcare Nurse, 23*(7), 441–451.

Glassman, A., Shapiro, P. A., Ford, D. E., et al. (2003). Cardiovascular health and depression. *Journal of Psychiatric Practice, 9*(4), 409–421.

Gordon, C., & Rempher, K. J. (2003). Brain (B-type) natriuretic peptide. Implications for heart failure management. *AACN Clinical Issues, 14*(4), 532–542.

Grundy, S., Howard, B., Smith, S., et al. (2002). Prevention Conference VI: Diabetes and cardiovascular disease executive summary: Conference proceeding for healthcare professionals from a special writing group of the American Heart Association. *Circulation, 105*(18), 2231–2239.

Hirsch, J. A., Reddy, S. A., Capasso, W. E., et al. (2003). Non-invasive hemostatic closure devices: "Patches and pads." *Techniques in Vascular & Interventional Radiology, 6*(2), 92–95.

Hoffer, E. K., & Block, R. D. (2003). Percutaneous arterial closure devices. *Journal of Vascular Interventional Radiology, 14*(7), 865–885.

*Kim, C. K., Bartholomew, B. A., Mastin, S. M., et al. (2003). Detection and reproducibility of mental stress–induced myocardial ischemia with Tc-99m sestamibi SPECT in normal and coronary artery disease populations. *Journal of Nuclear Cardiology, 10*(1), 56–62.

Koenig, W. (2005). Predicting risk and treatment benefit in atherosclerosis: The role of C-reactive protein. *International Journal of Cardiology, 98*(2), 199–206.

Leon, A. S., Franklin, B. A., Costa, F., et al. (2005). Cardiac rehabilitation and secondary prevention of coronary heart disease: An American Heart Association scientific statement from the Council on Clinical Cardiology (Subcommittee on Exercise, Cardiac Rehabilitation, and Prevention) and the Council on Nutrition, Physical Activity, and Metabolism (Subcommittee on Physical Activity), in collaboration with the American Association of Cardiovascular and Pulmonary Rehabilitation. *Circulation, 111*(3), 369–376.

*McSweeney, J. C., Cody, M., O'Sullivan, P., et al. (2003). Women's early warning symptoms of acute myocardial infarction. *Circulation, 108*(21), 2619–2623.

Mosca, L., Appel, L. J., Benjamin, E. J., et al. (2004). Evidence-based guidelines for cardiovascular disease prevention in women. *Journal of the American College of Cardiology, 43*(5), 900–921.

Pearson, T. A., Blair, S. W., Daniel, S. R., et al. (2002). AHA guidelines for primary prevention of cardiovascular disease and stroke: 2002 update. Consensus panel guide to comprehensive risk reduction for adult patients without coronary or other atherosclerotic vascular diseases. *Circulation, 106*(3), 388–391.

Ryan, C. J., DeVon, H. A., & Zerwic, J. J. (2005). Typical and atypical symptoms: Diagnosing acute coronary syndromes accurately. *American Journal of Nursing, 105*(2), 34–36.

Smith, S. C., Allen, G., Blair, S. N., et al. (2006). AHA/ACC guidelines for secondary prevention for patients with coronary and other atherosclerotic vascular disease. *Journal of the American College of Cardiology, 47*(10), 2130–2139.

*Steinke, E. E., & Swan, J. H. (2004). Effectiveness of a videotape for sexual counseling after myocardial infarction. *Research in Nursing & Health, 27*(4), 69–80.

Tachakra, S., Wang, X. H., Istepanian, R. S., et al. (2003). Mobile e-health: The unwired evolution of telemedicine. *Telemedicine Journal & E-Health, 9*(3), 247–257.

Zerwic, J. J., & Ryan, C. J. (2004). Delays in seeking MI treatment. *American Journal of Nursing, 104*(1), 81–83.

RESOURCES

American Heart Association, 7272 Greenville Avenue, Dallas, TX 75231; 1-800-242-8721; http://www.americanheart.org. Accessed May 30, 2006.

New York Cardiac Center, 467 Sylvan Avenue, Englewood Cliffs, NJ 07632, 201-569-8180; http://nycardiaccenter.org. Accessed May 30, 2006.

Nurse-Beat: Cardiac Nursing Electronic Journal; http://www.nurse-beat.com. Accessed May 30, 2006.

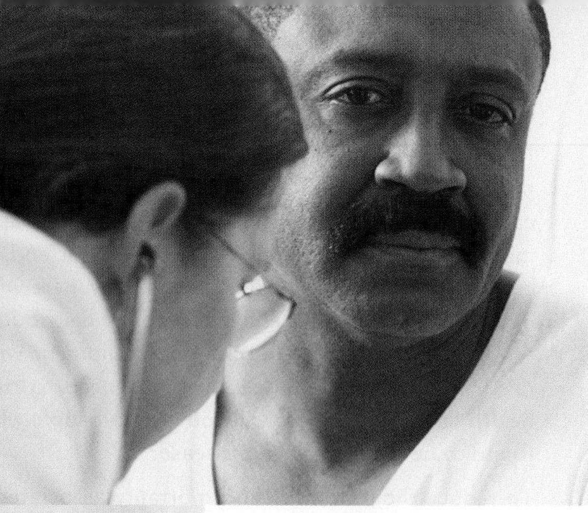

CHAPTER 27

Management of Patients With Dysrhythmias and Conduction Problems

Learning Objectives

On completion of this chapter, the learner will be able to:

1. Correlate the components of the normal electrocardiogram (ECG) with physiologic events of the heart.
2. Define the ECG as a waveform that represents the cardiac electrical event in relation to the lead depicted (placement of electrodes).
3. Analyze elements of an ECG rhythm strip: ventricular and atrial rate, ventricular and atrial rhythm, QRS complex and shape, QRS duration, P wave and shape, PR interval, and P:QRS ratio.
4. Identify the ECG criteria, causes, and management of several dysrhythmias, including conduction disturbances.
5. Use the nursing process as a framework for care of patients with dysrhythmias.
6. Compare the different types of pacemakers, their uses, possible complications, and nursing implications.
7. Use the nursing process as a framework for care of patients with implantable cardiac devices.
8. Describe the key points of using a defibrillator.
9. Describe the purpose of an implantable cardioverter defibrillator, the types available, and the nursing implications.
10. Describe invasive methods to diagnose and treat recurrent dysrhythmias and discuss the nursing implications.

Without a regular rate and rhythm, the heart may not perform efficiently as a pump to circulate oxygenated blood and other life-sustaining nutrients to all of the body's tissues and organs (including the heart itself). With an irregular or erratic rhythm, the heart is considered to be dysrhythmic (sometimes called arrhythmic). This has the potential to be a dangerous condition.

Dysrhythmias

Dysrhythmias are disorders of the formation or conduction (or both) of the electrical impulse within the heart. These disorders can cause disturbances of the heart rate, the heart rhythm, or both. Dysrhythmias may initially be evidenced by the hemodynamic effect they cause (eg, a change in conduction may change the pumping action of the heart and cause decreased blood pressure). Dysrhythmias are diagnosed by analyzing the electrocardiographic (ECG) waveform. They are named according to the site of origin of the impulse and the mechanism of formation or conduction involved (Chart 27-1). For example, an impulse that originates in the sinoatrial (SA) node and that has a slow rate is called sinus bradycardia.

CHART 27-1

Identifying Dysrhythmias

Sites of Origin

- Sinus (SA) node
- Atria
- Atrioventricular (AV) node or junction
- Ventricles

Mechanisms of Formation or Conduction

- Normal (idio) rhythm
- Bradycardia
- Tachycardia
- Dysrhythmia
- Flutter
- Fibrillation
- Premature complexes
- Conduction Blocks

Glossary

ablation: purposeful destruction of heart muscle cells, usually in an attempt to control a dysrhythmia

antiarrhythmic: a medication that suppresses or prevents a dysrhythmia

automaticity: ability of the cardiac cells to initiate an electrical impulse

cardioversion: electrical current administered in synchrony with the patient's own QRS complex to stop a dysrhythmia

chronotropy: rate of impulse formation

conduction: transmission of electrical impulses from one cell to another

defibrillation: electrical current administered to stop a dysrhythmia, not synchronized with the patient's QRS complex

depolarization: process by which cardiac muscle cells change from a more negatively charged to a more positively charged intracellular state

dromotropy: conduction velocity

dysrhythmia (also referred to as arrhythmia): disorder of the formation or conduction (or both) of the electrical impulse within the heart, altering the heart rate, heart rhythm, or both and potentially causing altered blood flow

implantable cardioverter defibrillator (ICD): a device implanted into the chest to treat dysrhythmias

inhibited: in reference to pacemakers, term used to describe the pacemaker withholding an impulse (not firing)

inotropy: force of myocardial contraction

P wave: the part of an electrocardiogram (ECG) that reflects conduction of an electrical impulse through the atrium; atrial depolarization

paroxysmal: a dysrhythmia that has a sudden onset and/or termination and is usually of short duration

PP interval: the duration between the beginning of one P wave and the beginning of the next P wave; used to calculate atrial rate and rhythm

PR interval: the part of an ECG that reflects conduction of an electrical impulse from the sinoatrial (SA) node through the atrioventricular (AV) node

proarrhythmic: an agent (eg, a medication) that causes or exacerbates a dysrhythmia

QRS complex: the part of an ECG that reflects conduction of an electrical impulse through the ventricles; ventricular depolarization

QT interval: the part of an ECG that reflects the time from ventricular depolarization through repolarization

repolarization: process by which cardiac muscle cells return to a more negatively charged intracellular condition, their resting state

sinus rhythm: electrical activity of the heart initiated by the sinoatrial (SA) node

ST segment: the part of an ECG that reflects the end of the QRS complex to the beginning of the T wave

supraventricular tachycardia (SVT): a rhythm that originates in the conduction system above the ventricles

TP interval: the part of an ECG that reflects the time between the end of the T wave and the beginning of the next P wave; used to identify the isoelectric line

T wave: the part of an ECG that reflects repolarization of the ventricles

triggered: in reference to pacemakers, term used to describe the release of an impulse in response to some stimulus

U wave: the part of an ECG that may reflect Purkinje fiber repolarization; usually it is not seen unless a patient's serum potassium level is low

ventricular tachycardia (VT): a rhythm that originates in the ventricles

Normal Electrical Conduction

The electrical impulse that stimulates and paces the cardiac muscle normally originates in the sinus (SA) node, an area located near the superior vena cava in the right atrium. Usually, the electrical impulse occurs at a rate of 60 to 100 times a minute in the adult. The electrical impulse quickly travels from the sinus node through the atria to the atrioventricular (AV) node (Fig. 27-1). The electrical stimulation of the muscle cells of the atria causes them to contract. The structure of the AV node slows the electrical impulse, which allows time for the atria to contract and fill the ventricles with blood. This part of atrial contraction is frequently referred to as the "atrial kick" and accounts for nearly one third of the volume ejected during ventricular contraction. The electrical impulse then travels very quickly through the bundle of His to the right and left bundle branches and the Purkinje fibers, located in the ventricular muscle. The electrical stimulation of the muscle cells of the ventricles in turn causes the mechanical contraction of the ventricles (systole). The cells repolarize and the ventricles then relax (diastole). The electrical impulse causes the mechanical contraction of the heart muscle that follows.

The electrical stimulation is called **depolarization**, and the mechanical contraction is called systole. Electrical relaxation is called **repolarization**, and mechanical relaxation is called

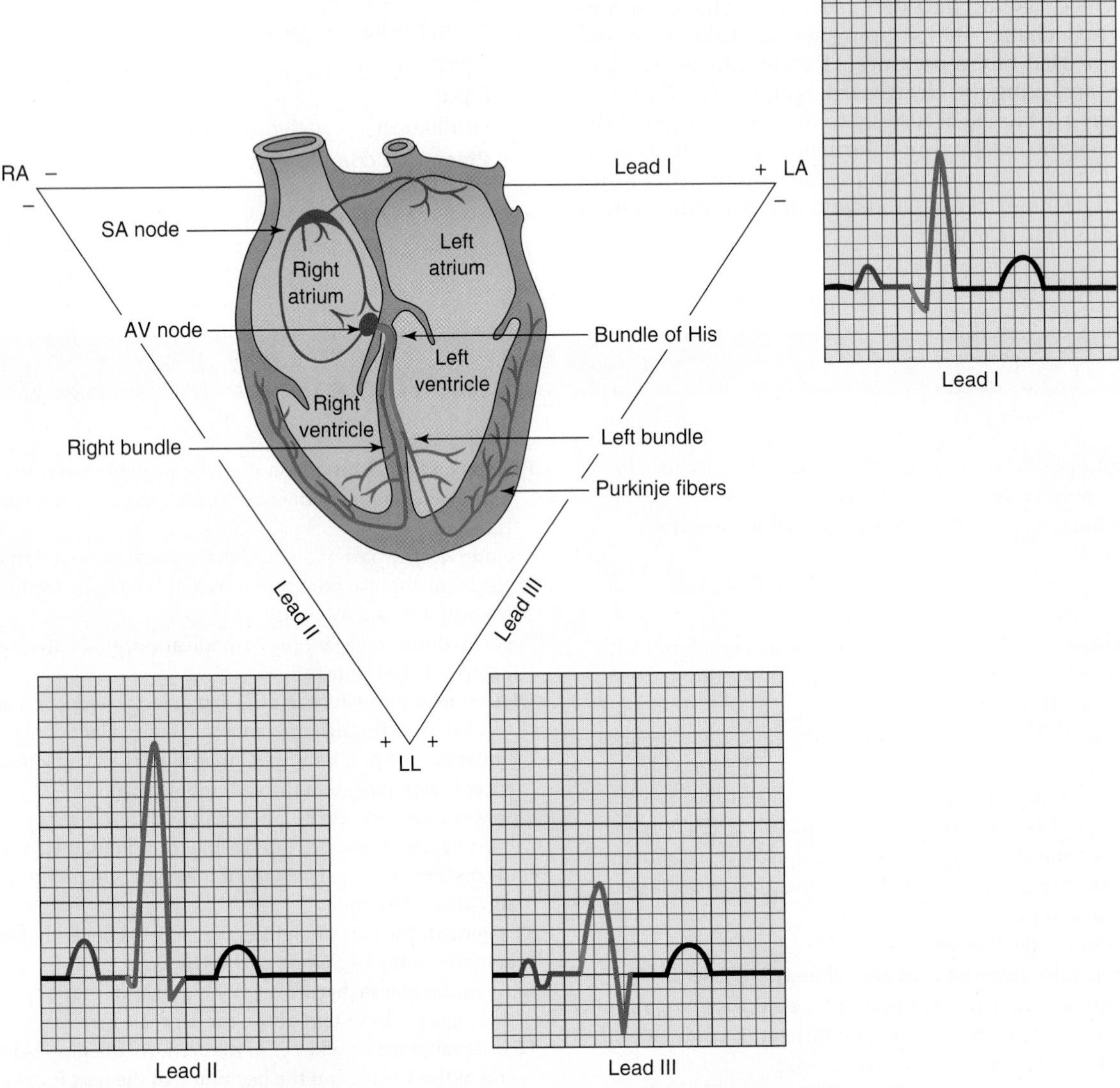

FIGURE 27-1. Relationship of electrocardiogram (ECG) complex, lead system, and electrical impulse. The heart conducts electrical activity, which the ECG measures and shows. The configurations of electrical activity displayed on the ECG vary depending on the lead (or view) of the ECG and on the rhythm of the heart. Therefore, the configuration of a normal rhythm tracing from lead I will differ from the configuration of a normal rhythm tracing from lead II, lead II will differ from lead III, and so on. The same is true for abnormal rhythms and cardiac disorders. To make an accurate assessment of the heart's electrical activity or to identify where, when, and what abnormalities occur, the ECG needs to be evaluated from every lead, not just from lead II. Here the different areas of electrical activity are identified by color. RA, right arm; LA, left arm; SA, sinoatrial; AV, atrioventricular; LL, left arm.

diastole. The process from sinus node electrical impulse generation through ventricular repolarization completes the electromechanical circuit, and the cycle begins again. See Chapter 26 for a more complete explanation of cardiac function.

Influences on Heart Rate and Contractility

The heart rate is influenced by the autonomic nervous system, which consists of sympathetic and parasympathetic fibers. Sympathetic nerve fibers (also referred to as adrenergic fibers) are attached to the heart and arteries as well as several other areas in the body. Stimulation of the sympathetic system increases heart rate (positive **chronotropy**), conduction through the AV node (positive **dromotropy**), and the force of myocardial contraction (positive **inotropy**). Sympathetic stimulation also constricts peripheral blood vessels, therefore increasing blood pressure. Parasympathetic nerve fibers are also attached to the heart and arteries. Parasympathetic stimulation reduces the heart rate (negative chronotropy), AV conduction (negative dromotropy), and the force of atrial myocardial contraction. The decreased sympathetic stimulation results in dilation of arteries, thereby lowering blood pressure.

Manipulation of the autonomic nervous system may increase or decrease the incidence of dysrhythmias. Increased sympathetic stimulation (eg, caused by exercise, anxiety, fever, or administration of catecholamines, such as dopamine [Intropin], aminophylline, or dobutamine [Dobutrex]) may increase the incidence of dysrhythmias. Decreased sympathetic stimulation (eg, with rest, anxiety-reduction methods such as therapeutic communication or meditation, or administration of beta-adrenergic blocking agents) may decrease the incidence of dysrhythmias.

The Electrocardiogram

The electrical impulse that travels through the heart can be viewed by means of electrocardiography, the end product of which is an electrocardiogram (ECG). Each phase of the cardiac cycle is reflected by specific waveforms on the screen of a cardiac monitor or on a strip of ECG graph paper.

An ECG is obtained by slightly abrading the skin with a clean dry gauze pad and placing electrodes on the body at specific areas. Electrodes come in various shapes and sizes, but all have two components: (1) an adhesive substance that attaches to the skin to secure the electrode in place and (2) a substance that reduces the skin's electrical impedance and promotes detection of the electrical current.

The number and placement of the electrodes depend on the type of ECG needed. Most continuous monitors use two to five electrodes, usually placed on the limbs and the chest. These electrodes create an imaginary line, called a lead, that serves as a reference point from which the electrical activity is viewed. A lead is like an eye of a camera: it has a narrow peripheral field of vision, looking only at the electrical activity directly in front of it. Therefore, the ECG waveforms that appear on the paper or cardiac monitor represent the electrical current in relation to the lead (see Fig. 27-1). A change in the waveform can be caused by a change in the electrical current (where it originates or how it is conducted) or by a change in the lead.

Obtaining an Electrocardiogram

Electrodes are attached to cable wires, which are connected to one of the following:

- An ECG machine placed at the patient's side for an immediate recording (standard 12-lead ECG)
- A cardiac monitor at the patient's bedside for continuous reading; this kind of monitoring, usually called hardwire monitoring, is associated with intensive care units
- A small box that the patient carries and that continuously transmits the ECG information by radiowaves to a central monitor located elsewhere (called telemetry)
- A small, lightweight tape recorder–like machine (called a Holter monitor) that the patient wears and that continuously records the ECG on a tape, which is later viewed and analyzed with a scanner

The placement of electrodes for continuous monitoring, telemetry, or Holter monitoring varies with the type of technology that is appropriate and available, the purpose of monitoring, and the standards of the institution. For a standard 12-lead ECG, 10 electrodes (6 on the chest and 4 on the limbs) are placed on the body (Fig. 27-2). To prevent interference from the electrical activity of skeletal muscle, the limb electrodes are usually placed on areas that are not bony and that do not have significant movement. These limb electrodes provide the first six leads: leads I, II, III, aVR, aVL, and aVF. The six chest electrodes are attached to the chest at very specific areas. The chest electrodes provide the V or precordial leads, V_1 through V_6. To locate the fourth intercostal space and the placement of V_1, the sternal angle and then the sternal notch, which is about 1 or 2 inches below the sternal angle, are located. When the fingers are moved to the patient's immediate right, the second rib can be palpated. The second intercostal space is the indentation felt just below the second rib.

Locating the specific intercostal space is critical for correct chest electrode placement. Errors in diagnosis can occur if electrodes are incorrectly placed. Sometimes, when the patient is in the hospital and needs to be monitored closely for ECG changes, the chest electrodes are left in place to ensure the same placement for follow-up ECGs.

A standard 12-lead ECG reflects the electrical activity primarily in the left ventricle. Placement of additional electrodes for other leads may be needed to obtain more complete information. For example, in patients with suspected right-sided heart damage, right-sided precordial leads are required to evaluate the right ventricle (see Fig. 27-2).

Interpreting the Electrocardiogram

The ECG waveform represents the function of the heart's conduction system, which normally initiates and conducts the electrical activity, in relation to the lead. When analyzed accurately, the ECG offers important information about the electrical activity of the heart. ECG waveforms are printed on graph paper that is divided by light and dark vertical and horizontal lines at standard intervals (Fig. 27-3). Time and rate are measured on the horizontal axis of the graph, and amplitude or voltage is measured on the vertical axis. When an ECG waveform moves toward the top of the paper, it is called a positive deflection. When it moves toward the bottom of the paper, it is called a negative deflection. When

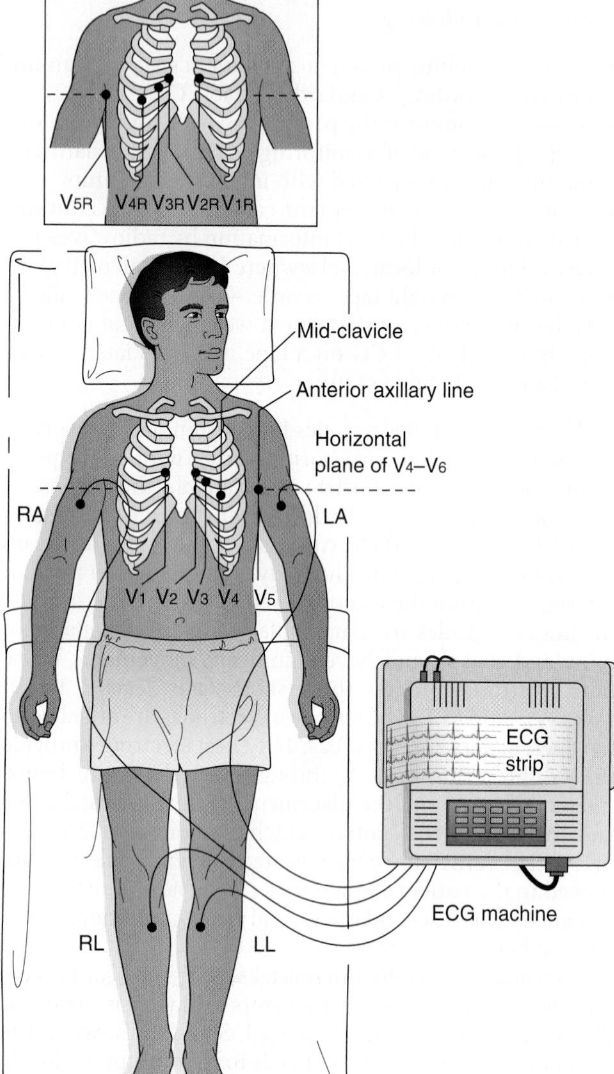

FIGURE 27-2. ECG electrode placement. The standard left precordial leads are V_1—4th intercostal space, right sternal border; V_2—4th intercostal space, left sternal border; V_3—diagonally between V_2 and V_4; V_4—5th intercostal space, left midclavicular line; V_5—same level as V_4, anterior axillary line; V_6 (not illustrated)—same level as V_4 and V_5, midaxillary line. The right precordial leads, placed across the right side of the chest, are the mirror opposite of the left leads. RA, right arm; LA, left arm; RL, right leg; LL, left leg. Adapted from Molle, E. A., Kronenberger, J., West-Stack, C., & Durham, L. S. (2005). *Lippincott Williams & Wilkins's pocket guide to medical assisting* (2nd ed.). Philadelphia: Lippincott Williams & Wilkins.

reviewing an ECG, each waveform should be examined and compared with the others.

WAVES, COMPLEXES, AND INTERVALS

The ECG is composed of waveforms (including the P wave, the QRS complex, the T wave, and possibly a U wave) and of segments or intervals (including the PR interval, the ST segment, and the QT interval) (see Fig. 27-3).

The **P wave** represents the electrical impulse starting in the sinus node and spreading through the atria. Therefore, the P wave represents atrial depolarization. It is normally 2.5 mm or less in height and 0.11 seconds or less in duration.

The **QRS complex** represents ventricular depolarization. Not all QRS complexes have all three waveforms. The Q wave is the first negative deflection after the P wave. The Q wave is normally less than 0.04 seconds in duration and less than 25% of the R-wave amplitude. The R wave is the first positive deflection after the P wave, and the S wave is the first negative deflection after the R wave. When a wave is less than 5 mm in height, small letters (q, r, s) are used; when a wave is taller than 5 mm, capital letters (Q, R, S) are used. The QRS complex is normally less than 0.12 seconds in duration.

The **T wave** represents ventricular repolarization (when the cells regain a negative charge; also called the resting state). It follows the QRS complex and is usually the same direction as the QRS complex. Atrial repolarization also occurs but is not visible on the ECG because it occurs at the same time as the QRS.

The **U wave** is thought to represent repolarization of the Purkinje fibers, but it sometimes is seen in patients with hypokalemia (low potassium levels), hypertension, or heart disease. If present, the U wave follows the T wave and is usually smaller than the P wave. If tall, it may be mistaken for an extra P wave.

The **PR interval** is measured from the beginning of the P wave to the beginning of the QRS complex and represents the time needed for sinus node stimulation, atrial depolarization, and conduction through the AV node before ventricular depolarization. In adults, the PR interval normally ranges from 0.12 to 0.20 seconds in duration.

The **ST segment**, which represents early ventricular repolarization, lasts from the end of the QRS complex to the beginning of the T wave. The beginning of the ST segment is usually identified by a change in the thickness or angle of the terminal portion of the QRS complex. The end of the ST segment may be more difficult to identify because it merges into the T wave. The ST segment is normally isoelectric (see discussion of TP interval). It is analyzed to identify whether it is above or below the isoelectric line, which may be, among other signs and symptoms, a sign of cardiac ischemia (see Chapter 28).

The **QT interval**, which represents the total time for ventricular depolarization and repolarization, is measured from the beginning of the QRS complex to the end of the T wave. The QT interval varies with heart rate, gender, and age, and the measured interval needs to be corrected for these variables through specific calculations. Several ECG interpretation books contain charts of these calculations. The QT interval is usually 0.32 to 0.40 seconds in duration if the heart rate is 65 to 95 beats per minute. If the QT interval becomes prolonged, the patient may be at risk for a lethal ventricular dysrhythmia called torsades de pointes.

The **TP interval** is measured from the end of the T wave to the beginning of the next P wave, an isoelectric period (see Fig. 27-3). When no electrical activity is detected, the line on the graph remains flat; this is called the isoelectric line. The ST segment is compared with the TP interval to detect changes from the line on the graph during the isoelectric period.

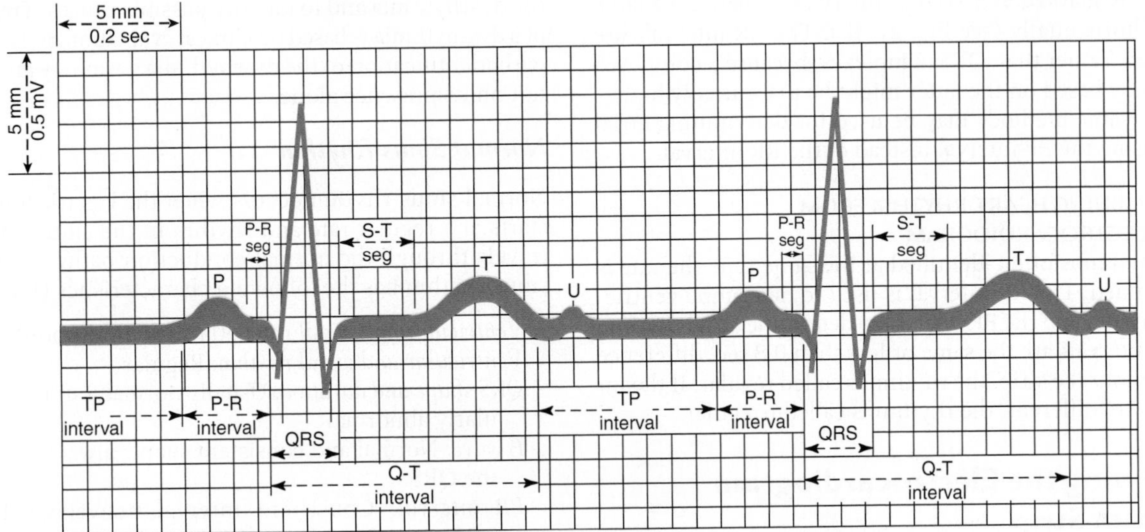

FIGURE 27-3. ECG graph and commonly measured components. Each small box represents 0.04 seconds on the horizontal axis and 1 mm or 0.1 millivolt on the vertical axis. The PR interval is measured from the beginning of the P wave to the beginning of the QRS complex; the QRS complex is measured from the beginning of the Q wave to the end of the S wave; the QT interval is measured from the beginning of the Q wave to the end of the T wave; and the TP interval is measured from the end of the T wave to the beginning of the next P wave.

The **PP interval** is measured from the beginning of one P wave to the beginning of the next. The PP interval is used to determine atrial rhythm and atrial rate. The RR interval is measured from one QRS complex to the next QRS complex. The RR interval is used to determine ventricular rate and rhythm (Fig. 27-4).

DETERMINING VENTRICULAR HEART RATE FROM THE ELECTROCARDIOGRAM

Heart rate can be obtained from the ECG strip by several methods. A 1-minute strip contains 300 large boxes and 1500 small boxes. Therefore, an easy and accurate method of determining heart rate with a regular rhythm is to count the number of small boxes within an RR interval and divide 1500 by that number. If, for example, there are 10 small boxes between two R waves, the heart rate is 1500/10, or 150; if there are 25 small boxes, the heart rate is 1500/25, or 60 (see Fig. 27-4A).

An alternative but less accurate method for estimating heart rate, which is usually used when the rhythm is irregular, is to count the number of RR intervals in 6 seconds and multiply that number by 10. The top of the ECG paper

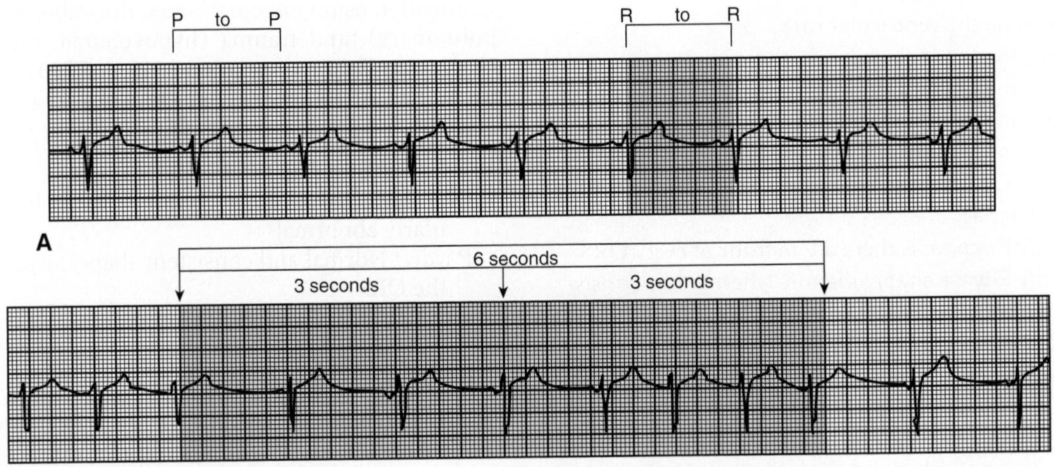

FIGURE 27-4. (**A**) Ventricular and atrial heart rate determination with a regular rhythm: 1500 divided by the number of small boxes between two P waves (atrial rate) or between two R waves (ventricular rate). In this example, there are 25 small boxes between both the R waves and the P waves, so the heart rate is 60 beats/minute. (**B**) Heart rate determination if the rhythm is irregular. There are approximately seven RR intervals in 6 seconds, so there are about 70 RR intervals in 60 seconds (7 × 10 = 70). The ventricular heart rate is 70 beats/minute.

is usually marked at 3-second intervals, which is 15 large boxes horizontally (see Fig. 27-4B). The RR intervals are counted, rather than QRS complexes, because a computed heart rate based on the latter might be inaccurately high.

The same methods may be used for determining atrial rate, using the PP interval instead of the RR interval.

DETERMINING HEART RHYTHM FROM THE ELECTROCARDIOGRAM

The rhythm is often identified at the same time the rate is determined. The RR interval is used to determine ventricular rhythm and the PP interval to determine atrial rhythm. If the intervals are the same or less than 0.8 sec. difference throughout the strip, the rhythm is called regular. If the intervals are different, the rhythm is called irregular.

Analyzing the Electrocardiogram Rhythm Strip

The ECG must be analyzed in a systematic manner to determine the patient's cardiac rhythm and to detect dysrhythmias and conduction disorders, as well as evidence of myocardial ischemia, injury, and infarction. Chart 27-2 is an example of a method that can be used to analyze the patient's rhythm.

Once the rhythm has been analyzed, the findings are compared with and matched to the ECG criteria for dysrhythmias to determine a diagnosis. It is important for the nurse to assess the patient to determine the physiologic effect of the dysrhythmia and to identify possible causes. Treatment of a dysrhythmia is based on clinical evaluation of the patient with identification of the dysrhythmia's etiology and effect, not on its presence alone.

CHART 27-2

Interpreting Dysrhythmias: Systematic Analysis of the Electrocardiogram

When examining an ECG rhythm strip to learn more about a patient's dysrhythmia, the nurse conducts the following assessment:

1. Determine the ventricular rate.
2. Determine the ventricular rhythm.
3. Determine QRS duration.
4. Determine whether the QRS duration is consistent throughout the strip. If not, identify other duration.
5. Identify QRS shape; if not consistent, then identify other shapes.
6. Identify P waves; is there a P in front of every QRS?
7. Identify P-wave shape; identify whether it is consistent or not.
8. Determine the atrial rate.
9. Determine the atrial rhythm.
10. Determine each PR interval.
11. Determine if the PR intervals are consistent, irregular but with a pattern to the irregularity, or just irregular.
12. Determine how many P waves for each QRS (P:QRS ratio).

In many cases, the nurse may use a checklist and document the findings next to the appropriate ECG criterion.

Normal Sinus Rhythm

Normal **sinus rhythm** occurs when the electrical impulse starts at a regular rate and rhythm in the sinus node and travels through the normal conduction pathway. Normal sinus rhythm has the following characteristics (Fig. 27-5):

Ventricular and atrial rate: 60 to 100 in the adult
Ventricular and atrial rhythm: Regular
QRS shape and duration: Usually normal, but may be regularly abnormal
P wave: Normal and consistent shape; always in front of the QRS
PR interval: Consistent interval between 0.12 and 0.20 seconds
P:QRS ratio: 1:1

Types of Dysrhythmias

Dysrhythmias include sinus, atrial, junctional, and ventricular dysrhythmias and their various subcategories.

SINUS NODE DYSRHYTHMIAS

Sinus Bradycardia. Sinus bradycardia occurs when the sinus node creates an impulse at a slower-than-normal rate. Causes include lower metabolic needs (eg, sleep, athletic training, hypothyroidism), vagal stimulation (eg, from vomiting, suctioning, severe pain, extreme emotions), medications (eg, calcium channel blockers, amiodarone, beta-blockers), increased intracranial pressure (ICP), and myocardial infarction (MI), especially of the inferior wall. Other possible contributing factors in clinically significant bradycardia include what are referred to as the H's and the T's: hypovolemia, hypoxia, hydrogen ion (acidosis), hypo- or hyperkalemia, hypoglycemia, and hypothermia; toxins, tamponade (cardiac), tension pneumothorax, thrombosis (coronary or pulmonary), and trauma (hypovolemia, increased ICP) (American Heart Association [AHA], 2005). Sinus bradycardia has the following characteristics (Fig. 27-6):

Ventricular and atrial rate: Less than 60 in the adult
Ventricular and atrial rhythm: Regular
QRS shape and duration: Usually normal, but may be regularly abnormal
P wave: Normal and consistent shape; always in front of the QRS
PR interval: Consistent interval between 0.12 and 0.20 seconds
P:QRS ratio: 1:1

All characteristics of sinus bradycardia are the same as those of normal sinus rhythm, except for the rate. The patient is assessed to determine the hemodynamic effect and the possible cause of the dysrhythmia. If the decrease in heart rate results from stimulation of the vagus nerve, such as with bearing down during defecation or vomiting, attempts are made to prevent further vagal stimulation. If the bradycardia is from a medication such as a beta-blocker, the medication may be withheld. If the slow heart rate causes significant

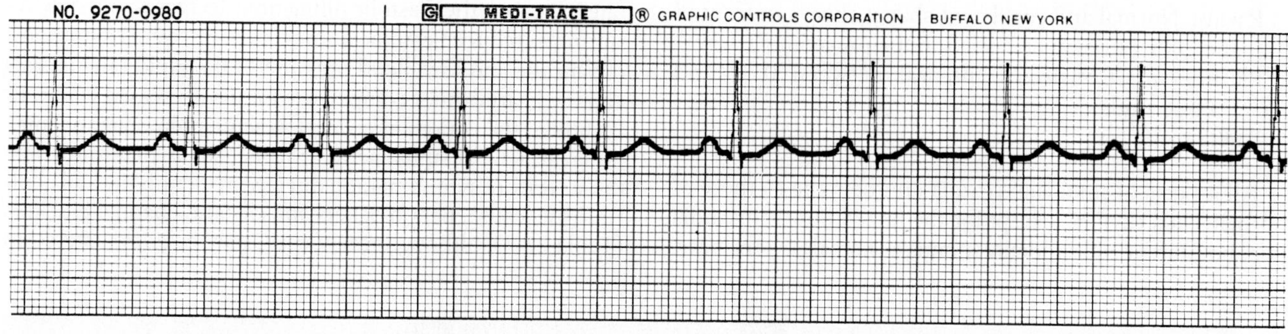

FIGURE 27-5. Normal sinus rhythm in lead II.

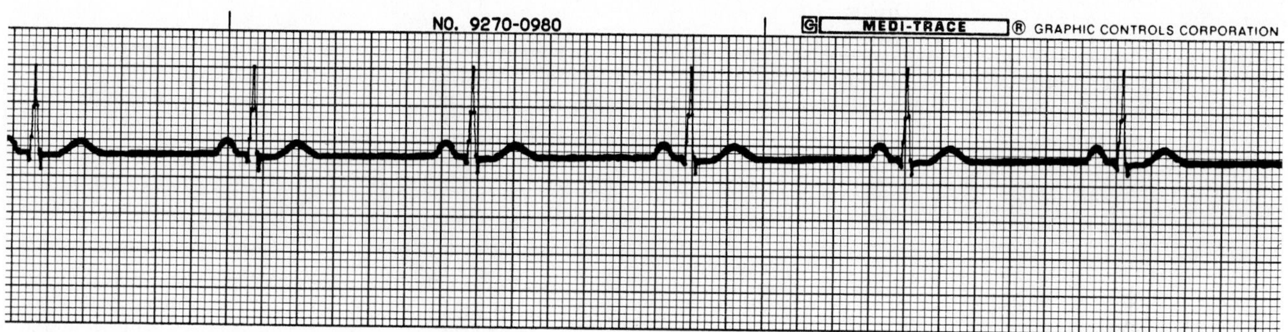

FIGURE 27-6. Sinus bradycardia in lead II.

hemodynamic changes, resulting in shortness of breath, acute alteration of mental status, angina, hypotension, ST-segment changes, or premature ventricular complexes, treatment is directed toward increasing the heart rate.

Atropine, 0.5 mg given rapidly as an intravenous (IV) bolus every 3 to 5 minutes to a maximum total dose of 3 mg, is the medication of choice in treating symptomatic sinus bradycardia. It blocks vagal stimulation, thus allowing a normal rate to occur. Rarely, catecholamines and emergency transcutaneous pacing also are implemented.

Sinus Tachycardia. Sinus tachycardia occurs when the sinus node creates an impulse at a faster-than-normal rate. Causes may include the following:

- Physiologic or psychological stress (eg, acute blood loss, anemia, shock, hypervolemia, hypovolemia, heart failure, pain, hypermetabolic states, fever, exercise, anxiety)
- Medications that stimulate the sympathetic response (eg, catecholamines, aminophylline, atropine), stimulants (eg, caffeine, alcohol, nicotine), and illicit drugs (eg, amphetamines, cocaine, Ecstasy)
- Enhanced automaticity of the SA node and/or excessive sympathetic tone with reduced parasympathetic tone, a condition called inappropriate sinus tachycardia (Blomström-Lundqvist, Scheinman, Aliot, et al., 2003)
- Autonomic dysfunction, which results in a type of sinus tachycardia called postural orthostatic tachycardia syndrome (POTS). Patients with POTS have tachycardia without hypotension within 5 to 10 minutes of standing or with head-upright tilt testing.

Sinus tachycardia has the following characteristics (Fig. 27-7):

Ventricular and atrial rate: Greater than 100 in the adult, but usually less than 120
Ventricular and atrial rhythm: Regular
QRS shape and duration: Usually normal, but may be regularly abnormal

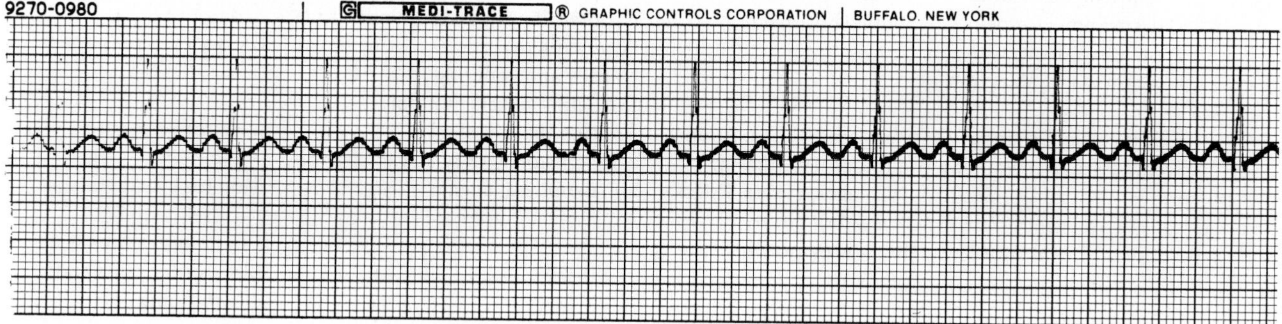

FIGURE 27-7. Sinus tachycardia in lead II.

P wave: Normal and consistent shape; always in front of the QRS, but may be buried in the preceding T wave
PR interval: Consistent interval between 0.12 and 0.20 seconds
P:QRS ratio: 1:1

All aspects of sinus tachycardia are the same as those of normal sinus rhythm, except for the rate. Sinus tachycardia does not start or end suddenly (nonparoxysmal). As the heart rate increases, the diastolic filling time decreases, possibly resulting in reduced cardiac output and subsequent symptoms of syncope and low blood pressure. If the rapid rate persists and the heart cannot compensate for the decreased ventricular filling, the patient may develop acute pulmonary edema.

Treatment of sinus tachycardia is usually determined by the severity of symptoms and directed at identifying and abolishing its cause. Beta-blockers and calcium channel blockers (Table 27-1), although rarely used, may be administered to

TABLE 27-1 Summary of Antiarrhythmic Medications*

Class	Action	Drugs: Generic (Trade) Names	Side Effects	Nursing Interventions
IA	Moderate depression of depolarization; prolongs repolarization Treats and prevents atrial and ventricular dysrhythmias	quinidine (Quinaglute, Quinidex, Cardioquin) procainamide (Pronestyl) disopyramide (Norpace)	Decreased cardiac contractility Prolonged QRS, QT Proarrhythmic Hypotension with IV administration Lupus-like syndrome with Pronestyl Anticholinergic effects: dry mouth, decreased urine output	Observe for HF Monitor BP with IV administration Monitor QRS duration for increase >50% from baseline Monitor for prolonged QT Monitor *N*-acetyl procainamide (NAPA) laboratory values during procainamide therapy
IB	Minimal depression of depolarization; shortened repolarization Treats ventricular dysrhythmias	lidocaine (Xylocaine) mexiletine (Mexitil) tocainide (Tonocard)	CNS changes (eg, confusion, lethargy)	Discuss with physician decreasing the dose in elderly patients and patients with cardiac/liver dysfunction
IC	Marked depression of depolarization; little effect on repolarization Treats atrial and ventricular dysrhythmias	flecainide (Tambocor) propafenone (Rythmol)	Proarrhythmic HF Bradycardia AV blocks	Discuss patient's left ventricular function with physician
II	Decreases automaticity and conduction Treats atrial and ventricular dysrhythmias	atenolol (Tenormin) bisoprolol/HCTZ (Ziac, Zebeta) esmolol (Brevibloc) labetalol (Trandate) metoprolol (Lopressor, Toprol) propranolol (Inderal, Innopran) sotalol (Betapace; Sorine; also has class III actions)	Bradycardia, AV block Decreased contractility Bronchospasm Hypotension with IV administration Masks hypoglycemia and thyrotoxicosis CNS disturbances	Monitor heart rate, PR interval, signs and symptoms of HF Monitor blood glucose level in patients with type 2 diabetes mellitus
III	Prolongs repolarization Treats and prevents ventricular and atrial dysrhythmias, especially in patients with ventricular dysfunction	amiodarone (Cordarone, Pacerone) dofetilide (Tikosyn) ibutilide (Corvert)	Pulmonary toxicity (amiodarone) Corneal microdeposits (amiodarone) Photosensitivity (amiodarone) Hypotension with IV administration Polymorphic ventricular dysrhythmias Nausea and vomiting See beta-blockers (sotalol)	Make sure patient is sent for baseline pulmonary function tests (amiodarone) Closely monitor patient
IV	Blocks calcium channel Treats atrial dysrhythmias	verapamil (Calan, Isoptin) diltiazem (Cardizem, Dilacor, Tiazac, Diltia, Cartia) bepridil (Vascor)	Bradycardia, AV blocks Hypotension with IV administration HF, peripheral edema	Monitor heart rate, PR interval Monitor blood pressure closely with IV administration Monitor for signs and symptoms of HF

*Based on Vaughn-Williams classification.
AV, atrioventricular; BP, blood pressure; CNS, central nervous system; HF, heart failure; IV, intravenous.

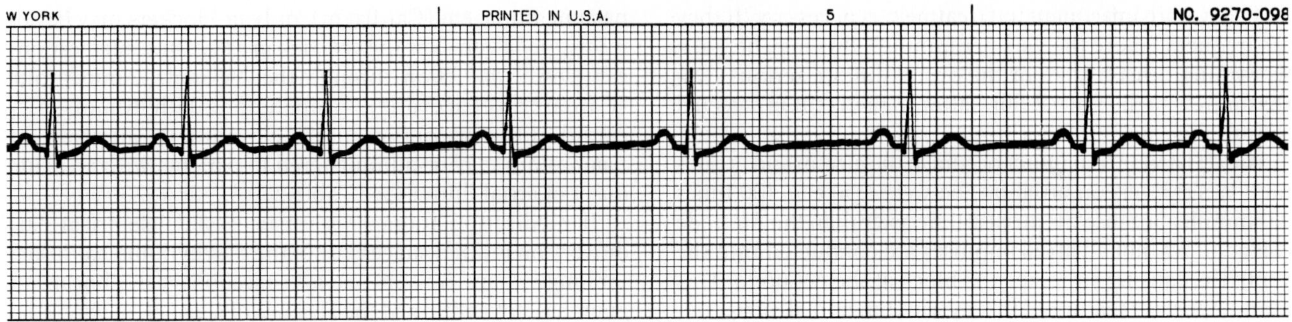

FIGURE 27-8. Sinus arrhythmia in lead II. Note irregular RR and PP intervals.

reduce the heart rate quickly. Catheter ablation (discussed later in this chapter) of the SA node may be used in cases of persistent inappropriate sinus tachycardia unresponsive to other treatments. Treatment for POTS may include increased fluid and sodium intake and use of compression stockings to prevent pooling of blood in the lower extremities.

Sinus Arrhythmia. Sinus arrhythmia occurs when the sinus node creates an impulse at an irregular rhythm; the rate usually increases with inspiration and decreases with expiration. Nonrespiratory causes include heart disease and valvular disease, but these are rare. Sinus arrhythmia has the following characteristics (Fig. 27-8):

Ventricular and atrial rate: 60 to 100 in the adult
Ventricular and atrial rhythm: Irregular
QRS shape and duration: Usually normal, but may be regularly abnormal
P wave: Normal and consistent shape; always in front of the QRS
PR interval: Consistent interval between 0.12 and 0.20 seconds
P:QRS ratio: 1:1

Sinus arrhythmia does not cause any significant hemodynamic effect and usually is not treated.

ATRIAL DYSRHYTHMIAS

Premature Atrial Complex. A premature atrial complex (PAC) is a single ECG complex that occurs when an electrical impulse starts in the atrium before the next normal impulse of the sinus node. The PAC may be caused by caffeine, alcohol, nicotine, stretched atrial myocardium (eg, as in hypervolemia), anxiety, hypokalemia (low potassium level), hypermetabolic states (eg, with pregnancy), or atrial ischemia, injury, or infarction. PACs are often seen with sinus tachycardia. PACs have the following characteristics (Fig. 27-9):

Ventricular and atrial rate: Depends on the underlying rhythm (eg, sinus tachycardia)
Ventricular and atrial rhythm: Irregular due to early P waves, creating a PP interval that is shorter than the others. This is sometimes followed by a longer-than-normal PP interval, but one that is less than twice the normal PP interval. This type of interval is called a noncompensatory pause.
QRS shape and duration: The QRS that follows the early P wave is usually normal, but it may be abnormal (aberrantly conducted PAC). It may even be absent (blocked PAC).
P wave: An early and different P wave may be seen or may be hidden in the T wave; other P waves in the strip are consistent.
PR interval: The early P wave has a shorter-than-normal PR interval, but still between 0.12 and 0.20 seconds.
P:QRS ratio: usually 1:1

PACs are common in normal hearts. The patient may say, "My heart skipped a beat." A pulse deficit (a difference between the apical and radial pulse rate) may exist.

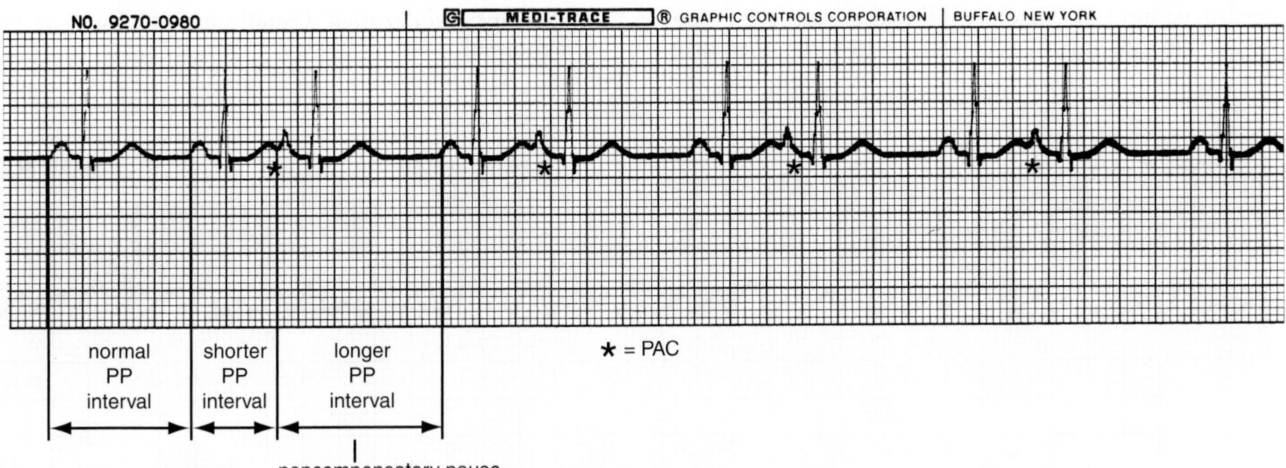

FIGURE 27-9. Premature atrial complexes (PACs) in lead II. Note that the pause following the PAC is longer than the normal PP interval but shorter than twice the normal PP interval.

If PACs are infrequent, no treatment is necessary. If they are frequent (more than six per minute), this may herald a worsening disease state or the onset of more serious dysrhythmias, such as atrial fibrillation. Treatment is directed toward the cause.

Atrial Flutter. Atrial flutter occurs in the atrium and creates impulses at a regular atrial rate between 250 and 400 times per minute. Because the atrial rate is faster than the AV node can conduct, not all atrial impulses are conducted into the ventricle, causing a therapeutic block at the AV node. This is an important feature of this dysrhythmia. If all atrial impulses were conducted to the ventricle, the ventricular rate would also be 250 to 400, which would result in ventricular fibrillation, a life-threatening dysrhythmia. Causes are similar to those of atrial fibrillation. Atrial flutter has the following characteristics (Fig. 27-10):

Ventricular and atrial rate: Atrial rate ranges between 250 and 400; ventricular rate usually ranges between 75 and 150.

Ventricular and atrial rhythm: The atrial rhythm is regular; the ventricular rhythm is usually regular but may be irregular because of a change in the AV conduction.

QRS shape and duration: Usually normal, but may be abnormal or may be absent

P wave: Saw-toothed shape; these waves are referred to as F waves

PR interval: Multiple F waves may make it difficult to determine the PR interval.

P:QRS ratio: 2:1, 3:1, or 4:1

Atrial flutter can cause serious signs and symptoms, such as chest pain, shortness of breath, and low blood pressure. If the patient is unstable, electrical cardioversion (discussed later) is usually indicated. In addition, rapid atrial pacing, also called overdrive atrial pacing, in which the atrium is paced at a faster rate than that in atrial flutter, may be considered as an alternative to cardioversion, especially in patients who have undergone cardiac surgery. If the patient is stable, the QRS is narrow, and the RR interval is regular, 6 mg adenosine (Adenocard, Adenoscan) may be rapidly administered IV, followed by a 20-mL saline flush and elevation of the arm to promote rapid circulation of the medication. If the rhythm does not convert to sinus rhythm within 1 to 2 minutes, a 12-mg bolus may be administered and repeated, if needed, within 1 to 2 minutes. If the adenosine fails to convert the rhythm or if the RR interval is irregular, then magnesium, diltiazem (Cardizem), or beta-blockers may be administered IV to slow the ventricular rate. These medications can slow conduction through the AV node. Amiodarone (Cardarone, Pacerone), propafenone (Rhythmol), flecainide (Tambocor), digoxin, clonidine (Catapres), or magnesium may be administered to patients with an acute onset of atrial flutter (see Table 27-1) (AHA, 2005).

If medication therapy is unsuccessful, electrical cardioversion is often successful. If the dysrhythmia has lasted for longer than 48 hours and a transesophageal echocardiogram has not confirmed the absence of atrial clots, then adequate anticoagulation may be indicated before cardioversion (electrical or chemical or ablation). Once conversion has occurred, flecainide, propafenone, amiodarone, or a beta-blocker may be given to prevent a recurrence (see Table 27-1) (AHA, 2005).

Atrial Fibrillation. Atrial fibrillation causes a rapid, disorganized, and uncoordinated twitching of atrial musculature. It has been linked to stroke, heart failure, dementia, and premature death and is considered a growing health problem in developed countries (Stewart, 2004). Atrial fibrillation may be transient, starting and stopping suddenly and occurring for a very short time (**paroxysmal**), or it may be persistent, requiring treatment to terminate the rhythm or to control the ventricular rate. Atrial fibrillation is usually associated with advanced age, valvular heart disease, coronary artery disease, hypertension, heart failure, diabetes, hyperthyroidism, pulmonary disease, acute moderate to heavy ingestion of alcohol ("holiday heart" syndrome), or the aftermath of open heart surgery (Stewart, 2004). Atrial fibrillation occurs in 11% to 64% of patients after coronary artery bypass, valvular replacements, and heart transplantation, and it increases the length and cost of the hospital stay and increases the risk for stroke (Kern, 2004). Its onset can also occur after hospital discharge without producing symptoms (Funk, Richards, Desjardins, et al., 2003). Sometimes atrial fibrillation occurs in people without any underlying pathophysiology (termed lone atrial fibrillation).

Atrial fibrillation has the following characteristics (Fig. 27-11):

Ventricular and atrial rate: Atrial rate is 300 to 600; ventricular rate is usually 120 to 200 in untreated atrial fibrillation.

Ventricular and atrial rhythm: Highly irregular

QRS shape and duration: Usually normal, but may be abnormal

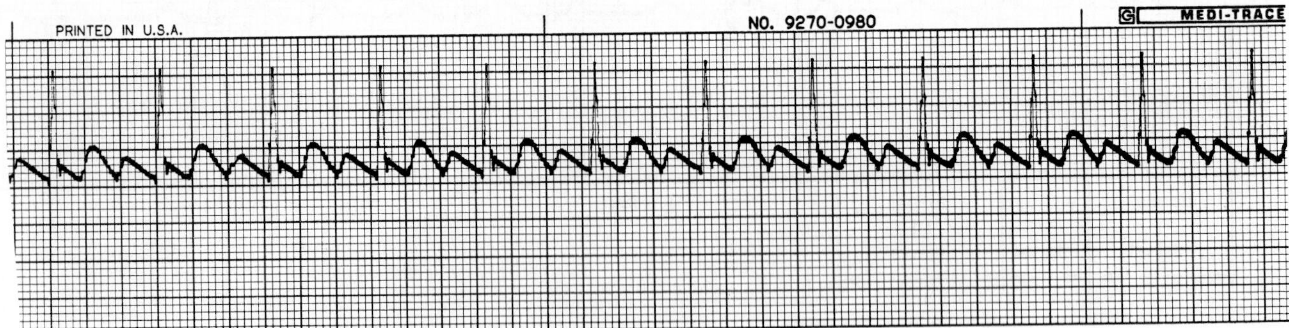

FIGURE 27-10. Atrial flutter in lead II.

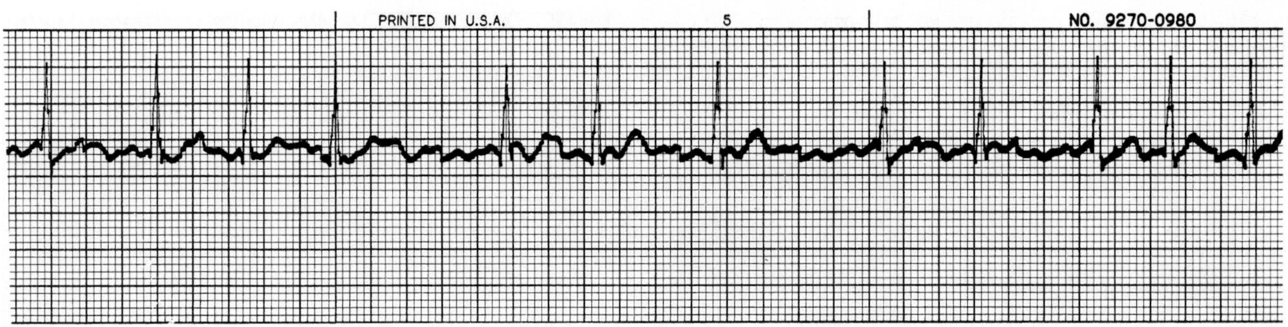

FIGURE 27-11. Atrial fibrillation in lead II.

P wave: No discernible P waves; irregular undulating waves are seen and are referred to as fibrillatory or f waves
PR interval: Cannot be measured
P:QRS ratio: Many:1

A rapid ventricular response reduces the time for ventricular filling, resulting in a smaller stroke volume. Because atrial fibrillation causes the atria and ventricles to contract at different times, the atrial kick (the last part of diastole and ventricular filling, which accounts for 25% to 30% of the cardiac output) is also lost. This leads to symptoms of irregular palpitations, fatigue, and malaise. There is usually a pulse deficit, a numeric difference between apical and radial pulse rates. The shorter time in diastole reduces the time available for coronary artery perfusion, thereby increasing the risk for myocardial ischemia. The erratic atrial contraction promotes the formation of a thrombus within the atria, increasing the risk for an embolic event. There is a two- to five-fold increase in the risk of stroke (brain attack).

Treatment of atrial fibrillation depends on its cause and duration and the patient's symptoms, age, and comorbidities. In many patients, atrial fibrillation converts to sinus rhythm within 24 hours and without treatment. Electrical cardioversion is indicated for atrial fibrillation that is hemodynamically unstable. Because of the high risk for embolization of atrial thrombi, cardioversion of atrial fibrillation that has lasted longer than 48 hours should be avoided unless the patient has received anticoagulants.

For atrial fibrillation of acute onset (usually defined as that with an onset within 48 hours), IV adenosine (Adenocard, Adenoscan) has been used to achieve cardioversion to sinus rhythm as well as to assist in the diagnosis. Other medications that may be administered to achieve cardioversion to sinus rhythm include amiodarone (Cardarone), flecainide (Tambocor), ibutilide (Corvert), digoxin, propafenone (Rythmol), clonidine (Catapres), or magnesium (AHA, 2005).

If the QRS is wide and the ventricular rhythm is irregular, atrial fibrillation with an accessory pathway should be suspected. An accessory pathway is congenital tissue between the atrial and ventricular myocardium. Electrical impulses conducted over these pathways bypass the slower-conducting AV node, causing early or pre-excited ventricular depolarization. Medications that block AV conduction (eg, adenosine [Adenocard], digoxin, diltiazem [Cardizem], and verapamil [Calan]) should be avoided.

If prevention of recurrence and maintenance of sinus rhythm are warranted to maintain quality of life, disopyramide, flecainide, propafenone, sotalol, or amiodarone may be prescribed (Kellen, 2004). Angiotensin-converting enzyme (ACE) inhibitors and angiotensin receptor blockers, which block the renin–angiotensin system, have also been found to be effective in preventing the recurrence of atrial fibrillation after cardioversion (Madrid, Bueno, Rebollo, et al., 2002; Ueng, Tsai, Yu, et al., 2003). Calcium channel blockers (diltiazem [Cardizem, Dilacor, Tiazac] and verapamil [Calan, Isoptin, Verelan]) and beta-blockers (see Table 27-1) are used to control the ventricular rate in atrial fibrillation (Kellen, 2004). However, verapamil should not be given to patients with impaired ventricular function. Digoxin may be used as a second-line agent to control the ventricular rate, especially in patients with poor cardiac function (ejection fraction less than 40%) (Snow, Weiss, LeFevre, et al., 2003).

Although control of the rhythm has been the initial treatment of choice, a recent study found that controlling the heart rate (resting heart rate less than 80) is equal to controlling the rhythm in terms of mortality (AFFIRM Investigators, 2002). The study also showed a trend toward increased hospitalization in the rhythm-control group compared to the rate-control group, but this difference was not significant. In a follow-up to the AFFIRM study, beta-blockers were found to be the most effective treatment in promoting adequate rate control (Olshansky, Rosenfeld, Warner, et al., 2004).

Warfarin is indicated if the patient with atrial fibrillation is at high risk for stroke (ie, older than 75 years of age or has hypertension, diabetes, heart failure, or history of stroke). If immediate anticoagulation is necessary, the patient may be placed on heparin until the warfarin level is therapeutic. Aspirin may be substituted for warfarin in patients with contraindications to warfarin and those who are at a lower risk for stroke (without the above stroke risk factors and younger than 75 years of age). Pacemaker implantation or surgery is sometimes indicated for patients who are unresponsive to medications. Several approaches are effective in preventing the occurrence of postoperative atrial fibrillation, including preoperative administration of a beta-blocker, immediate postoperative administration of IV amiodarone, and prophylactic atrial pacing (Kern, 2004).

JUNCTIONAL DYSRHYTHMIAS

Premature Junctional Complex. A premature junctional complex is an impulse that starts in the AV nodal area before the next normal sinus impulse reaches the AV node. Premature junctional complexes are less common than PACs.

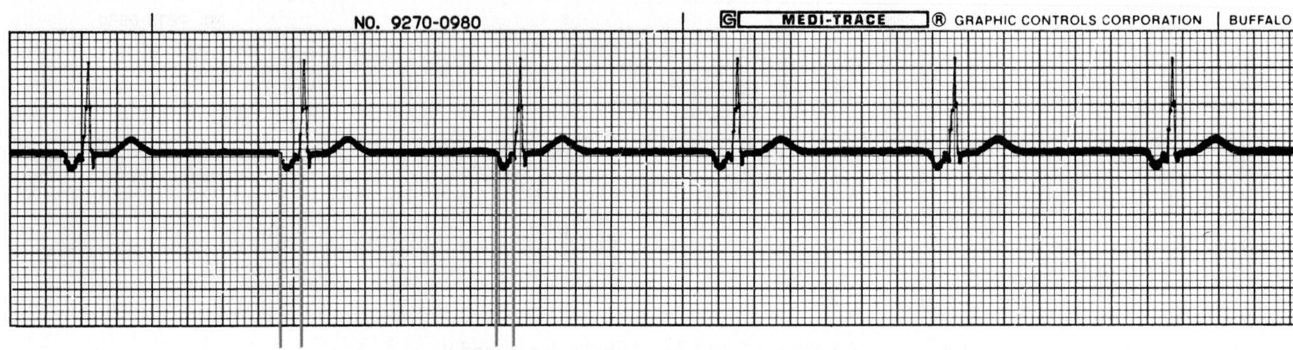

FIGURE 27-12. Junctional rhythm in lead II; note short PR intervals.

Causes of premature junctional complex include digitalis toxicity, heart failure, and coronary artery disease. The ECG criteria for premature junctional complex are the same as for PACs, except for the P wave and the PR interval. The P wave may be absent, may follow the QRS, or may occur before the QRS but with a PR interval of less than 0.12 seconds. Premature junctional complexes rarely produce significant symptoms. Treatment for frequent premature junctional complexes is the same as for frequent PACs.

Junctional Rhythm. Junctional or idionodal rhythm occurs when the AV node, instead of the sinus node, becomes the pacemaker of the heart. When the sinus node slows (eg, from increased vagal tone) or when the impulse cannot be conducted through the AV node (eg, because of complete heart block), the AV node automatically discharges an impulse. Junctional rhythm not caused by complete heart block has the following characteristics (Fig. 27-12):

Ventricular and atrial rate: Ventricular rate 40 to 60; atrial rate also 40 to 60 if P waves are discernible
Ventricular and atrial rhythm: Regular
QRS shape and duration: Usually normal, but may be abnormal
P wave: May be absent, after the QRS complex, or before the QRS; may be inverted, especially in lead II
PR interval: If the P wave is in front of the QRS, the PR interval is less than 0.12 seconds.
P:QRS ratio: 1:1 or 0:1

Junctional rhythm may produce signs and symptoms of reduced cardiac output. If this occurs, the treatment is the same as for sinus bradycardia. Emergency pacing may be needed.

Nonparoxysmal Junctional Tachycardia. Junctional tachycardia is caused by enhanced automaticity in the junctional area, resulting in a rhythm similar to junctional rhythm, except at a rate of 70 to 120. Although this rhythm generally does not have any detrimental hemodynamic effect, it may indicate a serious underlying condition, such as digitalis toxicity, myocardial ischemia, hypokalemia, or chronic obstructive pulmonary disease. Because junctional tachycardia is caused by increased automaticity, cardioversion is not an effective treatment; in fact, it causes an increase in the ventricular rate (AHA, 2005).

Atrioventricular Nodal Reentry Tachycardia. Atrioventricular nodal reentry tachycardia (AVNRT) occurs when an impulse is conducted to an area in the AV node that causes the impulse to be rerouted back into the same area over and over again at a very fast rate. Each time the impulse is conducted through this area, it is also conducted down into the ventricles, causing a fast ventricular rate. AVNRT that has an abrupt onset and an abrupt cessation with a QRS of normal duration has been termed paroxysmal atrial tachycardia (PAT). AVNRT also occurs when the duration of the QRS complex is 0.12 seconds or greater and a block in the bundle branch is known to be present. Factors associated with the development of AVNRT include caffeine, nicotine, hypoxemia, and stress. Underlying pathologies include coronary artery disease and cardiomyopathy; however, it occurs more often in females and not in association with underlying structural heart disease (Blomström-Lundqvist et al., 2003). AVNRT has the following characteristics (Fig. 27-13):

Ventricular and atrial rate: Atrial rate usually 150 to 250; ventricular rate usually 75 to 250

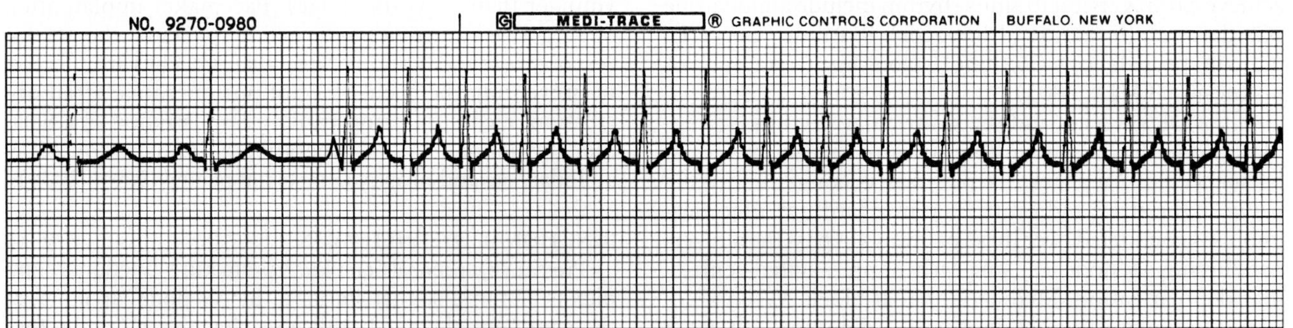

FIGURE 27-13. AV nodal reentry tachycardia in lead II.

Ventricular and atrial rhythm: Regular; sudden onset and termination of the tachycardia
QRS shape and duration: Usually normal, but may be abnormal
P wave: Usually very difficult to discern
PR interval: If the P wave is in front of the QRS, the PR interval is less than 0.12 seconds
P:QRS ratio: 1:1, 2:1

The clinical symptoms vary with the rate and duration of the tachycardia and the patient's underlying condition. The tachycardia usually is of short duration, resulting only in palpitations. A fast rate may also reduce cardiac output, resulting in significant signs and symptoms such as restlessness, chest pain, shortness of breath, pallor, hypotension, and loss of consciousness.

Treatment is aimed at breaking the reentry of the impulse. Vagal maneuvers, such as carotid sinus massage (Fig. 27-14), gag reflex, breath holding, and immersing the face in ice water, increase parasympathetic stimulation, causing slower conduction through the AV node and blocking the reentry of the rerouted impulse. Some patients have learned to use some of these methods to terminate the episode on their own. Because of the risk of a cerebral embolic event, carotid sinus massage is contraindicated in patients with carotid bruits. If the vagal maneuvers are ineffective, the patient may then receive a bolus of adenosine to correct the rhythm or diltiazem or a beta-blocker to control the rate. If the patient is unstable or does not respond to the medications, cardioversion is the treatment of choice. The unstable patient may be given adenosine while preparations for cardioversion are being made. For recurrent sustained AVNRT, the patient may be treated with verapamil, diltiazem, amiodarone, a beta-blocker, or digitalis to prevent a recurrence. Catheter ablation may be used to eliminate the area that permits the rerouting of the impulse that causes the tachycardia. If the rhythm is infrequent and there is no underlying cardiac structural disorder, the patient may be instructed to take a single oral dose of flecainide or a combination of diltiazem and propranolol during an episode of tachycardia.

If P waves cannot be identified, the rhythm may be called **supraventricular tachycardia (SVT)**, or paroxysmal supraventricular tachycardia (PSVT) if it had an abrupt onset, until the underlying rhythm and resulting diagnosis is determined. SVT and PSVT indicate only that the rhythm is not **ventricular tachycardia (VT).** SVT could be atrial fibrillation, atrial flutter, or AVNRT, among others. Vagal maneuvers and adenosine are used to convert the rhythm or at least slow conduction in the AV node to allow visualization of the P waves. If the ECG does not assist in the differentiation of the dysrhythmia, invasive electrophysiology testing may be necessary to make the diagnosis.

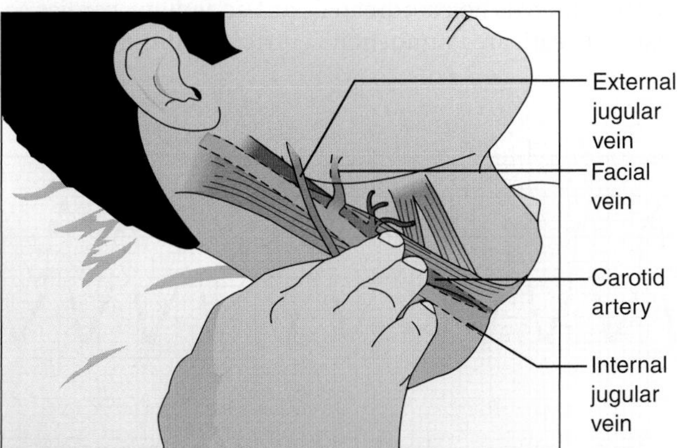

FIGURE 27-14. Carotid sinus massage.

VENTRICULAR DYSRHYTHMIAS

Premature Ventricular Complex. A premature ventricular complex (PVC) is an impulse that starts in a ventricle and is conducted through the ventricles before the next normal sinus impulse. PVCs can occur in healthy people, especially with intake of caffeine, nicotine, or alcohol. They are also caused by cardiac ischemia or infarction, increased workload on the heart (eg, exercise, fever, hypervolemia, heart failure, tachycardia), digitalis toxicity, hypoxia, acidosis, or electrolyte imbalances, especially hypokalemia.

In the absence of disease, PVCs usually are not serious. In the patient with an acute MI, PVCs may indicate the need for more aggressive therapy. In the past, PVCs were considered to be indicative of an increased risk for ensuing VT. However, PVCs that (1) are more frequent than six per minute, (2) are multifocal or polymorphic (having different shapes and rhythms), (3) occur two in a row (pair), and (4) occur on the T wave (the vulnerable period of ventricular depolarization) have not been found to be precursors of VT in patients without structural heart disease (Cardiac Arrhythmia Suppression Trial Investigators, 1989). These PVCs are no longer considered as warning or complex PVCs.

In a rhythm called bigeminy, every other complex is a PVC. In trigeminy, every third complex is a PVC, and in quadrigeminy, every fourth complex is a PVC. PVCs have the following characteristics (Fig. 27-15):

Ventricular and atrial rate: Depends on the underlying rhythm (eg, sinus rhythm)
Ventricular and atrial rhythm: Irregular due to early QRS, creating one RR interval that is shorter than the others. PP interval may be regular, indicating that the PVC did not depolarize the sinus node.
QRS shape and duration: Duration is 0.12 seconds or longer; shape is bizarre and abnormal
P wave: Visibility of P wave depends on the timing of the PVC; may be absent (hidden in the QRS or T wave) or in front of the QRS. If the P wave follows the QRS, the shape of the P wave may be different.
PR interval: If the P wave is in front of the QRS, the PR interval is less than 0.12 seconds.
P:QRS ratio: 0:1; 1:1

The patient may feel nothing or may say that the heart "skipped a beat." The effect of a PVC depends on its timing in the cardiac cycle and how much blood was in the ventricles when they contracted. Initial treatment is aimed at correcting the cause. Long-term pharmacotherapy for only PVCs is not indicated.

Ventricular Tachycardia. VT is defined as three or more PVCs in a row, occurring at a rate exceeding 100 beats per minute. The causes are similar to those of PVC. VT is usually associated with coronary artery disease and may precede ventricular fibrillation. VT is an emergency because

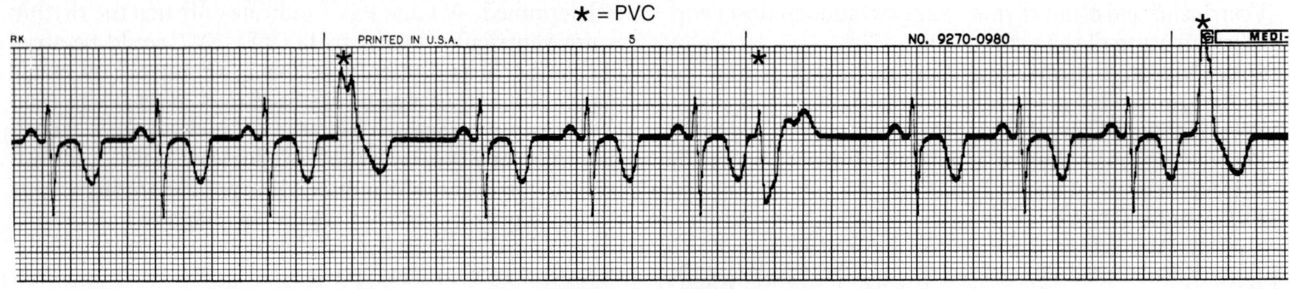

FIGURE 27-15. Multifocal premature ventricular complexes (PVCs) in quadrigeminy in lead V_1. Note regular PP interval (P wave within PVC).

the patient is usually (although not always) unresponsive and pulseless. VT has the following characteristics (Fig. 27-16):

Ventricular and atrial rate: Ventricular rate is 100 to 200 beats per minute; atrial rate depends on the underlying rhythm (eg, sinus rhythm)
Ventricular and atrial rhythm: Usually regular; atrial rhythm may also be regular
QRS shape and duration: Duration is 0.12 seconds or more; bizarre, abnormal shape
P wave: Very difficult to detect, so atrial rate and rhythm may be indeterminable
PR interval: Very irregular, if P waves are seen
P:QRS ratio: Difficult to determine, but if P waves are apparent, there are usually more QRS complexes than P waves

The patient's tolerance or lack of tolerance for this rapid rhythm depends on the ventricular rate and underlying disease. Several factors determine the initial treatment, including the following: identifying the rhythm as monomorphic (having a consistent QRS shape and rate) or polymorphic (having varying QRS shapes and rhythms); determining the existence of a prolonged QT interval before the initiation of VT; and ascertaining the patient's heart function (normal or decreased). If the patient is stable, continuing the assessment, especially obtaining a 12-lead ECG, may be the only action necessary. Amiodarone administered IV is the antidysrhythmic medication of choice for a stable patient with VT. Other medications that may be used are procainamide (Pronestyl) and sotalol (Betapace). Although lidocaine (Xylocaine) has been the medication most commonly used for immediate, short-term therapy, it has no proven short- or long-term efficacy in cardiac arrest (AHA, 2005). Cardioversion is the treatment of choice for monophasic VT in a symptomatic patient. Atrial fibrillation should be suspected as the cause of a VT with an irregular rhythm, and it should be treated appropriately. Torsades de pointes is a polymorphic VT preceded by a prolonged QT interval. Because this rhythm is likely to cause the patient to deteriorate and become pulseless, immediate treatment is required: correction of any electrolyte imbalance, administration of isoproterenol (Isuprel) IV, or initiation of ventricular pacing. Magnesium has frequently been used to treat torsades, but its use has not been proven effective (AHA, 2005). Any type of VT in a patient who is unconscious and without a pulse is treated in the same manner as ventricular fibrillation: immediate **defibrillation** is the action of choice.

Ventricular Fibrillation. Ventricular fibrillation is a rapid, disorganized ventricular rhythm that causes ineffective quivering of the ventricles. No atrial activity is seen on the ECG. Causes of ventricular fibrillation are the same as for VT; it may also result from untreated or unsuccessfully treated VT. Other causes include electrical shock and Brugada syndrome, in which the patient (frequently of Asian descent) has a structurally normal heart, few or no risk factors for coronary artery disease, and a family history of sudden cardiac death. Ventricular fibrillation has the following characteristics (Fig. 27-17):

Ventricular rate: Greater than 300 per minute
Ventricular rhythm: Extremely irregular, without a specific pattern
QRS shape and duration: Irregular, undulating waves without recognizable QRS complexes

This dysrhythmia is always characterized by the absence of an audible heartbeat, a palpable pulse, and respirations. Because there is no coordinated cardiac activity, cardiac arrest and death are imminent if ventricular fibrillation is not

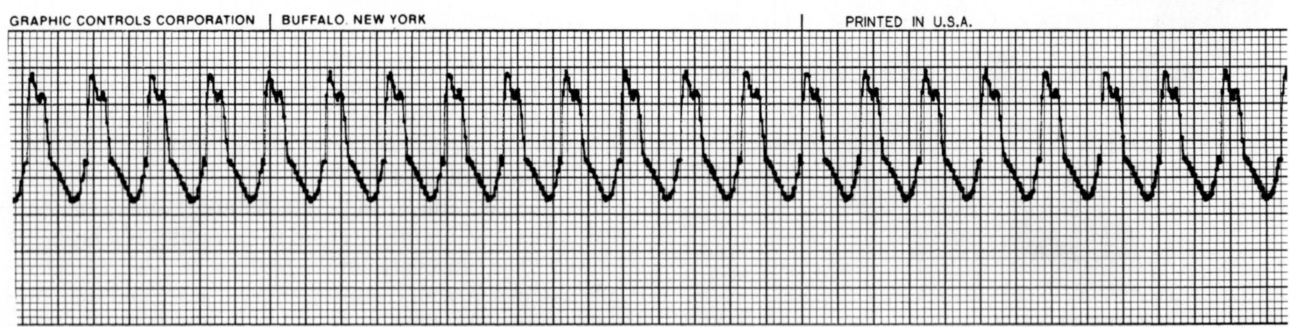

FIGURE 27-16. Ventricular tachycardia in lead V_1.

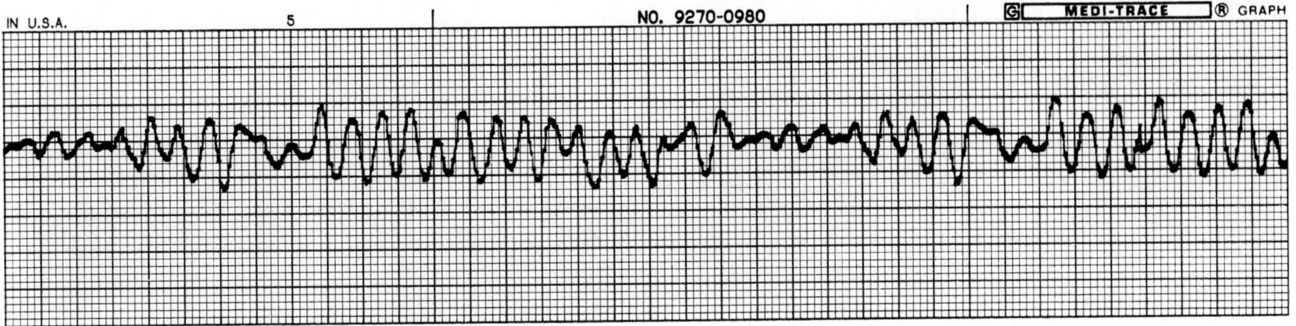

FIGURE 27-17. Ventricular fibrillation in lead II.

corrected. Treatment of choice is immediate bystander cardiopulmonary resuscitation (CPR), defibrillation as soon as possible, and activation of emergency services. If the arrest was not witnessed or there was more than a 4-minute delay in emergency services response, five cycles of CPR may be given prior to defibrillation (AHA, 2005). After the initial defibrillation, five cycles of CPR alternating with a rhythm check and defibrillation are the treatments used to convert ventricular fibrillation to an electrical rhythm that produces a pulse. Vasoactive medications (epinephrine, vasopressin, or both) should be administered as soon as possible after the second rhythm check (immediately before or after the second defibrillation). Antidysrhythmic medications (amiodarone, lidocaine, or possibly magnesium) should be administered as soon as possible after the third rhythm check (immediately before or after the third defibrillation). However, once the patient is intubated, CPR should be given continuously, not in cycles, and the rhythm check and medication administration occur every 2 minutes. In addition, underlying and contributing factors are identified and eliminated throughout the event (AHA, 2005).

Inducing hypothermia after a cardiac arrest from ventricular fibrillation was found to be beneficial to neurological outcomes in a select subset of patients. Therefore, current AHA guidelines now recommend inducing mild hypothermia for 12–24 hours in unconscious adults who experience cardiac arrest due to ventricular fibrillation. Hypothermia is defined as a core body temperature of 32°C–34°C (89.6°F–93.2°F). Further studies are needed to determine if hypothermia may be beneficial to other subsets of patients, as well as if the use of other methods of cooling may make this type of therapy more widely beneficial (American Heart Association, 2005).

A nurse caring for a patient with hypothermia (passive or induced) needs to monitor for its complications: pneumonia, sepsis, hyperglycemia, dysrhythmias, and coagulopathy, especially if the temperature drops below the intended goal.

Idioventricular Rhythm. Idioventricular rhythm, also called ventricular escape rhythm, occurs when the impulse starts in the conduction system below the AV node. When the sinus node fails to create an impulse (eg, from increased vagal tone) or when the impulse is created but cannot be conducted through the AV node (eg, due to complete AV block), the Purkinje fibers automatically discharge an impulse. When idioventricular rhythm is not caused by AV block, it has the following characteristics (Fig. 27-18):

Ventricular rate: 20 and 40; if the rate exceeds 40, the rhythm is known as accelerated idioventricular rhythm (AIVR)
Ventricular rhythm: Regular
QRS shape and duration: Bizarre, abnormal shape; duration is 0.12 seconds or more

Idioventricular rhythm commonly causes the patient to lose consciousness and experience other signs and symptoms of reduced cardiac output. In such cases, the treatment is the same as for asystole and pulseless electrical activity (PEA) if the patient is in cardiac arrest or for bradycardia if the patient is not in cardiac arrest. Interventions include identifying the underlying cause, administering IV atropine and vasopressor medications, and initiating emergency transcutaneous pacing. In some cases, idioventricular rhythm may cause no symptoms of reduced cardiac output. However, bed rest is prescribed so as not to increase the cardiac workload.

Ventricular Asystole. Commonly called flatline, ventricular asystole (Fig. 27-19) is characterized by absent QRS complexes confirmed in two different leads, although P waves may be apparent for a short duration. There is no heartbeat,

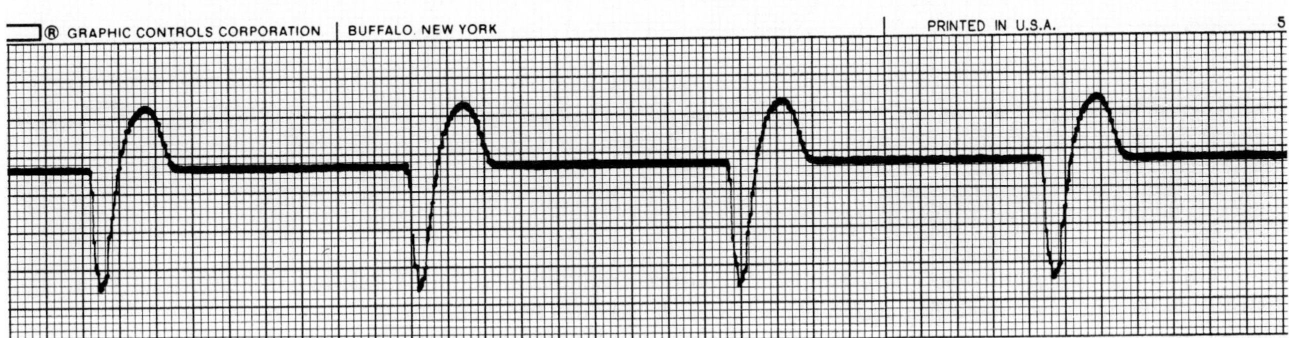

FIGURE 27-18. Idioventricular rhythm in lead V_1.

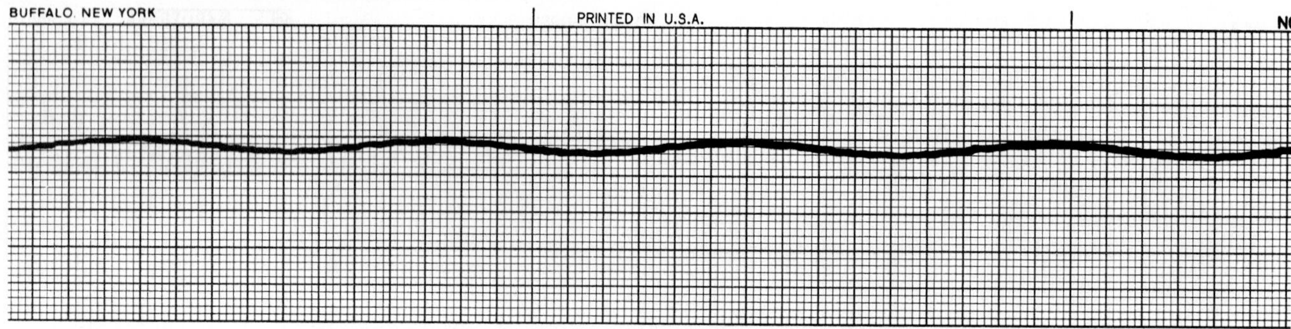

FIGURE 27-19. Asystole. Always check two different leads to confirm rhythm.

no palpable pulse, and no respiration. Without immediate treatment, ventricular asystole is fatal. Ventricular asystole is treated the same as PEA, focusing on high-quality CPR with minimal interruptions and identifying underlying and contributing factors. The guidelines for advanced cardiac life support (AHA, 2005) state that the key to successful treatment is rapid assessment to identify a possible cause, which may be hypoxia, acidosis, severe electrolyte imbalance, drug overdose, hypovolemia, cardiac tamponade, tension pneumothorax, coronary or pulmonary thrombosis, trauma, or hypothermia. After the initiation of CPR, intubation and establishment of IV access are the next recommended actions, with no or minimal interruptions in chest compressions. After 2 minutes or five cycles of CPR, a bolus of IV epinephrine is administered and repeated at 3- to 5-minute intervals. One dose of vasopressin may be administered for the first or second dose of epinephrine. A 1-mg bolus of IV atropine may also be administered as soon as possible after the rhythm check (AHA, 2005). Because of the poor prognosis associated with asystole, if the patient does not respond to these actions and others aimed at correcting underlying causes, resuscitation efforts are usually ended ("the code is called") unless special circumstances (eg, hypothermia, transportation to a hospital is required) exist.

CONDUCTION ABNORMALITIES

When assessing the rhythm strip, the underlying rhythm is first identified (eg, sinus rhythm, sinus arrhythmia). Then the PR interval is assessed for the possibility of an AV block. AV blocks occur when the conduction of the impulse through the AV nodal area is decreased or stopped. These blocks can be caused by medications (eg, digitalis, calcium channel blockers, beta-blockers), myocardial ischemia and infarction, valvular disorders, or myocarditis. If the AV block is caused by increased vagal tone (eg, suctioning, pressure above the eyes or on large vessels, anal stimulation), it is commonly accompanied by sinus bradycardia.

The clinical signs and symptoms of a heart block vary with the resulting ventricular rate and the severity of any underlying disease processes. Whereas first-degree AV block rarely causes any hemodynamic effect, the other blocks may result in decreased heart rate, causing a decrease in perfusion to vital organs, such as the brain, heart, kidneys, lungs, and skin. A patient with third-degree AV block caused by digitalis toxicity may be stable; another patient with the same rhythm caused by acute MI may be unstable. Health care providers must always keep in mind the need to treat the patient, not the rhythm. The treatment is based on the hemodynamic effect of the rhythm.

First-Degree Atrioventricular Block. First-degree AV block occurs when all the atrial impulses are conducted through the AV node into the ventricles at a rate slower than normal. This conduction disorder has the following characteristics (Fig. 27-20):

Ventricular and atrial rate: Depends on the underlying rhythm
Ventricular and atrial rhythm: Depends on the underlying rhythm
QRS shape and duration: Usually normal, but may be abnormal
P wave: In front of the QRS complex; shows sinus rhythm, regular shape

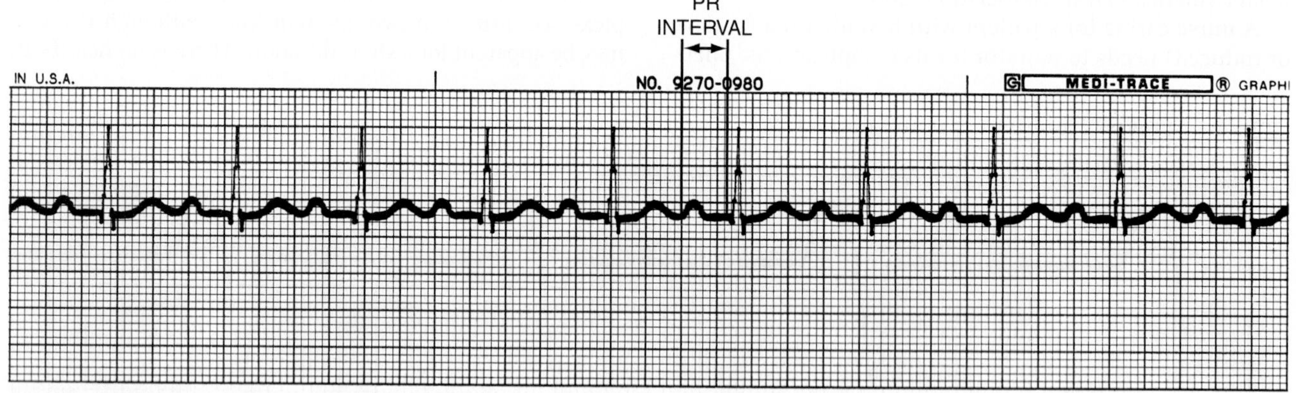

FIGURE 27-20. Sinus rhythm with first-degree AV block in lead II. Note that PR is constant but greater than 0.20 seconds.

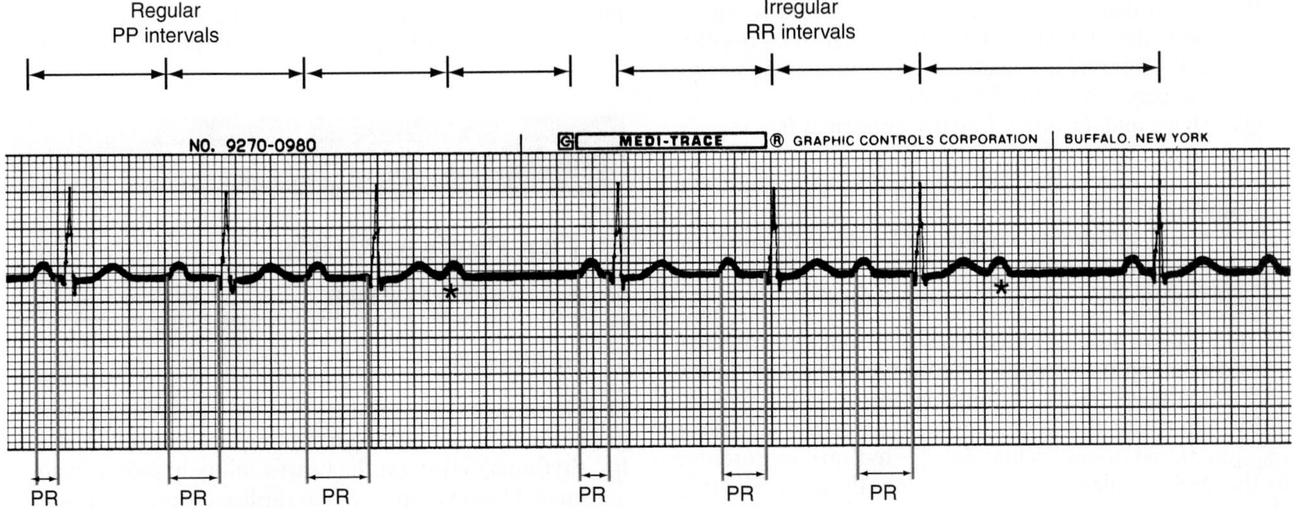

FIGURE 27-21. Sinus rhythm with second-degree AV block, type I in lead II. Note progressively longer PR durations until there is a nonconducted P wave, indicated by the asterisk.

PR interval: Greater than 0.20 seconds; PR interval measurement is constant

P:QRS ratio: 1:1

Second-Degree Atrioventricular Block, Type I. Second-degree AV block, type I, occurs when there is a repeating pattern in which all but one of a series of atrial impulses are conducted through the AV node into the ventricles (eg, every four of five atrial impulses are conducted). Each atrial impulse takes a longer time for conduction than the one before, until one impulse is fully blocked. Because the AV node is not depolarized by the blocked atrial impulse, the AV node has time to fully repolarize, so that the next atrial impulse can be conducted within the shortest amount of time. Second-degree AV block, type I, has the following characteristics (Fig. 27-21):

Ventricular and atrial rate: Depends on the underlying rhythm

Ventricular and atrial rhythm: The PP interval is regular if the patient has an underlying normal sinus rhythm; the RR interval characteristically reflects a pattern of change. Starting from the RR that is the longest, the RR interval gradually shortens until there is another long RR interval.

QRS shape and duration: Usually normal but may be abnormal

P wave: In front of the QRS complex; shape depends on underlying rhythm

PR interval: PR interval becomes longer with each succeeding ECG complex until there is a P wave not followed by a QRS. The changes in the PR interval are repeated between each "dropped" QRS, creating a pattern in the irregular PR interval measurements.

P:QRS ratio: 3:2, 4:3, 5:4, and so forth

Second-Degree Atrioventricular Block, Type II. Second-degree AV block, type II, occurs when only some of the atrial impulses are conducted through the AV node into the ventricles. Second-degree AV block, type II, has the following characteristics (Fig. 27-22):

Ventricular and atrial rate: Depends on the underlying rhythm

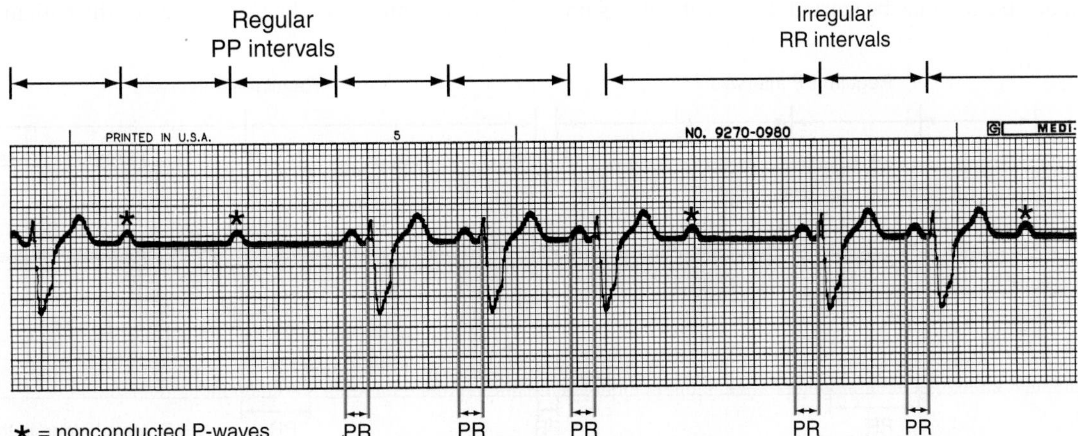

FIGURE 27-22. Sinus rhythm with second-degree AV block, type II in lead V_1; note constant PR interval and presence of more P waves than QRS complexes.

Ventricular and atrial rhythm: The PP interval is regular if the patient has an underlying normal sinus rhythm. The RR interval is usually regular but may be irregular, depending on the P:QRS ratio.
QRS shape and duration: Usually abnormal but may be normal
P wave: In front of the QRS complex; shape depends on underlying rhythm
PR interval: PR interval is constant for those P waves just before QRS complexes.
P:QRS ratio: 2:1, 3:1, 4:1, 5:1, and so forth

Third-Degree Atrioventricular Block. Third-degree AV block occurs when no atrial impulse is conducted through the AV node into the ventricles. In third-degree AV block, two impulses stimulate the heart: one stimulates the ventricles (eg, junctional or ventricular escape rhythm), represented by the QRS complex, and one stimulates the atria (eg, sinus rhythm, atrial fibrillation), represented by the P wave. P waves may be seen, but the atrial electrical activity is not conducted down into the ventricles to cause the QRS complex, the ventricular electrical activity. This is called AV dissociation. Complete block (third-degree AV block) has the following characteristics (Fig. 27-23):

Ventricular and atrial rate: Depends on the escape and underlying atrial rhythm
Ventricular and atrial rhythm: The PP interval is regular and the RR interval is regular, but the PP interval is not equal to the RR interval.
QRS shape and duration: Depends on the escape rhythm; in junctional escape, QRS shape and duration are usually normal, and in ventricular escape, QRS shape and duration are usually abnormal
P wave: Depends on underlying rhythm
PR interval: Very irregular
P:QRS ratio: More P waves than QRS complexes

Based on the cause of the AV block and the stability of the patient, treatment is directed toward increasing the heart rate to maintain a normal cardiac output. If the patient is stable and has no symptoms, no treatment is indicated other than decreasing or eliminating the cause (eg, withholding the medication or treatment). If the patient is short of breath or has chest pain, lightheadedness, or low blood pressure, an IV bolus of atropine is the initial treatment of choice. If the patient does not respond to atropine or has had an acute MI, transcutaneous pacing may be started. If the patient has no pulse, treatment is the same as for ventricular asystole. A permanent pacemaker may be necessary if the block persists.

Nursing Process

The Patient With a Dysrhythmia

Assessment

Major areas of assessment include possible causes of the dysrhythmia, contributing factors, and the dysrhythmia's effect on the heart's ability to pump an adequate blood volume. When cardiac output is reduced, the amount of oxygen reaching the tissues and vital organs is diminished. This diminished oxygenation produces the signs and symptoms associated with dysrhythmias. If these signs and symptoms are severe or if they occur frequently, the patient may experience significant distress and disruption of daily life.

A health history is obtained to identify any previous occurrences of decreased cardiac output, such as syncope (fainting), lightheadedness, dizziness, fatigue, chest discomfort, and palpitations. Coexisting conditions that could be a possible cause of the dysrhythmia (eg, heart disease, chronic obstructive pulmonary disease) may also be identified. All medications, prescribed and over-the-counter (including herbs and nutritional supplements), as well as the route of administration, are reviewed. Some medications (eg, digoxin) can cause dysrhythmias. Laboratory results are reviewed to assess levels of medications as well as factors that could contribute to the dysrhythmia (eg, anemia). A thorough psychosocial assessment is performed to identify the possible effects of the dysrhythmia, the patient's perception of the dysrhythmia, and whether anxiety is a significant contributing factor.

The nurse conducts a physical assessment to confirm the data obtained from the history and to observe for signs of diminished cardiac output during the dysrhythmic event, especially changes in level of consciousness. The nurse assesses the patient's skin,

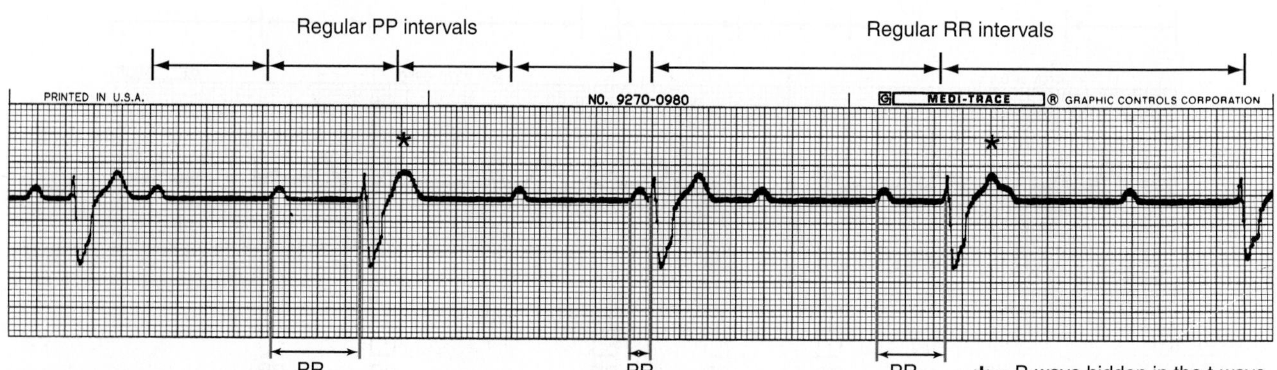

FIGURE 27-23. Sinus rhythm with third-degree AV block and idioventricular rhythm in lead V_1; note irregular PR intervals.

which may be pale and cool. Signs of fluid retention, such as neck vein distention and crackles and wheezes auscultated in the lungs, may be detected. The rate and rhythm of apical and peripheral pulses are also assessed, and any pulse deficit is noted. The nurse auscultates for extra heart sounds (especially S_3 and S_4) and for heart murmurs, measures blood pressure, and determines pulse pressures. A declining pulse pressure indicates reduced cardiac output. Just one assessment may not disclose significant changes in cardiac output; therefore, the nurse compares multiple assessment findings over time, especially those that occur with and without the dysrhythmia.

Diagnosis

Nursing Diagnoses

Based on assessment data, major nursing diagnoses of the patient may include:

- Decreased cardiac output
- Anxiety related to fear of the unknown
- Deficient knowledge about the dysrhythmia and its treatment

Collaborative Problems/ Potential Complications

Based on the assessment data, potential complications that may develop include the following:

- Cardiac arrest (see Chapter 30)
- Heart failure (see Chapter 30)
- Thromboembolic event, especially with atrial fibrillation (see Chapter 30)

Planning and Goals

The major goals for the patient may include eliminating or decreasing the occurrence of the dysrhythmia (by decreasing contributory factors) to maintain cardiac output, minimizing anxiety, and acquiring knowledge about the dysrhythmia and its treatment.

Nursing Interventions

Monitoring and Managing the Dysrhythmia

The nurse regularly evaluates the patient's blood pressure, pulse rate and rhythm, rate and depth of respirations, and breath sounds to determine the dysrhythmia's hemodynamic effect. The nurse also asks the patient about episodes of lightheadedness, dizziness, or fainting as part of the ongoing assessment. If a patient with a dysrhythmia is hospitalized, the nurse may obtain a 12-lead ECG, continuously monitor the patient, and analyze rhythm strips to track the dysrhythmia.

Control of the occurrence or the effect of the dysrhythmia, or both, is often achieved by the use of **antiarrhythmic** medications. The nurse assesses and observes for the beneficial and adverse effects of each medication. The nurse also manages medication administration carefully so that a constant serum blood level of the medication is maintained. The nurse may also administer a 6-minute walk test, which is used to identify the patient's ventricular rate in response to exercise. The patient is asked to walk for 6 minutes, covering as much distance as possible. The nurse monitors the patient for symptoms. At the end, the nurse records the distance covered and the pre- and postexercise heart rate as well as the patient's response (Kellen, 2004).

In addition to medication, the nurse assesses for factors that contribute to the dysrhythmia (eg, caffeine, stress, nonadherence to the medication regimen) and assists the patient in developing a plan to make lifestyle changes that eliminate or reduce these factors.

Minimizing Anxiety

When the patient experiences episodes of dysrhythmia, the nurse maintains a calm and reassuring attitude. This assists in reducing anxiety (reducing the sympathetic response) and fosters a trusting relationship with the patient. Successes are emphasized with the patient to promote a sense of self-management of the dysrhythmia. For example, if a patient is experiencing episodes of dysrhythmia and a medication is administered that begins to reduce the incidence of the dysrhythmia, the nurse communicates that information to the patient. In addition, the nurse can help the patient develop a system to identify possible causative, influencing, and alleviating factors (eg, keeping a diary). The nursing goal is to maximize the patient's control and to make the episode less threatening.

Promoting Home and Community-Based Care

TEACHING PATIENTS SELF-CARE

When teaching patients about dysrhythmias, the nurse presents the information in terms that are understandable and in a manner that is not frightening or threatening. The nurse explains the importance of maintaining therapeutic serum levels of antiarrhythmic medications so that the patient understands why medications should be taken regularly each day. In addition, the relationship between a dysrhythmia and cardiac output is explained so that the patient understands the rationale for the medical regimen. If the patient has a potentially lethal dysrhythmia, it is also important to establish with the patient and family a plan of action to take in case of an emergency. The patient and family should also be taught about potential effects of the dysrhythmia and their signs and symptoms. For example, the patient with chronic atrial fibrillation should be taught about the possibility of an embolic event. This information allows the patient and family to feel more in control and better prepared for possible events.

CONTINUING CARE

A referral for home care usually is not necessary for the patient with a dysrhythmia unless the patient is hemodynamically unstable and has significant symptoms of decreased cardiac output. Home care is also warranted if the patient has significant comorbidities, socioeconomic issues, or limited self-management skills that could increase the risk for nonadherence to the therapeutic regimen.

Evaluation

Expected Patient Outcomes

Expected patient outcomes may include:

1. Maintains cardiac output
   a. Demonstrates heart rate, blood pressure, respiratory rate, and level of consciousness within normal ranges
   b. Demonstrates no or decreased episodes of dysrhythmia
2. Experiences reduced anxiety
   a. Expresses a positive attitude about living with the dysrhythmia
   b. Expresses confidence in ability to take appropriate actions in an emergency
3. Expresses understanding of the dysrhythmia and its treatment
   a. Explains the dysrhythmia and its effects
   b. Describes the medication regimen and its rationale
   c. Explains the need to maintain a therapeutic serum level of the medication
   d. Describes a plan to eliminate or limit factors that contribute to the dysrhythmia
   e. States actions to take in the event of an emergency

Adjunctive Modalities and Management

Dysrhythmia treatments depend on whether the disorder is acute or chronic as well as on the cause of the dysrhythmia and its actual or potential hemodynamic effects.

Acute dysrhythmias may be treated with medications or with external electrical therapy (emergency defibrillation, cardioversion, or pacing). Many antiarrhythmic medications are used to treat atrial and ventricular tachydysrhythmias (see Table 27-1). The choice of medication depends on the specific dysrhythmia and its duration, the presence of heart failure and other diseases, and the patient's response to previous treatment. The nurse is responsible for monitoring and documenting the patient's responses to the medication and for ensuring that the patient has the knowledge and ability to manage the medication regimen.

If medications alone are ineffective in eliminating or decreasing the dysrhythmia, certain adjunctive mechanical therapies are available. The most common are elective cardioversion and defibrillation for acute tachydysrhythmia, and implantable devices (pacemakers for bradycardias and internal cardiodefibrillators for chronic tachydysrhythmias). Surgical treatments, although less common, are also available. The nurse is responsible for assessing the patient's understanding of and response to mechanical therapy, as well as the patient's self-management abilities. The nurse explains that the purpose of the device is to help the patient lead an active and productive life as his or her overall health allows.

Cardioversion and Defibrillation

Cardioversion and defibrillation are used to treat tachydysrhythmias by delivering an electrical current that depolarizes a critical mass of myocardial cells. When the cells repolarize, the sinus node is usually able to recapture its role as the heart's pacemaker. One major difference between cardioversion and defibrillation is the timing of the delivery of electrical current. In cardioversion, the delivery of the electrical current is synchronized with the patient's electrical events; in defibrillation, the delivery of the current is immediate and unsynchronized.

The electrical current may be delivered externally through the skin with the use of paddles or with conductor pads. Both paddles may be placed on the front of the chest (Fig. 27-24) (standard paddle placement), or one paddle may be placed on the front of the chest and the other connected to an adapter with a long handle and placed under the patient's back (anteroposterior placement) (Fig. 27-25).

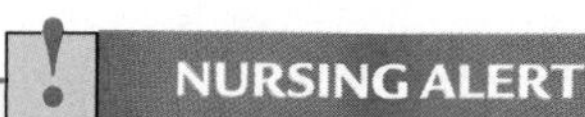

When using paddles, the appropriate conductant is applied between the paddles and the patient's skin. Any other type of conductant, such as ultrasound gel, should not be substituted.

Instead of paddles, defibrillator multifunction conductor pads may be used (Fig. 27-26). The pads, which contain a conductive medium, are placed in the same position as the paddles. They are connected to the defibrillator and allow for hands-off defibrillation. This method reduces the risk of touching the patient during the procedure and increases electrical safety. Automatic external defibrillators (AEDs), which are now found in public areas such as airports and grocery stores, use this type of delivery for the electrical current.

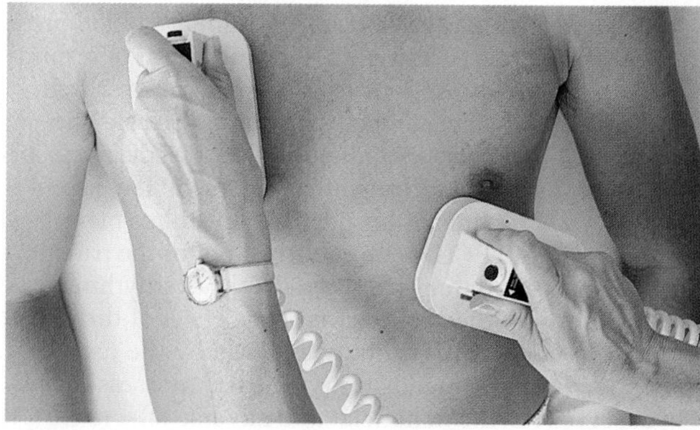

FIGURE 27-24. Standard paddle placement for defibrillation.

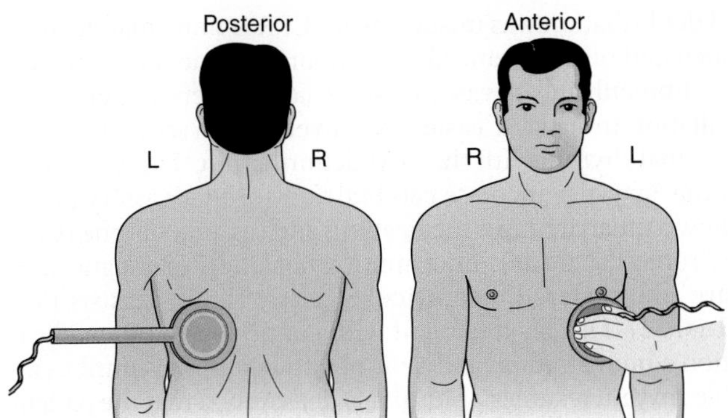

FIGURE 27-25. Anteroposterior paddle placement for defibrillation.

Whether using pads or paddles, the nurse must observe two safety measures. First, good contact must be maintained between the pads or paddles and the patient's skin (with a conductive medium in between them) to prevent electrical current from leaking into the air (arcing) when the defibrillator is discharged. Second, no one is to be in contact with the patient or with anything that is touching the patient when the defibrillator is discharged, to minimize the chance that electrical current will be conducted to anyone other than the patient.

When assisting with external defibrillation or cardioversion, the nurse should remember these key points:

- Use multifunction conductor pads or paddles with a conducting medium between the paddles and the skin (the conducting medium is available as a sheet, gel, or paste). Do not use gels or pastes with poor electrical conductivity (eg, ultrasound gel) (AHA, 2005).
- Place paddles or pads so that they do not touch the patient's clothing or bed linen and are not near medication patches or direct oxygen flow.
- If cardioverting, ensure that the monitor leads are attached to the patient and that the defibrillator is in the synchronized mode ("in sync"). If defibrillating, ensure that the defibrillator is *not* in the synchronized mode (most machines default to the "not-sync" mode).
- If using paddles, exert 20 to 25 pounds of pressure to ensure good skin contact.
- If using a manual discharge device, do not charge the device until ready to shock; then keep thumbs and fingers off the discharge buttons until paddles or pads are on the chest and ready to deliver the electrical charge.
- Before pressing the discharge button, call "Clear!" three times: As "Clear" is called the first time, ensure that you are not touching the patient, bed, or equipment; as "Clear" is called the second time, ensure that no one is touching the bed, the patient, or equipment, including the endotracheal tube or adjuncts; and as "Clear" is called the third time, perform a final visual check to ensure that you and everyone else are clear of the patient and anything touching the patient.
- Record the delivered energy.
- After the defibrillation, immediately resume CPR, starting with chest compressions.
- After five cycles (about 2 minutes) of CPR, check the cardiac rhythm and deliver another shock if indicated. Administer a vasoactive or antidysrhythmic medication as soon as possible after the rhythm check.
- After the event is complete, inspect the skin under the pads or paddles for burns; if any are detected, consult with the physician or a wound care nurse about treatment.

Electrical Cardioversion

Electrical **cardioversion** involves the delivery of a "timed" electrical current to terminate a tachydysrhythmia. In cardioversion, the defibrillator is set to synchronize with the ECG on a cardiac monitor so that the electrical impulse discharges during ventricular depolarization (QRS complex). The synchronization prevents the discharge from occurring during the vulnerable period of repolarization (T wave), which could result in VT or ventricular fibrillation. The ECG monitor connected to the external defibrillator usually displays a mark or line that indicates sensing of a QRS complex. Sometimes the lead and the electrodes must be changed for the monitor to recognize the patient's QRS complex. When the synchronizer is on, no electrical current is delivered if the defibrillator does not discern a QRS complex. Because there may be a short delay until recognition of the

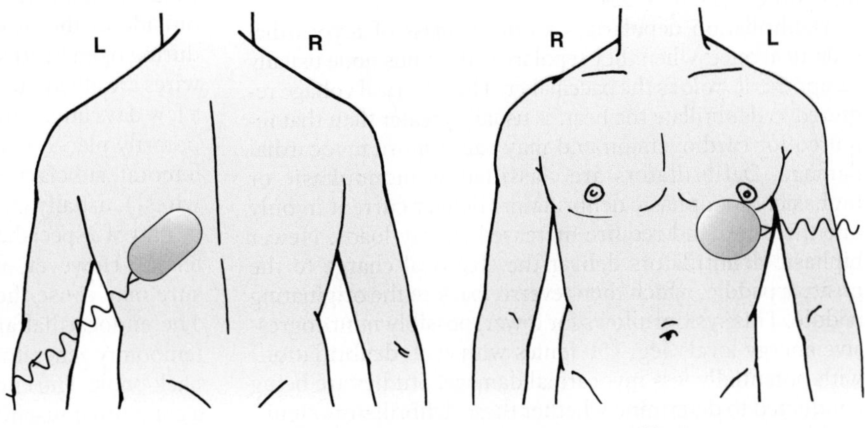

FIGURE 27-26. Multifunction pads for defibrillation.

QRS, the discharge buttons of an external defibrillator must be held down until the shock has been delivered.

If the cardioversion is elective and the dysrhythmia has lasted longer than 48 hours, anticoagulation for a few weeks before cardioversion may be indicated. Digoxin is usually withheld for 48 hours before cardioversion to ensure the resumption of sinus rhythm with normal conduction. The patient is instructed not to eat or drink for at least 4 hours before the procedure. Gel-covered paddles or conductor pads are positioned front and back (anteroposteriorly) for cardioversion. Before cardioversion, the patient receives IV moderate sedation as well as an analgesic medication or anesthesia. Respiration is then supported with supplemental oxygen delivered by a bag-mask-valve device with suction equipment readily available. Although patients rarely require intubation, equipment is nearby if it is needed. The amount of voltage used varies from 50 to 360 joules, depending on the defibrillator's technology and the type of dysrhythmia. If ventricular fibrillation occurs after cardioversion, the defibrillator is used to defibrillate the patient (sync mode is *not* used).

Indications of a successful response are conversion to sinus rhythm, adequate peripheral pulses, and adequate blood pressure. Because of the sedation, airway patency must be maintained and the patient's state of consciousness assessed. Vital signs and oxygen saturation are monitored and recorded until the patient is stable and recovered from sedation and analgesic medications or anesthesia. ECG monitoring is required during and after cardioversion.

Defibrillation

Defibrillation is used in emergency situations as the treatment of choice for ventricular fibrillation and pulseless VT, the most common cause of abrupt loss of cardiac function and sudden cardiac death. Defibrillation is not used on patients who are conscious or have a pulse. The sooner defibrillation is used, the better the survival rate: if it is used within 1 minute of the onset of VT or fibrillation, the survival rate is 90%; if it is delayed for 12 minutes, the survival rate is only 2% to 5%. A recent study demonstrated that early defibrillation performed by laypeople in a community setting can increase the survival rate (Hallstrom, Ornato, Weisfeldt, et al., 2004). If immediate CPR is provided and defibrillation is performed within 5 minutes, many adults in ventricular fibrillation may survive with intact neurologic function (AHA, 2005).

Defibrillation depolarizes a critical mass of myocardial cells all at once; when they repolarize, the sinus node usually recaptures its role as the pacemaker. The electrical voltage required to defibrillate the heart is usually greater than that required for cardioversion and may cause more myocardial damage. Defibrillators are classified as monophasic or biphasic. Monophasic defibrillators deliver current in only one direction and require increased energy loads. Newer biphasic defibrillators deliver the electrical charge to the positive paddle, which then reverses back to the originating paddle. This system allows for lower, possibly nonprogressive energy levels (eg, 150 joules with each defibrillation) with potentially less myocardial damage. Studies are being conducted to determine whether these defibrillators significantly improve outcomes (Adgey, Spence, & Walsh, 2005).

If defibrillation was unsuccessful, CPR is immediately initiated and other advanced life support treatments are begun.

Epinephrine or vasopressin is administered after defibrillation to make it easier to convert the dysrhythmia to a normal rhythm with the next defibrillation. These medications may also increase cerebral and coronary artery blood flow. Antiarrhythmic medications such as amiodarone (Cordarone, Pacerone), lidocaine (Xylocaine), or magnesium are administered if ventricular dysrhythmia persists (see Table 27-1). This treatment with continuous CPR, medication administration, and defibrillation continues until a stable rhythm resumes or until it is determined that the patient cannot be revived.

Pacemaker Therapy

A pacemaker is an electronic device that provides electrical stimuli to the heart muscle. Pacemakers are usually used when a patient has a slower-than-normal impulse formation or a symptomatic AV or ventricular conduction disturbance. They may also be used to control some tachydysrhythmias that do not respond to medication. Biventricular (both ventricles) pacing may be used to treat advanced heart failure that does not respond to medication. Pacemaker technology also may be used in an implantable cardioverter defibrillator (eg, in patients with coronary artery disease and a reduced ejection fraction). (See Chapter 30 for further discussion of heart failure.)

Pacemakers can be permanent or temporary. Temporary pacemakers are used to support patients until they improve or receive a permanent pacemaker (eg, after acute MI or during open heart surgery).

Pacemaker Design and Types

Pacemakers consist of two components: an electronic pulse generator and pacemaker electrodes, which are located on leads or wires. The generator contains the circuitry and batteries that determine the rate (measured in beats per minute) and the strength or output (measured in milliamperes [mA]) of the electrical stimulus delivered to the heart. The generator also can detect the heart's electrical activity to cause an appropriate response; this component of pacing is called sensitivity and is measured in millivolts (mV). Leads can be threaded through a major vein into the right ventricle (endocardial leads), or they can be lightly sutured onto the outside of the heart and brought through the chest wall during open heart surgery (epicardial wires). The epicardial wires are always temporary and are removed by a gentle tug a few days after surgery. The endocardial leads may be temporarily placed with catheters through a vein (usually the femoral, subclavian, or internal jugular vein [transvenous wires]), usually guided by fluoroscopy. The leads may also be part of a specialized pulmonary artery catheter (see Chapter 30). However, obtaining a pulmonary artery wedge pressure may cause the leads to move out of pacing position. The endocardial and epicardial wires are connected to a temporary generator, which is about the size of a small paperback book. The energy source for a temporary generator is a common household battery. This type of pacemaker therapy necessitates short-term hospitalization of the patient.

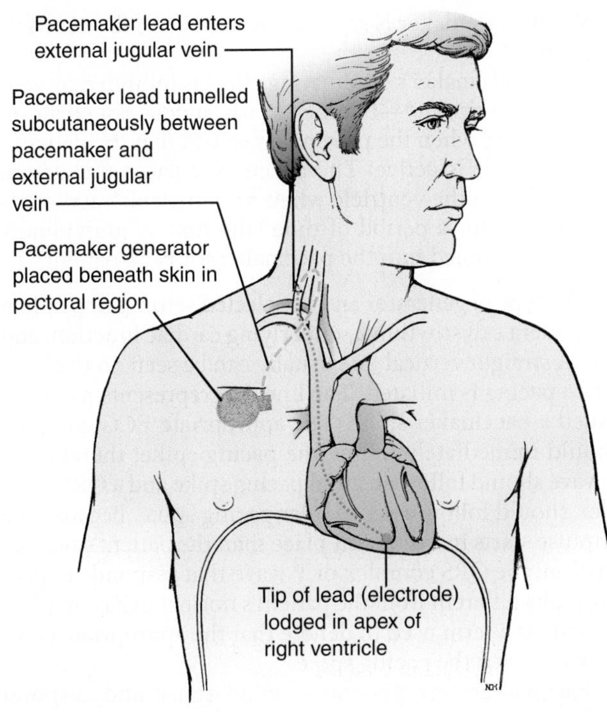

FIGURE 27-27. Implanted transvenous pacing lead (with electrode) and pacemaker generator.

Monitoring for pacemaker malfunctioning and battery failure is a nursing responsibility.

The endocardial leads also may be placed permanently, usually through the external jugular vein, and connected to a permanent generator. The generator, which often weighs less than 1 oz, is usually implanted in a subcutaneous pocket created in the pectoral region or below the clavicle (Fig. 27-27). Sometimes an abdominal site is selected. This procedure usually takes about 1 hour, and it is performed in a cardiac catheterization laboratory using a local anesthetic. Permanent pacemaker generators are insulated to protect against body moisture and warmth. While several different energy sources for permanent generators have been used and others have been investigated, lithium cell units are most often used today, and they last approximately 10 years. Some batteries are rechargeable. If the battery is not rechargeable and failure is impending, the leads are disconnected, the old generator is removed, and the new generator is reconnected to the existing leads and reimplanted in the already existing subcutaneous pocket. Battery replacement also is usually performed using a local anesthetic. Hospitalization is necessary for implantation or battery replacement; the patient usually can be discharged the next day.

If a patient suddenly develops a bradycardia, is symptomatic but has a pulse, and is unresponsive to atropine, emergency pacing may be started with transcutaneous pacing, which most defibrillators are now equipped to perform. Automatic external defibrillators (AEDs) are not able to do transcutaneous pacing. Large pacing ECG electrodes (sometimes the same conductive pads used for cardioversion and defibrillation) are placed on the patient's chest and back. The electrodes are connected to the defibrillator, which is the temporary pacemaker generator (Fig. 27-28). Because the impulse must travel through the patient's skin and tissue before reaching the heart, transcutaneous pacing can cause significant discomfort and is intended to be used only in emergencies. This type of pacing necessitates hospitalization. If the patient is alert, sedation and analgesia may be administered. Transcutaneous pacing is not indicated for pulseless bradycardia.

Pacemaker Generator Functions

Because of the sophistication and wide use of pacemakers, a universal code has been adopted to provide a means of safe communication about their function. The coding is referred to as the NASPE-BPEG code because it is sanctioned by the North American Society of Pacing and Electrophysiology (now called the Heart Rhythm Society) and the British Pacing and Electrophysiology Group. The complete code consists of five letters and was revised in 2002 (Bernstein et al., 2002):

- The first letter of the code identifies the chamber or chambers being paced (ie, the chamber containing a pacing

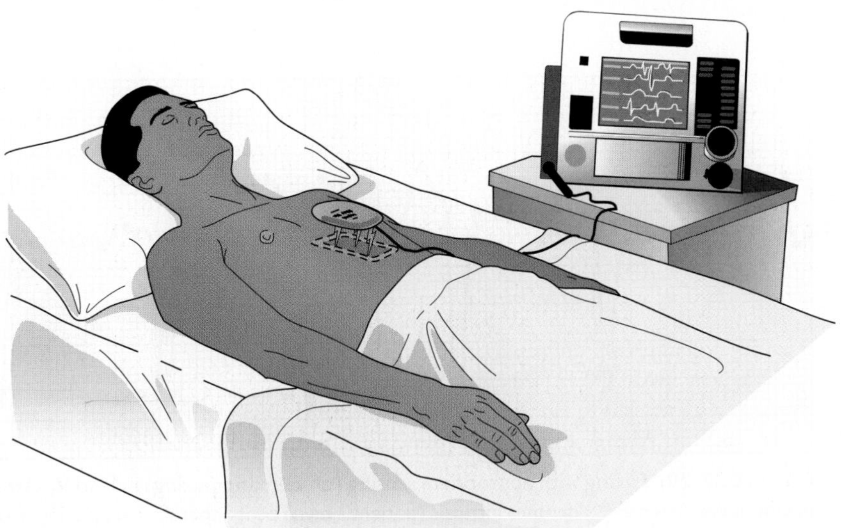

FIGURE 27-28. Transcutaneous pacemaker with electrode pads connected to the anterior and posterior chest walls.

electrode). The letter characters for this code are A (atrium), V (ventricle), or D (dual, meaning both A and V).

- The second letter identifies the chamber or chambers being sensed by the pacemaker generator. Information from the electrode within the chamber is sent to the generator for interpretation and action by the generator. The letter characters are A (atrium), V (ventricle), D (dual), and O (indicating that the sensing function is turned off).
- The third letter of the code describes the type of response that will be made by the pacemaker to what is sensed. The letter characters used to describe this response are I (**inhibited**), T (**triggered**), D (dual, inhibited and triggered), and O (none). Inhibited response means that the response of the pacemaker is controlled by the activity of the patient's heart; that is, when the patient's heart beats the pacemaker will not function, but when the heart does not beat, the pacemaker will function. In contrast, triggered response means that the pacemaker will respond (pace the heart) when it senses intrinsic heart activity.
- The fourth and fifth letters are used only with permanent pacemakers. The fourth letter of the code is related to a permanent generator's ability to vary the heart rate. The possible letters are O, indicating no rate responsiveness, or R, indicating that the generator has rate modulation (ie, the pacemaker has the ability to automatically adjust the pacing rate from moment to moment based on parameters such as physical activity, acid–base changes, temperature, rate and depth of respirations, or oxygen saturation). A pacemaker with rate-responsive ability is capable of improving cardiac output during times of increased cardiac demand, such as exercise. Research has shown that this mode of pacing reduces the incidence of recurrent atrial fibrillation (Glotzer, Hellkamp, Zimmerman, et al., 2003).
- The fifth letter of the code indicates that the permanent generator has multisite pacing capability. The letters are A (atrium), V (ventricle), D (dual), and O (none).

Commonly, only the first three letters are used for a pacing code. An example of a NASPE-BPEG code is DVI:

D: Both the atrium and the ventricle have a pacing electrode in place.

V: The pacemaker is sensing the activity of the ventricle only.

I: The pacemaker's stimulating effect is inhibited by ventricular activity—in other words, it does not create an impulse when the pacemaker senses that the patient's ventricle is active. The pacemaker paces the atrium and then the ventricle when no ventricular activity is sensed for a period of time (the time is individually programmed into the pacemaker for each patient).

The type of generator and its selected settings depend on the patient's dysrhythmia, underlying cardiac function, and age. A straight vertical line usually can be seen on the ECG when pacing is initiated. The line that represents pacing is called a pacemaker spike. The appropriate ECG complex should immediately follow the pacing spike; therefore, a P wave should follow an atrial pacing spike and a QRS complex should follow a ventricular pacing spike. Because the impulse starts in a different place than the patient's normal rhythm, the QRS complex or P wave that responds to pacing looks different from the patient's normal ECG complex. *Capture* is a term used to denote that the appropriate complex followed the pacing spike.

Pacemakers are generally set to sense and respond to intrinsic activity, which is called on-demand pacing (Fig. 27-29). If the pacemaker is set to pace but not to sense, it is called a fixed or asynchronous pacemaker (Fig. 27-30); this is written in pacing code as AOO or VOO. The pacemaker paces at a constant rate, independent of the patient's intrinsic rhythm. Because AOO pacing stimulates only the atrium, it may be used in a patient who has undergone open heart surgery and develops sinus bradycardia. AOO pacing ensures synchrony between atrial stimulation and ventricular stimulation (and therefore contraction), as long as the patient has no conduction disturbances in the AV node. VOO is rare because of the risk that the pacemaker may deliver an impulse during the vulnerable repolarization phase, leading to VT.

VVI (V, paces the ventricle; V, senses ventricular activity; I, paces only if the ventricles do not depolarize) pacing causes loss of AV synchrony and atrial kick, which may cause a decrease in cardiac output and an increase in atrial

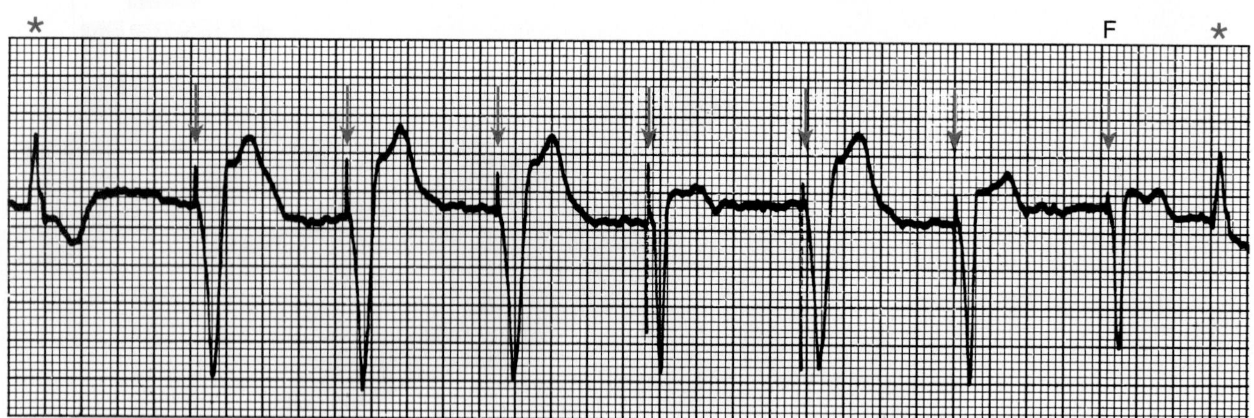

FIGURE 27-29. Pacing with appropriate sensing (on-demand pacing) in lead V_1. Arrows denote pacing spike. Asterisk (*) denotes intrinsic (patient's own) beats, therefore no pacing. F denotes a fusion beat, which is a combination of an intrinsic beat and a paced beat occurring at the same time.

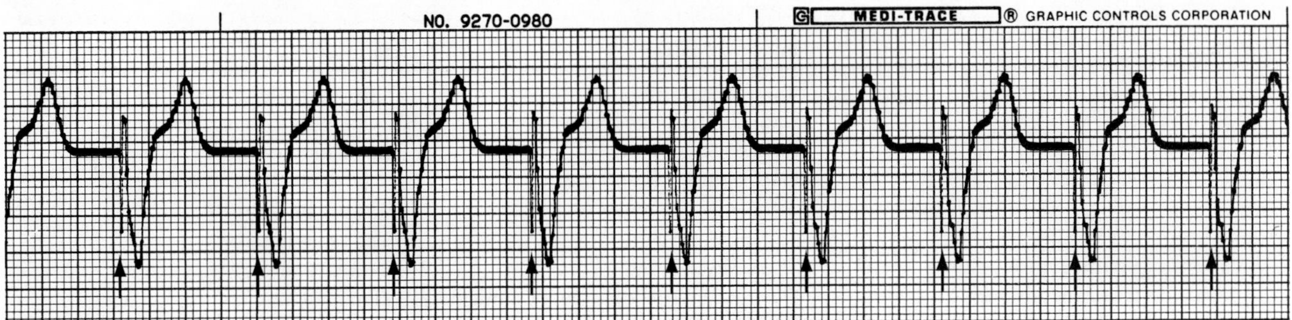

FIGURE 27-30. Fixed pacing or total loss of sensing pacing in lead V_1; arrows denote pacing spikes.

distention and venous congestion. This can lead to pacemaker syndrome, causing symptoms such as chest discomfort, shortness of breath, fatigue, activity intolerance, and postural hypotension. In addition, atrial pacing and dual chamber pacing have been found to reduce the incidence of atrial fibrillation; however, this reduction has not yet been proven to decrease the incidence of stroke, heart failure, or mortality (Troyman, Kim, & Pinski, 2004).

Synchronized biventricular pacing, also called cardiac resynchronized therapy (CRT), has recently been found to modify the intraventricular, interventricular, and atrial-ventricular conduction defects identified with symptomatic moderate to severe (New York Heart Association Functional Class III and IV) left ventricular dysfunction and heart failure. The generator for biventricular pacing has three leads: one for the right atrium; one for the right ventricle, as with most standard pacemaker generators; and one for the left ventricle, usually placed in the left lateral wall. Recent studies have shown that this therapy improves cardiac function, resulting in decreased heart failure symptoms and an improved quality of life (Trupp, 2004). Biventricular pacing may be used with an implantable cardioverter defibrillator.

Complications of Pacemaker Use

Complications associated with pacemakers relate to their presence within the body and improper functioning. The following complications may arise from a pacemaker:

- Local infection at the entry site of the leads for temporary pacing, or at the subcutaneous site for permanent generator placement
- Bleeding and hematoma at the lead entry sites for temporary pacing, or at the subcutaneous site for permanent generator placement
- Hemothorax from puncture of the subclavian vein or internal mammary artery
- Ventricular ectopy and tachycardia from irritation of the ventricular wall by the endocardial electrode
- Movement or dislocation of the lead placed transvenously (perforation of the myocardium)
- Phrenic nerve, diaphragmatic (hiccuping may be a sign), or skeletal muscle stimulation if the lead is dislocated or if the delivered energy (mA) is set high
- Rarely, cardiac tamponade from bleeding following removal of epicardial wires used for temporary pacing

In the initial hours after a temporary or permanent pacemaker is inserted, the most common complication is dislodgment of the pacing electrode. Minimizing patient activity can help prevent this complication. If a temporary electrode is in place, the extremity through which the catheter has been advanced is immobilized. With a permanent pacemaker, the patient is instructed initially to restrict activity on the side of the implantation.

The ECG is monitored very carefully to detect pacemaker malfunction. Improper pacemaker function, which can arise from failure in one or more components of the pacing system, is outlined in Table 27-2. The following data should be noted on the patient's record:

- Model of pacemaker
- Type of generator
- Date and time of insertion
- Location of pulse generator
- Stimulation threshold
- Pacer settings (eg, rate, energy output [mA], sensitivity [mV], and duration of interval between atrial and ventricular impulses [AV delay])

This information is important for identifying normal pacemaker function and diagnosing pacemaker malfunction.

A patient experiencing pacemaker malfunction may develop bradycardia as well as signs and symptoms of decreased cardiac output. The degree to which these symptoms become apparent depends on the severity of the malfunction, the patient's level of dependency on the pacemaker, and the patient's underlying condition. Pacemaker malfunction is diagnosed by analyzing the ECG. Manipulating the electrodes, changing the generator's settings, or replacing the pacemaker generator or leads (or both) may be necessary.

Inhibition of permanent pacemakers or reversion to asynchronous fixed rate pacing can occur with exposure to strong electromagnetic fields (electromagnetic interference [EMI]). The incidence of EMI is highest in dual-chambered pacemakers because of their programmed higher sensitivity to electrical stimuli (Yeo & Berg, 2004). However, recent pacemaker technology allows patients to safely use most household electronic appliances and devices (eg, microwave ovens, electric tools). Gas-powered engines should be turned off

TABLE 27-2 Assessing Pacemaker Malfunction

Problem	Possible Cause	Intervention
Loss of capture—complex does *not* follow pacing spike	Inadequate stimulus Catheter malposition Battery depletion Electronic insulation break	Check security of all connections; increase milliamperage. Reposition extremity; turn patient to left side. Change battery. Change generator.
Undersensing—pacing spike occurs at preset interval despite patient's intrinsic rhythm	Sensitivity too high Electrical interference (eg, by a magnet) Faulty generator	Decrease sensitivity. Eliminate interference. Replace generator.
Oversensing—loss of pacing artifact; pacing does *not* occur at preset interval despite lack of intrinsic rhythm	Sensitivity too low Electrical interference Battery depletion	Increase sensitivity. Eliminate interference. Change battery.
Loss of pacing—total absence of pacing spikes	Battery depletion Loose or disconnected wires Perforation	Change battery. Check security of all connections. Obtain 12-lead ECG and portable chest x-ray. Assess for murmur. Contact physician.
Change in pacing QRS shape	Septal perforation	Obtain 12-lead ECG and portable chest x-ray. Assess for murmur. Contact physician.
Rhythmic diaphragmatic or chest wall twitching or hiccuping	Output too high Myocardial wall perforation	Decrease milliamperage. Turn pacer off. Contact physician at once. Monitor closely for decreased cardiac output.

before working on them. Objects that contain magnets (eg, the earpiece of a phone; large stereo speakers; magnet therapy products such as mattresses, jewelry, and wraps) should not be near the generator for longer than a few seconds. Patients are advised to keep digital cellular phones at least 6 to 12 inches away from (or on the side opposite of) the pacemaker generator and not to carry them in a shirt pocket. Large electromagnetic fields, such as those produced by magnetic resonance imaging, radio and TV transmitter towers and lines, transmission power lines (these are different from the distribution lines that bring electricity into a home), and electrical substations may cause EMI (electromagnetic interference). Patients should be cautioned to avoid such situations or to simply move farther away from the area if they experience dizziness or a feeling of rapid or irregular heartbeats (palpitations). Welding and the use of a chain saw should be avoided. If such tools are used, precautionary steps such as limiting the welding current to a 60- to 130-ampere range or using electric rather than gasoline-powered chain saws are advised.

In addition, the metal of the pacemaker generator may trigger store and library anti-theft devices as well as airport and building security alarms; however, these alarm systems generally do not interfere with the pacemaker function. Patients should walk through them quickly and avoid standing in or near these devices. The handheld screening devices used in airports may interfere with the pacemaker. Patients should be advised to ask security personnel to perform a hand search instead of using the handheld screening device. Patients also should be instructed to wear or carry medical identification to alert personnel to the presence of the pacemaker.

Pacemaker Surveillance

Pacemaker clinics have been established to monitor patients and to test pulse generators for impending pacemaker battery failure. A computerized device is held over the generator to "interrogate" it with painless radio signals; it detects the generator's settings, battery status, pacing threshold, sensing function, lead integrity, and other stored information. Several factors, such as lead fracture, muscle inhibition, and insulation disruption, also may be assessed depending on the type of pacemaker and the equipment available. If indicated, the pacemaker is turned off for a few seconds, using a magnet or a programmer, while the ECG is recorded to assess the patient's underlying cardiac rhythm. Transtelephonic transmission of the generator's information is another follow-up method. Special equipment is used to transmit information about the patient's pacemaker over the telephone to a receiving system at a pacemaker clinic. The information is converted into tones; equipment at the clinic converts these tones to an electronic signal and records them on an ECG strip. The pacemaker rate and other data concerning pacemaker function are obtained and evaluated by a cardiologist. This simplifies the diagnosis of a failing generator, reassures the patient, and improves management when the patient is physically remote from pacemaker testing facilities. The frequency of the pacemaker checks varies with the patient's age and underlying condition, the degree of pacemaker dependency, the age and type of the device, and the results from previous pacemaker checks.

Implantable Cardioverter Defibrillator

The **implantable cardioverter defibrillator (ICD)** is a device that detects and terminates life-threatening episodes of tachycardia or fibrillation, especially those that are ventricular in origin. Patients at high risk of VT or ventricular fibrillation are those who have survived sudden cardiac death syndrome, usually caused by ventricular fibrillation, or have experienced symptomatic VT (syncope secondary to VT). Other people at risk of sudden cardiac death include those with dilated cardiomyopathy, hypertrophic cardiomyopathy, arrhythmogenic right ventricular dysfunction, and prolonged QT syndrome. In addition, patients with moderate to severe left ventricular dysfunction, with or without nonsustained VT, are at high risk for cardiac arrest; therefore, prophylactic implantation may be indicated (Bardy, Lee, Mark, et al., 2005; Moss, Zareba, Hall, et al., 2002). ICDs may also be implanted in patients with symptomatic, recurrent, medication-refractory atrial fibrillation.

An ICD consists of a generator and at least one lead that can sense intrinsic electrical activity and deliver an electrical impulse. The device is usually implanted much like a pacemaker (Fig. 27-31). ICDs are designed to respond to two criteria: a rate that exceeds a predetermined level, and a change in the isoelectric line segments. When a dysrhythmia occurs, rate sensors require a set duration of time to sense the dysrhythmia. Then the device automatically charges and delivers the programmed charge through the lead to the heart. However, in an ICD that has the capability of providing atrial therapies, the device may be programmed to be activated by the patient, giving the patient time to activate the charge at a time and place of his or her choosing. Battery life is about 5 years but varies depending on use of the ICD. ICD surveillance is similar to that of the pacemaker; however, it includes information about the number and frequency of shocks that have been delivered.

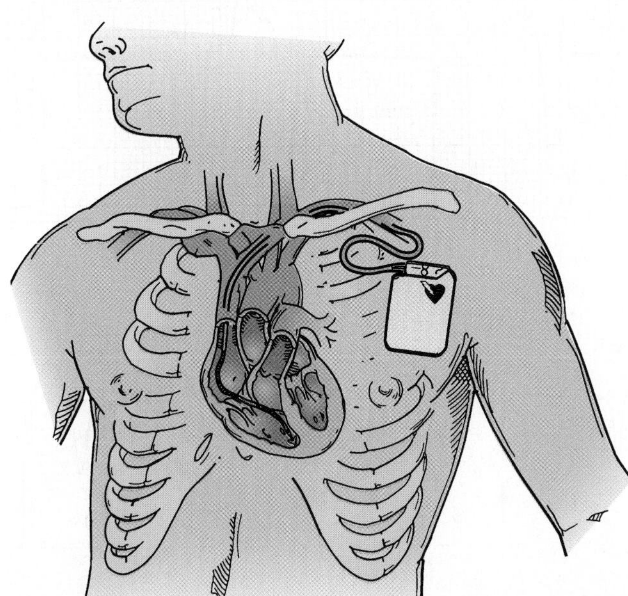

FIGURE 27-31. The implantable cardioverter defibrillator (ICD) consists of a generator and a sensing/pacing/defibrillating electrode.

Antiarrhythmic medication usually is administered with this technology to minimize the occurrence of the tachydysrhythmia and to reduce the frequency of ICD discharge.

The first defibrillator, which was implanted in 1980 at Johns Hopkins University, simply defibrillated the heart; it was called the automatic internal cardiodefibrillator (AICD). Today, several types of devices are available and may be programmed for multiple treatments (Fuster, Ryden, Asinger, et al., 2001). ICD, the generic name, is now used as the abbreviation for these various devices. Each device offers a different delivery sequence, but all are capable of delivering high-energy (high-intensity) defibrillation to treat a tachycardia (atrial or ventricular). The device may deliver up to six shocks if necessary.

Some ICDs can respond with antitachycardia pacing, in which the device delivers electrical impulses at a fast rate in an attempt to disrupt the tachycardia, by low-energy (low-intensity) cardioversion, by defibrillation, or all three (Fuster, Alexander, & O'Rourke, 2004). Antitachycardia pacing is used to terminate tachycardias caused by a conduction disturbance called reentry, which is repetitive restimulation of the heart by the same impulse. An impulse or a series of impulses is delivered to the heart by the pacemaker at a fast rate to collide with and stop the heart's reentry conduction impulses, and therefore to stop the tachycardia. Some ICDs also have pacemaker capability if the patient develops bradycardia, which sometimes occurs after treatment of the tachycardia. Usually the mode is VVI (V, paces the ventricle; V, senses ventricular activity; I, paces only if the ventricles do not depolarize). Some ICDs also deliver low-energy cardioversion, and some also treat atrial fibrillation (Daoud, Timmermans, Fellows, et al., 2000; Fuster et al., 2004).

Which device is used and how it is programmed depend on the patient's dysrhythmia. As with pacemakers, there is a NASPE-BPEG code for communicating the functions of the ICDs (Berstein, Daubert, Fletcher, et al., 2002). The first letter represents the chamber or chambers shocked (O = none, A = atrium, V = ventricle, D = both atrium and ventricle). The second letter represents the chamber that can be antitachycardia paced (O, A, V, D, meaning the same as the first letter). The third letter indicates the method used by the generator to detect a tachycardia (E = electrogram, H = hemodynamics). The last letter represents the chambers that have antibradycardia pacing (O, A, V, D, meaning the same as the first and second letters of the ICD code).

Complications are similar to those associated with pacemaker insertion. The primary complication associated with the ICD is surgery-related infection. There are a few complications associated with the technical aspects of the equipment, such as premature battery depletion and dislodged or fractured leads.

Nursing Process

The Patient with an Implantable Cardiac Device

Assessment

After a permanent electronic device (pacemaker or ICD) is inserted, the patient's heart rate and rhythm are monitored by ECG. The device's settings are noted and compared with the ECG recordings to assess the device's function. For example, pacemaker malfunction is detected by examining the pacemaker spike and its relationship to the surrounding ECG complexes (Fig. 27-32). In addition, cardiac output and hemodynamic stability are assessed to identify the patient's response to pacing and the adequacy of pacing. The appearance or increasing frequency of dysrhythmia is observed and reported to the physician. If the patient has an ICD implanted and develops VT or ventricular fibrillation, the ECG should be recorded to note the time between the onset of the dysrhythmia and the onset of the device's shock or antitachycardia pacing.

The incision site where the generator was implanted is observed for bleeding, hematoma formation, or infection, which may be evidenced by swelling, unusual tenderness, drainage, and increased heat. The patient may complain of continuous throbbing or pain. These symptoms are reported to the physician.

The patient should be assessed for anxiety, depression, or anger, which may be symptoms of ineffective coping with the implantation. In addition, the level of knowledge and learning needs of the patient and family and the history of adherence to the therapeutic regimen should be identified. It is especially important to include the family when providing education and support.

Diagnosis

Nursing Diagnoses

Based on assessment data, the patient's major nursing diagnoses may include the following:

- Risk for infection related to lead or generator insertion
- Risk for ineffective coping
- Deficient knowledge regarding self-care program

Collaborative Problems/ Potential Complications

Based on the assessment findings, potential complications that may develop include decreased cardiac output related to device malfunction.

Planning and Goals

The major goals for the patient may include absence of infection, adherence to a self-care program, effective coping, and maintenance of device function.

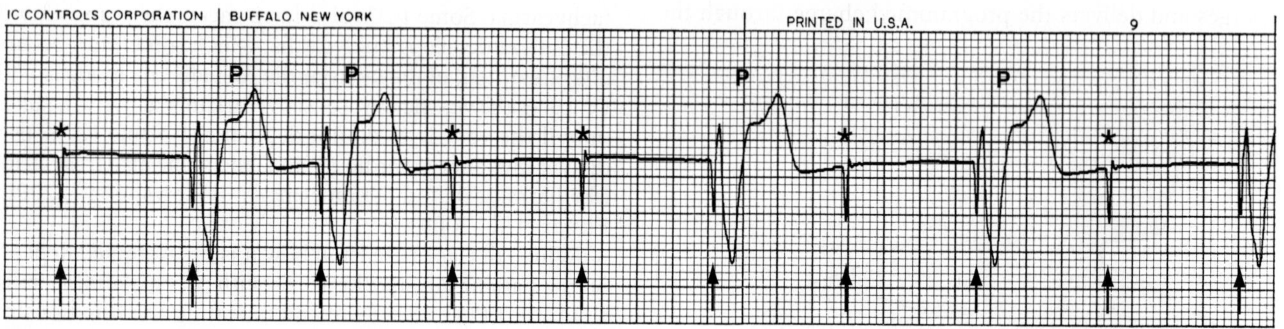

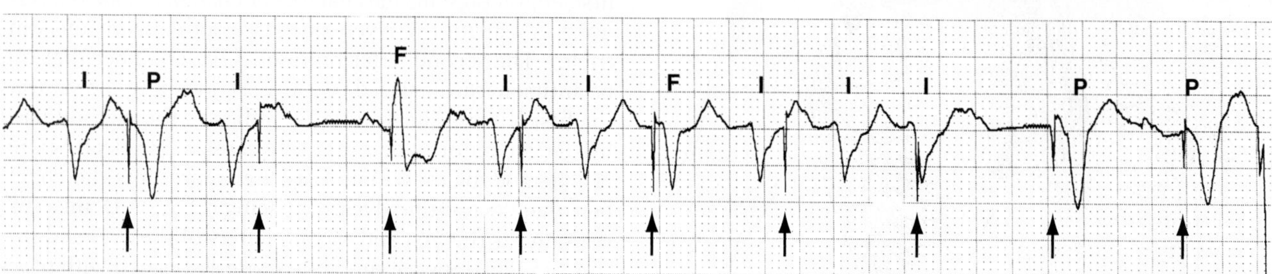

FIGURE 27-32. (**A**) Ventricular pacing with intermittent loss of capture (a pacing spike not followed by a QRS complex). (**B**) Ventricular pacing with loss of sensing (a pacing spike occurring at an inappropriate time). ↑ = pacing spike; * = loss of capture; P = pacemaker-induced QRS complex; I = patient's intrinsic QRS complex; F = fusion (a QRS complex formed by a merging of the patient's intrinsic QRS complex and the pacemaker-induced QRS complex). Both in lead V_1.

Nursing Interventions

Nursing interventions for the patient with an implantable cardiac device are provided throughout the preoperative, perioperative, and postoperative phases. In addition to providing the patient and family with explanations regarding implantation of the device in the preoperative phase, the nurse may need to manage acute episodes of life-threatening dysrhythmias. In the perioperative and postoperative phases, the nurse carefully observes the patient's responses to the device and provides the patient and family with further teaching as needed (Chart 27-3). The nurse also assists the patient and family in addressing concerns and in making decisions about self-care and lifestyle changes necessitated by the dysrhythmia and resulting device implantation (Dougherty, Pyper, & Benoliel, 2004; Dougherty, Pyper, & Fransz, 2004).

Preventing Infection

The nurse changes the dressing as needed and inspects the insertion site for redness, swelling, soreness, or any unusual drainage. An increase in the patient's temperature should be reported to the physician. Changes in wound appearance are also reported to the physician.

Promoting Effective Coping

The patient treated with an electronic device experiences not only lifestyle and physical changes but also emotional changes. At different times during the healing process, the patient may feel angry, depressed, fearful, anxious, or a combination of these emotions. Although each patient uses individual coping strategies (eg, humor, prayer, communication with a significant other) to manage emotional distress, some strategies may work better than others. Signs that may indicate ineffective coping include social isolation, increased or prolonged irritability or depression, and difficulty in relationships.

To promote effective coping strategies, the nurse must recognize the patient's as well as the family's emotional state and assist them to explore their feelings. Because of the unpredictable and painful ICD discharge, patients with ICDs are most vulnerable to feelings of helplessness, leading to depression (Edelman, Lemon, & Kidman, 2003). The nurse may help the patient identify perceived changes (eg, loss of ability to participate in contact sports), the emotional response to the change (eg, anger), and how the patient responds to that emotion (eg, quickly becomes angry when talking with spouse). The nurse reassures the patient that the responses are normal and then helps the patient identify realistic goals (eg, develop interest in another activity) and develop a plan to attain these goals. The patient and family should be encouraged to talk about their experiences and emotions with each other and the health care team. The nurse may refer the patient and family to a hospital, community, or online support group. The nurse may also teach the patient easy-to-use stress reduction techniques (eg, deep-breathing exercises) to facilitate coping. Instructing the patient about the ICD may help the patient to cope with changes that occur as a result of device implantation (Chart 27-4).

Promoting Home and Community-Based Care

TEACHING PATIENTS SELF-CARE

After device insertion, the patient's hospital stay may be 1 day or less, and follow-up in an outpatient clinic or office is common. The patient's anxiety and feelings of vulnerability may interfere with the ability to learn information provided. The nurse needs to include caregivers in the teaching and provide printed materials for use by the patient and caregiver. The nurse establishes priorities for learning with the patient and caregiver. Teaching may include the importance of periodic device monitoring, promoting safety, avoiding infection, and avoiding EMI (see Chart 27-3). In addition, the educational plan should include information about activities that are safe and those that may be dangerous. The nurse discusses with the patient and family what they are to do when a shock is delivered. They may wish to learn CPR.

Evaluation

Expected Patient Outcomes

Expected patient outcomes may include:

1. Remains free of infection
   a. Has normal temperature
   b. Has white blood cell count within normal range (5000 to 10,000/mm^3)
   c. Exhibits no redness or swelling of pacemaker insertion site
2. Adheres to a self-care program
   a. Responds appropriately when queried about the signs and symptoms of infection
   b. Identifies when to seek medical attention (as demonstrated in responses to signs and symptoms)
   c. Adheres to monitoring schedule
   d. Describes appropriate methods to avoid EMI
   e. Identifies activities that are safe and those to avoid
   f. For those with an ICD, describes how they will manage an ICD shock event
3. Maintains device function (see Chart 27-3)
   a. Measures and records pulse rate at regular intervals
   b. For those with pacemakers, experiences no abrupt changes in pulse rate or rhythm
4. Demonstrates and/or describes an effective coping strategy

Electrophysiologic Studies

An electrophysiology (EP) study is an invasive procedure used to evaluate and treat various dysrhythmias that have caused cardiac arrest or significant symptoms. It also is indicated for patients with symptoms that suggest a dysrhythmia

CHART 27-3

HOME CARE CHECKLIST • The Patient With an ICD Implantable Cardioverter Defibrillator

At the completion of home care instructions, the patient and significant other will be able to:	Patient	Caregiver
Avoid infection at the ICD insertion site.		
• Observe incision site daily for redness, swelling, and heat.	✔	✔
• Take temperature; report any increase.	✔	✔
• Avoid tight restrictive clothing that may cause friction over the insertion site.	✔	✔
Adhere to activity restrictions.		
• Restrict movement of arm until incision heals if the ICD was implanted in pectoral region.	✔	
• Avoid heavy lifting.	✔	
• Discuss safety of activities (eg, driving) with physician.	✔	✔
• Avoid contact sports.	✔	
Electromagnetic interference: Understand the importance of the following:		
• Avoid large magnetic fields such as those created by magnetic resonance imaging, large motors, arc welding, electrical substations, and so forth. Magnetic fields may deactivate the ICD, negating any effect on a dysrhythmia.	✔	
• At security gates at airports, government buildings, or other secured areas, show identification card and request a hand (not handheld device) search.	✔	
• Some electrical and small motor devices, as well as products that contain magnets (eg, cellular phones), may interfere with the functioning of the ICD if placed very close to the ICD. Avoid leaning directly over devices, or ensure contact is of brief duration; place cellular phone on opposite side of ICD.	✔	
• Household appliances (eg, microwave ovens) should not cause any concern.	✔	✔
Promote safety.		
• Describe what to do if symptoms occur and notify physician if any discharges seem unusual.	✔	✔
• Maintain a log that records discharges. Record events that precipitate the sensation of shock. This provides important data for the physician to use in readjusting the medical regimen.	✔	✔
• Encourage family members to attend a CPR class.		✔
• Call 911 for emergency assistance if feeling of dizziness occurs.	✔	✔
• Wear medical identification (eg, Medic-Alert) that includes physician information.	✔	
• Avoid frightening family or friends with unexpected shocks, which will not harm them. Inform family and friends that in the event they are in contact with the patient when a shock is delivered, they may also feel the shock. It is especially important to warn sexual partners that this may occur.	✔	✔
Follow-up care		
• Discuss psychological responses to the ICD implantation, such as changes in self-image, depression due to loss of mobility secondary to driving restrictions, fear of shocks, increased anxiety, concerns that sexual activity may trigger the ICD, and changes in partner relationship.	✔	✔
• Adhere to appointments that are scheduled to test electronic performance of ICD. Remember to take log of ICD discharges to review with physician.	✔	✔
• Attend an ICD support group within the area.	✔	

that has gone undetected and undiagnosed by other methods. An EP study is used to do the following:

- Identify the impulse formation and propagation through the cardiac electrical conduction system
- Assess the function or dysfunction of the SA and AV nodal areas
- Identify the location (called mapping) and mechanism of dysrhythmogenic foci
- Assess the effectiveness of antiarrhythmic medications and devices for the patient with a dysrhythmia
- Treat certain dysrhythmias through the destruction of the causative cells (**ablation**)

An EP procedure is a type of cardiac catheterization that is performed in a specially equipped cardiac catheterization laboratory by an electrophysiologist, who is a cardiologist with specialized training, assisted by other EP laboratory personnel. The patient is conscious but lightly sedated. Usually a catheter with multiple electrodes is inserted through a small incision in the femoral vein, threaded through the inferior vena cava, and advanced into the heart; however, a catheter may also be inserted into the femoral artery, depending on the type of study and the information needed. The electrodes are positioned within the heart at specific locations—for instance, in the right atrium near the sinus node, in the coronary sinus, near the tricuspid valve, and at the apex of

CHART 27-4

HOME CARE CHECKLIST • The Patient With an Implantable Cardiac Device

At the completion of home care instructions, the patient and significant other will be able to:	Patient	Caregiver
Monitor pacemaker function.		
• Describe the importance of reporting to physician or pacemaker clinic periodically as prescribed, so that the pacemaker's rate and function can be monitored. This is especially important during the first month after implantation.	✔	
• Adhere to monitoring schedule as instructed after implantation.	✔	
• Check pulse daily. Report *immediately* any sudden slowing or increasing of the pulse rate. This may indicate pacemaker malfunction.	✔	✔
• Resume more frequent monitoring when battery depletion is anticipated. (The time for reimplantation depends on the type of battery in use.)	✔	
Promote safety and avoid infection.		
• Wear loose-fitting clothing around the area of the pacemaker.	✔	
• State the reason for the slight bulge over the pacemaker implant.	✔	✔
• Notify physician if the pacemaker area becomes red or painful.	✔	✔
• Avoid trauma to the area of the pacemaker generator.	✔	
• Study the manufacturer's instructions and become familiar with the pacemaker.	✔	✔
• Recognize that physical activity does not usually have to be curtailed, with the exception of contact sports.	✔	
• Carry medical identification indicating physician's name, type and model number of pacemaker, manufacturer's name, pacemaker rate, and hospital where pacemaker was inserted.	✔	
Electromagnetic interference: Understand the importance of the following:		
• Avoid large magnetic fields such as those surrounding magnetic resonance imaging, large motors, arc welding, electrical substations. Magnetic fields can deactivate the pacemaker.	✔	
• Some electrical and small motor devices, as well as products that contain magnets (eg, cellular phones), may interfere with pacemaker function if placed very close to the generator. Avoid leaning directly over devices, or ensure that contact is brief; place cellular phone on opposite side of generator and do not carry in a shirt pocket.	✔	✔
• Household items, such as microwave ovens, should not cause any concern.	✔	✔
• When going through security gates (eg, at airports, government buildings) show identification card and request hand (not handheld device) search.	✔	✔
• Hospitalization may be necessary periodically to change battery or replace pacemaker unit.	✔	✔

the right ventricle. The number and placement of electrodes depend on the type of study being conducted. These electrodes allow the electrical signal to be recorded from within the heart (intracardiogram).

The electrodes also allow the clinician to introduce a pacing stimulus to the intracardiac area at a precisely timed interval and rate, thereby stimulating the area (programmed stimulation). An area of the heart may be paced at a rate much faster than the normal rate of **automaticity**, the rate at which impulses are spontaneously formed (eg, in the sinus node). This allows the pacemaker to become an artificial focus of automaticity and to assume control (overdrive suppression). Then the pacemaker is stopped suddenly, and the time it takes for the sinus node to resume control is assessed. A prolonged time indicates dysfunction of the sinus node.

One of the main purposes of programmed stimulation is to assess the ability of the area surrounding the electrode to cause a reentry dysrhythmia. One or a series of premature impulses is delivered to an area in an attempt to cause the tachydysrhythmia. Because the precise location of the suspected area and the specific timing of the pacing needed are unknown, the electrophysiologist uses several different techniques to cause the dysrhythmia during the study. If the dysrhythmia can be reproduced by programmed stimulation, it is called inducible. Once a dysrhythmia is induced, a treatment plan is determined and implemented. If, on the follow-up EP study, the tachydysrhythmia cannot be induced, then the treatment is determined to be effective. Different medications may be administered and combined with electrical devices (pacemaker, ICD) to determine the most effective treatment to suppress the dysrhythmia.

Patient care, patient teaching, and associated complications of an EP study are the same as those associated with cardiac catheterization (see Chapter 26). The study is usually about 2 hours in length; however, if the electrophysiologist conducts not only a diagnostic procedure but also treatment, the study can take up to 6 hours. During the procedure, patients benefit from a calm, reassuring approach.

Patients who are to undergo an EP study may be anxious about the procedure and its outcome. A detailed discussion involving the patient, the family, and the electrophysiologist usually occurs to ensure that the patient can give informed consent and to reduce the patient's anxiety about the procedure. Before the procedure, the patient should receive instructions about the procedure and its usual duration, the environment where the procedure is performed, and what to expect. Although an EP study is not painful, it does cause discomfort and can be tiring. It may also cause feelings that were experienced when the dysrhythmia occurred in the past. In addition, patients are taught what will be expected of them (eg, lying very still during the procedure, reporting symptoms or concerns).

The patient should also know that the dysrhythmia may occur during the procedure. It often stops on its own; if it does not, treatment is given to restore the patient's normal rhythm. The dysrhythmia may have to be terminated using cardioversion or defibrillation, but this is performed under more controlled circumstances than if performed in an emergency.

Postprocedural care is similar to that for cardiac catheterization, including restriction of activity to promote hemostasis at the insertion site. To identify any complications and to ensure healing, the patient's vital signs and the appearance of the insertion site are assessed frequently. Because an artery is not always used, there is a lower incidence of vascular complications than with other catheterization procedures. Cardiac arrest may occur, but the incidence is low (less than 1%) (Fuster et al., 2004).

Cardiac Conduction Surgery

Atrial tachycardias and ventricular tachycardias that do not respond to medications and are not suitable for antitachycardia pacing may be treated by methods that include a maze procedure and ablation. Hospitalization is required for both procedures.

Maze Procedure

The maze procedure is an open heart surgical procedure for refractory atrial fibrillation. Small transmural incisions are made throughout the atria. The resulting formation of scar tissue prevents reentry conduction of the electrical impulse. Although the procedure has been found to be about 95% effective, it usually requires significant time and cardiopulmonary bypass (Gaynor, Diodato, Prasad, et al., 2004). In addition, some patients need a permanent pacemaker after the surgery. Use of catheter ablation to perform the maze procedure using minimally invasive surgery is being studied. This less invasive procedure does not require cardiopulmonary bypass and is performed with catheters inserted through small sternal keyhole-type incisions.

Catheter Ablation Therapy

Catheter ablation destroys specific cells that are the cause or central conduction route of a tachydysrhythmia. It is performed with or after an EP study. Usual indications for ablation are AVNRT, a recurrent atrial dysrhythmia (especially atrial fibrillation), or VT unresponsive to previous therapy (or for which the therapy produced significant side effects).

Ablation is also indicated to eliminate accessory AV pathways or bypass tracts that exist in the hearts of patients with preexcitation syndromes such as Wolff-Parkinson-White (WPW) syndrome. During normal embryonic development, all connections between the atrium and ventricles disappear, except for that between the AV node and the bundle of His. In some people, embryonic connections of normal heart muscle between the atrium and ventricles remain, providing an accessory pathway or a tract through which the electrical impulse can bypass the AV node. These pathways can be located in several different areas. If the patient develops atrial fibrillation, the impulse may be conducted into the ventricle at a rate of 300 times per minute or more, which can lead to ventricular fibrillation and sudden cardiac death. Preexcitation syndromes are identified by specific ECG findings. For example, in WPW syndrome there is a shortened PR interval, slurring (called a delta wave) of the initial QRS deflection, and prolonged QRS duration (Fig. 27-33).

Ablation is most often accomplished by using radiofrequency, which involves placing a special catheter at or near the origin of the dysrhythmia. High-frequency, low-energy sound waves are passed through the catheter, causing thermal injury and cellular changes that result in localized de-

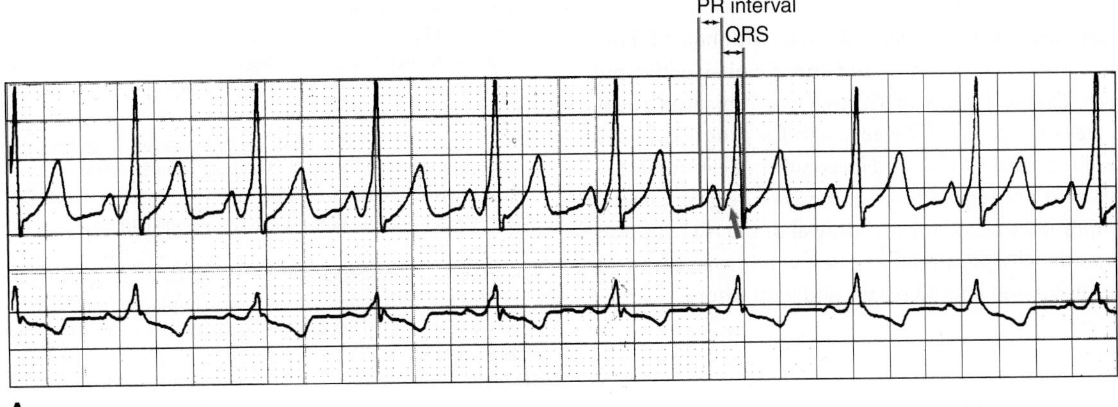

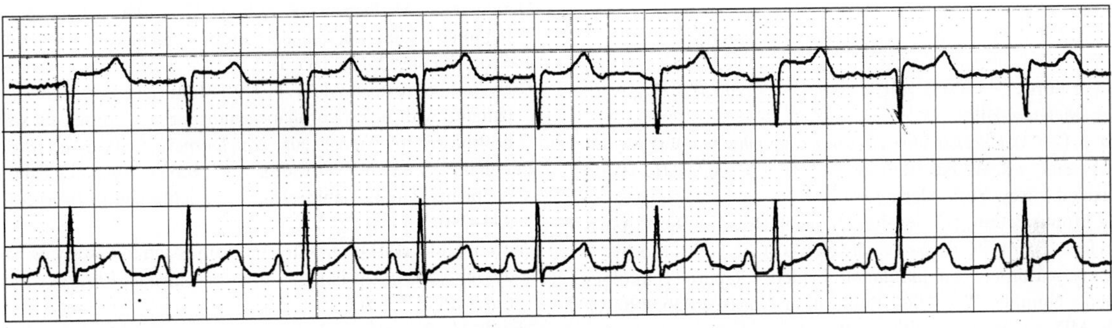

FIGURE 27-33. Wolff-Parkinson-White syndrome. (**A**) Sinus rhythm. Note the short PR interval, slurred initial upstroke of the QRS complex (delta wave, at the arrow), and prolonged QRS duration, upper lead II, lower lead V_1. (**B**) Rhythm strip of same patient following ablation, upper lead V_1, lower lead II. ECG strips courtesy of Linda Ardini and Catherine Berkmeyer, Inova Fairfax Hospital, Falls Church, VA.

struction and scarring. The tissue damage is more specific to the dysrhythmic tissue, with less trauma to the surrounding cardiac tissue than occurs with cryoablation or electrical ablation.

During the ablation procedure, defibrillation pads, an automatic blood pressure cuff, and a pulse oximeter are used, and an indwelling urinary catheter is inserted. The patient is usually given moderate sedation. An EP study is performed and attempts to induce the dysrhythmia are made. The ablation catheter is placed at the origin of the dysrhythmia, and the ablation procedure is performed. Multiple ablations may be necessary. Successful ablation is achieved when the dysrhythmia can no longer be induced. The patient is monitored for another 30 to 60 minutes and then retested to ensure that the dysrhythmia will not recur.

Postprocedural care on a step-down unit is similar to that for an EP study, except that the patient is monitored more closely, depending on the time needed for recovery from sedation.

Critical Thinking Exercises

1 ebp You are caring for a 79-year-old woman who had coronary artery bypass surgery 3 days ago. Her recovery had been uneventful until today, when her heart rate increased and the heart rhythm became irregular. Your analysis of the ECG strip indicates that she has developed sinus tachycardia with frequent PACs. What are some of the possible causes of this dysrhythmia? Identify some of the key factors that would need to be included in your assessment to assist in identification of the cause of the dysrhythmia. What nursing interventions are needed? What is the evidence base that supports these nursing interventions? Discuss the strength of the evidence and the criteria used to evaluate the strength of the evidence.

2 You are caring for a 40-year-old man who recently had an AV sequential pacemaker inserted, with the rate set at 72 beats per minute. When taking his pulse, you note that his heart rate is 66 beats per minute. Describe the possible causes of this difference in heart rates and the nursing actions that are needed.

3 ebp The wife of this same patient tells you that her husband has informed her that now that he has a pacemaker, they must get rid of their microwave oven. What would you say to the wife? How would you discuss this with the patient? What other education would you provide to this patient and his wife about safety in relation to the pacemaker? What is the evidence base that supports this education? Discuss the strength of the evidence and the criteria used to evaluate the strength of the evidence.

4 You are caring for a 65-year-old man with heart failure, chronic renal insufficiency, and chronic obstructive pulmonary disease. He has an ICD that was implanted 5 years ago. He was admitted 2 weeks ago for progressive dyspnea, peripheral edema, and intermittent delirium. He requests that only comfort measures now be given; he and his family have asked for withdrawal of the ICD support. Is this ethically permissible? How would you respond? What discussion should occur, and with whom?

REFERENCES AND SELECTED READINGS

BOOKS

Chulay, M., & Burns, S. (2005). *AACN essentials of critical care nursing.* New York: McGraw-Hill.

Conover, M. B. (2003). *Understanding electrocardiography.* St. Louis: Mosby.

Fuster, V., Alexander R. W., & O'Rourke, R. A. (Eds.). (2004). *Hurst's the heart* (11th ed.). New York: McGraw-Hill.

Kinney, M., Brooks-Brunn, J. A., Molter, N., et al. (Eds.). (1998). *AACN clinical reference for critical care nursing* (4th ed.). St. Louis: Mosby.

Management of new onset atrial fibrillation. Evidence Report/Technology Assessment: Number 12. AHRQ Publication No. 01-E026. (2001). Rockville, MD: Agency for Healthcare Research and Quality.

Marriott, H. J., & Conover, M. B. (1998). *Advanced concepts in arrhythmias.* St. Louis: Mosby.

McEvoy, G. K. (Ed.). (2005). *AHFS drug information.* Bethesda, MD: American Society of Health System Pharmacists.

McNamara, R. L., Bass, E. B., Miller, M. R., et al. (2001). *Management of new onset atrial fibrillation.* Evidence Report/Technology Assessment No. 12 (prepared by the Johns Hopkins University Evidence-Based Practice Center in Baltimore, MD, under Contract No. 290-97-0006). AHRQ Publication Number 01-E026. Rockville, MD: Agency for Healthcare Research and Quality.

Zipes, D. P., Libby, P., Bonow, R. O., et al. (Eds.). (2005). *Braunwald's heart disease: A textbook of cardiovascular medicine* (7th ed.) Philadelphia: W. B. Saunders.

JOURNALS

**Asterisks indicate nursing research articles.*

Adgey, A. A., Spence, M. S., & Walsh, S. J. (2005). Theory and practice of defibrillation: Defibrillation for ventricular fibrillation. *Heart, 9*(1), 118–125.

American Heart Association (2005). 2005 American Heart Association guidelines for cardiopulmonary resuscitation and emergency cardiovascular care. *Circulation, 112*(24 Supplement), 1–211.

Atrial Fibrillation Follow-up Investigation of Rhythm Management (AFFIRM) Investigators. (2002). A comparison of rate control and rhythm control in patients with atrial fibrillation. *New England Journal of Medicine, 347*(23), 1825–1833.

Bardy, G. H., Lee, K. L., Mark, D. B., et al. (2005). Amiodarone or an implantable cardioverter–defibrillator for congestive heart failure. *New England Journal of Medicine, 352*(3), 225–237.

Bernstein, A. D., Daubert, J-C., Fletcher, R. D., et al. (2002) The Revised NASPE/BPEG Generic Code for antibradycardia, adaptive-rate, and multisite pacing. *Journal of Pacing and Clinical Electrophysiology, 25*(2), 260–264.

Blomström-Lundqvist, C., Scheinman, M. M, Aliot, E. M., et al. (2003). ACC/AHA/ESC guidelines for the management of patients with supraventricular arrhythmias: A report of the American College of Cardiology/American Heart Association Task Force on Practice Guidelines and the European Society of Cardiology Committee for Practice Guidelines. (Writing Committee to Develop Guidelines for the Management of Patients with Supraventricular Arrhythmias. American College of Cardiology Web Site: Available at: http://www.acc.org/clinical/guidelines/arrhythmias/sva_index.pdf. Accessed June 2, 2006).

Cardiac Arrhythmia Suppression Trial Investigators. (1989). The Cardiac Arrhythmia Suppression Trial. *New England Journal of Medicine, 321*(25), 1754–1756.

Daoud, E. G., Timmermans, C., Fellows, C., et al. (2000). Initial clinical experience with ambulatory use of an implantable atrial defibrillator for conversion of atrial fibrillation. Metrix Investigators. *Circulation, 102*(12), 1407–1413.

*Dougherty, C. M., Pyper, G. P., & Benoliel, J. Q. (2004). Domains of concern of intimate partners of sudden cardiac arrest survivors after ICD implantation. *Journal of Cardiovascular Nursing, 19*(1), 21–31.

Dougherty, C. M., Pyper, G. P., & Frasz, H. A. (2004). Description of a nursing intervention program after an implantable cardioverter defibrillator. *Heart & Lung, 33*(3), 183–190.

Drew, B. J., & Krucoff, M. W. (1999). Multilead ST-segment monitoring in patients with acute coronary syndromes: A consensus statement for healthcare professionals. *American Journal of Critical Care, 8*(6), 372–386.

Edelman, S., Lemon, J., & Kidman, A. (2003). Psychological therapies for recipients of implantable cardioverter defibrillators. *Heart & Lung, 32*(4), 234–240.

Fenton, J. M. (2001). The clinician's approach to evaluating patients with dysrhythmias. *AACN Clinical Issues: Advanced Practice Acute Critical Care, 12*(1), 72–86.

*Funk, M., Richards, S. B., Desjardins J., et al. (2003). Incidence, timing, symptoms, and risk factors for atrial fibrillation after cardiac surgery. *American Journal of Critical Care, 12*(5), 424–435.

Fuster, V., Rydén, A., Asinger, R. W., et al (2001). ACC/AHA/ESC Guidelines for the management of patients with atrial fibrillation. *Journal of American College of Cardiology, 38,* 2118–2150.

Gaynor, S. L., Diodato, M. D., Prasad, S. M., et al. (2004). A prospective, single-center clinical trial of a modified Cox maze procedure with bipolar radiofrequency ablation. *Journal of Thoracic & Cardiovascular Surgery, 128*(4), 535–542.

Glotzer, T. V., Hellkamp, A. S., Zimmerman, J., et al. (2003). Atrial high rate episodes detected by pacemaker diagnostics predict death and stroke: Report of the Atrial Diagnostics Ancillary Study of the Mode Selection Trial (MOST). *Circulation, 107*(12), 1614–1619.

Gregoratos, G., Abrams, J., Epstein, A. E., et al. (2002). ACC/AHA/NASPE 2002 guideline update for implantation of cardiac pacemakers and antiarrhythmia devices: A report of the American College of Cardiology/American Heart Association Task Force on Practice Guidelines (ACC/AHA/NASPE). Committee to Pacemaker Implantation. *Circulation, 106*(16), 2145–2161.

Hallstrom, A. P., Ornato, J. P., Weisfeldt, M., et al. Public Access Defibrillation Trial Investigators (2004). Public-access defibrillation and survival after out-of-hospital cardiac arrest. *New England Journal of Medicine, 351*(7), 637–646.

Hirsh, J., Fuster, V., Ansell, J., et al. (2003). American Heart Association/American College of Cardiology Foundation guide to warfarin therapy. *Circulation, 107*(12), 1692–1711.

Kellen, J. C. (2004). Implications for nursing care of patients with atrial fibrillation. *Journal of Cardiovascular Nursing, 19*(2), 128–137.

Kellen, J. C., Ettinger, A., Todd, L., et al. (1996). The Cardiac Arrhythmia Suppression Trial: Implications for nursing practice. *American Journal of Critical Care, 5*(1), 19–25.

Kern, L. (2004). Postoperative atrial fibrillation: New directions in prevention and treatment. *Journal of Cardiovascular Nursing, 19*(2), 103–115.

Knight, B. P., Gersh, B. J., Carlson, M. D., et al. for the AHA Writing Group. (2005). Role of permanent pacing to prevent atrial fibrillation. *Circulation, 111*(2), 240–243.

Madrid, A. H., Bueno, M. G., Rebollo, J. M. G, et al. (2002). Use of irbesartan to maintain sinus rhythm in patients with long-lasting persistent

atrial fibrillation: A prospective and randomized study. *Circulation, 106*, 331–336.

Moss, A. J., Zareba, W., Hall, J., et al. for the Multicenter Automatic Defibrillator Implantation Trial II Investigators (2002). Prophylactic implantation of a defibrillator in patients with myocardial infarction and reduced ejection fraction. *New England Journal of Medicine, 346*(8), 877–883.

Obias-Manno, D., & Wijetunga, M. (2004). Risk stratification and primary prevention of sudden cardiac death: Sudden death prevention. *AACN Clinical Issues, 15*(3), 404–418.

Ocampo, C. M. (2000). Living with an implantable cardioverter defibrillator: Impact on the patient, family and society. *Nursing Clinics of North America, 35*(4), 1019–1030.

Olshansky, B., Rosenfeld, L. E., Warner, A. L., et al. (2004). The Atrial Fibrillation Follow-up Investigation of RhMthm management (AFFIRM) study: Approaches to control rate in atrial fibrillation. *Journal of American College of Cardiology, 43*(7), 1201–1208.

Shaffer, R. S. (2002). ICD therapy: The patient's perspective. *American Journal of Nursing, 102*(2), 46–49.

Snow, V., Weiss, K. B., LeFevre, M., et al. AAFP Panel on Atrial Fibrillation. ACP Panel on Atrial Fibrillation. (2003). Management of newly detected atrial fibrillation: A clinical practice guideline from the American Academy of Family Physicians and the American College of Physicians. *Annals of Internal Medicine. 139*(12), 1009–1017.

Stevenson, W. G., Chaitman, B. R., Ellenbogen, K. A., et al. for the Subcommittee on Electrocardiography and Arrhythmias of the American Heart Association Council on Clinical Cardiology, in collaboration with the Heart Rhythm Society. (2004). Clinical assessment and management of patients with implanted cardioverter-defibrillators presenting to nonelectrophysiologists. *Circulation, 110*(25), 3866–3869.

Stewart, S. (2004). Epidemiology and economic impact of atrial fibrillation. *Journal of Cardiovascular Nursing, 19*(2), 94–102.

Thomas, S. A., Friedmann, E., & Kelley, F. J. (2001). Living with an implantable cardioverter-defibrillator: A review of the current literature related to psychosocial factors. *AACN Clinical Issues: Advanced Practice Acute Critical Care, 12*(1), 156–163.

Troyman, R. G., Kim, M. H., & Pinski, S. L. (2004) Cardiac pacing: The state of the art. *Lancet, 364*(9446), 1701–1719.

Trupp, R. J. (2004). Cardiac resynchronization therapy: Optimizing the device, optimizing the patient. *Journal of Cardiovascular Nursing, 19*(4), 223–233.

Ueng, K. C., Tsai, T. P., Yu, W. C., et al. (2003). Use of enalapril to facilitate sinus rhythm maintenance after external cardioversion of long-standing persistent atrial fibrillation. Results of a prospective and controlled study. *European Heart, 24*(23), 2090–2098.

Yeo, T. P., & Berg, N. C. (2004). Counseling patients with implanted cardiac devices. *Nurse Practitioner, 29*(12), 58–65.

RESOURCES

American Association of Critical Care Nurses, 101 Columbia, Aliso Viejo, CA 92656-4109; 800-899-2226; http://www.aacn.org. Accessed June 2, 2006.

American College of Cardiology, 911 Old Georgetown Road, Bethesda, MD 20814; 800-253-4636; http://www.acc.org. Accessed June 2, 2006.

American Heart Association, National Center, 7272 Greenville Ave., Dallas, TX 75231; 1-800-242-8721; http://www.americanheart.org. Accessed June 2, 2006.

Heart Rhythm Society, 1400 K Street, N.W., Suite 500, Washington D.C. 20005; 202-464-3400; http://www.hrsonline.org. Accessed June 2, 2006.

National Heart, Lung, Blood Institute, Health Information Center, National Institutes of Health, PO Box 30105, Bethesda, MD 20824; 301-592-8573; http://www.nhlbi.nih.gov. Accessed June 2, 2006.

National Institute on Aging, Building 31, Room 5C27, 31 Center Drive, MSC 2292, Bethesda, MD 20892; 301-496-1752; http://www.nia.nih.gov. Accessed June 2, 2006.

CHAPTER 28

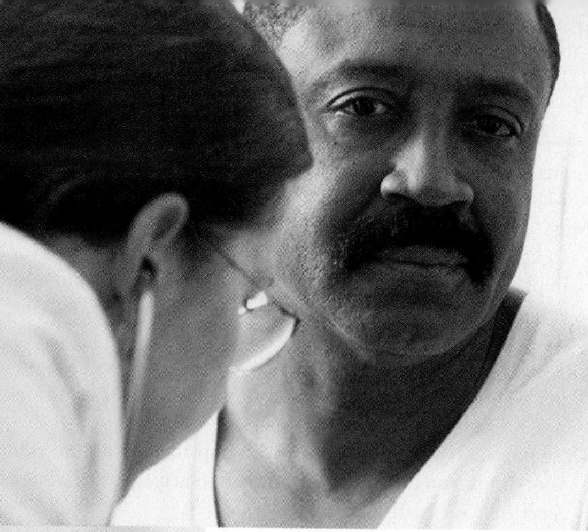

Management of Patients With Coronary Vascular Disorders

Learning Objectives

On completion of this chapter, the learner will be able to:

1. Describe the pathophysiology, clinical manifestations, and treatment of coronary atherosclerosis.
2. Describe the pathophysiology, clinical manifestations, and treatment of angina pectoris.
3. Use the nursing process as a framework for care of patients with angina pectoris.
4. Describe the pathophysiology, clinical manifestations, and treatment of myocardial infarction.
5. Use the nursing process as a framework for care of a patient with acute coronary syndrome.
6. Describe percutaneous coronary interventional and coronary artery revascularization procedures.
7. Describe the nursing care of a patient who has had a percutaneous coronary interventional procedure for treatment of coronary artery disease.
8. Describe the nursing care of a patient who has undergone cardiac surgery.

Cardiovascular disease is the leading cause of death in the United States for men and women of all racial and ethnic groups (American Heart Association [AHA], 2004). Research related to the identification and treatment of cardiovascular disease now includes all segments of the population affected by cardiac conditions, including women, children, and people of diverse racial and ethnic backgrounds.

Coronary Artery Disease

Coronary artery disease (CAD) is the most prevalent type of cardiovascular disease in adults. For this reason, it is important for nurses to become familiar with various manifestations of coronary artery conditions and methods for assessing, preventing, and treating these disorders medically and surgically.

Coronary Atherosclerosis

The most common cause of cardiovascular disease in the United States is **atherosclerosis**, an abnormal accumulation of lipid, or fatty, substances and fibrous tissue in the lining of arterial blood vessel walls. These substances create blockages and narrow the coronary vessels in a way that reduces blood flow to the myocardium. It is now known that atherosclerosis involves a repetitious inflammatory response to injury to the artery wall and subsequent alteration in the structural and biochemical properties of the arterial walls. New information that relates to the development of atherosclerosis has increased understanding of treatment and prevention of this progressive and potentially life-threatening process.

Pathophysiology

Atherosclerosis is thought to begin as fatty streaks of lipids that are deposited in the intima of the arterial wall. These lesions commonly begin early in life, perhaps even in childhood. Not all fatty streaks later develop into more advanced lesions. Genetics and environmental factors are involved in the progression of these lesions. The continued development of atherosclerosis involves an inflammatory response, which begins with injury to the vascular endothelium. The injury may be initiated by smoking, hypertension, and other factors. The presence of inflammation has multiple effects on the arterial wall, including the attraction of inflammatory cells (including macrophages) (Moustapha & Anderson, 2003). The macrophages infiltrate the injured vascular endothelium and ingest lipids, which turns them into what are called foam cells. Activated macrophages also

Glossary

acute coronary syndrome (ACS): signs and symptoms that indicate unstable angina or acute myocardial infarction

angina pectoris: chest pain brought about by myocardial ischemia

angiotensin-converting enzyme (ACE) inhibitors: medications that inhibit the angiotensin-converting enzyme

atherosclerosis: abnormal accumulation of lipid deposits and fibrous tissue within arterial walls and lumen

atheroma: fibrous cap composed of smooth muscle cells that forms over lipid deposits within arterial vessels and that protrudes into the lumen of the vessel, narrowing the lumen and obstructing blood flow; also called plaque

contractility: ability of the cardiac muscle to shorten in response to an electrical impulse

coronary artery bypass graft (CABG): a surgical procedure in which a blood vessel from another part of the body is grafted onto the occluded coronary artery below the occlusion in such a way that blood flow bypasses the blockage

creatine kinase (CK): an enzyme found in human tissues; one of the three types of CK is specific to heart muscle and may be used as an indicator of heart muscle injury

high-density lipoprotein (HDL): a protein-bound lipid that transports cholesterol to the liver for excretion in the bile; composed of a higher proportion of protein to lipid than low-density lipoprotein; exerts a beneficial effect on the arterial wall

ischemia: insufficient tissue oxygenation

low-density lipoprotein (LDL): a protein-bound lipid that transports cholesterol to tissues in the body; composed of a lower proportion of protein to lipid than high-density lipoprotein; exerts a harmful effect on the arterial wall

metabolic syndrome: a cluster of metabolic abnormalities including insulin resistance, obesity, dyslipidemia, and hypertension that increase the risk of cardiovascular disease

myocardial infarction (MI): death of heart tissue caused by lack of oxygenated blood flow; if acute, abbreviated as AMI

percutaneous coronary intervention (PCI): an invasive procedure in which a catheter is placed in a coronary artery, and one of several methods is employed to remove or reduce a blockage within the artery

percutaneous transluminal coronary angioplasty (PTCA): a type of percutaneous coronary intervention in which a balloon is inflated within a coronary artery to break an atheroma and open the vessel lumen, improving coronary artery blood flow

primary prevention: interventions taken to prevent the development of coronary artery disease

secondary prevention: interventions taken to prevent the advancement of existing coronary artery disease

stent: a woven mesh that provides structural support to a coronary vessel, preventing its closure

sudden cardiac death: immediate cessation of effective heart activity

thrombolytic: an agent or process that breaks down blood clots

troponin: myocardial protein; measurement is used to assess heart muscle injury

release biochemical substances that can further damage the endothelium, attracting platelets and initiating clotting.

Smooth muscle cells within the vessel wall subsequently proliferate and form a fibrous cap over a core filled with lipid and inflammatory infiltrate. These deposits, called **atheromas** or plaques, protrude into the lumen of the vessel, narrowing it and obstructing blood flow (Fig. 28-1). Plaque may be stable or unstable, depending on the degree of inflammation and consequent thickness of the fibrous cap. If the fibrous cap of the plaque is thick and the lipid pool remains relatively stable, it can resist the stress from blood flow and vessel movement. If the cap is thin and inflammation is ongoing, the lipid core may grow, causing it to rupture and hemorrhage into the plaque. A ruptured plaque is a focus for thrombus formation. The thrombus may then obstruct blood flow, leading to sudden cardiac death or an acute **myocardial infarction (MI)**, which is the death of a portion of the heart muscle.

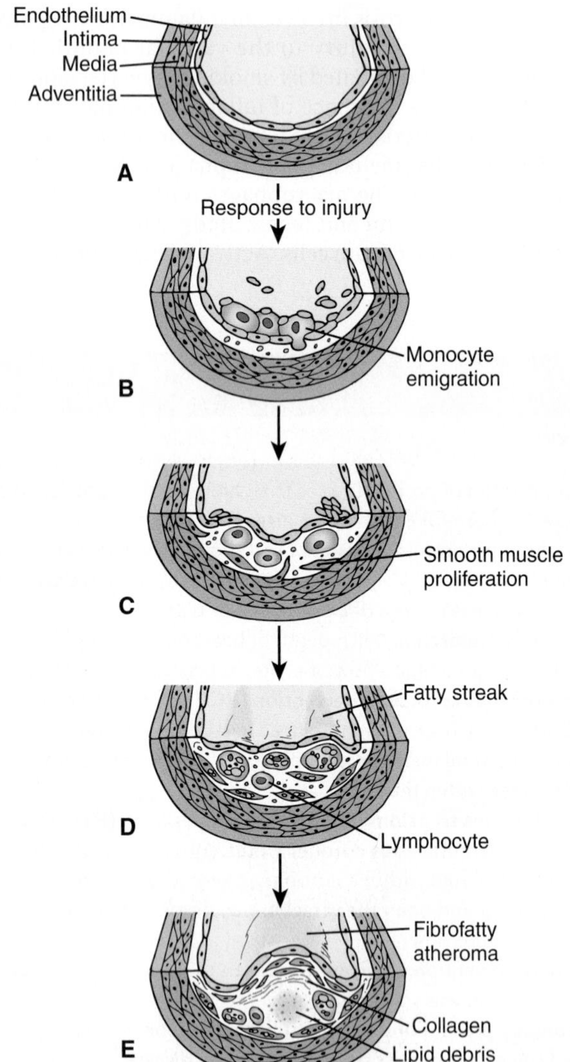

FIGURE 28-1. Atherosclerosis begins as monocytes and lipids enter the intima of an injured vessel (**A, B**). Smooth muscle cells proliferate within the vessel wall (**C**) contributing to the development of fatty accumulations and atheroma (**D**). As the plaque enlarges, the vessel narrows and blood flow decreases (**E**). The plaque may rupture and a thrombus might form, obstructing blood flow.

The anatomic structure of the coronary arteries makes them particularly susceptible to the mechanisms of atherosclerosis. As Figure 28-2 shows, the three major coronary arteries have multiple branches. Atherosclerotic lesions most often form where the vessels branch, suggesting a hemodynamic component that favors their formation (Porth, 2005). Although heart disease is most often caused by atherosclerosis of the coronary arteries, other phenomena may also decrease blood flow to the heart. Examples include vasospasm (sudden constriction or narrowing) of a coronary artery, myocardial trauma from internal or external forces, structural disease, congenital anomalies, decreased oxygen supply (eg, from acute blood loss, anemia, or low blood pressure), and increased oxygen demand (eg, from rapid heart rate, thyrotoxicosis, or use of cocaine).

Clinical Manifestations

Coronary atherosclerosis produces symptoms and complications according to the location and degree of narrowing of the arterial lumen, thrombus formation, and obstruction of blood flow to the myocardium. This impediment to blood flow is usually progressive, causing an inadequate blood supply that deprives the cardiac muscle cells of oxygen needed for their survival. The condition is known as **ischemia. Angina pectoris** refers to chest pain that is brought about by myocardial ischemia. Angina pectoris usually is caused by significant coronary atherosclerosis. If the decrease in blood supply is great enough, of long enough duration, or both, irreversible damage and death of myocardial cells, or MI, may result. Over time, irreversibly damaged myocardium undergoes degeneration and is replaced by scar tissue, causing various degrees of myocardial dysfunction. Significant myocardial damage may result in persistently low cardiac output, and the heart cannot support the body's needs for blood, which is called heart failure. A decrease in blood supply from CAD may even cause the heart to abruptly stop beating (**sudden cardiac death**).

The most common manifestation of myocardial ischemia is acute onset of chest pain. However, the classic epidemiologic study of the people in Framingham, Massachusetts, showed that nearly 15% of men and women who had MIs were totally asymptomatic (Kannel, 1986). Patients with myocardial ischemia may present to an emergency department or clinic with a variety of symptoms other than chest pain. Patients who are older or have a history of diabetes or heart failure may report symptoms such as shortness of breath. Many women have been found to have atypical symptoms, including dyspnea, nausea, and weakness (DeVon & Zerwic, 2003). Prodromal symptoms may occur (ie, angina a few hours to days before the acute episode), or a major cardiac event may be the first indication of coronary atherosclerosis.

Risk Factors

Epidemiologic studies point to several factors that increase the probability that heart disease will develop in a person.

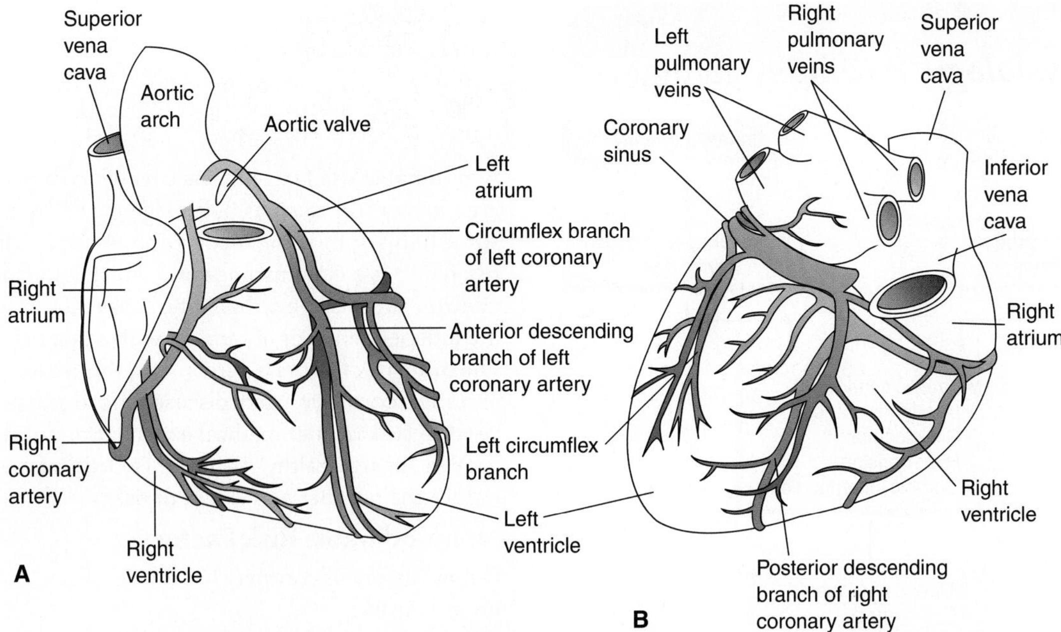

FIGURE 28-2. The coronary arteries supply the heart muscle with oxygenated blood, adjusting the flow according to metabolic needs. (**A**) Anterior view, and (**B**) posterior view of heart.

Major risk factors include elevated blood lipid levels, smoking, hypertension, diabetes mellitus, obesity, family history of premature cardiovascular disease (first-degree relative with cardiovascular disease at 55 years of age or younger for men and at 65 years of age or younger for women), and age (more than 45 years for men; more than 55 years for women). Some people do not have classic risk factors. The Third Report of the Expert Panel on Detection, Evaluation, and Treatment of High Blood Cholesterol in Adults (ATP III; Expert Panel, 2001) lists the clinical guidelines for cholesterol testing and management. ATP III guidelines address **primary prevention** (preventing the occurrence of CAD) and **secondary prevention** (preventing the progression of CAD). Elevated **low-density lipoprotein (LDL)** cholesterol, also known as the "bad cholesterol," is the primary target of cholesterol-lowering therapy. Those at highest risk for having a cardiac event within 10 years are those with existing CAD or those with diabetes, peripheral arterial disease, abdominal aortic aneurysm, or carotid artery disease. The latter diseases are called CAD risk equivalents, because patients with these diseases have the same risk for a cardiac event as patients with CAD (Chart 28-1). The possibility of having a cardiac event within 10 years is also determined by factors such as age, systolic blood pressure, smoking history, level of total cholesterol, level of LDL, and level of **high-density lipoprotein (HDL)**, also known as the "good cholesterol."

In addition, a cluster of metabolic abnormalities known as **metabolic syndrome** has emerged as a major risk factor for cardiovascular disease (Haffner & Taegtmeyer, 2003; Wilson & Grundy, 2003). A diagnosis of this syndrome includes three of the following conditions:

- Insulin resistance (fasting glucose more than 100 mg/dL or abnormal glucose tolerance test)
- Abdominal obesity (waist circumference more than 35 inches in women, more than 40 inches in men)
- Dyslipidemia (triglycerides more than 150 mg/dL, HDL less than 50 mg/dL in women, less than 40 mg/dL in men)
- Hypertension
- Proinflammatory state (high levels of C-reactive protein)
- Prothrombotic state (high fibrinogen)

Many people with type 2 diabetes mellitus fit this clinical picture. It is theorized that in obese patients, excessive adipose tissue may secrete mediators that lead to metabolic changes (Reilly & Rader, 2003). Immune mechanisms are activated and contribute to atherogenic changes in the cardiovascular system (Fig. 28-3).

Measurement of lipoprotein(a) [Lp(a)] and homocysteine (an amino acid associated with cardiac disease)

CHART 28-1

Coronary Artery Disease Risk Equivalents

Individuals at highest risk for a cardiac event within 10 years are those with existing coronary artery disease (CAD) and those with any of the following diseases, which are called CAD risk equivalents:

- Diabetes
- Peripheral arterial disease
- Abdominal aortic aneurysm
- Carotid artery disease

From Expert Panel on Detection, Evaluation, and Treatment of High Blood Cholesterol in Adults. (2001). Executive summary of the third report of the National Cholesterol Education Program (NCEP) Expert Panel on Detection, Evaluation, and Treatment of High Blood Cholesterol in Adults (Adult Treatment Panel III). *Journal of the American Medical Association, 285*(19), 2486–2497.

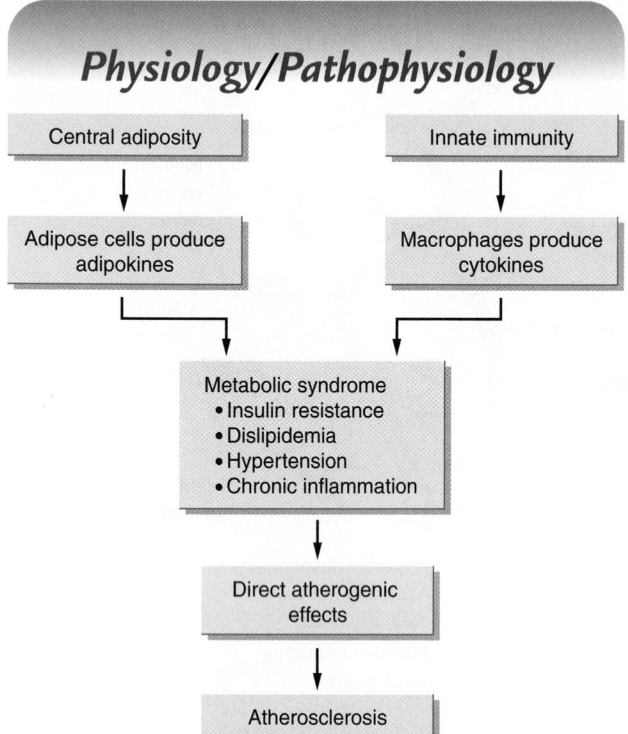

FIGURE 28-3. Pathophysiology of cardiovascular disease in metabolic syndrome. Both central adiposity and the immune system play a role in the development of metabolic syndrome. Adipokines (such as leptin) and cytokines (such as tumor necrosis factor) are thought to contribute to the development of metabolic abnormalities. The eventual effect of these processes is the promotion of atherosclerosis. Adapted from Reilly, M. P., & Rader, D. J. (2003). The metabolic syndrome: More than the sum of its parts? *Circulation, 108*(13), 1546–1551.

CHART 28-2

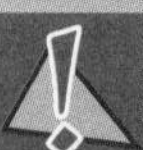

Risk Factors for Coronary Artery Disease

A modifiable risk factor is one over which a person may exercise control, such as by changing a lifestyle or personal habit or by using medication. A nonmodifiable risk factor is a circumstance over which a person has no control, such as age or heredity. A risk factor may operate independently or in tandem with other risk factors. The more risk factors a person has, the greater the likelihood of coronary artery disease. Those at risk are advised to seek regular medical examinations and to engage in "heart-healthy" behavior (a deliberate effort to reduce the number and extent of risks).

Nonmodifiable Risk Factors

Family history of coronary heart disease
Increasing age
Gender (men develop CAD at an earlier age than women)
Race (higher incidence of heart disease in African Americans than in Caucasians)

Modifiable Risk Factors

Hyperlipidemia
Cigarette smoking, tobacco use
Hypertension
Diabetes mellitus
Lack of estrogen in women
Obesity
Physical inactivity

may also be appropriate in some people (Pearson, Mensah, & Alexander, 2003).

Prevention

Four modifiable risk factors—cholesterol abnormalities, tobacco use, hypertension, and diabetes mellitus—have been cited as major risk factors for CAD and its complications. As a result, they receive much attention in health promotion programs (Chart 28-2).

Controlling Cholesterol Abnormalities

The association of a high blood cholesterol level with heart disease is well established. The metabolism of fats is an important contributor to the development of heart disease. Fats, which are insoluble in water, are encased in water-soluble lipoproteins that allow them to be transported within the circulatory system. The various lipoproteins are categorized by their protein content, which is measured in density. The density increases when more protein is present. Four elements of fat metabolism—total cholesterol, LDL, HDL, and triglycerides—affect the development of heart disease. Cholesterol is processed by the gastrointestinal tract into lipoprotein globules called chylomicrons. These are reprocessed by the liver as lipoproteins (Fig. 28-4). This is a physiologic process necessary for the formation of lipoprotein-based cell membranes and other important metabolic processes. When an excess of LDL is produced, LDL particles adhere to vulnerable points in the arterial endothelium. Here macrophages ingest them, leading to the formation of foam cells and the beginning of plaque formation.

All adults 20 years of age or older should have a fasting lipid profile (total cholesterol, LDL, HDL, and triglyceride) performed at least once every 5 years and more often if the profile is abnormal. Patients who have had an acute event (eg, MI), a **percutaneous coronary intervention (PCI)**, or a **coronary artery bypass graft (CABG)** require assessment of the LDL cholesterol level within a few months of the event or procedure, because LDL levels may be low immediately after the acute event or procedure. Subsequently, lipids should be monitored every 6 weeks until the desired level is achieved and then every 4 to 6 months (ATP III, 2001).

LDL exerts a harmful effect on the coronary vasculature because the small LDL particles can be easily transported into the vessel lining. In contrast, HDL promotes the use of total cholesterol by transporting LDL to the liver, where it is biodegraded and then excreted. The goal is to have low LDL values and high HDL values. The desired level of LDL depends on the patient:

- Less than 160 mg/dL for patients with one or no risk factors

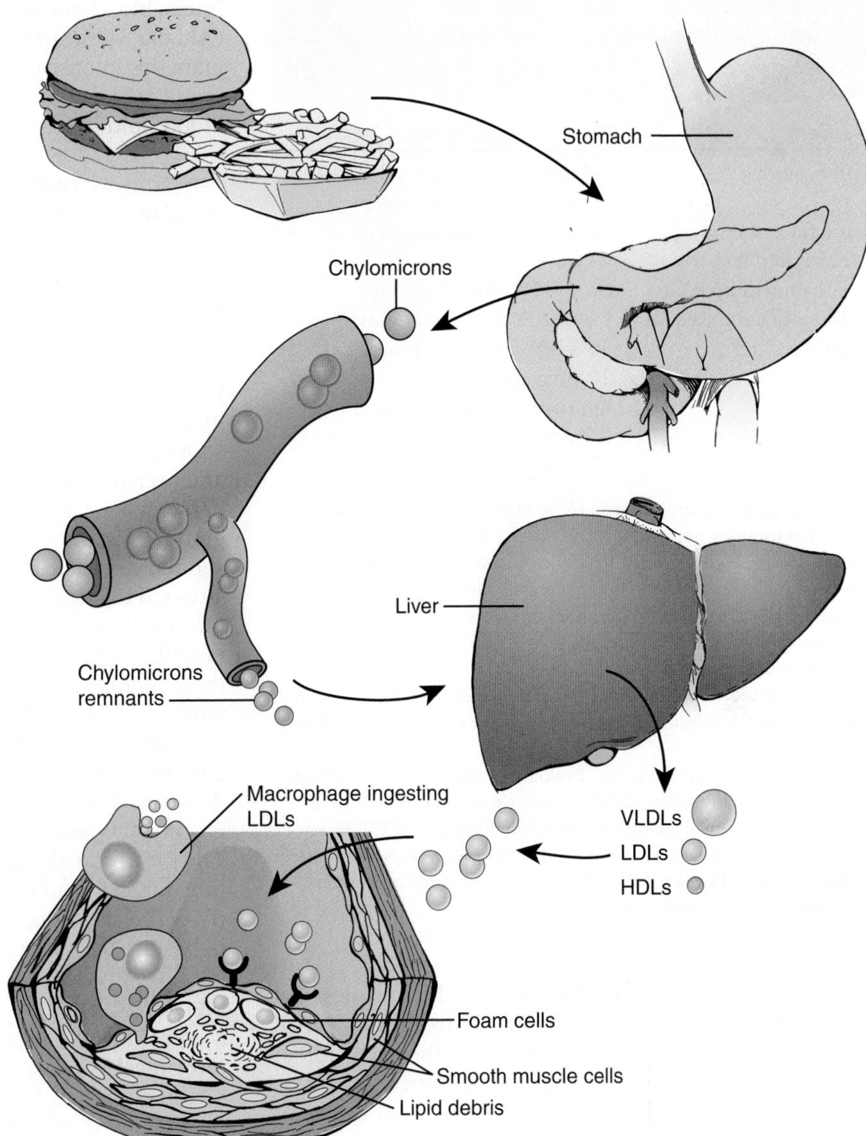

FIGURE 28-4. Lipoproteins and the development of atherosclerosis. As dietary cholesterol and saturated fat are processed by the gastrointestinal tract, chylomicrons enter the blood. They are broken down into chylomicron remnants in the capillaries. The liver processes them into lipoproteins. When these are released into the circulation, excess low-density lipoproteins (LDLs) adhere to receptors on the intimal wall. Macrophages also ingest LDLs and transport them into the vessel wall, beginning the process of plaque formation (Porth, 2005). HDLs, high-density lipoproteins; VLDL, very low density lipoprotein.

- Less than 130 mg/dL for patients with two or more risk factors
- Less than 100 mg/dL for patients with CAD or at high risk for CAD. Less than 70 mg/dL is desirable for patients at very high risk for an acute coronary event (Grundy, Cleeman, Merz, et al., 2004).

Serum cholesterol and LDL levels can often be controlled by diet and physical activity. Depending on the patient's LDL level and risk of CAD, medication may also be prescribed.

The level of HDL should exceed 40 mg/dL and should ideally be more than 60 mg/dL. A high HDL level is a strong negative risk factor for heart disease (ie, it protects against disease).

Triglyceride is another fatty substance, made up of fatty acids, that is transported through the blood by a lipoprotein. Although an elevated triglyceride level (more than 200 mg/dL) may be genetic in origin, it also can be caused by obesity, physical inactivity, excessive alcohol intake, high-carbohydrate diets, diabetes mellitus, kidney disease, and certain medications, such as oral contraceptives, corticosteroids, and beta-adrenergic blockers when given in higher doses. Management of an elevated triglyceride level focuses on weight reduction and increased physical activity. Medications such as nicotinic acid and fibric acids (eg, fenofibrate [Tricor], clofibrate [Atromid-S]) may also be prescribed, especially if the triglyceride level is greater than 500 mg/dL (ATP III, 2001).

DIETARY MEASURES

Table 28-1 provides recommendations of the Therapeutic Lifestyle Changes (TLC) diet (ATP III, 2001). These general recommendations may need to be adjusted for the individual patient who has other nutritional needs, such as the patient who is pregnant or has diabetes. To assist in following the appropriate TLC diet, the patient should be referred to a registered dietitian. Other TLC recommendations include weight loss, cessation of tobacco use, and increased physical activity.

TABLE 28-1 Nutrient Content of the Therapeutic Lifestyle Changes (TLC) Diet

Nutrient	Recommended Intake
Total calories*	Balance intake and expenditure to maintain desirable weight
Total fat	25%–35% of total calories
Saturated fat†	<7% of total calories
Polyunsaturated fat	Up to 10% of total calories
Monounsaturated fat	Up to 20% of total calories
Carbohydrate‡	50%–60% of total calories
Fiber	20–30 g/day
Protein	Approximately 15% of total calories
Cholesterol	<200 mg/day

*Daily energy expenditure should include at least moderate physical activity (contributing approximately 200 kcal per day).

†Trans-fatty acids are formed from the processing (manufacturing, hydrogenation) of vegetable oils into a more solid form. The effects of trans-fatty acids are similar to saturated fats (ie, raising low-density lipoprotein and lowering high-density lipoprotein). Intake of trans-fatty acids should be minimized.

‡Carbohydrates should be derived predominately from foods rich in complex carbohydrates, including grains, especially whole grains, fruits, and vegetables.

From Expert Panel on Detection, Evaluation, and Treatment of High Blood Cholesterol in Adults. (2001). Executive summary of the third report of the National Cholesterol Education Program (NCEP) Expert Panel on Detection, Evaluation, and Treatment of High Blood Cholesterol in Adults (Adult Treatment Panel III). *Journal of the American Medical Association, 285*(19), 2486–2497.

Soluble dietary fiber may also help reduce cholesterol levels. Soluble fibers, which are found in fresh fruit, cereal grains, vegetables, and legumes, enhance the excretion of metabolized cholesterol. The ability of fiber to reduce serum cholesterol continues to be investigated. Intake of at least 20 to 30 grams of fiber each day is recommended (ATP III, 2001).

Many resources are available to assist people to control their cholesterol levels. The National Heart, Lung, and Blood Institute (NHLBI) and its National Cholesterol Education Program (NCEP), the AHA, and the American Diabetes Association, as well as CAD support groups and reliable Internet sources, are a few examples of the available resources. Cookbooks and recipes that include the nutritional contents of foods can be included as resources for patients. Dietary control has been made easier because food manufacturers are required to provide comprehensive nutritional data on product labels. The label information of interest to a person attempting to eat a heart-healthy diet is as follows:

- Serving size, expressed in household measures
- Amount of total fat per serving
- Amount of saturated fat and trans fat per serving
- Amount of cholesterol per serving
- Amount of fiber per serving

Patients who adopt strict vegetarian dietary guidelines, such as those recommended by the Ornish Heart Disease Reversing Program, have significant reduction in blood lipids, blood glucose, body mass index, and blood pressure (Aldana, Whitmer, Greenlaw, et al., 2003). However, a program this intensive is not acceptable to all people who should modify risk factors. The effects of low-carbohydrate diets on blood lipid levels are under study.

PHYSICAL ACTIVITY

Regular, moderate physical activity increases HDL levels and reduces triglyceride levels. The goal for the average person is a total of 30 minutes of moderate exercise (such as brisk walking) on most days (Mosca, 2004). The nurse helps the patient set realistic goals for physical activity. For example, the inactive patient can start with activity that lasts 3 minutes, such as parking farther from a building to increase daily walking time. For sustained activity, patients should begin with a 5-minute warm-up period to stretch and prepare the body for exercise. They should end the exercise with a 5-minute cool-down period in which they gradually reduce the intensity of the activity to prevent a sudden decrease in cardiac output. Patients should be instructed to engage in an activity or variety of activities that interest them, to maintain motivation. They should also be taught to exercise to an intensity that does not preclude their ability to talk; if they cannot have a conversation while exercising, they should slow down or switch to a less intensive activity. When the weather is hot and humid, the patient should exercise during the early morning, or indoors, and wear loose-fitting clothing. When the weather is cold, the patient should layer clothing and wear a hat. The nurse can also suggest walking in large stores or shopping malls in bad weather. The patient should stop any activity if chest pain, unusual shortness of breath, dizziness, lightheadedness, or nausea occurs.

MEDICATIONS

Medications are used in some instances to control cholesterol levels (Table 28-2). If diet alone cannot normalize serum cholesterol levels, medications can have a synergistic effect with the prescribed diet. Lipid-lowering medications can reduce CAD mortality in patients with elevated lipid levels and in at-risk patients with normal lipid levels. The lipid-lowering agents affect the different lipid components and are usually grouped into four types:

- 3-Hydroxy-3-methylglutaryl coenzyme A (HMG-CoA) reductase inhibitors or statins (eg, atorvastatin [Lipitor], simvastatin [Zocor]; see Table 28-2) block cholesterol synthesis, lower LDL and triglyceride levels, and increase HDL levels. These medications are frequently the initial medication therapy for significantly elevated cholesterol and LDL levels. Because of their effect on the liver, results of hepatic function tests are monitored.
- Nicotinic acids (niacin [Niacor, Niaspan]; see Table 28-2) decrease lipoprotein synthesis, lower LDL and triglyceride levels, and increase HDL levels. The dose of niacin needs to be titrated weekly to achieve therapeutic dosage. Niacin may be used for minimally elevated cholesterol and LDL levels or as an adjunct to a statin when the lipid goal has not been achieved and triglycerides are elevated. Side effects include gastrointestinal upset, gout, and flushing. Because of the effect of niacin on the liver, hepatic function is monitored.

TABLE 28-2 Medications Affecting Lipoprotein Metabolism

Medication and Daily Dosage	Lipid/Lipoprotein Effects	Side Effects	Contraindications
HMG-CoA Reductase Inhibitors (statins)			
Lovastatin (Mevacor) Prevastatin (Pravachol) Simvastatin (Zocor) Fluvastatin (Lescol) Atorvastatin calcium (Lipitor) Rosuvastatin (Crestor)	LDL ↓ 18–55% HDL ↑ 5–15% TG ↓ 7–30%	Myopathy, increased liver enzyme levels	Absolute: active or chronic liver disease Relative: concomitant use of certain drugs*
Nicotinic Acid			
Niacin (Niacor, Niaspan) Immediate-release nicotinic acid Extended-release nicotinic acid Sustained-release nicotinic acid	LDL ↓ 5–25% HDL ↑ 15–35% TG ↓ 20–50%	Flushing, hyperglycemia, hyperuricemia (or gout), upper gastrointestinal distress, hepatotoxicity	Absolute: chronic liver disease, severe gout Relative: diabetes, hyperuricemia, peptic ulcer disease
Fibric Acids			
Fenofibrate (Tricor) Clofibrate (Atromid-S)	LDL ↓ 5–20% (may be increased in patients with high TG) HDL ↑ 10–20% TG ↓ 20–50%	Dyspepsia, gallstones, myopathy, unexplained non-CHD deaths	Absolute: severe renal disease, severe hepatic disease
Bile Acid Sequestrants			
Cholestyramine (LoCholest, Questran, Prevalite) Colesevelam (Welchol) Colestipol HCl (Colestid)	LDL ↓ 15–30% HDL ↑ 3–5% TG no change or increase	Gastrointestinal distress, constipation, decreased absorption of other drugs	Absolute: dysbetalipoproteinemia, TG >400 mg/dL Relative: TG >200 mg/dL

HMG-CoA, 3-hydroxy-3-methylglutaryl coenzyme A; LDL, low-density lipoprotein; HDL, high-density lipoprotein; TG, triglycerides; ↓ decrease, ↑ increase; CHD, coronary heart disease

*Cyclosporine (Neoral, Sandimmune, SangCya); macrolide antibiotics (azithromycin [Zithromax], clarithromycin [Biaxin]; dirithromycin [Dynabac]; erythromycin [Aknemycin, E-mycin, Ery-Tab]; various antifungal agents and cytochrome P-450 inhibitors; fibrates; and niacin should be used with appropriate caution).

From Expert Panel on Detection, Evaluation, and Treatment of High Blood Cholesterol in Adults. (2001). Executive summary of the third report of the National Cholesterol Education Program (NCEP) Expert Panel on Detection, Evaluation, and Treatment of High Blood Cholesterol in Adults (Adult Treatment Panel III). *Journal of the American Medical Association, 285*(19), 2486–2497.

- Fibric acid or fibrates (eg, clofibrate [Atromid-S], fenofibrate [Tricor]; see Table 28-2) decrease the synthesis of cholesterol, reduce triglyceride levels, and increase HDL levels. They have the potential to increase LDLs and may be used in patients with triglyceride levels above 400 mg/dL. Because of the risk of myopathy and acute renal failure, fibrates should be used with caution in patients who are also taking a statin.
- Bile acid sequestrants or resins (eg, cholestyramine [LoCholest, Questran, Prevalite]; see Table 28-2) bind cholesterol in the intestine, increase its breakdown, and lower LDL levels with minimal effect on HDLs and no effect (or minimal increase) on triglyceride levels. These medications are more often used as adjunct therapy when statins alone have not been effective in controlling lipid levels and triglyceride levels are less than 200 mg/dL. Significant side effects, such as gastric distention and constipation, can occur with use of these medications.

Medication therapy is reserved for at-risk patients and is not regarded as a substitute for dietary modification. All of these medications have been shown to reduce major coronary events (ATP III, 2001).

Patients with elevated cholesterol levels should be monitored for adherence to the therapeutic plan, the effect of cholesterol-lowering medications, and the development of side effects. Lipid levels are obtained and adjustments made to the diet and medication every 6 weeks until the lipid goal or maximum dose is achieved and then every 6 months thereafter.

Promoting Cessation of Tobacco Use

Cigarette smoking contributes to the development and severity of CAD in the following three ways:

- First, the inhalation of smoke increases the blood carbon monoxide level, and hemoglobin, the oxygen-carrying component of blood, combines more readily with carbon monoxide than with oxygen. A decreased amount of available oxygen may decrease the heart's ability to pump.
- Second, the nicotinic acid in tobacco triggers the release of catecholamines, which raise the heart rate and blood pressure. Nicotinic acid can also cause the coronary arteries to constrict. Smokers have a tenfold increase in risk for sudden cardiac death. The increase in catecholamines may be a factor in sudden cardiac death.
- Third, use of tobacco causes a detrimental vascular response and increases platelet adhesion, leading to a higher probability of thrombus formation.

A person with increased risk for heart disease is encouraged to stop tobacco use through any means possible: educational programs, counseling, consistent motivation and reinforcement messages, support groups, and medications. Some people have found complementary therapies (eg, acupuncture, guided imagery, hypnosis) to be helpful. People who stop smoking reduce their risk of heart disease by 30% to 50% within the first year, and the risk continues to decline as long as they refrain from smoking.

Exposure to other smokers' smoke (passive or secondhand smoke) is believed to cause heart disease in nonsmokers. Oral contraceptive use by women who smoke is inadvisable because these medications significantly increase the risk for CAD and sudden cardiac death.

Use of medications such as the nicotine patch (Nicotrol, NicoDerm CQ, Habitrol) or the antidepressant bupropion (Zyban) may assist with stopping use of tobacco. Products containing nicotine have some of the same effects as smoking: catecholamine release (increasing heart rate and blood pressure) and increased platelet adhesion. These medications should be used for a short time and at the lowest effective doses.

Managing Hypertension

Hypertension is defined as blood pressure measurements that repeatedly exceed 140/90 mm Hg. The risk of cardiovascular disease increases as blood pressure increases, and people with a blood pressure greater than 120/80 mm Hg are considered prehypertensive and at risk (Chobanian, Bakris, Cushman, et al., 2003). Long-standing elevated blood pressure may result in increased stiffness of the vessel walls, leading to vessel injury and a resulting inflammatory response within the intima. Inflammatory mediators then lead to the release of growth-promoting factors that cause vessel hypertrophy and hyperresponsiveness. These changes result in acceleration and aggravation of atherosclerosis. Hypertension also increases the work of the left ventricle, which must pump harder to eject blood into the arteries. Over time, the increased workload causes the heart to enlarge and thicken (ie, hypertrophy) and may eventually lead to cardiac failure.

Early detection of high blood pressure and adherence to a therapeutic regimen can prevent the serious consequences associated with untreated elevated blood pressure. Hypertension is discussed in detail in Chapter 32.

Controlling Diabetes Mellitus

The relationship between diabetes mellitus and heart disease has been confirmed. For 65% to 75% of patients with diabetes, cardiovascular disease is identified as the cause of death (Zipes, Libby, Bonow, et al., 2005). Hyperglycemia fosters dyslipidemia, increased platelet aggregation, and altered red blood cell function, which can lead to thrombus formation. It has been suggested that these metabolic alterations impair endothelial cell–dependent vasodilation and smooth muscle function. Treatment with insulin (eg, Humalog, Humulin, Novolin) and metformin (Glucophage) has shown improvement in endothelial function and improved endothelial-dependent dilation (Gaenzer, Neumayr, Marschang, et al., 2002). Diabetes is considered equivalent to existing CAD as a risk factor for a cardiac event within 10 years (ATP III, 2001). Diabetes is discussed in detail in Chapter 41.

Gender

Because heart disease had been considered to primarily affect Caucasian men, the disease has not been as readily recognized and treated in women. However, in the United States, it is reported that more than 500,000 women die of cardiovascular disease each year, a number that exceeds that for men and is higher than the next seven causes of death combined (AHA, 2004). For women, cardiovascular events occur an average of 10 years later in life than in men, but overall, women tend to have a higher incidence of complications from cardiovascular disease and a higher mortality. African-American women have a mortality rate nearly twice that of Caucasian women (AHA, 2004). Women tend not to recognize the symptoms as early as men and to wait longer to report their symptoms and seek medical assistance (Nabel & Selker, 2004). In the past, women were less likely than men to be referred for coronary artery diagnostic procedures, to receive medical therapy (eg, **thrombolytic** therapy to break down the blood clots that cause acute MI, or nitroglycerin), and to be treated with invasive interventions (eg, angioplasty) (Sheifer, Escarce, & Schulman, 2000). With better education of health care professionals and the general public, gender differences now have less influence on diagnosis and treatment. A recent analysis of procedures used for acute MI found that women were as likely as men to undergo cardiac catheterization and PCIs but were less likely to undergo coronary bypass surgery (Bertoni, Bonds, Lovato, et al., 2004).

In women younger than 55 years of age, the incidence of CAD is significantly lower than in men. However, in women older than 55 years of age, the incidence of CAD is approximately equal to that in men. The age difference between women and men newly diagnosed with CAD was traditionally thought to be related to estrogen. It is now recognized that menopause is a milestone in the aging process during which risk factors tend to accumulate. Cardiovascular disease may be well developed by the time of menopause, despite the supposed protective effects of estrogen (Mosca, 2004). Although hormone therapy (HT)—formerly referred to as hormone replacement therapy (HRT)—for menopausal women was once promoted as preventive therapy for CAD, research studies do not support HT as an effective means of prevention. HT decreases menopausal symptoms and the risk for osteoporosis-related bone fractures, but HT also has been associated with an increased incidence of CAD, breast cancer, deep vein thrombosis, stroke, and pulmonary embolism. The Women's Health Initiative demonstrated that long-term HT use may have more risks than benefits, and that HT should not be initiated or continued for primary prevention of CAD. The U.S. Preventive Services Task Force (2003) concurred with these recommendations.

Behavior Patterns

Many clinicians believe that stress and certain behaviors contribute to the pathogenesis of CAD and cardiac events. Psychological and epidemiologic studies have identified behaviors that characterize people who are prone to heart disease: excessive competitiveness, a sense of time urgency or impatience, aggressiveness, and hostility. A person with these behaviors is classified as having a type A personality.

The type A personality may not be as significant as was once thought; evidence of its precise role remains inconclusive. Current predictors of coronary events focus on physiologic factors (Moustapha & Anderson, 2003). However, it has long been recognized that emotional stress can lead to a release of catecholamines and subsequent coronary ischemia. Thus, people with type A traits are advised to alter behaviors and responses to triggering events and to reduce other risk factors. Nurses can assist by teaching cognitive restructuring and relaxation techniques. Because depression is associated with negative outcomes, patients should also be assessed for depression and appropriately treated.

CHART 28-3

Types of Angina

- **Stable angina:** predictable and consistent pain that occurs on exertion and is relieved by rest
- **Unstable angina** (also called preinfarction angina or crescendo angina): symptoms occur more frequently and last longer than stable angina. The threshold for pain is lower, and pain may occur at rest.
- **Intractable or refractory angina:** severe incapacitating chest pain
- **Variant angina** (also called Prinzmetal's angina): pain at rest with reversible ST-segment elevation; thought to be caused by coronary artery vasospasm
- **Silent ischemia:** objective evidence of ischemia (such as ECG changes with a stress test), but patient reports no symptoms

Angina Pectoris

Angina pectoris is a clinical syndrome usually characterized by episodes or paroxysms of pain or pressure in the anterior chest. The cause is insufficient coronary blood flow, resulting in a decreased oxygen supply when there is increased myocardial demand for oxygen in response to physical exertion or emotional stress. In other words, the need for oxygen exceeds the supply. The severity of angina is based on the precipitating activity and its effect on activities of daily living.

Pathophysiology

Angina is usually caused by atherosclerotic disease. Almost invariably, angina is associated with a significant obstruction of a major coronary artery. Normally, the myocardium extracts a large amount of oxygen from the coronary circulation to meet its continuous demands. When there is an increase in demand, flow through the coronary arteries needs to be increased. When there is blockage in a coronary artery, flow cannot be increased, and ischemia results. The types of angina are listed in Chart 28-3. Several factors are associated with typical anginal pain:

- Physical exertion, which can precipitate an attack by increasing myocardial oxygen demand
- Exposure to cold, which can cause vasoconstriction and elevated blood pressure, with increased oxygen demand
- Eating a heavy meal, which increases the blood flow to the mesenteric area for digestion, thereby reducing the blood supply available to the heart muscle. In a severely compromised heart, shunting of blood for digestion can be sufficient to induce anginal pain.
- Stress or any emotion-provoking situation, causing the release of catecholamines, which increases blood pressure, heart rate, and myocardial workload

Atypical angina is not associated with these listed factors. It may occur at rest.

Clinical Manifestations

Ischemia of the heart muscle may produce pain or other symptoms, varying in severity from mild indigestion to a choking or heavy sensation in the upper chest that ranges from discomfort to agonizing pain accompanied by severe apprehension and a feeling of impending death. The pain is often felt deep in the chest behind the sternum (retrosternal area). Typically, the pain or discomfort is poorly localized and may radiate to the neck, jaw, shoulders, and inner aspects of the upper arms, usually the left arm. The patient often feels tightness or a heavy, choking, or strangling sensation that has a viselike, insistent quality. The patient with diabetes mellitus may not have severe pain with angina because diabetic neuropathy can blunt nociceptors' transmission, dulling the perception of pain. A woman may have different symptoms than a man, because coronary disease in women tends to be more diffuse and affects long segments of the artery rather than discrete segments.

A feeling of weakness or numbness in the arms, wrists, and hands, as well as shortness of breath, pallor, diaphoresis, dizziness or lightheadedness, and nausea and vomiting, may accompany the pain. Anxiety may occur with angina. An important characteristic of angina is that it subsides with

NURSING RESEARCH PROFILE

Recognizing the Symptoms of Unstable Angina

DeVon, H. A., & Zerwic, J. J. (2003). The symptoms of unstable angina—do women and men differ? *Nursing Research, 52*(2), 108–118.

Purpose

Previous research has identified differences in the epidemiology, presentation, and outcomes of women and men with coronary artery disease. The purpose of this study was to determine whether there are gender differences in the symptoms of unstable angina, and if so, whether these differences remain after controlling for age, diabetes, anxiety, depression, and functional status.

Design

A convenience sample of 50 women and 50 men hospitalized with unstable angina was recruited from two medical centers. A quantitative, nonexperimental design was used. Subjects were interviewed in their hospital rooms. Three instruments (the Unstable Angina Symptoms Questionnaire [UASQ], the Canadian Cardiovascular Society [CCS] classification of angina, and the Hospital Anxiety and Depression Scale [HADS]) were used to assess anginal symptoms, anxiety, and depression.

Findings

The most frequently reported symptoms for both genders were chest pain and shortness of breath. More women than men experienced shortness of breath (74% versus 60%), weakness (74% versus 48%), difficulty breathing (66% versus 38%), nausea (42% versus 22%), and loss of appetite (40% versus 10%). Women also experienced more back pain, stabbing pain, and depression. The researchers concluded that during episodes of unstable angina, women have similar symptoms to those of men, but a higher proportion of women also have symptoms considered to be less typical, including upper back pain, stabbing pain, and knife-like pain.

Nursing Implications

The results of this study are consistent with previous studies that focused on gender differences in symptoms of acute myocardial infarction. Nurses should be aware that women with unstable angina frequently present with typical symptoms but may also present with a number of less typical symptoms. Patient assessment should include a careful history to elicit these symptoms. In addition, women should be educated about both typical and atypical symptoms of acute coronary events.

rest or nitroglycerin. In many patients, anginal symptoms follow a stable, predictable pattern.

Unstable angina is characterized by attacks that increase in frequency and severity and are not relieved by rest and nitroglycerin. Patients with unstable angina require medical intervention.

Gerontologic Considerations

The elderly person with angina may not exhibit the typical pain profile because of the diminished responses of neurotransmitters that occur with aging. Often, the presenting symptom in the elderly is dyspnea. If pain occurs, it is atypical pain that radiates to both arms rather than just the left arm. Sometimes, there are no symptoms ("silent" CAD), making recognition and diagnosis a clinical challenge. Elderly patients should be encouraged to recognize their chest pain–like symptom (eg, weakness) as an indication that they should rest or take prescribed medications. Pharmacologic stress testing may be used to diagnose CAD in elderly patients because other conditions (eg, peripheral vascular disease, arthritis, degenerative disk disease, physical disability, foot problems) may limit the patient's ability to exercise (Chart 28-4).

Assessment and Diagnostic Findings

The diagnosis of angina begins with the patient's history related to the clinical manifestations of ischemia. A 12-lead electrocardiogram (ECG) and blood laboratory values help in making the diagnosis. The patient may undergo an exercise or pharmacologic stress test in which the heart is monitored by ECG, echocardiogram, or both. The patient may also be referred for a nuclear scan or invasive procedure (eg, cardiac catheterization, coronary artery angiography).

Because CAD is believed to result from inflammation of the arterial endothelium, C-reactive protein (CRP), a marker for inflammation of vascular endothelium, may be measured. High blood levels of CRP have been associated with increased coronary artery calcification and risk of an acute cardiovascular event (eg, MI) in seemingly healthy people (Ridker, Rifai, Rose, et al., 2002). There is interest in using CRP levels as an additional risk factor for cardiovascular disease in clinical evaluation and research, but the predictive value of CRP levels has not yet been fully established (Pearson et al., 2003).

Medical Management

The objectives of the medical management of angina are to decrease the oxygen demand of the myocardium and to increase the oxygen supply. Medically, these objectives are met through pharmacologic therapy and control of risk factors. Alternatively, reperfusion procedures may be used to restore the blood supply to the myocardium. These include PCI procedures (eg, **percutaneous transluminal coronary angioplasty** [**PTCA**], intracoronary stents, and atherectomy) and CABG.

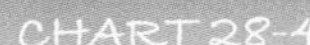

CHART 28-4

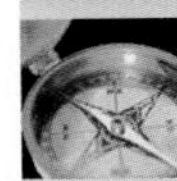

Ethics and Related Issues

Should Aggressive Treatment be Recommended for the Elderly With Acute Coronary Syndrome (ACS)?

SITUATION

Many patients who present with acute coronary events are elderly. They often have chronic conditions such as diabetes or arthritis. Elderly patients have traditionally been managed conservatively with medications, but currently interventions such as cardiac catheterization may be recommended. These patients look to their family members for help with treatment decisions.

DILEMMA

An 80-year-old woman is hospitalized with unstable angina. The cardiologist discusses the situation with her two adult sons. He recommends cardiac catheterization with possible PTCA and stent placement. The patient is oriented but lethargic. She defers to her sons regarding treatment decisions. One son worries that she will be subjected to an invasive procedure that is potentially high risk, painful, expensive, and possibly futile. The second son feels that if there is hope of success, she should have the procedure.

DISCUSSION

Research on the risks and benefits of treatment for ACS now includes the elderly as a subgroup. One study reports that the elderly may benefit as much, if not more, than younger patients from coronary reperfusion procedures in terms of reduction of death or myocardial infarction (Bach, Cannon, Weintraub, et al., 2004)

1. What arguments would you offer that support or discourage aggressive treatment for ACS in the elderly?
2. What assistance can you offer to enhance the patient and family's autonomy regarding decision making as well as their sense of justice regarding the allocation of resources?

Pharmacologic Therapy

NITROGLYCERIN

Nitrates remain the mainstay for treatment of angina pectoris. A vasoactive agent, nitroglycerin (Nitrostat, Nitrol, Nitro-Bid) is administered to reduce myocardial oxygen consumption, which decreases ischemia and relieves pain. Nitroglycerin dilates primarily the veins and, in higher doses, also the arteries. Dilation of the veins causes venous pooling of blood throughout the body. As a result, less blood returns to the heart, and filling pressure (preload) is reduced. If the patient is hypovolemic (does not have adequate circulating blood volume), the decrease in filling pressure can cause a significant decrease in cardiac output and blood pressure.

Nitrates in higher doses also relax the systemic arteriolar bed, lowering blood pressure and decreasing afterload. These effects decrease myocardial oxygen requirements and increase oxygen supply, bringing about a more favorable balance between supply and demand.

Nitroglycerin may be given by several routes: sublingual tablet or spray, oral capsule, topical agent, and intravenous (IV) administration. Sublingual nitroglycerin is generally placed under the tongue or in the cheek (buccal pouch) and alleviates the pain of ischemia within 3 minutes. Chart 28-5 provides more information on self-administration of sublingual nitroglycerin. Oral preparations and topical patches are used to provide sustained effects. The patches are often applied in the morning and removed at bedtime. This regimen allows for a nitrate-free period to prevent the development of tolerance.

A continuous or intermittent IV infusion of nitroglycerin may be administered to the hospitalized patient with recurring signs and symptoms of ischemia or after a revascularization procedure. The amount of nitroglycerin administered is based on the patient's symptoms while avoiding side effects such as hypotension. It usually is not administered if the systolic blood pressure is 90 mm Hg or less. Generally, after the patient is symptom-free, the nitroglycerin may be switched to a topical preparation within 24 hours.

BETA-ADRENERGIC BLOCKING AGENTS

Beta-blockers such as metoprolol (Lopressor, Toprol) and atenolol (Tenormin) reduce myocardial oxygen consumption by blocking beta-adrenergic sympathetic stimulation to the heart. The result is a reduction in heart rate, slowed conduction of impulses through the conduction system, decreased blood pressure, and reduced myocardial **contractility** (force of contraction) to balance the myocardial oxygen needs (demands) and the amount of oxygen available (supply). This helps control chest pain and delays the onset of ischemia during work or exercise. Beta-blockers reduce the incidence of recurrent angina, infarction, and cardiac mortality. The dose can be titrated to achieve a resting heart rate of 50 to 60 beats per minute.

Cardiac side effects and possible contraindications include hypotension, bradycardia, advanced atrioventricular block, and decompensated heart failure. If a beta-blocker is given IV for an acute cardiac event, the ECG, blood pressure, and heart rate are monitored closely after the medication has been administered. Because some beta-blockers also affect the beta-adrenergic receptors in the bronchioles, causing bronchoconstriction, they are contraindicated in patients with significant pulmonary obstructive diseases, such as asthma. Other side effects include depression, fatigue, decreased libido, and masking of symptoms of hypoglycemia. Patients taking beta-blockers are cautioned not to stop taking them abruptly, because angina may worsen and MI may develop. Beta-blocker therapy should be decreased gradually over several days before being discontinued. Patients with

CHART 28-5

℞ PHARMACOLOGY · Self-Administration of Nitroglycerin

Most patients with angina pectoris must self-administer nitroglycerin on an as-needed basis. A key nursing role in such cases is educating patients about the medication and how to take it. Sublingual nitroglycerin comes in tablet and spray forms.

- Instruct the patient to make sure the mouth is moist, the tongue is still, and saliva is not swallowed until the nitroglycerin tablet dissolves. If the pain is severe, the patient can crush the tablet between the teeth to hasten sublingual absorption.
- Advise the patient to carry the medication at all times as a precaution. However, because nitroglycerin is very unstable, it should be carried securely in its original container (eg, capped dark glass bottle); tablets should never be removed and stored in metal or plastic pillboxes.
- Explain that nitroglycerin is volatile and is inactivated by heat, moisture, air, light, and time. Instruct the patient to renew the nitroglycerin supply every 6 months.
- Inform the patient that the medication should be taken in anticipation of any activity that may produce pain. Because nitroglycerin increases tolerance for exercise and stress when taken prophylactically (ie, before angina-producing activity, such as exercise, stair-climbing, or sexual intercourse), it is best taken before pain develops.
- Recommend that the patient note how long it takes for the nitroglycerin to relieve the discomfort. Advise the patient that if pain persists after taking three sublingual tablets at 5-minute intervals, emergency medical services should be called.
- Discuss possible side effects of nitroglycerin, including flushing, throbbing headache, hypotension, and tachycardia.
- Advise the patient to sit down for a few minutes when taking nitroglycerin to avoid hypotension and syncope.

diabetes who take beta-blockers are instructed to monitor their blood glucose levels often and to observe for signs and symptoms of hypoglycemia.

CALCIUM CHANNEL BLOCKING AGENTS

Calcium channel blockers (calcium ion antagonists) have a variety of effects. These agents decrease sinoatrial node automaticity and atrioventricular node conduction, resulting in a slower heart rate and a decrease in the strength of the heart muscle contraction (negative inotropic effect). These effects decrease the workload of the heart. Calcium channel blockers also relax the blood vessels, causing a decrease in blood pressure and an increase in coronary artery perfusion. Calcium channel blockers increase myocardial oxygen supply by dilating the smooth muscle wall of the coronary arterioles; they decrease myocardial oxygen demand by reducing systemic arterial pressure and the workload of the left ventricle.

The calcium channel blockers most commonly used are amlodipine (Norvasc) and diltiazem (Cardizem, Tiazac). They may be used by patients who cannot take beta-blockers, who develop significant side effects from beta-blockers or nitrates, or who still have pain despite beta-blocker and nitroglycerin therapy. Calcium channel blockers are also used to prevent and treat vasospasm, which commonly occurs after an invasive interventional procedure.

First-generation calcium channel blockers such as nifedipine should be avoided or used with great caution in people with heart failure, because they decrease myocardial contractility. Amlodipine and felodipine (Plendil) are the calcium channel blockers of choice for patients with heart failure. Hypotension may occur after the IV administration of any of the calcium channel blockers. Other side effects may include atrioventricular block, bradycardia, constipation, and gastric distress.

ANTIPLATELET AND ANTICOAGULANT MEDICATIONS

Antiplatelet medications are administered to prevent platelet aggregation and subsequent thrombosis, which impedes blood flow.

Aspirin. Aspirin prevents platelet activation and reduces the incidence of MI and death in patients with CAD. A 160- to 325-mg dose of aspirin should be given to the patient with angina as soon as the diagnosis is made (eg, in the emergency department or physician's office) and then continued with 81 to 325 mg daily. Although aspirin may be one of the most important medications in the treatment of CAD, it may be overlooked because of its low cost and common use. Patients should be advised to continue aspirin even if they concurrently take nonsteroidal anti-inflammatory drugs (NSAIDs) or other analgesics. Because aspirin may cause gastrointestinal upset and bleeding, the use of H_2-blockers (eg, famotidine [Pepcid], ranitidine [Zantac]) or proton pump inhibitors (eg, omeprazole [Prilosec]) should be considered to allow continued aspirin therapy.

Clopidogrel and Ticlopidine. Clopidogrel (Plavix) or ticlopidine (Ticlid) is given to patients who are allergic to aspirin or given in addition to aspirin in patients at high risk for MI. Unlike aspirin, these medications take a few days to achieve their antiplatelet effect. They also cause gastrointestinal upset.

Heparin. IV unfractionated heparin prevents the formation of new blood clots. Treating patients with unstable angina with heparin reduces the occurrence of MI. If the patient's signs and symptoms indicate a significant risk for a cardiac event, the patient is hospitalized and may be given an IV bolus of heparin and started on a continuous infusion. The amount of heparin administered is based on the results of the activated partial thromboplastin time (aPTT). Heparin therapy is usually considered therapeutic when the aPTT is 2 to 2.5 times the normal aPTT value.

A subcutaneous injection of low-molecular-weight heparin (LMWH; enoxaparin [Lovenox] or dalteparin [Fragmin]) may be used instead of IV unfractionated heparin to treat patients with unstable angina or non–ST-segment elevation MIs (Antman, Anbe, Armstrong, et al., 2004). LMWH provides effective and stable anticoagulation, potentially reducing the risk of rebound ischemic events, and it eliminates the need to monitor aPTT results. LMWH may be beneficial before and during PCIs and for ST-segment elevation MIs.

Because unfractionated heparin and LMWH increase the risk of bleeding, the patient is monitored for signs and symptoms of external and internal bleeding, such as low blood pressure, increased heart rate, and decreased serum hemoglobin and hematocrit. The patient receiving heparin is placed on bleeding precautions, which include:

- Applying pressure to the site of any needle puncture for a longer time than usual
- Avoiding intramuscular (IM) injections
- Avoiding tissue injury and bruising from trauma or use of constrictive devices (eg, continuous use of an automatic blood pressure cuff)

A decrease in platelet count or evidence of thrombosis may indicate heparin-induced thrombocytopenia (HIT), an antibody-mediated reaction to heparin that may result in thrombosis (Cleveland, 2003). Patients who have received heparin within the past 3 months and those who have been receiving unfractionated heparin for 5 to 15 days are at high risk for HIT.

Glycoprotein IIb/IIIa Agents. IV administration of glycoprotein *(GP) IIb/IIIa agents* (abciximab [ReoPro], tirofiban [Aggrastat], eptifibatide [Integrilin]) is indicated for hospitalized patients with unstable angina and as adjunct therapy for PCI. These agents prevent platelet aggregation by blocking the GPIIb/IIIa receptors on the platelets, preventing adhesion of fibrinogen and other factors that crosslink platelets to each other and thereby allow platelets to form a thrombus (clot). As with heparin, bleeding is the major side effect, and bleeding precautions should be initiated.

OXYGEN ADMINISTRATION

Oxygen therapy is usually initiated at the onset of chest pain in an attempt to increase the amount of oxygen delivered to the myocardium and to decrease pain. The therapeutic effectiveness of oxygen is determined by observing the rate and rhythm of respirations. Blood oxygen saturation is monitored by pulse oximetry; the normal oxygen saturation (SpO_2) level is greater than 93%.

Nursing Process

The Patient With Angina Pectoris

Assessment

The nurse gathers information about the patient's symptoms and activities, especially those that precede and precipitate attacks of angina pectoris. Appropriate questions are listed in Chart 28-6, using a PQRST format. Other helpful questions may be asked: How long

CHART 28-6

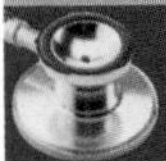

Assessing for Symptoms Associated With Angina

ACRONYM	FACTORS ABOUT PAIN THAT NEED TO BE ASSESSED	ASSESSMENT QUESTIONS
P	Position/Location	"Where is the pain? Can you point to it?"
	Provocation	"What were you doing when the pain began?"
Q	Quality	"How would you describe the pain?" "Is it like the pain you had before?"
	Quantity	"Has the pain been constant?"
R	Radiation	"Can you feel the pain anywhere else?"
	Relief	"Did anything make the pain better?"
S	Severity	"How would you rate the pain on a 0–10 scale with 0 being no pain and 10 being the most amount of pain?" (or use visual analog scale or adjective rating scale)
	Symptoms	"Did you notice any other symptoms with the pain?"
T	Timing	"How long ago did the pain start?"

Jarvis, C. (2004) *Physical examination and health assessment* (4th ed.) St. Louis: Saunders.

does the angina usually last? Does nitroglycerin relieve the angina? If so, how many tablets or sprays are needed to achieve relief? How long does it takes for relief to occur?

The answers to these questions form a basis for designing an effective program of treatment and prevention. In addition to assessing angina pectoris or its equivalent, the nurse also assesses the patient's risk factors for CAD, the patient's response to angina, the patient's and family's understanding of the diagnosis, and adherence to the current treatment plan.

Diagnosis

Nursing Diagnoses

Based on the assessment data, major nursing diagnoses may include:

- Ineffective cardiac tissue perfusion secondary to CAD, as evidenced by chest pain or equivalent symptoms
- Death anxiety
- Deficient knowledge about the underlying disease and methods for avoiding complications
- Noncompliance, ineffective management of therapeutic regimen related to failure to accept necessary lifestyle changes

Collaborative Problems/ Potential Complications

Potential complications that may develop include the following, which are discussed in the chapters indicated:

- Acute pulmonary edema (see Chapter 30)
- Heart failure (see Chapter 30)
- Cardiogenic shock (see Chapter 30)
- Dysrhythmias and cardiac arrest (see Chapters 27 and 30)
- MI (described later in this chapter)

Planning and Goals

Major patient goals include immediate and appropriate treatment when angina occurs, prevention of angina, reduction of anxiety, awareness of the disease process and understanding of the prescribed care, adherence to the self-care program, and absence of complications.

Nursing Interventions

Treating Angina

If the patient reports pain (or the person's equivalent to pain), the nurse takes immediate action. When a patient experiences angina, the nurse directs the patient to stop all activities and sit or rest in bed in a semi-Fowler's position to reduce the oxygen requirements of the ischemic myocardium. The nurse assesses the patient's angina, asking questions to determine whether the angina is the same as the patient typically experiences. A change may indicate a worsening of the disease or a different cause. The nurse then continues to assess the patient, measuring vital signs and observing for signs of respiratory distress. If the patient is in the hospital, a 12-lead ECG is usually obtained and scrutinized for ST-segment and T-wave changes. If the patient has been placed on cardiac monitoring with continuous ST-segment monitoring, the ST segment is assessed for changes.

Nitroglycerin is administered sublingually, and the patient's response is assessed (relief of chest pain and effect on blood pressure and heart rate). If the chest pain is unchanged or is lessened but still present, nitroglycerin administration is repeated up to three doses. Each time blood pressure, heart rate, and the ST segment (if the patient is on a monitor with ST-segment monitoring capability) are assessed. The nurse administers oxygen therapy if the patient's respiratory rate is increased or if the oxygen saturation level is decreased. Oxygen is usually administered at 2 L/min by nasal cannula, even without evidence of respiratory distress, although there is no documentation of its effect on outcome. If the pain is significant and continues after these interventions, the patient is further evaluated for acute MI and may be transferred to a higher-acuity nursing unit.

Reducing Anxiety

Patients with angina often fear loss of their roles within society and the family. They may also fear that the pain may lead to an MI or death. Exploring the implications that the diagnosis has for the patient and providing information about the illness, its treatment, and methods of preventing its progression are important nursing interventions. Various stress reduction methods should be explored with the patient. For example, music therapy, in which patients listen to selected music through headphones, has been shown to reduce anxiety in patients who are in a coronary care unit and may serve as an adjunct to therapeutic communication (Evans, 2002). Addressing the spiritual needs of the patient and family may also assist in allaying anxieties and fears.

Preventing Pain

The nurse reviews the assessment findings, identifies the level of activity that causes the patient's pain, and plans the patient's activities accordingly. If the patient has pain frequently or with minimal activity, the nurse alternates the patient's activities with rest periods. Balancing activity and rest is an important aspect of the educational plan for the patient and family.

Promoting Home and Community-Based Care

TEACHING PATIENTS SELF-CARE

Learning about the modifiable risk factors that contribute to the development of CAD and resulting angina is essential. Exploring what the patient and family see as their priorities in managing the disease and developing a plan based on those priorities can assist with patient adherence to the therapeutic regimen. It is important to explore with the patient methods to avoid, modify, or adapt the triggers for anginal pain. The teaching program for the patient with angina is designed so that the patient and family understand the illness, identify the symptoms of myocardial ischemia, state the actions to take when symptoms develop, and discuss methods to prevent chest pain and the advancement of CAD. The goals of the educational program are to reduce the frequency and severity of anginal attacks, to delay the progress of the underlying disease if possible, and to prevent complications. The factors outlined in Chart 28-7 are important in educating the patient with angina pectoris.

The self-care program is prepared in collaboration with the patient and family or friends. Activities should be planned to minimize the occurrence of angina episodes. The patient needs to understand that any pain unrelieved within 15 minutes by the usual methods, including nitroglycerin (see Chart 28-5), should be treated at the closest emergency center; the patient should call 911 for assistance.

CONTINUING CARE

Arrangements are made for a home care nurse when appropriate. The home care nurse assists the patient with scheduling and keeping follow-up appointments. The patient may need reminders about follow-up monitoring, including periodic blood laboratory testing and ECGs. In addition, the home care nurse may monitor the patient's adherence to dietary restrictions and to prescribed antianginal medications, including nitroglycerin. If the patient has severe anginal symptoms, the nurse may assess the home environment and recommend modifications that diminish the occurrence of anginal episodes. For instance, if a patient cannot climb stairs without experiencing ischemia, the home care nurse may help the patient plan daily activities that minimize stair climbing. Some patients may benefit from moving the bedroom to a lower level in the home.

Evaluation

Expected Patient Outcomes

Expected patient outcomes may include:

1. Reports that pain is relieved promptly
   a. Recognizes symptoms
   b. Takes immediate action
   c. Seeks medical assistance if pain persists or changes in quality
2. Reports decreased anxiety
   a. Expresses acceptance of diagnosis
   b. Expresses control over choices within medical regimen
   c. Does not exhibit signs and symptoms that indicate a high level of anxiety

CHART 28-7

HOME CARE CHECKLIST • Managing Angina Pectoris

At the completion of home care instructions, the patient and significant other will be able to:	Patient	Caregiver
• Reduce the probability of an episode of anginal pain by balancing rest with activity:		
- Participate in a regular daily program of activities that do not produce chest discomfort, shortness of breath, or undue fatigue.	✔	
- Avoid exercises requiring sudden bursts of activity; avoid isometric exercise.	✔	
- State that temperature extremes (particularly cold) may induce anginal pain; therefore, avoid exercise in temperature extremes.	✔	
- Alternate activity with periods of rest.	✔	
- Use appropriate resources for support during emotionally stressful times (eg, counselor, nurse, clergy, physician).	✔	✔
• Avoid using medications or any over-the-counter substances (eg, diet pills, nasal decongestants) that can increase the heart rate and blood pressure without first discussing with a health care provider.	✔	✔
• Stop smoking and other use of tobacco, and avoid second-hand smoke (because smoking increases the heart rate, blood pressure, and blood carbon monoxide levels).	✔	✔
• Eat a diet low in saturated fat, high in fiber, and if indicated, lower in calories.	✔	✔
• Achieve and maintain normal blood pressure.	✔	
• Achieve and maintain normal blood glucose levels.	✔	
• Take medications, especially aspirin and beta-blockers, as prescribed.	✔	
• Carry nitroglycerin at all times; state when and how to use it; identify its side effects.	✔	✔

3. Understands ways to avoid complications and is free of complications
   a. Describes the process of angina
   b. Explains reasons for measures to prevent complications
   c. Exhibits normal ECG and cardiac biomarkers
   d. Experiences no signs and symptoms of acute MI
4. Adheres to self-care program
   a. Takes medications as prescribed
   b. Keeps health care appointments
   c. Implements plan to reduce risk factors

CHART 28-8

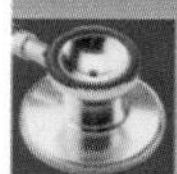

Assessing for Acute Myocardial Infarction (MI) or Acute Coronary Syndrome (ACS)

Be on the alert for the following signs and symptoms:

Cardiovascular

- Chest pain or discomfort, palpitations. Heart sounds may include S_3, S_4, and new onset of a murmur.
- Increased jugular venous distention may be seen if the MI has caused heart failure.
- Blood pressure may be elevated because of sympathetic stimulation or decreased because of decreased contractility, impending cardiogenic shock, or medications.
- Pulse deficit may indicate atrial fibrillation.
- In addition to ST-segment and T-wave changes, ECG may show tachycardia, bradycardia, or dysrhythmias.

Respiratory

Shortness of breath, dyspnea, tachypnea, and crackles if MI has caused pulmonary congestion. Pulmonary edema may be present.

Gastrointestinal

Nausea and vomiting.

Genitourinary

Decreased urinary output may indicate cardiogenic shock.

Skin

Cool, clammy, diaphoretic, and pale appearance due to sympathetic stimulation may indicate cardiogenic shock.

Neurologic

Anxiety, restlessness, and light-headedness may indicate increased sympathetic stimulation or a decrease in contractility and cerebral oxygenation. The same symptoms may also herald cardiogenic shock.

Psychological

Fear with feeling of impending doom, or patient may deny that anything is wrong.

Myocardial Infarction (MI)

Pathophysiology

In an MI, an area of the myocardium is permanently destroyed. MI is usually caused by reduced blood flow in a coronary artery due to rupture of an atherosclerotic plaque and subsequent occlusion of the artery by a thrombus. In unstable angina, the plaque ruptures but the artery is not completely occluded. Because unstable angina and acute MI are considered to be the same process but different points along a continuum, the term **acute coronary syndrome** (ACS) may be used in lieu of these diagnoses. Other causes of MI include vasospasm (sudden constriction or narrowing) of a coronary artery, decreased oxygen supply (eg, from acute blood loss, anemia, or low blood pressure), and increased demand for oxygen (eg, from a rapid heart rate, thyrotoxicosis, or ingestion of cocaine). In each case, a profound imbalance exists between myocardial oxygen supply and demand.

Coronary occlusion, heart attack, and MI are terms used synonymously, but the preferred term is MI. The area of infarction develops over minutes to hours. As the cells are deprived of oxygen, ischemia develops, cellular injury occurs, and the lack of oxygen results in infarction, or the death of cells. The expression "time is muscle" reflects the urgency of appropriate treatment to improve patient outcomes. Each year in the United States, nearly 900,000 people have acute MIs; one fourth of these people die of MI (AHA, 2004). Half of those who die never reach a hospital.

Various descriptions are used to further identify an MI: the type of MI (ST-segment elevation, non–ST-segment elevation), the location of the injury to the ventricular wall (anterior, inferior, posterior, or lateral wall), and the point in time within the process of infarction (acute, evolving, or old).

The ECG usually identifies the type and location, and other ECG indicators such as a Q wave and patient history identify the timing. Regardless of the location of the infarction of cardiac muscle, the goal of medical therapy is to prevent or minimize myocardial tissue death and to prevent complications. The pathophysiology of heart disease and the risk factors involved were discussed earlier in this chapter.

Clinical Manifestations

Chest pain that occurs suddenly and continues despite rest and medication is the presenting symptom in most patients with an MI (Chart 28-8). Some of these patients have prodromal symptoms or a previous diagnosis of CAD, but about half report no previous symptoms (AHA, 2004). Patients may present with a combination of symptoms, including chest pain, shortness of breath, indigestion, nausea, and anxiety. They may have cool, pale, and moist skin. Their heart rate and respiratory rate may be faster than normal. These signs and symptoms, which are caused by stimulation of the sympathetic nervous system, may be present for only a short time or may persist. In many cases, the signs and symptoms of MI cannot be distinguished from those of unstable angina.

Assessment and Diagnostic Findings

The diagnosis of MI is generally based on the presenting symptoms, the ECG, and laboratory test results (eg, serial cardiac biomarker values). The prognosis depends on the severity of coronary artery obstruction and the extent of myocardial damage. Physical examination is always conducted, but the examination alone does not confirm the diagnosis.

Patient History

The patient history has two parts: the description of the presenting symptom (eg, pain) and the history of previous illnesses and family history of heart disease. Previous history should also include information about the patient's risk factors for heart disease.

Electrocardiogram

The ECG provides information that assists in diagnosing acute MI. It should be obtained within 10 minutes from the time a patient reports pain or arrives in the emergency department. By monitoring serial ECG changes over time, the location, evolution, and resolution of an MI can be identified and monitored.

The ECG changes that occur with an MI are seen in the leads that view the involved surface of the heart. The classic ECG changes are T-wave inversion, ST-segment elevation, and development of an abnormal Q wave (Fig. 28-5). Because infarction evolves over time, the ECG also changes over time. The first ECG signs of an acute MI occur as a result of myocardial ischemia and injury. Myocardial injury causes the T wave to become enlarged and symmetric. As the area of injury becomes ischemic, myocardial repolarization is altered and delayed, causing the T wave to invert. The ischemic region may remain depolarized while adjacent areas of the myocardium return to the resting state. Myocardial injury also causes ST-segment changes. The injured myocardial cells depolarize normally but repolarize more rapidly than normal cells, causing the ST segment to rise at least 1 mm above the isoelectric line (area between the T wave and the next P wave is used as the reference for the isoelectric line) when measured 0.06 to 0.08 seconds after the end of the QRS, a point called the J point (Fig. 28-6). This elevation in the ST segment in two contiguous leads is a key diagnostic indicator for MI.

The appearance of abnormal Q waves is another indication of MI. Q waves develop within 1 to 3 days because there is no depolarization current conducted from necrotic tissue. The lead system then views the flow of current from other parts of the heart. An abnormal Q wave is 0.04 seconds or longer, 25% of the R-wave depth (provided the R wave exceeds a depth of 5 mm), or did not exist before the event. An acute MI may also cause a significant decrease in the height of the R wave. During an acute MI, injury and ischemic changes are usually present. An abnormal Q wave may be present without ST-segment and T-wave changes, which indicates an old, not acute, MI. For some patients, there are no persistent ECG changes, and the MI is diagnosed by blood levels of cardiac biomarkers.

Using the above information, patients are diagnosed with one of the following forms of ACS:

- Unstable angina: The patient has clinical manifestations of coronary ischemia, but ECG or cardiac biomarkers show no evidence of acute MI.
- ST-segment elevation MI: The patient has ECG evidence of acute MI with characteristic changes in two contiguous leads on a 12-lead ECG. In this type of MI, there is significant damage to the myocardium.
- Non–ST-segment elevation MI: The patient has elevated cardiac biomarkers but no definite ECG evidence of acute MI.

During recovery from an MI, the ST segment often is the first ECG indicator to return to normal (1 to 6 weeks). The T wave becomes large and symmetric for 24 hours, and it then inverts within 1 to 3 days for 1 to 2 weeks. Q-wave alterations are usually permanent. An old ST-segment elevation MI is usually indicated by an abnormal Q wave or decreased height of the R wave without ST-segment and T-wave changes.

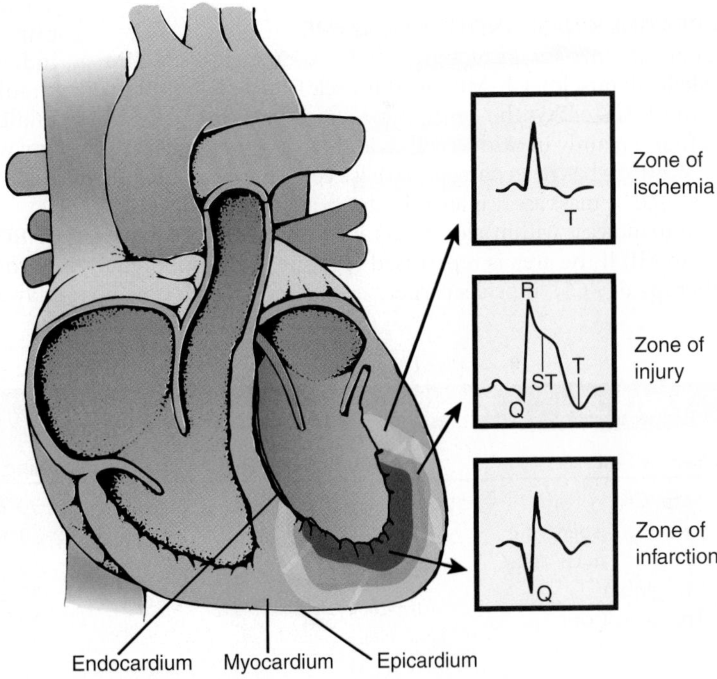

FIGURE 28-5. Effects of ischemia, injury, and infarction on an ECG recording. Ischemia causes inversion of the T wave because of altered repolarization. Cardiac muscle injury causes elevation of the ST segment and tall, symmetrical T waves. Later, Q waves develop because of the absence of depolarization current from the necrotic tissue and opposing currents from other parts of the heart.

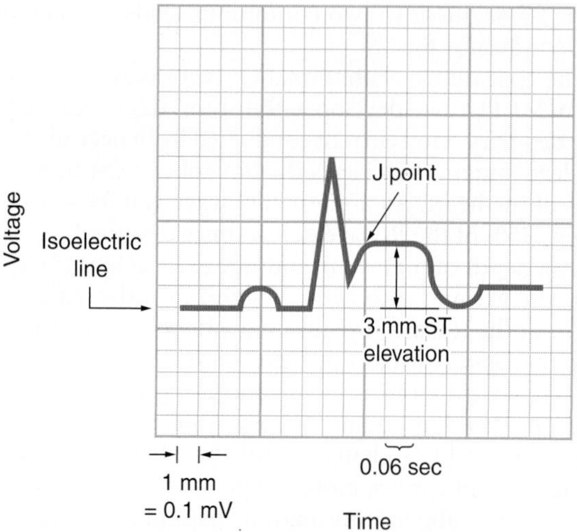

FIGURE 28-6. Using the ECG to diagnose acute myocardial infarction (MI). (ST-segment elevation is measured 0.06 to 0.08 seconds after the J point. An elevation of more than 1 mm in contiguous leads is indicative of acute MI.)

Echocardiogram

The echocardiogram is used to evaluate ventricular function. It may be used to assist in diagnosing an MI, especially when the ECG is nondiagnostic. The echocardiogram can detect hypokinetic and akinetic wall motion and can determine the ejection fraction (see Chapter 26).

Laboratory Tests

Laboratory tests called cardiac biomarkers are used to diagnose an MI. Newer laboratory tests with faster results, resulting in earlier diagnosis, include myoglobin and troponin analysis. These tests are based on the release of cellular contents into the circulation when myocardial cells die. Table 28-3 shows the time courses of cardiac biomarkers.

CREATINE KINASE AND ITS ISOENZYMES

There are three **creatine kinase** (CK) isoenzymes: CK-MM (skeletal muscle), CK-MB (heart muscle), and CK-BB (brain tissue). CK-MB is the cardiac-specific isoenzyme; CK-MB is found mainly in cardiac cells and therefore increases only when there has been damage to these cells. Elevated CK-MB assessed by mass assay is an indicator of acute MI; its level begins to increase within a few hours and peaks within 24 hours of an MI. If the area is reperfused (eg, due to thrombolytic therapy or PCI), it peaks earlier.

MYOGLOBIN

Myoglobin is a heme protein that helps transport oxygen. Like CK-MB enzyme, myoglobin is found in cardiac and skeletal muscle. The myoglobin level starts to increase within 1 to 3 hours and peaks within 12 hours after the onset of symptoms. An increase in myoglobin is not very specific in indicating an acute cardiac event; however, negative results are an excellent parameter for ruling out an acute MI.

TROPONIN

Troponin, a protein found in the myocardium, regulates the myocardial contractile process. There are three isomers of troponin: C, I, and T. Troponins I and T are specific for cardiac muscle, and these tests are currently recognized as reliable and critical markers of myocardial injury. An increase in the level of troponin in the serum can be detected within a few hours during acute MI. It remains elevated for a long period, often as long as 3 weeks, and it therefore can be used to detect recent myocardial damage.

Medical Management

The goal of medical management is to minimize myocardial damage, preserve myocardial function, and prevent complications. These goals are facilitated by the use of guidelines developed by the American College of Cardiology and American Heart Association (Chart 28-9). These goals may be achieved by reperfusing the area with the emergency use of thrombolytic medications or by PCI. Minimizing myocardial damage is also accomplished by reducing myocardial oxygen demand and increasing oxygen supply with medications, oxygen administration, and bed rest. The resolution of pain and ECG changes indicate that demand and supply are in equilibrium; they may also indicate reperfusion. Visualization of blood flow through an open vessel in the catheterization laboratory is evidence of reperfusion.

Pharmacologic Therapy

The patient with suspected MI is given aspirin, nitroglycerin, morphine, a beta-blocker, and other medications as indicated while the diagnosis is being confirmed. Patients should receive a beta-blocker initially, throughout the hospitalization, and after hospital discharge. Long-term therapy with beta-blockers can decrease the incidence of future cardiac events.

THROMBOLYTICS

Thrombolytics are usually administered IV, although some may also be given directly into the coronary artery in the

TABLE 28-3 Biomarkers of Acute Myocardial Infarction

Serum Test	Earliest Increase (hr)	Test Running Time (min)	Peak (hr)	Return to Normal
Total CK	3–6	30–60	24–36	3 days
CK-MB: isoenzyme	4–8	30–60	12–24	3–4 days
mass assay	2–3	30–60	10–18	3–4 days
Myoglobin	1–3	30–60	4–12	12 hr
Troponin T or I	3–4	30–60	4–24	1–3 wk

CHART 28-9

Medical Treatment Guidelines for Acute Myocardial Infarction

Use rapid transit to the hospital.

Obtain 12-lead ECG to be read within 10 minutes.

Obtain laboratory blood specimens of cardiac biomarkers, including troponin.

Obtain other diagnostics to clarify the diagnosis.

Begin routine medical interventions:

- Supplemental oxygen
- Nitroglycerin
- Morphine
- Aspirin 162–325 mg
- Beta-blocker
- Angiotensin-converting enzyme inhibitor within 24 hours

Evaluate for indications for reperfusion therapy:

- Percutaneous coronary intervention
- Thrombolytic therapy

Continue therapy as indicated:

- Intravenous heparin or low-molecular-weight heparin
- Clopidogrel (Plavix) or ticlopidine (Ticlid)
- Glycoprotein IIb/IIIa inhibitor
- Bed rest for a minimum of 12 to 24 hours

Antman, E. M. et al. (2004). ACC/AHA Guidelines for the management of patients with ST-elevation myocardial infarction. *Circulation, 110*(5), 1–49.

cardiac catheterization laboratory (Chart 28-10). The purpose of thrombolytics is to dissolve and lyse the thrombus in a coronary artery (thrombolysis), allowing blood to flow through the coronary artery again (reperfusion), minimizing the size of the infarction, and preserving ventricular function. Even though thrombolytics may dissolve the thrombus, they do not affect the underlying atherosclerotic lesion. The patient may be referred for a cardiac catheterization and other invasive interventions.

Thrombolytics dissolve all clots, not just the one in the coronary artery. Thus they should not be used if the patient has formed a protective clot elsewhere, such as after major surgery or hemorrhagic stroke. Because thrombolytics reduce the patient's ability to form a clot, the patient is at risk for bleeding. Thrombolytics should not be used if the patient is bleeding or has a bleeding disorder. All patients who receive thrombolytic therapy are placed on bleeding precautions to minimize the risk for bleeding. This means minimizing the number of punctures for inserting IV lines, avoiding IM injections, preventing tissue trauma, and applying pressure for longer than usual after any puncture.

To be effective, thrombolytics must be administered as early as possible after the onset of symptoms that indicate an acute MI, generally within 3 to 6 hours. They are given to patients with ECG evidence of acute MI. Hospitals monitor their ability to administer these medications within 30 minutes from the time the patient arrives in the emergency department. This is called *door-to-needle time*. The thrombolytic agents used most often are alteplase (t-PA, Activase) and reteplase (r-PA, TNKase).

Alteplase is a tissue plasminogen activator (t-PA) that activates the plasminogen present on the blood clot. An IV bolus dose is given and followed by an infusion. Aspirin and unfractionated heparin or LMWH may be used with t-PA to prevent another clot from forming at the same lesion site.

Reteplase, a newer recombinant thrombolytic, is very similar to alteplase and has similar effects. It is administered in two bolus doses, followed with a heparin infusion.

ANALGESICS

The analgesic of choice for acute MI is morphine sulfate administered in IV boluses to reduce pain and anxiety. It reduces preload and afterload, which decreases the workload of the heart. Morphine also relaxes bronchioles to enhance oxygenation. The cardiovascular response to morphine is monitored carefully, particularly the blood pressure, which can decrease, and the respiratory rate, which can be depressed. Because morphine decreases the sensation of pain, ST-segment monitoring may be a better indicator of subsequent ischemia than assessment of pain.

ANGIOTENSIN-CONVERTING ENZYME INHIBITORS

Angiotensin-converting enzyme (ACE) inhibitors prevent the conversion of angiotensin I to angiotensin II. In the absence of angiotensin II, the blood pressure decreases and the kidneys excrete sodium and fluid (diuresis), decreasing the oxygen demand of the heart. Use of ACE inhibitors in patients after MI decreases mortality rates and prevents remodeling of myocardial cells that is associated with the onset of heart failure. It is important to ensure that the patient is not hypotensive, hyponatremic, hypovolemic, or hyperkalemic before administering ACE inhibitors. Blood pressure, urine output, and serum sodium, potassium, and creatinine levels need to be monitored closely.

Emergent Percutaneous Coronary Intervention

The patient in whom an acute MI is suspected may be referred for an immediate PCI. PCI may be used to open the occluded coronary artery in an acute MI and promote reperfusion to the area that has been deprived of oxygen. Superior outcomes have been reported with use of PCI compared to thrombolytics (Antman, Anbe, Armstrong, et al., 2004). Early PCI has been shown to be effective in patients of all ages, including those older than 75 years (Bach, Cannon, Weintraub, et al., 2004). PCI treats the underlying atherosclerotic lesion. Because the duration of oxygen deprivation is directly related to the number of cells that die, the time from the patient's arrival in the emergency department to the time PCI is performed should be less than 60 minutes (time is muscle). This is frequently referred to as *door-to-balloon time*. A cardiac catheterization laboratory and staff must be available if an emergent PCI is to be performed within this short time.

Cardiac Rehabilitation

After the MI patient is free of symptoms, an active rehabilitation program is initiated. Cardiac rehabilitation is a program

CHART 28-10

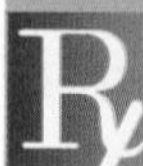

PHARMACOLOGY · Administration of Thrombolytic Therapy

Indications

- Chest pain for longer than 20 minutes, unrelieved by nitroglycerin
- ST-segment elevation in at least two leads that face the same area of the heart
- Less than 6 hours from onset of pain

Absolute Contraindications

- Active bleeding
- Known bleeding disorder
- History of hemorrhagic stroke
- History of intracranial vessel malformation
- Recent major surgery or trauma
- Uncontrolled hypertension
- Pregnancy

Nursing Considerations

- Minimize the number of times the patient's skin is punctured.
- Avoid intramuscular injections.
- Draw blood for laboratory tests when starting the IV line.
- Start IV lines before thrombolytic therapy; designate one line to use for blood draws.
- Avoid continual use of noninvasive blood pressure cuff.
- Monitor for acute dysrhythmias and hypotension.
- Monitor for reperfusion: resolution of angina or acute ST-segment changes.
- Check for signs and symptoms of bleeding: decrease in hematocrit and hemoglobin values, decrease in blood pressure, increase in heart rate, oozing or bulging at invasive procedure sites, back pain, muscle weakness, changes in level of consciousness, complaints of headache
- Treat major bleeding by discontinuing thrombolytic therapy and any anticoagulants; apply direct pressure and notify the physician immediately.
- Treat minor bleeding by applying direct pressure if accessible and appropriate; continue to monitor.

that targets risk reduction by means of education, individual and group support, and physical activity. Most insurance programs, including Medicare, cover the cost of cardiac rehabilitation, although only 8% to 39% of patients who are candidates for cardiac rehabilitation services participate in these programs (Williams, Fleg, Ades, et al., 2002).

The goals of rehabilitation for the patient who has had an MI are to extend life and improve the quality of life. The immediate objectives are to limit the effects and progression of atherosclerosis, return the patient to work and pre-illness lifestyle, enhance the psychosocial and vocational status of the patient, and prevent another cardiac event. These objectives are accomplished by encouraging physical activity and physical conditioning, educating the patient and family, and providing counseling and behavioral interventions.

Throughout all phases of rehabilitation, the goals of activity and exercise tolerance are achieved through gradual physical conditioning, aimed at improving cardiac efficiency over time. Cardiac efficiency is achieved when work and activities of daily living can be performed at a lower heart rate and lower blood pressure, thereby reducing the heart's oxygen requirements and reducing cardiac workload.

Physical conditioning is achieved gradually over time. It is not unusual for patients to "overdo it" in an attempt to achieve their goals too rapidly. Patients are observed for chest pain, dyspnea, weakness, fatigue, and palpitations and are instructed to stop exercise if any of these develop. In a monitored program, they are also monitored for an increase in heart rate above the target heart rate, an increase in systolic or diastolic blood pressure of more than 20 mm Hg, a decrease in systolic blood pressure, onset or worsening of dysrhythmias, or ST-segment changes on the ECG.

The target heart rate during hospitalization is an increase of less than 10% from the resting heart rate, or 120 beats per minute. Following discharge, the target heart rate is based on the patient's stress test results (usually 60% to 85% of the heart rate at which symptoms occurred), medications, and underlying condition. Oxygen saturation may also be assessed through pulse oximetry to ensure that it remains higher than 93%. If signs or symptoms occur, the patient is instructed to slow down or stop exercising. If the patient is exercising in an unmonitored program, he or she is cautioned to cease activity immediately if signs or symptoms occur and to seek appropriate medical attention.

Patients who are able to walk at 3 to 4 miles per hour can usually resume sexual activities. The nurse recommends that the patient be well rested and in a familiar setting, wait at least 1 hour after eating or drinking alcohol, and use a comfortable position. Sexual dysfunction or cardiac symptoms should be reported to the health care provider.

Phases of Cardiac Rehabilitation

Cardiac rehabilitation occurs along the continuum of the disease. It is typically categorized in three phases.

Phase I begins with the diagnosis of atherosclerosis, which may occur when the patient is admitted to the hospital for ACS (eg, unstable angina or acute MI). It consists of low-level activities and initial education for the patient and family. Because of today's brief hospital stays, mobilization occurs earlier and patient teaching focuses on the essentials of self-care, rather than instituting behavioral changes for risk reduction. Priorities for in-hospital teaching include the signs and symptoms that indicate the need to call 911 (seek emergency assistance), the medication regimen, rest–activity balance, and follow-up appointments with the physician. The nurse needs to reassure the patient that although CAD is a lifelong disease and must be treated as such, most patients can resume a normal life after an MI. This positive approach while in the hospital helps to motivate and teach the patient to continue the education and lifestyle changes that are usually needed after discharge. The amount of activity recommended at discharge depends on the age of the patient, his or her condition before the cardiac event, the extent of the disease, the course of the hospital stay, and the development of any complications.

Phase II occurs after the patient has been discharged. It usually lasts for 4 to 6 weeks but may last as long as 6 months. This outpatient program consists of supervised, often ECG-monitored, exercise training that is individualized based on the results of an exercise stress test. Support and guidance related to the treatment of the disease and teaching and counseling related to lifestyle modification for risk factor reduction are a part of this phase. Short-term and long-range goals are collaboratively determined based on the patient's needs. At each session, the patient is assessed for the effectiveness of and adherence to the medical plan. To prevent complications and another hospitalization, the cardiac rehabilitation staff alerts the referring physician to any problems.

Outpatient cardiac rehabilitation programs are designed to encourage patients and families to support each other. Many programs offer support sessions for spouses and significant others while the patients exercise. The programs involve group educational sessions for both patients and families that are given by cardiologists, exercise physiologists, dietitians, nurses, and other health care professionals. These sessions may take place outside a traditional classroom setting. For instance, a dietitian may take a group of patients and their families to a grocery store to examine labels and meat selections or to a restaurant to discuss menu offerings for a "heart-healthy" diet.

Phase III focuses on maintaining cardiovascular stability and long-term conditioning. The patient is usually self-directed during this phase and does not require a supervised program, although it may be offered. The goals of each phase build on the accomplishments of the previous phase.

Nursing Process

The Patient With Myocardial Infarction

Assessment

One of the most important aspects of care of the patient with an MI is the assessment. It establishes the baseline for the patient so that any deviations may be identified, systematically identifies the patient's needs, and helps determine the priority of those needs. Systematic assessment includes a careful history, particularly as it relates to symptoms: chest pain or discomfort, difficulty breathing (dyspnea), palpitations, unusual fatigue, faintness (syncope), or sweating (diaphoresis). Each symptom must be evaluated with regard to time, duration, and the factors that precipitate the symptom and relieve it, and in comparison with previous symptoms. A precise and complete physical assessment is critical to detect complications and any change in patient status. Chart 28-8 identifies important assessments and possible findings.

IV sites are examined frequently. Two IV lines are typically placed for any patient with ACS to ensure that access is available for administering emergency medications. Medications are administered IV to achieve rapid onset and to allow for timely adjustment. After the patient's condition stabilizes, IV lines may be changed to a saline lock to maintain IV access.

Diagnosis

Nursing Diagnoses

Based on the clinical manifestations, history, and diagnostic assessment data, major nursing diagnoses may include:

- Ineffective cardiac tissue perfusion related to reduced coronary blood flow from coronary thrombus and atherosclerotic plaque
- Risk for imbalanced fluid volume
- Risk for ineffective peripheral tissue perfusion related to decreased cardiac output from left ventricular dysfunction
- Death anxiety
- Deficient knowledge about post-MI self-care

Collaborative Problems/ Potential Complications

Based on the assessment data, potential complications that may develop include the following:

- Acute pulmonary edema (see Chapter 30)
- Heart failure (see Chapter 30)
- Cardiogenic shock (see Chapter 30)
- Dysrhythmias and cardiac arrest (see Chapters 27 and 30)
- Pericardial effusion and cardiac tamponade (see Chapter 30)

Planning and Goals

The major goals for the patient include relief of pain or ischemic signs and symptoms (eg, ST-segment changes), prevention of further myocardial damage, absence of respiratory dysfunction, maintenance or attainment of adequate tissue perfusion by decreasing the heart's workload, reduced anxiety, adherence to the self-care program, and absence or early recognition of complications. Care of the patient with an uncomplicated MI is summarized in the Plan of Nursing Care (Chart 28-11).

(text continues on page 883)

CHART 28-11

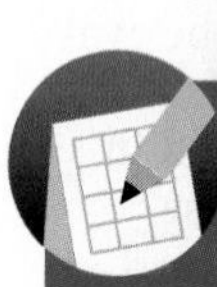

Plan of Nursing Care Care of the Patient With an Uncomplicated Myocardial Infarction

Nursing Diagnosis: Ineffective cardiac tissue perfusion related to reduced coronary blood flow.
Goal: Relief of chest pain/discomfort

NURSING INTERVENTIONS	RATIONALE	EXPECTED OUTCOMES
1. Initially assess, document, and report to the physician the following:	1. These data assist in determining the cause and effect of the chest discomfort and provide a baseline with which post-therapy symptoms can be compared.	• Reports beginning relief of chest discomfort and symptoms • Appears comfortable and is free of pain and other signs or symptoms: Respiratory rate, cardiac rate, and blood pressure return to prediscomfort level Skin warm and dry
a. The patient's description of chest discomfort, including location, intensity, radiation, duration, and factors that affect it. Other symptoms such as nausea, diaphoresis, or complaints of unusual fatigue.	a. There are many conditions associated with chest discomfort. There are characteristic clinical findings of ischemic pain and symptoms.	• Adequate cardiac output as evidenced by: stable/improving ECG Heart rate and rhythm Blood pressure Mentation Urine output Serum BUN and creatinine Skin color, temperature, and moisture
b. The effect of chest discomfort on cardiovascular perfusion—to the heart (eg, change in blood pressure, heart sounds), to the brain (eg, changes in LOC), to the kidneys (eg, decrease in urine output), and to the skin (eg, color, temperature).	b. MI decreases myocardial contractility and ventricular compliance and may produce dysrhythmias. Cardiac output is reduced, resulting in reduced blood pressure and decreased organ perfusion. The heart rate may increase as a compensatory mechanism to maintain cardiac output.	
2. Obtain a 12-lead ECG recording during the symptomatic event, as prescribed, to determine extension of infarction.	2. An ECG during symptoms may be useful in the diagnosis of an extension of MI.	
3. Administer oxygen as prescribed.	3. Oxygen therapy increases the oxygen supply to the myocardium if actual oxygen saturation is less than normal.	
4. Administer medication therapy as prescribed and evaluate the patient's response continuously.	4. Medication therapy (nitroglycerin, morphine, beta blocker, aspirin) is the first line of defense in preserving myocardial tissue. The side effects of these medications can be hazardous and the patient's status must be assessed.	
5. Ensure physical rest: use of the bedside commode with assistance; backrest elevated to promote comfort; diet as tolerated; arms supported during upper extremity activity; use of stool	5. Physical rest reduces myocardial oxygen consumption. Fear and anxiety precipitate the stress response; this results in increased levels of endogenous catecholamines, which increase myo-	

CHART 28-11

Plan of Nursing Care — Care of the Patient With an Uncomplicated Myocardial Infarction (Continued)

NURSING INTERVENTIONS	RATIONALE	EXPECTED OUTCOMES
softener to prevent straining at stool. Provide a restful environment, and allay fears and anxiety by being supportive, calm, and competent. Individualize visitation, based on patient response.	cardial oxygen consumption. Also, with increased epinephrine, the pain threshold is decreased, and pain increases myocardial oxygen consumption.	

Nursing Diagnosis: Potential impaired gas exchange related to fluid overload
Goal: Absence of respiratory difficulties

NURSING INTERVENTIONS	RATIONALE	EXPECTED OUTCOMES
1. Initially, every 4 hours, and with chest discomfort or symptoms, assess, document, and report to the physician abnormal heart sounds (particularly S_3 and S_4 gallops and the holosystolic murmur of left ventricular papillary muscle dysfunction), abnormal breath sounds (particularly crackles), and patient intolerance to specific activities.	1. These data are useful in diagnosing left ventricular failure. Diastolic filling sounds (S_3 and S_4 gallop) result from decreased left ventricular compliance associated with MI. Papillary muscle dysfunction (from infarction of the papillary muscle) can result in mitral regurgitation and a reduction in stroke volume, leading to left ventricular failure. The presence of crackles (usually at the lung bases) may indicate pulmonary congestion from increased left heart pressures. The association of symptoms and activity can be used as a guide for activity prescription and a basis for patient teaching.	• No shortness of breath, dyspnea on exertion, orthopnea, or paroxysmal nocturnal dyspnea • Respiratory rate less than 20 breaths/min with physical activity and 16 breaths/min with rest • Skin color normal • PaO_2 and $PaCO_2$ within normal range • Heart rate less than 100 beats/min and greater than 60 beats/min, with blood pressure within patient's normal limits • Chest x-ray normal • Relief of chest discomfort • Appears comfortable: Appears rested Respiratory rate, cardiac rate, and blood pressure return to prediscomfort level Skin warm and dry
2. Teach patient:	2.	
a. To adhere to the diet prescribed (for example, explain low-sodium, low-calorie diet)	a. Low-sodium diet may reduce extracellular volume, thus reducing preload and afterload, and thus myocardial oxygen consumption. In the obese patient, weight reduction may decrease cardiac work and improve tidal volume.	
b. To adhere to activity prescription	b. The activity prescription is determined individually to maintain the heart rate and blood pressure within safe limits.	

continued >

CHART 28-11

Plan of Nursing Care Care of the Patient With an Uncomplicated Myocardial Infarction (Continued)

Nursing Diagnosis: Risk for ineffective peripheral tissue perfusion related to decreased cardiac output
Goal: Maintenance/attainment of adequate tissue perfusion

NURSING INTERVENTIONS	RATIONALE	EXPECTED OUTCOMES
1. Initially, every 4 hours, and with chest discomfort, assess, document, and report to the physician the following: a. Hypotension b. Tachycardia and other dysrhythmia c. Activity intolerance d. Mentation changes (use family input) e. Reduced urine output (less than 200 mL per 8 hours) f. Cool, moist, cyanotic extremities	1. These data are useful in determining a low cardiac output state. An ECG with pain may be useful in the diagnosis of an extension of myocardial ischemia, injury, and infarction, and of variant angina.	• Blood pressure within the patient's normal range • Ideally, normal sinus rhythm without dysrhythmia is maintained, or patient's baseline rhythm is maintained between 60 and 100 beats/min without further dysrhythmia. • No complaints of fatigue with prescribed activity • Remains fully alert and oriented and without cognitive or behavioral change • Appears comfortable • Urine output greater than 30 mL/hr • Extremities warm and dry with normal color

Nursing Diagnosis: Death anxiety
Goal: Reduction of anxiety

NURSING INTERVENTIONS	RATIONALE	EXPECTED OUTCOMES
1. Assess, document, and report to the physician the patient's and family's level of anxiety and coping mechanisms.	1. These data provide information about the psychological well-being and a baseline so that post-therapy symptoms can be compared. Causes of anxiety are variable and individual, and may include acute illness, hospitalization, pain, disruption of activities of daily living at home and at work, changes in role and self-image due to illness, and financial concerns. Because anxious family members can transmit anxiety to the patient, the nurse must also identify strategies to reduce the family's fear and anxiety.	• Reports less anxiety • Patient and family discuss their anxieties and fears about death • Patient and family appear less anxious • Appears restful, respiratory rate less than 16/min, heart rate less than 100/min without ectopic beats, blood pressure within patient's normal limits, skin warm and dry • Participates actively in a progressive rehabilitation program • Practices stress reduction techniques
2. Assess the need for spiritual counseling and refer as appropriate.	2. If a patient finds support in a religion, spiritual counseling may assist in reducing anxiety and fear.	
3. Assess the need for social service referral.	3. Social services can assist with post-hospital care and financial concerns.	

CHART 28-11

Plan of Nursing Care — **Care of the Patient With an Uncomplicated Myocardial Infarction (Continued)**

NURSING INTERVENTIONS	RATIONALE	EXPECTED OUTCOMES
4. Allow patient (and family) to express anxiety and fear: a. By showing genuine interest and concern b. By facilitating communication (listening, reflecting, guiding) c. By answering questions	4. Unresolved anxiety (the stress response) increases myocardial oxygen consumption.	
5. Use of flexible visiting hours allows the presence of a supportive family to assist in reducing the patient's level of anxiety.	5. The presence of supportive family members may reduce both patient's and family's anxiety.	
6. Encourage active participation in a cardiac rehabilitation program.	6. Prescribed cardiac rehabilitation may help reduce anxiety, enhance feelings of well-being, and facilitate compliance with risk factor recommendations.	
7. Teach stress reduction techniques.	7. Stress reduction may help to reduce myocardial oxygen consumption and may enhance feelings of well-being.	

Nursing Diagnosis: Deficient knowledge about post-MI self-care
Goal: Adheres to the home health care program
Chooses lifestyle consistent with heart-healthy recommendations.

(See Chart 28-12, Promoting Health After MI)

Nursing Interventions

Relieving Pain and Other Signs and Symptoms of Ischemia

Balancing myocardial oxygen supply with demand (eg, as evidenced by the relief of chest pain) is the top priority in the care of the patient with an acute MI. Although medication therapy is required to accomplish this goal, nursing interventions are also important. Collaboration among the patient, nurse, and physician is critical in assessing the patient's response to therapy and in altering the interventions accordingly.

The recommended treatment for acute MI is reperfusion with thrombolytic therapy or emergent PCI for patients who present to the health care facility immediately and who have no major contraindications. These therapies are important because, in addition to relieving symptoms, they aid in minimizing or avoiding permanent injury to the myocardium. With or without reperfusion, administration of aspirin, an IV beta-blocker, and nitroglycerin is indicated. Use of a GPIIb/IIIa agent or heparin may also be indicated. The nurse administers morphine to relieve pain and anxiety and to promote vasodilation, reducing preload and afterload.

Oxygen should be administered along with medication therapy to assist with relief of symptoms. Administration of oxygen even in low doses raises the circulating level of oxygen to reduce pain associated with low levels of myocardial oxygen. The route of administration, usually by nasal cannula, and the oxygen flow rate are documented. A flow rate of 2 to 4 L/min is usually adequate to maintain oxygen saturation levels of 96% to 100% if no other disease is present.

Vital signs are assessed frequently as long as the patient is experiencing pain and other signs or symptoms of acute ischemia. Physical rest in bed with the backrest elevated or in a cardiac chair helps decrease chest discomfort and dyspnea. Elevation of the head and torso is beneficial for the following reasons:

- Tidal volume improves because of reduced pressure from abdominal contents on the diaphragm and better lung expansion and gas exchange.
- Drainage of the upper lung lobes improves.
- Venous return to the heart (preload) decreases, reducing the work of the heart.

Improving Respiratory Function

Regular and careful assessment of respiratory function can help the nurse detect early signs of pulmonary complications. Scrupulous attention to fluid volume status prevents overloading the heart and lungs. Encouraging the patient to breathe deeply and change position frequently helps keep fluid from pooling in the bases of the lungs.

Promoting Adequate Tissue Perfusion

Limiting the patient to bed or chair rest during the initial phase of treatment is particularly helpful in reducing myocardial oxygen consumption. This limitation should remain until the patient is pain-free and hemodynamically stable. Checking skin temperature and peripheral pulses frequently is important to monitor tissue perfusion. Oxygen may be administered.

Reducing Anxiety

Alleviating anxiety and decreasing fear are important nursing functions that reduce the sympathetic stress response. Decreased sympathetic stimulation decreases the workload of the heart, which may relieve pain and other signs and symptoms of ischemia.

Developing a trusting and caring relationship with the patient is critical in reducing anxiety. Providing information to the patient and family in an honest and supportive manner encourages the patient to be a partner in care and greatly assists in developing a positive relationship. Ensuring a quiet environment, preventing interruptions that disturb sleep, using a caring and appropriate touch, teaching the patient relaxation techniques, using humor and encouraging laughter, and providing the appropriate prayer book and helping the patient pray if consistent with the patient's beliefs are other nursing interventions that can be used to reduce anxiety. Frequent opportunities are provided for the patient to privately share concerns and fears. An atmosphere of acceptance helps the patient know that these concerns and fears are both realistic and normal. Music therapy is an effective method of reducing anxiety and managing stress (Evans, 2002). Pet therapy, in which animals are brought to the patient, appears to provide emotional support and reduce anxiety. Hospitals may have a procedure that has been developed based on research and infection control standards pertaining to the animals and their animal handlers and the patients who are eligible for pet therapy.

Monitoring and Managing Potential Complications

Complications that can occur after acute MI are caused by the damage that occurs to the myocardium and to the conduction system as a result of the reduced coronary blood flow. Because these complications can be life-threatening, close monitoring for and early identification of their signs and symptoms are critical (see the Plan of Nursing Care in Chart 28-11).

The nurse monitors the patient closely for changes in cardiac rate and rhythm, heart sounds, blood pressure, chest pain, respiratory status, urinary output, skin color and temperature, sensorium, ECG changes, and laboratory values. Any changes in the patient's condition are reported promptly to the physician, and emergency measures are instituted when necessary.

Promoting Home and Community-Based Care

TEACHING PATIENTS SELF-CARE

The most effective way to increase the probability that the patient will implement a self-care regimen after discharge is to identify the priorities as perceived by the patient, provide adequate education about heart-healthy living, and facilitate the patient's involvement in a cardiac rehabilitation program. Working with patients in developing plans to meet their specific needs further enhances the potential for an effective treatment plan (Chart 28-12).

CONTINUING CARE

Depending on the patient's condition and the availability of family assistance, a home care referral may be indicated. The home care nurse assists the patient with scheduling and keeping follow-up appointments and with adhering to the prescribed cardiac rehabilitation regimen. The patient may need reminders about follow-up monitoring, including periodic blood laboratory testing and ECGs. In addition, the home care nurse may monitor the patient's adherence to dietary restrictions and to prescribed medications. If the patient is receiving home oxygen, the nurse ensures that the patient is using the oxygen as prescribed and that appropriate home safety measures are maintained. If the patient has evidence of heart failure secondary to the myocardial infarction, appropriate home care guidelines for the patient with heart failure are followed (see Chapter 30, Continuing Care section).

Evaluation

Expected Patient Outcomes

Expected patient outcomes may include the following:

1. Relief of angina
2. No signs of respiratory difficulties
3. Adequate tissue perfusion
4. Decreased anxiety
5. Adherence to a self-care program
6. Absence of complications

CHART 28-12

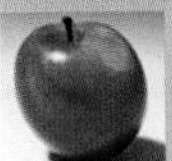

Health Promotion

Promoting Health After Myocardial Infarction and Other Acute Coronary Syndromes

To extend and improve the quality of life, a patient who has had an MI must learn to adjust his or her lifestyle to promote heart-healthy living. With this in mind, the nurse and patient develop a program to help the patient achieve desired outcomes.

Changing Lifestyle During Convalescence and Healing

Adaptation to an MI is an ongoing process and usually requires some modification of lifestyle. Some specific modifications include:

- Avoiding any activity that produces chest pain, extreme dyspnea, or undue fatigue
- Avoiding extremes of heat and cold and walking against the wind
- Losing weight, if indicated
- Stopping smoking and use of tobacco; avoiding second-hand smoke
- Using personal strengths to support lifestyle changes
- Developing heart-healthy eating patterns and avoiding large meals and hurrying while eating
- Modifying meals to align with the Therapeutic Lifestyle Changes (TLC) or the Dietary Approaches to Stopping Hypertension (DASH) diet
- Adhering to medical regimen, especially in taking medications
- Following recommendations that ensure blood pressure and blood glucose are in control
- Pursuing activities that relieve and reduce stress

Adopting an Activity Program

Additionally, the patient needs to undertake an *orderly* program of increasing activity and exercise for long-term rehabilitation as follows:

- Engaging in a regimen of physical conditioning with a gradual increase in activity duration and then a gradual increase in activity intensity
- Walking daily, increasing distance and time as prescribed
- Monitoring pulse rate during physical activity until the maximum level of activity is attained
- Avoiding activities that tense the muscles: isometric exercise, weight-lifting, any activity that requires sudden bursts of energy
- Avoiding physical exercise immediately after a meal
- Alternating activity with rest periods (some fatigue is normal and expected during convalescence)
- Participating in a daily program of exercise that develops into a program of regular exercise for a lifetime

Managing Symptoms

The patient must learn to recognize and take appropriate action for possible recurrences of symptoms as follows:

- Call 911 if chest pressure or pain (or anginal equivalent) is not relieved in 15 minutes by nitroglycerin
- Contacting the physician if any of the following occur: shortness of breath, fainting, slow or rapid heartbeat, swelling of feet and ankles

Invasive Coronary Artery Procedures

Percutaneous Coronary Interventions (PCIs)

Invasive interventional procedures to treat angina and CAD include PTCA, intracoronary stent implantation, atherectomy, and brachytherapy. All of these procedures are classified as PCIs.

Percutaneous Transluminal Coronary Angioplasty (PTCA)

In PTCA, an invasive interventional procedure, a balloon-tipped catheter is used to open blocked coronary vessels and resolve ischemia. It is used in patients with angina and as an intervention for acute MI. Catheter-based interventions can also be used to open blocked CABGs. The purpose of PTCA is to improve blood flow within a coronary artery by compressing and "cracking" the atheroma. The procedure is attempted when the cardiologist believes that PTCA can improve blood flow to the myocardium.

PTCA is carried out in the cardiac catheterization laboratory. Hollow catheters called sheaths are inserted, usually in the femoral artery (and sometimes femoral vein), providing a conduit for other catheters. Catheters are then threaded through the femoral artery, up through the aorta, and into the coronary arteries. Angiography is performed using injected radiopaque contrast agents (commonly called dye) to identify the location and extent of the blockage. A balloon-tipped dilation catheter is passed through the sheath and positioned over the lesion. The physician determines the catheter position by examining markers on the balloon that can be seen with fluoroscopy. When the catheter is properly positioned, the balloon is inflated with high pressure for several seconds and then deflated. The pressure compresses and possibly "cracks" the atheroma (Fig. 28-7). The media and adventitia of the coronary artery are also stretched.

Several inflations and several balloon sizes may be required to achieve the goal, usually defined as an improvement in blood flow and a residual stenosis of less than 20%. Other measures of the success of a PTCA are an increase in the artery's lumen, a difference of less than 20 mm Hg in blood pressure from one side of the lesion to the other, and no clinically obvious arterial trauma. Because the blood supply to the coronary artery decreases while the balloon is inflated, the patient may complain of chest pain and the ECG may display significant ST-segment changes. Intracoronary stents are usually positioned in the intima of the vessel to maintain patency after the balloon is withdrawn.

Coronary Artery Stent

After PTCA, the area that has been treated may close off partially or completely, a process called restenosis. The intima of the coronary artery has been injured and responds by initiating an acute inflammatory process. This process may include release of mediators that lead to vasoconstriction, clotting, and scar tissue formation. A coronary artery stent is placed to overcome these risks. A **stent** is a metal mesh that provides structural support to a vessel at risk of acute closure. The stent is positioned over the angioplasty balloon. When the balloon is inflated, the mesh expands and presses against the vessel wall, holding the artery open. The balloon is withdrawn, but the stent is left permanently in place within the artery (see Fig. 28-7). Eventually, endothelium covers the stent and it is incorporated into the vessel wall. Because of the risk of thrombus formation in the stent, the patient receives antiplatelet medications (eg, clopidogrel [Plavix] and aspirin). These medications are routinely continued for at least 3 to 6 months to decrease the risk of thrombus formation (Schwertz & Vaitkus, 2003). Some stents are coated with medications, such as sirolimus or paclitaxel, which may minimize the formation of thrombi or scar tissue within the stent. These drug-eluting stents have increased the success of PCI (Schwertz & Vaitkus, 2003).

Atherectomy

Atherectomy is an invasive interventional procedure that involves the removal of the atheroma, or plaque, from a coronary artery by cutting, shaving, or grinding (Fink, Abraham, Vincent, et al., 2005). It may be used in conjunction with PTCA. Directional coronary atherectomy and transluminal extraction catheter procedures involve the use of a catheter that removes the lesion and its fragments. Another procedure called rotational atherectomy uses a catheter with diamond chips impregnated on the tip (called a bur) that rotates like a dentist's drill at 130,000 to 180,000 rpm, pulverizing the lesion. Usually, several passes of these catheters are needed to achieve satisfactory results. Postprocedural patient care is the same as for a patient after PTCA.

Brachytherapy

PTCA and stent implantation cause a cellular reaction in the coronary artery that promotes proliferation of the intima of the artery, increasing the possibility of arterial obstruction. Brachytherapy reduces the recurrence of obstruction, preventing vessel restenosis by inhibiting smooth muscle cell proliferation. Brachytherapy (from the Greek word *brachys,* meaning *short*) involves the delivery of gamma or beta radiation by placing a radioisotope close to the lesion. The radioisotope may be delivered by a catheter or implanted with the stent. Long-term studies are needed to determine

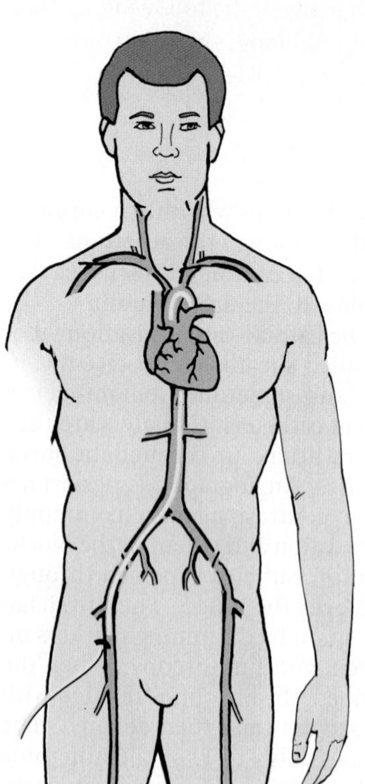

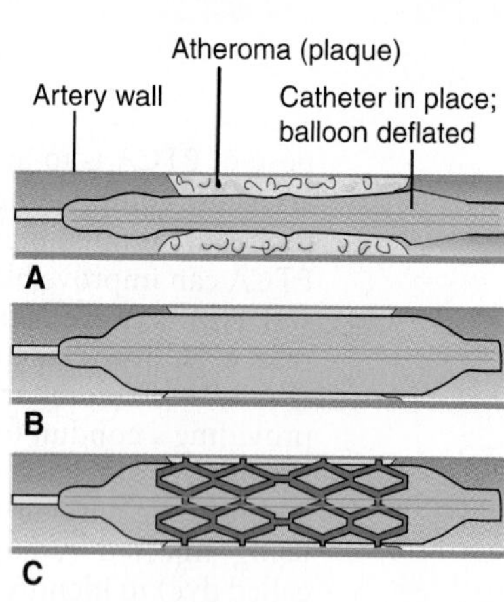

FIGURE 28-7. Percutaneous transluminal coronary angioplasty. **(A)** A balloon-tipped catheter is passed into the affected coronary artery and placed across the area of the atheroma (plaque). **(B)** The balloon is then rapidly inflated and deflated with controlled pressure. **(C)** A stent is placed to maintain patency of the artery, and the balloon is removed.

(1) whether the beneficial effects of radiation therapy are sustained and (2) the optimal dose and type of isotope to use for brachytherapy.

Complications

Complications that can occur during a PCI procedure include dissection, perforation, abrupt closure, or vasospasm of the coronary artery, acute MI, acute dysrhythmias (eg, ventricular tachycardia), and cardiac arrest. These may require emergency surgical treatment. Complications after the procedure may include abrupt closure of the coronary artery and vascular complications, such as bleeding at the insertion site, retroperitoneal bleeding, hematoma, pseudoaneurysm, arteriovenous fistula, or arterial thrombosis and distal embolization, as well as acute renal failure (Table 28-4) (Thompson & King, 2003).

Postprocedure Care

Patient care is similar to that for a cardiac catheterization (see Chapter 26). Many patients are admitted to the hospital the day of the PCI. Those with no complications go home the next day. When the PCI is performed emergently to relieve ACS, the patient will usually go to a critical care unit and stay in the hospital for a few days. During the PCI, patients receive IV heparin and are monitored closely for signs of bleeding. Patients may also receive a GPIIb/IIIa agent (eg, eptifibatide [Integrilin]) for several hours following the PCI to prevent platelet aggregation and thrombus formation in the coronary artery. Hemostasis is achieved, and femoral sheaths may be removed at the end of the procedure by using a vascular closure device (eg, Angio-Seal, VasoSeal) or a device that sutures the vessels. Hemostasis after sheath removal may also be achieved by direct manual pressure, a mechanical compression device (eg, C-shaped clamp), or a pneumatic compression device (eg, FemoStop).

The patient may return to the nursing unit with the large peripheral vascular access sheaths in place. The sheaths are then removed after blood studies (eg, activated clotting time) indicate that the heparin is no longer active and the clotting time is within an acceptable range. This usually takes a few hours, depending on the amount of heparin given during the procedure. The patient must remain flat in bed and keep the affected leg straight until the sheaths are removed and then for a few hours afterward to maintain hemostasis. Because the immobility and bed rest may cause discomfort, treatment may include analgesics and sedation. Sheath removal and the application of pressure on the vessel insertion site may cause the heart rate to slow and the blood pressure to decrease (vasovagal response). An IV bolus of atropine is usually given to treat this response.

Some patients with unstable lesions and at high risk for abrupt vessel closure are restarted on heparin after sheath removal, or they receive an IV infusion of a GPIIb/IIIa inhibitor. These patients are monitored more closely and may recover more slowly.

After hemostasis is achieved, a pressure dressing is applied to the site. Patients resume self-care and ambulate unassisted

TABLE 28-4 Complications After Percutaneous Transluminal Coronary Angioplasty (PTCA)

Complication	Signs and Symptoms	Possible Causes	Nursing Actions
Bleeding or hematoma	Hard lump or bluish tinge at sheath insertion site	Anticoagulant therapy, coughing, vomiting, bending leg or hip, obesity, bladder distention, high blood pressure	Keep the patient on bedrest. Apply manual pressure at site of sheath insertion. Outline extent of hematoma with a marking pen. If bleeding does not stop, notify physician or nurse practitioner.
Lost or weakened pulse distal to sheath insertion site	Extremity cool, cyanotic, pale, or painful	Arterial thrombus or embolus	Notify physician or nurse practitioner. Anticipate surgery and anticoagulation or thrombolytic therapy.
Pseudoaneurysm and arteriovenous fistula	Pulsatile mass felt or bruit heard near sheath insertion site	Vessel trauma during procedure	Notify physician or nurse practitioner. Anticipate ultrasound-guided compression. Prepare patient for surgery to close fistula.
Retroperitoneal bleeding	Back or flank pain Low blood pressure Tachycardia Restlessness and agitation Decreased hematocrit	Arterial tear causing bleeding into flank area	Notify physician or nurse practitioner immediately. Stop any anticoagulation medication. Anticipate need for intravenous fluids and/or administration of blood.
Acute renal failure	Decreased urine output Elevated BUN, creatinine	Nephrotoxic contrast agent	Monitor urine output. Monitor BUN and creatinine. Provide adequate hydration. Administer renal protective agents (eg acetylcysteine) before and after procedure as prescribed.

Adapted from Washington Adventist Hospital. Care of the interventional cardiology patient nursing protocol, based on communication from Amy Dukovic, Cardiac Interventional Nurse Practitioner.

within a few hours of the procedure. The duration of immobilization depends on the size of the sheath inserted, the amount of anticoagulant administered, the method of hemostasis, the patient's underlying condition, and the physician's preference. On the day after the procedure, the site is inspected and the dressing replaced with an adhesive bandage. The nurse teaches the patient to monitor the site for bleeding or development of a hard mass indicative of hematoma.

Surgical Procedures: Coronary Artery Revascularization

Advances in diagnostics, medical management, surgical and anesthesia techniques, as well as the care provided in critical care and surgical units, home care, and rehabilitation programs, have continued to make surgery a viable treatment option for patients with CAD. CAD has been treated by myocardial revascularization since the 1960s, and the most common CABG techniques have been performed for approximately 35 years. CABG is a surgical procedure in which a blood vessel is grafted to the occluded coronary artery so that blood can flow beyond the occlusion; it is also called a bypass graft.

The major indications for CABG are as follows (Eagle & Guyton, 2004; Rihal, Raco, Gersh, et al., 2003):

- Alleviation of angina that cannot be controlled with medication or PCI
- Treatment of left main coronary artery stenosis or multi-vessel CAD
- Prevention and treatment of MI, dysrhythmias, or heart failure
- Treatment for complications from an unsuccessful PCI

The recommendation for CABG is determined by a number of factors, including the number of diseased coronary vessels, the degree of left ventricular dysfunction, the presence of other health problems, the patient's symptoms, and any previous treatment. Studies have shown that CABG may be the preferred treatment for high-risk patients such as those with severe triple-vessel CAD, ventricular dysfunction, and diabetes (Rihal et al., 2003). Studies continue to compare clinical outcomes of CABG and PCI in patients with CAD (Berger, Sketch, & Califf, 2004).

For a patient to be considered for CABG, the coronary arteries to be bypassed must have approximately a 70% occlusion (60% if in the left main coronary artery). If significant blockage is not present, the flow through the artery will compete with the flow through the bypass, and circulation to the ischemic area of myocardium may not be improved. It is also necessary that the artery be patent beyond the area of blockage, or the flow through the bypass will be impeded.

A vessel commonly used for CABG is the greater saphenous vein, followed by the lesser saphenous vein (Fig. 28-8). Cephalic and basilic veins are used also. The vein is removed from the leg (or arm) and grafted to the ascending aorta and to the coronary artery distal to the lesion. The saphenous veins are used in emergency CABG procedures because they can be obtained quickly by one surgeon while another performs the chest surgery. A common adverse effect of vein removal is edema in the extremity from which the vein was taken. The degree of edema varies and usually diminishes over time. Within 5 to 10 years, atherosclerotic changes often develop in saphenous vein grafts.

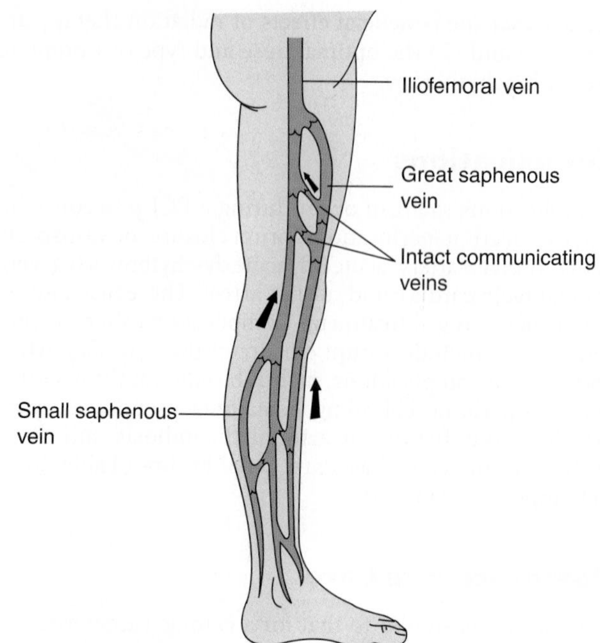

FIGURE 28-8. The greater and lesser saphenous veins are commonly used in bypass graft procedures.

The right and left internal mammary arteries and occasionally the radial arteries are also used for CABG. Arterial grafts are preferred to venous grafts because they do not develop atherosclerotic changes as quickly and remain patent longer. The surgeon leaves the proximal end of the mammary artery intact and detaches the distal end of the artery from the chest wall. This end of the artery is then grafted to the coronary artery distal to the occlusion. The internal mammary arteries may not be long enough to use for multiple bypasses. Because of this, many CABG procedures are performed with a combination of venous and arterial grafts.

Traditional Coronary Artery Bypass Graft

The traditional CABG procedure is performed with the patient under general anesthesia. The surgeon makes a median sternotomy incision and connects the patient to the cardiopulmonary bypass (CPB) machine. Next, a blood vessel from another part of the patient's body (eg, saphenous vein, left internal mammary artery) is grafted distal to the coronary artery lesion, bypassing the obstruction (Fig. 28-9). CPB is then discontinued, chest tubes and epicardial pacing wires are placed, and the incision is closed. The patient then is admitted to a critical care unit.

Cardiopulmonary Bypass

Many cardiac surgical procedures are possible because of CPB (ie, extracorporeal circulation). The procedure me-

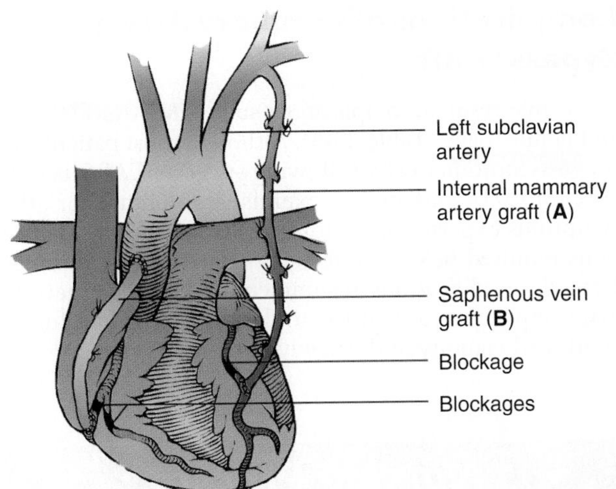

FIGURE 28-9. Coronary artery bypass grafts. One or more procedures may be performed using various veins and arteries. (**A**) Left internal mammary artery, used frequently because of its functional longevity. (**B**) Saphenous vein, also used as bypass graft.

chanically circulates and oxygenates blood for the body while bypassing the heart and lungs. CPB maintains perfusion to body organs and tissues and allows the surgeon to complete the anastomoses in a motionless, bloodless surgical field.

CPB is accomplished by placing a cannula in the right atrium, vena cava, or femoral vein to withdraw blood from the body. The cannula is connected to tubing filled with an isotonic crystalloid solution (usually 5% dextrose in lactated Ringer's solution). Venous blood removed from the body by the cannula is filtered, oxygenated, cooled or warmed by the machine, and then returned to the body. The cannula used to return the oxygenated blood is usually inserted in the ascending aorta, or it may be inserted in the femoral artery (Fig. 28-10). The heart is stopped by the injection of cardioplegia solution, which is high in potassium, into the coronary arteries. The patient receives heparin to prevent clotting and thrombus formation in the bypass circuit when blood comes in contact with the foreign surfaces of the tubing. At the end of the procedure when the patient is disconnected from the bypass machine, protamine sulfate is administered to reverse the effects of heparin.

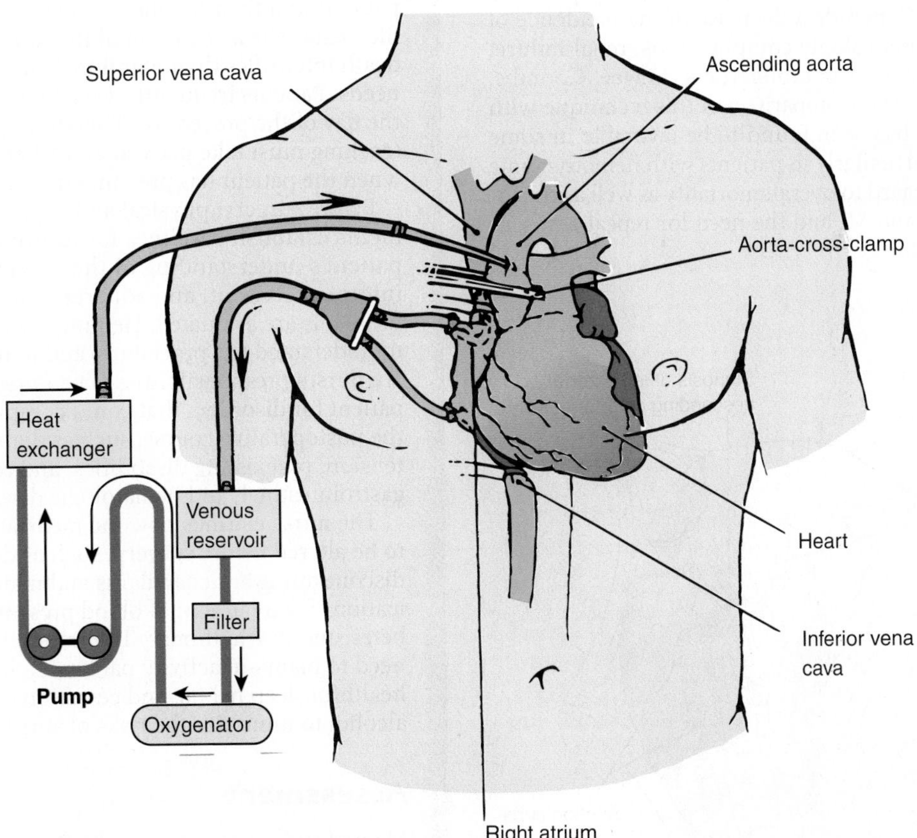

FIGURE 28-10. The cardiopulmonary bypass (CPB)system, in which cannulas are placed through the right atrium into the superior and inferior vena cavae to divert blood from the body and into the bypass system. The pump system creates a vacuum, pulling blood into the venous reservoir. The blood is cleared of air bubbles, clots, and particulates by the filter and then is passed through the oxygenator, releasing carbon dioxide and obtaining oxygen. Next, the blood is pulled to the pump and pushed out to the heat exchanger, where its temperature is regulated. The blood is then returned to the body via the ascending aorta.

During the procedure, hypothermia is maintained, usually 28°C to 32°C (82.4°F to 89.6°F). The blood is cooled during CPB and returned to the body. The cooled blood slows the body's basal metabolic rate, thereby decreasing the demand for oxygen. Cooled blood usually has a higher viscosity, but the crystalloid solution used to prime the bypass tubing dilutes the blood. When the surgical procedure is completed, the blood is rewarmed as it passes through the CPB circuit. Urine output, arterial blood gases, electrolytes, and coagulation studies are monitored to assess the patient's status during CPB.

Alternative Coronary Artery Bypass Graft Techniques

A number of alternative CABG techniques have been developed that may have fewer complications for some groups of patients. Off-pump CABG (OPCAB) surgery has been used successfully in many patients since the 1990s. OPCAB involves a standard median sternotomy incision, but the surgery is performed without CPB. A beta-adrenergic blocker may be used to slow the heart rate. The surgeon also uses a myocardial stabilization device to hold the site still for the anastomosis of the bypass graft into the coronary artery while the heart continues to beat (Fig. 28-11). The potential benefits of OPCAB include a decrease in the incidence of stroke and other neurologic complications, renal failure, and other postoperative complications (Magee, Coombs, Peterson, et al., 2003). Comparison of this technique with traditional CABG has been found to be favorable in some patient groups, particularly in patients with hemodynamic instability, with regard to overall mortality as well as the incidence of stroke and MI and the need for repeat revascularization (Rose, 2003).

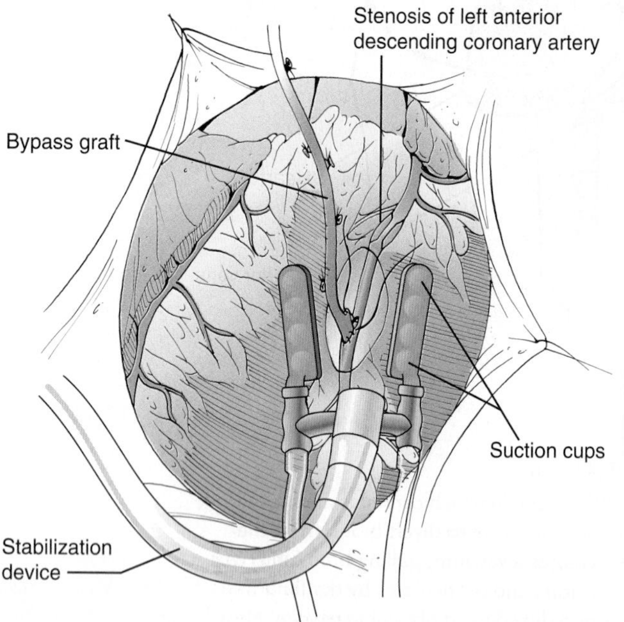

FIGURE 28-11. Stabilizer device for off-pump coronary artery bypass surgery.

Complications of Coronary Artery Bypass Graft

CABG may result in complications such as MI, dysrhythmias, and hemorrhage (Table 28-5). Although most patients improve symptomatically following surgery, CABG is not a cure for CAD, and angina, exercise intolerance, or other symptoms experienced before CABG may recur. Medications required before surgery may need to be continued. Lifestyle modifications recommended before surgery remain important to treat the underlying CAD and for the continued viability of the newly implanted grafts.

Nursing Process

The Preoperative Cardiac Surgery Patient

Cardiac surgery patients have many of the same needs and require the same perioperative care as other surgical patients (see Chapters 18 through 20). These patients and their families are experiencing a major life crisis. The association of the heart with life and death intensifies their emotional and psychological needs. Patients frequently are admitted to the hospital the day of the procedure. Therefore, preoperative teaching must take place at an earlier time, usually when the patient has preadmission testing.

Before surgery, physical and psychological assessments establish baselines for future reference. The patient's understanding of the surgical procedure, informed consent, and adherence to treatment protocols are evaluated. Helping the patient to cope, to understand the procedure, and to maintain dignity are nursing responsibilities. The nurse assesses the patient for disorders that could complicate or affect the postoperative course, such as diabetes, hypertension, preexisting disabilities, and respiratory, gastrointestinal, and hematologic diseases.

The nurse clarifies how the medication regimen is to be altered before surgery, such as decreasing or discontinuing anticoagulants and maintaining medications for treatment of blood pressure, angina, diabetes, and dysrhythmias. The nurse also clarifies the need to maintain activity patterns, a healthy diet, healthful sleep habits, and cessation of smoking and alcohol to minimize the risks of surgery.

Assessment

Most of the preoperative evaluation is completed before the patient enters the hospital. Many surgeons' offices or hospitals mail an information packet to the patient's home.

A history and physical examination are performed by nursing and medical personnel. A chest x-ray, ECG, laboratory tests, blood typing and cross-matching, and

(text continues on page 894)

TABLE 28-5 Potential Complications of Cardiac Surgery

Complication	Description	Assessment and Management
Cardiac Complications (The patient may require interventions for more than one complication at a time. Collaboration among nurses, physicians, pharmacists, respiratory therapists, and dietitians is necessary to achieve the desired patient outcomes.)		
Decreased Cardiac Output		
Hypovolemia (most common cause of decreased cardiac output after cardiac surgery)	• Net loss of blood and intravascular volume • Surgical hypothermia (As the reduced body temperature rises after surgery, blood vessels dilate, and more volume is needed to fill the vessels.) • Intravenous fluid loss to the interstitial spaces because surgery and anesthesia make capillary beds more permeable • Increased heart rate, arterial hypotension, low pulmonary artery wedge pressure (PAWP), and low central venous pressures (CVP) often are seen	• Fluid replacement may be prescribed. Replacement fluids include: colloid (albumin, hetastarch), packed red blood cells, or crystalloid solution (normal saline, lactated Ringer's solution).
Persistent bleeding	• Cardiopulmonary bypass may cause platelet dysfunction, and hypothermia alters clotting mechanisms • Surgical trauma causing tissues and blood vessels to ooze bloody drainage • Intraoperative anticoagulant (heparin) therapy • Postoperative coagulopathy may also result from liver dysfunction and depletion of clotting components	• Accurate measurement of wound bleeding and chest tube blood is essential. Bloody drainage should not exceed 200 mL/h for the first 4 to 6 hours. Drainage should decrease and stop within a few days, while progressing from sanguineous to serosanguineous and serous drainage. • Protamine sulfate may be administered to neutralize unfractionated heparin; vitamin K and blood products may be used to treat hematologic deficiencies. • If bleeding persists, the patient may return to the operating room.
Cardiac tamponade	• Fluid and clots accumulate in the pericardial sac, which compresses the heart, preventing blood from filling the ventricles. • Signs and symptoms include arterial hypotension, tachycardia, muffled heart sounds, decreasing urine output, and ↑ CVP. Additional signs and symptoms: arterial pressure waveform demonstrating a pulsus paradoxus (decrease of more than 10 mm Hg during inspiration) and decreased chest tube drainage (suggesting that the drainage is trapped or clotted in the mediastinum).	• The chest drainage system is checked to eliminate possible kinks or obstructions in the tubing. • Drainage system patency may be reestablished by milking the tubing (taking care not to strip the tubing, creating negative pressure within the chest, which may harm the surgical repair or trigger a dysrhythmia). • Chest x-ray may show a widening mediastinum. • Emergency medical management is required; may include pericardiocentesis or return to surgery.
Fluid overload	• High PAWP, CVP, and pulmonary artery diastolic pressures as well as crackles indicate fluid overload.	• Diuretics are prescribed and the rate of IV fluid administration is reduced. • Alternative treatments include continuous renal replacement therapy and dialysis.
Hypothermia	• Low body temperature leads to vasoconstriction, shivering, and arterial hypertension.	• Patient is rewarmed gradually after surgery, decreasing vasoconstriction
Hypertension	• Results from postoperative vasoconstriction. It may stretch suture lines and cause postoperative bleeding. The condition may be transient.	• Vasodilators (nitroglycerin [Tridil], nitroprusside [Nipride, Nitropress]) may be used to treat hypertension. Administer cautiously to avoid hypotension.

continued >

TABLE 28-5 Potential Complications of Cardiac Surgery (Continued)

Complication	Description	Assessment and Management
Tachydysrhythmias	• Increased heart rate is common with perioperative volume changes. Uncontrolled atrial fibrillation commonly occurs during the first few days postoperatively.	• If a tachydysrhythmia is the primary problem, the heart rhythm is assessed and medications (eg, adenosine [Adenocard, Adenoscan], amiodarone [Cordarone], digoxin [Lanoxin], diltiazem [Cardizem], esmolol [Brevibloc], lidocaine [Xylocaine], procainamide [Pronestyl]), may be prescribed. Patients may be prescribed antiarrhythmics before CABG to minimize the risk of postoperative tachydysrhythmias. • Carotid massage may be performed by a physician to assist with diagnosing or treating the dysrhythmia. • Cardioversion and defibrillation are alternatives for symptomatic tachydysrhythmias. • For patients who cannot attain normal sinus rhythm, an alternate goal may be to establish a stable rhythm that produces a sufficient cardiac output.
Bradycardias	• Decreased heart rate	• Many postoperative patients will have temporary pacer wires that can be attached to a pulse generator (pacemaker) to stimulate the heart to beat faster. Less commonly, atropine, epinephrine, or isoproterenol may be used to increase heart rate.
Cardiac failure	• Myocardial contractility may be decreased perioperatively.	• The nurse observes for and reports falling mean arterial pressure; rising PAWP, pulmonary artery diastolic pressure, and CVP; increasing tachycardia; restlessness and agitation; peripheral cyanosis; venous distention; labored respirations; and edema. • Medical management includes diuretics, digoxin, and IV inotropic agents.
Myocardial infarction (may occur intraoperatively or postoperatively)	• Portion of the cardiac muscle dies; therefore, contractility decreases. Impaired ventricular wall motion further decreases cardiac output. Symptoms may be masked by the postoperative surgical discomfort or the anesthesia–analgesia regimen.	• Careful assessment to determine the type of pain the patient is experiencing; MI suspected if the mean blood pressure is low with normal preload. • Serial ECGs and cardiac biomarkers assist in making the diagnosis (alterations may be due to the surgical intervention). Analgesics are prescribed in small amounts while the patient's blood pressure and respiratory rate are monitored (because vasodilation secondary to analgesics or decreasing pain may occur and compound the hypotension). • Activity progression depends on the patient's activity tolerance.

TABLE 28-5 Potential Complications of Cardiac Surgery (Continued)

Complication	Description	Assessment and Management
Pulmonary Complications		
Impaired gas exchange	• During and after anesthesia, patients require mechanical assistance to breathe. • Potential for postoperative atelectasis. • Anesthetic agents stimulate production of mucus and chest incision pain may decrease the effectiveness of ventilation.	• Pulmonary complications are often detected during assessment of breath sounds, oxygen saturation levels, arterial blood gases, and when monitoring peak pressure and exhaled tidal volumes on the ventilator. • Extended periods of mechanical ventilation may be required while complications are treated.
Fluid Volume Complications		
Hemorrhage	• Untoward and excessive bleeding may be life-threatening.	• Serial hemoglobin, hematocrit, and coagulation studies are performed to guide therapy. • Administration of fluids, colloids, and blood products: packed red blood cells, fresh frozen plasma, platelet concentrate. • Administration of aprotinin (Trasylol) perioperatively to reduce blood transfusion needs. • Administration of desmopressin acetate (DDAVP) to enhance platelet function.
Neurologic Complications		
Neurologic changes; stroke	• Inability to follow simple command within 6 hours of recovery from anesthetic; different capabilities on right or left side of body	• Neurologically, most patients begin to recover from anesthesia in the operating room. • Patients who are elderly or who have renal or hepatic failure may take longer to recover. • Patient should be evaluated for stroke when neurologic changes are evident.
Pain (see Chapter 13)		
Renal Failure and Electrolyte Imbalance		
Renal failure	• Usually acute and resolves within 3 months, but may become chronic and require ongoing dialysis	• May respond to diuretics or may require continuous renal replacement therapy (CRRT) or dialysis
Acute tubular necrosis	• Often results from hypoperfusion of the kidneys or from injury to the renal tubules by nephrotoxic medications	• Fluids, electrolytes, and urine output are monitored frequently.
Electrolyte imbalance	• Postoperative imbalances in potassium, magnesium, sodium, calcium, and blood glucose are related to surgical losses, metabolic changes, and the administration of medications and IV fluids.	• Monitor electrolytes and basic metabolic studies frequently. • Implement treatment to correct electrolyte imbalance promptly (see Chart 28-13).

continued >

TABLE 28-5 Potential Complications of Cardiac Surgery (Continued)

Complication	Description	Assessment and Management
Other Complications		
Hepatic failure	• Most common in patients with cirrhosis, hepatitis, or prolonged right-sided heart failure	• Use of medications metabolized by the liver must be minimized. • Bilirubin, albumin, and amylase levels are monitored, and nutritional support must be provided.
Infection	• Surgery and anesthesia alter the patient's immune system. Many invasive devices are used to monitor and support the patient's recovery and may serve as a source of infection.	• The following must be monitored to detect signs of possible infection: body temperature, white blood cell counts and differential counts, incision and puncture sites, cardiac output and systemic vascular resistance, urine (clarity, color, and odor), bilateral breath sounds, sputum (color, odor, amount), as well as nasogastric secretions. • Antibiotic therapy may be expanded or modified as necessary. • Invasive devices must be discontinued as soon as they are no longer required. Institutional protocols for maintaining and replacing invasive lines and devices must be followed to minimize the patient's risk for infection.

autologous blood donation (patient's own blood) may also be performed. The health assessment focuses on obtaining baseline physiologic, psychological, and social information. The patient's and family's learning needs are identified and addressed as necessary. Of particular importance are the patient's usual functional level, coping mechanisms, and support systems. These are important because the support of the family or significant others affects the patient's postoperative course and rehabilitation. Discharge plans are influenced by the lifestyle demands of the home situation and the physical environment of the home.

Health History

The preoperative history and health assessment should be thorough and well documented because they provide a basis for postoperative comparison. A systematic assessment of all systems is performed, with emphasis on cardiovascular functioning.

The functional status of the cardiovascular system is determined by reviewing the patient's symptoms, including past and present experiences with chest pain, hypertension, palpitations, cyanosis, breathing difficulty (dyspnea), leg pain that occurs with walking (intermittent claudication), orthopnea, paroxysmal nocturnal dyspnea, and peripheral edema. Because alterations in cardiac output can affect renal, respiratory, gastrointestinal, integumentary, hematologic, and neurologic functioning, a history of these systems is also reviewed. The patient's history of major illnesses, previous surgeries, medication therapies, and use of drugs, alcohol, and tobacco is also obtained.

Particular attention is paid to blood glucose control in patients with diabetes, because there is a higher incidence of postoperative complications when glycemic control is poor (Goldrick, 2003).

Physical Assessment

A complete physical examination is performed, with special emphasis on the following:

- General appearance and behavior
- Vital signs
- Nutritional and fluid status, weight, and height
- Inspection and palpation of the heart, noting the point of maximal impulse, abnormal pulsations, and thrills
- Auscultation of the heart, noting pulse rate, rhythm, and quality; S_3 and S_4, snaps, clicks, murmurs, and friction rub
- Jugular venous pressure
- Peripheral pulses
- Peripheral edema

Psychosocial Assessment

The psychosocial assessment and the assessment of the patient's and family's learning needs are as important as the physical examination. Anticipation of cardiac surgery is a source of great stress to the patient and family. They are anxious and fearful and often have many unanswered questions. Their anxiety usually increases with the patient's admission to the hospital and the immediacy of surgery. An assessment of the level of anxiety is important. If it is low, it may indicate denial. If it is extremely high, it may interfere with the use of effective coping mechanisms and with preoperative teaching. Questions may be asked to obtain the following information:

- Meaning of the surgery to the patient and family
- Coping mechanisms that are being used
- Measures used in the past to deal with stress
- Anticipated changes in lifestyle
- Support systems in effect
- Fears regarding the present and the future
- Knowledge and understanding of the surgical procedure, postoperative course, and long-term rehabilitation

The nurse allows adequate time for the patient and family to express their fears. Those most often expressed are fear of the unknown, fear of pain, fear of body image change, and fear of dying. During the assessment, the nurse determines how much the patient and family know about the impending surgery and the expected postoperative events. They are encouraged to ask questions and to indicate how much information they wish to receive. Some patients prefer not to have detailed information, whereas others want to know as much as possible. Patients are approached as unique individuals with their own specific learning needs, learning styles, and levels of understanding.

Patients requiring emergency heart surgery may have cardiac catheterization and surgery within several hours of admission. The nurse has little opportunity to assess and meet their emotional and learning needs before surgery. As a result, patients require extra help after surgery to adjust to the situation.

Diagnosis

Preoperative Nursing Diagnoses

Nursing diagnoses for patients awaiting cardiac surgery vary according to each patient's cardiac disease and symptoms. Preoperative nursing diagnoses may include:

- Fear related to the surgical procedure, its uncertain outcome, and the threat to well-being
- Deficient knowledge regarding the surgical procedure and the postoperative course
- Ineffective cardiac tissue perfusion related to reduced coronary blood flow

Collaborative Problems/ Potential Complications

The stress of impending cardiac surgery may precipitate complications that require collaborative management with the physician. Based on the assessment data, potential complications that may develop include:

- Angina
- Severe anxiety requiring an anxiolytic (anxiety-reducing) medication
- Cardiac dysrhythmias

Planning and Goals

The major goals for the patient may include reducing fear, learning about the surgical procedure and postoperative course, and avoiding perioperative complications.

Nursing Interventions

During the preoperative phase of cardiac surgery, the nurse develops a plan of care that includes emotional support and teaching for the patient and family. Establishing rapport, answering questions, listening to fears and concerns, clarifying misconceptions, and providing information about what to expect are interventions the nurse uses to prepare the patient and family emotionally for the surgery and the postoperative events.

Reducing Fear

The patient and family are given time and opportunities to express their fears. If there is fear of the unknown, other surgical experiences that the patient has had can be compared with the impending surgery. It is often helpful to describe to the patient the sensations that he or she can expect. If the patient has already had a cardiac catheterization, the similarities and differences between that procedure and the surgery may be compared. The patient is encouraged to talk about any concerns related to previous experiences.

A discussion of the patient's fears about pain is initiated. A comparison is made between the pain experienced with cardiac surgery and other pain experiences. The preoperative sedation, the anesthetic, and the postoperative pain medications are described. The nurse reassures the patient that the fear of pain is normal, that some pain will be experienced, that medication to relieve pain will be provided, and that the patient will be closely observed. The patient is encouraged to take the analgesic medication before the pain becomes severe. Positioning and relaxation often make the pain more tolerable. Patients who have concern about scarring from surgery are encouraged to discuss this concern, and misconceptions are corrected. It may be helpful to indicate that the health care team members will keep the patient informed about the healing process.

The patient and family are encouraged to talk about their fear of the patient dying. They should be reassured that this fear is normal. For those who only hint about this concern despite efforts to encourage them to talk about it, coaching may be helpful (eg, "Are you worrying about not making it through surgery? Most people who have heart surgery at least think about the possibility of dying."). After the fear is expressed, the nurse can help the patient and family explore their feelings.

By alleviating undue anxiety and fear, preparing the patient emotionally for surgery decreases the chance of preoperative problems, promotes smooth anesthesia induction, and enhances the patient's involvement in care and recovery after surgery. Preparing the family for the usual postoperative events helps them to cope, support the patient, and participate in postoperative and rehabilitative care.

Monitoring and Managing Potential Complications

Angina may occur because of increased stress and anxiety related to the forthcoming surgery. The patient who develops angina usually responds to normal angina therapy, most commonly nitroglycerin. Some patients require oxygen and IV nitroglycerin infusions (see the Angina Pectoris section). Physiologically unstable patients may require management in a critical care unit preoperatively.

For patients with extreme anxiety or fear and for whom emotional support and education are not successful, medication therapy may be helpful. The anxiolytic agents most commonly used before cardiac surgery are lorazepam (Ativan) and diazepam (Valium).

Promoting Home and Community-Based Care

TEACHING PATIENTS SELF-CARE

Patient and family teaching is based on assessed learning needs. Teaching usually includes information about hospitalization, surgery (eg, preoperative and postoperative care, length of surgery, pain and discomfort that can be expected, visiting hours and procedures in the critical care unit), the recovery phase (eg, length of hospitalization, what to expect from home care and rehabilitation, when normal activities such as housework, shopping, and work can be resumed), and ongoing lifestyle habits. Any changes made in medical therapy and preoperative preparations need to be explained and reinforced.

The patient is informed that physical preparation usually involves showering with an antiseptic solution. A sedative may be prescribed the night before and the morning of surgery. Most cardiac surgical teams use prophylactic antibiotic therapy, and this is initiated immediately before surgery.

Teaching the patient and family together may be most effective. Anxiety often increases with the admission process and impending surgery. Teaching the patient and family together capitalizes on their established support relationship.

The patient may be offered a tour of the critical care unit, the postanesthesia care unit (PACU), or both. (In some hospitals, the patient initially goes to the PACU.) The patient recovering from anesthesia may be reassured by having already seen the surroundings and having met someone from the unit. The patient and family are informed about the equipment, tubes, and lines that will be present after surgery and their purposes. They should know to expect monitors, several IV lines, chest tubes, and a urinary catheter. Explaining the purpose and the approximate time that these devices will be in place helps to reassure the patient. Most patients remain intubated and on mechanical ventilation for 2 to 24 hours after surgery. They should be aware that this prevents them from talking, and they should be reassured that the staff will be able to assist them with other means of communication.

The nurse takes care to answer the patient's questions about postoperative care and procedures. Deep breathing and coughing, use of the incentive spirometer, and foot exercises are explained and practiced by the patient before surgery. The family's questions at this time usually focus on the length of the surgery, who will discuss the results of the procedure with them after surgery and when this may occur, where to wait during the surgery, the visiting procedures for the critical care unit, and how they can support the patient before surgery and in the critical care unit.

Evaluation

Expected Patient Outcomes

Expected patient outcomes may include:

1. Demonstrates reduced fear
   a. Identifies fears
   b. Discusses fears with family
   c. Uses past experiences as a focus for comparison
   d. Expresses positive attitude about outcome of surgery
   e. Expresses confidence in measures to be used to relieve pain
2. Learns about the surgical procedure and postoperative course
   a. Identifies the purposes of the preoperative preparation procedure
   b. Tours the critical care unit, if desired
   c. Identifies limitations expected after surgery
   d. Discusses expected immediate postoperative environment (eg, tubes, machines, nursing surveillance)
   e. Demonstrates expected activities after surgery (eg, deep breathing, coughing, early ambulation)
3. Shows no evidence of complications
   a. Reports anginal pain is relieved with medications and rest
   b. Takes medications as prescribed

Intraoperative Nursing Management

The perioperative nurse performs an assessment and prepares the patient for the operating room and recovery experience. Any changes in the patient's status and the need for changes in therapy are identified. Procedures are explained before they are performed, such as the application of electrodes and use of continuous monitoring, indwelling catheters, and an SpO_2 probe. IV lines are inserted to administer fluids, medications, and blood products. The patient receives general anesthesia, is intubated, and is placed on mechanical ventilation. In addition to assisting with the surgical procedures, perioperative nurses are responsible for the comfort and safety of the patient. Some of the areas of intervention include positioning, skin care, wound care, and emotional support of the patient and family.

Before the chest incision is closed, chest tubes are inserted to evacuate air and drainage from the mediastinum and the thorax. Temporary epicardial pacemaker electrodes may be implanted on the surface of the right atrium and the right ventricle. These epicardial electrodes can be connected to an external pacemaker if the patient has persistent bradycardia perioperatively. Possible intraoperative complications include low cardiac output, dysrhythmias, hemorrhage, MI, stroke, embolization, and organ failure from shock, embolus, or adverse drug reactions. Astute intraoperative patient assessment is critical to prevent, detect, and initiate prompt intervention for these complications.

Nursing Process

The Postoperative Cardiac Surgery Patient

Initial postoperative care focuses on achieving or maintaining hemodynamic stability and recovery from general anesthesia. Care may be provided in the PACU or intensive care unit. After the patient's cardiac status and respiratory status are stable, the patient is transferred to a surgical progressive care unit with telemetry. Care focuses on the monitoring of cardiopulmonary status, pain management, wound care, progressive activity, and nutrition. Education about medications and risk factor modification is emphasized. Discharge from the hospital may occur 3 to 5 days after CABG in patients without complications. Following recovery from the surgery, patients can expect fewer symptoms from CAD and an improved quality of life. CABG has been shown to increase the lifespan of high-risk patients, including those with left main artery blockages and left ventricular dysfunction with multivessel blockages (Magee et al., 2003).

The immediate postoperative period for the patient who has undergone cardiac surgery presents many challenges to the health care team. All efforts are made to facilitate the transition from the operating room to the critical care unit or PACU with minimal risk. Specific information about the surgical procedure and important factors about postoperative management are communicated by the surgical team and anesthesia personnel to the critical care nurse, who then assumes responsibility for the patient's care. Figure 28-12 presents an overview of the many aspects of postoperative care of the cardiac surgical patient.

Assessment

When the patient is admitted to the critical care unit or PACU, and hourly for at least every 12 hours thereafter, a complete assessment of all systems is performed to determine the postoperative status of the patient compared with the preoperative baseline and to identify anticipated changes since surgery. The following parameters are assessed:

Neurologic status: level of responsiveness, pupil size and reaction to light, reflexes, facial symmetry, movement of the extremities, and hand grip strength

Cardiac status: heart rate and rhythm, heart sounds, pacemaker status, arterial blood pressure, central venous pressure (CVP), pulmonary artery pressure, pulmonary artery wedge pressure (PAWP), waveforms from the invasive blood pressure lines, cardiac output or index, systemic and pulmonary vascular resistance, pulmonary artery oxygen saturation (SvO_2) (see Chapter 26 for a detailed description of hemodynamic monitoring)

Respiratory status: chest movement, breath sounds, ventilator settings (eg, rate, tidal volume, oxygen concentration, mode such as synchronized intermittent mandatory ventilation, positive end-expiratory pressure, pressure support), respiratory rate, peak inspiratory pressure, arterial oxygen saturation (SaO_2), percutaneous oxygen saturation (SpO_2), end-tidal CO_2, pleural chest tube drainage, arterial blood gases

Peripheral vascular status: peripheral pulses; color of skin, nail beds, mucosa, lips, and earlobes; skin temperature; edema; condition of dressings and invasive lines

Renal function: urinary output; urine specific gravity and osmolality may be assessed

Fluid and electrolyte status: intake, output from all drainage tubes, all cardiac output parameters, and indications of electrolyte imbalance

Pain: nature, type, location, and duration (incisional pain must be differentiated from anginal pain); apprehension; response to analgesics

Assessment also includes observing all equipment and tubes to determine whether they are functioning properly: endotracheal tube, ventilator, end-tidal CO_2 monitor, SpO_2 monitor, pulmonary artery catheter, SvO_2 monitor, arterial and IV lines, IV infusion devices and tubing, cardiac monitor, pacemaker, chest tubes, and urinary drainage system.

As the patient regains consciousness and progresses through the postoperative period, the nurse also assesses indicators of psychological and emotional status. The patient may exhibit behavior that reflects denial or depression or may experience postcardiotomy delirium. Characteristic signs of delirium include transient perceptual illusions, visual and auditory hallucinations, disorientation, and paranoid delusions.

It is also necessary to assess the family's needs. The nurse ascertains how family members are coping with the situation; determines their psychological, emotional, and spiritual needs; and finds out whether they are receiving adequate information about the patient's condition.

Nasogastric tube to decompress stomach.
Endotracheal tube for providing ventilatory assistance, suctioning, and use of end-tidal CO_2 monitor.
Swan-Ganz catheter for monitoring central venous pressure, pulmonary artery and pulmonary artery wedge pressures, temperature, SVO_2. Can be used for determining cardiac output, for venous and pulmonary artery blood sampling, and for medication administration. Venous lines can be used for fluid administration.
ECG electrodes for monitoring heart rate and rhythm.
SpO_2 monitor for measuring arterial oxygen saturation.
Assess peripheral pulses: radial, posterior tibial, dorsalis pedis.
Neurological assessment:
• Level of responsiveness
• Hand grasp
• Pupils
• Pain
• Movement
Assess skin color and temperature, color of lips, and color and capillary refill of nail beds.
Epicardial pacing electrodes to temporarily pace the heart.
Mediastinal and pleural chest tubes attached to suction; drainage and wound healing are monitored.
Radial arterial line; used for monitoring arterial blood pressure and for blood sampling.
Indwelling catheter to closed drainage system for accurate measurement of urine output; a temperature probe may be part of the indwelling catheter.

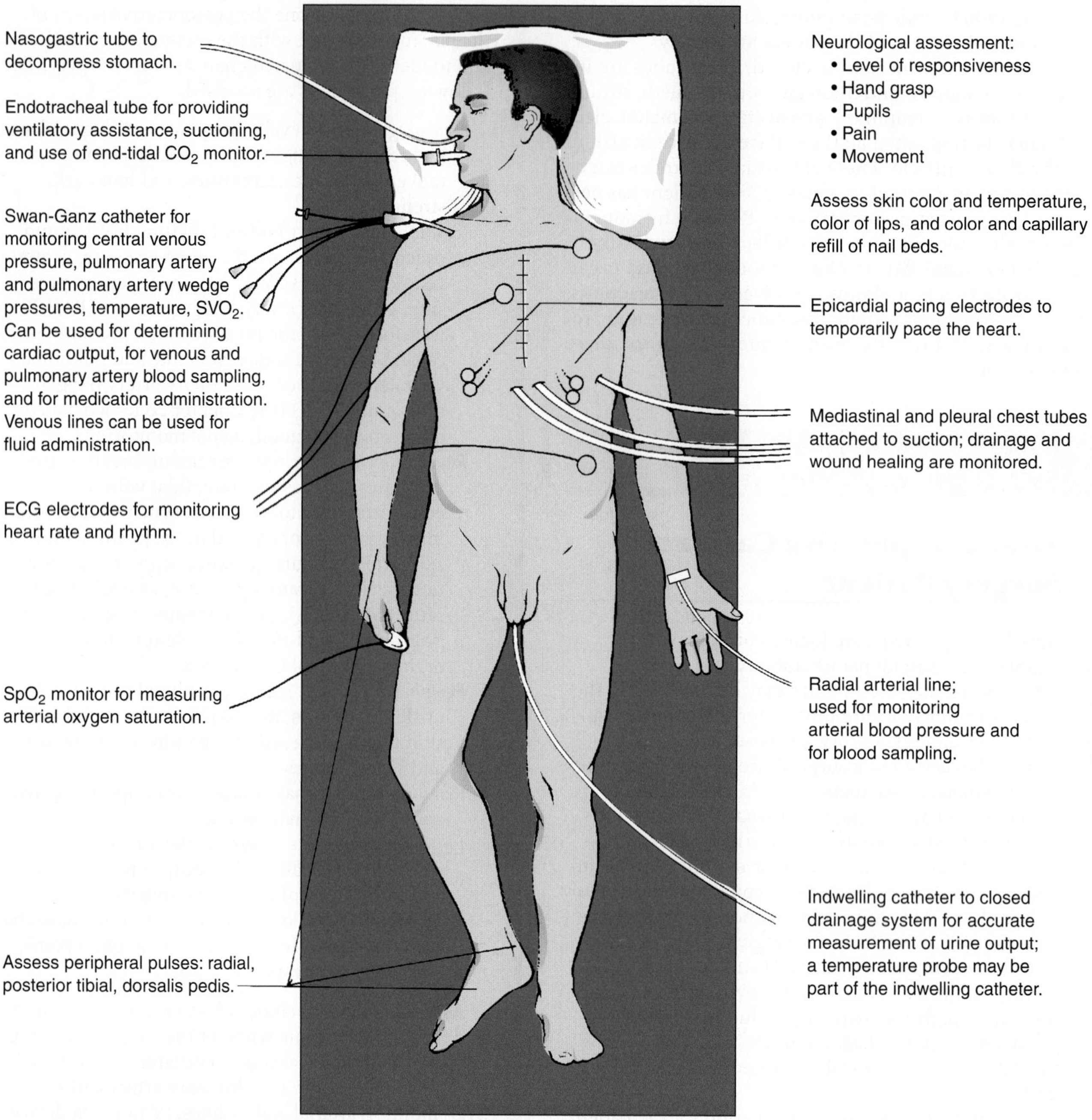

FIGURE 28-12. Postoperative care of the cardiac surgical patient requires the nurse to be proficient in interpreting hemodynamics, correlating physical assessments with laboratory results, sequencing interventions, and evaluating progress toward desired outcomes.

Assessing for Complications

The patient is continuously assessed for indications of impending complications (see Table 28-5). The nurse and the surgeon function collaboratively to prevent complications, to identify early signs and symptoms of complications, and to institute measures to reverse their progression.

DECREASED CARDIAC OUTPUT

A decrease in cardiac output is always a threat to the patient who has had cardiac surgery. It can have a variety of causes:

- Preload alterations: too little blood volume returning to the heart as a result of hypovolemia, persistent bleeding, or cardiac tamponade; or too much blood volume returning to the heart from fluid overload
- Afterload alteration: constricted arteries from postoperative hypertension or hypothermic vasoconstriction impede left ventricular emptying, increasing the workload of the heart
- Heart rate alterations: too fast, too slow, or dysrhythmias
- Contractility alterations: cardiac failure, MI, electrolyte imbalances, hypoxia

FLUID VOLUME AND ELECTROLYTE IMBALANCE

Fluid and electrolyte imbalance may occur after cardiac surgery. Nursing assessment for these complications includes monitoring of intake and output, weight, hemodynamic parameters, hematocrit levels, distention of neck veins, edema, liver size, breath sounds (eg, fine crackles, wheezing), and electrolyte levels. Changes in serum electrolytes are reported promptly so that treatment can be instituted. Especially important are dangerously high or dangerously low levels of potassium, magnesium, sodium, and calcium. Elevated blood glucose levels are common in the postoperative period. Administration of IV insulin may be required in patients both with and without diabetes to achieve the glycemic control necessary for promoting wound healing (Van den Berghe, Wouters, Bouillon, et al., 2003).

IMPAIRED GAS EXCHANGE

Impaired gas exchange is another possible complication after cardiac surgery. All body tissues require an adequate supply of oxygen for survival. To achieve this after surgery, an endotracheal tube with ventilator assistance may be used for 24 hours or more. The assisted ventilation is continued until the patient's blood gas measurements are acceptable and the patient demonstrates the ability to breathe independently. Patients who are stable after surgery may be extubated as early as 2 to 4 hours after surgery, which reduces their discomfort and anxiety regarding their limited ability to communicate.

The patient is continuously assessed for signs of impaired gas exchange: restlessness, anxiety, cyanosis of mucous membranes and peripheral tissues, tachycardia, and fighting the ventilator. Breath sounds are assessed often to detect fluid in the lungs and monitor lung expansion. Arterial blood gases, SpO_2, and end-tidal CO_2 are assessed for decreased oxygen and increased carbon dioxide. Following extubation, aggressive pulmonary interventions, such as turning, coughing, and deep breathing, are necessary to prevent atelectasis and pneumonia.

IMPAIRED CEREBRAL CIRCULATION

Brain function depends on a continuous supply of oxygenated blood. The brain does not have the capacity to store oxygen and must rely on adequate continuous perfusion by the heart. It is important to observe the patient for any symptoms of hypoxia: restlessness, headache, confusion, dyspnea, hypotension, and cyanosis. An assessment of the patient's neurologic status includes level of consciousness, response to verbal commands and painful stimuli, pupil size and reaction to light, facial symmetry, movement of the extremities, hand grip strength, presence of pedal and popliteal pulses, and temperature and color of extremities. Any indication of a change in status is documented, and abnormal findings are reported to the surgeon because they may signal the onset of a complication. Hypoperfusion or microemboli may produce central nervous system injury after cardiac surgery.

Diagnosis

Nursing Diagnoses

Based on the assessment data and the type of surgical procedure performed, major nursing diagnoses may include:

- Decreased cardiac output related to blood loss, compromised myocardial function, and dysrhythmias
- Impaired gas exchange related to the trauma of chest surgery
- Risk for imbalanced fluid volume (and electrolyte imbalance) related to alteration in circulating blood volume
- Disturbed sensory perception (visual or auditory) related to excessive environmental stimuli (critical care environment, surgical experience), insufficient sleep, psychological stress, altered sensory integration, and electrolyte imbalances
- Acute pain related to surgical trauma and pleural irritation caused by chest tubes
- Ineffective tissue perfusion (renal, cerebral, cardiopulmonary, gastrointestinal, peripheral) related to decreased cardiac output, hemolysis, vasopressor drug therapy, embolization, underlying atherosclerotic disease, or coagulation problems
- Ineffective thermoregulation related to infection or postpericardiotomy syndrome
- Deficient knowledge about self-care activities

Collaborative Problems/ Potential Complications

Based on the assessment data, potential complications that may develop include:

- Cardiac complications: heart failure, MI, stunned myocardium, dysrhythmias, tamponade, cardiac arrest
- Pulmonary complications: pulmonary edema, pulmonary emboli, pleural effusions, pneumothorax or hemothorax, respiratory failure, acute respiratory distress syndrome
- Hemorrhage/coagulopathy
- Neurologic complications: embolic or hemorrhagic stroke
- Renal failure
- Electrolyte imbalances
- Hepatic failure
- Infection/sepsis

Planning and Goals

The major goals for the patient include restoration of cardiac output, adequate gas exchange, maintenance of fluid and electrolyte balance, reduction of symptoms of sensory-perception alterations, relief of pain, maintenance of adequate tissue perfusion, maintenance of normal body temperature, learning self-care activities, and absence of complications.

Nursing Interventions

Restoring Cardiac Output

To evaluate the patient's cardiac status, the nurse primarily determines the effectiveness of cardiac output through clinical observations and routine measurements: serial readings of blood pressure, heart rate, CVP, arterial pressure, and pulmonary artery pressures.

Renal function is related to cardiac function, as blood pressure and heart rate drive glomerular filtration; therefore, urinary output is measured and recorded. Urine output of less than 30 mL/hr may indicate a decrease in cardiac output. Urine specific gravity may also be assessed (normal is 1.010 to 1.025), as may urine osmolality. Inadequate fluid volume may be manifested by low urinary output and high specific gravity, whereas overhydration is manifested by high urine output and low specific gravity.

Body tissues depend on adequate cardiac output to provide a continuous supply of oxygenated blood to meet the changing demands of the organs and body systems. Because the buccal mucosa, nail beds, lips, and earlobes are sites with rich capillary beds, they should be observed for cyanosis or duskiness as possible signs of reduced cardiac output. Moist or dry skin may indicate vasodilation or vasoconstriction, respectively. Distention of the neck veins or of the dorsal surface of the hand raised to heart level may signal right-sided heart failure. If cardiac output has decreased, the skin becomes cool, moist, and cyanotic or mottled.

Dysrhythmias may develop when perfusion of the heart is poor. The most common dysrhythmias encountered during the postoperative period are atrial fibrillation, bradycardias, tachycardias, and ectopic beats. Continuous observation of the cardiac monitor for dysrhythmias is essential.

Any indications of decreased cardiac output are reported promptly to the physician. These assessment data and results of diagnostic tests are used by the physician to determine the cause of the problem. After a diagnosis has been made, the physician and the nurse work collaboratively to restore cardiac output and prevent further complications. When indicated, the physician prescribes blood components, fluids, digitalis or other antidysrhythmics, diuretics, vasodilators, or vasopressors. If additional surgery is necessary, the patient and family are prepared for the procedure.

Promoting Adequate Gas Exchange

To ensure adequate gas exchange, the nurse assesses and maintains the patency of the endotracheal tube. The patient is suctioned when wheezes, coarse crackles, or rhonchi are present. Routinely, 100% oxygen is delivered to the patient from the ventilator or by a manual resuscitation bag (eg, Ambu-Bag) before and after suctioning to minimize the risk of hypoxia that can result from the suctioning procedure. Arterial blood gas determinations are compared with baseline data, and changes are reported to the physician promptly.

Because a patent airway is essential for oxygen and carbon dioxide exchange, the endotracheal tube must be secured to prevent it from slipping into the right mainstem bronchus and occluding the left bronchus. When the patient's condition stabilizes, body position is changed every 1 to 2 hours. Frequent changes of patient position provide for optimal pulmonary ventilation and perfusion by allowing the lungs to expand more fully. The nurse assesses breath sounds to detect crackles, wheezes, and fluid in the lungs.

The patient is usually weaned from the ventilator and extubated within 24 hours of CABG. Physical assessment and arterial blood gas results guide the process. Before being extubated, the patient should have cough and gag reflexes and stable vital signs; be able to lift the head off the bed or give firm hand grasps; have adequate vital capacity, negative inspiratory force, and minute volume appropriate for body size; and have acceptable arterial blood gas levels while breathing warmed humidified oxygen without the assistance of the ventilator.

During this time, the nurse assists with the weaning process and eventually with removal of the endotracheal tube. Deep breathing and coughing are encouraged at least every 1 to 2 hours after extubation to open the alveolar sacs and provide for increased ventilation, and to clear secretions.

Maintaining Fluid and Electrolyte Balance

To promote fluid and electrolyte balance, the nurse carefully assesses intake and output. Flow sheets are used to determine positive or negative fluid balance. All fluid intake is recorded, including IV, nasogastric tube, and oral fluids. All output is recorded, including urine, nasogastric drainage, and chest drainage.

Hemodynamic parameters (ie, blood pressure, CVP, PAWP) are correlated with intake, output, and weight to determine the adequacy of hydration and cardiac output. Serum electrolytes are monitored, and the patient is observed for signs of potassium, magnesium, sodium, or calcium imbalance.

Any indications of dehydration, fluid overload, or electrolyte imbalance are reported promptly, and the physician and nurse work collaboratively to restore fluid and electrolyte balance. The patient's response is monitored.

Minimizing Sensory-Perception Imbalance

Some patients exhibit abnormal behaviors that occur with varying intensity and duration. In the early years of cardiac surgery, this phenomenon occurred more frequently than it does today. Advances in surgical techniques and in the delivery of anesthetic agents have significantly decreased the incidence of postoperative delirium. When it occurs today, it is thought to be caused by anxiety, sleep deprivation, increased sensory input, medications, and physiologic problems such as hypoxemia (Marshall & Soucy, 2003). Delirium may appear after a 2- to 5-day stay in an intensive care environment.

Basic comfort measures are used in conjunction with prescribed analgesics and sedatives to promote rest. Because of safety concerns, lines and tubes are discontinued as soon as possible. Patient care is coordinated to provide undisturbed periods of rest. As the patient's condition stabilizes and the patient is disturbed less frequently for monitoring and therapeutic procedures, rest periods can be extended. As much uninterrupted sleep as possible is provided, especially during the patient's normal hours of sleep.

Careful explanations of all procedures and of the need for cooperation help keep the patient oriented throughout the postoperative course. Continuity of care is desirable; a familiar face and a nursing staff with a consistent approach help the patient feel safe. The patient's family should be welcomed at the bedside. A well-designed and individualized plan of nursing care can assist the nursing team in coordinating their efforts for the emotional well-being of the patient.

Relieving Pain

Deep pain may not be felt in the peri-incisional area but may occur in a broader, more diffuse area. Patients who have had cardiac surgery experience pain caused by the interruption of intercostal nerves along the incision route and irritation of the pleura by the chest catheters. Incisional pain may also be experienced from peripheral vein or artery graft harvest sites.

It is essential to observe and listen to the patient for verbal and nonverbal clues about pain. The nurse accurately records the nature, type, location, and duration of the pain (chest incisional pain must be differentiated from anginal pain). The patient is encouraged to use patient-controlled analgesia (PCA) or accept medication as often as it is prescribed to reduce the amount of pain. The addition of IV and oral NSAIDs (or other adjunctive pain relievers) to opioids has decreased the amount of opioids required for pain relief and increased patient comfort. Patients report the most pain during coughing, turning, and moving (Milgrom, Brooks, Qi, et al., 2004). Physical support of the incision with a folded bath blanket or small pillow during deep breathing and coughing helps to minimize pain. The patient should then be able to participate in respiratory exercises and to increase self-care progressively. Patient comfort improves after removal of the chest tubes.

Pain produces tension, which may stimulate the central nervous system to release catecholamines, resulting in constriction of the arterioles and increased heart rate. This can cause increased afterload and decreased cardiac output. Opioids alleviate pain and induce sleep and feelings of euphoria, which reduces the metabolic rate and oxygen demands. After the administration of opioids, any observations indicating relief of apprehension and pain are documented in the patient's record. The patient is observed for any adverse effects of opioids, which may include respiratory depression, hypotension, ileus, or urinary retention. If serious side effects occur, an opioid antagonist (eg, naloxone [Narcan]) may be used. However, continuous titration of low hourly doses of an opioid via either IV drip or PCA pump, as opposed to periodic IV or IM boluses, until the pain is tolerable decreases the occurrence of adverse effects.

Maintaining Adequate Tissue Perfusion

Peripheral pulses (eg, pedal, tibial, femoral, radial, brachial) are routinely palpated to assess for arterial obstruction. If a pulse is absent in any extremity, the cause may be prior catheterization of that extremity or chronic peripheral vascular disease. The newly identified absence of any pulse is immediately reported to the physician.

Thromboemboli formation also can result from injury to the intima of the blood vessels, dislodging a clot from a damaged valve, loosening of mural thrombi, or coagulation problems. Air embolism can result from CPB or central venous cannulation. Symptoms of embolization vary according to site. The usual embolic sites are the lungs, coronary arteries, mesentery, spleen, extremities, kidneys, and brain. The patient is observed for onset of the following:

- Chest pain and respiratory distress from pulmonary embolus or MI
- Abdominal or back pain from mesenteric emboli
- Pain, cessation of pulses, blanching, numbness, or coldness in an extremity
- Decreased urine output from renal emboli
- One-sided weakness and pupillary changes, as occur in stroke

All such symptoms are promptly reported to the physician.

After surgery, the following measures are taken to prevent venous stasis, which can cause deep venous thrombosis and subsequent pulmonary embolism:

- Applying elastic compression stockings or elastic bandage wraps and sequential pneumatic compression wraps
- Discouraging crossing of legs
- Avoiding use of the knee gatch on the bed
- Omitting pillows in the popliteal space
- Instituting passive exercises followed by active exercises to promote circulation and prevent venous stasis

Inadequate renal perfusion can occur as a complication of cardiac surgery. One possible cause is low cardiac output. Trauma to blood cells during CPB can cause hemolysis of red blood cells, which then occlude the renal glomeruli. Use of vasopressor agents to increase blood pressure may constrict the renal arterioles and reduce blood flow to the kidneys.

Nursing management includes accurate measurement of urine output. An output of less than 30 mL/hr may indicate hypovolemia or renal insufficiency. Urine specific gravity can be monitored to determine the kidneys' ability to concentrate urine in the renal tubules. Fluids may be prescribed to increase cardiac output and renal blood flow. IV diuretics may be administered to increase urine output. The nurse should be aware of the patient's blood urea nitrogen, serum creatinine, and urine and serum electrolyte levels. Abnormal levels are reported promptly because it may be necessary to adjust fluids and the dose or type of medication administered. If efforts to maintain renal perfusion are ineffective, the patient may require continuous renal replacement therapy or dialysis (see Chapter 44).

Maintaining Normal Body Temperature

Patients are usually hypothermic when admitted to the critical care unit following the cardiac surgical procedure. The patient must be gradually warmed to a normal temperature. This is accomplished partially by the patient's own basal metabolic processes and often with the assistance of warmed ventilator air, warm air or warm cotton blankets, or heat lamps. While the patient is hypothermic, the clotting process is less efficient, the heart is prone to dysrhythmias, and oxygen does not readily transfer from the hemoglobin to the tissues. Because anesthesia and hypothermia suppress normal basal metabolism, oxygen supply usually meets the cellular demand.

After cardiac surgery, the patient is at risk for developing elevated body temperature caused by infection or postpericardiotomy syndrome. The resultant increase in metabolic rate increases tissue oxygen demands and increases cardiac workload. Measures are taken to prevent this sequence of events or to halt it as soon as it is recognized.

Common sites of infection include the lungs, urinary tract, incisions, and intravascular catheters. Meticulous care is used to prevent contamination at the sites of catheter and tube insertions. Aseptic technique is used when changing dressings and when providing endotracheal tube and catheter care. Clearance of pulmonary secretions is accomplished by frequent repositioning of the patient, suctioning, and chest physical therapy, as well as teaching and encouraging the patient to breathe deeply and cough. Closed systems are used to maintain all IV and arterial lines. All invasive equipment is discontinued as soon as possible after surgery.

Postpericardiotomy syndrome may occur in patients who undergo cardiac surgery (Porth, 2005). The syndrome is characterized by fever, pericardial pain, pleural pain, dyspnea, pericardial effusion, pericardial friction rub, and arthralgia. These signs and symptoms may occur in combination. Leukocytosis occurs, along with elevation of the erythrocyte sedimentation rate. These signs frequently appear after the patient is discharged from the hospital.

It is necessary to differentiate postpericardiotomy syndrome from other postoperative complications (eg, infection, incisional pain, MI, pulmonary embolus, bacterial endocarditis, pneumonia, atelectasis). Treatment depends on the severity of the symptoms. Anti-inflammatory agents often produce a dramatic improvement in symptoms.

Promoting Home and Community-Based Care

TEACHING PATIENTS SELF-CARE

Depending on the type of surgery and postoperative progress, the patient may be discharged from the hospital a few days after surgery. Although the patient may be eager to return home, the patient and family usually are apprehensive about this transition. The family members often express the fear that they are not capable of caring for the patient at home. They often are concerned that complications will occur that they are unprepared to handle.

The nurse helps the patient and family set realistic, achievable goals. A teaching plan that meets the patient's individual needs is developed with the patient and family. This is started before admission and reviewed each shift through the hospital stay or with each home care and rehabilitation contact. Specific instructions are provided about incision care; signs and symptoms of infection; diet; activity progression and exercise; deep breathing, incentive spirometry, and smoking cessation; weight and temperature monitoring; the medication regimen; and follow-up visits with home care nurses, the rehabilitation personnel, the surgeon, and the cardiologist or internist.

Some patients have difficulty learning and retaining information after cardiac surgery. Many patients have difficulties in cognitive function after cardiac surgery that do not occur after other types of major surgery. The patient may experience recent memory loss, short attention span, difficulty with simple math, poor handwriting, and visual disturbances. Patients with these difficulties often become frustrated when they try to resume normal activities and learn how to care for themselves at home. The patient and family are reassured that the difficulty is almost always temporary and will subside, usually in 6 to 8 weeks. In the meantime, instructions are given to the patient at a much slower pace than normal, and a family member assumes responsibility for making sure that the prescribed regimen is followed. All information is provided in writing in the patient's primary language; alternate formats (eg, large print, Braille, audiotapes) are used if indicated.

NURSING RESEARCH PROFILE

Recovery of Women Following CABG

DiMattio, M. K., & Tulman, L. (2003). A longitudinal study of functional status and correlates following coronary artery bypass graft surgery in women. *Nursing Research, 52*(2), 98–107.

Purpose

Only limited information is available to help women gauge their functional status following coronary artery bypass grafts (CABGs). These women tend to be older and more likely to have age-related comorbidities than men. In addition, they have a greater frequency of symptoms related to the surgery and often have less social support than men. The purpose of this study was to describe women's functional recovery during the first 6 weeks at home following CABG procedures.

Design

This longitudinal study enrolled 81 participants in five medical centers, where they all had CABGs. Of this number, 61 completed the study. Participants who dropped out were more likely to be older and readmitted to the hospital. Data were collected by an initial face-to-face interview in the hospital followed by phone interviews at 2, 4, and 6 weeks after discharge. A number of scales and subscales were used to rate functional status, including the Inventory of Functional Status in the Elderly, select subscales of the Sickness Impact Profile, and the Energy/Fatigue and Pain Severity subscales of the Medical Outcomes Study Patient Assessment Questionnaire.

Findings

Women had significant gains in functional status over the 6 weeks, especially between weeks 2 and 4. They engaged most frequently in personal care and low-level household activity. None of the women recovered completely or regained their baseline functional status within 6 weeks. Although fatigue and pain decreased over time, these symptoms were still experienced at 6 weeks.

Nursing Implications

The study gives nurses valuable information to use with discharge planning and follow-up for women after CABGs. Women should not expect to be fully recovered at 6 weeks after discharge.

CONTINUING CARE

Arrangements are made for a home care nurse when appropriate. Because the hospital stay is relatively short, it is particularly important for the nurse to assess the patient's and family's ability to manage care in the home. Teaching is continued by the home care nurse. Vital signs and incisions are monitored, the patient is assessed for signs and symptoms of complications, and support for the patient and family is provided. Additional interventions may include dressing changes, IV antibiotic administration, diet counseling, and tobacco use cessation strategies. Patients and families need to know that cardiac surgery did not cure the patient's underlying heart disease. Lifestyle changes for risk factor reduction must be made, and medications taken before surgery may still be needed after surgery.

Patient teaching does not end at the time of discharge from home healthcare. The patient is encouraged to contact the surgeon, cardiologist, and nurse if he or she has problems or questions. This provides the patient and family with reassurance that professional support is available. The patient is expected to have at least one follow-up visit with the surgeon.

Many patients and families benefit from supportive programs such as the postcardiac surgery rehabilitation programs offered by many medical centers. These programs provide exercise monitoring; instructions about diet and stress reduction; information about resuming exercise, work, driving, and sexual activity; assistance with tobacco use cessation; and support groups for patients and families. The AHA sponsors the Mended Hearts Club, which provides information as well as an opportunity for families to share experiences.

Evaluation

Expected Patient Outcomes

Expected patient outcomes may include:

1. Maintains adequate cardiac output
2. Maintains adequate gas exchange
3. Maintains fluid (and electrolyte) balance
4. Experiences decreased symptoms of sensory-perception disturbances
5. Experiences relief of pain
6. Maintains adequate tissue perfusion
7. Maintains normal body temperature
8. Incisions are well healed
9. Performs self-care activities
10. Engages in follow-up care with health care providers and cardiac rehabilitation services
11. Adheres to recommendations for diet and lifestyle changes to maintain optimal future health
12. Exhibits no complications

A typical plan of postoperative nursing care and more detailed expected outcomes for the cardiac surgery patient are presented in Chart 28-13.

(text continues on page 912)

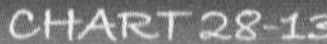

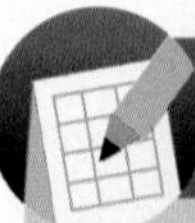

Plan of Nursing Care Care of the Patient After Cardiac Surgery

Nursing Diagnosis: Decreased cardiac output related to blood loss and compromised myocardial function
Goal: Restoration of cardiac output to maintain organ and tissue perfusion

NURSING INTERVENTIONS	RATIONALE	EXPECTED OUTCOMES
1. Monitor cardiovascular status. Serial readings of blood pressures (arterial, pulmonary artery, pulmonary artery wedge pressure [PAWP], central venous pressure [CVP]), cardiac output/index, systemic and pulmonary vascular resistance, and cardiac rhythm and rate are obtained, recorded, and correlated with the patient's condition.	1. Effectiveness of cardiac output is determined by hemodynamic monitoring.	The following parameters are within the patient's normal ranges: • Arterial pressure • PAWP • Pulmonary artery pressures • CVP • Heart sounds • Pulmonary and systemic vascular resistance • Cardiac output and cardiac index • Peripheral pulses • Cardiac rate and rhythm • Cardiac biomarkers • Urine output • Skin and mucosal color • Skin temperature
a. Assess arterial blood pressure every 15 minutes until stable; then arterial or cuff blood pressure every 1–4 hours × 24 hours; then every 8–12 hours until hospital discharge; then every visit.	a. Blood pressure is one of the most important physiologic parameters to follow; vasoconstriction after cardiopulmonary bypass may require treatment with an IV vasodilator.	
b. Auscultate for heart sounds and rhythm.	b. Auscultation provides evidence of cardiac tamponade (muffled distant heart sounds), pericarditis (precordial rub), dysrhythmias.	
c. Assess peripheral pulses (pedal, tibial, radial).	c. Presence or absence and quality of pulses provide data about cardiac output as well as obstructive lesions.	
d. Measure pulmonary artery diastolic (PAD) pressure and PAWP to determine left ventricular end-diastolic volume and to assess cardiac output.	d. Rising pressures may indicate congestive heart failure or pulmonary edema. Low pressures may indicate need for volume replacement.	
e. Monitor PAWP, PAD, and CVP to assess blood volume, vascular tone, and pumping effectiveness of the heart. *Trends are more important than isolated readings.* Mechanical ventilation may alter hemodynamics.	e. High PAWP, PAD, or CVP may result from hypervolemia, heart failure, or cardiac tamponade. If blood pressure drop is due to low blood volume, PAWP, PAD, and CVP will show corresponding drop.	
f. Monitor ECG pattern for cardiac dysrhythmias (see Chap. 27 for discussion of dysrhythmias).	f. Dysrhythmias may occur with coronary ischemia, hypoxia, alterations in serum potassium, edema, bleeding, acid-base or electrolyte disturbances, digitalis toxicity, cardiac failure. ST-segment	

CHART 28-13

Plan of Nursing Care — Care of the Patient After Cardiac Surgery (Continued)

NURSING INTERVENTIONS	RATIONALE	EXPECTED OUTCOMES
	changes may indicate myocardial ischemia. Pacemaker capture and antiarrhythmic medications are used to maintain a heart rate and rhythm and to support stable blood pressures.	
g. Assess cardiac biomarker results when available.	g. Elevations may indicate myocardial infarction.	
h. Measure urine output every ½ hour to 1 hour at first, then with vital signs.	h. Urine output less than 30 mL/h indicates decreased renal perfusion and may reflect decreased cardiac output.	
i. Observe buccal mucosa, nailbeds, lips, earlobes, and extremities.	i. Duskiness and cyanosis may indicate decreased cardiac output.	
j. Assess skin; note temperature and color.	j. Cool moist skin indicates vasoconstriction and decreased cardiac output.	
2. Observe for persistent bleeding: steady, continuous drainage of blood; hypotension; low CVP; tachycardia. Prepare to administer blood products, IV solutions.	2. Bleeding can result from cardiac incisions, tissue fragility, trauma to tissues, clotting defects.	• Less than 200 mL/hr of drainage through chest tubes during first 4 to 6 hours • Vital signs stable
3. Observe for cardiac tamponade: hypotension; rising PAWP, PAD, CVP, or pulsus paradoxus; muffled heart sounds; weak, thready pulse; jugular vein distention; decreasing urinary output. Check for diminished amount of blood in chest drainage collection system. Prepare for reoperation.	3. Cardiac tamponade results from bleeding into the pericardial sac or accumulation of fluid in the sac, which compresses the heart and prevents adequate filling of the ventricles. Decrease in chest drainage may indicate that fluid and clots are accumulating in the pericardial sac.	• CVP and other hemodynamic parameters within normal limits • Urinary output within normal limits • Skin color normal • Respirations unlabored, clear breath sounds • Pain limited to incision • ECG and cardiac biomarkers negative for ischemic changes
4. Observe for cardiac failure: hypotension, rising PAWP, PAD, CVP, tachycardia, restlessness, agitation, cyanosis, venous distention, dyspnea, moist crackles, ascites. Prepare to administer diuretics, digoxin, IV inotropic agents.	4. Cardiac failure results from decreased pumping action of the heart; can cause deficient perfusion to vital organs.	
5. Observe for myocardial infarction: ST-segment elevations, T-wave changes, decreased cardiac output in the presence of normal circulating volume and filling pressures. Monitor serial ECGs and cardiac biomarkers. Differentiate myocardial pain from incisional pain.	5. Symptoms may be masked by the patient's level of consciousness and pain medication.	

continued >

CHART 28-13

Plan of Nursing Care Care of the Patient After Cardiac Surgery (Continued)

Nursing Diagnosis: Impaired gas exchange related to trauma of extensive chest surgery
Goal: Adequate gas exchange

NURSING INTERVENTIONS	RATIONALE
1. Maintain mechanical ventilation until the patient is able to breathe independently.	1. Ventilatory support may be used to decrease work of the heart, to maintain effective ventilation, and to provide an airway in the event of complications.
2. Monitor arterial blood gases, tidal volume, peak inspiratory pressure, and extubation parameters.	2. ABGs and ventilator parameters indicate effectiveness of ventilator and changes that need to be made to improve gas exchange.
3. Auscultate chest for breath sounds.	3. Crackles indicate pulmonary congestion; decreased or absent breath sounds may indicate pneumothorax, hemothorax, dislodgement of tube.
4. Sedate patient adequately, as prescribed, and monitor respiratory rate and depth if ventilations are not "controlled" by ventilator.	4. Sedation helps the patient to tolerate the endotracheal tube and to cope with ventilatory sensations; sedatives can depress respiratory rate and depth.
5. Suction tracheobronchial secretions as needed, using strict aseptic technique.	5. Retention of secretions leads to hypoxia and possible infection.
6. Assist in weaning and endotracheal tube removal.	6. Decreased risk of pulmonary infections and enhanced ability of patient to communicate without an endotracheal tube.
7. After extubation, promote deep breathing, coughing, and turning. Encourage use of the incentive spirometer and compliance with breathing treatments. Teach incisional splinting with a "cough pillow" to decrease discomfort.	7. Aids in keeping airway patent, preventing atelectasis, and facilitating lung expansion.

EXPECTED OUTCOMES

- Airway patent
- ABGs within normal range
- Endotracheal tube correctly placed, as evidenced by x-ray
- Breath sounds clear
- Ventilator synchronous with respirations
- Breath sounds clear after suctioning/coughing
- Nailbeds and mucous membranes pink
- Mental acuity consistent with amount of sedatives and analgesics received
- Oriented to person; able to respond yes and no appropriately
- Able to be weaned successfully from ventilator

Nursing Diagnosis: Risk for imbalanced fluid volume and electrolyte imbalance related to alterations in blood volume
Goal: Fluid and electrolyte balance

NURSING INTERVENTIONS	RATIONALE
1. Maintain fluid and electrolyte balance.	1. Adequate circulating blood volume is necessary for optimal cellular activity; metabolic acidosis and electrolyte imbalance can occur after surgery.

EXPECTED OUTCOMES

- Fluid intake and output balanced
- Hemodynamic assessment parameters negative for fluid overload or hypovolemia
- Normal blood pressure with position changes
- Absence of dysrhythmia

CHART 28-13

Plan of Nursing Care — Care of the Patient After Cardiac Surgery (Continued)

NURSING INTERVENTIONS	RATIONALE	EXPECTED OUTCOMES
a. Keep intake and output flow sheets; record urine volume every ½ hour to 4 hours while in critical care unit; then every 8 to 12 hours while hospitalized.	a. Provides a method to determine positive or negative fluid balance and fluid requirements.	• Stable weight • Blood pH 7.35 to 7.45 • Serum potassium 3.5 to 5.0 mEq/L (3.5 to 5.0 mmol/L) • Serum magnesium 1.3 to 2.3 mg/dL (0.62 to 0.95 mmol/L) • Serum sodium 135 to 145 mEq/L (135 to 145 mmol/L) • Serum calcium 8.6 to 10.2 mg/dL (2.15 to 2.55 mmol/L) • Serum glucose <110mg/dL
b. Assess blood pressure, hemodynamic parameters, weight, electrolytes, hematocrit, jugular venous pressure, tissue turgor, breath sounds, urinary output, and nasogastric tube drainage.	b. Provides information about state of hydration.	
c. Measure postoperative chest drainage (should not exceed 200 mL/hr for first 4 to 6 hours); cessation of drainage may indicate kinked or blocked chest tube. Ensure patency and integrity of the drainage system. Maintain autotransfusion system if in use.	c. Excessive blood loss from chest cavity can cause hypovolemia.	
d. Weigh daily. Notify physician if weight gain of 2 lb or more in 24 hours.	d. Indicator of fluid balance.	
2. Be alert to changes in serum electrolyte levels.	2. A specific concentration of electrolytes is necessary in both extracellular and intracellular body fluids to sustain life.	
a. Hypokalemia (low potassium) *Effects:* dysrhythmias: PVCs, ventricular tachycardia Observe for specific ECG changes. Administer IV potassium replacement as prescribed.	a. *Causes:* inadequate intake, diuretics, vomiting, excessive nasogastric drainage, stress from surgery	
b. Hyperkalemia (high potassium) *Effects:* ECG changes, tall peaked T waves, wide QRS, brachycardia Be prepared to administer diuretic or an ion-exchange resin (sodium polystyrene sulfonate [Kayexalate]); IV sodium bicarbonate, or IV insulin and glucose.	b. *Causes:* increased intake, hemolysis from cardiopulmonary bypass/mechanical assist devices, acidosis, renal insufficiency, tissue necrosis, adrenal cortical insufficiency. The resin binds potassium and promotes intestinal excretion of it. IV sodium bicarbonate drives potassium into the cells from extracellular fluid.	

continued >

CHART 28-13

Plan of Nursing Care — Care of the Patient After Cardiac Surgery (Continued)

NURSING INTERVENTIONS	RATIONALE	EXPECTED OUTCOMES
	Insulin assists the cells with glucose and potassium absorption.	
c. Hypomagnesemia (low magnesium) *Effects:* dysrhythmias: PVCs, ventricular tachycardia, paresthesias, carpopedal spasm, muscle cramps, tetany, irritability, tremors, hyperexcitability, hyperreflexia, seizures. Be prepared to treat the cause. Magnesium supplements may be given (oral route preferred, IV administered with caution).	c. *Causes:* decreased intake, impaired absorption, increased excretion normal for 24 hours after major surgery and diuretic therapy.	
d. Hyponatremia (low sodium) *Effects:* weakness, fatigue, confusion, seizures, coma Administer sodium or diuretics as prescribed.	d. *Causes:* reduction of total body sodium, or increased water intake causing dilution of sodium	
e Hypocalcemia (low calcium) *Effects:* numbness and tingling; carpal spasm; muscle cramps; tetany, hypotension, dysrhythmias Administer oral or IV replacement therapy as prescribed.	e. *Causes:* alkalosis, multiple blood transfusions of citrated blood products	
f. Hypercalcemia (high calcium) *Effects:* dysrhythmias Institute treatment as prescribed.	f. *Causes:* diuretic therapy, prolonged immobility	
g. Hyperglycemia (high blood glucose) *Effects:* increased urine output, thirst, metabolic acidosis Administer insulin as prescribed.	g. *Cause:* stress response to surgery	

Nursing Diagnosis: Disturbed sensory perception related to excessive environmental stimulation, sleep deprivation, electrolyte imbalance
Goal: Reduction of symptoms of sensory perceptual imbalance; prevention of postcardiotomy delirium

NURSING INTERVENTIONS	RATIONALE	EXPECTED OUTCOMES
1. Use measures to prevent postcardiotomy delirium: a. Explain all procedures and the need for patient cooperation.	1. Postcardiotomy delirium may result from anxiety, sleep deprivation, increased sensory input, disorientation to night and day.	• Cooperates with procedures • Sleeps for long, uninterrupted intervals • Oriented to person, place, time

CHART 28-13

Plan of Nursing Care — Care of the Patient After Cardiac Surgery (Continued)

NURSING INTERVENTIONS	RATIONALE	EXPECTED OUTCOMES
b. Plan nursing care to provide for periods of uninterrupted sleep with patient's normal day–night pattern. c. Decrease sleep-preventing environmental stimuli as much as possible. d. Promote continuity of care. e. Orient to time and place frequently. Encourage family to visit. f. Assess for medications that may contribute to delirium. g. Teach relaxation techniques and diversions. h. Encourage self-care as much as tolerated to enhance self-control. Assess support systems and coping mechanisms 2. Observe for perceptual distortions, hallucinations, disorientation, and paranoid delusions.	Normally, sleep cycles are at least 50 min long. The first cycle may be as long as 90 to 120 min and then shorten during successive cycles. Sleep deprivation results when the sleep cycles are interrupted or inadequate in number.	• Experiences no perceptual distortions, hallucinations, disorientation, delusions

Nursing Diagnosis: Acute pain related to surgical trauma and pleural irritation caused by chest tubes
Goal: Relief of pain

NURSING INTERVENTIONS	RATIONALE	EXPECTED OUTCOMES
1. Record nature, type, location, intensity, and duration of pain.	1. Pain and anxiety increase pulse rate, oxygen consumption, and cardiac workload.	• States pain is decreasing in severity • Reports absence of pain • Restlessness decreased • Vital signs stable • Participates in deep-breathing and coughing exercises • Verbalizes fewer complaints of pain each day • Positions self; participates in care activities • Gradually increases activity
2. Assist patient to differentiate between surgical pain and anginal pain.	2. Anginal pain requires immediate assessment and treatment.	
3. Encourage routine pain medication dosing for the first 24 to 72 hours and observe for side effects of lethargy, hypotension, tachycardia, respiratory depression.	3. Analgesia promotes rest, decreases oxygen consumption caused by pain, and aids patient in performing deep-breathing and coughing exercises; pain medications is more effective when taken before pain is severe.	

continued >

CHART 28-13

Plan of Nursing Care — Care of the Patient After Cardiac Surgery (Continued)

Nursing Diagnosis: Ineffective renal tissue perfusion related to decreased cardiac output, hemolysis, or vasopressor drug therapy
Goal: Maintenance of adequate renal perfusion

NURSING INTERVENTIONS	RATIONALE	EXPECTED OUTCOMES
1. Assess renal function:	1. Renal injury can be caused by deficient perfusion, hemolysis, low cardiac output, and use of vasopressor agents to increase blood pressure.	• Urine output consistent with fluid intake; greater than 30 mL/hr • Urine specific gravity 1.003 to 1.030 • BUN, creatinine, electrolytes within normal limits
a. Measure urine output every ½ hour to 4 hours in critical care then every 8–12 hours until hospital discharge.	a. Less than 30 mL/h indicates decreased renal function.	
b. Measure urine specific gravity.	b. Indicates kidneys' ability to concentrate urine in renal tubules.	
c. Monitor and report lab results: BUN, serum creatinine, urine and serum electrolytes.	c. Indicate kidneys' ability to excrete waste products.	
2. Prepare to administer rapid-acting diuretics or inotropic drugs (eg, dobutamine).	2. Promote renal function and increase cardiac output and renal blood flow.	
3. Prepare patient for dialysis or continuous renal replacement therapy if indicated.	3. Provides patient with the opportunity to ask questions and prepare for the procedure.	

Nursing Diagnosis: Ineffective thermoregulation related to infection or postpericardiotomy syndrome
Goal: Maintenance of normal body temperature

NURSING INTERVENTIONS	RATIONALE	EXPECTED OUTCOMES
1. Assess temperature every hour.	1. Fever can indicate infectious or inflammatory process.	• Normal body temperature • Incisions are free of infection and are healing • Absence of symptoms of postpericardiotomy syndrome
2. Use aseptic technique when changing dressings, suctioning endotracheal tube; maintain closed systems for all intravenous and arterial lines and for indwelling urinary catheter.	2. Decreases risk of infection.	
3. Observe for symptoms of postpericardiotomy syndrome: fever, malaise, pericardial effusion, pericardial friction rub, arthralgia.	3. Occurs in approximately 10% of patients after cardiac surgery.	
4. Obtain cultures and other labwork (CBC, ESR); administer antibiotics as prescribed	4. Antibiotics treat documented infection.	

CHART 28-13

Plan of Nursing Care — Care of the Patient After Cardiac Surgery (Continued)

NURSING INTERVENTIONS	RATIONALE	EXPECTED OUTCOMES
5. Administer anti-inflammatory agents as directed.	5. Relieve symptoms of inflammation (eg, warm or flushed sensation, swelling, fullness, stiffness or aching sensation, and fatigue).	

Nursing Diagnosis: Deficient knowledge about self-care activities
Goal: Ability to perform self-care activities

NURSING INTERVENTIONS	RATIONALE	EXPECTED OUTCOMES
1. Develop teaching plan for patient and family. Provide specific instructions for the following: • Diet and daily weights • Activity progression • Exercise • Deep breathing, coughing, lung expansion exercises • Temperature monitoring • Medication regimen • Pulse taking • Access to the emergency medical system • Need for MedicAlert identification	1. Each patient will have unique learning needs.	• Patient and family members explain and comply with therapeutic regimen • Patient and family members identify necessary lifestyle changes • Has copy of discharge instructions (in the patient's primary language and at appropriate reading level; has an alternate format if indicated) • Keeps follow-up appointments
2. Provide verbal and written instructions; provide several teaching sessions for reinforcement and answering questions.	2. Repetition promotes learning by allowing for clarification of misinformation. After cardiac surgery, patients have short-term memory difficulty; information written in the patient's primary language and appropriate reading level is essential because it can be used as a resource after discharge.	
3. Involve family in teaching sessions.	3. Family members responsible for home care are usually anxious and require adequate time for learning.	
4. Provide contact information for surgeon and cardiologist and instructions about follow-up visit with surgeon.	4. Arrangements for contacts with health care personnel help to allay anxieties.	
5. Make appropriate referrals: home care agency, cardiac rehabilitation program, community support groups, Mended Hearts Club.	5. Learning and lifestyle changes continue after discharge from the hospital.	

Critical Thinking Exercises

1 [ebp] You are working in a cardiology office and you receive a phone call from a patient who had an MI 2 years ago. She reports that she is experiencing some shortness of breath and mild back pain. What evidence base is there to suggest that symptoms of an MI may be different for women than men? Discuss the strength of this evidence and its significance in determining assessment criteria to be used for women and men. What questions would you ask this patient? What would you instruct her to do? Provide rationale for your instructions.

2 You are taking over the care of a patient who returned from the catheterization laboratory 2 hours ago following a successful PCI. He was reported to be stable on bed rest, with no bleeding from the right femoral site. The patient appears very pale and complains of right flank pain. Identify the key parameters that need to be assessed. Describe the actions you would take and state why.

3 You are caring for a patient who has been hospitalized awaiting CABG surgery. As you deliver his morning medications, he states that he is feeling "pressure" in the lower sternal area, but he thinks it is just "nerves." What questions would you ask and what would you assess? What would your next actions be?

REFERENCES AND SELECTED READINGS

BOOKS

American Heart Association (2004). *Heart disease and stroke statistics—2004 update.* Dallas, TX: American Heart Association.

Carpenito, L. J. (2004). *Nursing diagnosis: Application to clinical practice* (10th ed.). Philadelphia: Lippincott Williams & Wilkins.

Cummins, R. O. (Ed.) (2003) *ACLS: Principles and practice.* Dallas, TX: American Heart Association.

Fink, M. P., Abraham, E., Vincent, J. L., et al. (2005). *Textbook of critical care* (5th ed.). Philadelphia: Elsevier.

Morton, P. G., Fontaine, D. K., Hudak, C. M., et al. (2005). *Critical care nursing* (8th ed.). Philadelphia: Lippincott Williams & Wilkins.

Porth, C. M. (2005). *Pathophysiology: Concepts of altered health states* (7th ed.). Philadelphia: Lippincott Williams & Wilkins.

Zipes, D. P., Libby, P., Bonow, R. D., et al. (2005). *Braunwald's heart disease* (10th ed.). Philadelphia: Saunders.

JOURNALS

**Asterisks indicate nursing research articles.*

Aldana, S. G., Whitmer, W. R., Greenlaw, R., et al. (2003). Cardiovascular risk reductions associated with aggressive lifestyle modification and cardiac rehabilitation. *Heart & Lung, 32*(6), 374–382.

American College of Cardiology Foundation and American Heart Association. (2002). ACC/AHA 2002 guideline update for exercise testing: A report of the American College of Cardiology/American Heart Association Task Force on Practice Guidelines (Committee on Exercise Testing). *Circulation, 106*(14), 1883–1892.

Antman, E. M., Anbe, D. T., Armstrong, P. W., et al. (2004). ACC/AHA Guidelines for the management of patients with ST-elevation myocardial infarction—executive summary. *Circulation, 110*(5), 1–49.

Bach, R. G., Cannon, C. P., Weintraub, W. S., et al. (2004). The effect of routine, early invasive management on outcome for elderly patients with non-ST-segment elevation acute coronary syndromes. *Annals of Internal Medicine, 141*(3), 186–195.

Berger, P. B., Sketch, M. H., & Califf, R. M. (2004). Choosing between percutaneous coronary intervention and coronary artery bypass grafting for patients with multivessel disease: What can we learn from the arterial revascularization therapy study (ARTS)? *Circulation, 109*(9), 1079–1081.

Bertoni, A. G., Bonds, D. E., Lovato, J., et al. (2004). Sex disparities in procedure use for acute myocardial infarction in the United States, 1995–2001. *American Heart Journal, 147*(6), 1054–1060.

Braunwald, E., Antman, E. M., Beasley, J. W., et al. (2002). ACC/AHA Guideline update for the management of patients with unstable angina and non-ST-segment elevation myocardial infarction—2002: Summary article. *Circulation, 106*(14), 1893–1900.

Chobanian, A. V., Bakris, G. L., Cushman, W. C., et al. (2003). The Seventh Report of the Joint National Committee on Prevention, Detection, Evaluation, and Treatment of High Blood Pressure: The JNC 7 Report. *Journal of the American Medical Association, 289*(19), 2560–2571.

Cleveland, K. W. (2003). Argatroban: A new treatment option for heparin-induced thrombocytopenia. *Critical Care Nurse, 23*(6), 61–69.

*DeVon, H. A., & Zerwic, J. J. (2003). The symptoms of unstable angina. Do women and men differ? *Nursing Research, 52*(2), 108–118.

*DeVon, H. A., & Zerwic, J. J. (2004) Differences in the symptoms associated with unstable angina and myocardial infarction. *Progress in Cardiovascular Nursing, 19*(1), 6–11.

*DiMattio, M. K., & Tulman, L. (2003). A longitudinal study of functional status and correlates following coronary artery bypass graft surgery in women. *Nursing Research, 52*(2), 98–107.

Eagle, K. A., & Guyton, R. A. (2004). ACC/AHA 2004 guideline update for coronary artery bypass graft surgery: Summary article. A report of the American College of Cardiology/American Heart Association Task Force on Practice Guidelines (Committee to update the 1999 Guidelines for Coronary Artery Bypass Graft Surgery). *Circulation, 110*(14), 1–9.

Evans, D. (2002). The effectiveness of music as an intervention for hospital patients: A systematic review. *Journal of Advanced Nursing, 37*(1), 8–18.

Expert Panel on Detection, Evaluation, and Treatment of High Blood Cholesterol in Adults. (2001). Executive summary of the third report of the National Cholesterol Education Program (NCEP) Expert Panel on Detection, Evaluation, and Treatment of High Blood Cholesterol in Adults (Adult Treatment Panel III). *JAMA, 285*(19), 2486–2497.

Gaenzer, H., Neumayr, G., Marschang, P., et al. (2002). Effects of insulin therapy on endothelium-dependent dilation in type 2 diabetes mellitus. *American Journal of Cardiology, 89*(4), 431–434.

Gibbons, R. J. (2003). ACC/AHA 2002 guideline update for the management of patients with chronic stable angina: A report of the American College of Cardiology/American Heart Association Task Force on Practice Guidelines. *Circulation, 107*(1), 149–158.

Goldrick, B. A. (2003). Surgical-site infections: Obesity, diabetes among risk factors for infections within 30 days of surgery. *American Journal of Nursing, 103*(4), 64AA.

Grundy, S. M., Cleeman, J. I., Merz, N. B., et al. (2004). Implications of recent clinical trials for the national cholesterol education program Adult Treatment Panel III guidelines. *Circulation, 110*(2), 227–239.

Haffner, S., & Taegtmeyer, H. (2003). Epidemic obesity and the metabolic syndrome. *Circulation 108*(13), 1541–1545.

Kannel, W. B. (1986). Silent myocardial ischemia and infarction: Insights from the Framingham Study. *Cardiology Clinics, 4*(4), 583–591.

Magee, M. J., Coombs, L. P., Peterson, E. D., et al. (2003). Patient selection and current practice for off-pump coronary artery bypass surgery. *Circulation, 108*(10, supp), II-9–II-14.

Marshall, M. C., & Soucy, M. D. (2003). Delirium in the intensive care unit. *Critical Care Nursing Quarterly, 26*(3), 172–178.

*Milgrom, L. B., Brooks, J. A., Qi, R., et al. (2004). Pain levels experienced with activities after cardiac surgery. *American Journal of Critical Care, 13*(2), 116–125.

Mosca, L. (2004). Evidence-based guidelines for cardiovascular disease prevention in women. *Circulation, 109*(5), 672–693.

Moustapha, A., & Anderson, V. (2003). Contemporary view of the acute coronary syndromes. *Journal of Invasive Cardiology, 15*(2), 71–79.

Nabel, E. G., & Selker, H. P. (2004). Women's ischemic syndrome evaluation. *Circulation, 109*(6), e50–e52.

Pearson, T., Mensah, G. A., & Alexander, R. W. (2003). Markers of inflammation and cardiovascular disease. A statement for health care professionals from the Centers for Disease Control and Prevention and the American Heart Association. *Circulation, 107*(3), 499–511.

Regar, E., Lemos, P. A., & Saia, F. (2004) Incidence of thrombotic stent occlusion during the first three months after sirolimus-eluting stent implantation in 500 consecutive patients. *American Journal of Cardiology, 93*(10), 1271–1275.

Reilly, M. P., & Rader, D. J. (2003). The metabolic syndrome: More than the sum of its parts? *Circulation, 108*(13), 1546–1551.

Ridker, P. M., Rifai, N., Rose, L., et al. (2002). Comparison of C-reactive protein and low-density lipoprotein cholesterol levels in the prediction of first cardiovascular events. *New England Journal of Medicine, 347*(20), 1557–1565.

Rihal, C. S., Raco, D. L., Gersh, B. J., et al. (2003). Indications for coronary artery bypass surgery and percutaneous coronary intervention in chronic stable angina: Review of the evidence and methodological considerations. *Circulation, 108*(20), 2439–2445.

Rose, E. S. (2003). Off-pump coronary artery bypass surgery. *New England Journal of Medicine, 348*(5), 379–380.

Schwertz, D. W., & Vaitkus, P. (2003). Drug-eluting stents to prevent reblockage of coronary arteries. *Journal of Cardiovascular Nursing, 18*(1), 11–16.

Sheifer, S. E., Escarce, J. J., & Schulman, K. A. (2000). Race and sex differences in the management of coronary artery disease. *American Heart Journal, 139*(5), 848–857.

Thompson, E. J., & King, S. L. (2003). Acetylcysteine and fenoldopam. *Critical Care Nurse, 23*(3), 39–46.

U.S. Preventive Services Task Force. (2003). Postmenopausal hormone replacement therapy for the primary prevention of chronic conditions: Recommendations and rationale. *American Journal of Nursing, 103*(6), 83–91.

Van den Berghe, G., Wouters, P. J., Bouillon, R., et al. (2003). Outcome benefit of intensive insulin therapy in the critically ill: Insulin dose versus glycemic control. *Critical Care Medicine, 31*(2), 359–366.

Williams, M. A., Fleg, J. L., Ades, P. A., & American Heart Association Council on Clinical Cardiology Subcommittee on Exercise, Cardiac Rehabilitation, and Prevention. (2002). Secondary prevention of coronary heart disease in the elderly (with emphasis on patients ≥75 years of age): An American Heart Association scientific statement from the Council on Clinical Cardiology Subcommittee on Exercise, Cardiac Rehabilitation, and Prevention. *Circulation, 105*(14), 1735–1743.

Wilson, P. W., & Grundy, S. M. (2003). The metabolic syndrome: Practical guide to origins and treatment: part I. *Circulation, 108*(12), 1422–1425.

RESOURCES

American Dietetic Association, 216 W. Jackson Blvd., Chicago, IL 60606; 1-800-366-1644; http://www.eatright.org. Accessed May 30, 2006.

American Heart Association, 7272 Greenville Ave., Dallas, TX 75231; 1-800-AHA-USA1 (1-800-242-8721); http://www.americanheart.org. Accessed May 30, 2006.

Healthy People 2010, Office of Disease Prevention and Health Promotion, U.S. Department of Health and Human Services, 200 Independence Ave., SW, Washington, DC 20201; 1-800-877-696-6775; http://www.health.gov/healthypeople. Accessed May 30, 2006.

Heartmates, P.O. Box 16202, Minneapolis, MN 55416; 952-929-3331; http://www.heartmates.com. Accessed May 30, 2006.

National Heart, Lung, and Blood Institute, National Institutes of Health, Building 31, Room 5A52, Bethesda, MD 20892; 301-592-8593; http://www.nhlbi.nih.gov. Accessed May 30, 2006.

CHAPTER 29

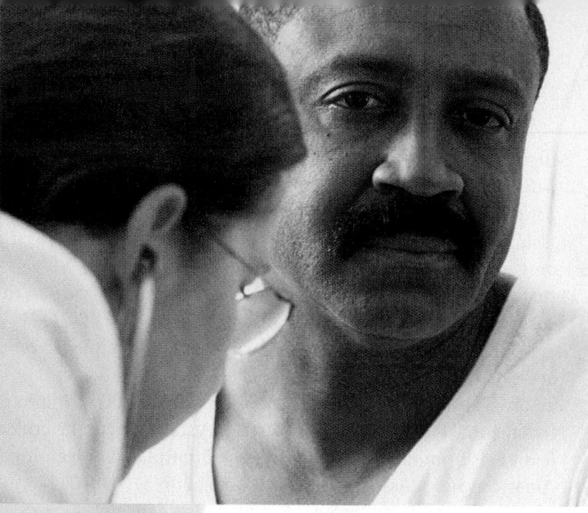

Management of Patients With Structural, Infectious, and Inflammatory Cardiac Disorders

Learning Objectives

On completion of this chapter, the learner will be able to:

1. Define valvular disorders of the heart and describe the pathophysiology, clinical manifestations, and management of patients with mitral and aortic disorders.
2. Describe types of cardiac valve repair and replacement procedures used to treat valvular problems and the care needed by patients who undergo these procedures.
3. Describe the pathophysiology, clinical manifestations, and management of patients with cardiomyopathies.
4. Describe the pathophysiology, clinical manifestations, and management of patients with infections of the heart.
5. Describe the rationale for prophylactic antibiotic therapy for patients with mitral valve prolapse, valvular heart disease, rheumatic endocarditis, infective endocarditis, and myocarditis.

Structural disorders of the heart present many challenges for the patient, family, and health care team, as do the conduction and vascular disorders discussed in Chapters 27 and 28. Problems with the heart valves, holes in the intracardiac septum, cardiomyopathies, and infectious diseases of the heart muscle alter cardiac output. Treatments for these disorders may be noninvasive, such as medication therapy and activity and dietary modification. Invasive treatments, such as valve repair or replacement, septal repair, ventricular assist devices, total artificial hearts, cardiac transplantation, and other procedures, may also be used. Nurses play an integral role in the care of patients with structural, infectious, and inflammatory cardiac conditions.

Valvular Disorders

The valves of the heart control the flow of blood through the heart into the pulmonary artery and aorta by opening and closing in response to the blood pressure changes as the heart contracts and relaxes through the cardiac cycle.

The atrioventricular valves separate the atria from the ventricles and include the **tricuspid valve**, which separates the right atrium from the right ventricle, and the **mitral valve**, which separates the left atrium from the left ventricle. The tricuspid valve has three leaflets; the mitral valve has two. Both valves have chordae tendineae that anchor the valve leaflets to the papillary muscles and ventricular wall.

The semilunar valves are located between the ventricles and their corresponding arteries. The **pulmonic valve** lies between the right ventricle and the pulmonary artery; the **aortic valve** lies between the left ventricle and the aorta. Figure 29-1 shows valves in the closed position.

When any of the heart valves do not close or open properly, blood flow is affected. When valves do not close completely, blood flows backward through the valve in a process called **regurgitation.** When valves do not open completely, a condition called **stenosis**, the flow of blood through the valve is reduced.

Disorders of the mitral valve fall into the following categories: mitral valve **prolapse** (ie, stretching of the valve leaflet into the atrium during systole), mitral regurgitation, and mitral stenosis. Disorders of the aortic valve are categorized as aortic regurgitation and aortic stenosis. These valvular disorders may require surgical repair or replacement of the valve to correct the problem, depending on severity of symptoms (Fig. 29-2). Tricuspid and pulmonic valve disorders also occur, usually with fewer symptoms and complications. Regurgitation and stenosis may occur at the same time in the same or different valves.

Mitral Valve Prolapse

Mitral valve prolapse, formerly known as mitral prolapse syndrome, is a deformity that usually produces no symptoms. Rarely, it progresses and can result in sudden death. Mitral valve prolapse occurs more frequently in women than in men, and it is now being diagnosed more frequently than it once was, probably because of improved diagnostic methods. The cause of mitral valve prolapse is usually an inherited connective tissue disorder resulting in enlargement of one or

Glossary

allograft: heart valve replacement made from a human heart valve (synonym: homograft)

annuloplasty: repair of a cardiac valve's outer ring

aortic valve: semilunar valve located between the left ventricle and the aorta

autograft: heart valve replacement made from the patient's own heart valve (eg, the pulmonic valve is excised and used as an aortic valve)

cardiomyopathy: disease of the heart muscle

chordoplasty: repair of the stringy, tendinous fibers that connect the free edges of the atrioventricular valve leaflets to the papillary muscles

commissurotomy: splitting or separating fused cardiac valve leaflets

heterograft: heart valve replacement made of tissue from an animal heart valve (synonym: xenograft)

homograft: heart valve replacement made from a human heart valve (synonym: allograft)

leaflet repair: repair of a cardiac valve's movable "flaps" (leaflets)

mitral valve: atrioventricular valve located between the left atrium and left ventricle

orthotopic transplantation: the recipient's heart is removed, and a donor heart is grafted into the same site; the patient has one heart

prolapse (of a valve): stretching of an atrioventricular heart valve leaflet into the atrium during systole

pulmonic valve: semilunar valve located between the right ventricle and the pulmonary artery

regurgitation: backward flow of blood through a heart valve

stenosis: narrowing or obstruction of a cardiac valve's orifice

total artificial heart: mechanical device used to aid a failing heart, assisting the right and left ventricles

tricuspid valve: atrioventricular valve located between the right atrium and right ventricle

valve replacement: insertion of a device at the site of a malfunctioning heart valve to restore blood flow in one direction through the heart

valvuloplasty: repair of a stenosed or regurgitant cardiac valve by commissurotomy, annuloplasty, leaflet repair, or chordoplasty (or a combination of procedures)

ventricular assist device: mechanical device used to aid a failing right or left ventricle

xenograft: heart valve replacement made of tissue from an animal heart valve (synonym: heterograft)

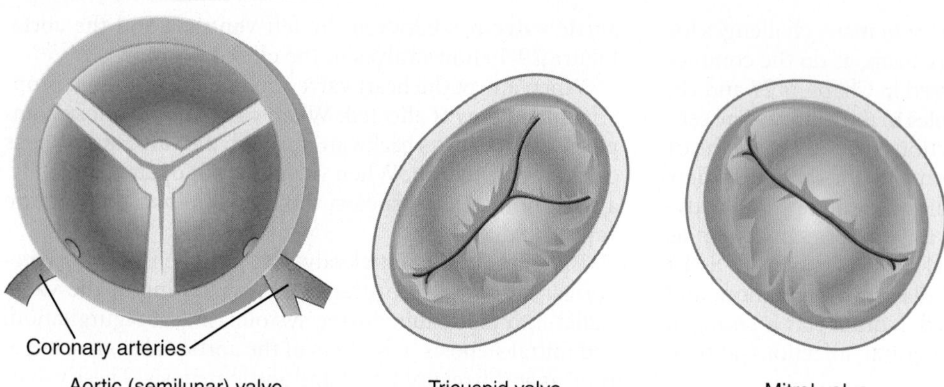

FIGURE 29-1. The valves of the heart (aortic or semilunar, tricuspid, and mitral) in the closed position.

both of the mitral valve leaflets. The annulus often dilates. The chordae tendineae and papillary muscles may elongate.

Pathophysiology

In mitral valve prolapse, a portion of one or both mitral valve leaflets balloons back into the atrium during systole. Rarely, the ballooning stretches the leaflet to the point that the valve does not remain closed during systole (ie, ventricular contraction). Blood then regurgitates from the left ventricle back into the left atrium. About 15% of patients who develop murmurs eventually experience heart enlargement, atrial fibrillation, pulmonary hypertension, or congestive heart failure (Zipes, Libby, Bonow, et al., 2005).

Physiology/Pathophysiology

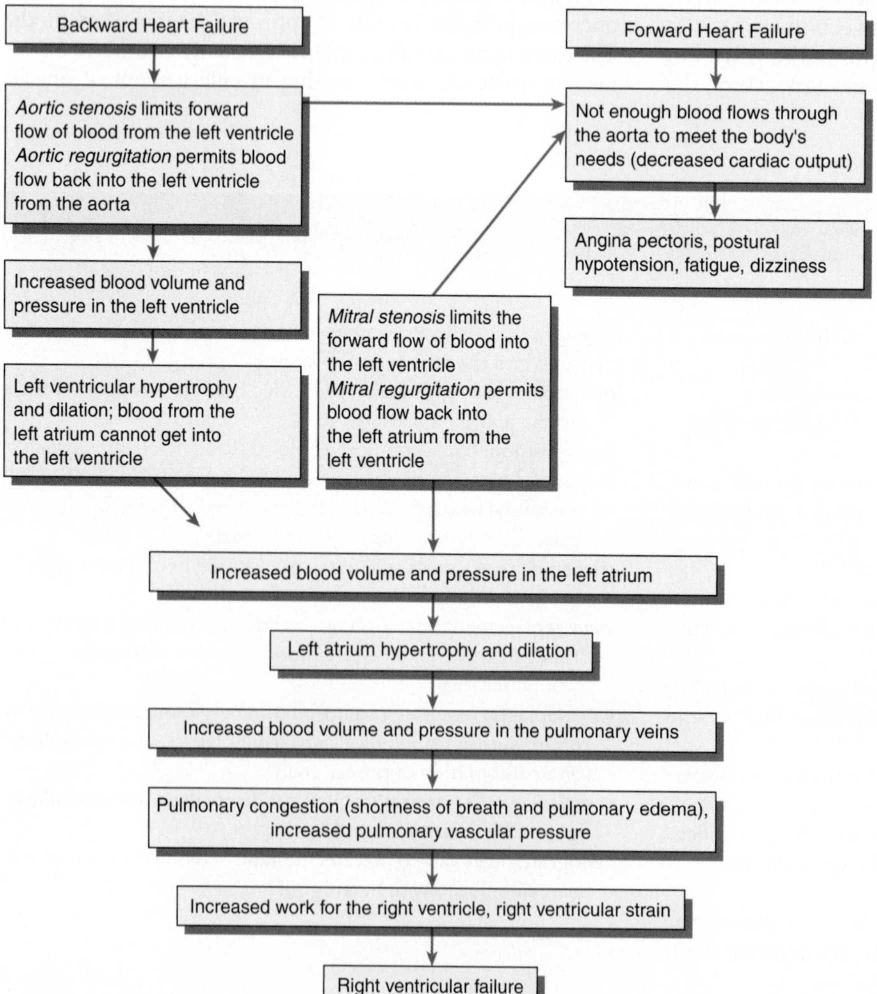

Backward Heart Failure

Aortic stenosis limits forward flow of blood from the left ventricle
Aortic regurgitation permits blood flow back into the left ventricle from the aorta

Increased blood volume and pressure in the left ventricle

Left ventricular hypertrophy and dilation; blood from the left atrium cannot get into the left ventricle

Mitral stenosis limits the forward flow of blood into the left ventricle
Mitral regurgitation permits blood flow back into the left atrium from the left ventricle

Forward Heart Failure

Not enough blood flows through the aorta to meet the body's needs (decreased cardiac output)

Angina pectoris, postural hypotension, fatigue, dizziness

Increased blood volume and pressure in the left atrium

Left atrium hypertrophy and dilation

Increased blood volume and pressure in the pulmonary veins

Pulmonary congestion (shortness of breath and pulmonary edema), increased pulmonary vascular pressure

Increased work for the right ventricle, right ventricular strain

Right ventricular failure

FIGURE 29-2. Pathophysiology: left-sided heart failure as a result of aortic and mitral valvular heart disease and the development of right ventricular failure.

Clinical Manifestations

Most people who have mitral valve prolapse never have symptoms. A few have symptoms of fatigue, shortness of breath, lightheadedness, dizziness, syncope, palpitations, chest pain, and anxiety (Fuster, Alexander, & O'Rourke, 2004; Woods, Froelicher, Motzer, et al., 2005; Zipes et al., 2005). Fatigue may occur regardless of activity level and amount of rest or sleep. Shortness of breath is not correlated with activity levels or pulmonary function. Atrial or ventricular dysrhythmias may produce the sensation of palpitations, but palpitations have been reported while the heart has been beating normally. Chest pain, which is often localized to the chest, is not correlated with activity and may last for days.

Anxiety may be a response to the symptoms; however, some patients report anxiety as the only symptom. Some clinicians speculate that the symptoms may be explained by dysautonomia (a dysfunction of the autonomic nervous system resulting in increased excretion of catecholamines), although no consensus exists about the cause of the symptoms experienced by some patients.

Assessment and Diagnostic Findings

Often, the first and only sign of mitral valve prolapse is identified when a physical examination of the heart reveals an extra heart sound, referred to as a mitral click. A systolic click is an early sign that a valve leaflet is ballooning into the left atrium. In addition to the mitral click, a murmur of mitral regurgitation may be heard if progressive valve leaflet stretching and regurgitation have occurred. A few patients experience signs and symptoms of heart failure if mitral regurgitation exists. Doppler echocardiography may be used to diagnose and monitor the progression of mitral valve prolapse.

Medical Management

Medical management is directed at controlling symptoms. If dysrhythmias are documented and cause symptoms, the patient is advised to eliminate caffeine and alcohol from the diet and to stop smoking, and antidysrhythmic medications may be prescribed.

Chest pain that does not respond to nitrates may respond to calcium channel blockers or beta-blockers. Heart failure is treated the same as it would be for any other case of heart failure (see Chapter 30). In advanced stages of disease, mitral valve repair or replacement may be necessary.

Nursing Management

The nurse educates the patient about the diagnosis and the possibility that the condition is hereditary. First-degree relatives (eg, parents, siblings) may be advised to have echocardiograms. Because most patients with mitral valve prolapse are asymptomatic, the nurse explains the need to inform the health care provider about any symptoms that may develop. The nurse also instructs the patient about the need for prophylactic antibiotic therapy before undergoing invasive procedures (eg, dental work, genitourinary or gastrointestinal procedures) that may introduce infectious agents systemically. This therapy is prescribed for symptomatic patients and for asymptomatic patients who have both a systolic click and murmur or mitral regurgitation. If the patient is in doubt about risk factors and the need for antibiotics, he or she should consult the physician. Women diagnosed with mitral valve prolapse without mitral regurgitation or other complications may complete pregnancies and have vaginal deliveries.

To minimize symptoms, the nurse teaches the patient to avoid caffeine and alcohol. The nurse encourages the patient to read product labels, particularly on over-the-counter products such as cough medicine, because these products may contain alcohol, caffeine, ephedrine, and epinephrine, which may produce dysrhythmias and other symptoms. Treatment of dysrhythmias, chest pain, heart failure, or other complications of mitral valve prolapse is described in Chapter 30. In addition, the nurse also explores possible diet, activity, sleep, and other lifestyle factors that may correlate with symptoms.

Mitral Regurgitation

Mitral regurgitation involves blood flowing back from the left ventricle into the left atrium during systole. Often, the margins of the mitral valve cannot close during systole. The leaflets cannot close because of the thickening and fibrosis of the leaflets and chordae tendineae, resulting in their contraction. The most common causes of mitral valve regurgitation in developed countries are degenerative changes of the mitral valve and ischemia of the left ventricle (Fuster et al., 2004). The most common causes in developing countries are rheumatic heart disease and its sequelae (Fuster et al., 2004).

Other conditions leading to mitral regurgitation include myxomatous changes, which enlarge and stretch the left atrium and ventricle, causing leaflets and chordae tendineae to stretch or rupture. Infective endocarditis may cause perforation of a leaflet, or the scarring following the infection may cause retraction of the leaflets or chordae tendineae. Collagen-vascular diseases (eg, systemic lupus erythematosus), cardiomyopathy, and ischemic heart disease may also result in changes in the left ventricle, causing the papillary muscles, chordae tendineae, or leaflets to stretch, shorten, or rupture.

Pathophysiology

Mitral regurgitation may result from problems with one or more of the leaflets, the chordae tendineae, the annulus, or the papillary muscles. As previously stated, a mitral valve leaflet may shorten or tear, and the chordae tendineae may elongate, shorten, or tear. The annulus may be stretched by heart enlargement or deformed by calcification. The papillary muscle may rupture, stretch, or be pulled out of position by changes in the ventricular wall (eg, scar from a myocardial infarction or ventricular dilation). The papillary muscles may be unable to contract because of ischemia. Regardless of the cause, blood regurgitates back into the atrium during systole.

With each beat of the left ventricle, some of the blood is forced back into the left atrium. Because this blood is added to the blood flowing in from the lungs, the left atrium must stretch. It eventually hypertrophies and dilates. The backward flow of blood from the ventricle diminishes the volume of blood flowing into the atrium from the lungs. As a result, the lungs become congested, eventually adding extra strain on the right ventricle. Mitral regurgitation ultimately involves the lungs and the right ventricle.

Clinical Manifestations

Chronic mitral regurgitation is often asymptomatic, but acute mitral regurgitation (eg, that resulting from a myocardial infarction) usually manifests as severe congestive heart failure. Dyspnea, fatigue, and weakness are the most common symptoms. Palpitations, shortness of breath on exertion, and cough from pulmonary congestion also occur.

Assessment and Diagnostic Findings

A systolic murmur is heard as a high-pitched, blowing sound at the apex. The pulse may be regular and of good volume, or it may be irregular as a result of extrasystolic beats or atrial fibrillation. Doppler echocardiography is used to diagnose and monitor the progression of mitral regurgitation. Transesophageal echocardiography (TEE) provides the best images of the mitral valve.

Medical Management

Management of mitral regurgitation is the same as that for congestive heart failure (see Chapter 30). Usually, patients with mitral regurgitation benefit from afterload reduction (arterial dilation) by treatment with angiotensin-converting enzyme (ACE) inhibitors, such as captopril (Capoten), enalapril (Vasotec), lisinopril (Prinivil, Zestril), ramipril (Altace), or hydralazine (Apresoline). Once symptoms of heart failure develop, the patient needs to restrict his or her activity level. Antibiotic prophylaxis therapy is instituted to prevent infectious endocarditis. Surgical intervention consists of mitral valvuloplasty (ie, surgical repair of the heart valve) or valve replacement.

Mitral Stenosis

Mitral stenosis is an obstruction of blood flowing from the left atrium into the left ventricle. It is most often caused by rheumatic endocarditis, which progressively thickens the mitral valve leaflets and chordae tendineae. The leaflets often fuse together. Eventually, the mitral valve orifice narrows and progressively obstructs blood flow into the ventricle.

Pathophysiology

Normally, the mitral valve opening is as wide as the diameter of three fingers. In cases of marked stenosis, the opening narrows to the width of a pencil. The left atrium has great difficulty moving blood into the ventricle because of the increased resistance of the narrowed orifice. The left atrium dilates (stretches) and hypertrophies (thickens) because of the increased blood volume it holds. Because there is no valve to protect the pulmonary veins from the backward flow of blood from the atrium, the pulmonary circulation becomes congested. As a result, the right ventricle must contract against an abnormally high pulmonary arterial pressure and is subjected to excessive strain. Eventually, the right ventricle fails. The enlarged left atrium may create pressure on the left bronchial tree, resulting in a dry cough or wheezing.

Clinical Manifestations

The first symptom of mitral stenosis is often breathing difficulty (ie, dyspnea) on exertion as a result of pulmonary venous hypertension. Symptoms usually develop after the valve opening is reduced by one-third to one-half its usual size. Patients are likely to show progressive fatigue as a result of low cardiac output. They may expectorate blood (ie, hemoptysis); cough; wheeze; and experience palpitations, orthopnea, paroxysmal nocturnal dyspnea (PND), and repeated respiratory infections.

Assessment and Diagnostic Findings

The pulse is weak and often irregular because of atrial fibrillation (caused by the strain on the atrium). A low-pitched, rumbling, diastolic murmur is heard at the apex. As a result of the increased blood volume and pressure, the atrium dilates, hypertrophies, and becomes electrically unstable, and patients experience atrial dysrhythmias. Doppler echocardiography is used to diagnose mitral stenosis. Electrocardiography (ECG) and cardiac catheterization with angiography may be used to help determine the severity of the mitral stenosis.

Medical Management

Congestive heart failure is treated as described in Chapter 30. Patients with mitral stenosis may benefit from anticoagulants to decrease the risk for developing atrial thrombus and may also require treatment for anemia. Antibiotic prophylaxis is instituted to prevent infectious endocarditis.

Patients with mitral stenosis are advised to avoid strenuous activities and competitive sports, both of which increase the heart rate. Mitral stenosis decreases the amount of blood that can flow from the left atrium to the left ventricle during diastole. When the heart rate increases, diastole is shortened, and thus the amount of time for the forward flow of blood is less. Therefore, as the heart rate increases, cardiac output decreases and pulmonary pressures increase with the backup of blood from the left atrium into the pulmonary veins.

Surgical intervention consists of valvuloplasty, usually a commissurotomy to open or rupture the fused commissures of the mitral valve. Percutaneous transluminal valvuloplasty or mitral valve replacement may be performed.

Aortic Regurgitation

Aortic regurgitation is the flow of blood back into the left ventricle from the aorta during diastole. It may be caused by inflammatory lesions that deform the leaflets of the aortic valve, preventing them from completely closing the aortic valve orifice. This valvular defect also may result from infective or rheumatic endocarditis, congenital abnormalities, diseases such as syphilis, a dissecting aneurysm that causes dilation or tearing of the ascending aorta, blunt chest trauma, or deterioration of an aortic valve replacement. In many cases, the cause is unknown and is classified as idiopathic.

Pathophysiology

Blood from the aorta returns to the left ventricle during diastole, in addition to the blood normally delivered by the left atrium. The left ventricle dilates in an attempt to accommodate the increased volume of blood. It also hypertrophies in an attempt to increase muscle strength to expel more blood with above-normal force, thus increasing systolic blood pressure. The arteries attempt to compensate for the higher pressures by reflex vasodilation; the peripheral arterioles relax, reducing peripheral resistance and diastolic blood pressure.

Clinical Manifestations

Aortic insufficiency develops without symptoms in most patients. Some patients are aware of a forceful heartbeat, especially in the head or neck. Marked arterial pulsations that are visible or palpable at the carotid or temporal arteries may be present as a result of the increased force and volume of the blood ejected from the hypertrophied left ventricle. Exertional dyspnea and fatigue follow. Progressive signs and symptoms of left ventricular failure include breathing difficulties (eg, orthopnea, PND).

Assessment and Diagnostic Findings

A diastolic murmur is heard as a high-pitched, blowing sound at the third or fourth intercostal space at the left sternal border. The pulse pressure (ie, difference between systolic and diastolic pressures) is considerably widened in patients with aortic regurgitation. One characteristic sign of the disease is the water-hammer (Corrigan's) pulse, in which the pulse strikes the palpating finger with a quick, sharp stroke and then suddenly collapses. The diagnosis may be confirmed by Doppler echocardiography (preferably transesophageal), radionuclide imaging, ECG, magnetic resonance imaging (MRI), and cardiac catheterization. Patients with symptoms usually have echocardiograms every 4 to 6 months, and those without symptoms have echocardiograms every 2 to 3 years.

Medical Management

Before the patient undergoes invasive or dental procedures, antibiotic prophylaxis is needed to prevent endocarditis. The patient is advised to avoid physical exertion, competitive sports, and isometric exercise. Dysrhythmias and heart failure are treated as described in Chapters 27 and 30.

The medications usually prescribed first for patients with symptoms of aortic regurgitation are vasodilators such as calcium channel blockers (eg, nifedipine [Adalat, Procardia]) and ACE inhibitors (eg, captopril [Capoten], enalapril [Vasotec], lisinopril [Prinivil, Zestril], ramipril [Altace]) or hydralazine (Apresoline). The treatment of choice is aortic valvuloplasty or valve replacement, preferably performed before left ventricular failure occurs. Surgery is recommended for any patient with left ventricular hypertrophy, regardless of the presence or absence of symptoms.

Aortic Stenosis

Aortic valve stenosis is narrowing of the orifice between the left ventricle and the aorta. In adults, the stenosis is often a result of degenerative calcifications. Calcifications begin on the flexion lines of the leaflets (cusps) at the base (ring, annulus) of the valve and progressively extend outward over the cusps. The calcification may be caused by inflammatory changes that occur in response to years of normal mechanical stress. Diabetes mellitus, hypercholesterolemia, hypertension, and low levels of high-density lipoprotein cholesterol may be risk factors for degenerative changes of the valve. Congenital leaflet malformations or an abnormal number of leaflets (ie, one or two rather than three) may be involved. Rarely, rheumatic endocarditis may cause adhesions or fusion of the commissures and valve ring, stiffening of the cusps, and calcific nodules on the cusps. However, the cause of cusp calcification may be unknown.

Pathophysiology

Progressive narrowing of the valve orifice occurs, usually over several years to several decades. The left ventricle overcomes the obstruction to circulation by contracting more slowly but with greater energy than normal, forcibly squeezing the blood through the smaller orifice. The obstruction to left ventricular outflow increases pressure on the left ventricle. The ventricular wall thickens, or hypertrophies. When these compensatory mechanisms of the heart begin to fail, clinical signs and symptoms develop.

Clinical Manifestations

Many patients with aortic stenosis are asymptomatic. When symptoms develop, patients usually first have exertional dyspnea, caused by increased pulmonary venous pressure due to left ventricular failure. Orthopnea, PND, and pulmonary edema may also occur. Other symptoms are dizziness and syncope because of reduced blood flow to the brain. Angina pectoris is a frequent symptom resulting from the increased oxygen demands of the hypertrophied left ventricle, the decreased time in diastole for myocardial perfusion, and the decreased blood flow into the coronary arteries. Blood pressure may be low but is usually normal. Pulse pressure may be low (30 mm Hg or less) because of diminished blood flow.

Assessment and Diagnostic Findings

On physical examination, a loud, rough systolic murmur may be heard over the aortic area. The sound to listen for is a systolic crescendo–decrescendo murmur, which may radiate into the carotid arteries and to the apex of the left ventricle. The murmur is low-pitched, rough, rasping, and vibrating. An S_4 sound may be heard. If the examiner rests a hand over the base of the heart (second intercostal space next to the sternum and above the suprasternal notch up along the carotid arteries), a vibration may be felt. The vibration is caused by turbulent blood flow across the narrowed valve orifice. By having the patient lean forward during auscultation and palpation, especially during exhalation, it is possible to accentuate the signs of aortic stenosis.

Doppler echocardiography is used to diagnose and monitor the progression of aortic stenosis. Patients with symptoms usually have echocardiograms every 6 to 12 months, and those without symptoms have echocardiograms every 2 to 5 years. Evidence of left ventricular hypertrophy may be seen on a 12-lead ECG and an echocardiogram. After stenosis progresses to the point that surgical intervention is considered, left-sided heart catheterization is necessary to measure the severity of the valvular abnormality and to evaluate the coronary arteries. Pressure tracings are taken from the left ventricle and from the base of the aorta. The systolic pressure in the left ventricle is considerably higher than that in the aorta during systole. Graded exercise studies (stress tests) are not usually prescribed for patients with aortic stenosis because of the high risk of precipitating ventricular tachycardia or fibrillation.

Medical Management

Antibiotic prophylaxis to prevent endocarditis is essential for anyone with aortic stenosis undergoing invasive procedures. After dysrhythmia or left ventricular failure occurs, medications are prescribed (see Chapters 27 and 30). Definitive treatment for aortic stenosis is surgical replacement of the aortic valve. Patients who are symptomatic and are not surgical candidates may benefit from one- or two-balloon percutaneous valvuloplasty procedures.

Nursing Management: Valvular Heart Disorders

The nurse teaches the patient with valvular heart disease about the diagnosis, the progressive nature of valvular heart disease, and the treatment plan. The patient is taught to report new symptoms or changes in symptoms to the health care provider. In addition, the nurse emphasizes the need for prophylactic antibiotic therapy before any invasive procedure (eg, dental work, genitourinary or gastrointestinal procedure) that may introduce infectious agents into the bloodstream. The nurse teaches the patient that the infectious agent, usually a bacterium, is able to adhere to the diseased heart valve more readily than to a normal valve. Once attached to the valve, the infectious agent multiplies, resulting in endocarditis and further damage to the valve.

The nurse measures the patient's heart rate, blood pressure, and respiratory rate, compares these results with previous data, and notes any changes. Heart and lung sounds are auscultated and peripheral pulses palpated. The nurse assesses the patient with valvular heart disease for the following conditions:

- Signs and symptoms of heart failure, such as fatigue, dyspnea on exertion, an increase in coughing, hemoptysis, multiple respiratory infections, orthopnea, and PND (see Chapter 30)
- Dysrhythmias, by palpating the patient's pulse for strength and rhythm (ie, regular or irregular) and asking whether the patient has experienced palpitations or felt forceful heartbeats (see Chapter 27)
- Symptoms such as dizziness, syncope, increased weakness, or angina pectoris (see Chapter 28)

The nurse collaborates with the patient to develop a medication schedule and teaches about the name, dosage, actions, adverse effects, and any drug–drug or drug–food interactions of the prescribed medications for heart failure, dysrhythmias, angina pectoris, or other symptoms. Particular precautions are emphasized, such as the risk to patients with aortic stenosis who experience angina pectoris and take nitroglycerin. The venous dilation that results from nitroglycerin decreases blood return to the heart, thus decreasing cardiac output and increasing the risk of syncope and decreased coronary artery blood flow. The nurse teaches the patient about the importance of attempting to relieve the symptoms of angina with rest and relaxation before taking nitroglycerin and to anticipate the potential adverse effects.

In addition, the nurse teaches the patient to weigh himself or herself daily and report gains of 2 pounds in 1 day or 5 pounds in 1 week to the health care provider. The nurse may assist the patient with planning activity and rest periods to achieve an acceptable lifestyle. The patient may need to be advised to rest and sleep sitting in a chair or bed with the head elevated when experiencing symptoms of pulmonary congestion. Care of patients treated with valvuloplasty or surgical valve replacement is described later in this chapter.

Valve Repair and Replacement Procedures

Valvuloplasty

The repair, rather than replacement, of a cardiac valve is referred to as **valvuloplasty**. In general, valves that undergo valvuloplasty function longer than prosthetic valve replacements, and patients do not require continuous anticoagulation. The type of valvuloplasty depends on the cause and type of valve dysfunction. Repair may be made to the commissures between the leaflets in a procedure known as **commissurotomy**, to the annulus of the valve by annuloplasty, to the leaflets, or to the chordae by chordoplasty. Transesophageal echocardiography (TEE) is usually performed at the conclusion of a valvuloplasty to evaluate the effectiveness of the procedure.

Most valvuloplasty procedures require general anesthesia and often require cardiopulmonary bypass. However, some procedures can be performed in the cardiac catheterization laboratory and do not always require general anesthesia or cardiopulmonary bypass. Percutaneous partial cardiopulmonary bypass is used in some cardiac catheterization laboratories. Cardiopulmonary bypass is achieved by inserting a large catheter (ie, cannula) into two peripheral blood vessels, usually a femoral vein and an artery. Blood is diverted from the body through the venous catheter to the cardiopulmonary bypass machine (see Chapter 28) and returned to the patient through the arterial catheter.

Commissurotomy

The most common valvuloplasty procedure is commissurotomy. Each valve has leaflets; the site where the leaflets meet is called the *commissure*. The leaflets may adhere to one another and close the commissure (ie, stenosis). Less commonly, the leaflets fuse in such a way that in addition to stenosis, the leaflets are also prevented from closing completely, resulting in a backward flow of blood (ie, regurgitation). A commissurotomy is the procedure performed to separate the fused leaflets.

Closed Commissurotomy

Closed commissurotomies do not require cardiopulmonary bypass. The valve is not directly visualized. The most common commissurotomy procedure is percutaneous balloon valvuloplasty. Some closed commissurotomies are performed using a surgical technique.

BALLOON VALVULOPLASTY

Balloon valvuloplasty (Fig. 29-3) is beneficial for mitral valve stenosis in younger patients, for aortic valve stenosis in elderly patients, and for patients with complex medical conditions that place them at high risk for the complications of more extensive surgical procedures. Most commonly used for mitral and aortic valve stenosis, balloon valvuloplasty also has been used for tricuspid and pulmonic valve stenosis. The procedure is contraindicated for patients with left atrial or ventricular thrombus, severe aortic root dilation, significant mitral valve regurgitation, thoracolumbar scoliosis, rotation of the great vessels, and other cardiac conditions that require open heart surgery.

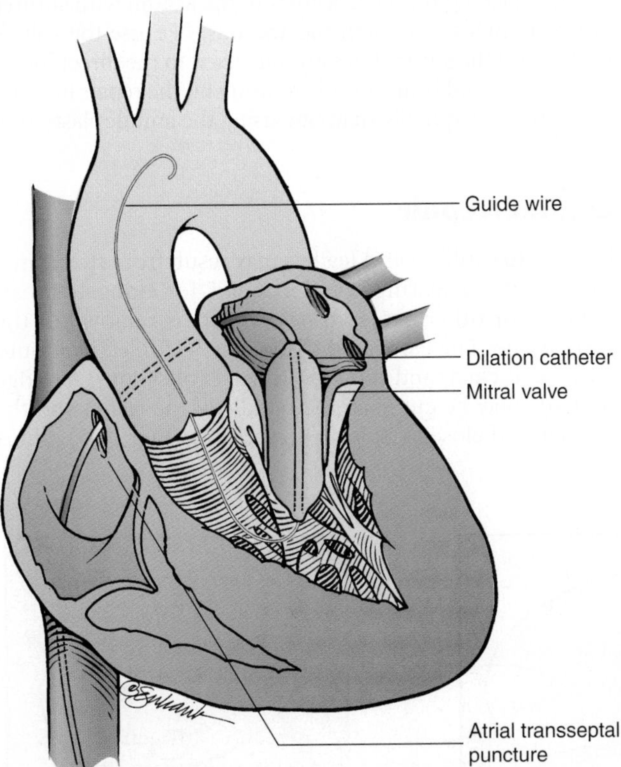

FIGURE 29-3. Balloon valvuloplasty: cross-section of heart illustrating the guide wire and dilation catheter placed through an atrial transseptal puncture and across the mitral valve. The guide wire is extended out from the aortic valve into the aorta for catheter support.

Balloon valvuloplasty is performed in the cardiac catheterization laboratory. The patient may receive light or moderate sedation or just a local anesthetic. Mitral balloon valvuloplasty involves advancing one or two catheters into the right atrium, through the atrial septum into the left atrium, across the mitral valve into the left ventricle, and out into the aorta. A guide wire is placed through each catheter, and the original catheter is removed. A large balloon catheter is then placed over the guide wire and positioned with the balloon across the mitral valve. The balloon is then inflated with a dilute angiographic solution. When two balloons are used, they are inflated simultaneously. The advantage of two balloons is that they are each smaller than the one large balloon often used, making smaller atrial septal defects. As the balloons are inflated, they usually do not completely occlude the mitral valve, thereby permitting some forward flow of blood during the inflation period. The balloons are usually inflated for 10 to 30 seconds. Multiple inflations are usually required to achieve the desired results.

All patients have some degree of mitral regurgitation after the procedure. Other possible complications include bleeding from the catheter insertion sites, emboli resulting in complications such as strokes, and rarely, left-to-right atrial shunts through an atrial septal defect caused by the procedure.

Aortic balloon valvuloplasty is performed most commonly by introducing a catheter through the aorta, across the aortic valve, and into the left ventricle, although it also may be performed by passing the balloon or balloons through the atrial septum. The one-balloon or the two-balloon technique can be used for treating aortic stenosis. Balloons are inflated for 15 to 60 seconds, and inflation is usually repeated multiple times. The aortic valve procedure is not as effective as the mitral valve procedure, and the rate of restenosis is 36% to 80% in the first 12 months after the procedure (Zipes et al., 2005). Possible complications include aortic regurgitation, emboli, ventricular perforation, rupture of the aortic valve annulus, ventricular dysrhythmia, mitral valve damage, and bleeding from the catheter insertion sites.

CLOSED SURGICAL VALVULOPLASTY

Closed surgical valvuloplasty has been performed for mitral, aortic, tricuspid, and pulmonary valve stenosis. The procedure is performed in the operating room with the patient under general anesthesia. A midsternal incision is made, a small hole is cut into the heart, and the surgeon's finger or a dilator is used to open the commissure.

Open Commissurotomy

Open commissurotomies are performed with direct visualization of the valve. The patient is under general anesthesia.

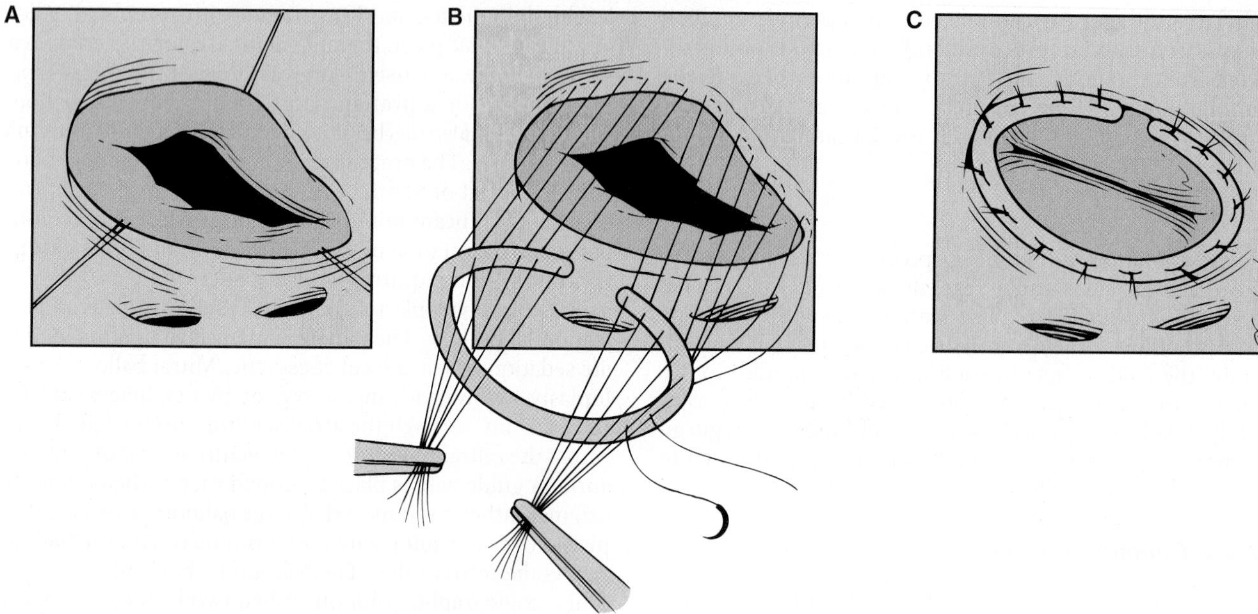

FIGURE 29-4. Annuloplasty ring insertion. (A) Mitral valve regurgitation; leaflets do not close. (B) Insertion of an annuloplasty ring. (C) Completed valvuloplasty; leaflets close.

A midsternal or left thoracic incision is made. Cardiopulmonary bypass is initiated, and an incision is made into the heart. The valve is exposed, and the surgeon uses a finger, scalpel, balloon, or dilator to open the commissures.

An added advantage of direct visualization of the valve is that thrombus and calcifications may be identified and removed. If the valve has chordae or papillary muscles, they may be inspected and surgically repaired as necessary (chordoplasty is discussed later in this chapter).

Annuloplasty

Annuloplasty is the repair of the valve annulus (ie, junction of the valve leaflets and the muscular heart wall). General anesthesia and cardiopulmonary bypass are required for all annuloplasties. The procedure narrows the diameter of the valve's orifice and is useful for the treatment of valvular regurgitation.

There are two annuloplasty techniques. One technique uses an annuloplasty ring (Fig. 29-4), which may be preshaped (rigid/semirigid) or flexible. The leaflets of the valve are sutured to a ring, creating an annulus of the desired size. When the ring is in place, the tension created by the moving blood and contracting heart is borne by the ring rather than by the valve or a suture line, and progressive regurgitation is prevented by the repair. The second technique involves tacking the valve leaflets to the atrium with sutures or taking tucks to tighten the annulus. Because the valve's leaflets and the suture lines are subjected to the direct forces of the blood and heart muscle movement, the repair may degenerate more quickly than one using the annuloplasty ring technique.

Leaflet Repair

Damage to cardiac valve leaflets may result from stretching, shortening, or tearing. **Leaflet repair** for elongated, ballooning, or other excess tissue leaflets is removal of the extra tissue. The elongated tissue may be folded over onto itself (ie, tucked) and sutured (ie, leaflet plication). A wedge of tissue may be cut from the middle of the leaflet and the gap sutured closed (ie, leaflet resection) (Fig. 29-5). Short

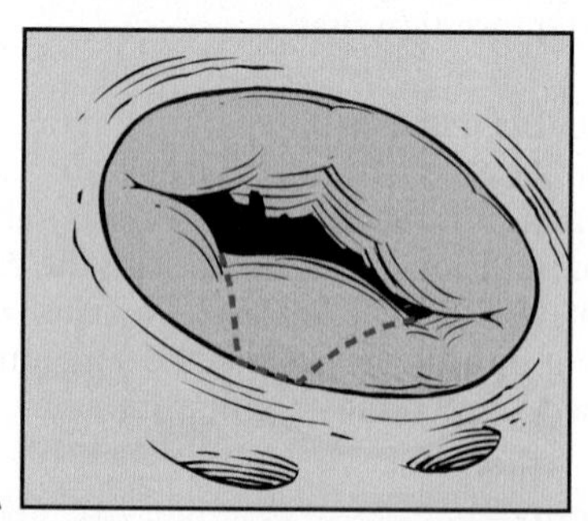

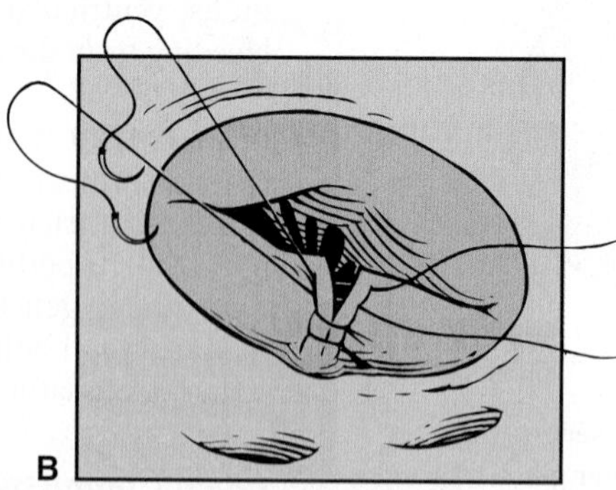

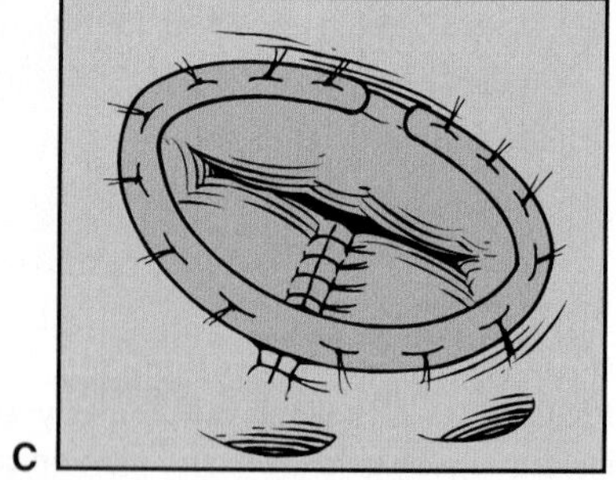

FIGURE 29-5. Valve leaflet resection and repair with a ring annuloplasty. (A) Mitral valve regurgitation; the section indicated by dashed lines is excised. (B) Approximation of edges and suturing. (C) Completed valvuloplasty, leaflet repair, and annuloplasty ring.

leaflets are most often repaired by chordoplasty. After the short chordae are released, the leaflets often unfurl and can resume their normal function (closing the valve during systole). A piece of pericardium may also be sutured to extend the leaflet. A pericardial or synthetic patch may be used to repair holes in the leaflets.

Chordoplasty

Chordoplasty is repair of the chordae tendineae. The mitral valve is involved with chordoplasty (because it has the chordae tendineae), and chordoplasty is seldom required for the tricuspid valve. Regurgitation may be caused by stretched, torn, or shortened chordae tendineae. Stretched chordae tendineae can be shortened, transposed to the other leaflet, or replaced with synthetic chordae. Torn chordae can be reattached to the leaflet and shortened chordae can be elongated. Regurgitation may also be caused by stretched papillary muscles, which can be shortened.

Valve Replacement

Prosthetic **valve replacement** began in the 1960s. When valvuloplasty or valve repair is not a viable alternative, such as when the annulus or leaflets of the valve are immobilized by calcifications, valve replacement is performed. General anesthesia and cardiopulmonary bypass are used for valve replacements. Most procedures are performed through a median sternotomy (ie, incision through the sternum), although the mitral valve may be approached through a right thoracotomy incision. Mitral, and more rarely aortic, valve replacements may be performed with minimally invasive techniques that do not involve cutting through the length of the sternum. Instead, incisions are made in only the upper or lower half of the sternum or between ribs; these incisions are only 2 to 4 inches long. Some of these minimally invasive procedures are robot-assisted; the surgical instruments are connected to a robot, and the surgeon, watching a video display, uses a joystick to control the robot and surgical instruments. With these procedures, patients have less bleeding, pain, risk for infection, and scarring. Hospital stays average 3 days, and recovery may be as short as 3 weeks (Aazami & Schafers, 2003; Fuster et al., 2004; Mitka, 2003).

After the valve is visualized, the leaflets of the aortic or pulmonic valve are removed, but some or all of the mitral valve structures (leaflets, chordae, and papillary muscles) are left in place to help maintain the shape and function of the left ventricle after mitral valve replacement. Sutures are placed around the annulus and then through the valve prosthesis. The replacement valve is slid down the suture into position and tied into place (Fig. 29-6). The incision is closed, and the surgeon evaluates the function of the heart and the quality of the prosthetic repair. The patient is weaned from cardiopulmonary bypass, the surgical repair is often assessed with color flow Doppler TEE, and surgery is completed.

Before surgery, the heart had gradually adjusted to the pathology, but the surgery abruptly "corrects" the way blood flows through the heart. Complications unique to

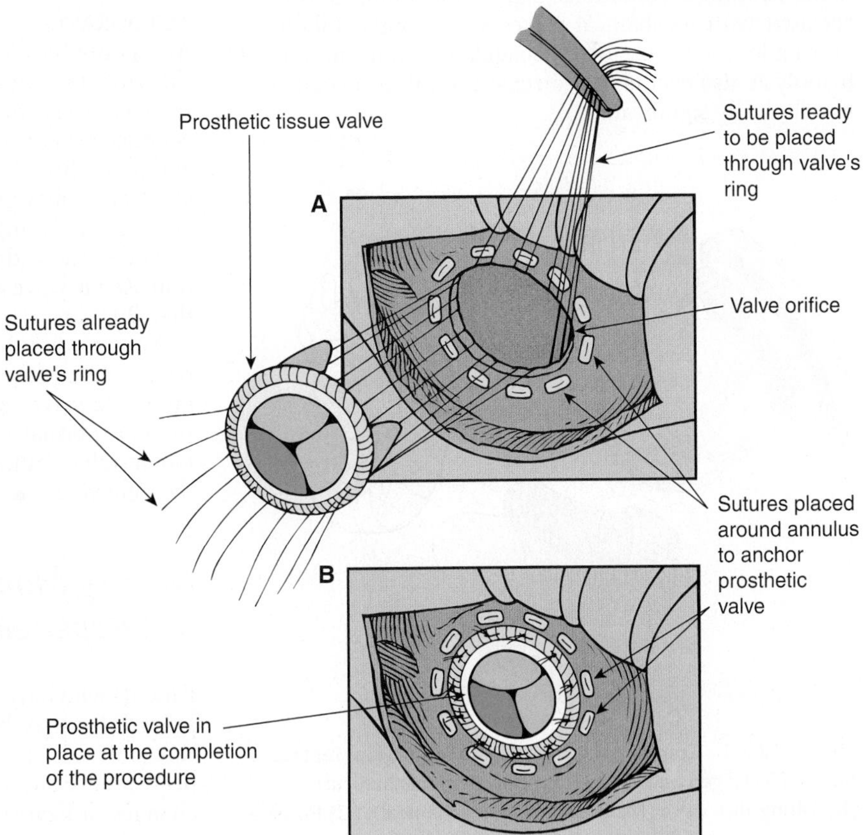

FIGURE 29-6. Valve replacement. **(A)** The native valve is trimmed, and the prosthetic valve is sutured in place. **(B)** Once all sutures are placed through the ring, the surgeon slides the prosthetic valve down the sutures and into the natural orifice. The sutures are then tied off and trimmed.

valve replacement are related to the sudden changes in intracardiac blood pressures. All prosthetic valve replacements create a degree of stenosis when they are implanted in the heart. Usually, the stenosis is mild and does not affect heart function. If valve replacement was for a stenotic valve, blood flow through the heart is often improved. The signs and symptoms of the backward heart failure resolve in a few hours or days. If valve replacement was for a regurgitant valve, it may take months for the chamber into which blood had been regurgitating to achieve its optimal postoperative function. The signs and symptoms of heart failure resolve gradually as the heart function improves. Patients are at risk for many postoperative complications, such as bleeding, thromboembolism, infection, congestive heart failure, hypertension, dysrhythmias, hemolysis, and mechanical obstruction of the valve.

Types of Valve Prostheses

Two types of valve prostheses may be used: mechanical and tissue (ie, biologic) valves (Fig. 29-7).

Mechanical Valves

Mechanical valves are of the ball-and-cage or disk design and are thought to be more durable than tissue prosthetic valves; therefore, they are often used for younger patients. Mechanical valves are used for patients with renal failure, hypercalcemia, endocarditis, or sepsis who require valve replacement. The mechanical valves do not deteriorate or become infected as easily as the tissue valves used for patients with these conditions. Significant complications associated with mechanical valves are thromboemboli requiring long-term use of anticoagulants. Some amount of hemolysis also occurs with mechanical valves; usually it is not clinically significant.

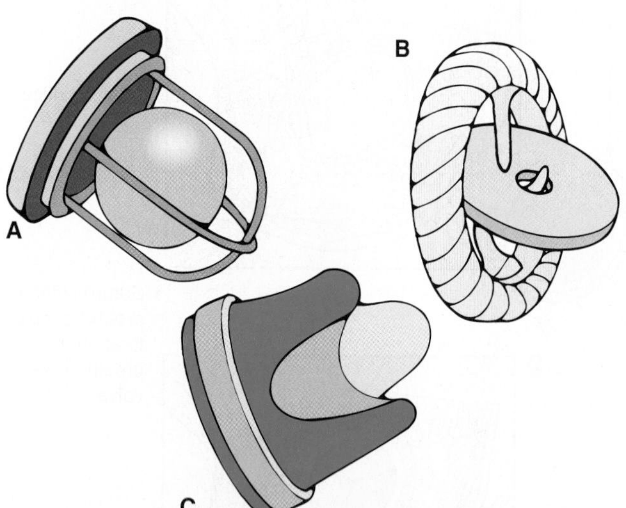

FIGURE 29-7. Common mechanical and tissue valve replacements. (**A**) Caged ball valve (Starr-Edwards, mechanical). (**B**) Tilting-disk valve (Medtronic-Hall, mechanical). (**C**) Porcine heterograft valve (Carpenter-Edwards, tissue).

Tissue (Biologic) Valves

Tissue (ie, biologic) valves are of three types: xenografts, homografts, and autografts. Tissue valves are less likely to generate thromboemboli, and long-term anticoagulation is not required. Tissue valves are not as durable as mechanical valves and require replacement more frequently.

XENOGRAFTS

Xenografts are tissue valves (eg, bioprostheses, **heterografts**) that are used for all tricuspid valve replacements. They are used for women of childbearing age because the potential complications of long-term anticoagulation associated with menses, placental transfer to a fetus, and delivery of a child do not exist. They also are used for patients older than 70 years of age, patients with a history of peptic ulcer disease, and others who cannot tolerate long-term anticoagulation. Most xenografts are from pigs (porcine), but valves from cows (bovine) may also be used. Viability is 7 to 10 years. Xenografts do not generate thrombi, thereby eliminating the need for long-term anticoagulation.

HOMOGRAFTS

Homografts, or **allografts** (ie, human valves), are obtained from cadaver tissue donations and are used for aortic and pulmonic valve replacement. The aortic valve and a portion of the aorta or the pulmonic valve and a portion of the pulmonary artery are harvested and stored cryogenically. Homografts are not always available and are very expensive. They last for about 10 to 15 years, somewhat longer than xenografts. They are not thrombogenic and are resistant to subacute bacterial endocarditis.

AUTOGRAFTS

Autografts (ie, autologous valves) are obtained by excising the patient's own pulmonic valve and a portion of the pulmonary artery for use as the aortic valve. Anticoagulation is unnecessary because the valve is the patient's own tissue and is not thrombogenic. The autograft is an alternative for children (it may grow as the child grows), women of childbearing age, young adults, patients with a history of peptic ulcer disease, and people who cannot tolerate anticoagulation. Aortic valve autografts have remained viable for more than 20 years.

Most aortic valve autograft procedures are double valve-replacement procedures; a homograft also is performed for pulmonic valve replacement. If pulmonary vascular pressures are normal, some surgeons elect not to replace the pulmonic valve. Patients can recover without a valve between the right ventricle and the pulmonary artery.

Nursing Management: Valvuloplasty and Replacement

Patients who have had percutaneous balloon valvuloplasty procedures may be admitted to a telemetry or intensive care unit. The nurse assesses for signs and symptoms of heart failure and emboli (see Chapter 30), listens for any changes in heart sounds at least every 4 hours, and provides the patient with the same care as for postprocedure cardiac catheterization or percutaneous transluminal coronary angioplasty (PTCA) (see Chapter 28). After undergoing percutaneous balloon valvuloplasty, the patient usually remains in the hospital for 24 to 48 hours.

Patients who have had surgical valvuloplasty or valve replacements are admitted to the intensive care unit. Care focuses on recovery from anesthesia and hemodynamic stability. Vital signs are assessed every 5 to 15 minutes and as needed until the patient recovers from anesthesia or sedation, and then are assessed every 2 to 4 hours and as needed. Intravenous (IV) medications to increase or decrease blood pressure and to treat dysrhythmias or altered heart rates are administered and their effects monitored. The medications are gradually decreased until they are no longer required or the patient can take the needed medication by another route (eg, oral, topical). Patient assessments are conducted every 1 to 4 hours and as needed, with particular attention to neurologic, respiratory, and cardiovascular systems. (See Chapter 28, Chart 28-13, which presents a plan of nursing care for a patient recovering from cardiac surgery.)

After the patient has recovered from anesthesia and sedation, is hemodynamically stable without IV medications, and has stable physical assessment parameters, he or she is usually transferred to a telemetry unit, typically within 24 to 72 hours of surgery. Nursing care continues as for most postoperative patients, including wound care and patient teaching regarding diet, activity, medications, and self-care.

The nurse educates the patient about long-term anticoagulant therapy, explaining the need for frequent follow-up appointments and blood laboratory studies. Patients who take warfarin (Coumadin) usually have individualized target International Normalized Ratios (INRs) between 2 and 3.5. Patients who have been treated with an annuloplasty ring or a tissue valve replacement usually require anticoagulation for only 3 months, unless there are other risk factors such as atrial fibrillation or a history of thromboembolism. Aspirin may be prescribed with warfarin for some patients. The nurse provides teaching about all prescribed medications: the name of the medication, dosage, its actions, prescribed schedule, potential adverse effects, and any drug–drug or drug–food interactions. Patients with a mechanical valve prosthesis (including annuloplasty rings and other prosthetic materials used in valvuloplasty) or a history of rheumatic heart disease require education to prevent infective endocarditis with antibiotic prophylaxis, which is prescribed before all dental and surgical procedures.

The patient is usually discharged from the hospital in 3 to 7 days. Home care and office or clinic nurses reinforce all new information and self-care instructions with patients and families for 4 to 8 weeks after the procedure. Doppler echocardiograms are usually performed 3 to 4 weeks after discharge from the hospital to further evaluate the effects and results of the surgery. The echocardiogram also provides a baseline for future comparison should cardiac symptoms or complications develop. Doppler echocardiograms are usually repeated every 1 to 2 years.

Septal Repair

The atrial or ventricular septum may have an abnormal opening between the right and left sides of the heart (ie, septal defect). Although most septal defects are congenital and are repaired during infancy or childhood, adults may not have undergone early repair or may develop septal defects as a result of myocardial infarctions or diagnostic and treatment procedures.

Repair of septal defects requires general anesthesia and cardiopulmonary bypass. The heart is opened, and a pericardial or synthetic (usually polyester or Dacron) patch is used to close the opening. Atrial septal defect repairs have low morbidity and mortality rates. When the mitral or tricuspid valve is involved, however, the procedure is more complicated because valve repair or replacement may be required and the heart failure may be more severe. Generally, ventricular septal defect repairs are uncomplicated, but close proximity of the defect to the intraventricular conduction system and the valves may make this repair more complex. (See Chapter 28, Chart 28-13, which presents a plan of nursing care for a patient recovering from cardiac surgery.) Patients should be taught the importance of infective endocarditis antibiotic prophylaxis for 6 months after the repair. If minimal or no hemodynamic abnormality is evident by Doppler echocardiography after 6 months, antibiotic prophylaxis may be discontinued.

Cardiomyopathy

Cardiomyopathy is a heart muscle disease associated with cardiac dysfunction. It is classified according to the structural and functional abnormalities of the heart muscle: dilated cardiomyopathy (DCM), hypertrophic cardiomyopathy (HCM), restrictive or constrictive cardiomyopathy (RCM), arrhythmogenic right ventricular cardiomyopathy (ARVC), and unclassified cardiomyopathy (Richardson, McKenna, Bristow, et al., 1996). The patient may have pathology representing more than one of these classifications, such as a patient with HCM developing dilation and symptoms of DCM. *Ischemic cardiomyopathy* is a term frequently used to describe an enlarged heart caused by coronary artery disease, which is usually accompanied by heart failure (see Chapter 30).

Regardless of type and cause, cardiomyopathy may lead to severe heart failure, lethal dysrhythmias, and death. The mortality rate is highest for African Americans and the elderly.

Pathophysiology

The pathophysiology of all cardiomyopathies is a series of events that culminate in impaired cardiac output. Decreased stroke volume stimulates the sympathetic nervous system and the renin–angiotensin–aldosterone response, resulting in increased systemic vascular resistance and increased sodium and fluid retention, which places an increased workload on the heart. These alterations can lead to heart failure (see Chapter 30).

Dilated Cardiomyopathy (DCM)

DCM is the most common form of cardiomyopathy, with an incidence of 5 to 8 cases per 100,000 people per year and increasing. DCM occurs more often in men and African

Americans, who also have higher mortality rates (Zipes et al., 2005). DCM is distinguished by significant dilation of the ventricles without simultaneous hypertrophy (ie, increased muscle wall thickness) and systolic dysfunction (Fig. 29-8). The ventricles have elevated systolic and diastolic volumes but a decreased ejection fraction (EF). DCM was formerly named *congestive cardiomyopathy,* but it may exist without signs and symptoms of congestion.

More than 75 conditions and diseases may cause DCM, including pregnancy, heavy alcohol intake, viral infection (eg, influenza), and Chagas disease. When the causative factor cannot be identified, the diagnosis is *idiopathic DCM*. Idiopathic DCM accounts for approximately 25% of all heart failure cases. Because genetic factors may be involved, echocardiography and ECG should be used to screen all first-degree blood relatives (eg, parents, siblings, children) for DCM (Zipes et al., 2005).

Microscopic examination of the muscle tissue shows diminished contractile elements (actin and myosin filaments) of the muscle fibers and diffuse necrosis of myocardial cells. The result is poor systolic function. The structural changes decrease the amount of blood ejected from the ventricle with systole, increasing the amount of blood remaining in the ventricle after contraction. Less blood is then able to enter the ventricle during diastole, increasing end-diastolic pressure and eventually increasing pulmonary and systemic venous pressures. Altered valve function, usually regurgitation, can result from an enlarged stretched ventricle. Poor blood flow through the ventricle may also cause ventricular or atrial thrombi, which may embolize to other locations in the body. Early diagnosis and treatment can prevent or delay significant symptoms and sudden death from DCM.

Hypertrophic Cardiomyopathy (HCM)

HCM is a rare autosomal dominant condition, occurring in men, women, and children (often detected after puberty) with an estimated prevalence rate of 0.05% to 0.2% (Berul & Zevitz, 2002). Echocardiograms may be performed every year from 12 to 18 years of age and then every 5 years from 18 to 70 years of age. HCM also may be idiopathic (ie, no known cause).

In HCM, the heart muscle asymmetrically increases in size and mass, especially along the septum (see Fig. 29-8). HCM often affects nonadjacent areas of the ventricle. The increased thickness of the heart muscle reduces the size of the ventricular cavities and causes the ventricles to take a longer time to relax after systole. During the first part of diastole it is more difficult for the ventricles to fill with blood. The atrial contraction at the end of diastole becomes critical for ventricular filling and systolic contraction.

HCM may be nonobstructive or obstructive. If the increased septal size causes misalignment of the papillary muscles of the left ventricle, the septum and mitral valve can obstruct the flow of blood from the left ventricle into the aorta during ventricular contraction. Because of the structural changes, HCM had also been called idiopathic hypertrophic subaortic stenosis (IHSS) and asymmetric septal hypertrophy (ASH). The structural changes that result in the smaller-than-normal ventricular cavity also create a higher-velocity flow of blood out of the left ventricle into the aorta. HCM may cause significant diastolic dysfunction, but systolic function is usually normal or high, resulting in a higher-than-normal ejection fraction. Doppler echocardiography is used to detect the HCM and blood flow alterations (Zipes et al., 2005).

Cardiac muscle cells normally lie parallel to and end-to-end with each other. The hypertrophied cardiac muscle cells are oblique and perpendicular to each other, decreasing the effectiveness of contractions and possibly increasing the risk for dysrhythmias such as ventricular tachycardia and ventricular fibrillation. In HCM the coronary arteriole walls are thickened, which decreases the internal diameter of the arterioles. The narrow arterioles restrict the blood supply to the myocardium, causing numerous small areas of ischemia and necrosis. The necrotic areas of the myocardium ultimately fibrose and scar, further impeding ventricular contraction.

Restrictive Cardiomyopathy

RCM is characterized by diastolic dysfunction caused by rigid ventricular walls that impair diastolic filling and ventricular stretch (see Fig. 29-8). Systolic function is usually normal. Because RCM is the least common cardiomyopathy, representing approximately 5% of cases of pediatric

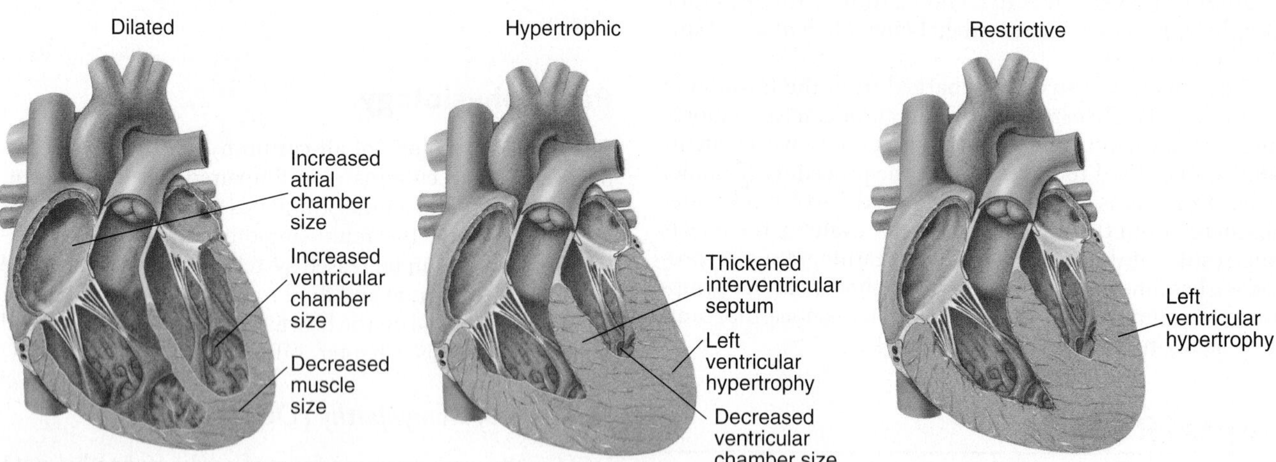

FIGURE 29-8. Cardiomyopathies that lead to congestive heart failure. From Anatomical Chart Company (2006). *Atlas of pathophysiology* (2nd ed.). Ambler, PA: Lippincott Williams & Wilkins.

cardiomyopathies, its pathogenesis is the least understood (Shaddy, 2004). RCM may be associated with amyloidosis (amyloid, a protein substance, is deposited within cells) and other such infiltrative diseases. However, the cause is unknown (ie, idiopathic) in most cases. Signs and symptoms are similar to constrictive pericarditis: dyspnea, nonproductive cough, and chest pain. Echocardiography is used to differentiate the two conditions. In addition, patients with RCM usually have pulmonary artery systolic (PAS) pressures of at least 50 mm Hg and pulmonary artery wedge pressures (PAWPs) at least 5 mm Hg greater than central venous pressures (CVPs), and computed tomography (CT) or MRI scans usually show normal thickness of the pericardium. Patients with constrictive pericarditis usually have PAS pressures less than 50 mm Hg and PAWP and CVP within 5 mm Hg of each other, and CT or MRI scans show thickening of the pericardium.

Arrhythmogenic Right Ventricular Cardiomyopathy

ARVC occurs when the myocardium of the right ventricle is progressively infiltrated and replaced by fibrous scar and adipose tissue. Initially, only localized areas of the right ventricle are affected, but as the disease progresses, the entire heart is affected. Eventually, the right ventricle dilates and develops poor contractility, right ventricular wall abnormalities, and dysrhythmias. The prevalence of ARVC is unknown because many cases are not recognized. Palpitations or syncope may develop between 15 and 40 years of age. ARVC should be suspected in patients with ventricular tachycardia originating in the right ventricle (ie, a left bundle branch block configuration on ECG) or sudden death, especially among previously symptom-free athletes (McRae, Chung, Asher et al., 2001). ARVC may be genetic (ie, autosomal dominant) (Richardson et al., 1996). First-degree blood relatives (eg, parents, siblings, children) should be screened for the disease with a 12-lead ECG, Holter monitor, and echocardiography.

Unclassified Cardiomyopathies

Unclassified cardiomyopathies are different from or have characteristics of more than one of the previously described types. Examples of unclassified cardiomyopathies include fibroelastosis, noncompacted myocardium, systolic dysfunction with minimal dilation, and mitochondrial involvement (Richardson et al., 1996).

Clinical Manifestations

Patients with cardiomyopathy may remain stable and without symptoms for many years. As the disease progresses, so do symptoms. Frequently, dilated or restrictive cardiomyopathy is first diagnosed when the patient presents with signs and symptoms of heart failure (eg, dyspnea on exertion, fatigue). Patients with cardiomyopathy may also report PND, cough (especially with exertion), and orthopnea, which may lead to a misdiagnosis of bronchitis or pneumonia. Other symptoms include fluid retention, peripheral edema, and nausea, which is caused by poor perfusion of the gastrointestinal system. The patient also may experience chest pain, palpitations, dizziness, nausea, and syncope with exertion. However, with HCM, cardiac arrest (ie, sudden cardiac death) may be the initial manifestation in young people, including athletes (Maron, McKenna, Danielson, et al., 2003).

Assessment and Diagnostic Findings

Physical examination in the early stage may reveal tachycardia and extra heart sounds (eg, S_3, S_4). Patients with DCM may have diastolic murmurs, and patients with DCM and HCM may have systolic murmurs. With disease progression, examination also reveals signs and symptoms of heart failure (eg, crackles on pulmonary auscultation, jugular vein distention, pitting edema of dependent body parts, enlarged liver).

Diagnosis is usually made from findings disclosed by the patient history and by ruling out other causes of heart failure such as myocardial infarction. The echocardiogram is one of the most helpful diagnostic tools because the structure and function of the ventricles can be observed easily. ECG demonstrates dysrhythmias (atrial fibrillation, ventricular dysrhythmias) and changes consistent with left ventricular hypertrophy (left axis deviation, wide QRS, ST changes, inverted T waves). In ARVC, there often is a small deflection, an epsilon wave, at the end of the QRS. The chest x-ray reveals heart enlargement and possibly pulmonary congestion. Cardiac catheterization is sometimes used to rule out coronary artery disease as a causative factor. Endomyocardial biopsy may be performed to analyze myocardial tissue cells.

Medical Management

Medical management is directed toward determining and managing possible underlying or precipitating causes; correcting the heart failure with medications, a low-sodium diet, and an exercise/rest regimen (see Chapter 30); and controlling dysrhythmias with antiarrhythmic medications and possibly with an implanted electronic device, such as an implantable cardioverter defibrillator (see Chapter 27). Infective endocarditis prophylaxis and systemic anticoagulation to prevent thromboembolic events are usually recommended. If the patient has signs and symptoms of congestion, fluid intake may be limited to 2 liters each day. Patients with HCM should avoid dehydration and may need beta-blockers [atenolol (Tenormin), metoprolol (Lopressor), nadolol (Corgard), propranolol (Inderal)] to maintain cardiac output and minimize the risk of left ventricular outflow tract obstruction during systole. Patients with HCM or RCM may need to limit physical activity to avoid a life-threatening dysrhythmia.

A pacemaker may be implanted to alter the electrical stimulation of the muscle and prevent the forceful hyperdynamic contractions that occur with HCM. Atrial-ventricular and biventricular pacing have been used to decrease symptoms and obstruction of the left ventricular outflow tract. For some patients with DCM and HCM, biventricular pacing increases the ejection fraction and reverses some of the structural changes in the myocardium.

Nonsurgical septal reduction therapy, also called alcohol septal ablation, has been used to treat obstructive HCM. In the cardiac catheterization laboratory, a percutaneous catheter is positioned in one or more of the septal coronary arteries. Once the position is verified, 2 to 5 mL of ethanol (ethyl alcohol) is injected at a rate of about 1 mL/minute to kill the myocardial cells; it is believed that the ethanol causes dehydration of the cardiac cells (Cruickshank, 2004; Maron, 2002). The slow rate of injection minimizes the risk of heart block and premature ventricular contractions (PVCs). The procedure produces a septal myocardial infarction. The resulting scar is thinner than the living myocardium would have been, so the obstruction is decreased. The patient may develop a left anterior hemibranch block or left bundle branch block. If the patient experiences pain, hydrocodone/acetaminophen (Vicodin) is usually administered. Nitrates and morphine are not used, because coronary artery dilation is contraindicated.

Surgical Management

When heart failure progresses and medical treatment is no longer effective, surgical intervention, including heart transplantation, is considered. However, because of the limited number of organ donors, many patients die waiting for transplantation. In some cases, a left ventricular assist device is implanted to support the failing heart until a suitable donor heart becomes available (mechanical assist devices and total artificial hearts are discussed later in this chapter).

LEFT VENTRICULAR OUTFLOW TRACT SURGERY

When patients with HCM become symptomatic despite medical therapy and a difference in pressure of 50 mm Hg or more exists between the left ventricle and the aorta, surgery is considered. The most common procedure is a myectomy (sometimes referred to as a myotomy-myectomy), in which some of the heart tissue is excised. Septal tissue approximately 1 cm wide and deep is cut from the enlarged septum below the aortic valve. The length of septum removed depends on the degree of obstruction caused by the hypertrophied muscle.

Instead of a septal myectomy, the surgeon may open the left ventricular outflow tract to the aortic valve by mitral valvuloplasty involving the leaflets, chordae, or papillary muscles, or the patient's mitral valve may be replaced with a low-profile disk valve. The space taken up by the mitral valve is substantially reduced by the valvuloplasty or prosthetic valve, allowing blood to move around the enlarged septum to the aortic valve through the area the mitral valve once occupied. The primary complication of all the procedures is dysrhythmias. Additional complications include postoperative surgical complications such as pain, ineffective airway clearance, deep vein thrombosis, risk for infection, and delayed surgical recovery.

LATISSIMUS DORSI MUSCLE WRAP

DCM may be treated with a latissimus dorsi muscle wrap, also called dynamic cardiomyoplasty (Rigatelli, Barbiero, Cotogni, et al., 2003; Woods et al., 2005; Zipes et al., 2005). The left latissimus dorsi muscle is dissected from the lateral side and back of the chest, leaving the medial end of the muscle and the blood supply intact, and the lateral end of the muscle is pulled through the pleural space into the pericardium. The latissimus dorsi muscle flap is then wrapped around the ventricles and sutured in place. Pacemaker leads are implanted into the muscle flap, and a pacemaker generator is implanted in the chest wall. For at least 2 weeks following surgery, the pacemaker remains turned off to facilitate the development of adhesions between the muscle wrap and the ventricles. Eventually, the pacemaker is turned on and used to stimulate latissimus dorsi muscle contraction. Several weeks of training, or conditioning, are necessary before this skeletal muscle functions effectively. The ultimate goal is for the latissimus dorsi muscle wrap to augment ventricular contraction and increase cardiac output. This skeletal muscle loses its contractility over time, and the patient may be evaluated for heart transplantation.

HEART TRANSPLANTATION

The first human-to-human heart transplant was performed in 1967. Since then, transplant procedures, equipment, and medications have continued to improve. In 1983, when cyclosporine became available, heart transplantation became a therapeutic option for patients with end-stage heart disease. Cyclosporine (Neoral, Sandimmune, SangCya) is an immunosuppressant that greatly decreases the body's rejection of foreign proteins, such as transplanted organs. Unfortunately, cyclosporine also decreases the body's ability to resist infections, and a satisfactory balance must be achieved between suppressing rejection and avoiding infection.

Cardiomyopathy, ischemic heart disease, valvular disease, rejection of previously transplanted hearts, and congenital heart disease are the most common indications for transplantation (Taylor, Edwards, Mohacsi, et al., 2003; Woods et al., 2005). Typical candidates have severe symptoms uncontrolled by medical therapy, no other surgical options, and a prognosis of less than 12 months to live. A multidisciplinary team screens the candidate before recommending the transplantation procedure. The person's age, pulmonary status, other chronic health conditions, psychosocial status, family support, infections, history of other transplantations, compliance, and current health status are considered.

When a donor heart becomes available, a computer generates a list of potential recipients on the basis of ABO blood group compatibility, the body sizes of the donor and the potential recipient, and the geographic locations of the donor and potential recipient. Distance is a factor, because postoperative function depends on the heart being implanted within 6 hours of harvest from the donor. Some patients are candidates for more than one organ transplant: (eg, heart–lung, heart–pancreas, heart–kidney, heart–liver).

Orthotopic Transplantation. Orthotopic transplantation is the most common surgical procedure for cardiac transplantation (Fig. 29-9). The recipient's heart is removed, and the donor heart is implanted at the vena cava and pulmonary veins. Some surgeons prefer to remove the recipient's heart leaving a portion of the recipient's atria (with the vena cava and pulmonary veins) in place. The donor heart, which usually has been preserved in ice, is prepared for implant by cutting away a small section of the atria that corresponds with the sections of the recipient's heart that were left in place. The donor heart is implanted by suturing the donor atria to the residual atrial tissue of the recipient's heart. After the venous or atrial anastomoses are complete, the recipient's pulmonary artery and aorta are sutured to those of the donor heart.

Postoperative Course. Patients who have had heart transplants are constantly balancing the risk of rejection with the risk of infection. They must adhere to a complex regimen of diet, medications, activity, follow-up laboratory studies, biopsies of the transplanted heart (to diagnose rejection),

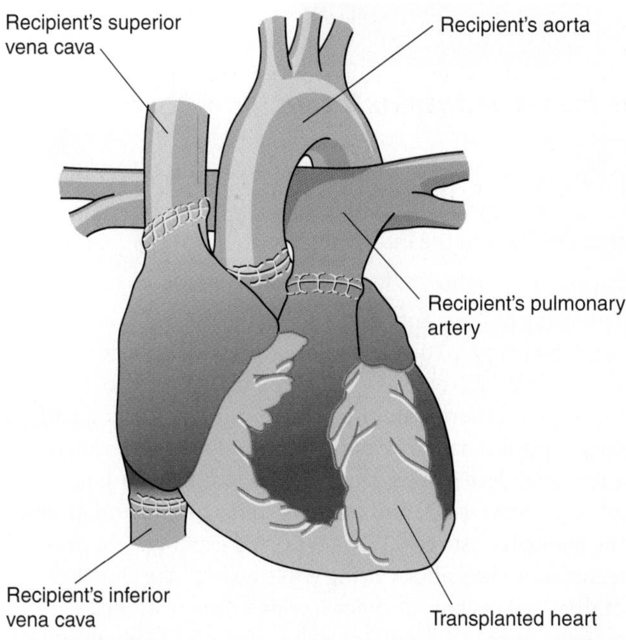

FIGURE 29-9. Orthotopic method of heart transplantation.

and clinic visits. Most commonly, patients receive cyclosporine or tacrolimus (Prograf), azathioprine (Imuran) or mycophenolate mofetil (CellCept), and corticosteroids (ie, prednisone) to minimize rejection.

The transplanted heart has no nerve connections to the recipient's body (ie, denervated heart), and the sympathetic and vagus nerves do not affect the transplanted heart. The resting rate of the transplanted heart is approximately 70 to 90 beats per minute, but it increases gradually if catecholamines are in the circulation. Patients must gradually increase and decrease their exercise (ie, extended warm-up and cool-down periods), because 20 to 30 minutes may be required to achieve the desired heart rate. Atropine does not increase the heart rate of transplanted hearts.

In addition to rejection and infection, complications may include accelerated atherosclerosis of the coronary arteries (ie, cardiac allograft vasculopathy or accelerated graft atherosclerosis). Both immunologic and nonimmunologic factors cause arterial injury and inflammation of the coronary arteries, which contribute to the accelerated atherosclerosis along the entire length of the coronary arteries (Deng, 2002; Woods et al., 2005). Hypertension may occur in patients taking cyclosporine or tacrolimus; the cause has not been identified. Osteoporosis frequently occurs as a side effect of the antirejection medications and pretransplantation dietary insufficiency and medications as well as the long-term sedentary lifestyle. Posttransplantation lymphoproliferative disease and cancer of the skin and lips are the most common malignancies after transplantation, possibly caused by immunosuppression. Weight gain; obesity; diabetes; dyslipidemias (eg, hypercholesterolemia); hypotension; renal failure; and central nervous system, respiratory, and gastrointestinal disturbances may be adverse effects of the corticosteroids or other immunosuppressants. Toxicity from immunosuppressant medications may occur. The 1-year survival rate for patients with transplanted hearts is approximately 80% to 90%, and the 5-year survival rate is approximately 60% to 70% (Deng, 2002; Fuster et al., 2004; Zipes, et al., 2005).

Patients respond to the psychosocial stresses imposed by organ transplantation in various ways. They may experience guilt that someone had to die for them to be able to live, have anxiety about the new heart, experience depression or fear about rejection, or have difficulty with family role changes before and after transplantation (Evangelista, Doering, & Dracup et al., 2003; Fuster et al., 2004; Woods et al., 2004).

MECHANICAL ASSIST DEVICES AND TOTAL ARTIFICIAL HEARTS

The use of cardiopulmonary bypass for cardiovascular surgery and the possibility of performing heart transplantation for end-stage cardiac disease have increased the need for mechanical assist devices. Patients who cannot be weaned from cardiopulmonary bypass and patients in cardiogenic shock may benefit from a period of mechanical heart assistance. The most commonly used device is the intra-aortic balloon pump (see Chapter 30). This pump decreases the work of the heart during contraction but does not perform the actual work of the heart.

Ventricular Assist Devices. More complex devices that actually perform some or all of the pumping function for the heart also are being used. These more sophisticated **ventricular assist devices** (VADs) can circulate as much blood per minute as the heart, if not more (Fig. 29-10). Each VAD is used to support one ventricle. Some VADs can be combined with an oxygenator; the combination is called extracorporeal membrane oxygenation (ECMO). The oxygenator–VAD combination is used for the patient whose heart cannot pump adequate blood through the lungs or the body.

There are two basic types of VADs: pneumatic and electric or electromagnetic. Pneumatic VADs are external or implanted pulsatile devices with a flexible reservoir housed in a rigid exterior. The reservoir usually fills with blood drained from the patient's atrium or ventricle. The device then forces pressurized air into the rigid housing, compressing the reservoir and returning the blood to the patient's circulation, usually into the aorta. Electric or electromagnetic VADs are similar to the pneumatic VADs, but instead of using pressurized air to return the blood to the patient's circulation, one or more flat metal plates are pushed against the reservoir.

Total Artificial Hearts. Total artificial hearts are designed to replace both ventricles. Some require the removal of the patient's heart to implant the total artificial heart, and others do not. All of these devices are experimental. Although there has been some short-term success, the long-term results have been disappointing. Researchers hope to develop a device that can be permanently implanted and that will eliminate the need for donated human heart transplantation for end-stage cardiac disease (Fuster et al., 2004; Kherani & Oz, 2004; Zipes et al., 2005).

Most VADs and total artificial hearts are temporary treatments while the patient's own heart recovers or until a donor heart becomes available for transplantation (ie, "bridge to transplant"). Some devices are being investigated for permanent use. Complications of VADs and total artificial hearts include bleeding disorders, hemorrhage, thrombus, emboli, hemolysis, infection, renal failure, right-sided heart failure, multisystem failure, and mechanical failure (Zipes et al., 2005). Nursing care for these patients focuses on assessing for and minimizing these complications and providing emotional support and education about the mechanical assist device and about the underlying cardiac disease.

NURSING RESEARCH PROFILE

Perspectives of Women After Heart Transplantation

Evangelista, L. S., Doering, L., & Dracup, K. (2003). Meaning and life purpose: The perspectives of post-transplant women. *Heart & Lung, 32*(4), 250–257.

Purpose

Studies have shown that psychological distress is experienced following heart transplant surgery. However, few studies have explored how heart transplant recipients have perceived their transplant experiences and how their lives have been affected by the transplant. The majority of studies that have been conducted have been limited to male subjects. The purpose of this descriptive, exploratory study was to examine women's perceptions and psychosocial responses to the experiences of end-stage heart failure and heart transplant surgery.

Design

Participants were women who had had a heart transplant. Thirty-three participants, who had a mean age of 62.3 years and who were a mean of 4.6 years since heart transplant, were recruited from an outpatient posttransplant clinic to complete two standardized questionnaires (Life Attitudes Profile; Multiple Affect Adjective Checklist) and participate in a semistructured interview with a researcher. The data collection took place in the participants' homes. The Life Attitudes Profile was used to measure the participants' perceptions of their life's meaning, goals, anxiety, fulfillment, and satisfaction with life. The Multiple Affect Adjective Checklist was used to measure participants' mood states of anxiety, depression, and hostility. During the interviews the participants were asked to describe their perceptions about their illness and health condition and how their lives had been affected by their health experiences, including their heart transplant surgery. Analysis of the data included correlations between life's meaning, life purpose, and psychological mood states. Content analysis was used to identify common themes that emerged in the interviews.

Findings

The study participants had an average meaning score of 30.64 (range, 10–43) and an average life purpose score of 40.12 (range, 17–63)—the higher the scores, the higher or better are the perceptions of meaning and life purpose. The participants reported that they experienced high levels of psychological distress, including anxiety, depression, and hostility, both before and after the transplant surgery. They reported experiencing pretransplant fears about dying while asleep, the shortage of donated organs, and not having enough strength to manage their conditions, and they reported experiencing posttransplant fears about physiologic rejection of the new heart and about the continuing possibility of dying. These data validated the results of previous studies.

The participants reported that they had experienced feelings of lack of control over their health and lives, and this lack of control caused some participants to become depressed or angry. The women's perceptions of lack of control were important findings among heart transplant patients. The majority of the women had positive attitudes about their transplant surgery.

Nursing Implications

Nurses need to provide psychological support and counseling to women before and after heart transplant surgery. The counseling should address individual concerns, promote positive meaning in life, and encourage optimistic behaviors. Discussions about life's meaning and purpose may decrease a woman's psychological distress. Women need to be assisted to identify their fears and develop strategies to retain a sense of control.

Nursing Process

The Patient with Cardiomyopathy

Assessment

Nursing assessment for the patient with cardiomyopathy begins with a detailed history of the presenting signs and symptoms. The nurse identifies possible etiologic factors, such as heavy alcohol intake, recent illness or pregnancy, or history of the disease in immediate family members. If the patient reports chest pain, a thorough review of the pain, including its precipitating factors, is warranted. The review of systems includes the presence of orthopnea, PND, and syncope or dyspnea with exertion. The number of pillows needed to sleep, usual weight, any weight change, and limitations on activities of daily living are assessed. The New York Heart Association Classification for heart failure is determined. The patient's usual diet is evaluated to determine whether alterations are needed to reduce sodium intake.

Because of the chronicity of cardiomyopathy, the nurse conducts a careful psychosocial history, exploring the impact of the disease on the patient's role within the family and community. Identification of per-

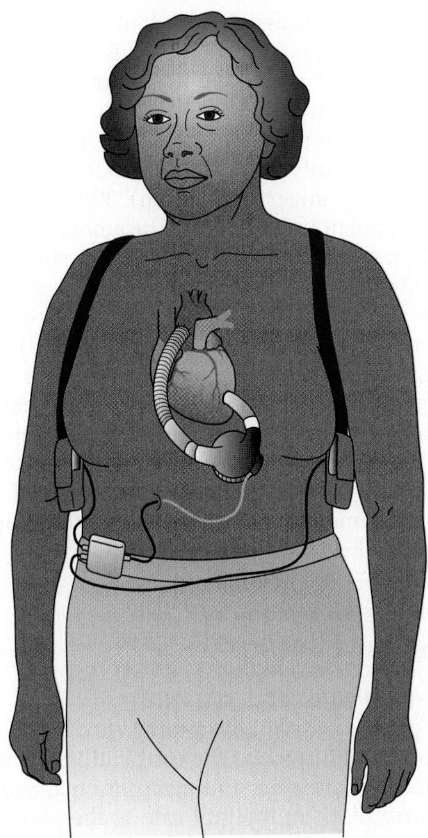

FIGURE 29-10. Left ventricular assist device.

ceived stressors helps the patient and the health care team to implement activities to relieve anxiety related to changes in health status. Very early on, the patient's support systems are identified, and members become involved in the patient's care and therapeutic regimen. The assessment addresses the effect the diagnosis has had on the patient and members of his or her support system and the patient's emotional status. Depression is not uncommon in a patient with cardiomyopathy who has developed heart failure.

The physical assessment focuses on signs and symptoms of heart failure. The baseline assessment includes such key components as:

- Vital signs
- Calculation of pulse pressure and identification of pulsus paradoxus
- Current weight and any weight gain or loss
- Detection by palpation of the point of maximal impulse, often shifted to the left
- Cardiac auscultation for a systolic murmur and S_3 and S_4 heart sounds
- Pulmonary auscultation for crackles
- Measurement of jugular vein distention
- Assessment of edema and its severity

Diagnosis

Nursing Diagnoses

Based on the assessment data, major nursing diagnoses may include:

- Decreased cardiac output related to structural disorders caused by cardiomyopathy or to dysrhythmia from the disease process and medical treatments
- Ineffective cardiopulmonary, cerebral, peripheral, and renal tissue perfusion related to decreased peripheral blood flow (resulting from decreased cardiac output)
- Impaired gas exchange related to pulmonary congestion caused by myocardial failure (resulting from decreased cardiac output)
- Activity intolerance related to decreased cardiac output or excessive fluid volume, or both
- Anxiety related to the change in health status and in role functioning
- Powerlessness related to disease process
- Noncompliance with medication and diet therapies

Collaborative Problems/ Potential Complications

Based on the assessment data, potential complications include:

- Congestive heart failure
- Ventricular dysrhythmias
- Atrial dysrhythmias
- Cardiac conduction defects
- Pulmonary or cerebral embolism
- Valvular dysfunction

These complications are discussed earlier in this chapter and in Chapters 27 and 30.

Planning and Goals

The major goals for patients include improvement or maintenance of cardiac output, increased activity tolerance, reduction of anxiety, adherence to the self-care program, increased sense of power with decision making, and absence of complications.

Nursing Interventions

Improving Cardiac Output

During a symptomatic episode, rest is indicated. Many patients with DCM find that sitting up with their legs down is more comfortable than lying down in a bed. This position is helpful in pooling venous blood in the periphery and reducing preload. Assessing the patient's oxygen saturation at rest and during activity may assist with determining a need for supplemental oxygen. Oxygen is usually administered through a nasal cannula when indicated.

Ensuring that medications are taken as prescribed is important to preserving adequate cardiac output. The nurse may assist the patient with planning a schedule for taking medications and identifying methods to remember to follow it, such as associating the time to take a medication with an activity (eg, eating a meal, brushing teeth). It is important to ensure that patients with DCM avoid verapamil (Calan, Isoptin), patients with HCM avoid diuretics, and patients with RCM avoid nifedipine (Adalat, Procardia) to maintain contractility. In patients with HCM, the inotropic action of digoxin may create or worsen left ventricular outflow track obstruction. Patients with RCM have increased sensitivity to digoxin, and the nurse must anticipate that low doses will be prescribed and assess for digoxin toxicity.

It is also important to ensure that the patient receives or chooses food selections that are appropriate for a low-sodium diet. One way to monitor a patient's response to treatment is to determine the patient's weight every day and identify any significant change. Another indication of the effect of treatment involves assessment of shortness of breath after activity and comparison to before treatment. Patients with low cardiac output may need assistance keeping warm and frequently changing position to stimulate circulation and reduce the possibility of skin breakdown. Patients with HCM must be taught to avoid dehydration. One guideline for patients to use for self-assessment is to anticipate the urge to void at least every 4 hours while awake; if the urge to void is not present or the urine is a deep yellow color, more fluid intake is necessary.

Increasing Activity Tolerance

The nurse plans the patient's activities so that they occur in cycles, alternating rest with activity periods. This benefits the patient's physiologic status, and it helps teach the patient about the need for planned cycles of rest and activity. For example, after taking a bath or shower, the patient should plan to sit and read a newspaper or engage in other relaxing activities. Suggesting that the patient sit while chopping vegetables, drying his or her hair, or shaving helps the patient identify methods to balance rest with activity. The nurse also makes sure that the patient recognizes the symptoms indicating the need for rest and actions to take when the symptoms occur. Patients with HCM or RCM must avoid strenuous activity, isometric exercises, and competitive sports.

Reducing Anxiety

Spiritual, psychological, and emotional support may be indicated for patients, families, and significant others. Interventions are directed toward eradicating or alleviating perceived stressors. Patients receive appropriate information about cardiomyopathy and self-management activities. It is important to provide an atmosphere in which patients feel free to verbalize concerns and receive assurance that their concerns are legitimate. If the patient is awaiting transplantation or facing death, it is necessary to allow time to discuss these issues. Providing the patient with realistic hope helps reduce anxiety while he or she awaits a donor heart. The nurse helps the patient, family, and significant others with anticipatory grieving.

Decreasing the Sense of Powerlessness

Patients must recognize that they go through a grieving process when given a diagnosis of cardiomyopathy. The patient is assisted in identifying the things in life that he or she has lost (eg, foods that the patient enjoyed eating but are high in sodium, the ability to engage in an active lifestyle, the ability to play sports, the ability to lift grandchildren). The patient also is assisted in identifying his or her emotional responses to the loss (eg, anger, depression). The nurse then assists the patient in identifying the amount of control that the patient has over his or her life, such as making food choices, managing medications, and working with health care providers to achieve the best possible outcomes. The use of tools that track behaviors with the resulting symptoms may be helpful. For example, a diary in which the patient records his or her food selections and weight may help the patient understand the relationship between sodium intake and weight gain. Some patients can manage a self-titrating diuretic regimen in which they adjust the dose of diuretic to their symptoms.

Promoting Home and Community-Based Care

TEACHING PATIENTS SELF-CARE

A key part of the plan of nursing care involves teaching patients about the medication regimen, symptom monitoring, and symptom management. The nurse plays an integral role as the patient learns to balance his or her lifestyle and work while accomplishing therapeutic activities. Helping patients cope with their disease status helps them adjust their lifestyles and implement a self-care program at home. Attainment of a goal, no matter how small, also promotes the patient's sense of well-being.

CONTINUING CARE

The nurse reinforces previous teaching and performs ongoing assessment of the patient's symptoms and progress. The nurse also assists the patient and family to adjust to lifestyle changes. It often helps to teach patients to read nutrition labels, to maintain a record of daily weights and symptoms, and to organize daily activities to increase activity tolerance. In addition, the nurse assesses the patient's response to recommendations about diet and fluid intake and to the medication regimen, and stresses the signs and symptoms that should be reported to the physician. Because of the risk of dysrhythmia, it may be necessary to teach the patient's family cardiopulmonary resuscitation. Women are often advised to avoid pregnancy, but each case is assessed individually. The nurse assesses the psychosocial needs of the patient and family on an ongoing basis. There may be concerns and fears about the prognosis, changes in lifestyle, effects of medications, and the possibility of others in the family having the same condition, and these often increase the patient's anxiety and interfere with effective coping strategies. Establishing trust is vital to the nurse's relationship with these chronically ill patients and their families. This is particularly significant when the nurse is involved with a patient and family in discussions about end-of-life decisions. Patients who have significant symptoms of heart failure or other complications of cardiomyopathy may need a home care referral.

Evaluation

Expected Patient Outcomes

Expected patient outcomes may include:

1. Maintains or improves cardiac function
   a. Exhibits heart and respiratory rates within normal limits
   b. Reports decreased dyspnea and increased comfort; maintains or improves gas exchange
   c. Reports no weight gain; appropriate weight for height
   d. Maintains or improves peripheral blood flow
2. Maintains or increases activity tolerance
   a. Carries out activities of daily living (eg, brushes teeth, feeds self)
   b. Reports increased tolerance to activity
3. Is less anxious
   a. Discusses prognosis freely
   b. Verbalizes fears and concerns
   c. Participates in support groups if appropriate
4. Decreases sense of powerlessness
   a. Identifies emotional response to diagnosis
   b. Discusses control that he or she has
5. Adheres to self-care program
   a. Takes medications according to prescribed schedule
   b. Modifies diet to accommodate sodium and fluid recommendations
   c. Modifies lifestyle to accommodate recommended activity and rest behaviors
   d. Identifies signs and symptoms to be reported to health care professionals

Infectious Diseases of the Heart

Any of the heart's three layers may be affected by an infectious process. The diseases are named for the layer of the heart most involved in the infectious process: infective endocarditis (endocardium), myocarditis (myocardium), and pericarditis (pericardium). Rheumatic endocarditis is a unique infective endocarditis syndrome. The diagnosis is made primarily on the basis of the patient's symptoms and echocardiography. The ideal management for all infectious diseases is prevention. IV antibiotics are usually necessary once an infection in the heart has developed.

Rheumatic Endocarditis

Acute rheumatic fever, which occurs most often in school-age children, may develop after an episode of group A beta-hemolytic streptococcal pharyngitis (Chart 29-1). Patients with rheumatic fever may develop rheumatic heart disease as evidenced by a new heart murmur, cardiomegaly, pericarditis, and heart failure. Prompt treatment of "strep" throat with antibiotics can prevent the development of rheumatic fever. The streptococcus is spread by direct contact with oral or respiratory secretions. Although the bacteria are the causative agents, malnutrition, overcrowding, and lower socioeconomic status may predispose individuals to rheumatic fever (Chin & Worley, 2003). The incidence of rheumatic fever in the United States and other developed countries is believed to have steadily decreased, but the exact incidence is difficult to determine because the infection may go unrecognized, and people may not seek treatment (Zipes et al., 2005). Clinical diagnostic criteria are not standardized, and autopsies are not routinely performed.

CHART 29-1

Rheumatic Fever

Rheumatic fever is a preventable disease. Diagnosing and treating streptococcal pharyngitis can prevent rheumatic fever and, therefore, rheumatic heart disease. Signs and symptoms of streptococcal pharyngitis include:

- Fever (38.9° to 40°C [101° to 104°F])
- Chills
- Sore throat (sudden in onset)
- Diffuse redness of throat with exudate on oropharynx (may not appear until after the first day)
- Enlarged and tender lymph nodes
- Abdominal pain (more common in children)
- Acute sinusitis and acute otitis media (may cause or result from streptococcal pharyngitis)

If signs and symptoms of streptococcal pharyngitis are present, a throat culture is necessary to make an accurate diagnosis. All patients with throat cultures positive for streptococcal pharyngitis must adhere to the prescribed antibiotic treatment. Penicillin is the most common antibiotic prescribed. Completing the course of prescribed antibiotics minimizes the risk of developing rheumatic fever (and subsequent rheumatic heart disease).

Pathophysiology

Rheumatic endocarditis is not infectious in the sense that tissues are not invaded and directly damaged by the streptococci. Injury is caused by an inflammatory or sensitivity reaction to streptococci. Leukocytes accumulate in the affected tissues and form nodules, which eventually are replaced by scar tissue. The myocardium is involved in the inflammatory process. Rheumatic myocarditis develops, which temporarily weakens the contractile power of the heart. The pericardium is affected, and rheumatic pericarditis occurs during the acute illness. Myocardial and pericardial involvement usually resolves without serious sequelae. However, rheumatic endocarditis results in permanent and often crippling adverse effects.

Rheumatic endocarditis first manifests anatomically as tiny translucent vegetations or growths, which resemble pinhead-sized beads arranged in a row along the free margins of the valve leaflets. These tiny beads look harmless and may disappear without injuring the leaflet. However, more often they have serious effects. They are the starting point of a process that gradually thickens the leaflets, causing them to shorten and thicken, preventing them from closing completely. As a result, blood flows backward through the valve; this is called *valvular regurgitation.* The most common site of valvular regurgitation is the mitral valve. In some patients, the inflamed margins of the valve leaflets become adherent or the chordae tendineae fuse, resulting in valvular stenosis, a narrowed or stenotic valvular orifice. Regurgitation and stenosis may occur in the same valve.

Clinical Manifestations

The Jones criteria are one set of diagnostic criteria for rheumatic fever. According to these criteria, patients who have had a group A beta-hemolytic streptococcal infection are diagnosed with rheumatic fever if they develop at least two of the following: carditis, polyarthritis, subcutaneous nodules, erythema marginatum, or chorea (Special Writing Group of the Committee on Rheumatic Fever, Endocarditis, and Kawasaki's Disease of the Council on Cardiovascular Disease in the Young of the American Heart Association, 1992). Carditis, the inflammatory process of the disease, affects all three layers of the heart and may also affect bone joints, producing polyarthritis that may last for up to 4 weeks. Round, firm, painless, free-moving, subcutaneous nodules may develop over bony surfaces and tendons. These nodules usually disappear after 1 to 2 weeks. Patients may also develop a macular or papular, nonitchy rash on the trunk and proximal extremities, called erythema marginatum. The rash blanches with pressure, is not indurated, and does not leave a scar. Individual lesions may come and go over a few minutes, moving from place to place on the body. Patients may develop chorea (rapid, purposeless, erratic, jerky, uncoordinated, involuntary movements of the extremities and face) during the acute phase and up to several months afterward. The chorea usually resolves completely within 6 months. Rheumatic heart disease may cause valvular insufficiency, heart failure, and death.

Most patients with rheumatic fever recover within 3 to 4 weeks. However, a few patients become critically ill with intractable heart failure, serious dysrhythmias, and pneumonia. Once the symptoms of rheumatic fever subside, residual effects of rheumatic endocarditis may lead to progressive valvular deformities. The existence and extent of cardiac damage may not be apparent in clinical examinations during the acute phase of the disease. However, eventually the heart murmurs characteristic of valvular regurgitation, stenosis, or both become audible on auscultation. In some patients, thrills are detectable on palpation. Usually, the myocardium can compensate for these valvular defects for a time, and the patient remains in good health. As the valvular pathology progresses, the myocardium is no longer able to compensate (see Fig. 29-2), and the signs and symptoms of heart failure develop (see Chapter 30).

Assessment and Diagnostic Findings

A sore throat, or a history of one within 5 weeks, is a first symptom of possible rheumatic fever. Other symptoms include those described in Clinical Manifestations as well as fever, headache, weight loss, fatigue, malaise, diaphoresis, and pallor. More rarely, chest pain, abdominal pain, or vomiting may also occur.

Throat cultures are necessary to diagnose the presence of a group A beta-hemolytic streptococcal infection. Results from a rapid antigen detection test for group A beta-hemolytic streptococci may be used until the throat culture results are available. Rapid antigen detection tests have a 95% specificity but only 60% to 90% sensitivity; thus, throat cultures are used in addition to the rapid antigen tests (Chin & Worley, 2003). (See Chapter 22 for additional information.)

During assessment for rheumatic heart disease, the nurse should keep in mind that no diagnostic studies are specific for rheumatic endocarditis and that symptoms may not develop until years after the rheumatic fever. The symptoms depend on which side of the heart is involved. The mitral valve is most often affected, producing symptoms of left-sided heart failure—shortness of breath with crackles and wheezes in the lungs (see Chapter 30 for a discussion of left-sided versus right-sided failure). The severity of the symptoms depends on the size and location of the lesion in the heart. The systemic symptoms are proportional to the virulence of the invading organism. When a new murmur is detected in a patient with a systemic infection, infectious endocarditis should be suspected. Patients are also at risk for sequelae associated with embolic phenomena of the lung, kidney, spleen, heart, brain, or peripheral vessels.

The ECG may show sinus tachycardia, sinus bradycardia, sinus dysrhythmia, first-degree heart block, and atrial fibrillation or atrial flutter. The erythrocyte sedimentation rate (ESR) or serum C-reactive protein level may be elevated.

Prevention

Rheumatic fever and rheumatic endocarditis may be prevented through early and adequate treatment of oropharyngeal streptococcal infections. A first-line approach in preventing initial attacks of rheumatic fever is recognition of oropharyngeal streptococcal infections, adequate treatment, and control of epidemics in the community. Every nurse should be familiar with the signs and symptoms of streptococcal pharyngitis: high fever (38.9°C to 40°C [101°F to 104°F]), chills, sore throat, redness of the throat with exudate, enlarged lymph nodes, abdominal pain, and acute rhinitis (see Chart 29-1).

Medical Management

The objectives of medical management for oropharyngeal infections are to identify and eradicate the causative organism and prevent additional complications, such as rheumatic fever and rheumatic endocarditis. Throat cultures are used to identify the causative organism, if any, for the pharyngitis. If group A beta-hemolytic streptococcus is suspected, a one-time intramuscular injection of penicillin or a 10-day course of oral penicillin is prescribed. Erythromycin or cephalosporin may be prescribed for patients who are allergic to penicillin.

Initially, patients diagnosed with rheumatic fever are treated like patients with oropharyngeal group A beta-hemolytic streptococcal infections. After the initial antibiotic treatment, the patient should receive a prophylactic intramuscular dose of penicillin every 3 to 4 weeks to prevent recurrence of rheumatic fever and rheumatic heart disease. Prophylactic antibiotics are prescribed for 5 years (or until age 21, whichever is longer) if the patient did not experience carditis, or for 10 years (or until age 40, whichever is longer) if the patient had carditis or develops valvular heart disease. Oral erythromycin is prescribed for patients who are allergic to penicillin. For other symptoms except chorea, anti-inflammatory medications (eg, salicylates [aspirin], corticosteroids [prednisone]) may be prescribed. Although the chorea usually does not require treatment, patients may be treated with diazepam (Valium) or phenobarbital if the condition is severe. Symptoms of heart failure are treated as described in Chapter 30.

Patients also require prophylactic antibiotics for invasive procedures. Clindamycin (Cleocin), azithromycin (Zithromax), and clarithromycin (Biaxin) are often prescribed because the bacteria may be resistant to the antibiotic used for recurrent rheumatic fever prophylaxis (Chin & Worley, 2003; Dajani, Taubert, Wilson, et al., 1997).

Nursing Management

A key nursing role in the care of patients with rheumatic fever and rheumatic endocarditis is teaching patients about the disease, its treatment, and the preventive steps needed to minimize recurrence and potential complications. After acute treatment with antibiotics, patients must take prophylactic antibiotics on a regular schedule and before invasive procedures. It is important to have long-term cardiac reevaluations, to maintain hydration, and to report any signs of thromboemboli or heart failure to health care providers.

Patients who have rheumatic endocarditis and whose valvular dysfunction is mild may require no further treatment. Nevertheless, the danger exists for recurrent attacks of acute rheumatic fever, bacterial endocarditis, embolism from vegetations or mural thrombi in the heart, and eventual cardiac failure. The nurse monitors the patient for signs and symptoms of valvular disease, heart failure, pulmonary hypertension, thromboemboli, and dysrhythmias.

CHART 29-2

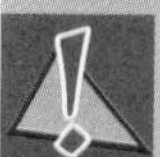

Risk Factors for Infective Endocarditis

High Risk

- Prosthetic cardiac valves
- History of bacterial endocarditis (even without heart disease)
- Complex cyanotic congenital malformations
- Surgically constructed systemic or pulmonary shunts or conduits
- Aortic valve disease
- Mitral regurgitation
- Combined mitral regurgitation and stenosis
- Patent ductus arteriosus
- Ventricular septal defect
- Coarctation of the aorta

Moderate Risk

- Mitral valve prolapse with valvular regurgitation or thickened leaflets
- Hypertrophic cardiomyopathy
- Acquired valvular dysfunction
- Most congenital cardiac malformations (other than those listed above)
- Atrial septal defect (unrepaired or repaired)
- Ventricular septal defect (repaired)
- Patent ductus arteriosus (repaired)
- Parenteral nutrition lines or IV lines into the right atrium
- Nonvalvular cardiac implants
- Degenerative valve disease

Infective Endocarditis

Infective endocarditis is a microbial infection of the endothelial surface of the heart. It usually develops in people with prosthetic heart valves, structural cardiac defects (eg, valve disorders, HCM) (Chart 29-2). It is more common in older people, who are more likely to have degenerative or calcific valve lesions, reduced immunologic response to infection, and the metabolic alterations associated with aging. Staphylococcal endocarditis infections of the valves in the right side of the heart are common among injection drug users (Miro, del Rio, & Mestres, 2003; Zipes et al., 2005). Hospital-acquired infective endocarditis occurs most often in patients with debilitating disease or indwelling catheters and in patients who are receiving prolonged IV fluid or antibiotic therapy. Patients taking immunosuppressive medications or corticosteroids are more susceptible to fungal endocarditis.

Invasive procedures, particularly those involving mucosal surfaces, can cause a bacteremia, which rarely lasts for more than 15 minutes. If a patient has any anatomic cardiac defects, however, bacteremia can cause bacterial endocarditis. From 1950 to the mid-1980s, the incidence of infective endocarditis remained steady at about 4.2 cases per 100,000 patients. The incidence then increased, partially attributed to increased IV/injection drug abuse (Zipes et al., 2005).

Pathophysiology

A deformity or injury of the endocardium leads to accumulation on the endocardium of fibrin and platelets and clot formation. Infectious organisms, usually streptococci, staphylococci, enterococci, or pneumococci, invade the clot and endocardial lesion. Other causative microorganisms include fungi (eg, *Candida, Aspergillus*) and Rickettsiae. The infection most frequently results in platelets, fibrin, blood cells, and microorganisms that cluster as vegetations on the endocardium. The vegetations may embolize to other tissues throughout the body. As the clot on the endocardium continues to expand, the infecting organism is covered by the new clot and concealed from the body's normal defenses. The infection may erode through the endocardium into the underlying structures (eg, valve leaflets), causing tears or other deformities of valve leaflets, dehiscence of prosthetic valves, deformity of the chordae tendineae, or mural abscesses.

A diagnosis of *acute* bacterial (infective) endocarditis (ABE) is made when the onset of infection and resulting valvular destruction is rapid, occurring within days to weeks. A diagnosis of *subacute* bacterial (infective) endocarditis (SBE) is made when the onset of infection and resulting valvular destruction takes 2 weeks to months to occur (Zipes et al., 2005).

Usually, the onset of infective endocarditis is insidious. The signs and symptoms develop from the toxic effect of the infection, from destruction of the heart valves, and from embolization of fragments of vegetative growths on the heart. Systemic emboli occur with left-sided heart infective endocarditis; pulmonary emboli occur with right-sided heart infective endocarditis (Crawford & Durack, 2003; Zipes et al., 2005).

Clinical Manifestations

The primary presenting symptoms of infective endocarditis are fever and a heart murmur. The fever may be intermittent or absent, especially in patients who are receiving antibiotics or corticosteroids, in those who are elderly, or those who have heart failure or renal failure. A heart murmur may be absent initially but develops in almost all patients. Murmurs that worsen over time indicate progressive damage from vegetations or perforation of the valve or the chordae tendineae.

In addition to the fever and heart murmur, clusters of petechiae may be found on the body. Small, painful nodules (Osler nodes) may be present in the pads of fingers or toes. Irregular, red or purple, painless, flat macules (Janeway lesions) may be present on the palms, fingers, hands, soles, and toes. Hemorrhages with pale centers (Roth spots) caused by emboli in the nerve fiber layer of the eye may be observed in the fundi of the eyes. Splinter hemorrhages (ie, reddish-brown lines and streaks) may be seen under the fingernails and toenails, and petechiae may appear in the conjunctiva and mucous membranes. There may be cardiomegaly, heart failure, tachycardia, or splenomegaly.

Central nervous system manifestations of infective endocarditis include headache; temporary or transient cerebral ischemia; and strokes, which may be caused by emboli to the cerebral arteries. Embolization may be a presenting symptom, and it may occur at any time and may involve other organ systems. Embolic phenomena may occur, as discussed in the previous section on rheumatic endocarditis.

Assessment and Diagnostic Findings

Although the previously described characteristics may indicate infective endocarditis, the signs and symptoms may indicate other diseases as well. Vague complaints of malaise, anorexia, weight loss, cough, and back and joint pain may be mistaken for influenza. A definitive diagnosis is made when a microorganism is found in two separate blood cultures, in a vegetation, or in an abscess. Three sets of blood cultures (with each set including one aerobic and one anaerobic culture) drawn 1 hour apart should be obtained before administration of any antimicrobial agents. Negative blood cultures do not definitely rule out infective endocarditis. Patients may have elevated white blood cell (WBC) counts. In addition, patients may be anemic and have an elevated ESR and a positive rheumatoid factor. Microscopic hematuria may be present on urinalysis.

Doppler echocardiography may assist in the diagnosis by demonstrating a mass on the valve, prosthetic valve, or supporting structures and by identification of vegetations, abscesses, new prosthetic valve dehiscence, or new regurgitation (Moss & Munt, 2003; Zipes et al., 2005). The echocardiogram may reveal the development of heart failure. TEE may provide better data than transthoracic imaging.

Prevention

Although rare, bacterial endocarditis may be life-threatening. A key strategy is primary prevention in moderate- and high-risk patients (ie, those with rheumatic heart disease, mitral valve prolapse, or prosthetic heart valves). Antibiotic prophylaxis is recommended for moderate- and high-risk patients immediately before and sometimes after the following procedures:

- Dental procedures that induce gingival or mucosal bleeding, including professional cleaning and placement of orthodontic bands (not brackets)
- Tonsillectomy or adenoidectomy
- Surgical procedures that involve intestinal or respiratory mucosa
- Bronchoscopy with a rigid bronchoscope
- Sclerotherapy for esophageal varices
- Esophageal dilation
- Endoscopic retrograde cholangiography with biliary obstruction
- Gallbladder surgery
- Cystoscopy
- Urethral dilation
- Urethral catheterization if urinary tract infection is present
- Urinary tract surgery if urinary tract infection is present
- Prostatic surgery
- Incision and drainage of infected tissue
- Vaginal hysterectomy

The type of antibiotic used for prophylaxis varies with the type of procedure and the degree of risk. Patients are usually instructed to take 2 g of amoxicillin (Amoxil) orally 1 hour before dental, oral, respiratory, or esophageal procedures. If patients are allergic to penicillin, clindamycin (Cleocin), cephalexin (Keflex), cefadroxil (Duricef), azithromycin (Zithromax), or clarithromycin (Biaxin) may be used. Antibiotic recommendations for gastrointestinal or genitourinary procedures are ampicillin and gentamicin (Garamycin) for high-risk patients, and amoxicillin or ampicillin for moderate-risk patients; only patients allergic to ampicillin or amoxicillin should receive vancomycin (Vancocin) as a substitute.

The severity of oral inflammation and infection is a significant factor in the incidence and degree of bacteremia.

Poor dental hygiene can lead to bacteremia, particularly in the setting of a dental procedure. Regular professional oral care combined with personal oral care may reduce the risk of bacteremia. Personal oral care includes using a soft toothbrush and toothpaste to brush the teeth, gums, tongue, and oral mucosa at least twice a day, as well as rinsing the mouth for 30 seconds intermittently between tooth brushing with an antiseptic mouthwash. Patients must be advised to avoid nail biting and to minimize outbreaks of acne and psoriasis. Female patients are advised not to use intrauterine devices (IUDs).

Increased vigilance is also required in patients with IV catheters and during invasive procedures. To minimize the risk of infection, nurses must ensure meticulous hand hygiene, site preparation, and aseptic technique during insertion and maintenance procedures. All catheters, tubes, drains, and other devices are removed as soon as they are no longer needed or no longer function.

Complications

Even if the patient responds to therapy, endocarditis can be destructive to the heart and other organs. Heart failure and cerebral vascular complications, such as stroke (i.e., cerebrovascular accident or brain attack), may occur before, during, or after therapy. Heart failure, which may result from perforation of a valve leaflet, rupture of chordae, blood flow obstruction due to vegetations, or intracardiac shunts from dehiscence of prosthetic valves, indicates a poor prognosis with medical therapy alone and a higher surgical risk (Zipes et al., 2005). Valvular stenosis or regurgitation, myocardial damage, and mycotic (fungal) aneurysms are potential cardiac complications. First-, second-, and third-degree atrioventricular blocks may occur and are often a sign of a valve ring abscess. Septic or nonseptic emboli, immunologic responses, abscess of the spleen, mycotic aneurysms, cerebritis, and hemodynamic deterioration may cause complications in other organs.

Medical Management

The causative organism may be identified by serial blood cultures. The objective of treatment is to eradicate the invading organism through adequate doses of an appropriate antimicrobial agent.

Pharmacologic Therapy

Antibiotic therapy is usually administered parenterally in a continuous IV infusion for 2 to 6 weeks. Parenteral therapy is administered in doses that produce a high serum concentration and for a significant period to ensure eradication of the dormant bacteria within the dense vegetations. This therapy is often delivered in the patient's home and is monitored by a home care nurse. Serum levels of the selected antibiotic are monitored. If the serum does not demonstrate bactericidal activity, increased dosages of the antibiotic are prescribed or a different antibiotic is used. Numerous antimicrobial regimens are in use, but penicillin is usually the medication of choice. Blood cultures are taken periodically to monitor the effect of therapy. In fungal endocarditis, an antifungal agent, such as amphotericin B (Abelcet, Amphocin, Fungizone), is the usual treatment.

The patient's temperature is monitored at regular intervals, because the course of the fever is one indication of the effectiveness of treatment. However, febrile reactions also may occur as a result of medication. After adequate antimicrobial therapy is initiated, the infective organism is usually eliminated. The patient should begin to feel better, regain an appetite, and have less fatigue. During this time, patients require psychosocial support, because although they feel well, they may find themselves confined to the hospital or home with restrictive IV therapy.

Surgical Management

Surgical interventions include valve débridement or excision, débridement of vegetations, débridement and closure of an abscess, and closure of a fistula. Aortic or mitral valve débridement, excision, or replacement is required in patients who develop congestive heart failure despite adequate medical treatment; those who have more than one serious systemic embolic episode, valve obstruction, a periannular (heart valve) or myocardial abscess, or aortic abscess; and those with uncontrolled infection, persistent or recurrent infection, or fungal endocarditis. Surgical valve replacement greatly improves the prognosis for patients with severe symptoms from damaged heart valves. The aortic valve may be best treated with an autograft, as previously described. Most patients who have prosthetic valve endocarditis (ie, infected valve replacements) require valve replacement.

Nursing Management

The nurse monitors the patient's temperature. The patient may have a fever for weeks. Heart sounds are assessed. A new or worsening murmur may indicate dehiscence of a prosthetic valve, rupture of an abscess, or injury to valve leaflets or chordae tendineae. The nurse monitors for signs and symptoms of systemic embolization, or, for patients with right-sided heart endocarditis, for signs and symptoms of pulmonary infarction and infiltrates. In addition, the nurse assesses signs and symptoms of organ damage such as stroke (ie, cerebrovascular accident or brain attack), meningitis, heart failure, myocardial infarction, glomerulonephritis, and splenomegaly.

Patient care is directed toward management of infection. The patient is started on antibiotics as soon as blood cultures have been obtained. Long-term IV antimicrobial therapy is often necessary; therefore, many patients have peripherally inserted central catheters or other long-term IV access. All invasive lines and wounds must be assessed daily for redness, tenderness, warmth, swelling, drainage, or other signs of infection. The patient and family are instructed about activity restrictions, medications, and signs and symptoms of infection. The nurse instructs the patient and family about the need for prophylactic antibiotics not only before, but possibly after, dental, respiratory, gastrointestinal, or genitourinary procedures. The home care nurse supervises and monitors IV antibiotic therapy delivered in the home setting and educates the patient and family about prevention and health promotion. The nurse provides the patient and family with emotional support and facilitates coping strategies during the prolonged course of the infection and antibiotic treatment. If the patient has undergone surgical treatment, the nurse provides postoperative care and instructions.

Myocarditis

Myocarditis, an inflammatory process involving the myocardium, can cause heart dilation, thrombi on the heart wall (mural thrombi), infiltration of circulating blood cells around the coronary vessels and between the muscle fibers, and degeneration of the muscle fibers themselves. Mortality varies with the severity of symptoms. Most patients with mild symptoms recover completely, but some patients develop cardiomyopathy and heart failure.

Pathophysiology

Myocarditis usually results from viral (coxsackievirus A and B), rickettsial, fungal, parasitic, metazoal, protozoal, or spirochetal infection. It also may occur after acute systemic infections such as rheumatic fever or Chagas disease; in patients receiving immunosuppressive therapy; or in patients with infective endocarditis, Crohn disease, or systemic lupus erythematosus. Myocarditis may result from an immune reaction to pharmacologic agents used in the treatment of other diseases or radiation (especially to the left chest or upper back). It may begin in one small area of the myocardium and then spread throughout the myocardium. The degree of myocardial involvement determines the degree of hemodynamic effect and the resulting signs and symptoms. It is theorized that DCM is a latent manifestation of myocarditis (Calabrese & Thiene, 2003; Zipes et al., 2005).

Clinical Manifestations

The symptoms of acute myocarditis depend on the type of infection, the degree of myocardial damage, and the capacity of the myocardium to recover. Patients may be asymptomatic, and the infection resolves on its own. However, they may develop mild to moderate symptoms and seek medical attention, often reporting fatigue and dyspnea, palpitations, and occasional discomfort in the chest and upper abdomen. The most common symptoms are flu-like. Patients may also sustain sudden cardiac death or quickly develop severe congestive heart failure.

Assessment and Diagnostic Findings

Assessment of the patient may reveal no detectable abnormalities; as a result, the entire illness can go undiagnosed. Patients may be tachycardic or may report chest pain (with a subsequent cardiac catheterization demonstrating normal coronary arteries). Endocardial biopsies may be diagnostic for an organism, immune process, or radiation reaction causing the myocarditis. Patients without any abnormal heart structure (at least initially) may suddenly develop dysrhythmias or ST-T wave changes. If the patient has structural heart abnormalities (eg, systolic dysfunction), a clinical assessment may disclose cardiac enlargement, faint heart sounds (especially S_1), a gallop rhythm, or a systolic murmur. The WBC count and ESR may be elevated.

Prevention

Prevention of infectious diseases by means of appropriate immunizations (eg, influenza, hepatitis) and early treatment appears to be important in decreasing the incidence of myocarditis (Zipes et al., 2005).

Medical Management

Patients are given specific treatment for the underlying cause if it is known (eg, penicillin for hemolytic streptococci) and are placed on bed rest to decrease cardiac workload. Bed rest also helps decrease myocardial damage and the complications of myocarditis. In young patients with myocarditis, activities, especially athletics, should be limited for a 6-month period or at least until heart size and function have returned to normal. Physical activity is increased slowly, and the patient is instructed to report any symptoms that occur with increasing activity, such as a rapidly beating heart. The use of corticosteroids in treating myocarditis remains controversial (Zipes et al., 2005). Nonsteroidal anti-inflammatory drugs (NSAIDs) such as aspirin and ibuprofen should not be used during the acute phase or if heart failure develops, because these medications can cause further myocardial damage. If heart failure or dysrhythmia develops, management is essentially the same as for all causes of heart failure and dysrhythmias (see Chapters 27 and 30), except that beta-blockers are avoided because they decrease the strength of ventricular contraction (have a negative inotropic effect).

Nursing Management

The nurse assesses for resolution of tachycardia, fever, and any other clinical manifestations. The cardiovascular assessment focuses on signs and symptoms of heart failure and dysrhythmias. Patients with dysrhythmias should have continuous cardiac monitoring with personnel and equipment readily available to treat life-threatening dysrhythmias.

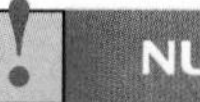

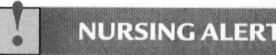

NURSING ALERT

Patients with myocarditis are sensitive to digitalis. Nurses must closely monitor these patients for digitalis toxicity, which is evidenced by dysrhythmia, anorexia, nausea, vomiting, headache, and malaise.

Elastic compression stockings and passive and active exercises should be used because embolization from venous thrombosis and mural thrombi can occur, especially in patients on bed rest.

Pericarditis

Pericarditis refers to an inflammation of the pericardium, the membranous sac enveloping the heart. It may be a primary illness or it may develop during various medical and surgical disorders. For example, pericarditis may occur after pericardectomy (opening of the pericardium) following cardiac surgery. Pericarditis also may occur 10 days to 2 months after acute myocardial infarction (Dressler syndrome). Pericarditis may be subacute, acute, or chronic. It is classified either as adhesive (or constrictive) because the layers of the pericardium become attached to each other and restrict ventricular filling, or by what accumulates in the pericardial sac: serous (serum), purulent (pus), calcific (calcium deposits), fibrinous (clotting proteins), or sanguinous (blood). Pericarditis also may be described as exudative or noneffusive.

Pathophysiology

Causes underlying or associated with pericarditis are listed in Chart 29-3. Pericarditis may lead to an accumulation of fluid in the pericardial sac (pericardial effusion) and increased pressure on the heart, leading to cardiac tamponade (see Chapter 30). Frequent or prolonged episodes of pericarditis may also lead to thickening and decreased elasticity of the pericardium, or scarring may fuse the visceral and parietal pericardium. These conditions restrict the heart's ability to fill with blood (constrictive pericarditis). The pericardium may become calcified, further restricting ventricular expansion during ventricular filling (diastole). With less filling, the ventricles pump less blood, leading to decreased cardiac output and signs and symptoms of heart failure. Restricted diastolic filling may result in increased systemic venous pressure, causing peripheral edema and hepatic failure.

CHART 29-3

Causes of Pericarditis

- Idiopathic or nonspecific causes
- Infection: usually viral (eg, human immunodeficiency virus, coxsackievirus, influenza); rarely bacterial (eg, streptococci, staphylococci, meningococci, gonococci, gram-negative rods); and mycotic (fungal)
- Disorders of connective tissue: systemic lupus erythematosus, rheumatic fever, rheumatoid arthritis, polyarteritis, scleroderma
- Hypersensitivity states: immune reactions, medication reactions, serum sickness
- Disorders of adjacent structures: myocardial infarction, dissecting aneurysm, pleural and pulmonary disease (pneumonia)
- Neoplastic disease: caused by metastasis from lung cancer or breast cancer, leukemia, and primary (mesothelioma) neoplasms
- Radiation therapy of chest and upper torso (peak occurrence 5–9 months after treatment)
- Trauma: chest injury, cardiac surgery, cardiac catheterization, implantation of pacemaker or implantable cardioverter defibrillator (ICD)
- Renal failure and uremia
- Tuberculosis

Clinical Manifestations

Pericarditis may be asymptomatic. The most characteristic symptom of pericarditis is chest pain, although pain also may be located beneath the clavicle, in the neck, or in the left trapezius (scapula) region. The pain or discomfort usually remains fairly constant, but it may worsen with deep inspiration and when lying down or turning. It may be relieved with a forward-leaning or sitting position. The most characteristic sign of pericarditis is a creaky or scratchy friction rub heard most clearly at the left lower sternal border. Other signs may include a mild fever, increased WBC count, anemia, and an elevated ESR or C-reactive protein level. Patients may have a nonproductive cough. Dyspnea and other signs and symptoms of heart failure may occur as the result of pericardial compression due to constrictive pericarditis or cardiac tamponade.

Assessment and Diagnostic Findings

The diagnosis is most often made on the basis of the history, signs, and symptoms. An echocardiogram may detect inflammation, pericardial effusion or tamponade, and heart failure. It may help confirm the diagnosis and may be used to guide pericardiocentesis (needle or catheter drainage of the pericardium). TEE may be useful in diagnosis but may underestimate the extent of pericardial effusions. CT may be the best diagnostic tool for determining the size, shape, and location of pericardial effusions and may be used to guide pericardiocentesis. MRI may assist with detection of inflammation and adhesions. Occasionally, a video-assisted pericardioscope-guided biopsy of the pericardium or epicardium is performed to obtain tissue samples for culture and microscopic examination. Because the pericardial sac surrounds the heart, a 12-lead ECG may show concave ST elevations in many, if not all, leads (with no reciprocal changes) and may show depressed PR segments or atrial dysrhythmias.

Medical Management

The objectives of management of pericarditis are to determine the cause, administer therapy for treatment and symptom relief, and detect signs and symptoms of cardiac tamponade. When cardiac output is impaired, the patient is placed on bed rest until the fever, chest pain, and friction rub have subsided.

Analgesics and NSAIDs such as aspirin or ibuprofen (Motrin) may be prescribed for pain relief during the acute phase. These agents also hasten the reabsorption of fluid in patients with rheumatic pericarditis. Indomethacin (Indocin) is contraindicated, because it may decrease coronary blood flow. Corticosteroids (eg, prednisone) may be prescribed if the pericarditis is severe or if the patient does not respond to NSAIDs. Colchicine may also be used as alternative therapy.

Pericardiocentesis, a procedure in which some of the pericardial fluid is removed, is rarely necessary. It may be performed to assist in the identification of the cause or relieve symptoms, especially if there are signs and symptoms of heart failure or tamponade. Pericardial fluid is cultured if bacterial, tubercular, or fungal disease is suspected, and a sample is sent for cytology if neoplastic disease is suspected. A pericardial window, a small opening made in the pericardium, may be performed to allow continuous drainage into the chest cavity. Surgical removal of the tough encasing pericardium (pericardiectomy) may be necessary to release both ventricles from the constrictive and restrictive inflammation and scarring.

Nursing Management

Patients with acute pericarditis require pain management with analgesics, positioning, and psychological support. Patients with chest pain often benefit from education and reassurance that the pain is not a heart attack. To minimize complications, the nurse helps the patient with activity restrictions until the pain and fever subside. As the patient's condition improves, the nurse encourages gradual increases of activity. However, if pain, fever, or friction rub reappear, activity restrictions must be resumed. The nurse educates the patient and family about a healthy lifestyle to enhance the patient's immune system.

Nurses caring for patients with pericarditis must be alert to cardiac tamponade (see Chapter 30). The nurse monitors the patient for heart failure. Patients with hemodynamic instability or pulmonary congestion are treated as they would be if they had heart failure (see Chapter 30).

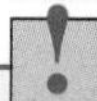

NURSING ALERT

A pericardial friction rub is diagnostic of pericarditis. It has a creaky or scratchy sound and is louder at the end of exhalation. Nurses should search diligently for the pericardial friction rub by placing the diaphragm of the stethoscope tightly against the thorax and auscultating the left sternal edge in the fourth intercostal space, the site where the pericardium comes into contact with the left chest wall. The rub may be heard best when a patient is sitting and leaning forward.

Nursing Process

The Patient With Pericarditis

Assessment

The primary symptom of the patient with pericarditis is pain, which is assessed by evaluating the patient in various positions. The nurse tries to identify whether the pain is influenced by respiratory movements, while holding an inhaled breath or holding an exhaled breath; by flexion, extension, or rotation of the spine, including the neck; by movements of the shoulders and arms; by coughing; or by swallowing. Recognizing the events that precipitate or intensify pain may help establish a diagnosis and differentiate the pain of pericarditis from the pain of myocardial infarction.

A pericardial friction rub occurs when the pericardial surfaces lose their lubricating fluid because of inflammation. The rub is audible on auscultation and is synchronous with the heartbeat. However, it may be elusive and difficult to detect.

If there is difficulty in distinguishing a pericardial friction rub from a pleural friction rub, the patient is asked to hold his or her breath; a pericardial friction rub will continue.

The patient's temperature is monitored frequently. Pericarditis may cause an abrupt onset of fever in a patient who has been afebrile.

Diagnosis

Nursing Diagnosis

Based on the assessment data, the major nursing diagnosis may be:

- Acute pain related to inflammation of the pericardium

Collaborative Problems/ Potential Complications

Based on the assessment data, potential complications that may develop include:

- Pericardial effusion
- Cardiac tamponade

Planning and Goals

The patient's major goals may include relief of pain and absence of complications.

Nursing Interventions

Relieving Pain

Relief of pain is achieved by rest. Because sitting upright and leaning forward is the posture that tends to relieve pain, chair rest may be more comfortable. It is important to instruct the patient to restrict activity until the pain subsides. As the chest pain and friction rub abate, activities of daily living may be resumed gradually. If the patient is taking analgesics, antibiotics, or corticosteroids for the pericarditis, his or her responses are monitored and recorded. Patients taking NSAIDs are assessed for gastrointestinal adverse effects. If chest pain and friction rub recur, bed rest or chair rest is resumed.

Monitoring and Managing Potential Complications

PERICARDIAL EFFUSION

Fluid may accumulate between the pericardial linings or in the pericardial sac, a condition called *pericardial effusion* (see Chapter 30). The fluid can constrict the myocardium and impair its ability to pump. Cardiac output declines further with each contraction. Failure to identify and treat this problem can lead to the development of cardiac tamponade and possible sudden death.

CARDIAC TAMPONADE

The signs and symptoms of cardiac tamponade may begin with the patient reporting shortness of breath, chest tightness, or dizziness. The nurse may observe that the patient is becoming progressively more restless. Assessment of blood pressure may reveal a decrease of 10 mm Hg or more in the systolic blood pressure during inspiration (pulsus paradoxus). Usually, the systolic pressure decreases and the diastolic pressure remains stable; hence, the pulse pressure narrows. The patient may have tachycardia, and the ECG voltage may be decreased or the QRS complexes may alternate in height (electrical alternans). Heart sounds may progress from distant to imperceptible. Neck vein distention and other signs of rising central venous pressure develop. These signs and symptoms occur because as the fluid-filled pericardial sac compresses the myocardium. Blood continues to return to the heart from the periphery but cannot flow into the heart to be pumped back into the circulation.

In such situations, the nurse notifies the physician immediately and prepares to assist with diagnostic echocardiography and pericardiocentesis (see Chapter 30). The nurse stays with the patient and continues to assess and record signs and symptoms while intervening to decrease patient anxiety.

Evaluation

Expected Patient Outcomes

Expected patient outcomes may include:

1. Freedom from pain
   a. Performs activities of daily living without pain, fatigue, or shortness of breath
   b. Temperature returns to normal range
   c. Exhibits no pericardial friction rub
2. Absence of complications
   a. Sustains blood pressure in normal range
   b. Has heart sounds that are strong and can be auscultated
   c. Shows absence of neck vein distention

Critical Thinking Exercises

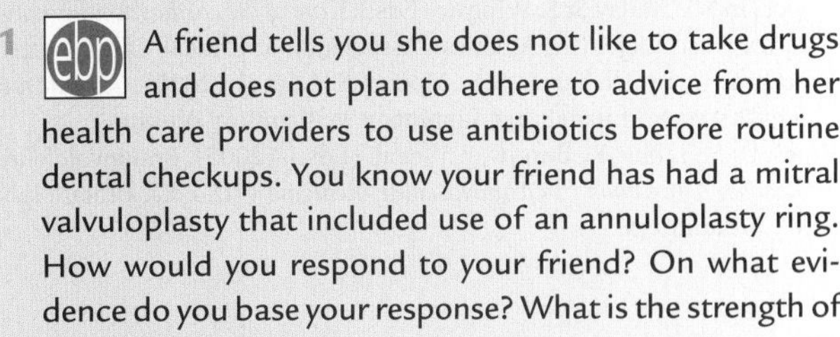

1 ebp A friend tells you she does not like to take drugs and does not plan to adhere to advice from her health care providers to use antibiotics before routine dental checkups. You know your friend has had a mitral valvuloplasty that included use of an annuloplasty ring. How would you respond to your friend? On what evidence do you base your response? What is the strength of that evidence?

2 A 19-year-old man with hypertrophic cardiomyopathy is being discharged from the hospital. He lives alone and states he really needs to get back to the gym to resume his weight training. Based on your knowledge about the developmental tasks of 19-year-olds, what do you anticipate his psychosocial needs would be? His family came to the hospital during the first 2 days of his hospital stay, but they live out of town and have returned home. Should they be included in the plan of care? The cardiologist has requested a consult with transplant services. How will this consult be included in the plan of care?

3 A 68-year-old man with atrial fibrillation, who is recovering from an aortic valve replacement for aortic stenosis and three coronary artery bypass grafts, has been prescribed a beta-blocker, an ACE inhibitor, digoxin, and warfarin. The cardiologist advises the patient to continue to carry nitroglycerin spray for treatment of angina, should it occur. What are this patient's teaching and discharge planning needs? As you care for the patient on the third postoperative day, you assess that the patient has short-term memory deficits. What are your plans to achieve discharge as expected on postoperative day 5 to 7?

4 You are caring for a 34-year-old man with infective endocarditis. He reports difficulty breathing. As you enter the room, you find a very anxious patient sitting upright in bed, breathing very rapidly with audible moist/bubbling respiratory sounds. Perspiration on his face is noticeable. Describe the actions you would take and explain why.

REFERENCES AND SELECTED READINGS

BOOKS

American Heart Association. (2004). *Heart and stroke statistical update.* Dallas, TX: American Heart Association.

Beers, M. H., Berkow, R., & Burs, M. (Eds.) (1999). *The Merck manual of diagnosis and therapy* (17th ed.). Whitehouse Station, NJ: Merck & Co.

Bickley, L. S., & Szilagyi, P. G. (2003). *Bates's guide to physical examination and history taking* (8th ed.). Philadelphia: Lippincott Williams & Wilkins.

Fuster, V., Alexander, R. W., & O'Rourke, R. A. (Eds.). (2004). *Hurst's the heart* (11th ed.). New York: McGraw-Hill.

Lynn-McHale Wiegand, D. J., & Carlson, K. K. (2005). *AACN procedure manual for critical care* (5th ed.). Philadelphia: Elsevier.

Morton, P. G., Fontaine, D. K., Hudak, C. M., & Gallo, B. M. (2005). *Critical care nursing: A holistic approach* (8th ed.). Philadelphia: Lippincott Williams & Wilkins.

Schakenbach, L. H. (2001). Care of the patient with a ventricular assist device. In M. Chulay & S. Wingate (Eds.), *Care of the cardiovascular patient series.* Aliso Viejo, CA: American Association of Critical-Care Nurses.

Woods, S. L., Froelicher, E. S. S., Motzer, S. A., et al. (2005). *Cardiac nursing* (5th ed.). Philadelphia: Lippincott Williams & Wilkins.

Zipes, D. P., Libby, P., Bonow, E.T, et al. (Eds.). (2005). *Braunwald's heart disease: A textbook of cardiovascular medicine* (7th ed.). Philadelphia: W. B. Saunders.

JOURNALS

**Asterisks indicate nursing research articles.*

Aazami, M., & Schafers, H. J. (2003). Advances in heart valve surgery. *Journal of Interventional Cardiology, 16*(6), 535–541.

Avery, R. K. (2003). Cardiac allograft vasculopathy. *New England Journal of Medicine, 349*(9), 829–830.

Bahruth, A. J. (2004). What every patient should . . . pretransplantation and posttransplantation. *Critical Care Nursing Quarterly, 27*(1), 31–60.

Baptiste, M. M. (2001). Aortic valve replacement. *RN, 64*(1), 58–64.

Berul, C., & Zevitz, M. E. (2004). Cardiomyopathy, hypertrophic. *eMedicine.* Retrieved from http://www.emedicine.com/PED/topic1102.htm. Accessed June 11, 2006.

Bond, A. E., Nelson, K., Germany, C. L., et al. (2003). The left ventricular assist device. *American Journal of Nursing, 103*(1), 32–40.

Borer, J. S., & Bonow, R. O. (2003). Contemporary approach to aortic and mitral regurgitation. *Circulation, 108*(20), 2432–2438.

Braunwald, E., Seidman, C. E., & Sigwart, U. (2003). Contemporary evaluation and management of hypertrophic cardiomyopathy. *Circulation, 106*(11), 1312–1316.

Calabrese, F., & Thiene, G. (2003). Myocarditis and inflammatory cardiomyopathy: Microbiological and molecular biological aspects. *Cardiovascular Research, 60*(1), 11–25.

Camp, D. (2000). The left ventricular assist device (LVAD). *Critical Care Nursing Clinics of North America, 12*(1), 61–68.

Cheitlin, M. D., Armstrong, W. F., Aurigemma, G. P., et al. (2003). ACC/AHA/ASE 2003 guideline update for the clinical application of echocardiography: Summary article: A report of the American College of Cardiology/American Heart Association Task Force on Practice Guidelines (ACC/AHA/ASE Committee to Update the 1997 Guidelines for the Clinical Application of Echocardiography). *Circulation, 108*(9), 1146–1162.

Chin, T. K., & Worley, C. (2003). Rheumatic fever. *eMedicine.* Retrieved from http://www.emedicine.com/ped/topic2006.htm. Accessed June 11, 2006.

Christensen, D. M. (2000). The ventricular assist device: An overview. *Nursing Clinics of North America, 35*(4), 945–959.

Christensen, T. D., Andersen, N. T., Attermann, J., et al. (2003). Mechanical heart valve patients can manage oral anticoagulant therapy themselves. *European Journal of Cardio-Thoracic Surgery, 23*(3), 292–298.

Cilliers, A. M., Manyemba, J., & Saloojee, H. (2004). Anti-inflammatory treatment for carditis in acute rheumatic fever. *Cochrane Database of Systematic Reviews, 2.*

Crawford, M. H., & Durack, D. T. (2003). Clinical presentation of infective endocarditis. *Cardiology Clinics, 21*(2), 159–166.

Cruickshank, S. (2004). Cardiomyopathy. *Nursing Standard, 18*(23), 46–55.

Dajani, A. S., Taubert, K. A., Wilson, W., et al. (1997). Prevention of bacterial endocarditis. *Circulation, 96*(1), 358–366.

Deng, M. C. (2002). Cardiac transplantation. *Heart, 87*(2), 177–184.

Deng, M. C., Edwards, L. B., Hertz, M. I., et al. (2003). Mechanical circulatory support device database of the International Society for Heart and Lung Transplantation: First annual report, 2003. *Journal of Heart & Lung Transplantation, 22*(6), 653–662.

Dhawan, V. K. (2003). Infective endocarditis. *Topics in Emergency Medicine, 25*(2), 123–133.

Durack, D., Lukes, A. S., & Bright, D. K. (1994). New criteria for diagnosis of infective endocarditis: Utilization of specific echocardiographic findings. *American Journal of Medicine, 96*(3), 200–209.

*Evangelista, L. S., Doering, L., & Dracup, K. (2003). Meaning and life purpose: Perspectives of post-transplant women. *Heart & Lung, 32*(4), 250–257.

Freed, L. A., Levy, D., Levine, R. A., et al. (1999). Prevalence and clinical outcome of mitral-valve prolapse. *New England Journal of Medicine, 34*(1), 1–7.

Freedman, R. (2001). Use of implantable pacemakers and implantable defibrillators in hypertrophic cardiomyopathy. *Current Opinion in Cardiology, 16*(1), 58–65.

Goldsmith, I., Alexander, G. G., & Lip, G. Y. H. (2002). Valvar heart disease and prosthetic heart valves. *British Medical Journal, 325*(7374), 1228–1231.

Granowitz, E. V. (2003). Risk stratification and bedside prognostication in infective endocarditis. *Journal of the American Medical Association, 289*(15), 1991–1993.

Gulbins, H., Kreuzer, E., & Reichart, B. (2003). Homografts: A review. *Expert Review of Cardiovascular Therapy, 1*(4), 533–539.

Haley, J. H., Tajik, A. J., Danielson, G. K., et al. (2004). Transient constrictive pericarditis: Causes and natural history. *Journal of the American College of Cardiology, 43*(2), 271–275.

Hasbun, R., Vikram, H. R., Barakat, L. A., et al. (2003). Complicated left-sided native valve endocarditis in adults: Risk classification for mortality. *Journal of the American Medical Association, 289*(15), 1933–1940.

Kherani, A. R., & Oz, M. C. (2004). Ventricular assistance to bridge to transplantation. *Surgical Clinics of North America, 84*(1), 75–89, viii–ix.

Lewis, P. S., Boyd, C. M., Hubert, N. E., et al. (2001). Ethanol-induced therapeutic myocardial infarction to treat hypertrophic obstructive cardiomyopathy. *Critical Care Nurse, 21*(2), 20–34.

Maron, B., Estes, N. A. M., III, Maron, M., et al. (2003). Primary prevention of sudden death as a novel treatment strategy in hypertrophic cardiomyopathy. *Circulation, 107*(23), 2872–2875.

Maron, B. J. (2002). Hypertrophic cardiomyopathy: A systematic review. *Journal of the American Medical Association, 287*(10), 1308–1320.

Maron, B. J., McKenna, W. J., Danielson, G. K., et al. (2003). American College of Cardiology/European Society of Cardiology clinical expert consensus document on hypertrophic cardiomyopathy: A report of the American College of Cardiology Foundation Task Force on Clinical Expert Consensus Documents and the European Society of Cardiology Committee for Practice Guidelines. *Journal of the American College of Cardiology, 42*(9), 1687–1713.

Mason, J. W. (2003). Myocarditis and dilated cardiomyopathy: An inflammatory link. *Cardiovascular Research, 60*(1), 5–10.

Mason, V. F., & Konicki, A. J. (2003). Left ventricular assist devices as destination therapy. *AACN Clinical Issues, 14*(4), 488–497.

McKenna, W., & Behr, E. (2002). Hypertrophic cardiomyopathy: Management, risk stratification, and prevention of sudden death. *Heart, 87*(2), 169–176.

McRae, A. I., Chung, M. K., & Asher, C. R. (2001). Arrhythmogenic right ventricular cardiomyopathy: A cause of sudden death in young people. *Cleveland Clinic Journal of Medicine, 68*(5), 459–467.

Miro, J. M., del Rio, A., & Mestres, C. A. (2003). Infective endocarditis and cardiac surgery in IV drug abusers and HIV-1 infected patients. *Cardiology Clinics, 21*(2), 167–184.

Mitka, M. (2003). Trials planned for testing nonsurgical approach to replacing heart valves. *Journal of the American Medical Association, 289*(11), 1366–1367.

Moreillon, P., & Que, Y. A. (2004). Infective endocarditis. *Lancet, 363*(9403), 139–149.

Morse, C. J. (2001). Advanced practice nursing in heart transplantation. *Progress in Cardiovascular Nursing, 16*(1), 21–24, 38.

Moss, R., & Munt, B. (2003). Injection drug use and right sided endocarditis. *Heart, 89*(5), 577–581.

Murtagh, B., Frazier, O. H. & Letsou, G. V. (2003). Diagnosis and management of bacterial endocarditis in 2003. *Current Opinions in Cardiology, 18*(2), 106–110.

Nauer, K. A., Schouchoff, B., & Demitras, K. (2000). Minimally invasive aortic valve surgery. *Critical Care in Nursing Quarterly, 23*(1), 66–71.

Neuner, J. M., Hamel, M. B., Phillips, R. S., et al. (2003). Diagnosis and management of adults with pharyngitis. A cost-effectiveness analysis. *Annals of Internal Medicine, 139*(2), 113–122.

Nishimura, R. A., & Holmes, D. R., Jr. (2004). Hypertrophic obstructive cardiomyopathy. *New England Journal of Medicine, 350*(13), 1320–1327.

Olaison, L., & Pettersson, G. (2003). Current best practices and guidelines. Indications for surgical intervention in infective endocarditis. *Cardiology Clinics, 21*(2), 235–251, vii.

Poston, R. S., & Griffith, B. P. (2004). Heart transplantation. *Journal of Intensive Care Medicine, 19*(1), 3–12.

Rahimtoola, S. H. (2003). Choice of prosthetic heart valve for adult patients. *Journal of the American College of Cardiology, 41*(6), 893–904.

Rhodes, L. R. (2004). Cardiac allograft vasculopathy. *Critical Care Nursing Quarterly, 27*(1), 10–16.

Richardson, P., McKenna, W., Bristow, M., et al. (1996). Report of the 1995 World Health Organization/International Society and Federation of Cardiology Task Force on the Definition and Classification of Cardiomyopathies. *Circulation, 93*(5), 841–842.

Rigatelli, G., Rigatelli, G., Barbiero, M., et al. (2003). "Demand" stimulation of latissimus dorsi heart wrap: Experience in humans and comparison with adynamic girdling. *Annals of Thoracic Surgery, 76*(5), 1587–1592.

Rose, E. A., Gelijns, A. S., Moskowitz, A. J., et al. (2001). Long-term use of a left ventricular assist device for end-stage heart failure. *New England Journal of Medicine, 345*(20), 1435–1443.

Rosenhek, R., Binder, T., & Maurer, G. (2002). Intraoperative transesophageal echocardiography in valve replacement surgery. *Echocardiography, 19*(8), 701–707.

Savage, L. (2003). Quality of life among patients with a left ventricular assist device: What is new? *AACN Clinical Issues: Advanced Practice in Acute Critical Care, 14*(1), 64–72.

Schmid, M. W. (2000). Risks and complications of peripherally and centrally inserted IV catheters. *Critical Care Nursing Clinics of North America, 12*(2), 165–174.

Sexton, D. J., & Spelman, D. (2003). Current best practices and guidelines. Assessment and management of complications in infective endocarditis. *Cardiology Clinics, 21*(2), 273–282, vii–viii.

Shaddy, R. E. (2004). Cardiomyopathy, restrictive. *eMedicine.* Retrieved from http://www.emedicine.com/PED/topic2503.htm. Accessed June 11, 2006.

Soler, R., Rodriguez, E., Remuinan, C., et al. (2003). Magnetic resonance imaging of primary cardiomyopathies. *Journal of Computer Assisted Tomography, 27*(5), 724–734.

Special Writing Group of the Committee on Rheumatic Fever, Endocarditis, and Kawasaki's Disease of the Council on Cardiovascular Disease in the Young of the American Heart Association. (1992). Guidelines for the diagnosis of rheumatic fever. Jones Criteria, 1992 update. *Journal of the American Medical Association, 268*(15), 2069–2973.

Starr, A., Fessler, C. L., Grunkemeier, G., et al. (2002). Heart valve replacement surgery: Past, present and future. *Clinical & Experimental Pharmacology & Physiology, 29*(8), 735–738.

Stewart, K. J., Badenhop, D., Brubaker, P. H., et al. (2003). Cardiac rehabilitation following percutaneous revascularization, heart transplant, heart valve surgery, and for chronic heart failure. *Chest, 123*(6), 2104–2111.

Tam, J., Shaikh, N., & Sutherland, E. (2002). Echocardiographic assessment of patients with hypertrophic and restrictive cardiomyopathy: Imaging and echocardiography. *Current Opinion in Cardiology, 17*(5), 470–477.

Taylor, D. O., Edwards, L. B., Mohacsi, P. J., et al. (2003). The registry of the International Society for Heart and Lung Transplantation: Twentieth official adult heart transplant report—2003. *Journal of Heart and Lung Transplantation, 22*(6), 616–624.

Wade, C. R., Reith, K. K., Sikora, J. H., et al. (2004). Postoperative nursing care of the cardiac transplant recipient. *Critical Care Nursing Quarterly, 27*(1), 17–28.

Wiegand, D. L. (2003). Cardiovascular surgery. Advances in cardiac surgery: Valve repair. *Critical Care Nurse, 23*(2), 72–91.

RESOURCES

American Heart Association, National Center, 7272 Greenville Avenue, Dallas, TX 75231; 1-800-242-8721; http://www.americanheart.org. Accessed June 2, 2006.

Cardiomyopathy Association, 40 Metro Center, Tolpits Lane, Watford, Herts, WD18 9SB, United Kingdom; 44-(0)-1923-249-977; www.cardiomyopathy.org. Accessed June 2, 2006.

Heartmates, Inc., P.O. Box 16202, Minneapolis, MN 55416; 612-558-3331; http://www.heartmates.com. Accessed June 2, 2006.

National Heart, Lung, and Blood Institute, Health Information Center, National Institutes of Health, P.O. Box 30105, Bethesda, MD 20824-0105; 301-592-8573; http://www.nhlbi.nih.gov. Accessed June 2, 2006.

CHAPTER 30

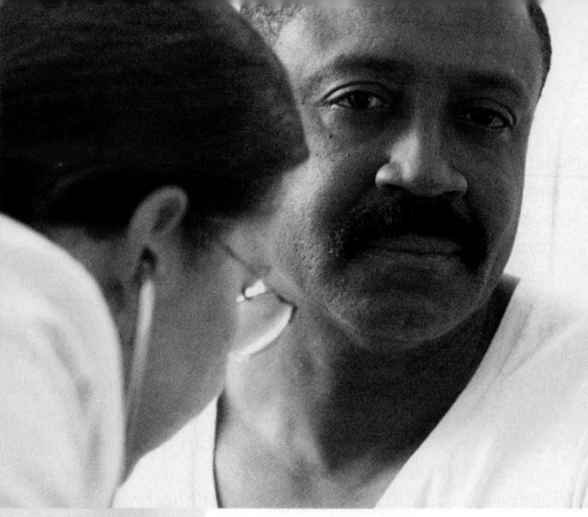

Management of Patients With Complications From Heart Disease

Learning Objectives

On completion of this chapter, the learner will be able to:

1. Describe the management of patients with heart failure (HF).
2. Use the nursing process as a framework for care of patients with HF.
3. Develop a teaching plan for patients with HF.
4. Describe the management of patients with pulmonary edema and cardiogenic shock.
5. Describe the management of patients with thromboembolism, pericardial effusion, and sudden cardiac death.

Today, the patient with heart disease can be assisted to live longer and achieve a higher quality of life than even a decade ago. Through advances in diagnostic procedures that allow earlier and more accurate diagnoses, treatment can begin well before significant debilitation occurs. Newer treatments, technologies, and pharmacotherapies are being developed rapidly. However, heart disease remains a chronic condition, and complications may develop. This chapter presents the complications most often resulting from heart diseases and the treatments provided by the health care team for these complications.

Cardiac Hemodynamics

The basic function of the heart is to pump blood. The heart's ability to pump is measured by **cardiac output (CO)**, the amount of blood pumped per minute. CO is determined by measuring the heart rate (HR) and multiplying it by the **stroke volume (SV)**, the amount of blood pumped out of the ventricle with each contraction. CO usually is calculated using the equation CO = HR × SV.

The HR is primarily controlled by the autonomic nervous system. When SV decreases, the nervous system is stimulated to increase HR and thereby maintain adequate CO. HR is easily measured, but SV is more difficult to measure precisely. SV depends on three factors: preload, afterload, and contractility (Fig. 30-1). Precise measurement of these factors requires hemodynamic monitoring.

Preload is the amount of blood presented to the ventricle just before systole. It increases pressure in the ventricle, which stretches the ventricular wall. Like a rubber band, the ventricular muscle fibers need to be stretched (by blood volume) to produce optimal ejection of blood. Too little or too much muscle fiber stretch decreases the volume of blood ejected. The major factor that determines preload is venous return, the volume of blood that enters the ventricle during diastole. Another factor that determines preload is ventricular **compliance**, the elasticity or amount of "give" when blood enters the ventricle. Elasticity is decreased when the muscle thickens, as in hypertrophic cardiomyopathy (see Chapter 29) or when there is increased fibrotic tissue within the ventricle. Fibrotic tissue replaces dead myocardial cells, such as after a myocardial infarction (MI) (see Chapter 28). Fibrotic tissue has little compliance, making the ventricle stiff. Given the same volume of blood, a noncompliant ventricle has a higher intraventricular pressure than a compliant one. Higher pressure increases the workload of the heart and can lead to **heart failure (HF)** if it is sustained.

Glossary

afterload: the amount of resistance to ejection of blood from a ventricle

anuria: urine output of less than 50 mL per 24 hours

ascites: an accumulation of serous fluid in the peritoneal cavity

cardiac output (CO): the amount of blood pumped out of the heart in 1 minute

cardiac resynchronization therapy (CRT): a treatment for heart failure in which a device paces both ventricles to synchronize contractions

compliance: the elasticity or amount of "give" when blood enters the ventricle

congestive heart failure (CHF): a fluid overload condition (congestion) associated with heart failure

contractility: the force of ventricular contraction; related to the number and state of myocardial cells

diastolic heart failure: the inability of the heart to pump sufficiently because of an alteration in the ability of the heart to fill; current term used to describe a type of heart failure

dyspnea on exertion (DOE): shortness of breath that occurs with exertion

ejection fraction (EF): percentage of blood volume in the ventricles at the end of diastole that is ejected during systole; a measurement of contractility

heart failure (HF): the inability of the heart to pump sufficient blood to meet the needs of the tissues for oxygen and nutrients; signs and symptoms of pulmonary and systemic congestion may or may not be present

implantable cardioverter defibrillator (ICD): a device implanted in patients with ventricular dysrhythmias that detects and treats dysrhythmias

left-sided heart failure (left ventricular failure): inability of the left ventricle to fill or pump (empty) sufficient blood to meet the needs of the tissues for oxygen and nutrients; traditional term used to describe patient's symptoms of heart failure

oliguria: diminished urine output; less than 400 mL per 24 hours

orthopnea: shortness of breath when lying flat

paroxysmal nocturnal dyspnea (PND): shortness of breath that occurs suddenly during sleep

pericardiocentesis: procedure that involves aspiration of fluid from the pericardial sac

pericardiotomy: surgically created opening of the pericardium

preload: the amount of myocardial stretch just before systole caused by the volume of blood presented to the ventricle

pulmonary edema: abnormal accumulation of fluid in the interstitial spaces or in the alveoli of the lungs

pulseless electrical activity (PEA): condition in which electrical activity is present but there is not an adequate pulse or blood pressure because of ineffective cardiac contraction or circulating blood volume

pulsus paradoxus: systolic blood pressure of more than 10 mm Hg higher during exhalation than during inspiration; difference is normally less than 10 mm Hg

right-sided heart failure (right ventricular failure): inability of the right ventricle to fill or pump (empty) sufficient blood to the pulmonary circulation

stroke volume (SV): amount of blood pumped out of the ventricle with each contraction

systolic heart failure: inability of the heart to pump sufficiently because of an alteration in the ability of the heart to contract; current term used to describe a type of heart failure

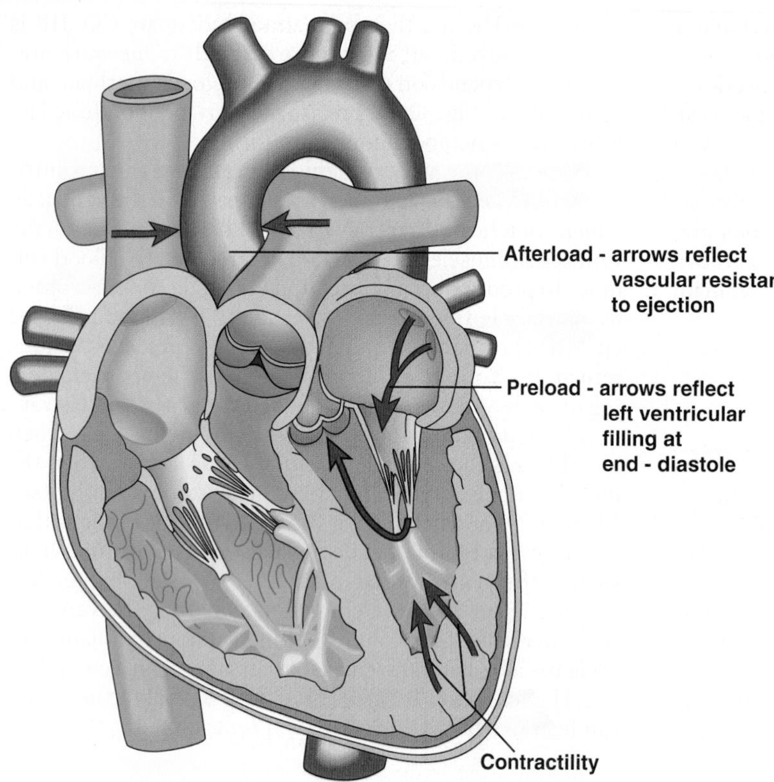

FIGURE 30-1. The determinants of stroke volume (SV). The SV is determined by the amount of preload presented to the ventricle, the amount of afterload or resistance to ventricular ejection, and the strength of cardiac contractility. The cardiac output is the product of SV and heart rate. Redrawn from Porth, C. M. (2005). *Pathophysiology: Concepts of altered health states* (7th ed.). Philadelphia: Lippincott Williams & Wilkins.

Afterload refers to the amount of resistance to the ejection of blood from the ventricle. To eject blood, the ventricle must overcome the resistance caused by tension in the aorta and systemic vessels. Afterload is inversely related to SV, and an increase in afterload causes the ventricle to work harder and may decrease the amount of blood ejected. The major factors that determine afterload are the diameter and distensibility of the great vessels (aorta and pulmonary artery) and the opening and competence of the semilunar valves (pulmonic and aortic valves). When the valves open easily, resistance is lower. If the patient has significant vasoconstriction, hypertension, or a narrowed valvular opening from stenosis, resistance (afterload) increases. When afterload increases, the workload of the heart must increase to overcome the resistance and eject blood.

Contractility, the force of contraction, is related to the status of the myocardium. Catecholamines, released by sympathetic stimulation during exercise or from administration of positive inotropic medications, can increase contractility and SV. MI causes necrosis and subsequent fibrosis of some myocardial cells, shifting the workload to the remaining cells. Significant loss of myocardial cells can decrease contractility and cause HF. Afterload can be reduced by medications to match the lower contractility and maintain adequate CO.

Noninvasive Assessment of Cardiac Hemodynamics

Several noninvasive assessment findings can indicate cardiac hemodynamic status, although the findings do not directly correlate to preload, afterload, or contractility. Right ventricular preload may be estimated by measuring jugular venous distention (JVD). Elevated left ventricular preload may be identified by a positive hepatojugular test. Mean arterial blood pressure is an approximate indicator of left ventricular afterload. Activity tolerance may be used as an indicator of overall cardiac functioning. These assessments are described in more detail later in this chapter.

Invasive Assessment of Cardiac Hemodynamics

An important tool for evaluating the components of SV in a hemodynamically unstable patient is the pulmonary artery catheter, which is used to obtain the hemodynamic data essential for diagnosis and treatment (see Chapter 26). Measurements of intracardiac pressures, pulmonary artery pressures, and cardiac output are made at intervals. Therapy, especially intravenous (IV) medication, is adjusted based on the assessment and diagnostic findings. The patient with an invasive hemodynamic catheter is usually managed in an intensive care environment because of the need for frequent nursing assessments and interventions.

Heart Failure

HF is the inability of the heart to pump sufficient blood to meet the needs of the tissues for oxygen and nutrients. In the past, HF was often referred to as **congestive heart failure (CHF)**, because many patients experience pulmonary or peripheral congestion. Currently HF is recognized as a clinical syndrome characterized by signs and symptoms of fluid overload or of inadequate tissue perfusion. Fluid overload and decreased tissue perfusion result when the heart cannot generate a CO sufficient to meet the body's demands. The term HF indicates myocardial disease in which there is a problem with contraction of the heart (systolic dysfunction) or filling of the heart (diastolic dysfunction) that may or may not cause pulmonary or systemic congestion. Some cases of HF are reversible, depending on the cause. Most often, HF is a progressive, life-long diagnosis that is managed with lifestyle changes and medications to prevent acute congestive episodes.

Chronic Heart Failure

As with coronary artery disease, the incidence of HF increases with age. At least 5 million people in the United States have HF, and 550,000 new cases are diagnosed each year (American Heart Association [AHA], 2004). Although HF can affect people of all ages, the prevalence in people older than 75 years of age is about 10%, and as the U.S. population ages, HF has become an epidemic that challenges the country's health care resources (AHA, 2004). HF is the most common reason for hospitalization of people older than 65 years of age and the second most common reason for visits to a physician's office. The rate of hospital readmission remains staggeringly high. The economic burden caused by HF is estimated to be more than $25 billion in direct and indirect costs and is expected to increase (AHA, 2004).

The increase in the incidence of HF reflects the increased number of elderly people and improvements in treatment of cardiac diseases, resulting in increased survival rates. Many hospitalizations could be prevented by appropriate outpatient care. Prevention and early intervention to arrest the progression of HF are major health initiatives in the United States.

There are two types of HF, which are identified by assessment of left ventricular functioning, usually by echocardiogram. The more common type is an alteration in ventricular contraction called **systolic heart failure**, which is characterized by a weakened heart muscle. The less common alteration is **diastolic heart failure**, which is characterized by a stiff and noncompliant heart muscle, making it difficult for the ventricle to fill. An assessment of the **ejection fraction (EF)** is performed to assist in determining the type of HF. EF, an indication of the volume of blood ejected with each contraction, is calculated by subtracting the amount of blood at the end of systole from the amount at the end of diastole and calculating the percentage of blood that is ejected. A normal EF is 55% to 65% of the ventricular volume; the ventricle does not completely empty between contractions. The EF is normal in diastolic HF but severely reduced in systolic HF.

Although a low EF is a hallmark of HF, the severity of HF is frequently classified according to the patient's symptoms. The New York Heart Association (NYHA) Classification is described in Table 30-1, and the causes are explained in subsequent sections of this chapter. The American College of Cardiology and the American Heart Association (ACC/AHA) have proposed a new HF classification system (Institute for Clinical Systems Improvement [ICSI], 2004). This system (Table 30-2) takes into consideration the natural history and progressive nature of HF. Treatment guidelines have been developed for each stage.

TABLE 30-1 New York Heart Association (NYHA) Classification of Heart Failure

Classification	Symptoms	Prognosis
I	Ordinary physical activity does not cause undue fatigue, dyspnea, palpitations, or chest pain No pulmonary congestion or peripheral hypotension Patient is considered asymptomatic Usually no limitations of activities of daily living (ADLs)	Good
II	Slight limitation on ADLs Patient reports no symptoms at rest but increased physical activity will cause symptoms Basilar crackles and S_3 murmur may be detected	Good
III	Marked limitation on ADL Patient feels comfortable at rest but less than ordinary activity will cause symptoms	Fair
IV	Symptoms of cardiac insufficiency at rest	Poor

Pathophysiology

HF results from a variety of cardiovascular conditions, including chronic hypertension, coronary artery disease, and valvular disease. These conditions can result in decreased contraction (systole), decreased filling (diastole), or both. Significant myocardial dysfunction most often occurs before the patient experiences signs and symptoms of HF such as shortness of breath, edema, or fatigue.

As HF develops, the body activates neurohormonal compensatory mechanisms. These mechanisms represent the

TABLE 30-2 American College of Cardiology and American Heart Association (ACC/AHA) Classification of Heart Failure

Classification	Symptoms
Stage A	Patients at high risk of developing left ventricular dysfunction
Stage B	Patients with left ventricular dysfunction who have not developed symptoms
Stage C	Patients with left ventricular dysfunction with current or prior symptoms
Stage D	Patients with refractory end-stage heart failure

body's attempt to cope with the HF and are responsible for the signs and symptoms that eventually develop. Understanding these mechanisms is important because the treatment of HF is aimed at relieving them.

Systolic HF results in decreased blood volume being ejected from the ventricle. The decreased ventricular stretch is sensed by baroreceptors in the aortic and carotid bodies (Piano & Prasun, 2003). The sympathetic nervous system is then stimulated to release epinephrine and norepinephrine (Fig. 30-2). The purpose of this initial response is to increase heart rate and contractility and support the failing myocardium, but the continued response has multiple negative effects. Sympathetic stimulation causes vasoconstriction of the skin, gastrointestinal tract, and kidneys. A decrease in renal perfusion due to low CO and vasoconstriction then causes the release of renin by the kidney. Renin promotes the formation of angiotensin I, a benign, inactive substance. Angiotensin-converting enzyme (ACE) in the lumen of pulmonary blood vessels converts angiotensin I to angiotensin II, a potent vasoconstrictor, which then increases the blood pressure and afterload. Angiotensin II also stimulates the release of aldosterone from the adrenal cortex, resulting in sodium and fluid retention by the renal tubules and stimulating the thirst center. This leads to the fluid volume overload commonly seen in HF. Angiotensin, aldosterone, and other neurohormones (eg, endothelin, prostacyclin) lead to an increase in preload and afterload, which increases stress on the ventricular wall, causing an increase in the workload of the heart. A counterregulatory mechanism is attempted through the release of natriuretic peptides. Atrial natriuretic peptide (ANP) and B-type natriuretic peptide (BNP) are released from the overdistended cardiac chambers. These substances promote vasodilation and diuresis. However, their effect is usually not strong enough to overcome the negative effects of the other mechanisms.

As the heart's workload increases, contractility of the myocardial muscle fibers decreases. Decreased contractility results in an increase in end-diastolic blood volume in the ventricle, stretching the myocardial muscle fibers and increasing the size of the ventricle (ventricular dilation). The increased size of the ventricle further increases the stress on the ventricular wall, adding to the workload of the heart. One way the heart compensates for the increased workload is to increase the thickness of the heart muscle (ventricular hypertrophy). However, hypertrophy results in an abnormal proliferation of myocardial cells, a process known as ventricular remodeling. Under the influence of neurohormones (eg, angiotensin II), large myocardial cells are produced that are dysfunctional and die early, leaving the other normal myocardial cells to struggle to maintain CO (Ammon, 2001). The compensatory mechanisms of HF have been called the "vicious cycle of HF" because the heart does not pump sufficient blood to the body, which causes the body to stimulate the heart to work harder; the heart cannot respond and failure becomes worse.

Diastolic HF develops because of continued increased workload on the heart, which responds by increasing the number and size of myocardial cells (ie, ventricular hypertrophy and altered cellular functioning). These responses cause resistance to ventricular filling, which increases ventricular filling pressures despite a normal or reduced blood volume. Less blood in the ventricles causes decreased CO. The low CO and high ventricular filling pressures can cause the same neurohormonal responses as described for systolic HF.

Etiology

Myocardial dysfunction is most often caused by coronary artery disease, cardiomyopathy, hypertension, or valvular disorders. Patients with diabetes mellitus are also at high risk for HF. Atherosclerosis of the coronary arteries is the primary cause of HF, and coronary artery disease is found in more than 60% of the patients with HF (Zipes, Libby, & Bonow, 2005). Ischemia causes myocardial dysfunction because of resulting hypoxia and acidosis from the accumulation of lactic acid. MI causes focal heart muscle necrosis, the death of myocardial cells, and a loss of contractility; the extent of the infarction correlates with the severity of HF. Revascularization of the coronary artery by a percutaneous coronary intervention or by coronary artery bypass surgery may improve myocardial oxygenation and ventricular function.

Cardiomyopathy is a disease of the myocardium. There are three types: dilated, hypertrophic, and restrictive (see Chapter 29). Dilated cardiomyopathy, the most common type of cardiomyopathy, causes diffuse cellular necrosis and fibrosis, leading to decreased contractility (systolic failure). Dilated cardiomyopathy can be idiopathic (unknown cause), or it can result from an inflammatory process, such as myocarditis, or from a cytotoxic agent, such as alcohol or doxorubicin (Adriamycin). Hypertrophic cardiomyopathy and restrictive cardiomyopathy lead to decreased distensibility and ventricular filling (diastolic failure). Usually, HF due to cardiomyopathy becomes chronic and progressive. However, cardiomyopathy and HF may resolve following removal of the causative agent, such as with the cessation of alcohol ingestion.

Systemic or pulmonary hypertension increases afterload (resistance to ejection), which increases the workload of the heart and leads to hypertrophy of myocardial muscle fibers; this can be considered a compensatory mechanism because it increases contractility. However, the hypertrophy may impair the heart's ability to fill properly during diastole, and the hypertrophied ventricle may eventually fail.

Valvular heart disease is also a cause of HF. The valves ensure that blood flows in one direction. With valvular dysfunction, blood has increasing difficulty moving forward, increasing pressure within the heart and increasing cardiac workload, leading to HF. Chapter 29 discusses the effects of valvular heart disease.

Several systemic conditions contribute to the development and severity of HF, including increased metabolic rate (eg, fever, thyrotoxicosis), iron overload (eg, from hemochromatosis), hypoxia, and severe anemia (serum hematocrit less than 25%). All of these conditions require an increase in CO to satisfy the systemic oxygen demand. Hypoxia or anemia also may decrease the supply of oxygen to the myocardium. Cardiac dysrhythmias may cause HF or may be a result of HF; either way, the altered electrical stimulation impairs myocardial contraction and decreases the overall efficiency of myocardial function. Other factors, such as acidosis (respiratory or metabolic), electrolyte abnormalities, and antiarrhythmic medications, can worsen myocardial function.

Physiology/Pathophysiology

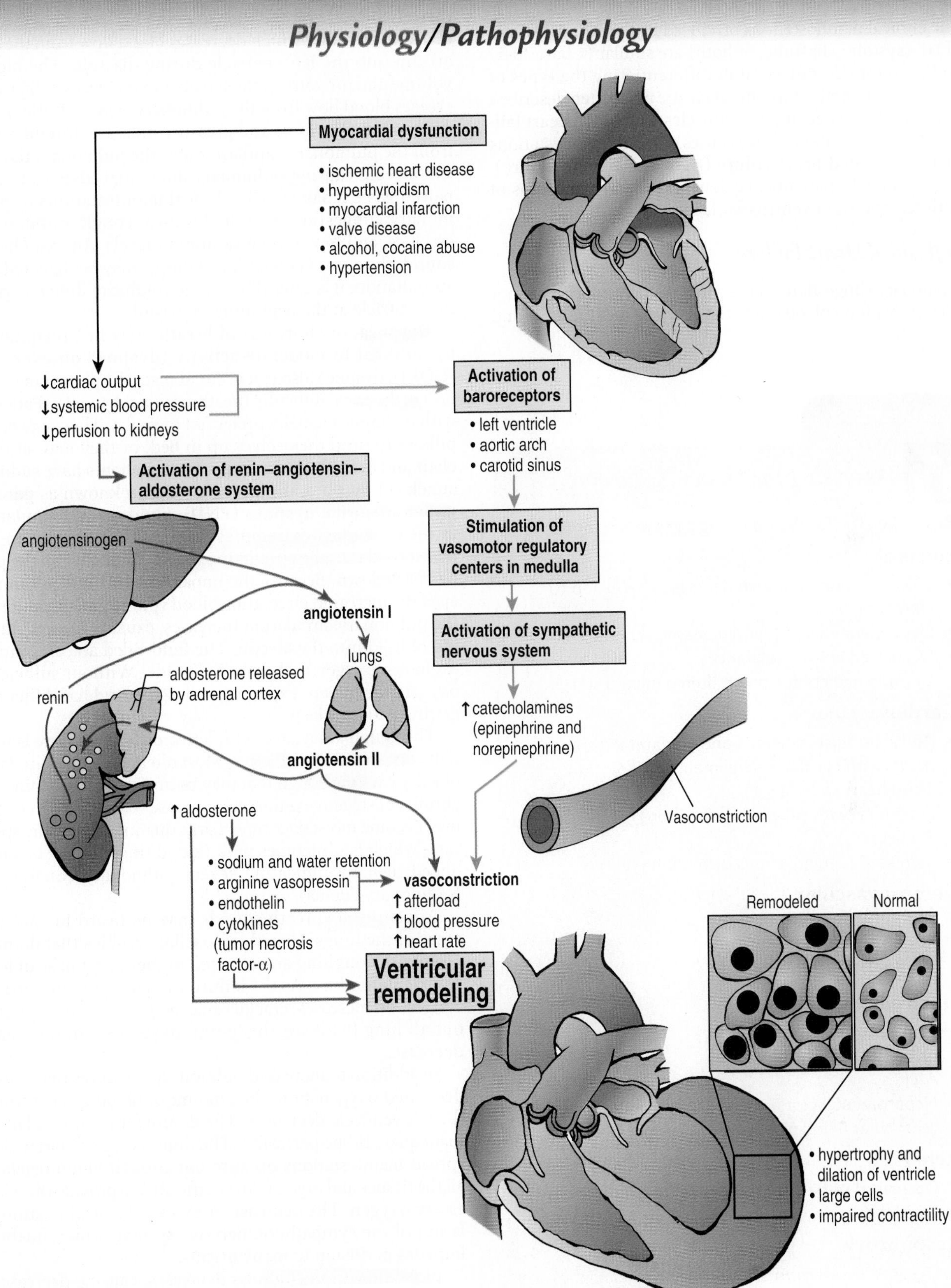

FIGURE 30-2. The pathophysiology of heart failure. A decrease in cardiac output activates multiple neurohormonal mechanisms that ultimately result in the signs and symptoms of heart failure.

Clinical Manifestations

The clinical manifestations produced by the different types of HF (systolic, diastolic, or both) are similar (Chart 30-1) and therefore do not assist in differentiating the types of HF. The signs and symptoms of HF are most often described in terms of the effect on the ventricles. **Left-sided heart failure (left ventricular failure)** causes different manifestations than **right-sided heart failure (right ventricular failure)**. In chronic HF, patients may have signs and symptoms of both left and right ventricular failure.

Left-Sided Heart Failure

Pulmonary congestion occurs when the left ventricle cannot effectively pump blood out of the ventricle into the aorta and the systemic circulation. The increased left ventricular end-diastolic blood volume increases the left ventricular end-diastolic pressure, which decreases blood flow from the left atrium into the left ventricle during diastole. The blood volume and pressure in the left atrium increases, which decreases blood flow from the pulmonary vessels. Pulmonary venous blood volume and pressure increase, forcing fluid from the pulmonary capillaries into the pulmonary tissues and alveoli, causing pulmonary interstitial edema and impaired gas exchange. The clinical manifestations of pulmonary congestion include dyspnea, cough, pulmonary crackles, and low oxygen saturation levels. An extra heart sound, the S_3, or ventricular "gallop," may be detected on auscultation. It is caused by a large volume of fluid entering the ventricle at the beginning of diastole.

Dyspnea, or shortness of breath, may be precipitated by minimal to moderate activity (**dyspnea on exertion [DOE]**); dyspnea also can occur at rest. The patient may report **orthopnea**, difficulty breathing when lying flat. Patients with orthopnea usually prefer not to lie flat. They may need pillows to prop themselves up in bed, or they may sit in a chair and even sleep sitting up. Some patients have sudden attacks of dyspnea at night, a condition known as **paroxysmal nocturnal dyspnea (PND)**. Fluid that accumulated in the dependent extremities during the day begins to be reabsorbed into the circulating blood volume when the patient lies down. Because the impaired left ventricle cannot eject the increased circulating blood volume, the pressure in the pulmonary circulation increases, causing further shifting of fluid into the alveoli. The fluid-filled alveoli cannot exchange oxygen and carbon dioxide. Without sufficient oxygen, the patient experiences dyspnea and has difficulty getting enough sleep.

The cough associated with left ventricular failure is initially dry and nonproductive. Most often, patients complain of a dry hacking cough that may be mislabeled as asthma or chronic obstructive pulmonary disease (COPD). The cough may become moist over time. Large quantities of frothy sputum, which is sometimes pink (blood-tinged), may be produced, usually indicating severe pulmonary congestion (pulmonary edema).

Adventitious breath sounds may be heard in various areas of the lungs. Usually, bibasilar crackles that do not clear with coughing are detected in the early phase of left ventricular failure. As the failure worsens and pulmonary congestion increases, crackles may be auscultated throughout all lung fields. At this point, oxygen saturation may decrease.

In addition to increased pulmonary pressures that cause decreased oxygenation, the amount of blood ejected from the left ventricle decreases. The dominant feature in HF is inadequate tissue perfusion. The diminished CO has widespread manifestations because not enough blood reaches all the tissues and organs (low perfusion) to provide the necessary oxygen. The decrease in SV can also lead to stimulation of the sympathetic nervous system, which further impedes perfusion to many organs.

Blood flow to the kidneys decreases, causing decreased perfusion and reduced urine output (**oliguria**). Renal perfusion pressure falls, which results in the release of renin from the kidney. Release of renin leads to aldosterone secretion and increased intravascular volume. However, when the patient is sleeping, the cardiac workload is decreased,

CHART 30-1

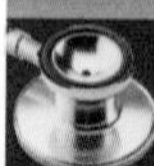

Assessing for Heart Failure

Be on the alert for the following signs and symptoms:

General
- Pale, cyanotic skin (with decreased perfusion to extremities)
- Dependent edema (with increased venous pressure)
- Decreased activity tolerance
- Unexplained confusion or altered mental status

Cardiovascular
- Apical impulse, enlarged and left lateral displacement (with cardiac enlargement)
- Third heart sound (S_3)
- Murmurs (with valvular dysfunction)
- Tachycardia
- Increased jugular venous distention (JVD)

Cerebrovascular
- Lightheadedness
- Dizziness
- Confusion

Gastrointestinal
- Nausea and anorexia
- Enlarged liver
- Ascites
- Hepatojugular test, increased (with increased right ventricular filling pressure)

Renal
- Decreased urinary frequency during the day
- Nocturia

Respiratory
- Dyspnea on exertion
- Orthopnea
- Paroxysmal nocturnal dyspnea
- Bilateral crackles that do not clear with cough
- Cough on exertion or when supine

improving renal perfusion, which may then lead to frequent urination at night (nocturia).

As HF progresses, decreased CO may cause other symptoms. Decreased gastrointestinal perfusion causes altered digestion. Decreased brain perfusion causes dizziness, lightheadedness, confusion, restlessness, and anxiety due to decreased oxygenation and blood flow. As anxiety increases, so does dyspnea, increasing anxiety and creating a vicious cycle. Stimulation of the sympathetic system also causes the peripheral blood vessels to constrict, so the skin appears pale or ashen and feels cool and clammy.

Decreases in ejected ventricular volume cause the sympathetic nervous system to increase the heart rate (tachycardia), often causing the patient to complain of palpitations. The pulses become weak and thready. Without adequate CO, the body cannot respond to increased energy demands, and the patient becomes easily fatigued and has decreased activity tolerance. Fatigue also results from the increased energy expended in breathing and the insomnia that results from respiratory distress, coughing, and nocturia.

Right-Sided Heart Failure

When the right ventricle fails, congestion in the peripheral tissues and the viscera predominates. This occurs because the right side of the heart cannot eject blood and cannot accommodate all the blood that normally returns to it from the venous circulation. Increased venous pressure leads to JVD and increased hydrostatic pressure throughout the venous system.

The systemic clinical manifestations include edema of the lower extremities (dependent edema), hepatomegaly (enlargement of the liver), **ascites** (accumulation of fluid in the peritoneal cavity), anorexia and nausea, and weakness and weight gain due to retention of fluid.

Edema usually affects the feet and ankles and worsens when the patient stands or dangles the legs. The edema decreases when the patient elevates the legs. The edema can gradually progress up the legs and thighs and eventually into the external genitalia and lower trunk. Edema in the abdomen, as evidenced by increased abdominal girth, may be the only edema present. Sacral edema is not uncommon in patients who are on bed rest, because the sacral area is dependent. Pitting edema, in which indentations in the skin remain after even slight compression with the fingertips (Fig. 30-3), is obvious only after retention of at least 4.5 kg (10 lb) of fluid (4.5 L).

Hepatomegaly and tenderness in the right upper quadrant of the abdomen result from venous engorgement of the liver. The increased pressure may interfere with the liver's ability to function (secondary liver dysfunction). As hepatic dysfunction progresses, increased pressure within the portal vessels may force fluid into the abdominal cavity, a condition known as ascites. Ascites may increase pressure on the stomach and intestines and cause gastrointestinal distress. Hepatomegaly may also increase pressure on the diaphragm, causing respiratory distress.

Anorexia (loss of appetite) and nausea or abdominal pain results from the venous engorgement and venous stasis within the abdominal organs. The weakness that accompanies right-sided HF results from reduced CO, impaired circulation, and inadequate removal of catabolic waste products from the tissues.

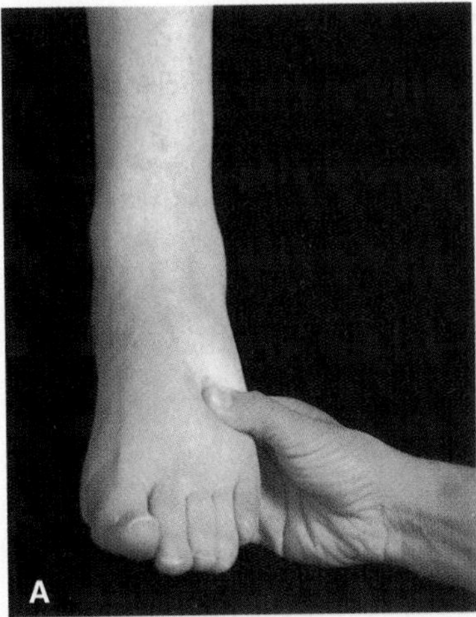

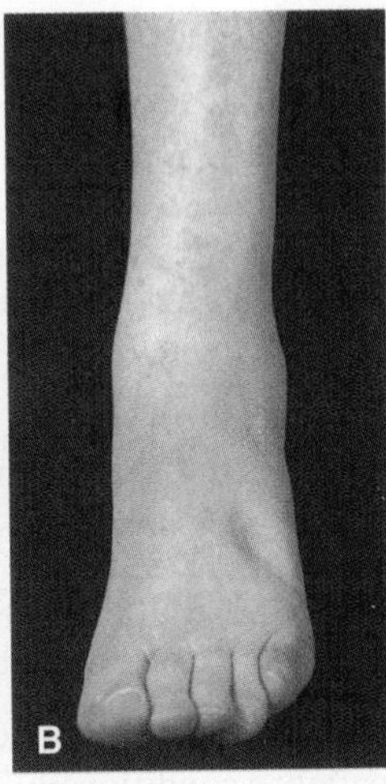

FIGURE 30-3. Example of pitting edema. (**A**) The nurse applies finger pressure to an area near the ankle. (**B**) When the pressure is released, an indentation remains in the edematous tissue. From Bickley, L. S. & Szilagyi, P. G. (2005). *Bates' guide to physical examination and history taking* (9th ed). Philadelphia: Lippincott Williams & Wilkins.

Assessment and Diagnostic Findings

HF may go undetected until the patient presents with signs and symptoms of pulmonary and peripheral edema. However, the physical signs that suggest HF may also occur with other diseases, such as renal failure, liver failure, oncologic conditions, and COPD. If further assessment and evaluation are not completed, these patients may be treated for HF inappropriately. Assessment of ventricular function is an essential part of the initial diagnostic workup.

An echocardiogram is usually performed to confirm the diagnosis of HF, help identify the underlying cause, and determine the EF, which helps identify the type and severity of HF. This information may also be obtained noninvasively by radionuclide ventriculography or invasively by ventriculography as part of a cardiac catheterization procedure. A chest x-ray and an electrocardiogram (ECG) are obtained to assist in the diagnosis and to determine the underlying cause of HF. Laboratory studies usually completed in the initial workup include serum electrolytes, blood urea nitrogen (BUN), creatinine, thyroid-stimulating hormone, complete blood cell count, B-type natriuretic peptide (BNP), and routine urinalysis. The BNP level is a key diagnostic indicator of HF. High levels of BNP are a sign of high cardiac filling pressure and can aid in the diagnosis of HF (ICSI, 2004). The results of these laboratory studies assist in determining the underlying cause and can also be used to establish a baseline to assess effects of treatment. Exercise testing or cardiac catheterization may be performed to determine whether coronary artery disease and cardiac ischemia are causing the HF.

In patients with acute MI who are at risk for HF, ventricular function is assessed before discharge from the hospital. Quantifying the degree of left-ventricular dysfunction is important to determine appropriate medical management. Evaluation of ventricular function may also be performed if the initial assessment of HF suggested noncardiac causes but treatment failed to produce a response.

Medical Management

The overall goals of management of HF are to relieve patient symptoms, to improve functional status and quality of life, and to extend survival. Medical management is based on the type, severity, and cause of HF. Specific objectives of medical management include the following:

- Eliminate or reduce any etiologic contributory factors, especially those that may be reversible (eg, atrial fibrillation, excessive alcohol ingestion)
- Reduce the workload on the heart by reducing afterload and preload
- Optimize all therapeutic regimens
- Prevent exacerbations of HF

Treatment options vary according to the severity of the patient's condition and may include basic lifestyle changes, oral and IV pharmacologic management, supplemental oxygen, implantation of assistive devices, and surgical approaches, including cardiac transplantation.

Managing the patient with HF includes providing general education and counseling to the patient and family. It is important that the patient and family understand the nature of HF and the importance of their participation in the treatment regimen. Lifestyle recommendations include restriction of dietary sodium; avoidance of excessive fluid intake, alcohol, and smoking; weight reduction when indicated; and regular exercise. The patient must know how to recognize signs and symptoms that need to be reported to the health care professional.

Pharmacologic Therapy

Several medications are routinely prescribed for systolic HF, including ACE inhibitors, beta-blockers, diuretics, and digitalis. Medications for diastolic failure depend on the underlying condition, such as hypertension (see Chapter 32) or valvular dysfunction (see Chapter 29).

ANGIOTENSIN-CONVERTING ENZYME INHIBITORS

ACE inhibitors play a pivotal role in the management of HF due to systolic dysfunction. They have been found to relieve the signs and symptoms of HF and significantly decrease mortality and morbidity. ACE inhibitors slow the progression of HF, improve exercise tolerance, and decrease the number of hospitalizations for HF (Moser & Biddle, 2003). Available as oral and IV medications, ACE inhibitors promote vasodilation and diuresis by decreasing afterload and preload. By doing so, they decrease the workload of the heart. Vasodilation reduces resistance to left ventricular ejection of blood, diminishing the heart's workload and improving ventricular emptying. In promoting diuresis, ACE inhibitors decrease the secretion of aldosterone, a hormone that causes the kidneys to retain sodium and water. ACE inhibitors stimulate the kidneys to excrete sodium and fluid (while retaining potassium), thereby reducing left ventricular filling pressure and decreasing pulmonary congestion. ACE inhibitors may be the first medication prescribed for patients in mild failure—patients with fatigue or DOE but without signs of fluid overload and pulmonary congestion.

ACE inhibitors are started at a low dose that is increased every 2 weeks until the optimal dose is achieved and the patient is hemodynamically stable. The final maintenance dose depends on the patient's blood pressure, fluid status, and renal status and on the severity of the HF.

Patients receiving ACE inhibitors are monitored for hypotension, hypovolemia, hyperkalemia, and alterations in renal function, especially if they are also receiving diuretics. When to observe for these effects and for how long depends on the onset, peak, and duration of the medication. Table 30-3 identifies several types of ACE inhibitors and their pharmacokinetics. Hypotension is most likely to develop from ACE inhibitor therapy in patients older than 75 years of age and in those with a systolic blood pressure of 100 mm Hg or less, a serum sodium level of lower than 135 mEq/L, or severe heart failure. Adjusting the dose or type of diuretic in response to the patient's blood pressure and renal function may allow for continued increases in the dosage of ACE inhibitors.

Because ACE inhibitors cause the kidneys to retain potassium, the patient who is also receiving a diuretic may not need to take oral potassium supplements. However, patients receiving potassium-sparing diuretics (which do not cause potassium loss with diuresis) must be carefully monitored for hyperkalemia, an increased level of potassium in the

℞ TABLE 30-3 Angiotensin-Converting Enzyme (ACE) Inhibitors

ACE Inhibitor	Pharmacokinetics: *Onset*	*Peak (hr)*	*Duration (hr)*	Nursing Considerations
benazepril (Lotensin)	within 1 hr	2–4	24	Monitor blood pressure, urine output, and electrolyte levels.
captopril (Capoten)	15–60 min	1–1.5	6–12*	Monitor serum creatinine and urine creatinine clearance.
enalapril (Vasotec)	1 hr	4–6	24	Monitor for development of cough that is resistant to cough suppressants.
enalaprilat (Vasotec I.V.)	15 min	1–4	6	Teach patient to change positions gradually and to report signs of dizziness or lethargy.
fosinopril (Monopril)	within 1 hr	2–6	24	Instruct patient to weigh self daily and to report rapid weight gain and significant feet and hand swelling.
lisinopril (Prinival, Zestril)	1 hr	6	24	
moexipril (Univasc)	1 hr	3–6	24	
quinapril (Accupril)	within 1 hr	2–4	up to 24*	
ramipril (Altace)	1–2 hr	4–6	24	
trandolapril (Mavik)	within 30 min	2–4	> 8 days	

*Duration of effect is related to the dose.

blood. Before the initiation of the ACE inhibitor, hyperkalemic and hypovolemic states must be corrected. ACE inhibitors may be discontinued if the potassium level remains greater than 5.0 mEq/L or if the serum creatinine is 3.0 mg/dL or more.

Other side effects of ACE inhibitors include a dry, persistent cough that may not respond to cough suppressants. However, the cough could also indicate a worsening of ventricular function and failure. Rarely, the cough indicates angioedema. If angioedema affects the oropharyngeal area and impairs breathing, the ACE inhibitor must be stopped immediately.

If the patient cannot continue taking an ACE inhibitor because of development of cough, an elevated creatinine level, or hyperkalemia, an angiotensin II receptor blocker (ARB) or hydralazine (Apresoline) and isosorbide dinitrate (Dilatrate SR, Isordil, Sorbitrate) are prescribed.

ANGIOTENSIN II RECEPTOR BLOCKERS

Although the action of ARBs is different than that of ACE inhibitors, ARBs (eg, valsartan [Diovan]) have similar hemodynamic effects: decreased blood pressure, decreased systemic vascular resistance, and improved cardiac output (ICSI, 2004). Whereas ACE inhibitors block the conversion of angiotensin I to angiotensin II, ARBs block the effects of angiotensin II at the angiotensin II receptor. ACE inhibitors and ARBs also have similar side effects: hyperkalemia, hypotension, and renal dysfunction. ARBs are usually prescribed as an alternative to ACE inhibitors, especially when patients cannot tolerate ACE inhibitors because of cough.

HYDRALAZINE AND ISOSORBIDE DINITRATE

A combination of hydralazine (Apresoline) and isosorbide dinitrate (Dilatrate SR, Isordil, Sorbitrate) may be another alternative for patients who cannot take ACE inhibitors. Nitrates (eg, isosorbide dinitrate) cause venous dilation, which reduces the amount of blood return to the heart and lowers preload. Hydralazine lowers systemic vascular resistance and left ventricular afterload. This combination of medications is usually used when patients cannot tolerate ACE inhibitors.

BETA-BLOCKERS

Beta-blockers, such as carvedilol (Coreg) and metoprolol (Lopressor, Toprol), have been found to reduce mortality and morbidity in patients with NYHA Class II or III HF by reducing the adverse effects from the constant stimulation of the sympathetic nervous system. Beta-blockers are routinely prescribed in addition to ACE inhibitors, diuretics, and digitalis (ICSI, 2004) and have also been recommended for patients with asymptomatic systolic dysfunction, such as those with a decreased EF, to prevent the onset of symptoms of HF.

Beta-blockers may produce many side effects and may exacerbate symptoms of HF. Side effects are most common in the initial few weeks of treatment. The most frequent side effects are dizziness, hypotension, and bradycardia. Because of these side effects, beta-blockers are started only after the patient is stabilized and euvolemic (eg, state of normal volume). The dose is titrated slowly (every 2 weeks), with close monitoring at each increase. If symptoms of HF increase during the titration phase, treatment options include increasing the dose of the diuretic, reducing the dose of the ACE inhibitor, or decreasing the dose of the beta-blocker.

An important nursing role during titration is educating the patient about the potential worsening of symptoms during the early phase of treatment and stressing that improvement may take several weeks. It is very important for nurses to provide support to patients going through this symptom-provoking phase of treatment. Because beta-blockade can cause bronchiole constriction, a beta-1–selective beta-blocker (ie, one that primarily blocks the beta-adrenergic receptor sites in the heart) such as metoprolol (Lopressor, Toprol) is recommended for patients with well-controlled, mild to moderate asthma. Patients need to be monitored closely for increased asthma symptoms nonetheless, as even cardioselective beta-blockers retain some modest beta-2 effects. Any type of beta-blocker is contraindicated in patients with severe or uncontrolled asthma.

DIURETICS

Diuretics are prescribed to remove excess extracellular fluid by increasing the rate of urine produced in patients with signs and symptoms of fluid overload. Of the types of diuretics prescribed for patients with edema from HF, three are most common: thiazide, loop, and potassium-sparing diuretics. These medications are classified according to their site of action in the kidney and their effects on renal electrolyte excretion and reabsorption.

Thiazide diuretics, such as metolazone (Zaroxolyn), inhibit sodium and chloride reabsorption mainly in the early distal tubules. They also increase potassium and bicarbonate excretion. Loop diuretics, such as furosemide (Lasix), inhibit sodium and chloride reabsorption mainly in the ascending loop of Henle. Both of these types of diuretics may be used for patients in severe HF who are unresponsive to a single diuretic. Diuretics may be most effective if the patient assumes a supine position for 1 or 2 hours after taking them. These medications may not be necessary if the patient responds to activity recommendations, avoids excessive fluid intake (eg, more than 2 quarts/day), and adheres to a low-sodium diet (eg, less than 2 g/day).

Spironolactone (Aldactone) is a potassium-sparing diuretic that inhibits sodium reabsorption in the late distal tubule and collecting duct. It has been found to be effective in reducing mortality and morbidity in patients with moderate to severe HF when taken along with ACE inhibitors, loop diuretics, and digoxin (ICSI, 2004). Serum creatinine and potassium levels are monitored frequently (eg, within the first week and then every 4 weeks) when this medication is first administered.

Side effects of diuretics include electrolyte imbalances, symptomatic hypotension (especially with overdiuresis), hyperuricemia (causing gout), and ototoxicity. The dose depends on the indications, patient age, clinical signs and symptoms, and renal function. Table 30-4 lists commonly used diuretics and their recommended doses and pharmacokinetic properties. Careful patient monitoring and dose adjustments are necessary to balance the effectiveness of these medications with the side effects (Chart 30-2). Diuretics are administered IV for exacerbations of HF when rapid diuresis is necessary. Diuretics tend to improve the patient's symptoms, provided that renal function is adequate (ICSI, 2004).

TABLE 30-4 Diuretic Medications Used to Treat Heart Failure

Diuretic	Usual Adult Dose	Onset (hr)	Peak (hr)	Duration (hr)
Thiazide Diuretics				
bendroflumethiazide (Naturetin)	2.5–20 mg in single or divided dose, once a day, once every other day, or once a day for 3–5 days per week	2	4	12–16
benzthiazide (Exna)	12.5–200 mg in single or divided dose	2	4–6	16–18
chlorothiazide (Diuril)	Oral: 0.25–2 g as single or divided dose; may be given on alternate days	2	4	16–18
	IV: 0.5–1 g in single or divided dose (note: avoid extravasation)	15 min	30 min	
chlorthalidone (Hygroton)	12.5–200 mg once a day, once every other day, or once a day for 3 days per week	2	2–6	24–72
hydrochlorothiazide (HydroDIURIL, Esidrix, Oretic)	12.5–200 mg as single or divided dose once a day, once every other day, or once a day for 3–5 days per week	2	4–6	12–16
hydroflumethiazide (Diucardin, Saluron)	25–200 mg as single or divided dose once a day, once every other day, or once a day for 3–5 days per week	2	4	12–16
methyclothiazide (Enduron)	2.5–10 mg once a day	2	6	24
metolazone (Zaroxolyn, Mykrox)	Zaroxolyn: 2.5–20 mg once a day Mykrox: 0.5–1 mg once a day	1	2	12–24
polythiazide (Renese)	1–4 mg once a day, once every other day, or once a day for 3–5 days per week	2	6	24–28
quinethazone (Hydromox)	25–100 mg as single or divided dose; rarely, 200 mg once a day	2	6	18–24
trichlormethiazide (Metahydrin, Naqua)	1–4 mg once or twice a day	2	6	24
Loop Diuretics				
bumetanide (Bumex)	0.5–2 mg once, twice, or three times a day; may be given on alternate days or once every 3 days	30–60 min	1–2	4–6
	0.5–1 mg over 2 min; repeat every 2–3 h; a continuous infusion may be given at a rate of 1 mg/h	5–10 min	15–30 min	½–1
ethacrynic acid (Edecrin)	50–400 mg as single or divided dose	<30 min	2	6–8
	0.5–1 mg/kg (max 100 mg) over several min; may be repeated within 2–6 h; repeat every hour in emergencies	<5 min	15–30 min	2
furosemide (Lasix)	20–600 mg as single daily dose, divided daily dose, as a dose given every other day or given once a day for 2–4 days per week	<1	1–2	6–8
	20–200 mg (max 6 mg/kg) given at a rate of 4 mg/min; after response obtained, given once or twice a day	<5 min	30 min	2
torsemide (Demadex)	5–200 mg as a daily single dose	<1	1–2	6–8
	IV and oral doses are equivalent; give IV over 2 min.	<10 min	<1	6–8
Potassium-Sparing Diuretics				
amiloride (Midamor)	5–20 mg daily as single dose	2	6–10	24
spironolactone (Aldactone)	25–400 mg as single dose or divided up to 4 doses	24–48	48–72	48–72
triamterene (Dyrenium)	50–300 mg as single dose	2–4	6–8	12–16

DIGITALIS

The most commonly prescribed form of digitalis for patients with HF is digoxin (Lanoxin). This medication increases the force of myocardial contraction and slows conduction through the atrioventricular node. It improves contractility, increasing left ventricular output, which also results in enhanced diuresis. The effect of a given dose of digoxin depends on the state of the myocardium, electrolyte and fluid balance, and renal function. Although the use of digitalis does not result in decreased mortality rates among patients with HF, it is effective in decreasing the symptoms of systolic HF and in increasing the patient's ability to perform activities of daily living (Spencer, 2003).

A key concern associated with digitalis therapy is digitalis toxicity. Chart 30-3 summarizes the actions and uses of digoxin along with the nursing surveillance required when it is administered. The patient is observed for indications that digitalis therapy is effective: lessening dyspnea and orthopnea, decrease in pulmonary crackles on auscultation, relief of peripheral edema, weight loss, and increase in activity tolerance. The serum potassium level is measured at

CHART 30-2

PHARMACOLOGY · Administering and Monitoring Diuretic Therapy

When nursing care involves diuretic therapy for conditions such as heart failure, the nurse needs to administer the medication and monitor the patient's response carefully, as follows:

- Administer the diuretic at a time conducive to the patient's lifestyle; for example, early in the day to avoid nocturia.
- Give supplementary potassium with thiazide and loop diuretics as prescribed to replace potassium loss.
- Check laboratory results for electrolyte depletion, especially potassium, magnesium, and sodium; and for electrolyte elevation, especially potassium with potassium-sparing agents.
- Monitor daily weights, intake and output to assess response. Monitor serum blood urea nitrogen and creatinine. Notify health care provider if renal impairment is suspected.
- Assess lung sounds, jugular vein distention, daily weight, and peripheral, abdominal, or sacral edema to identify response to therapy.
- Monitor for adverse reactions, such as nausea and gastrointestinal distress, vomiting, diarrhea, weakness, headache, fatigue, anxiety or agitation, and cardiac dysrhythmias.
- Assess for signs of volume depletion, such as postural hypotension, dizziness, and balance problems.
- Monitor for glucose intolerance in patients with and without diabetes mellitus who are receiving thiazide diuretics.
- Monitor for potential ototoxicity in patients, especially those with renal failure, who are receiving a loop diuretic.
- Advise patients to avoid prolonged exposure to the sun because of the risk of photosensitivity.
- Monitor for elevated serum uric acid levels and the development of gout.
- Implement nursing actions to facilitate effect of medication, such as positioning patient supine after dose is taken.

intervals because diuresis may cause hypokalemia. The effect of digoxin is enhanced in the presence of hypokalemia, so digoxin toxicity may occur. Serum digoxin levels are obtained if there have been changes in the patient's medications, renal function, or symptoms.

CALCIUM CHANNEL BLOCKERS

First-generation calcium channel blockers, such as verapamil (Calan, Isoptin), nifedipine (Adalat, Procardia), and diltiazem (Cardizem, Tiazac), are contraindicated in patients with systolic dysfunction, although they may be used in patients with diastolic dysfunction. Amlodipine (Norvasc) and felodipine (Plendil), which are dihydropyridine calcium channel blockers, cause vasodilation, reducing systemic vascular resistance. They may be used to improve symptoms, especially in patients with nonischemic cardiomyopathy.

INTRAVENOUS INFUSIONS

Nesiritide. Nesiritide (Natrecor), a BNP made using recombinant technology, is indicated for patients with acutely decompensated HF. BNPs are produced by the myocardium to mount a compensatory response in the presence of the myocardial demands, including increased ventricular end-diastolic pressure, myocardial wall stress, and increased release of neurohormones (eg, norepinephrine, renin, aldosterone), that occur with HF. Specifically, BNP binds to vascular smooth muscle and endothelial cells, causing dilation of arteries and veins. It also suppresses the neurohormones responsible for fluid retention, thus promoting diuresis. The result is reduced preload and afterload and increased SV (Hachey & Smith, 2003).

Nesiritide causes rapid improvement in the symptoms of HF. It may be used to treat hospitalized patients with acute exacerbations or to prevent exacerbations in outpatients when given as a series of intermittent IV infusions. The most common side effect is dose-related hypotension.

Milrinone. Milrinone (Primacor) is a phosphodiesterase inhibitor that delays the release of calcium from intracellular reservoirs and prevents the uptake of extracellular calcium by the cells. This promotes vasodilation, resulting in decreased preload and afterload and reduced cardiac workload. Milrinone is administered IV if the patient has not responded to other therapies. The major side effects are hypotension (usually asymptomatic), gastrointestinal dysfunction, increased ventricular dysrhythmias, and, rarely, decreased platelet counts. Blood pressure is monitored closely.

Dobutamine. Dobutamine (Dobutrex) is an IV medication administered to patients with significant left ventricular dysfunction. A catecholamine, dobutamine stimulates the beta-1–adrenergic receptors. Its major action is to increase cardiac contractility. However, at high doses, it also increases the heart rate and the incidence of ectopic beats and tachydysrhythmias. Because it also increases atrioventricular conduction, care must be taken in patients who have underlying atrial fibrillation.

Patients receiving continuous IV infusions of any of these vasoactive medications are routinely monitored continuously via ECG, and their vital signs are assessed frequently.

MEDICATIONS FOR DIASTOLIC DYSFUNCTION

Patients with predominant diastolic dysfunction may be treated with different pharmacologic agents than indicated for patients with systolic dysfunction. After contributing causes such as hypertension and ischemic heart disease are evaluated and treated, patients may be started on ACE inhibitors and diuretics. Beta-blockers are also used in

CHART 30-3

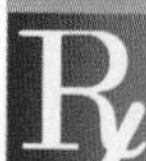

PHARMACOLOGY · Digoxin Use and Toxicity in Heart Failure

Digoxin, a cardiac glycoside derived from digitalis, is used for patients with systolic HF, atrial fibrillation, and atrial flutter. Digoxin improves cardiac function as follows:

- Increases the force of myocardial contraction
- Slows cardiac conduction through the AV node and therefore slows the ventricular rate in instances of supraventricular dysrhythmias
- Increases cardiac output by enhancing the force of ventricular contraction
- Promotes diuresis by increasing cardiac output.

The therapeutic level is usually 0.5 to 2.0 ng/mL. Blood samples are usually obtained and analyzed to determine digitalis concentration at least 6 to 10 hours after the last dose. Toxicity may occur despite normal serum levels, and recommended dosages vary considerably.

Preparations

DIGOXIN

- Tablets: 0.125, 0.25, 0.5 mg (Lanoxin)
- Capsules: 0.05, 0.1, 0.2 mg (Lanoxicaps)
- Elixir: 0.05 mg/mL (Lanoxin Pediatric elixir)
- Injection: 0.25 mg/mL, 0.1 mg/mL (Lanoxin)

Digoxin Toxicity

A serious complication of digoxin therapy is toxicity. Diagnosis of digoxin toxicity is based on the patient's clinical symptoms, which include the following:

- Anorexia, nausea, vomiting, fatigue, depression, and malaise (early effects of digitalis toxicity)
- Changes in heart rate or rhythm; onset of irregular rhythm.
- ECG changes indicating SA or AV block; new onset of irregular rhythm indicating ventricular dysrhythmias; and atrial tachycardia with block, junctional tachycardia, and ventricular tachycardia

Reversal of Toxicity

Digoxin toxicity is treated by holding the medication while monitoring the patient's symptoms and serum digoxin level. If the toxicity is severe, digoxin immune FAB (Digibind) may be prescribed. Digibind binds with digoxin and makes it unavailable for use. The Digibind dosage is based on the digoxin level and the patient's weight. Serum digoxin values are not accurate for several days after administration of Digibind because they do not differentiate between bound and unbound digoxin. Because Digibind quickly decreases the amount of available digoxin, an increase in ventricular rate due to atrial fibrillation and worsening of symptoms of HF may ensue shortly after its administration.

Nursing Considerations and Actions

1. Assess the patient's clinical response to digoxin therapy by evaluating relief of symptoms such as dyspnea, orthopnea, crackles, hepatomegaly, and peripheral edema.
2. Monitor the patient for factors that increase the risk of toxicity:
   - Decreased potassium level (hypokalemia), which may be caused by diuretics. Hypokalemia increases the action of digoxin and predisposes patients to digoxin toxicity and dysrhythmias.
   - Use of medications that enhance the effects of digoxin, including oral antibiotics and cardiac drugs that slow AV conduction and can further decrease heart rate
   - Impaired renal function, particularly in patients age 65 and older. Because digoxin is eliminated by the kidneys, renal function (serum creatinine) is monitored and doses of digoxin are adjusted accordingly.
3. Before administering digoxin, it is standard nursing practice to assess apical heart rate. When the patient's rhythm is atrial fibrillation and the heart rate is less than 60, or the rhythm becomes regular, the nurse may withhold the medication and notify the physician, because these signs indicate the development of AV conduction block. Although withholding digoxin is a common practice, the medication does not need to be withheld for a heart rate of less than 60 if the patient is in sinus rhythm because digoxin does not affect sinoatrial node automaticity. Measuring the PR interval for a patient with cardiac monitoring is more important than the apical pulse in determining whether digoxin should be held.
4. Monitor for gastrointestinal side effects: anorexia, nausea, vomiting, abdominal pain and distention.
5. Monitor for neurologic side effects: headache, malaise, nightmares, forgetfulness, social withdrawal, depression, agitation, confusion, paranoia, hallucinations, decreased visual acuity, yellow or green halo around objects (especially lights), or "snowy" vision.

these patients if they have concomitant atrial fibrillation (ICSI, 2004).

OTHER MEDICATIONS

Anticoagulants may be prescribed, especially if the patient has a history of an embolic event or atrial fibrillation or a mural thrombus is present. Other medications, such as antianginal medications, may be administered to treat the underlying cause of HF. Nonsteroidal anti-inflammatory drugs (NSAIDs) such as ibuprofen (Advil, Motrin) should be avoided, because they increase systemic vascular resistance and decrease renal perfusion, especially in the elderly. For similar reasons, use of decongestants should be avoided.

Nutritional Therapy

A low-sodium (2 to 3 g/day) diet and avoidance of excessive amounts of fluid are usually recommended. Dietary restriction of sodium reduces fluid retention and the symptoms of peripheral and pulmonary congestion. The purpose of sodium restriction is to decrease the amount of circulating blood volume, which would decrease the need for the heart to pump that volume. A balance needs to be achieved between the ability of the patient to comply with the diet and the recommended dietary restriction. Any change in diet needs to be made with consideration of good nutrition as well as the patient's likes, dislikes, and cultural food patterns. Patient compliance is important because dietary indiscretions may result in severe exacerbations of HF requiring hospitalization. However, behavioral changes in this area are difficult for many patients (Sneed & Paul, 2003).

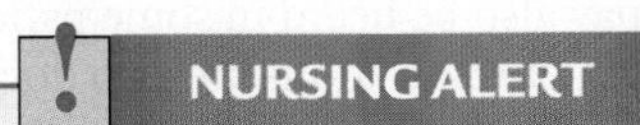

NURSING ALERT

The sources of sodium should be specified in describing the regimen, rather than simply saying "low-salt" or "salt-free," and the quantity should be indicated in milligrams. Salt is not 100% sodium; there are 393 mg of sodium in 1 g (1000 mg) of salt.

Additional Therapy

SUPPLEMENTAL OXYGEN

Oxygen therapy may become necessary as heart failure progresses. The need is based on the degree of pulmonary congestion and resulting hypoxia. Some patients require supplemental oxygen only during activity.

OTHER INTERVENTIONS

A number of procedures and surgical approaches may benefit patients with HF. If the patient has underlying coronary artery disease, coronary artery revascularization with percutaneous coronary intervention or coronary artery bypass surgery (see Chapter 28) may be considered. Ventricular function may improve in some patients when coronary flow is increased (Albert, 2003b).

Patients with HF are at high risk for dysrhythmias. Sudden cardiac death accounts for half of all deaths from heart failure (Young, Abraham, & Smith, 2003). In patients with life-threatening dysrhythmias, placement of an **implantable cardioverter defibrillator (ICD)** can prevent sudden cardiac death and extend survival.

In the patient with HF who does not improve with standard therapy, **cardiac resynchronization therapy (CRT)** is another treatment that may be beneficial. CRT involves the use of a biventricular pacemaker to treat electrical conduction defects. Left bundle branch block is a feature of delayed conduction that is frequently seen in patients with HF that results in dyssynchronous conduction and contraction of the right and left ventricles, which can further decrease EF (Albert, 2003a). Use of a pacing device with leads placed in the right atrium, right ventricle, and left ventricular cardiac vein can synchronize the contractions of the right and left ventricles. This intervention has been shown to improve cardiac output, optimize myocardial energy consumption, reduce mitral regurgitation, and slow the ventricular remodeling process. For selected patients, this results in fewer symptoms and increased functional status (Bradley, Bradley, & Baughman, 2003). For patients who require CRT and an ICD, combination devices are available.

For some patients with end-stage HF, cardiac transplantation is the only option for long-term survival (Tokarczyk, 2003). Some of these patients require mechanical circulatory assistance with an implanted ventricular assist device as a bridge therapy to cardiac transplantation (see Chapter 29). Research continues toward perfection of a totally implantable artificial heart that may be used as an alternative to transplantation.

Nursing Management

Despite advances in medical and surgical approaches to HF, mortality remains high. Nurses can make a major difference in promoting positive outcomes. In both inpatient and outpatient settings, nursing interventions for the patient with HF include the following:

- Administering medications and assessing the patient's response to the pharmacologic regimen
- Assessing fluid balance, including intake and output, with a goal of optimizing volume status
- Weighing the patient daily at the same time and on the same scale, usually in the morning after urination; monitoring for a 2- to 3-lb gain in a day or 5-lb gain in a week
- Auscultating lung sounds to detect an increase or decrease in pulmonary crackles
- Determining the degree of jugular venous distention (JVD)
- Identifying and evaluating the severity of dependent edema
- Monitoring pulse rate and blood pressure; checking for postural hypotension due to dehydration
- Examining skin turgor and mucous membranes for signs of dehydration
- Assessing for symptoms of fluid overload (eg, orthopnea, PND, DOE)

Monitoring and Managing Potential Complications

Many potential problems associated with HF therapy relate to the use of diuretics:

- Profuse and repeated diuresis can lead to hypokalemia (ie, potassium depletion). Signs include ventricular dysrhythmias, hypotension, muscle weakness, diminished deep tendon reflexes, and generalized weakness. Hypokalemia poses problems for the patient with HF because it markedly weakens cardiac contractions. In patients receiving digoxin, hypokalemia can lead to digitalis toxicity. Digitalis toxicity and hypokalemia increase the likelihood of dangerous dysrhythmias (see Chart 30-3). Patients with HF may also develop low levels of magnesium, which can add to the risk of dysrhythmias.

- Hyperkalemia may occur, especially with the use of ACE inhibitors, ARBs, or spironolactone.
- Prolonged diuretic therapy may produce hyponatremia (deficiency of sodium in the blood), which results in disorientation, apprehension, weakness, fatigue, malaise, and muscle cramps.
- Other problems associated with diuretic administration are hyperuricemia (excessive uric acid in the blood) and gout, plus volume depletion from excessive fluid loss.

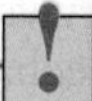

NURSING ALERT

Grapefruit (fresh and juice) is a good dietary source of potassium but has serious drug–food interactions. Patients are advised to consult their physician or pharmacist before including grapefruit in their diet.

Gerontologic Considerations

Several normal changes that occur with aging increase the frequency of HF: increased systolic blood pressure, increased ventricular wall thickness, increased atrial size, and increased myocardial fibrosis. Elderly people may present with atypical signs and symptoms: fatigue, weakness, and somnolence. Decreased renal function makes the elderly patient resistant to diuretics and more sensitive to changes in volume, especially with diastolic dysfunction. The administration of diuretics to elderly men requires nursing surveillance for bladder distention caused by urethral obstruction from an enlarged prostate gland. The bladder may be assessed with an ultrasound scanner, or the suprapubic area palpated for an oval mass and percussed for dullness, indicative of bladder fullness. Frequency and urgency from diuretics may be particularly stressful to the elderly patient.

Nursing Process

The Patient With Heart Failure

Assessment

The nursing assessment for the patient with HF focuses on observing for effectiveness of therapy and for the patient's ability to understand and implement self-management strategies. Signs and symptoms of pulmonary and systemic fluid overload are recorded and reported immediately so that adjustments can be made in therapy. The nurse also explores the patient's emotional response to the diagnosis of HF, a chronic and often progressive condition.

Health History

The health history focuses on the signs and symptoms of HF, such as dyspnea, shortness of breath, and cough. Sleep disturbances, particularly sleep suddenly interrupted by shortness of breath, may be reported. The nurse also asks about the number of pillows needed for sleep (an indication of orthopnea), edema, abdominal symptoms, altered mental status, activities of daily living, and the activities that cause fatigue. The nurse explores the patient's understanding of HF, self-management strategies, and the desire to adhere to those strategies. The nurse helps patients identify the impact the illness has had on their quality of life and successful coping skills that they have used. Family and significant others are often included in these discussions.

Physical Examination

The lungs are auscultated to detect crackles and wheezes. Crackles, which are produced by the sudden opening of edematous small airways and alveoli that have adhered together by exudate, may be heard at the end of inspiration and are not cleared with coughing. Wheezing may also be heard in some patients. The rate and depth of respirations are also documented.

The heart is auscultated for an S_3 heart sound, a sign that the heart is beginning to fail and that increased blood volume fills the ventricle with each beat. HR and rhythm are also documented. When the heart rate is rapid, the SV decreases because the ventricle has less time to fill. This in turn produces increased pressure in the atria and eventually in the pulmonary vascular bed.

JVD is also assessed; distention greater than 3 cm above the sternal angle is considered abnormal. This is an estimate, not a precise measurement, of central venous pressure.

Sensorium and level of consciousness must be evaluated. As the volume of blood ejected by the heart decreases, so does the amount of oxygen transported to the brain.

The nurse assesses dependent parts of the patient's body for perfusion and edema. With significant decreases in SV, there is a decrease in perfusion to the periphery, causing the skin to feel cool and appear pale or cyanotic. If the patient is sitting upright, the feet and lower legs are examined for edema; if the patient is supine in bed, the sacrum and back are also assessed for edema. Fingers and hands may also become edematous.

The liver is assessed for hepatojugular reflux. The patient is asked to breathe normally while manual pressure is applied over the right upper quadrant of the abdomen for 30 to 60 seconds. If neck vein distention increases more than 1 cm, the finding is positive for increased venous pressure.

If the patient is hospitalized, the nurse measures output carefully to establish a baseline against which to assess the effectiveness of diuretic therapy. Intake and output records are rigorously maintained. It is important to know whether the patient has ingested more fluid than he or she has excreted (positive fluid balance), which is then correlated with a gain in weight. The patient must be monitored for oliguria (diminished urine output, less than 400 mL/24 hours) or **anuria** (urine output less than 50 mL/24 hours).

The patient is weighed daily in the hospital or at home, at the same time of day, with the same type of clothing, and on the same scale. If there is a significant change in weight (ie, 2- to 3-lb increase in a day or 5-lb increase in a week), the patient is instructed to notify the physician or to adjust the medications (eg, increase the diuretic dose).

Diagnosis

Nursing Diagnoses

Based on the assessment data, major nursing diagnoses for the patient with HF may include the following:

- Activity intolerance and fatigue related to imbalance between oxygen supply and demand because of decreased CO
- Excess fluid volume related to excess fluid or sodium intake, and retention of fluid related to the HF syndrome
- Anxiety related to breathlessness and restlessness from inadequate oxygenation
- Powerlessness related to inability to perform role responsibilities because of chronic illness and hospitalizations
- Noncompliance related to lack of knowledge

Collaborative Problems/ Potential Complications

Based on the assessment data, potential complications that may develop include the following:

- Cardiogenic shock (see also Chapter 15)
- Dysrhythmias (see Chapter 27)
- Thromboembolism (see Chapter 31)
- Pericardial effusion and cardiac tamponade (see Chapter 29)

Planning and Goals

Major goals for the patient may include promoting activity and reducing fatigue, relieving fluid overload symptoms, decreasing the incidence of anxiety or increasing the patient's ability to manage anxiety, encouraging the patient to verbalize his or her ability to make decisions and influence outcomes, and teaching the patient about the self-care program.

Nursing Interventions

Promoting Activity Tolerance

Although prolonged bed rest and even short periods of recumbency promote diuresis by improving renal perfusion, they also decrease activity tolerance. Prolonged bed rest, which may be self-imposed, should be avoided because of its deconditioning effects and risks such as pressure ulcers (especially in edematous patients), venous thrombosis, and pulmonary embolism. An acute illness that exacerbates HF symptoms or that requires hospitalization may be an indication for temporary bed rest. Otherwise, a total of 30 to 45 minutes of physical activity every day should be encouraged (Pina, Apstein, Balady, et al., 2003). Exercise training has many favorable effects for HF, including increasing functional capacity and decreasing dyspnea. The exercise regimen should include 10 to 15 minutes of warm-up activities, followed by about 30 minutes of exercise at the prescribed intensity level. A typical program for a patient with HF might include a daily walking regimen, with duration increased over a 6-week period. The physician, nurse, and patient collaborate to develop a schedule that promotes pacing and prioritization of activities. The schedule should alternate activities with periods of rest and avoid having two significant energy-consuming activities occur on the same day or in immediate succession.

Before undertaking physical activity, the patient should be given the following safety guidelines:

- Begin with a few minutes of warm-up activities.
- Avoid performing physical activities outside in extreme hot, cold, or humid weather.
- Ensure that you are able to talk during the physical activity; if you cannot do so, decrease the intensity of activity.
- Wait 2 hours after eating a meal before performing the physical activity.
- Stop the activity if severe shortness of breath, pain, or dizziness develops.
- End with cool-down activities and a cool-down period.

Because some patients may be severely debilitated, they may need to limit physical activities to only 3 to 5 minutes at a time, one to four times per day. The patient should increase the duration of the activity, then the frequency, before increasing the intensity of the activity.

Barriers to performing other activities are identified, and methods of adjusting an activity are discussed. For example, vegetables can be chopped or peeled while sitting at the kitchen table rather than standing at the kitchen counter. Small, frequent meals decrease the amount of energy needed for digestion while providing adequate nutrition. The nurse helps the patient identify peak and low periods of energy, planning energy-consuming activities for peak periods. For example, the patient may prepare the meals for the entire day in the morning. Pacing and prioritizing activities help maintain the patient's energy to allow participation in regular physical activity.

The patient's response to activities needs to be monitored. If the patient is hospitalized, vital signs and oxygen saturation level are monitored before, during, and immediately after an activity to identify whether they are within the desired range. HR should return to baseline within 3 minutes following the activity. If the patient is at home, the degree of fatigue felt after the activity can be used to assess the response. If the patient tolerates the activity, short-term and long-term

NURSING RESEARCH PROFILE

Readiness for Behavioral Changes in Patients with Heart Failure

Sneed, N. V., & Paul., S. C. (2003). Readiness for behavioral changes in patients with heart failure. *American Journal of Critical Care, 12*(5), 444–453.

Purpose

Patient education for patients with heart failure (HF) focuses on the lifestyle changes that are necessary to control signs and symptoms. Important changes include avoiding sodium, alcohol, and tobacco; regular exercise; and weight loss. However, education does not guarantee changes in behavior. The purpose of this study was to identify stages of readiness for change pertaining to six important behaviors and to determine self-reported differences in patients who made the changes and in those who did not.

Design

A total of 178 patients with HF completed a survey rating their readiness for change. The survey questions were based on the five stages of change described by the Transtheoretical Model for Change (ie, whether patients planned to make a change, had already made the change). The survey also assessed patients' knowledge of the signs and symptoms of HF, as well as their adherence to recommendations for sodium restriction, fluid restriction, exercise, and (if applicable) weight loss, smoking cessation, and alcohol cessation. Participants were also asked to report their signs and symptoms of HF, such as shortness of breath and fatigue.

Findings

Participants generally reported adherence to the major lifestyle recommendations. However, only 38% reported engaging in a regular exercise program, and 92% had eaten foods high in sodium within the preceding 24 hours. Knowledge about HF was low and did not differ by the stage of change. The findings did not support the hypothesis that patients who had made the recommended lifestyle changes would report fewer signs and symptoms of HF.

Nursing Implications

Actual patient behaviors did not demonstrate that patients adhered to the recommended lifestyle changes, even when patients thought they were following them. The authors suggest that the scale for rating readiness for change may not work well in patients with HF. The lack of knowledge identified by patients may be related to the number of changes these patients are asked to make. Nurses continue to be challenged to find effective ways to educate patients with HF.

goals can be developed to gradually increase the intensity, duration, and frequency of activity.

Adherence to exercise training is essential if the patient is to benefit from it, but it may be difficult for patients with multiple other conditions (eg, arthritis) and longer duration of heart failure (Corvera-Tindel, Doering, Gomez, et al., 2004). Referral to a cardiac rehabilitation program may be needed, especially for HF patients with recent myocardial infarction, recent open heart surgery, or increased anxiety. A supervised program may also benefit those who need a structured environment, significant educational support, regular encouragement, and interpersonal contact.

Managing Fluid Volume

Patients with severe HF may receive IV diuretic therapy, but patients with less severe symptoms may receive oral diuretic medication (see Table 30-4 for a summary of common diuretics). Oral diuretics should be administered early in the morning so that diuresis does not interfere with the patient's nighttime rest. Discussing the timing of medication administration is especially important for elderly patients who may have urinary urgency or incontinence. A single dose of a diuretic may cause the patient to excrete a large volume of fluid shortly after its administration.

The nurse monitors the patient's fluid status closely, auscultating the lungs, monitoring daily body weights, and assisting the patient to adhere to a low-sodium diet by reading food labels and avoiding high-sodium foods such as canned, processed, and convenience foods (Chart 30-4). If the diet includes fluid restriction, the nurse can assist the patient to plan fluid intake throughout the day while respecting the patient's dietary preferences. If the patient is receiving IV fluids, the amount of fluid needs to be monitored closely, and the physician or pharmacist can be consulted about the possibility of maximizing the amount of medication in the same amount of IV fluid (eg, double-concentrating to decrease the fluid volume administered).

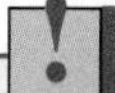

NURSING ALERT

Periodic assessment of the patient's electrolyte levels alerts health team members to hypokalemia, hypomagnesemia, and hyponatremia. Serum levels are assessed frequently when the patient starts diuretic therapy and then usually every 3 to 12 months. It is important to remember that serum potassium levels do not always indicate the total amount of potassium within the body.

CHART 30-4

Facts About Dietary Sodium

Although the major source of sodium in the average American diet is salt, many types of natural foods contain varying amounts of sodium. Even if no salt is added in cooking and if salty foods are avoided, the daily diet will still contain about 2000 mg of sodium.

Additives in Food

In general, food prepared at home is lower in sodium than restaurant or processed foods. Added food substances (additives), such as sodium alginate, which improves food texture; sodium benzoate, which acts as a preservative; and disodium phosphate, which improves cooking quality in certain foods, increase the sodium intake when included in the daily diet. Therefore, patients on low-sodium diets should be advised to check labels carefully for such words as "salt" or "sodium," especially on canned foods. For example, without looking at the sodium content per serving found on the nutrition labels, when given a choice between a serving of potato chips and a cup of canned cream of mushroom soup, most would think that soup is lower in sodium. However, when the labels are examined, the lower sodium choice is found to be the chips. Although potato chips are *not* recommended in a low sodium diet, this example illustrates that it is important to read food labels to determine both sodium content and serving size.

Nonfood Sodium Sources

Sodium is also contained in municipal water. Patients on sodium-restricted diets should be cautioned against using nonprescription medications such as antacids, cough syrups, and laxatives. Salt substitutes may be allowed, but it is recognized that they are high in potassium. Over-the-counter medications should not be used without first consulting the physician.

Promoting Dietary Adherence

If patients find food unpalatable because of the dietary sodium restrictions and/or the taste disturbances caused by the medications, they may refuse to eat or to comply with the dietary regimen. For this reason, severe sodium restrictions should be avoided and the amount of medication should be balanced with the patient's ability to restrict dietary sodium. A variety of flavorings, such as lemon juice, vinegar, and herbs, may be used to improve the taste of the food and increase acceptance of the diet. The patient's food preferences should be taken into account—diet counseling and educational handouts can be geared to individual and ethnic preferences. It is very important to involve the family in the dietary teaching.

The nurse positions the patient or teaches the patient how to assume a position that facilitates breathing. The number of pillows may be increased, the head of the bed may be elevated, or the patient may sit in a comfortable armchair. In this position, the venous return to the heart (preload) is reduced, pulmonary congestion is alleviated, and pressure on the diaphragm is minimized. The lower arms are supported with pillows to eliminate the fatigue caused by the constant pull of their weight on the shoulder muscles.

Because decreased circulation in edematous areas increases the risk of skin injury, the nurse assesses for skin breakdown and institutes preventive measures. Frequent changes of position, positioning to avoid pressure, the use of elastic compression stockings, and leg exercises may help prevent skin injury.

Controlling Anxiety

Because patients with HF have difficulty maintaining adequate oxygenation, they are likely to be restless and anxious and feel overwhelmed by breathlessness. These symptoms tend to intensify at night. Emotional stress stimulates the sympathetic nervous system, which causes vasoconstriction, elevated arterial pressure, and increased heart rate. This sympathetic response increases the cardiac workload. By decreasing anxiety, the patient's cardiac workload also is decreased. Oxygen may be administered during an acute event to diminish the work of breathing and to increase the patient's comfort.

When the patient exhibits anxiety, the nurse takes steps to promote physical comfort and psychological support. In many cases, a family member's presence provides reassurance. To help decrease the patient's anxiety, the nurse should speak in a slow, calm, and confident manner and maintain eye contact.

Once the patient is comfortable, the nurse can begin teaching ways to control anxiety and to avoid anxiety-provoking situations. The nurse explains how to use relaxation techniques and helps the patient identify factors that contribute to anxiety. Lack of sleep may increase anxiety, which may prevent adequate rest. Other contributing factors may include misinformation, lack of information, or poor nutritional status. Promoting physical comfort, providing accurate information, and teaching the patient to perform relaxation techniques and to avoid anxiety-triggering situations may relax the patient.

In cases of confusion and anxiety reactions that affect the patient's safety, the use of restraints should be avoided. Restraints are likely to be resisted, and resistance inevitably increases the cardiac workload. The patient who insists on getting out of bed at night can be seated comfortably in an armchair. As cerebral and systemic circulation improves, the degree of anxiety decreases and the quality of sleep improves.

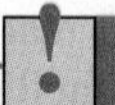

NURSING ALERT

Cerebral hypoxia with superimposed carbon dioxide retention may be a problem in HF, causing the patient to react to sedative–hypnotic medications with confusion and increased anxiety. Hepatic congestion may slow the liver's metabolism of medication, leading to toxicity. Sedative–hypnotic medications must be administered with caution.

In addition to anxiety, patients with HF have a high incidence of depression and should be screened for this condition (Artinian, 2003).

Minimizing Powerlessness

Patients need to recognize that they are not helpless and that they can influence the direction of their lives and the outcomes of treatment. The nurse assesses for factors that contribute to a sense of powerlessness and intervenes accordingly. Contributing factors may include lack of knowledge and lack of opportunities to make decisions, particularly if health care providers and family members behave in maternalistic or paternalistic ways. If the patient is hospitalized, hospital policies may promote standardization and limit the patient's ability to make decisions (eg, what time to have meals or to take medications).

Taking time to listen actively to patients often encourages them to express their concerns and ask questions. Other strategies include providing the patient with decision-making opportunities, such as when activities are to occur or where objects are to be placed, and increasing the frequency and significance of those opportunities over time; providing encouragement while identifying the patient's progress; and assisting the patient to differentiate between factors that can be controlled and those that cannot. In some cases, the nurse may want to review hospital policies and standards that tend to promote powerlessness and advocate for their elimination or change (eg, limited visiting hours, prohibition of food from home).

Promoting Home and Community-Based Care

TEACHING PATIENTS SELF-CARE

The nurse provides patient education and involves the patient in the therapeutic regimen to promote understanding and adherence to the plan. When the patient recognizes that the diagnosis of HF can be successfully managed with lifestyle changes and medications, recurrences of acute HF lessen, unnecessary hospitalizations decrease, and life expectancy increases. Patients and their families are taught to follow the medication regimen as prescribed, maintain a low-sodium diet, perform and record daily weights, engage in routine physical activity, and recognize and report symptoms that indicate worsening HF. Although noncompliance is not well understood, interventions that may promote adherence include teaching to ensure accurate understanding. A summary of teaching points for the patient with HF is presented in Chart 30-5.

The patient and family members are supported and encouraged to ask questions so that information can be clarified and understanding enhanced. The nurse should be aware of cultural factors and adapt the teaching plan accordingly. Patients and their families need to be informed that the progression of the disease is influenced in part by choices made about health care and the decisions about following the treatment plan. They also need to be informed that health care providers are there to assist them in reaching their health care goals. Patients and family members need to make the decisions about the treatment plan and need to understand the possible outcomes of those decisions. The treatment plan then will be based on the patient's goals rather than on what health care providers think is needed. The nurse conveys that monitoring symptoms and daily weights, restricting sodium intake, avoiding excess fluids, preventing infection through influenza and pneumococcal immunizations, avoiding noxious agents (eg, alcohol, tobacco), and participating in regular exercise all aid in preventing exacerbations of HF.

CONTINUING CARE

Success in management of HF requires a complex medical regimen and multiple lifestyle changes that the patient may find difficult. Assistance may be provided through home health care, a heart failure clinic, or telehealth management.

Depending on the patient's physical status and the availability of family assistance, a home care referral may be indicated for a patient who has been hospitalized. Elderly patients and those who have longstanding heart disease with compromised physical stamina often require assistance with the transition to home after hospitalization for an acute episode of HF. It is important for the home care nurse to assess the physical environment of the home. Suggestions for adapting the home environment to meet the patient's activity limitations are important. If stairs are a concern, the patient can plan the day's activities so that stair climbing is minimized; for some patients, a temporary bedroom may be set up on the main level of the home. The home care nurse works with the patient and family to maximize the benefits of these changes.

The home care nurse also reinforces and clarifies information about dietary changes and fluid restrictions, the need to monitor symptoms and daily body weights, and the importance of obtaining follow-up health care. Assistance may be given in scheduling and keeping appointments as well. The patient is encouraged to gradually increase his or her self-care and responsibility for accomplishing the therapeutic regimen.

Heart failure clinics offer disease management strategies for patients with HF. Referral to a heart failure

CHART 30-5

HOME CARE CHECKLIST • The Patient With Heart Failure

At the completion of the home care instruction, the patient or caregiver will be able to:	Patient	Caregiver
• Identify heart failure as a chronic disease that can be managed with medications and specific self-management behaviors.	✔	✔
• Take or administer medications daily, exactly as prescribed.	✔	✔
• Monitor effects of medication.	✔	✔
• Know signs and symptoms of orthostatic hypotension and how to prevent it.	✔	✔
• Weigh self daily. - Obtain weight at the same time each day (eg, every morning after urination).	✔	
• Restrict sodium intake to 2–3 g daily: adapt diet by examining nutrition labels to check sodium content per serving; avoid canned or processed foods; eat fresh or frozen foods; consult the written diet plan and the list of permitted and restricted foods; avoid salt use; and avoid excesses in eating and drinking.	✔	✔
• Review activity program. - Participate in a daily exercise program. - Increase walking and other activities gradually, provided they do not cause unusual fatigue or dyspnea. - Conserve energies by balancing activity with rest periods. - Avoid activity in extremes of heat and cold, which increase the work of the heart. - Recognize that air conditioning may be essential in a hot, humid environment.	✔	
• Develop methods to manage and prevent stress. - Avoid tobacco. - Avoid alcohol. - Engage in meditation, guided imagery, or music therapy.	✔	
• Keep regular appointments with physician or clinic.	✔	✔
• Be alert for symptoms that may indicate recurring heart failure. - Know how to reach healthcare provider.	✔	✔
• Report immediately to the physician or clinic any of the following: - Gain in weight of ≥ 2–3 lb (0.9–1.4 kg) in 1 day, or 5 lb (2.3 kg) in 1 week - Loss of appetite - Unusual shortness of breath with activity - Swelling of ankles, feet, or abdomen - Persistent cough - Development of restless sleep; increase in number of pillows needed to sleep	✔	✔

clinic gives the patient access to education, professional staff, and individualized treatment regimens. Research has shown that patients managed through HF clinics have fewer exacerbations of HF, fewer hospitalizations, decreased costs of medical care, and increased quality of life (Silver, Pisano, & Cianci, 2004).

Telehealth management can provide the frequent contact necessary to manage HF without requiring frequent visits to health care providers. A variety of techniques ranging from simple telephone monitoring to sophisticated computer and video connections that monitor daily weight, vital signs, and symptoms may be used. Studies have shown that telehealth management decreases costs and hospitalizations for exacerbations of HF (Gramsky, Josephson, Langford, et al., 2003).

Evaluation

Expected Patient Outcomes

Expected patient outcomes may include the following:

1. Demonstrates tolerance for increased activity
   a. Describes adaptive methods for usual activities
   b. Stops any activity that causes symptoms of intolerance
   c. Maintains vital signs (pulse, blood pressure, respiratory rate, and pulse oximetry) within the targeted range
   d. Identifies factors that contribute to activity intolerance and takes actions to avoid them
   e. Establishes priorities for activities
   f. Schedules activities to conserve energy and to reduce fatigue and dyspnea

2. Maintains fluid balance
   a. Exhibits decreased peripheral and sacral edema
   b. Demonstrates methods for preventing edema
3. Is less anxious
   a. Avoids situations that produce stress
   b. Sleeps comfortably at night
   c. Reports decreased stress and anxiety
4. Makes decisions regarding care and treatment
   a. States ability to influence outcomes
5. Adheres to self-care regimen
   a. Performs and records daily weights
   b. Ensures dietary intake includes no more than 2 to 3 g of sodium per day
   c. Takes medications as prescribed
   d. Reports any unusual symptoms or side effects

Acute Heart Failure (Pulmonary Edema)

Pulmonary edema is the abnormal accumulation of fluid in the lungs. The fluid may accumulate in the interstitial spaces and in the alveoli.

Pathophysiology

Pulmonary edema is an acute event that results from HF. It can occur acutely, such as with MI, or it can occur as an exacerbation of chronic HF. Myocardial scarring as a result of ischemia can limit the distensibility of the ventricle and render it vulnerable to a sudden increase in workload. With increased resistance to left ventricular filling, blood backs up into the pulmonary circulation. The patient quickly develops pulmonary edema, sometimes called flash pulmonary edema, from the blood volume overload in the lungs. Pulmonary edema can also be caused by noncardiac disorders, such as renal failure, liver failure, and oncologic conditions that cause the body to retain fluid. The pathophysiology is similar to that seen in HF, in that the left ventricle cannot handle the volume overload and blood volume and pressure build up in the left atrium. The rapid increase in atrial pressure results in an acute increase in pulmonary venous pressure, which produces an increase in hydrostatic pressure that forces fluid out of the pulmonary capillaries into the interstitial spaces and alveoli.

Impaired lymphatic drainage also contributes to the accumulation of fluid in the lung tissues. The fluid within the alveoli mixes with air, creating "bubbles" that are expelled from the mouth and nose, producing the classic symptom of pulmonary edema: frothy pink (blood-tinged) sputum. Because of the fluid within the alveoli, air cannot enter, and gas exchange is impaired. The result is hypoxemia, which is often severe. The onset may be preceded by premonitory symptoms of pulmonary congestion, but it also may develop quickly in the patient with a ventricle that has little reserve to meet increased oxygen needs.

Clinical Manifestations

As a result of decreased cerebral oxygenation, the patient becomes increasingly restless and anxious. Along with a sudden onset of breathlessness and a sense of suffocation, the patient's hands become cold and moist, the nail beds become cyanotic (bluish), and the skin turns ashen (gray). The pulse is weak and rapid, and the neck veins are distended. Incessant coughing may occur, producing increasing quantities of mucoid sputum. As pulmonary edema progresses, the patient's anxiety and restlessness increase; the patient becomes confused, then stuporous. Breathing is rapid, noisy, and moist-sounding. The patient's oxygen saturation is significantly decreased. The patient, nearly suffocated by the blood-tinged, frothy fluid filling the alveoli, is literally drowning in secretions. The situation demands immediate action.

Assessment and Diagnostic Findings

The diagnosis is made by evaluating the clinical manifestations resulting from pulmonary congestion. A chest x-ray may be obtained to confirm that the pulmonary veins are engorged. Abrupt onset of signs of left-sided HF (eg, crackles on auscultation of the lungs, flash pulmonary edema) may occur without evidence of right-sided HF (eg, no JVD, no dependent edema).

Prevention

Like most complications, pulmonary edema is easier to prevent than to treat. To recognize it in its early stages, the nurse auscultates the lung fields and heart sounds, measures JVD, and assesses the degree of peripheral edema and the severity of breathlessness. A dry, hacking cough; fatigue; weight gain; development or worsening of edema; and decreased activity tolerance may be early indicators of developing pulmonary edema.

In an early stage, the condition may be alleviated by placing the patient in an upright position with the feet and legs dependent, eliminating overexertion, and minimizing emotional stress to reduce the left ventricular load. The treatment regimen and the patient's understanding of and adherence to it are re-examined. The long-range approach to preventing pulmonary edema must be directed at identifying its precipitating factors.

Medical Management

Clinical management of a patient with acute pulmonary edema due to left ventricular failure is directed toward reducing volume overload, improving ventricular function, and increasing respiratory exchange. These goals are accomplished through a combination of oxygen and ventilatory support, IV medications, and nursing interventions.

Oxygen Therapy

Oxygen is administered in concentrations adequate to relieve hypoxemia and dyspnea. Usually, a face mask or nonrebreathing mask is initially used. If respiratory failure is severe or persists, continuous positive airway pressure may be delivered by a face mask with a tight seal. For some patients, endotracheal intubation and mechanical ventilation are required. The ventilator can provide positive end-expiratory pressure, which is effective in reducing venous return, decreasing fluid movement from the pulmonary capillaries to the alveoli, and improving oxygenation. Oxygenation is monitored by pulse oximetry and by measurement of arterial blood gases.

Morphine

Morphine is titrated IV in small doses (2 to 5 mg) to reduce peripheral resistance and venous return so that blood can be redistributed from the pulmonary circulation to other parts of the body. This decreases pressure in the pulmonary capillaries and seepage of fluid into the lung tissue. The effect of morphine in decreasing anxiety is also beneficial.

Diuretics

Diuretics promote the excretion of sodium and water by the kidneys. Furosemide (Lasix), for example, is administered IV to produce a rapid diuretic effect. Furosemide also causes vasodilation and pooling of blood in peripheral blood vessels, which reduces the amount of blood returned to the heart. Some physicians prescribe bumetanide (Bumex) and metolazone (Zaroxolyn) in place of furosemide.

Intravenous Infusions

As described earlier in this chapter, continuous IV infusions of nesiritide, dobutamine, and milrinone may be indicated for the patient with acutely decompensated heart function.

Nursing Management

Positioning the Patient to Promote Circulation

Proper positioning can help reduce venous return to the heart. The patient is positioned upright, preferably with the legs dangling over the side of the bed. This has the immediate effect of decreasing venous return, lowering the output of the right ventricle, and decreasing lung congestion. Patients who cannot sit with the lower extremities dependent may be placed in an upright position in bed.

Providing Psychological Support

As the ability to breathe decreases, the patient's fear and anxiety rise proportionately, making the condition more severe. Reassuring the patient and providing skillful anticipatory nursing care are integral parts of the therapy. Because the patient feels a sense of impending doom and has an unstable condition, the nurse must remain with the patient. The nurse gives the patient simple, concise information in a reassuring voice about what is being done to treat the condition and the expected results. The nurse also identifies any anxiety-inducing factors (eg, a pet left alone at home, presence of an unwelcome family member at the bedside, unpaid household bills) and initiates strategies to eliminate the concern or reduce its effect.

Monitoring Medications

The patient receiving morphine is observed for respiratory depression, hypotension, and vomiting; a morphine antagonist, such as naloxone hydrochloride (Narcan), is kept available and given to the patient who exhibits any serious side effects.

The patient receiving diuretic therapy may excrete a large volume of urine within minutes after a potent diuretic is administered. A bedside commode may be used to decrease the energy required by the patient and to reduce the resultant increase in cardiac workload induced by getting on and off a bedpan. If necessary, an indwelling urinary catheter may be inserted.

The patient receiving continuous IV infusions of vasoactive drugs requires ECG monitoring and frequent measurement of vital signs.

Other Complications

Cardiogenic Shock

Cardiogenic shock occurs when decreased CO leads to inadequate tissue perfusion and initiation of the shock syndrome. Cardiogenic shock may occur following MI when a large area of myocardium becomes ischemic, necrotic, and hypokinetic. It also can occur as a result of end-stage HF, cardiac tamponade, pulmonary embolism, cardiomyopathy, and dysrhythmias. Cardiogenic shock is a life-threatening condition with a high mortality rate (for further information see Chapter 15).

Pathophysiology

The signs and symptoms of cardiogenic shock reflect the circular nature of the pathophysiology of HF. The degree of shock is proportional to the extent of left ventricular dysfunction. The heart muscle loses its contractile power, resulting in a marked reduction in SV and CO. The decreased CO in turn reduces arterial blood pressure and tissue perfusion in the vital organs (heart, brain, lung, kidneys). Flow to the coronary arteries is reduced, resulting in decreased oxygen supply to the myocardium, which increases ischemia and further reduces the heart's ability to pump. Inadequate emptying of the ventricle also leads to increased pulmonary pressures, pulmonary congestion, and pulmonary edema, exacerbating the hypoxia, causing ischemia of vital organs, and setting a vicious cycle in motion (Fig. 30-4).

Clinical Manifestations

The classic signs of cardiogenic shock are those of tissue hypoperfusion and result from HF and the overall shock state. They include cerebral hypoxia (restlessness, confusion, agitation), low blood pressure, rapid and weak pulse, cold and clammy skin, tachypnea with respiratory crackles, and decreased urinary output. Initially, arterial blood gas analysis may show respiratory alkalosis. Dysrhythmias are common and result from myocardial ischemia.

Assessment and Diagnostic Findings

The patient with cardiogenic shock is managed in an intensive care unit. A pulmonary artery catheter may be inserted

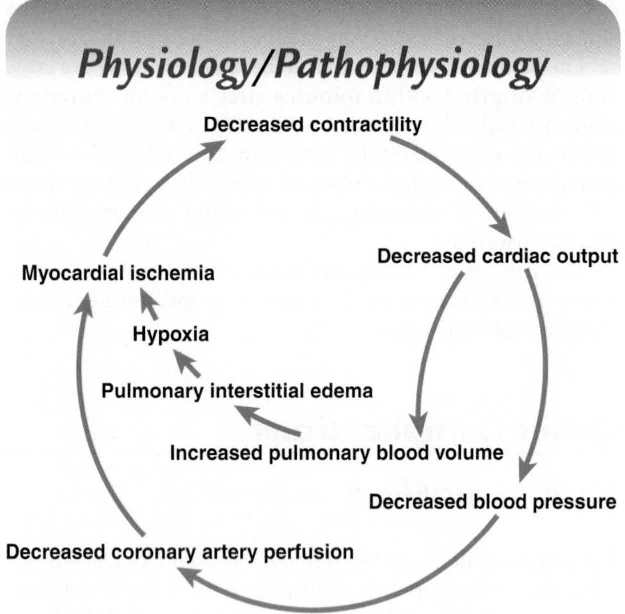

FIGURE 30-4. Pathophysiology of cardiogenic shock.

to measure CO and other hemodynamic parameters that are used to assess the severity of the problem and to guide patient management. The pulmonary artery wedge pressure is elevated and the CO is decreased as the left ventricle loses its ability to pump. The systemic vascular resistance is elevated because of the sympathetic nervous system stimulation that occurs as a compensatory response to the decrease in blood pressure. The decreased blood flow to the kidneys causes a hormonal response (ie, activation of the renin–angiotensin–aldosterone system) that causes fluid retention and further vasoconstriction. Increases in HR, circulating volume, and vasoconstriction occur to maintain circulation to the brain, heart, kidneys, and lungs, but at a cost: an increase in the workload of the heart.

The reduction in blood volume delivered to the tissues results in an increase in the amount of oxygen extracted from the blood that is delivered to the tissues (to try to meet the cellular demand for oxygen). The increased systemic oxygen extraction results in decreased venous (mixed and central) oxygen saturation. When the cellular oxygen needs cannot be met, anaerobic metabolism and buildup of lactic acid occur. Continuous central venous oximetry and measurement of blood lactic acid levels may help assess the severity of the shock as well as the effectiveness of treatment.

Continued cellular hypoperfusion eventually results in organ failure. The patient becomes unresponsive, severe hypotension ensues, and the patient develops shallow respirations and cold, cyanotic, or mottled skin. Arterial blood gas analysis shows metabolic acidosis, and all laboratory test results indicate organ dysfunction. Chapter 15 presents more detail about the pathophysiology and management of cardiogenic shock.

Medical Management

The most important approach to treating cardiogenic shock is to correct the underlying problem, reduce any further demand on the heart, improve oxygenation, and restore tissue perfusion. For example, if the ventricular failure is the result of an acute MI, emergency percutaneous coronary intervention may be indicated. Major dysrhythmias are corrected because they may have caused or contributed to the shock. If the patient has hypervolemia, diuresis is indicated. Diuretics, vasodilators, and mechanical therapies, such as continuous renal replacement therapy, have been used to reduce the circulating blood volume. If hypovolemia (low intravascular volume) is suspected or detected through hemodynamic pressure readings, the patient is given IV volume expanders (eg, normal saline solution, lactated Ringer's solution, albumin) to increase the amount of circulating fluid. The patient is placed on strict bed rest to conserve energy. If the patient has hypoxemia, as detected by pulse oximetry or arterial blood gas analysis, oxygen administration is increased, often under positive pressure when regular flow is insufficient to meet tissue demands. Intubation and sedation may be necessary to maintain oxygenation. The settings for mechanical ventilation are adjusted according to the patient's oxygenation status and the need for conserving energy.

Pharmacologic Therapy

Medication therapy is selected and guided according to CO, other cardiac parameters, and mean arterial blood pressure. Because of the decreased perfusion to the gastrointestinal system and the need to adjust the dosage quickly, most medications are administered IV.

Diuretics may be administered to decrease preload and afterload, reducing the workload of the heart. They are administered carefully to avoid worsening tissue hypoperfusion. Vasodilators such as milrinone (Primacor), sodium nitroprusside (Nipride), and nitroglycerin (Tridil) reduce the volume returning to the heart, decrease blood pressure, and decrease cardiac workload. They cause the arteries and veins to dilate, thereby shunting much of the intravascular volume to the periphery and causing a reduction in preload and afterload.

Positive inotropic medications are administered to increase myocardial contractility. Dobutamine (Dobutrex), dopamine (Intropin), and epinephrine (Adrenalin) can each cause tachydysrhythmias because they increase automaticity with increasing dosage. Therefore, monitoring baseline HR is important. As the baseline HR increases, so does the risk of developing tachydysrhythmias.

Vasopressors, or pressor agents, are used to increase blood pressure and increase CO. Many pressor medications are catecholamines, such as norepinephrine (Levophed) and high-dose dopamine (Intropin). Their purpose is to promote perfusion to the heart and brain, but they compromise circulation to other organs (eg, kidney). They also tend to increase the workload of the heart by increasing oxygen demand; thus, they are not administered early in cardiogenic shock.

Other Treatments

Other therapeutic modalities for cardiogenic shock include use of circulatory assist devices. The most frequently used mechanical support device is the intra-aortic balloon pump (IABP). The IABP is a catheter with an inflatable balloon at the end. The catheter is usually inserted through the femoral artery, and the balloon is positioned in the descending thoracic aorta (Fig. 30-5). The IABP uses internal counterpulsation through the regular inflation and deflation of the balloon to augment the pumping action of the heart. It inflates during diastole, increasing the pressure in the aorta during diastole and therefore increasing blood flow through the coronary and peripheral arteries. It deflates just before systole, lessening the pressure within the aorta before left ventricular contraction, decreasing the amount of resistance the heart has to overcome to eject blood and therefore decreasing the amount of work the heart must put forth to eject blood. The device is connected to a console that synchronizes the inflation and deflation of the balloon with the ECG or the arterial pressure (as indicators for systole and diastole). Hemodynamic monitoring is essential to determine the patient's response to the IABP.

Other ventricular assist devices for long-term support of the failing heart are described in Chapter 29.

Nursing Management

The patient in cardiogenic shock requires constant monitoring. Because of the frequency of nursing interventions and the technology required for effective patient management, the patient is treated in an intensive care unit. The critical care nurse must carefully assess the patient, observe the cardiac rhythm, monitor hemodynamic parameters, monitor fluid status, and adjust medications and therapies based on the assessment data. The patient is continuously evaluated for responses to the medical interventions and for the development of complications, so that problems can be addressed immediately.

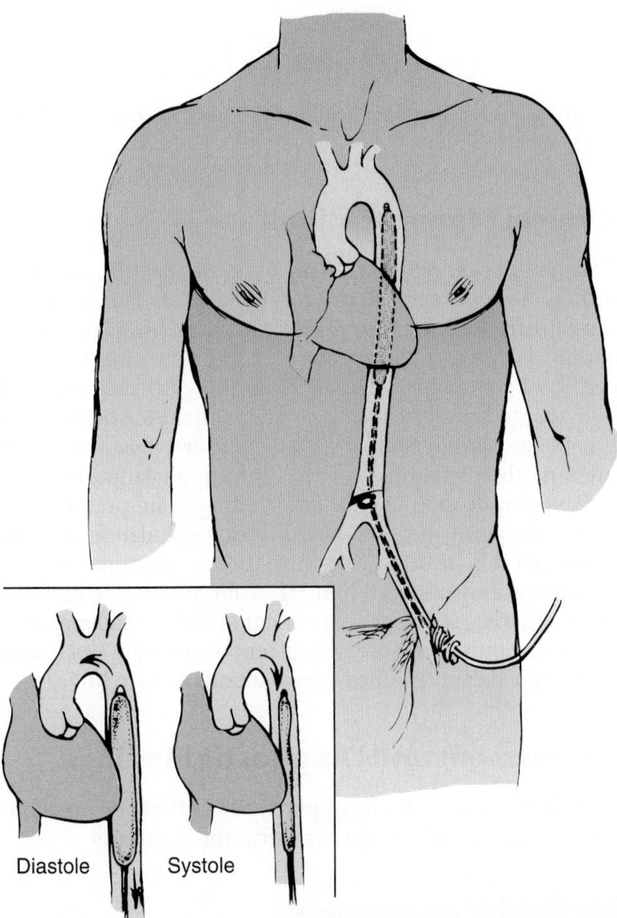

FIGURE 30-5. The intra-aortic balloon pump inflates at the beginning of diastole, which results in increased perfusion of the coronary and peripheral arteries. It deflates just before systole, which results in a decrease in afterload (resistance to ejection) and in the left ventricular workload.

Thromboembolism

The decreased mobility of the patient with cardiac disease and the impaired circulation that accompany these disorders contribute to the development of intracardiac and intravascular thrombosis. Intracardiac thrombus is especially common in patients with atrial fibrillation, because the atria do not contract forcefully and blood flows slowly and turbulently, increasing the likelihood of thrombus formation. Intracardiac thrombus is detected by an echocardiogram and treated with anticoagulants, such as heparin and warfarin (Coumadin). Adverse effects of thromboemboli are discussed in detail in Chapter 31.

Pulmonary Embolism

Pulmonary embolism is the most common thromboembolic problem among patients with HF. It poses a particular threat to people with cardiovascular disease (Koschel, 2004). Blood clots may form in the deep veins of the legs and embolize to the pulmonary vasculature, causing a life-threatening embolic event. Emboli mechanically obstruct the pulmonary vessels, cutting off the blood supply to sections of the lung (Fig. 30-6).

Clinical indicators of pulmonary embolism can vary but typically include dyspnea, chest pain, hemoptysis, tachycardia, and symptoms of deep venous thrombosis. Diagnostic tests often include a chest x-ray, ventilation–perfusion lung scan, or high-resolution helical computed tomography. A blood D-dimer assay is helpful to determine whether fibrinolysis of clots is taking place somewhere in the body.

Patient management begins with cardiopulmonary assessment and intervention. Emboli can cause hypoxic vasoconstriction and the release of inflammatory mediators in the pulmonary vessels, which can ultimately lead to right heart failure and respiratory failure (Goldhaber & Elliott, 2003). Anticoagulant therapy with unfractionated IV heparin or low-molecular-weight heparin is started when pulmonary embolism is suspected. Thrombolytic therapy may be used in patients with massive pulmonary emboli accompanied by hypotension and shock. Following initial therapy, patients are placed on warfarin (Coumadin) for at least 6 months. Prevention of deep vein thrombosis and pulmonary emboli is an important aspect of patient management. Both pharmacologic and mechanical means (eg, pneumatic compression devices) have proven effective in at-risk patients. Care for patients with pulmonary embolism is further discussed in Chapter 23.

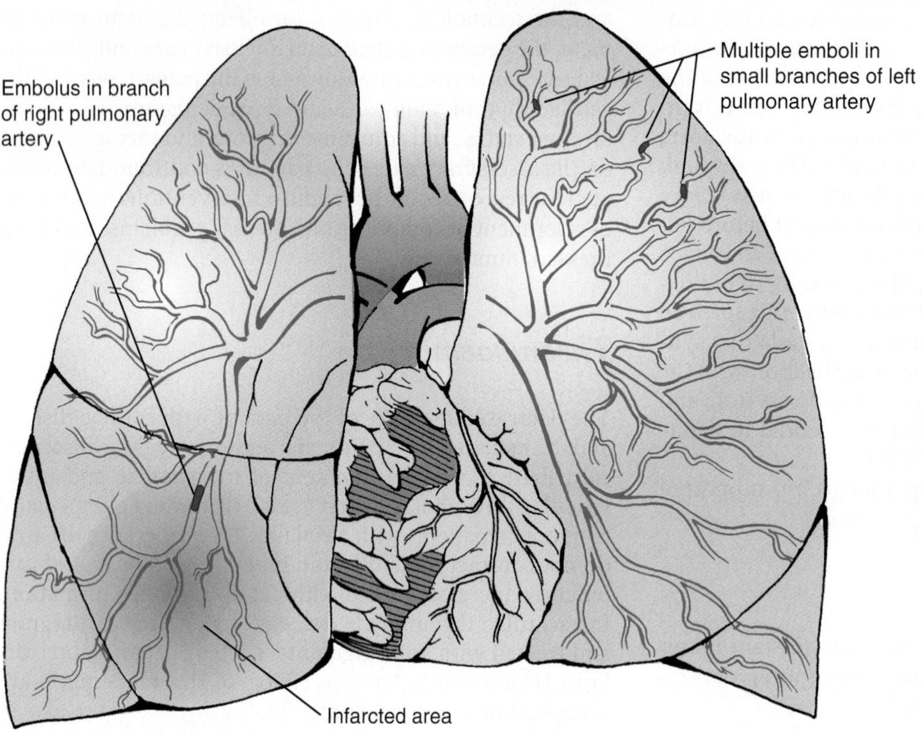

FIGURE 30-6. Pulmonary emboli may be single or multiple.

Pericardial Effusion and Cardiac Tamponade

Pathophysiology

Pericardial effusion (accumulation of fluid in the pericardial sac) may accompany pericarditis (see Chapter 29), advanced HF, metastatic carcinoma, cardiac surgery, or trauma.

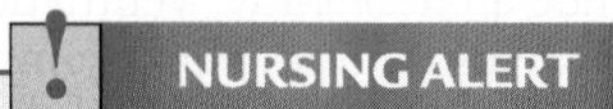

NURSING ALERT

Cardiac tamponade is a life-threatening situation, demanding immediate intervention.

Normally, the pericardial sac contains less than 50 mL of fluid, which is needed to decrease friction for the beating heart. An increase in pericardial fluid raises the pressure within the pericardial sac and compresses the heart. This has the following effects:

- Increased right and left ventricular end-diastolic pressures
- Decreased venous return
- Inability of the ventricles to distend and fill adequately

Pericardial fluid may accumulate slowly without causing noticeable symptoms until a large amount accumulates. However, a rapidly developing effusion can stretch the pericardium to its maximum size and, because of increased pericardial pressure, reduce venous return to the heart and decrease CO. The result is cardiac tamponade (eg, compression of the heart).

Clinical Manifestations

The patient may report a feeling of fullness within the chest or may have substantial or ill-defined pain. The feeling of pressure in the chest may result from stretching of the pericardial sac. Because of increased pressure within the pericardium, venous pressure tends to increase, as evidenced by engorged neck veins. Other signs include shortness of breath and labile or low blood pressure. Systolic blood pressure that is markedly lower during inhalation is called **pulsus paradoxus**. The difference in systolic pressure between the point that it is heard during exhalation and the point that it is heard during inhalation is measured. Pulsus paradoxus exceeding 10 mm Hg is abnormal. The cardinal signs of cardiac tamponade are falling systolic blood pressure, narrowing pulse pressure, rising venous pressure (increased JVD), and distant (muffled) heart sounds (Chart 30-6).

Assessment and Diagnostic Findings

A chest x-ray shows a large pericardial effusion. An echocardiogram is performed to confirm the diagnosis.

Medical Management

Pericardiocentesis

If cardiac function becomes seriously impaired, **pericardiocentesis** (puncture of the pericardial sac to aspirate pericardial fluid) is performed to remove fluid from the peri-

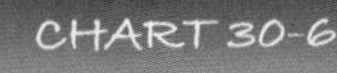

CHART 30-6

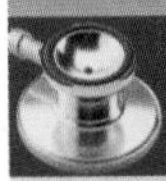

Assessing for Cardiac Tamponade

Assessment findings in cardiac tamponade resulting from pericardial effusion include feelings of faintness, shortness of breath, anxiety, and pain from decreased cardiac output, cough from pressure created in the trachea from swelling of the pericardial sac, distended neck veins from rising venous pressure, paradoxical pulse, and muffled or distant heart sounds.

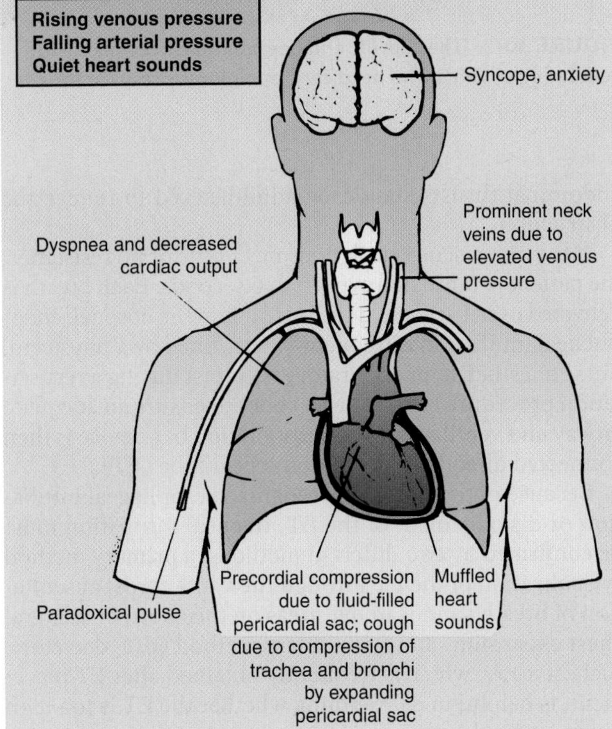

cardial sac. The major goal is to prevent cardiac tamponade, which restricts normal heart filling and contraction.

During the procedure, the patient is monitored by ECG and hemodynamic pressure measurements. Emergency resuscitation equipment should be readily available. The head of the bed is elevated to 45 to 60 degrees, placing the heart in proximity to the chest wall so that the needle can be inserted into the pericardial sac more easily. If a peripheral IV line is not already in place, one is inserted, and a slow IV infusion is started in case it becomes necessary to administer emergency medications or blood products.

The pericardial aspiration needle is attached to a 50-mL syringe by a three-way stopcock. Several possible sites are used for pericardial aspiration. Typically, ultrasound imaging is used to guide placement of the needle into the pericardial space. The needle is advanced slowly until it has entered the pericardium and fluid is obtained.

A resulting decrease in central venous pressure and an associated increase in blood pressure after withdrawal of pericardial fluid indicate that the cardiac tamponade has been relieved. The patient almost always feels immediate relief. If there is a substantial amount of pericardial fluid, a small catheter may be left in place to drain recurrent accumulation of blood or fluid. Pericardial fluid is sent to the laboratory for examination for tumor cells, bacterial culture, chemical and serologic analysis, and differential blood cell count.

Complications of pericardiocentesis include ventricular or coronary artery puncture, dysrhythmias, pleural laceration, gastric puncture, and myocardial trauma. After pericardiocentesis, the patient's heart rhythm, blood pressure, venous pressure, and heart sounds are monitored to detect possible recurrence of cardiac tamponade. If it recurs, repeated aspiration is necessary. Cardiac tamponade may require treatment by open pericardial drainage (pericardiotomy) (see Chapter 23).

Pericardiotomy

Recurrent pericardial effusions, usually associated with neoplastic disease, may be treated by a **pericardiotomy** (pericardial window). Under general anesthesia, a portion of the pericardium is excised to permit the pericardial fluid to drain into the lymphatic system. The nursing care is the same as that for other cardiac surgery (see Chapter 28).

Cardiac Arrest

Cardiac arrest occurs when the heart ceases to produce an effective pulse and circulate blood. It may be caused by a cardiac electrical event such as ventricular fibrillation, progressive profound bradycardia, or when there is no heart rhythm at all (asystole). Cardiac arrest may follow respiratory arrest; it may also occur when electrical activity is present but there is ineffective cardiac contraction or circulating volume, which is called **pulseless electrical activity (PEA).** Formerly called electrical-mechanical dissociation (EMD), PEA can be caused by hypovolemia (eg, with excessive bleeding), hypoxia, hypothermia, hyperkalemia, massive pulmonary embolism, myocardial infarction, and medication overdose (eg, beta-blockers, calcium channel blockers).

Clinical Manifestations

In cardiac arrest, consciousness, pulse, and blood pressure are lost immediately. Ineffective respiratory gasping may occur. The pupils of the eyes begin dilating within 45 seconds. Seizures may or may not occur.

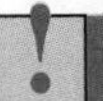

NURSING ALERT

The most reliable sign of cardiac arrest is the absence of a pulse. In the adult and the child, the carotid pulse is assessed. In an infant, the brachial pulse is assessed. Valuable time should not be wasted taking the blood pressure, listening for the heartbeat, or checking proper contact of electrodes.

The risk of irreversible brain damage and death increases with every minute from the time that circulation ceases. The interval varies with the age and underlying condition of the patient. During this period, the diagnosis of cardiac arrest must be made and measures must be taken immediately to restore circulation.

Emergency Management: Cardiopulmonary Resuscitation

Cardiopulmonary resuscitation (CPR) provides blood flow to vital organs until effective circulation can be re-established. The ABCDs of basic CPR are *a*irway, *b*reathing, *c*irculation, and *d*efibrillation (AHA, 2005). Once loss of consciousness has been established, the resuscitation priority for the adult in most cases is placing a phone call to activate the code team or the emergency medical system (EMS). Exceptions to this include near drowning, drug or medication overdose, and respiratory arrest situations, for which 2 minutes of CPR should be performed before activating the EMS. Because the underlying cause of arrest in an infant or child is usually respiratory, the priority is to begin CPR and then activate the EMS after 2 minutes of CPR. Because the care of the pediatric patient is individualized, the following discussion on the care of a cardiac arrest patient applies mainly to adults.

Resuscitation consists of the following steps:

1. Airway: maintaining an open airway
2. Breathing: providing artificial ventilation by rescue breathing
3. Circulation: promoting artificial circulation by external cardiac compression; administer medication therapy (eg, epinephrine for asystole)
4. Defibrillation with standard defibrillator or automatic external defibrillator (AED) for ventricular tachycardia and ventricular fibrillation

If the patient is already being monitored or is immediately placed on the monitor using the multifunction pads or the quick-look paddles (found on most defibrillators) and the ECG shows ventricular tachycardia or ventricular fibrillation, immediate defibrillation rather than CPR is the treatment of choice. In this scenario, CPR is performed initially only if the defibrillator is not immediately available. The survival rate decreases for every minute that defibrillation is delayed (AHA, 2005). If the patient has not been defibrillated within 10 minutes, the chance of survival is close to zero. More information on defibrillation can be found in Chapter 27.

Maintaining Airway and Breathing

The first step in CPR is to establish an open airway. Any obvious material in the mouth or throat should be removed. The airway should be opened using a head-tilt chin-lift maneuver. The rescuer "looks, listens, and feels" for air movement. An oropharyngeal airway is inserted if available. Two rescue ventilations are provided using a bag-mask or mouth-mask device (Fig. 30-7). An obstructed airway should be suspected when the rescuer cannot give the initial ventilations, and the Heimlich maneuver or abdominal thrusts should be administered to relieve the obstruction.

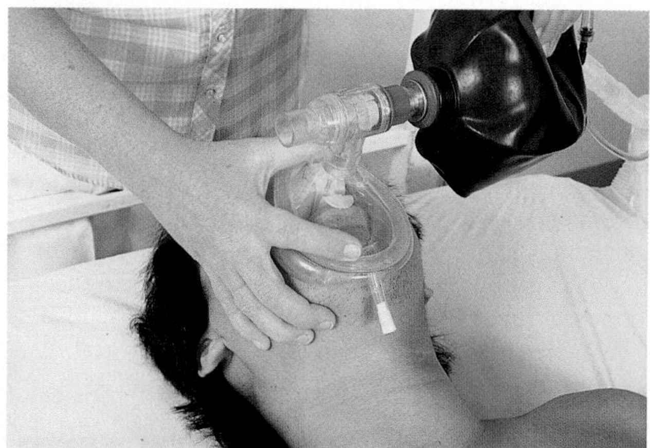

FIGURE 30-7. The chin lift and bag-and-mask technique for ventilating patients who need cardiopulmonary resuscitation.

If the first rescue ventilations meet little or no resistance, the patient is ventilated every 5 to 6 seconds. Each breath is delivered over 1 second. If the patient is in the hospital, endotracheal intubation is frequently performed by a physician, nurse anesthetist, or respiratory therapist during a resuscitation procedure (also called a code) to ensure an adequate airway and ventilation. The resuscitation bag device is then connected directly to the endotracheal tube (ET).

Because of the risk of unrecognized esophageal intubation or dislodgement of the ET, tracheal intubation must be confirmed by two different methods: a primary method (visualization of the ET through the vocal cords, auscultation of breath sounds in five areas on the chest, or bilateral chest expansion) and a secondary method (CO_2 detector). A chest x-ray, which is frequently obtained after ET placement, is helpful in determining whether the ET is too high or too low in the trachea. However, a chest x-ray cannot definitively confirm placement of an ET: an ET in the esophagus or the trachea produces the same appearance on the x-ray. Arterial blood gas levels are measured to guide oxygen therapy.

Restoring Circulation

After performing ventilation, the carotid pulse is assessed, and external cardiac compressions are provided if no pulse is detected. If a defibrillator is not yet available but a process has been put into place to obtain one, chest compressions are initiated. Compressions are performed with the patient on a firm surface, such as the floor, a cardiac board, or a meal tray. The rescuer (facing the patient's side) places the heel of one hand on the lower half of the sternum, two fingerwidths (3.8 cm [1.5 inches]) from the tip of the xiphoid, and positions the other hand on top of the first hand (Fig. 30-8). The fingers should not touch the chest wall (AHA, 2003).

Using the force of body weight while keeping the elbows straight, the rescuer presses quickly downward from the shoulder area to deliver a forceful compression to the victim's lower sternum about 3.8 to 5 cm (1.5 to 2 inches) toward the

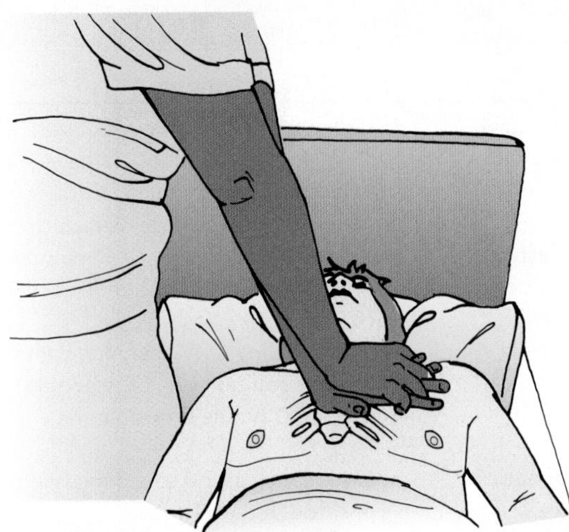

FIGURE 30-8. Chest compressions in cardiopulmonary resuscitation (CPR) are performed by placing the heel of one hand on the lower half of the sternum and the other hand on top of the first hand. Elbows are kept straight and body weight is used to apply quick, forceful compressions to the lower sternum. For the most effective hand placement and outcome, the patient's chest should be bare.

spine. The chest compression rate is approximately 100 times per minute. A compression to ventilation ratio of 30 to 2 is recommended without pause for ventilations.

When the code team or emergency medical personnel arrive, the patient is quickly assessed to determine cardiac rhythm and respiratory status, as well as possible causes of the arrest. The specific subsequent advanced life support interventions depend on the assessment results. For example, after the patient is placed on a cardiac monitor and ventricular fibrillation is detected, the patient is defibrillated up to three times, and then CPR is resumed. However, if asystole is detected on the monitor, CPR is resumed immediately while trying to identify the underlying cause, such as hypovolemia, hypothermia, or hypoxia. CPR may be stopped when the patient responds and begins to breathe, rescuers are too exhausted or at risk (eg, a building is at risk of collapsing) to continue CPR, or signs of death are obvious. If the patient does not respond to therapies given during the arrest, the resuscitation effort may be stopped or "called" by the physician. The decision to terminate resuscitation is based on medical considerations and takes into account the underlying condition of the patient and the chances for survival.

Follow-Up Monitoring and Care

Once resuscitated, the patient is transferred to an intensive care unit for close monitoring. Continuous ECG monitoring and frequent blood pressure assessments are essential until hemodynamic stability is re-established. Etiologic factors that precipitated the arrest, such as metabolic or rhythm abnormalities, must be identified and treated. Possible contributing factors, such as electrolyte or acid–base imbalances, need to be identified and corrected. Selected medications (Table 30-5) may be used during and after resuscitation.

NURSING RESEARCH PROFILE

Family Presence During Cardiopulmonary Resuscitation

MacLean, S. L., Guzzetta, C. E., White, C., et al. (2003). Family presence during cardiopulmonary resuscitation and invasive procedures: Practices of critical care and emergency nurses. *Journal of Emergency Nursing, 29*(3), 208–221.

Purpose

In hospitals and urgent care facilities, there is a growing trend to allow families to be present during CPR and invasive procedures. Among nurses there is variable support and controversy regarding this change in practice. The purpose of this study was to identify facility policies and nurse preferences and practices related to allowing family members to be present at the bedside during CPR and invasive procedures.

Design

A 30-item survey was randomly mailed to critical care and emergency department nurses who belong to various national specialty organizations. The survey included questions about written policies and the nurses' preferences as to whether there should be written policies. Nurses were also asked about their personal experiences with family presence. A total of 984 surveys were returned, for a response rate of 32.8%.

Findings

Only 5% of the nurses worked on units with written policies allowing family presence during CPR and invasive procedures. About 50% worked on units that permitted the presence of family members during these events but did not have written policies. Many nurses reported that they had taken family members to the bedside for CPR and other procedures (36% and 44%, respectively) or would do so in the future. They also reported that family members had requested to be present for CPR and invasive procedures (31% and 61%, respectively).

Nursing Implications

Most critical care and emergency department nurses support the option of family presence, provided that staff members are available to guide, educate, and support families. This reflects the trend toward family-centered care and the desire to meet the holistic needs of patients and family members. Written policies or guidelines are recommended.

TABLE 30-5 Medications Used in Cardiopulmonary Resuscitation

Agent and Action	Indications	Nursing Considerations
Oxygen—improves tissue oxygenation and corrects hypoxemia	Administered to all patients with acute cardiac ischemia or suspected hypoxemia, including those with COPD	• Use 100% FiO_2 during resuscitation. • Recognize that no lung damage occurs when used for less than 24 hours. • Monitor dose by pulse oximeter.
Epinephrine (Adrenalin)—increases systemic vascular resistance and blood pressure; improves coronary and cerebral perfusion and myocardial contractility	Given to patients in cardiac arrest, especially caused by asystole or pulseless electrical activity; may be given if caused by ventricular tachycardia or ventricular fibrillation	• Administer 1 mg every 3–5 minutes by IV push or through the endotracheal (ET) tube. • Avoid adding to IV lines that contain alkaline solution (eg, bicarbonate).
Vasopressin (Pitressin)—increases systemic vascular resistance and blood pressure	An alternative to epinephrine	• Give 40 U IV one time only.
Atropine—blocks parasympathetic action; increases SA node automaticity and AV conduction	Given to patients with symptomatic bradycardia (hemodynamically unstable, frequent premature ventricular contractions and symptoms of ischemia)	• Give rapidly as 2.0 to 2.5 mg IV push or through the ET tube. • Be aware that less than 0.5 mg in the adult can cause the heart rate to decrease to a worse bradycardia. • Monitor patient for reflexive tachycardia.
Sodium bicarbonate ($NaHCO_3$)—corrects metabolic acidosis	Given to correct metabolic acidosis that is refractory to standard advanced cardiac life support interventions (cardiopulmonary resuscitation, intubation, and respiratory management)	• Administer initial dose of 1 mEq/kg IV; then administer the dose based on the base deficit calculated from arterial blood gas values. • Recognize that to prevent development of rebound metabolic alkalosis, complete correction of acidosis is not indicated
Magnesium—promotes adequate functioning of the cellular sodium–potassium pump	Given to patients with torsades de pointes	• May give diluted over 1–2 min or intravenous push. • Monitor for hypotension, asystole, bradycardia, respiratory paralysis.

COPD, chronic obstructive pulmonary disease

Critical Thinking Exercises

1 You are assessing a 72-year-old woman with a 3-year history of HF. Her medications include carvedilol, valsartan, furosemide, and potassium. She reports two episodes of severe dizziness. What are possible causes of dizziness in this patient? What questions would you include in your assessment? What medical and nursing interventions would be appropriate for each possible cause?

2 ebp On an inpatient progressive care unit, you are assigned to care for a 60-year-old man who has been readmitted for the third time with severe HF and widespread edema. According to the patient's chart, he has a history of noncompliance with diet and medications. What are your immediate priorities and short-term goals for this patient? What medical interventions are indicated? Develop an evidence-based plan of care for this patient in the future. Describe your planned interaction with the patient (ie, communication technique, behaviors) that would encourage the patient to participate in the plan.

3 ebp On an inpatient progressive care unit, you receive a 55-year-old man who just been transferred from the cardiac intensive care unit. You realize that he is at risk of complications after a large anterior wall MI, which was treated with emergent cardiac catheterization and percutaneous coronary intervention. His medications include aspirin, clopidogrel, metoprolol, and lisinopril. During your initial assessment, you notice that the patient appears weak and pale. You have trouble hearing his blood pressure, but think you hear a systolic pressure of about 80 mm Hg. List the possible complications this patient may be experiencing. What assessment parameters would you check next? Discuss the strength of the evidence that supports priority nursing interventions and expected outcomes. Describe your communication with the patient during the interventions.

REFERENCES AND SELECTED READINGS

BOOKS

American Heart Association. (2004). *2004 Heart and stroke statistics.* Dallas, TX: Author.

Carpenito, L. J. (2004). *Nursing diagnosis: Application to clinical practice* (10th ed.). Philadelphia: Lippincott Williams & Wilkins.

Fink, M. P., Abraham, E., Vincent, J. L., et al. (Eds.). (2005). *Textbook of critical care* (5th ed.). Philadelphia: Elsevier.

Morton, P. G., Fontaine, D. K., Hudak, C. M., et al. (Eds.). (2005). *Critical care nursing* (8th ed.). Philadelphia: Lippincott Williams & Wilkins.

Porth, C. M. (2005). *Pathophysiology: Concepts of altered health states* (7th ed.). Philadelphia: Lippincott Williams & Wilkins.

Silver, M. A., Pisano, C., & Cianci, P. (2004). *Outpatient management of heart failure.* Littleton, CO: Postgraduate Institute for Medicine.

Zipes, D. P., Libby, P., & Bonow, R. D. (Eds.). (2005). *Braunwald's heart disease* (7th ed.). Philadelphia: Saunders.

JOURNALS

**Asterisks indicate nursing research articles.*

Albert, N. M. (2003a). Cardiac resynchronization therapy through biventricular pacing in patients with heart failure and ventricular dyssynchrony. *Critical Care Nurse, 23*(Supp), 2–13.

Albert, N. M. (2003b). Surgical management of heart failure. *Critical Care Nursing Clinics of North America, 15*(4), 477–487.

American Heart Association. (2005). Guidelines for cardiopulmonary resuscitation and emergency cardiovascular care. *Circulation, 112*(24), 1–203.

Ammon, S. (2001). Managing patients with heart failure. *American Journal of Nursing, 101*(12), 34–40.

Artinian, N. T. (2003). The psychosocial aspects of heart failure. *American Journal of Nursing, 103*(12), 32–43.

Bradley, D. J., Bradley, E. A., & Baughman, K. L. (2003). Cardiac resynchronization and death from progressive heart failure: A meta-analysis of randomized controlled trials. *Journal of the American Medical Association, 289*(6), 730–740.

*Corvera-Tindel, T., Doering, L. V., Gomez, T., et al. (2004). Predictors of noncompliance to exercise training in heart failure. *Journal of Cardiovascular Nursing, 19*(4), 269–277.

Goldhaber, S. Z., & Elliott, C. G. (2003). Acute pulmonary embolism. Part I: Epidemiology, pathophysiology, and diagnosis. *Circulation, 108*(22), 2726–2729.

Gramsky, C., Josephson, S., Langford, M., et al. (2003). Outpatient management of heart failure. *Critical Care Nursing Clinics of North America, 15*(4), 501–509.

Hachey, D. M., & Smith, T. (2003). Use of neseritide to treat acute decompensated heart failure. *Critical Care Nurse, 23*(1), 53–55.

Hunt, S. A., Baker, D. W., Chin, M. H., et al., American College of Cardiology/American Heart Association Task Force on Practice Guidelines (Committee to Revise the 1995 Guidelines for the Evaluation and Management of Heart Failure), International Society for Heart and Lung Transplantation, & Heart Failure Society of America. (2001). ACC/AHA guidelines for the evaluation and management of chronic heart failure in the adult: A report of the American College of Cardiology/American Heart Association Task Force on Practice Guidelines (Committee to Revise the 1995 Guidelines for the Evaluation and Management of Heart Failure). *Journal of the American College of Cardiology, 38*(7), 2101–2113.

Institute for Clinical Systems Improvement (ICSI) (2004). *Heart failure in adults.* Bloomington, MN: ICSI. Available at http://www.AHRQ.gov/summary/summary.aspx?doc_id=7657+ss=1. Accessed May 31, 2006.

Koschel, M. J. (2004). Pulmonary embolism. *American Journal of Nursing, 104*(6), 46–50.

*MacLean, S. L., Guzzetta, C. E., White, C., et al. (2003). Family presence during cardiopulmonary resuscitation and invasive procedures: Practices of critical care and emergency nurses. *Journal of Emergency Nursing, 29*(3), 208–221.

Moser, D. K., & Biddle, M. J. (2003). Angiotensin-converting enzyme inhibitors and angiotensin II receptor blockers. *Critical Care Nursing Clinics of North America, 15*(4), 423–437.

Piano, M. R., & Prasun, M. (2003). Neurohormone activation. *Critical Care Nursing Clinics of North America, 15*(4), 413–421.

Pina, I. L., Apstein, C. S., Balady, G. J., et al. (2003). Exercise and heart failure. *Circulation, 107*(8), 1210.

Smith, A. L., & Brown, C. S. (2003). New advances and novel treatments in heart failure. *Critical Care Nurse, 23*(Supp), 11–18.

*Sneed, N. V., & Paul, S. C. (2003). Readiness for behavioral changes in patients with heart failure. *American Journal of Critical Care, 12*(5), 444–453.

Spencer, A. P. (2003). Digoxin in heart failure. *Critical Care Nursing Clinics of North America, 15*(4), 447–452.

Tokarczyk, T. R. (2003). Cardiac transplantation as a treatment option for the heart failure patient. *Critical Care Nursing Quarterly, 26*(1), 61–68.

Trypp, R. J., Abraham, W. T., & Lamba, S. (2003). Future therapies for heart failure. *Critical Care Nursing Clinics of North America, 15*(4), 525–530.

Young, J. B., Abraham, W. T., & Smith, A. L. (2003). Combined cardiac resynchronization and implantable cardioversion defibrillation in advanced chronic heart failure. *Journal of the American Medical Association, 289*(20), 2685–2694.

RESOURCES

American Heart Association, 7320 Greenville Ave., Dallas, TX 75231; 1-800-242-8721; http://www.americanheart.org. Accessed May 31, 2006.

Heart Failure Society of America, Court International, Suite 238-N, 2550 University Avenue West, Saint Paul, MN 55144; 651-642-1633; http://www.abouthf.org. Accessed May 31, 2006.

Heartmates, Inc., P.O. Box 16202, Minneapolis, MN 55416; 952-929-3331; http://www.heartmates.com. Accessed May 31, 2006.

National Heart, Lung, and Blood Institute, National Institutes of Health, Building 31, Room 5A52, Bethesda, MD 20892; 301-592-8573; http://www.nhlbi.nih.gov. Accessed May 31, 2006.

CHAPTER 31

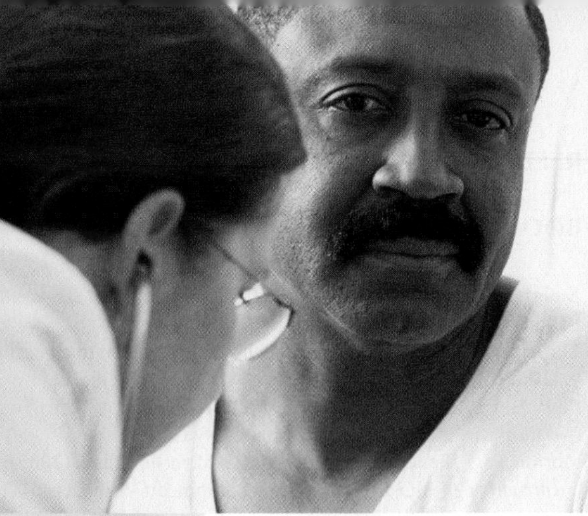

Assessment and Management of Patients With Vascular Disorders and Problems of Peripheral Circulation

Learning Objectives

On completion of this chapter, the learner will be able to:

1. Identify anatomic and physiologic factors that affect peripheral blood flow and tissue oxygenation.
2. Use appropriate parameters for assessment of peripheral circulation.
3. Use the nursing process as a framework of care for patients with vascular insufficiency of the extremities.
4. Compare the various diseases of the arteries and their causes, pathologic and physiologic changes, clinical manifestations, management, and prevention.
5. Describe the prevention and management of venous thrombosis.
6. Compare strategies to prevent venous insufficiency, leg ulcers, and varicose veins.
7. Use the nursing process as a framework of care for patients with leg ulcers.
8. Describe nursing and medical management of cellulitis.
9. Describe the relationship between lymphangitis and lymphedema.

Adequate perfusion ensures oxygenation and nourishment of body tissues, and it depends in part on a properly functioning cardiovascular system. Adequate blood flow depends on the efficiency of the heart as a pump, the patency and responsiveness of the blood vessels, and the adequacy of circulating blood volume. Nervous system activity, blood viscosity, and the metabolic needs of tissues influence the rate and adequacy of blood flow.

Anatomic and Physiologic Overview

The vascular system consists of two interdependent systems. The right side of the heart pumps blood through the lungs to the pulmonary circulation, and the left side of the heart pumps blood to all other body tissues through the systemic circulation. The blood vessels in both systems channel the blood from the heart to the tissues and back to the heart (Fig. 31-1). Contraction of the ventricles is the driving force that moves blood through the vascular system.

Arteries distribute oxygenated blood from the left side of the heart to the tissues, whereas the veins carry deoxygenated blood from the tissues to the right side of the heart. Capillary vessels located within the tissues connect the arterial and venous systems. These vessels permit the exchange of nutrients and metabolic wastes between the circulatory system and the tissues. Arterioles and venules immediately adjacent to the capillaries, together with the capillaries, make up the microcirculation.

The lymphatic system complements the function of the circulatory system. Lymphatic vessels transport lymph (a fluid similar to plasma) and tissue fluids (containing proteins, cells, and cellular debris) from the interstitial space to systemic veins.

Anatomy of the Vascular System

Arteries and Arterioles

Arteries are thick-walled structures that carry blood from the heart to the tissues. The aorta, which has a diameter of approximately 25 mm (1 inch) in the average-sized adult, gives rise to numerous branches, which continue to divide into progressively smaller arteries that are 4 mm (0.16 inch) in diameter. The vessels divide further, diminishing in size to approximately 30 μm in diameter. These smallest arteries, called the arterioles, are generally embedded within the tissues.

The walls of the arteries and arterioles are composed of three layers: the intima, an inner endothelial cell layer; the media, a middle layer of smooth muscle and elastic tissue; and the adventitia, an outer layer of connective tissue. The intima, a very thin layer, provides a smooth surface for contact with the flowing blood. The media makes up most of the vessel wall in the aorta and other large arteries of the body. This layer is composed chiefly of elastic and connective tissue fibers that give the vessels considerable strength and allow them to constrict and dilate to accommodate the blood ejected from the heart during each cardiac cycle (stroke volume) and maintain an even, steady flow of blood. The adventitia is a layer of connective tissue that anchors the vessel to its surroundings. There is much less elastic tissue in the smaller arteries and arterioles, and the media in these vessels is composed primarily of smooth muscle (Porth, 2005).

Smooth muscle controls the diameter of the vessels by contracting and relaxing. Chemical, hormonal, and neuronal factors influence the activity of smooth muscle. Because arterioles offer resistance to blood flow by altering their diameter, they are often referred to as *resistance vessels.* Arterioles regulate the volume and pressure in the arterial system and the rate of blood flow to the capillaries. Because

Glossary

anastomosis: junction of two vessels

aneurysm: a localized sac or dilation of an artery formed at a weak point in the vessel wall

ankle-brachial index (ABI) or ankle-arm index (AAI): ratio of the ankle systolic pressure to the arm systolic pressure; an objective measurement of arterial disease that provides quantification of the degree of stenosis

angioplasty: an invasive procedure that uses a balloon-tipped catheter to dilate a stenotic area of a blood vessel

arteriosclerosis: diffuse process whereby the muscle fibers and the endothelial lining of the walls of small arteries and arterioles thicken

atherosclerosis: disease process involving the accumulation of lipids, calcium, blood components, carbohydrates, and fibrous tissue on the intimal layer of a large or medium-sized artery

bruit: sound produced by turbulent blood flow through an irregular, tortuous, stenotic, or dilated vessel

dissection: separation of the weakened elastic and fibromuscular elements in the medial layer of an artery

duplex ultrasonography: combines B-mode gray-scale imaging of tissue, organs, and blood vessels with capabilities of estimating velocity changes by use of a pulsed Doppler

intermittent claudication: a muscular, cramp-like pain in the extremities consistently reproduced with the same degree of exercise or activity and relieved by rest

international normalized ratio (INR): method of measuring anticoagulation levels, such as warfarin (Coumadin); devised to bring a universal standard to monitoring of anticoagulation achieved by oral medications

ischemia: deficient blood supply

rest pain: persistent pain in the foot or digits when the patient is resting, indicating a severe degree of arterial insufficiency

rubor: reddish blue discoloration of the extremities; indicative of severe peripheral arterial damage in vessels that remain dilated and unable to constrict

stenosis: narrowing or constriction of a vessel

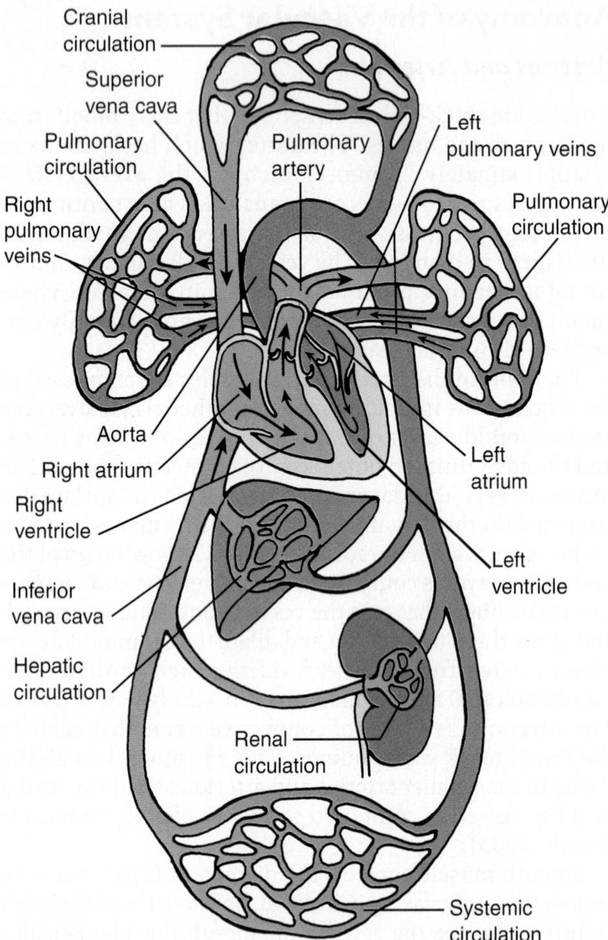

FIGURE 31-1. Systemic and pulmonary circulation. Oxygen-rich blood from the pulmonary circulation is pumped from the left heart into the aorta and the systemic arteries to the capillaries, where the exchange of nutrients and waste products takes place. The deoxygenated blood returns to the right heart by way of the systemic veins and is pumped into the pulmonary circulation. From *Stedman's Medical Dictionary* (28th ed.). (2006). Philadelphia: Lippincott Williams & Wilkins.

of the large amount of smooth muscle in the media, the walls of the arteries are relatively thick, accounting for approximately 25% of the total diameter of the artery.

The intima and the inner third of the smooth muscle layer of the media are in such close contact with the blood that the blood vessel receives its nourishment by direct diffusion. The adventitia and the outer media layers have a limited vascular system for nourishment and require their own blood supply to meet metabolic needs.

Capillaries

The walls of the capillaries, which lack smooth muscle and adventitia, are composed of a single layer of endothelial cells. This thin-walled structure permits rapid and efficient transport of nutrients to the cells and removal of metabolic wastes. The diameter of capillaries ranges from 5 to 10 μm; this means that red blood cells must alter their shape to pass through these vessels. Changes in a capillary's diameter are passive and are influenced by contractile changes in the blood vessels that carry blood to and from a capillary. The capillary's diameter also changes in response to chemical stimuli. In some tissues, a cuff of smooth muscle, called the precapillary sphincter, is located at the arteriolar end of the capillary and is responsible, along with the arteriole, for controlling capillary blood flow (Porth, 2005).

Some capillary beds, such as those in the fingertips, contain arteriovenous anastomoses, through which blood passes directly from the arterial to the venous system. These vessels are believed to regulate heat exchange between the body and the external environment.

The distribution of capillaries varies with the type of tissue. For example, skeletal tissue, which has high metabolic requirements, has a denser capillary network than cartilage, which has low metabolic needs.

Veins and Venules

Capillaries join to form larger vessels called venules, which join to form veins. The venous system is therefore structurally analogous to the arterial system; venules correspond to arterioles, veins to arteries, and the vena cava to the aorta. Analogous types of vessels in the arterial and venous systems have approximately the same diameters (see Fig. 31-1).

The walls of the veins, in contrast to those of the arteries, are thinner and considerably less muscular. In most veins, the wall makes up only 10% of the diameter, in contrast to 25% in most arteries. In veins, the walls are composed of three layers, like those of arteries, although in veins, these layers are not as well defined.

The thin, less muscular structure of the vein wall allows these vessels to distend more than arteries. Greater distensibility and compliance permit large volumes of blood to remain in the veins under low pressure. For this reason, veins are referred to as *capacitance vessels*. Approximately 75% of total blood volume is contained in the veins. The sympathetic nervous system, which innervates the vein musculature, can stimulate the veins to constrict (venoconstriction), thereby reducing venous volume and increasing the volume of blood in the general circulation. Contraction of skeletal muscles in the extremities creates the primary pumping action to facilitate venous blood flow back to the heart (Porth, 2005).

Some veins, unlike arteries, are equipped with valves. In general, veins that transport blood against the force of gravity, as in the lower extremities, have one-way bicuspid valves that prevent blood from seeping backward as it is propelled toward the heart. Valves are composed of endothelial leaflets, the competency of which depends on the integrity of the vein wall.

Lymphatic Vessels

The lymphatic vessels are a complex network of thin-walled vessels similar to the blood capillaries. This network collects lymphatic fluid from tissues and organs and transports the fluid to the venous circulation. The lymphatic vessels converge into two main structures: the thoracic duct and the right lymphatic duct. These ducts empty into the junction of the subclavian and the internal jugular veins. The right lymphatic duct conveys lymph primarily from the right side of the head, neck, thorax, and upper arms. The thoracic duct conveys lymph from the remainder of the body.

Peripheral lymphatic vessels join larger lymph vessels and pass through regional lymph nodes before entering the venous circulation. The lymph nodes play an important role in filtering foreign particles.

The lymphatic vessels are permeable to large molecules and provide the only means by which interstitial proteins can return to the venous system. With muscular contraction, lymph vessels become distorted to create spaces between the endothelial cells, allowing protein and particles to enter. Muscular contraction of the lymphatic walls and surrounding tissues aids in propelling the lymph toward the venous drainage points (Porth, 2005).

Function of the Vascular System

Circulatory Needs of Tissues

The amount of blood flow needed by body tissues constantly changes. The percentage of blood flow received by individual organs or tissues is determined by the rate of tissue metabolism, the availability of oxygen, and the function of the tissues. When metabolic requirements increase, blood vessels dilate to increase the flow of oxygen and nutrients to the tissues. When metabolic needs decrease, vessels constrict and blood flow to the tissues decreases. Metabolic demands of tissues increase with physical activity or exercise, local heat application, fever, and infection. Reduced metabolic requirements of tissues accompany rest or decreased physical activity, local cold application, and cooling of the body. If the blood vessels fail to dilate in response to the need for increased blood flow, tissue **ischemia** (deficient blood supply to a body part) results. The mechanism by which blood vessels dilate and constrict to adjust for metabolic changes ensures that normal arterial pressure is maintained (Porth, 2005).

As blood passes through tissue capillaries, oxygen is removed and carbon dioxide is added. The amount of oxygen extracted by each tissue differs. For example, the myocardium tends to extract about 50% of the oxygen from arterial blood in one pass through its capillary bed, whereas the kidneys extract only about 7% of the oxygen from the blood that passes through them. The average amount of oxygen removed collectively by all of the body tissues is about 25%. This means that the blood in the vena cava contains about 25% less oxygen than aortic blood. This is known as the *systemic arteriovenous oxygen difference* (Porth, 2005). This difference becomes greater when less oxygen is delivered to the tissues than they need.

Blood Flow

Blood flow through the cardiovascular system always proceeds in the same direction: left side of the heart to the aorta, arteries, arterioles, capillaries, venules, veins, vena cava, and right side of the heart. This unidirectional flow is caused by a pressure difference that exists between the arterial and venous systems. Because arterial pressure (approximately 100 mm Hg) is greater than venous pressure (approximately 40 mm Hg) and fluid always flows from an area of higher pressure to an area of lower pressure, blood flows from the arterial to the venous system.

The pressure difference (ΔP) between the two ends of the vessel propels the blood. Impediments to blood flow offer the opposing force, which is known as resistance (R). The rate of blood flow is determined by dividing the pressure difference by the resistance:

$$\text{Flow rate} = \Delta P/R$$

This equation clearly shows that when resistance increases, a greater driving pressure is required to maintain the same degree of flow (Porth, 2005). In the body, an increase in driving pressure is accomplished by an increase in the force of contraction of the heart. If arterial resistance is chronically elevated, the myocardium hypertrophies (enlarges) to sustain the greater contractile force.

In most long smooth blood vessels, flow is laminar or streamlined, with blood in the center of the vessel moving slightly faster than the blood near the vessel walls. Laminar flow becomes turbulent when the blood flow rate increases, when blood viscosity increases, when the diameter of the vessel becomes greater than normal, or when segments of the vessel are narrowed or constricted (Porth, 2005). Turbulent blood flow creates a sound, called a **bruit**, that can be heard with a stethoscope.

Blood Pressure

Chapters 26 and 32 provide more information on the physiology and measurement of blood pressure.

Capillary Filtration and Reabsorption

Fluid exchange across the capillary wall is continuous. This fluid, which has the same composition as plasma without the proteins, forms the interstitial fluid. The equilibrium between hydrostatic and osmotic forces of the blood and interstitium, as well as capillary permeability, determines the amount and direction of fluid movement across the capillary. Hydrostatic force is a driving pressure that is generated by the blood pressure. Osmotic pressure is the pulling force created by plasma proteins. Normally, the hydrostatic pressure at the arterial end of the capillary is relatively high compared with that at the venous end. This high pressure at the arterial end of the capillaries tends to drive fluid out of the capillary and into the tissue space. Osmotic pressure tends to pull fluid back into the capillary from the tissue space, but this osmotic force cannot overcome the high hydrostatic pressure at the arterial end of the capillary. However, at the venous end of the capillary, the osmotic force predominates over the low hydrostatic pressure, and there is a net reabsorption of fluid from the tissue space back into the capillary (Porth, 2005).

Except for a very small amount, fluid that is filtered out at the arterial end of the capillary bed is reabsorbed at the venous end. The excess filtered fluid enters the lymphatic circulation. These processes of filtration, reabsorption, and lymph formation aid in maintaining tissue fluid volume and removing tissue waste and debris. Under normal conditions, capillary permeability remains constant.

Under certain abnormal conditions, the fluid filtered out of the capillaries may greatly exceed the amounts reabsorbed and carried away by the lymphatic vessels. This imbalance can result from damage to capillary walls and subsequent increased permeability, obstruction of lymphatic drainage, elevation of venous pressure, or decrease in plasma protein osmotic force. Accumulation of excess interstitial fluid that results from these processes is known as *edema.*

Hemodynamic Resistance

The most important factor that determines resistance in the vascular system is the vessel radius. Small changes in vessel radius lead to large changes in resistance. The predominant sites of change in the caliber or width of blood vessels, and therefore in resistance, are the arterioles and the precapillary sphincter. Peripheral vascular resistance is the opposition to blood flow provided by the blood vessels. This resistance is proportional to the viscosity or thickness of the blood and the length of the vessel and is influenced by the diameter of the vessels. Under normal conditions, blood viscosity and vessel length do not change significantly, and these factors do not usually play an important role in blood flow. However, a large increase in hematocrit may increase blood viscosity and reduce capillary blood flow.

Peripheral Vascular Regulating Mechanisms

Even at rest, the metabolic needs of body tissues are continuously changing. Therefore, an integrated and coordinated regulatory system is necessary so that blood flow to individual tissues is maintained in proportion to the needs of those tissues. This regulatory mechanism is complex and consists of central nervous system influences, circulating hormones and chemicals, and independent activity of the arterial wall itself.

Sympathetic (adrenergic) nervous system activity, mediated by the hypothalamus, is the most important factor in regulating the caliber and therefore the blood flow of peripheral blood vessels. All vessels are innervated by the sympathetic nervous system except the capillary and precapillary sphincters. Stimulation of the sympathetic nervous system causes vasoconstriction. The neurotransmitter responsible for sympathetic vasoconstriction is norepinephrine (Porth, 2005). Sympathetic activation occurs in response to physiologic and psychological stressors. Diminution of sympathetic activity by medications or sympathectomy results in vasodilation.

Other hormonal substances affect peripheral vascular resistance. Epinephrine, released from the adrenal medulla, acts like norepinephrine in constricting peripheral blood vessels in most tissue beds. However, in low concentrations, epinephrine causes vasodilation in skeletal muscles, the heart, and the brain. Angiotensin I, which is formed from the interaction of renin (synthesized by the kidney) and angiotensinogen, a circulating serum protein, is then converted to angiotensin II by an enzyme secreted by the pulmonary vasculature, called angiotensin-converting enzyme (ACE). Angiotensin II is a potent vasoconstrictor, particularly of the arterioles. Although the amount of angiotensin II concentrated in the blood is usually small, its profound vasoconstrictive effects are important in certain abnormal states, such as heart failure and hypovolemia (Porth, 2005).

Alterations in local blood flow are influenced by various circulating substances that have vasoactive properties. Potent vasodilators include nitric oxide, prostacyclin, histamine, bradykinin, prostaglandin, and certain muscle metabolites. A reduction in available oxygen and nutrients and changes in local pH also affect local blood flow. Thromboxane A_2 and serotonin are substances liberated from platelets that aggregate at the site of damaged vessels, causing arteriolar vasoconstriction and continued platelet aggregation at the site of injury (Porth, 2005). The application of heat to parts of the body surface causes local vasodilation, whereas the application of cold causes vasoconstriction.

Pathophysiology of the Vascular System

Reduced blood flow through peripheral blood vessels characterizes all peripheral vascular diseases. The physiologic effects of altered blood flow depend on the extent to which tissue demands exceed the supply of oxygen and nutrients available. If tissue needs are high, even modestly reduced blood flow may be inadequate to maintain tissue integrity. Tissues then fall prey to ischemia, become malnourished, and ultimately die unless adequate blood flow is restored.

Pump Failure

Inadequate peripheral blood flow occurs when the heart's pumping action becomes inefficient. Left-sided heart failure (left ventricular failure) causes an accumulation of blood in the lungs and a reduction in forward flow or cardiac output, which results in inadequate arterial blood flow to the tissues. Right-sided heart failure (right ventricular failure) causes systemic venous congestion and a reduction in forward flow (see Chapter 30).

Alterations in Blood and Lymphatic Vessels

Intact, patent, and responsive blood vessels are necessary to deliver adequate amounts of oxygen to tissues and to remove metabolic wastes. Arteries can become damaged or obstructed as a result of atherosclerotic plaque, thromboemboli, chemical or mechanical trauma, infections or inflammatory processes, vasospastic disorders, and congenital malformations. A sudden arterial occlusion causes profound and often irreversible tissue ischemia and tissue death. When arterial occlusions develop gradually, there is less risk of sudden tissue death because collateral circulation may develop, giving that tissue the opportunity to adapt to gradually decreased blood flow.

Venous blood flow can be reduced by a thromboembolus obstructing the vein, by incompetent venous valves, or by a reduction in the effectiveness of the pumping action of surrounding muscles. Decreased venous blood flow results in increased venous pressure, a subsequent increase in capillary hydrostatic pressure, net filtration of fluid out of the capillaries into the interstitial space, and subsequent edema. Edematous tissues cannot receive adequate nutrition from the blood and consequently are more susceptible to breakdown, injury, and infection. Obstruction of lymphatic vessels also results in edema. Lymphatic vessels can become obstructed by a tumor or by damage from mechanical trauma or inflammatory processes.

Circulatory Insufficiency of the Extremities

Although many types of peripheral vascular diseases exist, most result in ischemia and produce some of the same symptoms: pain, skin changes, diminished pulse, and possible edema. The type and severity of symptoms depend in part on the type, stage, and extent of the disease process and on the speed with which the disorder develops. Table 31-1 highlights the distinguishing features of arterial and venous insufficiency. In this chapter, peripheral vascular disease is categorized as arterial, venous, or lymphatic.

Gerontologic Considerations

Aging produces changes in the walls of the blood vessels that affect the transport of oxygen and nutrients to the tissues. The intima thickens as a result of cellular proliferation and fibrosis. Elastin fibers of the media become calcified, thin, and fragmented, and collagen accumulates in the intima and the media. These changes cause the vessels to stiffen, which results in increased peripheral resistance, impaired blood flow, and increased left ventricular workload.

Assessment and Diagnostic Evaluation

Health History and Clinical Manifestations

An in-depth description from the patient of any pain and its precipitating factors, a thorough assessment of the patient's skin color and temperature, and the character of the peripheral pulses are all important in the diagnosis of arterial disorders.

Intermittent Claudication

A muscular, cramp-type pain in the extremities consistently reproduced with the same degree of exercise or activity and relieved by rest is experienced by patients with peripheral arterial insufficiency. Referred to as **intermittent claudication,** this pain is caused by the inability of the arterial system to provide adequate blood flow to the tissues in the face of increased demands for nutrients and oxygen during exercise. As the tissues are forced to complete the energy cycle without adequate nutrients and oxygen, muscle metabolites and lactic acid are produced. Pain is experienced as the metabolites aggravate the nerve endings of the surrounding tissue. Typically, about 50% of the arterial lumen or 75% of the cross-sectional area must be obstructed before intermittent claudication is experienced. When the patient rests and thereby decreases the metabolic needs of the muscles, the pain subsides. The progression of the arterial disease can be monitored by documenting the amount of exercise or the distance the patient can walk before pain is produced. Persistent pain in the forefoot (ie, the anterior portion of the foot) when the patient is resting indicates a severe degree of arterial insufficiency and a critical state of ischemia. Known as **rest pain,** this discomfort is often worse at night and may interfere with sleep. This pain frequently requires that the extremity be lowered to a dependent position to improve perfusion to the distal tissues.

The site of arterial disease can be deduced from the location of claudication, because pain occurs in muscle groups distal to the diseased vessel. Calf pain may accompany reduced blood flow through the superficial femoral or popliteal artery, whereas pain in the hip or buttock may result from reduced blood flow in the abdominal aorta or the common iliac or hypogastric arteries.

Changes in Skin Appearance and Temperature

Adequate blood flow warms the extremities and gives them a rosy coloring. Inadequate blood flow results in cool and pale extremities. Further reduction of blood flow to these tissues, which occurs when the extremity is elevated, for example, results in an even whiter or more blanched appearance

TABLE 31-1 Characteristics of Arterial and Venous Insufficiency

Characteristic	Arterial	Venous
Pain	Intermittent claudication to sharp, unrelenting, constant	Aching, cramping
Pulses	Diminished or absent	Present, but may be difficult to palpate through edema
Skin characteristics	Dependent rubor—elevation pallor of foot, dry, shiny skin, cool-to-cold temperature, loss of hair over toes and dorsum of foot, nails thickened and ridged	Pigmentation in gaitor area (area of medial and lateral malleolus), skin thickened and tough, may be reddish blue, frequently with associated dermatitis
Ulcer characteristics		
Location	Tip of toes, toe webs, heel or other pressure areas if confined to bed	Medial malleolus; infrequently lateral malleolus or anterior tibial area
Pain	Very painful	Minimal pain if superficial or may be very painful
Depth of ulcer	Deep, often involving joint space	Superficial
Shape	Circular	Irregular border
Ulcer base	Pale to black and dry gangrene	Granulation tissue—beefy red to yellow fibrinous in chronic long-term ulcer
Leg edema	Minimal unless extremity kept in dependent position constantly to relieve pain	Moderate to severe

(eg, pallor). **Rubor**, a reddish-blue discoloration of the extremities, may be observed within 20 seconds to 2 minutes after the extremity is placed in the dependent position. Rubor suggests severe peripheral arterial damage in which vessels that cannot constrict remain dilated. Even with rubor, the extremity begins to turn pale with elevation. Cyanosis, a bluish tint of the skin, is manifested when the amount of oxygenated hemoglobin contained in the blood is reduced.

Additional changes resulting from a chronically reduced nutrient supply include loss of hair, brittle nails, dry or scaling skin, atrophy, and ulcerations. Edema may be apparent bilaterally or unilaterally and is related to the affected extremity's chronically dependent position because of severe rest pain. Gangrenous changes appear after prolonged, severe ischemia and represent tissue necrosis. In elderly patients who are inactive, gangrene may be the first sign of disease. These patients may have adjusted their lifestyle to accommodate the limitations imposed by the disease and may not walk far enough to develop symptoms of claudication. Circulation is decreased, but this is not apparent to the patient until trauma occurs. At this point, gangrene develops when minimal arterial flow is impaired further by edema formation resulting from the traumatic event.

Pulses

Determining the presence or absence, as well as the quality, of peripheral pulses is important in assessing the status of peripheral arterial circulation (Fig. 31-2). Absence of a pulse may indicate that the site of **stenosis** (narrowing or constriction) is proximal to that location. Occlusive arterial disease impairs blood flow and can reduce or obliterate palpable pulsations in the extremities. Pulses should be palpated bilaterally and simultaneously, comparing both sides for symmetry in rate, rhythm, and quality.

Gerontologic Considerations

In elderly people, symptoms of peripheral arterial disease may be more pronounced than in younger people. Intermittent claudication may occur after walking only a few blocks or after walking up a slight incline. Any prolonged pressure on the foot can cause pressure areas that become ulcerated, infected, and gangrenous. The outcomes of arterial insufficiency can include reduced mobility and activity as well as a loss of independence.

Diagnostic Evaluation

Various tests may be performed to identify and diagnose abnormalities that can affect the vascular structures (arteries, veins, and lymphatics).

Doppler Ultrasound Flow Studies

Palpation of pulses is subjective, and the examiner may mistake his or her own pulse for that of the patient. To prevent

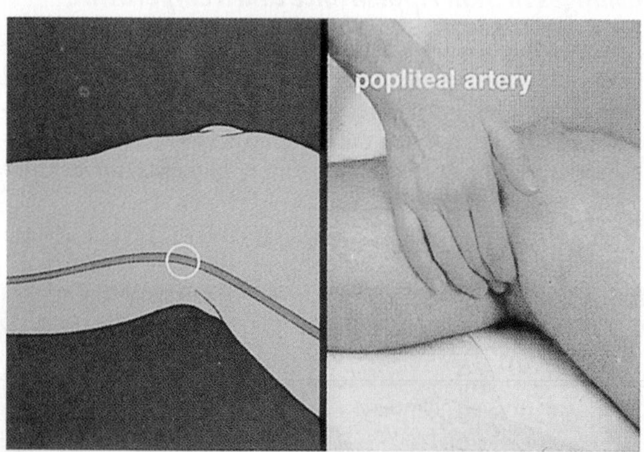

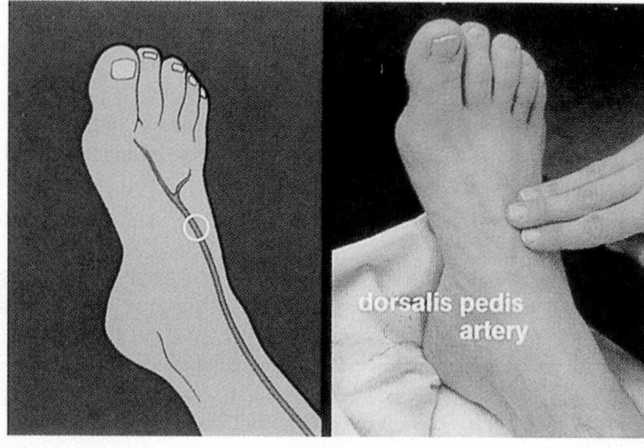

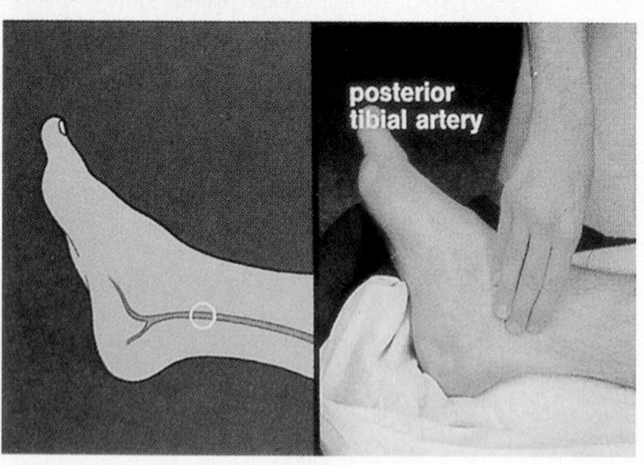

FIGURE 31-2. Assessing peripheral pulses. (*Left*) Popliteal pulse. (*Right*) Dorsalis pedis pulse. (*Bottom*) Posterior tibial pulse.

this, the examiner should use light touch and avoid using only the index finger for palpation because this finger has the strongest arterial pulsation of all the fingers. The thumb should not be used for the same reason. When pulses cannot be reliably palpated, a hand-held continuous wave (CW) Doppler ultrasound device may be used to hear (insonate) the blood flow in vessels. This hand-held device emits a continuous signal through the patient's tissues. The signals are reflected by ("echo off") the moving blood cells and are received by the device. The filtered-output Doppler signal is then transmitted to a loudspeaker or headphones, where it can be heard for interpretation. Because CW Doppler emits a continuous signal, all vascular structures in the path of the sound beam are insonated, and differentiating arterial from venous flow and detecting the site of a stenosis may be difficult. The depth at which blood flow can be detected by Doppler is determined by the frequency (in megahertz [MHz]) it generates. The lower the frequency, the deeper the tissue penetration; a 5- to 10-MHz probe may be used to evaluate the peripheral arteries.

To evaluate the lower extremities, the patient is placed in the supine position with the head of the bed elevated 20 to 30 degrees; the legs are externally rotated, if possible, to permit adequate access to the medial malleolus. Acoustic gel is applied to the patient's skin to permit uniform transmission of the ultrasound wave (electrocardiogram gel is not used because it contains sodium, which may dissolve the epoxy that covers the transducer's tip). The tip of the Doppler transducer is positioned at a 45- to 60-degree angle over the expected location of the artery and angled slowly to identify arterial blood flow. Excessive pressure is avoided because severely diseased arteries can collapse with even minimal pressure.

Because the transducer can detect blood flow in advanced arterial disease states, especially if collateral circulation has developed, identifying a signal documents only the presence of blood flow. The patient's primary care provider must be notified of the absence of a signal if one had been detected previously.

CW Doppler is more useful as a clinical tool when combined with ankle blood pressures, which are used to determine the **ankle-brachial index (ABI)**, also called the **ankle-arm index (AAI)** (Fig. 31-3). The ABI is the ratio of the systolic blood pressure in the ankle to the systolic blood pressure in the arm. It is an objective indicator of arterial disease that allows the examiner to quantify the degree of stenosis. With increasing degrees of arterial narrowing, there is a progressive decrease in systolic pressure distal to the involved sites.

The first step in determining the ABI is to have the patient rest in a supine position (not seated) for at least 5 minutes. An appropriate-sized blood pressure cuff (typically, a 10-cm cuff) is applied to the patient's ankle above the malleolus. After identifying an arterial signal at the posterior tibial and dorsalis pedis arteries, the systolic pressures are obtained in both ankles. Diastolic pressures in the ankles cannot be measured with a Doppler. If pressure in these arteries cannot be measured, pressure can be measured in the peroneal artery, which can also be assessed at the ankle (Fig. 31-4).

Doppler ultrasonography is used to measure brachial pressures in both arms. Both arms are evaluated because the patient may have an asymptomatic stenosis in the subclavian artery, causing brachial pressure on the affected side to be 20 mm Hg or more lower than systemic pressure. The abnormally low pressure should not be used for assessment.

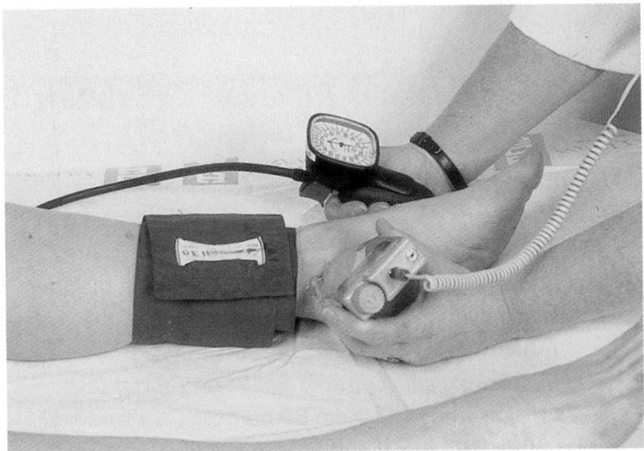

FIGURE 31-3. Continuous-wave (CW) Doppler ultrasound detects blood flow in peripheral vessels. Combined with computation of ankle or arm pressures, this diagnostic technique helps health care providers characterize the nature of peripheral vascular disease. Photograph reprinted with permission from Cantwell-Gab, K. (1996). Identifying chronic PAD. *American Journal of Nursing, 96*(7), 40–46.

To calculate ABI, the ankle systolic pressure for each foot is divided by the higher of the two brachial systolic pressures (Chart 31-1). The ABI can be computed for a patient with the following systolic pressures:

Right brachial: 160 mm Hg
Left brachial: 120 mm Hg
Right posterior tibial: 80 mm Hg
Right dorsalis pedis: 60 mm Hg
Left posterior tibial: 100 mm Hg
Left dorsalis pedis: 120 mm Hg

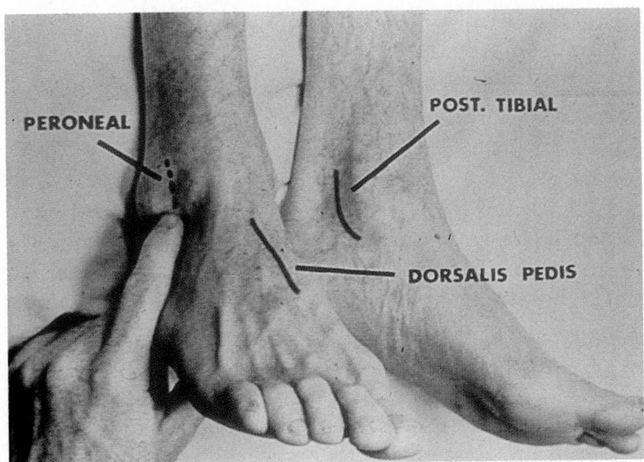

FIGURE 31-4. Location of peroneal artery; lateral malleolus. Photograph reprinted with permission from Cantwell-Gab, K. (1996). Identifying chronic PAD. *American Journal of Nursing, 96*(7), 40–46.

CHART 31-1

Avoiding Common Errors in Calculating Ankle-Brachial Index (ABI)

Take the following precautions to ensure an accurate ABI calculation:

- *Use the correctly sized blood pressure (BP) cuffs.* To obtain accurate BP measurements, use a cuff with a bladder width at least 40% and length at least 80% of the limb circumference.
- *On the nursing plan of care, document the BP cuff sizes used* (for example, "12-cm BP cuff used for brachial pressures; 10-cm BP cuff used for ankle pressures"). This minimizes the risk of shift-to-shift discrepancies in ABIs.
- *Use sufficient BP cuff inflation.* To ensure complete closure of the artery and the most accurate measurements, inflate cuffs 20 to 30 mm Hg beyond the point at which the last arterial signal is detected.
- *Do not deflate BP cuffs too rapidly.* Try to maintain a deflation rate of 2 to 4 mm Hg/second for patients without dysrhythmias and 2 mm Hg/second or slower for patients with dysrhythmias. Deflating the cuff more rapidly may miss the patient's highest pressure and result in recording an erroneous (low) BP measurement.
- *Be suspicious of arterial pressures recorded at less than 40 mm Hg.* This may mean the venous signal has been mistaken for the arterial signal. If the arterial pressure, which is normally 120 mm Hg, is measured at less than 40 mm Hg, ask a colleague to double-check the findings before recording this as an arterial pressure.
- *Suspect medial calcific sclerosis anytime an ABI is 1.3 or greater or ankle pressure is more than 300 mm Hg.* Medial calcific sclerosis is associated with diabetes mellitus, chronic renal failure, and hyperparathyroidism. It produces falsely elevated ankle pressures by hardening the media of the arteries, making the vessels noncompressible.

(From Cantwell-Gab, K. [1996]. Identifying chronic PAD. *American Journal of Nursing*, 96[1] 40–46, with permission.)

The highest systolic pressure for each ankle (80 mm Hg for the right, 120 mm Hg for the left) would be divided by the highest brachial pressure (160 mm Hg).

Right: 80/160 mm Hg = 0.50 ABI
Left: 120/160 mm Hg = 0.75 ABI

In general, systolic pressure in the ankle of a healthy person is the same or slightly higher than the brachial systolic pressure, resulting in an ABI of about 1.0 (no arterial insufficiency). Patients with claudication usually have an ABI of 0.95 to 0.50 (mild to moderate insufficiency); patients with ischemic rest pain have an ABI of less than 0.50; patients with severe ischemia or tissue loss have an ABI of 0.25 or less.

Exercise Testing

Exercise testing is used to determine how long a patient can walk and to measure the ankle systolic blood pressure in response to walking. The patient walks on a treadmill at 1.5 mph with a 10% incline for a maximum of 5 minutes. Most patients can complete the test unless they have severe cardiac, pulmonary, or orthopedic problems or a physical disability. A normal response to the test is little or no drop in ankle systolic pressure after exercise. However, in a patient with true claudication, ankle pressure drops. Combining this hemodynamic information with the walking time helps the physician determine whether intervention is necessary.

Duplex Ultrasonography

Duplex ultrasonography involves B-mode gray-scale imaging of the tissue, organs, and blood vessels (arterial and venous) and permits estimation of velocity changes by use of a pulsed Doppler (Fig. 31-5). Color flow techniques, which can identify vessels, may be used to shorten the examination time. The procedure primarily helps determine the level and extent of venous disease. The technique makes it possible to image and assess blood flow, evaluate flow of the distal vessels, locate the disease (stenosis versus occlusion), and determine anatomic morphology and the hemodynamic significance of plaque causing stenosis. Duplex ultrasound findings help in planning therapy and monitoring its outcomes. The test is noninvasive and usually requires no patient preparation. The equipment is portable, making it useful anywhere for initial diagnosis, screening, or follow-up evaluations.

Computed Tomography

Computed tomography (CT) provides cross-sectional images of soft tissue and visualizes the area of volume changes to an extremity and the compartment where changes take place. CT of a lymphedematous arm or leg, for example,

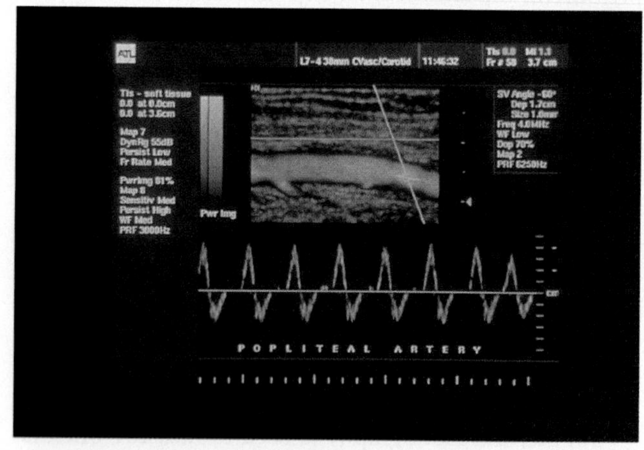

FIGURE 31-5. Color flow duplex image of popliteal artery with normal triphasic Doppler flow.

demonstrates a characteristic honeycomb pattern in the subcutaneous tissue.

In spiral (also called helical) CT, the scan head moves circumferentially around the patient as the patient passes through the scanner, creating a series of overlapping images that are connected to one another in a continuous spiral. In 1998, multidetector CT (MDCT) scanners capable of providing four "slices" or visual pictures per x-ray tube rotation became available. Currently, 9- and 16-slice scanners are available in some imaging centers and hospitals; these provide improved volume coverage speed and/or longitudinal spatial resolution, resulting in improved images (Fishman & Jeffrey, 2004). Scan times are short; however, the patient is exposed to x-rays, and a contrast agent usually must be injected to adequately visualize the blood vessels. Using computer software, the slice-like images are reconstructed into three-dimensional images that can be rotated and viewed from multiple angles.

Computed Tomography Angiography

In computed tomography angiography (CTA), a spiral CT scanner and rapid intravenous (IV) infusion of contrast agent are used to image very thin (between 1.0 and 1.25 mm) sections of the target area, and the results are configured in three dimensions so that the image closely resembles a regular angiogram. CTA shows the aorta and main arteries better than it shows smaller vessels. Scan times are usually between 20 and 30 seconds. The high volume of contrast agent injected into a peripheral vein limits the usefulness of this study in children and in patients with significantly impaired renal function (Fishman & Jeffrey, 2004).

Magnetic Resonance Angiography

Magnetic resonance angiography is performed with a standard magnetic resonance imaging (MRI) scanner, but with image-processing software specifically programmed to isolate the blood vessels. The images are reconstructed to resemble a standard angiogram, but because the images are reassembled in three dimensions, they can be rotated and viewed from multiple angles. Because a contrast agent may not be necessary, this study is useful in patients with poor renal function or allergy to contrast agent. The scan time can be long, and motion artifacts are common, requiring postprocessing methods and display techniques not available at every facility (Haaga, Lanziere, & Gilkeson, 2003).

Angiography

An arteriogram produced by angiography may be used to confirm the diagnosis of occlusive arterial disease when considering surgery or other interventions. It involves injecting a radiopaque contrast agent directly into the vascular system to visualize the vessels. The location of a vascular obstruction or an **aneurysm** (abnormal dilation of a blood vessel) and the collateral circulation can be demonstrated. Typically, the patient experiences a temporary sensation of warmth as the contrast agent is injected, and local irritation may occur at the injection site. Infrequently, a patient may have an immediate or delayed allergic reaction to the iodine contained in the contrast agent. Manifestations include dyspnea, nausea and vomiting, sweating, tachycardia, and numbness of the extremities. Any such reaction must be reported to the physician at once; treatment may include the administration of epinephrine, antihistamines, or corticosteroids. Additional risks include vessel injury, bleeding, and cerebrovascular accident (CVA, brain attack, stroke).

Air Plethysmography

Air plethysmography is used to quantify venous reflux and calf muscle pump ejection. Changes in leg volumes are measured with the patient's legs elevated, with the patient supine and standing, and after the patient performs toe-ups (the patient extends the ankle while standing; stands on his or her toes) by an air-filled device wrapped around the feet and legs. Air plethysmography provides information about venous filling time, functional venous volume, ejected volume, and residual volume. It is useful in evaluating patients with suspected valvular incompetence or chronic venous insufficiency.

Contrast Phlebography

Also known as venography, contrast phlebography involves injecting a radiopaque contrast agent into the venous system. If a thrombus exists, the x-ray image reveals an unfilled segment of vein in an otherwise completely filled vein. Injection of the contrast agent may cause brief but painful inflammation of the vein. The test is generally performed if the patient is to undergo thrombolytic therapy, but duplex ultrasonography is now accepted as the standard for diagnosing venous thrombosis.

Lymphangiography

Lymphangiography provides a way of detecting lymph node involvement resulting from metastatic carcinoma, lymphoma, or infection in sites that are otherwise inaccessible to the examiner except by surgery. In this test, a lymphatic vessel in each foot (or hand) is injected with contrast agent. A series of x-rays are taken at the conclusion of the injection, 24 hours later, and periodically thereafter, as indicated. The failure to identify subcutaneous lymphatic collection of contrast agent and the persistence of contrast agent in the tissue for days afterward help confirm a diagnosis of lymphedema.

Lymphoscintigraphy

Lymphoscintigraphy is a reliable alternative to lymphangiography. A radioactively labeled colloid is injected subcutaneously in the second interdigital space. The extremity is then exercised to facilitate the uptake of the colloid by the lymphatic system, and serial images are obtained at preset intervals.

Arterial Disorders

Arteriosclerosis and Atherosclerosis

Arteriosclerosis is the most common disease of the arteries; the term means "hardening of the arteries." It is a diffuse process whereby the muscle fibers and the endothelial lining of the walls of small arteries and arterioles become thickened. **Atherosclerosis** involves a different process, affecting the intima of the large and medium-sized arteries. These changes consist of the accumulation of lipids, calcium, blood components, carbohydrates, and fibrous tissue on the intimal layer of the artery. These accumulations are referred to as atheromas or plaques.

Although the pathologic processes of arteriosclerosis and atherosclerosis differ, rarely does one occur without the other, and the terms are often used interchangeably. Atherosclerosis is a generalized disease of the arteries, and when it is present in the extremities, it is usually present elsewhere in the body.

Pathophysiology

The most common direct results of atherosclerosis in arteries include narrowing (stenosis) of the lumen, obstruction by thrombosis, aneurysm, ulceration, and rupture. Its indirect results are malnutrition and the subsequent fibrosis of the organs that the sclerotic arteries supply with blood. All actively functioning tissue cells require an abundant supply of nutrients and oxygen and are sensitive to any reduction in the supply of these nutrients. If such reductions are severe and permanent, the cells undergo ischemic necrosis (death of cells due to deficient blood flow) and are replaced by fibrous tissue, which requires much less blood flow.

Atherosclerosis can develop at any point in the body, but certain sites are more vulnerable, such as regions where arteries bifurcate or branch areas. In the proximal lower extremity, these include the distal abdominal aorta, the common iliac arteries, the orifice of the superficial femoral and profunda femoris arteries, and the superficial femoral artery in the adductor canal, which is particularly narrow. Distal to the knee, atherosclerosis can occur anywhere along the artery.

Although many theories exist about the development of atherosclerosis, no single theory explains the pathogenesis completely; however, tenets of several theories are incorporated into the reaction-to-injury theory. According to this theory, vascular endothelial cell injury results from prolonged hemodynamic forces, such as shearing stresses and turbulent flow, irradiation, chemical exposure, or chronic hyperlipidemia. Injury to the endothelium increases the aggregation of platelets and monocytes at the site of the injury. Smooth muscle cells migrate and proliferate, allowing a matrix of collagen and elastic fibers to form. Multiple processes may be involved (Moore, 2002).

Atherosclerotic lesions are of two types: fatty streaks and fibrous plaque:

- Fatty streaks are yellow and smooth, protrude slightly into the lumen of the artery, and are composed of lipids and elongated smooth muscle cells. These lesions have been found in the arteries of people of all age groups, including infants. It is not clear whether fatty streaks predispose a person to the formation of fibrous plaques or whether they are reversible. They do not usually cause clinical symptoms.
- Fibrous plaques are composed of smooth muscle cells, collagen fibers, plasma components, and lipids. They are white to white-yellow and protrude in various degrees into the arterial lumen, sometimes completely obstructing it. These plaques are found predominantly in the abdominal aorta and the coronary, popliteal, and internal carotid arteries, and they are believed to be progressive, irreversible lesions (Fig. 31-6).

Gradual narrowing of the arterial lumen stimulates the development of collateral circulation (Fig. 31-7). Collateral circulation arises from preexisting vessels that enlarge to reroute blood flow around a hemodynamically significant stenosis or occlusion. Collateral flow allows continued per-

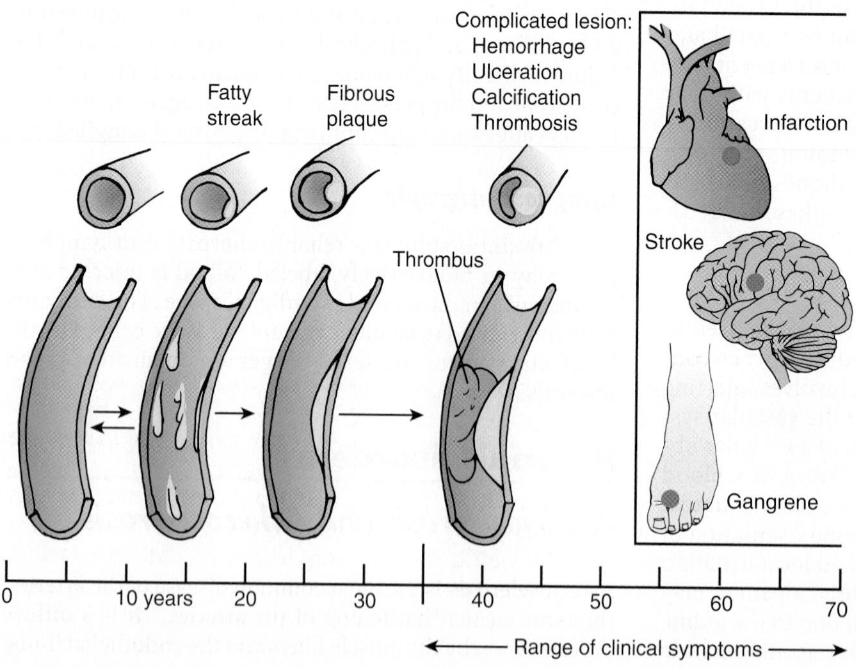

FIGURE 31-6. Schematic concept of the progression of atherosclerosis. Fatty streaks constitute one of the earliest lesions of atherosclerosis. Many fatty streaks regress, whereas others progress to fibrous plaques and eventually to atheroma, which may be complicated by hemorrhage, ulceration, calcification, or thrombosis and may produce myocardial infarction, stroke, or gangrene.

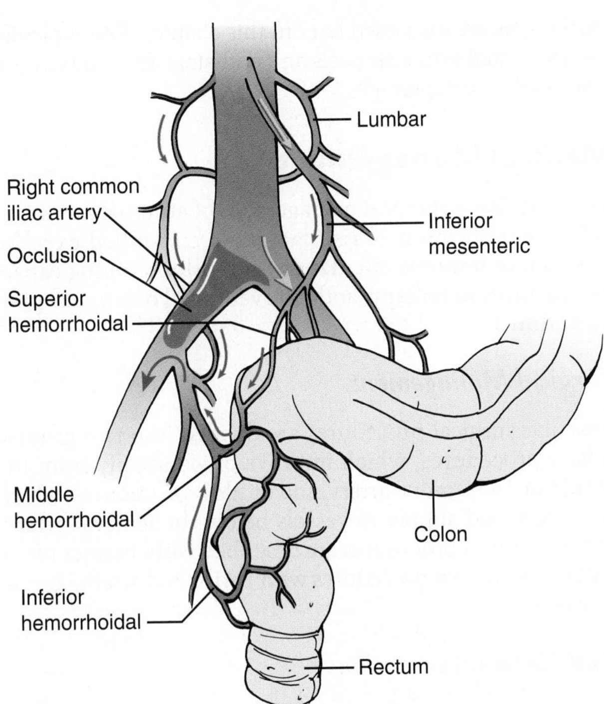

FIGURE 31-7. Development of channels for collateral blood flow in response to occlusion of the right common iliac artery and the terminal aortic bifurcation.

fusion to the tissues, but it is often inadequate to meet increased metabolic demand, and ischemia results.

Risk Factors

Many risk factors are associated with atherosclerosis (Chart 31-2). Although it is not entirely clear whether modification of these risk factors prevents the development of cardiovascular disease, evidence indicates that it may slow the disease process. Some risk factors, such as age, gender, and genetics, cannot be modified (Moore, 2002).

The use of tobacco products may be one of the most important risk factors in the development of atherosclerotic lesions. Nicotine in tobacco decreases blood flow to the extremities and increases heart rate and blood pressure by stimulating the sympathetic nervous system, causing vasoconstriction. It also increases the risk for clot formation by increasing the aggregation of platelets. Carbon monoxide, a toxin produced by burning tobacco, combines more readily with hemoglobin than oxygen does, depriving the tissues of oxygen. The amount of tobacco used is directly related to the extent of the disease, and cessation of tobacco use reduces the risks. Many other factors, such as obesity, stress, and lack of exercise, have been identified as contributing to the disease process.

C-reactive protein (CRP) is a sensitive marker of cardiovascular inflammation, both systemically and locally. Slight increases in serum CRP levels are associated with an increased risk of damage in the vasculature, especially if these increases are accompanied by other risk factors, including increasing age, female gender, hypertension, hypercholesterolemia, obesity, elevated blood glucose levels, smoking, or a positive family history of cardiovascular disease (Stuveling, Hillege, Bakker, et al., 2004).

Hyperhomocysteinemia has been demonstrated in patients with peripheral, cerebrovascular, and coronary artery disease and is now considered an independent risk factor for atherosclerosis. Homocysteine is a protein that promotes coagulation by increasing factor V and factor XI activity while depressing protein C activation and increasing the binding of lipoprotein (a) in fibrin. These processes increase thrombin formation and increase the propensity for thrombosis (Kohlman-Trigoboff, 2003). Some patients may benefit from the combined supplementation of vitamins B_6 and B_{12} as well as folate, which may lower homocysteine levels (Fletcher & Fairfield, 2005). However, it is not yet known whether this therapy changes the risk for atherosclerosis associated with hyperhomocysteinemia.

CHART 31-2

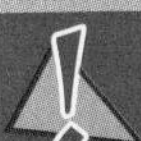

Risk Factors for Atherosclerosis and Peripheral Arterial Disease

Modifiable Risk Factors

- Nicotine use (ie, tobacco smoking or chewing)
- Diet (contributing to hyperlipidemia)
- Hypertension
- Diabetes mellitus (speeds the atherosclerotic process by thickening the basement membranes of both large and small vessels)
- Obesity
- Stress
- Sedentary lifestyle
- Elevated C-reactive protein
- Hyperhomocysteinemia

Nonmodifiable Risk Factors

- Age
- Gender
- Familial predisposition/genetics

Prevention

Intermittent claudication is a symptom of generalized atherosclerosis and may be a marker of occult coronary artery disease. Because it is suspected that a high-fat diet contributes to atherosclerosis, it is reasonable to measure serum cholesterol and to begin disease prevention efforts that include diet modification. The American Heart Association recommends reducing the amount of fat ingested in a healthy diet, substituting unsaturated fats for saturated fats, and decreasing cholesterol intake to reduce the risk of cardiovascular disease.

Certain medications that supplement dietary modification and exercise are used to reduce blood lipid levels. The National Cholesterol Education Program (NCEP) has established guidelines for treating hyperlipidemia, with the primary goal of low-density lipoprotein (LDL) levels of less than 100 mg/dL. LDL levels of less than 70 mg/dL are recommended for patients with a history of diabetes, cigarette smoking, atherosclerosis, or hypertension (Grundy, Cleeman, Berz, et al., 2004). Secondary goals include achieving total cholesterol levels of less than 200 mg/dL and triglyceride levels less than 150 mg/dL. Medications classified as HMG-CoA reductase inhibitors or "statins," including atorvastatin (Lipitor), lovastatin (Mevacor), pravastatin (Pravachol), and simvastatin (Zocor), are currently first-line treatment and reduce the incidence of major cardiovascular events (Cote, Ligeti, Cutler, et al., 2003). Several other classes of medications used to reduce lipid levels include bile acid sequestrants (cholestyramine [Questran, Prevalite], colesevelam [Welchol], colestipol [Colestid]), nicotinic acid (niacin [Niacor, Niaspan]), fibric acid inhibitors (gemfibrozil [Lopid]), and cholesterol absorption inhibitors (ezetimibe [Zetia]). Patients receiving long-term therapy with these medications require close medical supervision.

Hypertension, which may accelerate the rate at which atherosclerotic lesions form in high-pressure vessels, can lead to CVA (brain attack, stroke), ischemic renal disease, severe peripheral arterial disease, or coronary artery disease. Hypertension is a major risk factor for the development of peripheral arterial disease (PAD), resulting in a twofold risk of development of claudication. All patients with PAD should achieve blood pressure control consistent with the Seventh Report of the Joint National Committee on Prevention, Detection, Evaluation and Treatment of High Blood Pressure (JNC 7) guidelines (systolic blood pressure less than 130 mm Hg; diastolic blood pressure less than 90 mm Hg) (Chobanian, Bakris, Black, et al., 2003).

Although no single risk factor has been identified as the primary contributor to the development of atherosclerotic cardiovascular disease, it is clear that the greater the number of risk factors, the greater the risk of atherosclerosis. Elimination of all controllable risk factors, particularly the use of tobacco products, is strongly recommended.

Clinical Manifestations

The clinical signs and symptoms resulting from atherosclerosis depend on the organ or tissue affected. Coronary atherosclerosis (heart disease), angina, and acute myocardial infarction are discussed in Chapter 28. Cerebrovascular diseases, including transient cerebral ischemic attacks and stroke, are discussed in Chapter 62. Atherosclerosis of the aorta, including aneurysm, and atherosclerotic lesions of the extremities are discussed later in this chapter. Renovascular disease (renal artery stenosis and end-stage renal disease) is discussed in Chapter 45.

Medical Management

The traditional medical management of atherosclerosis involves modification of risk factors, a controlled exercise program to improve circulation and its functioning capacity, medication therapy, and interventional or surgical graft procedures.

Surgical Management

Vascular surgical procedures are divided into two groups: inflow procedures, which improve blood supply from the aorta into the femoral artery, and outflow procedures, which provide blood supply to vessels below the femoral artery. Inflow surgical procedures are described with diseases of the aorta and outflow procedures with peripheral arterial occlusive disease.

Radiologic Interventions

Several interventional radiologic techniques are important adjunctive therapies to surgical procedures. If an isolated lesion or lesions are identified during the arteriogram, **angioplasty**, also called percutaneous transluminal angioplasty (PTA), may be performed. After the patient receives a local anesthetic, a balloon-tipped catheter is maneuvered across the area of stenosis. Although some clinicians theorize that PTA improves blood flow by overstretching (and thereby dilating) the elastic fibers of the nondiseased arterial segment, most believe that the procedure widens the arterial lumen by "cracking" and flattening the plaque against the vessel wall (see Chapter 28). Complications from PTA include hematoma formation, embolus, **dissection** (separation of the intima) of the vessel, and bleeding. To decrease the risk of reocclusion, stents (small, mesh tubes made of nitinol, titanium, or stainless steel) may be inserted to support the walls of blood vessels and prevent collapse immediately after balloon inflation (Fig. 31-8). A variety of stents and stent-grafts may be used for short-segment stenoses. Complications associated with stent or stent-graft use include

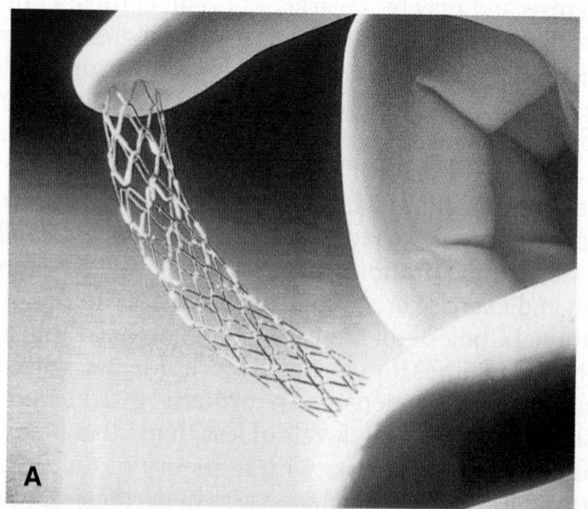

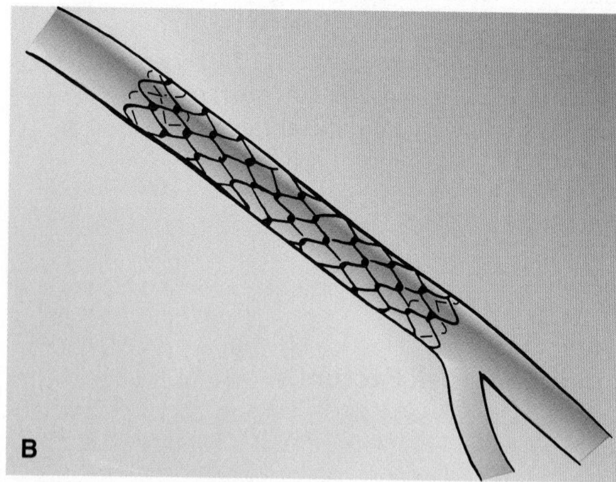

FIGURE 31-8. (**A**) Flexible stent. Courtesy of Medtronics, Peripheral Division, Santa Rosa, California. (**B**) Representation of a common iliac artery with a Wallstent (Boston Scientific).

distal embolization, intimal damage (dissection), and dislodgment. The advantage of angioplasty, stents, and stent-grafts is the decreased length of hospital stay required for the treatment; many of the procedures are performed on an outpatient basis.

Nursing Process

The Patient With Peripheral Arterial Insufficiency of the Extremities

Assessment

The nursing assessment includes a complete health and medication history and identification of risk factors for PAD. Signs and symptoms detected during the nursing assessment may include claudication pain; rest pain in the forefoot; pallor, rubor, or cyanosis; weak or absent peripheral pulses; and skin breakdown or ulcerations.

Nursing Diagnosis

Based on assessment data, major nursing diagnoses for the patient may include the following:

- Altered peripheral tissue perfusion related to compromised circulation
- Chronic pain related to impaired ability of peripheral vessels to supply tissues with oxygen
- Risk for impaired skin integrity related to compromised circulation
- Deficient knowledge regarding self-care activities

Planning and Goals

The major goals for the patient may include increased arterial blood supply to the extremities, promotion of vasodilation, prevention of vascular compression, relief of pain, attainment or maintenance of tissue integrity, and adherence to the self-care program. An overview of the care of a patient with peripheral arterial problems is provided in the Plan of Nursing Care: The Patient With Peripheral Vascular Problems (Chart 31-3).

Nursing Interventions

Improving Peripheral Arterial Circulation

Arterial blood supply to a body part can be enhanced by positioning the part below the level of the heart. For the lower extremities, this is accomplished by elevating the head of the patient's bed on 15-cm (6-inch) blocks or by having the patient use a reclining chair or sit with the feet resting on the floor.

The nurse can assist the patient with walking or other moderate or graded isometric exercises that may be prescribed to promote blood flow and encourage the development of collateral circulation. The nurse instructs the patient to walk to the point of pain, rest until the pain subsides, and then resume walking so that endurance can be increased as collateral circulation develops. Pain can serve as a guide in determining the amount of exercise appropriate for a person. The onset of pain indicates that the tissues are not receiving adequate oxygen, signaling the patient to rest before continuing activity. However, a regular exercise program can result in increased walking distance before the onset of claudication. The amount of exercise a patient can tolerate before the onset of pain is determined to provide a baseline for evaluation.

Not all patients with peripheral vascular disease should exercise. Before recommending any exercise program, the primary health care provider should be consulted. Conditions that worsen with exercise include leg ulcers, cellulitis, gangrene, or acute thrombotic occlusions.

Promoting Vasodilation and Preventing Vascular Compression

Arterial dilation promotes increased blood flow to the extremities and is therefore a goal for patients with PAD. However, if the arteries are severely sclerosed, inelastic, or damaged, dilation is not possible. For this reason, measures to promote vasodilation, such as medications or surgery, may be only minimally effective.

Nursing interventions may involve applications of warmth to promote arterial flow and instructions to the patient to avoid exposure to cold temperatures, which causes vasoconstriction. Adequate clothing and warm temperatures protect the patient from chilling. If chilling occurs, a warm bath or drink is helpful. A hot water bottle or heating pad may be applied to the patient's abdomen, causing vasodilation throughout the lower extremities.

In patients with vasospastic disorders (eg, Raynaud's disease), heat may be applied directly to ischemic extremities using a warmed or electric blanket; however, the temperature of the heat source must not exceed body temperature. Even at low temperatures, trauma to the tissues can occur in ischemic extremities. Excess heat may increase the metabolic rate of the extremities and increase the need for oxygen beyond that provided by the reduced arterial flow through the diseased artery.

NURSING ALERT

Patients are instructed to test the temperature of bath water and to avoid using hot water bottles and heating pads on the extremities. Applying a hot water bottle or a heating pad to the abdomen can cause reflex vasodilation in the extremities and is safer than direct application of heat to affected extremities.

(text continues on page 990)

CHART 31-3

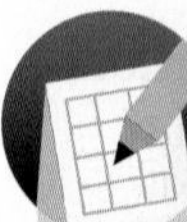

Plan of Nursing Care — The Patient With Peripheral Vascular Problems

Nursing Diagnosis: Ineffective peripheral tissue perfusion related to compromised circulation

Goal: Increased arterial blood supply to extremities

NURSING INTERVENTIONS	RATIONALE	EXPECTED OUTCOMES
1. Lower the extremities below the level of the heart (if condition is arterial in nature).	1. Dependency of lower extremities enhances arterial blood supply.	• Extremities warm to touch • Color of extremities improved • Experiences decreased muscle pain with exercise
2. Encourage moderate amount of walking or graded extremity exercises if no contraindications exist	2. Muscular exercise promotes blood flow and the development of collateral circulation.	

Goal: Decrease in venous congestion

NURSING INTERVENTIONS	RATIONALE	EXPECTED OUTCOMES
1. Elevate extremities above heart level (if condition is venous in nature).	1. Elevation of extremities counteracts gravity, promotes venous return, and prevents venous stasis.	• Elevates lower extremities as prescribed • Decreased edema of extremities • Avoids prolonged standing still or sitting • Gradually increases walking time daily
2. Discourage standing still or sitting for prolonged periods.	2. Prolonged standing still or sitting promotes venous stasis.	
3. Encourage walking.	3. Walking promotes venous return by activating the "muscle pump."	

Goal: Promotion of vasodilation and prevention of vascular compression

NURSING INTERVENTIONS	RATIONALE	EXPECTED OUTCOMES
1. Maintain warm temperature and avoid chilling.	1. Warmth promotes arterial flow by preventing the vasoconstriction effects of chilling.	• Protects extremities from exposure to cold • Avoids all tobacco products • Uses stress-management program to minimize emotional upset • Avoids constricting clothing and accessories • Avoids leg crossing • Takes medication as prescribed
2. Discourage use of tobacco products.	2. Nicotine in all tobacco products causes vasospasm, which impedes peripheral circulation.	
3. Counsel in ways to avoid emotional upsets; stress management.	3. Emotional stress causes peripheral vasoconstriction by stimulating the sympathetic nervous system.	
4. Encourage avoidance of constrictive clothing and accessories.	4. Constrictive clothing and accessories impede circulation and promote venous stasis.	
5. Encourage avoidance of leg crossing.	5. Leg crossing causes compression of vessels with subsequent impediment of circulation, resulting in venous stasis.	
6. Administer vasodilator medications and adrenergic blocking agents as prescribed, with appropriate nursing considerations.	6. Vasodilators relax smooth muscle; adrenergic blocking agents block the response to sympathetic nerve impulses or circulating catecholamines.	

CHART 31-3

Plan of Nursing Care — The Patient With Peripheral Vascular Problems (Continued)

Nursing Diagnosis: Chronic pain related to impaired ability of peripheral vessels to supply tissues with oxygen
Goal: Relief of pain

NURSING INTERVENTIONS	RATIONALE	EXPECTED OUTCOMES
1. Promote increased circulation.	1. Enhancement of peripheral circulation increases the oxygen supplied to the muscle and decreases the accumulation of metabolites that cause muscle spasms.	• Uses measures to increase arterial blood supply to extremities • Uses analgesics as prescribed
2. Administer analgesics as prescribed, with appropriate nursing considerations.	2. Analgesics help to reduce pain and allow the patient to participate in activities and exercises that promote circulation.	

Nursing Diagnosis: Risk for impaired skin integrity related to compromised circulation
Goal: Attainment/maintenance of tissue integrity

NURSING INTERVENTIONS	RATIONALE	EXPECTED OUTCOMES
1. Instruct in ways to avoid trauma to extremities.	1. Poorly nourished tissues are susceptible to trauma and bacterial invasion; healing of wounds is delayed or inhibited due to poor tissue perfusion.	• Inspects skin daily for evidence of injury or ulceration • Avoids trauma and irritation to skin • Wears protective shoes • Adheres to meticulous hygiene regimen • Eats a healthy diet that contains adequate protein and vitamins A and C
2. Encourage wearing protective shoes and padding for pressure areas.	2. Protective shoes and padding prevent foot injuries and blisters.	
3. Encourage meticulous hygiene; bathing with neutral soaps, applying lotions, carefully trimming nails.	3. Neutral soaps and lotions prevent drying and cracking of skin.	
4. Caution to avoid scratching or vigorous rubbing.	4. Scratching and rubbing can cause skin abrasions and bacterial invasion.	
5. Promote good nutrition; adequate intake of vitamins A and C, protein, and zinc; control of obesity.	5. Good nutrition promotes healing and prevents tissue breakdown.	

Nursing Diagnosis: Deficient knowledge regarding self-care activities
Goal: Adherence to the self-care program

NURSING INTERVENTIONS	RATIONALE	EXPECTED OUTCOMES
1. Include family/significant others in teaching program.	1. Adherence to the self-care program is enhanced when the patient receives support from family and from appropriate self-help groups and agencies.	• Practices frequent position changes as prescribed • Practices postural exercises as prescribed • Takes medications as prescribed

continued >

CHART 31-3

Plan of Nursing Care — The Patient With Peripheral Vascular Problems (Continued)

NURSING INTERVENTIONS	RATIONALE	EXPECTED OUTCOMES
2. Provide written instructions about foot care, leg care, and exercise program.	2. Written instructions serve as reminder and reinforcement of information.	• Avoids vasoconstrictors • Uses measures to prevent trauma • Uses stress management program • Accepts condition as chronic but amenable to therapies that will decrease symptoms
3. Assist to obtain properly fitting clothing, shoes, stockings.	3. Constrictive clothing and accessories impede circulation and promote venous stasis.	
4. Refer to self-help groups as indicated, such as smoking cessation clinics, stress management, weight management, and exercise program.	4. Reducing risk factors may reduce symptoms or slow disease progression.	

Nicotine from tobacco products causes vasospasm and can thereby dramatically reduce circulation to the extremities. Tobacco smoke also impairs transport and cellular use of oxygen and increases blood viscosity. Patients with arterial insufficiency who use tobacco (ie, smoke, chew) must be fully informed of the effects of nicotine on circulation and encouraged to stop using tobacco.

Emotional upsets stimulate the sympathetic nervous system, resulting in peripheral vasoconstriction. Emotional stress can be minimized to some degree by avoiding stressful situations when possible or by consistently following a stress-management program. Counseling services or relaxation training may be indicated for people who cannot cope effectively with situational stressors.

Constrictive clothing and accessories such as tight socks, panty girdles, and shoelaces impede circulation to the extremities and promote venous stasis and therefore should be avoided. Crossing the legs should be discouraged because it compresses vessels in the legs.

Relieving Pain

Frequently, the pain associated with peripheral arterial insufficiency is chronic, continuous, and disabling. It limits activities, affects work and responsibilities, disturbs sleep, and alters the patient's sense of well-being. Patients are often depressed, irritable, and unable to exert the energy necessary to execute prescribed therapies, making pain relief even more difficult. Analgesics such as oxycodone plus acetylsalicylic acid (Percodan) or oxycodone plus acetaminophen (Percocet) may be helpful in reducing pain so that the patient can participate in therapies that can increase circulation and ultimately relieve pain more effectively.

Maintaining Tissue Integrity

Poorly perfused tissues are susceptible to damage and infection. When lesions develop, healing may be delayed or inhibited because of the poor blood supply to the area. Infected, nonhealing ulcerations of the extremities can be debilitating and may require prolonged and often expensive treatments. Amputation of an ischemic limb may eventually be necessary. Measures to prevent these complications must be a high priority and vigorously implemented.

Trauma to the extremities must be avoided. Advising the patient to wear sturdy, well-fitting shoes or slippers to prevent foot injury and blisters may be helpful, and recommending neutral soaps and body lotions may prevent drying and cracking of skin. Scratching and vigorous rubbing can abrade skin and create sites for bacterial invasion; therefore, feet should be patted dry. Stockings should be clean and dry. Fingernails and toenails should be carefully trimmed straight across and sharp corners filed to follow the contour of the nail. If nails are thick and brittle and cannot be trimmed safely, a podiatrist must be consulted. Corns and calluses need to be removed by a health care professional. Special shoe inserts may be needed to prevent calluses from recurring. All signs of blisters, ingrown toenails, infection, or other problems should be reported to health care professionals for treatment and follow-up. Patients with diminished vision and those with disorders that limit mobility of the arms or legs may require assistance in periodically examining the lower extremities for trauma or evidence of inflammation or infection.

Good nutrition promotes healing and prevents tissue breakdown and is therefore included in the overall therapeutic program for patients with peripheral vascular disease. Eating a well-balanced diet that contains adequate protein and vitamins is necessary for patients with arterial insufficiency. Key nutrients play specific roles in wound healing. Vitamin C is essential for collagen synthesis and capillary development. Vitamin A enhances epithelialization. Zinc is necessary for cell mitosis and cell proliferation. Obesity strains the heart, increases venous congestion, and reduces circulation;

therefore, a weight-reduction plan may be necessary for some patients. A diet low in lipids may be indicated for patients with atherosclerosis.

Promoting Home and Community-Based Care

The self-care program is planned with the patient so that activities that promote arterial and venous circulation, relieve pain, and promote tissue integrity are acceptable. The patient and family are helped to understand the reasons for each aspect of the program, the possible consequences of nonadherence, and the importance of keeping follow-up appointments. Long-term care of the feet and legs is of prime importance in the prevention of trauma, ulceration, and gangrene. Chart 31-3 describes nursing care for patients with peripheral vascular disease. Chart 31-4 provides detailed patient instructions for foot and leg care.

Evaluation

Expected Patient Outcomes

Expected patient outcomes may include:

1. Demonstrates an increase in arterial blood supply to extremities
   a. Exhibits extremities warm to touch
   b. Has improved color of extremities (ie, free of rubor or cyanosis)

CHART 31-4

HOME CARE CHECKLIST • Foot and Leg Care in Peripheral Vascular Disease

At the completion of the home care instruction, the patient or caregiver will be able to:	Patient	Caregiver
• Demonstrate daily foot bathing: Wash between toes with mild soap and lukewarm water, then rinse thoroughly and pat rather than rub dry.	✔	✔
• Recognize the dangers of thermal injury: - Wear clean, loose, soft cotton socks (they are comfortable, allow air to circulate, and absorb moisture) - In cold weather, wear extra socks in extra-large shoes. - Avoid heating pads, whirlpools, and hot tubs. - Avoid sunburn.	✔	
• Identify safety concerns: - Inspect feet daily with a mirror for redness, dryness, cuts, blisters, etc. - Always wear soft shoes or slippers when out of bed. - Trim nails straight across after showering. - Consult podiatrist to trim nails if vision is decreased; also for care of corns, blisters, ingrown nails. - Clear pathways in house to prevent injury. - Avoid wearing thong sandals. - Use lamb's wool between toes if they overlap or rub each other.	✔	✔
• Demonstrate use of comfort measures: - Wear leather shoes with an extra-depth toebox. Synthetic shoes do not allow air to circulate. - If feet become dry and scaly, use cream with lanolin. Never put cream between toes. - If feet perspire, especially between toes, use powder daily and/or lamb's wool between toes to promote drying.	✔	
• Demonstrate strategies to decrease risk of constricting blood vessels: - Avoid circular compression around feet or knees—for example, by applying knee-high stockings or tight socks. - Do not cross legs at knees. - Stop using all tobacco products (ie, smoking or chewing) because nicotine causes vasoconstriction and vasospasm. - Avoid applying tight, constricting bandages. - Participate in a regular walking exercise program to stimulate circulation.	✔	
• Recognize when to seek medical attention: - Contact health care provider at the onset of skin breakdown such as abrasions, blisters, fungus infection (athlete's foot), or pain. - Do not use any medication on feet or legs unless prescribed. - Avoid using iodine, alcohol, corn/wart-removing compound, or adhesive products before checking with health care provider.	✔	✔

c. Experiences decreased muscle pain with exercise
d. Demonstrates an increase in walking distance or duration
2. Promotes vasodilation; prevents vascular compression
a. Protects extremities from exposure to cold
b. Avoids use of tobacco
c. Uses stress-management strategies to minimize emotional upset
d. Wears nonconstricting clothing
e. Avoids leg crossing
f. Takes medications as prescribed
3. Has decrease in severity and duration of pain
4. Attains or maintains tissue integrity
a. Avoids trauma and irritation to skin
b. Wears protective shoes
c. Adheres to meticulous hygiene regimen
d. Eats a healthy diet that contains adequate protein, vitamins A and C, and zinc
e. Performs self-care activities

Peripheral Arterial Occlusive Disease

Arterial insufficiency of the extremities occurs most often in men and is a common cause of disability. The legs are most frequently affected; however, the upper extremities may be involved. The age of onset and the severity are influenced by the type and number of atherosclerotic risk factors (see Chart 31-2). In PAD, obstructive lesions are predominantly confined to segments of the arterial system extending from the aorta below the renal arteries to the popliteal artery (Fig. 31-9). Distal occlusive disease is frequently seen in patients with diabetes mellitus and in elderly patients.

Clinical Manifestations

The hallmark symptom is intermittent claudication. This pain may be described as aching, cramping, or inducing fatigue or weakness that occurs with the same degree of exercise or activity and is relieved with rest. The pain commonly occurs in muscle groups distal to the area of stenosis or occlusion. As the disease progresses, the patient may have a decreased ability to walk the same distance as previously or may notice increased pain with ambulation. When the arterial insufficiency becomes severe, the patient has rest pain. This pain is associated with critical ischemia of the distal extremity and is persistent, aching, or boring; it may be so excruciating that it is unrelieved by opioids and is disabling. Ischemic rest pain is usually worse at night and often wakes the patient. Elevating the extremity or placing it in a horizontal position increases the pain, whereas placing the extremity in a dependent position reduces the pain. Some patients sleep with the affected leg hanging over the side of the bed. Some patients sleep in a reclining chair in an attempt to prevent or relieve the pain.

Assessment and Diagnostic Findings

A sensation of coldness or numbness in the extremities may accompany intermittent claudication and is a result of reduced arterial flow. The extremity is cool and pale when elevated or ruddy and cyanotic when placed in a dependent position. Skin and nail changes, ulcerations, gangrene, and muscle atrophy may be evident. Bruits may be auscultated with a stethoscope. Peripheral pulses may be diminished or absent.

Examination of the peripheral pulses is an important part of assessing arterial occlusive disease. Unequal pulses between extremities or the absence of a normally palpable pulse is a sign of PAD.

The presence, location, and extent of arterial occlusive disease are determined by a careful history of the symptoms and by physical examination. The color and temperature of the extremity are noted and the pulses palpated. The nails may be thickened and opaque, and the skin may be shiny, atrophic, and dry, with sparse hair growth. The assessment includes comparison of the right and left extremities.

The diagnosis of peripheral arterial occlusive disease may be made using CW Doppler and ABIs, treadmill testing for claudication, duplex ultrasonography, or other imaging studies previously described.

Medical Management

Generally, patients feel better with some type of exercise program. If this program is combined with weight reduction and cessation of tobacco use, patients often can improve their activity tolerance. Patients should not be promised that their symptoms will be relieved if they stop tobacco use, because claudication may persist, and they may lose their motivation to stop using tobacco.

Pharmacologic Therapy

Pentoxifylline (Trental) and cilostazol (Pletal) are the only medications specifically indicated for the treatment of claudication. Pentoxifylline increases erythrocyte flexibility, lowers blood fibrinogen concentrations, and has antiplatelet effects. However, recent meta-analyses have questioned the overall efficacy of this medication (Treat-Jacobson & Walsh, 2003). Cilostazol is a phosphodiesterase III inhibitor that is a vasodilator and that thwarts platelet aggregation.

Antiplatelet agents such as aspirin or clopidogrel (Plavix) help prevent the formation of thromboemboli, which can lead to myocardial infarction and stroke. Aspirin has been shown to reduce the risk of myocardial infarction, stroke, and death in patients with vascular disease; however, adverse events associated with aspirin use include gastrointestinal upset or bleeding. Clopidogrel is indicated for the prevention of cardiovascular ischemic events in patients with PAD but not for the treatment of claudication symptoms.

Surgical Management

In most patients, when intermittent claudication becomes severe and disabling or when the limb is at risk for amputation because of tissue necrosis, vascular grafting or endarterectomy is the treatment of choice. The choice of the surgical procedure depends on the degree and location of the stenosis or occlusion. Other important considerations are the overall health of the patient and the length of the procedure that can be tolerated. It is sometimes necessary

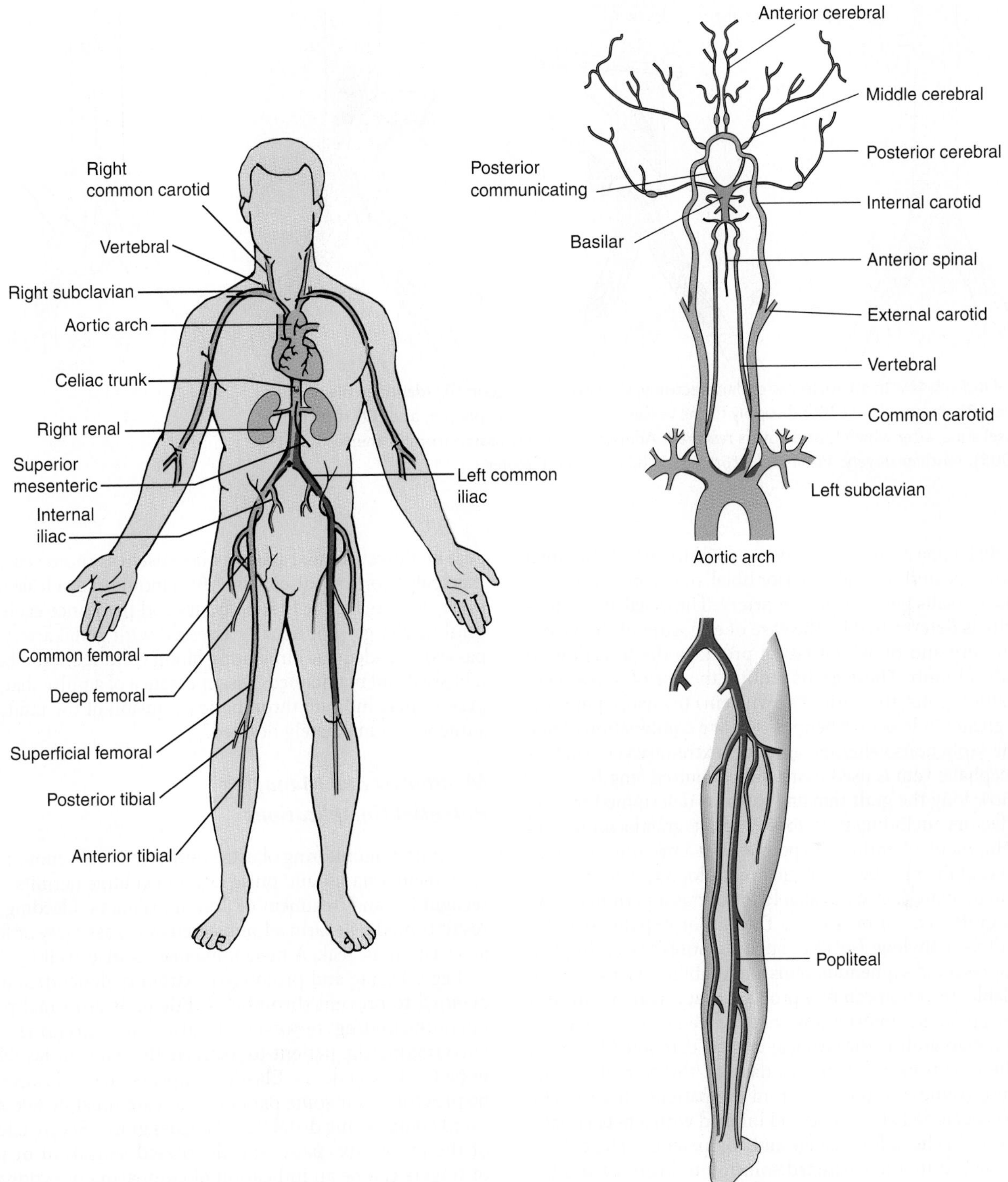

FIGURE 31-9. Common sites of atherosclerotic obstruction in major arteries.

to provide the palliative therapy of primary amputation rather than an arterial bypass. If endarterectomy is performed, an incision is made into the artery and the atheromatous obstruction is removed (Fig. 31-10).

Bypass grafts are performed to reroute the blood flow around the stenosis or occlusion. Before bypass grafting, the surgeon determines where the distal **anastomosis** (site where the vessels are surgically joined) will be placed. The distal outflow vessel must be at least 50% patent for the graft to remain patent. A higher bypass graft patency rate is associated with keeping the length of the bypass as short as possible (Rutherford, 2005).

If the atherosclerotic occlusion is below the inguinal ligament in the superficial femoral artery, the surgical procedure of choice is the femoral-to-popliteal graft. This procedure is further classified as above-knee and below-knee grafts, referring to the location of the distal anastomosis.

Lower leg or ankle vessels with occlusions may also require grafts. Occasionally, the popliteal artery is completely occluded and only collateral vessels maintain perfusion.

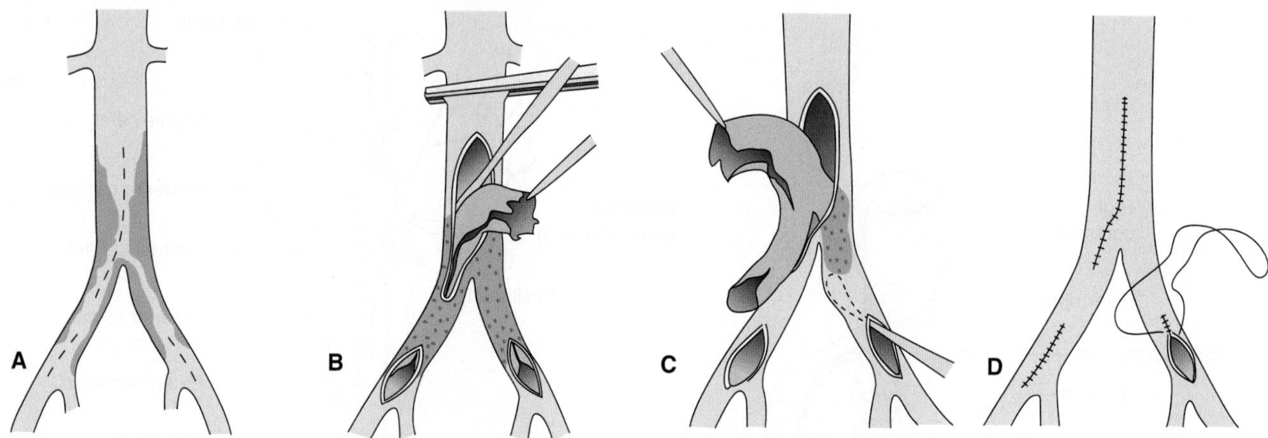

FIGURE 31-10. In an aortoiliac endarterectomy, the vascular surgeon (**A**) identifies the diseased area, (**B**) clamps off the blood supply to the vessel, (**C**) removes the plaque, and (**D**) sutures the vessel shut, after which blood flow is restored. Adapted with permission from Rutherford, R. B. (2005). *Vascular surgery: Vol. 1 and 2* (6th ed.). Philadelphia: Elsevier.

The distal anastomosis may be made onto any of the tibial arteries (posterior tibial, anterior tibial, or peroneal arteries) or the dorsalis pedis or plantar artery. The distal anastomosis site is determined by the ease of exposure of the vessel in surgery and by which vessel provides the best flow to the distal limb. These grafts require the use of native vein (ie, autologous; the patient's own vein) to ensure patency. The greater or lesser saphenous vein or a combination of one of the saphenous veins and an upper extremity vein such as the cephalic vein is used to meet the required length.

How long the graft remains patent is determined by several factors, including the size of the graft, graft location, and development of intimal hyperplasia at anastomosis sites. Bypass grafts may be synthetic or autologous vein. Several synthetic materials are available for use as a peripheral bypass graft: woven or knitted Dacron or expanded polytetrafluoroethylene (ePTFE, such as Gore-Tex or Impra). Cryopreserved saphenous veins and umbilical veins are also available. Infection can be a problem that threatens survival of the graft and almost always requires removal of the graft.

If a vein graft is the surgical choice, care must be taken in the operating room not to damage the vein after harvesting (removing the vein from the patient's body). The vein is occluded at one end and inflated with a heparinized solution to check for leakage and competency. The graft is then placed in a heparinized solution to keep it from becoming dry and brittle.

Nursing Management

Maintaining Circulation

The primary objective in the postoperative period is to maintain adequate circulation through the arterial repair. Pulses, Doppler assessment, color and temperature, capillary refill, and sensory and motor function of the affected extremity are checked and compared with those of the other extremity; these values are recorded every hour for the first 8 hours and then every 2 hours for 24 hours. Doppler evaluation of the vessels distal to the bypass graft should be performed for all postoperative vascular patients because it is more sensitive than palpation for pulses. The ABI is monitored at least once every 8 hours for the first 24 hours and then once each day until discharge (not usually assessed with pedal artery bypasses). An adequate circulating blood volume should be established and maintained. Disappearance of a pulse that was present may indicate thrombotic occlusion of the graft; the surgeon is immediately notified.

Monitoring and Managing Potential Complications

Continuous monitoring of urine output, central venous pressure, mental status, and pulse rate and volume permits early recognition and treatment of fluid imbalances. Bleeding can result from the heparin administered during surgery or from an anastomotic leak. A hematoma may form as well.

Leg crossing and prolonged extremity dependency are avoided to prevent thrombosis. Edema is a normal postoperative finding; however, elevating the extremities and encouraging the patient to exercise the extremities while in bed reduces edema. Elastic compression stockings may be prescribed for some patients, but care must be taken to avoid compressing distal vessel bypass grafts. Severe edema of the extremity, pain, and decreased sensation of toes or fingers can be an indication of compartment syndrome (see Chapter 69).

Promoting Home and Community-Based Care

Discharge planning includes assessing the patient's ability to manage activities of daily living (ADLs) independently. The nurse determines whether the patient has a network of family and friends to assist with ADLs. The patient is encouraged to make the lifestyle changes necessitated by the onset of a chronic disease, including pain management and modifications in diet, activity, and hygiene (skin care). The nurse ensures that the patient has the knowledge and ability to assess for any postoperative complications such as infection, occlusion of the artery or graft, and decreased blood flow.

The nurse assists the patient in developing and implementing a plan to stop using tobacco. Nursing care for patients with peripheral vascular disease is described in Chart 31-3.

Upper Extremity Arterial Occlusive Disease

Arterial occlusions occur less frequently in the upper extremities (arms) than in the legs and cause less severe symptoms because the collateral circulation is significantly better in the arms. The arms also have less muscle mass and are not subjected to the workload of the legs.

Clinical Manifestations

Stenosis and occlusions in the upper extremity result from atherosclerosis or trauma. The stenosis usually occurs at the origin of the vessel proximal to the vertebral artery, setting up the vertebral artery as the major contributor of flow. The patient typically complains of arm fatigue and pain with exercise (forearm claudication) and inability to hold or grasp objects (eg, painting, combing hair, placing objects on shelves above the head) and occasionally difficulty driving.

The patient may develop a "subclavian steal" syndrome characterized by reverse flow in the vertebral and basilar artery to provide blood flow to the arm. This syndrome may cause vertebrobasilar (cerebral) symptoms, including vertigo, ataxia, syncope, or bilateral visual changes.

Assessment and Diagnostic Findings

Assessment findings include coolness and pallor of the affected extremity, decreased capillary refill, and a difference in arm blood pressures of more than 20 mm Hg. Noninvasive studies performed to evaluate for upper extremity arterial occlusions include upper and forearm blood pressure determinations and duplex ultrasonography to identify the anatomic location of the lesion and to evaluate the hemodynamics of the blood flow. Transcranial Doppler evaluation is performed to evaluate the intracranial circulation and to detect any siphoning of blood flow from the posterior circulation to provide blood flow to the affected arm. If a surgical or interventional procedure is planned, an arteriogram may be necessary.

Medical Management

If a short, focal lesion is identified in an upper extremity artery, a PTA may be performed. If the lesion involves the subclavian artery with documented siphoning of blood flow from the intracranial circulation, several surgical procedures are available: carotid–to–subclavian artery bypass, axillary–to–axillary artery bypass, and autogenous reimplantation of the subclavian to the carotid artery.

Nursing Management

Nursing assessment involves bilateral comparison of upper arm blood pressures (obtained by stethoscope and Doppler); radial, ulnar, and brachial pulses; motor and sensory function; temperature; color changes; and capillary refill every 2 hours. Disappearance of a pulse or Doppler flow that had been present may indicate an acute occlusion of the vessel, and the physician is notified immediately.

After surgery, the arm is kept at heart level or elevated, with the fingers at the highest level. Pulses are monitored with Doppler assessment of the arterial flow every hour for 8 hours and then every 2 hours for 24 hours. Blood pressure (obtained by stethoscope and Doppler) is also assessed every hour for 8 hours and then every 2 hours for 24 hours. Motor and sensory function, warmth, color, and capillary refill are monitored with each arterial flow (pulse) assessment.

NURSING ALERT

Before and for 24 hours after surgery, the patient's arm is kept at heart level and protected from cold, venipunctures or arterial sticks, tape, and constrictive dressings.

Discharge planning includes assessing the patient's ability to manage ADLs independently. The nurse determines whether the patient has a network of family and friends to assist with ADLs. The patient may need to make the lifestyle changes necessary to accommodate a chronic disease, including pain management and modifications in diet, activity, and hygiene (skin care). The nurse ensures that the patient has the knowledge and ability to assess for any postoperative complications such as infection, reocclusion of the artery or occlusion of the graft, and decreased blood flow. The patient is assisted in developing and implementing a plan to stop using tobacco. Chart 31-3 describes nursing care for patients with peripheral vascular disease.

Thromboangiitis Obliterans (Buerger's Disease)

Buerger's disease is characterized by recurring inflammation of the intermediate and small arteries and veins of the lower and (in rare cases) upper extremities. It results in thrombus formation and occlusion of the vessels. It is differentiated from other vessel diseases by its microscopic appearance. In contrast to atherosclerosis, Buerger's disease is believed to be an autoimmune disease that results in occlusion of distal vessels.

The cause of Buerger's disease is unknown, but it is believed to be an autoimmune vasculitis. It occurs most often in men between 20 and 35 years of age, and it has been reported in all races and in many areas of the world. There is considerable evidence that heavy smoking or chewing of tobacco is a causative or an aggravating factor (Mills, 2003). Generally, the lower extremities are affected, but arteries in the upper extremities or viscera can also be involved. Buerger's disease is generally bilateral and symmetric with focal lesions. Superficial thrombophlebitis may be present.

Clinical Manifestations

Pain is the outstanding symptom of Buerger's disease. The patient complains of foot cramps, especially of the arch (instep claudication), after exercise. The pain is relieved by rest; often, a burning pain is aggravated by emotional disturbances, nicotine, or chilling. Cold sensitivity of the Raynaud type is found in half the patients and is frequently confined to the hands. Digital rest pain is constant, and the characteristics of the pain do not change between activity and rest.

Physical signs include intense rubor (reddish-blue discoloration) of the foot and absence of the pedal pulse, but with normal femoral and popliteal pulses. Radial and ulnar artery pulses are absent or diminished. Various types of paresthesias may develop.

As the disease progresses, definite redness or cyanosis of the part appears when the extremity is in a dependent position. Involvement is generally bilateral, but color changes may affect only one extremity or only certain digits. Color changes may progress to ulceration, and ulceration with gangrene eventually occurs.

Assessment and Diagnostic Findings

Segmental limb blood pressures are taken to demonstrate the distal location of the lesions or occlusions. Duplex ultrasonography is used to document patency of the proximal vessels and to visualize the extent of distal disease. Contrast angiography is used to identify the diseased portion of the anatomy.

Gerontologic Considerations

Although Buerger's disease is different from atherosclerosis, it may be accompanied by atherosclerosis of the larger vessels. The patient's ability to walk may be severely limited. Patients are at higher risk for nonhealing wounds because of impaired circulation.

Medical Management

The treatment of Buerger's disease is essentially the same as that for atherosclerotic peripheral arterial disease. The main objectives are to improve circulation to the extremities, prevent the progression of the disease, and protect the extremities from trauma and infection. Treatment of ulceration and gangrene is directed toward minimizing infection and conservative débridement of necrotic tissue. Tobacco use is highly detrimental, and patients are strongly advised to completely stop using tobacco. Symptoms are often relieved by cessation of tobacco use.

Vasodilators are rarely prescribed because these medications cause dilation of only healthy vessels; vasodilators may divert blood away from the partially occluded vessels, thus exacerbating the manifestations of the disease. A regional sympathetic block or ganglionectomy may be useful in some instances to produce vasodilation and increase blood flow.

If gangrene of a toe develops as a result of arterial occlusive disease in the leg, it is unlikely that toe amputation or even transmetatarsal amputation will be sufficient; often, a below-knee amputation or occasionally an above-knee amputation is necessary. The indications for amputation include gangrene, especially if the infected area is moist; severe rest pain; or fulminating sepsis.

Nursing Management

The patient is assisted in developing and implementing a plan to stop using tobacco and to manage pain. The patient may need to be encouraged to make the lifestyle changes necessary to adequately manage a chronic disease, including modifications in diet, activity, and hygiene (skin care). The nurse determines whether the patient has a network of family and friends to assist with ADLs. The nurse ensures that the patient has the knowledge and ability to assess for any postoperative complications such as infection and decreased blood flow. Chart 31-3 describes nursing care for patients with peripheral vascular disease. Nursing management during the immediate postoperative phase after amputation and through the rehabilitation phase is described in Chapter 69.

Aortitis

The aorta, which is the main trunk of the arterial system, is divided into the ascending aorta (contained in the pericardium), the aortic arch (extending upward, backward, and downward), and the descending aorta. The thoracic aorta is located above the diaphragm; the abdominal aorta is located below the diaphragm. The abdominal aorta is further designated as suprarenal (above renal artery level), perirenal level (at renal artery level), and infrarenal (below renal artery level).

Aortitis is inflammation of the aorta, particularly of the aortic arch. Two types are known to occur: Takayasu's disease (occlusive thromboaortopathy) and syphilitic aortitis. Both are rare.

Takayasu's disease, a chronic inflammatory disease of the aortic arch and its branches, primarily affects young or middle-aged women and is more common in those of Asian descent. It is nonatherosclerotic; the exact pathologic mechanism is unknown but is thought to be immune complex mediated. It progresses from a systemic inflammatory response with localized arteritis to end-organ ischemia because of large vessel stenosis or obstruction. Magnetic resonance angiography (MRA), CT, duplex ultrasonography, or arteriography is used to diagnose and evaluate the lesions, which are typically long, smooth areas of narrowing with or without aneurysms. The primary goal of treatment is to suppress the vascular inflammatory response. This may be achieved by administering a corticosteroid such as prednisone (Deltasone), 45 to 60 mg orally daily. Selective PTA and surgical revascularization may be performed after suppression of the systemic vascular inflammation.

Aortoiliac Disease

If collateral circulation has developed, patients with a stenosis or occlusion of the aortoiliac segment may be asymptomatic, or they may complain of buttock or low back discomfort associated with walking. Men may experience impotence. These patients may have decreased or absent femoral pulses.

Medical Management

The treatment of aortoiliac disease is essentially the same as that for atherosclerotic peripheral arterial occlusive disease. The surgical procedure of choice is the aortoiliac graft. If possible, the distal graft is anastomosed to the iliac artery, and the entire surgical procedure is performed within the abdomen. If the iliac vessels are diseased, the distal anastomosis is made to the femoral arteries (aortobifemoral graft). Bifurcated woven or knitted Dacron grafts are preferred for this surgical procedure.

Nursing Management

Preoperative assessment, in addition to the standard parameters (see Chapter 18), includes evaluating the brachial, radial, ulnar, femoral, posterior tibial, and dorsalis pedis pulses to establish a baseline for follow-up after arterial lines are placed and postoperatively. Patient teaching includes an overview of the procedure to be performed, the preparation for surgery, and the anticipated postoperative plan of care. Sights, sounds, and sensations that the patient may experience are discussed.

Postoperative care includes monitoring for signs of thrombosis in arteries distal to the surgical site. The nurse assesses color and temperature of the extremity, capillary refill time, sensory and motor function, and pulses by palpation and Doppler every hour for the first 8 hours and then every 2 hours for the first 24 hours. Any dusky or bluish discoloration, coolness, capillary refill time greater than 2 seconds, decrease in sensory or motor function, or decrease in pulse quality is reported immediately to the physician.

Postoperative care also includes monitoring urine output and ensuring that output is at least 30 mL/hour. Renal function may be impaired as a result of hypoperfusion from hypotension, ischemia to the renal arteries during the surgical procedure, hypovolemia, or embolization of the renal artery or renal parenchyma. Vital signs, pain, and intake and output are monitored with the pulse and extremity assessments. Results of laboratory tests are monitored and reported to the physician. Abdominal assessment for bowel sounds and paralytic ileus is performed at least every 8 hours. Bowel sounds may not return before the third postoperative day. The absence of bowel sounds, absence of flatus, and abdominal distention are indications of paralytic ileus. Manual manipulation of the bowel during surgery may have caused bruising, resulting in decreased peristalsis. Nasogastric suction may be necessary to decompress the bowel until peristalsis returns. A liquid bowel movement before the third postoperative day may indicate bowel ischemia, which may occur when the mesenteric blood supply (celiac, superior mesenteric, or inferior mesenteric arteries) is occluded. Ischemic bowel usually causes increased pain and a markedly elevated white blood cell count (20,000 to 30,000 cells/mm^3).

Aneurysm

An aneurysm is a localized sac or dilation formed at a weak point in the wall of the artery (Fig. 31-11). It may be classified by its shape or form. The most common forms of aneurysms are saccular and fusiform. A saccular aneurysm projects from one side of the vessel only. If an entire arterial segment becomes dilated, a fusiform aneurysm develops. Very small aneurysms due to localized infection are called mycotic aneurysms.

Historically, the cause of abdominal aortic aneurysm, the most common type of degenerative aneurysm, has been attributed to atherosclerotic changes in the aorta. Other causes of aneurysm formation are listed in Chart 31-5. Aneurysms are serious because they can rupture, leading to hemorrhage and death.

Thoracic Aortic Aneurysm

Approximately 85% of all cases of thoracic aortic aneurysm are caused by atherosclerosis. They occur most frequently in men between the ages of 40 and 70 years. The thoracic area is the most common site for a dissecting aneurysm. About one third of patients with thoracic aneurysms die of rupture of the aneurysm (Rutherford, 2005).

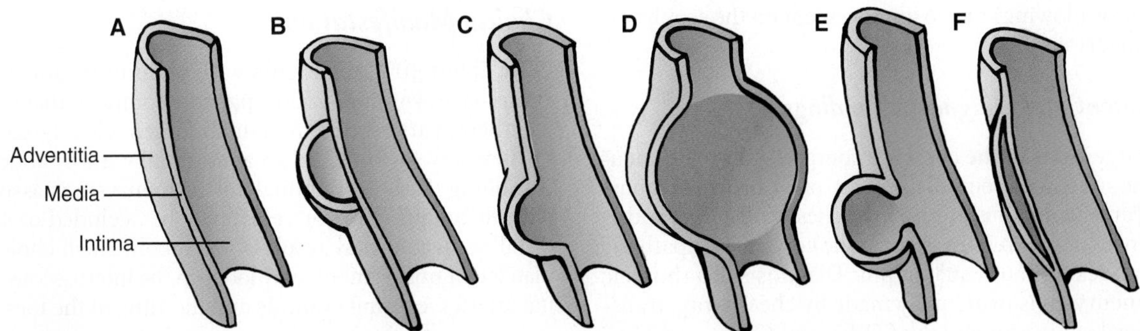

FIGURE 31-11. Characteristics of arterial aneurysm. (**A**) Normal artery. (**B**) False aneurysm—actually a pulsating hematoma. The clot and connective tissue are outside the arterial wall. (**C**) True aneurysm. One, two, or all three layers of the artery may be involved. (**D**) Fusiform aneurysm—symmetric, spindle-shaped expansion of entire circumference of involved vessel. (**E**) Saccular aneurysm—a bulbous protrusion of one side of the arterial wall. (**F**) Dissecting aneurysm—this usually is a hematoma that splits the layers of the arterial wall.

CHART 31-5

Etiologic Classification of Arterial Aneurysms

Congenital: Primary connective tissue disorders (Marfan's syndrome, Ehlers-Danlos syndrome) and other diseases (focal medial agenesis, tuberous sclerosis, Turner's syndrome, Menkes' syndrome)
Mechanical (hemodynamic): Poststenotic and arteriovenous fistula and amputation-related
Traumatic (pseudoaneurysms): Penetrating arterial injuries, blunt arterial injuries, pseudoaneurysms
Inflammatory (noninfectious): Associated with arteritis (Takayasu's disease, giant cell arteritis, systemic lupus erythematosus, Behçet's syndrome, Kawasaki's disease) and periarterial inflammation (ie, pancreatitis)
Infectious (mycotic): Bacterial, fungal, spirochetal infections
Pregnancy-related degenerative: Nonspecific, inflammatory variant
Anastomotic (postarteriotomy) and graft aneurysms: Infection, arterial wall failure, suture failure, graft failure

Adapted with permission from Rutherford, R. B. (2005). *Vascular surgery* (Vols. 1 and 2, 6th ed.). Philadelphia: W. B. Saunders.

Clinical Manifestations

Symptoms are variable and depend on how rapidly the aneurysm dilates and how the pulsating mass affects surrounding intrathoracic structures. Some patients are asymptomatic. In most cases, pain is the most prominent symptom. The pain is usually constant and boring but may occur only when the person is supine. Other conspicuous symptoms are dyspnea, the result of pressure of the aneurysm sac against the trachea, a main bronchus, or the lung itself; cough, frequently paroxysmal and with a brassy quality; hoarseness, stridor, or weakness or complete loss of the voice (aphonia), resulting from pressure against the laryngeal nerve; and dysphagia (difficulty in swallowing) due to impingement on the esophagus by the aneurysm.

Assessment and Diagnostic Findings

When large veins in the chest are compressed by the aneurysm, the superficial veins of the chest, neck, or arms become dilated, and edematous areas on the chest wall and cyanosis are often evident. Pressure against the cervical sympathetic chain can result in unequal pupils. Diagnosis of a thoracic aortic aneurysm is principally made by chest x-ray, transesophageal echocardiography (TEE), and CT.

Medical Management

In most cases, an aneurysm is treated by surgical repair. General measures such as controlling blood pressure and correcting risk factors may be helpful. It is important to control blood pressure in patients with dissecting aneurysms. Systolic pressure is maintained at about 100 to 120 mm Hg with antihypertensive medications (eg, hydralazine [Apresoline], or a beta-blocker such as esmolol [Brevibloc] or metoprolol [Lopressor]). Sodium nitroprusside (Nipride) may be used by continuous IV drip to emergently lower the blood pressure. The goal of surgery is to repair the aneurysm and restore vascular continuity with a vascular graft (Fig. 31-12). Intensive monitoring is usually required after this type of surgery, and the patient is cared for in the critical care unit. Repair of thoracic aneurysms using endovascular grafts implanted (deployed) percutaneously in an interventional suite (eg, interventional radiology, cardiac catheterization laboratory) or an operating room may decrease postoperative recovery time and decrease complications compared with traditional surgical techniques. Thoracic endografts are made of similar materials as in aortic endografts, such as Gore-Tex or PTFE material reinforced with stents (nitinol, titanium). These endovascular grafts are inserted into the thoracic aorta via various vascular access routes, including the femoral or iliac artery. Because a large operative incision is not necessary to gain vascular access, the overall patient recovery time tends to be shorter than if the patient had open surgical repair.

Abdominal Aortic Aneurysm

The most common cause of abdominal aortic aneurysm is atherosclerosis. The condition, which is more common among Caucasians, affects men four times more often than women and is most prevalent in elderly patients (Rutherford, 2005). Most of these aneurysms occur below the renal arteries (infrarenal aneurysms). Untreated, the eventual outcome may be rupture and death.

Pathophysiology

All aneurysms involve a damaged media layer of the vessel. This may be caused by congenital weakness, trauma, or disease. After an aneurysm develops, it tends to enlarge. Risk factors include genetic predisposition, tobacco use, and hypertension; more than half of patients with aneurysms have hypertension.

Clinical Manifestations

Only about 40% of patients with abdominal aortic aneurysms have symptoms. Some patients complain that they can feel their heart beating in their abdomen when lying down, or they may say they feel an abdominal mass or abdominal throbbing. If the abdominal aortic aneurysm is associated with thrombus, a major vessel may be occluded or smaller distal occlusions may result from emboli. Small cholesterol, platelet, or fibrin emboli may lodge in the interosseous or digital arteries, causing cyanosis and mottling of the toes.

Assessment and Diagnostic Findings

The most important diagnostic indication of an abdominal aortic aneurysm is a pulsatile mass in the middle and upper abdomen. About 80% of these aneurysms can be palpated. A systolic bruit may be heard over the mass. Duplex ultra-

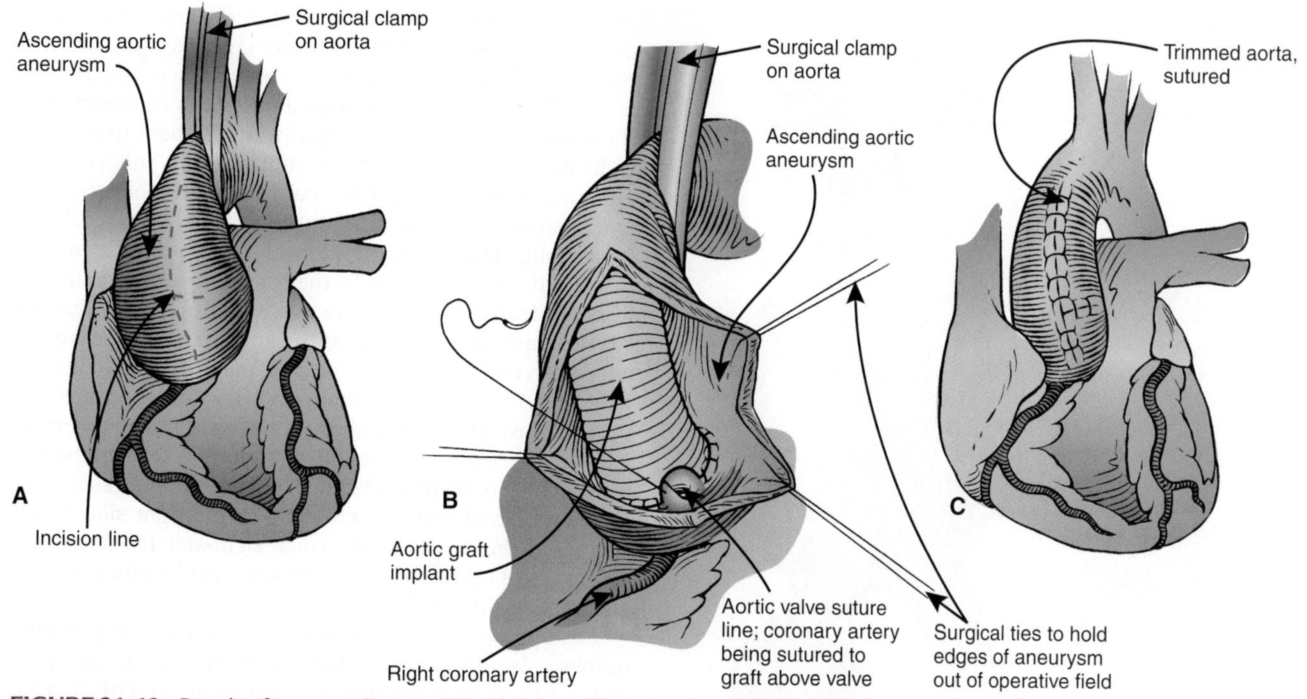

FIGURE 31-12. Repair of an ascending aortic aneurysm and aortic valve replacement. (**A**) Incision into aortic aneurysm. (**B**) Aortic valve replacement with aortic graft implant to repair ascending aortic aneurysm. (**C**) Aortic aneurysm trimmed and closed over graft.

sonography or CT is used to determine the size, length, and location of the aneurysm (Fig. 31-13). When the aneurysm is small, ultrasonography is conducted at 6-month intervals until the aneurysm reaches a size so that surgery to prevent rupture is of more benefit than the possible complications of a surgical procedure. Some aneurysms remain stable over many years of observation.

GERONTOLOGIC CONSIDERATIONS

Most abdominal aortic aneurysms occur in patients between 60 and 90 years of age. Rupture is likely with coexisting hypertension and with aneurysms more than 6 cm wide. In most cases at this point, the chances of rupture are greater than the chance of death during surgical repair. If the elderly patient is considered at moderate risk of complications related to surgery or anesthesia, the aneurysm is not repaired until it is at least 5.5 cm (2 inches) wide.

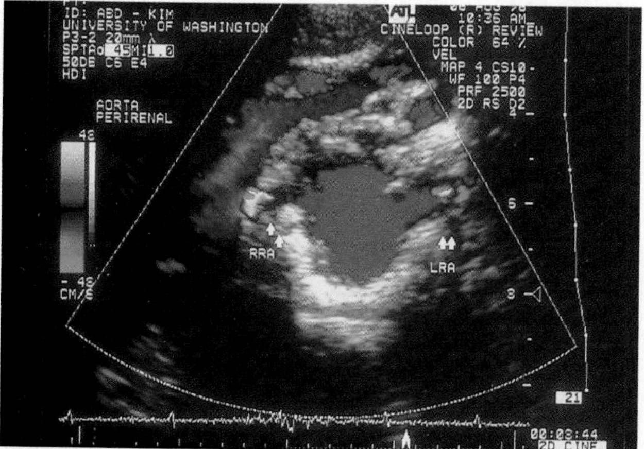

FIGURE 31-13. Duplex ultrasonic image of abdominal aortic aneurysm at the perirenal level. Cross-sectional image documents the location of right and left renal arteries.

Medical Management

PHARMACOLOGIC THERAPY

If the aneurysm is stable in size based on serial duplex ultrasound scans, the blood pressure is closely monitored over time, because there is an association between increased diastolic blood pressure (above 100 mm Hg) and aneurysm rupture (Rutherford, 2005). Antihypertensive agents, including diuretics, beta-blockers, ACE inhibitors, angiotensin II receptor antagonists, and calcium channel blockers, are frequently prescribed to maintain the patient's blood pressure within acceptable limits (see Chapter 32).

SURGICAL MANAGEMENT

An expanding or enlarging abdominal aortic aneurysm is likely to rupture. Surgery is the treatment of choice for abdominal aortic aneurysms more than 5.5 cm (2 inches) wide or those that are enlarging; the standard treatment has been open surgical repair of the aneurysm by resecting the vessel and sewing a bypass graft in place. The mortality rate associated with elective aneurysm repair, a major surgical procedure, is reported to be 1% to 4%. The prognosis for a patient with a ruptured aneurysm is poor, and surgery is performed immediately (Rutherford, 2005).

An alternative for treating an infrarenal abdominal aortic aneurysm is endovascular grafting, which involves the transluminal placement and attachment of a sutureless aortic graft prosthesis across an aneurysm (Fig. 31-14).

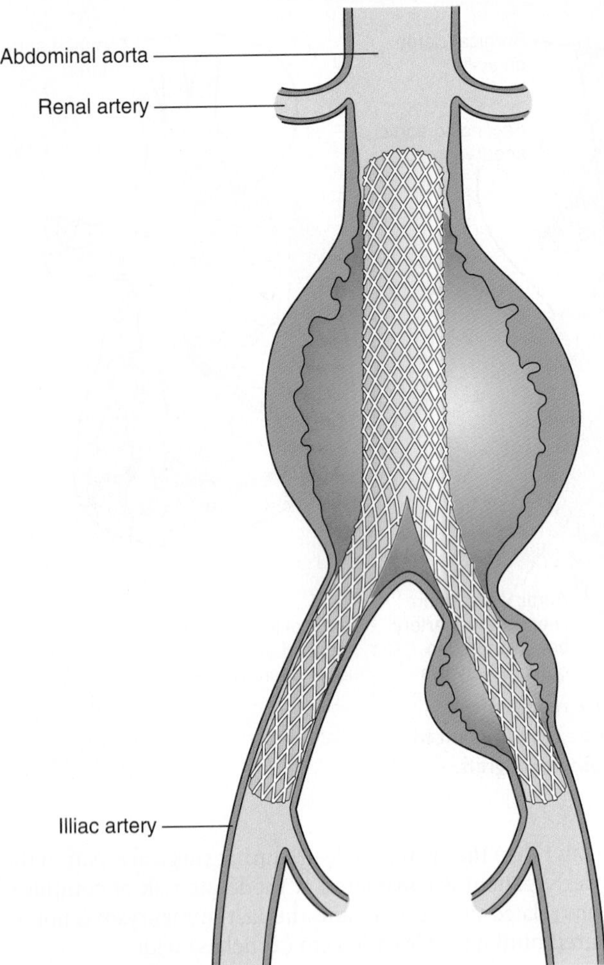

FIGURE 31-14. AneuRx Endograft repair of an abdominal aortic aneurysm (Medtronic).

This procedure can be performed under local or regional anesthesia. Endovascular grafting of abdominal aortic aneurysms may be performed if the patient's abdominal aorta and iliac arteries are not extremely tortuous and if the aneurysm does not begin at the level of the renal arteries. Clinical trials are being conducted to evaluate endograft treatment of abdominal aortic aneurysms at or above the level of the renal arteries and the thoracic aorta. Potential complications include bleeding, hematoma, or wound infection at the femoral insertion site; distal ischemia or embolization; dissection or perforation of the aorta; graft thrombosis or infection; break of the attachment system; graft migration; proximal or distal graft leaks; delayed rupture; and bowel ischemia.

Nursing Management

Before surgery, nursing assessment is guided by anticipating a rupture and by recognizing that the patient may have cardiovascular, cerebral, pulmonary, and renal impairment from atherosclerosis. The functional capacity of all organ systems should be assessed. Medical therapies designed to stabilize physiologic function should be promptly implemented.

Signs of impending rupture include severe back or abdominal pain, which may be persistent or intermittent. Abdominal pain is often localized in the middle or lower abdomen to the left of the midline. Low back pain may be present because of pressure of the aneurysm on the lumbar nerves. This is a significant symptom, usually indicating that the aneurysm is expanding rapidly and is about to rupture. Indications of a rupturing abdominal aortic aneurysm include constant, intense back pain; falling blood pressure; and decreasing hematocrit. Rupture into the peritoneal cavity is rapidly fatal. A retroperitoneal rupture of an aneurysm may result in hematomas in the scrotum, perineum, flank, or penis. Signs of heart failure or a loud bruit may suggest a rupture into the vena cava. If the aneurysm adheres to the adjacent vena cava, the vena cava may become damaged when rupture or leak of the aneurysm occurs. Rupture into the vena cava results in higher-pressure arterial blood entering the lower-pressure venous system and causing turbulence, which is heard as a bruit. The high blood pressure and increased blood volume returning to the right side of the heart from the vena cava may cause right-sided heart failure. The overall surgical mortality rate associated with a ruptured aneurysm is 50% to 75%.

Postoperative care requires intense monitoring of pulmonary, cardiovascular, renal, and neurologic status. Possible complications of surgery include arterial occlusion, hemorrhage, infection, ischemic bowel, renal failure, and impotence.

Other Aneurysms

Aneurysms may also arise in the peripheral vessels, most often as a result of atherosclerosis. These may involve such vessels as the subclavian artery, renal artery, femoral artery, or (most frequently) popliteal artery. Between 50% and 60% of popliteal aneurysms are bilateral and may be associated with abdominal aortic aneurysms.

The aneurysm produces a pulsating mass and disturbs peripheral circulation distal to it. Pain and swelling develop because of pressure on adjacent nerves and veins. Diagnosis is made by duplex ultrasonography and CT to determine the size, length, and extent of the aneurysm. Arteriography may be performed to evaluate the level of proximal and distal involvement.

Medical Management

Surgical repair is performed with replacement grafts or endovascular repair using a stent-graft or wall graft, which is a Dacron or PTFE graft with external structures made from a variety of materials (nitinol, titanium, stainless steel) for additional support.

Nursing Management

The patient who has had an endovascular repair must lie supine for 6 hours; the head of the bed may be elevated up to 45 degrees after 2 hours. The patient needs to use a bedpan or urinal while on bed rest, or an indwelling urinary catheter may be used. Vital signs and Doppler assessment of peripheral pulses are performed every 15 minutes for four times, then every 30 minutes for four times, then every hour for four times, and then as directed by the physician or agency policy. The access site (usually the femoral or iliac artery) is assessed when vital signs and pulses are monitored. The nurse assesses for bleeding, pulsation, swelling, pain, and hematoma formation. Skin changes of the lower extremity, lumbar area, or buttocks that might indicate signs of embolization, such as extremely tender, irregularly shaped, cyanotic areas, as well as any changes in vital signs, pulse quality, bleeding, swelling, pain, or hematoma, are immediately reported to the physician.

The patient's temperature should be monitored every 4 hours, and any signs of postimplantation syndrome should be reported. Postimplantation syndrome typically begins within 24 hours of stent-graft placement and consists of a spontaneously occurring fever, leukocytosis, and, occasionally, transient thrombocytopenia. The exact etiology is unknown, but the symptoms are thought to be related to the activation of cytokines, which results from thrombosis in the repaired aneurysm that occurs because of the release of coagulation proteins and platelets (Latessa, 2002). These symptoms can be managed with mild analgesics or anti-inflammatory agents, such as acetaminophen or ibuprofen, and usually subside within a week.

Because of the increased risk for hemorrhage, the physician is also notified of persistent coughing, sneezing, vomiting, or systolic blood pressure greater than 180 mm Hg. Most patients can resume their preprocedure diet and are encouraged to drink fluids. An IV infusion may be continued until the patient can drink normally. Fluids are important to maintain blood flow through the arterial repair site and to assist the kidneys with excreting IV contrast agent and other medications used during the procedure. Six hours after the procedure, the patient may be able to roll from side to side and may be able to ambulate with assistance to the bathroom. After the patient can take adequate fluids orally, the IV infusion may be discontinued and the IV access converted to a saline lock.

Dissecting Aorta

Occasionally, in an aorta diseased by arteriosclerosis, a tear develops in the intima or the media degenerates, resulting in a dissection (see Fig. 31-11). Arterial dissections are three times more common in men than in women and occur most commonly in the 50- to 70-year-old age group (Rutherford, 2005).

Pathophysiology

Arterial dissections (separations) are commonly associated with poorly controlled hypertension, blunt chest trauma, and cocaine use. The profound increase in sympathetic response caused by cocaine use creates an increase in the force of left ventricular contraction that causes heightened shear forces upon the aortic wall (Rutherford, 2005). Dissection is caused by rupture in the intimal layer. A rupture may occur through adventitia or into the lumen through the intima, allowing blood to re-enter the main channel and resulting in chronic dissection (eg, pseudoaneurysm) or occlusion of branches of the aorta.

As the separation progresses, the arteries branching from the involved area of the aorta shear and occlude. The tear occurs most commonly in the region of the aortic arch, with the highest mortality rate associated with ascending aortic dissection. The dissection of the aorta may progress backward in the direction of the heart, obstructing the openings to the coronary arteries or producing hemopericardium (effusion of blood into the pericardial sac) or aortic insufficiency, or it may extend in the opposite direction, causing occlusion of the arteries supplying the gastrointestinal tract, kidneys, spinal cord, and legs.

Clinical Manifestations

Onset of symptoms is usually sudden. Severe and persistent pain, described as tearing or ripping, may be reported. The pain is in the anterior chest or back and extends to the shoulders, epigastric area, or abdomen. Aortic dissection may be mistaken for an acute myocardial infarction, which could confuse the clinical picture and initial treatment. Cardiovascular, neurologic, and gastrointestinal symptoms are responsible for other clinical manifestations, depending on the location and extent of the dissection. The patient may appear pale. Sweating and tachycardia may be detected. Blood pressure may be elevated or markedly different from one arm to the other if dissection involves the orifice of the subclavian artery on one side. Because of the variable clinical picture associated with this condition, early diagnosis is usually difficult.

Assessment and Diagnostic Findings

Arteriography, CT, transesophageal echocardiography, duplex ultrasonography, and MRI aid in the diagnosis.

Medical Management

The medical or surgical treatment of a dissecting aorta depends on the type of dissection present and follows the general principles outlined for the treatment of thoracic aortic aneurysms.

Nursing Management

A patient with a dissecting aorta requires the same nursing care as a patient with an aortic aneurysm requiring surgical intervention, as described earlier in this chapter. Interventions described in Chart 31-3 are also appropriate.

Arterial Embolism and Arterial Thrombosis

Acute vascular occlusion may be caused by an embolus or acute thrombosis. Acute arterial occlusions may result from iatrogenic injury, which can occur during insertion of invasive catheters such as those used for arteriography, PTA or stent placement, or an intra-aortic balloon pump. Other causes include trauma from a fracture, crush injury, and penetrating wounds that disrupt the arterial intima. The accurate diagnosis of an arterial occlusion as embolic or thrombotic in origin is necessary to initiate appropriate treatment.

Pathophysiology

Arterial emboli arise most commonly from thrombi that develop in the chambers of the heart as a result of atrial fibrillation, myocardial infarction, infective endocarditis, or chronic heart failure. These thrombi become detached and are carried from the left side of the heart into the arterial system, where they lodge in and obstruct an artery that is smaller than the embolus. Emboli may also develop in advanced aortic atherosclerosis because the atheromatous plaques ulcerate or become rough. Acute thrombosis frequently occurs in patients with preexisting ischemic symptoms.

Clinical Manifestations

The symptoms of arterial emboli depend primarily on the size of the embolus, the organ involved, and the state of the collateral vessels. The immediate effect is cessation of distal blood flow. The blockage can progress distal and proximal to the site of the obstruction. Secondary vasospasm can contribute to the ischemia. The embolus can fragment or break apart, resulting in occlusion of distal vessels. Emboli tend to lodge at arterial bifurcations and areas narrowed by atherosclerosis. Cerebral, mesenteric, renal, and coronary arteries are often involved in addition to the large arteries of the extremities.

The symptoms of acute arterial embolism in extremities with poor collateral flow are acute, severe pain and a gradual loss of sensory and motor function. The six *P*s associated with acute arterial embolism are *p*ain, *p*allor, *p*ulselessness, *p*aresthesia, *p*oikilothermia (coldness), and *p*aralysis. Eventually, superficial veins may collapse because of decreased blood flow to the extremity. Because of ischemia, the part of the extremity distal to the occlusion is markedly colder and paler than the part proximal to the occlusion.

Arterial thrombosis can also acutely occlude an artery. A thrombosis is a slowly developing clot that usually occurs where the arterial wall has become damaged, generally as a result of atherosclerosis. Thrombi may also develop in an arterial aneurysm. The manifestations of an acute thrombotic arterial occlusion are similar to those described for embolic occlusion. However, treatment is more difficult with a thrombus because the arterial occlusion has occurred in a degenerated vessel and requires more extensive reconstructive surgery to restore flow than is required with an embolic event.

Assessment and Diagnostic Findings

An arterial embolus is usually diagnosed on the basis of the sudden nature of the onset of symptoms and an apparent source for the embolus. Two-dimensional transthoracic echocardiography or transesophageal echocardiography (TEE), chest x-ray, and electrocardiography may reveal underlying cardiac disease. Noninvasive duplex and Doppler ultrasonography can determine the presence and extent of underlying atherosclerosis, and arteriography may be performed.

Medical Management

Management of arterial thrombosis depends on its cause. Management of acute embolic occlusion usually requires surgery because time is of the essence. Because the onset of the event is acute, collateral circulation has not developed, and the patient quickly moves through the list of six *P*s to paralysis, the most advanced stage. Heparin therapy is initiated immediately to prevent further development of emboli and to hamper the extension of existing thrombi. Typically, an initial IV bolus of 5000 to 10,000 units is administered, followed by a continuous infusion of 1000 units per hour until the patient undergoes surgery.

Surgical Management

Emergency embolectomy is the procedure of choice if the involved extremity is viable (Fig. 31-15). Arterial emboli are usually treated by insertion of an embolectomy catheter. The catheter is passed through a groin incision into the affected artery and advanced past the occlusion. The catheter balloon is inflated with sterile saline solution, and the thrombus is extracted as the catheter is withdrawn. This procedure involves incising the vessel and removing the clot.

Endovascular Management

Percutaneous thrombectomy devices may also be used for the treatment of an acute thrombosis. All endovascular devices necessitate obtaining access to the patient's arterial system and inserting a catheter into the patient's artery to obtain access to the thrombus. The approach is similar to that used for angiograms in that it is made through the groin to the femoral artery. Some devices require that a small incision be made into the patient's artery. Available endovascular devices include:

- The AngioJet, which uses a backward-pointing jet of fluid flow to disrupt the thrombus. It then aspirates the particles into the device's catheter and deposits them in a collection device. Use of this device typically results in

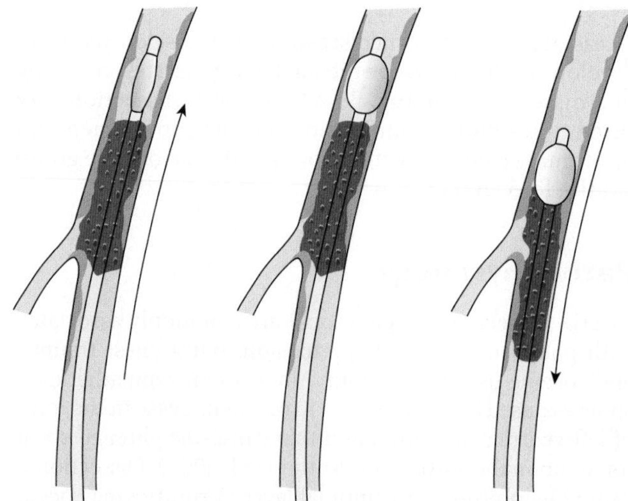

FIGURE 31-15. Extraction of an embolus by balloon-tipped embolectomy catheter. The deflated balloon-tipped catheter is advanced past the embolus, inflated, and then gently withdrawn, carrying the embolic material with it. Adapted with permission from Rutherford, R. B. (2005). *Vascular surgery: Vol. 1 and 2* (6th ed.). Philadelphia: Elsevier.

only 50% to 70% patency of the vessel, so many patients require additional thrombolytic therapy for dissolving the residual thrombus.
- The Bacchus Trellis device, which uses pharmacologic thrombolysis to produce clot dissolution. This device is placed into the patient's artery, with the tip at the location where the thrombus has occurred. A rotating, sinusoidal-shaped wire mixes the thrombolytic agent and simultaneously dissolves the clot, and the resultant particles are aspirated through the catheter into a collection device to prevent distal embolization.
- Therapeutic ultrasonic devices, which are inserted into the patient's artery through a catheter (eg, OmniSonics, Ekos catheter), use high-frequency, low-energy ultrasound to dissolve an occlusive thrombus. The thrombus is dissolved into particles small enough to traverse the distal capillary bed without causing further obstructive embolization. Clinical trials are underway to determine the long-term efficacy of these devices (Ouriel, 2003).

Complications arising from the use of any of the endovascular devices may include arterial dissection or distal artery embolization.

Pharmacologic Therapy

When the patient has collateral circulation, treatment may include IV anticoagulation with heparin, which can prevent the thrombus from spreading and reduce muscle necrosis. Intra-arterial thrombolytic medications are used to dissolve the embolus. Fibrin-specific thrombolytic medications (eg, tissue plasminogen activator [t-PA, Alteplase, Activase] and single-chain urokinase-type plasminogen activator [scu-PA, prourokinase]) do not deplete circulating fibrinogen and plasminogen, which prevents the development of systemic fibrinolysis. Other thrombolytic medications are reteplase (r-PA, Retavase), tenecteplase (TNKase), and staphylokinase (Moore, 2002). Although these agents differ in their pharmacokinetics, they are administered in a similar manner: a catheter is advanced under x-ray visualization to the clot, and the thrombolytic agent is infused.

Thrombolytic therapy should not be used when there are known contraindications to therapy or when the extremity cannot tolerate the several additional hours of ischemia that it takes for the agent to lyse (disintegrate) the clot. Contraindications to thrombolytic therapy include active internal bleeding, CVA (brain attack, stroke), recent major surgery, uncontrolled hypertension, and pregnancy.

Nursing Management

Before surgery, the patient remains on bed rest with the affected extremity level or slightly dependent (15 degrees). The affected part is kept at room temperature and protected from trauma. Heating and cooling pads are contraindicated because ischemic extremities are easily traumatized by alterations in temperature. If possible, tape and electrocardiogram electrodes should not be used on the extremity; sheepskin and foot cradles are used to protect an affected leg from mechanical trauma.

If the patient is treated with thrombolytic therapy, the dose of thrombolytic therapy is based on the patient's weight. The patient is admitted to a critical care unit for continuous monitoring. Vital signs are taken every 15 minutes for 2 hours, then every 30 minutes for the next 6 hours, and then every hour for 16 hours. Bleeding is the most common side effect of thrombolytic therapy, and the patient is closely monitored for any signs of bleeding. The nurse minimizes the number of punctures for inserting IV lines and obtaining blood samples, avoids intramuscular injections, prevents any possible tissue trauma, and applies pressure at least twice as long as usual after any puncture that is performed. If t-PA is used for the treatment, heparin is usually administered to prevent another thrombus from forming at the site of the lesion. The t-PA activates plasminogen on the thrombus more than circulating plasminogen, but it does not decrease the clotting factors as much as other thrombolytic therapies, so patients receiving t-PA can make new thrombi more readily than with some of the other thrombolytics.

During the postoperative period, the nurse collaborates with the surgeon about the patient's appropriate activity level based on the patient's condition. Generally, every effort is made to encourage the patient to move the extremity to stimulate circulation and prevent stasis. Anticoagulant therapy may be continued after surgery to prevent thrombosis of the affected artery and to diminish the development of subsequent thrombi at the initiating site. The nurse assesses for evidence of local and systemic hemorrhage, including mental status changes, which can occur when anticoagulants are administered. Pulses, Doppler signals, ABI, and motor and sensory function are assessed every hour for the first 24 hours, because significant changes may indicate reocclusion. Metabolic abnormalities, renal failure, and compartment syndrome may be complications after an acute arterial occlusion.

Raynaud's Disease

Raynaud's disease is a form of intermittent arteriolar vasoconstriction that results in coldness, pain, and pallor of the fingertips or toes. The cause is unknown, although many patients with the disease have immunologic disorders. Symptoms may result from a defect in basal heat production that eventually decreases the ability of cutaneous vessels to dilate. Episodes may be triggered by emotional factors or by unusual sensitivity to cold. The disease is most common in women between the ages of 16 and 40 years, and it occurs more frequently in cold climates and during the winter.

The term *Raynaud's phenomenon* is used to refer to localized, intermittent episodes of vasoconstriction of small arteries of the feet and hands that cause color and temperature changes. Generally unilateral and affecting only one or two digits, the phenomenon is always associated with underlying systemic disease. It may occur with scleroderma, systemic lupus erythematosus, rheumatoid arthritis, obstructive arterial disease, or trauma.

The prognosis for patients with Raynaud's disease varies; some slowly improve, some become progressively worse, and others show no change. Ulceration and gangrene are rare; however, chronic disease may cause atrophy of the skin and muscles. With appropriate patient teaching and lifestyle modifications, the disorder is generally benign and self-limiting.

Clinical Manifestations

The classic clinical picture reveals pallor brought on by sudden vasoconstriction. The skin then becomes bluish (cyanotic) due to pooling of deoxygenated blood during vasospasm. As a result of exaggerated reflow (hyperemia) due to vasodilation, a red color (rubor) is produced when oxygenated blood returns to the digits after the vasospasm stops. The characteristic sequence of color change of Raynaud's phenomenon is described as white, blue, and red. Numbness, tingling, and burning pain occur as the color changes. The involvement tends to be bilateral and symmetric.

Medical Management

Avoiding the particular stimuli (eg, cold, tobacco) that provoke vasoconstriction is a primary factor in controlling Raynaud's disease. Calcium channel blockers (nifedipine [Procardia, Adalat]) may be effective in relieving symptoms. Sympathectomy (interrupting the sympathetic nerves by removing the sympathetic ganglia or dividing their branches) may help some patients.

Nursing Management

The nurse teaches the patient to avoid situations that may be stressful or unsafe. Stress-management classes may be helpful. Exposure to cold must be minimized, and in areas where the fall and winter months are cold, the patient should remain indoors as much as possible and wear layers of clothing when outdoors. Hats and mittens or gloves should be worn at all times when outside. Fabrics specially designed for cold climates (eg, Thinsulate) are recommended. Patients should warm up their vehicles before getting in so that they can avoid touching a cold steering wheel or door handle, which could elicit an attack. During summer, a sweater should be available when entering air-conditioned rooms.

Patients are often concerned about serious complications, such as gangrene and amputation, but these complications are uncommon. Patients should avoid all forms of nicotine; the nicotine gum or patches used to help people quit smoking may induce attacks.

Patients should be cautioned to handle sharp objects carefully to avoid injuring the fingers. Patients should be informed about the postural hypotension that may result from medications, such as calcium channel blockers, used to treat Raynaud's disease. The nurse also discusses safety precautions related to alcohol, exercise, and hot weather.

Venous Disorders

Venous Thrombosis, Deep Vein Thrombosis, Thrombophlebitis, and Phlebothrombosis

Although the terms *venous thrombosis, deep vein thrombosis (DVT), thrombophlebitis,* and *phlebothrombosis* do not necessarily reflect identical disease processes, for clinical purposes they are often used interchangeably.

Pathophysiology

Superficial veins, such as the greater saphenous, lesser saphenous, cephalic, basilic, and external jugular veins, are thick-walled muscular structures that lie just under the skin. Deep veins are thin-walled and have less muscle in the media. They run parallel to arteries and bear the same names as the arteries. Deep and superficial veins have valves that permit unidirectional flow back to the heart. The valves lie at the base of a segment of the vein that is expanded into a sinus. This arrangement permits the valves to open without coming into contact with the wall of the vein, permitting rapid closure when the blood starts to flow backward. Other kinds of veins are known as perforating veins. These vessels have valves that allow one-way blood flow from the superficial system to the deep system.

Although the exact cause of venous thrombosis remains unclear, three factors, known as Virchow's triad, are believed to play a significant role in its development: stasis of blood (venous stasis), vessel wall injury, and altered blood coagulation (Chart 31-6). Venous stasis occurs when blood

CHART 31-6

Risk Factors for Deep Vein Thrombosis (DVT) and Pulmonary Embolism

Endothelial Damage

- Trauma
- Surgery
- Pacing wires
- Central venous catheters
- Dialysis access catheters
- Local vein damage
- Repetitive motion injury

Venous Stasis

- Bed rest or immobilization
- Obesity
- History of varicosities
- Spinal cord injury
- Age (greater than 65 years)

Altered Coagulation

- Cancer
- Pregnancy
- Oral contraceptive use
- Proteins C deficiency
- Protein S deficiency
- Antiphospholipid antibody syndrome
- Factor V Leiden defect
- Prothrombin 20210A defect
- Hyperhomocysteinemia
- Elevated factors II, VIII, IX, XI
- Antithrombin III deficiency
- Polycythemia
- Septicemia

flow is reduced, as in heart failure or shock; when veins are dilated, as with some medication therapies; and when skeletal muscle contraction is reduced, as in immobility, paralysis of the extremities, or anesthesia. Moreover, bed rest reduces blood flow in the legs by at least 50% (Porth, 2005). Damage to the intimal lining of blood vessels creates a site for clot formation. Direct trauma to the vessels, as with fractures or dislocation, diseases of the veins, and chemical irritation of the vein from IV medications or solutions, can damage veins. Increased blood coagulability occurs most commonly in patients for whom anticoagulant medications have been abruptly withdrawn. Oral contraceptive use and several blood dyscrasias (abnormalities) also can lead to hypercoagulability.

Formation of a thrombus frequently accompanies thrombophlebitis, which is an inflammation of the vein walls. When a thrombus develops initially in the veins as a result of stasis or hypercoagulability but without inflammation, the process is referred to as phlebothrombosis. Venous thrombosis can occur in any vein, but it occurs more in the veins of the lower extremities. The superficial and deep veins of the extremities may be affected.

Upper extremity venous thrombosis is not as common as lower extremity thrombosis. Upper extremity venous thrombosis is more common in patients with IV catheters or in patients with an underlying disease that causes hypercoagulability. Internal trauma to the vessels may result from pacemaker leads, chemotherapy ports, dialysis catheters, or parenteral nutrition lines. The lumen of the vein may be decreased as a result of the catheter or from external compression, such as by neoplasms or an extra cervical rib. Effort thrombosis of the upper extremity is caused by repetitive motion (as in competitive swimmers, tennis players, and construction workers) that irritates the vessel wall, causing inflammation and subsequent thrombosis.

Venous thrombi are aggregates of platelets attached to the vein wall that have a tail-like appendage containing fibrin, white blood cells, and many red blood cells. The "tail" can grow or can propagate in the direction of blood flow as successive layers of the thrombus form. A propagating venous thrombosis is dangerous because parts of the thrombus can break off and produce an embolic occlusion of the pulmonary blood vessels. Fragmentation of the thrombus can occur spontaneously as it dissolves naturally, or it can occur in association with an elevation in venous pressure, as occurs when a person stands suddenly or engages in muscular activity after prolonged inactivity. After an episode of acute DVT, recanalization (ie, reestablishment of the lumen of the vessel) typically occurs. The time required for complete recanalization is an important determinant of venous valvular incompetence, which is one complication of venous thrombosis (Tran & Meissner, 2002). Other complications of venous thrombosis are listed in Chart 31-7.

CHART 31-7

Complications of Venous Thrombosis

Chronic venous occlusion
Pulmonary emboli from dislodged thrombi
Valvular destruction
- Chronic venous insufficiency
- Increased venous pressure
- Varicosities
- Venous ulcers

Venous obstruction
- Increased distal pressure
- Fluid stasis
- Edema
- Venous gangrene

Clinical Manifestations

A major problem associated with recognizing DVT is that the signs and symptoms are nonspecific. The exception is phlegmasia cerulea dolens (massive iliofemoral venous thrombosis), in which the entire extremity becomes massively swollen, tense, painful, and cool to the touch. Despite this variability, clinical signs should always be investigated.

Deep Veins

With obstruction of the deep veins comes edema and swelling of the extremity because the outflow of venous blood is inhibited. The amount of swelling can be determined by measuring the circumference of the affected extremity at various levels with a tape measure and comparing one extremity with the other at the same level to determine size differences. If both extremities are swollen, a size difference may be difficult to detect. The affected extremity may feel warmer than the unaffected extremity, and the superficial veins may appear more prominent.

Tenderness, which usually occurs later, is produced by inflammation of the vein wall and can be detected by gently palpating the affected extremity. Homans' sign (pain in the calf after the foot is sharply dorsiflexed) is not specific for DVT because it can be elicited in any painful condition of the calf. In some cases, signs and symptoms of a pulmonary embolus are the first indication of DVT.

Superficial Veins

Thrombosis of superficial veins produces pain or tenderness, redness, and warmth in the involved area. The risk of the superficial venous thrombi becoming dislodged or fragmenting into emboli is very low because most of them dissolve spontaneously. This condition can be treated at home with bed rest, elevation of the leg, analgesics, and possibly anti-inflammatory medication.

Assessment and Diagnostic Findings

Careful assessment is invaluable in detecting early signs of venous disorders of the lower extremities. Patients with a history of varicose veins, hypercoagulation, neoplastic disease, cardiovascular disease, or recent major surgery or injury are at high risk. Other patients at high risk include those who are obese or elderly and women taking oral contraceptives.

When performing the nursing assessment, key concerns include limb pain, a feeling of heaviness, functional impairment, ankle engorgement, and edema; differences in leg circumference bilaterally from thigh to ankle; increase in the surface temperature of the leg, particularly the calf or ankle; and areas of tenderness or superficial thrombosis (ie, cord-like venous segment). Although Homans' sign has been used historically to assess for DVT, it is not a reliable or valid sign and has no clinical value in assessment for DVT (Gupta & Stouffer, 2001).

Prevention

Venous thrombosis, thrombophlebitis, and DVT can be prevented, especially if patients who are considered at high risk are identified and preventive measures are instituted without delay. Preventive measures include the application of elastic compression stockings, the use of intermittent pneumatic compression devices, and special body positioning and exercise (discussed later in the section on nursing management). An additional method to prevent venous thrombosis in surgical patients is administration of subcutaneous unfractionated or low-molecular-weight heparin (LMWH).

Medical Management

The objectives of treatment for DVT are to prevent the thrombus from growing and fragmenting (risking pulmonary embolism) and to prevent recurrent thromboemboli. Anticoagulant therapy (administration of a medication to delay the clotting time of blood, prevent the formation of a thrombus in postoperative patients, and forestall the extension of a thrombus after it has formed) can meet these objectives, although anticoagulants cannot dissolve a thrombus that has already formed.

Pharmacologic Therapy

Measures for preventing or reducing blood clotting within the vascular system are indicated in patients with thrombophlebitis, recurrent embolus formation, and persistent leg edema from heart failure. They are also indicated in elderly patients with a hip fracture that may result in lengthy immobilization. Contraindications for anticoagulant therapy are noted in Chart 31-8.

UNFRACTIONATED HEPARIN

Unfractionated heparin is administered subcutaneously to prevent development of DVT, or by intermittent or continuous IV infusion for 5 to 7 days to prevent the extension of a thrombus and the development of new thrombi. Oral anticoagulants, such as warfarin (Coumadin), are administered with heparin therapy. Medication dosage is regulated by monitoring the activated partial thromboplastin time (aPTT), the **international normalized ratio** (INR), and the platelet count.

LOW-MOLECULAR-WEIGHT HEPARIN

Subcutaneous LMWHs that may include medications such as dalteparin (Fragmin) and enoxaparin (Lovenox) are effective treatments for some cases of DVT. These agents have longer half-lives than unfractionated heparin, so doses can be given in one or two subcutaneous injections each day. Doses are adjusted according to weight. LMWHs prevent the extension of a thrombus and development of new thrombi, and they are associated with fewer bleeding complications and lower risks of heparin-induced thrombocytopenia (HIT) than unfractionated heparin. Because there are several preparations, the dosing schedule must be based on the product used and the protocol at each institution. The cost of LMWH is higher than that of unfractionated heparin; however, LMWH may be used safely in pregnant women, and patients who take it may be more mobile and have an improved quality of life.

THROMBOLYTIC THERAPY

Unlike the heparins, thrombolytic (fibrinolytic) therapy lyses and dissolves thrombi in 50% of patients. Thrombolytic therapy (eg, t-PA [Alteplase, Activase], reteplase [r-PA, Retavase], tenecteplase [TNKase], staphylokinase, urokinase, streptokinase) is given within the first 3 days after acute thrombosis. Therapy initiated beyond 5 days after the onset of symptoms is significantly less effective (Moore, 2002). The advantages of thrombolytic therapy include less long-term damage to the venous valves and a reduced incidence of postthrombotic syndrome and chronic venous insufficiency. However, thrombolytic therapy results in a threefold greater incidence of bleeding than heparin. If bleeding occurs and cannot be stopped, the thrombolytic agent is discontinued.

CHART 31-8

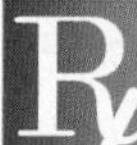

PHARMACOLOGY · Contraindications to Anticoagulant Therapy

- Lack of patient cooperation
- Bleeding from the following systems:
  - Gastrointestinal
  - Genitourinary
  - Respiratory
  - Reproductive
- Hemorrhagic blood dyscrasias
- Aneurysms
- Severe trauma
- Alcoholism
- Recent or impending surgery of:
  - Eye
  - Spinal cord
  - Brain
- Severe hepatic or renal disease
- Recent cerebrovascular hemorrhage
- Infections
- Open ulcerative wounds
- Occupations that involve a significant hazard for injury
- Recent delivery of a baby

FACTOR XA INHIBITOR

Fondaparinux (Arixtra) selectively inhibits factor Xa. This agent is given daily subcutaneously at a fixed dose, has a half-life of 17 hours, and is excreted unchanged via the kidneys (and therefore must be used with caution in patients with renal insufficiency). Fondaparinux has no effect on routine tests of coagulation, such as the aPTT or activated clotting time (ACT), so routine coagulation monitoring is unnecessary (Weitz, 2004). Fondaparinux is approved for prophylaxis during major orthopedic surgery, such as hip or knee arthroplasties.

ORAL ANTICOAGULANTS

Warfarin (Coumadin) is a vitamin K antagonist that is frequently used for extended therapy. Routine coagulation monitoring is essential to ensure that a therapeutic response is obtained and maintained over time. Interactions with a range of other medications can reduce or enhance the anticoagulant effects of warfarin, as can variable intake of foods containing vitamin K (see Chapter 33, Chart 33-15, for a review of agents that interact with warfarin). Warfarin has a narrow therapeutic window, and there is a slow onset of action. Treatment is initially supported with concomitant parenteral anticoagulation with heparin until the warfarin demonstrates anticoagulant effectiveness.

Surgical Management

Surgery is necessary for DVT when anticoagulant or thrombolytic therapy is contraindicated (see Chart 31-8), the danger of pulmonary embolism is extreme, or the venous drainage is so severely compromised that permanent damage to the extremity is likely. A thrombectomy (removal of the thrombosis) is the procedure of choice. A vena cava filter may be placed at the time of the thrombectomy; this filter traps large emboli and prevents pulmonary emboli (see Chapter 23). Balloon angioplasty and stent placement are being used in the iliac veins of patients with acute and chronic venous disease.

Nursing Management

If the patient is receiving anticoagulant therapy, the nurse must frequently monitor the aPTT, prothrombin time (PT), INR, ACT, hemoglobin and hematocrit values, platelet count, and fibrinogen level, depending on which medication is being given. Close observation is also required to detect bleeding; if bleeding occurs, it must be reported immediately and anticoagulant therapy discontinued.

Assessing and Monitoring Anticoagulant Therapy

To prevent inadvertent infusion of large volumes of unfractionated heparin, which could cause hemorrhage, continuous IV infusion by an electronic infusion device is the preferred method of administering unfractionated heparin. Dosage calculations are based on the patient's weight, and any possible bleeding tendencies are detected by a pretreatment clotting profile. If renal insufficiency exists, lower doses of heparin are required. Periodic coagulation tests and hematocrit levels are obtained. Heparin is in the effective, or therapeutic, range when the aPTT is 1.5 times the control.

Oral anticoagulants, such as warfarin (Coumadin), are monitored by the PT or the INR. Because the full anticoagulant effect of warfarin is delayed for 3 to 5 days, it is usually administered concurrently with heparin until desired anticoagulation has been achieved (ie, when the PT is 1.5 to 2 times normal or the INR is 2.0 to 3.0).

Monitoring and Managing Potential Complications

BLEEDING

The principal complication of anticoagulant therapy is spontaneous bleeding anywhere in the body. Bleeding from the kidneys is detected by microscopic examination of the urine and is often the first sign of excessive dosage. Bruises, nosebleeds, and bleeding gums are also early signs. To promptly reverse the effects of heparin, IV injections of protamine sulfate may be administered. Risks of protamine administration include bradycardia and hypotension, which can be minimized by slow administration. Protamine sulfate can be used in patients receiving LMWH, but it is less effective with LMWH than with unfractionated heparin. Reversing the anticoagulation effects of warfarin is more difficult, but effective measures that may be prescribed include administration of vitamin K and/or infusion of fresh-frozen plasma or prothrombin concentrate. Oral vitamin K significantly reduces the INR within 24 hours. Low-dose IV vitamin K is also effective.

THROMBOCYTOPENIA

Another complication of therapy may be HIT, which is defined as a sudden decrease in the platelet count by at least 30% of baseline levels in patients receiving heparin. Patients at greatest risk are those who receive unfractionated heparin for a long period of time (ie, several days or weeks). Therefore, it is preferable not to anticoagulate patients with unfractionated heparin over the long term. Beginning warfarin concomitantly with heparin can provide a stable INR or PT by day 5 of heparin treatment, at which time the heparin may be discontinued.

The administration of LMWH is less frequently associated with HIT. The thrombocytopenia is thought to result from an autoimmune mechanism that causes destruction of platelets. If the process is not arrested, platelets may aggregate, initiating inappropriate clotting, and thrombosis may occur. This serious complication results in thromboembolic manifestations known as HIT with thrombosis, and the prognosis is extremely guarded.

Prevention of thrombocytopenia depends on regular monitoring of platelet counts. Early signs include a decreasing platelet count, the need for increasing doses of heparin to maintain the therapeutic level, and thromboembolic or hemorrhagic complications (appearance of skin necrosis, either at the site of injection or at distal sites where thromboses occur; skin discoloration consisting of large hemorrhagic areas; hematomas; purpura; and blistering) (Miller, 2003). If thrombocytopenia does occur, platelet aggregation studies are conducted, the heparin is discontinued, and alternate anticoagulant therapy is rapidly initiated because the continued prothrombotic state poses an ongoing threat of continuous clot development.

Lepirudin (Refludan) and argatroban are direct thrombin inhibitors approved for treatment of HIT. Lepirudin has a half-life of 1.3 hours, is excreted by the kidneys, and can be monitored using the aPTT. An initial IV bolus infusion followed by a continuous infusion with subsequent adjustments to maintain the aPTT between 1.5 and 2.5 times baseline has been recommended. Strict dosage adjustment in renal failure is required, because the clearance of lepirudin is proportional to the patient's creatinine clearance. Argatroban has a half-life of 30 to 45 minutes, is metabolized by the liver, and is unaffected by renal function. The anticoagulant effect of argatroban is predictable, with low variability between patients, but it is dose-dependent and requires monitoring with either the aPTT or ACT.

There is no safe, rapidly acting antidote if the patient develops bleeding complications from direct thrombin inhibitors. Recombinant factor VIIa may reverse the anticoagulant effects, but it may not be available in all hospitals, and it is very expensive. The safety profile of the direct thrombin inhibitors is not known in patients with cancer or in women who are pregnant (Weitz, 2004).

DRUG INTERACTIONS

Because oral anticoagulants interact with many other medications and herbal and nutritional supplements, close monitoring of the patient's medication schedule is necessary. Many medications and supplements potentiate or inhibit oral anticoagulants; it is always wise to check to see if any medications or supplements are contraindicated with warfarin (see Chapter 33, Chart 33-15). Contraindications to anticoagulant therapy are summarized in Chart 31-8.

Providing Comfort

Bed rest, elevation of the affected extremity, elastic compression stockings, and analgesics for pain relief are adjuncts to therapy. They help improve circulation and increase comfort. Depending on the extent and location of a venous thrombosis, bed rest may be required for 5 to 7 days after diagnosis. This is approximately the time necessary for the thrombus to adhere to the vein wall, preventing embolization.

Warm, moist packs applied to the affected extremity reduce the discomfort associated with DVT, as do mild analgesics prescribed for pain control. When the patient begins to ambulate, elastic compression stockings are used. Walking is better than standing or sitting for long periods. Bed exercises, such as repetitive dorsiflexion of the foot, are also recommended.

Compression Therapy

STOCKINGS

Elastic compression stockings usually are prescribed for patients with venous insufficiency. These stockings exert a sustained, evenly distributed pressure over the entire surface of the calves, reducing the caliber of the superficial veins in the legs and resulting in increased flow in the deeper veins. The stockings may be knee-high, thigh-high, or panty hose. Thigh-high stockings are difficult for the patient to wear because they tend to roll down. The roll of the stocking further restricts blood flow rather than providing evenly distributed pressure over the thigh.

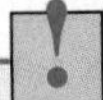

NURSING ALERT

Any type of stocking, including the elastic type, can inadvertently become a tourniquet if applied incorrectly (ie, rolled tightly at the top). In such instances, the stockings produce stasis rather than prevent it. For ambulatory patients, elastic compression stockings are removed at night and reapplied before the legs are lowered from the bed to the floor in the morning.

When the stockings are off, the skin is inspected for signs of irritation, and the calves are examined for tenderness. Any skin changes or signs of tenderness are reported. Stockings are contraindicated in patients with severe pitting edema because they can produce severe pitting at the knee.

Gerontologic Considerations. Because of decreased strength and manual dexterity, elderly patients may be unable to apply elastic compression stockings properly. If this is the case, a family member or friend should be taught to assist the patient to apply the stockings so that they do not cause undue pressure on any part of the feet or legs.

WRAPS

Short stretch elastic wraps may be applied from the toes to the knee in a 50% spiral overlap. These wraps are available in a two-layer system, which includes an inner layer of soft padding. These wraps are rectangular and become squares on stretching, indicating the appropriate degree of stretch and reducing the possibility of wrapping a leg too loosely or too tightly. Three- and four-layer systems are also available (Profore, Dynacare), but these may be used only once compared to the two-wrap system, which can be used multiple times.

Other types of compression are available. The Unna boot, which consists of a paste bandage impregnated with zinc oxide, glycerin, gelatin, and sometimes calamine, is applied without tension in a circular fashion from the base of the toes to the tibial tuberosity with a 50% spiral overlap. It is important to keep the foot dorsiflexed at a 90-degree angle to the leg, thus avoiding excess pressure or trauma to the anterior ankle area. This type of compression may remain in place for as long as 1 week. The CirCaid, a nonelastic leg wrap with a series of overlapping, interlocking Velcro straps, augments the effect of the muscle pump while the patient is walking. The CirCaid is usually worn during the day. Patients may find the CirCaid easier to apply and wear than the Unna boot.

INTERMITTENT PNEUMATIC COMPRESSION DEVICES

These devices can be used with elastic compression stockings to prevent DVT. They consist of an electric controller that is attached by air hoses to plastic knee-high or thigh-high sleeves. The leg sleeves are divided into compartments,

NURSING RESEARCH PROFILE

What is the Evidence for Choosing Either Below-Knee or Thigh-Length Graduated Compression Stockings to Prevent DVT?

Byrne, B. (2002). Deep vein thrombosis prophylaxis: The effectiveness and implications of using below-knee or thigh-length graduated compression stockings. *Journal of Vascular Nursing, 20*(2), 53–59.

Purpose

Patients with DVTs have an increased incidence of recurrent DVTs as well as chronic limb ischemia, venous insufficiency, and ulceration. Ambulation is well known as an effective way to prevent DVT, but for those who cannot walk, graduated compression stockings reduce the incidence of DVT. Thigh-length and below-knee graduated compression stockings are the lengths most commonly used in clinical practice. Thigh-length graduated compression stockings tend to be associated with less patient comfort and compliance, cost more, and are more difficult to apply. This review examined published research-based evidence for choosing one length of graduated compression stocking over the other in terms of DVT prophylaxis. In addition, it examined nursing implications of stocking length.

Design

A literature review was conducted using Medline, Cumulative Index to Nursing and Allied Health Literature (CINAHL), School of Health and Related Research, and the Cochrane Library databases with English and human subject restrictions. Thirty-two of 428 research articles were identified that studied graduated compression stockings in the prevention of DVT. Of these articles, only 10 specifically studied the benefits of the lengths of the stockings in DVT prophylaxis.

In addition to these methods, telephone interviews of nurse managers, clinical nurse teachers, or charge nurses employed in the intensive care units of 10 tertiary care hospitals in Victoria, Australia, were conducted to determine whether graduated compression stockings were routinely used in these units, and if so, to identify the preferred length of stockings used in these units and the rationale for the length chosen. Furthermore, two companies that produce graduated compression stockings in Australia were contacted and asked to provide the literature-based evidence that they used when making purchase recommendations.

Findings

Nine out of the 10 selected research articles reported that there was no difference in overall efficacy between below-knee and thigh-length stockings in preventing DVTs. These research studies used small samples that represented groups with specific diagnoses. Thus, findings from these studies were limited in terms of their generalizability.

Findings yielded from interviewing the nurses revealed that 5 of the 10 hospitals routinely used graduated compression stockings. When these facilities used the stockings (routinely or otherwise), 4 used thigh-length, 5 used below-knee, and 1 never used them. None of the nurses interviewed was able to refer to evidence on which their units' practices were based.

The two companies that manufactured graduated compression stockings provided either outdated references (eg, 25 years old) to support the use of their products or references already identified via the literature search independently conducted by this study's author.

Nursing Implications

Nursing care of patients determined to be "at risk" for DVT should include prevention, which includes wearing graduated compression stockings. The evidence in the literature to date suggests that below-knee stockings and thigh-length stockings are equally effective in DVT prophylaxis. Although more studies are needed to draw generalizable conclusions, it seems prudent to recommend that below-knee graduated compression stockings should be included in nursing DVT prophylaxis manuals as the standard of care, because they are easier to apply, more tolerable, and less costly than thigh-length graduated compression stockings.

which sequentially fill to apply pressure to the ankle, calf, and thigh at 35 to 55 mm Hg of pressure. These devices can increase blood velocity beyond that produced by the stockings. Nursing measures include ensuring that prescribed pressures are not exceeded and assessing for patient comfort.

Positioning the Body and Encouraging Exercise

When the patient is on bed rest, the feet and lower legs should be elevated periodically above the level of the heart. This position allows the superficial and tibial veins to empty rapidly and to remain collapsed. Active and passive leg exercises, particularly those involving calf muscles, should be performed to increase venous flow. Early ambulation is most effective in preventing venous stasis. Deep-breathing exercises are beneficial because they produce increased negative pressure in the thorax, which assists in emptying the large veins. Once ambulatory, the patient is instructed to avoid sitting for more than 2 hours at a time. The goal is to walk at least 10 minutes every 1 to 2 hours. The patient is also instructed to perform active and passive leg exercises as frequently as necessary when he or she cannot ambulate, such as during long car, train, and plane trips.

Promoting Home and Community-Based Care

In addition to teaching the patient how to apply elastic compression stockings and explaining the importance of elevating the legs and exercising adequately, the nurse teaches about the medication, its purpose, and the need to take the correct amount at the specific times prescribed (Chart 31-9). The patient should also be aware that periodic blood tests are necessary to determine if a change in medication or dosage is required. If the patient fails to adhere to the therapeutic regimen, continuation of the medication therapy should be questioned. A person who refuses to discontinue the use of alcohol should not receive anticoagulants because chronic alcohol use decreases their effectiveness. In patients with liver disease, the potential for bleeding may be exacerbated by anticoagulant therapy.

Chronic Venous Insufficiency

Venous insufficiency results from obstruction of the venous valves in the legs or a reflux of blood through the valves. Superficial and deep leg veins can be involved. Resultant venous hypertension can occur whenever there has been a prolonged increase in venous pressure, such as occurs with DVT. Because the walls of veins are thinner and more elastic than the walls of arteries, they distend readily when venous pressure is consistently elevated. In this state, leaflets of the venous valves are stretched and prevented from closing completely, allowing a backflow or reflux of blood in the veins. Duplex ultrasonography confirms the obstruction and identifies the level of valvular incompetence.

Clinical Manifestations

When the valves in the deep veins become incompetent after a thrombus has formed, postthrombotic syndrome may develop (Fig. 31-16). This disorder is characterized by chronic venous stasis, resulting in edema, altered pigmentation, pain, and stasis dermatitis. The patient may notice the symptoms less in the morning and more in the evening. Obstruction or poor calf muscle pumping in addition to valvular reflux must be present for the development of severe postthrombotic syndrome and stasis ulcers. Superficial veins may be dilated. The disorder is longstanding, difficult to treat, and often disabling.

Stasis ulcers develop as a result of the rupture of small skin veins and subsequent ulcerations. When these vessels rupture, red blood cells escape into surrounding tissues and then degenerate, leaving a brownish discoloration of the tissues. The pigmentation and ulcerations usually occur in the lower part of the extremity, in the area of the medial malleolus of the ankle. The skin becomes dry, cracks, and itches; subcutaneous tissues fibrose and atrophy. The risk for injury and infection of the extremities is increased.

CHART 31-9

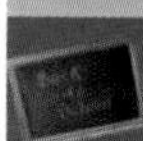

Patient Education

Taking Anticoagulant Medications

- Take the anticoagulant at the same time each day, usually between 8:00 and 9:00 am.
- Wear or carry identification indicating the anticoagulant being taken.
- Keep all appointments for blood tests.
- Because other medications affect the action of the anticoagulant, do not take any of the following medications or supplements without consulting with the primary health care provider: vitamins, cold medicines, antibiotics, aspirin, mineral oil, and anti-inflammatory agents, such as ibuprofen (Motrin) and similar medications or herbal or nutritional supplements. The primary health care provider should be contacted before taking any over-the-counter drugs.
- Avoid alcohol, because it may change the body's response to an anticoagulant.
- Avoid food fads, crash diets, or marked changes in eating habits.
- Do not take warfarin (Coumadin) unless directed.
- Do not stop taking Coumadin (when prescribed) unless directed.
- When seeking treatment from physician, a dentist, a podiatrist, or another health care provider, be sure to inform the caregiver that you are taking an anticoagulant.
- Contact your primary health care provider before having dental work or elective surgery.
- If any of the following signs appear, report them immediately to the primary health care provider:
  - Faintness, dizziness, or increased weakness
  - Severe headaches or abdominal pain
  - Reddish or brownish urine
  - Any bleeding—for example, cuts that do not stop bleeding
  - Bruises that enlarge, nosebleeds, or unusual bleeding from any part of the body
  - Red or black bowel movements
  - Rash
- Avoid injury that can cause bleeding.
- For women: Notify the primary health care provider if you suspect pregnancy.

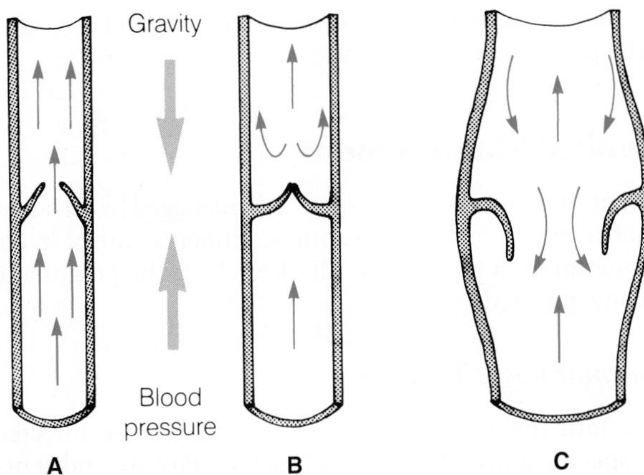

FIGURE 31-16. Competent valves showing blood flow patterns when the valve is open (A) and closed (B), allowing blood to flow against gravity. (C) With faulty or incompetent valves, the blood cannot move toward the heart.

Complications

Venous ulceration is the most serious complication of chronic venous insufficiency and can be associated with other conditions affecting the circulation of the lower extremities. Cellulitis or dermatitis may complicate the care of chronic venous insufficiency and venous ulcerations.

Management

Management of the patient with venous insufficiency is directed at reducing venous stasis and preventing ulcerations. Measures that increase venous blood flow are antigravity activities, such as elevating the leg, and compression of superficial veins with elastic compression stockings.

Elevating the legs decreases edema, promotes venous return, and provides symptomatic relief. The legs should be elevated frequently throughout the day (at least 15 to 30 minutes every 2 hours). At night, the patient should sleep with the foot of the bed elevated about 15 cm (6 inches). Prolonged sitting or standing in one position is detrimental; walking should be encouraged. When sitting, the patient should avoid placing pressure on the popliteal spaces, as occurs when crossing the legs or sitting with the legs dangling over the side of the bed. Constricting garments such as panty girdles or socks that are too tight at the top or that leave marks on the skin should be avoided.

Compression of the legs with elastic compression stockings reduces the pooling of venous blood and enhances venous return to the heart. Elastic compression stockings are recommended for people with venous insufficiency. The stocking should fit so that pressure is greater at the foot and ankle and then gradually declines to a lesser pressure at the knee or groin. If the top of the stocking is too tight or becomes twisted, a tourniquet effect is created, which worsens venous pooling. Stockings should be applied after the legs have been elevated for a period, when the amount of blood in the leg veins is at its lowest.

Extremities with venous insufficiency must be carefully protected from trauma; the skin is kept clean, dry, and soft. Signs of ulceration are immediately reported to the health care provider for treatment and follow-up.

Leg Ulcers

A leg ulcer is an excavation of the skin surface that occurs when inflamed necrotic tissue sloughs off. About 75% of all leg ulcers result from chronic venous insufficiency. Lesions due to arterial insufficiency account for approximately 20%; the remaining 5% are caused by burns, sickle cell anemia, and other factors (Gloviczki & Yao, 2001).

Pathophysiology

Inadequate exchange of oxygen and other nutrients in the tissue is the metabolic abnormality that underlies the development of leg ulcers. When cellular metabolism cannot maintain energy balance, cell death (necrosis) results. Alterations in blood vessels at the arterial, capillary, and venous levels may affect cellular processes and lead to the formation of ulcers.

Clinical Manifestations

The characteristics of leg ulcers are determined by the cause of the ulcer. Most ulcers, especially in elderly patients, have more than one cause. The symptoms depend on whether the problem is arterial or venous in origin (see Table 31-1). The severity of the symptoms depends on the extent and duration of the vascular insufficiency. The ulcer itself appears as an open, inflamed sore. The area may be draining or covered by eschar (dark, hard crust).

Arterial Ulcers

Chronic arterial disease is characterized by intermittent claudication, which is pain caused by activity and relieved after a few minutes of rest. The patient may also complain of digital or forefoot pain at rest. If the onset of arterial occlusion is acute, ischemic pain is unrelenting and rarely relieved even with opioid analgesics. Typically, arterial ulcers are small, circular, deep ulcerations on the tips of toes or in the web spaces between the toes. Ulcers often occur on the medial side of the hallux or lateral fifth toe and may be caused by a combination of ischemia and pressure (Fig. 31-17).

Arterial insufficiency may result in gangrene of the toe (digital gangrene), which usually is caused by trauma. The toe is stubbed and then turns black (see Fig. 31-17). Usually, patients with this problem are elderly people without adequate circulation to provide revascularization. Débridement is contraindicated in these instances. Although the toe is gangrenous, it is dry. Managing dry gangrene is preferable to débriding the toe and causing an open wound that will not heal because of insufficient circulation. If the toe were to be amputated, the lack of adequate circulation would prevent healing and might make further amputation necessary—a below-knee or an above-knee amputation. A higher-level amputation in an elderly person could result in a loss of independence and possibly the need for institutional care. Dry gangrene of the toe in an elderly person with poor cir-

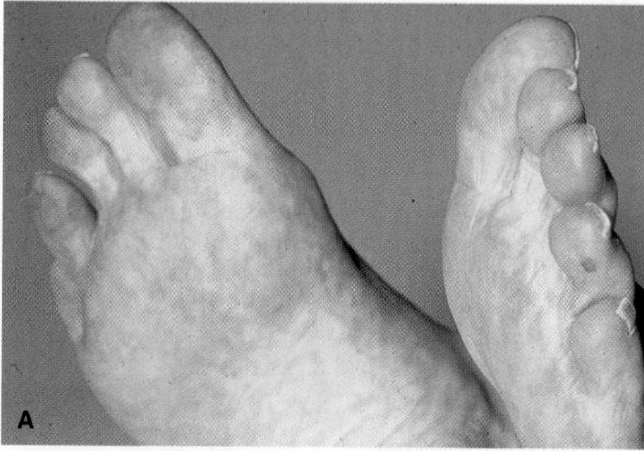

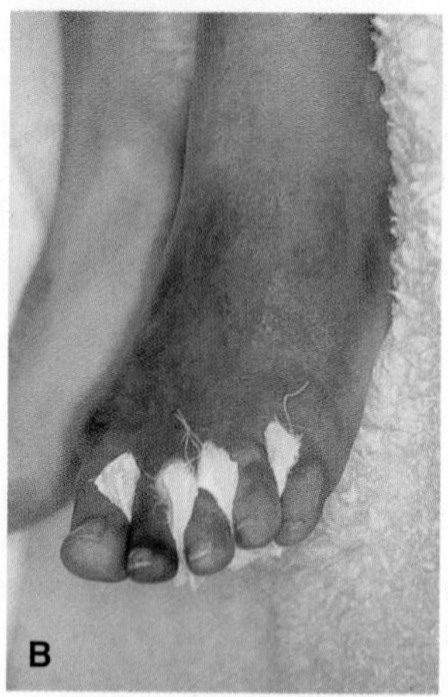

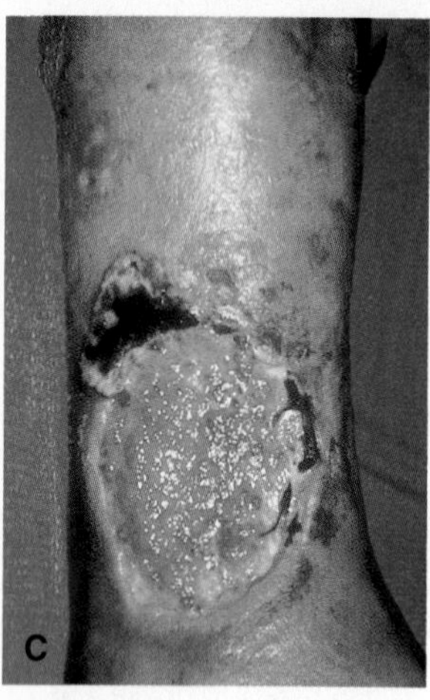

FIGURE 31-17. (**A**) Ulcers resulting from arterial emboli. (**B**) Gangrene of the toes resulting from severe arterial ischemia. (**C**) Ulcer from venous stasis.

culation is usually left undisturbed. The nurse keeps the toe clean and dry until it separates (without creating an open wound).

Venous Ulcers

Chronic venous insufficiency is characterized by pain described as aching or heaviness. The foot and ankle may be edematous. Ulcerations are in the area of the medial or lateral malleolus (gaiter area) and are typically large, superficial, and highly exudative. Venous hypertension causes extravasation of blood, which discolors the area (see Fig. 31-17). Patients with neuropathy frequently have ulcerations on the side of the foot over the metatarsal heads. These ulcers are painless and are described in further detail in Chapter 41.

Assessment and Diagnostic Findings

Because ulcers have many causes, the cause of each ulcer needs to be identified so appropriate therapy can be prescribed. The history of the condition is important in determining venous or arterial insufficiency. The pulses of the lower extremities (femoral, popliteal, posterior tibial, and dorsalis pedis) are carefully examined. More conclusive diagnostic aids are Doppler and duplex ultrasound studies, arteriography, and venography. Cultures of the ulcer bed may be necessary to determine whether an infecting agent is the primary cause of the ulcer.

Medical Management

Patients with ulcers can be effectively managed by advanced practice nurses or wound-ostomy-continence nurses in collaboration with physicians. All ulcers have the potential to become infected.

Pharmacologic Therapy

Antibiotic therapy is prescribed when the ulcer is infected; the specific antibiotic agent is based on culture and sensitivity test results. Oral antibiotics usually are prescribed because topical antibiotics have not proven to be effective for leg ulcers.

Compression Therapy

Adequate compression therapy involves the application of external or counter pressure to the lower extremity to facilitate venous return to the heart. The pressure should be applied in a gradient or graduated fashion with the pressure being somewhat higher at the ankle. One form is the compression stocking; some of these are custom-made to the patient's anatomic specifications. The patient should be instructed to wear the stockings at all times except at night and to reapply the stockings in the morning before getting out of bed. Short stretch elastic wraps, Unna boots, and CirCaids may be other effective options. (See previous section on Compression Therapy.)

Débridement

To promote healing, the wound is kept clean of drainage and necrotic tissue. The usual method is to flush the area with normal saline solution or clean it with a noncytotoxic wound-cleansing agent (Saf-Clens, Biolex, Restore). If this is unsuccessful, débridement may be necessary. Débridement is the removal of nonviable tissue from wounds. Removing the dead tissue is important, particularly in instances of infection. Débridement can be accomplished by several different methods:

- Surgical débridement is the fastest method and can be performed by a physician, skilled advanced practice nurse, or wound-ostomy-continence nurse in collaboration with the physician.
- Nonselective débridement can be accomplished by applying isotonic saline dressings of fine-mesh gauze to the ulcer. When the dressing dries, it is removed (dry), along with the debris adhering to the gauze. Pain management is usually necessary.
- Enzymatic débridement with the application of enzyme ointments may be prescribed to treat the ulcer. The ointment is applied to the lesion but not to normal surrounding skin. Most enzymatic ointments are covered with saline-soaked gauze that has been thoroughly wrung out. A dry gauze dressing and a loose bandage are then applied. The enzymatic ointment is discontinued when the necrotic tissue has been débrided, and an appropriate wound dressing is applied.

- Calcium alginate dressings (Kaltostat, Sorbsan, Aquacel Hydrofiber) may be used for débridement when absorption of exudate is needed. These dressings are changed when the exudate seeps through the cover dressing or at least every 7 days. The dressing can also be used on areas that are bleeding, because the material helps stop the bleeding. As the dry fibers absorb exudate, they become a gel that is painlessly removed from the ulcer bed. Calcium alginate dressings should not be used on dry or nonexudative wounds.

Topical Therapy

A variety of topical agents can be used in conjunction with cleansing and débridement therapies to promote healing of leg ulcers. The goals of treatment are to remove devitalized tissue and to keep the ulcer clean and moist while healing takes place. The treatment should not destroy developing tissue. For topical treatments to be successful, adequate nutritional therapy must be maintained.

Wound Dressing

After the circulatory status has been assessed and determined to be adequate for healing (ABI of more than 0.5), surgical dressings can be used to promote a moist environment. The simplest method is to use a wound contact material next to the wound bed and cover it with gauze. Other available options that promote the growth of granulation tissue and re-epithelialization include the hydrocolloids (eg, Comfeel, DuoDerm CGF, Restore, Tegasorb). These materials also provide a barrier for protection because they adhere to the wound bed and surrounding tissue. However, these dressings may not be effective treatment for deep wounds and infected wounds.

Knowledge deficit, frustration, fear, and depression can result in the patient's and family's decreased compliance with the prescribed therapy; therefore, patient and family education is necessary before beginning and throughout the wound care program.

Stimulated Healing

Tissue-engineered human skin equivalent (Apligraf [Graftskin]) is a skin product cultured from human dermal fibroblasts and keratinocytes used in combination with therapeutic compression. When applied, it seems to react to factors in the wound and may interact with the patient's cells to stimulate the production of growth factors. Application is not difficult, no suturing is involved, and the procedure is painless.

Hyperbaric Oxygenation

Hyperbaric oxygenation (HBO) may be beneficial as an adjunct treatment in patients with diabetes who evidence no signs of wound healing after 30 days of standard wound treatment. HBO is accomplished by placing the patient into a chamber that increases barometric pressure while the patient is breathing 100% oxygen. The process by which HBO is thought to work involves several factors. The edema in the wound area is decreased because high oxygen tension facilitates vasoconstriction and enhances the ability of leukocytes to phagocytize and kill bacteria. In addition, HBO is thought to increase diffusion of oxygen to the hypoxic wound, thereby enhancing epithelial migration and improving collagen production. The two most common adverse effects of HBO are middle ear barotrauma and confinement anxiety (Broussard, 2004).

Nursing Process

The Patient With Leg Ulcers

Assessment

A careful nursing history and assessment of symptoms are important. The extent and type of pain are carefully assessed, as are the appearance and temperature of the skin of both legs. The quality of all peripheral pulses is assessed, and the pulses in both legs are compared. The legs are checked for edema. If the extremity is edematous, the degree of edema is determined. Any limitation of mobility and activity that results from vascular insufficiency is identified. The patient's nutritional status is assessed, and a history of diabetes, collagen disease, or varicose veins is obtained.

Diagnosis

Nursing Diagnoses

Based on the assessment data, major nursing diagnoses for the patient may include:

- Impaired skin integrity related to vascular insufficiency
- Impaired physical mobility related to activity restrictions of the therapeutic regimen and pain
- Imbalanced nutrition: less than body requirements, related to increased need for nutrients that promote wound healing

Collaborative Problems/ Potential Complications

Based on the assessment data, potential complications that may develop include:

- Infection
- Gangrene

Planning and Goals

The major goals for the patient may include restoration of skin integrity, improved physical mobility, adequate nutrition, and absence of complications.

Nursing Interventions

The nursing challenge in caring for these patients is great, whether the patient is in the hospital, in a long-term care facility, or at home. The physical problem is often a long-term and disabling one that causes a substantial drain on the patient's physical, emotional, and economic resources.

Restoring Skin Integrity

To promote wound healing, measures are used to keep the area clean. Cleansing requires very gentle handling, a mild soap, and lukewarm water. Positioning of the legs depends on whether the ulcer is of arterial or venous origin. If there is arterial insufficiency, the patient should be referred to be evaluated for vascular reconstruction. If there is venous insufficiency, dependent edema can be avoided by elevating the lower extremities. A decrease in edema promotes the exchange of cellular nutrients and waste products in the area of the ulcer, promoting healing.

Avoiding trauma to the lower extremities is imperative in promoting skin integrity. Protective boots may be used (eg, Rooke Vascular boot); they are soft and provide warmth and protection from injury and displace tissue pressure to prevent ulcer formation. If the patient is on bed rest, it is important to relieve pressure on the heels to prevent pressure ulcerations. When the patient is in bed, a bed cradle can be used to relieve pressure from bed linens and to prevent anything from touching the legs. When the patient is ambulatory, all obstacles are moved from the patient's path so that the patient's legs will not be bumped. Heating pads, hot water bottles, or hot baths are avoided, because they increase the oxygen demands and thus the blood flow demands of the already compromised tissue. The patient with diabetes mellitus suffers from neuropathy with decreased sensation, and heating pads may produce injury before the patient is aware of being burned.

Improving Physical Mobility

Generally, physical activity is initially restricted to promote healing. When infection resolves and healing begins, ambulation should resume gradually and progressively. Activity promotes arterial flow and venous return and is encouraged after the acute phase of the ulcer process. Until full activity is resumed, the patient is encouraged to move about when in bed, to turn from side to side frequently, and to exercise the upper extremities to maintain muscle tone and strength. Meanwhile, diversional activities are encouraged. Consultation with an occupational therapist may be helpful if prolonged immobility and inactivity are anticipated.

If pain limits the patient's activity, analgesics may be prescribed by the physician. The pain of peripheral vascular disease is typically chronic and often disabling. Analgesics may be taken before scheduled activities to help the patient participate more comfortably.

Promoting Adequate Nutrition

Nutritional deficiencies are common, requiring dietary alterations to remedy deficiencies. A diet that is high in protein, vitamins C and A, iron, and zinc is encouraged to promote healing. Many patients with peripheral vascular disease are elderly. Particular consideration should be given to their iron intake, because many elderly people are anemic. After a dietary plan has been developed that meets the patient's nutritional needs and promotes healing, diet instruction is provided to the patient and family.

Promoting Home and Community-Based Care

The self-care program is planned with the patient so that activities that promote arterial and venous circulation, relieve pain, and promote tissue integrity are encouraged. Reasons for each aspect of the program are explained to the patient and family. Leg ulcers are often chronic and difficult to heal; they frequently recur, even when the patient rigorously follows the plan of care. Long-term care of the feet and legs to promote healing of wounds and prevent recurrence of ulcerations is the primary goal. Leg ulcers increase the patient's risk of infection, may be painful, and may limit mobility, necessitating lifestyle changes. Participation of family members and home health care providers may be necessary for treatments such as dressing changes, reassessments, reinforcement of instruction, and evaluation of the effectiveness of the plan of care. Regular follow-up with a primary health care provider is necessary.

Evaluation

Expected Patient Outcomes

Expected patient outcomes may include:

1. Demonstrates restored skin integrity
   a. Exhibits absence of inflammation
   b. Exhibits absence of drainage; negative wound culture
   c. Avoids trauma to the legs
2. Increases physical mobility
   a. Progresses gradually to optimal level of activity
   b. Reports that pain does not impede activity
3. Attains adequate nutrition
   a. Selects foods high in protein, vitamins, iron, and zinc
   b. Discusses with family members dietary modifications that need to be made at home
   c. Plans, with the family, a diet that is nutritionally sound

Varicose Veins

Varicose veins (varicosities) are abnormally dilated, tortuous, superficial veins caused by incompetent venous valves (see Fig. 31-16). Most commonly, this condition occurs in the lower extremities, the saphenous veins, or the lower trunk, but it can occur elsewhere in the body, such as the esophagus (eg, esophageal varices; see Chapter 39).

It is estimated that varicose veins occur in up to 60% of the adult population in the United States, with an increased incidence correlated with increased age (Johnson, 1997). The condition is most common in women and in people whose occupations require prolonged standing, such as salespeople, hair stylists, teachers, nurses and ancillary medical personnel, and construction workers. A hereditary weakness of the vein wall may contribute to the development of varicosities, and it commonly occurs in several members of the same family. Varicose veins are rare before puberty. Pregnancy may cause varicosities because of hormonal effects related to distensibility, increased pressure by the gravid uterus, and increased blood volume (Johnson, 1997).

Pathophysiology

Varicose veins may be primary (without involvement of deep veins) or secondary (resulting from obstruction of deep veins). A reflux of venous blood in the veins results in venous stasis. If only the superficial veins are affected, the person may have no symptoms but may be troubled by their appearance.

Clinical Manifestations

Symptoms, if present, may include dull aches, muscle cramps, increased muscle fatigue in the lower legs, ankle edema, and a feeling of heaviness of the legs. Nocturnal cramps are common. When deep venous obstruction results in varicose veins, the patient may develop the signs and symptoms of chronic venous insufficiency: edema, pain, pigmentation, and ulcerations. Susceptibility to injury and infection is increased.

Assessment and Diagnostic Findings

Diagnostic tests for varicose veins include the duplex scan, which documents the anatomic site of reflux and provides a quantitative measure of the severity of valvular reflux. Air plethysmography measures the changes in venous blood volume. Venography is not routinely performed to evaluate for valvular reflux. However, when it is used, it involves injecting a radiopaque contrast agent into the leg veins so that the vein anatomy can be visualized by x-ray studies during various leg movements.

Prevention

The patient should avoid activities that cause venous stasis, such as wearing a constricting panty girdle or socks that are too tight at the top or that leave marks on the skin; crossing the legs at the thighs; and sitting or standing for long periods. Changing position frequently, elevating the legs when they are tired, and getting up to walk for several minutes of every hour promote circulation. The patient is encouraged to walk 1 or 2 miles each day if there are no contraindications. Walking up the stairs rather than using the elevator or escalator is helpful, and swimming is good exercise.

Elastic compression stockings, especially knee-high stockings, are useful. The overweight patient should be encouraged to begin a weight-reduction plan.

Medical Management

Ligation and Stripping

Surgery for varicose veins requires that the deep veins be patent and functional. The saphenous vein is ligated and divided. The vein is ligated high in the groin, where the saphenous vein meets the femoral vein. Also, the vein may be removed (stripped). After the vein is ligated, an incision is made 2 to 3 cm below the knee, and a metal or plastic wire is passed the full length of the vein to the point of ligation. The wire is then withdrawn, pulling (removing, stripping) the vein as it is removed. Pressure and elevation minimize bleeding during surgery.

Thermal Ablation

Thermal ablation is a nonsurgical approach using thermal energy. Radiofrequency ablation uses an electrical contact inside the vein. As the device is withdrawn, the vein is sealed. Laser ablation uses a laser fiber tip that seals the vein (decompressed). Topical gel may be used first to numb the skin along the course of the saphenous vein. To protect the surrounding tissue, a series of small punctures are made along the vein, and 100 to 200 mL of dilute lidocaine is delivered to the perivenous space using ultrasound guidance. The goal of this tumescent anesthesia (ie, anesthesia that causes localized swelling) is to provide analgesia, thermal protection (the cuff of fluid surrounds the veins and accompanying nerves), and extrinsic compression of the vein. The saphenous vein is entered percutaneously near the knee using ultrasound guidance. A catheter is introduced into the saphenous vein and advanced to the saphenofemoral junction. The device is then activated and withdrawn, sealing the vein. Small bandages and compression stockings are applied after the procedure. The patient is asked not to remove the stockings for at least 48 hours and then to rewrap the legs and wear the compression stockings while ambulatory for at least 3 weeks. Patients are ambulatory prior to being discharged from the outpatient facility and have no activity restrictions, except that swimming is discouraged for 3 weeks. Nonsteroidal anti-inflammatory drugs such as acetaminophen (Tylenol) or ibuprofen (Motrin) are used as needed for pain. The patient is informed that he or she may bruise along the course of the saphenous vein, may experience leg cramps for a few days, and may find it difficult to straighten the knees for up to 1.5 weeks.

Sclerotherapy

Sclerotherapy involves injection of an irritating chemical into a vein to produce localized phlebitis and fibrosis, thereby obliterating the lumen of the vein. This treatment may be performed alone for small varicosities or may follow vein ablation, ligation, or stripping. Sclerosing is palliative rather than curative. Sclerotherapy is typically performed in an examination or procedure room and does not require any sedation. After the sclerosing agent is injected, elastic compression bandages are applied to the leg and are worn for approximately 5 days after the procedure. Elastic compression stockings are then worn for an additional 5 weeks. After sclerotherapy, walking activities are encouraged as prescribed to maintain blood flow in the leg and to dilute the sclerosing agent.

Nursing Management

Ligation and stripping can be performed in an outpatient setting, or the patient can be admitted to the hospital on the day of surgery and discharged the next day if a bilateral procedure is to be performed and the patient is at high risk for postoperative complications. If the procedure is performed in an outpatient setting, nursing measures are the same as if the patient were hospitalized. Bed rest is discouraged and the patient is encouraged to become ambulatory as soon as sedation has worn off. The patient is instructed to walk every hour for 5 to 10 minutes while awake for the first 24 hours if he or she can tolerate the discomfort, and then to increase walking and activity as tolerated. Elastic compression stockings are worn continuously for about 1 week after vein stripping. The nurse assists the patient to perform exercises and move the legs. The foot of the bed should be elevated. Standing and sitting are discouraged.

Promoting Comfort and Understanding

Analgesics are prescribed to help the patient move the affected extremities more comfortably. Dressings are inspected for bleeding, particularly at the groin, where the risk of bleeding is greatest. The nurse is alert for reported sensations of "pins and needles." Hypersensitivity to touch in the involved extremity may indicate a temporary or permanent nerve injury resulting from surgery, because the saphenous vein and nerve are close to each other in the leg.

Usually, the patient may shower after the first 24 hours. The patient is instructed to dry the incisions well with a clean towel using a patting technique, rather than rubbing. Alternatively, the patient may be instructed to dry the area using a blow-dryer. Application of skin lotion is avoided until the incisions are completely healed to avoid infection. The patient is instructed to apply sunscreen or zinc oxide to the incisional area prior to sun exposure; otherwise, hyperpigmentation of the incision, scarring, or both may occur.

If the patient underwent sclerotherapy, a burning sensation in the injected leg may be experienced for 1 or 2 days. The nurse may encourage the use of a mild analgesic as prescribed and walking to provide relief.

Promoting Home and Community-Based Care

Long-term leg elastic support is essential after discharge, and the patient needs to obtain adequate supplies of elastic compression stockings or bandages. Exercise of the legs is necessary; the development of an individualized plan requires consultation with the patient and the health care team.

Lymphatic Disorders

The lymphatic system consists of a set of vessels that spread throughout most of the body. These vessels start as lymph capillaries that drain unabsorbed plasma from the interstitial spaces (spaces between the cells). The lymphatic capillaries unite to form the lymph vessels, which pass through the lymph nodes and then empty into the large thoracic duct that joins the jugular vein on the left side of the neck.

The fluid drained from the interstitial space by the lymphatic system is called lymph. The flow of lymph depends on the intrinsic contractions of the lymph vessels, the contraction of muscles, respiratory movements, and gravity. The lymphatic system of the abdominal cavity maintains a steady flow of digested fatty food (chyle) from the intestinal mucosa to the thoracic duct. In other parts of the body, the lymphatic system's function is regional; the lymphatic vessels of the head, for example, empty into clusters of lymph nodes located in the neck, and those of the extremities empty into nodes of the axillae and the groin.

Lymphangitis and Lymphadenitis

Lymphangitis is an acute inflammation of the lymphatic channels. It arises most commonly from a focus of infection in an extremity. Usually, the infectious organism is a hemolytic streptococcus. The characteristic red streaks that extend up the arm or the leg from an infected wound outline the course of the lymphatic vessels as they drain.

The lymph nodes located along the course of the lymphatic channels also become enlarged, red, and tender (acute lymphadenitis). They can also become necrotic and form an abscess (suppurative lymphadenitis). The nodes involved most often are those in the groin, axilla, or cervical region.

Because these infections are nearly always caused by organisms that are sensitive to antibiotics, it is unusual to see abscess formation. Recurrent episodes of lymphangitis are often associated with progressive lymphedema. After acute attacks, an elastic compression stocking or sleeve should be worn on the affected extremity for several months to prevent long-term edema.

Lymphedema and Elephantiasis

Lymphedemas are classified as primary (congenital malformations) or secondary (acquired obstructions). Tissue swelling occurs in the extremities because of an increased quantity of lymph that results from obstruction of lymphatic vessels. It is especially marked when the extremity is in a dependent position. Initially, the edema is soft and pitting. As the condition progresses, the edema becomes firm, nonpitting, and unresponsive to treatment. The most common type is congenital lymphedema (lymphedema praecox), which is caused by hypoplasia of the lymphatic system of the lower extremity. This disorder is usually seen in women and first appears between 15 and 25 years of age.

The obstruction may be in the lymph nodes and the lymphatic vessels. Sometimes, it is seen in the arm after an axillary node dissection (eg, for breast cancer) and in the leg in association with varicose veins or chronic thrombophlebitis. In the latter case, the lymphatic obstruction usually is caused by chronic lymphangitis. Lymphatic obstruction caused by a parasite (filaria) is seen frequently in the tropics. When chronic swelling is present, there may be frequent bouts of acute infection characterized by high fever and chills and increased residual edema after the inflammation has resolved. These lead to chronic fibrosis, thickening of the subcutaneous tissues, and hypertrophy of the skin. This condition, in which chronic swelling of the extremity recedes only slightly with elevation, is referred to as elephantiasis.

Medical Management

The goal of therapy is to reduce and control the edema and prevent infection. Active and passive exercises assist in moving lymphatic fluid into the bloodstream. External compression devices milk the fluid proximally from the foot to the hip or from the hand to the axilla. When the patient is ambulatory, custom-fitted elastic compression stockings or sleeves are worn; those with the highest compression strength (exceeding 40 mm Hg) are required. When the leg is affected, continuous bed rest with the leg elevated may aid in mobilizing the fluids. Manual lymphatic drainage is a highly specialized massage technique designed to direct or shift the congested lymph through functioning lymphatics that have preserved drainage. Manual lymphatic drainage is incorporated in a sequential treatment approach used in combination with compression bandages, exercises, skin care, pressure gradient sleeves, and pneumatic pumps, depending on the severity and stage of the lymphedema (Cheville, McGarvery, Petrek, et al., 2003).

Pharmacologic Therapy

As initial therapy, the diuretic furosemide (Lasix) may be prescribed to prevent fluid overload due to mobilization of extracellular fluid. Diuretics have also been used along with elevation of the leg and the use of elastic compression stockings or sleeves. However, the use of diuretics alone has little benefit, because their main action is to limit capillary filtration by decreasing the circulating blood volume. If lymphangitis or cellulitis is present, antibiotic therapy is initiated. The patient is taught to inspect the skin for evidence of infection.

Surgical Management

Surgery is performed if the edema is severe and uncontrolled by medical therapy, if mobility is severely compromised, or if infection persists. One surgical approach involves the excision of the affected subcutaneous tissue and fascia, with skin grafting to cover the defect. Another procedure involves the surgical relocation of superficial lymphatic vessels into the deep lymphatic system by means of a buried dermal flap to provide a conduit for lymphatic drainage.

Nursing Management

After surgery, the management of skin grafts and flaps is the same as when these therapies are used for other conditions. Antibiotics may be prescribed for 5 to 7 days. Constant elevation of the affected extremity and observation for complications are essential. Complications may include flap necrosis, hematoma or abscess under the flap, and cellulitis. The nurse instructs the patient or caregiver to inspect the dressing daily. Unusual drainage or any inflammation around the wound margin suggests infection and should be reported to the physician. The patient is informed that there may be a loss of sensation in the skin graft area. The patient is also instructed to avoid the application of heating pads or exposure to sun to prevent burns or trauma to the area.

Cellulitis

Cellulitis is the most common infectious cause of limb swelling. Cellulitis can occur as a single isolated event or a series of recurrent events. It is often misdiagnosed, usually as recurrent thrombophlebitis or chronic venous insufficiency.

Pathophysiology

Cellulitis occurs when an entry point through normal skin barriers allows bacteria to enter and release their toxins in the subcutaneous tissues.

Clinical Manifestations

The acute onset of swelling, localized redness, and pain is frequently associated with systemic signs of fever, chills, and sweating. The redness may not be uniform and often skips areas. Regional lymph nodes may also be tender and enlarged.

Medical Management

Mild cases of cellulitis can be treated on an outpatient basis with oral antibiotic therapy. If the cellulitis is severe, the patient is treated with IV antibiotics for at least 7 to 14 days. The key to preventing recurrent episodes of cellulitis lies in adequate antibiotic therapy for the initial event and in identifying the site of bacterial entry. The most commonly overlooked areas are the cracks and fissures that occur in the skin between the toes. Other possible locations are drug use injection sites, contusions, abrasions, ulcerations, ingrown toenails, and hangnails.

Nursing Management

The patient is instructed to elevate the affected area above heart level and apply warm, moist packs to the site every 2 to 4 hours. Patients with sensory and circulatory deficits, such as those caused by diabetes and paralysis, should use caution when applying warm packs because burns may occur; it is advisable to use a thermometer or have a caregiver ensure that the temperature is not more than lukewarm. Education should focus on preventing a recurrent episode. The patient with peripheral vascular disease or diabetes mellitus should receive education or reinforcement about skin and foot care.

Critical Thinking Exercises

1 Your 75-year-old patient has been diagnosed with a stenosis of his external iliac artery and is scheduled for an angiogram with a possible balloon angioplasty and stent placement. What factors would you consider when planning his postprocedure care, continuing care, and home care? If the patient is taking warfarin (Coumadin) for

atrial fibrillation and has renal insufficiency (creatinine of 1.8 mg/dL) as a complication of diabetes, how would you address these factors in the plan of care?

2 Your 96-year-old patient presents with a 2-year history of chronic stasis ulceration of the left lower extremity requiring weekly placement of an Unna boot. The patient lives alone, six blocks from any mass transit or shopping area, and no longer drives a vehicle. The patient wants to continue living at his current location. What options and plan of care would you discuss with the patient?

3 ebp Your patient has been diagnosed with a recurrent DVT of the femoral vein. The patient has been treated previously with unfractionated heparin and developed HIT. What is the strength of the evidence that promotes the efficacy of alternative anticoagulants (eg, pharmacologic agents other than unfractionated heparin) in treating his DVT? Discuss strategies for DVT prophylaxis that you will include in your teaching plan with this patient. What is the strength of the evidence for each of these preventive strategies?

REFERENCES AND SELECTED READINGS

BOOKS

Ascher, E., & Haimovici, H. (2004). *Haimovici's vascular surgery* (5th ed). Malden, MA: Blackwell Publishers.

Bickley, L. S., & Szilagyi, P. G. (2003). *Bates' guide to physical examination and history taking* (8th ed.). Philadelphia: Lippincott Williams & Wilkins.

Coleman, R. W., Hirsch, J., Marder, V. J., et al. (2001). *Hemostasis and thrombosis: Basic principles and clinical practice* (4th ed.). Philadelphia: Lippincott Williams & Wilkins.

Fahey, V. (1999). *Vascular nursing* (3rd ed.). Philadelphia: W. B. Saunders.

Fishman, E. K., & Jeffrey, R. B. (2004). *Multidetector CT—Principles, techniques, and clinical applications.* Philadelphia: Lippincott Williams & Wilkins.

Gloviczki, P., & Yao, J. T. (2001). *Handbook of venous disorders—Guidelines of the American Venous Forum* (2nd ed.). New York: Oxford University Press.

Guyton, A., & Hall, J. (2005). *Textbook of medical physiology* (11th ed.). Philadelphia: Elsevier.

Haaga, J. R., Lanziere, C. F., & Gilkeson, R. C. (2003). *CT and MR imaging of the whole body* (Vol. 1, 4th ed.). St. Louis: Mosby.

Jarvis, C. (2004). *Physical examination and health assessment* (4th ed.). St. Louis: W. B. Saunders.

Lynn-McHale Wiegand, D. J. & Carlson, K. K. (2005). *AACN procedure manual for critical care nurses* (5th ed.). St. Louis: Mosby.

Moore, W. S. (2002). *Vascular surgery: A comprehensive review* (6th ed.). Philadelphia: W. B. Saunders.

Parodi, J. C., Veith, F. J., & Marin, M. (1999). *Endovascular grafting techniques.* Baltimore: Williams & Wilkins.

Porth, C. M. (2005). *Pathophysiology: Concepts of altered health states* (7th ed.). Philadelphia: Lippincott Williams & Wilkins.

Rutherford, R. B. (2005). *Vascular surgery* (6th ed., Vols. I and II). Philadelphia: Elsevier.

Strandness, D. E. (2002). *Duplex scanning in vascular disorders* (3rd ed.). Philadelphia: Lippincott Williams & Wilkins.

White, R. A., & Fogarty, T. J. (1999). *Peripheral endovascular interventions* (2nd ed.). New York: Springer-Verlag.

Yao, J. T., & Pearce, W. H. (1999). *Practical vascular surgery.* Stamford, CT: Appleton & Lange.

JOURNALS

**Asterisk indicates nursing research article.*

Bonham, P. A. (2003). Assessment and management of patients with venous, arterial and diabetic/neurotrophic lower extremity wounds. *AACN Clinical Issues, 14*(4), 442–456.

Brady, A. R., Thompson, S. G., Fowkes, G. R., et al. (2004). Abdominal aortic aneurysm: Expansion risk factors and time intervals for surveillance. *Circulation, 110*(1), 16–21.

Brem, H., Kirsner, R. S., & Falanga, V. (2004). Protocol for the successful treatment of venous ulcers. *American Journal of Surgery, 188*(1), 1–8.

Broussard, C. L. (2004). Hyperbaric oxygenation and wound healing. *Journal of Vascular Nursing, 22*(2), 42–48.

*Byrne, B. (2002). Deep vein thrombosis prophylaxis: The effectiveness and implications of using below-knee or thigh-high graduated compression stockings. *Journal of Vascular Nursing, 20*(2), 53–59.

Caprini, J. A., Glase C. J., Anderson, C. B., et al. (2004). Laboratory markers in the diagnosis of venous thromboembolism. *Circulation, 109*(12) [suppl I]:I-4–I-8.

Cheanvechai, V., Harthum, N. L., Graham, L. M., et al. (2004). Incidence of peripheral vascular disease in women: Is it different from that in men? *Journal of Thoracic and Cardiovascular Surgery, 127*(2), 314–317.

Cheville, A. L., McGarvery, C. L., Petrek, J. A., et al. (2003). Lymphedema management. *Seminars in Radiation Oncology, 13*(3), 290–301.

Chobanian, A. V., Bakris, G. L., Black, H. R., et al. (2003). The seventh report of the Joint National Committee on Prevention, Detection, Evaluation, and Treatment of High Blood Pressure: The JNC 7 report. *Journal of the American Medical Association, 289*(19), 2560–2572.

Cote, M. C., Ligeti, R., Cutler, B. S., et al. (2003). Management of hyperlipidemia in patients with vascular disease. *Journal of Vascular Nursing, 21*(2), 63–67.

Fletcher, R. H., & Fairfield, K. M. (2005). Vitamin supplementation in disease prevention. Available at http://www.UpToDate.com. Accessed January 30, 2006.

Grundy, S. M., Cleeman, C. N., Berz, B., et al. (2004). National Cholesterol Education Program (NCEP) Report: Implications of recent clinical trials for National Cholesterol Education Program Adult Treatment Panel III Guidelines. *Circulation, 110*(2), 227–239.

Gupta, R., & Stouffer, G. A. (2001). Deep venous thrombosis: A review of the pathophysiology, clinical features, and diagnostic modalities. *American Journal of the Medical Sciences, 322*(6), 358–364.

Johnson, M. T. (1997). Treatment and prevention of varicose veins. *Journal of Vascular Nursing, 15*(3), 97–103.

Kohlman-Trigoboff, D. (2003). Hyperhomcysteinemia and vascular disease. *Journal of Vascular Nursing, 21*(1), 30–31.

Kohlman-Trigoboff, D. (2004). Hypertension management in patients with vascular disease. *Journal of Vascular Nursing, 22*(2), 53–56.

Latessa, V. (2002). Endovascular stent-graft repair of descending thoracic aortic aneurysms: The nursing implications of care. *Journal of Vascular Nursing, 20*(2), 86–93.

Markel, A., Meissner, M., Manzo, R. A., et al. (2003). Deep venous thrombosis: Rate of spontaneous lysis and thrombus extension. *International Angiology, 22*(4), 376–382.

Miller, P. L. (2003). Heparin-induced thrombocytopenia—Recognition and treatment. *AORN Journal, 78*(1), 79–89.

Mills, J. L. (2003). Buerger's disease in the 21st century: Diagnosis, clinical features and therapy. *Seminars in Vascular Surgery, 16*(3), 179–189.

Ouriel, K. (2003). Endovascular techniques in the treatment of acute limb ischemia: Thrombolytic agents, trials, and percutaneous mechanical thrombectomy techniques. *Seminars in Vascular Surgery, 16*(4), 270–279.

Rutherford, R. B., & Krupski, W. C. (2004). Current status of open versus endovascular stent-graft repair of abdominal aortic aneurysm. *Journal of Vascular Surgery, 39*(5), 1129–1139.

Selvin, E., & Erlinger, T. P. (2004). Prevalence of and risk factors for peripheral arterial disease in the United States: Results from the National Health and Nutrition Examination Survey, 1999–2000. *Circulation, 110*(6), 738–743.

Stuveling, E. M., Hillege, H. L., Bakker, S. L., et al. (2004). C-reactive protein and microalbuminuria differ in their associations with various domains of vascular disease. *Atherosclerosis, 172*(1), 107–114.

Tran, N. T., & Meissner, M. H. (2002). Epidemiology, pathophysiology and natural history of chronic venous disease. *Seminars in Vascular Surgery, 15*(1), 5–12.

Treat-Jacobson, D., & Walsh, M. E. (2003). Treating patients with peripheral arterial disease and claudication. *Journal of Vascular Nursing, 21*(1), 5–14.

Weitz, J. I. (2004). New anticoagulants for treatment of venous thromboembolism. *Circulation, 110*(9 suppl I), I-19–I-26.

RESOURCES

Agency for Healthcare Research and Quality, 540 Gaither Road, Rockville, MD 20850; 301-427-1364; http://www.ahrq.gov. Accessed May 31, 2006.

American Venous Forum, 900 Cummings Center, #221-U, Beverly, MA 01915; 978-927-8330; http://www.venous-info.com. Accessed May 31, 2006.

National Heart, Lung, and Blood Institute, Health Information Center, P.O. Box 30105, Bethesda, MD 20824-0105; 301-592-8573; http://www.nhlbi.nih.gov. Accessed May 31, 2006.

Society for Vascular Surgery, 633 N. St. Clair, 24th Floor, Chicago, IL 60611; 1-800-258-7188; http://www.vascularweb.org. Accessed May 31, 2006.

Society of Vascular Nursing, 7794 Grow Drive, Pensacola, FL 32514; 888-536-4786; http://www.svnnet.org. Accessed May 31, 2006.

Society of Vascular Ultrasound, 4601 Presidents Drive, Suite 260, Lanham, MD 20706-4831; 1-800-788-8346; http://www.svunet.org. Accessed May 31, 2006.

Vascular Disease Foundation, 3333 S. Wadsworth Boulevard, #B104-37, Lakewood, CO 80227; 1-866-723-4636; http://www.vdf.org. Accessed May 31, 2006.

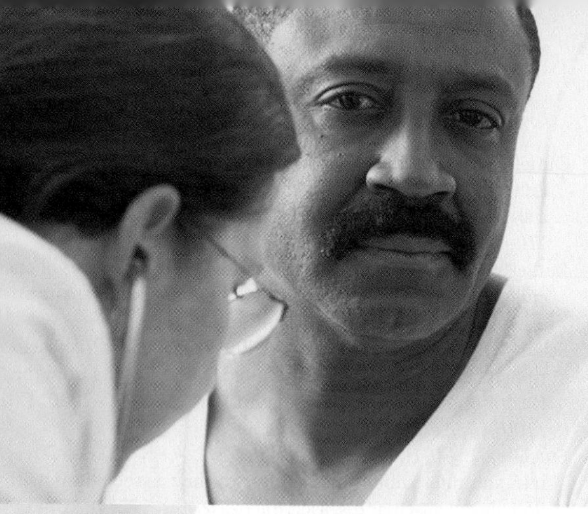

CHAPTER 32

Assessment and Management of Patients With Hypertension

Learning Objectives

On completion of this chapter, the learner will be able to:

1. Define normal blood pressure and categories of abnormal pressures.
2. Identify risk factors for hypertension.
3. Explain the differences between normal blood pressure and hypertension and discuss the significance of hypertension.
4. Describe treatment approaches for hypertension, including lifestyle changes and medication therapy.
5. Use the nursing process as a framework for care of the patient with hypertension.
6. Describe hypertensive crises and their treatment.

Blood pressure is the product of cardiac output multiplied by peripheral resistance. *Cardiac output* is the product of the heart rate multiplied by the stroke volume. In normal circulation, pressure is exerted by the flow of blood through the heart and blood vessels. High blood pressure, known as *hypertension,* can result from a change in cardiac output, a change in peripheral resistance, or both. The medications used for treating hypertension decrease peripheral resistance, blood volume, or the strength and rate of myocardial contraction.

Hypertension is defined by the Seventh Report of the Joint National Committee on Prevention, Detection, Evaluation, and Treatment of High Blood Pressure (JNC 7) as a systolic blood pressure greater than 140 mm Hg and a diastolic pressure greater than 90 mm Hg based on the average of two or more accurate blood pressure measurements taken during two or more contacts with a health care provider (Chobanian, Bakris, Black, et al., 2003). Table 32-1 shows the classification of blood pressure established by JNC 7 in 2003. The categories of blood pressure, from normal to stage 2 hypertension, emphasize the direct relationship between the risk of morbidity and mortality from increasing levels of blood pressure and the specific levels of both the systolic and diastolic blood pressures. The higher either the systolic or diastolic pressure, the greater the health risk (Lewington, Clark, Qizilbash, et al., 2002).

JNC 7 defines a blood pressure of less than 120/80 mm Hg diastolic as normal, 120 to 129/80 to 89 mm Hg as prehypertension, and 140/90 mm Hg or higher as hypertension (see Table 32-1) (Chobanian et al., 2003). The term *stage* is used to define two levels of hypertension so that it is similar to the terms used to describe cancer progression; thus, the public and health care professionals will understand that consistently higher elevations in blood pressure from stage 1 to stage 2 are associated with greater health risks. JNC 7 introduced a new category, *prehypertension,* into the categorization of blood pressure levels to emphasize that people whose blood pressure begins to rise above 120/80 mm Hg are more likely to become hypertensive. To prevent or delay progression to hypertension, JNC 7 urged health care providers to encourage people with blood pressures in the prehypertension category to begin lifestyle modifications such as nutritional changes and exercise. JNC 7 recommended that people with stage 1 hypertension be treated with drugs and be seen by their health care provider about every month until their blood pressure goal is reached and subsequently about every 3 to 6 months. People with stage 2 hypertension or with other complicating conditions need to be seen more frequently.

TABLE 32-1 Classification of Blood Pressure for Adults Age 18 and Older*

BP Classification*	Systolic BP (mm Hg)		Diastolic BP (mm Hg)
Normal	<120	and	<80
Prehypertension	120–139	or	or 80–89
Stage 1 hypertension	140–159	or	90–99
Stage 2 hypertension	≥160	or	≥100

* Based on the average of two or more properly measured, seated readings taken on each of two or more office visits.

From the Seventh Report of the Joint National Committee on Prevention, Detection, Evaluation, and Treatment of High Blood Pressure. (2003). *Hypertension, 42*(6), 1206–1252.

Hypertension

Between 28% and 31% of the adults in the United States have hypertension (Fields, Burt, Cutler, et al., 2004). Of this population, 90% to 95% have **primary hypertension,** high blood pressure from an unidentified cause (Oparil, Zaman, & Calhoun, 2003). The remaining 5% to 10% of this group have **secondary hypertension,** high blood pressure related to identified causes. These causes include narrowing of the renal arteries, renal parenchymal disease, hyperaldosteronism (mineralocorticoid hypertension), certain medications, pregnancy, and coarctation of the aorta (Kaplan, Lieberman, & Neal, 2002).

Glossary

BMI: body mass index, which is calculated by dividing body weight (in kilograms) by height (in meters) squared; a body mass index of greater than 30 is considered to indicate obesity

dyslipidemia: abnormal blood lipid levels, including high total, LDL, and triglyceride levels as well as low HDL levels

GFR: glomerular filtration rate, an indicator of renal function

HDL: high-density lipoprotein

hypertensive emergency: a situation in which blood pressure is severely elevated and there is evidence of actual or probable target organ damage

hypertensive urgency: a situation in which blood pressure is severely elevated but there is no evidence of target organ damage

JNC 7: Seventh Joint National Committee on the Prevention, Detection, Evaluation and Treatment of High Blood Pressure; committee established to study and make recommendations about hypertension in the United States; findings and recommendations of JNC 7 are contained in an extensive report published in 2003

LDL: low-density lipoprotein

monotherapy: medication therapy with a single medication

primary hypertension: also called essential hypertension; denotes high blood pressure from an unidentified cause

rebound hypertension: pressure that is controlled with therapy and that becomes uncontrolled (abnormally high) with the discontinuation of therapy

secondary hypertension: high blood pressure from an identified cause, such as renal disease

Hypertension is sometimes called "the silent killer" because people who have it are often symptom-free. In a national survey conducted from 1999 to 2000, 31% of people who had pressures exceeding 140/90 mm Hg were unaware of their elevated blood pressure (Hajjar & Kotchen, 2003). Once identified, elevated blood pressure should be monitored at regular intervals, because hypertension is a lifelong condition.

Hypertension often accompanies other risk factors for atherosclerotic heart disease, such as **dyslipidemia** (abnormal blood fat levels), obesity, diabetes mellitus, metabolic syndrome, and a sedentary lifestyle. The incidence of hypertension is higher in the southeastern United States, particularly among African Americans (Casper, Barnett, Williams, et al., 2003). Cigarette smoking does not cause high blood pressure; however, if a person with hypertension smokes, his or her risk of dying from heart disease or related disorders increases significantly.

High blood pressure can be viewed in three ways: as a sign, a risk factor for atherosclerotic cardiovascular disease, or a disease. As a sign, nurses and other health care professionals use blood pressure to monitor a patient's clinical status. Elevated pressure may indicate an excessive dose of vasoconstrictive medication or other problems. As a risk factor, hypertension contributes to the rate at which atherosclerotic plaque accumulates within arterial walls. As a disease, hypertension is a major contributor to death from cardiac, renal, and peripheral vascular disease.

Prolonged blood pressure elevation eventually damages blood vessels throughout the body, particularly in target organs such as the heart, kidneys, brain, and eyes. The usual consequences of prolonged, uncontrolled hypertension are myocardial infarction, heart failure, renal failure, strokes, and impaired vision. Hypertrophy (enlargement) of the left ventricle of the heart may occur as it works to pump blood against the elevated pressure. An echocardiogram is the recommended method of determining whether hypertrophy has occurred.

Pathophysiology

CONCEPTS in action ANIMATION

Although no precise cause can be identified for most cases of hypertension, it is understood that hypertension is a multifactorial condition. Because hypertension is a sign, it is most likely to have many causes, just as fever has many causes. For hypertension to occur, there must be a change in one or more factors affecting peripheral resistance or cardiac output (Fig. 32-1). In addition, there must also be a problem with the body's control systems that monitor or regulate pressure. Single gene mutations have been identified for a few rare types of hypertension, but most

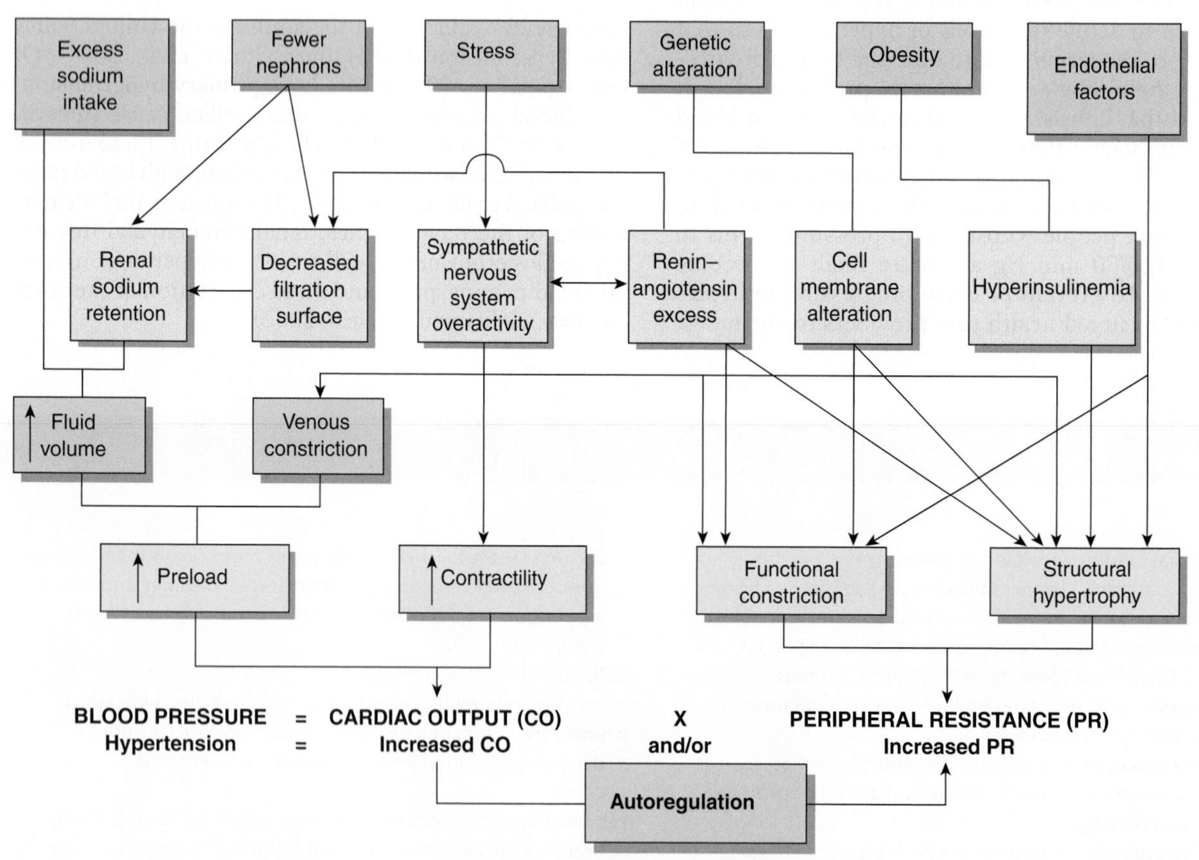

FIGURE 32-1. Factors involved in control of blood pressure. Adapted from Kaplan, N. M., Lieberman, E., & Neal, W. (2002). *Kaplan's clinical hypertension* (8th ed.). Philadelphia: Lippincott Williams & Wilkins.

types of high blood pressure are thought to be polygenic (mutations in more than one gene) (Dominiczak, Negrin, Clark, et al., 2000).

Many factors have been implicated as causes of hypertension:

- Increased sympathetic nervous system activity related to dysfunction of the autonomic nervous system
- Increased renal reabsorption of sodium, chloride, and water related to a genetic variation in the pathways by which the kidneys handle sodium
- Increased activity of the renin-angiotensin-aldosterone system, resulting in expansion of extracellular fluid volume and increased systemic vascular resistance
- Decreased vasodilation of the arterioles related to dysfunction of the vascular endothelium
- Resistance to insulin action, which may be a common factor linking hypertension, type 2 diabetes mellitus, hypertriglyceridemia, obesity, and glucose intolerance

Gerontologic Considerations

Structural and functional changes in the heart and blood vessels contribute to increases in blood pressure that occur with age. These changes include accumulation of atherosclerotic plaque, fragmentation of arterial elastins, increased collagen deposits, and impaired vasodilation. The result of these changes is a decrease in the elasticity of the major blood vessels. Consequently, the aorta and large arteries are less able to accommodate the volume of blood pumped out by the heart (stroke volume), and the energy that would have stretched the vessels instead elevates the systolic blood pressure. Isolated systolic hypertension is more common in older adults and is associated with significant cardiovascular and cerebrovascular morbidity and mortality.

Clinical Manifestations

Physical examination may reveal no abnormalities other than high blood pressure. Occasionally, retinal changes such as hemorrhages, exudates (fluid accumulation), arteriolar narrowing, and cotton-wool spots (small infarctions) occur. In severe hypertension, papilledema (swelling of the optic disc) may be seen. People with hypertension may be asymptomatic and remain so for many years. However, when specific signs and symptoms appear, they usually indicate vascular damage, with specific manifestations related to the organs served by the involved vessels. Coronary artery disease with angina or myocardial infarction is a common consequence of hypertension. Left ventricular hypertrophy occurs in response to the increased workload placed on the ventricle as it contracts against higher systemic pressure. When heart damage is extensive, heart failure follows. Pathologic changes in the kidneys (indicated by increased blood urea nitrogen [BUN] and serum creatinine levels) may manifest as nocturia. Cerebrovascular involvement may lead to a stroke or transient ischemic attack (TIA), manifested by alterations in vision or speech, dizziness, weakness, a sudden fall, or temporary paralysis on one side (hemiplegia). Cerebral infarctions account for most of the strokes and TIAs in patients with hypertension.

Assessment and Diagnostic Evaluation

A thorough health history and physical examination are necessary. The retinas are examined and laboratory studies are performed to assess possible target organ damage. Routine laboratory tests include urinalysis, blood chemistry (ie, analysis of sodium, potassium, creatinine, fasting glucose, and total and high density lipoprotein [**HDL**] cholesterol levels), and a 12-lead electrocardiogram (ECG). Left ventricular hypertrophy can be assessed by echocardiography. Renal damage may be suggested by elevations in BUN and creatinine levels or by microalbuminuria or macroalbuminuria. Additional studies, such as creatinine clearance, renin level, urine tests, and 24-hour urine protein, may be performed.

A risk factor assessment, as advocated by JNC 7, is needed to classify and guide the treatment of hypertensive people at risk for cardiovascular damage. Risk factors and cardiovascular problems related to hypertension are presented in Chart 32-1.

CHART 32-1

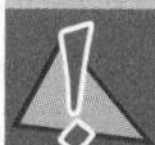

Risk Factors for Cardiovascular Problems in Hypertensive Patients

Major Risk Factors (in Addition to Hypertension)

- Smoking
- Dyslipidemia (elevated **LDL** [or total] cholesterol and/or low HDL cholesterol)*
- Diabetes mellitus*
- Impaired renal function (GFR < 60 mL/min and/or microalbuminuria)
- Obesity (body mass index [**BMI**] ≥ 30 kg/m^2)*
- Physical inactivity
- Age (older than 55 years for men, 65 years for women)
- Family history of cardiovascular disease (in female relative younger than 65 years or male relative younger than 55 years)

Target Organ Damage or Clinical Cardiovascular Disease

- Heart disease (left ventricular hypertrophy, angina or previous myocardial infarction, previous coronary revascularization, heart failure)
- Stroke (cerebrovascular accident, brain attack) or TIA
- Chronic kidney disease
- Peripheral arterial disease
- Retinopathy

* These risk factors plus hypertension, elevated triglyceride levels, and abdominal obesity are components of the metabolic syndrome.

Adapted from Table 6 of the Seventh Report of the Joint National Committee on Prevention, Detection, Evaluation, and Treatment of High Blood Pressure. (2003). *Hypertension, 42*(6), 1206–1252.

Medical Management

The goal of hypertension treatment is to prevent complications and death by achieving and maintaining the arterial blood pressure at 140/90 mm Hg or lower. JNC 7 specifies a lower goal pressure of 130/80 mm Hg for people with diabetes mellitus or chronic kidney disease, which is defined as either a reduced glomerular filtration rate (**GFR**) resulting in a serum creatinine of greater than 1.3 mg per dL in women or greater than 1.5 mg per dL in men, or albuminuria of greater than 300 mg per day (Chobanian et al., 2003). The optimal management plan would be one that is inexpensive and simple and causes the least possible disruption in the patient's life.

The management options for hypertension are summarized in the treatment algorithm issued by JNC 7 (Fig. 32-2). Table 32-2 summarizes recommended lifestyle modifications. The clinician uses the algorithm with the risk factor assessment data and the patient's blood pressure category to choose the initial and subsequent treatment plans for the

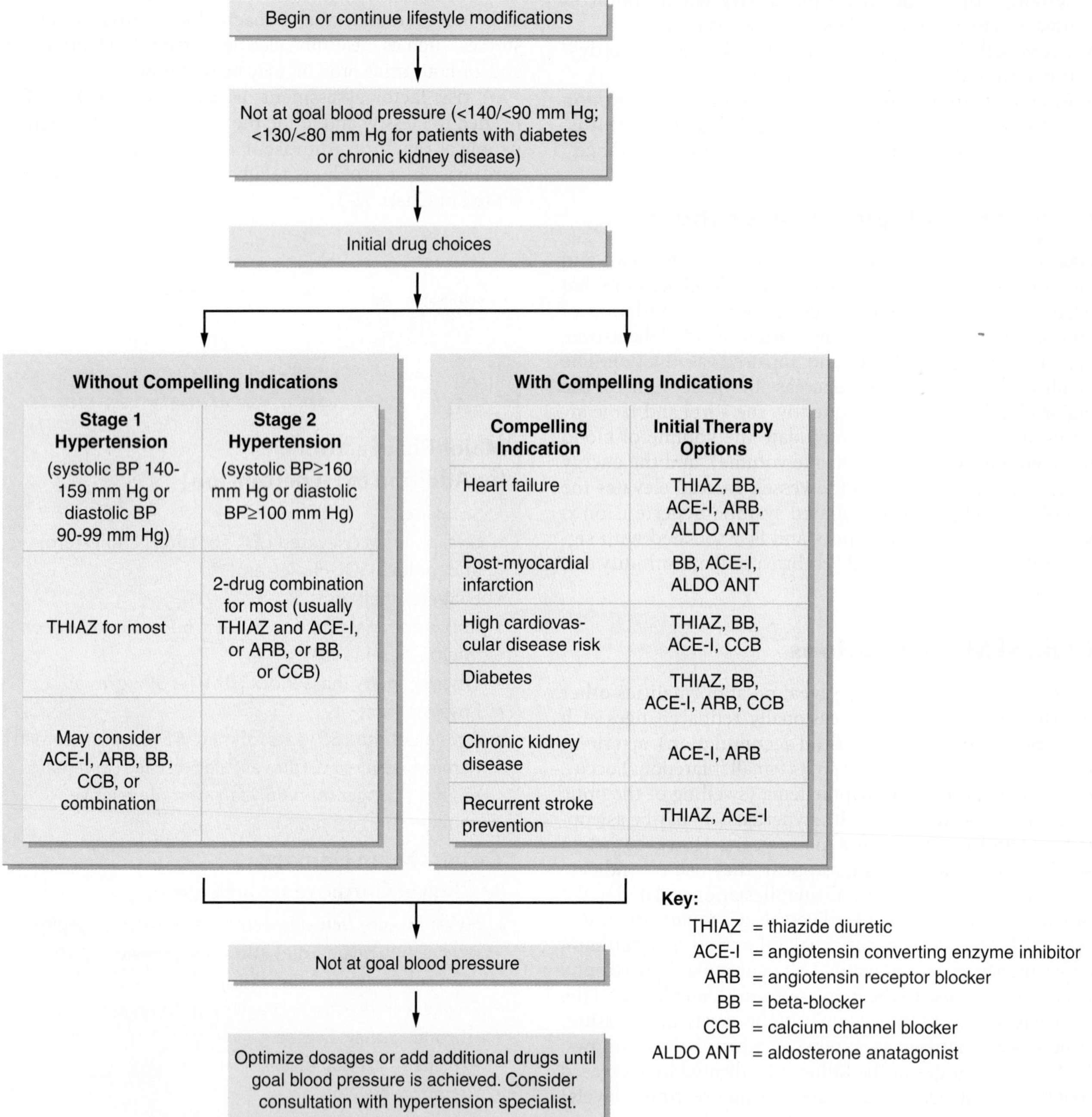

FIGURE 32-2. Algorithm of hypertension treatment. Treatment begins with lifestyle modifications and continues with various medication regimens. From the Seventh Report of the Joint National Committee on Prevention, Detection, Evaluation, and Treatment of High Blood Pressure (JNC 7). Reference card available from the National, Heart, Lung, and Blood Institute (NHLBI), available at http://www.nhlbi.nih.gov.

TABLE 32-2 Lifestyle Modifications To Prevent and Manage Hypertension*

Modification	Recommendation	Goal of SBP† Reduction (Range)‡
Weight reduction	Maintain normal body weight (body mass index 18.5–24.9 kg/m^2).	5–20 mm Hg/10 kg
Adopt DASH (Dietary Approaches to Stop Hypertension) eating plan	Consume a diet rich in fruits, vegetables, and low-fat dairy products with a reduced content of saturated and total fat.	8–14 mm Hg
Dietary sodium reduction	Reduce dietary sodium intake to no more than 100 mmol per day (2.4 g sodium or 6 g sodium chloride).	2–8 mm Hg
Physical activity	Engage in regular aerobic physical activity such as brisk walking (at least 30 minutes per day, most days of the week).	4–9 mm Hg
Moderation of alcohol consumption	Limit consumption to no more than 2 drinks (eg, 24 oz beer, 10 oz wine, or 3 oz 80-proof whiskey) per day in most men and to no more than 1 drink per day in women and lighter-weight people.	2–4 mm Hg

* For overall cardiovascular risk reduction, stop smoking.
† SBP = Systolic blood pressure.
‡ The effects of implementing these modifications are dose- and time-dependent and could be greater for some individuals.
From the Seventh Report of the Joint National Committee on Prevention, Detection, Evaluation, and Treatment of High Blood Pressure. (2003). *Hypertension, 42*(6), 1206–1252.

patient. Research findings demonstrate that weight loss, reduced alcohol and sodium intake, and regular physical activity are effective lifestyle adaptations to reduce blood pressure (Appel, Champagne, Harsha, et al., 2003; Appel, Espeland, Easter, et al., 2001; Cushman, Cutler, Hanna, et al., 1998; Hagberg, Park, & Brown, 2000; Sacks, Svetkey, & Vollmer, 2001; Stranges, Wu, Dorn, et al., 2004). Studies also show that diets high in fruits, vegetables, and low-fat dairy products can prevent the development of hypertension and can lower elevated blood pressure (Sacks et al., 2001). Table 32-3 shows the Dietary Approaches to Stop Hypertension (DASH) diet, which has been shown to lower blood pressure in people who follow it (Appel et al., 2003).

Pharmacologic Therapy

For patients with uncomplicated hypertension and no specific indications for another medication, the recommended initial medications include diuretics, beta-blockers, or both. Patients are first given low doses of medication. If blood pressure does not fall to less than 140/90 mm Hg, the dose is increased gradually, and additional medications are included as necessary to achieve control. Table 32-4 describes the various pharmacologic agents that are recommended for the treatment of hypertension. When the blood pressure is less than 140/90 mm Hg for at least 1 year, gradual reduction of the types and doses of medication is indicated. To promote compliance, clinicians try to prescribe the simplest treatment schedule possible, ideally one pill once each day.

Gerontologic Considerations

Hypertension, particularly elevated systolic blood pressure, increases the risk of death and complications in people older than 50 years (Chobanian et al., 2003). Treatment reduces this risk. Like younger patients, older patients should begin treatment with lifestyle modifications. If medications are needed to achieve the blood pressure goal of less than 140/90 mm Hg, the starting dose should be half that used in younger patients.

TABLE 32-3 The DASH (Dietary Approaches to Stop Hypertension) Diet

Food Group	Number of Servings Per Day
Grains and grain products	7 or 8
Vegetables	4 or 5
Fruits	4 or 5
Low-fat or fat-free dairy foods	2 or 3
Meat, fish, and poultry	2 or fewer
Nuts, seeds, and dry beans	4 or 5 weekly

The diet is based on 2,000 calories per day.
Source: www.nhlbi.nih.gov/health/public/heart/hbp/dash/index.htm

Nursing Process

The Patient With Hypertension

Assessment

When hypertension is initially detected, nursing assessment involves carefully monitoring the blood pressure at frequent intervals and then,

(text continues on page 1030)

TABLE 32-4 Medication Therapy for Hypertension

Medications	Major Action	Advantages and Contraindications	Effects and Nursing Considerations
Diuretics and Related Drugs			
Thiazide Diuretics			
chlorthalidone (Hygroton) chlorothiazide (Diuril) hydrochlorothiazide (Esidrix; HydroDIURIL) indapamide (Lozol) methyclothiazide (Enduron) metolazone (Mylerox, Zaroxolyn)	Decrease of blood volume, renal blood flow, and cardiac output Depletion of extracellular fluid Negative sodium balance (from natriuresis), mild hypokalemia Directly affect vascular smooth muscle	Relatively Inexpensive Effective orally Effective during long-term administration Mild side effects Enhance other antihypertensive medications Counter sodium retention effects of other antihypertensive medications *Contraindications:* Gout, known sensitivity to sulfonamide-derived medications, severely impaired kidney function, and history of hyponatremia	Side effects include dry mouth, thirst, weakness, drowsiness, lethargy, muscle aches, muscular fatigue, tachycardia, GI disturbance. Postural hypotension may be potentiated by alcohol, barbiturates, opioids, or hot weather. Because thiazides cause loss of sodium, potassium, and magnesium, monitor for signs of electrolyte imbalance. Encourage intake of potassium-rich foods (eg, fruits). *Gerontologic Considerations:* Risk of postural hypotension is significant because of volume depletion; measure blood pressure in three positions; caution patient to rise slowly.
Loop Diuretics			
furosemide (Lasix) bumetanide (Bumex) forsemide (Demadex)	Volume depletion Blocks reabsorption of sodium, chloride, and water in kidney	Action rapid Potent Used when thiazides fail or patient needs rapid diuresis *Contraindications:* Same as for thiazides	Risk of volume and electrolyte depletion from the profound diuresis that can occur Fluid and electrolyte replacement may be required *Gerontologic Considerations:* Same as for thiazides.
Potassium-Sparing Diuretics			
amiloride (Midamor) triamterene (Dyrenium)	Blocks sodium reabsorption Acts on distal tubule independently of aldosterone	Causes potassium retention *Contraindications:* Renal disease, azotemia, severe hepatic disease, hyperkalemia	Drowsiness, lethargy, headache Monitor for hyperkalemia if given with ACE inhibitor or angiotensin receptor blocker. Diarrhea and other GI symptoms—administer medication after meals.
Aldosterone Receptor Blockers			
eplerenone (Inspra) spironolactone (Aldactone)	Competitive inhibitors of aldosterone binding	Indicated for patients with a history of myocardial infarction or symptomatic ventricular dysfunction *Contraindications:* Hyperkalemia and impaired renal function Epleronone is contraindicated in diabetes mellitus with microalbuminuria	Drowsiness, lethargy, headache Monitor for hyperkalemia if given with ACE inhibitor or angiotensin receptor blocker (ARB) Diarrhea and other GI symptoms—administer medication after meals. Avoid use of potassium supplements or salt substitutes. Teach patients, families, and caregivers signs and symptoms of hyperkalemia. Spironolactone may cause gynecomastia.

TABLE 32-4 Medication Therapy for Hypertension (Continued)

Medications	Major Action	Advantages and Contraindications	Effects and Nursing Considerations
Central Alpha$_2$-Agonists and Other Centrally Acting Drugs			
reserpine (Serpasil)	Impairs synthesis and re-uptake of norepinephrine	Slows pulse, which counteracts tachycardia of hydralazine *Contraindications:* History of depression, psychosis, obesity, chronic sinusitis, peptic ulcer	May cause severe depression; report manifestations, as this may require that drug be omitted. Nasal congestion. Use with caution if history of gallbladder, renal, or cardiac disease, or seizure disorder. *Gerontologic Considerations:* Depression and postural hypotension common in elderly
methyldopa (Aldomet)	Dopa-decarboxylase inhibitor; displaces norepinephrine from storage sites	Drug of choice for pregnant women with hypertension Useful in patients with renal failure or prostate disease Does not decrease cardiac output or renal blood flow Does not induce oliguria *Contraindications:* Liver disease	Drowsiness, dizziness Dry mouth; nasal congestion (troublesome at first but then tends to disappear) Use with caution with renal disease. *Gerontologic Considerations:* May produce mental and behavioral changes in the elderly.
clonidine (Catapres) clonidine patch (Catapres-TTs)	Exact mode of action not understood, but acts through the central nervous system, apparently through centrally mediated alpha-adrenergic stimulation in the brain, producing blood pressure reduction	Little or no orthostatic effect. Moderately potent, and sometimes is effective when other medications fail to lower blood pressure. *Contraindications:* Severe coronary artery disease, pregnancy; contraindicated in children	Dry mouth, drowsiness, sedation, and occasional headaches and fatigue. Anorexia, malaise, and vomiting with mild disturbance of liver function have been reported. Rebound or withdrawal hypertension is relatively common; monitor blood pressure when stopping medication.
guanfacine (Tenex)	Stimulates central alpha-2 adrenergic receptors	Reduces heart rate and causes vasodilation. Serious adverse reactions are uncommon. Use with caution in persons with diminished liver function, recent myocardial infarction, or known cardiovascular disease.	Common side effects include dry mouth, dizziness, sleepiness, fatigue, headache, constipation, and impotence.
Beta Blockers			
atenolol (Tenormin) betaxolol (Kerlone) bisoprolol (Zebeta) propranolol (Inderal) propranolol long-acting (Inderal LA) metoprolol (Lopressor) metoprolol extended-release (Toprol XL) nadolol (Corgard) timolol (Blocadren)	Block the sympathetic nervous system (beta-adrenergic receptors), especially the sympathetics to the heart, producing a slower heart rate and lowered blood pressure	Reduce pulse rate in patients with tachycardia and blood pressure elevation Indicated for patients who also have stable angina pectoris and silent ischemia *Contraindications:* Bronchial asthma, allergic rhinitis, right ventricular failure from pulmonary hypertension, heart failure, depression, diabetes mellitus, dyslipidemia, heart block, peripheral vascular disease, heart rate less than 60 bpm	Mental depression manifested by insomnia, lassitude, weakness, and fatigue Avoid sudden discontinuation. Lightheadedness and occasional nausea, vomiting, and epigastric distress Check heart rate before giving. *Gerontologic Considerations:* Risk of toxicity is increased for elderly patients with decreased renal and liver function. Take blood pressure in three positions and observe for hypotension.

continued >

TABLE 32-4 Medication Therapy for Hypertension (Continued)

Medications	Major Action	Advantages and Contraindications	Effects and Nursing Considerations
Beta-Blockers with Intrinsic Sympathomimetic Activity			
acebutolol (Sectral) penbutolol (Levatrol) pindolol (Visken)	Block both cardiac $beta_1$ and $beta_2$ receptors Also have antiarrhythmic activity by slowing atrioventricular conduction	*Advantages:* Similar to beta-blockers *Contraindications:* Similar to beta-blockers	Avoid sudden discontinuation. Withhold if bradycardia or heart block is present. Use with caution with COPD, diabetes mellitus. Similar to beta-blockers.
$Alpha_1$-Blockers			
doxazosin (Cardura) prazosin hydrochloride (Minipress) terazosin (Hytrin)	Peripheral vasodilator acting directly on the blood vessel; similar to hydralazine	Act directly on the blood vessels and are effective agents in patients with adverse reactions to hydralazine *Contraindications:* Angina pectoris and coronary artery disease. Induces tachycardia if not preceded by administration of propranolol and a diuretic.	Occasional vomiting and diarrhea, urinary frequency, and cardiovascular collapse, especially if given in addition to hydralazine without lowering the dose of the latter. Patients occasionally experience drowsiness, lack of energy, and weakness.
Combined Alpha and Beta Blockers			
carvedilol (Coreg) labetalol hydrochloride (Normodyne, Trandate)	Block alpha- and beta-adrenergic receptors; cause peripheral dilation and decrease peripheral vascular resistance	Fast-acting No decrease in renal blood flow *Contraindications:* Asthma, cardiogenic shock, severe tachycardia, heart block	Orthostatic hypotension, tachycardia
Vasodilators			
fenoldopam mesylate (Corlopam)	Stimulates dopamine and $alpha_2$-adrenergic receptors	Given intravenously for hypertensive emergencies. Use with caution in patients with glaucoma, recent stroke (brain attack), asthma, hypokalemia, or diminished liver function.	Headache, flushing, hypotension, sweating, tachycardia caused by vasodilation Observe for local reactions at the injection site.
hydralazine (Apresoline)	Decreases peripheral resistance but concurrently elevates cardiac output Acts directly on smooth muscle of blood vessels	Not used as initial therapy; used in combination with other medications. Used also in pregnancy-induced hypertension *Contraindications:* Angina or coronary disease, heart failure, hypersensitivity	Headache, tachycardia, flushing, and dyspnea may occur—can be prevented by pretreating with reserpine Peripheral edema may require diuretics. May produce lupus erythematosus-like syndrome
minoxidil (Loniten)	Direct vasodilating action on arteriolar vessels, causing decreased peripheral vascular resistance; reduces systolic and diastolic pressures	Hypotensive effect more pronounced than with hydralazine No effect on vasomotor reflexes so does not cause postural hypotension *Contraindications:* Pheochromocytoma	Tachycardia, angina pectoris, ECG changes, edema Take blood pressure and apical pulse before administration. Monitor intake and output and daily weights. Causes hirsutism
sodium nitroprusside (Nipride, Nitropress) nitroglycerin (NitroBid IV, Tridil)	Peripheral vasodilation by relaxation of smooth muscle	Fast-acting Used only in hypertensive emergencies *Contraindications:* Sepsis, azotemia, high intracranial pressure	Dizziness, headache, nausea, edema, tachycardia, palpitations Can cause thiocyanate and cyanide intoxication.

Rx TABLE 32-4 Medication Therapy for Hypertension (Continued)

Medications	Major Action	Advantages and Contraindications	Effects and Nursing Considerations
Angiotensin-Converting Enzyme (ACE) Inhibitors			
benazepril (Lotensin) captopril (Capoten) enalaprilat (Vasotec IV) enalapril (Vasotec) fosinopril (Monopril) lisinopril (Prinivil, Zestril) moexipril (Univasc) perindopril (Accon) quinapril (Accupril) ramipril (Altace) trandolapril (Mavik)	Inhibit conversion of angiotensin I to angiotensin II Lower total peripheral resistance	Fewer cardiovascular side effects Can be used with thiazide diuretic and digitalis Hypotension can be reversed by fluid replacement. Angioedema is a rare but potentially life-threatening complication. *Contraindications:* Renal impairment, pregnancy	*Gerontologic Considerations:* Require reduced dosages and the addition of loop diuretics when there is renal dysfunction
Angiotensin II Receptor Blockers (ARBs)			
candesartan (Atacand) eprosartan (Teveten) irbesartan (Avapro) losartan (Cozaar) olmesartan (Benicar) telmisartan (Micardis) valsartan (Diovan)	Block the effects of angiotensin II at the receptor Reduce peripheral resistance	Minimal side effects *Contraindications:* Pregnancy, renovascular disease	Monitor for hyperkalemia.
Calcium Channel Blockers			
Nondihydropyridines			
diltiazem extended release (Cardizem CV, Dilacor XT, Tiazac) diltiazem long-acting (Cardizem LA)	Inhibit calcium ion influx Reduce cardiac afterload	Inhibit coronary artery spasm not controlled by beta-blockers or nitrates *Contraindications:* Sick sinus syndrome; AV block; hypotension; heart failure	Do not discontinue suddenly. Observe for hypotension. Report irregular heartbeat, dizziness, edema. Instruct on regular dental care because of potential gingivitis.
verapamil immediate release (Calan, Isoptin) verapamil long-acting (Calan SR, Isoptin SR) verapamil (Covera HS, Verelan PM)	Inhibits calcium ion influx Slows velocity of conduction of cardiac impulse	Effective antiarrhythmic Rapid IV onset Blocks SA and AV node channels *Contraindications:* Sinus or AV node disease; severe heart failure; severe hypotension	Administer on empty stomach or before meal. Do not discontinue suddenly. Depression may subside when medication is discontinued. To relieve headaches, reduce noise, monitor electrolytes. Decrease dose for patients with liver or renal failure.
Dihydropyridines			
amlodipine (Norvasc) felodipine (Plendil) isradipine (Dynacirc CR) nicardipine (Cardene) nifedipine long-acting (Procardia XL, Adalat CC) nisoldipine (Sular)	Inhibit calcium ion influx across membranes Vasodilating effects on coronary and peripheral arteriole Decrease cardiac work and energy consumption, increase delivery of oxygen to myocardium	Rapid action Effective by oral or sublingual route No tendency to slow SA nodal activity or prolong AV node conduction Isolated systolic hypertension *Contraindications:* None (except heart failure for nifedipine)	Administer on empty stomach. Use with caution in diabetic patients with diabetes. Small frequent meals if nausea Muscle cramps, joint stiffness, sexual difficulties may disappear when dose decreased. Report irregular heartbeat, constipation, shortness of breath, edema. May cause dizziness

after diagnosis, at routinely scheduled intervals. The American Heart Association has defined the standards for blood pressure measurement, including conditions required before measurements are made, equipment specifications, and techniques for measuring blood pressure to obtain accurate and reliable readings (Chart 32-2) (Pickering, Hall, Appel, et al., 2005). When the patient begins an antihypertensive treatment regimen, blood pressure assessments are needed to determine the effectiveness of medication therapy and to detect any changes in blood pressure that indicate the need for a change in the treatment plan.

A complete history is obtained to assess for signs and symptoms that indicate target organ damage (ie, whether specific tissues are damaged by the elevated blood pressure). Such manifestations may include anginal pain; shortness of breath; alterations in speech, vision, or balance; nosebleeds; headaches; dizziness; or nocturia.

During the physical examination, the nurse must also pay specific attention to the rate, rhythm, and character of the apical and peripheral pulses to detect effects of hypertension on the heart and blood vessels. A thorough assessment can yield valuable information about the extent to which the hypertension has affected the body and about any other personal, social, or financial factors related to the condition. For example, some patients' ability to adhere to an antihypertensive medication regimen may be thwarted if they lack the financial resources to buy the medication.

Diagnosis

Nursing Diagnoses

Based on the assessment data, nursing diagnoses for the patient may include the following:

- Deficient knowledge regarding the relation between the treatment regimen and control of the disease process
- Noncompliance with therapeutic regimen related to side effects of prescribed therapy

Collaborative Problems/ Potential Complications

Based on the assessment data, potential complications that may develop include the following:

- Left ventricular hypertrophy
- Myocardial infarction

CHART 32-2

Measuring Blood Pressure (BP)

EQUIPMENT

For the Patient at Home

- Automatic or semiautomatic device with digital display of readings

For the Practitioner

- Mercury sphygmomanometer, recently calibrated aneroid manometer, or validated electronic device
- Cuff

INSTRUCTIONS FOR THE PATIENT

- Avoid smoking cigarettes or drinking caffeine for 30 minutes before BP is measured.
- Sit quietly for 5 minutes before the measurement.
- Sit comfortably with the forearm supported at heart level on a firm surface, with both feet on the ground; avoid talking while the measurement is being taken.

INSTRUCTIONS FOR THE PRACTITIONER

- Select the size of the cuff based upon the size of the patient. (The cuff size should have a bladder width of at least 40% of limb circumference and length at least 80% of limb circumference.) The average adult cuff is 12 to 14 cm wide and 30 cm long. Using a cuff that is too small will give a higher BP measurement, and using a cuff that is too large results in a lower BP measurement compared to one taken with a properly sized cuff.
- Routinely calibrate the sphygmomanometer.
- Wrap the cuff firmly around the arm. Center the cuff bladder directly over the brachial artery.
- Position the patient's arm at the level of the heart.
- Palpate the systolic pressure before auscultating. This technique helps to detect the presence of an auscultatory gap more readily.
- Ask the patient to sit quietly while the BP is measured because the BP can increase when the patient is engaged in conversation.
- Initially, record BP results of both arms and take subsequent measurements from the arm with the higher BP. Normally, the BP should vary by no more than 5 mm Hg between arms.
- Record the site where the BP was measured and the position of the patient (eg, right arm).
- Inform the patient of his or her BP value and what it means. Emphasize the need for periodic reassessment, and encourage patients who measure BP at home to keep a written record of readings.

INTERPRETATION

Assessment is based on the average of at least two readings. (If two readings differ by more than 5 mm Hg, additional readings are taken and an average reading is calculated from the results.)

- Heart failure
- TIAs
- Cerebrovascular accident (stroke or brain attack)
- Renal insufficiency and failure
- Retinal hemorrhage

Planning and Goals

The major goals for the patient include understanding of the disease process and its treatment, participation in a self-care program, and absence of complications.

Nursing Interventions

The objective of nursing care for hypertensive patients focuses on lowering and controlling the blood pressure without adverse effects and without undue cost. To achieve these goals, the nurse must support and teach the patient to adhere to the treatment regimen by implementing necessary lifestyle changes, taking medications as prescribed, and scheduling regular follow-up appointments with the health care provider to monitor progress or identify and treat any complications of disease or therapy.

Increasing Knowledge

The patient needs to understand the disease process and how lifestyle changes and medications can control hypertension. The nurse needs to emphasize the concept of controlling hypertension rather than curing it. The nurse can encourage the patient to consult a dietitian to help develop a plan for weight loss. The program usually consists of restricting sodium and fat intake, increasing intake of fruits and vegetables, and implementing regular physical activity. Explaining that it takes 2 to 3 months for the taste buds to adapt to changes in salt intake may help the patient adjust to reduced salt intake. The patient should be advised to limit alcohol intake (see Table 32-2 for specific recommendations) and tobacco should be avoided—not because smoking is related to hypertension, but because anyone with high blood pressure is already at increased risk for heart disease, and smoking amplifies this risk. Support groups for weight control, smoking cessation, and stress reduction may be beneficial for some patients; others can benefit from the support of family and friends. The nurse assists the patient to develop and adhere to an appropriate exercise regimen, because regular activity is a significant factor in weight reduction and a blood pressure–reducing intervention in the absence of any loss in weight (Chobanian et al., 2003).

Promoting Home and Community-Based Care

Blood pressure screenings with the sole purpose of case finding are not recommended by the National High Blood Pressure Education Program because approximately 70% of people with hypertension are already aware of their blood pressure levels (Chobanian et al., 2003). If asked to participate in a blood pressure screening, the nurse should be sure that proper blood pressure measurement technique is being used (see Chart 32-2), that the manometers used are calibrated (Pickering et al., 2005), and that provision has been made to provide follow-up for any person identified as having an elevated blood pressure level. Adequate time should also be allowed to teach people what the blood pressure numbers mean. Each person should be given a written record of his or her blood pressure at the screening.

TEACHING PATIENTS SELF-CARE

The therapeutic regimen is the responsibility of the patient in collaboration with the health care provider. The nurse can help the patient achieve blood pressure control through education about high blood pressure and how to manage it through medication, lifestyle changes of diet, weight control, and exercise (see Table 32-2), setting goal blood pressures, and providing assistance with social support. Involving family members in education programs enables them to support the patient's efforts to control hypertension. The American Heart Association and the National Heart, Lung, and Blood Institute provide printed and electronic patient education materials.

Providing written information about the expected effects and side effects of medications is important. When side effects occur, patients need to understand the importance of reporting them and to whom they should be reported. Patients need to be informed that **rebound hypertension** can occur if antihypertensive medications are suddenly stopped. Both female and male patients should be informed that some medications, such as beta-blockers, may cause sexual dysfunction and that other medications are available if a problem with sexual function or satisfaction occurs. The nurse can encourage and teach patients to measure their blood pressure at home. This practice involves patients in their own care and emphasizes that failing to take medications may result in an identifiable rise in blood pressure. Patients need to know that blood pressure varies continuously and that the range within which their pressure varies should be monitored.

GERONTOLOGIC CONSIDERATIONS

Compliance with the therapeutic program may be more difficult for elderly people. The medication regimen can be difficult to remember, and the expense can be a problem. **Monotherapy** (treatment with a single agent), if appropriate, may simplify the medication regimen and make it less expensive. Special care must be taken to ensure that the elderly patient understands the regimen and can see and read instructions, open the medication container, and get the prescription refilled. The elderly person's family or caregivers should be included in the teaching program so that they understand the patient's needs, encourage adherence to the treatment plan, and know when and whom to call if problems arise or information is needed.

CONTINUING CARE

Regular follow-up care is imperative so that the disease process can be assessed and treated, depending on whether control or progression is found, as shown in Table 32-5. A history and physical examination should be completed at each clinic visit. The history should include all data pertaining to any potential problem, specifically medication-related problems such as postural (orthostatic) hypotension (experienced as dizziness or lightheadedness).

Deviation from the therapeutic program is a significant problem for people with hypertension and other chronic conditions requiring lifetime management. An estimated 50% of patients discontinue their medications within 1 year of beginning to take them. Blood pressure control is achieved by only 34% (Chobanian et al., 2003). Compliance increases, however, when patients actively participate in self-care, including self-monitoring of blood pressure and diet—possibly because patients receive immediate feedback and have a greater sense of control.

Patients with hypertension must make considerable effort to adhere to recommended lifestyle modifications and to take regularly prescribed medications. The effort needed to follow the therapeutic plan may seem unreasonable to some, particularly when they have no symptoms without medications but do have side effects with medications. The recommended lifestyle changes are listed in Table 32-2. Continued education and encouragement are usually needed to enable patients to formulate an acceptable plan that helps them live with their hypertension and adhere to the treatment plan. Compromises may have to be made about some aspects of therapy to achieve higher-priority goals.

The nurse can assist with behavior change by supporting patients in making small changes with each visit that move them toward their goals. Another important factor is following up at each visit to see how the patient has progressed with the plans made at the prior visit. If the patient has had difficulty with a particular aspect of the plan, the patient and nurse can work together to develop an alternative or modification to the plan that the patient believes will be more successful.

Monitoring and Managing Potential Complications

Symptoms suggesting that hypertension is progressing to the extent that target organ damage is occurring must be detected early so that appropriate treatment can be initiated. When the patient returns for follow-up care, all body systems must be assessed to detect any evidence of vascular damage. An eye examination with an ophthalmoscope is particularly important because retinal blood vessel damage indicates similar damage elsewhere in the vascular system. The patient is questioned about blurred vision, spots in front of the eyes, and diminished visual acuity. The heart, nervous system, and kidneys are also carefully assessed. Any significant findings are promptly reported to determine whether additional diagnostic studies are required. Based on the findings, medications may be changed to improve blood pressure control.

NURSING ALERT

The patient and caregivers should be cautioned that antihypertensive medications can cause hypotension. Low blood pressure or postural hypotension should be reported immediately. Elderly people have impaired cardiovascular reflexes and thus are more sensitive to the extracellular volume depletion caused by diuretics and to the sympathetic inhibition caused by adrenergic antagonists. The nurse teaches patients to change positions slowly when moving from a lying or sitting position to a standing position. The nurse also counsels elderly patients to use supportive devices such as hand rails and walkers as necessary to prevent falls that could result from dizziness.

TABLE 32-5 Recommendations for Follow-Up Based on Initial Blood Pressure Measurements for Adults Without Acute End Organ Damage

Initial BP (mm Hg)*	Follow-Up Recommended†
Normal	Recheck in 2 years
Prehypertension	Recheck in 1 year‡
Stage 1 hypertension	Confirm within 2 months‡
Stage 2 hypertension	Evaluate or refer to source of care within 1 month For those with higher pressures (eg, >180/100 mm Hg), evaluate and treat immediately or within 1 week, depending on clinical situation and complications.

* If systolic and diastolic values fall into different categories, follow recommendations for shorter follow-up (eg, 160/86 mm Hg should be evaluated or referred to source of care within 1 month).

† Modify the scheduling of follow-up according to reliable information about past blood pressure measurements, other cardiovascular risk factors, or target organ disease.

‡ Provide advice about lifestyle modifications.

From the Seventh Report of the Joint National Committee on Prevention, Detection, Evaluation, and Treatment of High Blood Pressure. (2003). *Hypertension, 42*(6), 1206–1252.

Evaluation

EXPECTED PATIENT OUTCOMES

Expected patient outcomes may include the following:

1. Maintains adequate tissue perfusion:
   a. Maintains blood pressure at less than 140/90 mm Hg (or less than 130/80 mm Hg for people with diabetes mellitus or chronic kidney disease) with lifestyle modifications, medications, or both
   b. Demonstrates no symptoms of angina, palpitations, or vision changes
   c. Has stable BUN and serum creatinine levels
   d. Has palpable peripheral pulses
2. Complies with the self-care program:
   a. Adheres to the dietary regimen as prescribed: reduces calorie, sodium, and fat intake; increases fruit and vegetable intake
   b. Exercises regularly
   c. Takes medications as prescribed and reports any side effects
   d. Measures blood pressure routinely
   e. Abstains from tobacco and excessive alcohol intake
   f. Keeps follow-up appointments
3. Has no complications:
   a. Reports no changes in vision
   b. Exhibits no retinal damage on vision testing
   c. Maintains pulse rate and rhythm and respiratory rate within normal ranges
   d. Reports no dyspnea or edema
   e. Maintains urine output consistent with intake
   f. Has renal function test results within normal range
   g. Demonstrates no motor, speech, or sensory deficits
   h. Reports no headaches, dizziness, weakness, changes in gait, or falls

Hypertensive Crises

JNC 7 describes two classes of hypertensive crisis that require immediate intervention: hypertensive emergency and hypertensive urgency (Chobanian et al., 2003). Hypertensive emergencies and urgencies may occur in patients whose hypertension has been poorly controlled or in those who have abruptly discontinued their medications. Once the hypertensive crisis has been managed, a complete evaluation is performed to review the patient's ongoing treatment plan and strategies to minimize the occurrence of subsequent hypertensive crises. The current recommendations for management of both hypertensive emergencies and urgencies are based on expert opinions because there are not clinical trial data comparing treatment options or identifying the impact of treatment on morbidity and mortality (Cherney & Straus, 2002).

Hypertensive emergency is a situation in which blood pressure is extremely elevated (more than 180/120 mm Hg) and must be lowered immediately (not necessarily to less than 140/90 mm Hg) to halt or prevent damage to the target organs (Chobanian et al., 2003). Assessment will reveal actual or developing clinical dysfunction of the target organ. Conditions associated with hypertensive emergency include hypertension of pregnancy, acute myocardial infarction, dissecting aortic aneurysm, and intracranial hemorrhage. Hypertensive emergencies are acute, life-threatening blood pressure elevations that require prompt treatment in an intensive care setting because of the serious target organ damage that may occur. The therapeutic goals are reduction of the mean blood pressure by up to 25% within the first hour of treatment, a further reduction to a goal pressure of about 160/100 mm Hg over a period of up to 6 hours, and then a more gradual reduction in pressure over a period of days. The exceptions to these goals are the treatment of ischemic stroke (in which there is no evidence of benefit from immediate pressure reduction) and treatment of aortic dissection (in which the goal is to lower systolic pressure to less than 100 mm Hg if the patient can tolerate the reduction) (Chobanian et al., 2003).

The medications of choice in hypertensive emergencies are those that have an immediate effect. Intravenous vasodilators, including sodium nitroprusside (Nipride, Nitropress), nicardipine hydrochloride (Cardene), fenoldopam mesylate (Corlopam), enalaprilat (Vasotec), and nitroglycerin (Nitro-Bid, Tridil) have immediate actions that are short-lived (minutes to 4 hours), and they are therefore used for initial treatment. For more information about these medications, see Table 32-4.

Hypertensive urgency describes a situation in which blood pressure is very elevated but there is no evidence of impending or progressive target organ damage (Chobanian et al., 2003). Elevated blood pressures associated with severe headaches, nosebleeds, or anxiety are classified as urgencies. Oral doses of fast-acting agents such as beta-adrenergic blocking agents (eg, labetalol [Normodyne, Trandate]), angiotensin-converting enzyme inhibitors (eg, captopril [Capoten]), or alpha$_2$-agonists (eg, clonidine [Catapres]) are recommended for the treatment of hypertensive urgencies (see Table 32-4).

Extremely close hemodynamic monitoring of the patient's blood pressure and cardiovascular status is required during treatment of hypertensive emergencies and urgencies (see Chapter 26). The exact frequency of monitoring is a matter of clinical judgment and varies with the patient's condition. Taking vital signs every 5 minutes is appropriate if the blood pressure is changing rapidly; taking vital signs at 15- or 30-minute intervals in a more stable situation may be sufficient. A precipitous drop in blood pressure can occur that would require immediate action to restore blood pressure to an acceptable level.

Critical Thinking Exercises

1 ebp You are a charge nurse in an emergency department. A 72-year-old man arrives one evening with a laceration of his right forearm from a minor gardening injury. The laceration will require suturing. When you take the patient's blood pressure on his left arm, you note that it is 164/78. You tell the patient his blood pressure and

express concern that his systolic blood pressure is high. He shrugs and tells you, "The top number is always elevated, but it's nothing to worry about." What is the evidence base that indicates that untreated isolated systolic hypertension can cause disability and death? What other information do you plan to gather from this patient? What plan of action might you initiate?

2 ebp You are volunteering at a church-sponsored blood pressure screening clinic that is being offered after Sunday services, in tandem with a fund-raising buffet breakfast. The pastor approaches you and notes that the breakfast buffet serves a variety of egg dishes, hash browns, sausage patties, bacon, and pastries. He asks you what effects, if any, this food may have on his parishioners' blood pressures. What effect might this type of diet have on the parishioners' blood pressures today? Discuss the strength of the evidence that supports specific dietary strategies aimed at preventing and treating hypertension.

REFERENCES AND SELECTED READINGS

BOOKS

Kaplan, N., Lieberman, E., & Neal, W. (2002). *Kaplan's clinical hypertension* (8th ed.). Philadelphia: Lippincott Williams & Wilkins.

Zipes, D. P., Libby, P., Bonow, R. O., et al. (Eds.) (2005). *Heart disease: A textbook of cardiovascular medicine* (7th ed.). Philadelphia: W. B. Saunders.

JOURNALS

Appel, L. J., Champagne, C. M., Harsha, D. W., et al. (2003). Effects of comprehensive lifestyle modification on blood pressure control: Main results of the premier clinical trial. *Journal of the American Medical Association, 289*(16), 2083–2093.

Appel, L. J., Espeland, M. A., Easter, L., et al. (2001). Effects of reduced sodium intake on hypertension control in older individuals: Results from the trial of nonpharmacologic interventions in the elderly (TONE). *Archives of Internal Medicine, 161*(5), 685–693.

Casper, M. L., Barnett, E., Williams, G. I., et al. Atlas of stroke mortality: Racial, ethnic, and geographic disparities in the United States. www.cdc.gov/cvh/maps/strokeatlas/index.htm. Accessed March 24, 2005.

Cherney, D., & Straus, S. (2002). Management of patients with hypertensive urgencies and emergencies: A systematic review of the literature. *Journal of General Internal Medicine, 17*(12), 937–945.

Chobanian, A. V., Bakris, G. L., Black, H. R., et al. (2003). The Seventh Report of the Joint National Committee on Prevention, Detection, Evaluation, and Treatment of High Blood Pressure: The JNC 7 Report (erratum in: *Journal of the American Medical Association,* 2003; 290(2):197). *Journal of the American Medical Association, 289*(19), 2560–2572.

Cushman, W. C., Cutler, J. A., Hanna, E., et al. (1998). Prevention and treatment of hypertension study (PATHS): Effects of an alcohol treatment program on blood pressure. *Archives of Internal Medicine, 158*(11), 1197–1207.

Dominiczak, A. F., Negrin, D. C., Clark, J. S., et al. (2000). Genes and hypertension: From gene mapping in experimental models to vascular gene transfer strategies. *Hypertension, 35*(1 Pt 2), 164–172.

Fields, L. E., Burt, V. L., Cutler, J. A., et al. (2004). The burden of adult hypertension in the United States 1999 to 2000: A rising tide. *Hypertension, 44*(4), 398–404.

Hagberg, J. M., Park, J. J., & Brown, M. D. (2000). The role of exercise training in the treatment of hypertension: An update. *Sports Medicine, 30*(3), 193–206.

Hajjar, I., & Kotchen, T. A. (2003). Trends in prevalence, awareness, treatment, and control of hypertension in the United States, 1988–2000. *JAMA, 290*(2), 199–206.

Lewington, S., Clarke, R., Qizilbash, N., et al. (2002). Age-specific relevance of usual blood pressure to vascular mortality: A meta-analysis of individual data for one million adults in 61 prospective studies. *Lancet, 360*(9349), 1903–1913.

Oparil, S., Zaman, M. A., & Calhoun, D. A. (2003). Pathogenesis of hypertension. *Annals of Internal Medicine, 139*(9), 761–776.

Pickering, T. G., Hall, J. E., Appel, L. J., et al. (2005). Recommendations for blood pressure measurement in humans and experimental animals: Part 1: Blood pressure measurement in humans: A statement for professionals from the Subcommittee of Professional and Public Education of the American Heart Association Council on High Blood Pressure Research. *Hypertension, 45*(1), 142–161.

Sacks, F. M., Svetkey, L. P., Vollmer, W. M., et al. (2001). Effects on blood pressure of reduced dietary sodium and the Dietary Approaches to Stop Hypertension (DASH) diet. DASH-Sodium Collaborative Research Group. *New England Journal of Medicine, 344*(1), 3–10.

Stranges, S., Wu, T., Dorn, J. M., et al. (2004). Relationship of alcohol drinking pattern to risk of hypertension: A population-based study. *Hypertension, 44*(6), 813–819.

RESOURCES

American Heart Association National Center, 7272 Greenville Ave., Dallas, TX 75231-4596; 1-214-373-6300; fax, 1-214-706-1191; http://www.americanheart.org/. Accessed April 1, 2006.

Centers for Disease Control and Prevention (CDC), 600 Clifton Rd., Atlanta, GA 30333; Cardiovascular Health Program: 1-404-639-3534 or 1-800-311-3435; http://www.cdc.gov/cvh. Accessed April 1, 2006.

Heart and Stroke Foundation of Canada, 222 Queen St., Suite 1402, Ottawa, Ontario K1P5V9, 1-613-569-4361; fax 1-613-569-3278; http://www.heartandstroke.ca/. Accessed April 1, 2006.

National Heart, Lung, and Blood Institute, NHLBI Information Center, P.O. Box 30105, Bethesda, MD 20824-0105; http://www.nhlbi.nih.gov. Accessed April 1, 2006.

World Health Association (WHO), Avenue Appia 20, 1211 Geneva, 27 Switzerland; Cardiovascular Disease Information: http://www.who.int/entity/cardiovascular_diseases/en. Accessed April 1, 2006.

CHAPTER 33

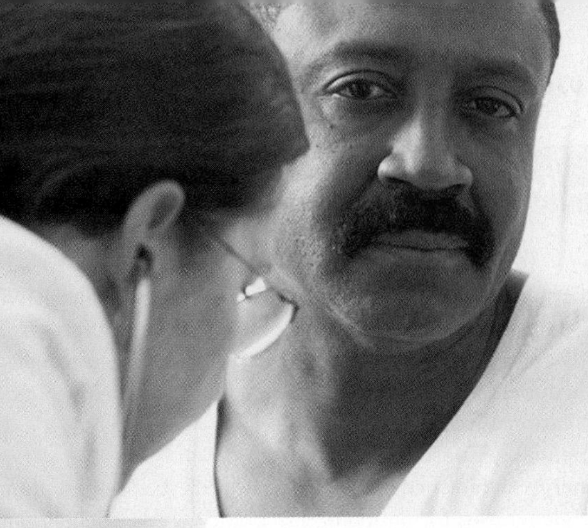

Assessment and Management of Patients With Hematologic Disorders

Learning Objectives

On completion of this chapter, the learner will be able to:

1. Describe the process of hematopoiesis.
2. Describe the processes involved in maintaining hemostasis.
3. Differentiate between the hypoproliferative and the hemolytic anemias and compare and contrast the physiologic mechanisms, clinical manifestations, medical management, and nursing interventions for each.
4. Use the nursing process as a framework for care of patients with anemia.
5. Compare the leukemias in terms of their incidence, physiologic alterations, clinical manifestations, management, and prognosis.
6. Use the nursing process as a framework for care of patients with acute leukemia.
7. Use the nursing process as a framework for care of patients with lymphoma or multiple myeloma.
8. Use the nursing process as a framework for care of patients with bleeding or thrombotic disorders.
9. Identify therapies for blood disorders, including the nursing implications for the administration of blood components.

Glossary

absolute neutrophil count (ANC): a mathematical calculation of the actual number of neutrophils in the circulation, derived from the total WBCs and the percentage of neutrophils counted in a microscope's visual field; provides a rough indication of infection risk
anemia: decreased RBC count
anergy: diminished reactivity to antigens (transient or complete)
angiogenesis: formation of new blood vessels, such as in a healing wound or in a malignant tumor
angular cheilosis: cracking sore at corner of mouth
aplasia: lack of cellular development (eg, of cells within the bone marrow)
apoptosis: complex process of programmed cell death
band cell: slightly immature neutrophil
blast cell: primitive WBC
cytokines: hormones produced by leukocytes that are vital to regulation of hematopoiesis, apoptosis, and immune responses
D-dimer: test that measures fibrin breakdown; considered to be more specific than fibrin degradation products in the diagnosis of disseminated intravascular coagulation (DIC)
differentiation: development of functions and characteristics that are different from those of the parent stem cell
dysplasia: abnormal development (eg, of blood cells); size, shape and appearance of cells are altered
ecchymosis: bruise
erythrocyte: see RBC
erythrocyte sedimentation rate (ESR): laboratory test that measures the rate of settling of RBCs; elevation is indicative of inflammation; also called the "sed rate"
erythroid cells: broad term used in reference to any cell that is or will become a mature RBC
erythropoiesis: process of formation of RBCs
erythropoietin: hormone produced primarily by the kidney; necessary for erythropoiesis
fibrin: filamentous protein; basis of thrombus and blood clot
fibrinogen: protein converted into fibrin to form thrombus and clot
fibrinolysis: process of breakdown of fibrin clot
granulocyte: granulated WBC (neutrophil, eosinophil, basophil); sometimes used synonymously with neutrophil
granulocytopenia: fewer than normal granulocytes
hematocrit: percentage of total blood volume consisting of RBCs
hematopoiesis: complex process of the formation and maturation of blood cells
hemoglobin: iron-containing protein of RBCs; delivers oxygen to tissues
hemolysis: destruction of RBCs; can occur within or outside of the vasculature
hemosiderin: iron-containing pigment derived from breakdown of hemoglobin
hemostasis: intricate balance between clot formation and clot dissolution
histiocytes: cells present in all loose connective tissue, capable of phagocytosis; part of the RES
hyperplasia: abnormally increased proliferation of normal cells
hypochromia: pallor within the RBC caused by decreased hemoglobin content
left shift, or shift to the left: increased release of immature forms of WBCs from the bone marrow in response to need
leukocyte: see WBC
leukemia: uncontrolled proliferation of WBCs, often immature
leukopenia: less than normal amount of WBCs in circulation
lymphoid: pertaining to lymphocytes
lymphocyte: form of WBC involved in immune functions
lysis: destruction of cells
macrocytosis: larger than normal RBCs
macrophage: cells of the RES that are capable of phagocytosis
mast cell: cells found in connective tissue involved in defense of the body and coagulation
microcytosis: smaller than normal RBCs
monocyte: large WBC that becomes a macrophage when it leaves the circulation and moves into body tissues
myeloid: pertaining to nonlymphoid blood cells that differentiate into RBCs, platelets, monocytes and macrophages, neutrophils, eosinophils, basophils, and mast cells
myelopoiesis: formation and maturation of cells derived from myeloid stem cell
neutropenia: lower than normal number of neutrophils
neutrophil: fully mature WBC capable of phagocytosis; primary defense against bacterial infection
normochromic: normal RBC color, indicating normal amount of hemoglobin
normocytic: normal size of RBC
nucleated RBC: immature form of RBC; portion of nucleus remains within the red cell; not normally seen in circulating blood
oxyhemoglobin: combined form of oxygen and hemoglobin; found in arterial blood
pancytopenia: abnormal decrease in WBCs, RBCs, and platelets
petechiae: tiny capillary hemorrhages
phagocytosis: process of ingestion and digestion of bacteria by cells
plasma: liquid portion of blood
plasminogen: protein that is converted to plasmin to dissolve thrombi and clots
platelet: thrombocyte; a cellular component of blood involved in blood coagulation
poikilocytosis: variation in shape of RBCs
polycythemia: excess RBCs
RBC: red blood cell, erythrocyte; a cellular component of blood involved in the transport of oxygen and carbon dioxide
red blood cell: see RBC
reticulocytes: slightly immature RBCs, usually only 1% of total circulating RBCs
reticuloendothelial system (RES): complex system of cells throughout body capable of phagocytosis
serum: portion of blood remaining after coagulation occurs
stem cell: primitive cell, capable of self-replication and differentiation into myeloid or lymphoid stem cell
thrombin: enzyme necessary to convert fibrinogen into fibrin clot
thrombocyte: see platelet
thrombocytopenia: lower than normal platelet count
thrombocytosis: higher than normal platelet count
WBC: white blood cells, leukocytes; cellular components of blood involved in defense of the body; subtypes include neutrophils, eosinophils, basophils, monocytes, and lymphocytes
white blood cell: see WBC

Unlike many other body systems, the hematologic system truly encompasses the entire human body. Patients with hematologic disorders often have significant abnormalities in blood tests but few or no symptoms. Therefore, the nurse must have a good understanding of the pathophysiology of the patient's condition and the ability to make a thorough assessment that relies heavily on the interpretation of laboratory tests. It is equally important for the nurse to anticipate potential patient needs and to target nursing interventions accordingly. Because it is so important to the understanding of most hematologic diseases, a basic appreciation of blood cells and bone marrow function is necessary.

Anatomic and Physiologic Overview

The hematologic system consists of the blood and the sites where blood is produced, including the bone marrow and the **reticuloendothelial system** (RES). Blood is a specialized organ that differs from other organs in that it exists in a fluid state. Blood is composed of plasma and various types of cells. **Plasma** is the fluid portion of blood; it contains various proteins, such as albumin, globulin, **fibrinogen**, and other factors necessary for clotting, as well as electrolytes, waste products, and nutrients. About 55% of blood volume is plasma.

Blood

The cellular component of blood consists of three primary cell types (Table 33-1): **erythrocytes (red blood cells [RBCs]**, red cells), **leukocytes (white blood cells [WBCs]**), and **thrombocytes (platelets).** These cellular components of blood normally make up 40% to 45% of the blood volume. Because most blood cells have a short life span, the need for the body to replenish its supply of cells is continuous; this process is termed **hematopoiesis.** The primary site for hematopoiesis is the bone marrow. During embryonic development and in other conditions, the liver and spleen may also be involved.

Under normal conditions, the adult bone marrow produces about 175 billion erythrocytes, 70 billion **neutrophils** (a mature type of WBC), and 175 billion platelets each day. When the body needs more blood cells, as in infection (when neutrophils are needed to fight the invading pathogen) or in bleeding (when more RBCs are required), the marrow increases its production of the cells required. Thus, under normal conditions, the marrow responds to increased demand and releases adequate numbers of cells into the circulation.

Blood makes up approximately 7% to 10% of the normal body weight and amounts to 5 to 6 L of volume. Circulating through the vascular system and serving as a link between body organs, blood carries oxygen absorbed from the lungs and nutrients absorbed from the gastrointestinal (GI) tract to the body cells for cellular metabolism. Blood also carries hormones, antibodies, and other substances to their sites of action or use. In addition, blood carries waste products produced by cellular metabolism to the lungs, skin, liver, and kidneys, where they are transformed and eliminated from the body.

TABLE 33-1 Blood Cells

Cell Type	Major Function
WBC (Leukocyte)	Fights infection
Neutrophil	Essential in preventing or limiting bacterial infection via phagocytosis
Monocyte	Enters tissue as macrophage; highly phagocytic, especially against fungus; immune surveillance
Eosinophil	Involved in allergic reactions (neutralizes histamine); digests foreign proteins
Basophil	Contains histamine; integral part of hypersensitivity reactions
Lymphocyte	Integral component of immune system
T lymphocyte	Responsible for cell-mediated immunity; recognizes material as "foreign" (surveillance system)
B lymphocyte	Responsible for humoral immunity; many mature into plasma cells to form antibodies
Plasma cell	Secretes immunoglobulin (Ig, antibody); most mature form of B lymphocyte
RBC (Erythrocyte)	Carries hemoglobin to provide oxygen to tissues; average life span is 120 days
Platelet (Thrombocyte)	Fragment of megakaryocyte; provides basis for coagulation to occur; maintains hemostasis; average life span is 10 days

Blood is fluid; therefore, the danger always exists that trauma can lead to loss of blood from the vascular system. To prevent this, an intricate clotting mechanism is activated when necessary to seal any leak in the blood vessels. Excessive clotting is equally dangerous, because it can obstruct blood flow to vital tissues. To prevent this, the body has a fibrinolytic mechanism that eventually dissolves clots (thrombi) formed within blood vessels. The balance between these two systems, clot (thrombus) formation and clot (thrombus) dissolution or **fibrinolysis**, is called **hemostasis.**

Bone Marrow

The bone marrow is the site of hematopoiesis, or blood cell formation (Fig. 33-1). All skeletal bones are involved in children, but as children age, marrow activity decreases. Marrow activity is usually limited to the pelvis, ribs, vertebrae, and sternum in adults.

Marrow is one of the largest organs of the body, making up 4% to 5% of total body weight. It consists of islands of cellular components (red marrow) separated by fat (yellow marrow). As the adult ages, the proportion of active marrow

Physiology/Pathophysiology

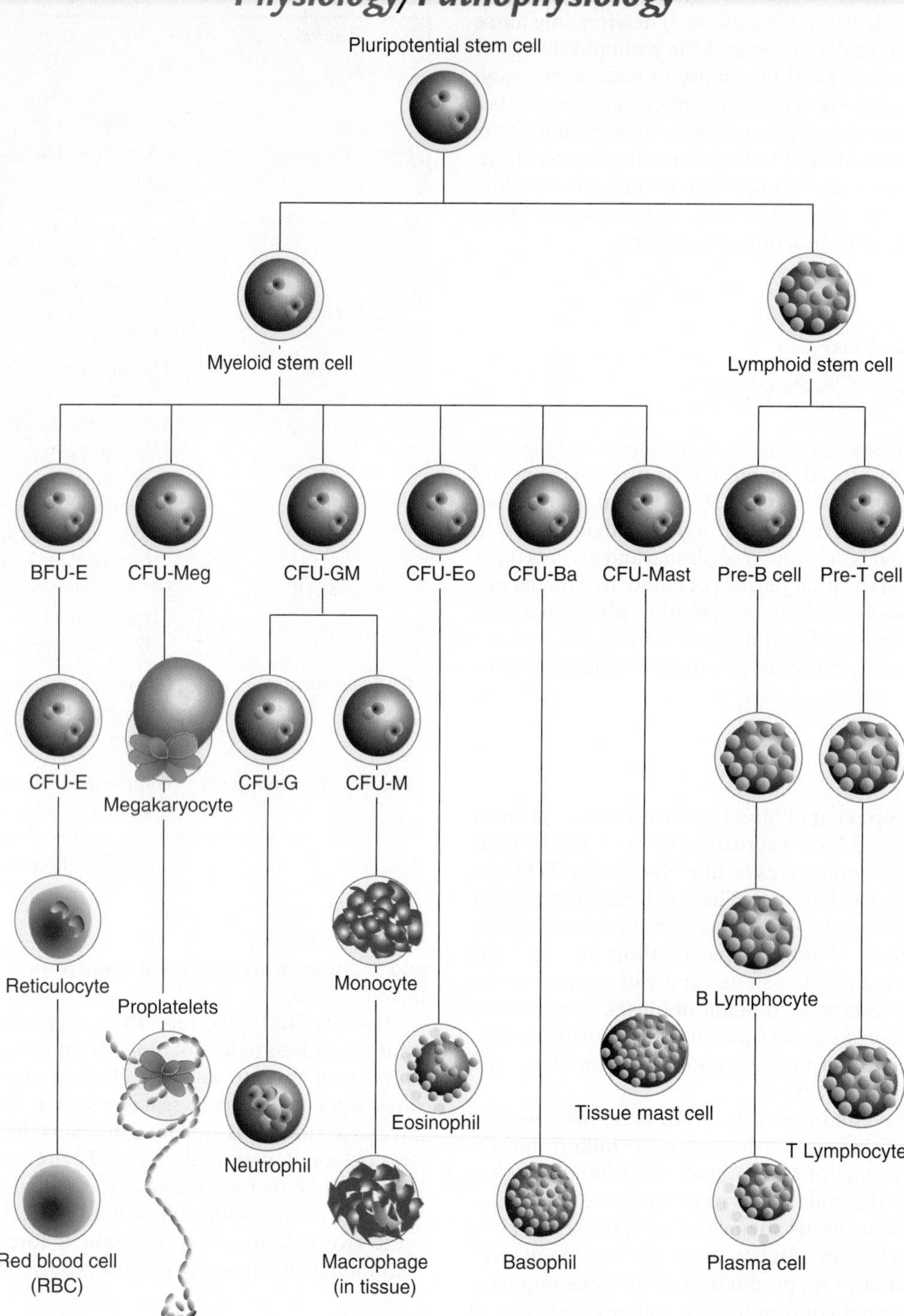

FIGURE 33-1. Hematopoiesis. Uncommitted (pluripotent) stem cells can differentiate into myeloid or lymphoid stem cells. These stem cells then undergo a complex process of differentiation and maturation into normal cells that are released into the circulation. The myeloid stem cell is responsible not only for all nonlymphoid white blood cells (WBCs) but also for the production of red blood cells (RBCs) and platelets. Each step of the differentiation process depends in part on the presence of specific growth factors for each cell type. When the stem cells are dysfunctional, they may respond inadequately to the need for more cells, or they may respond excessively, sometimes uncontrollably, as in leukemia. Adapted from Amgen, Inc., 1995, Thousand Oaks, CA.

is gradually replaced by fat; however, in the healthy person, the fat can again be replaced by active marrow when more blood cell production is required. In adults with disease that causes marrow destruction, fibrosis, or scarring, the liver and spleen can also resume production of blood cells by a process known as extramedullary hematopoiesis.

The marrow is highly vascular. Within it are primitive cells called **stem cells.** The stem cells have the ability to self-replicate, thereby ensuring a continuous supply of stem cells throughout the life cycle. When stimulated to do so, stem cells can begin a process of **differentiation** into either **myeloid** or **lymphoid** stem cells. These stem cells are committed to produce specific types of blood cells. Lymphoid stem cells produce either T or B **lymphocytes.** Myeloid stem cells differentiate into three broad cell types: erythrocytes, leukocytes, and platelets. Thus, with the exception of lymphocytes, all blood cells are derived from myeloid stem cells. A defect in a myeloid stem cell can cause problems with erythrocyte, leukocyte, and platelet production. Many complex mechanisms are involved in hematopoiesis, often at the molecular level. A thorough description of these processes is beyond the scope of this textbook; however, some mechanisms against which a specific treatment is targeted are briefly described in the relevant disease-specific sections of this chapter.

Blood Cells

Erythrocytes (Red Blood Cells)

The normal erythrocyte is a biconcave disk that resembles a soft ball compressed between two fingers (Fig. 33-2). It has a diameter of about 8 μm and is so flexible that it can pass easily through capillaries that may be as small as 2.8 μm in diameter. The membrane of the red cell is very thin so that gases, such as oxygen and carbon dioxide, can easily diffuse across it; the disk shape provides a large surface area that facilitates the absorption and release of oxygen molecules.

Mature erythrocytes consist primarily of **hemoglobin,** which contains iron and makes up 95% of the cell mass. Mature erythrocytes have no nuclei, and they have many fewer metabolic enzymes than do most other cells. The presence of a large amount of hemoglobin enables the red cell to perform its principal function, the transport of oxygen between the lungs and tissues. Occasionally the marrow releases slightly immature forms of erythrocytes, called **reticulocytes,** into the circulation. This occurs as a normal response to an increased demand for erythrocytes (as in bleeding) or in some disease states.

The oxygen-carrying hemoglobin molecule is made up of four subunits, each containing a heme portion attached to a globin chain. Iron is present in the heme component of the molecule. An important property of heme is its ability to bind to oxygen loosely and reversibly. Oxygen readily binds to hemoglobin in the lungs and is carried as **oxyhemoglobin** in arterial blood. Oxyhemoglobin is a brighter red than hemoglobin that does not contain oxygen (reduced hemoglobin), which is why arterial blood is a brighter red than venous blood. The oxygen readily dissociates (detaches) from hemoglobin in the tissues, where the oxygen is needed for cellular metabolism. In venous blood, hemoglobin combines with hydrogen ions produced by cellular metabolism and thus buffers excessive acid. Whole blood normally contains about 15 g of hemoglobin per 100 mL of blood.

ERYTHROPOIESIS

Erythroblasts arise from the primitive myeloid stem cells in bone marrow. The erythroblast is an immature nucleated cell that accumulates hemoglobin and then gradually loses its nucleus. At this stage, the cell is known as a reticulocyte. Further maturation into an erythrocyte entails the loss of the dark-staining material within the cell and slight shrinkage. The mature erythrocyte is then released into the circulation. Under conditions of rapid **erythropoiesis** (erythrocyte production), reticulocytes and other immature cells (eg, **nucleated RBCs**) may be released prematurely into the circulation. This is often seen when the liver or spleen takes over as the site of erythropoiesis and more nucleated red cells are seen within the circulation.

Differentiation of the primitive myeloid stem cell of the marrow into an erythroblast is stimulated by **erythropoietin,** a hormone produced primarily by the kidney. If the kidney detects low levels of oxygen (as would occur in **anemia,** in which fewer red cells are available to bind oxygen, or in people living at high altitudes), the release of erythropoietin is increased. The increased erythropoietin then stimulates the marrow to increase production of erythrocytes. The entire process typically takes 5 days.

For normal erythrocyte production, the bone marrow also requires iron, vitamin B_{12}, folic acid, pyridoxine (vitamin B_6), protein, and other factors. A deficiency of these factors during erythropoiesis can result in decreased red cell production and anemia.

Iron Stores and Metabolism. The average daily diet in the United States contains 10 to 15 mg of elemental iron, but only 0.5 to 1 mg of ingested iron is normally absorbed from the small intestine. The rate of iron absorption is regulated by the amount of iron already stored in the body and by the rate of erythrocyte production. Additional amounts of iron, up to 2 mg daily, must be absorbed by women of childbearing age to replace that lost during menstruation. Total body iron content in the average adult is approximately 3 g, most of which is present in hemoglobin or in one of its breakdown products. Iron is stored in the small intestine as ferritin and in reticuloendothelial cells. When required, the iron is released into the plasma, binds to transferrin, and is transported into the membranes of the normoblasts (erythrocyte precursor cells) within the marrow, where it is incorporated into hemoglobin. Iron is lost in the feces, either in bile, blood, or mucosal cells from the intestine.

The concentration of iron in blood is normally about 75 to 175 μg/dL (13 to 31 μmol/L) for men and 65 to 165 μg/dL (11 to 29 μmol/L) for women. With iron deficiency, bone marrow iron stores are rapidly depleted; hemoglobin synthesis is depressed, and the erythrocytes produced by the marrow are small and low in hemoglobin. Iron deficiency in the adult generally indicates that blood has been lost from the body (eg, from bleeding in the GI tract or heavy menstrual flow). In the adult, lack of dietary iron is rarely the sole cause of iron deficiency anemia. The source of iron deficiency should be investigated promptly, because iron deficiency in an adult may be a sign of bleeding in the GI tract or colon cancer.

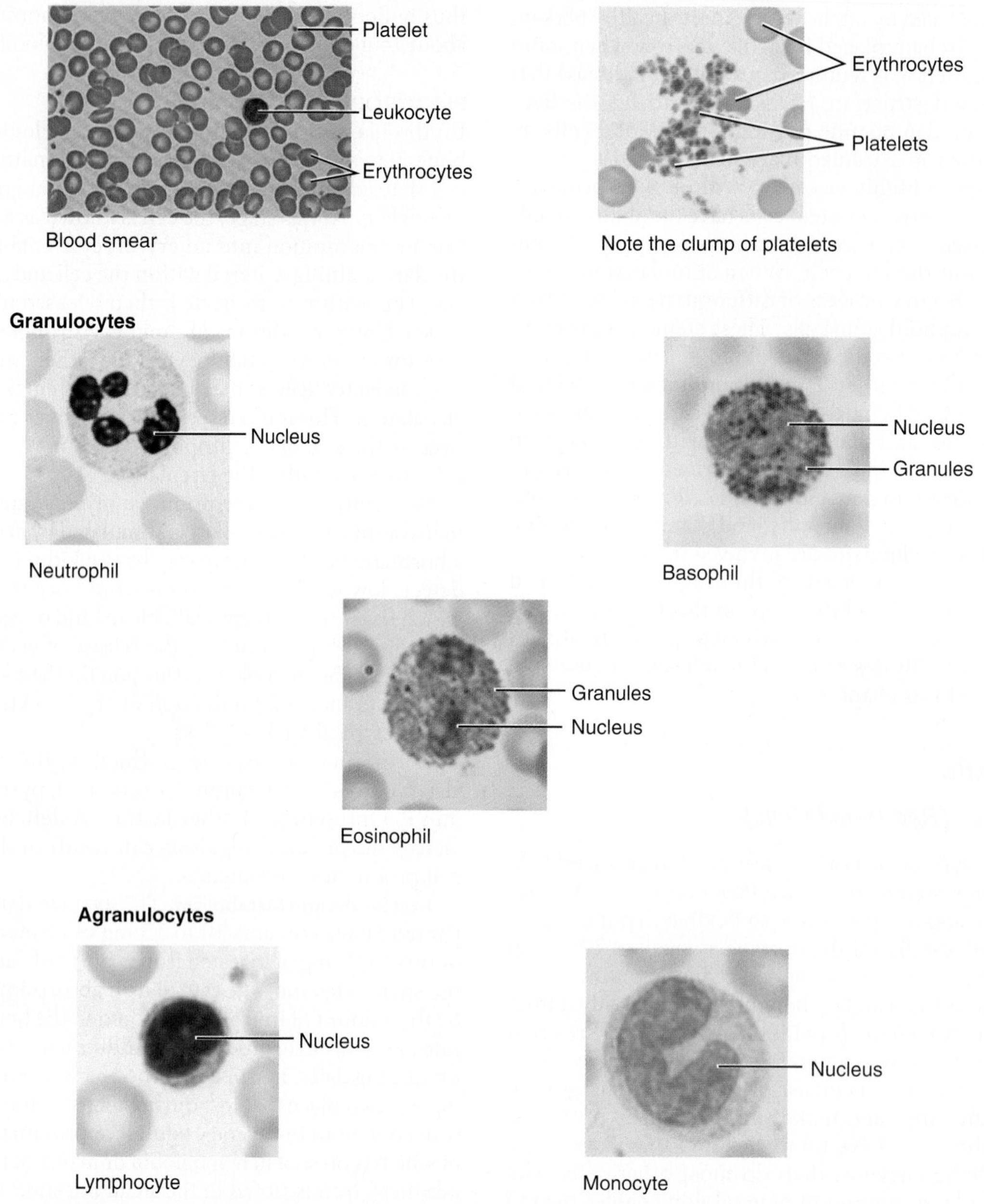

FIGURE 33-2. Normal types of blood cells. From Cohen, B. J. (2005). *Memmler's the human body in health and disease* (10th ed.). Philadelphia: Lippincott Williams & Wilkins.

Vitamin B_{12} and Folic Acid Metabolism. Vitamin B_{12} and folic acid are required for the synthesis of DNA in many tissues, but deficiencies of either of these vitamins have the greatest effect on erythropoiesis. Both vitamin B_{12} and folic acid are derived from the diet. Folic acid is absorbed in the proximal small intestine, but only small amounts are stored within the body. If the diet is deficient in folic acid, stores within the body quickly become depleted. Because vitamin B_{12} is found only in foods of animal origin, strict vegetarians may ingest little vitamin B_{12}. Vitamin B_{12} combines with intrinsic factor produced in the stomach. The vitamin B_{12}–intrinsic factor complex is absorbed in the distal ileum. People who have had a partial or total gastrectomy may have limited amounts of intrinsic factor, and therefore the absorption of vitamin B_{12} may be diminished. The effects of either decreased absorption or decreased intake of vitamin B_{12} are not apparent for 2 to 4 years.

Vitamin B_{12} and folic acid deficiencies are characterized by the production of abnormally large erythrocytes called megaloblasts. Because these cells are abnormal, many are sequestered (trapped) while still in the bone marrow, and their rate of release is decreased. Some of these cells actually die in the marrow before they can be released into the circulation. This results in megaloblastic anemia.

RED BLOOD CELL DESTRUCTION

The average life span of a normal circulating erythrocyte is 120 days. Aged erythrocytes lose their elasticity and become trapped in small blood vessels and the spleen. They are removed from the blood by the reticuloendothelial cells, particularly in the liver and the spleen. As the erythrocytes are destroyed, most of their hemoglobin is recycled. Some hemoglobin also breaks down to form bilirubin and is secreted in the bile. Most of the iron is recycled to form new hemoglobin molecules within the bone marrow; small amounts are lost daily in the feces and urine and monthly in menstrual flow.

Leukocytes (White Blood Cells)

Leukocytes are divided into two general categories: granulocytes and lymphocytes. In normal blood, the total leukocyte count is 5,000 to 10,000 cells per cubic millimeter. Of these, approximately 60% to 70% are granulocytes and 30% to 40% are lymphocytes. Both of these types of leukocytes primarily protect the body against infection and tissue injury.

GRANULOCYTES

Granulocytes are defined by the presence of granules in the cytoplasm of the cell. Granulocytes are divided into three main subgroups, which are characterized by the staining properties of these granules (see Fig. 33-2). Eosinophils have bright-red granules in their cytoplasm, whereas the granules in basophils stain deep blue. The third and by far the most numerous cell in this class is the neutrophil, with granules that stain a pink to violet hue. Neutrophils are also called polymorphonuclear neutrophils (PMNs, or polys) or segmented neutrophils (segs).

The nucleus of the mature neutrophil has multiple lobes (usually two to five) that are connected by thin filaments of nuclear material, or a "segmented" nucleus; it is usually twice the size of an erythrocyte. The somewhat less mature granulocyte has a single-lobed, elongated nucleus and is called a **band cell.** Ordinarily, band cells account for only a small percentage of circulating granulocytes, although their percentage can increase greatly under conditions in which neutrophil production increases, such as infection. An increased number of band cells is sometimes called a **left shift** or **shift to the left.** (Traditionally, the diagram of neutrophil maturation showed the myeloid stem cell on the left with progressive maturation stages toward the right, ending with a fully mature neutrophil on the far right side. A shift to the left indicates that more immature cells are present in the blood than normal.)

Fully mature neutrophils result from the gradual differentiation of myeloid stem cells, specifically myeloid **blast cells.** The process, called **myelopoiesis,** is highly complex and depends on many factors. These factors, including specific **cytokines** such as growth factors, are normally present within the marrow itself. As the blast cell matures, the cytoplasm of the cell changes in color (from blue to violet) and granules begin to form with the cytoplasm. The shape of the nucleus also changes. The entire process of maturation and differentiation takes about 10 days (see Fig. 33-1). Once the neutrophil is released into the circulation from the marrow, it stays there for only about 6 hours before it migrates into the body tissues to perform its function of **phagocytosis** (ingestion and digestion of bacteria and particles) (Fig. 33-3). Here, neutrophils last no more than 1 to 2 days before they die. The number of circulating granulocytes found in the healthy person is relatively constant, but in infection large numbers of these cells are rapidly released into the circulation.

AGRANULOCYTES

Monocytes. Monocytes (also called mononuclear leukocytes) are leukocytes with a single-lobed nucleus and a granule-free cytoplasm—hence the term *agranulocyte* (see Fig. 33-2). In normal adult blood, monocytes account for

Physiology/Pathophysiology

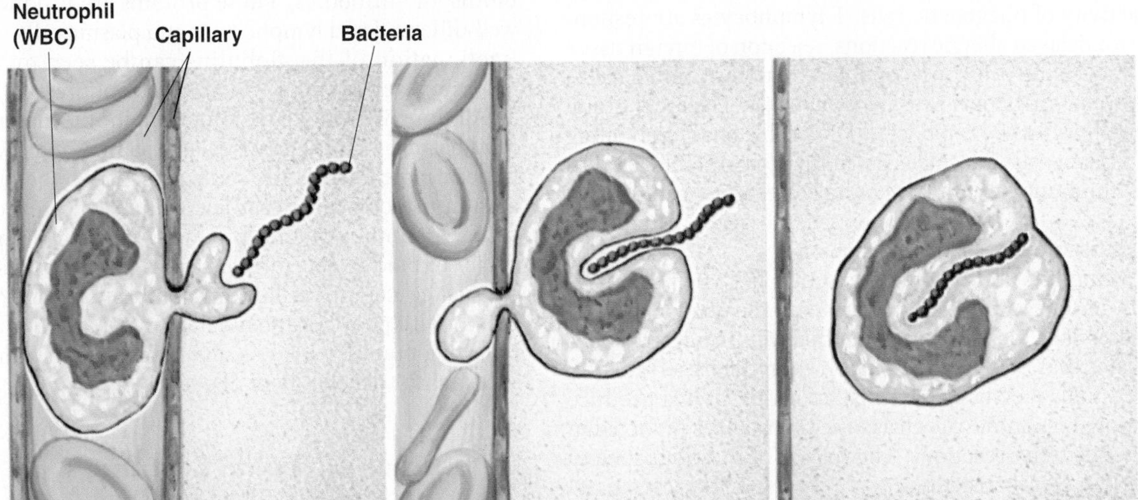

FIGURE 33-3. Phagocytosis. When foreign matter (eg, bacteria or dead tissue) comes in contact with the cell membrane of the neutrophil, the membrane surrounds and pinches off the area, leaving the membrane intact. Thus, the engulfed material is left in a vacuole within the neutrophil, where enzymes within the cell destroy the foreign material.

approximately 5% of the total leukocytes. Monocytes are the largest of the leukocytes. Produced by the bone marrow, they remain in the circulation for a short time before entering the tissues and transforming into **macrophages.** Macrophages are particularly active in the spleen, liver, peritoneum, and the alveoli; they remove debris from these areas and phagocytize bacteria within the tissues.

Lymphocytes. Mature lymphocytes are small cells with scanty cytoplasm (see Fig. 33-2). Immature lymphocytes are produced in the marrow from the lymphoid stem cells. A second major source of production is the cortex of the thymus. Cells derived from the thymus are known as T lymphocytes (or T cells); those derived from the marrow can also be T cells but are more commonly B lymphocytes (or B cells). Lymphocytes complete their differentiation and maturation primarily in the lymph nodes and in the lymphoid tissue of the intestine and spleen after exposure to a specific antigen. Mature lymphocytes are the principal cells of the immune system, producing antibodies and identifying other cells and organisms as "foreign."

FUNCTION OF LEUKOCYTES

Leukocytes protect the body from invasion by bacteria and other foreign entities. The major function of neutrophils is phagocytosis (see Fig. 33-3). Neutrophils arrive at a given site within 1 hour after the onset of an inflammatory reaction and initiate phagocytosis, but they are short-lived. An influx of monocytes follows; these cells continue their phagocytic activities for long periods as macrophages. This process constitutes a second line of defense for the body against inflammation and infection. Although neutrophils can often work adequately against bacteria without the help of macrophages, macrophages are particularly effective against fungi and viruses. Macrophages also digest senescent (aging or aged) blood cells, such as erythrocytes, primarily within the spleen.

The primary function of lymphocytes is to produce substances that aid in attacking foreign material. One group of lymphocytes (T lymphocytes) kills foreign cells directly or releases a variety of lymphokines, substances that enhance the activity of phagocytic cells. T lymphocytes are responsible for delayed allergic reactions, rejection of foreign tissue (eg, transplanted organs), and destruction of tumor cells. This process is known as *cellular immunity*. The other group of lymphocytes (B lymphocytes) is capable of differentiating into plasma cells. Plasma cells, in turn, produce antibodies called immunoglobulin (Ig), which are protein molecules that destroy foreign material by several mechanisms. This process is known as *humoral immunity*.

Eosinophils and basophils function in hypersensitivity reactions. Eosinophils are important in the phagocytosis of parasites. The increase in eosinophil levels in allergic states indicates that these cells are involved in the hypersensitivity reaction; they neutralize histamine. Basophils produce and store histamine as well as other substances involved in hypersensitivity reactions. The release of these substances provokes allergic reactions.

Platelets (Thrombocytes)

Platelets, or thrombocytes, are not technically cells; rather, they are granular fragments of giant cells in the bone marrow called megakaryocytes. Platelet production in the marrow is regulated in part by the hormone thrombopoietin, which stimulates the production and differentiation of megakaryocytes from the myeloid stem cell.

Platelets play an essential role in the control of bleeding. They circulate freely in the blood in an inactive state, where they nurture the endothelium of the blood vessels, maintaining the integrity of the vessel. When vascular injury occurs, platelets collect at the site and are activated. They adhere to the site of injury and to each other, forming a platelet plug that temporarily stops bleeding. Substances released from platelet granules activate coagulation factors in the blood plasma and initiate the formation of a stable clot composed of **fibrin**, a filamentous protein. Platelets have a normal life span of 7 to 10 days.

Plasma and Plasma Proteins

After cellular elements are removed from blood, the remaining liquid portion is called plasma. More than 90% of plasma is water. The remainder consists primarily of plasma proteins, clotting factors (particularly fibrinogen), and small amounts of other substances such as nutrients, enzymes, waste products, and gases. If plasma is allowed to clot, the remaining fluid is called **serum.** Serum has essentially the same composition as plasma, except that fibrinogen and several clotting factors have been removed in the clotting process.

Plasma proteins consist primarily of albumin and the globulins. The globulins can be separated into three main fractions (alpha, beta, and gamma), each of which consists of distinct proteins that have different functions. Important proteins in the alpha and beta fractions are the transport globulins and the clotting factors that are made in the liver. The transport globulins carry various substances in bound form in the circulation. For example, thyroid-binding globulin carries thyroxin, and transferrin carries iron. The clotting factors, including fibrinogen, remain in an inactive form in the blood plasma until activated by the clotting cascade. The gamma globulin fraction refers to the immunoglobulins, or antibodies. These proteins are produced by the well-differentiated lymphocytes and plasma cells. The actual fractionation of the globulins can be seen on a specific laboratory test (serum protein electrophoresis).

Albumin is particularly important for the maintenance of fluid balance within the vascular system. Capillary walls are impermeable to albumin, so its presence in the plasma creates an osmotic force that keeps fluid within the vascular space. Albumin, which is produced by the liver, has the capacity to bind to several substances that are transported in plasma (eg, certain medications, bilirubin, some hormones). People with poor hepatic function may have low concentrations of albumin, with a resultant decrease in osmotic pressure and the development of edema.

Reticuloendothelial System

The reticuloendothelial system (RES) is composed of special tissue macrophages, which are derived from monocytes. When released from the marrow, monocytes spend a short time in the circulation (about 24 hours) and then enter the body tissues. Within the tissues, the monocytes continue to differentiate into macrophages, which can survive for months. Macrophages have a variety of important functions. They defend the body against foreign invaders (ie, bacteria and other pathogens) via phagocytosis. They remove old or damaged cells from the circulation. They stimulate the inflammatory process and present antigens to the immune system (see Chapter 50). Macrophages give rise to tissue **histiocytes**, including Kupffer cells of the liver, peritoneal macrophages, alveolar macrophages, and other components of the RES. Thus, the RES is a component of many other organs within the body, particularly the spleen, lymph nodes, lungs, and liver.

The spleen is the site of activity for most macrophages. Most of the spleen (75%) is made of red pulp; here the blood enters the venous sinuses through capillaries that are surrounded by macrophages. Within the red pulp are tiny aggregates of white pulp, consisting of B and T lymphocytes. The spleen sequesters newly released reticulocytes from the marrow, removing nuclear fragments and other materials (eg, denatured hemoglobin, iron) before the now fully mature erythrocyte returns to the circulation. Although a minority of erythrocytes (less than 5%) is pooled in the spleen, a significant proportion of platelets (20% to 40%) is pooled here. If the spleen is enlarged, a greater proportion of red cells and platelets can be sequestered. The spleen is a major source of hematopoiesis in fetal life. It can resume hematopoiesis later in adulthood if necessary, particularly when marrow function is compromised (eg, in bone marrow fibrosis). The spleen has important immunologic functions as well. It forms substances called opsonins that promote the phagocytosis of neutrophils; it also forms the antibody IgM after exposure to an antigen.

Hemostasis

Hemostasis is the process of preventing blood loss from intact vessels and of stopping bleeding from a severed vessel. The prevention of blood loss from intact vessels requires adequate numbers of functional platelets. Platelets nurture the endothelium and thereby maintain the structural integrity of the vessel wall. Two processes are involved in arresting bleeding: primary and secondary hemostasis (Fig. 33-4).

In primary hemostasis, the severed blood vessel constricts. Circulating platelets aggregate at the site and adhere to the vessel and to one another. An unstable hemostatic plug is formed. For the coagulation process to be correctly activated, circulating inactive coagulation factors must be converted to active forms. This process occurs on the surface of the aggregated platelets at the site of vessel injury. The end result is the formation of fibrin, which reinforces the platelet plug and anchors it to the injury site. This process is termed secondary hemostasis. The process of blood coagulation is highly complex. It can be activated by the intrinsic or the extrinsic pathway. Both pathways are needed for maintenance of normal hemostasis.

Many factors are involved in the reaction cascade that forms fibrin. When tissue is injured, the extrinsic pathway is activated by the release of thromboplastin from the tissue. As the result of a series of reactions, prothrombin is converted to **thrombin**, which in turn catalyzes the conversion of fibrinogen to fibrin. Clotting by the intrinsic pathway is activated when the collagen that lines blood vessels is exposed. Clotting factors are activated sequentially until, as with the extrinsic pathway, fibrin is ultimately formed. Although the intrinsic pathway is slower, this sequence is probably most often responsible for clotting in vivo.

As the injured vessel is repaired and again covered with endothelial cells, the fibrin clot is no longer needed. The fibrin is digested via two systems: the plasma fibrinolytic system and the cellular fibrinolytic system. The substance **plasminogen** is required to lyse (break down) the fibrin. Plasminogen, which is present in all body fluids, circulates with fibrinogen and is therefore incorporated into the fibrin clot as it forms. When the clot is no longer needed (eg, after an injured blood vessel has healed), the plasminogen is activated to form plasmin. Plasmin digests the fibrinogen and fibrin. The breakdown particles of the clot, called fibrin degradation products, are released into the circulation. Through this system, clots are dissolved as tissue is repaired, and the vascular system returns to its normal baseline state.

Gerontologic Considerations

In elderly patients, the bone marrow's ability to respond to the body's need for blood cells (erythrocytes, leukocytes, and platelets) may be decreased. This decreased ability is a result of many factors, including diminished production of the growth factors necessary for hematopoiesis by stromal cells within the marrow or a diminished response to the growth factors (in the case of erythropoietin). In addition, in elderly patients, the bone marrow may be more susceptible to the myelosuppressive effects of medications. As a result of these factors, when an elderly person needs more blood cells (eg, leukocytes in infection, erythrocytes in anemia), the bone marrow may not be able to increase production of these cells adequately. **Leukopenia** (a decreased number of circulating leukocytes) or anemia can result.

Anemia is the most common hematologic condition affecting elderly patients; with each successive decade of life, the incidence of anemia increases. Anemia frequently results from iron deficiency (in the case of blood loss) or from a nutritional deficiency, particularly folate or vitamin B_{12} deficiency or protein-calorie malnutrition; it may also result from inflammation or chronic disease. Management of the disorder varies depending on the etiology. Therefore, it is important to identify the cause of the anemia rather than to consider it an inevitable consequence of aging. Elderly people with concurrent cardiac or pulmonary problems may not tolerate anemia very well, and a prompt, thorough evaluation is warranted.

Assessment of Hematologic Disorders

Most hematologic diseases reflect a defect in the hematopoietic, hemostatic, or reticuloendothelial system. The defect can be quantitative (eg, increased or decreased production of cells), qualitative (eg, the cells that are produced are defective in their normal functional capacity), or both.

Initially, many hematologic conditions cause few symptoms. Therefore, extensive laboratory tests are often required to diagnose a hematologic disorder. For most hematologic

Physiology/Pathophysiology

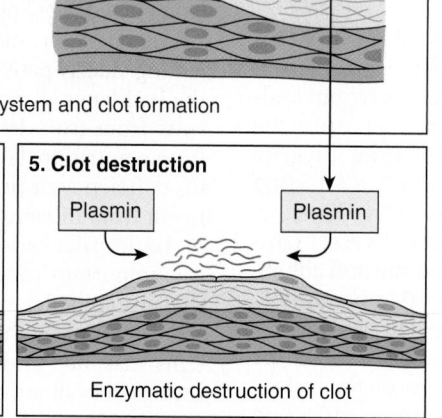

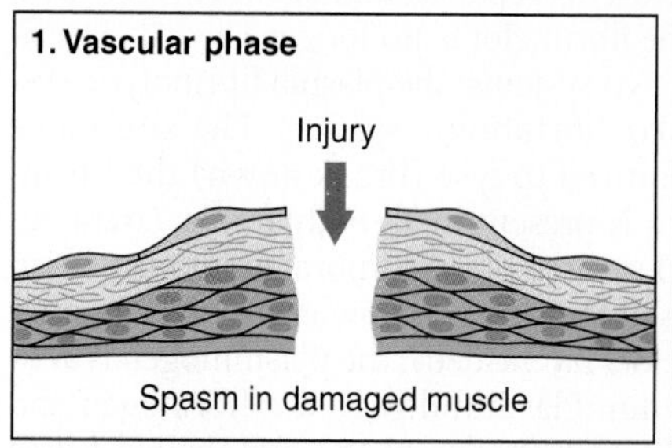

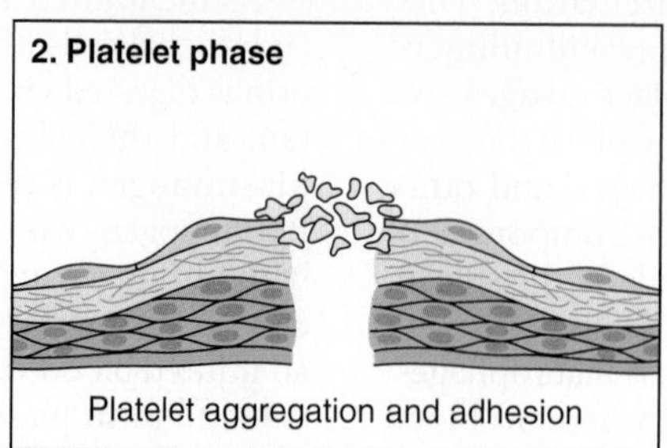

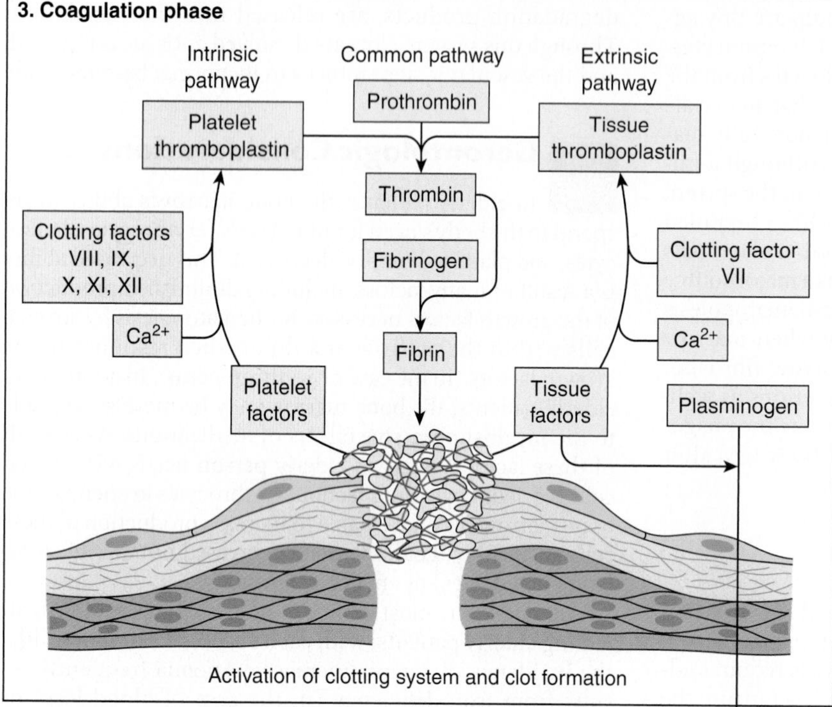

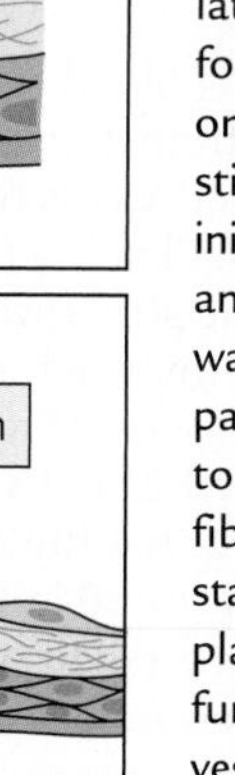

FIGURE 33-4. Hemostasis. When the endothelial surface of a blood vessel is injured, several processes occur. In primary hemostasis, platelets within the circulation are attracted to the exposed layer of collagen at the site of injury. They adhere to the site of injury, releasing factors that stimulate other platelets to aggregate at the site, forming an unstable platelet plug. In secondary hemostasis, based on the type of stimulus, one of two clotting pathways is initiated—the intrinsic or extrinsic pathway—and the clotting factors within that pathway are activated. The end result from either pathway is the conversion of prothrombin to thrombin. Thrombin is necessary for fibrinogen to be converted into fibrin, the stabilizing protein that anchors the fragile platelet plug to the site of injury to prevent further bleeding and permit the injuring vessel or site to heal. Modified from www.irvingcrowley.com/cls/clotting.gif.

conditions, continued monitoring via specific blood tests is required because it is very important to assess for changes in test results over time. In general, it is important to assess trends in blood counts because these trends help the clinician decide whether the patient is responding appropriately to interventions.

Hematologic Studies

The most common tests used are the complete blood count (CBC) and the peripheral blood smear (see Appendix A). The CBC identifies the total number of blood cells (leukocytes, erythrocytes, and platelets) as well as the hemoglobin, **hematocrit** (percentage of blood volume consisting of erythrocytes), and RBC indices. Because cellular morphology (shape and appearance of the cells) is particularly important in most hematologic disorders, the blood cells involved must be examined. This process is referred to as the manual examination of the peripheral smear, which may be part of the CBC. In this test, a drop of blood is spread on a glass slide, stained, and examined under a microscope. The shape and size of the erythrocytes and platelets, as well as the actual appearance of the leukocytes, provide useful information in identifying hematologic conditions. Blood for the CBC is typically obtained by venipuncture.

Bone Marrow Aspiration and Biopsy

The bone marrow aspiration and biopsy are crucial when additional information is needed to assess how a person's blood cells are being formed and to assess the quantity and quality of each type of cell produced within the marrow. These tests are also used to document infection or tumor within the marrow.

Normal bone marrow is in a semifluid state and can be aspirated through a special large needle. In adults, bone marrow is usually aspirated from the iliac crest and occasionally from the sternum. The aspirate provides only a sample of cells. Aspirate alone may be adequate for evaluating certain conditions, such as anemia. However, when more information is required, a biopsy is also performed. Biopsy samples are taken from the posterior iliac crest; occasionally, an anterior approach is required. A marrow biopsy shows the architecture of the bone marrow as well as its degree of cellularity.

Most patients need no more preparation than a careful explanation of the procedure, but for some very anxious patients, an antianxiety agent may be useful. It is always important for the physician or nurse to describe and explain to the patient the procedure and the sensations that will be experienced. The risks, benefits, and alternatives are also discussed. A signed informed consent is needed before the procedure is performed.

Before aspiration, the skin is cleansed as for any minor surgery, using aseptic technique. Then a small area is anesthetized with a local anesthetic through the skin and subcutaneous tissue to the periosteum of the bone. It is not possible to anesthetize the bone itself. The bone marrow needle is introduced with a stylet in place. When the needle is felt to go through the outer cortex of bone and enter the marrow cavity, the stylet is removed, a syringe is attached, and a small volume (0.5 mL) of blood and marrow is aspirated. Patients typically feel a pressure sensation as the needle is advanced into position. The actual aspiration always causes sharp but brief pain, resulting from the suction exerted as the marrow is aspirated into the syringe; the patient should be warned about this. Taking deep breaths or using relaxation techniques often helps ease the discomfort.

If a bone marrow biopsy is necessary, it is best performed after the aspiration and in a slightly different location, because the marrow structure may be altered after aspiration. A special biopsy needle is used. Because these needles are large, the skin is punctured first with a surgical blade to make a 3- or 4-mm incision. The biopsy needle is advanced well into the marrow cavity. When the needle is properly positioned, a portion of marrow is cored out, using a twisting or gentle rocking motion to free the sample and permit its removal within the biopsy needle. The patient feels a pressure sensation but should not feel actual pain. The nurse should instruct the patient to inform the physician if pain occurs so that an additional anesthetic can be administered.

Hazards of either bone marrow aspiration or biopsy include bleeding and infection. The risk for bleeding is somewhat increased if the patient's platelet count is low or if the patient has been taking a medication (eg, aspirin) that alters platelet function. After the marrow sample is obtained, pressure is applied to the site for several minutes. The site is then covered with a sterile dressing. Most patients have no discomfort after a bone marrow aspiration, but the site of a biopsy may ache for 1 or 2 days. Warm tub baths and a mild analgesic (eg, acetaminophen) may be useful. Aspirin-containing analgesics should be avoided because they can aggravate or potentiate bleeding.

Anemia

Overview

Anemia, a condition in which the hemoglobin concentration is lower than normal, reflects the presence of fewer than normal erythrocytes within the circulation. As a result, the amount of oxygen delivered to body tissues is also diminished. Anemia is not a specific disease state per se but a sign of an underlying disorder. It is by far the most common hematologic condition (Table 33-2). A common

TABLE 33-2 Classification of Anemias

Type of Anemia	Laboratory Findings
Hypoproliferative (Resulting From Defective RBC Production)	
Iron deficiency	Decreased reticulocytes, iron, ferritin, iron saturation, MCV; increased TIBC
Vitamin B_{12} deficiency (megaloblastic)	Decreased vitamin B_{12} level; increased MCV
Folate deficiency (megaloblastic)	Decreased folate level; increased MCV
Decreased erythropoietin production (eg, from renal dysfunction)	Decreased erythropoietin level; normal MCV and MCH; increased creatinine level
Cancer/inflammation	Normal MCV, MCH, normal or decreased erythropoietin level; increased % of iron saturation, ferritin level; decreased iron, TIBC
Bleeding (Resulting From RBC Loss)	
Bleeding from gastrointestinal tract, menorrhagia (excessive menstrual flow), epistaxis (nosebleed), trauma	Increased reticulocyte level; normal Hgb and Hct if measured soon after bleeding starts, but levels decrease thereafter; normal MCV initially but later decreases; decreased ferritin and iron levels (later)
Hemolytic (Resulting From RBC Destruction)	
Altered erythropoiesis (sickle cell anemia, thalassemia, other hemoglobinopathies)	Decreased MCV; fragmented RBCs; increased reticulocyte level
Hypersplenism (hemolysis)	Increased MCV
Drug-induced anemia	Increased spherocyte level
Autoimmune anemia	Increased spherocyte level
Mechanical heart valve–related anemia	Fragmented red cells

Hct, hematocrit; Hgb, hemoglobin concentration; MCH, mean corpuscular hemoglobin; MCV, mean corpuscular volume; RBCs, red blood cells; TIBC, total iron-binding capacity.

occurrence among all age groups, it is particularly prevalent among the elderly. A recent study documented the prevalence of anemia in elderly residents of skilled nursing facilities to be 48% (Artz et al., 2004).

Classification of Anemias

Anemia may be classified in several ways. A physiologic approach classifies anemia according to whether the deficiency in erythrocytes is caused by a defect in their production (hypoproliferative anemia), by their destruction (hemolytic anemia), or by their loss (bleeding).

In hypoproliferative anemias, the marrow cannot produce adequate numbers of erythrocytes. Decreased erythrocyte production is reflected by an inappropriately normal or low reticulocyte count. Inadequate production of erythrocytes may result from marrow damage due to medications (eg, chloramphenicol) or chemicals (eg, benzene) or from a lack of factors (eg, iron, vitamin B_{12}, folic acid, erythropoietin) necessary for erythrocyte formation.

In hemolytic anemias, premature destruction of erythrocytes results in the liberation of hemoglobin from the erythrocytes into the plasma. The increased erythrocyte destruction leads to tissue hypoxia, which in turn stimulates erythropoietin production. This increased production is reflected in an increased reticulocyte count as the bone marrow responds to the loss of erythrocytes. The released hemoglobin is converted in large part to bilirubin; therefore, the bilirubin concentration rises. **Hemolysis** can result from an abnormality within the erythrocyte itself (eg, sickle cell anemia, glucose-6-phosphate dehydrogenase [G-6-PD] deficiency) or within the plasma (eg, immune hemolytic anemias), or from direct injury to the erythrocyte within the circulation (eg, hemolysis caused by mechanical heart valve). Chart 33-1 identifies the causes of hemolytic anemia.

It is usually possible to determine whether the presence of anemia in a given patient is caused by destruction or by inadequate production of erythrocytes on the basis of the following factors:

- The marrow's ability to respond to decreased erythrocytes (as evidenced by an increased reticulocyte count in the circulating blood)
- The degree to which young erythrocytes proliferate in the bone marrow and the manner in which they mature (as observed on bone marrow biopsy)
- The presence or absence of end products of erythrocyte destruction within the circulation (eg, increased bilirubin level, decreased haptoglobin level)

CHART 33-1

Causes of Hemolytic Anemias

Inherited Hemolytic Anemia

- Abnormal hemoglobin
  - Sickle cell anemia*
  - Thalassemia*
- Red blood cell membrane abnormality
  - Hereditary spherocytosis*
  - Hereditary elliptocytosis
  - Acanthocytosis
  - Stomatocytosis
- Enzyme deficiencies
  - Glucose-6-phosphate dehydrogenase (G-6-PD) deficiency*

Acquired Hemolytic Anemia

- Antibody-related
  - Iso-antibody/transfusion reaction*
  - Autoimmune hemolytic anemia (AIHA)*
  - Cold agglutinin disease*
- Not antibody-related
  - Red blood cell membrane defects
  - Paroxysmal nocturnal hemoglobinuria (PNH)
  - Liver disease
  - Uremia
  - Trauma
  - Mechanical heart valve
  - Microangiopathic hemolytic anemia
  - Infection
    - Bacterial
    - Parasitic
  - Disseminated intravascular coagulation (DIC)*
  - Toxins
  - Hypersplenism*

*Discussed in text.

Clinical Manifestations

Aside from the severity of the anemia itself, several factors influence the development of anemia-associated symptoms:

- The rapidity with which the anemia has developed
- The duration of the anemia (ie, its chronicity)
- The metabolic requirements of the patient
- Other concurrent disorders or disabilities (eg, cardiopulmonary disease)
- Special complications or concomitant features of the condition that produced the anemia

In general, the more rapidly an anemia develops, the more severe its symptoms. An otherwise healthy person can often tolerate as much as a 50% gradual reduction in hemoglobin without pronounced symptoms or significant incapacity, whereas the rapid loss of as little as 30% may precipitate profound vascular collapse in the same person. A person who has become gradually anemic, with hemoglobin levels between 9 and 11 g/dL, usually has few or no symptoms other than slight tachycardia on exertion and fatigue.

People who customarily are very active or who have significant demands on their lives (eg, a single, working mother of small children) are more likely to have symptoms, and those symptoms are more likely to be pronounced than in more sedentary people. Patients with hypothyroidism with decreased oxygen needs may be completely asymptomatic, without tachycardia or increased cardiac output, at a hemoglobin level of 10 g/dL. Similarly, patients with coexistent cardiac, vascular, or pulmonary disease may develop more pronounced symptoms of anemia (eg, dyspnea, chest pain, muscle pain or cramping) at a higher hemoglobin level than those without these concurrent health problems.

Finally, some anemic disorders are complicated by various other abnormalities that do not result from the anemia but are inherently associated with these particular diseases. These abnormalities may give rise to symptoms that completely overshadow those of the anemia, as in the painful crises of sickle cell anemia.

Assessment and Diagnostic Findings

A variety of hematologic studies are performed to determine the type and cause of the anemia. In an initial evaluation, the hemoglobin, hematocrit, reticulocyte count, and RBC indices, particularly the mean corpuscular volume (MCV) and red cell distribution width (RDW), are particularly useful. Iron studies (serum iron level, total iron-binding capacity [TIBC], percent saturation, and ferritin), as well as serum vitamin B_{12} and folate levels, are also frequently obtained. Other tests include haptoglobin and erythropoietin levels. The remaining CBC values are useful in determining whether the anemia is an isolated problem or part of another hematologic condition, such as **leukemia** or myelodysplastic syndrome (MDS). Bone marrow aspiration may be performed. In addition, other diagnostic studies may be performed to determine the presence of underlying chronic illness, such as malignancy, or the source of any blood loss, such as polyps or ulcers within the GI tract.

Complications

General complications of severe anemia include heart failure, paresthesias, and confusion. At any given level of anemia, patients with underlying heart disease are far more likely to have angina or symptoms of heart failure than those without heart disease. Complications associated with specific types of anemia are included in the description of each type.

Medical Management

Management of anemia is directed toward correcting or controlling the cause of the anemia; if the anemia is severe, the erythrocytes that are lost or destroyed may be replaced with a transfusion of packed red blood cells (PRBCs). The management of the various types of anemia is covered in the discussions that follow.

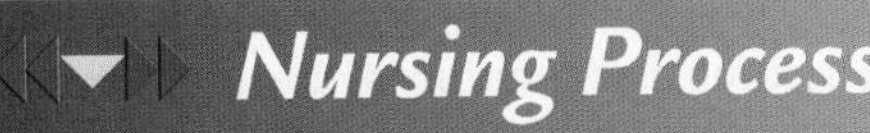

The Patient With Anemia

Assessment

The health history and physical examination provide important data about the type of anemia involved, the extent and type of symptoms it produces, and the impact of those symptoms on the patient's life. Weakness, fatigue, and general malaise are common, as are pallor of the skin and mucous membranes (conjunctivae, oral mucosa).

Jaundice may be present in patients with megaloblastic anemia or hemolytic anemia. The tongue may be smooth and red (in iron deficiency anemia) or beefy red and sore (in megaloblastic anemia); the corners of the mouth may be ulcerated (**angular cheilosis**) in both types of anemia. People with iron deficiency anemia may crave ice, starch, or dirt; this craving is known as pica. The nails may be brittle, ridged, and concave.

The health history should include a medication history, because some medications can depress bone marrow activity, induce hemolysis, or interfere with folate metabolism. An accurate history of alcohol intake, including the amount and duration, should be obtained. Family history is important, because certain anemias are inherited. Athletic endeavors should be assessed, because extreme exercise can decrease erythropoiesis and erythrocyte survival.

A nutritional assessment is important, because it may indicate deficiencies in essential nutrients such as iron, vitamin B_{12}, and folic acid. Children of indigent families may be at higher risk for anemia because of nutritional deficiencies. Strict vegetarians are also at risk for megaloblastic types of anemia if they do not supplement their diet with vitamin B_{12}.

Cardiac status should be carefully assessed. When the hemoglobin level is low, the heart attempts to compensate by pumping faster and harder in an effort to deliver more blood to hypoxic tissue. This increased cardiac workload can result in such symptoms as tachycardia, palpitations, dyspnea, dizziness, orthopnea, and exertional dyspnea. Heart failure may eventually develop, as evidenced by an enlarged heart (cardiomegaly) and liver (hepatomegaly) and by peripheral edema.

Assessment of the GI system may disclose complaints of nausea, vomiting (with specific questions about the appearance of any emesis [eg, looks like "coffee grounds"]), melena or dark stools, diarrhea, anorexia, and glossitis (inflammation of the tongue). Stools should be tested for occult blood. Women should be questioned about their menstrual periods (eg, excessive menstrual flow, other vaginal bleeding) and the use of iron supplements during pregnancy.

The neurologic examination is also important because of the effect of pernicious anemia on the central and peripheral nervous systems. Assessment should include the presence and extent of peripheral numbness and paresthesias, ataxia, poor coordination, and confusion. Finally, it is important to monitor relevant laboratory test results and to note any changes over time.

Diagnosis

Nursing Diagnoses

Based on the assessment data, major nursing diagnoses for the patient with anemia may include:

- Fatigue related to decreased hemoglobin and diminished oxygen-carrying capacity of the blood

- Altered nutrition, less than body requirements, related to inadequate intake of essential nutrients
- Altered tissue perfusion related to inadequate blood volume or hematocrit
- Noncompliance with prescribed therapy

Collaborative Problems/ Potential Complications

Based on the assessment data, potential complications that may develop include:

- Heart failure
- Angina
- Paresthesias
- Confusion

Planning and Goals

The major goals for the patient may include decreased fatigue, attainment or maintenance of adequate nutrition, maintenance of adequate tissue perfusion, compliance with prescribed therapy, and absence of complications.

Nursing Interventions

Managing Fatigue

The most common symptom and complication of anemia is fatigue. This distressing symptom is too often minimized by health care providers. Fatigue is often the symptom that has the greatest negative impact on a patient's level of functioning and consequent quality of life. Patients often describe the fatigue from anemia as oppressive. Fatigue can be significant, yet the anemia may not be severe enough to warrant transfusion. Fatigue can interfere with a person's ability to work, both inside and outside the home. It can harm relationships with family and friends. Patients often lose interest in hobbies and activities, including sexual activity. The distress from fatigue is often related to a person's responsibilities and life demands as well as the amount of assistance and support received from others.

Nursing interventions can focus on assisting the patient to prioritize activities and to establish a balance between activity and rest that is realistic and feasible from the patient's perspective. Patients with chronic anemia need to maintain some physical activity and exercise to prevent the deconditioning that results from inactivity.

Maintaining Adequate Nutrition

Inadequate intake of essential nutrients, such as iron, vitamin B_{12}, folic acid, and protein, can cause some anemias. The symptoms associated with anemia (eg, fatigue, anorexia) can in turn interfere with maintaining adequate nutrition. A healthy diet should be encouraged. The nurse should inform the patient that alcohol interferes with the utilization of essential nutrients and should advise the patient to avoid alcoholic beverages or to limit their intake. Dietary teaching sessions should be individualized and include cultural aspects related to food preferences and food preparation. The involvement of family members enhances compliance with dietary recommendations. Dietary supplements (eg, vitamins, iron, folate, protein) may be prescribed as well.

Equally important, the patient and family must understand the role of nutritional supplements in the proper context, because many forms of anemia are not the result of a nutritional deficiency. In such cases, even an excessive intake of nutritional supplements will not improve the anemia. A potential problem in patients with chronic transfusion requirements occurs with the indiscriminate use of iron supplements. Unless an aggressive program of chelation therapy is implemented, these people are at risk for iron overload from their transfusions. The addition of an iron supplement only exacerbates the situation.

Maintaining Adequate Perfusion

Patients with acute blood loss or severe hemolysis may have decreased tissue perfusion from decreased blood volume or reduced circulating erythrocytes (decreased hematocrit). Lost volume is replaced with transfusions or intravenous (IV) fluids, based on the symptoms and the laboratory test results. Supplemental oxygen may be necessary, but it is rarely needed on a long-term basis unless there is underlying severe cardiac or pulmonary disease. The nurse monitors the patient's vital signs and pulse oximeter readings closely; other medications, such as antihypertensive agents, may need to be adjusted or withheld.

Promoting Compliance With Prescribed Therapy

For patients with anemia, medications or nutritional supplements are often prescribed to alleviate or correct the condition. These patients need to understand the purpose of the medication, how to take the medication and over what time period, and how to manage any side effects of therapy. To enhance compliance, the nurse assists the patient to develop ways to incorporate the therapeutic plan into everyday activities, rather than merely giving the patient a list of instructions. For example, many patients have difficulty taking iron supplements because of related GI effects. Rather than seeking assistance from a health care provider in managing the problem, some patients simply stop taking the iron.

Abruptly stopping some medications can have serious consequences, as in the case of high-dose corticosteroids to manage hemolytic anemias. Some medications, such as growth factors, are extremely expensive. Patients receiving these medications may need assistance to obtain needed insurance coverage or to explore alternative ways to obtain these medications.

Monitoring and Managing Potential Complications

A significant complication of anemia is heart failure from chronic diminished blood volume and the heart's compensatory effort to increase cardiac output. Patients with anemia should be assessed for signs and symptoms of heart failure. A daily record of body weight can be more useful and accurate than a record of intake and output. Diuretics may be required if fluid retention results from heart failure.

In megaloblastic forms of anemia, the significant potential complications are neurologic. A neurologic assessment should be performed for patients with known or suspected megaloblastic anemia. Patients may initially complain of paresthesias in their lower extremities. These paresthesias are usually manifested as numbness and tingling on the bottom of the foot, and they gradually progress. As the anemia progresses, other signs become apparent. Position and vibration sense may be diminished; difficulty maintaining balance is not uncommon, and some patients have gait disturbances as well. Initially mild confusion may develop; it may become severe.

Evaluation

Expected Patient Outcomes

Expected patient outcomes may include:

1. Reports less fatigue
   a. Follows a progressive plan of rest, activity, and exercise
   b. Prioritizes activities
   c. Paces activities according to energy level
2. Attains and maintains adequate nutrition
   a. Eats a healthy diet
   b. Develops a meal plan that promotes optimal nutrition
   c. Maintains adequate amounts of iron, vitamins, and protein from diet or supplements
   d. Adheres to nutritional supplement therapy when prescribed
   e. Verbalizes understanding of rationale for using recommended nutritional supplements
   f. Verbalizes understanding of rationale for avoiding nonrecommended nutritional supplements
3. Maintains adequate perfusion
   a. Has vital signs within baseline for patient
   b. Has pulse oximetry (arterial oxygenation) value within normal limits
4. Absence of complications
   a. Avoids or limits activities that cause dyspnea, palpitations, dizziness, or tachycardia
   b. Uses rest and comfort measures to alleviate dyspnea
   c. Has vital signs within baseline for patient
   d. Has no signs of increasing fluid retention (eg, peripheral edema, decreased urine output, neck vein distention)
   e. Remains oriented to time, place, and situation
   f. Ambulates safely, using assistive devices as necessary
   g. Remains free of injury
   h. Verbalizes understanding of importance of serial CBC measurements
   i. Maintains safe home environment; obtains assistance as necessary

Hypoproliferative Anemias

Iron Deficiency Anemia

Iron deficiency anemia typically results when the intake of dietary iron is inadequate for hemoglobin synthesis. The body can store about one fourth to one third of its iron, and it is not until those stores are depleted that iron deficiency anemia actually begins to develop. Iron deficiency anemia is the most common type of anemia in all age groups, and it is the most common anemia in the world. It is particularly prevalent in developing countries, where inadequate iron stores can result from inadequate intake of iron (seen with vegetarian diets) or from blood loss (eg, from intestinal hookworm). Iron deficiency is also common in the United States. In children, adolescents, and pregnant women, the cause is typically inadequate iron in the diet to keep up with increased growth. However, for most adults with iron deficiency anemia, the cause is blood loss. In fact, in adults, the cause of iron deficiency anemia should be considered to be bleeding until proven otherwise.

The most common cause of iron deficiency anemia in men and postmenopausal women is bleeding (from ulcers, gastritis, inflammatory bowel disease, or GI tumors). The most common cause of iron deficiency anemia in premenopausal women is menorrhagia (excessive menstrual bleeding) and pregnancy with inadequate iron supplementation. Patients with chronic alcoholism often have chronic blood loss from the GI tract, which causes iron loss and eventual anemia. Other causes include iron malabsorption, as is seen after gastrectomy or with celiac disease.

Clinical Manifestations

Patients with iron deficiency primarily have the symptoms of anemia. If the deficiency is severe or prolonged, they may also have a smooth, sore tongue; brittle and ridged nails; and angular cheilosis (an ulceration of the corner of the mouth). These signs subside after iron replacement therapy. The health history may be significant for multiple pregnancies, gastrointestinal bleeding, and pica (a craving for unusual substances).

Assessment and Diagnostic Findings

The definitive method of establishing the diagnosis of iron deficiency anemia is bone marrow aspiration. The aspirate is stained to detect iron, which is at a low level or even absent. However, few patients with suspected iron deficiency anemia undergo bone marrow aspiration. In many patients, the diagnosis can be established with other tests, particularly in patients with a history of conditions that predispose them to this type of anemia.

There is a strong correlation between laboratory values that measure iron stores and hemoglobin levels. After iron stores are depleted (as reflected by low serum ferritin levels), the hemoglobin level falls. The diminished iron stores cause small erythrocytes to be produced by the marrow. Therefore, as the anemia progresses, the MCV, which measures the size of the erythrocytes, also decreases. Hematocrit and RBC levels are also low in relation to the hemoglobin level. Other laboratory tests that measure iron stores are useful but are not as consistent indicators as a low ferritin level, which reflects low iron stores. Typically, patients with iron deficiency anemia have a low serum iron level and an elevated TIBC, which measures the transport protein supplying the marrow with iron as needed (also referred to as transferrin). However, other disease states, such as infection and inflammatory conditions, can also cause a low serum iron level and TIBC, as well as an elevated ferritin level. Currently, the most reliable and clinically useful laboratory findings in evaluating iron deficiency anemia are the ferritin and hemoglobin values.

Medical Management

Except in the case of pregnancy, the cause of iron deficiency should be investigated. Anemia may be a sign of a curable GI cancer or of uterine fibroid tumors. Stool specimens should be tested for occult blood. People 50 years of age or older should have periodic colonoscopy, endoscopy, or x-ray examination of the GI tract to detect ulcerations, gastritis, polyps, or cancer. Several oral iron preparations—ferrous sulfate, ferrous gluconate, and ferrous fumarate—are available for treating iron deficiency anemia. The hemoglobin level may increase in only a few weeks, and the anemia can be corrected in a few months. Iron store replenishment takes much longer, so it is important that the patient continue taking the iron for as long as 6 to 12 months. Vitamin C facilitates the absorption of iron.

In some cases, oral iron is poorly absorbed or poorly tolerated, or iron supplementation is needed in large amounts. In these situations, IV or intramuscular (IM) administration of iron dextran may be needed. Before parenteral administration of a full dose, a small test dose should be administered parenterally to avoid the risk of anaphylaxis with either IV or IM injections. Emergency medications (eg, epinephrine) should be close at hand. If no signs of allergic reaction have occurred after 30 minutes, the remaining dose of iron may be administered. Several doses are required to replenish the patient's iron stores.

Nursing Management

Preventive education is important, because iron deficiency anemia is common in menstruating and pregnant women. Food sources high in iron include organ meats (beef or calf's liver, chicken liver), other meats, beans (black, pinto, and garbanzo), leafy green vegetables, raisins, and molasses. Taking iron-rich foods with a source of vitamin C (eg, orange juice) enhances the absorption of iron.

The nurse helps the patient select a healthy diet. Nutritional counseling can be provided for those whose usual diet is inadequate. Patients with a history of eating fad diets or strict vegetarian diets are counseled that such diets often contain inadequate amounts of absorbable iron. The nurse encourages the patient to continue iron therapy as long as it is prescribed, although the patient may no longer feel fatigued.

Because iron is best absorbed on an empty stomach, the patient is instructed to take the supplement an hour before meals. Iron supplements are usually given in the oral form, typically as ferrous sulfate. Most patients can use the less expensive, more standard forms of ferrous sulfate. Tablets with enteric coating may be poorly absorbed and should be avoided. Many patients have difficulty tolerating iron supplements because of GI side effects (primarily constipation, but also cramping, nausea, and vomiting). Some iron formulations are designed to limit GI side effects by the addition of a stool softener or use of sustained-release formulations to limit nausea or gastritis. Specific patient teaching aids (Chart 33-2) can assist patients with the use of iron supplements.

If taking iron on an empty stomach causes gastric distress, the patient may need to take it with meals. However, doing so diminishes iron absorption by as much as 50%, thus prolonging the time required to replenish iron stores. Antacids or dairy products should not be taken with iron, because they greatly diminish its absorption. Polysaccharide iron complex forms that have less GI toxicity are also available, but they are more expensive.

Liquid forms of iron that cause less GI distress are available. However, they can stain the teeth; the patient should be instructed to take this medication through a straw, to rinse the mouth with water, and to practice good oral hygiene

CHART 33-2

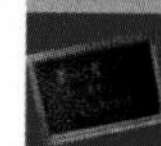

Patient Education

Taking Oral Iron Supplements

- Take iron on an empty stomach (1 hour before or 2 hours after a meal). Iron absorption is reduced with food, especially dairy products.
- To prevent gastrointestinal distress, the following schedule may work better if more than one tablet a day is prescribed: Start with only one tablet per day for a few days, then increase to two tablets per day, then three tablets per day. This method permits the body to adjust gradually to the iron.
- Increase the intake of vitamin C (citrus fruits and juices, strawberries, tomatoes, broccoli), to enhance iron absorption.
- Eat foods high in fiber to minimize problems with constipation.
- Remember that stools will become dark in color.
- To prevent staining the teeth with a liquid preparation, use a straw or place a spoon at the back of the mouth to take the supplement. Rinse the mouth thoroughly afterward.

after taking this medication. Finally, the patient should be informed that iron salts may color the stool dark green or black. However, iron replacement therapy does not cause a false-positive result on stool analyses for occult blood.

IV supplementation may be used when the patient's iron stores are completely depleted, the patient cannot tolerate oral forms of iron supplementation (see Medical Management), or both. IM supplementation is used infrequently. The volume of iron required when administered IM may be excessive. The IM injection causes some local pain and can stain the skin. These side effects are minimized by using the Z-track technique for administering iron dextran deep into the gluteus maximus muscle (buttock). The nurse avoids vigorously rubbing the injection site after the injection. Because of the problems with IM administration, the IV route is preferred for administration of iron dextran.

Anemias in Renal Disease

The degree of anemia in patients with end-stage renal disease varies greatly, but in general patients do not become significantly anemic until the serum creatinine level exceeds 3 mg/100 mL. The symptoms of anemia are often the most disturbing of the patient's symptoms. If untreated, the hematocrit usually falls to between 20% and 30%, although in rare cases it may fall to less than 15%. The erythrocytes appear normal on the peripheral smear.

This anemia is caused by both a mild shortening of erythrocyte life span and a deficiency of erythropoietin (necessary for erythropoiesis). As renal function decreases, erythropoietin, which is produced by the kidney, also decreases. Because erythropoietin is also produced outside the kidney, some erythropoiesis continues, even in patients whose kidneys have been removed. However, the number of red blood cells produced is small and the degree of erythropoiesis is inadequate.

Patients undergoing long-term hemodialysis lose blood into the dialyzer and therefore may become iron deficient. Folic acid deficiency develops because this vitamin passes into the dialysate. Therefore, patients who receive hemodialysis and who have anemia should be evaluated for iron and folate deficiency and treated appropriately.

The availability of recombinant erythropoietin (epoetin alfa [Epogen, Procrit]; darbepoetin alfa [Aranesp]) has dramatically altered the management of anemia in end-stage renal disease by decreasing the need for RBC transfusion, with its associated risks. Erythropoietin, in combination with oral iron supplements, can raise and maintain hematocrit levels to between 33% and 38%. This treatment has been successful with dialysis patients. Hypertension is the most serious side effect in this patient population when the hematocrit rapidly increases to a high level. Therefore, the hematocrit should be checked frequently when a patient with renal disease begins erythropoietin therapy. The dose of erythropoietin should be titrated to the hematocrit. In some patients, the elevated hematocrit and associated hypertension may necessitate antihypertensive therapy.

Anemia of Chronic Disease

The term "anemia of chronic disease" is a misnomer in that only the chronic diseases of inflammation, infection, and malignancy cause this type of anemia. Many chronic inflammatory diseases are associated with a **normochromic, normocytic** anemia (ie, the erythrocytes are normal in color and size). These disorders include rheumatoid arthritis; severe, chronic infections; and many cancers. It is therefore imperative that the "chronic disease" be diagnosed when this form of anemia is identified so that it can be appropriately managed.

The anemia is usually mild to moderate and nonprogressive. It develops gradually over 6 to 8 weeks and then stabilizes at a hematocrit seldom less than 25%. The hemoglobin level rarely falls below 9 g/dL, and the bone marrow has normal cellularity with increased stores of iron as the iron is diverted from the serum. Erythropoietin levels are low, perhaps because of decreased production, and iron use is blocked by **erythroid cells** (cells that are or will become mature erythrocytes). A moderate shortening of erythrocyte survival also occurs.

Most of these patients have few symptoms and do not require treatment for the anemia. With successful treatment of the underlying disorder, the bone marrow iron is used to make erythrocytes and the hemoglobin level rises.

Aplastic Anemia

Aplastic anemia is a rare disease caused by a decrease in or damage to marrow stem cells, damage to the microenvironment within the marrow, and replacement of the marrow with fat. The precise etiology is unknown, but it is hypothesized that the body's T cells mediate an inappropriate attack against the bone marrow (Bevans & Shalabi, 2004), resulting in bone marrow **aplasia** (markedly reduced hematopoiesis). Therefore, in addition to severe anemia, significant **neutropenia** and thrombocytopenia (a deficiency of platelets) are also seen.

Pathophysiology

Aplastic anemia can be congenital or acquired, but most cases are idiopathic (ie, without apparent cause). Infections and pregnancy can trigger it, or it may be caused by certain medications, chemicals, or radiation damage. Agents that regularly produce marrow aplasia include benzene and benzene derivatives (eg, airplane glue). Certain toxic materials, such as inorganic arsenic and several pesticides (including dichlorodiphenyltrichloroethane [DDT], which is no longer used or available in the United States), have also been implicated as potential causes.

Clinical Manifestations

The manifestations of aplastic anemia are often insidious. Complications resulting from bone marrow failure may occur before the diagnosis is established. Typical complications are infection and symptoms of anemia (eg, fatigue, pallor, dyspnea). Purpura (bruising) may develop later and should trigger a CBC and hematologic evaluation if these were not performed initially. If the patient has had repeated throat infections, cervical lymphadenopathy may be seen. Other lymphadenopathies and splenomegaly sometimes occur. Retinal hemorrhages are common.

Assessment and Diagnostic Findings

In many situations, aplastic anemia occurs when a medication or chemical is ingested in toxic amounts. However, in a few people, it develops after a medication has been taken at the recommended dosage. This may be considered an idiosyncratic reaction in those who are highly susceptible, possibly caused by a genetic defect in the medication biotransformation or elimination process. A bone marrow aspirate shows an extremely hypoplastic or even aplastic (very few to no cells) marrow replaced with fat.

Medical Management

It is presumed that the lymphocytes of patients with aplastic anemia destroy the stem cells and consequently impair the production of erythrocytes, leukocytes, and platelets. Despite its severity, aplastic anemia can be treated in most people. Those who are younger than 60 years, who are otherwise healthy, and who have a compatible donor can be cured of the disease by a bone marrow transplant (BMT) or peripheral blood stem cell transplant (PBSCT). In others, the disease can be managed with immunosuppressive therapy, commonly using a combination of antithymocyte globulin (ATG) and cyclosporine. ATG, a purified gamma globulin solution, is obtained from horses or rabbits immunized with human T lymphocytes (Bevans & Shalabi, 2004). Side effects during the infusion are common and may include fever and chills. The sudden onset of a rash or bronchospasm may herald anaphylaxis and requires prompt management (see Chapters 53 and 71). Serum sickness, as evidenced by fever, rash, arthralgias, and pruritus, may develop in some patients; it may take weeks to resolve. A recent study showed that 122 patients receiving this immunosuppressive treatment had a 55% 7-year survival rate (Rosenfeld et al., 2003).

Immunosuppressants prevent the patient's lymphocytes from destroying the stem cells. If relapse occurs (ie, the patient becomes pancytopenic again), reinstitution of the same immunologic agents may induce another remission. Corticosteroids are not very useful as immunosuppressive agents, because patients with aplastic anemia are particularly susceptible to the development of bone complications from corticosteroids (ie, aseptic necrosis of the head of the femur).

Supportive therapy plays a major role in the management of aplastic anemia. Any offending agent is discontinued. The patient is supported with transfusions of PRBCs and platelets as necessary. Death usually is caused by hemorrhage or infection.

Nursing Management

Patients with aplastic anemia are vulnerable to problems related to erythrocyte, leukocyte, and platelet deficiencies. They should be assessed carefully for signs of infection and bleeding. Specific interventions are delineated in the sections on neutropenia and thrombocytopenia.

Megaloblastic Anemias

In the anemias caused by deficiencies of vitamin B_{12} or folic acid, identical bone marrow and peripheral blood changes occur because both vitamins are essential for normal DNA synthesis. In either anemia, the erythrocytes that are produced are abnormally large and are called megaloblastic red cells. Other cells derived from the myeloid stem cell (nonlymphoid leukocytes, platelets) are also abnormal. A bone marrow analysis reveals **hyperplasia** (abnormal increase in the number of cells), and the precursor erythroid and myeloid cells are large and bizarre in appearance. However, many of these abnormal erythroid and myeloid cells are destroyed within the marrow, so the mature cells that do leave the marrow are actually fewer in number. Thus, **pancytopenia** (a decrease in all myeloid-derived cells) can develop. In advanced stages of disease, the hemoglobin value may be as low as 4 to 5 g/dL, the leukocyte count 2,000 to 3,000/mm^3, and the platelet count less than 50,000/mm^3. Those cells that are released into the circulation are often abnormally shaped. The neutrophils are hypersegmented. The platelets may be abnormally large. The erythrocytes are abnormally shaped, and the shapes may vary widely (**poikilocytosis**). Because the erythrocytes are very large, the MCV is very high, usually exceeding 110 μm^3.

Pathophysiology

FOLIC ACID DEFICIENCY

Folic acid is stored as compounds referred to as folates. The folate stores in the body are much smaller than those of vitamin B_{12}, and they are quickly depleted when the dietary intake of folate is deficient (within 4 months). Folate is found in green vegetables and liver. Folate deficiency occurs in people who rarely eat uncooked vegetables. Alcohol increases folic acid requirements, and at the same time patients with alcoholism usually have a diet that is deficient in the vitamin. Folic acid requirements are also increased in patients with chronic hemolytic anemias and in women who are pregnant, because the need for erythrocyte production is increased in these conditions. Some patients with malabsorptive diseases of the small bowel, such as sprue, may not absorb folic acid normally.

VITAMIN B_{12} DEFICIENCY

A deficiency of vitamin B_{12} can occur in several ways. Inadequate dietary intake is rare but can develop in strict vegetarians who consume no meat or dairy products. Faulty absorption from the GI tract is more common. This occurs in conditions such as Crohn's disease, or after ileal resection or gastrectomy. Another cause is the absence of intrinsic factor, as in pernicious anemia. Intrinsic factor is normally secreted by cells within the gastric mucosa; normally it binds with the dietary vitamin B_{12} and travels with it to the ileum, where the vitamin is absorbed. Without intrinsic factor, orally consumed vitamin B_{12} cannot be absorbed, and erythrocyte production is eventually diminished. Even if adequate vitamin B_{12} and intrinsic factor are present, a deficiency may occur if disease involving the ileum or pancreas impairs absorption. Pernicious anemia, which tends to run in families, is primarily a disorder of adults, particularly the elderly. The abnormality is in the gastric mucosa: the stomach wall atrophies and fails to secrete intrinsic factor. Therefore, the absorption of vitamin B_{12} is significantly impaired.

The body normally has large stores of vitamin B_{12}, so years may pass before the deficiency results in anemia. Because the body compensates so well, the anemia can be severe before the patient becomes symptomatic. For unknown reasons, patients with pernicious anemia have a higher incidence of gastric cancer than the general population; these patients should have endoscopies at regular intervals (every 1 to 2 years) to screen for early gastric cancer.

Clinical Manifestations

Symptoms of folic acid and vitamin B_{12} deficiencies are similar, and the two anemias may coexist. However, the neurologic manifestations of vitamin B_{12} deficiency do not occur with folic acid deficiency, and they persist if vitamin B_{12} is not replaced. Therefore, careful distinction between the two anemias must be made. Serum levels of both vitamins can be measured. In the case of folic acid deficiency, even small amounts of folate increase the serum folate level, sometimes to normal. Measuring the amount of folate within the red cell itself (red cell folate) is therefore a more sensitive test in determining true folate deficiency.

After the body stores of vitamin B_{12} are depleted, the patient may begin to show signs and symptoms of the anemia. However, because the onset and progression of the anemia are so gradual, the body can compensate very well until the anemia is severe, so that the typical manifestations of anemia (weakness, listlessness, fatigue) may not be apparent initially. The hematologic effects of deficiency are accompanied by effects on other organ systems, particularly the GI tract and nervous system. Patients with pernicious anemia develop a smooth, sore, red tongue and mild diarrhea. They are extremely pale, particularly in the mucous membranes. They may become confused; more often they have paresthesias in the extremities (particularly numbness and tingling in the feet and lower legs). They may have difficulty maintaining their balance because of damage to the spinal cord, and they also lose position sense (proprioception). These symptoms are progressive, although the course of illness may be marked by spontaneous partial remissions and exacerbations. Without treatment, patients can die after several years, usually from heart failure secondary to anemia.

Assessment and Diagnostic Findings

The classic method of determining the cause of vitamin B_{12} deficiency is the Schilling test, in which the patient receives a small oral dose of radioactive vitamin B_{12}, followed in a few hours by a large, nonradioactive parenteral dose of vitamin B_{12} (this aids in renal excretion of the radioactive dose). If the oral vitamin is absorbed, more than 8% will be excreted in the urine within 24 hours; therefore, if no radioactivity is present in the urine (ie, the radioactive vitamin B_{12} stays within the GI tract), the cause is GI malabsorption of the vitamin B_{12}. Conversely, if radioactivity is detected in the urine, the cause of the deficiency is not ileal disease or pernicious anemia. Later, the same procedure is repeated, but this time intrinsic factor is added to the oral radioactive vitamin B_{12}. If radioactivity is now detected in the urine (ie, the vitamin B_{12} was absorbed from the GI tract in the presence of intrinsic factor), the diagnosis of pernicious anemia can be made. The Schilling test is useful only if the urine collections are complete; therefore, the nurse must promote the patient's understanding and compliance with this collection.

Other methods of establishing the diagnosis are more frequently used. Although it is possible to measure methylmalonic acid levels in vitamin B_{12} deficiency, these levels also increase in the setting of renal insufficiency. Furthermore, it is expensive to measure these levels, which also limits the utility of the test. A more useful, easier test is the intrinsic factor antibody test. A positive test indicates the presence of antibodies that bind the vitamin B_{12}–intrinsic factor complex and prevent it from binding to receptors in the ileum, thus preventing its absorption. Unfortunately, this test is not specific for pernicious anemia alone, but it can aid in the diagnosis.

Medical Management

Folate deficiency is treated by increasing the amount of folic acid in the diet and administering 1 mg of folic acid daily. Folic acid is administered IM only to people with malabsorption problems. With the exception of the vitamins administered during pregnancy, most proprietary vitamin preparations do not contain folic acid, so it must be administered as a separate tablet. After the hemoglobin level returns to normal, the folic acid replacement can be stopped. However, patients with alcoholism should continue receiving folic acid as long as they continue to consume alcohol.

Vitamin B_{12} deficiency is treated by vitamin B_{12} replacement. Vegetarians can prevent or treat deficiency with oral supplements with vitamins or fortified soy milk. When the deficiency is due to the more common defect in absorption or the absence of intrinsic factor, replacement is by monthly IM injections of vitamin B_{12}. Even in the absence of intrinsic factor, a small amount of an oral dose of vitamin B_{12} can be absorbed by passive diffusion, but large doses (2 mg/day) are required if vitamin B_{12} is to be replaced orally.

As vitamin B_{12} is replaced, the reticulocyte count rises within 1 week, and in several weeks the blood counts are all normal. The tongue feels better and appears less red in several days. However, the neurologic manifestations require more time for recovery; if there is severe neuropathy, the patient may never recover fully. To prevent recurrence of pernicious anemia, vitamin B_{12} therapy must be continued for life.

NURSING ALERT

Even when the megaloblastic anemia is severe, RBC transfusions may not be used because the patient's body has compensated over time by expanding the total blood volume. Administration of blood transfusions to such patients, particularly those who are elderly or who have cardiac dysfunction, can precipitate pulmonary edema. If transfusions are required, the RBCs should be transfused slowly, with careful attention to signs and symptoms of fluid overload.

Nursing Management

Assessment of patients who have or are at risk of megaloblastic anemia includes inspection of the skin and mucous membranes. Mild jaundice may be apparent and is best seen in the sclera without using fluorescent lights. Vitiligo (patchy loss of skin pigmentation) and premature graying of the hair are often seen in patients with pernicious anemia. The tongue is smooth, red, and sore. Because of the neurologic complications associated with these anemias, a careful neurologic assessment is important, including tests of position and vibration sense.

The nurse needs to pay particular attention to ambulation and should assess the patient's gait and stability as well as the need for assistive devices (eg, canes, walkers) and for assistance in managing daily activities. Of particular concern is ensuring safety when position sense, coordination, and gait are affected. Physical and occupational therapy referrals may be needed. If sensation is altered, the patient needs to be instructed to avoid excessive heat and cold.

Because mouth and tongue soreness may restrict nutritional intake, the nurse advises the patient to eat small amounts of bland, soft foods frequently. The nurse also may explain that other nutritional deficiencies, such as alcohol-induced anemia, can induce neurologic problems.

PROMOTING HOME AND COMMUNITY-BASED CARE

The patient must be taught about the chronicity of the disorder and the need for monthly vitamin B_{12} injections or daily oral vitamin B_{12} even in the absence of symptoms. If parenteral replacement is used, many patients can be taught to self-administer their injections. The gastric atrophy associated with pernicious anemia increases the risk for gastric carcinoma, so the patient needs to understand that ongoing medical follow-up and screening are important.

Myelodysplastic Syndrome (MDS)

Myelodysplastic syndrome (MDS) is a group of disorders of the myeloid stem cell that causes **dysplasia** (abnormal development) in one or more types of cell lines. The most common feature of MDS—dysplasia of the erythrocytes—is manifested as a macrocytic anemia; however, the leukocytes (myeloid cells, particularly neutrophils) and platelets can also be affected. Although the bone marrow is actually hypercellular, many of the cells within it die before being released into the circulation. Therefore, the actual number of cells in the circulation is typically lower than normal. In addition to the quantitative defect (ie, fewer cells than normal), there is also a qualitative defect: the cells are not as functional as normal. The neutrophils have diminished ability to destroy bacteria by phagocytosis; platelets are less able to aggregate and are less adhesive than usual. The result of these qualitative defects is an increased risk of infection and bleeding, even when the actual number of circulating cells may not be excessively low. A significant proportion of MDS cases evolve into acute myeloid leukemia (AML); this type of leukemia tends to be nonresponsive to standard therapy.

Primary MDS tends to be a disease of the elderly: more than 80% of patients with MDS are older than 60 years. Secondary MDS may occur at any age and results from prior toxic exposure to chemicals, including chemotherapeutic medications (particularly alkylating agents). Secondary MDS tends to have a poorer prognosis than does primary MDS.

Clinical Manifestations

The manifestations of MDS can vary widely. Many patients are asymptomatic, with the illness being discovered incidentally when a CBC is performed for other purposes. Other patients have profound symptoms and complications from the illness. Fatigue is often present, at varying levels. Neutrophil dysfunction puts the person at risk for infection; recurrent pneumonias are common. Because platelet function can also be altered, bleeding can occur. These problems may persist in a fairly steady state for months, even years. They may also progress over time; as the dysplasia evolves into a leukemic state, the complications increase in severity.

Assessment and Diagnostic Findings

The CBC typically reveals a macrocytic anemia; leukocyte and platelet counts may be diminished as well. Serum erythropoietin levels may be inappropriately low, as is the reticulocyte count. As the disease evolves into AML, more immature blast cells are noted on the CBC.

Medical Management

With the exception of allogeneic bone marrow transplant (BMT), there is no known cure for MDS. Chemotherapy has been used, particularly in patients with more aggressive forms of the illness, but typically with disappointing results (Giralt, 2004). Recently, new agents, 5-azacytadine, lenolidomide, and decifibine, were approved by the U.S. Food and Drug Administration (FDA) for use in patients with MDS. Research studies indicated that patients who responded to these agents had decreased transfusion requirements, decreased evolution toward AML, and improved quality of life (Estey, 2004; Foss, 2004; List, Kurtin, Roe, et al., 2005; Silverman, 2004).

However, patients with mild cytopenias (low blood counts) often require no therapy. For most patients with MDS, transfusions of red cells may be required to control the anemia and its symptoms. These patients can develop significant problems with iron overload from the repeated transfusions; this problem can be diminished with prompt initiation of chelation therapy to remove the excess iron (see Nursing Management). In some patients, the use of erythropoietin can be successful in reducing the need for transfusions and their attendant complications. Some patients may require ongoing platelet transfusions to prevent significant bleeding. Over time, these patients often develop iso-sensitization to donor platelets, resulting in suboptimal increases in the platelet count after platelets are transfused. Infections need to be managed aggressively and promptly. Administration of growth factors, particularly granulocyte colony-stimulating factor (G-CSF), erythropoietin, or both, has been successful in increasing neutrophils and diminishing anemia in certain patients; however, these agents are expensive and the effect is lost if the medications are stopped.

Because MDS tends to occur in elderly people, other chronic conditions may limit treatment options. Secondary MDS and MDS that evolves into AML tend to be much more refractory to conventional therapy for leukemia.

Nursing Management

Caring for patients with MDS can be challenging because the illness is unpredictable. As with other hematologic conditions, some patients (especially those with no symptoms) have difficulty perceiving that they have a serious illness that can place them at risk of life-threatening complications. At the other extreme, many patients have tremendous difficulty coping with the uncertain trajectory of the illness and fear that the illness will evolve into AML at a time when they are feeling very well physically.

Patients with MDS need extensive instruction about infection risk, measures to avoid it, signs and symptoms of developing infection, and appropriate actions to take should such symptoms occur. Instruction should also be given regarding the risk of bleeding. Patients with MDS who are hospitalized may require neutropenic precautions.

Laboratory values need to be monitored closely to anticipate the need for transfusion and to determine response to treatment with growth factors. Patients with chronic transfusion requirements usually benefit from the insertion of a vascular access device for this purpose. Patients receiving growth factors or chelation therapy need instruction about these medications, their side effects, and administration techniques.

Chelation therapy is a process that is used to remove excess iron acquired from chronic transfusions. Iron is bound to a substance, the chelating agent, and then excreted in the urine. Oral forms of chelating agents have not previously been successful (due to either diminished efficacy or excessive toxicity), but new formulations are now available (Vanorden & Hagemann, 2006). Chelation therapy is most effective as a subcutaneous infusion administered over 8 to 12 hours; most patients prefer to do this at night. Because chelation therapy removes only a small amount of iron with each treatment, patients with chronic transfusion requirements (and iron overload) need to continue chelation therapy as long as the iron overload exists, potentially for the rest of their lives. Patients who are embarking on chelation therapy must be highly motivated and need instruction in the subcutaneous infusion technique, infusion pump maintenance, and side effect management. Local erythema at the injection site is the most common reaction and typically requires no intervention. Patients should have baseline and annual auditory and eye examinations, because hearing loss and visual changes can occur with chelation treatment.

Hemolytic Anemias

In hemolytic anemias, the erythrocytes have a shortened life span; thus, their number in the circulation is reduced. Fewer erythrocytes result in decreased available oxygen, causing hypoxia, which in turn stimulates an increase in erythropoietin release from the kidney. The erythropoietin stimulates the bone marrow to compensate by producing new erythrocytes and releasing some of them into the circulation somewhat prematurely as reticulocytes. If the red cell destruction persists, the hemoglobin is broken down excessively; about 80% of the heme is converted to bilirubin, conjugated in the liver, and excreted in the bile.

The mechanism of erythrocyte destruction varies, but all types of hemolytic anemia share certain laboratory features: the reticulocyte count is elevated, the fraction of indirect (unconjugated) bilirubin is increased, and the supply of haptoglobin (a binding protein for free hemoglobin) is depleted as more hemoglobin is released. As a result, the plasma haptoglobin level is low. If the marrow cannot compensate to replace the erythrocytes (indicated by a decreased reticulocyte count), the anemia will progress.

Hemolytic anemia has various forms. Among the inherited forms are sickle cell anemia, thalassemia and thalassemia major, G-6-PD deficiency, and hereditary spherocytosis. Acquired forms include autoimmune hemolytic anemia, nonimmune-mediated paroxysmal nocturnal hemoglobinuria, microangiopathic hemolytic anemia, and heart valve hemolysis, as well as anemias associated with hypersplenism.

Sickle Cell Anemia

Sickle cell anemia is a severe hemolytic anemia that results from inheritance of the sickle hemoglobin gene. This gene causes the hemoglobin molecule to be defective. The sickle hemoglobin (HbS) acquires a crystal-like formation when exposed to low oxygen tension. The oxygen level in venous blood can be low enough to cause this change; consequently, the erythrocyte containing HbS loses its round, pliable, biconcave disk shape and becomes deformed, rigid, and sickle-shaped (Fig. 33-5). These long, rigid erythrocytes can adhere to the endothelium of small vessels; when they adhere to each other, blood flow to a region or an organ may be reduced. If ischemia or infarction results, the patient may have pain, swelling, and fever. The sickling process takes time; if the erythrocyte is again exposed to adequate amounts of oxygen (eg, when it travels through the pulmonary circulation) before the membrane becomes too rigid, it can revert to a normal shape. For this reason, the "sickling crises" are intermittent. Cold can aggravate the sickling process, because vasoconstriction slows the blood flow. Oxygen delivery can also be impaired by an increased

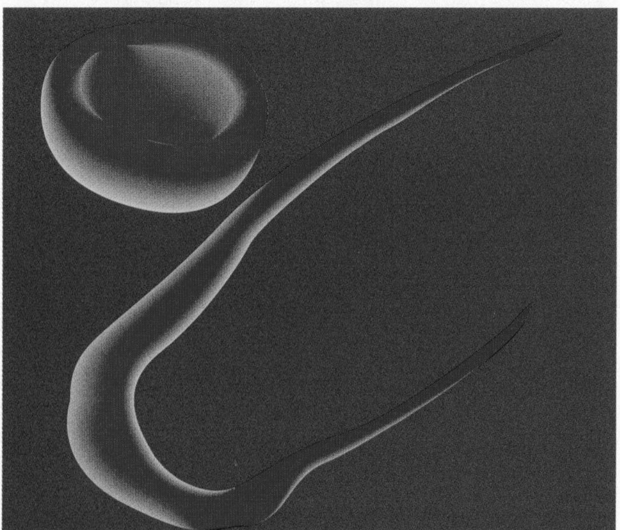

FIGURE 33-5. A normal red blood cell (*upper left*) and a sickled red blood cell.

blood viscosity, with or without occlusion due to adhesion of sickled cells; in this situation, the effects are seen in larger vessels, such as arterioles.

The *HbS* gene is inherited in people of African descent and to a lesser extent in people from the Middle East, the Mediterranean area, and aboriginal tribes in India. Sickle cell anemia is the most severe form of sickle cell disease. Less severe forms include sickle cell hemoglobin C (SC) disease, sickle cell hemoglobin D (SD) disease, and sickle cell beta-thalassemia. The clinical manifestations and management are the same as for sickle cell anemia. The term "sickle cell trait" refers to the carrier state for SC diseases; it is the most benign type of SC disease, in that less than 50% of the hemoglobin within an erythrocyte is HbS. However, in terms of genetic counseling, it is still an important condition. If two people with sickle cell trait have children, the children may inherit two abnormal genes. These children will produce only HbS and therefore will have sickle cell anemia. (Refer to Chapter 9 for additional discussion of genetic diseases.)

Clinical Manifestations

Symptoms of sickle cell anemia vary and are only somewhat based on the amount of HbS. Symptoms and complications result from chronic hemolysis or thrombosis. The sickled erythrocytes have a shortened life span. Anemia is always present; usually hemoglobin values are 7 to 10 g/dL. Jaundice is characteristic and is usually obvious in the sclerae. The bone marrow expands in childhood in a compensatory effort to offset the anemia, sometimes leading to enlargement of the bones of the face and skull. The chronic anemia is associated with tachycardia, cardiac murmurs, and often an enlarged heart (cardiomegaly). Dysrhythmias and heart failure may occur in adults.

Virtually any organ may be affected by thrombosis, but the primary sites involve those areas with normally slower circulation, such as the spleen, lungs, and central nervous system. All the tissues and organs are constantly vulnerable to microcirculatory interruptions by the sickling process and therefore are susceptible to hypoxic damage or true ischemic necrosis. Patients with sickle cell anemia are unusually susceptible to infection, particularly pneumonia and osteomyelitis. Complications of sickle cell anemia include infection, stroke, renal failure, impotence, heart failure, and pulmonary hypertension (Table 33-3).

SICKLE CELL CRISIS

There are three types of sickle cell crisis in the adult population. The most common is the very painful *sickle crisis,* which results from tissue hypoxia and necrosis due to inadequate blood flow to a specific region of tissue or organ. *Aplastic crisis* results from infection with the human parvovirus. The hemoglobin level falls rapidly and the marrow cannot compensate, as evidenced by an absence of reticulocytes. *Sequestration crisis* results when other organs pool the sickled cells. Although the spleen is the most common organ responsible for sequestration in children, most children with sickle cell anemia have had a splenic infarction by 10 years of age, and the spleen is then no longer functional (autosplenectomy). In adults, the common organs involved in sequestration are the liver and, more seriously, the lungs.

TABLE 33-3 Complications in Sickle Cell Anemia*

Organ Involved	Mechanisms*	Diagnostic Findings	Signs and Symptoms
Spleen	Primary site of sickling → infarctions → ↓ phagocytic function of macrophages	Autosplenectomy; ↑ infection (esp. pneumonia, osteomyelitis)	Abdominal pain; fever, signs of infection
Lungs	Infection Infarction → ↑ pulmonary pressure → pulmonary hypertension	Pulmonary infiltrate ↑ $sPLA_2$†	Chest pain; dyspnea
Central Nervous System	Infarction	Cerebral vascular accident (stroke, brain attack)	Weakness (if severe); learning difficulties (if mild)
Kidney	Sickling → damage to renal medulla	Hematuria; inability to concentrate urine; renal failure	Dehydration
Heart	Anemia	Tachycardia; cardiomegaly → heart failure	Weakness, fatigue, dyspnea
Bone	↑ Erythroid production	Widening of medullary spaces and cortical thinning	Ache, arthralgias
	Infarction of bone	Osteosclerosis → avascular necrosis	Bone pain, especially hips
Liver	Hemolysis	Jaundice and gallstone formation; hepatomegaly	Abdominal pain
Skin and peripheral vasculature	↑ Viscosity/stasis → infarction → skin ulcers	Skin ulcers; ↓ wound healing	Pain
Eye	Infarction	Scarring, hemorrhage, retinal detachment	↓ Vision; blindness
Penis	Sickling → vascular thrombosis	Priapism → impotence	Pain, impotence

*Problems encountered in sickle cell anemia vary and are the result of a variety of mechanisms, as depicted in this table. Common physical findings and symptoms are also variable.

†$sPLA_2$: Secretory phospholipase A_2, a laboratory test that can predict impending acute chest syndrome (see text).

ACUTE CHEST SYNDROME

Acute chest syndrome is manifested by a rapidly decreasing hemoglobin level, tachycardia, fever, and bilateral infiltrates seen on the chest x-ray. These signs often mimic infection, but in fact the most common cause appears to be infarction within the pulmonary vasculature (Hammerman & Faber, 2004). Another common cause is pulmonary fat embolism. Increased secretory phospholipase A_2 concentration has been identified as a predictor of impending acute chest syndrome; the increased amounts of free fatty acids can cause increased permeability of the pulmonary endothelium and leakage of the pulmonary capillaries (Hammerman & Faber, 2004). Although this syndrome is potentially lethal, prompt intervention can result in a favorable outcome.

PULMONARY HYPERTENSION

Pulmonary hypertension is a common sequela of sickle cell disease. Patients with sickle cell anemia are most likely to die of either pulmonary hypertension or chronic lung disease (Vichinsky, 2004). Unfortunately, diagnosing pulmonary hypertension is difficult because clinical symptoms rarely occur until damage is irreversible. Although changes are not evident on chest x-ray, high-resolution computed tomography (CT) of the chest often demonstrates microvascular occlusion and diminished perfusion of the lung. Pulse oximetry measurements are typically normal, and breath sounds are clear to auscultation until the disease has progressed to later stages (Vichinsky, 2004). A recent study demonstrated an improvement in diagnosis of pulmonary hypertension by screening patients with sickle cell disease with Doppler echocardiography (Gladwin, Sachdev, & Jison, 2004).

Assessment and Diagnostic Findings

The patient with sickle cell trait usually has a normal hemoglobin level, a normal hematocrit, and a normal blood smear. In contrast, the patient with sickle cell anemia has a low hematocrit and sickled cells on the smear. The diagnosis is confirmed by hemoglobin electrophoresis.

Prognosis

Patients with sickle cell anemia are usually diagnosed in childhood, because they become anemic in infancy and begin to have sickle cell crises at 1 or 2 years of age. Some children die in the first years of life, typically of infection, but antibiotic use and parent teaching strategies have greatly improved the outcomes for these children. However, with current management strategies, the average life expectancy is still suboptimal, at 42 to 48 years. Young adults are often forced to live with multiple, often severe, complications from their disease. In some patients, the symptoms and complications diminish by 30 years of age; these patients live into the sixth decade or longer. Currently, there is no way to predict which patients will fall into this subgroup.

Medical Management

Treatment for sickle cell anemia is the focus of continued research (Cao, 2004; Stuart & Nagel, 2004). Many trials of medications that have antisickling properties are being conducted, as is research using antiadhesion treatment for vasoocclusive crises. However, aside from the equally important aggressive management of symptoms and complications, currently there are only four primary treatment modalities for sickle cell diseases: bone marrow transplant (BMT), hydroxyurea, arginine, and long-term RBC transfusion.

BMT offers the potential for cure for this disease. However, this treatment modality is available to only a small subset of affected patients, because of either the lack of a compatible donor or the severe organ damage (eg, renal, liver, lung) already present in the patient.

PHARMACOLOGIC THERAPY

Hydroxyurea (Hydrea), a chemotherapy agent, has been shown to be effective in increasing hemoglobin F levels in patients with sickle cell anemia, thereby decreasing the permanent formation of sickled cells. Patients who receive hydroxyurea appear to have fewer painful episodes of sickle cell crisis, a lower incidence of acute chest syndrome, and less need for transfusions. However, whether hydroxyurea can prevent or reverse actual organ damage remains unknown. Side effects of hydroxyurea include chronic suppression of leukocyte formation, teratogenesis, and potential for later development of a malignancy. Patient response to this agent varies significantly. The incidence and severity of side effects are also highly variable within a dose range. Some patients have toxicity with a very small dose (5 mg/kg per day), whereas others have little toxicity with a much higher dose (35 mg/kg per day). More research is needed to identify specific patient subgroups that are more likely to respond to this medication.

Arginine has antisickling properties and can enhance the availability of nitric oxide, a potent vasodilator, resulting in decreased pulmonary artery pressure. Arginine is synergistic with hydroxyurea and can be useful as combination therapy for managing pulmonary hypertension (Vichinsky, 2004).

TRANSFUSION THERAPY

Chronic RBC transfusions have been shown to be highly effective in several situations: in an acute exacerbation of anemia (eg, aplastic crisis), in the prevention of severe complications from anesthesia and surgery, and in improving the response to infection (when it results in exacerbated anemia). Chronic transfusions have also been shown to be effective in diminishing episodes of sickle cell crisis in pregnant women, but these transfusions have not been shown to improve fetal survival. Transfusion therapy may be effective in preventing complications from sickle cell disease. Although controversial, some data support the use of chronic transfusions in patients with cerebral ischemic injury (as seen on magnetic resonance imaging [MRI] or Doppler studies) to prevent more severe injury (eg, cerebrovascular accident [CVA, brain attack, or stroke]) (Adams et al., 2004). More than 50% of asymptomatic patients have some cerebral ischemia documented by MRI. In a pivotal study, chronic transfusion with packed red blood cells (PRBCs) resulted in a 90% reduction of stroke in children at risk of this complication, defined by elevated blood viscosity on transcranial Doppler ultrasonography (Gebreyohanns & Adams, 2004). Transfusions may also be useful in the management of severe cases of acute chest syndrome (Liem et al., 2004).

The risk of complications from transfusion is important to consider. These risks include iron overload, which necessitates chronic chelation therapy (see Myelodysplastic Syndrome, Nursing Management); poor venous access, which necessitates a vascular access device (and its attendant risk of infection or thrombosis); infections (hepatitis, human immunodeficiency virus [HIV]); and alloimmunization (an immune response to antigens from donor cells) from repeated transfusions. Another complication from transfusion is increased blood viscosity without reduction in the concentration of hemoglobin S. Exchange transfusion (in which the patient's own blood is removed and replaced via transfusion) may be performed to diminish the risk of increasing the viscosity excessively; the objective is to reduce the hematocrit to less than 30%, with transfusions supplying more than 80% of the patient's blood volume. Finally, it is important to consider the significant financial cost of an aggressive transfusion and chelation program.

Patients with sickle cell anemia require daily folic acid replacements to maintain the supply required for increased erythropoiesis from hemolysis. Infections must be treated promptly with appropriate antibiotics; infection, particularly pneumococcal infection, remains a major cause of death. These patients should receive pneumococcal vaccines (Davies et al., 2004).

Acute chest syndrome is managed by prompt initiation of antibiotic therapy. Incentive spirometry has been shown to decrease the incidence of pulmonary complications significantly. In severe cases, bronchoscopy may be required to identify the source of pulmonary disease. Fluid restriction may be more beneficial than aggressive hydration. Corticosteroids may also be useful. Transfusions reverse the hypoxia and decrease the level of secretory phospholipase A_2. Pulmonary function should be monitored regularly to detect pulmonary hypertension early, when therapy (hydroxyurea, arginine, transfusions, or BMT) may have a positive impact.

Because repeated blood transfusions are necessary, patients may develop multiple autoantibodies, making cross-matching difficult. In this patient population, a hemolytic transfusion reaction (see later discussion) may mimic the signs and symptoms of a sickle cell crisis. The classic distinguishing factor is that with a hemolytic transfusion reaction, the patient becomes *more* anemic after being transfused. These patients need very close observation. Further transfusion is avoided if possible until the hemolytic process abates. If possible, the patient is supported with corticosteroids (prednisone), IV immunoglobulin (IVIG; Gammagard, Sandoglobulin, Venoglobulin), and erythropoietin (Epogen, Procrit).

SUPPORTIVE THERAPY

Supportive care is equally important. Pain management is a significant issue. The incidence of painful sickle cell crises is highly variable; many patients have pain on a daily basis. The severity of the pain may not be enough to cause the patient to seek assistance from health care providers but severe enough to interfere with the ability to work and function within the family unit. Acute pain episodes tend to be self-limited, lasting hours to days. If the patient cannot manage the pain at home, intervention is frequently sought in the acute care setting, usually at an urgent care facility or emergency department. Adequate hydration is important during a painful sickling episode. Oral hydration is acceptable if the patient can maintain adequate amounts of fluids; IV hydration with dextrose 5% in water (D_5W) or dextrose 5% in 0.25 normal saline solution (3 L/m^2/24 hours) is usually required for sickle crisis. Supplemental oxygen may also be needed.

The use of medication to relieve pain is important (see Chapter 13 for a discussion of pain management). Aspirin is very useful in diminishing mild to moderate pain; it also diminishes inflammation and potential thrombosis (due to its ability to diminish platelet adhesion). Nonsteroidal anti-inflammatory drugs (NSAIDs) are useful for moderate pain or in combination with opioid analgesics. Although no tolerance develops with NSAIDs, a "ceiling effect" does develop whereby an increase in dosage does not increase analgesia. NSAID use must be carefully monitored, because these medications can precipitate renal dysfunction. When opioid analgesics are used, morphine is the medication of choice for acute pain. Patient-controlled analgesia (PCA) is frequently used. A recent study of 40 adults with sickle cell disease found that PCA was beneficial in managing pain due to sickling crises because it restored the patient's control over analgesia during hospitalization, provided quicker pain relief, and provided increased independence from health care providers (Johnson, 2003).

Chronic pain increases in incidence as the patient ages. Here, the pain is caused by complications (eg, avascular necrosis of the hip) from the sickling. With chronic pain management, the principal goal is to maximize functioning; pain may not be completely eliminated without sacrificing function. This concept may be difficult for patients to accept; they may need repeated explanations and support from nonjudgmental health care providers. Nonpharmacologic approaches to pain management are crucial in this setting. Examples include physical and occupational therapy, physiotherapy (including the use of heat, massage, and exercise), cognitive and behavioral intervention (including distraction, relaxation, and motivational therapy), and support groups.

Working with patients who have multiple episodes of severe pain can be challenging. It is important for health care providers to realize that patients with sickle cell disease must face a lifelong experience with severe and unpredictable pain. Such pain is disruptive to the person's level of functioning, including social functioning, and may result in a feeling of helplessness. Patients with inadequate social support systems may have more difficulty coping with chronic pain.

Nursing Process

The Patient With Sickle Cell Crisis

A patient in sickle cell crisis should be assessed for factors that could have precipitated the crisis, such as symptoms of infection or dehydration, or situations that promote fatigue or emotional stress.

Assessment

The patient is asked to recall factors that precipitated previous crises and measures he or she uses to prevent and manage crises. Pain levels should always be monitored using a pain intensity scale, such as a 0-to-10 scale. The quality of the pain (eg, sharp, dull, burning), the frequency of the pain (constant versus intermittent), and factors that aggravate or alleviate the pain are included in this assessment. If a sickle cell crisis is suspected, the nurse needs to determine whether the pain currently experienced is the same as or different from the pain typically encountered in crisis.

Because the sickling process can interrupt circulation in any tissue or organ, with resultant hypoxia and ischemia, a careful assessment of all body systems is necessary. Particular emphasis is placed on pain, swelling, and fever. All joint areas are carefully examined for pain and swelling. The abdomen is assessed for pain and tenderness because of the possibility of splenic infarction.

The respiratory system must be assessed carefully, including auscultation of breath sounds, measurement of oxygen saturation levels, and signs of cardiac failure, such as the presence and extent of dependent edema, an increased point of maximal impulse (PMI), and cardiomegaly (as seen on a chest x-ray). The patient is assessed for signs of dehydration by a history of fluid intake and careful examination of mucous membranes, skin turgor, urine output, and serum creatinine and blood urea nitrogen values.

A careful neurologic examination is important to elicit symptoms of cerebral hypoxia. However, ischemic findings on MRI or Doppler studies may significantly precede the findings on the physical examination. MRI and Doppler studies are used for early diagnosis and may result in improved patient outcome because therapy can be initiated more promptly.

Because patients with sickle cell anemia are so susceptible to infections, they are assessed for the presence of any infectious process. Particular attention is given to examination of the chest, long bones, and femoral head, because pneumonia and osteomyelitis are especially common. Leg ulcers, which may be infected and are slow to heal, are common.

The extent of anemia (as measured by the hemoglobin level and the hematocrit) and the ability of the marrow to replenish erythrocytes (as measured by the reticulocyte count) are monitored and compared with the patient's baseline values. The patient's current and past history of medical management is also obtained, particularly chronic transfusion therapy, hydroxyurea use, and prior treatment for infection.

Diagnosis

Nursing Diagnoses

Based on the assessment data, major nursing diagnoses for the patient with sickle cell crisis may include:

- Acute pain related to tissue hypoxia due to agglutination of sickled cells within blood vessels
- Risk for infection
- Risk for powerlessness related to illness-induced helplessness
- Deficient knowledge regarding sickle crisis prevention

Collaborative Problems/ Potential Complications

Based on the assessment data, potential complications may include:

- Hypoxia, ischemia, infection, and poor wound healing leading to skin breakdown and ulcers
- Dehydration
- Cerebrovascular accident (CVA, brain attack, stroke)
- Anemia
- Renal dysfunction
- Heart failure, pulmonary hypertension, and acute chest syndrome
- Impotence
- Poor compliance
- Substance abuse related to poorly managed chronic pain

Planning and Goals

The major goals for the patient are relief of pain, decreased incidence of crisis, enhanced sense of self-esteem and power, and absence of complications.

Nursing Interventions

Managing Pain

Acute pain during a sickle cell crisis can be severe and unpredictable. The patient's subjective description and rating of pain on a pain scale must guide the use of analgesics, which are valuable in controlling the acute pain of a sickle crisis. Any joint that is acutely swollen should be supported and elevated until the swelling diminishes. Relaxation techniques, breathing exercises, and distraction are helpful for some patients. After the acute painful episode has diminished, aggressive measures should be implemented to preserve function. Physical therapy, whirlpool baths, and transcutaneous nerve stimulation (TENS) are examples of such modalities.

Preventing and Managing Infection

Nursing care focuses on monitoring the patient for signs and symptoms of infection. Prescribed antibiotics should be initiated promptly, and the patient should be assessed for signs of dehydration. If the patient is to take prescribed oral antibiotics at home, he or she must understand the need to complete the entire course of antibiotic therapy and must be able to identify a feasible administration schedule.

Promoting Coping Skills

This illness frequently leaves the patient feeling powerless and with decreased self-esteem because its acute exacerbations often result in chronic health problems. These feelings can be exacerbated by inadequate pain management, and enhancing pain management can be extremely useful in establishing a therapeutic relationship based on mutual trust. Nursing care that focuses on the patient's strengths rather than deficits can enhance effective coping skills. Providing the patient with opportunities to make decisions about daily care may increase the patient's feelings of control.

Minimizing Deficient Knowledge

Patients with sickle cell anemia benefit from understanding what situations can precipitate a sickle cell crisis and the steps they can take to prevent or diminish such crises. Keeping warm and maintaining adequate hydration can be very effective in diminishing the occurrence and severity of attacks. Avoiding stressful situations is more challenging. Group education may be more effective if it is carried out by members of the community who are from the same ethnic group as those with the disease.

Monitoring and Managing Potential Complications

Management measures for many of the potential complications were delineated in previous sections. Other measures follow.

LEG ULCERS

Leg ulcers require careful management and protection from trauma and contamination. Referral to a wound-ostomy-continence nurse may facilitate healing and assist with prevention. If leg ulcers fail to heal, skin grafting may be necessary. Scrupulous aseptic technique is warranted to prevent nosocomial infections.

PRIAPISM LEADING TO IMPOTENCE

Male patients may develop sudden, painful episodes of priapism (persistent penile erection). The patient is taught to empty his bladder at the onset of the attack, exercise, and take a warm bath. If an episode persists longer than 3 hours, medical attention, which consists of IV hydration, administration of analgesics, and possible penile intracavernosal aspiration, is recommended. Repeated episodes may lead to extensive vascular thrombosis, resulting in impotence.

CHRONIC PAIN AND SUBSTANCE ABUSE

Many patients have considerable difficulty coping with chronic pain and repeated episodes of sickle cell crisis. Those who feel they have little control over their health and the physical complications that result from this illness may find it difficult to adhere to a prescribed treatment plan. Being nonjudgmental and actively seeking involvement from the patient in establishing a treatment plan are useful strategies.

Some patients with sickle cell anemia develop problems with substance abuse. For many, this abuse results from inadequate management of acute pain during episodes of crisis. Some clinicians suggest that abuse may result from prescribing insufficient amounts of opioid analgesics. The patient's pain may never be adequately relieved, promoting mistrust of the health care system and (from the patient's perspective) the need to seek care from a variety of sources when the pain is not severe. This cycle is best managed by prevention. Receiving care from a single provider over time is much more beneficial than receiving care from rotating physicians and staff in an emergency department. When crises occur, the staff in the emergency department should be in contact with the patient's primary health care provider so that optimal management can be achieved. Once a pattern of substance abuse is established, it is very difficult to manage, but continuity of care and establishing written contracts with the patient can be useful management strategies.

Promoting Home and Community-Based Care

TEACHING PATIENTS SELF-CARE

Because patients with sickle cell anemia are typically diagnosed as children, parents participate in the initial education. Based on the parents' knowledge, socioeconomic level, and interest, teaching focuses on the disease process (including some pathophysiology), treatment, and the assessment and monitoring skills needed to identify potential complications. As the child ages, educational interventions prepare the child to assume more responsibility for self-care.

Vascular access device management and chelation therapy can be taught to most families. Follow-up care for patients with vascular access devices may also need to be provided by nurses in an outpatient facility or by a home care nurse.

CONTINUING CARE

The illness trajectory of sickle cell anemia is highly varied, with unpredictable episodes of complications and crises. Care is often provided on an emergency basis, especially for some patients with pain management problems (see previous section). All health care providers who provide services to patients with sickle cell disease and their families need to communicate regularly with each other. Patients need to learn which parameters are important for them to monitor and how to monitor them. Guidelines should also be given regarding when it is appropriate to seek urgent care.

Evaluation

Expected Patient Outcomes

Expected patient outcomes may include:

1. Control of pain
   a. Acute pain is controlled with analgesics
   b. Uses relaxation techniques, breathing exercises, distraction to help relieve pain

2. Is free of infection
   a. Has normal temperature
   b. Leukocyte count within normal range (5000 to 10,000/mm^3)
   c. Identifies importance of continuing antibiotics at home (if applicable)
3. Expresses improved sense of control
   a. Participates in goal setting and in planning and implementing daily activities
   b. Participates in decisions about care
4. Increases knowledge about disease process
   a. Identifies situations and factors that can precipitate sickle cell crisis
   b. Describes lifestyle changes needed to prevent crisis
   c. Describes the importance of warmth, adequate hydration, and prevention of infection in preventing crisis
5. Absence of complications

Thalassemia

The thalassemias are a group of hereditary anemias characterized by **hypochromia** (an abnormal decrease in the hemoglobin content of erythrocytes), extreme **microcytosis** (smaller-than-normal erythrocytes), destruction of blood elements (hemolysis), and variable degrees of anemia. The thalassemias occur worldwide, but the highest prevalence is found in people of Mediterranean, African, and Southeast Asian ancestry.

Thalassemias are associated with defective synthesis of the hemoglobin chain; the production of one or more globulin chains within the hemoglobin molecule is reduced. When this occurs, the imbalance in the configuration of the hemoglobin causes it to precipitate in the erythroid precursors or the erythrocytes themselves. This increases the rigidity of the erythrocytes and thus the premature destruction of these cells.

Thalassemias are classified into two major groups according to which hemoglobin chain is diminished: alpha or beta. The alpha-thalassemias occur mainly in people from Asia and the Middle East, and the beta-thalassemias are most prevalent in people from Mediterranean regions but also occur in those from the Middle East or Asia. The alpha-thalassemias are milder than the beta forms and often occur without symptoms; the erythrocytes are extremely microcytic, but the anemia, if present, is mild.

The severity of beta-thalassemia varies depending on the extent to which the hemoglobin chains are affected. Patients with mild forms have a microcytosis and mild anemia. If left untreated, severe beta-thalassemia (thalassemia major, or Cooley's anemia) can be fatal within the first few years of life. Bone marrow transplant (BMT) offers a chance of cure, but when this is not possible, the disease is usually treated with transfusion of PRBCs. Patients may survive into their 20s and 30s. Patient teaching during the reproductive years should include preconception counseling about the risk of thalassemia major.

Thalassemia Major

Thalassemia major (Cooley's anemia) is characterized by severe anemia, marked hemolysis, and ineffective erythropoiesis (production of erythrocytes). With early regular transfusion therapy, growth and development through childhood are facilitated. Organ dysfunction due to iron overload results from the excessive amounts of iron in multiple PRBC transfusions. Regular chelation therapy (eg, subcutaneous deferoxamine) has reduced the complications of iron overload and prolonged the life of these patients. This disease is potentially curable by BMT if the procedure can be performed before liver damage occurs (ie, during childhood).

Glucose-6-Phosphate Dehydrogenase Deficiency

The G-6-PD gene is the source of the abnormality in this disorder; this gene produces an enzyme within the erythrocyte that is essential for membrane stability. A few patients have inherited an enzyme so defective that they have a chronic hemolytic anemia; however, the most common type of defect results in hemolysis only when the erythrocytes are stressed by certain situations, such as fever or the use of certain medications. The disorder came to the attention of researchers during World War II, when some soldiers developed hemolysis while taking primaquine, an antimalarial agent. African Americans and people of Greek or Italian origin are those primarily affected by this disorder. The type of deficiency found in the Mediterranean population is more severe than that in the African Caribbean population, resulting in greater hemolysis and sometimes in life-threatening anemia. All types of G-6-PD deficiency are inherited as X-linked defects; therefore, many more men are at risk than women. In the United States, about 12% of African American males are affected. The deficiency is also common in those of Asian ancestry and in certain Jewish populations.

Oxidant drugs have hemolytic effects for people with G-6-PD deficiency. These medications include antimalarial agents (eg, chloroquine [Aralen]), sulfonamides (eg, trimethoprim/sulfamethoxazole [Bactrim, Septra]), nitrofurantoin (eg, Macrodantin), common coal tar analgesics (including aspirin in high doses), thiazide diuretics (eg, hydrochlorothiazide [HydroDIURIL], chlorothiazide [Diuril]), oral hypoglycemic agents (eg, glyburide [Micronase], metformin [Glucophage]), chloramphenicol (Chloromycetin), and vitamin K (phytonadione [AquaMEPHYTON]). In affected people, a severe hemolytic episode can also result from ingestion of fava beans.

Clinical Manifestations

Patients are asymptomatic and have normal hemoglobin levels and reticulocyte counts most of the time. However, several days after exposure to an offending medication, they may develop pallor, jaundice, and hemoglobinuria (hemoglobin in the urine). The reticulocyte count increases, and symptoms of hemolysis develop. Special stains of the peripheral blood may then disclose Heinz bodies (degraded hemoglobin) within the erythrocytes. Hemolysis is often mild and self-limited. However, in the more severe Mediterranean type of G-6-PD deficiency, spontaneous recovery may not occur, and transfusions may be necessary.

Assessment and Diagnostic Findings

The diagnosis is made by a screening test or by a quantitative assay of G-6-PD.

Medical Management

The treatment is to stop the offending medication. Transfusion is necessary only in the severe hemolytic state, which is more commonly seen in the Mediterranean variety of G-6-PD deficiency.

Nursing Management

The patient is educated about the disease and given a list of medications to avoid. If hemolysis does develop, nursing interventions are the same as for hemolysis from other causes. Patients should be instructed to wear MedicAlert bracelets that identify that they have G-6-PD deficiency.

Hereditary Spherocytosis

Hereditary spherocytosis is a relatively common (1 in 5000 people) hemolytic anemia characterized by an abnormal permeability of the erythrocyte membrane; this causes the cells to change into a spherical shape. These erythrocytes are destroyed prematurely in the spleen. The severity of this hemolytic anemia varies; jaundice can be intermittent, and splenomegaly (enlarged spleen) also can occur. Surgical removal of the spleen is the principal treatment for this disorder.

Immune Hemolytic Anemia

Hemolytic anemias can result from exposure of the erythrocyte to antibodies. Alloantibodies (ie, antibodies against the host, or "self") result from the immunization of a person with foreign antigens (eg, the immunization of an Rh-negative person with Rh-positive blood). Alloantibodies tend to be large (IgM type) and cause immediate destruction of the sensitized erythrocytes, either within the blood vessel (intravascular hemolysis) or within the liver. The most common type of alloimmune hemolytic anemia in adults results from a hemolytic transfusion reaction.

Autoantibodies may develop for many reasons. In many instances, the person's immune system is dysfunctional, so that it falsely recognizes its own erythrocytes as foreign and produces antibodies against them. This mechanism is seen in people with chronic lymphocytic leukemia (CLL). Another mechanism is a deficiency in suppressor lymphocytes, which normally prevent antibody formation against a person's own antigens. Autoantibodies tend to be of the IgG type. The erythrocytes are sequestered in the spleen and destroyed by the macrophages outside the blood vessel (extravascular hemolysis).

Autoimmune hemolytic anemias can be classified based on the body temperature involved when the antibodies react with the red blood cell antigen. Warm-body antibodies bind to erythrocytes most actively in warm conditions (37°C); cold-body antibodies react in cold conditions (0°C). Most autoimmune hemolytic anemias are the warm-body type. Autoimmune hemolytic anemia is associated with other disorders in most cases (eg, medication exposure, lymphoma, CLL, other malignancy, collagen vascular disease, autoimmune disease, infection). In idiopathic autoimmune hemolytic states, the reason why the immune system produces the antibodies is not known. All ages and both genders are equally vulnerable to this form, whereas the incidence of secondary forms is greater in people older than 45 years of age and in females.

Clinical Manifestations

Clinical manifestations can vary, and they usually reflect the degree of anemia. The hemolysis may be very mild, so that the patient's marrow compensates adequately and the patient is asymptomatic. At the other extreme, the hemolysis can be so severe that the resultant anemia is life-threatening. Most patients complain of fatigue and dizziness. Splenomegaly is the most common physical finding, occurring in more than 80% of patients; hepatomegaly, lymphadenopathy, and jaundice are also common.

Assessment and Diagnostic Findings

Laboratory tests show a low hemoglobin level and hematocrit, most often with an accompanying increase in the reticulocyte count. Erythrocytes appear abnormal; spherocytes are common. The serum bilirubin level is elevated, and if the hemolysis is severe, the haptoglobin level is low or absent. The Coombs test (also referred to as the direct antiglobulin test [DAT]), which detects antibodies on the surface of erythrocytes, shows a positive result.

Medical Management

Any possible offending medication should be immediately discontinued. The treatment consists of high doses of corticosteroids until hemolysis decreases. Corticosteroids decrease the macrophage's ability to clear the antibody-coated erythrocytes. If the hemoglobin level returns toward normal, usually after several weeks, the corticosteroid dose can be lowered or, in some cases, tapered and discontinued. However, corticosteroids rarely produce a lasting remission. In severe cases, blood transfusions may be required. Because the antibody may react with all possible donor cells, careful blood typing is necessary, and the transfusion should be administered slowly and cautiously.

Splenectomy (removal of the spleen) removes the major site of erythrocyte destruction; therefore, splenectomy may be performed if corticosteroids do not produce a remission. If neither corticosteroid therapy nor splenectomy is successful, immunosuppressive agents may be administered. The two immunosuppressive agents most frequently used are cyclophosphamide (Cytoxan), which has a more rapid effect but more toxicity, and azathioprine (Imuran), which has a less rapid effect but less toxicity. The synthetic androgen danazol can be useful in some patients, particularly in combination with corticosteroids. The mechanism for this success is unclear. If corticosteroids or immunosuppressive agents are used, the taper must be very gradual to prevent a rebound "hyperimmune" response and exacerbation of the hemolysis. Immunoglobulin administration is effective in about one third of patients, but the effect is transient and the medication is expensive. Transfusions may be necessary if the anemia is severe; it may be extremely difficult to cross-match samples of available units of PRBCs with that of the patient.

For patients with cold-antibody hemolytic anemia, no treatment may be required other than to advise the patient to keep warm; relocation to a warm climate may be necessary.

Nursing Management

Patients may have great difficulty understanding the pathologic mechanisms underlying the disease and may need repeated explanations in terms they can understand. Patients who have had a splenectomy should be vaccinated against pneumococcal infections (eg, Pneumovax) and informed that they are permanently at greater risk for infection. Patients receiving long-term corticosteroid therapy, particularly those with concurrent diabetes or hypertension, need careful monitoring. They must understand the need for the medication and the importance of never abruptly discontinuing it. A written explanation and a tapering schedule should be provided, and adjustments based on hemoglobin levels should be emphasized. Similar teaching should be provided when immunosuppressive agents are used. Corticosteroid therapy is not without significant risk, and patients need to be monitored closely for complications. The short- and long-term complications of corticosteroid therapy are presented in Chart 33-3 and in Chapter 42.

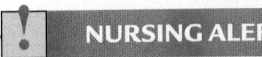

It can be difficult to cross-match blood when antibodies are present. If imperfectly cross-matched RBCs must be transfused, the nurse should begin the infusion very slowly (10 to 15 mL over 20 to 30 minutes) and monitor the patient very closely for signs and symptoms of a hemolytic transfusion reaction.

Hereditary Hemochromatosis

Hemochromatosis is a genetic condition in which iron is abnormally (excessively) absorbed from the GI tract. Normally the GI tract absorbs 1 to 2 mg of iron/day, but in those with hereditary hemochromatosis, this rate increases to 8 to 10 mg/day (Pietrangelo, 2004). The excessive iron is deposited in various organs, particularly the liver, myocardium, testes, thyroid, and pancreas. Eventually, the affected organs become dysfunctional. Although hereditary hemochromatosis is diagnosed in 0.5% of the population in the United States (ie, 1 million people), the actual prevalence is unknown because it is not always diagnosed. However, the genetic defect associated with hemochromatosis is most commonly seen as a specific mutation (C282Y homozygosity) of the *HFE* gene, with a prevalence of 5:1000 people of northern European descent (Pietrangelo, 2004). Women are less affected than men because of the natural loss of iron through menses.

Often there is no evidence of tissue damage until middle age, because the accumulation of iron in body organs occurs gradually. Symptoms of weakness, lethargy, arthralgia, weight loss, and loss of libido are common and occur earlier in the illness trajectory. The skin may be hyperpigmented with melanin deposits (occasionally **hemosiderin**, an iron-containing pigment) and appears bronze in color. Cardiac dysrhythmias and cardiomyopathy can occur, with resulting dyspnea and edema. Endocrine dysfunction is manifested as hypothyroidism, diabetes mellitus, and hypogonadism (testicular atrophy, diminished libido, and impotence). Cirrhosis is very common; thus, hemochromatosis should be considered in patients with cirrhosis who also have diabetes (Beutler et al., 2003). Development of hepatocellular carcinoma in one third of patients is a significant effect of the hemochromatosis.

The most useful laboratory findings are an elevated serum iron level and high transferrin saturation (more than 60% in men, more than 50% in women). CBC values are typically normal. The definitive diagnostic test for hemochromatosis has been liver biopsy, but testing for the *HFE* gene mutation is now more commonly used. Patients who are homozygous for the gene are at high risk for the disorder (Pietrangelo, 2004).

Medical Management

Therapy involves the removal of excess iron via therapeutic phlebotomy (removal of whole blood from a vein). Each unit of blood removed results in a decrease of 200 to 250 mg of iron. The objective is to reduce the serum ferritin to less than 50 μg/L and the transferrin saturation to 30% or less. To achieve this, frequent phlebotomy is required (1 to 2 units weekly), with a gradual reduction in frequency of phlebotomies over a 1- to 3-year period. After 1 to 3 years, the frequency of phlebotomy can be reduced to 1 unit of blood every several months to prevent reaccumulation of iron deposits. The goal is to maintain an iron saturation of less than 50% and a serum ferritin of less than 100 μg/L. Aggressive removal of excess iron can prevent end-organ dysfunction. However, if end-organ damage has already occurred (ie, destructive arthritis, cirrhosis, hypogonadism, type 1 diabetes mellitus), phlebotomy slows rather than reverses organ dysfunction (Pietrangelo, 2004).

Nursing Management

Patients with hemochromatosis often limit their dietary intake of iron, although this is not effective and is not encouraged. However, it is important for these patients to avoid any additional insults to the liver, such as alcohol abuse. Serial screening tests for hepatoma (ie, alpha-fetoprotein) are important. Other body systems should be monitored for signs of organ dysfunction, particularly the endocrine and cardiac systems, so that appropriate management can be implemented quickly. Because patients with hemochromatosis require frequent phlebotomies,

CHART 33-3

PHARMACOLOGY · Complications Associated with Corticosteroid Therapy

Whenever a patient begins a course of corticosteroid therapy, the potential for complications is great. Dosing regimens vary widely, depending on the underlying hematologic condition and the patient's response to the medication. For example, several chemotherapy protocols include high doses of corticosteroids for a period of several days. After that time, the medication is stopped abruptly without tapering the dosage. In other conditions, such as idiopathic thrombocytopenic purpura or hemolytic anemias, the corticosteroids are very carefully tapered to prevent a flare up of the underlying disease. With the exception of patients with preexisting conditions such as diabetes, hypertension, and osteoporosis, it is difficult to predict which complications will occur in a given patient. Patients who receive high doses of corticosteroids for longer than a few weeks should be screened for symptoms related to the potential complications listed here. If at all possible, patients who require long-term corticosteroid use should be switched to an alternate-day dosing schedule; this method may diminish the severity of complications that arise.

Short-Term Complications

Fluid and Electrolyte Complications
Fluid retention
Sodium retention
Potassium loss
Hypokalemic alkalosis
Hypertension

Endocrine Complications
Decreased carbohydrate tolerance
Diabetes mellitus
Persistent hyperglycemia in diabetes mellitus

Neurologic Complications
Headache

Musculoskeletal Complications
Muscle weakness

Psychological Complications
Depression
Euphoria
Mood swings
Insomnia
Psychosis

Long-Term Complications

Endocrine Complications
Decreased adrenocortical activity
Decreased ability to respond to stress
Decreased carbohydrate tolerance
Decreased growth rate (children)
Cushingoid state
Menstrual irregularities
Increased sweating

Metabolic Complications
Protein catabolism causing negative nitrogen balance

Gastrointestinal Complications
Gastritis
Ulcerative esophagitis
Peptic ulcer
Pancreatitis

Musculoskeletal Complications
Decreased muscle mass
Osteoporosis
Vertebral compression fracture
Pathologic fracture
Aseptic necrosis of femoral and humeral heads

Neurologic Complications
Vertigo
Increased intracranial pressure
Seizures

Ophthalmic Complications
Cataract formation
Glaucoma
Exophthalmos

Dermatologic Complications
Impaired wound healing
Ecchymoses
Increased skin fragility
Decreased skin thickness
Petechiae

Immunologic Complications
Decreased response to infection
Masked signs of early stages of infection
Suppressed reaction to skin tests
Increased risk for opportunistic infection (eg, *Pneumocystis*, herpes zoster)

problems with venous access are common. All children of patients who are homozygous for the *HFE* gene mutation should be screened for the mutation as well. Patients who are heterozygous for the *HFE* do not develop the disease but need to be counseled that they can transmit the gene to their children.

Polycythemia

Polycythemia, literally meaning "too many cells in the blood," refers to an increased volume of erythrocytes. It is a term used when the hematocrit is elevated (to more than 55% in males, more than 50% in females). Dehydration (decreased volume of plasma) can cause an elevated hematocrit, but not typically to the level to be considered polycythemia. Polycythemia is classified as either primary or secondary (Prchal, 2003).

Polycythemia Vera

Polycythemia vera, or primary polycythemia, is a proliferative disorder in which the myeloid stem cells seem to have escaped normal control mechanisms. The bone marrow is hypercellular, and the erythrocyte, leukocyte, and platelet counts in the peripheral blood are elevated. However, the erythrocyte elevation is predominant; the hematocrit can exceed 60%. This phase can last for an extended period (10 years or longer). Over time, the spleen resumes its embryonic function of hematopoiesis and enlarges. Eventually, the bone marrow may become fibrotic, with a resultant inability to produce as many cells ("burnt out" or spent phase). The disease evolves into myeloid metaplasia with myelofibrosis, MDS, or AML in a significant proportion of patients; this form of AML is usually refractory to standard treatments (Chomienne et al., 2004). The incidence of polycythemia has been estimated at 2.3 per 100,000 people. The median age at onset is 60 years (Prchal, 2003). Median survival exceeds 10 years with treatment but is only 6 to 18 months without treatment (Terreri, 2004).

Clinical Manifestations

Patients typically have a ruddy complexion and splenomegaly (enlarged spleen). Symptoms result from increased blood volume (headache, dizziness, tinnitus, fatigue, paresthesias, and blurred vision) or from increased blood viscosity (angina, claudication, dyspnea, and thrombophlebitis), particularly if the patient has atherosclerotic blood vessels. For this reason, blood pressure is often elevated. Uric acid may be elevated, resulting in gout and renal stone formation. Another common and bothersome problem is generalized pruritus, which may be caused by histamine release due to the increased number of basophils. Erythromelalgia, a burning sensation in the fingers and toes, may be reported and is only partially relieved by cooling.

Assessment and Diagnostic Findings

Diagnosis is based on an elevated erythrocyte mass (a nuclear medicine procedure), a normal oxygen saturation level, and often an enlarged spleen. Other factors useful in establishing the diagnosis include elevated leukocyte and platelet counts. The erythropoietin level is not as low as would be expected with an elevated hematocrit; it is normal or only slightly low. Causes of secondary erythrocytosis should not be present (see later discussion).

Complications

Patients with polycythemia vera are at increased risk for thromboses resulting in a CVA (brain attack, stroke) or myocardial infarction (MI); thrombotic complications are the most common cause of death. Bleeding is also a complication, possibly because the platelets (often very large) are somewhat dysfunctional. The bleeding can be significant and can occur in the form of nosebleeds, ulcers, frank GI bleeding, hematuria, and intracranial hemorrhage.

Medical Management

The objective of management is to reduce the high blood cell mass. Phlebotomy is an important part of therapy. It involves removing enough blood (initially 500 mL once or twice weekly) to diminish the blood viscosity and to deplete the patient's iron stores, thereby rendering the patient iron deficient and consequently unable to continue to manufacture erythrocytes excessively. Many patients are managed by routine phlebotomy on an intermittent basis. Radioactive phosphorus (^{32}P) or chemotherapeutic agents (eg, hydroxyurea [Hydrea]) can be used to suppress marrow function, but this may increase the risk for leukemia. Patients receiving hydroxyurea appear to have a lower incidence of thrombotic complications than those treated by phlebotomy alone; this may result from a more controlled platelet count. Anagrelide (Agrylin), which inhibits platelet aggregation, can also be useful in controlling the thrombocytosis associated with polycythemia vera. However, many patients have difficulty tolerating the medication; it can cause significant side effects, including headache, fluid retention, cardiac dysrhythmias, and heart failure. Furthermore, anagrelide is now considered leukemogenic (ie, may cause leukemia) (Berlin, 2003). Interferon alfa-2b (Intron-A) is the most effective treatment for managing the pruritus associated with polycythemia vera (Berlin, 2003) but may be difficult for patients to tolerate because of its frequent side effects (eg, flu-like syndrome, depression). Antihistamines, including histamine-2 blockers, are not particularly effective in controlling itching. Allopurinol (Zyloprim) is used to prevent gouty attacks in patients with elevated uric acid concentrations.

The use of aspirin to prevent thrombotic complications is controversial. A recent study comparing low-dose aspirin (100 mg) to placebo in 518 patients with polycythemia vera found that aspirin decreased the risk for significant thrombotic complications (deep vein thrombosis [DVT], pulmonary embolism, MI, stroke) (Landolfi et al., 2004). Low-dose aspirin is frequently used in patients with cardiovascular disease, but even this dose may be avoided in patients with prior bleeding, especially bleeding from the GI tract. Aspirin is also useful in reducing the pain associated with erythromelalgia.

Nursing Management

The nurse's role is primarily that of educator. Risk factors for thrombotic complications, particularly smoking, obesity, and poorly controlled hypertension, should be assessed, and the patient should be instructed about the signs and symptoms of thrombosis. To reduce the likelihood of DVT, avoidance of tight or restrictive clothing (particularly stockings), crossing the legs, and sedentary behavior should be encouraged. Patients with a history of bleeding are usually advised to avoid aspirin and aspirin-containing medications, because these medications alter platelet function. Minimizing alcohol intake should also be emphasized to further diminish the risk of bleeding. The patient needs to be instructed to avoid iron supplements, including those within multivitamin supplements, because the iron can further stimulate RBC production. For pruritus, the nurse may recommend bathing in tepid or cool water and avoiding vigorous toweling-off after bathing. Sodium bicarbonate dissolved in bath water may also be effective (Golden, 2003), along with applications of cocoa butter– or oatmeal-based lotions and bath products.

Secondary Polycythemia

Secondary polycythemia is caused by excessive production of erythropoietin. This may occur in response to a reduced amount of oxygen, which acts as a hypoxic stimulus, as in cigarette smoking, chronic obstructive pulmonary disease, or cyanotic heart disease, or in nonpathologic conditions such as living at a high altitude. It can also result from certain hemoglobinopathies (eg, hemoglobin Chesapeake), in which the hemoglobin has an abnormally high affinity for oxygen. Secondary polycythemia can also occur from neoplasms (eg, renal cell carcinoma) that stimulate erythropoietin production.

Medical Management

Management of secondary polycythemia may not be necessary; when it is, it involves treating the primary conditions. If the cause cannot be corrected (eg, by treating the renal cell carcinoma or improving pulmonary function), therapeutic phlebotomy may be necessary in symptomatic patients to reduce blood viscosity and volume.

Leukopenia

Leukopenia, a condition in which there are fewer leukocytes than normal, results from neutropenia (diminished neutrophils) or lymphopenia (diminished lymphocytes). Even if other types of leukocytes (eg, monocytes, basophils) are diminished, their numbers are too few to reduce the total leukocyte count significantly.

Neutropenia

Neutropenia (a neutrophil count of less than 2,000/mm^3) results from decreased production of neutrophils or increased destruction of these cells (Chart 33-4). Neutrophils are essential in preventing and limiting bacterial infection. A patient with neutropenia is at increased risk for infection from both exogenous and endogenous sources. (The GI tract and skin are common endogenous sources.) The risk of infection is based not only on the severity of the neutropenia (low neutrophil count) but also on the duration of the neutropenia. The actual number of neutrophils, known as the **absolute neutrophil count** (ANC), is determined by a simple mathematical calculation using data obtained from the CBC and differential (Chart 33-5). The risk for infection increases proportionately with the decrease in neutrophil count. The risk is significant when the ANC is less than 1000/mm^3, is high when it is less than 500/mm^3, and is almost certain when it is less than 100/mm^3. The risk of developing infection also increases with the length of time during which neutropenia persists, even if it is fairly mild. Conversely, even a severe neutropenia may not result in infection if the duration of the neutropenia is brief, as is often seen after chemotherapy (Chart 33-6).

CHART 33-4

Causes of Neutropenia

Decreased Production of Neutrophils
- Aplastic anemia, due to medications or toxins
- Metastatic cancer, lymphoma, leukemia
- Myelodysplastic syndromes
- Chemotherapy
- Radiation therapy

Ineffective Granulocytopoiesis
- Megaloblastic anemia

Increased Destruction of Neutrophils
- Hypersplenism
- Medication-induced*
- Immunologic disease (eg, systemic lupus erythematosus)
- Viral disease (eg, infectious hepatitis, mononucleosis)
- Bacterial infections

*Formation of antibody to medication, leading to a rapid decrease in neutrophils.

Clinical Manifestations

There are no definite symptoms of neutropenia until the patient becomes infected. A routine CBC with differential, as obtained after chemotherapy treatment, can reveal neutropenia before the onset of infection.

Medical Management

Treatment of the neutropenia varies depending on its cause. If the neutropenia is medication-induced, the offending agent is stopped immediately, if possible. Treatment of an underlying neoplasm can temporarily make the neutropenia worse, but with bone marrow recovery, treatment may actually improve it. Corticosteroids may be used if the cause is an immunologic disorder. The use of growth factors such as G-CSF or granulocyte-macrophage colony-stimulating factor (GM-CSF) can be effective in increasing neutrophil production when the cause of the neutropenia is decreased production. Withholding or reducing the dose of chemotherapy or radiation therapy may be required when the neutropenia is caused by these treatments; however, in the case of potentially curative therapy, administration of growth

CHART 33-5

Calculating the Absolute Neutrophil Count (ANC)

$$ANC = \frac{\text{Total WBC count} \times (\% \text{ neutrophils} + \% \text{ bands})}{100}$$

Normally, the neutrophil count is greater than 2000/mm^3. The actual (or absolute) neutrophil count (ANC) is calculated using the above formula.

For example, if the total white blood cell (WBC) count is 3000/mm^3 with 72% neutrophils and 3% bands, the ANC would be calculated as follows:

$$ANC = \frac{3000(72+3)}{100} = 2250$$

This result is not indicative of neutropenia, because the ANC is greater than 2000 despite the low total WBC count (3000/mm^3).

Conversely, in the following example, neutropenia is evident despite a normal WBC count (5500/mm^3) with 8% neutrophils and 0% bands:

$$ANC = \frac{5500(8+0)}{100} = 440$$

Here, the ANC is severely low (440) despite the normal total WBC count (5500/mm^3).

When evaluating neutropenia, it is important to calculate the ANC and not to rely solely on the total WBCs and percentage of neutrophils alone.

factor is considered to be preferable, so that the maximum antitumor effect can be achieved by maintaining the chemotherapy regimen as originally planned.

If the neutropenia is accompanied by fever, the patient is considered to have an infection and usually is admitted to the hospital. Cultures of blood, urine, and sputum and a chest x-ray are obtained. To ensure adequate therapy against the infectious organisms, broad-spectrum antibiotics are initiated as soon as the cultures are obtained, although the antibiotics may be changed after culture and sensitivity results are available.

Nursing Management

Nurses in all settings have a crucial role in assessing the severity of neutropenia and in preventing and managing complications, which most often include infections. Patient teaching is equally important, particularly in the outpatient setting, so that the patient can implement appropriate self-care measures and know when and how to seek medical care (Chart 33-7). Patients at risk of neutropenia should have blood drawn for a CBC with differential; the frequency is based on the suspected severity and duration of the neutropenia. Nurses need to be able to calculate the ANC (see Chart 33-5) and to assess the severity of neutropenia and the risk of infection. Chart 33-8 identifies nursing interventions related to neutropenia.

Lymphopenia

Lymphopenia (a lymphocyte count less than 1500/mm^3) can result from ionizing radiation, long-term use of corticosteroids, uremia, some neoplasms (eg, breast and lung cancers, advanced Hodgkin's disease), and some protein-losing enteropathies (in which the lymphocytes within the intestines are lost).

Leukemia

The term *leukocytosis* refers to an increased level of leukocytes in the circulation. Typically, only one specific cell type is increased. Usually, because the proportions of several types of leukocytes (eg, eosinophils, basophils, monocytes) are small, only an increase in neutrophils or lymphocytes can be great enough to elevate the total leukocyte count. Although leukocytosis can be a normal response to increased need (eg, in acute infection), the elevation in leukocytes should decrease as the physiologic need decreases. A prolonged or progressively increasing elevation in leukocytes is abnormal and should be evaluated. A significant cause for persistent leukocytosis is malignancy.

Hematopoiesis is characterized by a rapid, continuous turnover of cells. Normally, production of specific blood cells from their stem cell precursors is carefully regulated according to the body's needs. If the mechanisms that control the production of these cells are disrupted, the cells can proliferate excessively. Hematopoietic malignancies are often classified by the cells involved. **Leukemia**, literally "white blood," is a neoplastic proliferation of one particular cell type (granulocytes, monocytes, lymphocytes, or infrequently erythrocytes or megakaryocytes). The defect originates in the hematopoietic stem cell, the myeloid, or the lymphoid stem cell. The lymphomas are neoplasms of lymphoid tissue, usually derived from B lymphocytes. Multiple myeloma is a malignancy of the most mature form of B lymphocyte, the plasma cell.

The common feature of the leukemias is an unregulated proliferation of leukocytes in the bone marrow. In acute forms (or late stages of chronic forms), the proliferation of leukemic cells leaves little room for normal cell production. There can also be a proliferation of cells in the liver and spleen (extramedullary hematopoiesis). With acute forms, there can be infiltration of other organs, such as the meninges, lymph nodes, gums, and skin. The cause of leukemia is not fully known, but there is some evidence that genetic influences and viral pathogenesis may be involved. Bone marrow damage from radiation exposure or from chemicals such as benzene and alkylating agents (eg, melphalan [Alkeran]) can cause leukemia.

(text continues on page 1071)

CHART 33-6

Risk Factors for Development of Infection and Bleeding in Patients with Hematologic Disorders

Risk for Infection

- *Severity of neutropenia:* Risk of infection is proportional to duration and severity of neutropenia
- *Duration of neutropenia:* Increased duration leads to increased risk of infection
- *Nutritional status:* Decreased protein stores lead to decreased immune response and anergy
- *Deconditioning:* Decreased mobility leads to decreased respiratory effort, leading to increased pooling of secretions
- *Lymphocytopenia; disorders of lymphoid system (chronic lymphocytic leukemia [CLL], lymphoma, myeloma):* Decreased cell-mediated and humoral immunity
- *Invasive procedures:* Break in skin integrity leads to increased opportunity for organisms to enter blood system
- *Hypogammaglobulinemia:* Decreased antibody formation
- *Poor hygiene:* Increased organisms on skin and mucous membranes
- *Poor dentition; mucositis:* Decreased endothelial integrity leads to increased opportunity for organisms to enter blood system
- *Antibiotic therapy:* Increased risk for superinfection, often fungal
- *Certain medications:* See text

Risk for Bleeding

- *Severity of thrombocytopenia:* Risk increases when platelet count decreases; usually not a significant risk until platelet count is lower than 20,000/mm^3 or lower than 50,000/mm^3 when invasive procedure performed
- *Duration of thrombocytopenia:* Risk increases when duration increases (eg, risk is less when duration is transient after chemotherapy than when duration is permanent with poor marrow production)
- *Sepsis:* Mechanism unknown; appears to cause increased platelet consumption
- *Increased intracranial pressure:* Increased blood pressure leads to rupture of blood vessels
- *Liver dysfunction:* Decreased synthesis of clotting factors
- *Renal dysfunction:* Decreased platelet function
- *Dysproteinemia:* Protein coats surface of platelet, leading to decreased platelet function; protein causes increased viscosity, which leads to increased stretching of capillaries and thus increased bleeding
- *Alcohol abuse:* Suppressive effect on marrow leads to decreased platelet production and decreased ability to function; decreased liver function results in decreased production of clotting factors
- *Splenomegaly:* Increased platelet destruction; spleen traps circulating platelets
- *Concurrent medications:* See text

CHART 33-7

HOME CARE CHECKLIST • The Patient at Risk for Infection

At the completion of the home care instruction, the patient or caregiver will be able to:	Patient	Caregiver
• Describe consequences of alterations in neutrophils, lymphocytes, immunoglobulins, or their sources.	✔	✔
• Verbalize the reason for being at risk for infection.	✔	✔
• Identify signs and symptoms of infection.	✔	✔
• Demonstrate how to monitor for signs of infection.	✔	✔
• Describe to whom, how, and when to report signs of infection.	✔	✔
• Identify appropriate behaviors to take to prevent infection: –Maintain good hand hygiene technique, total body hygiene, and skin integrity. –Avoid fresh flowers, plants, garden work (soil), bird cages, and litter boxes. –Avoid fresh salads and unpeeled fruits or vegetables. –Maintain a high-calorie, high-protein diet, with fluid intake of 3,000 mL daily (unless fluids are restricted). –Avoid people with infections, crowds. –Perform deep breathing, use incentive spirometer every 4 hr while awake. –Provide adequate lubrication with gentle vaginal manipulation during sexual intercourse; avoid anal intercourse.	✔	✔
• Describe appropriate actions to take should infection occur.	✔	✔

CHART 33-8

Neutropenia Precautions

Nursing Diagnosis

Risk for infection secondary to impaired immunocompetence due to:

- Diminished neutrophil count (see below) secondary to bone marrow invasion or hypocellularity secondary to treatment
- Dysfunctional neutrophils (eg, secondary to myelodysplastic syndrome [MDS])
- Dysfunctional or diminished lymphocytes
- Hypogammaglobulinemia
- Diminished immune response or anergy
- Malnutrition
- Surgery or invasive procedures
- Antibiotic therapy (increased risk for superimposed infection)
  - –Neutropenic, infected patients often do *not* exhibit the classic signs of inflammation/infection (ie, redness, cloudiness of any drainage); the only initial sign may be fever (and it often occurs later in the infectious process with neutropenia).
  - –Skin and mucous membranes are the body's first line of defense against infection; loss of endothelial cell integrity allows organisms to enter the blood and lymph systems.

Assessment

PATIENT

Assess the following areas thoroughly every shift or visit (with spot checks throughout shift if the patient is hospitalized) and notify physician of any signs of infection or worsening of status:

- *Skin:* Check for tenderness, edema, breaks in skin integrity, moisture, drainage, lesions (especially under breasts, axillae, groin, skin folds, bony prominences, perineum); check all puncture sites (eg, intravenous sites) for signs and symptoms of inflammation/infection.
- *Oral mucosa:* Check for moisture, lesions, color (check palate, tongue, buccal mucosa, gums, lips, oropharynx).
- *Respiratory:* Check for presence of cough, sore throat; auscultate breath sounds.
- *Gastrointestinal:* Check for abdominal discomfort/distention, nausea, change in bowel pattern; auscultate bowel sounds.
- *Genitourinary:* Check for dysuria, urgency, frequency; check urine for color, clarity, odor.
- *Neurologic:* Check for complaints of headache, neck stiffness, visual disturbances; assess level of consciousness, orientation, behavior.
- *Temperature:* Check every 4 hr or every visit; call primary health care provider if temperature is >38°C (>101°F), fever is unresponsive to acetaminophen, or patient shows a decline in hemodynamic status.

DIAGNOSTIC STUDIES

- Monitor complete blood count (CBC) and differential daily (especially absolute neutrophil count [ANC], lymphocyte count).
- Call physician if ANC is <1,000, significantly different from previous count, or whenever patient becomes symptomatic (eg, febrile).
- Monitor globulin, albumin, total protein levels.
- Monitor all culture and sensitivity reports.
- Monitor x-ray reports.

Nursing Interventions

ENVIRONMENT AND STAFF

- **Thorough hand hygiene must be performed by everyone before entering patient's room each and every time**.
- Allow no one with a cold or sore throat to care for the patient or to enter room, or come in contact with patient at home.
- Care for neutropenic patients before caring for other patients (as much as possible).
- Use private room for patient if ANC is <1,000.
- Allow no fresh flowers (stagnant water).
- Change water in containers every shift (include O_2 humidification systems every 24 hr).
- Ensure room is cleaned daily.

DIETARY

- Provide low microbial diet.
- Eliminate fresh salads and unpeeled fresh fruits or vegetables.

PATIENT

- Avoid suppositories, enemas, rectal temperatures.
- Practice deep breathing (with incentive spirometer) every 4 hr while awake.
- Ambulate; wear high-efficiency particulate air (HEPA) filter mask if neutropenia is severe.
- Prevent skin dryness with water-soluble lubricants, especially in high-risk areas (eg, lips, corners of mouth, elbows, feet, bony prominences).

HYGIENE

- Provide meticulous total body hygiene daily (preferably with antimicrobial solution), including perineal care after every bowel movement.

continued >

CHART 33-8 Neutropenia Precautions, continued

- Provide thorough oral hygiene after meals and every 4 hr while awake; warm saline, or salt and soda solution, is effective; avoid use of lemon-glycerine swabs, commercial mouthwashes, and hydrogen peroxide.

INTRAVENOUS (IV) THERAPY

- Do not use plastic cannulas for peripheral IVs when ANC is <500; a central vascular access device is preferred for long-term or intensive IV therapy.
- Inspect IV sites every shift; monitor closely for any discomfort; erythema may not be present.
- Maintain meticulous IV site care.
- Cleanse skin with antimicrobial solution before venipuncture (unless patient is allergic).
- Moisture-vapor–permeable dressings are permissible with strict adherence to institutional protocol.
- Change IV tubing per institution policy, using aseptic technique.
- Administer antimicrobial agents on time.

Expected Patient Outcomes

- Patient demonstrates an absence of infection as evidenced by an absence of fever, chills, inflammation, drainage, cough, dyspnea, sore throat, dysuria, or urinary frequency.
- Patient demonstrates an absence of infection as evidenced by the presence of vital signs within normal limits, including intact neurologic status and intact skin.

Duration of Evaluation

Until patient is no longer neutropenic and any infection is resolved.

NURSING RESEARCH PROFILE

Timeliness of Antimicrobial Administration in Emergency Departments for Patients With Cancer and Febrile Neutropenia

Niremberg, A., Mulhearn, L., Lin, S., et al. (2004). Emergency department waiting times for patients with cancer and febrile neutropenia: A pilot study. *Oncology Nursing Forum, 31*(4), 711–715.

Purpose

Fever and neutropenia are potentially serious complications of chemotherapy treatment for cancer. Prompt initiation of antimicrobial therapy may diminish the risk of developing a serious outcome (eg, sepsis or septic shock). Because most patients require prompt treatment when clinics are closed, they typically use the emergency department (ED) for evaluation of these complications and initiation of antimicrobial therapy. The purpose of this study was to determine the length of time involved in the evaluation and treatment of febrile neutropenia among cancer patients in the ED.

Design

This prospective, descriptive study had a convenience sample of 19 adults with cancer and febrile neutropenia who sought ED treatment. Patients who presented to the ED during the night, weekends, or holidays (eg, times when the ambulatory unit was closed) were eligible to participate. There were 10 male (53%) and 9 female (47%) participants, who were mostly middle-aged (mean age 56 years), had family support for assistance (74%), had mostly private insurance coverage (79%), and most often received chemotherapy for multiple myeloma or lymphoma (53%). Participants were interviewed and their medical records examined to determine the time lapsed between initiation of the fever to arrival at the ED; the time of triage, or initial patient assessment; the time that laboratory results were completed; the time to initiation of antimicrobial therapy; and the time of admission to the hospital.

Findings

Thirty-three episodes of febrile neutropenia in the 19 study participants were evaluated. On average, participants had a fever for 21 hours (range, 1 to 72 hours) prior to entering the ED. Forty-eight percent had an indwelling vascular access device, and 17% had other indwelling devices (eg, stent). Thirty percent had oral mucositis. Both invasive devices and oral mucositis are risk factors for bacterial infection in patients with neutropenia.

The median waiting time in the ED was 75 minutes for evaluation and 210 minutes for administration of antimicrobial agents. The average time spent in the ED until hospital admission was 5.5 hours (range, 2 to 11.6 hours).

Nursing Implications

Patients receiving chemotherapy, particularly for hematologic malignancies, are typically taught about infection and the importance of seeking prompt medical care if they become febrile. Nurses are responsible for providing this education. Results of this study suggest that current educational interventions may be inadequate.

Nurses in the ED are responsible for the initial triage of patients and need to facilitate a thorough and expedient workup of patients with cancer and febrile neutropenia who have received chemotherapy. Nurses must serve as advocates for these patients so that antimicrobial therapy is initiated promptly.

The leukemias are commonly classified according to the stem cell line involved, either lymphoid or myeloid. They are also classified as either acute or chronic, based on the time it takes for symptoms to evolve and the phase of cell development that is halted (ie, with few leukocytes differentiating beyond that phase).

In acute leukemia, the onset of symptoms is abrupt, often occurring within a few weeks. Leukocyte development is halted at the blast phase, so that most leukocytes are undifferentiated cells or are blasts. Acute leukemia progresses very rapidly; death occurs within weeks to months without aggressive treatment.

In chronic leukemia, symptoms evolve over a period of months to years, and the majority of leukocytes produced are mature. Chronic leukemia progresses more slowly; the disease trajectory can extend for years.

Acute Myeloid Leukemia

Acute myeloid leukemia (AML) results from a defect in the hematopoietic stem cell that differentiates into all myeloid cells: monocytes, granulocytes (neutrophils, basophils, eosinophils), erythrocytes, and platelets. All age groups are affected; the incidence rises with age, with a peak incidence at age 60 years. AML is the most common nonlymphocytic leukemia.

The prognosis is highly variable. Patient age may be a factor; patients who are younger may survive for 5 years or more after diagnosis of AML. However, patients who are older or have a more undifferentiated form of AML tend to have a worse prognosis. Those who have leukemia stemming from preexisting MDS or who previously received alkylating agents for cancer (secondary AML) have a much worse prognosis; the leukemia tends to be more resistant to treatment, resulting in a much shorter duration of remission. With treatment, patients with secondary AML survive an average of less than 1 year, with death usually a result of infection or hemorrhage. Patients receiving supportive care also usually survive less than 1 year, dying of infection or bleeding. The 5-year survival rate for patients with AML who are 65 years or younger is 33%; it drops to 4% for those older than 65 years (American Cancer Society, 2006).

Clinical Manifestations

Most signs and symptoms of AML result from insufficient production of normal blood cells. Fever and infection result from neutropenia, weakness and fatigue from anemia, and bleeding tendencies from thrombocytopenia. The proliferation of leukemic cells within organs leads to a variety of additional symptoms: pain from an enlarged liver or spleen, hyperplasia of the gums, and bone pain from expansion of marrow.

Assessment and Diagnostic Findings

AML develops without warning, with symptoms occurring over a period of weeks to months. The CBC shows a decrease in both erythrocytes and platelets. Although the total leukocyte count can be low, normal, or high, the percentage of normal cells is usually vastly decreased. A bone marrow analysis shows an excess of immature blast cells (more than 30%). AML can be further classified into seven different subgroups, based on cytogenetics, histology, and morphology (appearance) of the blasts. The actual prognosis varies somewhat between subgroups, but the clinical course and treatment differ substantially. Patients with acute promyelocytic leukemia (APL, or AML-M3) often have significantly more problems with bleeding, in that they have underlying coagulopathy and a higher incidence of disseminated intravascular coagulation (DIC).

Complications

Complications of AML include bleeding and infection, the major causes of death. The risk of bleeding correlates with the level of platelet deficiency (thrombocytopenia). The low platelet count can result in **ecchymoses** (bruises) and **petechiae** (pinpoint red or purple hemorrhagic spots on the skin). Major hemorrhages also may develop when the platelet count drops to less than 10,000/mm^3. The most common sites of bleeding are GI, pulmonary, and intracranial. For undetermined reasons, fever and infection also increase the likelihood of bleeding.

Because of the lack of mature and normal granulocytes, patients with leukemia are always threatened by infection. The likelihood of infection increases with the degree and duration of neutropenia; neutrophil counts that persist at less than 100/mm^3 make the chances of systemic infection extremely high. As the duration of severe neutropenia increases, the patient's risk of developing fungal infection also increases.

Medical Management

The overall objective of treatment is to achieve complete remission, in which there is no evidence of residual leukemia in the bone marrow. Attempts are made to achieve remission by the aggressive administration of chemotherapy, called induction therapy, which usually requires hospitalization for several weeks. Induction therapy typically involves high doses of cytarabine (Cytosar, Ara-C) and daunorubicin (Cerubidine) or mitoxantrone (Novantrone) or idarubicin (Idamycin); sometimes etoposide (VP-16, VePesid) is added to the regimen. The choice of agents is based on the patient's physical status and history of prior antineoplastic treatment.

The aim of induction therapy is to eradicate the leukemic cells, but this is often accompanied by the eradication of normal types of myeloid cells. Thus, the patient becomes severely neutropenic (an ANC of 0 is not uncommon), anemic, and thrombocytopenic (a platelet count of less than 10,000/mm^3 is common). During this time, the patient is typically very ill, with bacterial, fungal, and occasionally viral infections, bleeding, and severe mucositis, which causes diarrhea and a marked decline in the ability to maintain adequate nutrition. Supportive care consists of administering blood products (PRBCs and platelets) and promptly treating infections. The use of granulocytic growth factors, either G-CSF (filgrastim [Neupogen]) or GM-CSF (sargramostim [Leukine]), can shorten the period of significant neutropenia by stimulating the bone marrow to produce leukocytes more quickly; these agents do not appear to increase the risk of producing more leukemic cells.

When the patient has recovered from the induction therapy (ie, the neutrophil and platelet counts have returned to normal and any infection has resolved), he or she typically receives consolidation therapy (postremission therapy) to eliminate any residual leukemia cells that are not clinically detectable and to reduce the chance for recurrence. Multiple treatment cycles of various agents are used, usually containing some form of cytarabine (eg, Cytosar, Ara-C). Frequently, the patient receives one cycle of treatment that is almost the same, if not identical, to the induction treatment but at lower dosages, therefore resulting in less toxicity.

Another aggressive treatment option is BMT or PBSCT. When a suitable tissue match can be obtained, the patient embarks on an even more aggressive regimen of chemotherapy (sometimes in combination with radiation therapy), with the treatment goal of destroying the hematopoietic function of the patient's bone marrow. The patient is then "rescued" with the infusion of the donor stem cells to reinitiate blood cell production. Patients who undergo PBSCT have a significant risk for infection, graft-versus-host disease (GVHD, in which the donor's lymphocytes [graft] recognize the patient's body as "foreign" and set up reactions to attack the "foreign" host), and other complications. The most appropriate use and timing of PBSCT remain unclear. Patients with a poorer prognosis may benefit from early PBSCT; those with a good prognosis may not need transplant at all. (See Chapter 16 for a discussion of nursing management in bone marrow transplantation.)

Another important option for the patient to consider is supportive care alone. In fact, supportive care may be the only option if the patient has significant comorbidity, such as extremely poor cardiac, pulmonary, renal, or hepatic function. In such cases, aggressive antileukemia therapy is not used; occasionally, hydroxyurea (Hydrea) may be used briefly to control the increase of blast cells. Patients are more commonly supported with antimicrobial therapy and transfusions as needed. This treatment approach provides the patient with some additional time at home; however, death frequently occurs within months, typically from infection or bleeding. (Refer to Chapter 17 for a discussion of end-of-life care.)

Complications of Treatment

Massive leukemic cell destruction from chemotherapy results in the release of intracellular electrolytes and fluids into the systemic circulation. Increases in uric acid levels, potassium, and phosphate are seen; this process is referred to as tumor **lysis** syndrome (see Chapter 16). The increased uric acid and phosphorus levels make the patient vulnerable to renal stone formation and renal colic, which can progress to acute renal failure. Hyperkalemia and hypocalcemia can lead to cardiac dysrhythmias; hypotension; neuromuscular effects such as muscle cramps, weakness, and spasm/tetany; confusion; and seizures. Patients require a high fluid intake, alkalization of the urine, and prophylaxis with allopurinol to prevent crystallization of uric acid and subsequent stone formation. GI problems may result from the infiltration of abnormal leukocytes into the abdominal organs and from the toxicity of the chemotherapeutic agents. Anorexia, nausea, vomiting, diarrhea, and severe mucositis are common. Because of the profound myelosuppressive effects of chemotherapy, significant neutropenia and thrombocytopenia typically result in serious infection and increased risk of bleeding.

Nursing Management

Nursing management of the patient with acute leukemia is presented at the end of the leukemia section in this chapter.

Chronic Myeloid Leukemia

Chronic myeloid leukemia (CML) arises from a mutation in the myeloid stem cell. Normal myeloid cells continue to be produced, but there is a pathologic increase in the production of forms of blast cells. Therefore, a wide spectrum of cell types exists within the blood, from blast forms through mature neutrophils. Because there is an uncontrolled proliferation of cells, the marrow expands into the cavities of long bones (eg, the femur), and cells are also formed in the liver and spleen (extramedullary hematopoiesis), resulting in enlargement of these organs that is sometimes painful. In 90% to 95% of patients with CML, a section of DNA is missing from chromosome 22 (the Philadelphia chromosome [Ph1]); it is translocated onto chromosome 9. The specific location of these changes is on the *BCR* gene of chromosome 22 and the *ABL* gene on chromosome 9. When these two genes fuse (*BCR-ABL* gene), they produce an abnormal protein (a tyrosine kinase protein) that causes leukocytes to divide rapidly. This *BCR-ABL* gene is present in virtually all patients with this disease.

CML is uncommon in people younger than 20 years; the incidence increases with age (median age, 55 to 60 years) (Cortes, 2004). Patients diagnosed with CML in the chronic phase have an overall median life expectancy of 3 to 5 years. During that time, they have few symptoms and complications from the disease itself. Problems with infections and bleeding are rare. However, once the disease transforms to the acute phase (blast crisis), the overall survival rarely exceeds several months.

Clinical Manifestations

The clinical picture of CML varies. Many patients are asymptomatic, and leukocytosis is detected by a CBC performed for some other reason. The leukocyte count commonly exceeds 100,000/mm^3. Patients with extremely high leukocyte counts may be somewhat short of breath or slightly confused due to decreased capillary perfusion to the lungs and brain from leukostasis (the excessive volume of leukocytes inhibits blood flow through the capillaries). The patient may have an enlarged, tender spleen. The liver may also be enlarged. Some patients have insidious symptoms, such as malaise, anorexia, and weight loss. Lymphadenopathy is rare. There are three stages in CML: chronic, transformation, and accelerated or blast crisis. Patients develop more symptoms and complications as the disease progresses.

Medical Management

Advances in understanding of the pathology of CML at a molecular level have led to dramatic changes in its treatment. An oral formulation of a tyrosine kinase inhibitor, imatinib mesylate (Gleevec), works by blocking signals within the leukemia cells that express the *BCR-ABL* protein, thus preventing a series of chemical reactions that cause the cell to grow and divide. Imatinib appears to be more useful in the chronic phase of the illness; clinical trials are in process to determine combination strategies with imatinib and other agents to improve response rates in the accelerated phase and blast crisis (Giles et al., 2004). Antacids and grapefruit juice may limit drug absorption, and large doses of acetaminophen can cause hepatotoxicity. The long-term effects of imatinib, its impact on survival, and the optimal length of treatment are being studied.

Other therapy depends on the stage of disease. In the chronic phase, the expected outcome is correction of the chromosomal abnormality (ie, conversion of the malignant stem cell population back to normal). Agents that have been used successfully for this purpose are interferon-alfa (Roferon-A) and cytosine, often in combination. These agents are administered daily as subcutaneous injections. This therapy is not benign; many patients cannot tolerate the profound fatigue, depression, anorexia, mucositis, and inability to concentrate. A less aggressive therapeutic approach focuses on reducing the leukocyte count to a more normal level but does not alter cytogenetic changes. This goal can be achieved by using oral chemotherapeutic agents, typically hydroxyurea (Hydrea) or busulfan (Myleran). In the case of an extreme leukocytosis at diagnosis (eg, leukocyte count greater than 300,000/mm^3), a more emergent treatment may be required. In this instance, leukapheresis (in which the patient's blood is removed and separated, with the leukocytes withdrawn, and the remaining blood returned to the patient) can temporarily reduce the number of leukocytes. An anthracycline chemotherapeutic agent (eg, daunomycin) may also be used to bring the leukocyte count down quickly to a safer level, where more conservative therapy can be instituted.

The transformation phase can be insidious or rapid; it marks the process of evolution (or transformation) to the acute form of leukemia (blast crisis). In the transformation phase, the patient may complain of bone pain and may report fevers (without any obvious sign of infection) and weight loss. Even with chemotherapy, the spleen may continue to enlarge. The patient may become more anemic and thrombocytopenic; an increased basophil level is detected by the CBC.

In the acute form of CML (blast crisis), treatment may resemble induction therapy for acute leukemia, using the same medications as for AML or ALL. Patients whose disease evolves into a "lymphoid" blast crisis are more likely to be able to reenter a chronic phase after induction therapy. For those whose disease evolves into AML, therapy is largely ineffective in achieving a second chronic phase. Life-threatening infections and bleeding occur frequently in this phase.

CML is a disease that can potentially be cured with BMT or PBSCT. Patients who receive such transplants while still in the chronic phase of the illness tend to have a greater chance for cure than those who receive them in the acute phase. The transplantation procedure may be considered for otherwise healthy patients who are younger than 65 years. More recently, research has shown that nonmyeloablative types of transplantation are effective and have diminished morbidity (Qazilbash et al., 2004). The use of imatinib therapy may decrease the need for transplantation in CML; however, the long-term efficacy of imatinib as well as its effects on transplant morbidity, mortality, and risk of relapse remain unknown (Radich et al., 2004).

Acute Lymphocytic Leukemia

Acute lymphocytic leukemia (ALL) results from an uncontrolled proliferation of immature cells (lymphoblasts) derived from the lymphoid stem cell. The cell of origin is the precursor to the B lymphocyte in approximately 75% of ALL cases; T-lymphocyte ALL occurs in approximately 25% of ALL cases. The *BCR-ABL* translocation (see earlier discussion) is found in 20% of ALL blast cells. ALL is most common in young children, with boys affected more often than girls; the peak incidence is 4 years of age. After 15 years of age, ALL is relatively uncommon. Increasing age appears to be associated with diminished survival; the 5-year event-free survival rate is almost 80% for children with ALL but drops to 40% for adults (Larson, 2004; Pui et al., 2004). Yet even if relapse occurs, resumption of induction therapy can often achieve a second complete remission. Moreover, BMT may be successful even after a second relapse, particularly in certain subsets of patients (eg, those with Philadelphia chromosome–positive ALL [Ph+ ALL]) (Larson, 2004).

Clinical Manifestations

Immature lymphocytes proliferate in the marrow and impede the development of normal myeloid cells. As a result, normal hematopoiesis is inhibited, resulting in reduced numbers of leukocytes, erythrocytes, and platelets. Leukocyte counts may be either low or high, but there is always a high proportion of immature cells. Manifestations of leukemic cell infiltration into other organs are more common with ALL than with other forms of leukemia and include pain from an enlarged liver or spleen and bone pain. The central nervous system is frequently a site for leukemic cells; thus, patients may exhibit headache and vomiting because of meningeal involvement.

Medical Management

The expected outcome of treatment is complete remission. Lymphoid blast cells are typically very sensitive to corticosteroids and to vinca alkaloids; therefore, these medications are an integral part of the initial induction therapy. Because ALL frequently invades the central nervous system, prophylaxis with cranial irradiation or intrathecal chemotherapy (eg, methotrexate) or both is also a key part of the treatment plan.

Treatment protocols for ALL tend to be complex, using a wide variety of chemotherapeutic agents. They often include a maintenance phase, when lower doses of medications are given for up to 3 years. Despite the complexity, treatment can be provided in the outpatient setting in some circumstances until severe complications develop. Imatinib appears effective in those with Philadelphia chromosome–positive ALL. Monoclonal antibodies, in which the antibody specific for the antigen expressed on the ALL blast cell is selected, are also being studied (Larson, 2004). For example, the CD52 antigen is expressed on approximately 70% of ALL cells; thus, alemtuzumab (Campath), a monoclonal antibody with specific affinity for the CD52 antigen, may be effective therapy for this subset of patients.

Infections, especially viral infections, are common. The use of corticosteroids to treat ALL increases the patient's susceptibility to infection. Patients with ALL tend to have a better response to treatment than do patients with AML. BMT or PBSCT offers a chance for prolonged remission, or even cure, if the illness recurs after therapy.

Nursing Management

Nursing management of the patient with acute leukemia is presented at the end of the leukemia section in this chapter.

Chronic Lymphocytic Leukemia

Chronic lymphocytic leukemia (CLL) is a common malignancy of older adults; two thirds of all patients with CLL are older than 60 years at diagnosis. It is the most common form of leukemia in the United States and Europe, affecting more than 120,000 people, but it is rarely seen in Asia. The average survival for patients with CLL ranges from 14 years (early stage) to 2 years (late stage) (Rai et al., 2004). CLL occurs more often in males (1.5:1 male–female ratio), and survival tends to be shorter in males (Rai et al., 2004).

Pathophysiology

CLL is typically derived from a malignant clone of B lymphocytes (T-lymphocyte CLL is rare). In contrast to the acute forms of leukemia, most of the leukemia cells in CLL are fully mature. It appears that these cells can escape **apoptosis** (programmed cell death), resulting in an excessive accumulation of the cells in the marrow and circulation. The antigen CD52 is prevalent on the surface of many of these leukemic B cells. The disease is classified into three or four stages (two classification systems are in use). In the early stage, an elevated lymphocyte count is seen; it can exceed 100,000/mm^3. Because the lymphocytes are small, they can easily travel through the small capillaries within the circulation, and the pulmonary and cerebral complications of leukocytosis (as seen with myeloid leukemias) typically are not found in CLL.

Lymphadenopathy occurs as the lymphocytes are trapped within the lymph nodes. The nodes can become very large and are sometimes painful. Hepatomegaly and splenomegaly then develop.

In later stages, anemia and thrombocytopenia may develop. Treatment is typically initiated in the later stages; earlier treatment does not appear to increase survival (Zent & Kay, 2004). Autoimmune complications can also occur at any stage, as either autoimmune hemolytic anemia or idiopathic thrombocytopenic purpura (ITP). In the autoimmune process, the reticuloendothelial system (RES) destroys the body's own erythrocytes or platelets.

Clinical Manifestations

Many patients are asymptomatic and are diagnosed incidentally during routine physical examinations or during treatment for another disease. An increased lymphocyte count (lymphocytosis) is always present. The erythrocyte and platelet counts may be normal or, in later stages of the illness, decreased. Enlargement of lymph nodes (lymphadenopathy) is common; this can be severe and sometimes painful. The spleen can also be enlarged (splenomegaly).

Patients with CLL can develop "B symptoms," a constellation of symptoms including fevers, drenching sweats (especially at night), and unintentional weight loss. Patients with CLL have defects in their humoral and cell-mediated immune systems; therefore, infections are common. The defect in cellular immunity is evidenced by an absent or decreased reaction to skin sensitivity tests (eg, *Candida*, mumps), which is known as **anergy.** Life-threatening infections are common. Viral infections, such as herpes zoster, can become widely disseminated.

Medical Management

In early stages, CLL may require no treatment. When symptoms are severe (drenching night sweats, painful lymphadenopathy) or when the disease progresses to later stages (with resultant anemia and thrombocytopenia), chemotherapy with fludarabine (Fludara) or corticosteroids and chlorambucil (Leukeran) is often used. The major side effect of fludarabine is prolonged bone marrow suppression, manifested by prolonged periods of neutropenia, lymphopenia, and thrombocytopenia. Patients are then at risk of such infections as *Pneumocystis jiroveci, Listeria,* mycobacteria, herpes viruses, and cytomegalovirus (CMV). Other useful agents include cyclophosphamide (Cytoxan), vincristine (Oncovin), and doxorubicin (Adriamycin).

The use of monoclonal antibodies is gaining popularity; these are effective and less toxic agents (Zent & Kay, 2004). The monoclonal antibody rituximab (Rituxan) has efficacy in CLL therapy and is often used in combination with other chemotherapeutic medications. The monoclonal antibody alemtuzumab (Campath) targets the CD52 antigen commonly found on CLL cells and is effective in clearing the marrow and circulation of these cells without affecting the stem cells. Because CD52 is present on both B and T lymphocytes, patients receiving alemtuzumab are at significant risk for infection; prophylactic use of antiviral agents and antibiotics (eg, trimethoprim/sulfamethoxazole [Bactrim, Septra]) is important and needs to continue for at least 2 months after treatment ends. Bacterial infections are common in patients with CLL, and IV treatment with immunoglobulin may be given to selected patients.

The disease trajectory of CLL is variable; thus, it is difficult to determine the best time to initiate treatment. Patients with early-stage disease are often monitored without treatment. In contrast, patients with signs of more aggressive disease or those who have developed an associated autoimmune disorder (autoimmune hemolytic anemia or ITP) are treated promptly (Ferrajoli & Keating, 2004).

Nursing Process

The Patient With Acute Leukemia

Assessment

Although the clinical picture varies with the type of leukemia as well as the treatment implemented, the health history may reveal a range of subtle symptoms reported by the patient before the problem is detectable on physical examination. Weakness and fatigue are common manifestations, not only of the leukemia, but also of the resulting complications of anemia and infection. If the patient is hospitalized, the assessments should be performed daily, or more frequently as warranted. Because the physical findings may be subtle initially, a thorough, systematic assessment incorporating all body systems is essential. For example, a dry cough, mild dyspnea, and diminished breath sounds may indicate a pulmonary infection. However, the infection may not be seen initially on the chest x-ray; the absence of neutrophils delays the inflammatory response against the pulmonary infection, and it is the inflammatory response that produces the x-ray changes. The platelet count can become dangerously low, leaving the patient at risk for significant bleeding. The specific body system assessments are delineated in the neutropenic precautions and bleeding precautions found in Charts 33-8 and 33-9, respectively. When serial assessments are performed, current findings are compared with previous findings to evaluate improvement or worsening.

The nurse also must closely monitor the results of laboratory studies. Flow sheets and spreadsheets are particularly useful in tracking the leukocyte count, ANC, hematocrit, platelet, creatinine and electrolyte levels, and hepatic function tests. Culture results need to be reported immediately so that appropriate antimicrobial therapy can begin or be modified.

Diagnosis

Nursing Diagnoses

Based on the assessment data, major nursing diagnoses for the patient with acute leukemia may include:

- Risk for infection and bleeding
- Risk for impaired skin integrity related to toxic effects of chemotherapy, alteration in nutrition, and impaired mobility
- Impaired gas exchange
- Impaired mucous membranes due to changes in epithelial lining of the GI tract from chemotherapy or prolonged use of antimicrobial medications
- Imbalanced nutrition, less than body requirements, related to hypermetabolic state, anorexia, mucositis, pain, and nausea
- Acute pain and discomfort related to mucositis, leukocyte infiltration of systemic tissues, fever, and infection
- Hyperthermia related to tumor lysis or infection
- Fatigue and activity intolerance related to anemia or infection
- Impaired physical mobility due to anemia and protective isolation
- Risk for excess fluid volume related to renal dysfunction, hypoproteinemia, need for multiple IV medications and blood products
- Diarrhea due to altered GI flora, mucosal denudation
- Risk for deficient fluid volume related to potential for diarrhea, bleeding, infection, and increased metabolic rate
- Self-care deficit due to fatigue, malaise, and protective isolation
- Anxiety due to knowledge deficit and uncertainty about future
- Disturbed body image related to change in appearance, function, and roles
- Grieving related to anticipatory loss and altered role functioning
- Potential for spiritual distress
- Deficient knowledge about disease process, treatment, complication management, and self-care measures

Collaborative Problems/ Potential Complications

Based on the assessment data, potential complications that may develop include:

- Infection
- Bleeding
- Renal dysfunction
- Tumor lysis syndrome
- Nutritional depletion
- Mucositis
- Depression

Planning and Goals

The major goals for the patient may include absence of complications and pain, attainment and maintenance of adequate nutrition, activity tolerance, ability to provide self-care and to cope with the diagnosis and prognosis, positive body image, and an understanding of the disease process and its treatment.

Nursing Interventions

Preventing or Managing Infection and Bleeding

The nursing interventions related to diminishing the risk of infection and for bleeding are delineated in Charts 33-8 and 33-9.

CHART 33-9

Bleeding Precautions

Nursing Diagnosis

Risk for injury/bleeding secondary to thrombocytopenia/ altered coagulation due to:

- Malignant invasion in bone marrow
- Bone marrow suppression resulting from chemotherapy (particularly alkylators, antitumor antibiotics, antimetabolites) and radiation therapy
- Hypersplenism
- Disseminated intravascular coagulation (DIC)
- Altered coagulation

Assessment

PATIENT

Assess the following areas thoroughly every shift (with spot checks throughout the shift if patient is hospitalized), and notify physician if there is new onset of the following and/or worsening of status:

- *Integument:* Petechiae (usually located on trunk, legs), ecchymoses or hematomas, conjunctival hemorrhages, bleeding gums, bleeding at puncture sites (venipuncture, lumbar puncture, bone marrow)
- *Cardiovascular:* Hypotension, tachycardia, dizziness, epistaxis
- *Pulmonary:* Respiratory distress, tachypnea
- *Gastrointestinal:* Hemoptysis, abdominal distention, rectal bleeding
- *Genitourinary:* Vaginal or urethral bleeding
- *Neurologic:* Headache, blurred vision, mental status changes

Laboratory Tests

- Monitor complete blood count (CBC), platelets daily (at least); coagulation panel.
- Notify physician if platelet count is <10,000/mm^3 or if count has changed significantly from previous count (including coagulation), or whenever patient becomes symptomatic.
- Ensure patient's blood was human leukocyte antigen (HLA) typed before transfusions or chemotherapy begins if admitted for induction therapy (eg, for acute leukemia).
- Obtain 1-hour posttransfusion platelet count if prescribed.
- Test all urine, emesis, stools for occult blood.

Nursing Interventions

PREVENT COMPLICATIONS

- Avoid aspirin and aspirin-containing medications or other medications known to inhibit platelet function, if possible.
- Do not give intramuscular injections.
- Do not insert indwelling catheters.
- Take no rectal temperatures; do not give suppositories, enemas.
- Use stool softeners, oral laxatives to prevent constipation.
- Use smallest possible needles when performing venipuncture.
- Apply pressure to venipuncture sites for 5 min or until bleeding has stopped.
- Permit no flossing of teeth and no commercial mouthwashes.
- Use only soft-bristled toothbrush for mouth care.
- Use only toothettes for mouth care if platelet count is <10,000/mm^3, or if gums bleed.
- Lubricate lips with water-soluble lubricant every 2 hr while awake.
- Avoid suctioning if at all possible; if unavoidable, use only gentle suctioning.
- Discourage vigorous coughing or blowing of the nose.
- Use only electric razor for shaving.
- Pad side rails as needed.
- Prevent falls by ambulating with patient as necessary.

CONTROL BLEEDING

- Apply direct pressure.
- For epistaxis, position patient in high Fowler's position; apply ice pack to back of neck and direct pressure to nose.
- Notify physician for prolonged bleeding (eg, unable to stop within 10 min).
- Administer platelets, fresh frozen plasma, packed red blood cells, as prescribed.

Evaluation and Expected Patient Outcomes

- Patient demonstrates an absence of bleeding as evidenced by absence of spontaneous petechiae, ecchymoses, epistaxis, hemoptysis, bleeding gums, conjunctival hemorrhage, vaginal bleeding, hematuria, guaiac positive stool, blurred vision, orthostatic hypotension, and prolonged bleeding from puncture sites.
- Patient demonstrates an absence of bleeding as evidenced by the presence of vital signs within normal limits and intact neurologic status.

*Serious hemorrhage is unusual in mildly thrombocytopenic patients in absence of local lesions (peptic ulcer, bleeding from hemorrhoids, cystitis).

Managing Mucositis

Although emphasis is placed on the oral mucosa, the entire GI mucosa can be altered, not only by the effects of chemotherapy but also from prolonged administration of antibiotics. Assessment of the oral mucosa must be thorough; therefore, dentures must be removed. Areas to assess include the palate, buccal mucosa, tongue, gums, lips, oropharynx, and the area under the tongue. In addition to identifying and describing lesions, the color and moisture of the mucosa should be noted.

Oral hygiene is very important to diminish the bacteria within the mouth, maintain moisture, and provide comfort. Soft-bristled toothbrushes should be used until the neutrophil and platelet counts become very low; at that time, sponge-tipped applicators may be substituted if necessary. Lemon-glycerin swabs and commercial mouthwashes should never be used because the glycerin and alcohol in them are extremely drying to the tissues. Simple rinses with saline (or saline and baking soda) solutions are inexpensive but effective in cleaning and moistening the oral mucosa. Because the risk for yeast or fungal infection in the mouth is great, other medications are often prescribed, such as chlorhexidine rinses (Peridex), clotrimazole troches (Mycelex), or fluconazole (Diflucan). The nurse reminds the patient about the importance of these medications to enhance adherence to the therapeutic regimen. Rinsing with chlorhexidine may discolor the teeth, and its efficacy is unclear.

To diminish perineal–rectal complications, it is important to cleanse this area thoroughly after each bowel movement. Women are instructed to cleanse the perineum from front to back. Sitz baths are a comfortable method of cleansing; the perineal–anal region and buttocks must be carefully dried afterward to minimize the chance of excoriation. Stool softeners should be used to increase the moisture of bowel movements; however, the stool texture must be monitored so that the softeners can be decreased or stopped if the stool becomes too loose.

Improving Nutritional Intake

The disease process can increase the patient's metabolic rate and nutritional requirements. (Sepsis further increases them.) Nutritional intake is often reduced because of pain and discomfort associated with stomatitis. Mouth care before and after meals and the administration of analgesics before eating can help increase intake. If oral anesthetics are used, the patient must be warned to chew with extreme care to avoid inadvertently biting the tongue or buccal mucosa.

Nausea should not be a major contributing factor, because recent advances in antiemetic therapy are highly effective. However, nausea can result from antimicrobial therapy, so some antiemetic therapy may still be required after the chemotherapy has been completed.

Small, frequent feedings of foods that are soft in texture and moderate in temperature may be better tolerated. Low-microbial diets are typically prescribed (avoiding uncooked fruits or vegetables and those without a peelable skin). Nutritional supplements are frequently used. Daily body weights (as well as intake and output measurements) are useful in monitoring fluid status. Both calorie counts and more formal nutritional assessments are useful. Parenteral nutrition is often required to maintain adequate nutrition.

Easing Pain and Discomfort

Recurrent fevers are common in acute leukemia; at times, they are accompanied by shaking chills (rigors), which can be severe. Myalgias and arthralgias can result. Acetaminophen is typically given to decrease fever, but it does so by increasing diaphoresis. Sponging with cool water may be useful, but cold water or ice packs should be avoided because the heat cannot dissipate from constricted blood vessels. Bedclothes need frequent changing as well. Gentle back and shoulder massage may provide comfort.

Stomatitis can also cause significant discomfort. In addition to oral hygiene practices, PCA can be effective in controlling the pain (see Chapter 13). With the exception of severe mucositis, less pain is associated with acute leukemia than with many other forms of cancer. However, the amount of psychological suffering that the patient must endure can be immense. Patients greatly benefit from active listening.

Because patients with acute leukemia require hospitalization for extensive nursing care (either during induction or consolidation therapy or during resultant complications), sleep deprivation frequently results. Nurses need to implement creative strategies that permit uninterrupted sleep for at least a few hours while still administering necessary medications on time.

Decreasing Fatigue and Deconditioning

Fatigue is a common and oppressive problem. Nursing interventions should focus on assisting the patient to establish a balance between activity and rest. Patients with acute leukemia need to maintain some physical activity and exercise to prevent the deconditioning that results from inactivity. Use of a high-efficiency particulate air (HEPA) filter mask can permit the patient to ambulate outside the room despite severe neutropenia. Although many patients lack the motivation or energy to use them, stationary bicycles within the room can also be used. At a minimum, patients should be encouraged to sit up in a chair while awake rather than staying in bed; even this simple activity can improve the patient's tidal volume and enhance circulation. Physical therapy can also be beneficial.

Maintaining Fluid and Electrolyte Balance

Febrile episodes, bleeding, and inadequate or overly aggressive fluid replacement can alter the patient's fluid status. Similarly, persistent diarrhea, vomiting, and long-term use of certain antimicrobial agents can cause significant deficits in electrolytes. Intake and output need to be measured accurately, and daily weights should also be monitored. The patient should be assessed for signs of dehydration as well as fluid overload, with particular attention to pulmonary status and the development of dependent edema. Laboratory test results, particularly electrolytes, blood urea nitrogen, creatinine, and hematocrit, should be monitored and compared with previous results. Replacement of electrolytes, particularly potassium and magnesium, is commonly required. Patients receiving amphotericin or certain antibiotics are at increased risk for electrolyte depletion.

Improving Self-Care

Because hygiene measures are so important in this patient population, they must be performed by the nurse when the patient cannot do so. However, the patient should be encouraged to do as much as possible to preserve mobility and function as well as self-esteem. Patients may have negative feelings, even disgust, because they can no longer care for themselves. Empathetic listening is helpful, as is realistic reassurance that these deficits are temporary. As the patient recovers, it is important to assist him or her to resume more self-care. Patients are usually discharged from the hospital with a central vascular access device (eg, Hickman catheter, peripherally inserted central catheter [PICC]), and most patients can care for the catheter with adequate instruction and practice under observation.

Managing Anxiety and Grief

Being diagnosed with acute leukemia can be extremely frightening. In many instances, the need to begin treatment is emergent, and the patient has little time to process the fact that he or she has the illness before making decisions about therapy. Providing emotional support and discussing the uncertain future are crucial. The nurse also needs to assess how much information the patient wants to have regarding the illness, its treatment, and potential complications. This desire should be reassessed at intervals, because needs and interest in information change throughout the course of the disease and treatment. Priorities must be identified so that procedures, assessments, and self-care expectations are adequately explained even to those who do not wish extensive information.

Many patients become depressed and begin to grieve for the losses they feel, such as normal family functioning, professional roles and responsibilities, and social roles, as well as physical functioning. The nurse can assist the patient to identify the source of the grief and encourage him or her to allow time to adjust to the major life changes produced by the illness. Role restructuring, in both family and professional life, may be required. Again, when possible, encouraging the patient to identify options and to take time making significant decisions regarding such restructuring is helpful.

Discharge from the hospital can also provoke anxiety. Although most patients are extremely eager to go home, they may lack confidence in their ability to manage potential complications and to resume their normal activity. Close communication between nurses across care settings can reassure patients that they will not be abandoned.

Encouraging Spiritual Well-Being

Because acute leukemia is a serious, potentially life-threatening illness, the nurse may offer support to enhance the patient's spiritual well-being. The patient's spiritual and religious practices should be assessed and pastoral services offered. Throughout the patient's illness, it is important that the nurse assist the patient to maintain hope. However, that hope should be realistic and will certainly change over the course of the illness. For example, the patient may initially hope to be cured, but with repeated relapses and a change to hospice or palliative care the same patient may hope for a quiet, dignified death. (Refer to Chapter 17 for a discussion of end-of-life care.)

Monitoring and Managing Potential Complications

Nursing interventions for potential complications were described previously.

Promoting Home and Community-Based Care

TEACHING PATIENTS SELF-CARE

Most patients cope better when they have an understanding of what is happening to them. Based on their education, literacy level, and interest, teaching of patient and family should focus on the disease (including some pathophysiology), its treatment, and certainly the significant risk for infection and bleeding (see Charts 33-8 and 33-9) that results.

Management of a vascular access device can be taught to most patients or family members. Follow-up and care for the devices may also need to be provided by nurses in an outpatient facility or by a home care agency.

CONTINUING CARE

Shortened hospital stays and outpatient care have significantly altered care for patients with acute leukemia. In many instances, when the patient is clinically stable but still requires parenteral antibiotics or blood products, these procedures can be performed in an outpatient setting. Nurses in these various settings must communicate regularly. The patient needs to learn which parameters are important to monitor and how to monitor them. Specific instructions need to be given about when the patient should seek care from the physician or other health care provider.

The patient and family need to have a clear understanding of the disease and the prognosis. The nurse acts as an advocate to ensure that this information is provided. When the patient no longer responds to therapy, it is important to respect the patient's choices about treatment, including measures to prolong life and other end-of-life measures. Advance directives, including living wills, provide patients with some measure of control during terminal illness.

Many patients in this stage still choose to be cared for at home, and families often need support when considering this option. Coordination of home care services and instruction can help alleviate anxiety about managing the patient's care in the home. As the patient becomes weaker, the caregivers must assume more of the patient's care. In addition, caregivers often need to be encouraged to take care of themselves, allowing time for rest and accepting emotional support. Hospice staff can assist in providing respite for family members as well as care for the patient. Patients and families also need assistance to cope with changes in their roles and responsibilities. Anticipatory grieving is an essential task during this time (see Chapter 17).

In patients with acute leukemia, death typically occurs from infection or bleeding. Family members need to have information about these complications and the measures to take should either occur. Many family members cannot cope with the care required when a patient begins to bleed actively. It is important to delineate alternatives to keeping the patient at home, such as inpatient hospice units. Should another option be sought, family members who may feel guilty that they could not keep the patient at home will require support from the nurse.

Evaluation

Expected Patient Outcomes

Expected patient outcomes may include:

1. Shows no evidence of infection
2. Experiences no bleeding
3. Has intact oral mucous membranes
   a. Participates in oral hygiene regimen
   b. Reports no discomfort in mouth
4. Attains optimal level of nutrition
   a. Maintains weight with increased food and fluid intake
   b. Maintains adequate protein stores (albumin)
5. Reports satisfaction with pain and comfort levels
6. Has less fatigue and increased activity
7. Maintains fluid and electrolyte balance
8. Participates in self-care
9. Copes with anxiety and grief
   a. Discusses concerns and fears
   b. Uses stress management strategies appropriately
   c. Participates in decisions regarding end-of-life care
   d. Discusses hope for peaceful death
10. Absence of complications

Agnogenic Myeloid Metaplasia

Agnogenic myeloid metaplasia (AMM), also known as myelofibrosis, is a chronic myeloproliferative disorder that arises from neoplastic transformation of an early hematopoietic stem cell. The disease is characterized by marrow fibrosis or scarring, splenomegaly, extramedullary hematopoiesis (typically spleen, liver, or both), leukocytosis and thrombocytosis, and anemia. Some patients have suppressed leukocyte and platelet counts as well as anemia (pancytopenia). Patients with AMM have increased **angiogenesis** (formation of new blood vessels) within the marrow. Early forms of blood cells (including nucleated RBCs and megakaryocyte fragments) are frequently found in the circulation.

AMM is a disease of the elderly, with a median age at diagnosis of 60 to 65 years. Survival varies from as little as 1 year to more than 30 years; the average is 3.5 to 5.5 years (Barosi, 2003). Heart failure, complications of marrow failure, and transformation to AML are the common causes of death.

Medical Management

For those unable to undergo stem cell transplant, medical management is directed toward palliation, reducing symptoms related to cytopenias, splenomegaly, and hypermetabolic state. Although one third of anemic patients respond to the combination of an androgen plus a corticosteroid, the primary treatment remains PRBC transfusion. Because of the prolonged requirement for these transfusions, iron overload is a common problem. Iron chelation therapy should be initiated in patients in whom survival is expected to exceed a few years. Hydroxyurea is often used to control high leukocyte and platelet counts and to reduce the size of the spleen. Splenic irradiation or splenectomy may also be used to control the significant splenomegaly that can develop. However, both modalities render the patient at significant risk of development of infection. Alpha-interferon has been useful in controlling the disease, particularly in younger patients. Thalidomide (Thalomid) has been tried in an attempt to diminish the angiogenesis within the marrow; unfortunately, most patients cannot tolerate the drug for more than several months (Barosi, 2003). BMT or PBSCT may be a useful treatment modality in younger, otherwise healthy people.

Nursing Management

Splenomegaly can be profound in patients with AMM, with enlargement of the spleen that extends to the pelvic rim. This condition is extremely uncomfortable and can severely limit nutritional intake. Analgesics are often ineffective. Methods to reduce the size of the spleen are usually more effective in controlling pain. Splenomegaly, coupled with a hypermetabolic state, results in weight loss (often severe) and muscle wasting. Patients benefit from very small, frequent meals of foods that are high in calories and protein. Weakness, fatigue, and altered body image are other significant problems. Energy conservation methods and active listening are important nursing interventions. The patient needs to be educated about signs and symptoms of infection as well as appropriate interventions when an infection is suspected.

Lymphoma

The lymphomas are neoplasms of cells of lymphoid origin. These tumors usually start in lymph nodes but can involve lymphoid tissue in the spleen, the GI tract (eg, the wall of the stomach), the liver, or the bone marrow. They are often classified according to the degree of cell differentiation and the origin of the predominant malignant cell. Lymphomas can be broadly classified into two categories: Hodgkin's disease and non-Hodgkin's lymphoma (NHL).

Hodgkin's Disease

Hodgkin's disease is a relatively rare malignancy that has an impressive cure rate. It is somewhat more common in men than women and has two peaks of incidence: one in the early 20s and the other after 50 years of age. Disease occurrence has a familial pattern: first-degree relatives have a higher-than-normal frequency of disease, but the actual incidence of this pattern is low. No increased incidence for non-blood relatives (eg, spouses) has been documented. Hodgkin's disease is seen more commonly in patients receiving chronic immunosuppressive therapy (eg, for renal transplant) and in woodworkers. It is also seen in veterans of the military who were exposed to the herbicide Agent Orange.

Pathophysiology

Unlike other lymphomas, Hodgkin's disease is unicentric in origin in that it initiates in a single node. The disease spreads by contiguous extension along the lymphatic system. The malignant cell of Hodgkin's disease is the Reed-Sternberg cell, a gigantic tumor cell that is morphologically unique and is thought to be of immature lymphoid origin. It is the pathologic hallmark and essential diagnostic criterion for Hodgkin's disease. However, the tumor is very heterogeneous and may actually contain few Reed-Sternberg cells. Repeated biopsies may be required to establish the diagnosis.

The cause of Hodgkin's disease is unknown but a viral etiology is suspected. In fact, fragments of the Epstein-Barr virus have been found in some Reed-Sternberg cells.

Hodgkin's disease is customarily classified into five subgroups based on pathologic analyses that reflect the natural history of the malignancy and suggest the prognosis. For example, when lymphocytes predominate, with few Reed-Sternberg cells and minimal involvement of the lymph nodes, the prognosis is much more favorable than when the lymphocyte count is low and the lymph nodes are virtually replaced by tumor cells of the most primitive type. Most patients with Hodgkin's disease have the types currently designated "nodular sclerosis" or "mixed cellularity." The nodular sclerosis type tends to occur more often in young women, at an earlier stage but with a worse prognosis than the mixed cellularity subgroup, which occurs more commonly in men and causes more constitutional symptoms but has a better prognosis.

Clinical Manifestations

Hodgkin's disease usually begins as a painless enlargement of one or more lymph nodes on one side of the neck. The individual nodes are painless and firm but not hard. The most common sites for lymphadenopathy are the cervical, supraclavicular, and mediastinal nodes; involvement of the iliac or inguinal nodes or spleen is much less common. A mediastinal mass may be seen on chest x-ray; occasionally, the mass is large enough to compress the trachea and cause dyspnea. Pruritus is common; it can be extremely distressing, and the cause is unknown. Some patients experience brief but severe pain after drinking alcohol, usually at the site of the tumor. Again, the cause of this is unknown.

All organs are vulnerable to invasion by Hodgkin's disease. The symptoms result from compression of organs by the tumor, such as cough and pulmonary effusion (from pulmonary infiltrates), jaundice (from hepatic involvement or bile duct obstruction), abdominal pain (from splenomegaly or retroperitoneal adenopathy), or bone pain (from skeletal involvement). Herpes zoster infections are common. A cluster of constitutional symptoms has important prognostic implications. Referred to as "B symptoms," they include fever (without chills), drenching sweats (particularly at night), and unintentional weight loss of more than 10%. "B symptoms" are found in 40% of patients and are more common in advanced disease.

A mild anemia is the most common hematologic finding. The leukocyte count may be elevated or decreased. The platelet count is typically normal, unless the tumor has invaded the bone marrow, suppressing hematopoiesis. The **erythrocyte sedimentation rate** (ESR) and the serum copper level are used by some clinicians to assess disease activity. Patients with Hodgkin's disease have impaired cellular immunity, as evidenced by an absent or decreased reaction to skin sensitivity tests (eg, *Candida,* mumps).

Assessment and Diagnostic Findings

Because many manifestations are similar to those occurring with infection, diagnostic studies are performed to rule out an infectious origin for the disease. The diagnosis is made by means of an excisional lymph node biopsy and the finding of the Reed-Sternberg cell. Once the diagnosis is confirmed and the histologic type is established, it is necessary to assess the extent of the disease, a process referred to as staging.

During the health history, the patient is assessed for any "B symptoms." Physical examination requires a careful, systematic evaluation of the lymph node chains, as well as the size of the spleen and liver. A chest x-ray and a CT scan of the chest, abdomen, and pelvis are crucial to identify the extent of lymphadenopathy within these regions. A positron emission tomography (PET) scan may be the most sensitive imaging test in identifying residual disease. Laboratory tests include CBC, platelet count, ESR, and liver and renal function studies. A bone marrow biopsy is performed if there are signs of marrow involvement, and some physicians routinely perform bilateral biopsies. Bone scans may be performed to identify any involvement in these areas. A staging laparotomy and lymphangiography are no longer considered mandatory, primarily because of the accuracy of CT and PET.

Medical Management

The general goal in treatment of Hodgkin's disease, regardless of stage, is cure. Treatment is determined primarily by the stage of the disease, not the histologic type; however, extensive research is ongoing to target treatment regimens to histologic subtypes or prognostic features. Traditionally, early Hodgkin's disease was treated by a staging laparotomy followed by radiation therapy. This treatment method has commonly been replaced by a short course (2 to 4 months) of chemotherapy followed by radiation therapy in certain subsets of early-stage disease (IA and IIA) (Bonadonna et al., 2004; Diehl et al., 2004). Some patients with early-stage disease and good prognostic features may receive radiation therapy alone. Combination chemotherapy, for example with doxorubicin (Adriamycin), bleomycin (Blenoxane), vinblastine (Velban), and dacarbazine (DTIC), referred to as ABVD, is now the standard treatment for more advanced disease (stages III and IV and all B stages).

Radiation therapy is still very useful for patients with extensive adenopathy (often termed bulky disease). In this group, residual disease often persists after the chemotherapy treatment is finished; radiation therapy to the areas of remaining adenopathy has been shown to improve survival.

Even when Hodgkin's disease does recur, the use of high doses of chemotherapeutic agents, followed by autologous BMT or stem cell transplantation, can be very effective in controlling the disease and extending survival time.

Long-Term Complications of Therapy

Much is now known about the long-term effects of chemotherapy and radiation therapy, primarily from the large numbers of people who were cured of Hodgkin's disease by these treatments. The various complications of treatment are listed in Chart 33-10. Risk factors for other cancers should be assessed, and long-term surveillance is crucial. Lung cancer is the most common type of second malignancy in patients with Hodgkin's disease, particularly following combination chemotherapy and radiation (Mauch, Aleman, Carde, et al., 2003). Breast cancer appears to be more common in women, particularly in those who were treated before age 30 years, and in those who received radiation therapy alone (Mauch et al., 2003). The potential development of a second malignancy is obviously of concern to the patient, and this potential should be addressed with the patient when treatment decisions are made. However, it is important to consider that Hodgkin's disease is curable. Patients should be encouraged to reduce other factors that increase the risk of developing second cancers, such as use of tobacco and alcohol and exposure to environmental carcinogens. Revised treatment approaches are aimed at diminishing the risk for complications without sacrificing the potential for cure.

CHART 33-10

Potential Long-Term Complications of Therapy for Hodgkin's Disease

Immune dysfunction
Herpes infections (zoster and varicella)
Pneumococcal sepsis
Acute myeloid leukemia (AML)
Myelodysplastic syndromes (MDS)
Non-Hodgkin's lymphoma
Solid tumors
Thyroid cancer
Thymic hyperplasia
Hypothyroidism
Pericarditis (acute or chronic)
Cardiomyopathy
Pneumonitis (acute or chronic)
Avascular necrosis
Growth retardation
Infertility
Decreased libido
Dental caries

Non-Hodgkin's Lymphomas (NHLs)

The NHLs are a heterogeneous group of cancers that originate from the neoplastic growth of lymphoid tissue. As in CLL, the neoplastic cells are thought to arise from a single clone of lymphocytes; however, in NHL, the cells may vary morphologically. Most NHLs involve malignant B lymphocytes; only 5% involve T lymphocytes. In contrast to Hodgkin's disease, the lymphoid tissues involved are largely infiltrated with malignant cells. The spread of these malignant lymphoid cells occurs unpredictably, and true localized disease is uncommon. Lymph nodes from multiple sites may be infiltrated, as may sites outside the lymphoid system (extranodal tissue).

There has been a threefold increase in incidence of NHL in recent years (Lister, 2004). It is now the sixth most common type of cancer diagnosed in the United States and the sixth most common cause of cancer death (Jemal, Siegal, Ward, et al., 2006). The incidence increases with each decade of life; the average age at diagnosis is 50 to 60 years. Although no common etiologic factor has been identified, the incidence of NHL has increased in people with immunodeficiencies or autoimmune disorders; prior treatment for cancer; prior organ transplant; viral infections (including Epstein-Barr virus and HIV); and exposure to pesticides, solvents, dyes, or defoliating agents, including Agent Orange. Prognosis varies greatly among the various types of NHL. Long-term survival (more than 10 years) is commonly achieved in low-grade, localized lymphomas. Even with aggressive disease forms, cure is possible in at least one third of patients who receive aggressive treatment.

Clinical Manifestations

Symptoms are highly variable, reflecting the diverse nature of the NHLs. Lymphadenopathy is most common (66%); however, in more indolent (less aggressive) types of lymphomas, the lymphadenopathy can wax and wane (Freedman, 2004).

With early-stage disease, or with the types that are considered more indolent, symptoms may be virtually absent or very minor, and the illness typically is not diagnosed until it progresses to a later stage, when the patient is symptomatic. At these stages (III or IV), lymphadenopathy is distinctly noticeable. One third of patients with NHLs have "B symptoms" (recurrent fever, drenching night sweats, and unintentional weight loss of 10% or more). Lymphomatous masses can compromise organ function. For example, a mass in the mediastinum can cause respiratory distress; abdominal masses can compromise the ureters, leading to renal dysfunction; and splenomegaly can cause abdominal discomfort, nausea, early satiety, anorexia, and weight loss. Involvement of the central nervous system with lymphoma is increasing in frequency (Freedman, 2004).

Assessment and Diagnostic Findings

The actual diagnosis of NHL is categorized into a highly complex classification system based on histopathology, immunophenotyping, and cytogenetic analyses of the malignant cells. The specific histopathologic type of the disease has important prognostic implications. Treatment also varies and is based on these features. Indolent types tend to have small cells that are distributed in a follicular pattern. Aggressive types tend to have large or immature cells distributed through the nodes in a diffuse pattern. Staging, also an important factor, is typically based on data obtained from CT and PET scans, bone marrow biopsies, and occasionally cerebrospinal fluid analysis. The stage is based on the site of disease and its spread to other sites. For example, in stage I disease, only one area of involvement is detected; thus, stage I disease is highly localized and may respond well to localized therapy (eg, radiation therapy). In contrast, in stage IV disease at least one extranodal site is detected.

Low-grade lymphomas may not require treatment until the disease progresses to a later stage, but historically they have also been relatively unresponsive to treatment, and in most cases, use of therapeutic modalities did not improve overall survival. More aggressive types of NHL (eg, lymphoblastic lymphoma, Burkitt's lymphoma) require prompt initiation of chemotherapy; however, these types tend to be more responsive to treatment.

Medical Management

Treatment is based on the actual classification of disease, the stage of disease, prior treatment (if any), and the patient's ability to tolerate therapy. If the disease is not an aggressive form and is truly localized, radiation alone may be the treatment of choice. With aggressive types of NHL, aggressive combinations of chemotherapeutic agents are given even in early stages. More intermediate forms are commonly treated with combination chemotherapy and radiation therapy for stage I and II disease. The biologic agent interferon has been approved for the treatment of follicular low-grade lymphomas, and an antibody to CD20, rituximab (Rituxan), has been effective in achieving partial responses in patients with recurrent low-grade lymphoma. In fact, the combination of rituximab with conventional chemotherapy (Cytoxan, doxorubicin, vincristine, and prednisone [CHOP]) is now considered standard treatment for common, aggressive lymphomas (Lister, 2004). Unfortunately, in most situations, relapse is commonly seen in patients with low-grade lymphomas. A recent study documented the effectiveness of maintenance therapy with rituximab in reducing progression of disease (Hochster et al., 2004). Central nervous system involvement is common with some aggressive forms of NHL; in this situation, cranial radiation or intrathecal chemotherapy is used in addition to systemic chemotherapy.

Treatment after relapse is controversial. BMT or PBSCT may be considered for patients younger than 60 years (see Chapter 16). Other treatment options include yttrium 90 ibritumomab tiuxetan (Zevalin) (Riley & Byar, 2004) or proteasome inhibitors (eg, bortezomib [Velcade]) (Goy et al., 2004).

Nursing Management

Lymphoma is a highly complex constellation of diseases. When caring for patients with lymphoma, it is extremely important to know the specific disease type, stage of disease, treatment history, and current treatment plan. Most of the care for patients with Hodgkin's disease or NHL takes place in the outpatient setting, unless complications occur (eg, infection, respiratory compromise due to mediastinal mass). The most commonly used treatment methods are chemotherapy and radiation therapy. Chemotherapy causes systemic side effects (eg, myelosuppression, nausea, hair loss, risk of infection), whereas radiation therapy causes specific effects that are limited to the area being irradiated. For example, patients receiving abdominal radiation therapy may experience nausea and diarrhea but not hair loss. Regardless of the type of treatment, all patients may experience fatigue.

The risk for infection is significant for these patients, not only from treatment-related myelosuppression but also from the defective immune response that results from the disease itself. Patients need to be taught to minimize the risks of infection, to recognize signs of possible infection, and to contact the health care professional should such signs develop (see Chart 33-7).

Additional complications depend on the location of the lymphoma. Therefore, it is important for the nurse to know the tumor location so that assessments can be targeted appropriately. For example, patients with lymphomatous masses in the upper chest should be assessed for superior vena cava obstruction or airway obstruction, if the mass is near the bronchus or trachea.

Many lymphomas can be cured with current treatments. However, as survival rates increase, the incidence of second malignancies, particularly AML or MDS, also increases. Therefore, survivors should be screened regularly for the development of second malignancies.

Multiple Myeloma

Multiple myeloma is a malignant disease of the most mature form of B lymphocyte, the plasma cell. It is not classified as a lymphoma. Plasma cells secrete immunoglobulins, proteins necessary for antibody production to fight infection.

Median survival time for patients with multiple myeloma is 3 to 5 years. Death usually results from infection.

Pathophysiology

In multiple myeloma, the malignant plasma cells produce an increased amount of a specific immunoglobulin that is nonfunctional. Functional types of immunoglobulin are still produced by nonmalignant plasma cells, but in lower-than-normal quantity. The specific immunoglobulin secreted by the myeloma cells is detectable in the blood or urine and is referred to as the monoclonal protein, or M protein. This protein serves as a useful marker to monitor the extent of disease and the patient's response to therapy. It is commonly measured by serum or urine protein electrophoresis. Moreover, the patient's total protein level is typically elevated, again due to the production of M protein. Malignant plasma cells also secrete certain substances to stimulate the creation of new blood vessels to enhance the growth of these clusters of plasma cells; this process is referred to as angiogenesis. Occasionally the plasma cells infiltrate other tissue, in which case they are referred to as plasmacytomas. Plasmacytomas can occur in the sinuses, spinal cord, and soft tissues.

Clinical Manifestations

The classic presenting symptom of multiple myeloma is bone pain, usually in the back or ribs. Bone pain is reported by two thirds of all patients at diagnosis. Unlike arthritic pain, the bone pain associated with myeloma increases with movement and decreases with rest; patients may report that they have less pain on awakening but the pain intensity increases during the day. In myeloma, a substance secreted by the plasma cells, osteoclast activating factor, and other substances (eg, interleukin-6 [IL-6]) are involved in stimulating osteoclasts. Both mechanisms appear to be involved in the process of bone breakdown. Thus, lytic lesions as well as osteoporosis may be seen on bone x-rays. (They are not well visualized on bone scans.) The bone destruction can be severe enough to cause vertebral collapse and fractures, including spinal fractures, which can impinge on the spinal cord and result in spinal cord compression. It is this bone destruction that causes significant pain.

If the bone destruction is fairly extensive, excessive ionized calcium is lost from the bone and enters the serum; hypercalcemia may therefore develop (frequently manifested by excessive thirst, dehydration, constipation, altered mental status, confusion, and perhaps coma). Renal failure may also occur; the configuration of the circulating immunoglobulin molecule (particularly the shape of lambda light chains) can damage the renal tubules.

NURSING ALERT

Any elderly patient whose chief complaint is back pain and who has an elevated total protein level should be evaluated for possible myeloma.

As more and more malignant plasma cells are produced, the marrow has less space for erythrocyte production, and anemia may develop. This anemia is also caused to a great extent by a diminished production of erythropoietin (a glycoprotein necessary for erythrocyte production) by the kidney. The patient may complain of fatigue and weakness due to the anemia. In the late stage of the disease, a reduced number of leukocytes and platelets may also be seen because the bone marrow is infiltrated by malignant plasma cells.

When plasma cells secrete excessive amounts of immunoglobulin, the serum viscosity can increase. Hyperviscosity may be manifested by bleeding from the nose or mouth, headache, blurred vision, paresthesias, or heart failure.

Assessment and Diagnostic Findings

Finding an elevated monoclonal protein spike in the serum (via serum protein electrophoresis) or urine (via urine protein electrophoresis) or light chain in the urine (sometimes referred to as Bence Jones protein) is considered to be a major criterion in the diagnosis of multiple myeloma. The presence of lytic bone lesions on x-ray studies aids in the diagnosis, as does the presence of anemia or hypercalcemia. The diagnosis of myeloma can be confirmed by bone marrow biopsy; the presence of sheets of plasma cells is the hallmark diagnostic criterion. Because the infiltration of the marrow by these malignant plasma cells is not uniform, the plasma cells may not be increased in a given sample (a false-negative result).

Medical Management

There is no cure for multiple myeloma. Even BMT or PBSCT is considered to extend remission rather than provide a cure. However, for many patients, it is possible to control the illness and maintain their level of functioning quite well for several years or longer. Chemotherapy is the primary treatment; corticosteroids, particularly dexamethasone (Decadron), are especially effective and are often combined with other agents (eg, melphalan [Alkeran], cyclophosphamide [Cytoxan], doxorubicin [Adriamycin], vincristine [Oncovin], and carmustine [BCNU]).

Radiation therapy is very useful in strengthening the bone at a specific lesion, particularly one at risk for bone fracture or spinal cord compression. It is also useful in relieving bone pain and reducing the size of plasma cell tumors that occur outside the skeletal system. However, because it is a nonsystemic form of treatment, it does not diminish the source of the bone conditions (ie, the production of malignant plasma cells). Therefore, radiation therapy is typically used in combination with systemic treatment such as chemotherapy.

When lytic lesions result in vertebral compression fractures, vertebroplasty is often performed. This procedure is performed under fluoroscopy. A hollow needle is positioned within the fractured vertebra, and when the precise location is confirmed, an orthopedic cement is infiltrated into the vertebra to stabilize the fracture and strengthen the vertebra. For most patients, relief from pain is almost immediate. This procedure has been enhanced by concomitant kyphoplasty, the use of a special inflatable balloon inserted into the vertebra to increase the height of the vertebra prior to injecting the cement.

Newer forms of bisphosphonates, such as pamidronate (Aredia) and zoledronic acid (Zometa), have been shown to strengthen bone in multiple myeloma by diminishing the secretion of osteoclast activating factor, thus controlling bone pain and potentially preventing bone fracture. These agents are also effective in managing and preventing hypercalcemia. Some evidence suggests that bisphosphonates may actually have activity against the myeloma cells themselves by inhibiting a growth factor necessary for myeloma cell survival (Lipton, 2004; Terpos & Rahemtulla, 2004). Recently, an increased incidence of osteonecrosis of the jaw has been found in people with and without multiple myeloma receiving long-term bisphosphonate therapy (Lugassy et al., 2004; Ruggiero et al., 2004). This association between bisphosphonates and osteonecrosis has not yet been proved, and the incidence of osteonecrosis appears to be very low. Nonetheless, careful assessment for this complication should be performed, and it may be prudent to warn patients to have any necessary invasive dental procedure performed prior to initiating bisphosphonate therapy.

When patients have signs and symptoms of hyperviscosity, plasmapheresis may be used to lower the immunoglobulin level. Symptoms may be more useful than serum viscosity levels in determining the need for this intervention.

Recent advances in the understanding of the process of angiogenesis have resulted in new therapeutic options. The sedative thalidomide (Thalomid), initially used as an antiemetic, has significant antimyeloma effects. It inhibits cytokines necessary for new vascular generation, such as vascular endothelial growth factor, and for myeloma cell growth and survival, such as IL-6 and tumor necrosis factor, by boosting the body's immune response against the tumor and by creating favorable conditions for apoptosis (programmed cell death) of the myeloma cells. Thalidomide is effective in refractory myeloma and in "smoldering" disease states and may prevent progression to a more active state. Thalidomide is not a typical chemotherapeutic agent and has a unique side effect profile. Fatigue, dizziness, constipation, rash, and peripheral neuropathy are commonly encountered; myelosuppression is not. There is also an increased incidence of DVT; prophylactic anticoagulation may be prescribed to prevent this complication (Kyle & Rajkumar, 2004). Thalidomide is contraindicated in pregnancy because of associated severe birth defects. Thus, the patient must be counseled and agree to use approved methods of birth control prior to taking this drug.

More recently, the use of a proteasome inhibiting agent, bortezomib (Velcade), has been approved by the FDA for use in refractory disease (Devenney, 2004). Side effects include transient thrombocytopenia, orthostatic hypotension, nausea and vomiting, skin rash, and neuropathy.

Further research has documented the efficacy of a thalidomide analogue, known as CC-5013, or Revlimid (lenalidomide). This agent inhibits angiogenesis and promotes apoptosis and cytotoxicity (Kyle & Rajkuman, 2004). The side effect profile is quite different from thalidomide: myelosuppression is common, whereas sedation, neuropathy, and constipation are not.

Nursing Management

Pain management is very important in patients with multiple myeloma. NSAIDs can be very useful for mild pain or can be administered in combination with opioid analgesics. Because NSAIDs can cause gastritis and renal dysfunction, renal function must be carefully monitored. The patient needs to be educated about activity restrictions (eg, lifting no more than 10 pounds, use of proper body mechanics). Braces are occasionally needed to support the spinal column.

The patient also needs to be instructed about the signs and symptoms of hypercalcemia. Maintaining mobility and hydration is important to diminish exacerbations of this complication; however, the primary cause is the disease itself. Renal function should also be monitored closely. Renal failure can become severe, and dialysis may be needed. Maintaining high urine output (3 L/day) can be very useful in preventing or limiting this complication.

Because antibody production is impaired, infections, particularly bacterial infections, are common and can be life-threatening. The patient needs to be instructed in appropriate infection prevention measures (see Chart 33-7) and should be advised to contact the health care provider immediately if he or she has a fever or other signs and symptoms of infection. The patient should receive pneumonia (Pneumovax) and influenza vaccines. Prophylactic antibiotics are sometimes used. IV immune globulin (IVIG) can be useful for patients with recurrent infections.

Gerontologic Considerations

The incidence of multiple myeloma increases with age; the disease rarely occurs in patients younger than 40 years of age. Because of the increasing older population, more patients are seeking treatment for this disease. Back pain, which is often a presenting symptom in this disease, should be closely investigated in older patients. BMT or PBSCT is an option that can prolong remission and potentially cure some patients, but it is unavailable to most older people because of age limitations.

Bleeding Disorders

Overview

Normal hemostatic mechanisms can control bleeding from vessels and prevent spontaneous bleeding. The bleeding vessel constricts and platelets aggregate at the site, forming an unstable hemostatic plug. Circulating coagulation factors are activated on the surface of these aggregated platelets, forming fibrin, which anchors the platelet plug to the site of injury.

The failure of normal hemostatic mechanisms can result in bleeding, which is severe at times. This bleeding is commonly provoked by trauma, but in certain circumstances it can occur spontaneously. When the source is platelet or coagulation factor abnormalities, the site of bleeding can be anywhere in the body. When the source is vascular abnormalities, the site of bleeding may be more localized. Some patients have defects in more than one hemostatic mechanism simultaneously.

In a variety of situations, the bone marrow may be stimulated to increase platelet production (thrombopoiesis). The increased production may be a reactive response, as in a compensatory response to significant bleeding, or a more general response to increased hematopoiesis, as in iron deficiency anemia. Sometimes, the increase in platelets does not result from increased production but from a loss in platelet pooling within the spleen. The spleen typically holds about one third of the circulating platelets at any time. If the spleen is absent (eg, splenectomy), the platelet reservoir is also lost, and an abnormally high number of platelets enters the circulation. In time, the rate of thrombopoiesis slows to reestablish a more normal platelet level.

Clinical Manifestations

Signs and symptoms of bleeding disorders vary depending on the type of defect. A careful history and physical examination can be very useful in determining the source of the hemostatic defect. Abnormalities of the vascular system give rise to local bleeding, usually into the skin. Because platelets are primarily responsible for stopping bleeding from small vessels, patients with platelet defects develop petechiae, often in clusters; these are seen on the skin and mucous membranes but also occur throughout the body. Bleeding from platelet disorders can be severe. Unless the platelet disorder is severe, bleeding can often be stopped promptly when local pressure is applied; it does not typically recur when the pressure is released.

In contrast, coagulation factor defects do not tend to cause superficial bleeding, because the primary hemostatic mechanisms are still intact. Instead, bleeding occurs deeper within the body (eg, subcutaneous or IM hematomas, hemorrhage into joint spaces). External bleeding diminishes very slowly when local pressure is applied; it often recurs several hours after pressure is removed. For example, severe bleeding may start several hours after a tooth extraction. Risk factors for bleeding are listed in Chart 33-6.

Medical Management

Management varies based on the underlying cause of the bleeding disorder. If bleeding is significant, transfusions of blood products are indicated. The specific blood product used is determined by the underlying defect. If fibrinolysis is excessive, hemostatic agents such as aminocaproic acid (Amicar) can be used to inhibit this process. This agent must be used with caution, because excessive inhibition of fibrinolysis can result in thrombosis.

Nursing Management

Patients who have bleeding disorders or who have the potential for development of such disorders as a result of disease or therapeutic agents must be taught to observe themselves carefully and frequently for bleeding (Chart 33-11). They need to understand the importance of avoiding activities that increase the risk of bleeding, such as contact sports. The skin is observed for petechiae and ecchymoses (bruises) and the nose and gums for bleeding. Hospitalized patients may be monitored for bleeding by testing all drainage and excreta (feces, urine, emesis, and gastric drainage) for occult as well as obvious blood. Outpatients are often given fecal occult blood screening cards to detect occult blood in stools.

Primary Thrombocythemia

Primary thrombocythemia (also called essential thrombocythemia) is a stem cell disorder within the bone marrow. A marked increase in platelet production occurs, with the platelet count consistently greater than 600,000/mm^3. Platelet size may be abnormal, but platelet survival is typically normal. Occasionally, the platelet increase is accompanied by an increase in erythrocytes, leukocytes, or both; however, these cells are not increased to the extent that they are in polycythemia vera, CML, or myelofibrosis. Although

CHART 33-11

HOME CARE CHECKLIST • The Patient at Risk for Bleeding

At the completion of the home care instruction, the patient or caregiver will be able to:	Patient	Caregiver
• Describe the source and function of platelets and clotting factors.	✔	✔
• Verbalize the rationale for being at risk for bleeding.	✔	✔
• Identify medications and other substances to avoid (eg, aspirin-containing medications, alcohol).	✔	✔
• Demonstrate how to monitor for signs of bleeding.	✔	✔
• Describe to whom, how, and when to report signs of bleeding.	✔	✔
• Notify health care professional before having dental work.	✔	✔
• Describe appropriate ways to prevent bleeding (avoid use of suppositories, enemas, tampons; avoid constipation, vigorous sexual intercourse, anal sex; use only electric razor for shaving and a soft-bristled toothbrush for teeth).	✔	✔
• Demonstrate appropriate actions to take should bleeding occur.	✔	✔

the exact cause is unknown, primary thrombocythemia is similar to other myeloproliferative disorders, particularly polycythemia vera. However, unlike the other myeloproliferative disorders, it rarely evolves into acute leukemia.

Primary thrombocythemia, which affects men and women equally, tends to occur in late middle age. The median survival exceeds 10 years.

Clinical Manifestations

Many patients with primary thrombocythemia are asymptomatic; the illness is diagnosed as the result of finding an elevated platelet count on a CBC. Symptoms, when they do occur, result primarily from hemorrhage or vasoocclusion in the microvasculature. Symptoms occur most often when the platelet count exceeds 1 million/mm^3. However, symptoms do not always correlate with the extent to which the platelet count is elevated. Thrombosis is common and can be either arterial or venous; arterial thrombosis is more common (Harrison & Green, 2003). Because these platelets can be dysfunctional, minor or major hemorrhage can also occur. Bleeding from the mucous membranes of the nose and mouth is common, and significant GI bleeding is also possible. Bleeding typically does not occur unless the platelet count exceeds 1.5 million/mm^3.

Vasoocclusive manifestations are most frequently seen in the form of erythromelalgia. The toxic effects of platelet substances include painful burning, warmth, and redness in a localized distal area of the extremities. Neurologic manifestations occur in 25% of patients (Schafer, 2004). Numbness, tingling, chronic headache, and visual disturbance may be seen; these occlusive manifestations can progress to stroke and seizure and, less commonly, to MI. More common forms of venous thrombosis include DVT and pulmonary embolism. The spleen may be enlarged but usually not to a significant extent.

Assessment and Diagnostic Findings

The diagnosis of primary thrombocythemia is made by ruling out other potential disorders—either other myeloproliferative disorders or underlying illnesses that cause a reactive or secondary thrombocytosis (see below). Iron deficiency should be excluded, because a reactive increase in the platelet count often accompanies this deficiency. Occult malignancy should be excluded. The CBC shows markedly large and abnormal platelets. Analysis of the bone marrow (by aspiration and biopsy) may not be particularly useful.

No data reliably predict the development of complications. Risk factors for the development of thrombotic complications are age older than 60 years, prior thrombotic or bleeding events, and preexisting cardiovascular risk factors (Schafer, 2004). Major bleeding tends to occur when the platelet count is very high.

Medical Management

The management of primary thrombocythemia is highly controversial. The risk for significant thrombotic or hemorrhagic complications may not be increased until the platelet count exceeds 1.5 million/mm^3 (Schafer, 2004). A careful assessment of other risk factors, such as history of peripheral vascular disease, history of tobacco use, atherosclerosis, and prior thrombotic events, should be used in making the decision as to when to initiate therapy.

In younger patients with no risk factors, low-dose aspirin therapy may be sufficient to prevent thrombotic complications. However, the use of aspirin can increase the risk of hemorrhagic complications and is typically a contraindication in patients with a history of GI bleeding. Aspirin can relieve the neurologic symptoms (eg, headache), erythromelalgia, and visual symptoms of primary thrombocythemia.

In older patients and in those with concurrent risk factors, more aggressive measures may be necessary. Hydroxyurea (Hydrea), a chemotherapeutic medication, is effective in lowering the platelet count. This agent is taken orally and causes minimal side effects other than dose-related leukopenia. (However, its potential for leukogenesis diminishes its efficacy in younger patients with risk factors.) The medication anagrelide (Agrylin) is more specific in lowering the platelet count than hydroxyurea but has more side effects. Severe headaches cause many patients to stop taking the medication. Tachycardia and chest pain may also occur, and anagrelide is contraindicated in patients with concurrent cardiac problems. Interferon-alfa-2b (Intron-A) has been shown to lower platelet counts by an unknown mechanism. The medication is administered subcutaneously at varying frequency, commonly three times per week. Significant side effects, such as fatigue, weakness, memory deficits, dizziness, anemia, and liver dysfunction, limit its usefulness.

Rarely, the occlusive symptoms are so great that the platelet count must be reduced immediately. When necessary, platelet pheresis (see later discussion) can reduce the amount of circulating platelets, but only transiently. The extent to which symptoms and complications (eg, thromboses) are reduced by pheresis remains unclear.

Nursing Management

Patients with primary thrombocythemia need to be instructed about the accompanying risks of hemorrhage and thrombosis. The patient is informed about signs and symptoms of thrombosis, particularly the neurologic manifestations, such as visual changes, numbness, tingling, and weakness. Risk factors for thrombosis are assessed, and measures to diminish risk factors (particularly cessation of tobacco use) are encouraged. Patients receiving aspirin therapy should be informed about the increased risk of bleeding. Patients who are at risk for bleeding should be instructed about medications (eg, aspirin, NSAIDs) and other substances (eg, alcohol) that can alter platelet function. Patients receiving interferon therapy are taught to self-administer the medication and manage side effects.

Secondary Thrombocytosis

Increased platelet production is the primary mechanism of secondary, or reactive, **thrombocytosis.** The platelet count is above normal, but, in contrast to primary thrombocythemia, an increase to more than 1 million/mm^3 is rare. Platelet function is normal; the platelet survival time is normal or decreased. Consequently, symptoms associated with hemorrhage or thrombosis are rare. Many disorders or conditions can cause a reactive increase in platelets, including infection, chronic inflammatory disorders, iron deficiency, malignant disease, acute hemorrhage, and splenectomy (see previous discussion of primary thrombocythemia). Treatment is aimed at the underlying disorder. With successful management, the platelet count usually returns to normal.

Thrombocytopenia

Thrombocytopenia (low platelet level) can result from various factors: decreased production of platelets within the bone marrow, increased destruction of platelets, or increased consumption of platelets. Causes and treatments are summarized in Table 33-4.

TABLE 33-4 Causes and Management of Thrombocytopenia

Cause	Management
Decreased Platelet Production	
Hematologic malignancy, especially acute leukemias	Treat leukemia; platelet transfusion
Myelodysplastic syndromes (MDS)	Treat MDS; platelet transfusion
Metastatic involvement of bone marrow from solid tumors	Treat solid tumor
Aplastic anemia	Treat underlying condition
Megaloblastic anemia	Treat underlying anemia
Toxins	Remove toxin
Medications	Stop medication
Infection (esp. septicemia, viral infection, tuberculosis)	Treat infection
Alcohol	Refrain from alcohol consumption
Chemotherapy	Delay or decrease dose; growth factor; platelet transfusion
Increased Platelet Destruction	
Due to antibodies:	Treat condition
Idiopathic thrombocytopenic purpura (ITP)	
Lupus erythematosus	
Malignant lymphoma	
Chronic lymphocytic leukemia (CLL)	Treat CLL and/or treat as ITP
Medications	Stop medication
Due to infection:	Treat infection
Bacteremia	
Postviral infection	
Sequestration of platelets in an enlarged spleen	If thrombocytopenia is severe, splenectomy may be needed
Increased Platelet Consumption	
Disseminated intravascular coagulation (DIC)	Treat underlying condition triggering DIC; administer heparin, EACA, blood products

Clinical Manifestations

Bleeding and petechiae usually do not occur with platelet counts greater than 50,000/mm^3, although excessive bleeding can follow surgery or other trauma. When the platelet count drops to less than 20,000/mm^3, petechiae can appear, along with nasal and gingival bleeding, excessive menstrual bleeding, and excessive bleeding after surgery or dental extractions. When the platelet count is less than 5000/mm^3, spontaneous, potentially fatal central nervous system or GI hemorrhage can occur. If the platelets are dysfunctional due to disease (eg, MDS) or medications (eg, aspirin), the risk for bleeding may be much greater even when the actual platelet count is not significantly reduced.

Assessment and Diagnostic Findings

A platelet deficiency that results from decreased production (eg, leukemia, MDS) can usually be diagnosed by examining the bone marrow via aspiration and biopsy. Infections, either viral or bacterial, as well as alcoholism can also suppress platelet production. When platelet destruction is the cause of thrombocytopenia, the marrow shows increased megakaryocytes (the cells from which the platelets originate) and normal or even increased platelet production as the body attempts to compensate for the decreased platelets in circulation. Another cause of thrombocytopenia is sequestration. Approximately one third of the circulating platelets are within the spleen, and a greatly enlarged spleen results in increased sequestration of platelets. Many medications (eg, sulfa drugs, methotrexate) can either decrease platelet production or shorten their life span. Numerous genetic causes of thrombocytopenia have been discovered, including autosomal dominant, autosomal recessive, and X-linked mutations (Drachman, 2004).

An important cause to exclude is "pseudothrombocytopenia." Here, platelets aggregate and clump in the presence of ethylenediamine tetra-acetic acid (EDTA), the anticoagulant present in the tube used for CBC collection. This clumping accounts for up to 20% of instances of isolated thrombocytopenia (Drachman, 2004). A manual examination of the peripheral smear can easily determine platelet clumping as the cause of thrombocytopenia; newer cell counter machines can also detect this.

Medical Management

The management of secondary thrombocytopenia is usually treatment of the underlying disease. If platelet production is impaired, platelet transfusions may increase the platelet count and stop bleeding or prevent spontaneous hemorrhage. If excessive platelet destruction occurs, transfused platelets are also destroyed, and the platelet count does not increase. The most common cause of excessive platelet destruction is ITP (see the following discussion). In some instances splenectomy can be a useful therapeutic intervention, but often it is not an option; for example, in patients in whom the enlarged spleen is due to portal hypertension related to cirrhosis, splenectomy may cause more bleeding disorders.

Nursing Management

The interventions for a patient with thrombocytopenia are listed in Chart 33-9.

Idiopathic Thrombocytopenic Purpura

ITP is a disease that affects people of all ages, but it is more common among children and young women. There are two forms of ITP: acute and chronic. Acute ITP, which occurs predominantly in children, often appears 1 to 6 weeks after a viral illness. This form is self-limited; remission often occurs spontaneously within 6 months. Chronic ITP is often diagnosed by exclusion of other causes of thrombocytopenia.

Pathophysiology

Although the precise cause of ITP remains unknown, viral infections sometimes precede the disease in children. Occasionally medications such as sulfa drugs can induce ITP. Other conditions, such as systemic lupus erythematosus or pregnancy, can also induce ITP. Antiplatelet autoantibodies that bind to the patient's platelets are found in the blood of patients with ITP. When the platelets are bound by the antibodies, the RES or tissue macrophage system ingests the platelets, destroying them. The body attempts to compensate for this destruction by increasing platelet production within the marrow.

Clinical Manifestations

Many patients have no symptoms, and the low platelet count (often less than 20,000/mm^3; less than 5000/mm^3 is not uncommon) is an incidental finding. Common physical manifestations are easy bruising, heavy menses, and petechiae on the extremities or trunk. Patients with simple bruising or petechiae ("dry purpura") tend to have fewer complications from bleeding than those with bleeding from mucosal surfaces, such as the GI tract (including the mouth) and pulmonary system (eg, hemoptysis), which is termed "wet purpura." Patients with wet purpura have a greater risk of intracranial bleeding than do those with dry purpura. Despite low platelet counts, the platelets are young and very functional. They adhere to endothelial surfaces and to one another, so spontaneous bleeding does not always occur. Thus, treatment may not be initiated unless bleeding becomes severe or life-threatening, or the platelet count is extremely low (less than 10,000/mm^3) (Stasi & Provan, 2004).

Assessment and Diagnostic Findings

Patients may have an isolated decrease in platelets (less than 20,000/mm^3 is common), but they may also have an increase in megakaryocytes (platelet precursors) within the marrow, as detected on bone marrow aspirate. Although many patients are found to be infected with *Helicobacter pylori*, it is currently unknown whether treatment of this infection will improve platelet counts (Franchini & Veneri, 2004). It is unclear why *H. pylori* and ITP are correlated. It is thought that *H. pylori* may cause an autoimmune reaction or that it binds von Willebrand factor (vWF), both of which may result in accelerated platelet demise.

Medical Management

The primary goal of treatment is a "safe" platelet count. Because the risk for bleeding typically does not increase until the platelet count is less than 10,000/mm^3, a patient whose count exceeds 30,000/mm^3 to 50,000/mm^3 may be carefully observed without additional intervention. However, if the count is less than 20,000/mm^3 or if bleeding occurs, the goal is to improve the patient's platelet count rather than to cure the disease. The decision to treat should not be made merely on the basis of the patient's platelet count, but also on his or her lifestyle and activity level. A person with a sedentary lifestyle can tolerate a low platelet count more safely than one with a more active lifestyle.

Treatment for ITP usually involves several approaches. If the patient is taking a medication known to cause ITP (eg, quinine, sulfa-containing medications), that medication must be stopped immediately. The mainstay of short-term therapy is the use of immunosuppressive agents. These agents block the binding receptors on macrophages so that the platelets are not destroyed. Prednisone is the agent typically used, and it is effective in about 80% of patients (Zimmer et al., 2004). Cyclophosphamide (Cytoxan) and azathioprine (Imuran) can also be used, and dexamethasone (Decadron) may be effective. Platelet counts typically begin to rise within a few days after institution of corticosteroid therapy; this effect takes longer with azathioprine. Because of the associated side effects, patients cannot take high doses of corticosteroids indefinitely. It is not unusual for the platelet count to drop once the corticosteroid dose is tapered. Some patients can be successfully maintained on low doses of prednisone.

IV immune globulin (IVIG) is also commonly used to treat ITP. It is effective in binding the receptors on the macrophages; however, high doses are required, the drug is very expensive, and the effect is transient. Splenectomy is an alternative treatment but results in a sustained normal platelet count only 50% of the time; however, many patients can maintain a "safe" platelet count of more than 30,000/mm^3 after removal of the spleen. Even those who do respond to splenectomy may have recurrences of severe thrombocytopenia months or years later. Patients who have undergone splenectomy are permanently at risk for sepsis; these patients should receive pneumonia (Pneumovax), *Haemophilus influenzae* B, and meningococcal vaccines, preferably 2 to 3 weeks before the splenectomy is performed. The Pneumovax vaccine should be repeated at 5- to 10-year intervals.

Other management options include the chemotherapy agent vincristine (Oncovin). Vincristine appears to work by blocking the receptors on the macrophages and therefore inhibiting platelet destruction; it may also stimulate thrombopoiesis. Some data support the efficacy of certain monoclonal antibodies (eg, rituximab) in increasing platelet counts, but more research on their effects is needed (Robak, 2004).

Another approach to the management of chronic ITP involves the use of anti-D (WinRho) in patients who are Rh(D)-positive. The actual mechanism of action is unknown. One theory is that the anti-D binds to the patient's erythrocytes, which are in turn destroyed by the body's macrophages. The receptors in the RES may become saturated with the sensitized erythrocytes, diminishing removal of antibody-coated platelets. Anti-D produces a transient decreased hematocrit and increased platelet count in many, but not all, patients with ITP. Anti-D appears to be most effective in children with ITP and least effective in patients who have undergone splenectomy.

Despite the extremely low platelet count, platelet transfusions are usually avoided. Transfusions tend to be ineffective because the patient's antiplatelet antibodies bind with the transfused platelets, causing them to be destroyed. Platelet counts can actually drop after platelet transfusion. Occasionally, transfusion of platelets may protect against catastrophic bleeding in patients with severe wet purpura. Aminocaproic acid (EACA, Amicar), a fibrinolytic enzyme inhibitor that slows the dissolution of clots, may be useful for patients with significant mucosal bleeding refractory to other treatments.

Nursing Management

Nursing care includes an assessment of the patient's lifestyle to determine the risk of bleeding from activity. A careful medication history is also obtained, including use of over-the-counter medications, herbs, and nutritional supplements. The nurse must be alert for sulfa-containing medications and others that alter platelet function (eg, aspirin-based or other NSAIDs). The nurse assesses for any history of recent viral illness and reports of headache or visual disturbances, which could be initial symptoms of intracranial bleeding. Patients who are admitted to the hospital with wet purpura and low platelet counts should have a neurologic assessment incorporated into their routine vital sign measurements. All injections or rectal medications should be avoided, and rectal temperature measurements should not be performed, because they can stimulate bleeding.

Patient teaching addresses signs of exacerbation of disease (petechiae, ecchymoses); how to contact appropriate health care personnel; the name and type of medication inducing ITP (if appropriate); current medical treatment (medications, tapering schedule if relevant, side effects); and the frequency of monitoring the platelet count. The patient is instructed to avoid all agents that interfere with platelet function. The patient should avoid constipation, the Valsalva maneuver (eg, straining at stool), and flossing of the teeth. Electric razors should be used for shaving, and soft-bristled toothbrushes should replace stiff-bristled ones. The patient is also counseled to refrain from vigorous sexual intercourse when the platelet count is less than 10,000/mm^3. Patients who are receiving corticosteroids long term are at risk for complications including osteoporosis, proximal muscle wasting, cataract formation, and dental caries (see Chart 33-3). Bone mineral density should be monitored, and these patients may benefit from calcium and vitamin D supplementation and bisphosphonate therapy to prevent significant bone disease.

Platelet Defects

Quantitative platelet defects are relatively common (thrombocytopenia), but qualitative defects can also occur. With qualitative defects, the number of platelets may be normal, but the platelets do not function normally. In the past, platelet function was most commonly evaluated by the bleeding time; however, this test was a crude measurement. Now other tests using a platelet function analyzer exist; this method is particularly valuable for rapid and simple screening (Harrison & Green, 2003).

An important functional platelet disorder is that induced by aspirin. Even small amounts of aspirin reduce normal platelet aggregation, and the prolonged bleeding time lasts for several days after aspirin ingestion. Although this does not cause bleeding in most people, patients with a coagulation disorder (eg, hemophilia) or thrombocytopenia can have significant bleeding after taking aspirin, particularly if invasive procedures or trauma has occurred.

NSAIDs can also inhibit platelet function, but the effect is not as prolonged as with aspirin (about 5 days versus 7 to 10 days). Other causes of platelet dysfunction include end-stage renal disease, possibly from metabolic products affecting platelet function; MDS; multiple myeloma (due to abnormal protein interfering with platelet function); cardiopulmonary bypass; and other medications (Chart 33-12).

Clinical Manifestations

Bleeding may be mild or severe. Its extent is not necessarily correlated with the platelet count or with tests that measure coagulation (prothrombin time [PT], partial thromboplastin time [PTT]). Ecchymoses are common, particularly on the extremities. Patients with platelet dysfunction may be at risk for significant bleeding after trauma or invasive procedures (eg, biopsy, dental extraction).

Medical Management

If the platelet dysfunction is caused by medication, use of the offending medication should be stopped, if possible, particularly when bleeding occurs. If platelet dysfunction is marked, bleeding can often be prevented by transfusion of normal platelets before invasive procedures. Aminocaproic acid (EACA, Amicar) may be required to prevent significant bleeding after such procedures.

Nursing Management

Patients with significant platelet dysfunction need to be instructed to avoid substances that can diminish platelet function, such as certain over-the-counter medications, herbs, nutritional supplements, and alcohol. They also need to serve as their own advocates and to inform their health care providers (including dentists) of the underlying condition before any invasive procedure is performed, so that appropriate steps can be initiated to diminish the risk of bleeding. Bleeding precautions should be initiated as appropriate (see Chart 33-9).

CHART 33-12

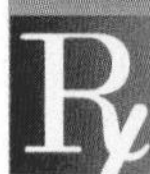

PHARMACOLOGY · Medications and Substances That Impair Platelet Function

Anesthetic Agents
Local anesthetics
Halothane

Antibiotics
Beta-lactam antibiotics
- Penicillins
- Cephalosporins

Nitrofurantoin
Sulfonamides

Anticoagulation Agents
Heparin
Fibrinolytic agents

Anti-inflammatory Agents (Nonsteroidal)
Aspirin
Ibuprofen
Naproxen

Antineoplastic Agents
Carmustine
Daunorubicin
Mithramycin

Cardiovascular Drugs
Beta-blockers
Calcium channel blockers
Isosorbide
Nitroglycerine
Nitroprusside
Quinidine

Medications That Increase Platelet cAMP
Dipyridamole
Prostacycline
Theophylline

Food and Food Additives
Caffeine
Chinese black tree fungus
Clove
Cumin
Ethanol
Fish oils
Garlic
Onion extract
Turmeric

Plasma Expanders
Dextrans
Hydroxyethyl starch

Psychotropic Agents
Tricyclic antidepressants
Phenothiazines

Miscellaneous
Antihistamines
Clofibrate
Furosemide
Heroin
Contrast agents
Ticlopidine
Vitamin E

Herbal Supplements
Feverfew
Ginger
Gingko
Ginseng
Kava kava

Hemophilia

Two inherited bleeding disorders—hemophilia A and hemophilia B—are clinically indistinguishable, although they can be distinguished by laboratory tests. Hemophilia A is caused by a genetic defect that results in deficient or defective factor VIII. Hemophilia B (also called Christmas disease) stems from a genetic defect that causes deficient or defective factor IX. Hemophilia is a relatively rare disease; hemophilia A, which occurs in 1 of every 10,000 births, is three times more common than hemophilia B. Both types of hemophilia are inherited as X-linked traits, so almost all affected people are males; females can be carriers but are almost always asymptomatic. The disease is recognized in early childhood, usually in the toddler age group. However, patients with mild hemophilia may not be diagnosed until they experience severe trauma (eg, a high-school football injury) or surgery. Hemophilia occurs in all ethnic groups.

Clinical Manifestations

Hemophilia, which can be severe, is manifested by hemorrhages into various parts of the body. Hemorrhage can occur even after minimal trauma. The frequency and severity of the bleeding depend on the degree of factor deficiency as well as the intensity of the precipitating trauma. For example, patients with a mild factor VIII deficiency (ie, 6% to 50% of normal levels) rarely develop hemorrhage spontaneously; hemorrhage tends to occur secondary to trauma. In contrast, spontaneous hemorrhages, particularly hemarthroses and hematomas, can frequently occur in patients with severe factor VIII deficiency (ie, less than 1% of normal levels). These patients require frequent factor VIII replacement therapy.

About 75% of all bleeding in patients with hemophilia occurs into joints. The most commonly affected joints are the knees, elbows, ankles, shoulders, wrists, and hips. Patients often note pain in a joint before they are aware of swelling and limitation of motion. Recurrent joint hemorrhages can result in damage so severe that chronic pain or ankylosis (fixation) of the joint occurs. Many patients with severe factor deficiency are crippled by the joint damage before they become adults. Hematomas can be superficial or deep hemorrhages into muscle or subcutaneous tissue. With severe factor VIII deficiency, hematomas can occur without known trauma and progressively extend in all directions. When the hematomas occur within muscle, particularly in the extremities, peripheral nerves can be compressed. Over time, this compression results in decreased sensation, weakness, and atrophy of the area involved.

Bleeding is not limited to the joint areas. Spontaneous hematuria and GI bleeding can occur. Bleeding is also common in other mucous membranes, such as the nasal passages. The most dangerous site of hemorrhage is in the head (intracranial or extracranial). Any head trauma requires prompt evaluation and treatment. Surgical procedures typically result in excessive bleeding at the surgical site. Because clot formation is poor, wound healing is also poor. Such bleeding is most commonly associated with dental extraction.

Medical Management

In the past, the only treatment for hemophilia was infusion of fresh frozen plasma, which had to be administered in such large quantities that patients experienced fluid volume overload. Now factor VIII and factor IX concentrates are available to all blood banks. Recombinant forms of these factors have been made available and may diminish the use of factor concentrates. Patients are given concentrates when they are actively bleeding or as a preventive measure before traumatic procedures (eg, lumbar puncture, dental extraction, surgery). The patient and family are taught how to administer the concentrate by IV at home at the first sign of bleeding. It is crucial to initiate treatment as soon as possible so that bleeding complications can be avoided. A few patients eventually develop antibodies to the concentrates, so their factor levels cannot be increased. Recombinant factor VIIa is approved by the FDA for patients with acquired antibodies to factors VIII and IX (Carr & Martin, 2004), but treatment is often unsuccessful.

Aminocaproic acid (EACA, Amicar) is very effective as an adjunctive measure after oral surgery. It is also useful in treating mucosal bleeding. Another agent, desmopressin (DDAVP), induces a transient rise in factor VIII levels; the mechanism for this response is unknown. In patients with mild forms of hemophilia A, desmopressin is extremely useful, significantly reducing the amount of blood products required. However, desmopressin is not effective in patients with severe factor VIII deficiency.

Nursing Management

Most patients with hemophilia are diagnosed as children. They often require assistance in coping with the condition because it is chronic, places restrictions on their lives, and is an inherited disorder that can be passed to future generations. From childhood, patients are helped to cope with the disease and to identify the positive aspects of their lives. They are encouraged to be self-sufficient and to maintain independence by preventing unnecessary trauma that can cause acute bleeding episodes and temporarily interfere with normal activities. As they work through their feelings about the condition and progress to accepting it, they can assume more and more responsibility for maintaining optimal health.

Patients with mild factor deficiency may not be diagnosed until adulthood if they do not experience significant trauma or surgery as children. These patients need extensive teaching about activity restrictions and self-care measures to diminish the chance of hemorrhage and complications of bleeding. The nurse should emphasize safety at home and in the workplace.

Patients with hemophilia are instructed to avoid any agents that interfere with platelet aggregation, such as aspirin, NSAIDs, herbs, nutritional supplements, and alcohol. This restriction applies to over-the-counter medications such as cold remedies. Dental hygiene is very important as a preventive measure because dental extractions are so hazardous. Applying pressure may be sufficient to control bleeding resulting from minor trauma if the factor deficiency is not severe. Nasal packing should be avoided, because bleeding frequently resumes when the packing is removed. Splints and other orthopedic devices may be useful in patients with joint or muscle hemorrhages. All injections should be avoided; invasive procedures (eg, endoscopy, lumbar puncture) should be minimized or performed after administration of appropriate factor replacement. Patients with hemophilia should be encouraged to carry or wear medical identification.

During hemorrhagic episodes, the extent of bleeding must be assessed carefully. Patients who are at risk for significant compromise (eg, bleeding into the respiratory tract or brain) warrant close observation and systematic assessment for emergent complications (eg, respiratory distress, altered level of consciousness). If the patient has had recent surgery, the nurse frequently and carefully assesses the surgical site for bleeding. Frequent vital sign monitoring is needed until the nurse is certain that there is no excessive postoperative bleeding.

Analgesics are commonly required to alleviate the pain associated with hematomas and hemorrhage into joints. Many patients report that warm baths promote relaxation, improve mobility, and lessen pain. However, during bleeding episodes, heat, which can accentuate bleeding, is avoided; applications of cold are used instead.

Although recent technology (ie, the formulation of heat-solvent or detergent-treated factor concentrates) has rendered factor VIII and IX preparations free of viruses such as HIV and hepatitis, many patients have already been exposed to these infections through previous transfusions. These patients and their families may need assistance in coping with the diagnosis and the consequences of these infections.

Between 20% and 30% of patients with hemophilia A and between 1% and 3% of patients with hemophilia B develop antibodies (inhibitors) to factor concentrates (Chehab, 2002). Although one third of such inhibitors are transient, their effects can be significant and induce partial or complete refractoriness to factor replacement and result in increased risk of bleeding. Patients may require plasmapheresis or concurrent immunosuppressive therapy, particularly in the setting of significant bleeding. Factor VIIa can be administered, although it is very expensive and requires frequent administration because of its short half-life. Occasionally, tolerance to the antibody can be induced by repeated daily exposure to factor VIII. Patients receiving daily administration of factor VIII can take months or longer for tolerance to develop; however, it can be successful 60% to 80% of the time (Key, 2004). Patients with severe factor deficiency should be screened for antibodies, particularly before major surgery.

Von Willebrand's Disease

Von Willebrand's disease, a common bleeding disorder affecting males and females equally, is usually inherited as a dominant trait. The prevalence of this disease is estimated to be 1%; thus, it is 50 times more prevalent than hemophilia (Tarantino & Aledort, 2004). The disease is caused by a deficiency of vWF, which is necessary for factor VIII activity. vWF is also necessary for platelet adhesion at the site of vascular injury. Although synthesis of factor VIII is normal, its half-life is shortened; therefore, factor VIII levels commonly are mildly low (15% to 50% of normal).

There are three types of von Willebrand's disease (Mannucci, 2004). Type 1, the most common, is characterized by decreases in structurally normal vWF. Type 2 shows variable qualitative defects based on the specific vWF subtype involved. Type 3 is very rare and is characterized by a severe vWF deficiency as well as significant deficiency of factor VIII.

Clinical Manifestations

Patients commonly have nosebleeds, heavy menses, prolonged bleeding from cuts, and postoperative bleeding, although they do not have massive soft tissue or joint hemorrhages. As the laboratory values fluctuate (see Assessment and Diagnostic Findings), so does the bleeding. For example, a careful history of prior bleeding may show little problem with postoperative bleeding on one occasion but significant bleeding from a dental extraction at another time.

Assessment and Diagnostic Findings

Laboratory test results show a normal platelet count but a prolonged bleeding time and a slightly prolonged PTT. These defects are not static, and laboratory test results can vary widely within the same patient over time. More important tests include the ristocetin cofactor, or vWF collagen binding assay, which measures vWF activity. Other tests include vWF antigen, factor VIII, and, for patients with suspected type 2 defects, vWF multimers (Paper, 2003).

Medical Management

The goal of treatment is to replace the deficient protein (eg, vWF or factor VIII) at the time of spontaneous bleeding or prior to an invasive procedure. Replacement products include Humate-P, a commercial concentrate of vWF and factor VIII, and Alphanate, which contains similar amounts of these factors (Mannucci, 2004). Replacement continues for several days to ensure correction of the factor VIII deficiency. Up to 7 to 10 days of treatment may be necessary after major surgery, and the dosage and frequency of administration depend on factor VIII levels. Antibody (inhibitor) formation is usually seen only in patients with type 3 von Willebrand's disease, when large amounts of replacement products have been administered. Desmopressin (DDAVP), a synthetic vasopressin analogue, can be used to prevent bleeding associated with dental or surgical procedures or to manage mild bleeding after surgery. Desmopressin provides a transient increase in factor VIII coagulant activity and may also correct the bleeding time. It can be administered as an IV infusion or intranasally. With major surgery or invasive procedures, IV administration is preferable. DDAVP is contraindicated in patients with unstable coronary artery disease, because it can induce platelet aggregation and cause MI. Side effects include headache, facial flushing, tachycardia, hyponatremia, and rarely seizures.

Other agents may be effective in reducing the bleeding. Aminocaproic acid (EACA, Amicar) is useful in managing mild forms of mucosal bleeding. Estrogen–progesterone compounds may diminish the extent of menses. Platelet transfusions are useful when there is significant bleeding.

Acquired Coagulation Disorders

Liver Disease

With the exception of factor VIII, most blood coagulation factors are synthesized in the liver. Therefore, hepatic dysfunction (due to cirrhosis, tumor, or hepatitis; see Chapter 39) can result in diminished amounts of the factors needed to maintain coagulation and hemostasis. Prolongation of the PT, unless it is caused by vitamin K deficiency, may indicate severe hepatic dysfunction. Although minor bleeding is common (eg, ecchymoses), these patients are also at risk for significant bleeding, related especially to trauma or surgery. Transfusion of fresh frozen plasma may be required to replace clotting factors and to prevent or stop bleeding. Patients may also have life-threatening hemorrhage from peptic ulcers or esophageal varices. In these cases, replacement with fresh frozen plasma, PRBCs, and platelets is usually required.

Vitamin K Deficiency

The synthesis of many coagulation factors depends on vitamin K. Vitamin K deficiency is common in malnourished patients, and some antibiotics decrease the intestinal flora that produce vitamin K, depleting vitamin K stores. Administration of vitamin K (phytonadione [Mephyton], either orally or as a subcutaneous injection) can correct the deficiency quickly; adequate synthesis of coagulation factors is reflected by normalization of the PT.

Complications of Anticoagulant Therapy

Anticoagulants are used in the treatment or prevention of thrombosis. These agents, particularly warfarin or heparin, can cause bleeding. If the PT or PTT is longer than desired and bleeding has not occurred, the medication can be stopped or the dose decreased. Vitamin K is administered as an antidote for warfarin toxicity. Protamine sulfate is rarely needed for heparin toxicity, because the half-life of heparin is very short. With significant bleeding, fresh frozen plasma is needed to replace the vitamin K–dependent coagulation factors. Other complications of anticoagulant therapy are discussed in Chapter 31.

Disseminated Intravascular Coagulation (DIC)

Disseminated intravascular coagulation (DIC), formerly termed disseminated intravascular coagulopathy, is not a disease but a sign of an underlying condition. DIC may be triggered by sepsis, trauma, cancer, shock, abruptio placentae, toxins, or allergic reactions. The severity of DIC is variable, but it is potentially life-threatening.

Pathophysiology

Normal hemostatic mechanisms are altered in DIC so that a massive amount of tiny clots forms in the microcirculation. Initially, the coagulation time is normal. However, as the platelets and clotting factors are consumed to form the microthrombi, coagulation fails. Thus, the paradoxical result of excessive clotting is bleeding. The clinical manifestations of DIC are reflected in the organs, which are affected either by excessive clot formation (with resultant ischemia to all or part of the organ) or by bleeding. The excessive clotting triggers the fibrinolytic system to release fibrin degradation products, which are potent anticoagulants, furthering the bleeding. The bleeding is characterized by low platelet and fibrinogen levels; prolonged PT, PTT, and thrombin time; and elevated fibrin degradation products (**D-dimers**) (Table 33-5).

The mortality rate can exceed 80% of patients who develop severe DIC with ischemic thrombosis and frank hemorrhage. Identification of patients who are at risk for DIC and recognition of the early clinical manifestations of this syndrome can result in earlier medical intervention, which may improve the prognosis. However, the primary prognostic factor is the ability to treat the underlying condition that precipitated DIC.

Clinical Manifestations

Patients with frank DIC may bleed from mucous membranes, venipuncture sites, and the GI and urinary tracts. The bleeding can range from minimal occult internal bleeding to profuse hemorrhage from all orifices. The patient may also develop organ dysfunction, such as renal failure and pulmonary and multifocal central nervous system infarctions, as a result of microthromboses, macrothromboses, or hemorrhages.

During the initial process of DIC, the patient may have no new symptoms, the only manifestation being a progressive decrease in the platelet count. As the thrombosis becomes more extensive, the patient exhibits signs and symptoms of thrombosis in the organs involved. Then, as the clotting factors and platelets are consumed to form these thrombi, bleeding occurs. Initially the bleeding is subtle, but it can develop into frank hemorrhage. Signs and symptoms, which depend on the organs involved, are listed in Chart 33-13.

Medical Management

The most important management factor in DIC is treating the underlying cause; until the cause is controlled, the DIC will persist. Correcting the secondary effects of tissue ischemia by improving oxygenation, replacing fluids, correcting electrolyte imbalances, and administering vasopressor medications is also important. If serious hemorrhage occurs, the depleted coagulation factors and platelets may be replaced to reestablish the potential for normal hemostasis and thereby diminish bleeding. Cryoprecipitate is given to replace fibrinogen and factors V and VII; fresh frozen plasma is administered to replace other coagulation factors.

A controversial treatment strategy is to interrupt the thrombosis process through the use of heparin infusion. Heparin may inhibit the formation of microthrombi and thus permit perfusion of the organs (skin, kidneys, or brain) to resume. Heparin use was traditionally reserved for patients in whom thrombotic manifestations predom-

TABLE 33-5 Laboratory Values Commonly Found in Disseminated Intravascular Coagulation (DIC)*

Test	Function Evaluated	Normal Range	Changes in DIC
Platelet count	Platelet number	150,000–450,000/mm_3	↓
Prothrombin time (PT)	Extrinsic pathway	11–12.5 sec	↑
Partial thromboplastin time (PTT)	Intrinsic pathway	23–35 sec	↑
Thrombin time (TT)	Clot formation	8–11 sec	↑
Fibrinogen	Amount available for coagulation	170–340 mg/dL	↓
D-dimer	Local fibrinolysis	0–250 ng/mL	↑
Fibrin degradation products (FDPs)	Fibrinolysis	0–5 µg/mL	↑
Euglobulin clot lysis	Fibrinolytic activity	≥2 hours	≤1 hour

*Because DIC is a dynamic condition, the laboratory values measured will change over time. Therefore, a progressive increase or decrease in a given laboratory value is likely to be more important than the actual value of a test at a single point in time.

CHART 33-13

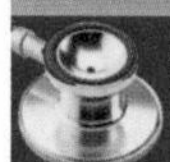

Assessing for Recognizing Thrombosis and Bleeding in Disseminated Intravascular Coagulation (DIC)*

SYSTEM	SIGNS AND SYMPTOMS OF MICROVASCULAR THROMBOSIS	SIGNS AND SYMPTOMS OF MICROVASCULAR AND FRANK BLEEDING
Integumentary system (skin)	↓ Temperature, sensation; ↑ pain; cyanosis in extremities, nose, earlobes; focal ischemia, superficial gangrene	Petechiae, including periorbital and oral mucosa; bleeding: gums, oozing from wounds, previous injection sites, around catheters (IVs, tracheostomies); epistaxis; diffuse ecchymoses; subcutaneous hemorrhage; joint pain
Circulatory system	↓ Pulses; capillary filling time > 3 sec	Tachycardia
Respiratory system	Hypoxia (secondary to clot in lung); dyspnea; chest pain with deep inspiration; ↓ breath sounds over areas of large embolism	High-pitched bronchial breath sounds; tachypnea; ↑ consolidation; signs and symptoms of acute respiratory distress syndrome
Gastrointestinal system	Gastric pain; "heartburn"	Hematemesis (heme⊕[†] NG output) melena (heme⊕ stools → tarry stools → bright-red blood from rectum) retroperitoneal bleeding (abdomen firm and tender to palpation; distended; ↑ abdominal girth)
Renal system	↓ Urine output; ↑ creatinine, ↑ blood urea nitrogen	Hematuria
Neurologic system	↓ Alertness and orientation; ↓ pupillary reaction; ↓ response to commands; ↓ strength and movement ability	Anxiety; restlessness; ↓ mentation, altered level of consciousness; headache; visual disturbances; conjunctival hemorrhage

*Note: Signs of microvascular thrombosis are the result of an inappropriate activation of the coagulation system, causing thrombotic occlusion of small vessels within all body organs. As the clotting factors and platelets are consumed, signs of microvascular bleeding appear. This bleeding can quickly extend into frank hemorrhage. Treatment must be aimed at the disorder underlying the DIC; otherwise, the stimulus for the syndrome will persist.

[†]heme⊕, positive for hemoglobin

inated or in whom extensive blood component replacement failed to halt the hemorrhage or increased fibrinogen and other clotting levels. Heparin is now considered also applicable for use in less acute forms of DIC (Leung, 2004). The effectiveness of heparin can best be determined by observing for normalization of the plasma fibrinogen concentration and diminishing signs of bleeding. Fibrinolytic inhibitors, such as aminocaproic acid (EACA, Amicar), may be used with heparin.

Other therapies include recombinant activated protein C (APC; drotrecogin alfa [Xigris]), which is effective in diminishing inflammatory responses on the surface of the vessels as well as having anticoagulant properties (Aird, 2004). Bleeding is common, can occur at any site, and can be significant. Antithrombin (AT) infusions can also be used for their anticoagulant and anti-inflammatory properties. Bleeding can be significant, particularly when administered in association with heparin.

Nursing Process

The Patient With Disseminated Intravascular Coagulation

Assessment

Nurses need to be aware of which patients are at risk of DIC. Sepsis and acute promyelocytic leukemia are the most common causes of DIC. Patients need to be assessed thoroughly and frequently for signs and symptoms of thrombi and bleeding and monitored for any progression of these signs (see Chart 33-13).

Diagnosis

Nursing Diagnoses

Based on the assessment data, major nursing diagnoses for the patient with DIC may include the following:

- Risk for deficient fluid volume related to bleeding
- Risk for impaired skin integrity related to ischemia or bleeding
- Risk for imbalanced fluid volume related to excessive blood/factor component replacement
- Ineffective tissue perfusion related to microthrombi
- Death anxiety

Collaborative Problems/ Potential Complications

Collaborative problems include the clinical conditions that precipitated the DIC. Based on the assessment data, potential complications may include:

- Renal failure
- Gangrene
- Pulmonary embolism or hemorrhage
- Altered level of consciousness
- Acute respiratory distress syndrome
- Stroke

Planning and Goals

Major patient goals include maintenance of hemodynamic status, maintenance of intact skin and oral mucosa, maintenance of fluid balance, maintenance of tissue perfusion, enhanced coping, and absence of complications, as described in the Plan of Nursing Care for the Patient with DIC (Chart 33-14).

Nursing Interventions

See Chart 33-14.

Monitoring and Managing Potential Complications

Assessment and interventions should target potential sites of end-organ damage. As organs are inadequately perfused from the microthrombi, organ function diminishes; the kidneys, lungs, brain, and skin are particularly vulnerable, and renal dysfunction is common. Lack of renal perfusion may result in acute tubular necrosis and renal failure, sometimes requiring dialysis. Placement of a large-bore dialysis catheter is extremely hazardous for this patient population and should be accompanied by adequate platelet and plasma transfusions. Hepatic dysfunction is also relatively common, reflected in altered liver function tests, depleted albumin stores, and diminished synthesis of clotting factors. Respiratory function warrants careful monitoring and aggressive measures to diminish alveolar compromise, such as incentive spirometry. Suctioning should be performed as gently as possible to diminish the risk for additional bleeding. Central nervous system involvement can be manifested as headache, visual changes, and alteration in level of consciousness.

Evaluation

See Chart 33-14 for evaluation and expected outcomes for the patient with DIC.

Thrombotic Disorders

As in many bleeding disorders, several conditions can alter the balance within the normal hemostasis process and cause excessive thrombosis. Abnormalities that predispose a person to thrombotic events include decreased clotting inhibitors within the circulation (which enhances coagulation), altered hepatic function (which may decrease production of clotting factors or clearance of activated coagulation factors), lack of fibrinolytic enzymes, and tortuous vessels (which promote platelet aggregation). Thrombosis can be caused by more than one predisposing factor. Several conditions can result from thrombosis, such as MI (see Chapter 28), CVA (brain attack or stroke; see Chapter 62), and peripheral arterial occlusion (see Chapter 31). Several inherited or acquired deficiency conditions, including hyperhomocysteinemia, AT III deficiency, protein C deficiency, APC resistance, factor V Leiden, and protein S deficiency can predispose a patient to repeated episodes of thrombosis; they are referred to as hypercoagulable states or thrombophilia. Table 33-6 lists these disorders, their abnormal laboratory values, and the need for family testing.

Thrombosis requires anticoagulation therapy. The duration of therapy varies with the location and extent of the thrombosis, precipitating events (eg, trauma, immobilization), and concurrent risk factors (eg, use of oral contraceptives, tortuous blood vessels, history of thrombotic events). With some conditions, lifelong anticoagulant therapy is necessary.

Hyperhomocysteinemia

Increased plasma levels of homocysteine are a significant risk factor not only for venous thrombosis (eg, DVT, pulmonary embolism) but also for arterial thrombosis (eg, stroke, MI). Hyperhomocysteinemia can be hereditary, or it can result from a nutritional deficiency of folic acid and, to a lesser extent, of vitamins B_{12} and B_6, because these vitamins are cofactors in homocysteine metabolism. For unknown reasons, people who are elderly, those with renal failure, and smokers may also have elevated levels of homocysteine in the absence of nutritional deficiencies of these vitamins. Although a simple fasting measurement of plasma homocysteine can serve as a useful screening test, people with genetically inherited hyperhomocysteinemia and those who are vitamin B_6 deficient may have normal or minimally elevated levels. A much more sensitive method involves obtaining a second measurement 4 hours after the patient consumes methionine; the hyperhomocysteinemia is found twice as often when this method is used. In hyperhomocys-

(text continues on page 1098)

CHART 33-14

Plan of Nursing Care — The Patient With Disseminated Intravascular Coagulation (DIC) (Continued)

NURSING INTERVENTIONS	RATIONALE	EXPECTED OUTCOMES
1. Assess neurologic, pulmonary, integumentary systems. 2. Monitor response to heparin therapy. 3. Assess extent of bleeding.	1. Initial signs of thrombosis can be subtle. 2. Response to heparin is most accurately reflected in fibrinogen level. 3. Objective measurements of all sites of bleeding are crucial to accurately assess extent of blood loss.	• Arterial blood gases, O_2 saturation, pulse oximetry, LOC within normal limits. • Breath sounds clear • Absence of edema • Intake does not exceed output • Weight stable
4. Monitor fibrinogen levels.	4. Response to heparin is most accurately reflected in fibrinogen level.	
5. Stop aminocaproic acid (EACA) if symptoms of thrombosis occur (see Table 33-7).	5. EACA should be used only in setting of extensive hemorrhage not responding to replacement therapy.	

Nursing Diagnosis: Death anxiety
Goals: Fears verbalized/identified; realistic hope maintained

NURSING INTERVENTIONS	RATIONALE	EXPECTED OUTCOMES
1. Identify previous coping mechanisms, if possible; encourage patient to use them as appropriate. 2. Explain all procedures and rationale for these in terms patient and family can understand.	1. Identifying previous stressful situations can aid in recall of successful coping mechanisms. 2. Decreased knowledge and uncertainty can increase anxiety.	• Previously used coping strategies identified and tried, to extent patient is able to do so • Patient indicates understanding of procedures and situation as condition permits
3. Assist family in supporting patient.	3. Family can be useful in assisting patient to use coping strategies and to maintain hope.	
4. Use services from behavioral medicine, chaplain as needed.	4. Additional professional intervention may be necessary, particularly if previous coping mechanisms are maladaptive or ineffective. Spiritual dimension should be supported.	

teinemia, the endothelial lining of the vessel walls is denuded; this can precipitate thrombus formation. Patients who are found to have hyperhomocysteinemia should receive folic acid, vitamin B_6, and/or vitamin B_{12} supplements and should understand the rationale for their use.

Antithrombin (AT) Deficiency

AT is a protein that inhibits thrombin and certain coagulation factors, and AT deficiency is a hereditary condition that can cause venous thrombosis, particularly when the AT level is less than 60% of normal. Patients with AT deficiency can develop venous thrombosis as young adults; by 50 years of age, two thirds of patients with AT deficiency have venous thrombosis. The most common sites for thrombosis are the deep veins of the leg and the mesentery. Recurrent thrombosis often occurs. There is an increased resistance to heparin anticoagulation, which means that these patients may require greater amounts of heparin to achieve adequate anticoagulation. Patients with AT deficiency should be encouraged to have their family members tested for the deficiency.

AT deficiency can also be acquired by four mechanisms: accelerated consumption of AT (as in DIC), re-

TABLE 33-6 Hypercoagulable States

Disorder	Abnormal Laboratory Value*
Inherited Disorders (Family Testing Necessary)	
Hyperhomocysteinemia	Homocysteine ↑ after methionine load
Antithrombin III (AT III) deficiency	AT III ↓
Protein C deficiency	Protein C activity ↓ (must be measured off warfarin [Coumadin])
Activated protein C (APC) resistance	Must be measured off anticoagulant; <2× prolongation of PTT when APC added. Patients with APC resistance have a smaller increase in clotting time than normal (ie, the prolongation of clotting time is less than normal).
Factor V Leiden	Positive
Protein S deficiency	Protein S activity ↓; must be measured off warfarin (Coumadin)
Dysfibrinogenemia	↑ thrombin time; ↑ reptilase time; ↓ functional fibrinogen; often requires special fibrinogen assays
Acquired Disorders (Family Testing Unnecessary)	
Anticardiolipin antibody	Positive
Cancer	Varied, depending on disorder
Lupus anticoagulant	Positive
Hyperhomocysteinemia	Homocystine ↑ after methionine load
AT III deficiency	AT III ↓
Paroxysmal nocturnal hemoglobinuria	+ Hamm's test; acid hemolysis
Myeloproliferative disorders	Varied, depending on disorder
Nephrotic syndrome	Varied, depending on disorder
Cancer chemotherapy	Varied, depending on disorder

*Protein C and protein S are vitamin K–dependent proteins. Warfarin (Coumadin) interferes with the hepatic synthesis of vitamin K-dependent factors, which may decrease levels of protein C or protein S; therefore, protein C and protein S should be measured while the patient is off warfarin.

duced synthesis of AT (as in hepatic dysfunction), increased excretion of AT (as in nephrotic syndrome), and medication-inducted (eg, estrogens, L-asparaginase) (Bauer, 2004).

Protein C Deficiency

Protein C is an enzyme that, when activated, inhibits coagulation. When levels of protein C are deficient, the risk for thrombosis increases, and thrombosis can often occur spontaneously. Protein C deficiency is at least as prevalent as AT deficiency, and people who are deficient in protein C can develop thrombosis early in life, as early as 15 years of age. A rare but significant complication of anticoagulation management in patients with protein C deficiency is warfarin-induced skin necrosis. This complication appears to result from progressive thrombosis in the capillaries within the skin; the extent of the necrosis can be extreme.

Activated Protein C (APC) Resistance and Factor V Leiden Mutation

APC resistance is a common condition that can occur with other hypercoagulable states. APC is an anticoagulant, and resistance to APC increases the risk for venous thrombosis. A molecular defect in the factor V gene has been identified in most (90%) of those with APC resistance; this defect is called factor V Leiden mutation. It has been identified as the most common cause of inherited hypercoagulability in Caucasians, but its incidence appears to be much lower in other ethnic groups. Factor V Leiden mutation synergistically increases the risk of thrombosis in patients with other risk factors (eg, use of oral contraceptives, hyperhomocysteinemia, increased age). It does not appear that the use of postmenopausal hormone therapy in women increases the risk of thrombotic events as does the use of oral contraceptives; the dose of estrogen in the former situation is much lower than in the latter. People who are homozygous for the factor V Leiden mutation are at extremely high risk of thrombosis and need life-long anticoagulation.

Protein S Deficiency

Protein S is another natural anticoagulant normally produced in the liver. APC requires protein S to inactivate certain clotting factors. When the level of protein S is deficient, this inactivation process is diminished, and the risk of thrombosis can be increased. Like patients with protein C deficiency, those with protein S deficiency have a greater risk of recurrent venous thrombosis at a young age, as young as 15 years.

Acquired Thrombophilia

Antibodies to phospholipids are common acquired causes for thrombophilia (hypercoagulable states). The most common antibodies present against phospholipids are either lupus or anticardiolipin antibodies. Both of these antibodies can be transient, resulting from infection or certain medications. Most thrombotic events are venous, but arterial thrombosis can occur in up to one third of the cases. Patients who persistently test positive for either antibody and who have had a thrombotic event are at significant risk of recurrent thrombosis (greater than 50%). Recurrent thromboses tend to be of the same type—that is, venous thrombosis after an initial venous thrombosis, arterial thrombosis after an initial arterial thrombosis. Thrombi typically occur in larger vessels.

Another common acquired cause of thrombophilia is cancer. Specific types of stomach, pancreatic, lung, and ovarian cancers are most commonly associated with thrombophilia. The type of thrombosis that results is unusual. Rather than DVT or pulmonary embolism, the thrombosis occurs in unusual sites, such as the portal, hepatic, or renal vein or the inferior vena cava. Migratory superficial thrombophlebitis or nonbacterial thrombotic endocarditis can also occur. In these patients, anticoagulation can be difficult to manage and the thrombosis can progress despite standard doses of anticoagulants.

Medical Management

The primary method of treating thrombotic disorders is anticoagulation. However, in thrombophilic conditions, when to treat (prophylaxis or not) and how long to treat (lifelong or not) can be controversial. Anticoagulation therapy is not without risks; the most significant risk is bleeding. Risks of anticoagulation therapy are identified in Chapter 31. The most common anticoagulant medications are identified in the following section.

Pharmacologic Therapy

Along with administering anticoagulant therapy, concerns include minimizing any risk factors that predispose a patient to thrombosis. When risk factors (eg, immobility after surgery, pregnancy) cannot be avoided, prophylactic anticoagulation may be necessary.

UNFRACTIONATED HEPARIN THERAPY

Heparin is a naturally occurring anticoagulant that enhances AT III and inhibits platelet function. To prevent thrombosis, heparin is typically given as a subcutaneous injection, two or three times daily. To treat thrombosis, heparin is usually administered IV. The therapeutic effect of heparin is monitored by serial measurements of the activated PTT; the dose is adjusted to maintain the range at 1.5 to 2.5 times the laboratory control. Oral forms are being evaluated in clinical trials (Nutescu et al., 2004).

Heparin-induced Thrombocytopenia. Heparin-induced thrombocytopenia (HIT) is a significant complication of heparin-based therapy, and any patient beginning heparin therapy should have the platelet count monitored. In HIT, antibodies are formed against the heparin complex. The actual incidence of HIT is unknown, but it has been shown to occur in as many as 5% of orthopedic patients receiving heparin (Warkentin, 2003). The type of heparin used and the duration of therapy appear to be risk factors for developing HIT: bovine preparations are more likely to lead to HIT than porcine preparations, and low-molecular-weight heparin (LMWH) formulations carry a lower risk. Prolonged use of heparin (beyond 4 days) and immobility are also risk factors (Warkentin, 2003). Neither the dose nor the route of administration (IV versus subcutaneous) is a risk (McIntosh, 2004). A decline in platelet count is a hallmark sign which typically occurs after 4 to 14 days of heparin therapy. The platelet count can drop significantly, usually by 50% of baseline. Interestingly, affected patients are at increased risk for thrombosis, either venous or arterial, and the thrombosis can range from DVT, MI, CVA (brain attack, stroke), to ischemic damage to an extremity necessitating amputation. The risk for fatal thrombosis is 4% to 5% (Warkentin, 2003). A mild form of HIT, HIT-1, is actually more common than HIT; HIT-1 results only in a mild decline in platelet count and usually occurs 1 to 4 days after heparin is initiated (Viale & Schwartz, 2004).

Treatment of HIT includes prompt cessation of heparin and initiation of an alternative means of anticoagulation. If the heparin is stopped without providing additional anticoagulation, the patient is at increased risk for developing new thrombi (McIntosh, 2004). Two inhibitors of thrombin, lepirudin (Refludan) and argatroban, are FDA-approved anticoagulants for the treatment of HIT.

LOW-MOLECULAR-WEIGHT HEPARIN THERAPY

LMWHs (eg, Dalteparin [Fragmin], Enoxaparin [Lovenox]) are special forms of heparin that have more selective effects on coagulation. Based on their biochemical properties, LMWHs have a longer half-life and a less variable anticoagulant response than standard heparin. These differences permit LMWHs to be safely administered only once or twice daily, without the need for laboratory monitoring for dose adjustments. The incidence of HIT is much lower when a LMWH is used; however, LMWH is 100% cross-reactive with HIT antibodies and therefore contraindicated in HIT (McIntosh, 2004). In certain conditions, the use of a LMWH has allowed anticoagulation therapy to be moved entirely to the outpatient setting. Many cases of uncomplicated DVT are being managed outside the hospital. LMWHs are also being increasingly used as "bridge therapy" when patients receiving anticoagulation therapy (warfarin) require an invasive procedure (eg, biopsy, surgery) (Spyropoulos et al., 2004). In this situation, warfarin is stopped and an LMWH is used in its place until the procedure is completed. After the procedure, warfarin therapy is resumed. The LMWH is discontinued after a therapeutic level of warfarin is achieved.

WARFARIN (COUMADIN) THERAPY

Coumarin anticoagulants (warfarin [Coumadin]) are antagonists of vitamin K and therefore interfere with the synthesis of vitamin K–dependent clotting factors. Coumarin anticoagulants bind to albumin, are metabolized in the liver, and have an extremely long half-life. Typically, a patient with a venous thromboembolus is initially treated with both heparin (either the unfractionated form or LMWH) and warfarin. When the international normalized ratio (INR), which is a standard method of reporting prothrombin time (PT), reaches the desired therapeutic range, the heparin is stopped. The dosage required to maintain the therapeutic range (typically an INR of 2.0 to 3.0) varies widely among patients and even within the same patient, depending on the diagnosis and the rationale for anticoagulation. Frequent monitoring of the INR is extremely important so that the dosage of warfarin can be adjusted as needed. Warfarin is affected by many medications; consultation with a pharmacist is important to assess the extent to which concurrently administered medications, herbs, and nutritional supplements may interact with warfarin. It is also affected by many foods, so patients need dietary instruction and may benefit from consultation with a dietitian. In particular, foods with high vitamin K content antagonize the effects of warfarin. Some of these foods include spinach, asparagus, and yogurt. Chart 33-15 lists agents that interact with warfarin.

Nursing Management

Patients with thrombotic disorders should avoid activities that promote circulatory stasis (eg, immobility, crossing the legs). Exercise, especially ambulation, should be per-

CHART 33-15

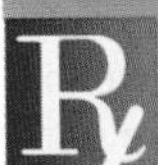

PHARMACOLOGY · Agents That Interact with Warfarin (Coumadin)

Although warfarin (Coumadin), an anticoagulant medication, is commonly used to treat and prevent thrombosis, many drug–drug and drug–food interactions are associated with its use. A careful medication history (including over-the-counter medications, herbs, and other substances, such as vitamins and minerals) is important when oral anticoagulation therapy is prescribed. Consultation with a pharmacist is recommended to assess the extent to which concurrent medications may affect the anticoagulant and for appropriate dosage adjustments. The following list contains a few examples of agents that interact with warfarin.

Agents That Inhibit Warfarin Function

Barbiturates
Carbamazepine
Cholestyramine
Corticosteroids
Digitalis
Estrogens
Ethanol
Glutethimide
Griseofulvin
Haloperidol
Oral contraceptives
Phenytoin
Rifampin
Spironolactone

Agents That Potentiate Warfarin Function

Acetaminophen
Allopurinol
Amiodarone
Anabolic steroids
Anti-inflammatory agents
Antimalarial agents
Aspirin
Broad-spectrum antibiotics
Chloral hydrate
Chloramphenicol
Cimetidine
Colchicine
Clofibrate
Chlorpromazine
Danazol
Disulfiram
Ethacrynic acid
Feprazone
Herbal medicines:
feverfew, garlic, gingko, ginseng
Vitamin C (in very large doses)
Vitamin E (in very large doses)
Isoniazid
Mefenamic acid
Methotrexate
Metronidazole
Oral hypoglycemic agents
Oxyphenbutazone
Phenytoin
Probenecid
Propylthiouracil
Quinidine
Quinine
Salicylates
Sulfinpyrazone
Sulfonamides (long-acting)
Thyroxine
Triclofos
Tricyclic antidepressants

formed frequently throughout the day, particularly during long trips by car or plane. Surgery further increases the risk for thrombosis. Medications that alter platelet aggregation, such as low-dose aspirin, may be prescribed. Some patients require life-long therapy with anticoagulants such as warfarin (Coumadin).

In addition, patients with thrombotic disorders, particularly those with thrombophilia, should be assessed for concurrent risk factors for thrombosis and should avoid concomitant risk factors if possible. For example, use of tobacco and nicotine products exacerbates the problem and should be avoided. Just as for other conditions, patients should know the name of their specific condition and understand its significance. In many instances, younger patients with thrombophilia may not require prophylactic anticoagulation; however, with concomitant risk factors (eg, pregnancy), increasing age, or subsequent thrombotic events, prophylactic or long-term anticoagulation therapy may be required. Being able to provide the health care provider with an accurate health history can be extremely useful and can help guide the selection of appropriate therapeutic interventions. Patients with hereditary disorders should encourage their siblings and children to be tested for the disorder.

When a patient with a thrombotic disorder is hospitalized, frequent assessments should be performed for signs and symptoms of beginning thrombus formation, particularly in the legs (DVT) and lungs (pulmonary embolism). Ambulation or range-of-motion exercises as well as the use of elastic compression stockings should be initiated promptly to decrease stasis. Prophylactic anticoagulants are commonly prescribed.

Therapies for Blood Disorders

Splenectomy

The surgical removal of the spleen (splenectomy) is sometimes necessary after trauma to the abdomen. Because the spleen is very vascular, severe hemorrhage can result if the spleen is ruptured. Under such circumstances, splenectomy becomes an emergency procedure.

Splenectomy is also a possible treatment for other hematologic disorders. For example, an enlarged spleen may be the site of excessive destruction of blood cells. If the destruction is life-threatening, surgery may be lifesaving. This is the case in autoimmune hemolytic anemia and ITP when these disorders do not respond to more conservative measures, such as corticosteroid therapy. Some patients with grossly enlarged spleens develop severe thrombocytopenia due to the platelets being sequestered in the spleen; splenectomy removes the "trap," and platelet counts may normalize over time.

In general, the mortality rate after splenectomy is low. Laparoscopic splenectomy can be performed in selected patients, with a resultant decrease in postoperative morbidity. Complications that may result from surgery are atelectasis, pneumonia, abdominal distention, and abscess formation. Although young children are at the highest risk after splenectomy, all age groups are vulnerable to overwhelming lethal infections and should receive the pneumonia vaccine (Pneumovax) before undergoing splenectomy, if possible.

The patient is instructed to seek prompt medical attention if even relatively minor symptoms of infection occur. Often, patients with high platelet counts have even higher counts after splenectomy (more than 1 million/mm^3), which can predispose them to serious thrombotic or hemorrhagic problems. However, this increase is transient and usually does not warrant additional treatment.

Therapeutic Apheresis

Apheresis is a Greek word meaning separation. In therapeutic apheresis (or pheresis), blood is taken from the patient and passed through a centrifuge, where a specific component is separated from the blood and removed (Table 33-7). The remaining blood is then returned to the patient. The entire system is closed, so the risk of bacterial contamination is extremely low. When platelets or leukocytes are removed, the decrease in these cells within the circulation is temporary. However, the temporary decrease provides a window of time until suppressive medications (eg, chemotherapy) can have therapeutic effects. Sometimes plasma is removed rather than blood cells—typically so that specific, abnormal proteins within the plasma are transiently lowered until a long-term therapy can be initiated.

Apheresis is also used to obtain larger amounts of platelets from a donor than can be provided from a single unit of whole blood. A unit of platelets obtained in this way is equivalent to six to eight units of platelets obtained from six to eight separate donors via standard blood donation methods. Platelet donors can have their platelets apheresed as often as every 14 days. Leukocytes can be obtained similarly, typically after the donor has received growth factors (G-CSF, GM-CSF) to stimulate the formation of additional leukocytes and thereby increase the leukocyte count. The use of these growth factors also stimulates the release of stem cells within the circulation. Apheresis is used to harvest these stem cells (typically over a period of several days) for use in PBSCT.

Therapeutic Phlebotomy

Therapeutic phlebotomy is the removal of a certain amount of blood under controlled conditions. Patients with elevated hematocrits (eg, those with polycythemia vera) or excessive iron absorption (eg, hemochromatosis) can usually be managed by periodically removing 1 unit (about 500 mL) of

TABLE 33-7 Types of Apheresis*

Procedure	Purpose	Examples of Clinical Use
Platelet pheresis	Remove platelets	Extreme thrombocytosis, essential thrombocythemia (temporary measure); single-donor platelets transfusion
Leukapheresis	Remove WBCs (can be specific to neutrophils or lymphocytes)	Extreme leukocytosis (eg, AML, CML) (very temporary measure); harvest WBCs for transfusion
Erythrocytapheresis (RBC exchange)	Remove RBCs	RBC dyscrasias (eg, sickle cell disease); RBCs replaced via transfusion
Plasmapheresis (plasma exchange)	Remove plasma proteins	Hyperviscosity syndromes; treatment for some renal and neurologic diseases (eg, Goodpasture's syndrome, Guillain-Barré, myasthenia gravis)
Stem cell harvest	Remove circulating stem cells	Transplantation (donor harvest or autologous)

*Therapeutic apheresis can be used to treat a wide variety of conditions. When it is used to treat a disease that causes an increase in a specific cell type with a short life in circulation (ie, WBCs, platelets), the reduction in those cells is temporary. However, this temporary reduction permits a margin of safety while waiting for a longer-lasting treatment modality (eg, chemotherapy) to take effect. Apheresis can also be used to obtain stem cells for transplantation, either from a matched donor (allogenic) or from the patient (autologous).

AML, acute myeloid leukemia; CML, chronic myeloid leukemia; RBC, red blood cell; WBC, white blood cell.

whole blood (Parker et al., 2004). Eventually this process can produce iron deficiency, leaving the patient unable to produce as many erythrocytes. The actual procedure for therapeutic phlebotomy is similar to that for blood donation (see later discussion).

Blood Component Therapy

A single unit of whole blood contains 450 mL of blood and 50 mL of an anticoagulant. A unit of whole blood can be processed and dispensed for administration. However, it is more appropriate, economical, and practical to separate that unit of whole blood into its primary components: erythrocytes, platelets, and plasma (leukocytes are rarely used; see later discussion). Because the plasma is removed, a unit of PRBCs is very concentrated (hematocrit approximately 70%). Each component must be processed and stored differently to maximize the longevity of the viable cells and factors within it; each individual blood component has a different storage life. PRBCs are stored at 4°C. With special preservatives, they can be stored safely for up to 42 days before they must be discarded. In contrast, platelets must be stored at room temperature because they cannot withstand cold temperatures, and they last for only 5 days before they must be discarded. To prevent clumping, platelets are gently agitated while stored. Plasma is immediately frozen to maintain the activity of the clotting factors within; it lasts for 1 year if it remains frozen. Alternatively, plasma can be further pooled and processed into blood derivatives, such as albumin, immune globulin, factor VIII, and factor IX. Table 33-8 describes each blood component and how it is commonly used.

TABLE 33-8 Blood and Blood Components Commonly Used in Transfusion Therapy*

	Composition	Indications and Considerations
Whole blood	Cells and plasma, hematocrit about 40%	Volume replacement and oxygen-carrying capacity; usually used only in significant bleeding (>25% blood volume lost)
Packed red blood cells (PRBCs)	RBCs with little plasma (hematocrit about 75%); some platelets and WBCs remain	↑ RBC mass Symptomatic anemia: platelets in the unit are not functional; WBCs in the unit may cause reaction and are not functional
Platelets—random	Platelets (5.5×10^{10} platelets/unit) Plasma; some RBCs, WBCs	Bleeding due to severe ↓ platelets Prevent bleeding when platelets <5,000–10,000/mm^3 Survival ↓ in presence of fever, chills, infection Repeated treatment → ↓ survival due to alloimmunization
Platelets—single donor	Platelets (3×10^{11} platelets/unit) 1 unit is equivalent to 6–8 units of random platelets	Used for repeated treatment: ↓ alloimmunization risk by limiting exposure to multiple donors
Plasma	Plasma; all coagulation factors Complement	Bleeding in patients with coagulation factor deficiencies; plasmapheresis
Granulocytes	Neutrophils (>1×10^{10}/unit); lymphocytes; some RBCs and platelets	Severe neutropenia in selected patients; controversial
Lymphocytes (WBCs)	Lymphocytes (number varies)	Stimulate graft-versus-disease effect
Cryoprecipitate	Fibrinogen ≥150 mg/bag, AHF (VIII:C) 80–110 units/bag, von Willebrand factor; fibronectin	von Willebrand's disease Hypofibrinogenemia Hemophilia A
Antihemophilic factor (AHF)	Factor VIII	Hemophilia A
Factor IX concentrate	Factor IX	Hemophilia B (Christmas disease)
Factor IX complex	Factors II, VII, IX, X	Hereditary factor VII, IX, X deficiency; hemophilia A with factor VII inhibitors
Albumin	Albumin 5%, 25%	Hypoproteinemia; burns; volume expansion by 5% to ↑ blood volume; 25% → ↓ hematocrit
Intravenous gamma globulin	IgG antibodies	Hypogammaglobulinemia (in CLL, recurrent infections); ITP; primary immunodeficiency states
Antithrombin III concentrate (AT III)	AT III (trace amounts of other plasma proteins)	AT III deficiency with or at risk for thrombosis

*The composition of each type of blood component is described as well as the most common indications for using a given blood component. RBCs, platelets, and fresh frozen plasma are the blood products most commonly used. When transfusing these blood products, it is important to realize that the individual product is always "contaminated" with very small amounts of other blood products (eg, WBCs mixed in a unit of platelets). This contamination can cause some difficulties, particularly isosensitization, in certain patients.

AHF, antihemophilic factor; CLL, chronic lymphocytic leukemia; ITP, idiopathic thrombocytopenic purpura.

Special Preparations

Factor VIII concentrate (antihemophilic factor) is a lyophilized, freeze-dried concentrate of pooled fractionated human plasma. It is used in treating hemophilia A. Factor IX concentrate (prothrombin complex) is similarly prepared and contains factors II, VII, IX, and X. It is used primarily for treatment of factor IX deficiency (hemophilia B). Factor IX concentrate is also useful in treating congenital factor VII and factor X deficiencies. Recombinant forms of factor VIII, such as Humate-P or Alphanate, are also useful. Because they contain vWF, these agents are used in von Willebrand's disease as well as in hemophilia A, particularly when patients develop acquired factor VIII inhibitors (eg, antibodies).

Plasma albumin is a large protein molecule that usually stays within vessels and is a major contributor to plasma oncotic pressure. This protein is used to expand the blood volume of patients in hypovolemic shock and, rarely, to increase the concentration of circulating albumin in patients with hypoalbuminemia.

Immune globulin is a concentrated solution of the antibody IgG; it contains very little IgA or IgM. It is prepared from large pools of plasma. The IV form (IVIG) is used in various clinical situations to replace inadequate amounts of IgG in patients who are at risk for recurrent bacterial infection (eg, those with CLL, those receiving BMT or PBSCT). It is also used in certain autoimmune disorders, such as ITP. IVIG, in contrast to all other fractions of human blood, cells, or plasma, can survive being subjected to heating at 60°C (140°F) for 10 hours to free it of the viral contaminants that may be present (Chart 33-16).

CHART 33-16

Diseases Transmitted by Blood Transfusion

Hepatitis (Viral Hepatitis B, C)

- Greater risk from pooled blood products and blood of paid donors than from volunteer donors
- Screening test detects most hepatitis B and C
- Transmittal risk estimated at 1:10,000

AIDS (HIV and HTLV)

- Donated blood screened for antibodies to HIV
- Transmittal risk estimated at 1:670,000
- People with high-risk behaviors (multiple sex partners, anal sex, IV/injection drug use) and people with signs and symptoms that suggest AIDS should not donate blood

Cytomegalovirus (CMV)

- Transmittal risk greater for premature newborns with CMV antibody-negative mothers and for immunocompromised recipients who are CMV-negative (eg, those with acute leukemia, organ or tissue transplant recipients).
- Blood products rendered "leukocyte-reduced" help reduce transmission of virus.

Graft-Versus-Host Disease (GVHD)

- Occurs only in severely immunocompromised recipients (eg, Hodgkin's disease, bone marrow transplantation).
- Transfused lymphocytes engraft in recipient and attack host lymphocytes or body tissues; signs and symptoms are fever, diffuse reddened skin rash, nausea, vomiting, diarrhea.
- Preventive measures include irradiating blood products to inactivate donor lymphocytes (no known radiation risks to transfusion recipient) and processing donor blood with leukocyte reduction filters.

Creutzfeldt-Jakob Disease (CJD)

- Rare, fatal disease causing irreversible brain damage
- No evidence of transmittal by transfusion, but hemophiliacs and others are concerned that transmittal is possible
- All blood donors must be screened for positive family history of CJD.
- Potential donors who spent 6 months or more in the United Kingdom (or Europe) from 1980 to 1996 cannot donate blood; blood products from a donor who develops CJD are recalled.

Procuring Blood and Blood Products

Blood Donation

To protect both the donor and the recipients, all prospective donors are examined and interviewed before they are allowed to donate their blood. The intent of the interview is to assess the general health status of the donor and to identify risk factors that might harm a recipient of the donor's blood. Donors should be in good health and without any of the following:

- A history of viral hepatitis at any time in the past, or a history of close contact with a patient who had hepatitis or was undergoing dialysis within 6 months
- A history of receiving a blood transfusion or an infusion of any blood derivative (other than serum albumin) within 12 months. (People previously transfused in the United Kingdom, Gibraltar, or Falkland Islands are not allowed to donate blood in the United States because they have an increased likelihood of transmitting Creutzfeldt-Jakob disease.)
- A history of untreated syphilis or malaria, because these diseases can be transmitted by transfusion even years later. A person who has been free of symptoms and off therapy for 3 years after malaria may be a donor.
- A history or evidence of drug abuse in which illicit drugs were self-injected, because many IV/injection drug abusers are carriers of hepatitis and because the risk of HIV is high in this group
- A history of possible exposure to HIV; the population at risk includes people who engage in anal sex, people with multiple sexual partners, IV drug abusers, sexual partners of people at risk of HIV, and people with hemophilia

- A skin infection, because of the possibility of contaminating the phlebotomy needle, and subsequently the blood itself
- A recent history of asthma, urticaria, or allergy to medications, because hypersensitivity can be transferred passively to the recipient
- Pregnancy, because of the nutritional demands of pregnancy on the mother
- A history of tooth extraction or oral surgery within 72 hours, because such procedures are frequently associated with transient bacteremia
- A history of untreated exposure to infectious disease within the past 3 weeks, because of the risk of transmission to the recipient
- Recent immunizations, because of the risk of transmitting live organisms (2-week waiting period for live, attenuated organisms; 1 month for rubella, mumps, varicella; 1 year for rabies)
- A history of recent tattoo, because of the risk of blood-borne infections (eg, hepatitis, HIV)
- Cancer, because of the uncertainty about transmission of the disease. People who have a history of a nonhematologic cancer treated with surgery or radiation and who are without evidence of recurrence for at least 5 years are eligible to donate.
- A diagnosis of hemochromatosis (although this exclusion is under debate)
- A history of whole blood donation within the past 56 days

Potential donors should be asked whether they have consumed any aspirin or aspirin-containing medications within the past 3 days. Although aspirin use does not render the donor ineligible, the platelets obtained would be dysfunctional and therefore not useful; aspirin usage within 48 to 72 hours contraindicates platelet donation. Aspirin does not affect the erythrocytes or plasma obtained from the donor.

All donors are expected to meet the following minimal requirements:

- Body weight should exceed 50 kg (110 pounds) for a standard 450-mL donation. Donors weighing less than 50 kg donate proportionately less blood. People younger than 17 years of age are disqualified from donation.
- The oral temperature should not exceed 37.5°C (99.6°F).
- The pulse rate should be regular and between 50 and 100 beats per minute.
- The systolic arterial blood pressure should be 90 to 180 mm Hg, and the diastolic pressure should be 50 to 100 mm Hg.
- The hemoglobin level should be at least 12.5 g/dL for women and 13.5 g/dL for men.

Directed Donation

At times, friends and family of a patient wish to donate blood for that person. These blood donations are termed directed donations. These donations are not any safer than those provided by random donors, because directed donors may not be as willing to identify themselves as having a history of any of the risk factors that disqualify a person from donating blood.

Standard Donation

Phlebotomy consists of venipuncture and blood withdrawal. Standard precautions are used. Donors are placed in a semi-recumbent position. The skin over the antecubital fossa is carefully cleansed with an antiseptic preparation, a tourniquet is applied, and venipuncture is performed. Withdrawal of 450 mL of blood usually takes less than 15 minutes. After the needle is removed, donors are asked to hold the involved arm straight up, and firm pressure is applied with sterile gauze for 2 to 3 minutes or until bleeding stops. A firm bandage is then applied. The donor remains recumbent until he or she feels able to sit up, usually within a few minutes. Donors who experience weakness or faintness should rest for a longer period. The donor then receives food and fluids and is asked to remain another 15 minutes.

The donor is instructed to leave the dressing on and to avoid heavy lifting for several hours, to avoid smoking for 1 hour, to avoid drinking alcoholic beverages for 3 hours, to increase fluid intake for 2 days, and to eat healthy meals for 2 weeks. Specimens from this donated blood are tested to detect infections and to identify the specific blood type (see later discussion).

Autologous Donation

A patient's own blood may be collected for future transfusion; this method is useful for many elective surgeries where the potential need for transfusion is high (eg, orthopedic surgery). Preoperative donations are ideally collected 4 to 6 weeks before surgery. Iron supplements are prescribed during this period to prevent depletion of iron stores. Occasionally, erythropoietin (epoetin-alfa [Epogen, Procrit]) is given to stimulate erythropoiesis so that the donor's hematocrit remains high enough to be eligible for donation. Typically, 1 unit of blood is drawn each week; the number of units obtained varies with the type of surgical procedure to be performed (ie, the amount of blood anticipated to be transfused). Phlebotomies are not performed within 72 hours of surgery. Individual blood components can also be collected.

The primary advantage of autologous transfusions is the prevention of viral infections from another person's blood. Other advantages include safe transfusion for patients with a history of transfusion reactions, prevention of alloimmunization, and avoidance of complications in patients with alloantibodies. It is the policy of the American Red Cross that autologous blood be transfused only to the donor. If the blood is not required, it can be frozen until the donor needs it in the future (for up to 10 years). The blood is never returned to the general donor supply of blood products to be used by another person.

The disadvantage of autologous donation is that it may be performed even when the likelihood that the anticipated procedure will necessitate a transfusion is small. Needless autologous donation is expensive, takes time, and uses resources inappropriately. Moreover, in an emergency situation, the autologous units available may be inadequate, and the patient may still require additional units from the general donor supply. Furthermore, although autologous transfusion can eliminate the risk of viral contamination, the risk for bacterial contamination is the same as that in transfusion from random donors.

Contraindications to donation of blood for autologous transfusion are acute infection, severely debilitating chronic disease, hemoglobin level less than 12.5 g/dL, hematocrit less than 38%, unstable angina, and acute cardiovascular or cerebrovascular disease. A history of poorly controlled epilepsy may be considered a contraindication in some centers. Patients with cancer may donate for themselves.

Intraoperative Blood Salvage

This transfusion method provides replacement for patients who cannot donate before surgery and for those undergoing vascular, orthopedic, or thoracic surgery. During a surgical procedure, blood lost into a sterile cavity (eg, hip joint) is suctioned into a cell-saver machine. The whole blood or PRBCs are washed, often with saline solution, filtered, and then returned to the patient as an IV infusion. Salvaged blood cannot be stored, because bacteria cannot be completely removed from the blood and it cannot be used when it is contaminated with bacteria (Kirschman, 2004).

Hemodilution

This transfusion method may be initiated before or after induction of anesthesia. About 1 to 2 units of blood are removed from the patient through a venous or arterial line and simultaneously replaced with a colloid or crystalloid solution. The blood obtained is then reinfused after surgery. The advantage of this method is that the patient loses fewer erythrocytes during surgery, because the added IV solutions dilute the concentration of erythrocytes and lower the hematocrit. However, patients who are at risk of myocardial injury should not be further stressed by hemodilution.

Complications of Blood Donation

Excessive bleeding at the donor's venipuncture site is sometimes caused by a bleeding disorder in the donor but more often results from a technique error: laceration of the vein, excessive tourniquet pressure, or failure to apply enough pressure after the needle is withdrawn.

Fainting is common after blood donation and may be related to emotional factors, a vasovagal reaction, or prolonged fasting before donation. Because of the loss of blood volume, hypotension and syncope may occur when the donor assumes an erect position. A donor who appears pale or complains of faintness should immediately lie down or sit with the head lowered below the knees. He or she should be observed for another 30 minutes.

Anginal chest pain may be precipitated in patients with unsuspected coronary artery disease. Seizures can occur in donors with epilepsy, although the incidence is very low. Both angina and seizures require further medical evaluation.

Many people have the misconception that donating blood can cause acquired immunodeficiency syndrome (AIDS) and other infections. Potential donors need to be educated that the equipment used in donation is sterile, a closed system, and not reusable; they are at no risk for acquiring infections such as AIDS from donating blood.

Blood Processing

Samples of the unit of blood are always taken immediately after donation so that the blood can be typed and tested. Each donation is tested for antibodies to HIV 1 and 2, hepatitis B core antibody (anti-HBc), hepatitis C virus (HCV), and human T-cell lymphotropic virus, type I (anti-HTLV-I/II). The blood is also tested for hepatitis B surface antigen (HbsAG) and for syphilis. Negative reactions are required for the blood to be used, and each unit of blood is labeled to certify the results. A new testing method, nucleic acid amplification testing, has increased the ability to detect the presence of HCV, HIV, and West Nile virus infection, because it directly tests for genomic nucleic acids of the viruses rather than for the presence of antibodies to the viruses. This testing significantly shortens the "window" of inability to detect HIV and HCV from a donated unit, further ensuring the safety of the blood; the risk of transmission of HIV or HCV is now estimated at 1 in 2 million blood units (Goodman, 2004). Blood is also screened for CMV; if it tests positive for CMV, it can still be used, except in recipients who are negative for CMV and who are immunocompromised (eg, BMT or PBSCT recipients).

Equally important to viral testing is accurate determination of the blood type. More than 200 antigens have been identified on the surface of RBC membranes. Of these, the most important for safe transfusion are the ABO and Rh systems. The ABO system identifies which sugars are present on the membrane of a person's erythrocytes: A, B, both A and B, or neither A nor B (type O). To prevent a significant reaction, the same type of PRBCs should be transfused. Previously, it was thought that in an emergency situation in which the patient's blood type was not known, type O blood could be safely transfused. This practice is no longer advised by the American Red Cross.

The Rh antigen (also called D) is present on the surface of erythrocytes in 85% of the population (Rh-positive). Those who lack the D antigen are called Rh-negative. PRBCs are routinely tested for the D antigen as well as ABO. Patients should receive PRBCs with a compatible Rh type.

The majority of transfusion reactions (other than those due to procedural error) are due to the presence of donor leukocytes within the blood component unit (PRBCs or platelets); the recipient may form antibodies to the antigens present on these leukocytes. PRBC components typically have 1 to 3×10^9 leukocytes remaining in each unit. Leukocytes from the blood product are frequently filtered to diminish the likelihood of developing reactions and refractoriness to transfusions, particularly in patients who have chronic transfusion needs. The process of leukocyte filtration renders the blood component "leukocyte-poor" (leukopoor). Filtration can occur at the time the unit is collected from the donor and processed, which achieves better results but is more expensive, or at the time the blood component is transfused by attaching a leukocyte filter to the blood administration tubing. Many centers advocate routinely using leukopoor filtered blood components for people who have or are likely to develop chronic transfusion requirements.

When a patient is extremely immunocompromised, as in the case of bone or stem cell transplant, any donor lymphocytes must be removed from the blood components. In this situation, the blood component is exposed to low amounts of radiation (25 Gy) that kill any lymphocytes within the blood component. Irradiated blood products are highly effective in preventing transfusion-associated GVHD, which is fatal in most cases. Irradiated blood products have a shorter shelf life.

Transfusion

Administration of blood and blood components requires knowledge of correct administration techniques and possible complications. It is very important to be familiar with the agency's policies and procedures for transfusion therapy. Methods for transfusing blood components are presented in Charts 33-17 and 33-18.

Setting

Although most blood transfusions are performed in the acute care setting, patients with chronic transfusion requirements often can receive transfusions in other settings. Free-standing infusion centers, ambulatory care clinics, physicians' offices, and even patients' homes may be appropriate settings for transfusion. Typically, patients who need chronic transfusions but are otherwise stable physically are appropriate candidates for outpatient therapy. Verification and administration of the blood product are performed as in a hospital setting. Although most blood products can be transfused in the outpatient setting, the home is typically

CHART 33-17

Transfusion of Packed Red Blood Cells (PRBCs)

Preprocedure

1. Confirm that the transfusion has been prescribed.
2. Check that patient's blood has been typed and cross-matched.
3. Verify that patient has signed a written consent form per institution or agency policy.
4. Explain the procedure to the patient. Instruct patient in signs and symptoms of transfusion reaction (itching, hives, swelling, shortness of breath, fever, chills).
5. Take patient's temperature, pulse, respiration, and blood pressure to establish a baseline for comparing vital signs during transfusion.
6. Use hand hygiene and wear gloves in accordance with Standard Precautions.
7. Use a 20-gauge or larger needle for insertion in a large vein. Use special tubing that contains a blood filter to screen out fibrin clots and other particulate matter. Do not vent the blood container.

Procedure

1. Obtain the PRBCs from the blood bank *after* the intravenous line is started. (Institution policy may limit release to only 1 unit at a time.)
2. Double-check the labels with another nurse or physician to make sure that the ABO group and Rh type agree with the compatibility record. Check to see that the number and type on the donor blood label and on the patient's chart are correct. Check the patient's identification by asking the patient's name and checking the identification wristband.
3. Check the blood for gas bubbles and any unusual color or cloudiness. (Gas bubbles may indicate bacterial growth. Abnormal color or cloudiness may be a sign of hemolysis.)
4. Make sure PRBC transfusion is initiated within 30 min after removal of the PRBCs from the blood bank refrigerator.
5. For first 15 minutes, run the transfusion slowly—no faster than 5 mL/min. Observe the patient carefully for adverse effects. If no adverse effects occur during the first 15 min, increase the flow rate unless the patient is at high risk for circulatory overload.
6. Monitor closely for 15–30 min to detect signs of reaction. Monitor vital signs at regular intervals per institution or agency policy; compare results with baseline measurements. Increase frequency of measurements based on patient's condition. Observe the patient frequently throughout the transfusion for any signs of adverse reaction, including restlessness, hives, nausea, vomiting, torso or back pain, shortness of breath, flushing, hematuria, fever, or chills. Should any adverse reaction occur, stop infusion immediately, notify physician, and follow the agency's transfusion reaction standard.
7. Note that administration time does not exceed 4 hr because of the increased risk for bacterial proliferation.
8. Be alert for signs of adverse reactions: circulatory overload, sepsis, febrile reaction, allergic reaction, and acute hemolytic reaction.
9. Change blood tubing after every 2 units transfused, to decrease chance of bacterial contamination.

Postprocedure

1. Obtain vital signs and compare with baseline measurements.
2. Dispose of used materials properly.
3. Document procedure in patient's medical record, including patient assessment findings and tolerance to procedure.
4. Monitor patient for response to and effectiveness of the procedure.

Note: Never add medications to blood or blood products; if blood is too thick to run freely, normal saline may be added to the unit. If blood must be warmed, use an in-line blood warmer with a monitoring system.

CHART 33-18

Transfusion of Platelets or Fresh Frozen Plasma (FFP)

Preprocedure

1. Confirm that the transfusion has been prescribed.
2. Verify that patient has signed a written consent form per institution policy.
3. Explain the procedure to the patient. Instruct patient in signs and symptoms of transfusion reaction (itching, hives, swelling, shortness of breath, fever, chills).
4. Take patient's temperature, pulse, respiration, and blood pressure to establish a baseline for comparing vital signs during transfusion.
5. Use hand hygiene and wear gloves in accordance with Standard Precautions.
6. Use a 22-gauge or larger needle for placement in a large vein, if possible. Use appropriate tubing per institution policy (platelets often require different tubing from that used for other blood products).

Procedure

1. Obtain the platelets or FFP from the blood bank (only *after* the intravenous line is started.)
2. Double-check the labels with another nurse or physician to make sure that the ABO group matches the compatibility record (not usually necessary for platelets; here only if compatible platelets are ordered). Check to see that the number and type on the donor blood label and on the patient's chart are correct. Check the patient's identification by asking the patient's name and checking the identification wristband.
3. Check the blood product for any unusual color or clumps (excessive redness indicates contamination with larger amounts of red blood cells).
4. Make sure platelets or FFP units are administered immediately after they are obtained.
5. Infuse each unit as fast as patient can tolerate to diminish platelet clumping during administration. Observe the patient carefully for adverse effects, including circulatory overload. Decrease rate of infusion if necessary.
6. Observe the patient closely throughout the transfusion for any signs of adverse reaction, including restlessness, hives, nausea, vomiting, torso or back pain, shortness of breath, flushing, hematuria, fever, or chills. Should any adverse reaction occur, stop infusion immediately, notify physician, and follow the agency's transfusion reaction standard.
7. Monitor vital signs at end of transfusion per institution policy; compare results with baseline measurements.
8. Flush line with saline after transfusion to remove blood component from tubing.

Postprocedure

1. Obtain vital signs and compare with baseline measurements.
2. Dispose of used materials properly.
3. Document procedure in patient's medical record, including patient assessment findings and tolerance to procedure.
4. Monitor patient for response to and effectiveness of procedure. A platelet count may be ordered 1 hr after platelet transfusion to facilitate this evaluation.

Note: FFP requires ABO but not Rh compatibility. Platelets are not typically cross-matched for ABO compatibility. Never add medications to blood or blood products.

limited to transfusions of PRBCs and factor components (eg, factor VIII for patients with hemophilia).

Pretransfusion Assessment

Patient History

Patient history is an important component of the pretransfusion assessment to determine the history of previous transfusions as well as previous reactions to transfusion. The history should include the type of reaction, its manifestations, the interventions required, and whether any preventive interventions were used in subsequent transfusions. It is important to assess the number of pregnancies a woman has had, because a high number can increase her risk for reaction due to antibodies developed from exposure to fetal circulation. Other concurrent health problems should be noted, with careful attention to cardiac, pulmonary, and vascular disease.

Physical Assessment

A systematic physical assessment and measurement of baseline vital signs are important before transfusing any blood product. The respiratory system should be assessed, including careful auscultation of the lungs and the patient's use of accessory muscles. Cardiac system assessment should include careful inspection for any edema as well as other signs of cardiac failure (eg, jugular venous distention). The skin should be observed for rashes, petechiae, and ecchymoses. The sclera should be examined for icterus. In the event of a transfusion reaction, a comparison of findings can help differentiate between types of reactions.

Patient Teaching

Reviewing the signs and symptoms of a transfusion reaction is crucial for patients who have not received a transfusion before. Even for patients who have received prior transfusions, a brief review of the signs and symptoms of transfusion reactions is advised. Signs and symptoms of a reaction include fever, chills, respiratory distress, low back pain, nausea, pain at the IV site, or anything "unusual." Although a thorough review is very important, it is also important to reassure the patient that the blood is carefully tested against the patient's own blood (cross-matched) to diminish the likelihood of any untoward reaction. Such assurance can be extremely beneficial in allaying anxiety. Similarly, the patient can be reassured about the very low possibility of contracting HIV from the transfusion; this fear persists among many people.

Complications

Any patient who receives a blood transfusion may develop complications from that transfusion. When explaining the reasons for the transfusion, it is important to include the risks and benefits and what to expect during and after the transfusion. Patients must be informed that the supply of blood is not completely risk-free, although it has been tested carefully. Nursing management is directed toward preventing complications, promptly recognizing complications if they develop, and promptly initiating measures to control complications. The following sections describe the most common or potentially severe transfusion-related complications.

Febrile Nonhemolytic Reaction

A febrile nonhemolytic reaction is caused by antibodies to donor leukocytes that remain in the unit of blood or blood component; it is the most common type of transfusion reaction, accounting for more than 90% of reactions. It occurs more frequently in patients who have had previous transfusions (exposure to multiple antigens from previous blood products) and in Rh-negative women who have borne Rh-positive children (exposure to an Rh-positive fetus raises antibody levels in the mother). These reactions occur in 1% of PRBC transfusions and 20% of platelet transfusions. More than 10% of patients with chronic transfusion requirements develop this type of reaction.

The diagnosis of a febrile nonhemolytic reaction is made by excluding other potential causes, such as a hemolytic reaction or bacterial contamination of the blood product. The signs and symptoms of a febrile nonhemolytic transfusion reaction are chills (minimal to severe) followed by fever (more than 1°C elevation). The fever typically begins within 2 hours after the transfusion is begun. Although the reaction is not life-threatening, the fever, and particularly the chills and muscle stiffness, can be frightening to the patient.

This reaction can be diminished, even prevented, by further depleting the blood component of donor leukocytes; this is accomplished by a leukocyte reduction filter. Antipyretics can be given to prevent fever, but routine premedication is not advised because it can mask the beginning of a more serious transfusion reaction.

Acute Hemolytic Reaction

The most dangerous, and potentially life-threatening, type of transfusion reaction occurs when the donor blood is incompatible with that of the recipient. Antibodies already present in the recipient's plasma rapidly combine with antigens on donor erythrocytes, and the erythrocytes are hemolyzed (destroyed) in the circulation (intravascular hemolysis). The most rapid hemolysis occurs in ABO incompatibility. This reaction can occur after transfusion of as little as 10 mL of PRBCs. Rh incompatibility often causes a less severe reaction. The most common causes of acute hemolytic reaction are errors in blood component labeling and patient identification that result in the administration of an ABO-incompatible transfusion.

Symptoms consist of fever, chills, low back pain, nausea, chest tightness, dyspnea, and anxiety. As the erythrocytes are destroyed, the hemoglobin is released from the cells and excreted by the kidneys; therefore, hemoglobin appears in the urine (hemoglobinuria). Hypotension, bronchospasm, and vascular collapse may result. Diminished renal perfusion results in acute renal failure, and DIC may also occur.

The reaction must be recognized promptly and the transfusion discontinued immediately. Blood and urine specimens must be obtained and analyzed for evidence of hemolysis. Treatment goals include maintaining blood volume and renal perfusion and preventing and managing DIC.

Acute hemolytic transfusion reactions are preventable. Meticulous attention to detail in labeling blood samples and blood components and accurately identifying the recipient cannot be overemphasized.

Allergic Reaction

Some patients develop urticaria (hives) or generalized itching during a transfusion. The cause of these reactions is thought to be a sensitivity reaction to a plasma protein within the blood component being transfused. Symptoms of an allergic reaction are urticaria, itching, and flushing. The reactions are usually mild and respond to antihistamines. If the symptoms resolve after administration of an antihistamine (eg, diphenhydramine [Benadryl]), the transfusion may be resumed. Rarely, the allergic reaction is severe, with bronchospasm, laryngeal edema, and shock. These reactions are managed with epinephrine, corticosteroids, and pressor support, if necessary.

Giving the patient antihistamines before the transfusion may prevent future reactions. For severe reactions, future blood components are washed to remove any remaining plasma proteins. Leukocyte filters are not useful to prevent such reactions, because the offending plasma proteins can pass through the filter.

Circulatory Overload

If too much blood is infused too quickly, hypervolemia can occur. This condition can be aggravated in patients who already have increased circulatory volume (eg, those with heart failure). PRBCs are safer to use than whole blood. If the administration rate is sufficiently slow, circulatory overload may be prevented. For patients who are at risk of, or already in, circulatory overload, diuretics are administered after the transfusion or between units of PRBCs. Patients receiving fresh frozen plasma or even platelets may also develop circulatory overload. The infusion rate of these blood components must also be titrated to the patient's tolerance.

Signs of circulatory overload include dyspnea, orthopnea, tachycardia, and sudden anxiety. Jugular vein distention, crackles at the base of the lungs, and an increase in blood pressure can also occur. If the transfusion is continued, pulmonary edema can develop, as manifested by severe dyspnea and coughing of pink, frothy sputum.

If fluid overload is mild, the transfusion can often be continued after slowing the rate of infusion and administering diuretics. However, if the overload is severe, the patient is placed in an upright position with the feet in a dependent position, the transfusion is discontinued, and the physician is notified. The IV line is kept patent with a very slow infusion of normal saline solution or a saline or heparin lock device to maintain access to the vein in case IV medications are necessary. Oxygen and morphine may be needed to treat severe dyspnea.

Bacterial Contamination

The incidence of bacterial contamination of blood components is very low; however, administration of contaminated products puts the patient at great risk. Contamination can occur at any point during procurement or processing but is usually due to organisms on the donor's skin (Goodman, 2004). Many bacteria cannot survive in the cold temperatures used to store PRBCs, but some organisms can survive cold temperatures. Platelets are at greater risk of contamination because they are stored at room temperature. Recently, blood centers have developed rapid methods of culturing the platelet unit (Goodman, 2004), thereby diminishing the risk of using a contaminated platelet unit for transfusion.

Preventive measures include meticulous care in the procurement and processing of blood components. When PRBCs or whole blood is transfused, it should be administered within a 4-hour period, because warm room temperatures promote bacterial growth. A contaminated unit of blood product may appear normal, or it may have an abnormal color.

The signs of bacterial contamination are fever, chills, and hypotension. These signs may not occur until the transfusion is complete, occasionally not until several hours after the transfusion. If the condition is not treated immediately with fluids and broad-spectrum antibiotics, shock can occur. Even with aggressive management, including vasopressor support, the mortality rate is high.

As soon as the reaction is recognized, any remaining transfusion is discontinued, and the IV line is kept open with normal saline solution. The physician and the blood bank are notified, and the blood container is returned to the blood bank for testing and culture. Septicemia is treated with IV fluids and antibiotics; corticosteroids and vasopressors are often also necessary.

Transfusion-Related Acute Lung Injury

This potentially fatal, idiosyncratic reaction occurs in fewer than 1 in 5000 transfusions. Antibodies (usually in the donor's plasma) that are present in the blood component stimulate the recipient's leukocytes; aggregates of these leukocytes form and occlude the microvasculature within the lungs or damage the endothelium in the lungs (Kopko, 2004). The precise pathologic mechanism is not yet completely understood, but the lung injury is manifested as pulmonary edema that can occur within 4 hours after the transfusion.

Signs and symptoms include fever, chills, acute respiratory distress (in the absence of other signs of left ventricular failure, such as elevated central venous pressure), and bilateral pulmonary infiltrates. Aggressive supportive therapy (oxygen, intubation, diuretics) may prevent death.

Delayed Hemolytic Reaction

Delayed hemolytic reactions usually occur within 14 days after transfusion, when the level of antibody has been increased to the extent that a reaction can occur. The hemolysis of the erythrocytes is extravascular via the RES and occurs gradually.

Signs and symptoms of a delayed hemolytic reaction are fever, anemia, increased bilirubin level, decreased or absent haptoglobin, and possibly jaundice. Rarely is there hemoglobinuria. Generally, these reactions are not dangerous, but it is useful to recognize them, because subsequent transfusions with blood products containing these antibodies may cause a more severe hemolytic reaction. However, recognition is also difficult, because the patient may not be in a health care setting to be tested for this reaction, and even if the patient is hospitalized, the reaction may be too mild to be recognized clinically. Because the amount of antibody present can be too low to detect, it is difficult to prevent delayed hemolytic reactions. Fortunately, the reaction is usually mild and requires no intervention.

Disease Acquisition

Despite advances in donor screening and blood testing, certain diseases can still be transmitted by transfusion of blood components (see Chart 33-16).

Complications of Long-Term Transfusion Therapy

The complications that have been described represent a real risk to any patient any time a blood component is administered. However, patients with long-term transfusion requirements (eg, those with MDS, thalassemia, aplastic anemia, sickle cell anemia) are at greater risk for infection transmission and for becoming more sensitized to donor antigens, simply because they are exposed to more units of blood and, consequently, more donors. A summary of complications associated with long-term transfusion therapy is given in Table 33-9.

Iron overload is a complication unique to people who have had long-term PRBC transfusions. One unit of PRBCs contains 250 mg of iron. Patients with chronic transfusion requirements can quickly acquire more iron than they can use, leading to iron overload. Over time, the excess iron deposits in body tissues and can cause organ damage, particularly in the liver, heart, testes, and pancreas. Promptly initiating a program of iron chelation therapy (eg, with deferoxamine [Desferal]) can prevent end-organ damage from iron toxicity (see Myelodysplastic Syndrome, Nursing Management, and Hereditary Hemochromatosis, Nursing Management). Chelation is a cumbersome process for the patient, necessitating chronic infusions, most often subcutaneously, at least several times per week. An oral formulation of chelating agents is now available.

TABLE 33-9 Common Complications Resulting from Long-Term PRBC Transfusion Therapy*

	Manifestation	Management
Infection	Hepatitis (B,C)	May immunize against hepatitis B; give alpha-interferon for hepatitis C; monitor hepatic function
	Cytomegalovirus (CMV)	WBC filters to protect against CMV
Iron overload	Heart failure Endocrine failure (diabetes, hypothyroidism, hypoparathyroidism, hypogonadism)	Prevent by chelation therapy
Transfusion reaction	Sensitization	Diminish by RBC phenotyping, using WBC-filtered products
	Febrile reactions	Diminish by using WBC-filtered products

*Patients with long-term transfusion therapy requirements are at risk not only for the transfusion reactions discussed in the text but also for the complications noted above. In many cases, the use of WBC-filtered (eg, leukocyte-poor) blood products is standard for patients who receive long-term PRBC transfusion therapy. An aggressive chelation program initiated early in the course of therapy can prevent problems with iron overload.

PRBC, packed red blood cells; WBC, white blood cell; RBC, red blood cell.

Nursing Management for Transfusion Reactions

If a transfusion reaction is suspected, the transfusion must be immediately stopped and the physician notified. A thorough patient assessment is crucial, because many complications have similar signs and symptoms. The following steps are taken to determine the type and severity of the reaction:

- Stop the transfusion. Maintain the IV line with normal saline solution through new IV tubing, administered at a slow rate.
- Assess the patient carefully. Compare the vital signs with baseline. Assess the patient's respiratory status carefully. Note the presence of adventitious breath sounds, use of accessory muscles, extent of dyspnea, and changes in mental status, including anxiety and confusion. Note any chills, diaphoresis, jugular vein distention, and reports of back pain or urticaria.
- Notify the physician of the assessment findings, and implement any treatments prescribed. Continue to monitor the patient's vital signs and respiratory, cardiovascular, and renal status.
- Notify the blood bank that a suspected transfusion reaction has occurred.
- Send the blood container and tubing to the blood bank for repeat typing and culture. The identifying tags and numbers are verified.

If a hemolytic transfusion reaction or bacterial infection is suspected, the nurse does the following:

- Obtain appropriate blood specimens from the patient.
- Collect a urine sample as soon as possible for a hemoglobin determination.
- Document the reaction according to the institution's policy.

Pharmacologic Alternatives to Blood Transfusions

Pharmacologic agents that stimulate production of one or more types of blood cells by the marrow are commonly used (Chart 33-19).

Researchers continue to seek a blood substitute that is practical and safe (Klein, 2005). Manufacturing artificial blood is problematic, given the myriad functions of blood components. Recent research has focused on the role of blood in oxygen transport or its role as an oxygen carrier and the manufacturing of a suitable RBC substitute. Current artificial RBC products undergoing clinical trials have distinct advantages and disadvantages compared with human RBCs. These products can be rendered essentially

CHART 33-19

Pharmacologic Alternatives to Blood Transfusions

Growth Factors

Recombinant technology has provided a means to produce hematopoietic growth factors necessary for the production of blood cells within the bone marrow. By increasing the body's production of blood cells, transfusions and complications resulting from diminished blood cells (eg, infection from neutropenia or transfusions) may be avoided. However, the successful use of growth factors requires functional bone marrow.

Erythropoietin

Erythropoietin (epoetin alpha [eg, Epogen, Procrit]) is an effective alternative treatment for patients with chronic anemia secondary to diminished levels of erythropoietin, as in chronic renal disease. This medication stimulates erythropoiesis. It also has been used for patients who are anemic from chemotherapy or zidovudine (AZT) therapy and for those who have diseases involving bone marrow suppression, such as myelodysplastic syndrome (MDS). The use of erythropoietin can also enable a patient to donate several units of blood for future use (eg, preoperative autologous donation). The medication can be administered intravenously or subcutaneously, although plasma levels are better sustained with the subcutaneous route. Side effects are rare, but erythropoietin can cause or exacerbate hypertension. If the anemia is corrected too quickly or is overcorrected, the elevated hematocrit can cause headache and, potentially, seizures. These adverse effects are rare except for patients with renal failure. Serial complete blood counts (CBCs) should be performed to evaluate the response to the medication. The dose and frequency of administration are titrated to the hematocrit.

Granulocyte-Colony Stimulating Factor (G-CSF)

G-CSF (filgrastim [Neupogen]) is a cytokine that stimulates the proliferation and differentiation of myeloid stem cells; a rapid increase in neutrophils is seen within the circulation. G-CSF is effective in improving transient but severe neutropenia after chemotherapy or in some forms of MDS. It is particularly useful in preventing bacterial infections that would be likely to occur with neutropenia. G-CSF is administered subcutaneously on a daily basis. The primary side effect is bone pain; this probably reflects the increase in hematopoiesis within the marrow. Serial CBCs should be performed to evaluate the response to the medication and to ensure that the rise in white blood cells is not excessive. The effect of G-CSF on myelopoiesis is short; the neutrophil count drops once the medication is stopped.

Granulocyte-Macrophage Colony Stimulating Factor (GM-CSF)

GM-CSF (sargramostim [Leukine]) is a cytokine that is naturally produced by a variety of cells, including monocytes and endothelial cells. It works either directly or synergistically with other growth factors to stimulate myelopoiesis. GM-CSF is not as specific to neutrophils as is G-CSF; thus, an increase in erythroid (RBC) and megakaryocytic (platelet) production may also be seen. GM-CSF serves the same purpose as G-CSF. However, it may have a greater effect on macrophage function and therefore may be more useful against fungal infections, whereas G-CSF may be better used to fight bacterial infections. GM-CSF is also administered subcutaneously. Side effects include bone pain, fevers, and myalgias.

Thrombopoietin

Thrombopoietin (TPO) is a cytokine that is necessary for the proliferation of megakaryocytes and subsequent platelet formation. Unfortunately, clinical studies have not consistently demonstrated effectiveness of TPO in the setting of chemotherapy-induced thrombocytopenia, but it is effective in facilitating platelet collection via apheresis (Vadhan-Raj, Cohen, & Bueso-Ramos, 2005). Further studies are ongoing to assess the efficacy of TPO in other, more chronic conditions associated with thrombocytopenia (Vadhan-Raj et al., 2005).

sterile, resulting in fewer immunity-related transfusion problems. They require no refrigeration, have approximately 12 times the shelf-life of PRBCs, and require no cross-matching. Their most significant disadvantage is their short half-life: approximately 1 day, versus the normal 120-day lifespan of a normal erythrocyte. Therefore, the usefulness of these products would likely be limited to situations where the need is short term (eg, surgery or trauma).

Peripheral Blood Stem Cell Transplantation and Bone Marrow Transplantation

PBSCT and BMT are therapeutic modalities that offer the possibility of cure for some patients with hematologic disorders such as severe aplastic anemia, some forms of leukemia, and thalassemia. Because most hematologic disease states arise from some form of bone marrow dysfunction, an autologous transplantation (receiving one's own stem cells) is not as common an option as is allogeneic transplantation. A patient receives intensive chemotherapy (sometimes with radiation therapy as well), with the goal being complete ablation of the patient's bone marrow. Stem cells from the donor (ideally, from a matched sibling) or actual marrow from the donor are then infused into the patient using a process similar to a PRBC transfusion. The stem cells travel to the marrow and slowly begin the process of resuming hematopoiesis. The advantage of autologous transplantation is the reduced likelihood of complications and mortality; however, the risk for relapse is also higher.

A relatively new strategy is based on transplantation for adoptive cell therapy using certain immune mechanisms derived from the donor's lymphocytes (Baron & Storb, 2004). In nonmyeloablative stem cell or marrow transplantation, also referred to as a "minitransplant," the conditioning regimen involves much less myelosuppression than in conventional regimens, rendering the patient immunosuppressed but for a shorter period of time. Consequently, the procedure is less toxic to the patient, and there is a significant decrease in morbidity.

After the deconditioning regimen (ie, during the time the patient is immunosuppressed), the allogeneic transplantation is performed, using either marrow or stem cells. The goal is for the donor's lymphocytes to react against any residual malignant cells within the patient and destroy them. This process is typically augmented by infusion of the donor's lymphocytes as well (referred to as donor lymphocyte infusion [DLI]). If relapse occurs, repeated DLI has been effective in reestablishing remission in many patients. This approach has great promise, particularly in the setting of hematologic malignancy, and may increase the utility of transplantation for more patients than is possible with conventional methods.

Recent research has focused on improving methods to utilize stem cells from cord blood as a source for allogeneic transplantation (Chao et al., 2004). These techniques have proved useful in children, but the amount of stem cells obtained from cord blood has been too small for use in adults. Methods to expand the stem cells harvested are being studied. An important advantage to using stem cells from cord blood is that precise tissue matching is not required because the donor's immune system is immature—yet it is that immaturity of immune function (ie, T-cell development) that renders the recipient more prone to infection and other complications.

The success of transplantation depends on tissue compatibility and the patient's tolerance of the immunosuppression that results from the ablative therapy. Patients require intensive nursing care that is directed toward preventing infection and assessing for early signs and symptoms of complications. One common complication involves the activation of donor T lymphocytes; these lymphocytes respond to their new host (ie, the patient) as foreign and mount a reaction against the body. This process (GVHD) can involve the skin, GI tract, and liver and can be life-threatening. Acute GVHD occurs in about 60% of patients receiving a matched related donor transplant; mortality can be as high as 50% (Bolanos-Meade & Vogelsang, 2004). GVHD is a significant complication in nonmyeloablative transplantation therapy as well as in conventional allotransplantation. In hematologic malignancies, some GVHD is actually desirable in that the donor lymphocytes can also mount a reaction against any lingering tumor cells; this process is referred to as graft-versus-disease effect. Late complications (occurring more than 100 days after transplantation) are common; these patients, particularly those who receive an allogeneic transplant, require careful follow-up for years after transplantation. (Refer to Chapter 16 for further discussion.)

Critical Thinking Exercises

1 You are working in a hematology-oncology clinic. The laboratory reports a critical laboratory result for one of your patients with possible MDS: the leukocyte count is 1200/mm^3 with 40% neutrophils. What other laboratory results would be important to review or consider? The patient is also anemic (hemoglobin 8.2 mg/dL) and platelets are 110,000/mm^3. What observations will you include in your assessment of this patient? Determine the extent to which this patient is neutropenic. What medical treatments would you anticipate? How would you educate the patient about neutropenia precautions? What information do you need to obtain about the patient's home setting that will assist you in determining the patient's risk of developing an infection at home? How will you modify this education if the patient has mild dementia? Lives alone? Does not understand or speak English well?

2 ebp You are caring for a 22-year-old-man who has had repeated hospitalizations for sickle cell crisis. What is the evidence base that indicates which factors should be assessed to determine the patient's educational, coping, and pain management needs? Identify the evidence base that supports concepts that you will incorporate into the patient's discharge plan.

3 You are caring for a man with a chronic transfusion requirement (typically 2 to 3 units of PRBCs each month). He asks you how he should modify his diet so that "I don't need so much blood." How would you respond? What role do iron supplements play in patients with chronic transfusion needs? How would you assess this patient for iron overload?

4 You are caring for a patient who is septic and is now receiving a transfusion of 2 units of PRBCs. The patient's temperature spikes to 101.3°F (38.5°C) after half of the second unit has been transfused. What are the possible causes of the fever? What are the appropriate nursing interventions?

REFERENCES AND SELECTED READINGS

BOOKS

Abrams, A. C. (2003). *Clinical drug therapy: Rationales for nursing practice* (7th ed.). Philadelphia: Lippincott Williams & Wilkins.

Anderson, K. C., & Ness, P. M. (2000). *Scientific basis of transfusion medicine: Implications for clinical practice.* Philadelphia: W. B. Saunders.

Berger, A., Portenoy, R., & Weissman, D. (2002). *Principles and practice of palliative care and supportive oncology* (2nd ed.). Philadelphia: Lippincott Williams & Wilkins.

Beutler, E., Lichtman, M. A., Coller, B. S., et al. (2005). *Williams hematology* (7th ed.). New York: McGraw Hill.

Bick, R. (2002). *Disorders of thrombosis and hemostasis: Clinical and laboratory practice* (3rd ed.). Philadelphia: Lippincott Williams & Wilkins.

Blumenthal, M., Goldberg, A., & Brinkman, J. (Eds.). (2000). *Herbal medicine.* Newton, MA: Integrative Medicine Communications.

Coleman, R. W., Hirsh, J., Marder, V. J., et al. (2000). *Hemostasis and thrombosis: Basic principles and clinical practice* (3rd ed.). Baltimore: Lippincott Williams & Wilkins.

Fisch, M. J., & Bruera, E. (2003). *Handbook of advanced cancer care.* New York: Cambridge.

Fischer, D., Knobf, M. T., Durivgage, H. J., et al. (2003). *The cancer chemotherapy handbook* (6th ed.). St. Louis: Mosby.

Greer, J., Foerster J., Lukens, J., et al. (2003). *Wintrobe's clinical hematology* (11th ed.). Philadelphia: Lippincott Williams & Wilkins.

Hoffman, R., Benz, E. J., Shattil, S. J., et al. (Eds.). (2005). *Hematology: Basic principles and practice* (4th ed.). New York: Churchill Livingstone.

McCullough, J. (2005). *Transfusion medicine* (2nd ed.). London, UK: Churchill Livingstone.

Mintz, P. D. (2005). *Transfusion therapy: Clinical principles and practice* (2nd ed.). Bethesda, MD: American Association of Blood Banks Press.

Skeel, R. (2003). *Handbook of cancer chemotherapy* (6th ed.). Philadelphia: Lippincott Williams & Wilkins.

Triulzi, D. J. (2002). *Blood transfusion therapy: A physician's handbook* (7th ed.). Bethesda, MD: American Association of Blood Banks.

Wilkes, G. M., & Barton-Burke, M. (2004). *2005 oncology nursing drug handbook.* Boston: Jones and Bartlett.

Winningham, M. L., & Barton-Burke, M. (2000). *Fatigue in cancer: A multidimensional approach.* Boston: Jones and Bartlett.

JOURNALS

**Asterisks indicate nursing research articles.*

Anemia

Adams, R. J., Brambilla, D. J., & Granger, S. (2004). Stroke and conversion to high risk in children screened with transcranial Doppler ultrasound during the STOP study. *Blood, 103*(10), 3689–3694.

Artz, A. S., Fergusson, D., Drink, P., et al. (2004). Prevalence of anemia in skilled-nursing home residents. *Archives in Gerontology and Geriatrics, 39*(3), 201–206.

Cao, H. (2004). Pharmacological induction of fetal hemoglobin synthesis using histone deacetylase inhibitors. *Hematology, 9*(3), 223–233.

Davies, E. G., Riddington, C. Lottenberg, R., et al. (2004). Pneumococcal vaccines for sickle cell disease. *Cochrane Database Systematic Review (1)*, CD003885.

Gebreyohanns, M., & Adams, R. J. (2004). Sickle cell disease: Primary stroke prevention. *CNS Spectrums, 9*(6), 445–449.

Gladwin, M., Sachdev, V., & Jison, M. (2004). Pulmonary hypertension as a risk factor for death in patients with sickle cell disease. *New England Journal of Medicine, 350*(9), 886–895.

Hammerman, S. I., & Faber, H. W. (2004). Pulmonary complications of sickle cell disease. Available at http://www.UpToDate.com. Accessed June 1, 2006.

*Johnson, L. (2003). Sickle cell disease patients and patient-controlled analgesia. *British Journal of Nursing, 12*(3), 144–153.

Liem, R. I., O'Gorman, M. K., & Brown, D. L. (2004). Effect of red cell exchange transfusion on plasma levels of inflammatory mediators in sickle cell patients with acute chest syndromes. *American Journal of Hematology, 76*(1), 19–25.

Rosenfeld, S., Follmann, D. Nunez, O., et al. (2003). Antithymocyte globulin and cyclosporine for severe aplastic anemia: association between hematologic response and long-term outcome. *Journal of the American Medical Association, 289*(9), 1130–1135.

Stuart, M. J., & Nagel, R. L. (2004). Sickle-cell disease. *Lancet, 364*(9442), 1343–1360.

Vichinsky, E. P. (2004). Pulmonary hypertension in sickle cell disease. *New England Journal of Medicine, 350*(9), 857–859.

Hemochromatosis

Beutler, E., Hoffbrand, V., & Cook, J. D. (2003). Iron deficiency and overload. *Hematology (American Society of Hematology Educational Program)*, 40–61.

Parker, D. M., Deel, P. C., & Arner, S. S. (2004). Iron out the details of therapeutic phlebotomy. *Nursing, 34*(2), 46–47.

Pietrangelo, A. (2004). Hereditary hemochromatosis: A new look at an old disease. *New England Journal of Medicine, 350*(23), 2383–2397.

Myelodysplastic Syndromes

Bevans, M. F., & Shalabi, R. A. (2004). Management of patients receiving antithymocyte globulin for aplastic anemia and myelodysplastic syndrome. *Clinical Journal of Oncology Nursing, 8*(4), 377–382.

Estey, E. H. (2004). Modulation of angiogenesis in patients with myelodysplastic syndrome. *Best Practice and Research. Clinical Haematology, 17*(4), 623–639.

Foss, F. M. (2004). Nucleoside analogs and antimetabolite therapies for myelodysplastic syndrome. *Best Practice and Research: Clinical Haematology, 17*(4), 573–584.

Giralt, S. A. (2004). Bone marrow transplant in myelodysplastic syndromes: New technologies, same questions. *Current Hematology Reports, 3*(3), 165–172.

Kantarjan, H., Issa, J. P., Rosenfeld, C. S., et al. (2006). Decitibine improves patient outcomes in myelodysplastic syndromes: Results of a phase III randomized study. *Cancer, 106*(8), 1794–1803.

List, A., Kurtin, S., Roe, D., et al. (2005). Efficacy of lenalidomide in myelodysplastic syndromes. *New England Journal of Medicine, 352*(6), 549–557.

Silverman, L. R. (2004). DNA methyltransferase inhibitors in myelodysplastic syndrome. *Best Practice and Research: Clinical Haematology, 17*(4), 585–594.

Vanorden, H. E., & Hagemann, T. M. (2006). Deferasirox—an oral agent for chronic iron overload. *Annals of Pharmacotherapy*, in press.

Polycythemia Vera

Berlin, N. I. (2003). Polycythemia vera. *Hematology/Oncology Clinics of North America, 17*(5), 1191–1210.

Chomienne, C., Rain, J. D., Briere, J., et al. (2004). Risk of leukemic transformation in PV and ET patients. *Pathologie Biologie, 52*(5), 289–293.

Golden, C. (2003). Polycythemia vera: A review. *Clinical Journal of Oncology Nursing, 7*(5), 553–556.

Landolfi, R., Marchioli, R., Kutti, J., et al. (2004). Efficacy and safety of low-dose aspirin in polycythemia vera. *New England Journal of Medicine, 350*(2), 114–124.

Prchal, J. T. (2003). Classification and molecular biology of polycythemias (erythrocytoses) and thrombocytosis. *Hematology/Oncology Clinics of North America, 17*(5), 1151–1158.

Terreri, A. (2004). Diagnostic approach to the patient with suspected polycythemia vera, Available at http://www.UptoDate.com. Accessed June 1, 2006.

Leukopenia/Neutropenia

Larson, E., & Nirenberg, A. (2004). Evidence-based nursing practice to prevent infection in hospitalized neutropenic patients with cancer. *Oncology Nursing Forum, 31*(4), 717–723.

*Nirenberg, A., Mulhearn, L., Lin, S., et al. (2004). Emergency department waiting times for patients with cancer with febrile neutropenia: A pilot study. *Oncology Nursing Forum, 31*(4), 711–715.

Leukemia/Myelofibrosis

American Cancer Society (2006). *What are the key statistics about acute myeloid leukemia?* Available at http://www.cancer.org/docroot/CRI/content/CRI_2_4_1x_What_Are_the_Key_Statistics_About_Acute_Myeloid_Leukemia_AML.asp?sitearea=. Accessed June 1, 2006.

Barosi, G. (2003). Myelofibrosis with myeloid metaplasia. *Hematology/Oncology Clinics of North America, 17*(5), 1211–1226.

Cortes, J. (2004). Natural history and staging of chronic myelogenous leukemia. *Hematology/Oncology Clinics of North America, 18*(3), 569–584.

Ferrajoli, A., & Keating, M. J. (2004). Current guidelines in defining therapeutic strategies. *Hematology/Oncology Clinics of North America, 18*(4), 881–893.

Giles, F. J., Cortes, E., Kantarjian, H. M., et al. (2004). Accelerated and blastic phases of chronic myelogenous leukemia. *Hematology/Oncology Clinics of North America, 18*(3), 753–774.

Iovino, C. S., & Camacho, L. H. (2003). Acute myeloid leukemia: A classification and treatment update. *Clinical Journal of Oncology Nursing, 7*(5), 535–540.

Larson, R. A. (2004). Adult ALL: Where are we and where are we going? *Clinical Advances in Hematology & Oncology, 2*(6), 342–344.

*Molassiotis, A. (2003). Research in brief: Anorexia and weight loss in long-term survivors of haematological malignancies. *Journal of Clinical Nursing, 12*(6), 925–927.

Pui, C. H., Relling, M. V., & Downing, J. R. (2004). Acute lymphoblastic leukemia. *New England Journal of Medicine, 350*(15), 1135–1148.

Qazilbash, M. H., Giralt, S. A., & Champlin, R. E. (2004). Nonmyeloblative stem cell transplantation for chronic myeloid leukemia. *Hematology/Oncology Clinics of North America, 18*(3), 703–713.

Radich, J. P., Olavarria, E., & Apperley, J. F. (2004). Allogeneic hematopoietic stem cell transplantation for chronic myeloid leukemia. *Hematology/Oncology Clinics of North America, 18*(3), 685–702.

Rai, K. R., Wasil, T., Iqbal, U., et al. (2004). Clinical staging and prognostic markers in chronic lymphocytic leukemia. *Hematology/Oncology Clinics of North America, 18*(4), 795–805.

Zent, C. S., & Kay, N. E. (2004). Update on monoclonal antibody therapy in chronic lymphocytic leukemia. *Clinical Advances in Hematology & Oncology, 2*(2), 107–113.

Lymphoma/Myeloma

Bonadonna, G., Bonfante, V., Viviani, S., et al. (2004). ABVD plus subtotal nodal versus involved-field radiotherapy in early-stage Hodgkin's disease: Long-term results. *Journal of Clinical Oncology, 22*(14), 2835–2841.

Devenney, B. (2004). Multiple myeloma: An overview. *Clinical Journal of Oncology Nursing, 8*(4), 401–405.

Diehl, V., Thomas, R. K., & Re, D. (2004). Part II: Hodgkin's lymphoma—diagnosis and treatment. *Lancet Oncology, 5*(1), 19–26.

Freedman, A. S. (2004). Approach to the diagnosis, staging, and prognosis of non-Hodgkin's lymphoma. Available at http://www.UptoDate.com. Accessed June 1, 2006.

Goy, A., Younces, A., McLaughlin, P., et al. (2004). Update on a phase II study of bortezomib in patients with relapsed or refractory indolent or aggressive non-Hodgkin's lymphomas. *Clinical Advances in Hematology & Oncology, 2*(10), 4–6.

Hochster, H. S., Weller, E., Ryan, T., et al. (2004). Results of E1496: A phase III trial of CVP with or without maintenance rituximab in advanced indolent lymphoma. Paper presented at the 40th ASCO Annual Meeting, New Orleans, American Society of Clinical Oncology.

Jemal, A., Siegal, R., Ward, E., et al. (2006). Cacer statistics. *CA: A Cancer Journal for Clinicians, 56*(2), 106–130.

Kyle, R. A., & Rajkumar, S. V. (2004). Multiple myeloma. *New England Journal of Medicine, 351*(18), 1860–1873.

Lipton, A. (2004). Pathophysiology of bone metastases: How this knowledge may lead to therapeutic intervention. *Journal of Supportive Oncology, 2*(3), 205–213.

Lister, T. A. (2004). Who should receive myeloablative therapy for lymphoma? *New England Journal of Medicine, 350*(13), 1277–1278.

Lugassy, G., Shaham, R., Nemets, A., et al. (2004). Severe osteomyelitis of the jaw in long-term survivors of multiple myeloma: A new clinical entity. *American Journal of Medicine, 117*(6), 440–441.

Mauch, P., Aleman, B., Carde, P., et al. (2003). Report from the Rockefeller Foundation–sponsored international workshop on reducing mortality and improving quality of life in long-term survivors of Hodgkin's disease. *European Journal of Haemotology, 66*(Suppl.), 68–76.

Riley, M. B., & Byar, K. (2004). The rationale for and background of radioimmunotherapy: An emerging therapy for B-cell non-Hodgkin's lymphoma. *Seminars in Oncology Nursing, 20*(suppl 1), 1–8.

Ruggiero, S. L., Mehrotra, B., Rosenberg, T. J., et al. (2004). Osteonecrosis of the jaw associated with the use of bisphosphonates: A review of 63 cases. *Journal of Oral Maxillofacial Surgery, 62*(5), 527–534.

Terpos, E., & Rahemtulla A. (2004). Bisphosphonate treatment for multiple myeloma. *Drugs Today, 40*(1), 29–40.

Platelet Disorders

Chomienne, C., Rain, J. D., Briere, J., et al. (2004). Risk of leukemic transformation in PV and ET patients. *Pathologie Biologie, 52*(5), 289–293.

Drachman, J. G. (2004). Inherited thrombocytopenia: When a low platelet count does not mean ITP. *Blood, 103*(2), 390–398.

Franchini, M., & Veneri D. (2004). *Helicobacter pylori* infection and immune thrombocytopenic purpura: An update. *Helicobacter, 9*(4), 342–346.

Harrison, C. N., & Green, A. R. (2003). Essential thrombocytopenia. *Hematology/Oncology Clinics of North America, 17*(5), 1175–1190.

Robak, T. (2004). Monoclonal antibodies in the treatment of autoimmune cytopenias. *European Journal of Haematology, 72*(2), 79–88.

Schafer, A. I. (2004). Thrombocytosis. *New England Journal of Medicine, 350*(12), 1211–1219.

Stasi, R., & Provan D. (2004). Management of immune thrombocytopenic purpura in adults. *Mayo Clinic Proceedings, 79*(4), 504–522.

Vadhan-Raj, S., Cohen, V., & Bueso-Ramos, C. (2005). Thrombotic growth factors and cytokines. *Current Hematology Reports, 4*(2), 137–144.

Zimmer, J., Andres, E., Noel, E., et al. (2004). Current management of adult idiopathic thrombocytopenia purpura in practice: A cohort study of 201 patients from a single center. *Clinical Laboratory, Haematology, 26*(2), 137–142.

Bleeding Disorders

Aird, W. C. (2004). Natural anticoagulant inhibitors: Activated protein C. *Clinical Haematology, 17*(1), 161–182.

Carr, M. E., & Martin, E. J. (2004). Recombinant factor VIIa: Clinical applications for an intravenous hemostatic agent with broad-spectrum potential. *Expert Review of Cardiovascular Therapy, 2*(5), 661–674.

Chehab, N. (2002). *A review of coagulation products used in the treatment of hemophilia.* The Cleveland Clinic Center for Continuing Education. Available at http://www.clevelandclinicmeded.com. Accessed June 1, 2006.

Harrison, P. (2003). Platelet function testing. Available at http://www.UpToDate.com. Accessed June 1, 2006.

Key, N. S. (2004). Inhibitors in congenital coagulation disorders. *British Journal of Hematology, 127*(4), 379–391.

Leung, L. (2004). Clinical features, diagnosis, and treatment of disseminated intravascular coagulation. Available at http://www.UpToDate.com. Accessed June 1, 2006.

Mannucci, P. M. (2004). Treatment of von Willebrand's disease. *New England Journal of Medicine, 351*(7), 683–694.

Paper, R. (2003). Can you recognize and respond to von Willebrand disease? *Nursing, 33*(7), 54–56.

Tarantino, M. D., & Aledort, L. M. (2004). Advances in clotting factor treatment for congenital hemorrhagic disorders. *Clinical Advances in Hematology & Oncology, 2*(6), 363–368.

Thrombotic Disorders

Bauer, K. A. (2004). Antithrombin (ATIII) deficiency. Available at http://www.UpToDate.com. Accessed June 1, 2006.

*Christian, J. B., Lapane, K. L., & Toppa, R. S. (2003). Racial disparities in receipt of secondary stroke prevention agents among US nursing home residents. *Stroke, 34*(11), 2693–2697.

Linkins, L. A., & Weitz, J. I. (2005). New anticoagulant therapy. *Annual Review of Medicine, 56*(1), 63–72.

McIntosh, B. A. (2004). Developing an algorithm for treating heparin-induced thrombocytopenia. *Clinical Advances in Hematology & Oncology, 2*(4), 216–222.

Nutescu, E. A., Helgason, C. M., Briller, J., et al. (2004). New blood thinner offers first potential alternative in 50 years: Ximelagatran. *Journal of Cardiovascular Nursing, 19*(6), 374–383.

Spyropoulos, A. C., Jenkins, P., & Bornikova, L. (2004). A disease management protocol for outpatient perioperative bridge therapy with enoxaparin in patients requiring temporary interruption of long-term oral anticoagulation. *Pharmacotherapy, 24*(5), 649–658.

Viale, P., & Schwartz, R. (2004). Venous thromboembolism in patients with cancer part II: Current treatment strategies. *Clinical Journal of Oncology Nursing, 8*(5), 465–469.

Warkentin, T. E. (2003). New approaches to the diagnosis of heparin-induced thrombocytopenia. *Chest, 127*(suppl. 2), 35S–45S.

*Wilson, F. L., Racine, E., Tekieli, V., et al. (2003). Literacy, readability and cultural barriers: Critical factors to consider when educating older African Americans about anticoagulation therapy. *Journal of Clinical Nursing, 12*(2), 275–282.

Bone Marrow/Stem Cell Transplantation

Baron, F., & Storb S. (2004). Allogeneic hematopoietic cell transplantation as treatment for hematological malignancies: A review. *Springer Seminars in Immunopathology, 26*(1–2), 71–94.

Bolanos-Meade, J., & Vogelsang, G. B. (2004). Acute graft-versus-host disease. *Clinical Advances in Hematology/Oncology, 2*(10), 672–682.

Chao, N. J., Emerson, S. G., & Weinberg, K. I. (2004). Stem cell transplantation (cord blood transplants). *Hematology, 9*(4), 354–371.

*El-Banna, M. N., Berger, A. M., Farr, L., et al. (2004). Fatigue and depression in patients with lymphoma undergoing autologous peripheral blood stem cell transplantation. *Oncology Nursing Forum, 31*(5), 937–944.

*Hacker, E. D. (2003). Quantitative measurement of quality of life in adult patients undergoing bone marrow transplant or peripheral blood stem cell transplant: A decade review. *Oncology Nursing Forum, 30*(4), 613–631.

*Larsen, J., Nordstrom, G., Bjorkstrand, B., et al. (2003). Symptom distress, functional status and health-related quality of life before high-dose chemotherapy with stem-cell transplantation. *European Journal of Cancer Care, 12*(1), 71–80.

Transfusion

Goodman, J. L. (2004). The safety and availability of blood and tissues: Progress and challenges. *New England Journal of Medicine, 351*(8), 819–822.

Kirschman, R. A. (2004). Finding alternatives to blood transfusion. *Nursing, 34*(6), 58–62.

Klein, H. G. (2005). Blood substitutes: How close to a solution? *Developmental Biology, 120*(1), 45–52.

Kopko, P. M. (2004). Leukocyte antibodies and biologically active mediators in the pathogenesis of transfusion-related acute lung injury. *Current Hematology Reports, 3*(6), 456–461.

Simmons, P. (2003). A primer for nurses who administer blood products. *MedSurg Nursing, 12*(3), 184–190.

General References

*Bulsara, C., Ward, A., & Joske, D. (2004). Haematological cancer patients: Achieving a sense of empowerment by use of strategies to control illness. *Journal of Clinical Nursing, 13*(2), 251–258.

Hessig, R. E., Arcand, L. L., & Frost, M. H. (2004). The effects of an educational intervention on oncology nurses' attitude, perceived knowledge, and self-reported application of complementary therapies. *Oncology Nursing Forum, 31*(1), 71–78.

RESOURCES

Alternative Medicine Foundation, Inc., 5411 W. Cedar Lane, Suite 205A, Bethesda, MD 20814; 301-340-1960; http://www.amfoundation.org. Accessed June 1, 2006.

American Association of Blood Banks (AABB), 8101 Glenbrook Road, Bethesda, MD 20814; 301-907-6977; http://www.aabb.org. Accessed June 1, 2006.

American Cancer Society, 1599 Clifton Rd., N.E., Atlanta, GA 30329; 800-227-2345; http://www.cancer.org. Accessed June 1, 2006.

American Hemochromatosis Society, 777 E. Atlantic Ave., PMB Z-363, Delray Beach, FL 33483; 1-888-655-4766; http://www.americanhs.org. Accessed June 1, 2006.

American Pain Society, 4700 W. Lake Ave., Glenview, IL 60025; 1-847-375-4715; http://www.ampainsoc.org. Accessed June 1, 2006.

American Red Cross, 1730 E Street NW, Washington, DC 20006; 1-202-639-3520; http://www.redcross.org. Accessed June 1, 2006.

American Society of Clinical Oncology (ASCO), 1900 Duke Street, Suite 200, Alexandria, VA, 22314; 1-703-299-0150; http://www.asco.org. Accessed June 1, 2006.

Aplastic Anemia and MDS International Foundation, P.O. Box 613, Annapolis, MD 21404; 1-800-747-2820; http://www.aplastic.org. Accessed June 1, 2006.

Blood and Marrow Transplant Newsletter, 1985 Spruce Ave., Highland Park, IL 60036.

International Myeloma Foundation, 12650 Riverside Drive, Suite 206, North Hollywood, CA 91607; 1-800-452-2873; http://www.myeloma.org. Accessed June 1, 2006.

Leukemia and Lymphoma Society, 1311 Mamaroneck Ave. White Plains, NY 10605; 1-800-955-4572; http://www.leukemia-lymphoma.org. Accessed June 1, 2006.

Myelodysplastic Syndromes Foundation, P.O. Box 477, 464 Main St., Crosswicks, NJ 08515; 1-800-637-0839; http://www.mds-foundation.org. Accessed June 1, 2006.

National Association of Vascular Access Networks, 11417 S. 700 East, Suite 205, Draper, UT 84020; 1-888-576-2826; http://www.navannet.org. Accessed June 1, 2006.

National Cancer Institute Cancer Information Service, 31 Center Drive, MSC 2580, Building 31, Room 10A16, Bethesda, MD 20892-2580; 1-800-4-CANCER; http://cis.nci.nih.gov. Accessed June 1, 2006.

National Center for Complementary and Alternative Medicine (NCCAM), National Institute of Health, Bethesda, MD, 20892, 1-888-644-6226; http://www.nccam.nih.gov. Accessed June 1, 2006.

National Hemophilia Foundation, 116 W. 32nd St., 11th Floor, New York, NY 10001; 1-800-424-2634; http://www.hemophilia.org. Accessed June 1, 2006.

National Library of Medicine, Health Information for Consumers, 8600 Rockville Pike, Bethesda, MD, 20894; 1-888-346-3656; http://www.nlm.nih.gov. Accessed June 1, 2006.

National Marrow Donor Program, Suite 500, 3001 Broadway St. N.E., Minneapolis, MN 55413; 1-800-627-7692; http://www.marrow.org. Accessed June 1, 2006.

Office of Dietary Supplements, National Institutes of Health, 6100 Executive Blvd., Rm 3B01, MSC 7517, Bethesda, MD 20892; 301-435-2920; http://ods.od.nih.gov. Accessed June 1, 2006.

Oncology Nursing Society, 501 Holiday Dr., Pittsburgh, PA 15220; http://www.ons.org. Accessed June 1, 2006.

Platelet Disorder Support Association, P.O. Box 61533, Potomac, MD 20859; 1-977-528-3538; http://www.pdsa.org. Accessed June 1, 2006.

Sickle Cell Disease Association of America, Inc., 200 Corporate Pointe, Suite 495, Culver City, CA 90230; http://www.sicklecelldisease.org. Accessed June 1, 2006.

UNIT 7

Digestive and Gastrointestinal Function

Case Study

Applying Concepts from NANDA, NIC, and NOC

A Patient With Nausea, Vomiting, and Diarrhea

Mr. Doyle is a 32-year-old man who has had several episodes of bloody diarrhea with severe cramping, nausea, and vomiting after attending a party 12 hours earlier where he drank eggnog and ate foods from a buffet table. Vital signs are: Temp 103°F; HR 108; B/P 118/80; Resp 20. Because Mr. Doyle is a kidney transplant recipient and is on immunosuppressive medications, he is admitted to the hospital; his diagnosis is salmonellosis.

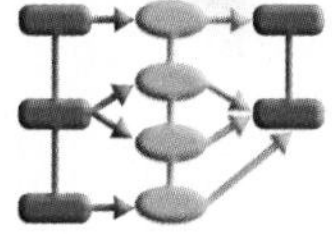

Turn to Appendix C to see a concept map that illustrates the relationships that exist between the nursing diagnoses, interventions, and outcomes for the patient's clinical problems.

Nursing Classifications and Languages

NANDA Nursing Diagnoses	NIC Nursing Interventions	NOC Nursing Outcomes Return to functional baseline status, stabilization of, or improvement in:
Nausea—Unpleasant wavelike sensation in the back of the throat, epigastrium, or abdomen that may lead to the urge or need to vomit	**Nausea Management**—Prevention and alleviation of nausea	**Symptom Severity**—Severity of perceived adverse changes in physical, emotional, and social functioning
Diarrhea—Passage of loose, unformed stools	**Diarrhea Management**—Prevention and alleviation of diarrhea	**Comfort Level**—Extent of physical and psychological ease
Risk for Deficient Fluid Volume—At risk for experiencing vascular, cellular, or intracellular dehydration	**Fluid/Electrolyte Management**—Regulation and prevention of complications from altered fluid and/or electrolyte levels **Vomiting Management**—Prevention and alleviation of vomiting	**Hydration**—Adequate water in the intracellular and extracellular compartments of the body

NANDA International (2005). *Nursing diagnoses: Definitions & classification 2005–2006.* Philadelphia: North American Nursing Diagnosis Association.
Dochterman, J. M., & Bulechek, G. M. (2004). *Nursing Interventions Classification (NIC)* (4th ed.). St. Louis: Mosby.
Iowa Outcomes Project, 2004. In S. Moorhead, M. Johnson, & M. Maas, M. (2004). *Nursing outcomes classification (NOC)* (3rd ed.). St. Louis: Mosby.
Dochterman, J. M., & Jones, D. A. (2003). *Unifying nursing languages: The harmonization of NANDA, NIC, and NOC.* Washington, D.C.: American Nurses Association.

CHAPTER 34

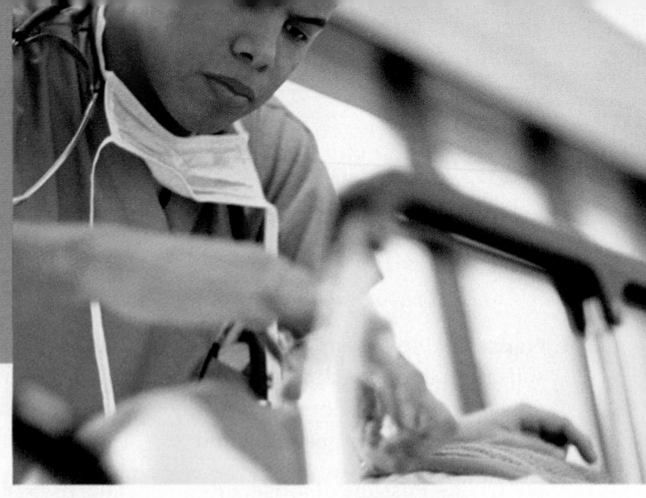

Assessment of Digestive and Gastrointestinal Function

Learning Objectives

On completion of this chapter, the learner will be able to:

1. Describe the structure and function of the organs of the gastrointestinal (GI) tract.
2. Describe the mechanical and chemical processes involved in digesting and absorbing foods and eliminating waste products.
3. Use assessment parameters appropriate for determining the status of GI function.
4. Describe the appropriate preparation, teaching, and follow-up care for patients who are undergoing diagnostic testing of the GI tract.

Anatomic and Physiologic Overview

Anatomy of the Gastrointestinal Tract

The gastrointestinal (GI) tract is a 23- to 26-foot-long pathway that extends from the **mouth** to the esophagus, stomach, small and large intestines, and rectum, to the terminal structure, the anus (Fig. 34-1). The **esophagus** is located in the mediastinum anterior to the spine and posterior to the trachea and heart. This hollow muscular tube, which is approximately 25 cm in length, passes through the diaphragm at an opening called the diaphragmatic hiatus.

The remaining portion of the GI tract is located within the peritoneal cavity. The **stomach** is situated in the left upper portion of the abdomen under the left lobe of the liver and the diaphragm, overlaying most of the pancreas (see Fig. 34-1). A hollow muscular organ with a capacity of approximately 1500 mL, the stomach stores food during eating, secretes digestive fluids, and propels the partially digested food, or chyme, into the small intestine. The gastroesophageal junction is the inlet to the stomach. The stomach has four anatomic regions: the cardia (entrance), fundus, body, and pylorus (outlet). Circular smooth muscle in the wall of the pylorus forms the pyloric sphincter and controls the opening between the stomach and the small intestine.

The **small intestine** is the longest segment of the GI tract, accounting for about two thirds of the total length. It folds back and forth on itself, providing approximately 7000 cm of surface area for secretion and **absorption**, the process by which nutrients enter the bloodstream through the intestinal walls. It has three sections: the most proximal section is the duodenum, the middle section is the jejunum, and the distal section is the ileum. They terminate at the ileocecal valve. This valve, or sphincter, controls the flow of digested material from the ileum into the cecal portion of the large intestine and prevents reflux of bacteria into the small intestine. Attached to the cecum is the vermiform appendix, an appendage that has little or no physiologic function. Emptying into the duodenum at the ampulla of Vater is the common bile duct, which allows for the passage of both bile and pancreatic secretions.

The **large intestine** consists of an ascending segment on the right side of the abdomen, a transverse segment that extends from right to left in the upper abdomen, and a descending segment on the left side of the abdomen. Completing the terminal portion of the large intestine are the sigmoid colon, the rectum, and the anus. Regulating the anal outlet is a network of striated muscle that forms both the internal and the external anal sphincters.

The GI tract receives blood from arteries that originate along the entire length of the thoracic and abdominal aorta and veins that return blood from the digestive organs and the spleen. This portal venous system is composed of five large veins: the superior mesenteric, inferior mesenteric, gastric, splenic, and cystic veins, which eventually form the vena portae that enters the liver. Once in the liver, the blood is distributed throughout and collected into the hepatic veins that then terminate in the inferior vena cava. Of particular importance are the gastric artery and the superior and inferior mesenteric arteries. Oxygen and nutrients are supplied to the stomach by the gastric artery and to the intestine by the

Glossary

absorption: phase of the digestive process that occurs when small molecules, vitamins, and minerals pass through the walls of the small and large intestine and into the bloodstream

amylase: an enzyme that aids in the digestion of starch

anus: last section of the GI tract; outlet for waste products from the system

chyme: mixture of food with saliva, salivary enzymes, and gastric secretions that is produced as the food passes through the mouth, esophagus, and stomach

digestion: phase of the digestive process that occurs when digestive enzymes and secretions mix with ingested food and when proteins, fats, and sugars are broken down into their component smaller molecules

elimination: phase of digestive process that occurs after digestion and absorption, when waste products are evacuated from the body

esophagus: collapsible tube connecting the mouth to the stomach, through which food passes as it is ingested

fibroscopy (gastrointestinal): intubation of a part of the GI system with a flexible, lighted tube to assist in diagnosis and treatment of diseases of that area

hydrochloric acid: acid secreted by the glands in the stomach; mixes with chyme to break it down into absorbable molecules and to aid in the destruction of bacteria

ingestion: phase of the digestive process that occurs when food is taken into the GI tract via the mouth and esophagus

intrinsic factor: a gastric secretion that combines with vitamin B_{12} so that the vitamin can be absorbed

large intestine: the portion of the GI tract into which waste material from the small intestine passes as absorption continues and elimination begins; consists of several parts—ascending segment, transverse segment, descending segment, sigmoid colon, and rectum

lipase: an enzyme that aids in the digestion of fats

mouth: first portion of the GI tract, through which food is ingested

pepsin: a gastric enzyme that is important in protein digestion

small intestine: longest portion of the GI tract, consisting of three parts—duodenum, jejunum, and ileum—through which food mixed with all secretions and enzymes passes as it continues to be digested and begins to be absorbed into the bloodstream

stomach: distensible pouch into which the food bolus passes to be digested by gastric enzymes

trypsin: enzyme that aids in the digestion of protein

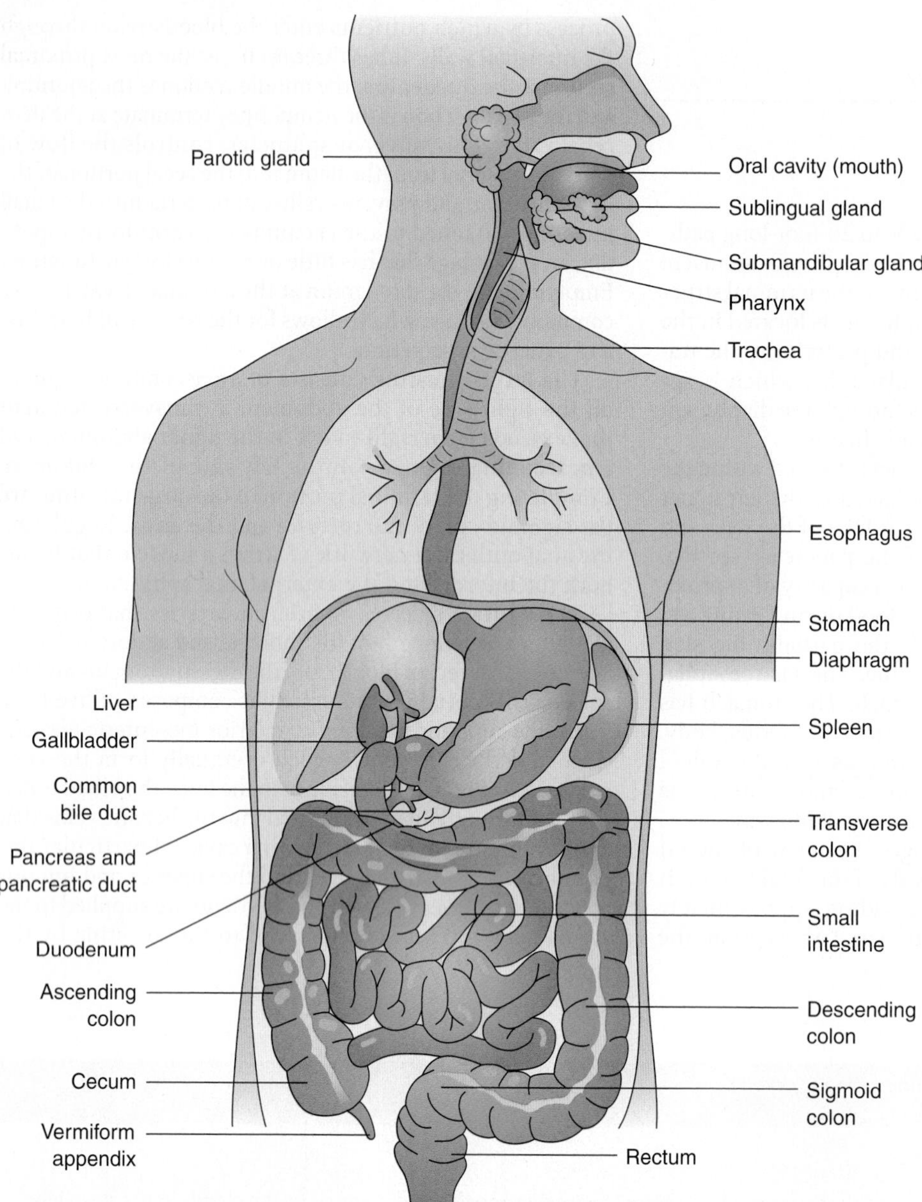

FIGURE 34-1. Organs of the digestive system and associated structures.

mesenteric arteries (Fig. 34-2). Venous blood is returned from the small intestine, cecum, and the ascending and transverse portions of the colon by the superior mesenteric vein, which corresponds with the distribution of the branches of the superior mesenteric artery. Blood flow to the GI tract is about 20% of the total cardiac output and increases significantly after eating.

Both the sympathetic and parasympathetic portions of the autonomic nervous system innervate the GI tract. In general, sympathetic nerves exert an inhibitory effect on the GI tract, decreasing gastric secretion and motility and causing the sphincters and blood vessels to constrict. Parasympathetic nerve stimulation causes peristalsis and increases secretory activities. The sphincters relax under the influence of parasympathetic stimulation except for the sphincter of the upper esophagus and the external anal sphincter, which are under voluntary control.

Functions of the Digestive System

All cells of the body require nutrients. These nutrients are derived from the intake of food that contains proteins, fats, carbohydrates, vitamins, minerals, and cellulose fibers and other vegetable matter, some of which has no nutritional value. Primary functions of the GI tract are the following:

- The breakdown of food particles into the molecular form for **digestion**
- The absorption into the bloodstream of small nutrient molecules produced by digestion
- The **elimination** of undigested unabsorbed foodstuffs and other waste products

After food is ingested, it is propelled through the GI tract, coming into contact with a wide variety of secretions that aid in its digestion, absorption, or elimination from the GI tract.

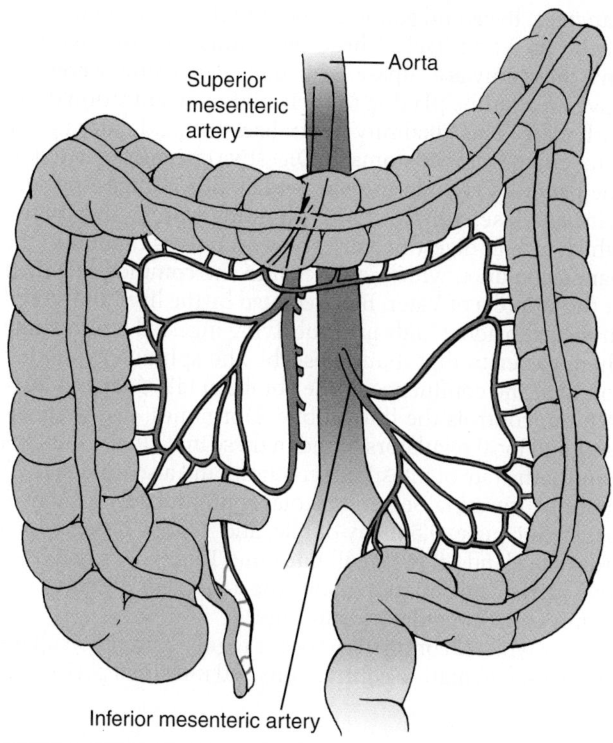

FIGURE 34-2. Anatomy and blood supply of the large intestine.

Chewing and Swallowing

The process of digestion begins with the act of chewing, in which food is broken down into small particles that can be swallowed and mixed with digestive enzymes. Eating—or even the sight, smell, or taste of food—can cause reflex salivation. Approximately 1.5 L of saliva is secreted daily from the parotid, the submaxillary, and the sublingual glands. Ptyalin, or salivary amylase, is an enzyme that begins the digestion of starches. Water and mucus, also contained in saliva, help lubricate the food as it is chewed, thereby facilitating swallowing.

Swallowing begins as a voluntary act that is regulated by the swallowing center in the medulla oblongata of the central nervous system (CNS). As a bolus of food is swallowed, the epiglottis moves to cover the tracheal opening and prevent aspiration of food into the lungs. Swallowing, which propels the bolus of food into the upper esophagus, thus ends as a reflex action. The smooth muscle in the wall of the esophagus contracts in a rhythmic sequence from the upper esophagus toward the stomach to propel the bolus of food along the tract. During this process of esophageal peristalsis, the lower esophageal sphincter relaxes and permits the bolus of food to enter the stomach. Subsequently, the lower esophageal sphincter closes tightly to prevent reflux of stomach contents into the esophagus.

Gastric Function

The stomach, which stores and mixes food with secretions, secretes a highly acidic fluid in response to the presence or anticipated **ingestion** of food. This fluid, which can total 2.4 L/day, can have a pH as low as 1 and derives its acidity from **hydrochloric acid** (HCl) secreted by the glands of the stomach. The function of this gastric secretion is twofold: to break down food into more absorbable components and to aid in the destruction of most ingested bacteria. **Pepsin**, an important enzyme for protein digestion, is the end product of the conversion of pepsinogen from the chief cells (Table 34-1). **Intrinsic factor**, also secreted by the gastric mucosa, combines with dietary vitamin B_{12} so that the

TABLE 34-1 The Major Digestive Enzymes and Secretions

Enzyme/Secretion	Enzyme Source	Digestive Action
Action of Enzymes That Digest Carbohydrates		
Ptyalin (salivary amylase)	Salivary glands	Starch→dextrin, maltose, glucose
Amylase	Pancreas and intestinal mucosa	Starch→dextrin, maltose, glucose Dextrin→maltose, glucose
Maltase	Intestinal mucosa	Maltose→glucose
Sucrase	Intestinal mucosa	Sucrose→glucose, fructose
Lactase	Intestinal mucosa	Lactose→glucose, galactose
Action of Enzymes/Secretions That Digest Protein		
Pepsin	Gastric mucosa	Protein→polypeptides
Trypsin	Pancreas	Proteins and polypeptides→polypeptides, dipeptides, amino acids
Aminopeptidase	Intestinal mucosa	Polypeptides→dipeptides, amino acids
Dipeptidase	Intestinal mucosa	Dipeptides→amino acids
Hydrochloric acid	Gastric mucosa	Protein→polypeptides, amino acids
Action of Enzymes Secretions That Digest Fat (Triglyceride)		
Pharyngeal lipase	Pharynx mucosa	Triglycerides→fatty acids, diglycerides, monoglycerides
Steapsin	Gastric mucosa	Triglycerides→fatty acids, diglycerides, monoglycerides
Pancreatic lipase	Pancreas	Triglycerides→fatty acids, diglycerides, monoglycerides
Bile	Liver and gallbladder	Fat emulsification

vitamin can be absorbed in the ileum. In the absence of intrinsic factor, vitamin B_{12} cannot be absorbed, and pernicious anemia results (see Chapter 33).

Peristaltic contractions in the stomach propel the stomach's contents toward the pylorus. Because large food particles cannot pass through the pyloric sphincter, they are churned back into the body of the stomach. In this way, food in the stomach is agitated mechanically and broken down into smaller particles. Food remains in the stomach for a variable length of time, from 30 minutes to several hours, depending on the volume, osmotic pressure, and chemical composition of the gastric contents. Peristalsis in the stomach and contractions of the pyloric sphincter allow the partially digested food to enter the small intestine at a rate that permits efficient absorption of nutrients. This partially digested food mixed with gastric secretions is called **chyme.** Hormones, neuroregulators, and local regulators found in the gastric secretions control the rate of gastric secretions and influence gastric motility (Table 34-2).

Small Intestine Function

The digestive process continues in the duodenum. Duodenal secretions come from the accessory digestive organs—the pancreas, liver, and gallbladder—and the glands in the wall of the intestine itself. These secretions contain digestive enzymes: amylase, lipase, and bile. Pancreatic secretions have an alkaline pH due to their high concentration of bicarbonate. This alkalinity neutralizes the acid entering the duodenum from the stomach. Digestive enzymes secreted by the pancreas include **trypsin**, which aids in digesting protein; **amylase**, which aids in digesting starch; and **lipase**, which aids in digesting fats. These secretions drain into the pancreatic duct, which empties into the common bile duct at the ampulla of Vater. Bile, secreted by the liver and stored in the gallbladder, aids in emulsifying ingested fats, making them easier to digest and absorb. The sphincter of Oddi, found at the confluence of the common bile duct and duodenum, controls the flow of bile. Hormones, neuroregulators, and local regulators found in these intestinal secretions control the rate of intestinal secretions and also influence GI motility. Intestinal secretions total approximately 1 L/day of pancreatic juice, 0.5 L/day of bile, and 3 L/day of secretions from the glands of the small intestine. Tables 34-1 and 34-2 give further information about the actions of digestive enzymes and GI regulatory substances.

Two types of contractions occur regularly in the small intestine: segmentation contractions and intestinal peristalsis.

TABLE 34-2 The Major Gastrointestinal Regulatory Substances

Substance	Stimulus for Production	Target Tissue	Effect on Secretions	Effect on Motility
Neuroregulators				
Acetylcholine	Sight, smell, chewing food, stomach distention	Gastric glands, other secretory glands, gastric and intestinal muscle	Increased gastric acid	Generally increased; decreased sphincter tone
Norepinephrine	Stress, other various stimuli	Secretory glands, gastric and intestinal muscle	Generally inhibitory	Generally decreased; increased sphincter tone
Hormonal Regulators				
Gastrin	Stomach distention with food	Gastric glands	Increased secretion of gastric juice, which is rich in HCl	Increased motility of stomach, decreased time required for gastric emptying Relaxation of ileocecal sphincter Excitation of colon Constriction of gastroesophageal sphincter
Cholecystokinin	Fat in duodenum	Gallbladder	Release of bile into duodenum	
		Pancreas	Increased production of enzyme-rich pancreatic secretions	
		Stomach	Inhibits gastric secretion somewhat	
Secretin	pH of chyme in duodenum below 4–5	Stomach	Inhibits gastric secretion somewhat	Inhibits stomach contractions
		Pancreas	Increased production of bicarbonate-rich pancreatic juice	
Local Regulator				
Histamine	Unclear; substances in food	Gastric glands	Increased gastric acid production	

Segmentation contractions produce mixing waves that move the intestinal contents back and forth in a churning motion. *Intestinal peristalsis* propels the contents of the small intestine toward the colon. Both movements are stimulated by the presence of chyme.

Food, initially ingested in the form of fats, proteins, and carbohydrates, is broken down into absorbable particles (constituent nutrients) by the process of digestion. Carbohydrates are broken down into disaccharides (eg, sucrose, maltose, and galactose) and monosaccharides (eg, glucose, fructose). Glucose is the major carbohydrate that tissue cells use as fuel. Proteins are a source of energy after they are broken down into amino acids and peptides. Ingested fats become monoglycerides and fatty acid by the process of emulsification, which makes them smaller and therefore easier to absorb. Chyme stays in the small intestine for 3 to 6 hours, allowing for continued breakdown and absorption of nutrients.

Small, finger-like projections called villi are present throughout the entire intestine and function to produce digestive enzymes as well as to absorb nutrients. Absorption is the primary function of the small intestine. Vitamins and minerals are not digested but rather absorbed essentially unchanged. The process of absorption begins in the jejunum and is accomplished by both active transport and diffusion across the intestinal wall into the circulation. Nutrients are absorbed at specific locations throughout the small intestine and duodenum, whereas fats, proteins, carbohydrates, sodium, and chloride are absorbed in the jejunum. Vitamin B_{12} and bile salts are absorbed in the ileum. Magnesium, phosphate, and potassium are absorbed throughout the small intestine.

Colonic Function

Within 4 hours after eating, residual waste material passes into the terminal ileum and slowly into the proximal portion of the right colon through the ileocecal valve. With each peristaltic wave of the small intestine, the valve opens briefly and permits some of the contents to pass into the colon.

Bacteria, which make up a major component of the contents of the large intestine, assist in completing the breakdown of waste material, especially of undigested or unabsorbed proteins and bile salts. Two types of colonic secretions are added to the residual material: an electrolyte solution and mucus. The electrolyte solution is chiefly a bicarbonate solution that acts to neutralize the end products formed by the colonic bacterial action, whereas the mucus protects the colonic mucosa from the interluminal contents and provides adherence for the fecal mass.

Slow, weak peristaltic activity moves the colonic contents along the tract. This slow transport allows for efficient reabsorption of water and electrolytes, which is the primary purpose of the colon. Intermittent strong peristaltic waves propel the contents for considerable distances. This generally occurs after another meal is eaten, when intestine-stimulating hormones are released. The waste materials from a meal eventually reach and distend the rectum, usually in about 12 hours. As much as one fourth of the waste materials from a meal may still be in the rectum 3 days after the meal was ingested.

Waste Products of Digestion

Feces consist of undigested foodstuffs, inorganic materials, water, and bacteria. Fecal matter is about 75% fluid and 25% solid material. The composition is relatively unaffected by alterations in diet because a large portion of the fecal mass is of nondietary origin, derived from the secretions of the GI tract. The brown color of the feces results from the breakdown of bile by the intestinal bacteria. Chemicals formed by intestinal bacteria are responsible in large part for the fecal odor. Gases formed contain methane, hydrogen sulfide, and ammonia, among others. The GI tract normally contains approximately 150 mL of these gases, which are either absorbed into the portal circulation and detoxified by the liver or expelled from the rectum as flatus.

Elimination of stool begins with distention of the rectum, which reflexively initiates contractions of the rectal musculature and relaxes the normally closed internal anal sphincter. The internal sphincter is controlled by the autonomic nervous system; the external sphincter is under the conscious control of the cerebral cortex. During defecation, the external anal sphincter voluntarily relaxes to allow colonic contents to be expelled. Normally, the external anal sphincter is maintained in a state of tonic contraction. Thus, defecation is seen to be a spinal reflex (involving the parasympathetic nerve fibers) that can be inhibited voluntarily by keeping the external anal sphincter closed. Contracting the abdominal muscles (straining) facilitates emptying of the colon. The average frequency of defecation in humans is once daily, but this varies among people.

Gerontologic Considerations

Although an increased prevalence of several common GI disorders occurs in the elderly population, aging per se appears to have minimal direct effect on most GI functions, in large part because of the functional reserve of the GI tract. Normal physiologic changes of the GI system that occur with aging are identified in Chart 34-1. Careful assessment and monitoring of signs and symptoms related to these changes are imperative.

Age-related changes in the mouth include loss of teeth, diminished number of taste buds, decreased production of saliva, and atrophy of gingival tissue. These changes cause difficulty in chewing and swallowing. Changes in the esophagus include decreased muscle tone and weakness in the lower esophageal sphincter, leading to reflux and heartburn.

Although irritable bowel symptoms decrease with aging, there seems to be an increase in many GI disorders of function and motility. The gastroenterologist frequently encounters elderly patients who have complaints of dysphagia, anorexia, dyspepsia, and disorders of colonic function (Prather, 2002). Decreased gastric motility leads to delayed gastric emptying. Atrophy of the mucosa causes a decrease in HCl production, and this can lead to food intolerances, malabsorption, or decrease in vitamin B_{12} absorption. Changes in the small and large intestine are evidenced largely by decreased motility and decreased transit time, which lead to complaints of indigestion and constipation. Other changes lead to decreased absorption of nutrients (dextrose, fats, calcium, and iron) in the large intestine. Fecal incontinence can result from decrease or loss of sphincter control.

CHART 34-1

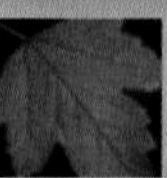

Gerontologic Considerations

Age-Related Changes of the Gastrointestinal System

Oral Cavity and Pharynx
- Injury/loss or decay of teeth
- Atrophy of taste buds
- Decreased saliva production
- Reduced ptyalin and amylase in saliva

Esophagus
- Decreased motility and emptying
- Weakened gag reflex
- Decreased resting pressure of lower esophageal sphincter

Stomach
- Degeneration and atrophy of gastric mucosal surfaces with decreased production of HCl
- Decreased secretion of gastric acids and most digestive enzymes
- Decreased motility and emptying

Small Intestine
- Atrophy of muscle and mucosal surfaces
- Thinning of villi and epithelial cells

Large Intestine
- Decrease in mucus secretion
- Decrease in elasticity of rectal wall
- Decreased tone of internal anal sphincter
- Slower and duller nerve impulses in rectal area

Assessment

Health History and Clinical Manifestations

A focused GI assessment begins with a complete history. Information about abdominal pain, dyspepsia, gas, nausea and vomiting, diarrhea, constipation, fecal incontinence, jaundice, and previous GI disease is investigated. Past and current medication use and any previous diagnostic studies, treatments, or surgery are noted. Current nutritional status is ascertained via history, and serum values (complete metabolic panel including liver function studies, triglyceride, iron studies, and complete blood count [CBC]) are obtained. Questioning about the use of tobacco and alcohol includes details about type, amount, length of use, and the date of discontinuation, if any. The nurse and patient discuss changes in appetite or eating patterns and any unexplained weight gain or loss over the past year. It is also important to include questions about psychosocial, spiritual, or cultural factors that may be affecting the patient.

Pain

Pain can be a major symptom of GI disease. The character, duration, pattern, frequency, location, distribution of referred pain (Fig. 34-3), and time of the pain vary greatly depending on the underlying cause. Other factors such as meals, rest, activity, and defecation patterns may directly affect this pain.

Dyspepsia

Dyspepsia, upper abdominal discomfort, or distress associated with eating (commonly called *indigestion*) is the most common symptom of patients with GI dysfunction.

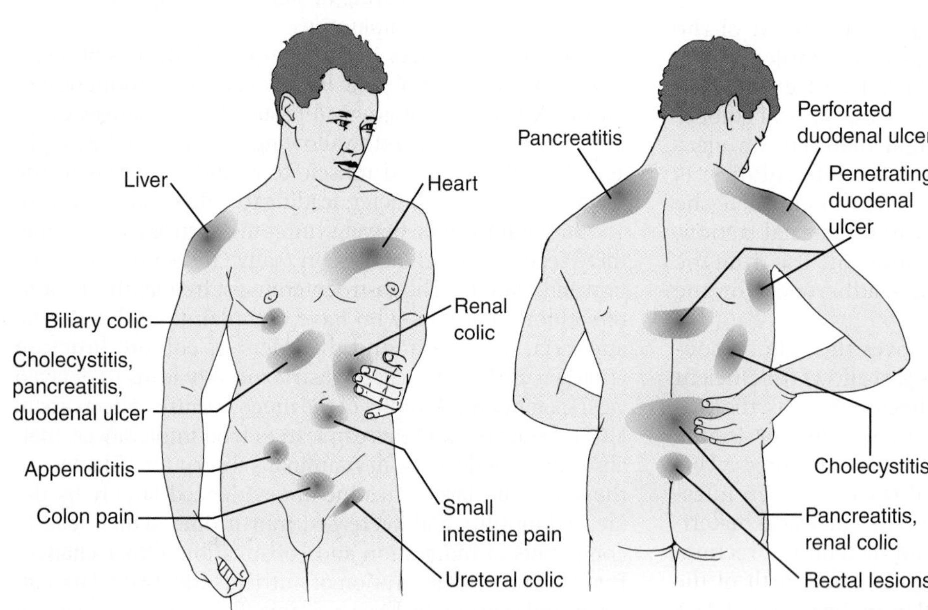

FIGURE 34-3. Common sites of referred abdominal pain.

Indigestion is an imprecise term that refers to a host of upper abdominal or epigastric symptoms such as pain, discomfort, fullness, bloating, early satiety, belching, heartburn, or regurgitation; it occurs in approximately 25% of the adult population. Typically, fatty foods cause the most discomfort because they remain in the stomach for digestion longer than proteins or carbohydrates. Salads and coarse vegetables as well as highly seasoned foods may also cause considerable GI distress.

Intestinal Gas

The accumulation of gas in the GI tract may result in belching (expulsion of gas from the stomach through the mouth) or flatulence (expulsion of gas from the rectum). Usually, gases in the small intestine pass into the colon and are released as flatus. Patients often complain of bloating, distention, or feeling "full of gas" with excessive flatulence as a symptom of food intolerance or gallbladder disease.

Nausea and Vomiting

Nausea is a vague, intensely unsettling sensation of sickness or "queasiness" that may or may not be followed by vomiting. It can be triggered by odors, activity, medications, or food intake. The emesis, or vomitus, may vary in color and content and may contain undigested food particles, blood (hematemesis), or bilious material mixed with gastric juices. The causes of nausea and vomiting are many; they may result from (1) visceral afferent stimulation (ie, dysmotility, peritoneal irritation, infections, hepatobiliary or pancreatic disorders, mechanical obstruction); (2) CNS disorders (ie, vestibular disorders, increased intracranial pressure, infections, psychogenic); and/or (3) irritation of the chemoreceptor trigger zone from radiation therapy, systemic disorders, and antitumor chemotherapy medications.

Change in Bowel Habits and Stool Characteristics

Changes in bowel habits may signal colonic dysfunction or disease. Diarrhea, an abnormal increase in the frequency and liquidity of the stool or in daily stool weight or volume, commonly occurs when the contents move so rapidly through the intestine and colon that there is inadequate time for the GI secretions and oral contents to be absorbed. This physiologic function is typically associated with abdominal pain or cramping and nausea or vomiting. Constipation, a decrease in the frequency of stool, or stools that are hard, dry, and of smaller volume than normal, may be associated with anal discomfort and rectal bleeding. See Chapter 38 for further discussion of diarrhea and constipation.

The characteristics of the stool can vary greatly. Stool is normally light to dark brown; however, specific disease processes and ingestion of certain foods and medications may change the appearance of stool (Table 34-3). Blood in the stool can present in various ways and must be investigated. If blood is shed in sufficient quantities into the upper GI tract, it produces a tarry-black color (melena), whereas blood entering the lower portion of the GI tract or passing rapidly through it will appear bright or dark red. Lower rectal or anal bleeding is suspected if there is streaking of blood on the surface of the stool or if blood is noted on toilet tissue. Other common abnormalities in stool characteristics described by the patient may include:

- Bulky, greasy, foamy stools that are foul in odor and may or may not float
- Light-gray or clay-colored stool, caused by a decrease or absence of conjugated bilirubin
- Stool with mucus threads or pus that may be visible on gross inspection of the stool
- Small, dry, rock-hard masses occasionally streaked with blood
- Loose, watery stool that may or may not be streaked with blood

TABLE 34-3 Foods and Medications That Alter Stool Color

Altering Substance	Color
Meat protein	Dark brown
Spinach	Green
Carrots and beets	Red
Cocoa	Dark red or brown
Senna	Yellow
Bismuth, iron, licorice, and charcoal	Black
Barium	Milky white

Physical Assessment

The physical examination includes assessment of the mouth, abdomen, and rectum and requires a good source of light, full exposure of the abdomen, warm hands with short fingernails, and a comfortable, relaxed patient with an empty bladder. The mouth, tongue, buccal mucosa, teeth, and gums are inspected, noting any ulcers, nodules, swelling, discoloration, or inflammation. Dentures should be removed to allow good visualization of the entire oral cavity.

The patient lies supine with knees flexed slightly for inspection, auscultation, palpation, and percussion of the abdomen (Fig. 34-4). For the purposes of examination and documentation, the abdomen can be divided into either four quadrants or nine regions (Fig. 34-5). Choosing one of these mapping methods and using it consistently results in a thorough evaluation of the abdomen and appropriate corresponding documentation. The four-quadrant method involves the use of an imaginary line drawn vertically from the sternum to the pubis through the umbilicus and a second line drawn perpendicular to the first horizontally across the abdomen through the umbilicus. Inspection is performed first, noting skin changes, nodules, lesions, scarring, discolorations, inflammation, bruising, or striae. Lesions are of particular importance, because GI diseases often produce skin changes. The contour and symmetry of the abdomen are noted and any localized bulging, distention, or peristaltic waves are identified. Expected contours of the anterior abdominal wall can be described as flat, rounded, or scaphoid.

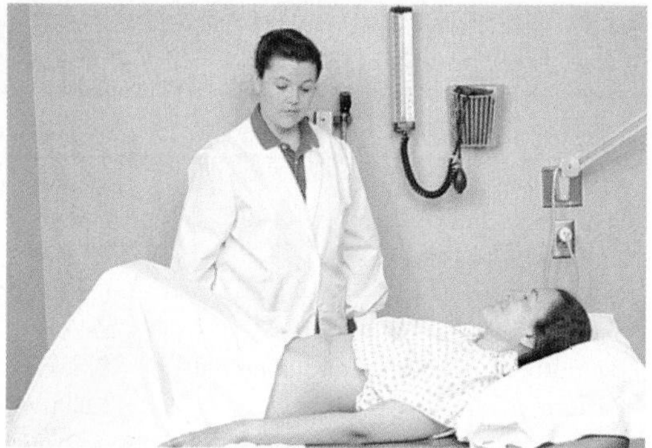

Inspecting the abdomen

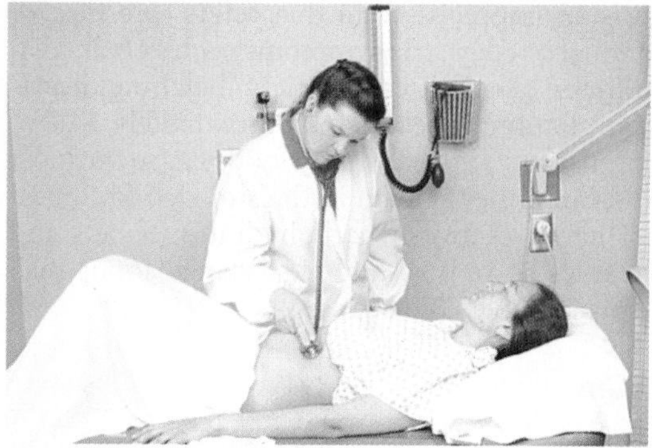

Auscultating the abdomen

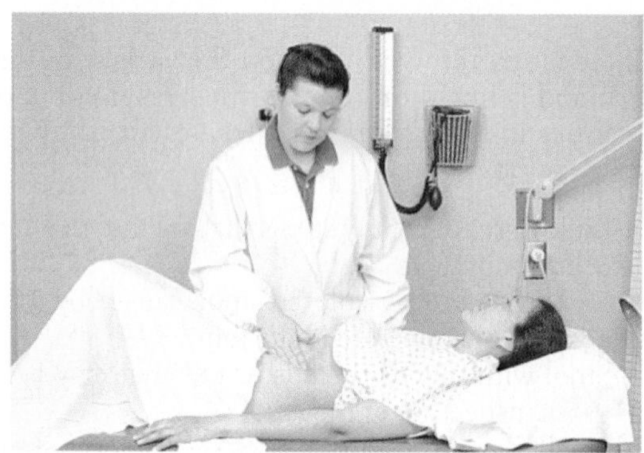

Palpating the abdomen

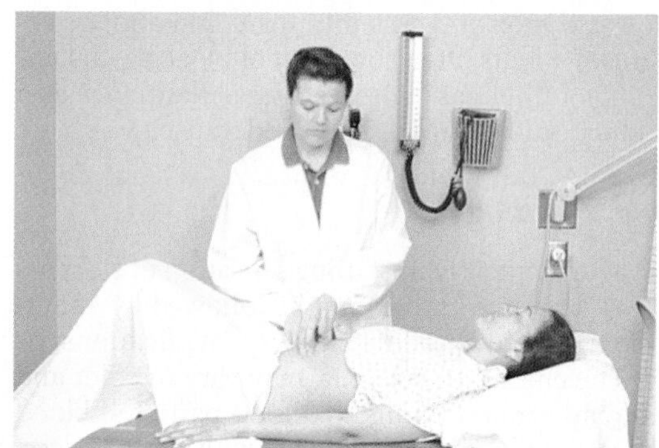

Percussing the abdomen

FIGURE 34-4. Examination of the abdomen includes inspection, auscultation, palpation, and percussion.

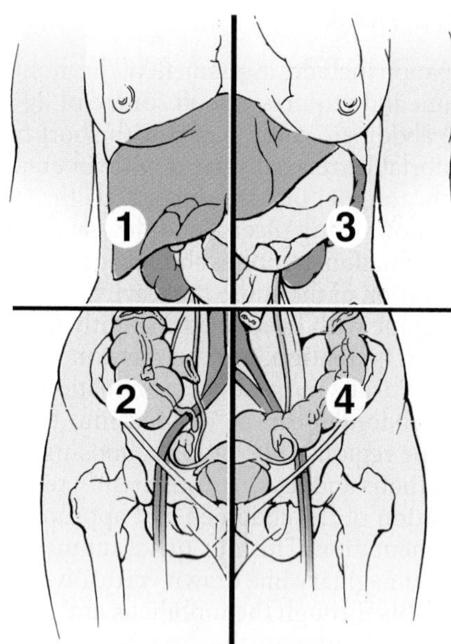

A. Four quadrants

1 - right upper quadrant (RUQ)
2 - right lower quadrant (RLQ)
3 - left upper quadrant (LUQ)
4 - left lower quadrant (LLQ)

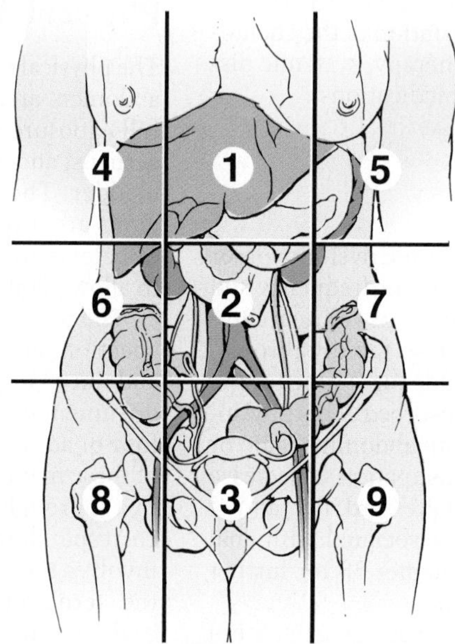

B. Nine regions

1 - epigastric region
2 - umbilical region
3 - hypogastric or suprapubic region
4 - right hypochondriac region
5 - left hypochondriac region
6 - right lumbar region
7 - left lumbar region
8 - right inguinal region
9 - left inguinal region

FIGURE 34-5. Division of the abdomen into (**A**) four quadrants or (**B**) nine regions.

Auscultation, which always precedes percussion and palpitation, is used to determine the character, location, and frequency of bowel sounds and to identify vascular sounds. Bowel sounds are assessed in all four quadrants using the diaphragm of the stethoscope, which affords greatest auscultation of high-pitched and gurgling sounds. The frequency and character of the sounds are usually heard as clicks and gurgles that occur irregularly and range from 5 to 35 per minute. The terms *normal* (sounds heard about every 5 to 20 seconds), *hypoactive* (one or two sounds in 2 minutes), *hyperactive* (5 to 6 sounds heard in less than 30 seconds), or *absent* (no sounds in 3 to 5 minutes) are frequently used in documentation, but these assessments are highly subjective. Using the bell of the stethoscope, any bruits in the aortic, renal, iliac, and femoral arteries are noted. Friction rubs are high-pitched and can be heard over the liver and spleen during respiration. Borborygmi or "stomach growling" is heard as a loud prolonged gurgle.

Percussion is used to assess the size and density of the abdominal organs and to detect the presence of air-filled, fluid-filled, or solid masses. Percussion is used either independently or concurrently with palpation because it can validate palpation findings. Use of light palpation is appropriate for identifying areas of tenderness or muscular resistance, and deep palpation is used to identify masses. All quadrants are percussed for a sense of overall tympani and dullness. Tympani is the predominant sound that results from the presence of air in the stomach and small intestines; dullness is heard over organs and solid masses. Testing for rebound tenderness is not performed by many examiners because it can cause severe pain; light percussion is used instead to produce a mild localized response when peritoneal irritation is present.

The final part of the examination is evaluation of the terminal portions of the GI tract, the rectum, perianal region, and anus. The anal canal is approximately 2.5 to 4 cm in length and opens into the perineum. Concentric rings of muscle, the internal and external sphincters, normally keep the anal canal securely closed. Gloves, water-soluble lubrication, a penlight, and drapes are necessary tools for the evaluation. Although the rectal examination is generally uncomfortable and often embarrassing for the patient, it is a mandatory part of every thorough examination. For women, the rectal examination may be part of the gynecologic examination. Positions for the rectal examination include knee-chest, left lateral with hips and knees flexed, or standing with hips flexed and upper body supported by the examination table. Most patients are comfortable on the right side with knees brought up to the chest. External examination includes inspection for lumps, rashes, inflammation, excoriation, tears, scars, pilonidal dimpling, and tufts of hair at the pilonidal area. The discovery of tenderness, inflammation, or both should alert the examiner to the possibility of a pilonidal cyst, perianal abscess, or anorectal fistula or fissure. The patient's buttocks are carefully spread and visually inspected until the patient has relaxed the external sphincter control. The patient is asked to bear down, thus allowing the ready appearance of fistulas, fissures, rectal prolapse, polyps, and internal hemorrhoids. Internal examination is performed with a lubricated index finger inserted into the anal canal while the patient bears down. The tone of the sphincter is noted, as are any nodules or irregularities of the anal ring. Because this is an uncomfortable part of the examination for most patients, the patient is encouraged to focus on deep breathing and visualization of a pleasant setting during the brief examination.

Diagnostic Evaluation

Initial diagnostic tests begin with serum laboratory studies, including but not limited to CBC, complete metabolic panel, prothrombin time/partial thromboplastin time, triglycerides, liver function tests, amylase, and lipase, with the possibility of more specific studies such as carcinoembryonic antigen (CEA), cancer antigen (CA) 19-9, and alpha-fetoprotein, indicating sensitivity and specificity for colorectal and hepatocellular carcinomas, respectively. CEA is a protein that is normally not detected in the blood of a healthy person; therefore, when detected it indicates that cancer is present, but not what type of cancer is present. Practitioners can use CEA results to determine the stage and extent of the disease and the prognosis for patients with cancer, especially GI and in particular colorectal cancer (Porth, 2005). CA 19-9 is also a protein that exists on the surface of certain cells and is shed by tumor cells, making it useful as a tumor marker to follow the course of the cancer. CA 19-9 levels are elevated in most patients with advanced pancreatic cancer, but it may also be elevated in other conditions such as colorectal, lung, and gallbladder cancers, gallstones, pancreatitis, cystic fibrosis, and liver disease.

Many other modalities are available for diagnostic assessment of the GI tract. The majority of these tests and procedures are performed on an outpatient basis in special settings designed for this purpose (eg, endoscopy suite or GI laboratory). In the past, patients who required such tests frequently were elderly; however, within the past 5 years, in part due to heightened media exposure and early diagnosis of colorectal cancer, the median age of patients evaluated for colorectal cancer has decreased significantly. Preparation for many of these studies includes clear liquid diets, fasting, ingestion of a liquid bowel preparation, the use of laxatives or enemas, and ingestion or injection of a contrast agent or a radiopaque dye. These measures are poorly tolerated by some patients and are especially problematic in the elderly population or patients with comorbidities because bowel preparations significantly alter the internal fluid and electrolyte balance. If further assessment or treatment is needed after any outpatient procedure, the patient may be admitted to the hospital.

Specific nursing interventions for each test are provided later in this chapter. General nursing interventions for the patient who is undergoing a GI diagnostic evaluation include:

- Establishing the nursing diagnosis
- Providing needed information about the test and the activities required of the patient
- Providing instructions about postprocedure care and activity restrictions
- Providing health information and procedural teaching to patients and significant others
- Helping the patient cope with discomfort and alleviating anxiety

- Informing the physician or nurse practitioner of known medical conditions or abnormal laboratory values that may affect the procedure
- Assessing for adequate hydration before, during, and immediately after the procedure, and providing education about maintenance of hydration

Stool Tests

Basic examination of the stool includes inspecting the specimen for consistency, color, and occult (not visible) blood. Additional studies, including fecal urobilinogen, fecal fat, nitrogen, *Clostridium difficile,* fecal leukocytes, calculation of stool osmolar gap, parasites, pathogens, food residues, and other substances, require laboratory evaluation.

Stool samples are usually collected on a random basis unless a quantitative study (eg, fecal fat, urobilinogen) is to be performed. Random specimens should be sent promptly to the laboratory for analysis; however, the quantitative 24- to 72-hour collections must be kept refrigerated until transported to the laboratory. Some stool collections require the patient to follow a specific diet or refrain from taking certain medications before the collection. Thorough and accurate patient education regarding a specific stool study prior to collection greatly increases the accuracy of study results.

Fecal occult blood testing (FOBT) is one of the most commonly performed stool tests. It can be useful in initial screening for several disorders, although it is used most frequently in early cancer detection programs. FOBT can be performed at the bedside, in the laboratory, or at home.

Probably the most widely used in-office or at-home occult blood test is the Hemoccult II. It is inexpensive, noninvasive, and carries minimal risk to the patient. However, it should not be performed when there is hemorrhoidal bleeding. In addition, red meats, aspirin, nonsteroidal anti-inflammatory drugs, turnips, and horseradish should be avoided for 72 hours prior to the study, because they may cause a false-positive result. Also, ingestion of vitamin C from supplements or foods can cause a false-negative result. Therefore, a careful assessment of the patient's diet and medication regimen is essential to avoid incorrect interpretation of results. A small amount of the specimen is applied to the guaiac-impregnated paper slide. If the test is performed at home, the patient mails the slide to the physician in an envelope provided for that purpose. Other occult blood tests that may yield more specific and more sensitive readings include Hematest II SENSA and HemoQuant.

Immunologic tests are more specific to human hemoglobin and decrease the problem of dietary interference. Hemoporphyrin assays detect the broadest range of blood derivatives, but a strict dietary protocol is essential. Immunochemical tests that use antihuman antibodies extremely sensitive to human hemoglobin are also available.

Breath Tests

The hydrogen breath test was developed to evaluate carbohydrate absorption, in addition to aiding in the diagnosis of bacterial overgrowth in the intestine and short bowel syndrome. This test determines the amount of hydrogen expelled in the breath after it has been produced in the colon (on contact of galactose with fermenting bacteria) and absorbed into the blood.

Urea breath tests detect the presence of *Helicobacter pylori,* the bacteria that can live in the mucosal lining of the stomach and cause peptic ulcer disease. After the patient ingests a capsule of carbon-labeled urea, a breath sample is obtained 10 to 20 minutes later. Because *H. pylori* metabolizes urea rapidly, the labeled carbon is absorbed quickly; it can then be measured as carbon dioxide in the expired breath to determine whether *H. pylori* is present. The patient is instructed to avoid antibiotics or loperamide (Pepto Bismol) for 1 month before the test; sucralfate (Carafate) and omeprazole (Prilosec) for 1 week before the test; and cimetidine (Tagamet), famotidine (Pepcid), and ranitidine (Zantac) for 24 hours before urea breath testing. *H. pylori* also can be detected by assessing serum antibody levels.

Abdominal Ultrasonography

Ultrasonography is a noninvasive diagnostic technique in which high-frequency sound waves are passed into internal body structures and the ultrasonic echoes are recorded on an oscilloscope as they strike tissues of different densities. It is particularly useful in the detection of an enlarged gallbladder or pancreas, the presence of gallstones, an enlarged ovary, an ectopic pregnancy, or appendicitis. Most recently this technique has proven useful in diagnosing acute colonic diverticulitis.

Advantages of abdominal ultrasonography include an absence of ionizing radiation, no noticeable side effects, relatively low cost, and almost immediate results. A disadvantage is that it cannot be used to examine structures that lie behind bony tissue because bone prevents sound waves from traveling into deeper structures. Gas and fluid in the abdomen or air in the lungs also prevent transmission of ultrasound. An ultrasound has no dangers; there have been no substantiated ill effects of ultrasound documented in studies in either humans or animals. However, some patients, typically pregnant women, have concerns regarding the energy emitted by the probe.

Endoscopic ultrasonography (EUS) is a specialized enteroscopic procedure that aids in the diagnosis of GI disorders by providing direct imaging of a target area. A small high-frequency ultrasonic transducer is mounted at the tip of the fiberoptic scope, which displays an image that enables tumor staging and visualization of marginal structures. This procedure delivers results with higher-quality resolution and definition in comparison with regular ultrasound imaging. EUS may be used for evaluating submucosal lesions, specifically determining their location and depth of penetration. In addition, EUS may aid in the evaluation of Barrett's esophagus, portal hypertension, chronic pancreatitis, suspected pancreatic neoplasm, biliary tract disease, and changes in the bowel wall that occur in ulcerative colitis. Intestinal gas, bone, and thick layers of adipose tissue (all of which hamper conventional ultrasonography) are not problems when EUS is used.

Nursing Interventions

The patient is instructed to fast for 8 to 12 hours before the test to decrease the amount of gas in the bowel. If gallbladder studies are being performed, the patient should eat a fat-free meal the evening before the test. If barium studies are to be performed, they should be scheduled after ultrasonography; otherwise, the barium could interfere with the transmission of the sound waves.

DNA Testing

Researchers have refined methods for genetics risk assessment, preclinical diagnosis, and prenatal diagnosis to identify people who are at risk for certain GI disorders (eg, gastric cancer, lactose deficiency, inflammatory bowel disease, colon cancer). In some cases, DNA testing allows physicians to prevent (or minimize) disease, by intervening before its onset, and to improve therapy; however, it is imperative to educate all genetics counselors routinely, given the exponential growth of genetics information (Beery & Hern, 2004). People who are identified as at risk of certain GI disorders may choose to undergo genetic counseling to learn about the disease, to understand options for preventing and treating the disease, and to receive support in coping with the situation. There are ethical and legal issues involved in genetic testing, and there are legal protections for patients against discrimination (Lowrey, 2004). For instance, false-positive results can create unnecessary worry, alarm, and further testing, typically at the expense of the patient and the family, with potential effects on health-related quality of life (McGovern, Gross, Krueger, et al., 2004). The nurse considers the questions, "How will the results—whether positive or negative—affect the patient? Do I have the resources to help the patient with the outcome?" Family members may receive genetic test results in different ways depending on the following: (1) how people at risk understand and communicate test results, (2) the dynamics of family relationships and communication, (3) familial obligations, and (4) the biologic meaning of family (Hamilton, Bowers, & Williams, 2004). The effects on the person doing the disclosing, the family members receiving the information, and most importantly the perceptions of the person tested are important factors in the testing and counseling process.

GENETICS IN NURSING PRACTICE

Digestive and Gastrointestinal Disorders

Several digestive and gastrointestinal disorders are associated with genetic abnormalities. Some examples are:

- Cleft lip and/or palate
- Familial adenomatous polyposis
- Hereditary nonpolyposis colorectal cancer (HNPCC)
- Hirschsprung disease (aganglionic megacolon)
- Inflammatory bowel disease (eg, Crohn's disease)
- Pyloric stenosis

NURSING ASSESSMENTS

Family History Assessment

- Careful family history assessment for other family members with a similar condition (eg, cleft lip/palate, pyloric stenosis)
- Assess for other family members in several generations with early-onset colorectal cancer
- Inquire about other family members with inflammatory bowel disease
- Assess family history for other cancers (eg, endometrial, ovarian, renal)

Patient Assessment

Assess for presence of other clinical symptoms:

- With clefting—congenital heart defect, mental retardation, other birth defects suggestive of a genetic syndrome
- With familial adenomatous polyposis—congenital hypertrophy of retinal pigment epithelium (CHRPE)

MANAGEMENT ISSUES SPECIFIC TO GENETICS

- Inquire whether any affected family member has had DNA mutation testing
- If indicated, refer for further genetic counseling and evaluation so that family members can discuss inheritance, risk to other family members, availability of genetics testing, and gene-based interventions
- Offer appropriate genetics information and resources
- Assess patients' understanding of genetics information
- Provide support to families with newly diagnosed genetic digestive disorders
- Participate in management and coordination of care for patients with genetic conditions and for those who are predisposed to develop or pass on a genetic condition

GENETICS RESOURCES

American Cancer Society—offers general information about cancer and support resources for families, http:/www.cancer.org

Gene Clinics—a listing of common genetic disorders with up-to-date clinical summaries and genetics counseling and testing information, http://www.geneclinics.org

Genetic Alliance—a directory of support groups for patients and families with genetic conditions, http://www.geneticalliance.org

National Cancer Institute—current information about cancer research, treatment, resources for health providers, individuals, and families, http://www.nci.nih.gov

National Organization of Rare Disorders—a directory of support groups and information for patients and families with rare genetic disorders, http://www.rarediseases.org

Online Mendelian Inheritance in Man (OMIM)—a complete listing of inherited genetic conditions, http://www.ncbi.nlm.nih.gov/omim/stats/html

Imaging Studies

Numerous minimally invasive and noninvasive imaging studies, including x-ray and contrast studies, computed tomography (CT), three-dimensional CT, magnetic resonance imaging (MRI), positron emission tomography (PET), and scintigraphy (radionuclide imaging), are available today. Advances in technology are made daily.

Upper Gastrointestinal Tract Study

An upper GI study delineates the entire GI tract after the introduction of a contrast agent. A radiopaque liquid (eg, barium sulfate) is commonly used; however, thin barium, Hypaque, and at times water are used due to their low associated risks. The GI series enables the examiner to detect or exclude anatomic or functional derangement of the upper GI organs or sphincters. It also aids in the diagnosis of ulcers, varices, tumors, regional enteritis, and malabsorption syndromes. The procedure may be extended to examine the duodenum and small bowel (small bowel follow-through). As the barium descends into the stomach, the position, patency, and caliber of the esophagus are visualized, enabling the examiner to detect or exclude any anatomic or functional derangement of that organ. Fluoroscopic examination next extends to the stomach as its lumen fills with barium, allowing observation of stomach motility, thickness of the gastric wall, the mucosal pattern, patency of the pyloric valve, and the anatomy of the duodenum. Multiple x-ray films are obtained during the procedure, and additional images may be taken at intervals for up to 24 hours to evaluate the rate of gastric emptying. Small bowel x-rays taken while the barium is passing through that area allow for observation of the motility of the small bowel. Obstructions, ileitis, and diverticula can be detected if present.

Variations of the upper GI study include double-contrast studies and enteroclysis. The double-contrast method of examining the upper GI tract involves administration of a thick barium suspension to outline the stomach and esophageal wall, after which tablets that release carbon dioxide in the presence of water are administered. This technique has the advantage of showing the esophagus and stomach in finer detail, permitting signs of early superficial neoplasms to be noted.

Enteroclysis is a very detailed, double-contrast study of the entire small intestine that involves the continuous infusion, through a duodenal tube, of 500 to 1000 mL of a thin barium sulfate suspension; after this, methylcellulose is infused through the tube. The barium and methylcellulose fill the intestinal loops and are observed continuously by fluoroscopy and viewed at frequent intervals as they progress through the jejunum and the ileum. This process (even with normal motility) can take up to 6 hours and can be quite uncomfortable for the patient. The procedure aids in the diagnosis of partial small-bowel obstructions or diverticula.

NURSING INTERVENTIONS

Education regarding dietary changes prior to the study should include a clear liquid diet, with nothing by mouth (NPO) from midnight the night before the study; however, each physician may prefer a specific bowel preparation for specific studies. When a patient with insulin-dependent diabetes is NPO, his or her insulin requirements will need to be adjusted accordingly. Smoking, chewing gum, and using mints can stimulate gastric motility, so the nurse advises against these practices. Typically, oral medications are withheld on the morning of the study and resumed that evening, but each patient's medication regimen should be evaluated on an individual basis.

Follow-up care is provided after the upper GI procedure to ensure that the patient has eliminated most of the ingested barium. Fluids may be increased to facilitate evacuation of stool and barium.

Lower Gastrointestinal Tract Study

Visualization of the lower GI tract is obtained after rectal installation of barium. The barium enema can be used to detect the presence of polyps, tumors, or other lesions of the large intestine and demonstrate any anatomic abnormalities or malfunctioning of the bowel. After proper preparation and evacuation of the entire colon, each portion of the colon may be readily observed. The procedure usually takes about 15 to 30 minutes, during which time x-ray images are obtained.

Other means for visualizing the colon include double-contrast studies and a water-soluble contrast study. A double-contrast or air-contrast barium enema involves the instillation of a thicker barium solution, followed by the instillation of air. The patient may feel some cramping or discomfort during this process. This test provides a contrast between the air-filled lumen and the barium-coated mucosa, allowing easier detection of smaller lesions.

If active inflammatory disease, fistulas, or perforation of the colon is suspected, a water-soluble iodinated contrast agent (eg, Gastrografin) can be used. The procedure is the same as for a barium enema, but the patient must be assessed for allergy to iodine or contrast agent. The contrast agent is eliminated readily after the procedure, so there is no need for postprocedure laxatives. Some diarrhea may occur in a few patients until the contrast agent has been totally eliminated.

NURSING INTERVENTIONS

Preparation of the patient includes emptying and cleansing the lower bowel. This often necessitates a low-residue diet 1 to 2 days before the test (the preparation required by different radiology departments may vary); a clear liquid diet and a laxative the evening before; NPO after midnight; and cleansing enemas until returns are clear the following morning. The nurse makes sure that barium enemas are scheduled before any upper GI studies. If the patient has active inflammatory disease of the colon, enemas are contraindicated. Barium enemas also are contraindicated in patients with signs of perforation or obstruction; instead, a water-soluble contrast study may be performed. Active GI bleeding may prohibit the use of laxatives and enemas.

Postprocedural patient education includes information about increasing fluid intake; evaluating bowel movements for evacuation of barium; and noting increased number of bowel movements, because barium, due to its high osmolarity, may draw fluid into the bowel, thus increasing the intraluminal contents and resulting in greater output.

Computed Tomography

CT provides cross-sectional images of abdominal organs and structures. Multiple x-ray images are taken from numerous angles, digitized in a computer, reconstructed, and then viewed on a computer monitor. As the sensitivity and specificity of CT have increased tremendously in the past 5 years, so has the frequency with which the study is performed. CT is a valuable tool for detecting and localizing many inflammatory conditions in the colon, such as appendicitis, diverticulitis, regional enteritis, and ulcerative colitis, as well as evaluating the abdomen for diseases of the liver, spleen, kidney, pancreas, and pelvic organs, and structural abnormalities of the abdominal wall. Because the adequacy of detail in the test depends on the presence of fat, this diagnostic tool is not useful for very thin, cachectic patients. The procedure is completely painless, but radiation doses are considerable. New continuous-motion (helical or spiral), three-dimensional CT that provides very detailed pictures of the GI organs and vasculature has been developed.

NURSING INTERVENTIONS

CT may be performed with or without oral or intravenous (IV) contrast, but the enhancement of the study is far superior with the administration of a contrast agent. Any allergies to contrast agents, iodine, or shellfish, the patient's current serum creatinine level, and urine human chorionic gonadotropin must be determined before administration of a contrast agent. Patients allergic to the contrast agent may be premedicated with IV prednisone 24 hours, 12 hours, and 1 hour before the scan.

In addition, renal protective measures include the administration of IV sodium bicarbonate 1 hour before and 6 hours after IV contrast and oral acetylcysteine (Mucomyst) before or after the study. Both sodium bicarbonate and Mucomyst are free radical scavengers that sequester the contrast byproducts that are destructive to renal cells.

Magnetic Resonance Imaging

MRI is used in gastroenterology to supplement ultrasonography and CT. This noninvasive technique uses magnetic fields and radio waves to produce an image of the area being studied. The use of oral contrast agents to enhance the image has increased the application of this technique for the diagnosis of GI diseases. It is useful in evaluating abdominal soft tissues as well as blood vessels, abscesses, fistulas, neoplasms, and other sources of bleeding.

The physiologic artifacts of heartbeat, respiration, and peristalsis may create a less-than-clear image; however, newer, fast-imaging MRI techniques help eliminate these physiologic motion artifacts. MRIs are not totally safe for all people. Any ferromagnetic objects (metals that contain iron) can be attracted to the magnet and cause injury. Items that can be problematic or dangerous include jewelry, pacemakers, dental implants, paperclips, pens, keys, IV poles, clips on patient gowns, and oxygen tanks. MRI is contraindicated for patients with permanent pacemakers, artificial heart valves and defibrillators, implanted insulin pumps, or implanted transcutaneous electrical nerve stimulation devices, because the magnetic field could cause malfunction. MRI is also contraindicated for patients with internal metal devices (eg, aneurysm clips) or intraocular metallic fragments. Foil-backed skin patches (eg, NicoDerm, nitroglycerine [Transderm-Nitro], scopolamine [Transderm-Scop], clonidine [Catapres-TTS]) should be removed before an MRI because of the risk of burns; however, the patient's physician should be consulted before the patch is removed to determine whether an alternate form of the medication should be provided.

NURSING INTERVENTIONS

Prestudy patient education includes NPO status 6 to 8 hours before the study and removal of all jewelry and other metals. The patient and family are informed that the study may take 60 to 90 minutes; during this time, the technician will instruct the patient to take deep breaths at specific intervals. The close-fitting scanners used in many MRI facilities may induce feelings of claustrophobia, and the machine will make a knocking sound during the procedure. Patients may choose to wear a headset and listen to music or to wear a blindfold during the procedure. Open MRIs that are less close-fitting eliminate the claustrophobia that many patients experience.

Positron Emission Tomography (PET)

PET scans produce images of the body by detecting the radiation emitted from radioactive substances. The radioactive substances are injected into the body IV and are usually tagged with a radioactive atom, such as carbon-11, fluorine-18, oxygen-15, or nitrogen-13. The atoms decay quickly, do not harm the body, have lower radiation levels than a typical x-ray or CT scan, and are eliminated in the urine or feces. The scanner essentially "captures" where the radioactive substances are in the body, transmits information to a scanner, and produces a scan with "hot spots" for evaluation by the radiologist or oncologist.

Scintigraphy

Scintigraphy (radionuclide testing) relies on the use of radioactive isotopes (ie, technetium, iodine, and indium) to reveal displaced anatomic structures, changes in organ size, and the presence of neoplasms or other focal lesions, such as cysts or abscesses. Scintigraphic scanning is also used to measure the uptake of tagged red blood cells and leukocytes. Tagging of red blood cells and leukocytes by injection of a radionuclide is performed to define areas of inflammation, abscess, blood loss, or neoplasm. A sample of blood is removed, mixed with a radioactive substance, and reinjected into the patient. Abnormal concentrations of blood cells are then detected at 24- and 48-hour intervals. Tagged red cell studies are useful in determining the source of internal bleeding when all other studies have returned a negative result.

Gastrointestinal Motility Studies

Radionuclide testing also is used to assess gastric emptying and colonic transit time. During gastric emptying studies, the liquid and solid components of a meal (typically scrambled eggs) are tagged with radionuclide markers. After ingestion of the meal, the patient is positioned under a scintiscanner, which measures the rate of passage of the radioactive substance from the stomach. This is useful in diagnosing disorders of gastric motility, diabetic gastroparesis, and dumping syndrome.

Colonic transit studies are used to evaluate colonic motility and obstructive defecation syndromes. This is usually an outpatient study. The patient is given a capsule containing 20 radionuclide markers and instructed to follow a regular diet and normal daily activities. Abdominal x-rays are taken every 24 hours until all markers are passed. This process usually takes 4 to 5 days, but in the presence of severe constipation it may take as long as 10 days. Patients with chronic diarrhea may be evaluated at 8-hour intervals. The amount of time that it takes for the radioactive material to move through the colon indicates colonic motility.

Endoscopic Procedures

Endoscopic procedures used in GI tract assessment include fibroscopy/esophagogastroduodenoscopy (EGD), small-bowel enteroscopy, colonoscopy, sigmoidoscopy, proctoscopy, anoscopy, and endoscopy through an ostomy.

Upper Gastrointestinal Fibroscopy/ Esophagogastroduodenoscopy

Fibroscopy of the upper GI tract allows direct visualization of the esophageal, gastric, and duodenal mucosa through a lighted endoscope (gastroscope) (Fig. 34-6). EGD is especially valuable when esophageal, gastric, or duodenal abnormalities or inflammatory, neoplastic, or infectious processes are suspected. This procedure also can be used to evaluate esophageal and gastric motility and to collect secretions and tissue specimens for further analysis.

In esophagogastroduodenoscopy (EGD), the gastroenterologist views the GI tract through a viewing lens and can take still or video photographs through the scope to document findings. Electronic video endoscopes also are available that attach directly to a video processor, converting the electronic signals into pictures on a television screen. This allows larger and continuous viewing capabilities, as well as the simultaneous recording of the procedure.

Recently, PillCam ESO, a pill-sized instrument equipped with two cameras, has become available. Each camera takes seven photographs per second and transmits them wirelessly to a nearby storage device (Eliakim, Sharma, & Yassin, 2005). This technique is gaining popularity with patients and practitioners alike as a comfortable, convenient alternative to endoscopy. Two major drawbacks to this method of endoscopy are that it evaluates only the esophagus and that it may become lodged in a previously anastomosed section of bowel and require further endoscopic or surgical intervention for removal.

Side-viewing flexible scopes are used to visualize the common bile duct and the pancreatic and hepatic ducts through the ampulla of Vater in the duodenum. This procedure, called endoscopic retrograde cholangiopancreatography (ERCP), uses the endoscope in combination with x-ray techniques to view the ductal structures of the biliary tract (Hibberts & Barnes, 2003). ERCP is helpful in evaluating jaundice, pancreatitis, pancreatic tumors, common bile duct stones, and biliary tract disease. ERCP is described further in Chapter 40.

Upper GI fibroscopy also can be a therapeutic procedure when it is combined with other procedures. Therapeutic endoscopy can be used to remove common bile duct stones, dilate strictures, and treat gastric bleeding and esophageal varices. Laser-compatible scopes can be used to provide laser therapy for upper GI neoplasms. Sclerosing solutions can be injected through the scope in an attempt to control upper GI bleeding.

After the patient is sedated, the endoscope is lubricated with a water-soluble lubricant and passed smoothly and slowly along the back of the mouth and down into the esophagus. The gastroenterologist views the gastric wall and the sphincters, and then advances the endoscope into the duodenum for further examination. Biopsy forceps to obtain tissue specimens or cytology brushes to obtain cells for microscopic study can be passed through the scope. The procedure usually takes about 30 minutes.

The patient may experience nausea, gagging, or choking. Use of topical anesthetics and moderate sedation makes it important to monitor and maintain the patient's oral airway during and after the procedure. Finger or ear oximeters are

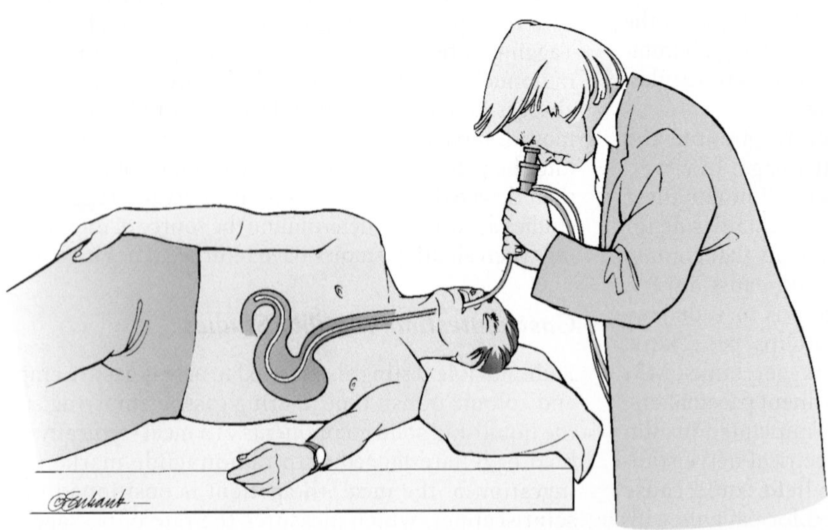

FIGURE 34-6. Patient undergoing gastroscopy.

used to monitor oxygen saturation, and supplemental oxygen may be administered if needed. Precautions must be taken to protect the scope, because the fiberoptic bundles can be broken if the scope is bent at an acute angle. The patient wears a mouth guard to keep from biting the scope.

NURSING INTERVENTIONS

Studies indicate that preoperative or preprocedure patient education is a cost-effective intervention in enhancing patient cooperation and satisfaction during ERCP (Ratanalert, Soontrapornchai, & Ovartlarnporn, 2002; vanVliet, Grypdonck, vanZuuren, et al., 2004). The patient should be NPO for 8 hours prior to the examination. Before the introduction of the endoscope, the patient is given a local anesthetic gargle or spray. Midazolam (Versed), a sedative that provides moderate sedation and relieves anxiety during the procedure, may be administered at the initiation of the study. Atropine may be administered to reduce secretions, and glucagon may be administered to relax smooth muscle. The patient is positioned in the left lateral position to facilitate clearance of pulmonary secretions and provide smooth entry of the scope.

After gastroscopy, assessment includes level of consciousness, vital signs, oxygen saturation, pain level, and monitoring for signs of perforation (ie, pain, bleeding, unusual difficulty swallowing, and rapidly elevated temperature). After the patient's gag reflex has returned, lozenges, saline gargle, and oral analgesics may be offered to relieve minor throat discomfort. Patients who were sedated for the procedure must remain in bed until fully alert. After moderate sedation, the patient must be transported home with a family member or friend if the procedure was performed on an outpatient basis. Someone should stay with the patient until the morning after the procedure. One study found that 69% of discharged patients could not recite postprocedure instructions to a nurse the morning following the procedure (Gall & Bull, 2003). For this reason, discharge instructions are provided to the person accompanying the patient home, as well as to the patient. In addition, many endoscopy suites have a program in which a nurse telephones the patient the morning after the procedure to find out if the patient has any concerns or questions related to the procedure.

Fiberoptic Colonoscopy

Historically, direct visualization of the bowel was the only means to evaluate the colon, but virtual colonoscopy (also known as CT colonography) has brought a more patient-friendly approach to this study. First described by Vining in 1994, virtual colonoscopy provides a computer-simulated endoluminal perspective of the air-filled distended colon using conventional spiral or helical CT scanning (Fletcher, Booya, & Johnson, 2005).

Direct visual inspection of the large intestine (anus, rectum, sigmoid, transcending and ascending colon) is possible by means of a flexible fiberoptic colonoscope (Fig. 34-7). These scopes have the same capabilities as those used for EGD but are larger in diameter and longer. Still and video recordings can be used to document the procedure and findings.

This procedure is used commonly as a diagnostic aid and screening device. It is most frequently used for cancer screening (Chart 34-2) and for surveillance in patients with previous colon cancer or polyps. In addition, tissue biopsies can be obtained as needed, and polyps can be removed and evaluated. Other uses of colonoscopy include the evaluation of patients with diarrhea of unknown cause, occult bleeding, or anemia; further study of abnormalities detected on barium enema; and diagnosis, clarification, and determination of the extent of inflammatory or other bowel disease.

Therapeutically, the procedure can be used to remove all visible polyps with a special snare and cautery through the colonoscope. Many colon cancers begin with adenomatous polyps of the colon; therefore, one goal of colonoscopic polypectomy is early detection and prevention of colorectal cancer. This procedure also can be used to treat

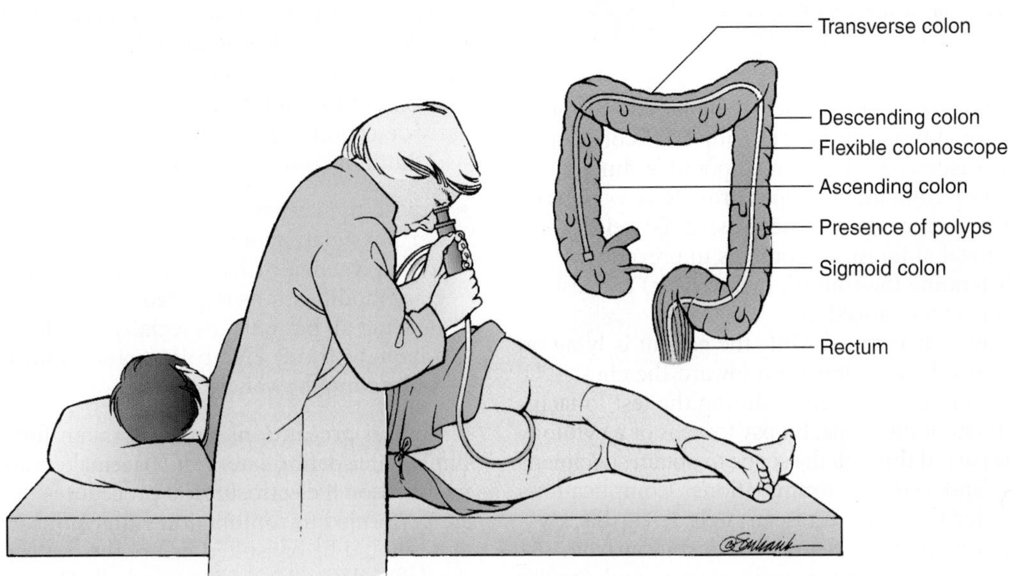

FIGURE 34-7. Colonoscopy. The flexible scope is passed through the rectum and sigmoid colon into the descending, transverse, and ascending colon.

CHART 34-2

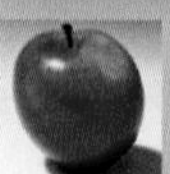

Health Promotion

Guidelines for Colon and Rectal Cancer Screening

Beginning at age 50, both men and women should follow one of these five testing schedules:

- Yearly fecal occult blood test (FOBT)* or fecal immunochemical test (FIT)
- Flexible sigmoidoscopy every 5 years
- Yearly FOBT* or FIT, plus flexible sigmoidoscopy every 5 years†
- Double-contrast barium enema every 5 years
- Colonoscopy every 10 years

All positive tests should be followed up with colonoscopy.

People should talk to their doctor about starting colorectal cancer screening earlier and/or undergoing screening more often if they have any of the following colorectal cancer risk factors:

- A personal history of colorectal cancer or adenomatous polyps
- A strong family history of colorectal cancer or polyps (cancer or polyps in a first-degree relative younger than 60 or in two first-degree relatives of any age)‡
- A personal history of chronic inflammatory bowel disease
- A family history of an hereditary colorectal cancer syndrome (familial adenomatous polyposis or hereditary non-polyposis colon cancer)

*For FOBT, the take-home multiple sample method should be used.

†The combination of yearly FOBT or FIT flexible sigmoidoscopy every 5 years is preferred over either of these options alone.

‡A first-degree relative is defined as a parent, sibling, or child.

areas of bleeding or stricture. Use of bipolar and unipolar coagulators, use of heater probes, and injections of sclerosing agents or vasoconstrictors are all possible during this procedure. Laser-compatible scopes provide laser therapy for bleeding lesions or colonic neoplasms. Bowel decompression (removal of intestinal contents to prevent gas and fluid from distending the coils of the intestine) can also be completed during the procedure.

Colonoscopy is performed while the patient is lying on the left side with the legs drawn up toward the chest. The patient's position may be changed during the test to facilitate advancement of the scope. Biopsy forceps or a cytology brush may be passed through the scope to obtain specimens for histology and cytology examinations. Complications during and after the procedure can include cardiac dysrhythmias and respiratory depression resulting from the medications administered, vasovagal reactions, and circulatory overload or hypotension resulting from overhydration or underhydration during bowel preparation. Therefore, it is important to monitor the patient's cardiac and respiratory function and oxygen saturation continuously, with supplemental oxygen used as necessary. Typically the procedure takes about 1 hour, and postprocedure discomfort results from instillation of air to expand the colon and insertion and movement of the scope during the procedure.

NURSING INTERVENTIONS

The success of the procedure depends on how well the colon is prepared. Adequate colon cleansing provides optimal visualization and decreases the time needed for the procedure. Cleansing of the colon can be accomplished in various ways. The physician may prescribe a laxative for two nights before the examination and a Fleet's or saline enema until the return is clear the morning of the test. However, more commonly, polyethylene glycol electrolyte lavage solutions (Go-LYTELY, CoLyte, and Nu-Lytely) are used as intestinal lavages for effective cleansing of the bowel. The patient maintains a clear liquid diet starting at noon the day before the procedure. Then the patient ingests the lavage solution orally at intervals over 3 to 4 hours. Surprisingly, patient compliance with this oral portion of the bowel prep is the same for the use of flavored and unflavored lavage solutions (Hayes, Buffum, & Fuller, 2003). If necessary, the nurse can give the solution through a feeding tube if the patient cannot swallow. Patients with a colostomy can receive this same bowel preparation. The use of lavage solutions is contraindicated in patients with intestinal obstruction or inflammatory bowel disease.

With the use of lavage solutions, bowel cleansing is fast (rectal effluent is clear in about 4 hours) and is tolerated fairly well by most patients. Side effects of the electrolyte solutions include nausea, bloating, cramps or abdominal fullness, fluid and electrolyte imbalance, and hypothermia (patients are often told to drink the preparation as cold as possible to make it more palatable). The side effects are especially problematic for elderly patients, and sometimes they have difficulty ingesting the required volume of solution. Monitoring elderly patients after a bowel prep is especially important because their physiologic ability to compensate for fluid loss is diminished. Many elderly people take multiple medications each day; therefore, the nurse's knowledge of their daily medication regimen can prompt assessment for and prevention of potential problems and early detection of physiologic changes.

Additional nursing actions include the following:

- Advise the patient with diabetes to consult with his or her physician about medication adjustment to prevent hyperglycemia or hypoglycemia resulting from the dietary modifications required in preparing for the test.
- Instruct all patients, especially the elderly, to maintain adequate fluid, electrolyte, and caloric intake while undergoing bowel cleansing.

Special precautions must be taken for some patients. Implantable defibrillators and pacemakers are at high risk of malfunction if electrosurgical procedures (ie, polypectomy) are performed in conjunction with colonoscopy. A cardiologist should be consulted before the test is performed, and the defibrillator should be turned off. These patients require careful cardiac monitoring during the procedure.

Colonoscopy cannot be performed if there is a suspected or documented colon perforation, acute severe diverticulitis, or fulminant colitis. Patients with prosthetic heart valves or a history of endocarditis require prophylactic antibiotics before the procedure.

Informed consent is obtained by the practitioner before the patient is sedated. Before the examination, an opioid analgesic or sedative (eg, midazolam) is administered to provide moderate sedation and relieve anxiety during the procedure. Glucagon may be administered, if needed, to relax the colonic musculature and to reduce spasm during the test. Elderly or debilitated patients may require a reduced dosage of the analgesic or sedative to decrease the risks of oversedation and cardiopulmonary complications.

During the procedure, the nurse monitors for changes in the patient's oxygen saturation, vital signs, color and temperature of the skin, level of consciousness, abdominal distention, vagal response, and pain intensity. After the procedure, patients who were sedated are maintained on bed rest until fully alert. Some patients have abdominal cramps caused by increased peristalsis stimulated by the air insufflated into the bowel during the procedure.

Immediately after the test, the nurse observes the patient for signs and symptoms of bowel perforation (eg, rectal bleeding, abdominal pain or distention, fever, focal peritoneal signs). If midazolam was used, the nurse explains its amnesic effects. It is important to provide written instructions, because the patient may be unable to recall verbal information. If the procedure is performed on an outpatient basis, someone must transport the patient home. After a therapeutic procedure, the nurse instructs the patient to report any bleeding to the physician.

Anoscopy, Proctoscopy, and Sigmoidoscopy

Endoscopic examination of the anus, rectum, and sigmoid and descending colon is used to evaluate chronic diarrhea, fecal incontinence, ischemic colitis, and lower GI hemorrhage and to observe for ulceration, fissures, abscesses, tumors, polyps, or other pathologic processes.

Flexible scopes have largely replaced the rigid scopes used in the past for routine examinations. The flexible fiberoptic sigmoidoscope (Fig. 34-8) permits the colon to be examined up to 40 to 50 cm (16 to 20 inches) from the anus, much more than the 25 cm (10 inches) that can be visualized with the rigid sigmoidoscope. It has many of the same capabilities as the scopes used for the upper GI study, including the use of still or video images to document findings.

For flexible scope procedures, the patient assumes a comfortable position on the left side with the right leg bent and placed anteriorly. It is important to keep the patient informed throughout the examination and to explain the sensations associated with the examination. Biopsies and polypectomies can be performed during this procedure. Biopsy is performed with small biting forceps introduced through the endoscope; one or more small pieces of tissue may be removed. If rectal or sigmoid polyps are present, they may be removed with a wire snare, which is used to grasp the pedicle, or stalk. An electrocoagulating current is then used to sever the polyp and prevent bleeding. It is extremely important that all excised tissue be placed immediately in moist gauze or in an appropriate receptacle, labeled correctly, and delivered without delay to the pathology laboratory for examination.

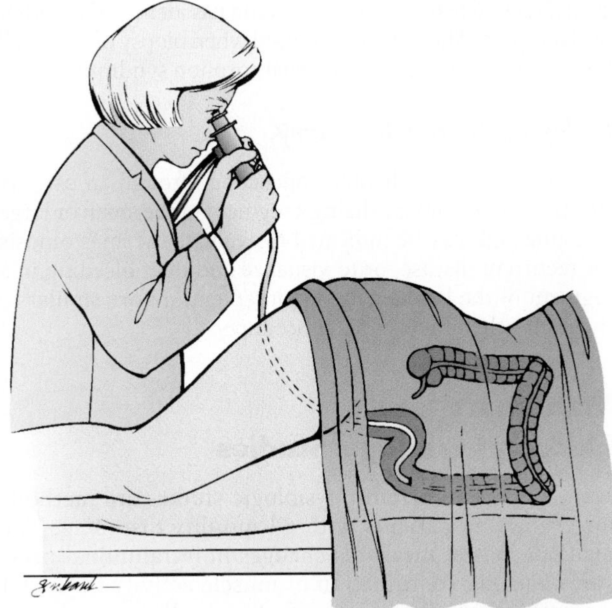

FIGURE 34-8. Flexible fiberoptic sigmoidoscopy. The flexible scope is advanced past the proximal sigmoid and then into the descending colon.

NURSING INTERVENTIONS

These examinations require only limited bowel preparation, including a warm tap water or Fleet's enema until returns are clear. Soap-suds and tap water enemas that were used in the past produced significantly greater returns, but patients were more uncomfortable. In addition, rectal biopsies showed surface epithelium loss after soap-suds and tap water enemas but not after Fleet's enema. Dietary restrictions usually are not necessary, and sedation usually is not required. During the procedure, the nurse monitors vital signs, skin color and temperature, pain tolerance, and vagal response. After the procedure, the nurse monitors the patient for rectal bleeding and signs of intestinal perforation (ie, fever, rectal drainage, abdominal distention, and pain). On completion of the examination, the patient can resume his or her regular activities and diet.

Small-Bowel Enteroscopy

Technology for the use of the small-caliber transnasal endoscope to allow direct inspection of the wall of the small intestine continues to improve. Two methods are being used at this time: the "push" and the "pull" endoscope methods. The "pull" endoscope is very long and flexible and has a balloon at its tip. When inflated, the balloon tip advances the scope by peristalsis through the small intestine. Metoclopramide (Reglan) may be administered IV to assist passage, and the procedure may take up to 10 hours to complete. The patient may stay in the recovery area or go home during this period. Once the scope has entered the distal ileum, the balloon is deflated and the tube is retracted slowly while the endoscopist examines the intestinal wall. "Push" endoscopes have been designed to be smaller in caliber and longer in length, while still allowing the use of biopsy forceps and probes. These two methods are especially useful in the evaluation of patients who have continued bleeding even after extensive diagnostic testing has identified no other problem area. They can also be used when biopsy of the small bowel is needed to diagnose malabsorption syndromes.

Endoscopy Through Ostomy

Endoscopy using a flexible endoscope through an ostomy stoma is useful for visualizing a segment of the small or large intestine and may be indicated to evaluate the anastomosis for recurrent disease, or to visualize and treat bleeding in a segment of the bowel. Nursing interventions are similar to those for other endoscopic procedures.

Manometry and Electrophysiologic Studies

Manometry and electrophysiologic studies are methods for evaluating patients with GI motility disorders. The manometry test measures changes in intraluminal pressures and the coordination of muscle activity in the GI tract with the pressures recorded manually, on a physiograph, or on a computer.

Esophageal manometry is used to detect motility disorders of the esophagus and the upper and lower esophageal sphincter. Also known as esophageal motility studies, these studies are very helpful in the diagnosis of achalasia, diffuse esophageal spasm, scleroderma, and other esophageal motor disorders. The patient must refrain from eating or drinking for 8 to 12 hours before the test. Medications that could have a direct affect on motility (eg, calcium channel blockers, anticholinergic agents, sedatives) are withheld for 24 to 48 hours. A pressure-sensitive catheter is inserted through the nose and is connected to a transducer and a video recorder. The patient then swallows small amounts of water while the resultant pressure changes are recorded. Evaluation of a patient for gastroesophageal reflux disease (GERD) typically includes esophageal manometry.

Gastroduodenal, small intestine, and colonic manometry procedures are used to evaluate delayed gastric emptying and gastric and intestinal motility disorders such as irritable bowel syndrome or atonic colon. This is often an ambulatory outpatient procedure lasting 24 to 72 hours. Anorectal manometry measures the resting tone of the internal anal sphincter and the contractibility of the external anal sphincter. It is helpful in evaluating patients with chronic constipation or fecal incontinence and is useful in biofeedback for the treatment of fecal incontinence. It can be performed in conjunction with rectal sensory functioning tests. Phospho-Soda or a saline cleansing enema is administered 1 hour before the test, and positioning for the test is either the prone or the lateral position.

Rectal sensory function studies are used to evaluate rectal sensory function and neuropathy. A catheter and balloon are passed into the rectum, with increasing balloon inflation until the patient feels distention. Then the tone and pressure of the rectum and anal sphincter are measured. The results are especially helpful in the evaluation of patients with chronic constipation, diarrhea, or incontinence.

Electrogastrography, an electrophysiologic study, also may be performed to assess gastric motility disturbances and can be useful in detecting motor or nerve dysfunction in the stomach. Electrodes are placed over the abdomen, and gastric electrical activity is recorded for up to 24 hours. Patients may exhibit rapid, slow, or irregular waveform activity.

Defecography

Defecography measures anorectal function and is performed with very thick barium paste instilled into the rectum. Fluoroscopy is used to assess the function of the rectum and anal sphincter while the patient attempts to expel the barium. The test requires no preparation.

Gastric Analysis, Gastric Acid Stimulation Test, and pH Monitoring

Analysis of the gastric juice yields information about the secretory activity of the gastric mucosa and the presence or degree of gastric retention in patients thought to have pyloric or duodenal obstruction. It is also useful for diagnosing Zollinger-Ellison syndrome, or atrophic gastritis.

The patient is NPO for 8 to 12 hours before the procedure. Any medications that affect gastric secretions are withheld for 24 to 48 hours before the test. Smoking is not allowed on the morning of the test, because it increases gastric secretions. A small nasogastric tube with a catheter tip marked at various points is inserted through the nose. When the tube is at a point slightly less than 50 cm (21 inches), it should be within the stomach, lying along the greater curvature. Once in place, the tube is secured to the patient's cheek and the patient is placed in a semireclining position. The entire stomach contents are aspirated by gentle suction into a syringe, and gastric samples are collected every 15 minutes for the next hour.

The gastric acid stimulation test usually is performed in conjunction with gastric analysis. Histamine or pentagastrin is administered subcutaneously to stimulate gastric secretions. It is important to inform the patient that this injection may produce a flushed feeling. The nurse monitors the patient's blood pressure and pulse frequently to detect hypotension. Gastric specimens are collected after the injection every 15 minutes for 1 hour and are labeled to indicate the time of specimen collection after histamine injection. The volume and pH of the specimen are measured; in certain instances, cytologic study by the Papanicolaou technique may be used to determine the presence or absence of malignant cells.

Important diagnostic information to be gained from gastric analysis includes the ability of the mucosa to secrete HCl. This ability is altered in various disease states, including:

- Pernicious anemia—patients with this disease secrete no acid under basal conditions or after stimulation
- Severe chronic atrophic gastritis or gastric cancer—patients with these diseases secrete little or no acid
- Peptic ulcer—patients with this disease secrete some acid
- Duodenal ulcers—patients with this disease usually secrete an excess amount of acid

Esophageal reflux of gastric acid may be diagnosed by ambulatory pH monitoring. The patient is NPO for 6 hours before the test, and all medications affecting gastric secretions are withheld for 24 to 36 hours before the test. A probe that measures pH is inserted through the nose and into position about 5 inches above the lower esophageal sphincter. It is connected to an external recording device and is worn for 24 hours while the patient continues his or her normal daily activities. The end result is a computer analysis and graphic display of the results. This test allows for the direct correlation between chest pain and reflux episodes (Wolfe, 2000).

A Bernstein test may be performed to evaluate complaints of acid-related chest or epigastric pain. HCl is instilled through a small feeding tube positioned in the esophagus to try to elicit the reported chest pain. Resultant signs and symptoms are compared with the patient's usual symptoms. However, since the advent of ambulatory pH monitoring, this previously popular evaluation tool is used infrequently (Wolfe, 2000).

Laparoscopy (Peritoneoscopy)

With the tremendous advances in minimally invasive surgery, diagnostic laparoscopy is efficient, cost-effective, and useful in the diagnosis of GI disease. After creating a pneumoperitoneum (injecting carbon dioxide into the peritoneal cavity, to separate the intestines from the pelvic organs), a small incision is made lateral to the umbilicus, allowing for the insertion of the fiberoptic laparoscope. This permits direct visualization of the organs and structures within the abdomen, permitting visualization and identification of any growths, anomalies, and inflammatory processes. In addition, biopsy samples can be taken from the structures and organs as necessary. This procedure can be used to evaluate peritoneal disease, chronic abdominal pain, abdominal masses, and gallbladder and liver disease. However, laparoscopy has not become an important diagnostic modality in patients with acute abdominal pain, because less invasive tools (ie, CT and MRI) are readily available. Laparoscopy usually requires general anesthesia and sometimes requires that the stomach and bowel be decompressed. Gas (usually carbon dioxide) is insufflated into the peritoneal cavity to create a working space for visualization. One of the benefits of this procedure is that after visualization of a problem, excision (eg, removal of the gallbladder) can then be performed at the same time, if appropriate.

Pathophysiologic and Psychological Considerations

Abnormalities of the GI tract are numerous and represent every type of major pathology that can affect other organ systems, including bleeding, perforation, obstruction, inflammation, and cancer. Congenital, inflammatory, infectious, traumatic, and neoplastic lesions have been encountered in every portion, and at every site, along the length of the GI tract. As with all other organ systems, the GI tract is subject to circulatory disturbances, faulty nervous system control, and aging.

Apart from the many organic diseases to which the GI tract is susceptible, many extrinsic factors can interfere with its normal function and produce symptoms. Stress and anxiety, for example, often find their chief expression in indigestion, anorexia, or motor disturbances of the intestines, sometimes producing constipation or diarrhea. In addition to the state of mental health, physical factors such as fatigue and an inadequate or abruptly changed dietary intake can markedly affect the GI tract. When assessing and instructing the patient, the nurse should consider the variety of mental and physical factors that affect the function of the GI tract.

GI diagnostic studies can confirm, rule out, stage, or diagnose disease. It is well documented that receiving a diagnosis of a serious condition (e.g., cancer) brings psychological distress, an emotional burden, a feeling of loss of personal control, and a threat to survival and self-image (Costelloe, 2004). Time should be allotted after the diagnosis for discussion with the patient, in addition to offering resource materials for information.

Critical Thinking Exercises

1 You are caring for a 45-year-old man who presents to the emergency department complaining of a 12-hour history of mid-epigastric pain. He denies nausea and vomiting and states that the pain worsens when he moves. He is lying flat on his back with his knees flexed, appearing hesitant to move. On palpation, his abdomen is firm and rigid with rebound tenderness in the mid-epigastrium. Bowel sounds are absent. What laboratory tests would you expect to be ordered? He is scheduled for an abdominal x-ray, a CT scan, and a sonogram of the abdomen. What are the purposes of these diagnostic studies, and what preparation is needed for these tests? What preprocedure teaching is needed?

2 ebp You are working in an endoscopy suite and are often assigned to care for patients who are scheduled to have screening fiberoptic colonoscopy. There are a variety of ways that cleansing of the colon can be accomplished prior to colonoscopy, with various periods of time for food and fluid restriction; laxatives; enemas; and electrolyte lavage solutions. You have found that the preparation prescribed varies from physician to physician. What is the evidence base that supports the use of each of the preparations? Discuss the strength of the evidence for the effectiveness of each of the preparations. Identify the criteria used to evaluate the strength of the evidence.

REFERENCES AND SELECTED READINGS

Bickley, L. S., & Szilagyi, P. G. (2003). *Bates' guide to physical examination and history taking* (8th ed.). Philadelphia: Lippincott Williams & Wilkins.

Eliopoulos, C. (2001). *Gerontological nursing* (5th ed.). Philadelphia: Lippincott Williams & Wilkins.

Kirsner, J. (Ed.). (2000). *Inflammatory bowel disease* (5th ed.). Philadelphia: W. B. Saunders.

Levine, M. (Ed.). (2000). *Double contrast gastrointestinal radiology*. Philadelphia: W. B. Saunders.

Ogilvie, J., Norwitz, J., & Kalloo, A. (2002). *Johns Hopkins manual for gastrointestinal endoscopy nursing*. Thorofare, NJ: Slack Incorporated.

Porth, C. M. (2005). *Pathophysiology. Concepts of altered health states.* Philadelphia: Lippincott Williams & Wilkins.

Society of Gastroenterologic Nursing and Associates. (2003). *Core curriculum* (3rd ed.). St. Louis: Mosby.

Wolfe, M. M. (Ed). (2000). *Therapy of digestive disorders.* Philadelphia: W. B. Saunders.

JOURNALS

**Asterisks indicate nursing research articles.*

Beery, T. A., & Hern, M. J. (2004). Genetic practice, education, and research: An overview for advanced practice nurses. *Clinical Nurse Specialist, 18*(3), 126–132.

Costelloe, M. N. (2004). The needs of recently diagnosed cancer patients. *Nursing Standard, 19*(13), 42–44.

Delgados-Aros, S., Locke, R., Camilleri, M., et al. (2004). Obesity is associated with increased risk of gastrointestinal symptoms: A population-based study. *American Journal of Gastroenterology, 99*(9), 1801.

Eliakim, R., Sharma, V. K., & Yassin, K. (2005). A prospective study of the diagnostic accuracy of PillCam ESO esophageal capsule endoscopy versus conventional upper endoscopy in patients with chronic gastroesophageal reflux diseases. *Journal of Clinical Gastroenterology, 39*(7), 572–578.

Fletcher, J. G., Booya, F., & Johnson, C. D. (2005). CT colonography: Unraveling the twists and turns. *Current Opinion in Gastroenterology, 21*(1), 90–98.

*Gall, S., & Bull, J. (2003). Discharging patients with no one at home. *Gastroenterology Nursing, 27*(3), 111–114.

Gavaghan, M. (1999). Anatomy and physiology of the esophagus. *AORN Journal, 69*(2), 370–374.

*Hamilton, R. J., Bowers, B. J., & Williams, J. K. (2004). Disclosing genetic test results to family members. *Journal of Nursing Scholarship, 37*(1), 18–24.

*Hayes, A., Buffum, M., & Fuller, D. (2003). Bowel preparation comparison: Flavored versus unflavored Colyte. *Gastroenterology Nursing, 26*(3), 106–109.

Hibberts, F., & Barnes, E. (2003). Use of ERCP. *Nursing Times, 99*(20), 26–37.

Lowrey, K. M. (2004). Legal and ethical issues in cancer genetics nursing. *Seminars in Oncology Nursing, 20*(3), 203–208.

McGovern, P. M., Gross, C. R., Krueger, R. A., et al. (2004). False-positive cancer screens and health-related quality of life. *Cancer Nursing, 27*(5), 347–352.

Prather, F. M. (2002). Gastrointestinal motility problems in the elderly patient. *Gastroenterology, 122*(6), 688–700.

*Ratanalert, S., Soontrapornchai, P., & Ovartlarnporn, B. (2002). Preoperative education improves quality of patient care for endoscopic retrograde cholangiopancreatography. *Gastroenterology Nursing, 26*(1), 21–25.

VanVliet, M., Grypdonck, M., VanZuuren, F., et al. (2004). Preparing patients for gastrointestinal endoscopy: The influence of information in medical situations. *Patient Education and Counseling, 52*(1), 23–30.

CHAPTER 35

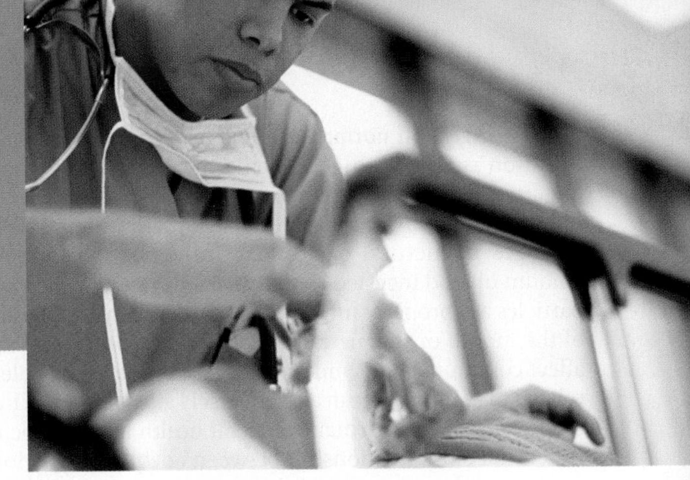

Management of Patients With Oral and Esophageal Disorders

Learning Objectives

On completion of this chapter, the learner will be able to:

1. Use the nursing process as a framework for care of patients with conditions of the oral cavity.
2. Describe the relationship of dental hygiene and dental problems to nutrition.
3. Describe the nursing management of patients with abnormalities of the lips, gums, teeth, mouth, and salivary glands.
4. Use the nursing process as a framework for care of patients with cancer of the oral cavity.
5. Identify the physical and psychosocial long-term needs of patients with oral cancer.
6. Use the nursing process as a framework for care of patients undergoing neck dissection.
7. Use the nursing process as a framework for care of patients with various conditions of the esophagus.
8. Describe the various conditions of the esophagus and their clinical manifestations and management.

Because digestion normally begins in the mouth, adequate nutrition is related to good dental health and the general condition of the mouth. Any discomfort or adverse condition in the oral cavity can affect a person's nutritional status. Changes in the oral cavity may influence the type and amount of food ingested as well as the degree to which food particles are properly mixed with salivary enzymes. Disease of the mouth or tongue can interfere with speech and thus affect communication and self-image. Esophageal problems related to swallowing can also adversely affect food and fluid intake, thereby jeopardizing general health and well-being. Given the close relationship between adequate nutritional intake and the structures of the upper gastrointestinal tract (lips, mouth, teeth, pharynx, esophagus), health teaching can help prevent disorders associated with these structures.

Oral health is a very important component of a person's physical and psychological sense of well-being. Severe periodontal disease affects approximately 14% of adults 45 to 64 years of age and 23% of adults 65 to 74 years of age (U.S. Department of Health and Human Services, 2000). Table 35-1 reviews common abnormalities of the oral cavity, their possible causes, and nursing management.

Disorders of the Teeth

Dental Plaque and Caries

Tooth decay is an erosive process that begins with the action of bacteria on fermentable carbohydrates in the mouth, which produces acids that dissolve tooth enamel. Although tooth enamel is the hardest substance in the human body, a recent study found that both regular and diet versions of popular soft drinks caused dental erosion by directly attacking the enamel. Soft drink consumption has increased sharply in the United States. In 1947, the average person drank about one hundred 12-ounce soft drinks per year, or two per week. Fifty years later, that number climbed to 600 annually, or two per day (von Fraunhofer & Rogers, 2004).

The extent of damage to the teeth depends on the following:

- The presence of dental plaque. Dental plaque is a gluey, gelatin-like substance that adheres to the teeth. The initial action that causes damage to a tooth occurs under dental plaque.
- The strength of the acids and the ability of the saliva to neutralize them
- The length of time the acids are in contact with the teeth
- The susceptibility of the teeth to decay

Dental decay begins with a small hole, usually in a fissure (a break in the tooth's enamel) or in an area that is hard to clean. Left unchecked, the decay extends into the dentin. Because dentin is not as hard as enamel, decay progresses more rapidly and in time reaches the pulp of the tooth. When the blood, lymph vessels, and nerves are exposed, they become infected and an abscess may form, either within the tooth or at the tip of the root. Soreness and pain usually occur with an abscess. As the infection continues, the patient's face may swell, and there may be pulsating pain.

Dentists can determine the extent of damage and the type of treatment needed using x-ray studies. Treatment for dental caries includes fillings, dental implants, and extraction, if necessary. In general, dental decay is associated with young people, but older adults are subject to decay as well, particularly from drug-induced or age-related oral dryness (Chart 35-1).

Prevention

Measures used to prevent and control dental caries include practicing effective mouth care, reducing the intake of starches and sugars (refined carbohydrates), applying fluoride to the teeth or drinking fluoridated water, refraining from smoking, controlling diabetes, and using pit and fissure sealants (Chart 35-2).

Mouth Care

Healthy teeth must be conscientiously and effectively cleaned on a daily basis. Brushing and flossing are particularly

Glossary

achalasia: absent or ineffective peristalsis (wavelike contraction) of the distal esophagus accompanied by failure of the esophageal sphincter to relax in response to swallowing
dysphagia: difficulty swallowing
dysplasia: abnormal change in cells
esophagogastroduodenoscopy (EGD): passage of a fiberoptic tube through the mouth and throat into the digestive tract for visualization of the esophagus, stomach, and small intestine; biopsies can be performed
gastroesophageal reflux: back-flow of gastric or duodenal contents into the esophagus
hernia: protrusion of an organ or part of an organ through the wall of the cavity that normally contains it
lithotripsy: use of shock waves to break up or disintegrate stones
odynophagia: pain on swallowing
parotitis: inflammation of the parotid gland
pyrosis: heartburn
periapical abscess: abscessed tooth
sialadenitis: inflammation of the salivary glands
stomatitis: inflammation of the oral mucosa
temporomandibular disorders: a group of conditions that cause pain or dysfunction of the temporomandibular joint (TMJ) and surrounding structures
vagotomy syndrome: dumping syndrome; gastrointestinal symptoms, such as diarrhea and abdominal cramping, resulting from rapid gastric emptying
xerostomia: dry mouth

TABLE 35-1 Disorders of the Lips, Mouth, and Gums

Condition	Signs and Symptoms	Possible Causes and sequelae	Nursing Considerations
Abnormalities of the Lips			
Actinic cheilitis	Irritation of lips associated with scaling, crusty, fissure; white overgrowth of horny layer of epidermis (hyperkeratosis) Considered a premalignant squamous cell skin cancer	Exposure to sun; more common in fair-skinned people and in those whose occupations involve sun exposure, such as farmers May lead to squamous cell cancer	Teach patient importance of protecting lips from the sun by using protective ointment such as sun block Instruct patient to have a periodic checkup by physician
Herpes simplex 1 (cold sore or fever blister)	Symptoms may be delayed up to 20 days after exposure; singular or clustered painful vesicles that may rupture	An opportunistic infection; frequently seen in immunosuppressed patients; very contagious May recur with menstruation, fever, or sun exposure	Use acyclovir (Zovirax) ointment or systemic medications as prescribed Administer analgesics as prescribed Instruct patient to avoid irritating foods
Chancre	Reddened circumscribed lesion that ulcerates and becomes crusted	Primary lesion of syphilis; very contagious	Comfort measures: cold soaks to lip, mouth care Administer antibiotics as prescribed Instruct patient regarding contagion
Contact dermatitis	Red area or rash; itching	Allergic reaction to lipstick, cosmetic ointments, or toothpaste	Instruct patient to avoid possible causes Administer corticosteroids as prescribed
Abnormalities of the Mouth			
Leukoplakia	White patches; may be hyperkeratotic; usually in buccal mucosa; usually painless	Fewer than 2% are malignant, but may progress to cancer Common among tobacco users	Instruct patient to see a physician if leukoplakia persists longer than 2 weeks Eliminate risk factors, such as tobacco
Hairy leukoplakia	White patches with rough hair-like projections; typically found on lateral border of the tongue	Possibly viral; smoking and use of tobacco Often seen in people who are HIV positive	Instruct patient to see a physician if condition persists longer than 2 weeks
Lichen planus	White papules at the intersection of a network of interlacing lesions; usually ulcerated and painful	Recurrences are common May lead to a malignant process Unknown cause	Apply topical corticosteroids such as fluocinolone acetonide oral base gel Avoid foods that irritate Administer corticosteroids systemically or intralesionally as prescribed Instruct the patient of need for follow-up if condition is chronic
Candidiasis (moniliasis/thrush)	Cheesy white plaque that looks like milk curds; when rubbed off, it leaves an erythematous and often bleeding base	*Candida albicans* fungus; predisposing factors include diabetes, antibiotic therapy, and immunosuppression	Antifungal medications such as nystatin (Mycostatin), amphotericin B, clotrimazole, or ketoconazole may be prescribed; these may be taken in pill form or as a suspension; when used as a suspension, instruct the patient to swish vigorously for at least 1 minute and then swallow
Aphthous stomatitis (canker sore)	Shallow ulcer with a white or yellow center and red border; seen on the inner side of the lip and cheek or on the tongue; it begins with a burning or tingling sensation and slight swelling; painful; usually lasts 7–10 days and heals without a scar	Associated with emotional or mental stress, fatigue, hormonal factors, minor trauma (such as biting), allergies, acidic foods and juices, and dietary deficiencies Associated with HIV infection May recur	Instruct the patient in comfort measures, such as saline rinses, and a soft or bland diet Antibiotics or corticosteroids may be prescribed

continued >

TABLE 35-1 Disorders of the Lips, Mouth, and Gums (Continued)

Condition	Signs and Symptoms	Possible Causes and sequelae	Nursing Considerations
Nicotine stomatitis (smoker's patch)	Two stages—begins as a red stomatitis; over time the tongue and mouth become covered with a creamy, thick, white mucous membrane, which may slough, leaving a beefy red base	Chronic irritation by tobacco	Cessation of tobacco use; if condition exists for longer than 2 weeks a physician should be consulted and a biopsy may be needed
Krythoplakia	Red patch on the oral mucous membrane	Nonspecific inflammation; more frequently seen in the elderly	
Kaposi's sarcoma	Appears first on the oral mucosa as a red, purple, or blue lesion; may be singular or multiple; may be flat or raised	HIV infection	Instruct patient regarding side effects of planned treatment
Stomatitis	Mild redness (erythema) and edema; if severe, painful ulcerations, bleeding, and secondary infection	Chemotherapy; radiation therapy; severe drug allergy; myelosuppression (bone marrow depression)	Prophylactic mouth care, including brushing, flossing, and rinsing, for any patient receiving chemotherapy or radiation therapy Teach patient proper oral hygiene, including the use of a soft-bristled toothbrush and nonabrasive toothpaste; for painful ulcers, oral swabs with sponge-like applicators can be used in place of a toothbrush; avoid alcohol-based mouth rinses and hot or spicy foods Apply topical anti-inflammatory, antibiotic, and anesthetic agents as prescribed
Abnormalities of the Gums			
Gingivitis	Painful, inflamed, swollen gums; usually the gums bleed in response to light contact	Poor oral hygiene: food debris, bacterial plaque, and calculus (tartar) accumulate; the gums may also swell in response to normal processes such as puberty and pregnancy	Teach patient proper oral hygiene; see Chart 35-2
Necrotizing gingivitis (trench mouth)	Gray-white pseudomembranous ulcerations affecting the edges of the gums, mucosa of the mouth, tonsils, and pharynx; foul breath; painful, bleeding gums; swallowing and talking are painful	Poor oral hygiene; bacterial infection, inadequate rest, overwork, emotional stress, smoking, and poor nutrition may contribute to development	Teach patient proper oral hygiene; see Chart 35-2 Irrigate with 2% to 3% hydrogen peroxide or normal saline solution Avoid irritants such as smoking and spicy foods
Herpetic gingivostomatitis	Burning sensation with the appearance of small vesicles 24–48 hours later; vesicles may rupture, forming sore, shallow ulcers covered with a gray membrane	Herpes simplex virus; occurs most frequently in people who are immunosuppressed; may occur in other infectious processes such as streptococcal pneumonia, meningococcal meningitis, and malaria	Apply topical anesthetics as prescribed; may need opioids if pain is severe Saline or 2% to 3% hydrogen peroxide irrigations Antiviral agents such as acyclovir may be prescribed
Periodontitis	Little discomfort at onset; may have bleeding, infection, gum recession, and loosening of teeth; later in the disease tooth loss may occur	May result from untreated gingivitis Poor or inadequate dental hygiene and inadequate diet contribute to development	Instruct patient in proper oral hygiene Instruct patient to consult a dentist

CHART 35-1

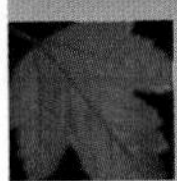

Gerontologic Considerations

Oral Conditions in the Older Adult

Many medications taken by the elderly cause dry mouth, which is uncomfortable, impairs communication, and increases the risk of oral infection. These medications include the following:

- Diuretics
- Antihypertensive medications
- Anti-inflammatory agents
- Antidepressant medications

Poor dentition can exacerbate problems of aging, such as:

- Decreased food intake
- Loss of appetite
- Social isolation
- Increased susceptibility to systemic infection (from periodontal disease)
- Trauma to the oral cavity secondary to thinner, less vascular oral mucous membranes

effective in mechanically breaking up the bacterial plaque that collects around teeth.

Normal mastication (chewing) and the normal flow of saliva also aid greatly in keeping the teeth clean. Because many ill patients do not eat adequate amounts of food, they produce less saliva, which in turn reduces this natural tooth cleaning process. The nurse may need to assume the responsibility for brushing the patient's teeth. Merely wiping the patient's mouth and teeth with a swab is ineffective. The most effective method is mechanical cleansing (brushing). If brushing is impossible, it is better to wipe the teeth with a gauze pad, then have the patient swish an antiseptic mouthwash several times before expectorating into an emesis basin. A soft-bristled toothbrush is more effective than a sponge or foam stick. To prevent drying, the lips may be coated with a water-soluble gel.

CHART 35-2

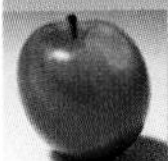

Health Promotion

Preventive Oral Hygiene

- Brush teeth using a soft toothbrush at least two times daily. Hold toothbrush at a 45-degree angle between the brush and the gums and teeth. A small brush is better than a large brush. Gums and tongue surface should be brushed.
- Floss at least once daily.
- Use an antiplaque mouth rinse.
- Visit a dentist at least every 6 months, or when you have a chipped tooth, a lost filling, an oral sore that persists longer than 2 weeks, or a toothache.
- Avoid alcohol and tobacco products, including smokeless tobacco.
- Maintain adequate nutrition and avoid sweets.
- Replace toothbrush at first signs of wear, usually every 2 months.

Diet

Dental caries may be prevented by decreasing the amount of sugar and starch in the diet. Patients who snack should be encouraged to choose less cariogenic alternatives, such as fruits, vegetables, nuts, cheeses, or plain yogurt. In addition, frequent brushing, especially after meals, is necessary. Flossing should be performed daily.

Fluoridation

Fluoridation of public water supplies has been found to decrease dental caries. Some areas of the country have natural fluoridation; other communities have added fluoride to public water supplies. Fluoridation may be achieved also by having a dentist apply a concentrated gel or solution to the teeth; adding fluoride to home water supplies; using fluoridated toothpaste or mouth rinse; or using sodium fluoride tablets, drops, or lozenges.

Pit and Fissure Sealants

The occlusal surfaces of the teeth have pits and fissures, areas that are prone to caries. Some dentists apply a special coating to fill and seal these areas from potential exposure to cariogenic processes. These sealants can last 5 to 10 years, depending on how dry the tooth surface is prior to application.

Dentoalveolar Abscess or Periapical Abscess

Periapical abscess, more commonly referred to as an abscessed tooth, involves a collection of pus in the apical dental periosteum (fibrous membrane supporting the tooth structure) and the tissue surrounding the apex of the tooth (where it is suspended in the jaw bone). The abscess may be acute or chronic. Acute periapical abscess is usually secondary to a suppurative pulpitis (a pus-producing inflammation of the dental pulp) that arises from an infection extending from dental caries. The infection of the dental pulp extends through the apical foramen of the tooth to form an abscess around the apex.

Chronic dentoalveolar abscess is a slowly progressive infectious process. In contrast to the acute form, a fully formed abscess may occur without the patient's knowledge. The infection eventually leads to a "blind dental abscess," which is actually a periapical granuloma. It may enlarge to as much as 1 cm in diameter. It is often discovered on x-ray films and is treated by extraction or root canal therapy, often with apicectomy (excision of the apex of the tooth root).

Clinical Manifestations

The abscess produces a dull, gnawing, continuous pain, often with a surrounding cellulitis and edema of the adjacent facial structures, and mobility of the involved tooth. The gum opposite the apex of the tooth is usually swollen on the cheek side. Swelling and cellulitis of the facial structures may make it difficult for the patient to open the mouth. There may also be a systemic reaction, fever, and malaise.

Management

In the early stages of an infection, a dentist or oral surgeon may perform a needle aspiration or drill an opening into the pulp chamber to relieve pressure and pain and to provide drainage. Usually, the infection will have progressed to a periapical abscess. Drainage is provided by an incision through the gingiva down to the jawbone. Pus (purulent material) escapes under pressure. This procedure may be performed in the dentist's office, an outpatient surgery center, or a same-day surgery department. After the inflammatory reaction has subsided, the tooth may be extracted or root canal therapy performed. Antibiotics may be prescribed.

Nursing Management

The nurse assesses the patient for bleeding after treatment and instructs the patient to use a warm saline or warm water mouth rinse to keep the area clean. The patient is also instructed to take antibiotics and analgesics as prescribed, to advance from a liquid diet to a soft diet as tolerated, and to keep follow-up appointments.

Malocclusion

Malocclusion is a misalignment of the teeth of the upper and lower dental arcs when the jaws are closed. Malocclusion can be inherited or acquired (from thumb-sucking, trauma, or some medical conditions). Malocclusion makes the teeth difficult to clean and can lead to decay, gum disease, and excess wear on supporting bone and gum tissues. About 50% of the population has some form of malocclusion. Correction of malocclusion requires an orthodontist, a patient who is motivated and cooperative, and adequate time. Most treatments begin when the patient has shed the last primary tooth and the last permanent successor has erupted, usually at about 12 or 13 years of age, but treatment may occur in adulthood. Preventive orthodontics may be started in children as early as 5 years of age if malocclusion is diagnosed early. The need for teeth straightening in adolescents is reduced if preventive orthodontics is started with the primary teeth.

Management

People with malocclusion have an obviously misaligned bite or crooked, crowded, widely spaced, or protruding teeth. To realign the teeth, the orthodontist gradually forces the teeth into a new location by using wires or plastic bands (braces). These devices may be unattractive, but this psychological burden must be overcome if good results are to be achieved. In the final phase of treatment, a retaining device is worn for several hours each day to support the tissues as they adjust to the new alignment of the teeth.

Nursing Management

The patient must practice meticulous oral hygiene, and the nurse encourages the patient to continue this important part of the treatment. An adolescent or adult undergoing orthodontic correction who is admitted to the hospital for some other problem may have to be reminded to continue wearing the retainer (if it does not interfere with the problem requiring hospitalization).

Disorders of the Jaw

Abnormal conditions affecting the mandible (jaw) and of the temporomandibular joint (which connects the mandible to the temporal bone at the side of the head in front of the ear) include congenital malformation, fracture, chronic dislocation, cancer, and syndromes characterized by pain and limited motion. Temporomandibular disorders and jaw surgery (a treatment common in many structural abnormalities or cancer of the jaw) are presented in this section.

Temporomandibular Disorders

Temporomandibular disorders are categorized as follows (U.S. Department of Health and Human Services, 2000):

- Myofascial pain—a discomfort in the muscles controlling jaw function and in neck and shoulder muscles
- Internal derangement of the joint—a dislocated jaw, a displaced disc, or an injured condyle
- Degenerative joint disease—rheumatoid arthritis or osteoarthritis in the jaw joint

Diagnosis and treatment of temporomandibular disorders remain somewhat ambiguous, but the condition is thought to affect about 10 million people in the United States. Misalignment of the joints in the jaw and other problems associated with the ligaments and muscles of mastication are thought to result in tissue damage and muscle tenderness. Suggested causes include arthritis of the jaw, head injury, trauma or injury to the jaw or joint, stress, and malocclusion (although research does not support malocclusion as a cause).

Clinical Manifestations

Patients have pain ranging from a dull ache to throbbing, debilitating pain that can radiate to the ears, teeth, neck muscles, and facial sinuses. They often have restricted jaw motion and locking of the jaw. There also may be a sudden change in the way the upper and lower teeth fit together. The patient may hear clicking and grating noises, and chewing and swallowing may be difficult. Symptoms such as headaches, earaches, dizziness, and hearing problems may sometimes be related to temporomandibular disorders (National Institute of Dental & Craniofacial Research, 2004).

Assessment and Diagnostic Findings

Diagnosis is based on the patient's report of pain, limitations in range of motion, dysphagia, difficulty chewing, difficulty with speech, or hearing difficulties. Magnetic resonance imaging, x-ray studies, and an arthrogram may be performed.

Management

Although some practitioners think the role of stress in temporomandibular joint disorders is overrated, patient education in stress management may be helpful (to reduce grinding and clenching of teeth). The patient may also benefit from range-of-motion exercises. Pain management measures may include nonsteroidal anti-inflammatory drugs (NSAIDs), with the possible addition of opioids, muscle relaxants, or mild antidepressants. Occasionally, intra-oral orthotics (a plastic guard worn over the upper and lower teeth) may be worn to reposition the condyle head in the joint space to a more normal position, which in turn relieves the stress and pressure on the tissues of the joint. This allows the tissues to heal. Conservative and reversible treatment is recommended. If irreversible surgical options are recommended, the patient is encouraged to seek a second opinion.

Jaw Disorders Requiring Surgical Management

Correction of mandibular structural abnormalities may require surgery involving repositioning or reconstruction of the jaw. Simple fractures of the mandible without displacement, resulting from a blow on the chin, and planned surgical interventions, as in the correction of long or short jaw syndrome, may require treatment by these means. Jaw reconstruction may be necessary in the aftermath of trauma from a severe injury or cancer, both of which can cause tissue and bone loss.

Mandibular fractures are usually closed fractures. Rigid plate fixation (insertion of metal plates and screws into the bone to approximate and stabilize the bone) is the current treatment of choice in many cases of mandibular fracture and in some mandibular reconstructive surgery procedures. Bone grafting may be performed to replace structural defects using bones from the patient's own ilium, ribs, or cranial sites. Rib tissue may also be harvested from cadaver donors.

Nursing Management

The patient who has had rigid fixation should be instructed not to chew food in the first 1 to 4 weeks after surgery. A liquid diet is recommended, and dietary counseling should be obtained to ensure optimal caloric and protein intake.

Promoting Home and Community-Based Care

The patient needs specific guidelines for mouth care and feeding. Any irritated areas in the mouth should be reported to the physician. The importance of keeping scheduled appointments to assess the stability of the fixation appliance is emphasized.

Consultation with a dietitian may be indicated so that the patient and family can learn about foods that are high in essential nutrients and ways in which these foods can be prepared so that they can be consumed through a straw or spoon while remaining palatable. Nutritional supplements may be recommended.

Disorders of the Salivary Glands

The salivary glands consist of the parotid glands, one on each side of the face below the ear; the submandibular and sublingual glands, both in the floor of the mouth; and the buccal gland, beneath the lips. About 1200 mL of saliva are produced daily and swallowed. The glands' primary functions are lubrication, protection against harmful bacteria, and digestion.

Parotitis

Parotitis (inflammation of the parotid gland) is the most common inflammatory condition of the salivary glands, although inflammation can occur in the other salivary glands as well. Mumps (epidemic parotitis), a communicable disease caused by viral infection and most commonly affecting children, is an inflammation of a salivary gland, usually the parotid.

Elderly, acutely ill, or debilitated people with decreased salivary flow from general dehydration or medications are at high risk for parotitis. The infecting organisms travel from the mouth through the salivary duct. The organism is usually *Staphylococcus aureus* (except in mumps). The onset of this complication is sudden, with an exacerbation of both the fever and the symptoms of the primary condition. The gland swells and becomes tense and tender. The patient feels pain in the ear, and swollen glands interfere with swallowing. The swelling increases rapidly, and the overlying skin soon becomes red and shiny.

Medical management includes maintaining adequate nutritional and fluid intake, good oral hygiene, and discontinuing medications (eg, tranquilizers, diuretics) that can diminish salivation. Antibiotic therapy is necessary, and analgesics may be prescribed to control pain. If antibiotic therapy is not effective, the gland may need to be drained by a surgical procedure known as parotidectomy. This procedure may be necessary to treat chronic parotitis. The patient is advised to have any necessary dental work performed prior to surgery.

Sialadenitis

Sialadenitis (inflammation of the salivary glands) may be caused by dehydration, radiation therapy, stress, malnutrition, salivary gland calculi (stones), or improper oral hygiene. The inflammation is associated with infection by *S. aureus*, *Streptococcus viridans*, or pneumococci. In hospitalized or institutionalized patients, the infecting organism may be methicillin-resistant *S. aureus* (MRSA). Symptoms include pain, swelling, and purulent discharge. Antibiotics are used to treat infections. Massage, hydration, warm compresses, and corticosteroids frequently cure the problem. Chronic sialadenitis with uncontrolled pain is treated by surgical drainage of the gland or excision of the gland and its duct.

Salivary Calculus (Sialolithiasis)

Sialolithiasis, or salivary calculi (stones), usually occurs in the submandibular gland. Salivary gland ultrasonography or sialography (x-ray studies filmed after the injection of a radiopaque substance into the duct) may be required to demonstrate obstruction of the duct by stenosis. Salivary calculi are formed mainly from calcium phosphate. If located within the gland, the calculi are irregular and vary in diameter from 3 to 30 mm. Calculi in the duct are small and oval.

Calculi within the salivary gland itself cause no symptoms unless infection arises; however, a calculus that obstructs the gland's duct causes sudden, local, and often colicky pain, which is abruptly relieved by a gush of saliva. This characteristic symptom is often disclosed in the patient's health history. On physical assessment, the gland is swollen and quite tender, the stone itself can be palpable, and its shadow may be seen on x-ray films.

The calculus can be extracted fairly easily from the duct in the mouth. Sometimes, enlargement of the ductal orifice permits the stone to pass spontaneously. Occasionally **lithotripsy**, a procedure that uses shock waves to disintegrate the stone, may be used instead of surgical extraction for parotid stones and smaller submandibular stones. Lithotripsy requires no anesthesia, sedation, or analgesia. Side effects can include local hemorrhage and swelling. Surgery may be necessary to remove the gland if symptoms and calculi recur repeatedly.

Neoplasms

Although they are uncommon, neoplasms (tumors or growths) of almost any type may develop in the salivary gland. Tumors occur more often in the parotid gland. The incidence of salivary gland tumors is similar in men and women. Risk factors include prior exposure to radiation to the head and neck. Diagnosis is based on the health history and physical examination and the results of fine-needle aspiration biopsy.

Management of salivary gland tumors may involve partial excision of the gland, along with the tumor and a wide margin of surrounding tissue. Dissection is carefully performed to preserve the seventh cranial nerve (facial nerve), although it may not be possible to do so if the tumor is extensive. If the tumor is malignant, radiation therapy may follow surgery. Radiation therapy alone may be a treatment choice for tumors that are thought to be localized or if there is risk of facial nerve damage from surgical intervention. Chemotherapy is usually used for palliative purposes. Local recurrences are common, and the recurrent tumors usually are more aggressive than the original. Patients with salivary gland tumors have an increased incidence of second primary cancers (Bull, 2001).

Cancer of the Oral Cavity

Cancers of the oral cavity, which can occur in any part of the mouth or throat, are curable if discovered early. If the cancer is detected before it has spread to the lymph nodes, the 5-year survival rate is approximately 80% (American Cancer Society, 2005). Oral cancers are often associated with the use of alcohol and tobacco, which if used together have a synergistic carcinogenic effect. About 95% of oral cancers occur in people older than 40 years of age, but the incidence is increasing in men younger than 30 years because of the use of smokeless tobacco, especially snuff (Centers for Disease Control and Prevention, 2004). Men are more likely to use smokeless tobacco than women, and Caucasian men have the highest percentage of smokeless tobacco use, at 18% (American Cancer Society, 2005).

Cancer of the oral cavity affects men more often than women; however, the incidence of oral cancer in women is increasing, possibly because they use tobacco and alcohol more frequently than they did in the past. Cancers of the oral cavity and oropharynx occur more often in African Americans than in Caucasians.

Approximately 30,000 new cases of oral cavity and oropharyngeal cancer occur annually in the United States (American Cancer Society, 2005). For the past 20 years, the number of new cases has been decreasing; it has decreased by 5% per year for the past 2 years. In addition, since the late 1970s, the death rate has been decreasing. Eighty-one percent of patients with cancer of the oral cavity and oropharynx survive at least 1 year after diagnosis. Regardless of the stage of cancer at diagnosis, the 5-year relative survival rate is 56% and the 10-year survival rate is 41%.

Chronic irritation by a warm pipe stem or prolonged exposure to the sun and wind may predispose a person to lip cancer. Predisposing factors for other oral cancers are exposure to tobacco (including smokeless tobacco), ingestion of alcohol, dietary deficiency, and ingestion of smoked meats.

Pathophysiology

Malignancies of the oral cavity are usually squamous cell cancers. Any area of the oropharynx can be a site of malignant growths, but the lips, the lateral aspects of the tongue, and the floor of the mouth are most commonly affected.

Clinical Manifestations

Many oral cancers produce few or no symptoms in the early stages. Later, the most frequent symptom is a painless sore or mass that will not heal. A typical lesion in oral cancer is a painless indurated (hardened) ulcer with raised edges. Tissue from any ulcer of the oral cavity that does not heal in 2 weeks should be examined through biopsy. As the cancer progresses, the patient may complain of tenderness; difficulty in chewing, swallowing, or speaking; coughing of blood-tinged sputum; or enlarged cervical lymph nodes.

Assessment and Diagnostic Findings

Diagnostic evaluation consists of an oral examination as well as an assessment of the cervical lymph nodes to detect possible metastases. Biopsies are performed on suspicious lesions (those that have not healed in 2 weeks). High-risk areas include the buccal mucosa and gingiva in people who use snuff or smoke cigars or pipes. For those who smoke cigarettes and drink alcohol, high-risk areas include the floor of the mouth, the ventrolateral tongue, and the soft palate complex (soft palate, anterior and posterior tonsillar area, uvula, and the area behind the molar and tongue junction).

Medical Management

Management varies with the nature of the lesion, the preference of the physician, and patient choice. Surgical resection, radiation therapy, chemotherapy, or a combination of these therapies may be effective.

In cancer of the lip, small lesions are usually excised liberally. Radiation therapy may be more appropriate for larger lesions involving more than one third of the lip because of superior cosmetic results. The choice depends on the extent of the lesion and what is necessary to cure the patient while preserving the best appearance. Tumors larger than 4 cm often recur.

In cancer of the tongue, treatment with radiation therapy and chemotherapy may preserve organ function and maintain quality of life. A combination of radioactive interstitial implants (surgical implantation of a radioactive source into the tissue adjacent to or at the tumor site) and external beam radiation may be used. Surgical procedures include hemiglossectomy (surgical removal of half of the tongue) and total glossectomy (removal of the tongue).

Often cancer of the oral cavity has metastasized through the extensive lymphatic channel in the neck region (Fig. 35-1), requiring a neck dissection and reconstructive surgery of the oral cavity. A common reconstructive technique involves use of a radial forearm free flap (a thin layer of skin from the forearm along with the radial artery).

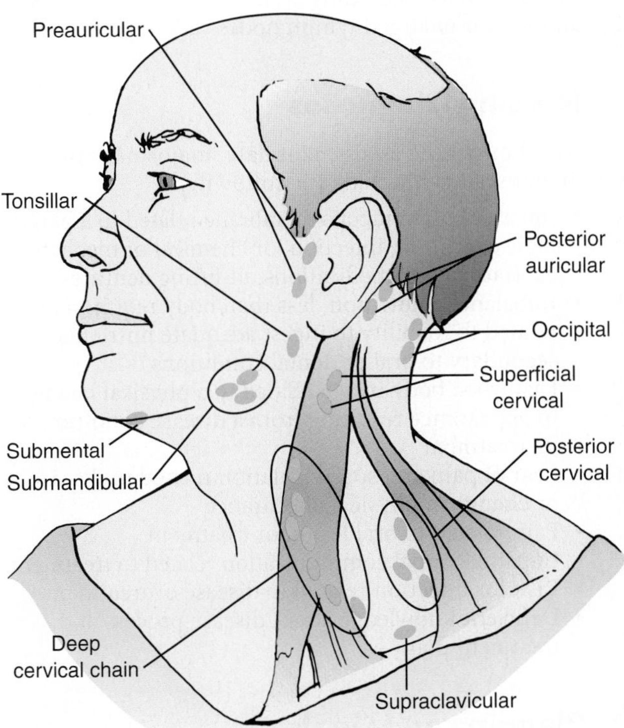

FIGURE 35-1. Lymphatic drainage of the head and neck.

Nursing Management

The nurse assesses the patient's nutritional status preoperatively, and a dietary consultation may be necessary. The patient may require enteral (through the gastrointestinal tract) or parenteral (intravenous [IV]) feedings before and after surgery to maintain adequate nutrition. If a radial graft is to be performed, an Allen test on the donor arm must be performed to ensure that the ulnar artery is patent and can provide blood flow to the hand after removal of the radial artery. The Allen test is performed by asking the patient to make a fist and then manually compressing the ulnar artery. The patient is then asked to open the hand into a relaxed, slightly flexed position. The palm will be pale. Pressure on the ulnar artery is released. If the ulnar artery is patent, the palm will flush within about 3 to 5 seconds.

Postoperatively, the nurse assesses for a patent airway. The patient may be unable to manage oral secretions, making suctioning necessary. If grafting was part of the surgery, suctioning must be performed with care to prevent damage to the graft. The graft is assessed postoperatively for viability. Although color should be assessed (white may indicate arterial occlusion, and blue mottling may indicate venous congestion), it can be difficult to assess the graft by looking into the mouth. A Doppler ultrasound device may be used to locate the radial pulse at the graft site and to assess graft perfusion.

Nursing Process

The Patient With Conditions of the Oral Cavity

Assessment

Obtaining a health history allows the nurse to determine the patient's learning needs concerning preventive oral hygiene and to identify symptoms requiring medical evaluation. The history addresses the patient's normal brushing and flossing routine; frequency of dental visits; awareness of any lesions or irritated areas in the mouth, tongue, or throat; recent history of sore throat or bloody sputum; discomfort caused by certain foods; daily food intake; use of alcohol and tobacco, including smokeless chewing tobacco; and the need to wear dentures or a partial plate. For more information about dentures, see Chart 35-3.

A careful physical assessment follows the health history. Both the internal and the external structures of the mouth and throat are inspected and palpated. Dentures and partial plates are removed to ensure a thorough inspection of the mouth. In general, the examination can be accomplished by using a bright light source (penlight) and a tongue depressor. Gloves are worn to palpate the tongue and any abnormalities.

Lips

The examination begins with inspection of the lips for moisture, hydration, color, texture, symmetry, and

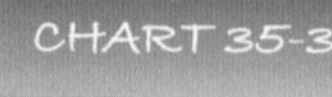
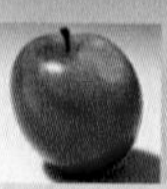

Health Promotion

Denture Care

- Brush dentures twice a day.
- Remove dentures at night and soak them in water or a denture product. (Never put dentures in hot water, because they may warp.)
- Rinse mouth with warm salt water in the morning, after meals, and at bedtime.
- Clean well under partial dentures, where food particles tend to get caught.
- Consume nonsticky foods that have been cut into small pieces; chew slowly.
- See dentist regularly to assess and adjust fit.

the presence of ulcerations or fissures. The lips should be moist, pink, smooth, and symmetric. The patient is instructed to open the mouth wide; a tongue blade is then inserted to expose the buccal mucosa for an assessment of color and lesions. Stensen's duct of each parotid gland is visible as a small red dot in the buccal mucosa next to the upper molars.

Gums

The gums are inspected for inflammation, bleeding, retraction, and discoloration. The odor of the breath is also noted. The hard palate is examined for color and shape.

Tongue

The dorsum (back) of the tongue is inspected for texture, color, and lesions. A thin white coat and large, vallate papillae in a "V" formation on the distal portion of the dorsum of the tongue are normal findings. The patient is instructed to protrude the tongue and move it laterally. This provides the examiner with an opportunity to estimate the tongue's size as well as its symmetry and strength (to assess the integrity of the 12th cranial nerve [hypoglossal]).

Further inspection of the ventral surface of the tongue and the floor of the mouth is accomplished by asking the patient to touch the roof of the mouth with the tip of the tongue. Any lesions of the mucosa or any abnormalities involving the frenulum or superficial veins on the undersurface of the tongue are assessed for location, size, color, and pain. This is a common area for oral cancer, which presents as a white or red plaque, an indurated ulcer, or a warty growth.

A tongue blade is used to depress the tongue for adequate visualization of the pharynx. It is pressed firmly beyond the midpoint of the tongue; proper placement avoids a gagging response. The patient is told to tip the head back, open the mouth wide, take a deep breath, and say "ah." Often this flattens the posterior tongue and briefly allows a full view of the tonsils, uvula, and posterior pharynx (Fig. 35-2). These structures are inspected for color, symmetry, and evidence of exudate, ulceration, or enlargement. Normally, the uvula and soft palate rise symmetrically with a deep inspiration or "ah"; this indicates an intact vagus nerve (10th cranial nerve).

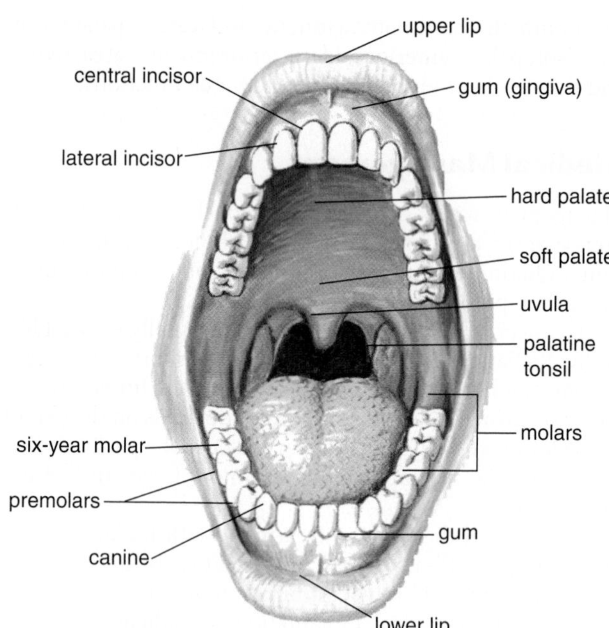

FIGURE 35-2. Structures of the mouth, including the tongue and palate.

A complete assessment of the oral cavity is essential because many disorders, such as cancer, diabetes, and immunosuppressive conditions resulting from medication therapy or acquired immunodeficiency syndrome (AIDS), may be manifested by changes in the oral cavity, including stomatitis. The neck is examined for enlarged lymph nodes (adenopathy).

Nursing Diagnoses

Based on all the assessment data, major nursing diagnoses may include the following:

- Impaired oral mucous membrane related to a pathologic condition, infection, or chemical or mechanical trauma (eg, medications, ill-fitting dentures)
- Imbalanced nutrition, less than body requirements, related to inability to ingest adequate nutrients secondary to oral or dental conditions
- Disturbed body image related to a physical change in appearance resulting from a disease condition or its treatment
- Fear of pain and social isolation related to disease or change in physical appearance
- Pain related to oral lesion or treatment
- Impaired verbal communication related to treatment
- Risk for infection related to disease or treatment
- Deficient knowledge about disease process and treatment plan

Planning and Goals

The major goals for the patient may include improved condition of the oral mucous membrane, improved nutritional intake, attainment of a positive self-image, relief of pain, identification of alternative communication methods, prevention of infection, and understanding of the disease and its treatment.

Nursing Interventions

Promoting Mouth Care

The nurse instructs the patient in the importance and techniques of preventive mouth care. If a patient cannot tolerate brushing or flossing, an irrigating solution of 1 teaspoon of baking soda to 8 ounces of warm water, half-strength hydrogen peroxide, or normal saline solution is recommended. The nurse reinforces the need to perform oral care and provides such care to patients who cannot provide it for themselves.

If a bacterial or fungal infection is present, the nurse administers the appropriate medications and instructs the patient in how to administer the medications at home. The nurse monitors the patient's physical and psychological response to treatment.

Xerostomia, dryness of the mouth, is a frequent sequela of oral cancer, particularly when the salivary glands have been exposed to radiation or major surgery. It is also seen in patients who are receiving psychopharmacologic agents, patients with human immunodeficiency virus (HIV) infection, and patients who cannot close the mouth and as a result become mouth-breathers. To minimize this problem, the patient is advised to avoid dry, bulky, and irritating foods and fluids, as well as alcohol and tobacco. The patient is also encouraged to increase intake of fluids (when not contraindicated) and to use a humidifier during sleep. The use of synthetic saliva, a moisturizing antibacterial gel such as Oral Balance, or a saliva production stimulant such as Salagen may be helpful.

Stomatitis, or mucositis, which involves inflammation and breakdown of the oral mucosa, is often a side effect of chemotherapy or radiation therapy. Prophylactic mouth care is started when the patient begins receiving treatment; however, mucositis may become so severe that a break in treatment is necessary. If a patient receiving radiation therapy has poor dentition, extraction of the teeth before radiation treatment in the oral cavity is often initiated to prevent infection. Many radiation therapy centers recommend the use of fluoride treatments for patients receiving radiation to the head and neck. (See Chapter 16 for more information about stomatitis.)

Ensuring Adequate Food and Fluid Intake

The patient's weight, age, and level of activity are recorded to determine whether nutritional intake is adequate. A daily calorie count may be necessary to determine the exact quantity of food and fluid ingested. The frequency and pattern of eating are recorded to determine whether any psychosocial or physiologic factors are affecting ingestion. Based on the disorder and the patient's preferences, the nurse recommends changes in the consistency of foods and the frequency of eating. Consultation with a dietitian may be helpful. The goal is to help the patient attain and maintain desirable body weight and level of energy, as well as to promote the healing of tissue.

Supporting a Positive Self-Image

A patient who has a disfiguring oral condition or has undergone disfiguring surgery may experience an alteration in self-image. The patient is encouraged to verbalize the perceived change in body appearance and to realistically discuss actual changes or losses. The nurse offers support while the patient verbalizes fears and negative feelings (withdrawal, depression, anger). The nurse listens attentively and determines the patient's needs and individualizes the plan of care. The patient's strengths, achievements, and positive attributes are reinforced.

The nurse should determine the patient's anxieties concerning relationships with others. Referral to support groups, a psychiatric liaison nurse, a social worker, or a spiritual advisor may be useful in helping the patient to cope with anxieties and fears. The patient's progress toward development of positive self-esteem is documented. The nurse should be alert to signs of grieving and should document emotional changes. By providing acceptance and support, the nurse encourages the patient to verbalize feelings.

Minimizing Pain and Discomfort

Oral lesions can be painful. Strategies to reduce pain and discomfort include avoiding foods that are spicy, hot, or hard (eg, pretzels, nuts). The patient is instructed about mouth care. It may be necessary to provide the patient with an analgesic such as viscous lidocaine (Xylocaine Viscous 2%) or opioids, as prescribed. The nurse can reduce the patient's fear of pain by providing information about pain control methods.

Promoting Effective Communication

Verbal communication may be impaired by radical surgery for oral cancer. It is therefore vital to assess the patient's ability to communicate in writing before surgery. Pen and paper are provided postoperatively to patients who can use them to communicate. A communication board with commonly used words or pictures is obtained preoperatively and given after surgery to patients who cannot write so that they may point to needed items. A speech therapist is also consulted postoperatively.

Preventing Infection

Leukopenia (a decrease in white blood cells) may result from radiation, chemotherapy, AIDS, and some medications used to treat HIV infection. Leukopenia reduces defense mechanisms, increasing the risk for infections. Malnutrition, which is also common among these patients, may further decrease resistance to infection. If the patient has diabetes, the risk for infection is further increased.

Laboratory results should be evaluated frequently and the patient's temperature checked every 4 to 8 hours for an elevation that may indicate infection. Visitors who might transmit microorganisms are prohibited if the patient's immunologic system is depressed. Sensitive skin tissues are protected from trauma to maintain skin integrity and prevent infection. Aseptic technique is necessary when changing dressings. Desquamation (shedding of the epidermis) is a reaction to radiation therapy that causes dryness and itching and can lead to a break in skin integrity and subsequent infection.

As previously described, adequate nutrition is helpful in preventing infection. Signs of wound infection (redness, swelling, drainage, tenderness) are reported to the physician. Antibiotics may be prescribed prophylactically.

Promoting Home and Community-Based Care

TEACHING PATIENTS SELF-CARE

The patient who is recovering from treatment of an oral condition is instructed about mouth care, nutrition, prevention of infection, and signs and symptoms of complications (Chart 35-4). Methods of preparing nutritious foods that are seasoned according to the patient's preference and at the preferred temperature are explained. For some patients, it may be more convenient to use commercial baby foods than to prepare liquid and soft diets. The patient who cannot take foods orally may receive enteral or parenteral nutrition; the administration of these feedings is explained and demonstrated to the patient and the caregiver.

For patients with cancer, instructions are provided in the use and care of any dentures. The importance of keeping dressings clean and the need for conscientious oral hygiene are emphasized.

CONTINUING CARE

The need for ongoing care in the home depends on the patient's condition. The patient, the family members or others responsible for home care, the nurse, and other health care professionals (eg, speech therapist, nutritionist, psychologist) work together to prepare an individual plan of care.

If suctioning of the mouth or tracheostomy tube is required, the necessary equipment is obtained and the patient and caregivers are taught how to use it. Considerations include the control of odors and humidification of the home to keep secretions moist. The patient and caregivers are taught how to assess for obstruction, hemorrhage, and infection and what actions to take if they occur. The home care nurse may provide physical care, monitor for changes in the patient's physical status (eg, skin integrity, nutritional status, respiratory function), and assess the adequacy of pain control measures. The nurse also assesses the patient's and family's ability to manage incisions, drains, and feeding tubes and the use of recommended strategies for communication. The ability of the patient and family to accept physical, psychological, and role changes is assessed and addressed.

Follow-up visits to the physician are important to monitor the patient's condition and to determine the need for modifications in treatment and general care. The nurse reinforces instructions in an effort to promote the patient's self-care and comfort.

Because patients and their family members and health care providers tend to focus on the most obvious needs and issues, the nurse reminds the patient and family about the importance of continuing health promotion and screening practices. Patients who have not been involved in these practices in the past are educated about their importance and are referred to appropriate health care providers.

Evaluation

Expected Patient Outcomes

Expected patient outcomes may include:

1. Shows evidence of intact oral mucous membranes
   a. Is free of pain and discomfort in the oral cavity
   b. Has no visible alteration in membrane integrity
   c. Identifies and avoids foods that are irritating (eg, nuts, pretzels, spicy foods)
   d. Describes measures that are necessary for preventive mouth care

CHART 35-4

HOME CARE CHECKLIST • The Patient With an Oral Condition

At the completion of the home care instruction, the patient or caregiver will be able to:	Patient	Caregiver
• Demonstrate use of suction equipment if indicated.	✔	✔
• State rationale for humidification.	✔	✔
• Identify foods necessary to meet caloric needs and dietary needs (ie, change in consistency, seasoning limitations, supplements).	✔	✔
• Demonstrate effective oral hygiene.	✔	✔
• Demonstrate care of incision.	✔	✔
• State when next medical/dental follow-up appointment will be scheduled.	✔	✔

   e. Complies with medication regimen
   f. Limits or avoids use of alcohol and tobacco (including smokeless tobacco)
2. Attains and maintains desirable body weight
3. Has a positive self-image
   a. Verbalizes anxieties
   b. Is able to accept change in appearance and modify self-concept accordingly
4. Attains an acceptable level of comfort
   a. Verbalizes that pain is absent or under control
   b. Avoids foods and liquids that cause discomfort
   c. Adheres to medication regimen
5. Has decreased fears related to pain, isolation, and the inability to cope
   a. Accepts that pain will be managed if not eliminated
   b. Freely expresses fears and concerns
6. Is free of infection
   a. Exhibits normal laboratory values
   b. Is afebrile
   c. Performs oral hygiene after every meal and at bedtime
7. Acquires information about disease process and course of treatment

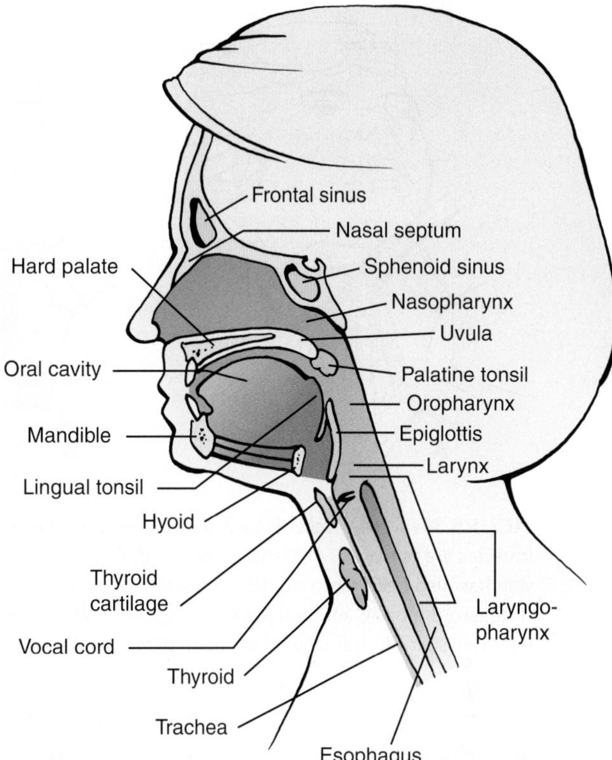

FIGURE 35-3. Anatomy of the head and neck.

Neck Dissection

Malignancies of the head and neck include those of the oral cavity, oropharynx, hypopharynx, nasopharynx, nasal cavity, paranasal sinus, and larynx (Fig. 35-3). (Laryngeal cancer is presented in Chapter 22.) These cancers account for fewer than 5% of all cancers. Depending on the location and stage, treatment may consist of radiation therapy, chemotherapy, surgery, or a combination of these modalities. Deaths from malignancies of the head and neck are primarily attributable to local-regional metastasis to the cervical lymph nodes in the neck. This often occurs by way of the lymphatics before the primary lesion has been treated. This local-regional metastasis is not amenable to surgical resection and responds poorly to chemotherapy and radiation therapy.

A radical neck dissection involves removal of all cervical lymph nodes from the mandible to the clavicle and removal of the sternocleidomastoid muscle, internal jugular vein, and spinal accessory muscle on one side of the neck. The associated complications include shoulder drop and poor cosmesis (visible neck depression). Modified radical neck dissection, which preserves one or more of the nonlymphatic structures, is used more often. A selective neck dissection (in comparison to a radical dissection) preserves one or more of the lymph node groups, the internal jugular vein, the sternocleidomastoid muscle, and the spinal accessory nerve (Fig. 35-4).

Reconstructive techniques may be performed with a variety of grafts. A cutaneous flap (skin and subcutaneous tissue), such as the deltopectoral flap, may be used. A myocutaneous flap (subcutaneous tissue, muscle and skin) is a more frequently used graft; the pectoralis major muscle is usually used. For large grafts, a microvascular free flap may be used. This involves the transfer of muscle, skin, or bone with an artery and vein to the area of reconstruction, using microinstrumentation. Areas used for a free flap include the scapula, the radial area of the forearm, or the fibula. The fibula, which provides a larger bone area, may be used if mandibular reconstruction is involved.

Nursing Process

The Patient Undergoing a Neck Dissection

Assessment

Preoperatively, the patient's physical and psychological preparation for major surgery is assessed, along with his or her knowledge of the preoperative and postoperative procedures. Postoperatively, the patient is assessed for complications such as altered respiratory status, wound infection, and hemorrhage. As healing occurs, neck range of motion is assessed to determine whether there has been a decrease in range of motion due to nerve or muscle damage.

Diagnosis

Nursing Diagnoses

Based on all the assessment data, major nursing diagnoses may include the following:

- Deficient knowledge about preoperative and postoperative procedures

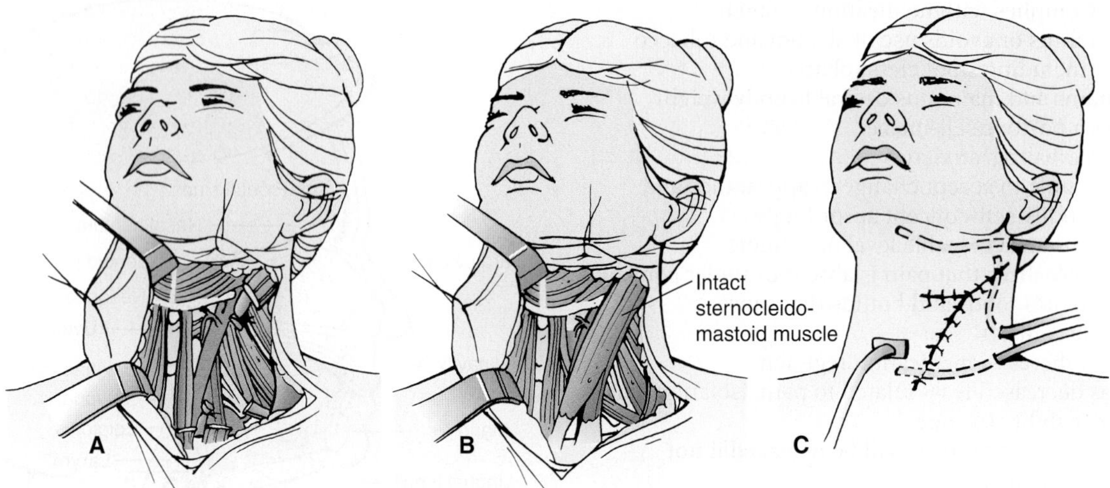

FIGURE 35-4. (**A**) A classic radical neck dissection in which the sternocleidomastoid and smaller muscles are removed. All tissue is removed, from the ramus of the jaw to the clavicle. The jugular vein has also been removed. (**B**) The selective neck dissection is similar but preserves the sternocleidomastoid muscle, internal jugular vein, and spinal accessory nerve. The wound is closed (**C**), and portable suction drainage tubes are in place.

- Ineffective airway clearance related to obstruction by mucus, hemorrhage, or edema
- Acute pain related to surgical incision
- Risk for infection related to surgical intervention secondary to decreased nutritional status, or immunosuppression from chemotherapy or radiation therapy
- Impaired tissue integrity secondary to surgery and grafting
- Imbalanced nutrition, less than body requirements, related to disease process or treatment
- Situational low self-esteem related to diagnosis or prognosis
- Impaired verbal communication secondary to surgical resection
- Impaired physical mobility secondary to nerve injury

Collaborative Problems/ Potential Complications

Potential postoperative complications that may develop include the following:

- Hemorrhage
- Chyle fistula
- Nerve injury

Planning and Goals

The major goals for the patient include participation in the treatment plan, maintenance of respiratory status, attainment of comfort, absence of infection, viability of the graft, maintenance of adequate intake of food and fluids, effective coping strategies, effective communication, maintenance of shoulder and neck motion, and absence of complications.

Nursing Interventions

Providing Preoperative Patient Education

Before surgery, the patient should be informed about the nature and extent of the surgery, and what the postoperative period will be like. The patient is encouraged to ask questions and to express concerns about the upcoming surgery and the expected results. During this exchange, the nurse has an opportunity to assess the patient's coping abilities, answer questions, and develop a plan for offering assistance. A sense of mutual understanding and rapport make the postoperative experience less traumatic for the patient. The patient's expressions of concern, anxieties, and fears guide the nurse in providing support postoperatively.

Providing General Postoperative Care

The general postoperative nursing interventions are similar to those presented in Chapter 20. For the patient who has had extensive neck surgery, specific postoperative interventions include maintenance of a patent airway and continuous assessment of respiratory status, wound care and oral hygiene, maintenance of adequate nutrition, and observation for hemorrhage or nerve injury.

Maintaining the Airway

After the endotracheal tube or airway has been removed and the effects of the anesthesia have worn off, the patient may be placed in Fowler's position to facilitate breathing and promote comfort. This position also increases lymphatic and venous drainage, facilitates swallowing, and decreases venous pressure on the skin flaps.

In the immediate postoperative period, the nurse assesses for stridor (coarse, high-pitched sound on inspiration) by listening frequently over the trachea with a stethoscope. This finding must be reported immediately because it indicates obstruction of the airway. Signs of respiratory distress, such as dyspnea, cyanosis, changes in mental status, and changes in vital signs, are assessed because they may suggest edema, hemorrhage, inadequate oxygenation, or inadequate drainage.

Pneumonia may occur in the postoperative phase if pulmonary secretions are not removed. To aid in the removal of secretions, coughing and deep breathing are encouraged. The patient should assume a sitting position, with the nurse supporting the neck so that the patient can bring up excessive secretions. If this is ineffective, the patient's respiratory tract may have to be suctioned. Care is taken to protect the suture lines during suctioning. If a tracheostomy tube is in place, suctioning is performed through the tube. The patient may also be instructed on use of Yankauer suction (tonsil tip suction) to remove oral secretions. Temperature should not be taken orally.

Relieving Pain

Pain and the patient's fear of pain are assessed and managed. Patients with head and neck cancer often report less pain than patients with other types of cancer; however, the nurse needs to be aware that each person's pain experience is individual. The nurse administers analgesics as prescribed and assesses their effectiveness.

Providing Wound Care

Wound drainage tubes are usually inserted during surgery to prevent the collection of fluid subcutaneously. The drainage tubes are connected to a portable suction device (eg, Jackson-Pratt), and the container is emptied periodically. Between 80 and 120 mL of serosanguineous secretions may drain over the first 24 hours. Excessive drainage may be indicative of a chyle fistula or hemorrhage (see later discussion). If dressings are present, they may need to be reinforced periodically. Dressings are observed for evidence of hemorrhage and constriction, which impairs respiration and perfusion of the graft. A graft, if present, is assessed for color and temperature, and for the presence of a pulse if applicable, to determine viability. The graft should be pale pink and warm to the touch. The surgical incisions are also assessed for infection, which is reported immediately. Prophylactic antibiotics may be prescribed.

Maintaining Adequate Nutrition

Nutritional status is assessed preoperatively; early intervention to correct nutritional imbalances may decrease the risk of postoperative complications. Frequently, nutrition is less than optimal because of inadequate intake, and the patient often requires enteral or parenteral supplements preoperatively and postoperatively to attain and maintain a positive nitrogen balance. Supplements (eg, Ensure, Sustacal) that are nutritionally dense may help reestablish a positive nitrogen balance. They may be taken enterally by mouth, by nasogastric feeding tube, or by gastrostomy feeding tube. (See the Plan of Nursing Care in Chart 35-5 for further discussion.)

The patient who can chew may take food by mouth; the level of the patient's chewing ability determines whether some diet modification (eg, soft, puréed, or liquid foods) is necessary. Food preferences should also be discussed with the patient. Oral care before eating may enhance the patient's appetite, and oral care after eating is important to prevent infection and dental caries. Most patients can maintain and gain weight.

Supporting Coping Measures

Preoperatively, information about the planned surgery is given to the patient and family. Postoperatively, psychological nursing interventions are aimed at supporting the patient who has had a change in body image or who has major concerns regarding the prognosis. The patient may have difficulty communicating and may be concerned about his or her ability to breathe and swallow normally. The nurse supports the patient's family and friends in encouraging and reassuring the patient that adjusting to the results of this surgery will take time.

The person who has had extensive neck surgery often is sensitive about his or her appearance. This can occur when the operative area is covered by bulky dressings, when the incision line is visible, or later after healing has occurred and the appearance of the neck and possibly the lower face has been significantly altered. If the nurse accepts the patient's appearance and expresses a positive, optimistic attitude, the patient is more likely to be encouraged. The patient also needs an opportunity to express concerns regarding the success of the surgery and the prognosis. The American Cancer Society may be a resource to provide a volunteer to meet with the patient either preoperatively or postoperatively.

People with cancer of the head and neck frequently have used alcohol or tobacco before surgery; postoperatively, the patient is encouraged to abstain from these substances. Alternative methods of coping need to be explored. A referral to Alcoholics Anonymous may be appropriate.

Promoting Effective Communication

If a laryngectomy was performed, the nurse explores other methods of communicating with the patient and obtains a consultation with a speech/language therapist. Alternatives to verbal communication may include use of a pencil and paper or pointing to needed items on a picture pad. Alternative speech techniques, such as an electrolarynx (a mechanical device held against the neck) or esophageal speech, may be taught by a speech/language therapist.

(text continues on page 1159)

CHART 35-5

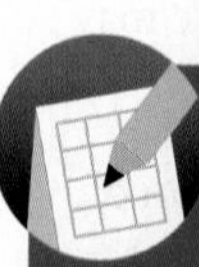

Plan of Nursing Care: The Patient Who Has Undergone Neck Dissection

Nursing Diagnosis: Ineffective airway clearance related to obstruction secondary to edema, hemorrhage, or inadequate wound drainage
Goal: Maintenance of normal respiratory function

NURSING INTERVENTIONS	RATIONALE	EXPECTED OUTCOMES
1. Place the patient in Fowler's position.	1. Fowler's position facilitates expansion of the lungs because the diaphragm is pulled downward and the abdominal viscera are pulled away from the lungs. Breathing is promoted. This position also increases lymphatic and venous drainage, and decreases venous pressure on the graft. Regurgitation and aspiration of stomach contents are prevented postoperatively.	• Achieves a normal respiratory rate • Breathes comfortably • Avoids use of accessory muscles of respiration • Maintains vital signs within patient's normal range • Shows evidence of normal breath sounds • Coughs effectively • Maintains a patent airway • Does not develop a mucus plug
2. Monitor vital signs according to postoperative routine.	2. Edema, hemorrhage, or inadequate drainage will alter heart rate and respirations. Tachypnea and restlessness may indicate respiratory distress.	
3. Auscultate breath sounds as needed. In the immediate postoperative period, place the stethoscope over the trachea to assess for stridor.	3. Abnormal breath sounds may indicate ineffective ventilation, decreased perfusion, and fluid accumulation. Stridor, a harsh, high-pitched sound primarily heard on inspiration, indicates airway obstruction.	
4. Encourage deep breathing and coughing. Place the patient in a sitting position and support the neck area with both hands.	4. Deep breathing before coughing promotes expansion of the airways and a more forceful cough. The coughing mechanism assists airway cilia with removal of secretions. Splinting the incision during coughing reduces strain and promotes the expulsion of secretions by allowing deeper inspirations.	
5. Suction the airway as needed using sterile technique and a soft catheter.	5. Suctioning assists in removal of secretions that the patient may be unable to cough up, thereby assisting with maintaining a patent airway.	
6. Provide humidified air or oxygen if the patient has a tracheostomy.	6. Keeps secretions thin.	

CHART 35-5

Plan of Nursing Care: The Patient Who Has Undergone Neck Dissection (Continued)

Nursing Diagnosis: Risk for infection
Goal: Absence of infection

NURSING INTERVENTIONS	RATIONALE	EXPECTED OUTCOMES
1. Instruct the patient in preoperative and postoperative oral hygiene using slightly alkaline solutions such as 8 oz of water mixed with 1 teaspoon of baking soda, or normal saline solution, every 4 hours.	1. Oral care decreases oral bacteria, thereby decreasing the risk of bacterial infection postoperatively. Hydrogen peroxide should not be used, because it may break down fresh granulation tissue.	• Patient performs oral hygiene preoperatively and postoperatively every 4 hours • Mouth remains clean • Wound drains less than 200 mL of serosanguineous drainage on the first postoperative day • No hematoma at skin graft • Serosanguineous drainage is within normal limits • Dressing remains intact with no constriction of airway or blood flow • Wound and surrounding skin remain clean and free of infection • Patient is afebrile with normal respirations and a normal heart rate • Patient is alert and aware of surroundings
2. Monitor wound suction drainage.	2. Suction drainage negates the need for pressure dressings because the skin flaps are pulled down tightly. Drainage should be 80–120 mL of serosanguineous secretions for the first 24 hours; then the secretions should decrease daily. Continuous bloody drainage indicates small vessel oozing.	
3. Note drainage quantity and odor.	3. Purulent, malodorous drainage indicates an infection. Drainage greater than 300 mL in the first 24 hours is considered abnormal.	
4. Assess condition of dressing and reinforce pressure dressings as needed. Assess for any possible constrictions that would affect respirations or decrease blood flow to graft.	4. If portable wound suction is not used, pressure dressings may be applied to obliterate dead spaces and provide immobilization. These dressings are reinforced, not changed, as needed.	
5. Use aseptic technique to cleanse skin around the drains; change the dressings as ordered by surgeon (usually the second through fifth postoperative days).	5. Aseptic technique prevents wound contamination. Sterile saline effectively cleans the skin around the drains.	
6. Monitor vital signs. Assess for symptoms of infection: chills, diaphoresis, altered level of consciousness.	6. An elevated temperature, tachypnea, and tachycardia may indicate an infection.	

Nursing Diagnosis: Impaired skin integrity
Goal: Maintenance of intact skin and viability of graft

NURSING INTERVENTIONS	RATIONALE	EXPECTED OUTCOMES
1. Assess condition of graft for viability.	1. Cyanotic, cool graft indicates possible necrosis. Pale graft indicates arterial thrombosis; purple graft indicates venous congestion.	• Graft is pale pink in color and warm to touch • Tissue blanches to gentle touch

continued >

CHART 35-5

Plan of Nursing Care — The Patient Who Has Undergone Neck Dissection (Continued)

NURSING INTERVENTIONS	RATIONALE	EXPECTED OUTCOMES
2. Assess wound for signs and symptoms of infection.	2. Infected wound interferes with healing and threatens the viability of the graft.	• Graft has pulse via Doppler ultrasound • Patient does not have wound infection

Nursing Diagnosis: Imbalanced nutrition, less than body requirements, related to anorexia and dysphagia
Goal: Attainment/maintenance of adequate nutrition

NURSING INTERVENTIONS	RATIONALE	EXPECTED OUTCOMES
1. Assess nutritional status preoperatively, consult with dietitian.	1. Poor nutritional status preoperatively impairs wound healing and increases potential for infection.	• Does not have weight loss greater than 10% of body weight. (If weight loss is greater than 10%, supplements are given to maintain/increase weight and obtain positive nitrogen balance.) • Tolerates tube feedings • No signs of aspiration • No sign of fistula • Expresses a desire for food • Swallows food easily • Is comfortable eating alone or with others
2. Administer tube feedings as prescribed. Keep head of bed elevated during feeding to prevent aspiration. Monitor for signs of tracheoesophageal fistula (feeding in tracheal secretions).	2. A nasogastric tube may be in place for several days to administer enteral feedings.	
3. Provide oral hygiene before and after meals.	3. Oral hygiene enhances appetite.	
4. Assist with oral intake: a. Offer easily chewed foods; mash or blenderize if necessary. b. Suggest that the head be tilted to the unaffected side when swallowing. c. Inquire whether privacy is desired when eating. d. Provide altered eating utensils as needed.	4. Soft-textured foods facilitate swallowing. Passage of food may be tolerated better when the head is tilted to the unaffected side. Self-feeding difficulties may cause embarrassment and interfere with intake.	

Nursing Diagnosis: Situational low self-esteem and body image related to changes in appearance and alterations in communication
Goal: Attainment of positive self-image

NURSING INTERVENTIONS	RATIONALE	EXPECTED OUTCOMES
1. Assist the patient to communicate effectively: a. Provide materials for writing messages. b. Make certain that the call bell is readily accessible.	1. Temporary hoarseness is common after neck surgery. A tracheostomy may be performed, and verbal communication may not be possible. Communication with head movement may be impossible because of incisional pain and need to maintain position of	• Recognizes that hoarseness is temporary • Develops alternative forms of communication • Willingly conveys fears and concerns • Accepts prognosis with realistic limitations

CHART 35-5

Plan of Nursing Care — The Patient Who Has Undergone Neck Dissection (Continued)

NURSING INTERVENTIONS	RATIONALE	EXPECTED OUTCOMES
c. Develop nonverbal ways to communicate (eg, finger-tapping, sign language, sign board). d. Consult speech/language therapist.	neck for graft. A speech/language therapist may assist with other forms of communication, such as esophageal speech or electrolarynx.	• Accepts support as offered • Absence of facial paralysis • Absence of drooling and dysphagia • Maintains normal shoulder function • Verbalizes methods to enhance physical appearance
2. Encourage verbalization of fears: a. Provide time to listen. b. Project a positive, optimistic attitude. c. Reinforce reality. d. Collaborate with family members to elicit their support and encouragement. e. Consult support groups such as New Voice Club through the American Cancer Society.	2. Listening conveys acceptance and encourages further verbalization. An optimistic approach conveys interest and hope. Honesty will promote a trusting relationship. This includes confirming cosmetic and functional limitations. Family members or significant others can provide valuable support to the patient.	
3. Observe for facial paralysis.	3. Injury to facial nerve will cause lower facial paralysis.	
4. Observe for excessive drooling.	4. Damage to the hypoglossal nerve will result in excessive drooling and decreased ability to swallow.	
5. Check for normal shoulder position and function.	5. Damage to the spinal accessory nerve will result in drooping of the shoulder. Rehabilitation exercises are begun after the incision is healed.	
6. Provide information on clothing/cosmetics to deemphasize physical defects (offer information on "Look Good, Feel Better" program through American Cancer Society).	6. Physical appearance may be enhanced through use of cosmetics or clothing.	

Maintaining Physical Mobility

Excision of muscles and nerves results in weakness at the shoulder that can cause shoulder drop, a forward curvature of the shoulder. Many problems can be avoided with a conscientious exercise program. These exercises are usually begun after the drains have been removed and the neck incision is sufficiently healed. The purpose of the exercises depicted in Figure 35-5 is to promote maximal shoulder function and neck motion after surgery. Physical therapists and occupational therapists can assist patients in performing these exercises.

Monitoring and Managing Potential Complications

HEMORRHAGE

Hemorrhage may occur from carotid artery rupture as a result of necrosis of the graft or damage to the artery itself from tumor or infection. The following measures are indicated:

- Vital signs are assessed. Tachycardia, tachypnea, and hypotension may indicate hemorrhage and impending hypovolemic shock.
- The patient is instructed to avoid the Valsalva maneuver to prevent stress on the graft and carotid artery.

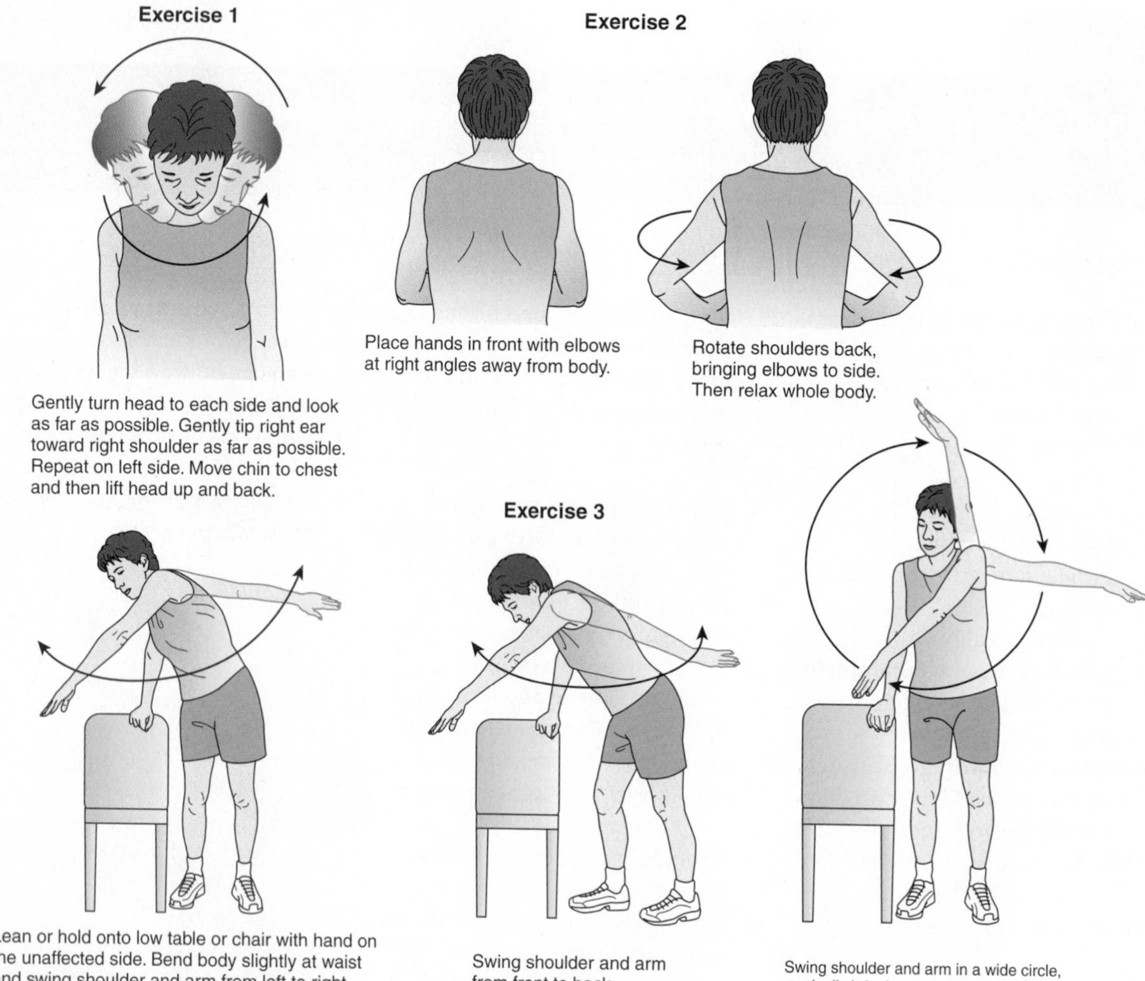

FIGURE 35-5. Three rehabilitation exercises after head and neck surgery. The objective is to regain maximum shoulder function and neck motion after neck surgery. From *Exercise for radical neck surgery patients.* Head and Neck Service, Department of Surgery, Memorial Hospital, New York, NY.

- Signs of impending rupture, such as high epigastric pain or discomfort, are reported.
- Dressings and wound drainage are observed for excessive bleeding.
- If hemorrhage occurs, assistance is summoned immediately.
- Hemorrhage requires the continuous application of pressure to the bleeding site or major associated vessel.
- Although some advocate placing the patient in the modified Trendelenburg position to maintain blood pressure, others recommend that the head of the patient's bed be elevated to maintain airway patency and prevent aspiration.
- A controlled, calm manner allays the patient's anxiety.
- The surgeon is notified immediately, because a vascular or ligature tear requires surgical intervention.

CHYLE FISTULA

A chyle fistula (milk-like drainage from the thoracic duct into the thoracic cavity) may develop as a result of damage to the thoracic duct during surgery. The diagnosis is made if there is excess drainage that has a 3% fat content and a specific gravity of 1.012 or greater. Treatment of a small leak (500 mL or less) includes application of a pressure dressing and a diet of medium-chain fatty acids or parenteral nutrition. Surgical intervention to repair the damaged duct is necessary for larger leaks.

NERVE INJURY

Nerve injury can occur if the cervical plexus or spinal accessory nerves are severed during surgery. Because lower facial paralysis may occur as a result of injury to the facial nerve, this complication is observed for and reported. Likewise, if the superior laryngeal nerve is damaged, the patient may have difficulty swallowing liquids and food because of the partial lack of sensation of the glottis. Speech therapy may be indicated to assist with the problems related to nerve injury.

Promoting Home and Community-Based Care

TEACHING PATIENTS SELF-CARE

The patient and caregiver require instructions about management of the wound, the dressing, and any drains that remain in place. Patients who require oral suctioning or who have a tracheostomy may be very anxious about their care at home; the transition to home can be eased if the caregiver is given several opportunities to demonstrate the ability to meet the patient's needs (Chart 35-6). The patient and caregiver are also instructed about possible complications such as bleeding and respiratory distress and when to notify the health care provider of signs and symptoms of these complications.

If the patient cannot take food by mouth, detailed instructions and demonstration of enteral or parenteral feedings will be required. Education in techniques of effective oral hygiene is also important.

CONTINUING CARE

A referral for home care nursing may be necessary in the early period after discharge. The nurse assesses healing, ensures that feedings are being administered properly, and monitors for any complications. The home care nurse assesses the patient's adjustment to changes in physical appearance and status, and ability to communicate and to eat normally. Physical and speech therapy also may be continued at home.

The patient is given information regarding local support groups such as "I Can Cope" or "New Voice Club," if indicated. The local chapter of the American Cancer Society may be contacted for information and equipment needed for the patient.

Evaluation

Expected Patient Outcomes

Expected patient outcomes may include:

1. Discusses expected course of treatment
2. Demonstrates good respiratory exchange
   a. Lungs are clear to auscultation
   b. Breathes easily with no shortness of breath
   c. Demonstrates ability to use suction effectively
3. Remains free of infection
   a. Maintains normal laboratory values
   b. Is afebrile
4. Graft is pink and warm to touch
5. Maintains adequate intake of foods and fluids
   a. Accepts altered route of feeding
   b. Is well hydrated
   c. Maintains or gains weight
6. Demonstrates ability to cope
   a. Discusses emotional responses to the diagnosis
   b. Attends support group meetings
7. Verbalizes comfort
8. Attains maximal mobility
   a. Adheres to physical therapy exercises
   b. Attains maximal range of motion
9. Exhibits no complications
   a. Vital signs stable
   b. No excessive bleeding or discharge
   c. Able to move muscles of lower face

The Plan of Nursing Care in Chart 35-5 presents an overview of the care of a patient undergoing a neck dissection.

CHART 35-6

HOME CARE CHECKLIST • Recovering From Neck Surgery

At the completion of the home care instruction, the patient or caregiver will be able to:	Patient	Caregiver
• Demonstrate use of suction equipment.	✔	✔
• State rationale for humidification.	✔	✔
• State dietary modifications needed to meet caloric needs.	✔	✔
• Demonstrate enteral or parenteral feeding techniques.	✔	✔
• Demonstrate care of incision and drains.	✔	✔
• Identify signs and symptoms (eg, bleeding, respiratory distress, drainage) to be reported to health care provider.	✔	✔
• State when next checkup is needed.	✔	✔
• Demonstrate exercises.	✔	
• Identify available support groups.	✔	✔

Disorders of the Esophagus

The esophagus is a mucus-lined, muscular tube that carries food from the mouth to the stomach. It begins at the base of the pharynx and ends about 4 cm below the diaphragm. Its ability to transport food and fluid is facilitated by two sphincters. The upper esophageal sphincter, also called the hypopharyngeal sphincter, is located at the junction of the pharynx and the esophagus. The lower esophageal sphincter, also called the gastroesophageal sphincter or cardiac sphincter, is located at the junction of the esophagus and the stomach. An incompetent lower esophageal sphincter allows reflux (backward flow) of gastric contents. There is no serosal layer of the esophagus; therefore, if surgery is necessary, it is more difficult to perform suturing or anastomosis.

Disorders of the esophagus include motility disorders (achalasia, diffuse spasm), hiatal hernias, diverticula, perforation, foreign bodies, chemical burns, gastroesophageal reflux disease, Barrett's esophagus, benign tumors, and carcinoma. **Dysphagia** (difficulty swallowing), the most common symptom of esophageal disease, may vary from an uncomfortable feeling that a bolus of food is caught in the upper esophagus to acute pain on swallowing (**odynophagia**). Obstruction of food (solid and soft) and even liquids may occur anywhere along the esophagus. Often the patient can indicate that the problem is located in the upper, middle, or lower third of the esophagus.

Achalasia

Achalasia is absent or ineffective peristalsis of the distal esophagus, accompanied by failure of the esophageal sphincter to relax in response to swallowing. Narrowing of the esophagus just above the stomach results in a gradually increasing dilation of the esophagus in the upper chest. Achalasia may progress slowly and occurs most often in people 40 years or older.

Clinical Manifestations

The primary symptom is difficulty in swallowing both liquids and solids. The patient has a sensation of food sticking in the lower portion of the esophagus. As the condition progresses, food is commonly regurgitated either spontaneously or intentionally by the patient to relieve the discomfort produced by prolonged distention of the esophagus by food that will not pass into the stomach. The patient may also report chest pain and heartburn (**pyrosis**) that may or may not be associated with eating. Secondary pulmonary complications may result from aspiration of gastric contents.

Assessment and Diagnostic Findings

X-ray studies show esophageal dilation above the narrowing at the gastroesophageal junction. Barium swallow, CT of the chest, and endoscopy may be used for diagnosis; however, manometry, a process in which the esophageal pressure is measured by a radiologist or gastroenterologist, confirms the diagnosis.

Management

The patient is instructed to eat slowly and to drink fluids with meals. As a temporary measure, calcium channel blockers and nitrates have been used to decrease esophageal pressure and improve swallowing. Injection of botulinum toxin (Botox) to quadrants of the esophagus via endoscopy has been helpful because it inhibits the contraction of smooth muscle. Periodic injections are required to maintain remission.

Achalasia may be treated conservatively by pneumatic dilation to stretch the narrowed area of the esophagus (Fig. 35-6). Pneumatic dilation has a high success rate. Although perforation is a potential complication, its incidence is low. The procedure can be painful; therefore, moderate sedation in the form of an analgesic or tranquilizer, or both, is administered for the treatment. The patient is monitored for perforation. Abdominal tenderness and fever may indicate perforation (see later discussion).

Achalasia may be treated surgically by esophagomyotomy. The procedure usually is performed laparoscopically, either with a complete lower esophageal sphincter myotomy and an antireflux procedure, or without an antireflux procedure. The esophageal muscle fibers are separated to relieve the lower esophageal stricture.

Diffuse Spasm

Diffuse spasm is a motor disorder of the esophagus. The cause is unknown, but stress may be a factor. It is more common in women and usually manifests in middle age.

Clinical Manifestations

Diffuse spasm is characterized by difficulty (dysphagia) or pain (odynophagia) on swallowing and by chest pain similar to that of coronary artery spasm.

Assessment and Diagnostic Findings

Esophageal manometry, which measures the motility of the esophagus and the pressure within the esophagus, indicates that simultaneous contractions of the esophagus occur irregularly. Diagnostic x-ray studies after ingestion of barium show separate areas of spasm.

Management

Conservative therapy includes administration of sedatives and long-acting nitrates to relieve pain. Calcium channel blockers (eg, nifedipine [Procardia], verapamil [Calan]) have also been used to manage diffuse spasm. Small, frequent feedings and a soft diet are usually recommended to decrease the esophageal pressure and irritation that lead to spasm. Dilation performed by bougienage (use of progressively sized flexible dilators), pneumatic dilation, or esophagomyotomy may be necessary if the pain becomes intolerable.

If none of the conservative approaches is successful in managing symptoms, surgery may be considered. An esophageal Heller myotomy by a minimally invasive ap-

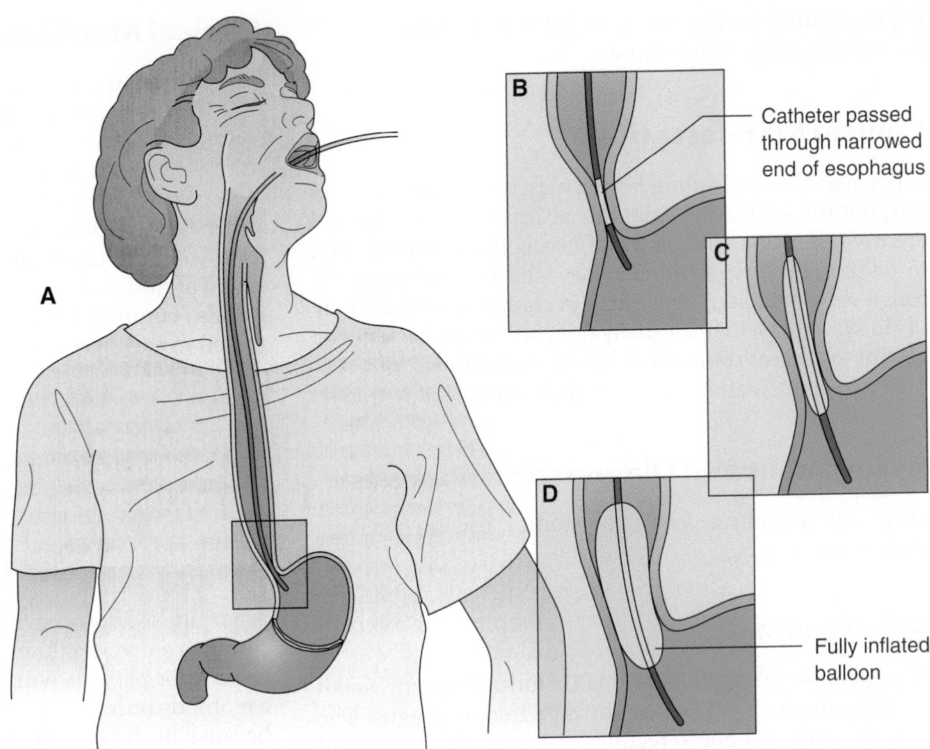

FIGURE 35-6. Treatment of achalasia by pneumatic dilation. (**A–C**) The dilator is passed, guided by a previously inserted guide wire. (**D**) When the balloon is in proper position, it is distended by pressure sufficient to dilate the narrowed area of the esophagus.

proach is considered first and has shown positive results. If an open surgical approach is required, then a transhiatal esophagectomy is performed (see discussion in Cancer of the Esophagus).

Hiatal Hernia

In the condition known as hiatus (or hiatal) **hernia**, the opening in the diaphragm through which the esophagus passes becomes enlarged, and part of the upper stomach tends to move up into the lower portion of the thorax. Hiatal hernia occurs more often in women than in men. There are two types of hiatal hernias: sliding and paraesophageal. Sliding, or type I, hiatal hernia occurs when the upper stomach and the gastroesophageal junction are displaced upward and slide in and out of the thorax (Fig. 35-7A). About 90% of patients with esophageal hiatal hernia have a sliding hernia. A paraesophageal hernia occurs when all or part of the stomach pushes through the diaphragm beside the esophagus (see Fig. 35-7B). Paraesophageal hernias are further classified as types II, III, or

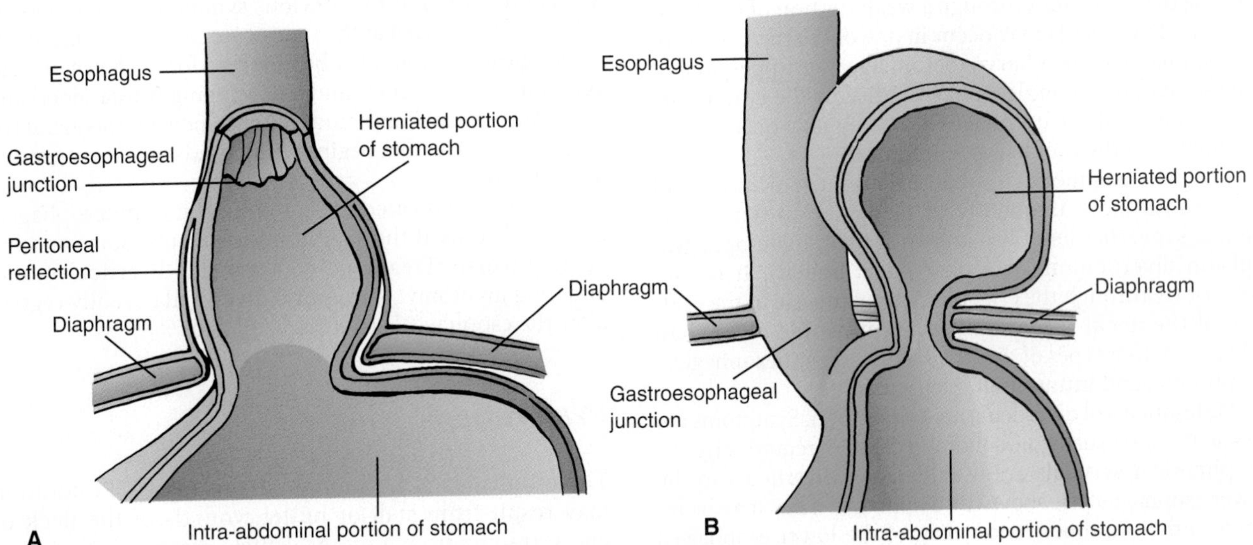

FIGURE 35-7. (**A**) Sliding esophageal hernia. The upper stomach and gastroesophageal junction have moved upward and slide in and out of the thorax. (**B**) Paraesophageal hernia. All or part of the stomach pushes through the diaphragm next to the gastroesophageal junction.

IV, depending on the extent of herniation, with type IV having the greatest herniation.

Clinical Manifestations

The patient with a sliding hernia may have heartburn, regurgitation, and dysphagia, but at least 50% of patients are asymptomatic. Sliding hiatal hernia is often implicated in reflux. The patient with a paraesophageal hernia usually feels a sense of fullness after eating or chest pain, or there may be no symptoms. Reflux usually does not occur, because the gastroesophageal sphincter is intact. Hemorrhage, obstruction, and strangulation can occur with any type of hernia.

Assessment and Diagnostic Findings

Diagnosis is confirmed by x-ray studies, barium swallow, and fluoroscopy.

Management

Management for an axial hernia includes frequent, small feedings that can pass easily through the esophagus. The patient is advised not to recline for 1 hour after eating, to prevent reflux or movement of the hernia, and to elevate the head of the bed on 4- to 8-inch (10- to 20-cm) blocks to prevent the hernia from sliding upward. Surgery is indicated in about 15% of patients. Medical and surgical management of a paraesophageal hernia is similar to that for gastroesophageal reflux; however, people with paraesophageal hernias may require emergency surgery to correct torsion (twisting) of the stomach or other body organ that leads to restriction of blood flow to that area.

Diverticulum

A diverticulum is an outpouching of mucosa and submucosa that protrudes through a weak portion of the musculature. Diverticula may occur in one of the three areas of the esophagus—the pharyngoesophageal or upper area of the esophagus, the midesophageal area, or the epiphrenic or lower area of the esophagus—or they may occur along the border of the esophagus intramurally.

The most common type of diverticulum, which is found three times more frequently in men than in women, is Zenker's diverticulum (also known as pharyngoesophageal pulsion diverticulum or a pharyngeal pouch). It occurs posteriorly through the cricopharyngeal muscle in the midline of the neck. It is usually seen in people older than 60 years. Other types of diverticula include midesophageal, epiphrenic, and intramural diverticula.

Midesophageal diverticula are uncommon. Symptoms are less acute, and usually the condition does not require surgery. Epiphrenic diverticula are usually larger diverticula in the lower esophagus just above the diaphragm. They may be related to the improper functioning of the lower esophageal sphincter or to motor disorders of the esophagus. Intramural diverticulosis is the occurrence of numerous small diverticula associated with a stricture in the upper esophagus.

Clinical Manifestations

Symptoms experienced by the patient with a pharyngoesophageal pulsion diverticulum include difficulty swallowing, fullness in the neck, belching, regurgitation of undigested food, and gurgling noises after eating. The diverticulum, or pouch, becomes filled with food or liquid. When the patient assumes a recumbent position, undigested food is regurgitated, and coughing may be caused by irritation of the trachea. Halitosis and a sour taste in the mouth are also common because of the decomposition of food retained in the diverticulum.

Symptoms produced by midesophageal diverticula are less acute. One third of patients with epiphrenic diverticula are asymptomatic, and the remaining two thirds report dysphagia and chest pain. Dysphagia is the most common symptom of patients with intramural diverticulosis.

Assessment and Diagnostic Findings

A barium swallow may determine the exact nature and location of a diverticulum. Manometric studies are often performed for patients with epiphrenic diverticula to rule out a motor disorder. Esophagoscopy usually is contraindicated because of the danger of perforation of the diverticulum, with resulting mediastinitis (inflammation of the organs and tissues that separate the lungs). Blind insertion of a nasogastric tube should be avoided.

Management

Because pharyngoesophageal pulsion diverticulum is progressive, the only means of cure is surgical removal of the diverticulum. During surgery, care is taken to avoid trauma to the common carotid artery and internal jugular veins. The sac is dissected free and amputated flush with the esophageal wall. In addition to a diverticulectomy, a myotomy of the cricopharyngeal muscle is often performed to relieve spasticity of the musculature, which otherwise seems to contribute to a continuation of the previous symptoms. A nasogastric tube may be inserted at the time of surgery. Postoperatively, the surgical incision must be observed for evidence of leakage from the esophagus and a developing fistula. Food and fluids are withheld until x-ray studies show no leakage at the surgical site. The diet begins with liquids and is progressed as tolerated.

Surgery is indicated for epiphrenic and midesophageal diverticula only if the symptoms are troublesome and becoming worse. Treatment consists of a diverticulectomy and long myotomy. Intramural diverticula usually regress after the esophageal stricture is dilated.

Perforation

The esophagus is a common site of injury. Perforation may result from stab or bullet wounds of the neck or chest, trauma from a motor vehicle crash, caustic injury from a chemical burn, or inadvertent puncture by a surgical instrument during examination or dilation such as endoscopy.

Clinical Manifestations

The patient has persistent pain followed by dysphagia. Infection, fever, leukocytosis, and severe hypotension may be noted. In some instances, signs of pneumothorax are observed.

Assessment and Diagnostic Findings

X-ray studies and fluoroscopy by either a barium swallow or esophagram are used to identify the site of the injury.

Management

Because of the high risk of infection, broad-spectrum antibiotic therapy is initiated. If the perforation is small enough and without symptoms, medical intervention may not be necessary. Nothing is given by mouth; nutritional needs are met by parenteral or enteral nutrition. The type of nutritional support depends on the location of the injury. The enteral or parenteral nutrition lasts for at least 1 month to give the esophagus a chance to heal. A repeat barium swallow study is performed, and the involved area is reevaluated. If there is no evidence of perforation, foods are reintroduced, beginning with liquids and then slowly progressing to solids as tolerated.

Surgery may be necessary to close the wound; in such cases, postoperative nutritional support becomes a primary concern. Depending on the incision site and the nature of surgery, the postoperative nursing management is similar to that for patients who have had thoracic or abdominal surgery.

Foreign Bodies

Many swallowed foreign bodies pass through the gastrointestinal tract without the need for medical intervention. However, some swallowed foreign bodies (eg, dentures, fish bones, pins, small batteries, items containing mercury or lead) may injure the esophagus or obstruct its lumen and must be removed. Pain and dysphagia may be present, and dyspnea may occur as a result of pressure on the trachea. The foreign body may be identified by x-ray. Perforation may have occurred (see earlier discussion).

Glucagon, because of its relaxing effect on the esophageal muscle, may be injected intramuscularly. An endoscope (with a covered hood or overtube) may be used to remove the impacted food or object from the esophagus. A mixture consisting of sodium bicarbonate and tartaric acid may be prescribed to increase intraluminal pressure by the formation of a gas. Caution must be used with this treatment because there is risk of perforation.

Chemical Burns

Chemical burns of the esophagus occur most often when a patient, either intentionally or unintentionally, swallows a strong acid or base (eg, lye). This patient is emotionally distraught as well as in acute physical pain. Chemical burns of the esophagus may also be caused by undissolved medications in the esophagus. This occurs more frequently in the elderly than it does among the general adult population. A chemical burn may also occur after swallowing of a battery, which may release a caustic alkaline. An acute chemical burn of the esophagus may be accompanied by severe burns of the lips, mouth, and pharynx, with pain on swallowing. There may be difficulty in breathing due to either edema of the throat or a collection of mucus in the pharynx.

The patient, who may be profoundly toxic, febrile, and in shock, is treated immediately for shock, pain, and respiratory distress. Esophagoscopy and barium swallow are performed as soon as possible to determine the extent and severity of damage. The patient is given nothing by mouth, and IV fluids are administered. A nasogastric tube may be inserted by the physician. Vomiting and gastric lavage are avoided to prevent further exposure of the esophagus to the caustic agent. The use of corticosteroids to reduce inflammation and minimize subsequent scarring and stricture formation is of questionable value. Prophylactic antibiotics should be prescribed only if there is documented infection (Hostetler, 2004).

After the acute phase has subsided, the patient may need nutritional support via enteral or parenteral feedings. The patient may require further treatment to prevent or manage strictures of the esophagus. Dilation by bougienage may be sufficient but may need to be repeated periodically. (In bougienage, cylindrical rubber tubes of different sizes, called bougies, are advanced into the esophagus via the oral cavity. Progressively larger bougies are used to dilate the esophagus. The procedure usually is performed in the endoscopy suite or clinic by the gastroenterologist.) For strictures that do not respond to dilation, surgical management is necessary. Reconstruction may be accomplished by esophagectomy and colon interposition to replace the portion of esophagus removed.

Gastroesophageal Reflux Disease

Some degree of **gastroesophageal reflux** (back-flow of gastric or duodenal contents into the esophagus) is normal in both adults and children. Excessive reflux may occur because of an incompetent lower esophageal sphincter, pyloric stenosis, or a motility disorder. The incidence of reflux seems to increase with aging.

Clinical Manifestations

Symptoms of gastroesophageal reflux disease (GERD) may include pyrosis (burning sensation in the esophagus), dyspepsia (indigestion), regurgitation, dysphagia or odynophagia (pain on swallowing), hypersalivation, and esophagitis. The symptoms may mimic those of a heart attack. The patient's history aids in obtaining an accurate diagnosis.

Assessment and Diagnostic Findings

Diagnostic testing may include an endoscopy or barium swallow to evaluate damage to the esophageal mucosa. Ambulatory 12- to 36-hour esophageal pH monitoring is used to evaluate the degree of acid reflux. Bilirubin monitoring (Bilitec) is used to measure bile reflux patterns. Exposure to bile can cause mucosal damage.

Management

Management begins with teaching the patient to avoid situations that decrease lower esophageal sphincter pressure or cause esophageal irritation. The patient is instructed to eat a low-fat diet; to avoid caffeine, tobacco, beer, milk, foods containing peppermint or spearmint, and carbonated beverages; to avoid eating or drinking 2 hours before bedtime; to maintain normal body weight; to avoid tight-fitting clothes; to elevate the head of the bed on 6- to 8-inch (15- to 20-cm) blocks; and to elevate the upper body on pillows. If reflux persists, the patient may be given antacids or H_2 receptor antagonists, such as famotidine (Pepcid), nizatidine (Axid), or ranitidine (Zantac). Proton pump inhibitors (medications that decrease the release of gastric acid, such as lansoprazole [Prevacid], rabeprazole [AciPhex], esomeprazole [Nexium]) may be used; however, these products may increase intragastric bacterial growth and the risk for infection. In addition, the patient may receive prokinetic agents, which accelerate gastric emptying. These agents include bethanechol (Urecholine), domperidone (Motilium), and metoclopramide (Reglan). Metoclopramide can have extrapyramidal side effects that are increased in certain neuromuscular disorders, such as Parkinson's disease. These patients should be carefully monitored.

If medical management is unsuccessful, surgical intervention may be necessary. Surgical management involves a Nissen fundoplication (wrapping of a portion of the gastric fundus around the sphincter area of the esophagus). A Nissen fundoplication can be performed by the open method or by laparoscopy.

Barrett's Esophagus

Barrett's esophagus is a condition in which the lining of the esophageal mucosa is altered. It typically occurs in association with GERD; indeed, longstanding untreated GERD may lead to Barrett's esophagus. Reflux eventually causes changes in the cells lining the lower esophagus. The cells that are laid to cover the exposed area are no longer squamous in origin. These precancerous cells initiate the healing process and can be a precursor to esophageal cancer.

Clinical Manifestations

The patient complains of symptoms of GERD, notably frequent heartburn. The patient may also complain of symptoms related to peptic ulcers or esophageal stricture, or both.

Assessment and Diagnostic Findings

An **esophagogastroduodenoscopy (EGD)** is performed. This usually reveals an esophageal lining that is red rather than pink. Biopsies are performed, and high-grade **dysplasia** (HGD) is evidenced by the squamous mucosa of the esophagus replaced by columnar epithelium that resembles that of the stomach or intestines (Porth, 2005).

Management

Monitoring varies depending on the extent of cell changes. Some physicians recommend a repeat EGD in 6 to 12 months if there are minor cell changes.

Photodynamic therapy (PDT) may be an alternative for the patient who is considered an operative risk (eg, 70 years or older, significant cardiac risk). PDT is a type of laser thermal ablation of the esophageal mucosa that is used to destroy the metaplastic cells once the patient has received a photosensitizing agent, such as Photofrin. Early studies suggest that this therapy shows promise for the patient with early-stage disease; however, it is not recommended for the patient with late-stage disease accompanied by nodal disease (Overholt, Panjehpour, & Teffetellar, 1995). There have been no long-term follow-up studies of patients who have undergone ablation therapy. Therefore, PDT should be reserved for patients who are not surgical candidates for prophylactic esophagectomy.

Research suggests that prophylactic transhiatal esophagectomy is a recommended therapy for patients with Barrett's esophagus and HGD. Patients with Barrett's esophagus and HGD who have had prophylactic esophagectomy have shown a significant reduction in invasive adenocarcinoma following the procedure. A significant number of these patients who did not have a preoperative diagnosis of cancer have been found to have invasive adenocarcinoma during surgery. Furthermore, researchers have found that only patients with dysplasia develop invasive adenocarcinoma and that persistent HGD is a reliable histopathologic marker for the subsequent development of adenocarcinoma (Heitmiller et al., 1996). These results suggest that esophageal surgery was the best option for patients with Barrett's esophagus with HGD. Updated results continue to support the performance of a prophylactic esophagectomy in the presence of HGD. Five-year survival was 88%, and Barrett's esophagus with HGD continues to be an indication for prophylactic esophagectomy (Tseng, Wu, Yeo, et al., 2003).

Benign Tumors of the Esophagus

Benign tumors can arise anywhere along the esophagus. The most common lesion is a leiomyoma (tumor of the smooth muscle), which can occlude the lumen of the esophagus. Most benign tumors are asymptomatic and are distinguished from cancerous lesions by a biopsy. Small lesions are excised during esophagoscopy; lesions that occur within the wall of the esophagus may require treatment via a thoracotomy.

Cancer of the Esophagus

In the United States, carcinoma of the esophagus occurs more than three times as often in men as in women. It is seen more frequently in African Americans than in Caucasians and usually occurs in the fifth or sixth decade of life. Cancer of the esophagus has a much higher incidence (10 to 100 times higher) in other parts of the world, including China and northern Iran (American Cancer Society, 2005).

Chronic irritation is a risk factor for esophageal cancer. In the United States, cancer of the esophagus has been associated with ingestion of alcohol and the use of tobacco.

There seems to be an association between GERD and adenocarcinoma of the esophagus. People with Barrett's esophagus (which is caused by chronic irritation of the mucous membranes due to reflux of gastric and duodenal contents) have a higher incidence of esophageal cancer (Stein et al., 1999).

Pathophysiology

Esophageal cancer can be of two cell types: adenocarcinoma and squamous cell carcinoma. The rate of adenocarcinoma is rapidly increasing in the United States as well as in other Western countries. It is found primarily in the distal esophagus and gastroesophageal junction (Quinn & Reedy, 1999).

Risk factors for adenocarcinoma of the esophagus include GERD. GERD may progress to Barrett's esophagus that can be either low-grade or high-grade dysplasia (see section on Barrett esophagus for more details).

Risk factors for squamous cell carcinoma of the esophagus include chronic ingestion of hot liquids or foods, nutritional deficiencies, poor oral hygiene, exposure to nitrosamines in the environment or food, cigarette smoking or chronic alcohol exposure (especially in Western cultures), and some esophageal medical conditions such as caustic injury.

Tumor cells of adenocarcinoma and of squamous cell carcinoma may spread beneath the esophageal mucosa or directly into, through, and beyond the muscle layers into the lymphatics. In the latter stages, obstruction of the esophagus is noted, with possible perforation into the mediastinum and erosion into the great vessels.

Clinical Manifestations

Many patients have an advanced ulcerated lesion of the esophagus before symptoms are manifested. Symptoms include dysphagia, initially with solid foods and eventually with liquids; a sensation of a mass in the throat; painful swallowing; substernal pain or fullness; and, later, regurgitation of undigested food with foul breath and hiccups. The patient first becomes aware of intermittent and increasing difficulty in swallowing. As the tumor grows and the obstruction becomes nearly complete, even liquids cannot pass into the stomach. Regurgitation of food and saliva occurs, hemorrhage may take place, and progressive loss of weight and strength occurs from starvation. Later symptoms include substernal pain, persistent hiccup, respiratory difficulty, and foul breath.

The delay between the onset of early symptoms and the time when the patient seeks medical advice is often 12 to 18 months. Any person having swallowing difficulties should be encouraged to consult a physician immediately.

Assessment and Diagnostic Findings

Currently, diagnosis is confirmed most often by EGD with biopsy and brushings. The biopsy can be used to determine the presence of disease and cell differentiation. At presentation, most patients have moderately differentiated tumors.

Several imaging techniques may provide useful diagnostic information. CT of the chest and abdomen is beneficial for detecting any metastatic disease, especially of the lungs, liver, and kidney. Positron emission tomography (PET) may help detect metastasis with more sensitivity than CT. Endoscopic ultrasound is used to determine whether the cancer has spread to the lymph nodes and other mediastinal structures; it can also determine the size and invasiveness of the tumor. Exploratory laparoscopy is the best method for finding positive lymph nodes in patients with distal lesions.

Future diagnostic techniques that may serve as predictors for dysplastic progression in patients with Barrett's esophagus involve molecular markers. The usefulness of molecular markers in treating esophageal cancer is being researched. Research also includes the development of medications that target the pathways of various molecular markers (Lau, Moore, Brooks, et al., 2002).

Medical Management

If esophageal cancer is detected at an early stage, treatment goals may be directed toward cure; however, it is often detected in late stages, making relief of symptoms the only reasonable goal of therapy. Treatment may include surgery, radiation, chemotherapy, or a combination of these modalities, depending on the type of cell, the extent of the disease, and the patient's condition. A standard treatment plan for a person who is newly diagnosed with esophageal cancer includes the following: preoperative combination chemotherapy/radiation therapy for 4 to 6 weeks; followed by a period of no medical intervention for 4 weeks; and, lastly, surgical resection of the esophagus.

Standard surgical management includes a total resection of the esophagus (esophagectomy) with removal of the tumor plus a wide tumor-free margin of the esophagus and the lymph nodes in the area. The surgical approach may be through the thorax or the abdomen, depending on the location of the tumor. When tumors occur in the cervical or upper thoracic area, esophageal continuity may be maintained by a free jejunal graft transfer, in which the tumor is removed and the area is replaced with a portion of the jejunum (Fig. 35-8). A segment of the colon may be used, or the stomach can be elevated into the chest and the proximal section of the esophagus anastomosed to the stomach.

Tumors of the lower thoracic esophagus are more amenable to surgery than are tumors located higher in the esophagus. Gastrointestinal tract integrity is maintained by anastomosing the lower esophagus to the stomach (Fig. 35-9).

Surgical resection of the esophagus has a relatively high mortality rate because of infection, pulmonary complications, or leakage through the anastomosis. Postoperatively, the patient has a nasogastric tube in place that should not be manipulated. The patient is given nothing by mouth until x-ray studies confirm that the anastomosis is free from an esophageal leak, there is no obstruction, and there is no evidence of pulmonary aspiration.

Palliative treatment may be necessary to keep the esophagus open, to assist with nutrition, and to control saliva. Palliation may be accomplished with dilation of the esophagus, laser therapy, placement of an endoprosthesis (stent), radiation, or chemotherapy.

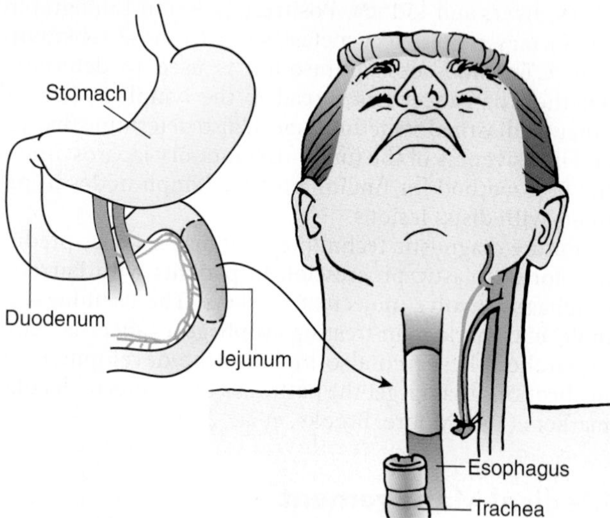

FIGURE 35-8. Esophageal reconstruction with free jejunal transfer. A portion of the jejunum is grafted between the esophagus and pharynx to replace the abnormal portion of the esophagus. The vascular structures are also anastomosed. A portion of the graft may be externalized through the neck wound to evaluate graft viability.

Nursing Management

Intervention is directed toward improving the patient's nutritional and physical status in preparation for surgery, radiation therapy, or chemotherapy. A program to promote weight gain based on a high-calorie and high-protein diet, in liquid or soft form, is provided if adequate food can be taken by mouth. If this is not possible, parenteral or enteral nutrition is initiated. Nutritional status is monitored throughout treatment. The patient is informed about the nature of the postoperative equipment that will be used, including that required for closed chest drainage, nasogastric suction, parenteral fluid therapy, and gastric intubation.

Immediate postoperative care is similar to that provided for patients undergoing thoracic surgery. It is not uncommon for patients to be placed in an intensive care unit or step-down unit. After recovering from the effects of anesthesia, the patient is placed in a low Fowler's position, and later in a Fowler's position, to help prevent reflux of gastric secretions. The patient is observed carefully for regurgitation and dyspnea. A common postoperative complication is aspiration pneumonia. Therefore, the patient is placed on a vigorous pulmonary plan of care that includes incentive spirometry, sitting up in a chair, and, if necessary, nebulizer treatments. Chest physiotherapy is avoided due to the risk for aspiration. The patient's temperature is monitored to detect any elevation that may indicate aspiration or seepage of fluid through the operative site into the mediastinum, which would indicate an esophageal leak. Drainage from the cervical neck wound, usually saliva, is evidence of an early esophageal leak. Typically, no treatment other than nothing by mouth and parenteral or enteral support is warranted.

Cardiac complications include atrial fibrillation, which occurs due to irritation of the vagus nerve at the time of surgery. Typical medical management includes digitalization or beta blockade, depending on the patient's response. Rarely, cardioversion may be used.

During surgery, a nasogastric tube is inserted and taped in place. It is connected to low intermittent suction. The nasogastric tube is not manipulated; if displacement occurs, it is not replaced, because damage to the anastomosis may occur. The nasogastric tube is removed 5 to 7 days after surgery; before the patient is allowed to eat, a barium swallow is performed to assess for any anastomotic leak.

Once feeding begins, the nurse encourages the patient to swallow small sips of water. Eventually, the diet is advanced as tolerated to a soft, mechanical diet. When the patient can increase his or her food and fluid intake to an adequate amount, parenteral fluids are discontinued. After each meal, the patient remains upright for at least 2 hours to allow the food to move through the gastrointestinal tract. It is a challenge to encourage the patient to eat, because the appetite

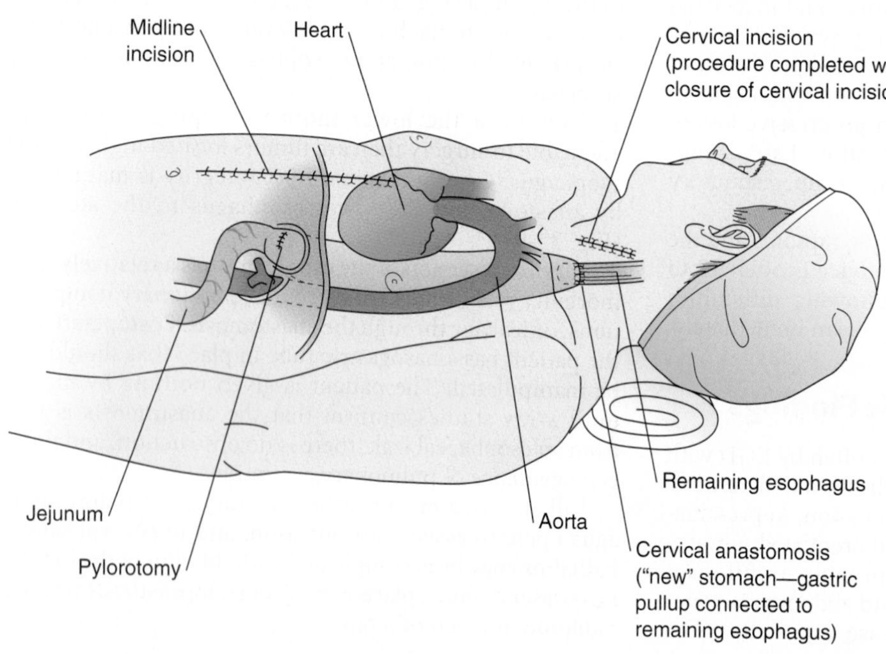

FIGURE 35-9. Transhiatal esophagectomy: surgical removal of tumor of the lower esophagus with anastomosis of the remaining esophagus to the stomach. Redrawn with permission from *Operative Techniques in Thoracic and Cardiovascular Surgery, 4*(3), 263 © 1999 Elsevier Inc.

CONTINUING CARE

Patients with chronic esoph... quire an individualized app... ment at home. Foods may n... special way (blenderized foo... the patient may need to eat n... (eg, six to eight small servings p... medication schedule is adjusted to ... daily activities as much as possible. Anal... medications and antacids can usually be take... needed every 3 to 4 hours.

Postoperative home health care focuses on nutritional support, management of pain, and respiratory function. Some patients are discharged from the hospital with enteral feeding by means of a gastrostomy or jejunostomy tube or parenteral nutrition. The patient and caregiver need specific instructions regarding management of the equipment and treatments. Home care visits by a nurse may be necessary to assess the patient and the caregiver's ability to provide the necessary care. (See Chapter 36 for more information about parenteral nutrition and management of the patient with a gastrostomy.) For some patients, a multidisciplinary team that includes a dietitian, a social worker, and family members is helpful. Hospice care and consideration of end-of-life issues are appropriate for some patients.

Evaluation

Expected Patient Outcomes

Expected patient outcomes may include:

1. Achieves an adequate nutritional intake
   a. Eats small, frequent meals
   b. Drinks small sips of water with small servings of food
   c. Avoids irritants (alcohol, tobacco, very hot beverages)
   d. Maintains desired weight
2. Does not aspirate or develop pneumonia
   a. Maintains upright position during feeding
   b. Uses oral suction equipment effectively
3. Is free of pain or able to control pain within a tolerable level
   a. Avoids large meals and irritating foods
   b. Takes medications as prescribed and with adequate fluids (at least 4 ounces), and remains upright for at least 10 minutes after taking medications
   c. Maintains an upright position after meals for 1 to 4 hours
   d. Reports that there is less eructation and chest pain
4. Increases knowledge level of esophageal condition, treatment, and prognosis
   a. States cause of condition
   b. Discusses rationale for medical or surgical management and diet or medication regimen
   c. Describes treatment program
   d. Practices preventive measures so injuries are avoided

...itical Thinking Exercises

...rviewing a man in the medical clinic. During ...history, the patient describes his symp-...ss, vague chest pain, and occasional ... solid foods only. Explain what other ... ask this patient to rule out the ...eal mass and to determine what ... most helpful. What instruc-

2 You ar... and have b... who has underg...out preparation for these ... form of nutritional su... the intensive care unit being used, and why? What ...toperative patient used to facilitate breathing a... ...ssection. Which Describe the potential complication... most likely see ...es would be dissection and the assessment parameters ... comfort? ...al neck to detect the earliest signs and symptoms of th... ...used co... plications.

3 ebp An elderly woman is brought to the emergency department by the rescue squad. Her daughter found her on the kitchen floor. A bottle of cleaning fluid with a poison label was open next to the kitchen sink. On admission the patient was in respiratory distress. Burns were observed around her mouth. What emergency care would be provided for this patient to prevent further trauma to the gastrointestinal and respiratory tracts? Identify the evidence that supports this care and evaluate the strength of the evidence.

REFERENCES AND SELECTED READINGS

BOOKS

American Cancer Society (2005). *Cancer Facts and Figures*. Atlanta, GA: Author.

Bickley, L. S., & Szilagyi, P. G. (2005). *Bates' guide to physical examination and history taking* (9th ed.). Philadelphia: Lippincott Williams & Wilkins.

Brandt, L. J. (Ed.). (1999). *Clinical practice of gastroenterology* (Vols. I & II). Philadelphia: Churchill-Livingstone.

Castell, D. O., & Richter, J. E. (2003). *The esophagus* (4th ed.). Philadelphia: Lippincott Williams & Wilkins.

DeVita, V. T., Hellman, S., & Rosenberg, S. A. (Eds.). (2005). *Cancer: Principles and practice of oncology* (7th ed.). Philadelphia: Lippincott Williams & Wilkins.

Fonseca, R. J. (Ed.). (2000). *Oral and maxillofacial surgery*. Philadelphia: W. B. Saunders.

Garber, T. M. (Ed.). (2000). *Orthodontics: Current principles and techniques*. St. Louis: Mosby.

Harris, N. O., & Garcia-Godoy, F. (2003). *Primary preventive dentistry* (6th ed.). Norwalk, CT: Appleton & Lange.

Harrison, L. B., Sessions, R. B., Hong, W. … bro- cancer: A multidisciplinary approach (2… Williams & Wilkins.

McEvoy, G. R. (Ed.). (2004). Am… aparoscopic … Bethesda, MD: American Society…

Murray, J. (1999). Manual of dys… Singular Publishing.

National Institute of Dental &… mandibular disorders. Bethe… …ered health states

Pappas, T. N., Eubanks, S., … surgery (2nd ed.). Norw… Wilkins.

Porth, C. M. (2005). P… (7th ed.). Philadelphi…

Proffit, W. R., & Field… …ary orthodontics. St. Louis: Mosby.

U.S. Department … Services. (2000). Oral health in America: A re… …neral. Executive summary. Rockville, MD: Nation… …tal and Craniofacial Research, National Institutes…

Yamada, T…, Laine, L., et al. (2003). Textbook of gastro-enterol… Vols. I & II). Philadelphia: Lippincott Williams & Wilk…

…URNALS

…onditions and Cancer of the Oral Cavity

…ova, R., Ian, C., & Coman, W. (2004). Total glossectomy: Is it justified? *Australian and New Zealand Journal of Surgery, 74*(3), 134–138.

Brown, L. G., Wall, T. P., & Lazar, V. (2002). Trends in caries among adults 18 to 45 years old. *Journal of the American Dental Association, 133*(7), 827–834.

Bull, P. D. (2001). Salivary gland stones: Diagnosis and treatment. *Hospital Medicine, 62*(7), 396–399.

Capaccio, P., Ottaviani, F., Manzo, R., et al. (2004). Extracorporeal lithotripsy for salivary calculi: A long-term clinical experience. *Laryngoscope, 114*(6), 1069–1073.

Centers for Disease Prevention and Control. (2004). Oral cancer: Deadly to ignore. Fact sheet. Available at: http://www.cdc.gov/OralHealth/factsheet/oc-facts.htm. Accessed June 8, 2006.

Jemal, A., Taylor, M., Ward, E., et al. (2005). Cancer statistics, 2005. *CA Cancer Journal for Clinicians, 55*(1), 10–30.

McQuone, S. J. (1999). Acute viral and bacterial infections of the salivary glands. *Otolaryngology Clinics of North America, 32*(5), 793–811.

Moynihan, P., & Petersen, P. E. (2004). Diet, nutrition and the prevention of dental diseases. *Public Health Nutrition, 7*(1), 201–226.

Rice, D. H. (1999). Chronic inflammatory disorders of the salivary glands. *Otolaryngology Clinics of North America, 32*(5), 813–818.

Rice, D. H. (1999). Noninflammatory, non-neoplastic disorders of the salivary gland. *Otolaryngology Clinics of North America, 32*(5), 835–843.

Sessons, D. G., et al. (2000). Analysis of treatment results for floor-of-mouth cancer. *Laryngoscope, 110*(10 Pt. 1), 1764–1772.

Von Fraunhofer, J. Q., & Rogers, M. M. (2004). Dissolution of dental enamel in soft drinks. *General Dentistry, 15*(4), 308–312.

Wright, E. F. (2000). Referred craniofacial pain patterns in patients with temporomandibular disorder. *Journal of the American Dental Association, 131*(9), 1307–1315.

Conditions and Treatment of the Esophagus

Farshad, A., Modlin, I., Kidd, M., et al. (2004). Surgical treatment of achalasia: Current status and controversies. *Digestive Surgery, 21*(1), 165–176.

…. (2005). Genetics and prevention of esophageal adeno-…a. *Recent Results of Cancer Research, 155*(1), 35–46.

…, Siersema, P. D., vanDekken, H., et al. (2004). Esophageal can-… incidence and mortality in patients with long-segment Barrett's esophagus after a mean follow-up of 12.7 years. *Scandinavian Journal of Gastroenterology, 39*(12), 1175–1179.

Heitmiller, R. F., Redmond, M., & Hamilton, S. R. (1996). Barrett's esophagus with high grade dysplasia: An indication for prophylactic esophagectomy. *Annals of Surgery, 224*(1), 66–71.

Hemminger, L. L. (2002). Photodynamic therapy for Barrett's esophagus and high-grade dysplasia: Results of a patient satisfaction survey. *Gastroenterology Nursing, 25*(4), 139–141.

Hostetler, M. A. (2004). Chemical burns. Available at: http://www.emedicine.com/ped/topic2735.htm. Accessed June 5, 2006.

Lau, C. L., Moore, M. B., Brooks, K. R., et al. (2002). Molecular staging of lung and esophageal cancer. *Surgical Clinics of North America, 82*(3), 497–523.

May, A., Gossner, L., Pech, O., et al. (2002). Intraepithelial high-grade neoplasia and early adenocarcinoma in short-segment Barrett's esophagus (SSBE): Curative treatment using local endoscopic treatment techniques. *Endoscopy, 34*(4), 604–610.

Overholt, B. F., Panjehpour, M., & Teffetellar, E. (1995). Photodynamic therapy for treatment of early adenocarcinoma in Barrett's esophagus. *Gastrointestinal Endoscopy, 49*(1), 73–76.

Para, M. (2002). Epidemiology of esophageal cancer, especially adenocarcinoma of the esophagus and esophagogastric junction. *Recent Results in Cancer Research, 155*, 1–14.

Quinn, K. L., & Reedy, A. (1999). Esophageal cancer: Therapeutic approaches and nursing care. *Seminars in Oncology Nursing, 15*(1), 17–25.

Qureshi, W. (2002). Gastrointestinal uses of botulinum toxin. *Journal of Clinical Gastroenterology, 34*(2), 126–128.

Shenfine, J., McNamee, P., Steer, N., et al. (2005). A pragmatic randomised controlled trial of the cost-effectiveness of palliative therapies for patients with inoperable esophageal cancer. *Health Technology Assessment, 9*(5), 1–136.

Sifrim, D., Castell, D., Dent, J., et al. (2004). Gastro-oesophageal reflux monitoring: Review and consensus report on detection and definitions of acid, non-acid, and gas reflux. *Gut, 53*(7), 1024–1031.

Stein, H. J., Kauer, W. K. H., Feussoner, H., et al. (1999). Bile acids as components of the duodenogastric refluate: Detection, relationship to bilirubin, mechanism of injury, and clinical relevance. *Hepatogastroenterology, 46*, 66–73.

Tseng, E. E., Wu, T. T., Yeo, C. J., et al. (2003). Barrett's esophagus with high-grade dysplasia: Surgical results and long-term outcome—an update. *Journal of Gastrointestinal Surgery, 7*(2), 164–171.

Watson, D. (2004). Laparoscopic treatment of gastro-oesophageal reflux disease. *Best Practice & Research Clinical Gastroenterology, 18*(1), 19–35.

Wolfsen, H. (2005). Present status of photodynamic therapy for high-grade dysplasia in Barrett's esophagus. *Journal of Clinical Gastroenterology, 39*(3), 189–202.

Conditions and Treatment of the Head and Neck

ElGhani, F., van den Brekel, M. W., DeGoede, C. J., et al. (2002). Shoulder function and patient well-being after various types of neck dissections. *Clinical Otolaryngology, 27*(5), 403–408.

Garden, A. S., Harris, J., Vokes, E. E., et al. (2004). Preliminary results of radiation therapy oncology group 97-03: A randomized phase II trial of concurrent radiation and chemotherapy for advanced squamous cell carcinomas of the head and neck. *Journal of Clinical Oncology, 22*(7), 2856–2864.

Girling, D. J. (2004). Surgical resection with or without preoperative chemotherapy in oesophageal cancer: A randomised controlled trial. *Lancet*. March 10, 2005. Available at: http://www.thelancet.com/search/search.isa. Accessed June 5, 2006.

Pre-operative chemotherapy appears to improve survival in esophageal cancer. (2004). Cancer Consultants.com. Available at: http://patient.cancerconsultants.com/esophageal_cancer_news.aspx?id=17597. Accessed June 2, 2006.

Robbins, K. D., Clayman, G., Levine, P. A., et al. (2002). Neck dissection classification update: Revisions proposed by the American Head and Neck Society and the American Academy of Otolaryngology-Head and Neck Surgery. *Archives of Otolaryngology Head and Neck Surgery, 128*(7), 751–758.

Terrell, J. E., Ronis, D. L., Fowler, K. E., et al. (2004). Clinical predictors of quality of life in patients with head and neck cancer. *Archives of Otolaryngology Head Neck Surgery, 130*(1), 401–408.

RESOURCES

American Cancer Society, 1599 Clifton Rd. NE, Atlanta, GA 30329; 1-800-ACS-2345; http://www.cancer.org. Accessed June 2, 2006.

American Dental Association, 211 E. Chicago Ave., Chicago, IL 60611; 312-440-2806; http://www.ada.org. Accessed June 2, 2006.

Centers for Disease Control and Prevention, 1600 Clifton Rd., Atlanta, GA 30333; 404-639-7000; http://www.cdc.gov/health. Accessed June 2, 2006.

National Institute of Dental and Craniofacial Research, National Institutes of Health, 900 Rockville Pike, Bethesda, MD 20892; 301-496-4261; http://www.nidr.nih.gov. Accessed June 2, 2006.

CHAPTER 36

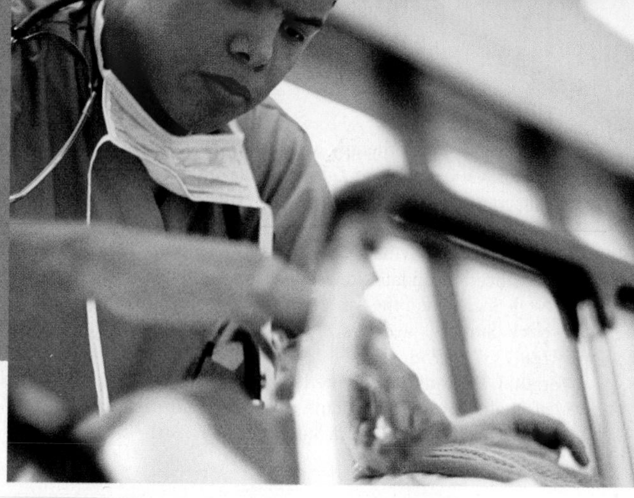

Gastrointestinal Intubation and Special Nutritional Modalities

Learning Objectives

On completion of this chapter, the learner will be able to:

1. Describe the purposes and types of gastrointestinal intubation.
2. Discuss nursing management of the patient who has a nasogastric or nasoenteric tube.
3. Use the nursing process as a framework for care of the patient receiving an enteral feeding.
4. Explain the preoperative and postoperative care of the patient with a gastrostomy.
5. Use the nursing process as a framework for care of the patient with a gastrostomy.
6. Identify the purposes and uses of parenteral nutrition.
7. Use the nursing process as a framework for care of the patient receiving parenteral nutrition.
8. Describe the nursing measures used to prevent complications from parenteral nutrition.

This chapter presents several topics related to gastrointestinal (GI) intubation. Nursing management topics relate to managing the care of patients with **nasogastric** (NG) and nasoenteric tubes and gastrostomies, providing tube feedings, and teaching points concerning home health care and nutritional therapy. In addition, parenteral nutrition is presented, including general indications for this nutritional modality and nursing care of patients receiving these support measures.

Gastrointestinal Intubation

GI intubation is the insertion of a flexible tube into the stomach beyond the pylorus into the **duodenum** (the first section of the small intestine) or the **jejunum** (the second section of the small intestine). The tube may be inserted through the mouth, the nose, or the abdominal wall. The tubes are of various lengths, depending on their intended use. GI intubation may be performed for the following reasons:

- To decompress the stomach and remove gas and fluid
- To lavage the stomach and remove ingested toxins
- To diagnose disorders of GI motility and other disorders
- To administer medications and feedings
- To treat an obstruction
- To compress a bleeding site
- To aspirate gastric contents for analysis

A variety of tubes are used for decompression, aspiration, and **lavage.** Orogastric tubes are large-bore tubes with wide proximal outlets for removal of gastric contents; they are primarily used in emergency departments or in intensive care settings (see Chapter 71). The Sengstaken-Blakemore tube is a type of NG tube used to treat bleeding esophageal varices (see Chapter 39). Various other tubes are used to administer feedings and medications. The tubes are made of various materials (rubber, polyurethane, silicone); polyurethane catheters are more resistant to deterioration (Sartori, Trevisani, Neilsen, et al., 2003). They also vary in length (90 cm to 3 m [3 to 10 ft]), in size (6 to 18 French [Fr]), in purpose, and in placement in the GI tract (stomach, duodenum, jejunum) (Table 36-1). Any solution administered through a tube is poured through a syringe or delivered by a drip mechanism by gravity or regulated by an electric pump. **Aspiration** (suctioning) to remove gas and fluids is accomplished with the use of a syringe, an electric suction machine, or a wall suction outlet.

Gastric Tubes

An NG tube is introduced through the nose into the stomach, often before or during surgery. Commonly used gastric tubes include the Levin tube and the gastric sump tube. Gastric tubes are used in adults primarily to remove fluid and gas from the upper GI tract; this is called **decompression.** They are occasionally used for the short-term (3 to 4 weeks) administration of medications or feedings.

Glossary

antireflux valve: valve that prevents return or backward flow of fluid

aspiration: removal of substance by suction; breathing of fluids or foods into the trachea and lungs

bolus: a feeding administered into the stomach in large amounts and at designated intervals

central venous access device (CVAD): a device designed and used for long-term administration of medications and fluids into central veins

cyclic feeding: periodic feeding/infusion given over a short period (8 to 12 hours)

decompression (intestinal): removal of intestinal contents to prevent gas and fluid from distending the coils of the intestine

dumping syndrome: rapid emptying of the stomach contents into the small intestine; characterized by sweating and weakness

duodenum: the first part of the small intestine, which connects with the pylorus of the stomach and extends to the jejunum

gastrostomy: surgical creation of an opening into the stomach for the purpose of administering foods and fluids

intravenous fat emulsion (IVFE, Intralipids): an oil-in-water emulsion of oils, egg phospholipids, and glycerin

jejunum: second portion of the small intestine, extending from the duodenum to the ileum

lavage: flushing of the stomach via the gastric tube with water or other fluids to clear it

low-profile gastrostomy device (LPGD, G-button): an enteral feeding access device that is flush with the skin and is used for long-term feeding

nasoduodenal tube: tube inserted through the nose into the beginning of the small intestine (duodenum)

nasogastric (NG) tube: tube inserted through the nose into the stomach

nasojejunal tube: tube inserted through the nose into the second portion of the small intestine (jejunum)

osmolality: ionic concentration of fluid

osmosis: passage of solvent through a semipermeable membrane; the solvent, usually water, passes through the membrane from a region of low concentration of solute to that of a higher concentration of solute

parenteral nutrition (PN): method of supplying nutrients to the body by an intravenous route

percutaneous endoscopic gastrostomy (PEG): an endoscopic procedure for inserting a feeding tube into the stomach in order to provide long-term nutritional support

peristalsis: wavelike movement that occurs involuntarily in the alimentary canal

pH: the degree of acidity or alkalinity of a substance or solution

peripherally inserted central catheter (PICC): a device used for intermediate-term intravenous therapy

stoma: artificially created opening between a body cavity (eg, intestine) and the body surface

total nutrient admixture (TNA): an admixture of lipid emulsions, proteins, carbohydrates, electrolytes, vitamins, trace minerals, and water

TABLE 36-1 Nasogastric and Nasoenteric Feeding Tubes

Tube Type	Length (cm)	Size (French)	Lumen	Other Characteristics
Nasogastric Tubes				
Levin (plastic or rubber)	125	14–18	Single	Circular markings at intervals along the tube serve as guidelines for insertion
Gastric sump or Salem (plastic)	120	12–18	Double	Smaller lumen acts as a vent
Moss	90	12–16	Triple	Contains both a gastric decompression lumen and a duodenal lumen for postoperative feedings
Sengstaken-Blakemore (rubber)			Triple	Two lumens are used to inflate the gastric and esophageal balloons, and one tube is reserved for suction or drainage
Nasoenteric Feeding Tubes				
Dobbhoff or EnteraFlo (polyurethane or silicone rubber)	160–175	8–12	Single	Tungsten-weighted tip, radiopaque, stylet

Levin Tube

The Levin tube has a single lumen (the hollow part of the tube), ranges from 14 to 18 Fr in size, and is made of plastic or rubber with openings near its tip. It is 125 cm (50 in) long. Circular markings at specific points on the tube serve as guides for insertion. A marking is made on the tube to indicate the midpoint. The tube is advanced cautiously until this marking reaches the patient's nostril, suggesting that the tube is in the stomach. Placement is checked by observing the characteristics of the aspirate and by testing the **pH** (which varies according to the source of the aspirate). Visualizing the tube's placement on x-ray is the only definitive way to verify its location. The Levin tube is connected to low intermittent suction (30 to 40 mm Hg). Intermittent suction is used to avoid erosion or tearing of the stomach lining, which can result from constant adherence of the tube's lumen to the mucosal lining of the stomach.

Gastric Sump

The gastric sump (Salem) tube is a radiopaque, clear plastic, double-lumen NG tube used to decompress the stomach and keep it empty. It is 120 cm (48 in) long and is passed into the stomach in the same way as the Levin tube. The inner, smaller tube vents the larger suction-drainage tube to the atmosphere by means of an opening at the distal end of the tube. The sump tube can protect gastric suture lines because, when used properly, it maintains the force of suction at the drainage openings, or outlets, at less than 25 mm Hg, the level of capillary fragility. The small vent tube (known as the blue pigtail or port) controls this action. Gastric sump tubes are connected to low continuous suction. The suction lumen is irrigated as prescribed to maintain patency.

To prevent reflux of gastric contents through the vent lumen (blue pigtail), the vent lumen is kept above the patient's waist; otherwise it will act as a siphon. A one-way **antireflux valve** seated in the blue pigtail can prevent the reflux of gastric contents out the vent lumen (Fig. 36-1). The valve is removed after irrigation of the suction lumen, and 20 mL of air is injected to reestablish a buffer of air between the gastric contents and the valve.

Enteric Tubes

Nasoenteric tubes are used for feeding. Feeding tubes placed in the duodenum are 160 cm (60 in) long and called **nasoduodenal tubes**; feeding tubes placed in the jejunum (the portion of the small intestine distal to the duodenum) are 175 cm (66 in) long. They can be inserted before or dur-

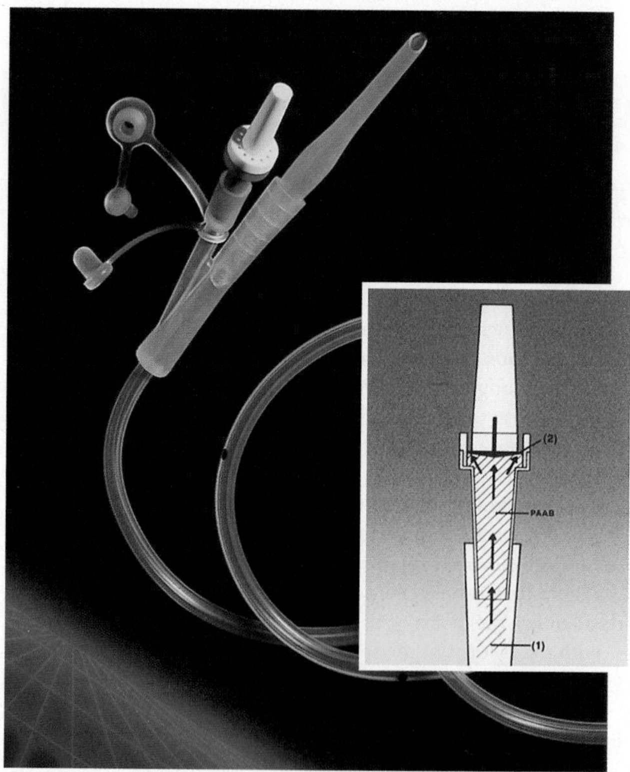

FIGURE 36-1. Gastric sump tube (Salem) equipped with a one-way valve that allows air to enter and can prevent reflux of gastric contents. The antireflux valve is designed with a pressure-activated air buffer (PAAB). The buffer is activated (1) and the valve closes (2) when pressure from gastric contents enters the tubing. Argyle Silicone Salem Sump Tube with preattached Argyle Salem Sump Anti-Reflux Valve courtesy of Sherwood Medical, St. Louis, Missouri.

ing surgery, by interventional radiologists assisted by fluoroscopy, or at the bedside. If the tube is inserted at the bedside, placement is verified by x-ray study. After insertion, the tip of the tube is initially placed in the stomach; it usually takes 24 hours for the tube to pass through the stomach and into the intestines by **peristalsis.** Surgically placed enteric tubes are inserted directly into the jejunum.

Polyurethane or silicone rubber feeding tubes have narrow diameters (6 to 12 Fr) and tungsten tips (rather than mercury-filled bags), and some have a water-activated lubricant that makes it easier to insert the tube. The tubing may kink when a stylet is not used, particularly if the patient is uncooperative or unable to swallow. Feeding tubes with a stylet are inserted with caution in patients predisposed to esophageal puncture, such as patients who are elderly or frail or who have thin tissues. These tubes are advanced in the same way as an NG tube (ie, with the patient in Fowler's position). If this is not possible, the patient is placed on the right side.

Nursing Management

Nursing interventions include the following:

- Explaining to the patient the purpose of the tube and the procedure required for inserting and advancing it
- Describing the sensations to be expected during tube insertion
- Inserting the NG tube and assisting with insertion of the nasoenteric tube
- Confirming the placement of the NG tube
- Advancing the nasoenteric tube
- Monitoring the patient and maintaining tube function
- Providing oral and nasal hygiene and care
- Monitoring for potential complications
- Removing the tube

Preparing the Patient

Before the patient is intubated, the nurse explains the purpose of the tube; this information may assist the patient to be cooperative and tolerant of what is often an unpleasant procedure. The general activities related to inserting the tube are then reviewed, including the fact that the patient may have to breathe through the mouth and that the procedure may cause gagging until the tube has passed the area of the gag reflex.

Inserting the Tube

Before inserting the tube, the nurse determines the length of tubing that will be needed to reach the stomach or the small intestine. A mark is made on the tube to indicate the desired length. This length is determined by (1) measuring the distance from the tip of the nose to the earlobe and from the earlobe to the xiphoid process, and (2) adding 6 inches for NG placement or 8 to 10 inches for intestinal placement (Fig. 36-2).

While the tube is being inserted, the patient usually sits upright with a towel or some type of protective barrier spread bib-fashion over the chest. Tissue wipes are made

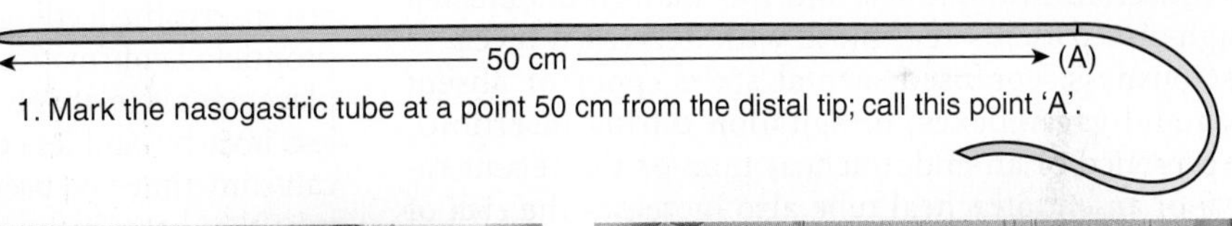

50 cm
(A)
1. Mark the nasogastric tube at a point 50 cm from the distal tip; call this point 'A'.

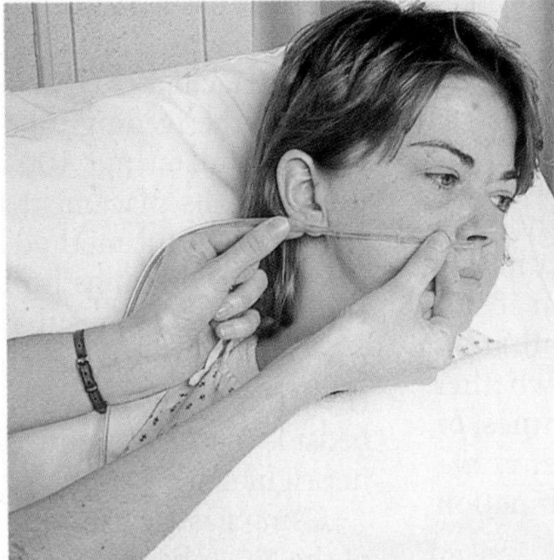

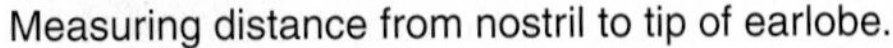

Measuring distance from nostril to tip of earlobe.

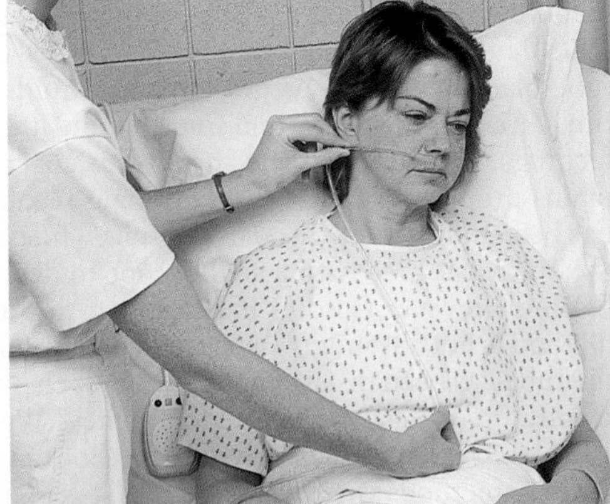

Measuring distance from earlobe to tip of xiphoid process.

2. Have the patient sit in a neutral position with head facing forward. Place the distal tip of the tubing at the tip of the patient's nose (N); extend tube to the tragus (tip) of the ear (E), and then extend the tube straight down to the tip of the xiphoid (X). Mark this point 'B' on the tubing.

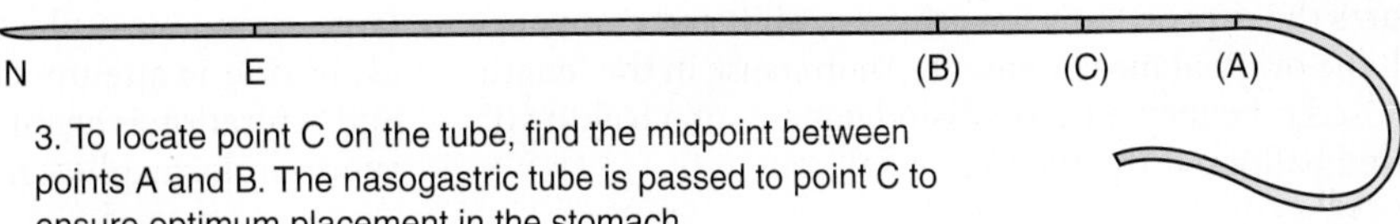

N
E
(B)
(C)
(A)
3. To locate point C on the tube, find the midpoint between points A and B. The nasogastric tube is passed to point C to ensure optimum placement in the stomach.

FIGURE 36-2. Measuring length of nasogastric tube for placement into stomach.

available. Privacy and adequate light are provided. The physician may swab the nostril and spray the oropharynx with tetracaine/benzocaine (Cetacaine) to numb the nasal passage and suppress the gag reflex. This makes the entire procedure more tolerable. Having the patient gargle with a liquid anesthetic or hold ice chips in the mouth for a few minutes can have a similar effect. Encouraging the patient to breathe through the mouth or to pant often helps, as does swallowing water, if permitted.

A polyurethane tube may need to be warmed to make it more pliable. To make the tube easier to insert, it should be lubricated with a water-soluble lubricant unless it has a dry coating (called hydromer), which, when moistened, provides its own lubrication. The nurse wears gloves during the procedure.

The patient is placed in Fowler's position, and the nostrils are inspected for any obstruction. The more patent nostril is selected for use. The tip of the patient's nose is tilted, and the tube is aligned to enter the nostril. When the tube reaches the nasopharynx, the patient is instructed to lower the head slightly and to begin to swallow as the tube is advanced. The patient may also sip water through a straw to facilitate advancement of the tube. The oropharynx is inspected to ensure that the tube has not coiled in the pharynx or mouth.

Confirming Placement

To ensure patient safety, it is essential to confirm that the tube has been placed correctly: the tube may be inadvertently inserted in the lungs, and this may go undetected in high-risk patients (eg, those with decreased levels of consciousness, confused mental states, poor or absent cough and gag reflexes, or agitation during insertion). The presence of an endotracheal tube or the recent removal of an endotracheal tube also increases the risk of inadvertent placement of the tube in the lung (Metheny, 1998). Initially, an x-ray study should be used to confirm tube placement. However, each time liquids or medications are administered, and once a shift for continuous feedings, the tube must be checked to ensure that it remains properly placed. The traditional recommendation has been to inject air through the tube while auscultating the epigastric area with a stethoscope to detect air insufflation. However, studies indicate that this auscultatory method is not absolutely accurate in determining whether the tube has been inserted into the stomach, intestines, or respiratory tract (Metheny, McSweeney, Wehrle, et al., 1990). Instead of the auscultation method, a combination of three methods is recommended:

- Measurement of tube length
- Visual assessment of aspirate
- pH measurement of aspirate

After the tube is inserted, the exposed portion of the tube is measured and the length is documented. The nurse measures the exposed tube length every shift and compares it with the original measurement. An increase in the length of exposed tube may indicate dislodgement, or a leaking or ruptured balloon if the tube has a balloon.

Visual assessment of the color of the aspirate may help identify tube placement. Gastric aspirate is most frequently cloudy and green, tan or off-white, or bloody or brown. Intestinal aspirate is primarily clear and yellow to bile-colored. Pleural fluid is usually pale yellow and serous, and tracheobronchial secretions are usually tan or off-white mucus. The appearance of the aspirate may be helpful in distinguishing between gastric and intestinal placement but is of little value in ruling out respiratory placement. Visual inspection is less helpful when the patient is receiving continuous tube feedings, because the gastric or intestinal aspirate often looks like the formula being used for the feeding (Metheny & Titler, 2001).

Determining the pH of the tube aspirate is a more accurate method of confirming tube placement than maintaining tube length or visually assessing tube aspirate. The pH method can also be used to monitor the advancement of the tube into the small intestine. The pH of gastric aspirate is acidic (1 to 5). The pH of intestinal aspirate is approximately 6 or higher, and the pH of respiratory aspirate is more alkaline (7 or greater). pH testing is best suited for distinguishing between gastric and intestinal placement. A pH sensor enteral tube that does not require fluid aspirate to obtain pH values is available and can be useful in distinguishing gastric from small intestinal placement of the tube. The pH method is less helpful with continuous feedings, because tube feedings have a pH value of 6.6 and neutralize the GI pH (Metheny & Titler, 2001).

Ensuring bedside placement of postpyloric feeding tubes into the duodenum can be a challenge. If a gastroenterologist inserts the feeding tube using fiberoptic endoscopy, appropriate confirmation is ensured. However, this method of placement is relatively costly. Other placement methods are less invasive and less costly. For instance, external magnets can sometimes be used to help guide a postpyloric feeding tube that has a magnet inserted in the tip. Metoclopramide (Reglan), a prokinetic agent, is administered intravenously (IV) and facilitates GI peristalsis, thereby encouraging movement of the feeding tube into the duodenum. Insufflating (eg, administering) 100 to 500 mL of air into the feeding tube once its placement in the stomach is confirmed may also be a useful method of ensuring eventual postpyloric placement. Findings from research suggest that the air insufflation method results in quicker postpyloric placement, particularly among patients who also receive opioid agents (Lenart & Polissar, 2003). Typical guidelines for all of these bedside methods require that the patient be placed on his or her right side.

Using gastric aspiration to verify the correct placement of the NG tube may be a problem because of the characteristic properties and diameter of the tubes. Aspiration may be performed more easily with polyurethane tubes and tubes with a size 10 Fr diameter or larger. If it is difficult to aspirate fluid from small-bore or large-bore feeding tubes, 20 mL of air is injected through the tube with a large syringe (30 to 60 mL), and then the plunger is pulled back. If this is ineffective, another 20 mL of air is injected, the large syringe is replaced with a smaller one (10 mL), and aspiration is attempted. The patient's position is changed and aspiration is again attempted. If these measures are unsuccessful, the physician is notified.

NURSING RESEARCH PROFILE

Postpyloric Placement of Enteral Feeding Tubes

Lenart, S., & Polissar, N. (2003). Comparison of 2 methods for post-pyloric placement of enteral feeding tubes. *American Journal of Critical Care, 12*(4), 357–360.

Purpose

Multiple bedside techniques are used to facilitate placement of postpyloric enteral tubes. A study was conducted to determine which of two techniques, prokinetic metoclopramide (Reglan) or gastric insufflation of air, was superior in ensuring placement of these feeding tubes beyond the gastric pylorus.

Design

Sixty patients from cardiac care and intensive care units were prospectively randomized to two groups. Patients with basilar skull or facial fractures, esophageal varices or tears, pyloric stenosis, and ileus or recent gastrointestinal surgery were excluded. Patients in group 1 received metoclopramide 10 mg 10 minutes prior to feeding tube insertion into the stomach. Patients in group 2 had 350 mL of air insufflated via syringe through the tube immediately after tube placement into the stomach. Patients in both groups were placed on their right sides to facilitate migration of the tubes beyond the pylorus into the small bowel. Abdominal x-ray studies were used to confirm tube tip location in the duodenum.

Findings

Demographic and clinical data did not vary significantly between groups. Overall, success of tube placement was significantly greater in patients who had air insufflation than in those who received metoclopramide. Moreover, patients who were receiving opioids achieved better placement success than with metoclopramide.

Nursing Implications

Both metoclopramide administration and air insufflation are performed by the nurse at the bedside when prescribed. Although endoscopically assisted and fluoroscopically guided insertions of postpyloric feeding tubes are fairly common practices in critical care units, these procedures are more costly than bedside placement procedures in terms of time and manpower resources. Verifying an effective bedside technique facilitates more successful placement and earlier nutrition support. The results of this study suggest that there is decreased financial cost and clinical risk when air insufflation, rather than metoclopramide administration, is used to facilitate postpyloric tube placement. In addition, the possible effects of opioids should be considered when attempting to place postpyloric tubes using either air insufflation or metoclopramide.

Cola and cranberry juice have historically been recommended as effective, noninvasive means of declogging tubes, but evidence indicates that a mixture of pancreatic enzymes and water is superior in restoring the patency of feeding tubes (Keithley & Swanson, 2004). However, correct placement of the NG tube must be confirmed before any mixture is injected to declog the tube.

Securing the Tube

After the correct position of the tip of the tube has been confirmed, the NG tube is secured to the nose (Fig. 36-3). A liquid skin barrier should be applied to the skin where the NG tube will be secured. The prepared area is covered with a strip of hypoallergenic tape or Op-Site, and the tube is then placed over the tape and secured with a second piece of tape. Instead of tape, a feeding tube attachment device (Hollister) can be used to secure the tube. This device adheres to the nose and uses an adjustable clip to hold the tube in place (Fig. 36-4).

Monitoring the Patient and Maintaining Tube Function

If the NG tube is used for decompression, it is attached to suction. If it is used for enteral nutrition, the end of the tube is plugged between feedings. The nurse confirms tube placement by measuring tube length and comparing the length to the baseline before any fluids or medications are instilled and once a shift for continuous feedings. Displacement of the tube may be caused by tension on the tube (when the patient moves around in the bed or room), coughing, tracheal or nasotracheal suctioning, or airway intubation. If the NG tube is removed inadvertently in a patient who has undergone esophageal or gastric surgery, it is usually replaced under fluoroscopy by the physician to avoid trauma to the suture line.

It is important to keep an accurate record of all fluid intake, feedings, and irrigation. To maintain patency, the tube is irrigated every 4 to 6 hours with water or normal saline to avoid electrolyte loss through gastric drainage. The nurse records the amount, color, and type of all drainage every 8 hours.

When double- or triple-lumen tubes are used, each lumen is labeled according to its intended use: aspiration, feeding, or balloon inflation. To avoid tension on the tube, the portion of the tube from the nose to the drainage unit is fixed in position, either with a safety pin or with adhesive tape loops that are pinned to the patient's pajamas or gown. The tube must be looped loosely to prevent tension and dislodgement (see Fig. 36-3).

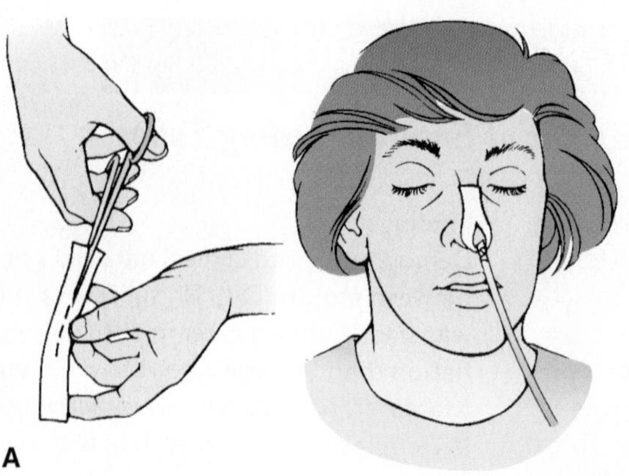

A

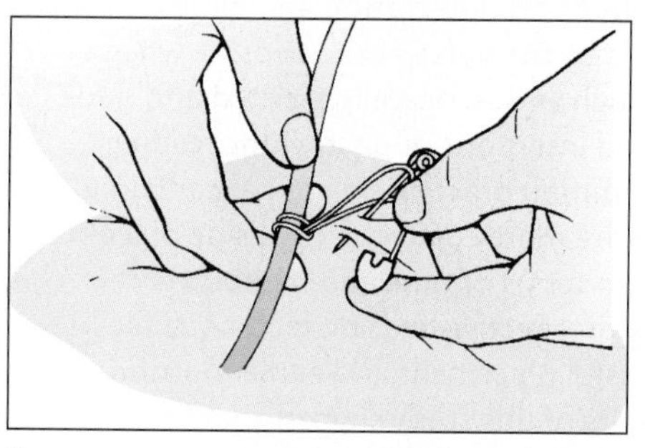

B

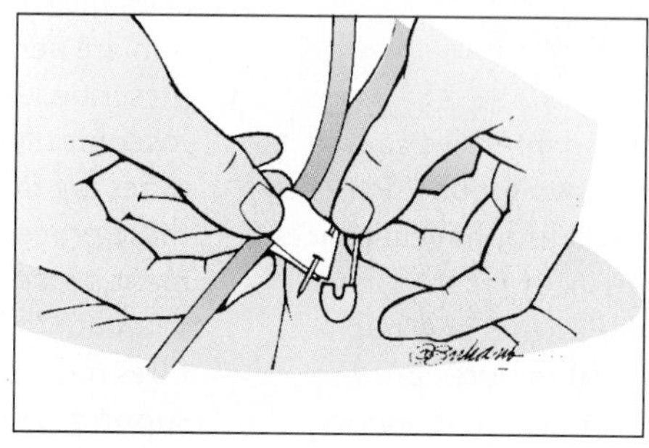

C

FIGURE 36-3. Securing nasogastric (NG) tubes. (**A**) The NG tube is secured to the nose with tape to prevent injury to the nasopharyngeal passages. (**B,C**) The tubing is secured to the patient's gown with either an elastic band or tape attached to a safety pin to prevent tension on the line during movement of the patient.

Providing Oral and Nasal Hygiene

Regular and conscientious oral and nasal hygiene is a vital part of patient care, because the tube causes discomfort and pressure and may be in place for several days. Moistened cotton-tipped swabs can be used to clean the nose, followed by cleansing with a water-soluble lubricant. Frequent mouth care is comforting for the patient. The nasal tape is changed every 2 to 3 days, and the nose is inspected for skin irritation. If the nasal and pharyngeal mucosa are excessively dry, steam or cool vapor inhalations may be beneficial. Throat lozenges, an ice collar, chewing gum, or sucking on hard candies (if permitted) and limiting talking also assist in relieving patient discomfort. These activities keep the mucous membranes moist and help prevent inflammation of the parotid glands.

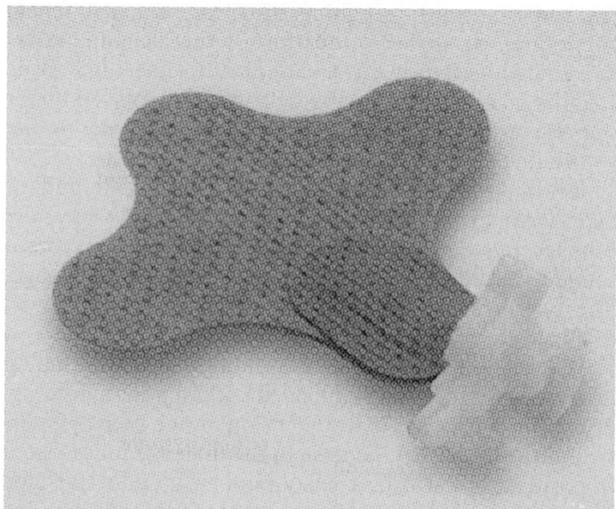

FIGURE 36-4. Feeding tube attachment device. Courtesy of Hollister, Incorporated.

Monitoring and Managing Potential Complications

Patients with NG or nasoenteric intubation are susceptible to a variety of problems, including fluid volume deficit, pulmonary complications, and tube-related irritations. These potential complications require careful ongoing assessment.

Symptoms of fluid volume deficit include dry skin and mucous membranes, decreased urinary output, lethargy, and increased heart rate. Assessment of fluid volume deficit involves maintaining an accurate record of intake and output. This includes measuring NG drainage, fluid instilled by irrigation of the NG tube, water taken by mouth, vomitus, water administered with tube feedings, and IV fluids. Laboratory values, particularly blood urea nitrogen and creatinine, are monitored. The nurse assesses 24-hour fluid balance and reports negative fluid balance, increased NG output, interruption of IV therapy, or any other disturbance in fluid intake or output.

Pulmonary complications from NG intubation occur because coughing and clearing of the pharynx are impaired, because gas buildup can irritate the phrenic nerve, and because tubes may become dislodged, retracting the distal end above the esophagogastric sphincter (which places the patient at risk for **aspiration**, or breathing fluids or foods into the trachea and lungs). Medications (eg, antacids, simethicone [Gaviscon], and metoclopramide [Reglan]) can be administered to decrease potential problems. Signs and symptoms of complications include coughing during the administration of foods or medications, difficulty clearing the airway, tachypnea, and fever. Assessment includes regular auscultation of lung sounds and routine assessment of vital signs. It is important to encourage the patient to cough and to take deep breaths regularly. The nurse also carefully confirms the proper placement of the tube by assessing tube length before instilling any fluids or medications.

Irritation of the mucous membranes is a common complication of NG intubation. The nostrils, oral mucosa, esophagus, and trachea are susceptible to irritation and necrosis. Visible areas are inspected frequently, and the adequacy of hydration is assessed. When providing oral hygiene, the nurse carefully inspects the mucous membranes for signs of irritation or excessive dryness. The nurse palpates the area around the parotid glands to detect any tenderness or enlarged nodes, indicating parotitis, and observes for any irritation or necrosis at the insertion site (eg, nares) or of the mucous membranes. In addition, it is important to assess the patient for esophagitis and tracheitis; symptoms include sore throat and hoarseness.

Removing the Tube

Before removing a tube, the nurse may intermittently clamp and unclamp it for a trial period of several hours to ensure that the patient does not experience nausea, vomiting, or distention. Before the tube is removed, it is flushed with 10 mL of water or normal saline to ensure that it is free of debris and away from the gastric lining; then the balloon (if present) is deflated. Gloves are worn to remove the tube. The tube is withdrawn gently and slowly for 15 to 20 cm (6 to 8 in) until the tip reaches the esophagus; the remainder is withdrawn rapidly from the nostril. If the tube does not come out easily, force should not be used, and the problem should be reported to the physician. As the tube is withdrawn, it is concealed in a towel to prevent secretions from soiling the patient or nurse. After the tube is removed, the nurse provides oral hygiene.

Tube Feedings With Nasogastric and Nasoenteric Devices

Tube feedings are given to meet nutritional requirements when oral intake is inadequate or not possible and the GI tract is functioning normally. Tube feedings have several advantages over parenteral nutrition: they are low in cost, safe, well tolerated by the patient, and easy to use both in extended care facilities and in the patient's home. Tube feedings have other advantages:

- They preserve GI integrity by delivery of nutrients and medications intraluminally.
- They preserve the normal sequence of intestinal and hepatic metabolism.
- They maintain fat metabolism and lipoprotein synthesis.
- They maintain normal insulin/glucagon ratios.

Tube feedings are delivered to the stomach (in the case of NG intubation or gastrostomy) or to the distal duodenum or proximal jejunum (in the case of nasoduodenal or **nasojejunal tube** feeding). Nasoduodenal or nasojejunal feeding is indicated when the esophagus and stomach need to be bypassed or when the patient is at risk for aspiration. For long-term feedings (longer than 4 weeks), gastrostomy or jejunostomy tubes are preferred for administration of medications or food. The numerous conditions requiring enteral nutrition are summarized in Table 36-2.

Osmosis and Osmolality

Osmolality is an important consideration for patients receiving tube feedings through the duodenum or jejunum because feeding formulas with a high osmolality may lead to undesirable effects, such as dumping syndrome (described below).

Fluid balance is maintained by **osmosis**, the process by which water moves through membranes from a dilute solution of lower **osmolality** (ionic concentration) to a more concentrated solution of higher osmolality until both solutions are of nearly equal osmolality. The osmolality of normal body fluids is approximately 300 mOsm/kg. The body attempts to keep the osmolality of the contents of the stomach and intestines at approximately this level.

Highly concentrated solutions and certain foods can upset the normal fluid balance in the body. Individual

TABLE 36-2 Conditions Requiring Enteral Therapy

Condition or Need	Examples
Preoperative bowel preparation	—
Gastrointestinal problems	Fistula, short-bowel syndrome, mild pancreatitis, Crohn's disease, ulcerative colitis, nonspecific maldigestion or malabsorption
Cancer therapy	Radiation, chemotherapy
Convalescent care	Surgery, injury, severe illness
Coma, semi-consciousness*	Stroke, head injury, neurologic disorder, neoplasm
Hypermetabolic conditions	Burns, trauma, multiple fractures, sepsis, AIDS, organ transplantation
Alcoholism, chronic depression, anorexia nervosa*	Chronic illness, psychiatric or neurologic disorder
Debilitation*	Disease or injury
Maxillofacial or cervical surgery	Disease or injury
Oropharyngeal or esophageal paralysis*	Disease or injury, neoplasm, inflammation, trauma, respiratory failure

*Because some of these patients are at risk for regurgitating or vomiting and aspirating administered formula, each condition must be considered individually.

amino acids and carbohydrates are small particles that have great osmotic effect. Proteins are extremely large particles and therefore have less osmotic effect. Fats are not water-soluble and do not enter into a solution in water; thus, they have no osmotic effect. Electrolytes, such as sodium and potassium, are comparatively small particles; they have a great effect on osmolality and consequently on the patient's ability to tolerate a given solution.

When a concentrated solution of high osmolality is taken in large amounts, water moves to the stomach and intestines from fluid surrounding the organs and the vascular compartment. The patient has a feeling of fullness, nausea, and diarrhea; this causes dehydration, hypotension, and tachycardia, collectively termed the **dumping syndrome**. It is generally believed that starting with a more dilute commercial formula and increasing the concentration over several days may alleviate this problem. However, there is a lack of research data supporting the dilution of formula with water to relieve dumping syndrome (Parrish, 2003). Patients vary in the degree to which they tolerate the effects of high osmolality; usually debilitated patients are less tolerant. The nurse needs to be knowledgeable about the osmolality of the patient's formula and needs to observe for and take steps to prevent undesired effects.

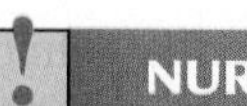

NURSING ALERT

Commercial formulas frequently present problems because the composition is fixed and some patients cannot tolerate certain ingredients, such as sodium, protein, or potassium. Modular products may be substituted, and the critical constituents of sodium, potassium, and fat can be added. Attention is given to including all essential minerals and vitamins. Total intake of calories, nutrients, and fluids must be assessed when there is a reduction in total intake or excessive dilution of feedings.

Tube Feeding Formulas

The choice of formula to be delivered by tube feeding is influenced by the status of the GI tract and the nutritional needs of the patient. The formula characteristics that are considered prior to selection include the chemical composition of the nutrient source (protein, carbohydrates, fat), caloric density, osmolality, residue, bacteriologic safety, vitamins, minerals, and cost.

Various major formula types for tube feedings are available commercially. Blenderized formulas can be made by the patient's family or obtained in a ready-to-use form that is carefully prepared according to directions. Commercially prepared polymeric formulas (formulas with high molecular weight) are composed of protein, carbohydrates, and fats in a high-molecular-weight form (eg, Boost Plus, TwoCal HN, Isosource). Chemically defined formulas (eg, Peptomen 1.5 or Vivonex) contain predigested and easy-to-absorb nutrients. Modular products contain only one major nutrient, such as protein (Beneprotein). Disease-specific formulas are available for various conditions. For patients with renal failure, a formula such as Nepro that is high in calories and low in electrolytes is ideal because it is formulated to maintain electrolyte and fluid balance. For patients with severe chronic obstructive pulmonary disease, a formula such as Pulmocare may be selected because it is high in fat and low in carbohydrates, has a high density (1.5 calories/mL) that helps maintain fluid restriction, and reduces carbon dioxide production. Fiber is added to some formulas (eg, Jevity) to decrease the occurrence of diarrhea in some at-risk patients. Some feedings are given as supplements, and others are designed to meet the patient's total nutritional needs. Dietitians collaborate with physicians and nurses to determine the best formula for the individual patient.

Tube Feeding Administration Methods

Many patients do not tolerate NG and nasoenteric tube feedings well. Often a medium- or fine-bore Silastic nasoenteric tube is better tolerated than a plastic or rubber tube. The finer-bore tube requires a finely dispersed formula to ensure that the tube remains patent. For long-term tube feeding therapy, a gastrostomy or jejunostomy tube is often used (see later discussion).

The tube feeding method chosen depends on the location of the tube in the GI tract, patient tolerance, convenience, and cost. Intermittent bolus feedings are administered into the stomach (usually by gastrostomy tube) in large amounts at designated intervals and may be given four to eight times per day. The intermittent gravity drip, another method for administering tube feedings into the stomach, is commonly used when the patient is at home. In this instance, the tube feeding is administered over 30 minutes at designated intervals. Both of these tube feeding methods are practical and inexpensive. However, the feedings delivered at variable rates may be poorly tolerated and time-consuming.

The continuous infusion method is used when feedings are administered into the small intestine. This method is preferred for patients who are at risk for aspiration or who tolerate tube feedings poorly (Shang, Geiger, Sturm, et al., 2004). The feedings are given continuously at a constant rate by means of a pump. This method decreases abdominal distention, gastric residuals, and the risk of aspiration. However, pumps are expensive, and they allow the patient less flexibility than intermittent feedings.

An alternative to the continuous infusion method is **cyclic feeding**. The infusion is given at a faster rate over a shorter time (usually 8 to 12 hours). Feedings may be infused at night to avoid interrupting the patient's lifestyle. Cyclic continuous infusions may be appropriate for patients who are being weaned from tube feedings to an oral diet, as supplements for patients who cannot eat enough, and for patients at home who need daytime hours free from the pump.

Tube feeding solutions vary in terms of required preparation, consistency, and the number of calories and vitamins they contain. The choice of solution depends on the size and location of the tube in the GI tract, the patient's nutrient needs, the type of nutritional supplement, the method of delivery, and the convenience for the patient at home. A wide variety of containers, feeding tubes and catheters, delivery systems, and pumps are available for use with tube feedings.

Nursing Process

The Patient Receiving a Tube Feeding

Assessment

A preliminary assessment of the patient who requires a tube feeding includes several considerations:

- What is the patient's nutritional status, as judged by current physical appearance, dietary history, and history of recent weight loss?
- Are there any existing chronic illnesses or factors that will increase metabolic demands on the body (eg, surgical stress, fever)?
- What is the patient's hydration status? Are fluid requirements (ie, 30 to 40 mL/kg body weight) being met?
- Is the patient's digestive tract functioning?
- Are the patient's kidneys functioning normally? What are the patient's electrolyte levels?
- What medications and other therapies is the patient receiving that may affect nutritional intake and function of the digestive system?
- Does the dietary prescription fulfill the patient's needs?

In addition, a more elaborate assessment is performed for patients who require extensive nutritional therapy. A team that includes the nurse, advanced practice nurse, physician, and dietitian conducts this assessment. In addition to the history and physical examination (which includes anthropometric measurements), a nutritional assessment is performed. This consists of recording any weight change; determining albumin, prealbumin, and transferrin levels; measuring total lymphocyte count; and evaluating muscle function. (See Chapter 5 for a detailed description of nutritional assessment.)

Diagnosis

Nursing Diagnoses

Based on the assessment data, the major nursing diagnoses may include the following:

- Imbalanced nutrition, less than body requirements, related to inadequate intake of nutrients
- Risk for diarrhea related to the dumping syndrome or to tube feeding intolerance
- Risk for ineffective airway clearance related to aspiration of tube feeding
- Risk for deficient fluid volume related to hypertonic dehydration
- Risk for ineffective coping related to discomfort imposed by the presence of the NG or nasoenteric tube
- Risk for ineffective therapeutic regimen management
- Deficient knowledge about home tube feeding regimen

Collaborative Problems/ Potential Complications

Complications of NG and nasoenteric tube feeding therapy are classified into three types—GI, mechanical, and metabolic. Table 36-3 summarizes complications, possible causes, and appropriate interventions.

Planning and Goals

The major goals for the patient may include nutritional balance, normal bowel elimination pattern, reduced risk of aspiration, adequate hydration, individual coping, knowledge and skill in self-care, and prevention of complications.

Nursing Interventions

Maintaining Feeding Equipment and Nutritional Balance

The temperature and volume of the feeding, the flow rate, and the patient's total fluid intake are important factors to be considered when tube feedings are administered. The schedule of tube feedings, including the correct quantity and frequency, is maintained. The nurse must carefully monitor the drip rate and avoid administering fluids too rapidly.

Feedings are administered by gravity (drip), bolus, or continuous controlled pump (mL/hour). Gravity feedings are placed above the level of the stomach, with the speed of administration determined by gravity. **Bolus** feedings are given in large volumes (300 to 400 mL every 4 to 6 hours). Continuous feeding is the preferred method; delivery of the feeding in small amounts over long periods reduces the incidence of aspiration, distention, nausea, vomiting, and diarrhea. Continuous administration rates vary depending on the caloric density of the formula and the energy needs of the patient. The overall goal is to achieve positive nitrogen balance and weight maintenance or gain without producing abdominal cramps and diarrhea. If the feeding is intermittent, 200 to 350 mL is given over a span of 10 to 15 minutes.

Enteral pumps are mechanical devices that control the delivery rate of feeding formula (Fig. 36-5). Pumps allow for a constant flow rate and can infuse a viscous formula through a small-diameter feeding tube. These pumps are relatively heavy and must be attached to an IV pole. For home use, there are portable lightweight enteral pumps available that weigh about 4 pounds and are easy to handle.

Residual gastric content is measured before each intermittent feeding and every 4 to 8 hours during

TABLE 36-3 Complications of Enteral Therapy

Complications	Causes	Selected Nursing Interventions: Treatment	Selected Nursing Interventions: Prevention
Gastrointestinal			
Diarrhea (most common)	Hyperosmolar feedings Rapid infusion/bolus feedings Bacteria-contaminated feedings Lactase deficiency Medications/antibiotic therapy Decreased serum osmolality level Food allergies Cold formula	Assess fluid balance and electrolyte levels; report findings Implement changes in tube feeding formula or rate	Assess rate of infusion and temperature of formula Replace formula every 4 hours; change tube feeding container and tubing daily
Nausea/vomiting	Change in formula or rate Hyperosmolar formula Inadequate gastric emptying	Review medications	Check residuals; if ≥200 mL for NG or >100 mL for gastrostomy, continue feeding and recheck; report if residual is still high
Gas/bloating/cramping	Air in tube	Notify physician if persistent	Keep tubing free of air
Dumping syndrome	Bolus feedings/rapid rate Cold formula	Check fiber and water content; report findings Check rate and temperature of formula	Avoid rapid infusion of feeding Administer feeding at or near room temperature
Constipation	High milk (lactose) content Lack of fiber Inadequate fluid intake/dehydration Opioid use	Check fiber and water content; report findings	Administer adequate amount of hydration as flushes
Mechanical			
Aspiration pneumonia	Improper tube placement Vomiting with aspiration of tube feeding Flat in bed Use of large tube	Assess respiratory status and notify physician	Implement reliable method for checking small-bore enteral tube placement (ie, measuring length of exposed tube) Keep head of bed elevated 30 degrees continuously
Tube displacement	Excessive coughing/vomitus Tension on the tube or unsecured tube Tracheal suctioning Airway intubation	Stop feeding and notify physician	Check tube placement before administering feeding
Tube obstruction	Inadequate flushing/formula rate	Follow policy for declogging feeding tubes	Obtain liquid medications when possible
Residue	Inadequate crushing of medications and flushing after administration		Flush tube and crush medications adequately
Nasopharyngeal irritation	Tube position/improper taping Use of large tubes	Assess nasopharyngeal mucous membranes every 4 hours	Tape tube to prevent pressure on nares
Metabolic			
Hyperglycemia	Glucose intolerance High carbohydrate content of the feeding	Check blood glucose levels periodically Request dietary consult to reevaluate choice of feeding product	
Dehydration and azotemia (excessive urea in the blood)	Hyperosmolar feedings with insufficient fluid intake	Report signs and symptoms of dehydration Implement changes in tube feeding formula, rate, or ratio to water	Provide adequate hydration through flushes

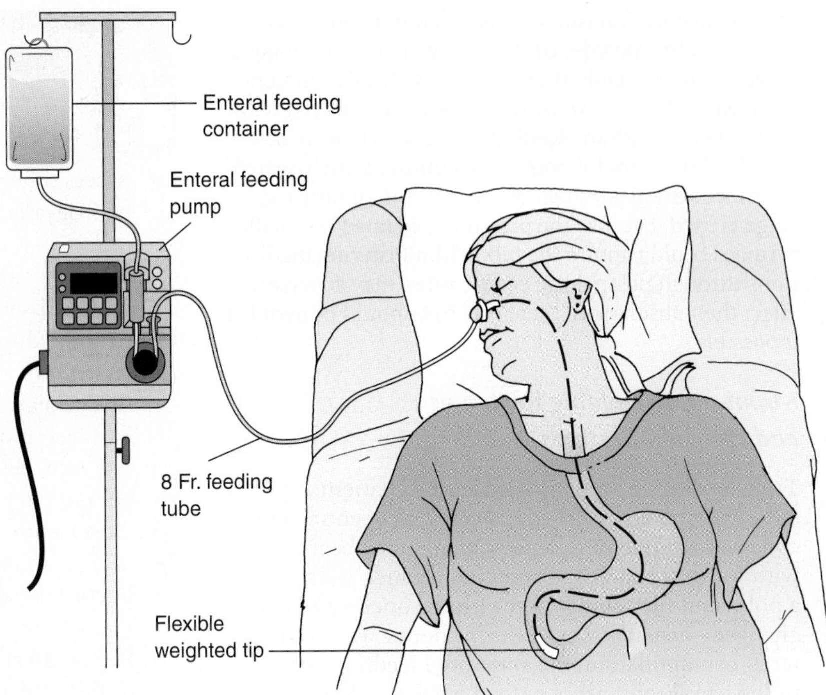

FIGURE 36-5. Nasoenteric tube feeding by continuous controlled pump. The head of the bed should be elevated to prevent aspiration.

continuous feedings. (This aspirated fluid is readministered to the patient.) In a recent systematic review of the literature, it was found that there was little correlation between residual volumes and tube feeding tolerance (Keithley & Swanson, 2004). Although a residual volume of 200 mL or greater is generally considered a cause for concern in patients at high risk for aspiration, feedings do not necessarily need to be withheld in all patients. Tube feedings may be continued with close monitoring of gastric residual volume, x-ray study results, and the patient's physical status. If excessive residual volumes (eg, more than 200 mL) occur twice, the nurse notifies the physician.

Maintaining tube function is an ongoing responsibility of the nurse, patient, or primary caregiver. To ensure patency and to decrease the chance of bacterial growth, crusting, or occlusion of the tube, at least 30 to 50 mL of water or normal saline is administered in each of the following instances:

- Before and after each dose of medication and each tube feeding
- After checking for gastric residuals and gastric pH
- Every 4 to 6 hours with continuous feedings
- If the tube feeding is discontinued or interrupted for any reason
- When the tube is not being used, twice-daily administration is recommended.

Any water or normal saline used to irrigate these tubes must be recorded as fluid intake. One study has shown that tap water may injure the small bowel and supports the practice of flushing postpyloric nasoduodenal or jejunostomy tubes with normal saline (Schloerb, Wood, Casillan, et al., 2004).

Providing Medications By Tube

When different types of medications are administered, each type is given separately, using a bolus method that is compatible with the medication's preparation (Table 36-4). The tube is flushed with 30 to 50 mL of water after each dose, and this fluid is recorded as intake. If a liquid form of a medication is not available

TABLE 36-4 Preparing Medication for Delivery by Feeding Tube

Medication Form	Preparation
Liquid	None
Simple compressed tablets	Crush and dissolve in water
Buccal or sublingual tablets	Administer as prescribed
Soft gelatin capsules filled with liquid	Make an opening in capsule and squeeze out contents
Enteric-coated tablets	Do not crush; change in form is required
Timed-release tablets	Do not crush tablets because doing so may release too much drug too quickly (overdose); check with pharmacist for alternative formulation
Timed-release capsules or sustained-release capsules	Some can be opened and contents added to tube-feeding formula; *always* check with pharmacist before doing this

and the medication can be crushed, it must first be reduced to a fine powder or the tube will become clogged. Devices are available that crush and dissolve tablets with water (Fig. 36-6). Medications are not mixed with each other or with the feeding formula. When small-bore feeding tubes for continuous infusion are irrigated after medication administration, a 30-mL or larger syringe is used, because the pressure generated by smaller syringes could rupture the tube. Administering medications through postpyloric enteric tubes may adversely affect their absorption; therefore, this should be avoided if possible.

Maintaining Feeding Regimens and Delivery Systems

Tube feeding formula is delivered to patients by either an open or a closed system. The open system comes as a liquid or as a powder and may be mixed with water. The feeding container (which is hung on a pole) and the tubing used with the open system are changed—usually every 24 to 72 hours. To avoid bacterial contamination, the amount of feeding formula in the bag should never exceed what should be infused in a 4-hour period.

Closed delivery systems use a prefilled, sterile container that is spiked with enteral tubing. The bag holding the feeding formula for the closed system can be hung safely for 24 to 48 hours.

The tube feeding regimen must be assessed frequently to evaluate its effectiveness and avoid complications (Chart 36-1).

Maintaining Normal Bowel Elimination Pattern

Patients receiving NG or nasoenteric tube feedings commonly have diarrhea (watery stools occurring three or more times in 24 hours). Pasty, unformed stool is expected with enteral therapy, because many formulas have little or no residue. The dumping syndrome also leads to diarrhea; however, to confirm dumping syndrome as the cause of diarrhea, other possible causes must be excluded, such as:

- Contaminated formula
- Malnutrition—A decrease in the intestinal absorptive area resulting from malnutrition can cause diarrhea
- Medication therapy—Antibiotics, such as clindamycin (Cleocin); antiarrhythmics, such as quinidine (Quinaglute) and propranolol (Inderal); and aminophylline (Phyllocontin), theophylline (Theobid), and digitalis (digoxin [Lanoxin]) have been found to increase the frequency of diarrhea in some patients. Elixir-based medications often contain sorbitol, which can act as a cathartic (Dickerson et al., 2003).

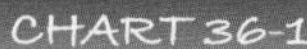

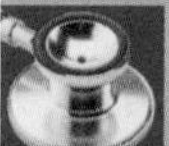

Assessing for Tube Feeding Regimens

- Assess tube placement, patient's position (head of bed elevated 30 to 45 degrees), and formula flow rate.
- Determine the patient's ability to tolerate the formula. Observe for fullness, bloating, distention, urticaria, nausea, vomiting, and stool pattern and character.
- Check clinical responses, as noted in laboratory findings (blood urea nitrogen, serum protein, prealbumin, electrolytes, renal function, hemoglobin, hematocrit).
- Observe for signs of dehydration (dry mucous membranes, thirst, decreased urine output).
- Record the amount of formula actually taken in by the patient.
- Report an elevated blood glucose level, decreased urinary output, sudden weight gain, and periorbital or dependent edema.
- Replace any formula administered by an open system every 4 hours with fresh formula. Formula should be at room temperature or cool (not cold).
- Change tube feeding container and tubing every 24 to 72 hours.
- Assess residual volume before each feeding or, in the case of continuous feedings, every 4 hours. Return the aspirate to the stomach.
- Monitor intake and output.
- Weigh the patient twice weekly.
- Consult the dietitian regularly.

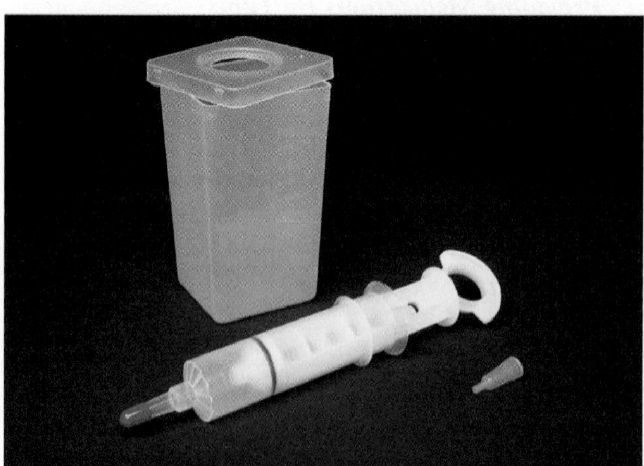

FIGURE 36-6. The Pill Crusher™ Syringe (from Welcon, Inc.) crushes medications to a fine powder and then allows them to be administered to patients with feeding tubes. The Pill Crusher™ is also used to irrigate the feeding tube and assists in hydrating the patient. Courtesy of Welcon, Inc., Fort Worth, TX (www.welcon.com).

- *Clostridium difficile* colitis infection—This infection can result in significant diarrhea, especially in hospitalized patients (Carroll, 2003).

The dumping syndrome results from rapid distention of the jejunum when hypertonic solutions are administered rapidly (over 10 to 20 minutes). Foods high in carbohydrates and electrolytes draw extracellular fluid from the vascular system into the jejunum so that dilution and absorption can occur. Measures for managing the GI symptoms (diarrhea, nausea) associated with the dumping syndrome are presented in Chart 36-2.

Reducing the Risk for Aspiration

Aspiration pneumonia occurs when stomach contents or enteral feedings are regurgitated and aspirated, or when an NG tube is improperly positioned and feedings are instilled into the pharynx or the trachea. Feeding patients through nasoenteric tubes placed beyond the pylorus has helped decrease the frequency of regurgitation and aspiration.

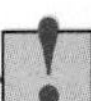

NURSING ALERT

To prevent aspiration, the nurse must verify the correct tube placement before every feeding, each time medications are administered, and once every shift if the tube feeding is continuous.

Feedings and medications should always be administered with the patient in the proper position to prevent regurgitation. The semi-Fowler's position is necessary for an NG feeding, with the patient's head elevated at least 30 to 45 degrees to reduce the risk for reflux and pulmonary aspiration. This position is maintained at least 1 hour after completion of an intermittent tube feeding and is maintained at all times for patients receiving continuous tube feedings. Another prevention strategy is to monitor the residual volume and notify the physician and stop the feedings if the residual volume is excessive, as discussed previously.

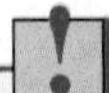

NURSING ALERT

If aspiration is suspected, the feeding is stopped immediately, the pharynx and trachea are suctioned, and the patient is placed on the right side with the head of the bed down. The physician is notified immediately.

Maintaining Adequate Hydration

The nurse carefully monitors hydration because in many cases the patient cannot communicate the need for water. Water is given every 4 to 6 hours and after feedings to prevent hypertonic dehydration. At the beginning of administration, the feeding is given in continuous drip administration. This gradual administration allows assessment of residual volume and helps the patient develop tolerance, especially for hyperosmolar solutions. Key nursing interventions include observing for signs of dehydration (eg, dry mucous membranes, thirst, decreased urine output); administering water routinely and as needed; and monitoring intake, output, residual volume, and fluid balance (24-hour intake versus output).

Promoting Coping Ability

The psychosocial goal of nursing care is to support and encourage the patient to accept physical changes and to convey hope that daily progressive improvement is possible. If the patient is having difficulty adjusting to the treatment, the nurse intervenes by encouraging self-care (eg, recording daily weight and intake and output), within the parameters of the patient's activity level. In addition, the nurse reinforces an optimistic approach by identifying indicators of progress (daily weight trends, electrolyte balance, absence of nausea and diarrhea).

Promoting Home and Community-Based Care

TEACHING PATIENTS SELF-CARE

Patients who require long-term tube feedings in the home care setting have conditions such as obstruction of the upper GI tract, malabsorption syndrome, surgery of the GI tract or of the head or neck region, or decreased level of consciousness. For a patient to be considered for tube feeding at home, the following

CHART 36-2

Preventing Symptoms of Dumping Syndrome

The following strategies may help prevent some of the uncomfortable symptoms of dumping syndrome related to tube feeding:

- Slow the formula instillation rate to provide time for carbohydrates and electrolytes to be diluted.
- Administer feedings at room temperature, because temperature extremes stimulate peristalsis.
- Administer feeding by continuous drip (if tolerated) rather than by bolus, to prevent sudden distention of the intestine.
- Advise the patient to remain in semi-Fowler's position for 1 hour after the feeding; this position prolongs intestinal transit time by decreasing the effect of gravity.
- Instill the minimal amount of water needed to flush the tubing before and after a feeding, because fluid given with a feeding increases intestinal transit time.

criteria should be met (Ireton-Jones, DeLegge, Epperson, et al., 2003):

- The patient should be medically stable and should have successfully completed a tube feeding trial (tolerated 70% of feeding).
- The patient must be capable of self-care or have a caregiver willing to assume the responsibility.
- The patient or caregiver must have access to supplies and interest in learning how to administer tube feedings at home.

Preparation of the patient for home administration of enteral feedings begins while the patient is still hospitalized. Ideally, the nurse teaches while administering the feedings so that the patient and/or caregiver can observe the mechanics of the procedure, participate in the procedure, ask questions, and express any concerns. Before discharge, the nurse provides information about the equipment needed, formula purchase and storage, and administration of the feedings (frequency, quantity, rate of instillation).

Family members who will be active in the patient's home care are encouraged to participate in all teaching sessions. Available printed information about the equipment, the formula, and the procedure is reviewed. The nurse encourages the patient and caregiver to learn the basic process with the supervision of the nurse. Arrangements are made for the caregiver to obtain the equipment and formula and have it ready for use before the patient's discharge.

CONTINUING CARE

Referral to a home care agency is important so that a nurse can supervise and provide support during the first feeding at home. Additional visits will depend on the skill and comfort of the patient or caregiver in administering the feedings. During all visits, the nurse monitors the patient's physical status (weight, vital signs, activity level) and the ability of the patient and family to administer the tube feedings correctly. In addition, the nurse assesses for any complications (dumping syndrome, nausea or vomiting, weight loss, lethargy, confusion, excessive thirst). The patient or caregiver is encouraged to keep a diary to record times and amounts of feedings and any symptoms that occur. The nurse can review the diary with the patient and caregiver during home visits.

Evaluation

Expected Patient Outcomes

Expected patient outcomes may include:

1. Attains or maintains nutritional balance
   a. Has a positive nitrogen balance
   b. Maintains laboratory values within normal limits (ie, blood urea nitrogen, hemoglobin, hematocrit, prealbumin, serum protein)
   c. Attains or maintains hydration of body tissue
   d. Attains or maintains desired body weight
2. Is free of episodes of diarrhea
   a. Has fewer than three watery stools a day
   b. Does not have a bowel movement after a bolus feeding
   c. Reports no intestinal cramping
   d. Has normal bowel sounds
3. Avoids aspiration
   a. Lungs are clear to auscultation
   b. Exhibits normal heart rate and respiratory rate
4. Attains or maintains hydration of body tissue
   a. Has a balanced fluid intake and output every 24 hours
   b. Does not have dry skin or dry mucous membranes
5. Copes effectively with tube feeding regimen
6. Demonstrates skill in managing tube feeding regimen
7. Experiences no complications
   a. Has no GI disturbances
   b. Tube remains intact and patent for duration of therapy
   c. Maintains metabolic balance within normal limits

Gastrostomy

A **gastrostomy** is a surgical procedure in which an opening is created into the stomach for the purpose of administering foods and fluids via a feeding tube. In some instances, a gastrostomy is preferred for prolonged enteral nutrition support (longer than 4 weeks) (Roche, 2003). Gastrostomy is also preferred over NG feedings in the patient who is comatose because the gastroesophageal sphincter remains intact. Regurgitation and aspiration are less likely to occur with a gastrostomy than with NG feedings.

Different types of feeding gastrostomies may be used, including the Stamm (temporary and permanent), Janeway (permanent), and percutaneous endoscopic gastrostomy (temporary) systems. The Stamm and Janeway gastrostomies require either an upper abdominal midline incision or a left upper quadrant transverse incision. The Stamm procedure requires the use of concentric purse-string sutures to secure the tube to the anterior gastric wall. To create the gastrostomy, an exit wound is created in the left upper abdomen. The Janeway procedure necessitates the creation of a tunnel (called a gastric tube) that is brought out through the abdomen to form a permanent **stoma.**

Insertion of a **percutaneous endoscopic gastrostomy (PEG)** requires the services of two physicians (or a physician and a nurse with specialty skills). After administering a local anesthetic, one physician inserts a cannula into the stomach through an abdominal incision and then threads a nonabsorbable suture through the cannula; the second physician inserts an endoscope via the patient's upper GI tract and uses the endoscopic snare to grasp the end of the suture and guide it up through the patient's mouth. The suture is knotted to the dilator tip at the end of the PEG tube. The endoscopist then advances the dilator tip through the patient's mouth while the first physician pulls the suture through the cannula site. The attached PEG tube is guided down the esophagus, into the stomach, and out through the abdominal in-

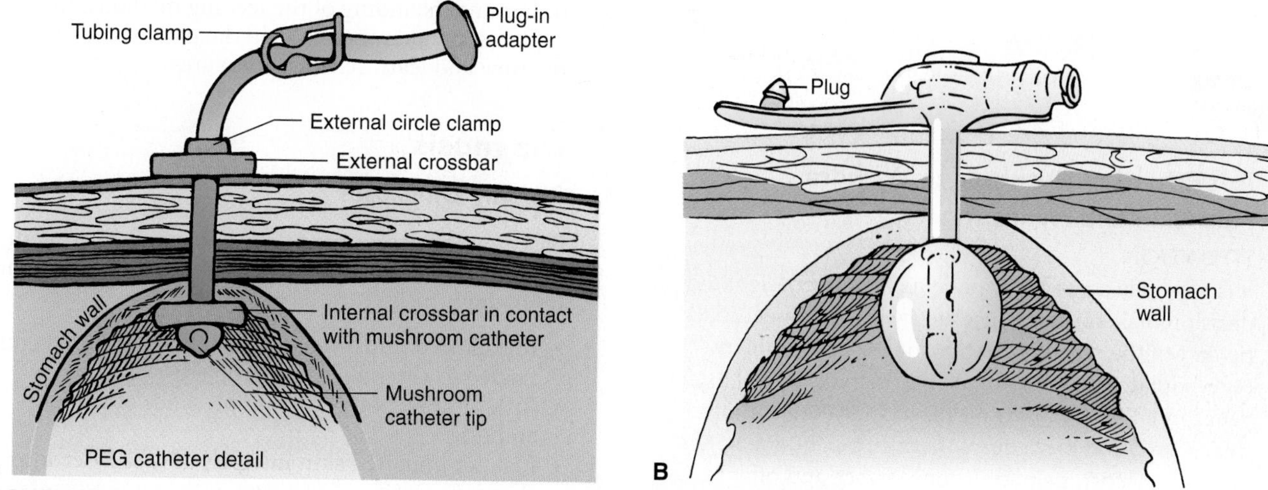

FIGURE 36-7. (**A**) A detail of the abdomen and the percutaneous endoscopic gastrostomy (PEG) tube, showing catheter fixation. (**B**) A detail of the abdomen and the nonobturated low-profile gastrostomy device (LPGD), showing balloon fixation.

cision (Fig. 36-7A). The mushroom catheter tip and internal crossbar secure the tube against the stomach wall. An external crossbar or bumper keeps the catheter in place. A tubing adaptor is in place between feedings, and a clamp or plug is used to close or open the tubing. If an endoscope cannot be passed through the esophagus, then the gastrostomy can be performed under x-ray guidance through the abdominal wall (Neef, Crowder, McIvor, et al., 2003).

The initial PEG device can be removed and replaced once the tract is well established (10 to 14 days after insertion). Replacement of the PEG device is indicated to provide long-term nutritional support, to replace a clogged or migrated tube, or to enhance patient comfort. The PEG replacement device should be fitted securely to the stoma to prevent leakage of gastric acid and is maintained in place through traction between the internal and anchoring devices.

An alternative to the PEG device is a **low-profile gastrostomy device (LPGD)** (see Fig. 36-7B). The LPGD may be inserted 3 to 6 months after initial gastrostomy tube placement. These devices are inserted flush with the skin; they eliminate the possibility of tube migration and obstruction and have antireflux valves to prevent gastric reflux. Two types of devices may be used—obturated or nonobturated. The obturated devices (G-button) have a dome tip that acts as an internal stabilizer. Only a physician may obturate (insert a tube that is larger than the actual stoma). The nonobturated device (MIC-KEY) has an external skin disk and is inserted into the stoma without force; a balloon is inflated to secure placement. A nurse in the home setting may insert these nonobturated devices. The drawbacks of both types of LPGDs are the inability to assess residual volumes (one-way valve) and the need for a special adaptor to connect the device to the feeding container.

Reflux from stomach feedings can result in aspiration pneumonia. Therefore, patients at risk for aspiration pneumonia are not ideal candidates for a gastrostomy. A jejunostomy is preferred, or jejunal feeding through a nasojejunal tube may be recommended.

Nursing Process

The Patient With a Gastrostomy

Assessment

The focus of the preoperative assessment is to determine the patient's ability both to understand and cope with the impending surgical experience. The nurse assesses the patient's ability to adjust to a change in body image and to participate in self-care, along with the patient's and the family's psychological status. There are multiple medical and ethical issues that the patient, the caregivers, and the physician should discuss together (Angus & Burakoff, 2003) (Chart 36-3).

The purpose of the operative procedure is explained so that the patient has a better understanding of the expected postoperative course. The patient needs to know that the purpose of the procedure is to bypass the mouth and esophagus so that liquid feedings can be administered directly into the stomach by means of a rubber or plastic tube or a prosthesis. If the prosthesis is to be permanent, the patient should be made aware of this. Psychologically, this is often difficult for the patient to accept. If the procedure is being performed to relieve discomfort, prolonged vomiting, debilitation, or an inability to eat, the patient may find it more acceptable.

The nurse evaluates the patient's skin condition and determines whether a delay in healing at the tube insertion site may be anticipated because of a systemic disorder (eg, diabetes mellitus, ascites, cancer).

In the postoperative period, the patient's fluid and nutritional needs are assessed to ensure proper intake of food and fluids. The nurse inspects the tube for proper maintenance and the incision for signs of infection. At the same time, the nurse evaluates the patient's response to the change in body image and his

CHART 36-3

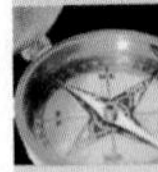

Ethics and Related Issues

Is It Ethical to Withhold or Withdraw Nutrition and Hydration?

SITUATION

It is generally agreed that patients (or their designated decision makers) can refuse life-saving treatment, particularly if the means of treatment are extraordinary (eg, ventilators, dialysis machines, extracorporeal oxygenators). Extraordinary means include medications, treatments, and procedures that can be obtained only at excessive cost, pain, or inconvenience and offer no reasonable hope of benefit. Nutrition and hydration therapy, however, are perceived as ordinary means by many.

Ordinary means are those medications, treatments, and procedures that offer a reasonable hope of benefit and can be obtained without excessive expense, pain, or inconvenience. Additionally, withdrawing or withholding nutrition and hydration can in and of itself cause death. Thus, some have argued that nutrition and hydration should always be provided to every patient, regardless of the patient's preference or condition.

DILEMMA

The patient's desire to have nutrition or hydration withdrawn or withheld may conflict with the reluctance of others to harm the patient by withdrawing the food and water needed for survival (autonomy versus nonmaleficence).

DISCUSSION

Answer the following questions using as an example a patient in a persistent vegetative state (ie, unable to express his or her wishes).

- What arguments would you offer *against* the withholding and withdrawing of nutrition and hydration?
- What arguments would you offer *in favor of* withholding and withdrawing of nutrition and hydration?
- Are foods and fluids always "ordinary means," or are there instances in which they might be considered "extraordinary"? Support your answer.
- What are some of the religious, cultural, and financial issues that can complicate family and caregiver decisions?
- Should an attempt be made to involve critically ill or sedated patients in their own end-of-life decisions when their death is clearly imminent? How does one balance the issues of patient autonomy versus beneficence in this situation?

or her understanding of the feeding methods. Interventions are identified to help the patient cope with the tube and learn self-care measures.

Diagnosis

Nursing Diagnoses

Based on the assessment data, the major nursing diagnoses in the postoperative period may include the following:

- Imbalanced nutrition, less than body requirements, related to enteral feeding problems
- Risk for infection related to presence of wound and tube
- Risk for impaired skin integrity at tube insertion site
- Ineffective coping related to inability to eat normally
- Disturbed body image related to presence of tube
- Risk for ineffective therapeutic regimen management related to knowledge deficit about home care and the feeding procedure

Collaborative Problems/ Potential Complications

Potential complications that may develop include the following (Roche, 2003):

- Wound infection, cellulitis, leakage, and abdominal wall abscess
- GI bleeding
- Premature removal of the tube
- Aspiration
- Constipation or diarrhea

Planning and Goals

The major goals for the patient may include attaining an optimal level of nutrition, preventing infection, maintaining skin integrity, enhancing coping, adjusting to changes in body image, acquiring knowledge of and skill in self-care, and preventing complications.

Nursing Interventions

Meeting Nutritional Needs

The first fluid nourishment is administered soon after surgery and usually consists of tap water and 10% dextrose. At first, only 30 to 60 mL (1 to 2 oz) is given at one time, but the amount administered is increased gradually. By the second day, 180 to 240 mL (6 to 8 oz) may be given at one time, provided it is tolerated and no leakage of fluid occurs around the tube. Water and enteral feeding can be infused after 24 hours for a permanent gastrostomy.

Blenderized foods can be added gradually to clear liquids until a full diet is achieved. Powdered feedings that are easily liquefied are commercially available. The patient who receives blenderized tube feedings typically is not forced to give up usual dietary patterns, which may prove to be psychologically more acceptable. In addition, near-normal bowel function is promoted because the fiber and residue are similar to those of a normal diet.

Providing Tube Care and Preventing Infection

A small dressing can be applied over the tube insertion site, and the gastrostomy tube can be held in place by a thin strip of adhesive tape that is first placed around the tube and then firmly attached to the abdomen. The dressing protects the skin around the incision from seepage of gastric acid and spillage of feedings (Fig. 36-8).

The nurse verifies the tube's placement, assesses residuals, and gently manipulates the tube or stabilizing disk once daily to prevent skin breakdown. Some gastrostomy tubes have balloons that are inflated with water to anchor the tube in the stomach. Balloon integrity is checked weekly by deflating and reinflating the balloon using a Luer-tip syringe.

Providing Skin Care

The skin surrounding a gastrostomy requires special care because it may become irritated from the enzymatic action of gastric juices that leak around the tube. Left untreated, the skin becomes macerated, red, raw, and painful. The nurse washes the area around the tube with soap and water daily, removes any encrustation with saline solution, rinses the area well with water, and pats it dry. A long-term gastrostomy may require a special dressing or stabilization device to protect the skin around the tube from gastric secretions and to help secure the tube in place (see Fig. 36-8).

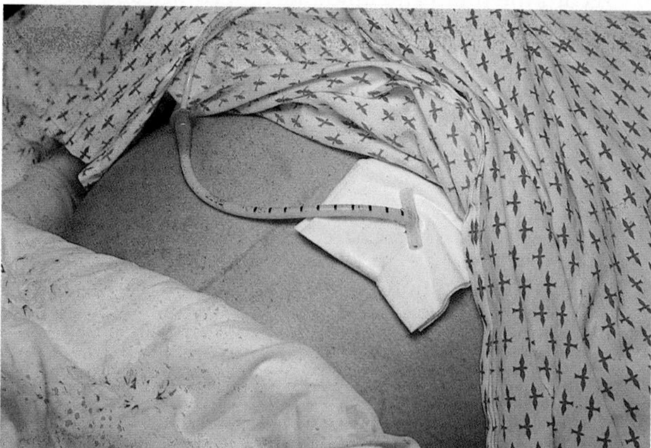

FIGURE 36-8. Protection at the gastrostomy site. A PEG tube may be protected by a dressing that allows access to the tube but covers the exit site. Typically, the tube is stabilized with tape over the dressing. From Craven, R., & Hirnle, C. (2006). *Fundamentals of nursing: Human health and function* (5th ed.). Philadelphia: Lippincott Williams & Wilkins.

Skin at the exit site is evaluated daily for signs of breakdown, irritation, excoriation, and the presence of drainage or gastric leakage. The nurse encourages the patient and family members to participate in this evaluation and in hygiene activities. If skin problems do occur, an enterostomal therapist or wound ostomy continence nurse can be of assistance.

Enhancing Body Image

The patient with a gastrostomy has experienced a major assault to body image. Eating, a physiologic and social function, can no longer be taken for granted. The patient is also aware that gastrostomy as a therapeutic intervention is performed only in the presence of a major, chronic, or perhaps terminal illness.

Calm discussion of the purposes and routines of gastrostomy feeding can help keep the patient from feeling overwhelmed. Talking with a person who has had a gastrostomy can also help the patient accept the expected changes. Adjusting to a change in body image takes time and requires family support and acceptance. Evaluating the existing family support system is necessary.

Monitoring and Managing Potential Complications

During the postoperative course, the nurse monitors the patient for potential complications. The most common complications are wound infection and other wound problems, including cellulitis at the exit site and abscesses in the abdominal wall. Because many patients who receive tube feedings are debilitated and have compromised nutritional status, any signs of infection are promptly reported to the physician so that appropriate therapy can be instituted.

Bleeding from the insertion site in the stomach may also occur. The nurse closely monitors the patient's vital signs and observes all drainage from the operative site, vomitus, and stool for evidence of bleeding. Any signs of bleeding are reported promptly.

Premature removal of the tube, whether it is done inadvertently by the patient or by the caregiver, is another complication. If the tube is removed prematurely, the skin is cleansed and a sterile dressing is applied; the nurse immediately notifies the physician. The tract will close within 4 to 6 hours if the tube is not replaced promptly.

Promoting Home and Community-Based Care

TEACHING PATIENTS SELF-CARE

The patient who is to receive gastrostomy tube feedings in the home setting must be capable of, and responsible for, administering the tube feedings or have a caregiver who can do so. There must also be the physical, financial, and social resources to maintain care.

The nurse assesses the patient's level of knowledge, interest in learning about the tube feeding, and ability to understand and apply the information before providing detailed instructions about how to prepare the formula and manage the tube feeding. Written materials for patients and caregivers are designed to outline the care instructions. To facilitate self-care, the nurse encourages the patient to participate in the tube feedings during hospitalization and to establish as normal a routine as possible.

Demonstration of the tube feeding begins by showing the patient how to check for residual gastric contents before the feeding. The patient then learns how to check and maintain the patency of the tube by administering room-temperature water before and after the feeding. This establishes patency before the feeding and then clears the tube of food particles, which could decompose if allowed to remain in the tube. All feedings are given at room temperature or near body temperature.

For a bolus feeding, the nurse shows the patient how to introduce the liquid into the catheter by using a funnel or the barrel of a syringe. The receptacle is tilted to allow air to escape while the liquid is being instilled initially. As the funnel or syringe fills with liquid, the feeding is allowed to flow into the stomach by gravity by holding the barrel or syringe perpendicular to the abdomen (Fig. 36-9). Raising or lowering the receptacle to no higher than 45 cm (18 in) above the abdominal wall regulates the rate of flow.

A bolus feeding of 300 to 500 mL usually is given for each meal and requires 10 to 15 minutes to complete. The amount is often determined by the patient's reaction. If the patient feels full, it may be desirable to give smaller amounts more frequently.

The patient and caregiver must understand that keeping the head of the bed elevated a minimum of 45 degrees for at least 1 hour after feeding facilitates digestion and decreases the risk of aspiration. Any obstruction requires that the feeding be stopped and the physician notified.

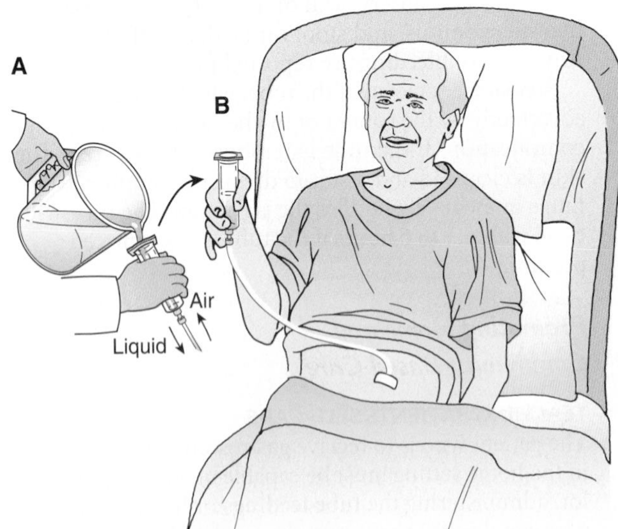

FIGURE 36-9. Bolus gastrostomy feeding by gravity. (**A**) Feeding is instilled at an angle so that air does not enter the stomach. (**B**) Syringe is raised perpendicular to the abdomen so that feeding can enter by gravity.

The patient or caregiver is instructed to flush the tube with 30 to 50 mL of water after each bolus or medication administration and to also flush the tube daily to keep it patent. Adaptors are available that can be secured to the end of the tube to create a "Y" site for ease of flushing or medication delivery. The flushing equipment is cleaned with warm, soapy water and rinsed after each use.

The patient and caregiver are made aware that the tube is marked at skin level to provide the patient with a baseline for later comparison. They are advised to monitor the tube's length and to notify the physician or home care nurse if the segment of the tube outside the body becomes shorter or longer.

If the patient is to use an intermittent or continuous-pressure feeding pump at home, instruction in the use of the particular type of pump is essential. Most feeding pumps have built-in alarms that signal when the bag is empty, when the battery is low, or when the tube is occluded. The patient and caregiver need to be aware of these alarms and how to troubleshoot the pump.

CONTINUING CARE

Referral to a home care agency is important to ensure initial supervision and support for the patient and caregiver. The home care nurse assesses the patient's status and progress and evaluates the techniques used in administering the tube feeding. Further instruction and supervision in the home setting may be required to help the patient and caregiver adapt to a physical environment and equipment that are different from the hospital setting. The nurse also reviews with the patient and caregiver complications to report (eg, dumping syndrome, nausea and vomiting, infection of the skin at the insertion site of the tube).

The home care nurse assists the patient and family in establishing as normal a routine as possible. The patient or caregiver is encouraged to keep a diary to record the times and amounts of feedings and any symptoms that occur. The nurse reviews the diary during home visits. In addition, the patient or caregiver must be taught how to replace the tube.

Evaluation

Expected Patient Outcomes

Expected patient outcomes may include the following:

1. Achieves an adequate intake of nutrients
   a. Tolerates quantity and frequency of tube feedings
   b. Has 100 mL or less of residual gastric content before each feeding
   c. Has no diarrhea
   d. Maintains or gains weight
   e. Has normal electrolyte values
2. Is free from infection and skin breakdown
   a. Is afebrile
   b. Has no drainage from the incision

   c. Demonstrates intact skin surrounding the exit site
   d. Inspects exit site daily
3. Adjusts to change in body image
   a. Is able to discuss expected changes
   b. Verbalizes concerns
4. Demonstrates skill in managing feeding regimen
   a. Helps prepare prescribed formula or blenderized feeding
   b. Handles equipment competently
   c. Helps administer the feeding or does so independently
   d. Demonstrates how to maintain tube patency
   e. Cleans tubing as needed
   f. Keeps an accurate record of intake
   g. If indicated, can remove and reinsert the tube as appropriate and needed for feedings
5. Avoids complications
   a. Exhibits adequate wound healing
   b. Has no abnormal bleeding from puncture site
   c. Tube remains intact for the duration of therapy

Parenteral Nutrition

Parenteral nutrition (PN) is a method of providing nutrients to the body by an IV route. The nutrients are a very complex admixture containing proteins, carbohydrates, fats, electrolytes, vitamins, trace minerals, and sterile water in a single container. The goals of PN are to improve nutritional status, establish a positive nitrogen balance, maintain muscle mass, promote weight maintenance or gain, and enhance the healing process.

Establishing Positive Nitrogen Balance

When a patient's intake of protein and nutrients is significantly less than that required by the body to meet energy expenditures, a state of negative nitrogen balance results. In response, the body begins to convert the protein found in muscles into carbohydrates to be used to meet energy needs. The result is muscle wasting, weight loss, fatigue, and, if left uncorrected, death. The goal for patients receiving nutrition support is to achieve positive nitrogen balance (Huckleberry, 2004).

The average postoperative adult patient requires approximately 1500 calories per day to keep the body from using its own store of protein. Traditional IV fluids do not provide sufficient calories or nitrogen to meet the body's daily requirements. PN solutions, which supply nutrients such as dextrose, amino acids, electrolytes, vitamins, minerals, and fat emulsions, provide enough calories and nitrogen to meet the patient's daily nutritional needs. In general, PN usually provides 25 to 35 kcal/kg of ideal body weight and 1.0 to 1.5 g of protein/kg of ideal body weight.

The patient with fever, trauma, burns, major surgery, or hypermetabolic disease requires additional daily calories. The volume of fluid necessary to provide these calories would surpass fluid tolerance and lead to pulmonary edema or heart failure. To provide the required calories in a small volume, it is necessary to increase the concentration of nutrients and use a route of administration (ie, a large, high-flow vein such as the subclavian) that rapidly dilutes incoming nutrients to the proper levels of body tolerance.

When highly concentrated dextrose is administered, caloric requirements are satisfied and the body uses amino acids for protein synthesis rather than for energy. Additional potassium is added to the solution to maintain proper electrolyte balance and to transport glucose and amino acids across cell membranes. To prevent deficiencies and fulfill requirements for tissue synthesis, other elements, such as calcium, phosphorus, magnesium, and sodium chloride, are added.

Clinical Indications

The indications for PN include a 10% deficit in body weight (compared with pre-illness weight), an inability to take oral food or fluids within 7 days after surgery, and hypercatabolic situations such as major infection with fever. Enteral nutrition should be considered before parenteral support since it assists in maintaining gut mucosal integrity (Huckleberry, 2004). In both the home and hospital setting, PN is indicated in the following situations:

- The patient's intake is insufficient to maintain an anabolic state (eg, severe burns, malnutrition, short bowel syndrome, acquired immunodeficiency syndrome [AIDS], sepsis, cancer).
- The patient's ability to ingest food orally or by tube is impaired (eg, paralytic ileus, Crohn's disease with obstruction, post-radiation enteritis, severe hyperemesis gravidarum in pregnancy).
- The patient is unwilling or unable to ingest adequate nutrients (eg, anorexia nervosa, postoperative elderly patients).
- The underlying medical condition precludes being fed orally or by tube (eg, acute pancreatitis, high enterocutaneous fistula).
- Preoperative and postoperative nutritional needs are prolonged (eg, extensive bowel surgery).

Formulas

A total of 2 to 3 L of solution is administered over a 24-hour period using a filter (1.2-micron particulate filter). Before administration, the PN infusion must be inspected for clarity and any precipitate. The label is compared with the physician's order, noting the expiration date. **Intravenous fat emulsions** (IVFEs, Intralipids) may be infused simultaneously with PN through a Y-connector close to the infusion site and should not be filtered. Before administration, the IVFE is inspected for frothiness, separation, or oily appearance. If any of these are present, the solution is not used. Usually 500 mL of a 10% emulsion or 250 mL of 20% emulsion is administered over 6 to 12 hours, one to three times a week. IVFEs can provide up to 30% of the total daily calorie intake.

IVFEs can be admixed with other components of PN to create a "three-in-one formulation" commonly called a **total nutrient admixture** (TNA). All the parenteral nutrient components are mixed in one container and administered to the patient over a 24-hour period. A special final filter (1.5-micron filter) is used with this solution. Before administration, the solution is observed for oil droplets that have separated from the solution, forming a noticeable layer ("cracking of lipid emulsion"); such a solution should be discarded. Advantages of the TNA over PN are cost savings in preparation and equipment, decreased risk of catheter or nutrient contamination, decreased pharmacy preparation time, less nursing time, and increased patient convenience and satisfaction. Ideally, the pharmacist, nutritionist, and physician collaborate to determine the specific formula needed.

Initiating Therapy

PN solutions are initiated slowly and advanced gradually each day to the desired rate as the patient's fluid and glucose tolerance permits. The patient's laboratory test results and response to PN therapy are monitored on an ongoing basis by the physician and licensed nutrition provider. Standing orders are initiated for weighing the patient; monitoring intake, output, and blood glucose; and baseline and periodic monitoring of complete blood count, platelet count, and chemistry panel, including serum carbon dioxide, magnesium, phosphorus, triglycerides, and prealbumin. A 24-hour urine nitrogen determination may be performed for analysis of nitrogen balance. In most hospitals, the physician prescribes PN solutions on a daily standard PN order form. The formulation of the PN solutions is calculated carefully each day to meet the complete nutritional needs of the individual patient.

Administration Methods

Various vascular access devices are used to administer PN solutions in clinical practice. PN may be administered through either peripheral or central IV lines, depending on the patient's condition and the anticipated length of therapy.

Peripheral Method

To supplement oral intake when complete bowel rest is not indicated and NG or nasoenteric suction is not required, a peripheral parenteral nutrition (PPN) formula may be prescribed. PPN is administered through a peripheral vein; this is possible because the solution is less hypertonic than PN solution. PPN formulas are not nutritionally complete: there is typically less dextrose content. Dextrose concentrations of more than 10% should not be administered through peripheral veins because they irritate the intima (innermost walls) of small veins, causing chemical phlebitis. Lipids are administered simultaneously to buffer the PPN and to protect the peripheral vein from irritation. The usual length of therapy using PPN is 5 to 7 days (Correia, Guimaraes, de Mattos, et al., 2004).

Central Method

Because PN solutions have five or six times the solute concentration of blood (and exert an osmotic pressure of about 2000 mOsm/L), they are injurious to the intima of peripheral veins. Therefore, to prevent phlebitis and other venous complications, these solutions are administered into the vascular system through a catheter inserted into a high-flow, large blood vessel (the subclavian vein). Concentrated solutions are then very rapidly diluted to isotonic levels by the blood in this vessel.

Four types of **central venous access devices (CVADs)** are available—nontunneled (or percutaneous) central catheters, peripherally inserted central catheters, tunneled catheters, and implanted ports. Whenever one of these catheters is inserted, catheter tip placement should be confirmed by x-ray studies before PN therapy is initiated. The optimal position is the midproximal third of the superior vena cava at the junction of the right atrium (see Chapter 16).

NONTUNNELED CENTRAL CATHETERS

Nontunneled central catheters are used for short-term (less than 6 weeks) IV therapy in acute care, long-term care, and home care settings. The physician inserts these catheters. Examples of nontunneled central catheters are Vas Cath, percutaneous subclavian Arrow, and Hohn catheters. The subclavian vein is the most common vessel used, because the subclavian area provides a stable insertion site to which the catheter can be anchored, allows the patient freedom of movement, and provides easy access to the dressing site. The jugular vein should only be used as a last resort and then only for 1 to 2 days. Single-, double-, and triple-lumen central catheters are available for central lines, but the Centers for Disease Control and Prevention (CDC) recommends that single-lumen catheters be used for TNA whenever practicable (CDC, 2002). To ensure accessibility in a patient with limited IV access, a triple-lumen subclavian catheter can be used, because it offers three ports for various uses (Fig. 36-10). The 16-gauge distal lumen can be used to infuse blood or other viscous fluids. The 18-gauge middle lumen is reserved for PN infusion. The 18-gauge proximal port can be used for administration of blood or medications. A port not being used for fluid administration can be used for obtaining blood specimens if indicated.

If a single-lumen central catheter is used for administering PN, various restrictions apply. Blood cannot be drawn from the catheter and transfusions of blood products cannot be given through the main line, because red blood cells may coat the lumen of the catheter, thereby reducing the flow of the nutritional solution. Medications also cannot be administered through it, because the medication may be incompatible with the components of the nutritional solution (insulin is an exception). If medications must be given, they must be infused through a separate peripheral IV line, not by piggyback into the PN line.

Insertion. The procedure is explained so that the patient understands the importance of not touching the catheter insertion site and is aware of what to expect during the insertion procedure. The patient is placed supine in the Trendelenburg position (to produce dilation of neck and shoulder vessels, which makes entry easier and prevents air embolus). The area is shaved if necessary, and the skin is prepared with acetone and alcohol to remove surface oils. Final skin preparation includes cleaning with tincture of 2% iodine or chlorhexidine. To afford maximal accuracy in the placement of the catheter, the patient is instructed to turn the head away from the site of venipuncture and to remain motionless while the catheter is inserted and the wound is dressed. The preferred insertion route is the subclavian vein,

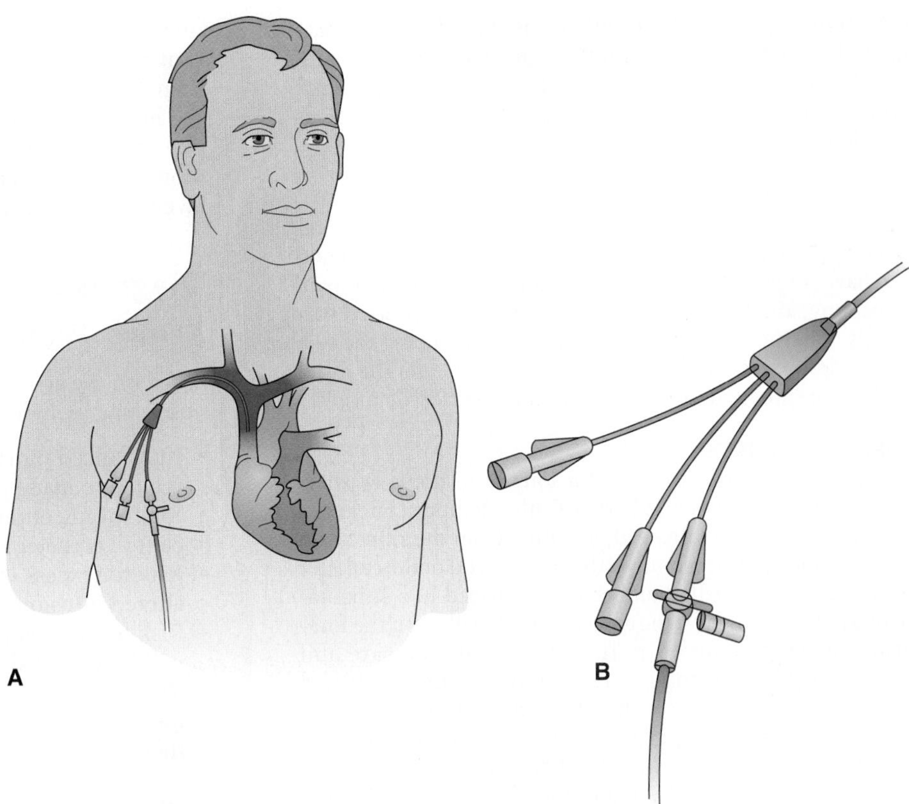

FIGURE 36-10. Subclavian triple-lumen catheter used for parenteral nutrition and other adjunctive therapy. (**A**) The catheter is threaded through the subclavian vein into the vena cava. (**B**) Each lumen is an avenue for solution administration. The lumens are secured with threaded needleless adapters or Luer-Lok–type caps when the device is not in use.

which leads into the superior vena cava. The external jugular route can be used, but usually only in emergency situations. Because a nontunneled central catheter is always a potential source of serious infection, the insertion site should be changed every 4 to 6 weeks, or as recommended by the latest CDC guidelines.

Full-length sterile drapes are applied. Procaine or lidocaine is injected to anesthetize the skin and underlying tissues. The target area is the inferior border at the midpoint of the clavicle. A large-bore needle on a syringe is inserted and moved parallel to and beneath the clavicle until it enters the vein. The syringe is then detached and a radiopaque wire is inserted through the needle into the vein. The catheter is then advanced over the wire, the needle is withdrawn, and the hub of the catheter is attached to the IV tubing. Until the syringe is detached from the needle and the catheter is inserted, the patient may be asked to perform the Valsalva maneuver. (To do this, the patient is instructed to take a deep breath, hold it, and bear down with mouth closed. Compression of the abdomen may also accomplish the maneuver.) The Valsalva maneuver is performed to produce a positive phase in central venous pressure, thereby lessening the possibility of air being drawn into the circulatory system (air embolism). The physician sutures the catheter to the skin to avoid inadvertent removal.

The catheter insertion site is swabbed with either tincture of 2% iodine or a chlorhexidine solution. A gauze or transparent dressing is applied using strict sterile technique (CDC, 2002). An isotonic IV solution, such as dextrose 5% in water (D5W), is administered to keep the vein patent.

The position of the tip of the catheter is checked with x-ray or fluoroscopy to confirm its location in the superior vena cava and to rule out a pneumothorax resulting from inadvertent puncture of the pleura. Once the catheter's position is confirmed, the prescribed PN solution is started. The initial rate of infusion is usually 50 mL/hour, and the rate is gradually increased to the maintenance rate or predetermined dose (eg, 100 to 125 mL/hour). An infusion pump is always used for administration of PN.

An injection site cap is attached to the end of each central catheter lumen, creating a closed system. IV infusion tubing is connected to the insertion site cap of the central catheter with a threaded needleless adapter or Luer-Lok device. Each lumen is labeled according to location (proximal, middle, distal). To ensure patency, all lumens are flushed with a diluted heparin flush initially, daily when not in use, after each intermittent infusion, after blood drawing, and whenever an infusion is disconnected. Force is never used to flush the catheter. If resistance is met, aspiration may restore lumen patency; if this is not effective, the physician is notified. Low-dose tissue plasminogen activator (alteplase) may be prescribed to dissolve a clot or fibrin sheath. If attempts to clear the lumen are ineffective, the lumen is labeled as "clotted off" and not used again.

PERIPHERALLY INSERTED CENTRAL CATHETERS

Peripherally inserted central catheters (PICCs) are used for intermediate-term (several days to months) IV therapy in the hospital, long-term care, or home setting. These catheters may be inserted at the bedside or in the outpatient setting by a specially trained nurse (Philpot & Griffiths, 2003). The basilic or cephalic vein is accessed through the antecubital space, and the catheter is threaded to a designated location, depending on the type of solution to be infused (superior vena cava for PN). Taking of blood pressure and blood specimens from the extremity with the PICC is avoided (see Chapter 14 and Chapter 16, Fig. 16-6).

TUNNELED CENTRAL CATHETERS

Tunneled central catheters are for long-term use and may remain in place for many years. These catheters are cuffed and can have single or double lumens; examples are the Hickman, Groshong, and Permacath. These catheters are inserted surgically. They are threaded under the skin (reducing the risk of ascending infection) to the subclavian vein, and the distal end of the catheter is advanced into the superior vena cava.

IMPLANTED PORTS

Implanted ports are also used for long-term home IV therapy; examples include the Port-A-Cath, Mediport, Hickman Port, and P.A.S. Port. Instead of exiting from the skin, as do the Hickman and Groshong catheters, the end of the catheter is attached to a small chamber that is placed in a subcutaneous pocket, either on the anterior chest wall or on the forearm. The subcutaneous port requires minimal care and allows the patient complete freedom of activity. Implanted ports are more expensive than the external catheters, and access requires passing a special non-coring needle (Huber-tipped) through the skin into the chamber to initiate IV therapy (see Chapter 16). Taking of blood pressure and blood specimens from the extremity with the port system should be avoided.

Discontinuing Parenteral Nutrition

The PN solution is discontinued gradually to allow the patient to adjust to decreased levels of glucose. If the PN solution is abruptly terminated, isotonic dextrose is administered for 1 to 2 hours to protect against rebound hypoglycemia. Providing oral carbohydrates shortens the tapering time. Specific symptoms of rebound hypoglycemia include weakness, faintness, sweating, shakiness, feeling cold, confusion, and increased heart rate. Once all IV therapy is completed, the nurse (with a physician's order) removes the nontunneled central venous catheter or PICC and applies an occlusive dressing to the exit site. Tunneled catheters and implanted ports are removed only by the physician.

In cases of serious illness when death is imminent, some patients or families may request that PN be discontinued. This situation poses many ethical questions, some of which are discussed in Chart 36-3.

Nursing Process

The Patient Receiving Parenteral Nutrition

Assessment

The nurse assists in identifying patients who may be candidates for PN. Indicators include any significant weight loss (10% or more of usual weight), a decrease in oral food intake for more than 1 week, any significant sign of protein loss (serum albumin levels less than 3.2 g/dL [32 g/L], muscle wasting, decreased tissue healing, or abnormal urea nitrogen excretion), and persistent vomiting and diarrhea. The nurse carefully monitors the patient's hydration status, electrolyte levels, and calorie intake.

Diagnosis

Nursing Diagnoses

Based on the assessment data, the major nursing diagnoses may include the following:

- Imbalanced nutrition, less than body requirements, related to inadequate oral intake of nutrients
- Risk for infection related to contamination of the central catheter site or infusion line
- Risk for excess or deficient fluid volume related to altered infusion rate
- Risk for immobility related to fear that the catheter will become dislodged or occluded
- Risk for ineffective therapeutic regimen management related to knowledge deficit about home PN therapy

Collaborative Problems/ Potential Complications

The most common complications are pneumothorax, air embolism, a clotted or displaced catheter, sepsis, hyperglycemia, rebound hypoglycemia, and fluid overload. These problems and the associated collaborative interventions are described in Table 36-5.

Planning and Goals

The major goals for the patient may include optimal level of nutrition, absence of infection, adequate fluid volume, optimal level of activity (within individual limitations), knowledge of and skill in self-care, and absence of complications.

Nursing Interventions

Maintaining Optimal Nutrition

A continuous, uniform infusion of PN solution over a 24-hour period is desired. However, in some cases (eg, home care patients), cyclic PN may be appropriate. With cyclic PN, there is a set time during a 24-hour period when PN is infused and a set time when it is not. The time periods for infusion are sufficient to meet the patient's nutritional and pharmacologic needs. Ideally, cyclic PN is infused over a 10- to 15-hour period during the night.

The patient is weighed daily (this may be decreased to two or three times per week) at the same time of the day under the same conditions for accurate comparison. Under the PN regimen (without additional energy expenditure), satisfactory weight maintenance

TABLE 36-5 Complications of Parental Nutrition

Complications	Cause	Nursing Actions and Collaborative Interventions: *Treatment*	Nursing Actions and Collaborative Interventions: *Prevention*
Pneumothorax	Improper catheter placement and inadvertent puncture of the pleura	Place patient in Fowler's position.	Assist patient to remain still in Trendelenburg position during catheter insertion.
		Offer reassurance. Monitor vital signs. Prepare for thoracentesis or chest tube insertion.	
Air embolism	Disconnected tubing	Replace tubing immediately and notify physician.	Tape all tubing connection sites securely.
	Cap missing from port	Replace cap and notify physician.	
	Blocked segment of vascular system	Turn patient on left side and place in the head-low position. Notify physician.	
Clotted catheter line	Inadequate/infrequent heparin flushes Disruption of infusion	On *rare* occasions, flush with thrombolytic declotting medication as prescribed.	Administer heparin flush in unused lines twice a day. Monitor infusion rate hourly and inspect the integrity of the line.
Catheter displacement and contamination	Excessive movement, possibly with a nonsecured catheter Separation of tubing and contamination	Stop the infusion and notify the physician.	Tape all tubing connection sites. Avoid interrupting the main line or piggybacking other lines.
Sepsis	Separation of dressings	Reinforce or change dressing quickly using aseptic technique.	Maintain sterile technique when changing tubing, dressing, or total nutrient admixture bag.
	Contaminated solution	Discard. Notify pharmacist.	
	Infection at insertion site of catheter	Notify physician. Monitor vital signs every 4 hours.	
Hyperglycemia	Glucose intolerance	Notify physician; addition of insulin to PN solution may be prescribed.	Monitor glucose levels (blood and urine). Monitor urine output. Observe for stupor, confusion, or lethargy.
Fluid overload	Fluid infusing rapidly	Decrease infusion rate. Monitor vital signs. Notify physician. Treat respiratory distress by sitting patient upright and administering oxygen as needed, if prescribed.	Use infusion pump. Verify correct infusion rate ordered.
Rebound hypoglycemia	Feedings stopped too abruptly	Monitor for symptoms (weakness, tremors, diaphoresis, headache, hunger, and apprehension); notify physician.	Gradually wean patient from PN.

or gain is usually achieved. It is important to keep accurate intake and output records and calculations of fluid balance. A calorie count is kept of any oral nutrients. Trace elements (copper, zinc, chromium, manganese, and selenium) are included in PN solutions and are individualized for each patient. The PN solutions are prescribed daily by the physician on a standard PN order form based on laboratory results and patient tolerance.

Preventing Infection

The high glucose content of PN solutions makes these solutions ideal culture media for bacterial and fungal growth, and CVADs provide a port of entry. Gram-negative cocci and gram-negative bacilli, including *Staphylococcus aureus, S. epidermidis,* and *Klebsiella pneumoniae,* are the most common infectious organisms (Alberti, Brun-Buisson, Burchardi, et al., 2002). Other infectious organisms can be fungal, including *Candida albicans.* Meticulous technique is essential to prevent infection.

The primary sources of microorganisms for catheter-related infections are the skin and the catheter hub. The catheter site is covered with an occlusive gauze dressing that is usually changed every other day. Alternatively, a transparent dressing may be used and changed weekly. The CDC (2002) recommends changing CVAD dressings only if they are damp, bloody, loose, or soiled. The dressings are changed using sterile technique. The nurse and patient wear masks during dressing changes to reduce the possibility of airborne contamination. The area is checked for leakage; bloody or purulent drainage; a kinked catheter; and skin reactions such as inflammation, redness, swelling, or tenderness. The nurse wears sterile gloves and cleanses the area with tincture of 2% iodine or a chlorhexidine solution on a sterile gauze. The site is cleaned thoroughly using a circular motion from the site outward to approximately 3 inches; this procedure is repeated two times. Then the same cleaning procedure is performed, using 2 × 2-inch gauze pads moistened with sterile water or saline solution (alcohol is used to remove iodine). Next the catheter ports are cleaned from the exit site to the distal end with an alcohol wipe. The insertion site is covered with an occlusive gauze pad or transparent dressing centered over the area.

The advantages of using a transparent dressing instead of a gauze pad are that it allows frequent examination of the catheter site without changing the dressing, it adheres well, and it is more comfortable for the patient. When an extension set is used with a central catheter, it is considered an extension of the catheter itself. It is not routinely changed with dressing or tubing changes. The connection (hub) between the catheter and extension tubing is secured with adhesive tape to prevent separation and exposure to air. Mainline IV tubing and filters are changed every 72 to 96 hours, and all connections are taped securely to avoid breaks in the integrity of the system (CDC, 2002). The dressing and tubing are labeled with the date, time of insertion, time of dressing change, and initials of the person who carried out the procedure; this information is also documented in the patient's medical record.

The catheter is another major source of colonization and infection. Studies have been conducted on the use of catheters with antiseptic coatings, antimicrobial coatings, and impregnated antimicrobial cuffs with varying conclusions (Bong, Kite, Wilco, et al., 2003). Prophylactic antibiotic therapy, antibiotic locks, use of antithrombolytics, various exit-site dressings, and the use of various disinfectants for cleansing catheter exit sites have also been proposed (Peterson, 2003).

Maintaining Fluid Balance

An infusion pump is necessary for PN to maintain an accurate rate of administration. A designated rate is set in milliliters per hour, and the rate is checked every 3 to 4 hours. An alarm signals a problem. The infusion rate should not be increased or decreased to compensate for fluids that have infused too quickly or too slowly. If the solution runs out, 10% dextrose and water is infused until the next PN solution is available from the pharmacy.

If the rate is too rapid, hyperosmolar diuresis occurs. Excess glucose is excreted by the renal tubules, pulling large volumes of water into the tubules via osmosis, resulting in higher-than-normal urine output and intravascular fluid volume deficit. If the hyperosmolar diuresis is severe enough, it can cause dehydration of brain cells resulting in intractable seizures, coma, and death. Symptoms of rapid hypertonic fluid intake include headache, nausea, fever, chills, and increasing lethargy.

If the flow rate is too slow, the patient does not receive the maximal benefit of calories and nitrogen. Intake and output are recorded every 8 hours so that fluid imbalance can be readily detected. The patient is weighed two or three times a week; ideally, the patient shows neither weight loss nor significant weight gain. The nurse assesses for signs of dehydration (eg, thirst, decreased skin turgor, decreased central venous pressure) and reports these findings to the physician immediately. It is essential to monitor blood glucose levels, because hyperglycemia can cause diuresis and excessive fluid loss.

Encouraging Activity

Activities and ambulation are encouraged when the patient is physically able. With a catheter in the subclavian vein, the patient is free to move the extremities, and activity should be encouraged to maintain good muscle tone. If applicable, the teaching and exercise program initiated in the occupational and physical therapy departments is reinforced.

Promoting Home and Community-Based Care

TEACHING PATIENTS SELF-CARE

Successful home PN requires teaching the patient and family specialized skills using an intensive training program and follow-up supervision in the home. This is best accomplished through a team effort (Ireton-Jones et al., 2003). The financial costs of such programs, although high, are less than those incurred in a hospital. Initiation of a home program may be the only way the patient can be discharged from the hospital (Evans, Steinhart, Cohen, et al., 2003).

Ideal candidates for home PN are patients who have a reasonable life expectancy after return home, have a limited number of illnesses other than the one that has resulted in the need for PN, and are highly motivated and fairly self-sufficient. In addition, ability to learn, availability of family interest and support, adequate finances, and the physical plan of the home are factors that must be assessed when the decision about home PN is made (Chart 36-4).

Home health care agencies sponsoring home PN programs have developed teaching brochures and videos for every aspect of treatment, including catheter and dressing care, use of an infusion pump, administration of fat emulsions, and instillation of heparin flushes (Smith, Curtas, Kleinbeck, et al., 2003). Teaching begins in the hospital and continues in the home or in an ambulatory infusion center. If the patient or assisting family member has a disability (motor or sensory deficit, vision or hearing loss), alternate formats of educational materials are needed to ensure adequate preparation and self-management.

CONTINUING CARE

The home care nurse should be aware that the typical patient needs several instruction sessions for assessment of learning and reinforcement. For more information about home patient education, see Charts 36-5 and 36-6. Special considerations for elderly patients who go home with nutrition support are presented in Chart 36-7.

CHART 36-4

Discharge Planning: Home Assessment for Nutrition Support

The following aspects of the home setting must be assessed before making a decision that a patient can return home with parenteral nutrition:

- Water: necessary for hand washing and cleaning of work areas
- Electricity: reliable power source is needed to provide proper lighting and charging of pumps
- Refrigeration: must be adequate for accommodation of several bags of total nutrient admixture solution
- Telephone: necessary for contacting home health personnel, arranging for prompt delivery of supplies, and for emergency purposes
- Environment:
  - Should be free of rodents and insects
  - Should have storage that is not accessible to pets and small children
  - Should be assessed for stairs, carpets, and inaccessible areas, which can limit mobility with infusion pumps if the patient has a disability
  - Should be assessed for bathroom access

Adapted from Ireton-Jones, C., DeLegge, M., Epperson, L., et al. (2003). Management of the home parenteral nutrition patient. *Nutrition in Clinical Practice, 18*(4), 310–317.

CHART 36-5

Teaching Patients About Home Parenteral Nutrition

An effective home care teaching program prepares the patient to manage the appropriate form of PN: how to store solutions, set up the infusion, flush the line with heparin, change the dressings, and troubleshoot for problems. The most common complication is sepsis. Strict aseptic technique is taught for hand hygiene, handling equipment, changing the dressing, and preparing the solution.

Troubleshooting Mechanical Difficulties

Mechanical problems usually arise from technical complications in the infusion pump or catheter site. The patient needs to know how to measure the length of the external portion of the catheter; this measurement is used as a comparison if the line is pulled or if dislodgement is suspected. The patient also needs to know how to recognize catheter problems (eg, leakage, loose cap, blood clot, dislodgement) and should receive a list of instructions explaining what to do for each problem.

Recognizing Metabolic Complications

The patient is given a list of signs and symptoms that indicate metabolic complications (neuropathies, mentation changes, diarrhea, nausea, skin changes, decreased urine output) and directions on how to contact the home health care nurse or physician if any of these complications occurs. The patient is instructed to have routine serum chemistry and hematology tests as well.

Obtaining Psychosocial Support

The psychosocial aspects of home PN are as important as the physiologic and technical concerns. Patients must cope with the loss of eating and with changes in lifestyle brought on by sleep disturbances (frequent urination during infusions, usually two or three times during the night).

Major psychosocial reactions include depression, anger, withdrawal, anxiety, and impaired self-image. A successful home PN program depends on the patient's and family's motivation, emotional stability, and technical competence. Patients and families need to know which support groups are available in the community to help them cope with the transition and to minimize disruption of lifestyle.

Evaluation

Expected Patient Outcomes

Expected patient outcomes may include the following:

1. Attains or maintains nutritional balance
2. Is free of infection at the catheter site
   a. Is afebrile

CHART 36-6

HOME CARE CHECKLIST • The Patient Receiving Parenteral Nutrition

At the completion of the home care instruction, the patient or caregiver will be able to:	Patient	Caregiver
• Discuss goal and purpose of PN therapy.	✔	✔
• Discuss basic components of PN solution.	✔	✔
• List emergency phone numbers.	✔	✔
• Demonstrate how to handle PN solutions and medications correctly.	✔	✔
• Demonstrate how to operate infusion pump.	✔	✔
• Demonstrate how to prime tubing and filter.	✔	✔
• Demonstrate how to connect and disconnect PN infusion.	✔	✔
• Demonstrate how to perform catheter dressing changes.	✔	✔
• Demonstrate how to heparinize central line.	✔	✔
• Identify possible PN complications and interventions.	✔	✔

CHART 36-7

Gerontologic Considerations

Home Parenteral and Enteral Nutrition

Age-related conditions that affect home nutrition support goals include the following:

- Arthritis: possible decreased hand dexterity and fine motor coordination
- Sensory impairment: inability to hear pump alarms; vision loss may affect ability to see pump menus or fill syringes
- Constipation: decreased overall bowel tone, which can cause intolerance of enteral feedings; increasing water flushes and assessing fiber needs may help
- Dehydration: decreased sensation of thirst, which may require close clinical management of fluid needs
- Obesity: decreased basal metabolic rate increases tendency toward weight gain; may require a reduction in overall kilocalorie intake to compensate
- Diabetes mellitus: increased insulin resistance, which makes glucose control during parenteral nutrition infusion more challenging
- Depression/dementia: mood and memory disorders, which may present as low motivation to learn and adhere to the nutrition support regimen
- Multiple medications: conversion to an appropriate intravenous or enteral route, if possible, is required

Adapted from White, J., Brewer, D., Stockton, M., et al. (2003). Nutrition in chronic disease management in the elderly. *Nutrition in Clinical Practice, 18*(1), 3–11.

   b. Has no purulent drainage from the catheter insertion site
   c. Has intact IV access
3. Is hydrated, as evidenced by good skin turgor
4. Achieves an optimal level of activity, within limitations
5. Demonstrates skill in managing PN regimen
6. Prevents complications
   a. Maintains proper catheter and equipment function
   b. Has no symptoms of sepsis
   c. Maintains metabolic balance within normal limits
   d. Shows improved and stabilized nutritional status

Critical Thinking Exercises

1 You prepare to administer a patient's scheduled bolus enteral tube feeding, and he states that he feels too full for another feeding. It has been 4 hours since his last feeding. His stomach is somewhat distended but he has bowel sounds. What are some of the causes of abdominal fullness and distention? How would current medications and patterns of elimination affect these signs and symptoms? Whom should you consult?

2 ebp A patient who is receiving gastrostomy tube feedings is to be discharged from the hospital to return home within the next few days. The patient has many questions regarding the equipment that he will need. What is the strength of the evidence that leads you to espouse the advantages of a simple bolus regimen of tube

feeding versus around-the-clock pump feeding? For this ambulatory patient, what is the evidence base that assists you in advising him to select an optimal regimen of administration?

3 A patient has just been diagnosed with small bowel strictures from Crohn's disease and requires preoperative total nutrient admixture (TNA) for at least 1 week. The patient does not want a central access catheter placed and prefers to continue with simple IV fluids. What can you tell her about the nutritional advantages of TNA when compared with simple hydration fluids? With strict adherence to protocols for IV line management and dressing care, what complications can be avoided?

4 ebp You are preparing to administer a gravity bolus enteral tube feeding to a patient assigned to your care on a general medicine inpatient unit. You find the patient lying on his side in the bed with the tape no longer around the tube but still adhered to his outer nares. Before proceeding with the feeding, what is the strength of the evidence you will consider when you determine optimal positioning of this patient to prevent complications such as regurgitation and aspiration? What is the evidence base that guides you in determining appropriate placement of the feeding tube?

REFERENCES AND SELECTED READINGS

BOOKS

Buchman, A. (2004). *Practical nutrition support techniques* (2nd ed.). Thorofare, NJ: Slack International.

Gottschlich, M., Fuhrman, M., & Hammond, K., et al. (Eds.). (2000). *The science and practice of nutrition support: A case-based core curriculum.* American Society of Parenteral and Enteral Nutrition (ASPEN). Dubuque, Iowa: Kendall/Hunt.

Josephson, D. (2003). *Intravenous infusion therapy for nurses* (2nd ed.). Clifton Park, NY: Delmar Thomas Learning.

Latifi, R., & Dudrick, S. (2003). *The biology and practice of nutritional support* (2nd ed.). Georgetown, TX: Landes Bioscience.

Rolandelli, R., Bankhead, R., Boulatta, J., et al. (Eds.). (2004). *Clinical nutrition: Enteral and tube feeding* (4th ed.). Philadelphia: W. B. Saunders.

Worthington, P. (2004). *Practical aspects of nutritional support: An advanced practice guide.* Philadelphia: W. B. Saunders.

Yamada, T., & Alpers, D. H. (Eds.). (2003). *Textbook of gastroenterology* (4th ed.). Philadelphia: Lippincott Williams & Wilkins.

JOURNALS

**Asterisks indicate nursing research articles.*

Gastrostomies, Nasogastric and Nasoenteric Intubation and Feeding

Angus, F., & Burakoff, R. (2003). The percutaneous endoscopic gastrostomy tube. Medical and ethical issues in placement. *American Journal of Gastroenterology, 98*(2), 272–277.

Carroll, D. (2003). Moxifloxacin-induced *Clostridium difficile*-associated diarrhea. *Pharmacotherapy, 23*(11), 1517–1519.

Dickerson, R., Tidwell, A., & Brown, R. (2003). Adverse effects from inappropriate medication administration via a jejunostomy tube. *Nutrition in Clinical Practice, 18*(5), 402–405.

Keithley, J., & Swanson, B. (2004). Enteral nutrition: An update on practice recommendations. *MedSurg Nursing, 13*(2), 131–134.

*Lenart, S., & Polissar, N. (2003). Comparison of two methods for postpyloric placement of enteral feeding tubes. *American Journal of Critical Care, 12*(4), 357–360.

Metheny, N. A. (1998). Detection of improperly positioned feeding tubes. *Journal of Health Care Risk Management, 18*(3), 37–45.

*Metheny, N. A., Dettenmeier, P., Hampton, K., et al. (1990). Determinant of inadvertent respiratory placement of small-bore feeding tubes. A report of 10 cases. *Heart and Lung, 19*(6), 631–638.

*Metheny, N. A., McSweeney, M., Wehrle, M. A., et al. (1990). Effectiveness of the auscultatory method in predicting feeding tube location. *Nursing Research, 39*(5), 282–287.

*Metheny, N. A., Smith, L., Stewart, B. J., et al. (2000). Development of a reliable and valid bedside test for bilirubin and its utility for predicting feeding tube location. *Nursing Research, 49*(6), 302–309.

*Metheny, N. A., Stewart, B. J., Smith, L., et al. (1999). pH and concentration of bilirubin in feeding tube aspirates as predictors of tube placement. *Nursing Research, 48*(3), 189–197.

Metheny, N. A., & Titler, M. G. (2001). Assessing placement of feeding tubes. *American Journal of Nursing, 101*(5), 36–46.

Neef, M., Crowder, V., McIvor, N., et al. (2003). Comparison of the use of endoscopic and radiological gastrostomy in a single head and neck cancer unit. *Australian and New Zealand Journal of Surgery, 73*(1), 590–593.

Parrish, C. (2003). Enteral feeding: The art and the science. *Nutrition in Clinical Practice, 18*(1), 76–84.

Roche, V. (2003). Percutaneous endoscopic gastrostomy: Clinical care of PEG tubes in older adults. *Geriatrics, 58*(11), 22–29.

Sartori, S., Trevisani, L., Neilsen, I., et al. (2003). Longevity of silicone and polyurethane catheters in long-term enteral feeding via percutaneous endoscopic gastrostomy. *Alimentary Pharmacology and Therapeutics, 17*(6), 853–856.

Schloerb, P., Wood, J., Casillan, A., et al. (2004). Bowel necrosis caused by water in jejunal feeding, (2004). *Journal of Parenteral and Enteral Nutrition, 28*(1), 27–29.

Shang, E., Geiger, N., Sturm, J., et al. (2004). Pump-assisted enteral nutrition can prevent aspiration in bedridden endoscopic gastrostomy patients. *Journal of Parenteral and Enteral Nutrition, 28*(3), 180–183.

Tonelli, M. (2005). Waking the dying: Must we always attempt to involve critically ill patients in end-of-life decisions? *Chest, 127*(2), 637–642.

White, J., Brewer, D., Stockton, M., et al. (2003). Nutrition in chronic disease management in the elderly. *Nutrition in Clinical Practice, 18*(1), 3–11.

Parenteral Nutrition

Alberti, C., Brun-Buisson, C., Burchardi, H., et al. (2002). Epidemiology of sepsis and infection in ICU patients from an international multicentre cohort study. *Intensive Care Medicine, 28*(4), 108–121.

American Society of Parenteral and Enteral Nutrition (ASPEN). (1998). Special report: Safe practices for parenteral nutrition formulas. Available at: http://www.nutritioncare.org. Accessed June 13, 2006.

Bong, J., Kite, P., Wilco, M., et al. (2003). Prevention of catheter-related bloodstream infection by silver iontophoretic central venous catheters: A randomized controlled trial. *Journal of Clinical Pathology, 56*(10), 731–735.

Centers for Disease Control and Prevention (2002). Guidelines for the prevention of intravascular catheter-related infections. *Morbidity and Mortality Weekly Report,* 51 (RR-10), 1–36.

Correia, M., Guimaraes, J., de Mattos, L., et al. (2004). Peripheral parenteral nutrition: An option for patients with an indication for short-term parenteral nutrition. *Nutricion Hospitalaria, 19*(1), 14–18.

Evans, J., Steinhart, A., Cohen, Z., et al. (2003). Home total parenteral nutrition: An alternative to early surgery for complicated inflammatory bowel disease. *Journal of Gastrointestinal Surgery, 7*(4), 562–566.

Huckleberry, Y. (2004). Nutritional support and the surgical patient. *American Journal of Health System Pharmacy, 61*(7), 671–682.

Ireton-Jones, C., DeLegge, M., Epperson, L., et al. (2003). Management of the home parenteral nutrition patient. *Nutrition in Clinical Practice, 18*(4), 310–317.

Peterson, K. (2003). Central line sepsis. *Clinical Journal in Oncology Nursing, 7*(2), 218–221.

Philpot, P., & Griffiths, V. (2003). The peripherally-inserted central catheter. *Nursing Standard, 17*(44), 39–46.

Smith, C., Curtas, S., Kleinbeck, S., et al. (2003). Clinical trial of interactive and videotaped educational interventions reduce infection, reactive depression and rehospitalizations for sepsis in patients on home parenteral nutrition. *Journal of Parenteral and Enteral Nutrition, 27*(2), 137–145.

Teitelbaum, D., Guenter, P., Howel, W., et al. (2005). Definition of terms, style and conventions used in A.S.P.E.N. guidelines and standards. *Nutrition in Clinical Practice, 20*(2), 281–285.

RESOURCES

American Cancer Society, 1599 Clifton Rd. N.E., Atlanta, GA 30329; 1-404-320-3333; http://www.cancer.org. Accessed June 3, 2006.

American Society for Clinical Nutrition, 9650 Rockville Pike, Bethesda, MD 20814; http://www.ascn.org. Accessed June 3, 2006.

American Society for Gastrointestinal Endoscopy, 13 Elm St., Manchester, MA 01944; http://www.asge.org. Accessed June 3, 2006.

American Society for Parenteral and Enteral Nutrition (ASPEN), 8630 Fenton St., #412, Silver Spring, MD 20910-3805; http://www.nutritioncare.org. Accessed June 3, 2006.

Oley Foundation for Home Parenteral and Enteral Nutrition, 214 Hun Memorial, A-23, New Scotland Ave., Albany, NY 12208; http://www.iffgd.org/oley.html. Accessed June 3, 2006.

Society of Gastroenterology Nurses & Associates, Inc., 140 North Michigan Ave., Chicago, IL, 60611; 800-245-7462; in Illinois, 312-321-5165; http://www.sgna.org. Accessed June 3, 2006.

CHAPTER 37

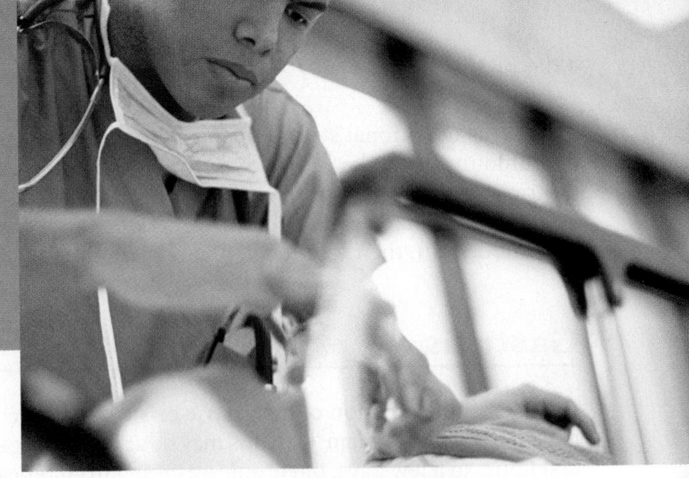

Management of Patients With Gastric and Duodenal Disorders

Learning Objectives

On completion of this chapter, the learner will be able to:

1. Compare the etiology, clinical manifestations, and management of acute gastritis, chronic gastritis, and peptic ulcer.
2. Use the nursing process as a framework for care of patients with gastritis.
3. Use the nursing process as a framework for care of patients with peptic ulcer.
4. Describe the dietary, pharmacologic, and surgical treatment of peptic ulcer.
5. Describe the nursing management of patients who undergo surgical procedures to treat obesity.
6. Use the nursing process as a framework for care of patients with gastric cancer.
7. Use the nursing process as a framework for care of patients undergoing gastric surgery.
8. Identify the complications of gastric surgery and their prevention and management.
9. Describe the home health care needs of the patient who has had gastric surgery.

A person's nutritional status depends not only on the type and amount of intake but also on the functioning of the gastric and intestinal portions of the gastrointestinal (GI) system. This chapter describes disorders of the stomach and duodenum, their treatment, and related nursing care.

Gastritis

Gastritis (inflammation of the **gastric** or stomach mucosa) is a common GI problem. Gastritis may be acute, lasting several hours to a few days, or chronic, resulting from repeated exposure to irritating agents or recurring episodes of acute gastritis.

Acute gastritis is often caused by dietary indiscretion—the person eats food that is irritating, too highly seasoned, or contaminated with disease-causing microorganisms. Other causes of acute gastritis include overuse of aspirin and other nonsteroidal anti-inflammatory drugs (NSAIDs), excessive alcohol intake, bile reflux, and radiation therapy. A more severe form of acute gastritis is caused by the ingestion of strong acid or alkali, which may cause the mucosa to become gangrenous or to perforate. Scarring can occur, resulting in **pyloric stenosis** or obstruction. Acute gastritis also may develop in acute illnesses, especially when the patient has had major traumatic injuries; burns; severe infection; hepatic, renal, or respiratory failure; or major surgery. Gastritis may be the first sign of an acute systemic infection.

Chronic gastritis and prolonged inflammation of the stomach may be caused either by benign or malignant ulcers of the stomach or by the bacteria *Helicobacter pylori* (*H. pylori*). Chronic gastritis is sometimes associated with autoimmune diseases such as pernicious anemia; dietary factors such as caffeine; the use of medications such as NSAIDs, bisphosphonate (eg, alendronate [Fosamax], or risedronate [Actonel]); alcohol; smoking; or chronic reflux of pancreatic secretions and bile into the stomach.

Pathophysiology

In gastritis, the gastric mucous membrane becomes edematous and hyperemic (congested with fluid and blood) and undergoes superficial erosion (Fig. 37-1). It secretes a scanty amount of gastric juice, containing very little acid but much mucus. Superficial ulceration may occur and can lead to hemorrhage.

Clinical Manifestations

The patient with acute gastritis may have a rapid onset of symptoms, such as abdominal discomfort, headache, lassitude, nausea, anorexia, vomiting, and hiccupping, which can last from a few hours to a few days. The patient with chronic gastritis may complain of anorexia, heartburn after eating, belching, a sour taste in the mouth, or nausea and vomiting. Some patients may have only mild epigastric discomfort or report intolerance to spicy or fatty foods or slight pain that is relieved by eating. Patients with chronic gastritis from vitamin deficiency usually have evidence of malabsorption of vitamin B_{12} caused by the production of antibodies that interfere with the binding of vitamin B_{12} to intrinsic factor. However, some patients with chronic gastritis have no symptoms.

Glossary

achlorhydria: lack of hydrochloric acid in digestive secretions of the stomach

antrectomy: removal of the pyloric (antrum) portion of the stomach with anastomosis (surgical connection) to the duodenum (gastroduodenostomy or Billroth I) or anastomosis to the jejunum (gastrojejunostomy or Billroth II)

bariatric: term that comes from two Greek words meaning "weight" and "treatment"

dumping syndrome: physiologic response to rapid emptying of gastric contents into the jejunum, manifested by nausea, weakness, sweating, palpitations, syncope, and possibly diarrhea; occurs in patients who have had partial gastrectomy and gastrojejunostomy

duodenum: first portion of the small intestine, between the stomach and the jejunum

enteroclysis: fluoroscopic x-ray of the small intestine; a tube is placed from the nose or mouth through the esophagus and the stomach to the duodenum, a barium-based liquid contrast material is infused through the tube, and x-rays are taken as it travels through the duodenum

gastric: refers to the stomach

gastric outlet obstruction (GOO): any condition that mechanically impedes normal gastric emptying; there is obstruction of the channel of the pylorus and duodenum through which the stomach empties

gastritis: inflammation of the stomach

hematemesis: vomiting of blood

ligament of Treitz: suspensory ligament of the duodenum; important anatomic landmark used to divide the gastrointestinal tract into an upper and a lower portion

melena: tarry or black stools; indicative of blood in stools

morbid obesity: more than twice ideal body weight, 100 pounds or more over ideal body weight, or body mass index (BMI) exceeding 30 kg/m^2

omentum: fold of the peritoneum that surrounds the stomach and other organs of the abdomen

peritoneum: thin membrane that lines the inside of the wall of the abdomen and covers all the abdominal organs

pyloroplasty: surgical procedure to increase the opening of the pyloric orifice

pylorus: opening between the stomach and the duodenum

pyrosis: heartburn

serosa: thin membrane that forms the outer layer of the stomach

stenosis: narrowing or tightening of an opening or passage in the body

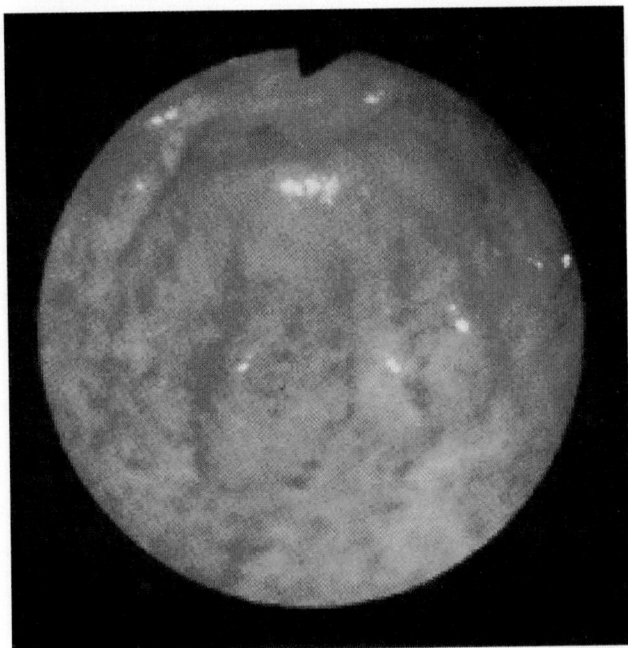

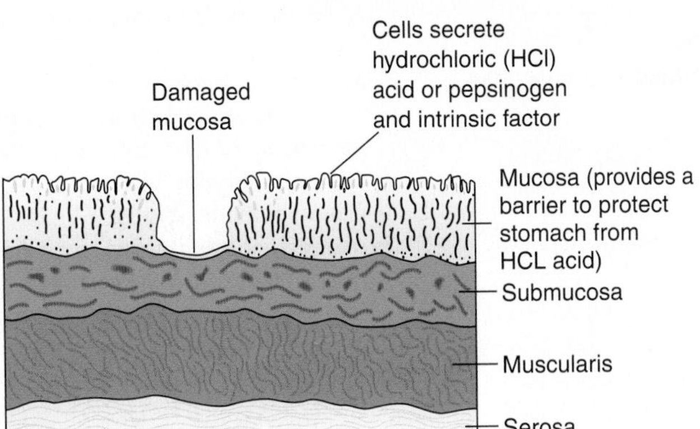

FIGURE 37-1. Endoscopic view of erosive gastritis (*left*). Damage from irritants (*right*) results in increased intracellular pH, impaired enzyme function, disrupted cellular structures, ischemia, vascular stasis, and tissue death. Reproduced with permission from Porth, C. (2005). *Pathophysiology: Concepts of altered health states* (7th ed.). Philadelphia: Lippincott Williams & Wilkins. © 2005, Lippincott Williams & Wilkins.

Assessment and Diagnostic Findings

Gastritis is sometimes associated with **achlorhydria** or hypochlorhydria (absence or low levels of hydrochloric acid [HCl]) or with hyperchlorhydria (high levels of HCl). Diagnosis can be determined by an upper GI x-ray series or endoscopy and histologic examination of a tissue specimen obtained by biopsy. Diagnostic measures for detecting *H. pylori* infection may be used and are discussed in the section on peptic ulcers.

Medical Management

The gastric mucosa is capable of repairing itself after a bout of gastritis. As a rule, the patient recovers in about 1 day, although the appetite may be diminished for an additional 2 or 3 days. Acute gastritis is also managed by instructing the patient to refrain from alcohol and food until symptoms subside. When the patient can take nourishment by mouth, a nonirritating diet is recommended. If the symptoms persist, intravenous (IV) fluids may need to be administered. If bleeding is present, management is similar to the procedures used to control upper GI tract hemorrhage discussed later in this chapter.

If gastritis is caused by ingestion of strong acids or alkalis, emergency treatment consists of diluting and neutralizing the offending agent. To neutralize acids, common antacids (eg, aluminum hydroxide) are used; to neutralize an alkali, diluted lemon juice or diluted vinegar is used. If corrosion is extensive or severe, emetics and lavage are avoided because of the danger of perforation and damage to the esophagus.

Therapy is supportive and may include nasogastric (NG) intubation, analgesic agents and sedatives, antacids, and IV fluids. Fiberoptic endoscopy may be necessary. In extreme cases, emergency surgery may be required to remove gangrenous or perforated tissue. A gastric resection or a gastrojejunostomy (anastomosis of jejunum to stomach to detour around the pylorus) may be necessary to treat pyloric obstruction, a narrowing of the pyloric orifice that cannot be relieved by medical management.

Chronic gastritis is managed by modifying the patient's diet, promoting rest, reducing stress, recommending avoidance of alcohol and NSAIDs, and initiating pharmacotherapy. *H. pylori* may be treated with selected drug combinations (Table 37-1).

Nursing Process

The Patient With Gastritis

Assessment

When obtaining the history, the nurse asks about the patient's presenting signs and symptoms. Does the patient have heartburn, indigestion, nausea, or vomiting? Do the symptoms occur at any specific time of the day, before or after meals, after ingesting spicy or irritating foods, or after the ingestion of certain drugs or alcohol? Has there been recent weight gain or loss? Are the

TABLE 37-1 Pharmacotherapy for Peptic Ulcer Disease and Gastritis

Pharmacologic Agent	Major Action	Nursing Considerations
Antibiotics		
Amoxicillin (Amoxil)	A bactericidal antibiotic that assists with eradicating *H. pylori* bacteria in the gastric mucosa	• May cause diarrhea • Should not be used in patients allergic to penicillin
Clarithromycin (Biaxin)	Exerts bactericidal effects to eradicate *H. pylori* bacteria in the gastric mucosa	• May cause GI upset, headache, altered taste • Many drug–drug interactions (eg, cisapride, colchicine, lovastatin, warfarin [Coumadin])
Metronidazole (Flagyl)	A synthetic antibacterial and antiprotozoal agent that assists with eradicating *H. pylori* bacteria in the gastric mucosa when administered with other antibiotics and proton pump inhibitors	• Should be administered with meals to decrease GI upset; may cause anorexia and metallic taste • Patient should avoid alcohol; Flagyl increases blood-thinning effects of warfarin (Coumadin)
Tetracycline	Exerts bacteriostatic effects to eradicate *H. pylori* bacteria in the gastric mucosa	• May cause photosensitivity reaction; warn patient to use sunscreen • May cause GI upset • Must be used with caution in patients with renal or hepatic impairment • Milk or dairy products may reduce effectiveness
Antidiarrheal		
Bismuth subsalicylate (Pepto-Bismol)	Suppresses *H. pylori* bacteria in the gastric mucosa and assists with healing of mucosal ulcers	• Given concurrently with antibiotics to eradicate *H. pylori* infection • Should be taken on empty stomach
Histamine-2 (H_2) receptor antagonists		
Cimetidine (Tagamet)	Decreases amount of HCl produced by stomach by blocking action of histamine on histamine receptors of parietal cells in the stomach	• Least expensive of H_2 receptor antagonists • May cause confusion, agitation, or coma in the elderly or those with renal or hepatic insufficiency • Long-term use may cause diarrhea, dizziness, gynecomastia • Many drug–drug interactions (eg, amiodarone, amitriptyline, benzodiazepines, metoprolol, nifedipine, phenytoin, warfarin [Coumadin])
Famotidine (Pepcid)	Same as for cimetidine	• Best choice for critically ill patient, because it is known to have the least risk of drug–drug interactions; does not alter liver metabolism • Prolonged half-life in patients with renal insufficiency • Short-term relief for GERD
Nizatidine (Axid)	Same as for cimetidine	• Used for treatment of ulcers and GERD • Prolonged half-life in patients with renal insufficiency • May cause headache, dizziness, diarrhea, nausea/vomiting, GI upset as well as urticaria
Ranitidine (Zantac)	Same as for cimetidine	• Prolonged half-life in patients with renal and hepatic insufficiency • Causes fewer side effects than cimetidine • May cause headache, dizziness, constipation, nausea and vomiting, or abdominal discomfort
Proton pump inhibitors of gastric acid (PPIs)		
Esomeprazole (Nexium)	Decreases gastric acid secretion by slowing the hydrogen-potassium adenosine triphosphatase (H^+, K^+-ATPase) pump on the surface of the parietal cells of the stomach	• Used mainly for treatment of duodenal ulcer disease and *H. pylori* infection • A delayed-release capsule that is to be swallowed whole and taken before meals
Lansoprazole (Prevacid)	Decreases gastric acid secretion by slowing the H^+, K^+-ATPase pump on the surface of the parietal cells	• A delayed-release capsule that is to be swallowed whole and taken before meals

TABLE 37-1 Pharmacotherapy for Peptic Ulcer Disease and Gastritis (Continued)

Pharmacologic Agent	Major Action	Nursing Considerations
Omeprazole (Prilosec)	Decreases gastric acid secretion by slowing the H^+, K^+-ATPase pump on the surface of the parietal cells	• A delayed-release capsule that is to be swallowed whole and taken before meals • May cause diarrhea, nausea, constipation, abdominal pain, vomiting, headache, or dizziness
Pantoprazole (Protonix)	Decreases gastric acid secretion by slowing the H^+, K^+-ATPase pump on the surface of the parietal cells	• A delayed-release capsule that is to be swallowed whole and taken before meals • May cause diarrhea and hyperglycemia, headache, abdominal pain, and abnormal liver function tests
Rabeprazole (AcipHex)	Decreases gastric acid secretion by slowing the H^+, K^+-ATPase pump on the surface of the parietal cells	• A delayed-release tablet to be swallowed whole • May cause abdominal pain, diarrhea, nausea, and headache • Drug–drug interactions with digoxin, iron, and warfarin (Coumadin)
Prostaglandin E_1 analog		
Misoprostol (Cytotec)	Synthetic prostaglandin; protects the gastric mucosa from agents that cause ulcers; also increases mucous production and bicarbonate levels	• Used to prevent ulceration in patients using NSAIDs • Administer with food • May cause diarrhea and cramping (including uterine cramping)
Sucralfate (Carafate)	Creates a viscous substance in the presence of gastric acid that forms a protective barrier, binding to the surface of the ulcer, and prevents digestion by pepsin	• Used mainly for the treatment of duodenal ulcers • Should be taken without food but with water • Other medications should be taken 2 hours before or after this medication • May cause constipation or nausea

GI, gastrointestinal; NSAID, nonsteroidal anti-inflammatory drug; GERD, gastroesophageal reflux disease.

symptoms related to anxiety, stress, allergies, eating or drinking too much, or eating too quickly? How are the symptoms relieved? Is there a history of previous gastric disease or surgery? A diet history plus a 72-hour dietary recall (a list of everything the patient has eaten and drunk in the past 72 hours) may be helpful.

A thorough history is important because it helps the nurse identify whether known dietary excesses or other indiscretions are associated with the current symptoms, whether others in the patient's environment have similar symptoms, whether the patient is vomiting blood, and whether any known caustic element has been ingested. The nurse also identifies the duration of the current symptoms, any methods used by the patient to treat these symptoms, and whether the methods are effective.

Signs to note during the physical examination include abdominal tenderness, dehydration, and evidence of any systemic disorder that might be responsible for the symptoms of gastritis.

Nursing Diagnoses

Based on the assessment data, the patient's major nursing diagnoses may include the following:

- Anxiety related to treatment
- Imbalanced nutrition, less than body requirements, related to inadequate intake of nutrients
- Risk for imbalanced fluid volume related to insufficient fluid intake and excessive fluid loss subsequent to vomiting
- Deficient knowledge about dietary management and disease process
- Acute pain related to irritated stomach mucosa

Planning and Goals

The major goals for the patient may include reduced anxiety, avoidance of irritating foods, adequate intake of nutrients, maintenance of fluid balance, increased awareness of dietary management, and relief of pain.

Nursing Interventions

Reducing Anxiety

If the patient has ingested acids or alkalis, emergency measures may be necessary. The nurse offers supportive therapy to the patient and family during treatment and after the ingested acid or alkali has been neutralized or diluted. In some cases, the nurse may need to prepare the patient for additional diagnostic studies (endoscopies) or surgery. The patient may be anxious because of pain and planned treatment modalities. The nurse uses a calm approach to assess the patient and to answer all questions as completely as possible. It is important to explain all procedures and treatments based on the patient's level of understanding.

Promoting Optimal Nutrition

For acute gastritis, the nurse provides physical and emotional support and helps the patient manage the symptoms, which may include nausea, vomiting, heartburn, and fatigue. The patient should take no foods or fluids by mouth—possibly for a few days—until the acute symptoms subside, thus allowing the gastric mucosa to heal. If IV therapy is necessary, the nurse monitors fluid intake and output along with serum electrolyte values. After the symptoms subside, the nurse may offer the patient ice chips followed by clear liquids. Introducing solid food as soon as possible may provide adequate oral nutrition, decrease the need for IV therapy, and minimize irritation to the gastric mucosa. As food is introduced, the nurse evaluates and reports any symptoms that suggest a repeat episode of gastritis.

The nurse discourages the intake of caffeinated beverages, because caffeine is a central nervous system stimulant that increases gastric activity and pepsin secretion. It also is important to discourage alcohol use. Discouraging cigarette smoking is important because nicotine reduces the secretion of pancreatic bicarbonate, which inhibits the neutralization of gastric acid in the duodenum (Wu & Cho, 2004). When appropriate, the nurse initiates and refers the patient for alcohol counseling and smoking cessation programs.

Promoting Fluid Balance

Daily fluid intake and output are monitored to detect early signs of dehydration (minimal urine output of 30 mL/hour, minimal intake of 1.5 L/day). If food and oral fluids are withheld, IV fluids (3 L/day) usually are prescribed and a record of fluid intake plus caloric value (1 L of 5% dextrose in water = 170 calories of carbohydrate) needs to be maintained. Electrolyte values (sodium, potassium, chloride) are assessed every 24 hours to detect any imbalance.

The nurse must always be alert for any indicators of hemorrhagic gastritis, which include **hematemesis** (vomiting of blood), tachycardia, and hypotension. If these occur, the physician is notified and the patient's vital signs are monitored as the patient's condition warrants. Guidelines for managing upper GI tract bleeding are discussed later in this chapter.

Relieving Pain

Measures to help relieve pain include instructing the patient to avoid foods and beverages that may be irritating to the gastric mucosa and instructing the patient about the correct use of medications to relieve chronic gastritis. The nurse must regularly assess the patient's level of pain and the extent of comfort attained from the use of medications and avoidance of irritating substances.

Promoting Home and Community-Based Care

TEACHING PATIENTS SELF-CARE

The nurse evaluates the patient's knowledge about gastritis and develops an individualized teaching plan that includes information about stress management, diet, and medications (Chart 37-1). Dietary instructions take into account the patient's daily caloric needs, food preferences, and pattern of eating. The nurse and patient review foods and other substances to be avoided (eg, spicy, irritating, or highly seasoned foods; caffeine; nicotine; alcohol). Consultation with a dietitian may be recommended.

Providing information about prescribed antibiotics, bismuth salts, medications to decrease gastric secretion, and medications to protect mucosal cells from gastric secretions may help the patient to better understand why these medications assist in recovery and prevent recurrence. The importance of completing the medication regimen as prescribed to eradicate *H. pylori* infection must be reinforced to the patient and any caregivers.

CONTINUING CARE

The nurse reinforces previous teaching and conducts ongoing assessment of the patient's symptoms and progress. Patients with pernicious anemia need information about lifelong vitamin B_{12} injections; the nurse may instruct a family member or caregiver how to administer the injections or make arrangements for the patient to receive the injections from a health care provider. Finally, the nurse emphasizes the

CHART 37-1

HOME CARE CHECKLIST • The Patient With Gastritis

At the completion of the home care instruction, the patient or caregiver will be able to:	Patient	Caregiver
• Identify foods and other substances that may cause gastritis.	✔	✔
• Report inability to ingest adequate solids and liquids.	✔	✔
• Describe medication regimen.	✔	✔
• State need for vitamin B_{12} injections if patient has pernicious anemia.	✔	✔
• State schedule of follow-up appointments with health care provider.	✔	✔

importance of keeping follow-up appointments with health care providers.

Evaluation

Expected Patient Outcomes

Expected patient outcomes may include the following:

1. Exhibits low level of anxiety
2. Avoids eating irritating foods or drinking caffeinated beverages or alcohol
3. Maintains fluid balance
   a. Has oral fluid intake of at least 1.5 L daily
   b. Drinks six to eight glasses of water daily
   c. Has urinary output of approximately 1 L daily
   d. Displays adequate skin turgor
4. Adheres to medical regimen
   a. Selects nonirritating foods and beverages
   b. Takes medications as prescribed
5. Maintains appropriate weight
6. Reports less pain

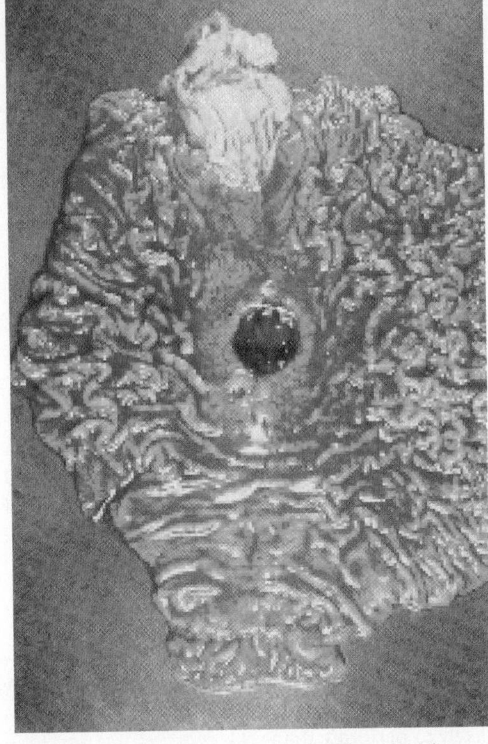

FIGURE 37-2. Deep peptic ulcer. Reproduced with permission from Porth, C. (2005). *Pathophysiology: Concepts of altered health states* (7th ed.). Philadelphia: Lippincott Williams & Wilkins. © 2005, Lippincott Williams & Wilkins.

Peptic Ulcer Disease

A peptic ulcer may be referred to as a gastric, duodenal, or esophageal ulcer, depending on its location. A person who has a peptic ulcer has peptic ulcer disease. A peptic ulcer is an excavation (hollowed-out area) that forms in the mucosal wall of the stomach, in the **pylorus** (the opening between the stomach and duodenum), in the **duodenum** (the first part of small intestine), or in the esophagus. Erosion of a circumscribed area of mucous membrane is the cause (Fig. 37-2). This erosion may extend as deeply as the muscle layers or through the muscle to the **peritoneum**.

Peptic ulcers are more likely to be in the duodenum than in the stomach. As a rule they occur alone, but they may occur in multiples. Chronic gastric ulcers tend to occur in the lesser curvature of the stomach, near the pylorus. Table 37-2 compares the features of gastric and duodenal ulcers. Esophageal ulcers occur as a result of the backward flow of HCl from the stomach into the esophagus (gastroesophageal reflux disease [GERD]).

Peptic ulcer disease occurs with the greatest frequency in people between 40 and 60 years of age. It is relatively uncommon in women of childbearing age, but it has been observed in children and even in infants. After menopause, the incidence of peptic ulcers in women is almost equal to that in men. Peptic ulcers in the body of the stomach can occur without excessive acid secretion.

In the past, stress and anxiety were thought to be causes of ulcers, but research has documented that peptic ulcers result from infection with the gram-negative bacteria *H. pylori*, which may be acquired through ingestion of food and water. Person-to-person transmission of the bacteria also occurs through close contact and exposure to emesis. Although *H. pylori* infection is common in the United States, most infected people do not develop ulcers. It is not known why *H. pylori* infection does not cause ulcers in all people, but most likely the predisposition to ulcer formation depends on certain factors, such as the type of *H. pylori* and other as yet unknown factors (Moss & Sood, 2003).

In addition, excessive secretion of HCl in the stomach may contribute to the formation of peptic ulcers, and stress may be associated with its increased secretion. The ingestion of milk and caffeinated beverages, smoking, and alcohol also may increase HCl secretion. Stress and eating spicy foods may make peptic ulcers worse.

Familial tendency also may be a significant predisposing factor. People with blood type O are more susceptible to peptic ulcers than are those with blood type A, B, or AB; this is another genetic link. There also is an association between peptic ulcers and chronic pulmonary disease or chronic renal disease. Other predisposing factors associated with peptic ulcer include chronic use of NSAIDs, alcohol ingestion, and excessive smoking.

Peptic ulcers are found in rare cases in patients with tumors that cause secretion of excessive amounts of the hormone gastrin. The Zollinger-Ellison syndrome (ZES) consists of severe peptic ulcers, extreme gastric hyperacidity, and gastrin-secreting benign or malignant tumors of the pancreas.

Pathophysiology

Peptic ulcers occur mainly in the gastroduodenal mucosa because this tissue cannot withstand the digestive action of

TABLE 37-2 Comparison of Duodenal and Gastric Ulcers

Duodenal Ulcer	Gastric Ulcer
Incidence	
Age 30–60	Usually 50 and over
Male: female = 2–3:1	Male: female = 1:1
80% of peptic ulcers are duodenal	15% of peptic ulcers are gastric
Signs, Symptoms, and Clinical Findings	
Hypersecretion of stomach acid (HCl)	Normal—hyposecretion of stomach acid (HCl)
May have weight gain	Weight loss may occur
Pain occurs 2–3 hours after a meal; often awakened 1–2 AM; ingestion of food relieves pain	Pain occurs ½ to 1 hour after a meal; rarely occurs at night; may be relieved by vomiting; ingestion of food does not help, sometimes increases pain
Vomiting uncommon	Vomiting common
Hemorrhage less likely than with gastric ulcer, but if present, melena more common than hematemesis	Hemorrhage more likely to occur than with duodenal ulcer; hematemesis more common than melena
More likely to perforate than gastric ulcers	
Malignancy Possibility	
Rare	Occasionally
Risk Factors	
H. pylori, alcohol, smoking, cirrhosis, stress	*H. pylori*, gastritis, alcohol, smoking, use of NSAIDs, stress

gastric acid (HCl) and pepsin. The erosion is caused by the increased concentration or activity of acid-pepsin, or by decreased resistance of the mucosa. A damaged mucosa cannot secrete enough mucus to act as a barrier against HCl. The use of NSAIDs inhibits the secretion of mucus that protects the mucosa. Patients with duodenal ulcer disease secrete more acid than normal, whereas patients with gastric ulcer tend to secrete normal or decreased levels of acid. Damage to the gastroduodenal mucosa allows for decreased resistance to bacteria, and thus infection from *H. pylori* bacteria may occur.

ZES is suspected when a patient has several peptic ulcers or an ulcer that is resistant to standard medical therapy. It is identified by the following: hypersecretion of gastric juice, duodenal ulcers, and gastrinomas (islet cell tumors) in the pancreas. Ninety percent of tumors are found in the "gastric triangle," which encompasses the cystic and common bile ducts, the second and third portions of the duodenum, and the junction of the head and body of the pancreas. Approximately one third of gastrinomas are malignant. Diarrhea and steatorrhea (unabsorbed fat in the stool) may be evident. The patient may have coexisting parathyroid adenomas or hyperplasia and may therefore exhibit signs of hypercalcemia. The most common symptom is epigastric pain. *H. pylori* is not a risk factor for ZES.

Stress ulcer is the term given to the acute mucosal ulceration of the duodenal or gastric area that occurs after physiologically stressful events, such as burns, shock, severe sepsis, and multiple organ traumas. These ulcers, which are clinically different from peptic ulcers, are most common in ventilator-dependent patients after trauma or surgery. Fiberoptic endoscopy within 24 hours of trauma or surgery reveals shallow erosions of the stomach wall; by 72 hours, multiple gastric erosions are observed. As the stressful condition continues, the ulcers spread. When the patient recovers, the lesions are reversed. This pattern is typical of stress ulceration.

Differences of opinion exist as to the actual cause of mucosal ulceration in stress ulcers. Usually, the ulceration is preceded by shock; this leads to decreased gastric mucosal blood flow and to reflux of duodenal contents into the stomach. In addition, large quantities of pepsin are released. The combination of ischemia, acid, and pepsin creates an ideal climate for ulceration.

Stress ulcers should be distinguished from Cushing's ulcers and Curling's ulcers, two other types of gastric ulcers. Cushing's ulcers are common in patients with head injury and brain trauma. They may occur in the esophagus, stomach, or duodenum and are usually deeper and more penetrating than stress ulcers. Curling's ulcer is frequently observed about 72 hours after extensive burns and involves the antrum of the stomach or the duodenum.

Clinical Manifestations

Symptoms of an ulcer may last for a few days, weeks, or months and may disappear only to reappear, often without an identifiable cause. Many people with ulcers have no symptoms, and perforation or hemorrhage may occur in 20% to 30% of patients who had no preceding manifestations.

As a rule, the patient with an ulcer complains of dull, gnawing pain or a burning sensation in the midepigastrium or in the back. It is believed that the pain occurs when the increased acid content of the stomach and duodenum erodes the lesion and stimulates the exposed nerve endings. Another theory suggests that contact of the lesion with acid stimulates a local reflex mechanism that initiates contraction of the adjacent smooth muscle. Pain is usually relieved by eating, because food neutralizes the acid, or by taking alkali; however, once the stomach has emptied or the alkali's effect has decreased, the pain returns. Sharply localized tenderness can be elicited by applying gentle pressure to the epigastrium at or slightly to the right of the midline.

Other symptoms include **pyrosis** (heartburn), vomiting, constipation or diarrhea, and bleeding. Pyrosis is a burning sensation in the esophagus and stomach that moves up to the mouth. Heartburn is often accompanied by sour eructation, or burping, which is common when the patient's stomach is empty.

Although vomiting is rare in uncomplicated duodenal ulcer, it may be a symptom of a complication of an ulcer. It results from obstruction of the pyloric orifice, caused by either muscular spasm of the pylorus or mechanical obstruction from scarring or acute swelling of the inflamed mucous membrane adjacent to the ulcer. Vomiting may or may not be preceded by nausea; usually it follows a bout of severe pain and bloating, which is relieved by ejection of the gastric contents. Emesis often contains undigested food eaten many hours earlier. Constipation or diarrhea may occur, probably as a result of diet and medications.

Fifteen percent of patients with peptic ulcer experience bleeding. Patients may present with GI bleeding as evidenced by the passage of **melena** (tarry stools). A small portion of patients who bleed from an acute ulcer have only very mild symptoms or none at all (Yamada & Alpers, 2003).

Assessment and Diagnostic Findings

A physical examination may reveal pain, epigastric tenderness, or abdominal distention. A barium study of the upper GI tract may show an ulcer; however, endoscopy is the preferred diagnostic procedure because it allows direct visualization of inflammatory changes, ulcers, and lesions. Through endoscopy, a biopsy of the gastric mucosa and of any suspicious lesions can be obtained. Endoscopy may reveal lesions that, because of their size or location, are not evident on x-ray studies.

Stools may be tested periodically until they are negative for occult blood. Gastric secretory studies are of value in diagnosing achlorhydria and ZES. *H. pylori* infection may be determined by endoscopy and histologic examination of a tissue specimen obtained by biopsy, or a rapid urease test of the biopsy specimen. Other less invasive diagnostic measures for detecting *H. pylori* include serologic testing for antibodies against the *H. pylori* antigen, stool antigen test, and urea breath test.

Medical Management

Once the diagnosis is established, the patient is informed that the condition can be controlled. Recurrence may develop; however, peptic ulcers treated with antibiotics to eradicate *H. pylori* have a lower recurrence rate than those not treated with antibiotics. The goals are to eradicate *H. pylori* and to manage gastric acidity. Methods used include medications, lifestyle changes, and surgical intervention.

Pharmacologic Therapy

Currently, the most commonly used therapy for peptic ulcers is a combination of antibiotics, proton pump inhibitors, and bismuth salts that suppress or eradicate *H. pylori*.

Recommended therapy for 10 to 14 days includes triple therapy with two antibiotics (eg, metronidazole [Flagyl] or amoxicillin [Amoxil] and clarithromycin [Biaxin]) plus a proton pump inhibitor (eg, lansoprazole [Prevacid] or omeprazole [Prilosec]), or quadruple therapy with two antibiotics (metronidazole [Flagyl] and tetracycline) plus a proton pump inhibitor and bismuth salts (Pepto-Bismol). Research is being conducted to develop a vaccine against *H. pylori* (Sutton & Doidge, 2003).

Histamine-2 (H_2) receptor antagonists and proton pump inhibitors are used to treat NSAID-induced ulcers and other ulcers not associated with *H. pylori* infection. Table 37-3 provides information about the drug regimens used

TABLE 37-3 Drug Regimens for Peptic Ulcer Disease

Indications	Drug Regimen	Comments
Ulcer healing	**H_2 receptor antagonists** Ranitidine 150 mg bid or 300 mg at bedtime Cimetidine 400 mg bid or 800 mg at bedtime Famotidine 20 mg bid or 40 mg at bedtime Nizatidine 150 mg bid or 300 mg at bedtime	Should be used for 6 weeks for duodenal ulcer; 8 weeks for gastric ulcer
	Proton pump inhibitors (PPIs) Omeprazole 20 mg daily Lansoprazole 30 mg daily Rabeprazole 20 mg daily Pantoprazole 40 mg daily Esomeprazole 40 mg daily	Should be used for 4 weeks for duodenal ulcer and 6 weeks for gastric ulcer Healing occurs in 90% of patients who are compliant with therapy
Initial *Helicobacter pylori* therapy	**First-line therapy:** PPI twice a day plus clarithromycin 500 mg twice a day plus amoxicillin 1000 mg twice a day *or* metronidazole 500 mg twice a day for 10–14 days	Efficacy of therapy is approximately 85%
	Second-line therapy: Pepto-Bismol 2 tabs four times a day plus tetracycline 250 mg four times a day plus metronidazole 250 mg four times a day (optional: add PPI daily) for 14 days	QID dosing may decrease compliance
Therapy for retreatment of *H. pylori* therapy failure	Repeat first-line therapy, substitute metronidazole for amoxicillin (or vice versa) for 14 days; may add Pepto-Bismol. Add second-line *H. pylori* therapy.	Efficacy of retreatment not known; success of more than 2 courses of treatment is very low
Prophylactic therapy for NSAID ulcers	Peptic ulcer healing doses of PPIs (above) Misoprostol 200 mcg twice a day	Prevents recurrent ulceration in approximately 80%–90% of patients

NSAID, nonsteroidal anti-inflammatory drug

for peptic ulcer disease. (Table 37-1 presents details about medications that can be used to treat peptic ulcer disease.)

The patient is advised to adhere to and complete the medication regimen to ensure complete healing of the ulcer. Because most patients become symptom-free within a week, it is a nursing responsibility to stress to the patient the importance of following the prescribed regimen so that the healing process can continue uninterrupted and the return of chronic ulcer symptoms can be prevented. Rest, sedatives, and tranquilizers may be added for the patient's comfort and are prescribed as needed. Maintenance dosages of H_2 receptor antagonists are usually recommended for 1 year.

For patients with ZES, hypersecretion of acid may be controlled with high doses of H_2 receptor antagonists. These patients may require twice the normal dose, and dosages usually need to be increased with prolonged use. Octreotide (Sandostatin), a medication that suppresses gastrin levels, also may be prescribed.

Patients at risk for stress ulcers (eg, patients with head injury or extensive burns) may be treated prophylactically with IV H_2 receptor antagonists and cytoprotective agents (eg, misoprostol, sucralfate) because of the risk for upper GI tract hemorrhage.

Stress Reduction and Rest

Reducing environmental stress requires physical and psychological modifications on the patient's part as well as the aid and cooperation of family members and significant others. The nurse assists the patient to identify situations that are stressful or exhausting. A rushed lifestyle and an irregular schedule may aggravate symptoms and interfere with regular meals taken in relaxed settings along with the regular administration of medications. The patient may benefit from regular rest periods during the day, at least during the acute phase of the disease. Biofeedback, hypnosis, behavior modification, massage, or acupuncture may be helpful.

Smoking Cessation

Studies have shown that smoking decreases the secretion of bicarbonate from the pancreas into the duodenum, resulting in increased acidity of the duodenum. Research indicates that continued smoking may significantly inhibit ulcer repair (Konturek, Bielanski, Plenka, et al., 2003). Therefore, the patient is strongly encouraged to stop smoking. Smoking cessation support groups and other smoking cessation approaches should be offered to patients.

Dietary Modification

The intent of dietary modification for patients with peptic ulcers is to avoid oversecretion of acid and hypermotility in the GI tract. These can be minimized by avoiding extremes of temperature of food and beverage and overstimulation from consumption of meat extracts, alcohol, coffee (including decaffeinated coffee, which also stimulates acid secretion) and other caffeinated beverages, and diets rich in milk and cream (which stimulate acid secretion). In addition, an effort is made to neutralize acid by eating three regular meals a day. Small, frequent feedings are not necessary as long as an antacid or a histamine blocker is taken. Diet compatibility becomes an individual matter: the patient eats foods that are tolerated and avoids those that produce pain.

Surgical Management

The introduction of antibiotics to eradicate *H. pylori* and of H_2 receptor antagonists as treatment for ulcers has greatly reduced the need for surgical intervention. However, surgery is usually recommended for patients with intractable ulcers (those that fail to heal after 12 to 16 weeks of medical treatment), life-threatening hemorrhage, perforation, or obstruction and for those with ZES not responding to medications (Yamada & Alpers, 2003). Surgical procedures include vagotomy, with or without pyloroplasty, and the Billroth I and Billroth II procedures (Table 37-4; see also the section on gastric surgery later in this chapter).

Patients who require surgery may have had a long illness. They may be discouraged and have had interruptions in their work role and pressures in their family life that affect their outlook on surgery and resolution of their disease.

Follow-up Care

Recurrence of peptic ulcer disease within 1 year may be prevented with the prophylactic use of H_2-receptor antagonists taken at a reduced dose. Not all patients require maintenance therapy; it may be prescribed only for those with two or three recurrences per year, those who have had a complication such as bleeding or gastric outlet obstruction, or those who are candidates for gastric surgery but for whom it poses too high a risk. The likelihood of recurrence is reduced if the patient avoids smoking, coffee (including decaffeinated coffee) and other caffeinated beverages, alcohol, and ulcerogenic medications (eg, NSAIDs).

Nursing Process

The Patient With Peptic Ulcer Disease

Assessment

The nurse asks the patient to describe the pain and the methods used to relieve it (eg, food, antacids). The patient usually describes peptic ulcer pain as burning or gnawing; it occurs about 2 hours after a meal and frequently awakens the patient between midnight and 3 AM. Taking antacids, eating, or vomiting often relieves the pain. If the patient reports a recent history of vomiting, the nurse determines how often emesis has occurred and notes important characteristics of the vomitus: Is it bright red, does it resemble coffee grounds, or is there undigested food from previous meals? Has the patient noted any bloody or tarry stools?

The nurse also asks the patient to list his or her usual food intake for a 72-hour period and to

TABLE 37-4 Surgical Procedures for Peptic Ulcer Disease

Operation	Description	Comments
Vagotomy Vagotomy 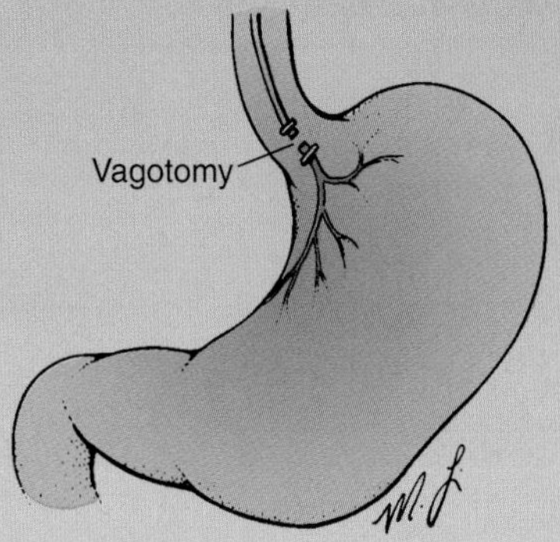	Severing of the vagus nerve. Decreases gastric acid by diminishing cholinergic stimulation to the parietal cells, making them less responsive to gastrin. May be performed via open surgical approach, laparoscopy, or thoracoscopy	May be performed to reduce gastric acid secretion. A drainage type of procedure (see pyloroplasty) is usually performed to assist with gastric emptying (because there is total denervation of the stomach). Some patients experience problems with feeling of fullness, dumping syndrome, diarrhea, and gastritis.
Truncal vagotomy	Severs the right and left vagus nerves as they enter the stomach at the distal part of the esophagus	This type of vagotomy is most commonly used to decrease acid secretions and reduce gastric and intestinal motility. Recurrence rate of ulcer is 10%–15%.
Selective vagotomy	Severs vagal innervation to the stomach but maintains innervation to the rest of the abdominal organs	
Proximal (parietal cell) gastric vagotomy without drainage	Denervates acid-secreting parietal cells but preserves vagal innervation to the gastric antrum and pylorus	No dumping syndrome. No need for drainage procedure. Recurrence rate of ulcer is 10%–15%.
Pyloroplasty 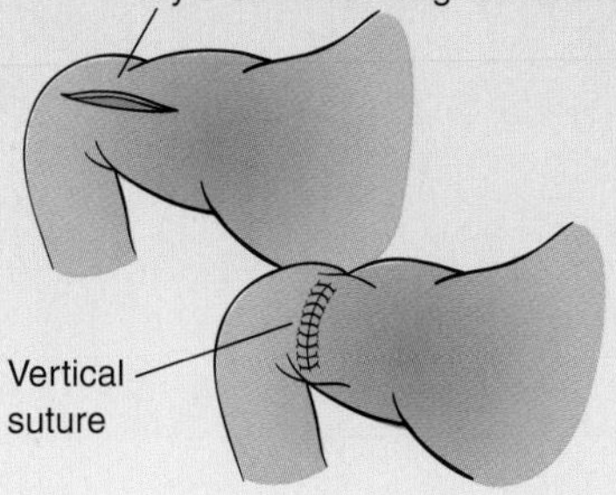 Pylorus—note longitudinal incision Vertical suture	A surgical procedure in which a longitudinal incision is made into the pylorus and transversely sutured closed to enlarge the outlet and relax the muscle	Usually accompanies truncal and selective vagotomies, which produce delayed gastric emptying due to decreased innervation.

continued >

TABLE 37-4 Surgical Procedures for Peptic Ulcer Disease (Continued)

Operation	Description	Comments
Antrectomy		
Billroth I (Gastroduodenostomy) Fundus Body Antrectomy Duodenum Duodenal anastomosis Billroth I	Removal of the lower portion of the antrum of the stomach (which contains the cells that secrete gastrin) as well as a small portion of the duodenum and pylorus. The remaining segment is anastomosed to the duodenum (Billroth I)	May be performed in conjunction with a truncal vagotomy. The patient may have problems with feeling of fullness, dumping syndrome, and diarrhea. Recurrence rate of ulcer is <1%.
Billroth II (Gastrojejunostomy) 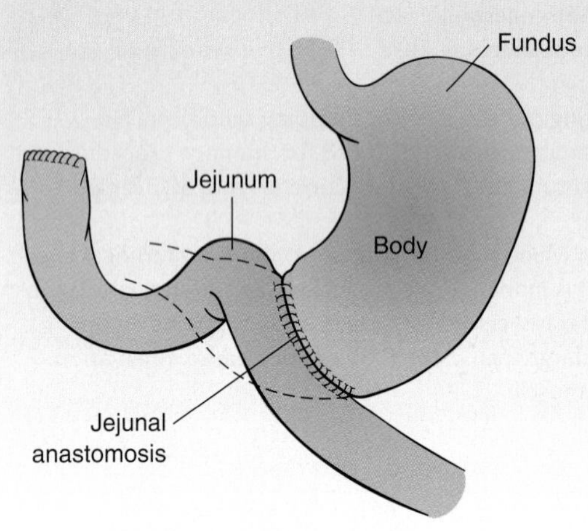 Billroth II (Gastrojejunostomy)	Removal of lower portion (antrum) of stomach with anastomosis to jejunum. Dotted lines show portion removed (antrectomy). A duodenal stump remains and is oversewn.	Dumping syndrome, anemia, malabsorption, weight loss. Recurrence rate of ulcer is 10%–15%.

describe food habits (eg, speed of eating, regularity of meals, preference for spicy foods, use of seasonings, use of caffeinated beverages and decaffeinated coffee). Lifestyle and other habits are a concern as well. Does the patient use irritating substances? For example, does he or she smoke cigarettes? If yes, how many? Does the patient ingest alcohol? If yes, how much and how often? Are NSAIDs used? The nurse inquires about the patient's level of anxiety and his or her perception of current stressors. How does the patient express anger or cope with stressful situations? Is the patient experiencing occupational stress or problems within the family? Is there a family history of ulcer disease?

The nurse assesses the patient's vital signs and reports tachycardia and hypotension, which may indicate anemia from GI bleeding. The stool is tested for occult blood, and a physical examination, including palpation of the abdomen for localized tenderness, is performed.

Diagnosis

Nursing Diagnoses

Based on the assessment data, the patient's nursing diagnoses may include the following:

- Acute pain related to the effect of gastric acid secretion on damaged tissue
- Anxiety related to an acute illness
- Imbalanced nutrition related to changes in diet
- Deficient knowledge about prevention of symptoms and management of the condition

Collaborative Problems/ Potential Complications

Potential complications may include the following:

- Hemorrhage
- Perforation
- Penetration
- Pyloric obstruction (gastric outlet obstruction)

Planning and Goals

The goals for the patient may include relief of pain, reduced anxiety, maintenance of nutritional requirements, knowledge about the management and prevention of ulcer recurrence, and absence of complications.

Nursing Interventions

Relieving Pain

Pain relief can be achieved with prescribed medications. The patient should avoid aspirin, foods and beverages that contain caffeine, and decaffeinated coffee. In addition, meals should be eaten at regularly paced intervals in a relaxed setting. Some patients benefit from learning relaxation techniques to help manage stress and pain.

Reducing Anxiety

The nurse assesses the patient's level of anxiety. Patients with peptic ulcers are usually anxious, but their anxiety is not always obvious. Appropriate information is provided at the patient's level of understanding, all questions are answered, and the patient is encouraged to express fears openly. Explaining diagnostic tests and administering medications as scheduled also help to reduce anxiety. The nurse interacts with the patient in a relaxed manner, helps identify stressors, and explains various coping techniques and relaxation methods, such as biofeedback, hypnosis, or behavior modification. The patient's family is also encouraged to participate in care and to provide emotional support.

Maintaining Optimal Nutritional Status

The nurse assesses the patient for malnutrition and weight loss. After recovery from an acute phase of peptic ulcer disease, the patient is advised about the importance of complying with the medication regimen and dietary restrictions.

Monitoring and Managing Potential Complications

HEMORRHAGE

Gastritis and hemorrhage from peptic ulcer are the two most common causes of upper GI tract bleeding (which may also occur with esophageal varices, as discussed in Chapter 39). Hemorrhage, the most common complication, occurs in 10% to 20% of patients with peptic ulcers. Bleeding may be manifested by hematemesis or melena (Yamada & Alpers, 2003). The vomited blood can be bright red, or it can have a dark "coffee grounds" appearance from the oxidation of hemoglobin to methemoglobin. When the hemorrhage is large (2000 to 3000 mL), most of the blood is vomited. Because large quantities of blood may be lost quickly, immediate correction of blood loss may be required to prevent hemorrhagic shock. When the hemorrhage is small, much or all of the blood is passed in the stools, which appear tarry black because of the digested hemoglobin. Management depends on the amount of blood lost and the rate of bleeding.

The nurse assesses the patient for faintness or dizziness and nausea, which may precede or accompany bleeding. It is important to monitor vital signs frequently and to evaluate the patient for tachycardia, hypotension, and tachypnea. Other nursing interventions include monitoring the hemoglobin and hematocrit, testing the stool for gross or occult blood, and recording hourly urinary output to detect anuria or oliguria (absence of or decreased urine production).

Many times the bleeding from a peptic ulcer stops spontaneously; however, the incidence of recurrent bleeding is high. Because bleeding can be fatal, the cause and severity of the hemorrhage must be identified quickly and the blood loss treated to prevent hemorrhagic shock. Management of upper GI tract bleeding consists of quickly estimating the amount of blood lost and the rate of bleeding, rapidly replacing the blood that has been lost, stopping the bleeding, stabilizing the patient, and diagnosing and treating the cause. Related nursing and collaborative interventions include the following:

- Inserting a peripheral IV line for the infusion of saline or lactated Ringer's solution and blood products. The nurse may need to assist with the placement of a central venous catheter for rapid infusion of large amounts of blood and fluids as well as hemodynamic monitoring. Blood component therapy is initiated if there are signs of shock (eg, tachycardia, sweating, coldness of the extremities).
- Monitoring the hemoglobin and hematocrit to assist in evaluating blood loss
- Inserting an NG tube to distinguish fresh blood from "coffee grounds" material, to aid in the removal of clots and acid, to prevent nausea and vomiting, and to provide a means of monitoring further bleeding
- Administering an NG lavage of saline solution. The temperature of the solution (cold or room temperature) is a topic of controversy (Yamada & Alpers, 2003).
- Inserting an indwelling urinary catheter and monitoring urinary output
- Monitoring vital signs and oxygen saturation and administering oxygen therapy
- Placing the patient in the recumbent position with the legs elevated to prevent hypotension, or placing the patient on the left side to prevent aspiration from vomiting
- Treating hemorrhagic shock (described in Chapter 15)

If bleeding cannot be managed by the measures described, other treatment modalities may be used. Transendoscopic coagulation by laser, heat probe, medication, a sclerosing agent, or a combination of these therapies can halt bleeding and avoid surgical intervention. There is debate regarding how soon endoscopy should be performed. Some clinicians believe endoscopy should be performed within the first 24 hours after hemorrhage has been stabilized. Others believe endoscopy may be performed during acute bleeding, as long as the esophageal or gastric area can be visualized (blood may decrease visibility) (Yamada & Alpers, 2003).

For patients who are unable to undergo surgery, selective embolization may be used. This procedure involves forcing emboli of autologous blood clots with or without Gelfoam (absorbable gelatin sponge) through a catheter in the artery to a point above the bleeding lesion. This procedure is performed by an interventional radiologist.

Rebleeding may occur and often warrants surgical intervention. The nurse monitors the patient carefully so that bleeding can be detected quickly. Signs of bleeding include tachycardia, tachypnea, hypotension, mental confusion, thirst, and oliguria. If bleeding recurs within 48 hours after medical therapy has begun, or if more than 6 to 10 units of blood are required within 24 hours to maintain blood volume, the patient is likely to require surgery. Some physicians recommend surgical intervention if a patient hemorrhages three times. Other criteria for surgery are the patient's age (massive hemorrhaging is three times more likely to be fatal in those older than 60 years of age), a history of chronic duodenal ulcer, and a coincidental gastric ulcer. The area of the ulcer is removed or the bleeding vessels are ligated. Many patients also undergo procedures (eg, vagotomy and pyloroplasty, gastrectomy) aimed at controlling the underlying cause of the ulcers (see Table 37-4).

PERFORATION AND PENETRATION

Perforation is the erosion of the ulcer through the gastric **serosa** into the peritoneal cavity without warning. It is an abdominal catastrophe and requires immediate surgery. Penetration is erosion of the ulcer through the gastric serosa into adjacent structures such as the pancreas, biliary tract, or gastrohepatic **omentum.** Symptoms of penetration include back and epigastric pain not relieved by medications that were effective in the past. Like perforation, penetration usually requires surgical intervention.

Signs and symptoms of perforation include the following:

- Sudden, severe upper abdominal pain (persisting and increasing in intensity); pain may be referred to the shoulders, especially the right shoulder, because of irritation of the phrenic nerve in the diaphragm
- Vomiting and collapse (fainting)
- Extremely tender and rigid (boardlike) abdomen
- Hypotension and tachycardia, indicating shock

Because chemical peritonitis develops within a few hours after perforation and is followed by bacterial peritonitis, the perforation must be closed as quickly as possible and the abdominal cavity lavaged of stomach or intestinal contents. In select patients, it may be safe and advisable to perform surgery to treat the ulcer disease in addition to suturing the perforation.

Postoperatively, the stomach contents are drained by means of an NG tube. The nurse monitors fluid and electrolyte balance and assesses the patient for localized infection or peritonitis (increased temperature, abdominal pain, paralytic ileus, increased or absent bowel sounds, abdominal distention). Antibiotic therapy is administered parenterally as prescribed.

PYLORIC OBSTRUCTION

Pyloric obstruction, also called **gastric outlet obstruction** (GOO), occurs when the area distal to the pyloric sphincter becomes scarred and stenosed from spasm or edema or from scar tissue that forms when an ulcer alternately heals and breaks down. The patient may have nausea and vomiting, constipation, epigastric fullness, anorexia, and, later, weight loss.

In treating the patient with pyloric obstruction, the first consideration is to insert an NG tube to decompress the stomach. Confirmation that obstruction is the cause of the discomfort is accomplished by assessing the amount of fluid aspirated from the NG tube. A residual of more than 400 mL strongly suggests obstruction. Usually an upper GI study or endoscopy is performed to confirm pyloric obstruction. Decompression of the stomach and management of extracellular fluid volume and electrolyte balances may improve the patient's condition and avert the need for surgical intervention. A balloon dilation of the pylorus via endoscopy may be beneficial. If the obstruction is unrelieved by medical management, surgery (in the form of a vagotomy and **antrectomy** or gastrojejunostomy and vagotomy) may be required.

Promoting Home and Community-Based Care

TEACHING PATIENTS SELF-CARE

The nurse instructs the patient about the factors that will relieve and those that will aggravate the condition (Chart 37-2). The nurse reviews information about medications to be taken at home, including name, dosage, frequency, and possible side effects, stressing the importance of continuing to take medications even after signs and symptoms have decreased or subsided. The nurse instructs the patient to avoid certain medications and foods that exacerbate symptoms as well as substances that have acid-producing potential (eg, alcohol; caffeinated and decaffeinated beverages such as coffee, tea, and colas). It is important to counsel the patient to eat meals at regular times and in a relaxed setting, and to avoid overeating. If relevant, the nurse also informs the patient about the irritant effects of smoking on the ulcer and provides information about smoking cessation programs.

CHART 37-2

HOME CARE CHECKLIST • The Patient With Peptic Ulcer Disease

At the completion of the home care instruction, the patient or caregiver will be able to:	Patient	Caregiver
• State the medication regimen and importance of complying with medication schedule.	✔	✔
• State dietary restrictions and foods that may exacerbate condition (caffeinated and decaffeinated products, milk).	✔	✔
• Identify smoking cessation groups.	✔	
• Identify methods to reduce stress.	✔	✔
• State signs and symptoms of complications: Hemorrhage—cool skin, confusion, increased heart rate, labored breathing, blood in stool Penetration and perforation—severe abdominal pain, rigid and tender abdomen, vomiting, elevated temperature, increased heart rate Pyloric obstruction—nausea and vomiting, distended abdomen, abdominal pain	✔	✔
• State need for follow-up medical care.	✔	✔

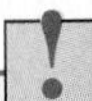

NURSING ALERT

The nurse reviews with the patient and family the signs and symptoms of complications to be reported. These complications include hemorrhage (cool skin, confusion, increased heart rate, labored breathing, and blood in the stool), penetration and perforation (severe abdominal pain, rigid and tender abdomen, vomiting, elevated temperature, and increased heart rate), and pyloric obstruction (nausea, vomiting, distended abdomen, and abdominal pain).

CONTINUING CARE

The nurse reinforces the importance of follow-up care for approximately 1 year, the need to report recurrence of symptoms, and the need for treating possible problems that occur after surgery, such as intolerance to dairy products and sweet foods. The nurse also reminds the patient and family of the importance of participating in health promotion activities and recommended health screening.

Evaluation

Expected Patient Outcomes

Expected patient outcomes may include the following:

1. Reports freedom from pain between meals
2. Reports feeling less anxiety
3. Complies with therapeutic regimen
   a. Avoids irritating foods and beverages
   b. Eats regularly scheduled meals
   c. Takes medications as prescribed
   d. Uses coping mechanisms to deal with stress
4. Maintains weight
5. Exhibits no complications

Morbid Obesity

Morbid obesity is a term applied to people who are more than two times their ideal body weight or whose body mass index (BMI) exceeds 30 kg/m^2 (see Chapter 5). Another definition of morbid obesity is body weight that is more than 100 pounds greater than the ideal body weight (Blackwood, 2004). In the United States, where morbid obesity is a rapidly growing problem, approximately 65% of the people are overweight (O'Brien, Dixon, & Brown, 2004).

Patients with morbid obesity are at higher risk for health complications, such as diabetes, heart disease, stroke, hypertension, gallbladder disease, osteoarthritis, sleep apnea and other breathing problems, and some forms of cancer (uterine, breast, colorectal, kidney, and gallbladder). They frequently suffer from low self-esteem, impaired body image, and depression.

Medical Management

Conservative management of obesity consists of placing the person on a weight loss diet in conjunction with behavioral modification and exercise; however, dietary and behavioral approaches to obesity have had limited success. Depression may be a contributing factor to weight gain, and treatment of the depression with an antidepressant may be helpful (Appolinario, Bueno, & Coutinho, 2004; Rosmond, 2004).

Pharmacologic Management

Several medications are approved for obesity, including sibutramine HCl (Meridia) and orlistat (Xenical). Sibutramine decreases appetite by inhibiting the reuptake of serotonin and norepinephrine. Orlistat reduces caloric intake by binding to gastric and pancreatic lipase to prevent digestion of fats. Both medications require a prescription from a licensed health care provider. Sibutramine may increase blood pressure and should not be taken by people with a history of coronary artery disease, angina pectoris, dysrhythmias, or kidney disease; by those taking antidepressants or monoamine oxidase inhibitors; or by pregnant or nursing women. Other side effects of sibutramine may include dry mouth, insomnia, headache, diaphoresis, and increased heart rate. Side effects of orlistat may include increased frequency of bowel movements, gas with oily discharge, decreased food absorption, decreased bile flow, and decreased absorption of some vitamins. A multivitamin is usually recommended for patients taking orlistat. Orlistat should not be taken by pregnant or nursing women.

Unfortunately, these medications rarely result in loss of more than 10% of total body weight (Arterburn, Crane, & Veenstra, 2004). Furthermore, studies are needed to evaluate their long-term efficacy and risks.

Surgical Management

Bariatric surgery, or surgery for morbid obesity, is performed only after other nonsurgical attempts at weight control have failed. Bariatric surgical procedures work by (1) restricting a patient's ability to eat (restrictive procedure), (2) interfering with ingested nutrient absorption (malabsorptive procedures), or both. Different bariatric surgical procedures entail different lifestyle modifications, and patients must be well informed about the specific lifestyle changes, eating habits, and bowel habits that may result from a particular procedure. Recent studies have shown that the average weight loss after bariatric surgery in the majority of patients is approximately 61% of previous body weight; comorbid conditions such as diabetes mellitus, hypertension, and sleep apnea resolve; and dyslipidemia improves (Buchwald, Avidor, Braunwald, et al., 2004). Although controversial, bariatric surgery has been extended to carefully selected adolescents because of its results in adults (Rosemurgy, 2003).

Patient selection is critical, and the preliminary process may necessitate 6 to 12 months of counseling, education, and evaluation by a multidisciplinary team, including social workers, dietitians, a nurse counselor, psychologist or psychiatrist, as well as a surgeon (Chart 37-3). Because bariatric surgery involves such a drastic change in the functioning of the digestive system, patients need extensive counseling before and after the surgery. Guidelines have been developed to assist physicians and nurses in the care of patients having bariatric surgery (AORN Bariatric Surgery Guideline, 2004). After bariatric surgery, all patients require lifelong monitoring of weight loss, comorbidities, metabolic and nutritional status, and dietary and activity behaviors because they are at risk for developing malnutrition or weight gain (Ferraro, 2004). Women of childbearing age who have bariatric surgery are advised to use contraceptives for approximately 2 years after surgery to avoid pregnancy until their weight stabilizes.

The first surgical procedure used to treat morbid obesity was jejunoileal bypass. This procedure, which resulted in significant complications, has been largely replaced by gastric restriction procedures. Roux-en-Y gastric bypass, gastric banding, vertical-banded gastroplasty, and biliopancreatic diversion with duodenal switch are the current procedures of choice. These procedures may be performed by laparoscopy or by an open surgical technique.

The Roux-en-Y gastric bypass is recommended for long-term weight loss. It is a combined restrictive and malabsorptive procedure. In this procedure, a small pouch (20 to 30 mL) is isolated from the rest of the stomach by a horizontal row of staples across the fundus of the stomach. The jejunum is divided distal to the **ligament of Treitz.** The distal end of the jejunum is anastomosed to the new pouch and the other open end of the jejunum is reanastomosed to the lower jejunum (Fig. 37-3A).

Gastric banding and vertical-banded gastroplasty are restrictive procedures. Gastric banding uses a prosthetic device to restrict oral intake by creating a small pouch of 10 to 15 mL at the fundus of the stomach. This small gastric pouch then empties through the narrow outlet to the remainder of the stomach. During laparoscopic adjustable gastric banding, a silicone band is placed around the upper stomach, and the band is connected by a catheter to a subcutaneous reservoir into which saline solution can be injected to adjust the diameter of the band (see Fig. 37-3B). Vertical-banded gastroplasty involves placement of a vertical row of staples along the lesser curvature of the stomach, creating a new, small (10 to 15 mL) gastric pouch (see Fig. 37-3C).

Biliopancreatic diversion with duodenal switch combines gastric restriction with intestinal malabsorption. Half of the stomach is removed to create a small pouch that can hold about 60 mL. The entire jejunum is excluded from the rest of the GI tract to create a shorter small intestine to absorb fewer calories. The duodenum is disconnected, and the end is closed. The small bowel (ileum) is divided approximately 300 cm above the ileocecal junction, and the

CHART 37-3

Factors Considered in the Selection of Patients for Bariatric Surgery

- Body weight
  - Body weight ≥ 45 kg/m² or 100% above ideal weight
  - BMI > 40 kg/m²
  - BMI > 35 kg/m² with medical comorbidities (eg, severe sleep apnea, hypertension, cardiomyopathy related to obesity, severe diabetes mellitus; serious musculoskeletal or neurologic disorders)
- Long-standing history of obesity
- Failure of multiple nonsurgical attempts to lose weight
- Absence of endocrine disorders that cause morbid obesity
- Psychological stability
  - Absence of alcohol and drug use
  - Understanding of how surgery causes weight loss
  - Realization that surgery itself does not guarantee good results
  - Ability to comply with dietary and behavioral changes as recommended by the weight management team

Source: National Institutes of Health Publication No. 98-4083, 1998: *Society of American Gastrointestinal Endoscopic Surgeons (SAGES) guidelines for laparoscopic and conventional surgical treatment of morbid obesity,* May 2000; and American Society for Bariatric Surgery, 2001.

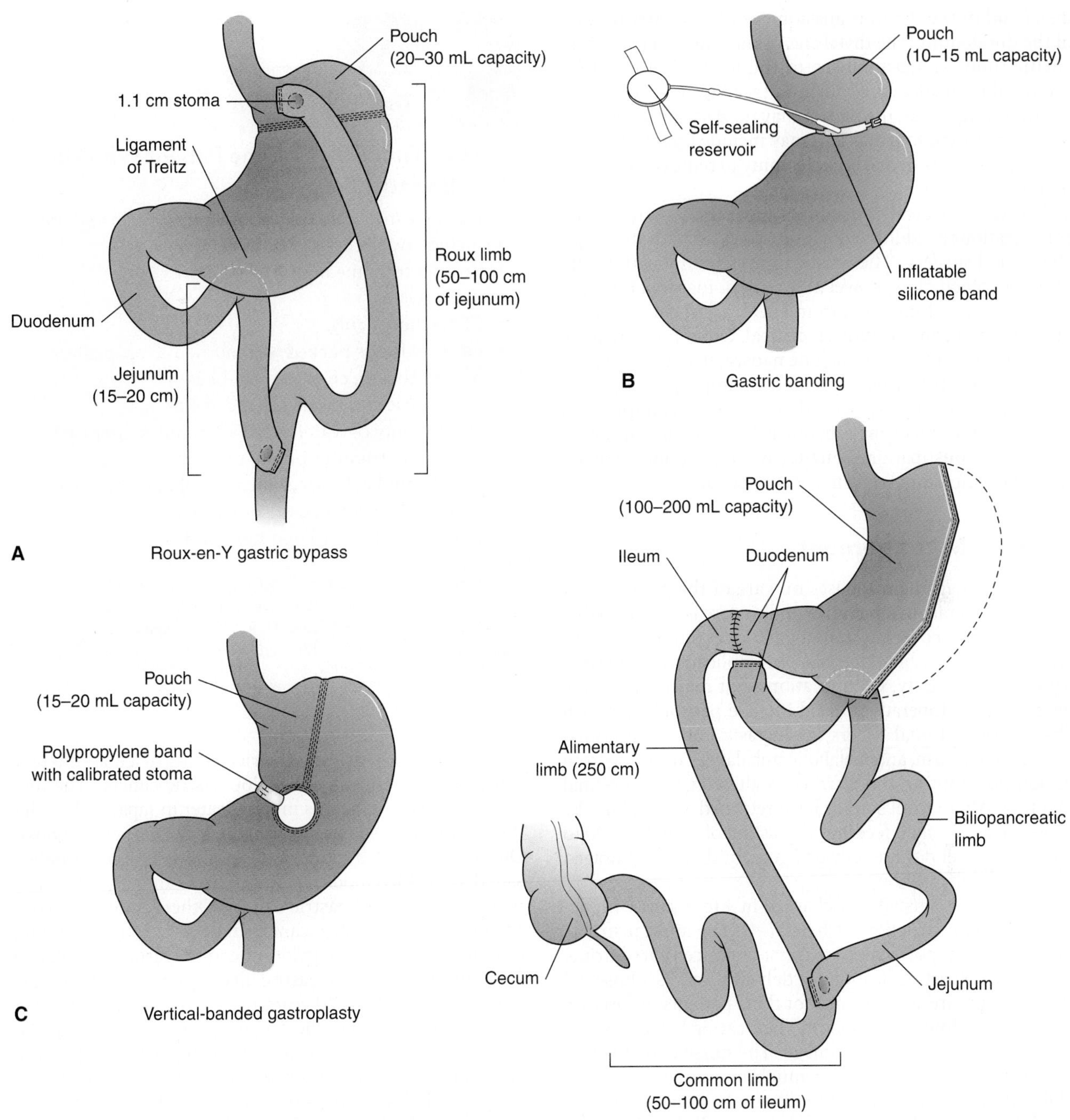

FIGURE 37-3. Surgical procedures for morbid obesity. (**A**) Roux-en-Y gastric bypass. A horizontal row of staples across the fundus of the stomach creates a pouch with a capacity of 20 to 30 mL. The jejunum is divided distal to the ligament of Trietz and the distal end is anastomosed to the new pouch. The proximal segment is anastomosed to the jejunum. (**B**) Gastric banding. A prosthetic device is used to restrict oral intake by creating a small pouch of 10 to 15 mL that empties through the narrow outlet into the remainder of the stomach. (**C**) Vertical-banded gastroplasty. A vertical row of staples along the lesser curvature of the stomach creates a new, smaller stomach pouch of 10 to 15 mL. (**D**) Biliopancreatic diversion with duodenal switch. Half of the stomach is removed, leaving a small area that holds about 60 mL. The entire jejunum is excluded from the rest of the GI tract. The duodenum is disconnected and sealed off. The ileum is divided above the ileocecal junction and the distal end of the jejunum is anastomosed to the first portion of the duodenum. The distal end of the biliopancreatic limb is anastomosed to the ileum.

distal end of the ileum is anastomosed to the first portion of the duodenum. The distal end of the jejunum (biliopancreatic limb) is anastomosed to the ileum 50 to 100 cm proximal to the ileocecal junction (see Fig. 37-3D).

After weight loss, the patient may need surgical intervention for body contouring. This may include lipoplasty to remove fat deposits or a panniculectomy to remove excess abdominal skinfolds.

Bariatric surgical procedures have their own unique complications in addition to those associated with any major abdominal surgery. The most common complications are bleeding, blood clots, bowel obstruction, incisional or ventral hernias, and infection from a leak at the anastomosis. Prevention of complications is critical. Other postoperative problems that may occur include nausea, usually as a result of overfilling the stomach pouch or improper chewing; dumping syndrome associated with the consumption of simple sugars; and changes in bowel function, including diarrhea and constipation. Long-term complications that are related to nutritional deficiency may occur.

CHART 37-4

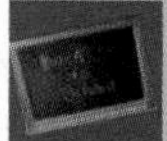

Patient Education

Dietary Guidelines for the Patient Who Has Had Bariatric Surgery

- Eat three meals per day (containing protein and fiber).
- Include two protein snacks per day.
- Restrict total meal size to less than 1 cup.
- Eat slowly.
- Chew thoroughly.
- Eat only foods packed with nutrients (eg, peanut butter, cheese, chicken, fish, beans).
- Do not eat and drink at the same time.
- Drink plenty of water, from 90 minutes after each meal to 15 minutes before the next meal.
- Avoid liquid calories, such as alcoholic beverages, fruit drinks, and regular soda (cola).
- Walk for at least 30 minutes per day.

From Favretti, F., O'Brien, P. E., & Dixon, J. B. (2002). Patient management after LAP-BAND placement. *American Journal of Surgery, 184*(6B), 38S–41S, and Ferraro, D. R. (2003). Laparoscopic adjustable gastric banding for morbid obesity. *AORN Journal, 77*(5), 923–940.

Nursing Management

Nursing management focuses on care of the patient after surgery. General postoperative nursing care is similar to that for a patient recovering from a gastric resection, but with great attention given to the risks of complications associated with morbid obesity. Complications that may occur in the immediate postoperative period include peritonitis, stomal obstruction, stomal ulcers, atelectasis and pneumonia, thromboembolism, and metabolic imbalances resulting from prolonged vomiting and diarrhea or altered gastrointestinal function. After bowel sounds have returned and oral intake is resumed, six small feedings consisting of a total of 600 to 800 calories per day are provided, and fluids are encouraged to prevent dehydration.

The patient is usually discharged in 4 to 5 days with detailed dietary instructions (Chart 37-4). The nurse instructs the patient to report excessive thirst or concentrated urine, both of which are indications of dehydration. Psychosocial interventions are also essential for these patients. Efforts are directed at helping them modify their eating behaviors and cope with changes in body image. The nurse explains that noncompliance by eating too much or too fast or eating high-calorie liquids and soft foods results in vomiting and painful esophageal distention. The nurse discusses dietary instructions before discharge and emphasizes the importance of routine follow-up outpatient appointments. Long-term side effects may include increased risk of gallstones, nutritional deficiencies, and potential to regain weight.

Gastric Cancer

The incidence of gastric or stomach cancer continues to decrease in the United States; however, it still accounts for almost 12,000 deaths annually (American Cancer Society, 2005). The typical patient with gastric cancer is between 40 and 70 years of age, but gastric cancer can occur in people younger than 40 years of age. Men have a higher incidence of gastric cancer than women. Native Americans, Hispanic Americans, and African Americans are twice as likely as Caucasian Americans to develop gastric cancer. The incidence of gastric cancer is much greater in Japan, which has instituted mass screening programs for earlier diagnosis. Diet appears to be a significant factor: a diet high in smoked, salted, or pickled foods and low in fruits and vegetables may increase the risk of gastric cancer. Other factors related to the incidence of gastric cancer include chronic inflammation of the stomach, *H. pylori* infection, pernicious anemia, smoking, achlorhydria, gastric ulcers, previous subtotal gastrectomy (more than 20 years ago), and genetics. The prognosis is generally poor: the diagnosis is usually made late because most patients are asymptomatic during the early stages of the disease. Most cases of gastric cancer are discovered only after local invasion has advanced or metastases are present (Layke & Lopez, 2004).

Pathophysiology

Most gastric cancers are adenocarcinomas; they can occur anywhere in the stomach. The tumor infiltrates the surrounding mucosa, penetrating the wall of the stomach and adjacent organs and structures. The liver, pancreas, esophagus, and duodenum are often affected at the time of diagnosis. Metastasis through lymph to the peritoneal cavity occurs later in the disease.

Clinical Manifestations

Symptoms of early disease, such as pain relieved by antacids, resemble those of benign ulcers and are seldom definitive, because most gastric tumors begin on the lesser curvature of the stomach, where they cause little disturbance of gastric function. Symptoms of progressive disease include dyspepsia (indigestion), early satiety, weight loss, abdominal pain just above the umbilicus, loss or decrease in appetite, bloating after meals, nausea and vomiting, and symptoms similar to those of peptic ulcer disease.

Assessment and Diagnostic Findings

Usually the physical examination is not helpful in detecting the cancer because most early gastric tumors are not palpable. Advanced gastric cancer may be palpable as a mass. Ascites and hepatomegaly (enlarged liver) may be apparent if the cancer cells have metastasized to the liver. Palpable nodules around the umbilicus, called Sister Mary Joseph's nodule, are a sign of a GI malignancy, usually a gastric cancer. Esophagogastroduodenoscopy for biopsy and cytologic washings is the diagnostic study of choice, and a barium x-ray examination of the upper GI tract may also be performed. Endoscopic ultrasound is an important tool to assess tumor depth and any lymph node involvement. Computed tomography (CT) completes the diagnostic studies, particularly to assess for surgical resectability of the tumor before surgery is scheduled. CT of the chest, abdomen, and pelvis is valuable in staging gastric cancer because it determines the existence of metastases.

Medical Management

There is no successful treatment for gastric carcinoma except removal of the tumor. If the tumor can be removed while it is still localized to the stomach, the patient may be cured. If the tumor has spread beyond the area that can be excised, cure is less likely. In many patients, effective palliation to prevent discomfort caused by obstruction or dysphagia may be obtained by resection of the tumor (see Gastric Surgery). A diagnostic laparoscopy may be the initial surgical approach to evaluate the gastric tumor, obtain tissue for pathologic diagnosis, and detect metastasis. The patient with a tumor that is deemed resectable would undergo an open surgical procedure to resect the tumor and appropriate lymph nodes. The patient with an unresectable tumor and advanced disease would undergo chemotherapy. Palliative rather than radical surgery may be performed if there is metastasis to other vital organs, such as the liver.

A total gastrectomy may be performed for a resectable cancer in the midportion or body of the stomach. The entire stomach is removed along with duodenum, the section of esophagus attached to the stomach, supporting mesentery, and lymph nodes. Reconstruction of the GI tract is performed by anastomosing the end of the jejunum to the end of the esophagus, a procedure called an esophagojejunostomy.

A radical subtotal gastrectomy is performed for a resectable tumor in the middle and distal portions of the stomach. A Billroth I or Billroth II operation (see Table 37-4) is performed. The Billroth I involves a limited resection and offers a lower cure rate than the Billroth II. The Billroth II procedure is a wider resection that involves removing approximately 75% of the stomach and decreases the possibility of lymph node spread or metastatic recurrence.

A proximal subtotal gastrectomy may be performed for a resectable tumor located in the proximal portion of the stomach or cardia. A total gastrectomy or an esophagogastrectomy is usually performed in place of this procedure to achieve a more extensive resection. A palliative surgical procedure may be required for patients with gastric cancer to achieve a better quality of life.

Common problems of advanced gastric cancer that often require surgery include pyloric obstruction, bleeding, and severe pain. Gastric perforation is an emergency situation requiring surgical intervention. A gastric resection may be the most effective palliative procedure for advanced gastric cancer. Palliative procedures such as gastric or esophageal bypass, gastrostomy, or jejunostomy may temporarily alleviate symptoms such as nausea and vomiting.

If surgical treatment does not offer cure, treatment with chemotherapy may offer further control of the disease or palliation. Commonly used single-agent chemotherapeutic medications include 5-fluorouracil (5-FU), cisplatin, doxorubicin (Adriamycin), etoposide, and mitomycin-C. For improved response rates it is more common to administer combination therapy, primarily 5-FU–based therapy, with other agents. Studies are being conducted to assess the use of chemotherapy before surgery. Radiation therapy is mainly used for palliation in patients with obstruction, GI bleeding secondary to tumor, and significant pain. Assessment of tumor markers (blood analysis for antigens indicative of cancer) such as carcinoembryonic antigen (CEA), carbohydrate antigen (CA 19-9), and CA 50 may help determine the effectiveness of treatment. If these values were elevated before treatment, they should decrease if the tumor is responding to the treatment (Mihmanli, Dilege, Demir, et al., 2004).

Nursing Process

The Patient With Gastric Cancer

Assessment

The nurse obtains a dietary history from the patient, focusing on recent nutritional intake and status. Has the patient lost weight? If so, how much and over what period of time? Can the patient tolerate a full diet? If not, what foods can he or she eat? What other changes in eating habits have occurred? Does the patient have an appetite? Does the patient feel full after eating a small amount of food? Is the patient in pain? Do foods, antacids, or medications relieve the pain, make no difference, or worsen the pain? Is there a history of infection with *H. pylori*? Other health information to obtain includes the patient's smoking and alcohol history and family history (eg, any first- or second-degree relatives with gastric or other cancer). A psychosocial assessment, including questions about social support, individual and family coping skills, and financial resources, helps the nurse plan for care in acute and community settings.

After the interview, the nurse performs a complete physical examination, carefully assesses the patient's abdomen for tenderness or masses, as well as palpates and percusses the abdomen to detect ascites.

Nursing Diagnosis

Based on the assessment data, the patient's major nursing diagnoses may include the following:

- Anxiety related to the disease and anticipated treatment
- Imbalanced nutrition, less than body requirements, related to early satiety or anorexia
- Pain related to tumor mass
- Anticipatory grieving related to the diagnosis of cancer
- Deficient knowledge regarding self-care activities

Planning and Goals

The major goals for the patient may include reduced anxiety, optimal nutrition, relief of pain, and adjustment to the diagnosis and anticipated lifestyle changes.

Nursing Interventions

Reducing Anxiety

A relaxed, nonthreatening atmosphere is provided so the patient can express fears, concerns, and possibly anger about the diagnosis and prognosis. The nurse encourages the family or significant other to support the patient, offering reassurance and supporting positive coping measures. The nurse advises the patient about any procedures and treatments so that the patient knows what to expect. The nurse also may suggest talking with a support person (eg, social worker, spiritual advisor), if the patient desires.

Promoting Optimal Nutrition

The nurse encourages the patient to eat small, frequent portions of nonirritating foods to decrease gastric irritation. Food supplements should be high in calories, as well as vitamins A and C and iron, to enhance tissue repair. If the patient is unable to eat adequately prior to surgery to meet nutritional requirements, parenteral nutrition may be necessary. Because the patient may develop dumping syndrome when enteral feeding resumes after gastric resection, the nurse explains ways to prevent and manage it (six small feedings daily that are low in carbohydrates and sugar; fluids between meals rather than with meals) and informs the patient that symptoms often resolve after several months. If a total gastrectomy is performed, injection of vitamin B_{12} will be required for life, because dietary vitamin B_{12} is absorbed in the stomach. The nurse monitors the IV therapy and nutritional status and records intake, output, and daily weights to ensure that the patient is maintaining or gaining weight. The nurse assesses for signs of dehydration (thirst, dry mucous membranes, poor skin turgor, tachycardia, decreased urine output) and reviews the results of daily laboratory studies to note any metabolic abnormalities (sodium, potassium, glucose, blood urea nitrogen). Antiemetics are administered as prescribed.

Relieving Pain

The nurse administers analgesics as prescribed. A continuous IV infusion of an opioid may be necessary for postoperative or severe pain. The nurse routinely assesses the frequency, intensity, and duration of the pain to determine the effectiveness of the analgesic. The nurse works with the patient to help manage pain by suggesting nonpharmacologic methods for pain relief, such as position changes, imagery, distraction, relaxation exercises (using relaxation audiotapes), backrubs, massage, and periods of rest and relaxation.

Providing Psychosocial Support

The nurse helps the patient express fears, concerns, and grief about the diagnosis. It is important to answer the patient's questions honestly and to encourage the patient to participate in treatment decisions. Some patients mourn the loss of a body part and perceive their surgery as a type of mutilation. Some express disbelief and need time and support to accept the diagnosis.

The nurse offers emotional support and involves family members and significant others whenever possible. This includes recognizing mood swings and defense mechanisms (eg, denial, rationalization, displacement, regression) and reassuring the patient, family members, and significant others that emotional responses are normal and expected. The services of clergy, psychiatric clinical nurse specialists, psychologists, social workers, and psychiatrists are made available, if needed. The nurse projects an empathetic attitude and spends time with the patient. Many patients may begin to participate in self-care activities after they have acknowledged their loss.

Promoting Home and Community-Based Care

TEACHING PATIENTS SELF-CARE

Self-care activities depend on the type of treatments used—surgery, chemotherapy, radiation, or palliative care. Patient and family teaching will include information about diet and nutrition, treatment regimens, activity and lifestyle changes, pain management, and possible complications (Chart 37-5). Consultation with a dietitian is essential to determine how the patient's nutritional needs can best be met at home. The nurse teaches the patient or caregiver about administration of enteral or parenteral nutrition. If chemotherapy or radiation is prescribed, the nurse provides explanations to the patient and family about what to expect, including the length of treatments, the expected side effects (eg, nausea, vomiting, anorexia, fatigue, neutropenia), and the need for transportation

CHART 37-5

HOME CARE CHECKLIST • The Patient With Gastric Cancer

At the completion of the home care instruction, the patient or caregiver will be able to:	Patient	Caregiver
• Demonstrate safe management of enteral or parenteral feedings, if applicable.	✔	✔
• Describe dietary restrictions.	✔	✔
• Identify potential side effects of chemotherapy or radiation therapy, if applicable	✔	✔
• Identify signs and symptoms of wound infection.	✔	✔
• State signs and symptoms of obstruction or perforation.	✔	✔
• Describe follow-up needs.	✔	✔
• Make decisions about end-of-life care as appropriate.	✔	✔

to appointments for treatment. Psychological counseling may also be helpful.

CONTINUING CARE

The need for ongoing care in the home depends on the patient's condition and treatment. The home care nurse reinforces nutritional counseling and supervises the administration of any enteral or parenteral feedings; the patient or caregiver must become skillful in administering the feedings and in detecting and preventing untoward effects or complications related to the feedings (see Chapter 36 to review management of enteral and parenteral feedings). The nurse teaches the patient or a caregiver to record the patient's daily intake, output, and weight and explains strategies to manage pain, nausea, vomiting, or other symptoms. The nurse also teaches the patient or caregiver to recognize and report signs and symptoms of complications that require immediate attention, such as bleeding, obstruction, perforation, or any symptoms that become progressively worse. It is important to explain the chemotherapy or radiation therapy regimen. The patient and family or significant other need to understand the care that will be needed during and after treatments (see Chapter 16). Because the prognosis for gastric cancer is poor, the nurse may need to assist the patient, the family, or significant other with decisions regarding end-of-life care and make referrals as warranted.

Evaluation

Expected Patient Outcomes

Expected patient outcomes may include the following:

1. Reports less anxiety
   a. Expresses fears and concerns about surgery
   b. Seeks emotional support
2. Attains optimal nutrition
   a. Eats small, frequent meals high in calories, iron, and vitamins A and C
   b. Complies with enteral or parenteral nutrition as needed
3. Has decreased pain
4. Performs self-care activities and adjusts to lifestyle changes
   a. Resumes normal activities within 3 months
   b. Alternates periods of rest and activity
   c. Manages enteral feedings
5. Prepares for the dying process
   a. Acknowledges disease process
   b. Reports control of symptoms
   c. Verbalizes fears and concerns about dying; involves family/caregiver in discussions
   d. Completes advance directives, and other appropriate documents

Gastric Surgery

Gastric surgery may be performed on patients with peptic ulcers who have life-threatening hemorrhage, obstruction, perforation, or penetration or whose condition does not respond to medication. It also may be indicated for patients with gastric cancer or trauma. Surgical procedures include a vagotomy and **pyloroplasty** (transecting nerves that stimulate acid secretion and opening the pylorus), a partial gastrectomy, or a total gastrectomy (see Table 37-4).

Nursing Process

The Patient Undergoing Gastric Surgery

Assessment

Before surgery, the nurse assesses the patient's and family's knowledge of preoperative and postoperative surgical routines and the rationale for surgery. The nurse also assesses the patient's nutritional status: Has the patient lost weight? How much? Over how much time? Does the patient have nausea and vomiting? Has the patient had hematemesis? The nurse assesses for the presence of bowel sounds and palpates the abdomen to detect masses or tenderness.

After surgery, the nurse assesses the patient for complications secondary to the surgical intervention, such as hemorrhage, infection, abdominal distention, atelectasis, or impaired nutritional status (see Chapters 20 and 25).

Diagnosis

Nursing Diagnoses

Based on the assessment data, the patient's major nursing diagnoses may include the following:

- Anxiety related to surgical intervention
- Acute pain related to surgical incision
- Deficient knowledge about surgical procedure and postoperative course
- Imbalanced nutrition, less than body requirements, related to poor nutrition before surgery and altered GI system after surgery

Collaborative Problems/ Potential Complications

In addition to the complications to which all postoperative patients are subject, the patient undergoing gastric surgery is at increased risk for:

- Hemorrhage
- Dietary deficiencies
- Bile reflux
- Dumping syndrome

Planning and Goals

The major goals for the patient undergoing gastric surgery may include reduced anxiety, increased knowledge and understanding about the surgical procedure and postoperative course, optimal nutrition and management of the complications that can interfere with nutrition, relief of pain, avoidance of hemorrhage and steatorrhea, and enhanced self-care skills at home. General postoperative care guidelines for the patient who has received general anesthesia, as discussed in Chapter 20, should be followed.

Nursing Interventions

Reducing Anxiety

An important part of the preoperative nursing care involves allaying the patient's fears and anxieties about the impending surgery and its implications. The nurse encourages the patient to verbalize fears and concerns and answers the patient's and family's questions. If the patient has an acute obstruction, a perforated bowel, or an active GI hemorrhage, adequate psychological preparation may not be possible. In this event, the nurse caring for the patient after surgery should anticipate the concerns, fears, and questions that are likely to surface and should be available for support and further explanations.

Relieving Pain

After surgery, analgesics may be administered as prescribed to relieve pain and discomfort. It is important to provide adequate pain relief so the patient can perform pulmonary care activities (deep breathing and coughing) and leg exercises, turn from side to side, and ambulate. The nurse assesses the effectiveness of analgesic intervention and consults with other members of the health care team if pain is not adequately controlled. Positioning the patient in Fowler's position promotes comfort and allows emptying of the stomach after gastric surgery.

The nurse maintains functioning of the NG tube to prevent distention and secures the tube to prevent dislocation, which may result in increased pain and tension on the suture line. Normally, the amount of NG drainage after a total gastrectomy is minimal, as there is no reservoir where secretions can collect.

Increasing Knowledge

The nurse explains routine preoperative and postoperative procedures to the patient, which include preoperative medications, NG intubation, IV fluids, abdominal dressings, the possible need for a feeding tube, pain management, and pulmonary care. These explanations need to be reinforced after surgery, especially if the patient had emergency surgery.

Resuming Enteral Intake

The patient's nutritional status is evaluated before surgery. If surgery is performed for gastric cancer, the patient is often malnourished and may require preoperative enteral or, more often, parenteral nutrition (see Chapter 36). After surgery, parenteral nutrition may be continued to meet caloric needs, to replace fluids lost through drainage and vomiting, and to support the patient metabolically until oral intake is adequate.

After the return of bowel sounds and removal of the NG tube, the nurse may give fluids, followed by food in small portions. Foods are gradually added until the patient is able to eat six small meals a day and drink 120 mL of fluid between meals. The key to increasing the dietary content is to offer food and fluids gradually as tolerated and to recognize that each patient's tolerance is different.

Recognizing Obstacles to Adequate Nutrition

DYSPHAGIA AND GASTRIC RETENTION

Dysphagia may occur in patients who have had a truncal vagotomy, a surgical procedure that may result in trauma to the lower esophagus. Gastric retention may be evidenced by abdominal distention, nau-

NURSING RESEARCH PROFILE

Assessment of Life After Gastric Surgery

Hicks, F. D., & Spector, N. M. (2004). The Life After Gastric Surgery Index—Conceptual basis and initial psychometric assessment. *Gastroenterology Nursing, 27*(2), 50–54.

Purpose

The purpose of this methodological study was to better understand the influence of postoperative symptoms on a person's life. The researchers developed the Life After Gastric Surgery Index (LAGSI) to assist health care providers in assessing the frequency, intensity, or bothersomeness of symptoms that may occur after gastrointestinal surgery.

Design

Initial development and testing of the LAGSI was undertaken to estimate the tool's reliability and validity. In the first version, only a scale that assessed the frequency of symptoms made up the survey, and it was administered to a sample of 27 people who had either a total gastrectomy or a Roux-en-Y procedure. In the second version, severity and bothersomeness dimensions were added to the scale, and it was administered to 36 people participating in a study examining life satisfaction and health-related quality of life after gastroesophageal surgery for cancer. A total of 92 LAGSI surveys were then mailed to subjects identified from a cancer data bank of a Midwestern medical center. Thirty-six of the indexes were returned (39% return rate). Participants also completed the Gastrointestinal Quality of Life Index (GQLI), an instrument designed to measure disease-specific aspects of quality of life in persons with general gastrointestinal conditions, and the Cantril Life Satisfaction Ladder, an instrument designed to measure general life satisfaction. The following psychometric analyses were conducted: estimation of internal consistency reliability (Cronbach's alpha) of each of the scales, and determination of inter-item, item-to-item, and scale-to-scale correlations. Validity was examined by correlating the scores on the LAGSI with those of the GQLI and with the Cantril Life Satisfaction Ladder.

Findings

Internal consistency reliability for the LAGSI was determined to be acceptable for a new tool, at 0.87 for the frequency scale and 0.90 for both the severity scale and the bothersomeness scale. Likewise, the validity of the tool was determined to be acceptable, with positive correlations with the GQLI and the Cantril Life Satisfaction Ladder. The LAGSI shares common characteristics with these other valid and reliable tools, and it also appears to measure different underlying constructs, namely frequency, severity, and bothersomeness. However, sample sizes were small, and further study is needed.

Nursing Implications

The LASGI is only one page in length, is easily understandable, and is easily administered and scored. The instrument allows for multidimensional assessment of significant gastrointestinal symptoms in patients who have undergone gastric surgery. This assessment could help understand the symptoms that patients are experiencing and how these symptoms are affecting their quality of life. This could in turn suggest nursing interventions that would be most appropriate and helpful for patients.

---

sea, and vomiting. Regurgitation may also occur if the patient has eaten too much or too quickly. It also may indicate that edema along the suture line is preventing fluids and food from moving into the intestinal tract. If gastric retention occurs, it may be necessary to reinstate NPO status and NG suction; pressure must be low in the remaining portion of the stomach to avoid disrupting the sutures.

BILE REFLUX

Bile reflux gastritis and esophagitis may occur with the removal of the pylorus, which acts as a barrier to the reflux of duodenal contents. Burning epigastric pain and vomiting of bilious material manifest this condition. Eating or vomiting does not relieve the situation. Agents that bind with bile acid, such as cholestyramine (Questran), may be helpful. Aluminum hydroxide gel (an antacid) and metoclopramide hydrochloride (Reglan) have been used with limited success.

DUMPING SYNDROME

Dumping syndrome is an unpleasant set of vasomotor and GI symptoms that sometimes occur in patients who have had gastric surgery or a form of vagotomy. It may be the mechanical result of surgery in which a small gastric remnant is connected to the jejunum through a large opening. Foods high in carbohydrates and electrolytes must be diluted in the jejunum before absorption can take place, but the passage of food from the stomach remnant into the jejunum is too rapid to allow this to happen. The hypertonic intestinal contents draw extracellular fluid from the circulating blood volume into the jejunum to dilute the high concentration of electrolytes and sugars. The ingestion of fluid at mealtime is another factor that causes the stomach contents to empty rapidly into the jejunum.

Early symptoms include a sensation of fullness, weakness, faintness, dizziness, palpitations, diaphoresis, cramping pains, and diarrhea. These symptoms resolve once the intestine has been evacuated. Later, there is a rapid elevation of blood glucose, followed by increased insulin secretion. This results in a reactive hypoglycemia, which also is unpleasant for the patient. Vasomotor symptoms that occur 10 to 90 minutes after eating are pallor, perspiration, palpitations, headache, and feelings of warmth, dizziness, and even drowsiness. Anorexia may also be a result of the dumping syndrome, as the person may be reluctant to eat.

Steatorrhea also may occur in the patient with gastric surgery. It is partially the result of rapid gastric emptying, which prevents adequate mixing with pancreatic and biliary secretions. In mild cases, reducing the intake of fat and administering an antimotility medication (eg, loperamide [Imodium]) may control steatorrhea.

VITAMIN AND MINERAL DEFICIENCIES

Other dietary deficiencies that the nurse should be aware of include malabsorption of organic iron, which may require supplementation with oral or parenteral iron, and a low serum level of vitamin B_{12}, which may require supplementation by the intramuscular route. Total gastrectomy results in lack of intrinsic factor, a gastric secretion required for the absorption of vitamin B_{12} from the GI tract. Unless this vitamin is supplied by parenteral injection after gastrectomy, the patient inevitably will suffer vitamin B_{12} deficiency, which eventually leads to a condition identical to pernicious anemia. All manifestations of pernicious anemia, including macrocytic anemia and combined system disease (neurologic disorders of the central and peripheral nervous systems), may be expected to develop within a period of 5 years or less; they progress in severity thereafter and, in the absence of therapy, are fatal. This complication is avoided by the regular monthly intramuscular injection of vitamin B_{12}. This regimen should be started without delay after gastrectomy. Weight loss is a common long-term problem because the patient experiences early fullness, which suppresses the appetite.

Teaching Dietary Self-Management

Because the patient may experience any of the described conditions affecting nutrition, nursing intervention includes proper dietary instruction. The following teaching points are emphasized:

- To delay stomach emptying and dumping syndrome, the patient should assume a low Fowler's position during mealtime, and after the meal the patient should lie down for 20 to 30 minutes.
- Antispasmodics, as prescribed, also may aid in delaying the emptying of the stomach.
- Fluid intake with meals is discouraged; instead, fluids may be consumed up to 1 hour before or 1 hour after mealtime.
- Meals should contain more dry items than liquid items.
- The patient can eat fat as tolerated but should keep carbohydrate intake low and avoid concentrated sources of carbohydrates.
- The patient should eat smaller but more frequent meals.
- Dietary supplements of vitamins and medium-chain triglycerides and injections of vitamin B_{12} and iron may be prescribed.

The nurse also gives instructions regarding enteral or parenteral supplementation if it is needed.

Monitoring and Managing Potential Complications

Occasionally hemorrhage complicates gastric surgery. The patient has the usual signs of rapid blood loss and shock (see Chapter 15) and may vomit considerable amounts of bright-red blood. The nurse assesses NG drainage for type and amount; some bloody drainage for the first 12 hours is expected, but excessive bleeding should be reported. The nurse also assesses the abdominal dressing for bleeding. Because this situation is upsetting to the patient and family, the nurse should remain calm. The nurse performs emergency measures, such as NG lavage and administration of blood and blood products, along with vigilant hemodynamic monitoring.

Promoting Home and Community-Based Care

TEACHING PATIENTS SELF-CARE

Patient teaching is based on the assessment of the patient's physical and psychological readiness to participate in self-care. The nurse provides information about nutrition, enteral or parenteral nutrition if required, nutritional supplements, pain management, and the symptoms of dumping syndrome and measures to prevent or minimize these symptoms (Chart 37-6). It is important to emphasize the continued need for vitamin B_{12} injections.

CONTINUING CARE

The patient and caregivers benefit from a team approach to discharge planning. The team members include the patient and caregiver along with the nurse, physician, dietitian, and social worker. Written or video instructions about meals, activities, medications, and follow-up care are helpful. After the patient is discharged from the hospital, the home care nurse helps with the transition to home by supervising the administration of any enteral or parenteral feedings, emphasizing information about detection and prevention of untoward effects or complications related to feedings. Information about community support groups and end-of-life care is provided to the patient, family, or significant other when indicated.

Evaluation

Expected Patient Outcomes

Expected patient outcomes may include:

1. Reports decreased anxiety; expresses fears and concerns about surgery

CHART 37-6

HOME CARE CHECKLIST • The Patient With Gastric Resection

At the completion of the home care instruction, the patient or caregiver will be able to:	Patient	Caregiver
• Demonstrate enteral or parenteral feedings as applicable.	✔	✔
• State necessary dietary changes.	✔	✔
• Use nutritional supplements as appropriate.	✔	
• Relieve pain with pharmacologic or nonpharmacologic interventions.	✔	✔
• Identify available support groups.	✔	✔
• Explain medication regimen.	✔	✔
• Identify the need for continued vitamin B_{12} injections.	✔	✔
• Identify signs and symptoms of complications.	✔	✔
• State schedule of follow-up appointments.	✔	✔

2. Demonstrates knowledge regarding postoperative course by discussing the surgical procedure and postoperative course
3. Attains optimal nutrition
   a. Maintains a reasonable weight
   b. Does not have excessive diarrhea
   c. Tolerates six small meals a day
   d. Does not experience dysphagia, gastric retention, bile reflux, dumping syndrome, or vitamin and mineral deficiencies
4. Attains optimal level of comfort
5. Exhibits no complications

Duodenal Tumors

Tumors of the duodenum are uncommon and are usually benign and asymptomatic. They are most often discovered at autopsy. Malignant tumors are more likely to cause specific signs and symptoms leading to diagnosis. Unfortunately, malignant tumors are often not discovered until they have metastasized to distant sites. Benign tumors may place patients at an increased risk for malignancy. The relative rarity of tumors of the duodenum and the nonspecific nature of their manifestations complicate their diagnosis and treatment.

Clinical Manifestations

Duodenal tumors often present insidiously with vague, nonspecific symptoms. Most benign tumors are discovered incidentally on an x-ray study, during surgery, or at autopsy. When the patient is symptomatic, benign tumors often present with intermittent pain. The next most common presentation is occult bleeding. Malignant tumors often result in symptoms that lead to their diagnosis, although these symptoms may reflect advanced disease. Most patients have sustained weight loss and are malnourished at diagnosis. Bleeding and pain are common. Perforation of the bowel occurs in approximately 10% of patients (Kummar, Ciesielski, & Fogarasi, 2002).

Assessment and Diagnostic Findings

An upper GI x-ray series with small bowel follow-through using oral water-insoluble contrast with frequent and detailed x-rays to follow the contrast through the small bowel is the traditional approach to diagnosis. A more sensitive examination is an **enteroclysis**, in which a nasogastric tube is advanced into the small bowel to a position above the area in question; the area is then studied by single-contrast and double-contrast techniques. Abdominal CT is used to determine the extent of disease outside the lumen of the duodenum.

Management

Benign tumors of the duodenum include adenomas, lipomas, hemangiomas, and hamartomas (a focal malformation that resembles a neoplasm, but unlike a neoplasm does not result in compression of adjacent tissue). These tumors may be treated endoscopically by excision/resection or electrocautery if the patient is symptomatic. Routine surveillance may be recommended to assess for malignant transformation.

The most common primary malignant tumor of the duodenum is adenocarcinoma; the second and third portions of the duodenum are most often involved. These tumors may present with bleeding or duodenal obstruction. If the tumor is located at the ampulla of Vater, obstructive jaundice is likely. Other rare malignant tumors of the duodenum include carcinoid tumors, lymphoma, and gastrointestinal stromal tumors. Specialized abdominal surgery may be required to remove these rare tumors. Chemotherapy and radiation therapy may also be part of the treatment regimen.

The nursing process related to the care of the patient with a duodenal tumor is similar to that of the patient with gastric cancer. Each patient requires specialized care, astute assessment for complications, prompt interventions, and individualized teaching for self-care.

Critical Thinking Exercises

1 A 45-year-old woman with a history of rheumatoid arthritis and gastritis related to her medication is admitted with abdominal discomfort, headache, lassitude, and nausea and vomiting. What questions should you ask the patient? What signs should be noted during the physical examination? What diagnostic studies should you anticipate for this patient? Describe your nursing interventions, including teaching. How would you modify teaching for this patient if she does not understand English?

2 ebp A 27-year-old morbidly obese woman has tried conservative medical management (weight loss diet, behavior modification, exercise, medications for obesity) of her weight condition. She is scheduled for a vertical-banded gastroplasty. Describe the dietary modifications along with nutritional needs for this patient during the immediate postoperative period, after discharge from the hospital, and for long-term maintenance. What is the evidence base that supports the use of specific dietary modifications to meet her nutritional needs after surgical procedures to treat obesity? Describe the strength of this evidence and identify the criteria used to evaluate the strength of the evidence that supports the appropriateness of the dietary modifications.

3 You are caring for a 60-year-old man who has been diagnosed with gastric cancer and is scheduled for a total gastrectomy. The patient has been reluctant to discuss his diagnosis and proposed surgery. What should you do to prepare your patient for this surgery, both physically and emotionally? What nutritional needs do you anticipate for this patient preoperatively, immediately postoperatively, and after discharge from the hospital?

4 A 54-year-old business executive has been admitted with the diagnosis of peptic ulcer disease. As you enter his room, he is vomiting bright-red blood. What are the nursing interventions for managing and monitoring this complication? If the bleeding cannot be controlled, what invasive measures may need to be performed? How would you prepare your patient for these? What other complications may occur with a peptic ulcer and how should they be managed? What teaching interventions are warranted for this patient?

REFERENCES AND SELECTED READINGS

BOOKS

American Cancer Society. (2005). *Cancer facts and figures*. Atlanta: Author.

Cameron, J. L. (Ed.). (2004). *Current surgical therapy*. Philadelphia: Elsevier Mosby.

Cotton, P., & Williams, C. (2003). *Practical gastrointestinal endoscopy*. Massachusetts: Blackwell Publishing Ltd.

DeVita, V. T., Hellman, S., & Rosenberg, S. A. (Eds.). (2004). *Cancer: Principles and practice of oncology* (7th ed.). Philadelphia: Lippincott Williams & Wilkins.

Friedman, S. L., McQuaid, K. R., & Grendell, J. H. (Eds.). (2003). *Current diagnosis and treatment in gastroenterology*. New York: McGraw-Hill.

McEvoy, G. R. (Ed.). (2004). *American Hospital Formulary drug information service*. Bethesda, MD: American Society of Health-System Pharmacists.

Macfadyen, B. V., Arrequi, M. E., Eubanks, S., et al. (Eds.). (2003). *Laparoscopic surgery of the abdomen*. New York: Springer.

National Institutes of Health. (2000). *The practical guide: Identification, evaluation and treatment of overweight and obesity in adults*. Bethesda, MD: National Institutes of Health, National Heart, Lung and Blood Institute and North American Association for the Study of Obesity; 2000. NIH publication 00-4084.

Shelton, B. K., Ziegfeld, C. R., & Olsen, M. M. (Eds.). (2004). *The Sidney Kimmel Comprehensive Cancer Center at Johns Hopkins manual of cancer nursing*. Philadelphia: Lippincott Williams & Wilkins.

U.S. Department of Health and Human Services. (2001). *The Surgeon General's call to action to prevent and decrease overweight and obesity*. Rockville, MD: Author.

Yamada, T., & Alpers, D. H. (2003). *Textbook of gastroenterology*. Philadelphia: Lippincott Williams & Wilkins.

Yarbro, C. H., Frogge, M. H., Goodman, M., et al. (Eds.). (2005). *Cancer nursing: Principles and practice*. Boston: Jones & Bartlett.

JOURNALS

Asterisks indicate nursing research articles.

Gastric Cancer

Asao, T., Kuwano, H., & Mochiki, E. (2004). Laparoscopic surgery update for gastrointestinal malignancy. *Journal of Gastroenterology, 39*(4), 309–318.

Ba-Ssalamah, A., Prokop, M., Uffmann, M., et al. (2003). Dedicated multidetector CT of the stomach: Spectrum of diseases. *RadioGraphics, 23*(3), 625–644.

Enzinger, P. C., & Mayer, R. J. (2004). Gastrointestinal cancer in older patients. *Seminars in Oncology, 31*(2), 206–219.

Genta, R. M. (2003). The gastritis connection: Prevention and early detection of gastric neoplasms. *Journal of Clinical Gastroenterology, 36*(Suppl. 1), S44–S49.

Gonzalez, C. A., Sala, N., & Capella, G. (2002). Genetic susceptibility and gastric cancer risk. *International Journal of Cancer, 100*(3), 249–260.

Hicks, F. D., & Spector, N. M. (2004). The life after gastric surgery index—Conceptual basis and initial psychometric assessment. *Gastroenterology Nursing, 27*(2), 50–54.

Jemal, A., Murray, T., Ward, E. et al. (2005). Cancer statistics, 2005. *CA: A Cancer Journal for Clinicians, 55*(1), 10–30.

Kelley, J. R., & Duggan, J. M. (2003). Gastric cancer epidemiology and risk factors. *Journal of Clinical Epidemiology, 56*, 1–9.

Layke, J. C., & Lopez, P. P. (2004). Gastric cancer: Diagnosis and treatment options. *American Family Physician, 69*(5), 1133–1146.

Louhimo, J., Kokkola, A., Alfthan, H., et al. (2004). Preoperative hCG beta and CA 72-4 are prognostic factors in gastric cancer. *International Journal of Cancer, 111*(6), 929–933.

Macdonald, J. S. (2004). Treatment of localized gastric cancer. *Seminars in Oncology, 31*(4), 566–573.

Macdonald, J. S. (2004). Clinical overview: Adjuvant therapy of gastrointestinal cancer. *Cancer Chemotherapy and Pharmacology, 54*(Suppl 1), S4–S11.

Mihmanli, M., Dilege, E., Demir, U., et al. (2004). The use of tumor markers as predictors of prognosis in gastric cancer. *Hepatogastroenterology, 51*(9), 1544–1547.

Moreto, M. (2003). Diagnosis of esophagogastric tumors. *Endoscopy, 35*(1), 36–42.

Suerbaum, S., & Michetti, P. (2002). Medical progress: *Helicobacter pylori* infection. *New England Journal of Medicine, 347*(15), 1175–1186

Ushijima, T., & Sasako, M. (2004). Focus on gastric cancer. *Cancer Cell, 5*(2), 121–125.

Wong, B. C., Lam, S. K., Wong, W. M., et al. (2004). *Helicobacter pylori* eradication to prevent gastric cancer in a high-risk region of China: A randomized controlled study. *Journal of the American Medical Association, 291*(2), 187–194.

Yasui, W., Oue, N., Ito, R., et al. (2004). Search for new biomarkers of gastric cancer through serial analysis of gene expression and its clinical implications. *Cancer Science, 95*(5), 385–392.

Morbid Obesity

Abir, F., & Bell, R. (2004). Assessment and management of the obese patient. *Critical Care Medicine, 32*(Suppl)(4), S87–S91.

American Society for Bariatric Surgery. (2001). Rationale for the surgical treatment of morbid obesity. Available at: http://www.asbs.org/html/rationale/rationale.html. Accessed June 29, 2006.

AORN Bariatric Surgery Guideline. (2004). *AORN Journal, 79*(5), 1026–1052.

Appolinario, J. C., Bueno, J. R., & Coutinho, W. (2004). Psychotropic drugs in the treatment of obesity: What promise? *CNS Drugs,* 18(10), 629–651.

Arterburn, D. E., Crane, P. K., & Veenstra, D. L. (2004). The efficacy and safety of sibutramine for weight loss: A systematic review. *Archives of Internal Medicine, 163*(9), 994–1003.

Baltasar, A., Bou, R., Bengochea, M., et al. (2001). Duodenal switch: An effective therapy for morbid obesity: Intermediate results. *Obesity Surgery, 11*(1), 54–58.

Blackwood, H. S. (2004). Obesity: A rapidly expanding challenge. *Nursing Management, 35*(5), 27–36.

Brody, F. (2004). Minimally invasive surgery for morbid obesity. *Cleveland Clinic Journal of Medicine, 71*(4), 289–298.

Brolin, R. E. (2002). Bariatric surgery and long-term control of morbid obesity. *Journal of the American Medical Association, 288*(22), 2793–2796.

Buchwald, H., Avidor, Y., Braunwald, E., et al. (2004). Bariatric surgery: A systematic review and meta-analysis. *Journal of the American Medical Association, 292*(14), 1724–1737.

Chapman, A. E., Kiroff, G., Game, P., et al. (2004). Laparoscopic adjustable gastric banding in the treatment of obesity: A systematic literature review. *Surgery, 135*(3), 326–351.

Choban, P. S., Jackson, B., Poplawski, S., et al. (2002). Bariatric surgery for morbid obesity: Why, who, when, how, where, and what? *Cleveland Clinic Journal of Medicine, 69*(11), 897–903.

Collene, A. L., & Hertzler, S. (2003). Metabolic outcomes of gastric bypass. *Nutrition in Clinical Practice, 18*(2), 136–139.

Cottam, D. R., Mattar, S. G., & Schauer, P. R. (2003). Laparoscopic era of operations for morbid obesity. *Archives of Surgery, 13*(4), 367–375.

Damcott, C. M., Sack, P., & Shuldiner, A. R. (2003). The genetics of obesity. *Endocrinology and Metabolism Clinics of North America, 32*(4), 761–786.

Davidson, J. E., Kruse, M. W., Cox, D. H., et al. (2003). Critical care of the morbidly obese. *Critical Care Nurse Quarterly, 26*(2), 105–116.

Deitel, M., & Shikora, S. (2002). The development of the surgical treatment of morbid obesity. *Journal of the American College of Nutrition, 21*(5), 365–371.

Dressel, A., Kuhn, J. A., & McCarty, T. M. (2004). Laparoscopic Roux-en-Y gastric bypass in morbidly obese patients. *American Journal of Surgery, 187*(2), 230–232.

Elliot, K. (2003). Nutritional considerations after bariatric surgery. *Critical Care Nursing Quarterly, 26*(2), 133–138.

Favretti, F., O'Brien, P. E., & Dixon, J. B. (2002). Patient management after LAP-BAND placement. *American Journal of Surgery, 184*(6B), 38S–41S.

Ferraro, D. R. (2003). Laparoscopic adjustable gastric banding for morbid obesity. *AORN Journal, 77*(5), 923–940.

Ferraro, D. R. (2004). Preparing patients for bariatric surgery: The clinical considerations. *Clinician Reviews, 14*(1), 58–63.

Ferraro, D. R. (2004). Management of the bariatric surgery patient: Lifelong postoperative care. *Clinician Reviews, 14*(2), 74–79.

Fobi, M. A. (2004). Surgical treatment of obesity: A review. *Journal of National Medical Association, 96*(1), 61–75.

Herron, D. M. (2004). The surgical management of severe obesity. *Mount Sinai Journal of Medicine, 71*(1), 63–71.

Hurst, S., Blanco, K., Boyle, D., et al. (2004). Bariatric implications of critical care nursing. *Dimensions of Critical Care Nursing, 23*(2), 76–83.

Jacob, B. P., & Gagner, M. (2003). New developments in gastric bypass procedures and physiologic mechanisms. *Surgical Technology International, 11,* 119–126.

Jones, K. B. (2004). Bariatric surgery—where do we go from here? *International Surgery, 89*(1), 51–57.

Kim, J., Tarnoff, M., & Shikora, S. (2003). Surgical treatment for extreme obesity: evolution of a rapidly growing field. *Nutrition in Clinical Practice, 18*(2), 109–123.

Lamvu, G., Zolnoun, D., Boggess, J., et al. (2004). Obesity: Physiologic changes and challenges during laparoscopy. *American Journal of Obstetrics and Gynecology, 191*(2), 669–674.

Livingston, E. H., & Fink, A. S. (2003). Quality of life: Cost and future of bariatric surgery. *Archives of Surgery, 138*(4), 383–388.

McGohan, L. D., & Caflisch, A. J. (2004). Bariatric surgery. *Journal of Continuing Education in Nursing, 35*(5), 198–199.

Miller, K., & Hell, E. (2003). Laparoscopic surgical concepts of morbid obesity. *Archives of Surgery, 388*(6), 375–384.

Nguyen, N., Goldman, C., Rosenquist, C., et al. (2001). Laparoscopic versus open gastric bypass: A randomized study of outcomes, quality of life, and costs. *Annals of Surgery, 234*(3), 279–899.

O'Brien, P. E., Dixon, J. B., & Brown, W. (2004). Obesity is a surgical disease: Overview of obesity and bariatric surgery. *Australia and New Zealand Journal of Surgery, 74*(4), 200–204.

O'Donnell, K. (2004). Bariatric surgery: Nutritional concerns on the weigh down. *Practical Gastroenterology, 28*(2), 33–46.

Padwal, R., Li, S. K., & Lau, D. C. (2004). Long-term pharmacology for obesity and overweight. *Cochrane Database of Systematic Reviews,* 3, CD004094.

Raftopoulos, I., Ercole, J., Udekwu, A. O., et al. (2005). Outcomes of Roux-en-Y gastric bypass stratified by a body mass index of 70 kg/m^2: A comparative analysis of 825 procedures. *Journal of Gastrointestinal Surgery, 9*(1), 44–52.

Rosmond, R. (2004). Obesity and depression: Same disease, different name? *Medical Hypotheses, 62*(6), 976–979.

Rosemurgy, A. S. (2003). What's new in surgery: Gastrointestinal conditions. *Journal of the American College of Surgeons, 197*(5), 792–801.

Sammons, D. (2002). Roux-en-Y gastric bypass. *American Journal of Nursing, 102*(10), 24A–24D.

Schauer, P. R., Ilramuddin, S., Gourash, W., et al. (2000). Outcomes after laparoscopic Roux-en-Y gastric bypass for morbid obesity. *Annals of Surgery, 232*(4), 515–529.

Sjostrom, L., Lindroos, A. K., Petonen, M., et al. (2004). Lifestyle, diabetes, and cardiovascular risk factors 10 years after bariatric surgery. *New England Journal of Medicine, 351*(26), 2683–2693.

Sogg, S., & Mori, D. L. (2004). The Boston interview for gastric bypass: Determining the psychological suitability of surgical candidates. *Obesity Surgery, 14*(3), 370–380.

Ukleja, A., & Stone, R. L. (2004). Medical and gastroenterologic management of the post-bariatric surgery patient. *Journal of Clinical Gastroenterology, 38*(4), 312–321.

Woodward, B. G. (2003). Bariatric surgery options. *Critical Care Nurse Quarterly, 26*(2), 89–100.

Peptic Ulcers and Gastritis

Aihara, T., Nakamura, E., & Amagase, K. (2003). Pharmacological control of gastric acid secretion for the treatment of acid-related peptic disease: Past, present, and future. *Pharmacology & Therapeutics, 98*(1), 109–127.

Allen, M. E., Kopp, B. J., & Erstad, B. L. (2004). Stress ulcer prophylaxis in the postoperative period. *American Journal of Health System-Pharmacy, 61*(6), 588–596.

Basset, C., Holton, J., Gatta, L., et al. (2004). *Helicobacter pylori* infection: Anything new we should know? *Alimentary Pharmacology & Therapeutics, 20*(Suppl 2), 31–41.

Dore, M. P., & Graham, D. Y. (2004). Ulcers and gastritis. *Endoscopy, 36*(1), 42–47.

Der, G. (2003). An overview of proton pump inhibitors. *Gastroenterology Nursing, 26*(5), 1182–1190.

Ford, A., Delaney, B., Forman, D., et al. (2003). Eradication therapy for peptic ulcer disease in *Helicobacter pylori*-positive patients. *Cochrane Database System Review,* 4:CD003840.

Garnett, W. R. (2003). History of acid suppression: Focus on the hospital setting. *Pharmacotherapy, 23*(10), 56S–60S.

Gene, E., Calvet X., Azagra, R., et al. (2003). Triple vs. quadruple therapy for treating *Helicobacter pylori* infection: A meta-analysis. *Alimentary Pharmacology & Therapeutics, 17*(9), 1137–1143.

Goto, H. (2003). *Helicobacter pylori* and gastric diseases. *Nagoya Journal of Medical Science, 66*(3-4), 77–85.

Greenwald, D. A. (2004). Aging, the gastrointestinal tract, and risk of acid-related disease. *American Journal of Medicine, 117*(Suppl 5A), 8S–13S.

Hawkey, C. J., & Langman, M. J. S. (2002). Non-steroidal anti-inflammatory drugs: Overall risks and management. Complementary roles for COX-2 inhibitors and proton pump inhibitors. *Gut, 52*(4), 600–608.

Hellstrom, P. M., & Vitols, S. (2004). The choice of proton pump inhibitor: Does it matter? *Basic & Clinical Pharmacology & Toxicology, 94*(3), 106–111.

Hirschowitz, B. I. (2003). Usual and unusual causes of duodenal ulcer. *Digestive and Liver Disease, 35*(8), 519–522.

Holtmann, G., & Howden, C. W. (2004). Management of peptic ulcer bleeding: The roles of proton pump inhibitors and *Helicobacter pylori* eradication. *Alimentary Pharmacology & Therapeutics, 19*(Suppl 1), 66–70.

Horton, K. M., & Fishman, E. K. (2003). Current role of CT in imaging of the stomach. *Radiographics, 23*(1), 75–87.

Konturek, S. J., Bielanski, W., Plenka, M., et al. (2003). *Helicobacter pylori* nonsteroidal anti-inflammatory drugs and smoking in risk pattern of gastroduodenal ulcers. *Scandanavian Journal of Gastroenterology, 38*(9), 923–930.

Laine, L. (2003). Gastrointestinal effects of NSAIDs and coxibs. *Journal of Pain and Symptom Management, 25*(2), 32–40.

Laine, L. (2003). The role of proton pump inhibitors in NSAID-associated gastropathy and upper gastrointestinal symptoms. *Reviews in Gastroenterological Disorders, 3*(Suppl 4), S30.

Lehman, F., Hildebrand, P., & Beglinger, C. (2003). New molecular targets for treatment of peptic ulcer disease. *Drugs, 63*(17), 1785–1797.

Meurer, L. N., & Bower, D. J. (2002). Management of *Helicobacter pylori* infection. *American Family Physician, 65*(7), 1327–1336.

Moss, S. F., & Sood, S. (2003). *Helicobacter pylori. Current Opinions in Infectious Disease, 16,* 445–451.

Mukherjee, D., Nissen, S. E., & Topol, E. J. (2001). Risk of cardiovascular events associated with selective COX-2 inhibitors. *Journal of the American Medical Association, 286*(8), 954–959.

Robinson, M., & Horn, J. (2004). Clinical pharmacology of proton pump inhibitors: What the practicing physician needs to know. *Drugs, 63*(24), 2739–2754.

Scheiman, J. M. (2003). Gastroduodenal safety of cyclooxygenase-2 inhibitors. *Current Pharmaceutical Design,* (27), 2197–2206.

Sharma, P., & Vakil, N. (2003). *Helicobacter pylori* and reflux disease. *Alimentary Pharmacology & Therapeutics, 17*(3), 297–305.

Spirt, M. J. (2004). Stress-related mucosal disease: Risk factors and prophylactic therapy. *Clinical Therapeutics, 26*(2), 197–213.

Suerbaum, S., & Michetti, P. (2002). *Helicobacter pylori. New England Journal of Medicine, 347,* 1175–1186.

Sung, J. J. (2003). The role of acid suppression in the management and prevention of gastrointestinal hemorrhage associated with gastroduodenal ulcers. *Gastroenterology Clinics of North America, 32*(3 Suppl), S11–S23.

Sutton, P., & Doidge, C. (2003). *Helicobacter pylori* vaccines spiral into the new millennium. *Digestive and Liver Disease, 35*(10), 675–687.

Thomopoulos, K. C., Vagenas, K. A., & Vagianos, E. C. (2004). Changes in etiology and clinical outcome of acute upper gastrointestinal bleeding during the last 15 years. *European Journal of Gastroenterology and Hepatology, 16*(2), 177–182.

Tytgat, G. (2000). *Helicobacter pylori:* Past, present and future. *Journal of Gastroenterology and Hepatology, 15*(Suppl.), G30–G33.

Van Rensburg, O. (2004). *Helicobacter pylori* in peptic ulcer disease. *Journal of the South African Dental Association, 59*(8), 334–335.

Wolfe, M. M. (2003). Risk factors associated with the development of gastroduodenal ulcers due to the use of NSAIDs. *International Journal of Clinical Practice Supplement,* (135), 32–37.

Wu, W. K. K., & Cho, C. H. (2004). The pharmacological actions of nicotine on the gastrointestinal tract. *Journal of Pharmacological Sciences, 94*(4), 348–358.

Duodenal Tumors

Kummar, S., Ciesielski, T. E., & Fogarasi, M. (2002). Management of small bowel adenocarcinoma. *Oncology, 16*(10), 1364–1370.

Wei, C., Chiang, J., Lin, W., et al. (2003). Tumor and tumor-like lesions of the duodenum: CT and barium imaging features. *Journal of Clinical Imaging, 27*(2), 89–96.

RESOURCES

American Cancer Society, 1599 Clifton Rd., N.E., Atlanta, GA 30329; 1-800-ACS-2345; http://www.cancer.org. Accessed June 29, 2006.

American Gastroenterological Association, 4930 Del Ray Avenue, Bethesda, MD 20814; 301-654-2005l; http://www.gastro.org. Accessed June 29, 2006.

Cancer Source, 263 Summer St., Boston, MA 02210-1506; http://www.cancerSource.com. Accessed June 29, 2006.

Agency for Healthcare Research and Quality, 540 Gaither Road, Rockville, MD 20850; 301-427-1364; http://www.ahrq.gov. Accessed June 29, 2006.

American Society for Bariatric Surgery, 100 SW 75th Street, Suite 201, Gainesville, FL 32607; 352-331-4900; http://www.asbs.org. Accessed June 29, 2006.

Centers for Disease Control and Prevention, 1600 Clifton Rd., Atlanta, GA 30333; 404-639-3311; http://www.cdc.gov/nchs/products/pubs/pubd/hestats/obese/obese99.htm. Accessed June 29, 2006.

National Comprehensive Cancer Network (NCCN) Clinical Practice Guidelines, 5000 Old York Road, Suite 250, Jenkintown, PA 19046; 215-690-0300; http://www.nccn.org. Accessed June 29, 2006.

National Digestive Diseases Information Clearinghouse (NDDIC), 2 Information Way, Bethesda, MD 20892; 1-800-891-5389; http://digestive.niddk.nih.gov/ (NDDIC is a service of the National Institute of Diabetes and Digestive and Kidney Diseases [NIDDK]). Accessed June 29, 2006.

Obesity Law and Advocacy Center, 1392 East Palomar Street, Suite 403-233, Chula Vista, CA 91913; 619-656-5251; http://www.obesitylaw.com. Accessed June 29, 2006.

Society of American Gastrointestinal Endoscopic Surgeons (SAGES), 11300 West Olympic Boulevard, Suite 600, Los Angeles, CA 90064; 310-437-0544; http://www.sages.org/sg pub30.html. Accessed June 29, 2006.

Weight loss surgery information: http://weightlossurgeryinfo.com. Accessed June 29, 2006.

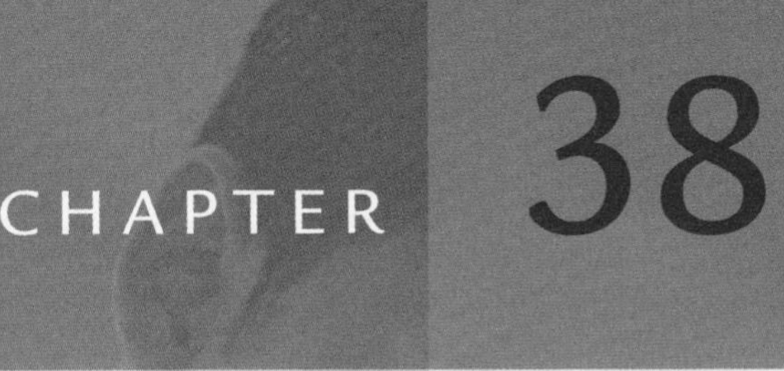
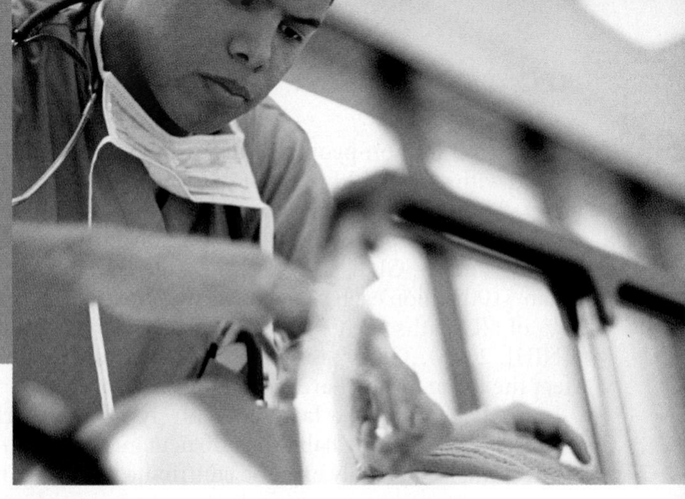

CHAPTER 38

Management of Patients With Intestinal and Rectal Disorders

Learning Objectives

On completion of this chapter, the learner will be able to:

1. Identify the health care learning needs of patients with constipation or diarrhea.
2. Compare the conditions of malabsorption with regard to their pathophysiology, clinical manifestations, and management.
3. Use the nursing process as a framework for care of patients with diverticulitis.
4. Compare regional enteritis and ulcerative colitis with regard to their pathophysiology; clinical manifestations; diagnostic evaluation; and medical, surgical, and nursing management.
5. Use the nursing process as a framework for care of the patient with inflammatory bowel disease.
6. Describe the responsibilities of the nurse in meeting the needs of the patient with an ileostomy.
7. Describe the various types of intestinal obstructions and their management.
8. Use the nursing process as a framework for care of the patient with cancer of the colon or rectum.
9. Use the nursing process as a framework for care of the patient with an anorectal condition.

At least 60 million people in the United States are diagnosed with some type of disease of the gastrointestinal (GI) tract. These diseases account for more than 45 million office visits and approximately 14 million hospital admissions annually. GI diseases cost the American public more than $100 billion each year and account for approximately 9% of all deaths each year (National Institutes of Health [NIH], 2005). The types of diseases and disorders that affect the lower GI tract are many and varied.

In all age groups, a fast-paced lifestyle, high levels of stress, irregular eating habits, insufficient intake of fiber and water, and lack of daily exercise contribute to GI disorders. There is a growing understanding of the biopsychosocial implications of GI disease. Nurses can have an impact on these GI disorders by identifying behavior patterns that put patients at risk, by educating the public about prevention and management, and by helping those affected to improve their condition and prevent complications.

Abnormalities of Fecal Elimination

Changes in patterns of fecal elimination are symptoms of functional disorders or diseases of the GI tract. The most common changes seen are constipation, diarrhea, and fecal incontinence. The nurse should be aware of the causes and therapeutic management of these disorders and of nursing management techniques. Education is important for patients with these conditions.

Constipation

Constipation is an abnormal infrequency or irregularity of defecation, abnormal hardening of stools that makes their passage difficult and sometimes painful, a decrease in stool volume, or retention of stool in the rectum for a prolonged period. Any variation from normal habits may be considered a problem. It is estimated that 4.5 million Americans are clinically constipated at any time and that women and adults older than 65 years are disproportionately constipated (Stessman, 2003).

Constipation can be caused by certain medications (ie, tranquilizers, anticholinergics, antidepressants, antihypertensives, bile acid sequestrants, opioids, aluminum-based antacids, iron preparations); rectal or anal disorders (eg, hemorrhoids, fissures); obstruction (eg, bowel tumors); metabolic, neurologic, and neuromuscular conditions (eg, diabetes mellitus, Hirschsprung's disease, Parkinson's disease, multiple sclerosis); endocrine disorders (eg, hypothyroidism, pheochromocytoma); lead poisoning; and connective tissue disorders (eg, scleroderma, systemic lupus erythematosus). Constipation is a major problem for patients

Glossary

abscess: localized collection of purulent material surrounded by inflamed tissues, typically associated with signs of infection

borborygmus: rumbling noise caused by the movement of gas through the intestines

colostomy: surgical opening into the colon by means of a stoma to allow drainage of bowel contents; one type of fecal diversion

constipation: subjectively described infrequency or irregularity of defecation, with or without an abnormal hardening of feces that makes their passage difficult and sometimes painful, with or without a decrease in fecal volume

diverticulitis: inflammation of a diverticulum from obstruction (by fecal matter), resulting in abscess formation

diverticulosis: presence of several diverticula in the intestine; common in middle age

diverticulum: saclike outpouching of the lining of the bowel protruding through the muscle of the intestinal wall, usually caused by high intraluminal pressure

enterostomal therapist: nurse specially educated in the appropriate use of fecal and urinary diversions; guides patients, their families, surgeons, and nurses by recommending appropriate use of skin, wound, ostomy, and continence products; often referred to as a wound-ostomy-continence nurse (WOCN)

fecal incontinence: involuntary passage of feces

fissure: normal or abnormal fold, groove, or crack in body tissue

fistula: anatomically abnormal tract that arises between two internal organs or between an internal organ and the body surface

hemorrhoids: dilated portions of the anal veins; can occur internal or external to the anal sphincter

ileostomy: surgical opening into the ileum by means of a stoma to allow drainage of bowel contents; one type of fecal diversion

inflammatory bowel disease (IBD): group of chronic disorders (most common are ulcerative colitis and regional enteritis [Crohn's disease]) that result in inflammation or ulceration (or both) of the bowel lining; associated with abdominal pain, diarrhea, fever, and weight loss

irritable bowel syndrome (IBS): functional disorder that affects frequency of defecation and consistency of stool; associated with crampy abdominal pain and bloating

Kock pouch: type of continent ileal reservoir created surgically by making an internal pouch with a portion of the ileum and placing a nipple valve flush with the stoma

malabsorption: impaired transport across the mucosa

peritonitis: inflammation of the lining of the abdominal cavity, usually as a result of a bacterial infection of an area in the gastrointestinal tract with leakage of contents into the abdominal cavity

steatorrhea: excess of fatty wastes in the feces or the urine

tenesmus: ineffective and sometimes painful straining to eliminate either feces or urine

Valsalva maneuver: forcible exhalation against a closed glottis followed by a rise in intrathoracic pressure and subsequent possible dramatic rise in arterial pressure; may occur during straining at stool

taking opioids for pain. Diseases of the colon commonly associated with constipation include irritable bowel syndrome and diverticular disease. Constipation can also occur with an acute disease process in the abdomen (eg, appendicitis).

Other causes of constipation may include weakness, immobility, debility, fatigue, and an inability to increase intra-abdominal pressure to facilitate the passage of stools, as may occur in patients with emphysema, for instance. Many people develop constipation because they do not take the time to defecate or they ignore the urge to defecate. Constipation is also a result of dietary habits (ie, low consumption of fiber and inadequate fluid intake), lack of regular exercise, and a stress-filled life.

Perceived constipation can also be a problem. This subjective problem occurs when a person's bowel elimination pattern is not consistent with what he or she perceives as normal. Chronic laxative use may contribute to this problem and is a major health concern in the United States.

Pathophysiology

The pathophysiology of constipation is poorly understood, but it is thought to include interference with one of three major functions of the colon: mucosal transport (ie, mucosal secretions facilitate the movement of colon contents), myoelectric activity (ie, mixing of the rectal mass and propulsive actions), or the processes of defecation. Any of the causative factors previously identified can interfere with any of these three processes.

The urge to defecate is stimulated normally by rectal distention, which initiates a series of four actions: stimulation of the inhibitory rectoanal reflex, relaxation of the internal sphincter muscle, relaxation of the external sphincter muscle and muscles in the pelvic region, and increased intra-abdominal pressure. Interference with any of these processes can lead to constipation.

If all organic causes are eliminated, idiopathic constipation is diagnosed. When the urge to defecate is ignored, the rectal mucous membrane and musculature become insensitive to the presence of fecal masses, and consequently a stronger stimulus is required to produce the necessary peristaltic rush for defecation. The initial effect of fecal retention is to produce irritability of the colon, which at this stage frequently goes into spasm, especially after meals, giving rise to colicky midabdominal or low abdominal pains. After several years of this process, the colon loses muscular tone and becomes essentially unresponsive to normal stimuli. Atony or decreased muscle tone occurs with aging. This also leads to constipation because the stool is retained for longer periods.

Clinical Manifestations

Clinical manifestations of constipation include fewer than three bowel movements per week; abdominal distention; pain and pressure; decreased appetite; headache; fatigue; indigestion; a sensation of incomplete evacuation; straining at stool; and the elimination of small-volume, lumpy, hard, dry stools.

Assessment and Diagnostic Findings

Chronic constipation is usually considered idiopathic, but secondary causes should be excluded. In patients with severe, intractable constipation, further diagnostic testing is needed (Stessman, 2003). The diagnosis of constipation is based on the patient's history, physical examination, possibly the results of a barium enema or sigmoidoscopy, and stool testing for occult blood. These tests are used to determine whether this symptom results from spasm or narrowing of the bowel. Anorectal manometry (ie, pressure studies) may be performed to determine malfunction of the sphincter. Defecography and colonic transit studies can also assist in the diagnosis (see Chapter 34).

Complications

Complications of constipation include hypertension, fecal impaction, **hemorrhoids** (dilated portions of anal veins), **fissures** (tissue folds), and megacolon. Increased arterial pressure can occur with defecation. Straining at stool, which results in the **Valsalva maneuver** (ie, forcibly exhaling with the glottis closed), has a striking effect on arterial blood pressure. During active straining, the flow of venous blood in the chest is temporarily impeded because of increased intrathoracic pressure. This pressure tends to collapse the large veins in the chest. The atria and the ventricles receive less blood, and consequently less blood is ejected by the left ventricle. Cardiac output is decreased, and there is a transient drop in arterial pressure. Almost immediately after this period of hypotension, an increase in arterial pressure occurs; the pressure is elevated momentarily to a point far exceeding the original level (ie, rebound phenomenon). In patients with hypertension, this compensatory reaction may be exaggerated greatly, and the peak pressure attained may be dangerously high—sufficient to rupture a major artery in the brain or elsewhere.

Fecal impaction occurs when an accumulated mass of dry feces cannot be expelled. The mass may be palpable on digital examination, may produce pressure on the colonic mucosa that results in ulcer formation, and frequently causes seepage of liquid stools.

Hemorrhoids and anal fissures can develop as a result of constipation. Hemorrhoids develop as a result of perianal vascular congestion caused by straining. Anal fissures may result from the passage of the hard stool through the anus, tearing the lining of the anal canal.

Megacolon is a dilated and atonic colon caused by a fecal mass that obstructs the passage of colon contents. Symptoms include constipation, liquid fecal incontinence, and abdominal distention. Megacolon can lead to perforation of the bowel.

Gerontologic Considerations

Physician visits for constipation are more common in people 65 years and older (Stessman, 2003). The most common complaint they voice is the need to strain at stool. People who have loose-fitting dentures or have lost their teeth have difficulty chewing and frequently choose soft, processed foods that are low in fiber. Older adults tend to have decreased food intake, reduced mobility, and weak abdominal and pelvic muscles, and they are more likely to have multiple chronic illnesses requiring medications (eg, calcium channel blockers, bile acid sequestrants, opioids) that often cause constipation. Low-fiber convenience foods are widely used by people who have lost interest in eating. Some older people reduce their fluid intake if they are not eating regular meals. Depression, weakness, or prolonged bed rest also contribute to constipation by decreasing intestinal motility and anal sphincter tone. Nerve impulses are dulled, and there is a decreased urge to defecate. Many older people overuse laxatives in an attempt to have a daily bowel movement and become dependent on them.

Medical Management

Treatment is aimed at the underlying cause of constipation and includes education, bowel habit training, increased fiber and fluid intake, and judicious use of laxatives. Management may also include discontinuing laxative abuse. Routine exercise to strengthen abdominal muscles is encouraged. Biofeedback is a technique that can be used to help patients learn to relax the sphincter mechanism to expel stool (Stessman, 2003). Daily dietary intake of 6 to 12 teaspoonfuls of unprocessed bran is recommended, especially for the treatment of constipation in the elderly. If laxative use is necessary, one of the following may be prescribed: bulk-forming agents, saline and osmotic agents, lubricants, stimulants, or fecal softeners. The physiologic action and patient education information related to these laxatives are given in Table 38-1. Enemas and rectal suppositories are generally not recommended for treating constipation; they should be reserved for the treatment of impaction. If long-term laxative use is necessary, a bulk-forming agent may be prescribed in combination with an osmotic laxative.

Specific medications may be prescribed to enhance colonic transit by increasing propulsive motor activity. These may include cholinergic agents (eg, bethanechol [Urecholine]), cholinesterase inhibitors (eg, neostigmine [Prostigmin]), or prokinetic agents (eg, metoclopramide [Reglan]).

Nursing Management

The nurse elicits information about the onset and duration of constipation, current and past elimination patterns, the

℞ TABLE 38-1 Laxatives: Classification, Agent, Action, and Patient Education

Classification	Sample Agent	Action	Patient Education
Bulk forming	Psyllium hydrophilic mucilloid (Metamucil)	Polysaccharides and cellulose derivatives mix with intestinal fluids, swell, and stimulate peristalsis.	Take with 8 oz water and follow with 8 oz water; do not take dry. Report abdominal distention or unusual amount of flatulence.
Saline agent	Magnesium hydroxide (Milk of Magnesia)	Nonabsorbable magnesium ions alter stool consistency by drawing water into the intestines by osmosis; peristalsis is stimulated. Action occurs within 2 h.	The liquid preparation is more effective than the tablet form. Only short-term use is recommended because of toxicity (CNS or neuromuscular depression, electrolyte imbalance). Magnesium laxatives should not be taken by patients with renal insufficiency.
Lubricant	Mineral oil	Nonabsorbable hydrocarbons soften fecal matter by lubricating the intestinal mucosa; the passage of stool is facilitated. Action occurs within 6–8 h.	Do not take with meals, because mineral oils can impair the absorption of fat-soluble vitamins and delay gastric emptying. Swallow carefully, because drops of oil that gain access to the pharynx can produce a lipid pneumonia.
Stimulant	Bisacodyl (Dulcolax)	Irritates the colon epithelium by stimulating sensory nerve endings and increasing mucosal secretions. Action occurs within 6–8 h.	Catharsis may cause fluid and electrolyte imbalance, especially in the elderly. Tablets should be swallowed, not crushed or chewed. Avoid milk or antacids within 1 hour of taking the medication, because the enteric coating may dissolve prematurely.
Fecal softener	Dioctyl sodium sulfosuccinate (Colace)	Hydrates the stool by its surfactant action on the colonic epithelium (increases the wetting efficiency of intestinal water); aqueous and fatty substances are mixed. Does not exert a laxative action.	Can be used safely by patients who should avoid straining (cardiac patients, patients with anorectal disorders)
Osmotic agent	Polyethylene glycol and electrolytes (Colyte)	Cleanses colon rapidly and induces diarrhea	This is a large-volume product. It takes time to consume it safely. It can cause considerable nausea and bloating.

patient's expectation of normal bowel elimination, and lifestyle information (eg, exercise and activity level, occupation, food and fluid intake, and stress level) during the health history interview. Past medical and surgical history, current medications, and laxative and enema use are important, as is information about the sensation of rectal pressure or fullness, abdominal pain, excessive straining at defecation, and flatulence.

Patient education and health promotion are important functions of the nurse (Chart 38-1). After the health history is obtained, the nurse sets specific goals for teaching. Goals for the patient include restoring or maintaining a regular pattern of elimination by responding to the urge to defecate, ensuring adequate intake of fluids and high-fiber foods, learning about methods to avoid constipation, relieving anxiety about bowel elimination patterns, and avoiding complications.

Diarrhea

Diarrhea is an increased frequency of bowel movements (more than three per day), an increased amount of stool (more than 200 g per day), and altered consistency (ie, looseness) of stool. It is usually associated with urgency, perianal discomfort, incontinence, or a combination of these factors. Any condition that causes increased intestinal secretions, decreased mucosal absorption, or altered motility can produce diarrhea. Irritable bowel syndrome, inflammatory bowel disease, and lactose intolerance are frequently the underlying disease processes that cause diarrhea.

Diarrhea can be acute or chronic. Acute diarrhea is most often associated with infection and is usually self-limiting; chronic diarrhea persists for a longer period and may return sporadically. Diarrhea can be caused by certain medications (eg, thyroid hormone replacement, stool softeners and laxatives, antibiotics, chemotherapy, magnesium-based antacids), certain tube-feeding formulas, metabolic and endocrine disorders (eg, diabetes, Addison's disease, thyrotoxicosis), and viral or bacterial infectious processes (eg, dysentery, shigellosis, food poisoning). Other disease processes associated with diarrhea include nutritional and malabsorptive disorders (eg, celiac disease), anal sphincter defect, Zollinger-Ellison syndrome, paralytic ileus, intestinal obstruction, and acquired immunodeficiency syndrome (AIDS).

CHART 38-1

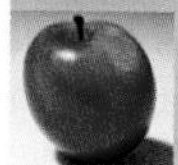

Health Promotion

Preventing Constipation

- Describe the physiology of defecation.
- Emphasize the importance of responding to the urge to defecate.
- Discuss normal variations in patterns of defecation.
- Teach how to establish a bowel routine, and explain that having a regular time for defecation (eg, best time is after breakfast) may aid in initiating the reflex.
- Provide dietary information; suggest eating high-residue, high-fiber foods, adding bran daily (must be introduced gradually), and increasing fluid intake (unless contraindicated).
- Explain how an exercise regimen, increased ambulation, and abdominal muscle toning will increase muscle strength and help propel colon contents.
- Describe abdominal toning exercises (contracting abdominal muscles 4 times daily and leg-to-chest lifts 10 to 20 times each day).
- Explain that the normal position (semisquatting) maximizes use of abdominal muscles and force of gravity.

Pathophysiology

Types of diarrhea include secretory, osmotic, and mixed diarrhea. Secretory diarrhea is usually high-volume diarrhea and is caused by increased production and secretion of water and electrolytes by the intestinal mucosa into the intestinal lumen. Osmotic diarrhea occurs when water is pulled into the intestines by the osmotic pressure of unabsorbed particles, slowing the reabsorption of water. Mixed diarrhea is caused by increased peristalsis (usually from inflammatory bowel disease) and a combination of increased secretion and decreased absorption in the bowel. The pathophysiology of diarrhea related to infection is discussed in Chapter 70.

Clinical Manifestations

In addition to the increased frequency and fluid content of stools, the patient usually has abdominal cramps, distention, intestinal rumbling (ie, **borborygmus**), anorexia, and thirst. Painful spasmodic contractions of the anus and ineffective straining (ie, **tenesmus**) may occur with defecation. Other symptoms depend on the cause and severity of the diarrhea but are related to dehydration and to fluid and electrolyte imbalances.

Watery stools are characteristic of disorders of the small bowel, whereas loose, semisolid stools are associated more often with disorders of the large bowel. Voluminous, greasy stools suggest intestinal malabsorption, and the presence of mucus and pus in the stools suggests inflammatory enteritis or colitis. Oil droplets on the toilet water are almost always diagnostic of pancreatic insufficiency. Nocturnal diarrhea may be a manifestation of diabetic neuropathy.

Assessment and Diagnostic Findings

When the cause of the diarrhea is not obvious, the following diagnostic tests may be performed: complete blood cell count; serum chemistries; urinalysis; routine stool examination; and stool examinations for infectious or parasitic organisms, bacterial toxins, blood, fat, and electrolytes. Endoscopy or barium enema may assist in identifying the cause.

Complications

Complications of diarrhea include the potential for cardiac dysrhythmias because of significant fluid and electrolyte loss (especially loss of potassium). Urinary output of less than 30 mL per hour for 2 to 3 consecutive hours, muscle weakness, paresthesia, hypotension, anorexia, and drowsiness with a potassium level of less than 3.5 mEq/L (3.5 mmol/L) must be reported.

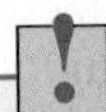

NURSING ALERT

Decreased potassium levels cause cardiac dysrhythmias (ie, atrial and ventricular tachycardia, ventricular fibrillation, premature ventricular contractions) that can lead to death.

Gerontologic Considerations

Elderly patients can become dehydrated quickly and develop low potassium levels (ie, hypokalemia) as a result of diarrhea. The nurse observes for clinical manifestations of muscle weakness, dysrhythmias, or decreased peristaltic motility that may lead to paralytic ileus. The older patient taking digitalis (eg, digoxin [Lanoxin]) must be aware of how quickly dehydration and hypokalemia can occur with diarrhea. The nurse teaches the patient to recognize the symptoms of hypokalemia because low levels of potassium intensify the action of digitalis, leading to digitalis toxicity.

Medical Management

Primary management is directed at controlling symptoms, preventing complications, and eliminating or treating the underlying disease. Certain medications (eg, antibiotics, anti-inflammatory agents) may be used to reduce the severity of the diarrhea and treat the underlying disease.

Nursing Management

The nurse's role includes assessing and monitoring the characteristics and pattern of diarrhea. A health history should address the patient's medication therapy, medical and surgical history, and dietary patterns and intake. Reports of recent exposure to an acute illness or recent travel to another geographic area are important. Assessment includes abdominal auscultation and palpation for abdominal tenderness. Inspection of the abdomen, mucous membranes, and skin is important to determine hydration status. Stool samples are obtained for testing.

During an episode of acute diarrhea, the nurse encourages bed rest and intake of liquids and foods low in bulk until the acute attack subsides. When the patient is able to tolerate food intake, the nurse recommends a bland diet of semisolid and solid foods. The patient should avoid caffeine, carbonated beverages, and very hot and very cold foods, because they stimulate intestinal motility. It may be necessary to restrict milk products, fat, whole-grain products, fresh fruits, and vegetables for several days. The nurse administers antidiarrheal medications such as diphenoxylate (Lomotil) or loperamide (Imodium) as prescribed. Intravenous (IV) fluid therapy may be necessary for rapid rehydration in some patients, especially in elderly patients and in patients with preexisting GI conditions (eg, inflammatory bowel disease). It is important to monitor serum electrolyte levels closely. The nurse immediately reports evidence of dysrhythmias or a change in a patient's level of consciousness.

The perianal area may become excoriated because diarrheal stool contains digestive enzymes that can irritate the skin. The patient should follow a perianal skin care routine to decrease irritation and excoriation (see Chapter 56). The skin of an older person is very sensitive because of decreased turgor and reduced subcutaneous fat layers.

Fecal Incontinence

Fecal incontinence describes the involuntary passage of stool from the rectum. Factors that influence fecal continence include the ability of the rectum to sense and accommodate stool, the amount and consistency of stool, the integrity of the anal sphincters and musculature, and rectal motility.

Pathophysiology

Fecal incontinence can result from trauma (eg, after surgical procedures involving the rectum), neurologic disorders (eg, stroke, multiple sclerosis, diabetic neuropathy, dementia), inflammation, infection, chemotherapy, radiation treatment, fecal impaction, pelvic floor relaxation, laxative abuse, medications, or advancing age (ie, weakness or loss of anal or rectal muscle tone). It is an embarrassing and socially incapacitating problem that requires a many-tiered approach to treatment and much adaptation on the patient's part.

Clinical Manifestations

Patients may have minor soiling, occasional urgency and loss of control, or complete incontinence. Patients may also experience poor control of flatus, diarrhea, or constipation.

Assessment and Diagnostic Findings

Diagnostic studies are necessary because the treatment of fecal incontinence depends on the cause. A rectal examination and other endoscopic examinations such as a flexible sigmoidoscopy are performed to rule out tumors, inflammation, or fissures. X-ray studies such as barium enema, computed tomography (CT), anorectal manometry, and transit studies may be helpful in identifying alterations in intestinal mucosa and muscle tone or in detecting other structural or functional problems.

Medical Management

Although there is no known cause or cure for fecal incontinence, specific management techniques can help the patient achieve a better quality of life. If fecal incontinence is related to diarrhea, the incontinence may disappear when diarrhea is successfully treated. Fecal incontinence is frequently a symptom of a fecal impaction. After the impaction is removed and the rectum is cleansed, normal functioning of the anorectal area can resume. If the fecal incontinence is related to a more permanent condition, other treatments are initiated. Biofeedback therapy can be of assistance if the problem is decreased sensory awareness or sphincter control. Bowel training programs can also be effective. Surgical procedures include surgical reconstruction, sphincter repair, or fecal diversion.

Nursing Management

The nurse obtains a thorough health history, including information about previous surgical procedures, chronic illnesses, dietary patterns, bowel habits and problems, and current medication regimen. The nurse also completes an examination of the rectal area.

The nurse initiates a bowel-training program that involves setting a schedule to establish bowel regularity. The goal is to help the patient achieve fecal continence. If this is not possible, the goal should be to manage the problem so the person can have predictable, planned elimination. Sometimes, it is necessary to use suppositories to stimulate the anal reflex. After the patient has achieved a regular schedule, the suppository can be discontinued. Biofeedback can be used in conjunction with these therapies to help the patient improve sphincter contractility and rectal sensitivity.

Fecal incontinence can also cause problems with perineal skin integrity. Maintaining skin integrity is a priority, especially in the debilitated or elderly patient. Incontinence briefs, although helpful in containing the fecal material, allow for increased skin contact with the feces and may cause excoriation of the skin. The nurse encourages and teaches meticulous skin hygiene.

Continence sometimes cannot be achieved, and the nurse assists the patient and family to accept and cope with this chronic situation. The patient can use fecal incontinence devices, which include external collection devices and internal drainage systems. External devices are special pouches that are drainable. They are attached to a synthetic adhesive skin barrier specially designed to conform to the buttocks. Internal drainage systems can be used to eliminate fecal skin contact and are especially useful when there is extensive excoriation or skin breakdown. A large catheter is inserted into the rectum and is connected to a drainage system.

Irritable Bowel Syndrome

Irritable bowel syndrome (IBS) is one of the most common GI conditions. Approximately 12% of adults in the United States report classic symptoms of IBS (Mertz, 2003). It occurs more commonly in women than in men, and the cause remains unknown (Motzer, Hertig, Jarrett, et al., 2003). Although no anatomic or biochemical abnormalities have been found that account for the common symptoms, various factors are associated with the syndrome: heredity, psychological stress or conditions such as depression and anxiety, a diet high in fat and stimulating or irritating foods, alcohol consumption, and smoking. The diagnosis is made only after tests confirm the absence of structural or other disorders.

Pathophysiology

IBS results from a functional disorder of intestinal motility. The change in motility may be related to neuroendocrine dysregulation, infection or irritation, or a vascular or metabolic disturbance. The peristaltic waves are affected at specific segments of the intestine and in the intensity with which they propel the fecal matter forward. There is no evidence of inflammation or tissue changes in the intestinal mucosa.

Clinical Manifestations

There is a wide variability in symptom presentation. Symptoms range in intensity and duration from mild and infrequent to severe and continuous. The primary symptom is an alteration in bowel patterns—constipation, diarrhea, or a combination of both. Pain, bloating, and abdominal distention often accompany changes in bowel pattern. The abdominal pain is sometimes precipitated by eating and is frequently relieved by defecation.

Assessment and Diagnostic Findings

A definite diagnosis of IBS requires tests that confirm the absence of structural or other disorders. Stool studies, contrast x-ray studies, and proctoscopy may be performed to rule out other colon diseases. Barium enema and colonoscopy may reveal spasm, distention, or mucus accumulation in the intestine (Fig. 38-1). Manometry and electromyography

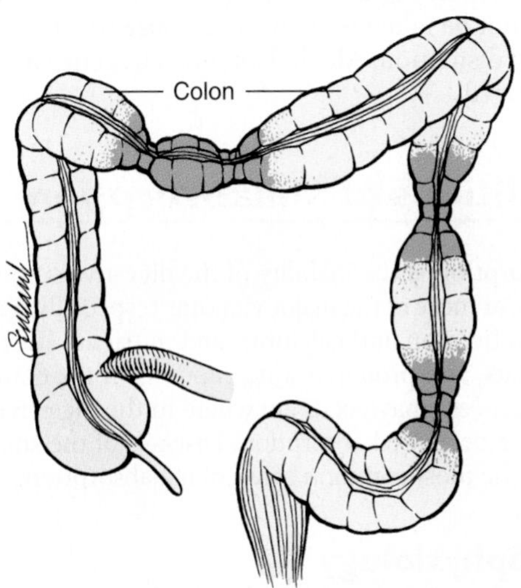

FIGURE 38-1. In irritable bowel syndrome (IBS), the spastic contractions of the bowel can be seen on x-ray contrast studies.

(EMG) are used to study intraluminal pressure changes generated by spasticity.

Medical Management

The goals of treatment are relieving abdominal pain, controlling the diarrhea or constipation, and reducing stress. Restriction and then gradual reintroduction of foods that are possibly irritating may help determine what types of food are acting as irritants (eg, beans, caffeinated products, fried foods, alcohol, spicy foods). A high-fiber diet is prescribed to help control the diarrhea and constipation. Exercise can assist in reducing anxiety and increasing intestinal motility. Patients often find it helpful to participate in a stress reduction or behavior modification program. Hydrophilic colloids (ie, bulk) and antidiarrheal agents (eg, loperamide [Imodium]) may be given to control the diarrhea and fecal urgency. Antidepressants can assist in treating underlying anxiety and depression. Anticholinergics (eg, propantheline [Pro-Banthine]) may be taken to decrease smooth muscle spasm, decreasing cramping and constipation.

Tegaserod (Zelnorm) may be prescribed to treat women with IBS whose chief complaint is chronic constipation. Tegaserod increases the effects of serotonin in the intestines, thereby increasing intestinal motility. The most commonly reported side effect of this medication is diarrhea, which typically subsides after the first week of treatment. Research has shown that some women with IBS who take tegaserod develop diarrhea with hypovolemia and hypotension (Aschenbrenner, 2004). Thus, women who take tegaserod must be taught to discontinue the drug and contact their primary health care provider if they develop severe diarrhea, particularly if it is accompanied by dizziness or orthostasis.

Nursing Management

The nurse's role is to provide patient and family education. The nurse emphasizes teaching and reinforces good dietary habits. Patients are encouraged to eat at regular times and to chew food slowly and thoroughly. They should understand that although adequate fluid intake is necessary, fluid should not be taken with meals because this results in abdominal distention. Alcohol use and cigarette smoking are discouraged.

Conditions of Malabsorption

Malabsorption is the inability of the digestive system to absorb one or more of the major vitamins (especially A and B_{12}), minerals (ie, iron and calcium), and nutrients (ie, carbohydrates, fats, and proteins). Interruptions in the complex digestive process may occur anywhere in the digestive system and cause decreased absorption. Diseases of the small intestine are the most common cause of malabsorption.

Pathophysiology

The conditions that cause malabsorption can be grouped into the following categories:

- Mucosal (transport) disorders causing generalized malabsorption (eg, celiac sprue, regional enteritis, radiation enteritis)
- Infectious diseases causing generalized malabsorption (eg, small bowel bacterial overgrowth, tropical sprue, Whipple's disease)
- Luminal disorders causing malabsorption (eg, bile acid deficiency, Zollinger-Ellison syndrome, pancreatic insufficiency)
- Postoperative malabsorption (eg, after gastric or intestinal resection)
- Disorders that cause malabsorption of specific nutrients (eg, disaccharidase deficiency leading to lactose intolerance)

Table 38-2 lists the clinical and pathologic aspects of malabsorptive diseases.

Clinical Manifestations

The hallmarks of malabsorption syndrome from any cause are diarrhea or frequent, loose, bulky, foul-smelling stools that have increased fat content and are often grayish. Patients often have associated abdominal distention, pain, increased flatus, weakness, weight loss, and a decreased sense of well-being. The chief result of malabsorption is malnutrition, manifested by weight loss and other signs of vitamin and mineral deficiency (eg, easy bruising, osteoporosis, anemia). Patients with a malabsorption syndrome, if untreated, become weak and emaciated because of starvation and dehydration. Failure to absorb the fat-soluble vitamins A, D, and K causes a corresponding avitaminosis.

Assessment and Diagnostic Findings

Several diagnostic tests may be prescribed, including stool studies for quantitative and qualitative fat analysis, lactose tolerance tests, D-xylose absorption tests, and Schilling tests. The hydrogen breath test that is used to evaluate carbohydrate absorption (see Chapter 34) is performed if carbohydrate malabsorption is suspected. Endoscopy with biopsy of the mucosa is the best diagnostic tool. Biopsy of the small intestine is performed to assay enzyme activity or to identify infection or destruction of mucosa. Ultrasound studies, CT scans, and x-ray findings can reveal pancreatic or intestinal tumors that may be the cause. A complete blood cell count is used to detect anemia. Pancreatic function tests can assist in the diagnosis of specific disorders.

Medical Management

Intervention is aimed at avoiding dietary substances that aggravate malabsorption and at supplementing nutrients that have been lost. Common supplements are water-soluble vitamins (eg, B_{12}, folic acid), fat-soluble vitamins (ie, A, D, and K), and minerals (eg, calcium, iron). Primary disease states may be managed surgically or nonsurgically. Dietary therapy is aimed at reducing gluten intake in patients with celiac sprue. Folic acid supplements are prescribed for patients with tropical sprue. Antibiotics (eg, tetracycline [Tetracap, Tetracyn], ampicillin [Polycillin]) are sometimes

NURSING RESEARCH PROFILE

Quality of Life in Women with Irritable Bowel Syndrome

Motzer, S. A., Hertig, V., Jarrett, M., et al. (2003). Sense of coherence and quality of life in women with and without irritable bowel syndrome. *Nursing Research, 52*(5), 329–337.

Purpose

Irritable bowel syndrome (IBS) disproportionately affects women, and its onset occurs most commonly during adolescence or early adulthood. It is thought that IBS symptoms are negatively associated with feelings of confidence that life is manageable and meaningful, which is referred to as a sense of coherence (SOC). It is also believed that IBS has detrimental effects on quality of life (QOL) because of its chronic, relapsing nature, its refractoriness to effective treatment, and its associated psychological distress. The aims of this study were to compare the SOC and QOL in women with and without IBS and to examine the relationships between IBS and SOC, QOL, and psychological distress.

Design

The sample consisted of 342 women participants between 18 and 49 years of age, 235 of whom self-reported IBS and 89 of whom did not report IBS or similar gastrointestinal (GI) symptoms. Participants completed several surveys, including the following:

- Antonovsky's SOC Questionnaire, to measure SOC
- Flanagan's Modified Quality of Life Scale (MQOLS), to measure QOL
- Bowel Disease Questionnaire (BDQ), to measure GI symptoms
- Global Severity Index (GSI) and the subscales for depression, anxiety, and somatization from Derogatis's Symptom Checklist-90-R, to measure general and select psychological symptoms

Independent sample *t* tests were analyzed to determine whether there was a difference in SOC, QOL, GI symptoms, and psychological symptoms between women with and without IBS. Pearson's correlation coefficients were also analyzed to identify the relationships among these variables of interest.

Findings

Women with IBS reported significantly lower SOC and QOL than women without IBS. In addition, women with IBS reported significantly more global distress, somatization with and without GI symptoms, depression, and anxiety than did women without IBS. Low SOC and low QOL were both correlated with increased feelings of global distress, depression, anxiety, somatization without GI symptoms, and the GI symptom of alternating constipation and diarrhea.

Nursing Implications

Findings from this study confirm that women with IBS report a decreased SOC and QOL compared with women without IBS. Moreover, women with IBS report having more psychological symptoms of global distress, somatization, depression, and anxiety than women without IBS. It remains unknown whether symptoms of IBS cause psychological distress or whether psychological distress exacerbates symptoms of the syndrome. Nursing interventions targeted at enhancing SOC and QOL should be developed to determine whether they improve the psychological distress associated with IBS.

needed in the treatment of tropical sprue and bacterial overgrowth syndromes. Antidiarrheal agents may be used to decrease intestinal spasms. Parenteral fluids may be necessary to treat dehydration.

Gerontologic Considerations

The older patient may have more subtle symptoms of malabsorption that may be extraintestinal, including fatigue and confusion. Medical management may include the administration of corticosteroids, which may cause a host of adverse effects such as hypertension, hypokalemia, and confusion. Antibiotics may reduce vitamin K–producing intestinal flora, resulting in a prolonged prothrombin time (PT) and international normalized ratio (INR) if the patient is concurrently taking warfarin (Coumadin). Urinary retention, altered mental status, or glaucoma may occur as adverse effects of anticholinergic drug therapy in older people.

Nursing Management

The nurse provides patient and family education regarding diet and the use of nutritional supplements (Chart 38-2). It is important to monitor patients with diarrhea for fluid and electrolyte imbalances. The nurse conducts ongoing assessments to determine whether the clinical manifestations related to the nutritional deficits have abated. Patient education includes information about the risk of osteoporosis related to malabsorption of calcium.

Acute Inflammatory Intestinal Disorders

Any part of the lower GI tract is susceptible to acute inflammation caused by bacterial, viral, or fungal infection. Two such conditions are appendicitis and diverticulitis,

TABLE 38-2 Characteristics of Diseases of Malabsorption

Diseases/Disorders	Physiologic Pathology	Clinical Features
Gastric resection with gastrojejunostomy	Decreased pancreatic stimulation because of duodenal bypass; poor mixing of food, bile, pancreatic enzymes; decreased intrinsic factor	Weight loss, moderate steatorrhea, anemia (combination of iron deficiency, vitamin B_{12} malabsorption, folate deficiency)
Pancreatic insufficiency (chronic pancreatitis, pancreatic carcinoma, pancreatic resection, cystic fibrosis)	Reduced intraluminal pancreatic enzyme activity, with maldigestion of lipids and proteins	History of abdominal pain followed by weight loss; marked steatorrhea, azotorrhea (excess of nitrogenous matter in the feces or urine); also frequent glucose intolerance (70% in pancreatic insufficiency)
Ileal dysfunction (resection or disease)	Loss of ileal absorbing surface leads to reduced bile-salt pool size and reduced vitamin B_{12} absorption; bile in colon inhibits fluid absorption	Diarrhea, weight loss with steatorrhea, especially when greater than 100 cm resection, decreased vitamin B_{12} absorption
Stasis syndromes (surgical strictures, blind loops, enteric fistulas, multiple jejunal diverticula, scleroderma)	Overgrowth of intraluminal intestinal bacteria, especially anaerobic organisms, to greater than 10^6/mL results in deconjugation of bile salts, leading to decreased effective bile-salt pool size, also bacterial utilization of vitamin B_{12}	Weight loss, steatorrhea; low vitamin B_{12} absorption; may have low D-xylose absorption
Zollinger-Ellison syndrome	Hyperacidity in duodenum inactivates pancreatic enzymes	Ulcer diathesis, steatorrhea
Lactose intolerance	Deficiency of intestinal lactase results in high concentration of intraluminal lactose with osmotic diarrhea	Varied degrees of diarrhea and cramps after ingestion of lactose-containing foods; positive lactose intolerance test, decreased intestinal lactase
Celiac disease (gluten enteropathy)	Toxic response to a gluten fraction by surface epithelium results in destruction of absorbing surface	Weight loss, diarrhea, bloating, anemia (low iron, folate), osteomalacia, steatorrhea, azotorrhea, low D-xylose absorption; folate and iron malabsorption
Tropical sprue	Unknown toxic factor results in mucosal inflammation, partial villous atrophy	Weight loss, diarrhea, anemia (low folate, vitamin B_{12}); steatorrhea; low D-xylose absorption, low vitamin B_{12} absorption
Whipple's disease	Bacterial invasion of intestinal mucosa	Arthritis, hyperpigmentation, lymphadenopathy, serous effusions, fever, weight loss, steatorrhea, azotorrhea
Certain parasitic diseases (giardiasis, strongyloidiasis, coccidiosis, capillariasis)	Damage to or invasion of surface mucosa	Diarrhea, weight loss; steatorrhea; organism may be seen on jejunal biopsy or recovered in stool
Immunoglobulinopathy	Decreased local intestinal defenses, lymphoid hyperplasia, lymphopenia	Frequent association with *Giardia:* hypogammaglobulinemia or isolated IgA deficiency

both of which may lead to **peritonitis**, an inflammation of the lining of the abdominal cavity.

Appendicitis

The appendix is a small, finger-like appendage about 10 cm (4 in) long that is attached to the cecum just below the ileocecal valve. The appendix fills with food and empties regularly into the cecum. Because it empties inefficiently and its lumen is small, the appendix is prone to obstruction and is particularly vulnerable to infection (ie, appendicitis).

Appendicitis, the most common cause of acute abdomen in the United States, is the most common reason for emergency abdominal surgery. Although it can occur at any age, it more commonly occurs between the ages of 10 and 30 years (NIH, 2005).

Pathophysiology

The appendix becomes inflamed and edematous as a result of becoming kinked or occluded by a fecalith (ie, hardened mass of stool), tumor, or foreign body. The inflammatory process increases intraluminal pressure, initiating a progressively severe, generalized or periumbilical pain that becomes localized to the right lower quadrant of the abdomen within a few hours. Eventually, the inflamed appendix fills with pus.

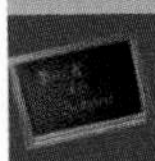

CHART 38-2

Patient Education

Managing Lactose Intolerance

- Deficiency of lactase, a digestive enzyme essential for the absorption of lactose from the intestines, results in an intolerance to milk.
- Elimination of milk and milk substances can prevent symptoms.
- Many processed foods have fillers, such as dried milk, added to them.
- Pretreatment of foods with lactase preparations (eg, LactAid drops) before ingestion can reduce symptoms.
- Ingestion of lactase enzyme tablets with the first bite of food can reduce symptoms.
- Most people can tolerate 1 to 2 cups of milk or milk products daily without major problems; they are best tolerated if ingested in small amounts during the day.
- Lactase activity of yogurt with "active cultures" helps the digestion of lactose within the intestine better than lactase preparations do.
- Milk and milk products are rich sources of calcium and vitamin D; elimination of milk from the diet may result in calcium and vitamin D deficiencies; decreased intake without supplements can lead to osteoporosis.

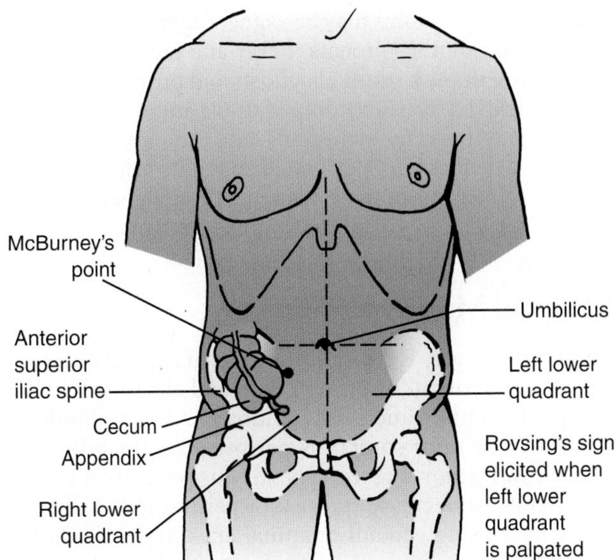

FIGURE 38-2. When the appendix is inflamed, tenderness can be noted in the right lower quadrant at McBurney's point, which is between the umbilicus and the anterior superior iliac spine. Rovsing's sign is pain felt in the right lower quadrant after the left lower quadrant has been palpated.

Clinical Manifestations

Vague epigastric or periumbilical pain progresses to right lower quadrant pain and is usually accompanied by a low-grade fever and nausea and sometimes by vomiting. Loss of appetite is common. In up to 50% of presenting cases, local tenderness is elicited at McBurney's point when pressure is applied (Fig. 38-2). Rebound tenderness (ie, production or intensification of pain when pressure is released) may be present. The extent of tenderness and muscle spasm and the existence of constipation or diarrhea depend not so much on the severity of the appendiceal infection as on the location of the appendix. If the appendix curls around behind the cecum, pain and tenderness may be felt in the lumbar region. If its tip is in the pelvis, these signs may be elicited only on rectal examination. Pain on defecation suggests that the tip of the appendix is resting against the rectum; pain on urination suggests that the tip is near the bladder or impinges on the ureter. Some rigidity of the lower portion of the right rectus muscle may occur. Rovsing's sign may be elicited by palpating the left lower quadrant; this paradoxically causes pain to be felt in the right lower quadrant (see Fig. 38-2). If the appendix has ruptured, the pain becomes more diffuse; abdominal distention develops as a result of paralytic ileus, and the patient's condition worsens.

Constipation can also occur with an acute process such as appendicitis. Laxatives administered in this instance may result in perforation of the inflamed appendix. In general, a laxative or cathartic should never be given when a person has fever, nausea, or pain.

Assessment and Diagnostic Findings

Diagnosis is based on results of a complete physical examination and on laboratory findings and imaging studies. The complete blood cell count demonstrates an elevated white blood cell count with an elevation of the neutrophils. Abdominal x-ray films, ultrasound studies, and CT scans may reveal a right lower quadrant density or localized distention of the bowel. A diagnostic laparoscopy may be used to rule out acute appendicitis in equivocal cases.

Complications

The major complication of appendicitis is perforation of the appendix, which can lead to peritonitis, **abscess** formation (collection of purulent material), or portal pylephlebitis, which is septic thrombosis of the portal vein caused by vegetative emboli that arise from septic intestines. Perforation generally occurs 24 hours after the onset of pain. Symptoms include a fever of 37.7°C (100°F) or greater, a toxic appearance, and continued abdominal pain or tenderness.

Gerontologic Considerations

Acute appendicitis is uncommon in the elderly population. When it does occur, classic signs and symptoms are altered and may vary greatly. Pain may be absent or minimal. Symptoms may be vague, suggesting bowel obstruction or another process. Fever and leukocytosis may not be present. As a result, diagnosis and prompt treatment may be delayed, causing complications and mortality. The patient may have no symptoms until the appendix ruptures. The incidence of perforated appendix is higher in the elderly population because many of these patients do not seek health care as quickly as younger patients.

Medical Management

Immediate surgery is typically indicated if appendicitis is diagnosed. To correct or prevent fluid and electrolyte imbalance, dehydration, and sepsis, antibiotics and IV fluids are administered until surgery is performed. Appendectomy (ie, surgical removal of the appendix) is performed as soon as possible to decrease the risk of perforation. It may be performed using general or spinal anesthesia with a low abdominal incision (laparotomy) or by laparoscopy. Both laparotomy and laparoscopy are safe and effective in the treatment of appendicitis with perforation. However, recovery after laparoscopic surgery is generally quicker.

When perforation of the appendix occurs, an abscess may form. If this occurs, the patient may be initially treated with antibiotics, and the surgeon may place a drain in the abscess. After the abscess is drained and there is no further evidence of infection, an appendectomy is then typically performed.

Nursing Management

Goals include relieving pain, preventing fluid volume deficit, reducing anxiety, eliminating infection due to the potential or actual disruption of the GI tract, maintaining skin integrity, and attaining optimal nutrition.

The nurse prepares the patient for surgery, which includes an IV infusion to replace fluid loss and promote adequate renal function and antibiotic therapy to prevent infection. If there is evidence or likelihood of paralytic ileus, a nasogastric tube is inserted. An enema is not administered because it can lead to perforation.

After surgery, the nurse places the patient in a high-Fowler position. This position reduces the tension on the incision and abdominal organs, helping to reduce pain. An opioid, usually morphine sulfate, is prescribed to relieve pain. When tolerated, oral fluids are administered. Any patient who was dehydrated before surgery receives IV fluids. Food is provided as desired and tolerated on the day of surgery when normal bowel sounds are present.

The patient may be discharged on the day of surgery if the temperature is within normal limits, there is no undue discomfort in the operative area, and the appendectomy was uncomplicated. Discharge teaching for the patient and family is imperative. The nurse instructs the patient to make an appointment to have the surgeon remove the sutures between the fifth and seventh days after surgery. Incision care and activity guidelines are discussed; normal activity can usually be resumed within 2 to 4 weeks.

If there is a possibility of peritonitis, a drain is left in place at the area of the incision. Patients at risk for this complication may be kept in the hospital for several days and are monitored carefully for signs of intestinal obstruction or secondary hemorrhage. Secondary abscesses may form in the pelvis, under the diaphragm, or in the liver, causing elevation of the temperature, pulse rate, and white blood cell count.

When the patient is ready for discharge, the nurse teaches the patient and family to care for the incision and perform dressing changes and irrigations as prescribed. A home care nurse may be needed to assist with this care and to monitor the patient for complications and wound healing. Other complications of appendectomy are listed in Table 38-3.

Diverticular Disease

A **diverticulum** is a saclike herniation of the lining of the bowel that extends through a defect in the muscle layer. Diverticula may occur anywhere in the small intestine or colon but most commonly occur in the sigmoid colon (at least 95%) (Beitz, 2004).

Diverticulosis exists when multiple diverticula are present without inflammation or symptoms. Diverticular disease of the colon is very common in developed countries, and its prevalence increases with age: more than 50% of Americans older than 80 years have diverticulosis (Beitz, 2004). A low intake of dietary fiber is considered a predisposing factor, but the exact cause has not been identified. Most patients with diverticular disease are asymptomatic, so its exact prevalence is unknown.

TABLE 38-3 Potential Complications and Nursing Interventions After Appendectomy

Complication	Nursing Interventions
Peritonitis	Observe for abdominal tenderness, fever, vomiting, abdominal rigidity, and tachycardia. Employ constant nasogastric suction. Correct dehydration as prescribed. Administer antibiotic agents as prescribed.
Pelvic abscess	Evaluate for anorexia, chills, fever, and diaphoresis. Observe for diarrhea, which may indicate pelvic abscess. Prepare patient for rectal examination. Prepare patient for surgical drainage procedure.
Subphrenic abscess (abscess under the diaphragm)	Assess patient for chills, fever, and diaphoresis. Prepare for x-ray examination. Prepare for surgical drainage of abscess.
Ileus (paralytic and mechanical)	Assess for bowel sounds. Employ nasogastric intubation and suction. Replace fluids and electrolytes by intravenous route as prescribed. Prepare for surgery, if diagnosis of mechanical ileus is established.

Diverticulitis results when food and bacteria retained in a diverticulum produce infection and inflammation that can impede drainage and lead to perforation or abscess formation. At least 10% of patients with diverticulosis have diverticulitis at some point. A congenital predisposition is suspected when the disorder occurs in those younger than 40 years. Diverticulitis may occur as an acute attack or may persist as a continuing, smoldering infection. The symptoms manifested generally result from complications: abscess, **fistula** (abnormal tract) formation, obstruction, perforation, peritonitis, and hemorrhage.

Pathophysiology

Diverticula form when the mucosa and submucosal layers of the colon herniate through the muscular wall because of high intraluminal pressure, low volume in the colon (ie, fiber-deficient contents), and decreased muscle strength in the colon wall (ie, muscular hypertrophy from hardened fecal masses). Bowel contents can accumulate in the diverticulum and decompose, causing inflammation and infection. The diverticulum can also become obstructed and then inflamed if the obstruction continues. The inflammation of the weakened colonic wall of the diverticulum can cause it to perforate, giving rise to irritability and spasticity of the colon (ie, diverticulitis). In addition, abscesses develop and may eventually perforate, leading to peritonitis and erosion of the arterial blood vessels, resulting in bleeding.

Clinical Manifestations

Chronic constipation often precedes the development of diverticulosis by many years. Frequently, no problematic symptoms occur with diverticulosis. Signs and symptoms of diverticulosis are relatively mild and include bowel irregularity with intervals of diarrhea, nausea and anorexia, and bloating or abdominal distention. With repeated local inflammation of the diverticula, the large bowel may narrow with fibrotic strictures, leading to cramps, narrow stools, and increased constipation or at times intestinal obstruction. Weakness, fatigue, and anorexia are common symptoms. With diverticulitis, the patient reports an acute onset of mild to severe pain in the lower left quadrant, accompanied by nausea, vomiting, fever, chills, and leukocytosis. The condition, if untreated, can lead to septicemia.

Assessment and Diagnostic Findings

Diverticulosis is typically diagnosed by colonoscopy, which permits visualization of the extent of diverticular disease and allows the clinician to biopsy tissue to rule out other diseases as needed. Until recently, barium enema had been the preferred diagnostic test, but it is now used less frequently than colonoscopy. If there are symptoms of peritoneal irritation when the diagnosis is diverticulitis, barium enema is contraindicated because of the potential for perforation.

CT is the diagnostic test of choice if the suspected diagnosis is diverticulitis; it can also reveal abscesses. Abdominal x-rays may demonstrate free air under the diaphragm if a perforation has occurred from the diverticulitis. Laboratory tests that assist in diagnosis include a complete blood cell count, revealing an elevated white blood cell count, and elevated erythrocyte sedimentation rate (ESR).

Complications

Complications of diverticulitis include peritonitis, abscess formation, and bleeding. If an abscess develops, the associated findings are tenderness, a palpable mass, fever, and leukocytosis. An inflamed diverticulum that perforates results in abdominal pain localized over the involved segment, usually the sigmoid; local abscess or peritonitis follows. Abdominal pain, a rigid board-like abdomen, loss of bowel sounds, and signs and symptoms of shock occur with peritonitis. Noninflamed or slightly inflamed diverticula may erode areas adjacent to arterial branches, causing massive rectal bleeding.

Gerontologic Considerations

The incidence of diverticular disease increases with age because of degeneration and structural changes in the circular muscle layers of the colon and because of cellular hypertrophy. The symptoms are less pronounced in the elderly than in other adults. The elderly may not have abdominal pain until infection occurs. They may delay reporting symptoms because they fear surgery or are afraid that they may have cancer. Blood in the stool is overlooked frequently, especially in the elderly, because of a failure to examine the stool or the inability to see changes if vision is impaired.

Medical Management

Dietary and Medication Management

Diverticulitis can usually be treated on an outpatient basis with diet and medication. When symptoms occur, rest, analgesics, and antispasmodics are recommended. Initially, the diet is clear liquid until the inflammation subsides; then a high-fiber, low-fat diet is recommended. This type of diet helps increase stool volume, decrease colonic transit time, and reduce intraluminal pressure. Antibiotics are prescribed for 7 to 10 days. A bulk-forming laxative also is prescribed.

In acute cases of diverticulitis with significant symptoms, hospitalization is required. Hospitalization is often indicated for those who are elderly, immunocompromised, or taking corticosteroids. Withholding oral intake, administering IV fluids, and instituting nasogastric suctioning if vomiting or distention occurs are used to rest the bowel. Broad-spectrum antibiotics are prescribed for 7 to 10 days. An opioid (eg, meperidine [Demerol]) is prescribed for pain relief. Morphine is contraindicated because it can increase intraluminal pressure in the colon, exacerbating symptoms. Oral intake is increased as symptoms subside. A low-fiber diet may be necessary until signs of infection decrease.

Antispasmodics such as propantheline bromide (Pro-Banthine) and oxyphencyclimine (Daricon) may be prescribed. Often it is not possible for patients to consume the 20 to 30 g of daily fiber that is recommended. Normal stools can be achieved by supplementing dietary fiber by using bulk preparations (psyllium [Metamucil]) or stool softeners (docusate [Colace]), by instilling warm oil into the rectum, or by inserting an evacuant suppository (bisacodyl [Dulcolax]). Such a prophylactic plan can reduce the bacterial flora of the bowel, diminish the bulk of the stool, and soften the fecal mass so that it moves more easily through the area of inflammatory obstruction.

Surgical Management

Although acute diverticulitis usually subsides with medical management, immediate surgical intervention is necessary if complications (eg, perforation, peritonitis, hemorrhage, obstruction) occur. In cases of abscess formation without peritonitis, hemorrhage, or obstruction, CT-guided percutaneous drainage may be performed to drain the abscess, and IV antibiotics are administered. After the abscess is drained and the acute episode of inflammation has subsided (after approximately 6 weeks), surgery may be recommended to prevent repeated episodes. Two types of surgery are typically considered either to treat acute complications or prevent further episodes of inflammation:

- One-stage resection, in which the inflamed area is removed and a primary end-to-end anastomosis is completed
- Multiple-stage procedures for complications such as obstruction or perforation (Fig. 38-3)

The type of surgery performed depends on the extent of complications found during surgery. When possible, the area of diverticulitis is resected and the remaining bowel is joined end-to-end (ie, primary resection and end-to-end anastomosis). This is performed through traditional surgical or laparoscopically assisted colectomy. A two-stage resection may be performed in which the diseased colon is resected (as in a one-stage procedure) but no anastomosis is performed; both ends of the bowel are brought out onto the abdomen as stomas. This "double-barrel" temporary colostomy is then reanastomosed in a later procedure. Fecal diversion procedures are discussed later in this chapter.

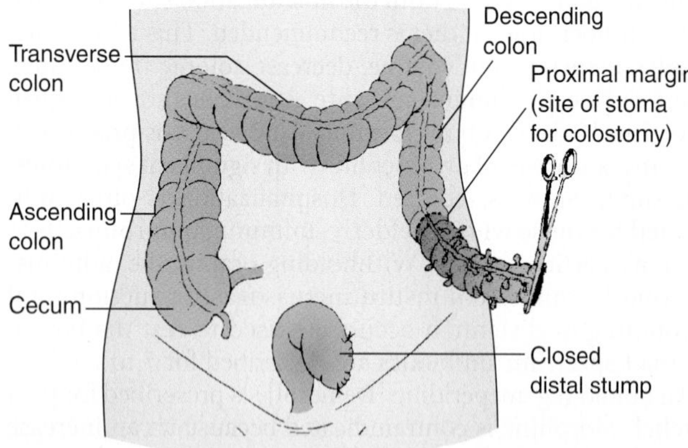

FIGURE 38-3. The Hartmann procedure for diverticulitis: primary resection for diverticulitis of the colon. The affected segment (*clamp attached*) has been divided at its distal end. In a primary anastomosis, the proximal margin (*dotted line*) is transected and the bowel attached end-to-end. In a two-stage procedure, a colostomy is constructed at the proximal margin with the distal stump oversewn (Hartmann procedure, as shown) or brought to the outer surface as a mucous fistula. The second stage consists of colostomy takedown and anastomosis.

Nursing Process

The Patient With Diverticulitis

Assessment

During the health history, the nurse asks the patient about the onset and duration of pain and about past and present elimination patterns. The nurse reviews dietary habits to determine fiber intake and asks the patient about straining at stool, history of constipation with periods of diarrhea, tenesmus, abdominal bloating, and distention.

Assessment includes auscultation for the presence and character of bowel sounds and palpation for lower left quadrant pain, tenderness, or firm mass. The stool is inspected for pus, mucus, or blood. Temperature, pulse, and blood pressure are monitored for abnormal variations.

Diagnosis

Nursing Diagnoses

Based on the assessment data, the nursing diagnoses may include the following:

- Constipation related to narrowing of the colon from thickened muscular segments and strictures
- Acute pain related to inflammation and infection

Collaborative Problems/ Potential Complications

Potential complications that may develop include the following:

- Peritonitis
- Abscess formation
- Bleeding

Planning and Goals

The major goals for the patient may include attainment and maintenance of normal elimination patterns, pain relief, and absence of complications.

Nursing Interventions

Maintaining Normal Elimination Patterns

The nurse recommends a fluid intake of 2 L per day (within limits of the patient's cardiac and renal reserve) and suggests foods that are soft but have increased fiber, such as prepared cereals or soft-cooked vegetables, to increase the bulk of the stool and facilitate peristalsis, thereby promoting defecation. An individualized exercise program is encouraged to improve abdominal muscle tone. It is important to review the patient's daily routine to establish a schedule for meals and a set time for defecation and to assist in identifying habits that may have suppressed the urge to defecate. The nurse encourages daily intake of bulk laxatives such as psyllium (Metamucil), which helps propel feces through the colon. Stool softeners are administered as prescribed to decrease straining at stool, which decreases intestinal pressure. Oil retention enemas may be prescribed to soften the stool, making it easier to pass.

Relieving Pain

Opioid analgesics (eg, meperidine [Demerol]) to relieve the pain of diverticulitis and antispasmodic agents to decrease intestinal spasm are administered as prescribed. The nurse records the intensity, duration, and location of pain to determine whether the inflammatory process worsens or subsides.

Monitoring and Managing Potential Complications

The major nursing focus is to prevent complications by identifying patients at risk and managing their symptoms as needed. The nurse assesses for the following signs and symptoms of perforation:

- Increased abdominal pain and tenderness accompanied by abdominal rigidity
- Elevated white blood cell count
- Elevated ESR
- Increased temperature
- Tachycardia
- Hypotension

Perforation is a surgical emergency. The clinical manifestations of perforation and peritonitis and the care of the patient with peritonitis are presented in the next section. The nurse monitors vital signs and urine output and administers IV fluids to replace volume loss as needed.

Promoting Home and Community-Based Care

Because patients and their family members and health care providers tend to focus on the most obvious needs and issues, the nurse reminds the patient and family about the importance of continuing health promotion and screening practices. The nurse educates patients who have not been involved in these practices in the past about their importance and refers the patients to appropriate health care providers.

Evaluation

Expected Patient Outcomes

Expected patient outcomes may include the following:

1. Attains a normal pattern of elimination
   a. Reports less abdominal cramping and pain
   b. Reports the passage of soft, formed stool without pain
   c. Adds unprocessed bran to foods
   d. Drinks at least 10 glasses of fluid each day (if fluid intake is tolerated)
   e. Exercises daily
2. Reports decreased pain
   a. Requests analgesics as needed
   b. Adheres to a low-fiber diet during acute episodes
3. Recovers without complications
   a. Is afebrile
   b. Has normal blood pressure
   c. Has a soft, nontender abdomen with normal bowel sounds
   d. Maintains adequate urine output
   e. Has no blood in the stool

Peritonitis

Peritonitis is inflammation of the peritoneum, the serous membrane lining the abdominal cavity and covering the viscera. Usually, it is a result of bacterial infection; the organisms come from diseases of the GI tract or, in women, from the internal reproductive organs. Peritonitis can also result from external sources such as injury or trauma (eg, gunshot wound, stab wound) or an inflammation that extends from an organ outside the peritoneal area, such as the kidney. The most common bacteria implicated are *Escherichia coli, Klebsiella, Proteus,* and *Pseudomonas.* Inflammation and paralytic ileus are the direct effects of the infection. Other common causes of peritonitis are appendicitis, perforated ulcer, diverticulitis, and bowel perforation (Fig. 38-4). Peritonitis may also be associated with abdominal surgical procedures and peritoneal dialysis.

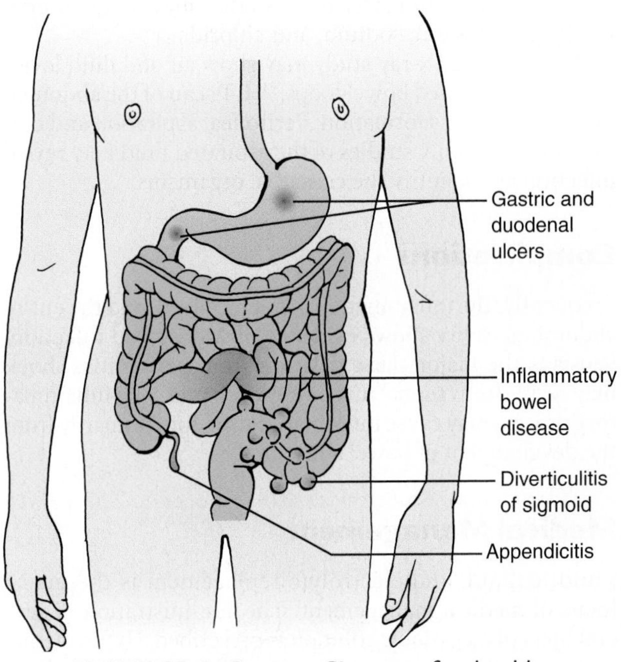

FIGURE 38-4. Common GI causes of peritonitis.

Pathophysiology

Peritonitis is caused by leakage of contents from abdominal organs into the abdominal cavity, usually as a result of inflammation, infection, ischemia, trauma, or tumor perforation. Bacterial proliferation occurs. Edema of the tissues results, and exudation of fluid develops in a short time. Fluid in the peritoneal cavity becomes turbid with increasing amounts of protein, white blood cells, cellular debris, and blood. The immediate response of the intestinal tract is hypermotility, soon followed by paralytic ileus with an accumulation of air and fluid in the bowel.

Clinical Manifestations

Symptoms depend on the location and extent of the inflammation. The early clinical manifestations of peritonitis frequently are the symptoms of the disorder causing the condition. At first, a diffuse type of pain is felt. The pain tends to become constant, localized, and more intense near the site of the inflammation. Movement usually aggravates it. The affected area of the abdomen becomes extremely tender and distended, and the muscles become rigid. Rebound tenderness and paralytic ileus may be present. Diminished perception of pain in peritonitis can occur in people receiving corticosteroids or analgesics. Patients with diabetes who have symptoms of advanced neuropathy and patients with cirrhosis who have signs of ascites may not experience pain during an acute bacterial episode. Usually, nausea and vomiting occur and peristalsis is diminished. A temperature of 100° to 101°F (37.8° to 38.3°C) can be expected, along with an increased pulse rate.

Assessment and Diagnostic Findings

The white blood cell count is almost always elevated. The hemoglobin and hematocrit levels may be low if blood loss has occurred. Serum electrolyte studies may reveal altered levels of potassium, sodium, and chloride.

An abdominal x-ray study may show air and fluid levels as well as distended bowel loops. A CT scan of the abdomen may show abscess formation. Peritoneal aspiration and culture and sensitivity studies of the aspirated fluid may reveal infection and identify the causative organisms.

Complications

Frequently, the inflammation is not localized, and the entire abdominal cavity shows evidence of widespread infection. Sepsis is the major cause of death from peritonitis. Shock may result from septicemia or hypovolemia. The inflammatory process may cause intestinal obstruction, primarily from the development of bowel adhesions.

Medical Management

Fluid, colloid, and electrolyte replacement is the major focus of medical management. The administration of several liters of an isotonic solution is prescribed. Hypovolemia occurs because massive amounts of fluid and electrolytes move from the intestinal lumen into the peritoneal cavity and deplete the fluid in the vascular space.

Analgesics are prescribed for pain. Antiemetics are administered as prescribed for nausea and vomiting. Intestinal intubation and suction assist in relieving abdominal distention and in promoting intestinal function. Fluid in the abdominal cavity can cause pressure that restricts expansion of the lungs and causes respiratory distress. Oxygen therapy by nasal cannula or mask generally promotes adequate oxygenation, but airway intubation and ventilatory assistance occasionally are required.

Antibiotic therapy is initiated early in the treatment of peritonitis. Large doses of a broad-spectrum antibiotic are administered IV until the specific organism causing the infection is identified and appropriate antibiotic therapy can be initiated.

Surgical objectives include removing the infected material and correcting the cause. Surgical treatment is directed toward excision (ie, appendix), resection with or without anastomosis (ie, intestine), repair (ie, perforation), and drainage (ie, abscess). With extensive sepsis, a fecal diversion may need to be created.

The two most common postoperative complications are wound evisceration and abscess formation. Any suggestion from the patient that an area of the abdomen is tender or painful or "feels as if something just gave way" must be reported. The sudden occurrence of serosanguineous wound drainage strongly suggests wound dehiscence (see Chapter 20).

Nursing Management

Intensive care is often needed. The blood pressure is monitored by arterial line if shock is present. The central venous pressure or pulmonary artery wedge pressure and urine output are monitored frequently. In addition, ongoing assessment of pain, GI function, and fluid and electrolyte balance is important. The nurse reports the nature of the pain, its location in the abdomen, and any changes in location. Administering analgesic medication and positioning the patient for comfort are helpful in decreasing pain. The patient is placed on the side with knees flexed; this position decreases tension on the abdominal organs. Accurate recording of all intake and output and central venous pressures and/or pulmonary artery pressures assist in calculating fluid replacement. The nurse administers and closely monitors IV fluids.

Signs that indicate that peritonitis is subsiding include a decrease in temperature and pulse rate, softening of the abdomen, return of peristaltic sounds, passing of flatus, and bowel movements. The nurse increases fluid and food intake gradually and reduces parenteral fluids as prescribed. A worsening clinical condition may indicate a complication, and the nurse must prepare the patient for emergency surgery.

Drains are frequently inserted during the surgical procedure, and the nurse must observe and record the character of the drainage postoperatively. Care must be taken when moving and turning the patient to prevent the drains from being dislodged. It is also important for the nurse to prepare the patient and family for discharge by teaching the patient to care for the incision and drains if the patient will be sent home with the drains still in place. Referral for home care may be indicated for further monitoring and patient and family teaching.

Inflammatory Bowel Disease

Inflammatory bowel disease (IBD) refers to two chronic inflammatory GI disorders: regional enteritis (ie, Crohn's disease) and ulcerative colitis. Both disorders have striking similarities but also several differences. Table 38-4 compares regional enteritis and ulcerative colitis.

The incidence of IBD in the United States has increased in the past century: over 30,000 new cases occur annually. People between 15 and 30 years of age are at the greatest risk of developing IBD, followed by people between 50 and 70 years of age. Women and men tend to be equally affected, and family history appears to predispose people to develop IBD, particularly if a first-degree relative has the disease. Although it was previously believed that psychological symptoms such as anxiety or depression predisposed certain people to IBD, this theory has been discarded (NIH, 2005).

Despite extensive research, the cause of IBD is still unknown. Researchers theorize that it is triggered by environmental agents such as pesticides, food additives, tobacco, and radiation (Green, Morris, & Lin, 2005; NIH, 2005). Nonsteroidal anti-inflammatory drugs (NSAIDs) have been found to exacerbate IBD. Allergies and immune

TABLE 38-4 Comparison of Regional Enteritis and Ulcerative Colitis

Factor	Regional Enteritis (Crohn's)	Ulcerative Colitis
Course	Prolonged, variable	Exacerbations, remissions
Pathology		
Early	Transmural thickening	Mucosal ulceration
Late	Deep, penetrating granulomas	Minute, mucosal ulcerations
Clinical Manifestations		
Location	Ileum, ascending colon (usually)	Rectum, descending colon
Bleeding	Usually not, but if it occurs, tends to be mild	Common—severe
Perianal involvement	Common	Rare—mild
Fistulas	Common	Rare
Rectal involvement	About 20%	Almost 100%
Diarrhea	Less severe	Severe
Diagnostic Study Findings		
Barium series	Regional, discontinuous lesions Narrowing of colon Thickening of bowel wall Mucosal edema Stenosis, fistulas	Diffuse involvement No narrowing of colon No mucosal edema Stenosis rare Shortening of colon
Sigmoidoscopy	May be unremarkable unless accompanied by perianal fistulas	Abnormal inflamed mucosa
Colonoscopy	Distinct ulcerations separated by relatively normal mucosa in ascending colon	Friable mucosa with pseudopolyps or ulcers in descending colon
Therapeutic Management	Corticosteroids, sulfonamides (sulfasalazine [Azulfidine]) Antibiotics Parenteral nutrition Partial or complete colectomy, with ileostomy or anastomosis Rectum can be preserved in some patients Recurrence common	Corticosteroids, sulfonamides; sulfasalazine useful in preventing recurrence Bulk hydrophilic agents Antibiotics Proctocolectomy, with ileostomy Rectum can be preserved in only a few patients "cured" by colectomy
Systemic Complications	Small bowel obstruction Right-sided hydronephrosis Nephrolithiasis Cholelithiasis Arthritis Retinitis, iritis Erythema nodosum	Toxic megacolon Perforation Hemorrhage Malignant neoplasms Pyelonephritis Nephrolithiasis Cholangiocarcinoma Arthritis Retinitis, iritis Erythema nodosum

disorders have also been suggested as causes. Abnormal response to dietary or bacterial antigens has been studied extensively, and genetic factors also are being studied. There is a high prevalence of coexistent IBS, which complicates the overall symptom presentation.

Types of Chronic Inflammatory Bowel Disease

Regional Enteritis (Crohn's Disease)

Regional enteritis is usually first diagnosed in adolescents or young adults but can appear at any time of life. Histopathologic changes consistent with regional enteritis most commonly occur in the distal ileum and colon but can occur anywhere along the GI tract. The incidence of regional enteritis has risen over the past 30 years (NIH, 2005). Regional enteritis is seen more often in smokers than in nonsmokers (Colwell, Goldberg, & Carmel, 2004).

Pathophysiology

Regional enteritis is a subacute and chronic inflammation of the GI tract wall that extends through all layers (ie, transmural lesion). Although it can occur anywhere in the GI tract, it most commonly occurs in the distal ileum and, to a lesser degree, the ascending colon. It is characterized by periods of remission and exacerbation. The disease process begins with edema and thickening of the mucosa. Ulcers begin to appear on the inflamed mucosa. These lesions are not in continuous contact with one another and are separated by normal tissue. Hence, these clusters of ulcers tend to take on a classic "cobblestone" appearance. Fistulas, fissures, and abscesses form as the inflammation extends into the peritoneum. Granulomas occur in 50% of patients. As the disease advances, the bowel wall thickens and becomes fibrotic, and the intestinal lumen narrows. Diseased bowel loops sometimes adhere to other loops surrounding them.

Clinical Manifestations

The onset of symptoms is usually insidious in regional enteritis, with prominent lower right quadrant abdominal pain and diarrhea unrelieved by defecation. Scar tissue and the formation of granulomas interfere with the ability of the intestine to transport products of the upper intestinal digestion through the constricted lumen, resulting in crampy abdominal pains. There is abdominal tenderness and spasm. Because eating stimulates intestinal peristalsis, the crampy pains occur after meals. To avoid these bouts of crampy pain, the patient tends to limit food intake, reducing the amounts and types of food to such a degree that normal nutritional requirements are often not met. As a result, weight loss, malnutrition, and secondary anemia occur. Ulcers in the membranous lining of the intestine and other inflammatory changes result in a weeping, edematous intestine that continually empties an irritating discharge into the colon. Disrupted absorption causes chronic diarrhea and nutritional deficits. The result is a person who is thin and emaciated from inadequate food intake and constant fluid loss. In some patients, the inflamed intestine may perforate, leading to intra-abdominal and anal abscesses. Fever and leukocytosis occur. Chronic symptoms include diarrhea, abdominal pain, **steatorrhea** (ie, excessive fat in the feces), anorexia, weight loss, and nutritional deficiencies.

Abscesses, fistulas, and fissures are common. Manifestations may extend beyond the GI tract and commonly include joint disorders (eg, arthritis), skin lesions (eg, erythema nodosum), ocular disorders (eg, conjunctivitis), and oral ulcers. The clinical course and symptoms can vary; in some patients, periods of remission and exacerbation occur, but in others, the disease follows a fulminating course.

Assessment and Diagnostic Findings

A proctosigmoidoscopy is usually performed initially to determine whether the rectosigmoid area is inflamed. A stool examination is also performed; the result may be positive for occult blood and steatorrhea. The most conclusive diagnostic aid for regional enteritis is a barium study of the upper GI tract that shows the classic "string sign" on an x-ray film of the terminal ileum, indicating the constriction of a segment of intestine. Endoscopy, colonoscopy, and intestinal biopsies may be used to confirm the diagnosis. A barium enema may show ulcerations (the cobblestone appearance described earlier), fissures, and fistulas. A CT scan may show bowel wall thickening and fistula formation.

A complete blood cell count is performed to assess hematocrit and hemoglobin levels (usually decreased) as well as the white blood cell count (may be elevated). The ESR is usually elevated. Albumin and protein levels may be decreased, indicating malnutrition.

Complications

Complications of regional enteritis include intestinal obstruction or stricture formation, perianal disease, fluid and electrolyte imbalances, malnutrition from malabsorption, and fistula and abscess formation. The most common type of small bowel fistula caused by regional enteritis is the enterocutaneous fistula (ie, an abnormal opening between the small bowel and the skin). Abscesses can be the result of an internal fistula that results in fluid accumulation and infection. Patients with regional enteritis are also at increased risk of colon cancer.

Ulcerative Colitis

Ulcerative colitis is a recurrent ulcerative and inflammatory disease of the mucosal and submucosal layers of the colon and rectum. The prevalence of ulcerative colitis is highest in Caucasians and people of Jewish heritage (Johnson & Chan, 2004). It is a serious disease, accompanied by systemic complications and a high mortality rate. Approximately 5% of patients with ulcerative colitis develop colon cancer (NIH, 2005).

Pathophysiology

Ulcerative colitis affects the superficial mucosa of the colon and is characterized by multiple ulcerations, diffuse inflammations, and desquamation or shedding of the colonic epithelium. Bleeding occurs as a result of the ulcerations.

The mucosa becomes edematous and inflamed. The lesions are contiguous, occurring one after the other. Abscesses form, and infiltrate is seen in the mucosa and submucosa, with clumps of neutrophils found in the lumens of the crypts (ie, crypt abscesses) that line the intestinal mucosa (Porth, 2005). The disease process usually begins in the rectum and spreads proximally to involve the entire colon. Eventually, the bowel narrows, shortens, and thickens because of muscular hypertrophy and fat deposits.

Clinical Manifestations

The clinical course is usually one of exacerbations and remissions. The predominant symptoms of ulcerative colitis include diarrhea, lower left quadrant abdominal pain, intermittent tenesmus, and rectal bleeding. The bleeding may be mild or severe, and pallor, anemia, and fatigue result. The patient may have anorexia, weight loss, fever, vomiting, and dehydration, as well as cramping, the feeling of an urgent need to defecate, and the passage of 10 to 20 liquid stools each day. The disease is classified as mild, severe, or fulminant, depending on the severity of the symptoms. Hypocalcemia and anemia frequently develop. Rebound tenderness may occur in the right lower quadrant. Extra-intestinal manifestations include skin lesions (eg, erythema nodosum), eye lesions (eg, uveitis), joint abnormalities (eg, arthritis), and liver disease.

Assessment and Diagnostic Findings

The patient should be assessed for tachycardia, hypotension, tachypnea, fever, and pallor. Other assessments address level of hydration and nutritional status. The abdomen is examined for bowel sounds, distention, and tenderness. These findings assist in determining the severity of the disease.

The stool is positive for blood, and laboratory test results reveal low hematocrit and hemoglobin levels in addition to an elevated white blood cell count, low albumin levels, and an electrolyte imbalance. Abdominal x-ray studies are useful for determining the cause of symptoms. Free air in the peritoneum and bowel dilation or obstruction should be excluded as a source of the presenting symptoms. Sigmoidoscopy or colonoscopy and barium enema are valuable in distinguishing this condition from other diseases of the colon with similar symptoms. A barium enema may show mucosal irregularities, focal strictures or fistulas, shortening of the colon, and dilation of bowel loops. Colonoscopy may reveal friable, inflamed mucosa with exudate and ulcerations. This procedure assists in defining the extent and severity of the disease. CT scanning, magnetic resonance imaging (MRI), and ultrasound studies can identify abscesses and perirectal involvement. Leukocyte scanning (see Chapter 34) is useful when severe colitis prohibits the use of colonoscopy to determine the extent of inflammation.

Careful stool examination for parasites and other microbes is performed to rule out dysentery caused by common intestinal organisms, especially *Entamoeba histolytica* and *Clostridium difficile*.

Complications

Complications of ulcerative colitis include toxic megacolon, perforation, and bleeding as a result of ulceration, vascular engorgement, and highly vascular granulation tissue. In toxic megacolon, the inflammatory process extends into the muscularis, inhibiting its ability to contract and resulting in colonic distention. Symptoms include fever, abdominal pain and distention, vomiting, and fatigue. If the patient with toxic megacolon does not respond within 24 to 72 hours to medical management with nasogastric suction, IV fluids with electrolytes, corticosteroids, and antibiotics, surgery is required. Total colectomy is then indicated. For many patients, surgery becomes necessary to relieve the effects of the disease and to treat these serious complications; an ileostomy usually is performed. The surgical procedures involved and the care of patients with this type of fecal diversion are discussed later in this chapter.

Patients with IBD also have a significantly increased risk of osteoporotic fractures due to decreased bone mineral density. Corticosteroid therapy may also contribute to the diminished bone density.

Medical Management of Chronic Inflammatory Bowel Disease

Medical treatment for regional enteritis and ulcerative colitis is aimed at reducing inflammation, suppressing inappropriate immune responses, providing rest for a diseased bowel so that healing may take place, improving quality of life, and preventing or minimizing complications. Most patients have long periods of well-being interspersed with short intervals of illness (Lederman & Winshall, 2004). Management depends on the disease location, severity, and complications.

Nutritional Therapy

Oral fluids and a low-residue, high-protein, high-calorie diet with supplemental vitamin therapy and iron replacement are prescribed to meet nutritional needs, reduce inflammation, and control pain and diarrhea. Fluid and electrolyte imbalances from dehydration caused by diarrhea are corrected by IV therapy as necessary if the patient is hospitalized or by oral fluids if the patient is managed at home. Any foods that exacerbate diarrhea are avoided. Milk may contribute to diarrhea in those with lactose intolerance. Cold foods and smoking are avoided because both increase intestinal motility. Parenteral nutrition may be indicated (see Chapter 36).

Pharmacologic Therapy

Sedatives and antidiarrheal and antiperistaltic medications are used to minimize peristalsis to rest the inflamed bowel. They are continued until the patient's stools approach normal frequency and consistency.

Aminosalicylate formulations such as sulfasalazine (Azulfidine) are often effective for mild or moderate inflammation and are used to prevent or reduce recurrences in long-term maintenance regimens. Sulfa-free aminosalicylates (eg, mesalamine [Asacol, Pentasa]) are effective in preventing and treating recurrence of inflammation.

Antibiotics (eg, metronidazole [Flagyl]) are used for secondary infections, particularly for purulent complications such as abscesses, perforation, and peritonitis.

Corticosteroids are used to treat severe and fulminant disease and can be administered orally (eg, prednisone [Deltasone]) in outpatient treatment or parenterally (eg, hydrocortisone [Solu-Cortef]) in hospitalized patients. Topical (ie, rectal administration) corticosteroids (eg, hydrocortisone enema, budesonide [Entocort]) are also widely used in the treatment of distal colon disease. When the dosage of corticosteroids is reduced or stopped, the symptoms of disease may return. If corticosteroids are continued, adverse sequelae such as hypertension, fluid retention, cataracts, hirsutism (ie, abnormal hair growth), adrenal suppression, poor wound healing, and loss of bone density may occur.

Immunomodulators (eg, azathioprine [AZA], 6-mercaptopurine [6-MP], methotrexate, cyclosporine) have been used to alter the immune response. The exact mechanism of action of these medications in treating IBD is unknown. They are used for patients with severe disease who have not responded favorably to other therapies. These medications are useful in maintenance regimens to prevent relapses. Newer biologic therapies using monoclonal antibodies are being studied, including natalizumab (Tysabri) for treating Crohn's disease (Sandborn, Colombel, Enns, et al., 2005) and infliximab (Remicade) for treating ulcerative colitis (Rutgeerts, Sandborn, Feagan, et al., 2005). Initial reports from clinical trials appear promising for both these agents (Rutgeerts et al., 2005; Sandborn et al., 2005), although the adverse effects of natalizumab may seriously limit its therapeutic usefulness.

Surgical Management

When nonsurgical measures fail to relieve the severe symptoms of IBD, surgery may be necessary. More than 50% of all patients with regional enteritis require surgery within 5 years of diagnosis (Colwell et al., 2004). The most common indications for surgery are medically intractable disease, poor quality of life, or complications from the disease or its treatment. Recurrence of inflammation and disease after surgery in regional enteritis is inevitable. The rate of recurrence after surgery is approximately 28% in the first 5 years (Colwell et al., 2004).

A common procedure performed for strictures of the small intestines is laparoscope-guided strictureplasty, in which the blocked or narrowed sections of the intestines are widened, leaving the intestines intact. In some cases, a small bowel resection is performed and diseased segments of the small intestines are resected and the remaining portions of the intestines are anastomosed. Surgical removal of up to 50% of the small bowel usually can be tolerated. In cases of severe regional enteritis of the colon, a total colectomy and ileostomy may be the procedure of choice.

A newer surgical procedure developed for patients with severe regional enteritis is intestinal transplant. This technique is now available to children and to young and middle-aged adults who have lost intestinal function from disease. Although this procedure is not a cure, it may eventually provide improvement in quality of life for some patients. The associated technical and immunologic problems remain formidable, and the costs and mortality rates remain high.

At least 25% of patients with ulcerative colitis eventually have total colectomies (NIH, 2005). When the colon is surgically removed, the patient is considered "cured" in that extra-intestinal manifestations subside and the disease process is otherwise limited to the colon. Indications for surgery include lack of improvement and continued deterioration, profuse bleeding, perforation, continued stricture formation, and cancer. Surgical excision usually improves quality of life. Proctocolectomy with ileostomy (ie, complete excision of colon, rectum, and anus) is recommended when the rectum is severely diseased. If the rectum can be preserved, restorative proctocolectomy with ileal pouch anal anastomosis (IPAA) is the procedure of choice.

Other types of surgical procedures, known as fecal diversions, are discussed later in this chapter.

Total Colectomy With Ileostomy

An **ileostomy**, the surgical creation of an opening into the ileum or small intestine (usually by means of an ileal stoma on the abdominal wall), is commonly performed after a total colectomy (ie, excision of the entire colon). It allows for drainage of fecal matter (ie, effluent) from the ileum to the outside of the body. The drainage is very mushy and occurs at frequent intervals. Nursing management of the patient with an ileostomy is discussed later in this chapter.

Continent Ileostomy

Another procedure involves the creation of a continent ileal reservoir (ie, **Kock pouch**) by diverting a portion of the distal ileum to the abdominal wall and creating a stoma. This procedure eliminates the need for an external fecal collection bag. Approximately 30 cm of the distal ileum is reconstructed to form a reservoir with a nipple valve that is created by pulling a portion of the terminal ileal loop back into the ileum. GI effluent can accumulate in the pouch for several hours and then be removed by means of a catheter inserted through the nipple valve. In many patients, a total colectomy is also performed with the Kock pouch. Possible indications for a total colectomy with Kock pouch placement (rather than a restorative proctocolectomy with IPAA) include a badly diseased rectum, lack of rectal sphincter tone, or inability to achieve fecal continence post-IPAA.

The major problem with the Kock pouch is malfunction of the nipple valve. Surgical research is currently focused on developing valves that may slip less frequently than the nipple valve.

Restorative Proctocolectomy With Ileal Pouch Anal Anastomosis

A restorative proctocolectomy with IPAA is the surgical procedure of choice in cases where the rectum can be preserved, in that it eliminates the need for a permanent ileostomy. It establishes an ileal reservoir, and anal sphincter control of elimination is retained. The procedure involves connecting a portion of the ileum to the anus (ie, ileoanal anastomosis) in conjunction with removal of the colon and the rectal mucosa (ie, total abdominal colectomy and mucosal proctectomy) (Fig. 38-5). A temporary diverting loop ileostomy is constructed at the time of surgery and closed about 3 months later.

With ileoanal anastomosis, the diseased colon and rectum are removed, voluntary defecation is maintained, and anal continence is preserved. The ileal reservoir decreases the number of bowel movements by 50%, from approximately 14 to 20 per day to 7 to 10 per day. Nighttime elimination is gradually reduced to one bowel movement. Complications of ileoanal anastomosis include irritation of the perianal skin from leakage of fecal contents, stricture formation at the anastomosis site, and small bowel obstruction.

Nursing Management of Chronic Inflammatory Bowel Disease

Nursing management of patients with IBD may be medical, surgical, or both. Patients in the community setting or those recently diagnosed may require education about diet and medications and referral to support groups. Hospitalized patients with long-standing or severe disease also require careful monitoring, parenteral nutrition, fluid replacement, and possibly emergent surgery. The surgical procedures may involve a fecal diversion, with attendant needs for physical care, emotional support, and extensive teaching about management of the ostomy.

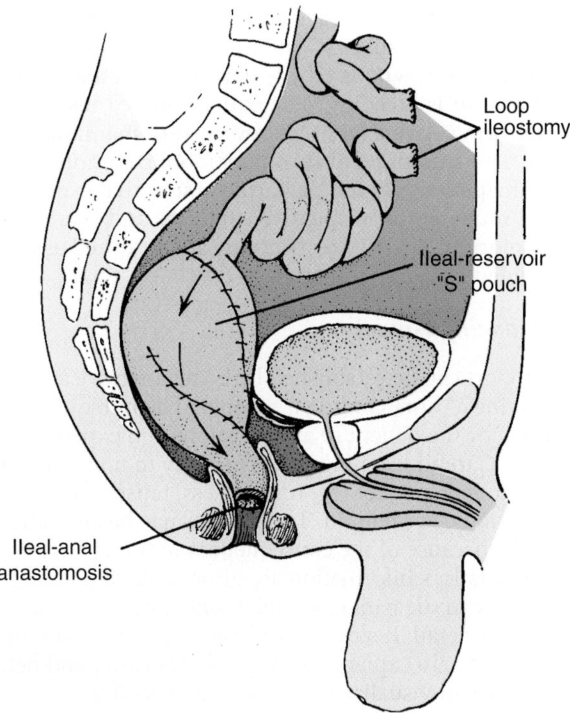

FIGURE 38-5. A mucosal proctectomy precedes anastomosis of the ileal reservoir. A temporary loop ileostomy diverts effluent for several months to allow healing.

Nursing Process

Management of the Patient With Inflammatory Bowel Disease

Assessment

The nurse obtains a health history to identify the onset, duration, and characteristics of abdominal pain; the presence of diarrhea or fecal urgency, straining at stool (tenesmus), nausea, anorexia, or weight loss; and family history of IBD. It is important to discuss dietary patterns, including the amounts of alcohol, caffeine, and nicotine-containing products used daily and weekly. The nurse asks about patterns of bowel elimination, including character, frequency, and presence of blood, pus, fat, or mucus. It is important to note allergies and food intolerance, especially milk (lactose) intolerance. The patient may identify sleep disturbances if diarrhea or pain occurs at night.

Assessment includes auscultating the abdomen for bowel sounds and their characteristics; palpating the abdomen for distention, tenderness, or pain; and inspecting the skin for evidence of fistulas or signs of dehydration. The stool is inspected for blood and mucus.

Pain is usually localized in the right lower quadrant in regional enteritis, where hyperactive bowel sounds can be heard because of borborygmus and increased peristalsis. Abdominal tenderness is present with palpation. The most prominent symptom is intermittent pain that occurs with diarrhea but does not decrease after defecation. Pain in the periumbilical region usually indicates involvement of the terminal ileum. With ulcerative colitis, the abdomen may be distended, and rebound tenderness may be present. Rectal bleeding is a significant sign.

Diagnosis

Nursing Diagnoses

Based on the assessment data, the nursing diagnoses may include the following:

- Diarrhea related to the inflammatory process
- Acute pain related to increased peristalsis and GI inflammation
- Deficient fluid volume related to anorexia, nausea, and diarrhea
- Imbalanced nutrition, less than body requirements, related to dietary restrictions, nausea, and malabsorption
- Activity intolerance related to fatigue
- Anxiety related to impending surgery
- Ineffective coping related to repeated episodes of diarrhea
- Risk for impaired skin integrity related to malnutrition and diarrhea

- Risk for ineffective therapeutic regimen management related to insufficient knowledge concerning the process and management of the disease

Collaborative Problems/ Potential Complications

Potential complications that may develop include the following:

- Electrolyte imbalance
- Cardiac dysrhythmias related to electrolyte depletion
- GI bleeding with fluid volume loss
- Perforation of the bowel

Planning and Goals

The major goals for the patient include attainment of normal bowel elimination patterns, relief of abdominal pain and cramping, prevention of fluid volume deficit, maintenance of optimal nutrition and weight, avoidance of fatigue, reduction of anxiety, promotion of effective coping, absence of skin breakdown, increased knowledge about the disease process and therapeutic regimen, and avoidance of complications.

Nursing Interventions

Maintaining Normal Elimination Patterns

The nurse determines if there is a relationship between diarrhea and certain foods, activities, or emotional stressors. Identifying precipitating factors, the frequency of bowel movements, and the character, consistency, and amount of stool passed is important. The nurse provides ready access to a bathroom, commode, or bedpan and keeps the environment clean and odor-free. It is important to administer antidiarrheal medications as prescribed, to record the frequency and consistency of stools after therapy is initiated, and to encourage bed rest to decrease peristalsis.

Relieving Pain

The character of the pain is described as dull, burning, or crampy. It is important to ask about its onset. Does it occur before or after meals, during the night, or before elimination? Is the pattern constant or intermittent? Is it relieved with medications? The nurse administers anticholinergic medications 30 minutes before a meal as prescribed to decrease intestinal motility and administers analgesics as prescribed for pain. Position changes, local application of heat (as prescribed), diversional activities, and prevention of fatigue also are helpful for reducing pain.

Maintaining Fluid Intake

To detect fluid volume deficit, the nurse keeps an accurate record of oral and IV fluids and maintains a record of output (ie, urine, liquid stool, vomitus, wound or fistula drainage). The nurse monitors daily weights for fluid gains or losses and assesses the patient for signs of fluid volume deficit (ie, dry skin and mucous membranes, decreased skin turgor, oliguria, exhaustion, decreased temperature, increased hematocrit, elevated urine specific gravity, and hypotension). It is important to encourage oral intake of fluids and to monitor the IV flow rate. The nurse initiates measures to decrease diarrhea (eg, dietary restrictions, stress reduction, antidiarrheal agents).

Maintaining Optimal Nutrition

Parenteral nutrition is used when the symptoms of IBD are severe. With parenteral nutrition, the nurse maintains an accurate record of fluid intake and output as well as the patient's daily weight. The patient should gain 0.5 kg daily during parenteral nutrition therapy. Because parenteral nutrition is very high in glucose and can cause hyperglycemia, blood glucose levels are monitored every 6 hours. Once the symptoms of IBD exacerbation have diminished and the patient has gained or stabilized weight, parenteral nutrition is stopped and the patient is advanced on oral elemental feedings. Elemental feedings are high in protein and low in fat and residue. They are digested primarily in the jejunum, do not stimulate intestinal secretions, and allow the bowel to continue to rest. The nurse notes intolerance if the patient exhibits nausea, vomiting, diarrhea, or abdominal distention.

If oral foods are tolerated, small, frequent, low-residue feedings are given to avoid overdistending the stomach and stimulating peristalsis. It is important that the patient restrict activity to conserve energy, reduce peristalsis, and reduce calorie requirements.

Promoting Rest

The nurse recommends intermittent rest periods during the day and schedules or restricts activities to conserve energy and reduce the metabolic rate. It is important to encourage activity within the limits of the patient's capacity. The nurse suggests bed rest for a patient who is febrile, has frequent diarrheal stools, or is bleeding. The patient on bed rest should perform active exercises, however, to maintain muscle tone and prevent thromboembolic complications. If the patient cannot perform these active exercises, the nurse performs passive exercises and joint range of motion. Activity restrictions are modified as needed on a day-to-day basis.

Reducing Anxiety

Rapport can be established by being attentive and displaying a calm, confident manner. The nurse allows time for the patient to ask questions and express feelings. Careful listening and sensitivity to nonverbal indicators of anxiety (eg, restlessness, tense facial expressions) are helpful. The patient may be emotionally labile because of the consequences of the disease; the nurse tailors information about possible impending surgery to the patient's level of understanding and desire for detail. If surgery is planned, pictures and illustrations help explain the surgical procedure and help the patient visualize what a stoma looks like.

Enhancing Coping Measures

Because the patient may feel isolated, helpless, and out of control, understanding and emotional support are essential. The patient may respond to stress in a variety of ways that may alienate others (eg, anger, denial, social self-isolation).

The nurse needs to recognize that the patient's behavior may be affected by a number of factors unrelated to inherent emotional characteristics. Any patient suffering the discomforts of frequent bowel movements and rectal soreness is anxious, discouraged, and depressed. It is important to develop a relationship with the patient that supports all attempts to cope with these stressors. It is also important to communicate that the patient's feelings are understood by encouraging the patient to talk and express his or her feelings and to discuss any concerns. Stress reduction measures that may be used include relaxation techniques, visualization, breathing exercises, and biofeedback. Professional counseling may be needed to help the patient and family manage issues associated with chronic illness and resulting disability.

Preventing Skin Breakdown

The nurse examines the patient's skin frequently, especially the perianal skin. Perianal care, including the use of a skin barrier (eg, petroleum ointment [Vaseline]), is important after each bowel movement. The nurse gives immediate attention to reddened or irritated areas over bony prominences and uses pressure-relieving devices to prevent skin breakdown. Consultation with an **enterostomal therapist** (a nurse specially trained in the use of a variety of fecal and urinary diversions) otherwise known as wound-ostomy-continence nurse (WOCN) is often helpful.

Monitoring and Managing Potential Complications

Serum electrolyte levels are monitored daily, and electrolyte replacements are administered as prescribed. It is important to report evidence of dysrhythmias or changes in level of consciousness immediately.

The nurse closely monitors rectal bleeding and administers blood component therapy and volume expanders as prescribed to prevent hypovolemia. It is important to monitor the blood pressure for hypotension and to obtain coagulation profiles and hemoglobin and hematocrit levels frequently. Vitamin K may be prescribed to increase clotting factors.

The nurse closely monitors the patient for indications of perforation (ie, acute increase in abdominal pain, rigid abdomen, vomiting, or hypotension) and obstruction and toxic megacolon (ie, abdominal distention, decreased or absent bowel sounds, change in mental status, fever, tachycardia, hypotension, dehydration, and electrolyte imbalances).

Promoting Home and Community-Based Care

TEACHING PATIENTS SELF-CARE

The nurse assesses the patient's understanding of the disease process and his or her need for additional information about medical management (eg, medications, diet) and surgical interventions. The nurse provides information about nutritional management; a bland, low-residue, high-protein, high-calorie, and high-vitamin diet relieves symptoms and decreases diarrhea. It is important to explain the rationale for the use of corticosteroids and anti-inflammatory, antibacterial, antidiarrheal, and antispasmodic medications. The nurse emphasizes the importance of taking medications as prescribed and not abruptly discontinuing them (especially corticosteroids) to avoid development of serious medical problems (Chart 38-3). The nurse reviews ileostomy care as necessary (see Nursing Management of the Patient with an Ileostomy). Patient education information can be obtained from the National Foundation for Ileitis and Colitis.

CHART 38-3

HOME CARE CHECKLIST • Inflammatory Bowel Disease

At the completion of the home care instruction, the patient or caregiver will be able to:	Patient	Caregiver
• Verbalize an understanding of the disease process.	✔	✔
• Discuss nutritional management: bland, low-residue, high-protein, high-vitamin diet; identify foods to include and foods to be avoided.	✔	✔
• Describe medication regimen; identify medications by name, use, route, and frequency.	✔	✔
• Identify measures to be used to treat exacerbation of symptoms, to include rest, dietary modifications, and medications.	✔	✔
• Identify measures to be used to promote fluid and electrolyte balance during acute exacerbations	✔	✔
• Demonstrate management of parenteral nutrition therapy, if applicable; identify possible complications and interventions	✔	✔
• Incorporate stress reduction measures into lifestyle	✔	

CONTINUING CARE

Patients with chronic IBD are managed at home with follow-up care by their physician or through an outpatient clinic. Those whose nutritional status is compromised and who are receiving parenteral nutrition need home care nursing to ensure that their nutritional requirements are being met and that they or their caregivers can follow through with the instructions for parenteral nutrition. Patients who are medically managed need to understand that their disease can be controlled and that they can lead a healthy life between exacerbations. Control implies management based on an understanding of the disease and its treatment. Patients in the home setting need information about their medications (ie, name, dose, side effects, and frequency of administration) and need to take medications on schedule. Medication reminders such as containers that separate pills according to day and time or daily checklists are helpful.

During a flare-up, the nurse encourages the patient to rest as needed and to modify activities according to his or her energy level. Patients should limit tasks that impose strain on the lower abdominal muscles. They should sleep in a room close to the bathroom because of the frequent diarrhea (10 to 20 times per day); quick access to a toilet helps alleviate worry about having an "accident." Room deodorizers help control odors.

Dietary modifications can control but do not cure the disease; the nurse recommends a low-residue, high-protein, high-calorie diet, especially during an acute phase. It is important to encourage the patient to keep a record of the foods that irritate the bowel and to avoid them and to drink at least eight glasses of water each day.

The prolonged nature of the disease has an impact on the patient and often strains his or her family life and financial resources. Family support is vital; however, some family members may be resentful, guilty, and tired and feel unable to cope with the emotional demands of the illness and the physical demands of providing care. Some patients with IBD do not socialize for fear of being embarrassed. Many prefer to eat alone. Because they have lost control over elimination, they may fear losing control over other aspects of their lives. They need time to express their fears and frustrations. Individual and family counseling may be helpful.

Evaluation

Expected Patient Outcomes

Expected patient outcomes may include the following:

1. Reports a decrease in the frequency of diarrheal stools
   a. Complies with dietary restrictions; maintains bed rest
   b. Takes medications as prescribed
2. Has reduced pain
3. Maintains fluid volume balance
   a. Drinks 1 to 2 L of oral fluids daily
   b. Has normal body temperature
   c. Displays adequate skin turgor and moist mucous membranes
4. Attains optimal nutrition; tolerates small, frequent feedings without diarrhea
5. Avoids fatigue
   a. Rests periodically during the day
   b. Adheres to activity restrictions
6. Is less anxious
7. Copes successfully with diagnosis
   a. Verbalizes feelings freely
   b. Uses appropriate stress reduction behaviors
8. Maintains skin integrity
   a. Cleans perianal skin after defecation
   b. Uses lotion or ointment as skin barrier
9. Acquires an understanding of the disease process
   a. Modifies diet appropriately to decrease diarrhea
   b. Adheres to medication regimen as prescribed
10. Recovers without complications
    a. Electrolytes within normal ranges
    b. Normal sinus or baseline cardiac rhythm
    c. Maintains fluid balance
    d. Experiences no perforation or rectal bleeding

Nursing Management of the Patient Requiring an Ileostomy

Some patients with IBD eventually require a permanent fecal diversion with creation of an ileostomy to manage symptoms and to treat or prevent complications. The Plan of Nursing Care summarizes care for the patient requiring an ostomy (Chart 38-4).

Providing Preoperative Care

A period of preparation with intensive replacement of fluid, blood, and protein is necessary before surgery is performed. Antibiotics may be prescribed. If the patient has been taking corticosteroids, they will be continued during the surgical phase to prevent steroid-induced adrenal insufficiency. Usually, the patient is given a low-residue diet, provided in frequent, small feedings. All other preoperative measures are similar to those for general abdominal surgery. The abdomen is marked for the proper placement of the stoma by the surgeon or the enterostomal therapist. Care is taken to ensure that the stoma is conveniently placed—usually in the right lower quadrant about 2 inches below the waist, in an area away from previous scars, bony prominences, skin folds, or fistulas.

The patient must have a thorough understanding of the surgery to be performed and what to expect after surgery. Information about an ileostomy is presented to the patient by means of written materials, models, and discussion. Preoperative teaching includes management of drainage from the stoma; the nature of drainage; and the need for nasogastric intubation, parenteral fluids, and possibly perineal packing.

Providing Postoperative Care

General abdominal surgery wound care is required. The nurse observes the stoma for color and size. It should be

(text continues on page 1258)

CHART 38-4

Plan of Nursing Care — The Patient Undergoing Ostomy Surgery

Nursing Diagnosis: Deficient knowledge about the surgical procedure and preoperative preparation
Goal: Understands the surgical process and the necessary preoperative preparations

NURSING INTERVENTIONS	RATIONALE	EXPECTED OUTCOMES
Preoperative Care 1. Ascertain whether the patient has had a previous surgical experience and ask for recollections of positive and negative impressions.	1. Fear of a repeated negative experience increases anxiety. Talking about the experience with a nurse helps clarify misconceptions and helps the patient ventilate any repressed emotions. Positive experiences are reinforced.	• Expresses anxieties and fears about the surgical process • Projects a positive attitude toward the surgical procedure • Repeats in own words information given by the surgeon • Identifies normal anatomy and physiology of gastrointestinal tract and how it will be altered; can point to expected location of abdominal wound and stoma; describes stoma appearance and size • Adheres to "bowel prep" regimen of antimicrobials or mechanical cleansing • Tolerates the presence of nasogastric/nasoenteric tube
2. Determine what information the surgeon gave the patient and family and whether it was understood. Clarify and elaborate as necessary. Determine whether the stoma is permanent or temporary. Be aware of the patient's prognosis if carcinoma exists.	2. Clarification prevents misunderstandings and alleviates anxiety.	
3. Use pictures or drawings to illustrate the location and appearance of the surgical wounds (abdominal, perineal) and the stoma if the patient is receptive.	3. Knowledge, for some, alleviates anxiety because fear of the unknown is decreased. Others choose not to know because it makes them more anxious.	
4. Explain that oral/parenteral antimicrobials will be administered to cleanse the bowel preoperatively. Mechanical cleansing may also be required.	4. Antimicrobials and mechanical cleansing reduce intestinal bacterial flora.	
5. Assist the patient during nasogastric/nasoenteric intubation. Measure drainage from the tube.	5. Nasoenteral intubation is used for decompression and drainage of gastrointestinal contents before surgery.	

Nursing Diagnosis: Disturbed body image
Goal: Attainment of a positive self-concept

NURSING INTERVENTIONS	RATIONALE	EXPECTED OUTCOMES
1. Encourage the patient to verbalize feelings about the stoma. Offer to be present when the stoma is first viewed and touched.	1. Free expression of feelings allows the patient the opportunity to verbalize and identify concerns. Expressed concerns can be therapeutically addressed by health care team members.	• Freely expresses concerns and fears • Accepts support • Seeks help as needed • States is willing to talk with an ostomate
2. Suggest that the spouse or significant other view the stoma.	2. Helps patient to overcome fears about partner's response.	
3. Offer counseling, if desired.	3. Provides opportunity for additional support.	
4. Arrange for a visit with an ostomate.	4. Ostomates can offer support and share mutual feelings and experiences.	

continued >

CHART 38-4

Plan of Nursing Care — The Patient Undergoing Ostomy Surgery (Continued)

Nursing Diagnosis: Anxiety related to the loss of bowel control
Goal: Reduction of anxiety

NURSING INTERVENTIONS	RATIONALE	EXPECTED OUTCOMES
Postoperative Care 1. Provide information about expected bowel function: a. Characteristics of effluent b. Frequency of discharge	1. Emotional adjustment is facilitated if adequate information is provided at the level of the learner.	• Expresses interest in learning about altered bowel function • Handles equipment correctly • Changes the appliance unassisted • Irrigates colostomy successfully • Progresses toward a regular schedule of elimination
2. Teach the patient how to prepare the appliance for an adequate fit.	2. Adequate fit is necessary for successful use of the appliance.	
a. Choose the drainage appliance that will provide a secure fit around the stoma. Measure the stoma size with a measuring guide provided by the ostomy equipment manufacturer and compare with the opening on the pouch. About 3-mm (⅛-in) clearance should be provided around the stoma.	a. The appliance opening should be larger than the stoma for an adequate fit. Available brands come in different sizes to fit the stoma. Adjustments are made as necessary.	
b. Remove any plastic covering that protects the appliance adhesive. *Note:* The pouch is applied by pressing the adhesive for 30 seconds to the skin or skin barrier.	b. The appliance is ready to apply directly to the skin or skin protector.	
3. Demonstrate how to change the appliance before leakage occurs. Be aware that the elderly person may have diminished vision and difficulty handling equipment.	3. Manipulation of the appliance is a learned motor skill that requires practice and positive reinforcement.	
4. When appropriate, demonstrate how to irrigate the colostomy (usually on the 4th–5th day). Recommend that irrigation be performed at a consistent time, depending on the type of colostomy.	4. Colostomy irrigation is used to regulate the passage of fecal material; alternatively the bowel can be allowed to evacuate naturally.	

Nursing Diagnosis: Risk for impaired skin integrity related to irritation of the peristomal skin by the effluent
Goal: Maintenance of skin integrity

NURSING INTERVENTIONS	RATIONALE	EXPECTED OUTCOMES
1. Provide information about signs and symptoms of irritated or inflamed skin. Use pictures if possible.	1. Peristomal skin should be slightly pink without abrasions and similar to that of the entire abdomen.	• Describes appearance of healthy skin • Correctly cleanses the skin • Successfully applies a skin barrier

CHART 38-4

Plan of Nursing Care — The Patient Undergoing Ostomy Surgery (Continued)

NURSING INTERVENTIONS	RATIONALE	EXPECTED OUTCOMES
2. Teach patient how to cleanse the peristomal skin gently.	2. Mild friction with warm water and a gentle soap cleanses the skin and minimizes irritation and possible abrasions. Patting the skin dry prevents tissue trauma.	• Gently removes the drainage appliance without skin damage
3. Demonstrate how to apply a skin barrier (powder, gel, paste, wafer).	3. Skin barriers protect the peristomal skin from enzymes and bacteria.	• Demonstrates intact skin around the colostomy stoma
4. Demonstrate how to remove the pouch.	4. Gently separate adhesive from the skin to avoid irritation. Never pull!	

Nursing Diagnosis: Potential imbalanced nutrition, less than body requirements, related to avoidance of foods that may cause GI discomfort
Goal: Achievement of an optimal nutritional intake

NURSING INTERVENTIONS	RATIONALE	EXPECTED OUTCOMES
1. Conduct a complete nutritional assessment to identify any foods that may increase peristalsis by irritating the bowel.	1. Patients react differently to certain foods because of individual sensitivity.	• Modifies diet to avoid offensive foods yet maintains adequate nutritional intake
2. Advise the patient to avoid food products with a cellulose or hemicellulose base (nuts, seeds).	2. Cellulose food products are the nondigestible residue of plant foods. They hold water, provide bulk, and stimulate elimination.	• Avoids cellulose-based foods such as peanuts
3. Recommend moderation in intake of certain irritating fruits such as prunes, grapes, and bananas.	3. These fruits tend to increase the quantity of effluent.	• Modifies intake of certain fruits

Nursing Diagnosis: Sexual dysfunction related to altered body image
Goal: Attainment of satisfactory sexual performance

NURSING INTERVENTIONS	RATIONALE	EXPECTED OUTCOMES
1. Encourage the patient to verbalize concerns and fears. The sexual partner is welcomed to participate in the discussion.	1. Expressed needs help the therapist develop a plan of care.	• Expresses fears and concerns
2. Recommend alternative sexual positions.	2. Avoid patient embarrassment with the visual appearance of the stoma. Avoid peristomal skin irritation secondary to friction.	• Discusses alternative sexual positions
3. Seek assistance from a sexual therapist, enterostomal therapist, or advanced practice nurse.	3. Some patients need professional sexual counseling.	• Accepts services of a professional counselor

continued >

CHART 38-4

Plan of Nursing Care — The Patient Undergoing Ostomy Surgery (Continued)

Nursing Diagnosis: Risk for deficient fluid volume related to anorexia and vomiting and increased loss of fluids and electrolytes from GI tract
Goal: Attainment of fluid balance

NURSING INTERVENTIONS	RATIONALE	EXPECTED OUTCOMES
1. Estimate fluid intake and output:	1. Provides indication of fluid balance.	• Maintains fluid balance
a. Strict intake and output	a. An early indicator of fluid imbalance is a daily, significant difference between intake and output. The average person ingests (food, fluids) and loses (urine, feces, lungs) about 2 L of fluid every 24 h.	
b. Daily weights	b. A gain/loss of 1 L of fluid is reflected in a body weight change of 2.2 lb.	
2. Assess serum and urinary values of sodium and potassium.	2. Sodium is the major electrolyte regulating water balance. Vomiting results in decreased urinary and serum sodium levels. Urinary sodium values, in contrast to serum values, reflect early, sensitive changes in sodium balance. Sodium works in conjunction with potassium, which is also decreased with vomiting. A significant deficiency in potassium is associated with a decrease in intracellular potassium bicarbonate, which leads to acidosis and compensatory hyperventilation.	• Maintains normal serum and urinary values for sodium and potassium
3. Observe and record skin turgor and the appearance of the tongue.	3. Adequate hydration is reflected by the skin's ability to return to its normal shape after being grasped between the fingers. *Note:* In the older person, it is normal for the return to be delayed. Changes in the mucous membrane covering the tongue are accurate and early indicators of hydration status.	• Normal skin turgor • Surface of tongue is pink, with a moist mucous membrane

pink to bright red and shiny. Typically, a temporary plastic bag with an adhesive facing is placed over the ileostomy in the operating room and firmly pressed onto the surrounding skin. The nurse monitors the ileostomy for fecal drainage, which should begin about 72 hours after surgery. The drainage is a continuous liquid from the small intestine because the stoma does not have a controlling sphincter. The contents drain into the plastic bag and are thus kept from coming into contact with the skin. They are collected and measured when the bag becomes full. If a continent ileal reservoir was created, as described for the Kock pouch, continuous drainage is provided by an indwelling reservoir catheter for 2 to 3 weeks after surgery. This allows the suture lines to heal.

As with other patients undergoing abdominal surgery, the nurse encourages those with an ileostomy to engage in early ambulation. It is important to administer prescribed pain medications as required.

Because these patients lose much fluid in the early postoperative period, an accurate record of fluid intake, urinary output, and fecal discharge is necessary to help gauge the fluid needs of the patient. There may be 1000 to 2000 mL of fluid lost each day in addition to expected fluid loss through urine, perspiration, respiration, and other sources. With this loss, sodium and potassium are depleted. The nurse monitors laboratory values and administers electrolyte replacements as prescribed. Fluids are administered IV for 4 to 5 days to replace lost fluids.

Nasogastric suction is also a part of immediate postoperative care, with the tube requiring frequent irrigation, as prescribed. The purpose of nasogastric suction is to prevent a buildup of gastric contents. After the tube is removed, the nurse offers sips of clear liquids and gradually progresses the diet. It is important to report nausea and abdominal distention, which may indicate intestinal obstruction, immediately.

By the end of the first week, rectal packing is removed. Because this procedure may be uncomfortable, the nurse may administer an analgesic an hour before its removal. After the packing is removed, the perineum is irrigated two or three times daily until full healing takes place.

PROVIDING EMOTIONAL SUPPORT

The patient may think that everyone is aware of the ileostomy and may view the stoma as a mutilation compared with other abdominal incisions that heal and are hidden. Because there is loss of a body part and a major change in anatomy and function, the patient often goes through the various phases of grieving—shock, disbelief, denial, rejection, anger, and restitution. Nursing support through these phases is important, and understanding of the patient's emotional outlook in each instance should determine the approach taken. For example, teaching may be ineffective until the patient is ready to learn. Concern about body image may lead to questions related to family relationships, sexual function, and, for women, the ability to become pregnant and to deliver a baby normally. Patients need to know that someone understands and cares about them. A calm, nonjudgmental attitude exhibited by the nurse aids in gaining the patient's confidence. It is important to recognize the dependency needs of these patients. Their prolonged illness can make them irritable, anxious, and depressed. The nurse can coordinate patient care through meetings attended by consultants such as the physician, psychologist, psychiatrist, social worker, enterostomal therapist, and dietitian. The team approach is important in facilitating the often complex care of the patient.

Conversely, a surgical procedure to create an ileostomy can produce dramatic positive changes in patients who have suffered from IBD for several years. After the discomfort of the disease has decreased and the patient learns how to take care of the ileostomy, he or she often develops a more positive outlook. Until the patient progresses to this phase, an empathetic and tolerant approach by the nurse plays an important part in recovery. The sooner the patient masters the physical care of the ileostomy, the sooner he or she will psychologically accept it.

Support from other people with ostomies is also helpful. The United Ostomy Association is dedicated to the rehabilitation of people with ostomies. This organization gives patients useful information about living with an ostomy through an educational program of literature, lectures, and exhibits. Local associations offer visiting services by qualified members who provide hope and rehabilitation services to patients with new ostomies. Hospitals and other health care agencies may have an enterostomal therapist on staff who can serve as a valuable resource person for the patient with an ileostomy.

MANAGING SKIN AND STOMA CARE

The patient with a traditional ileostomy cannot establish regular bowel habits because the contents of the ileum are fluid and are discharged continuously. The patient must wear a pouch at all times. Stomal size and pouch size vary initially; the stoma should be rechecked 3 weeks after surgery, when the edema has subsided. The final size and type of appliance is selected in 3 months, after the patient's weight has stabilized and the stoma shrinks to a stable shape.

The location and length of the stoma are significant in the management of the ileostomy by the patient. The surgeon positions the stoma as close to the midline as possible and at a location where even an obese patient with a protruding abdomen can care for it easily. Usually, the ileostomy stoma is about 2.5 cm (1 in) long, which makes it convenient for the attachment of an appliance.

Skin excoriation around the stoma can be a persistent problem. Peristomal skin integrity may be compromised by several factors, such as an allergic reaction to the ostomy appliance, skin barrier, or paste; chemical irritation from the effluent; mechanical injury from the removal of the appliance; and infection. If irritation and yeast growth occur, nystatin powder (Mycostatin) is dusted lightly on the peristomal skin.

CHANGING AN APPLIANCE

A regular schedule for changing the pouch before leakage occurs must be established for those with a traditional ileostomy. The patient can be taught to change the pouch in a manner similar to that described in Chart 38-5.

The amount of time a person can keep the appliance sealed to the body surface depends on the location of the stoma and on body structure. The usual wearing time is 5 to 7 days. The appliance is emptied every 4 to 6 hours, or at the same time the patient empties the bladder. An emptying spout at the bottom of the appliance is closed with a special clip made for this purpose.

Most pouches are disposable and odor-proof. Foods such as spinach and parsley act as deodorizers in the intestinal tract; foods that cause odors include cabbage, onions, and fish. Bismuth subcarbonate tablets, which may be prescribed and taken orally three or four times each day, are effective in reducing odor. Oral diphenoxylate (Lomotil) can also be prescribed to diminish intestinal motility, thereby thickening the stool and assisting in odor control.

IRRIGATING A CONTINENT ILEOSTOMY

For a continent ileostomy (ie, Kock pouch), the nurse teaches the patient to drain the pouch, as described in Chart 38-6. A catheter is inserted into the reservoir to drain

CHART 38-5 Guidelines for Changing an Ileostomy Appliance

Changing an ileostomy appliance is necessary to prevent leakage (the bag is usually changed every 5 to 7 days), to allow for examination of the skin around the stoma, and to assist in controlling odor if this becomes a problem. The appliance should be changed at any time that the patient complains of burning or itching under the disk or pain in the area of the stoma; routine changes should be performed early in the morning before breakfast or 2 to 4 hours after a meal, when the bowel is least active.

NURSING ACTION	RATIONALE
1. Promote patient comfort and involvement in the procedure. a. Have the patient assume a relaxed position. b. Provide privacy. c. Explain details of the procedure. d. Expose the ileostomy area; remove the ileostomy belt (if worn).	1. Providing a relaxed atmosphere and adequate explanations help the patient to become an active participant in the procedure.
2. Remove the appliance. a. Have the patient sit on the toilet or on a chair facing the toilet. A patient who prefers to stand should face the toilet. b. The appliance (pouch) can be removed by gently pushing the skin away from the adhesive.	2. These positions facilitate disposal or drainage.

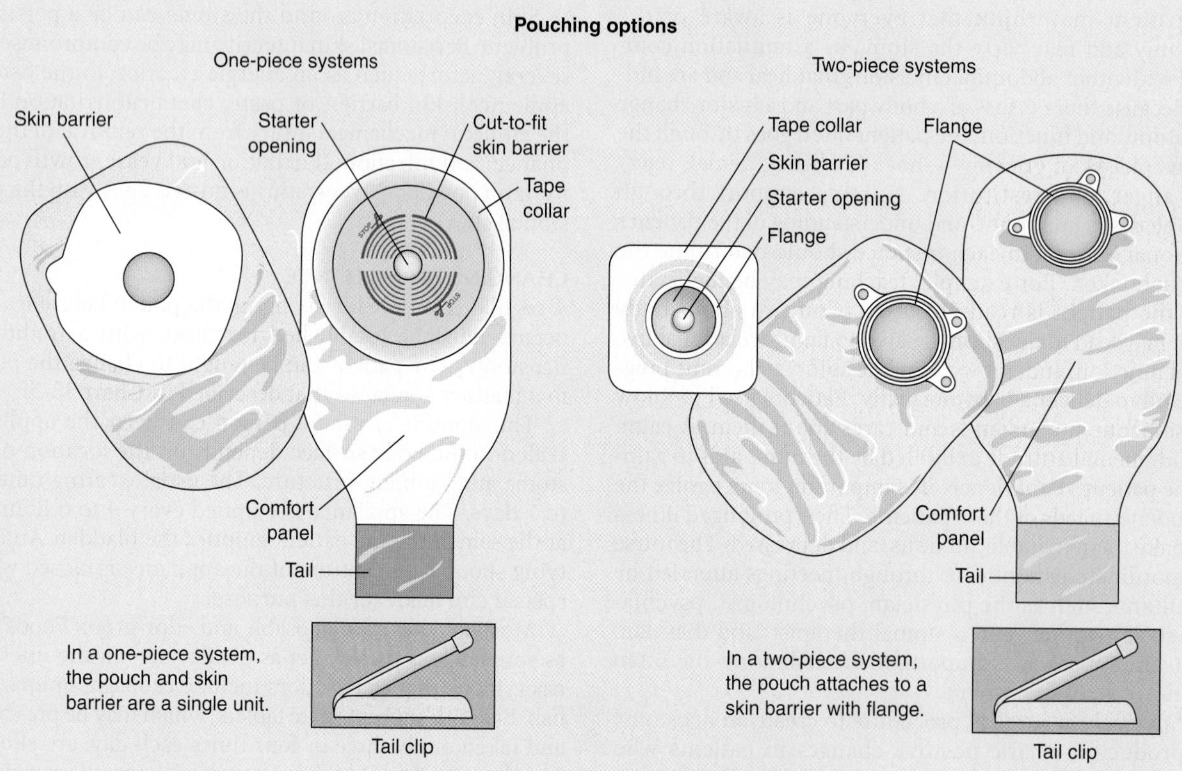

NURSING ACTION	RATIONALE
3. Cleanse the skin: a. Wash the skin gently with a soft cloth moistened with tepid water and mild soap; the patient may prefer to bathe before putting on a clean appliance.	3. The patient may shower with or without the pouch. a. Micropore or waterproof tape applied to the sides of the faceplate will keep it secure during bathing.

CHART 38-5 Guidelines for Changing an Ileostomy Appliance, continued

NURSING ACTION	RATIONALE
b. Rinse and dry the skin thoroughly after cleansing.	b. Moisture or soap residue will interfere with appliance adhesion.
4. Apply appliance (when there is *no* skin irritation): a. An appropriate skin barrier is applied to the peristomal skin before the appliance is applied. b. Remove cover from adherent surface of disk of disposable plastic appliance and apply directly to the skin. c. Press firmly in place for 30 seconds to ensure adherence.	4. Many appliances have a built-in skin barrier. The skin should be thoroughly dried before applying the appliance. 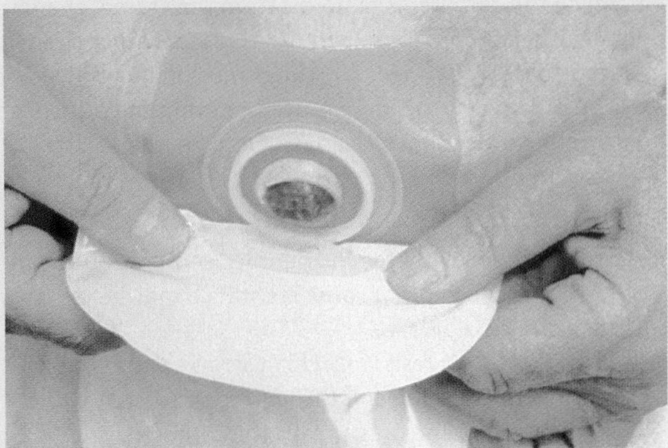 Pressing the appliance into place. Courtesy of Convatec, a Squibb Company.
5. Apply appliance (when there is skin irritation): a. Cleanse the skin thoroughly but gently; pat dry. b. Apply Kenalog spray; blot excess moisture with a cotton pledget and dust lightly with nystatin (Mycostatin) powder. OR Apply as an alternative a wafer of Stomahesive (Squibb), which is commercially available. The stomal opening should be cut the same size as the stoma; use a cutting guide (supplied with Stomahesive). The wafer is applied directly to the skin. c. Another alternative is to moisten a karaya gum washer and apply when it is tacky. If the skin is moist, karaya powder may be applied first and any excess dusted off gently. d. The pouch is then applied to the treated skin.	5. a. To remove debris b. The corticosteroid preparation (Kenalog) helps to decrease inflammation. The antifungal agent (nystatin) treats those types of infections that are common around stomas. A prescription is required for either medication. Stomahesive is a substance that facilitates healing of excoriated skin. It adheres well even to moist, irritated skin. c. Karaya also facilitates skin healing. Tackiness promotes adherence. d. This will allow skin to heal while the appliance is in place.
6. Check the pouch bottom for closure; use the rubber band or clip provided.	6. Proper closure controls leakage.

the fluid. The length of time between drainage periods is gradually increased until the reservoir needs to be drained only every 4 to 6 hours and irrigated once each day. A pouch is not necessary; instead, most patients wear a small dressing over the opening.

When the fecal discharge is thick, water can be injected through the catheter to loosen and soften it. The consistency of the effluent is affected by food intake. At first, drainage is only 60 to 80 mL, but as time goes on, the amount increases significantly. The internal Kock pouch stretches, eventually accommodating 500 to 1000 mL. The patient learns to use the sensation of pressure in the pouch as a gauge to determine how often the pouch should be drained.

CHART 38-6 Guidelines for Draining a Continent Ileostomy (Kock Pouch)

A continent ileostomy is the surgical creation of a pouch of small intestine that can serve as an internal receptacle for fecal discharge; a nipple valve is constructed at the outlet. Postoperatively, a catheter extends from the stoma and is attached to a closed drainage suction system. To ensure patency of the catheter, 10 to 20 mL of normal saline is instilled gently into the pouch usually every 3 hours; return flow is not aspirated but is allowed to drain by gravity.

After approximately 2 weeks, when the healing process has progressed to the point at which the catheter is removed from the stoma, the patient is taught to drain the pouch. The equipment required includes a catheter, tissues, water-soluble lubricant, gauze squares, a syringe, irrigating solution in a bowl, and an emesis or receiving basin.

The following procedure is used to drain the pouch; the patient is helped to participate in this procedure to learn to perform it unassisted.

NURSING ACTION	RATIONALE
1. Lubricate the catheter and gently insert it about 5 cm (2 in), at which point some resistance may be felt at the valve or nipple.	1. When gentle pressure is used, the catheter usually will enter the pouch.
2. If there is much resistance, fill a syringe with 20 mL of air or water and inject it through the catheter, while still exerting some pressure on the catheter.	2. This will permit the catheter to enter the pouch.
3. Place the other end of the catheter in a drainage basin held below the level of the stoma. Later this process can be carried out at the toilet with drainage delivered into the toilet bowl.	3. Gravity facilitates drainage. Drainage may include flatus as well as effluent.
4. After drainage, the catheter is removed and the area around the stoma is gently washed with warm water. Pat dry and apply an absorbent pad over the stoma. Fasten the pad with hypoallergenic tape.	4. The entire procedure requires about 5 to 10 min; at first it is performed every 3 h. The time between procedures is gradually lengthened to three times daily.

MANAGING DIETARY AND FLUID NEEDS

A low-residue diet is followed for the first 6 to 8 weeks. Strained fruits and vegetables are given. These foods are important sources of vitamins A and C. Later, there are few dietary restrictions, except for avoiding foods that are high in fiber or hard-to-digest kernels, such as celery, popcorn, corn, poppy seeds, caraway seeds, and coconut. Foods are reintroduced one at a time. The nurse assesses the patient's tolerance for these foods and reminds him or her to chew food thoroughly.

Fluids may be a problem during the summer, when fluid lost through perspiration adds to the fluid loss through the ileostomy. Fluids such as Gatorade are helpful in maintaining electrolyte balance. If the fecal discharge is too watery, fibrous foods (eg, whole-grain cereals, fresh fruit skins, beans, corn, nuts) are restricted. If the effluent is excessively dry, salt intake is increased. Increased intake of water or fluid does not increase the effluent, because excess water is excreted in the urine.

PREVENTING COMPLICATIONS

Monitoring for complications is an ongoing activity for the patient with an ileostomy. Peristomal skin irritation, which results from leakage of effluent, is the most common complication of an ileostomy. A drainable pouching system that does not fit well is often the cause. Components of the drainable pouching system include the pouch, a solid skin barrier, and adhesive. The enterostomal therapist typically recommends the appropriate drainable pouching system. The solid skin barrier is the component of this system that is most important in ensuring healthy peristomal skin. Solid skin barriers are typically shaped as rectangular or elliptical wafers and are composed of polymers and hydrocolloids. They protect the skin around the stoma from effluent from the stoma and provide a stable interface between the stoma and the pouch.

Other common complications include diarrhea, stomal stenosis, urinary calculi, and cholelithiasis. Even in the presence of a properly fitted drainable pouching system, diarrhea can be problematic. Diarrhea, manifested by very irritating effluent that rapidly fills the pouch (every hour or sooner), can quickly lead to dehydration and electrolyte losses. Supplemental water, sodium, and potassium are administered to prevent hypovolemia and hypokalemia. Antidiarrheal agents are administered. Stenosis is caused by circular scar tissue that forms at the stoma site. The scar tissue must be surgically released. Urinary calculi may occur in patients with ileostomies and are at least partly attributed to dehydration from decreased fluid intake. Intense lower abdominal pain that radiates to the legs, hematuria, and signs of dehydration indicate that the urine should be strained. Fluid intake is encouraged. Sometimes, small stones are passed during urination; otherwise, treatment is necessary to crush or remove the calculi (see Chapter 45).

Cholelithiasis (ie, gallstones) occurs more commonly in patients with an ileostomy than in the general population because of changes in the absorption of bile acids that occur postoperatively. Spasm of the gallbladder causes severe upper right abdominal pain that can radiate to the back and right shoulder (see Chapter 40).

PROMOTING HOME AND COMMUNITY-BASED CARE

Teaching Patients Self-Care. The spouse and family should be familiar with the adjustments that will be necessary when the patient returns home. They need to know why it is necessary for the patient to occupy the bathroom for 10 minutes or more at certain times of the day and why certain equipment is needed. Their understanding is necessary to reduce tension; a relaxed patient tends to have fewer problems. Visits from an enterostomal therapist may be arranged to ensure that the patient is progressing as expected and to provide additional guidance and teaching as needed.

Continuing Care. The patient needs to know the commercial name of the drainable pouching system to be used so that he or she can obtain a ready supply and should know how to obtain other supplies. The names and contact information of a local enterostomal therapist and local self-help groups are often helpful. Any restrictions on driving or working also need to be reviewed. The nurse teaches the patient about common postoperative complications and how to recognize and report them (Chart 38-7).

Intestinal Obstruction

Intestinal obstruction exists when blockage prevents the normal flow of intestinal contents through the intestinal tract. Two types of processes can impede this flow:

- *Mechanical obstruction:* An intraluminal obstruction or a mural obstruction from pressure on the intestinal wall occurs. Examples are intussusception, polypoid tumors and neoplasms, stenosis, strictures, adhesions, hernias, and abscesses.
- *Functional obstruction:* The intestinal musculature cannot propel the contents along the bowel. Examples are amyloidosis, muscular dystrophy, endocrine disorders such as diabetes mellitus, or neurologic disorders such as Parkinson's disease. The blockage also can be temporary and the result of the manipulation of the bowel during surgery.

The obstruction can be partial or complete. Its severity depends on the region of bowel affected, the degree to which the lumen is occluded, and especially the degree to which the vascular supply to the bowel wall is disturbed.

Most bowel obstructions occur in the small intestine. Adhesions are the most common cause of small bowel obstruction, followed by hernias and neoplasms. Other causes include intussusception, volvulus (ie, twisting of the bowel), and paralytic ileus. Most obstructions in the large bowel occur in the sigmoid colon. The most common causes are carcinoma, diverticulitis, inflammatory bowel disorders, and benign tumors. Table 38-5 and Figure 38-6 list mechanical causes of obstruction and describe how they occur.

Small Bowel Obstruction

Pathophysiology

Intestinal contents, fluid, and gas accumulate above the intestinal obstruction. The abdominal distention and retention of fluid reduce the absorption of fluids and stimulate more gastric secretion. With increasing distention, pressure within the intestinal lumen increases, causing a decrease in venous and arteriolar capillary pressure. This causes edema, congestion, necrosis, and eventual rupture or perforation of the intestinal wall, with resultant peritonitis.

Reflux vomiting may be caused by abdominal distention. Vomiting results in loss of hydrogen ions and potassium from the stomach, leading to reduction of chlorides

CHART 38-7

HOME CARE CHECKLIST • Managing Ostomy Care

At the completion of the home care instruction, the patient or caregiver will be able to:	Patient	Caregiver
• Demonstrate ostomy care, including wound cleansing, irrigation, and appliance changing.	✔	✔
• Describe the importance of maintaining peristomal skin integrity.	✔	✔
• Identify sources for obtaining additional dressing and appliance supplies.	✔	✔
• Identify dietary restrictions (foods that can cause diarrhea and constipation).	✔	✔
• Identify measures to be used to promote fluid and electrolyte balance	✔	✔
• Describe medication regimen: identify medications by name, use, route, and frequency.	✔	✔
• Describe potential complications and necessary actions to be taken if complications occur.	✔	✔
• Identify how to contact enterostomal therapist or home health nurse.	✔	✔

TABLE 38-5 Mechanical Causes of Intestinal Obstruction

Cause	Course of Events	Result
Adhesions	Loops of intestine become adherent to areas that heal slowly or scar after abdominal surgery.	After surgery, adhesions produce a kinking of an intestinal loop.
Intussusception	One part of the intestine slips into another part located below it (like a telescope shortening).	The intestinal lumen becomes narrowed.
Volvulus	Bowel twists and turns on itself.	Intestinal lumen becomes obstructed. Gas and fluid accumulate in the trapped bowel.
Hernia	Protrusion of intestine through a weakened area in the abdominal muscle or wall.	Intestinal flow may be completely obstructed. Blood flow to the area may be obstructed as well.
Tumor	A tumor that exists within the wall of the intestine extends into the intestinal lumen, or a tumor outside the intestine causes pressure on the wall of the intestine.	Intestinal lumen becomes partially obstructed; if the tumor is not removed, complete obstruction results.

and potassium in the blood and to metabolic alkalosis. Dehydration and acidosis develop from loss of water and sodium. With acute fluid losses, hypovolemic shock may occur.

Clinical Manifestations

The initial symptom is usually crampy pain that is wavelike and colicky. The patient may pass blood and mucus but no fecal matter and no flatus. Vomiting occurs. If the obstruction is complete, the peristaltic waves initially become extremely vigorous and eventually assume a reverse direction, with the intestinal contents propelled toward the mouth instead of toward the rectum. If the obstruction is in the ileum, fecal vomiting takes place. First, the patient vomits the stomach contents, then the bile-stained contents of the duodenum and the jejunum, and finally, with each paroxysm of pain, the darker, fecal-like contents of the ileum. The signs of dehydration become evident: intense thirst, drowsiness, generalized malaise, aching, and a parched tongue and mucous membranes. The abdomen becomes distended. The lower the obstruction is in the GI tract, the more marked the abdominal distention. If the obstruction continues uncorrected, hypovolemic shock occurs from dehydration and loss of plasma volume.

Assessment and Diagnostic Findings

Diagnosis is based on the symptoms described previously and on imaging studies. Abdominal x-ray and CT findings include abnormal quantities of gas, fluid, or both in the intestines. Laboratory studies (ie, electrolyte studies and a complete blood cell count) reveal a picture of dehydration, loss of plasma volume, and possible infection.

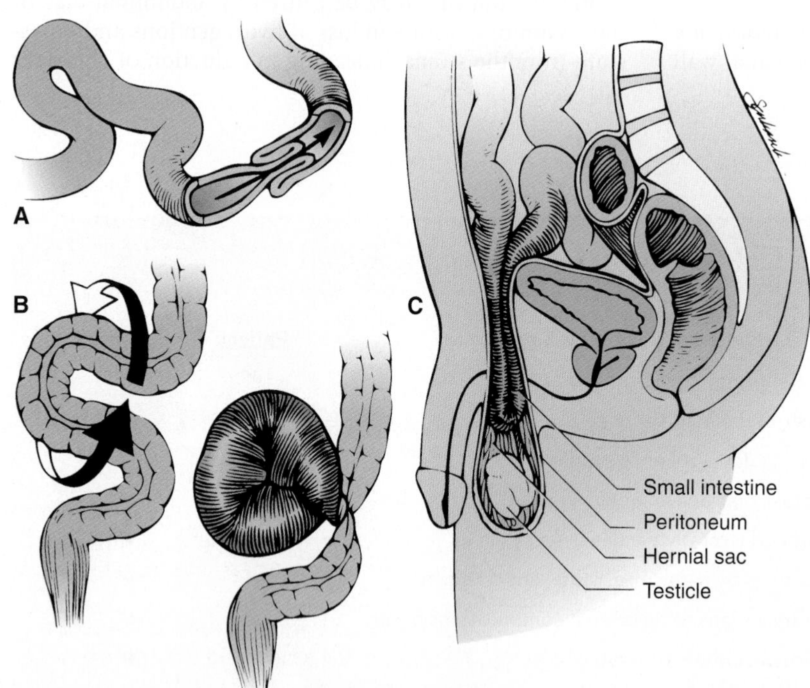

FIGURE 38-6. Three causes of intestinal obstruction. **(A)** Intussusception invagination or shortening of the colon caused by the movement of one segment of bowel into another. **(B)** Volvulus of the sigmoid colon; the twist is counterclockwise in most cases. Note the edematous bowel. **(C)** Hernia (inguinal). The sac of the hernia is a continuation of the peritoneum of the abdomen. The hernial contents are intestine, omentum, or other abdominal contents that pass through the hernial opening into the hernial sac.

Medical Management

Decompression of the bowel through a nasogastric tube (see Chapter 36) is successful in most cases. When the bowel is completely obstructed, the possibility of strangulation warrants surgical intervention. Before surgery, IV therapy is necessary to replace the depleted water, sodium, chloride, and potassium.

The surgical treatment of intestinal obstruction depends largely on the cause of the obstruction. In the most common causes of obstruction, such as hernia and adhesions, the surgical procedure involves repairing the hernia or dividing the adhesion to which the intestine is attached. In some instances, the portion of affected bowel may be removed and an anastomosis performed. The complexity of the surgical procedure for intestinal obstruction depends on the duration of the obstruction and the condition of the intestine.

Nursing Management

Nursing management of the nonsurgical patient with a small bowel obstruction includes maintaining the function of the nasogastric tube, assessing and measuring the nasogastric output, assessing for fluid and electrolyte imbalance, monitoring nutritional status, and assessing improvement (eg, return of normal bowel sounds, decreased abdominal distention, subjective improvement in abdominal pain and tenderness, passage of flatus or stool). The nurse reports discrepancies in intake and output, worsening of pain or abdominal distention, and increased nasogastric output. If the patient's condition does not improve, the nurse prepares him or her for surgery. The exact nature of the surgery depends on the cause of the obstruction. Nursing care of the patient after surgical repair of a small bowel obstruction is similar to that for other abdominal surgeries (see Chapter 20).

Large Bowel Obstruction

Pathophysiology

As in small bowel obstruction, large bowel obstruction results in an accumulation of intestinal contents, fluid, and gas proximal to the obstruction. Obstruction in the large bowel can lead to severe distention and perforation unless some gas and fluid can flow back through the ileal valve. Large bowel obstruction, even if complete, may be undramatic if the blood supply to the colon is not disturbed. However, if the blood supply is cut off, intestinal strangulation and necrosis (ie, tissue death) occur; this condition is life threatening. In the large intestine, dehydration occurs more slowly than in the small intestine because the colon can absorb its fluid contents and can distend to a size considerably beyond its normal full capacity.

Adenocarcinoid tumors account for the majority of large bowel obstructions. Most tumors occur beyond the splenic flexure, making them accessible with a flexible sigmoidoscope.

Clinical Manifestations

Large bowel obstruction differs clinically from small bowel obstruction in that the symptoms develop and progress relatively slowly. In patients with obstruction in the sigmoid colon or the rectum, constipation may be the only symptom for months. The shape of the stool is altered as it passes the obstruction that is gradually increasing in size. Blood in the stool may result in iron deficiency anemia. The patient may experience weakness, weight loss, and anorexia. Eventually, the abdomen becomes markedly distended, loops of large bowel become visibly outlined through the abdominal wall, and the patient has crampy lower abdominal pain. Finally, fecal vomiting develops. Symptoms of shock may occur.

Assessment and Diagnostic Findings

Diagnosis is based on symptoms and on imaging studies. Abdominal x-ray and abdominal CT or MRI findings reveal a distended colon and pinpoint the site of the obstruction. Barium studies are contraindicated.

Medical Management

Restoration of intravascular volume, correction of electrolyte abnormalities, and nasogastric aspiration and decompression are instituted immediately. A colonoscopy may be performed to untwist and decompress the bowel. A cecostomy, in which a surgical opening is made into the cecum, may be performed in patients who are poor surgical risks and urgently need relief from the obstruction. The procedure provides an outlet for releasing gas and a small amount of drainage. A rectal tube may be used to decompress an area that is lower in the bowel. However, the usual treatment is surgical resection to remove the obstructing lesion. A temporary or permanent colostomy may be necessary. An ileoanal anastomosis may be performed if it is necessary to remove the entire large bowel.

Nursing Management

The nurse's role is to monitor the patient for symptoms that indicate that the intestinal obstruction is worsening and to provide emotional support and comfort. The nurse administers IV fluids and electrolytes as prescribed. If the patient's condition does not respond to nonsurgical treatment, the nurse prepares the patient for surgery. This preparation includes preoperative teaching as the patient's condition indicates. After surgery, general abdominal wound care and routine postoperative nursing care are provided.

Colorectal Cancer

Tumors of the colon and rectum are relatively common; the colorectal area (the colon and rectum combined) is now the third most common site of new cancer cases and deaths in the United States. Colorectal cancer is a disease of Western cultures. Almost 150,000 new cases and 56,000 deaths from colorectal cancer occur annually (American Cancer Society [ACS], 2006).

The incidence increases with age (the incidence is highest in people older than 85 years) and is higher in people with a family history of colon cancer and those with IBD or polyps. The exact cause of colon and rectal cancer is still unknown, but risk factors have been identified (Chart 38-8).

Improved screening strategies have helped reduce the number of deaths from colon cancer in recent years. Of the approximately 150,000 people diagnosed each year, fewer than half that number die annually (ACS, 2006). Early diagnosis and prompt treatment could save almost three of every four people. If the disease is detected and treated at an early stage, the 5-year survival rate is 90%; however, only 34% of colorectal cancers are detected at an early stage (ACS, 2006). Survival rates after late diagnosis are very low. Most people are asymptomatic for long periods and seek health care only when they notice a change in bowel habits or rectal bleeding. Prevention and early screening are key to detection and reduction of mortality rates.

Pathophysiology

Cancer of the colon and rectum is predominantly (95%) adenocarcinoma (ie, arising from the epithelial lining of the intestine) (ACS, 2006). It may start as a benign polyp but may become malignant, invade and destroy normal tissues, and extend into surrounding structures. Cancer cells may migrate away from the primary tumor and spread to other parts of the body (most often to the liver).

Clinical Manifestations

The symptoms are greatly determined by the location of the cancer, the stage of the disease, and the function of the intestinal segment in which it is located. The most common presenting symptom is a change in bowel habits. The passage of blood in the stools is the second most common symptom. Symptoms may also include unexplained anemia, anorexia, weight loss, and fatigue.

The symptoms most commonly associated with right-sided lesions are dull abdominal pain and melena (ie, black, tarry stools). The symptoms most commonly associated with left-sided lesions are those associated with obstruction (ie, abdominal pain and cramping, narrowing stools, constipation, distention), as well as bright-red blood in the stool. Symptoms associated with rectal lesions are tenesmus (ie, ineffective, painful straining at stool), rectal pain, the feeling of incomplete evacuation after a bowel movement, alternating constipation and diarrhea, and bloody stool.

CHART 38-8

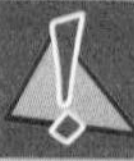

Risk Factors for Colorectal Cancer

- Increasing age
- Family history of colon cancer or polyps
- Previous colon cancer or adenomatous polyps
- History of inflammatory bowel disease
- High-fat, high-protein (with high intake of beef), low-fiber diet
- Genital cancer (eg, endometrial cancer, ovarian cancer) or breast cancer (in women)

Assessment and Diagnostic Findings

Along with an abdominal and rectal examination, the most important diagnostic procedures for cancer of the colon are fecal occult blood testing, barium enema, proctosigmoidoscopy, and colonoscopy (see Chapter 34). The majority of colorectal cancer cases can be identified by colonoscopy with biopsy or cytology smears.

Carcinoembryonic antigen (CEA) studies may also be performed. Although CEA may not be a highly reliable indicator in diagnosing colon cancer because not all lesions secrete CEA, studies show that CEA levels are reliable prognostic predictors. With complete excision of the tumor, the elevated levels of CEA should return to normal within 48 hours. Elevations of CEA at a later date suggest recurrence.

Complications

Tumor growth may cause partial or complete bowel obstruction. Extension of the tumor and ulceration into the surrounding blood vessels result in hemorrhage. Perforation, abscess formation, peritonitis, sepsis, and shock may occur.

Gerontologic Considerations

The incidence of carcinoma of the colon and rectum increases with age. These cancers are considered common malignancies in advanced age. In men, only the incidence of prostate cancer and lung cancer exceeds that of colorectal cancer. In women, only the incidence of breast cancer exceeds that of colorectal cancer. Symptoms are often insidious. Patients with colorectal cancer usually report fatigue, which is caused primarily by iron deficiency anemia. In early stages, minor changes in bowel patterns and occasional bleeding may occur. The later symptoms most commonly reported by the elderly are abdominal pain, obstruction, tenesmus, and rectal bleeding.

Colon cancer in the elderly has been closely associated with dietary carcinogens. Lack of fiber is a major causative factor because the passage of feces through the intestinal tract is prolonged, which extends exposure to possible carcinogens. Excess dietary fat, high alcohol consumption, and smoking all increase the incidence of colorectal tumors. Physical activity and dietary folate have protective effects (Varricchio, Ades, Hinds, et al., 2004).

Medical Management

The patient with symptoms of intestinal obstruction is treated with IV fluids and nasogastric suction. If there has been significant bleeding, blood component therapy may be required.

Treatment for colorectal cancer depends on the stage of the disease (Chart 38-9) and consists of surgery to remove the tumor, supportive therapy, and adjuvant therapy. Patients

CHART 38-9

Staging of Colorectal Cancer: Dukes' Classification–Modified Staging System

Class A: Tumor limited to muscular mucosa and submucosa
Class B_1: Tumor extends into mucosa
Class B_2: Tumor extends through entire bowel wall into serosa or pericolic fat, no nodal involvement
Class C_1: Positive nodes, tumor is limited to bowel wall
Class C_2: Positive nodes, tumor extends through entire bowel wall
Class D: Advanced and metastasis to liver, lung, or bone

Another staging system, the TNM (tumor, nodal involvement, metastasis) classification, may be used to describe the anatomic extent of the primary tumor, depending on:

- Size, invasion depth, and surface spread
- Extent of nodal involvement
- Presence or absence of metastasis

Rudy, D. R., & Zdon, M. J. (2000). Update on colorectal cancer. *American Family Physician, 61*(6), 1759–1774.

who receive some form of adjuvant therapy, which may include chemotherapy, radiation therapy, immunotherapy, or multimodality therapy, typically demonstrate delays in tumor recurrence and increases in survival time.

Adjuvant Therapy

The standard adjuvant therapy administered to patients with Dukes' class C colon cancer is the 5-fluorouracil plus levamisole regimen. Patients with Dukes' class B or C rectal cancer are given 5-fluorouracil and high doses of pelvic irradiation. Mitomycin is also used. Radiation therapy is used before, during, and after surgery to shrink the tumor, to achieve better results from surgery, and to reduce the risk of recurrence. For inoperative or unresectable tumors, radiation is used to provide significant relief from symptoms. Intracavitary and implantable devices are used to deliver radiation to the site. The response to adjuvant therapy varies.

Surgical Management

Surgery is the primary treatment for most colon and rectal cancers. It may be curative or palliative. Advances in surgical techniques can enable the patient with cancer to have sphincter-saving devices that restore continuity of the GI tract. The type of surgery recommended depends on the location and size of the tumor. Cancers limited to one site can be removed through the colonoscope. Laparoscopic colotomy with polypectomy minimizes the extent of surgery needed in some cases. A laparoscope is used as a guide in making an incision into the colon; the tumor mass is then excised. Use of the neodymium/yttrium-aluminum-garnet (Nd:YAG) laser has proved effective with some lesions as well. Bowel resection is indicated for most class A lesions and all class B and C lesions. Surgery is sometimes recommended for class D colon cancer, but the goal of surgery in this instance is palliative; if the tumor has spread and involves surrounding vital structures, it is considered nonresectable.

Surgical procedures include the following:

- Segmental resection with anastomosis (ie, removal of the tumor and portions of the bowel on either side of the growth, as well as the blood vessels and lymphatic nodes) (Fig. 38-7)
- Abdominoperineal resection with permanent sigmoid colostomy (ie, removal of the tumor and a portion of the sigmoid and all of the rectum and anal sphincter) (Fig. 38-8)
- Temporary colostomy followed by segmental resection and anastomosis and subsequent reanastomosis of the colostomy, allowing initial bowel decompression and bowel preparation before resection
- Permanent colostomy or ileostomy for palliation of unresectable obstructing lesions
- Construction of a coloanal reservoir called a colonic J pouch, which is performed in two steps. A temporary loop ileostomy is constructed to divert intestinal flow, and the newly constructed J pouch (made from 6 to 10 cm of colon) is reattached to the anal stump. About 3 months after the initial stage, the ileostomy is reversed and intestinal continuity is restored. The anal sphincter and therefore continence are preserved.

A **colostomy** is the surgical creation of an opening (ie, stoma) into the colon. It can be created as a temporary or permanent fecal diversion. It allows the drainage or evacuation of colon contents to the outside of the body. The consistency of the drainage is related to the placement of the colostomy, which is dictated by the location of the tumor and the extent of invasion into surrounding tissues (Fig. 38-9). With improved surgical techniques, colostomies are performed in fewer than one third of patients with colorectal cancer.

GERONTOLOGIC CONSIDERATIONS

The elderly are at increased risk of complications after surgery and may have difficulty managing colostomy care. Some elderly patients may have decreased vision, impaired hearing, and difficulty with fine motor coordination. It may be helpful for patients to handle ostomy equipment and simulate cleaning the peristomal skin and irrigating the stoma before surgery. Skin care is a major concern in older patients with a colostomy because of the skin changes that occur with aging—the epithelial and subcutaneous fatty layers become thin, and the skin is irritated easily. To prevent skin breakdown, special attention is paid to skin cleansing and the proper fit of an appliance. Arteriosclerosis causes decreased blood flow to the wound and stoma site. As a result, transport of nutrients is delayed, and healing time may be prolonged. Some patients have delayed elimination after irrigation because of decreased peristalsis and mucus production. Most patients require 6 months before they feel comfortable with their ostomy care.

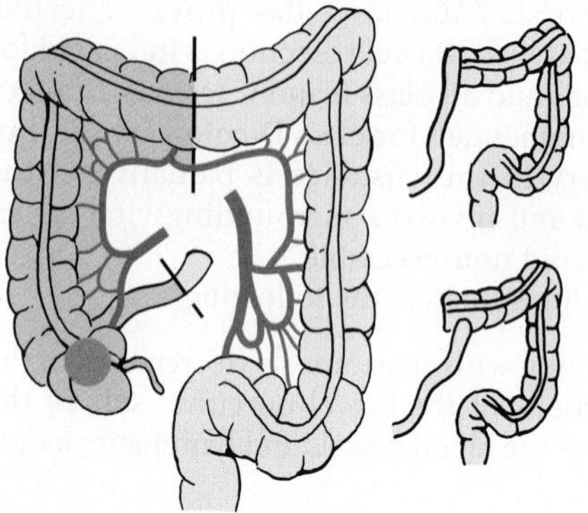
Cecum and lower ascending colon

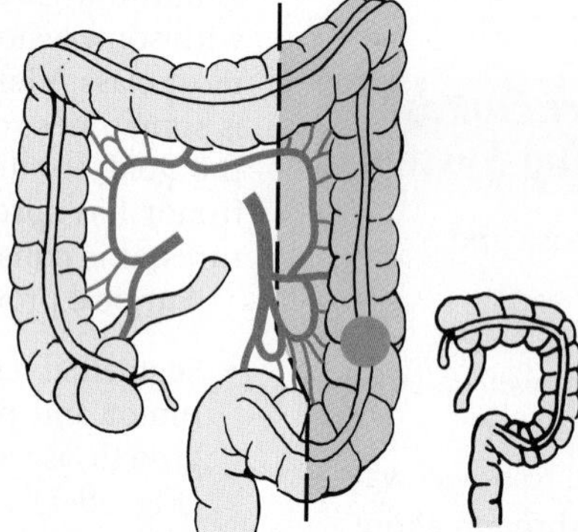
Descending colon and upper sigmoid

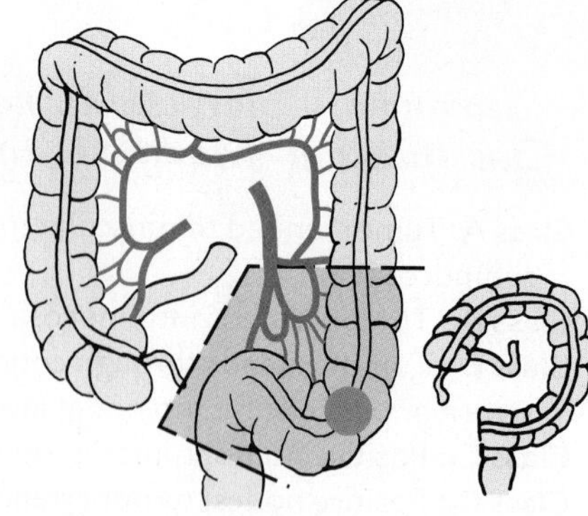
Low sigmoid and upper rectum

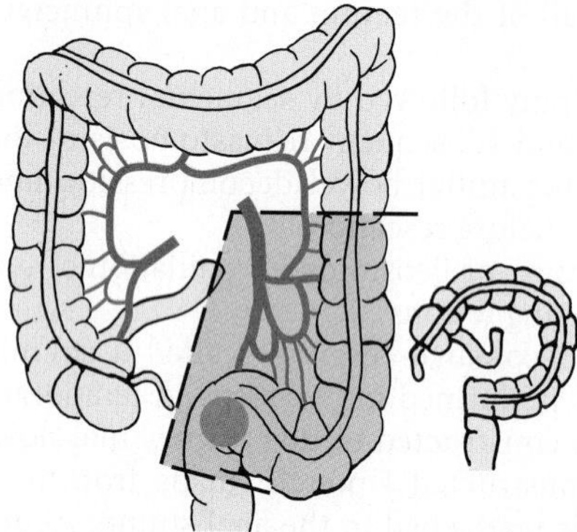
Rectal sigmoid resection

FIGURE 38-7. Examples of areas where cancer can occur, the area that is removed, and how the anastomosis is performed (*small diagrams*).

Nursing Process

The Patient With Colorectal Cancer

Assessment

The nurse obtains a health history about the presence of fatigue, abdominal or rectal pain (eg, location, frequency, duration, association with eating or defecation), past and present elimination patterns, and characteristics of stool (eg, color, odor, consistency, presence of blood or mucus). Additional information includes a history of IBD or colorectal polyps, a family history of colorectal disease, and current medication therapy. The nurse identifies dietary habits, including fat and fiber intake, as well as amounts of alcohol consumed and history of smoking. The nurse describes and documents a history of weight loss and feelings of weakness and fatigue.

Assessment includes auscultation of the abdomen for bowel sounds and palpation of the abdomen for areas of tenderness, distention, and solid masses. Stool specimens are inspected for character and presence of blood.

Diagnosis

Nursing Diagnoses

Based on the assessment data, the major nursing diagnoses may include the following:

- Imbalanced nutrition, less than body requirements, related to nausea and anorexia
- Risk for deficient fluid volume related to vomiting and dehydration
- Anxiety related to impending surgery and the diagnosis of cancer
- Risk for ineffective therapeutic regimen management related to knowledge deficit concerning the diagnosis, the surgical procedure, and self-care after discharge
- Impaired skin integrity related to the surgical incisions (abdominal and perianal), the formation of a stoma, and frequent fecal contamination of peristomal skin
- Disturbed body image related to colostomy
- Ineffective sexuality patterns related to presence of ostomy and changes in body image and self-concept

Collaborative Problems/ Potential Complications

Potential complications that may develop include the following:

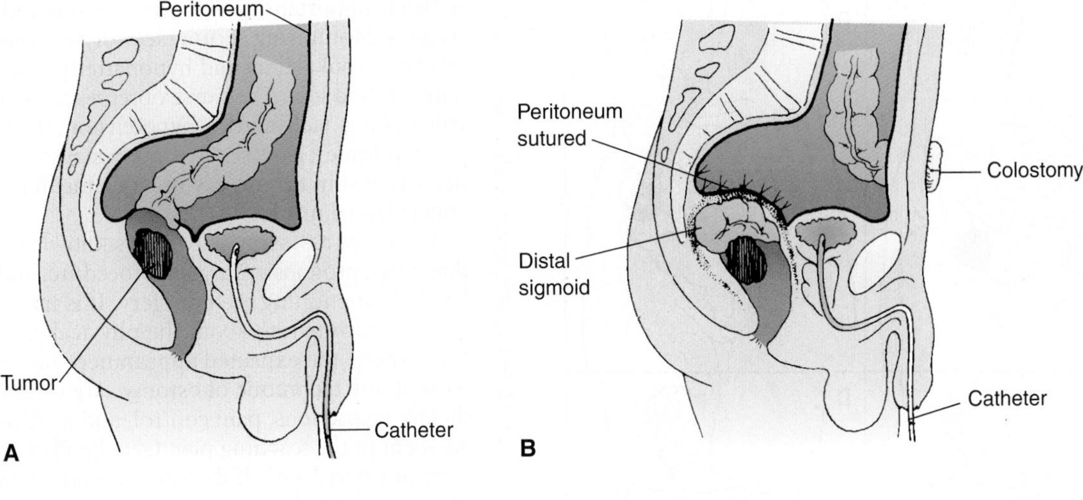

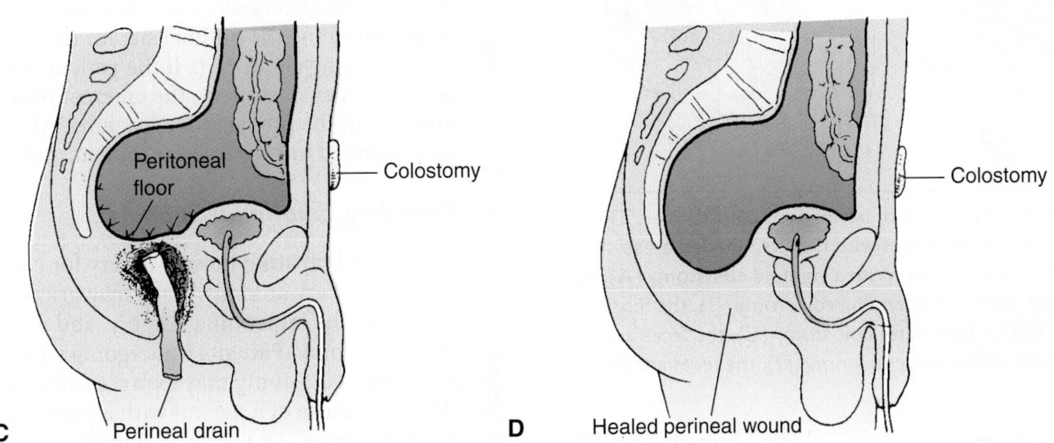

FIGURE 38-8. Abdominoperineal resection for carcinoma of the rectum. (**A**) Prior to surgery. Note tumor in rectum. (**B**) During surgery, the sigmoid is removed and the colostomy is established. The distal bowel is dissected free to a point below the pelvic peritoneum, which is sutured over the closed end of the distal sigmoid and rectum. (**C**) Perineal resection includes removal of the rectum and free portion of the sigmoid from below. A perineal drain is inserted. (**D**) The final result after healing. Note the healed perineal wound and the permanent colostomy.

- Intraperitoneal infection
- Complete large bowel obstruction
- GI bleeding
- Bowel perforation
- Peritonitis, abscess, and sepsis

Planning and Goals

The major goals for the patient may include attainment of optimal level of nutrition; maintenance of fluid and electrolyte balance; reduction of anxiety; learning about the diagnosis, surgical procedure, and self-care after discharge; maintenance of optimal tissue healing; protection of peristomal skin; learning how to irrigate the colostomy and change the appliance; expressing feelings and concerns about the colostomy and the impact on himself or herself; and avoidance of complications.

Nursing Interventions

Preparing the Patient for Surgery

The patient awaiting surgery for colorectal cancer has many concerns, needs, and fears. He or she may be physically debilitated and emotionally distraught with concerns about lifestyle changes after surgery, prognosis, ability to perform in established roles, and finances. Priorities for nursing care include preparing the patient physically for surgery; providing information about postoperative care, including stoma care if a colostomy is to be created; and supporting the patient and family emotionally.

Physical preparation for surgery involves building the patient's stamina in the days preceding surgery and cleansing and sterilizing the bowel the day before surgery. If the patient's condition permits, the nurse

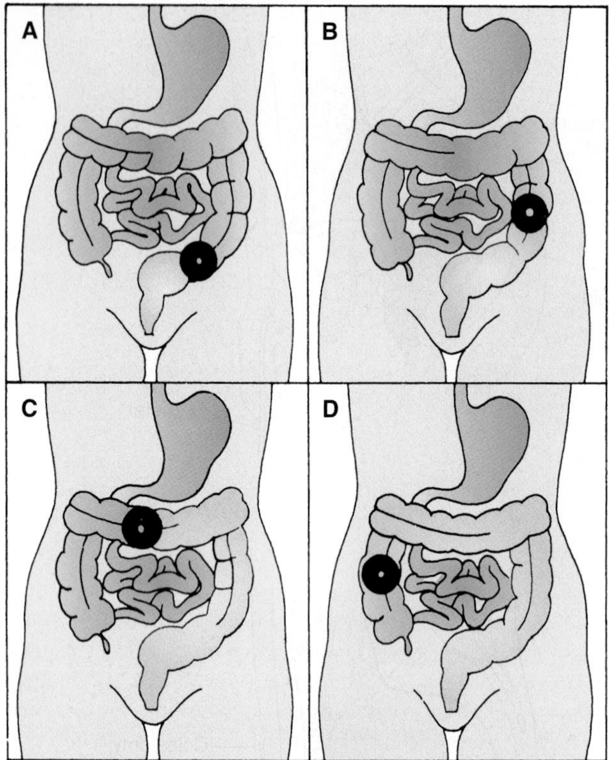

FIGURE 38-9. Placement of permanent colostomies. The nature of the discharge varies with the site. Shaded areas show sections of bowel removed. With a sigmoid colostomy (**A**), the feces are solid. With a descending colostomy (**B**), the feces are semimushy. With a transverse colostomy (**C**), the feces are mushy. With an ascending colostomy (**D**), the feces are fluid.

recommends a diet high in calories, protein, and carbohydrates and low in residue for several days before surgery to provide adequate nutrition and minimize cramping by decreasing excessive peristalsis. A full liquid diet may be prescribed 24 to 48 hours before surgery to decrease bulk. If the patient is hospitalized in the days preceding surgery, parenteral nutrition may be required to replace depleted nutrients, vitamins, and minerals. In some instances, parenteral nutrition is administered at home before surgery. Antibiotics such as kanamycin (Kantrex), neomycin (Mycifradin), and cephalexin (Keflex) are administered orally the day before surgery to reduce intestinal bacteria. The bowel is cleansed with laxatives, enemas, or colonic irrigations the evening before and the morning of surgery.

For the patient who is very ill and hospitalized, the nurse measures and records intake and output, including vomitus, to provide an accurate record of fluid balance. The patient's intake of oral food and fluids may be restricted to prevent vomiting. The nurse administers antiemetics as prescribed. Full or clear liquids may be tolerated, or the patient may be allowed nothing by mouth. A nasogastric tube may be inserted to drain accumulated fluids and prevent abdominal distention. The nurse monitors the abdomen for increasing distention, loss of bowel sounds, and pain or rigidity, which may indicate obstruction or perforation.

It also is important to monitor IV fluids and electrolytes. Monitoring serum electrolyte levels can detect the hypokalemia and hyponatremia that occur with GI fluid loss. The nurse observes for signs of hypovolemia (eg, tachycardia, hypotension, decreased pulse volume); assesses hydration status; and reports decreased skin turgor, dry mucous membranes, and concentrated urine.

The nurse assesses the patient's knowledge about the diagnosis, prognosis, surgical procedure, and expected level of functioning after surgery. It is important to include information about the physical preparation for surgery, the expected appearance and care of the wound, the technique of ostomy care (if applicable), dietary restrictions, pain control, and medication management in the teaching plan (see the Plan of Nursing Care in Chart 38-4). If the patient is admitted the day of surgery, the physician's office may arrange for the patient to be seen by an enterostomal therapist in the days preceding surgery. The enterostomal therapist helps determine the optimal site for the stoma and provides teaching about care. If the patient is hospitalized before the day of surgery, the enterostomal therapist is involved in the preoperative teaching. All procedures are explained in language the patient understands.

Providing Emotional Support

Patients anticipating bowel surgery for colorectal cancer may be very anxious. They may grieve about the diagnosis, the impending surgery, and possible permanent colostomy. Patients undergoing surgery for a temporary colostomy may express fears and concerns similar to those of a person with a permanent stoma. All members of the health care team, including the enterostomal therapist, should be available for assistance and support. The nurse's role is to assess the patient's anxiety level and coping mechanisms and suggest methods for reducing anxiety, such as deep-breathing exercises and visualizing a successful recovery from surgery and cancer. Other supportive measures include providing privacy and teaching relaxation techniques to the patient. Time is set aside to listen to the patient who wishes to talk, cry, or ask questions. The nurse can arrange a meeting with a spiritual advisor if the patient desires or with the physicians if the patient wishes to discuss the treatment or prognosis. To promote patient comfort, the nurse projects a relaxed, professional, and empathetic attitude.

The patient undergoing a colostomy may find the anticipated changes in body image and lifestyle profoundly disturbing. Because the stoma is located on the abdomen, the patient may think that everyone will be aware of the ostomy. The nurse helps reduce this fear by presenting facts about the surgical procedure and the creation and management of the ostomy. If the patient is receptive, the nurse can use diagrams, photographs, and appliances to explain and clarify. Because the patient is experiencing emotional stress, the nurse may need to repeat some of the information. The nurse provides time for the patient and family to ask questions; the nurse's acceptance and understanding of the patient's concerns and feelings convey a caring, competent attitude that promotes confidence and cooperation. Consultation with an enterostomal therapist during the preoperative period can be extremely helpful, as can speaking with a person who is successfully managing a colostomy. The United Ostomy Association provides useful information about living with an ostomy through literature, lectures, and exhibits. Visiting services by qualified members and rehabilitation services for patients with new ostomies are provided.

Providing Postoperative Care

Postoperative nursing care for patients undergoing colon resection or colostomy is similar to nursing care for any abdominal surgery patient (see Chapter 20), including pain management during the immediate postoperative period. The nurse also monitors the patient for complications such as leakage from the site of the anastomosis, prolapse of the stoma, perforation, stoma retraction, fecal impaction, skin irritation, and pulmonary complications associated with abdominal surgery. The nurse assesses the abdomen for returning peristalsis and assesses the initial stool characteristics. It is important to help patients with a colostomy out of bed on the first postoperative day and encourage them to begin participating in managing the colostomy.

Maintaining Optimal Nutrition

The nurse teaches all patients undergoing surgery for colorectal cancer about the health benefits to be derived from consuming a healthy diet. The diet is individualized as long as it is nutritionally sound and does not cause diarrhea or constipation. The return to normal diet is rapid.

A complete nutritional assessment is important for the patient with a colostomy. The patient avoids foods that cause excessive odor and gas, including foods in the cabbage family, eggs, fish, beans, and high-cellulose products such as peanuts. It is important to determine whether the elimination of specific foods is causing any nutritional deficiency. Nonirritating foods are substituted for those that are restricted so that deficiencies are corrected. The nurse advises the patient to experiment with an irritating food several times before restricting it, because an initial sensitivity may decrease with time. The nurse can help the patient identify any foods or fluids that may be causing diarrhea, such as fruits, high-fiber foods, soda, coffee, tea, or carbonated beverages. Diphenoxylate with atropine (Lomotil) may be prescribed as needed to control the diarrhea. For constipation, prune or apple juice or a mild laxative is effective. The nurse suggests fluid intake of at least 2 L per day.

Providing Wound Care

The nurse frequently examines the abdominal dressing during the first 24 hours after surgery to detect signs of hemorrhage. It is important to help the patient splint the abdominal incision during coughing and deep breathing to lessen tension on the edges of the incision. The nurse monitors temperature, pulse, and respiratory rate for elevations, which may indicate an infectious process. If the patient has a colostomy, the stoma is examined for swelling (slight edema from surgical manipulation is normal), color (a healthy stoma is pink or red), discharge (a small amount of oozing is normal), and bleeding (an abnormal sign).

If the malignancy has been removed using the perineal route, the perineal wound is observed for signs of hemorrhage. This wound may contain a drain or packing, which is removed gradually. Bits of tissue may slough off for a week. This process is hastened by mechanical irrigation of the wound or with sitz baths performed two or three times each day initially. The condition of the perineal wound and any bleeding, infection, or necrosis are documented.

Monitoring and Managing Complications

The patient is observed for signs and symptoms of complications. It is important to frequently assess the abdomen, including decreasing or changing bowel sounds and increasing abdominal girth, to detect bowel obstruction. The nurse monitors vital signs for increased temperature, pulse, and respirations and for decreased blood pressure, which may indicate an intra-abdominal infectious process. It is important to report rectal bleeding immediately because it indicates hemorrhage. The nurse monitors hemoglobin and hematocrit levels and administers blood component therapy as prescribed. Any abrupt change in abdominal pain is reported promptly. Elevated white blood cell counts and temperature or symptoms of shock are reported because they may indicate sepsis. The nurse administers antibiotics as prescribed.

Pulmonary complications are always a concern with abdominal surgery; patients older than 50 years are at risk, especially if they are or have been receiving sedatives or are being maintained on bed rest for a prolonged period. Two major pulmonary complications are pneumonia and atelectasis. Frequent activity (eg, turning the patient from side to side every 2 hours), deep breathing, coughing, and early ambulation can reduce the risk for these complications. Table 38-6 lists postoperative complications.

The incidence of complications related to the colostomy is about half that of an ileostomy. Some common complications are prolapse of the stoma (usually from obesity), perforation (from improper stoma irrigation), stoma retraction, fecal impaction, and skin irritation. Leakage from an anastomotic site can occur if the remaining bowel segments are diseased or weakened. Leakage from an intestinal anastomosis causes peritonitis with abdominal distention and rigidity, temperature elevation, and signs of shock. Surgical repair is necessary.

Removing and Applying the Colostomy Appliance

The colostomy begins to function 3 to 6 days after surgery. The nurse manages the colostomy and

TABLE 38-6 Potential Complications and Nursing Interventions After Intestinal Surgery

Complication	Nursing Interventions
General Complications	
Paralytic ileus	Initiate or continue nasogastric intubation as prescribed. Prepare patient for x-ray study. Ensure adequate fluid and electrolyte replacement. Administer prescribed antibiotics if patient has symptoms of peritonitis.
Mechanical obstruction	Assess patient for intermittent colicky pain, nausea, and vomiting.
Intra-abdominal Septic Conditions	
Peritonitis	Evaluate patient for nausea, hiccups, chills, spiking fever, tachycardia. Administer antibiotics as prescribed. Prepare patient for drainage procedure. Administer parenteral fluid and electrolyte therapy as prescribed. Prepare patient for surgery if condition deteriorates.
Abscess formation	Administer antibiotics as prescribed. Apply warm compresses as prescribed. Prepare for surgical drainage.
Surgical Wound Complications	
Infection	Monitor temperature; report temperature elevation. Observe for redness, tenderness, and pain around the surgical wound. Assist in establishing local drainage. Obtain specimen of drainage material for culture and sensitivity studies.
Wound disruption	Observe for sudden drainage of profuse serous fluid from wound. Cover wound area with sterile towels held in place with binder. Prepare patient immediately for surgery.
Intraperitoneal infection and abdominal wound infection	Monitor for evidence of constant or generalized abdominal pain, rapid pulse, and elevation of temperature. Prepare for tube decompression of bowel. Administer fluids and electrolytes by IV route as prescribed. Administer antibiotics as prescribed.
Anastomotic Complications	
Dehiscence of anastomosis	Prepare patient for surgery.
Fistulas	Assist in bowel decompression. Administer parenteral fluids as prescribed to correct fluid and electrolyte deficits.

teaches the patient about its care until the patient can take over its management. The nurse teaches skin care and how to apply and remove the drainage pouch. Care of the peristomal skin is an ongoing concern because excoriation or ulceration can develop quickly. The presence of such irritation makes adhering the ostomy appliance difficult, and adhering the ostomy appliance to irritated skin can worsen the skin condition. The effluent discharge and the degree to which it is irritating vary with the type of ostomy. With a transverse colostomy, the stool is soft and mushy and irritating to the skin. With a descending or sigmoid colostomy, the stool is fairly solid and less irritating to the skin. Other skin problems include yeast infections and allergic dermatitis.

If the patient wants to bathe or shower before putting on the clean appliance, micropore tape applied to the sides of the pouch will keep it secure during bathing. To remove the appliance, the patient assumes a comfortable sitting or standing position and gently pushes the skin down from the faceplate while pulling the pouch up and away from the stoma. Gentle pressure prevents the skin from being traumatized and any liquid fecal contents from spilling out. The nurse advises the patient to protect the peristomal skin by then washing the area gently with a moist, soft cloth and a mild soap. Soap acts as a mild abrasive agent to remove enzyme residue from fecal spillage. The patient should remove any excess skin barrier. While the skin is being cleansed, a gauze dressing can cover the stoma, or a vaginal tampon can be inserted gently to absorb excess drainage. After cleansing the skin, the patient pats the skin completely dry with a gauze pad, taking care not to rub the area. The patient can lightly dust nystatin (Mycostatin) powder on the peristomal skin if irritation or yeast growth is present.

Smoothly applying the drainage appliance for a secure fit requires practice and a well-fitting appliance. Patients can choose from a wide variety of appliances, depending on their individual needs. The stoma is measured to determine the correct size for the pouch; the pouch opening should be about 0.3 cm (1/8 in) larger than the stoma. After the skin is cleansed according to the previously described procedure, the patient applies the peristomal skin barrier (ie, wafer, paste, or powder). Mild skin irritation may require dusting the skin with karaya or Stomahesive powder before attaching the pouch. The patient removes the backing from the adherent surface of the appliance and applies pressure over the adhesive backing for approximately 30 seconds to ensure adherence over the stoma. The patient empties or changes the drainage appliance when it is one-third to one-fourth full so that the weight of its contents does not cause the appliance to separate from the adhesive disk and spill the contents. Most appliances are disposable and odor-resistant; commercially prepared deodorizers are available.

For some patients, colostomy appliances are not always necessary. As soon as the patient has learned a routine for evacuation, bags may be dispensed with, and a closed ostomy appliance or a simple dressing of disposable tissue (often covered with plastic wrap) is used, held in place by an elastic belt. Except for gas and a slight amount of mucus, nothing escapes from the colostomy opening between irrigations. Colostomy plugs that expand on insertion to prevent passage of flatus and feces are available.

Irrigating the Colostomy

The purpose of irrigating a colostomy is to empty the colon of gas, mucus, and feces so that the patient can go about social and business activities without fear of fecal drainage. A stoma does not have voluntary muscular control and may empty at irregular intervals. Regulating the passage of fecal material is achieved by irrigating the colostomy or allowing the bowel to evacuate naturally without irrigations. The choice often depends on the person and the type of the colostomy. By irrigating the stoma at a regular time, there is less gas and retention of the irrigant. The time for irrigating the colostomy should be consistent with the schedule the person will follow after leaving the hospital. Chart 38-10 describes the irrigating procedure.

Supporting a Positive Body Image

The patient is encouraged to verbalize feelings and concerns about altered body image and to discuss the surgery and the stoma (if one was created). A supportive environment and a supportive attitude on the nurse's part are crucial in promoting the patient's adaptation to the changes brought about by the surgery. If applicable, the patient must learn colostomy care and begin to plan for incorporating stoma care into daily life. The nurse helps the patient overcome aversion to the stoma or fear of self-injury by providing care and teaching in an open, accepting manner and by encouraging the patient to talk about his or her feelings about the stoma. The nurse's positive, supportive facial expression and other nonverbal cues help the patient develop a positive attitude toward independent stoma care.

Discussing Sexuality Issues

The nurse encourages the patient to discuss feelings about sexuality and sexual function. Some patients may initiate questions about sexual activity directly or give indirect clues about their fears. Some may view the surgery as mutilating and a threat to their sexuality; some fear impotence. Others may express worry about odor or leakage from the pouch during sexual activity. Although the appliance presents no deterrent to sexual activity, some patients wear silk or cotton covers and smaller pouches during sex. Alternative sexual positions are recommended, as well as alternative methods of stimulation to satisfy sexual drives. The nurse assesses the patient's needs and attempts to identify specific concerns. If the nurse is uncomfortable with this or if the patient's concerns seem complex, it is appropriate for the nurse to seek assistance from an enterostomal therapist, sex counselor or therapist, or advanced practice nurse.

Promoting Home and Community-Based Care

TEACHING PATIENTS SELF-CARE

Patient education and discharge planning require the combined efforts of the physician, nurse, enterostomal therapist, social worker, and dietitian. Patients are given specific information, individualized to their needs, about ostomy care and signs and symptoms of potential complications. Dietary instructions are essential to help patients identify and eliminate irritating foods that can cause diarrhea or constipation. It is important to teach patients about their prescribed medications (ie, action, purpose, and possible side and toxic effects).

The nurse reviews treatments (eg, irrigations, wound cleansing) and dressing changes and encourages the family to participate. Because the hospital stay is short, the patient may not be able to become proficient in stoma care techniques before discharge home. Many patients need referral to a home care agency and the telephone number of the local chapter of the American Cancer Society. The home care nurse goes to the home to provide further care and teaching and to assess how well the patient and family are adjusting to the colostomy. The home environment is assessed for adequacy of resources that allow the patient to manage self-care activities. A family member may assume responsibility for purchasing the equipment and supplies needed at home.

Patients need very specific directions about when to call the physician. They need to know which complications require prompt attention (ie, bleeding, abdominal distention and rigidity, diarrhea, fever, wound drainage, and disruption of suture line). If radiation therapy is planned, the possible side effects (ie, anorexia, vomiting, diarrhea, fatigue) are reviewed.

CHART 38-10 Guidelines for Irrigating a Colostomy

A colostomy is irrigated to empty the colon of feces, gas, or mucus, cleanse the lower intestinal tract, and establish a regular pattern of evacuation so that normal life activities may be pursued. A suitable time for the irrigation is selected that is compatible with the patient's posthospital pattern of activity (preferably after a meal). Irrigation should be performed at the same time each day.

Before the procedure, the patient sits on a chair in front of the toilet or on the toilet itself. An irrigating reservoir containing 500 to 1500 mL of lukewarm tapwater is hung 45 to 50 cm (18 to 20 in) above the stoma (shoulder height when the patient is seated). The dressing or pouch is removed. The following procedure is used; the patient is helped to participate in the procedure so he or she can learn to perform it unassisted.

NURSING ACTION	RATIONALE
1. Apply an irrigating sleeve or sheath to the stoma. Place the end in the commode.	1. This helps to control odor and splashing and allows feces and water to flow directly into the commode.

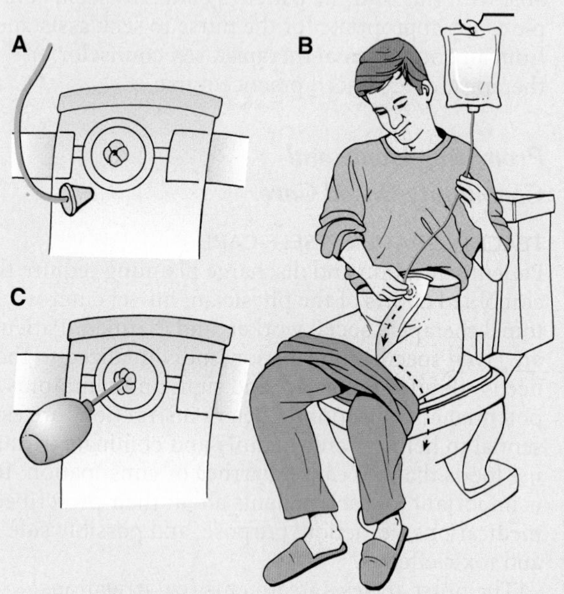

Colostomy irrigation. (**A**) Irrigating catheter has a cone attachment to prevent injury to stomal tissue. (**B**) Irrigating fluid is instilled with sleeve in place. Drainage contents empty into toilet. (**C**) The bulb syringe method can be used to stimulate fecal drainage. Note that a portion of the hard nozzle is removed and a catheter attached to minimize stomal irritation.

NURSING ACTION	RATIONALE
2. Allow some of the solution to flow through the tubing and catheter/cone.	2. Air bubbles in the setup are released so that air is not introduced into the colon, which would cause crampy pain.
3. Lubricate the catheter/cone and gently insert it into the stoma. Insert the catheter no more than 8 cm (3 in). Hold the shield/cone gently, but firmly, against the stoma to prevent backflow of water.	3. Lubrication permits ease of insertion of the catheter/cone.
4. If the catheter does not advance easily, allow water to flow slowly while advancing catheter. *Never force the catheter!*	4. A slow rate of flow helps to relax the bowel and facilitates passage of the catheter.
5. Allow tepid fluid to enter the colon slowly. If cramping occurs, clamp off the tubing and allow the patient to rest before progressing. Water should flow in over a 5- to 10-minute period.	5. Painful cramps usually are caused by too rapid a flow or by too much solution; 300 mL of fluid may be all that is needed to stimulate evacuation. Volume may be increased with subsequent irrigations to 500, 1000, or 1500 mL as needed by the patient for effective results.
6. Hold the shield/cone in place 10 seconds after the water has been instilled; then gently remove it.	6. This minimizes or eliminates spillage of water.

CHART 38-10 **Guidelines for Irrigating a Colostomy, continued**

NURSING ACTION	RATIONALE
7. Allow 10 to 15 minutes for most of the return; then dry the bottom of the sleeve/sheath and attach it to the top, or apply the appropriate clamp to the bottom of the sleeve.	7. Most of the water, feces, and flatus will be expelled in 10 to 15 minutes.
8. Leave the sleeve/sheath in place for 30 to 45 minutes while the patient gets up and moves around.	8. Ambulation stimulates peristalsis and completion of the irrigation return.
9. Cleanse the area with a mild soap and water; pat the area dry.	9. Cleanliness and dryness will provide the patient with hours of comfort.
10. Replace the colostomy dressing or appliance.	10. The patient should use an appliance until the colostomy is sufficiently controlled. Then a dressing may be all that is needed.

CONTINUING CARE

Ongoing care of the patient with cancer and a colostomy often extends well beyond the initial hospital stay. Home care nurses manage ostomy follow-up care, manage the assessment and care of the debilitated patient, and coordinate adjuvant therapy. The home visits also provide the nurse with opportunities to assess the patient's physical and emotional status and the patient's and family's ability to carry out recommended management strategies. Visits from an enterostomal therapist are available to the patient and family as they learn to care for the ostomy and work through their feelings about it, the diagnosis of cancer, and the future. Some patients are interested in and can benefit from involvement in an ostomy support group.

Evaluation

Expected Patient Outcomes

Expected patient outcomes may include the following:

1. Consumes a healthy diet
   a. Avoids foods and fluids that cause diarrhea
   b. Substitutes nonirritating foods and fluids for those that are restricted
2. Maintains fluid balance
   a. Experiences no vomiting or diarrhea
   b. Experiences no signs or symptoms of dehydration
3. Feels less anxious
   a. Expresses concerns and fears freely
   b. Uses coping measures to manage stress
4. Acquires information about diagnosis, surgical procedure, preoperative preparation, and self-care after discharge
   a. Discusses the diagnosis, surgical procedure, and postoperative self-care
   b. Demonstrates techniques of ostomy care
5. Maintains clean incision, stoma, and perineal wound
6. Expresses feelings and concerns about self
   a. Gradually increases participation in stoma and peristomal skin care
   b. Discusses feelings related to changed appearance
7. Discusses sexuality in relation to ostomy and to changes in body image
8. Recovers without complications
   a. Is afebrile
   b. Regains normal bowel activity
   c. Exhibits no signs and symptoms of perforation or bleeding
   d. Identifies signs and symptoms that should be reported to health care provider

Polyps of the Colon and Rectum

A polyp is a mass of tissue that protrudes into the lumen of the bowel. Polyps can occur anywhere in the intestinal tract and rectum. They can be classified as neoplastic (ie, adenomas and carcinomas) or non-neoplastic (ie, mucosal and hyperplastic). Non-neoplastic polyps, which are benign epithelial growths, are common in the Western world. They occur more commonly in the large intestine than in the small intestine. Although most polyps do not develop into invasive neoplasms, they must be identified and followed closely. Adenomatous polyps are more common in men. The proportion of these polyps arising in the proximal part of the colon increases with age (after 50 years of age). Prevalence rates vary from 25% to 60%, depending on age. Non-neoplastic polyps occur in 80% of the population, and their frequency increases with age. Up to two thirds of people older than 65 years are at risk for colonic adenomas (Tierney, 2004).

Clinical manifestations depend on the size of the polyp and the amount of pressure it exerts on intestinal tissue. The most common symptom is rectal bleeding. Lower abdominal pain may also occur. If the polyp is large enough, symptoms of obstruction occur. The diagnosis is based on history and digital rectal examination, barium enema studies, sigmoidoscopy, or colonoscopy.

After a polyp is identified, it should be removed. There are several methods: colonoscopy with the use of special equipment (ie, biopsy forceps and snares), laparoscopy, or colonoscopic excision with laparoscopic visualization. The latter technique enables immediate detection of potential problems and allows laparoscopic resection and repair of the major complications of perforation and bleeding that may occur with polypectomy. Microscopic examination of the polyp then identifies the type of polyp and indicates what further surgery is required, if any.

Diseases of the Anorectum

Anorectal disorders are common, and the majority of the population will experience one at some time during their lives. Patients with anorectal disorders seek medical care primarily because of pain, rectal bleeding, or change in bowel habits. Other common complaints are protrusion of hemorrhoids, anal discharge, perianal itching, swelling, anal tenderness, stenosis, and ulceration. Constipation results from delaying defecation because of anorectal pain.

There has been a steady increase in the prevalence of sexually transmitted diseases (STDs; also called sexually transmitted infections, or STIs) in recent decades, leading to the identification of new anorectal syndromes. The prevalence of these conditions is increasing. These syndromes include venereal infections such as syphilis, gonorrhea, herpes, chlamydia, and candidiasis, and they are most commonly seen in male homosexuals who practice anorectal intercourse.

Anorectal Abscess

An anorectal abscess is caused by obstruction of an anal gland, resulting in retrograde infection. People with regional enteritis or immunosuppressive conditions such as AIDS are particularly susceptible to these infections. Many of these abscesses result in fistulas.

An abscess may occur in a variety of spaces in and around the rectum. It often contains a quantity of foul-smelling pus and is painful. If the abscess is superficial, swelling, redness, and tenderness are observed. A deeper abscess may result in toxic symptoms, lower abdominal pain, and fever.

Palliative therapy consists of sitz baths and analgesics. However, prompt surgical treatment to incise and drain the abscess is the treatment of choice. When a deeper infection exists with the possibility of a fistula, the fistulous tract must be excised. If possible, the fistula is excised when the abscess is incised and drained, or a second procedure may be necessary to do so. The wound may be packed with gauze and allowed to heal by granulation.

Anal Fistula

An anal fistula is a tiny, tubular, fibrous tract that extends into the anal canal from an opening located beside the anus (Fig. 38-10A). Fistulas usually result from an infection. They may also develop from trauma, fissures, or regional enteritis. Pus or stool may leak constantly from the cutaneous opening. Other symptoms may be the passage of flatus or feces from the vagina or bladder, depending on the fistula tract. Untreated fistulas may cause systemic infection with related symptoms.

Surgery is always recommended, because few fistulas heal spontaneously. A fistulectomy (ie, excision of the fistulous tract) is the recommended surgical procedure. The lower bowel is evacuated thoroughly with several prescribed enemas. The fistula is dissected out or laid open by an incision from its rectal opening to its outlet. The wound is packed with gauze.

Anal Fissure

An anal fissure is a longitudinal tear or ulceration in the lining of the anal canal (see Fig. 38-10B). Fissures are usually caused by the trauma of passing a large, firm stool or from persistent tightening of the anal canal because of stress and

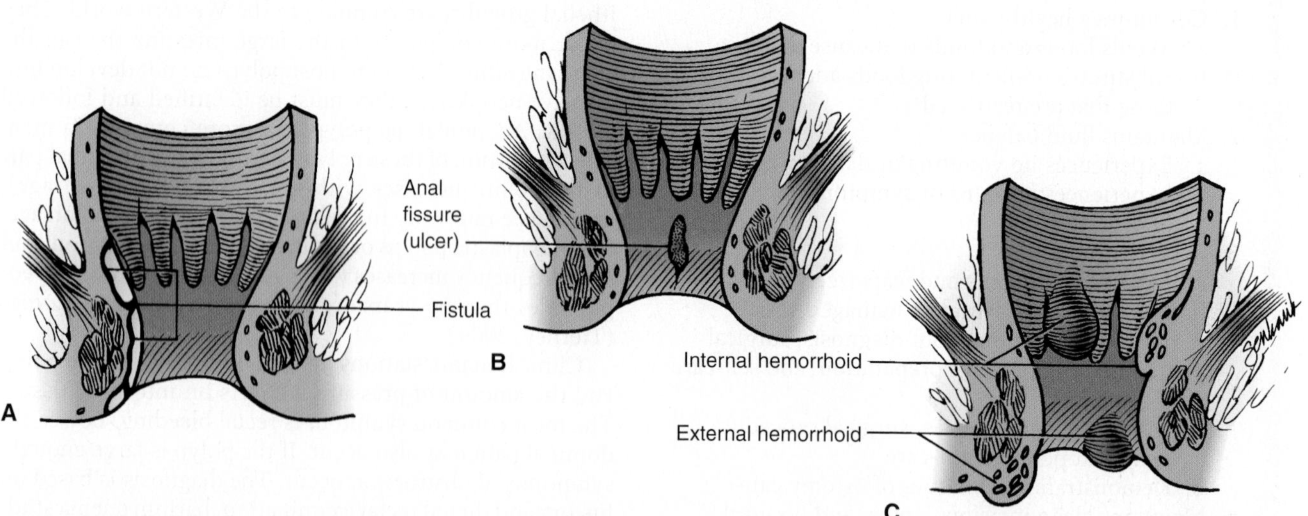

FIGURE 38-10. Various types of anal lesions. (A) Fistula. (B) Fissure. (C) External and internal hemorrhoids.

anxiety (leading to constipation). Other causes include childbirth, trauma, and overuse of laxatives.

Extremely painful defecation, burning, and bleeding characterize fissures. Bright-red blood may be seen on the toilet tissue after a bowel movement. Most of these fissures heal if treated by conservative measures, which include dietary modification with addition of fiber supplements, stool softeners and bulk agents, an increase in water intake, sitz baths, and emollient suppositories. A suppository combining an anesthetic with a corticosteroid helps relieve the discomfort. Anal dilation under anesthesia may be required.

If fissures do not respond to conservative treatment, surgery is indicated. Most surgeons consider the procedure of choice to be the lateral internal sphincterotomy with excision of the fissure.

Hemorrhoids

Hemorrhoids are dilated portions of veins in the anal canal. They are very common: by 50 years of age, about 50% of people have hemorrhoids (NIH, 2005). Shearing of the mucosa during defecation results in the sliding of the structures in the wall of the anal canal, including the hemorrhoidal and vascular tissues. Increased pressure in the hemorrhoidal tissue due to pregnancy may initiate hemorrhoids or aggravate existing ones. Hemorrhoids are classified as one of two types: those above the internal sphincter are called internal hemorrhoids, and those appearing outside the external sphincter are called external hemorrhoids (see Fig. 38-10C).

Hemorrhoids cause itching and pain and are the most common cause of bright-red bleeding with defecation. External hemorrhoids are associated with severe pain from the inflammation and edema caused by thrombosis (ie, clotting of blood within the hemorrhoid). This may lead to ischemia of the area and eventual necrosis. Internal hemorrhoids are not usually painful until they bleed or prolapse when they become enlarged.

Hemorrhoid symptoms and discomfort can be relieved by good personal hygiene and by avoiding excessive straining during defecation. A high-residue diet that contains fruit and bran along with an increased fluid intake may be all the treatment that is necessary to promote the passage of soft, bulky stools to prevent straining. If this treatment is not successful, the addition of hydrophilic bulk-forming agents such as psyllium (Metamucil) may help. Warm compresses, sitz baths, analgesic ointments and suppositories, astringents (eg, witch hazel), and bed rest allow the engorgement to subside.

There are several types of nonsurgical treatments for hemorrhoids. Infrared photocoagulation, bipolar diathermy, and laser therapy are used to affix the mucosa to the underlying muscle. Injection of sclerosing agents is also effective for small, bleeding hemorrhoids. These procedures help prevent prolapse.

A conservative surgical treatment of internal hemorrhoids is the rubber-band ligation procedure. The hemorrhoid is visualized through the anoscope, and its proximal portion above the mucocutaneous lines is grasped with an instrument. A small rubber band is then slipped over the hemorrhoid. Tissue distal to the rubber band becomes necrotic after several days and sloughs off. Fibrosis occurs; the result is that the lower anal mucosa is drawn up and adheres to the underlying muscle. Although this treatment has been satisfactory for some patients, it has proven painful for others and may cause secondary hemorrhage. It has also been known to cause perianal infection.

Cryosurgical hemorrhoidectomy, another method for removing hemorrhoids, involves freezing the hemorrhoid for a sufficient time to cause necrosis. Although it is relatively painless, this procedure is not widely used because the discharge is very foul-smelling and wound healing is prolonged. The Nd:YAG laser is useful in excising hemorrhoids, particularly external hemorrhoidal tags. The treatment is quick and relatively painless. Hemorrhage and abscess are rare postoperative complications.

The previously described methods of treating hemorrhoids are not effective for advanced thrombosed veins, which must be treated by more extensive surgery. Hemorrhoidectomy, or surgical excision, can be performed to remove all the redundant tissue involved in the process. During surgery, the rectal sphincter is usually dilated digitally and the hemorrhoids are removed with a clamp and cautery or are ligated and then excised. After the surgical procedures are completed, a small tube may be inserted through the sphincter to permit the escape of flatus and blood; pieces of Gelfoam or Oxycel gauze may be placed over the anal wounds.

Sexually Transmitted Anorectal Diseases

Three infectious syndromes that are related to STDs have been identified: proctitis, proctocolitis, and enteritis. Proctitis involves the rectum. It is commonly associated with recent anal-receptive intercourse with an infected partner. Symptoms include a mucopurulent discharge or bleeding, pain in the area, and diarrhea. The pathogens most frequently involved are *Neisseria gonorrhoeae, Chlamydia,* herpes simplex virus, and *Treponema pallidum.* Proctocolitis involves the rectum and lowest portion of the descending colon. Symptoms are similar to proctitis but may also include watery or bloody diarrhea, cramps, pain, and bloating. Enteritis involves more of the descending colon, and symptoms include watery, bloody diarrhea; abdominal pain; and weight loss. The most common pathogens causing enteritis are *E. histolytica, Giardia lamblia, Shigella,* and *Campylobacter.*

Sigmoidoscopy is performed to identify portions of the anorectum involved. Samples are taken with rectal swabs, and cultures are obtained to identify the pathogens involved. Antibiotics (ie, cefixime [Suprax], doxycycline [Vibramycin], and penicillin G) are the treatment of choice for bacterial infections. Acyclovir [Zovirax] is given to patients with viral infections. Antiamebic therapy (ie, metronidazole [Flagyl]) is appropriate for infections with *E. histolytica* and *G. lamblia.* Ciprofloxacin (Cipro) is effective for *Shigella.* The antibiotics erythromycin (E-Mycin) and ciprofloxacin are the treatment of choice for *Campylobacter* infection.

Pilonidal Sinus or Cyst

A pilonidal sinus or cyst is found in the intergluteal cleft on the posterior surface of the lower sacrum (Fig. 38-11). Current theories suggest that it results from local trauma, causing the penetration of hairs into the epithelium and subcutaneous tissue. It may also be formed congenitally by

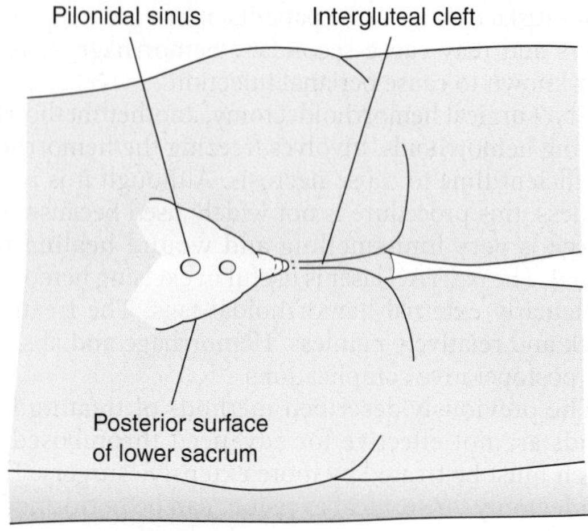

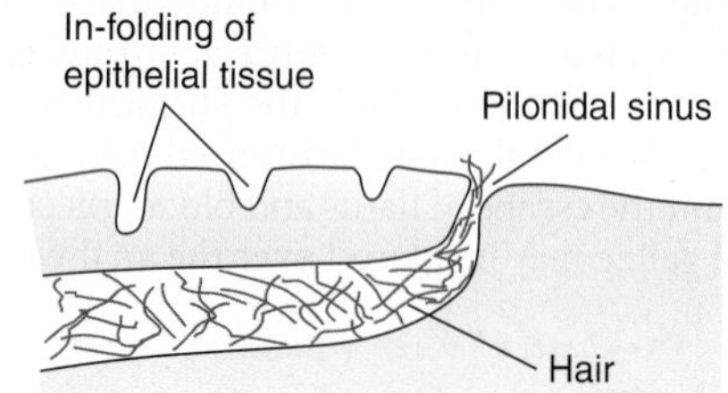

FIGURE 38-11. (**A**) Pilonidal sinus on lower sacrum about 5 cm (2 in) above the anus in the intergluteal cleft. (**B**) Hair particles emerge from the sinus tract, and localized indentations (pits) can appear on the skin near the sinus openings.

an infolding of epithelial tissue beneath the skin, which may communicate with the skin surface through one or several small sinus openings. Hair frequently is seen protruding from these openings, and this gives the cyst its name, *pilonidal* (ie, a nest of hair). The cysts rarely cause symptoms until adolescence or early adult life, when infection produces an irritating drainage or an abscess. Perspiration and friction easily irritate this area.

In the early stages of the inflammation, the infection may be controlled by antibiotic therapy, but after an abscess has formed, surgery is indicated. The abscess is incised and drained under local anesthesia. After the acute process resolves, further surgery is performed to excise the cyst and the secondary sinus tracts. The wound is allowed to heal by granulation. Gauze dressings are placed in the wound to keep its edges separated while healing occurs.

Nursing Process

The Patient With an Anorectal Condition

Assessment

The nurse obtains a health history to determine the presence and characteristics of pruritus, burning, or anorectal pain. Other questions included in the medical history include the following: Do these symptoms occur during bowel movements? How long do they last? Is any abdominal pain associated with them? Does any bleeding occur from the rectum? How much? How frequently? Is it bright red? Is there any other discharge, such as mucus or pus? Other questions relate to elimination patterns and laxative use, diet history (including fiber intake), amount of exercise, activity levels, and occupation (especially one that involves prolonged sitting or standing). Assessment also includes inspection of the stool for blood or mucus and the perianal area for hemorrhoids, fissures, irritation, or purulent drainage.

Diagnosis

Nursing Diagnoses

Based on the assessment data, the major nursing diagnoses may include the following:

- Constipation related to ignoring the urge to defecate because of pain during elimination
- Anxiety related to impending surgery and embarrassment
- Acute pain related to irritation, pressure, and sensitivity in the anorectal area from anorectal disease and sphincter spasms after surgery
- Urinary retention related to postoperative reflex spasm and fear of pain
- Risk for ineffective therapeutic regimen management

Collaborative Problems/ Potential Complications

Potential complications that may develop include the following:

- Hemorrhage

Planning and Goals

The major goals for the patient may include adequate elimination patterns, reduction of anxiety, pain relief, promotion of urinary elimination, managing the therapeutic regimen, and absence of complications.

Nursing Interventions

Relieving Constipation

The nurse encourages intake of at least 2 L of water daily to provide adequate hydration and recommends high-fiber foods to promote bulk in the stool and to make it easier to pass fecal matter through the rectum. Bulk laxatives such as psyllium (Metamucil) and stool softeners (eg, docusate [Colace]) are administered as prescribed. The patient is advised to set aside a time for bowel movements and to heed the urge to defecate as promptly as possible. It may be helpful to have the patient perform relaxation exercises before defecating to relax the abdominal and perineal muscles, which may be constricted or in spasm. Administering an analgesic before a bowel movement is beneficial.

Reducing Anxiety

Patients facing rectal surgery may be upset and irritable because of discomfort, pain, and embarrassment. The nurse identifies specific psychosocial needs and individualizes the plan of care. The nurse maintains the patient's privacy while providing care and limits visitors, if the patient desires. Soiled dressings are removed from the room promptly to prevent unpleasant odors; room deodorizers may be needed if dressings are foul-smelling.

Relieving Pain

During the first 24 hours after rectal surgery, painful spasms of the sphincter and perineal muscles may occur. Control of pain is a prime consideration. The patient is encouraged to assume a comfortable position. Flotation pads under the buttocks when sitting help decrease the pain, as may ice and analgesic ointments. Warm compresses may promote circulation and soothe irritated tissues. Sitz baths taken three or four times each day can relieve soreness and pain by relaxing sphincter spasm. Twenty-four hours after surgery, topical anesthetic agents may be beneficial in relieving local irritation and soreness. Medications may include topical anesthetics (ie, suppositories), astringents, antiseptics, tranquilizers, and antiemetics. Patients are more compliant and less apprehensive if they are free of pain.

Wet dressings saturated with equal parts of cold water and witch hazel help relieve edema. When wet compresses are being used continuously, petrolatum is applied around the anal area to prevent skin maceration. The patient is instructed to assume a prone position at intervals because this position reduces edema of the tissue.

Promoting Urinary Elimination

Voiding may be a problem after surgery because of a reflex spasm of the sphincter at the outlet of the bladder and a certain amount of muscle guarding from apprehension and pain. The nurse tries all methods to encourage voluntary voiding (ie, increasing fluid intake, listening to running water, and pouring warm water over the urinary meatus) before resorting to catheterization. After rectal surgery, urinary output is closely monitored.

Monitoring and Managing Complications

The operative site is examined frequently for rectal bleeding. The nurse assesses the patient for systemic indicators of excessive bleeding (ie, tachycardia, hypotension, restlessness, and thirst). After hemorrhoidectomy, hemorrhage may occur from the veins that were cut. If a tube has been inserted through the sphincter after surgery, blood may be visible on the dressings. If bleeding is obvious, direct pressure is applied to the area, and the physician is notified. It is important to avoid using moist heat because it encourages vessel dilation and bleeding.

Promoting Home and Community-Based Care

TEACHING PATIENTS SELF-CARE

Most patients with anorectal conditions are not hospitalized. Those who undergo surgical procedures to correct the condition often are discharged directly from the outpatient surgical center. If they are hospitalized, it is for a short time, usually only 24 hours. Patient teaching is essential to facilitate recovery at home.

The nurse instructs the patient to keep the perianal area as clean as possible by gently cleansing with warm water and then drying with absorbent cotton wipes. The patient should avoid rubbing the area with toilet tissue. Instructions are provided about how to take a sitz bath and how to test the temperature of the water.

CONTINUING CARE

Sitz baths may be given in the bathtub or plastic sitz bath unit three or four times each day. Sitz baths should follow each bowel movement for 1 to 2 weeks after surgery. The nurse encourages the patient to respond quickly to the urge to defecate to prevent constipation. The diet is modified to increase fluids and fiber. Moderate exercise is encouraged, and the patient is taught about the prescribed diet, the significance of proper eating habits and exercise, and the laxatives that can be taken safely.

Evaluation

Expected Patient Outcomes

Expected patient outcomes may include the following:

1. Attains a normal pattern of elimination
   a. Sets aside a time for defecation, usually after a meal or at bedtime
   b. Responds to the urge to defecate and takes the time to sit on the toilet and try to defecate
   c. Uses relaxation exercises as needed
   d. Increases fluid intake to 2 L per day
   e. Adds high-fiber foods to diet
   f. Reports passage of soft, formed stools
   g. Reports decreased abdominal discomfort
2. Is less anxious
3. Has less pain
   a. Modifies body position and activities to minimize pain and discomfort
   b. Applies warmth or cold to anorectal area
   c. Takes sitz baths three or four times each day
4. Voids without difficulty
5. Adheres to the therapeutic regimen
   a. Keeps perianal area dry
   b. Eats bulk-forming foods
   c. Has a soft, formed stool on a regular basis
6. Exhibits no evidence of complications
   a. Has a clean incision
   b. Has normal vital signs
   c. Shows no signs of hemorrhage

Critical Thinking Exercises

1 As a community health nurse you are conducting a regularly scheduled blood pressure clinic in a suburban community. In talking with an apparently well 74-year-old woman, you ask her if she has any questions regarding her health. She whispers to you that she has noticed some blood on the toilet tissue after bowel movements but has been too embarrassed to tell anyone about it. Consider what additional questions you might ask her during your initial nursing assessment. Analyze these findings, indicate what you think the possible causes may be, and explain the actions you would take and why. Explain the implications of this woman's age on likely subsequent referrals and treatments.

2 ebp A 22-year-old graduate student presents to the student health center of a local university with complaints of a five-day episode of watery diarrhea, lethargy, poor sleep patterns, and nervousness. She reports a recent weight loss of 15 pounds. Her social history reveals that she is preparing for her comprehensive final examinations and is very anxious about her examinations and her current health status. Her family history reveals that her father has had Crohn's disease for many years. What is the strength of the evidence that suggests her risk of having Crohn's disease? Prioritize your nursing plan and actions. What further data would be helpful? What specific nursing actions should be taken? Identify the evidence base for each aspect of your care.

3 You are the charge nurse in the emergency department of a large urban teaching hospital. A 53-year-old man presents with an acute onset of severe abdominal pain. Your physical examination of his abdomen reveals involuntary guarding and a rigid abdomen. The CT scan confirms intra-abdominal findings of purulent peritonitis. Intraperitoneal free air is evident. He is to be admitted to the hospital with an apparent perforation of diverticulitis into the peritoneal cavity. Both he and his wife are extremely upset. The operating room is put on call for an immediate surgical intervention. Identify priority nursing measures that must be initiated to meet the urgent physical needs of this man, what steps must be initiated to prepare him for surgery, and how to offer appropriate emotional support for him and his wife.

4 A 34-year-old attorney is admitted to the outpatient surgical center for drainage of an anorectal abscess. You are the admitting nurse and take his history, which includes a 6-week episode of swelling, throbbing, continuous perirectal pain accompanied by purulent drainage from his anus. He is scheduled for an incision and drainage within the next hour but asks why he must have surgery; he asks you, "Why can't I just get an antibiotic?" Considering the pathophysiologic implications of his diagnosis, what would you say to him? Make a judgment regarding essential actions you must take before he is taken to the operating room.

After your interventions, this man decided to undergo surgery. Later that afternoon, he is prepared for discharge. Design a discharge plan for him for the next 2 weeks, and include the principles of care that you will teach him so that he may understand the reasons for his home care routine.

REFERENCES AND SELECTED READINGS

BOOKS

American Cancer Society. (2006). *Cancer facts and figures 2006*. Atlanta, GA: Author.

Andreoli, T., Carpenter, D. J., Griggs, R. C., et al. (2003). *Cecil essentials of medicine* (6th ed.). Philadelphia: W. B. Saunders.

Chan, P. D., Safani, M., & Winkle, P. (2005). *Medicine*. Laguna Hills, CA: Current Clinical Strategies Publishing.

Colwell, J. C., Goldberg, M. T., & Carmel, J. E. (2004). *Fecal and urinary diversions: Management principles*. St. Louis, MO: Mosby.

Friedman, S., McQuaid, R., & Grendell, J. (2003). *Current diagnosis and treatment in gastroenterology*. New York: McGraw-Hill Companies.

Gilbert, D. M., Moellering, R., Eliopoulos, G., et al. (2005). *The Sanford guide to antimicrobial therapy*. Spercyville, VA: Antimicrobial Therapy.

Green, G., Morris, J., & Lin, G. (2005). *Washington manual of medical therapeutics* (31st ed.). Philadelphia: Lippincott Williams & Wilkins.

Johnson, M., & Chan, P. (2004). *Treatment guidelines for medicine and primary care, 2004*. Laguna Hills, CA: Current Clinical Strategies Publishing.

Kasper, D., Braunwald, E., Fauci, A., et al. (2004). *Harrison's principles of internal medicine* (16th ed.). New York: McGraw-Hill Professional.

Lederman, R., & Winshall, J. (2004). *Tarascon internal medicine & critical care pocketbook* (3rd ed.). Loma Linda, CA: Tarascon Publishing.

National Institutes of Health: National Institute of Diabetes and Digestive and Kidney Diseases (2005). *National digestive diseases information clearinghouse*. Bethesda, MD: National Institutes of Health.

Porth, C. (2005). *Pathophysiology: Concepts of altered health states* (7th ed.). Philadelphia: Lippincott Williams & Wilkins.

Rothrock, S. (2004). *Tarascon adult emergency handbook* (3rd ed.). Loma Linda, CA: Tarascon Publishing.

Tierney, L. (2004). *Current medical diagnosis and treatment, 2005* (44th ed.). New York: McGraw-Hill Medical.

Townsend, C., Beauchamp, D., Evers, M., et al. (2004) *Sabiston textbook of surgery: The biological basis of modern surgical practice* (17th ed.). Philadelphia: W. B. Saunders.

Varricchio, C., Ades, T., Hinds, P., et al. (2004). *A cancer sourcebook for nurses*. Atlanta, GA: American Cancer Society and Jones & Bartlett Publishers.

JOURNALS

**Asterisk indicates nursing research article*

General

Beitz, J. (2004). Diverticulosis and diverticulitis: Spectrum of a modern malady. *Journal of Wound, Ostomy and Continence Nursing*, 31(2), 75–84.

*Gall, S., & Bull, J. (2004). Clinical risk: Discharging patients with no one at home. *Gastroenterology Nursing, 27*(3), 111–114.

*Li, H., Melnyk, B. M., & McCann, R. (2004). Review of intervention studies of families with hospitalized elderly relatives. *Journal of Nursing Scholarship, 36*(1), 54–59.

Mick, D. J., & Ackerman, M. H. (2004). Critical care nursing for older adults: Pathophysiological and functional considerations. *Nursing Clinics of North America, 39*(3), 473–493.

*Reilly, T., & Walker, G. (2004). Reasons for poor colonic preparation with inpatients. *Gastroenterology Nursing, 27*(3), 115–117.

*Scible, L., & Anwer, M. B. (2004). Detecting a small bowel tumor via wireless capsule endoscopy: A clinical case study. *Gastroenterology Nursing, 27*(3), 118–120.

Smith, C., Hellebusch, S. J., & Mandel, K. G. (2003). Patient and physician evaluation of a new bulk fiber laxative tablet. *Gastroenterology Nursing, 26*(1), 31–37.

Steffen, K. A. (2003) When your trauma patient is over 65. *Nursing, 33*(4), 53–56.

Stessman, M. (2003). Biofeedback: Its role in the treatment of chronic constipation. *Gastroenterology Nursing, 26*(6), 251–260.

*Zalon, M. (2004). Correlates of recovery among older adults after major abdominal surgery. *Nursing Research, 53*(2), 99–106.

Cancer of the Colon and Rectum

Banks, N., & Razor, B. (2003). Preoperative stoma site assessment and marking. *American Journal of Nursing, 103*(3), 64A–64E.

Feingold, D., Addona, T., Forde, K. A., et al. (2004). Safety and reliability of tattooing colorectal neoplasm prior to laparoscopic resection. *Journal of Gastrointestinal Surgery, 8*(5), 543–546.

Lynch, H. T., Coronel, S. M., Okimoto, R., et al. (2004). A founder mutation of the *MSH2* gene and hereditary nonpolyposis colorectal cancer in the United States. *Journal of the American Medical Association, 291*(6), 718–724.

Madoff, R. D. (2004). Chemoradiotherapy for rectal cancer: When, why, and how? *New England Journal of Medicine, 351*(17), 1790–1791.

Morrin, M., & LaMont, T. (2003). Screening virtual colonoscopy: Ready for prime time? *New England Journal of Medicine, 349*(13), 2261–2264.

Rudy, D. R., & Zdon, M. J. (2000). Update on colorectal cancer. *American Family Physician, 61*(6), 1759–1774.

Sauer, R., Becker, H., Hohenberger, W., et al. (2004). Preoperative versus postoperative chemoradiotherapy for rectal cancer. *New England Journal of Medicine, 351*(17), 1731–1740.

Sargent, C., & Murphy, D. (2003). What you need to know about colorectal cancer. *Nursing, 33*(2), 36–41.

Inflammatory Bowel Disease

Rutgeerts, P., Sandborn, W. J., Feagan, B. G., et al. (2005). Infliximab for induction and maintenance therapy for ulcerative colitis. *New England Journal of Medicine, 353*(23), 2462–2476.

Sandborn, W. J., Colombel, J. F., Enns, R., et al. (2005). Natalizumab induction and maintenance therapy for Crohn's disease. *New England Journal of Medicine, 353*(18), 1912–1925.

Irritable Bowel Syndrome

Aschenbrenner, D. (2004). Risks have been newly associated with a drug taken for IBS: Changes to labeling of tegaserod. *American Journal of Nursing, 104*(7), 33–34.

Kupecz, D., & Berardinelli, C. (2003). Drug news: New therapy for women with irritable bowel syndrome. *Nurse Practitioner, 28*(4), 48–50.

Mertz, H. (2003). Drug therapy: Irritable bowel syndrome. *New England Journal of Medicine, 349*(22), 2136.

*Motzer, S., Hertig, V., Jarrett, M., et al. (2003). Sense of coherence and quality of life in women with and without irritable bowel syndrome. *Nursing Research, 52*(5), 329–337.

RESOURCES

American Cancer Society, 1599 Clifton Rd., N.E., Atlanta, GA 30329; 1-800-277-2345; http://www.cancer.org. Accessed June 20, 2006.

Colon Cancer Alliance, 175 Ninth Ave., New York, NY 10011; 1-212-627-7451; http://www.ccalliance.org. Accessed June 20, 2006.

Crohn's & Colitis Foundation of America, 386 Park Avenue South, New York, NY 10016; 1-800-932-2423; http://www.ccfa.org. Accessed June 20, 2006.

International Foundation for Functional Gastrointestinal Disorders, P.O. Box 17864, Milwaukee, WI 17864; 1-888-964-2001; http://www.iffgd.org. Accessed June 20, 2006.

Medicine Online: Colon Cancer Information Library: http://www.meds.com/colon/colon.html. Accessed June 20, 2006.

National Association for Continence, P.O. Box 544, Union, SC 29379; 1-803-585-8789; http://www.nafc.org/site2/index.html. Accessed June 20, 2006.

STOP Colon/Rectal Cancer Foundation, P.O. Box 1616, Barrington, IL 60010; 1-312-782-4828; http://www.coloncancerprevention.org. Accessed June 20, 2006.

United Ostomy Association, 19772 MacArthur Blvd., Suite 200, Irvine, CA 92612; 1-800-826-0826; http://www.uoa.org. Accessed June 20, 2006.

UNIT 8

Metabolic and Endocrine Function

Case Study

Applying Concepts from NANDA, NIC, and NOC

A Patient With Complications of Diabetes

Mr. Johansen is a 58-year-old man with type 2 diabetes, peripheral vascular disease, hyperlipidemia, and peripheral neuropathy. He is also 50 lb over his ideal body weight. He takes an oral antidiabetic agent twice daily and lovastatin for elevated cholesterol levels. Mr. Johansen comes to the clinic for treatment of an unrelated respiratory infection. While there, he tells the nurse that he has numbness and tingling of his feet and has burning pain in his legs if he stands for long periods of time. The nurse assesses his feet and notes decreased sensory function in both feet. Mr. Johansen states that he has not seen his doctor for more than 1 year and only comes to the clinic if he feels sick.

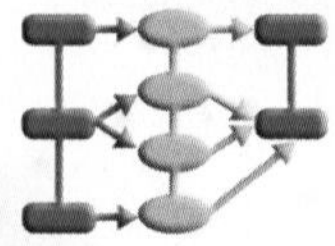

Turn to Appendix C to see a concept map that illustrates the relationships that exist between the nursing diagnoses, interventions, and outcomes for the patient's clinical problems.

Nursing Classifications and Languages

NANDA Nursing Diagnoses	NIC Nursing Interventions	NOC Nursing Outcomes Return to functional baseline status, stabilization of, or improvement in:
Ineffective Tissue Perfusion (all types)—Decrease in oxygen resulting in the failure to nourish tissues at the capillary level	**Circulatory Care: Arterial Insufficiency**—Promotion of arterial circulation	**Circulation Status**—Extent to which blood flows unobstructed, unidirectionally, and at an appropriate pressure through large vessels of the systemic and pulmonary circuits
Disturbed Tactile Sensory Perception—Change in the amount or patterning of incoming stimuli accompanied by a diminished, exaggerated, distorted, or impaired response to such stimuli	**Circulatory Precautions**—Protection of localized area with limited perfusion	**Sensory Function: Cutaneous**—Extent to which stimulation of the skin is correctly sensed
Ineffective Therapeutic Regimen Management—Pattern of regulating and integrating into daily living a program for treatment of illness and the sequelae of illness that is unsatisfactory for meeting specific health goals	**Teaching: Foot Care**—Preparing an at-risk patient and/or a significant other to provide preventive foot care	**Tissue Integrity: Skin and Mucous Membranes**—Structural intactness and normal physiologic function of skin and mucous membranes
	Skin Surveillance—Collection and analysis of patient data to maintain skin and mucous membrane integrity	**Knowledge: Diabetes Management**—Extent of understanding conveyed about diabetes mellitus and its control
	Teaching: Individual—Planning, implementation, and evaluation of a teaching program designed to address a patient's particular needs	

NANDA International (2005). *Nursing diagnoses: Definitions & Classification 2005–2006.* Philadelphia: North American Nursing Diagnosis Association.
Dochterman, J. M., & Bulechek, G. M. (2004). *Nursing interventions classification (NIC)* (4th ed.). St. Louis: Mosby.
Iowa Outcomes Project (2004). In Moorhead, S., Johnson, M. & Maas, M. (2004). *Nursing outcomes classification (NOC)* (3rd ed.). St. Louis: Mosby.
Dochterman, J. M. & Jones, D. A. (2003). *Unifying nursing languages: The harmonization of NANDA, NIC, and NOC.* Washington D.C.: American Nurses Association.

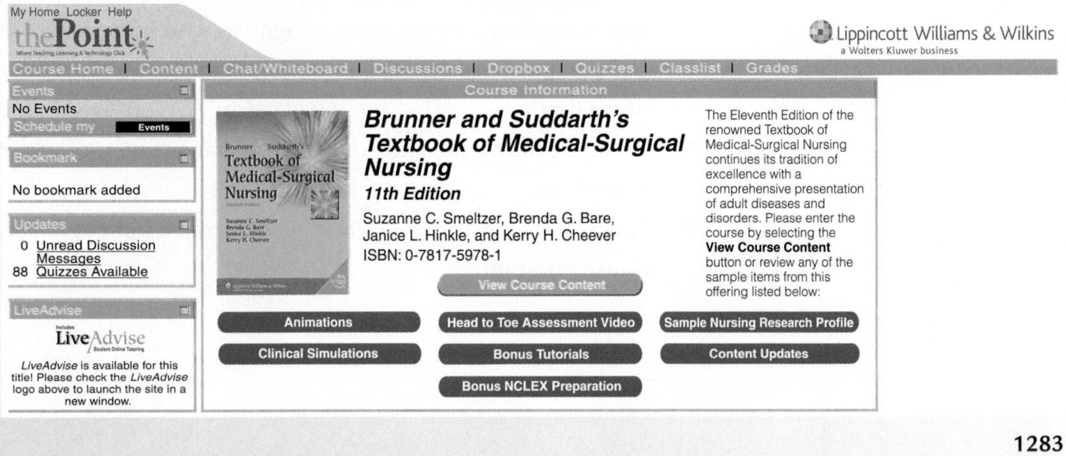

CHAPTER 39

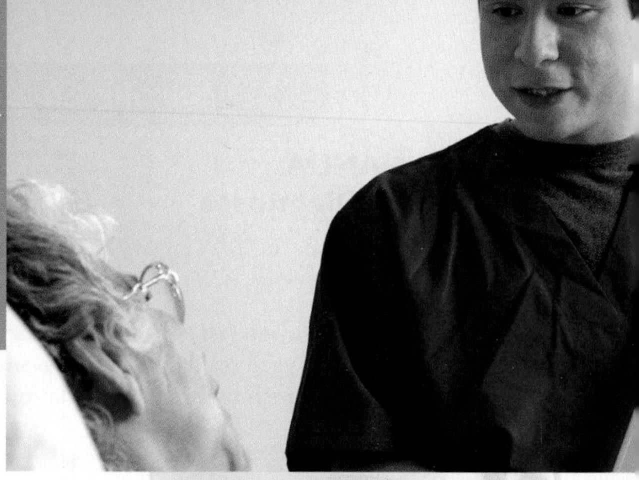

Assessment and Management of Patients With Hepatic Disorders

Learning Objectives

On completion of this chapter, the learner will be able to:

1. Identify the metabolic functions of the liver and the alterations in these functions that occur with liver disease.
2. Explain liver function tests and the clinical manifestations of liver dysfunction in relation to pathophysiologic alterations of the liver.
3. Relate jaundice, portal hypertension, ascites, varices, nutritional deficiencies, and hepatic coma to pathophysiologic alterations of the liver.
4. Describe the medical, surgical, and nursing management of patients with esophageal varices.
5. Compare the various types of hepatitis and their causes, prevention, clinical manifestations, management, prognosis, and home health care needs.
6. Use the nursing process as a framework for care of the patient with cirrhosis of the liver.
7. Compare the nonsurgical and surgical management of patients with cancer of the liver.
8. Describe the postoperative nursing care of the patient undergoing liver transplantation.

Liver function is complex, and liver dysfunction affects all body systems. For this reason, the nurse must understand how the liver functions and must have expert clinical assessment and management skills to care for patients undergoing complex diagnostic and treatment procedures. The nurse also must understand technologic advances in the management of liver disorders. Liver disorders are common and may result from a virus, exposure to toxic substances such as alcohol, or tumors.

Anatomic and Physiologic Overview

The liver, the largest gland of the body, can be considered a chemical factory that manufactures, stores, alters, and excretes a large number of substances involved in metabolism. The location of the liver is essential in this function, because it receives nutrient-rich blood directly from the gastrointestinal (GI) tract and then either stores or transforms these nutrients into chemicals that are used elsewhere in the body for metabolic needs. The liver is especially important in the regulation of glucose and protein metabolism. The liver manufactures and secretes bile, which has a major role in the digestion and absorption of fats in the GI tract. The liver removes waste products from the bloodstream and secretes them into the bile. The bile produced by the liver is stored temporarily in the gallbladder until it is needed for digestion, at which time the gallbladder empties and bile enters the intestine (Fig. 39-1).

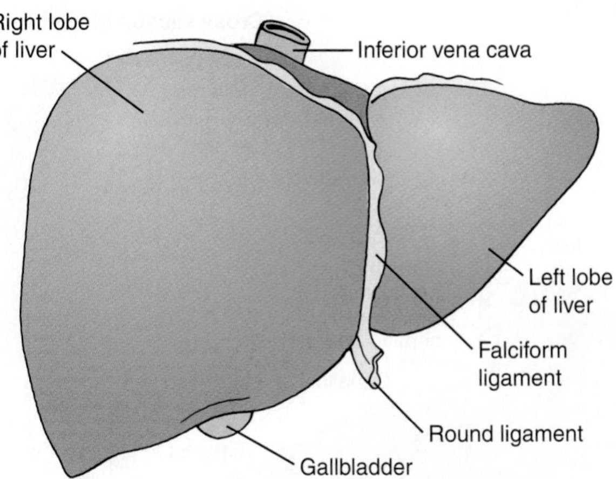

FIGURE 39-1. The liver and biliary system.

Anatomy of the Liver

The liver is located behind the ribs in the upper right portion of the abdominal cavity. It weighs about 1800 g in men and 1400 g in women and is divided into four lobes. A thin layer of connective tissue surrounds each lobe, extending into the lobe itself and dividing the liver mass into small, functional units called lobules (Zakim & Boyer, 2003).

The circulation of the blood into and out of the liver is of major importance to liver function. The blood that perfuses the liver comes from two sources. Approximately 75% of the blood supply comes from the portal vein, which drains the GI tract and is rich in nutrients. The remainder of the blood supply enters by way of the hepatic artery and is rich in oxygen. Terminal branches of these two blood vessels join to form common capillary beds, which constitute the sinusoids of the liver (Fig. 39-2). Thus, a mixture of venous and arterial blood bathes the liver cells (hepatocytes). The sinusoids empty into venules that occupy the center of each liver lobule and are called the central veins. The central veins join to form the hepatic vein, which constitutes the venous drainage from the liver and empties into the inferior vena cava, close to the diaphragm. Thus, there

Glossary

asterixis: involuntary flapping movements of the hands associated with metabolic liver dysfunction

balloon tamponade: use of balloons placed within the esophagus and proximal portion of the stomach and inflated to compress bleeding vessels (esophageal and gastric varices)

Budd-Chiari syndrome: hepatic vein thrombosis resulting in noncirrhotic portal hypertension

cirrhosis: a chronic liver disease characterized by fibrotic changes and the formation of dense connective tissue within the liver, subsequent degenerative changes, and loss of functioning cells

constructional apraxia: inability to draw figures in two or three dimensions

cryoablation: method of treating malignant hepatic lesions that involves exposing the tumor to temperatures lower than −20°C and subsequent thawing. This surgical intervention is performed via a probe through which liquid nitrogen flows.

fetor hepaticus: sweet, slightly fecal odor to the breath, presumed to be of intestinal origin; prevalent with the extensive collateral portal circulation in chronic liver disease

fulminant hepatic failure: sudden, severe onset of acute liver failure that occurs within 8 weeks after the first symptoms of jaundice

hepatic encephalopathy: central nervous system dysfunction resulting from liver disease; frequently associated with elevated ammonia levels that produce changes in mental status, altered level of consciousness, and coma

orthotopic liver transplantation (OLT): grafting of a donor liver into the normal anatomic location, with removal of the diseased native liver

portal hypertension: elevated pressure in the portal circulation resulting from obstruction of venous flow into and through the liver

sclerotherapy: the injection of substances into or around esophagogastric varices to cause constriction, thickening, and hardening of the vessel and thus to stop bleeding

variceal banding: procedure that involves the endoscopic placement of a rubber band-like device over esophageal varices to ligate the area and stop bleeding

xenograft: transplantation of organs from one species to another

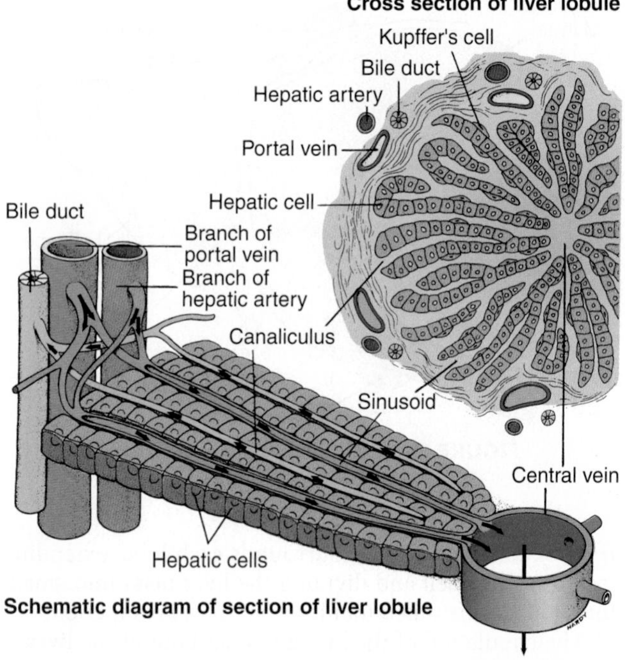

FIGURE 39-2. A section of liver lobule showing the location of hepatic veins, hepatic cells, liver sinusoids, and branches of the portal vein and hepatic artery.

are two sources of blood flowing into the liver and only one exit pathway (MacSween, Burt, Portmann, et al., 2002).

In addition to hepatocytes, phagocytic cells belonging to the reticuloendothelial system are present in the liver. Other organs that contain reticuloendothelial cells are the spleen, bone marrow, lymph nodes, and lungs. In the liver, these cells are called Kupffer cells. As the most common phagocyte in the human body, their main function is to engulf particulate matter (eg, bacteria) that enters the liver through the portal blood.

The smallest bile ducts, called canaliculi, are located between the lobules of the liver. The canaliculi receive secretions from the hepatocytes and carry them to larger bile ducts, which eventually form the hepatic duct. The hepatic duct from the liver and the cystic duct from the gallbladder join to form the common bile duct, which empties into the small intestine. The sphincter of Oddi, located at the junction where the common bile duct enters the duodenum, controls the flow of bile into the intestine. Disorders of the gallbladder are described in Chapter 40.

Functions of the Liver

Glucose Metabolism

The liver plays a major role in the metabolism of glucose and the regulation of blood glucose concentration. After a meal, glucose is taken up from the portal venous blood by the liver and converted into glycogen, which is stored in the hepatocytes. Subsequently, the glycogen is converted back to glucose (glycogenolysis) and released as needed into the bloodstream to maintain normal levels of blood glucose. This process, however, provides a limited amount of glucose. Additional glucose can be synthesized by the liver through a process called gluconeogenesis. For this process, the liver uses amino acids from protein breakdown or lactate produced by exercising muscles (Zakim & Boyer, 2003).

Ammonia Conversion

Use of amino acids from protein for gluconeogenesis results in the formation of ammonia as a byproduct. The liver converts this metabolically generated ammonia into urea. Ammonia produced by bacteria in the intestines is also removed from portal blood for urea synthesis. In this way, the liver converts ammonia, a potential toxin, into urea, a compound that is excreted in the urine (Porth, 2005).

Protein Metabolism

The liver also plays an important role in protein metabolism. It synthesizes almost all of the plasma proteins (except gamma-globulin), including albumin, alpha- and beta-globulins, blood clotting factors, specific transport proteins, and most of the plasma lipoproteins. Vitamin K is required by the liver for synthesis of prothrombin and some of the other clotting factors. Amino acids are used by the liver for protein synthesis (Porth, 2005).

Fat Metabolism

The liver is also active in fat metabolism. Fatty acids can be broken down for the production of energy and the production of ketone bodies (acetoacetic acid, beta-hydroxybutyric acid, and acetone). Ketone bodies are small compounds that can enter the bloodstream and provide a source of energy for muscles and other tissues. Breakdown of fatty acids into ketone bodies occurs primarily when the availability of glucose for metabolism is limited, as in starvation or in uncontrolled diabetes. Fatty acids and their metabolic products are also used for the synthesis of cholesterol, lecithin, lipoproteins, and other complex lipids (Porth, 2005).

Under some conditions, lipids may accumulate in the hepatocytes, resulting in the abnormal condition called fatty liver.

Vitamin and Iron Storage

Vitamins A, B, and D and several of the B-complex vitamins are stored in large amounts in the liver. Certain substances, such as iron and copper, are also stored in the liver. Because the liver is rich in these substances, liver extracts have been used for therapy for a wide range of nutritional disorders.

Drug Metabolism

The liver metabolizes many medications, such as barbiturates, opioids, sedative agents, anesthetics, and amphetamines. Metabolism generally results in inactivation of the medication, although in some cases activation of the medication may occur. One of the important pathways for medication metabolism involves conjugation (binding) of the medication with a variety of compounds, such as glucuronic acid or acetic acid, to form more soluble substances. The conjugated products may be excreted in the feces or urine, similar to bilirubin excretion. Bioavailability is the fraction of the administered medication that actually reaches the systemic circulation. The bioavailability of an oral medication (absorbed from the GI tract) can be decreased if the medication is metabolized to a great extent by the liver before it reaches the systemic circulation; this is known as "first-pass effect." Some medications have such a large first-pass effect that their use is essentially limited to the parenteral route, or oral doses must be substantially larger than parenteral doses to achieve the same effect.

Bile Formation

Bile is continuously formed by the hepatocytes and collected in the canaliculi and bile ducts. It is composed mainly of water and electrolytes such as sodium, potassium, calcium, chloride, and bicarbonate, and it also contains significant amounts of lecithin, fatty acids, cholesterol, bilirubin, and bile salts. Bile is collected and stored in the gallbladder and is emptied into the intestine when needed for digestion. The functions of bile are excretory, as in the excretion of bilirubin; bile also serves as an aid to digestion through the emulsification of fats by bile salts.

Bile salts are synthesized by the hepatocytes from cholesterol. After conjugation or binding with amino acids (taurine and glycine), bile salts are excreted into the bile. The bile salts, together with cholesterol and lecithin, are required for emulsification of fats in the intestine, which is necessary for efficient digestion and absorption. Bile salts are then reabsorbed, primarily in the distal ileum, into portal blood for return to the liver and are again excreted into the bile. This pathway from hepatocytes to bile to intestine and back to the hepatocytes is called the enterohepatic circulation. Because of the enterohepatic circulation, only a small fraction of the bile salts that enter the intestine are excreted in the feces. This decreases the need for active synthesis of bile salts by the liver cells (Porth, 2005).

Bilirubin Excretion

Bilirubin is a pigment derived from the breakdown of hemoglobin by cells of the reticuloendothelial system, including the Kupffer cells of the liver. Hepatocytes remove bilirubin from the blood and chemically modify it through conjugation to glucuronic acid, which makes the bilirubin more soluble in aqueous solutions. The conjugated bilirubin is secreted by the hepatocytes into the adjacent bile canaliculi and is eventually carried in the bile into the duodenum.

In the small intestine, bilirubin is converted into urobilinogen, which is partially excreted in the feces and partially absorbed through the intestinal mucosa into the portal blood. Much of this reabsorbed urobilinogen is removed by the hepatocytes and secreted into the bile once again (enterohepatic circulation). Some of the urobilinogen enters the systemic circulation and is excreted by the kidneys in the urine. Elimination of bilirubin in the bile represents the major route of its excretion.

The bilirubin concentration in the blood may be increased in the presence of liver disease, if the flow of bile is impeded (eg, by gallstones in the bile ducts), or if there is excessive destruction of red blood cells. With bile duct obstruction, bilirubin does not enter the intestine; as a consequence, urobilinogen is absent from the urine and decreased in the stool (Porth, 2005).

Biliary tract disorders are discussed in Chapter 40.

Gerontologic Considerations

Chart 39-1 summarizes age-related changes in the liver. In the elderly, the most common change in the liver is a decrease in size and weight, accompanied by a decrease in total hepatic blood flow. In general, however, these decreases are proportional to the decreases in body size and weight seen in normal aging. Results of liver function tests do not normally change in the elderly; abnormal results in an elderly patient indicate abnormal liver function and are not a result of the aging process itself.

The immune system is altered in the aged. A less responsive immune system may be responsible for the increased incidence and severity of hepatitis B among elderly persons and the increased incidence of liver abscesses secondary to decreased phagocytosis by the Kupffer cells. With the advent of hepatitis B vaccine as the standard for prevention, the incidence of hepatic diseases may decrease in the future.

Metabolism of medications by the liver decreases in the elderly, but such changes are usually accompanied by changes in intestinal absorption, renal excretion, and altered body distribution of some medications secondary to changes in fat deposition. These alterations necessitate careful medication administration and monitoring; if appropriate, reduced dosages may be needed to prevent medication toxicity.

Assessment

Health History

If liver function test results are abnormal, the patient is evaluated for liver disease. In such cases, the health history focuses on previous exposure of the patient to hepatotoxic substances or infectious agents. The patient's

CHART 39-1

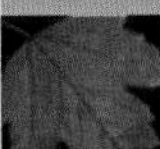

Age-Related Changes of the Hepatobiliary System

- Steady decrease in size and weight of the liver, particularly in women
- Decrease in blood flow
- Decrease in replacement/repair of liver cells after injury
- Reduced drug metabolism
- Slow clearance of hepatitis B surface antigen
- More rapid progression of hepatitis C infection and lower response rate to therapy
- Decline in drug clearance capability
- Increased prevalence of gallstones due to the increase in cholesterol secretion in bile
- Decreased gallbladder contraction after a meal
- Atypical clinical presentation of biliary disease
- More severe complications of biliary tract disease

occupational, recreational, and travel history may assist in identifying exposure to hepatotoxins (eg, industrial chemicals, other toxins). The patient's history of alcohol and drug use, including but not limited to the use of intravenous (IV)/injection drugs, provides additional information about exposure to toxins and infectious agents. Many medications (including acetaminophen, ketoconazole, and valproic acid) are responsible for hepatic dysfunction and disease. A thorough medication history to assess hepatic dysfunction should address all current and past prescription medications, over-the-counter medications, herbal remedies, and dietary supplements.

Lifestyle behaviors that increase the risk for exposure to infectious agents are identified. IV/injection drug use, sexual practices, and a history of foreign travel are all potential risk factors for liver disease. The amount and type of alcohol consumption are identified using screening tools (questionnaires) that have been developed for this purpose (see Chapter 5). Men who consume 60 to 80 g of alcohol per day (approximately four glasses of beer, wine, or mixed drinks) and women whose alcohol intake is 40 to 60 g/day are estimated to be at high risk for cirrhosis.

The history also includes an evaluation of the patient's past medical history to identify risk factors for the development of liver disease. Current and past medical conditions, including those of a psychological or psychiatric nature, are identified. The family history includes questions about familial liver disorders that may have their origin in alcohol abuse or gallstone disease, as well as other familial or genetic diseases, such as hemochromatosis, Wilson's disease, or $alpha_1$-antitrypsin disease (see "Genetics in Nursing Practice" in Chapter 42).

The history also addresses symptoms that suggest liver disease. Symptoms that may have their origin in liver disease but are not specific to hepatic dysfunction include jaundice, malaise, weakness, fatigue, pruritus, abdominal pain, fever, anorexia, weight gain, edema, increasing abdominal girth, hematemesis, melena, hematochezia (passage of bloody stools), easy bruising, changes in mental acuity, personality changes, sleep disturbances, and decreased libido in men and secondary amenorrhea in women.

Physical Examination

The nurse assesses the patient for physical signs that may occur with liver dysfunction, including the pallor often seen with chronic illness and jaundice. The skin, mucosa, and sclerae are inspected for jaundice, and the extremities are assessed for muscle atrophy, edema, and skin excoriation secondary to scratching. The nurse observes the skin for petechiae or ecchymotic areas (bruises), spider angiomas, and palmar erythema. The male patient is assessed for unilateral or bilateral gynecomastia and testicular atrophy due to hormonal changes. The patient's cognitive status (recall, memory, abstract thinking) and neurologic status are assessed. The nurse observes for general tremor, asterixis, weakness, and slurred speech. These symptoms are discussed later.

The nurse assesses for the presence of an abdominal fluid wave (discussed later). The abdomen is palpated to assess liver size and to detect any tenderness over the liver. The liver may be palpable in the right upper quadrant. A palpable liver presents as a firm, sharp ridge with a smooth surface (Fig. 39-3). The nurse estimates the size of the liver by percussing its upper and lower borders. If the liver is not palpable but tenderness is suspected, tapping the lower right thorax briskly may elicit tenderness. For comparison, the nurse then performs a similar maneuver on the left lower thorax (Bickley & Szilagyi, 2003).

If the liver is palpable, the examiner notes and records its size, its consistency, any tenderness, and whether its outline is regular or irregular. If the liver is enlarged, the degree to which it descends below the right costal margin is recorded to provide some indication of its size. The examiner determines whether the liver's edge is sharp and smooth or blunt, and whether the enlarged liver is nodular or smooth. The liver of a patient with cirrhosis is small and hard, whereas the liver of a patient with acute hepatitis is soft, and the hand easily moves the edge.

Tenderness of the liver indicates recent acute enlargement with consequent stretching of the liver capsule. The absence of tenderness may imply that the enlargement is of longstanding duration. The liver of a patient with viral hepatitis is tender, whereas that of a patient with alcoholic hepatitis is not. Enlargement of the liver is an abnormal finding that requires evaluation (Bickley & Szilagyi, 2003).

Diagnostic Evaluation

Liver Function Tests

More than 70% of the parenchyma of the liver may be damaged before liver function test results become abnormal. Function is generally measured in terms of serum enzyme activity (ie, serum aminotransferases, alkaline phosphatase, lactic dehydrogenase) and serum concentrations of proteins (albumin and globulins), bilirubin, ammonia, clotting fac-

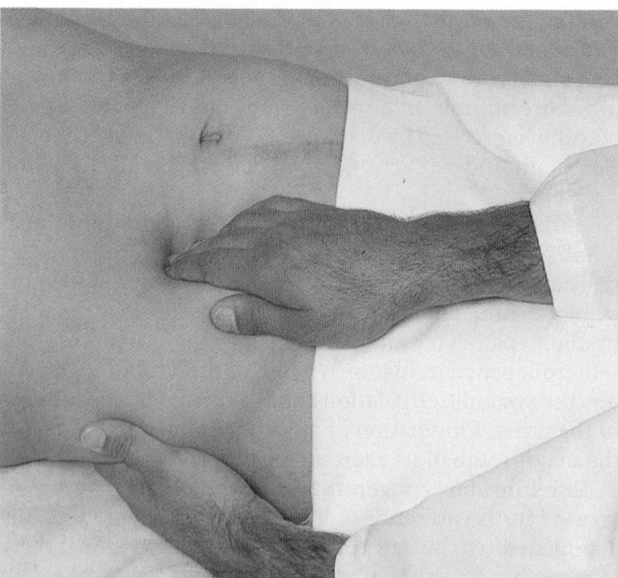

FIGURE 39-3. Technique for palpating the liver. The examiner places one hand under the right lower rib cage and presses downward with light pressure with the other hand.

tors, and lipids. Several of these tests may be helpful for assessing patients with liver disease. However, the nature and extent of hepatic dysfunction cannot be determined by these tests alone, because other disorders can affect test results.

Serum aminotransferases (also called transaminases) are sensitive indicators of injury to the liver cells and are useful in detecting acute liver disease such as hepatitis. Alanine aminotransferase (ALT), aspartate aminotransferase (AST), and gamma-glutamyl transferase (GGT) (also called G-glutamyl transpeptidase) are the most frequently used tests of liver damage. ALT levels increase primarily in liver disorders and may be used to monitor the course of hepatitis or cirrhosis or the effects of treatments that may be toxic to the liver. AST is present in tissues that have high metabolic activity; therefore, the level may be increased if there is damage to or death of tissues of organs such as the heart, liver, skeletal muscle, and kidney. Although not specific to liver disease, levels of AST may be increased in cirrhosis, hepatitis, and liver cancer. Increased GGT levels are associated with cholestasis but can also be due to alcoholic liver disease. Although the kidney has the highest level of the enzyme, the liver is considered the source of normal serum activity. The test determines liver cell dysfunction and is a sensitive indicator of cholestasis. Its main value in liver disease is confirming the hepatic origin of an elevated alkaline phosphatase level. Common liver function tests are summarized in Table 39-1.

Liver Biopsy

Liver biopsy is the removal of a small amount of liver tissue, usually through needle aspiration. It permits examination of liver cells. The most common indication is to evaluate diffuse disorders of the parenchyma and to diagnose space-occupying lesions. Liver biopsy is especially useful when clinical findings and laboratory tests are not diagnostic. Bleeding and bile peritonitis after liver biopsy are the major complications; therefore, coagulation studies are obtained, their values are noted, and abnormal results are treated before liver biopsy is performed. Other techniques for liver biopsy are preferred if ascites or coagulation abnormalities exist. A liver biopsy can be performed percutaneously with ultrasound guidance or transvenously through the right internal jugular vein to right hepatic vein under fluoroscopic control. Liver biopsy can also be performed laparoscopically. Nursing responsibilities related to percutaneous liver biopsy are summarized in Chart 39-2.

Other Diagnostic Tests

Ultrasonography, computed tomography (CT), and magnetic resonance imaging (MRI) are used to identify normal structures and abnormalities of the liver and biliary tree. A radioisotope liver scan may be performed to assess liver size and hepatic blood flow and obstruction.

Laparoscopy (insertion of a fiberoptic endoscope through a small abdominal incision) is used to examine the liver and other pelvic structures. It is also used to perform guided liver biopsy, to determine the cause of ascites, and to diagnose and stage tumors of the liver and other abdominal organs.

Manifestations of Hepatic Dysfunction

Hepatic dysfunction results from damage to the liver's parenchymal cells, directly from primary liver diseases or indirectly from either obstruction of bile flow or derangements of hepatic circulation. Liver dysfunction may be acute or chronic; the latter is far more common.

Chronic liver disease, including **cirrhosis**, is the ninth most common cause of death in the United States among young and middle-aged adults. At least 40% of those deaths are associated with alcohol use. The rate of chronic liver disease for men is twice that for women, and chronic liver disease is more common among African Americans than among Caucasians (Friedman, McQuaid & Grendell, 2003).

Disease processes that lead to hepatocellular dysfunction may be caused by infectious agents such as bacteria and viruses and by anoxia, metabolic disorders, toxins and medications, nutritional deficiencies, and hypersensitivity states. The most common cause of parenchymal damage is malnutrition, especially that related to alcoholism.

The parenchymal cells respond to most noxious agents by replacing glycogen with lipids, producing fatty infiltration with or without cell death or necrosis. This is commonly associated with inflammatory cell infiltration and growth of fibrous tissue. Cell regeneration can occur if the disease process is not too toxic to the cells. The result of chronic parenchymal disease is the shrunken, fibrotic liver seen in cirrhosis.

The consequences of liver disease are numerous and varied. Their ultimate effects are often incapacitating or life-threatening, and their presence is ominous. Treatment often is difficult. Among the most common and significant symptoms of liver disease are the following:

- Jaundice, resulting from increased bilirubin concentration in the blood
- Portal hypertension, ascites, and varices, resulting from circulatory changes within the diseased liver and producing severe GI hemorrhages and marked sodium and fluid retention
- Nutritional deficiencies, which result from the inability of the damaged liver cells to metabolize certain vitamins (responsible for impaired functioning of the central and peripheral nervous systems and for abnormal bleeding tendencies and to synthesize proteins)
- Hepatic encephalopathy or coma, reflecting accumulation of ammonia in the serum due to impaired protein metabolism by the diseased liver

Jaundice

When the bilirubin concentration in the blood is abnormally elevated, all the body tissues, including the sclerae and the skin, become tinged yellow or greenish-yellow, a condition called jaundice. Jaundice becomes clinically evident when the serum bilirubin level exceeds 2.5 mg/dL (43 fmol/L). Increased serum bilirubin levels and jaundice may result from impairment of hepatic uptake, conjugation of bilirubin,

TABLE 39-1 Liver Function Studies

Test	Normal	Clinical Functions
Pigment Studies		
Serum bilirubin, direct	0–0.3 mg/dL (0–5.1 μmol/L)	These studies measure the ability of the liver to conjugate and excrete bilirubin. Results are abnormal in liver and biliary tract disease and are associated with jaundice clinically.
Serum bilirubin, total	0–0.9 mg/dL (1.7–20.5 μmol/L)	
Urine bilirubin	0(0)	
Urine urobilinogen	0.05–2.5 mg/24 h (0.09–4.23 μmol/24 h)	
Fecal urobilinogen (infrequently used)	40–200 mg/24 h (0.068–0.34 mmol/24 h)	
Protein Studies		
Total serum protein	7.0–7.5 g/dL (70–75 g/L)	Proteins are manufactured by the liver. Their levels may be affected in a variety of liver impairments: albumin is affected in cirrhosis, chronic hepatitis, edema and ascites, globulins are affected in cirrhosis, liver disease, chronic obstructive jaundice, and viral hepatitis.
Serum albumin	4.0–5.5 g/dL (40–55 g/L)	
Serum globulin	1.7–3.3 g/dL (17–33 g/L)	
Serum protein electrophoresis		
Albumin	4.0–5.5 g/dL (40–55 g/L)	
α_1-Globulin	0.15–0.25 g/dL (1.5–2.5 g/L)	
α_2-Globulin	0.43–0.75 g/dL (4.3–7.5 g/L)	
β-Globulin	0.5–1.0 g/dL (5–10 g/L)	
γ-Globulin	0.6–1.3 g/dL (6–13 g/L)	
Albumin/globulin (A/G) ratio	A > G or 1.5:1–2.5:1	A/G ratio is reversed in chronic liver disease (decreased albumin and increased globulin).
Prothrombin Time	100% or 12–16 seconds	Prothrombin time may be prolonged in liver disease. It will not return to normal with vitamin K in severe liver cell damage.
Serum Alkaline Phosphatase	Varies with method: 2–5 Bodansky units 30–50 U/L at 34°C (17–142 U/L at 30°C) (20–90 U/L at 30°C)	Serum alkaline phosphatase is manufactured in bones, liver, kidneys, and intestine and excreted through biliary tract. In absence of bone disease, it is a sensitive measure of biliary tract obstruction.
Serum Aminotransferase Studies		
AST	10–40 units (4.8–19 U/L)	The studies are based on release of enzymes from damaged liver cells. These enzymes are elevated in liver cell damage.
ALT	5–35 units (2.4–17 U/L)	
GGT, GGTP	10–48 IU/L	Elevated in alcohol abuse. Marker for biliary cholestasis.
LDH	100–200 units (100–225 U/L)	
Ammonia (plasma)	15–45 μg/dL (11–32 μmol/L)	Liver converts ammonia to urea. Ammonia level rises in liver failure.
Cholesterol		
Ester	60% of total (fraction of total cholesterol: 0.60)	Cholesterol levels are elevated in biliary obstruction and decreased in parenchymal liver disease.
HDL (high-density lipoprotein)	HDL Male: 35–70 mg/dL, Female: 35–85 mg/dL	
LDL (low-density lipoprotein)	LDL < 130 μg/dL	

Additional Studies	Clinical Functions
Barium study of esophagus	To identify varices, which indicate increased portal blood pressure
Abdominal x-ray	To determine gross liver size
Liver scan with radiotagged iodinated rose bengal, gold, technetium, or gallium	To show size and shape of liver; to show replacement of liver tissue with scars, cysts, or tumor
Cholecystogram and cholangiogram	To visualize gallbladder and bile duct visualization
Celiac axis arteriography	To visualize liver and pancreas visualization
Splenoportogram (splenic portal venography)	To determine adequacy of portal blood flow
Laparoscopy	To directly visualize anterior surface of liver, gallbladder, and mesentery through a trocar
Liver biopsy (percutaneous or transjugular)	To determine anatomic changes in liver tissue
Measurement of portal pressure	To detect increased portal pressure which occurs with cirrhosis of the liver
Esophagoscopy/endoscopy	To search for esophageal varices and other abnormalities

TABLE 39-1 Liver Function Studies (Continued)

Additional Studies	Clinical Functions
Electroencephalogram	To detect abnormalities that occur with hepatic coma
Ultrasonography	To show size of abdominal organs and presence of masses
Computed tomography (CT scan)	To detect hepatic neoplasms; diagnose cysts, abscesses, and hematomas; and distinguish between obstructive and nonobstructive jaundice. Detects cerebral atrophy in hepatic encephalopathy.
Angiography	To visualize hepatic circulation and detect presence and nature of hepatic masses
Magnetic resonance imaging (MRI)	To detect hepatic neoplasms; diagnose cysts, abscesses, and hematomas. Detects cerebral atrophy in encephalopathy.
Endoscopic retrograde cholangiopancreatography (ERCP)	To visualize biliary structures via endoscopy

or excretion of bilirubin into the biliary system. There are several types of jaundice: hemolytic, hepatocellular, and obstructive jaundice, and jaundice due to hereditary hyperbilirubinemia. Hepatocellular and obstructive jaundice are the two types commonly associated with liver disease.

Hemolytic Jaundice

Hemolytic jaundice is the result of an increased destruction of the red blood cells, the effect of which is to flood the plasma with bilirubin so rapidly that the liver, although functioning normally, cannot excrete the bilirubin as quickly as it is formed. This type of jaundice is encountered in patients with hemolytic transfusion reactions and other hemolytic disorders. In these patients, the bilirubin in the blood is predominantly unconjugated or free. Fecal and urine urobilinogen levels are increased, but the urine is free of bilirubin. Patients with this type of jaundice, unless their hyperbilirubinemia is extreme, do not experience symptoms or complications as a result of the jaundice per se. However, prolonged jaundice, even if mild, predisposes to the formation of pigment stones in the gallbladder, and extremely severe jaundice (levels of free bilirubin exceeding 20 to 25 mg/dL) poses a risk for brain stem damage.

Hepatocellular Jaundice

Hepatocellular jaundice is caused by the inability of damaged liver cells to clear normal amounts of bilirubin from the blood. The cellular damage may be caused by hepatitis viruses (eg, hepatitis A, B, C, D, or E), other viruses that affect the liver (eg, yellow fever virus, Epstein-Barr virus), medications or chemical toxins (eg, carbon tetrachloride, chloroform, phosphorus, arsenicals, certain medications), or alcohol. Cirrhosis of the liver is a form of hepatocellular disease that may produce jaundice. It is usually associated with excessive alcohol intake, but it may also be a late result of liver cell necrosis caused by viral infection. In prolonged obstructive jaundice, cell damage eventually develops, so that both types of jaundice (ie, obstructive and hepatocellular jaundice) appear together.

Patients with hepatocellular jaundice may be mildly or severely ill, with lack of appetite, nausea, malaise, fatigue, weakness, and possible weight loss. In some cases of hepatocellular disease, jaundice may not be obvious. The serum bilirubin concentration and the urine urobilinogen level may be elevated. In addition, AST and ALT levels may be increased, indicating cellular necrosis. The patient may report headache, chills, and fever if the cause is infectious. Depending on the cause and extent of the liver cell damage, hepatocellular jaundice may be completely reversible.

Obstructive Jaundice

Obstructive jaundice resulting from extrahepatic obstruction may be caused by occlusion of the bile duct from a gallstone, an inflammatory process, a tumor, or pressure from an enlarged organ (eg, liver, gallbladder). The obstruction may also involve the small bile ducts within the liver (ie, intrahepatic obstruction); this may be caused, for example, by pressure on these channels from inflammatory swelling of the liver or by an inflammatory exudate within the ducts themselves. Intrahepatic obstruction resulting from stasis and inspissation (thickening) of bile within the canaliculi may occur after the ingestion of certain medications, which are referred to as cholestatic agents. These agents include phenothiazines, antithyroid medications, sulfonylureas, tricyclic antidepressant agents, nitrofurantoin, androgens and estrogens, propylthiouracil, amoxicillin-clavulanic acid, and erythromycin estolate.

Regardless of whether the obstruction is intrahepatic or extrahepatic, and regardless of its cause, bile cannot flow normally into the intestine and becomes backed up into the liver substance. It is then reabsorbed into the blood and carried throughout the entire body, staining the skin, mucous membranes, and sclerae. It is excreted in the urine, which becomes deep orange and foamy. Because of the decreased amount of bile in the intestinal tract, the stools become light or clay-colored. The skin may itch intensely, requiring repeated soothing baths. Dyspepsia and intolerance to fatty foods may develop because of impaired fat digestion in the absence of intestinal bile. In general, AST, ALT, and GGT levels rise only

CHART 39-2 Guidelines for Assisting With Percutaneous Liver Biopsy

NURSING INTERVENTIONS	RATIONALE
Preprocedure	
1. Ascertain that results of coagulation tests (prothrombin time, partial thromboplastin time, and platelet count) are available and that compatible donor blood is available.	1. Many patients with liver disease have clotting defects and are at risk for bleeding.
2. Check for signed consent; confirm that informed consent has been provided.	2. Ensures that the patient consents to this invasive procedure.
3. Measure and record the patient's pulse, respirations, and blood pressure immediately before biopsy.	3. Prebiopsy values provide a basis on which to compare the patient's vital signs and evaluate status after the procedure.
4. Describe to the patient in advance: steps of the procedure; sensations expected; after-effects anticipated; restrictions of activity and monitoring procedures to follow.	4. Explanations allay fears and ensure cooperation.
During Procedure	
1. Support the patient during the procedure.	1. Encouragement and support of the nurse enhance comfort and promote a sense of security.
2. Expose the right side of the patient's upper abdomen (right hypochondriac).	2. The skin at the site of penetration will be cleansed and a local anesthetic will be infiltrated.
3. Instruct the patient to inhale and exhale deeply several times, finally to exhale, and to hold breath at the end of expiration. The physician promptly introduces the biopsy needle by way of the transthoracic (intercostal) or transabdominal (subcostal) route, penetrates the liver, aspirates, and withdraws.	3. Holding the breath immobilizes the chest wall and the diaphragm; penetration of the diaphragm thereby is avoided, and the risk of lacerating the liver is minimized.
4. Instruct the patient to resume breathing.	4. The patient often continues holding his or her breath because of anxiety.

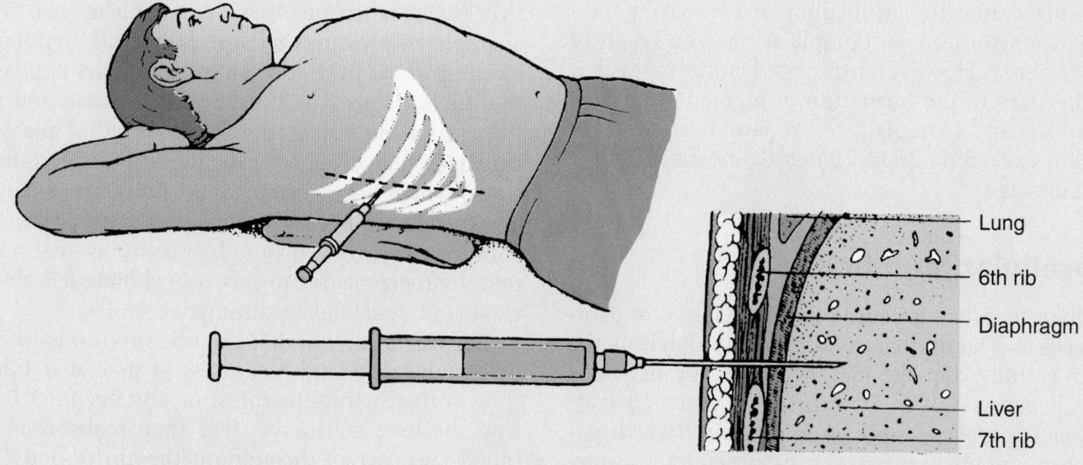

CHART 39-2 **Guidelines for Assisting With Percutaneous Liver Biopsy, continued**

NURSING INTERVENTIONS	RATIONALE
Postprocedure	
1. Immediately after the biopsy, assist the patient to turn onto the right side; place a pillow under the costal margin, and caution the patient to remain in this position, recumbent and immobile, for several hours. Instruct the patient to avoid coughing or straining.	1. In this position, the liver capsule at the site of penetration is compressed against the chest wall, and the escape of blood or bile through the perforation is prevented.
2. Measure and record the patient's pulse, respiratory rate, and blood pressure at 10- to 15-minute intervals for the first hour, then every 30 minutes for the next 1 to 2 hours or until the patient's condition stabilizes.	2. Changes in vital signs may indicate bleeding, severe hemorrhage, or bile peritonitis, the most frequent complications of liver biopsy.
3. If the patient is discharged after the procedure, instruct the patient to avoid heavy lifting and strenuous activity for 1 week.	3. Activity restriction reduces the risk of bleeding at the biopsy puncture site.

moderately, but bilirubin and alkaline phosphatase levels are elevated.

Hereditary Hyperbilirubinemia

Increased serum bilirubin levels (hyperbilirubinemia) resulting from any of several inherited disorders can also produce jaundice. Gilbert's syndrome is a familial disorder characterized by an increased level of unconjugated bilirubin that causes jaundice. Although serum bilirubin levels are increased, liver histology and liver function test results are normal, and there is no hemolysis. This syndrome affects 3% to 8% of the population, predominantly males (Yamada, 2003).

Other conditions that are probably caused by inborn errors of biliary metabolism include Dubin–Johnson syndrome (chronic idiopathic jaundice, with pigment in the liver) and Rotor's syndrome (chronic familial conjugated hyperbilirubinemia without pigment in the liver); the "benign" cholestatic jaundice of pregnancy, with retention of conjugated bilirubin, probably secondary to unusual sensitivity to the hormones of pregnancy; and benign recurrent intrahepatic cholestasis.

Portal Hypertension

Obstructed blood flow through the damaged liver results in increased pressure throughout the portal venous system (**portal hypertension**). Portal hypertension is commonly associated with hepatic cirrhosis, but it can also occur with noncirrhotic liver disease. Although splenomegaly (enlarged spleen) with possible hypersplenism is a common manifestation of portal hypertension, the two major consequences of portal hypertension are ascites and varices.

In ascites, fluid accumulates in the peritoneal cavity. Although ascites is often a result of liver damage, it may also occur with disorders such as cancer, kidney disease, and heart failure. Varices are varicosities that develop from elevated pressure in the veins that drain into the portal system. They are prone to rupture and often are the source of massive hemorrhages from the upper GI tract and the rectum. In addition, blood clotting abnormalities, often seen in patients with severe liver disease, increase the likelihood of bleeding and significant blood loss.

Ascites

Pathophysiology

The mechanisms responsible for the development of ascites are not completely understood. Portal hypertension and the resulting increase in capillary pressure and obstruction of venous blood flow through the damaged liver are contributing factors. The vasodilation that occurs in the splanchnic circulation is also a suspected causative factor. The failure of the liver to metabolize aldosterone increases sodium and water retention by the kidney. Sodium and water retention, increased intravascular fluid volume, increased lymphatic flow and decreased synthesis of albumin by the damaged liver all contribute to the movement of fluid from the vascular system into the peritoneal space. The process becomes self-perpetuating as loss of fluid into the peritoneal space causes further sodium and water retention by the kidney in an effort to maintain the vascular fluid volume.

As a result of liver damage, large amounts of albumin-rich fluid, 15 L or more, may accumulate in the peritoneal cavity as ascites. With the movement of albumin from the serum to the peritoneal cavity, the osmotic pressure of the serum decreases. This, combined with increased portal pressure, results in movement of fluid into the peritoneal cavity (Fig. 39-4).

Clinical Manifestations

Increased abdominal girth and rapid weight gain are common presenting symptoms of ascites. The patient may be short of breath and uncomfortable from the enlarged abdomen, and

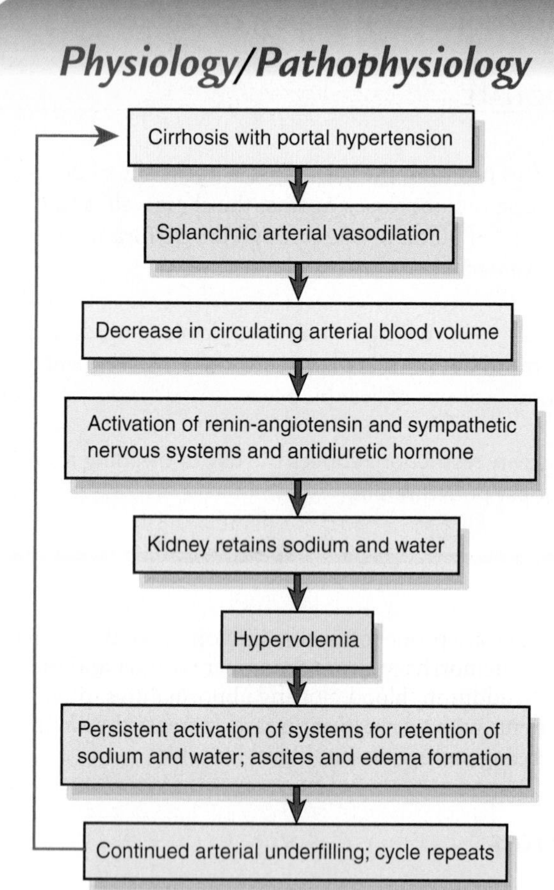

FIGURE 39-4. Pathogenesis of ascites (arterial vasodilation theory).

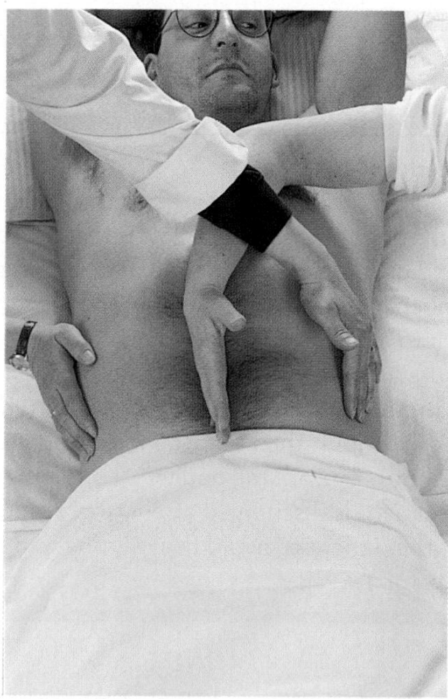

FIGURE 39-5. Assessing for abdominal fluid wave. The examiner places the hands along the sides of the patient's flanks, then strikes one flank sharply, detecting any fluid wave with the other hand. An assistant's hand is placed (ulnar side down) along the patient's midline to prevent the fluid wave from being transmitted through the tissues of the abdominal wall.

striae and distended veins may be visible over the abdominal wall. Umbilical hernias also occur frequently in those patients with cirrhosis. Fluid and electrolyte imbalances are common.

Assessment and Diagnostic Evaluation

The presence and extent of ascites are assessed by percussion of the abdomen. When fluid has accumulated in the peritoneal cavity, the flanks bulge when the patient assumes a supine position. The presence of fluid can be confirmed either by percussing for shifting dullness or by detecting a fluid wave (Fig. 39-5). A fluid wave is likely to be found only if a large amount of fluid is present. Daily measurement and recording of abdominal girth and body weight are essential to assess the progression of ascites and its response to treatment.

Medical Management

Dietary Modification

The goal of treatment for the patient with ascites is a negative sodium balance to reduce fluid retention. Table salt, salty foods, salted butter and margarine, and all ordinary canned and frozen foods that are not specifically prepared for low-sodium (2-g sodium) diets should be avoided. It may take 2 to 3 months for the patient's taste buds to adjust to unsalted foods. In the meantime, the taste of unsalted foods can be improved by using salt substitutes such as lemon juice, oregano, and thyme. Commercial salt substitutes need to be approved by the physician, because those that contain ammonia could precipitate hepatic coma. Most salt substitutes contain potassium and should be avoided if the patient has impaired renal function. The patient should make liberal use of powdered, low-sodium milk and milk products. If fluid accumulation is not controlled with this regimen, the daily sodium allowance may be reduced further to 500 mg, and diuretics may be administered.

Dietary control of ascites via strict sodium restriction is difficult to achieve at home. The likelihood that the patient will follow even a 2-g sodium diet increases if the patient and the person preparing meals understand the rationale for the diet and receive periodic guidance about selecting and preparing appropriate foods. Approximately 10% of patients with ascites respond to these measures alone. Nonresponders and those who find sodium restriction difficult require diuretic therapy.

Diuretics

Use of diuretics along with sodium restriction is successful in 90% of patients with ascites. Spironolactone (Aldactone), an aldosterone-blocking agent, is most often the first-line therapy in patients with ascites from cirrhosis. When used with other diuretics, spironolactone helps prevent potassium loss. Oral diuretics such as furosemide (Lasix) may be added but should be used cautiously, because long-term use may induce severe sodium depletion (hyponatremia).

Ammonium chloride and acetazolamide (Diamox) are contraindicated because of the possibility of precipitating hepatic coma. Daily weight loss should not exceed 1 to 2 kg (2.2 to 4.4 lb) in patients with ascites and peripheral edema or 0.5 to 0.75 kg (1.1 to 1.65 lb) in patients without edema. Fluid restriction is not attempted unless the serum sodium concentration is very low.

Possible complications of diuretic therapy include fluid and electrolyte disturbances (including hypovolemia, hypokalemia, hyponatremia, and hypochloremic alkalosis) and encephalopathy. Encephalopathy may be precipitated by dehydration and hypovolemia. In addition, when potassium stores are depleted, the amount of ammonia in the systemic circulation increases, which may cause impaired cerebral functioning and encephalopathy.

Bed Rest

In patients with ascites, an upright posture is associated with activation of the renin–angiotensin–aldosterone system and sympathetic nervous system (Porth, 2005). This causes reduced renal glomerular filtration and sodium excretion and a decreased response to loop diuretics. Therefore, bed rest may be a useful therapy, especially for patients whose condition is refractory to diuretics.

Paracentesis

Paracentesis is the removal of fluid (ascites) from the peritoneal cavity through a puncture or a small surgical incision through the abdominal wall under sterile conditions. Ultrasound guidance may be indicated in some patients who are at high risk for bleeding because of an abnormal coagulation profile and in those who have had previous abdominal surgery and may have adhesions. Paracentesis was once considered a routine form of treatment for ascites. However, it is now performed primarily for diagnostic examination of ascitic fluid, for treatment of massive ascites that is resistant to nutritional and diuretic therapy and that is causing severe problems to the patient, and as a prelude to diagnostic imaging studies, peritoneal dialysis, or surgery. A sample of the ascitic fluid may be sent to the laboratory for cell count, albumin and total protein levels, culture, and other tests.

Large-volume (5 to 6 L) paracentesis has been shown to be a safe method for treating patients with severe ascites. This technique, in combination with the IV infusion of salt-poor albumin or other colloid, has become a standard management strategy yielding an immediate effect. Refractive, massive ascites is unresponsive to multiple diuretics and sodium restriction for 2 weeks or more and can result in severe sequelae such as respiratory distress, which requires rapid intervention. Albumin infusions help to correct decreases in effective arterial blood volume that lead to sodium retention. Use of this colloid reduces the incidence of hyponatremia and renal dysfunction associated with decreased effective arterial volume (Friedman et al., 2003). The beneficial effects of albumin administration on hemodynamic stability and renal functional status may be related to an improvement in cardiac function as well as a decrease in the degree of arterial vasodilation (Fernandez, Drebin, Lineham, et al., 2004). Although the patient with cirrhosis has a greatly increased extracellular blood volume, the kidney incorrectly senses that the effective volume has decreased. The renin–angiotensin–aldosterone axis is stimulated, and sodium is reabsorbed. In addition, antidiuretic hormone (ADH) secretion increases, which leads to increased retention of free water and sometimes to the development of dilutional hyponatremia (Fishman, Hoffman, Klauser, et al., 2004). Therapeutic paracentesis provides only temporary removal of fluid; ascites rapidly recurs, necessitating repeated fluid removal. Nursing care of the patient undergoing paracentesis is presented in Chart 39-3.

Transjugular Intrahepatic Portosystemic Shunt (TIPS)

Transjugular intrahepatic portosystemic shunt (TIPS) is a method of treating ascites in which a cannula is threaded into the portal vein by the transjugular route (Fig. 39-6). To reduce portal hypertension, an expandable stent is inserted to serve as an intrahepatic shunt between the portal circulation and the hepatic vein. TIPS is the treatment of choice for refractive ascites. It is extremely effective in decreasing sodium retention, improving the renal response to diuretic therapy, and preventing recurrence of fluid accumulation (Gines, Cardenas, Arroyo, et al., 2004).

Because the development of ascites in patients with cirrhosis is associated with a 50% mortality rate, any patient who is considered a candidate for liver transplantation should be referred for TIPS.

Other Methods of Treatment

Ascites can also be treated by the insertion of a peritoneovenous shunt to redirect ascitic fluid from the peritoneal cavity into the systemic circulation. However, this procedure is seldom used because of the high complication rate and high incidence of shunt failure. In fact, use of this shunt has virtually been abandoned, except for patients who are not candidates for liver transplantation.

Nursing Management

If a patient with ascites from liver dysfunction is hospitalized, nursing measures include assessment and documentation of intake and output, abdominal girth, and daily weight to assess fluid status. The nurse monitors serum ammonia and electrolyte levels to assess electrolyte balance, response to therapy, and indicators of encephalopathy.

Promoting Home and Community-Based Care

TEACHING PATIENTS SELF-CARE

The patient treated for ascites is likely to be discharged with some ascites still present. Before hospital discharge, the nurse teaches the patient and family about the treatment plan, including the need to avoid all alcohol intake, adhere to a low-sodium diet, take medications as prescribed, and check with the physician before taking any new medications (Chart 39-4). Additional patient and family teaching addresses skin care and the need to weigh the

CHART 39-3 Guidelines for Assisting With a Paracentesis

NURSING INTERVENTIONS	RATIONALE
Preprocedure	
1. Check for signed consent form.	1. Ensures that patient has agreed to procedure.
2. Prepare the patient by providing the necessary information and instructions and by offering reassurance.	2. Having information increases the patient's understanding of the procedure and the reason for it.
3. Instruct the patient to void.	3. An empty bladder minimizes the risk of inadvertent puncture of the bladder and minimizes discomfort from a full bladder.
4. Gather appropriate sterile equipment and collection receptacles.	4. Sterility of equipment is essential to minimize risk of infection; having equipment available enables the procedure to be performed smoothly.
5. Place the patient in upright position on the edge of the bed or in a chair with feet supported on a stool. Fowler's position should be used by the patient confined to bed.	5. An upright position results in movement of the peritoneal fluid close to the abdominal wall and promotes easier puncture and removal of fluid.
6. Place the sphygmomanometer cuff around patient's arm.	6. This allows the nurse to monitor the patient's blood pressure during procedure.
Procedure	
1. The physician, using aseptic technique, inserts the trocar through a puncture below the umbilicus. The trocar or needle is connected to a drainage tube, the end of which is inserted into a collecting receptacle.	1. Sterile technique minimizes the risk of infection. Bleeding at the puncture site is minimal at this location. The fluid drains by gravity or mild siphon into the container.
2. Help the patient maintain position throughout the procedure.	2. The patient who is fatigued or weak may have difficulty maintaining an optimal position for drainage of fluid.
3. Measure and record blood pressure at frequent intervals throughout the procedure.	3. Decreased blood pressure may occur with vascular collapse, which can result from removal of the fluid from the peritoneal cavity and fluid shifts.
4. Monitor the patient closely for signs of vascular collapse: pallor, increased pulse rate, or decreased blood pressure.	4. Vascular collapse (hypovolemia) may occur as fluid moves from the vascular system to replace fluid drained from peritoneal cavity.

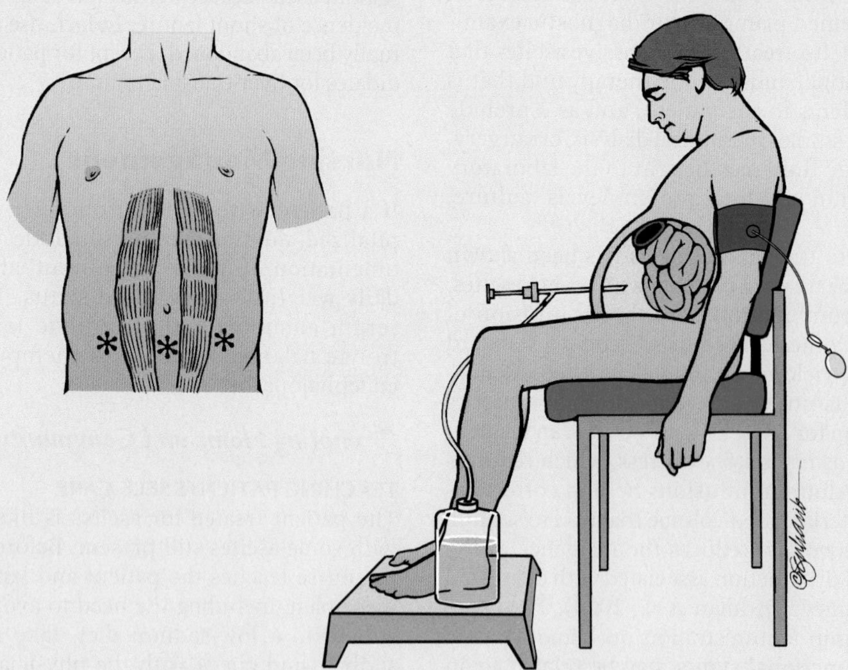

Figure on left shows possible sites for insertion of trocar.

CHART 39-3 Guidelines for Assisting With a Paracentesis, continued

NURSING ACTION	RATIONALE
Postprocedure	
1. Return the patient to bed or to a comfortable sitting position.	1. The weak or fatigued patient may have difficulty resuming a comfortable position without assistance.
2. Measure, describe, and record the fluid collected.	2. The volume of fluid removed may range from small to very large, and its removal may affect fluid and vascular status; volume should be included in input and output records. The characteristics of the fluid (clear vs. cloudy, red vs. colorless) may be helpful in diagnostic evaluation.
3. Label samples of fluid and send to laboratory.	3. Peritoneal fluid is analyzed as part of the diagnostic workup.
4. Monitor vital signs every 15 min for 1 h, every 30 min for 2 h, every hour for 2 h, and then every 4 h.	4. Vital signs (blood pressure, pulse rate) may change as fluid shifts occur after removal of fluid, especially if a large volume of fluid has been removed.
5. Measure the patient's temperature.	5. An elevated temperature is a sign of infection and should be reported to the patient's physician.
6. Assess for hypovolemia, electrolyte shifts, changes in mental status, and encephalopathy.	6. Changes in fluid and electrolyte states and mental and cognitive status may occur with removal of fluid and fluid shifts, and should be reported.
7. When taking vital signs, check puncture site for leakage or bleeding.	7. Leakage of fluid may occur because of changes in abdominal pressure and may contribute to further loss of fluid if undetected. Leakage suggests a possible site for infection, and bleeding may occur in patients with altered clotting secondary to liver disease.
8. Provide patient teaching regarding need to monitor for bleeding or excessive drainage from puncture site, importance of avoiding heavy lifting or straining, the need to change position slowly, and frequency of monitoring for fever.	8. The patient (or family members) need to monitor the patient and puncture site for bleeding and excessive drainage if the patient is discharged home after the procedure. Heavy lifting or straining is avoided to enable the puncture site to close. Slow changes in position are recommended because of the risk of hypovolemia related to fluid removal. Monitoring for fever is needed to detect infection.

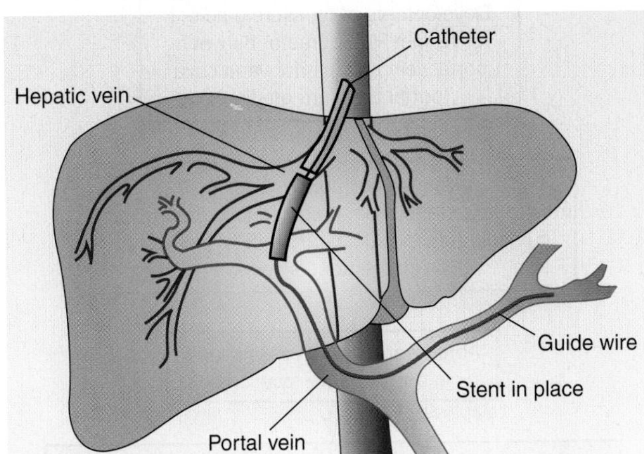

FIGURE 39-6. Transjugular intrahepatic portosystemic shunt (TIPS). A stent is inserted via catheter to the portal vein to divert blood flow and reduce portal hypertension.

patient daily and to watch for and report signs and symptoms of complications.

CONTINUING CARE

A referral for home care may be warranted, especially if the patient lives alone or cannot provide self-care. The home visit enables the nurse to assess changes in the patient's condition and weight, abdominal girth, skin, and cognitive and emotional status. The home care nurse assesses the home environment and the availability of resources needed to adhere to the treatment plan (eg, a scale to obtain daily weights, facilities to prepare and store appropriate foods, resources to purchase needed medications). It is important to assess the patient's adherence to the treatment plan and the ability to buy, prepare, and eat appropriate foods. The nurse reinforces previous teaching and emphasizes the need for regular follow-up and the importance of keeping scheduled health care appointments.

CHART 39-4

HOME CARE CHECKLIST • Management of Ascites

At the completion of the home care instruction, the patient or caregiver will be able to:	Patient	Caregiver
• Make appropriate dietary choices consistent with dietary prescription and recommendations.	✔	✔
• State the importance of weighing self daily and keeping a daily record of weight.	✔	✔
• Maintain record of daily weight and identify daily weight-loss goals.	✔	✔
• List weight changes (loss or gain) that should be reported to the primary health care provider.	✔	✔
• Explain the rationale for monitoring and recording daily intake and output.	✔	✔
• Identify changes in output that should be reported to primary health care provider (eg, decreasing urine output).	✔	✔
• Identify rationale for fluid restrictions (if needed), and comply with fluid restriction.	✔	✔
• Discuss importance of avoiding nonsteroidal anti-inflammatory agents, medications (eg, cough mixtures) containing alcohol, antibiotics or antacids containing salt.	✔	✔
• Describe effects, side effects, and monitoring parameters for diuretic therapy.	✔	✔
• Identify need to stop all alcohol intake as critical to well-being.	✔	✔
• Explain how to contact Alcoholics Anonymous or alcohol counselors in related organizations.	✔	✔
• Demonstrate how to care for skin, alleviate pressure over bony prominences by turning when in bed or chair, and decrease edema by position changes.	✔	✔
• Identify early signs and symptoms of complications (encephalopathy, spontaneous bacterial peritonitis, dehydration, electrolyte abnormalities, azotemia).	✔	✔

Esophageal Varices

Bleeding or hemorrhage from esophageal varices occurs in approximately one third of patients with cirrhosis and varices. The first bleeding episode has a mortality rate of 30% to 50% and is one of the major causes of death in patients with cirrhosis (Friedman et al., 2003). The mortality rate increases with each subsequent bleeding episode.

Pathophysiology

Esophageal varices are dilated, tortuous veins that are usually found in the submucosa of the lower esophagus but may develop higher in the esophagus or extend into the stomach. This condition is almost always caused by portal hypertension, which results from obstruction of the portal venous circulation within the damaged liver.

Because of increased obstruction of the portal vein, venous blood from the intestinal tract and spleen seeks an outlet through collateral circulation (new pathways for return of blood to the right atrium). The effect is increased pressure, particularly in the vessels in the submucosal layer of the lower esophagus and upper part of the stomach. These collateral vessels are not very elastic; rather, they are tortuous and fragile, and they bleed easily (Fig. 39-7). Less common causes of varices are abnormalities of the circulation in the splenic vein or superior vena cava and hepatic venothrombosis.

Physiology/Pathophysiology

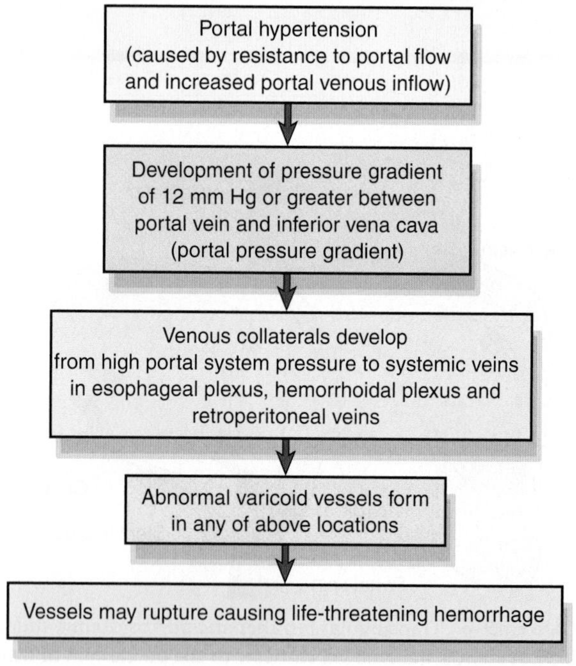

Portal hypertension (caused by resistance to portal flow and increased portal venous inflow)

↓

Development of pressure gradient of 12 mm Hg or greater between portal vein and inferior vena cava (portal pressure gradient)

↓

Venous collaterals develop from high portal system pressure to systemic veins in esophageal plexus, hemorrhoidal plexus and retroperitoneal veins

↓

Abnormal varicoid vessels form in any of above locations

↓

Vessels may rupture causing life-threatening hemorrhage

FIGURE 39-7. Pathogenesis of bleeding esophageal varices.

Bleeding esophageal varices are life-threatening and can result in hemorrhagic shock that produces decreased cerebral, hepatic, and renal perfusion. In turn, there is an increased nitrogen load from bleeding into the GI tract and an increased serum ammonia level, increasing the risk for encephalopathy. Usually the dilated veins cause no symptoms. However, if the portal pressure increases sharply and the mucosa or supporting structures become thin, massive hemorrhaging occurs.

Factors that contribute to hemorrhage are muscular exertion from lifting heavy objects; straining at stool; sneezing, coughing, or vomiting; esophagitis; irritation of vessels by poorly chewed foods or irritating fluids; and reflux of stomach contents (especially alcohol). Salicylates and any medication that erodes the esophageal mucosa or interferes with cell replication also may contribute to bleeding.

Clinical Manifestations

The patient with bleeding esophageal varices may present with hematemesis, melena, or general deterioration in mental or physical status and often has a history of alcohol abuse. Signs and symptoms of shock (cool clammy skin, hypotension, tachycardia) may be present.

Assessment and Diagnostic Findings

Endoscopy is used to identify the bleeding site, along with barium swallow, ultrasonography, CT, and angiography. Because the incidence of varices is 50% in patients with cirrhosis, it is recommended that these patients undergo screening endoscopy every 2 years in an effort to identify and treat large varices, which are the ones most likely to bleed (Zakim & Boyer, 2003).

Endoscopy

Immediate endoscopy (see Chapter 34) is indicated to identify the cause and the site of bleeding; at least 30% of patients with suspected bleeding from esophageal varices are actually bleeding from another source (gastritis, ulcer). Nursing support can be effective in relieving anxiety during this often stressful experience. Careful monitoring can detect early signs of cardiac dysrhythmias, perforation, and hemorrhage.

After the examination, fluids are not given until the gag reflex returns. Lozenges and gargles may be used to relieve throat discomfort if the patient's physical condition and mental status permit. If the patient is actively bleeding, oral intake will not be permitted, and the patient will be prepared for further diagnostic and therapeutic procedures.

Portal Hypertension Measurements

Portal hypertension may be suspected if dilated abdominal veins and hemorrhoids are detected. A palpable enlarged spleen (splenomegaly) and ascites may also be present. Portal venous pressure can be measured directly or indirectly. Indirect measurement of the hepatic vein pressure gradient is the most common procedure. The measurement requires insertion of a catheter with a balloon into the antecubital or femoral vein. The catheter is advanced under fluoroscopy to a hepatic vein. Fluid is infused once the catheter is in position to inflate the balloon. A "wedged" pressure (similar to pulmonary artery wedge pressure) is obtained by occluding the blood flow in the blood vessel; pressure in the unoccluded vessel is also measured. Although the values obtained may underestimate portal pressure, this measurement may be taken several times to evaluate the results of therapy.

Direct measurement of portal vein pressure can be obtained by several methods. During laparotomy, a needle may be introduced into the spleen; a manometer reading of more than 20 mL saline is abnormal. Another direct measurement requires insertion of a catheter into the portal vein or one of its branches. Endoscopic measurement of pressure within varices is used only in conjunction with endoscopic sclerotherapy.

Laboratory Tests

Laboratory tests may include various liver function tests, such as serum aminotransferases, bilirubin, alkaline phosphatase, and serum proteins. Splenoportography, which involves serial or segmental x-rays, is used to detect extensive collateral circulation in esophageal vessels, which would indicate varices. Other tests are hepatoportography and celiac angiography. These are usually performed in the operating room or radiology department.

Medical Management

Bleeding from esophageal varices is an emergency that can quickly lead to hemorrhagic shock. The patient is critically ill, requiring aggressive medical care and expert nursing care, and is usually transferred to the intensive care unit (ICU) for close monitoring and management. See Chapter 15 for a discussion of care of the patient in shock.

The extent of bleeding is evaluated, and vital signs are monitored continuously if hematemesis and melena are present. Signs of potential hypovolemia are noted, such as cold clammy skin, tachycardia, a drop in blood pressure, decreased urine output, restlessness, and weak peripheral pulses. The volume of circulating blood is estimated and monitored with a central venous catheter or pulmonary artery catheter. Blood pressure is monitored via an arterial catheter. Oxygen is administered to prevent hypoxia and to maintain adequate blood oxygenation.

Because patients with bleeding esophageal varices have intravascular volume depletion and are subject to electrolyte imbalance, IV fluids with electrolytes and volume expanders are provided to restore fluid volume and replace electrolytes. Transfusion of blood components also may be required.

Caution must be taken with volume resuscitation so that overhydration does not occur, because this would raise portal pressure and increase bleeding. An indwelling urinary catheter is usually inserted to permit frequent monitoring of urine output.

Although a variety of pharmacologic, endoscopic, and surgical approaches are used to treat bleeding esophageal varices, none is ideal, and most are associated with considerable risk to the patient. Nonsurgical treatment of bleeding esophageal varices is preferable because of the high mortality rate of emergency surgery to control bleeding esophageal varices and because of the poor physical condition that is typical of the patient with severe liver dysfunction.

Pharmacologic Therapy

In an actively bleeding patient, medications are administered initially because they can be obtained and administered quicker than other therapies, which take longer to initiate. Vasopressin (Pitressin) may be the initial mode of therapy, because it produces constriction of the splanchnic arterial bed and decreases portal pressure. It may be administered by IV or intra-arterial infusion (Zakim & Boyer, 2003). Either method requires close monitoring by the nurse. Vital signs and the presence or absence of blood in the gastric aspirate indicate the effectiveness of vasopressin. Monitoring of fluid intake and output and electrolyte levels is necessary, because hyponatremia may develop and vasopressin may have an antidiuretic effect.

Coronary artery disease is a contraindication to the use of vasopressin, because coronary vasoconstriction is a side effect that may precipitate myocardial infarction. The combination of vasopressin with nitroglycerin (administered by the IV, sublingual, or transdermal route) has been effective in reducing or preventing the side effects (constriction of coronary vessels and angina) caused by vasopressin alone.

Somatostatin and octreotide (Sandostatin) have been reported to be more effective than vasopressin in decreasing bleeding from esophageal varices, and they lack the vasoconstrictive effects of vasopressin. These medications cause selective splanchnic vasoconstriction. Propranolol (Inderal) and nadolol (Corgard), beta-blocking agents that decrease portal pressure, have been shown to prevent bleeding from esophageal varices in some patients; however, it is recommended that they be used only in combination with other treatment modalities such as variceal band ligation or sclerotherapy. Beta-blockers should not be used in acute variceal hemorrhage, but they are effective prophylaxis against such an episode. Nitrates such as isosorbide (Isordil) lower portal pressure by venodilation and decreased cardiac output and may be used in combination with beta-blockers. Further studies of these and other medications are necessary to evaluate their use in the treatment and prevention of bleeding episodes (Friedman et al., 2003).

Balloon Tamponade

To control hemorrhage in certain patients, **balloon tamponade** may be used. In this procedure, pressure is exerted on the cardia (upper orifice of the stomach) and against the bleeding varices by a double-balloon tamponade (Sengstaken-Blakemore tube) (Fig. 39-8). The tube has four openings, each with a specific purpose: gastric aspiration, esophageal aspiration, gastric balloon inflation, and esophageal balloon inflation.

The balloon in the stomach is inflated with 100 to 200 mL of air. An x-ray confirms proper positioning of the gastric balloon. The tube is pulled gently to exert a force against the gastric cardia. The preferred method for applying traction may be with weights suspended from an overbed trapeze. Attachment of the balloon tamponade tube to the face shield of a football helmet is a method that has also been used to obtain the necessary traction. Irrigation of the tubing is performed to detect bleeding; if returns are clear, the esophageal balloon is not used. If bleeding continues, the esophageal balloon is inflated. The desired pressure in the esophageal and gastric balloons is 25 to 40 mm Hg, as measured by the manometer. On inflation of the esophageal balloon, there is a possibility of injury or rupture of the esophagus, so constant nursing surveillance is necessary.

Gastric suction is provided by connecting the gastric catheter outlet to low suction (80 to 100 mm Hg). The tubing is irrigated hourly, and the color of the drainage indicates whether bleeding has been controlled. Room-temperature lavage or irrigation may be used in the gastric balloon. The pressure within the esophageal balloon is measured and recorded every 2 to 4 hours via the manometer to detect underinflation (which can allow bleeding to continue) or prevent overinflation (which can cause esophageal injury). When it appears that bleeding has stopped, the balloons are deflated carefully and sequentially. The esophageal balloon is deflated first, and the patient is monitored for recurrent bleeding. After several hours without bleeding, the gastric balloon can be deflated safely. If there is still no bleeding, the tamponade tube is removed. The therapy is used for as short a time as possible to control bleeding while emergency treatment is completed and definitive therapies are instituted (no longer than 24 hours).

Although balloon tamponade has been fairly successful, there are some inherent dangers. Displacement of the tube and the inflated balloon into the oropharynx can cause life-threatening obstruction of the airway and asphyxiation. This may occur if the patient pulls on the tube because of confusion or discomfort. It may also result from rupture of the gastric balloon, which causes the esophageal balloon to move into the oropharynx. Sudden rupture of the balloon causes airway obstruction and aspiration of gastric contents into the lungs. Therefore, the tube must be tested before insertion to minimize this risk by ensuring that the balloons can attain and maintain inflation. Aspiration of blood and secretions into the lungs is frequently associated with balloon tamponade, especially in the stuporous or comatose patient. Endotracheal intubation before insertion of the tube protects the airway and minimizes the risk of aspiration. Ulceration and necrosis of the nose, the mucosa of the stomach, or the esophagus may occur if the tube is left in place too long, inflated too long, or inflated at too high a pressure.

NURSING ALERT

The patient being treated with balloon tamponade must remain under close observation in the intensive care unit because of the risk for serious complications. The patient must be monitored closely and continuously. Precautions must be taken to ensure that the patient does not pull on or inadvertently displace the tube.

These potential complications necessitate intensive, expert care. A confused or restless patient requires close monitoring to prevent displacement of the tube and inflated balloons. Nursing measures include frequent mouth and nasal care. For secretions that accumulate in the mouth, tissues

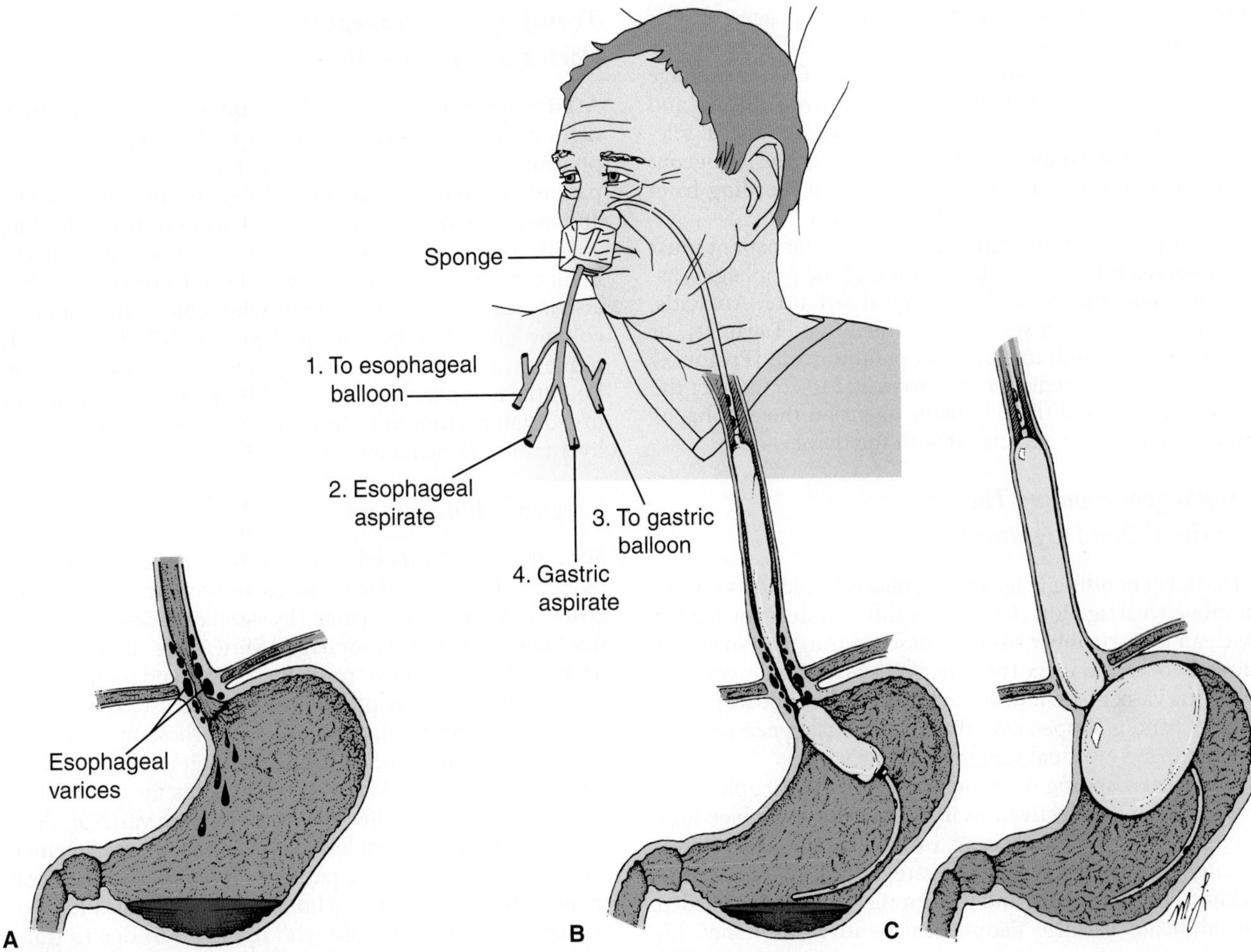

FIGURE 39-8. Balloon tamponade to treat esophageal varices. (**A**) Dilated, bleeding esophageal veins (varices) of the lower esophagus. (**B**) A four-lumen esophageal tamponade tube with balloons (uninflated) in place. (**C**) Compression of bleeding esophageal varices by inflated esophageal and gastric balloons. The gastric and esophageal outlets permit the nurse to aspirate secretions.

should be within easy reach of the patient. Oral suction may be necessary to remove oral secretions. Because of the many potential complications, balloon tamponade tubes are used only as a temporary measure.

The patient with esophageal hemorrhage is usually extremely anxious and frightened. Knowing that the nurse is nearby and ready to respond immediately can help alleviate some of this anxiety. Tube insertion is uncomfortable and never pleasant. Careful explanation during the procedure and while the tube is in place may be reassuring to the patient. Sedation may be prescribed.

Although balloon tamponade stops the bleeding in 90% of patients, bleeding recurs in 60% to 70%, necessitating other treatment modalities, such as sclerotherapy or banding (Friedman et al., 2003). Once the balloons are deflated or the tube is removed, the patient must be assessed frequently because of the high risk for recurrent bleeding.

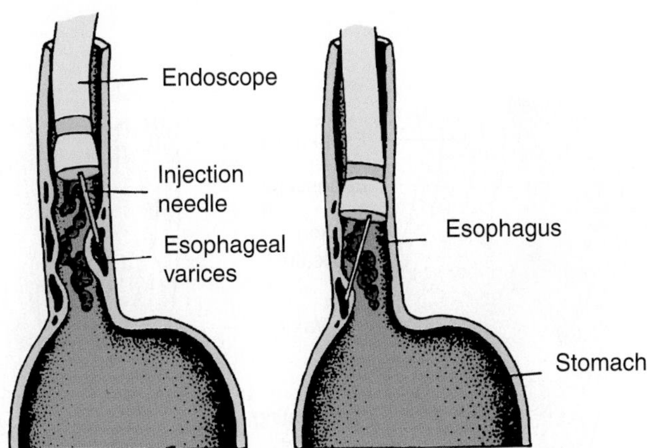

FIGURE 39-9. Endoscopic or injection sclerotherapy. Injection of sclerosing agent into esophageal varices through an endoscope promotes thrombosis and eventual sclerosis, thereby obliterating the varices.

Endoscopic Therapies

In endoscopic **sclerotherapy** (Fig. 39-9), also referred to as injection sclerotherapy, a sclerosing agent is injected through a fiberoptic endoscope into the bleeding esophageal varices to promote thrombosis and eventual sclerosis. The procedure has been used successfully to treat acute GI hemorrhage (Zakim & Boyer, 2003). Because of unproven efficacy and a high incidence of complications, endoscopic variceal sclerotherapy is used only to treat active bleeding and is not considered an appropriate method to prevent bleeding from esophageal varices (Zakim & Boyer, 2003).

After treatment for acute hemorrhage, the patient must be observed for bleeding, perforation of the esophagus, aspiration pneumonia, and esophageal stricture. Antacids, histamine-2 antagonists such as cimetidine [Tagamet], or proton pump inhibitors such as pantoprazole [Protonix] may be administered after the procedure to counteract the chemical effects of the sclerosing agent on the esophagus and the acid reflux associated with the therapy.

Esophageal Banding Therapy (Variceal Band Ligation)

In **variceal banding** (Fig. 39-10), also referred to as esophageal variceal ligation (EVL), a modified endoscope loaded with an elastic rubber band is passed through an overtube directly onto the varix (or varices) to be banded. After the bleeding varix is suctioned into the tip of the endoscope, the rubber band is slipped over the tissue, causing necrosis, ulceration, and eventual sloughing of the varix.

Variceal banding is comparable to endoscopic sclerotherapy in its effectiveness in controlling acute bleeding. Compared with sclerotherapy, variceal banding also significantly reduces the rebleeding rate, mortality, procedure-related complications, and the number of sessions needed to eradicate varices. Esophageal band ligation has replaced sclerotherapy as the treatment of choice in the management of esophageal varices. Complications include superficial ulceration and dysphagia, transient chest discomfort, and, rarely, esophageal strictures. Band ligation in combination with pharmacologic therapy may be more effective than monotherapy (ie, a single mode of therapy) in the treatment of acute hemorrhage. EVL is recommended for patients who have experienced variceal bleeding while receiving beta-blocker therapy and for those who cannot tolerate beta-blocking agents.

Transjugular Intrahepatic Portosystemic Shunting

A TIPS procedure (see Fig. 39-6) is indicated for the treatment of an acute episode of variceal bleeding refractory to pharmacologic or endoscopic therapy. In 10% to 20% of patients for whom urgent band ligation or sclerotherapy and medications are not successful in eradicating bleeding, a TIPS procedure can effectively control acute variceal hemorrhage by rapidly lowering portal pressure. TIPS is also indicated for those patients who rebleed after pharmacologic or endoscopic prophylaxis has failed. This technique is also used as a bridge to liver transplantation. Potential complications include bleeding, sepsis, heart failure, organ perforation, shunt thrombosis, and progressive liver failure (Friedman et al., 2003).

Surgical Management

Several surgical procedures have been developed to treat esophageal varices and to minimize rebleeding, but these procedures are often accompanied by significant risk. Procedures that may be used for esophageal varices are direct surgical ligation of varices; splenorenal, mesocaval, and portacaval venous shunts to relieve portal pressure; and esophageal transection with devascularization. Use of these procedures is controversial, and studies regarding their effectiveness and outcomes continue. What is known thus far is that these procedures are very effective in controlling variceal bleeding. They may be considered as second-line management (rescue therapy) for those patients for whom all other treatments have failed, those who are not candidates for liver transplantation, and those who require a bridge to transplantation. There is a high incidence of encephalopathy after these procedures, and morbidity and mortality statistics remain high (Zakim & Boyer, 2003). The TIPS procedure has largely replaced the use of surgical decompressive shunts and ligation procedures.

SURGICAL BYPASS PROCEDURES

Surgical decompression of the portal circulation can prevent variceal bleeding if the shunt remains patent (Zakim & Boyer, 2003). One of the various surgical shunting pro-

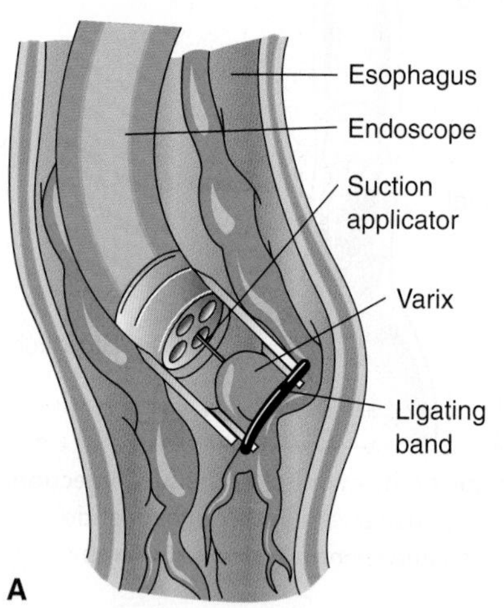

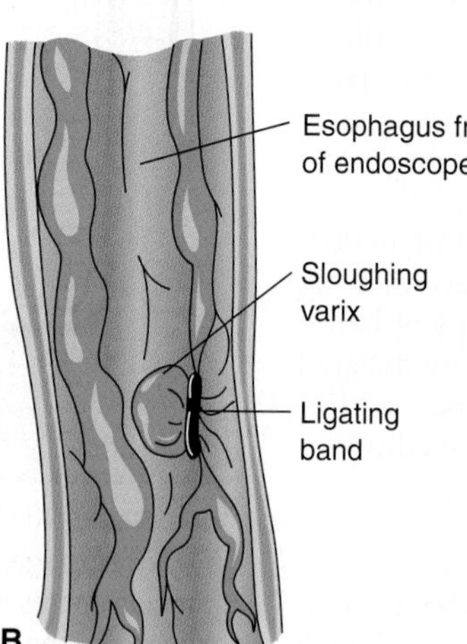

FIGURE 39-10. Esophageal banding. **(A)** A rubber band–like ligature is slipped over an esophageal varix via an endoscope. **(B)** Necrosis results, and the varix eventually sloughs off.

cedures (Fig. 39-11) is the distal splenorenal shunt, which is made between the splenic vein and the left renal vein after splenectomy. A mesocaval shunt is created by anastomosing the superior mesenteric vein to the proximal end of the vena cava or to the side of the vena cava using grafting material. The goal of distal splenorenal and mesocaval shunts is to decrease portal pressure by draining only a portion of venous blood from the portal bed; therefore, they are considered selective shunts. The liver continues to receive some portal flow, and the incidence of encephalopathy may be reduced. Portacaval shunts are considered nonselective shunts because they divert all portal flow to the vena cava via end-to-side or side-to-side approaches.

These procedures are extensive and are not always successful because of secondary thrombosis in the veins used for the shunt and because of complications (eg, encephalopathy, accelerated liver failure). The effectiveness of these procedures has been studied extensively. All shunt procedures are equally effective in preventing recurrent variceal bleeding but may cause further impairment of liver function and encephalopathy. Partial portacaval shunts with interposition grafts are as effective as other shunts but are associated with a lower rate of encephalopathy (Zakim & Boyer, 2003). The severity of the disease (by a classification such as the Child-Pugh system, discussed later) and the potential for future liver transplantation guide the treatment decision.

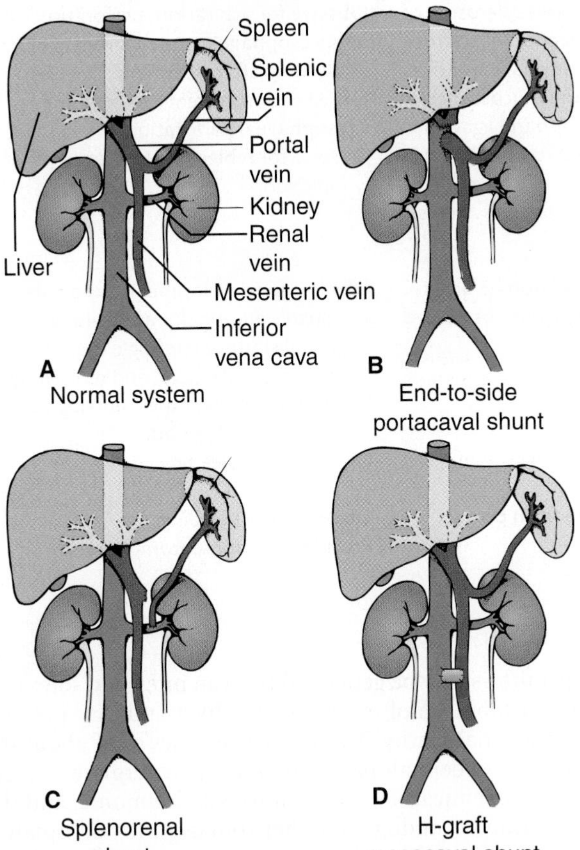

FIGURE 39-11. Portal systemic shunts. (**A**) Normal portal system. (**B** through **D**) Examples of portal shunts to reduce portal pressure.

If the cause of portal hypertension is the rare **Budd-Chiari syndrome** or other venous obstructive disease, a portacaval or a mesoatrial shunt may be performed (see Fig. 39-11). The mesoatrial shunt is required when the infrahepatic vena cava is thrombosed and must be bypassed.

DEVASCULARIZATION AND TRANSECTION

Devascularization and staple-gun transection procedures to separate the bleeding site from the high-pressure portal system have been used in the emergency management of variceal bleeding. The lower end of the esophagus is reached through a small gastrostomy incision; a staple gun permits anastomosis of the transected ends of the esophagus. Rebleeding is a risk, and the outcomes of these procedures vary among patient populations.

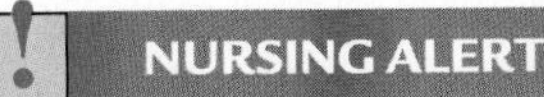

NURSING ALERT

Postoperative care is similar to that for any abdominal surgery, but the risk for complications (hypovolemic or hemorrhagic shock, hepatic encephalopathy, electrolyte imbalance, metabolic and respiratory alkalosis, alcohol withdrawal syndrome, and seizures) is high. The surgical procedures do not alter the course of the progressive liver disease, and bleeding may recur as new collateral vessels develop.

Nursing Management

Overall nursing assessment includes monitoring the patient's physical condition and evaluating emotional responses and cognitive status. The nurse monitors and records vital signs and assesses the patient's nutritional and neurologic status. This assessment assists in identifying hepatic encephalopathy, which results from the breakdown of blood in the GI tract and a rising serum ammonia level. Manifestations range from drowsiness to encephalopathy and coma.

If complete rest of the esophagus is indicated because of bleeding, parenteral nutrition is initiated. Gastric suction usually is initiated to keep the stomach as empty as possible and to prevent straining and vomiting. The patient often complains of severe thirst, which may be relieved by frequent oral hygiene and moist sponges to the lips. The nurse closely monitors the blood pressure. Vitamin K therapy and multiple blood transfusions often are indicated because of blood loss. A quiet environment and calm reassurance may help to relieve the patient's anxiety and reduce agitation.

Bleeding anywhere in the body is anxiety-provoking, resulting in a crisis for the patient and family. If the patient has been a heavy user of alcohol, delirium secondary to alcohol withdrawal can complicate the situation. The nurse provides support and explanations about medical and nursing interventions. Close monitoring of the patient helps in detecting and managing complications. Management modalities and nursing care of the patient with bleeding esophageal varices are summarized in Table 39-2.

TABLE 39-2 Management Modalities and Nursing Care for the Patient With Bleeding Esophageal Varices

Treatment Modality*	Action	Nursing Priorities
Nonsurgical Modalities		
Pharmacologic agents		
Vasopressin (Pitressin)	Reduces portal pressure by constricting splanchnic arteries	Observe response to therapy. Monitor for side effects: *vasopressin*—angina; nitroglycerin may be prescribed to prevent or treat angina.
Propranolol (Inderal)/nadolol (Corgard)	Reduces portal pressure by β-adrenergic blocking action	*propranolol* and *nadolol*—decreased pulse pressure, impaired cardiovascular response to hemorrhage.
Somatostatin/octreotide (Sandostatin)	Reduces portal pressure by selective vasodilation of portal system	Support patient during treatment.
Balloon tamponade	Exerts pressure directly to bleeding sites in esophagus and stomach	Explain procedure to patient briefly to obtain cooperation with insertion and maintenance of esophageal/gastric tamponade tube and reduce patient's fear of the procedure. Monitor closely to prevent inadvertent removal or displacement of tube, subsequent airway obstruction, and aspiration. Provide frequent oral hygiene.
Room-temperature saline lavage	Clears blood and secretions before endoscopy and other procedures	Ensure patency of the nasogastric tube to prevent aspiration. Observe gastric aspirate for blood and cessation of bleeding.
Injection sclerotherapy	Promotes thrombosis and sclerosing of bleeding sites by injection of sclerosing agent into the esophageal varices	Observe for aspiration, perforation of the esophagus, and recurrence of bleeding after treatment.
Variceal banding	Provides thrombosis and mucosal necrosis of bleeding sites by band ligation	Observe for recurrence of bleeding, esophageal perforation.
Transjugular intrahepatic portosystemic shunt (TIPS)	Reduces portal pressure by creating a shunt within the liver between the portal and systemic venous systems.	Observe for rebleeding and signs of infection.
Surgical Modalities		
Portal-systemic shunt	Reduces portal hypertension by diverting blood flow away from obstructed portal system	Observe for development of portal-systemic encephalopathy (altered mental status, neurologic dysfunction), hepatic failure, and rebleeding. Requires intensive, expert nursing care for prolonged period.
Surgical ligation of varices	Ties off blood vessels at the site of bleeding	Observe for rebleeding.
Esophageal transection and devascularization	Separates bleeding site from portal system	Observe for rebleeding. Provide postthoracotomy care.

*Several modalities may be used concurrently or in sequence.

Hepatic Encephalopathy and Coma

Hepatic encephalopathy, a life-threatening complication of liver disease, occurs with profound liver failure and may result from the accumulation of ammonia and other toxic metabolites in the blood. Hepatic coma represents the most advanced stage of hepatic encephalopathy. Although the exact cause is not fully understood, false or weak neurotransmitters have been suggested as a cause. These neurotransmitters may be generated from an intestinal source or from metabolism of protein by the liver and may precipitate encephalopathy. Many other theories exist about the causes of encephalopathy, including synergistic effects of other chemicals (ie, serotonin) with ammonia, and the generation of endogenous benzodiazepines or opiates. Benzodiazepine-like chemicals (compounds) have been detected in the plasma and cerebrospinal fluid of patients with hepatic encephalopathy due to cirrhosis (MacSween et al., 2002).

Portal-systemic encephalopathy, the most common type of hepatic encephalopathy, occurs primarily in patients with cirrhosis who have portal hypertension and portal-systemic shunting.

Pathophysiology

Ammonia, which is constantly entering the bloodstream, accumulates because damaged liver cells fail to detoxify and convert the ammonia to urea. Ammonia enters the bloodstream as a result of its absorption from the GI tract and its liberation from kidney and muscle cells. The increased ammonia concentration in the blood causes brain dysfunction and damage, resulting in hepatic encephalopathy.

Circumstances that increase serum ammonia levels tend to aggravate or precipitate hepatic encephalopathy. The largest source of ammonia is the enzymatic and bacterial digestion of dietary and blood proteins in the GI tract. Ammonia from these sources increases as a result of GI bleeding (ie, bleeding esophageal varices, chronic GI bleeding), a high-protein diet, bacterial infection, or uremia. The ingestion of ammonium salts also increases the blood ammonia level. In the presence of alkalosis or hypokalemia, increased amounts of ammonia are absorbed from the GI tract and from the renal tubular fluid. Conversely, serum ammonia is decreased by elimination of protein from the diet and by the administration of antibiotic agents, such as neomycin sulfate, that reduce the number of intestinal bacteria capable of converting urea to ammonia (Dudek, 2006).

Other factors unrelated to increased serum ammonia levels that can cause hepatic encephalopathy in susceptible patients include excessive diuresis, dehydration, infections, surgery, fever, and some medications (sedatives, tranquilizers, analgesics, and diuretics that cause potassium loss). Table 39-3 presents the stages of hepatic encephalopathy, common signs and symptoms, and potential nursing diagnoses for each stage.

Clinical Manifestations

The earliest symptoms of hepatic encephalopathy include minor mental changes and motor disturbances. The patient appears slightly confused and unkempt and has alterations in mood and sleep patterns. The patient tends to sleep during the day and have restlessness and insomnia at night. As hepatic encephalopathy progresses, the patient may become difficult to awaken.

Asterixis (flapping tremor of the hands) may occur (Fig. 39-12). Simple tasks, such as handwriting, become difficult. A handwriting or drawing sample (eg, star figure), taken daily, may provide graphic evidence of progression or reversal of hepatic encephalopathy. Inability to reproduce a simple figure (Fig. 39-13) is referred to as **constructional apraxia.** In the early stages of hepatic encephalopathy, the deep tendon reflexes are hyperactive; with worsening of the encephalopathy, these reflexes disappear and the extremities may become flaccid.

Assessment and Diagnostic Findings

The electroencephalogram (EEG) shows generalized slowing, an increase in the amplitude of brain waves, and characteristic triphasic waves. Occasionally, **fetor hepaticus,** a sweet, slightly fecal odor to the breath that is presumed to be of intestinal origin, may be noticed. The odor has also been described as similar to that of freshly mowed grass, acetone, or old wine. Fetor hepaticus is prevalent with extensive collateral portal circulation in chronic liver disease. In a more advanced stage, there are gross disturbances of consciousness and the patient is completely disoriented with respect to time and place. With further progression of the disorder, the patient lapses into frank coma and may have seizures. The survival rate after a first episode of overt hepatic encephalopathy in patients with cirrhosis is approximately 40% at 1 year. Patients should be referred for liver transplantation after a first episode of encephalopathy (Friedman et al., 2003).

Medical Management

Medical management of hepatic encephalopathy focuses on identifying and eliminating the precipitating cause if possible. Lactulose (Cephulac) is administered to reduce

TABLE 39-3 Stages of Hepatic Encephalopathy and Possible Nursing Diagnoses*

Stage	Clinical Symptoms	Clinical Signs and EEG Changes	Selected Potential Nursing Diagnoses
1	Normal level of consciousness with periods of lethargy and euphoria; reversal of day–night sleep patterns	Asterixis; impaired writing and ability to draw line figures. Normal EEG.	Activity intolerance Self-care deficit Disturbed sleep pattern
2	Increased drowsiness; disorientation; inappropriate behavior; mood swings; agitation	Asterixis; fetor hepaticus. Abnormal EEG with generalized slowing.	Impaired social interaction Ineffective role performance Risk for injury
3	Stuporous; difficult to rouse; sleeps most of time; marked confusion; incoherent speech	Asterixis; increased deep tendon reflexes; rigidity of extremities. EEG markedly abnormal.	Imbalanced nutrition Impaired mobility Impaired verbal communication
4	Comatose; may not respond to painful stimuli	Absence of asterixis; absence of deep tendon reflexes; flaccidity of extremities. EEG markedly abnormal.	Risk for aspiration Impaired gas exchange Impaired tissue integrity Disturbed sensory perception

*Nursing diagnoses are likely to progress, so that most nursing diagnoses present at earlier stages will occur during later stages as well.

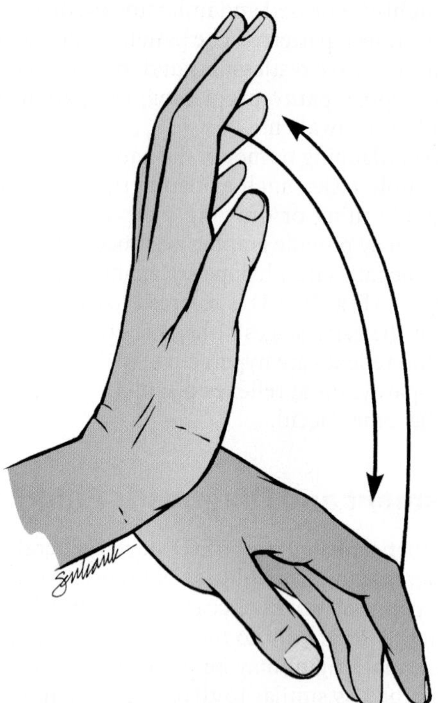

FIGURE 39-12. Asterixis or "liver flap" may occur in hepatic encephalopathy. The patient is asked to hold the arm out with the hand held upward (dorsiflexed). Within a few seconds, the hand falls forward involuntarily and then quickly returns to the dorsiflexed position.

serum ammonia levels. It acts by several mechanisms that promote the excretion of ammonia in the stool: (1) ammonia is kept in the ionized state, resulting in a decrease in colon pH, reversing the normal passage of ammonia from the colon to the blood; (2) evacuation of the bowel takes place, which decreases the ammonia absorbed from the colon; and (3) the fecal flora are changed to organisms that do not produce ammonia from urea. Two or three soft stools per day are desirable; this indicates that lactulose is performing as intended.

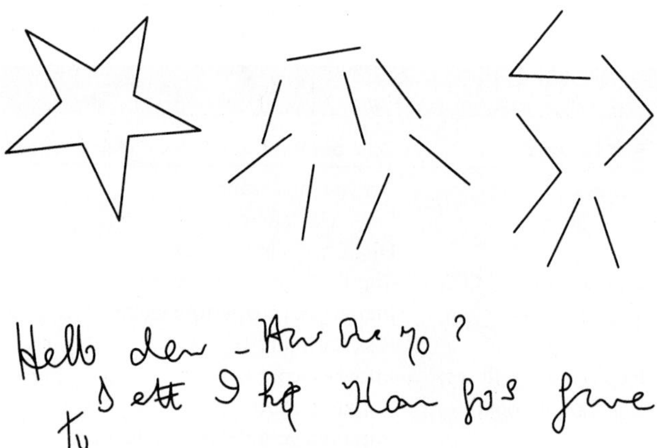

FIGURE 39-13. Effects of constructional apraxia. Deterioration of handwriting and inability to draw a simple star figure occurs with progressive hepatic encephalopathy. With permission from Sherlock, S. & Dooley, J. (2002). *Diseases of the liver and biliary system* (11th ed.). Oxford, UK: Blackwell Scientific Ltd.

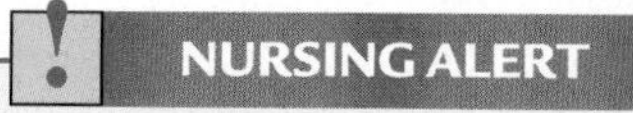

NURSING ALERT

The patient receiving lactulose is monitored closely for the development of watery diarrheal stools, because they indicate a medication overdose.

Possible side effects include intestinal bloating and cramps, which usually disappear within a week. To mask the sweet taste, which some patients dislike, lactulose can be diluted with fruit juice. The patient is closely monitored for hypokalemia and dehydration. Other laxatives are not prescribed during lactulose administration, because their effects disturb dosage regulation. Lactulose may be administered by nasogastric tube or enema for patients who are comatose or for those in whom oral administration is contraindicated or impossible.

Other aspects of management include IV administration of glucose to minimize protein breakdown, administration of vitamins to correct deficiencies, and correction of electrolyte imbalances (especially potassium). Additional principles of management of hepatic encephalopathy include the following:

- Therapy is directed toward treating or removing the cause.
- Neurologic status is assessed frequently.
- Mental status is monitored by keeping a daily record of handwriting and arithmetic performance.
- Fluid intake and output and body weight are recorded each day.
- Vital signs are measured and recorded every 4 hours.
- Potential sites of infection (peritoneum, lungs) are assessed frequently, and abnormal findings are reported promptly.
- Serum ammonia level is monitored daily.
- Protein intake is moderately restricted in patients who are comatose or who have encephalopathy that is refractory to lactulose and antibiotic therapy (Chart 39-5).
- Reduction in the absorption of ammonia from the GI tract is accomplished by the use of gastric suction, enemas, or oral antibiotics.
- Electrolyte status is monitored and corrected if abnormal.
- Sedatives, tranquilizers, and analgesic medications are discontinued.
- Benzodiazepine antagonists such as flumazenil (Romazicon) may be administered to improve encephalopathy, whether or not the patient has previously taken benzodiazepines.

Nursing Management

The nurse is responsible for maintaining a safe environment to prevent injury, bleeding, and infection. The nurse administers the prescribed treatments and monitors the patient for the numerous potential complications. The nurse also communicates with the patient's family, to inform them

CHART 39-5

Nutritional Management of Hepatic Encephalopathy

- Prevent the formation and absorption of toxins, principally ammonia, from the intestine.
- Keep daily protein intake between 1.0 and 1.5 g/kg, depending on the degree of decompensation.
- Avoid protein restriction if possible, even in those with encephalopathy. If necessary, implement temporary restriction of 0.5 to 0.8 g/kg.
- For patients who are truly protein-intolerant, provide additional nitrogen in the form of an amino acid supplement. Use of branched-chain amino acids is still controversial.
- Provide small, frequent meals and an evening snack of complex carbohydrates to avoid protein loading.
- Substitute vegetable protein for animal protein in as high a percentage as possible.

about the patient's status, and supports them by explaining the procedures and treatments that are part of the patient's care. If the patient recovers from hepatic encephalopathy and coma, rehabilitation is likely to be prolonged. Therefore, the patient and family will require assistance to understand the causes of this severe complication and to recognize that it may recur.

Promoting Home and Community-Based Care

TEACHING PATIENTS SELF-CARE

If the patient has recovered from hepatic encephalopathy and is to be discharged home, the nurse instructs the family to watch for subtle signs of recurrent encephalopathy. In the acute phase of hepatic encephalopathy, dietary protein may be reduced for a brief period to 0.8 to 1.0 g/kg per day. During recovery and in the home situation, it is important to instruct the patient in maintenance of a moderate-protein, high-calorie diet. Protein may then be added in 10-g increments every 3 to 5 days. Any relapse is treated by returning protein intake to the previous level. The limits of tolerance are usually 40 to 60 g/day (1.0 to 1.5 g/kg per day). Continued use of lactulose in the home environment is not uncommon, and the patient and family should closely monitor its efficacy and side effects. They should also be cautioned that constipation can precipitate encephalopathy and should be prevented through the prescribed use of lactulose, which is crucial in preventing constipation. Use of vegetable rather than animal protein may be indicated in patients whose total daily protein tolerance is less than 1 g/kg. Vegetable protein intake may result in improved nitrogen balance without precipitating or advancing hepatic encephalopathy (Zakim & Boyer, 2003).

CONTINUING CARE

Referral for home care is warranted for the patient who returns home after recovery from hepatic encephalopathy. The home care nurse assesses the patient's physical and mental status and collaborates closely with the physician. The home visit also provides an opportunity for the nurse to assess the home environment and the ability of the patient and family to monitor signs and symptoms and to follow the treatment regimen. The safety of the home environment is also assessed closely to identify areas of risk for falls and other injuries. Home care visits are especially important if the patient lives alone, because encephalopathy may affect the patient's ability to remember or follow the treatment regimen. The nurse reinforces previous teaching and reminds the patient and family about the importance of dietary restrictions, close monitoring, and follow-up.

Other Manifestations of Hepatic Dysfunction

Edema and Bleeding

Many patients with liver dysfunction develop generalized edema caused by hypoalbuminemia resulting from decreased hepatic production of albumin. The production of blood clotting factors by the liver is also reduced, leading to an increased incidence of bruising, epistaxis, bleeding from wounds, and, as described previously, GI bleeding.

Vitamin Deficiency

Decreased production of several clotting factors may be partially due to deficient absorption of vitamin K from the GI tract. This probably is caused by the inability of liver cells to use vitamin K to make prothrombin. Absorption of the other fat-soluble vitamins (vitamins A, D, and E) as well as dietary fats may also be impaired because of decreased secretion of bile salts into the intestine.

Another group of problems common to patients with severe chronic liver dysfunction results from inadequate intake of sufficient vitamins. These include the following:

- Vitamin A deficiency, resulting in night blindness and eye and skin changes
- Thiamine deficiency, leading to beriberi, polyneuritis, and Wernicke-Korsakoff psychosis
- Riboflavin deficiency, resulting in characteristic skin and mucous membrane lesions
- Pyridoxine deficiency, resulting in skin and mucous membrane lesions and neurologic changes
- Vitamin C deficiency, resulting in the hemorrhagic lesions of scurvy
- Vitamin K deficiency, resulting in hypoprothrombinemia, characterized by spontaneous bleeding and ecchymoses
- Folic acid deficiency, resulting in macrocytic anemia

Because of these avitaminoses, the diet of every patient with chronic liver disease (especially if alcohol-related) is supplemented with ample quantities of vitamins A, B complex, C, and K and folic acid.

Metabolic Abnormalities

Abnormalities of glucose metabolism also occur; the blood glucose level may be abnormally high shortly after a meal (a diabetic-type glucose tolerance test result), but hypoglycemia may occur during fasting because of decreased hepatic glycogen reserves and decreased gluconeogenesis. Medications must be used cautiously and in reduced dosages, because the ability to metabolize medications is decreased in the patient with liver failure.

Many endocrine abnormalities also occur with liver dysfunction, because the liver cannot properly metabolize hormones, including androgens and sex hormones. Failure of the damaged liver to inactivate estrogens normally can cause gynecomastia, amenorrhea, testicular atrophy, loss of pubic hair in the male, menstrual irregularities in the female, and other disturbances of sexual function and sex characteristics.

Pruritus and Other Skin Changes

Patients with liver dysfunction resulting from biliary obstruction commonly develop severe pruritus due to retention of bile salts. Patients may develop vascular (or arterial) spider angiomas (Fig. 39-14) on the skin, usually above the waistline. These are numerous small vessels resembling a spider's legs. They are most often associated with cirrhosis, especially in alcoholic liver disease. Patients may also develop reddened palms ("liver palms" or palmar erythema).

Viral Hepatitis

Viral hepatitis is a systemic, viral infection in which necrosis and inflammation of liver cells produce a characteristic cluster of clinical, biochemical, and cellular changes. To date, five definitive types of viral hepatitis have been identified: hepatitis A, B, C, D, and E. Hepatitis A and E are similar in mode of transmission (fecal–oral route), whereas hepatitis B, C, and D share many other characteristics. Terms associated with viral hepatitis are listed in Chart 39-6. The increasing incidence of viral hepatitis is a public health concern; some 200,000 to 700,000 new cases are identified in the United States each year (Edmundowicz, 2002). It is easily transmitted and causes high morbidity and prolonged loss of time from school or employment.

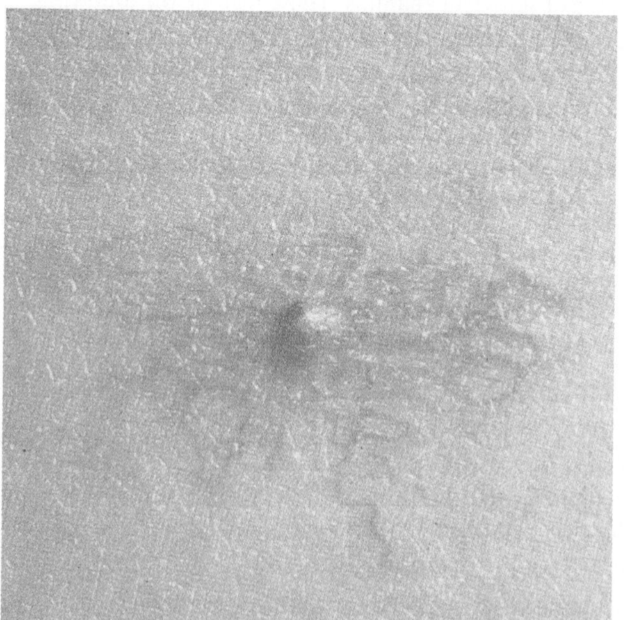

FIGURE 39-14. Spider angioma. This vascular (arterial) spider appears on the skin. Beneath the elevated center and radiating branches, the blood vessels are looped and tortuous.

It is estimated that 60% to 90% of viral hepatitis cases go unreported. The occurrence of subclinical cases, failure to recognize mild cases, and misdiagnosis are thought to contribute to the underreporting. In the United States, hepatitis A is seen mainly in the adult population. Fewer than 25% of children have antibodies to hepatitis A virus (HAV). The prevalence of HAV antibody increases with age, and most people older than 50 years of age have evidence of prior exposure (Fishman et al., 2004). Table 39-4 compares the major forms of viral hepatitis.

Hepatitis A Virus

HAV accounts for 20% to 25% of cases of clinical hepatitis in developed countries. Hepatitis A, formerly called infectious hepatitis, is caused by an RNA virus of the Enterovirus family. This disease is transmitted primarily through the fecal–oral route, by the ingestion of food or liquids infected by the virus. It is more prevalent in developing countries and in areas with overcrowding and poor sanitation. The virus has been found in the stool of infected patients before the onset of symptoms and during the first few days of illness.

Typically, a child or a young adult acquires the infection at school through poor hygiene, hand-to-mouth contact, or close contact during play. The virus is carried home, where haphazard sanitary habits spread it through the family. An infected food handler can spread the disease, and people can contract it by consuming water or shellfish from sewage-contaminated waters. Outbreaks have occurred in day care centers and institutions as a result of poor hygiene among people with developmental disabilities. Hepatitis A can be transmitted during sexual activity; this is more likely with oral–anal contact or anal intercourse and with multiple sex partners (Centers for Disease Control and Prevention [CDC], 2002). It is rarely, if ever, transmitted by blood transfusions.

The incubation period is estimated to be between 15 and 50 days, with a mean of 28 to 30 days (Zakim & Boyer, 2003). The illness may be prolonged, lasting 4 to 8 weeks. It usually lasts longer and is more severe in those older than 40 years of age. Most patients recover from hepatitis A; it rarely progresses to acute liver necrosis or fulminant hepatitis resulting in cirrhosis of the liver or death. The mortality rate of hepatitis A is approximately 0.5% for those younger than 40 years of age and 1% to 2% for older people. In patients with underlying chronic liver disease, morbidity and mortality are increased in the presence of an acute hepatitis A infection. No carrier state exists, and no chronic hepatitis is associated with hepatitis A. The virus is present only briefly in the serum; by the time jaundice occurs, the patient is likely to be noninfectious. Although

CHART 39-6

Hepatitis Terms and Abbreviations

HEPATITIS A	
HAV	Hepatitis A virus; etiologic agent of hepatitis A (formerly infectious hepatitis)
Anti-HAV	Antibody to hepatitis A virus; appears in serum soon after onset of symptoms; disappears after 3–12 mo.
IgM anti-HAV	IgM antibody to HAV; indicates recent infection with HAV; positive up to 6 mo. after infection
HEPATITIS B	
HBV	Hepatitis B virus; etiologic agent of hepatitis B (formerly serum hepatitis)
HBsAG	Hepatitis B surface antigen (Australian antigen); indicates acute or chronic hepatitis B or carrier state; indicates infectious state
Anti-HBs	Antibody to hepatitis B surface antigen; indicates prior exposure and immunity to hepatitis; may indicate passive antibody from HBIG or immune response from hepatitis B vaccine
HBeAg	Hepatitis B e-antigen; present in serum early in course; indicates highly infectious stage of hepatitis B; persistence in serum indicates progression to chronic hepatitis
Anti-HBe	Antibody to hepatitis B e-antigen; suggests low titer of HBV
HBcAg	Hepatitis B core antigen; found in liver cells; not easily detected in serum
Anti-HBc	Antibody to hepatitis B core antigen; most sensitive indicator of hepatitis B; appears late in the acute phase of the disease; indicates infection of HBV at some time in the past
IgM anti-HBc	IgM antibody to HBcAg; present for up to 6 mo. after HBV infection
HEPATITIS C	
HCV	Hepatitis C virus (formerly non-A, non-B virus); may be more than one virus
HEPATITIS D	
HDV	Hepatitis D virus (delta agent); etiologic agent to hepatitis D; HBV required for replication
HDAg	Hepatitis delta antigen; detectable in early acute HDV infection
Anti-HDV	Antibody to HDV; indicates past or present infection with HDV
HEPATITIS E	
HEV	Hepatitis E virus; etiologic agent of hepatitis E
HEPATITIS G	
HGV	Hepatitis G virus; also known as GB virus C or GB-C

hepatitis A confers immunity against itself, the person may contract other forms of hepatitis.

Clinical Manifestations

Many patients are anicteric (without jaundice) and symptomless. When symptoms appear, they resemble those of a mild, flu-like upper respiratory tract infection, with low-grade fever. Anorexia, an early symptom, is often severe. It is thought to result from release of a toxin by the damaged liver or from failure of the damaged liver cells to detoxify an abnormal product. Later, jaundice and dark urine may become apparent. Indigestion is present in varying degrees, marked by vague epigastric distress, nausea, heartburn, and flatulence. The patient may also develop a strong aversion to the taste of cigarettes or the presence of cigarette smoke and other strong odors. These symptoms tend to clear as soon as the jaundice reaches its peak, perhaps 10 days after its initial appearance. Symptoms may be mild in children; in adults, they may be more severe, and the course of the disease prolonged.

Assessment and Diagnostic Findings

The liver and spleen are often moderately enlarged for a few days after onset; other than jaundice, there are few other physical signs. Hepatitis A antigen may be found in the stool 7 to 10 days before illness and for 2 to 3 weeks after symptoms appear. HAV antibodies are detectable in the serum, but usually not until symptoms appear. Analysis of subclasses of immunoglobulins can help determine whether the antibody represents acute or past infection.

Prevention

A number of strategies exist to prevent transmission of HAV. Patients and their families should be taught these strategies and encouraged to consider them if recommended by their primary health care provider. There are many general precautions that can prevent transmission of the virus. Scrupulous handwashing, safe water supplies, and proper control of sewage disposal are just a few of these prevention strategies.

TABLE 39-4 Comparison of Major Forms of Viral Hepatitis

	Hepatitis A	Hepatitis B	Hepatitis C	Hepatitis D	Hepatitis E
Previous names	Infectious hepatitis	Serum hepatitis	Non-A, non-B hepatitis		
Epidemiology					
Cause	Hepatitis A virus (HAV)	Hepatitis B virus (HBV)	Hepatitis C virus (HCV)	Hepatitis D virus (HDV)	Hepatitis E virus (HEV)
Mode of transmission	Fecal–oral route; poor sanitation. Person-to-person contact. Water-borne; food-borne. Transmission possible with oral–anal contact during sex.	Parenterally; by intimate contact with carriers or those with acute disease; sexual and oral–oral contact. Perinatal transmission from mothers to infants. An important occupational hazard for health care personnel.	Transfusion of blood and blood products; exposure to contaminated blood through equipment or drug paraphernalia. Transmission possible with sex with infected partner; risk increased with STD.	Same as HBV. HBV surface antigen necessary for replication; pattern similar to that of hepatitis B.	Fecal–oral route; person to person contact may be possible, although risk appears low
Incubation (days)	15–50 days Average: 30 days	28–160 days Average: 70–80 days	15–160 days Average: 50 days	21–140 days Average: 35 days	15–65 days Average: 42 days
Immunity	Homologous	Homologous	Second attack may indicate weak immunity or infection with another agent.	Homologous	Unknown
Nature of Illness					
Signs and symptoms	May occur with or without symptoms; flulike illness *Preicteric phase:* Headache, malaise, fatigue, anorexia, fever *Icteric phase:* Dark urine, jaundice of sclera and skin, tender liver	May occur without symptoms May develop arthralgias, rash	Similar to HBV; less severe and anicteric	Similar to HBV	Similar to HAV. Very severe in pregnant women.
Outcome	Usually mild with recovery. Fatality rate: <1%. No carrier state or increased risk of chronic hepatitis, cirrhosis, or hepatic cancer.	May be severe. Fatality rate: 1–10%. Carrier state possible. Increased risk of chronic hepatitis, cirrhosis, and hepatic cancer.	Frequent occurrence of chronic carrier state and chronic liver disease. Increased risk of hepatic cancer.	Similar to HBV but greater likelihood of carrier state, chronic active hepatitis, and cirrhosis	Similar to HAV except very severe in pregnant women

In February 1995, the U.S. Food and Drug Administration (FDA) approved the first vaccine against hepatitis A for use in the United States. Effective (94% to 100% after two to three doses) and safe HAV vaccines include Havrix and Vagta (Edmundowicz, 2002; Koff, 2001). It is recommended that the two-dose vaccine be given to adults 18 years of age or older, with the second dose given 6 to 12 months after the first. Protection against hepatitis A develops within several weeks after the first dose of the vaccine. Children and adolescents 2 to 18 years of age receive three doses; the second dose is given 1 month after the first, and the third dose is given 6 to 12 months later. It is believed that vaccines for immunization against hepatitis A may confer 6 to 7 years of protection against infection (Yamada, 2003). Currently, no country recommends universal vaccination against hepatitis A, but it is a mandatory vaccination for infants in many states in the United States. Hepatitis A vaccine is recommended for people traveling to locations where sanitation and hygiene are unsatisfactory. Vaccination is also recommended for those from high-risk groups, such as homosexual men, IV/injection drug users, staff of day care centers, and health care personnel (CDC, 2002). The vaccine has also been used to interrupt community-wide outbreaks. As with other vaccinations, precautions must be taken to ensure prevention, detection, and treatment of hypersensitivity reactions to the vaccine.

For people who have not been previously vaccinated, hepatitis A can be prevented by intramuscular administration of globulin during the incubation period, if given within 2 weeks of exposure. This bolsters the person's antibody production and provides 6 to 8 weeks of passive immunity. Immune globulin may suppress overt symptoms of the disease; the resulting subclinical case of hepatitis A would produce immunity to subsequent episodes of the virus.

Immune globulin is also recommended for household members and sexual contacts of people with hepatitis A. Susceptible people in the same household as the patient are usually also infected by the time the diagnosis is made and should receive immune globulin. Day care center and restaurant workers with exposure to or infection by hepatitis A should also receive immune globulin to provide passive immunity (Reddy & Long, 2004). Although they are rare, systemic reactions to immune globulin do occur. Caution is required when anyone who has previously had angioedema, hives, or other allergic reactions is treated with any human immune globulin. Epinephrine should be available in case of systemic, anaphylactic reaction.

Pre-exposure prophylaxis is recommended for those traveling to developing countries or settings with poor or uncertain sanitation conditions who do not have sufficient time to acquire protection by administration of hepatitis A vaccine (Friedman et al., 2003). Community interventions for preventing hepatitis A are outlined in Chart 39-7.

Medical Management

Bed rest during the acute stage and a diet that is both acceptable to the patient and nutritious are part of the treatment and nursing care. During the period of anorexia, the patient should receive frequent small feedings, supplemented if necessary by IV fluids with glucose. Because the patient often has an aversion to food, gentle persistence and creativity may be required to stimulate appetite. Optimal food and fluid levels are necessary to counteract weight loss and to speed recovery. Even before the icteric phase, however, many patients recover their appetites (Chart 39-8).

The patient's sense of well-being and laboratory test results are generally appropriate guides to bed rest and restriction of physical activity. Gradual but progressive ambulation seems to hasten recovery, provided the patient rests after activity and does not participate in activities to the point of fatigue.

Nursing Management

Management usually occurs in the home unless symptoms are severe. Therefore, the nurse assists the patient and family in coping with the temporary disability and fatigue that are common in hepatitis and instructs them to seek additional health care if the symptoms persist or worsen. The patient and family also need specific guidelines about diet, rest, follow-up blood work, and the importance of avoiding alcohol, as well as sanitation and hygiene measures (particularly handwashing) to prevent spread of the disease to other family members.

Specific teaching to patients and families about reducing the risk for contracting hepatitis A includes good personal hygiene, stressing careful handwashing (after bowel movements and before eating) and environmental sanitation (safe food and water supply, effective sewage disposal).

CHART 39-7

Community Prevention of Hepatitis A

- Proper community and home sanitation
- Conscientious individual hygiene
- Safe practices for preparing and dispensing food
- Effective health supervision of schools, dormitories, extended care facilities, barracks, and camps
- Community health education programs
- Mandatory reporting of viral hepatitis to local health departments
- Vaccination for travelers to developing countries, illegal drug users (injection and noninjection drug users), men who have sex with men, and persons with chronic liver disease
- Vaccination to interrupt community-wide outbreaks

CHART 39-8

Dietary Management of Viral or Drug-Related Hepatitis

- Recommend small, frequent meals.
- Provide intake of 2000 to 3000 kcal/d during acute illness.
- Although early studies indicate that a high-protein, high-calorie diet may be beneficial, advise patient not to force food and to restrict fat intake.
- Carefully monitor fluid balance.
- If anorexia and nausea and vomiting persist, enteral feedings may be necessary.
- Instruct patient to abstain from alcohol during acute illness and for at least 6 mo. after recovery.
- Advise patient to avoid substances (medications, herbs, illicit drugs, and toxins) that may affect liver function.

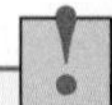

NURSING ALERT

The FDA (CDC, 2002) has approved a combined hepatitis A and B vaccine (Twinrix) for vaccination of people 18 years of age and older with indications for both hepatitis A and B vaccination. Vaccination consists of three doses, on the same schedule as that used for single-antigen hepatitis B vaccine (Yamada, 2003).

Hepatitis B Virus

Unlike HAV, which is transmitted primarily by the fecal–oral route, the hepatitis B virus (HBV) is transmitted primarily through blood (percutaneous and permucosal routes). HBV can be found in blood, saliva, semen, and vaginal secretions and can be transmitted through mucous membranes and breaks in the skin. HBV is also transferred from carrier mothers to their babies, especially in areas with a high incidence (eg, Southeast Asia). The infection usually is not transmitted via the umbilical vein but from the mother at the time of birth and during close contact afterward.

HBV has a long incubation period. It replicates in the liver and remains in the serum for relatively long periods, allowing transmission of the virus. Those at risk for development of hepatitis B include surgeons, clinical laboratory workers, dentists, nurses, and respiratory therapists. Staff and patients in hemodialysis and oncology units, sexually active homosexual and bisexual men, and IV/injection drug users are also at increased risk. Screening of blood donors has greatly reduced the occurrence of hepatitis B after blood transfusion. Risk factors for HBV infection are summarized in Chart 39-9.

CHART 39-9

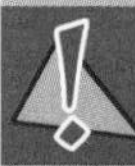

Risk Factors for Hepatitis B

- Frequent exposure to blood, blood products, or other body fluids
- Health care workers: hemodialysis staff, oncology and chemotherapy nurses, personnel at risk for needlesticks, operating room staff, respiratory therapists, surgeons, dentists
- Hemodialysis
- Male homosexual and bisexual activity
- IV/injection drug use
- Close contact with carrier of HBV
- Travel to or residence in area with uncertain sanitary conditions
- Multiple sexual partners
- Recent history of sexually transmitted disease
- Receipt of blood or blood products (eg, clotting factor concentrate)

Most people (more than 90%) who contract HBV infection develop antibodies and recover spontaneously in 6 months. The mortality rate from hepatitis B has been reported to be as high as 10%. Another 10% of patients who have hepatitis B progress to a carrier state or develop chronic hepatitis with persistent HBV infection and hepatocellular injury and inflammation. It remains a major worldwide cause of cirrhosis and hepatocellular carcinoma.

The elderly patient who contracts hepatitis B has a serious risk of severe liver cell necrosis or fulminant hepatic failure, particularly if other illnesses are present. Because the patient is seriously ill and the prognosis is poor, efforts should be undertaken to eliminate other factors (eg, medications, alcohol) that may affect liver function.

Clinical Manifestations

Clinically, the disease closely resembles hepatitis A, but the incubation period is much longer (1 to 6 months). Signs and symptoms of hepatitis B may be insidious and variable. Fever and respiratory symptoms are rare; some patients have arthralgias and rashes. The patient may have loss of appetite, dyspepsia, abdominal pain, generalized aching, malaise, and weakness. Jaundice may or may not be evident. If jaundice occurs, light-colored stools and dark urine accompany it. The liver may be tender and enlarged to 12 to 14 cm vertically. The spleen is enlarged and palpable in a few patients; the posterior cervical lymph nodes may also be enlarged. Subclinical episodes also occur frequently.

Assessment and Diagnostic Findings

HBV is a DNA virus composed of the following antigenic particles:

- HBcAg—hepatitis B core antigen (antigenic material in an inner core)
- HBsAg—hepatitis B surface antigen (antigenic material on the viral surface, a marker of active replication and infection)
- HBeAg—an independent protein circulating in the blood
- HBxAg—gene product of X gene of HBV DNA

Each antigen elicits its specific antibody and is a marker for different stages of the disease process:

- anti-HBc—antibody to core antigen of HBV; persists during the acute phase of illness; may indicate continuing HBV in the liver
- anti-HBs—antibody to surface determinants on HBV; detected during late convalescence; usually indicates recovery and development of immunity
- anti-HBe—antibody to hepatitis B e-antigen; usually signifies reduced infectivity
- anti-HBxAg—antibody to the hepatitis B x-antigen; may indicate ongoing replication of HBV

HBsAg appears in the circulation in 80% to 90% of infected patients 1 to 10 weeks after exposure to HBV and 2 to 8 weeks before the onset of symptoms or an increase in transferase levels. Patients with HBsAg that persists for 6 months or longer after acute infection are considered to be HBsAg carriers (Friedman et al., 2003; Zakim & Boyer,

2003). HBeAg is the next antigen of HBV to appear in the serum. It usually appears within 1 week of the appearance of HBsAg but before changes in aminotransferase levels; it disappears from the serum within 2 weeks. HBV DNA, detected by polymerase chain reaction testing, appears in the serum at about the same time as HBeAg. HBcAg is not always detected in the serum in HBV infection.

About 15% of American adults are positive for anti-HBs, which indicates that they have had hepatitis B. Anti-HBs may be positive in as many as two-thirds of IV/injection drug users.

Prevention

The goals of prevention are to interrupt the chain of transmission, to protect people who are at high risk by active immunization through the use of hepatitis B vaccine, and to use passive immunization for unprotected people exposed to HBV.

Preventing Transmission

Continued screening of blood donors for the presence of hepatitis B antigens will further decrease the risk of transmission by blood transfusion. The use of disposable syringes, needles, and lancets and the introduction of needleless IV administration systems have reduced the risk of spreading this infection from one patient to another or to health care personnel during the collection of blood samples or the administration of parenteral therapy. Good personal hygiene is fundamental to infection control. In the clinical laboratory, work areas should be disinfected daily. Gloves are worn when handling all blood and body fluids, as well as HBAg-positive specimens, or when there is potential exposure to blood (eg, blood drawing) or to patients' secretions. Eating and smoking are prohibited in the laboratory and in other areas exposed to secretions, blood, or blood products. Patient education regarding the nature of the disease, its infectiousness, and prognosis is a critical factor in preventing transmission and protecting contacts.

Active Immunization: Hepatitis B Vaccine

Active immunization is recommended for individuals who are at high risk for hepatitis B (eg, health care personnel, hemodialysis patients). In addition, individuals with hepatitis C and other chronic liver diseases should receive the vaccine (Yamada, 2003). A yeast-recombinant hepatitis B vaccine (Recombivax HB) is used to provide active immunity and has shown rates of protection greater than 90% in healthy individuals (Friedman et al., 2003). Although antibody levels may become low or undetectable, immunologic memory may remain intact for at least 5 to 10 years. Measurable levels of antibodies may not be essential for protection. In general, in those with normal immune systems, booster doses are not required. Presently, the CDC (2002) does not recommend booster doses, except for patients on hemodialysis and some immunocompromised patients. The need for booster doses may be revisited if reports of hepatitis B increase or an increased prevalence of the carrier state develops, indicating that protection is declining.

A hepatitis B vaccine prepared from plasma of humans chronically infected with HBV is used only rarely, in patients who are immunodeficient or allergic to recombinant yeast-derived vaccines.

Both forms of the hepatitis B vaccine are administered intramuscularly in three doses; the second and third doses are given 1 and 6 months after the first dose. The third dose is very important in producing prolonged immunity. Hepatitis B vaccination should be administered to adults in the deltoid muscle. Antibody response may be measured by anti-HBs levels 1 to 3 months after completion of the basic course of vaccine, but this testing is not routine and is not currently recommended. Individuals who do not respond may benefit from one to three additional doses (Yamada, 2003).

People who are at high risk, including nurses and other health care personnel exposed to blood or blood products, should receive active immunization. Health care workers who have had frequent contact with blood are screened for anti-HBs to determine whether immunity is already present from previous exposure. The vaccine produces active immunity to HBV in 90% of healthy people (Yamada, 2003). It does not provide protection to those already exposed to HBV, and it provides no protection against other types of viral hepatitis. Side effects of immunization are infrequent; soreness and redness at the injection site are the most common complaints.

Because hepatitis B infection is frequently transmitted sexually, hepatitis B vaccination is recommended for all unvaccinated people being evaluated for a sexually transmitted disease (STD). It is also recommended for those with a history of an STD, people with multiple sex partners, people who have sex with IV/injection drug users, and sexually active men who have sex with other men (CDC, 2002).

Universal childhood vaccination for hepatitis B prevention has been instituted in the United States. Vaccination was initially targeted at select high-risk populations, but the U.S. Public Health Service has endorsed universal vaccination of all infants. Catch-up vaccination is also recommended for all children and prepubertal adolescents up to the age of 19 years who were not previously immunized (Friedman et al., 2003). Universal vaccination of all newborns in endemic areas has dramatically reduced the carrier rate among children and the incidence of childhood hepatocellular carcinoma. Development of chronic carrier states has not been reported in adult responders to the vaccine.

Passive Immunity: Hepatitis B Immune Globulin

Hepatitis B immune globulin (HBIG) provides passive immunity to hepatitis B and is indicated for people exposed to HBV who have never had hepatitis B and have never received hepatitis B vaccine. Specific indications for postexposure vaccine with HBIG include (1) inadvertent exposure to HBAg-positive blood through percutaneous (needlestick) or transmucosal (splashes in contact with mucous membrane) routes, (2) sexual contact with people positive for HBAg, and (3) perinatal exposure (babies born to HBV-infected mothers should receive HBIG within 12 hours after delivery). HBIG is prepared from plasma selected for high titers of anti-HBs. Prompt immunization with HBIG (within hours to a few days after exposure to hepatitis B) increases the likelihood of protection. Both active and passive immunization are recommended for people who have been exposed to hepatitis B through sexual contact or through the percutaneous or transmucosal routes. If HBIG and hepatitis B vaccine are administered at the same time, separate sites and separate syringes should be used. There has been no evidence that HIV infection can be transmitted by HBIG (Friedman et al., 2003).

Medical Management

The goals of treatment are to minimize infectivity and liver inflammation and decrease symptoms. Of all the agents that have been used to treat chronic type B viral hepatitis, alpha-interferon as the single modality of therapy that offers the most promise. A regimen of 5 million units daily or 10 million units three times weekly for 4 to 6 months results in remission of disease in approximately one third of patients (Friedman et al., 2003). A prolonged course of treatment may also have additional benefits and is currently under study. Interferon must be administered by injection and has significant side effects, including fever, chills, anorexia, nausea, myalgias, and fatigue. Delayed side effects are more serious and may necessitate dosage reduction or discontinuation. These include bone marrow suppression, thyroid dysfunction, alopecia, and bacterial infections.

Two antiviral agents, lamivudine (Epivir) and adefovir (Hepsera), oral nucleoside analogues, have been approved for use in chronic hepatitis B in the United States. Studies have revealed improved seroconversion rates, loss of detectable virus, improved liver function, and reduced progression to cirrhosis with lamivudine. It can be used for patients with decompensated cirrhosis who are awaiting liver transplantation (Friedman et al., 2003). Adefovir may be effective in people who are resistant to lamivudine.

Bed rest may be recommended, regardless of other treatment, until the symptoms of hepatitis have subsided. Activities are restricted until the hepatic enlargement and elevated levels of serum bilirubin and liver enzymes have disappeared. Gradually increased activity is then allowed.

Adequate nutrition should be maintained. Proteins are restricted if symptoms indicate that the liver's ability to metabolize protein byproducts is impaired. Measures to control the dyspeptic symptoms and general malaise include the use of antacids and antiemetics, but all medications should be avoided if vomiting occurs. If vomiting persists, the patient may require hospitalization and fluid therapy. Because of the mode of transmission, the patient is evaluated for other bloodborne diseases (eg, human immunodeficiency virus [HIV] infection).

Nursing Management

Convalescence may be prolonged, with complete symptomatic recovery sometimes requiring 3 to 4 months or longer. During this stage, gradual resumption of physical activity is encouraged after the jaundice has resolved.

The nurse identifies psychosocial issues and concerns, particularly the effects of separation from family and friends if the patient is hospitalized during the acute and infective stages. Even if not hospitalized, the patient will be unable to work and must avoid sexual contact. Planning is required to minimize social isolation. Planning that includes the family helps to reduce their fears and anxieties about the spread of the disease.

Promoting Home and Community-Based Care

TEACHING PATIENTS SELF-CARE

Because of the prolonged period of convalescence, the patient and family must be prepared for home care. Provision for adequate rest and nutrition must be ensured. The nurse informs family members and friends who have had intimate contact with the patient about the risks of contracting hepatitis B and makes arrangements for them to receive hepatitis B vaccine or hepatitis B immune globulin as prescribed. Those at risk must be made aware of the early signs of hepatitis B and of ways to reduce risk by avoiding all modes of transmission. Patients with all forms of hepatitis should avoid drinking alcohol and eating raw shellfish.

CONTINUING CARE

Follow-up visits by a home care nurse may be needed to assess the patient's progress and answer family members' questions about disease transmission. During a home visit, the nurse assesses the patient's physical and psychological status and confirms that the patient and family understand the importance of adequate rest and nutrition. The nurse also reinforces previous instructions. Because of the risk of transmission through sexual intercourse, strategies to prevent exchange of body fluids are advised, such as abstinence or the use of condoms. The nurse emphasizes the importance of keeping follow-up appointments and participating in other health promotion activities and recommended health screenings.

Hepatitis C Virus

A significant proportion of cases of viral hepatitis are neither hepatitis A, hepatitis B, nor hepatitis D, and are classified as hepatitis C. Whereas blood transfusions and sexual contact once accounted for most cases of hepatitis C in the United States, other parenteral means, such as sharing of contaminated needles by IV/injection drug users and unintentional needlesticks and other injuries in health care workers, now account for a significant number of cases. Approximately 35,000 new cases of hepatitis C are reported in the United States each year. About 4 million people (1.8% of the United States population) have been infected with the hepatitis C virus (HCV), making it the most common chronic bloodborne infection nationally. A fourfold increase in the number of adults diagnosed with HCV infection is projected from 1990 to 2015. The highest prevalence of hepatitis C is in adults 40 to 59 years of age, and in this age group its prevalence is highest among African Americans. There are 10,000 to 12,000 deaths each year in the United States due to hepatitis C, and it has been suggested that deaths from this cause are underestimated. HCV is the underlying cause of about one third of cases of hepatocellular carcinoma, and it is the most common reason for liver transplantation (Aspinal & Taylor-Robinson, 2002; National Institutes of Health, 2002).

Individuals who are at special risk for hepatitis C include IV/injection drug users, sexually active people with multiple partners, patients receiving frequent transfusions, those who require large volumes of blood, and health care personnel (Chart 39-10). The incubation period is variable and may range from 15 to 160 days. The clinical course of acute hepatitis C is similar to that of hepatitis B; symptoms are usually mild. A chronic carrier state occurs frequently, however, and there is an increased risk of chronic liver disease, including cirrhosis or liver cancer, after hepatitis C. Small amounts of alcohol taken regularly appear to encourage progression of the disease. Therefore, alcohol and medications that may affect the liver should be avoided.

There is no benefit from rest, diet, or vitamin supplements. Studies have demonstrated that a combination of two antiviral agents, interferon (Intron-A) and ribavirin (Rebetol), is effective in producing improvement in patients with hepatitis C and in treating relapses. Some patients experience complete remission with combination therapy (Fishman et al., 2004; Friedman et al., 2003). Hemolytic anemia, the most frequent side effect, may be severe enough to require discontinuation of treatment. Ribavirin must be used with caution in women of childbearing age. The molecule polyethylene glycol moiety (PEG) is added to the interferon to keep it in the body longer without reducing its efficacy; this extends the dosing interval to once a week. Pegylated interferon (Pegasys) is now available, and some studies have shown it to have a somewhat improved virologic response rate compared with interferon (Friedman et al., 2003).

Screening of blood has reduced the incidence of hepatitis C associated with blood transfusion, and public health programs are helping to reduce the number of cases associated with shared needles in illicit drug use.

Hepatitis D Virus

Hepatitis D virus (delta agent) infection occurs in some cases of hepatitis B. Because the virus requires hepatitis B surface antigen for its replication, only individuals with hepatitis B are at risk for hepatitis D. Anti-delta antibodies in the presence of HBAg on testing confirm the diagnosis.

CHART 39-10

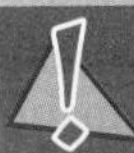

Risk Factors for Hepatitis C

- Recipient of blood products or organ transplant before 1992 or clotting factor concentrates before 1987
- Health care and public safety workers after needle-stick injuries or mucosal exposure to blood
- Children born to women infected with hepatitis C virus
- Past/current illicit IV/injection drug use
- Past treatment with chronic hemodialysis
- Multiple sex partners, history of sexually transmitted disease, unprotected sex

Hepatitis D is common among IV/injection drug users, hemodialysis patients, and recipients of multiple blood transfusions. Sexual contact with those with hepatitis B is considered to be an important mode of transmission of hepatitis B and D. The incubation period varies between 21 and 140 days (MacSween et al., 2002).

The symptoms of hepatitis D are similar to those of hepatitis B, except that patients are more likely to develop fulminant hepatitis and to progress to chronic active hepatitis and cirrhosis. Treatment is similar to that of other forms of hepatitis; interferon as a specific treatment for hepatitis D is under investigation.

Hepatitis E Virus

It is believed that hepatitis E virus (HEV) is transmitted by the fecal–oral route, principally through contaminated water in areas with poor sanitation. The incubation period is variable, estimated to range between 15 and 65 days. In general, hepatitis E resembles hepatitis A. It has a self-limited course with an abrupt onset. Jaundice is almost always present. Chronic forms do not develop.

Avoiding contact with the virus through good hygiene, including handwashing, is the major method of prevention of hepatitis E. The effectiveness of immune globulin in protecting against hepatitis E virus is uncertain.

Hepatitis G Virus and GB Virus-C

It has long been believed that there is another non-A–E agent causing hepatitis in humans. The incubation period for post-transfusion hepatitis is 14 to 145 days, too long for hepatitis B or C. In the United States, about 5% of chronic liver disease remains cryptogenic (ie, does not appear to be autoimmune or viral in origin), and 50% of these patients have received blood transfusions before developing disease. Therefore, another form of hepatitis, called hepatitis G virus (HGV) or GB virus-C (GBV-C) has been described; these are thought to be two different isolates of the same virus identified at the CDC. Autoantibodies are absent.

The clinical significance of this virus remains uncertain. Risk factors are similar to those for hepatitis C. There is no clear relationship between HGV/GBV-C infection and progressive liver disease. Persistent infection does occur but does not affect the clinical course.

Nonviral Hepatitis

Certain chemicals have toxic effects on the liver and produce acute liver cell necrosis or toxic hepatitis when taken by mouth, inhaled, or injected parenterally. The chemicals most commonly implicated in this disease are carbon tetrachloride, phosphorus, chloroform, and gold compounds. These substances are true hepatotoxins. Many medications can induce hepatitis but are only sensitizing rather than toxic. Drug-induced hepatitis is similar to acute viral hepatitis, but parenchymal destruction tends to be more

NURSING RESEARCH PROFILE

The Experience of Fatigue in Patients Living With Hepatitis C

Glacken, M., Coates, V., Kernohan, G., et al. (2003). The experience of fatigue for people living with hepatitis C. *Journal of Clinical Nursing, 12(2),* 244–252.

Purpose

Worldwide, hepatitis C affects approximately 3% of the population. The fatigue that accompanies hepatitis C (and the other hepatitis viral infections) is often recognized and discussed, but there is little information about the nature of this fatigue and its impact on quality of life of the individuals affected. This study was conducted to describe the fatigue associated with hepatitis C and the ways in which it affects an infected person's life.

Design

The qualitative approach of grounded theory was used. The theoretical sampling process generated 28 participants with hepatitis C for in-depth interviews to elicit processes and changes over time. Data analysis consisted of three coding processes, each with its own purpose and method. Twenty of the 28 participants were female, with participants ranging in age from 36 to 64 years. The primary goal of the interviews was to give authentic insight into participants' experiences. The majority of the interviews were tape recorded and followed by unrecorded debriefing sessions for each participant. Constant comparison was used to analyze the qualitative data.

Findings

The majority of participants were unable to share their experience except in the form of metaphors, comparing what they believed was the norm with how they were feeling at the time of the interview. Although they had difficulty articulating the nature of their fatigue, participants described feeling as if they were having concrete poured over them, coming out of anesthesia, or trying to grasp the normal world from another world. The major description of the fatigue given by people with hepatitis C was that it was a pernicious experience in onset, duration, dimensions, and severity. Some participants could isolate a time frame for when and how their fatigue began; others experienced the onset as a more insidious process. The fatigue was described as arresting, aging, impregnable, invincible, and like "night and day" compared with "normal fatigue." Two types of fatigue emerged—chronic and idiopathic—which appeared to be universal. Overall, the fatigue was described as multidimensional and multifactorial, with physical, cognitive, and affective components.

Nursing Implications

It is important to recognize the issues shared by those living with hepatitis C or any hepatitis infection. This study provides a beginning understanding of the fatigue experience of people living with hepatitis C. Knowledge about the effects of this fatigue is crucial in helping nurses and other members of the health care team develop appropriate interventions to help those affected live with this disabling symptom. A fatigue management program using data from this and related studies may enhance the quality of life of people living with hepatitis C.

extensive. Medications that can lead to hepatitis include isoniazid, halothane, acetaminophen, methyldopa, and certain antibiotics, antimetabolites, and anesthetic agents.

Toxic Hepatitis

At the onset of disease, toxic hepatitis resembles viral hepatitis. Obtaining a history of exposure to hepatotoxic chemicals, medications, botanical agents, or other toxic agents assists in early treatment and removal of the causative agent. Anorexia, nausea, and vomiting are the usual symptoms; jaundice and hepatomegaly are noted on physical assessment. Symptoms are more intense for the more severely toxic patient.

Recovery from acute toxic hepatitis is rapid if the hepatotoxin is identified early and removed or if exposure to the agent has been limited. Recovery is unlikely if there is a prolonged period between exposure and onset of symptoms. There are no effective antidotes. The fever rises; the patient becomes toxic and prostrated. Vomiting may be persistent, with the emesis containing blood. Clotting abnormalities may be severe, and hemorrhages may appear under the skin. The severe GI symptoms may lead to vascular collapse. Delirium, coma, and seizures develop, and within a few days the patient may die of fulminant hepatic failure (discussed later) unless he or she receives a liver transplant.

Short of liver transplantation, few treatment options are available. Therapy is directed toward restoring and maintaining fluid and electrolyte balance, blood replacement, and comfort and supportive measures. A few patients recover from acute toxic hepatitis only to develop chronic liver disease. If the liver heals, there may be scarring, followed by postnecrotic cirrhosis.

Drug-Induced Hepatitis

Drug-induced liver disease is the most common cause of acute liver failure, accounting for more than 50% of all cases in the United States and United Kingdom (Friedman et al., 2003). Manifestations of sensitivity to a medication may occur on the first day of its use or not until several months later, depending on the medication. Usually the onset is abrupt, with chills, fever, rash, pruritus, arthralgia, anorexia, and nausea. Later, there may be jaundice, dark urine, and an enlarged and tender liver. After the offending medication is withdrawn, symptoms may gradually subside. However, reactions can be severe, or even fatal, even if the medication is stopped. If fever, rash, or pruritus occurs from any medication, its use should be stopped immediately.

Although any medication can affect liver function, use of acetaminophen (found in many over-the-counter medications used to treat fever and pain) has been identified as the leading cause of acute liver failure (Ostapowicz, Fontana, Schiodt, et al., 2002). Other mechanisms commonly associated with liver injury include anesthetic agents, medications used to treat rheumatic and musculoskeletal disease, antidepressants, psychotropic medications, anticonvulsants, and antituberculosis agents.

Inhalational agents of the halothane family (halokanes) are metabolized by the liver and excreted in bile. These volatile anesthetics may also decrease hepatic blood flow. Halothane hepatitis is a dreaded but rare complication of halothane administration. Sevoflurane and desflurane may have less hepatotoxic effects than halokanes. Nitrous oxide, an adjunct to halokanes, is not hepatotoxic.

Although its efficacy is uncertain, a short course of high-dose corticosteroids may be used in patients with severe hypersensitivity. Liver transplantation is an option for drug-induced hepatitis, but outcomes may not be as successful as with other causes of liver failure.

Fulminant Hepatic Failure

Fulminant hepatic failure is the clinical syndrome of sudden and severely impaired liver function in a previously healthy person. According to the original and generally accepted definition, fulminant hepatic failure develops within 8 weeks after the first symptoms of jaundice (Zakim & Boyer, 2003). Patterns of the progression from jaundice to encephalopathy have been identified and have led to proposals of time-based classifications. However, no agreement as to these classifications has been reached. Three categories are frequently cited: hyperacute, acute, and subacute liver failure. In hyperacute liver failure, the duration of jaundice before the onset of encephalopathy is 0 to 7 days; in acute liver failure, it is 8 to 28 days; and in subacute liver failure, it is 28 to 72 days. The prognosis for fulminant hepatic failure is much worse than for chronic liver failure. However, in fulminant failure, the hepatic lesion is potentially reversible, and survival rates are approximately 50% to 85% (depending greatly on the cause of liver failure). Those who do not survive die of massive hepatocellular injury and necrosis (Friedman et al., 2003).

Viral hepatitis is a common cause of fulminant hepatic failure; other causes include toxic medications (eg, acetaminophen) and chemicals (eg, carbon tetrachloride), metabolic disturbances (eg, Wilson's disease, a hereditary syndrome with deposition of copper in the liver), and structural changes (eg, Budd-Chiari syndrome, an obstruction to outflow in major hepatic veins).

Jaundice and profound anorexia may be the initial reasons the patient seeks health care. Fulminant hepatic failure is often accompanied by coagulation defects, renal failure and electrolyte disturbances, cardiovascular abnormalities, infection, hypoglycemia, encephalopathy, and cerebral edema.

The key to optimized treatment is rapid recognition of acute liver failure and intensive intervention. Supporting the patient in the ICU and assessing the indications for and feasibility of liver transplantation are hallmarks of management of this population. The use of antidotes for certain conditions may be indicated such as N-acetylcysteine for acetaminophen toxicity and penicillin for mushroom poisoning. Treatment modalities may include plasma exchanges (plasmapheresis) to correct coagulopathy and to stabilize the patient awaiting liver transplantation and prostaglandin therapy to enhance hepatic blood flow; however, more clinical trials are needed to determine the effects or outcomes of these treatments. Hepatocytes within synthetic fiber columns have been tested as liver support systems (liver assist devices) to provide a bridge to transplantation.

Research into interventions for acute liver failure has begun to focus on techniques that combine the efficacy of a whole liver with the convenience and biocompatibility of hemodialysis. The acronyms ELAD (extracorporeal liver assist devices) and BAL (bioartificial liver) have been used to describe these hybrid devices. These short-term devices, which remain experimental, may help patients to survive until transplantation is possible. The BAL device exposes separated plasma to a cartridge containing porcine liver cells after the plasma has flowed through a charcoal column that removes substances toxic to hepatocytes. The ELAD exposes whole blood to cartridges containing human hepatoblastoma cells, resulting in removal of toxic substances. In the near future, similar extracorporeal circuits using **xenografts** will likely be studied as a bridge to liver transplantation (Friedman et al., 2003). These approaches appear promising and have had success in animal studies. In human clinical application, the use of various BAL systems has resulted in improved neurologic and biochemical parameters. To fully determine the clinical applicability of such systems on outcomes and survival rates, controlled, randomized clinical trials in large patient groups are required (van de Kerkhove, Hoekstra, Chamuleau, et al., 2004).

In patients who have fulminant liver failure with stage 4 encephalopathy, there is a high risk for cerebral edema, a life-threatening complication. The cause is not fully understood, although disruption of the blood–brain barrier and plasma leakage into the cerebrospinal fluid has been proposed as one theory (Friedman et al., 2003; Sherlock & Dooley, 2002). These patients require intracranial pressure monitoring. Measures to promote adequate cerebral perfusion include careful fluid balance and hemodynamic assessments, a quiet environment, and diuresis with mannitol, an osmotic diuretic.

Use of barbiturate anesthesia or pharmacologic paralysis and sedation is indicated to prevent surges in intracranial pressure related to agitation. Other support measures include monitoring for and treating hypoglycemia, coagulopathies, and infection. Despite these treatment modalities, the mortality rate remains high. Consequently, liver transplantation (discussed later) has become the treatment of choice for fulminant hepatic failure.

Hepatic Cirrhosis

Cirrhosis is a chronic disease characterized by replacement of normal liver tissue with diffuse fibrosis that disrupts the structure and function of the liver. There are three types of cirrhosis or scarring of the liver:

- Alcoholic cirrhosis, in which the scar tissue characteristically surrounds the portal areas. This is most frequently caused by chronic alcoholism and is the most common type of cirrhosis.
- Postnecrotic cirrhosis, in which there are broad bands of scar tissue. This is a late result of a previous bout of acute viral hepatitis.
- Biliary cirrhosis, in which scarring occurs in the liver around the bile ducts. This type of cirrhosis usually results from chronic biliary obstruction and infection (cholangitis); it is much less common than the other two types.

The portion of the liver chiefly involved in cirrhosis consists of the portal and the periportal spaces, where the bile canaliculi of each lobule communicate to form the liver bile ducts. These areas become the sites of inflammation, and the bile ducts become occluded with inspissated (thickened) bile and pus. The liver attempts to form new bile channels; hence, there is an overgrowth of tissue made up largely of disconnected, newly formed bile ducts and surrounded by scar tissue.

Clinical manifestations include intermittent jaundice and fever. Initially the liver is enlarged, hard, and irregular, but eventually it atrophies.

Pathophysiology

Although several factors have been implicated in the etiology of cirrhosis, alcohol consumption is considered the major causative factor. Cirrhosis occurs with greatest frequency among people with alcoholism. Although nutritional deficiency with reduced protein intake contributes to liver destruction in cirrhosis, excessive alcohol intake is the major causative factor in fatty liver and its consequences. However, cirrhosis has also occurred in people who do not consume alcohol and in those who consume a normal diet and have a high alcohol intake.

Some people appear to be more susceptible than others to this disease, whether or not they have alcoholism or are malnourished. Other factors may play a role, including exposure to certain chemicals (carbon tetrachloride, chlorinated naphthalene, arsenic, or phosphorus) or infectious schistosomiasis. Twice as many men as women are affected, although, for unknown reasons, women are at greater risk for development of alcohol-induced liver disease. Most patients are between 40 and 60 years of age. Each year more than 27,000 people die of chronic liver diseases and cirrhosis in the United States (MacSween et al., 2002).

Alcoholic cirrhosis is characterized by episodes of necrosis involving the liver cells, which sometimes occur repeatedly throughout the course of the disease. The destroyed liver cells are gradually replaced by scar tissue. Eventually, the amount of scar tissue exceeds that of the functioning liver tissue. Islands of residual normal tissue and regenerating liver tissue may project from the constricted areas, giving the cirrhotic liver its characteristic hobnail appearance. The disease usually has an insidious onset and a protracted course, occasionally proceeding over a period of 30 or more years.

The prognoses for different forms of cirrhosis caused by various liver diseases have been investigated in several studies. Of the many prognostic indicators, the Child-Pugh classification seems most useful in predicting the outcome of patients with liver disease (Table 39-5). It is also used in choosing management approaches.

Clinical Manifestations

Signs and symptoms of cirrhosis increase in severity as the disease progresses. The severity of the manifestations helps to categorize the disorder as compensated or decompensated cirrhosis (Chart 39-11). Compensated cirrhosis, with its less severe, often vague symptoms, may be discovered secondarily at a routine physical examination. The hallmarks of decompensated cirrhosis result from failure of the liver to synthesize proteins, clotting factors, and other substances and manifestations of portal hypertension (see earlier sections of this chapter for clinical manifestations and management of portal hypertension, ascites, varices, and hepatic encephalopathy).

Liver Enlargement

Early in the course of cirrhosis, the liver tends to be large and the cells are loaded with fat. The liver is firm and has a sharp edge that is noticeable on palpation. Abdominal pain may be present because of recent, rapid enlargement of the liver, which produces tension on the fibrous covering of the liver (Glisson's capsule). Later in the disease, the liver decreases in size as scar tissue contracts the liver tissue. The liver edge, if palpable, is nodular.

Portal Obstruction and Ascites

Portal obstruction and ascites, late manifestations of cirrhosis, are caused partly by chronic failure of liver function and partly by obstruction of the portal circulation. Almost all of the blood from the digestive organs is collected in the portal veins and carried to the liver. Because

TABLE 39-5 Modified Child-Pugh Classification of the Severity of Liver Disease*

	Points Assigned		
Parameter	**1**	**2**	**3**
Ascites	Absent	Slight	Moderate
Bilirubin (mg/dL)	≤ 2	2–3	> 3
Albumin (g/dL)	> 3.5	2.8–3.5	< 2.8
Prothrombin time (seconds over control)	1–3	4–6	> 6
Encephalopathy	None	Grade 1–2	Grade 3–4

*Total score of 1–6, grade A; 7–9, grade B; 10–15, grade C.
Schiff, E.R., Somell, M.F. & Maddrey, W.C. (Eds.) (2003). *Schiff's diseases of the liver* (9th ed.). Philadelphia: Lippincott Williams & Wilkins.

CHART 39-11

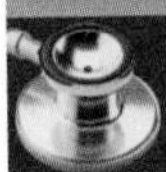

Assessing for Cirrhosis

Be on the alert for the following signs and symptoms:

COMPENSATED

- Intermittent mild fever
- Vascular spiders
- Palmar erythema (reddened palms)
- Unexplained epistaxis
- Ankle edema
- Vague morning indigestion
- Flatulent dyspepsia
- Abdominal pain
- Firm, enlarged liver
- Splenomegaly

DECOMPENSATED

- Ascites
- Jaundice
- Weakness
- Muscle wasting
- Weight loss
- Continuous mild fever
- Clubbing of fingers
- Purpura (due to decreased platelet count)
- Spontaneous bruising
- Epistaxis
- Hypotension
- Sparse body hair
- White nails
- Gonadal atrophy

a cirrhotic liver does not allow free blood passage, blood backs up into the spleen and the GI tract, and these organs become the seat of chronic passive congestion; that is, they are stagnant with blood and therefore cannot function properly. Indigestion and altered bowel function result. Fluid rich in protein may accumulate in the peritoneal cavity, producing ascites. This can be detected through percussion for shifting dullness or a fluid wave (see Fig. 39-5).

Infection and Peritonitis

Bacterial peritonitis may develop in patients with cirrhosis and ascites in the absence of an intra-abdominal source of infection or an abscess. This condition is referred to as spontaneous bacterial peritonitis (SBP). Bacteremia due to translocation of intestinal flora is believed to be the most likely route of infection. Clinical signs may be absent, necessitating paracentesis for diagnosis. Antibiotic therapy is effective in the treatment and prevention of recurrent episodes of SBP. The most severe complication of SBP is hepatorenal syndrome, a functional renal failure unresponsive to administration of fluid or diuretics. This type of renal failure is characterized by a lack of pathologic changes in the kidney; there is no evidence of dehydration or obstruction of the urinary tract or any other renal disorder.

Gastrointestinal Varices

The obstruction to blood flow through the liver caused by fibrotic changes also results in the formation of collateral blood vessels in the GI system and shunting of blood from the portal vessels into blood vessels with lower pressures. As a result, the patient with cirrhosis often has prominent, distended abdominal blood vessels, which are visible on abdominal inspection (caput medusae), and distended blood vessels throughout the GI tract. The esophagus, stomach, and lower rectum are common sites of collateral blood vessels. These distended blood vessels form varices or hemorrhoids, depending on their location (see Fig. 39-6).

Because these vessels were not intended to carry the high pressure and volume of blood imposed by cirrhosis, they may rupture and bleed. Therefore, assessment must include observation for occult and frank bleeding from the GI tract.

Edema

Another late symptom of cirrhosis is edema, which is attributed to chronic liver failure. A reduced plasma albumin concentration predisposes the patient to the formation of edema. Although edema is generalized, it often affects the lower extremities, the upper extremities, and the presacral area. Facial edema is not typical. Overproduction of aldosterone occurs, causing sodium and water retention and potassium excretion.

Vitamin Deficiency and Anemia

Because of inadequate formation, use, and storage of certain vitamins (notably vitamins A, C, and K), signs of deficiency are common, particularly hemorrhagic phenomena associated with vitamin K deficiency. Chronic gastritis and impaired GI function, together with inadequate dietary intake and impaired liver function, account for the anemia that is often associated with cirrhosis. The patient's anemia, poor nutritional status, and poor state of health result in severe fatigue, which interferes with the ability to carry out routine activities of daily living (ADLs).

Mental Deterioration

Additional clinical manifestations include deterioration of mental and cognitive function with impending hepatic encephalopathy and hepatic coma. Neurologic assessment is indicated, including assessment of the patient's general behavior, cognitive abilities, orientation to time and place, and speech patterns.

Assessment and Diagnostic Findings

The extent of liver disease and the type of treatment are determined after review of the laboratory findings. Because the functions of the liver are complex, there are many diagnostic tests that provide information about liver function (see Table 39-1). The patient needs to know why these tests are being performed and how to cooperate.

In severe parenchymal liver dysfunction, the serum albumin level tends to decrease, and the serum globulin level rises. Enzyme tests indicate liver cell damage: serum alkaline phosphatase, AST, ALT, and GGT levels increase, and the serum cholinesterase level may decrease. Bilirubin tests are performed to measure bile excretion or retention; increased levels of bilirubin can occur with cirrhosis and other liver disorders. Prothrombin time is prolonged.

Ultrasound scanning is used to measure the difference in density of parenchymal cells and scar tissue. CT, MRI, and radioisotope liver scans give information about liver size and hepatic blood flow and obstruction. Diagnosis is confirmed by liver biopsy. Arterial blood gas analysis may reveal a ventilation–perfusion imbalance and hypoxia.

Medical Management

The management of the patient with cirrhosis is usually based on the presenting symptoms. For example, antacids or H_2 antagonists are prescribed to decrease gastric distress and minimize the possibility of GI bleeding. Vitamins and nutritional supplements promote healing of damaged liver cells and improve the patient's general nutritional status. Potassium-sparing diuretics such as spironolactone (Aldactone) or triamterene (Dyrenium) may be indicated to decrease ascites, if present; these diuretics are preferred because they minimize the fluid and electrolyte changes commonly seen with other agents. An adequate diet and avoidance of alcohol are essential. Although the fibrosis of the cirrhotic liver cannot be reversed, its progression may be halted or slowed by such measures.

Preliminary studies indicate that colchicine, an anti-inflammatory agent used to treat the symptoms of gout, may increase survival time in patients with mild to moderate cirrhosis. Although colchicine therapy has not been widely used, its use is associated with improved survival in patients with alcoholic liver disease (Friedman et al., 2003).

Many patients who have end-stage liver disease (ESLD) with cirrhosis use the herb milk thistle (*Silybum marianum*) to treat jaundice and other symptoms. This herb has been used for centuries because of its healing and regenerative properties for liver disease. Silymarin from milk thistle has anti-inflammatory and antioxidant properties that may have beneficial effects, especially in hepatitis. The natural compound, SAM-e (adenosylmethione), may improve outcomes in liver disease by improving liver function, possibly through enhancing antioxidant function. Primary biliary cirrhosis has been treated with ursodeoxycholic acid to improve liver function.

Nursing Process

The Patient With Hepatic Cirrhosis

Assessment

Nursing assessment focuses on the onset of symptoms and the history of precipitating factors, particularly long-term alcohol abuse, as well as dietary intake and changes in the patient's physical and mental status. The patient's past and current patterns of alcohol use (duration and amount) are assessed and documented. It is also important to document any exposure to toxic agents encountered in the workplace or during recreational activities. The nurse documents and reports exposure to potentially hepatotoxic substances, including medications, illicit IV/injection drugs, inhalants, and general anesthetic agents.

The nurse assesses the patient's mental status during the interview and other interactions with the patient; orientation to person, place, and time is noted. The patient's ability to carry out a job or household activities provides some information about physical and mental status. The patient's relationships with family, friends, and coworkers may give some indication about incapacitation secondary to alcohol abuse and cirrhosis. Abdominal distention and bloating, GI bleeding, bruising, and weight changes are noted.

The nurse assesses nutritional status, which is of major importance in cirrhosis, by obtaining daily weights and monitoring plasma proteins, transferrin, and creatinine levels.

Diagnosis

Nursing Diagnoses

Based on all the assessment data, the patient's major nursing diagnoses may include the following:

- Activity intolerance related to fatigue, general debility, muscle wasting, and discomfort
- Imbalanced nutrition, less than body requirements, related to chronic gastritis, decreased GI motility, and anorexia
- Impaired skin integrity related to compromised immunologic status, edema, and poor nutrition
- Risk for injury and bleeding related to altered clotting mechanisms

Collaborative Problems/ Potential Complications

Based on assessment data, potential complications may include the following:

- Bleeding and hemorrhage
- Hepatic encephalopathy
- Fluid volume excess

Planning and Goals

The goals for the patient may include increased participation in activities, improvement of nutritional status, improvement of skin integrity, decreased potential for injury, improvement of mental status, and absence of complications.

Nursing Interventions

Promoting Rest

The patient with active liver disease requires rest and other supportive measures to permit the liver to reestablish its functional ability. If the patient is hospitalized, weight and fluid intake and output are measured and recorded daily. The nurse adjusts the patient's position in bed for maximal respiratory efficiency, which is especially important if ascites is marked, because it interferes with adequate thoracic excursion. Oxygen therapy may be required in liver failure to oxygenate the damaged cells and prevent further cell destruction.

Rest reduces the demands on the liver and increases the liver's blood supply. Because the patient is susceptible to the hazards of immobility, efforts to prevent respiratory, circulatory, and vascular disturbances are initiated. These measures may help prevent such problems as pneumonia, thrombophlebitis, and pressure ulcers. After nutritional status improves and strength increases, the nurse encourages the patient to increase activity gradually. Activity and mild exercise, as well as rest, are planned.

Improving Nutritional Status

The patient with cirrhosis who has no ascites or edema and exhibits no signs of impending hepatic coma should receive a nutritious, high-protein diet, if tolerated, supplemented by vitamins of the B complex and others as indicated (including vitamins A, C, K and folic acid). Because proper nutrition is so important, the nurse makes every effort to encourage the patient to eat. Proper nutrition is as important as any medication. Often small, frequent meals are better tolerated than three large meals because of the abdominal pressure exerted by ascites. Protein supplements may also be indicated.

Patient preferences are considered. Patients with prolonged or severe anorexia and those who are vomiting or eating poorly for any reason may receive nutrients by the enteral or parenteral route.

Patients with fatty stools (steatorrhea) should receive water-soluble forms of fat-soluble vitamins—A, D, and E (Aquasol A, D, and E). Folic acid and iron are prescribed to prevent anemia. If the patient shows signs of impending or advancing coma, the amount of protein in the diet is decreased temporarily. In the absence of hepatic encephalopathy, a moderate-protein, high-calorie intake is provided, with protein foods of high biologic value. A diet containing 1 to 1.5 g of protein per kilogram of body weight per day is required unless the patient is malnourished. Protein is restricted if encephalopathy develops. Incorporating vegetable protein to meet protein needs may decrease the risk for encephalopathy. Sodium restriction is also indicated to prevent ascites.

A high-calorie intake should be maintained, and supplemental vitamins and minerals should be provided (eg, oral potassium if the serum potassium level is normal or low and renal function is normal).

Providing Skin Care

Providing careful skin care is important because of subcutaneous edema, the patient's immobility, jaundice, and increased susceptibility to skin breakdown and infection. Frequent changes in position are necessary to prevent pressure ulcers. It is important to avoid irritating soaps and the use of adhesive tape, to prevent trauma to the skin. Lotion may be soothing to irritated skin; the nurse takes measures to minimize scratching by the patient.

Reducing Risk of Injury

The nurse protects the patient with cirrhosis from falls and other injuries. The side rails should be in place and padded with blankets or other materials in case the patient becomes agitated or restless. To minimize agitation, the nurse orients the patient to time and place and explains all procedures. The nurse instructs the patient to ask for assistance to get out of bed. The nurse carefully evaluates any injury because of the possibility of internal bleeding.

Because of the risk for bleeding from abnormal clotting, the patient should use an electric razor rather than a safety razor. A soft-bristled toothbrush helps minimize bleeding gums, and pressure applied to all venipuncture sites helps minimize bleeding.

Monitoring and Managing Potential Complications

BLEEDING AND HEMORRHAGE

The patient is at increased risk for bleeding and hemorrhage because of decreased production of prothrombin and decreased ability of the diseased liver to synthesize the necessary substances for blood coagulation. Precautionary measures include protecting the patient with padded side rails, applying pressure to injection sites, and avoiding injury from sharp objects. The nurse observes for melena and assesses stools for blood (signs of possible internal bleeding). Vital signs are monitored regularly. Precautions are taken to minimize rupture of esophageal varices by avoiding further increases in portal pressure (see earlier discussion). Dietary modification and appropriate use of stool softeners may help prevent straining during defecation. The nurse closely monitors the patient for GI bleeding and keeps the following readily available: equipment (eg, Sengstaken-Blakemore or other balloon tamponade tube), IV fluids, and medications needed to treat hemorrhage from esophageal and gastric varices.

If hemorrhage occurs, the nurse helps the physician initiate measures to halt the bleeding and administers fluid and blood component therapy and medications. The patient with massive hemorrhage from bleeding esophageal or gastric varices is transferred to the ICU and requires emergency surgery or other treatment modalities. The patient and family require explanations about the event and the necessary treatment.

HEPATIC ENCEPHALOPATHY

Hepatic encephalopathy and coma, possible complications of cirrhosis, may manifest as deteriorating mental status and dementia or as physical signs such as abnormal voluntary and involuntary movements. Hepatic encephalopathy is mainly caused by the accumulation of ammonia in the blood and its effect on cerebral metabolism. Many factors predispose the patient with cirrhosis to hepatic encephalopathy. Therefore, the patient may require extensive diagnostic testing to identify hidden sources of bleeding and ammonia production.

Treatment may include the use of lactulose and nonabsorbable intestinal tract antibiotics to decrease ammonia levels, modification of medications to eliminate those that may precipitate or worsen hepatic encephalopathy, and bed rest to minimize energy expenditure.

Monitoring is an essential nursing function to identify early deterioration in mental status. The nurse monitors the patient's mental status closely and reports changes so that treatment of encephalopathy can be initiated promptly. Because electrolyte disturbances can contribute to encephalopathy, serum electrolyte levels are carefully monitored and corrected if abnormal. Oxygen is administered if oxygen desaturation occurs. The nurse monitors for fever or abdominal pain, which may signal the onset of bacterial peritonitis or other infection (see earlier discussion of hepatic encephalopathy).

FLUID VOLUME EXCESS

Patients with advanced chronic liver disease develop cardiovascular abnormalities. These occur due to an increased cardiac output and decreased peripheral vascular resistance, possibly resulting from the release of vasodilators. A hyperdynamic circulatory state develops in patients with cirrhosis, and plasma volume increases. This increase in circulating plasma volume is probably multifactorial, but some studies have implicated excess production of nitrous oxide, like that seen in sepsis, as one causative factor (Zakim & Boyer, 2003). The greater the degree of hepatic decompensation, the more severe the hyperdynamic state. Close assessment of cardiovascular and respiratory status is of key importance for the care of patients with this disorder. Pulmonary compromise, which is always a potential complication of ESLD because of plasma volume excess, makes prevention of pulmonary complications an important role for the nurse. Administering diuretics, implementing fluid restrictions, and enhancing patient positioning can optimize pulmonary function. Fluid retention may be noted in the development of ascites, lower extremity swelling, and dyspnea. Monitoring of intake and output, daily weight changes, changes in abdominal girth, and edema formation is part of nursing assessment in the hospital or in the home setting. Patients are also monitored for nocturia and, later, for oliguria, because these states indicate increasing severity of liver dysfunction (Zakim & Boyer, 2003).

Promoting Home and Community-Based Care

TEACHING PATIENTS SELF-CARE

During the hospital stay, the nurse and other health care providers prepare the patient with cirrhosis for discharge, focusing on dietary instruction. Of greatest importance is the exclusion of alcohol from the diet. The patient may need referral to Alcoholics Anonymous, psychiatric care, or counseling or may benefit from support from a spiritual advisor. The patient should also avoid the consumption of raw shellfish.

Sodium restriction will continue for a considerable time, if not permanently. The patient will require written instructions, teaching, reinforcement, and support from the staff as well as family members.

Successful treatment depends on convincing the patient of the need to adhere completely to the therapeutic plan. This includes rest, lifestyle changes, adequate dietary intake, and the elimination of alcohol. The nurse also instructs the patient and family about symptoms of impending encephalopathy, possible bleeding tendencies, and susceptibility to infection.

Recovery is neither rapid nor easy; there are frequent setbacks and apparent lack of improvement. Many patients find it difficult to refrain from using alcohol for comfort or escape. The nurse has a significant role in offering support and encouragement to the patient.

CONTINUING CARE

Referral for home care may assist the patient in dealing with the transition from hospital to home. The use of alcohol may have been an important part of normal home and social life in the past. The home care nurse assesses the patient's progress at home and the manner in which the patient and family are coping with the elimination of alcohol and the dietary restrictions. The nurse also reinforces previous teaching and answers questions that may not have occurred to the patient or family until the patient was back home and trying to establish new patterns of eating, drinking, and lifestyle. The plan of nursing care in Chart 39-12 provides an overall view of nursing management for the patient with impaired liver function.

Evaluation

Expected Patient Outcomes

Expected patient outcomes may include the following:

1. Participates in activities
   a. Plans activities and exercises to allow alternating periods of rest and activity
   b. Reports increased strength and well-being
   c. Participates in hygiene care
2. Increases nutritional intake
   a. Demonstrates intake of appropriate nutrients and avoidance of alcohol as reflected by diet log

(text continues on page 1333)

CHART 39-12

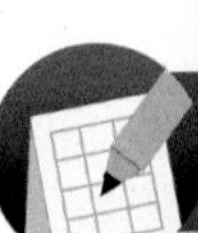

Plan of Nursing Care — The Patient With Impaired Liver Function

Nursing Diagnosis: Activity intolerance related to fatigue, lethargy, and malaise
Goal: Patient reports decrease in fatigue and reports increased ability to participate in activities

NURSING INTERVENTIONS	RATIONALE
1. Assess level of activity tolerance and degree of fatigue, lethargy, and malaise when performing routine ADLs.	1. Provides baseline for further assessment and criteria for assessment of effectiveness of interventions
2. Assist with activities and hygiene when fatigued.	2. Promotes exercise and hygiene within patient's level of tolerance
3. Encourage rest when fatigued or when abdominal pain or discomfort occurs.	3. Conserves energy and protects the liver
4. Assist with selection and pacing of desired activities and exercise.	4. Stimulates patient's interest in selected activities
5. Provide diet high in carbohydrates with protein intake consistent with liver function.	5. Provides calories for energy and protein for healing
6. Administer supplemental vitamins (A, B complex, C, and K).	6. Provides additional nutrients

EXPECTED OUTCOMES

- Exhibits increased interest in activities and events
- Participates in activities and gradually increases exercise within physical limits
- Reports increased strength and well-being
- Reports absence of abdominal pain and discomfort
- Plans activities to allow ample periods of rest
- Takes vitamins as prescribed

Nursing Diagnosis: Imbalanced nutrition: less than body requirements, related to abdominal distention and discomfort and anorexia
Goal: Positive nitrogen balance, no further loss of muscle mass; meets nutritional requirements

NURSING INTERVENTIONS	RATIONALE
1. Assess dietary intake and nutritional status through diet history and diary, daily weight measurements and laboratory data.	1. Identifies deficits in nutritional intake and adequacy of nutritional state
2. Provide diet high in carbohydrates with protein intake consistent with liver function.	2. Provides calories for energy, sparing protein for healing
3. Assist patient in identifying low-sodium foods.	3. Reduces edema and ascites formation
4. Elevate the head of the bed during meals.	4. Reduces discomfort from abdominal distention and decreases sense of fullness produced by pressure of abdominal contents and ascites on the stomach
5. Provide oral hygiene before meals and pleasant environment for meals at meal time.	5. Promotes positive environment and increased appetite; reduces unpleasant taste
6. Offer smaller, more frequent meals (6 per day).	6. Decreases feeling of fullness, bloating

EXPECTED OUTCOMES

- Exhibits improved nutritional status by increased weight (without fluid retention) and improved laboratory data.
- States rationale for dietary modifications
- Identifies foods high in carbohydrates and within protein requirements (moderate to high protein in cirrhosis and hepatitis, low protein in hepatic failure)
- Reports improved appetite
- Participates in oral hygiene measures
- Reports increased appetite; identifies rationale for smaller, frequent meals
- Demonstrates intake of high-calorie diet; adheres to protein restriction

continued >

CHART 39-12

Plan of Nursing Care The Patient With Impaired Liver Function (Continued)

NURSING INTERVENTIONS	RATIONALE
7. Encourage patient to eat meals and supplementary feedings.	7. Encouragement is essential for the patient with anorexia and gastrointestinal discomfort.
8. Provide attractive meals and an aesthetically pleasing setting at meal time.	8. Promotes appetite and sense of well-being
9. Eliminate alcohol.	9. Eliminates "empty calories" and further damage from alcohol
10. Apply an ice collar for nausea.	10. May reduce incidence of nausea
11. Administer medications prescribed for nausea, vomiting, diarrhea, or constipation.	11. Reduces gastrointestinal symptoms and discomforts that decrease the appetite and interest in food
12. Encourage increased fluid intake and exercise if the patient reports constipation.	12. Promotes normal bowel pattern and reduces abdominal discomfort and distention

EXPECTED OUTCOMES

- Identifies foods and fluids that are nutritious and permitted on diet
- Gains weight without increased edema or ascites formation
- Reports increased appetite and well-being
- Excludes alcohol from diet
- Takes medications for gastrointestinal disorders as prescribed
- Reports normal gastrointestinal function with regular bowel function

Nursing Diagnosis: Impaired skin integrity related to pruritus from jaundice and edema

Goal: Decrease potential for pressure ulcer development; breaks in skin integrity

NURSING INTERVENTIONS	RATIONALE
1. Assess degree of discomfort related to pruritus and edema.	1. Assists in determining appropriate interventions
2. Note and record degree of jaundice and extent of edema.	2. Provides baseline for detecting changes and evaluating effectiveness of interventions
3. Keep patient's fingernails short and smooth.	3. Prevents skin excoriation and infection from scratching
4. Provide frequent skin care; avoid use of soaps and alcohol-based lotions.	4. Removes waste products from skin while preventing dryness of skin
5. Massage every 2 h with emollients; turn every 2 h	5. Promotes mobilization of edema
6. Initiate use of alternating-pressure mattress or low air loss bed.	6. Minimizes prolonged pressure on bony prominences susceptible to breakdown
7. Recommend avoiding use of harsh detergents.	7. May decrease skin irritation and need for scratching
8. Assess skin integrity every 4–8 h. Instruct patient and family in this activity.	8. Edematous skin and tissue have compromised nutrient supply and are vulnerable to pressure and trauma
9. Restrict sodium as prescribed.	9. Minimizes edema formation
10. Perform range of motion exercises every 4 h; elevate edematous extremities whenever possible.	10. Promotes mobilization of edema

EXPECTED OUTCOMES

- Exhibits intact skin without redness, excoriation, or breakdown
- Reports relief from pruritus
- Exhibits no skin excoriation from scratching
- Uses nondrying soaps and lotions. States rationale for use of nondrying soaps and lotions.
- Turns self periodically. Exhibits reduced edema of dependent parts of the body.
- Exhibits no areas of skin breakdown
- Exhibits decreased edema; normal skin turgor

CHART 39-12

Plan of Nursing Care — The Patient With Impaired Liver Function (Continued)

Nursing Diagnosis: High risk for injury related to altered clotting mechanisms and altered level of consciousness
Goal: Reduced risk of injury

NURSING INTERVENTIONS	RATIONALE
1. Assess level of consciousness and cognitive level.	1. Assists in determining patient's ability to protect self and comply with required self-protective actions; may detect deterioration of hepatic function
2. Provide safe environment (pad side rails, remove obstacles in room, prevent falls).	2. Minimizes falls and injury if falls occur
3. Provide frequent surveillance to orient patient and avoid use of restraints.	3. Protects patient from harm while stimulating and orienting patient; use of restraints may disturb patient further
4. Replace sharp objects (razors) with safer items.	4. Avoids cuts and bleeding
5. Observe each stool for color, consistency, and amount.	5. Permits detection of bleeding in gastrointestinal tract
6. Be alert for symptoms of anxiety, epigastric fullness, weakness, and restlessness.	6. May indicate early signs of bleeding and shock
7. Test each stool and emesis for occult blood.	7. Detects early evidence of bleeding
8. Observe for hemorrhagic manifestations: ecchymosis, epistaxis, petechiae, and bleeding gums.	8. Indicates altered clotting mechanisms
9. Record vital signs at frequent intervals, depending on patient acuity (every 1–4 h).	9. Provides baseline and evidence of hypovolemia, and hemorrhagic shock
10. Keep patient quiet and limit activity.	10. Minimizes risk of bleeding and straining
11. Assist physician in passage of tube for esophageal balloon tamponade, if its insertion is indicated.	11. Promotes nontraumatic insertion of tube in anxious and combative patient for immediate treatment of bleeding
12. Observe during blood transfusions.	12. Permits detection of transfusion reactions (risk is increased with multiple blood transfusions needed for active bleeding from esophageal varices)
13. Measure and record nature, time, and amount of vomitus.	13. Assists in evaluating extent of bleeding and blood loss

EXPECTED OUTCOMES

- Is oriented to time, place, and person
- Exhibits no hallucinations, and demonstrates no efforts to get up unassisted or to leave hospital
- Exhibits no ecchymoses (bruises), cuts, or hematoma
- Uses electric razor rather than sharp-edged razor
- Exhibits absence of frank bleeding from gastrointestinal tract
- Exhibits absence of restlessness, epigastric fullness, and other indicators of hemorrhage and shock
- Exhibits negative results of test for occult gastrointestinal bleeding
- Is free of ecchymotic areas or hematoma formation
- Exhibits normal vital signs
- Maintains rest and remains quiet if active bleeding occurs
- Identifies rationale for blood transfusions and measures to treat bleeding
- Uses measures to prevent trauma (eg, uses soft toothbrush, blows nose gently, avoids bumps and falls, avoids straining during defecation)
- Experiences no side effects of medications
- Takes all medications as prescribed
- Identifies rationale for precautions with use of all medications
- Cooperates with treatment modalities

continued >

CHART 39-12

Plan of Nursing Care — The Patient With Impaired Liver Function (Continued)

NURSING INTERVENTIONS	RATIONALE	EXPECTED OUTCOMES
14. Maintain patient in fasting state, if indicated.	14. Reduces risk of aspiration of gastric contents and minimizes risk of further trauma to esophagus and stomach by preventing vomiting	
15. Administer vitamin K as prescribed.	15. Promotes clotting by providing fat-soluble vitamin necessary for clotting.	
16. Remain with patient during episodes of bleeding.	16. Reassures anxious patient and permits monitoring and detection of further needs of the patient	
17. Offer cold liquids by mouth when bleeding stops (if prescribed).	17. Minimizes risk of further bleeding by promoting vasoconstriction of esophageal and gastric blood vessels	
18. Institute measures to prevent trauma:	18. Promotes safety of patient	
a. Maintain safe environment.	a. Minimizes risk of trauma and bleeding by avoiding falls and cuts, etc.	
b. Encourage *gentle* blowing of nose.	b. Reduces risk of nosebleed (epistaxis) secondary to trauma and decreased clotting	
c. Provide soft toothbrush and avoid use of toothpicks.	c. Prevents trauma to oral mucosa while promoting good oral hygiene	
d. Encourage intake of foods with high content of vitamin C.	d. Promotes healing	
e. Apply cold compresses where indicated.	e. Minimizes bleeding into tissues by promoting local vasoconstriction	
f. Record location of bleeding sites.	f. Permits detection of new bleeding sites and monitoring of previous sites of bleeding	
g. Use small-gauge needles for injections.	g. Minimizes oozing and blood loss from repeated injections	
19. Administer medications carefully; monitor for side effects.	19. Reduces risk of side effects secondary to damaged liver's inability to detoxify (metabolize) medications normally	

CHART 39-12

Plan of Nursing Care — The Patient With Impaired Liver Function (Continued)

Nursing Diagnosis: Disturbed body image related to changes in appearance, sexual dysfunction, and role function
Goal: Patient verbalizes feelings consistent with improvement of body image and self-esteem

NURSING INTERVENTIONS	RATIONALE	EXPECTED OUTCOMES
1. Assess changes in appearance and the meaning these changes have for patient and family.	1. Provides information for assessing impact of changes in appearance, sexual function, and role on the patient and family	• Verbalizes concerns related to changes in appearance, life, and lifestyle • Shares concerns with significant others • Identifies past coping strategies that have been effective • Uses past effective coping strategies to deal with changes in appearance, life, and lifestyle • Maintains good grooming and hygiene • Identifies short-term goals and strategies to achieve them • Takes an active role in decision making about self and care • Identifies resources that are not harmful • Verbalizes that some of previous lifestyle practices have been harmful • Uses healthy expressions of frustration, anger, anxiety
2. Encourage patient to verbalize reactions and feelings about these changes.	2. Enables patient to identify and express concerns; encourages patient and significant others to share these concerns	
3. Assess patient's and family's previous coping strategies.	3. Permits encouragement of those coping strategies that are familiar to patient and have been effective in the past	
4. Assist and encourage patient to maximize appearance and explore alternatives to previous sexual and role functions.	4. Encourages patient to continue safe roles and functions while encouraging exploration of alternatives	
5. Assist patient in identifying short-term goals.	5. Accomplishing these goals serves as positive reinforcement and increases self-esteem.	
6. Encourage and assist patient in decision making about care.	6. Promotes patient's control of life and improves sense of well-being and self-esteem	
7. Identify with patient resources to provide additional support (counselor, spiritual advisor).	7. Assists patient in identifying resources and accepting assistance from others when indicated	
8. Assist patient in identifying previous practices that may have been harmful to self (alcohol and drug abuse).	8. Recognition and acknowledgment of the harmful effects of these practices are necessary for identifying a healthier lifestyle.	

Nursing Diagnosis: Chronic pain and discomfort related to enlarged tender liver and ascites
Goal: Increased level of comfort

NURSING INTERVENTIONS	RATIONALE	EXPECTED OUTCOMES
1. Maintain bed rest when patient experiences abdominal discomfort.	1. Reduces metabolic demands and protects the liver	• Reports pain and discomfort if present • Maintains bed rest and decreases activity in presence of pain • Takes antispasmodic and analgesics as indicated and as prescribed
2. Administer antispasmodic and analgesic agents as prescribed.	2. Reduces irritability of the gastrointestinal tract and decreases abdominal pain and discomfort	

continued >

CHART 39-12

Plan of Nursing Care The Patient With Impaired Liver Function (Continued)

NURSING INTERVENTIONS	RATIONALE	EXPECTED OUTCOMES
3. Observe, record, and report presence and character of pain and discomfort. 4. Reduce sodium and fluid intake if prescribed. 5. Prepare patient and assist with paracentesis.	3. Provides baseline to detect further deterioration of status and to evaluate interventions 4. Minimizes further formation of ascites 5. Removal of ascites fluid may decrease abdominal discomfort	• Reports decreased pain and abdominal discomfort • Reduces sodium and fluid intake to prescribed levels if indicated to treat ascites • Exhibits decreased abdominal girth and appropriate weight changes • Reports decreased discomfort after paracentesis

Nursing Diagnosis: Fluid volume excess related to ascites and edema formation
Goal: Restoration of normal fluid volume

NURSING INTERVENTIONS	RATIONALE	EXPECTED OUTCOMES
1. Restrict sodium and fluid intake if prescribed. 2. Administer diuretics, potassium, and protein supplements as prescribed. 3. Record intake and output every 1 to 8 h depending on response to interventions and on patient acuity. 4. Measure and record abdominal girth and weight daily. 5. Explain rationale for sodium and fluid restriction. 6. Prepare patient and assist with paracentesis.	1. Minimizes formation of ascites and edema 2. Promotes excretion of fluid through the kidneys and maintenance of normal fluid and electrolyte balance 3. Indicates effectiveness of treatment and adequacy of fluid intake 4. Monitors changes in ascites formation and fluid accumulation 5. Promotes patient's understanding of restriction and cooperation with it 6. Paracentesis will temporarily decrease amount of ascites present.	• Consumes diet low in sodium and within prescribed fluid restriction • Takes diuretics, potassium, and protein supplements as indicated without experiencing side effects • Exhibits increased urine output • Exhibits decreasing abdominal girth • Exhibits no rapid increase in weight • Identifies rationale for sodium and fluid restriction • Shows a decrease in ascites with decreased weight

Nursing Diagnosis: Disturbed thought processes related to deterioration of liver function and increased serum ammonia level
Goal: Improved mental status; safety maintained

NURSING INTERVENTIONS	RATIONALE	EXPECTED OUTCOMES
1. Restrict dietary protein as prescribed. 2. Give frequent, small feedings of carbohydrates. 3. Protect from infection. 4. Keep environment warm and draft-free.	1. Reduces source of ammonia (protein foods) 2. Promotes consumption of adequate carbohydrates for energy requirements and spares protein from breakdown for energy 3. Minimizes risk for further increase in metabolic requirements 4. Minimizes shivering, which would increase metabolic requirements	• Adheres to protein restriction • Demonstrates an interest in events and activities in environment • Demonstrates normal attention span • Follows and participates in conversation appropriately • Is oriented to person, place, and time

CHART 39-12

Plan of Nursing Care: The Patient With Impaired Liver Function (Continued)

NURSING INTERVENTIONS	RATIONALE	EXPECTED OUTCOMES
5. Pad the side rails of the bed.	5. Provides protection for the patient should hepatic coma and seizure activity occur	• Remains in bed when indicated • Reports no urinary or fecal incontinence • Experiences no seizures
6. Limit visitors.	6. Minimizes patient's activity and metabolic requirements	
7. Provide careful nursing surveillance to ensure patient's safety.	7. Provides close monitoring of new symptoms and minimizes trauma to the confused patient	
8. Avoid opioids and barbiturates.	8. Prevents masking of symptoms of hepatic coma and prevents drug overdose secondary to reduced ability of the damaged liver to metabolize opioids and barbiturates	
9. Awaken at intervals (every 2–4 h) to assess cognitive status.	9. Provides stimulation to the patient and opportunity for observing the patient's level of consciousness	

Nursing Diagnosis: Risk for imbalanced body temperature: hyperthermia related to inflammatory process of cirrhosis or hepatitis
Goal: Maintenance of normal body temperature, free from infection

NURSING INTERVENTIONS	RATIONALE	EXPECTED OUTCOMES
1. Record temperature regularly (every 4 h).	1. Provides baseline to detect fever and to evaluate interventions	• Exhibits normal temperature and reports absence of chills or sweating • Demonstrates adequate intake of fluids • Exhibits no evidence of local or systemic infection
2. Encourage fluid intake.	2. Corrects fluid loss from perspiration and fever and increases patient's level of comfort	
3. Apply cool sponges or icebag for elevated temperature.	3. Promotes reduction of fever and increases patient's comfort	
4. Administer antibiotics as prescribed.	4. Ensures appropriate serum concentration of antibiotics to treat infection	
5. Avoid exposure to infections.	5. Minimizes risk of further infection and further increases in body temperature and metabolic rate	
6. Keep patient at rest while temperature is elevated.	6. Reduces metabolic rate	
7. Assess for abdominal pain, tenderness.	7. May occur with bacterial peritonitis	

continued >

CHART 39-12

Plan of Nursing Care — The Patient With Impaired Liver Function (Continued)

Nursing Diagnosis: Ineffective breathing pattern related to ascites and restriction of thoracic excursion secondary to ascites, abdominal distention, and fluid in the thoracic cavity
Goal: Improved respiratory status

NURSING INTERVENTIONS	RATIONALE	EXPECTED OUTCOMES
1. Elevate head of bed to at least 30 degrees.	1. Reduces abdominal pressure on the diaphragm and permits fuller thoracic excursion and lung expansion	• Experiences improved respiratory status • Reports decreased shortness of breath • Reports increased strength and sense of well-being • Exhibits normal respiratory rate (12–18/min) with no adventitious sounds • Exhibits full thoracic excursion without shallow respirations • Exhibits normal arterial blood gases • Exhibits adequate oxygen saturation by pulse oximetry • Experiences absence of confusion or cyanosis
2. Conserve patient's strength by providing rest periods and assisting with activities.	2. Reduces metabolic and oxygen requirements	
3. Change position every 2 h.	3. Promotes expansion and oxygenation of all areas of the lungs	
4. Assist with paracentesis or thoracentesis.	4. Paracentesis and thoracentesis (performed to remove fluid from the abdominal and thoracic cavities, respectively) may be frightening to the patient.	
a. Explain procedure and its purpose to patient.	a. Helps obtain patient's cooperation with procedures	
b. Have patient void before paracentesis.	b. Prevents inadvertent bladder injury	
c. Support and maintain position during procedure.	c. Prevents inadvertent organ or tissue injury	
d. Record both the amount and the character of fluid aspirated.	d. Provides record of fluid removed and indication of severity of limitation of lung expansion by fluid	
e. Observe for evidence of coughing, increasing dyspnea, or pulse rate.	e. Indicates irritation of the pleural space and evidence of pneumothorax or hemothorax.	

Collaborative Problem: Gastrointestinal bleeding and hemorrhage
Goal: Absence of episodes of gastrointestinal bleeding and hemorrhage

NURSING INTERVENTIONS	RATIONALE	EXPECTED OUTCOMES
1. Assess patient for evidence of gastrointestinal bleeding or hemorrhage. If bleeding does occur: a. Monitor vital signs (blood pressure, pulse, respiratory rate) every 4 h or more frequently, depending on acuity. b. Assess skin temperature, level of consciousness every 4 hours or more frequently, depending on acuity.	1. Allows early detection of signs and symptoms of bleeding and hemorrhage	• Experiences no episodes of bleeding and hemorrhage • Vital signs are within acceptable range for patient • No evidence of bleeding from gastrointestinal tract • Hematocrit and hemoglobin levels within acceptable limits • Turns and moves without straining and increasing intra-abdominal pressure

CHART 39-12

Plan of Nursing Care The Patient With Impaired Liver Function (Continued)

NURSING INTERVENTIONS	RATIONALE	EXPECTED OUTCOMES
c. Monitor gastrointestinal secretions and output (emesis, stool for occult or obvious bleeding). Test emesis for blood once per shift and with any color change. Hematest each stool. d. Monitor hematocrit and hemoglobin for trends and changes.		• No straining with bowel movements • No further bleeding episodes if aggressive treatment of bleeding and hemorrhage was needed • Patient and family state rationale for treatments • Patient and family identify supports available to them • Patient and family describe signs and symptoms of a recurrent bleeding episode and identify needed action
2. Avoid activities that increase intra-abdominal pressure (straining, turning). a. Avoid coughing/sneezing. b. Assist patient to turn. c. Keep all needed items within easy reach. d. Use measures to prevent constipation such as adequate fluid intake; stool softeners. e. Ensure small meals.	2. Minimizes increases in intra-abdominal pressure that could lead to rupture and bleeding of esophageal or gastric varices	
3. Have equipment (Blakemore tube, medications, IV fluids) available if indicated.	3. Equipment, medications, and supplies will be readily available if patient experiences bleeding from ruptured esophageal or gastric varices.	
4. Assist with procedures and therapy needed to treat gastrointestinal bleeding and hemorrhage.	4. Gastrointestinal bleeding and hemorrhage require emergency measures (eg, insertion of Blakemore tube, administration of fluids and medications).	
5. Monitor respiratory status every hour and minimize risk of respiratory complications if balloon tamponade is needed.	5. The patient is at high risk for respiratory complications, including asphyxiation if gastric balloon of tamponade tube ruptures or migrates upward.	
6. Prepare patient physically and psychologically for other treatment modalities if needed.	6. The patient who experiences hemorrhage is very anxious and fearful; minimizing anxiety assists in control of hemorrhage.	
7. Monitor patient for recurrence of bleeding and hemorrhage.	7. Risk of rebleeding is high with all treatment modalities used to halt gastrointestinal bleeding.	
8. Keep family informed of patient's status.	8. Family members are likely to be anxious about the patient's status; providing information will reduce their anxiety level and promote more effective coping.	

continued >

CHART 39-12

Plan of Nursing Care — The Patient With Impaired Liver Function (Continued)

NURSING INTERVENTIONS	RATIONALE	EXPECTED OUTCOMES
9. Once recovered from bleeding episode, provide patient and family with information regarding signs and symptoms of gastrointestinal bleeding.	9. Risk of rebleeding is high. Subtle signs may be more quickly identified.	

Collaborative Problem: Hepatic encephalopathy
Goal: Absence of changes in cognitive status and of injury

NURSING INTERVENTIONS	RATIONALE	EXPECTED OUTCOMES
1. Assess cognitive status every 4–8 h: a. Assess patient's orientation to person, place, and time. b. Monitor patient's level of activity, restlessness, and agitation. Assess for presence of flapping hand tremors (asterixis). c. Obtain and record daily sample of patient's handwriting or ability to construct a simple figure (eg, star). d. Assess neurologic signs (deep tendon reflexes, ability to follow instructions).	1. Data will provide baseline of patient's cognitive status and enable detection of changes.	• Remains awake, alert, and aware of surroundings • Is oriented to time, place, and person • Exhibits no restlessness or agitation • Record of handwriting demonstrates no deterioration in cognitive function • States rationale for treatment used to prevent or treat hepatic encephalopathy • Demonstrates stable serum ammonia level within acceptable limits • Consumes adequate caloric intake and adheres to protein restriction • Takes medications as prescribed • Breath sounds are normal without adventitious sounds • Skin and tissue intact without evidence of pressure or breaks in integrity
2. Monitor medications to prevent administration of those that may precipitate hepatic encephalopathy (sedatives, hypnotics, analgesics).	2. Medications are a common precipitating factor in development of hepatic encephalopathy in patients at risk.	
3. Monitor laboratory data, especially serum ammonia level.	3. Increases in serum ammonia level are associated with hepatic encephalopathy and coma.	
4. Notify physician of even subtle changes in patient's neurologic status and cognitive function.	4. Allows early initiation of treatment of hepatic encephalopathy and prevention of hepatic coma	
5. Limit sources of protein from diet if indicated.	5. Reduces breakdown and conversion of protein to ammonia	
6. Administer medications prescribed to reduce serum ammonia level (eg, lactulose, antibiotics, glucose, benzodiazepine antagonist [Flumazenil] if indicated).	6. Reduces serum ammonia level	
7. Assess respiratory status and initiate measures to prevent complications.	7. The patient who develops hepatic coma is at risk for respiratory complications (ie, pneumonia, atelectasis, infection).	
8. Protect patient's skin and tissue from pressure and breakdown.	8. The patient in coma is at risk for skin breakdown and pressure ulcer formation.	

   b. Gains weight without increased edema and ascites formation
   c. Reports decrease in GI disturbances and anorexia
   d. Identifies foods and fluids that are nutritious and allowed on or restricted from the diet
   e. Adheres to vitamin therapy regimen
   f. Describes the rationale for small, frequent meals
3. Exhibits improved skin integrity
   a. Has intact skin without evidence of breakdown, infection, or trauma
   b. Demonstrates normal turgor of skin of the extremities and trunk, without edema
   c. Changes position frequently and inspects bony prominences daily
   d. Uses lotions to decrease pruritus
4. Avoids injury
   a. Is free of ecchymotic areas or hematoma formation
   b. States rationale for side rails and asks for assistance to get out of bed
   c. Uses measures to prevent trauma (eg, uses electric razor and soft toothbrush, blows nose gently, arranges furniture to prevent bumps and falls, avoids straining during defecation)
5. Is free of complications
   a. Reports absence of frank bleeding from the GI tract (ie, absence of melena and hematemesis)
   b. Is oriented to time, place, and person and demonstrates normal attention span
   c. Has a serum ammonia level within normal limits
   d. Identifies early, reportable signs of impaired thought processes

Cancer of the Liver

Hepatic tumors may be malignant or benign. Benign liver tumors were uncommon until the widespread use of oral contraceptives. With the use of oral contraceptives, benign tumors of the liver occur most frequently in women in their reproductive years.

Primary Liver Tumors

Few cancers originate in the liver. Primary liver tumors usually are associated with chronic liver disease, hepatitis B and C infections, and cirrhosis. Hepatocellular carcinoma (HCC) is by far the most common type of primary liver cancer, accounting for up to 50% of cancer deaths in other parts of the world. It is rare in the United States, accounting for 0.5% to 2.0% of all cancers (Kelly, Sarr & Hinder, 2004; Zakim & Boyer, 2003). HCC is usually nonresectable because of rapid growth and metastasis. Other types of primary liver cancer include cholangiocellular carcinoma and combined hepatocellular and cholangiocellular carcinoma. If found early, resection of primary liver cancer may be possible, but early detection is unlikely. Cirrhosis, chronic infection with hepatitis B and C, and exposure to certain chemical toxins (eg, vinyl chloride, arsenic) have been implicated as causes of HCC. Cigarette smoking has also been identified as a risk factor, especially when combined with alcohol use. Some evidence suggests that aflatoxin, a metabolite of the fungus *Aspergillus flavus*, may be a risk factor for HCC. This is especially true in areas where HCC is endemic (ie, Asia and Africa). Aflatoxin and other similar toxic molds can contaminate food such as ground nuts and grains and may act as co-carcinogens with hepatitis B. The risk of contamination is greatest when these foods are stored unrefrigerated in tropical or subtropical climates.

Liver Metastases

Metastases from other primary sites are found in the liver in 36% to 42% of those patients dying as a result of advanced cancer (Friedman et al., 2003). Malignant tumors are likely to reach the liver eventually, by way of the portal system or lymphatic channels, or by direct extension from an abdominal tumor. Moreover, the liver apparently is an ideal place for these malignant cells to thrive. Often the first evidence of cancer in an abdominal organ is the appearance of liver metastases; unless exploratory surgery or an autopsy is performed, the primary tumor may never be identified.

Clinical Manifestations

The early manifestations of malignancy of the liver include pain—a continuous dull ache in the right upper quadrant, epigastrium, or back. Weight loss, loss of strength, anorexia, and anemia may also occur. The liver may be enlarged and irregular on palpation. Jaundice is present only if the larger bile ducts are occluded by the pressure of malignant nodules in the hilum of the liver. Ascites develops if such nodules obstruct the portal veins or if tumor tissue is seeded in the peritoneal cavity.

Assessment and Diagnostic Findings

The diagnosis of liver cancer is based on clinical signs and symptoms, the history and physical examination, and the results of laboratory and x-ray studies. Increased serum levels of bilirubin, alkaline phosphatase, AST, GGT, and lactic dehydrogenase may occur. Leukocytosis (increased white blood cells), erythrocytosis (increased red blood cells), hypercalcemia, hypoglycemia, and hypocholesterolemia may also be seen on laboratory assessment.

The serum level of alpha-fetoprotein (AFP), which serves as a tumor marker, is elevated in 30% to 40% of patients with primary liver cancer. The level of carcinoembryonic antigen (CEA), a marker of advanced cancer of the digestive tract, may be elevated. These two markers together are useful to distinguish between metastatic liver disease and primary liver cancer.

Many patients have metastases from the primary liver tumor to other sites by the time the diagnosis is made; metastases occur primarily to the lung but may also occur to regional lymph nodes, adrenals, bone, kidneys, heart, pancreas, or stomach.

X-rays, liver scans, CT scans, ultrasound studies, MRI, arteriography, and laparoscopy may be part of the diagnostic workup and may be performed to determine the extent of the cancer. Positive emission tomograms (PET scans) are used to evaluate a wide range of metastatic tumors of the liver.

Confirmation of a tumor's histology can be made by biopsy under imaging guidance (CT scan or ultrasound) or laparoscopically. Local or systemic dissemination of the tumor by needle biopsy or fine-needle biopsy can occur but is rare. Some clinicians believe that these procedures should not be performed if the tumor is thought to be resectable; rather, primary HCC diagnosis should be confirmed by frozen section at the time of laparotomy in those patients with resectable lesions detected by imaging studies.

Medical Management

Although surgical resection of the liver tumor is possible in some patients, the underlying cirrhosis is so prevalent in cancer of the liver that it increases the risks associated with surgery. Radiation therapy and chemotherapy have been used to treat cancer of the liver with varying degrees of success. Although these therapies may prolong survival and improve quality of life by reducing pain and discomfort, their major effect is palliative.

Radiation Therapy

The use of external beam radiation for the treatment of liver tumors has been limited by the radiosensitivity of normal hepatocytes. More effective methods of delivering radiation to tumors of the liver include (1) IV or intra-arterial injection of antibodies tagged with radioactive isotopes that specifically attack tumor-associated antigens and (2) percutaneous placement of a high-intensity source for interstitial radiation therapy (delivery of radiation directly to the tumor cells).

Chemotherapy

Chemotherapy has been used to improve quality of life and prolong survival; it also may be used as adjuvant therapy after surgical resection of hepatic tumors. Systemic chemotherapy and regional infusion chemotherapy are two methods used to administer antineoplastic agents to patients with primary and metastatic hepatic tumors. Embolization of tumor vessels with chemotherapy (a process known as chemoembolization) produces anoxic necrosis with high concentrations of trapped chemotherapeutic agents. This therapy has begun to show some promising results (Jang, Lee, Kim, et al., 2004; Huang, Chen, & Chang, 2004). An implantable pump has been used to deliver a high concentration of chemotherapy by constant infusion to the liver through the hepatic artery. This method has shown a moderate response rate (Abbruzzese, Evans, Willett, et al., 2004; Friedman et al., 2003).

Percutaneous Biliary Drainage

Percutaneous biliary or transhepatic drainage is used to bypass biliary ducts obstructed by liver, pancreatic, or bile duct tumors in patients who have inoperable tumors or are considered poor surgical risks. Under fluoroscopy, a catheter is inserted through the abdominal wall and past the obstruction into the duodenum. Such procedures are used to reestablish biliary drainage, relieve pressure and pain from the buildup of bile behind the obstruction, and decrease pruritus and jaundice. As a result, the patient is made more comfortable and quality of life and survival are improved.

For several days after its insertion, the catheter is opened to external drainage. The bile is observed closely for amount, color, and presence of blood and debris. Complications of percutaneous biliary drainage include sepsis, leakage of bile, hemorrhage, and reobstruction of the biliary system by debris in the catheter or by encroaching tumor. Therefore, the patient is observed for fever and chills, bile drainage around the catheter, changes in vital signs, and evidence of biliary obstruction, including increased pain or pressure, pruritus, and recurrence of jaundice.

Other Nonsurgical Treatments

Laser hyperthermia has been used to treat hepatic metastases. Heat has been directed to tumors through several methods to cause necrosis of the tumor cells while sparing normal tissue. In radiofrequency thermal ablation, a needle electrode is inserted into the liver tumor under imaging guidance. Radiofrequency energy passes through to the noninsulated needle tip, causing heat and tumor cell death from coagulation necrosis.

Immunotherapy is another treatment modality under investigation. In this therapy, lymphocytes with antitumor reactivity are administered to the patient with hepatic cancer. Tumor regression has been demonstrated in patients with metastatic cancer for whom standard treatment has failed.

Transcatheter arterial embolization interrupts the arterial blood flow to small tumors by injecting small particulate embolic or chemotherapeutic agents into the artery supplying the tumor. As a result, ischemia and necrosis of the tumor occur.

For multiple small lesions, ultrasound-guided injection of alcohol promotes dehydration of tumor cells and tumor necrosis (Friedman et al., 2003).

Surgical Management

Surgical resection is the treatment of choice when HCC is confined to one lobe of the liver and the function of the remaining liver is considered adequate for postoperative recovery. In the case of metastasis, hepatic resection can be performed if the primary site can be completely excised and the metastasis is limited. However, metastases to the liver are rarely limited or solitary. Capitalizing on the regenerative capacity of the liver cells, some surgeons have successfully removed 90% of the liver. However, the presence of cirrhosis limits the ability of the liver to regenerate. Staging of liver tumors aids in predicting the likelihood of surgical cure.

In preparation for surgery, the patient's nutritional, fluid, and general physical status are assessed, and efforts are undertaken to ensure the best physical condition possible. Support, explanation, and encouragement are provided to help the patient prepare psychologically for the surgery.

Extensive diagnostic studies may be performed. Specific studies may include liver scan, liver biopsy, cholangiography, selective hepatic angiography, percutaneous needle biopsy, peritoneoscopy, laparoscopy, ultrasound, CT scan, PET scan,

MRI, and blood tests, particularly determinations of serum alkaline phosphatase, AST, and GGT and its isoenzymes.

LOBECTOMY

Removal of a lobe of the liver is the most common surgical procedure for excising a liver tumor. If it is necessary to restrict blood flow from the hepatic artery and portal vein for longer than 15 minutes, it is likely that hypothermia will be used. For a right-liver lobectomy or an extended right lobectomy (including the medial left lobe), a thoracoabdominal incision is used. An extensive abdominal incision is made for a left lobectomy.

CRYOSURGERY

In cryosurgery (**cryoablation**), tumors are destroyed by liquid nitrogen at –196°C. To destroy the diseased tissue, two or three freeze-and-thaw cycles are administered via probes during open laparotomy. This technique may also be performed laparoscopically or under ultrasound guidance. It has been used alone or as an adjunct to hepatic resection in HCC and for colorectal metastases not amenable to radical surgical excision. The efficacy of cryosurgery is still being evaluated; indications and outcomes require further investigation.

LIVER TRANSPLANTATION

Removing the liver and replacing it with a healthy donor organ is another way to treat liver cancer. Studies have shown decreased recurrence rates of the primary liver malignancy after transplantation, with improvement in 5-year survival rates to consistently greater than 70% (Bruix & Llovet, 2002; Yamada, 2003). Metastasis and recurrence may be enhanced by the immunosuppressive therapy that is needed to prevent rejection of the transplanted liver. In patients with small (less than 5 cm), single lesions, liver transplantation has been shown to be beneficial, but its use is limited by organ shortages. The increasing use of living donor transplantation may improve this situation and decrease the waiting time and tumor proliferation that is characteristic of patients with liver cancer (see later discussion).

Nursing Management

If the patient has had surgery to treat liver cancer, potential problems related to cardiopulmonary involvement may include vascular complications and respiratory and liver dysfunction. Metabolic abnormalities require careful attention. A constant infusion of 10% glucose may be required in the first 48 hours to prevent a precipitous fall in the blood glucose level that results from decreased gluconeogenesis. Because extensive blood loss may occur as well, the patient receives infusions of blood and IV fluids. The patient requires constant, close monitoring and care for the first 2 or 3 days, similar to postsurgical abdominal and thoracic nursing care.

The patient undergoing cryosurgery is monitored closely for hypothermia, hemorrhage, or bile leak; myoglobinuria can occur as a result of tissue necrosis and is minimized by hydration.

If the patient is to receive chemotherapy or radiation therapy in an effort to relieve symptoms, he or she may be discharged home while still receiving one or both of these therapies. The patient may also go home with a biliary drainage system or hepatic artery catheter in place. In most cases, the hepatic artery catheter has been inserted surgically and has a prefilled infusion pump that delivers a continuous chemotherapeutic dose until completed. Although somewhat less desirable, a hepatic artery port may also be inserted to provide access for intermittent chemotherapy infusion (Abbruzzese et al., 2004). This port dwells under the skin, but, because it provides direct arterial access, it is not used for continuous infusion therapy in the home environment; the access line is discontinued once the chemotherapeutic agent has infused. The patient and family require teaching about care of the biliary catheter and the effects and side effects of hepatic artery chemotherapy. This teaching is necessary because of participation of the patient and family in patient care in the home setting.

Promoting Home and Community-Based Care

TEACHING PATIENTS SELF-CARE

The nurse instructs the patient to recognize and report the potential complications and side effects of the chemotherapy and the desirable and undesirable effects of the specific chemotherapy regimen. The nurse also emphasizes the importance of follow-up visits to assess the patient and the tumor's response to chemotherapy and radiation therapy.

If the patient is receiving chemotherapy on an outpatient basis, the nurse explains the patient's and family's role in managing the chemotherapy infusion and in assessing the infusion/insertion site. The nurse encourages the patient to resume routine activities as soon as possible, while cautioning about activities that may damage the infusion pump or site.

The family and the patient at home with a biliary drainage system in place typically fear that the catheter will become dislodged. Reassurance and instruction can help reduce their fear that the catheter will fall out easily. The patient and family also require instruction on catheter care. The family and the patient need to learn how to keep the catheter site clean and dry and how to assess the catheter and its insertion site. Irrigation of the catheter with sterile normal saline solution or water may be prescribed to keep the catheter patent and free of debris. The patient and caregivers are taught proper technique to avoid introducing bacteria into the biliary system or catheter during irrigation. They are instructed not to aspirate or draw back on the syringe during irrigation, to prevent entry of irritating duodenal contents into the biliary tree or catheter. The patient and caregivers are also instructed about the signs of complications and are encouraged to notify the nurse or physician if problems or questions arise.

Patients with implantable ports are instructed about the chemotherapy regimen, types of medications, effects and side effects that may occur, and appropriate management strategies if problems occur. If a hepatic artery port is inserted for intermittent chemotherapy, patients and their families are provided the same educational content. Such a port has an internal one-way valve; therefore, it not aspirated for a blood return before the infusion is initiated. The patient is instructed to assess the port site between infusions and to note and report any sign of infection or inflammation.

CONTINUING CARE

In many cases, referral for home care enables the patient with liver cancer to be at home in a familiar environment with family and friends. Because of the poor prognosis associated with liver cancer, the home care nurse serves a vital role in assisting the patient and family to cope with the symptoms that may occur and the prognosis. The home care nurse assesses the patient's physical and psychological status, adequacy of pain relief, nutritional status, and presence of symptoms indicating complications of treatment or progression of disease. During home visits, the nurse assesses the function of the chemotherapy pump, the infusion site, and the biliary drainage system, if indicated. The nurse collaborates with the other members of the health care team, the patient, and the family to ensure effective pain management and to manage potential problems, which include weakness, pruritus, inadequate dietary intake, jaundice, and symptoms associated with metastasis to other sites. The home care nurse also assists the patient and family in making decisions about hospice care and assists with initiation of referrals. The patient is encouraged to discuss preferences for end-of-life care with family members and health care providers (see Chapter 17).

Liver Transplantation

Liver transplantation is used to treat life-threatening ESLD for which no other form of treatment is available. The transplantation procedure involves total removal of the diseased liver and replacement with a healthy liver in the same anatomic location (**orthotopic liver transplantation** [OLT]). Removal of the liver creates a space for the new liver and permits anatomic reconstruction of the hepatic vasculature and biliary tract as close to normal as possible.

The success of liver transplantation depends on successful immunosuppression. Immunosuppressants currently used include cyclosporine (Neoral), tacrolimus (Prograf), corticosteroids, azathioprine (Imuran), mycophenolate mofetil (CellCept), OKT3 (a monoclonal antibody), sirolimus (formerly known as rapamycin [Rapamune]), Thymoglobulin, basiliximab, and daclizumab. Studies are underway to find the most effective combination of immunosuppressive agents and to identify new agents with fewer side effects (Friedman et al., 2003; Zakim & Boyer, 2003).

Despite the success of immunosuppression in reducing the incidence of rejection of transplanted organs, liver transplantation is not routine and may be accompanied by complications related to the lengthy surgical procedure, immunosuppressive therapy, infection, and the technical difficulties encountered in reconstructing the blood vessels and biliary tract. Long-standing systemic problems resulting from the primary liver disease may complicate the preoperative and postoperative course. Previous surgery of the abdomen, including procedures to treat complications of advanced liver disease (ie, shunt procedures used to treat portal hypertension and esophageal varices) increase the complexity of the transplantation procedure.

The indications for liver transplantation are not as limited today as they were when the procedure was first introduced, due to advances in immunosuppressive therapy, improvements in biliary tract reconstruction, and, in some cases, the use of venovenous bypass. General indications for liver transplantation include irreversible advanced chronic liver disease, fulminant hepatic failure, metabolic liver diseases, and some hepatic malignancies. Examples of disorders that are indications for liver transplantation include hepatocellular liver diseases (eg, viral hepatitis, drug- or alcohol-induced liver disease, Wilson's disease) and cholestatic diseases (primary biliary cirrhosis, sclerosing cholangitis, and biliary atresia).

The patient being considered for liver transplantation frequently has many systemic problems that influence preoperative and postoperative care. Because transplantation is more difficult if the patient has developed severe GI bleeding and hepatic coma, efforts are made to perform the procedure before the disease progresses to this stage. The patient must undergo a thorough evaluation of hepatic reserve and general health. Part of this evaluation includes classification of the degree of medical need, an objective determination known as the Model of End Stage Liver Disease (MELD) classification, which stratifies the level of illness of those awaiting a liver transplant. The MELD score is derived from a complex formula incorporating bilirubin levels, prothrombin time (reported as international normalized ratio [INR]), creatinine, and the cause of the liver disease (ie, cholestatic, alcoholic, or other). This system has replaced the Child-Pugh classification and other related scoring systems for prioritizing patients on the liver transplantation list (Rosemurgy, Zervos, Clarke, et al., 2004). Although the Child-Pugh score classifies the severity of liver disease and stratifies patients into levels for varied treatment regimens, the MELD score is an indicator of short-term mortality for those with ESLD. Organs are allocated using the MELD score in an effort to provide transplants to the most severely ill patients.

Because liver transplantation is now recognized as an established therapeutic modality, rather than an experimental procedure to treat these disorders, the number of liver transplantation centers is increasing. Patients requiring transplantation are often referred from distant hospitals to these sites. To prepare the patient and family for liver transplantation, nurses in all settings must understand the processes and procedures of liver transplantation.

Surgical Procedure

During the procedure, the donor liver is freed from other structures, the bile is flushed from the gallbladder to prevent damage to the walls of the biliary tract, and the liver is perfused with a preservative and cooled. Before the donor liver is placed in the recipient, it is flushed with cold lactated Ringer's solution to remove potassium and air bubbles. The presence of portal hypertension increases the difficulty of the procedure. To minimize this problem, many centers use venovenous bypass, which decompresses the venous system below the diaphragm by temporarily shunting blood to the superior vena cava via the axillary vein (Friedman et al., 2003).

Anastomoses (connections) of the blood vessels and bile duct are performed between the donor liver and the recipient liver. There are two types of biliary anastomoses. Biliary reconstruction is performed with an end-to-end anastomosis of the donor and recipient common bile ducts, with a stented T-tube inserted for external drainage of bile. If an end-to-end anastomosis is not possible because of diseased or absent bile ducts, an end-to-side anastomosis is made between the common bile duct of the graft and a loop (Roux-en-Y portion) of jejunum (Fig. 39-15A); in this case, bile drainage is internal, and a T-tube is not inserted (Kelly et al., 2004). Figure 39-15B and C illustrates the final appearance of the grafted liver and final closure and drain placement.

Several additional techniques have been developed to expand the donor pool for liver transplantation. In a split liver transplant, a single organ is used to provide grafts for two individuals with ESLD, with the smaller patient receiving the smaller left lobe. This procedure has resulted in a higher complication rate and lower survival rate than traditional liver transplantation. Auxiliary liver transplantation has been used in adults with fulminant hepatic failure until the patient's own liver recovers function. This procedure incorporates removal of a segment of diseased liver and implantation of a reduced-size graft. Living donor transplantation is being increasingly performed from adult to adult using full right lobes, although it is controversial because it is a major surgical procedure for the donor, and some donor deaths have been reported. The results thus far have indicated that this procedure is not appropriate for patients with severely decompensated liver disease (Friedman et al., 2003).

Liver transplantation is a long surgical procedure, partly because the patient with liver failure often has portal hypertension, requiring ligation of many venous collateral vessels. Blood loss during the surgical procedure may be extensive. If the patient has adhesions from previous abdominal surgery, lysis of adhesions is often necessary. If a shunt procedure was performed previously, it must be surgically reversed to permit adequate portal venous blood supply to the new liver. During the lengthy

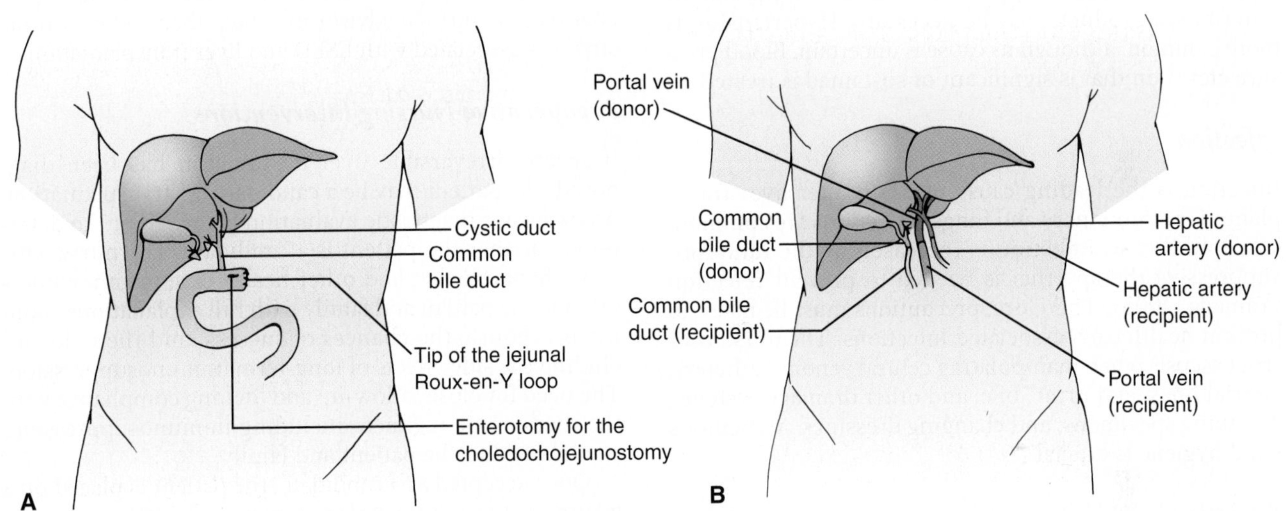

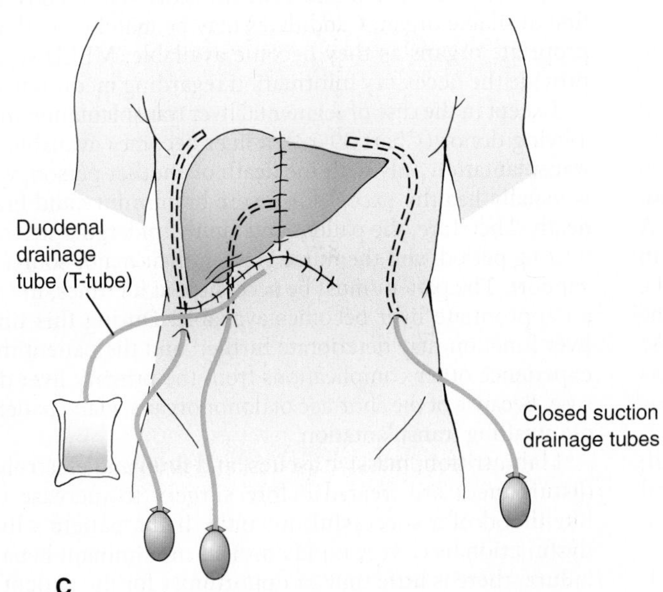

FIGURE 39-15. (A) Roux-en-Y hepatojejunostomy. (B) Final appearance of implanted liver graft. (C) Final closure and drain placement after liver transplantation.

surgery, it is helpful to provide regular updates to the family about the progress of the operation and the patient's status.

Complications

The postoperative complication rate is high, primarily because of technical complications or infection. Immediate postoperative complications may include bleeding, infection, and rejection. Disruption, infection, obstruction of the biliary anastomosis, and impaired biliary drainage may occur. Vascular thrombosis and stenosis are other potential complications.

Bleeding

Bleeding is common in the postoperative period and may result from coagulopathy, portal hypertension, and fibrinolysis caused by ischemic injury to the donor liver. Hypotension may occur in this phase, secondary to blood loss. Administration of platelets, fresh-frozen plasma, or other blood products may be necessary. Hypertension is more common, although its cause is uncertain. Blood pressure elevation that is significant or sustained is treated.

Infection

Infection is the leading cause of death after liver transplantation. Pulmonary and fungal infections are common; susceptibility to infection is increased by the immunosuppressive therapy that is needed to prevent rejection (Yamada, 2003). Therefore, precautions must be taken to prevent health care–associated infections. The nurse uses strict asepsis when manipulating central venous catheters, arterial lines, and urine, bile, and other drainage systems; obtaining specimens; and changing dressings. Meticulous hand hygiene is crucial.

Rejection

Rejection is a primary concern. A transplanted liver is perceived by the immune system as a foreign antigen. This triggers an immune response, leading to the activation of T lymphocytes that attack and destroy the transplanted liver. Immunosuppressive agents are used as long-term therapy to prevent this response and rejection of the transplanted liver. These agents inhibit the activation of immunocompetent T lymphocytes to prevent the production of effector T cells.

Although the 1- and 5-year survival rates have increased dramatically with the use of new immunosuppressive therapies, these advances are not without major side effects. A major side effect of cyclosporine, which is widely used in transplantation, is nephrotoxicity; this problem seems to be dose-related, and renal dysfunction can be reversed if the dose of cyclosporine is appropriately decreased or if its use is not initiated immediately. Cyclosporine-related side effects have caused many centers to use tacrolimus as first-line therapy because of its efficacy and lower side-effect profile.

Corticosteroids, azathioprine, mycophenolate mofetil, rapamycin, Thymoglobulin, basiliximab, daclizumab, and OKT3 are also used in various regimens of immunosuppression; they may be used as the initial therapy to prevent rejection or used later to treat rejection. Liver biopsy and ultrasound may be required to evaluate suspected episodes of rejection.

Retransplantation is usually attempted if the transplanted liver fails, but the success rate of retransplantation does not approach that of initial transplantation.

Nursing Management

The patient considering transplantation, together with the family, must make difficult choices about treatment, use of financial resources, and relocation to another area to be closer to the medical center. They must also cope with the patient's long-standing health problems and any social and family problems associated with behaviors that may have caused the patient's liver failure. As a result, considerable emotional stress occurs while the patient and family consider liver transplantation and wait for an available liver. The nurse must be aware of these issues and attuned to the emotional and psychological status of the patient and family. Referral to a psychiatric liaison nurse, psychologist, psychiatrist, or spiritual advisor may help them cope with the stressors associated with ESLD and liver transplantation.

Preoperative Nursing Interventions

If severe, irreversible liver dysfunction has been diagnosed, the patient may be a candidate for transplantation. An extensive diagnostic evaluation is carried out to determine whether the patient is a candidate. The nurse, surgeon, hepatologist, and other health care team members provide the patient and family with full explanations about the procedure, the chances of success, and the risks, including the side effects of long-term immunosuppression. The need for close follow-up and lifelong compliance with the therapeutic regimen, including immunosuppression, is explained to the patient and family.

Once accepted as a candidate, the patient is placed on a waiting list at the transplant center, and patient information is entered into the United Network for Organ Sharing (UNOS) computer system. The UNOS system uses the MELD score to determine organ allocation priorities so that the patient with the highest MELD score will receive the first available organ. Candidates may be matched with appropriate organs as they become available. MELD scores provide the necessary information regarding medical need.

Except in the case of segmental liver transplantation from a living donor (Chart 39-13), a liver becomes available for transplantation only with the death of another person, who is usually healthy except for severe brain injury and brain death. Therefore, the patient and family undergo a stressful waiting period, and the nurse is often their major source of support. The patient must be accessible at all times, in case an appropriate liver becomes available. During this time, liver function may deteriorate further, and the patient may experience other complications from the primary liver disease. Because of the shortage of donor organs, many patients die awaiting transplantation.

Malnutrition, massive ascites, and fluid and electrolyte disturbances are treated before surgery to increase the likelihood of a successful outcome. If the patient's liver dysfunction has a very rapid onset, as in fulminant hepatic failure, there is little time or opportunity for the patient to

CHART 39-13

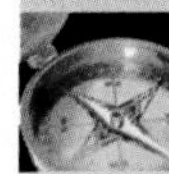

Ethics and Related Issues

What Ethical Principles Apply in Transplantation of a Segment of a Living Donor's Liver?

SITUATION

A 47-year-old patient has developed liver cancer following hepatitis C after 25 years of IV/injection drug use and alcohol abuse. His 45-year-old sister, to whom he is very close, has volunteered to donate part of her liver to her brother. The sister's husband and children are adamantly opposed to her donating a portion of her liver. They believe that the risks are too great for her when the patient's own behaviors were responsible for his health problems and that he is likely to resume his risky behaviors after the transplantation. The sister's husband asks the nurse her opinion about the risks to his wife if she donates part of her liver for segmental liver transplantation.

DILEMMA

There are surgical risks to the healthy sister if she donates part of her liver, and she has responsibilities to her family as a mother and a wife. The brother's own personal lifestyle and risky behaviors are responsible for his liver disease and liver cancer. The brother's previous lifestyle and risky behaviors may continue after transplantation and threaten his survival as well as that of the transplanted liver.

DISCUSSION

1. What ethical principles are involved in this situation?
2. How does the nurse respond when she knows about the risks to the patient's sister and also believes that the patient is likely to revert back to his previous risky behaviors after successful transplantation?

consider and weigh options and their consequences; often this patient is in a coma, and the decision to proceed with transplantation is made by the family.

The nurse coordinator is an integral member of the transplant team and plays an important role in preparing the patient for liver transplantation. The nurse serves as advocate for the patient and family and assumes the important role of liaison between the patient and the other members of the transplant team. The nurse also serves as a resource to other nurses and health care team members involved in evaluating and caring for the patient.

Postoperative Nursing Interventions

The patient is maintained in an environment as free from bacteria, viruses, and fungi as possible, because immunosuppressive medications reduce the body's natural defenses. In the immediate postoperative period, cardiovascular, pulmonary, renal, neurologic, and metabolic functions are monitored continuously. Mean arterial and pulmonary artery pressures are also monitored continuously. Cardiac output, central venous pressure, pulmonary capillary wedge pressure, arterial and mixed venous blood gases, oxygen saturation, oxygen demand and delivery, urine output, heart rate, and blood pressure are used to evaluate the patient's hemodynamic status and intravascular fluid volume. Liver function tests, electrolyte levels, the coagulation profile, chest x-ray, electrocardiogram, and fluid output (including urine, bile from the T-tube, and drainage from Jackson-Pratt tubes) are monitored closely. Because the liver is responsible for the storage of glycogen and the synthesis of protein and clotting factors, these substances need to be monitored and replaced in the immediate postoperative period.

There is a high risk for atelectasis and an altered ventilation–perfusion ratio, caused by insult to the diaphragm during the surgical procedure, prolonged anesthesia, immobility, and postoperative pain. Because of this risk, the patient will have an endotracheal tube in place and will require mechanical ventilation during the initial postoperative period. Suctioning is performed as required, and sterile humidification is provided.

As the vital signs and condition stabilize, efforts are made to assist the patient to recover from the trauma of this complex surgery. After removal of the endotracheal tube, the nurse encourages the patient to use an incentive spirometer to decrease the risk for atelectasis. Once the arterial lines and the urinary catheter are removed, the patient is assisted to get out of bed, to ambulate as tolerated, and to participate in self-care to prevent the complications associated with immobility. Close monitoring for signs and symptoms of liver dysfunction and rejection continue throughout the hospital stay. Plans are made for close follow-up after discharge as well. Teaching is initiated during the preoperative period and continues after surgery.

Promoting Home and Community-Based Care

TEACHING PATIENTS SELF-CARE

Teaching the patient and family about long-term measures to promote health is crucial for the success of transplantation and represents an important role of the nurse. The patient and family must understand why they need to adhere continuously to the therapeutic regimen, with special emphasis on the methods of administration, rationale, and side effects of the prescribed immunosuppressive agents. The nurse provides written as well as verbal instructions about how and when to take the medications. To avoid running out of medication or skipping a dose, the patient must make sure that an adequate supply of medication is available. Instructions are also provided about the signs and symptoms that indicate problems necessitating consultation with the transplant team. The patient with a T-tube in place must be taught how to manage the tube, drainage, and skin care.

CONTINUING CARE

The nurse emphasizes the importance of follow-up blood tests and appointments with the transplant team. Trough blood levels of immunosuppressive agents are obtained, along with other blood tests that assess the function of the liver and kidneys. During the first months, the patient is likely to require blood tests two or three times a week. As the patient's condition stabilizes, blood studies and visits to the transplant team are less frequent. The importance of routine ophthalmologic examinations is emphasized because of the increased incidence of cataracts and glaucoma associated with the long-term corticosteroid therapy used with transplantation. Regular oral hygiene and follow-up dental care, with administration of prophylactic antibiotics before dental examinations and treatments, are recommended because of the immunosuppression.

The nurse reminds the patient that preventing rejection and infection leads to a successful transplantation and increases the chances for survival and living a more normal life than before transplantation. Many patients have lived successful and productive lives after receiving a liver transplant. In fact, pregnancy can be considered 1 year after transplantation. Although successful outcomes have been reported, these pregnancies are considered high risk for both mother and infant (Sherlock & Dooley, 2002).

Liver Abscesses

Two categories of liver abscess have been identified: amebic and pyogenic. Amebic liver abscesses are most commonly caused by *Entamoeba histolytica.* Most amebic liver abscesses occur in the developing countries of the tropics and subtropics because of poor sanitation and hygiene. Pyogenic liver abscesses are much less common, but they are more common in developed countries than the amebic type.

Pathophysiology

Whenever an infection develops anywhere along the biliary or GI tract, infecting organisms may reach the liver through the biliary system, portal venous system, or hepatic arterial or lymphatic system. Most bacteria are destroyed promptly, but occasionally some gain a foothold. The bacterial toxins destroy the neighboring liver cells, and the resulting necrotic tissue serves as a protective wall for the organisms.

Meanwhile, leukocytes migrate into the infected area. The result is an abscess cavity full of a liquid containing living and dead leukocytes, liquefied liver cells, and bacteria. Pyogenic abscesses of this type may be either single or multiple and small. Examples of causes of pyogenic liver abscess include cholangitis (usually related to benign or malignant obstruction of the biliary tree) and abdominal trauma.

Clinical Manifestations

The clinical picture is one of sepsis with few or no localizing signs. Fever with chills and diaphoresis, malaise, anorexia, nausea, vomiting, and weight loss may occur. The patient may complain of dull abdominal pain and tenderness in the right upper quadrant of the abdomen. Hepatomegaly, jaundice, anemia, and pleural effusion may develop. Sepsis and shock may be severe and life-threatening. In the past, the mortality rate was 100% because of the vague clinical symptoms, inadequate diagnostic tools, and inadequate surgical drainage of the abscess. With the aid of ultrasound, CT, MRI, and liver scans, early diagnosis and surgical drainage of abscesses have greatly reduced the mortality rate.

Assessment and Diagnostic Findings

Although blood cultures are obtained, the organism may not be identified. Aspiration of the liver abscess, guided by ultrasound, CT, or MRI, may be performed to assist in diagnosis and to obtain cultures of the organism. Percutaneous drainage of pyogenic abscesses is carried out to evacuate the abscess material and promote healing. A catheter may be left in place for continuous drainage; the patient must be instructed about its management.

Medical Management

Treatment includes IV antibiotic therapy; the specific antibiotic used in treatment depends on the organism identified. Continuous supportive care is indicated because of the serious condition of the patient. Open surgical drainage may be required if antibiotic therapy and percutaneous drainage are ineffective.

Nursing Management

Although the manifestations of liver abscess vary with the type of abscess, most patients appear acutely ill. Others appear to be chronically ill and debilitated. The nursing management depends on the patient's physical status and the medical management that is indicated. For patients who undergo evacuation and drainage of an abscess, monitoring of the drainage and skin care are imperative. Strategies must be implemented to contain the drainage and to protect the patient from other sources of infection. Vital signs are monitored to detect changes in the patient's physical status. Deterioration in vital signs or the onset of new symptoms such as increasing pain, which may indicate rupture or extension of the abscess, is reported promptly. The nurse administers IV antibiotic therapy as prescribed. The white blood cell count and other laboratory test results are monitored closely for changes consistent with worsening infection. The nurse prepares the patient for discharge by providing instruction about symptom management, signs and symptoms that should be reported to the physician, management of drainage, and the importance of taking antibiotics as prescribed.

Critical Thinking Exercises

1 A 28-year-old African woman came to the United States from Nigeria 3 years ago to live with relatives. She is being treated for end-stage liver disease (ESLD) with cirrhosis related to hepatitis B and is undergoing evaluation for liver transplantation. The sequelae of ESLD that she was experiencing included encephalopathy and ascites. What would you anticipate this patient's treatment regimen to include? What medications would be most appropriate

for her? What would you include in your cultural assessment when you develop a preoperative teaching plan for this patient? What alternative therapies might be employed preoperatively? Once the patient receives a liver transplant, what medications would you expect to be prescribed for her in addition to an immunosuppressant regimen?

2 A 42-year-old executive with an accounting firm has just received unexpected notice that he must travel to Peru for a business meeting in 2 days. Is he a candidate for the hepatitis A vaccine before he leaves? What other prophylactic measures are available to him before he leaves for his trip? What guidelines would you provide him in terms of minimizing his risk for acquiring the hepatitis A virus? What, if anything, is available on his return to prevent him from developing hepatitis A? What signs and symptoms are important for him to watch for and to report to his health care provider? What modifications, if any, should be implemented for his close household contacts?

3 ebp A 64-year-old man is admitted to the hospital with end-stage liver disease (ESLD), ascites, and impending hepatic encephalopathy. Dietary modifications and lactulose (Cephulac) are prescribed to minimize hepatic encephalopathy. What is the evidence base for use of dietary measures and lactulose in reducing or reversing hepatic encephalopathy? What is the strength of that evidence? What are the nursing implications associated with prescribed dietary modifications, lactulose, and other measures to reduce the severity and progression of hepatic encephalopathy?

4 A 55-year-old man is admitted to the hospital with a diagnosis of bleeding esophageal varices. Describe the monitoring you would initiate. What possible management strategies to prevent bleeding and to treat active bleeding of the esophageal varices would you anticipate? What are the nursing implications for each of these strategies? How would medical management and nursing care be modified if the patient had chronic obstructive pulmonary disease in addition to esophageal varices? How would you explain treatment strategies to the patient and his family if one or more of them had hearing impairment?

REFERENCES AND SELECTED READINGS

BOOKS

Abbruzzese, J. L., Evans, D. B., Willett, C. G., et al. (Eds.). (2004). *Gastrointestinal oncology*. Oxford: Oxford University Press.

American Cancer Society. (2005). *Cancer facts and figures*. Atlanta: Author.

Aspinal, R. J. & Taylor-Robinson, S. D. (2002). *Mosby's color atlas and text of gastroenterology and liver disease*. New York: Mosby.

Bickley, L. S. & Szilagyi, P. G. (2003). *Bates' guide to physical examination and history taking*. (8th ed.). Philadelphia: Lippincott Williams & Wilkins.

Dudek, S. G. (2006). *Nutrition essentials for nursing practice* (5th ed.). Philadelphia: Lippincott Williams & Wilkins.

Edmundowicz, S. A. (2002). *20 common problems in gastroenterology*. New York: McGraw-Hill.

Feldman, M., Friedman, L. S. & Sleisenger, M. H. (2002). *Sleisenger and Fordtran's gastrointestinal and liver disease: Pathophysiology, diagnosis and management*. Philadelphia: Saunders.

Fishman, M. C., Hoffman, A. R., Klauser, R. D., et al. (2004). *Medicine* (5th ed.). Philadelphia: Lippincott Williams & Wilkins.

Friedman, S. L., McQuaid, K. R. & Grendell, J. H. (Eds.). (2003). *Current diagnosis and treatment in gastroenterology* (2nd ed.). New York: Lange Medical Books/McGraw-Hill.

Greene, F. L., Page, D. L., Fleming, I. D., et al. (Eds.). (2002). *AJCC cancer staging manual* (6th ed.). New York: Springer-Verlag.

Kaplowitz, N. (Ed.). (2003). *Drug-induced liver disease*. New York: Marcel Dekker.

Kelly, K. A., Sarr, M. G. & Hinder, R. A. (Eds.). (2004). *Mayo clinic gastrointestinal surgery*. Philadelphia: Saunders.

Kelsen, D. P. (Ed.). (2002). *Gastrointestinal oncology: Principles and practice*. Philadelphia: Lippincott Williams & Wilkins.

MacSween, R. N. M., Burt, A. D., Portmann, B. C., et al. (Eds.). (2002). *Pathology of the liver*. London: Churchill-Livingstone.

Manzarbeitia, C. (Ed.). (2002). *Practical manual of abdominal organ transplantation*. New York: Kluwer Academic.

Molmenti, E. P. & Kintmalm, G. B. (2002). *Atlas of liver transplantation*. Philadelphia: Saunders.

National Digestive Diseases Information Clearinghouse (NDDIC). (2004). *Cirrhosis of the liver*. NIH Publication No. 04-1134. Bethesda, MD: National Institutes of Health.

Odze, R. D., Goldblum, J. R. & Crawford, J. M. (2004). *Surgical pathology of the gastrointestinal tract: Liver, biliary tract and pancreas*. Philadelphia: Saunders.

Porth, C. M. (2005). *Pathophysiology: Concepts of altered health states* (7th ed.). Philadelphia: Lippincott Williams & Wilkins.

Reddy, K. J. & Long, W. B. (Eds.). (2004). *Hepatobiliary tract and pancreas*. Edinburgh: Mosby.

Rogiers, X. (Ed.). (2002). *Split liver transplantation: Theoretical and practical aspects*. Berlin: Springer.

Rustgi, A. S. & Crawford, J. (Eds.). (2003). *Gastrointestinal cancers: A companion to Sleisenger and Fordtran's gastrointestinal disease*. Philadelphia: Saunders.

Sherlock, S. & Dooley, J. (2002). *Diseases of the liver and biliary system*. Oxford, UK: Blackwell Science.

Wilmore, D. W., Cheung, L. Y. & Harken, A. H. (2004). *ACS surgery: Principles and practice 2004*. New York: Web MD Professional Publication.

Yamada, T. (Ed.). (2003). *Textbook of gastroenterology* (4th ed.). Philadelphia: Lippincott Williams & Wilkins.

Zakim, D. & Boyer, T. D. (2003). *Hepatology: A textbook of liver disease* (4th ed.). Philadelphia: Saunders.

JOURNALS

**Asterisks indicate nursing research articles.*

General

Angulo, P. (2002). Nonalcoholic fatty liver disease. *New England Journal of Medicine, 346*(16), 1221–1231.

Biancofiore, G., Bindi, L. M., Urbani, L., et al. (2003). Combined twice daily plasma exchange and continuous veno-veno hemodiafiltration for bridging severe acute liver failure. *Transplantation Proceedings, 35*(8), 3011–3014.

Fingerhood, M. (2000). Substance abuse in older people. *Journal of the American Geriatrics Society, 48*(8), 86–99.

Jonsen, P. L. (2002). Liver disease in the elderly. *Best Practice and Research in Clinical Gastroenterology, 16*(1), 149–158.

Kaplan, M. M. & Gershwin, M. E. (2005). Primary biliary cirrhosis. *New England Journal of Medicine, 353*(12), 1261–1273.

Kjaergard, L. L., Liu, J., Als-Nielsen, B., et al. (2003). Artificial and bioartificial support systems for acute and acute-on-chronic liver failure: A systematic review. *Journal of the American Medical Association, 289*(2), 217–222.

Lee, W. M. (2003). Medical progress: Drug-induced hepatotoxicity. *New England Journal of Medicine, 349*(5), 474–485.

Maddrey, W. C. (2000). Alcohol-induced liver disease. *Clinics in Liver Disease, 4*(1), 115–131.

Marrero, J., Martinez, F. J. & Hyzy, R. (2003). Advances in critical care hepatology. *American Journal of Respiratory and Critical Care Medicine, 168*(12), 1421–1426.

Menon, K. V., Shah, V. & Kamath, P. S. (2004). Current concepts: The Budd-Chiari syndrome. *New England Journal of Medicine, 350*(6), 578–585.

Rosado, B. & Kamath, P. S. (2003). Transjugular intrahepatic portosystemic shunts: An update. *Liver Transplantation, 9*(3), 207–217.

Rosemurgy, A. S., Zervos, E. E., Clark, W. C., et al. (2004). TIPS versus peritoneovenous shunt in the treatment of medically intractable ascites: A prospective randomized trial. *Annals of Surgery, 239*(6), 883–891.

Russo, M. W., Asheesh, S., Jacobsen, I. M., et al. (2003). Transjugular intrahepatic portosystemic shunt for refractory ascites: An analysis of the literature on efficacy, morbidity and mortality. *American Journal of Gastroenterology, 98*(11), 2521–2527.

Schiff, E. R. (2000). Update in hepatology. *Annals of Internal Medicine, 132*(6), 460–466.

Van de Kerkhove, M. P., Hoekstra, R., Chamuleau, R. A., et al. (2004). Clinical application of bioartificial liver support systems. *Annals of Surgery, 240*(2), 216–230.

Wiklund, R. A. (2004). Preoperative preparation of patients with advanced liver disease. *Critical Care Medicine, 32*(4 Suppl), S106–S115.

Cirrhosis and Esophageal Varices

Anonymous. (2000). Medical consequences of alcohol abuse. *Alcohol Research and Health: The Journal of the National Institute on Alcohol Abuse and Alcoholism, 24*(1), 27–31.

Benjaminov, F. S., Prentice, M., Sniderman, K. W., et al. (2003). Portopulmonary hypertension in decompensated cirrhosis with refractory ascites. *Gut, 52*(9), 1355–1362.

Gines, P., Cardenas, A., Arroyo, V., et al. (2004). Current concepts: Management of cirrhosis and ascites. *New England Journal of Medicine, 350*(16), 1646–1654.

Orloff, M. J., Orloff, M. S., Girard, B., et al. (2002). Bleeding esophageal varices from extrahepatic portal hypertension: 40 Year experience with portal systemic shunts. *Journal of American College of Surgeons, 194*(6), 717–728.

Prince, M. I., Chetwynd, A., Craig, W. L., et al. (2004). Asymptomatic primary biliary cirrhosis: Clinical features, prognosis and symptom progression in a large population based cohort. *Gut, 53*(6), 865–870.

Sorbi, D., Gostout, C. J., Peura, D., et al. (2003). An assessment of the management of acute bleeding varices: A multicenter prospective member-based study. *American Journal of Gastroenterology, 98*(11), 2424–2434.

Tripathi, D., Lui, H. F., Helmy, A., et al. (2004). Randomized controlled trial of long-term portographic follow-up versus variceal band ligation following transjugular portosystemic stent shunt for preventing variceal rebleeding. *Gut, 53*(3), 431–437.

Zaman, A., Hopke, R. J., Flora, K., et al. (2004). Changing compliance to the American College of Gastroenterology guidelines for the management of variceal hemorrhage: A regional survey. *American Journal of Gastroenterology, 99*(4), 645–659.

Hepatitis

Benvegnu, L., Gios, M., Boccato, S., et al. (2004). Natural history of compensated viral cirrhosis: A prospective study on the incidence and hierarchy of major complications. *Gut, 53*(5), 744–749.

Bialek, S. R., Thoroughman, D. A., Hu, D., et al. (2004). Hepatitis A incidence and hepatitis A vaccination among American Indians and Alaska natives 1990–2001. *American Journal of Public Health, 94*(6), 996–1001.

Centers for Disease Control and Prevention (CDC). (2002). Sexually transmitted diseases treatment guidelines 2002. *MMWR: Morbidity and Mortality Weekly Report, 51*(RR-6), 1–84.

Craig, A. S. & Schaffner, W. (2004). Prevention of hepatitis A with the hepatitis A vaccine. *New England Journal of Medicine, 350*(5), 476–481.

Davis, G. L., Wong, J. B., McHutchison, J. J., et al. (2003). Early virologic response to therapy with peginterferon alpha 2-b plus ribavirin with chronic hepatitis C. *Hepatology, 38*(3), 645–652.

Flamm S. K. (2003). Chronic hepatitis C virus infection. *Journal of American Medical Association, 289*(18), 2413–2417.

Ganem, D. & Prince, A. M. (2004). Mechanisms of disease: Hepatitis B virus infection—Natural history and clinical consequences. *New England Journal of Medicine, 350*(11), 1118–1129.

*Glacken, M., Coates, V., Kernohan, G., et al. (2003). The experience of fatigue for people living with hepatitis C. *Journal of Clinical Nursing, 12*(2), 244–252.

Goldrick, B. A. (2004). Hepatitis A. *American Journal of Nursing, 104*(3), 27–28.

Harkness, G. A. (2003). Hepatitis C: The "silent stalker." *American Journal of Nursing, 103*(9), 24–25.

Huang, M. A. & Lok, A. S. (2003). Natural history of hepatitis B and outcomes after liver transplantation. *Clinics in Liver Disease, 7*(3), 521–536.

Hui, A. Y., Chan, H. L., Leung, N. W., et al. (2002). Survival and prognostic indicators in patients with hepatitis B virus-related cirrhosis after onset of hepatic decompensation. *Journal of Clinical Gastroenterology, 34*(5), 569–572.

Jarrett, M. & Cox, P. (2004). Hepatitis C virus. *Nursing Clinics of North America, 39*(1), 219–229.

Koff, R. S. (2001). Hepatitis vaccines. *Infectious Disease Clinics of North America, 15*(1), 83–93.

Lok, A. S., Lai, C. L., Leung, N., et al. (2003). Long-term safety of lamivudine therapy in patients with chronic hepatitis B. *Gastroenterology, 125*(6), 1714–1722.

Lok, A. S. & McMahon, B. J. (2004). Practice Guidelines Committee, American Association of Liver Diseases (AASLD): Chronic hepatitis B—Update of recommendations. *Hepatology, 39*(3), 857–861.

Manns, M. P. (2004). Adherence to combination therapy: Influence on sustained virologic response and economic impact. *Gastroenterology Clinics of North America, 33*(1 Suppl), S11–S24.

Muir, A. J., Bornstein, J. D., Killenberg, P. G., et al. (2004). Peginterferon alfa-2b and ribavirin for the treatment of chronic hepatitis C in blacks and non-Hispanic whites. *New England Journal of Medicine, 350*(22), 2265–2271.

National Institutes of Health. (2002). Consensus statement on management of hepatitis C. *NIH Consensus and State-of-the-Science Statements, 19*(3), 1–46.

Ostapowicz, G., Fontana, R. J., Schiodt, F. V., et al. (2002). Results of a prospective study of acute liver failure at 17 tertiary care centers in the United States. *Annals of Internal Medicine, 137*(12), 947–954.

Shehab, T. M., Orrego, M., Chunduri, R., et al. (2003). Identification and management of hepatitis C patients in primary care clinics. *American Journal of Gastroenterology, 98*(3), 639–644.

Sjögren, M. (2003). Immunization and the decline of viral hepatitis as a cause of acute liver failure. *Hepatology, 38*(3), 554–556.

Wesley, A., Samandari, T., & Bell, B. P. (2005). Incidence of hepatitis A in the United States in the era of vaccination. *Journal of American Medical Association, 294*(2), 194–201.

Wiegand, J., Jackel, E., Cornberg, M., et al. (2004). Long-term follow up after successful interferon therapy of acute hepatitis C. *Hepatology, 40*(1), 98–107.

Yashida, H., Arakawa, Y., Sata, M., et al. (2002). Interferon therapy prolonged life expectancy among chronic hepatitis C patients. *Gastroenterology, 123*(2), 483–491.

Liver Cancer

Barber, F. D. & Febugais-Nazario, L. E. (2003). What's old is new again: Patients receiving hepatic arterial infusion chemotherapy. *Clinical Journal of Oncology Nursing, 7*(6), 647–652.

Barber, F. D., Mavligit, G. & Kurzrock, R. (2004). Hepatic arterial infusion chemotherapy for metastatic colorectal cancer: A concise review. *Cancer Treatment Reviews, 30*(5), 425–436.

Bruix, J. & Llovet, J. M. (2002). Prognostic prediction and treatment strategy in hepatocellular carcinoma. *Hepatology, 35*(3), 519–524.

Camma, C., Schepis, F., Orlando, A., et al. (2002). Transarterial chemoembolization for unresectable hepatocellular carcinoma: Meta-analysis of randomized controlled trials. *Radiology, 224*(1), 47–54.

Fernandez, F. G., Drebin, J. A., Lineham, D. C., et al. (2004). Five-year survival after resection of hepatic metastases from colorectal cancer in patients screened by positron emission tomography. *Annals of Surgery, 240*(3), 438–447.

Hayashi, P. H., Trotter, J. F., Kugelmas, M., et al. (2004). Impact of pretransplant diagnosis of hepatocellular carcinoma on cadaveric liver allocation in the era of MELD. *Liver Transplantation, 10*(1), 42–48.

Huang, Y., Chen, C. & Chang, T. (2004). The role of transcatheter arterial embolization in patients with resectable hepatocellular carcinoma: A nationwide multicenter study. *Liver International, 24*(5), 419–424.

Jang, M. K., Lee, H.C., Kim, I. S. et al. (2004). Role of additional angiography and chemoembolization in patients with hepatocellular carcinoma. *Journal of Gastroenterology & Hepatology, 19*(9), 1074–1080.

Nowak, A. K., Chow, P. K. & Findlay, M. (2004). Systemic therapy for advanced hepatocellular carcinoma: A review. *European Journal of Cancer, 40*(10), 1474–1484.

Oshowo, A., Gilliams, A., Harrison, E., et al. (2003). Comparison of resection and radiofrequency ablation for treatment of solitary colorectal liver metastases. *British Journal of Surgery, 90*(10), 1240–1243.

Sharma, P., Balan, V., Hernandez, J. L., et al. (2004). Liver transplantation for hepatocellular carcinoma: The MELD impact. *Liver Transplantation, 10*(1), 36–41.

Liver Transplantation

Biancofiore, G., Bindi, L. M., Urbani, L., et al. (2003). Combined twice-daily plasma exchange and continuous veno-venous hemodiafiltration for bridging severe acute liver failure. *Transplantation Proceedings, 35*(8), 3011–3014.

Brown, J., Sorrell, J.H., McClaren, J. et al. (2006). Waiting for a liver transplant. *Qualitative Health Research, 16*(1), 199–136.

Chouker, A., Martignoni, A., Dugas, M., et al. (2004). Estimation of liver size for liver transplantation: The impact of age and gender. *Liver Transplantation, 10*(5), 678–685.

Cowling, T., Jennings, L. W., Goldstein, R. M., et al. (2004). Liver transplantation and health-related quality of life: Scoring differences between men and women. *Liver Transplantation, 10*(1), 88–96.

Eghtesad, B., Jain, A. B., & Fung, J. J. (2003). Living donor liver transplantation: Ethics and safety. *Transplantation Proceedings, 35*(1), 51–52.

Hata, S., Sugawara, Y., Kishi, Y., et al. (2004). Volume regeneration after right lobe liver donation. *Liver Transplantation, 10*(1), 65–70.

Humar, A., Khwaja, K., Glessing, B., et al. (2004). Regionwide sharing for status 1 liver patients: Beneficial impact on waiting time and pre- and posttransplant survival. *Liver Transplantation, 10*(5), 661–665.

Montalbano, M., Neff, G. W., Yamashiki, N., et al. (2004). A retrospective review of liver transplant patients treated with sirolimus from a single center: An analysis of sirolimus-related complications. *Transplantation, 78*(2), 264–268.

Orug, T., Soonawalla, Z. F., Tekin, K., et al. (2004). Role of surgical portosystemic shunts in the era of interventional radiology and liver transplantation. *British Journal of Surgery, 91*(6), 769–773.

Surman, O. S. (2002). The ethics of partial-liver donation. *New England Journal of Medicine, 346*(14), 1038.

Trotter, J. F., Wachs, M., Everson, G. T., et al. (2002). Adult-to-adult transplantation of the right hepatic lobe from a living donor. *New England Journal of Medicine, 346*(14), 1074–1082.

Voight, M. D., Zimmerman, B., Katz, D. A., et al. (2004). New national liver transplant allocation policy: Is the regional review board process fair? *Liver Transplantation, 10*(5), 666–674.

Walter, W. M., Dammann, G., Papachristou, C., et al. (2003). Quality of life of living donors before and after living donor liver transplantation. *Transplantation Proceedings, 35*(8), 2961–2963.

RESOURCES

Al-Anon Family Group Headquarters, 1600 Corporate Landing Parkway, Virginia Beach, VA 23454-5617; for meetings, 800-344-2666 (8 AM to 6 PM, Monday through Friday); for information, 800-356-9996 (7 days a week, 24 hours); http://www.al-anon.alateen.org. Accessed May 15, 2006.

Alcoholics Anonymous World Services, 475 Riverside Drive, 11th Floor, New York, NY 10115; 212-870-3400; aa.org. Accessed May 15, 2006.

American Association for the Study of Liver Diseases, 1729 King Street, Suite 200, Alexandria, VA, 22314; 703-299-9766; http://www.aasld.org. Accessed May 15, 2006.

American College of Gastroenterology, Post Office Box 3099, Alexandria, VA, 22302; 703-820-7400; http://www.acg.gi.org. Accessed May 15, 2006.

American Liver Foundation, 75 Maiden Lane, Suite 603, New York, NY 10038; 800-465-4837; http://www.liverfoundation.org. Accessed May 15, 2006.

Hepatitis Foundation International, 504 Blick Drive, Silver Spring, MD 20904-2901; 800-891-0707; http://www.hepfi.org. Accessed May 15, 2006.

National Council on Alcoholism and Drug Dependence, 20 Exchange Place, Suite 2902, New York, NY 10005; 800-NCA-CALL or 212-269-7797; http://www.ncadd.org. Accessed May 15, 2006.

National Digestive Diseases Information Clearing House, 2 Information Way, Bethesda, MD 20892-3570; 301-654-3810; http://www.niddk.nih.gov. Accessed May 15, 2006.

National Institute on Alcohol Abuse and Alcoholism, 5635 Fishers Lane, MSC 9304, Bethesda, MD 20892-9304; 301-496-1993; http://www.niaaa.nih.gov. Accessed May 15, 2006.

United Network for Organ Sharing, Post Office Box 2484, Richmond, VA, 23218; 804-782-4800, 804-782-4876, or 888-894-6361; http://www.unos.org. Accessed May 15, 2006.

CHAPTER 40

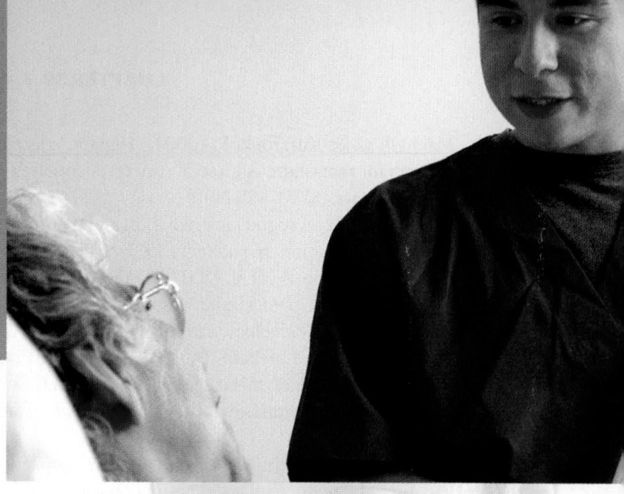

Assessment and Management of Patients With Biliary Disorders

Learning Objectives

On completion of this chapter, the learner will be able to:

1. Compare approaches to management of cholelithiasis.
2. Use the nursing process as a framework for care of patients with cholelithiasis and those undergoing laparoscopic or open cholecystectomy.
3. Differentiate between acute and chronic pancreatitis.
4. Use the nursing process as a framework for care of patients with acute pancreatitis.
5. Describe the nutritional and metabolic effects of surgical treatment of tumors of the pancreas.

Disorders of the biliary tract and pancreas are common and include gallbladder stones and pancreatic dysfunction. An understanding of the structure and function of the biliary tract and pancreas is essential, along with an understanding of how biliary tract disorders are closely linked with liver disease. Patients with acute or chronic biliary tract or pancreatic disease require care from nurses knowledgeable about the diagnostic procedures and interventions that are used in the management of gallbladder and pancreatic disorders.

Anatomic and Physiologic Overview

The Gallbladder

The gallbladder, a pear-shaped, hollow, saclike organ, 7.5 to 10 cm (3 to 4 in) long, lies in a shallow depression on the inferior surface of the liver, to which it is attached by loose connective tissue. The capacity of the gallbladder is 30 to 50 mL of bile. Its wall is composed largely of smooth muscle. The gallbladder is connected to the common bile duct by the cystic duct (Fig. 40-1).

The gallbladder functions as a storage depot for bile. Between meals, when the sphincter of Oddi is closed, bile produced by the hepatocytes enters the gallbladder. During storage, a large portion of the water in bile is absorbed through the walls of the gallbladder, so that gallbladder bile is five to ten times more concentrated than that originally secreted by the liver. When food enters the duodenum, the gallbladder contracts and the sphincter of Oddi (located at the junction of the common bile duct with the duodenum) relaxes. Relaxation of the sphincter of Oddi allows the bile to enter the intestine. This response is mediated by secretion of the hormone **cholecystokinin-pancreozymin** (**CCK-PZ**) from the intestinal wall. Bile is composed of water and electrolytes (sodium, potassium, calcium, chloride, and bicarbonate) along with significant amounts of lecithin, fatty acids, cholesterol, bilirubin, and bile salts. The bile salts, together with cholesterol, assist in emulsification of fats in the distal ileum. They are then reabsorbed into the portal blood for return to the liver, after which they are once again excreted into the bile. This pathway from hepatocytes to bile to intestine and back to the hepatocytes is called the enterohepatic circulation. Because of the enterohepatic circulation, only a small fraction of the bile salts that enter the intestine are excreted in the feces. This decreases the need for active synthesis of bile salts by the liver cells.

Approximately half of the bilirubin, a pigment derived from the breakdown of red blood cells, is converted by the intestinal flora into urobilinogen, a highly soluble substance. Urobilinogen is either excreted in the feces or returned to the portal circulation, where it is re-excreted into the bile. About 5% is normally absorbed into the general circulation and then excreted by the kidneys (Porth, 2005).

If the flow of bile is impeded (eg, by gallstones in the bile ducts), bilirubin does not enter the intestine. As a result, blood levels of bilirubin increase. This causes increased renal excretion of urobilinogen, which results from conversion of bilirubin in the small intestine, and decreased excretion in the stool. These changes produce many of the signs and symptoms seen in gallbladder disorders.

The Pancreas

The pancreas, located in the upper abdomen, has **endocrine** as well as **exocrine** functions (see Fig. 40-1). The exocrine

Glossary

amylase: pancreatic enzyme; aids in the digestion of carbohydrates
cholecystitis: inflammation of the gallbladder
cholecystokinin-pancreozymin (CCK-PZ): hormone; major stimulus for digestive enzyme secretion; stimulates contraction of the gallbladder
cholecystectomy: removal of the gallbladder
cholecystojejunostomy: anastomosis of the jejunum to the gallbladder to divert bile flow
cholecystostomy: opening and drainage of the gallbladder
choledocholithiasis: stones in the common duct
choledochostomy: opening into the common duct
cholelithiasis: calculi in the gallbladder
dissolution therapy: use of medications to break up/dissolve gallstones
endocrine: secreting internally; hormonal secretion of a ductless gland
endoscopic retrograde cholangiopancreatography (ERCP): an endoscopic procedure using fiberoptic technology to visualize the biliary system
enterostomal therapist: nurse specially educated in appropriate skin, wound, ostomy, and continence care; often referred to as wound-care specialist or wound-ostomy-continence nurse (WOCN)
exocrine: secreting externally; hormonal secretion from excretory ducts
laparoscopic cholecystectomy: removal of gallbladder through endoscopic procedure
lipase: pancreatic enzyme; aids in the digestion of fats
lithotripsy: disintegration of gallstones by shock waves
pancreaticojejunostomy: joining of the pancreatic duct to the jejunum by side-to-side anastomosis; allows drainage of the pancreatic secretions into the jejunum
pancreatitis: inflammation of the pancreas; may be acute or chronic
secretin: hormone responsible for stimulating secretion of pancreatic juice; also used as an aid in diagnosing pancreatic exocrine disease and in obtaining desquamated pancreatic cells for cytologic examination
steatorrhea: frothy, foul-smelling stools with a high fat content; results from impaired digestion of proteins and fats due to a lack of pancreatic juice in the intestine
trypsin: pancreatic enzyme; aids in digestion of proteins
Zollinger-Ellison tumor: hypersecretion of gastric acid that produces peptic ulcers as a result of a non-beta cell tumor of the pancreatic islets

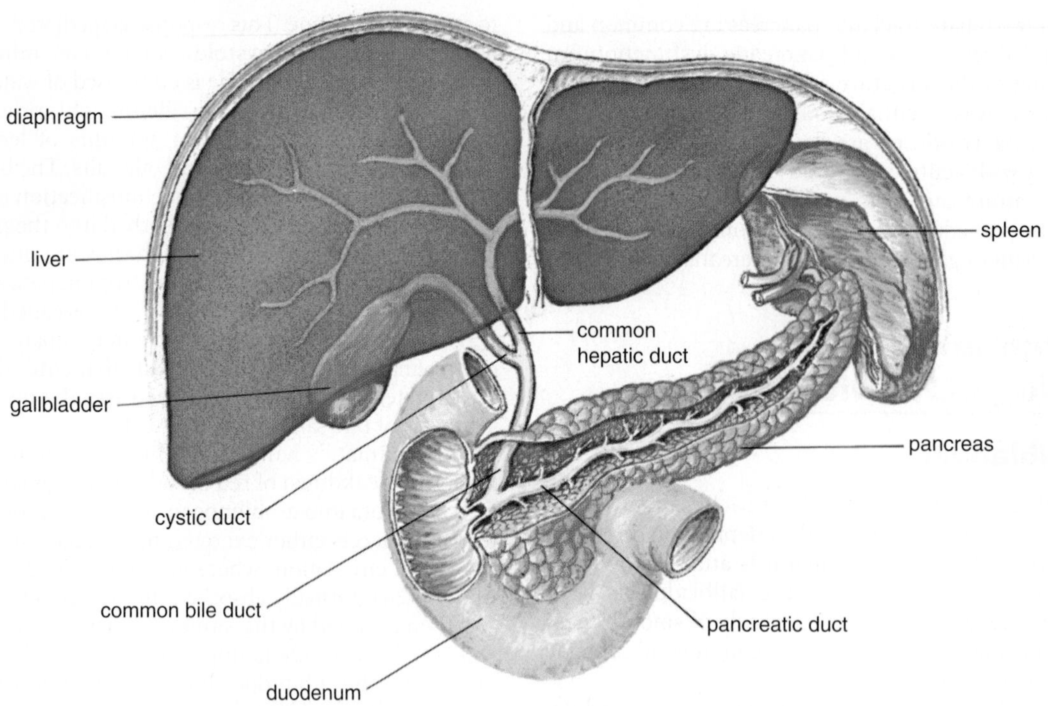

FIGURE 40-1. The liver, biliary system, and pancreas.

functions include secretion of pancreatic enzymes into the gastrointestinal tract through the pancreatic duct. The endocrine functions include secretion of insulin, glucagon, and somatostatin directly into the bloodstream.

The Exocrine Pancreas

The secretions of the exocrine portion of the pancreas are collected in the pancreatic duct, which joins the common bile duct and enters the duodenum at the ampulla of Vater. Surrounding the ampulla is the sphincter of Oddi, which partially controls the rate at which secretions from the pancreas and the gallbladder enter the duodenum.

The secretions of the exocrine pancreas are digestive enzymes high in protein content and an electrolyte-rich fluid. The secretions, which are very alkaline because of their high concentration of sodium bicarbonate, are capable of neutralizing the highly acid gastric juice that enters the duodenum. The enzyme secretions include **amylase**, which aids in the digestion of carbohydrates; **trypsin**, which aids in the digestion of proteins; and **lipase**, which aids in the digestion of fats. Other enzymes that promote the breakdown of more complex foodstuffs are also secreted.

Hormones originating in the gastrointestinal tract stimulate the secretion of these exocrine pancreatic juices. The hormone **secretin** is the major stimulus for increased bicarbonate secretion from the pancreas, and the major stimulus for digestive enzyme secretion is the hormone CCK-PZ. The vagus nerve also influences exocrine pancreatic secretion.

The Endocrine Pancreas

The islets of Langerhans, the endocrine part of the pancreas, are collections of cells embedded in the pancreatic tissue. They are composed of alpha, beta, and delta cells. The hormone produced by the beta cells is called insulin; the alpha cells secrete glucagon and the delta cells secrete somatostatin.

INSULIN

A major action of insulin is to lower blood glucose by permitting entry of glucose into the cells of the liver, muscle, and other tissues, where it is either stored as glycogen or used for energy. Insulin also promotes the storage of fat in adipose tissue and the synthesis of proteins in various body tissues. In the absence of insulin, glucose cannot enter the cells and is excreted in the urine. This condition, called diabetes mellitus, can be diagnosed by high levels of glucose in the blood. In diabetes mellitus, stored fats and protein are used for energy instead of glucose, causing loss of body mass. (Diabetes mellitus is discussed in detail in Chapter 41.) The level of glucose in the blood normally regulates the rate of insulin secretion from the pancreas.

GLUCAGON

The effect of glucagon (opposite to that of insulin) is chiefly to raise the blood glucose by converting glycogen to glucose in the liver. Glucagon is secreted by the pancreas in response to a decrease in the level of blood glucose.

SOMATOSTATIN

Somatostatin exerts a hypoglycemic effect by interfering with release of growth hormone from the pituitary and glucagon from the pancreas, both of which tend to raise blood glucose levels.

Endocrine Control of Carbohydrate Metabolism

Glucose required for energy is derived by metabolism of ingested carbohydrates and also from proteins by the process of gluconeogenesis. Glucose can be stored temporarily in the liver, muscles, and other tissues in the form of glycogen. The endocrine system controls the level of blood glucose by regulating the rate at which glucose is synthesized, stored, and moved to and from the bloodstream. Through the action of hormones, blood glucose is normally maintained at about 100 mg/dL (5.5 mmol/L). Insulin is the primary hormone that lowers the blood glucose level. Hormones that raise the blood glucose level are glucagon, epinephrine, adrenocorticosteroids, growth hormone, and thyroid hormone.

The endocrine and exocrine functions of the pancreas are interrelated. The major exocrine function is to facilitate digestion through secretion of enzymes into the proximal duodenum. Secretin and CCK-PZ are hormones from the gastrointestinal tract that aid in the digestion of food substances by controlling the secretions of the pancreas. Neural factors also influence pancreatic enzyme secretion. Considerable dysfunction of the pancreas must occur before enzyme secretion decreases and protein and fat digestion becomes impaired. Pancreatic enzyme secretion is normally 1500 to 2500 mL/day.

Gerontologic Considerations

There is little change in the size of the pancreas with age. There is, however, an increase in fibrous material and some fatty deposition in the normal pancreas in people older than 70 years of age. Some localized arteriosclerotic changes occur with age. There is also a decreased rate of pancreatic secretion (decreased lipase, amylase, and trypsin) and decreased bicarbonate output in older patients. Some impairment of normal fat absorption occurs with increasing age, possibly because of delayed gastric emptying and pancreatic insufficiency. Decreased calcium absorption may also occur. These changes require care in interpreting diagnostic test results in the normal elderly person and in providing dietary counseling.

Disorders of the Gallbladder

Several disorders affect the biliary system and interfere with normal drainage of bile into the duodenum. These disorders include inflammation of the biliary system and carcinoma that obstructs the biliary tree. Gallbladder disease with gallstones is the most common disorder of the biliary system. Although not all occurrences of gallbladder inflammation (**cholecystitis**) are related to gallstones (**cholelithiasis**), more than 90% of patients with acute cholecystitis have gallstones. However, most of the 15 million Americans with gallstones have no pain and are unaware of the presence of stones. For a guide to the terminology associated with biliary disorders and procedures, see Chart 40-1.

CHART 40-1

Biliary Terms

Cholecystitis: inflammation of the gallbladder
Cholelithiasis: the presence of calculi in the gallbladder
Cholecystectomy: removal of the gallbladder
Cholecystostomy: opening and drainage of the gallbladder
Choledochotomy: opening into the common duct
Choledocholithiasis: stones in the common duct
Choledocholithotomy: incision of common bile duct for removal of stones
Choledochoduodenostomy: anastomosis of common duct to duodenum
Choledochojejunostomy: anastomosis of common duct to jejunum
Lithotripsy: disintegration of gallstones by shock waves
Laparoscopic cholecystectomy: removal of gallbladder through endoscopic procedure
Laser cholecystectomy: removal of gallbladder using laser rather than scalpel and traditional surgical instruments

Cholecystitis

Acute inflammation (cholecystitis) of the gallbladder causes pain, tenderness, and rigidity of the upper right abdomen that may radiate to the midsternal area or right shoulder and is associated with nausea, vomiting, and the usual signs of an acute inflammation. An empyema of the gallbladder develops if the gallbladder becomes filled with purulent fluid (pus).

Calculous cholecystitis is the cause of more than 90% of cases of acute cholecystitis (Cuschieri, Steele & Moossa, 2002). In calculous cholecystitis, a gallbladder stone obstructs bile outflow. Bile remaining in the gallbladder initiates a chemical reaction; autolysis and edema occur; and the blood vessels in the gallbladder are compressed, compromising its vascular supply. Gangrene of the gallbladder with perforation may result. Bacteria play a minor role in acute cholecystitis; however, secondary infection of bile with *Escherichia coli* (60%), *Klebsiella* species (22%), or *Streptococcus* (18%) is identified with cultures obtained during surgery in a small percentage of surgically treated patients (Cuschieri et al., 2002).

Acalculous cholecystitis describes acute gallbladder inflammation in the absence of obstruction by gallstones. Acalculous cholecystitis occurs after major surgical procedures, severe trauma, or burns. Other factors associated with this type of cholecystitis include torsion, cystic duct obstruction, primary bacterial infections of the gallbladder, and multiple blood transfusions. It is speculated that acalculous cholecystitis is caused by alterations in fluids and electrolytes and alterations in regional blood flow in the visceral circulation. Bile stasis (lack of gallbladder contraction) and increased viscosity of the bile are also thought to play a role. The occurrence of acalculous cholecystitis with major surgical procedures or trauma makes its diagnosis difficult.

Cholelithiasis

Calculi, or gallstones, usually form in the gallbladder from the solid constituents of bile; they vary greatly in size, shape, and composition (Fig. 40-2). They are uncommon

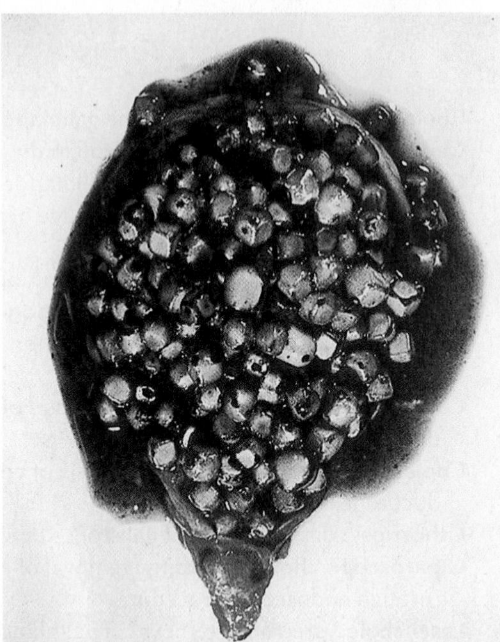
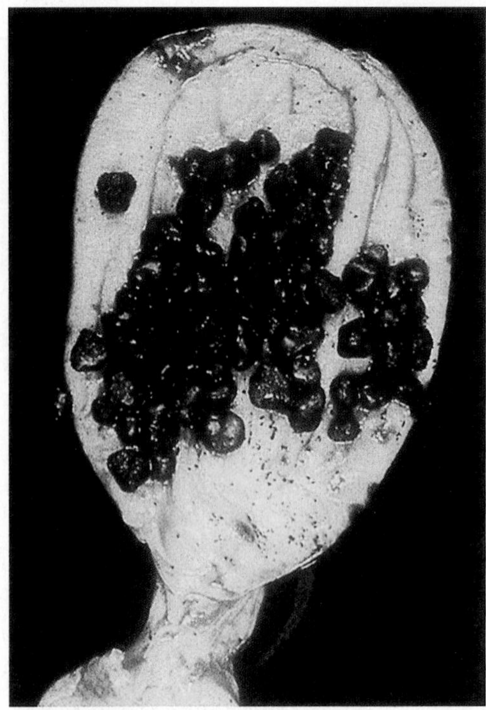

FIGURE 40-2. Examples of cholesterol gallstones (*left*) made up of a coalescence of multiple small stones and pigment gallstones (*right*) composed of calcium bilirubinate. From Rubin, E. & Farber, J. L. (2005). *Pathology* (4th ed.). Philadelphia: Lippincott Williams & Wilkins.

in children and young adults but become increasingly prevalent after 40 years of age, especially in women. The incidence of cholelithiasis increases after the age of 40 years, affecting 30% to 40% of the population by the age of 80 years.

Pathophysiology

There are two major types of gallstones: those composed predominantly of pigment and those composed primarily of cholesterol. Pigment stones probably form when unconjugated pigments in the bile precipitate to form stones; these stones account for about 25% of cases in the United States (Kelly, Sarr & Hinder, 2004). The risk of developing such stones is increased in patients with cirrhosis, hemolysis, and infections of the biliary tract. Pigment stones cannot be dissolved and must be removed surgically.

Cholesterol stones account for most of the remaining 75% of cases of gallbladder disease in the United States. Cholesterol, a normal constituent of bile, is insoluble in water. Its solubility depends on bile acids and lecithin (phospholipids) in bile. In gallstone-prone patients, there is decreased bile acid synthesis and increased cholesterol synthesis in the liver, resulting in bile supersaturated with cholesterol, which precipitates out of the bile to form stones. The cholesterol-saturated bile predisposes to the formation of gallstones and acts as an irritant that produces inflammatory changes in the gallbladder.

Two to three times more women than men develop cholesterol stones and gallbladder disease; affected women are usually older than 40 years of age, multiparous, and obese. The incidence of stone formation is greater among people who use oral contraceptives, estrogens, or clofibrate; these medications are known to increase biliary cholesterol saturation. The incidence of stone formation increases with age as a result of increased hepatic secretion of cholesterol and decreased bile acid synthesis. In addition, there is an increased risk due to malabsorption of bile salts in patients with gastrointestinal disease or T-tube fistula and in those who have undergone ileal resection or bypass. The incidence also increases in people with diabetes (Chart 40-2).

CHART 40-2

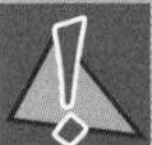

Risk Factors for Cholelithiasis

- Obesity
- Women, especially those who have had multiple pregnancies or who are of Native American or U.S. Southwestern Hispanic ethnicity
- Frequent changes in weight
- Rapid weight loss (leads to rapid development of gallstones and high risk of symptomatic disease)
- Treatment with high-dose estrogen (eg, in prostate cancer)
- Low-dose estrogen therapy—a small increase in the risk of gallstones
- Ileal resection or disease
- Cystic fibrosis
- Diabetes mellitus

Clinical Manifestations

Gallstones may be silent, producing no pain and only mild gastrointestinal symptoms. Such stones may be detected incidentally during surgery or evaluation for unrelated problems.

The patient with gallbladder disease resulting from gallstones may develop two types of symptoms: those due to disease of the gallbladder itself and those due to obstruction of the bile passages by a gallstone. The symptoms may be acute or chronic. Epigastric distress, such as fullness, abdominal distention, and vague pain in the right upper quadrant of the abdomen, may occur. This distress may follow a meal rich in fried or fatty foods.

Pain and Biliary Colic

If a gallstone obstructs the cystic duct, the gallbladder becomes distended, inflamed, and eventually infected (acute cholecystitis). The patient develops a fever and may have a palpable abdominal mass. The patient may have biliary colic with excruciating upper right abdominal pain that radiates to the back or right shoulder. Biliary colic is usually associated with nausea and vomiting, and is noticeable several hours after a heavy meal. The patient moves about restlessly, unable to find a comfortable position. In some patients the pain is constant rather than colicky.

Such a bout of biliary colic is caused by contraction of the gallbladder, which cannot release bile because of obstruction by the stone. When distended, the fundus of the gallbladder comes in contact with the abdominal wall in the region of the right ninth and tenth costal cartilages. This produces marked tenderness in the right upper quadrant on deep inspiration and prevents full inspiratory excursion.

The pain of acute cholecystitis may be so severe that analgesics are required. The use of morphine has traditionally been avoided because of concern that it could cause spasm of the sphincter of Oddi, and meperidine has been used instead. This is controversial, because morphine is the preferred analgesic agent for management of acute pain, and meperidine has metabolites that are toxic to the central nervous system (CNS). Furthermore, all opioids stimulate the sphincter of Oddi to some degree (Porth, 2005).

If the gallstone is dislodged and no longer obstructs the cystic duct, the gallbladder drains and the inflammatory process subsides after a relatively short time. If the gallstone continues to obstruct the duct, abscess, necrosis, and perforation with generalized peritonitis may result.

Jaundice

Jaundice occurs in a few patients with gallbladder disease, usually with obstruction of the common bile duct. The bile, which is no longer carried to the duodenum, is absorbed by the blood and gives the skin and mucous membranes a yellow color. This is frequently accompanied by marked pruritus (itching) of the skin.

Changes in Urine and Stool Color

The excretion of the bile pigments by the kidneys gives the urine a very dark color. The feces, no longer colored with bile pigments, are grayish, like putty, and usually described as clay-colored.

Vitamin Deficiency

Obstruction of bile flow also interferes with absorption of the fat-soluble vitamins A, D, E, and K. Patients may exhibit deficiencies of these vitamins if biliary obstruction has been prolonged. For example, a patient may have bleeding caused by vitamin K deficiency (vitamin K is necessary for normal blood clotting.)

Assessment and Diagnostic Findings

Table 40-1 identifies various procedures and their diagnostic uses.

Abdominal X-Ray

If gallbladder disease is suspected, an abdominal x-ray may be obtained to exclude other causes of symptoms. However, only 15% to 20% of gallstones are calcified sufficiently to be visible on such x-ray studies.

Ultrasonography

Ultrasonography has replaced cholecystography (discussed later) as the diagnostic procedure of choice, because it is rapid and accurate and can be used in patients with liver dysfunction and jaundice. It does not expose patients to ionizing radiation. The procedure is most accurate if the

TABLE 40-1 Studies Used in the Diagnosis of Biliary Tract and Pancreatic Disease

Studies	Diagnostic Uses
Cholecystogram, cholangiogram	To visualize gallbladder and bile duct
Celiac axis arteriography	To visualize liver and pancreas
Laparoscopy	To visualize anterior surface of liver, gallbladder, and mesentery through a trocar
Ultrasonography	To show size of abdominal organs and presence of masses
Magnetic resonance imaging (MRI) and computed tomography (CT scans)	To detect neoplasms; diagnose cysts, pseudocysts, abscess, and hematomas
Endoscopic retrograde cholangiopancreatography (ERCP)	To visualize biliary structures and pancreas via endoscopy
Serum alkaline phosphatase	In absence of bone disease, to measure biliary tract obstruction
Gamma-glutamyl (GGT), gamma-glutamyl transpeptidase (GGTP), lactate dehydrogenase (LDH)	Markers for biliary stasis; also elevated in alcohol abuse
Cholesterol levels	Elevated in biliary obstruction; decreased in parenchymal liver disease

patient fasts overnight so that the gallbladder is distended. Ultrasound studies are based on analysis of reflected sound waves. Ultrasonography can detect with 95% accuracy calculi in the gallbladder or a dilated common bile duct.

Radionuclide Imaging or Cholescintigraphy

Cholescintigraphy is used successfully in the diagnosis of acute cholecystitis or blockage of a bile duct. In this procedure, a radioactive agent is administered intravenously. It is taken up by the hepatocytes and excreted rapidly through the biliary tract. The biliary tract is then scanned, and images of the gallbladder and biliary tract are obtained. This test is more expensive than ultrasonography, takes longer to perform, exposes the patient to radiation, and cannot detect gallstones. It is often used when ultrasonography is not conclusive.

Cholecystography

Although cholecystography has been replaced by ultrasonography as the test of choice, it is still used if ultrasound equipment is not available or if the ultrasound results are inconclusive. Oral cholangiography may be performed to detect gallstones and to assess the ability of the gallbladder to fill, concentrate its contents, contract, and empty. An iodide-containing contrast agent that is excreted by the liver and concentrated in the gallbladder is administered to the patient. The normal gallbladder fills with this radiopaque substance. If gallstones are present, they appear as shadows on the x-ray film.

Contrast agents include iopanoic acid (Telepaque), iodipamide meglumine (Cholografin), and sodium ipodate (Oragrafin). These agents are administered orally 10 to 12 hours before the x-ray study. After the contrast agent is administered, the patient is permitted nothing by mouth, to prevent contraction and emptying of the gallbladder.

The patient is asked about allergies to iodine or seafood. If no allergy is identified, the patient receives the oral form of the contrast agent the evening before the x-rays are obtained. An x-ray of the right upper abdomen is obtained. If the gallbladder is found to fill and empty normally and to contain no stones, gallbladder disease is ruled out. If gallbladder disease is present, the gallbladder may not be visualized because of obstruction by gallstones. If the gallbladder is not visualized on the first attempt, a repeat of the oral cholecystogram with a second dose of the contrast agent may be necessary.

Cholecystography in the obviously jaundiced patient is not useful because the liver cannot excrete the radiopaque dye into the gallbladder in the presence of jaundice. Oral cholecystography is likely to continue to be used as part of the evaluation of the few patients who have been treated with gallstone **dissolution therapy** or lithotripsy.

Endoscopic Retrograde Cholangiopancreatography

Endoscopic retrograde cholangiopancreatography (ERCP) permits direct visualization of structures that previously could be seen only during laparotomy. The examination of the hepatobiliary system is carried out via a side-viewing flexible fiberoptic endoscope inserted through the esophagus to the descending duodenum (Fig. 40-3). Multiple position changes are required to pass the endoscope during the procedure, beginning in the left semiprone position.

Fluoroscopy and multiple x-rays are used during ERCP to evaluate the presence and location of ductal stones. Careful insertion of a catheter through the endoscope into the common bile duct is the most important step in sphincterotomy (division of the muscles of the biliary sphincter) for gallstone extraction via this technique (see later discussion).

NURSING IMPLICATIONS

The procedure requires a cooperative patient to permit insertion of the endoscope without damage to the gastrointestinal tract structures, including the biliary tree. Before the procedure, the patient is given an explanation of the procedure and his or her role in it. The patient takes nothing by mouth for several hours before the procedure. Moderate sedation is used, and the sedated patient must be monitored closely. Most endoscopists use a combination of an opioid and a benzodiazepine. It may be necessary to administer medications, such as glucagon or anticholinergics, to make cannulation easier by decreasing duodenal peristalsis. The nurse observes closely for signs of respiratory and central nervous system depression, hypotension, oversedation, and vomiting (if glucagon is administered). During ERCP, the nurse monitors intravenous (IV) fluids, administers medications, and positions the patient.

After the procedure, the nurse monitors the patient's condition, observing vital signs and monitoring for signs of perforation or infection. The nurse also monitors the patient for side effects of any medications received during the procedure and for return of the gag and cough reflexes after the use of local anesthetics.

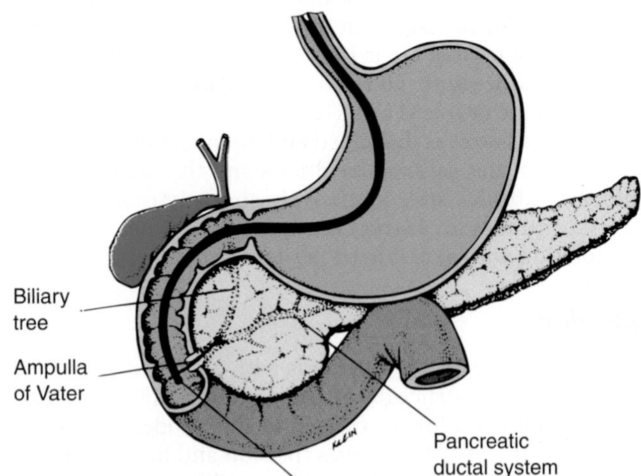

FIGURE 40-3. Endoscopic retrograde cholangiopancreatography (ERCP). A fiberoptic duodenoscope, with side-viewing apparatus, is inserted into the duodenum. The ampulla of Vater is catheterized, and the biliary tree is injected with contrast agent. The pancreatic ductal system is also assessed, if indicated. This procedure is of special value in visualizing neoplasms of the ampulla area and extracting a biopsy specimen.

Percutaneous Transhepatic Cholangiography

Percutaneous transhepatic cholangiography involves the injection of dye directly into the biliary tract. Because of the relatively large concentration of dye that is introduced into the biliary system, all components of the system, including the hepatic ducts within the liver, the entire length of the common bile duct, the cystic duct, and the gallbladder, are outlined clearly.

This procedure can be carried out even in the presence of liver dysfunction and jaundice. Percutaneous transhepatic cholangiography is useful for (1) distinguishing jaundice caused by liver disease (hepatocellular jaundice) from that caused by biliary obstruction, (2) investigating the gastrointestinal symptoms of a patient whose gallbladder has been removed, (3) locating stones within the bile ducts, and (4) diagnosing cancer involving the biliary system.

This sterile procedure is performed under moderate sedation on a patient who has been fasting; the patient receives local anesthesia and moderate sedation. Coagulation parameters and platelet count should be normal to minimize the risk for bleeding. Broad-spectrum antibiotics are administered during the procedure due to the high prevalence of bacterial colonization from obstructed biliary systems. After infiltration with a local anesthetic agent, a flexible needle is inserted into the liver from the right side in the midclavicular line immediately beneath the right costal margin. Successful entry of a duct is noted when bile is aspirated or on injection of a contrast agent. Ultrasound can be used to guide puncture of the duct. Bile is aspirated and samples are sent for bacteriology and cytology. A water-soluble contrast agent is injected to fill the biliary system. The fluoroscopy table is tilted and the patient repositioned to allow x-rays to be taken in multiple projections. Delayed x-ray views can identify abnormalities of more distant ducts and determine the length of a stricture or multiple strictures. Before the needle is removed, as much dye and bile as possible are aspirated to forestall subsequent leakage into the needle tract and eventually into the peritoneal cavity, thus minimizing the risk of bile peritonitis.

NURSING ALERT

Although the complication rate after this procedure is low, the nurse must closely observe the patient for symptoms of bleeding, peritonitis, and septicemia. The nurse assesses the patient for pain and indications of these complications and reports them promptly to the physician. Antibiotic agents are often prescribed to minimize the risk of sepsis and septic shock.

Medical Management

The major objectives of medical therapy are to reduce the incidence of acute episodes of gallbladder pain and cholecystitis by supportive and dietary management and, if possible, to remove the cause of cholecystitis by pharmacologic therapy, endoscopic procedures, or surgical intervention. Although nonsurgical approaches have the advantage of eliminating risks associated with surgery, these approaches are associated with persistent symptoms or recurrent stone formation. Most of the nonsurgical approaches, including lithotripsy and dissolution of gallstones, provide only temporary solutions to gallstone problems. They are therefore rarely used in the United States. In some instances, other treatment approaches may be indicated; these are described later.

Removal of the gallbladder (**cholecystectomy**) through traditional surgical approaches was considered the standard treatment for more than 100 years. However, dramatic changes have occurred in the surgical management of gallbladder disease. There is now widespread use of **laparoscopic cholecystectomy** (removal of the gallbladder through a small incision through the umbilicus). As a result, surgical risks have decreased, along with the length of hospital stay and the long recovery period required after standard surgical cholecystectomy.

Nutritional and Supportive Therapy

Approximately 80% of the patients with acute gallbladder inflammation achieve remission with rest, IV fluids, nasogastric suction, analgesia, and antibiotic agents. Unless the patient's condition deteriorates, surgical intervention is delayed until the acute symptoms subside and a complete evaluation can be performed.

The diet required immediately after an episode is usually limited to low-fat liquids. These can include powdered supplements high in protein and carbohydrate stirred into skim milk. Cooked fruits, rice or tapioca, lean meats, mashed potatoes, non–gas-forming vegetables, bread, coffee, or tea may be added as tolerated. The patient should avoid eggs, cream, pork, fried foods, cheese, rich dressings, gas-forming vegetables, and alcohol. It is important to remind the patient that fatty foods may bring on an episode of cholecystitis. Dietary management may be the major mode of therapy in patients who have had only dietary intolerance to fatty foods and vague gastrointestinal symptoms (Dudek, 2006).

Pharmacologic Therapy

Ursodeoxycholic acid (UDCA) and chenodeoxycholic acid (chenodiol or CDCA) have been used to dissolve small, radiolucent gallstones composed primarily of cholesterol. UDCA has fewer side effects than chenodiol and can be administered in smaller doses to achieve the same effect. It acts by inhibiting the synthesis and secretion of cholesterol, thereby desaturating bile. Treatment with UDCA can reduce the size of existing stones, dissolve small stones, and prevent new stones from forming. Six to 12 months of therapy is required in many patients to dissolve stones, and monitoring of the patient for recurrence of symptoms or the occurrence of side effects is required during this time. The effective dose of medication depends on body weight. This method of treatment is generally indicated for patients who refuse surgery or for whom surgery is considered too risky.

Patients with significant, frequent symptoms; cystic duct occlusion; or pigment stones are not candidates for this therapy. Laparoscopic or open cholecystectomy is more appropriate for symptomatic patients with acceptable operative risk.

Nonsurgical Removal of Gallstones

DISSOLVING GALLSTONES

Several methods have been used to dissolve gallstones by infusion of a solvent (mono-octanoin or methyl tertiary butyl ether [MTBE]) into the gallbladder. The solvent can be infused through the following routes: through a tube or catheter inserted percutaneously directly into the gallbladder; through a tube or drain inserted through a T-tube tract to dissolve stones not removed at the time of surgery; endoscopically with ERCP; or via a transnasal biliary catheter.

In the last procedure, the catheter is introduced through the mouth and inserted into the common bile duct. The upper end of the tube is then rerouted from the mouth to the nose and left in place. This enables the patient to eat and drink normally while passage of stones is monitored or chemical solvents are infused to dissolve the stones. This method of dissolution of stones is not widely used.

STONE REMOVAL BY INSTRUMENTATION

Several nonsurgical methods are used to remove stones that were not removed at the time of cholecystectomy or have become lodged in the common bile duct (Fig. 40-4A,B). A catheter and instrument with a basket attached are threaded through the T-tube tract or fistula formed at the time of T-tube insertion; the basket is used to retrieve and remove the stones lodged in the common bile duct.

A second procedure involves the use of the ERCP endoscope (see Fig. 40-4C). After the endoscope is inserted, a cutting instrument is passed through the endoscope into the ampulla of Vater of the common bile duct. It may be used to cut the submucosal fibers, or papilla, of the sphincter of Oddi, enlarging the opening, which may allow the lodged stones to pass spontaneously into the duodenum. Another instrument with a small basket or balloon at its tip may be inserted through the endoscope to retrieve the stones (see Fig. 40-4D–F). Although complications after this procedure are rare, the patient must be observed closely for bleeding, perforation, and the development of pancreatitis or sepsis.

The ERCP procedure is particularly useful in diagnosis and treatment of patients who have symptoms after biliary tract surgery, patients with intact gallbladders, and patients for whom surgery is particularly hazardous.

INTRACORPOREAL LITHOTRIPSY

Stones in the gallbladder or common bile duct may be fragmented by means of laser pulse technology. A laser pulse is directed under fluoroscopic guidance with the use of devices that can distinguish between stones and tissue. The laser pulse produces rapid expansion and disintegration of plasma on the stone surface, resulting in a mechanical shock wave. Electrohydraulic lithotripsy uses a probe with two electrodes that deliver electric sparks in rapid pulses, creating expansion of the liquid environment surrounding the gallstones. This results in pressure waves that cause stones to fragment. This technique can be employed percutaneously with the use of a basket or balloon catheter system or by direct visualization through an endoscope. Repeated procedures may be necessary because of stone size, local anatomy, bleeding, or technical difficulty. A nasobiliary tube can be inserted to allow for biliary decompression and to prevent stone impaction in the common

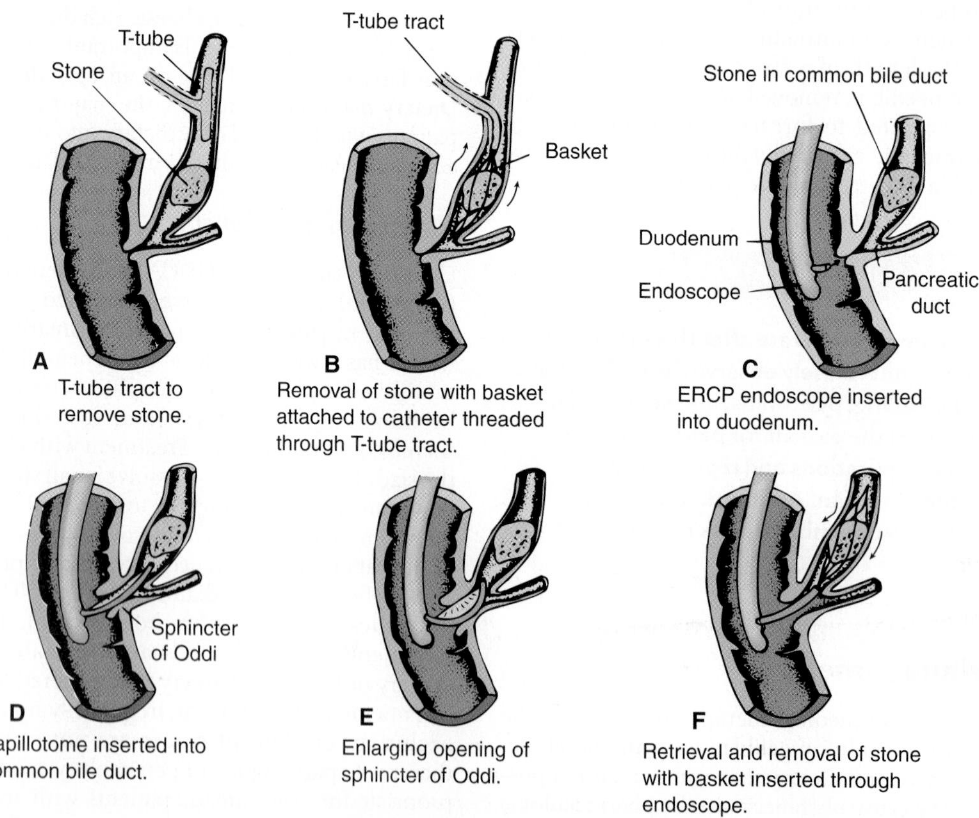
T-tube
Stone
A
T-tube tract to remove stone.
T-tube tract
Basket
B
Removal of stone with basket attached to catheter threaded through T-tube tract.
Stone in common bile duct
Duodenum
Endoscope
Pancreatic duct
C
ERCP endoscope inserted into duodenum.
Sphincter of Oddi
D
Papillotome inserted into common bile duct.
E
Enlarging opening of sphincter of Oddi.
F
Retrieval and removal of stone with basket inserted through endoscope.

FIGURE 40-4. Nonsurgical techniques for removing gallstones.

bile duct. This approach allows time for improvement in the patient's clinical condition until gallstones are cleared endoscopically, percutaneously, or surgically.

EXTRACORPOREAL SHOCK-WAVE LITHOTRIPSY

Extracorporeal shock-wave therapy (lithotripsy or ESWL) has been used for nonsurgical fragmentation of gallstones. **Lithotripsy**, a noninvasive procedure, uses repeated shock waves directed at the gallstones in the gallbladder or common bile duct to fragment the stones. The waves are transmitted to the body through a fluid-filled bag or by immersing the patient in a water bath. After the stones are gradually broken up, the stone fragments can be spontaneously passed from the gallbladder or common bile duct, removed by endoscopy, or dissolved with oral bile acid or solvents. Because the procedure requires no incision and no hospitalization, patients are usually treated as outpatients, but usually several sessions are necessary. This procedure has largely been replaced by laparoscopic cholecystectomy. ESWL is used in some centers for a small percentage of suitable patients (those with common bile duct stones who may not be surgical candidates), sometimes in combination with dissolution therapy.

Surgical Management

Surgical treatment of gallbladder disease and gallstones is carried out to relieve persistent symptoms, to remove the cause of biliary colic, and to treat acute cholecystitis. Surgery may be delayed until the patient's symptoms have subsided, or it may be performed as an emergency procedure, if necessitated by the patient's condition.

PREOPERATIVE MEASURES

Chest x-ray, electrocardiogram (ECG), and liver function tests may be performed in addition to x-ray studies of the gallbladder. Vitamin K may be administered if the prothrombin level is low. Nutritional requirements are considered, and, if the nutritional status is suboptimal, it may be necessary to provide IV glucose with protein hydrolysate supplements to aid wound healing and help prevent liver damage.

Preparation for gallbladder surgery is similar to that for any upper abdominal laparotomy or laparoscopy. Instructions and explanations are given before surgery with regard to turning and deep breathing. Pneumonia and atelectasis are possible postoperative complications that can be avoided by deep-breathing exercises and frequent turning. The patient should be informed that drainage tubes and a nasogastric tube and suction might be required during the immediate postoperative period if an open cholecystectomy is performed.

LAPAROSCOPIC CHOLECYSTECTOMY

Laparoscopic cholecystectomy (Fig. 40-5) has dramatically changed the approach to the management of cholecystitis. It has become the new standard for therapy of symptomatic gallstones. Approximately 500,000 patients in the United States require surgery each year for removal of the gallbladder, and 80% to 90% of them are candidates for laparoscopic cholecystectomy (Kelly et al., 2004). If the common bile duct is thought to be obstructed by a gallstone, an ERCP with sphincterotomy may be performed to explore the duct before laparoscopy.

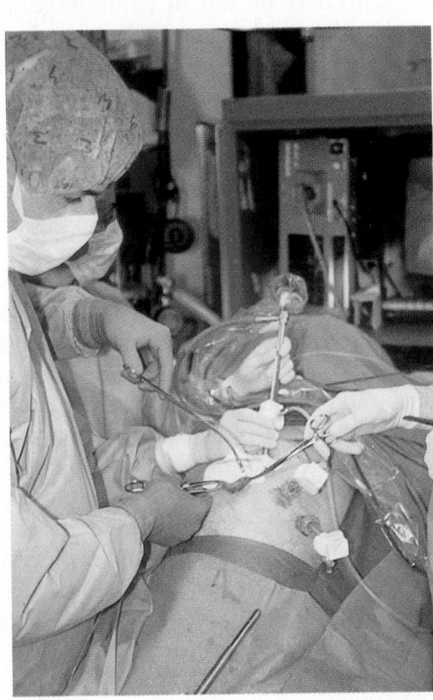

A

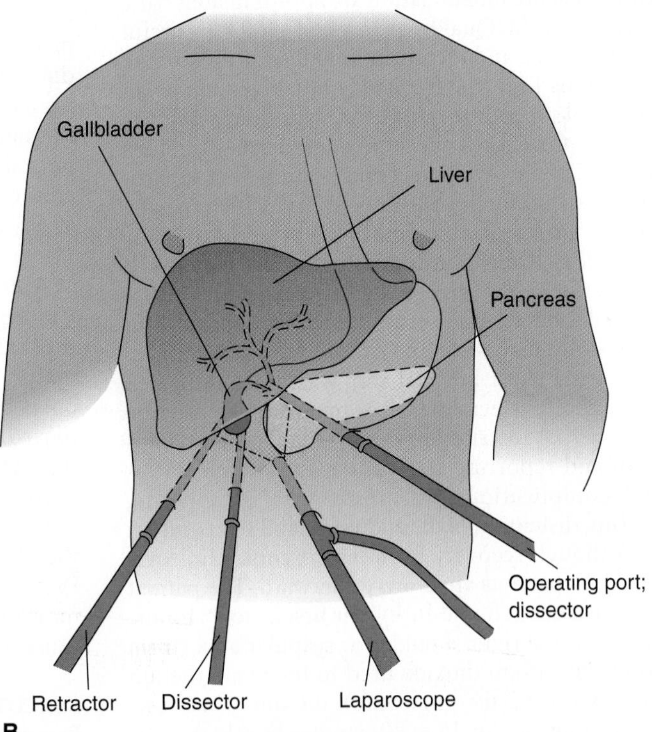

B

FIGURE 40-5. In laparoscopic cholecystectomy (**A**), the surgeon makes four small incisions (less than ½ inch each) in the abdomen (**B**) and inserts a laparoscope with a miniature camera through the umbilical incision. The camera apparatus displays the gallbladder and adjacent tissues on a screen, allowing the surgeon to visualize the sections of the organ for removal.

Before the procedure, the patient is informed that an open abdominal procedure may be necessary, and general anesthesia is administered. Laparoscopic cholecystectomy is performed through a small incision or puncture made through the abdominal wall at the umbilicus. The abdominal cavity is insufflated with carbon dioxide (pneumoperitoneum) to assist in inserting the laparoscope and to aid in visualizing the abdominal structures. The fiberoptic scope is inserted through the small umbilical incision. Several additional punctures or small incisions are made in the abdominal wall to introduce other surgical instruments into the operative field. The surgeon visualizes the biliary system through the laparoscope; a camera attached to the scope permits a view of the intra-abdominal field to be transmitted to a television monitor. After the cystic duct is dissected, the common bile duct can be visualized by ultrasound or cholangiography to evaluate the anatomy and identify stones. The cystic artery is dissected free and clipped. The gallbladder is separated from the hepatic bed and dissected. The gallbladder is then removed from the abdominal cavity after bile and small stones are aspirated. Stone forceps also can be used to remove or crush larger stones.

Advantages of the laparoscopic procedure are that the patient does not experience the paralytic ileus that occurs with open abdominal surgery and has less postoperative abdominal pain. The patient is often discharged from the hospital on the same day of surgery or within 1 or 2 days and can resume full activity and employment within 1 week after the surgery.

Conversion to a traditional abdominal surgical procedure may be necessary if problems are encountered during the laparoscopic procedure; this occurs in 3.5% to 5% of reported surgical cases (Edmundowicz, 2002). Conversion rates in cases of acute inflammation are approximately 10% higher (Friedman, McQuaid & Grendell, 2003). Careful screening of patients and identification of those at low risk for complications limit the frequency of conversion to an open abdominal procedure. However, with increasing use of laparoscopic procedures, the number of such conversions may increase. The most serious complication after laparoscopic cholecystectomy is a bile duct injury, which may be identified and corrected at the time of the procedure. A bile leak that develops from an unrecognized injury may result in fluid collections that can usually be managed by endoscopic stent placement. Bile peritonitis, a more serious but rare complication, may result in critical illness or death.

Because of the short hospital stay with uncomplicated laparoscopic cholecystectomies, it is important to provide written and verbal instructions about managing postoperative pain and reporting signs and symptoms of intra-abdominal complications, including loss of appetite, vomiting, pain, distention of the abdomen, and temperature elevation. Although recovery from laparoscopic cholecystectomy is rapid, patients are drowsy afterward. The patient must have assistance at home during the first 24 to 48 hours. If pain occurs in the right shoulder or scapular area (from migration of the carbon dioxide used to insufflate the abdominal cavity during the procedure), the nurse may recommend a heating pad for 15 to 20 minutes hourly.

CHOLECYSTECTOMY

In cholecystectomy, the gallbladder is removed through an abdominal incision (usually right subcostal) after the cystic duct and artery are ligated. The procedure is performed for acute and chronic cholecystitis. In some patients, a drain is placed close to the gallbladder bed and brought out through a puncture wound if there is a bile leak. The drain type is chosen based on the physician's preference. A small leak should close spontaneously in a few days, with the drain preventing accumulation of bile. Usually, only a small amount of serosanguineous fluid drains in the initial 24 hours after surgery; afterward, the drain is removed. The drain is typically maintained if there is excess oozing or bile leakage. Use of a T-tube inserted into the common bile duct during the open procedure is now uncommon; it is used only in the setting of a complication (ie, retained common bile duct stone). Bile duct injury is a serious complication of cholecystectomy, but it occurs less frequently than with the laparoscopic approach. At one time one of the most common surgical procedures in the United States, this procedure has largely been replaced by laparoscopic cholecystectomy.

MINI-CHOLECYSTECTOMY

Mini-cholecystectomy is a surgical procedure in which the gallbladder is removed through a small incision. If needed, the surgical incision is extended to remove larger gallbladder stones. Drains may or may not be used. The cost savings resulting from the short hospital stay have been identified as a major reason for pursuing this type of procedure. The procedure is controversial because it limits exposure to all the involved biliary structures.

CHOLEDOCHOSTOMY

Choledochostomy is reserved for the patient with acute cholecystitis who may be too ill to undergo a surgical procedure. It involves making an incision in the common duct, usually for removal of stones. After the stones have been evacuated, a tube is usually inserted into the duct for drainage of bile until edema subsides. This tube is connected to gravity drainage tubing; the patient is monitored closely, and a cholecystectomy is planned for a future date (Kelly et al., 2004).

SURGICAL CHOLECYSTOSTOMY

Cholecystostomy is performed when the patient's condition precludes more extensive surgery or when an acute inflammatory reaction is severe. The gallbladder is surgically opened, stones and the bile or the purulent drainage are removed, and a drainage tube is secured with a purse-string suture. The drainage tube is connected to a drainage system to prevent bile from leaking around the tube or escaping into the peritoneal cavity. After recovery from the acute episode, the patient may return for subsequent cholecystectomy. Despite its lower risk, surgical cholecystostomy has a high mortality rate (reported to be as high as 20% to 30%) because of the underlying disease process.

PERCUTANEOUS CHOLECYSTOSTOMY

Percutaneous cholecystostomy has been used in the treatment and diagnosis of acute cholecystitis in patients who are poor risks for any surgical procedure or for general anesthesia. These may include patients with sepsis or severe cardiac, renal, pulmonary, or liver failure. Under local anesthesia, a fine needle is inserted through the abdominal wall and liver edge into the gallbladder under the guidance of ultrasound or computed tomography (CT). Bile is aspirated to ensure adequate placement of the needle, and a catheter is inserted into the gallbladder to decompress the biliary tract. Almost immediate relief of pain and resolution of signs and symptoms of sepsis and cholecystitis have been reported with this procedure. Antibiotic agents are administered before, during, and after the procedure.

Gerontologic Considerations

Surgical intervention for disease of the biliary tract is the most common operative procedure performed in the elderly. Cholesterol saturation of bile increases with age because of increased hepatic secretion of cholesterol and decreased bile acid synthesis.

Although the incidence of gallstones increases with age, the elderly patient may not exhibit the typical symptoms of fever, pain, chills, and jaundice. Symptoms of biliary tract disease in the elderly may be accompanied or preceded by those of septic shock, which include oliguria, hypotension, changes in mental status, tachycardia, and tachypnea.

Although surgery in the elderly presents a risk because of preexisting associated diseases, the mortality rate from serious complications of biliary tract disease itself is also high. The risk of death and complications is increased in the elderly patient who undergoes emergency surgery for life-threatening disease of the biliary tract. Despite chronic illness in many elderly patients, elective cholecystectomy is usually well tolerated and can be carried out with low risk if expert assessment and care are provided before, during, and after the surgical procedure.

Because of recent changes in reimbursement for health care expenses, there has been a decrease in the number of elective surgical procedures performed, including cholecystectomies. As a result, patients requiring the procedure are seen in later stages of disease. At the same time, patients undergoing surgery are increasingly older than 60 years of age and may have complicated acute cholecystitis. The higher risk of complications and shorter hospital stay make it essential that older patients and their family members receive specific information about signs and symptoms of complications and measures to prevent them.

Nursing Process

The Patient Undergoing Surgery for Gallbladder Disease

Assessment

The patient who is to undergo surgical treatment of gallbladder disease is often admitted to the hospital or same-day surgery unit on the morning of surgery. Preadmission testing is often completed a week or longer before admission. At that time, the nurse instructs the patient about the need to avoid smoking, to enhance pulmonary recovery postoperatively and to avoid respiratory complications. It also is important to instruct the patient to avoid the use of aspirin and other agents (over-the-counter medications and herbal remedies) that can alter coagulation and other biochemical processes.

Assessment should focus on the patient's respiratory status. If a traditional surgical approach is planned, the high abdominal incision required during surgery may interfere with full respiratory excursion. The nurse notes a history of smoking, previous respiratory problems, shallow respirations, a persistent or ineffective cough, and the presence of adventitious breath sounds. Nutritional status is evaluated through a dietary history and a general examination performed at the time of preadmission testing. The nurse also reviews previously obtained laboratory results to obtain information about the patient's nutritional status.

Diagnosis

Nursing Diagnoses

Based on all the assessment data, the major postoperative nursing diagnoses for the patient undergoing surgery for gallbladder disease may include the following:

- Acute pain and discomfort related to surgical incision
- Impaired gas exchange related to the high abdominal surgical incision (if traditional surgical cholecystectomy was performed)
- Impaired skin integrity related to altered biliary drainage after surgical intervention (if a T-tube was inserted because of retained stones in the common bile duct or another drainage device was employed)
- Imbalanced nutrition, less than body requirements, related to inadequate bile secretion
- Deficient knowledge about self-care activities related to incision care, dietary modifications (if needed), medications, and reportable signs or symptoms (eg, fever, bleeding, vomiting)

Collaborative Problems/ Potential Complications

Based on assessment data, potential complications may include the following:

- Bleeding
- Gastrointestinal symptoms (may be related to biliary leak or injury to the bowel)

Planning and Goals

The goals for the patient include relief of pain, adequate ventilation, intact skin and improved biliary drainage, optimal nutritional intake, absence of complications, and understanding of self-care routines.

Postoperative Nursing Interventions

After recovery from anesthesia, the patient is placed in the low Fowler's position. Fluids may be administered intravenously, and nasogastric suction (a nasogastric tube was probably inserted immediately before surgery for a nonlaparoscopic procedure) may be instituted to relieve abdominal distention. Water and other fluids are administered within hours after laparoscopic procedures. A soft diet is started after bowel sounds return, which is usually the next day if the laparoscopic approach is used.

Relieving Pain

The location of the subcostal incision in nonlaparoscopic gallbladder surgery often causes the patient to avoid turning and moving, to splint the affected site, and to take shallow breaths to prevent pain. Because full expansion of the lungs and gradually increased activity are necessary to prevent postoperative complications, the nurse administers analgesic agents as prescribed to relieve the pain and to promote well-being in addition to helping the patient turn, cough, breathe deeply, and ambulate as indicated. Use of a pillow or binder over the incision may reduce pain during these maneuvers.

Improving Respiratory Status

Patients undergoing biliary tract surgery are especially prone to pulmonary complications, as are all patients with upper abdominal incisions. Therefore, the nurse reminds the patient to take deep breaths and cough every hour, to expand the lungs fully and prevent atelectasis. The early and consistent use of incentive spirometry also helps improve respiratory function. Early ambulation prevents pulmonary complications as well as other complications, such as thrombophlebitis. Pulmonary complications are more likely to occur in elderly patients, obese patients, and those with preexisting pulmonary disease.

Promoting Skin Care and Biliary Drainage

In patients who have undergone a cholecystostomy or choledochostomy, the drainage tube must be connected immediately to a drainage receptacle. The nurse should fasten tubing to the dressings or to the patient's gown, with enough leeway for the patient to move without dislodging or kinking it. Because a drainage system remains attached when the patient is ambulating, the drainage bag may be placed in a bathrobe pocket or fastened so that it is below the waist or common duct level. If a Penrose drain is used, the nurse changes the dressings as required.

After these surgical procedures, the patient is observed for indications of infection, leakage of bile into the peritoneal cavity, and obstruction of bile drainage. If bile is not draining properly, an obstruction is probably causing bile to be forced back into the liver and bloodstream. Because jaundice may result, the nurse should be particularly observant of the color of the sclerae. The nurse should also note and report right upper quadrant abdominal pain, nausea and vomiting, bile drainage around any drainage tube, clay-colored stools, and a change in vital signs.

Bile may continue to drain from the drainage tract in considerable quantities for some time, necessitating frequent changes of the outer dressings and protection of the skin from irritation (bile is corrosive to the skin).

To prevent total loss of bile, the physician may want the drainage tube or collection receptacle elevated above the level of the abdomen so that the bile drains externally only if pressure develops in the duct system. Every 24 hours, the nurse measures the bile collected and records the amount, color, and character of the drainage. After several days of drainage, the tube may be clamped for 1 hour before and after each meal to deliver bile to the duodenum to aid in digestion. Within 7 to 14 days, the drainage tube is removed. The patient who goes home with a drainage tube in place requires instruction and reassurance about the function and care of the tube.

In all patients with biliary drainage, the nurse (or the patient, if at home) observes the stools daily and notes their color. Specimens of both urine and stool may be sent to the laboratory for examination for bile pigments. In this way, it is possible to determine whether the bile pigment is disappearing from the blood and is draining again into the duodenum. Maintaining a careful record of fluid intake and output is important.

Improving Nutritional Status

The nurse encourages the patient to eat a diet that is low in fats and high in carbohydrates and proteins immediately after surgery. At the time of hospital discharge, there are usually no special dietary instructions other than to maintain a nutritious diet and avoid excessive fats. Fat restriction usually is lifted in 4 to 6 weeks, when the biliary ducts dilate to accommodate the volume of bile once held by the gallbladder and when the ampulla of Vater again functions effectively. After this time, when the patient eats fat, adequate bile will be released into the digestive tract to emulsify the fats and allow their digestion. This is in contrast to the condition before surgery, when fats may not be digested completely or adequately, and flatulence may occur. However, one purpose of gallbladder surgery is to allow a normal diet.

Monitoring and Managing Potential Complications

Bleeding may occur as a result of inadvertent puncture or nicking of a major blood vessel. Postoperatively, the nurse closely monitors vital signs and inspects the surgical incisions and drains, if any are in place, for evidence of bleeding. The nurse also periodically assesses the patient for increased tenderness and rigidity of the abdomen. If these signs and symptoms occur, they are reported to the surgeon. The nurse instructs the patient and family to report to the surgeon any change in the color of stools, because this may indicate complications. Gastrointestinal symptoms, although not common, may occur with manipulation of the intestines during surgery.

After laparoscopic cholecystectomy, the nurse assesses the patient for loss of appetite, vomiting, pain, distention of the abdomen, and temperature elevation. These may indicate infection or disruption of the gastrointestinal tract and should be reported to the surgeon promptly. Because the patient is discharged soon after laparoscopic surgery, the patient and family are instructed verbally and in writing about the importance of reporting these symptoms promptly.

Promoting Home and Community-Based Care

TEACHING PATIENTS SELF-CARE

The nurse instructs the patient about the medications that are prescribed (vitamins, anticholinergics, and antispasmodics) and their actions. It also is important to inform the patient and family about symptoms that should be reported to the physician, including jaundice, dark urine, pale-colored stools, pruritus, and signs of inflammation and infection, such as pain or fever.

Some patients report one to three bowel movements a day. This is the result of a continual trickle of bile through the choledochoduodenal junction after cholecystectomy. Usually, such frequency diminishes over a period of a few weeks to several months.

If a patient is discharged from the hospital with a drainage tube still in place, the patient and family need instructions about its management. The nurse instructs them in proper care of the drainage tube and the importance of reporting to the surgeon promptly any changes in the amount or characteristics of drainage. Assistance in securing the appropriate dressings reduces the patient's anxiety about going home with the drain or tube still in place. (See Chart 40-3 for more details.)

CONTINUING CARE

With sufficient support at home, most patients recover quickly from a cholecystectomy. However, elderly or frail patients and those who live alone may require a referral for home care. During home visits, the nurse assesses the patient's physical status, especially wound healing, and progress toward recovery. Assessing the patient for adequacy of pain relief and pulmonary exercises is also important. If the patient has a drainage system in place, the nurse assesses it for patency and appropriate management by the patient and family. Assessing for signs of infection and teaching the patient about the signs and symptoms of infection are also important nursing interventions. The patient's understanding of the therapeutic regimen (medications, gradual return to normal activities) is assessed, and previous teaching is reinforced. The nurse emphasizes the importance of keeping follow-up appointments and reminds the patient and family of the importance of participating in health promotion activities and recommended health screening.

Evaluation

Expected Patient Outcomes

Expected patient outcomes may include the following:

1. Reports decrease in pain
   a. Splints abdominal incision to decrease pain
   b. Avoids foods that cause pain
   c. Uses postoperative analgesia as prescribed

CHART 40-3

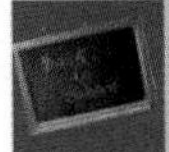

Patient Education

Managing Self-Care After Laparoscopic Cholecystectomy

RESUMING ACTIVITY

- Begin light exercise (walking) immediately.
- Take a shower or bath after 1 or 2 days.
- Drive a car after 3 or 4 days.
- Avoid lifting objects exceeding 5 pounds after surgery, usually for 1 week.
- Resume sexual activity when desired.

CARING FOR THE WOUND

- Check puncture site daily for signs of infection.
- Wash puncture site with mild soap and water.
- Allow special adhesive strips on the puncture site to fall off. Do not pull them off.

RESUMING EATING

- Resume your normal diet.
- If you had fat intolerance before surgery, gradually add fat back into your diet in small increments.

MANAGING PAIN

- You may experience pain or discomfort in your right shoulder from the gas used to inflate your abdominal area during surgery. Sitting upright in bed or a chair, walking, or use of a heating pad may ease the discomfort.
- Take analgesics as needed and as prescribed. Report to surgeon if pain is unrelieved even with analgesic use.

MANAGING FOLLOW-UP CARE

- Make an appointment with your surgeon for 7 to 10 days after discharge.
- Call your surgeon if you experience any signs or symptoms of infection at or around the puncture site: redness, tenderness, swelling, heat, or drainage.
- Call your surgeon if you experience a fever of 37.7°C (100°F) or more for 2 consecutive days.
- Call your surgeon if you develop nausea, vomiting, or abdominal pain.

2. Demonstrates appropriate respiratory function
   a. Achieves full respiratory excursion, with deep inspiration and expiration
   b. Coughs effectively, using pillow to splint abdominal incision
   c. Uses postoperative analgesia as prescribed
   d. Exercises as prescribed (eg, turns, ambulates)
3. Exhibits normal skin integrity around biliary drainage site (if applicable)
   a. Is free of fever, abdominal pain, change in vital signs, and presence of bile, foul-smelling drainage, or pus around drainage tube
   b. Demonstrates correct management of drainage tube (if applicable)
   c. Identifies signs and symptoms of biliary obstruction to be noted and reported
   d. Has serum bilirubin level within normal range
4. Obtains relief from dietary intolerance
   a. Maintains adequate dietary intake and avoids foods that cause gastrointestinal symptoms
   b. Reports decreased or absent nausea, vomiting, diarrhea, flatulence, and abdominal discomfort
5. Absence of complications
   a. Has normal vital signs (blood pressure, pulse, respiratory rate and pattern, and temperature)
   b. Reports absence of bleeding from gastrointestinal tract and from biliary drainage tube or catheter (if present) and no evidence of bleeding in stool
   c. Reports return of appetite and no evidence of vomiting, abdominal distention, or pain
   d. Lists symptoms that should be reported to surgeon promptly and demonstrates an understanding of self-care, including wound care

Disorders of the Pancreas

Pancreatitis (inflammation of the pancreas) is a serious disorder. The most basic classification system used to describe or categorize the various stages and forms of pancreatitis divides the disorder into acute and chronic forms. Acute pancreatitis can be a medical emergency associated with a high risk for life-threatening complications and mortality, whereas chronic pancreatitis often goes undetected until 80% to 90% of the exocrine and endocrine tissue is destroyed. Acute pancreatitis does not usually lead to chronic pancreatitis unless complications develop. However, chronic pancreatitis can be characterized by acute episodes. Typically, patients are men 40 to 45 years of age with a history of alcoholism or women 50 to 55 years of age with a history of gallstone pancreatitis (Swaroop, Chari & Clain, 2004).

Although the mechanisms causing pancreatic inflammation are unknown, pancreatitis is commonly described as autodigestion of the pancreas. It is believed that the pancreatic duct becomes temporarily obstructed, accompanied by hypersecretion of the exocrine enzymes of the pancreas. These enzymes enter the bile duct, where they are activated and, together with bile, back up (reflux) into the pancreatic duct, causing pancreatitis.

Acute Pancreatitis

Acute pancreatitis ranges from a mild, self-limited disorder to a severe, rapidly fatal disease that does not respond to any treatment. Mild acute pancreatitis is characterized by edema and inflammation confined to the pancreas. Minimal organ dysfunction is present, and return to normal function usually occurs within 6 months. Although this is considered the milder form of pancreatitis, the patient is acutely ill and at risk for hypovolemic shock, fluid and electrolyte disturbances, and sepsis. A more widespread and complete enzymatic digestion of the gland characterizes severe acute pancreatitis. Enzymes damage the local blood vessels, and bleeding and thrombosis can occur. The tissue may become necrotic, with damage extending into the retroperitoneal tissues. Local complications consist of pancreatic cysts or abscesses and acute fluid collections in or near the pancreas. Patients who develop systemic complications with organ failure, such as pulmonary insufficiency with hypoxia, shock, renal failure, and gastrointestinal bleeding, are also characterized as having severe acute pancreatitis. This disorder is seen in approximately 20% of all patients with acute pancreatitis and has a mortality rate of 15% to 20% (Reddy & Long, 2004).

Gerontologic Considerations

Acute pancreatitis affects people of all ages, but the mortality rate associated with acute pancreatitis increases with advancing age. In addition, the pattern of complications changes with age. Younger patients tend to develop local complications; the incidence of multiple organ failure increases with age, possibly as a result of progressive decreases in physiologic function of major organs with increasing age. Close monitoring of major organ function (ie, lungs, kidneys) is essential, and aggressive treatment is necessary to reduce mortality from acute pancreatitis in the elderly.

Pathophysiology

Self-digestion of the pancreas by its own proteolytic enzymes, principally trypsin, causes acute pancreatitis. Eighty percent of patients with acute pancreatitis have biliary tract disease; however, only a small percentage of patients with gallstones develop pancreatitis (Yamada, 2003). Gallstones enter the common bile duct and lodge at the ampulla of Vater, obstructing the flow of pancreatic juice or causing a reflux of bile from the common bile duct into the pancreatic duct, thus activating the powerful enzymes within the pancreas. Normally, these remain in an inactive form until the pancreatic secretions reach the lumen of the duodenum. Activation of the enzymes can lead to vasodilation, increased vascular permeability, necrosis, erosion, and hemorrhage (Reddy & Long, 2004).

Long-term use of alcohol is commonly associated with acute episodes of pancreatitis, but the patient usually has had undiagnosed chronic pancreatitis before the first episode of acute pancreatitis occurs. Other, less common causes of pancreatitis include bacterial or viral infection, with pancreatitis occasionally developing as a complication of mumps virus. Spasm and edema of the ampulla of Vater, caused by duodenitis, can probably produce pancreatitis. Blunt abdominal trauma, peptic ulcer disease, ischemic vascular disease, hyperlipidemia, hypercalcemia, and the use of corticosteroids, thiazide diuretics, oral contraceptives, and other medications have also been associated with an increased incidence of pancreatitis. Acute pancreatitis may develop after surgery on or near the pancreas or after instrumentation of the pancreatic duct. Acute idiopathic pancreatitis accounts for up to 20% of the cases of acute pancreatitis (Swaroop et al., 2004). In addition, there is a small incidence of hereditary pancreatitis.

The overall mortality rate of patients with acute pancreatitis is high (10%) because of shock, anoxia, hypotension, or fluid and electrolyte imbalances (Swaroop et al., 2004). Attacks of acute pancreatitis may result in complete recovery, may recur without permanent damage, or may progress to chronic pancreatitis. The patient who is admitted to the hospital with a diagnosis of pancreatitis is acutely ill and needs expert nursing and medical care.

The severity of acute alcoholic pancreatitis and its outcomes can be predicted based on clinical and laboratory data (Chart 40-4).

Clinical Manifestations

Severe abdominal pain is the major symptom of pancreatitis that causes the patient to seek medical care. Abdominal pain and tenderness and back pain result from irritation and edema of the inflamed pancreas, which stimulate the nerve endings. Increased tension on the pancreatic capsule and obstruction of the pancreatic ducts also contribute to the pain. Typically, the pain occurs in the midepigastrium. Pain is frequently acute in onset, occurring 24 to 48 hours after a very heavy meal or alcohol ingestion, and it may be diffuse and difficult to localize. It is generally more severe after meals and is unrelieved by antacids. Pain may be accompanied by abdominal distention; a poorly defined, palpable abdominal mass; and decreased peristalsis. Pain caused by pancreatitis is accompanied frequently by vomiting that fails to relieve the pain or nausea.

The patient appears acutely ill. Abdominal guarding is present. A rigid or board-like abdomen may develop and is generally an ominous sign; the abdomen may remain soft in the absence of peritonitis. Ecchymosis (bruising) in the flank or around the umbilicus may indicate severe pancreatitis. Nausea and vomiting are common in acute pancreatitis. The emesis is usually gastric in origin but may also be bile-stained. Fever, jaundice, mental confusion, and agitation may also occur.

Hypotension is typical and reflects hypovolemia and shock caused by the loss of large amounts of protein-rich fluid into the tissues and peritoneal cavity. In addition to hypotension, the patient may develop tachycardia, cyanosis, and cold, clammy skin. Acute renal failure is common.

Respiratory distress and hypoxia are common, and the patient may develop diffuse pulmonary infiltrates, dyspnea, tachypnea, and abnormal blood gas values. Myocardial depression, hypocalcemia, hyperglycemia, and disseminated intravascular coagulation (DIC) may also occur with acute pancreatitis.

CHART 40-4

*Criteria for Predicting Severity of Pancreatitis**

CRITERIA ON ADMISSION TO HOSPITAL

Age >55 years
WBC >16,000 mm^3
Serum glucose >200 mg/dL (>11.1 mmol/L)
Serum LDH >350 IU/L (>350 U/L)
AST >250 U/mL (120 U/L)

CRITERIA WITHIN 48 HOURS OF HOSPITAL ADMISSION

Fall in hematocrit >10% (>0.10)
BUN increase >5 mg/dL (>1.7 mmol/L)
Serum calcium <8 mg/dL (<2.0 mmol/L)
Base deficit >4 mEq/L (>4 mmol/L)
Fluid retention or sequestration >6 L
PO_2 <60 mm Hg

Two or fewer signs, 1% mortality; 3 or 4 signs, 15% mortality; 5 or 6 signs, 40% mortality; >6 signs, 100% mortality.

*Note: The more risk factors a patient has, the greater the severity and likelihood of complications or death.

Assessment and Diagnostic Findings

The diagnosis of acute pancreatitis is based on a history of abdominal pain, the presence of known risk factors, physical examination findings, and diagnostic findings. Serum amylase and lipase levels are used in making the diagnosis of acute pancreatitis. In 90% of the cases, serum amylase and lipase levels rise in excess of three times their normal upper limit within 24 hours (Reddy & Long, 2004). Serum amylase usually returns to normal within 48 to 72 hours, but serum lipase levels may remain elevated for 5 to 7 days (Fishman, Hoffman, Klausner, et al., 2004). Urinary amylase levels also become elevated and remain elevated longer than serum amylase levels. The white blood cell count is usually elevated; hypocalcemia is present in many patients and correlates well with the severity of pancreatitis. Transient hyperglycemia and glucosuria and elevated serum bilirubin levels occur in some patients with acute pancreatitis.

X-ray studies of the abdomen and chest may be obtained to differentiate pancreatitis from other disorders that can cause similar symptoms and to detect pleural effusions. Ultrasound and contrast-enhanced computed tomographic (CT) scans are used to identify an increase in the diameter of the pancreas and to detect pancreatic cysts, abscesses, or pseudocysts.

Hematocrit and hemoglobin levels are used to monitor the patient for bleeding. Peritoneal fluid, obtained through paracentesis or peritoneal lavage, may contain increased levels of pancreatic enzymes. The stools of patients with pancreatic disease are often bulky, pale, and foul-smelling. Fat content of stools varies between 50% and 90% in pancreatic disease; normally, the fat content is 20% (Yamada, 2003). ERCP is rarely used in the diagnostic evaluation of acute pancreatitis, because the patient is acutely ill; however, it may be valuable in the treatment of gallstone pancreatitis.

Medical Management

Management of acute pancreatitis is directed toward relieving symptoms and preventing or treating complications. All oral intake is withheld, to inhibit stimulation of the pancreas and its secretion of enzymes. Parenteral nutrition is usually an important part of therapy, particularly in debilitated patients, because of the extreme metabolic stress associated with acute pancreatitis (McIntyre, Steigmann & Eiseman, 2004). Ongoing research has shown positive outcomes with the use of enteral feedings (Reddy & Long, 2004). The current recommendation is that, whenever possible, the enteral route should be used to meet nutritional needs in patients with pancreatitis. This strategy also has been found to prevent infectious complications, safely and cost effectively (Swaroop et al., 2004). Patients who do not tolerate enteral feeding require parenteral nutrition. Nasogastric suction may be used to relieve nausea and vomiting and to decrease painful abdominal distention and paralytic ileus. Research data do not support the routine use of nasogastric tubes to remove stomach secretions in an effort to limit pancreatic secretion. Histamine-2 (H_2) antagonists such as cimetidine (Tagamet) and ranitidine (Zantac) may be prescribed to decrease pancreatic activity by inhibiting secretion of hydrogen chloride. Proton pump inhibitors such as pantoprazole (Protonix) may be used for patients who do not tolerate H_2 antagonists or for whom this therapy is ineffective.

Pain Management

Adequate administration of analgesia is essential during the course of acute pancreatitis to provide sufficient pain relief and to minimize restlessness, which may stimulate pancreatic secretion further. Pain relief may require parenteral opioids such as morphine. The use of morphine was avoided in the past because of concern that it could cause painful spasms of the sphincter of Oddi and worsen pancreatitis. However, there is no evidence that this affects the outcome of the disease. Meperidine (Demerol) had been the medication of choice, although all opioids stimulate the sphincter of Oddi to some degree. There is no clinical evidence to support the use of meperidine for pain relief in pancreatitis, and, in fact, accumulation of its metabolites can cause CNS irritability and possibly seizures. The current recommendation for pain management is the use of morphine (Reddy & Long, 2004; Swaroop et al., 2004). Hydromorphone (Dilaudid) may also be effective, but more research is needed to identify the best option for pain management in the patient with acute pancreatitis. Antiemetic agents may be prescribed to prevent vomiting.

Intensive Care

Correction of fluid and blood loss and low albumin levels is necessary to maintain fluid volume and prevent renal failure. The patient is usually acutely ill and is monitored in the intensive care unit, where hemodynamic monitoring and arterial blood gas monitoring are initiated. Antibiotic agents may be prescribed if infection is present. The role of prophylactic antibiotics is controversial and still under study. Insulin may be required if hyperglycemia occurs. Intensive insulin therapy (continuous infusion) in the critically ill patient has undergone much study and has shown promise in terms of positive patient outcomes when compared to intermittent insulin dosing (Van den Berghe, Wouters, Bouillon, et al., 2003).

Respiratory Care

Aggressive respiratory care is indicated because of the high risk for elevation of the diaphragm, pulmonary infiltrates and effusion, and atelectasis. Hypoxemia occurs in a significant number of patients with acute pancreatitis, even with normal x-ray findings. Respiratory care may range from close monitoring of arterial blood gases to use of humidified oxygen to intubation and mechanical ventilation (see Chapter 25 for further discussion).

Biliary Drainage

Placement of biliary drains (for external drainage) and stents (indwelling tubes) in the pancreatic duct through endoscopy has been performed to reestablish drainage of the pancreas. This has resulted in decreased pain and increased weight gain.

Surgical Intervention

Although surgery is often risky because the acutely ill patient is a poor surgical risk, it may be performed to assist in the diagnosis of pancreatitis (diagnostic laparotomy), to establish pancreatic drainage, or to resect or débride a necrotic pancreas. The patient who undergoes pancreatic surgery may have multiple drains in place postoperatively, as well as a surgical incision that is left open for irrigation and repacking every 2 to 3 days to remove necrotic debris (Fig. 40-6).

Postacute Management

Antacids may be used after acute pancreatitis begins to resolve. Oral feedings that are low in fat and protein are initiated gradually. Caffeine and alcohol are eliminated from the diet. If the episode of pancreatitis occurred during treatment with thiazide diuretics, corticosteroids, or oral contraceptives, these medications are discontinued. Follow-up may include ultrasound, x-ray studies, or ERCP to determine whether the pancreatitis is resolving and to assess for abscesses and pseudocysts. ERCP may also be used to identify the cause of acute pancreatitis if it is in question and for endoscopic sphincterotomy and removal of gallstones from the common bile duct.

Nursing Process

The Patient With Acute Pancreatitis

Assessment

The health history focuses on the presence and character of the abdominal pain and discomfort. The nurse assesses the patient for the presence of pain, its

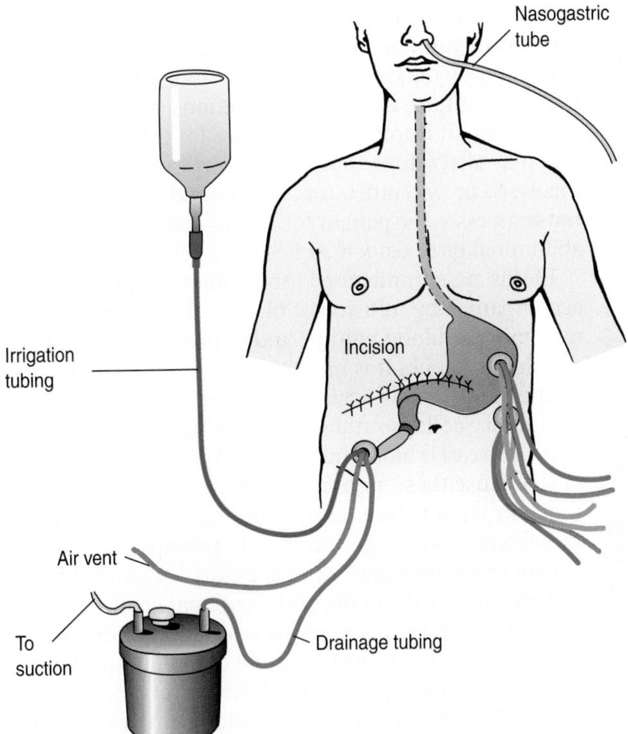

FIGURE 40-6. Multiple sump tubes are used after pancreatic surgery. Triple-lumen tubes consist of ports that provide tubing for irrigation, air venting, and drainage.

location, its relationship to eating and to alcohol consumption, and the effectiveness of pain relief measures. It also is important to assess the patient's nutritional and fluid status, history of gallbladder attacks, and alcohol use. The patient history is obtained for gastrointestinal problems, including nausea, vomiting, diarrhea, and passage of fatty stools. The nurse assesses the abdomen for pain, tenderness, guarding, and bowel sounds, noting the presence of a board-like or soft abdomen. It also is important to assess respiratory status, respiratory rate and pattern, and breath sounds. Normal and adventitious breath sounds and abnormal findings on chest percussion, including dullness at the bases of the lungs and abnormal tactile fremitus, are documented. The nurse assesses the emotional and psychological status of the patient and family, and, because of anxiety surrounding the severity of the symptoms and the acuteness of illness, notes their ability to cope.

Diagnosis

Nursing Diagnoses

Based on all the assessment data, the major nursing diagnoses of the patient with acute pancreatitis may include the following:

- Acute pain related to inflammation, edema, distention of the pancreas, and peritoneal irritation
- Ineffective breathing pattern related to severe pain, pulmonary infiltrates, pleural effusion, atelectasis, and elevated diaphragm
- Imbalanced nutrition, less than body requirements, related to reduced food intake and increased metabolic demands
- Impaired skin integrity related to poor nutritional status, bed rest, multiple drains, and surgical wound

Collaborative Problems/ Potential Complications

Based on assessment data, potential complications that may occur include the following:

- Fluid and electrolyte disturbances
- Necrosis of the pancreas
- Shock and multiple organ dysfunction syndrome (MODS)

Planning and Goals

The major goals for the patient include relief of pain and discomfort, improved respiratory function, improved nutritional status, maintenance of skin integrity, and absence of complications.

Nursing Interventions

Relieving Pain and Discomfort

Because the pathologic process responsible for pain is autodigestion of the pancreas, the objectives of therapy are to relieve pain and decrease secretion of pancreatic enzymes. The pain of acute pancreatitis is often very severe, necessitating the liberal use of analgesics. The current recommendation for pain management in this population is parenteral opioids, preferably morphine (Reddy & Long, 2004; Swaroop et al., 2004). Alternatively, hydromorphone may be used (Yamada, 2003). Oral feedings are withheld to decrease the formation and secretion of secretin. The patient is maintained on parenteral fluids and electrolytes to restore and maintain fluid balance. Nasogastric suction may be used to relieve nausea and vomiting or to treat abdominal distention and paralytic ileus. The nurse provides frequent oral hygiene and care to decrease discomfort from the nasogastric tube and relieve dryness of the mouth.

The acutely ill patient is maintained on bed rest to decrease the metabolic rate and reduce the secretion of pancreatic and gastric enzymes. If the patient experiences increasing severity of pain, the nurse reports this to the physician, because the patient may be experiencing hemorrhage of the pancreas or the dose of analgesic may be inadequate.

The patient with acute pancreatitis often has a clouded sensorium because of severe pain, fluid and electrolyte disturbances, and hypoxia. Therefore, the nurse provides frequent and repeated but simple explanations about the need for withholding fluids, maintenance of gastric suction, and bed rest.

Improving Breathing Pattern

The nurse maintains the patient in a semi-Fowler's position to decrease pressure on the diaphragm by a distended abdomen and to increase respiratory expansion. Frequent changes of position are necessary to prevent atelectasis and pooling of respiratory secretions. Pulmonary assessment and monitoring of pulse oximetry or arterial blood gases are essential to detect changes in respiratory status so that early treatment can be initiated. The nurse instructs the patient in techniques of coughing and deep breathing and in the use of incentive spirometry to improve respiratory function and encourages and assists the patient to perform these activities every hour.

Improving Nutritional Status

The patient with acute pancreatitis is not permitted food or oral fluid intake. However, it is important to assess the patient's nutritional status and to note factors that alter the patient's nutritional requirements (eg, temperature elevation, surgery, drainage). Laboratory test results and daily weights are useful to monitor the nutritional status.

Enteral or parenteral nutrition may be prescribed. In addition to administering enteral or parenteral nutrition, the nurse monitors serum glucose levels every 4 to 6 hours. As the acute symptoms subside, the nurse gradually reintroduces oral feedings. Between acute attacks, the patient receives a diet that is high in carbohydrates and low in fats and proteins. The patient should avoid heavy meals and alcoholic beverages.

Improving Skin Integrity

The patient is at risk for skin breakdown because of poor nutritional status, enforced bed rest, and restlessness, which may result in pressure ulcers and breaks in tissue integrity. In addition, the patient who has undergone surgery may have multiple drains or an open surgical incision and is at risk for skin breakdown and infection. The nurse carefully assesses the wound, drainage sites, and skin for signs of infection, inflammation, and breakdown. The nurse carries out wound care as prescribed and takes precautions to protect intact skin from contact with drainage. Consultation with an enterostomal therapist (also referred to as a wound care specialist or wound-ostomy-continence nurse) is often helpful in identifying appropriate skin care devices and protocols. It is important to turn the patient every 2 hours; use of specialty beds may be indicated to prevent skin breakdown.

Monitoring and Managing Potential Complications

Fluid and electrolyte disturbances are common complications because of nausea, vomiting, movement of fluid from the vascular compartment to the peritoneal cavity, diaphoresis, fever, and the use of gastric suction. The nurse assesses the patient's fluid and electrolyte status by noting skin turgor and moistness of mucous membranes. The nurse weighs the patient daily and carefully measures fluid intake and output, including urine output, nasogastric secretions, and diarrhea. In addition, it is important to assess for other factors that may affect fluid and electrolyte status, including increased body temperature and wound drainage. The nurse assesses the patient for ascites and measures abdominal girth daily if ascites is suspected.

Fluids are administered intravenously and may be accompanied by infusion of blood or blood products to maintain the blood volume and to prevent or treat hypovolemic shock. It is important to keep emergency medications readily available because of the risk for circulatory collapse and shock. The nurse promptly reports decreased blood pressure and reduced urine output, because these signs may indicate hypovolemia and shock or renal failure. Low serum calcium and magnesium levels may occur and require prompt treatment.

Pancreatic necrosis is a major cause of morbidity and mortality in patients with acute pancreatitis. The patient who develops necrosis is at risk for hemorrhage, septic shock, and multiple organ failure. The patient may undergo diagnostic procedures to confirm pancreatic necrosis; surgical débridement or insertion of multiple drains may be performed. The patient with pancreatic necrosis is usually critically ill and requires expert medical and nursing management, including hemodynamic monitoring in the intensive care unit.

In addition to carefully monitoring vital signs and other signs and symptoms, the nurse is responsible for administering prescribed fluids, medications, and blood products; assisting with supportive management, such as use of a ventilator; preventing additional complications; and attending to the patient's physical and psychological care.

Shock and multiple organ failure may occur with acute pancreatitis. Hypovolemic shock may occur as a result of hypovolemia and sequestering of fluid in the peritoneal cavity. Hemorrhagic shock may occur with hemorrhagic pancreatitis. Septic shock may occur with bacterial infection of the pancreas. Cardiac dysfunction may occur as a result of fluid and electrolyte disturbances, acid–base imbalances, and release of toxic substances into the circulation.

The nurse closely monitors the patient for early signs of neurologic, cardiovascular, renal, and respiratory dysfunction. The nurse must be prepared to respond quickly to rapid changes in the patient's status, treatments, and therapies. In addition, it is important to inform the family about the status and progress of the patient and to allow them to spend time with the patient. (Management of shock is discussed in detail in Chapter 15.)

Promoting Home and Community-Based Care

TEACHING PATIENTS SELF-CARE

The patient who has survived an episode of acute pancreatitis has been acutely ill. A prolonged period is needed to regain strength and return to the previous level of activity. The patient is often still weak and debilitated for weeks or months after an acute episode of pancreatitis. Because of the severity of the acute illness, the patient may not recall many of the explanations and instructions given during the acute phase. Teaching often needs to be repeated and reinforced. The nurse instructs the patient about the factors implicated in the onset of acute pancreatitis and about the need to avoid high-fat foods, heavy meals, and alcohol. It is important to give the patient and family verbal and written instructions about signs and symptoms of acute pancreatitis and possible complications that should be reported promptly to the physician.

If acute pancreatitis is a result of biliary tract disease, such as gallstones and gallbladder disease, additional explanations are needed about required dietary modifications. If the pancreatitis is a result of alcohol abuse, the nurse reminds the patient of the importance of eliminating all alcohol.

CONTINUING CARE

A referral for home care is often indicated. This enables the nurse to assess the patient's physical and psychological status and adherence to the therapeutic regimen. The nurse also assesses the home situation and reinforces instructions about fluid and nutrition intake and avoidance of alcohol. After the acute attack has subsided, some patients may be inclined to return to their previous drinking habits. The nurse provides specific information about resources and support groups that may be of assistance in avoiding alcohol in the future. Referral to Alcoholics Anonymous or other appropriate support groups is essential. (See the accompanying plan of nursing care in Chart 40-5 for the patient with acute pancreatitis.)

Evaluation

Expected Patient Outcomes

Expected patient outcomes may include the following:

1. Reports relief of pain and discomfort
   a. Uses analgesics and anticholinergics as prescribed, without overuse
   b. Maintains bed rest as prescribed
   c. Avoids alcohol to decrease abdominal pain
2. Experiences improved respiratory function
   a. Changes position in bed frequently
   b. Coughs, takes deep breaths, uses incentive spirometer at least every hour while awake
   c. Demonstrates normal respiratory rate and pattern, full lung expansion, normal breath sounds
   d. Demonstrates normal body temperature and absence of respiratory infection
3. Achieves nutritional and fluid and electrolyte balance
   a. Reports decrease in number of episodes of diarrhea
   b. Identifies and consumes high-carbohydrate, low-protein foods
   c. Explains rationale for eliminating alcohol intake
   d. Maintains adequate fluid intake within prescribed guidelines
   e. Exhibits adequate urine output
4. Exhibits intact skin
   a. Skin is without breakdown or infection
   b. Drainage is contained adequately
5. Exhibits absence of complications
   a. Demonstrates normal skin turgor, moist mucous membranes, normal serum electrolyte levels
   b. Exhibits stabilization of weight, with no increase in abdominal girth
   c. Exhibits normal neurologic, cardiovascular, renal, and respiratory function

Chronic Pancreatitis

Chronic pancreatitis is an inflammatory disorder that is characterized by progressive anatomic and functional destruction of the pancreas. As cells are replaced by fibrous tissue with repeated attacks of pancreatitis, pressure within the pancreas increases. The end result is mechanical obstruction of the pancreatic and common bile ducts and the duodenum. Additionally, there is atrophy of the epithelium of the ducts, inflammation, and destruction of the secreting cells of the pancreas.

Alcohol consumption in Western societies and malnutrition worldwide are the major causes of chronic pancreatitis. Excessive and prolonged consumption of alcohol accounts for approximately 70% to 80% of all cases of chronic pancreatitis (Reddy & Long, 2004). The incidence of pancreatitis is 50 times greater in people with alcoholism than in those who do not abuse alcohol. Long-term alcohol consumption causes hypersecretion of protein in pancreatic secretions, resulting in protein plugs and calculi within the pancreatic ducts. Alcohol also has a direct toxic effect on the cells of the pancreas. Damage to these cells is more likely to occur and to be more severe in patients whose diets are poor in protein content and either very high or very low in fat.

Clinical Manifestations

Chronic pancreatitis is characterized by recurring attacks of severe upper abdominal and back pain, accompanied by vomiting. Attacks are often so painful that opioids, even in large doses, do not provide relief. As the disease progresses, recurring attacks of pain are more severe, more frequent, and of longer duration. Some patients experience continuous severe pain; others have a dull, nagging constant pain. The risk of opioid dependence is increased in pancreatitis because of the chronic nature and severity of the pain. In some patients, chronic pancreatitis is painless. Approximately 20% of patients, even those with severe disease, report no pain (Reddy & Long, 2004).

Weight loss is a major problem in chronic pancreatitis: more than 75% of patients experience significant weight loss, usually caused by decreased dietary intake secondary to

(text continues on page 1368)

CHART 40-5

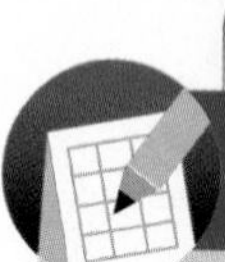

Plan of Nursing Care | Care of the Patient With Acute Pancreatitis

Nursing Diagnosis: Acute pain and discomfort related to edema, distention of the pancreas, and peritoneal irritation
Goal: Relief of pain and discomfort

NURSING INTERVENTIONS	RATIONALE	EXPECTED OUTCOMES
1. Administer morphine frequently, as prescribed, to achieve level of pain acceptable to patient based on patient's level of pain and discomfort.	1. Morphine acts by depressing the central nervous system and thereby increasing the patient's pain threshold. Meperidine (Demerol) is avoided because it has failed acute pain studies and it possesses toxic metabolites.	• Reports relief of pain • Moves and turns without increasing pain and discomfort • Rests comfortably and sleeps for increasing periods • Reports less frequent episodes of pain, discomfort, and cramping • Experiences enhanced pain relief • Reports increased feelings of well-being and security with the health care team
2. Using a pain scale, assess pain level before and after administration of analgesic.	2. Assessment and control of pain are important because restlessness increases body metabolism, which stimulates the secretion of pancreatic and gastric enzymes.	
3. Report unrelieved pain or increasing intensity of pain.	3. Pain may increase pancreatic enzymes and may also indicate pancreatic hemorrhage.	
4. Assist the patient to assume positions of comfort; turn and reposition every 2 hours.	4. Frequent turning relieves pressure and assists in preventing pulmonary and vascular complications.	
5. Use nonpharmacologic interventions for relieving pain (eg, relaxation, focused breathing, diversion).	5. Use of nonpharmacologic methods will enhance the effects of analgesics. Gate control theory suggests that cutaneous stimulation closes the pain pathways.	
6. Listen to patient's expression of pain experience.	6. Demonstration of caring can help to decrease anxiety.	

Goal: Relief of pain related to stimulation of the pancreas

NURSING INTERVENTIONS	RATIONALE	EXPECTED OUTCOMES
1. Administer anticholinergic medications as prescribed.	1. Anticholinergic medications reduce gastric and pancreatic secretion.	• Reports relief of pain, discomfort, and abdominal cramping • Consumes no fluid and food during acute phase • Maintains bed rest • Identifies rationale for fluid and dietary restrictions and use of nasogastric drainage • Cooperates with insertion of nasogastric tube and suction
2. Withhold oral intake.	2. Pancreatic secretion is increased by food and fluid intake.	
3. Maintain the patient on bed rest.	3. Bed rest decreases body metabolism and thus reduces pancreatic and gastric secretions.	
4. Maintain continuous nasogastric drainage if paralytic ileus or nausea and vomiting, abdominal distention are present. a. Measure gastric secretions at specified intervals.	4. Nasogastric suction relieves nausea, vomiting, and abdominal distention. Decompression of the intestines (if intestinal intubation is used) also assists in relieving respiratory distress.	

CHART 40-5

Plan of Nursing Care — Care of the Patient With Acute Pancreatitis (Continued)

NURSING INTERVENTIONS	RATIONALE	EXPECTED OUTCOMES
b. Observe and record color and viscosity of gastric secretions. c. Ensure that the nasogastric tube is patent to permit free drainage.		

Nursing Diagnosis: Discomfort related to nasogastric tube
Goal: Relief of discomfort associated with nasogastric intubation used to treat ileus, vomiting, distention

NURSING INTERVENTIONS	RATIONALE	EXPECTED OUTCOMES
1. Use water-soluble lubricant around external nares.	1. Prevents irritation of nares	• Exhibits intact skin and tissue of nares at site of nasogastric tube insertion • Reports no pain or irritation of nares or oropharynx • Exhibits moist, clean mucous membranes of mouth and nasopharynx • States that thirst is relieved by oral hygiene • Identifies rationale for nasogastric tube and suction
2. Turn patient at intervals; avoid pressure or tension on nasogastric tube	2. Relieves pressure of tube on esophageal and gastric mucosa	
3. Provide oral hygiene and gargling solutions without alcohol.	3. Relieves dryness and irritation of oropharynx	
4. Explain rationale for use of nasogastric drainage.	4. Assists patient to cooperate with the drainage, nasogastric tube, and suction.	

Nursing Diagnosis: Imbalanced nutrition: less than body requirements related to inadequate dietary intake, impaired pancreatic secretions, increased nutritional needs secondary to acute illness, and increased body temperature
Goal: Improvement in nutritional status

NURSING INTERVENTIONS	RATIONALE	EXPECTED OUTCOMES
1. Assess current nutritional status and increased metabolic requirements.	1. Alteration in pancreatic secretions interferes with normal digestive processes. Acute illness, infection, and fever increase metabolic needs.	• Maintains normal body weight • Demonstrates no additional weight loss • Maintains normal serum glucose levels • Reports decreasing episodes of vomiting and diarrhea • Reports return of normal stool characteristics and bowel pattern • Consumes foods high in carbohydrate, low in fat and protein • Explains rationale for high-carbohydrate, low-fat, low-protein diet • Eliminates alcohol from diet • Explains rationale for limiting coffee intake and avoiding spicy foods
2. Monitor serum glucose levels and administer insulin as prescribed.	2. Impairment of endocrine function of the pancreas leads to increased serum glucose levels.	
3. Administer intravenous fluid and electrolytes, enteral or parenteral nutrition as prescribed.	3. Parenteral administration of fluids and electrolytes, and enteral or parenteral nutrients are essential to provide fluids, calories, electrolytes, and nutrients when oral intake is prohibited.	
4. Provide high-carbohydrate, low-protein, low-fat diet when tolerated.	4. These foods increase caloric intake without stimulating pancreatic secretions beyond the ability of the pancreas to respond.	

continued >

CHART 40-5

Plan of Nursing Care — Care of the Patient With Acute Pancreatitis (Continued)

NURSING INTERVENTIONS	RATIONALE	EXPECTED OUTCOMES
5. Instruct patient to eliminate alcohol and refer to Alcoholics Anonymous if indicated.	5. Alcohol intake produces further damage to pancreas and precipitates attacks of acute pancreatitis.	• Participates in Alcoholics Anonymous or other counseling approach
6. Counsel patient to avoid excessive use of coffee and spicy foods.	6. Coffee and spicy foods increase pancreatic and gastric secretions.	• Returns to and maintains desirable weight
7. Monitor daily weights.	7. This provides a baseline and a means to measure weight gain or weight loss.	

Nursing Diagnosis: Ineffective breathing pattern related to splinting from severe pain, pulmonary infiltrates, pleural effusion, and atelectasis
Goal: Improvement in respiratory function

NURSING INTERVENTIONS	RATIONALE	EXPECTED OUTCOMES
1. Assess respiratory status (rate, pattern, breath sounds), pulse oximetry, and arterial blood gases.	1. Acute pancreatitis produces retroperitoneal edema, elevation of the diaphragm, pleural effusion, and inadequate lung ventilation. Intra-abdominal infection and labored breathing increase the body's metabolic demands, which further decreases pulmonary reserve and leads to respiratory failure.	• Demonstrates normal respiratory rate and pattern and full lung expansion • Demonstrates normal breath sounds and absence of adventitious breath sounds • Demonstrates normal arterial blood gases and pulse oximetry • Maintains semi-Fowler's position when in bed
2. Maintain semi-Fowler's position.	2. Decreases pressure on diaphragm and allows greater lung expansion.	• Changes position in bed frequently
3. Instruct and encourage patient to take deep breaths and to cough every hour.	3. Taking deep breaths and coughing will clear the airways and reduce atelectasis.	• Coughs and takes deep breaths at least every hour • Demonstrates normal body temperature
4. Assist patient to turn and change position every 2 hours.	4. Changing position frequently assists aeration and drainage of all lobes of the lungs.	• Exhibits no signs or symptoms of respiratory infection or impairment
5. Reduce the excessive metabolism of the body. a. Administer antibiotics as prescribed. b. Place patient in an air-conditioned room. c. Administer nasal oxygen as required for hypoxia. d. Use a hypothermia blanket if necessary.	5. Pancreatitis produces a severe peritoneal and retroperitoneal reaction that causes fever, tachycardia, and accelerated respirations. Placing the patient in an air-conditioned room and supporting the patient with oxygen therapy decrease the workload of the respiratory system and the tissue utilization of oxygen. Reduction of fever and pulse rate decreases the metabolic demands on the body.	• Is alert and responsive to environment

CHART 40-5

Plan of Nursing Care — Care of the Patient With Acute Pancreatitis (Continued)

Collaborative Problem: Fluid and electrolyte disturbances, hypovolemia, shock
Goal: Improvement in fluid and electrolyte status, prevention of hypovolemia and shock

NURSING INTERVENTIONS	RATIONALE	EXPECTED OUTCOMES
1. Assess fluid and electrolyte status (skin turgor, mucous membranes, urine output, vital signs, hemodynamic parameters).	1. The amount and type of fluid and electrolyte replacement are determined by the status of the blood pressure, the laboratory evaluations of serum electrolyte and blood urea nitrogen levels, the urinary volume, and the assessment of the patient's condition.	• Exhibits moist mucous membranes and normal skin turgor • Exhibits normal blood pressure without evidence of postural (orthostatic) hypotension • Excretes adequate urine volume • Exhibits normal, not excessive, thirst • Maintains normal pulse and respiratory rate • Remains alert and responsive • Exhibits normal arterial pressures and blood gases • Exhibits normal electrolyte levels • Exhibits no signs or symptoms of calcium deficit (eg, tetany, carpopedal spasm) • Exhibits no additional losses of fluids and electrolytes through vomiting, diarrhea, or diaphoresis • Reports stabilization of weight • Demonstrates no increase in abdominal girth • Demonstrates no fluid wave on palpation of the abdomen • Demonstrates stable organ function without manifestations of failure
2. Assess sources of fluid and electrolyte loss (vomiting, diarrhea, nasogastric drainage, excessive diaphoresis).	2. Electrolyte losses occur from nasogastric suctioning, severe diaphoresis, emesis, and as a result of the patient's being in a fasting state.	
3. Combat shock if present. a. Administer corticosteroids as prescribed if patient does not respond to conventional treatment. b. Evaluate the amount of urinary output. Attempt to maintain this at 50 mL/h.	3. Extensive acute pancreatitis may cause peripheral vascular collapse and shock. Blood and plasma may be lost into the abdominal cavity, and, therefore, there is a decreased blood and plasma volume. The toxins from the bacteria of a necrotic pancreas may cause shock.	
4. Administer blood products, fluids, and electrolytes (sodium, potassium, chloride) as prescribed.	4. Patients with hemorrhagic pancreatitis lose large amounts of blood and plasma, which decreases effective circulation and blood volume.	
5. Administer plasma and blood products as prescribed.	5. Replacement with blood, plasma or albumin assists in ensuring effective circulating blood volume.	
6. Keep a supply of intravenous calcium gluconate readily available.	6. Calcium may be prescribed to prevent or treat tetany, which may result from calcium losses into retroperitoneal (peri-pancreatic) exudate	
7. Assess abdomen for ascites formation: a. Measure abdominal girth daily. b. Weigh patient daily. c. Palpate abdomen for fluid wave.	7. During acute pancreatitis, plasma may be lost into the abdominal cavity, which diminishes the blood volume.	
8. Monitor for manifestations of multiple organ failure: neurologic, cardiovascular, renal, and respiratory dysfunction.	8. All body systems may fail if pancreatitis is severe and treatment is ineffective.	

anorexia or fear that eating will precipitate another attack. Malabsorption occurs late in the disease, when as little as 10% of pancreatic function remains (Friedman et al., 2003). As a result, digestion, especially of proteins and fats, is impaired. The stools become frequent, frothy, and foul-smelling because of impaired fat digestion, which results in stools with a high fat content. This is referred to as **steatorrhea.** As the disease progresses, calcification of the gland may occur, and calcium stones may form within the ducts.

Assessment and Diagnostic Findings

ERCP is the most useful study in the diagnosis of chronic pancreatitis. It provides detail about the anatomy of the pancreas and the pancreatic and biliary ducts. It is also helpful in obtaining tissue for analysis and differentiating pancreatitis from other conditions, such as carcinoma. Various imaging procedures, including magnetic resonance imaging (MRI), CT scans, and ultrasound, have been useful in the diagnostic evaluation of patients with suspected pancreatic disorders. A CT scan or ultrasound study is also helpful to detect pancreatic cysts.

A glucose tolerance test evaluates pancreatic islet cell function and provides necessary information for making decisions about surgical resection of the pancreas. An abnormal glucose tolerance test may indicate the presence of diabetes associated with pancreatitis. Acute exacerbations of chronic pancreatitis may result in increased serum amylase levels. Steatorrhea can be confirmed by laboratory analysis of fecal fat content (McIntyre et al., 2004).

Medical Management

The management of chronic pancreatitis depends on its probable cause in each patient. Treatment is directed toward preventing and managing acute attacks, relieving pain and discomfort, and managing exocrine and endocrine insufficiency of pancreatitis.

Nonsurgical Management

Nonsurgical approaches may be indicated for the patient who refuses surgery, who is a poor surgical risk, or whose disease and symptoms do not warrant surgical intervention. Endoscopy to remove pancreatic duct stones and strictures may be effective in selected patients to manage pain and relieve obstruction (Reddy & Long, 2004).

Management of abdominal pain and discomfort is similar to that of acute pancreatitis; however, the focus is usually on the use of nonopioid methods to manage pain. Persistent, unrelieved pain is often the most difficult aspect of management (Kelly et al., 2004; Reddy & Long, 2004). The physician, nurse, and dietitian emphasize to the patient and family the importance of avoiding alcohol and foods that have produced abdominal pain and discomfort in the past. The health care team stresses to the patient that no other treatment is likely to relieve pain if the patient continues to consume alcohol.

Diabetes mellitus resulting from dysfunction of the pancreatic islet cells is treated with diet, insulin, or oral antidiabetic agents. The hazard of severe hypoglycemia with alcohol consumption is stressed to the patient and family. Pancreatic enzyme replacement is indicated for the patient with malabsorption and steatorrhea. A proton pump inhibitor (omeprazole [Prilosec], lansoprazole [Prevacid]) is administered with enzyme therapy to reduce gastric acid inactivation of enzymes (Reddy & Long, 2004).

Surgical Management

Surgery is carried out to relieve abdominal pain and discomfort, restore drainage of pancreatic secretions, and reduce the frequency of acute attacks of pancreatitis. The type of surgery that is performed depends on the anatomic and functional abnormalities of the pancreas, including the location of disease within the pancreas, the presence of diabetes, exocrine insufficiency, biliary stenosis, and pseudocysts of the pancreas. Other considerations for surgery selection include the patient's likelihood for continued use of alcohol and the likelihood that the patient will be able to manage the endocrine or exocrine changes that are expected after surgery.

Pancreaticojejunostomy (also referred to as Roux-en-Y), with a side-to-side anastomosis or joining of the pancreatic duct to the jejunum, allows drainage of the pancreatic secretions into the jejunum. Pain relief occurs within 6 months in more than 80% of the patients who undergo this procedure, but pain returns in a substantial number of patients as the disease progresses (Friedman et al., 2003; Reddy & Long, 2004).

Other surgical procedures may be performed for different degrees and types of underlying disorders. These procedures include revision of the sphincter of the ampulla of Vater, internal drainage of a pancreatic cyst into the stomach (see later discussion), insertion of a stent, and wide resection or removal of the pancreas. A Whipple resection (pancreaticoduodenectomy) can be carried out to relieve the pain of chronic pancreatitis.

Autotransplantation or implantation of the patient's pancreatic islet cells has been attempted to preserve the endocrine function of the pancreas in patients who have undergone total pancreatectomy. Moving the pancreas to another location within the abdomen with revised vascular and enteric anastomoses may provide relief from pain and preserve endocrine function (Reddy & Long, 2004). Testing and refinement of these procedures continue in an effort to improve outcomes.

When chronic pancreatitis develops as a result of gallbladder disease, the obstruction is treated by surgery to explore the common duct and remove the stones; usually, the gallbladder is removed at the same time. In addition, an attempt is made to improve the drainage of the common bile duct and the pancreatic duct by dividing the sphincter of Oddi, a muscle that is located at the ampulla of Vater (this surgical procedure is known as a sphincterotomy). A T-tube usually is placed in the common bile duct, requiring a drainage system to collect the bile postoperatively. Nursing care after such surgery is similar to that indicated after other biliary tract surgery.

Endoscopic and laparoscopic procedures such as distal pancreatectomy, longitudinal decompression of the pancreatic duct, and nerve denervation have been performed and are being refined. Minimally invasive procedures to treat chronic pancreatitis may prove to be successful adjuncts in the management of this complex disorder (Kelly et al., 2004).

Patients who undergo surgery for chronic pancreatitis may experience weight gain and improved nutritional status; this may result from reduction in pain associated with eating rather than from correction of malabsorption. However, morbidity and mortality after these surgical procedures are high because of the poor physical condition of the patient before surgery and the concomitant presence of cirrhosis. Even after undergoing these surgical procedures, the patient is likely to continue to have pain and impaired digestion secondary to pancreatitis, unless alcohol is avoided completely.

Pancreatic Cysts

As a result of the local necrosis that occurs at the time of acute pancreatitis, collections of fluid may form close to the pancreas. These fluid collections become walled off by fibrous tissue and are called pancreatic pseudocysts. They are the most common type of pancreatic cyst. Less common cysts occur as a result of congenital anomalies or secondary to chronic pancreatitis or trauma to the pancreas.

Diagnosis of pancreatic cysts and pseudocysts is made by ultrasound, CT scan, and ERCP. ERCP may be used to define the anatomy of the pancreas and evaluate the patency of pancreatic drainage. Pancreatic pseudocysts may be of considerable size. When pancreatic pseudocysts enlarge, they impinge on and displace the adjacent stomach or the colon, because of the location of pseudocysts behind the posterior peritoneum. Eventually, through pressure or secondary infection, they produce symptoms and require drainage.

Drainage into the gastrointestinal tract or through the skin and abdominal wall may be established. In the latter instance, the drainage is likely to be profuse and destructive to tissue because of the enzyme contents. Hence, steps (including application of skin ointment) must be taken to protect the skin near the drainage site from excoriation. A suction apparatus may be used to continuously aspirate digestive secretions from the drainage tract, so that skin contact with the digestive enzymes is avoided. Expert nursing attention is required to ensure that the suction tube does not become dislodged and suction is not interrupted. Consultation with an enterostomal therapist (wound care specialist) is indicated to identify appropriate strategies for maintaining drainage and protecting the skin.

Cancer of the Pancreas

The incidence of pancreatic cancer has decreased slightly over the past 25 years among non-Caucasian men. It is the fourth leading cause of cancer death in men in the United States and the fifth leading cause of cancer death in women. Its incidence peaks in the seventh and eighth decades of life for both men and women (American Cancer Society, 2005). It is extremely rare before the age of 40 years (Reddy & Long, 2004). Cigarette smoking, exposure to industrial chemicals or toxins in the environment, and a diet high in fat, meat, or both are associated with pancreatic cancer, although their roles are not completely clear. The risk for pancreatic cancer increases as the extent of cigarette smoking increases. Diabetes mellitus, chronic pancreatitis, and hereditary pancreatitis are also associated with pancreatic cancer. The pancreas can also be the site of metastasis from other tumors.

Cancer may develop in the head, body, or tail of the pancreas; clinical manifestations vary depending on the location of the lesion and whether functioning, insulin-secreting pancreatic islet cells are involved. Approximately 75% of pancreatic cancers originate in the head of the pancreas and give rise to a distinctive clinical picture (Friedman et al., 2003; Reddy & Long, 2004). Functioning islet cell tumors, whether benign (adenoma) or malignant (carcinoma), are responsible for the syndrome of hyperinsulinism. With these exceptions, the symptoms are nonspecific, and patients usually do not seek medical attention until late in the disease; 80% to 85% of patients have advanced, unresectable tumor when first detected. In fact, pancreatic carcinoma has only a 4% survival rate at 5 years regardless of the stage of disease at diagnosis or treatment (American Cancer Society, 2005).

Clinical Manifestations

Pain, jaundice, or both are present in more than 80% of patients and, along with weight loss, are considered classic signs of pancreatic carcinoma (Reddy & Long, 2004). However, they often do not appear until the disease is far advanced. Other signs include rapid, profound, and progressive weight loss as well as vague upper or midabdominal pain or discomfort that is unrelated to any gastrointestinal function and is often difficult to describe. Such discomfort radiates as a boring pain in the midback and is unrelated to posture or activity. It is often progressive and severe, requiring the use of opioids. It is often more severe at night and is accentuated when lying supine. Relief may be obtained by sitting up and leaning forward.

Malignant cells from pancreatic cancer are often shed into the peritoneal cavity, increasing the likelihood of metastasis. The formation of ascites is common. An important sign, if it is present, is the onset of symptoms of insulin deficiency: glucosuria, hyperglycemia, and abnormal glucose tolerance. Therefore, diabetes may be an early sign of carcinoma of the pancreas. Meals often aggravate epigastric pain, which usually occurs before the appearance of jaundice and pruritus.

Assessment and Diagnostic Findings

Spiral (helical) CT has more than 90% accuracy in the diagnosis and staging of pancreatic cancer and is currently the most useful preoperative imaging technique (McIntyre et al., 2004; Reddy & Long, 2004). MRI may also be used. ERCP is also used in the diagnosis of pancreatic carcinoma. Cells obtained during ERCP are sent to the laboratory for histologic analysis. Gastrointestinal x-ray findings may demonstrate deformities in adjacent organs caused by the impinging pancreatic mass.

A histologic diagnosis is not usually required in patients who are candidates for surgery. The tissue diagnosis will be made at the time of the surgical procedure. Percutaneous fine-needle aspiration biopsy of the pancreas is used to diagnose pancreatic tumor. This type of biopsy is also used to confirm the diagnosis in patients whose tumors are not resectable so that a palliative plan of care can be determined. This may eliminate the stress and postoperative pain of ineffective surgery. In this procedure, a needle is inserted through the anterior abdominal wall into the pancreatic mass, guided by CT, ultrasound, ERCP, or other imaging techniques. The aspirated material is examined for malignant cells. Although percutaneous biopsy is a valuable diagnostic tool, it has some potential drawbacks: a false-negative result if small tumors are missed and the risk of seeding of cancer cells along the needle track. Low-dose radiation to the site may be used before the biopsy to reduce this risk.

Percutaneous transhepatic cholangiography is another procedure that may be performed to identify obstructions of the biliary tract by a pancreatic tumor. Several tumor markers (eg, CA 19-9, CEA, DU-PAN-2) may be used in the diagnostic workup, but they are nonspecific for pancreatic carcinoma. These tumor markers are useful as indicators of disease progression.

Angiography, CT scans, and laparoscopy may be performed to determine whether the tumor can be removed surgically. Intraoperative ultrasonography has been used to determine whether there is metastatic disease to other organs.

Medical Management

If the tumor is resectable and localized (typically tumors in the head of the pancreas), the surgical procedure to remove it is usually extensive (see later discussion). However, total excision of the lesion often is not possible. This is because tumors are not diagnosed until after extensive growth and because of the probable widespread metastases (especially to the liver, lungs, and bones). More often, treatment is limited to palliative measures.

Although pancreatic tumors may be resistant to standard radiation therapy, the patient may be treated with radiation and chemotherapy (fluorouracil, leucovorin, and gemcitabine). Newer biologic agents, including farnesyl transferase inhibitors and monoclonal antibodies, are currently under study for the treatment of metastatic pancreatic cancer (Choti, 2004). If the patient undergoes surgery, intraoperative radiation therapy may be used to deliver a high dose of radiation to the tumor with minimal injury to other tissues; this may also be helpful in relief of pain. Interstitial implantation of radioactive sources has also been used, although the rate of complications is high. A large biliary stent inserted percutaneously or by endoscopy may be used to relieve jaundice.

Nursing Management

Pain management and attention to nutritional requirements are important nursing measures that improve the level of patient comfort. Skin care and nursing measures are directed toward relief of pain and discomfort associated with jaundice, anorexia, and profound weight loss. Specialty mattresses are beneficial and protect bony prominences from pressure. Pain associated with pancreatic cancer may be severe and may require liberal use of opioids; patient-controlled analgesia should be considered for the patient with severe, escalating pain.

Because of the poor prognosis and likelihood of short survival, end-of-life preferences are discussed and honored. If appropriate, the nurse refers the patient to hospice care. (See Chapters 16 and 17 for care of the patient with cancer and end-of-life care, respectively.)

Promoting Home and Community-Based Care

TEACHING PATIENTS SELF-CARE

The specific teaching for the patient and family varies with the stage of disease and the treatment choices made by the patient. If the patient elects to receive chemotherapy, the nurse focuses teaching on prevention of side effects and complications of the agents used. If surgery is performed to relieve obstruction and establish biliary drainage, teaching addresses management of the drainage system and monitoring for complications. The nurse instructs the family about changes in the patient's status that should be reported to the physician.

CONTINUING CARE

A referral for home care is indicated to help the patient and family deal with the physical problems and discomforts associated with pancreatic cancer and the psychological impact of the disease. The home care nurse assesses the patient's physical status, fluid and nutritional status, and skin integrity and the adequacy of pain management. The nurse teaches the patient and family strategies to prevent skin breakdown and relieve pain, pruritus, and anorexia. It is important to discuss and arrange palliative care (hospice services) in an effort to relieve patient discomfort, assist with care, and comply with the patient's end-of-life decisions and wishes.

Tumors of the Head of the Pancreas

Sixty to eighty percent of pancreatic tumors occur in the head of the pancreas (Reddy & Long, 2004). Tumors in this region of the pancreas obstruct the common bile duct where the duct passes through the head of the pancreas to join the pancreatic duct and empty at the ampulla of Vater into the duodenum. The tumors producing the obstruction may arise from the pancreas, the common bile duct, or the ampulla of Vater.

Clinical Manifestations

The obstructed flow of bile produces jaundice, clay-colored stools, and dark urine. Malabsorption of nutrients and fat-soluble vitamins may result if the tumor obstructs the entry of bile to the gastrointestinal tract. Abdominal discomfort or pain and pruritus may be noted, along with anorexia, weight loss, and malaise. If these signs and symptoms are present, cancer of the head of the pancreas is suspected.

The jaundice of this disease must be differentiated from that due to a biliary obstruction caused by a gallstone in the common duct. Jaundice caused by a gallstone is usually intermittent and appears typically in obese patients, who are most often women, and who have had previous symptoms of gallbladder disease.

Assessment and Diagnostic Findings

Diagnostic studies may include duodenography, angiography by hepatic or celiac artery catheterization, pancreatic scanning, percutaneous transhepatic cholangiography, ERCP, and percutaneous needle biopsy of the pancreas. Results of a biopsy of the pancreas may aid in the diagnosis.

Medical Management

Before extensive surgery can be performed, a fairly long period of preparation is often necessary, because the patient's nutritional and physical condition is often quite compromised. Various liver and pancreatic function studies are performed. A diet high in protein along with pancreatic enzymes is often prescribed. Preoperative preparation includes adequate hydration, correction of prothrombin deficiency with vitamin K, and treatment of anemia to minimize postoperative complications. Parenteral nutrition and blood component therapy are frequently required.

A biliary-enteric shunt may be performed to relieve the jaundice and, perhaps, to provide time for a thorough diagnostic evaluation. Total pancreatectomy (removal of the pancreas) may be performed if there is no evidence of direct extension of the tumor to adjacent tissues or regional lymph nodes. A pancreaticoduodenectomy (Whipple's procedure or resection) is used for potentially resectable cancer of the head of the pancreas (Fig. 40-7). This procedure involves removal of the gallbladder, distal portion of the stomach, duodenum, head of the pancreas, and common bile duct and anastomosis of the remaining pancreas and stomach to the jejunum (Kelly et al., 2004; Reddy & Long, 2004). The result is removal of the tumor, allowing flow of bile into the jejunum. If the tumor cannot be excised, the jaundice may be relieved by diverting the bile flow into the jejunum by anastomosing the jejunum to the gallbladder, a procedure known as **cholecystojejunostomy.**

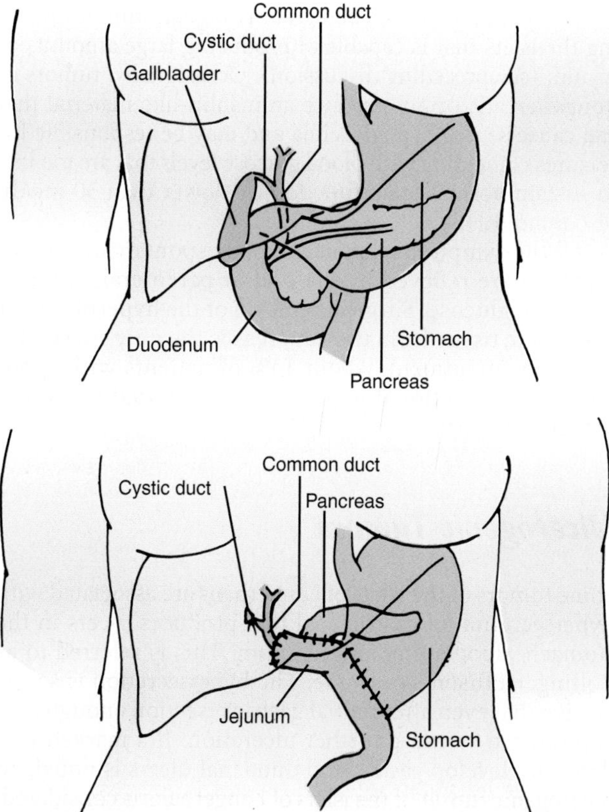

FIGURE 40-7. Pancreatoduodenectomy (Whipple's procedure or resection). End result of resection of carcinoma of the head of the pancreas or the ampulla of Vater. The common duct is sutured to the end of the jejunum, and the remaining portion of the pancreas and the end of the stomach are sutured to the side of the jejunum.

The postoperative management of patients who have undergone a pancreatectomy or a pancreaticoduodenectomy is similar to the management of patients after extensive gastrointestinal or biliary surgery. The patient's physical status is often suboptimal, increasing the risk for postoperative complications. Hemorrhage, vascular collapse, and hepatorenal failure remain the major complications of these extensive surgical procedures. The mortality rate associated with these procedures has improved because of advances in nutritional support and improved surgical techniques. A nasogastric tube with suction and parenteral nutrition allow the gastrointestinal tract to rest while promoting adequate nutrition.

Nursing Management

Preoperatively and postoperatively, nursing care is directed toward promoting patient comfort, preventing complications, and assisting the patient to return to and maintain as normal and comfortable a life as possible. The nurse closely monitors the patient in the intensive care unit after surgery; in the immediate postoperative period, multiple IV and arterial lines are used for fluid and blood replacement and hemodynamic monitoring, and a mechanical ventilator is used. It is important to note and report changes in vital signs, arterial blood gases and pressures, pulse oximetry, laboratory values, and urine output. The nurse must also consider the patient's compromised nutritional status and risk for bleeding. Depending on the type of surgical procedure performed, malabsorption syndrome and diabetes mellitus are likely; the nurse must address these issues during acute and long-term patient care.

Although the patient's physiologic status is the focus of the health care team in the immediate postoperative period, the patient's psychological and emotional state must be considered, along with that of the family. The patient has undergone a major high-risk surgery and is critically ill; anxiety and depression may affect recovery. The immediate and long-term outcomes of this extensive surgical resection are uncertain, and the patient and family require emotional support and understanding in the critical and stressful preoperative and postoperative periods.

Promoting Home and Community-Based Care

TEACHING PATIENTS SELF-CARE

The patient who has undergone this extensive surgery requires careful and thorough preparation for self-care at home. The nurse instructs the patient and family about the need for modifications in the diet because of malabsorption and hyperglycemia resulting from the surgery. It is important to instruct the patient and family about the continuing need for pancreatic enzyme replacement, a low-fat diet, and vitamin supplementation.

The nurse teaches the patient and family strategies to relieve pain and discomfort, along with strategies to manage drains, if present, and to care for the surgical incision. The patient and family members may require instruction about use of patient-controlled analgesia, parenteral nutrition, wound care, skin care, and management of drainage. It is important to describe, verbally and in writing, the signs and symptoms of complications, and to teach the patient and family about indicators of complications that should be reported promptly.

Discharge of the patient to a long-term care or rehabilitation facility may be warranted after surgery as extensive as pancreatectomy or pancreaticoduodenectomy, particularly if the patient's preoperative status was not optimal. Information about the teaching that has been provided is shared with the long-term care staff so that instructions can be clarified and reinforced. During the recovery or long-term phase of care, the patient and family receive further instructions about self-care in the home.

CONTINUING CARE

A referral for home care may be indicated when the patient returns home. The home care nurse assesses the patient's physical and psychological status and the ability of the patient and family to manage needed care. The home care nurse provides needed physical care and monitors the adequacy of pain management. In addition, it is important to assess the patient's nutritional status and monitor the use of parenteral nutrition. The nurse discusses the use of hospice services with the patient and family and makes a referral if indicated.

Pancreatic Islet Tumors

The pancreas contains the islets (islands) of Langerhans, small nests of cells that secrete hormones directly into the bloodstream and therefore are part of the endocrine system. The hormone insulin is essential for the metabolism of glucose. Diabetes mellitus (see Chapter 41) is the result of deficient insulin secretion. At least two types of tumors of the pancreatic islet cells are known: those that secrete insulin (insulinoma) and those in which insulin secretion is not increased ("nonfunctioning" islet cell cancer). Insulinomas produce hypersecretion of insulin and cause an excessive rate of glucose metabolism. The resulting hypoglycemia may produce symptoms of weakness, mental confusion, and seizures. These symptoms may be relieved almost immediately by oral or IV administration of glucose. The 5-hour glucose tolerance test is helpful to diagnose insulinoma and to distinguish this diagnosis from other causes of hypoglycemia.

Surgical Management

If a tumor of the islet cells has been diagnosed, surgical treatment with removal of the tumor is usually recommended (Kelly et al., 2004). The tumors may be benign adenomas, or they may be malignant. Complete removal usually results in almost immediate relief of symptoms. In some patients, symptoms may be produced by simple hypertrophy of this tissue rather than a tumor of the islet cells. In such cases, a partial pancreatectomy (removal of the tail and part of the body of the pancreas) is performed.

Nursing Management

In preparing the patient for surgery, the nurse must be alert for symptoms of hypoglycemia and be ready to administer glucose as prescribed if symptoms occur. Postoperatively, the nursing management is the same as after other upper abdominal surgical procedures, with special emphasis on monitoring serum glucose levels. Patient teaching is determined by the extent of surgery and alterations in pancreatic function.

Hyperinsulinism

Hyperinsulinism is caused by overproduction of insulin by the pancreatic islets. Symptoms resemble those of excessive doses of insulin and are attributable to the same mechanism: an abnormal reduction in blood glucose levels. Clinically, it is characterized by episodes during which the patient experiences unusual hunger, nervousness, sweating, headache, and faintness; in severe cases, seizures and episodes of unconsciousness may occur. The findings at the time of surgery or at autopsy may indicate hyperplasia (overgrowth) of the islets of Langerhans or a benign or malignant tumor involving the islets that is capable of producing large amounts of insulin (see preceding discussion). Occasionally, tumors of nonpancreatic origin produce an insulin-like material that can cause severe hypoglycemia and may be responsible for seizures coinciding with blood glucose levels that are too low to sustain normal brain function (ie, lower than 30 mg/dL [1.6 mmol/L]).

All the symptoms that accompany spontaneous hypoglycemia are relieved by the oral or parenteral administration of glucose. Surgical removal of the hyperplastic or neoplastic tissue from the pancreas is the only successful method of treatment. About 15% of patients with spontaneous or functional hypoglycemia eventually develop diabetes mellitus.

Ulcerogenic Tumors

Some tumors of the islets of Langerhans are associated with hypersecretion of gastric acid that produces ulcers in the stomach, duodenum, and jejunum. This is referred to as **Zollinger-Ellison syndrome.** The hypersecretion is so excessive that even after partial gastric resection enough acid is produced to cause further ulceration. If a marked tendency to develop gastric and duodenal ulcers is noted, an ulcerogenic tumor of the islets of Langerhans is considered.

These tumors, which may be benign or malignant, are treated by excision, if possible. Frequently, however, removal is not possible because of extension beyond the pancreas. In many patients, a total gastrectomy may be necessary to reduce the secretion of gastric acid sufficiently to prevent further ulceration.

Critical Thinking Exercises

1 A 34-year-old woman is scheduled for a cholecystectomy. Since undergoing bariatric surgery a year ago, she has lost 150 pounds. What postoperative care is indicated for this patient? What impact, if any, does her previous surgical procedure have on her postoperative recovery?

2 A 56-year-old man with a history of alcoholism and cirrhosis is admitted to your unit with a diagnosis of pancreatitis. He is complaining of severe epigastric pain, vomiting, and diarrhea. What medications and laboratory tests would you expect to see prescribed for this patient? What physical assessment findings will you see? Describe nursing care for this patient, and compare and contrast care with and without the diagnosis of cirrhosis. What issues would be of high priority in caring for this patient during his hospital stay? What issues would be of high priority in preparing him for hospital discharge?

3 A 78-year-old woman is being discharged home with a diagnosis of advanced pancreatic cancer. She has a biliary drain in place to relieve obstruction. She has been legally blind for 4 years. What teaching about management of the drainage system is needed for the patient and her family? How would the patient's vision loss affect your teaching? What other issues should be discussed with the patient and her family? How would you modify your discharge plans for her if she lives alone and has no family support available?

4 ebp A 54-year-old woman is scheduled for a laparoscopic cholecystectomy. She is being discharged on her first postoperative day. What information will you provide about expectations for postoperative pain, and what instructions will you provide to the patient about pharmacological and nonpharmacologic pain management strategies? What is the evidence base for the pain management strategies you provide to her, and what is the strength of that evidence?

5 Compare and contrast the nursing care of a 68-year-old patient with a diagnosis of acute pancreatitis with that of a 78-year-old patient with a diagnosis of chronic pancreatitis. Explain the rationale for differences in care for these two diagnoses.

REFERENCES AND SELECTED READINGS

BOOKS

Abbruzzese, J. L., Evans, D. B., Willet, C. G., et al. (Eds.). (2004). *Gastrointestinal cancer.* Oxford: Oxford University Press.
American Cancer Society. (2005). *Cancer facts and figures.* Atlanta: Author.
Aspinall, R. J. & Taylor-Robinson, S. D. (2002). *Mosby's color atlas and text of gastroenterology and liver disease.* Edinburgh: Mosby.
Cuschieri, A., Steele, R. J. C. & Moossa, A. R. (2002). *Essential surgical practice* (4th ed.). London: Arnold.
Dudek, S. (2006). *Nutrition essentials for nursing practice.* Philadelphia: Lippincott Williams & Wilkins.
Edmundowicz, S. A. (2002). *20 common problems in gastroenterology.* New York: McGraw-Hill.
Feldman, M., Friedman, L. S. & Sleisenger, M. H. (Eds.). (2002). *Sleisenger and Fordtran's gastrointestinal and liver disease: Pathophysiology, diagnosis, and management.* Philadelphia: Saunders.
Friedman, S. L., McQuaid, K. R. & Grendell, J. H. (Eds.). (2003). *Current diagnosis and treatment in gastroenterology* (2nd ed.). New York: Lange Medical Books/McGraw-Hill.
Fishman, M. C., Hoffman, A. R., Klausner, R. D., et al. (2004). *Medicine.* Philadelphia: Lippincott Williams & Wilkins.
Kelly, K. A., Sarr, M. G. & Hinder, R. A. (Eds.). (2004). *Mayo Clinic gastrointestinal surgery.* Philadelphia: Saunders.
McIntyre, R. C., Steigmann, G. V. & Eiseman, B. (Eds.). (2004). *Surgical decision making* (5th ed.). Philadelphia: Elsevier Saunders.
Odze, R. D., Goldblum, J. R. & Crawford, J. M. (2004). *Surgical pathology of the gastrointestinal tract, liver, biliary tract and pancreas.* Philadelphia: Saunders.
Porth, C. M. (2005). *Pathophysiology: Concepts of altered health states* (7th ed.). Philadelphia: Lippincott Williams & Wilkins.
Reddy, K. R. & Long, W. B. (Eds.). (2004). *Hepatobiliary tract and pancreas.* Edinburgh: Mosby.
Su, G. H. (Ed.). (2005). *Pancreatic cancer: Methods and protocols.* Totowa, NJ: Humana Press.
Yamada, T. (Ed.). (2003). *Textbook of gastroenterology* (4th ed.). Philadelphia: Lippincott Williams & Wilkins.
Zetka, J. R. (2003). *Surgeons and the scope.* Ithaca, NY: ILR Press.

JOURNALS

**Asterisks indicate nursing research articles.*

General

Ahmed, N., Ahmedzai, S., Vora, V., et al. (2004). Supportive care for patients with gastrointestinal cancer [review]. *Cochrane Database of Systematic Reviews, 3,* CD003445.
Scott-Conner, C. E. H. (2002). Laparoscopic gastrointestinal surgery. *Medical Clinics of North America, 86*(6), 1401–1422.

Gallbladder Disease

Collins, C., Maguire, D., Ireland, A., et al. (2004). A prospective study of common bile duct calculi in patients undergoing laparoscopic cholecystectomy: Natural history of choledocholithiasis revisited. *Annals of Surgery, 239*(1), 28–33.
Knight, J. S., Mercer, S. J., Somers, S. S., et al. (2004). Timing of urgent laparoscopic cholecystectomy does not influence conversion rate. *British Journal of Surgery, 91*(5), 601–604.
Larsen, J. F., Svendsen, F. M., & Pedersen, V. (2004). Randomized clinical trial of the effect of pneumoperitoneum on cardiac function and hemodynamics during laparoscopic cholecystectomy. *British Journal of Surgery, 91*(7), 848–854.
Leeder, P. C., Matthews, T., Krzeminska, K., et al. (2004). Routine day-case laparoscopic cholecystectomy. *British Journal of Surgery, 91*(3), 312–316.
Papi, C., Catarci, M., D'Ambrosio, L., et al. (2004). Timing of cholecystectomy for acute calculous cholecystitis: A meta-analysis. *American Journal of Gastroenterology, 99*(1), 147–155.
Pelinka, L. E., Schmidhammer, R., Hamid, L., et al. (2003). Acute acalculous cholecystitis after trauma: A prospective study. *Journal of Trauma: Injury and Critical Care, 55*(2), 323–329.
Quintana, J. M., Arostegui, I., Cabriada, J., et al. (2003). Predictors of improvement in health-related quality of life in patients undergoing cholecystectomy. *British Journal of Surgery, 90*(12), 1549–1555.

Rakesh, K., Barjesh, C. S., Jagdeep, S., et al. (2004). Endoscopic biliary drainage for severe acute cholangitis in biliary obstruction as a result of malignant and benign disease. *Journal of Gastroenterology and Hepatology, 19*(9), 994–997.

Susumu, T., Tomoji, N., Hidenori, O., et al. (2003). Treating gallstones in the elderly. *Journal of Gastroenterology and Hepatology, 18*(2), 157–161.

Walsh, R. M., Vogt, D. P., Brown, N., et al. (2004). Management of failed biliary repairs for major bile duct injuries after laparoscopic cholecystectomy. *Journal of the American College of Surgeons, 199*(2), 192–197.

*Watt-Watson, J., Chung, D., Chan, V. W. S., et al. (2004). Pain management following discharge after ambulatory same-day surgery. *Journal of Nursing Management, 12*(3), 153–161.

Young, E. J., Hyun-Soo, K., Sung-Kyu, C., et al. (2003). Case of mucinous adenocarcinoma with porcelain gallbladder. *Journal of Gastroenterology and Hepatology, 18*(8), 995–998.

Zacks, S. L., Sandler, R. S., Rutledge, R., et al. (2002). A population-based cohort study comparing laparoscopic cholecystectomy and open cholecystectomy. *American Journal of Gastroenterology, 97*(2), 334–340.

Pancreatic Disorders

Alexakis, N., Halloran, C., Raraty, M., et al. (2004). Current standards of surgery for pancreatic cancer. *British Journal of Surgery, 91*(11), 1410–1427.

Buter, A., Imrie, C. W., Carter, C. R., et al. (2002). Dynamic nature of early dysfunction determines outcome in acute pancreatitis. *British Journal of Surgery, 89*(3), 298–302.

Choti, M. A. (2004). Adjuvant therapy for pancreatic cancer-the debate continues. *New England Journal of Medicine, 350*(12), 1249–1251.

Diaz-Rubio, E. (2004). New advances in chemotherapeutic advances in pancreatic, colorectal, and gastric cancers. *Oncologist, 9*(3), 282–294.

Gavaghan, M. (2002). The pancreas: Hermit of the abdomen. *AORN Online 75*(6), 1109–1138.

Hughes, E. (2004). Understanding the care of patients with acute pancreatitis. *Nursing Standard, 18*(18), 45–52, 54–55.

Lightner, A. M., Glasgow, R. E., Jordan, T. H., et al. (2004). Pancreatic resection in the elderly. *Journal of the American College of Surgeons, 198*(5), 697–706.

Liu, T. H., Kwong, K. L., Tamm, E. P., et al. (2003). Acute pancreatitis in intensive care unit patients: Value of clinical and radiologic prognosticators at predicting clinical course and outcome. *Critical Care Medicine, 31*(4), 1026–1030.

Pennachio, D. L. (2002). The latest approaches to pancreatic disease. *Patient Care for the Nurse Practitioner, 4*(9), 41–44, 47–48.

Soichiro, U., Katsuhiro, G., Hiroshi, H., et al. (2003). Immune function in patients with acute pancreatitis. *Journal of Gastroenterology and Hepatology, 18*(4), 363–370.

Swaroop, V. S., Chari, S. T., & Clain, J. E. (2004). Severe acute pancreatitis. *Journal of the American Medical Association, 291*(23), 2865–2868.

Takaaki, M., Koji, O., Mitsuko, I., et al. (2004). Pancreatic enzyme supplement improves dysmotility in chronic pancreatitis patients. *Journal of Gastroenterology and Hepatology, 19*(9), 1005–1009.

Van den Berghe, G, Wouters, P. J., Bouillon, R., et al. (2003). Outcome benefit of intensive insulin therapy in the critically ill: Insulin dose versus glycemic control. *Critical Care Medicine, 31*(2), 359–366.

RESOURCES

American Gastroenterological Association, 4930 Del Ray Avenue, Bethesda, MD 20814; 301-654-2055; http://www.gastro.org. Accessed May 15, 2006.

National Digestive Diseases Information Clearing House, 2 Information Way, Bethesda, MD 20892-3570; 1-800-891-5389 or 301-654-3810; http://www.niddk.nih.gov. Accessed May 15, 2006.

National Endocrine Society, 8401 Connecticut Avenue, Suite 900, Chevy Chase, MD 20815; 1-888-363-6274 or 301-941-0200; http://www.endo-society.org. Accessed May 15, 2006.

National Pancreas Foundation, P.O. Box 15333, Boston, MA 02215; 1-866-726-2737 or 617-578-0382; http://www.pancreasfoundation.org. Accessed May 15, 2006.

CHAPTER 41

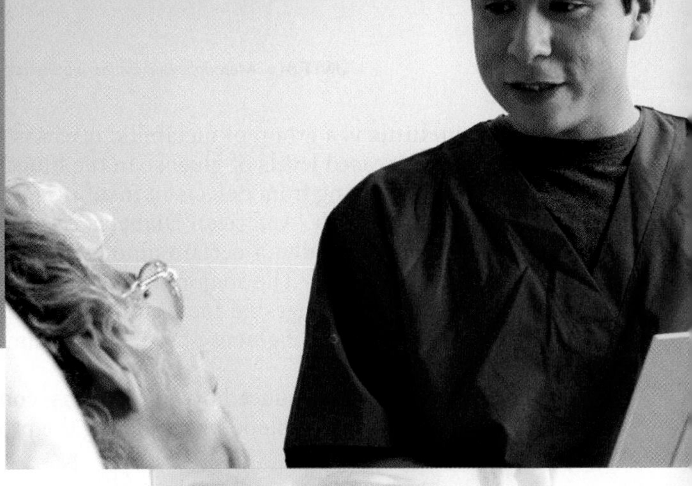

Assessment and Management of Patients With Diabetes Mellitus

Learning Objectives

On completion of this chapter, the learner will be able to:

1. Differentiate between type 1 and type 2 diabetes.
2. Describe etiologic factors associated with diabetes.
3. Relate the clinical manifestations of diabetes to the associated pathophysiologic alterations.
4. Identify the diagnostic and clinical significance of blood glucose test results.
5. Explain the dietary modifications used for management of people with diabetes.
6. Describe the relationships among diet, exercise, and medication (ie, insulin or oral antidiabetic agents) for people with diabetes.
7. Develop a plan for teaching insulin self-management.
8. Identify the role of oral antidiabetic agents in diabetic therapy.
9. Differentiate between hyperglycemia with diabetic ketoacidosis and hyperosmolar nonketotic syndrome.
10. Describe management strategies for a person with diabetes to use during "sick days."
11. Describe the major macrovascular, microvascular, and neuropathic complications of diabetes and the self-care behaviors that are important in their prevention.
12. Identify the teaching aids and community support groups available for people with diabetes.
13. Use the nursing process as a framework for care of patients with diabetes.

Diabetes mellitus is a group of metabolic diseases characterized by increased levels of glucose in the blood (**hyperglycemia**) resulting from defects in insulin secretion, insulin action, or both (American Diabetes Association [ADA], 2004r). Normally, a certain amount of glucose circulates in the blood. The major sources of this glucose are absorption of ingested food in the gastrointestinal tract and formation of glucose by the liver from food substances.

Insulin, a hormone produced by the pancreas, controls the level of glucose in the blood by regulating the production and storage of glucose. In diabetes, the cells may stop responding to insulin or the pancreas may stop producing insulin entirely. This leads to hyperglycemia, which may result in acute metabolic complications such as **diabetic ketoacidosis (DKA)** and **hyperglycemic hyperosmolar nonketotic syndrome (HHNS)**. Long-term effects of hyperglycemia contribute to macrovascular complications (coronary artery disease, cerebrovascular disease, and peripheral vascular disease), chronic microvascular complications (kidney and eye disease), and neuropathic complications (diseases of the nerves).

Glossary

alpha glucosidase inhibitor: a category of oral agents used to treat type 2 diabetes that delay the absorption of carbohydrate, resulting in lower postprandial blood glucose levels

continuous subcutaneous insulin infusion: a small device that delivers insulin on a 24-hour basis as basal insulin; it is also programmed by the patient to deliver a bolus dose before eating a meal in an attempt to mimic normal pancreatic function

continuous glucose monitoring system (CGMS): a device worn for 72 hours that continuously monitors blood glucose levels; the data are downloaded and analyzed for blood glucose patterns for that time period; presently used diagnostically to elicit patterns and tailor treatment

diabetes mellitus: a group of metabolic diseases characterized by hyperglycemia resulting from defects in insulin secretion, insulin action, or both

diabetic ketoacidosis (DKA): a metabolic derangement in type 1 diabetes that results from a deficiency of insulin. Highly acidic ketone bodies are formed, resulting in acidosis; usually requires hospitalization for treatment and is usually caused by nonadherence to the insulin regimen, concurrent illness, or infection.

fasting plasma glucose (FPG): blood glucose determination obtained in the laboratory after fasting for more than 8 hours. Although plasma levels are specified in diagnostic criteria, blood glucose levels, which are slightly higher than plasma levels, are more commonly used.

gestational diabetes mellitus (GDM): any degree of glucose intolerance with its onset during pregnancy

Glycated hemoglobin (glycosylated hemoglobin, Hgb A_{1C} or A1C): a long-term measure of glucose control that is a result of glucose attaching to hemoglobin for the life of the red blood cell (120 days). The goal of diabetes therapy is a normal to near-normal level of glycolated hemoglobin, the same as in the nondiabetic population.

hyperglycemia: elevated blood glucose level; fasting level greater than 110 mg/dL (6.1 mmol/L); 2-hour postprandial level greater than 140 mg/dL (7.8 mmol/L)

hyperglycemic hyperosmolar nonketotic syndrome (HHNS): a metabolic disorder of type 2 diabetes resulting from a relative insulin deficiency initiated by an intercurrent illness that raises the demand for insulin; associated with polyuria and severe dehydration

hypoglycemia: low blood glucose level (less than 60 mg/dL [less than 2.7 mmol/L])

impaired fasting glucose (IFG), impaired glucose tolerance (IGT): a metabolic stage intermediate between normal glucose homeostasis and diabetes; not clinical entities in their own right but risk factors for future diabetes and cardiovascular disease

insulin: a hormone secreted by the beta cells of the islets of Langerhans of the pancreas that is necessary for the metabolism of carbohydrates, proteins, and fats; a deficiency of insulin results in diabetes mellitus

insulin pump: see *continuous subcutaneous insulin infusion*

islet cell transplantation: an investigational procedure in which purified islet cells from cadaver donors are injected into the portal vein of the liver, with the goal of having these cells secrete insulin and cure type 1 diabetes.

ketone: a highly acidic substance formed when the liver breaks down free fatty acids in the absence of insulin. The result is diabetic ketoacidosis.

medical nutrition therapy (MNT): nutritional therapy prescribed by the physician for management of diabetes

nephropathy: a long-term complication of diabetes in which the kidney cells are damaged; characterized by microalbuminuria in early stages and progressing to end-stage renal disease

neuropathy: a long-term complication of diabetes resulting from damage to the nerve cell.

prediabetes: impaired glucose metabolism in which blood glucose concentrations fall between normal levels and those considered diagnostic for diabetes

retinopathy: a long-term complication of diabetes in which the microvascular system of the eye is damaged

self-monitoring of blood glucose (SMBG): a method of capillary blood glucose testing in which the patient pricks his or her finger and applies a drop of blood to a test strip that is read by a meter

sulfonylurea: a classification of oral antidiabetic medication for treating type 2 diabetes; stimulates insulin secretion and insulin action

thiazolidinedione: a class of oral antidiabetic medications that reduce insulin resistance in target tissues, enhancing insulin action without directly stimulating insulin secretion

type 1 diabetes: a metabolic disorder characterized by an absence of insulin production and secretion from autoimmune destruction of the beta cells of the islets of Langerhans in the pancreas. Formerly called insulin-dependent, juvenile, or type I diabetes.

type 2 diabetes: a metabolic disorder characterized by the relative deficiency of insulin production and a decreased insulin action and increased insulin resistance. Formerly called non–insulin-dependent, adult-onset, or type II diabetes.

Diabetes is becoming more common in the United States. From 1980 through 2002, the number of Americans with diabetes more than doubled. Currently, it is estimated that almost 21 million people in the United States have diabetes, although almost one third of these cases are undiagnosed (Centers for Disease Control and Prevention [CDC], 2005). By 2030, this figure is expected to exceed 30 million. In 2000, the worldwide estimate of the prevalence of diabetes was 171 million people, and by 2030, this is expected to increase to 366 million (Wild, Roglic, Green, et al., 2004). Diabetes is especially prevalent in the elderly; as many as 50% of people older than 65 years of age have some degree of glucose intolerance. People 65 years and older account for almost 40% of people with diabetes.

From 1980 through 2002, the prevalence of diagnosed diabetes increased in all age groups. People between 65 and 74 years of age had the highest prevalence, followed by people 75 years of age or older, people 45 to 64 years of age, and people younger than 45 years of age. In 2002, the prevalence of diagnosed diabetes among people 65 to 74 years of age (16.8%) was almost 14 times that of people younger than 45 years of age (1.2%). However, many people with diabetes are undiagnosed.

Minority populations are disproportionately affected by diabetes. From 1980 through 2002, the age-adjusted prevalence of diabetes increased among all gender and race groups. It was highest among African American women, and, overall, it was higher among African Americans than Caucasians. During this period, the age-adjusted prevalence of diabetes increased by 98% in Caucasian men, 54% in Caucasian women, and 66% in African American men and women. From 1997 through 2002, the age-adjusted prevalence of diabetes among Hispanic men and women was similar to that among African American men. Compared to Caucasians, African Americans and members of other racial and ethnic groups (Native Americans and persons of Hispanic origin) are more likely to develop diabetes, are at greater risk for many of the complications, and have higher death rates due to diabetes (CDC, 2004, 2005). Chart 41-1 summarizes risk factors for diabetes mellitus.

Diabetes has far-reaching and devastating physical, social, and economic consequences, including the following:

- In the United States, diabetes is the leading cause of nontraumatic amputations, blindness in working-age adults, and end-stage renal disease (U.S. Public Health Service [USPHS], 2000).
- Diabetes is the third leading cause of death from disease, primarily because of the high rate of cardiovascular disease (myocardial infarction, stroke, and peripheral vascular disease) among people with diabetes.
- Hospitalization rates for people with diabetes are 2.4 times greater for adults and 5.3 times greater for children than for the general population.

The economic cost of diabetes continues to increase because of increasing health care costs and an aging population. Half of all people who have diabetes and are older than 65 years of age are hospitalized each year, and severe and life-threatening complications often contribute to the increased rates of hospitalization. Costs related to diabetes are estimated to be almost $132 billion annually, including direct medical care expenses and indirect costs attributable to disability and premature death (CDC, 2005). It is estimated that these costs will increase to $156 billion by 2010 and to $192 billion by 2020 (Zhang, Engelgau, Norris, et al., 2004).

The primary goals of treatment for people with diabetes include controlling blood glucose levels and preventing acute and long-term complications. Nurses who care for patients with diabetes must help them develop self-care management skills.

CHART 41-1

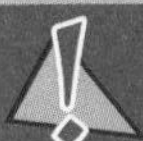

Risk Factors for Diabetes Mellitus

- Family history of diabetes (ie, parents or siblings with diabetes)
- Obesity (ie, ≥20% over desired body weight or BMI ≥27 kg/m^2)
- Race/ethnicity (eg, African Americans, Hispanic Americans, Native Americans, Asian Americans, Pacific Islanders)
- Age ≥45 y
- Previously identified impaired fasting glucose or impaired glucose tolerance
- Hypertension (≥140/90 mm Hg)
- HDL cholesterol level ≤35 mg/dL (0.90 mmol/L) and/or triglyceride level ≥250 mg/dL (2.8 mmol/L)
- History of gestational diabetes or delivery of babies over 9 lb

Used with permission of American Diabetes Association. (2004). Report of the Expert Committee on the Diagnosis and Classification of Diabetes Mellitus. *Diabetes Care, 27*(1), 5–10.

Diabetes and Its Classification

Diabetes has been classified in several ways. The different types of diabetes mellitus vary in cause, clinical course, and treatment.

Overview

The major classifications of diabetes are type 1 diabetes, type 2 diabetes, gestational diabetes (ADA, 2004r), and diabetes mellitus associated with other conditions or syndromes.

Table 41-1 summarizes the major classifications of diabetes, current terminology, old labels, and major clinical characteristics. This classification system is dynamic in two ways. First, research findings suggest many differences among individuals within each category. Second, except for people with type 1 diabetes, patients may move from one category to another. For example, a woman with gestational diabetes may, after delivery, move into the type 2 category.

The terms "insulin-dependent diabetes" and "non–insulin-dependent diabetes" and their acronyms (IDDM and NIDDM, respectively) are no longer used, because they resulted in classification of patients on the basis of the treatment of their diabetes rather than the underlying cause. Use of Roman numerals (type I and type II) to distinguish be-

NURSING RESEARCH PROFILE

Nurse-Directed Diabetes Care in a Minority Population

Davidson, M. B. (2003). Effect of nurse-directed diabetes care in a minority population. *Diabetes Care, 26*(8), 2281–2287.

Purpose

To prevent the complications of diabetes, the goal of health care for affected patients is to provide the standard of care recommended by the American Diabetes Association (ADA), which is based on the evidence of research findings. The purpose of this study was to compare the level of comprehensiveness of health care that patients received from a nurse-managed clinic with that of patients who attended a traditional diabetes clinic.

Specially trained nurses who followed algorithms and protocols delivered the care. Process and outcome measures (eg, number of visits, diabetes education, nutritional counseling, glycated hemoglobin (HbA_{1C}) lipid profiles, eye examinations, foot examinations, renal evaluations, and angiotensin-converting enzyme inhibitor therapy) were assessed and compared to determine compliance with ADA recommendations.

Design

In three Los Angeles County clinics, nurse-directed clinic care was provided to 252 patients, 92% of whom were Hispanic and 2% of whom were African American. These patients were matched as to type of diabetes, diabetes therapy, duration of diabetes, ethnicity, age, and gender to 252 patients with diabetes who received care in a traditional physician-directed clinic. Patients (n = 209) from a teaching clinic served as an additional control group for two of the variables of interest.

Findings

In the nurse-directed clinic, almost all process measures (receipt of recommended testing, examinations, and patient education) were carried out significantly more often ($p < .001$) than for control patients who were under usual physician-directed care. Glycated hemoglobin levels decreased from 10.1% to 8.5% in the group of patients who received care in the usual care diabetes clinics but decreased even further, to 7.1%, after a year of care in the nurse-directed clinic, indicating improved glycemic control.

Nursing Implications

Diabetes is a self-managed disease that requires many strategies to keep it under control and a system of care to monitor the prevention and provide early treatment of complications. Efforts should be directed to strategies that can be used to teach people with diabetes and a system in which care can be provided in a cost-effective way to reduce the occurrence of these costly complications. Nurses are ideal professionals to provide this care; patient education is a key component of nursing practice. Patients are often more comfortable with nurses, and nurses spend more time with patients and have the expertise to teach them to manage their diabetes properly. The provision of care in nurse-directed clinics may contribute to keeping patients with diabetes healthy and free of complications.

tween the two types has been changed to arabic numbers (type 1 and type 2) to reduce confusion (ADA, 2004r).

In **type 1 diabetes**, the insulin-producing pancreatic beta cells are destroyed by an autoimmune process. As a result, patients produce little or no insulin and require insulin injections to control their blood glucose levels. Type 1 diabetes affects approximately 5% to 10% of people with the disease. Type 1 diabetes is characterized by an acute onset, usually before 30 years of age (CDC, 2004).

In **type 2 diabetes**, people have decreased sensitivity to insulin (called insulin resistance) and impaired beta cell functioning resulting in decreased insulin production. Type 2 diabetes affects approximately 90% to 95% of people with the disease (CDC, 2005). It occurs more commonly among people who are older than 30 years of age and obese (National Institute of Diabetes and Digestive and Kidney Diseases, 2005), although its incidence is rapidly increasing in younger people because of the growing epidemic of obesity in children, adolescents, and young adults (CDC, 2004). Initially, type 2 diabetes is treated with diet and exercise. If elevated glucose levels persist, diet and exercise are supplemented with oral antidiabetic agents. In some people with type 2 diabetes, oral agents do not control hyperglycemia, and insulin injections are required. In addition, insulin injections may be necessary during periods of acute physiologic stress (eg, illness or surgery).

Diabetes complications can develop in anyone with type 1 or type 2 diabetes, not only in patients who take insulin. Some patients with type 2 diabetes who are treated with oral medications may have the impression that they do not *truly* have diabetes or that they simply have "borderline" diabetes. They may believe that, compared with patients who require insulin injections, their diabetes is not serious. It is important for nurses to emphasize to these patients that they *do* have diabetes, not a borderline problem with sugar (glucose) metabolism. **Prediabetes** is classified as **impaired glucose tolerance (IGT)** or **impaired fasting glucose (IFG)** and refers to a condition in which blood glucose concentrations fall between normal levels and those considered diagnostic for diabetes.

CONCEPTS in action ANIMATION

Pathophysiology

Insulin is secreted by beta cells, which are one of four types of cells in the islets of Langerhans in the pancreas. Insulin is

TABLE 41-1 Classification of Diabetes Mellitus and Related Glucose Intolerances

Current Classification	Previous Classifications	Clinical Characteristics and Clinical Implications
Type 1 (5–10% of all diabetes)	Juvenile diabetes Juvenile-onset diabetes Ketosis-prone diabetes Brittle diabetes Insulin-dependent diabetes mellitus (IDDM)	Onset any age, but usually young (<30 y) Usually thin at diagnosis; recent weight loss Etiology includes genetic, immunologic, and environmental factors (eg, virus). Often have islet cell antibodies Often have antibodies to insulin even before insulin treatment Little or no endogenous insulin Need insulin to preserve life Ketosis-prone when insulin absent Acute complication of hyperglycemia: diabetic ketoacidosis
Type 2 (90–95% of all diabetes: obese—80% of type 2; nonobese—20% of type 2)	Adult-onset diabetes Maturity-onset diabetes Ketosis-resistant diabetes Stable diabetes Non-insulin-dependent diabetes (NIDDM)	Onset any age, usually over 30 y Usually obese at diagnosis Causes include obesity, heredity, and environmental factors No islet cell antibodies Decrease in endogenous insulin, or increased with insulin resistance Most patients can control blood glucose through weight loss if obese Oral antidiabetic agents may improve blood glucose levels if dietary modification and exercise are unsuccessful May need insulin on a short- or long-term basis to prevent hyperglycemia Ketosis uncommon, except in stress or infection Acute complication: hyperglycemic hyperosmolar nonketotic syndrome
Diabetes mellitus associated with other conditions or syndromes	Secondary diabetes	Accompanied by conditions known or suspected to cause the disease: pancreatic diseases, hormonal abnormalities, medications such as corticosteroids and estrogen-containing preparations Depending on the ability of the pancreas to produce insulin, the patient may require treatment with oral antidiabetic agents or insulin
Gestational diabetes	Gestational diabetes	Onset during pregnancy, usually in the second or third trimester Due to hormones secreted by the placenta, which inhibit the action of insulin Above-normal risk for perinatal complications, especially macrosomia (abnormally large babies) Treated with diet and, if needed, insulin to strictly maintain normal blood glucose levels Occurs in about 2–5% of all pregnancies Glucose intolerance transitory but may recur: • In subsequent pregnancies • 30–40% will develop overt diabetes (usually type 2) within 10 years (especially if obese) Risk factors include obesity, age older than 30 y, family history of diabetes, previous large babies (>9 lb) Screening tests (glucose challenge test) should be performed on all pregnant women between 24 and 28 wk gestation
Impaired glucose tolerance	Borderline diabetes Latent diabetes Chemical diabetes Subclinical diabetes Asymptomatic diabetes	Oral glucose tolerance test value between 140 mg/dL (7.7 mmol/L) and 200 mg/dL (11 mmol/L) Impaired fasting glucose is defined as a fasting plasma glucose between 110 mg/dL (6 mmol/L) and 126 mg/dL (7 mmol/L) 29% eventually develop diabetes Above-normal susceptibility to atherosclerotic disease Renal and retinal complications usually not significant May be obese or nonobese; obese should reduce weight Should be screened for diabetes periodically
Prediabetes	Previous abnormality of glucose tolerance (PrevAGT)	Current normal glucose metabolism Previous history of hyperglycemia (eg, during pregnancy or illness) Periodic blood glucose screening after age 40 y if there is a family history of diabetes or if symptomatic Encourage ideal body weight, because loss of 10–15 lb may improve glycemic control

continued >

TABLE 41-1 Classification of Diabetes Mellitus and Related Glucose Intolerances (Continued)

Current Classification	Previous Classifications	Clinical Characteristics and Clinical Implications
Prediabetes	Potential abnormality of glucose tolerance (PotAGT)	No history of glucose intolerance Increased risk of diabetes if: • Positive family history • Obesity • Mother of babies over 9 lb at birth • Member of certain Native American (eg, Pima) tribes with high prevalence of diabetes Screening and weight advice as in PrevAGT

an anabolic, or storage, hormone. When a person eats a meal, insulin secretion increases and moves glucose from the blood into muscle, liver, and fat cells. In those cells, insulin

- Transports and metabolizes glucose for energy
- Stimulates storage of glucose in the liver and muscle (in the form of glycogen)
- Signals the liver to stop the release of glucose
- Enhances storage of dietary fat in adipose tissue
- Accelerates transport of amino acids (derived from dietary protein) into cells

Insulin also inhibits the breakdown of stored glucose, protein, and fat.

During fasting periods (between meals and overnight), the pancreas continuously releases a small amount of insulin (basal insulin); another pancreatic hormone called glucagon (secreted by the alpha cells of the islets of Langerhans) is released when blood glucose levels decrease and stimulates the liver to release stored glucose. The insulin and the glucagon together maintain a constant level of glucose in the blood by stimulating the release of glucose from the liver.

Initially, the liver produces glucose through the breakdown of glycogen (glycogenolysis). After 8 to 12 hours without food, the liver forms glucose from the breakdown of noncarbohydrate substances, including amino acids (gluconeogenesis).

Type 1 Diabetes

Type 1 diabetes is characterized by destruction of the pancreatic beta cells. Combined genetic, immunologic, and possibly environmental (eg, viral) factors are thought to contribute to beta cell destruction. Although the events that lead to beta cell destruction are not fully understood, it is generally accepted that a genetic susceptibility is a common underlying factor in the development of type 1 diabetes. People do not inherit type 1 diabetes itself but rather a genetic predisposition, or tendency, toward development of type 1 diabetes. This genetic tendency has been found in people with certain human leukocyte antigen (HLA) types. HLA refers to a cluster of genes responsible for transplantation antigens and other immune processes; a cluster is referred to as a haplotype. About 95% of Caucasians with type 1 diabetes exhibit specific HLA-DR3 or HLA-DR4. The risk of developing type 1 diabetes is increased three to five times in people who have one of these two HLA types. Compared with the general population, this risk is increased 10 to 20 times in people who have both DR3 and DR4 HLA haplotypes. Immune-mediated diabetes commonly develops during childhood and adolescence, but it can occur at any age (ADA, 2004r).

There is also evidence of an autoimmune response in type 1 diabetes. This is an abnormal response in which antibodies are directed against normal tissues of the body, responding to these tissues as if they were foreign. Autoantibodies against islet cells and against endogenous (internal) insulin have been detected in people at the time of diagnosis and even several years before the development of clinical signs of type 1 diabetes. In addition to genetic and immunologic components, environmental factors, such as viruses or toxins, that may initiate destruction of the beta cell are being investigated.

Regardless of the specific cause, the destruction of the beta cells results in decreased insulin production, unchecked glucose production by the liver, and fasting hyperglycemia. In addition, glucose derived from food cannot be stored in the liver but instead remains in the bloodstream and contributes to postprandial (after meals) hyperglycemia. If the concentration of glucose in the blood exceeds the renal threshold for glucose, usually 180 to 200 mg/dL (9.9 to 11.1 mmol/L), the kidneys may not reabsorb all of the filtered glucose; the glucose then appears in the urine (glycosuria). When excess glucose is excreted in the urine, it is accompanied by excessive loss of fluids and electrolytes. This is called osmotic diuresis.

Because insulin normally inhibits glycogenolysis (breakdown of stored glucose) and gluconeogenesis (production of new glucose from amino acids and other substrates), these processes occur in an unrestrained fashion in people with insulin deficiency and contribute further to hyperglycemia. In addition, fat breakdown occurs, resulting in an increased production of **ketone** bodies, which are the byproducts of fat breakdown.

NURSING ALERT

Ketone bodies are acids that disturb the acid–base balance of the body when they accumulate in excessive amounts. The resulting diabetic ketoacidosis (DKA) may cause signs and symptoms such as abdominal pain, nausea, vomiting, hyperventilation, a fruity breath odor, and, if left untreated, altered level of consciousness, coma, and death. Initiation of insulin treatment, along with fluid and electrolytes as needed, is essential to treat hyperglycemia and DKA and rapidly improves the metabolic abnormalities.

Type 2 Diabetes

The two main problems related to insulin in type 2 diabetes are insulin resistance and impaired insulin secretion. Insulin resistance refers to a decreased tissue sensitivity to insulin. Normally, insulin binds to special receptors on cell surfaces and initiates a series of reactions involved in glucose metabolism. In type 2 diabetes, these intracellular reactions are diminished, making insulin less effective at stimulating glucose uptake by the tissues and at regulating glucose release by the liver (Fig. 41-1). The exact mechanisms that lead to insulin resistance and impaired insulin secretion in type 2 diabetes are unknown, although genetic factors are thought to play a role.

To overcome insulin resistance and to prevent the buildup of glucose in the blood, increased amounts of insulin must be secreted to maintain the glucose level at a normal or slightly elevated level. However, if the beta cells cannot keep up with the increased demand for insulin, the glucose level rises, and type 2 diabetes develops.

Despite the impaired insulin secretion that is characteristic of type 2 diabetes, there is enough insulin present to prevent the breakdown of fat and the accompanying production of ketone bodies. Therefore, DKA does not typically occur in type 2 diabetes. However, uncontrolled type 2 diabetes may lead to another acute problem—HHNS (see later discussion).

Because type 2 diabetes is associated with a slow, progressive glucose intolerance, its onset may go undetected for many years. If the patient experiences symptoms, they are frequently mild and may include fatigue, irritability, polyuria, polydipsia, poorly healing skin wounds, vaginal infections, or blurred vision (if glucose levels are very high).

For most patients (approximately 75%), type 2 diabetes is detected incidentally (eg, when routine laboratory tests or ophthalmoscopic examinations are performed). One consequence of undetected diabetes is that long-term diabetes complications (eg, eye disease, peripheral neuropathy, peripheral vascular disease) may have developed before the actual diagnosis of diabetes is made (ADA, 2004r).

Because insulin resistance is associated with obesity, the primary treatment of type 2 diabetes is weight loss. Exercise is also important in enhancing the effectiveness of insulin. Oral antidiabetic agents may be added if meal planning (or medical nutrition therapy [MNT]) and exercise are not successful in controlling blood glucose levels. If maximum doses of a single category of oral agents fail to reduce glucose levels to satisfactory levels, additional oral agents may be used. Insulin may be added to oral agent therapy, or the patient may move to insulin therapy entirely. Some patients require insulin on an ongoing basis; others require insulin on a temporary basis during periods of acute physiologic stress, such as illness or surgery. A patient's treatment depends on the severity of the hyperglycemia at the time of diagnosis.

Recent studies have demonstrated that type 2 diabetes can be prevented or delayed in people at high risk for the disease through weight reduction and increased participation in moderate exercise (Diabetes Prevention Program Research Group, 2002). Metformin, one of the antidiabetic agents, also prevented or delayed the onset of type 2 diabetes, but to a lesser degree. These findings support the role that weight reduction and exercise play in the prevention of type 2 diabetes (Chart 41-2).

Physiology/Pathophysiology

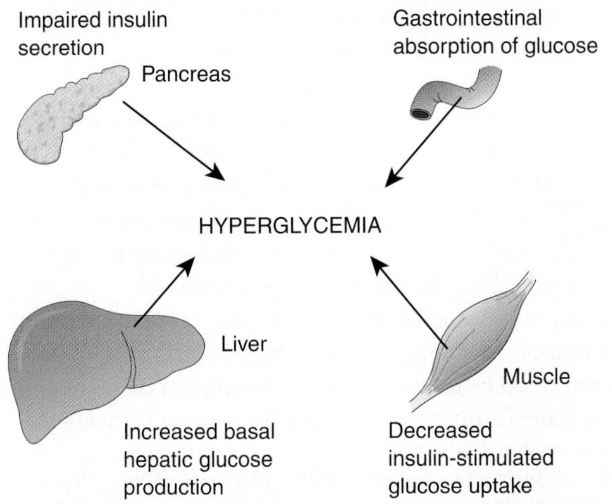

Impaired insulin secretion

Pancreas

Gastrointestinal absorption of glucose

HYPERGLYCEMIA

Liver

Muscle

Increased basal hepatic glucose production

Decreased insulin-stimulated glucose uptake

FIGURE 41-1. Pathogenesis of type 2 diabetes.

CHART 41-2

Prevention of Type 2 Diabetes

In 2002, the Diabetes Prevention Program Research Group reported that type 2 diabetes can be prevented with appropriate changes in lifestyle. Persons at high risk for type 2 diabetes (BMI ≥24, fasting and postprandial plasma glucose levels elevated but not to levels diagnostic of diabetes) received either standard lifestyle recommendations plus metformin, standard lifestyle recommendations plus placebo, or an intensive program of lifestyle modifications. The 16-lesson curriculum of the intensive program of lifestyle modifications focused on weight reduction of >7% of initial body weight and physical activity of moderate intensity. It also included behavior modification strategies designed to help patients achieve the goals of weight reduction and participation in exercise. The lifestyle intervention group had a 58% lower incidence of diabetes and the metformin group had a 31% lower incidence of diabetes compared to the placebo group. These findings were found in both genders and all racial and ethnic groups. These findings demonstrate that type 2 diabetes can be prevented or delayed in persons at high risk for the disease.

From Diabetes Prevention Program Research Group (2002). Reduction in the incidence of type 2 diabetes with lifestyle intervention or metformin. *New England Journal of Medicine, 346*(6), 393–403.

Gestational Diabetes

Gestational diabetes mellitus (GDM) is any degree of glucose intolerance with its onset during pregnancy. Hyperglycemia develops during pregnancy because of the secretion of placental hormones, which causes insulin resistance. Gestational diabetes occurs in as many as 14% of pregnant women and increases their risk for hypertensive disorders during pregnancy (ADA, 2004f).

Women who are considered to be at high risk for GDM and who should be screened by blood glucose testing at their first prenatal visit are those with marked obesity, a personal history of GDM, glycosuria, or a strong family history of diabetes. High-risk ethnic groups include Hispanic Americans, Native Americans, Asian Americans, African Americans, and Pacific Islanders. If these high-risk patients do not have GDM at initial screening, they should be retested between 24 and 28 weeks of gestation. Women of average risk should be tested at 24 to 28 weeks of gestation. Testing is not specifically recommended for women identified as being at low risk. Low-risk women are those who meet all of the following criteria: age younger than 25 years, normal weight before pregnancy, member of an ethnic group with low prevalence of GDM, no history of abnormal glucose tolerance, no known history of diabetes in first-degree relatives, and no history of poor obstetric outcome (ADA, 2004f). Women considered to be at high risk or average risk should have either an oral glucose tolerance test (OGTT) or a glucose challenge test (GCT) followed by OGTT in women who exceed the glucose threshold value of 140 mg/dL (7.8 mmol/L) (ADA, 2004f).

Initial management includes dietary modification and blood glucose monitoring. If hyperglycemia persists, insulin is prescribed. Goals for blood glucose levels during pregnancy are 105 mg/dL (5.8 mmol/L) or less before meals and 130 mg/dL (7.2 mmol/L) or less 2 hours after meals (ADA, 2004f).

After delivery, blood glucose levels in women with GDM usually return to normal. However, many women who have had GDM develop type 2 diabetes later in life. Therefore, a woman who has had GDM should be counseled to maintain her ideal body weight and to exercise regularly to reduce her risk for type 2 diabetes (ADA, 2004f).

Clinical Manifestations

Clinical manifestations depend on the patient's level of hyperglycemia. Classic clinical manifestations of all types of diabetes include the "three Ps": polyuria, polydipsia, and polyphagia. Polyuria (increased urination) and polydipsia (increased thirst) occur as a result of the excess loss of fluid associated with osmotic diuresis. Patients also experience polyphagia (increased appetite) resulting from the catabolic state induced by insulin deficiency and the breakdown of proteins and fats. Other symptoms include fatigue and weakness, sudden vision changes, tingling or numbness in hands or feet, dry skin, skin lesions or wounds that are slow to heal, and recurrent infections. The onset of type 1 diabetes may also be associated with sudden weight loss or nausea, vomiting, or abdominal pains, if DKA has developed.

Assessment and Diagnostic Findings

An abnormally high blood glucose level is the basic criterion for the diagnosis of diabetes. **Fasting plasma glucose (FPG)** levels of 126 mg/dL (7.0 mmol/L) or higher or random plasma glucose levels exceeding 200 mg/dL (11.1 mmol/L) on more than one occasion are diagnostic of diabetes. The OGTT and the intravenous (IV) glucose tolerance test are no longer recommended for routine clinical use. See Chart 41-3 for the ADA's diagnostic criteria for diabetes mellitus (ADA, 2004r).

Because laboratory methods measure plasma glucose, most blood glucose monitors approved for patients' use in the home and some test strips calibrate blood glucose readings to plasma values. Plasma glucose values are 10% to 15% higher than whole blood glucose values, and it is crucial for patients with diabetes to know whether their monitor and strips provide whole blood or plasma results (ADA, 2004w).

In addition to the assessment and diagnostic evaluation performed to diagnose diabetes, ongoing specialized assessment of patients with known diabetes and evaluation for complications in patients with newly diagnosed diabetes are important components of care. Parameters that should be regularly assessed are discussed in Chart 41-4.

Gerontologic Considerations

Elevated blood glucose levels appear to be age related and occur in both men and women throughout the world. Elevated blood glucose levels commonly appear in the fifth decade of life and increase in frequency with ad-

CHART 41-3

Criteria for the Diagnosis of Diabetes Mellitus

1. Symptoms of diabetes plus casual plasma glucose concentration equal to or greater than 200 mg/dL (11.1 mmol/L). Casual is defined as any time of day without regard to time since last meal. The classic symptoms of diabetes include polyuria, polydipsia, and unexplained weight loss.

or

2. Fasting plasma glucose greater than or equal to 126 mg/dL (7.0 mmol/L). Fasting is defined as no caloric intake for at least 8 hours.

or

3. Two-hour postload glucose equal to or greater than 200 mg/dL (11.1 mmol/L) during an oral glucose tolerance test. The test should be performed as described by the World Health Organization, using a glucose load containing the equivalent of 75 g anhydrous glucose dissolved in water.

In the absence of unequivocal hyperglycemia with acute metabolic decompensation, these criteria should be confirmed by repeat testing on a different day. The third measure is not recommended for routine clinical use.

Used with permission of American Diabetes Association. (2004). Report of the Expert Committee on the Diagnosis and Classification of Diabetes Mellitus, *Diabetes Care, 27*(1), 5–10.

CHART 41-4

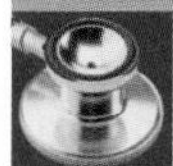

Assessing the Patient With Diabetes

HISTORY

- Symptoms related to the diagnosis of diabetes:
  - Symptoms of hyperglycemia
  - Symptoms of hypoglycemia
    - Frequency, timing, severity, and resolution
- Results of blood glucose monitoring
- Status, symptoms, and management of chronic complications of diabetes:
  - Eye; kidney; nerve; genitourinary and sexual, bladder, and gastrointestinal
  - Cardiac; peripheral vascular; foot complications associated with diabetes
- Adherence to/ability to follow prescribed dietary management plan
- Adherence to prescribed exercise regimen
- Adherence to/ability to follow prescribed pharmacologic treatment (insulin or oral antidiabetic agents)
- Use of tobacco, alcohol, and prescribed and over-the-counter medications/drugs
- Lifestyle, cultural, psychosocial, and economic factors that may affect diabetes treatment
- Effects of diabetes or its complications on functional status (eg, mobility, vision)

PHYSICAL EXAMINATION

- Blood pressure (sitting and standing to detect orthostatic changes)
- Body mass index (height and weight)
- Fundoscopic examination and visual acuity
- Foot examination (lesions, signs of infection, pulses)
- Skin examination (lesions and insulin-injection sites)
- Neurologic examination
  - Vibratory and sensory examination using monofilament
  - Deep tendon reflexes
- Oral examination

LABORATORY EXAMINATION

- $HgbA_{1C}$ (A1C)
- Fasting lipid profile
- Test for microalbuminuria
- Serum creatinine level
- Urinalysis
- Electrocardiogram

NEED FOR REFERRALS

- Ophthalmology
- Podiatry
- Dietitian
- Diabetes educator
- Others if indicated

vancing age. Approximately 10% to 30% of elderly people have age-related hyperglycemia, not counting those with overt diabetes. What causes age-related changes in carbohydrate metabolism is not known. Possibilities include poor diet, physical inactivity, a decrease in the lean body mass in which ingested carbohydrate may be stored, altered insulin secretion, and increase in fat tissue, which increases insulin resistance.

Overall Management of Diabetes

The main goal of diabetes treatment is to normalize insulin activity and blood glucose levels to reduce the development of vascular and neuropathic complications. The Diabetes Control and Complications Trial (DCCT), a 10-year prospective clinical trial conducted from 1983 to 1993, demonstrated the importance of tight blood glucose control. The trial investigated the impact of intensive glucose control on the development and progression of complications such as **retinopathy**, **nephropathy**, and **neuropathy**. A cohort of 1441 people with type 1 diabetes were randomly assigned to conventional treatment (one or two insulin injections per day) or intensive treatment (three or four insulin injections per day or **insulin pump** therapy plus frequent blood glucose monitoring and weekly contacts with diabetes educators). Results showed that the risk of developing retinopathy, neuropathy, and early signs of nephropathy (microalbuminuria and albuminuria) was dramatically reduced in the intensive treatment group. The reduction was attributed to control of blood glucose levels to normal or near-normal levels. The ADA now recommends that all patients with diabetes strive for glucose control to reduce their risk of complications (ADA, 2004j).

The DCCT trial showed that the major adverse effect of intensive therapy was a threefold increase in the incidence of severe **hypoglycemia** (severe enough to require assistance from another person), coma, or seizure. Because of these adverse effects, intensive therapy must be initiated with caution and must be accompanied by thorough education of the patient and family and by responsible behavior of the patient. Careful screening of patients is a key step in initiating intensive therapy. (For situations that preclude the initiation of very tight blood glucose control, see the discussion of insulin in this chapter.)

A study conducted in the United Kingdom and reported in 1998 supported the results of the DCCT in type 2 diabetes and demonstrated a decrease in complications among patients with type 2 diabetes receiving intensive therapy compared to those receiving conventional therapy (United Kingdom Prospective Diabetes Study Group [UKPDS], 1998; ADA, 2003c).

The results of the DCCT and UKPDS have been supported by follow-up studies, including the Epidemiology of

Diabetes Interventions and Complications (EDIC) study (Nathan, Cleary, Backlund, et al., 2005).

Therefore, the therapeutic goal for diabetes management is to achieve normal blood glucose levels (euglycemia) without hypoglycemia while maintaining a high quality of life. Diabetes management has five components (Fig. 41-2):

- Nutritional therapy
- Exercise
- Monitoring
- Pharmacologic therapy
- Education

Treatment varies because of changes in lifestyle and physical and emotional status as well as advances in treatment methods. Therefore, diabetes management involves constant assessment and modification of the treatment plan by health professionals and daily adjustments in therapy by the patient. Although the health care team directs the treatment, it is the individual patient who must manage the complex therapeutic regimen. For this reason, patient and family education is an essential component of diabetes treatment and is as important as all other components of the regimen.

Nutritional Therapy

Nutrition, meal planning, and weight control are the foundation of diabetes management. The most important objectives in the dietary and nutritional management of diabetes are control of total caloric intake to attain or maintain a reasonable body weight, control of blood glucose levels, and normalization of lipids and blood pressure to prevent heart disease. Success in this area alone is often associated with reversal of hyperglycemia in type 2 diabetes. However, achieving these goals is not always easy. Because medical nutrition therapy (MNT, nutritional management) of diabetes is complex, a registered dietitian who understands diabetes management has the major responsibility for designing and teaching this aspect of the therapeutic plan. Nurses and all other members of the health care team must be knowledgeable about nutritional therapy and supportive of patients who need to implement nutritional and lifestyle changes (ADA, 2004r). Nutritional management of diabetes includes the following goals (ADA, 2004e):

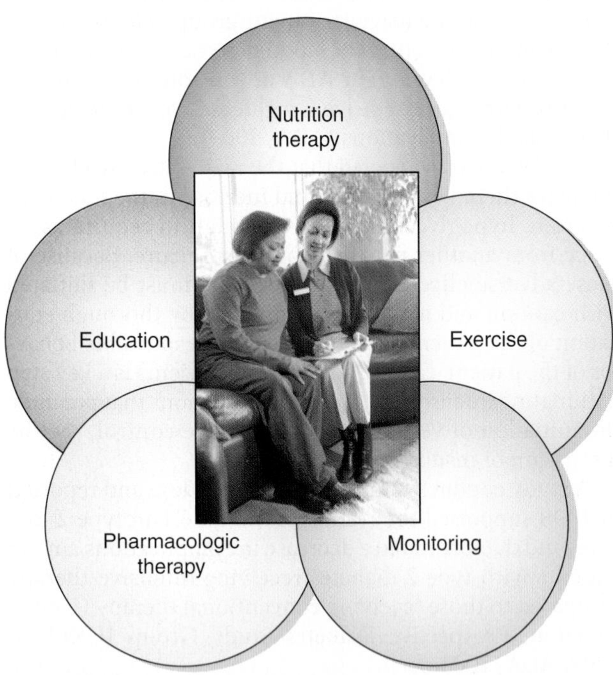

FIGURE 41-2. The five components of diabetes management.

- Providing all the essential food constituents (eg, vitamins, minerals) necessary for optimal nutrition
- Meeting energy needs
- Achieving and maintaining a reasonable weight
- Preventing wide daily fluctuations in blood glucose levels, with blood glucose levels as close to normal as is safe and practical to prevent or reduce the risk for complications
- Decreasing serum lipid levels, if elevated, to reduce the risk for macrovascular disease

For patients who require insulin to help control blood glucose levels, maintaining as much consistency as possible in the amount of calories and carbohydrates ingested at each meal is essential. In addition, consistency in the approximate time intervals between meals, with the addition of snacks if necessary, helps prevent hypoglycemic reactions and maintain overall blood glucose control. For patients who can master the insulin-to-carbohydrate calculations, lifestyle can be more flexible and diabetes control more predictable.

For obese patients with diabetes (especially those with type 2 diabetes), weight loss is the key to treatment. (It is also a major factor in preventing diabetes.) In general, overweight is considered to be a body mass index (BMI) of 25 to 29; obesity is defined as 20% above ideal body weight or a BMI equal to or greater than 30 (National Institutes of Health, 2000). BMI is a weight-to-height ratio calculated by dividing body weight (in kilograms) by the square of the height (in meters). Calculation of BMI is discussed in Chapter 5. Obesity is associated with an increased resistance to insulin; it is also a main factor in type 2 diabetes. Some obese patients who have type 2 diabetes and who require insulin or oral agents to control blood glucose levels may be able to reduce or eliminate the need for medication through weight loss. A weight loss as small as 10% of total weight may significantly improve blood glucose levels (Diabetes Prevention Program Research Group, 2002). For obese patients with diabetes who do not take insulin or sulfonylureas, consistent meal content or timing is important but not as critical. Rather, decreasing the overall caloric intake assumes more importance. However, meals should not be skipped. Pacing food intake throughout the day places more manageable demands on the pancreas.

Consistently following a meal plan is one of the most challenging aspects of diabetes management. For obese patients, it may be more realistic to restrict calories only moderately. For patients who have lost weight, maintaining the weight loss may be difficult. To help these patients incorporate new dietary habits into their lifestyles, diet education, behavioral therapy, group support, and ongoing nutrition counseling are encouraged.

Meal Planning and Related Teaching

For all patients with diabetes, the meal plan must consider the patient's food preferences, lifestyle, usual eating times, and ethnic and cultural background. For patients using intensive insulin therapy, there may be greater flexibility in the timing and content of meals by allowing adjustments in insulin dosage for changes in eating and exercise habits. Advances in insulin management (new insulin analogues, insulin algorithms, insulin pumps) permit greater flexibility of schedules than was previously possible. This contrasts with the older concept of maintaining a constant dose of insulin, which requires patients to adjust their schedule to the actions and duration of the insulin.

The first step in preparing a meal plan is a thorough review of the patient's diet history to identify his or her eating habits and lifestyle. A thorough assessment of the patient's need for weight loss, gain, or maintenance is also undertaken. In most instances, people with type 2 diabetes require weight reduction.

In teaching about meal planning, clinical dietitians use various educational tools, materials, and approaches. Initial education addresses the importance of consistent eating habits, the relationship of food and insulin, and the provision of an individualized meal plan. In-depth follow-up education then focuses on management skills, such as eating at restaurants, reading food labels, and adjusting the meal plan for exercise, illness, and special occasions. The nurse plays an important role in communicating pertinent information to the dietitian and reinforcing the patient's understanding.

For some patients, certain aspects of meal planning, such as the food exchange system, may be difficult to learn. This may be related to limitations in the patient's intellectual level or to emotional issues, such as difficulty accepting the diagnosis of diabetes or feelings of deprivation and undue restriction in eating. In any case, it helps to emphasize that using the exchange system (or any food classification system) provides a new way of thinking about food rather than a new way of eating. It is also important to simplify information as much as possible and to provide opportunities for the patient to practice and repeat activities and information.

CALORIC REQUIREMENTS

Calorie-controlled diets are planned by first calculating a person's energy needs and caloric requirements based on age, gender, height, and weight. An activity element is then factored in to provide the actual number of calories required for weight maintenance. To promote a 1- to 2-pound weight loss per week, 500 to 1000 calories are subtracted from the daily total. The calories are distributed into carbohydrates, proteins, and fats, and a meal plan is then developed, taking into account the patient's lifestyle and food preferences.

The 1995 Exchange Lists for Meal Planning (ADA, 1995) are presented to the patient using the appropriate amount of calories and setting realistic goals. Unfortunately, it is often confusing and difficult to comply with calorie-controlled diets, which require the patient to measure precise portions and to eat specific foods and amounts at each meal and snack. Development of a meal plan based on the patient's usual eating habits and lifestyle may be a more realistic approach to glucose control and weight loss or weight maintenance. In either instance, the patient needs to work closely with a registered dietitian to assess current eating habits and to achieve realistic, individualized goals.

For example, the priority for a young patient with type 1 diabetes should be a diet with enough calories to maintain normal growth and development. Some patients may be underweight at the onset of type 1 diabetes because of rapid weight loss from severe hyperglycemia. The goal with these patients initially may be to provide a higher-calorie diet to regain lost weight.

CALORIC DISTRIBUTION

A meal plan for diabetes also focuses on the percentages of calories that come from carbohydrates, proteins, and fats. In general, carbohydrate foods have the greatest effect on blood glucose levels, because they are more quickly digested than other foods and are converted into glucose rapidly. Several decades ago, it was recommended that diabetic diets contain more calories from protein and fat foods than from carbohydrates, to reduce postprandial increases in blood glucose levels. However, this resulted in a dietary intake inconsistent with the goal of reducing the cardiovascular disease commonly associated with diabetes (ADA, 2004e).

Carbohydrates. The caloric distribution currently recommended is higher in carbohydrates than in fat and protein. However, research into the appropriateness of a higher-carbohydrate diet in patients with decreased glucose tolerance is ongoing, and recommendations may change accordingly. Currently, the ADA and the American Dietetic Association recommend that, for all levels of caloric intake, 50% to 60% of calories should be derived from carbohydrates, 20% to 30% from fat, and the remaining 10% to 20% from protein. The majority of the selections for carbohydrates should come from whole grains. These recommendations are also consistent with those of the American Heart Association, American Cancer Society, and the U.S. Department of Agriculture (2000).

Carbohydrates consist of sugars and starches. Little scientific evidence supports the belief that sugars (eg, sucrose) promote a higher blood glucose level than starches (eg, rice, pasta, bread). Low glycemic index diets (described later) may reduce postprandial glucose levels. Therefore, the nutrition guidelines recommend that all carbohydrates should be eaten in moderation to avoid high postprandial blood glucose levels (ADA, 1995). Foods high in carbohydrates, such as sucrose, are not eliminated from the diet but should be eaten in moderation (up to 10% of total calories), because they are typically high in fat and lack vitamins, minerals, and fiber.

Carbohydrate counting is another nutritional tool used for blood glucose management, because carbohydrates are the main nutrients in food that influence blood glucose levels. This method provides flexibility in food choices, can be less complicated to understand than the diabetic food exchange list, and allows more accurate management with multiple daily injections (insulin before each meal). However, if carbohydrate counting is not used with other meal-planning techniques, weight gain can result. A variety of methods are used to count carbohydrates. When developing a diabetic meal plan using carbohydrate counting, all food sources should be considered. Once digested, 100% of carbohydrates are converted to glucose. However, approximately 50% of protein foods (meat, fish, and poultry) are also converted to glucose, but this has minimal effect on blood glucose levels.

One method of carbohydrate counting includes counting grams of carbohydrates. If target goals are not reached by counting carbohydrates alone, protein is factored into the calculations. This is especially true if the meal consists only of meat, fish, and nonstarchy vegetables.

An alternative to counting grams of carbohydrate is measuring servings or choices. This method is used more often by people with type 2 diabetes. It is similar to the food exchange list and emphasizes portion control of total servings of carbohydrate at meals and snacks. One carbohydrate serving is equivalent to 15 g of carbohydrate. Examples of one serving are an apple 2 inches in diameter and one slice of bread. Vegetables and meat are counted as one third of a carbohydrate serving.

Although carbohydrate counting is now commonly used for blood glucose management with type 1 and type 2 diabetes, it is not a perfect system. All carbohydrates affect the blood glucose level to different degrees, regardless of equivalent serving size. When carbohydrate counting is used, reading labels on food items is the key to success. Knowing what the "carbohydrate budget" for the meal is and knowing how many grams of carbohydrate are in a serving of a food, the patient can calculate the amount in one serving.

Fats. The recommendations regarding fat content of the diabetic diet include both reducing the total percentage of calories from fat sources to less than 30% of total calories and limiting the amount of saturated fats to 10% of total calories. Additional recommendations include limiting the total intake of dietary cholesterol to less than 300 mg/day. This approach may help reduce risk factors such as increased serum cholesterol levels, which are associated with the development of coronary artery disease, the leading cause of death and disability among people with diabetes.

The meal plan may include the use of some nonanimal sources of protein (eg, legumes, whole grains), to help reduce saturated fat and cholesterol intake. In addition, the amount of protein intake may be reduced in patients with early signs of renal disease.

Fiber. The use of fiber in diets for diabetes has received increased attention as researchers study the effects on diabetes of a high-carbohydrate, high-fiber diet. This type of diet plays a role in lowering total cholesterol and low-density lipoprotein cholesterol in the blood. Increased fiber in the diet may also improve blood glucose levels and decrease the need for exogenous insulin.

There are two types of dietary fibers: soluble and insoluble. Soluble fiber—in foods such as legumes, oats, and some fruits—plays more of a role in lowering blood glucose and lipid levels than does insoluble fiber, although the clinical significance of this effect is probably small (ADA, 2004r). Soluble fiber is thought to be related to the formation of a gel in the gastrointestinal tract. This gel slows stomach emptying and the movement of food through the upper digestive tract. The potential glucose-lowering effect of fiber may be caused by the slower rate of glucose absorption from foods that contain soluble fiber. Insoluble fiber is found in whole-grain breads and cereals and in some vegetables. This type of fiber plays more of a role in increasing stool bulk and preventing constipation. Both insoluble and soluble fibers increase satiety, which is helpful for weight loss. Ideally, 25 g of fiber should be ingested daily.

One risk involved in suddenly increasing fiber intake is that it may require adjusting the dosage of insulin or oral agents to prevent hypoglycemia. Other problems may include abdominal fullness, nausea, diarrhea, increased flatulence, and constipation if fluid intake is inadequate. If fiber is added to or increased in the meal plan, it should be done gradually and in consultation with a dietitian. The Exchange Lists for Meal Planning (ADA, 1995) is an excellent guide for increasing fiber intake. Fiber-rich food choices within the vegetable, fruit, and starch/bread exchanges are highlighted in the lists.

FOOD CLASSIFICATION SYSTEMS

To teach diet principles and to help patients in meal planning, several systems have been developed in which foods are organized into groups with common characteristics, such as number of calories, composition of foods (ie, amount of protein, fat, or carbohydrate in the food), or effect on blood glucose levels.

Exchange Lists. A commonly used tool for nutritional management is the Exchange Lists for Meal Planning (ADA, 1995). There are six main exchange lists: bread/starch, vegetable, milk, meat, fruit, and fat. Foods included on one list (in the amounts specified) contain equal numbers of calories and are approximately equal in grams of protein, fat, and carbohydrate. Meal plans (tailored to the patient's needs and preferences) are based on a recommended number of choices from each exchange list. Foods on one list may be interchanged with one another, allowing the patient to choose a variety while maintaining as much consistency as possible in the nutrient content of foods eaten. Table 41-2 presents three sample lunch menus that are interchangeable in terms of carbohydrate, protein, and fat content.

Exchange list information on combination foods such as pizza, chili, and casseroles, as well as convenience foods,

TABLE 41-2 Selected Sample Menus from Exchange Lists

Exchanges	Sample Lunch #1	Sample Lunch #2	Sample Lunch #3
2 starch	2 slices bread	Hamburger bun	1 cup cooked pasta
3 meat	2 oz sliced turkey and 1 oz lowfat cheese	3 oz lean beef patty	3 oz boiled shrimp
1 vegetable	Lettuce, tomato, onion	Green salad	½ cup plum tomatoes
1 fat	1 tsp mayonnaise	1 tbsp salad dressing	1 tsp olive oil
1 fruit	1 medium apple	1¼ cup watermelon	1¼ cup fresh strawberries
"Free" items (optional)	Unsweetened iced tea Mustard, pickle, hot pepper	Diet soda 1 tbsp catsup, pickle, onions	Ice water with lemon Garlic, basil

desserts, snack foods, and fast foods, is available from the ADA. Some food manufacturers and restaurants publish exchange lists that describe their products. For more nutrition information, contact the ADA (see Resources).

Nutrition Labels. Food manufacturers are required to have the nutrition content of foods listed on package labels, and reading food labels is an important skill for patients to learn and use when food shopping. The label provides information about how many grams of carbohydrate are in a serving of food. Some patients use this information to determine how much medication they need. For example, a patient who takes premeal insulin may use the algorithm, 1 unit of insulin for 15 g of carbohydrate. Patients can also be taught to have a "carbohydrate budget" per meal (eg, 45 to 60 g).

Food Guide Pyramid. The Food Guide Pyramid (ie, MyPyramid) is another tool used to develop meal plans. It is commonly used for patients with type 2 diabetes who have a difficult time following a calorie-controlled diet. The 2005 food pyramid consists of the following food groups: (1) grains, (2) vegetables, (3) fruits, (4) milk and other dairy products, and (5) meats and beans. Oils and other high-fat foods comprise another food group on the pyramid (see Chapter 5). Foods (starches, fruits, and vegetables) that are lowest in calories and fat and highest in fiber should make up the basis of the diet. For those with diabetes, as well as for the general population, 50% to 60% of the daily caloric intake should be from these three groups. Foods higher in fat (particularly saturated fat) should account for a smaller percentage of the daily caloric intake. Fats, oils, and sweets should be used sparingly by people with diabetes to obtain weight and blood glucose control and to reduce the risk for cardiovascular disease. Reliance on the MyPyramid may result in fluctuations in blood glucose levels, however, because high-carbohydrate foods may be grouped with low-carbohydrate foods. The pyramid is appropriately used only as a first-step teaching tool for patients who are learning how to control food portions and how to identify which foods contain carbohydrate, protein, and fat.

Glycemic Index. One of the main goals of diet therapy in diabetes is to avoid sharp, rapid increases in blood glucose levels after food is eaten. The term "glycemic index" is used to describe how much a given food increases the blood glucose level compared with an equivalent amount of glucose. The effects of use of the glycemic index on blood glucose levels and on long-term patient outcomes are unclear, but it may be beneficial (ADA, 2004r). Although more research is necessary, the following guidelines may be helpful when making dietary recommendations:

- Combining starchy foods with protein- and fat-containing foods tends to slow their absorption and lower the glycemic response.
- In general, eating foods that are raw and whole results in a lower glycemic response than eating chopped, puréed, or cooked foods.
- Eating whole fruit instead of drinking juice decreases the glycemic response, because fiber in the fruit slows absorption.
- Adding foods with sugars to the diet may result in a lower glycemic response if these foods are eaten with foods that are more slowly absorbed.

Patients can create their own glycemic index by monitoring their blood glucose level after ingestion of a particular food. This can help patients improve blood glucose control through individualized manipulation of the diet. Many patients who use frequent monitoring of blood glucose levels can use this information to adjust their insulin doses in accordance with variations in food intake.

Other Dietary Concerns

ALCOHOL CONSUMPTION

Patients with diabetes do not need to give up alcoholic beverages entirely, but patients and health care professionals must be aware of the potential adverse effects of alcohol specific to diabetes. Alcohol is absorbed before other nutrients and does not require insulin for absorption. Large amounts can be converted to fats, increasing the risk for DKA. In general, the same precautions regarding the use of alcohol by people without diabetes should be applied to patients with diabetes. Moderation is recommended. A major danger of alcohol consumption by the patient with diabetes is hypoglycemia, especially for patients who take insulin. Alcohol may decrease the normal physiologic reactions in the body that produce glucose (gluconeogenesis). Therefore, if a patient with diabetes consumes alcohol on an empty stomach, there is an increased likelihood of hypoglycemia. In addition, excessive alcohol intake may impair the patient's ability to recognize and treat hypoglycemia or to follow a prescribed meal plan to prevent hypoglycemia. To reduce the risk of hypoglycemia, the patient should be cautioned to consume food along with the alcohol (American Association of Diabetes Educators [AADE], 2004).

Alcohol consumption may lead to excessive weight gain (from the high caloric content of alcohol), hyperlipidemia, and elevated glucose levels (especially with mixed drinks and liqueurs). Patient teaching regarding alcohol intake must emphasize moderation in the amount of alcohol consumed. Moderate intake is considered to be one alcoholic beverage per day for women and two per day for men. Lower-calorie or less sweet drinks (eg, light beer, dry wine) and food intake along with alcohol consumption are advised. Especially for patients with type 2 diabetes who wish to control their weight, it is important to incorporate the calories from alcohol into the overall meal plan.

SWEETENERS

Use of sweeteners is acceptable for patients with diabetes, especially if it assists in overall dietary adherence. Moderation in the amount of sweetener used is encouraged, to avoid potential adverse effects. There are two main types of sweeteners: nutritive and non-nutritive. The nutritive sweeteners contain calories, and the non-nutritive sweeteners have few or no calories in the amounts normally used.

Nutritive sweeteners include fructose (fruit sugar), sorbitol, and xylitol. They are not calorie free; they provide calories in amounts similar to those in sucrose (table sugar). They cause less elevation in blood sugar levels than sucrose does and are often used in "sugar-free" foods. Sweeteners containing sorbitol may have a laxative effect.

Non-nutritive sweeteners have minimal or no calories. They are used in food products and are also available for table use. They produce minimal or no elevation in blood glucose levels and have been approved by the U.S. Food and Drug Administration (FDA) as safe for people with diabetes. Saccharin contains no calories. Aspartame (NutraSweet) is packaged with dextrose; it contains 4 calories per packet and loses sweetness with heat. Acesulfame-K (Sunnette) is also packaged with dextrose; it contains 1 calorie per packet. Sucralose (Splenda), a derivative of glucose, is a newer non-nutritive, high-intensity sweetener that is about 600 times sweeter than sugar. The FDA has approved it for use in baked goods, nonalcoholic beverages, chewing gum, coffee, confections, frostings, and frozen dairy products.

MISLEADING FOOD LABELS

Foods labeled "sugarless" or "sugar-free" may still provide calories equal to those of the equivalent sugar-containing products if they are made with nutritive sweeteners. Therefore, for weight loss, these products may not always be useful. In addition, patients must not consider them "free" foods to be eaten in unlimited quantity, because they can elevate blood glucose levels.

Foods labeled "dietetic" are not necessarily reduced-calorie foods. They may be lower in sodium or have other special dietary uses. Patients are advised that foods labeled "dietetic" may still contain significant amounts of sugar or fat.

Patients must also be taught to read the labels of "health foods"—especially snacks—because they often contain carbohydrates such as honey, brown sugar, and corn syrup. In addition, these supposedly healthy snacks frequently contain saturated vegetable fats (eg, coconut or palm oil), hydrogenated vegetable fats, or animal fats, which may be contraindicated in people with elevated blood lipid levels.

Exercise

Benefits

Exercise is extremely important in diabetes management because of its effects on lowering blood glucose and reducing cardiovascular risk factors. Exercise lowers blood glucose levels by increasing the uptake of glucose by body muscles and by improving insulin utilization. It also improves circulation and muscle tone. Resistance (strength) training, such as weight lifting, can increase lean muscle mass, thereby increasing the resting metabolic rate. These effects are useful in diabetes in relation to losing weight, easing stress, and maintaining a feeling of well-being. Exercise also alters blood lipid concentrations, increasing levels of high-density lipoproteins and decreasing total cholesterol and triglyceride levels. This is especially important for people with diabetes because of their increased risk of cardiovascular disease (Nathan et al., 2005). General precautions for exercise in diabetes are presented in Chart 41-5.

Exercise Precautions

Patients who have blood glucose levels exceeding 250 mg/dL (14 mmol/L) and who have ketones in their urine should not begin exercising until the urine test results are negative for ketones and the blood glucose level is closer to normal. Exercising with elevated blood glucose levels increases the secretion of glucagon, growth hormone, and catecholamines. The liver then releases more glucose, and the result is an increase in the blood glucose level (ADA, 2004n).

CHART 41-5

General Precautions for Exercise in People With Diabetes

- Use proper footwear and, if appropriate, other protective equipment.
- Avoid exercise in extreme heat or cold.
- Inspect feet daily after exercise.
- Avoid exercise during periods of poor metabolic control.

The physiologic decrease in circulating insulin that normally occurs with exercise cannot occur in patients treated with insulin. Initially, patients who require insulin should be taught to eat a 15-g carbohydrate snack (a fruit exchange) or a snack of complex carbohydrates with a protein before engaging in moderate exercise, to prevent unexpected hypoglycemia. If the patient is exercising to lose or control weight, a decrease in the insulin dose with exercise would be indicated. The exact amount of food needed varies from person to person and should be determined by blood glucose monitoring. Some patients find that they do not require a pre-exercise snack if they exercise within 1 to 2 hours after a meal. Other patients may require extra food regardless of when they exercise. If extra food is required, it need not be deducted from the regular meal plan.

Another potential problem for patients who take insulin is hypoglycemia that occurs many hours after exercise. To avoid postexercise hypoglycemia, especially after strenuous or prolonged exercise, the patient may need to eat a snack at the end of the exercise session and at bedtime and monitor the blood glucose level more frequently. In addition, it may be necessary to reduce the dosage of insulin that peaks at the time of exercise. Patients who are capable, knowledgeable, and responsible can learn to adjust their own insulin doses by working closely with a diabetes educator. Others need specific instructions on what to do when they exercise.

Patients participating in extended periods of exercise should test their blood glucose levels before, during, and after the exercise period, and they should snack on carbohydrates as needed to maintain blood glucose levels (ADA, 2004n). Other participants or observers should be aware that the person exercising has diabetes, and they should know what assistance to give if severe hypoglycemia occurs.

In obese people with type 2 diabetes, exercise in addition to dietary management both improves glucose metabolism and enhances loss of body fat. Exercise coupled with weight loss improves insulin sensitivity and may decrease the need for insulin or oral antidiabetic agents. Eventually, the patient's glucose tolerance may return to normal. Patients with type 2 diabetes who are not taking insulin or an oral agent may not need extra food before exercise.

Exercise Recommendations

Ideally, a person with diabetes should exercise at the same time (preferably when blood glucose levels are at their peak) and in the same amount each day. Regular daily exercise, rather than sporadic exercise, should be encouraged. Exercise recommendations must be altered as necessary for patients with diabetic complications such as retinopathy, autonomic neuropathy, sensorimotor neuropathy, and cardiovascular disease (ADA, 2004n). Increased blood pressure associated with exercise may aggravate diabetic retinopathy and increase the risk of a hemorrhage into the vitreous or retina. Patients with ischemic heart disease risk triggering angina or a myocardial infarction, which may be silent. Avoiding trauma to the lower extremities is especially important in patients with numbness related to neuropathy.

In general, a slow, gradual increase in the exercise period is encouraged. For many patients, walking is a safe and beneficial form of exercise that requires no special equipment (except for proper shoes) and can be performed anywhere. People with diabetes should discuss an exercise program with their health care providers and undergo a careful medical evaluation with appropriate diagnostic studies before beginning program (ADA, 2004n).

For patients who are older than 30 years and who have two or more risk factors for heart disease, an exercise stress test is recommended. Risk factors for heart disease include hypertension, obesity, high cholesterol levels, abnormal resting electrocardiogram (ECG), sedentary lifestyle, smoking, male gender, and a family history of heart disease. An abnormal stress test may indicate cardiac ischemia. Typically, an abnormal stress test is followed up with a cardiac catheterization and in some cases an intervention such as angioplasty, stent replacement, or cardiac surgery.

Gerontologic Considerations

Physical activity that is consistent and realistic is beneficial to elderly people with diabetes. Physical fitness in the elderly population with diabetes may lead to less chronic vascular disease and an improved quality of life (ADA, 2004n). Advantages of exercise in this population include a decrease in hyperglycemia, a general sense of well-being, and better use of ingested calories, resulting in weight reduction. Because there is an increased incidence of cardiovascular problems in the elderly, a physical examination and exercise stress test are usually warranted before an exercise program is initiated. A pattern of gradual, consistent exercise should be planned that does not exceed the patient's physical capacity. Physical impairment due to other chronic diseases must also be considered. In some cases, a physical therapy evaluation may be indicated, with the goal of determining exercises specific to the patient's needs and abilities. Tools such as the "Armchair Fitness" video may be helpful. For more information about age-related changes that affect diabetes management, see Chart 41-6.

CHART 41-6

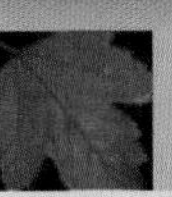

Gerontologic Considerations

Age-Related Changes That May Affect Diabetes and Its Management

SENSORY CHANGES

Decreased vision
Decreased smell
Taste changes
Decreased proprioception
Diminished thirst

GASTROINTESTINAL CHANGES

Dental problems
Appetite changes
Delayed gastric emptying
Decreased bowel motility

ACTIVITY/EXERCISE PATTERN CHANGES

More sedentary

RENAL FUNCTION CHANGES

Decreased function
Decreased drug clearance

AFFECTIVE/COGNITIVE CHANGES

Medications/meals omitted or taken erratically

SOCIOECONOMIC FACTORS

Fad diets
Loneliness/living alone
Lack of money/lack of support system

CHRONIC DISEASES

Hypertension
Arthritis
Neoplasms
Acute/chronic infections

POTENTIAL DRUG INTERACTIONS

Use of another person's medications
Consulting multiple physicians for different illnesses
Alcohol use/abuse

Monitoring Glucose Levels and Ketones

Self-Monitoring of Blood Glucose

Blood glucose monitoring is a cornerstone of diabetes management, and **self-monitoring of blood glucose (SMBG)** levels by patients has dramatically altered diabetes care. Using frequent SMBG and learning how to respond to the results enable people with diabetes to adjust their treatment regimen to obtain optimal blood glucose control. This allows for detection and prevention of hypoglycemia and hyperglycemia and plays a crucial role in normalizing blood glucose levels, which in turn may reduce the risk of long-term diabetic complications.

Various methods for SMBG are available. Most involve obtaining a drop of blood from the fingertip, applying the blood to a special reagent strip, and allowing the blood to stay on the strip for the amount of time specified by the manufacturer (usually 5 to 30 seconds). The meter gives a digital readout of the blood glucose value.

The meters available for SMBG offer various features and benefits. The test strip is placed in the meter first, before blood is applied to it. Once the blood is placed on the strip, it remains there for the duration of the test. The meter automatically displays the blood glucose level after a short time (less than 1 minute). Some meters are biosensors that can use blood obtained from alternative test sites, such as the forearm. They have a special lancing device that is useful for patients who have painful fingertips or experience pain with fingersticks.

Some meters can be used by patients with visual impairments. They have audio components that assist the patient in performing the test and obtaining the result. In addition, meters are available to check both blood glucose and blood ketone levels by those who are particularly susceptible to DKA.

ADVANTAGES AND DISADVANTAGES OF SMBG SYSTEMS

Methods for SMBG must match the skill level of patients. Factors affecting SMBG performance include visual acuity, fine motor coordination, cognitive ability, comfort with technology and willingness to use it, and cost.

The use of meters to monitor blood glucose is recommended, because meters have become much less expensive and less dependent on technique, making the results more accurate. Referral to a social worker may be warranted to assist a patient who is without the financial means to purchase a meter. Most insurance companies cover some or all of the costs of meters and strips.

A potential hazard of all methods of SMBG is that the patient may obtain and report erroneous blood glucose values as a result of using incorrect techniques. Some common sources of error include the following:

- Improper application of blood (eg, drop too small)
- Damage to the reagent strips caused by heat or humidity; use of outdated strips
- Improper meter cleaning and maintenance (eg, allowing dust or blood to accumulate on the optic window). This is not an issue in the biosensor type of meter.

Nurses play an important role in providing initial teaching about SMBG techniques. Equally important is evaluating the techniques of patients who are experienced in self-monitoring. Patients should be discouraged from purchasing SMBG products from stores or catalogs that do not provide direct education. Every 6 to 12 months, patients should conduct a comparison of their meter result with a simultaneous laboratory-measured blood glucose level in their physician's office. The accuracy of the meter and strips should also be assessed with control solutions specific to that meter whenever a new vial of strips is used and whenever the validity of the reading is in doubt.

CANDIDATES FOR SMBG

For everyone with diabetes, SMBG is a useful tool for managing self-care. It is a key component of treatment for any intensive insulin therapy regimen (ie, two to four injections per day or use of an insulin pump) and for diabetes management during pregnancy. It is also recommended for patients with the following conditions:

- Unstable diabetes (severe swings from very high to very low blood glucose levels within a 24-hour day)
- A tendency to develop severe ketosis or hypoglycemia
- Hypoglycemia without warning symptoms

For patients not taking insulin, SMBG is helpful for monitoring the effectiveness of exercise, diet, and oral antidiabetic agents. It can also help motivate patients to continue with treatment. For patients with type 2 diabetes, SMBG is recommended during periods of suspected hyperglycemia (eg, illness) or hypoglycemia (eg, unusual increased activity levels) and when the medication or dosage of medication is modified (ADA, 2004n).

FREQUENCY OF SMBG

For most patients who require insulin, SMBG is recommended two to four times daily (usually before meals and at bedtime). For patients who take insulin before each meal, SMBG is required at least three times daily before meals to determine each dose (ADA, 2004w). Patients not receiving insulin may be instructed to assess their blood glucose levels at least two or three times per week, including a 2-hour postprandial test. For all patients, testing is recommended whenever hypoglycemia or hyperglycemia is suspected. Patients should increase the frequency of SMBG with changes in medications, activity, or diet and with stress or illness.

RESPONDING TO SMBG RESULTS

Patients are asked to keep a record or logbook of blood glucose levels so that they can detect patterns. Testing is done at the peak action time of the medication to evaluate the need for dosage adjustments. To evaluate basal insulin and determine bolus insulin doses, testing is performed before meals. To determine bolus doses of regular or lispro insulin, testing is done 2 hours after meals. Patients with type 2 diabetes are encouraged to test before and 2 hours after the largest meal of the day. Patients who take insulin at bedtime or who use an insulin infusion pump should also test at 3 AM once a week to document that the blood glucose level is not decreasing during the night. If the patient is unwilling or cannot afford to test frequently, then once or twice a day may be sufficient if the time of testing is varied (eg, before breakfast one day and before lunch the next day).

A tendency to discontinue SMBG is more likely to occur if the patient does not receive instruction about using the results to alter the treatment regimen, if positive reinforcement is not given, and if costs of testing increase. Instructions vary according to the patient's understanding and the physician's philosophy of diabetes management. At the very least, the patient should be given parameters for contacting the physician. Patients using intensive insulin therapy regimens may be instructed in the use of algorithms (rules or decision trees) for changing the insulin doses based on patterns of values greater or less than the target range and the amount of carbohydrate to be consumed. Baseline patterns should be established by SMBG for 1 to 2 weeks.

Continuous Glucose Monitoring System

A **continuous glucose monitoring system (CGMS)** (Fig. 41-3) that can continuously monitor blood glucose is now available. A sensor attached to an infusion set, which is similar to an insulin pump infusion set, is inserted subcutaneously in the abdomen and connected to the device worn on a belt. After 72 hours, the data from the device are downloaded, and blood glucose readings are analyzed. Although the CGMS cannot be used for making decisions

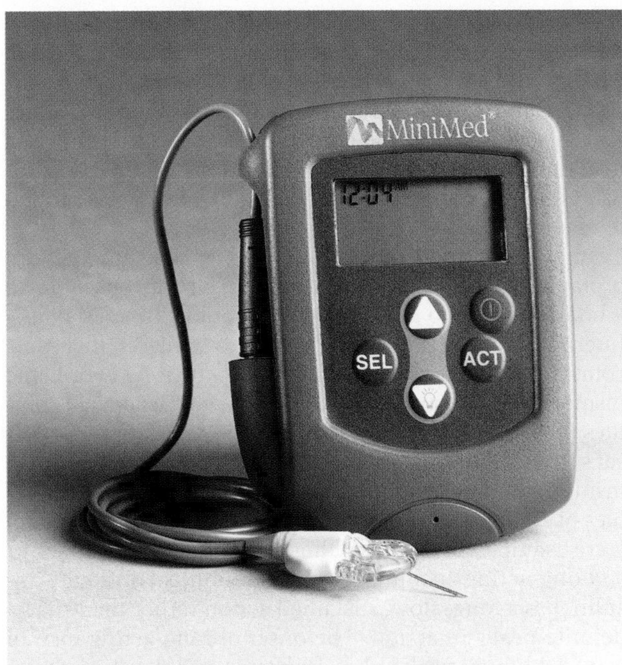

FIGURE 41-3. MiniMed CGMS System Gold Continuous Glucose Monitoring System (Medtronic, Northridge, CA).

about specific insulin doses, it can be used to determine whether treatment is adequate over a 24-hour period. This device will be refined in the future so that it can be used by patients to make daily treatment decisions.

Glycated Hemoglobin

Glycated hemoglobin (also referred to as **glycosylated hemoglobin, $HgbA_{1C}$, or A1C**) is a blood test that reflects average blood glucose levels over a period of approximately 2 to 3 months (ADA, 2004w). When blood glucose levels are elevated, glucose molecules attach to hemoglobin in red blood cells. The longer the amount of glucose in the blood remains above normal, the more glucose binds to hemoglobin and the higher the glycated hemoglobin level becomes. This complex (hemoglobin attached to the glucose) is permanent and lasts for the life of an individual red blood cell, approximately 120 days. If near-normal blood glucose levels are maintained, with only occasional increases, the overall value will not be greatly elevated. However, if the blood glucose values are consistently high, then the test result is also elevated. If the patient reports mostly normal SMBG results but the glycated hemoglobin is high, there may be errors in the methods used for glucose monitoring, errors in recording results, or frequent elevations in glucose levels at times during the day when the patient is not usually monitoring blood sugar levels. The normal values differ slightly from test to test and from laboratory to laboratory and typically range from 4% to 6%. Values within the normal range indicate consistently near-normal blood glucose concentrations, a goal made easier by SMBG.

Urine Glucose Testing

Before SMBG was available, urine glucose testing was the only way to monitor diabetes on a daily basis. Its advantages are that it is less expensive than SMBG and is not invasive. Urine glucose testing is no longer used for the following reasons:

- Results do not accurately reflect the blood glucose level at the time of the test.
- The renal threshold for glucose (the level of blood glucose at which glucose starts to appear in the urine) is 180 to 200 mg/dL (9.9 to 11.1 mmol/L), far above target blood glucose levels.
- Hypoglycemia cannot be detected because a "negative" urine glucose result may occur when the blood glucose level ranges from 0 to 180 mg/dL (9.9 mmol/L) or higher.
- Patients may have a false sense of being in good control when results are always negative.
- Various medications (eg, aspirin, vitamin C, some antibiotics) may interfere with test results.
- In elderly patients and patients with kidney disease, the renal threshold is increased; therefore, false-negative readings may occur at dangerously elevated glucose levels.

Testing for Ketones

Ketones (or ketone bodies) are byproducts of fat breakdown, and they accumulate in the blood and urine. Ketones in the urine signal that control of type 1 diabetes is deteriorating, and the risk of DKA is high. When there is almost no effective insulin available, the body starts to break down stored fat for energy. Urine testing is the most common method used for self-testing of ketone bodies by patients. A meter that enables testing of blood for ketones is available.

Most commonly, the patient uses a urine dipstick (Ketostix or Chemstrip uK) to detect ketonuria. The reagent pad on the strip turns purplish when ketones are present. (One of the ketone bodies is called acetone, and this term is frequently used interchangeably with the term "ketones.") Other strips are available for measuring both urine glucose and ketones (Keto-Diastix or Chemstrip uGK). Large amounts of ketones may depress the color response of the glucose test area.

Urine ketone testing should be performed whenever patients with type 1 diabetes have glycosuria or persistently elevated blood glucose levels (more than 240 mg/dL or 13.2 mmol/L for two testing periods in a row) and during illness, in pregnancy with preexisting diabetes, and in gestational diabetes (ADA, 2004w).

Pharmacologic Therapy

As previously stated, insulin is secreted by the beta cells of the islets of Langerhans and works to lower the blood glucose level after meals by facilitating the uptake and utilization of glucose by muscle, fat, and liver cells. In the absence of adequate insulin, pharmacologic therapy is essential.

Insulin Therapy and Insulin Preparations

In type 1 diabetes, exogenous insulin must be administered for life because the body loses the ability to produce insulin. In type 2 diabetes, insulin may be necessary on a long-term basis to control glucose levels if meal planning and oral agents are ineffective. In addition, some patients in whom type 2 diabetes is usually controlled by meal planning alone or by meal planning and an oral antidiabetic agent may require insulin temporarily during illness, infection, pregnancy, surgery, or some other stressful event. In many cases, insulin injections are administered two or more times daily to control the blood glucose level. Because the insulin dose required by the individual patient is determined by the level of glucose in the blood, accurate monitoring of blood glucose levels is essential; thus, SMBG has become a cornerstone of insulin therapy. A number of insulin preparations are available. They vary according to three main characteristics: time course of action, species (source), and manufacturer.

TIME COURSE OF ACTION

Insulins may be grouped into several categories based on the onset, peak, and duration of action (Table 41-3). Human insulin preparations have a shorter duration of action than insulin from animal sources because the presence of animal proteins triggers an immune response that results in the binding of animal insulin, which slows its availability.

Rapid-acting insulins such as insulin lispro (Humalog) and insulin aspart (NovoLog) produce a more rapid effect that is of shorter duration than regular insulin. These insulins have an onset of 5 to 15 minutes, a peak action of 60 to 90 minutes after injection, and a duration of 2 to 4 hours. Because of their rapid onset, the patient should be instructed to eat no more than 5 to 15 minutes after injection. Because of the short duration of action of these insulin analogues, patients with type 1 diabetes and some patients with type 2 or gestational diabetes also require a long-acting insulin to maintain glucose control. Basal insulin is necessary to maintain blood glucose levels irrespective of meals. A constant level of insulin is required at all times. Intermediate-acting insulins function as basal insulins but may have to be split into two injections to achieve 24-hour coverage.

Short-acting insulins, called regular insulin (marked R on the bottle), have an onset of 30 minutes to 1 hour; peak, 2 to 3 hours; and duration, 4 to 6 hours. Regular insulin is a clear solution and is usually administered 20 to 30 minutes before a meal, either alone or in combination with a longer-acting insulin. Regular insulin is the only insulin approved for IV use. Humulin R, Iletin Regular, and Novolin R are examples of regular insulin.

Intermediate-acting insulins, called NPH insulin (neutral protamine Hagedorn) or Lente insulin, have an onset of 3 to 4 hours; peak, 4 to 12 hours; and duration, 16 to 20 hours. Intermediate-acting insulins, which are similar in their time course of action, appear white and cloudy. If NPH or Lente insulin is taken alone, it is not crucial that it be taken 30 minutes before the meal. However, it is important that patients eat some food around the time of the onset and peak of these insulins. Humulin N, Iletin NPH, and Novolin N are examples of NPH insulins, and Humulin L, Iletin L, and Novolin L are examples of Lente insulins.

Long-acting insulin, such as Humulin Ultralente insulin, has a long, slow, sustained action rather than sharp, definite peaks in action. The onset of long-acting insulin is 6 to 8 hours; peak, 12 to 16 hours; and duration, 20 to 30 hours.

"Peakless" basal or very long-acting insulin (glargine [Lantus]) is approved for use as a basal insulin—that is, the insulin is absorbed very slowly over 24 hours and can be given once a day. Because the insulin is in a suspension with a pH of 4, it cannot be mixed with other insulins because this would cause precipitation. It was originally approved to be given once a day at bedtime; however, it has now been approved to be given once a day at any time of the day but must be given at the same time each day to prevent overlap of action. Many patients fall asleep, forgetting to take their bedtime insulin or may be wary of taking

TABLE 41-3 Categories of Insulin

Time Course	Agent	Onset	Peak	Duration	Indications
Rapid-acting	Lispro (Humalog) Aspart (Novolog)	10–15 min 5–15 min	1 h 40–50 min	2–4h 2–4 h	Used for rapid reduction of glucose level, to treat postprandial hyperglycemia, and/or to prevent nocturnal hypoglycemia
Short-acting	Regular (Humalog R, Novolin R, Iletin II Regular)	½–1 h	2–3 h	4–6 h	Usually administered 20–30 min before a meal; may be taken alone or in combination with longer-acting insulin
Intermediate-acting	NPH (neutral protamine Hagedorn)	2–4 h	4–12 h	16–20 h	Usually taken after food
	(Humulin N, Iletin II Lente, Iletin II NPH, Novolin L [Lente], Novolin N [NPH])	3–4 h	4–12 h	16–20 h	
Long-acting	Ultralente ("UL")	6–8 h	12–16 h	20–30 h	Used primarily to control fasting glucose level
Very long-acting	Glargine (Lantus)	1 h	Continuous (no peak)	24 h	Used for basal dose

insulin before going to sleep. Having these patients take their insulin in the morning ensures that the dose is taken.

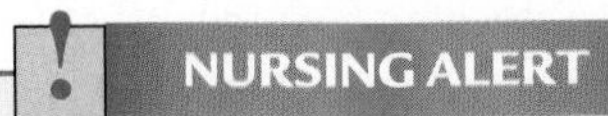

When administering insulin, it is very important to read the label carefully and to be sure that the correct type of insulin is administered. It is also important to avoid mistaking Lantus insulin for Lente insulin and vice versa.

Inhaled insulin was approved in 2005 by the FDA for use in people with type 2 diabetes. This insulin, called Exubera, is used as a pre-meal dose. It is not basal insulin, so basal insulin will be required by the patient who requires insulin to control blood glucose levels. The insulin is delivered through an inhaler device. The doses are in microgram increments. Before a meal the person puts a blister pack of Exubera in the device and inhales the drug. Particles of insulin are absorbed through the respiratory tract and enter the bloodstream. The advantages are that insulin enters the bloodstream quickly without the pain of injections, the doses are consistent, and the blood glucose level decreases. The disadvantages are that the device is big and bulky. Blister packs are available only in incremental doses, so there is less flexibility of dosing. Early studies indicated that inhaled insulin therapy used as initial single therapy may be a safe and effective method of treatment for patients whose type 2 diabetes is not adequately controlled through diet and exercise alone (Defronzo, Bergenstal, Cefalu, et al., 2005; Rosenstock, Zinman, Murphy, et al., 2005). There have been no adverse effects on the lungs during short-term use; however, the effects on the lungs with long-term use must be studied further. The FDA has recommended that people who smoke and people with some types of lung disease (eg, asthma) not use inhaled insulin.

The nurse should focus on which meals—and snacks—are being "covered" by which insulin doses. In general, the rapid- and short-acting insulins are expected to cover the increase in glucose levels after meals, immediately after the injection; the intermediate-acting insulins are expected to cover subsequent meals; and the long-acting insulins provide a relatively constant level of insulin and act as a basal insulin.

SPECIES (SOURCE)

In the past, all insulins were obtained from beef (cow) and pork (pig) pancreases. "Human insulins" are now widely available. They are produced by recombinant DNA technology and have largely replaced insulin from animal sources (ADA, 2004k). These insulins are largely preferable to animal source insulins because they are not antigenic and do not depend on sufficient animal sources.

Insulin Regimens

Insulin regimens vary from one to four injections per day. Usually there is a combination of a short-acting insulin and a longer-acting insulin. The normally functioning pancreas continuously secretes small amounts of insulin during the day and night. In addition, whenever blood glucose increases after ingestion of food, there is a rapid burst of insulin secretion in proportion to the glucose-raising effect of the food. The goal of all but the simplest, one-injection insulin regimens is to mimic this normal pattern of insulin secretion in response to food intake and activity patterns. Table 41-4 describes several insulin regimens and the advantages and disadvantages of each.

The patient can learn to use SMBG results and carbohydrate counting to vary the insulin doses. This allows the patient more flexibility in timing and content of meals and exercise periods. However, complex insulin regimens require a strong level of commitment, intensive education, and close follow-up by the health care team. In addition, patients aiming for normal blood glucose levels run the risk of more hypoglycemic reactions.

The type of regimen used by a particular patient varies. For example, patient knowledge, willingness, goals, health status, and finances all may affect decisions regarding insulin treatment. In addition, the physician's philosophy about blood glucose control and the availability of equipment and support staff may influence decisions regarding insulin therapy. There are two general approaches to insulin therapy: conventional and intensive.

CONVENTIONAL REGIMEN

One approach is to simplify the insulin regimen as much as possible, with the aim of avoiding the acute complications of diabetes (hypoglycemia and symptomatic hyperglycemia). With this type of simplified regimen (eg, one or more injections of a mixture of short- and intermediate-acting insulins per day), the patient should not vary meal patterns and activity levels. The simplified regimen would be appropriate for the terminally ill, the frail elderly with limited self-care abilities, or patients who are completely unwilling or unable to engage in the self-management activities that are part of a more complex insulin regimen. Otherwise, patients should be taught to adjust meal doses based on carbohydrate content and premeal blood glucose levels.

INTENSIVE REGIMEN

The second approach is to use a more complex insulin regimen to achieve as much control over blood glucose levels as is safe and practical. The results of the landmark DCCT study (1993) and the UKPDS study (1998) demonstrated that maintaining blood glucose levels as close to normal as possible prevents or slows the progression of long-term diabetic complications. These results were confirmed by the findings of the DCCT/EDIC study (Nathan et al., 2005). Another reason for using a more complex insulin regimen is to allow the patient more flexibility to change the insulin doses from day to day in accordance with changes in eating and activity patterns, with stress and illness, and as needed for variations in the prevailing glucose level.

Although the DCCT found that intensive treatment (three or four injections of insulin per day) reduced the risk of complications, not all people with diabetes are candidates for very tight control of blood glucose. The DCCT also found that the risk of severe hypoglycemia was increased threefold in patients receiving intensive treatment

(text continues on page 1396)

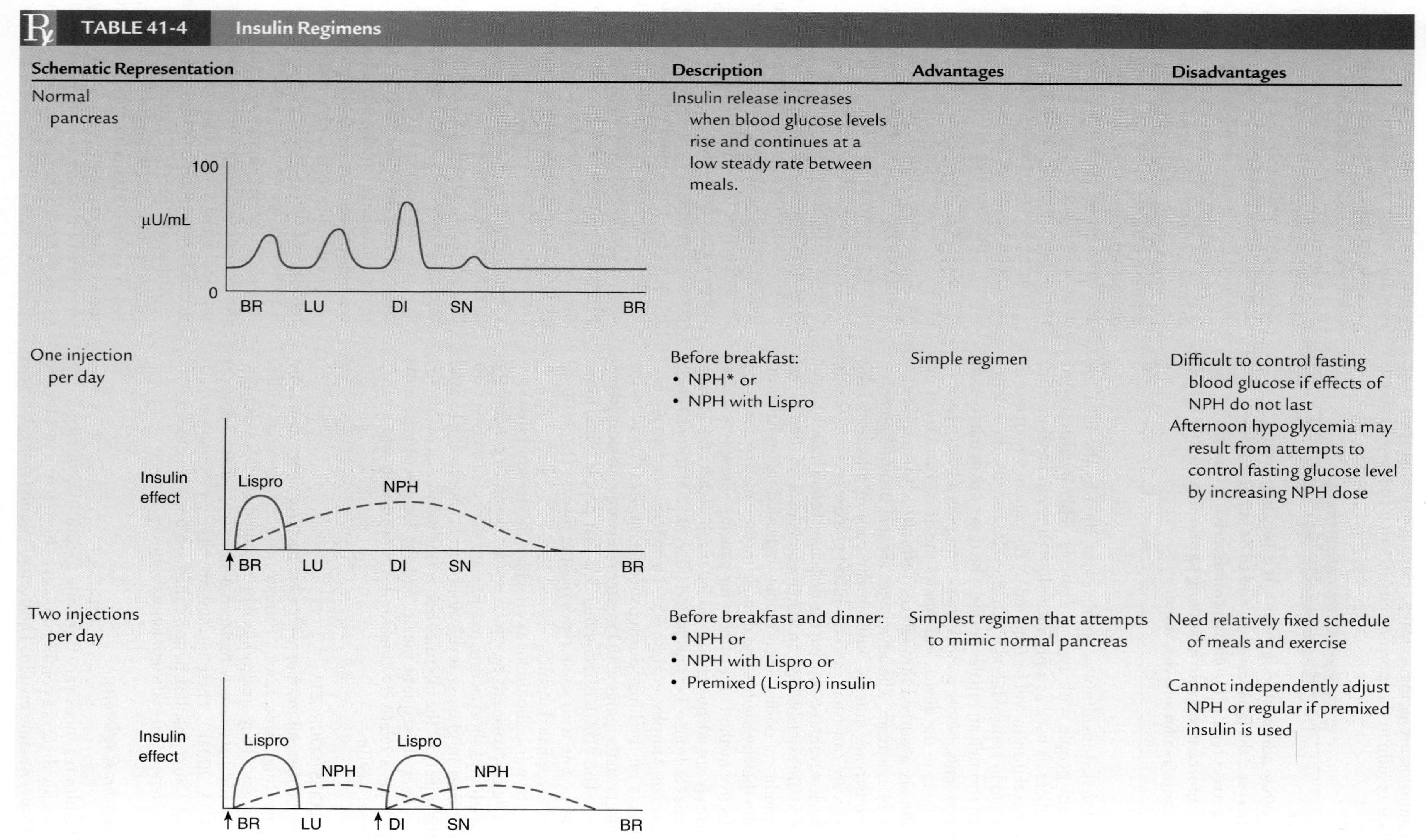

TABLE 41-4 Insulin Regimens

Schematic Representation	Description	Advantages	Disadvantages
Normal pancreas	Insulin release increases when blood glucose levels rise and continues at a low steady rate between meals.		
One injection per day	Before breakfast: • NPH* or • NPH with Lispro	Simple regimen	Difficult to control fasting blood glucose if effects of NPH do not last Afternoon hypoglycemia may result from attempts to control fasting glucose level by increasing NPH dose
Two injections per day	Before breakfast and dinner: • NPH or • NPH with Lispro or • Premixed (Lispro) insulin	Simplest regimen that attempts to mimic normal pancreas	Need relatively fixed schedule of meals and exercise Cannot independently adjust NPH or regular if premixed insulin is used

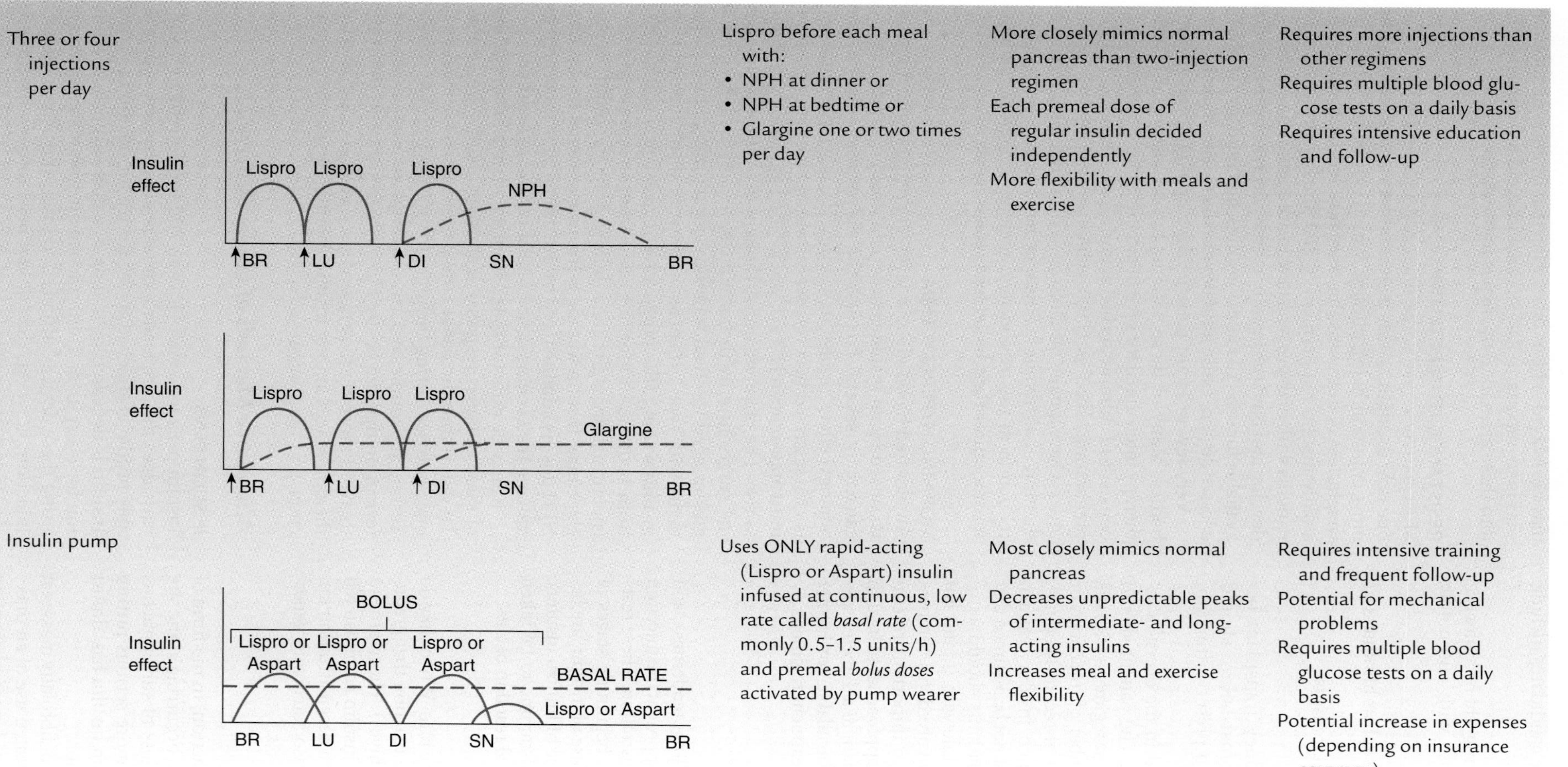

Three or four injections per day	Lispro before each meal with: • NPH at dinner or • NPH at bedtime or • Glargine one or two times per day	More closely mimics normal pancreas than two-injection regimen Each premeal dose of regular insulin decided independently More flexibility with meals and exercise	Requires more injections than other regimens Requires multiple blood glucose tests on a daily basis Requires intensive education and follow-up
Insulin pump	Uses ONLY rapid-acting (Lispro or Aspart) insulin infused at continuous, low rate called *basal rate* (commonly 0.5–1.5 units/h) and premeal *bolus doses* activated by pump wearer	Most closely mimics normal pancreas Decreases unpredictable peaks of intermediate- and long-acting insulins Increases meal and exercise flexibility	Requires intensive training and frequent follow-up Potential for mechanical problems Requires multiple blood glucose tests on a daily basis Potential increase in expenses (depending on insurance coverage)

BR, breakfast; LU, lunch; DI, dinner; SN, snack; REG, regular; ↑ indicates insulin injections.

(ADA, 2004j). Patients who may not be candidates include those with

- Nervous system disorders rendering them unaware of hypoglycemic episodes (eg, those with autonomic neuropathy)
- Recurring severe hypoglycemia
- Irreversible diabetic complications, such as blindness or end-stage renal disease
- Cerebrovascular and/or cardiovascular disease
- Ineffective self-care skills

Patients who have received a kidney transplant because of nephropathy and chronic renal failure should follow an intensive insulin regimen to preserve function of the new kidney.

The patient should be very involved in the decision regarding which insulin regimen to use. The patient should compare the potential benefits of different regimens with the potential costs (eg, time involved, number of injections or fingersticks for glucose testing, amount of record-keeping). There are no set guidelines as to which insulin regimen should be used for which patient. It must not be assumed that elderly patients or visually impaired patients should automatically be given a simplified regimen. Likewise, it must not be assumed that all people want to be involved in a complex treatment regimen. The nurse plays an important role in educating the patient about the various approaches to insulin therapy. The nurse should refer the patient to a diabetes specialist or a diabetes education center, if available, for further training and education in the insulin treatment regimens.

Complications of Insulin Therapy

LOCAL ALLERGIC REACTIONS

A local allergic reaction (redness, swelling, tenderness, and induration or a 2- to 4-cm wheal) may appear at the injection site 1 to 2 hours after the insulin administration. These reactions, which usually occur during the beginning stages of therapy and disappear with continued use of insulin, are becoming rare because of the increased use of human insulins. The physician may prescribe an antihistamine to be taken 1 hour before the injection if such a local reaction occurs.

SYSTEMIC ALLERGIC REACTIONS

Systemic allergic reactions to insulin are rare. When they do occur, there is an immediate local skin reaction that gradually spreads into generalized urticaria (hives). The treatment is desensitization, with small doses of insulin administered in gradually increasing amounts using a desensitization kit. These rare reactions are occasionally associated with generalized edema or anaphylaxis.

INSULIN LIPODYSTROPHY

Lipodystrophy refers to a localized reaction, in the form of either lipoatrophy or lipohypertrophy, occurring at the site of insulin injections. Lipoatrophy is loss of subcutaneous fat; it appears as slight dimpling or more serious pitting of subcutaneous fat. The use of human insulin has almost eliminated this disfiguring complication.

Lipohypertrophy, the development of fibrofatty masses at the injection site, is caused by the repeated use of an injection site. If insulin is injected into scarred areas, absorption may be delayed. This is one reason that rotation of injection sites is so important. Patients should avoid injecting insulin into these areas until the hypertrophy disappears.

RESISTANCE TO INJECTED INSULIN

Most patients have some degree of insulin resistance at one time or another. This may occur for various reasons, the most common being obesity, which can be overcome by weight loss. Clinical insulin resistance has been defined as a daily insulin requirement of 200 units or more. In most patients with diabetes who take insulin, immune antibodies develop and bind the insulin, thereby decreasing the insulin available for use. All animal insulins, and human insulins to a lesser degree, cause antibody production in humans.

Very few resistant patients develop high levels of antibodies. Many of these patients have a history of insulin therapy interrupted for several months or longer. Treatment consists of administering a more concentrated insulin preparation, such as U500, which is available by special order. Occasionally, prednisone is needed to block the production of antibodies. This may be followed by a gradual reduction in the insulin requirement. Therefore, patients must monitor their blood for hypoglycemia.

MORNING HYPERGLYCEMIA

An elevated blood glucose level on arising in the morning is caused by an insufficient level of insulin, which may be caused by several factors: the dawn phenomenon, the Somogyi effect, or insulin waning. The dawn phenomenon is characterized by a relatively normal blood glucose level until approximately 3 AM, when blood glucose levels begin to rise. The phenomenon is thought to result from nocturnal surges in growth hormone secretion, which create a greater need for insulin in the early morning hours in patients with type 1 diabetes. It must be distinguished from insulin waning (the progressive increase in blood glucose from bedtime to morning) and from the Somogyi effect (nocturnal hypoglycemia followed by rebound hyperglycemia). Insulin waning is frequently seen if the evening NPH dose is administered before dinner; it is prevented by moving the evening dose of NPH insulin to bedtime.

It may be difficult to tell from a patient's history which of these causes is responsible for morning hyperglycemia. To determine the cause, the patient must be awakened once or twice during the night to test blood glucose levels. Testing at bedtime, at 3 AM, and on awakening provides information that can be used to make adjustments in insulin to avoid morning hyperglycemia. Table 41-5 summarizes the differences among insulin waning, the dawn phenomenon, and the Somogyi effect.

Alternative Methods of Insulin Delivery

INSULIN PENS

Insulin pens use small (150- to 300-unit) prefilled insulin cartridges that are loaded into a penlike holder. A disposable needle is attached to the device for insulin injection. Insulin is delivered by dialing in a dose or pushing a button for every 1- or 2-unit increment administered. People using these devices still need to insert the needle for each injection; however, they do not need to carry insulin bottles or draw up insulin before each injection. These devices

TABLE 41-5 Causes of Morning Hyperglycemia

Characteristic	Treatment
Insulin Waning	
Progressive rise in blood glucose from bedtime to morning	Increase evening (predinner or bedtime) dose of intermediate- or long-acting insulin, or institute a dose of insulin before the evening meal if one is not already part of the treatment regimen.
Dawn Phenomenon	
Relatively normal blood glucose until about 3 AM, when the level begins to rise	Change time of injection of evening intermediate-acting insulin from dinnertime to bedtime.
Somogyi Effect	
Normal or elevated blood glucose at bedtime, a decrease at 2–3 AM to hypoglycemic levels, and a subsequent increase caused by the production of counterregulatory hormones	Decrease evening (predinner or bedtime) dose of intermediate-acting insulin, or increase bedtime snack.

are most useful for patients who need to inject only one type of insulin at a time (eg, premeal rapid-acting insulin three times a day and bedtime NPH insulin) or who can use the premixed insulins. These pens are convenient for those who administer insulin before dinner if eating out or traveling. They are also useful for patients with impaired manual dexterity, vision, or cognitive function that makes the use of traditional syringes difficult.

JET INJECTORS

As an alternative to needle injections, jet injection devices deliver insulin through the skin under pressure in an extremely fine stream. These devices are more expensive and require thorough training and supervision when first used. In addition, patients should be cautioned that absorption rates, peak insulin activity, and insulin levels may be different when changing to a jet injector. (Insulin administered by jet injector is usually absorbed faster.) Use of jet injectors has been associated with bruising in some patients.

INSULIN PUMPS

Continuous subcutaneous insulin infusion involves the use of small, externally worn devices that closely mimic the functioning of the normal pancreas (ADA, 2004c). Insulin pumps contain a 3-mL syringe attached to a long (24- to 42-in), thin, narrow-lumen tube with a needle or Teflon catheter attached to the end (Figs. 41-4 and 41-5). The patient inserts the needle or catheter into subcutaneous tissue (usually on the abdomen) and secures it with tape or a transparent dressing. The needle or catheter is changed at least every 3 days. The pump is then worn either on a belt

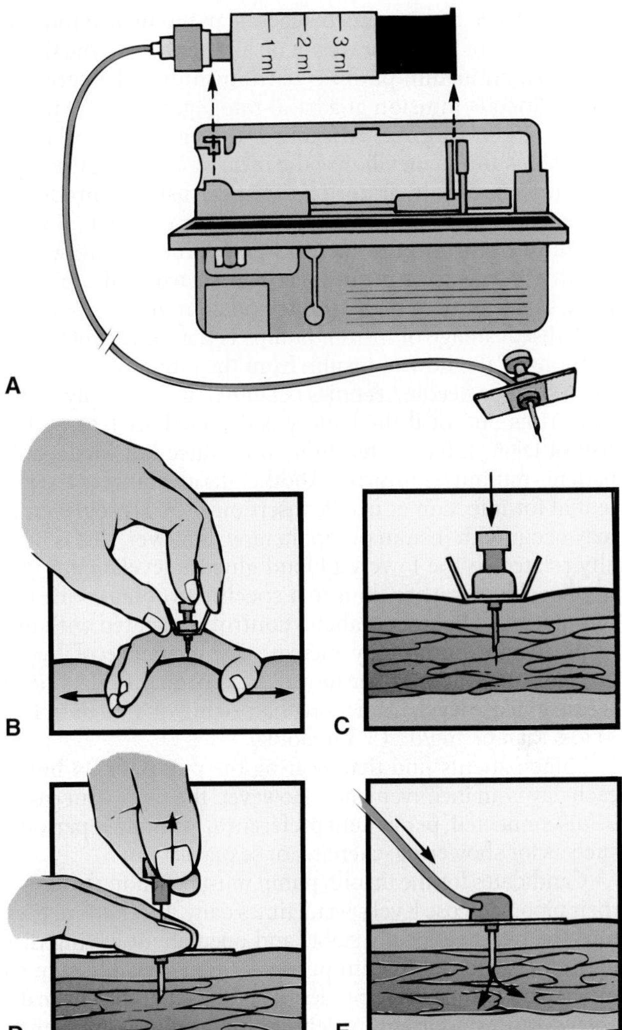

FIGURE 41-4. (**A**) Diagram of an insulin pump showing syringe in place inside pump and connection of pump via tubing to needle site. (**B–E**) Actual insertion site before, during, and after the needle and catheter have been inserted.

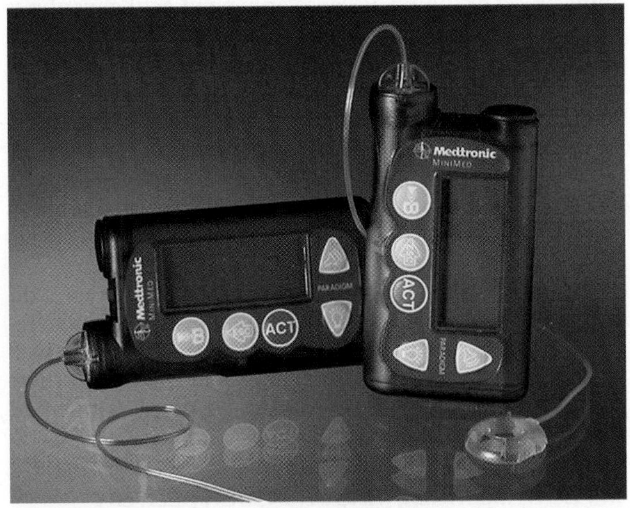

FIGURE 41-5. Medtronic (Northridge, CA) insulin pump system.

or in a pocket. Some women keep the pump tucked into the front or side of the bra or wear it on a garter belt on the thigh.

When an insulin pump is used, insulin is delivered by subcutaneous infusion at a basal rate (eg, 0.5 to 2.0 units/hour). When a meal is consumed, the patient calculates a dose of insulin to metabolize the meal by counting the total amount of carbohydrate for the meal using a predetermined insulin-to-carbohydrate ratio; for example, a ratio of 1 unit of insulin for every 15 g of carbohydrate would require 3 units for a meal with 45 g of carbohydrate. This allows flexibility of meal timing and content.

A disadvantage of insulin pumps is that unexpected disruptions in the flow of insulin from the pump may occur if the tubing or needle becomes occluded, if the supply of insulin runs out, or if the battery is depleted, increasing the risk of DKA. Effective teaching to produce knowledgeable patients minimizes this risk. Another disadvantage is the potential for infection at needle insertion sites. Hypoglycemia may occur with insulin pump therapy; however, this is usually related to the lowered blood glucose levels many patients achieve rather than to a specific problem with the pump itself. The tight diabetes control associated with use of an insulin pump may increase the incidence of hypoglycemia unawareness because of the very gradual decline in serum glucose level, from more than 70 mg/dL (3.9 mmol/L) to less than 60 mg/dL (3.3 mmol/L).

Some patients find that wearing the pump for 24 hours each day is an inconvenience. However, the pump can easily be disconnected, per patient preference, for limited periods, such as for showering, exercise, or sexual activity.

Candidates for the insulin pump must be willing to assess their blood glucose level several times daily. In addition, they must be psychologically stable and open about having diabetes, because the insulin pump is often a visible sign to others and a constant reminder to patients that they have diabetes. Most important, patients using insulin pumps must have extensive education in the use of the pump and in self-management of blood glucose and insulin doses. They must work closely with a team of health care professionals who are experienced in insulin pump therapy—specifically, a diabetologist/endocrinologist, a dietitian, and a certified diabetes educator.

The most common risk of insulin pump therapy is ketoacidosis, which may occur if there is an occlusion in the infusion set or tubing. Because only rapid-acting insulin is used in the pump, any interruption in the flow of insulin may rapidly cause the patient to be without insulin. The patient should be taught to administer insulin by manual injection if an insulin interruption is suspected (eg, no response in blood glucose level after a meal bolus).

Many insurance policies cover the cost of pump therapy. If not, the extra expense of the pump and associated supplies may be a deterrent for some patients. Medicare now covers insulin pump therapy for patients with type 1 diabetes.

Insulin pumps have been used in patients with type 2 diabetes whose beta cell function has diminished and who require insulin. Patients with a hectic lifestyle often do well with an insulin pump. There is no risk of DKA when there is an interruption of the flow of insulin in people with type 2 diabetes wearing an insulin pump.

IMPLANTABLE AND INHALANT INSULIN DELIVERY

Research into mechanical delivery of insulin has involved implantable insulin pumps that can be externally programmed according to blood glucose test results. Clinical trials with these devices are continuing. In addition, there is research into the development of implantable devices that both measure the blood glucose level and deliver insulin as needed. Methods of administering insulin by the oral route (oral spray or capsule), skin patch, and inhalation are undergoing intensive study.

TRANSPLANTATION OF PANCREATIC CELLS

Transplantation of the whole pancreas or a segment of the pancreas is being performed on a limited population (mostly patients with diabetes who are receiving a kidney transplantation simultaneously). One main issue is weighing the risks of antirejection medications against the advantages of pancreas transplantation. Implantation of insulin-producing pancreatic islet cells is another approach under investigation (ADA, 2004m). This latter approach involves a less extensive surgical procedure and a potentially lower incidence of immunogenic problems. However, thus far, independence from exogenous insulin has been limited to 2 years after transplantation of islet cells. Results of recent studies of patients with **islet cell transplants** using less toxic antirejection drugs have shown promise (Shapiro, Nanji & Lakey, 2003).

Oral Antidiabetic Agents

Oral antidiabetic agents may be effective for patients who have type 2 diabetes that cannot be treated effectively with MNT and exercise alone. In the United States, oral antidiabetic agents include first- and second-generation sulfonylureas, biguanides, alpha-glucosidase inhibitors, non-sulfonylurea insulin secretogogues (meglitinides and phenylalanine derivatives), and thiazolidinediones (glitazones) (Table 41-6). Sulfonylureas and meglitinides are considered insulin secretagogues because their action increases the secretion of insulin by the pancreatic beta cells.

Patients must understand that oral agents are prescribed as an addition to (not as a substitute for) other treatment modalities, such as MNT and exercise. Use of oral antidiabetic medications may need to be halted temporarily and insulin prescribed if hyperglycemia develops that is attributable to infection, trauma, or surgery.

In time, oral antidiabetic agents may no longer be effective in controlling the patient's diabetes because of decline of beta cells. In such cases, the patient is treated with insulin. Approximately half of all patients who initially use oral antidiabetic agents eventually require insulin. This is referred to as a secondary failure. Primary failure occurs when the blood glucose level remains high 1 month after initial medication use.

Because mechanisms of action vary (Fig. 41-6), effects may be enhanced with the use of multidose, multiple medications. Use of multiple medications with different mechanisms of action is very common today. A combination of oral agents with insulin, usually glargine at bedtime, has also been used frequently as a treatment for some patients with type 2 diabetes.

SULFONYLUREAS

The **sulfonylureas** exert their primary action by directly stimulating the pancreas to secrete insulin. Therefore, a functioning pancreas is necessary for these agents to be

TABLE 41-6 Oral Antidiabetic Agents

Generic (Trade) Name	Action/Indications	Side Effects	Implications
First-Generation Sulfonylureas			
Acetohexamide (Dymelor) Chlorpropamide (Diabinese) Tolazamide (Tolinase) Tolbutamide (Orinase)	Used infrequently in U.S. today Used in type 2 diabetes to control blood glucose levels Stimulate beta cells of the pancreas to secrete insulin; may improve binding between insulin and insulin receptors or increase the number of insulin receptors	Hypoglycemia Mild GI symptoms Weight gain Drug–drug interactions (NSAIDs, warfarin, sulfonamides) Sulfa allergy	Monitor patient for hypoglycemia Monitor blood glucose and urine ketone levels to assess effectiveness of therapy Patients at high risk for hypoglycemia: advanced age, renal insufficiency When taken with beta-adrenergic blocking agents may mask usual warning signs and symptoms of hypoglycemia Instruct patients to avoid use of alcohol
Second-Generation Sulfonylureas			
Glipizide (Glucatrol, Glucatrol XL) Glyburide (Micronase, Glynase, Dia-Beta) Glimepiride (Amaryl)	Stimulate beta cells of the pancreas to secrete insulin; may improve binding between insulin and insulin receptors or increase the number of insulin receptors Used in type 2 diabetes to control blood glucose levels Have more potent effects than first-generation sulfonylureas May be used in combination with metformin or insulin to improve glucose control	Hypoglycemia Mild GI symptoms Weight gain Drug–drug interactions (NSAIDs, warfarin, sulfonamides) Sulfa allergy	Monitor patient for hypoglycemia Monitor blood glucose and urine ketone levels to assess effectiveness of therapy Patients at high risk for hypoglycemia: advanced age, renal insufficiency When taken with beta-adrenergic blocking agents, may mask usual warning signs and symptoms of hypoglycemia Instruct patients to avoid use of alcohol
Biguanides			
Metformin (Glucophase, Glucophage XL, Fortamet) Metformin with glyburide (Glucovance)	Inhibit production of glucose by the liver Increase body tissues' sensitivity to insulin Decrease hepatic synthesis of cholesterol Used in type 2 diabetes to control blood glucose levels	Lactic acidosis Hypoglycemia if metformin is used in combination with insulin or other antidiabetic agents Drug–drug interaction GI disturbances Contraindicated in patients with impaired renal or liver function, respiratory insufficiency, severe infection, or alcohol abuse	Monitor for lactic acidosis and hypoglycemia Patients taking metformin are at increased risk of acute renal failure and lactic acidosis with use of iodinated contrast material for diagnostic studies; metformin should be stopped 48 h prior to and for 48 h after use of contrast agent or until renal function is evaluated and normal
Alpha-Glucosidase Inhibitors			
Acarbose (Precose) Miglitol (Glyset)	Delay absorption of complex carbohydrates in the intestine and slow entry of glucose into systemic circulation Do not increase insulin secretion Used in type 2 diabetes to control blood glucose levels Can be used alone or in combination with sulfonylureas, metformin, or insulin to improve glucose control	Hypoglycemia (risk increased if used with insulin or other antidiabetic agents) GI side effects (abdominal discomfort or distention, diarrhea, flatulence) Drug–drug interactions	Must be taken with first bite of food to be effective Monitor for GI side effects (diarrhea, abdominal distention) Monitor for blood glucose levels to assess effectiveness of therapy Monitor liver function studies every 3 mo for 1 y, then periodically Contraindicated in patients with GI or renal dysfunction, or cirrhosis

continued >

TABLE 41-6 Oral Antidiabetic Agents (Continued)

Generic (Trade) Name	Action/Indications	Side Effects	Implications
Non-Sulfonylurea Insulin Secretagogues			
Repaglinide (Prandin) categorized as a meglitinide Neteglide (Starlix) categorized as a D-phenylalanine derivative	Stimulate pancreas to secrete insulin Used in type 2 diabetes to control blood glucose levels Can be used alone or in combination with metformin or thiazolidinediones to improve glucose control	Hypoglycemia/weight gain less likely than sulfonylureas Drug-drug interactions (with ketoconazole, fluconazole, erythromycin, rifampin, isoniazid)	Monitor blood glucose levels to assess effectiveness of therapy Has rapid action and short half-life Monitor patients with impaired liver function and renal impairment Has no effect on plasma lipids Is taken before each meal
Thiazolidinediones (or glitazones)			
Pioglitazone (Actos) Rosiglitazone (Avandia)	Sensitize body tissue to insulin; stimulate insulin receptor sites to lower blood glucose and improve action of insulin May be used alone or in combination with sulfonylurea, metformin or insulin	Hypoglycemia (risk increased with use of insulin or other antidiabetic agents) Anemia Weight gain, edema Decrease effectiveness of oral contraceptives Possible liver dysfunction Drug–drug interactions Hyperlipidemia (has variable effect on lipids; pioglitazone may be preferred choice in patients with lipid abnormalities) Impaired platelet function	Monitor blood glucose levels to assess effectiveness of therapy Monitor liver function tests Arrange dietary teaching to establish weight control program

effective, and they cannot be used in patients with type 1 diabetes. These agents improve insulin action at the cellular level and may also directly decrease glucose production by the liver (see Table 41-6).

The most common side effects of sulfonylureas are gastrointestinal symptoms and dermatologic reactions. Hypoglycemia may occur when an excessive dose of a sulfonylurea is used or when a patient omits or delays meals, reduces food intake, or increases activity. Because of the prolonged hypoglycemic effects of these agents, some patients need to be hospitalized for treatment of oral agent–induced hypoglycemia. Some medications (eg, sulfonamides, chloramphenicol, clofibrate, phenylbutazone, bishydroxycoumarin) may directly interact with sulfonylureas, potentiating their

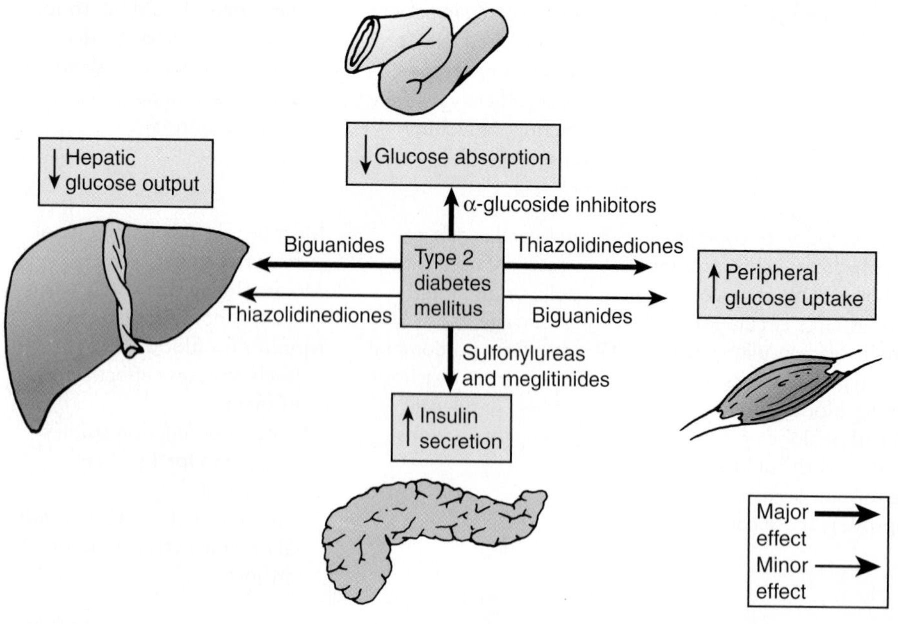

FIGURE 41-6. Sites of action of oral antidiabetic medications.

hypoglycemic effects. In addition, certain medications may independently affect blood glucose levels, thereby indirectly interfering with these agents. Medications that may increase glucose levels include potassium-losing diuretics, corticosteroids, estrogen compounds, and some antiseizure agents (phenytoin [Dilantin]). Medications that may cause hypoglycemia include salicylates, propranolol, monoamine oxidase inhibitors, and pentamidine.

Second-generation sulfonylureas have the advantage of a shorter half-life and excretion by both the kidney and the liver. This makes these medications safer to use in the elderly, in whom accumulation of the medication can cause recurring hypoglycemia. The first-generation sulfonylureas are seldom used today, because the second-generation drugs are a better option.

NON-SULFONYLUREA INSULIN SECRETAGOGUES

Repaglinide (Prandin), an oral glucose-lowering agent of the class of oral agents called non-sulfonylurea insulin secretagogues, lowers the blood glucose level by stimulating insulin release from the pancreatic beta cells. Its effectiveness depends on the presence of functioning beta cells. Therefore, repaglinide is contraindicated in patients with type 1 diabetes. Repaglinide has a fast action and a short duration. It should be taken before each meal to stimulate the release of insulin in response to that meal. It is also indicated for use in combination with metformin in patients whose hyperglycemia cannot be controlled by exercise, MNT, and either metformin or repaglinide alone. The principal side effect of repaglinide is hypoglycemia; however, this side effect is less severe and less frequent than for a sulfonylurea because repaglinide has a short half-life (approximately 1 hour). The patient must be taught the signs and symptoms of hypoglycemia and should understand that the medication should not be taken unless he or she is able to eat a meal. Repaglinide is supplied in 0.5-, 1-, and 2-mg tablets.

Naglitinide (Starlix), another secretagogue, is a derivative of phenylalanine; it has a very rapid onset and short duration. It should be taken with meals and should not be taken if the meal is skipped. Hypoglycemia risk is low if naglitinide is taken correctly.

BIGUANIDES

The biguanides are another type of oral antidiabetic agent. Metformin (Glucophage), the most commonly used biguanide, produces its antidiabetic effects by facilitating the action of insulin on peripheral receptor sites. Biguanides have no effect on pancreatic beta cells. Biguanides used with a sulfonylurea may enhance the glucose-lowering effect more than either medication used alone. Medications that may interact with biguanides include anticoagulants, corticosteroids, diuretics, and hormonal contraceptives. Metformin is contraindicated in patients with renal impairment (serum creatinine level greater than 1.4 mg/mL) and in those at risk for renal dysfunction (eg, patients with acute myocardial infarction or heart failure). Renal function studies should be performed periodically to ensure that function is not impaired. Metformin should not be administered for 2 days before any diagnostic testing that may require use of a contrast agent. These situations increase the risk for lactic acidosis. Lactic acidosis is a potential and serious complication of biguanide therapy; the patient must be monitored closely in these situations, as well as when therapy is initiated and when the dosage is changed.

An extended-release form and combination forms (Glucophage XR, Metaglip) combine metformin with a sulfonylurea, such as glyburide or glipizide. The combination provides two mechanisms of action and results in increased efficacy and improved patient compliance but increases the risk for hypoglycemia.

ALPHA-GLUCOSIDASE INHIBITORS

Acarbose (Precose) and miglitol (Glyset) are oral **alpha-glucosidase inhibitors** used in type 2 diabetes management. They work by delaying the absorption of glucose in the intestinal system, which results in a lower postprandial blood glucose level. As a consequence of plasma glucose reduction, hemoglobin A1C levels drop. Acarbose and miglitol, unlike the sulfonylureas, do not enhance insulin secretion. They can be used alone with MNT as monotherapy or in combination with sulfonylureas, thiazolidinediones, or meglitinides. If these medications are used in combination with sulfonylureas or meglitinides, hypoglycemia may occur.

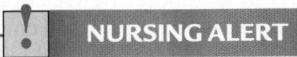

Patients taking alpha-glucosidase inhibitors must be advised that, if hypoglycemia occurs, sucrose absorption will be blocked, and treatment for hypoglycemia should be in the form of glucose, such as glucose tablets.

The advantage of oral alpha-glucosidase inhibitors is that they are not systemically absorbed and are safe to use. Side effects include diarrhea and flatulence. These effects may be minimized by starting at a very low dose and increasing the dose gradually. Because acarbose and miglitol affect food absorption, they must be taken immediately before a meal, making therapeutic adherence a potential problem.

THIAZOLIDINEDIONES

Rosiglitazone (Avandia) and pioglitazone (Actos) are oral antidiabetic medications categorized as **thiazolidinediones** (TZDs). They are indicated for patients with type 2 diabetes who take insulin injections and whose blood glucose control is inadequate (glycated hemoglobin level [A1C] greater than 8.5%). They have also been approved as first-line agents to treat type 2 diabetes, in combination with MNT. TZDs enhance insulin action at the receptor site without increasing insulin secretion from the beta cells of the pancreas. These medications may impair liver function; therefore, liver function studies must be performed at baseline and at frequent intervals (monthly for the first 12 months of treatment, and quarterly thereafter). Women should be informed that TZDs decrease the effectiveness of hormonal contraceptives and can cause resumption of ovulation in perimenopausal anovulatory women, making pregnancy a possibility.

OTHER PHARMACOLOGIC THERAPY

Two new medications were approved in 2005 by the FDA for use in the pharmacologic management of diabetes. Both are injectable medications; neither is a substitute for insulin if insulin is required to control diabetes.

Pramlintide (Symlin), a synthetic analogue of human amylin, a hormone that is secreted by the beta cells of the pancreas, has recently been approved for treatment of both type 1 and type 2 diabetes. It is used to control hyperglycemia in adults who have not achieved acceptable levels of glucose control despite the use of insulin at mealtimes. It is used with insulin, not in the place of insulin. Although pramlintide is not yet widely used, it is anticipated that it will be useful to minimize fluctuations in daily glucose levels and provide better glucose control. Risks associated with pramlintide include hypoglycemia; therefore, a source of glucose must be available if hypoglycemia occurs. Pramlintide must be injected into the abdomen or thigh because of variable absorption rates if it is injected into the arm. It should not be injected close to an insulin injection site. Caution must be exercised in preparing and administering pramlintide to avoid errors in dosing. Patients are instructed to monitor their blood glucose level before each meal, 2 hours afterward, and at bedtime during the initial period of use of pramlintide (FDA, 2005).

Exanatide (Byetta) is another newly approved medication for the treatment of type 2 diabetes in combination with metformin or sulfonylureas. It is derived from a hormone that is produced in the small intestine and has been found to be deficient in type 2 diabetes. It is normally released after food is ingested, to delay gastric emptying and enhance insulin secretion, resulting in dampening of the rise in blood glucose levels after meals and a feeling of satiety. The return of the blood glucose level to normal results in decreased production of the hormone. Hypoglycemia is not a side effect of exanatide if adjustments are made in the sulfonylurea dose. Exanatide has been shown to result in weight loss because of the increased satiety produced. Exanatide must be injected twice a day within 1 hour before breakfast and dinner. It is not a substitute for insulin in patients who require insulin to control their diabetes (FDA, 2005).

Nursing Management

Nursing management of patients with diabetes can involve treatment of a wide variety of physiologic disorders, depending on the patient's health status and whether the patient is newly diagnosed or seeking care for an unrelated health problem. Nursing management of newly diagnosed patients and of those with diabetes as a secondary diagnosis is discussed in subsequent sections of this chapter. Because all patients with diabetes must master the concepts and skills necessary for long-term management and avoidance of potential complications of diabetes, a solid educational foundation is necessary for competent self-care and is an ongoing focus of nursing care.

Patient Education

Diabetes mellitus is a chronic illness that requires a lifetime of special self-management behaviors. Because MNT, physical activity, and physical and emotional stress affect diabetic control, patients must learn to balance a multitude of factors. They must learn daily self-care skills to prevent acute fluctuations in blood glucose, and they must also incorporate into their lifestyle many preventive behaviors for avoidance of long-term diabetic complications. Patients must become knowledgeable about nutrition, medication effects and side effects, exercise, disease progression, prevention strategies, blood glucose monitoring techniques, and medication adjustment. In addition, they must learn the skills associated with monitoring and managing diabetes and must incorporate many new activities into their daily routines. An appreciation for the knowledge and skills that patients with diabetes must acquire can help nurses provide effective patient education and counseling.

Developing a Diabetic Teaching Plan

Changes in the health care system as a whole have had a major impact on diabetes education and training. Patients with new-onset type 1 diabetes are hospitalized for much shorter periods or may be managed completely on an outpatient basis. Patients with new-onset type 2 diabetes are rarely hospitalized for initial care. There has been a proliferation of outpatient diabetes education and training programs, with increasing support of third-party reimbursement. All encounters with patients with diabetes are opportunities for reinforcement of self-management skills, regardless of the setting.

Many hospitals employ nurses who specialize in diabetes education and management and who are certified by the National Certification Board of Diabetes Educators as Certified Diabetes Educators. However, because of the large number of patients with diabetes who are admitted to every unit of a hospital for reasons other than diabetes or its complications, staff nurses play a vital role in identifying patients with diabetes, assessing self-care skills, providing basic education, reinforcing the teaching provided by the specialist, and referring patients for follow-up care after discharge. Diabetes patient education programs that have been peer-reviewed by the ADA as meeting National Standards for Diabetes Education can be reimbursed for education.

Organizing Information

There are various strategies for organizing and prioritizing the vast amount of information that must be taught to patients with diabetes. In addition, many hospitals and outpatient diabetes centers have devised written guidelines, care plans, and documentation forms (often based on ADA guidelines) that may be used to document and evaluate teaching.

One approach is to organize education using the seven tips for managing diabetes identified and developed by the AADE (2004):

1. Healthy eating
2. Being active
3. Monitoring
4. Taking medicines
5. Problem solving
6. Reducing risks
7. Healthy coping

NURSING RESEARCH PROFILE

Diabetes Education

Izquierdo, R. E., Knudson, P. E., Meyer, S., et al. (2003). A comparison of diabetes education administered through telemedicine versus in person. *Diabetes Care, 26*(4), 1002–1007.

Purpose

Treatment goals such as glycemic control are important components of management to prevent and delay the complications of diabetes, including retinopathy, nephropathy, and neuropathy. The purpose of this study was to compare two types of diabetes education delivery to patients to determine whether there was any difference in achievement of the treatment goals. This study compared the outcomes of diabetes education provided by in-person consultation versus telephone consultations.

Design

The 46 patients who participated in this study were randomly assigned to either an in-person or a teleconference approach. The participants were middle-aged adults, both men and women, with type 1 or type 2 diabetes. Variables examined included glycemic control as measured by glycated hemoglobin and psychological variables. Psychological measures were assessed using validated instruments such as the Problem Areas in Diabetes scale, the Diabetes Quality of Life scale, and the Appraisal of Diabetes scale to determine whether there were differences in patients' quality and satisfaction with life with diabetes according to method of delivery of patient education. Education was provided in person in clinics or by telemedicine, through teleconferencing, to patients in the home.

Findings

There was significant improvement ($p < .001$) in metabolic control in both groups, as demonstrated by decreases in glycated hemoglobin levels after the program. However, there were no significant between-group differences, suggesting that both approaches are acceptable methods for teaching patients. With regard to the psychological measures, both groups positively appraised their diabetes management. There was no difference between the groups, and patients who received the teleconference education were satisfied with the approach.

Nursing Implications

Diabetes management requires daily self-care by affected people to prevent the devastating complications of blindness, kidney disease, and neuropathy leading to amputations. All people with diabetes must be taught how to properly manage their diabetes. This can be very labor intensive, and, because the incidence of diabetes is increasing, the skills of all sorts of health care professionals are required. However, people live in remote areas and do not have access to diabetes education in clinics and hospitals. Creative ways to provide diabetes education are necessary, and nurses can develop and implement innovative ways to teach patients in a cost-effective manner. Telemedicine makes diabetes care more accessible. Perhaps the novelty of receiving education in this way can spur patients' interest in learning.

The AADE can be contacted for additional information about assessment and documentation of outcomes of this approach to teaching.

Another general approach is to organize information and skills into two main types: basic, initial, or "survival" skills and information, and in-depth (advanced) or continuing education.

TEACHING SURVIVAL SKILLS

This information must be taught to all patients with newly diagnosed type 1 or type 2 diabetes and all patients receiving insulin for the first time. This basic information is literally what patients must know to survive (eg, to avoid severe hypoglycemic or acute hyperglycemic complications after discharge). An outline of survival information includes the following:

1. Simple pathophysiology
   a. Basic definition of diabetes (having a high blood glucose level)
   b. Normal blood glucose ranges and target blood glucose levels
   c. Effect of insulin and exercise (decrease glucose)
   d. Effect of food and stress, including illness and infections (increase glucose)
   e. Basic treatment approaches
2. Treatment modalities
   a. Administration of insulin and oral antidiabetes medications
   b. Meal planning (food groups, timing of meals)
   c. Monitoring of blood glucose and urine ketones
3. Recognition, treatment, and prevention of acute complications
   a. Hypoglycemia
   b. Hyperglycemia
4. Pragmatic information
   a. Where to buy and store insulin, syringes, and glucose monitoring supplies
   b. When and how to contact the physician

For patients with newly diagnosed type 2 diabetes, emphasis is initially placed on meal planning and exercise. Patients who are starting to take oral sulfonylureas or insulin secretagogues need to know about detecting, preventing, and treating hypoglycemia. If diabetes has gone undetected for many years, the patient may already be experiencing some chronic diabetic complications. Therefore, for some patients with newly diagnosed type 2 diabetes, basic diabetes teaching must include information on preventive skills, such as foot care and eye care (eg, planning yearly or more frequent complete [dilated eye] examinations by an ophthalmologist, understanding that retinopathy is largely asymptomatic until advanced stages).

Patients also need to realize that once they master the basic skills and information, further diabetes education must be pursued. Acquiring in-depth and advanced diabetes knowledge occurs throughout the patient's lifetime, both formally through programs of continuing education and informally through experience and sharing of information with other people with diabetes.

PLANNING IN-DEPTH AND CONTINUING EDUCATION

This education involves teaching more detailed information related to survival skills (eg, learning to vary food choices and insulin, preparing for travel) as well as learning preventive measures for avoiding long-term diabetic complications. Preventive measures include

- Foot care
- Eye care
- General hygiene (eg, skin care, oral hygiene)
- Risk factor management (eg, control of blood pressure and blood lipid levels, normalizing blood glucose levels)

More advanced continuing education may include alternative methods for insulin delivery, such as the insulin pump, and algorithms or rules for evaluating and adjusting insulin doses. For example, the patient can be taught to increase or decrease insulin doses based on a several-day pattern of blood glucose levels. The degree of advanced diabetes education to be provided depends on the patient's interest and ability. However, learning preventive measures (especially foot care and eye care) is mandatory for early detection and treatment to reduce the occurrence of amputations and blindness in patients with diabetes.

Assessing Readiness to Learn

Before initiating diabetes education, the nurse assesses the patient's (and family's) readiness to learn. When patients are first diagnosed with diabetes (or first told of their need for insulin), they often go through various stages of the grieving process. These stages may include shock and denial, anger, depression, negotiation, and acceptance. The amount of time it takes for the patient and family members to work through the grieving process varies from patient to patient. They may experience helplessness, guilt, altered body image, loss of self-esteem, and concern about the future. The nurse must assess the patient's coping strategies and reassure the patient and family that feelings of depression and shock are normal.

Asking the patient and family about their major concerns or fears is an important way to learn about any misinformation that may be contributing to anxiety. Some common misconceptions regarding diabetes and its treatment are listed in Table 41-7. Simple, direct information should be provided to dispel misconceptions. More information can be provided once the patient masters survival skills.

After dispelling misconceptions or answering the questions that concern the patient the most, the nurse focuses attention on concrete survival skills. Because of the immediate need for multiple new skills, teaching is initiated as soon as possible after diagnosis. Nurses whose patients are in the hospital rarely have the luxury of waiting until the patient feels ready to learn; short hospital stays necessitate initiation of survival skill education as early as possible. This gives the patient the opportunity to practice skills with supervision by the nurse before discharge. Follow-up by home health nurses is often necessary for reinforcement of survival skills.

A goal of patient teaching is training educated consumers—patients who are informed about the wide variations in the prices of medications and supplies and about the importance of comparing prices.

Determining Teaching Methods

Maintaining flexibility with regard to teaching approaches is important. Teaching skills and information in a logical sequence is not always the most helpful method for patients. For example, many patients fear self-injection. Before they learn how to prepare, purchase, store, and mix insulins, they should be taught to insert the needle and inject insulin (or practice with saline solution). Patients who observe numerous demonstrations by the nurse or practice injections before they themselves (or a family member) give the first injection may actually develop increased anxiety and fear of self-injection. Once patients have actually performed injections, most are more prepared to hear and to comprehend other information. (If they then want to practice further using a pillow, that would be appropriate.) Therefore, having the patient self-inject first or having the patient perform a fingerstick for glucose monitoring first may enhance learning to draw up the insulin or to operate the glucose meter. Ample opportunity should be provided for patients and families to practice skills under supervision (including self-injection, self-testing, meal selection, verbalization of symptoms, and treatment of hypoglycemia). Once skills have been mastered, participation in ongoing support groups may help the patient incorporate new habits and follow the treatment regimen consistently.

Various tools can be used to complement teaching. Many of the companies that manufacture products for diabetes self-care also provide booklets and videotapes to assist in patient teaching. Teaching/educational materials are also available from the AADE and the ADA. It is important to use a variety of written handouts that match the patient's learning needs (including different languages, low-literacy information, large print) and reading level and to ensure that these materials are technically accurate. Patients can continue learning about diabetes care by participating in activities sponsored by local hospitals and diabetes organizations. In addition, magazines with information on diabetes management are available for people with diabetes (see Resources).

TABLE 41-7 Misconceptions Related to Insulin Treatment

Misconception	Response
Once insulin injections are started (for treatment of type 2 diabetes), they can never be discontinued	During periods of acute stress (eg, illness, infection, surgery) or when receiving certain medications that cause elevations in blood glucose, some patients with type 2 diabetes require insulin. If the diabetes had previously been well controlled with diet alone or diet with oral antidiabetic agents, the patient should be able to resume previous methods for control of diabetes after the stress is resolved. In addition, insulin is sometimes used to control blood glucose levels in obese type 2 diabetic patients who have been unsuccessful at weight loss. If the patient can lose weight after insulin therapy is initiated, the insulin doses may be tapered and the patient may be able to switch to diet and exercise alone or with oral antidiabetic agents for control of blood glucose. (For patients with type 1 diabetes, insulin is needed on an ongoing basis. For thin patients with type 2 diabetes, once insulin has to be started, it is usually required permanently).
If increasing doses of insulin are needed to control the blood glucose, the diabetes must be getting "worse"	Explain to the patient that unlike other medications that are given in standard doses, there is not a standard dose of insulin that is effective for all patients. Rather, the dose must be adjusted according to blood glucose test results. If the initial insulin dose prescribed for the patient does not adequately decrease the glucose level, the patient may assume that he or she has a "bad" case of diabetes or that the diabetes is getting worse. It is important to instruct patients that many different factors may affect the ability of insulin to lower the glucose, including obesity, puberty, pregnancy, illness, and certain medications. In addition, to avoid hypoglycemia, physicians frequently initiate insulin therapy with smaller dosages than will eventually be needed. The doses are then increased in small increments until blood glucose levels are in the desired range.
Insulin causes blindness (or other diabetic complications)	If the patient has a diabetic acquaintance in whom the initiation of insulin therapy happened to coincide with the onset of diabetic complications, the patient may view insulin as the cause of complications such as blindness or amputation. In these situations, the acquaintance probably had type 2 diabetes that was no longer controllable with diet and oral hypoglycemic agents. It must be explained to the patient that factors such as elevated blood glucose (and not insulin therapy) contribute to some of the diabetic complications. Further, emphasize that insulin is a natural hormone that is present in every person's body, helps control blood glucose levels, and definitely does *not* cause long-term complications of diabetes.
Insulin must be injected directly into the vein	When patients first learn that one area used for insulin injections is on the arm, they may envision inserting the needle directly into a vein in the antecubital area, as in blood withdrawal. The patient must be reassured that insulin is injected into the fat tissue on the *back* of the arm (or on the abdomen, thigh, or hip) and that the needle is much shorter than that used for venipuncture.
There is extreme danger in injecting insulin if there are any air bubbles in the syringe	Patients may have a fear of dying if air bubbles are injected with a syringe. (This may be related to the misconception that insulin is injected directly into the vein.) Reassure patients that the main danger in having air bubbles in the insulin syringe is that the amount of insulin being injected is less than the required dose. It is often difficult to remove every small "champagne" bubble from the syringe. Thus, patients should be reassured that injection of insulin when these bubbles are present does not cause any harm.
Insulin always causes people to have bad (hypoglycemic) reactions	First, make sure that patients are aware that low blood sugar reactions are often related to an imbalance with the insulin, food, and activity and can often be avoided. Thus, before starting on insulin, patients should discuss their usual schedule of meals and activities as well as the content of meals with the health care team. Make sure that patients are aware that various different insulins and insulin schedules can be used to try to allow patients to maintain some of their usual lifestyle habits. Reassure patients that avoiding hypoglycemic reactions is a high priority for the diabetes team. In addition, tell patients of the importance of reporting any hypoglycemic reactions to the health care team immediately so that early adjustments can be made in the insulin dosage. Focus early insulin education on treatment and prevention of hypoglycemia.
People who take insulin must travel only where there is a refrigerator to store the insulin	Insulin bottles in use may be kept at room temperature. Therefore, for most business trips or vacations, keeping the insulin in a purse or briefcase (or special diabetes supply case) is acceptable. If a prolonged trip is planned (more than 2 to 3 months), patients may want to consult the pharmacist or insulin manufacturer for suggestions. Most importantly, emphasize with patients that taking insulin should never deter them from pursuing activities they enjoy.

Pearce, M. A., Rosenberg, C. S, & Davidson, M. B. (2003). Patient education. In Davidson, M. B. (Ed.). *Diabetes mellitus: Diagnosis and treatment* (4th ed.). New York: Churchill Livingstone. Reprinted with permission from Elsevier Science.

Implementing the Plan

Teaching Experienced Patients

Nurses should continue to assess the skills and self-care behaviors of patients who have had diabetes for many years, because it is estimated that as many as 50% of patients make errors in self-care. Assessment of these patients must include direct observation of skills, not just the patient's self-report of self-care behaviors. In addition, these patients must be fully aware of preventive measures related to foot care, eye care, and risk factor management. Patients experiencing long-term diabetic complications for the first time may go through the grieving process again. Some patients may have a renewed interest in diabetes self-care in the hope of delaying further complications. Others may be overwhelmed by feelings of guilt and depression. The patient is encouraged to discuss feelings and fears related to complications. Meanwhile, the nurse provides appropriate information regarding diabetic complications.

Teaching Patients to Self-Administer Insulin

Insulin injections are self-administered into the subcutaneous tissue with the use of special insulin syringes. A variety of syringes and injection-aid devices are available. Chart 41-7 provides important information to include and evaluate when teaching patients about insulin. Basic information includes explanations of the equipment, insulins, and syringes and how to mix insulin.

STORING INSULIN

Whether insulin is the short- or the long-acting preparation, vials not in use, including spare vials, should be refrigerated. Extremes of temperature should be avoided; insulin should not be allowed to freeze and should not be kept in direct sunlight or in a hot car. The insulin vial in use should be kept at room temperature to reduce local irritation at the injection site, which may occur if cold insulin is injected. If a vial of insulin will be used up within 1 month, it may be kept at room temperature. The patient should be instructed to always have a spare vial of the type or types of insulin he or she uses (ADA, 2004k). Cloudy insulins should be thoroughly mixed by gently inverting the vial or rolling it between the hands before drawing the solution into a syringe or a pen.

Bottles of intermediate-acting insulin should also be inspected for flocculation, which is a frosted, whitish coating inside the bottle. This occurs most commonly with human insulins that are exposed to extremes of temperature. If a frosted, adherent coating is present, some of the insulin is bound, and it should not be used.

SELECTING SYRINGES

Syringes must be matched with the insulin concentration (eg, U-100). Currently, three sizes of U-100 insulin syringes are available:

- 1-mL syringes that hold 100 units
- 0.5-mL syringes that hold 50 units
- 0.3-mL syringes that hold 30 units

The concentration of insulin used most often in the United States is U-100; that is, there are 100 units per milliliter (or cubic centimeter). Small syringes allow patients who require small amounts of insulin to measure and draw up the amount of insulin accurately. Patients who require large amounts of insulin use larger syringes. There is a U-500 (500 units/mL) concentration of insulin available by special order for patients who have severe insulin resistance and require massive doses of insulin. (To avoid dosing errors, people who travel outside the United States should be aware that insulin is available in U-40 concentration.)

Most insulin syringes have a disposable 27- to 29-gauge needle that is approximately 0.5 inch long. The smaller syringes are marked in 1-unit increments and may be easier to use for patients with visual deficits and those taking very small doses of insulin. The 1-mL syringes are marked in 1- and 2-unit increments. A small disposable insulin needle (31 gauge, 8 mm long) is available for very thin patients and children.

PREPARING THE INJECTION: MIXING INSULINS

When rapid- or short-acting insulins are to be given simultaneously with longer-acting insulins, they are usually mixed together in the same syringe; the longer-acting insulins must be mixed thoroughly before use. The most important issue is that patients be consistent in how they prepare their insulin injections from day to day.

There are varying opinions regarding which type of insulin (short- or longer-acting) should be drawn up into the syringe first when they are going to be mixed, but the ADA recommends that the regular insulin be drawn up first. Again, the most important issues are (1) that patients be consistent in technique, so as not to draw up the wrong dose in error or the wrong type of insulin, and (2) that patients not inject one type of insulin into the bottle containing a different type of insulin (ADA, 2004k). Injecting cloudy insulin into a vial of clear insulin contaminates the entire vial of clear insulin and alters its action.

For patients who have difficulty mixing insulins, two options are available: they may use a premixed insulin, or they may have prefilled syringes prepared (Fig. 41-7). Premixed insulins are available in several different ratios of NPH insulin to regular insulin. The ratio of 70/30 (70% NPH and 30% regular insulin in one bottle) is most common; this combination is available as Novolin 70/30 (Novo-Nordisk) and Humulin 70/30 (Lilly). Combinations with a ratio of 75% NPL and 25% insulin lispro are also available (ADA, 2004k). NPL is used only in the mix with Humalog; its action is the same as NPH. The appropriate initial dosage of premixed insulin must be calculated so that the ratio of NPH to regular insulin most closely approximates the separate doses needed.

For patients who can inject insulin but who have difficulty drawing up a single or mixed dose, syringes may be prefilled with the help of home care nurses or family and friends. A 3-week supply of insulin syringes may be prepared and kept in the refrigerator. The prefilled syringes should be stored with the needle in an upright position to avoid clogging of the needle (ADA, 2004k); they should be mixed thoroughly before the insulin is injected.

WITHDRAWING INSULIN

Most (if not all) of the printed materials available on insulin dose preparation instruct patients to inject air into

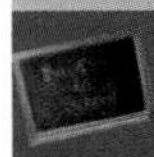

CHART 41-7

Patient Education

Self-Injection of Insulin

1. With one hand, stabilize the skin by spreading it or pinching up a large area.

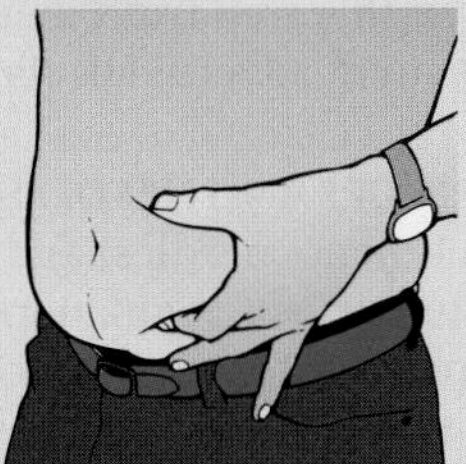

Pinching the skin

2. Pick up syringe with the other hand and hold it as you would a pencil. Insert needle straight into the skin.*

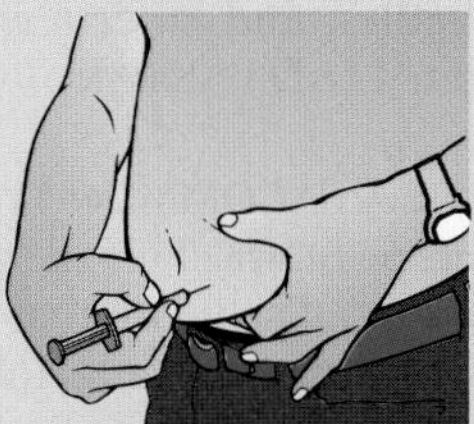

Inserting the needle into the skin

3. To inject the insulin, push the plunger all the way in.

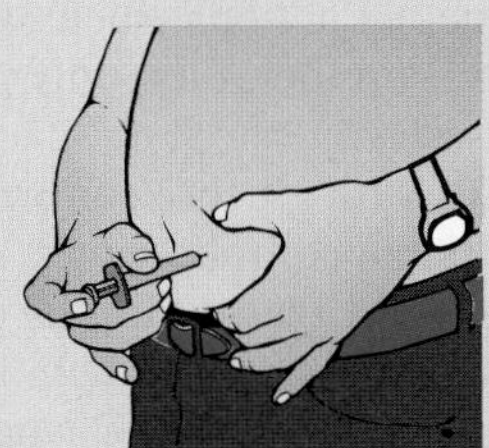

Injecting the insulin

4. Pull needle straight out of skin. Press cotton ball over injection site for several seconds.

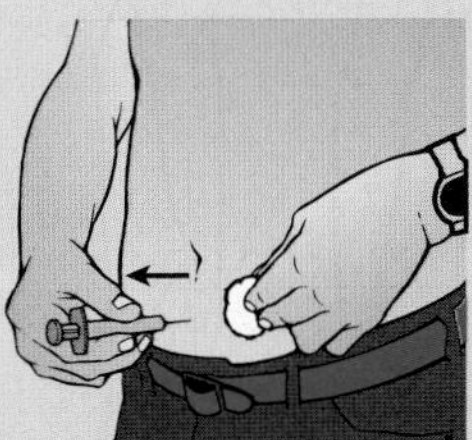

Removing the needle and holding cotton ball over site

5. Use disposable syringe *only once* and discard into hard plastic container (with a tight-fitting top) such as an empty bleach or detergent container.† Follow state regulations for disposal of syringes and needles.

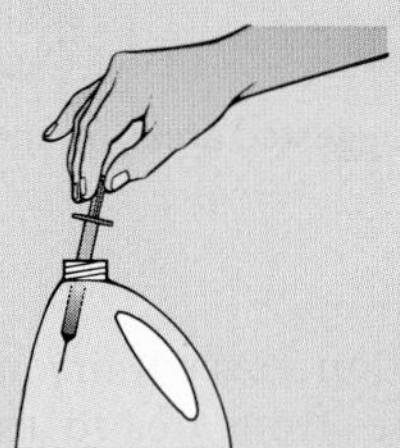

Disposing of syringe

*Some patients may be taught to insert the needle at a 45-degree angle.

†Although some studies suggest that reusing disposable syringes may be safe, it is recommended that this be done only in the absence of poor personal hygiene, an acute concurrent illness, open wounds on the hands, or decreased resistance to infection.

the bottle of insulin equivalent to the number of units of insulin to be withdrawn. The rationale for this is to prevent the formation of a vacuum inside the bottle, which would make it difficult to withdraw the proper amount of insulin.

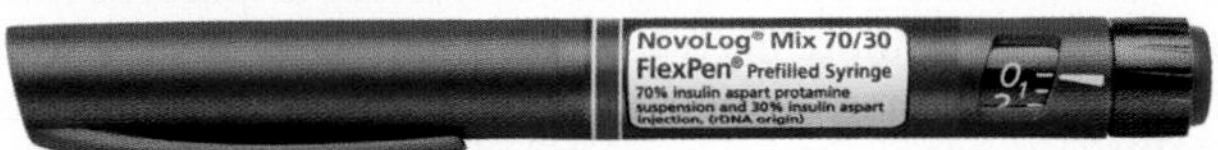

FIGURE 41-7. Prefilled insulin syringe.

SELECTING AND ROTATING THE INJECTION SITE

The four main areas for injection are the abdomen, upper arms (posterior surface), thighs (anterior surface), and hips (Fig. 41-8). Insulin is absorbed faster in some areas of the body than others. The speed of absorption is greatest in the abdomen and decreases progressively in the arm, thigh, and hip, respectively.

Systematic rotation of injection sites within an anatomic area is recommended to prevent localized changes in fatty tissue (lipodystrophy). In addition, to promote consistency in insulin absorption, the patient should be encouraged to

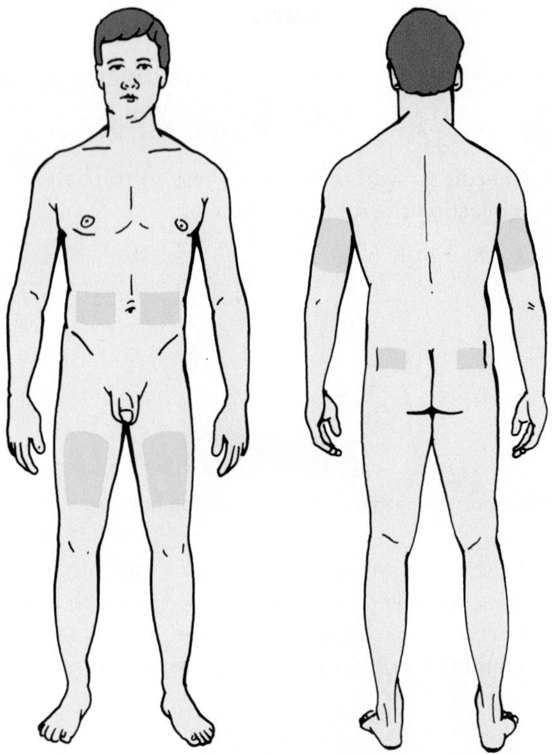

FIGURE 41-8. Suggested areas for insulin injection.

use all available injection sites within one area rather than randomly rotating sites from area to area (ADA, 2004k). For example, some patients almost exclusively use the abdominal area, administering each injection 0.5 to 1 inch away from the previous injection. Another approach to rotation is always to use the same area at the same time of day. For example, patients may inject morning doses into the abdomen and evening doses into the arms or legs.

A few general principles apply to all rotation patterns. First, the patient should try not to use the same site more than once in 2 to 3 weeks. In addition, if the patient is planning to exercise, insulin should not be injected into the limb that will be exercised because this will cause the drug to be absorbed faster, which may result in hypoglycemia.

In the past, patients were taught to rotate injections from one area to the next (eg, injecting once in the right arm, then once in the right abdomen, then once in the right thigh). Patients who still use this system must be taught to avoid repeated injections into the same site within an area. However, as previously stated, it is preferable for patients to use the same anatomic area at the same time of day consistently; this reduces day-to-day variation in blood glucose levels caused by different absorption rates.

PREPARING THE SKIN

Use of alcohol to cleanse the skin is not recommended, but patients who have learned this technique often continue to use it. They should be cautioned to allow the skin to dry after cleansing with alcohol. If the skin is not allowed to dry before the injection, the alcohol may be carried into the tissues, resulting in a localized reddened area and a burning sensation.

INSERTING THE NEEDLE

There are varying approaches to inserting the needle for insulin injections. The correct technique is based on the need for the insulin to be injected into the subcutaneous tissue. Injection that is too deep (eg, intramuscular) or too shallow may affect the rate of absorption of the insulin. Aspiration (inserting the needle and then pulling back on the plunger to assess for blood being drawn into the syringe) is generally not recommended with self-injection of insulin. Many patients who have been using insulin for an extended period have eliminated this step from their insulin injection routine with no apparent adverse effects.

DISPOSING OF SYRINGES AND NEEDLES

Insulin syringes and pens, needles, and lancets should be disposed of according to local regulations. Some areas have special needle disposal programs to prevent sharps from being discarded in the main waste disposal system. If community disposal programs are unavailable, used sharps should be placed in a puncture-resistant container. The patient should contact local trash authorities for instructions about proper disposal of filled containers, which should not be mixed with containers to be recycled. In areas with container-recycling programs, placement of containers of used syringes, needles, and lancets with materials to be recycled is prohibited (ADA, 2004k).

PROMOTING HOME AND COMMUNITY-BASED CARE

Teaching Patients Self-Care. The therapeutic plan is the most important aspect of self-care that patients must master. Patients who are having difficulty following the diabetes treatment plan must be approached with care and understanding. Using scare tactics (such as threats of blindness or amputation if a patient does not adhere to the treatment plan) or making a patient feel guilty is not productive and may interfere with establishing a trusting nurse–patient relationship. Judgmental actions, such as asking patients if they have "cheated" on their diet, only promote feelings of guilt and low self-esteem.

If problems exist with glucose control or with the development of preventable complications, it is the nurse's responsibility to assess the reasons for the patient's ineffective management of the treatment regimen. It should not be assumed that problems with diabetes management are related to the patient's willful decision to ignore self-management. The patient may have forgotten or never learned certain information. The problem may be correctable simply through providing complete information and ensuring that the patient understands the information. The focus of diabetes education should be patient empowerment. Patient education should address behavior change, self-efficacy, and health beliefs. Chart 41-8 details how to evaluate the effectiveness of self-injection of insulin education.

If knowledge deficit is not the problem, certain physical or emotional factors may be impairing the patient's ability to perform self-care skills. For example, decreased visual acuity may impair the patient's ability to administer insulin accurately, measure the blood glucose level, or inspect the skin and feet. In addition, decreased joint mobility (especially in the elderly) or preexisting disability may impair the patient's ability to inspect the bottom of the feet. Emotional factors such as denial of the diagnosis or depression may impair the

CHART 41-8

Outcome Criteria for Determining Effectiveness of Self-Injection of Insulin Education

EQUIPMENT

Insulin

1. Identifies information on label of insulin bottle:
   - Type (eg, NPH, regular, 70/30)
   - Species (human, biosynthetic, pork)
   - Manufacturer (Lilly, Novo Nordisk)
   - Concentration (eg, U-100)
   - Expiration date
2. Checks appearance of insulin:
   - Clear or milky white
   - Checks for flocculation (clumping, frosted appearance)
3. Identifies where to purchase and store insulin:
   - Indicates approximately how long bottle will last (1,000 units per bottle U-100 insulin)
   - Indicates how long opened bottles can be used

Syringes

1. Identifies concentration (U-100) marking on syringe
2. Identifies size of syringe (eg, 100-unit, 50-unit, 30-unit)
3. Describes appropriate disposal of used syringe

PREPARATION AND ADMINISTRATION OF INSULIN INJECTION

1. Draws up correct amount and type of insulin
2. Properly mixes two insulins if necessary
3. Inserts needle and injects insulin
4. Describes site rotation:
   - Demonstrates injection with all anatomic areas to be used
   - Describes pattern for rotation, such as using abdomen only or using certain areas at the same time of day
   - Describes system for remembering site locations, such as horizontal pattern across the abdomen as if drawing a dotted line

KNOWLEDGE OF INSULIN ACTION

1. Lists prescription:
   - Type and dosage of insulin
   - Timing of insulin injections
2. Describes approximate time course of insulin action:
   - Identifies long- and short-acting insulins by name.
   - States approximate time delay until onset of insulin action.
   - Identifies need to delay food until 5 to 15 min after injection of rapid-acting insulin (lispro, aspart).
   - Knows that longer time delays are safe when blood glucose level is high, and time delays may need to be shortened when blood glucose level is low.

INCORPORATION OF INSULIN INJECTIONS INTO DAILY SCHEDULE

1. Recites proper order of premeal diabetes activities:
   - May use mnemonic device such as the word "tie," which helps the patient remember the order of activities ("t" = test [blood glucose], "i" = insulin injection, "e" = eat).
   - Describes daily schedule, such as test, insulin, eat before breakfast and dinner; test and eat, before lunch and bedtime.
2. Describes information regarding hypoglycemia:
   - Symptoms: shakiness, sweating, nervousness, hunger, weakness
   - Causes: too much insulin, too much exercise, not enough food
   - Treatment: 15 g concentrated carbohydrate, such as two or three glucose tablets, 1 tube glucose gel, 0.5 cup juice
   - After initial treatment, follow with snack including starch and protein, such as cheese and crackers, milk and crackers, half sandwich.
3. Describes information regarding prevention of hypoglycemia:
   - Avoids delays in meal timing.
   - Eats a meal or snack approximately every 4 to 5 h (while awake).
   - Does not skip meals.
   - Increases food intake before exercise if blood glucose level is <100 mg/dL.
   - Checks blood glucose regularly.
   - Identifies safe modification of insulin doses consistent with management plan.
   - Carries a form of fast-acting sugar at all times.
   - Wears a medical identification bracelet.
   - Teaches family, friends, coworkers about signs and treatment of hypoglycemia.
   - Has family, roommates, traveling companions learn to use injectable glucagon for severe hypoglycemic reactions.
4. Maintains regular follow-up for evaluation of diabetes control:
   - Keeps written record of blood glucose, insulin doses, hypoglycemic reactions, variations in diet.
   - Keeps all appointments with health professionals.
   - Sees health care provider regularly (usually two to four times per year).
   - States how to contact health care provider in case of emergency.
   - States when to call health care provider to report variations in blood glucose levels.

patient's ability to carry out multiple daily self-care measures. In other circumstances, family, personal, or work problems may be of higher priority to the patient; the patient who is facing competing demands for time and attention may benefit from assistance in establishing priorities. It is also important to assess the patient for infection or emotional stress, which may lead to elevated blood glucose levels despite adherence to the treatment regimen.

The following nursing approaches are helpful for promoting self-care management skills:

- Address any underlying factors (eg, knowledge deficit, self-care deficit, illness) that may affect diabetic control.
- Simplify the treatment regimen if it is too difficult for the patient to follow.
- Adjust the treatment regimen to meet patient requests (eg, adjust diet or insulin schedule to allow increased flexibility in meal content or timing).
- Establish a specific plan or contract with each patient with simple, measurable goals.
- Provide positive reinforcement of self-care behaviors performed instead of focusing on behaviors that were neglected (eg, positively reinforce blood glucose tests that were performed instead of focusing on the number of missed tests).
- Help the patient identify personal motivating factors rather than focusing on wanting to please physicians or nurses.
- Encourage the patient to pursue life goals and interests, and discourage an undue focus on diabetes.

Continuing Care. As discussed, continuing care of patients with diabetes is critical in managing and preventing complications. The degree to which patients interact with health care providers to obtain ongoing care depends on many factors. Age, socioeconomic level, existing complications, type of diabetes, and comorbid conditions all may dictate the frequency of follow-up visits. Many patients with diabetes are seen by home health nurses for diabetes education, wound care, insulin preparation, or assistance with glucose monitoring. Even patients who achieve excellent glucose control and have no complications can expect to see their primary health care provider at least twice a year for ongoing evaluation and should receive routine nutrition updates. In addition, it is critical that the nurse remind the patient about the importance of participating in other health promotion activities (eg, immunizations) and recommended age-appropriate health screenings (eg, pelvic examinations, mammograms).

In addition to follow-up care with health professionals, participation in support groups is encouraged for patients who have had diabetes for many years as well as for those who are newly diagnosed. Such participation may help the patient and family cope with changes in lifestyle that occur with the onset of diabetes and its complications. People who participate in support groups often have an opportunity to share valuable information and experiences and to learn from others. Support groups provide an opportunity for discussion of strategies to deal with diabetes and its management and to clarify and verify information with nurses or other health care professionals. Participation in support groups may help the patient and family to become more knowledgeable about diabetes and its management and may promote healthy activities.

Acute Complications of Diabetes

There are three major acute complications of diabetes related to short-term imbalances in blood glucose levels: hypoglycemia, diabetic ketoacidosis (DKA), and hyperglycemic hyperosmolar nonketotic syndrome (HHNS), which is also called hyperglycemic hyperosmolar syndrome or state (HHS).

Hypoglycemia (Insulin Reactions)

Hypoglycemia (abnormally low blood glucose level) occurs when the blood glucose falls to less than 50 to 60 mg/dL (2.7 to 3.3 mmol/L). It can be caused by too much insulin or oral hypoglycemic agents, too little food, or excessive physical activity. Hypoglycemia may occur at any time of the day or night. It often occurs before meals, especially if meals are delayed or snacks are omitted. For example, midmorning hypoglycemia may occur when the morning regular insulin is peaking, whereas hypoglycemia that occurs in the late afternoon coincides with the peak of the morning NPH or Lente insulin. Middle-of-the-night hypoglycemia may occur because of peaking evening or predinner NPH or Lente insulins, especially in patients who have not eaten a bedtime snack.

Gerontologic Considerations

In elderly patients with diabetes, hypoglycemia is a particular concern for many reasons:

- Elderly people frequently live alone and may not recognize the symptoms of hypoglycemia.
- With decreasing renal function, it takes longer for oral hypoglycemic agents to be excreted by the kidneys.
- Skipping meals may occur because of decreased appetite or financial limitations.
- Decreased visual acuity may lead to errors in insulin administration.

Clinical Manifestations

The clinical manifestations of hypoglycemia may be grouped into two categories: adrenergic symptoms and central nervous system (CNS) symptoms.

In mild hypoglycemia, as the blood glucose level falls, the sympathetic nervous system is stimulated, resulting in a surge of epinephrine and norepinephrine. This causes symptoms such as sweating, tremor, tachycardia, palpitation, nervousness, and hunger.

In moderate hypoglycemia, the fall in blood glucose level deprives the brain cells of needed fuel for functioning. Signs of impaired function of the CNS may include inability to concentrate, headache, lightheadedness, confusion, memory lapses, numbness of the lips and tongue, slurred speech, impaired coordination, emotional changes, irrational or combative behavior, double vision, and drowsiness. Any combination of these symptoms (in addition to adrenergic symptoms) may occur with moderate hypoglycemia.

In severe hypoglycemia, CNS function is so impaired that the patient needs the assistance of another person for treatment of hypoglycemia. Symptoms may include disoriented behavior, seizures, difficulty arousing from sleep, or loss of consciousness.

Assessment and Diagnostic Findings

Symptoms of hypoglycemia may occur suddenly and unexpectedly and vary considerably from person to person. To some degree, this may be related to the actual level to which the blood glucose falls or to the rate at which it falls. For example, patients who usually have a blood glucose level in the hyperglycemic range (eg, 200 mg/dL or greater) may feel hypoglycemic (adrenergic) symptoms when their blood glucose falls rapidly to 120 mg/dL (6.6 mmol/L) or less. Conversely, patients who frequently have a glucose level in the low range of normal (eg, 80 to 100 mg/dL) may be asymptomatic when the blood glucose falls slowly to less than 50 mg/dL (2.7 mmol/L).

Decreased hormonal (adrenergic) response to hypoglycemia may also contribute to lack of symptoms of hypoglycemia. This occurs in some patients who have had diabetes for many years. It may be related to autonomic neuropathy, a chronic diabetic complication (see later discussion). As the blood glucose level falls, the normal surge in adrenalin does not occur, and the usual adrenergic symptoms, such as sweating and shakiness, do not take place. The hypoglycemia may not be detected until moderate or severe CNS impairment occurs. Affected patients must perform SMBG on a frequent regular basis, especially before driving or engaging in other potentially dangerous activities.

Management

Immediate treatment must be given when hypoglycemia occurs. The usual recommendation is for 15 g of a fast-acting concentrated source of carbohydrate such as the following, given orally:

- Three or four commercially prepared glucose tablets
- 4 to 6 oz of fruit juice or regular soda
- 6 to 10 hard candies
- 2 to 3 teaspoons of sugar or honey

It is not necessary to add sugar to juice, even if it is labeled as unsweetened juice: the fruit sugar in juice contains enough carbohydrate to raise the blood glucose level. Adding table sugar to juice may cause a sharp increase in the blood glucose level, and patients may experience hyperglycemia for hours after treatment.

The blood glucose level should be retested in 15 minutes and retreated if it is less than 70 to 75 mg/dL (3.8 to 4 mmol/L). If the symptoms persist for longer than 10 to 15 minutes after initial treatment, the treatment is repeated even if blood glucose testing is not possible. Once the symptoms resolve, a snack containing protein and starch (eg, milk or cheese and crackers) is recommended unless the patient plans to eat a regular meal or snack within 30 to 60 minutes.

Teaching Patients

It is important that patients with diabetes, especially those receiving insulin, learn to carry some form of simple sugar with them at all times (ADA, 2004k). There are many different commercially prepared glucose tablets and gels that the patient may find convenient to carry. If the patient has a hypoglycemic reaction and does not have any of the recommended emergency foods available, he or she should eat any available food (preferably a carbohydrate food).

Patients are advised to refrain from eating high-calorie, high-fat dessert foods (eg, cookies, cakes, doughnuts, ice cream) to treat hypoglycemia. The high fat content of these foods may slow the absorption of the glucose, and the hypoglycemic symptoms may not resolve as quickly as they would after the intake of carbohydrates. The patient may subsequently eat more of the foods when symptoms do not resolve rapidly; this in turn may cause very high blood glucose levels for several hours after the reaction and may also contribute to weight gain.

Patients who feel unduly restricted by their meal plan may view hypoglycemic episodes as a time to reward themselves with desserts. It may be more prudent to teach these patients to incorporate occasional desserts into the meal plan. This may make it easier for them to limit their treatment of hypoglycemic episodes to simple (low-calorie) carbohydrates such as juice or glucose tablets.

Initiating Emergency Measures

In emergency situations, for adult patients who are unconscious and cannot swallow, an injection of glucagon 1 mg can be administered either subcutaneously or intramuscularly. Glucagon is a hormone produced by the alpha cells of the pancreas that stimulates the liver to release glucose (through the breakdown of glycogen, the stored glucose). Injectable glucagon is packaged as a powder in 1-mg vials and must be mixed with a diluent before being injected. After injection of glucagon, the patient may take as long as 20 minutes to regain consciousness. A concentrated source of carbohydrate followed by a snack should be given to the patient on awakening to prevent recurrence of hypoglycemia (because the duration of the action of 1 mg of glucagon is brief—its onset is 8 to 10 minutes, and its action lasts 12 to 27 minutes) and to replenish liver stores of glucose. Some patients experience nausea after the administration of glucagon. If this occurs, the patient should be turned to the side to prevent aspiration in case the patient vomits.

Glucagon is sold by prescription only and should be part of the emergency supplies available to patients with diabetes who require insulin. Family members, friends, neighbors, and coworkers should be instructed in the use of glucagon, especially for patients who have little or no warning of hypoglycemic episodes. Patients should be instructed to notify their physician after severe hypoglycemia has occurred.

In hospitals and emergency departments, for patients who are unconscious or cannot swallow, 25 to 50 mL of 50% dextrose in water ($D_{50}W$) may be administered IV. The effect is usually seen within minutes. The patient may complain of a headache and of pain at the injection site. Assuring patency of the IV line used for injection of 50%

dextrose is essential, because hypertonic solutions such as 50% dextrose are very irritating to veins.

Promoting Home and Community-Based Care

TEACHING PATIENTS SELF-CARE

Hypoglycemia is prevented by a consistent pattern of eating, administering insulin, and exercising. Between-meal and bedtime snacks may be needed to counteract the maximum insulin effect. In general, the patient should cover the time of peak activity of insulin by eating a snack and by taking additional food when physical activity is increased. Routine blood glucose tests are performed so that changing insulin requirements may be anticipated and the dosage adjusted. Because unexpected hypoglycemia may occur, all patients treated with insulin should wear an identification bracelet or tag stating that they have diabetes.

Patients and family members must be instructed about the symptoms of hypoglycemia. Family members in particular must be made aware that any subtle (but unusual) change in behavior may be an indication of hypoglycemia. They should be taught to encourage and even insist that the person with diabetes assess blood glucose levels if hypoglycemia is suspected. When some patients are hypoglycemic, they become very resistant to testing or eating and become angry at family members who are trying to treat the hypoglycemia. Family members must be taught to persevere and to understand that the hypoglycemia can cause irrational behavior.

Some patients who have autonomic neuropathy or who are taking beta-blockers such as propranolol to treat hypertension or cardiac dysrhythmias may not experience the typical symptoms of hypoglycemia. It is very important that these patients perform blood glucose tests on a frequent and regular basis. Patients who have type 2 diabetes and who take oral sulfonylurea agents may also develop hypoglycemia, which can be prolonged and severe; this is a particular risk for elderly patients.

Diabetic Ketoacidosis (DKA)

DKA is caused by an absence or markedly inadequate amount of insulin. This deficit in available insulin results in disorders in the metabolism of carbohydrate, protein, and fat. The three main clinical features of DKA are

- Hyperglycemia
- Dehydration and electrolyte loss
- Acidosis

Pathophysiology

Without insulin, the amount of glucose entering the cells is reduced, and production and release of glucose by the liver is increased. Both factors lead to hyperglycemia. In an attempt to rid the body of the excess glucose, the kidneys excrete the glucose along with water and electrolytes (eg, sodium, potassium). This osmotic diuresis, which is characterized by excessive urination (polyuria), leads to dehydration and marked electrolyte loss. Patients with severe DKA may lose up to 6.5 L of water and up to 400 to 500 mEq each of sodium, potassium, and chloride over a 24-hour period.

Another effect of insulin deficiency or deficit is the breakdown of fat (lipolysis) into free fatty acids and glycerol. The free fatty acids are converted into ketone bodies by the liver. In DKA, there is excessive production of ketone bodies because of the lack of insulin that would normally prevent this from occurring. Ketone bodies are acids; their accumulation in the circulation leads to metabolic acidosis.

Three main causes of DKA are decreased or missed dose of insulin, illness or infection, and undiagnosed and untreated diabetes (DKA may be the initial manifestation of diabetes). An insulin deficit may result from an insufficient dosage of insulin prescribed or from insufficient insulin being administered by the patient. Errors in insulin dosage may be made by patients who are ill and who assume that if they are eating less or if they are vomiting, they must decrease their insulin doses. (Because illness, especially infections, can cause increased blood glucose levels, the patient does not need to decrease the insulin dose to compensate for decreased food intake when ill and may even need to increase the insulin dose.)

Other potential causes of decreased insulin include patient error in drawing up or injecting insulin (especially in patients with visual impairments), intentional skipping of insulin doses (especially in adolescents with diabetes who are having difficulty coping with diabetes or other aspects of their lives), or equipment problems (eg, occlusion of insulin pump tubing). Illness and infections are associated with insulin resistance. In response to physical (and emotional) stressors, there is an increase in the level of "stress" hormones—glucagon, epinephrine, norepinephrine, cortisol, and growth hormone. These hormones promote glucose production by the liver and interfere with glucose utilization by muscle and fat tissue, counteracting the effect of insulin. If insulin levels are not increased during times of illness and infection, hyperglycemia may progress to DKA.

Clinical Manifestations

The hyperglycemia of DKA leads to polyuria and polydipsia (increased thirst). In addition, the patient may experience blurred vision, weakness, and headache (Fig. 41-9). Patients with marked intravascular volume depletion may have orthostatic hypotension (drop in systolic blood pressure of 20 mm Hg or more on changing from a reclining to a standing position). Volume depletion may also lead to frank hypotension with a weak, rapid pulse.

The ketosis and acidosis of DKA lead to gastrointestinal symptoms such as anorexia, nausea, vomiting, and abdominal pain. The abdominal pain and physical findings on examination can be so severe that they resemble an acute abdominal disorder that requires surgery. The patient may have acetone breath (a fruity odor), which occurs with elevated ketone levels. In addition, hyperventilation (with very deep, but not labored, respirations) may occur. These Kussmaul respirations represent the body's attempt to decrease the acidosis, counteracting the effect of the ketone buildup. In addition, mental status changes in DKA vary widely. The patient may be alert, lethargic, or comatose, most likely depending on the plasma osmolarity (concentration of osmotically active particles).

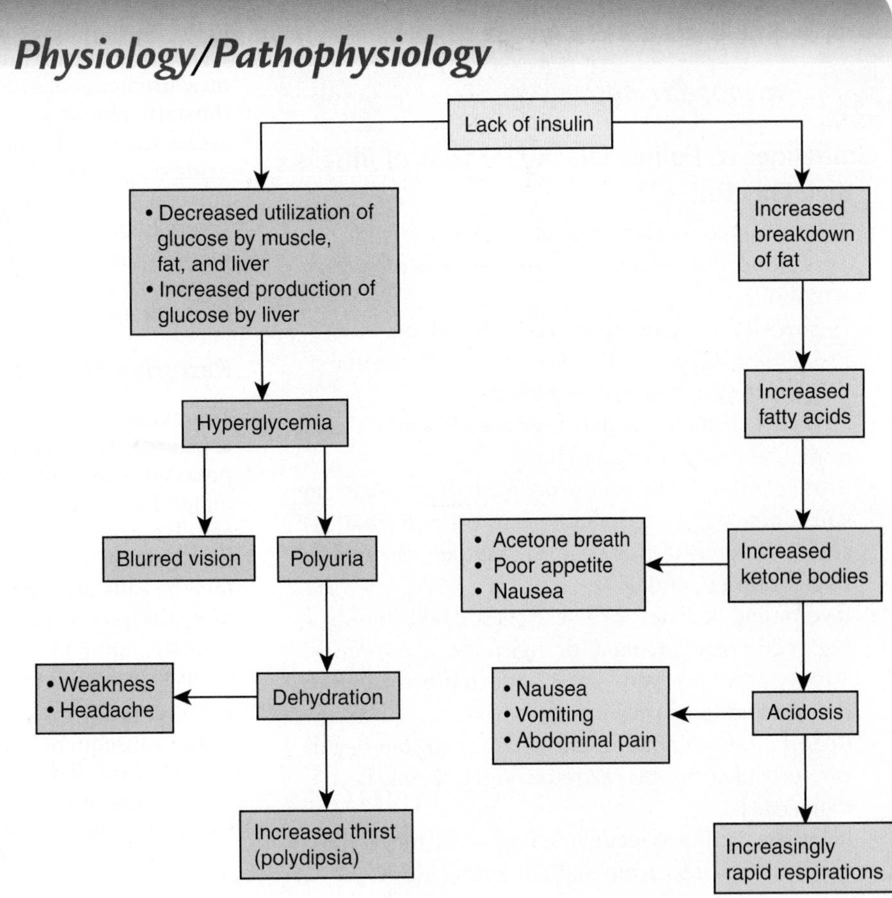

FIGURE 41-9. Abnormal metabolism that causes signs and symptoms of diabetic ketoacidosis. From Pearce, M. A., Rosenberg, C. S. & Davidson, M. D. (2003). Patient education. In Davidson, M. B. (Ed.). *Diabetes mellitus: Diagnosis and treatment.* New York: Churchill Livingstone.

Assessment and Diagnostic Findings

Blood glucose levels may vary between 300 and 800 mg/dL (16.6 to 44.4 mmol/L). Some patients have lower glucose values, and others have values of 1000 mg/dL (55.5 mmol/L) or higher (usually depending on the degree of dehydration). The severity of DKA is not necessarily related to the blood glucose level. Some patients have severe acidosis with modestly elevated blood glucose levels, whereas others have no evidence of DKA despite blood glucose levels of 400 to 500 mg/dL (22.2 to 27.7 mmol/L). Evidence of ketoacidosis is reflected in low serum bicarbonate (0 to 15 mEq/L) and low pH (6.8 to 7.3) values. A low partial pressure of carbon dioxide (PCO_2 10 to 30 mm Hg) reflects respiratory compensation (Kussmaul respirations) for the metabolic acidosis. Accumulation of ketone bodies (which precipitates the acidosis) is reflected in blood and urine ketone measurements.

Sodium and potassium concentrations may be low, normal, or high, depending on the amount of water loss (dehydration). Despite the plasma concentration, there has been a marked total body depletion of these (and other) electrolytes. Ultimately, these electrolytes will need to be replaced.

Increased levels of creatinine, blood urea nitrogen (BUN), and hematocrit may also be seen with dehydration. After rehydration, continued elevation in the serum creatinine and BUN levels is present in patients with underlying renal insufficiency.

Prevention

For prevention of DKA related to illness, patients must be taught "sick day" rules for managing their diabetes when ill (Chart 41-9). The most important concept to teach patients is not to eliminate insulin doses when nausea and vomiting occur. Instead, the patient should take the usual insulin dose (or previously prescribed special "sick day" doses) and then attempt to consume frequent small portions of carbohydrates (including foods usually avoided, such as juices, regular sodas, and gelatin). Drinking fluids every hour is important to prevent dehydration. Blood glucose and urine ketones must be assessed every 3 to 4 hours.

If the patient cannot take fluids without vomiting, or if elevated glucose or ketone levels persist, the physician must be contacted. Patients are taught to have foods available for use on sick days. In addition, a supply of urine test strips (for ketone testing) and blood glucose test strips should be available. The patient must know how to contact his or her physician 24 hours a day.

After the acute phase of DKA has resolved, the nurse should assess for underlying causes of DKA. If there are psychological reasons for the patient's deliberately missing

CHART 41-9

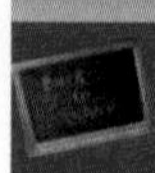

Patient Education

Guidelines to Follow During Periods of Illness ("Sick Day Rules")

- Take insulin or oral antidiabetic agents as usual.
- Test blood glucose and test urine ketones every 3 to 4 h.
- Report elevated glucose levels (>300 mg/dL [16.6 mmol/L] or as otherwise specified) or urine ketones to your health care provider.
- If you take insulin, you may need supplemental doses of regular insulin every 3 to 4 h.
- If you cannot follow your usual meal plan, substitute soft foods (eg, ⅓ cup regular gelatin, 1 cup cream soup, ½ cup custard, 3 squares graham crackers) six to eight times per day.
- If vomiting, diarrhea, or fever persists, take liquids (eg, ½ cup regular cola or orange juice, ½ cup broth, 1 cup Gatorade) every ½ to 1 hour to prevent dehydration and to provide calories.
- Report nausea, vomiting, and diarrhea to your health care provider, because extreme fluid loss may be dangerous.
- If you are unable to retain oral fluids, you may require hospitalization to avoid diabetic ketoacidosis and possibly coma.

insulin doses, the patient and family may be referred for evaluation and counseling or therapy.

Medical Management

In addition to treating hyperglycemia, management of DKA is aimed at correcting dehydration, electrolyte loss, and acidosis.

Rehydration

In dehydrated patients, rehydration is important for maintaining tissue perfusion. In addition, fluid replacement enhances the excretion of excessive glucose by the kidneys. The patient may need as much as 6 to 10 L of IV fluid to replace fluid losses caused by polyuria, hyperventilation, diarrhea, and vomiting.

Initially, 0.9% sodium chloride (normal saline) solution is administered at a rapid rate, usually 0.5 to 1 L/hour for 2 to 3 hours. Half-strength normal saline (0.45%) solution (also known as hypotonic saline solution) may be used for patients with hypertension or hypernatremia and those at risk for heart failure. After the first few hours, half-strength normal saline solution is the fluid of choice for continued rehydration, provided the blood pressure is stable and the sodium level is not low. Moderate to high rates of infusion (200 to 500 mL/hour) may continue for several more hours. When the blood glucose level reaches 300 mg/dL (16.6 mmol/L) or less, the IV solution may be changed to dextrose 5% in water (D_5W) to prevent a precipitous decline in the blood glucose level (ADA, 2004h).

Monitoring of fluid volume status involves frequent measurements of vital signs (including monitoring for orthostatic changes in blood pressure and heart rate), lung assessment, and monitoring of intake and output. Initial urine output lags behind IV fluid intake as dehydration is corrected. Plasma expanders may be necessary to correct severe hypotension that does not respond to IV fluid treatment. Monitoring for signs of fluid overload is especially important for patients who are older, have renal impairment, or are at risk for heart failure.

Restoring Electrolytes

The major electrolyte of concern during treatment of DKA is potassium. Although the initial plasma concentration of potassium may be low, normal, or even high, there is a major loss of potassium from body stores and an intracellular-to-extracellular shift of potassium. Furthermore, the serum level of potassium decreases as potassium reenters the cells during the course of treatment of DKA; therefore, the serum potassium level must be monitored frequently. Some of the factors related to treating DKA that reduce the serum potassium concentration include

- Rehydration, which leads to increased plasma volume and subsequent decreases in the concentration of serum potassium. Rehydration also leads to increased urinary excretion of potassium.
- Insulin administration, which enhances the movement of potassium from the extracellular fluid into the cells.

Cautious but timely potassium replacement is vital to avoid dysrhythmias that may occur with hypokalemia. As much as 40 mEq/hour may be needed for several hours. Because extracellular potassium levels decrease during DKA treatment, potassium must be infused even if the plasma potassium level is normal.

Frequent (every 2 to 4 hours initially) ECGs and laboratory measurements of potassium are necessary during the first 8 hours of treatment. Potassium replacement is withheld only if hyperkalemia is present or if the patient is not urinating.

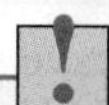

NURSING ALERT

Because a patient's serum potassium level may drop quickly as a result of rehydration and insulin treatment, potassium replacement must begin once potassium levels drop to normal.

Reversing Acidosis

Ketone bodies (acids) accumulate as a result of fat breakdown. The acidosis that occurs in DKA is reversed with insulin, which inhibits fat breakdown, thereby stopping acid buildup. Insulin is usually infused intravenously at a slow, continuous rate (eg, 5 units/hour). Hourly blood glucose values must be measured. IV fluid solutions with higher concentrations of glucose, such as normal saline (NS) solution (eg, D_5NS, $D_5.45NS$), are administered when blood glucose levels reach 250 to 300 mg/dL (13.8 to 16.6 mmol/L), to avoid too rapid a drop in the blood glucose level (ie, hypoglycemia) during treatment.

Regular insulin, the only type of insulin approved for IV use, may be added to IV solutions. The nurse must convert hourly rates of insulin infusion (frequently prescribed as "units per hour") to IV drip rates. For example, if 100 units of regular insulin are mixed into 500 mL of 0.9% NS, then 1 unit of insulin equals 5 mL; therefore, an initial insulin infusion rate of 5 units/hour would equal 25 mL/hour. The insulin is often infused separately from the rehydration solutions to allow frequent changes in the rate and content of the latter.

Insulin must be infused continuously until subcutaneous administration of insulin can be resumed. Any interruption in administration may result in the reaccumulation of ketone bodies and worsening acidosis. Even if blood glucose levels are decreasing and returning to normal, the insulin drip must not be stopped until subcutaneous insulin therapy has been started. Rather, the rate or concentration of the dextrose infusion should be increased. Blood glucose levels are usually corrected before the acidosis is corrected. Therefore, IV insulin may be continued for 12 to 24 hours, until the serum bicarbonate level improves (to at least 15 to 18 mEq/L) and until the patient can eat. In general, bicarbonate infusion to correct severe acidosis is avoided during treatment of DKA because it precipitates further, sudden (and potentially fatal) decreases in serum potassium levels. Continuous insulin infusion is usually sufficient for reversal of DKA.

NURSING ALERT

When mixing the insulin drip, it is important to flush the insulin solution through the entire IV infusion set and to discard the first 50 mL of fluid. Insulin molecules adhere to the inner surface of IV infusion sets; therefore, the initial fluid may contain a decreased concentration of insulin.

Nursing Management

Nursing care of patients with DKA focuses on monitoring fluid, electrolyte, and hydration status as well as blood glucose levels; administering fluids, insulin, and other medications; and preventing other complications such as fluid overload. Urine output is monitored to ensure adequate renal function before potassium is administered to prevent hyperkalemia. The ECG is monitored for dysrhythmias indicating abnormal potassium levels. Vital signs (especially blood pressure and pulse), arterial blood gases, breath sounds, and mental status are assessed every hour and recorded on a flow sheet. The nurse documents the patient's laboratory values and the frequent changes in fluids and medications that are prescribed and monitors the patient's responses. As DKA resolves and the potassium replacement rate is decreased, the nurse makes sure that

- There are no signs of hyperkalemia on the ECG (tall, peaked or tented T waves)
- Laboratory values of potassium are normal or approaching normal
- The patient is urinating (ie, no renal shutdown).

As the patient recovers, the nurse reassesses the factors that may have led to DKA and teaches the patient and family about strategies to prevent its recurrence. If indicated, the nurse initiates a referral for home care and outpatient diabetes education to ensure the patient's continued recovery.

Hyperglycemic Hyperosmolar Nonketotic Syndrome (HHNS)

HHNS is a serious condition in which hyperosmolarity and hyperglycemia predominate, with alterations of the sensorium (sense of awareness). At the same time, ketosis is usually minimal or absent. The basic biochemical defect is lack of effective insulin (ie, insulin resistance). Persistent hyperglycemia causes osmotic diuresis, which results in losses of water and electrolytes. To maintain osmotic equilibrium, water shifts from the intracellular fluid space to the extracellular fluid space. With glycosuria and dehydration, hypernatremia and increased osmolarity occur. Table 41-8 compares DKA and HHNS.

TABLE 41-8 Comparison of Diabetic Ketoacidosis (DKA) and Hyperglycemic Hyperosmolar Nonketotic Syndrome (HHNS)

Characteristics	DKA	HHNS
Patients most commonly affected	Can occur in type 1 or type 2 diabetes; more common in type 1 diabetes	Can occur in type 1 or type 2 diabetes; more common in type 2 diabetes, especially elderly patients with type 2 diabetes
Precipitating event	Omission of insulin; physiologic stress (infection, surgery, CVA, MI)	Physiologic stress (infection, surgery, CVA, MI)
Onset	Rapid (<24 h)	Slower (over several days)
Blood glucose levels	Usually >250 mg/dL (>13.9 mmol/L)	Usually >600 mg/dL (>33.3 mmol/L)
Arterial pH level	<7.3	Normal
Serum and urine ketones	Present	Absent
Serum osmolality	300–350 mOsm/L	>350 mOsm/L
Plasma bicarbonate level	<15 mEq/L	Normal
BUN and creatinine levels	Elevated	Elevated
Mortality rate	<5%	10–40%

CVA, cerebrovascular accident; MI, myocardial infarction.

HHNS occurs most often in older people (50 to 70 years of age) who have no known history of diabetes or who have type 2 diabetes. HHNS often can be traced to a precipitating event such as an acute illness (eg, pneumonia, CVA), medications (eg, thiazides) that exacerbate hyperglycemia, or treatments such as dialysis. The history includes days to weeks of polyuria with adequate fluid intake. What distinguishes HHNS from DKA is that ketosis and acidosis generally do not occur in HHNS, partly because of differences in insulin levels. In DKA, no insulin is present, and this promotes the breakdown of stored glucose, protein, and fat, which leads to the production of ketone bodies and ketoacidosis. In HHNS, the insulin level is too low to prevent hyperglycemia (and subsequent osmotic diuresis), but it is high enough to prevent fat breakdown. Patients with HHNS do not have the ketosis-related gastrointestinal symptoms that lead them to seek medical attention. Instead, they may tolerate polyuria and polydipsia until neurologic changes or an underlying illness (or family members or others) prompts them to seek treatment. Because of possible delays in therapy, hyperglycemia, dehydration, and hyperosmolarity may be more severe in HHNS.

Clinical Manifestations

The clinical picture of HHNS is one of hypotension, profound dehydration (dry mucous membranes, poor skin turgor), tachycardia, and variable neurologic signs (eg, alteration of sensorium, seizures, hemiparesis). The mortality rate ranges from 10% to 40%, usually related to an underlying illness, the vulnerability of the elderly patient, and the severity of HHNS.

Assessment and Diagnostic Findings

Diagnostic assessment includes a range of laboratory tests, including blood glucose, electrolytes, BUN, complete blood count, serum osmolality, and arterial blood gas analysis. The blood glucose level is usually 600 to 1200 mg/dL, and the osmolality exceeds 350 mOsm/kg. Electrolyte and BUN levels are consistent with the clinical picture of severe dehydration. Mental status changes, focal neurologic deficits, and hallucinations are common secondary to the cerebral dehydration that results from extreme hyperosmolality. Postural hypotension accompanies the dehydration (ADA, 2004h).

Medical Management

The overall approach to the treatment of HHNS is similar to that of DKA: fluid replacement, correction of electrolyte imbalances, and insulin administration. Because patients with HHNS are typically older, close monitoring of volume and electrolyte status is important for prevention of fluid overload, heart failure, and cardiac dysrhythmias. Fluid treatment is started with 0.9% or 0.45% NS, depending on the patient's sodium level and the severity of volume depletion. Central venous or hemodynamic pressure monitoring guides fluid replacement. Potassium is added to IV fluids when urinary output is adequate and is guided by continuous ECG monitoring and frequent laboratory determinations of potassium.

Extremely elevated blood glucose concentrations decrease as the patient is rehydrated. Insulin plays a less important role in the treatment of HHNS because it is not needed for reversal of acidosis, as in DKA. Nevertheless, insulin is usually administered at a continuous low rate to treat hyperglycemia, and replacement IV fluids with dextrose are administered (as in DKA) after the glucose level has decreased to the range of 250 to 300 mg/dL (13.8 to 16.6 mmol/L) (ADA, 2004h).

Other therapeutic modalities are determined by the underlying illness and the results of continuing clinical and laboratory evaluation. It may take 3 to 5 days for neurologic symptoms to clear, and treatment of HHNS usually continues well after metabolic abnormalities have resolved. After recovery from HHNS, many patients can control their diabetes with MNT alone or with MNT and oral antidiabetic medications. Insulin may not be needed once the acute hyperglycemic complication is resolved. Frequent SBGM is important in prevention of recurrence of HHNS.

Nursing Management

Nursing care of patients with HHNS includes close monitoring of vital signs, fluid status, and laboratory values. In addition, strategies are implemented to maintain safety and prevent injury related to changes in the sensorium secondary to HHNS. Fluid status and urine output are closely monitored because of the high risk of renal failure secondary to severe dehydration. In addition, the nurse must direct nursing care to the condition that may have precipitated the onset of HHNS. Because HHNS tends to occur in older patients, the physiologic changes that occur with aging should be noted. Careful assessment of cardiovascular, pulmonary, and renal function throughout the acute and recovery phases of HHNS is important.

Nursing Process

The Patient Newly Diagnosed With Diabetes Mellitus

Assessment

The history and physical assessment focus on the signs and symptoms of prolonged hyperglycemia and on physical, social, and emotional factors that may affect the patient's ability to learn and perform diabetes self-care activities. The patient is asked to describe symptoms that preceded the diagnosis of diabetes, such as polyuria, polydipsia, polyphagia, skin dryness, blurred vision, weight loss, vaginal itching, and nonhealing ulcers. Blood glucose levels are measured in patients with either type 1 or type 2 diabetes. In addition, urine ketone levels are measured, because the patient with type 1 diabetes may have ketones in the urine.

Patients diagnosed with type 1 diabetes are assessed for signs of DKA, including ketonuria, Kussmaul respirations, orthostatic hypotension, and lethargy. The patient is asked about symptoms of DKA, such as nausea, vomiting, and abdominal pain. Laboratory values are monitored for metabolic acidosis (ie, decreased pH and decreased bicarbonate level) and for electrolyte imbalance. Patients diagnosed with type 2 diabetes are assessed for signs of HHNS, including hypotension, altered sensorium, seizures, and decreased skin turgor. Laboratory values are monitored for hyperosmolality and electrolyte imbalance.

If the patient exhibits signs and symptoms of DKA or HHNS, nursing care first focuses on treatment of these acute complications, as outlined earlier. Once these complications are resolving, nursing care then focuses on long-term management of diabetes, as discussed in this section.

Then the patient is assessed for physical factors that may impair his or her ability to learn or perform self-care skills, such as

- Visual deficits (the patient is asked to read numbers or words on the insulin syringe, menu, newspaper, or written teaching materials)
- Deficits in motor coordination (the patient is observed eating or performing other tasks or handling a syringe or finger-lancing device)
- Neurologic deficits caused by stroke, other neurologic disorders, or other disabling conditions, from the history in the chart (the patient is assessed for aphasia or decreased ability to follow simple commands)

The nurse evaluates the patient's social situation for factors that may influence the diabetes treatment and education plan, such as

- Low literacy level (may be evaluated while assessing for visual deficits by having the patient read from teaching materials)
- Limited financial resources or lack of health insurance
- Presence or absence of family support
- Typical daily schedule (the patient is asked about timing and number of usual daily meals, work and exercise schedule, plans for travel)

The patient's emotional status is assessed by observing his or her general demeanor (eg, withdrawn, anxious) and body language (eg, avoids eye contact). The patient is asked about major concerns and fears about diabetes; this allows the nurse to assess for any misconceptions or misinformation regarding diabetes. Coping skills are assessed by asking how the patient has dealt with difficult situations in the past.

Diagnosis

Nursing Diagnoses

Based on the assessment data, major nursing diagnoses may include the following:

- Risk for fluid volume deficit related to polyuria and dehydration
- Imbalanced nutrition related to imbalance of insulin, food, and physical activity
- Deficient knowledge about diabetes self-care skills/information
- Potential self-care deficit related to physical impairments or social factors
- Anxiety related to loss of control, fear of inability to manage diabetes, misinformation related to diabetes, fear of diabetes complications

Collaborative Problems/ Potential Complications

Based on assessment data, potential complications may include the following:

- Fluid overload, pulmonary edema, and heart failure
- Hypokalemia
- Hyperglycemia and ketoacidosis
- Hypoglycemia
- Cerebral edema

Planning and Goals

The major goals for the patient may include maintenance of fluid and electrolyte balance, optimal control of blood glucose levels, reversal of weight loss, ability to perform diabetes survival skills and self-care activities, decreased anxiety, and absence of complications.

Nursing Interventions

Maintaining Fluid and Electrolyte Balance

Intake and output are measured. IV fluids and electrolytes are administered as prescribed, and oral fluid intake is encouraged when it is permitted. Laboratory values of serum electrolytes (especially sodium and potassium) are monitored. Vital signs are monitored hourly for signs of dehydration (tachycardia, orthostatic hypotension) along with assessment of breath sounds, level of consciousness, presence of edema, and cardiac status (ECG rhythm strips).

Improving Nutritional Intake

Meal planning is implemented, with the control of glucose as the primary goal. Planning must take into consideration the patient's lifestyle, cultural background, activity level, and food preferences. An appropriate caloric intake allows the patient to achieve and maintain the desired body weight. The patient is encouraged to eat full meals and snacks as prescribed in the diet prescription. Arrangements may be made with the dietitian for extra snacks before increased physical activity. It is important for the nurse to ensure that insulin orders are altered as needed to correspond to delays in eating caused by diagnostic and other procedures that affect timing of meals.

Reducing Anxiety

The nurse provides emotional support and sets aside time to talk with the patient who wishes to express feelings, cry, or ask questions about the new diagnosis.

Any misconceptions the patient or family may have regarding diabetes are dispelled (see Table 41-7). The patient and family are assisted to focus on learning self-care behaviors. The patient is encouraged to perform the skills that he or she fears most and must be reassured that once a skill such as self-injection or lancing a finger for glucose monitoring is performed for the first time, anxiety will decrease. Positive reinforcement is given for the self-care behaviors attempted, even if the technique is not yet completely mastered.

Improving Self-Care

As previously discussed, patient teaching is the major strategy used to prepare patients for self-care. Special equipment may be needed for instruction on diabetes survival skills, such as a magnifying glass for insulin preparation or an injection-aid device for insulin injection. Low-literacy information and literature in other languages can be obtained from the ADA. Families are also taught so that they can assist in diabetes management; for example, they can prefill syringes or monitor the patient's blood glucose level. The diabetes educator is consulted regarding various blood glucose monitors and other equipment for use by patients with physical impairments. The patient is assisted in identifying community resources for education and supplies as needed. Other members of the health care team are informed about variations in the timing of meals and the work schedule (eg, if the patient works at night or in the evenings and sleeps during the day) so that the diabetes treatment regimen can be adjusted accordingly.

Monitoring and Managing Potential Complications

FLUID OVERLOAD

Fluid overload can occur because of the administration of a large volume of fluid at a rapid rate, which is often required to treat patients with DKA or HHNS. This risk is increased in elderly patients and in those with preexisting cardiac or renal disease. To avoid fluid overload and resulting heart failure and pulmonary edema, the nurse monitors the patient closely during treatment by measuring vital signs and intake and output at frequent intervals. Central venous pressure monitoring and hemodynamic monitoring may be initiated to provide additional measures of fluid status. Physical examination focuses on assessment of cardiac rate and rhythm, breath sounds, venous distention, skin turgor, and urine output. The nurse monitors fluid intake and keeps careful records of IV and other fluid intake, along with urine output measurements.

HYPOKALEMIA

As previously described, hypokalemia is a potential complication during the treatment of DKA as potassium is lost from body stores. Low serum potassium levels may result from rehydration, increased urinary excretion of potassium, and movement of potassium from the extracellular fluid into the cells with insulin administration. Prevention of hypokalemia includes cautious replacement of potassium; however, before its administration, it is important to ensure that a patient's kidneys are functioning. Because of the adverse effects of hypokalemia on cardiac function, monitoring of the cardiac rate, cardiac rhythm, ECG, and serum potassium levels is essential.

HYPERGLYCEMIA AND KETOACIDOSIS

Although the hyperglycemia and ketoacidosis that may have led to the new diagnosis of diabetes may be resolved, patients are at risk for their subsequent recurrence. Therefore, blood glucose levels and urine ketones are monitored, and medications (insulin, oral antidiabetic agents) are administered as prescribed. The nurse monitors the concentrations of blood glucose and urine ketones and reports any value out of the target range. IV insulin and IV fluids may need to be administered again.

HYPOGLYCEMIA

Hypoglycemia may occur if the patient skips or delays meals, does not follow the prescribed meal plan, or greatly increases the amount of exercise without modifying food intake and insulin. In addition, hospitalized patients or outpatients who fast in preparation for diagnostic testing are at risk for hypoglycemia. Juice, milk, or glucose tablets are used for treatment of hypoglycemia. The patient is encouraged to eat full meals and snacks as prescribed in the meal plan. If hypoglycemia is a recurring problem, the total therapeutic regimen should be reevaluated.

Because of the risk of hypoglycemia, especially with intensive insulin regimens, it is important for the nurse to review with the patient the signs and symptoms, possible causes, and measures for prevention and treatment of hypoglycemia. The nurse should stress to the patient and family the importance of having information on diabetes at home for reference.

CEREBRAL EDEMA

Although the cause of cerebral edema is unknown, rapid correction of hyperglycemia, resulting in fluid shifts, is thought to be the cause. Cerebral edema, which occurs more often in children than in adults, can be prevented by gradual reduction in the blood glucose level (ADA, 2004h). An hourly flow sheet is used to enable close monitoring of the blood glucose level, serum electrolyte levels, urine output, mental status, and neurologic signs. Precautions are taken to minimize activities that could increase intracranial pressure.

Promoting Home and Community-Based Care

TEACHING PATIENTS SELF-CARE

The patient is taught survival skills, including treatment modalities (diet, insulin administration, monitoring of blood glucose, and, for type 1 diabetes, monitoring of urine ketones); recognition, treatment, and prevention of acute complications (hypoglycemia and hyperglycemia); practical information (where to obtain supplies, when to call the physician); and simple pathophysiology that the patient will understand. If the patient has signs of long-term diabetes complications at the time of diagnosis of diabetes, teaching about relevant preventive behaviors (eg, foot care, eye care) is appropriate at this time (Chart 41-10).

CONTINUING CARE

Follow-up education is arranged with a home care nurse and dietitian or an outpatient diabetes education center. This is particularly important for patients who have had difficulty coping with the diagnosis, patients who have limitations that may affect their ability to learn or to carry out the management plan, and patients who are without any family or social supports. Referral to social services and community resources (eg, centers for the visually impaired) may be needed, depending on the patient's financial circumstances and physical limitations. The importance of self-monitoring and of monitoring and follow-up by primary health care providers is reinforced, and the patient is reminded about the importance of keeping follow-up appointments. Patients who are newly diagnosed with diabetes are also reminded about the importance of participating in other health promotion activities and health screening. Chart 41-11 is a checklist of self-care skills.

Evaluation

Expected Patient Outcomes

Expected patient outcomes may include the following:

1. Achieves fluid and electrolyte balance
   a. Demonstrates intake and output balance
   b. Exhibits electrolyte values within normal limits
   c. Exhibits vital signs that remain stable, with resolution of orthostatic hypotension and tachycardia
2. Achieves metabolic balance
   a. Avoids extremes of glucose levels (hypoglycemia or hyperglycemia)
   b. Exhibits glucose levels within target range with minimal episodes of hypoglycemia
   c. Recognizes and treats hypoglycemia appropriately
   d. Demonstrates rapid resolution of hypoglycemic episodes
   e. Avoids further weight loss (if applicable) and begins to approach desired weight
3. Demonstrates/verbalizes diabetes survival skills
   a. Defines diabetes as a condition in which high blood glucose levels are present
   b. States normal and target blood glucose ranges
   c. Identifies factors that cause the blood glucose level to fall (insulin, exercise, some oral antidiabetic medications)
   d. Identifies factors that cause the blood glucose level to rise (food, illness, stress, and infections)
   e. Describes the major treatment modalities: nutrition therapy, exercise, monitoring, medication, education
   f. Demonstrates proper technique for drawing up and injecting insulin (including mixing two types of insulin, if necessary)

CHART 41-10

Patient Education

Foot Care Tips

1. Take care of your diabetes.
   - Work with your health care team to keep your blood glucose level within a normal range.
2. Inspect your feet every day.
   - Look at your bare feet every day for cuts, blisters, red spots, and swelling.
   - Use a mirror to check the bottoms of your feet or ask a family member for help if you have trouble seeing.
   - Check for changes in temperature.
3. Wash your feet every day.
   - Wash your feet in warm, not hot, water.
   - Dry your feet well. Be sure to dry between the toes.
   - Do not soak your feet.
   - Do not check water temperature with your feet; use a thermometer or elbow.
4. Keep the skin soft and smooth.
   - Rub a thin coat of skin lotion over the tops and bottoms of your feet, but not between your toes.
5. Smooth corns and calluses gently.
   - Use a pumice stone to smooth corns and calluses.
6. Trim your toenails each week or when needed.
   - Trim your toenails straight across and file the edges with an emery board or nail file.
7. Wear shoes and socks at all times.
   - Never walk barefoot.
   - Wear comfortable shoes that fit well and protect your feet.
   - Feel inside your shoes before putting them on each time to make sure the lining is smooth and there are no objects inside.
8. Protect your feet from hot and cold.
   - Wear shoes at the beach or on hot pavement.
   - Wear socks at night if your feet get cold.
9. Keep the blood flowing to your feet.
   - Put your feet up when sitting.
   - Wiggle your toes and move your ankles up and down for 5 minutes, 2 or 3 times a day.
   - Do not cross your legs for long periods of time.
   - Do not smoke.
10. Check with your health care provider.
    - Have your health care provider check your bare feet and find out whether you are likely to have serious foot problems. Remember that you may not feel the pain of an injury.
    - Call your health care provider right away if a cut, sore, blister, or bruise on your foot does not begin to heal after one day.
    - Follow your health care provider's advice about foot care.
    - Do not self-medicate or use home remedies or over-the-counter agents to treat foot problems.

CHART 41-11

HOME CARE CHECKLIST • The Person With Newly Diagnosed Diabetes

At the completion of the home care instruction, the patient or caregiver will be able to:	Patient	Caregiver
• State the importance of diabetes survival skills.	✔	✔
• Explain underlying pathology of diabetes.	✔	✔
• State target range for blood glucose.	✔	✔
• Identify factors that cause hyper- and hypoglycemia.	✔	✔
• Describe the major modalities used to control diabetes (meal planning, exercise, monitoring, medication, education).	✔	✔
• Demonstrate proper technique for drawing up and injecting insulin (including mixing two types of insulin if necessary).	✔	✔
• State dose and timing of injections, peak action and duration of insulin.	✔	✔
• Explain insulin injection rotation plan and its rationale.	✔	✔
• State dose, timing, peak action and duration of prescribed oral agents.	✔	✔
• Describe where to purchase and store insulin, syringes, and glucose monitoring supplies.	✔	✔
• Identify classification of food groups (depending on system used).	✔	✔
• State appropriate schedule for eating snacks and meals.	✔	✔
• Select appropriate foods on menus and identify foods that may be substituted for one another on the meal plan.	✔	
• Demonstrate proper technique for monitoring blood glucose.	✔	
• Describe strategies to be used to treat hypoglycemic episodes.	✔	✔
• Use proper technique for disposing of lancets used for blood glucose monitoring and equipment used for insulin injections.	✔	
• Demonstrate proper technique for urine ketone testing (for patients with type 1 diabetes), and verbalize appropriate times to assess for ketones.	✔	✔
• Identify community, outpatient resources for obtaining further diabetes education.	✔	✔
• Identify signs and symptoms of hypoglycemia.	✔	✔
• Describe appropriate treatment of hypoglycemia.	✔	✔
• Identify factors that may cause hypoglycemia.	✔	✔
• State strategies that minimize risk for hypoglycemia.	✔	✔
• State rationale for wearing medical identification and carrying a source of simple carbohydrate at all times.	✔	
• Identify signs and symptoms of hyperglycemia.	✔	✔
• Describe appropriate treatment of hyperglycemia.	✔	✔
• Identify factors that may cause hyperglycemia.	✔	✔
• Identify rules for sick-day management.	✔	✔
• Identify appropriate circumstances for contacting physician.	✔	✔

g. States dose and timing of injections, peak action, duration, and adverse effects of insulin
h. States dose, timing, peak action, and duration of prescribed oral antidiabetic agents
i. Verbalizes plan for rotating insulin injection sites
j. Verbalizes understanding of food group classifications (depending on system used)
k. Verbalizes appropriate schedule for eating snacks and meals; orders appropriate foods on menus; identifies foods that may be substituted for one another on the meal plan
l. Demonstrates proper technique for monitoring blood glucose, including using finger-lancing device; obtaining a drop of blood; applying

blood properly to strip; obtaining value of blood glucose; and recording blood glucose value. Also, is able to calibrate and clean meter, change batteries, identify alarms and warnings on meter, and use control solutions to validate strips.

m. Demonstrates proper technique for disposal of lancets and needles used for blood glucose monitoring and insulin injections (ie, discarding them into sharps container)
n. Demonstrates proper technique for urine ketone testing (for patients with type 1 diabetes) and verbalizes appropriate times to assess for ketones (when ill or when blood glucose test results are repeatedly and inexplicably greater than 250 to 300 mg/dL [13.8 to 16.6 mmol/L])
o. Identifies community, outpatient resources for obtaining further diabetes education
p. Identifies acute complications (hypoglycemia and hyperglycemia)
q. Verbalizes symptoms of hypoglycemia (shakiness, sweating, headache, hunger, numbness or tingling of lips or fingers, weakness, fatigue, difficulty concentrating, change of mood) and dangers of untreated hypoglycemia (seizures and coma)
r. Identifies appropriate treatment of hypoglycemia, including 15 g simple carbohydrate (eg, two to four glucose tablets, 4 to 6 oz juice or soda, 2 to 3 teaspoons sugar, 6 to 10 hard candies) followed by a snack of protein and carbohydrate (eg, cheese and crackers or milk) or by a regularly scheduled meal
s. States potential causes of hypoglycemia (too much insulin, delayed or decreased food intake, increased physical activity) and verbalizes preventive behaviors, such as frequent monitoring of blood glucose when daily schedule is changed and eating a snack before exercise
t. Verbalizes importance of wearing or carrying medical identification and carrying a source of simple carbohydrate at all times
u. Verbalizes symptoms of prolonged hyperglycemia (increased thirst and urination)
v. Verbalizes rules for sick day management
w. Describes where to purchase and store insulin, syringes, and glucose monitoring supplies
x. Identifies appropriate circumstances for calling the physician (when ill, when glucose levels repeatedly exceed a certain level [per physician guidelines], or when skin wounds fail to heal) and also identifies name of physician (or other health care team member) and 24-hour phone number

4. Absence of complications
   a. Exhibits normal cardiac rate and rhythm and normal breath sounds
   b. Exhibits no jugular venous distention
   c. Exhibits blood glucose and urine ketone levels within target range
   d. Exhibits no manifestations of hypoglycemia or hyperglycemia
   e. Shows improved mental status without signs of cerebral edema

Long-Term Complications of Diabetes

There has been a steady decline in the number of deaths attributable to ketoacidosis and infection in patients with diabetes but an alarming increase in the number of deaths from cardiovascular and renal complications. Long-term complications, which are becoming more common as more people live longer with diabetes, can affect almost every organ system of the body and are a major cause of disability. The general categories of long-term diabetic complications are macrovascular disease, microvascular disease, and neuropathy.

The specific causes and pathogenesis of each type of complication are still being investigated. However, it appears that increased levels of blood glucose may play a role in neuropathic disease, microvascular complications, and risk factors contributing to macrovascular complications. Hypertension may also be a major contributing factor, especially in macrovascular and microvascular diseases.

Long-term complications are seen in both type 1 and type 2 diabetes but usually do not occur within the first 5 to 10 years after diagnosis. However, evidence of these complications may be present at the time of diagnosis of type 2 diabetes, because patients may have had undiagnosed diabetes for many years. Renal (microvascular) disease is more prevalent in patients with type 1 diabetes, and cardiovascular (macrovascular) complications are more prevalent in older patients with type 2 diabetes.

Macrovascular Complications

Diabetic macrovascular complications result from changes in the medium to large blood vessels. Blood vessel walls thicken, sclerose, and become occluded by plaque that adheres to the vessel walls. Eventually, blood flow is blocked. These atherosclerotic changes tend to occur more often and at an earlier age in patients with diabetes and are unstable. Coronary artery disease, cerebrovascular disease, and peripheral vascular disease are the three main types of macrovascular complications that occur more frequently in the diabetic population.

Myocardial infarction is twice as common in men with diabetes and three times as common in women with diabetes, compared to people without diabetes. There is also an increased risk for complications resulting from myocardial infarction and an increased likelihood of a second myocardial infarction. Coronary artery disease may account for 50% to 60% of all deaths among patients with diabetes. One unique feature of coronary artery disease in patients with diabetes is that the typical ischemic symptoms may be absent. Therefore, the patient may not experience the early warning signs of decreased coronary blood flow and may have "silent" myocardial infarctions, which may be discovered only as changes on the ECG. However, ECG changes may not be apparent. This lack of ischemic symptoms may be secondary to autonomic neuropathy (see later discussion). Cardiac disease is discussed in detail in Chapter 28.

Cerebral blood vessels are similarly affected by accelerated atherosclerosis. Occlusive changes or the formation of an embolus elsewhere in the vasculature that lodges in a cerebral blood vessel can lead to transient ischemic attacks and strokes. People with diabetes have twice the risk of developing cerebrovascular disease, and studies suggest that there may be a greater likelihood of death from cerebrovascular disease in patients with diabetes. In addition, recovery from a stroke may be impaired in patients who have elevated blood glucose levels at the time of and immediately after a stroke. Because symptoms of cerebrovascular disease may be similar to symptoms of acute diabetic complications (HHNS or hypoglycemia), it is very important to assess the blood glucose level (and treat abnormal levels) rapidly in patients reporting these symptoms, so that testing and treatment of cerebrovascular disease (stroke) can be initiated promptly if indicated.

Atherosclerotic changes in the large blood vessels of the lower extremities are responsible for the increased incidence (two to three times higher than in nondiabetic people) of occlusive peripheral arterial disease in patients with diabetes. Signs and symptoms of peripheral vascular disease include diminished peripheral pulses and intermittent claudication (pain in the buttock, thigh, or calf during walking). The severe form of arterial occlusive disease in the lower extremities is largely responsible for the increased incidence of gangrene and subsequent amputation in patients with diabetes. Neuropathy and impairments in wound healing also play a role in diabetic foot disease (see later discussion).

Role of Diabetes in Macrovascular Diseases

Researchers continue to investigate the relationship between diabetes and macrovascular diseases. The main feature unique to diabetes is elevated blood glucose; however, a direct link has not been found between hyperglycemia and atherosclerosis. Although it may be tempting to attribute the increased prevalence of macrovascular diseases to the increased prevalence of certain risk factors (eg, obesity, increased triglyceride levels, hypertension) in patients with diabetes, there is a higher-than-expected rate of macrovascular diseases among patients with diabetes compared with patients without diabetes who have the same risk factors (ADA, 2004d). Therefore, diabetes itself is seen as an independent risk factor for accelerated atherosclerosis. Other potential factors that may play a role in diabetes-related atherosclerosis include platelet and clotting factor abnormalities, decreased flexibility of red blood cells, decreased oxygen release, changes in the arterial wall related to hyperglycemia, and possibly hyperinsulinemia.

Management

The focus of management is aggressive modification and reduction of risk factors. This involves prevention and treatment of the commonly accepted risk factors for atherosclerosis. MNT and exercise are important in managing obesity, hypertension, and hyperlipidemia. In addition, the use of medications to control hypertension and hyperlipidemia is indicated. Smoking cessation is essential. Control of blood glucose levels may reduce triglyceride concentrations and can significantly reduce the incidence of complications.

When macrovascular complications do occur, patients may require increased amounts of insulin or may need to switch from oral antidiabetic agents to insulin during illnesses.

Microvascular Complications

Diabetic microvascular disease (or microangiopathy) is characterized by capillary basement membrane thickening. The basement membrane surrounds the endothelial cells of the capillary. Researchers believe that increased blood glucose levels react through a series of biochemical responses to thicken the basement membrane to several times its normal thickness. Two areas affected by these changes are the retina and the kidneys.

Diabetic Retinopathy

Diabetic retinopathy is the leading cause of blindness among people between 20 and 74 years of age in the United States; it occurs in both type 1 and type 2 diabetes (ADA, 2004s).

People with diabetes are subject to many visual complications (Table 41-9). The eye pathology referred to as diabetic retinopathy is caused by changes in the small blood vessels in the retina, the area of the eye that receives images and sends information about the images to the brain (Fig. 41-10). The retina is richly supplied with blood vessels of all kinds: small arteries and veins, arterioles, venules, and capillaries. Retinopathy has three main stages: nonproliferative (background), preproliferative, and proliferative.

Almost all patients with type 1 diabetes and more than 60% of patients with type 2 diabetes have some degree of retinopathy after 20 years (ADA, 2004s). Changes in the microvasculature include microaneurysms, intraretinal hemorrhage, hard exudates, and focal capillary closure. Although most patients do not develop visual impairment, it can be devastating if it occurs. A complication of nonproliferative retinopathy, macular edema, occurs in approximately 10% of people with type 1 or type 2 diabetes and may lead to visual distortion and loss of central vision.

An advanced form of background retinopathy, preproliferative retinopathy, is considered to be a precursor to the more serious proliferative retinopathy. In preproliferative retinopathy, there are more widespread vascular changes and loss of nerve fibers. Epidemiologic evidence suggests that 10% to 50% of patients with preproliferative retinopathy will develop proliferative retinopathy within a short time (possibly as little as 1 year). As with background retinopathy, if visual changes occur during the preproliferative stage, they are usually caused by macular edema.

Proliferative retinopathy represents the greatest threat to vision and is characterized by the proliferation of new blood vessels growing from the retina into the vitreous. These new vessels are prone to bleeding. The visual loss associated with proliferative retinopathy is caused by this vitreous hemorrhage, retinal detachment, or both. The vitreous is normally clear, allowing light to be transmitted to the retina. When there is a hemorrhage, the vitreous becomes clouded and cannot transmit light, resulting in loss of vision. Another consequence of vitreous hemorrhage is that

TABLE 41-9 Ocular Complications of Diabetes

Eye Disorder	Characteristics
Retinopathy	Deterioration of the small blood vessels that nourish the retina
Background	Early stage, asymptomatic retinopathy. Blood vessels within the retina develop microaneurysms that leak fluid, causing swelling and forming deposits (exudates). In some cases, macular edema causes distorted vision.
Preproliferative	Represents increased destruction of retinal blood vessels
Proliferative	Abnormal growth of new blood vessels on the retina. New vessels rupture, bleeding into the vitreous and blocking light. Ruptured blood vessels in the vitreous form scar tissue, which can pull on and detach the retina.
Cataracts	Opacity of the lens of the eye; cataracts occur at an earlier age in patients with diabetes.
Lens changes	The lens of the eye can swell when blood glucose levels are elevated. For some patients, visual changes related to lens swelling may be the first symptoms of diabetes. It may take up to 2 months of improved blood glucose control before hyperglycemic swelling subsides and vision stabilizes. Therefore, patients are advised not to change eyeglass prescriptions during the 2 months after discovery of hyperglycemia.
Extraocular muscle palsy	This may occur as a result of diabetic neuropathy. The involvement of various cranial nerves responsible for ocular movements may lead to double vision. This usually resolves spontaneously.
Glaucoma	Results from occlusion of the outflow channels by new blood vessels. Glaucoma may occur with slightly higher frequency in the diabetic population.

resorption of the blood in the vitreous leads to the formation of fibrous scar tissue. This scar tissue may place traction on the retina, resulting in retinal detachment and subsequent visual loss.

Clinical Manifestations

Retinopathy is a painless process. In nonproliferative and preproliferative retinopathy, blurry vision secondary to macular edema occurs in some patients, although many patients are asymptomatic. Even patients with a significant degree of proliferative retinopathy and some hemorrhaging may not experience major visual changes. However, symptoms indicative of hemorrhaging include floaters or cobwebs in the visual field, sudden visual changes including spotty or hazy vision, or complete loss of vision.

Assessment and Diagnostic Findings

Diagnosis is by direct visualization of the retina through dilated pupils with an ophthalmoscope or with a technique known as fluorescein angiography. Fluorescein angiography can document the type and activity of the retinopathy. Dye is injected into an arm vein and is carried to various parts of the body through the blood, but especially through the vessels of the retina of the eye. This technique allows an ophthalmologist, using special instruments, to see the retinal vessels in bright detail and gives useful information that cannot be obtained with just an ophthalmoscope.

Side effects of this diagnostic procedure may include nausea during the dye injection; yellowish, fluorescent discoloration of the skin and urine lasting 12 to 24 hours; and occasionally allergic reactions, usually manifested by hives or itching. However, the diagnostic procedure is generally safe. Patient preparation involves explaining

- The steps of the procedure
- The fact that the procedure is painless
- The potential side effects
- The type of information the technique can provide
- That the flash of the camera may be slightly uncomfortable for a short time

Medical Management

The first focus of management of retinopathy is on primary and secondary prevention. The DCCT study demonstrated that in patients without preexisting retinopathy, maintenance of blood glucose to a normal or near-normal level in type 1 diabetes through intensive insulin therapy and patient education decreased the risk of retinopathy by 76%, compared with conventional therapy. The progression of retinopathy was decreased by 54% in patients with very mild to moderate nonproliferative retinopathy at the time of initiation of treatment. Similarly, the UKPDS study demonstrated that better control of blood glucose levels in patients with type 2 diabetes led to reduced risk of retinopathy (ADA, 2004s). Other strategies that may slow the progression of diabetic retinopathy include the following:

- Control of hypertension
- Control of blood glucose
- Cessation of smoking

For advanced cases of diabetic retinopathy, the main treatment is argon laser photocoagulation. The laser treatment destroys leaking blood vessels and areas of neovascularization. For patients who are at increased risk for hemorrhage, panretinal photocoagulation may significantly reduce the rate of progression to blindness. Panretinal photocoagulation involves the systematic application of multiple (more than 1000) laser burns throughout the retina (except in the macular region). This stops the widespread growth of new vessels and hemorrhaging of damaged vessels. The role of "mild" panretinal photocoagulation (with

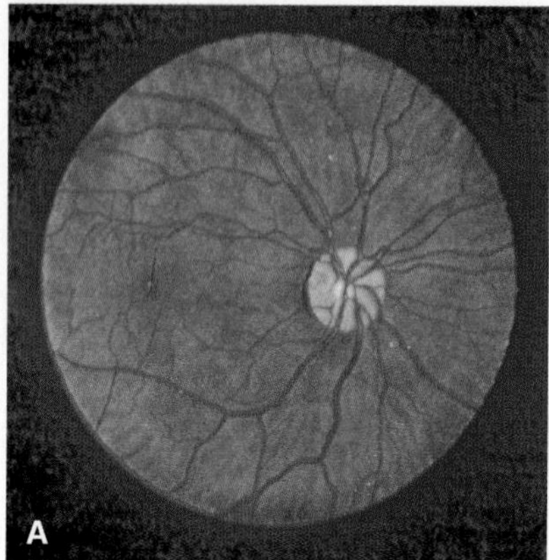

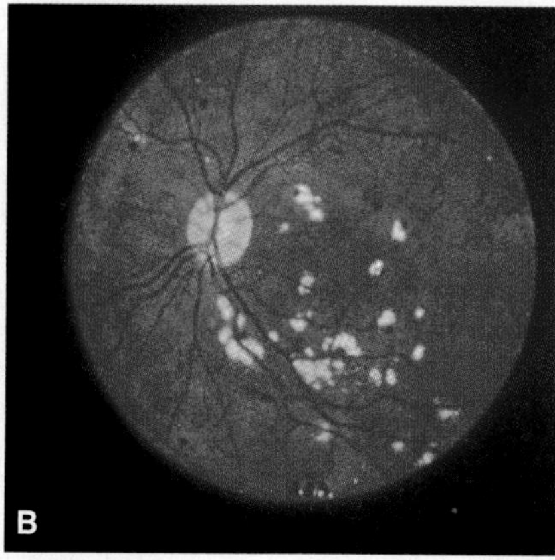

FIGURE 41-10. Diabetic retinopathy. (**A**) In the fundus photograph of a normal eye, the light circular area over which a number of blood vessels converge is the optic disc, where the optic nerve meets the back of the eye. (**B**) The fundus photograph of a patient with diabetic retinopathy shows characteristic waxy-looking retinal lesions, microaneurysms of the vessels, and hemorrhages. Courtesy of American Optometric Association.

only one-third to one-half as many laser burns) in the early stages of proliferative retinopathy or in patients with preproliferative changes is being investigated. For patients with macular edema, focal photocoagulation is used to apply smaller laser burns to specific areas of microaneurysms in the macular region. This may reduce the rate of visual loss from macular edema by 50% (ADA, 2004s).

Photocoagulation treatments are usually performed on an outpatient basis, and most patients can return to their usual activities by the next day. For some patients, limitations may be placed on activities involving weight bearing or bearing down. In most cases, the treatment does not cause intense pain, although patients may report varying degrees of discomfort. Usually an anesthetic eye drop is all that is needed during the treatment. A few patients may experience slight visual loss, loss of peripheral vision, or impairments in adaptation to the dark. However, for most patients, the risk of slight visual changes from the laser treatment itself is much less than the potential for loss of vision from progression of retinopathy.

A major hemorrhage into the vitreous may occur, with the vitreous fluid becoming mixed with blood, preventing light from passing through the eye; this can cause blindness. A vitrectomy is a surgical procedure in which vitreous humor filled with blood or fibrous tissue is removed with a special drill-like instrument and replaced with saline or another liquid. A vitrectomy is performed for patients who already have visual loss and in whom the vitreous hemorrhage has not cleared on its own after 6 months. The purpose is to restore useful vision; recovery to near-normal vision is not usually expected.

Nursing Management

Nursing management of patients with diabetic retinopathy or other eye disorders involves implementing the individual plan of care and providing patient education. Education focuses on prevention through regular ophthalmologic examinations and blood glucose control and self-management of eye care regimens. The effectiveness of early diagnosis and prompt treatment is emphasized in teaching the patient and family. If vision loss occurs, nursing care must also address the patient's adjustment to impaired vision and use of adaptive devices for diabetes self-care as well as activities of daily living. Nursing care for patients with low vision or loss of vision is discussed in detail in Chapter 58.

PROMOTING HOME AND COMMUNITY-BASED CARE

Teaching Patients Self-Care. In all forms of therapy for retinopathy, something is destroyed in the process of saving vision, and the facts must be presented to the patient and family as honestly as possible. The course of the retinopathy may be long and stressful. In teaching and counseling patients, it is important to stress the following:

- Retinopathy may appear after many years of diabetes, and its appearance does not necessarily mean that the diabetes is on a downhill course.
- The odds for maintaining vision are in the patient's favor, especially with adequate control of glucose levels and blood pressure.
- Frequent eye examinations are the best way to preserve vision, because they allow for the detection and prompt treatment of retinopathy.

Some additional points for the nurse to keep in mind when a patient with diabetes has some type of visual impairment include the following:

- Visual impairment can be a shock. A patient's response to vision loss depends on personality, self-concept, and coping mechanisms.
- As in any loss, acceptance of blindness occurs in stages; some patients may learn to accept blindness in a rather short period, and others may never do so.
- Although retinopathy occurs bilaterally, the severity may differ in the two eyes.
- Many of the chronic complications of diabetes occur simultaneously. For example, a patient who is blind due to diabetic retinopathy may also have peripheral neuropathy and may experience impairment of manual dexterity and tactile sensation.

The need for glycemic control persists despite diabetic retinopathy, to prevent other complications.

Continuing Care. Continuing care for a patient with impaired vision due to diabetic changes depends on the severity of the impairment and the effectiveness of the patient's coping in response to the impairment. The importance of careful diabetes management is emphasized as one means of slowing the progression of visual changes. The patient is reminded of the need to see an ophthalmologist regularly. If eye changes are progressive and unrelenting, the patient should be prepared for inevitable blindness. Therefore, consideration is given to making referrals for teaching the patient Braille and for training him or her with guide (ie, service) dogs. Referral to state agencies should be made to ensure that the patient receives services for the blind. Family members are also taught how to assist the patient to remain as independent as possible despite decreasing visual acuity.

Referral for home care may be indicated for some patients, particularly those who live alone, those who are not coping well, and those who have other health problems or complications of diabetes that may interfere with their ability to perform self-care. During home visits, the nurse can assess the patient's home environment and his or her ability to manage diabetes despite visual impairments. Medical management and nursing care of patients with visual disturbances are discussed in detail in Chapter 58.

Nephropathy

Nephropathy, or renal disease secondary to diabetic microvascular changes in the kidney, is a common complication of diabetes. In the United States each year, people with diabetes account for almost 50% of new cases of end-stage renal disease (ESRD) and about 25% of those requiring dialysis or transplantation. About 20% to 30% of people with type 1 or type 2 diabetes develop nephropathy, but fewer of those with type 2 diabetes progress to ESRD. Native American, Hispanic, and African American people with type 2 diabetes are at greater risk for ESRD than non-Hispanic whites (ADA, 2004l).

Patients with type 1 diabetes frequently show initial signs of renal disease after 10 to 15 years, whereas patients with type 2 diabetes develop renal disease within 10 years after the diagnosis of diabetes. Many patients with type 2 diabetes have had diabetes for many years before the diabetes is diagnosed and treated. Therefore, they may have evidence of nephropathy at the time of diagnosis.

If blood glucose levels are elevated consistently for a significant period of time, the kidney's filtration mechanism is stressed, allowing blood proteins to leak into the urine. As a result, the pressure in the blood vessels of the kidney increases. It is thought that this elevated pressure serves as the stimulus for the development of nephropathy. Various medications and diets are being tested to prevent these complications.

The DCCT results showed that intensive treatment of type 1 diabetes with a goal of achieving a hemoglobin A_{1C} level as close to the nondiabetic range as possible reduced the occurrence of early signs of nephropathy, such as microalbuminuria by 39% and albuminuria by 54%. Similarly, the UKPDS study demonstrated a reduced incidence of overt nephropathy in patients with type 2 diabetes who controlled their blood glucose levels (ADA, 2004l).

Clinical Manifestations

Most of the signs and symptoms of renal dysfunction in patients with diabetes are similar to those seen in patients without diabetes (see Chapter 44). In addition, as renal failure progresses, the catabolism (breakdown) of both exogenous and endogenous insulin decreases, and frequent hypoglycemic episodes may result. Insulin needs change as a result of changes in the catabolism of insulin, changes in diet related to the treatment of nephropathy, and changes in insulin clearance that occur with decreased renal function. The stress of renal disease affects self-esteem, family relationships, marital relations, and virtually all aspects of daily life. As renal function decreases, patients commonly have multiple-system failure (eg, declining visual acuity, impotence, foot ulcerations, heart failure, nocturnal diarrhea).

Assessment and Diagnostic Findings

Albumin is one of the most important blood proteins that leaks into the urine. Although small amounts may leak undetected for years, its leakage into the urine is among the earliest signs that can be detected. Clinical nephropathy eventually develops in more than 85% of people with microalbuminuria, but in fewer than 5% of people without microalbuminuria. The urine should be checked annually for the presence of microalbumin. If the microalbuminuria exceeds 30 mg/24 hours on two consecutive random urine tests, a 24-hour urine sample should be obtained and tested. If results are positive, treatment is indicated (see later discussion).

In addition to the urine test for microalbuminuria, tests for serum creatinine and BUN levels should be conducted annually. Diagnostic testing for cardiac or other systemic disorders may also be required with progression of other complications, and caution is indicated if contrast agents are used with these tests. Contrast agents and dyes used for some diagnostic tests may not be easily cleared by the damaged kidney, and the potential benefits of these diagnostic tests must be weighed against their potential risks.

Hypertension often develops in patients (with and without diabetes) who are in the early stages of renal disease. However, essential hypertension occurs in as many as 50% of all people with diabetes (for unknown reasons). Therefore, this symptom may or may not be due to renal disease; other diagnostic criteria must also be present.

Medical Management

In addition to achieving and maintaining near-normal blood glucose levels, management for all patients with diabetes should include careful attention to the following:

- Control of hypertension (the use of angiotensin-converting enzyme [ACE] inhibitors, such as captopril), because control of hypertension may also decrease or delay the onset of early proteinuria
- Prevention or vigorous treatment of urinary tract infections
- Avoidance of nephrotoxic substances (eg, antibiotics, other selected medications)
- Adjustment of medications as renal function changes
- Low-sodium diet
- Low-protein diet

If the patient has already developed microalbuminuria and its level exceeds 30 mg/24 hours on two consecutive tests, an ACE inhibitor should be prescribed. ACE inhibitors lower blood pressure and reduce microalbuminuria, thereby protecting the kidney. Alternatively, angiotensin-receptor blocking (ARB) agents may be prescribed. This preventive strategy should be part of the standard of care for all people with diabetes. Carefully designed low-protein diets also appear to reverse early leakage of small amounts of protein from the kidney.

In chronic or end-stage renal failure, two types of treatment are available: dialysis (hemodialysis or peritoneal dialysis) and transplantation from a relative or a cadaver. Hemodialysis for patients with diabetes is similar to that for patients without the disease (see Chapter 44). Because hemodialysis creates additional stress on patients with cardiovascular disease, it may not be appropriate for certain patients. In addition, it is extremely intrusive in the patient's life.

Continuous ambulatory peritoneal dialysis is being used by an increasing number of patients with diabetes, mainly because of the independence it allows. In addition, insulin can be mixed into the dialysate, which may result in better blood glucose control and end the need for insulin injections. However, these patients may require higher doses of insulin, because the dialysate contains glucose. Major risks of peritoneal dialysis are infection and peritonitis. The mortality rate for patients with diabetes undergoing dialysis is higher than that for patients without diabetes undergoing dialysis and is closely related to the severity of cardiovascular problems.

Renal disease is frequently accompanied by advancing retinopathy that may require laser treatments and surgery. Severe hypertension also worsens eye disease because of the additional stress it places on the blood vessels. Patients being treated with hemodialysis who require eye surgery may be changed to peritoneal dialysis and have their hypertension aggressively controlled for several weeks before surgery to prevent bleeding and damage to the retina. The rationale for this change is that hemodialysis requires anticoagulants that can increase the risk of bleeding after the surgery, and peritoneal dialysis minimizes pressure changes in the eyes.

The success rate for kidney transplantation in patients with diabetes has improved. In medical centers performing large numbers of transplantations, the chances are 75% to 80% that the transplanted kidney will continue to function in patients with diabetes for at least 5 years. Like the original kidneys, transplanted kidneys can eventually be damaged if blood glucose levels are consistently high after the transplantation. Therefore, monitoring blood glucose levels frequently and adjusting insulin levels in patients with diabetes is essential for long-term success of kidney transplantation.

Pancreas transplantation is sometimes attempted when kidney transplantation is performed in patients with diabetes, but it has not been successful enough to be performed alone because of the risks associated with immunosuppression.

Diabetic Neuropathies

Diabetic neuropathy refers to a group of diseases that affect all types of nerves, including peripheral (sensorimotor), autonomic, and spinal nerves. The disorders appear to be clinically diverse and depend on the location of the affected nerve cells. The prevalence increases with the age of the patient and the duration of the disease and may be as high as 50% in patients who have had diabetes for 25 years.

The etiology of neuropathy may involve elevated blood glucose levels over a period of years. The DCCT results showed that control of blood glucose levels to normal or near-normal levels decreased the incidence of neuropathy by 60%. The pathogenesis of neuropathy may be attributed to either a vascular or a metabolic mechanism or both. Capillary basement membrane thickening and capillary closure may be present. In addition, there may be demyelinization of the nerves, which is thought to be related to hyperglycemia. Nerve conduction is disrupted when there are aberrations of the myelin sheaths.

The two most common types of diabetic neuropathy are sensorimotor polyneuropathy and autonomic neuropathy. Sensorimotor polyneuropathy is also called peripheral neuropathy. It most commonly affects the distal portions of the nerves, especially the nerves of the lower extremities; it affects both sides of the body symmetrically and may spread in a proximal direction. Cranial mononeuropathies—those affecting the oculomotor nerve—also occur in diabetes, especially in the elderly.

Peripheral Neuropathy

CLINICAL MANIFESTATIONS

Although approximately half of patients with diabetic neuropathy do not have symptoms, initial symptoms may include paresthesias (prickling, tingling, or heightened sensation) and burning sensations (especially at night). As the neuropathy progresses, the feet become numb. In addition, a decrease in proprioception (awareness of posture and movement of the body and of position and weight of objects in relation to the body) and a decreased sensation of light touch may lead to an unsteady gait. Decreased sensations of pain and temperature place patients with neuropathy at increased risk for injury and undetected foot infections. Deformities of the foot may also occur; neuropathy-related joint changes produce Charcot joints. These joint deformities result from the abnormal weight distribution on joints resulting from lack of proprioception.

On physical examination, a decrease in deep tendon reflexes and vibratory sensation is found. For patients who have few or no symptoms of neuropathy, these physical findings may be the only indication of neuropathic changes. For patients with signs or symptoms of neuropathy, it is important to rule out other possible causes, including alcohol-induced and vitamin-deficiency neuropathies.

MANAGEMENT

The results of the DCCT study demonstrated that intensive insulin therapy and control of blood glucose levels delay the onset and slow the progression of neuropathy. Pain, particularly of the lower extremities, is a disturbing symptom in some people with neuropathy secondary to diabetes. For some patients, neuropathic pain spontaneously resolves within 6 months; for others, pain persists for many years. Various approaches to pain management can be tried. These include analgesics (preferably nonopioid); tricyclic antidepressants; phenytoin, carbamazepine, or gabapentin (antiseizure medications); mexiletine (an antiarrhythmic); and transcutaneous electrical nerve stimulation (TENS).

Duloxetine (Cymbalta), an antidepressant medication, has been approved for treatment of peripheral diabetic neuropathy.

Autonomic Neuropathies

Neuropathy of the autonomic nervous system results in a broad range of dysfunctions affecting almost every organ system of the body. Three manifestations of autonomic neuropathy are related to the cardiac, gastrointestinal, and renal systems. Cardiovascular symptoms range from a fixed, slightly tachycardic heart rate and orthostatic hypotension to silent, or painless, myocardial ischemia and infarction. Delayed gastric emptying may occur with the typical gastrointestinal symptoms of early satiety, bloating, nausea, and vomiting. "Diabetic" constipation or diarrhea (especially nocturnal diarrhea) may occur as a result. In addition, there may be unexplained wide swings in blood glucose levels related to inconsistent absorption of the glucose from ingested foods secondary to the inconsistent gastric emptying.

Urinary retention, a decreased sensation of bladder fullness, and other urinary symptoms of neurogenic bladder result from autonomic neuropathy. The patient with a neurogenic bladder is predisposed to development of urinary tract infections because of the inability to empty the bladder completely. This is especially true of patients with poorly controlled diabetes, because hyperglycemia impairs resistance to infection. Erectile dysfunction (ED, impotence) is another complication and is primarily caused by autonomic neuropathy.

HYPOGLYCEMIC UNAWARENESS

Autonomic neuropathy that affects the adrenal medulla is responsible for diminished or absent adrenergic symptoms of hypoglycemia. Patients may report that they no longer feel the typical shakiness, sweating, nervousness, and palpitations associated with hypoglycemia. Frequent blood glucose monitoring is recommended for these patients. Their inability to detect and treat these warning signs of hypoglycemia puts them at risk for development of dangerously low blood glucose levels. Therefore, their goals for blood glucose levels may need to be adjusted to reduce the risk for hypoglycemia. Patients and families need to be taught to recognize subtle and atypical symptoms of hypoglycemia, such as numbness around the mouth and impaired ability to concentrate (Tkacs, 2002).

SUDOMOTOR NEUROPATHY

The neuropathic condition called sudomotor neuropathy refers to a decrease or absence of sweating (anhidrosis) of the extremities, with a compensatory increase in upper body sweating. Dryness of the feet increases the risk for the development of foot ulcers.

SEXUAL DYSFUNCTION

Sexual dysfunction, especially ED in men, is a complication of diabetes. The effects of autonomic neuropathy on female sexual functioning are not well documented. Reduced vaginal lubrication has been mentioned as a possible neuropathic effect. Other possible changes in sexual function in women with diabetes include decreased libido and lack of orgasm. Vaginal infection, which increases in incidence in women with diabetes, may be associated with decreased lubrication and vaginal pruritus (itching) and tenderness. Urinary tract infections and vaginitis may also affect sexual function (Enzlin, 2002).

Impotence (inability of the penis to become rigid and sustain an erection adequate for penetration) occurs with greater frequency in men with diabetes than in other men of the same age. However, diabetic neuropathy is not the only cause of impotence in men with diabetes. Medications such as antihypertensive agents, psychological factors, and other medical conditions (eg, vascular insufficiency) that may affect other men also play a role in impotence in men with diabetes.

Some men with autonomic neuropathy have normal erectile function and can experience orgasm but do not ejaculate normally. Retrograde ejaculation occurs; seminal fluid is propelled backward through the posterior urethra and into the urinary bladder. Examination of the urine confirms the diagnosis because of the large number of active sperm present. Fertility counseling may be necessary for couples attempting conception.

MANAGEMENT

Management strategies depend on symptoms and focus also on modification and management of risk factors. The prognosis for painless cardiac ischemia is poor. However, detection is important, so that education about avoiding strenuous exercise can be provided. Orthostatic hypotension may respond to a diet high in sodium, discontinuation of medications that impede autonomic nervous system responses, use of sympathomimetics and other agents (eg, caffeine) that stimulate an autonomic response, mineralocorticoid therapy, and use of lower-body elastic garments that maximize venous return and prevent pooling of blood in the extremities.

Treatment of delayed gastric emptying includes a low-fat diet, frequent small meals, close blood glucose monitoring, and use of agents that increase gastric motility (eg, metoclopramide, bethanechol). Treatment of diabetic diarrhea may include bulk-forming laxatives or antidiarrheal agents. Constipation is treated with a high-fiber diet and adequate hydration; medications, laxatives, and enemas may be necessary if constipation is severe. Management of neurogenic bladder is discussed in Chapter 44.

Treatment of sudomotor dysfunction focuses on education about skin care and heat intolerance. ED is discussed in Chapter 49.

Foot and Leg Problems

Between 50% and 75% of lower extremity amputations are performed on people with diabetes. More than 50% of these amputations are thought to be preventable, provided patients are taught foot care measures and practice them on a daily basis (ADA, 2004q). Complications of diabetes that contribute to the increased risk of foot problems and infections include the following:

- Neuropathy—Sensory neuropathy leads to loss of pain and pressure sensation, and autonomic neuropathy leads to increased dryness and fissuring of the skin (secondary to decreased sweating). Motor neuropathy results in muscular atrophy, which may lead to changes in the shape of the foot.

- Peripheral vascular disease—Poor circulation of the lower extremities contributes to poor wound healing and the development of gangrene.
- Immunocompromise—Hyperglycemia impairs the ability of specialized leukocytes to destroy bacteria. Therefore, in poorly controlled diabetes, there is a lowered resistance to certain infections.

The typical sequence of events in the development of a diabetic foot ulcer begins with a soft tissue injury of the foot, formation of a fissure between the toes or in an area of dry skin, or formation of a callus (Fig. 41-11). Patients with an insensitive foot do not feel injuries, which may be thermal (eg, from using heating pads, walking barefoot on hot concrete, testing bath water with the foot), chemical (eg, burning the foot while using caustic agents on calluses, corns, or bunions), or traumatic (eg, injuring skin while cutting nails, walking with an undetected foreign object in the shoe, or wearing ill-fitting shoes and socks).

If the patient is not in the habit of thoroughly inspecting both feet on a daily basis, the injury or fissure may go unnoticed until a serious infection has developed. Drainage, swelling, redness of the leg (from cellulitis), or gangrene may be the first sign of foot problems that the patient notices. Treatment of foot ulcers involves bed rest, antibiotics, and débridement. In addition, controlling glucose levels, which tend to increase when infections occur, is important for promoting wound healing. In patients with peripheral vascular disease, foot ulcers may not heal because of the decreased ability of oxygen, nutrients, and antibiotics to reach the injured tissue. Amputation may be necessary to prevent the spread of infection.

Foot assessment and foot care instructions are most important when caring for patients who are at high risk for foot infections. Some of the high-risk characteristics include

- Duration of diabetes more than 10 years
- Age older than 40 years
- History of smoking
- Decreased peripheral pulses
- Decreased sensation
- Anatomic deformities or pressure areas (eg, bunions, calluses, hammer toes)
- History of previous foot ulcers or amputation

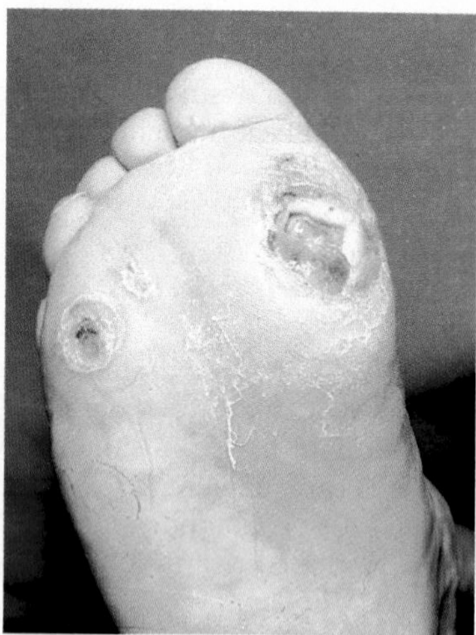

FIGURE 41-11. Neuropathic ulcers occur on pressure points in areas with diminished sensation in diabetic polyneuropathy. Because pain is absent, the ulcer may go unnoticed.

Management

Teaching patients proper foot care (see Chart 41-10) is a nursing intervention that can prevent costly and painful complications that result in disability. Preventive foot care begins with careful daily assessment of the feet. The feet must be inspected on a daily basis for any redness, blisters, fissures, calluses, ulcerations, changes in skin temperature, or development of foot deformities (hammer toes, bunions). For patients with visual impairment or decreased joint mobility (especially the elderly), use of a mirror to inspect the bottoms of both feet or the help of a family member in foot inspection may be necessary. The interior surfaces of shoes should also be inspected for any rough spots or foreign objects.

In addition to the daily visual and manual inspection of the feet, the feet should be examined during every health care visit or at least once per year (more often if there is an increase in risk) by a podiatrist, physician, or nurse (ADA, 2004q). Patients with neuropathy should also undergo evaluation of neurologic status by an experienced examiner using a monofilament device (Fig. 41-12). Patients with pressure areas, such as calluses, or thick toenails should see a podiatrist routinely for treatment of calluses and trimming of nails.

Additional aspects of preventive foot care that are taught to patients and families include the following:

- Properly bathing, drying, and lubricating the feet, taking care not to allow moisture (water or lotion) to accumulate between the toes
- Wearing closed-toe shoes that fit well. A podiatrist can provide the patient with inserts (orthotics) to remove pressure from pressure points on the foot. New shoes should be broken in slowly (ie, worn for 1 to 2 hours initially, with gradual increases in the length of time worn) to avoid blister formation. Patients with bony deformities may need shoes with extra width or depth. High-risk behaviors, such as walking barefoot, using heating pads on the feet, wearing open-toed shoes, soaking the feet, and shaving calluses, should be avoided.
- Trimming toenails straight across and filing sharp corners to follow the contour of the toe (AADE, 2004). If the patient has visual deficits, is unable to reach the feet because of disability, or has thickened toenails, a podiatrist should cut the nails.
- Reducing risk factors, such as smoking and elevated blood lipids, that contribute to peripheral vascular disease
- Avoiding home remedies, over-the-counter agents, and self-medicating to treat foot problems (ADA, 2004q)

Blood glucose control is important for avoiding decreased resistance to infections and for preventing diabetic neuropathy. The patient may be referred by the physician to a wound care center for management of persistent wounds of the feet or legs. Many wound care centers provide diabetes educa-

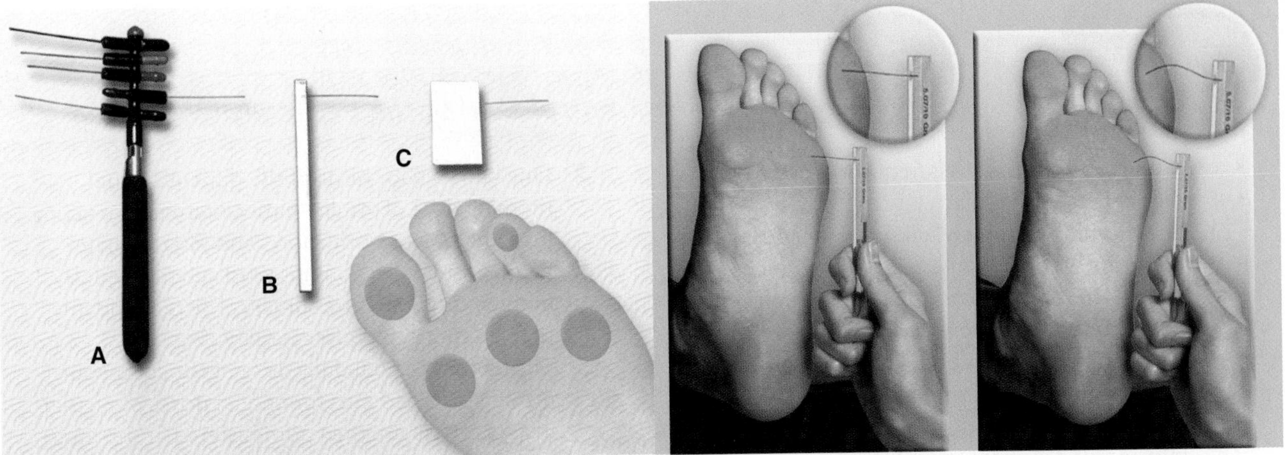

FIGURE 41-12. The monofilament test is used to assess the sensory threshold in patients with diabetes. The test instrument—a monofilament—is gently applied to about five pressure points on the foot (as shown in image on *left*). (**A**) Example of a monofilament used for advanced quantitative assessment. (**B**) Semmes-Weinstein monofilament used by clinicians. (**C**) Disposable monofilament used by patients. The examiner applies the monofilament to the test area to determine whether the patient feels the device. Adapted with permission from Cameron, B. L. (2002). Making diabetes management routine. *American Journal of Nursing, 102*(2), 26–32.

tion; however, the patient should discuss recommendations for treating wounds with his or her own physician, as well as any related issues about diabetes management.

Special Issues in Diabetes Care

Patients With Diabetes Who Are Undergoing Surgery

During periods of physiologic stress, such as surgery, blood glucose levels tend to increase, because levels of stress hormones (epinephrine, norepinephrine, glucagon, cortisol, and growth hormone) increase. If hyperglycemia is not controlled during surgery, the resulting osmotic diuresis may lead to excessive loss of fluids and electrolytes. Patients with type 1 diabetes also risk developing ketoacidosis during periods of stress.

Hypoglycemia is also a concern in patients with diabetes who are undergoing surgery. For example, this is a special concern during the preoperative period if surgery is delayed beyond the morning in a patient who received a morning injection of intermediate-acting insulin.

There are various approaches to managing glucose control during the perioperative period. Frequent blood glucose monitoring is essential throughout the preoperative and postoperative periods, regardless of the method used for glucose control. Examples of these approaches are described in Chart 41-12. The use of IV insulin and dextrose has become widespread with the increased availability of meters for intraoperative glucose monitoring.

During the postoperative period, patients with diabetes must also be closely monitored for cardiovascular complications because of the increased prevalence of atherosclerosis, wound infections, and skin breakdown (especially in patients with decreased sensation in the extremities due to neuropathy). Maintaining adequate nutrition and blood glucose control promotes wound healing.

Management of Hospitalized Patients With Diabetes

At any one time, 10% to 20% of hospitalized general medical-surgical patients have diabetes. This number may increase as elderly patients make up an increasing proportion of the hospitalized population. Although some hospitals have a specialized diabetic/metabolic unit, typically patients with diabetes are admitted throughout the hospital.

Often diabetes is not the primary medical diagnosis, yet problems with control of diabetes frequently result from changes in the patient's normal routine or from surgery or illness. Some of the main issues pertinent to nursing care of hospitalized patients with diabetes are presented in the following sections.

Self-Care Issues

All patients admitted to the hospital must relinquish control of some aspects of their daily care to the hospital staff. For patients with diabetes who are actively involved in diabetes self-management (especially insulin dose adjustment), relinquishing control over meal timing, insulin timing, and insulin dosage can be particularly difficult. The patient may fear hypoglycemia and express much concern over possible delays in receiving attention from the nurse if hypoglycemic symptoms occur.

It is important for the nurse to acknowledge the patient's concerns and involve the patient in the plan of care as much as possible. If the patient disagrees with certain aspects of the nursing or medical care related to diabetes, the nurse must communicate this to other members of the health care team and, where appropriate, make changes in the plan to

CHART 41-12

Approaches to Management of Glucose Control During the Perioperative Period

- Monitor blood glucose levels frequently (every 1 to 2 h).
- For patients taking insulin
  1. The morning of surgery, all subcutaneous insulin doses are withheld, unless the blood glucose level is elevated (eg, >200 mg/dL [11.1 mmol/L]), in which case a small dose of subcutaneous regular insulin may be prescribed. The blood glucose level is controlled during surgery with the IV infusion of regular insulin, which is balanced by an infusion of dextrose. The insulin and dextrose infusion rates are adjusted according to frequent (hourly) capillary glucose determinations. After surgery, the insulin infusion may be continued until the patient can eat. If IV insulin is discontinued, subcutaneous regular insulin may be administered at set intervals (every 4–6 h), or intermediate-acting insulin may be administered every 12 h with supplemental regular insulin as necessary until the patient is eating and the usual pattern of insulin dosing is resumed.
     - Carefully monitor the insulin infusion rate and blood glucose levels in a patient with diabetes who is receiving IV insulin. IV insulin has a much shorter duration of action than subcutaneous insulin. If the infusion is interrupted or discontinued, hyperglycemia will develop rapidly (within 1 h in type 1 diabetes and within a few hours in type 2 diabetes).
     - Ensure that subcutaneous insulin is administered 30 min before the IV insulin infusion is discontinued.
  2. One half to two thirds of the patient's usual morning dose of insulin (either intermediate-acting insulin alone or both short- and intermediate-acting insulins) is administered subcutaneously in the morning before surgery. The remainder is then administered after surgery.
  3. The patient's usual daily dose of subcutaneous insulin is divided into four equal doses of regular insulin. These are then administered at 6-h intervals. The last two approaches do not provide the control achieved by IV administration of insulin and dextrose.
- Patients with type 2 diabetes who do not usually take insulin may require insulin during the perioperative period to control blood glucose elevations. Patients who are taking metformin may be instructed to discontinue the oral agent 24 to 48 h before surgery, if possible. Some of these patients may resume their usual regimen of diet and oral agent during the recovery period. Other patients (whose diabetes is probably not well controlled with diet and an oral antidiabetic agent before surgery) need to continue with insulin injections after discharge.
- For patients with type 2 diabetes who are undergoing minor surgery but who do not normally take insulin, glucose levels may remain stable provided no dextrose is infused during the surgery. After surgery, these patients may require small doses of regular insulin until the usual diet and oral agent are resumed.

meet the patient's needs. Nurses and other health care providers must pay particular attention to patients who are successful in managing self-care; they should assess these patients' self-care management skills and encourage them to continue if their performance is correct and effective.

Hyperglycemia During Hospitalization

Hyperglycemia may occur in hospitalized patients as a result of the original illness that led to the need for hospitalization. In addition, a number of other factors may contribute to hyperglycemia; examples include

- Changes in the usual treatment regimen (eg, increased food, decreased insulin, decreased activity)
- Medications (eg, corticosteroids such as prednisone, which are used in the treatment of a variety of inflammatory disorders)
- IV dextrose, which may be part of the maintenance fluids or may be used for the administration of antibiotics and other medications, without adequate insulin therapy
- Overly vigorous treatment of hypoglycemia
- Inappropriate withholding of insulin or inappropriate use of "sliding scales"
- Mismatched timing of meals and insulin (eg, postmeal hyperglycemia may occur if short-acting insulin is administered immediately before or even after a meal)

Nursing actions to correct some of these factors are important for avoiding hyperglycemia. Assessment of the patient's usual home routine is important. The nurse should try to approximate as much as possible the home schedule of insulin, meals, and activities. Monitoring blood glucose levels has been identified by the ADA as an additional "vital sign" essential in assessment of patients (ADA, 2004b). The results of blood glucose monitoring provide information needed to obtain orders for extra doses of insulin (at times when insulin is usually taken), an important nursing function. Insulin doses must not be withheld when blood glucose levels are normal.

Short-acting insulin is usually needed to avoid postprandial hyperglycemia (even in patients with normal premeal glucose levels), and NPH insulin does not peak until many hours after the dose is given. IV antibiotics should be mixed in normal saline (if possible) to avoid excess infusion of dextrose (especially in patients who are eating). It is important to avoid overly vigorous treatment of hypoglycemia, which may lead to hyperglycemia. Treatment of hypoglycemia should be based on the established hospital protocol (usually 15 g carbohydrate in the form of juice, glucose tablets, or, if necessary, 0.5 to 1 ampule of 50% dextrose by IV). Extra sugar should not be added to the juice. If the initial treatment does not increase the glucose level adequately, the same treatment may be repeated after 15 minutes.

Hypoglycemia During Hospitalization

Hypoglycemia in hospitalized patients is usually the result of too much insulin or delays in eating. Specific examples include

- Overuse of "sliding scale" regular insulin, particularly as a supplement to regularly scheduled, twice-daily short- and intermediate-acting insulins
- Lack of change in insulin dosage when dietary intake is changed (eg, in the patient taking nothing by mouth [NPO])
- Overly vigorous treatment of hyperglycemia (eg, giving too-frequent successive doses of regular insulin before the time of peak insulin activity is reached) so that there is a cumulative effect
- Delayed meal after administration of lispro or aspart insulin (the patient should eat within 5 to 15 minutes after insulin administration)

The nurse must assess the pattern of glucose values and avoid giving doses of insulin that repeatedly lead to hypoglycemia. Successive doses of subcutaneous regular insulin should be administered no more frequently than every 3 to 4 hours. For patients receiving NPH or Lente insulin before breakfast and dinner, the nurse must use caution in administering supplemental doses of regular insulin at lunch and bedtime. Hypoglycemia may occur when two insulins peak at similar times (eg, morning NPH peaks with lunchtime regular insulin and may lead to late-afternoon hypoglycemia, dinnertime NPH peaks with bedtime regular insulin and may lead to nocturnal hypoglycemia). To avoid hypoglycemic reactions caused by delayed food intake, the nurse should arrange for snacks to be given to the patient if meals are going to be delayed because of procedures, physical therapy, or other activities.

Common Alterations in Diet

Dietary modifications commonly prescribed during hospitalization require special consideration for patients who have diabetes.

NOTHING BY MOUTH

For patients with diabetes who must be NPO in preparation for diagnostic or surgical procedures, the nurse must ensure that the usual insulin dosage has been changed. These changes may include eliminating the rapid-acting insulin and giving a decreased amount (eg, half the usual dose) of intermediate-acting NPH or Lente insulin. Another approach is to use frequent (every 3 to 4 hours) dosing of rapid-acting insulin only. IV dextrose may be administered to provide calories and to avoid hypoglycemia.

Even without food, glucose levels may increase as a result of hepatic glucose production, especially in patients with type 1 diabetes and lean patients with type 2 diabetes. Furthermore, in type 1 diabetes, elimination of the insulin dose may lead to the development of DKA. Therefore, administration of insulin to patients with type 1 diabetes who are NPO is an important nursing action.

For patients with type 2 diabetes who are taking insulin, DKA does not usually develop when insulin doses are eliminated because the patient's pancreas produces some insulin. Therefore, skipping the insulin dose altogether (when the patient is receiving IV dextrose) may be safe; however, close monitoring of blood glucose levels is essential.

For patients who are NPO for extended periods (24 hours), glucose testing and insulin administration should be performed at regular intervals, usually four times per day. Insulin regimens for the patient who is NPO for an extended period may include NPH insulin every 12 hours (with rapid-acting insulin added to the NPH, depending on the results of glucose testing) or rapid-acting insulin only every 4 to 6 hours. These patients should receive dextrose infusions to provide some calories and limit ketosis.

To prevent the problems that result from the need to withhold food, diagnostic tests and procedures and surgery should be scheduled early in the morning if possible.

CLEAR LIQUID DIET

When the diet is advanced to include clear liquids, patients with diabetes receive more simple carbohydrate foods, such as juice and gelatin desserts, than are usually included in the diabetic diet. It is important for hospitalized patients to maintain their nutritional status as much as possible to promote healing. Therefore, the use of reduced-calorie substitutes such as diet soda or diet gelatin desserts would not be appropriate when the only source of calories is clear liquids. Simple carbohydrates, if eaten alone, cause a rapid rise in blood glucose levels; therefore, it is important to try to match peak times of insulin effect with peaks in the blood glucose concentration. If the patient receives insulin at regular intervals while NPO, the scheduled times for glucose tests and insulin injections must match meal times.

ENTERAL TUBE FEEDINGS

Tube feeding formulas contain more simple carbohydrates and less protein and fat than the typical meal plan for diabetes. This results in increased levels of glucose in patients with diabetes who are receiving tube feedings. It is important that insulin doses be administered at regular intervals (eg, NPH every 12 hours or regular insulin every 4 to 6 hours) when continuous tube feedings are administered. If insulin is administered at routine (prebreakfast and predinner) times, hypoglycemia during the day may result (because the patient receives more insulin without more calories); and hyperglycemia may occur during the night if feedings continue but insulin action decreases.

A common cause of hypoglycemia in patients receiving both continuous tube feedings and insulin is inadvertent or purposeful discontinuation of the feeding. The nurse must discuss with the medical team any plans for temporarily discontinuing the tube feeding (eg, when the patient is away from the unit). Planning ahead may allow for alterations to be made in the insulin dose, or for administration of IV dextrose. In addition, if problems with the tube feeding develop unexpectedly (eg, the patient pulls out the tube, the tube clogs, the feeding is discontinued when residual gastric contents are found), the nurse must notify the physician, assess blood glucose levels more frequently, and administer IV dextrose if indicated.

PARENTERAL NUTRITION

Patients with diabetes receiving parenteral nutrition may receive both IV insulin (added to the parenteral nutrition container) and subcutaneous intermediate- or short-acting insulins. If the patient is receiving continuous parenteral nutrition, the blood glucose level should be monitored and insulin administered at regular intervals. If the parenteral nutrition is infused over a limited number of hours, subcutaneous insulin should be administered so that peak times of insulin action coincide with times of parenteral nutrition infusion.

Hygiene

Nurses caring for hospitalized patients with diabetes must focus attention on oral hygiene and skin care. Because these patients are at increased risk for periodontal disease, it is important for the nurse to assist the patient with daily dental care. The patient may also require assistance in keeping the skin clean and dry, especially in areas of contact between two skin surfaces (eg, groin, axilla, under the breasts), where chafing and fungal infections tend to occur.

For patients who are confined to bed, nursing care must emphasize the prevention of skin breakdown at pressure points. The heels are particularly susceptible to breakdown because of loss of sensation of pain and pressure associated with sensory neuropathy.

Feet should be cleaned, dried, lubricated with lotion (but not between the toes), and inspected frequently. If the patient is in the supine position, pressure on the heels can be alleviated by elevating the lower legs on a pillow, with the heels positioned over the edge of the pillow. When the patient is seated in a chair, the feet should be positioned so that pressure is not placed on the heels. If the patient has an ulcer on one foot, it is important to provide preventive care to the unaffected foot as well as special care of the affected foot.

As always, every opportunity should be taken to teach the patient about diabetes self-management, including daily oral, skin, and foot care. Female patients should also be instructed about measures for the avoidance of vaginal infections, which occur more frequently when blood glucose levels are elevated. Patients often take their cues from nurses and realize the importance of daily personal hygiene if this is emphasized during their hospitalization.

Stress

As mentioned earlier, physiologic stress, such as infections and surgery, contributes to hyperglycemia and may precipitate DKA or HHNS. Emotional stress can have a negative impact on diabetic control as well. An increase in stress hormones leads to an increase in glucose levels, especially if intake of food and insulin remains unchanged. In addition, during periods of emotional stress, people with diabetes may alter their usual pattern of meals, exercise, and medication. This can contribute to hyperglycemia or even hypoglycemia (eg, in the patient taking insulin or oral antidiabetic agents who stops eating in response to stress).

People with diabetes must be made aware of the potential deterioration in diabetic control that can accompany emotional stress. They must be encouraged to follow the diabetes treatment plan as much as possible during times of stress. In addition, learning strategies for minimizing stress and coping with stress when it does occur are important aspects of diabetes education. Healthy coping is one of the seven steps to managing diabetes identified by the AADE, 2004.

Gerontologic Considerations

Because people with diabetes are living longer, both type 1 and type 2 diabetes are being seen more frequently in the elderly population. Regardless of the type or duration of diabetes, the goals of diabetes treatment may need to be altered when caring for elderly patients. The focus is on quality-of-life issues, such as maintaining independent functioning and promoting general well-being. Although striving for strict control of blood glucose levels may not be safe or appropriate, prolonged hyperglycemia should be avoided.

Some elderly patients cannot manage a detailed diabetes treatment plan, but nurses must not assume that all patients older than a certain age can adhere to only the simplest regimen. Although the goal may be simply to avoid hypoglycemia and symptomatic hyperglycemia, certain patients may prefer more complex regimens that allow more flexibility in meals and daily schedule. As with all people with diabetes, individualization of the treatment plan with frequent follow-up by the health care team is important.

Some of the barriers to learning and self-care that may be seen in the elderly include decreased vision, hearing loss, memory deficits, decreased mobility and fine motor coordination, increased tremors, depression and isolation, decreased financial resources, and limitations related to disabilities and other medical disorders. Assessing patients for these barriers as well as discussing any misconceptions or folk beliefs regarding the cause and treatment of diabetes is important in planning diabetes treatment and educational activities. Presenting brief, simplified instructions with ample opportunity for practice of skills is important. The use of special devices such as a magnifier for the insulin syringe, an insulin pen, or a mirror for foot inspection is helpful. Frequent evaluation of self-care skills (insulin administration, blood glucose monitoring, foot care, diet planning) is essential, especially in patients with deteriorating vision and memory.

If appropriate, family members may be called on to assist with diabetes survival skills, and referral to community resources may be made. It is preferable to teach the patient or family members to test blood glucose at home; the choice of meter should be tailored to the patient's visual and cognitive status and dexterity.

Following a meal plan is difficult for some elderly patients because of decreased appetite, poor dentition, and decreased physical and financial ability to prepare meals.

In addition, the elderly patient may be unwilling to change long-standing dietary habits. Altering the meal plan to incorporate these eating habits or other limitations may be necessary.

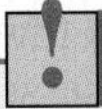

NURSING ALERT

Careful monitoring for diabetes complications must not be neglected in elderly patients. Hypoglycemia is especially dangerous, because it may go undetected and result in falls. Dehydration is a concern in patients who have chronically elevated blood glucose levels. Assessment for long-term complications, especially eye and foot problems, is important. Avoiding blindness and amputation through early detection and treatment of retinopathy and foot ulcers may mean the difference between placement in a long-term facility and continued independent living for the elderly person with diabetes.

Nursing Process

The Patient With Diabetes as a Secondary Diagnosis

Patients with diabetes frequently seek medical attention for problems not directly related to blood glucose control. However, during the course of treatment for the primary medical diagnosis, blood glucose control may worsen. In addition, the only opportunity for some patients with diabetes to update their knowledge about diabetes self-care and prevention of complications may be during hospitalization. Therefore, it is important for nurses caring for patients with diabetes to focus attention on the diabetes as well as the primary health issue. Furthermore, control of blood glucose levels is important, because hyperglycemia impairs resistance to certain infections and impedes wound healing.

Assessment

Assessment of patients with diabetes who have a primary problem such as cardiac disease, renal disease, cerebrovascular disease, peripheral vascular disease, surgery, or any other type of illness is the same as that for all patients and is described in other chapters. In addition to nursing assessment for the primary problem, assessment of the patient with diabetes must also focus on hypoglycemia and hyperglycemia, skin breakdown, and diabetes self-care skills, including survival skills and measures for prevention of long-term complications. In addition, the patient is asked about use of alternative and complementary therapies; studies have demonstrated that patients with diabetes are twice as likely as other patients to use these therapies, some of which may be harmful (Egede, Ye & Zheng, 2002).

Assessment for hypoglycemia and hyperglycemia involves frequent blood glucose monitoring (usually prescribed before meals and at bedtime) and monitoring for signs and symptoms of hypoglycemia or prolonged hyperglycemia (including DKA or HHNS), as described previously.

Careful assessment of the skin, especially at pressure points and on the lower extremities, is important. The skin is assessed for dryness, cracks, skin breakdown, and redness. The patient is asked about symptoms of neuropathy, such as tingling and pain or numbness of the feet. Deep tendon reflexes are assessed.

The nurse should assess the patient's diabetes self-care skills as soon as possible to determine whether further diabetes teaching is required. The nurse observes the patient preparing and injecting the insulin, monitoring blood glucose, and performing foot care. (Simply questioning the patient about these skills without actually observing performance of the skills is not sufficient.) The patient's knowledge about diet can be assessed with the help of a dietitian through direct questioning and review of the patient's menu choices. The patient is asked about signs and symptoms, treatment, and prevention of hypoglycemia and hyperglycemia. The patient's knowledge of risk factors for macrovascular disease, including hypertension, increased lipids, and smoking, is assessed. In addition, the patient is asked the date of his or her last eye examination (including dilation of the pupils). It is also important to assess the patient's use of preventive health measures, including annual influenza vaccination (flu shot), date of the most recent pneumonia vaccination (ADA, 2004k), and daily dose of aspirin (unless contraindicated) (ADA, 2004a).

Diagnosis

Nursing Diagnoses

Based on the assessment data, major nursing diagnoses may include the following:

- Imbalanced nutrition related to increase in stress hormones (caused by primary medical problem) and imbalances in insulin, food, and physical activity
- Risk for impaired skin integrity related to immobility and lack of sensation (caused by neuropathy)
- Deficient knowledge about diabetes self-care skills (caused by lack of basic diabetes education or lack of continuing in-depth diabetes education)

Collaborative Problems/ Potential Complications

Based on the assessment data, potential complications may include the following:

- Inadequate control of blood glucose levels (hyperglycemia, hypoglycemia)
- DKA and HHNS

Planning and Goals

The major goals for the patient may include improved nutritional status, maintenance of skin integrity (foot care), ability to perform basic diabetes self-care skills as well as preventive care for the avoidance of chronic diabetes complications, and absence of complications.

Nursing Interventions

Improving Nutritional Status

The patient's food intake is planned with the primary goal of glucose control; however, the dietary prescription must also consider the primary health problem in addition to lifestyle, cultural background, activity level, and food preferences. If alterations are needed in the patient's diet because of the primary health problem (eg, gastrointestinal problems), alternative strategies to ensure adequate nutritional intake must be implemented. The patient's nutritional intake is monitored carefully along with blood glucose, urine ketones, and daily weight.

Maintaining Skin Care

The skin is assessed daily for dryness or breaks. The feet are cleaned with warm water and soap. Excessive soaking of the feet (eg, to the point of wrinkling the skin) is avoided. The feet are dried thoroughly, especially between the toes, and lotion is applied to the entire foot except between the toes. For patients who are confined to bed (especially those with a history of neuropathy), the heels are elevated off the bed with a pillow placed under the lower legs and the heels resting over the edge of the pillow. A bed cradle may be used to keep the bed covers off the feet of the patient with diabetic neuropathy. Dermal ulcers are treated as indicated and prescribed. The nurse promotes optimal blood glucose control in the patient with skin breakdown.

Addressing Knowledge Deficits

Hospital admission of the patient with diabetes provides an ideal opportunity for the nurse to assess the patient's level of knowledge about diabetes and its management. The nurse uses this opportunity to assess the patient's understanding of diabetes management, including blood glucose monitoring, administration of medications (ie, insulin, oral agents), meal planning, exercise, and strategies to prevent long- and short-term complications of diabetes. The nurse also assesses the adjustment of the patient and family to diabetes and its management and identifies any misconceptions they have.

Monitoring and Managing Potential Complications

Inadequate control of blood glucose levels may hinder recovery from the primary health problem. Blood glucose levels are monitored, and insulin is administered as prescribed. It is important for the nurse to ensure that prescribed insulin dosage is modified as needed to compensate for changes in the patient's schedule or eating pattern. Treatment is given for hypoglycemia (with oral glucose) or hyperglycemia (with supplemental regular insulin no more often than every 3 to 4 hours). Blood glucose records are assessed for patterns of hypoglycemia and hyperglycemia at the same time of day, and findings are reported to the physician for modification in insulin orders. In the patient with prolonged elevations in blood glucose, laboratory values and the patient's physical condition are monitored for signs and symptoms of DKA or HHNS.

Development of acute complications of diabetes secondary to inadequate control of blood glucose levels may be associated with other health care problems because of changes in activity level and diet and physiologic alterations related to the primary health problem itself. Therefore, the patient must be monitored for acute complications (hyperglycemia, hypoglycemia), and measures must be implemented for their prevention and early treatment.

Promoting Home and Community-Based Care

TEACHING PATIENTS SELF-CARE

Even if the patient has had diabetes for many years, it is important to assess his or her knowledge and adherence to the plan of care. It may be necessary to plan and implement a teaching plan that includes basic information about diabetes, its cause and symptoms, and acute and chronic complications and their treatment. The nurse asks the patient to give repeated return demonstrations of skills that were not performed correctly during the initial assessment. The patient is taught self-care activities for the prevention of long-term complications, including foot care, eye care, and risk factor management. The nurse also reminds the patient and family about the importance of health promotion activities and recommended health screening.

CONTINUING CARE

A patient who is hospitalized for another health problem may require referral for home care for that problem or if gaps in knowledge about self-care are uncovered. In either case, the home care nurse can use this opportunity to assess the patient's knowledge about diabetes management and the patient's and family's ability to carry out that management. The nurse reinforces the teaching provided in the hospital, clinic, office, or diabetes education center and assesses the home care environment to determine its adequacy for self-care and safety.

During home care visits, the nurse assesses the patient for signs and symptoms of long-term complications and assesses the patient's and family's techniques in blood glucose monitoring, insulin administration, and food selection. In addition, the patient and family are reminded of the importance of keeping appointments with health care providers and participating in health promotion activities as well as recommended health screening.

Evaluation

Expected Patient Outcomes

Expected patient outcomes may include the following:

1. Achieves optimal control of blood glucose
   a. Avoids extremes of hypoglycemia and hyperglycemia
   b. Takes steps to resolve rapidly any hypoglycemic episodes
2. Maintains skin integrity
   a. Demonstrates intact skin without dryness and cracking
   b. Avoids ulcers caused by pressure and neuropathy
3. Demonstrates/verbalizes diabetes survival skills and preventive care
4. Understands treatment modalities
   a. Demonstrates correct technique for administering insulin or oral antidiabetic medications and assessing blood glucose
   b. Demonstrates appropriate knowledge of diet through proper menu selections and identification of pattern used for selecting foods at home
   c. Verbalizes signs, appropriate treatment, and prevention of hypoglycemia and hyperglycemia
5. Demonstrates proper foot care
   a. Inspects feet (using mirror if necessary to see the bottoms of both feet), including inspection for cracks or fungal infections between toes
   b. Washes feet with warm water and soap; dries feet thoroughly
   c. Applies lotion to entire foot except between toes
   d. Identifies strategies that decrease the risk of foot ulcers, including wearing shoes at all times; using hand or elbow, not foot, to test temperature of bath water; avoiding use of heating pad on feet; avoiding constrictive shoes; wearing new shoes for brief periods only; avoiding home remedies for treatment of corns and calluses; having feet examined at every appointment with the physician or nurse practitioner; and consulting a podiatrist for regular nail care if necessary
6. Takes steps to prevent eye disease
   a. Verbalizes need for yearly or more frequent thorough dilated eye examinations by an ophthalmologist (starting at 5 years after diagnosis for type 1 diabetes or the year of diagnosis for type 2 diabetes)
   b. Verbalizes that retinopathy usually does not cause change in vision until serious damage to the retina has occurred
   c. States that early laser treatment along with good control of blood glucose and blood pressure may prevent visual loss from retinopathy
   d. Identifies hypoglycemia and hyperglycemia as two causes of temporary blurred vision
7. States measures to control macrovascular risk factors
   a. Smoking cessation
   b. Limitation of fats and cholesterol
   c. Control of hypertension
   d. Exercise
   e. Regular monitoring of renal function
8. Reports absence of acute complications
   a. Maintains blood glucose and urine ketones within normal limits
   b. Experiences no signs or symptoms of hypoglycemia or hyperglycemia
   c. Identifies signs and symptoms of hypoglycemia or hyperglycemia
   d. Reports appearance of symptoms so that treatment can be initiated

Critical Thinking Exercises

1 A 65-year-old man with type 2 diabetes is scheduled for surgical repair of an abdominal aortic aneurysm. What modifications in nursing assessment and care before, during, and after surgery are indicated because of the diagnosis of type 2 diabetes? How would these differ if the patient had type 1 diabetes?

2 You are providing discharge instructions for a patient being discharged from the hospital after cardiac artery bypass surgery. The 52-year-old man was overweight before surgery and smoked 2 packs of cigarettes daily for 20 years. He states that he neglected his health and his type 2 diabetes for two reasons: (1) the stress of his work, and (2) his belief that he did not consider his diabetes serious because he never required insulin. Identify the areas of patient teaching you would provide for this patient and the rationale for each topic as it relates to the complications of diabetes.

3 A 28-year-old patient is newly diagnosed with type 1 diabetes. Identify the major nursing assessment issues and nursing interventions in each of the following situations: (1) the patient is in the first trimester of pregnancy; (2) the patient has a phobia about use of needles; (3) the patient has been blind from birth; and (4) the patient speaks very little English.

4 A 48-year-old woman is brought to the emergency department by her coworkers because she has become drowsy and has had slurred speech for the past hour. Her coworkers report that she lives alone and has no family nearby. They state that they think she has diabetes but can provide no additional information, including the type of diabetes or the name of her physician. What would be your initial actions? What assessment data would you initially obtain? What diagnostic tests and treatments would you anticipate? Provide the rationale for those tests and treatments.

5 A 45-year-old man who has three children has had diabetes for 5 years and has not followed the prescribed treatment regimen. He says, "My father and grandfather both died from diabetes. I don't see any point in modifying my life if I'm going to die from diabetes anyway." How would you approach this patient? What resources would you use? How would you alter your approach if your first efforts to convince him of the benefits of treatment were unsuccessful? How would you modify your teaching plan if the patient understands little English?

6 ebp You are caring for a patient with diabetes, and blood glucose monitoring is recommended. Identify teaching approaches to instruct the patient about blood glucose monitoring. What is the evidence base for the teaching approach or strategy that you selected? What is the strength of the evidence, and what criteria do you use to select the approach? How would you evaluate the effectiveness of your teaching to this patient? Explain how the results of monitoring are used in the management of type 1 and type 2 diabetes.

REFERENCES AND SELECTED READINGS

BOOKS

American Association of Diabetes Educators (AADE). (2004). *A core curriculum for diabetes educators* (5th ed.). Chicago: Author.

American Diabetes Association (ADA). (1995). *Exchange lists for meal planning.* Alexandria, VA: Author.

ADA. (2003a). *Diabetes education goals.* Alexandria, VA: Author.

ADA. (2003b). *Guide to medical nutrition therapy for diabetes.* Alexandria, VA: Author.

ADA. (2003d). *Medical management of pregnancy complicated by diabetes* (3rd ed.). Alexandria, VA: Author.

American Nurses Association and American Association of Diabetes Educators. (2003). *Scope and standards of diabetes nursing practice.* Washington, DC: American Nurses Publishing.

Centers for Disease Control and Prevention (CDC). (2005). *National diabetes fact sheet: National estimates on diabetes.* Atlanta: Author.

Davidson, M. B., Harmel., A. P. & Mathur, R. (2004). *Davidson's diabetes mellitus: Diagnosis and treatment* (5th ed.). Philadelphia: Saunders.

Guthrie, D. W. & Guthrie, R. A. (Eds.). (2002). *Nursing management of diabetes mellitus: A guide to the pattern approach* (5th ed.). New York: Springer.

National Institute of Diabetes and Digestive and Kidney Disease. (2005). National Diabetes Statistics fact sheet: general information and national estimates on diabetes in the United States, 2005. Bethesda, MD: U.S. Department of Health and Human Services, National Institutes of Health, NIH Publication No. 06-3892 Available at http://diabetes.niddk.nih.gov/dm/pubs/statistics/index.htm. Accessed July 2, 2006.

National Institutes of Health, National Heart, Lung and Blood Institute, North American Association for the Study of Obesity. (2000). *The practical guide: Identification, evaluation and treatment of overweight and obesity in adults.* NIH Publication Number 00-4084. Bethesda, MD: NIH.

Porth, C. M. (2005). *Pathophysiology: Concepts of altered health states* (7th ed.). Philadelphia: Lippincott Williams & Wilkins.

Tilton, M. C. (1997). Diabetes and amputation. In Sipski, M. L. & Alexander, C. J. (Eds.). *Sexual function in people with disability and chronic illness: A health professional's guide.* Gaithersburg, MD: Aspen Publishers.

U.S. Department of Agriculture. (2005). *Nutrition and your health: Dietary guidelines for Americans.* Washington, DC: U.S. Government Printing Office.

U.S. Department of Health and Human Services. (2000). *Healthy People 2010.* Washington, DC: U.S. Government Printing Office.

U.S. Food and Drug Administration (FDA). (2005). Available at http://www.fda.gov. Accessed July 2, 2006.

U.S. Public Health Service. (2000). *Healthy People 2010.* U.S. Department of Health and Human Services. Washington, D.C.

JOURNALS

**Asterisks indicate nursing research articles.*

General

American Diabetes Association (ADA). (2003c). Implications of the United Kingdom Prospective Diabetes Study [position statement]. *Diabetes Care, 26*(1), 28–32.

ADA. (2003e). Third-party reimbursement for diabetes care, self-management education and supplies [position statement]. *Diabetes Care, 26*(1), 143–144.

ADA. (2004j). Implications of the Diabetes Control and Complications Trial [position statement]. *Diabetes Care, 27*(1), 25–27.

ADA. (2004k). Influenza and pneumococcal immunization in diabetes. *Diabetes Care, 27*(Suppl 1), S111–S113.

ADA. (2004p). Prevention of type 1 diabetes. *Diabetes Care, 27*(Suppl 1), S133.

ADA. (2004r). Report of the Expert Committee on the Diagnosis and Classification of Diabetes Mellitus [position statement]. *Diabetes Care, 27*(1), 5–10.

ADA. (2004t). Screening for type 2 diabetes. *Diabetes Care, 27*(Suppl 1), S11–S14.

Bardsley, J. K. & Want, L. L. (2004). Overview of diabetes. *Critical Care Nursing Quarterly, 27*(2), 106–112.

Centers for Disease Control and Prevention (CDC). (2004). Diabetes Surveillance System. National diabetes fact sheet. Available at http://www.cdc.gov/diabetes/Statistics/. Accessed July 2, 2006.

Diabetes Prevention Program Research Group (2002). Reduction in the incidence of type 2 diabetes with lifestyle intervention or metformin. *New England Journal of Medicine, 346*(6), 393–403.

Dyck, B. (1998). Clinical update: Diabetes update with a cardiac perspective. *Progress in Cardiovascular Nursing, 13*(2), 28–36.

Egede, L. E., Ye, X., Zheng, D., et al. (2002). The prevalence and pattern of complementary and alternative medicine use in individuals with diabetes. *Diabetes Care, 25*(2), 324–329.

Enzlin, P., Mathieu, C., Van den Bruel, A. et al. (2002). Sexual dysfunction in women with type 1 diabetes: A controlled study. *Diabetes Care. 25*(4), 672–677.

Green, H., De Ruiter, H-P., Atkins, N., et al. (2002). Diabetes expertise: A subspecialty on a general medical unit. *MedSurg Nursing, 11*(6), 281–287.

Guthrie, R. A. & Guthrie, D. W. (2004). Pathophysiology of diabetes mellitus. *Critical Care Nursing Quarterly, 27*(2), 113–125.

*Izquierdo, R. E., Kearns, J., Knudson, P. E., et al. (2003). A comparison of diabetes education administered through telemedicine versus in person. *Diabetes Care, 26*(4), 1002–1007.

Martin, W. (1999). Oral health and the older diabetic. *Clinics in Geriatric Medicine, 15*(2), 339–350.

Mensing, C., Boucher, J., Cypress, M., et al. (2003). National standards for diabetes self-management education. *Diabetes Care, 27*(1), 143–150.

Quinn, L. (2002). Mechanisms in the development of type 2 diabetes mellitus. *Journal of Cardiovascular Nursing, 16*(2), 1–16.

Quinn, L. (2003). Behavior and biology: The prevention of type 2 diabetes. *Journal of Cardiovascular Nursing, 18*(1), 62–68.

Weiss, R. (1999). Communication strategies: Diabetics learn while they shop in disease-management program. *Health Progress, 80*(1), 68.

Wild, S., Roglic, G., Green, A., et al. (2004). Global prevalence of diabetes: Estimates for the year 2000 and projections for 2030. *Diabetes Care, 27*(5), 1047–1053.

Zhang, P., Engelgau, M. M., Norris, S. L., et al. (2004). Application of economic analysis to diabetes and diabetes care. *Annals of Internal Medicine, 140*(11), 972–977.

Complications

Aljahlan, M., Lee, K. C. & Toth, E. (1999). Limited joint mobility in diabetes. *Postgraduate Medicine, 105*(2), 99–106.

American Diabetes Association (ADA). (2004h). Hyperglycemic crisis in diabetes. *Diabetes Care, 27*(Suppl 1), S94–S102.

ADA. (2004l). Nephropathy in diabetes. *Diabetes Care,* 27(Suppl 1), S79–S83.

ADA. (2004s). Retinopathy in diabetes. *Diabetes Care, 27*(Suppl 1), S84–S87.

Boulton, A. J. M., Kisner, R. S. & Vileikyte, L. (2004). Neuropathic diabetic foot ulcers. *New England Journal of Medicine, 351*(1), 48–55.

Crispin, J. C. & Alcocer-Varela, J. (2003). Rheumatologic manifestations of diabetes mellitus. *American Journal of Medicine, 114*(9), 753–757.

Cryer, P. E., Davis, S. N. & Shamoon, H. (2003). Hypoglycemia in diabetes. *Diabetes Care, 26*(6), 1902–1912.

DCCT Research Group. (1993). The effect of intensive treatment of diabetes on the development and progression of long-term complications in insulin-dependent diabetes mellitus. Diabetes Control and Complications Trial. *New England Journal of Medicine, 329*(14), 977–986.

Diabetes Control and Complications Trial/Epidemiology of Diabetes Interventions and Complications Research Group Writing Team. (2002). Effect of intensive therapy on the microvascular complications of type 1 diabetes mellitus. *Journal of the American Medical Association, 287*(19), 2563–2569.

English, P. & Williams, G. (2004). Hyperglycaemic crises and lactic acidosis in diabetes mellitus. *Postgraduate Medical Journal, 80*(943), 253–261.

Fritschi, C. (2001). Preventive care of the diabetic foot. *Nursing Clinics of North America, 36*(2), 303–320.

Gæde, P., Vedel, P., Larsen, N., et al. (2003). Multifactorial intervention and cardiovascular disease in patients with type 2 diabetes. *New England Journal of Medicine, 348*(5), 383–393.

Goldberg, P. A. & Inzucchi, S. E. (2003). Critical issues in endocrinology. *Clinics in Chest Medicine, 24*(4), 583–606.

Goldstein, I., Young, J. M, Fischer, J., et al. (2003). Vardenafil, a new phosphodiesterase type 5 inhibitor, in the treatment of erectile dysfunction in men with diabetes: A multicenter double-blind placebo-controlled fixed-dose study. *Diabetes Care, 26*(3), 777–783.

Haas, R. M. & Hoffman, A. R. (2004). Treatment of diabetic ketoacidosis: Should mode of insulin administration dictate use of intensive care facilities? *American Journal of Medicine, 117*(5), 357–358.

Jayashree, M. & Singhi, S. (2004). Diabetic ketoacidosis: Predictors of outcome in a pediatric intensive care unit of a developing country. *Pediatric Critical Care Medicine, 5*(5), 427–433.

Magee, M. F. & Bhatt, B. A. (2001). Management of decompensated diabetes: Diabetic ketoacidosis and hyperglycemic hyperosmolar syndrome. *Critical Care Clinics, 17*(1), 75–106.

Pudner, R. (2002). Assessing diabetic patients at risk of foot ulceration. *Journal of Community Nursing, 16*(1), 18–22.

Rodriguez, B. (2002). Limited joint mobility. *Diabetes Self Management, 19*(5), 107–109.

Stuckey, B., Jadzinsky, M. N., Murphy, L. J, et al. (2003). Sildenafil citrate for treatment of erectile dysfunction in men with type 1 diabetes: Results of a randomized controlled trial. *Diabetes Care, 26*(2), 279–284.

Tesfaye, S., Chaturvedi, N., Eaton, S. E. M., et al. (2005). Vascular risk factors and diabetic neuropathy. *New England Journal of Medicine, 352*(4), 341–350.

Tkacs, N. C. (2002). Hypoglycemia unawareness: Your patients with diabetes won't always know when their blood sugar is low. *American Journal of Nursing, 102*(2), 34–40.

Management

American Diabetes Association (ADA). (2004a). Aspirin therapy in diabetes [position statement]. *Diabetes Care, 27*(1), 72–73.

ADA. (2004b). Bedside blood glucose monitoring in hospitals [position statement]. *Diabetes Care, 27*(1), 104.

ADA. (2004c). Continuous subcutaneous insulin infusion [position statement]. *Diabetes Care, 27*(1), 110.

ADA. (2004d). Dyslipidemia management in adults with diabetes [position statement]. *Diabetes Care, 27*(1), 68–71.

ADA. (2004e). Evidence-based nutrition principles and recommendations in diabetes [position statement]. *Diabetes Care, 27*(1), 36.

ADA. (2004g). Hospital admission guidelines for diabetes. *Diabetes Care, 27*(Suppl 1), S103.

ADA. (2004i). Hypertension management in adults with diabetes [position statement]. *Diabetes Care, 27*(1), 65–67.

ADA. (2004k). Insulin administration [position statement]. *Diabetes Care, 27*(1), 106–107.

ADA. (2004m). Pancreas transplantation for patients with type 1 diabetes [position statement]. *Diabetes Care, 27*(1), 105.

ADA. (2004n). Physical activity/exercise and diabetes mellitus [position statement]. *Diabetes Care, 27*(1), 58–62.

ADA. (2004q). Preventive foot care in adults with diabetes [position statement]. *Diabetes Care, 27*(1), 63–64.

ADA. (2004u). Smoking and diabetes [position statement]. *Diabetes Care, 27*(1), 74–75.

ADA. (2004v). Standards of medical care in diabetes. *Diabetes Care,* 27(Suppl 1), S15–S35.

ADA. (2004w). Tests of glycemia in diabetes. *Diabetes Care, 27*(Suppl 1), S91–S93.

ADA. (2004x). Translation of the diabetes nutrition recommendations for health care institutions [position statement]. *Diabetes Care, 27*(1), 55.

American Dietetic Association. (2004). Position of the American Dietetic Association: Integration of medical nutrition therapy and pharmacotherapy. *Journal of the American Dietetic Association, 103*(10), 1353–1370.

Aye, M. & Masson E. A. (2002). Dermatological care of the diabetic foot. *American Journal of Clinical Dermatology, 3*(7), 463–474.

Blonde, L., Klein, E. J., Han, J. et al. (2006). Interim analysis of the effects of exenatide treatment on A1C, weight and cardiovascular risk factors over 82 weeks in 314 overweight patients with type 2 diabetes. *Diabetes, Obesity and Metabolism, 8*(4), 436–447.

Butler, A. B., & Lawlor, M. T. (2004). It takes a village: Helping families live with diabetes. *Diabetes Spectrum, 17*(1), 26–31.

Capriotti, T. (2005). Type 2 diabetes epidemic increases use of oral antidiabetic agents. *MedSurg Nursing, 14*(5), 341–347.

Cunningham, M. A. (2001). Glucose monitoring in type 2 diabetes. *Nursing Clinics of North America, 36*(2), 361–374.

Davidson, M. B. (2003). Effect of nurse-directed diabetes care in a minority population. *Diabetes Care, 26*(8), 2281–2287.

Defronzo, R. A., Bergenstal, R. M., Cefalu, W. T., et al. (2005). Efficacy of inhaled insulin in patients with type 2 diabetes not controlled with diet and exercise: A 12-week, randomized, comparative trial. *Diabetes Care, 28*(8), 1922–1928.

DeWitt, D. E. & Dugdale, D. C. (2003). Using new insulin strategies in the outpatient treatment of diabetes: Clinical applications. *Journal of American Medical Association, 289*(17), 2265–2269.

DeWitt, D. E. & Hirsch, I. B. (2003). Outpatient insulin therapy in type 1 and type 2 diabetes mellitus [scientific review]. *Journal of American Medical Association, 289*(17), 2254–2264.

*Doyle, E. A., Ahern, J. H., Weinzimer, S. A., et al. (2004). A randomized, prospective trial comparing the efficacy of continuous subcutaneous insulin infusion with multiple daily injections using insulin glargine. *Diabetes Care, 27*(7), 1554–1558.

Durso, S. C. (2006). Using clinical guidelines designed for older adults with diabetes mellitus and complex health status. *Journal of the American Medical Association.* 295(6), 1935–1940.

*Durso, S. C., Wendel, I., Letzt, A. M., et al. (2003). Older adults using cellular telephones for diabetes management: A pilot study. *MedSurg Nursing, 12*(5), 313–317.

Flood, L. & Constance, A. (2002). Diabetes and exercise safety. *American Journal of Nursing, 102*(6), 47–55.

Funnell, M. M. & Anderson, R. M. (2004). Empowerment and self-management of diabetes. *Clinical Diabetes, 22*(3), 123–127.

Hirsch, I. B. (2005). Insulin analogues. *New England Journal of Medicine, 352*(2), 174–183.

Jacobson, A. F. (1999). Saving limbs with Semmes-Weinstein monofilament. *American Journal of Nursing, 99*(2), 76.

Keresztes, P. A. & Brick, K. (2003). Lantus: A new insulin. *MedSurg Nursing, 12*(6), 408–410.

Lachance, P. A. & Fisher, M. C. (2005). Reinvention of the food pyramid to promote health. *Advances in Food and Nutrition Research, 49*, 1–39.

McCormick, M., & Quinn, L. (2002). Treatment of type 2 diabetes mellitus: Pharmacologic intervention. *Journal of Cardiovascular Nursing, 16*(2), 55–67.

Nathan, D. M., Cleary, P. A., Backlund, J-Y C. et al. (2005). Intensive diabetes treatment and cardiovascular disease in patients with type 1 diabetes. *New England Journal of Medicine, 353*(25), 2643–2653.

Ramchandani, N. (2004). Type 2 diabetes in children. *American Journal of Nursing, 104*(3), 65–68.

Rosenstock, J., Zinman, B., Murphy, L. J., et al. (2005). Inhaled insulin improves glycemic control when substituted for or added to oral combination therapy in type 2 diabetes: A randomized, controlled trial. *Annals of Internal Medicine, 143*(8), 549–558.

Shapiro, A. M., Nanji, S. A. & Lakey, J. R. (2003). Clinical islet transplant: Current and future directions towards tolerance. *Immunology Review, 196*, 219–236.

Shapiro, A. M., Ricordi, C. & Hering, B. (2003). Edmonton's islet success has indeed been replicated elsewhere. *Lancet, 362*(9391), 1242.

United Kingdom Prospective Diabetes Study Group. (1998). Intensive blood glucose control with sulfonylureas or insulin compared with conventional treatment and risk of complications with type 2 diabetes. *Lancet, 352*(9131), 837–853.

Webb, K. E. (2006). Use of insulin pumps for diabetes management. *MedSurg Nursing, 15*(2), 61–68, 94.

White, J. R., Davis, S. N., Cooppan, R., et al. (2003). Clarifying the role of insulin in type 2 diabetes management. *Clinical Diabetes, 21*(1), 14–21.

Yeh, G., Eisenberg, D., Kaptchuk, T., et al. (2003). Systematic review of herbs and dietary supplements for glycemic control in diabetes. *Diabetes Care, 26*(4), 1277–1294.

Yki-Jävinen, H. (2004). Thiazolidinediones. *New England Journal of Medicine, 351*(11), 1106–1118.

Pregnancy and Gestational Diabetes

American Diabetes Association (ADA). (2004f). Gestational diabetes mellitus [position statement]. *Diabetes Care, 27*(1), 88–90.

ADA. (2004o). Preconception care of women with diabetes [position statement]. *Diabetes Care, 27*(1), 76–78.

RESOURCES

AGENCIES

American Association of Diabetes Educators, 444 N. Michigan Ave., Suite 1240, Chicago, IL 60611; 800-832-6874; http://www.aadenet.org/. Accessed May 15, 2006.

American Diabetes Association, 1660 Duke St., Alexandria, VA 22314; 800-232-3472; http://www.diabetes.org. Accessed May 15, 2006.

American Dietetic Association, 216 W. Jackson Boulevard, Chicago, IL 60606; 800-366-1655; http://www.eatright.org. Accessed May 15, 2006.

American Foundation for the Blind, 15 W. 16th St., New York, NY 10011; 800-232-5463; http://www.afb.org. Accessed May 15, 2006.

Centers for Disease Control and Prevention, 1600 Clifton Rd., Atlanta, GA 30333; 404-639-3311; http://www.cdc.gov/diabetes/pubs/factsheet.htm. Accessed May 15, 2006.

Juvenile Diabetes Research Foundation International, 120 Wall St., 19th Floor, New York, NY 10005; 800-533-CURE or 800-223-1138; http://www.jdrf.org. Accessed May 15, 2006.

MedicAlert Foundation International, 2323 Colorado St., Turlock, CA 95381-1009; 209-668-3333; http://www.medicalert.org. Accessed May 15, 2006.

National Library Services for the Blind and Physically Handicapped (NLS-BPH), Library of Congress, 1291 Taylor St., NW, Washington DC 20542; 202-287-5100 or 800-424-8567; http://www.loc.gov/nls/. Accessed May 15, 2006.

National Diabetes Information Clearinghouse, 1 Information Way, Bethesda, MD 20892; 800-GETWELL or 301-654-3327; http://www.niddk.nih.gov. Accessed May 15, 2006.

JOURNALS FOR PATIENTS

Diabetes Forecast, American Diabetes Association, Membership Center, P.O. Box 2055, Harlan, IA 51593-0238.

Diabetes Self-Management, P.O. Box 51125, Boulder, CO 80321-1125.

Living Well With Diabetes, Diabetes Center, 13911 Ridgedale Dr., Suite 250, Minnetonka, MN 55343.

CHAPTER 42

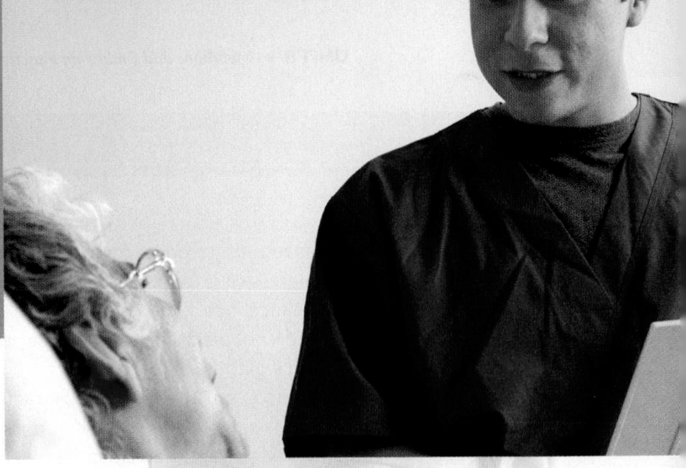

Assessment and Management of Patients With Endocrine Disorders

Learning Objectives

On completion of this chapter, the learner will be able to:

1. Describe the functions of each of the endocrine glands and their hormones.
2. Identify the diagnostic tests used to determine alterations in function of each of the endocrine glands.
3. Compare hypothyroidism and hyperthyroidism: their causes, clinical manifestations, management, and nursing interventions.
4. Develop a plan of nursing care for the patient undergoing thyroidectomy.
5. Compare hyperparathyroidism and hypoparathyroidism: their causes, clinical manifestations, management, and nursing interventions.
6. Compare Addison's disease with Cushing's syndrome: their causes, clinical manifestations, management, and nursing interventions.
7. Use the nursing process as a framework for care of patients with adrenal insufficiency.
8. Use the nursing process as a framework for care of patients with Cushing's syndrome.
9. Identify the teaching needs of patients requiring corticosteroid therapy.

Glossary

acromegaly: disease process resulting from excessive secretion of somatotropin; causes progressive enlargement of peripheral body parts, commonly the face, head, hands, and feet

Addison's disease: chronic adrenocortical insufficiency secondary to destruction of the adrenal glands

addisonian crisis: acute adrenocortical insufficiency; characterized by acute hypotension, cyanosis, fever, nausea and vomiting, and the classic signs of shock; precipitated by stress or abrupt withdrawal of therapeutic glucocorticoids

adrenalectomy: surgical removal of one or both adrenal glands.

adrenocorticotropic hormone (ACTH): hormone secreted by the anterior pituitary, essential for growth and development

androgens: hormones secreted by the adrenal cortex; stimulate activity of accessory male sex organs and development of male sex characteristics

adrenogenital syndrome: masculinization in women, feminization in men, or premature sexual development in children; result of abnormal secretion of adrenocortical hormones, especially androgens

basal metabolic rate: chemical reactions occurring when the body is at rest

calcitonin: hormone secreted by the parafollicular cells of the thyroid gland; participates in calcium regulation

Chvostek's sign: spasm of the facial muscles produced by sharply tapping over the facial nerve in front of the parotid gland and anterior to the ear; causes spasm or twitching of the mouth, nose, and eye; suggestive of latent tetany in patients with hypocalcemia

corticosteroids: hormones produced by the adrenal cortex or their synthetic equivalents; also referred to as adrenal-cortical hormone and adrenocorticosteroid; consist of glucocorticoids, mineralocorticoids, and androgens

cretinism: stunted body growth and mental development appearing during the first year of life as a result of congenital hypothyroidism

Cushing's syndrome: group of symptoms produced by an excess of free circulating cortisol from the adrenal cortex; characterized by truncal obesity, "moon face," acne, abdominal striae, and hypertension

diabetes insipidus: condition in which abnormally large volumes of dilute urine are excreted as a result of deficient production of vasopressin

dilutional hyponatremia: sodium deficiency that develops as a result of fluid retention; associated with excessive antidiuretic hormone secretion in patients with SIADH

dwarfism: generalized limited growth; condition caused by insufficient secretion of growth hormone during childhood

endocrine: secreting internally; hormonal secretion of a ductless gland

euthyroid: state of normal thyroid hormone production

exocrine: secreting externally; hormonal secretion from excretory ducts

exophthalmos: abnormal protrusion of one or both eyeballs; produces a startled expression; usually due to hyperthyroidism

glucocorticoids: steroid hormones (ie, cortisol, cortisone, and corticosterone) secreted by the adrenal cortex in response to ACTH; produce a rise of liver glycogen and blood glucose

Graves' disease: a form of hyperthyroidism; characterized by a diffuse goiter and exophthalmos

goiter: enlargement of the thyroid gland; usually caused by an iodine-deficient diet

Hashimoto's disease: thyroiditis characterized by high levels of antimicrosomal antibodies; most common cause of hypothyroidism in the United States; also known as chronic lymphocytic thyroiditis or autoimmune thyroiditis

hormones: chemical transmitter substances produced in one organ or part of the body and carried by the bloodstream to other cells or organs on which they have a specific regulatory effect; produced mainly by endocrine glands (eg, pituitary, thyroid, gonads)

hypophysectomy: surgical removal or destruction of all or part of the pituitary gland

mineralocorticoid: steroid of the adrenal cortex; influences sodium and potassium

myxedema: severe form of hypothyroidism characterized by an accumulation of mucopolysaccharides in subcutaneous and other interstitial tissues, a masklike expression, puffy eyelids, hair loss in the eyebrows, thick lips, and a broad tongue

negative feedback: regulating mechanism in which an increase or decrease in the level of a substance decreases or increases the function of the organ producing the substance

oxytocin: hormone secreted by the posterior pituitary; causes myometrial contraction at term and milk release during lactation

pheochromocytoma: chromaffin cell tumor, usually benign, located in the adrenal medulla; characterized by secretion of catecholamines resulting in hypertension, severe headache, profuse sweating, visual blurring, anxiety, and nausea

radioimmunoassay: measurement of hormone or other substance using radioisotope-labeled antigen

syndrome of inappropriate antidiuretic hormone (SIADH) secretion: excessive secretion of antidiuretic hormone (ADH) from the pituitary gland despite low serum osmolality level; occurs with oat cell carcinoma of the lung and other malignant tumors that produce ADH

thyroid-stimulating hormone (TSH): released from the pituitary gland; causes stimulation of the thyroid gland, resulting in release of T_3 and T_4

thyroid storm: severe life-threatening form of hyperthyroidism precipitated by stress; usually of abrupt onset; characterized by high fever, extreme tachycardia, and altered mental state

thyroidectomy: surgical removal of all or part of the thyroid gland

thyroiditis: inflammation of the thyroid gland; may lead to chronic hypothyroidism or may resolve spontaneously

thyrotoxicosis: condition produced by excessive endogenous or exogenous thyroid hormone

thyroxine (T_4) thyroid hormone: active iodine compound formed and stored in the thyroid; deiodinated in peripheral tissues to form triiodothyronine (T_3); maintains body metabolism in a steady state

triiodothyronine (T_3): thyroid hormone; formed and stored in the thyroid; released in smaller quantities, biologically more active and with faster onset of action than thyroxine (T_4); widespread effect on cellular metabolism, influences every major organ system

Trousseau's sign: carpopedal spasm induced when blood flow to the arm is occluded using a blood pressure cuff or tourniquet, causing ischemia to the distal nerves; suggestive sign for latent tetany in hypocalcemia

vasopressin: antidiuretic hormone (ADH) secreted by the posterior pituitary; causes contraction of smooth muscle, particularly blood vessels

The nervous system and the interconnected network of glands known as the endocrine system control body systems. Disorders of the endocrine system are common and have the potential to affect the function of every organ system in the body. Understanding the function of each of the endocrine glands and the consequences of hypofunction and hyperfunction of each gland enables the nurse to anticipate physiologic changes and to plan interventions to address them. Nursing interventions that are essential in managing endocrine disorders are carried out in every setting, from the intensive care unit to the outpatient setting and the home.

Anatomic and Physiologic Overview

The endocrine system has far-reaching effects in the human body because of its links with the nervous system and the immune system. The hormones secreted by the endocrine system are affected in large part by structures in the central nervous system, such as the hypothalamus. Other structures located in the brain, such as the pituitary gland, are endocrine glands that influence the function of a large number of other endocrine glands. Hormones secreted by the endocrine system affect the nervous system and are, in turn, mediated by the nervous system. The adrenal medulla, for example, secretes a number of substances (eg, norepinephrine, epinephrine) that act as neurotransmitters. The immune system also interacts closely with the endocrine system. It responds to the introduction of foreign agents by means of chemicals (eg, interleukins, interferons) and is regulated by hormones secreted by the adrenal cortex (Porth, 2005).

In addition to the hormones secreted by the major endocrine glands, other tissues produce hormones that are secreted into body fluids and act on nearby cells and tissues. The gastrointestinal mucosa produces hormones (eg, gastrin, enterogastrone, secretin, cholecystokinin) that are important in the digestive process. The kidneys produce erythropoietin, a hormone that stimulates the bone marrow to produce red blood cells. The white blood cells produce cytokines that actively participate in inflammatory and immune responses.

Hormones are important in regulation of the internal environment of the body and affect every aspect of life. Some hormones target specific tissues; for example, **adrenocorticotropic hormone (ACTH)**, or corticotrophin, is secreted by the anterior pituitary gland and targets the adrenal cortex to increase the secretion of the hormones of the adrenal cortex (ie, glucocorticoids, mineralocorticoids, androgens). Other hormones affect a wide variety of cells and tissues of the body. Thyroid hormone is one example; it affects metabolic activity of cells throughout the body.

Glands of the Endocrine System

The **endocrine** glands include the pituitary, thyroid, parathyroids, adrenals, pancreatic islets, ovaries, and testes (Fig. 42-1). Endocrine glands secrete their products directly into the bloodstream, which differentiates them from **exocrine** glands, such as sweat glands, which secrete their products through ducts onto epithelial surfaces or into the gastrointestinal tract. The hypothalamus is the link between the nervous system and the endocrine system. (Because of the unique endocrine and exocrine functions of the pancreas, pancreatic function and disorders are discussed in Chapters 40 and 41; reproductive structures, such as the ovaries and testes, are discussed in Chapters 47 and 49.)

Function and Regulation of Hormones

The chemical substances secreted by the endocrine glands are called **hormones.** Hormones help regulate organ function in concert with the nervous system. This dual regulatory system, in which rapid action by the nervous system is balanced by slower hormonal action, permits precise control of organ functions in response to varied changes within and outside the body. Table 42-1 lists the major hormones, their target tissue, and some of their properties.

The endocrine glands are composed of secretory cells arranged in minute clusters known as acini. No ducts are present, but the glands have a rich blood supply, so the hormones they produce enter the bloodstream rapidly. In the healthy physiologic state, hormone concentration in the bloodstream is maintained at a relatively constant level. When the hormone concentration increases, further production of that hormone is inhibited. When the hormone concentration decreases, the rate of production of that hormone increases. This mechanism for regulating hormone concentration in the bloodstream is called **negative feedback,** and it is important in the regulation of many biologic processes.

Classification and Action of Hormones

Hormones are classified as steroid hormones (eg, hydrocortisone), peptide or protein hormones (eg, insulin), amine hormones (eg, epinephrine), and fatty acid derivatives (eg, retinoids). These different classes of hormones act on the target tissues by different mechanisms. Hormones can alter the function of the target tissue by interacting with chemical receptors located either on the cell membrane or in the interior of the cell.

Peptide and protein hormones interact with receptor sites on the cell surface, which results in stimulation of the intracellular enzyme adenyl cyclase. This causes increased production of cyclic 3′,5′-adenosine monophosphate (cyclic AMP). The cyclic AMP inside the cell alters enzyme activity. Thus, cyclic AMP is the "second messenger" that links the peptide hormone at the cell surface to a change in the intracellular environment. Some of the protein and peptide hormones also act by changing membrane permeability. These hormones act within seconds or minutes. The mechanism of action for amine hormones is similar to that for peptide hormones.

Steroid hormones, because of their smaller size and higher lipid solubility, penetrate the cell membranes and interact with intracellular receptors. The steroid–receptor complex modifies cell metabolism and the formation of messenger ribonucleic acid (mRNA) from deoxyribonucleic acid (DNA). The mRNA then stimulates protein synthesis within the cell. Steroid hormones require several hours to exert their

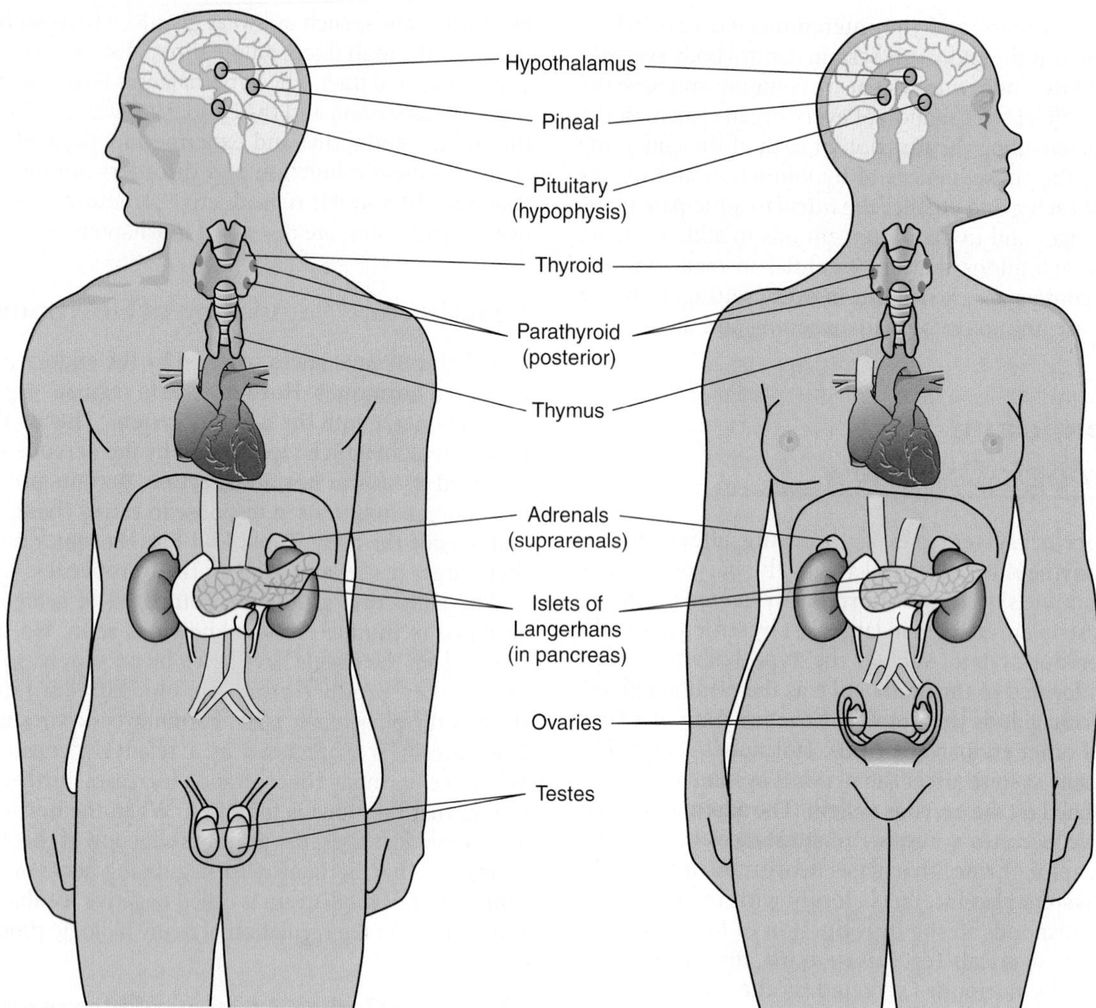

FIGURE 42-1. Major hormone-secreting glands of the endocrine system.

effects, because they exert their action by the modification of protein synthesis.

Assessment

Health History and Clinical Manifestations

Because of the widespread effects of the endocrine system on the body, a wide variety of signs and symptoms occur with endocrine disorders. Although specific endocrine disorders are often accompanied by specific clinical symptoms, more general manifestations may occur with a number of endocrine disorders. Changes in energy level and fatigue are common to many endocrine imbalances. During the health history, the nurse asks the patient about fatigue and changes in usual energy levels and about how the changes affect the patient's ability to carry out activities of daily life. The nurse also asks about changes in the patient's tolerance of heat and cold as well as recent changes in weight: increases or decreases may occur with changes in adrenal and thyroid disorders and may be a result of changes in fat distribution or fluid loss or retention.

Changes in sexual function and secondary sex characteristics may occur with any number of endocrine disorders and are assessed by obtaining a sexual history. Asking the patient or family about changes in mood, memory, and ability to concentrate and altered sleep patterns is important, because these changes are common in endocrine disorders. Other specific symptoms that occur with various endocrine disorders are discussed with each of those disorders.

Physical Assessment

The patient is observed for obvious changes in appearance that may indicate endocrine dysfunction. Changes in skin texture are common with both hypofunction and hyperfunction of the thyroid gland. Eye changes, such as exophthalmos, may occur with hyperthyroidism and Graves' disease. Changes in physical appearance (eg, appearance of facial hair in women, "moon face," "buffalo hump," thinning of the skin, obesity of the trunk and thinness of the extremities, increased size of the feet and hands, edema) may signify disorders of the thyroid, adrenal cortex, or pituitary gland.

Vital signs are measured and compared with previous values if known. Elevated blood pressure may occur with

TABLE 42-1 Major Action and Source of Selected Hormones

Source	Hormone	Major Action
Hypothalamus	Releasing and inhibiting hormones Corticotropin-releasing hormone (CRH) Thyrotropin-releasing hormone (TRH) Growth hormone-releasing hormone (GHRH) Gonadotropin-releasing hormone (GnRH)	Controls the release of pituitary hormones
	Somatostatin	Inhibits growth hormone and thyroid-stimulating hormone
Anterior pituitary	Growth hormone (GH)	Stimulates growth of bone and muscle, promotes protein synthesis and fat metabolism, decreases carbohydrate metabolism
	Adrenocorticotropic hormone (ACTH)	Stimulates synthesis and secretion of adrenal cortical hormones
	Thyroid-stimulating hormone (TSH)	Stimulates synthesis and secretion of thyroid hormone
	Follicle-stimulating hormone (FSH)	Female: stimulates growth of ovarian follicle, ovulation Male: stimulates sperm production
	Luteinizing hormone (LH)	Female: stimulates development of corpus luteum, release of oocyte, production of estrogen and progesterone Male: stimulates secretion of testosterone, development of interstitial tissue of testes
	Prolactin	Prepares female breast for breast-feeding
Posterior pituitary	Antidiuretic hormone (ADH)	Increases water reabsorption by kidney
	Oxytocin	Stimulates contraction of pregnant uterus, milk ejection from breasts after childbirth
Adrenal cortex	Mineralocorticosteroids, mainly aldosterone	Increases sodium absorption, potassium loss by kidney
	Glucocorticoids, mainly cortisol	Affects metabolism of all nutrients; regulates blood glucose levels, affects growth, has anti-inflammatory action, and decreases effects of stress
	Adrenal androgens, mainly dehydro-epiandrosterone (DHEA) and androstenedione	Have minimal intrinsic androgenic activity; they are converted to testosterone and dihydrotestosterone in the periphery
Adrenal medulla	Epinephrine Norepinephrine	Serve as neurotransmitters for the sympathetic nervous system
Thyroid (follicular cells)	Thyroid hormones: triiodothyronine (T_3), thyroxine (T_4)	Increase the metabolic rate; increase protein and bone turnover; increase responsiveness to catecholamines; necessary for fetal and infant growth and development
Thyroid C cells	Calcitonin	Lowers blood calcium and phosphate levels
Parathyroid glands	Parathormone (PTH, parathyroid hormone)	Regulates serum calcium
Pancreatic islet cells	Insulin	Lowers blood glucose by facilitating glucose transport across cell membranes of muscle, liver, and adipose tissue
	Glucagon	Increases blood glucose concentration by stimulation of glycogenolysis and glyconeogenesis
	Somatostatin	Delays intestinal absorption of glucose
Kidney	1,25-Dihydroxyvitamin D	Stimulates calcium absorption from the intestine
	Renin	Activates renin-angiotensin-aldosterone system
	Erythropoietin	Increases red blood cell production
Ovaries	Estrogen	Affects development of female sex organs and secondary sex characteristics
	Progesterone	Influences menstrual cycle; stimulates growth of uterine wall; maintains pregnancy
Testes	Androgens, mainly testosterone	Affect development of male sex organs and secondary sex characteristics; aid in sperm production

Reproduced with permission from Porth, C. (2005). *Pathophysiology: Concepts of altered health states* (7th ed.) Philadelphia: Lippincott Williams & Wilkins.

GENETICS IN NURSING PRACTICE

Metabolic Disorders

Some examples of metabolic and endocrine disorders influenced by genetic factors include the following:

- Alpha-1 antitrypsin deficiency
- Cystic fibrosis
- Diabetes mellitus type 1 and type 2
- Hereditary hemochromatosis
- Multiple endocrine neoplasia (MEN) type I and type II
- Von Hippel-Lindau syndrome
- Wilson's disease

NURSING ASSESSMENTS

Family History Assessment

- Assess family history for relatives with early-onset hepatic, pancreatic, or endocrine disease.
- Inquire about family members with diabetes and their ages at onset.
- Assess family history of other related genetic conditions such as cystic fibrosis, alpha-1 antitrypsin deficiency, and hereditary hemochromatosis.

Patient Assessment

- Assess for physical symptoms such as mucosal neuromas, hypertrophied lips, skeletal abnormalities, and marfanoid appearance.
- Assess for signs of arthritis and bronze pigmentation of the skin (hereditary hemochromatosis).

MANAGEMENT ISSUES SPECIFIC TO GENETICS

- Inquire whether DNA mutation testing has been performed on any affected family member.
- If indicated, refer for further genetics counseling and evaluation so that family members can discuss inheritance, risk to other family members, and availability of genetics testing and gene-based interventions.
- Offer appropriate genetics information and resources.
- Assess patient's understanding of genetics information.
- Provide support to families with newly diagnosed genetics-related metabolic and endocrine conditions.
- Participate in management and coordination of care of patients with genetic conditions and people predisposed to develop or pass on a genetic condition.

GENETICS RESOURCES FOR NURSES AND THEIR PATIENTS ON THE WEB

Genetic Alliance: www.geneticalliance.org—a directory of support groups for patients and families with genetic conditions

Gene Clinics: www.geneclinics.org—a listing of common genetics disorders with clinical summaries, genetic counseling and testing information

National Organization of Rare Disorders: www.rarediseases.org—a directory of support groups and information for patients and families with rare genetic disorders

OMIM: Online Mendelian Inheritance in Man: www.ncbi.nlm.nih.gov/projects/omim—a complete listing of inherited genetic conditions

hyperfunction of the adrenal cortex or tumor of the adrenal medulla. Decreased blood pressure may occur with hypofunction of the adrenal cortex. Other specific physical assessment findings are discussed with each endocrine disorder.

Diagnostic Evaluation

Although a wide variety of tests can be used in the diagnostic workup, three major categories of diagnostic tests are common: blood tests, urine tests, and stimulation and suppression tests. Specific tests are discussed with the specific endocrine disorders in this chapter.

Blood tests may be used to determine hormone blood levels. For example, if a patient is thought to have a thyroid disorder, serum levels of **thyroid-stimulating hormone (TSH)** and thyroid hormone provide information about the nature (hypofunction or hyperfunction) and site (thyroid, pituitary, or hypothalamus) of the disorder. Other blood tests are used to detect antibodies or to assess the effect of the hormone on other substances (eg, the effect of insulin on blood glucose levels). **Radioimmunoassays**, which are radioisotope-labeled antigen tests used to measure hormones or other substances, may be performed.

Urine tests may be used to measure the amount of hormone or the end products of hormones excreted by the kidneys. One-time specimens are obtained, or in some disorders 24-hour urine specimens are collected to measure hormones or their metabolites. For example, urinary levels of free catecholamines (norepinephrine, epinephrine, and dopamine) may be measured in patients with suspected tumors of the adrenal medulla (**pheochromocytoma**).

Stimulation and suppression tests may be used to diagnose endocrine disorders. Stimulation tests can determine how an endocrine gland responds to the administration of stimulating hormones that are normally produced or released by the hypothalamus or pituitary gland. If the endocrine gland responds to this stimulation, the specific disorder may be in the hypothalamus or pituitary. Failure of the endocrine gland to respond to this stimulation helps to identify the problem as being in the endocrine gland itself. Suppression tests may be used to determine whether negative feedback mechanisms that normally control secretion of hormones from the hypothalamus or pituitary gland are intact.

The Pituitary Gland

Anatomic and Physiologic Overview

The pituitary gland, or hypophysis, is a round structure about 1.27 cm (½ inch) in diameter located on the inferior aspect of the brain. Commonly referred to as the master gland, the pituitary secretes hormones that control the secretion of hormones by other endocrine glands (Fig. 42-2). The pituitary itself is controlled by the hypothalamus, an adjacent area of the brain that is connected to the pituitary by the pituitary stalk. The pituitary gland is divided into the anterior and posterior lobes.

Anterior Pituitary

The major hormones of the anterior pituitary gland are follicle-stimulating hormone (FSH), luteinizing hormone

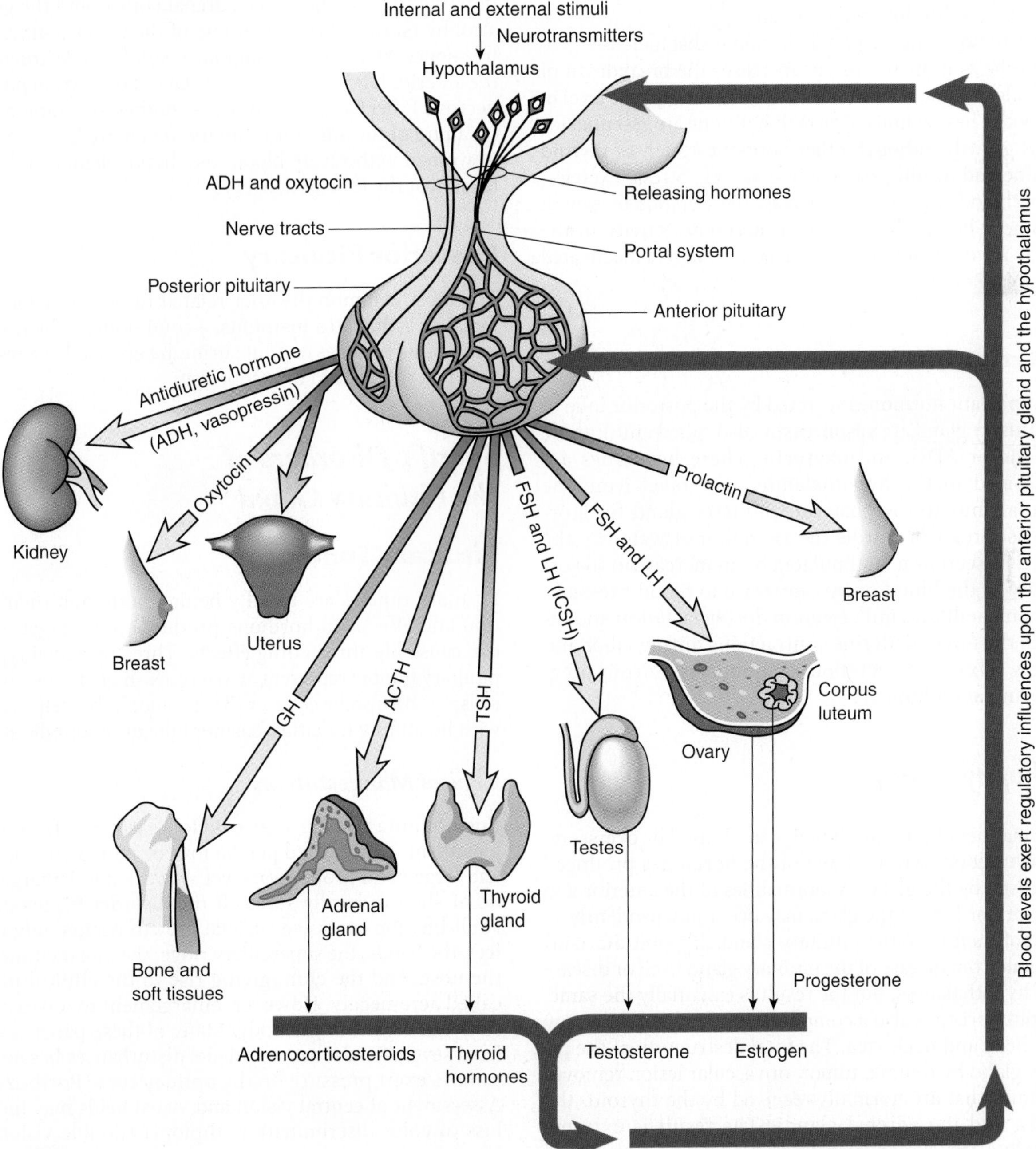

FIGURE 42-2. The pituitary gland, the relationship of the brain to pituitary action, and the hormones secreted by the anterior and posterior pituitary lobes.

(LH), prolactin, ACTH, TSH, and growth hormone (also referred to as somatotropin). The secretion of these major hormones is controlled by releasing factors secreted by the hypothalamus. These releasing factors reach the anterior pituitary by way of the bloodstream in a special circulation called the pituitary portal blood system. Other hormones include melanocyte-stimulating hormone and beta-lipotropin; the function of lipotropin is poorly understood.

The hormones released by the anterior pituitary enter the general circulation and are transported to their target organs. The main function of TSH, ACTH, FSH, and LH is the release of hormones from other endocrine glands. Prolactin acts on the breast to stimulate milk production. Hormones that stimulate other organs and tissues are discussed in conjunction with their target organs.

Growth hormone is a protein hormone that increases protein synthesis in many tissues, increases the breakdown of fatty acids in adipose tissue, and increases the glucose level in the blood. These actions of growth hormone are essential for normal growth, although other hormones, such as thyroid hormone and insulin, are required as well. Stress, exercise, and low blood glucose levels increase the secretion of growth hormone. The half-life of growth hormone activity in the blood is 20 to 30 minutes; the hormone is largely inactivated in the liver.

Posterior Pituitary

The important hormones secreted by the posterior lobe of the pituitary gland are **vasopressin**, also called antidiuretic hormone or ADH, and **oxytocin**. These hormones are synthesized in the hypothalamus and travel from the hypothalamus to the posterior pituitary gland for storage. Vasopressin controls the excretion of water by the kidney; its secretion is stimulated by an increase in the osmolality of the blood or by a decrease in blood pressure. Oxytocin facilitates milk ejection during lactation and increases the force of uterine contractions during labor and delivery. Oxytocin secretion is stimulated during pregnancy and at childbirth.

Pathophysiology

Abnormalities of pituitary function are caused by oversecretion or undersecretion of any of the hormones produced or released by the gland. Abnormalities of the anterior and posterior portions of the gland may occur independently.

Hypofunction of the pituitary gland (hypopituitarism) can result from disease of the pituitary gland itself or disease of the hypothalamus, but the result is essentially the same. Hypopituitarism is also a complication of radiation therapy to the head and neck area. The total destruction of the pituitary gland by trauma, tumor, or vascular lesion removes all stimuli that are normally received by the thyroid, the gonads, and the adrenal glands. The result is extreme weight loss, emaciation, atrophy of all endocrine glands and organs, hair loss, impotence, amenorrhea, hypometabolism, and hypoglycemia. Coma and death occur if the missing hormones are not replaced.

Anterior Pituitary

Oversecretion (hypersecretion) most commonly involves ACTH or growth hormone and results in **Cushing's syndrome** or **acromegaly**, respectively. Acromegaly, an excess of growth hormone in adults, results in bone and soft tissue deformities and enlargement of the viscera without an increase in height. In children, oversecretion of growth hormone results in gigantism, with a person reaching 7 or even 8 feet tall. Conversely, insufficient secretion of growth hormone during childhood results in generalized limited growth and **dwarfism** (Porth, 2005). Undersecretion (hyposecretion) commonly involves all of the anterior pituitary hormones and is termed *panhypopituitarism*. In this condition, the thyroid gland, the adrenal cortex, and the gonads atrophy (shrink) because of loss of the trophic-stimulating hormones. Hypopituitarism may result from destruction of the anterior lobe of the pituitary gland. Postpartum pituitary necrosis (Sheehan's syndrome) is another uncommon cause of failure of the anterior pituitary. It is more likely to occur in women with severe blood loss, hypovolemia, and hypotension at the time of delivery.

Posterior Pituitary

The most common disorder related to posterior lobe dysfunction is **diabetes insipidus**, a condition in which abnormally large volumes of dilute urine are excreted as a result of deficient production of vasopressin.

Specific Disorders of the Pituitary Gland

Pituitary Tumors

Pituitary tumors are usually benign, although their location and effects on hormone production by target organs can cause life-threatening effects. Three principal types of pituitary tumors represent an overgrowth of (1) eosinophilic cells, (2) basophilic cells, or (3) chromophobic cells (ie, cells with no affinity for either eosinophilic or basophilic stains).

Clinical Manifestations

Eosinophilic tumors that develop early in life result in gigantism. The affected person may be more than 7 feet tall and large in all proportions, yet so weak and lethargic that he or she can hardly stand. If the disorder begins during adult life, the excessive skeletal growth occurs only in the feet, the hands, the superciliary ridge, the molar eminences, the nose, and the chin, giving rise to the clinical picture called acromegaly. However, enlargement involves all tissues and organs of the body. Many of these patients suffer from severe headaches and visual disturbances because the tumors exert pressure on the optic nerves (Porth, 2005). Assessment of central vision and visual fields may indicate loss of color discrimination, diplopia (double vision), or blindness in a portion of a field of vision. Decalcification of the skeleton, muscular weakness, and endocrine disturbances, similar to those occurring in patients with hyperthyroidism, also are associated with this type of tumor.

Basophilic tumors give rise to Cushing's syndrome with features largely attributable to hyperadrenalism, including masculinization and amenorrhea in females, truncal obesity, hypertension, osteoporosis, and polycythemia.

Chromophobic tumors represent 90% of pituitary tumors. These tumors usually produce no hormones but destroy the rest of the pituitary gland, causing hypopituitarism. People with this disease are often obese and somnolent and exhibit fine, scanty hair; dry, soft skin; a pasty complexion; and small bones. They also experience headaches, loss of libido, and visual defects progressing to blindness. Other signs and symptoms include polyuria, polyphagia, a lowering of the **basal metabolic rate**, and a subnormal body temperature.

Assessment and Diagnostic Findings

Diagnostic evaluation requires a careful history and physical examination, including assessment of visual acuity and visual fields. Computed tomography (CT) and magnetic resonance imaging (MRI) are used to diagnose the presence and extent of pituitary tumors. Serum levels of pituitary hormones may be obtained along with measurements of hormones of target organs (eg, thyroid, adrenal) to assist in diagnosis if other information is inconclusive.

Medical Management

Surgical removal of the pituitary tumor through a transsphenoidal approach is the usual treatment. Stereotactic radiation therapy, which requires use of a neurosurgery-type stereotactic frame, may be used to deliver external-beam radiation therapy precisely to the pituitary tumor with minimal effect on normal tissue (see Chapter 16). Other treatments include conventional radiation therapy, bromocriptine (dopamine antagonist), and octreotide (Sandostatin, a synthetic analogue of growth hormone). These medications inhibit the production or release of growth hormone and may bring about marked improvement of symptoms. Octreotide may also be used preoperatively to improve the patient's clinical condition and to shrink the tumor.

SURGICAL MANAGEMENT

Hypophysectomy, or removal of the pituitary gland, may be performed to treat primary pituitary gland tumors. It is the treatment of choice in patients with Cushing's syndrome resulting from excessive production of ACTH by a tumor of the pituitary gland. Hypophysectomy may also be performed on occasion as a palliative measure to relieve bone pain secondary to metastasis of malignant lesions of the breast and prostate.

Several approaches are used to remove or destroy the pituitary gland, including surgical removal by transfrontal, subcranial, or oronasal–transsphenoidal approaches; irradiation; and cryosurgery. (The transsphenoidal approach and the nursing management of a patient undergoing cranial surgery are discussed in Chapter 61.) Even if surgery succeeds at removing the tumor, many of the features or symptoms of acromegaly will be unaffected.

The absence of the pituitary gland alters the function of many body systems. Menstruation ceases and infertility occurs after total or near-total ablation of the pituitary gland. Replacement therapy with corticosteroids and thyroid hormone is necessary; therefore, patient teaching is imperative (see later discussion).

Diabetes Insipidus

Diabetes insipidus is a disorder of the posterior lobe of the pituitary gland that is characterized by a deficiency of ADH (vasopressin). Excessive thirst (polydipsia) and large volumes of dilute urine characterize the disorder. It may occur secondary to head trauma, brain tumor, or surgical ablation or irradiation of the pituitary gland. It may also occur with infections of the central nervous system (meningitis, encephalitis, tuberculosis) or with tumors (eg, metastatic disease, lymphoma of the breast or lung). Another cause of diabetes insipidus is failure of the renal tubules to respond to ADH; this nephrogenic form may be related to hypokalemia, hypercalcemia, and a variety of medications (eg, lithium, demeclocycline [Declomycin]).

Clinical Manifestations

Without the action of ADH on the distal nephron of the kidney, an enormous daily output of very dilute, waterlike urine with a specific gravity of 1.001 to 1.005 occurs. The urine contains no abnormal substances such as glucose or albumin. Because of the intense thirst, the patient tends to drink 2 to 20 L of fluid daily and craves cold water. In the hereditary form of diabetes insipidus, the primary symptoms may begin at birth. In adults, the onset of diabetes insipidus may be abrupt or insidious.

The disease cannot be controlled by limiting fluid intake, because the high-volume loss of urine continues even without fluid replacement. Attempts to restrict fluids cause the patient to experience an insatiable craving for fluid and to develop hypernatremia and severe dehydration.

Assessment and Diagnostic Findings

The fluid deprivation test is carried out by withholding fluids for 8 to 12 hours or until 3% to 5% of the body weight is lost. The patient is weighed frequently during the test. Plasma and urine osmolality studies are performed at the beginning and end of the test. The inability to increase the specific gravity and osmolality of the urine is characteristic of diabetes insipidus. The patient continues to excrete large volumes of urine with low specific gravity and experiences weight loss, increasing serum osmolality, and elevated serum sodium levels. The patient's condition needs to be monitored frequently during the test, and the test is terminated if tachycardia, excessive weight loss, or hypotension develops.

Other diagnostic procedures include concurrent measurements of plasma levels of ADH and plasma and urine osmolality as well as a trial of desmopressin (synthetic vasopressin) therapy and intravenous (IV) infusion of hypertonic saline solution. If the diagnosis is confirmed and the cause (eg, head injury) is not obvious, the patient is carefully assessed for tumors that may be causing the disorder.

Medical Management

The objectives of therapy are (1) to replace ADH (which is usually a long-term therapeutic program), (2) to ensure adequate fluid replacement, and (3) to identify and correct the underlying intracranial pathology. Nephrogenic causes require different management approaches.

PHARMACOLOGIC THERAPY

Desmopressin (DDAVP), a synthetic vasopressin without the vascular effects of natural ADH, is particularly valuable because it has a longer duration of action and fewer adverse effects than other preparations previously used to treat the disease. It is administered intranasally; the patient sprays the solution into the nose through a flexible calibrated plastic tube. One or two administrations daily (ie, every 12 to 24 hours) usually control the symptoms (Tierney, McPhee, & Papadakis, 2005).

Intramuscular administration of ADH, vasopressin tannate in oil, is used if the intranasal route is not possible. The medication is administered every 24 to 96 hours. The vial of medication should be warmed or shaken vigorously before administration. The injection is administered in the evening so that maximum results are obtained during sleep. Abdominal cramps are a side effect of this medication. Rotation of injection sites is necessary to prevent lipodystrophy.

Clofibrate, a hypolipidemic agent, has been found to have an antidiuretic effect on patients with diabetes insipidus who have some residual hypothalamic vasopressin. Chlorpropamide (Diabinese) and thiazide diuretics are also used in mild forms of the disease because they potentiate the action of vasopressin. The patient receiving chlorpropamide should be warned of the possibility of hypoglycemic reactions.

If the diabetes insipidus is renal in origin, the previously described treatments are ineffective. Thiazide diuretics, mild salt depletion, and prostaglandin inhibitors (ibuprofen, indomethacin, and aspirin) are used to treat the nephrogenic form of diabetes insipidus.

Nursing Management

The patient with possible diabetes insipidus needs support while undergoing studies for a possible cranial lesion. The nurse needs to inform the patient and family about follow-up care and emergency measures. The nurse also needs to provide specific verbal and written instructions, show the patient how to administer the medications, and observe return demonstrations as appropriate. The nurse also advises the patient to wear a medical identification bracelet and to carry medication and information about this disorder at all times. Vasopressin must be administered with caution if the patient has coronary artery disease, because the medication causes vasoconstriction.

Syndrome of Inappropriate Antidiuretic Hormone Secretion

The **syndrome of inappropriate antidiuretic hormone (SIADH) secretion** includes excessive ADH secretion from the pituitary gland even in the face of subnormal serum osmolality. Patients with this disorder cannot excrete a dilute urine. They retain fluids and develop a sodium deficiency known as **dilutional hyponatremia.** SIADH is often of nonendocrine origin; for instance, the syndrome may occur in patients with bronchogenic carcinoma in which malignant lung cells synthesize and release ADH. SIADH has also occurred in patients with severe pneumonia, pneumothorax, and other disorders of the lungs, as well as malignant tumors that affect other organs (Porth, 2005).

Disorders of the central nervous system, such as head injury, brain surgery or tumor, and infection, are thought to produce SIADH by direct stimulation of the pituitary gland. Some medications (eg, vincristine, phenothiazines, tricyclic antidepressants, thiazide diuretics) and nicotine have been implicated in SIADH; they either directly stimulate the pituitary gland or increase the sensitivity of renal tubules to circulating ADH.

Eliminating the underlying cause, if possible, and restricting fluid intake are typical interventions for managing this syndrome. Because retained water is excreted slowly through the kidneys, the extracellular fluid volume contracts and the serum sodium concentration gradually increases toward normal. Diuretics such as furosemide (Lasix) may be used along with fluid restriction if severe hyponatremia is present.

Close monitoring of fluid intake and output, daily weight, urine and blood chemistries, and neurologic status is indicated for the patient at risk for SIADH. Supportive measures and explanations of procedures and treatments assist the patient to deal with this disorder.

The Thyroid Gland

The thyroid gland is a butterfly-shaped organ located in the lower neck, anterior to the trachea (Fig. 42-3). It consists of two lateral lobes connected by an isthmus. The gland is about 5 cm long and 3 cm wide and weighs about 30 g. The blood flow to the thyroid is very high (about 5 mL/min per gram of thyroid tissue), approximately five times the blood flow to the liver. This reflects the high metabolic activity of the thyroid gland. The thyroid gland produces three hormones: **thyroxine (T_4), triiodothyronine (T_3),** and **calcitonin.** T_4 and T_3 are referred to collectively as thyroid hormone.

Anatomic and Physiologic Overview

Various hormones and chemicals are responsible for normal thyroid function. Key among them are thyroid hormone, calcitonin, and iodine.

Thyroid Hormone

T_4 and T_3, the two separate hormones produced by the thyroid gland that make up thyroid hormone, are amino acids with the unique property of containing iodine molecules bound to the amino acid structure. T_4 contains four iodine atoms in each molecule, and T_3 contains three. These hor-

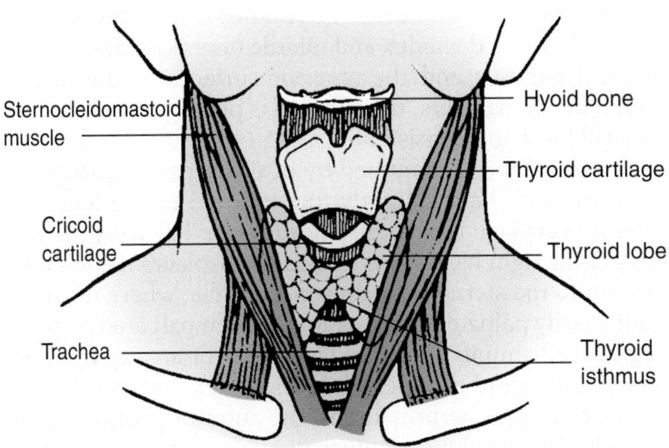

FIGURE 42-3. The thyroid gland and surrounding structures. From Weber, J. W. & Kelley, J. (2003). *Health assessment in nursing* (2nd ed.). Philadelphia: Lippincott Williams & Wilkins.

mones are synthesized and stored bound to proteins in the cells of the thyroid gland until needed for release into the bloodstream. About 75% of bound thyroid hormone is bound to thyroxine-binding globulin (TBG); the remaining bound thyroid hormone is bound to thyroid-binding prealbumin and albumin.

Synthesis of Thyroid Hormone

Iodine is essential to the thyroid gland for synthesis of its hormones. In fact, the major use of iodine in the body is by the thyroid, and the major derangement in iodine deficiency is alteration of thyroid function. Iodide is ingested in the diet and absorbed into the blood in the gastrointestinal tract. The thyroid gland is extremely efficient at taking up iodide from the blood and concentrating it within the cells, where iodide ions are converted to iodine molecules, which react with tyrosine (an amino acid) to form the thyroid hormones.

Regulation of Thyroid Hormone

The secretion of T_3 and T_4 by the thyroid gland is controlled by TSH (also called thyrotropin) from the anterior pituitary gland. TSH controls the rate of thyroid hormone release. In turn, the level of thyroid hormone in the blood determines the release of TSH. If the thyroid hormone concentration in the blood decreases, the release of TSH increases, which causes increased output of T_3 and T_4. This is an example of negative feedback. The term **euthyroid** refers to thyroid hormone production that is within normal limits.

Thyrotropin-releasing hormone (TRH), secreted by the hypothalamus, exerts a modulating influence on the release of TSH from the pituitary. Environmental factors, such as a decrease in temperature, may lead to increased secretion of TRH, resulting in elevated secretion of thyroid hormones. Figure 42-4 shows the hypothalamic–pituitary–thyroid axis, which regulates thyroid hormone production.

Function of Thyroid Hormone

The primary function of thyroid hormone is to control cellular metabolic activity. T_4, a relatively weak hormone, maintains body metabolism in a steady state. T_3 is about five times as potent as T_4 and has a more rapid metabolic action. These hormones accelerate metabolic processes by increasing the level of specific enzymes that contribute to oxygen consumption and altering the responsiveness of tissues to other hormones. The thyroid hormones influence cell replication and are important in brain development. Thyroid hormone is also necessary for normal growth. The thyroid hormones, through their widespread effects on cellular metabolism, influence every major organ system.

Calcitonin

Calcitonin, or thyrocalcitonin, is another important hormone secreted by the thyroid gland. It is secreted in response to high plasma levels of calcium, and it reduces the plasma level of calcium by increasing its deposition in bone.

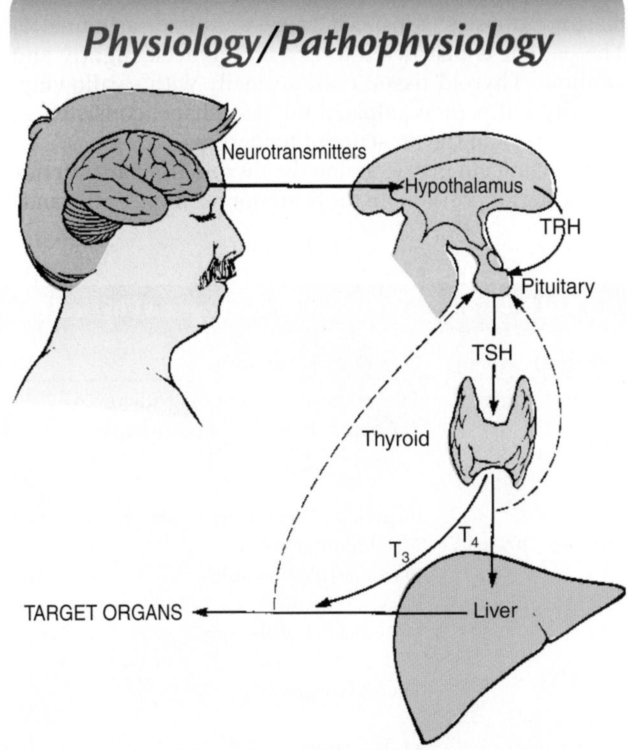

FIGURE 42-4. The hypothalamic–pituitary–thyroid axis. Thyroid-releasing hormone (TRH) from the hypothalamus stimulates the pituitary gland to secrete thyroid-stimulating hormone (TSH). TSH stimulates the thyroid to produce thyroid hormone (T_3 and T_4). High circulating levels of T_3 and T_4 inhibit further TSH secretion and thyroid hormone production through a negative feedback mechanism (*dashed lines*).

Pathophysiology

Inadequate secretion of thyroid hormone during fetal and neonatal development results in stunted physical and mental growth (**cretinism**) because of general depression of metabolic activity. In adults, hypothyroidism manifests as lethargy, slow mentation, and generalized slowing of body functions.

Oversecretion of thyroid hormones (hyperthyroidism) is manifested by a greatly increased metabolic rate. Many of the other characteristics of hyperthyroidism result from the increased response to circulating catecholamines (epinephrine and norepinephrine). Oversecretion of thyroid hormones is usually associated with an enlarged thyroid gland (**goiter**). Goiter also commonly occurs with iodine deficiency. In this latter condition, lack of iodine results in low levels of circulating thyroid hormones, which causes increased release of TSH; the elevated TSH causes overproduction of thyroglobulin (a precursor of T_3 and T_4) and hypertrophy of the thyroid gland.

Assessment and Diagnostic Findings

Physical Examination

The thyroid gland is inspected and palpated routinely in all patients. Inspection begins with identification of landmarks. The lower neck region between the sternocleidomastoid muscles is inspected for swelling or asymmetry. The patient is instructed to extend the neck slightly and swallow. Thyroid tissue rises normally with swallowing. The thyroid is then palpated for size, shape, consistency, symmetry, and the presence of tenderness.

The clinician may examine the thyroid from an anterior or a posterior position. In the posterior position, both hands encircle the patient's neck. The thumbs rest on the nape of the neck, while the index and middle fingers palpate for the thyroid isthmus and the anterior surfaces of the lateral lobes. When palpable, the isthmus is perceived as firm and of a rubber-band consistency.

The left lobe is examined by positioning the patient so that the neck flexes slightly forward and to the left. The thyroid cartilage is then displaced to the left with the fingers of the right hand. This maneuver displaces the left lobe deep into the sternocleidomastoid muscle, where it can be more easily palpated. The left lobe is then palpated by placing the left thumb deep into the posterior area of the sternocleidomastoid muscle, while the index and middle fingers exert opposite pressure in the anterior portion of the muscle. Having the patient swallow during the maneuver may assist the examiner to locate the thyroid as it ascends in the neck. The procedure is reversed to examine the right lobe. The isthmus is the only portion of the thyroid that is normally palpable. If a patient has a very thin neck, two thin, smooth, nontender lobes may also be palpable.

If palpation discloses an enlarged thyroid gland, both lobes are auscultated using the diaphragm of the stethoscope. Auscultation identifies the localized audible vibration of a bruit. This abnormal finding indicates increased blood flow through the thyroid gland and necessitates referral to a physician. Tenderness, enlargement, and nodularity within the thyroid also require referral for additional evaluation (Table 42-2) (Bickley & Szilagyi, 2003).

Laboratory and Diagnostic Studies

Assessment measures in addition to palpation and auscultation include thyroid function tests, such as laboratory measurement of thyroid hormones, thyroid scanning, biopsy, and ultrasonography. The most widely used tests are serum immunoassay for TSH and free T_4 (Tierney et al., 2005).

TABLE 42-2 Summary of Findings on Physical Examination of the Thyroid Gland

Physical Finding	Differential Diagnosis	Special Features
Single nodule	Autonomously functioning adenoma	Opposite lobe not palpable
	Adenoma or adenomatous nodule	Rubbery, firm; tenderness suggests recent hemorrhage or infarction
	Cancer	Usually hard; may have associated lymph node enlargement or vocal cord palsy
	Hyperplasia secondary to unilobar agenesis	Opposite lobe not palpable
Multiple nodules	Multinodular goiter Hashimoto's thyroiditis	Firm lobes or irregular surface may be misinterpreted as multiple nodules
Diffuse goiter	Graves' disease	Bruit or thrill; pyramidal lobe
	Hashimoto's thyroiditis	Irregular surface; pyramidal lobe; rubbery or firm; occasionally tender; fibrous variant may be hard
	Thyroid lymphoma	Rapidly growing goiter, particularly in setting of preexisting Hashimoto's thyroiditis
	Multinodular goiter	Nodules may be hidden within gland and may become apparent with thyroid hormone suppression
Tenderness	Subacute thyroiditis	Unilateral or bilateral; tenderness often severe
	Hemorrhagic or infarcted adenoma	Discrete nodule with tenderness
	Hashimoto's thyroiditis	Mild tenderness
	Cancer	Irregular, firm thyroid nodule with chronic tenderness

Measurement of TSH has a sensitivity of 98% and specificity of greater than 92% (U.S. Preventive Services Task Force, 2004). Free T_4 levels correlate with metabolic status; they are elevated in hyperthyroidism and decreased in hypothyroidism. Ultrasound, CT, and MRI may be used to clarify or confirm the results of other diagnostic studies.

Thyroid Tests

SERUM THYROID-STIMULATING HORMONE

Measurement of the serum TSH concentration is the single best screening test of thyroid function in outpatients because of its high sensitivity. The ability to detect minute changes in serum TSH makes it possible to distinguish subclinical thyroid disease from euthyroid states in patients with low or high normal values. Values greater than the normal range of 0.4 to 6.15 μU/mL indicate primary hypothyroidism, and low values indicate hyperthyroidism. If the TSH is normal, there is a 98% chance that the free T_4 is also normal. Measurement of TSH is also used for monitoring thyroid hormone replacement therapy and for differentiating between disorders of the thyroid gland itself and disorders of the pituitary or hypothalamus. Current recommendations suggest TSH screening for all adults beginning at 35 years of age, and every 5 years thereafter (U.S. Preventive Services Task Force, 2004).

SERUM FREE T_4

The test most commonly used to confirm an abnormal TSH result is free T_4. It is a direct measurement of free (unbound) thyroxine, the only metabolically active fraction of T_4. The range of free T_4 in serum is normally 0.9 to 1.7 ng/dL (11.5 to 21.8 pmol/L). When measured by the dialysis method, free T_4 is not affected by variations in protein binding and is the procedure of choice for monitoring the changes in T_4 secretion during treatment of hyperthyroidism. Measurement of free T_4 by the immunoassay technique is less reliable, because it can be affected by medication, illness, or changes in protein binding.

SERUM T_3 AND T_4

Measurement of total T_3 or T_4 includes protein-bound and free hormone levels that occur in response to TSH secretion. T_4 is 80% bound to TBG; T_3 is bound less firmly. Only 0.03% of T_4 and 0.3% of T_3 are unbound. Any factor that alters binding proteins also changes the T_3 and T_4 levels. Serious systemic illnesses, medications (eg, oral contraceptives, corticosteroids, phenytoin, salicylates), and protein wasting as a result of nephrosis or use of androgens may interfere with accurate test results. Normal range for T_4 is 4.5 to 11.5 μg/dL (58.5 to 150 nmol/L). Although serum T_3 and T_4 levels generally increase or decrease together, the T_3 level appears to be a more accurate indicator of hyperthyroidism, which causes a greater increase in T_3 than in T_4 levels. The normal range for serum T_3 is 70 to 220 ng/dL (1.15 to 3.10 nmol/L).

T_3 RESIN UPTAKE TEST

The T_3 resin uptake test is an indirect measure of unsaturated thyroxine-binding globulin (TBG). Its purpose is to determine the amount of thyroid hormone bound to TBG and the number of available binding sites. This provides an index of the amount of thyroid hormone already present in the circulation. Normally, TBG is not fully saturated with thyroid hormone, and additional binding sites are available to combine with radioiodine-labeled T_3 added to the blood specimen. The normal T_3 uptake value is 25% to 35% (relative uptake fraction, 0.25 to 0.35), which indicates that about one third of the available sites of TBG are occupied by thyroid hormone. If the number of free or unoccupied binding sites is low, as in hyperthyroidism, the T_3 uptake is greater than 35% (0.35). If the number of available sites is high, as occurs in hypothyroidism, the test result is less than 25% (0.25).

T_3 uptake is useful in the evaluation of thyroid hormone levels in patients who have received diagnostic or therapeutic doses of iodine. The test results may be altered by the use of estrogens, androgens, salicylates, phenytoin, anticoagulants, or corticosteroids.

THYROID ANTIBODIES

Autoimmune thyroid diseases include both hypothyroid and hyperthyroid conditions. Results of testing by immunoassay techniques for antithyroid antibodies, specifically antimicrosomal antibodies, are positive in chronic autoimmune thyroid disease (90%), Hashimoto's thyroiditis (100%), Graves' disease (80%), and other organ-specific autoimmune diseases, such as lupus erythematosus and rheumatoid arthritis. Antithyroid antibody titers are normally present in 5% to 10% of the population and increase with age.

RADIOACTIVE IODINE UPTAKE

The radioactive iodine uptake test measures the rate of iodine uptake by the thyroid gland. The patient is administered a tracer dose of iodine 123 (^{123}I) or another radionuclide, and a count is made over the thyroid gland with a scintillation counter, which detects and counts the gamma rays released from the breakdown of ^{123}I in the thyroid. It measures the proportion of the administered dose that is present in the thyroid gland at a specific time after its administration. It is a simple test and provides reliable results. It is affected by the patient's intake of iodide or thyroid hormone; therefore, a careful preliminary clinical history is essential in evaluating results. Normal values vary from one geographic region to another and with the intake of iodine. Patients with hyperthyroidism exhibit a high uptake of the ^{123}I (in some patients, as high as 90%), whereas patients with hypothyroidism exhibit a very low uptake.

FINE-NEEDLE ASPIRATION BIOPSY

Use of a small-gauge needle to sample the thyroid tissue for biopsy is a safe and accurate method of detecting malignancy. It is often the initial test for evaluation of thyroid masses. Results are reported as (1) negative (benign), (2) positive (malignant), (3) indeterminate (suspicious), and (4) inadequate (nondiagnostic).

THYROID SCAN, RADIOSCAN, OR SCINTISCAN

In a thyroid scan, a scintillation detector or gamma camera moves back and forth across the area to be studied in a series of parallel tracks, and a visual image is made of the distribution of radioactivity in the area being scanned. Although ^{123}I has been the most commonly used isotope, several other radioactive isotopes, including technetium 99m (^{99m}Tc) pertechnetate, thallium, and americium, are also used.

Scans are helpful in determining the location, size, shape, and anatomic function of the thyroid gland, particularly when thyroid tissue is substernal or large. Identifying areas of increased function ("hot" areas) or decreased function ("cold" areas) can assist in diagnosis. Although most areas of decreased function do not represent malignancies, lack of function increases the likelihood of malignancy, particularly if only one nonfunctioning area is present. Scanning of the entire body, to obtain the total body profile, may be carried out in a search for a functioning thyroid metastasis (ie, a lesion that produces thyroid hormones).

SERUM THYROGLOBULIN

Thyroglobulin (Tg) can be measured reliably in the serum by radioimmunoassay. Clinically, it is used to detect persistence or recurrence of thyroid carcinoma.

Nursing Implications

When thyroid tests are scheduled, it is necessary to determine whether the patient has taken medications or agents that contain iodine, because these may alter the test results. Iodine-containing medications include contrast agents and those used to treat thyroid disorders. Less obvious sources of iodine are topical antiseptics, multivitamin preparations, and food supplements frequently found in health food stores; cough syrups; and amiodarone, an antiarrhythmic agent. Other medications that may affect test results are estrogens, salicylates, amphetamines, chemotherapeutic agents, antibiotics, corticosteroids, and mercurial diuretics. The nurse asks the patient about the use of these medications and notes their use on the laboratory requisition. Chart 42-1 gives a partial list of agents that may interfere with accurate testing of thyroid gland function.

CHART 42-1

℞ PHARMACOLOGY • Partial List of Medications That May Alter Thyroid Test Results

Estrogens	Opioids
Sulfonylureas	Androgens
Corticosteroids	Salicylates
Iodine	Lithium
Propranolol	Amiodarone
Cimetidine	Clofibrate
5-Fluorouracil	Furosemide
Phenytoin	Diazepam
Heparin	Danazol
Chloral hydrate	Dopamine antagonists
X-ray contrast agents	Propylthiouracil

Specific Disorders of the Thyroid Gland

Hypothyroidism

Hypothyroidism results from suboptimal levels of thyroid hormone. Thyroid deficiency can affect all body functions and can range from mild, subclinical forms to **myxedema**, an advanced form. The most common cause of hypothyroidism in adults is autoimmune thyroiditis (**Hashimoto's disease**), in which the immune system attacks the thyroid gland. Symptoms of hyperthyroidism may later be followed by those of hypothyroidism and myxedema. Hypothyroidism also commonly occurs in patients with previous hyperthyroidism that has been treated with radioiodine or antithyroid medications or thyroidectomy. It occurs most frequently in older women. There is an increased incidence of thyroid cancer in men who have undergone radiation therapy for head and neck cancer. Therefore, testing of thyroid function is recommended for all patients who receive such treatment. Other causes of hypothyroidism are presented in Chart 42-2.

More than 95% of patients with hypothyroidism have primary or thyroidal hypothyroidism, which refers to dysfunction of the thyroid gland itself. If the cause of the thyroid dysfunction is failure of the pituitary gland, the hypothalamus, or both, the hypothyroidism is known as central hypothyroidism. If the cause is entirely a pituitary disorder, it may be referred to as pituitary or secondary hypothyroidism. if the cause is a disorder of the hypothalamus resulting in inadequate secretion of TSH due to decreased stimulation by TRH, it is referred to as hypothalamic or tertiary hypothyroidism. If thyroid deficiency is present at birth, the hypothyroidism is known as cretinism. In such instances, the mother may also have thyroid deficiency.

The term myxedema refers to the accumulation of mucopolysaccharides in subcutaneous and other interstitial

CHART 42-2

Causes of Hypothyroidism

- Autoimmune disease (Hashimoto's thyroiditis, post-Graves' disease)
- Atrophy of thyroid gland with aging
- Therapy for hyperthyroidism
  - Radioactive iodine (^{131}I)
  - Thyroidectomy
- Medications
  - Lithium
  - Iodine compounds
  - Antithyroid medications
- Radiation to head and neck for treatment of head and neck cancers, lymphoma
- Infiltrative diseases of the thyroid (amyloidosis, scleroderma, lymphoma)
- Iodine deficiency and iodine excess

tissues. Although myxedema occurs in long-standing hypothyroidism, the term is used appropriately only to describe the extreme symptoms of severe hypothyroidism.

Clinical Manifestations

Early symptoms of hypothyroidism are nonspecific, but extreme fatigue makes it difficult for the person to complete a full day's work or participate in usual activities. Reports of hair loss, brittle nails, and dry skin are common, and numbness and tingling of the fingers may occur. On occasion, the voice may become husky, and the patient may complain of hoarseness. Menstrual disturbances such as menorrhagia or amenorrhea occur, in addition to loss of libido. Hypothyroidism affects women five times more frequently than men and occurs most often between the ages of 30 and 60 years.

Severe hypothyroidism results in a subnormal temperature and pulse rate. The patient usually begins to gain weight even without an increase in food intake, although he or she may be cachectic. The skin becomes thickened because of an accumulation of mucopolysaccharides in the subcutaneous tissues (the origin of the term myxedema). The hair thins and falls out, and the face becomes expressionless and masklike. The patient often complains of being cold even in a warm environment.

At first, the patient may be irritable and may complain of fatigue, but as the condition progresses, the emotional responses are subdued. The mental processes become dulled, and the patient appears apathetic. Speech is slow, the tongue enlarges, and hands and feet increase in size. The patient frequently complains of constipation. Deafness may also occur.

Advanced hypothyroidism may produce personality and cognitive changes characteristic of dementia. Inadequate ventilation and sleep apnea can occur with severe hypothyroidism. Pleural effusion, pericardial effusion, and respiratory muscle weakness may also occur.

Severe hypothyroidism is associated with an elevated serum cholesterol level, atherosclerosis, coronary artery disease, and poor left ventricular function. The patient with advanced hypothyroidism is hypothermic and abnormally sensitive to sedatives, opioids, and anesthetic agents. Therefore, these medications are administered only with extreme caution.

Patients with unrecognized hypothyroidism who are undergoing surgery are at increased risk for intraoperative hypotension, postoperative heart failure, and altered mental status.

Myxedema coma describes the most extreme, severe stage of hypothyroidism, in which the patient is hypothermic and unconscious. Increasing lethargy may progress to stupor and then coma. Myxedema coma may also develop with undiagnosed hypothyroidism and may be precipitated by infection or other systemic disease or by use of sedatives or opioid analgesic agents. The patient's respiratory drive is depressed, resulting in alveolar hypoventilation, progressive carbon dioxide retention, narcosis, and coma. These symptoms, along with cardiovascular collapse and shock, require aggressive and intensive therapy if the patient is to survive. However, even with early vigorous therapy, the mortality rate is high.

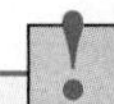

NURSING ALERT

In all patients with hypothyroidism, the effects of analgesic agents, sedatives, and anesthetic agents are prolonged; particular caution is necessary in administering these agents to elderly patients because of concurrent changes in liver and renal function.

Medical Management

The primary objective in the management of hypothyroidism is to restore a normal metabolic state by replacing the missing hormone.

PHARMACOLOGIC THERAPY

Synthetic levothyroxine (Synthroid or Levothroid) is the preferred preparation for treating hypothyroidism and suppressing nontoxic goiters. The dosage for hormone replacement is based on the patient's serum TSH concentration. Desiccated thyroid is used infrequently today, because it often results in transient elevated serum concentrations of T_3, with occasional symptoms of hyperthyroidism. If replacement therapy is adequate, the symptoms of myxedema disappear and normal metabolic activity is resumed.

Prevention of Cardiac Dysfunction. Any patient who has had hypothyroidism for a long period is almost certain to have elevated serum cholesterol, atherosclerosis, and coronary artery disease. As long as metabolism is subnormal and the tissues, including the myocardium, require relatively little oxygen, a reduction in blood supply is tolerated without overt symptoms of coronary artery disease. When thyroid hormone is administered, the oxygen demand increases, but oxygen delivery cannot be increased unless, or until, the atherosclerosis improves. This occurs very slowly, if at all. The occurrence of angina is the signal that the oxygen needs of the myocardium exceed its blood supply. Angina or dysrhythmias can occur when thyroid replacement is initiated because thyroid hormones enhance the cardiovascular effects of catecholamines.

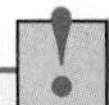

NURSING ALERT

The nurse must monitor for myocardial ischemia or infarction, which can occur in response to therapy in patients with severe, long-standing hypothyroidism or myxedema coma. The nurse must also be alert for signs of angina, especially during the early phase of treatment; if detected, it must be reported and treated at once to avoid a fatal myocardial infarction.

Obviously, if angina or dysrhythmias occur, thyroid hormone administration must be discontinued immediately. Later, when it can be resumed safely, thyroid hormone replacement should be prescribed cautiously at a lower dosage and under the close observation of the physician and the nurse.

Prevention of Medication Interactions. Precautions must be taken during the course of therapy because of the interaction of thyroid hormones with other medications. Thyroid hormones may increase blood glucose levels, which may necessitate adjustment in the dosage of insulin or oral antidiabetic agents in patients with diabetes. The effects of thyroid hormone may be increased by phenytoin (Dilantin) and by tricyclic antidepressant agents. Thyroid hormones may also increase the pharmacologic effects of digitalis glycosides, anticoagulant agents, and indomethacin, necessitating careful observation and assessment by the nurse for side effects. Bone loss and osteoporosis may also occur with thyroid therapy.

Even in small doses, hypnotic and sedative agents may induce profound somnolence, lasting far longer than anticipated. Furthermore, they are likely to cause respiratory depression, which can easily be fatal because of decreased respiratory reserve and alveolar hypoventilation. If their use is necessary, the dose should be one half or one third of that ordinarily prescribed in patients of similar age and weight with normal thyroid function. If these medications must be used, the patient must be monitored closely for signs of impending narcosis (stuporlike condition) or respiratory failure.

SUPPORTIVE THERAPY

In severe hypothyroidism and myxedema coma, management includes maintaining vital functions. Arterial blood gases may be measured to determine carbon dioxide retention and to guide the use of assisted ventilation to combat hypoventilation. Pulse oximetry may also be helpful in monitoring oxygen saturation levels. Fluids are administered cautiously because of the danger of water intoxication. Application of external heat (eg, heating pads) is avoided, because it increases oxygen requirements and may lead to vascular collapse. If hypoglycemia is evident, concentrated glucose may be prescribed to provide glucose without precipitating fluid overload. If myxedema has progressed to myxedema coma, thyroid hormone (usually Levothyroxine) is administered intravenously until consciousness is restored. Treatment then continues with oral thyroid hormone therapy. Because of an associated adrenocortical insufficiency, corticosteroid therapy may be necessary.

Nursing Management

Nursing care of the patient with hypothyroidism and myxedema is summarized in the plan of nursing care in Chart 42-3.

MODIFYING ACTIVITY

The patient with hypothyroidism experiences decreased energy and moderate to severe lethargy. As a result, the risk of complications from immobility increases. The patient's ability to exercise and to participate in activities is further limited by the changes in cardiovascular and pulmonary status that occur secondary to hypothyroidism. A major role of the nurse is assisting with care and hygiene while encouraging the patient to participate in activities within established tolerance levels, to prevent the complications of immobility.

MONITORING PHYSICAL STATUS

The nurse closely monitors the patient's vital signs and cognitive level to detect the following:

- Deterioration of physical and mental status
- Signs and symptoms indicating that treatment has resulted in a metabolic rate exceeding the ability of the cardiovascular and pulmonary systems to respond
- Continued limitations or complications of myxedema

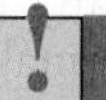
NURSING ALERT

Medications are administered to the patient with hypothyroidism with extreme caution because of the potential for altered metabolism and excretion and depressed metabolic rate and respiratory status.

PROMOTING PHYSICAL COMFORT

The patient often experiences chilling and extreme intolerance to cold, even if the room feels comfortable or hot to others. Extra clothing and blankets are provided, and the patient is protected from drafts. Use of heating pads and electric blankets is avoided because of the risk for peripheral vasodilation, further loss of body heat, and vascular collapse. In addition, the patient could be burned by these items without being aware of it because of delayed responses and decreased mental status.

ENHANCING COPING MEASURES

The patient with moderate to severe hypothyroidism may experience severe emotional reactions to changes in appearance and body image and the frequent delay in diagnosis. The nonspecific, early symptoms may have produced negative reactions by family members and friends, who may have labeled the patient mentally unstable, uncooperative, or unwilling to participate in self-care activities.

As hypothyroidism is treated successfully and symptoms subside, the patient may experience depression and guilt as a result of the progression and severity of symptoms that occurred. The nurse informs the patient and family that the symptoms and inability to recognize them are common and are part of the disorder itself. The patient and family may require assistance and counseling to deal with the emotional concerns and reactions that result.

PROMOTING HOME AND COMMUNITY-BASED CARE

Teaching Patients Self-Care. Because most hypothyroidism treatment takes place at home, the patient and family require

(text continues on page 1458)

CHART 42-3

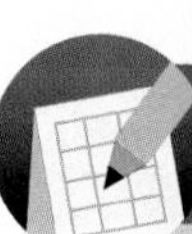

Plan of Nursing Care Care of the Patient With Hypothyroidism

Nursing Diagnosis: Activity intolerance related to fatigue and depressed cognitive process
Goal: Increased participation in activities and increased independence

NURSING INTERVENTIONS	RATIONALE	EXPECTED OUTCOMES
1. Promote independence in self-care activities.	1. Encouragement needed in fatigued, often depressed patient	• Participates in self-care activities • Reports decreased level of fatigue • Displays interest and awareness in environment • Participates in activities and events in environment • Participates in family events and activities • Reports no chest pain, increased fatigue, or breathlessness with increased level of activity
a. Space activities to promote rest and exercise as tolerated.	a. Encourages activities while allowing time for adequate rest	
b. Assist with self-care activities when patient is fatigued.	b. Permits patient to participate to the extent possible in self-care activities	
c. Provide stimulation through conversation and nonstressful activities.	c. Promotes interest without overly stressing the patient	
d. Monitor patient's response to increasing activities.	d. Guards against over- and underexertion by the patient	

Nursing Diagnosis: Risk for imbalanced body temperature
Goal: Maintenance of normal body temperature

NURSING INTERVENTIONS	RATIONALE	EXPECTED OUTCOMES
1. Provide extra layer of clothing or extra blanket.	1. Minimizes heat loss	• Experiences relief of discomfort and cold intolerance • Maintains baseline body temperature • Reports adequate feeling of warmth and lack of chilling • Uses extra layer of clothing or extra blanket • Explains rationale for avoiding external heat source
2. Avoid and discourage use of external heat source (eg, heating pads, electric or warming blankets).	2. Reduces risk of peripheral vasodilation and vascular collapse	
3. Monitor patient's body temperature and report decreases from patient's baseline value.	3. Detects decreased body temperature and onset of myxedema coma	
4. Protect from exposure to cold and drafts.	4. Increases patient's level of comfort and decreases further heat loss	

Nursing Diagnosis: Constipation related to depressed gastrointestinal function
Goal: Return of normal bowel function

NURSING INTERVENTIONS	RATIONALE	EXPECTED OUTCOMES
1. Encourage increased fluid intake within limits of fluid restriction.	1. Promotes passage of soft stools	• Reports normal bowel function • Identifies and consumes foods high in fiber • Drinks recommended amount of fluid each day • Participates in gradually increasing exercises
2. Provide foods high in fiber.	2. Increases bulk of stools and more frequent bowel movements	
3. Instruct patient about foods with high water content.	3. Provides rationale for patient to increase fluid intake	
4. Monitor bowel function.	4. Permits detection of constipation and return to normal bowel pattern	

continued >

CHART 42-3

Plan of Nursing Care — Care of the Patient With Hypothyroidism (Continued)

NURSING INTERVENTIONS	RATIONALE	EXPECTED OUTCOMES
5. Encourage increased mobility within patient's exercise tolerance. 6. Encourage patient to use laxatives and enemas sparingly.	5. Promotes evacuation of the bowel 6. Minimizes patient's dependence on laxatives and enemas and encourages normal pattern of bowel evacuation	• Uses laxatives as prescribed and avoids excessive dependence on laxatives and enemas

Nursing Diagnosis: Deficient knowledge about the therapeutic regimen for lifelong thyroid replacement therapy
Goal: Knowledge and acceptance of the prescribed therapeutic regimen

NURSING INTERVENTIONS	RATIONALE	EXPECTED OUTCOMES
1. Explain rationale for thyroid hormone replacement. 2. Describe desired effects of medication to patient. 3. Assist patient to develop schedule and checklist to ensure self-administration of thyroid replacement. 4. Describe signs and symptoms of over- and underdose of medication. 5. Explain the necessity for long-term follow-up to patient and family.	1. Provides rationale for patient to use thyroid hormone replacement as prescribed 2. Provides encouragement to patient by identifying improved physical status and well-being that will occur with thyroid hormone therapy and return to a euthyroid state 3. Increases chances that medication will be taken as prescribed 4. Serves as check for patient to determine if therapeutic goals are met 5. Increases likelihood that hypo- or hyperthyroidism will be detected and treated	• Describes therapeutic regimen correctly • Explains rationale for thyroid hormone replacement • Identifies positive outcomes of thyroid hormone replacement • Administers medication to self as prescribed • Identifies adverse side effects that should be reported promptly to physician: recurrence of symptoms of hypothyroidism and occurrence of symptoms of hyperthyroidism • Restates need for periodic/long-term follow-up visits to physician

Nursing Diagnosis: Ineffective breathing pattern related to depressed ventilation
Goal: Improved respiratory status and maintenance of normal breathing pattern

NURSING INTERVENTIONS	RATIONALE	EXPECTED OUTCOMES
1. Monitor respiratory rate, depth, pattern, pulse oximetry, and arterial blood gases. 2. Encourage deep breathing, coughing, and use of incentive spirometry. 3. Administer medications (hypnotics and sedatives) with caution.	1. Identifies patient's baseline to monitor further changes and evaluate effectiveness of interventions 2. Prevents atelectasis and promotes adequate ventilation 3. Patients with hypothyroidism are *very* susceptible to respiratory depression with use of hypnotics and sedatives.	• Shows improved respiratory status and maintenance of normal breathing pattern • Demonstrates normal respiratory rate, depth, and pattern • Takes deep breaths, coughs, and uses incentive spirometry when encouraged • Demonstrates normal breath sounds without adventitious sounds on auscultation

Plan of Nursing Care — Care of the Patient With Hypothyroidism (Continued)

NURSING INTERVENTIONS	RATIONALE	EXPECTED OUTCOMES
4. Maintain patent airway through suction and ventilatory support if indicated (see Chapter 25 for care of patients requiring mechanical ventilation).	4. Use of an artificial airway and ventilatory support may be necessary with respiratory depression.	• Explains rationale for cautious use of medications • Cooperates with suction procedure and ventilator support when necessary

Nursing Diagnosis: Disturbed thought processes related to depressed metabolism and altered cardiovascular and respiratory status
Goal: Improved thought processes

NURSING INTERVENTIONS	RATIONALE	EXPECTED OUTCOMES
1. Orient patient to time, place, date, and events around him or her.	1. Provides reality orientation to patient	• Shows improved cognitive functioning • Identifies time, place, date, and events correctly
2. Provide stimulation through conversation and nonthreatening activities.	2. Provides stimulation within patient's level of tolerance for stress	• Responds when stimulated • Responds spontaneously as treatment becomes effective
3. Explain to patient and family that change in cognitive and mental functioning is a result of disease process.	3. Reassures patient and family about the cause of the cognitive changes and that a positive outcome is possible with appropriate treatment	• Interacts spontaneously with family and environment • Explains that change in mental and cognitive processes is a result of disease processes
4. Monitor cognitive and mental processes and response of these to medication and other therapy.	4. Permits evaluation of the effectiveness of treatment	• Takes medications as prescribed to prevent decrease in cognitive processes

Collaborative Problem: Myxedema and myxedema coma
Goal: Absence of complications

NURSING INTERVENTIONS	RATIONALE	EXPECTED OUTCOMES
1. Monitor patient for increasing severity of signs and symptoms of hypothyroidism: a. Decreased level of consciousness; dementia b. Decreased vital signs (blood pressure, respiratory rate, temperature, pulse rate) c. Increasing difficulty in awakening or arousing patient	1. Extreme hypothyroidism may lead to myxedema, myxedema coma, and slowing of all body systems if untreated	• Exhibits reversal of myxedema and myxedema coma • Responds appropriately to questions and surroundings • Vital signs return to normal or near-normal ranges • Respiratory status improves with adequate spontaneous ventilatory effort
2. Assist in ventilatory support if respiratory depression and failure occur.	2. Ventilatory support is necessary to maintain adequate oxygenation and maintenance of airway	• Reports no episodes of angina or other indicators of cardiac insufficiency • Experiences minimal or no complications caused by immobility
3. Administer prescribed medications (eg, thyroxine) with extreme caution.	3. The slow metabolism and atherosclerosis of myxedema may result in angina with administration of thyroxine	

continued >

CHART 42-3

Plan of Nursing Care — Care of the Patient With Hypothyroidism (Continued)

NURSING INTERVENTIONS	RATIONALE	EXPECTED OUTCOMES
4. Turn and reposition patient at intervals.	4. Minimizes risks associated with immobility	
5. Avoid use of hypnotic, sedative, and analgesic agents.	5. Altered metabolism of these agents greatly increases the risks of their use in myxedema	

information and instruction that enable them to monitor the patient's condition and response to therapy. The nurse instructs the patient about the desired actions and side effects of medications and about how and when to take prescribed medications. In addition, the nurse also stresses the importance of continuing to take medications as prescribed even after symptoms improve. Because of the slowed mental processes that occur with hypothyroidism, it is also important to teach a family member about treatment goals, medication schedules, and side effects to be reported to the physician. The nurse provides written instructions and guidelines for the patient and family.

Dietary instruction is provided to promote weight loss once medication has been initiated and to promote return of normal bowel patterns. The patient and family are often very concerned about the changes they have observed as a result of the hypothyroid state. It is often reassuring for them to learn that many of the symptoms will disappear with effective treatment (Chart 42-4).

Continuing Care. The patient with hypothyroidism and myxedema coma needs considerable follow-up and health care. Before hospital discharge, arrangements are made to ensure that the patient returns to an environment that will promote adherence to the prescribed treatment plan. Assistance in devising a schedule or record ensures accurate and complete administration of medications. The nurse reinforces the importance of continued thyroid hormone replacement and periodic follow-up testing and instructs the patient and family members about the signs of overmedication and undermedication.

If indicated, a referral is made for home care. The home care nurse assesses the patient's progress toward recovery and ability to cope with the recent changes, along with the patient's physical and cognitive status and the patient's and

CHART 42-4

HOME CARE CHECKLIST • The Patient With Hypothyroidism (Myxedema)

At the completion of the home care instruction, the patient or caregiver will be able to:	Patient	Caregiver
• State present and potential effects of hypothyroidism on the body	✔	✔
• State precipitating factors and interventions for complications (hyperthyroidism, myxedema coma)	✔	✔
• Explain the purpose, dose, route, schedule, side effects, and precautions of prescribed medication (synthetic thyroid hormone)	✔	✔
• State that compliance with medical regimen is lifelong	✔	✔
• State the need to avoid extreme cold temperature until condition is stable	✔	✔
• State importance of regular follow-up visits with health care provider	✔	✔
• Identify dietary strategies to promote weight reduction and prevent constipation (high fiber, low calorie, adequate fluid intake)	✔	✔
• State potential for menstrual irregularities and potential for pregnancy for women	✔	✔
• State the importance of avoiding infection	✔	✔
• Identify changes in personality as related to hypothyroidism	✔	✔
• Identify areas of activity limitations and impact on lifestyle	✔	✔

family's understanding of the importance of prescribed long-term medication therapy and compliance with the medication schedule and recommended follow-up tests and appointments. The nurse documents, and reports to the patient's primary health care provider, subtle signs and symptoms that may indicate either inadequate or excessive thyroid hormone.

Gerontologic Considerations

Most patients with primary hypothyroidism are between the ages of 40 and 70 years and present with long-standing mild to moderate hypothyroidism. Subclinical disease is common among older women and can be asymptomatic or mistaken for other medical conditions (Li, 2002). Subtle symptoms of hypothyroidism, such as fatigue, muscle aches, and mental confusion, may be attributed to the normal aging process by the patient, family, and health care provider. The higher prevalence of hypothyroidism among elderly people may be related to alterations in immune function with age. Screening of TSH levels is recommended for women older than 50 years of age who have one or more symptoms, because they are at high risk for hypothyroidism (U.S. Preventive Services Task Force, 2004).

The signs and symptoms of hypothyroidism are often atypical in elderly people; the elderly patient may have few or no symptoms until the dysfunction is severe. Depression, apathy, and decreased mobility or activity may be the major initial symptoms and may be accompanied by significant weight loss. Constipation affects one fourth of elderly patients with hypothyroidism.

In the elderly patient with mild to moderate hypothyroidism, thyroid hormone replacement must be started with low dosages and increased gradually to prevent serious cardiovascular and neurologic side effects. Angina, for example, may occur with rapid thyroid replacement in the presence of coronary artery disease secondary to the hypothyroid state. Heart failure and tachydysrhythmias may worsen during the transition from the hypothyroid state to the normal metabolic state. Dementia may become more apparent during early thyroid hormone replacement in the elderly patient.

Elderly patients with severe hypothyroidism and atherosclerosis may become confused and agitated if their metabolic rate is increased too quickly. Marked clinical improvement follows the administration of hormone replacement; such medication must be continued for life, even though signs of hypothyroidism disappear within 3 to 12 weeks.

Myxedema and myxedema coma usually occur exclusively in patients older than 50 years of age. The high mortality rate of myxedema coma mandates immediate IV administration of high doses of thyroid hormone as well as supportive care.

The elderly patient requires periodic follow-up monitoring of serum TSH levels, because poor compliance with therapy may occur or the patient may take the medications erratically. A careful history can identify the need for further teaching about the importance of the medication.

Hyperthyroidism

Hyperthyroidism is the second most prevalent endocrine disorder, after diabetes mellitus. **Graves' disease**, the most common type of hyperthyroidism, results from an excessive output of thyroid hormones caused by abnormal stimulation of the thyroid gland by circulating immunoglobulins. It affects women eight times more frequently than men, with onset usually between the second and fourth decades (Tierney et al., 2005). It may appear after an emotional shock, stress, or an infection, but the exact significance of these relationships is not understood. Other common causes of hyperthyroidism include thyroiditis and excessive ingestion of thyroid hormone.

Clinical Manifestations

Patients with well-developed hyperthyroidism exhibit a characteristic group of signs and symptoms (sometimes referred to as **thyrotoxicosis**). The presenting symptom is often nervousness. These patients are often emotionally hyperexcitable, irritable, and apprehensive; they cannot sit quietly; they suffer from palpitations; and their pulse is abnormally rapid at rest as well as on exertion. They tolerate heat poorly and perspire unusually freely. The skin is flushed continuously, with a characteristic salmon color, and is likely to be warm, soft, and moist. However, elderly patients may report dry skin and diffuse pruritus. A fine tremor of the hands may be observed. Patients may exhibit **exophthalmos** (bulging eyes), which produces a startled facial expression.

Other manifestations include an increased appetite and dietary intake, progressive weight loss, abnormal muscular fatigability and weakness (difficulty in climbing stairs and rising from a chair), amenorrhea, and changes in bowel function. The pulse rate ranges constantly between 90 and 160 beats/min; the systolic, but characteristically not the diastolic, blood pressure is elevated; atrial fibrillation may occur; and cardiac decompensation in the form of heart failure is common, especially in elderly patients. Osteoporosis and fracture are also associated with hyperthyroidism.

Cardiac effects may include sinus tachycardia or dysrhythmias, increased pulse pressure, and palpitations; it has been suggested that these changes may be related to increased sensitivity to catecholamines or to changes in neurotransmitter turnover. Myocardial hypertrophy and heart failure may occur if the hyperthyroidism is severe and untreated.

The course of the disease may be mild, characterized by remissions and exacerbations and terminating with spontaneous recovery in a few months or years. Conversely, it may progress relentlessly, with the untreated person becoming emaciated, intensely nervous, delirious, and even disoriented; eventually, the heart fails.

Symptoms of hyperthyroidism may occur with the release of excessive amounts of thyroid hormone as a result of inflammation after irradiation of the thyroid or destruction of thyroid tissue by tumor. Such symptoms may also occur with excessive administration of thyroid hormone for treatment of hypothyroidism. Long-standing use of thyroid hormone in the absence of close monitoring may be a cause of symptoms of hyperthyroidism. It is also likely to result in premature osteoporosis, particularly in women.

Assessment and Diagnostic Findings

The thyroid gland invariably is enlarged to some extent. It is soft and may pulsate; a thrill often can be palpated, and a bruit is heard over the thyroid arteries. These are signs of greatly increased blood flow through the thyroid gland. In advanced cases, the diagnosis is made on the basis of the symptoms, a decrease in serum TSH, increased free T_4, and an increase in radioactive iodine uptake.

Medical Management

Appropriate treatment of hyperthyroidism depends on the underlying cause and often consists of a combination of therapies, including antithyroid agents, radioactive iodine, and surgery. Treatment of hyperthyroidism is directed toward reducing thyroid hyperactivity to relieve symptoms and preventing complications. Use of radioactive iodine is the most common form of treatment for Graves' disease in North America (Ginsberg, 2003). Beta-adrenergic blocking agents are used as adjunctive therapy for symptomatic relief, particularly in transient thyroiditis (Cooper, 2005). Surgical removal of most of the thyroid gland is a nonpharmacologic alternative.

No treatment for thyrotoxicosis is without side effects, and all three treatments (radioactive iodine therapy, antithyroid medications, and surgery) share the same complications: relapse or recurrent hyperthyroidism and permanent hypothyroidism. The rate of relapse increases in patients who have had very severe disease, a long history of dysfunction, ocular and cardiac symptoms, large goiter, or relapse after previous treatment. The relapse rate after radioactive iodine therapy depends on the dose used in treatment. Patients receiving a lower dose of radioactive iodine are more likely to require subsequent treatment than those being treated with a higher dose. The remission rate achieved with a single dose of radioactive iodine is 80% (Metso, Jaatinen, Huhtala, et al., 2004).

Although rates of relapse and the occurrence of hypothyroidism vary, relapse with antithyroid medications is about 45% 1 year after completion of therapy and almost 75% 5 years later (Larsen, Kronenberg, Melmed, et al., 2003). Discontinuation of antithyroid medications before therapy is complete usually results in relapse within 6 months. The incidence of relapse with subtotal thyroidectomy is 19% at 18 months; an incidence of hypothyroidism of 25% has been reported at 18 months after surgery. The risk of these complications illustrates the importance of long-term follow-up of patients treated for hyperthyroidism.

PHARMACOLOGIC THERAPY

Two forms of pharmacotherapy are available for treating hyperthyroidism and controlling excessive thyroid activity: (1) use of irradiation by administration of the radioisotope iodine 131 (^{131}I) for destructive effects on the thyroid gland and (2) antithyroid medications that interfere with the synthesis of thyroid hormones and other agents that control manifestations of hyperthyroidism.

Radioactive Iodine Therapy. The goal of radioactive iodine therapy (^{131}I) is to destroy the overactive thyroid cells. Almost all the iodine that enters and is retained in the body becomes concentrated in the thyroid gland. Therefore, the radioactive isotope of iodine is concentrated in the thyroid gland, where it destroys thyroid cells without jeopardizing other radiosensitive tissues. Over a period of several weeks, thyroid cells exposed to the radioactive iodine are destroyed, resulting in reduction of the hyperthyroid state and inevitably hypothyroidism.

The patient is instructed about what to expect with this tasteless, colorless radioiodine, which may be administered by the radiologist. Typically, a single dose is needed (Metso et al., 2004). About 95% of patients are cured by one dose of radioactive iodine. The additional 5% require two doses; rarely is a third dose necessary. Use of an ablative dose of radioactive iodine initially causes an acute release of thyroid hormone from the thyroid gland and may cause an increase of symptoms. The patient is observed for signs of **thyroid storm** (Chart 42-5); propranolol (Inderal) is useful in controlling these symptoms.

After treatment with radioactive iodine, the patient is monitored closely until the euthyroid state is reached. In 3 to 4 weeks, symptoms of hyperthyroidism subside. Close follow-up is required to evaluate thyroid function, because the incidence of hypothyroidism after this form of treatment is very high. Approximately 20% of patients become hypothyroid within 2 years after treatment, and another 3% to 5% of patients each year thereafter (Schori-Ahmed, 2003). Thyroid hormone replacement is necessary; small doses are usually prescribed, with the dose gradually increased over a period of months (up to about 1 year) until the free T_4 and TSH levels stabilize within normal ranges.

Radioactive iodine has been used to treat toxic adenomas, multinodular goiter, and most varieties of thyrotoxicosis (rarely with permanent success); it is preferred for treating patients beyond the childbearing years who have diffuse toxic goiter. Radioiodine treatment is contraindicated during pregnancy (because it crosses the placenta) and while breast-feeding (because it is secreted in breast milk) to prevent hypothyroidism in one infant (Blackwell, 2004). Pregnancy should be postponed for at least 6 months after treatment.

A major advantage of treatment with radioactive iodine is that it avoids many of the side effects associated with antithyroid medications. However, some patients and their families fear medications that are radioactive. For this reason, patients may elect to take antithyroid medications rather than radioactive iodine.

Antithyroid Medications. Antithyroid medications are summarized in Table 42-3. The objective of pharmacotherapy is to inhibit one or more stages in thyroid hormone synthesis or hormone release. Antithyroid agents block the utilization of iodine by interfering with the iodination of tyrosine and the coupling of iodotyrosines in the synthesis of thyroid hormones. This prevents the synthesis of thyroid hormone. Most commonly, propylthiouracil (PTU) or methimazole (Tapazole) is used until the patient is euthyroid (ie, neither hyperthyroid nor hypothyroid). These medications block extrathyroidal conversion of T_4 to T_3.

The therapeutic dose is determined on the basis of clinical criteria, including changes in pulse rate, pulse pressure, body weight, size of the goiter, and results of laboratory studies of thyroid function. Because antithyroid medications do not interfere with release or activity of previously formed thyroid hormones, it may take several weeks until relief of symptoms occurs. At that time, the maintenance dose is established, and a gradual withdrawal of the medication over the next several months follows.

CHART 42-5

Thyroid Storm (Thyrotoxic Crisis, Thyrotoxicosis)

Thyroid storm (thyrotoxic crisis) is a form of severe hyperthyroidism, usually of abrupt onset. Untreated, it is almost always fatal, but with proper treatment the mortality rate is reduced substantially. The patient with thyroid storm or crisis is critically ill and requires astute observation and aggressive and supportive nursing care during and after the acute stage of illness.

CLINICAL MANIFESTATIONS

Thyroid storm is characterized by

- High fever (hyperpyrexia) above 38.5°C (101.3°F)
- Extreme tachycardia (more than 130 beats/min)
- Exaggerated symptoms of hyperthyroidism with disturbances of a major system—for example, gastrointestinal (weight loss, diarrhea, abdominal pain), or cardiovascular (edema, chest pain, dyspnea, palpitations)
- Altered neurologic or mental state, which frequently appears as delirium psychosis, somnolence, or coma

Life-threatening thyroid storm is usually precipitated by stress, such as injury, infection, thyroid and nonthyroid surgery, tooth extraction, insulin reaction, diabetic ketoacidosis, pregnancy, digitalis intoxication, abrupt withdrawal of antithyroid medications, extreme emotional stress, or vigorous palpation of the thyroid. These factors can precipitate thyroid storm in the partially controlled or completely untreated patient with hyperthyroidism. Current methods of diagnosis and treatment for hyperthyroidism have greatly decreased the incidence of thyroid storm, making it uncommon today.

MANAGEMENT

Immediate objectives are reduction of body temperature and heart rate and prevention of vascular collapse. Measures to accomplish these objectives include:

- A hypothermia mattress or blanket, ice packs, a cool environment, hydrocortisone, and acetaminophen (Tylenol). Salicylates (eg, aspirin) are not used because they displace thyroid hormone from binding proteins and worsen the hypermetabolism.
- Humidified oxygen is administered to improve tissue oxygenation and meet the high metabolic demands. Arterial blood gas levels or pulse oximetry may be used to monitor respiratory status.
- Intravenous fluids containing dextrose are administered to replace liver glycogen stores that have been decreased in the hyperthyroid patient.
- PTU or methimazole is administered to impede formation of thyroid hormone and block conversion of T_4 to T_3, the more active form of thyroid hormone.
- Hydrocortisone is prescribed to treat shock or adrenal insufficiency.
- Iodine is administered to decrease output of T_4 from the thyroid gland. For cardiac problems such as atrial fibrillation, dysrhythmias, and heart failure, sympatholytic agents may be administered. Propranolol, combined with digitalis, has been effective in reducing severe cardiac symptoms.

Toxic complications of antithyroid medications are relatively uncommon; nevertheless, the importance of periodic follow-up is emphasized, because medication sensitization, fever, rash, urticaria, or even agranulocytosis and thrombocytopenia (decrease in granulocytes and platelets) may develop. With any sign of infection, especially pharyngitis and fever or the occurrence of mouth ulcers, the patient is advised to stop the medication, notify the physician immediately, and undergo hematologic studies. Rash, arthralgias, and fever occur in 1% to 5% of patients (Pearce, Farwell, & Braverman, 2004). Agranulocytosis, the most serious toxic side effect, occurs in approximately 0.5% of patients. Its incidence is higher in patients older than 40 years of age. It usually occurs within the first 3 months but may occur up to 1 year after therapy is started.

Patients taking antithyroid medications are instructed not to use decongestants for nasal stuffiness, because these agents are poorly tolerated. PTU is the treatment of choice during pregnancy. Once the thyrotoxicity is under control, the dose is decreased to prevent fetal hypothyroidism (Cooper, 2005). Antithyroid medications are contraindicated in late pregnancy, because they may produce goiter and cretinism in the fetus (Cooper, 2005).

Another goal of therapy is to reduce the amount of thyroid tissue, with resulting decreased thyroid hormone production. Thyroid hormone is occasionally administered with antithyroid medications to put the thyroid gland at rest. In this approach, hypothyroidism from excess antithyroid medication is avoided, as is stimulation of the thyroid gland by TSH. Levothyroxine sodium (Synthroid) is the most common thyroid hormone preparation used. It takes approximately 10 days of its administration to achieve full effect. Liothyronine sodium (Cytomel) has a more rapid onset, and its action is of short duration.

Antithyroid medications may also be used to normalize thyroid function before radioactive iodine is administered, to suppress symptoms of thyrotoxicosis that may occur with this therapy (Cooper, 2005).

Adjunctive Therapy. Iodine or iodide compounds, once the only therapy available for patients with hyperthyroidism, are no longer used as the sole method of treatment. Such compounds decrease the release of thyroid hormones from the

℞ TABLE 42-3 Pharmacologic Agents Used to Treat Hyperthyroidism

Agent	Action	Nursing Considerations
Propylthiouracil (PTU)	Blocks synthesis of hormones (conversion of T_3 to T_4)	Monitor cardiac parameters. Observe for conversion to hypothyroidism. Must be given by mouth. Watch for rash, nausea, vomiting, agranulocytosis, lupus syndrome.
Methimazole	Blocks synthesis of thyroid hormone	More toxic than PTU. Watch for rash and other symptoms as for PTU.
Sodium iodide	Suppresses release of thyroid hormone	Given 1 h after PTU or methimazole. Watch for edema, hemorrhage, gastrointestinal upset.
Potassium iodide	Suppresses release of thyroid hormone	Discontinue for rash. Watch for signs of toxic iodinism.
Saturated solution of potassium iodide (SSKI)	Suppresses release of thyroid hormone	Mix with juice or milk. Give by straw to prevent staining of teeth.
Dexamethasone	Suppresses release of thyroid hormone	Monitor input and output. Monitor glucose. May cause hypertension, nausea, vomiting, anorexia, infection.
Beta-blocker (eg, propranolol)	Beta-adrenergic blocking agent	Monitor cardiac status. Hold for bradycardia or decreased cardiac output. Use with caution in patients with heart failure.

Adapted from Morton, P. G., Fontaine, D. K., Hudak, C. M., & Gallo, B. M. (2005). *Critical care nursing: A holistic approach.* Philadelphia: Lippincott Williams & Wilkins.

thyroid gland and reduce the vascularity and size of the thyroid. Compounds such as potassium iodide (KI), Lugol's solution, and saturated solution of potassium iodide (SSKI) may be used in combination with antithyroid agents or beta-adrenergic blockers to prepare the patient with hyperthyroidism for surgery. These agents reduce the activity of the thyroid hormone and the vascularity of the thyroid gland, making the surgical procedure safer. Solutions of iodine and iodide compounds are more palatable in milk or fruit juice and are administered through a straw to prevent staining of the teeth. These compounds reduce the metabolic rate more rapidly than antithyroid medications do, but their action does not last as long.

NURSING ALERT

Patients receiving these medications should be observed for the development of goiter and should be cautioned against use of over-the-counter medications that contain iodides and can increase the response to iodide therapy. Cough medications, expectorants, bronchodilators, and salt substitutes may contain iodide and should be avoided by the patient receiving iodide therapy.

Beta-adrenergic blocking agents are important in controlling the sympathetic nervous system effects of hyperthyroidism. For example, propranolol is used to control nervousness, tachycardia, tremor, anxiety, and heat intolerance. The patient continues taking propranolol until the free T_4 is within the normal range and the TSH level approaches normal.

SURGICAL MANAGEMENT

Surgery to remove thyroid tissue was once the primary method of treating hyperthyroidism; today, surgery is reserved for special circumstances—for example, in pregnant women who are allergic to antithyroid medications, in patients with large goiters, or in patients who are unable to take antithyroid agents. Surgery for treatment of hyperthyroidism is performed soon after the thyroid function has returned to normal (4 to 6 weeks).

The surgical removal of about five sixths of the thyroid tissue (subtotal thyroidectomy) reliably results in a prolonged remission in most patients with exophthalmic goiter. Its use today is reserved for patients with obstructive symptoms, for pregnant women in the second trimester, and for patients with a need for rapid normalization of thyroid function (Pearce & Braverman, 2004). Before surgery, PTU is administered until signs of hyperthyroidism have disappeared. A beta-adrenergic blocking agent (propranolol) may be used to reduce the heart rate and other signs and symptoms of hyperthyroidism; however, this does not create a euthyroid state. Iodine (Lugol's solution or KI) may be prescribed in an effort to reduce blood loss; however, the effectiveness of this treatment is unknown. Medications that may prolong clotting (eg, aspirin) are stopped several weeks before surgery to reduce the risk of postoperative bleeding. Patients receiving iodine medication must be monitored for evidence of iodine toxicity (iodism), which requires immediate withdrawal of the medication. Symptoms of iodism include swelling of the buccal mucosa, excessive salivation, coryza, and skin eruptions.

Gerontologic Considerations

Although hyperthyroidism is much less common in elderly people than hypothyroidism, patients older than 60 years of age account for 10% to 15% of the cases of thyrotoxicosis. Some older patients develop typical signs and symptoms of thyrotoxicosis, but an atypical picture is not uncommon. The only presenting manifestations may be anorexia and weight loss, absence of ocular signs, or isolated atrial fibrillation. New or worsening heart failure or angina is more likely to occur in elderly than in younger patients. The elderly patient may experience a single manifestation (eg, anorexia, weight loss). These signs and symptoms may mask the underlying thyroid disease. Elderly patients also tend to have symptoms for longer periods of time and commonly present with vague and nonspecific signs and symptoms, making disorders difficult to detect (Ginsberg, 2003). Symptoms such as tachycardia, fatigue, mental confusion, weight loss, change in bowel habits, and depression can be attributed to age and other illnesses that are common in elderly people. In addition, patients may report cardiovascular symptoms and difficulty climbing stairs or rising from a chair because of muscle weakness.

Spontaneous remission of hyperthyroidism is rare in elderly patients. Measurement of TSH is indicated in elderly patients who have unexplained physical or mental deterioration. The use of radioactive iodine is generally recommended for treatment of thyrotoxicosis in elderly patients unless an enlarged thyroid gland is pressing on the airway. The hypermetabolic state of thyrotoxicosis must be controlled by antithyroid medications before radioactive iodine is administered, because radiation therapy may precipitate thyroid storm by increasing the release of hormone from the thyroid gland. Thyroid storm, if it occurs, has a mortality rate of 10% in elderly patients.

Antithyroid medications are not generally recommended for elderly patients because of the increased incidence of side effects, such as granulocytopenia, and the need for frequent monitoring. The dosage of other medications used to treat other chronic illnesses in elderly patients may need to be modified because of the altered rate of metabolism in hyperthyroidism. In addition, antithyroid medications are considered to be less effective in the treatment of toxic nodular goiter, the most common cause of thyrotoxicosis in the elderly.

Use of beta-adrenergic blocking agents (eg, propranolol) may be indicated to decrease the cardiovascular and neurologic signs and symptoms of thyrotoxicosis. These agents must be used with extreme caution in elderly patients to minimize adverse effects on cardiac function that may produce heart failure.

Nursing Process

The Patient With Hyperthyroidism

Assessment

The health history and examination focus on symptoms related to accelerated or exaggerated metabolism. These include the patient's and family's reports of irritability and increased emotional reaction and the impact these changes have had on the patient's interactions with family, friends, and coworkers. The history includes other stressors and the patient's ability to cope with stress.

The nurse assesses the patient's nutritional status and the presence of symptoms. Symptoms related to excessive nervous system output and changes in vision and appearance of the eyes are noted. The nurse periodically assesses and monitors the patient's cardiac status, including heart rate, blood pressure, heart sounds, and peripheral pulses.

Because emotional changes are associated with hyperthyroidism, the patient's emotional state and psychological status are evaluated, as well as such symptoms as irritability, anxiety, sleep disturbances, apathy, and lethargy, all of which may occur with hyperthyroidism. The family may also provide information about recent changes in the patient's emotional status.

Diagnosis

Nursing Diagnoses

Based on all the assessment data, the major nursing diagnoses of the patient with hyperthyroidism may include the following:

- Imbalanced nutrition, less than body requirements, related to exaggerated metabolic rate, excessive appetite, and increased gastrointestinal activity
- Ineffective coping related to irritability, hyperexcitability, apprehension, and emotional instability
- Low self-esteem related to changes in appearance, excessive appetite, and weight loss
- Altered body temperature

Collaborative Problems/ Potential Complications

Based on assessment data, potential complications may include the following:

- Thyrotoxicosis or thyroid storm
- Hypothyroidism

Planning and Goals

The goals for the patient may be improved nutritional status, improved coping ability, improved self-esteem, maintenance of normal body temperature, and absence of complications.

Nursing Interventions

Improving Nutritional Status

Hyperthyroidism affects all body systems, including the gastrointestinal system. The appetite is increased but may be satisfied by several well-balanced meals of small size, even up to six meals a day. Foods and fluids are selected to replace fluid lost through diarrhea and diaphoresis and to control the diarrhea that results from increased peristalsis. Rapid movement of food through the gastrointestinal tract may result in nutritional imbalance and further weight loss. To reduce diarrhea, highly seasoned foods and stimulants such as coffee, tea, cola, and alcohol are discouraged. High-calorie, high-protein foods are encouraged. A quiet atmosphere during mealtime may aid digestion. Weight and dietary intake are recorded to monitor nutritional status.

Enhancing Coping Measures

The patient with hyperthyroidism needs reassurance that the emotional reactions being experienced are a result of the disorder and that with effective treatment those symptoms will be controlled. Because of the negative effect these symptoms have on family and friends, they too need reassurance that the symptoms are expected to disappear with treatment.

It is important to use a calm, unhurried approach with the patient. Stressful experiences are minimized; therefore, if hospitalized, the patient is not placed in a room with very ill or talkative patients. The environment is kept quiet and uncluttered. Noises, such as loud music, conversation, and equipment alarms, are minimized. The nurse encourages relaxing activities if they do not overstimulate the patient.

If thyroidectomy is planned, the patient needs to know that pharmacologic therapy is necessary to prepare the thyroid gland for surgical treatment. The nurse instructs and reminds the patient to take the medications as prescribed. Because of hyperexcitability and shortened attention span, the patient may require repetition of this information and written instructions.

Improving Self-Esteem

The patient with hyperthyroidism is likely to experience changes in appearance, appetite, and weight. These factors, along with the patient's inability to cope well with family and the illness, may result in loss of self-esteem. The nurse conveys an understanding of the patient's concern about these problems and assists the patient to develop effective coping strategies. The patient and family need to know that these changes are a result of the thyroid dysfunction and are, in fact, out of the patient's control.

If changes in appearance are very disturbing to the patient, mirrors may be covered or removed. In addition, the nurse reminds family members and personnel to avoid bringing these changes to the patient's attention. The nurse explains to the patient and family that most of these changes are expected to disappear with effective treatment.

If the patient experiences eye changes secondary to hyperthyroidism, eye care and protection may be necessary. The patient may need instructions about instillation of eye drops or ointment prescribed to soothe the eyes and protect the exposed cornea.

The patient may be embarrassed by the need to eat large meals. Therefore, the nurse arranges for the patient to eat alone if desired and avoids commenting on the patient's large dietary intake while making sure that the patient receives sufficient food.

Maintaining Normal Body Temperature

The patient with hyperthyroidism frequently finds a normal room temperature too warm because of an exaggerated metabolic rate and increased heat production. If the patient is hospitalized, the nurse maintains the environment at a cool, comfortable temperature and changes bedding and clothing as needed. Instructions to the patient and family emphasize that cool baths and cool or cold fluids may provide relief. The reason for the patient's discomfort and the importance of providing a cool environment are explained to the family and staff.

Monitoring and Managing Potential Complications

The nurse closely monitors the patient with hyperthyroidism for signs and symptoms that may be indicative of thyroid storm. Cardiac and respiratory function are assessed by measuring vital signs and cardiac output, electrocardiographic (ECG) monitoring, arterial blood gases, and pulse oximetry. Assessment continues after treatment is initiated because of the potential effects of treatment on cardiac function. Oxygen is administered to prevent hypoxia, to improve tissue oxygenation, and to meet the high metabolic demands. IV fluids may be necessary to maintain blood glucose levels and to replace lost fluids. Antithyroid medications (PTU or methimazole) may be prescribed to reduce thyroid hormone levels. In addition, propranolol and digitalis may be prescribed to treat cardiac symptoms. If shock develops, treatment strategies must be implemented (see Chapter 15).

Hypothyroidism is likely to occur with any of the treatments used for hyperthyroidism. Therefore, the nurse periodically monitors the patient. Most patients report a greatly improved sense of well-being after treatment of hyperthyroidism, and some fail to continue to take prescribed thyroid replacement therapy. Therefore, part of patient and family teaching is instruction about the importance of continuing therapy indefinitely after discharge and a discussion of the consequences of failing to take medication.

Promoting Home and Community-Based Care

TEACHING PATIENTS SELF-CARE

The nurse teaches the patient with hyperthyroidism how and when to take prescribed medication and provides instruction about the essential role of the medication in the broader therapeutic plan. Because of the hyperexcitability and decreased attention span associated with hyperthyroidism, the nurse provides a written plan for the patient to use at home. The type and amount of information given depend on the patient's stress and anxiety levels. The patient and family members receive verbal and written information about the actions and possible side effects of the medications. The nurse identifies adverse effects that should be reported if they occur (Chart 42-6).

If a total or subtotal thyroidectomy is anticipated, the patient needs information about what to expect. This information is repeated as the time of surgery approaches. The nurse also advises the patient to avoid stressful situations that may precipitate thyroid storm.

CONTINUING CARE

Referral for home care, if indicated, allows the home care nurse to assess the home and family environment and the patient's and family's understanding of the importance of adhering to the therapeutic regimen and the recommended follow-up monitoring. The nurse reinforces to the patient and family the importance of long-term follow-up because of the risk for hypothyroidism after thyroidectomy or treatment with antithyroid medications or radioactive iodine. The nurse also assesses the patient for changes indicating return to normal thyroid function and signs and symptoms of hyperthyroidism and hypothyroidism. Furthermore, the nurse reminds the patient and family about the importance of health promotion activities and recommended health screening.

Evaluation

Expected Patient Outcomes

Expected patient outcomes may include the following:

1. Improves nutritional status
   a. Reports adequate dietary intake and decreased hunger
   b. Identifies high-calorie, high-protein foods; identifies foods to be avoided
   c. Avoids use of alcohol and other stimulants
   d. Reports decreased episodes of diarrhea
2. Demonstrates effective coping methods in dealing with family, friends, and coworkers
   a. Explains reasons for irritability and emotional instability
   b. Avoids stressful situations, events, and people
   c. Participates in relaxing, nonstressful activities
3. Achieves increased self-esteem
   a. Verbalizes feelings about self and illness
   b. Describes feelings of frustration and loss of control
   c. Describes reasons for increased appetite
4. Maintains normal body temperature
5. Absence of complications
   a. Has serum thyroid hormone and TSH levels within normal limits
   b. Identifies signs and symptoms of thyroid storm and hypothyroidism
   c. Has vital signs and results of ECG, arterial blood gases, and pulse oximetry within normal limits
   d. States importance of regular follow-up and lifelong maintenance of prescribed therapy

CHART 42-6

HOME CARE CHECKLIST • The Patient With Hyperthyroidism

At the completion of the home care instruction, the patient or caregiver will be able to:	Patient	Caregiver
• State present and potential effects of hyperthyroidism on the body	✔	✔
• State precipitating factors and interventions for complications (hypothyroidism, thyroid storm)	✔	✔
• State the purpose, dose, route, schedule, side effects, and precautions of prescribed medications (propylthiouracil, radioactive iodine)	✔	✔
• State the need to contact health care provider before taking over-the-counter medications	✔	✔
• State need for regular follow-up visits with health care provider	✔	✔
• Identify the need for planned rest periods and methods to improve sleep patterns	✔	✔
• Identify the need for increased dietary intake until weight stabilizes	✔	✔
• Identify areas of physical and emotional stress	✔	✔
• State that emotional lability is part of disease process	✔	✔
• Describe the potential benefits and risks of surgical intervention or radioactive iodine therapy	✔	✔
• Identify potential for menstrual irregularities, increased risk for osteoporosis, and potential for pregnancy for women	✔	✔
• State need to wear medical identification and carry medical information card	✔	✔

Thyroiditis

Thyroiditis, inflammation of the thyroid gland, can be acute, subacute, or chronic. Each type of thyroiditis is characterized by inflammation, fibrosis, or lymphocytic infiltration of the thyroid gland. Several forms of thyroiditis are characterized by autoimmune damage to the thyroid. The various forms of thyroiditis may cause thyrotoxicosis, hypothyroidism, or both (Pearce et al., 2003).

Acute Thyroiditis

Acute thyroiditis is a rare disorder caused by infection of the thyroid gland by bacteria, fungi, mycobacteria, or parasites. *Staphylococcus aureus* and other staphylococci are the most common causes. Infection typically causes anterior neck pain and swelling, fever, dysphagia, and dysphonia. Pharyngitis or pharyngeal pain is often present. Examination may reveal warmth, erythema (redness), and tenderness of the thyroid gland. Treatment of acute thyroiditis includes antimicrobial agents and fluid replacement. Surgical incision and drainage may be needed if an abscess is present.

Subacute Thyroiditis

Subacute thyroiditis may be subacute granulomatous thyroiditis (de Quervain's thyroiditis) or painless thyroiditis (silent thyroiditis or subacute lymphocytic thyroiditis). Subacute granulomatous thyroiditis is an inflammatory disorder of the thyroid gland that predominantly affects women between the ages of 40 and 50 years (Fatourechi, Aniszewski, Fatourechi, et al., 2003). The condition manifests as a painful swelling in the anterior neck that lasts 1 to 2 months and then disappears spontaneously without residual effect. It often follows a respiratory infection. The thyroid enlarges symmetrically and may be painful. The overlying skin is often reddened and warm. Swallowing may be difficult and uncomfortable. Irritability, nervousness, insomnia, and weight loss—manifestations of hyperthyroidism—are common, and many patients experience chills and fever as well.

Treatment aims to control the inflammation. In general, nonsteroidal anti-inflammatory drugs are used to relieve neck pain. Acetylsalicylic acid (aspirin) is avoided if symptoms of hyperthyroidism occur, because aspirin displaces thyroid hormone from its binding sites and increases the amount of circulating hormone. Beta-blocking agents (eg, propranolol) may be used to control symptoms of hyperthyroidism. Antithyroid agents, which block the synthesis of T_3 and T_4, are not effective in thyroiditis because the associated thyrotoxicosis results from the release of stored thyroid hormones rather than from their increased synthesis. In more severe cases, oral corticosteroids may be prescribed to reduce swelling and relieve pain; however, they do not usually affect the underlying cause. In some cases, temporary hypothyroidism may develop and may necessitate thyroid hormone therapy. Follow-up monitoring is necessary to document the patient's return to a euthyroid state.

Painless thyroiditis (subacute lymphocytic thyroiditis) often occurs in the postpartum period and is thought to be an autoimmune process. Symptoms of hyperthyroidism or hypothyroidism are possible. Treatment is directed at symptoms, and yearly follow-up is recommended to determine the patient's need for treatment of subsequent hypothyroidism.

Chronic Thyroiditis (Hashimoto's Disease)

Chronic thyroiditis, which occurs most frequently in women between the ages of 30 and 50 years, has been termed Hashimoto's disease, or chronic lymphocytic thyroiditis; its diagnosis is based on the histologic appearance of the inflamed thyroid gland. In contrast to acute thyroiditis, the chronic forms usually are not accompanied by pain, pressure symptoms, or fever, and thyroid activity usually is normal or low rather than increased. Cell-mediated immunity may play a significant role in the pathogenesis of chronic thyroiditis, and there may be a genetic predisposition to it. If untreated, the disease runs a slow, progressive course, leading eventually to hypothyroidism.

The objective of treatment is to reduce the size of the thyroid gland and prevent hypothyroidism. Thyroid hormone therapy is prescribed to reduce thyroid activity and the production of thyroglobulin. If hypothyroid symptoms are present, thyroid hormone therapy is prescribed. Surgery may be required if pressure symptoms persist.

Thyroid Tumors

Tumors of the thyroid gland are classified on the basis of being benign or malignant, the presence or absence of associated thyrotoxicosis, and the diffuse or irregular quality of the glandular enlargement. If the enlargement is sufficient to cause a visible swelling in the neck, the tumor is referred to as a goiter.

All grades of goiter are encountered, from those that are barely visible to those producing disfigurement. Some are symmetric and diffuse; others are nodular. Some are accompanied by hyperthyroidism, in which case they are described as toxic; others are associated with a euthyroid state and are called nontoxic goiters.

Endemic (Iodine-Deficient) Goiter

The most common type of goiter, once encountered chiefly in geographic regions where the natural supply of iodine is deficient (eg, the Great Lakes areas of the United States), is the so-called simple or colloid goiter. In addition to being caused by an iodine deficiency, simple goiter may be caused by an intake of large quantities of goitrogenic substances in patients with unusually susceptible glands. These substances include excessive amounts of iodine or lithium, which is used in treating bipolar disorders.

Simple goiter represents a compensatory hypertrophy of the thyroid gland, caused by stimulation by the pituitary gland. The pituitary gland produces thyrotropin or TSH, a hormone that controls the release of thyroid hormone from the thyroid gland. Its production increases if there is subnormal thyroid activity, as when insufficient iodine is available for production of the thyroid hormone. Such goiters usually cause no symptoms, except for the swelling in the neck, which may result in tracheal compression when excessive.

Many goiters of this type recede after the iodine imbalance is corrected. Supplementary iodine, such as SSKI, is prescribed to suppress the pituitary's thyroid-stimulating activity. When surgery is recommended, the risk of postoperative complications is minimized by ensuring a preoperative euthyroid state through treatment with antithyroid medications and iodide to reduce the size and vascularity of the goiter.

Providing children in iodine-poor regions with iodine compounds can prevent simple or endemic goiter. If the mean iodine intake is less than 40 fg/day, the thyroid gland hypertrophies. The World Health Organization recommends that salt be iodized to a concentration of 1 part in 100,000, which is adequate for the prevention of endemic goiter. In the United States, salt is iodized to 1 part in 10,000. The introduction of iodized salt has been the single most effective means of preventing goiter in at-risk populations.

Nodular Goiter

Some thyroid glands are nodular because of areas of hyperplasia (overgrowth). No symptoms may arise as a result of this condition, but not uncommonly these nodules slowly increase in size, with some descending into the thorax, where they cause local pressure symptoms. Some nodules become malignant, and some are associated with a hyperthyroid state. Therefore, the patient with many thyroid nodules may eventually require surgery.

Thyroid Cancer

Cancer of the thyroid is much less prevalent than other forms of cancer; however, it accounts for 90% of endocrine malignancies. According to the American Cancer Society (2005), an estimated 25,690 new cases of thyroid cancer are diagnosed each year, 19,190 in women and 6,500 in men. About 860 women and 630 men die annually from this malignancy. There are several types of cancer of the thyroid gland; the type determines the course and prognosis (Table 42-4).

External radiation of the head, neck, or chest in infancy and childhood increases the risk for thyroid carcinoma. Between 1940 and 1960, radiation therapy was occasionally used to shrink enlarged tonsillar and adenoid tissue, to treat acne, or to reduce an enlarged thymus. For people exposed to external radiation in childhood, there appears to be an increased incidence of thyroid cancer 5 to 40 years after irradiation. Consequently, people who underwent such treatment should consult a physician, request an isotope thyroid scan as part of the evaluation, follow recommended treatment of abnormalities of the gland, and continue with annual checkups (Chart 42-7).

ASSESSMENT AND DIAGNOSTIC FINDINGS

Lesions that are single, hard, and fixed on palpation or associated with cervical lymphadenopathy suggest malignancy. Thyroid function tests may be helpful in evaluating thyroid nodules and masses; however, results are rarely conclusive. Needle biopsy of the thyroid gland is used as an outpatient procedure to make a diagnosis of thyroid cancer, to differentiate cancerous thyroid nodules from noncancerous nodules, and to stage the cancer if detected. The procedure is safe and usually requires only a local anesthetic. However, patients who undergo the procedure are monitored closely, because cancerous tissues may be missed during the procedure. A second type of aspiration or biopsy uses a large-bore needle rather than the fine needle used in standard biopsy; it may be used when the results of the standard biopsy are inconclusive or with rapidly growing tumors. Additional diagnostic studies include ultrasound, MRI, CT, thyroid scans, radioactive iodine uptake studies, and thyroid suppression tests.

TABLE 42-4 Types of Thyroid Cancers

Type of Thyroid Cancer	Incidence (%)	Characteristics
Papillary adenocarcinoma	70	Most common and least aggressive Asymptomatic nodule in a normal gland Starts in childhood or early adult life, remains localized Metastasizes along the lymphatics if untreated More aggressive in the elderly
Follicular adenocarcinoma	15	Appears after 40 y of age Encapsulated; feels elastic or rubbery on palpation Spreads through the bloodstream to bone, liver, and lung Prognosis is not as favorable as for papillary adenocarcinoma
Medullary	5	Appears after 50 y of age Occurs as part of multiple endocrine neoplasia (MEN) Hormone-producing tumor causing endocrine dysfunction symptoms Metastasizes by lymphatics and bloodstream Moderate survival rate
Anaplastic	5	50% of anaplastic thyroid carcinomas occur in patients older than 60 y Hard, irregular mass that grows quickly and spreads by direct invasion to adjacent tissues May be painful and tender Survival for patients with anaplastic cancer is usually less than 6 mo
Thyroid lymphoma	5	Appears after age 40 y May have history of goiter, hoarseness, dyspnea, pain, and pressure Good prognosis

CHART 42-7

Radiation-Induced Thyroid Damage and Cancer

The thyroid gland has a very efficient mechanism to remove iodine from the bloodstream and concentrate or "trap" it for subsequent synthesis of thyroid hormone. The effectiveness of this mechanism to concentrate iodide is reflected in a concentration of iodide 20 to 40 times the concentration of iodide in the plasma.

If milk and other food sources become contaminated with radioactivity as a result of a nuclear detonation or a nuclear power plant incident or mishap, the radioactive iodide would become concentrated in the thyroid gland at a very high concentration and would irradiate the thyroid gland, increasing the risk for thyroid gland cancer. Therefore, in communities exposed to increased radioactivity, attempts have been made to block the uptake of radioactive iodide by flooding or saturating the thyroid gland with nonradioactive iodide.

Administration of potassium iodide (KI) or other iodide preparations as soon as possible after exposure almost completely inhibits thyroid absorption of the radioactive iodide and promotes rapid excretion of any that is absorbed. In 2001, the Food and Drug Administration (FDA) issued a statement recommending KI administration in advance of exposure to radioactive iodine—that is, when exposure is imminent (Thyroid Carcinoma Task Force, 2001).

MEDICAL MANAGEMENT

The treatment of choice for thyroid carcinoma is surgical removal. Total or near-total **thyroidectomy** is performed if possible. Modified neck dissection or more extensive radical neck dissection is performed if there is lymph node involvement.

Efforts are made to spare parathyroid tissue to reduce the risk of postoperative hypocalcemia and tetany. After surgery, ablation procedures are carried out with radioactive iodine to eradicate residual thyroid tissue if the tumor is radiosensitive. Radioactive iodine also maximizes the chance of discovering thyroid metastasis at a later date if total-body scans are carried out.

After surgery, thyroid hormone is administered in suppressive doses to lower the levels of TSH to a euthyroid state (Thyroid Carcinoma Task Force, 2001). If the remaining thyroid tissue is inadequate to produce sufficient thyroid hormone, thyroxine is required permanently.

Several routes are available for administering radiation to the thyroid or tissues of the neck, including oral administration of radioactive iodine and external administration of radiation therapy. The patient who receives external sources of radiation therapy is at risk for mucositis, dryness of the mouth, dysphagia, redness of the skin, anorexia, and fatigue (see Chapter 16). Chemotherapy is infrequently used to treat thyroid cancer.

Patients whose thyroid cancer is detected early and who are appropriately treated usually do very well. Patients who have had papillary cancer, the most common and least aggressive tumor, have a 10-year survival rate greater than 90%. Long-term survival is also common in follicular cancer, a more aggressive form of thyroid cancer (Tierney et al., 2005). However, continued thyroid hormone therapy and periodic follow-up and diagnostic testing are important to ensure the patient's well-being (Thyroid Carcinoma Task Force, 2001).

Postoperatively, the patient is instructed to take exogenous thyroid hormone to prevent hypothyroidism. Later follow-up includes clinical assessment for recurrence of nodules or masses in the neck and signs of hoarseness, dysphagia, or dyspnea. Total-body scans are performed 2 to 4 months after surgery to detect residual thyroid tissue or metastatic disease. Thyroid hormones are stopped for about 6 weeks before the tests. Care must be taken to avoid iodine-containing foods and contrast agents. A repeat scan is performed 1 year after the initial surgery. If measurements are stable, a final scan is obtained in 3 to 5 years.

Free T_4, TSH, and serum calcium and phosphorus levels are monitored to determine whether the thyroid hormone supplementation is adequate and to note whether calcium balance is maintained.

Although local and systemic reactions to radiation may occur and may include neutropenia or thrombocytopenia, these complications are rare when radioactive iodine is used. Patients who undergo surgery that is combined with radioactive iodine have a higher survival rate than those who undergo surgery alone. Patient teaching emphasizes the importance of taking prescribed medications and following recommendations for follow-up monitoring. The patient who is undergoing radiation therapy is also instructed in how to assess and manage side effects of treatment.

NURSING MANAGEMENT

Important preoperative goals are to gain the patient's confidence and reduce anxiety. Often, the patient's home life has become tense because of his or her restlessness, irritability, and nervousness secondary to hyperthyroidism. Efforts are necessary to protect the patient from such tension and stress to avoid precipitating thyroid storm. If the patient reports increased stress when with family or friends, suggestions are made to limit contact with them. Quiet and relaxing forms of recreation or occupational therapy may be helpful.

Providing Preoperative Care. The nurse instructs the patient about the importance of eating a diet high in carbohydrates and proteins. A high daily caloric intake is necessary because of the increased metabolic activity and rapid depletion of glycogen reserves. Supplementary vitamins, particularly thiamine and ascorbic acid, may be prescribed. The patient is reminded to avoid tea, coffee, cola, and other stimulants.

The nurse also informs the patient about the purpose of preoperative tests, if they are to be performed, and explains what preoperative preparations to expect. This information should help to reduce the patient's anxiety about the surgery. In addition, special efforts are made to ensure a good night's rest before surgery, although many patients are admitted to the hospital on the day of surgery.

NURSING RESEARCH PROFILE

Thyroid Cancer: Quality of Life

Huang, S., Lee, C., Chien, L., et al. (2004). Postoperative quality of life among patients with thyroid cancer. *Journal of Advanced Nursing, 47*(5), 492–499.

Purpose

Thyroid cancer is a fairly common form of cancer, and the overall long-term worldwide survival rate of patients is more than 90%. Although the goals of cancer treatment are to increase survival and to preserve the patient's quality of life (QOL), few studies have addressed QOL in thyroid cancer survivors. The purpose of this study was to examine and describe factors associated with quality of life among patients with thyroid cancer who are treated surgically.

Design

A cross-sectional design was used with a convenience sample that included 146 patients from one medical center in Taiwan. Patients who had undergone thyroidectomy 6 to 36 months previously to treat thyroid cancer participated in the study. Telephone interviews were used to obtain sociodemographic data, information on their disease and its treatment characteristics, and social support information from study participants. QOL was measured by the Chinese version of the Quality of Life Index. Multivariate analyses were performed using multiple linear regressions.

Findings

Symptoms such as temporary hoarseness, tetany, and tingling around the mouth were prevalent up to 6 months after surgery, and about 10% of respondents reported that these symptoms lasted longer than 6 months. Patients also experienced fatigue, chills, and insomnia. In addition, they were concerned about the effect of the surgical incision or scar on appearance and social relationships.

Factors associated with postoperative QOL included length of time since surgery, perceived impact of the surgical scar on activities, current fatigue, current chills, and social support from friends and family. These factors were negatively associated with QOL. Social support from family and friends and the support of health care providers were positively associated with QOL scores. The QOL of patients 19 to 36 months after thyroidectomy was lower than that of those within 18 months of thyroidectomy.

Nursing Implications

Nurses caring for patients who have undergone thyroidectomy to treat thyroid cancer should be aware that patients often have postoperative physical symptoms as well as emotional reactions to the surgical scar. Preparing patients for the occurrence of these symptoms by providing patient teaching in the preoperative period and psychosocial support in the postoperative period may improve the QOL in patients who have undergone surgical treatment for thyroid cancer.

Preoperative teaching includes demonstrating to the patient how to support the neck with the hands after surgery to prevent stress on the incision. This involves raising the elbows and placing the hands behind the neck to provide support and reduce strain and tension on the neck muscles and the surgical incision.

Providing Postoperative Care. The nurse periodically assesses the surgical dressings and reinforces them if necessary. When the patient is in a recumbent position, the nurse observes the sides and the back of the neck as well as the anterior dressing for bleeding. In addition to monitoring the pulse and blood pressure for any indication of internal bleeding, it is important to be alert for complaints of a sensation of pressure or fullness at the incision site. Such symptoms may indicate subcutaneous hemorrhage and hematoma formation and should be reported.

Difficulty in respiration can occur as a result of edema of the glottis, hematoma formation, or injury to the recurrent laryngeal nerve. This complication requires that an airway be inserted. Therefore, a tracheostomy set is kept at the bedside at all times, and the surgeon is summoned at the first indication of respiratory distress. If the respiratory distress is caused by hematoma, surgical evacuation is required.

The intensity of pain is assessed, and analgesic agents are administered as prescribed for pain. The nurse should anticipate apprehension in the patient and should inform the patient that oxygen will assist breathing. When moving and turning the patient, the nurse carefully supports the patient's head and avoids tension on the sutures. The most comfortable position is the semi-Fowler's position, with the head elevated and supported by pillows.

IV fluids are administered during the immediate postoperative period. Water may be given by mouth as soon as nausea subsides. Usually, there is a little difficulty in swallowing; initially, cold fluids and ice may be taken better than other fluids. Often, patients prefer a soft diet to a liquid diet in the immediate postoperative period.

The patient is advised to talk as little as possible to reduce edema to the vocal cords; however, when the patient does speak, any voice changes are noted, because they might indicate injury to the recurrent laryngeal nerve, which lies just behind the thyroid next to the trachea.

An overbed table may be used to provide easy access to items that are needed frequently, such as tissues, a water pitcher and glass, and a small emesis basin. These are kept within easy reach so that the patient does not need to turn the head to reach for them. It is also convenient to use this table when vapor-mist inhalations are prescribed for the relief of excessive mucus accumulation.

The patient is usually permitted out of bed as soon as possible and is encouraged to eat foods that are easily swallowed. A well-balanced, high-calorie diet may be prescribed to promote weight gain. Sutures or skin clips are usually removed on the second day. The patient is usually discharged from the hospital on the day of surgery or soon afterward if the postoperative course is uncomplicated.

Monitoring and Managing Potential Complications. Hemorrhage, hematoma formation, edema of the glottis, and injury to the recurrent laryngeal nerve are complications that have been reviewed previously in this chapter. Occasionally in thyroid surgery, the parathyroid glands are injured or removed, producing a disturbance in calcium metabolism. As the blood calcium level falls, hyperirritability of the nerves occurs, with spasms of the hands and feet and muscle twitching (see Chapter 14). This group of symptoms is termed tetany, and the nurse must immediately report its appearance, because laryngospasm, although rare, may occur and obstruct the airway. Tetany of this type is usually treated with IV calcium gluconate. This calcium abnormality is usually temporary after thyroidectomy unless all parathyroid tissue was removed.

Promoting Home and Community-Based Care. The patient is usually discharged within 1 or 2 days. Therefore, the patient and family need to be knowledgeable about the signs and symptoms of the complications that may occur and those that should be reported. Strategies are suggested for managing postoperative pain at home and for increasing humidification. The nurse explains to the patient and family the need for rest, relaxation, and nutrition. The patient is permitted to resume his or her former activities and responsibilities completely once recovered from surgery.

If indicated, a referral to home care is made. The home care nurse assesses the patient's recovery from surgery. The nurse also assesses the surgical incision and reinforces instruction about limiting activities that put strain on the incision and sutures. Family responsibilities and factors relating to the home environment that produce emotional tension have often been implicated as precipitating causes of thyrotoxicosis. A home visit provides an opportunity to evaluate these factors and to suggest ways to improve the home and family environment. The nurse gives specific instructions regarding follow-up visits to the physician or the clinic, which are important for monitoring the thyroid status.

The Parathyroid Glands

Anatomic and Physiologic Overview

The parathyroid glands (normally four) are situated in the neck and embedded in the posterior aspect of the thyroid gland (Fig. 42-5). Parathormone (parathyroid hormone), the protein hormone produced by the parathyroid glands, regulates calcium and phosphorus metabolism. Increased secretion of parathormone results in increased calcium absorption from the kidney, intestine, and bones, which raises the blood calcium level. Some actions of this hormone are increased by the presence of vitamin D. Parathormone also tends to lower the blood phosphorus level. The serum level of ionized calcium regulates the output of parathormone. Increased serum calcium results in decreased parathormone secretion, creating a negative feedback system.

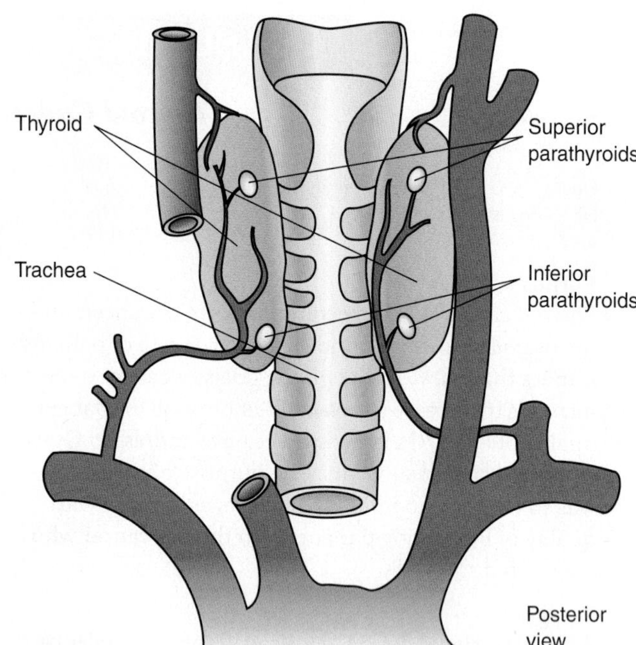

FIGURE 42-5. The parathyroid glands are located behind the thyroid gland. The parathyroids may be embedded in the thyroid tissue.

Pathophysiology

Excess parathormone can result in markedly increased levels of serum calcium, a potentially life-threatening situation. When the product of serum calcium and serum phosphorus (calcium × phosphorus) rises, calcium phosphate may precipitate in various organs of the body (eg, the kidneys) and cause tissue calcification.

Specific Disorders of the Parathyroid Glands

Hyperparathyroidism

Hyperparathyroidism, which is caused by overproduction of parathormone by the parathyroid glands, is characterized by bone decalcification and the development of renal calculi (kidney stones) containing calcium.

Primary hyperparathyroidism occurs two to four times more often in women than in men and is most common in people between 60 and 70 years of age. About 100,000 new cases of hyperparathyroidism are detected each year in the United States. The disorder is rare in children younger than

15 years of age, but the incidence increases tenfold between the ages of 15 and 65 years. Half of the people diagnosed with hyperparathyroidism do not have symptoms.

Secondary hyperparathyroidism, with manifestations similar to those of primary hyperparathyroidism, occurs in patients who have chronic renal failure and so-called renal rickets as a result of phosphorus retention, increased stimulation of the parathyroid glands, and increased parathormone secretion.

Clinical Manifestations

The patient may have no symptoms or may experience signs and symptoms resulting from involvement of several body systems. Apathy, fatigue, muscle weakness, nausea, vomiting, constipation, hypertension, and cardiac dysrhythmias may occur. All these signs and symptoms are attributable to the increased concentration of calcium in the blood. Psychological manifestations may vary from irritability and neurosis to psychoses caused by the direct effect of calcium on the brain and nervous system. An increase in calcium produces a decrease in the excitation potential of nerve and muscle tissue.

The formation of stones in one or both kidneys, related to the increased urinary excretion of calcium and phosphorus, is one of the important complications of hyperparathyroidism and occurs in 55% of patients with primary hyperparathyroidism. Renal damage results from the precipitation of calcium phosphate in the renal pelvis and parenchyma, which causes renal calculi (kidney stones), obstruction, pyelonephritis, and renal failure.

Musculoskeletal symptoms accompanying hyperparathyroidism may be caused by demineralization of the bones or by bone tumors composed of benign giant cells resulting from overgrowth of osteoclasts. The patient may develop skeletal pain and tenderness, especially of the back and joints; pain on weight bearing; pathologic fractures; deformities; and shortening of body stature. Bone loss attributable to hyperparathyroidism increases the risk for fracture.

The incidence of peptic ulcer and pancreatitis is increased with hyperparathyroidism and may be responsible for many of the gastrointestinal symptoms that occur.

Assessment and Diagnostic Findings

Primary hyperparathyroidism is diagnosed by persistent elevation of serum calcium levels and an elevated concentration of parathormone. Radioimmunoassays for parathormone are sensitive and differentiate primary hyperparathyroidism from other causes of hypercalcemia in more than 90% of patients with elevated serum calcium levels. An elevated serum calcium level alone is a nonspecific finding, because serum levels may be altered by diet, medications, and renal and bone changes. Bone changes may be detected on x-ray or bone scans in advanced disease. The double-antibody parathyroid hormone test is used to distinguish between primary hyperparathyroidism and malignancy as a cause of hypercalcemia. Ultrasound, MRI, thallium scan, and fine-needle biopsy have been used to evaluate the function of the parathyroids and to localize parathyroid cysts, adenomas, or hyperplasia.

Medical Management

The recommended treatment of primary hyperparathyroidism is the surgical removal of abnormal parathyroid tissue (parathyroidectomy). In some patients who are without symptoms and have only mildly elevated serum calcium concentrations and normal renal function, surgery may be delayed and the patient monitored closely for worsening of hypercalcemia, bone deterioration, renal impairment, or the development of kidney stones.

HYDRATION THERAPY

Because kidney involvement is possible, patients with hyperparathyroidism are at risk for renal calculi. Therefore, a daily fluid intake of 2000 mL or more is encouraged to help prevent calculus formation. Cranberry juice is suggested, because it may lower the urinary pH. It can be added to other juices or to ginger ale for variety. Cranberry extract tablets are an alternative to reduce urinary pH. The patient is instructed to report other manifestations of renal calculi, such as abdominal pain and hematuria. Thiazide diuretics are avoided, because they decrease the renal excretion of calcium and further elevate serum calcium levels. Because of the risk for hypercalcemic crisis (see later discussion), the patient is instructed to avoid dehydration and to seek immediate health care if conditions that commonly produce dehydration (eg, vomiting, diarrhea) occur.

MOBILITY

Mobility of the patient, with walking or use of a rocking chair for those with limited mobility, is encouraged as much as possible, because bones that are subjected to normal stress give up less calcium. Bed rest increases calcium excretion and the risk for renal calculi. Oral phosphates lower the serum calcium level in some patients; long-term use is not recommended because of the risk of ectopic calcium phosphate deposition in soft tissues.

DIET AND MEDICATIONS

Nutritional needs are met, but the patient is advised to avoid a diet with restricted or excess calcium. If the patient has a coexisting peptic ulcer, prescribed antacids and protein feedings are necessary. Because anorexia is common, efforts are made to improve the appetite. Prune juice, stool softeners, and physical activity, along with increased fluid intake, help to offset constipation, which is common postoperatively.

Nursing Management

The insidious onset and chronic nature of hyperparathyroidism and its diverse and commonly vague symptoms may result in depression and frustration. The family may have considered the patient's illness to be psychosomatic. An awareness of the course of the disorder and an understanding approach by the nurse may help the patient and family deal with their reactions and feelings.

The nursing management of the patient undergoing parathyroidectomy is essentially the same as that of a patient undergoing thyroidectomy. However, the previously described precautions about dehydration, immobility, and diet are particularly important in the patient who is awaiting or recovering from parathyroidectomy. Although not all parathyroid tissue is removed during surgery in an effort to control the calcium–phosphorus balance, the nurse closely monitors the patient to detect symptoms of tetany (which may be an early postoperative complication). Most patients quickly regain function of the remaining parathyroid tissue and experience only mild, transient postoperative hypocalcemia. In patients with significant bone disease or bone changes, a more prolonged period of hypocalcemia should be anticipated. The nurse reminds the patient and family about the importance of follow-up to ensure return of serum calcium levels to normal (Chart 42-8).

Complications: Hypercalcemic Crisis

Acute hypercalcemic crisis can occur with extreme elevation of serum calcium levels. Serum calcium levels greater than 15 mg/dL (3.7 mmol/L) result in neurologic, cardiovascular, and renal symptoms that can be life-threatening. Treatment includes rehydration with large volumes of IV fluids, diuretic agents to promote renal excretion of excess calcium, and phosphate therapy to correct hypophosphatemia and decrease serum calcium levels by promoting calcium deposition in bone and reducing the gastrointestinal absorption of calcium. Cytotoxic agents (eg, mithramycin), calcitonin, and dialysis may be used in emergency situations to decrease serum calcium levels quickly.

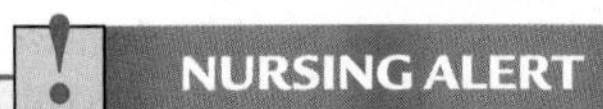

NURSING ALERT

The patient in acute hypercalcemic crisis requires close monitoring for life-threatening complications and prompt treatment to reduce serum calcium levels.

A combination of calcitonin and corticosteroids has been administered in emergencies to reduce the serum calcium level by increasing calcium deposition in bone. Other agents that may be administered to decrease serum calcium levels include bisphosphonates (eg, etidronate [Didronel], pamidronate [Aredia]).

Expert assessment and care are required to minimize complications and reverse the life-threatening hypercalcemia. Medications are administered with care, and attention is given to fluid balance to promote return of normal fluid and electrolyte balance. Supportive measures are necessary for the patient and family. (See Chapters 14 and 16 for further discussion of hypercalcemic crisis.)

Hypoparathyroidism

The most common cause of hypoparathyroidism is inadequate secretion of parathormone after interruption of the blood supply or surgical removal of parathyroid gland tissue during thyroidectomy, parathyroidectomy, or radical neck dissection. These small glands are easily overlooked and can be removed inadvertently during thyroid surgery. Atrophy of the parathyroid glands of unknown cause is a less common cause of hypoparathyroidism.

Deficiency of parathormone results in increased blood phosphate (hyperphosphatemia) and decreased blood calcium (hypocalcemia) levels. In the absence of parathormone, there is decreased intestinal absorption of dietary calcium and decreased resorption of calcium from bone and through the renal tubules. Decreased renal excretion of phosphate causes hypophosphaturia, and low serum calcium levels result in hypocalciuria.

Clinical Manifestations

Hypocalcemia causes irritability of the neuromuscular system and contributes to the chief symptom of hypopara-

CHART 42-8

HOME CARE CHECKLIST • The Patient With Hyperparathyroidism

At the completion of the home care instruction, the patient or caregiver will be able to:	Patient	Caregiver
• State present and potential effects of hyperparathyroidism on the body	✔	✔
• State precipitating factors and interventions for complications	✔	✔
• State importance of regular follow-up visits with health care provider	✔	✔
• Describe potential benefits and risks of parathyroidectomy	✔	✔
• State the purpose, dose, route, schedule, side effects, and precautions of prescribed medications (loop diuretics, phosphate, calcitonin, mithramycin)	✔	✔
• State the need to contact health care provider before taking over-the-counter medication containing calcium	✔	✔
• State need to take pain medications on a scheduled basis	✔	✔
• Describe nonpharmacologic methods of pain management	✔	✔
• Identify safety hazards and methods of injury prevention	✔	✔
• Identify areas of activity limitations and impact on lifestyle	✔	✔
• State need for increased fluid intake and diet low in calcium and vitamin D	✔	✔

thyroidism—tetany. Tetany is a general muscle hypertonia, with tremor and spasmodic or uncoordinated contractions occurring with or without efforts to make voluntary movements. Symptoms of latent tetany are numbness, tingling, and cramps in the extremities, and the patient complains of stiffness in the hands and feet. In overt tetany, the signs include bronchospasm, laryngeal spasm, carpopedal spasm (flexion of the elbows and wrists and extension of the carpophalangeal joints and dorsiflexion of the feet), dysphagia, photophobia, cardiac dysrhythmias, and seizures. Other symptoms include anxiety, irritability, depression, and even delirium. ECG changes and hypotension also may occur.

Assessment and Diagnostic Findings

A positive Trousseau's sign or a positive Chvostek's sign suggests latent tetany. **Trousseau's sign** is positive when carpopedal spasm is induced by occluding the blood flow to the arm for 3 minutes with a blood pressure cuff. **Chvostek's sign** is positive when a sharp tapping over the facial nerve just in front of the parotid gland and anterior to the ear causes spasm or twitching of the mouth, nose, and eye (see Chapter 14).

The diagnosis of hypoparathyroidism often is difficult because of the vague symptoms, such as aches and pains. Therefore, laboratory studies are especially helpful. Tetany develops at serum calcium levels of 5 to 6 mg/dL (1.2 to 1.5 mmol/L) or lower. Serum phosphate levels are increased, and x-rays of bone show increased density. Calcification is detected on x-rays of the subcutaneous or paraspinal basal ganglia of the brain.

Medical Management

The goal of therapy is to increase the serum calcium level to 9 to 10 mg/dL (2.2 to 2.5 mmol/L) and to eliminate the symptoms of hypoparathyroidism and hypocalcemia. When hypocalcemia and tetany occur after a thyroidectomy, the immediate treatment is administration of IV calcium gluconate. If this does not decrease neuromuscular irritability and seizure activity immediately, sedative agents such as pentobarbital may be administered.

Parenteral parathormone can be administered to treat acute hypoparathyroidism with tetany. However, the high incidence of allergic reactions to injections of parathormone limits its use to acute episodes of hypocalcemia. The patient receiving parathormone is monitored closely for allergic reactions and changes in serum calcium levels.

Because of neuromuscular irritability, the patient with hypocalcemia and tetany requires an environment that is free of noise, drafts, bright lights, or sudden movement. Tracheostomy or mechanical ventilation may become necessary, along with bronchodilating medications, if the patient develops respiratory distress.

Therapy for chronic hypoparathyroidism is determined after serum calcium levels are obtained. A diet high in calcium and low in phosphorus is prescribed. Although milk, milk products, and egg yolk are high in calcium, they are restricted because they also contain high levels of phosphorus. Spinach also is avoided because it contains oxalate, which would form insoluble calcium substances. Oral tablets of calcium salts, such as calcium gluconate, may be used to supplement the diet. Aluminum hydroxide gel or aluminum carbonate (Gelusil, Amphojel) also is administered after meals to bind phosphate and promote its excretion through the gastrointestinal tract.

Variable dosages of a vitamin D preparation—dihydrotachysterol (AT 10 or Hytakerol), ergocalciferol (vitamin D), or cholecalciferol (vitamin D)—are usually required and enhance calcium absorption from the gastrointestinal tract.

Nursing Management

Nursing management of the patient with possible acute hypoparathyroidism includes the following:

- Care of postoperative patients who have undergone thyroidectomy, parathyroidectomy, or radical neck dissection is directed toward detecting early signs of hypocalcemia and anticipating signs of tetany, seizures, and respiratory difficulties.
- Calcium gluconate is kept at the bedside, with equipment necessary for IV administration. If the patient has a cardiac disorder, is subject to dysrhythmias, or is receiving digitalis, calcium gluconate is administered slowly and cautiously.
- Calcium and digitalis increase systolic contraction and also potentiate each other; this can produce potentially fatal dysrhythmias. Consequently, the cardiac patient requires continuous cardiac monitoring and careful assessment.

An important aspect of nursing care is teaching about medications and diet therapy. The patient needs to know the reason for high calcium and low phosphate intake and the symptoms of hypocalcemia and hypercalcemia; he or she should know to contact the physician immediately if these symptoms occur (Chart 42-9).

The Adrenal Glands

Anatomic and Physiologic Overview

Each person has two adrenal glands, one attached to the upper portion of each kidney. Each adrenal gland is, in reality, two endocrine glands with separate, independent functions. The adrenal medulla at the center of the gland secretes catecholamines, and the outer portion of the gland, the adrenal cortex, secretes steroid hormones (Fig. 42-6). The secretion of hormones from the adrenal cortex is regulated by the hypothalamic–pituitary–adrenal axis. The hypothalamus secretes corticotropin-releasing hormone (CRH), which stimulates the pituitary gland to secrete ACTH, which in turn stimulates the adrenal cortex to secrete glucocorticoid hormone (cortisol). Increased levels of the adrenal hormone then inhibit the production or secretion of CRH and ACTH. This system is an example of a negative feedback mechanism.

Adrenal Medulla

The adrenal medulla functions as part of the autonomic nervous system. Stimulation of preganglionic sympathetic nerve fibers, which travel directly to the cells of the adrenal medulla, causes release of the catecholamine hormones epinephrine and norepinephrine. About 90% of the secretion of the human adrenal medulla is epinephrine (also called adrenaline). Catecholamines regulate metabolic pathways to promote catabolism of stored fuels to meet caloric needs from endogenous sources. The major effects of epinephrine

CHART 42-9

HOME CARE CHECKLIST • The Patient With Hypoparathyroidism

At the completion of the home care instruction, the patient or caregiver will be able to:	Patient	Caregiver
• State present and potential effects of hypoparathyroidism on the body	✔	✔
• State precipitating factors and interventions for complications (seizure, cardiac dysrhythmias, cardiac arrest)	✔	✔
• State necessary actions for seizure activity		✔
• State importance of regular follow-up visits with health care provider	✔	✔
• State purpose, dose, route, schedule, side effects, and precautions of prescribed medications (calcium, phosphate binders)	✔	✔
• State need to alternate activity and rest periods	✔	✔
• Identify areas of activity limitations and impact on lifestyle	✔	✔
• Identify foods high in calcium and vitamin D, low in phosphorus	✔	✔

release are to prepare to meet a challenge (fight-or-flight response). Secretion of epinephrine causes decreased blood flow to tissues that are not needed in emergency situations, such as the gastrointestinal tract, and increased blood flow to tissues that are important for effective fight or flight, such as cardiac and skeletal muscle. Catecholamines also induce the release of free fatty acids, increase the basal metabolic rate, and elevate the blood glucose level.

Adrenal Cortex

A functioning adrenal cortex is necessary for life; adrenocortical secretions make it possible for the body to adapt to stress of all kinds. The three types of steroid hormones produced by the adrenal cortex are **glucocorticoids**, the prototype of which is hydrocortisone; **mineralocorticoids**, mainly aldosterone; and sex hormones, mainly **androgens** (male sex hormones). Without the adrenal cortex, severe stress would cause peripheral circulatory failure, circulatory shock, and prostration. Survival in the absence of a functioning adrenal cortex is possible only with nutritional, electrolyte, and fluid replacement and appropriate replacement with exogenous adrenocortical hormones.

GLUCOCORTICOIDS

The glucocorticoids are so named because they have an important influence on glucose metabolism: increased hydro-

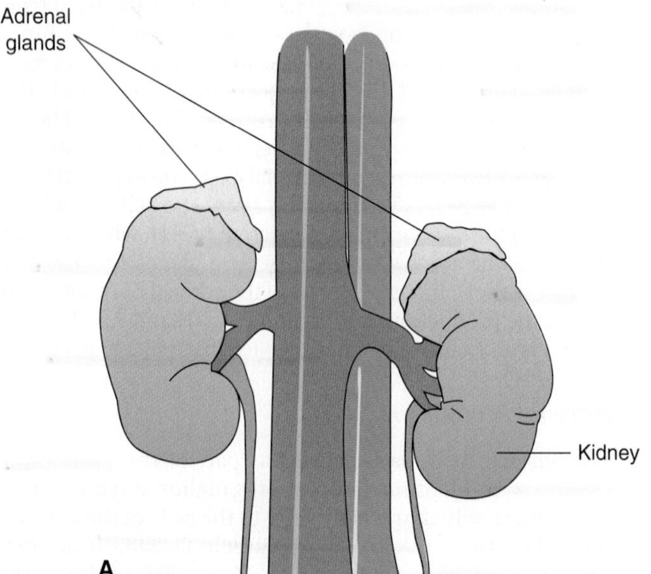

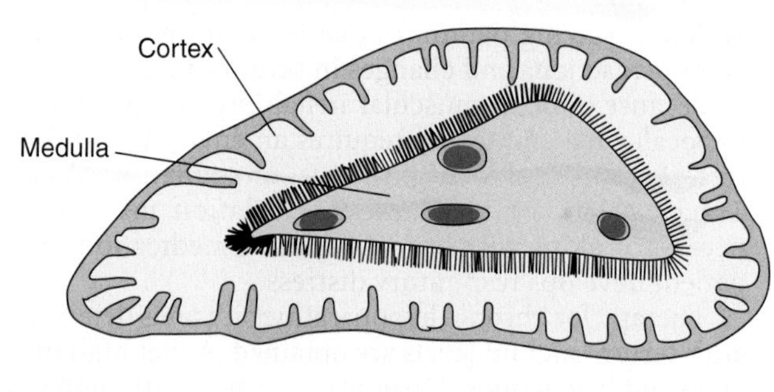

FIGURE 42-6. (**A**) The adrenal glands sit on top of the kidneys. (**B**) Each gland is composed of an outer cortex and an inner medulla. Each area secretes specific hormones. The adrenal medulla secretes catecholamines—epinephrine and norepinephrine; the adrenal cortex secretes glucocorticoids, mineralocorticoids, and sex hormones. Adapted from Porth, C. (2002). *Pathophysiology: Concepts of altered health states* (6th ed.). Philadelphia: Lippincott Williams & Wilkins.

cortisone secretion results in elevated blood glucose levels. However, the glucocorticoids have major effects on the metabolism of almost all organs of the body. Glucocorticoids are secreted from the adrenal cortex in response to the release of ACTH from the anterior lobe of the pituitary gland. This system represents an example of negative feedback. The presence of glucocorticoids in the blood inhibits the release of corticotropin-releasing factor (CRH) from the hypothalamus and also inhibits ACTH secretion from the pituitary. The resultant decrease in ACTH secretion causes diminished release of glucocorticoids from the adrenal cortex.

Glucocorticoids (in the form of **corticosteroids**) are administered frequently to inhibit the inflammatory response to tissue injury and to suppress allergic manifestations. Their side effects include the development of diabetes mellitus, osteoporosis, peptic ulcer, increased protein breakdown resulting in muscle wasting and poor wound healing, and redistribution of body fat. Large amounts of exogenously administered glucocorticoids in the blood inhibit the release of ACTH and endogenous glucocorticoids. Because of this, the adrenal cortex can atrophy. If exogenous glucocorticoid administration is discontinued suddenly, adrenal insufficiency results because of the inability of the atrophied cortex to respond adequately.

MINERALOCORTICOIDS

Mineralocorticoids exert their major effects on electrolyte metabolism. They act principally on the renal tubular and gastrointestinal epithelium to cause increased sodium ion absorption in exchange for excretion of potassium or hydrogen ions. ACTH only minimally influences aldosterone secretion. It is primarily secreted in response to the presence of angiotensin II in the bloodstream. Angiotensin II is a substance that elevates the blood pressure by constricting arterioles. Its concentration is increased when renin is released from the kidney in response to decreased perfusion pressure. The resultant increased aldosterone levels promote sodium reabsorption by the kidney and the gastrointestinal tract, which tends to restore blood pressure to normal. The release of aldosterone is also increased by hyperkalemia. Aldosterone is the primary hormone for the long-term regulation of sodium balance.

ADRENAL SEX HORMONES (ANDROGENS)

Androgens, the third major type of steroid hormones produced by the adrenal cortex, exert effects similar to those of male sex hormones. The adrenal gland may also secrete small amounts of some estrogens, or female sex hormones. ACTH controls the secretion of adrenal androgens. When secreted in normal amounts, the adrenal androgens probably have little effect, but when secreted in excess, as in certain inborn enzyme deficiencies, masculinization may result. This is termed the **adrenogenital syndrome**.

Specific Disorders of the Adrenal Glands

Pheochromocytoma

Pheochromocytoma is a tumor that is usually benign and originates from the chromaffin cells of the adrenal medulla. In 90% of patients (O'Connell, 2004), the tumor arises in the medulla; in the remaining patients, it occurs in the extra-adrenal chromaffin tissue located in or near the aorta, ovaries, spleen, or other organs. Pheochromocytoma may occur at any age, but its peak incidence is between 40 and 50 years of age (O'Connell, 2004). It affects men and women equally. Ten percent of the tumors are bilateral, and 10% are malignant. Because of the high incidence of pheochromocytoma in family members of affected people, the patient's family members should be alerted and screened for this tumor. Pheochromocytoma may occur in the familial form as part of multiple endocrine neoplasia type 2; therefore, it should be considered a possibility in patients who have medullary thyroid carcinoma and parathyroid hyperplasia or tumor.

Pheochromocytoma is the cause of high blood pressure in 0.1% of patients with hypertension (Bravo & Tagle, 2003). Although it is uncommon, it is one form of hypertension that is usually cured by surgery; however, without detection and treatment, it is usually fatal.

Clinical Manifestations

The nature and severity of symptoms of functioning tumors of the adrenal medulla depend on the relative proportions of epinephrine and norepinephrine secretion. The typical triad of symptoms is headache, diaphoresis, and palpitations in the patient with hypertension (Bravo & Tagle, 2003). Approximately 8% of patients are completely asymptomatic. Hypertension and other cardiovascular disturbances are common. The hypertension may be intermittent or persistent. However, only half of patients with pheochromocytoma have sustained or persistent hypertension. If the hypertension is sustained, it may be difficult to distinguish from other causes of hypertension. Other symptoms may include tremor, headache, flushing, and anxiety. Hyperglycemia may result from conversion of liver and muscle glycogen to glucose due to epinephrine secretion; insulin may be required to maintain normal blood glucose levels.

The clinical picture in the paroxysmal form of pheochromocytoma is usually characterized by acute, unpredictable attacks lasting seconds or several hours. Symptoms usually begin abruptly and subside slowly. During these attacks, the patient is extremely anxious, tremulous, and weak. The patient may experience headache, vertigo, blurring of vision, tinnitus, air hunger, and dyspnea. Other symptoms include polyuria, nausea, vomiting, diarrhea, abdominal pain, and a feeling of impending doom. Palpitations and tachycardia are common (Porth, 2005). Blood pressures exceeding 250/150 mm Hg have been recorded. Such blood pressure elevations are life-threatening and can cause severe complications, such as cardiac dysrhythmias, dissecting aneurysm, stroke, and acute renal failure. Postural hypotension (decrease in systolic blood pressure, lightheadedness, dizziness on standing) occurs in 70% of patients with untreated pheochromocytoma.

Assessment and Diagnostic Findings

Pheochromocytoma is suspected if signs of sympathetic nervous system overactivity occur in association with marked elevation of blood pressure. These signs can be associated with the "five Hs": hypertension, headache, hyperhidrosis (excessive sweating), hypermetabolism, and hyperglycemia. The presence of these signs has a 93.8% specificity and a 90.9% sensitivity for pheochromocytoma (Bravo & Tagle, 2003).

Paroxysmal symptoms of pheochromocytoma commonly develop in the fifth decade of life.

Measurements of urine and plasma levels of catecholamines and metanephrine (MN), a catecholamine metabolite, are the most direct and conclusive tests for overactivity of the adrenal medulla. A new test for detecting pheochromocytoma has recently been developed that measures free MN in plasma by high-pressure liquid chromatography and electrochemical detection (Bravo & Tagle, 2003; Lenders, Pacak, & Eisenhofer, 2002). A negative test result virtually excludes pheochromocytoma. However, increased levels of at least one catecholamine or MN can occur in 10% of patients with essential hypertension.

Measurements of catecholamine metabolites (MN and vanillylmandelic acid [VMA]) or free catecholamines have been extensively used in the clinical setting. In most cases, pheochromocytoma can be diagnosed or confirmed based on a properly collected 24-hour urine sample (Bravo & Tagle, 2003). Levels can be as high as two times the normal limit. A 24-hour specimen of urine is collected for determination of free catecholamines, MN, and VMA; the use of combined tests increases the diagnostic accuracy of testing. A number of medications and foods, such as coffee and tea (including decaffeinated varieties), bananas, chocolate, vanilla, and aspirin, may alter the results of these tests; therefore, careful instructions to avoid restricted items must be given to the patient. Urine collected over a 2- or 3-hour period after an attack of hypertension can be assayed for catecholamine content.

The total plasma catecholamine (epinephrine and norepinephrine) concentration is measured with the patient supine and at rest for 30 minutes. To prevent elevation of catecholamine levels resulting from the stress of venipuncture, a butterfly needle, scalp vein needle, or venous catheter may be inserted 30 minutes before the blood specimen is obtained.

Factors that may elevate catecholamine concentrations must be controlled to obtain valid results; these factors include consumption of coffee or tea (including decaffeinated varieties), use of tobacco, emotional and physical stress, and use of many prescription and over-the-counter medications (eg, amphetamines, nose drops or sprays, decongestant agents, bronchodilators).

Normal plasma values of epinephrine are 100 pg/mL (590 pmol/L); normal values of norepinephrine are generally less than 100 to 550 pg/mL (590 to 3240 pmol/L). Values of epinephrine greater than 400 pg/mL (2180 pmol/L) or norepinephrine values greater than 2000 pg/mL (11,800 pmol/L) are considered diagnostic of pheochromocytoma. Values that fall between normal levels and those diagnostic of pheochromocytoma indicate the need for further testing.

A clonidine suppression test may be performed if the results of plasma and urine tests of catecholamines are inconclusive. Clonidine (Catapres) is a centrally acting antiadrenergic medication that suppresses the release of neurogenically mediated catecholamines. The suppression test is based on the principle that catecholamine levels are normally increased through the activity of the sympathetic nervous system. In pheochromocytoma, increased catecholamine levels result from the diffusion of excess catecholamines into the circulation, bypassing normal storage and release mechanisms. Therefore, in patients with pheochromocytoma, clonidine does not suppress the release of catecholamines.

Imaging studies, such as CT, MRI, and ultrasonography, may also be carried out to localize the pheochromocytoma and to determine whether more than one tumor is present. Use of ^{131}I-metaiodobenzylguanidine (MIBG) scintigraphy may be required to determine the location of the pheochromocytoma and to detect metastatic sites outside the adrenal gland. MIBG is a specific isotope for catecholamine-producing tissue. It has been helpful in identifying tumors not detected by other tests or procedures. MIBG scintigraphy is a noninvasive, safe procedure that has increased the accuracy of diagnosis of adrenal tumors.

Other diagnostic studies may focus on evaluating the function of other endocrine glands because of the association of pheochromocytoma in some patients with other endocrine tumors.

Medical Management

During an episode or attack of hypertension, tachycardia, anxiety, and the other symptoms of pheochromocytoma, the patient is prescribed bed rest with the head of the bed elevated to promote an orthostatic decrease in blood pressure.

PHARMACOLOGIC THERAPY

The patient may be moved to the intensive care unit for close monitoring of ECG changes and careful administration of alpha-adrenergic blocking agents (eg, phentolamine [Regitine]) or smooth muscle relaxants (eg, sodium nitroprusside [Nipride]) to lower the blood pressure quickly.

Phenoxybenzamine (Dibenzyline), a long-acting alpha-blocker, may be used after the blood pressure is stable to prepare the patient for surgery. Calcium channel blockers such as nifedipine (Procardia) are usually well tolerated by patients and have reduced perioperative fluid requirements. They are also useful for prevention of cardiovascular complications, because they prevent catecholamine-induced coronary vasospasm and myocarditis (Bravo & Tagle, 2003). Beta-adrenergic blocking agents such as propranolol (Inderal) may be used in patients with cardiac dysrhythmias and in those not responsive to alpha-blockers. Alpha-adrenergic and beta-adrenergic blocking agents must be used with caution, because patients with pheochromocytoma may have increased sensitivity to them. Still other medications that may be used preoperatively are catecholamine synthesis inhibitors, such as alpha-methyl-*p*-tyrosine (metyrosine). These are occasionally used if adrenergic blocking agents do not reduce the effects of catecholamines.

SURGICAL MANAGEMENT

The definitive treatment of pheochromocytoma is surgical removal of the tumor, usually with **adrenalectomy**. Bilateral adrenalectomy may be necessary if tumors are present in both adrenal glands. Patient preparation includes control of blood pressure and blood volumes; usually this is carried out over 4 to 7 days. Nifedipine (Procardia) and nicardipine (Cardene) may be used safely without causing undue hypotension. For episodes of severe hypertension, nifedipine is a fast and effective treatment, because the capsules can be pierced and chewed. The patient needs to be well hydrated before, during, and after surgery to prevent hypotension.

Manipulation of the tumor during surgical excision may cause release of stored epinephrine and norepinephrine, with marked increases in blood pressure and changes in heart rate. Therefore, use of sodium nitroprusside (Nipride) and alpha-adrenergic blocking agents may be required during and after surgery. Exploration of other possible tumor sites is frequently undertaken to ensure removal of all tumor tissue. As a result, the patient is subject to the stress and effects of a long surgical procedure, which may increase the risk for hypertension postoperatively.

Corticosteroid replacement is required if bilateral adrenalectomy has been necessary. Corticosteroids may also be required for the first few days or weeks after removal of a single adrenal gland. IV administration of corticosteroids (methylprednisolone sodium succinate [Solu-Medrol]) may begin on the evening before surgery and continue during the early postoperative period to prevent adrenal insufficiency. Oral preparations of corticosteroids (prednisone) are prescribed after the acute stress of surgery diminishes.

Hypotension and hypoglycemia may occur in the postoperative period because of the sudden withdrawal of excessive amounts of catecholamines. Therefore, careful attention is directed toward monitoring and treating these changes. Blood pressure is expected to return to normal with treatment; however, one third of patients continue to be hypertensive after surgery. This may result if not all pheochromocytoma tissue was removed, if pheochromocytoma recurs, or if the blood vessels were damaged by severe and prolonged hypertension. Several days after surgery, urine and plasma levels of catecholamines and their metabolites are measured to determine whether the surgery was successful.

Nursing Management

The patient who has undergone surgery to treat pheochromocytoma has experienced a stressful preoperative and postoperative course and may remain fearful of repeated attacks. Although it is usually expected that all pheochromocytoma tissue has been removed, there is a possibility that other sites were undetected and that attacks may recur. The patient is monitored for several days in the intensive care unit with special attention given to ECG changes, arterial pressures, fluid and electrolyte balance, and blood glucose levels. Several IV lines are inserted for administration of fluids and medications.

PROMOTING HOME AND COMMUNITY-BASED CARE

Teaching Patients Self-Care. During the preoperative and postoperative phases of care, the nurse informs the patient about the importance of follow-up monitoring to ensure that pheochromocytoma does not recur undetected. After adrenalectomy, use of corticosteroids may be needed. Therefore, the nurse instructs the patient about their purpose, the medication schedule, and the risks of skipping doses or stopping their administration abruptly.

It is important to teach the patient and family how to measure the patient's blood pressure and when to notify the physician about changes in blood pressure. In addition, the nurse provides verbal and written instructions about the procedure for collecting 24-hour urine specimens to monitor urine catecholamine levels.

Continuing Care. A follow-up visit from a home care nurse may be indicated to assess the patient's postoperative recovery, surgical incision, and compliance with the medication schedule. This may help reinforce previous teaching about management and monitoring. The home care nurse also obtains blood pressure measurements and assists the patient in preventing or dealing with problems that may result from long-term use of corticosteroids.

Because of the risk for recurrence of hypertension, periodic checkups are required, especially in young patients and in those whose families have a history of pheochromocytoma. The patient is scheduled for periodic follow-up appointments to observe for return of normal blood pressure and plasma and urine levels of catecholamines.

Adrenocortical Insufficiency (Addison's Disease)

Addison's disease, or adrenocortical insufficiency, occurs when adrenal cortex function is inadequate to meet the patient's need for cortical hormones. Autoimmune or idiopathic atrophy of the adrenal glands is responsible for 80% to 90% of cases (Arlt & Allolio, 2003). Other causes include surgical removal of both adrenal glands and infection of the adrenal glands. Tuberculosis and histoplasmosis are the most common infections that destroy adrenal gland tissue. Although autoimmune destruction has replaced tuberculosis as the principal cause of Addison's disease, tuberculosis should be considered in the diagnostic workup because of its increasing incidence. Inadequate secretion of ACTH from the pituitary gland also results in adrenal insufficiency because of decreased stimulation of the adrenal cortex.

Therapeutic use of corticosteroids is the most common cause of adrenocortical insufficiency (Arlt & Allolio, 2003). The symptoms of adrenocortical insufficiency may also result from the sudden cessation of exogenous adrenocortical hormonal therapy, which suppresses the body's normal response to stress and interferes with normal feedback mechanisms. Treatment with daily administration of corticosteroids for 2 to 4 weeks may suppress function of the adrenal cortex; therefore, adrenal insufficiency should be considered in any patient who has been treated with corticosteroids.

Clinical Manifestations

Addison's disease is characterized by muscle weakness; anorexia; gastrointestinal symptoms; fatigue; emaciation; dark pigmentation of the mucous membranes and the skin, especially of the knuckles, knees, and elbows; hypotension; and low blood glucose, low serum sodium, and high serum potassium levels. Mental status changes such as depression, emotional lability, apathy, and confusion are present in 60% to 80% of patients. In severe cases, the disturbance of sodium and potassium metabolism may be marked by depletion of sodium and water and severe, chronic dehydration.

With disease progression and acute hypotension, **addisonian crisis** develops. This condition is characterized by cyanosis and the classic signs of circulatory shock: pallor, apprehension, rapid and weak pulse, rapid respirations, and low blood pressure. In addition, the patient may complain of headache, nausea, abdominal pain, and diarrhea and may show signs of confusion and restlessness. Even slight overexertion, exposure to cold, acute infection, or a decrease in salt intake may lead to circulatory collapse, shock, and death if untreated. The stress of surgery or dehydration resulting from preparation for diagnostic tests or surgery may precipitate an addisonian or hypotensive crisis.

Assessment and Diagnostic Findings

Although the clinical manifestations presented appear specific, the onset of Addison's disease usually occurs with nonspecific symptoms. The diagnosis is confirmed by laboratory test results. Combined measurements of early-morning serum cortisol and plasma ACTH are performed to differentiate patients with primary adrenal insufficiency from those with secondary adrenal insufficiency and from people who are healthy (Arlt & Allolio, 2003). Patients with primary insufficiency have a greatly increased plasma ACTH level (more than 22.0 pmol/L) and a serum cortisol concentration lower than the normal range (less than 165 nmol/L) or in the low-normal range. Other laboratory findings include decreased levels of blood glucose (hypoglycemia) and sodium (hyponatremia), an increased serum potassium concentration (hyperkalemia), and an increased white blood cell count (leukocytosis).

The diagnosis is confirmed by low levels of adrenocortical hormones in the blood or urine and decreased serum cortisol levels. If the adrenal cortex is destroyed, baseline values are low, and ACTH administration fails to cause the normal increase in plasma cortisol and urinary 17-hydroxycorticosteroids. If the adrenal gland is normal but not stimulated properly by the pituitary, a normal response to repeated doses of exogenous ACTH is seen, but no response occurs after the administration of metyrapone, which stimulates endogenous ACTH.

Medical Management

Immediate treatment is directed toward combating circulatory shock: restoring blood circulation, administering fluids and corticosteroids, monitoring vital signs, and placing the patient in a recumbent position with the legs elevated. Hydrocortisone (Solu-Cortef) is administered intravenously, followed by 5% dextrose in normal saline. Vasopressor amines may be required if hypotension persists.

Antibiotics may be administered if infection has precipitated adrenal crisis in a patient with chronic adrenal insufficiency. In addition, the patient is assessed closely to identify other factors, stressors, or illnesses that led to the acute episode.

Oral intake may be initiated as soon as tolerated. IV fluids are gradually decreased after oral fluid intake is adequate to prevent hypovolemia. If the adrenal gland does not regain function, the patient needs lifelong replacement of corticosteroids and mineralocorticoids to prevent recurrence of adrenal insufficiency. During stressful procedures or significant illnesses, additional supplementary therapy with glucocorticoids is required to prevent addisonian crisis. In addition, the patient may need to supplement dietary intake with added salt during gastrointestinal losses of fluids through vomiting and diarrhea.

Nursing Management

ASSESSING THE PATIENT

The health history and examination focus on the presence of symptoms of fluid imbalance and on the patient's level of stress. To detect inadequate fluid volume, the nurse monitors the blood pressure and pulse rate as the patient moves from a lying to a standing position. The nurse assesses the skin color and turgor for changes related to chronic adrenal insufficiency and hypovolemia. Other key assessments include checking for weight changes, muscle weakness, and fatigue and investigating any illness or stress that may have precipitated the acute crisis.

MONITORING AND MANAGING ADDISONIAN CRISIS

The patient at risk is monitored for signs and symptoms indicative of addisonian crisis. These symptoms are often the manifestations of shock: hypotension; rapid, weak pulse; rapid respiratory rate; pallor; and extreme weakness. The patient with addisonian crisis is at risk for circulatory collapse and shock (see Chapter 15); therefore, physical and psychological stressors must be avoided. These include exposure to cold, overexertion, infection, and emotional distress.

The patient with addisonian crisis requires immediate treatment with IV administration of fluid, glucose, and electrolytes, especially sodium; replacement of missing steroid hormones; and vasopressors. During acute addisonian crisis, the patient must avoid exertion; therefore, the nurse anticipates the patient's needs and takes measures to meet them.

Careful monitoring of symptoms, vital signs, weight, and fluid and electrolyte status is essential to assess the patient's progress and return to a precrisis state. To reduce the risk of future episodes of addisonian crisis, efforts are made to identify and reduce the factors that may have led to the crisis.

RESTORING FLUID BALANCE

To provide information about fluid balance and the adequacy of hormone replacement, the nurse assesses the patient's skin turgor, mucous membranes, and weight while instructing the patient to report increased thirst, which may indicate impending fluid imbalance. Lying, sitting, and standing blood pressure measurements also provide information about fluid status. A decrease in systolic pressure (20 mm Hg or more) may indicate depletion of fluid volume, especially if accompanied by symptoms. The nurse encourages the patient to consume foods and fluids that assist in restoring and maintaining fluid and electrolyte balance; along with the dietitian, the nurse helps the patient select foods high in sodium during gastrointestinal disturbances and in very hot weather.

The nurse instructs the patient and family to administer hormone replacement as prescribed and to modify the dosage during illness and other stressful situations. Written and verbal instructions are provided about the administration of mineralocorticoid (Florinef) or corticosteroid (prednisone) as prescribed.

IMPROVING ACTIVITY TOLERANCE

Until the patient's condition is stabilized, the nurse takes precautions to avoid unnecessary activity and stress that could precipitate another hypotensive episode. Efforts are made to detect signs of infection or the presence of other stressors. Even minor events or stressors may be excessive in patients with adrenal insufficiency. During the acute crisis, the nurse maintains a quiet, nonstressful environment and performs all activities (eg, bathing, turning) for the patient. Explaining all procedures to the patient and family reduces their anxiety. Explaining the rationale for minimizing stress during the acute crisis assists the patient to increase activity gradually.

PROMOTING HOME AND COMMUNITY-BASED CARE

Teaching Patients Self-Care. Because of the need for lifelong replacement of adrenal cortex hormones to prevent addisonian crises, the patient and family members receive explicit verbal and written instructions about the rationale for replacement therapy and proper dosage. In addition, they are instructed about how to modify the medication dosage and increase salt intake in times of illness, very hot weather, and other stressful situations. The patient also learns how to modify diet and fluid intake to help maintain fluid and electrolyte balance.

The patient and family are frequently prescribed preloaded, single-injection syringes of corticosteroid for use in emergencies. Specific instructions about how and when to use the injection are also provided. It is important to instruct the patient to inform other health care providers, such as dentists, about the use of corticosteroids, to wear a medical alert bracelet, and to carry information at all times about the need for corticosteroids. If the patient with Addison's disease requires surgery, careful administration of fluids and corticosteroids is necessary before, during, and after surgery to prevent addisonian crisis.

The patient and family need to know the signs of excessive or insufficient hormone replacement. The development of edema or weight gain may signify too high a dose of hormone; postural hypotension and weight loss frequently signify too low a dose (Chart 42-10).

Continuing Care. Although most patients can return to their job and family responsibilities soon after hospital discharge, others cannot do so because of concurrent illnesses or incomplete recovery from the episode of adrenal insufficiency. In these circumstances, a referral for home care enables the home care nurse to assess the patient's recovery, monitor hormone replacement, and evaluate stress in the home. The nurse assesses the patient's and family's knowledge about medication therapy and dietary modifications. A home visit also allows the nurse to assess the patient's plans for follow-up visits to the clinic or physician's office. The nurse reminds the patient and family about the importance of participating in health promotion activities and health screening.

Cushing's Syndrome

Cushing's syndrome results from excessive, rather than deficient, adrenocortical activity. Cushing's syndrome is commonly caused by use of corticosteroid medications and is infrequently due to excessive corticosteroid production secondary to hyperplasia of the adrenal cortex (Lionakis & Kontoyiannis, 2003). However, overproduction of endogenous corticosteroids may be caused by several mechanisms, including a tumor of the pituitary gland that produces ACTH and stimulates the adrenal cortex to increase its hormone secretion despite production of adequate amounts. Primary hyperplasia of the adrenal glands in the absence of a pituitary tumor is less common. Another less common cause of Cushing's syndrome is the ectopic production of ACTH by malignancies; bronchogenic carcinoma is the most common type of these malignancies. Regardless of the cause, the normal feedback mechanisms that control the function of the adrenal cortex become ineffective, and the usual diurnal pattern of cortisol is lost. The signs and symptoms of Cushing's syndrome are primarily a result of oversecretion of glucocorticoids and androgens (sex hormones), although mineralocorticoid secretion also may be affected.

CHART 42-10

HOME CARE CHECKLIST • The Patient With Adrenal Insufficiency (Addison's Disease)

At the completion of the home care instruction, the patient or caregiver will be able to:	Patient	Caregiver
• State present and potential effects of adrenal insufficiency on the body	✔	✔
• State warning signs of adrenal crisis and need for emergency care	✔	✔
• Explain components of an emergency kit and indications for their use; demonstrate how to use them	✔	✔
• State strategies for dealing with stress and avoiding adrenal crisis	✔	✔
• State the purpose, dose, route, schedule, side effects, and precautions of prescribed medications (corticosteroid replacement)	✔	✔
• State that compliance with medical regimen is lifelong	✔	✔
• State importance of regular follow-up visits with health care provider	✔	✔
• Recognize the need for dosage adjustment during times of stress	✔	✔
• State need to wear medical alert identification and carry medical information card	✔	✔
• State need to notify health care providers about disease before treatment or procedure	✔	✔
• State need to avoid strenuous activity in hot, humid weather	✔	✔
• State need for increased fluid intake and salt with excessive perspiration	✔	✔
• State need for high-carbohydrate, high-protein diet with adequate sodium intake	✔	✔
• Identify needed activity limitations and impact on lifestyle	✔	✔

Clinical Manifestations

When overproduction of the adrenal cortical hormone occurs, arrest of growth, obesity, and musculoskeletal changes occur along with glucose intolerance. The classic picture of Cushing's syndrome in the adult is that of central-type obesity, with a fatty "buffalo hump" in the neck and supraclavicular areas, a heavy trunk, and relatively thin extremities. The skin is thin, fragile, and easily traumatized; ecchymoses (bruises) and striae develop. The patient complains of weakness and lassitude. Sleep is disturbed because of altered diurnal secretion of cortisol.

Excessive protein catabolism occurs, producing muscle wasting and osteoporosis. Kyphosis, backache, and compression fractures of the vertebrae may result. Retention of sodium and water occurs as a result of increased mineralocorticoid activity, producing hypertension and heart failure.

The patient develops a "moon-faced" appearance and may experience increased oiliness of the skin and acne. There is increased susceptibility to infection. Hyperglycemia or overt diabetes may develop. The patient may also report weight gain, slow healing of minor cuts, and bruises.

Women between the ages of 20 and 40 years are five times more likely than men to develop Cushing's syndrome. In females of all ages, virilization may occur as a result of excess androgens. Virilization is characterized by the appearance of masculine traits and the recession of feminine traits. There is an excessive growth of hair on the face (hirsutism), the breasts atrophy, menses cease, the clitoris enlarges, and the voice deepens. Libido is lost in men and women.

Changes occur in mood and mental activity, and psychosis may develop. Distress and depression are common and are increased by the severity of the physical changes that occur with this syndrome. If Cushing's syndrome is a consequence of pituitary tumor, visual disturbances may occur because of pressure of the growing tumor on the optic chiasm. Chart 42-11 summarizes the changes associated with Cushing's syndrome.

CHART 42-11

Clinical Manifestations of Cushing's Syndrome

OPHTHALMIC
- Cataracts
- Glaucoma

CARDIOVASCULAR
- Hypertension
- Heart failure

ENDOCRINE/METABOLIC
- Truncal obesity
- Moon face
- Buffalo hump
- Sodium retention
- Hypokalemia
- Metabolic alkalosis
- Hyperglycemia
- Menstrual irregularities
- Impotence
- Negative nitrogen balance
- Altered calcium metabolism
- Adrenal suppression

IMMUNE FUNCTION
- Decreased inflammatory responses
- Impaired wound healing
- Increased susceptibility to infections

SKELETAL
- Osteoporosis
- Spontaneous fractures
- Aseptic necrosis of femur
- Vertebral compression fractures

GASTROINTESTINAL
- Peptic ulcer
- Pancreatitis

MUSCULAR
- Myopathy
- Muscle weakness

DERMATOLOGIC
- Thinning of skin
- Petechiae
- Ecchymoses
- Striae
- Acne

PSYCHIATRIC
- Mood alterations
- Psychoses

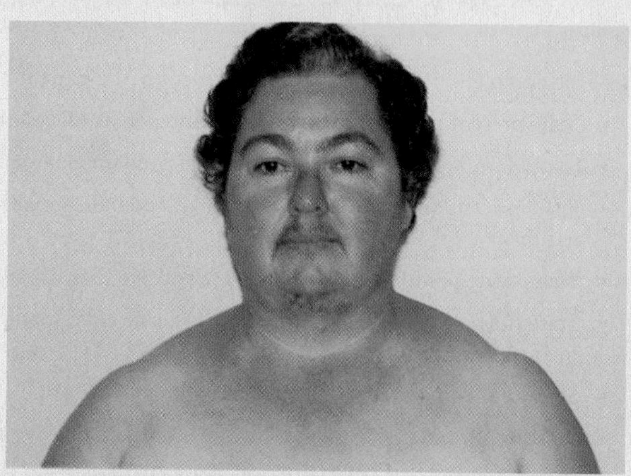

This woman with Cushing's syndrome has several classic signs, including facial hair, buffalo hump, and moon face. From Rubin, E., & Farber, J. L. (2005). *Pathology* (4th ed.). Philadelphia: Lippincott Williams & Wilkins.

Assessment and Diagnostic Findings

An overnight dexamethasone suppression test is the most widely used and most sensitive screening test for diagnosis of pituitary and adrenal causes of Cushing's syndrome (Raff & Findling, 2003). It can be performed on an outpatient basis. Dexamethasone (1 mg) is administered orally at 11 PM, and a plasma cortisol level is obtained at 8 AM the next morning. Suppression of cortisol to less than 5 mg/dL indicates that the hypothalamic–pituitary–adrenal axis is functioning properly. Stress, obesity, depression, and medications such as antiseizure agents, estrogen (during pregnancy or as oral medications), and rifampin can falsely elevate cortisol levels. Recent studies have shown that nighttime salivary cortisol levels show promise in screening for Cushing's syndrome (Raff & Findling, 2003).

Indicators of Cushing's syndrome include an increase in serum sodium and blood glucose levels and a decrease in serum potassium, a reduction in the number of blood eosinophils, and disappearance of lymphoid tissue. Measurements of plasma and urinary cortisol levels are obtained. Several blood samples may be collected to determine whether the normal diurnal variation in plasma levels is present; this variation is frequently absent in adrenal dysfunction. If several blood samples are required, they must be collected at the times specified, and the time of collection must be noted on the requisition slip. Other diagnostic studies include a 24-hour urinary free cortisol level and a low-dose dexamethasone suppression test. Low-dose suppression tests are similar to the overnight test but vary in dosage and timing.

Measurement of plasma ACTH by radioimmunoassay is used in conjunction with the high-dose suppression test to distinguish pituitary tumors from ectopic sites of ACTH production as the cause of Cushing's syndrome. Elevation of both ACTH and cortisol indicates pituitary or hypothalamic disease. A low ACTH with a high cortisol level indicates adrenal disease. CT, ultrasound, or MRI may be performed to localize adrenal tissue and detect tumors of the adrenal gland.

Medical Management

If Cushing's syndrome is caused by pituitary tumors rather than tumors of the adrenal cortex, treatment is directed at the pituitary gland. Surgical removal of the tumor by transsphenoidal hypophysectomy (see Chapter 61) is the treatment of choice and has an 80% success rate (Hammer, Tyrrell, Lamborn, et al., 2004). Radiation of the pituitary gland also has been successful, although it may take several months for control of symptoms. Adrenalectomy is the treatment of choice in patients with primary adrenal hypertrophy.

Postoperatively, symptoms of adrenal insufficiency may begin to appear 12 to 48 hours after surgery because of reduction of the high levels of circulating adrenal hormones. Temporary replacement therapy with hydrocortisone may be necessary for several months, until the adrenal glands begin to respond normally to the body's needs. If both adrenal glands have been removed (bilateral adrenalectomy), lifetime replacement of adrenal cortex hormones is necessary.

Adrenal enzyme inhibitors (eg, metyrapone, aminoglutethimide, mitotane, ketoconazole) may be used to reduce hyperadrenalism if the syndrome is caused by ectopic ACTH secretion by a tumor that cannot be eradicated. Close monitoring is necessary, because symptoms of inadequate adrenal function may result and because of possible side effects of these medications.

If Cushing's syndrome is a result of the administration of corticosteroids, an attempt is made to reduce or taper the medication to the minimum dosage needed to treat the underlying disease process (eg, autoimmune or allergic disease, rejection of a transplanted organ). Frequently, alternate-day therapy decreases the symptoms of Cushing's syndrome and allows recovery of the adrenal glands' responsiveness to ACTH.

Nursing Process

The Patient With Cushing's Syndrome

Assessment

The health history and examination focus on the effects on the body of high concentrations of adrenal cortex hormones and on the inability of the adrenal cortex to respond to changes in cortisol and aldosterone levels. The history includes information about the patient's level of activity and ability to carry out routine and self-care activities. The skin is observed and assessed for trauma, infection, breakdown, bruising, and edema. Changes in physical appearance are noted, and the patient's responses to these changes are elicited. The nurse assesses the patient's mental function, including mood, responses to questions, awareness of environment, and level of depression. The family is often a good source of information about gradual changes in the patient's physical appearance as well as emotional status.

Diagnosis

Nursing Diagnoses

Based on all the assessment data, the major nursing diagnoses of the patient with Cushing's syndrome include the following:

- Risk for injury related to weakness
- Risk for infection related to altered protein metabolism and inflammatory response
- Self-care deficit related to weakness, fatigue, muscle wasting, and altered sleep patterns
- Impaired skin integrity related to edema, impaired healing, and thin and fragile skin
- Disturbed body image related to altered physical appearance, impaired sexual functioning, and decreased activity level
- Disturbed thought processes related to mood swings, irritability, and depression

Collaborative Problems/ Potential Complications

Potential complications may include the following:

- Addisonian crisis
- Adverse effects of adrenocortical activity

Planning and Goals

The major goals for the patient include decreased risk of injury, decreased risk of infection, increased ability to carry out self-care activities, improved skin integrity, improved body image, improved mental function, and absence of complications.

Nursing Interventions

Decreasing Risk of Injury

Establishing a protective environment helps prevent falls, fractures, and other injuries to bones and soft tissues. The patient who is very weak may require assistance from the nurse in ambulating to avoid falling or bumping into sharp corners of furniture. Foods high in protein, calcium, and vitamin D are recommended to minimize muscle wasting and osteoporosis. Referral to a dietitian may assist the patient in selecting appropriate foods that are also low in sodium and calories.

Decreasing Risk of Infection

The patient should avoid unnecessary exposure to others with infections. The nurse frequently assesses the patient for subtle signs of infection, because the anti-inflammatory effects of corticosteroids may mask the common signs of inflammation and infection.

Preparing the Patient for Surgery

The patient is prepared for adrenalectomy, if indicated, and the postoperative course (see later discussion). If Cushing's syndrome is a result of a pituitary tumor, a transsphenoidal hypophysectomy may be performed (see Chapter 61). Diabetes mellitus and peptic ulcer are common in patients with Cushing's syndrome. Therefore, insulin therapy and medication to treat peptic ulcer will be initiated if needed. Before, during, and after surgery, blood glucose monitoring and assessment of stools for blood are carried out to monitor for these complications. If the patient has other symptoms of Cushing's syndrome, these are considered in the preoperative preparation. For example, if the patient has experienced weight gain, special instruction is given about postoperative breathing exercises.

Encouraging Rest and Activity

Weakness, fatigue, and muscle wasting make it difficult for the patient with Cushing's syndrome to carry out normal activities, yet the nurse should encourage moderate activity to prevent complications of immobility and promote increased self-esteem. Insomnia often contributes to the patient's fatigue. It is important to help the patient plan and space rest periods throughout the day. Efforts are made to promote a relaxing, quiet environment for rest and sleep.

Promoting Skin Integrity

Meticulous skin care is necessary to avoid traumatizing the patient's fragile skin. Use of adhesive tape is avoided, because it can irritate the skin and tear the fragile tissue when the tape is removed. The nurse frequently assesses the skin and bony prominences and encourages and assists the patient to change positions frequently to prevent skin breakdown.

Improving Body Image

If the cause of Cushing's syndrome can be treated successfully, the major physical changes disappear in time. The patient may benefit from discussion of the effect the changes have had on his or her self-concept and relationships with others. Weight gain and edema may be modified by a low-carbohydrate, low-sodium diet, and a high protein intake may reduce some of the other bothersome symptoms.

Improving Thought Processes

Explanations to the patient and family members about the cause of emotional instability are important in helping them cope with the mood swings, irritability, and depression that may occur. Psychotic behavior may occur in a few patients and should be reported. The nurse encourages the patient and family members to verbalize their feelings and concerns.

Monitoring and Managing Potential Complications

ADDISONIAN CRISIS

The patient with Cushing's syndrome whose symptoms are treated by withdrawal of corticosteroids, by adrenalectomy, or by removal of a pituitary tumor is at risk for adrenal hypofunction and addisonian crisis. If high levels of circulating adrenal hormones have suppressed the function of the adrenal cortex, atrophy of the adrenal cortex is likely. If the circulating hormone level is decreased rapidly because of surgery or abrupt cessation of corticosteroid agents, manifestations of adrenal hypofunction and addisonian crisis may develop. Therefore, the patient with Cushing's syndrome is monitored closely for hypotension; rapid, weak pulse; rapid respiratory rate; pallor; and extreme weakness. Efforts are made to identify factors that may have led to the crisis.

The patient with Cushing's syndrome who experiences highly stressful events, such as trauma or emergency surgery, is at increased risk for addisonian crisis because of long-term suppression of the adrenal cortex. The patient may require IV administration of fluid and electrolytes and corticosteroids before, during, and after treatment or surgery. If addisonian crisis occurs, the patient is treated for circulatory collapse and shock (see Chapter 15).

ADVERSE EFFECTS OF ADRENOCORTICAL ACTIVITY

The nurse assesses fluid and electrolyte status by monitoring laboratory values and daily weights. Because of the increased risk for glucose intolerance and hyperglycemia, blood glucose monitoring is initiated. The nurse reports elevated blood glucose levels to the physician so that treatment can be prescribed if indicated.

Promoting Home and Community-Based Care

TEACHING PATIENTS SELF-CARE

The patient with Cushing's syndrome and the patient's family require teaching and support to enable them to prevent problems associated with the syndrome and to manage those that cannot be prevented. The nurse presents information verbally and in writing. If the disorder is a result of corticosteroid use for treatment of a chronic disease, the patient and family need to understand that stopping the corticosteroid use abruptly and without medical supervision is likely to result in acute adrenal insufficiency as well as reappearance of the underlying symptoms of the chronic disease for which corticosteroids were prescribed. The nurse emphasizes the need to ensure an adequate supply of the corticosteroid, because running out of the medication or skipping doses can precipitate addisonian crisis (see Therapeutic Uses of Corticosteroids).

The nurse stresses the need for dietary modifications to ensure adequate calcium intake without increasing the risks for hypertension, hyperglycemia, and weight gain. The patient and family may be taught to monitor blood pressure, blood glucose levels, and weight. Wearing a medical alert bracelet and notifying other health care providers (eg, the patient's dentist) are important to alert others that the patient has Cushing's syndrome (Chart 42-12).

CONTINUING CARE

The need for follow-up depends on the origin and duration of the disease and its management. The patient who has been treated by adrenalectomy or removal of a pituitary tumor requires close monitoring to ensure that adrenal function has returned to normal and to ensure adequacy of circulating adrenal hormones. The patient who requires continued corticosteroid therapy is monitored to ensure understanding of the medications and the need for a dosage that treats the underlying disorder while minimizing the side effects. Home care referral may be indicated to ensure a safe environment that minimizes stress and risk of falls and other side effects. The home care nurse assesses the patient's physical and psychological status and reports changes to the physician. The nurse also assesses the patient's understanding of the medication regimen and his or her compliance with the regimen and reinforces previous teaching about the medications and the importance of taking them as prescribed. The nurse emphasizes the importance of regular medical follow-up, the side effects and toxic effects of medications, and the need to wear medical identification with Addison's and Cushing's disease. In addition, the nurse reminds the patient and family about the importance of health promotion activities and recommended health screening, including bone mineral density testing.

Evaluation

Expected Patient Outcomes

Expected patient outcomes may include the following:

1. Decreases risk of injury
   a. Is free of fractures or soft tissue injuries
   b. Is free of ecchymotic areas
2. Decreases risk of infection
   a. Experiences no temperature elevation, redness, pain, or other signs of infection or inflammation
   b. Avoids contact with others who have infections
3. Increases participation in self-care activities
   a. Plans activities and exercises to allow alternating periods of rest and activity
   b. Reports improved well-being
   c. Is free of complications of immobility
4. Attains/maintains skin integrity
   a. Has intact skin, without evidence of breakdown or infection
   b. Exhibits decreased edema in extremities and trunk

CHART 42-12

HOME CARE CHECKLIST • The Patient With Cushing's Syndrome

At the completion of the home care instruction, the patient or caregiver will be able to:	Patient	Caregiver
• State present and potential effects of Cushing's syndrome on the body	✔	✔
• Identify signs and symptoms of excessive and insufficient adrenal hormone	✔	✔
• State the relationship between adrenal hormones, emotional state, and stress	✔	✔
• Identify methods for managing labile emotions	✔	✔
• Describe protective skin care measures and use of protective devices and practices	✔	✔
• State the importance of regular follow-up visits with primary health care provider	✔	✔
• State the purpose, dose, route, schedule, side effects, and precautions for prescribed medications (adrenocortical inhibitors)	✔	✔
• Identify need to wear medical alert identification and carry medical information card	✔	✔
• State importance of compliance with medical regimen	✔	✔
• State the need to contact health care provider before taking over-the-counter medications	✔	✔
• Identify foods high in potassium and low in sodium, calories, and carbohydrates	✔	✔
• Identify areas of activity limitations and impact on lifestyle	✔	✔

   c. Changes position frequently and inspects bony prominences daily
5. Achieves improved body image
   a. Verbalizes feelings about changes in appearance, sexual function, and activity level
   b. States that physical changes are a result of excessive corticosteroids
6. Exhibits improved mental functioning
7. Exhibits absence of complications
   a. Exhibits normal vital signs and weight and is free of symptoms of addisonian crisis
   b. Identifies signs and symptoms of adrenocortical hypofunction that should be reported and measures to take in case of severe illness and stress
   c. Identifies strategies to minimize complications of Cushing's syndrome
   d. Complies with recommendations for follow-up appointments and health screening.

Primary Aldosteronism

The principal action of aldosterone is to conserve body sodium. Under the influence of this hormone, the kidneys excrete less sodium and more potassium and hydrogen. Excessive production of aldosterone, which occurs in some patients with functioning tumors of the adrenal gland, causes a distinctive pattern of biochemical changes and a corresponding set of clinical manifestations that are diagnostic of this condition.

Clinical Manifestations

Patients with aldosteronism exhibit a profound decline in the serum levels of potassium (hypokalemia) and hydrogen ions (alkalosis), as demonstrated by an increase in pH and serum bicarbonate concentration. The serum sodium level is normal or elevated, depending on the amount of water reabsorbed with the sodium. Hypertension is the most prominent and almost universal sign of aldosteronism and is present in up to 10% of individuals with hypertension (Mulatero, Dluhy, Giacchetti, et al., 2005).

Hypokalemia is responsible for the variable muscle weakness, cramping, and fatigue in patients with aldosteronism, as well as an inability on the part of the kidneys to acidify or concentrate the urine. Accordingly, the urine volume is excessive, leading to polyuria. Serum, by contrast, becomes abnormally concentrated, contributing to excessive thirst (polydipsia) and arterial hypertension. A secondary increase in blood volume and possible direct effects of aldosterone on nerve receptors, such as the carotid sinus, are other factors that result in hypertension.

Hypokalemic alkalosis may decrease the ionized serum calcium level and predispose the patient to tetany and paresthesias. Trousseau's and Chvostek's signs may be used to assess neuromuscular irritability before overt paresthesia and tetany occur. Glucose intolerance may occur, because hypokalemia interferes with insulin secretion from the pancreas.

Assessment and Diagnostic Findings

In addition to a high or normal serum sodium level and a low serum potassium level, diagnostic studies indicate high serum aldosterone and low serum renin levels. The measurement of the aldosterone excretion rate after salt loading is a useful diagnostic test for primary aldosteronism. The renin–aldosterone stimulation test and bilateral adrenal venous sampling are useful in differentiating the cause of primary aldosteronism. Antihypertensive medication may be discontinued up to 2 weeks before testing.

Medical Management

Treatment of primary aldosteronism usually involves surgical removal of the adrenal tumor through adrenalectomy. Hypokalemia resolves for all patients after surgery, but hypertension may persist. Spironolactone may be prescribed to control hypertension.

Adrenalectomy is performed through an incision in the flank or the abdomen. In general, the postoperative care resembles that for other abdominal surgery. However, the patient is susceptible to fluctuations in adrenocortical hormones and requires administration of corticosteroids, fluids, and other agents to maintain blood pressure and prevent acute complications. If the adrenalectomy is bilateral, replacement of corticosteroids will be lifelong; if one adrenal gland is removed, replacement therapy may be temporarily necessary because of suppression of the remaining adrenal gland by high levels of adrenal hormones. A normal serum glucose level is maintained with insulin, appropriate IV fluids, and dietary modifications.

Nursing Management

Nursing management in the postoperative period includes frequent assessment of vital signs to detect early signs and symptoms of adrenal insufficiency and crisis or hemorrhage. Explaining all treatments and procedures, providing comfort measures, and providing rest periods can reduce the patient's stress and anxiety level.

Corticosteroid Therapy

Corticosteroids are used extensively for adrenal insufficiency and are also widely used in suppressing inflammation and autoimmune reactions, controlling allergic reactions, and reducing the rejection process in transplantation. Commonly used corticosteroid preparations are listed in Table 42-5. Their anti-inflammatory and antiallergy actions make corticosteroids effective in treating rheumatic or connective tissue diseases, such as rheumatoid arthritis and systemic lupus erythematosus. They are also frequently used in the treatment of asthma, multiple sclerosis, and other autoimmune disorders.

High doses appear to allow patients to tolerate high degrees of stress. Such antistress action may be caused by the ability of corticosteroids to aid circulating vasopressor substances in keeping the blood pressure elevated; other effects, such as maintenance of the serum glucose level, also may keep blood pressure elevated.

Side Effects

Although the synthetic corticosteroids are safer for some patients because of relative freedom from mineralocorticoid activity, most natural and synthetic corticosteroids produce similar kinds of side effects. The dose required for

TABLE 42-5 Commonly Used Corticosteroid Preparations

Generic Names	Trade Names
Hydrocortisone	Cortisol, Cortef, Hydrocortone, Solu-Cortef
Cortisone	Cortone, Cortate, Cortogen
Dexamethasone	Decadron, Dexameth, Deronil, Delalone, Dexasone, Dexone, Hexadrol
Prednisone	Meticorten, Deltasone, Orasone, Panasol, Novo-prednisone
Prednisolone	Meticortelone, Delta-Cortef, Prelone, Predalone
Methylprednisolone	Medrol, Solu-Medrol, Meprolone
Triamcinolone	Aristocort, Kenacort, Kenalog, Cenocort, Azmacort, Aristospan
Beclomethasone	Beconase, Beclovent, Vanceril, Vancenase, Propaderm
Betamethasone	Celestone, Betameth, Betnesol, Betnelan

anti-inflammatory and antiallergy effects also produces metabolic effects, pituitary and adrenal gland suppression, and changes in the function of the central nervous system. Therefore, although corticosteroids are highly effective therapeutically, they may also be very dangerous. Dosages of these medications are frequently altered to allow high concentrations when necessary and then tapered in an attempt to avoid undesirable effects. This requires that patients be observed closely for side effects and that the dose be reduced when high doses are no longer required. Suppression of the adrenal cortex may persist up to 1 year after a course of corticosteroids of only 2 weeks' duration.

Therapeutic Uses of Corticosteroids

The dosage of corticosteroids is determined by the nature and chronicity of the illness as well as the patient's other medical conditions. Rheumatoid arthritis, bronchial asthma, and multiple sclerosis are chronic disorders that corticosteroids do not cure; however, these medications may be useful when other measures do not provide adequate control of symptoms. In addition, corticosteroids may be used to treat acute exacerbations of these disorders.

In such situations, the adverse effects of corticosteroids are weighed against the patient's current condition. These medications may be used for a period but then are gradually reduced or tapered as the symptoms subside. The nurse plays an important role in providing encouragement and understanding during times when the patient is experiencing (or is apprehensive about experiencing) recurrence of symptoms while taking smaller doses.

Treatment of Acute Conditions

Acute flare-ups and crises are treated with large doses of corticosteroids. Examples include emergency treatment for bronchial obstruction in status asthmaticus and for septic shock from septicemia caused by gram-negative bacteria. Other measures, such as anti-infective agents or medications, are also used with corticosteroids to treat shock and other major symptoms. At times, corticosteroids are continued past the acute flare-up stage to prevent serious complications.

Ophthalmologic Treatment

A different problem exists when corticosteroids are used to treat eye infections. Outer eye infection can be treated by topical application of eye drops, because the agents do not cause systemic toxicity. However, long-term application can cause an increase in intraocular pressure, which leads to glaucoma in some patients. In some patients, prolonged use of corticosteroids leads to cataract formation.

Dermatologic Disorders

Topical administration of corticosteroids in the form of creams, ointments, lotions, and aerosols is especially effective in many dermatologic disorders. It may be more effective in some conditions to use occlusive dressings around the affected part to achieve maximum absorption of the medication. Penetration and absorption are also increased if the medication is applied when the skin is hydrated or moist (eg, immediately after bathing).

Absorption of topical agents varies with body location. For example, absorption is greater through the layers of skin on the scalp, face, and genital area than on the forearm; as a result, use of topical agents on these sites increases the risk of side effects. The availability of over-the-counter topical corticosteroids increases the risk of side effects in patients who are unaware of their potential risks. Excessive use of these agents, especially on large surface areas of inflamed skin, can lead to decreased therapeutic effects and increased side effects.

Dosage

Attempts have been made to determine the best time to administer pharmacologic doses of steroids. If symptoms have been controlled on a 6-hour or 8-hour program, a once-daily or every-other-day schedule may be implemented. In keeping with the natural secretion of cortisol, the best time of day for the total corticosteroid dose is in the early morning, between 7 AM and 8 AM. Large-dose therapy at 8 AM., when the adrenal gland is most active, produces maximal suppression of the gland. A large 8 AM. dose is more physiologic because it allows the body to escape effects of the steroids from 4 PM to 6 AM, when serum levels are normally low, hence minimizing cushingoid effects. If symptoms of the disorder being treated are suppressed, alternate-day therapy is helpful in reducing pituitary–adrenal suppression in patients requiring prolonged therapy. Some patients report discomfort associated with symptoms of their primary illness on the second day; therefore, it is important to explain to patients that this regimen is necessary to minimize side effects and suppression of adrenal function.

Tapering

Corticosteroid dosages are reduced gradually (tapered) to allow normal adrenal function to return and to prevent

TABLE 42-6 Side Effects of Corticosteroid Therapy and Implications for Nursing Practice

Side Effects	Collaborative Interventions
Cardiovascular Effects	
Hypertension Thrombophlebitis Thromboembolism Accelerated atherosclerosis	Monitor for elevated blood pressure. Assess for signs and symptoms of DVT: redness, warmth, tenderness and edema of an extremity. Remind patient to avoid positions and situations that restrict blood flow (eg, crossing legs, prolonged sitting in same position). Encourage foot and leg exercises when recumbent. Encourage low sodium intake. Encourage limited intake of fat.
Immunologic Effects	
Increased risk of infection and masking of signs of infection	Assess for subtle signs of infection and inflammation. Encourage patient to avoid exposure to others with upper respiratory infection. Monitor patient for fungal infections. Encourage hand washing.
Ophthalmologic Changes	
Glaucoma Corneal lesions	Encourage frequent eye examinations. Refer patient to ophthalmologist if changes in visual acuity are detected.
Musculoskeletal Effects	
Muscle wasting Poor wound healing Osteoporosis with vertebral compression fractures, pathologic fractures of long bones, aseptic necrosis of head of the femur	Encourage high protein intake. Encourage high protein intake and vitamin C supplementation. Encourage diet high in calcium and vitamin D or calcium and vitamin D supplementation if indicated. Take measures to avoid falls and other trauma. Use caution in moving and turning patient. Encourage postmenopausal women on corticosteroids to consider bone mineral density testing and treatment, if indicated. Instruct patient to rise slowly from bed or chair to avoid falling due to postural hypotension.
Metabolic Effects	
Alterations in glucose metabolism Steroid withdrawal syndrome	Monitor blood glucose levels at periodic intervals. Instruct patient about medications, diet, and exercise prescribed to control blood glucose level. Report signs of adrenal insufficiency. Administer corticosteroids and mineralocorticoids as prescribed. Monitor fluid and electrolyte balance. Administer fluids and electrolytes as prescribed. Instruct patient about importance of taking corticosteroids as prescribed without abruptly stopping therapy. Encourage patient to obtain and wear a medical identification bracelet. Advise patient to notify all health care providers (eg, dentist) about need for corticosteroid therapy.
Changes in Appearance	
Moon face Weight gain Acne	Encourage low-calorie, low-sodium diet. Assure patient that most changes in appearance are temporary and will disappear if and when corticosteroid therapy is no longer necessary.

steroid-induced adrenal insufficiency. Up to 1 year or longer after use of corticosteroids, the patient is still at risk for adrenal insufficiency in times of stress. For example, if surgery for any reason is necessary, the patient is likely to require IV corticosteroids during and after surgery to reduce the risk for acute adrenal crisis. Patients receiving corticosteroids must have an adequate supply of medication on hand, so that they do not miss a scheduled dose and increase their risk of adrenal insufficiency. Table 42-6 provides an overview of the effects of corticosteroid therapy and their nursing implications.

Critical Thinking Exercises

1 **A 68-year-old woman has just been diagnosed with thyroid cancer. She is scheduled for a total thyroidectomy in 1 week. What preoperative and postoperative nursing care is important for her? What long-term follow-up would you anticipate and discuss with the patient and her family?**

2 A 70-year-old man has a diagnosis of bronchogenic carcinoma. He is being evaluated for possible syndrome of inappropriate antidiuretic hormone (SIADH) secretion. The patient and his family are asking for explanations about the syndrome and about methods of managing it. What nursing interventions and patient and family teaching are warranted when caring for this patient? Contrast the clinical picture and symptoms of SIADH with those of diabetes insipidus.

3 A 44-year-old woman with multiple sclerosis (MS) has received several courses of corticosteroids in the past year to treat MS exacerbations. She is scheduled for a hysterectomy to treat uterine fibroids. How will her history of corticosteroid use affect her preoperative and postoperative courses? What nursing observations are important during the postoperative period?

4 ebp Your neighbor is concerned about the possibility of a radiation-induced thyroid cancer in herself and her children in the event of a terrorist attack on the nearby nuclear power plant. She asks you about the use of potassium iodide to prevent thyroid cancer. What advice would you give to her? What is the evidence base for your advice? How strong is that evidence, and what criteria would you use to determine the strength of the evidence?

5 During a home visit to a postoperative patient, you are introduced to the patient's elderly mother. Although it is warm in the home, the elderly woman is wearing several sweaters to keep warm. She moves slowly, her verbal responses are very slow, and she appears apathetic. You suspect that she may have severe hypothyroidism. What assessment would you conduct, and what course of action would you take? What precautions are warranted for her before she is evaluated? What precautions are warranted if she is diagnosed with hypothyroidism and begins treatment for it?

6 A 24-year-old woman is undergoing diagnostic testing for possible pheochromocytoma. How would you explain this possible diagnosis to the patient? If pheochromocytoma is diagnosed and she is scheduled for an adrenalectomy, what preoperative and postoperative nursing care would you anticipate?

REFERENCES AND SELECTED READINGS

BOOKS

American Cancer Society. (2005). *Cancer facts and figures.* Atlanta: Author.

Bickley, L. S. & Szilagyi, P. G. (2003). *Bates' guide to physical examination and history taking* (8th ed.). Philadelphia: Lippincott Williams & Wilkins.

Ferri, F. (Ed). (2005). *Ferri clinical advisor: Instant diagnosis and treatment* (5th ed.). Philadelphia: Mosby.

Fink, M. P., Abraham, E., Kochanek, P., et al. (Eds.). (2005). *Textbook of critical care* (5th ed.). Philadelphia: W. B. Saunders.

Goldman, L. & Ausiello, D. (Eds.). (2004). *Cecil textbook of medicine* (22nd ed.). Philadelphia: W. B. Saunders.

Greenspan, F. S. & Gardner, D. G. (Eds.). (2003). *Basic and clinical endocrinology* (7th ed.). New York: McGraw-Hill.

Kasper, D. L., Braunwald, E., Fauci, A. S., et al. (Eds.). (2004). *Harrison's principles of internal medicine* (16th ed.). New York: McGraw-Hill.

Larsen, P. R., Kronenberg, H. M., Melmed, S. et al. (Eds.). (2003). *Williams textbook of endocrinology* (10th ed.). Philadelphia: W. B. Saunders.

Morton, P. G., Fontaine, D. K., Hudak, C. M., et al. (2005). *Critical care nursing: A holistic approach* (8th ed.). Philadelphia: Lippincott Williams & Wilkins.

O'Connell, D. T. (2004). The adrenal medulla, catecholamines, and pheochromocytoma. In Goldman, L. & Ausiello, D. (Eds.). *Cecil textbook of medicine* (22nd ed.). Philadelphia: W. B. Saunders.

Porth, C. M. (2005). *Pathophysiology: Concepts of altered health states* (7th ed.). Philadelphia: Lippincott Williams & Wilkins.

Rakel, R. E. & Bope, E. T. (Eds.). (2005). *Conn's current therapy 2005.* Philadelphia: W. B. Saunders.

Tierney, L. M., McPhee, S. J., & Papadakis, M. A. (Eds.). (2005). *Current medical diagnosis and treatment.* New York: Lange Medical Books/McGraw-Hill.

Weber, J., & Kelley, J. (2003). *Health assessment in nursing* (2nd ed.). Philadelphia: Lippincott Williams & Wilkins.

JOURNALS

**Asterisks indicate nursing research articles.*

Bauer, D. G. (2005). Review of the endocrine system. *MedSurg Nursing, 14*(5), 335–337.

National Institutes of Health. (2003). Endocrine-related resources from the National Institutes of Health. *Endocrinology, 144*(12), 5671–5673.

Pituitary Gland

Flounders, J. (2003). Oncology emergency modules: Syndrome of inappropriate antidiuretic hormone. *Oncology Nursing Forum Online, 30*(3), E63–E70.

Hanberg, A. (2005). Common disorders of the pituitary gland: Hyposecretion versus hypersecretion. *Journal of Infusion Nursing, 28*(1), 36–44.

Letournel, F., Menei, P. Gilles, G., et al. (2003). Transsphenoidal surgery in the elderly. *Journal of American Geriatrics Society, 51*(5), 729–730.

Prather, S. H., Forsyth, L. W., Russell, K. D., et al. (2003). Caring for the patient undergoing transsphenoidal surgery in the acute care setting: An alternative to critical care. *Journal of Neuroscience Nursing, 35*(5), 270–275.

Thyroid Gland

American Association of Clinical Endocrinologists (AACE) Thyroid Task Force. (2002). AACE medical guidelines for clinical practice for the evaluation and treatment of hyperthyroidism and hypothyroidism. *Endocrine Practice, 8*(6), 457–469.

Auer, J., Berent, R., Weber, T., et al. (2003). Hyperthyroidism. *Lancet, 362*(9395), 1584.

Blackwell, J. (2004). Evaluation and treatment of hyperthyroidism and hypothyroidism. *Journal of the American Academy of Nurse Practitioners, 16*(10), 422–425.

Col, N. F., Surks, M. I. & Daniels, G. H. (2004). Subclinical thyroid disease: Clinical applications. *Journal of the American Medical Association, 291*(2), 239–243.

Cooper, D. S. (2005). Drug therapy: Antithyroid drugs. *New England Journal of Medicine, 352*(9), 905–917.

Fatourechi, V., Aniszewski, J. P., Fatourechi, G. Z., et al. (2003). Clinical features and outcome of subacute thyroiditis in an incidence cohort: Olmsted County, Minnesota, study. *Journal of Endocrinology and Metabolism, 88*(5), 2100–2105.

Felicetta, J. V. (2002). Thyroid disease in the elderly: When to suspect, when to treat. *Consultant, 43*(13), 1597–1599, 1603–1606.

Franklyn, J. A., Sheppard, M. C. & Maisonneuve, P. (2005). Thyroid function and mortality in patients treated for hypertension. *Journal of the American Medical Association, 294*(1), 71–80.

Ginsberg, J. (2003). Diagnosis and management of Graves' disease. *Canadian Medical Association Journal, 168*(5), 575–585.

Grimes, C., Muniz, H., Montgomery, W., et al. (2004). Intraoperative thyroid storm: A case report. *AANA Journal, 72*(1), 53–55.

Hegedüs, L. (2004). The thyroid nodule. *New England Journal of Medicine, 351*(17), 1764–1771.

Helfand, M. (2004). Screening for subclinical thyroid dysfunction in non-pregnant adults: A summary of the evidence for the U.S. Preventive Services Task Force. *Annals of Internal Medicine, 140*(2), 128–141.

Holcomb, S. S. (2002). Thyroid diseases: A primer for the critical care nurse. *DCCN Dimensions of Critical Care Nursing, 21*(4), 127–133.

Holcomb, S. S. (2003a). Detecting thyroid disease, part 2: Learn about treatment and how to help your patient manage symptoms. *Nursing, 33*(9), 32cc1–32cc4.

Holcomb, S. S. (2003b). Detecting thyroid disease. *Nursing 2005, 35*(10 Suppl.), 4–8.

*Huang, S-M., Lee C-H., Chien, L-Y., et al. (2004). Postoperative quality of life among patients with thyroid cancer. *Journal of Advanced Nursing, 47*(5), 492–499.

Kumrow, D. & Dahlen, R. (2002). Thyroidectomy: Understanding the potential for complications. *MedSurg Nursing, 11*(5), 228–235.

Li, T-M. (2002). Hypothyroidism in elderly people. *Geriatric Nurse, 23*(2), 88–93.

Metso, S., Jaatinen, P., Huhtala, H., et al. (2004). Long-term follow-up study of radioiodine treatment of hyperthyroidism. *Clinical Endocrinology, 61*(5), 641–648.

Mohandas, R. & Gupta, K. L. (2003). Managing thyroid dysfunction in the elderly: Answers to seven common questions. *Postgraduate Medicine, 113*(5), 54–56, 65–68.

Pearce, E. N. & Braverman, L. E. (2004). Hyperthyroidism: Advantages and disadvantages of medical therapy. *Surgical Clinics of North America, 84*(3), 833–847.

Pearce, E. N., Farwell, A. P. & Braverman, L. E. (2003). Thyroiditis. *New England Journal of Medicine, 348*(26), 2646–2655.

Schori-Ahmed, D. (2003). Defenses gone awry: Thyroid disease. *RN, 66*(6), 38–44.

Stark, S. (2002). Clinical issues related to hyperthyroidism. *Clinical Excellence for Nurse Practitioners, 6*(4), 21–25.

Surks, M. I., Ortiz, E., Daniels, G. H., et al. (2004). Subclinical thyroid disease: Scientific review and guidelines for diagnosis and management. *Journal of the American Medical Association, 291*(2), 228–238.

Thyroid Carcinoma Task Force. (2001). AACE/AAES medical/surgical guidelines for clinical practice: Management of thyroid carcinoma. *Endocrine Practice, 7*(3), 202–220.

U.S. Preventive Services Task Force. (2004). Screening for thyroid disease: Recommendation statement. *Annals of Internal Medicine, 140*(2), 125–127.

Welker, M. J. & Orlov, D. (2003). Thyroid nodules. *American Family Physician, 67*(3), 559–566.

Parathyroid Glands

Bro, S. (2003). How abnormal calcium, phosphate, and parathyroid hormone relate to cardiovascular disease. *Nephrology Nursing Journal, 30*(3), 275–283.

Carroll, M. E. & Schade, D. S. (2003). A practical approach to hypercalcemia. *American Family Physician, 67*(9), 1959–1966.

Jorde, R., Szumlas, K., Haug, E., et al. (2002). The effects of calcium supplementation to patients with primary hyperparathyroidism and a low calcium intake. *European Journal of Nutrition, 41*(6), 358–363.

Michael, M. & Garcia, D. (2004). Secondary hyperparathyroidism in chronic kidney disease: Clinical consequences and challenges. *Nephrology Nursing Journal, 31*(2), 185–196.

Taniegra, E. D. (2004). Hyperparathyroidism. *American Family Physician, 69*(2), 333–339.

Updates: First treatment for serious complications of kidney disease, parathyroid cancer. *FDA Consumer, 38*(3), 6.

Westreich, R. W., Brandwein, M., Mechanick, J. I., et al. (2003). Preoperative parathyroid localization: Correlating false-negative technetium 99m sestamibi scans with parathyroid disease. *Laryngoscope, 113*(3), 567–572.

Adrenal Glands

Arlt, W. & Allolio, B. (2003). Adrenal insufficiency. *Lancet, 361*(9372), 1881–1893.

Barnard, C., Kanani, R. & Friedman (2004). Her tongue tipped us off. *Canadian Medical Association Journal, 171*(5), 451.

Bravo, E. & Tagle, R. (2003). Pheochromocytoma: State-of-the-art and future prospects. *Endocrine Review, 24*(4), 539–553.

Brender, E. (2005). Adrenal insufficiency [JAMA patient page]. *Journal of the American Medical Association, 294*(19), 2528.

Daub, K. F. (2002). Pheochromocytoma, up close and personal: A perceptive nurse's suggestion led my husband and me to a rare diagnosis. *Nursing, 32*(3), 32hn1–32hn4.

Dorin, R. I., Qualls, C. R. & Crapo, L. M. (2003). Diagnosis of adrenal insufficiency. *Annals of Internal Medicine, 139*(3), 194–206.

Findling, J. W. & Raff, H. (2005). Screening and diagnosis of Cushing's syndrome. *Endocrinology and Metabolism Clinics of North America, 34*(2), 385–402.

Hammer, G. D., Tyrrell, J. B., Lamborn, K. R., et al. (2004). Transsphenoidal microsurgery for Cushing's disease: Initial outcome and long-term results. *Journal of Clinical Endocrinology and Metabolism, 89*(12), 6348–6357.

Lenders, J. W., Pacak, K. & Eisenhofer, G. (2002). New advances in the biochemical diagnosis of pheochromocytoma: Moving beyond catecholamines. *Annals of the New York Academy of Sciences, 970*, 29–40.

Lionakis, M. S. & Kontoyiannis, D. P. (2003). Glucocorticoids and invasive fungal infections. *Lancet, 362*(9398), 1828–1838.

Mann, N. K. (2003). Cushing's syndrome. *Access, 17*(7), 25–29.

Marik, P. E. & Zaloga, G. P. (2002). Adrenal insufficiency in the critically ill: A new look at an old problem. *Chest, 122*(5), 1784–1795.

McConnell, E. (2002). About Addison's disease. *Nursing 2002, 32*(8), 79.

Mulatero, P., Dluhy, R. G., Giacchetti, G., et al. (2005). Diagnosis of primary aldosteronism: From screening to subtype differentiation. *Trends in Endocrinology and Metabolism, 16*(3), 114–119.

Poulin, E. C., Schlachta, C. M., Burpee, S. E., et al. (2003). Laparoscopic adrenalectomy: Pathologic features determine outcome. *Canadian Journal of Surgery, 46*(5), 340–344.

Raff, H. & Findling, J. W. (2003). A physiologic approach to diagnosis of the Cushing syndrome. *Annals of Internal Medicine, 17*(12), 980–991.

Raisbeck, E. (2002). Recognizing adrenal insufficiency. *Emergency Nurse, 10*(4), 24–26.

Rhen, T. & Cidlowski, J. A. (2005). Antiinflammatory action of glucocorticoids: New mechanisms for old drugs. *New England Journal of Medicine, 353*(16), 1711–1723.

Sabol, V. K. (2001). Addisonian crisis: The life-threatening condition may be triggered by a variety of stressors. *American Journal of Nursing, 101*(7), 24AAA–24DDD.

Salvatori, R. (2005). Adrenal insufficiency. *Journal of the American Medical Association, 294*(19), 2481–2488.

Stowasser, M. & Gordon, R. D. (2004). Primary aldosteronism: Careful investigation is essential and rewarding. *Molecular and Cellular Endocrinology, 217*(1), 33–39.

Stowasser, M. & Gordon, R. D. (2003). Primary aldosteronism: From genesis to genetics. *Trends in Endocrinology and Metabolism, 14*(7), 310–317.

Wilson, W. C. (2004). Preventing a fatal outcome in Addison's disease. *JAAPA, 17*(8), 35–38.

RESOURCES

American Association of Clinical Endocrinologists, 1000 Riverside Ave, Suite 205, Jacksonville, FL 32204; 904-353-7878; e-mail: Info@aace.com; http://www.aace.com. Accessed May 15, 2006.

American Thyroid Association, Inc., Montefiore Medical Center, 111 E. 210th St., Room 311, Bronx, NY 10467; 718-882-6047; http://www.thyroid.org. Accessed May 15, 2006.

Cushing's Support and Research Foundation, 65 East India Row, Suite 22B, Boston, MA 02110; 617-723-3674; http://world.std.com/~CSRF. Accessed May 15, 2006.

National Adrenal Disease Foundation, 505 Northern Boulevard, Suite 200, Great Neck, NY 11021; 516-487-4992; http://www.medhelp.org/nadf. Accessed May 15, 2006.

National Cancer Institute, CancerNet for Health Professionals; http://cancernet.nci.nih.gov/cancertopics. Accessed May 15, 2006.

The Endocrine Society, 4350 E. West Hwy, Suite 500, Bethesda, MD 20814-4410; 301-941-0200; e-mail: http://www.endo-society.org. Accessed May 15, 2006.

The Thyroid Society for Education and Research, 7515 S. Main St, Suite 545, Houston, TX 77030; 800-849-7643; http://www.the-thyroid-society.org. Accessed May 15, 2006.

UNIT 9

Renal and Urinary Tract Function

Case Study

Applying Concepts from NANDA, NIC, and NOC

A Patient With Involuntary Urine Loss During Physical Exertion and Ineffective Bladder Emptying

Mrs. Lopez is a 38-year-old woman with no significant past medical history. She has three children. During her annual physical examination, she tells the women's health nurse practitioner that when she jogs, coughs, or sneezes, she experiences an involuntary loss of small amounts of urine. The patient's urinalysis is normal. On physical examination, the nurse finds that Mrs. Lopez has a moderate cystocele and that her bladder feels mildly distended, although she had just voided to provide a urine sample. The nurse catheterizes Mrs. Lopez to check for postvoid residual urine and obtains 120 mL of clear urine.

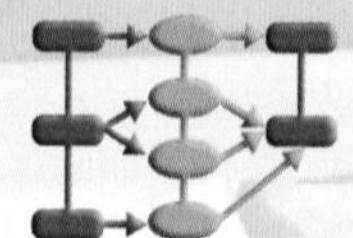

Turn to Appendix C to see a concept map that illustrates the relationships that exist among the nursing diagnoses, interventions, and outcomes for the patient's clinical problems.

Nursing Classifications and Languages

NANDA Nursing Diagnoses	NIC Nursing Interventions	NOC Nursing Outcomes Return to functional baseline status, stabilization of, or improvement in:
Stress Urinary Incontinence—Loss of less than 50 mL of urine occurring with increased abdominal pressure	**Pelvic Muscle Exercises**—Strengthening and training the levator ani and urogenital muscles through voluntary, repetitive contraction to decrease stress, urge, or mixed types of urinary incontinence	**Symptom Control**—Personal actions to minimize perceived changes in physical and emotional functioning
Urinary Retention—Incomplete emptying of the bladder	**Urinary Bladder Training**—Improving bladder function for those with urge incontinence by increasing the bladder's ability to hold urine and the patient's ability to suppress urination	**Urinary Continence**—Control of elimination of urine from the bladder **Infection Severity**—Severity of infection and associated symptoms
Risk for Infection—At increased risk for being invaded by pathogenic organisms	**Urinary Catheterization: Intermittent**—Regular periodic use of a catheter to empty the bladder **Infection Protection**—Prevention and early detection of infection in a patient at risk	

NANDA International (2005). *Nursing diagnoses: Definitions & Classification 2005–2006*. Philadelphia: North American Nursing Diagnosis Association.
*Dochterman, J. M. & Bulechek, G. M. (2004). *Nursing interventions classification (NIC)* (4th ed.). St. Louis: Mosby.
Iowa Outcomes Project (2004). In Moorhead, S., Johnson, M. & Maas, M. (2004). *Nursing outcomes classification (NOC)* (3rd ed.). St. Louis: Mosby.
Dochterman, J. M. & Jones, D. A. (2003). *Unifying nursing languages: The harmonization of NANDA, NIC, and NOC*. Washington D.C.: American Nurses Association.

CHAPTER 43

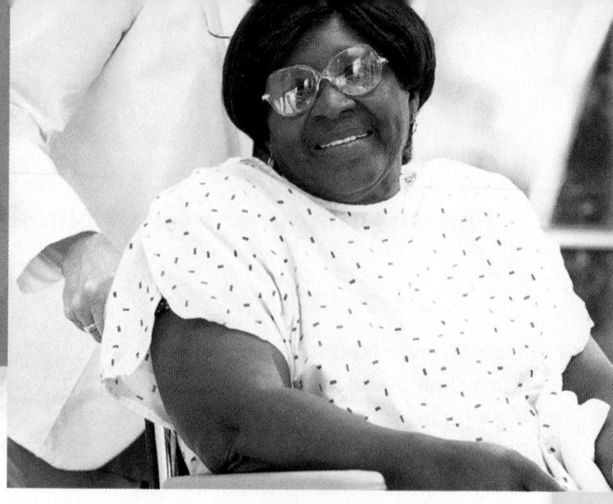

Assessment of Renal and Urinary Tract Function

Learning Objectives

On completion of this chapter, the learner will be able to:

1. Describe the anatomy and physiology of the renal and urinary systems.
2. Discuss the role of the kidney in regulating fluid and electrolyte balance, acid–base balance, and blood pressure.
3. Describe the diagnostic studies used to determine upper and lower urinary tract function.
4. Identify the assessment parameters used for determining the status of upper and lower urinary tract function.
5. Initiate education and preparation for patients undergoing assessment of the urinary system.

Proper function of the renal and urinary systems is essential to life. Dysfunction of the kidneys and lower urinary tract is common and may occur at any age and with varying degrees of severity. Assessment of upper and lower urinary tract function is part of every health examination and necessitates an understanding of the anatomy and physiology of the urinary system as well as the effects of changes in the system on other physiologic functions.

CHART 43-1

Functions of the Kidney

- Urine formation
- Excretion of waste products
- Regulation of electrolytes
- Regulation of acid–base balance
- Control of water balance
- Control of blood pressure
- Renal clearance
- Regulation of red blood cell production
- Synthesis of vitamin D to active form
- Secretion of prostaglandins
- Regulates calcium and phosphorus balance
- Activates growth hormone

Anatomic and Physiologic Overview

The primary function of the renal and urinary systems is to maintain the body's state of homeostasis by carefully regulating fluid and electrolytes, removing wastes, and providing hormones that are involved in red blood cell production, bone metabolism, and hypertension (Chart 43-1). Therefore, a thorough understanding of the renal and urinary systems is necessary for assessing people with acute or chronic dysfunction and implementing appropriate nursing care.

Anatomy of the Renal and Urinary Tract Systems

The renal and urinary systems include the kidneys, ureters, bladder, and urethra. Urine is formed by the kidney and flows through the other structures to be eliminated from the body.

Kidneys

The kidneys are a pair of bean-shaped, brownish-red structures located retroperitoneally (behind and outside the peritoneal cavity) on the posterior wall of the abdomen—from the twelfth thoracic vertebra to the third lumbar vertebra in the adult (Fig. 43-1A). The average adult kidney weighs approximately 113 to 170 g (about 4.5 oz), and is 10 to 12 cm long, 6 cm wide, and 2.5 cm thick (Porth, 2005). The right kidney is slightly lower than the left due to the location of the liver.

Externally, the kidneys are well protected by the ribs and by the muscles of the abdomen and back. Internally, fat deposits surround each kidney, providing protection against jarring. The kidneys and surrounding fat are suspended from the abdominal wall by renal fascia made of connective tissue. The fibrous connective tissue, blood vessels, and

Glossary

aldosterone: hormone synthesized and released by the adrenal cortex; causes the kidneys to reabsorb sodium

antidiuretic hormone (ADH): hormone secreted by the posterior pituitary gland; causes the kidneys to reabsorb more water; also called vasopressin

anuria: total urine output less than 50 mL in 24 h

bacteriuria: bacteria in the urine; bacterial count higher than 100,000 colonies/mL

creatinine: endogenous waste product of muscle energy metabolism

dysuria: painful or difficult urination

frequency: voiding more frequently than every 3 h

glomerulus: tuft of capillaries forming part of the nephron through which filtration occurs

glomerular filtration rate (GFR): volume of plasma filtered at the glomerulus into the kidney tubules each minute; normal rate is approximately 120 mL/min

hematuria: red blood cells in the urine

micturition: urination or voiding

nephron: structural and functional unit of the kidney responsible for urine formation

nocturia: awakening at night to urinate

oliguria: total urine output less than 400 mL in 24 h

proteinuria: protein in the urine

pyuria: white blood cells in the urine

renal clearance: volume of plasma that the kidneys can clear of a specific solute (eg, creatinine); expressed in milliliters per minute

renal glycosuria: recurring or persistent excretion of glucose in the urine

specific gravity: reflects the weight of particles dissolved in the urine; expression of the degree of concentration of the urine

tubular reabsorption: movement of a substance from the kidney tubule into the blood in the peritubular capillaries or vasa recta

tubular secretion: movement of a substance from the blood in the peritubular capillaries or vasa recta into the kidney tubule

urea nitrogen: nitrogenous end product of protein metabolism

urinary incontinence: involuntary loss of urine

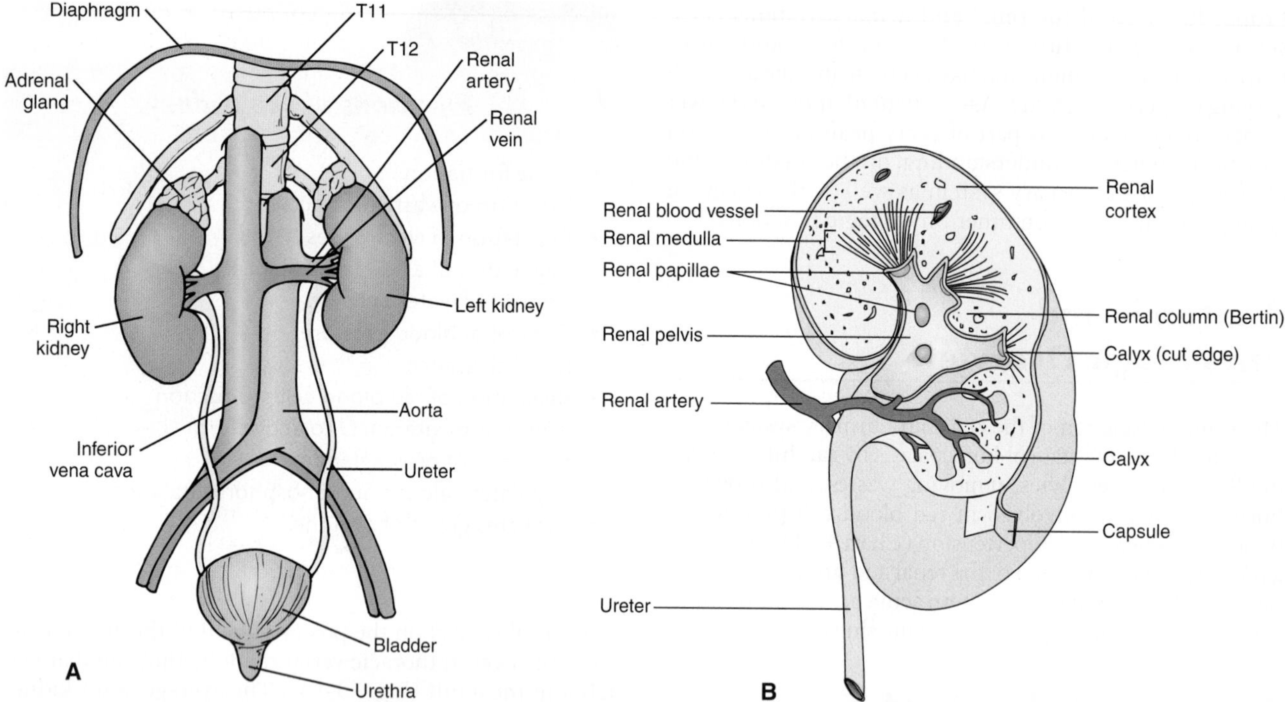

FIGURE 43-1. (**A**) Kidneys, ureters, and bladder. (The right kidney is usually lower than the left.) (**B**) Internal structure of the kidney. From Porth, C. M. (2005). *Pathophysiology: Concepts of altered health states* (7th ed.). Philadelphia: Lippincott Williams & Wilkins.

lymphatics surrounding each kidney are known as the renal capsule (Fig. 43-1B).

An adrenal gland lies on top of each kidney. Each organ is independent in terms of its function, blood supply, and innervation.

The renal parenchyma is divided into two parts: the cortex and the medulla. The medulla, which is approximately 5 cm wide, is the inner portion of the kidney. It contains the loops of Henle, the vasa recta, and the collecting ducts of the juxtamedullary nephrons. The collecting ducts from both the juxtamedullary and the cortical nephrons connect to the renal pyramids, which are triangular and are situated with the base facing the concave surface of the kidney and the point (papilla) facing the hilum, or pelvis. Each kidney contains approximately 8 to 18 pyramids. The pyramids drain into 4 to 13 minor calices, which drain into 2 to 3 major calices that open directly into the renal pelvis. The renal pelvis is the beginning of the collecting system and is composed of structures that are designed to collect and transport urine. Once the urine leaves the renal pelvis, the composition or amount of urine does not change.

The cortex, which is approximately 1 cm wide, is located farthest from the center of the kidney and around the outermost edges. It contains the **nephrons** (the functional units of the kidney), which are discussed below.

BLOOD SUPPLY TO THE KIDNEYS

The hilum, or pelvis, is the concave portion of the kidney through which the renal artery enters and the ureters and renal vein exit. The kidneys receive 20% to 25% of the total cardiac output, which means that all of the body's blood circulates through the kidneys approximately 12 times per hour. The renal artery (arising from the abdominal aorta) divides into smaller and smaller vessels, eventually forming the afferent arterioles. Each afferent arteriole branches to form a **glomerulus**, which is the capillary bed responsible for glomerular filtration. Blood leaves the glomerulus through the efferent arteriole and flows back to the inferior vena cava through a network of capillaries and veins.

NEPHRONS

Each kidney has 1 million nephrons, which usually allows for adequate renal function even if the opposite kidney is damaged or becomes nonfunctional. The nephrons are the structures located within the renal parenchyma that are responsible for the initial formation of urine. If the total number of functioning nephrons is less then 20% of normal, renal replacement therapy needs to be considered.

There are two kinds of nephrons. The cortical nephrons, which make up 80% to 85% of the total number, are located in the outermost part of the cortex, and the juxtamedullary nephrons, which make up the remaining 15% to 20%, are located deeper in the cortex. The juxtamedullary nephrons are distinguished by long loops of Henle, which are surrounded by long capillary loops called vasa recta that dip into the medulla of the kidney. The length of the tubular component of the nephron is directly related to its ability to concentrate urine.

Nephrons are made up of two basic components: a filtering element composed of an enclosed capillary network (the glomerulus) and the attached tubule (Fig. 43-2). The glomerulus is a unique network of capillaries suspended between the afferent and efferent blood vessels, which are enclosed in an epithelial structure called Bowman's cap-

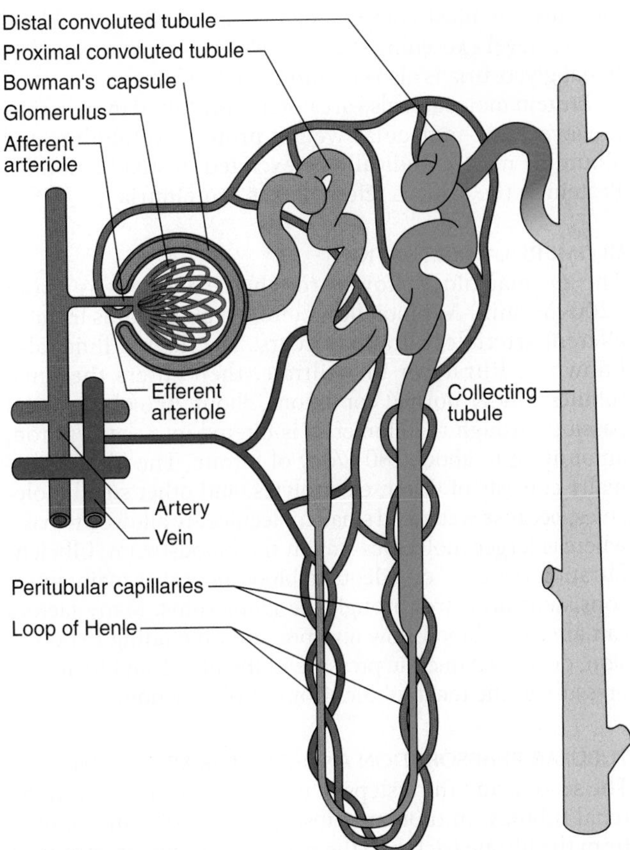

FIGURE 43-2. Representation of a nephron. Each kidney has about 1 million nephrons, which take two forms: cortical and juxtamedullary. Cortical nephrons are located in the cortex of the kidney; juxtamedullary nephrons are adjacent to the medulla.

sule. The glomerular membrane is composed of three filtering layers: the capillary endothelium, the basement membrane, and the epithelium. This membrane normally allows filtration of fluid and small molecules yet limits passage of larger molecules, such as blood cells and albumin. Pressure changes and the permeability of the glomerular membrane of Bowman's capsule facilitate the passage of fluids and various substances from the blood vessels, filling the space within Bowman's capsule with this filtered solution.

The tubular component of the nephron begins in the Bowman's capsule. The filtrate created in the Bowman's capsule travels first into the proximal tubule, then the loop of Henle, the distal tubule, and either the cortical or medullary collecting ducts. The structural arrangement of the tubule allows the distal tubule to lie in close proximity to where the afferent and efferent arteriole respectively enter and leave the glomerulus. The distal tubular cells located in this area, known as the macula densa, function with the adjacent afferent arteriole and create what is known as the juxtaglomerular apparatus. This is the site of renin production. Renin is a hormone directly involved in the control of arterial blood pressure; it is essential for proper functioning of the glomerulus (see later discussion).

The tubular component consists of the Bowman's capsule, the proximal tubule, the descending and ascending limbs of the loop of Henle, and the cortical and medullary collecting ducts. This portion of the nephron is responsible for making adjustments in the filtrate based on the body's needs. Changes are continually made as the filtrate travels through the tubules until it enters the collecting system and is expelled from the body (see Fig. 43-2).

Ureters, Bladder, and Urethra

The urine formed in the nephrons flows into the renal pelvis and then into the ureters, which are long fibromuscular tubes that connect each kidney to the bladder. These narrow tubes, each 24 to 30 cm long, originate at the lower portion of the renal pelvis and terminate in the trigone of the bladder wall.

The left ureter is slightly shorter than the right ureter. The lining of the ureters is made up of transitional cell epithelium called urothelium. The urothelium prevents reabsorption of urine. The movement of urine from each renal pelvis through the ureter into the bladder is facilitated by peristaltic contraction of the smooth muscles in the ureter wall. There are three narrowed areas of each ureter: the ureteropelvic junction, the ureteral segment near the sacroiliac junction, and the ureterovesical junction. These three areas of the ureters have a propensity for obstruction by renal calculi (kidney stones) or stricture. Obstruction of the ureteropelvic junction is the most serious because of its close proximity to the kidney and the risk of associated kidney dysfunction.

The urinary bladder is a muscular, hollow sac located just behind the pubic bone. The capacity of the adult bladder is about 300 to 500 mL. The bladder is characterized by its central, hollow area, called the vesicle, which has two inlets (the ureters) and one outlet (the urethra). The area surrounding the bladder neck is called the urethrovesical junction. The angling of the ureterovesical junction is the primary means of providing antegrade, or downward, movement of urine, also referred to as efflux of urine. This angling prevents vesicoureteral reflux (retrograde, or backward, movement of urine) from the bladder, up the ureter, toward the kidney.

The wall of the bladder contains four layers. The outermost layer is the adventitia, which is made up of connective tissue. Immediately beneath the adventitia is a smooth muscle layer known as the detrusor. Beneath the detrusor is a submucosal layer of loose connective tissue that serves as an interface between the detrusor and the innermost layer, a mucosal lining. The inner layer contains specialized transitional cell epithelium, a membrane that is impermeable to water and prevents reabsorption of urine stored in the bladder. The bladder neck contains bundles of involuntary smooth muscle that form a portion of the urethral sphincter known as the internal sphincter. An important portion of the sphincteric mechanism that helps maintain continence is the external urinary sphincter at the anterior urethra, the segment most distal from the bladder (Porth, 2005). During voiding (**micturition**), increased intravesical pressure keeps the ureterovesical junction closed and keeps urine within the ureters. As soon as micturition is completed, intravesical pressure returns to its normal low baseline value, allowing efflux of urine to resume. Therefore, the only time that the bladder is completely empty is in the last seconds of micturition, before efflux of urine resumes.

The urethra arises from the base of the bladder: In the male, it passes through the penis; in the female, it opens just anterior to the vagina. In the male, the prostate gland, which lies just below the bladder neck, surrounds the urethra posteriorly and laterally.

Physiology of the Upper and Lower Urinary Tracts

CONCEPTS in action ANIMATION *Urine Formation*

The healthy human body is composed of approximately 60% water. Water balance is regulated by the kidneys and results in the formation of urine. Urine is formed in the nephrons through a complex three-step process: glomerular filtration, **tubular reabsorption**, and **tubular secretion** (Fig. 43-3). The various substances normally filtered by the glomerulus, reabsorbed by the tubules, and excreted in the urine include sodium, chloride, bicarbonate, potassium, glucose, urea, creatinine, and uric acid. Within the tubule, some of these substances are selectively reabsorbed into the blood. Others are secreted from the blood into the filtrate as it travels down the tubule.

Amino acids and glucose are usually filtered at the level of the glomerulus and reabsorbed so that neither is excreted in the urine. Normally, glucose does not appear in the urine. However, **renal glycosuria** (recurring or persistent excretion of glucose in the urine) occurs if the amount of glucose in the blood and glomerular filtrate exceeds the amount that the tubules are able to reabsorb. Renal glycosuria occurs in diabetes, the most common clinical expression of a blood glucose level exceeding the kidney's reabsorption capacity. Renal glycosuria is also common in pregnancy.

Protein molecules also are not usually found in the urine; however, low-molecular-weight proteins (globulins and albumin) may periodically be excreted in small amounts. Protein in the urine is referred to as **proteinuria.**

GLOMERULAR FILTRATION

The normal blood flow through the kidneys is about 1200 mL/min. As blood flows into the glomerulus from an afferent arteriole, filtration occurs. The filtered fluid, also known as filtrate or ultrafiltrate, then enters the renal tubules. Under normal conditions, about 20% of the blood passing through the glomeruli is filtered into the nephron, amounting to about 180 L/day of filtrate. The filtrate normally consists of water, electrolytes, and other small molecules, because water and small molecules are allowed to pass, whereas larger molecules stay in the bloodstream. Efficient filtration depends on adequate blood flow that maintains a consistent pressure through the glomerulus. Many factors can alter this blood flow and pressure, including hypotension, decreased oncotic pressure in the blood, and increased pressure in the renal tubules from an obstruction.

TUBULAR REABSORPTION AND TUBULAR SECRETION

The second and third steps of urine formation occur in the renal tubules. In tubular reabsorption, a substance moves from the filtrate back into the peritubular capillaries or vasa recta. In tubular secretion, a substance moves from the peri-

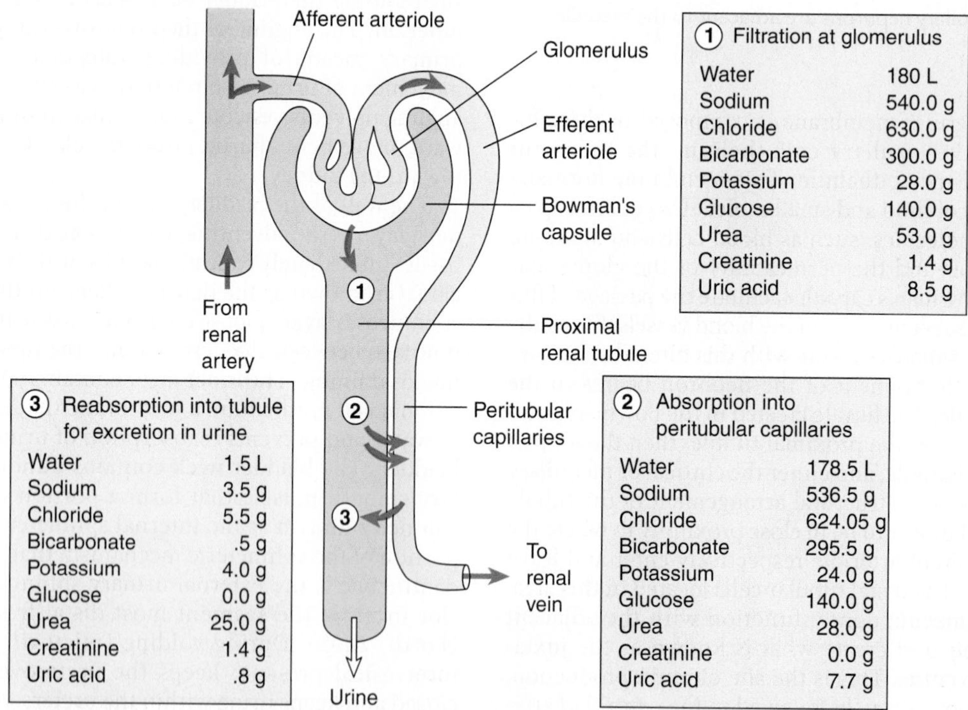

FIGURE 43-3. Urine is formed in the nephrons in a three-step process: filtration, reabsorption, and excretion. Water, electrolytes, and other substances, such as glucose and creatinine, are filtered by the glomerulus; varying amounts of these substances are reabsorbed in the renal tubule or excreted in the urine. Approximate normal volumes of these substances during the steps of urine formation are shown at the top. Wide variations may occur in these values depending on diet.

tubular capillaries or vasa recta into tubular filtrate. Of the 180 L (45 gallons) of filtrate that the kidneys produce each day, 99% is reabsorbed into the bloodstream, resulting in the formation of 1000 to 1500 mL of urine each day. Although most reabsorption occurs in the proximal tubule, reabsorption occurs along the entire tubule. Reabsorption and secretion in the tubule frequently involve passive and active transport and may require the use of energy. Filtrate becomes concentrated in the distal tubule and collecting ducts under hormonal influence and becomes urine, which then enters the renal pelvis.

Antidiuretic Hormone

Antidiuretic hormone (ADH), also known as vasopressin, is a hormone that is secreted by the posterior portion of the pituitary gland in response to changes in osmolality of the blood. With decreased water intake, blood osmolality tends to increase, stimulating ADH release. ADH then acts on the kidney, increasing reabsorption of water and thereby returning the osmolality of the blood to normal. With excess water intake, the secretion of ADH by the pituitary is suppressed; therefore, less water is reabsorbed by the kidney tubule. This latter situation leads to increased urine volume (**diuresis**).

A dilute urine with a fixed specific gravity (about 1.010) or fixed osmolality (about 300 mOsm/L) indicates an inability to concentrate and dilute the urine, a common early sign of kidney disease.

Osmolarity and Osmolality

Osmolarity refers to the ratio of solute to water. The regulation of salt and water is paramount for control of the extracellular volume and both serum and urine osmolarity. Controlling either the amount of water or the amount of solute can change osmolarity. Osmolarity and ionic composition are maintained by the body within very narrow limits. As little as a 1% to 2% change in the serum osmolarity can cause a conscious desire to drink and conservation of water by the kidneys (Candela & Yucha, 2004).

The degree of dilution or concentration of the urine is also measured in terms of osmolality, the number of osmoles (the standard unit of osmotic pressure) dissolved per kilogram of solution. The filtrate in the glomerular capillary normally has the same osmolality as the blood, 275 to 300 mOsm/kg. Serum and urine osmolality and osmolarity are discussed in more detail in Chapter 14.

Regulation of Water Excretion

Regulation of the amount of water excreted is an important function of the kidney. With high fluid intake, a large volume of dilute urine is excreted. Conversely, with a low fluid intake, a small volume of concentrated urine is excreted. A person normally ingests about 1300 mL of oral liquids and 1000 mL of water in food per day. Of the fluid ingested, approximately 900 mL is lost through the skin and lungs (called insensible loss), 50 mL through sweat, and 200 mL through feces (Candela & Yucha, 2004). It is important to consider all fluid gained and lost when evaluating total fluid status. Daily weight measurements are a reliable means of determining overall fluid status. One pound equals approximately 500 mL, so a weight change of as little as 1 lb could suggest an overall fluid gain or loss of 500 mL.

Regulation of Electrolyte Excretion

When the kidneys are functioning normally, the volume of electrolytes excreted per day is equal to the amount ingested. For example, the average American daily diet contains 6 to 8 g each of sodium chloride (salt) and potassium chloride, and approximately the same amounts are excreted in the urine.

SODIUM

Normal serum sodium levels are between 135 to 145 mmol/L, making sodium the most plentiful extracellular ion (see Chapter 14). Sodium plays an important role in controlling the fluid and electrolyte balance. It is the only cation that exerts significant osmotic pressure; where sodium goes, water quickly follows. Therefore, sodium is inseparably linked to both blood volume and blood pressure. The kidneys are responsible for regulating electrolyte loss, and approximately 90% of the sodium contained in the renal filtrate is reabsorbed in the proximal tubules and loops of Henle (Johnson & Criddle, 2004).

As water from the filtrate follows the reabsorbed sodium, the body's osmotic balance is maintained. If more sodium is excreted than ingested, dehydration results; if less sodium is excreted than ingested, fluid retention results.

The regulation of sodium volume excreted depends on **aldosterone**, a hormone synthesized and released from the adrenal cortex. With increased aldosterone in the blood, less sodium is excreted in the urine, because aldosterone fosters renal reabsorption of sodium. Release of aldosterone from the adrenal cortex is largely under the control of angiotensin II. Angiotensin II levels are in turn controlled by renin, an enzyme that is released from specialized cells in the kidneys (Fig. 43-4). This complex system is activated when pressure in the renal arterioles falls below normal levels, as occurs with shock, dehydration, or decreased sodium chloride delivery to the tubules. Activation of this system increases the retention of water and expansion of the intravascular fluid volume, thereby maintaining enough pressure within the glomerulus to ensure adequate filtration.

POTASSIUM

Potassium is the most abundant intracellular ion; about 98% of the total body potassium is located intracellularly. To maintain a normal serum potassium balance (see Chapter 14), the kidneys are responsible for excreting more than 90% of the total daily potassium intake. Several factors influence potassium loss through the kidneys. Aldosterone causes the kidneys to excrete potassium, in contrast to its effects on sodium described previously. The acid–base balance, the amount of dietary potassium intake, and the flow rate of the filtrate in the distal tubule also influence the amount of potassium secreted into the urine. Retention of potassium is the most life-threatening effect of renal failure.

Regulation of Acid–Base Balance

The normal serum pH is about 7.35 to 7.45 and must be maintained within this narrow range for optimal physio-

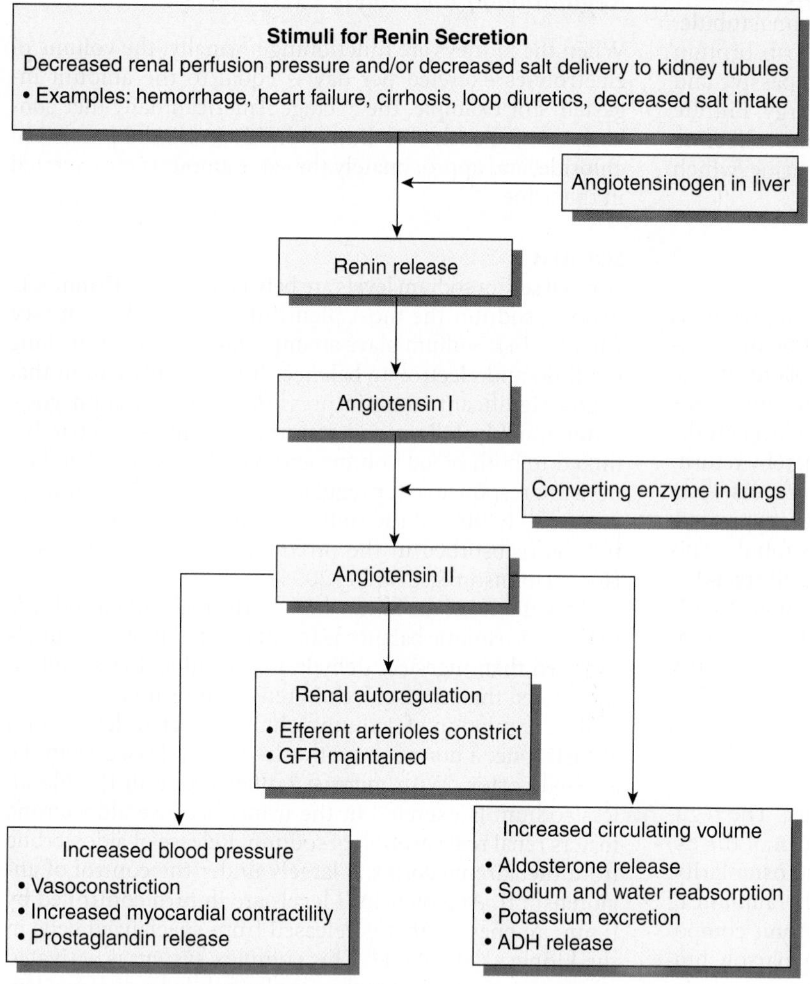

FIGURE 43-4. The renin–angiotensin system. ADH, antidiuretic hormone; GFR, glomerular filtration rate.

logic function (Yucha, 2004). The kidney performs two major functions to assist in this balance. The first is to reabsorb and return to the body's circulation any bicarbonate from the urinary filtrate; the second is to excrete acid in the urine. Because bicarbonate is a small ion, it is freely filtered at the glomerulus. The renal tubules actively reabsorb most of the bicarbonate in the urinary filtrate. To replace any lost bicarbonate, new bicarbonate is generated by the renal tubular cells through a variety of chemical reactions. This newly generated bicarbonate is then reabsorbed by the tubules and returned to the body.

The body's acid production is the result of catabolism, or breakdown, of proteins, which produces acid compounds, in particular phosphoric and sulfuric acids. The normal daily diet also includes a certain amount of acid materials. Unlike carbon dioxide (CO_2), phosphoric and sulfuric acids are nonvolatile and cannot be eliminated by the lungs. Because accumulation of these acids in the blood would lower its pH (making the blood more acidic) and inhibit cell function, they must be excreted in the urine. A person with normal kidney function excretes about 70 mEq of acid each day. The kidney is able to excrete some of this acid directly into the urine until the urine pH reaches 4.5, which is 1000 times more acidic than blood.

However, more acid usually needs to be eliminated from the body than can be secreted directly as free acid in the urine. These excess acids are bound to chemical buffers so that they can be excreted in the urine. Two important chemical buffers are phosphate ions and ammonia (NH_3). When buffered with acid, ammonia becomes ammonium (NH_4). Phosphate is present in the glomerular filtrate, and ammonia is produced by the cells of the renal tubules and secreted into the tubular fluid. Through the buffering process, the kidney is able to excrete large quantities of acid in a bound form, without further lowering the pH of the urine.

Autoregulation of Blood Pressure

Regulation of blood pressure is also a function of the kidney. Specialized vessels of the kidney, called the vasa recta, constantly monitor blood pressure as blood begins its passage into the kidney. When the vasa recta detect a decrease in blood pressure, specialized juxtaglomerular cells near the afferent arteriole, distal tubule, and efferent arteriole secrete the hormone renin. Renin converts angiotensinogen to angiotensin I, which is then converted to angiotensin II, the most powerful vasoconstrictor known; angiotensin II causes the blood pressure to increase (Goshorn, 2005). The adrenal cortex secretes aldosterone in response to stimulation by the pituitary gland, which occurs in response to poor perfusion or increasing serum osmolality. The result is an increase in blood pressure. When the vasa recta recognize the increase in blood pressure, renin secretion stops. Failure of this feedback mechanism is one of the primary causes of hypertension.

Renal Clearance

Renal clearance refers to the ability of the kidneys to clear solutes from the plasma. A 24-hour collection of urine is the primary test of renal clearance used to evaluate how well the kidney performs this important excretory function. Renal clearance depends on several factors: how quickly the substance is filtered across the glomerulus, how much of the substance is reabsorbed along the tubules, and how much of the substance is secreted into the tubules. It is possible to measure the renal clearance of any substance, but the one measure that is particularly useful is the creatinine clearance.

Creatinine is an endogenous waste product of skeletal muscle that is filtered at the glomerulus, passed through the tubules with minimal change, and excreted in the urine. Hence, creatinine clearance is a good measure of the **glomerular filtration rate (GFR).** To calculate creatinine clearance, a 24-hour urine specimen is collected. Midway through the collection, the serum creatinine level is measured. The following formula is then used to calculate the creatinine clearance:

$$\frac{(\text{Volume of urine } [\text{mL/min}] \times \text{urine creatinine } [\text{mL/dL}])}{\text{Serum creatinine } (\text{mg/dL})}$$

The adult GFR can vary from a normal of approximately 125 mL/min (1.67 to 2.0 mL/sec) to a high of 200 mL/min (Porth, 2005). Creatinine clearance is an excellent measure of renal function; as renal function declines, creatinine clearance decreases.

Regulation of Red Blood Cell Production

When the kidneys sense a decrease in the oxygen tension in renal blood flow, they release erythropoietin. Erythropoietin stimulates the bone marrow to produce red blood cells (RBCs), thereby increasing the amount of hemoglobin available to carry oxygen.

Vitamin D Synthesis

The kidneys are also responsible for the final conversion of inactive vitamin D to its active form, 1,25-dihydroxycholecalciferol. Vitamin D is necessary for maintaining normal calcium balance in the body.

Secretion of Prostaglandins

The kidneys also produce prostaglandin E and prostacyclin, which have a vasodilatory effect and are important in maintaining renal blood flow.

Excretion of Waste Products

The kidney functions as the body's main excretory organ, eliminating the body's metabolic waste products. The major waste product of protein metabolism is urea, of which about 25 to 30 g are produced and excreted daily. All of this urea must be excreted in the urine; otherwise it accumulates in body tissues. Other waste products of metabolism that must be excreted are creatinine, phosphates, and sulfates. Uric acid, formed as a waste product of purine metabolism, is also eliminated in the urine. The kidneys serve as the primary mechanism for excreting drug metabolites.

Urine Storage

The bladder is the reservoir for urine. Both filling and emptying of the bladder are mediated by coordinated sympathetic and parasympathetic nervous system control mechanisms involving the detrusor muscle and the bladder outlet. Conscious awareness of bladder filling occurs as a result of sympathetic neuronal pathways that travel via the spinal cord to the level of T10 through T12, where peripheral, hypogastric nerve innervation allows for continued bladder filling. As bladder filling continues, stretch receptors in the bladder wall are activated, coupled with the desire to void. This information from the detrusor muscle is relayed back to the cerebral cortex via the parasympathetic pelvic nerves at the level of S1 through S4 (Porth, 2005). Overall bladder pressure remains low due to the bladder's compliance (ability to expand or collapse) as urine volume changes.

Bladder compliance is due in part to the smooth muscle lining of the bladder and collagen deposits within the wall of the bladder, as well as to neuronal mechanisms that inhibit the detrusor muscle from contracting (specifically, adrenergic receptors that mediate relaxation). To maintain adequate kidney filtration rates, bladder pressure during filling must remain lower than 40 cm H_2O. This low pressure allows the urine to freely leave the renal pelvis and enter the ureters. The bladder is capable of holding 1500 to 2000 mL of urine. This is referred to as the "anatomic capacity" of the bladder. The sensation of bladder fullness is transmitted to the central nervous system when the bladder has reached about 150 to 200 mL in adults, and an initial desire to void occurs (Porth, 2005). A marked sense of fullness and discomfort with a strong desire to void usually occurs when the bladder contains 350 mL or more of urine, referred to as the "functional capacity." Neurologic changes to the bladder at the level of the supraspinal nerves, the spinal nerves, or the bladder wall itself can cause abnormally high volumes of urine to be stored due to a decreased or absent urge to void.

Under normal circumstances with average fluid intake of approximately 1500 to 2000 mL/day, the bladder should be able to store urine for periods of 2 to 4 hours at a time during the day. At night, the release of vasopressin in response to decreased fluid intake causes a decrease in the production of urine and makes it more concentrated. This phenomenon usually allows the bladder to continue filling for periods of 6 to 8 hours in adolescents and adults, making them able to sleep for longer periods before needing to void. In older people, decreasing bladder compliance and decreased vasopressin levels often cause **nocturia** (the need to wake up during the night to urinate).

Bladder Emptying

Micturition (voiding) normally occurs approximately eight times in a 24-hour period. It is activated via the micturition reflex arc within the sympathetic and parasympathetic nervous system, which causes a coordinated sequence of events. Initiation of voiding occurs when the efferent pelvic nerve, which originates in the S1 to S4 area, stimulates the bladder to contract, resulting in complete relaxation of the striated urethral sphincter. This is followed by a decrease in urethral pressure, contraction of the detrusor muscle, opening of the vesicle neck and proximal urethra, and flow of urine. This coordinated effort by the parasympathetic system is mediated by muscarinic and, to a lesser extent, cholinergic receptors within the detrusor muscle. The pressure generated in the bladder during micturition is about 20 to 40 cm H_2O in females. It is somewhat higher and more variable in males 45 years of age and older due to the normal hyperplasia of the cells of the middle lobes of the prostate gland, which surround the proximal urethra. Any obstruction of the bladder outlet, such as in advanced benign prostatic hyperplasia (BPH), results in a high voiding pressure. High voiding pressures make it more difficult to start urine flow and maintain it.

If the spinal pathways from the brain to the urinary system are destroyed (eg, after a spinal cord injury), reflex contraction of the bladder is maintained, but voluntary control over the process is lost. In both situations, the detrusor muscle can contract and expel urine, but the contractions are generally insufficient to empty the bladder completely, so residual urine (urine left in the bladder after voiding) remains. Normally, residual urine amounts to no more than 50 mL in the middle-aged adult and less than 50 to 100 mL in the older adult.

Gerontologic Considerations

Upper and lower urinary tract function changes with age (Stanley, Blair & Beare, 2005). The GFR decreases, starting between 35 and 40 years of age, and a yearly decline of about 1 mL/min continues thereafter. The elderly are more susceptible to acute and chronic renal failure due to the structural and functional changes in the kidney. Examples include sclerosis of the glomerulus and renal vasculature, decreased blood flow, decreased GFR, altered tubular function, and acid–base imbalance. Although renal function usually remains adequate despite these changes, renal reserve is decreased and may reduce the kidneys' ability to respond effectively to drastic or sudden physiologic changes. This steady decrease in glomerular filtration, combined with the use of multiple medications in which metabolites are cleared by the kidneys, puts the older person at higher risk for adverse drug effects and drug–drug interactions (Stanley et al., 2005).

The elderly are more prone to develop hypernatremia and fluid volume deficit, because increasing age is also associated with diminished osmotic stimulation of thirst (Stanley et al., 2005). Thirst is a subjective sensory symptom that is defined as an awareness of the desire to drink. The sense of thirst is so protective that hypernatremia almost never occurs in adults younger than 60 years of age.

Structural or functional abnormalities that occur with aging may also prevent complete emptying of the bladder. This may be due to decreased bladder wall contractility; secondary to myogenic or neurogenic factors; or it may be related to bladder outlet obstruction, such as in BPH or after prostatectomy (Joseph, 2003). Vaginal and urethral tissues atrophy (become thinner) in aging women due to decreased estrogen levels. This causes decreased blood supply to the urogenital tissues, resulting in urethral and vaginal irritation and urinary incontinence.

Urinary incontinence is the most common reason for admission to skilled nursing facilities. Many older people and their families are unaware that urinary incontinence stems from many causes. The nurse needs to inform the patient and family that, with appropriate evaluation, urinary incontinence can often be managed at home, and in many cases it can be eliminated. Many treatments are available for urinary incontinence in the elderly, including noninvasive, behavioral interventions that the patient or caregiver can carry out (Engberg, Bender & Stilley, 2003; Newman, 2003). Treatment modalities for urinary incontinence are described in further detail in Chapter 45.

Preparation of the elderly patient for diagnostic tests must be managed carefully to prevent dehydration, which might precipitate renal failure in a patient with marginal renal reserve. Limitations in mobility may affect an elderly patient's ability to void adequately or to consume an adequate volume of fluids. The patient may limit fluid intake to minimize the frequency of voiding or the risk of incontinence. Teaching the patient and family about the dangers of an inadequate fluid intake is an important role of the nurse caring for the elderly incontinent patient.

Assessment

Obtaining a comprehensive health history, which includes an assessment of risk factors, is the first step in assessing a patient with upper or lower urinary tract dysfunction. Various diseases or clinical situations can increase a patient's risk for renal and urinary tract dysfunction. Data collection about previous health problems or diseases provides the health care team with useful information for evaluating the patient's current urinary status. Risk factors for specific disorders and kidney and lower urinary tract dysfunction are summarized in Table 43-1 and discussed in Chapters 44 and 45.

Health History

Obtaining a urologic health history requires excellent communication skills, because many patients are embarrassed or uncomfortable discussing genitourinary function or symptoms (Cooper & Watt, 2003). It is important to use language the patient can understand and to avoid medical jargon. It is also important to review risk factors, particularly for those patients who are at high risk. For example, the nurse needs to be aware that multiparous women delivering their children vaginally have a high risk for stress **urinary incontinence**, which, if severe enough, can also lead to urge incontinence. Elderly women and people with neurologic

TABLE 43-1 Risk Factors for Selected Renal or Urologic Disorders

Risk Factor	Possible Renal or Urologic Disorder
Childhood diseases: "strep throat" impetigo, nephrotic syndrome	Chronic renal failure
Advanced age	Incomplete emptying of bladder, leading to urinary tract infection
Instrumentation of urinary tract, cystoscopy, catheterization	Urinary tract infection, incontinence
Immobilization	Kidney stone formation
Occupational, recreational, or environmental exposure to chemicals (plastics, pitch, tar, rubber)	Acute renal failure
Diabetes mellitus	Chronic renal failure, neurogenic bladder
Hypertension	Renal insufficiency, chronic renal failure
Multiple sclerosis	Incontinence, neurogenic bladder
Parkinson's disease	Incontinence
Systemic lupus erythematosus	Nephritis, chronic renal failure
Gout, hyperparathyroidism, Crohn's disease, ileostomy	Kidney stone formation
Sickle cell anemia, multiple myeloma	Chronic renal failure
Benign prostatic hyperplasia	Obstruction to urine flow, leading to frequency, oliguria, anuria
Radiation therapy to pelvis	Cystitis, fibrosis of ureter, or fistula in urinary tract
Recent pelvic surgery	Inadvertent trauma to ureters or bladder
Pregnancy	Proteinuria, frequent voiding
Obstetric injury, tumors	Incontinence
Spinal cord injury	Neurogenic bladder, urinary tract infection, incontinence

disorders such as diabetic neuropathy, multiple sclerosis (MS), or Parkinson's disease often have incomplete emptying of the bladder and urinary stasis, which may result in urinary tract infection or increasing bladder pressure, leading to overflow incontinence, hydronephrosis, pyelonephritis, or renal insufficiency.

People with a family history of urinary tract problems are at increased risk for renal disorders (Tierney & Henderson, 2005). People with diabetes who have consistent hypertension and those with primary hypertension are at risk for renal dysfunction (Brady & Wilcox, 2003). Older men are at risk for prostatic enlargement, which causes urethral obstruction and can result in urinary tract infections and renal failure. Furthermore, many people with a history of systemic lupus erythematosus (SLE) develop lupus nephritis (Brady & Wilcox, 2003). When obtaining the health history, the nurse should inquire about the following:

- The patient's chief concern or reason for seeking health care, the onset of the problem, and its effect on the patient's quality of life
- The location, character, and duration of pain, if present, and its relationship to voiding; factors that precipitate pain, and those that relieve it
- History of urinary tract infections, including past treatment or hospitalization for urinary tract infection
- Fever or chills
- Previous renal or urinary diagnostic tests or use of indwelling urinary catheters
- **Dysuria** and when during voiding (ie, at initiation or at termination of voiding) it occurs
- Hesitancy, straining, or pain during or after urination
- Urinary incontinence (stress incontinence, urge incontinence, overflow incontinence, or functional incontinence)
- Hematuria or change in color or volume of urine
- Nocturia and its date of onset
- Renal calculi (kidney stones), passage of stones or gravel in urine
- Female patients: number and type (vaginal or cesarean) of deliveries; use of forceps; vaginal infection, discharge, or irritation; contraceptive practices
- History of anuria (decreased urine production) or other renal problem
- Presence or history of genital lesions or sexually transmitted diseases
- Use of tobacco, alcohol, or recreational drugs
- Any prescription and over-the-counter medications (including those prescribed for renal or urinary problems)

Other key information to obtain while gathering the health history includes an assessment of the patient's psychosocial status, level of anxiety, perceived threats to body image, available support systems, and sociocultural patterns. Obtaining this information during the initial and subsequent nursing assessments enables the nurse to uncover special needs, misunderstandings, lack of knowledge, and need for patient teaching. Pain, changes in voiding, and gastrointestinal symptoms are particularly suggestive of urinary tract disease. Dysfunction of the kidney can produce a complex array of symptoms throughout the body.

Unexplained Anemia

Gradual kidney dysfunction can be insidious in its presentation, although fatigue is a common symptom. Fatigue, shortness of breath, and exercise intolerance all result from the condition known as "anemia of chronic disease." Although historically hematocrit has been the blood test of choice when assessing a patient for anemia, use of the hemoglobin level rather than hematocrit is currently recommended, because that measurement is a better assessment of the oxygen transport ability of the blood.

Pain

Genitourinary pain is usually caused by distention of some portion of the urinary tract as a result of obstructed urine flow or inflammation and swelling of tissues. Severity of pain is related to the sudden onset rather than the extent of distention.

GENETICS IN NURSING PRACTICE

Renal and Urinary Tract Disorders

Various conditions that affect the renal system and urinary tract function are influenced by genetic factors. Some examples of these genetic disorders are:

- Alport syndrome
- Congenital absence of the vas deferens (caused by *CFTR* gene mutation for cystic fibrosis)
- Cystic, dysplastic kidneys
- Fabry disease
- Familial Wilms' tumor
- Focal and segmental glomerulosis
- Horseshoe kidney
- Polycystic kidney (autosomal dominant gene)
- Nephrosis of later onset
- Renal cystic disease in tuberous sclerosis complex

NURSING ASSESSMENTS

Family History

- Inquire about other family members with renal and/or urinary tract malformations.
- Ask about family history of kidney disease with onset in third to fifth decade (polycystic kidney, autosomal dominant gene).
- Identify family history of male infertility and cystic fibrosis (congenital absence of vas deferens).
- Be alert for family members with history of early-onset renal (Wilms' tumor) or other cancers.

Physical Assessment

- Be alert for signs and symptoms of renal disease at an early age (hematuria, hypertension, abdominal mass).
- Assess for clinical findings suggesting that renal disease is a component of a genetic syndrome (eg, seizures, mental retardation, skin involvement).

MANAGEMENT ISSUES SPECIFIC TO GENETICS

- Inquire whether DNA mutation or other genetics testing has been performed on an affected family member.
- If indicated, refer for genetic counseling and evaluation so that the family can discuss concerns regarding inheritance, risks to other family members, availability of genetics testing, and gene-based interventions.
- Offer appropriate genetics information and resources (eg, Genetic Alliance web site).
- Provide support to families newly diagnosed with gene-related renal and/or kidney disease.

GENETICS RESOURCES FOR NURSES AND THEIR PATIENTS ON THE WEB

Genetic Alliance, www.geneticalliance.org—a directory of support groups for patients and families with genetic conditions

Gene Clinics, www.geneclinics.org—a listing of common genetic disorders with up-to-date clinical summaries, genetic counseling and testing information

National Organization of Rare Disorders, www.rarediseases.org—a directory of support groups and information for patients and families with rare genetic disorders

OMIM: Online Mendelian Inheritance in Man, www.ncbi.nlm.nih.gov/projects/omim—a complete listing of inherited genetic conditions

TABLE 43-2 Identifying Characteristics of Genitourinary Pain

Type	Location	Character	Associated Signs and Symptoms	Possible Etiology
Kidney	Costovertebral angle, may extend to umbilicus	Dull constant ache; if sudden distention of capsule, pain is severe, sharp, stabbing, and colicky in nature	Nausea and vomiting, diaphoresis, pallor, signs of shock	Acute obstruction, kidney stone, blood clot, acute pyelonephritis, trauma
Bladder	Suprapubic area	Dull, continuous pain, may be intense with voiding, may be severe if bladder full	Urgency, pain at end of voiding, painful straining	Overdistended bladder, infection, interstitial cystitis; tumor
Ureteral	Costovertebral angle, flank, lower abdominal area, testis, or labium	Severe, sharp, stabbing pain, colicky in nature	Nausea and vomiting, paralytic ileus	Ureteral stone, edema or stricture, blood clot
Prostatic	Perineum and rectum	Vague discomfort, feeling of fullness in perineum, vague back pain	Suprapubic tenderness, obstruction to urine flow; frequency, urgency, dysuria, nocturia	Prostatic cancer, acute or chronic prostatitis
Urethral	Male: along penis to meatus; female: urethra to meatus	Pain variable, most severe during and immediately after voiding	Frequency, urgency, dysuria, nocturia, urethral discharge	Irritation of bladder neck, infection of urethra, trauma, foreign body in lower urinary tract

Table 43-2 lists the various types of genitourinary pain, characteristics of the pain, associated signs and symptoms, and possible causes. However, kidney disease does not always involve pain. It tends to be diagnosed because of other symptoms that cause a patient to seek health care, such as pedal edema, shortness of breath, and changes in urine elimination (Stanley et al., 2005).

Changes in Voiding

Micturition (ie, voiding) is normally a painless function that occurs approximately eight times in a 24-hour period. The average person voids 1200 to 1500 mL of urine in 24 hours, although this amount varies depending on fluid intake, sweating, environmental temperature, vomiting, or diarrhea. Common problems associated with voiding include **frequency**, urgency, dysuria, hesitancy, incontinence, enuresis, polyuria, **oliguria**, and hematuria. These problems and others are described in Table 43-3. Increased urinary urgency and frequency coupled with decreasing urine volumes strongly suggest urine retention. Depending on the acuity of the onset of these symptoms, immediate bladder emptying via catheterization and evaluation are necessary to prevent kidney dysfunction (Newman, 2003).

Gastrointestinal Symptoms

Gastrointestinal symptoms may occur with urologic conditions because of shared autonomic and sensory innervation and renointestinal reflexes. The proximity of the right kidney to the colon, duodenum, head of the pancreas, common bile duct, liver, and gallbladder may cause gastrointestinal disturbances. The proximity of the left kidney to the colon (splenic flexure), stomach, pancreas, and spleen may also result in intestinal symptoms. The most common signs and symptoms are nausea, vomiting, diarrhea, abdominal discomfort, and abdominal distention. Urologic symptoms can mimic such disorders as appendicitis, peptic ulcer disease, and cholecystitis; this can make diagnosis difficult, especially in the elderly, who have decreased neurologic innervation to this area (Goshorn, 2005).

Gerontologic Considerations

Many age-related changes in the renal and urinary systems should be considered when obtaining a health history of an older adult. Examples include anatomic changes (eg, decreased glomerular surface area), decreased ability to concentrate the urine, and decreased bladder capacity. Urinary incontinence is not a normal age-related change,

TABLE 43-3 Problems Associated With Changes in Voiding

Problem	Definition	Possible Etiology
Frequency	Frequent voiding—more than every 3 h	Infection, obstruction of lower urinary tract leading to residual urine and overflow, anxiety, diuretics, benign prostatic hyperplasia, urethral stricture, diabetic neuropathy
Urgency	Strong desire to void	Infection, chronic prostatitis, urethritis, obstruction of lower urinary tract leading to residual urine and overflow, anxiety, diuretics, benign prostatic hyperplasia, urethral stricture, diabetic neuropathy
Dysuria	Painful or difficult voiding	Lower urinary tract infection, inflammation of bladder or urethra, acute prostatitis, stones, foreign bodies, tumors in bladder
Hesitancy	Delay, difficulty in initiating voiding	Benign prostatic hyperplasia, compression of urethra, outlet obstruction, neurogenic bladder
Nocturia	Excessive urination at night	Decreased renal concentrating ability, heart failure, diabetes mellitus, incomplete bladder emptying, excessive fluid intake at bedtime, nephrotic syndrome, cirrhosis with ascites
Incontinence	Involuntary loss of urine	External urinary sphincter injury, obstetric injury, lesions of bladder neck, detrusor dysfunction, infection, neurogenic bladder, medications, neurologic abnormalities
Enuresis	Involuntary voiding during sleep	Delay in functional maturation of central nervous system (bladder control usually achieved by 5 y of age), obstructive disease of lower urinary tract, genetic factors, failure to concentrate urine, urinary tract infection, psychological stress
Polyuria	Increased volume of urine voided	Diabetes mellitus, diabetes insipidus, use of diuretics, excess fluid intake, lithium toxicity, some forms of kidney disease (hypercalcemic and hypokalemic nephropathy)
Oliguria	Urine output less than 400 mL/d	Acute or chronic renal failure (see Chapter 44), inadequate fluid intake
Anuria	Urine output less than 50 mL/d	Acute or chronic renal failure (see Chapter 44), complete obstruction
Hematuria	Red blood cells in the urine	Cancer of genitourinary tract, acute glomerulonephritis, renal stones, renal tuberculosis, blood dyscrasia, trauma, extreme exercise, rheumatic fever, hemophilia, leukemia, sickle cell trait or disease
Proteinuria	Abnormal amounts of protein in the urine	Acute and chronic renal disease, nephrotic syndrome, vigorous exercise, heat stroke, severe heart failure, diabetic nephropathy, multiple myeloma

but it is common in older adults, especially women, because of loss of pelvic muscle tone (Stanley et al., 2005).

It is especially important to obtain a thorough medication history when assessing elderly patients, for whom the increased occurrence of chronic illness often leads to polypharmacy (concurrent use of multiple medications). Aging affects the way the body absorbs, metabolizes, and excretes drugs, placing the elderly patient at risk for adverse reactions. Aging also affects the genitourinary system, leading to compromise and dysfunction in the renal and urinary systems (Stern, 2005).

Physical Examination

Several body systems can affect upper and lower urinary tract dysfunction, and that dysfunction can affect several end organs; therefore, a head-to-toe assessment is indicated. Areas of emphasis include the abdomen, suprapubic region, genitalia, lower back, and lower extremities.

The kidneys are not usually palpable. However, palpation of the kidneys may detect an enlargement that could prove to be very important (Bickley & Szilagyi, 2003). The correct technique for palpation is illustrated in Figure 43-5. It may be possible to palpate the smooth, rounded lower pole of the kidney between the hands. The right kidney is easier to detect, because it is somewhat lower than the left one. In obese patients, palpation of the kidneys is more difficult.

Renal dysfunction may produce tenderness over the costovertebral angle, which is the angle formed by the lower border of the 12th, or bottom, rib and the spine (Fig. 43-6). The abdomen (just slightly to the right and left of midline in both upper quadrants) is auscultated to assess for bruits (low-pitched murmurs that indicate renal artery stenosis or an aortic aneurysm). The abdomen is also assessed for the presence of ascites (accumulation of fluid in the peritoneal cavity), which may occur with kidney as well as liver dysfunction.

To check for residual urine, the bladder should be percussed after the patient voids. Percussion of the bladder begins at the midline just above the umbilicus and proceeds downward. The sound changes from tympanic to dull when percussing over the bladder. The bladder, which can be palpated only if it is moderately distended, feels like a smooth, firm, round mass rising out of the abdomen, usually at midline (Fig. 43-7). Dullness to percussion of the bladder after voiding indicates incomplete bladder emptying.

In older men, BPH or prostatitis can cause difficulty with urination (Stanley et al., 2005). Because the signs and symptoms of prostate cancer can mimic those of BPH, the prostate gland is palpated by digital rectal examination (DRE) as part of the yearly physical examination in men 40 years of age and older (see Chapter 49). In addition, a blood specimen is obtained to test the prostate-specific antigen (PSA) level annually; the results of the DRE and PSA are then correlated. Blood is drawn for PSA before the DRE, because manipulation of the prostate can cause the PSA level to increase temporarily. The inguinal area is ex-

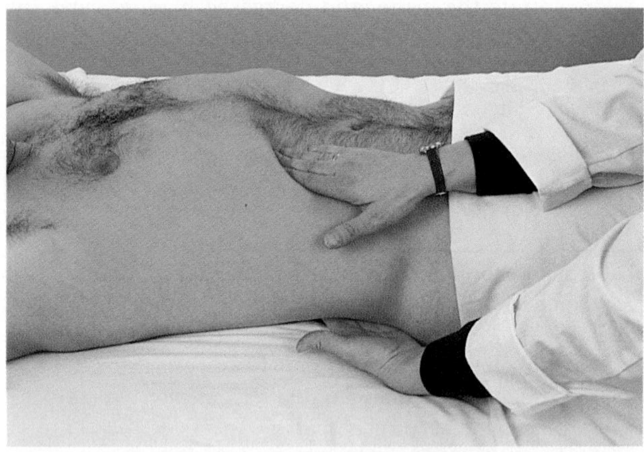

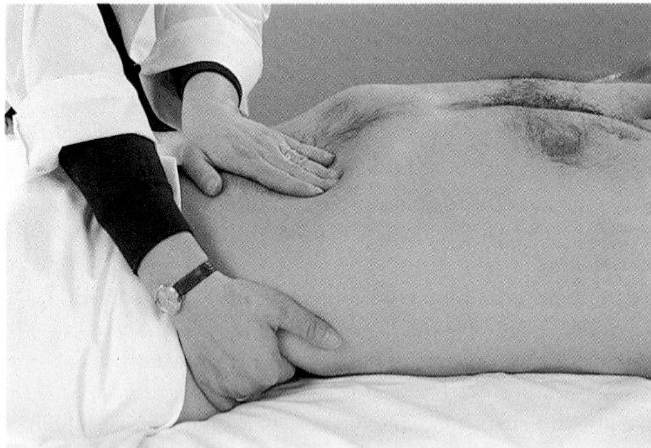

FIGURE 43-5. Technique for palpating the right kidney (*top*). Place one hand under the patient's back with the fingers under the lower rib. Place the palm of the other hand anterior to the kidney with fingers above the umbilicus. Push the hand on top forward as the patient inhales deeply. The left kidney (*bottom*) is palpated similarly by reaching over to the patient's left side and placing the right hand beneath the patient's lower left rib. From Weber, J. W., & Kelley, J. (2003). *Health assessment in nursing.* Philadelphia: Lippincott Williams & Wilkins.

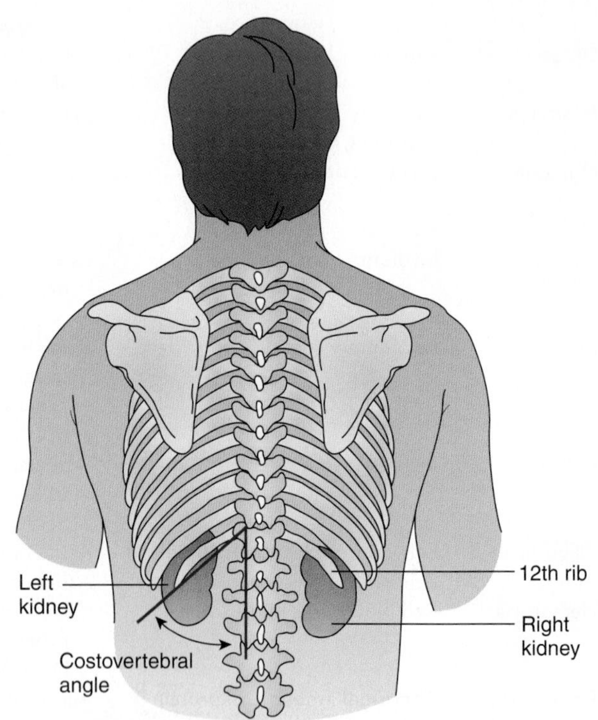

FIGURE 43-6. Location of the costovertebral angle.

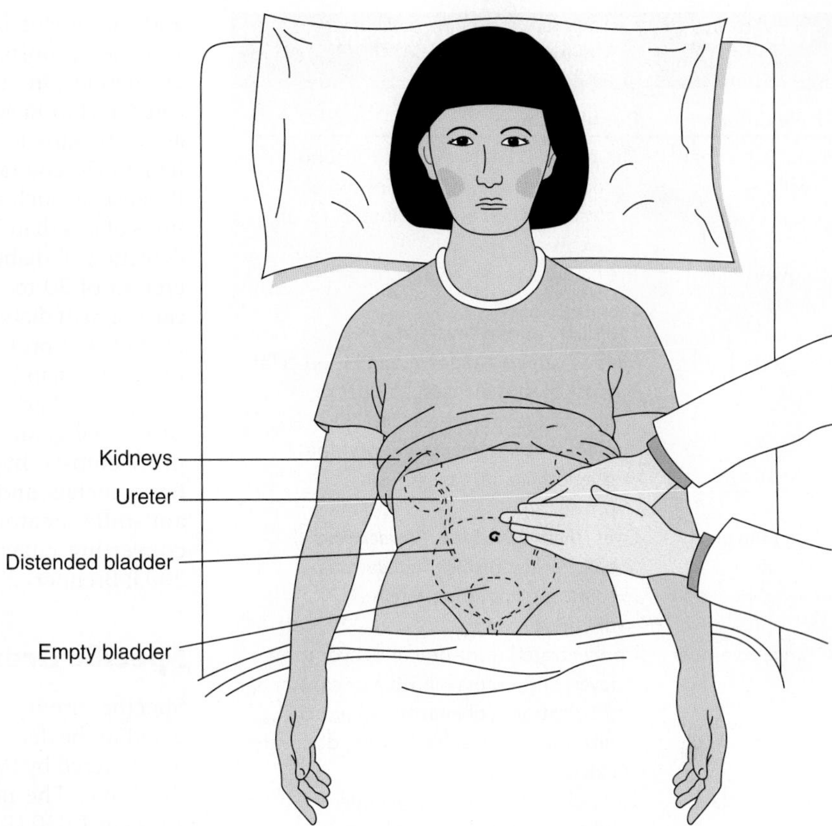

FIGURE 43-7. Palpation of the bladder.

amined for enlarged nodes, an inguinal or femoral hernia, and varicocele (varicose veins of the spermatic cord).

In women, the vulva, urethral meatus, and vagina are examined. The urethra is palpated for diverticula, and the vagina is assessed for adequate estrogen effect and any of five types of herniation (Newman, 2003). Urethrocele is the bulging of the anterior vaginal wall into the urethra. Cystocele is the herniation of the bladder wall into the vaginal vault. Pelvic prolapse is bulging of the cervix into the vaginal vault. Enterocele is herniation of the bowel into the posterior vaginal wall. Rectocele is herniation of the rectum into the vaginal wall. These prolapses are graded depending on the degree of herniation (see Chapter 47 for more information).

The woman is asked to cough and perform a Valsalva maneuver to assess the urethra's system of muscular and ligament support. If urine leakage occurs, the index and middle fingers of the examiner's gloved hand are used to support either side of the urethra as the woman is asked to repeat the Valsalva maneuvers; this is called the Marshall-Boney maneuver. If this produces urinary leakage, referral is suggested.

The patient is assessed for edema and changes in body weight. Edema may be observed, particularly in the face and dependent parts of the body, such as the ankles and sacral areas, and suggests fluid retention. An increase in body weight commonly accompanies edema. A 1-kg weight gain equals approximately 1000 mL of fluid (1 lb ≈ 500 mL).

The deep tendon reflexes of the knee are assessed for quality and symmetry. This is an important part of testing for neurologic causes of bladder dysfunction, because the sacral area, which innervates the lower extremities, is the same peripheral nerve area responsible for urinary continence. The gait pattern of the person with bladder dysfunction is also noted, as well as the patient's ability to walk toe-to-heel. These tests evaluate possible supraspinal causes for urinary incontinence.

Diagnostic Evaluation

A comprehensive health history is used to determine the appropriate laboratory and diagnostic tests. The following sections review some of the tests that might be used.

Urinalysis and Urine Culture

The urinalysis provides important clinical information about kidney function and helps diagnose other diseases, such as diabetes. The urine culture determines whether bacteria are present in the urine, as well as their strains and concentration. Urine culture and sensitivity also identify the antimicrobial therapy that is best suited for the particular strains identified, taking into consideration the antibiotics that have the best rate of resolution in that particular geographic region. Appropriate evaluation of any abnormality can assist in detecting serious underlying diseases.

Urine examination includes the following:

- Urine color (Table 43-4)
- Urine clarity and odor
- Urine pH and specific gravity
- Tests to detect protein, glucose, and ketone bodies in the urine (proteinuria, glycosuria, and ketonuria, respectively)

TABLE 43-4 Changes in Urine Color and Possible Causes

Urine Color	Possible Cause
Colorless to pale yellow	Dilute urine due to diuretics, alcohol consumption, diabetes insipidus, glycosuria, excess fluid intake, renal disease
Yellow to milky white	Pyuria, infection, vaginal cream
Bright yellow	Multiple vitamin preparations
Pink to red	Hemoglobin breakdown, red blood cells, gross blood, menses, bladder or prostate surgery, beets, blackberries, medications (phenytoin, rifampin, phenothiazine, cascara, senna products)
Blue, blue green	Dyes, methylene blue, *Pseudomonas* species organisms, medications (amitriptyline, triamterene, phenylsalicylate)
Orange to amber	Concentrated urine due to dehydration, fever, bile, excess bilirubin or carotene, medications (phenazopyridium HCl, nitrofurantoin, sulfasalazine, docusate calcium, thiamine)
Brown to black	Old red blood cells, urobilinogen, bilirubin, melanin, porphyrin, extremely concentrated urine due to dehydration, medications (cascara, metronidazole, iron preparations, quinine, senna products, methyldopa, nitrofurantoin)

- Microscopic examination of the urine sediment after centrifugation to detect RBCs (**hematuria**), white blood cells, casts (cylindruria), crystals (crystalluria), pus (**pyuria**), and bacteria (**bacteriuria**)

Significance of Findings

Several abnormalities, such as hematuria and proteinuria, produce no symptoms but may be detected during a routine urinalysis using a dipstick. Normally, about 1 million RBCs pass into the urine daily, which is equivalent to one to three RBCs per high-power field. Hematuria (more than three RBCs per high-power field) can develop from an abnormality anywhere along the genitourinary tract and is more common in women than in men. Common causes include acute infection (cystitis, urethritis, or prostatitis), renal calculi, and neoplasm. Other causes include systemic disorders, such as bleeding disorders; malignant lesions; and medications, such as warfarin (Coumadin) and heparin. Although hematuria may initially be detected using a dipstick test, further microscopic evaluation is necessary (Tierney & Henderson, 2005).

Proteinuria may be a benign finding, or it may signify serious disease (Burrows-Hudson, 2005). Occasional loss of up to 150 mg/day of protein in the urine, primarily albumin and Tamm-Horsfall protein (also known as uromodulin), is considered normal and usually does not require further evaluation (Brenner, 2004). A dipstick examination, which can detect from 30 to 1000 mg/dL of protein, should be used as a screening test only, because urine concentration, pH, hematuria, and radiocontrast materials all affect the results. Because dipstick analysis does not detect protein concentrations of less than 30 mg/dL, the test cannot be used for early detection of diabetic nephropathy. Microalbuminuria (excretion of 20 to 200 mg/dL of protein in the urine) is an early sign of diabetic nephropathy. Common benign causes of transient proteinuria are fever, strenuous exercise, and prolonged standing.

Causes of persistent proteinuria include glomerular diseases, malignancies, collagen diseases, diabetes mellitus, preeclampsia, hypothyroidism, heart failure, exposure to heavy metals, and use of medications, such as nonsteroidal anti-inflammatory drugs (NSAIDs) and angiotensin-converting enzyme (ACE) inhibitors (Brady & Wilcox, 2003; Brenner, 2004).

Specific Gravity

Specific gravity measures the density of a solution compared to the density of water, which is 1.000. Specific gravity is altered by the presence of blood, protein, and casts in the urine. The normal range of urine specific gravity is 1.003 to 1.030 (Brenner, 2004).

Methods for determination of specific gravity include the following:

- Multiple-test dipstick (most common method), with a specific reagent area for specific gravity
- Urinometer (least accurate method), in which urine is placed in a small cylinder, and the urinometer is floated in the urine; a specific gravity reading is obtained at the meniscus level of the urine
- Refractometer, an instrument used in a laboratory setting, which measures differences in the speed of light passing through air and the urine sample

Urine specific gravity depends largely on hydration status. When fluid intake decreases, specific gravity normally increases. With high fluid intake, specific gravity decreases. In patients with kidney disease, urine specific gravity does not vary with fluid intake, and the patient's urine is said to have a fixed specific gravity. Disorders or conditions that cause decreased urine specific gravity include diabetes insipidus, glomerulonephritis, and severe renal damage. Those that can cause increased specific gravity include diabetes mellitus, nephritis, and fluid deficit.

Osmolality

Osmolality is the most accurate measurement of the kidney's ability to dilute and concentrate urine. It measures the number of solute particles in a kilogram of water. Serum and urine osmolality are measured simultaneously to assess the body's fluid status. The normal range of serum osmolality is 275 to 300 mOsm/kg. The normal range of urine osmolality is 50 to 1200 mOsm/kg. For a 24-hour urine sample, the normal value is 300 to 900 mOsm/kg.

Renal Function Tests

Renal function tests are used to evaluate the severity of kidney disease and to assess the status of the patient's kidney function. These tests also provide information about the effectiveness of the kidney in carrying out its excretory function. Renal function test results may be within normal limits until the GFR is reduced to less than 50% of normal. Renal function can be assessed most accurately if several tests are performed and their results are analyzed together. Common tests of renal function include renal concentration tests, creatinine clearance, and serum creatinine and blood **urea nitrogen** levels. Table 43-5 describes the purpose and gives the normal range for each test. Other tests for evaluating renal function that may be helpful include serum electrolyte levels (see Chapter 14).

Imaging Modalities

Kidney, Ureter, and Bladder Studies

An x-ray study of the abdomen or kidneys, ureters, and bladder (KUB) may be performed to delineate the size, shape, and position of the kidneys and to reveal any abnormalities, such as calculi (stones) in the kidneys or urinary tract, hydronephrosis (distention of the pelvis of the kidney), cysts, tumors, or kidney displacement by abnormalities in surrounding tissues.

General Ultrasonography

Ultrasonography is a noninvasive procedure that uses sound waves passed into the body through a transducer to detect abnormalities of internal tissues and organs. Structures of the urinary system create characteristic ultrasonographic images. Abnormalities such as fluid accumulation, masses, congenital malformations, changes in organ size, and obstructions can be identified. During the test, the lower abdomen and genitalia may need to be exposed. Ultrasonography requires a full bladder; therefore, fluid intake should be encouraged before the procedure. Because of its sensitivity, ultrasonography has replaced many other tests as the initial diagnostic procedure (Burrow-Hudson, 2005).

Bladder Ultrasonography

Bladder ultrasonography is a noninvasive method of measuring urine volume in the bladder. It may be indicated for

TABLE 43-5 Renal Function Tests

Test	Purpose	Normal Values		
Renal Concentration Tests				
Specific gravity	Evaluates ability of kidneys to concentrate solutes in urine.	1.003–1.030		
Urine osmolality	Concentrating ability is lost early in kidney disease; hence, these test findings may disclose early defects in renal function.	300–900 mOsm/kg/24 h, 50–1200 mOsm/kg random sample		
24-Hour Urine Test				
Creatinine clearance	Detects and evaluates progression of renal disease. Test measures volume of blood cleared of endogenous creatinine in 1 min, which provides an approximation of the glomerular filtration rate. Sensitive indicator of renal disease used to follow progression of renal disease.	Measured in mL/min/1.73 m^2		
		Age	**Male**	**Female**
		Under 30	88–146	81–134
		30–40	82–140	75–128
		40–50	75–133	69–122
		50–60	68–126	64–116
		60–70	61–120	58–110
		70–80	55–113	52–105
Serum Tests				
Creatinine level	Measures effectiveness of renal function. Creatinine is end product of muscle energy metabolism. In normal function, level of creatinine, which is regulated and excreted by the kidneys, remains fairly constant in body.	0.6–1.2 mg/dL (50–110 mmol/L)		
Urea nitrogen (blood urea nitrogen [BUN])	Serves as index of renal function. Urea is nitrogenous end product of protein metabolism. Test values are affected by protein intake, tissue breakdown, and fluid volume changes.	7–18 mg/dL Patients >60 y: 8–20 mg/dL		
BUN to creatinine ratio	Evaluates hydration status. An elevated ratio is seen in hypovolemia; a normal ratio with an elevated BUN and creatinine is seen with intrinsic renal disease.	About 10:1		

urinary frequency, inability to void after removal of an indwelling urinary catheter, measurement of postvoiding residual urine volume, inability to void postoperatively, or assessment of the need for catheterization during the initial stages of an intermittent catheterization training program. Portable, battery-operated devices are available for bedside use. The scan head is placed on the patient's abdomen and directed toward the bladder. The device automatically calculates and displays urine volume.

Computed Tomography and Magnetic Resonance Imaging

Computed tomography (CT) scans and magnetic resonance imaging (MRI) are noninvasive techniques that provide excellent cross-sectional views of the kidney and urinary tract. They are used to evaluate genitourinary masses, nephrolithiasis, chronic renal infections, renal or urinary tract trauma, metastatic disease, and soft tissue abnormalities. Occasionally, an oral or IV radiopaque contrast agent is used in CT scanning to enhance visualization.

PREPARATION FOR MAGNETIC RESONANCE IMAGING

Patient preparation should include teaching relaxation techniques and informing the patient that he or she will be able to talk to the staff by means of a microphone located inside the scanner. Many MRI suites provide headphones so that patients can listen to the music of their choice during the procedure. Nursing care guidelines for patient preparation and test precautions for any imaging procedure that requires a contrast agent (contrast medium) are explained in Chart 43-2.

Before the patient enters the room where the MRI is to be performed, all metal objects and credit cards (the magnetic field can erase them) are removed. This includes medication patches (eg, nicotine and nitroglycerine) that have a metal backing, which can cause burns if they are not removed (Karch, 2004). No metal objects (eg, oxygen tanks, ventilators, stethoscopes) may be brought into the MRI room. The magnetic field is so strong that any metal-containing items will be pulled toward the magnet, causing severe injury and possible death. A patient history is obtained to determine the presence of any metal objects (eg, aneurysm clips, orthopedic hardware, pacemakers, artificial heart valves, intrauterine devices). These objects could malfunction, be dislodged, or heat up as they absorb energy. Cochlear implants are inactivated by MRI; therefore, other imaging procedures are considered. A sedative may be prescribed, because claustrophobia is a problem for some patients.

Nuclear Scans

Nuclear scans require injection of a radioisotope (a technetium 99m–labeled compound or iodine 123 hippurate) into the circulatory system; the isotope is then monitored as it moves through the blood vessels of the kidneys. A scintillation camera is placed behind the kidney with the patient in a supine, prone, or seated position. Hypersensitivity to the radioisotope is rare. The technetium scan provides information about kidney perfusion. The ^{123}I-hippurate renal scan provides information about kidney function, such as GFR.

Nuclear scans are used to evaluate acute and chronic renal failure, renal masses, and blood flow before and after kidney transplantation. The radioisotope is injected at a specified time before the study to achieve the proper concentration in the kidneys. After the procedure is completed, the patient is encouraged to drink fluids to promote excretion of the radioisotope by the kidneys.

CHART 43-2

Patient Care During Urologic Testing with Contrast Agents

For some patients, contrast agents are nephrotoxic and allergenic. The following guidelines can help the nurse and other health care providers respond quickly in the event of a problem.

NURSING ACTIONS FOR ROOM PREPARATION

- Have emergency equipment and medications available in case the patient has an anaphylactic reaction to the contrast agent. Emergency supplies include epinephrine, corticosteroids, vasopressors, oxygen, and airway and suction equipment.

NURSING ACTIONS FOR PATIENT PREPARATION

- Obtain the patient's allergy history with emphasis on allergy to iodine, shellfish, and other seafood, because many contrast agents contain iodine.
- Notify physician and radiologist if the patient is allergic or suspected to be allergic to iodine.
- Obtain health history. Contrast agents should be used with caution in older patients and patients who have diabetes mellitus, multiple myeloma, renal insufficiency, or volume depletion.
- Inform the patient that he or she may experience a temporary feeling of warmth, flushing of the face, and an unusual flavor (similar to that of seafood) in the mouth when the contrast agent is infused.
- Monitor patient closely for allergic reaction and monitor urine output.

Intravenous Urography

IV urography includes various tests such as excretory urography, intravenous pyelography (IVP), and infusion drip pyelography. A radiopaque contrast agent is administered intravenously. An IVP shows the kidneys, ureter, and bladder via x-ray imaging as the dye moves through the upper and then the lower urinary system. A nephrotomogram may be carried out as part of the study to visualize different layers of the kidney and the diffuse structures within each layer and to differentiate solid masses or lesions from cysts in the kidneys or urinary tract.

IV urography may be used as the initial assessment of many suspected urologic problems, especially lesions in the kidneys and ureters. It also provides an approximate estimate of renal function. After the contrast agent (sodium diatrizoate or meglumine diatrizoate) is administered intravenously, multiple x-rays are obtained to visualize drainage structures in the upper and lower urinary systems.

Infusion drip pyelography requires IV infusion of a large volume of a dilute contrast agent to opacify the renal parenchyma and fill the urinary tract. This examination method is useful when prolonged opacification of the drainage structures is desired so that tomograms (body-section radiography) can be made. Images are obtained at specified intervals after the start of the infusion. These images show the filled and distended collecting system. The patient preparation is the same as for excretory urography, except that fluids are not restricted.

Retrograde Pyelography

In retrograde pyelography, catheters are advanced through the ureters into the renal pelvis by means of cystoscopy. A contrast agent is then injected. Retrograde pyelography is usually performed if IV urography provides inadequate visualization of the collecting systems. It may also be used before extracorporeal shock-wave lithotripsy and in patients with urologic cancer who need follow-up and have an allergy to IV contrast agents. Possible complications include infection, hematuria, and perforation of the ureter. Retrograde pyelography is used infrequently because of improved techniques in excretory urography.

Cystography

Cystography aids in evaluating vesicoureteral reflux (backflow of urine from the bladder into one or both ureters) and in assessing for bladder injury. A catheter is inserted into the bladder, and a contrast agent is instilled to outline the bladder wall. The contrast agent may leak through a small bladder perforation stemming from bladder injury, but such leakage is usually harmless. Cystography can also be performed with simultaneous pressure recordings inside the bladder.

Voiding Cystourethrography

Voiding cystourethrography uses fluoroscopy to visualize the lower urinary tract and assess urine storage in the bladder. It is commonly used as a diagnostic tool to identify vesicoureteral reflux. A urethral catheter is inserted, and a contrast agent is instilled into the bladder. When the bladder is full and the patient feels the urge to void, the catheter is removed, and the patient voids. Retrograde urethrography, in which a contrast agent is injected retrograde into the urethra, is always performed before urethral catheterization if urethral trauma is suspected.

Renal Angiography

A renal angiogram, or renal arteriogram, provides an image of the renal arteries. The femoral (or axillary) artery is pierced with a needle, and a catheter is threaded up through the femoral and iliac arteries into the aorta or renal artery. A contrast agent is injected to opacify the renal arterial supply. Angiography is used to evaluate renal blood flow in suspected renal trauma, to differentiate renal cysts from tumors, and to evaluate hypertension. It is used preoperatively for renal transplantation. Before the procedure, a laxative may be prescribed to evacuate the colon so that unobstructed x-rays can be obtained. Injection sites (groin for femoral approach or axilla for axillary approach) may be shaved. The peripheral pulse sites (radial, femoral, and dorsalis pedis) are marked for easy access during post-procedural assessment. The patient is informed that there may be a brief sensation of heat along the course of the vessel when the contrast agent is injected.

After the procedure, vital signs are monitored until stable. If the axillary artery was the injection site, blood pressure measurements are taken on the opposite arm. The injection site is examined for swelling and hematoma. Peripheral pulses are palpated, and the color and temperature of the involved extremity are noted and compared with those of the uninvolved extremity. Cold compresses may be applied to the injection site to decrease edema and pain. Possible complications include hematoma formation, arterial thrombosis or dissection, false aneurysm formation, and altered renal function.

Urologic Endoscopic Procedures

Endourology, or urologic endoscopic procedures, can be performed in one of two ways: using a cystoscope inserted into the urethra, or percutaneously, through a small incision.

The cystoscopic examination is used to directly visualize the urethra and bladder. The cystoscope, which is inserted through the urethra into the bladder, has a self-contained optical lens system that provides a magnified, illuminated view of the bladder (Fig. 43-8). The use of a high-intensity light and interchangeable lenses allows excellent visualization and permits still and motion pictures to be taken. The cystoscope is manipulated to allow complete visualization of the urethra and bladder as well as the ureteral orifices and prostatic urethra. Small ureteral catheters can be passed through the cystoscope, allowing assessment of the ureters and the pelvis of each kidney.

The cystoscope also permits the urologist to obtain a urine specimen from each kidney to evaluate its function. Cup forceps can be inserted through the cystoscope for biopsy. Calculi may be removed from the urethra, bladder, and ureter using cystoscopy. If a lower tract cystoscopy is

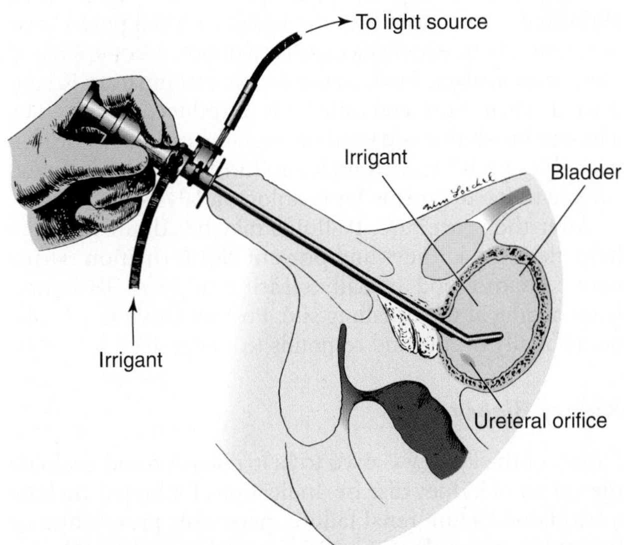

FIGURE 43-8. Cystoscopic examination. A rigid or semirigid cystoscope is introduced into the bladder. The upper cord is an electric line for the light at the distal end of the cystoscope. The lower tubing leads from a reservoir of sterile irrigant that is used to inflate the bladder.

performed, the patient is usually conscious, and the procedure is usually no more uncomfortable than a catheterization. To minimize post-test urethral discomfort, viscous lidocaine is administered several minutes before the study. If the cystoscopy includes examination of the upper tracts, a sedative may be administered before the procedure. General anesthesia is usually administered to ensure that there are no involuntary muscle spasms when the scope is being passed through the ureters or kidney.

The nurse describes the procedure to the patient and family to prepare them and to allay their fears. If an upper cystoscopy is to be performed, the patient is usually restricted to nothing by mouth (NPO) for several hours beforehand.

Postprocedural management is directed at relieving any discomfort resulting from the examination. Some burning on voiding, blood-tinged urine, and urinary frequency from trauma to the mucous membranes can be expected. Moist heat to the lower abdomen and warm sitz baths are helpful in relieving pain and relaxing the muscles.

After a cystoscopic examination, the patient with obstructive pathology may experience urine retention if the instruments used during the examination caused edema. The nurse carefully monitors the patient with prostatic hyperplasia for urine retention. Warm sitz baths and antispasmodic medication, such as flavoxate (Urispas), may be prescribed to relieve temporary urine retention caused by poor relaxation of the urinary sphincter; however, intermittent catheterization may be necessary for a few hours after the examination. The nurse monitors the patient for signs and symptoms of urinary tract infection. Because edema of the urethra secondary to local trauma may obstruct urine flow, the patient is also monitored for signs and symptoms of obstruction.

Biopsy

Renal and Ureteral Brush Biopsy

Brush biopsy techniques provide specific information when abnormal x-ray findings of the ureter or renal pelvis raise questions about whether a defect is a tumor, a stone, a blood clot, or an artifact. First, a cystoscopic examination is conducted. Then, a ureteral catheter is introduced, followed by a biopsy brush that is passed through the catheter. The suspected lesion is brushed back and forth to obtain cells and surface tissue fragments for histologic analysis.

After the procedure, IV fluids may be administered to help clear the kidneys and prevent clot formation. Urine may contain blood (usually clearing in 24 to 48 hours) from oozing at the brushing site. Postoperative renal colic occasionally occurs and responds to analgesics.

Kidney Biopsy

Biopsy of the kidney is used to help diagnose and evaluate the extent of kidney disease. Indications for biopsy include unexplained acute renal failure, persistent proteinuria or hematuria, transplant rejection, and glomerulopathies. A small section of renal cortex is obtained either percutaneously (needle biopsy) or by open biopsy through a small flank incision. Before the biopsy is carried out, coagulation studies are conducted to identify any risk of postbiopsy bleeding. Contraindications to kidney biopsy include bleeding tendencies, uncontrolled hypertension, a solitary kidney, and morbid obesity (Morton, Fontaine, Hudak, et al., 2005).

PROCEDURE

The patient may be prescribed a fasting regimen 6 to 8 hours before the test. An IV line is established. A urine specimen is obtained and saved for comparison with the postbiopsy specimen.

If a needle biopsy is to be performed, the patient is instructed to breathe in and hold that breath (to prevent the kidney from moving) while the needle is being inserted. The sedated patient is placed in a prone position with a sandbag under the abdomen. The skin at the biopsy site is infiltrated with a local anesthetic. The biopsy needle is introduced just inside the renal capsule of the outer quadrant of the kidney. The location of the needle may be confirmed by fluoroscopy or by ultrasound, in which case a special probe is used.

With open biopsy, a small incision is made over the kidney, allowing direct visualization. Preparation for an open biopsy is similar to that for any major abdominal surgery.

Nursing Implications

Most patients undergoing urologic testing or imaging studies are apprehensive, even those who have had these tests in the past. Patients frequently feel discomfort and embarrassment about such a private and personal function as voiding. Voiding in the presence of others can frequently cause guarding, a natural reflex that inhibits voiding due to situational anxiety. Because the outcomes of these studies determine the plan of care, the nurse must help the patient relax by providing as much privacy and explanation about the procedure as possible (Chart 43-3).

Nursing Diagnosis

Potential nursing diagnoses for the patient undergoing assessment of urinary or renal function include the following:

- Deficient knowledge about the procedures and diagnostic tests
- Acute pain related to renal infection, edema, obstruction, or bleeding along the urinary tract or to invasive diagnostic procedures
- Fear related to possible diagnosis of serious illness, altered renal function, and embarrassment secondary to discussion of urinary function and exposure and invasion of genitalia

Planning, Implementation, and Evaluation

The goals, nursing interventions and rationale, and expected outcomes of diagnostic testing are discussed in greater detail in the plan of nursing care in Chart 43-4. In preparing the patient for urodynamic testing, the nurse explains the urodynamic procedure to the patient and describes what sensations can be expected during and after the procedure. The nurse reassures the patient that staff will be present during the procedure but that privacy and comfort will be maintained. Patient and family education is essential to help the patient understand the purpose of the procedure

CHART 43-3

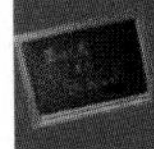

Patient Education

Before and After Urodynamic Testing

- A physician or nurse will conduct an in-depth interview. Questions related to your urologic symptoms and voiding habits will be asked.
- You will be asked to describe sensations felt during the procedure.
- During the procedure, you might be asked to change positions (for example, from supine to sitting or standing).
- You may be asked to cough or perform the Valsalva maneuver (bear down) during the procedure.
- You will probably need to have one or two urethral catheters inserted so that bladder pressure and bladder filling can be measured. Another catheter may be placed in the rectum or vagina to measure abdominal pressure.
- You may also have electrodes (surface, wire, or needle) placed in the perianal area for electromyography (EMG). This may be uncomfortable initially during insertion and later during position changes.
- Your bladder will be filled through the urethral catheter one or more times during the procedure.
- After the procedure, you may experience urinary frequency, urgency, or dysuria from the urethral catheters. Avoid caffeinated, carbonated, and alcoholic beverages after the procedure because these can further irritate the bladder. These symptoms usually decrease or subside by the day after the procedure.
- You might notice a slight hematuria (blood-tinged urine) right after the procedure (especially in men with benign prostatic hyperplasia). Drinking fluids will help to clear the hematuria.
- If the urinary meatus is irritated, a warm sitz bath may be helpful.
- Be alert for signs of a urinary tract infection after the procedure. Contact your physician if you experience fever, chills, lower back pain, or continued dysuria and hematuria.
- If you receive an antibiotic medication before the procedure, you should continue taking the complete course of medication after the procedure. This is a measure to prevent infection.

CHART 43-4

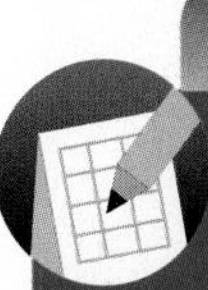

Plan of Nursing Care — Care of the Patient Undergoing Diagnostic Testing of the Renal-Urologic System

Nursing Diagnosis: Deficient knowledge about procedures and diagnostic tests
Goal: Patient demonstrates increased understanding of the procedure and tests and expected behaviors.

NURSING INTERVENTIONS	RATIONALE	EXPECTED OUTCOMES
1. Assess patient's level of understanding of planned diagnostic tests.	1. Provides basis for teaching and gives indication of patient's perception of tests	• States rationale for planned diagnostic tests and what tasks and behaviors are expected during the procedure
2. Provide a description of tests in language the patient can understand.	2. Understanding what is expected enhances patient compliance and cooperation.	• Complies with urine collection, fluid modifications, or other procedures required for diagnostic evaluation
3. Assess patient's understanding of test results after their completion.	3. Apprehension may interfere with patient's ability to understand information and results provided by health care team.	• Restates in own words results of diagnostic tests
4. Reinforce information provided to patient about test results and implications for follow-up care.	4. Provides opportunity for patient to clarify information and anticipate follow-up care	• Asks for clarification of terms and procedures • Explains rationale for follow-up care • Participates in follow-up care

continued >

CHART 43-4

Plan of Nursing Care | Care of the Patient Undergoing Diagnostic Testing of the Renal-Urologic System (Continued)

Nursing Diagnosis: Acute pain related to infection, edema, obstruction, or bleeding along urinary tract or to invasive diagnostic tests
Goal: Patient reports decrease in pain and absence of discomfort.

NURSING INTERVENTIONS	RATIONALE
1. Assess level of pain: dysuria, burning on urination, abdominal or flank pain, bladder spasm.	1. Provides baseline for evaluation of pain relief strategies and progression of dysfunction
2. Encourage fluid intake (unless contraindicated).	2. Promotes dilute urine and flushing of the lower urinary tract
3. Encourage warm sitz baths.	3. Relieves local discomfort and promotes relaxation
4. Report increased pain to physician.	4. May indicate progression or recurrence of dysfunction, or untoward signs (eg, bleeding, calculi)
5. Administer analgesics and antispasmodics for pain and spasm as prescribed.	5. Prescribed to relieve pain or spasm
6. Assess voiding patterns and hygiene practices and provide instructions about recommended voiding patterns and hygienic practices.	6. Delayed emptying of the bladder and poor hygiene may contribute to pain secondary to renal or urinary tract dysfunction.

EXPECTED OUTCOMES

- Reports decreasing levels of pain
- Reports absence of local symptoms
- States ability to start and stop urinary stream without discomfort
- Consumes increased fluid intake if indicated
- Uses sitz bath as indicated
- Identifies signs and symptoms to be reported to the health care provider
- Takes medications as prescribed
- Does not delay in emptying bladder
- Uses appropriate hygienic measures, avoids use of bubble bath, uses appropriate hygiene after bowel movements

Nursing Diagnosis: Fear related to potential alteration in renal function and embarrassment secondary to discussion of urinary function and invasion of genitalia
Goal: Patient appears relaxed and reports decreased fear and anxiety.

NURSING INTERVENTIONS	RATIONALE
1. Assess patient's level of fear and apprehension.	1. A high level of fear or apprehension can interfere with learning and cooperation.
2. Explain all procedures and tests to patient.	2. Knowledge about what is expected helps reduce fear and apprehension.
3. Provide privacy and respect patient's modesty by closing doors and keeping patient covered. Keep urinal and bedpan covered and out of sight.	3. Communicates that you are aware of and accept patient's need for privacy and modesty
4. Use correct terminology in a factual manner when questioning patient about urinary tract dysfunction.	4. Conveys that you are comfortable discussing patient's urinary dysfunction and symptoms with patient
5. Assess patient's fears about perceived changes associated with tests and other procedures.	5. May uncover fears and misconceptions of the patient that can be alleviated by correct understanding
6. Instruct patient in relaxation techniques.	6. Promotes relaxation and assists the patient in coping with uncertainty about outcomes

EXPECTED OUTCOMES

- Appears relaxed with a low level of fear or apprehension
- States rationale for tests and procedures in a calm, relaxed manner
- Maintains usual privacy and modesty
- Discusses own urinary tract dysfunction using correct terminology without overt indications of embarrassment or discomfort
- Relates fears and concerns
- Demonstrates correct understanding of procedures and possible outcomes
- Appears relaxed with low level of fear and apprehension

and what to expect before, during, and after it. Pertinent home care considerations can be discussed at this time.

PROMOTING HOME AND COMMUNITY-BASED CARE

Teaching Patients Self-Care. Many procedures and tests used to evaluate upper and lower urinary tract function are carried out in outpatient or short-procedure settings. Therefore, family members or other caregivers in the home may be called on to provide postprocedure care. They need clear explanations about the procedures and tests; how to prepare for them; and what precautions, if any, need to be taken afterward. The patient and family members are provided with verbal and written explanations about monitoring that may be necessary at home and are instructed about steps to take if complications occur.

Continuing Care. Follow-up telephone calls made to the patient and family at home provide an opportunity for them to ask questions and to report on the patient's status. Teaching is reinforced, and the patient is reminded of the importance of keeping follow-up appointments with primary health care providers.

Critical Thinking Exercises

1 ebp Following the removal of an indwelling catheter 2 days after a complete abdominal hysterectomy, your patient complains of abdominal pain. Describe the assessment techniques appropriate to evaluate her pain. Review the possible causes, describe the actions you would take and the rationale for each action, and identify the evidence base that supports the actions. What criteria would you use to evaluate the strength of the evidence?

2 A 76-year-old patient with a history of diabetes is admitted to the hospital for evaluation of a kidney mass and is scheduled for an MRI. Explain why the MRI is indicated for this patient and what, if any, precautions must be taken because the patient has diabetes. What nursing observations and assessments are indicated because of the history of diabetes? What patient teaching is appropriate before the MRI?

3 ebp You make a home visit to an elderly patient who is incontinent. Identify assessments and possible interventions you would use to evaluate and manage the incontinence. Identify the evidence for the assessments and interventions you chose and the strength of that evidence.

REFERENCES AND SELECTED READINGS

BOOKS

Brady, H. R. & Wilcox, C. S. (2003). *Therapy in nephrology and hypertension* (2nd ed.). St. Louis: Elsevier Saunders.

Brenner, B. M. (2004). *Brenner and Rector's the kidney* (7th ed.). Philadelphia: Saunders.

Bickley, L. S. & Szilagyi, P. G. (2003). *Bates' guide to physical examination and history taking* (8th ed.). Philadelphia: Lippincott Williams & Wilkins.

Diepenbrock, N. H. (2004). *Quick reference to critical care* (2nd ed.). Philadelphia: Lippincott Williams & Wilkins.

Dochterman, J. C. & Bulechek, G. M. (2004). *Nursing interventions classification (NIC)* (4th ed.). St. Louis: Mosby.

Fischbach, F. (2002). *Common laboratory and diagnostic tests* (3rd ed.). Philadelphia: Lippincott Williams & Wilkins.

Goshorn, J. (2005). Acute renal failure. In Sole, M. L., Klein, D. G. & Moseley, M. J. (Eds.). *Introduction to critical care nursing.* St. Louis: Elsevier Saunders.

Morton, P. G., Fontaine, D. K., Hudak, C. M., et al. (2005). *Critical care nursing: A holistic approach* (8th ed.). Philadelphia: Lippincott Williams & Wilkins.

Porth, C. M. (2005). *Pathophysiology: Concepts of altered health states* (7th ed.). Philadelphia: Lippincott Williams & Wilkins.

Stanley, M., Blair, K. A. & Beare, P. G. (2005). *Gerontological nursing: Promoting successful aging with older adults* (3rd ed.). Philadelphia: F. A. Davis.

Tierney, L. M. & Henderson, M. C. (2005). *The patient history: Evidence-based approach.* New York: Lange Medical Books.

Weber, J. & Kelley, J. (2003). *Health assessment in nursing* (2nd ed.). Philadelphia: Lippincott Williams & Wilkins.

JOURNALS

**Asterisks indicate nursing research articles.*

Burrows-Hudson, S. (2005). Chronic kidney disease. *American Journal of Nursing, 105*(2), 40–50.

Candela, L. & Yucha, C. (2004). Renal regulation of extracellular fluid volume and osmolarity. *Nephrology Nursing Journal: Journal of the American Nephrology Nurses' Association, 31*(4), 397–404.

Chmielewski, C. (2003). Renal anatomy and overview of nephron function. *Nephrology Nursing Journal: Journal of the American Nephrology Nurses' Association, 30*(2), 185–190.

*Cooper, G. & Watt, E. (2003). An exploration of acute care nurses' approach to assessment and management of people with urinary incontinence. *Journal of Wound Ostomy and Continence Nursing, 30*(6), 305–313.

Engberg, S. J., Bender, M. A. & Stilley, C. S. (2003). Kegels and communication. *American Journal of Nursing, 103*(7), 93–94.

Guthrie, D. & Yucha, C (2004). Urinary concentration and dilution. *Nephrology Nursing Journal: Journal of the American Nephrology Nurses' Association, 31*(3), 297–302.

Holechek, M. (2003). Glomerular filtration: An overview. *Nephrology Nursing Journal: Journal of the American Nephrology Nurses' Association, 30*(3), 285–291.

Johnson, A. & Criddle, L. (2004). Pass the salt: Indications for the implications of using hypertonic saline. *Critical Care Nurse, 24*(5), 36–46.

Joseph, A. C. (2003). Continence: The sixth vital sign? *American Journal of Nursing, 103*(7), 11.

Karch, A. M. (2004). Don't get burnt by the MRI. *American Journal of Nursing, 104*(8), 31.

Newman, D. (2003). Stress urinary incontinence in women. *American Journal of Nursing, 103*(8), 46–55.

Stern, M. (2005). Aging with multiple sclerosis. *Physical Medicine and Rehabilitation Clinics of North America, 16*(1), 219–234.

Yucha, C. (2004). Renal regulation of acid-base balance. *Nephrology Nursing Journal: Journal of the American Nephrology Nurses' Association, 31*(2), 201–208.

RESOURCES

American Association of Kidney Patients, 3505 E. Frontage Rd. Ste 315, Tampa, FL 33607; 800-749-2257; fax 813-636-8122; http://www.aakp.org. Accessed May 15, 2006.

National Kidney Foundation (NKF), 20 East 33rd Street, New York, NY 10016; 800-622-9010; http://www.kidney.org. Accessed May 15, 2006.

National Institute of Diabetes and Digestive and Kidney Diseases, National Institutes of Health, Bethesda, MD 20892; 301-654-4415; http://www.niddk.nih.gov. Accessed May 15, 2006.

CHAPTER 44

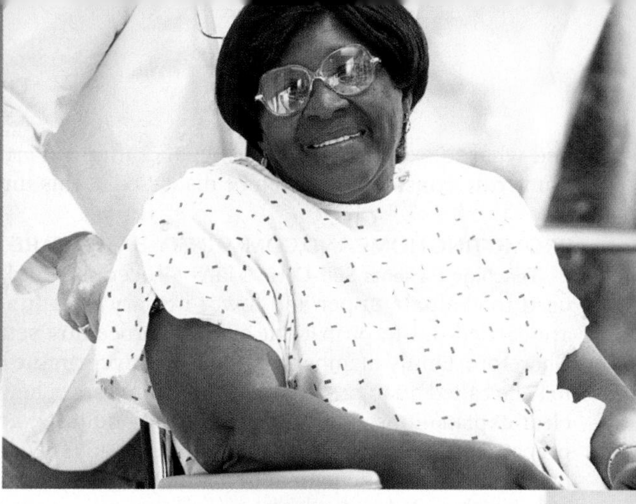

Management of Patients With Renal Disorders

Learning Objectives

On completion of this chapter, the learner will be able to:

1. Describe the clinical manifestations common to renal disorders.
2. Compare and contrast the pathophysiology, clinical manifestations, medical management, and nursing management of the glomerular diseases.
3. Describe the causes of acute and chronic renal failure and compare and contrast treatment options: hemodialysis, peritoneal dialysis, and continuous renal replacement therapy.
4. Describe the nursing management of the hospitalized patient on dialysis.
5. Use the nursing process as a framework for the care of patients with acute and chronic renal failure.
6. Develop a postoperative plan of nursing care and teaching plan for the patient undergoing kidney surgery and transplantation.
7. Describe the causes, treatment, and nursing care of the patient with renal cancer.

The renal system is an important regulator of the body's internal environment and is essential for the maintenance of life. Chronic kidney disease is an umbrella term that is used to describe kidney damage or a decrease in the glomerular filtration rate (GFR) for 3 or more months (Johnson, Levey, Coresh, et al., 2004; Thomas-Hawkins & Zazworsky, 2005). Patients with renal disorders often exhibit similar symptoms regardless of the specific underlying disorder. This chapter provides an overview of electrolyte imbalances that are common in patients with many renal conditions. The glomerular diseases, many of which result in chronic kidney disease, are addressed, together with their management strategies (eg, dialysis, transplantation, and kidney surgery). Care of the patient who has undergone kidney surgery, transplantation, or has renal cancer or trauma is also discussed.

Fluid and Electrolyte Imbalances in Renal Disorders

Patients with renal disorders commonly experience fluid and electrolyte imbalances and require careful assessment and close monitoring for signs of potential problems. The fluid intake and output record, a key monitoring tool, is used to document important fluid parameters, including the amount of fluid taken in (orally or parenterally), the volume of urine excreted, and other fluid losses (diarrhea, vomiting, diaphoresis). Patient weight is also important, and documenting trends in weight is a key assessment strategy essential for determining the daily fluid allowance and indicating signs of fluid overload or deficit. The patient whose fluid intake exceeds the ability of the kidneys to excrete fluid is said to have fluid overload. If fluid intake is inadequate, the patient is said to be volume-depleted and may show signs and symptoms of fluid volume deficit.

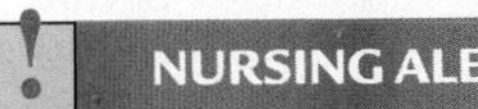

The most accurate indicator of fluid loss or gain in an acutely ill patient is weight. An accurate daily weight must be obtained and recorded. A 1-kg weight gain is equal to 1,000 mL of retained fluid.

Clinical Manifestations

The signs and symptoms of common fluid and electrolyte disturbances that can occur in patients with renal disorders and their general management strategies are listed in Table 44-1.

Glossary

acute tubular necrosis: type of acute renal failure in which there is actual damage to the kidney tubules

anuria: total urine output less than 50 mL in 24 hours

arteriovenous fistula: type of vascular access for dialysis; created by surgically connecting an artery to a vein

arteriovenous graft: type of surgically created vascular access for dialysis by which a piece of biologic, semibiologic, or synthetic graft material connects the patient's artery to a vein

azotemia: concentration of urea and other nitrogenous wastes in the blood

continuous ambulatory peritoneal dialysis (CAPD): method of peritoneal dialysis whereby a patient performs four or five complete exchanges or cycles throughout the day

continuous cyclic peritoneal dialysis (CCPD): method of peritoneal dialysis in which a peritoneal dialysis machine (cycler) automatically performs exchanges, usually while the patient sleeps

continuous renal replacement therapy (CRRT): variety of methods used to replace normal kidney function by circulating the patient's blood through a filter and returning it to the patient

continuous venovenous hemodialysis (CVVHD): form of continuous renal replacement therapy that results in removal of fluid and waste products; venous blood circulates through a hemofilter and returns to the patient

continuous venovenous hemofiltration (CVVH): form of continuous renal replacement therapy that primarily results in removal of fluid; venous blood circulates through a hemofilter and returns to the patient

dialysate: solution that circulates through the dialyzer in hemodialysis and through the peritoneal membrane in peritoneal dialysis

dialyzer: "artificial kidney" or dialysis machine; contains a semipermeable membrane through which particles of a certain size can pass

diffusion: movement of solutes (waste products) from an area of higher concentration to an area of lower concentration

end-stage renal disease (ESRD): progressive, irreversible deterioration in renal function that results in retention of uremic waste products

glomerulonephritis: inflammation of the glomerular capillaries

hemodialysis: procedure during which a patient's blood is circulated through a dialyzer to remove waste products and excess fluid

interstitial nephritis: inflammation within the renal tissue

nephrosclerosis: hardening of the renal arteries

osmosis: movement of water through a semipermeable membrane from an area of lower solute concentration to an area of higher solute concentration

peritoneal dialysis: procedure that uses the lining of the patient's peritoneal cavity as the semipermeable membrane for exchange of fluid and solutes

peritonitis: inflammation of the peritoneal membrane (lining of the peritoneal cavity)

pyelonephritis: inflammation of the renal pelvis

ultrafiltration: process whereby water is removed from the blood by means of a pressure gradient between the patient's blood and the dialysate

uremia: an excess of urea and other nitrogenous wastes in the blood

urinary casts: proteins secreted by damaged kidney tubules

TABLE 44-1 Common Fluid and Electrolyte Disturbances in Renal Disorders

Disturbance	Manifestations	General Management Strategies
Fluid volume deficit	Acute weight loss ≥5%, decreased skin turgor, dry mucous membranes, oliguria or anuria, increased hematocrit, blood urea nitrogen (BUN) level increased out of proportion to creatinine level, hypothermia	Fluid challenge, fluid replacement orally or parenterally
Fluid volume excess	Acute weight gain ≥5%, edema, crackles, shortness of breath, decreased BUN, decreased hematocrit, distended neck veins	Fluid and sodium restriction, diuretics, dialysis
Sodium deficit	Nausea, malaise, lethargy, headache, abdominal cramps, apprehension, seizures	Diet, normal saline or hypertonic saline solutions
Sodium excess	Dry, sticky mucous membranes, thirst, rough dry tongue, fever, restlessness, weakness, disorientation	Fluids, diuretics, dietary restriction
Potassium deficit	Anorexia, abdominal distention, paralytic ileus, muscle weakness, ECG changes, dysrhythmias	Diet, oral or parenteral potassium replacement therapy
Potassium excess	Diarrhea, colic, nausea, irritability, muscle weakness, ECG changes	Dietary restriction, diuretics, IV glucose, insulin and sodium bicarbonate, cation exchange resin, calcium gluconate, dialysis
Calcium deficit	Abdominal and muscle cramps, stridor, carpopedal spasm, hyperactive reflexes, tetany, positive Chvostek's or Trousseau's sign, tingling of fingers and around mouth, ECG changes	Diet, oral or parenteral calcium salt replacement
Calcium excess	Deep bone pain, flank pain, muscle weakness, depressed deep tendon reflexes, constipation, nausea and vomiting, confusion, impaired memory, polyuria, polydipsia, ECG changes	Fluid replacement, etidronate, pamidronate, mithramycin, calcitonin, glucocorticoids, phosphate salts
Bicarbonate deficit	Headache, confusion, drowsiness, increased respiratory rate and depth, nausea and vomiting, warm flushed skin	Bicarbonate replacement, dialysis
Bicarbonate excess	Depressed respirations, muscle hypertonicity, dizziness, tingling of fingers and toes	Fluid replacement if volume depleted; ensure adequate chloride
Protein deficit	Chronic weight loss, emotional depression, pallor, fatigue, soft flabby muscles	Diet, dietary supplements, hyperalimentation, albumin
Magnesium deficit	Dysphagia, muscle cramps, hyperactive reflexes, tetany, positive Chvostek's or Trousseau's sign, tingling of fingers, dysrhythmias, vertigo	Diet, oral or parenteral magnesium replacement therapy
Magnesium excess	Facial flushing, nausea and vomiting, sensation of warmth, drowsiness, depressed deep tendon reflexes, muscle weakness, respiratory depression, cardiac arrest	Calcium gluconate, mechanical ventilation, dialysis
Phosphorus deficit	Deep bone pain, flank pain, muscle weakness and pain, paresthesia, apprehension, confusion, seizures	Diet, oral or parenteral phosphorus supplementation therapy
Phosphorus excess	Tetany, tingling of fingers and around mouth, muscle spasms, soft tissue calcification	Diet restriction, phosphate binders, normal saline solution, IV dextrose solution, and insulin

The nurse continually assesses, monitors, and informs appropriate members of the health care team if the patient exhibits any of these signs (Goshorn, 2005). Management strategies for fluid and electrolyte disturbances in renal disease are discussed in greater depth later in this chapter (see also Chapter 14).

Gerontologic Considerations

Changes in kidney function with normal aging increase the susceptibility of elderly patients to kidney dysfunction and renal failure (Stanley, Blair, & Beare, 2005). In addition, the incidence of systemic diseases, such as atherosclerosis, hypertension, heart failure, diabetes, and cancer, increases with advancing age, predisposing older adults to renal disease associated with these disorders. Therefore, acute problems need to be prevented if possible or recognized and treated quickly to avoid kidney damage, and nurses in all settings need to be alert for signs and symptoms of renal dysfunction in elderly patients.

Elderly patients frequently take multiple prescription and over-the-counter medications. Because alterations in renal blood flow, glomerular filtration, and renal clearance increase the risk for medication-associated changes in renal function, precautions are indicated with all medications. When elderly patients undergo extensive diagnostic tests or when new medications (eg, diuretic agents) are added, precautions must be taken to prevent dehydration, which can compromise marginal renal function and lead to renal failure.

With aging, the kidney is less able to respond to acute fluid and electrolyte changes. Elderly patients may develop atypical and nonspecific signs and symptoms of disturbed renal function and fluid and electrolyte imbalances. Recognition of these problems is further hampered by their association with preexisting disorders and the misconception that they are normal changes of aging.

Primary Glomerular Diseases

A variety of diseases, including acute and chronic glomerulonephritis, rapidly progressive glomerulonephritis, and nephrotic syndrome, can affect the glomerular capillaries. In these disorders, the glomerular capillaries are primarily involved. Antigen–antibody complexes form in the blood and become trapped in the glomerular capillaries (the filtering portion of the kidney), inducing an inflammatory response. Immunoglobulin G (IgG), the major immunoglobulin (antibody) found in the blood, can be detected in the glomerular capillary walls. The major clinical manifestations of glomerular injury include proteinuria, hematuria, decreased GFR, and alterations in excretion of sodium (leading to edema and hypertension).

Acute Glomerulonephritis

Glomerulonephritis is an inflammation of the glomerular capillaries. Acute glomerulonephritis is more common in children older than 2 years of age, but it can occur at nearly any age.

Pathophysiology

Primary glomerulonephritis and primary glomerular diseases are disorders in which the glomerulus is the predominant or sole tissue involved (Mulzahn & Butera, 2006). Examples of primary diseases are postinfectious glomerulonephritis, rapidly progressive glomerulonephritis, membrane proliferative glomerulonephritis, and membranous glomerulonephritis. Postinfectious causes are group A beta-hemolytic streptococcal infection of the throat that precedes the onset of glomerulonephritis by 2 to 3 weeks (Fig. 44-1). It may also follow impetigo (infection of the skin) and acute viral infections (upper respiratory tract infections, mumps, varicella zoster virus, Epstein-Barr virus, hepatitis B, and human immunodeficiency virus [HIV] infection). In some patients, antigens outside the body (eg, medications, foreign serum) initiate the process, resulting in antigen–antibody complexes being deposited in the glomeruli. In other patients, the kidney tissue itself serves as the inciting antigen.

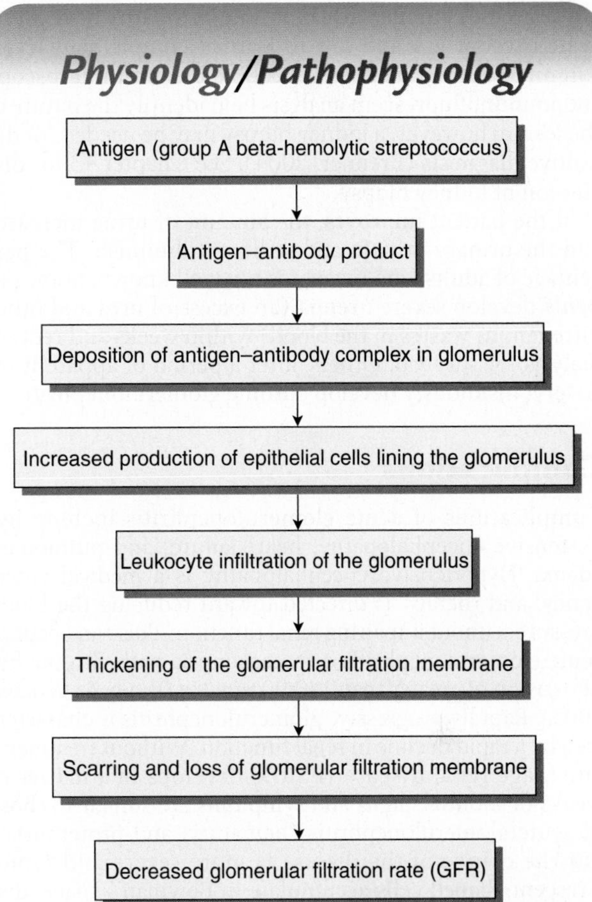

FIGURE 44-1. Sequence of events in acute glomerulonephritis.

Clinical Manifestations

The primary presenting features of acute glomerulonephritis are hematuria, edema, **azotemia** (concentration of urea and other nitrogenous wastes in the blood), and proteinuria (<3.0 g of proteinuria per day) (Hricik, Miller & Sedor, 2003). The hematuria may be microscopic (identifiable only through microscopic examination) or macroscopic (visible to the eye). The urine may appear cola-colored because of red blood cells (RBCs) and protein plugs or casts; RBC casts indicate glomerular injury. Glomerulonephritis may be mild and the hematuria discovered incidentally through a routine microscopic urinalysis, or the disease may be severe, with acute renal failure (ARF) and oliguria.

Some degree of edema and hypertension is present in most patients. Marked proteinuria due to the increased permeability of the glomerular membrane may also occur, with associated pitting edema, hypoalbuminemia, hyperlipidemia, and fatty casts in the urine. Blood urea nitrogen (BUN) and serum creatinine levels may increase as urine output decreases. In addition, anemia may be present.

In the more severe form of the disease, patients also complain of headache, malaise, and flank pain. Elderly patients may experience circulatory overload with dyspnea, engorged neck veins, cardiomegaly, and pulmonary edema. Atypical symptoms include confusion, somnolence, and seizures, which are often confused with the symptoms of a primary neurologic disorder.

Assessment and Diagnostic Findings

In acute glomerulonephritis, the kidneys become large, edematous, and congested. All renal tissues including the glomeruli, tubules, and blood vessels are affected to varying degrees. Patients with an IgA nephropathy have an elevated serum IgA and low to normal complement levels (Brenner, 2004; Hricik et al., 2003). Electron microscopy and immunofluorescent analysis help identify the nature of the lesion; however, a kidney biopsy may be needed for definitive diagnosis (Brenner, 2004). See Chapter 43 for discussion of kidney biopsy.

If the patient improves, the amount of urine increases and the urinary protein and sediment diminish. The percentage of adults who recover is not well known. Some patients develop severe **uremia** (an excess of urea and other nitrogenous wastes in the blood) within weeks and require dialysis for survival. Others, after a period of apparent recovery, insidiously develop chronic glomerulonephritis.

Complications

Complications of acute glomerulonephritis include hypertensive encephalopathy, heart failure, and pulmonary edema. Hypertensive encephalopathy is a medical emergency, and therapy is directed toward reducing the blood pressure without impairing renal function. This can occur in acute glomerulonephritis or preeclampsia with chronic hypertension of greater than 140/90 mm Hg (Brady & Wilcox, 2003). Rapidly progressive glomerulonephritis is characterized by a rapid decline in renal function. Without treatment, **end-stage renal disease (ESRD)** develops in a matter of weeks or months. Signs and symptoms are similar to those of acute glomerulonephritis (hematuria and proteinuria), but the course of the disease is more severe and rapid. Crescent-shaped cells accumulate in Bowman's space, disrupting the filtering surface. Plasma exchange (plasmapheresis) and treatment with high-dose corticosteroids and cytotoxic agents have been used to reduce the inflammatory response. Dialysis is initiated in acute glomerulonephritis if signs and symptoms of uremia are severe. The prognosis for patients with acute glomerulonephritis is favorable and approximately 60% recover completely (Porth, 2005).

Medical Management

Management consists primarily of treating symptoms, attempting to preserve kidney function, and treating complications promptly. Pharmacologic therapy depends on the cause of acute glomerulonephritis. If residual streptococcal infection is suspected, penicillin is the agent of choice; however, other antibiotic agents may be prescribed. Corticosteroids and immunosuppressant medications may be prescribed for patients with rapidly progressive acute glomerulonephritis.

Dietary protein is restricted when renal insufficiency and nitrogen retention (elevated BUN) develop. Sodium is restricted when the patient has hypertension, edema, and heart failure. Loop diuretic and antihypertensive medications may be prescribed to control hypertension. Prolonged bed rest has little value and does not alter long-term outcomes.

Nursing Management

Although most patients with acute uncomplicated glomerulonephritis are cared for as outpatients, nursing care is important in every setting. In a hospital setting, carbohydrates are given liberally to provide energy and reduce the catabolism of protein (Morton, Fontaine, Hudak, et al., 2005). Intake and output are carefully measured and recorded. Fluids are given according to the patient's fluid losses and daily body weight. Insensible fluid loss through the lungs (300 mL) and skin (600 mL) is considered when estimating fluid loss (see Table 14-2). Diuresis begins about 1 week after the onset of symptoms with a decrease in edema and blood pressure. Proteinuria and microscopic hematuria may persist for many months, and some patients may develop chronic glomerulonephritis (Brenner, 2004). Other nursing interventions focus on patient education about the disease process, explanations of laboratory and other diagnostic tests, and preparation for safe and effective self-care at home.

Promoting Home and Community-Based Care

TEACHING PATIENTS SELF-CARE

Patient education is directed toward symptom management and monitoring for complications. Fluid and diet restrictions must be reviewed with the patient to avoid worsening of edema and hypertension. The patient is instructed to notify the physician if symptoms of renal failure occur (eg, fatigue, nausea, vomiting, diminishing urine output) or at the first sign of any infection. Information is given verbally and in writing.

CONTINUING CARE

The importance of follow-up evaluations of blood pressure, urinalysis for protein, and BUN and serum creatinine levels to determine if the disease has progressed is stressed to the patient. A referral for home care may be indicated; a visit from a home care nurse provides an opportunity for careful assessment of the patient's progress and detection of early signs and symptoms of renal insufficiency. If corticosteroids, immunosuppressant agents, or antibiotic medications are prescribed, the home care nurse or nurse in the outpatient setting uses the opportunity to review the dosage, desired actions, and adverse effects of medications and the precautions to be taken.

Chronic Glomerulonephritis

Pathophysiology

Chronic glomerulonephritis may be due to repeated episodes of acute glomerulonephritis, hypertensive **nephrosclerosis** (hardening of the renal arteries), hyperlipidemia, chronic tubulointerstitial injury, or hemodynamically mediated glomerular sclerosis (Porth, 2005). Secondary glomerular diseases that can have systemic effects include lupus erythematosus, Goodpasture's syndrome (caused by antibodies to the glomerular basement membrane), diabetic glomerulosclerosis, and amyloidosis. The kidneys are reduced to as little as one-fifth their normal size (consisting largely of fibrous tissue). The cortex layer shrinks to 1 to 2 mm in thickness or less. Bands of scar tissue distort the remaining cortex, making the surface of the kidney rough and irregular. Numerous glomeruli and their tubules become scarred, and the branches of the renal artery are thickened. The result is severe glomerular damage that can result in ESRD.

Clinical Manifestations

The symptoms of chronic glomerulonephritis vary. Some patients with severe disease have no symptoms at all for many years. Their condition may be discovered when hypertension or elevated BUN and serum creatinine levels are detected. The diagnosis may be suggested during a routine eye examination when vascular changes or retinal hemorrhages are found. The first indication of disease may be a sudden, severe nosebleed, a stroke, or a seizure. Many patients report that their feet are slightly swollen at night. Most patients also have general symptoms, such as loss of weight and strength, increasing irritability, and an increased need to urinate at night (nocturia). Headaches, dizziness, and digestive disturbances are common.

As chronic glomerulonephritis progresses, signs and symptoms of chronic kidney disease and chronic renal failure may develop. The patient appears poorly nourished, with a yellow-gray pigmentation of the skin and periorbital and peripheral (dependent) edema. Blood pressure may be normal or severely elevated. Retinal findings include hemorrhage, exudate, narrowed tortuous arterioles, and papilledema. Mucous membranes are pale because of anemia. Cardiomegaly, a gallop rhythm, distended neck veins, and other signs and symptoms of heart failure may be present (Bickley & Szilagyi, 2003). Crackles can be heard in the lungs.

Peripheral neuropathy with diminished deep tendon reflexes and neurosensory changes occur late in the disease. The patient becomes confused and demonstrates a limited attention span. An additional late finding includes evidence of pericarditis with a pericardial friction rub and pulsus paradoxus (difference in blood pressure during inspiration and expiration of greater than 10 mm Hg).

Assessment and Diagnostic Findings

A number of laboratory abnormalities occur. Urinalysis reveals a fixed specific gravity of about 1.010, variable proteinuria, and **urinary casts** (proteins secreted by damaged kidney tubules). As renal failure progresses and the GFR falls below 50 mL/min, the following changes occur:

- Hyperkalemia due to decreased potassium excretion, acidosis, catabolism, and excessive potassium intake from food and medications
- Metabolic acidosis from decreased acid secretion by the kidney and inability to regenerate bicarbonate
- Anemia secondary to decreased erythropoiesis (production of RBCs)
- Hypoalbuminemia with edema secondary to protein loss through the damaged glomerular membrane
- Increased serum phosphorus level due to decreased renal excretion of phosphorus
- Decreased serum calcium level (calcium binds to phosphorus to compensate for elevated serum phosphorus levels)
- Mental status changes
- Impaired nerve conduction due to electrolyte abnormalities and uremia

Chest x-rays may show cardiac enlargement and pulmonary edema. The electrocardiogram (ECG) may be normal or may indicate left ventricular hypertrophy associated with hypertension and signs of electrolyte disturbances, such as tall, tented (or peaked) T waves associated with hyperkalemia. Computed tomography (CT) and magnetic resonance imaging (MRI) scans show a decrease in the size of the renal cortex.

Medical Management

Symptom management guides the course of treatment for the patient with chronic glomerulonephritis. If the patient has hypertension, efforts are made to reduce the blood pressure with sodium and water restriction, antihypertensive agents, or both. Weight is monitored daily, and diuretic medications are prescribed to treat fluid overload. Proteins of high biologic value (dairy products, eggs, meats) are provided to promote good nutritional status. Adequate calories are also important to spare protein for tissue growth and repair. Urinary tract infections (UTIs) must be treated promptly to prevent further renal damage.

Initiation of dialysis is considered early in the course of the disease to keep the patient in optimal physical condition, prevent fluid and electrolyte imbalances, and minimize the risk of complications of renal failure. The course of dialysis is smoother if treatment begins before the patient develops complications.

Nursing Management

Whether the patient is hospitalized or cared for in the home, the nurse observes the patient for common fluid and electrolyte disturbances in renal disease (see Table 44-1). Changes in fluid and electrolyte status and in cardiac and neurologic status are reported promptly to the physician. Anxiety levels are often extremely high for both the patient and family. Throughout the course of the disease and treatment, the nurse gives emotional support by providing opportunities for the patient and family to verbalize their concerns, have their questions answered, and explore their options.

Promoting Home and Community-Based Care

TEACHING PATIENTS SELF-CARE

The nurse has a major role in teaching the patient and family about the prescribed treatment plan and the risks associated with noncompliance. Instructions to the patient include explanations and scheduling for follow-up evaluations: blood pressure, urinalysis for protein and casts, and laboratory studies of BUN and serum creatinine levels. If long-term dialysis is needed, the patient and family are taught about the procedure, how to care for the access site, dietary restrictions, and other necessary lifestyle modifications. These topics are discussed later in this chapter.

Periodic hospitalization, visits to the outpatient clinic or office, and home care referrals provide the nurse in each setting with the opportunity for careful assessment of the patient's progress and continued education about changes to report to the primary health care provider (worsening signs and symptoms of renal failure, such as nausea, vomiting, and diminished urine output). Specific teaching may include explanations about recommended diet and fluid modifications and medications (purpose, desired effects, adverse effects, dosage, and administration schedule).

CONTINUING CARE

Periodic laboratory evaluations of creatinine clearance and BUN and serum creatinine levels are carried out to assess residual renal function and the need for dialysis or transplantation. If dialysis is initiated, the patient and family require considerable assistance and support in dealing with therapy and its long-term implications. The patient and family are reminded of the importance of participation in health promotion activities, including health screening. The patient is instructed to inform all health care providers about the diagnosis of glomerulonephritis so that all medical management, including pharmacologic therapy, is based on altered renal function.

Nephrotic Syndrome

Nephrotic syndrome is not a specific glomerular disease but a cluster of clinical findings, including:

- Marked increase in protein (particularly albumin) in the urine (proteinuria)
- Decrease in albumin in the blood (hypoalbuminemia)
- Edema
- High serum cholesterol and low-density lipoproteins (hyperlipidemia)

The syndrome is apparent in any condition that seriously damages the glomerular capillary membrane and results in increased glomerular permeability to plasma proteins (Porth, 2005). Although the liver is capable of increasing the production of albumin, it cannot keep up with the daily loss of albumin through the kidneys. Thus, hypoalbuminemia results (Fig. 44-2).

Pathophysiology

Nephrotic syndrome can occur with almost any intrinsic renal disease or systemic disease that affects the glomerulus. Although generally considered a disorder of childhood, nephrotic syndrome also occurs in adults, including the elderly. Causes include chronic glomerulonephritis, diabetes mellitus with intercapillary glomerulosclerosis, amyloidosis of the kidney, systemic lupus erythematosus, multiple myeloma, and renal vein thrombosis.

Clinical Manifestations

The major manifestation of nephrotic syndrome is edema (Brenner, 2004). It is usually soft, pitting, and commonly occurs around the eyes (periorbital), in dependent areas

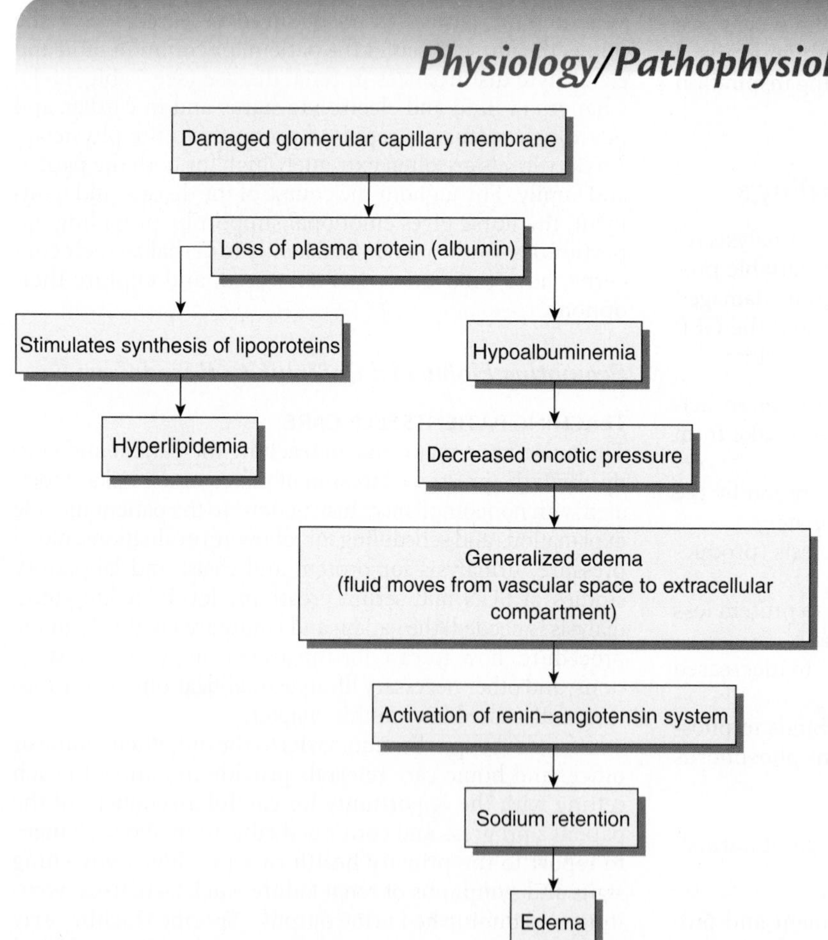

FIGURE 44-2. Sequence of events in nephrotic syndrome.

(sacrum, ankles, and hands), and in the abdomen (ascites). Patients may also exhibit irritability, headache, and malaise.

Assessment and Diagnostic Findings

Proteinuria (predominately albumin) exceeding 3.5 g/day is the hallmark of the diagnosis of nephrotic syndrome (Brenner, 2004). Protein electrophoresis and immunoelectrophoresis may be performed on the urine to categorize the type of proteinuria. The urine may also contain increased white blood cells (WBCs) as well as granular and epithelial casts. A needle biopsy of the kidney may be performed for histologic examination of renal tissue to confirm the diagnosis. Recent studies have confirmed the usefulness of serum markers as a means of assessing the disease process. Anti-C1q antibodies are the most reliable markers for assessing disease activity in lupus nephritis (Weening, D'Ageti, Schwartz, et al., 2004).

Complications

Complications of nephrotic syndrome include infection (due to a deficient immune response), thromboembolism (especially of the renal vein), pulmonary emboli, ARF (due to hypovolemia), and accelerated atherosclerosis (due to hyperlipidemia).

Medical Management

The objective of management is to preserve renal function and prevent complications. Diuretics may be prescribed for the patient with severe edema; however, caution must be used because of the risk of reducing the plasma volume to the point of impaired circulation with subsequent prerenal ARF. The use of angiotensin-converting enzyme (ACE) inhibitors in combination with loop diuretics often reduces the degree of proteinuria but may take 4 to 6 weeks to be effective. Problems of drug resistance also arise with long-term use of diuretics (Brady & Wilcox, 2003).

Other medications used in treating nephrotic syndrome include antineoplastic agents (cyclophosphamide [Cytoxan]) or immunosuppressant medications (azathioprine [Imuran], chlorambucil [Leukeran], or cyclosporine [Neoral]). It may be necessary to repeat treatment with corticosteroids if relapse occurs. Treatment of the associated hyperlipidemia is controversial. The usual medications used to treat hyperlipidemia are often ineffective or have serious consequences, including muscle injury.

The patient who does not have hyperkalemia may be placed on a low-sodium diet containing liberal amounts of potassium. This type of diet enhances the sodium–potassium pump mechanism and assists in elimination of sodium to reduce edema. Dietary restrictions of protein and cholesterol help lower lipidemia (Brady & Wilcox, 2003).

Nursing Management

In the early stages of nephrotic syndrome, nursing management is similar to that of the patient with acute glomerulonephritis, but as the condition worsens, management is similar to that of the patient with chronic renal failure (see the following section). The patient who is receiving corticosteroids or cyclosporine requires instructions about the medications and signs and symptoms that should be reported to the physician. Dietary instructions may also be necessary.

Patients with nephrotic syndrome need adequate instruction about the importance of following all medication and dietary regimens so that their condition can remain stable as long as possible. Patients must be made aware of the importance of communicating any health-related change to their health care providers as soon as possible so that appropriate medication and dietary changes can be made before further changes occur within the glomeruli. When indications of an acute infection, such as an acute respiratory tract infection, are first apparent, increased maintenance doses of corticosteroids have been found to decrease the risk of relapse.

Nephrosclerosis

Nephrosclerosis in the renal arteries is most often due to prolonged hypertension and diabetes, both of which can cause decreased blood flow to the kidney and patchy necrosis of the renal parenchyma (Brenner, 2004). Over time, fibrosis occurs and glomeruli are destroyed. Nephrosclerosis is a major cause of ESRD secondary to many disorders.

Pathophysiology

There are two forms of nephrosclerosis: malignant (accelerated) and benign. Malignant nephrosclerosis is often associated with malignant hypertension (diastolic blood pressure higher than 130 mm Hg). It usually occurs in young adults, and men are affected twice as often as women. The disease process progresses rapidly. Without dialysis, more than half of patients die from uremia in a few years. Benign nephrosclerosis is usually found in older adults and is often associated with atherosclerosis and hypertension.

Assessment and Diagnostic Findings

Symptoms are rare early in the disease, even though the urine usually contains protein and occasional casts. Renal insufficiency and associated signs and symptoms occur late in the disease.

Medical Management

Treatment of nephrosclerosis is aggressive antihypertensive therapy. In hypertensive nephrosclerosis, therapy containing an ACE inhibitor, alone or in combination with other antihypertensive medications, significantly reduces the incidence.

Renal Failure

Renal failure results when the kidneys cannot remove the body's metabolic wastes or perform their regulatory functions. The substances normally eliminated in the urine accumulate in the body fluids as a result of impaired renal excretion, leading to a disruption in endocrine and metabolic functions as well as fluid, electrolyte, and acid–base disturbances. Renal failure is a systemic disease and is a final common pathway of many different kidney and urinary tract diseases. Each year, the number of deaths from irreversible renal failure increases (U.S. Renal Data System, 2004).

Acute Renal Failure

Pathophysiology

Acute renal failure (ARF) is a reversible clinical syndrome where there is a sudden and almost complete loss of kidney function (decreased GFR) over a period of hours to days with failure to excrete nitrogenous waste products and to maintain fluid and electrolyte homeostasis (Porth, 2005). Although ARF is often thought of as a problem seen only in hospitalized patients, it may occur in the outpatient setting as well. ARF manifests as an increase in serum creatinine and BUN. Urine volume may be normal, or changes may occur. Possible changes include oliguria (less than 400 mL/day), nonoliguria (greater than 400 mL/day), or **anuria** (less than 50 mL/day) (Porth, 2005).

Although the exact pathogenesis of ARF and oliguria is not always known, many times there is a specific underlying problem. Some of the factors may be reversible if identified and treated promptly, before kidney function is impaired. This is true of the following conditions that reduce blood flow to the kidney and impair kidney function: (1) hypovolemia; (2) hypotension; (3) reduced cardiac output and heart failure; (4) obstruction of the kidney or lower urinary tract by tumor, blood clot, or kidney stone; and (5) bilateral obstruction of the renal arteries or veins. If these conditions are treated and corrected before the kidneys are permanently damaged, the increased BUN and creatinine levels, oliguria, and other signs associated with ARF may be reversed.

Although renal stones are not a common cause of ARF, some types may increase the risk for ARF. Some hereditary stone diseases (see Chapter 45), primary struvite stones, and infection-related urolithiasis associated with anatomic and functional urinary tract anomalies and spinal cord injury may cause recurrent bouts of obstruction as well as crystal-specific damage to tubular epithelial cells and interstitial renal cells (Brenner, 2004).

Categories of Acute Renal Failure

The major categories of ARF are prerenal (hypoperfusion of kidney), intrarenal (actual damage to kidney tissue), and postrenal (obstruction to urine flow). Common causes of each type of ARF are summarized in Chart 44-1.

- Prerenal ARF, which occurs in 60% to 70% of cases, is the result of impaired blood flow that leads to hypoperfusion of the kidney and a decrease in the GFR. Common clinical situations are volume-depletion states (hemorrhage or gastrointestinal [GI] losses), impaired cardiac performance (myocardial infarction, heart failure, or cardiogenic shock), and vasodilation (sepsis or anaphylaxis).
- Intrarenal ARF is the result of actual parenchymal damage to the glomeruli or kidney tubules. Nephrotoxic agents, such as aminoglycosides and radiocontrast agents, account for 30% of cases of **acute tubular necrosis** (ATN), and ischemia due to decreased renal perfusion accounts for more than 50% of cases of ATN. Characteristics of ATN are intratubular obstruction, tubular back leak (abnormal reabsorption of filtrate and decreased urine

CHART 44-1

Causes of Acute Renal Failure

PRERENAL FAILURE

- Volume depletion resulting from:
  - Hemorrhage
  - Renal losses (diuretics, osmotic diuresis)
  - Gastrointestinal losses (vomiting, diarrhea, nasogastric suction)
- Impaired cardiac efficiency resulting from:
  - Myocardial infarction
  - Heart failure
  - Dysrhythmias
  - Cardiogenic shock
- Vasodilation resulting from:
  - Sepsis
  - Anaphylaxis
  - Antihypertensive medications or other medications that cause vasodilation

INTRARENAL FAILURE

- Prolonged renal ischemia resulting from:
  - Pigment nephropathy (associated with the breakdown of blood cells containing pigments that in turn occlude kidney structures)
  - Myoglobinuria (trauma, crush injuries, burns)
  - Hemoglobinuria (transfusion reaction, hemolytic anemia)
- Nephrotoxic agents such as:
  - Aminoglycoside antibiotics (gentamicin, tobramycin)
  - Radiopaque contrast agents
  - Heavy metals (lead, mercury)
  - Solvents and chemicals (ethylene glycol, carbon tetrachloride, arsenic)
  - Nonsteroidal anti-inflammatory drugs (NSAIDs)
  - Angiotensin-converting enzyme inhibitors (ACE inhibitors)
- Infectious processes such as:
  - Acute pyelonephritis
  - Acute glomerulonephritis

POSTRENAL FAILURE

- Urinary tract obstruction, including:
  - Calculi (stones)
  - Tumors
  - Benign prostatic hyperplasia
  - Strictures
  - Blood clots

flow through the tubule), vasoconstriction, and changes in glomerular permeability (Hricik et al., 2003). These processes result in a decrease of GFR, progressive azotemia, and impaired fluid and electrolyte balance. Conditions such as burns, crush injuries, infections, and severe blood transfusion reactions can lead to intrarenal ARF and ultimately ATN. With burns and crush injuries, myoglobin (a protein released from muscle when injury occurs) and hemoglobin are liberated, causing obstruction, renal toxicity, and ischemia. Severe transfusion reactions may also cause intrarenal failure; hemoglobin is released through hemolysis, filters through the glomeruli, and becomes concentrated in the kidney tubules to such a degree that precipitation of hemoglobin occurs. Certain medications, especially nonsteroidal anti-inflammatory drugs (NSAIDs) and ACE inhibitors, may also predispose a patient to intrarenal damage. These medications interfere with the normal autoregulatory mechanisms of the kidney and may cause hypoperfusion and eventual ischemia.

- Postrenal ARF is usually the result of an obstruction somewhere distal to the kidney. Pressure rises in the kidney tubules and eventually, the GFR decreases.

Phases of Acute Renal Failure

There are four clinical phases of ARF: initiation, oliguria, diuresis, and recovery.

- The initiation period begins with the initial insult and ends when oliguria develops.
- The oliguria period is accompanied by an increase in the serum concentration of substances usually excreted by the kidneys (urea, creatinine, uric acid, organic acids, and the intracellular cations [potassium and magnesium]). The minimum amount of urine needed to rid the body of normal metabolic waste products is 400 mL. In this phase uremic symptoms first appear and life-threatening conditions such as hyperkalemia develop.

  Some patients have decreased renal function with increasing nitrogen retention, yet actually excrete normal amounts of urine (2 L/day or more). This is the nonoliguric form of renal failure and occurs predominantly after exposure of the patient to nephrotoxic agents; it may also occur with burns, traumatic injury, and the use of halogenated anesthetic agents.
- The diuresis period is marked by a gradual increase in urine output, which signals that glomerular filtration has started to recover. Laboratory values stop increasing and eventually decrease. Although the volume of urinary output may reach normal or elevated levels, renal function may still be markedly abnormal. Because uremic symptoms may still be present, the need for expert medical and nursing management continues. The patient must be observed closely for dehydration during this phase; if dehydration occurs, the uremic symptoms are likely to increase.
- The recovery period signals the improvement of renal function and may take 3 to 12 months. Laboratory values return to the patient's normal level. Although a permanent 1% to 3% reduction in the GFR is common, it is not clinically significant.

Clinical Manifestations

Almost every system of the body is affected when there is failure of the normal renal regulatory mechanisms. The patient may appear critically ill and lethargic. The skin and mucous membranes are dry from dehydration. Central nervous system signs and symptoms include drowsiness, headache, muscle twitching, and seizures. Table 44-2 summarizes common clinical findings in all three categories of ARF.

Assessment and Diagnostic Findings

Assessment of the patient with ARF includes evaluation for changes in the urine, diagnostic tests that evaluate the kidney contour, and a variety of laboratory values. See Chapter 43 for information about the normal characteristics of urine, diagnostic findings, and laboratory values in the renal system.

In ARF, urine output varies (scanty to normal volume), hematuria may be present, and the urine has a low specific gravity (compared with a normal value of 1.003 to 1.030). One of the earliest manifestations of tubular damage is the inability to concentrate the urine (Porth, 2005). Patients

TABLE 44-2 Comparing Categories of Acute Renal Failure

	Categories		
Characteristics	***Prerenal***	***Intrarenal***	***Postrenal***
Etiology	Hypoperfusion	Parenchymal damage	Obstruction
Blood urea nitrogen value	Increased (out of normal 20:1 proportion to creatinine)	Increased	Increased
Creatinine	Increased	Increased	Increased
Urine output	Decreased	Varies, often decreased	Varies, may be decreased, or sudden anuria
Urine sodium	Decreased to <20 mEq/L	Increased to >40 mEq/L	Varies, often decreased to 20 mEq/L or less
Urinary sediment	Normal, few hyaline casts	Abnormal casts and debris	Usually normal
Urine osmolality	Increased to 500 mOsm	About 350 mOsm similar to serum	Varies, increased or equal to serum
Urine specific gravity	Increased	Low normal	Varies

with prerenal azotemia have a decreased amount of sodium in the urine (less than 20 mEq/L) and normal urinary sediment. Patients with intrarenal azotemia usually have urinary sodium levels greater than 40 mEq/L with urinary casts and other cellular debris.

Ultrasonography is a critical component of the evaluation of patients with renal failure. A renal sonogram or a CT or MRI scan may show evidence of anatomical changes (Brenner, 2004).

The BUN level increases steadily at a rate dependent on the degree of catabolism (breakdown of protein), renal perfusion, and protein intake. Serum creatinine increases in conjunction with glomerular damage. Serum creatinine levels are useful in monitoring kidney function and disease progression.

With a decline in the GFR, the patient cannot excrete potassium normally. Patients with oliguria and anuria are at high risk for hyperkalemia. Protein catabolism results in the release of cellular potassium into the body fluids, causing severe hyperkalemia (high serum potassium levels). Hyperkalemia may lead to dysrhythmias, such as ventricular tachycardia and cardiac arrest. Sources of potassium include normal tissue catabolism, dietary intake, blood in the GI tract, or blood transfusion and other sources (eg, intravenous [IV] infusions, potassium penicillin, and extracellular shift in response to metabolic acidosis).

Progressive metabolic acidosis also accompanies renal failure because patients cannot eliminate the daily metabolic load of acid-type substances produced by the normal metabolic processes. In addition, normal renal buffering mechanisms fail. This is reflected by a decrease in the serum CO_2-combining power and blood pH.

There may be an increase in blood phosphate concentrations; calcium levels may be low in response to decreased absorption of calcium from the intestine and as a compensatory mechanism for the elevated blood phosphate levels. Anemia is another common laboratory finding in ARF, as a result of reduced erythropoietin production, uremic GI lesions, reduced RBC life span, and blood loss, usually from the GI tract.

CHART 44-2

Preventing Acute Renal Failure

1. Provide adequate hydration to patients at risk of dehydration:
   Surgical patients before, during, and after surgery
   Patients undergoing intensive diagnostic studies requiring fluid restriction and contrast agents (eg, barium enema, intravenous pyelograms), especially elderly patients who may have marginal renal reserve
   Patients with neoplastic disorders or disorders of metabolism (eg, gout) and those receiving chemotherapy
2. Prevent and treat shock promptly with blood and fluid replacement.
3. Monitor central venous and arterial pressures and hourly urine output of critically ill patients to detect the onset of renal failure as early as possible.
4. Treat hypotension promptly.
5. Continually assess renal function (urine output, laboratory values) when appropriate.
6. Take precautions to ensure that the appropriate blood is administered to the correct patient in order to avoid severe transfusion reactions, which can precipitate renal failure.
7. Prevent and treat infections promptly. Infections can produce progressive renal damage.
8. Pay special attention to wounds, burns, and other precursors of sepsis.
9. To prevent infections from ascending in the urinary tract, give meticulous care to patients with indwelling catheters. Remove catheters as soon as possible.
10. To prevent toxic drug effects, closely monitor dosage, duration of use, and blood levels of all medications metabolized or excreted by the kidneys.

Prevention

Management of ARF is expensive and complex, and even when optimal, the mortality rate can be as high as 60% to 80%, depending on etiology and comorbidities (Porth, 2005). Therefore, prevention of ARF is essential (Chart 44-2).

A careful history is obtained to determine whether the patient has been taking potentially nephrotoxic antibiotic agents or has been exposed to environmental toxins. The kidneys are especially susceptible to the adverse effects of medications because the kidneys are repeatedly exposed to substances in the blood. Patients taking potentially nephrotoxic medications (eg, aminoglycosides, gentamicin, tobramycin, colistimethate, polymyxin B, amphotericin B, vancomycin, amikacin, cyclosporine) should be monitored closely for changes in renal function. BUN and serum creatinine levels should be obtained at baseline within 24 hours after initiation of these medications and at least twice a week while the patient is receiving them.

Any agent that reduces renal blood flow (eg, long-term analgesic use) may cause renal insufficiency. Chronic use of analgesics, particularly NSAIDs, may cause **interstitial nephritis** (inflammation within the renal tissue) and papillary necrosis. Patients with heart failure or cirrhosis with ascites are at particular risk for NSAID-induced renal failure. Increased age, preexisting renal disease, and the administration of several nephrotoxic agents simultaneously increase the risk for kidney damage.

Radiocontrast-induced nephropathy is a major cause of hospital-acquired ARF (Brady & Wilcox, 2003). This is a potentially preventable condition if patients are identified as at risk before a procedure for which the radiocontrast is to be administered. Baseline levels of creatinine greater than 2 mg/dL identify the patient as being high risk. Preprocedure hydration and prescription of acetylcysteine (Mucomyst) the day prior to the test is effective in prevention. The action of acetylcysteine is not fully understood, but it is thought to be an antioxidant that works by scavenging free radicals (Brenner & Myer, 2003).

Medical Management

The kidneys have a remarkable ability to recover from insult. The objectives of treatment of ARF are to restore normal chemical balance and prevent complications until repair of renal tissue and restoration of renal function can occur. Management includes maintaining fluid balance, avoiding fluid excesses, or possibly performing dialysis. The underlying cause is identified, treated, and eliminated when possible (Singri, Ahya, & Levin, 2003). Prerenal azotemia is treated by optimizing renal perfusion, whereas postrenal failure is treated by relieving the obstruction. Intrarenal azotemia is treated with supportive therapy, with removal of causative agents, aggressive management of prerenal and postrenal failure, and avoidance of associated risk factors. Shock and infection, if present, are treated promptly (see Chapter 15).

Maintenance of fluid balance is based on daily body weight, serial measurements of central venous pressure, serum and urine concentrations, fluid losses, blood pressure, and the clinical status of the patient. The parenteral and oral intake and the output of urine, gastric drainage, stools, wound drainage, and perspiration are calculated and are used as the basis for fluid replacement. The insensible fluid produced through the normal metabolic processes and lost through the skin and lungs is also considered in fluid management.

Fluid excesses can be detected by the clinical findings of dyspnea, tachycardia, and distended neck veins. The patient's lungs are auscultated for moist crackles. Because pulmonary edema may be caused by excessive administration of parenteral fluids, extreme caution must be used to prevent fluid overload. The development of generalized edema is assessed by examining the presacral and pretibial areas several times daily. Mannitol (Osmitrol), furosemide (Lasix), or ethacrynic acid (Edecrin) may be prescribed to initiate diuresis and prevent complications.

Adequate blood flow to the kidneys in patients with prerenal causes of ARF may be restored by IV fluids or transfusions of blood products. If ARF is caused by hypovolemia secondary to hypoproteinemia, an infusion of albumin may be prescribed. Dialysis may be initiated to prevent serious complications of ARF, such as hyperkalemia, severe metabolic acidosis, pericarditis, and pulmonary edema. Dialysis corrects many biochemical abnormalities; allows for liberalization of fluid, protein, and sodium intake; diminishes bleeding tendencies; and may help wound healing. **Hemodialysis** (a procedure that circulates the patient's blood through a dialyzer to remove waste products and excess fluid), **peritoneal dialysis** (a procedure that uses the patient's peritoneal membrane [the lining of the peritoneal cavity] as the semipermeable membrane to exchange fluid and solutes), or a variety of **continuous renal replacement therapies (CRRTs)** (methods used to replace normal kidney function by circulating the patient's blood through a hemofilter) may be performed. These forms of dialysis and other treatment modalities for patients with renal dysfunction are discussed later in this chapter.

Pharmacologic Therapy

Hyperkalemia is the most life-threatening of the fluid and electrolyte changes that occur in patients with renal disturbances (Morton et al., 2005). Therefore, the patient is monitored for hyperkalemia through serial serum electrolyte levels (potassium value more than 5.5 mEq/L [5.5 mmol/L]), ECG changes (tall, tented, or peaked T waves), and changes in clinical status.

The elevated potassium levels may be reduced by administering cation-exchange resins (sodium polystyrene sulfonate [Kayexalate]) orally or by retention enema. Kayexalate works by exchanging sodium ions for potassium ions in the intestinal tract. Sorbitol may be administered in combination with Kayexalate to induce a diarrhea-type effect (it induces water loss in the GI tract). If a Kayexalate retention enema is administered (the colon is the major site of potassium exchange), a rectal catheter with a balloon may be used to facilitate retention if necessary. The patient should retain the Kayexalate for 30 to 45 minutes to promote potassium removal. Afterward, a cleansing enema may be prescribed to remove remaining medication as a precaution against fecal impaction.

If the patient is hemodynamically unstable (low blood pressure, changes in mental status, dysrhythmia), IV dextrose 50%, insulin, and calcium replacement may be administered to shift potassium back into the cells. Albuterol sulfate (Ventolin HFA) by nebulizer can lower plasma potassium concentration by 0.5 to 1.5 mEq/L (Schrier, 2005).

Many medications are eliminated through the kidneys; therefore, medication dosages must be reduced when a patient has ARF. Examples of commonly used agents that require adjustment are antibiotic medications (especially aminoglycosides), digoxin, ACE inhibitors, and magnesium-containing agents.

In addition, many medications have been used in patients with ARF in an attempt to improve patient outcomes. Diuretic agents are often used to control fluid volume, but they have not been shown to hasten the recovery from ARF.

In patients with severe acidosis, the arterial blood gases and serum bicarbonate levels (CO_2-combining power) must be monitored because the patient may require sodium bicarbonate therapy or dialysis. If respiratory problems develop, appropriate ventilatory measures must be instituted. The elevated serum phosphate level may be controlled with phosphate-binding agents (aluminum hydroxide). These agents help prevent a continuing rise in serum phosphate levels by decreasing the absorption of phosphate from the intestinal tract.

Nutritional Therapy

ARF causes severe nutritional imbalances (because nausea and vomiting contribute to inadequate dietary intake), impaired glucose use and protein synthesis, and increased tissue catabolism. The patient is weighed daily and can be expected to lose 0.2 to 0.5 kg (0.5 to 1 lb) daily if the nitrogen balance is negative (ie, caloric intake falls below caloric requirements). If the patient gains or does not lose weight or develops hypertension, fluid retention should be suspected.

The patient's nutritional support is based on the underlying cause of ARF, the catabolic response, the type and frequency of renal replacement therapy, comorbidities, and nutritional status. Dietary proteins are individualized to provide the maximum benefit (Morton et al., 2005). Caloric requirements are met with high-carbohydrate meals, because carbohydrates have a protein-sparing effect (ie, in a high-carbohydrate diet, protein is not used for meeting energy requirements but is "spared" for growth and tissue healing). Foods and fluids containing potassium or phosphorus (eg, bananas, citrus fruits and juices, coffee) are restricted. Potassium intake may be restricted, and the patient may require parenteral nutrition.

The oliguric phase of ARF may last 10 to 20 days and is followed by the diuretic phase, at which time urine output begins to increase, signaling that kidney function is returning. Results of blood chemistry tests are used to determine the amounts of sodium, potassium, and water needed for replacement, along with assessment for overhydration or underhydration. Following the diuretic phase, the patient is placed on a high-protein, high-calorie diet and is encouraged to resume activities gradually.

Nursing Management

The nurse has an important role in caring for the patient with ARF. The nurse monitors for complications, participates in emergency treatment of fluid and electrolyte imbalances, assesses the patient's progress and response to treatment, and provides physical and emotional support. Additionally, the nurse keeps family members informed about the patient's condition, helps them understand the treatments, and provides psychological support. Although the development of ARF may be the most serious problem, the nurse must continue to include in the plan of care those nursing measures indicated for the primary disorder (eg, burns, shock, trauma, obstruction of the urinary tract).

Monitoring Fluid and Electrolyte Balance

Because of the serious fluid and electrolyte imbalances that can occur with ARF, the nurse monitors the patient's serum electrolyte levels and physical indicators of these complications during all phases of the disorder. Hyperkalemia is the most immediate life-threatening imbalance seen in ARF. Parenteral fluids, all oral intake, and all medications are screened carefully to ensure that hidden sources of potassium are not inadvertently administered or consumed. IV solutions must be carefully selected according to the patient's fluid and electrolyte status. The patient's cardiac function and musculoskeletal status are monitored closely for signs of hyperkalemia.

The nurse monitors fluid status by paying careful attention to fluid intake (IV medications should be administered in the smallest volume possible), urine output, apparent edema, distention of the jugular veins, alterations in heart sounds and breath sounds, and increasing difficulty in breathing. Accurate daily weights, as well as intake and output records, are essential.

Indicators of deteriorating fluid and electrolyte status are reported immediately to the physician, and preparation is made for emergency treatment. Hyperkalemia is treated with dextrose 50%, insulin, calcium gluconate, sodium polystyrene sulfonate (Kayexalate), or dialysis (Morton et al., 2005). Fluid and other electrolyte disturbances are often treated with hemodialysis, peritoneal dialysis, or other CRRTs.

Reducing Metabolic Rate

The nurse also attends to reducing the patient's metabolic rate. Bed rest may be indicated to reduce exertion and the metabolic rate during the most acute stage of the disorder. Fever and infection, both of which increase the metabolic rate and catabolism, are prevented or treated promptly.

Promoting Pulmonary Function

Attention is given to pulmonary function, and the patient is assisted to turn, cough, and take deep breaths frequently to prevent atelectasis and respiratory tract infection. Drowsiness and lethargy may prevent the patient from moving and turning without encouragement and assistance.

Preventing Infection

Asepsis is essential with invasive lines and catheters to minimize the risk of infection and increased metabolism. An indwelling urinary catheter is avoided whenever possible because of the high risk of UTI associated with its use.

Providing Skin Care

The skin may be dry or susceptible to breakdown as a result of edema; therefore, meticulous skin care is important. Additionally, excoriation and itching of the skin may result from the deposit of irritating toxins in the patient's tissues. Turning the patient frequently, bathing him or her with cool water, and keeping the skin clean and well moisturized and the fingernails trimmed to avoid excoriation are often comforting and prevent skin breakdown (Morton et al., 2005).

Providing Support

The patient with ARF may require treatment with hemodialysis, peritoneal dialysis, or CRRT to prevent serious complications. The length of time that these treatments are necessary varies with the cause and extent of damage to the kidneys. The patient and family need assistance, explanation, and support during this period. The purpose and rationale of the treatments are explained to the patient and family by the physician. However, high levels of anxiety and fear may necessitate repeated explanation and clarification by the nurse. The family members may initially be afraid to touch and talk to the patient during these procedures but should be encouraged and assisted to do so.

In an intensive care setting, many of the nurse's functions are devoted to the technical aspects of patient care; however, it is essential that the psychological needs and other concerns of the patient and family be addressed.

Continued assessment of the patient for complications of ARF and precipitating causes is essential.

Gerontologic Considerations

The incidence of ARF is increasing in older, hospitalized patients. About half of all patients who develop ARF during hospitalization for a medical or surgical problem are older than 60 years. Evidence also demonstrates that ARF is often seen in the community setting. Nurses in the ambulatory setting need to be aware of the risk of ARF in elderly patients, especially those undergoing diagnostic testing or procedures that can result in dehydration. The mortality rate is slightly higher for ARF in elderly patients than for their younger counterparts.

The etiology of ARF in older adults includes prerenal causes, such as dehydration, intrarenal causes such as nephrotoxic agents (eg, medications, contrast agents), and complications of major surgery (Brenner, 2004). Diabetes mellitus increases the risk for contrast agent-induced renal failure because of preexisting renal insufficiency and the imposed fluid restriction needed for many tests. Suppression of thirst, enforced bed rest, lack of access to drinking water, and confusion all contribute to the older patient's failure to consume adequate fluids, and this may lead to dehydration and compromise of already decreased renal function.

Chronic Renal Failure (End-Stage Renal Disease)

Chronic renal failure, or ESRD, is a progressive, irreversible deterioration in renal function in which the body's ability to maintain metabolic and fluid and electrolyte balance fails, resulting in uremia or azotemia. The incidence of ESRD has increased by almost 8% per year for the past 5 years. In the United States, more than 280,000 patients with chronic renal failure (65%) are receiving hemodialysis; more than 120,000 (28%) have functioning renal transplants, and more than 24,000 (7%) are receiving peritoneal dialysis (United States Renal Data System [USRDS], 2004).

Conditions that cause ESRD include systemic diseases, such as diabetes mellitus (leading cause); hypertension; chronic glomerulonephritis; **pyelonephritis** (inflammation of the renal pelvis); obstruction of the urinary tract; hereditary lesions, as in polycystic kidney disease; vascular disorders; infections; medications; or toxic agents. Comorbid conditions that develop during chronic renal insufficiency contribute to the high morbidity and mortality among patients with ESRD (Burrows-Hudson, 2005).

Environmental and occupational agents that have been implicated in chronic renal failure include lead, cadmium, mercury, and chromium. Dialysis or kidney transplantation eventually becomes necessary for patient survival. Dialysis is an effective means of correcting metabolic toxicities at any age.

Pathophysiology

As renal function declines, the end products of protein metabolism (which are normally excreted in urine) accumulate in the blood. Uremia develops and adversely affects every system in the body. The greater the buildup of waste products, the more severe the symptoms (Chart 44-3).

The rate of decline in renal function and progression of chronic renal failure is related to the underlying disorder, the urinary excretion of protein, and the presence of hypertension. The disease tends to progress more rapidly in patients who excrete significant amounts of protein or have elevated blood pressure than in those without these conditions.

Clinical Manifestations

Because virtually every body system is affected by the uremia of chronic renal failure, patients exhibit a number of signs and symptoms. The severity of these signs and symptoms depends in part on the degree of renal impairment, other underlying conditions, and the patient's age.

- **Cardiovascular manifestations.** Hypertension (due to sodium and water retention or from activation of the renin–angiotensin–aldosterone system), heart failure and pulmonary edema (due to fluid overload), and pericarditis (due to irritation of the pericardial lining by uremic toxins) are among the cardiovascular problems manifested in ESRD. Cardiovascular disease is the predominant cause of death in patients with ESRD. In patients receiving chronic hemodialysis, approximately 45% of overall mortality is attributable to cardiac disease, and about 20% of these cardiac deaths are due to acute myocardial infarction (USRDS, 2004).

CHART 44-3

Stages of Chronic Kidney Disease

Stages are based on the glomerular filtration rate (GFR). The normal GFR is 125 mL/min/1.73 m^2.

STAGE 1
GFR ≥ 90 mL/min/1.73 m^2
Kidney damage with normal or increased GFR

STAGE 2
GFR = 60–89 mL/min/1.73 m^2
Mild decrease in GFR

STAGE 3
GFR = 30–59 mL/min/1.73 m^2
Moderate decrease in GFR

STAGE 4
GFR = 15–29 mL/min/1.73 m^2
Severe decrease in GFR

STAGE 5
GFR <15 mL/min/1.73 m^2
Kidney failure

Adapted from Levy, J., Morgan, J. & Brown, E. (2004). *Oxford handbook of dialysis* (2nd ed.). Oxford University Press.

- **Dermatologic manifestations.** Severe pruritus (itching) is common. Uremic frost, the deposit of urea crystals on the skin, is uncommon today because of early and aggressive treatment of ESRD with dialysis.
- **Gastrointestinal manifestations.** GI signs and symptoms are common and include anorexia, nausea, vomiting, and hiccups. The patient's breath may have the odor of urine (uremic fetor); this may be associated with inadequate dialysis.
- **Neurologic manifestations.** Neurologic changes, including altered level of consciousness, inability to concentrate, muscle twitching, agitation, confusion, and seizures, have been observed. Peripheral neuropathy, a disorder of the peripheral nervous system, is present in some patients. Patients complain of severe pain and discomfort (Parker, 2006). Restless leg syndrome and burning feet can occur in the early stage of uremic peripheral neuropathy (Brenner, 2004).

The precise mechanisms for many of these diverse signs and symptoms have not been identified. However, it is generally thought that the accumulation of uremic waste products is the probable cause. Chart 44-4 summarizes the signs and symptoms often seen in chronic renal failure.

Assessment and Diagnostic Findings

Glomerular Filtration Rate

The GFR is the amount of plasma filtered through the glomeruli per unit of time. Creatinine clearance is measured by obtaining a 24-hour urine, obtaining a serum cre-

CHART 44-4

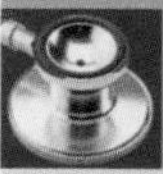

Assessing for Signs and Symptoms of Chronic Renal Failure

NEUROLOGIC
- Weakness and fatigue
- Confusion
- Inability to concentrate
- Disorientation
- Tremors
- Seizures
- Asterixis
- Restlessness of legs
- Burning of soles of feet
- Behavior changes

INTEGUMENTARY
- Gray-bronze skin color
- Dry, flaky skin
- Pruritus
- Ecchymosis
- Purpura
- Thin, brittle nails
- Coarse, thinning hair

CARDIOVASCULAR
- Hypertension
- Pitting edema (feet, hands, sacrum)
- Periorbital edema
- Pericardial friction rub
- Engorged neck veins
- Pericarditis
- Pericardial effusion
- Pericardial tamponade
- Hyperkalemia
- Hyperlipidemia

PULMONARY
- Crackles
- Thick, tenacious sputum
- Depressed cough reflex
- Pleuritic pain
- Shortness of breath
- Tachypnea
- Kussmaul-type respirations
- Uremic pneumonitis

GASTROINTESTINAL
- Ammonia odor to breath ("uremic fetor")
- Metallic taste
- Mouth ulcerations and bleeding
- Anorexia, nausea, and vomiting
- Hiccups
- Constipation or diarrhea
- Bleeding from gastrointestinal tract

HEMATOLOGIC
- Anemia
- Thrombocytopenia

REPRODUCTIVE
- Amenorrhea
- Testicular atrophy
- Infertility
- Decreased libido

MUSCULOSKELETAL
- Muscle cramps
- Loss of muscle strength
- Renal osteodystrophy
- Bone pain
- Bone fractures
- Foot drop

atinine, and using a formula to estimate the amount of creatinine the kidneys are able to clear in a 24-hour period (Goshorn, 2005). Normal values differ in men and women. Calculation of GFR is discussed in Chapter 43, and the stages of chronic kidney disease based on GFR can be found in Chart 44-3.

As glomerular filtration decreases (due to nonfunctioning glomeruli), the creatinine clearance value decreases, whereas the serum creatinine and BUN levels increase. Serum creatinine is the more sensitive indicator of renal function because of its constant production in the body. The BUN is affected not only by renal disease but also by protein intake in the diet, catabolism (tissue and RBC breakdown), parenteral nutrition, and medications such as corticosteroids.

Sodium and Water Retention

The kidney cannot concentrate or dilute the urine normally in ESRD. Appropriate responses by the kidney to changes in the daily intake of water and electrolytes, therefore, do not occur. Some patients retain sodium and water, increasing the risk for edema, heart failure, and hypertension. Hypertension may also result from activation of the renin–angiotensin–aldosterone axis and the concomitant increased aldosterone secretion. Other patients have a tendency to lose sodium and run the risk of developing hypotension and hypovolemia. Episodes of vomiting and diarrhea may cause sodium and water depletion, which worsens the uremic state.

Acidosis

In advanced renal disease, metabolic acidosis occurs because the kidneys are unable to excrete increased loads of acid. Decreased acid secretion results from the inability of the kidney tubules to excrete ammonia (NH_3^-) and to reabsorb sodium bicarbonate (HCO_3^-). There is also decreased excretion of phosphates and other organic acids.

Anemia

Anemia develops as a result of inadequate erythropoietin production, the shortened life span of RBCs, nutritional deficiencies, and the patient's tendency to bleed, particularly from the GI tract. Erythropoietin, a substance normally produced by the kidneys, stimulates bone marrow to produce RBCs. In renal failure, erythropoietin production decreases and profound anemia results, producing fatigue, angina, and shortness of breath.

Calcium and Phosphorus Imbalance

Another major abnormality seen in chronic renal failure is a disorder in calcium and phosphorus metabolism. Serum calcium and phosphate levels have a reciprocal relationship in the body: as one increases, the other decreases. With a decrease in filtration through the glomerulus of the kidney, there is an increase in the serum phosphate level and a reciprocal or corresponding decrease in the serum calcium level. The decreased serum calcium level causes increased secretion of parathormone from the parathyroid glands. However, in renal failure, the body does not respond normally to the increased secretion of parathormone; as a result, calcium leaves the bone, often producing bone changes and bone disease as well as calcification of major blood vessels in the body. In addition, the active metabolite of vitamin D (1,25-dihydroxycholecalciferol) normally manufactured by the kidney decreases as renal failure progresses. Uremic bone disease, often called renal osteodystrophy, develops from the complex changes in calcium, phosphate, and parathormone balance. There is also evidence of calcification of blood vessels (Schrier, 2005).

Complications

Potential complications of chronic renal failure that concern the nurse and necessitate a collaborative approach to care include the following:

- Hyperkalemia due to decreased excretion, metabolic acidosis, catabolism, and excessive intake (diet, medications, fluids)
- Pericarditis, pericardial effusion, and pericardial tamponade due to retention of uremic waste products and inadequate dialysis
- Hypertension due to sodium and water retention and malfunction of the renin–angiotensin–aldosterone system
- Anemia due to decreased erythropoietin production, decreased RBC life span, bleeding in the GI tract from irritating toxins and ulcer formation, and blood loss during hemodialysis
- Bone disease and metastatic and vascular calcifications due to retention of phosphorus, low serum calcium levels, abnormal vitamin D metabolism, and elevated aluminum levels

Medical Management

The goal of management is to maintain kidney function and homeostasis for as long as possible. All factors that contribute to ESRD and all factors that are reversible (eg, obstruction) are identified and treated. Management is accomplished primarily with medications and diet therapy, although dialysis may also be needed to decrease the level of uremic waste products in the blood and to control electrolyte balance.

Pharmacologic Therapy

Complications can be prevented or delayed by administering prescribed phosphate-binding agents, calcium supplements, antihypertensive and cardiac medications, antiseizure medications, and erythropoietin (Epogen).

CALCIUM AND PHOSPHORUS BINDERS

Hyperphosphatemia and hypocalcemia are treated with medications that bind dietary phosphorus in the GI tract. Binders such as calcium carbonate (Os-Cal), or calcium acetate (PhosLo) are prescribed, but there is a risk of hypercalcemia. If calcium is high or the calcium–phosphorus product exceeds 55 mg/dL, a polymeric phosphate binder such as sevelamer hydrochloride (Renagel) may be used (Zonderman & Doyle, 2006). These medications bind dietary phosphorus in the intestinal tract. All binding agents must be administered with food to be effective. Magnesium-based antacids are avoided to prevent magnesium toxicity.

ANTIHYPERTENSIVE AND CARDIOVASCULAR AGENTS

Hypertension is managed by intravascular volume control and a variety of antihypertensive agents. Heart failure and pulmonary edema may also require treatment with fluid restriction, low-sodium diets, diuretic agents, inotropic agents such as digoxin (Lanoxin) or dobutamine (Dobutrex), and dialysis. The metabolic acidosis of chronic renal failure usually produces no symptoms and requires no treatment; however, sodium bicarbonate supplements or dialysis may be needed to correct the acidosis if it causes symptoms (Molzahn & Butera, 2006).

ANTISEIZURE AGENTS

Neurologic abnormalities may occur, so the patient must be observed for early evidence of slight twitching, headache, delirium, or seizure activity. If seizures occur, the onset of the seizure is recorded along with the type, duration, and general effect on the patient. The physician is notified immediately. IV diazepam (Valium) or phenytoin (Dilantin) is usually administered to control seizures. The side rails of the bed should be raised and padded to protect the patient. The nursing management of the patient with seizures is discussed in Chapter 61.

ERYTHROPOIETIN

Anemia associated with chronic renal failure is treated with recombinant human erythropoietin (Epogen). Patients with anemia (hematocrit less than 30%) present with nonspecific symptoms, such as malaise, general fatigability, and decreased activity tolerance. Erythropoietin therapy is initiated to achieve a hematocrit of 33% to 38% and a target hemoglobin of 12 g/dL, which generally alleviates the symptoms of anemia.

Erythropoietin is administered intravenously or subcutaneously three times a week in ESRD. It may take 2 to 6 weeks for the hematocrit to increase; therefore, the medication is not indicated for patients who need immediate correction of severe anemia. Adverse effects seen with erythropoietin therapy include hypertension (especially during early stages of treatment), increased clotting of vascular access sites, seizures, and depletion of body iron stores (Zonderman & Doyle, 2006). Patients may experience influenza-like symptoms with initiation of therapy; these tend to subside with repeated doses.

Management involves adjustment of heparin to prevent clotting of the lines during hemodialysis treatments, frequent monitoring of hemoglobin and hematocrit, and periodic assessment of serum iron and transferrin levels. Because adequate stores of iron are necessary for an adequate response to erythropoietin, supplementary iron may be prescribed. Common iron supplements include iron sucrose (Venofer) and ferric gluconate (Ferrlecit). In addition, the patient's blood pressure and serum potassium level are monitored to detect hypertension and increasing serum potassium levels, which may occur with therapy and the increasing RBC mass. The occurrence of hypertension requires initiation or adjustment of the patient's antihypertensive therapy. Hypertension that cannot be controlled is a contraindication to recombinant erythropoietin therapy.

Patients who have received erythropoietin therapy have reported decreased levels of fatigue, increased feelings of well-being, better tolerance of dialysis, higher energy levels, and improved exercise tolerance. Additionally, this therapy has decreased the need for transfusion and its associated risks, including bloodborne infectious disease, antibody formation, and iron overload.

Nutritional Therapy

Dietary intervention is necessary with deterioration of renal function and includes careful regulation of protein intake, fluid intake to balance fluid losses, sodium intake to balance sodium losses, and some restriction of potassium. At the same time, adequate caloric intake and vitamin supplementation must be ensured. Protein is restricted because urea, uric acid, and organic acids—the breakdown products of dietary and tissue proteins—accumulate rapidly in the blood when there is impaired renal clearance. The allowed protein must be of high biologic value (dairy products, eggs, meats). High-biologic-value proteins are those that are complete proteins and supply the essential amino acids necessary for growth and cell repair.

Usually, the fluid allowance per day is 500 mL to 600 mL more than the previous day's 24-hour urine output. Calories are supplied by carbohydrates and fat to prevent wasting. Vitamin supplementation is necessary because a protein-restricted diet does not provide the necessary complement of vitamins. Additionally, the patient on dialysis may lose water-soluble vitamins during the dialysis treatment.

Hyperkalemia is usually prevented by ensuring adequate dialysis treatments with potassium removal and careful monitoring of diet, medications, and fluids for their potassium content. Sodium polystyrene sulfonate (Kayexalate), a cation-exchange resin, may be needed for acute hyperkalemia.

Dialysis

The patient with increasing symptoms of chronic renal failure is referred to a dialysis and transplantation center early in the course of progressive renal disease. Dialysis is usually initiated when the patient cannot maintain a reasonable lifestyle with conservative treatment.

Nursing Management

The patient with chronic renal failure requires astute nursing care to avoid the complications of reduced renal function and the stresses and anxieties of dealing with a life-threatening illness. Examples of potential nursing diagnoses for these patients include the following:

- Excess fluid volume related to decreased urine output, dietary excesses, and retention of sodium and water
- Imbalanced nutrition: less than body requirements related to anorexia, nausea and vomiting, dietary restrictions, and altered oral mucous membranes
- Deficient knowledge regarding condition and treatment regimen
- Activity intolerance related to fatigue, anemia, retention of waste products, and dialysis procedure
- Risk for situational low self-esteem related to dependency, role changes, changes in body image, and sexual dysfunction

Nursing care is directed toward assessing fluid status and identifying potential sources of imbalance, implementing a dietary program to ensure proper nutritional intake within the limits of the treatment regimen, and promoting positive feelings by encouraging increased self-care and greater independence. It is extremely important to provide explanations and information to the patient and family concerning ESRD, treatment options, and potential complications. A great deal of emotional support is needed by the patient and family because of the numerous changes experienced. Specific interventions, along with rationale and evaluation criteria, are presented in more detail in the plan of nursing care for the patient with chronic renal failure (Chart 44-5).

Promoting Home and Community-Based Care

TEACHING PATIENTS SELF-CARE

The nurse plays an important role in teaching the patient with ESRD. Because of the extensive teaching needed, the home care nurse, dialysis nurse, and nurses in the hospital and outpatient settings all provide ongoing education and reinforcement while monitoring the patient's progress and compliance with the treatment regimen.

A nutritional referral and explanations of nutritional needs are helpful because of the numerous dietary changes required. The patient is taught how to check the vascular access device for patency and appropriate precautions, such as avoiding venipuncture and blood pressure measurements on the arm with the access device.

Additionally, the patient and family need to know what problems to report to the health care provider. These include the following:

- Worsening signs and symptoms of renal failure (nausea, vomiting, change in usual urine output [if any], ammonia odor on breath)
- Signs and symptoms of hyperkalemia (muscle weakness, diarrhea, abdominal cramps)
- Signs and symptoms of access problems (clotted fistula or graft, infection)

These signs and symptoms of decreasing renal function, in addition to increasing BUN and serum creatinine levels, may indicate a need to alter the dialysis prescription. The dialysis nurses also provide ongoing education and support at each treatment visit.

CONTINUING CARE

The importance of follow-up examinations and treatment is stressed to the patient and family because of changing physical status, renal function, and dialysis requirements. Referral for home care provides the home care nurse with the opportunity to assess the patient's environment, emotional status, and the coping strategies used by the patient and family to deal with the changes in family roles often associated with chronic illness.

The home care nurse also assesses the patient for further deterioration of renal function and signs and symptoms of complications resulting from the primary renal disorder, the resulting renal failure, and effects of treatment strategies (eg, dialysis, medications, dietary restrictions). Many patients need ongoing education and reinforcement on the multiple dietary restrictions required, including fluid, sodium, potassium, and protein restriction. Reminders about the need for health promotion activities and health screening are an important part of nursing care for the patient with renal failure.

Gerontologic Considerations

Historically, the age of patients developing ESRD has increased steadily each year, but since 2001, it appears to have stabilized at approximately 65 years (USRDS, 2004). In the past, rapidly progressive glomerulonephritis, membranous glomerulonephritis, and nephrosclerosis were the most common causes of chronic renal failure in the elderly. Today, however, long-standing diabetes, hypertension, and chronic glomerulonephritis are the leading causes of chronic renal failure in this population (Brenner, 2004). Other common causes of chronic renal failure in the elderly population are interstitial nephritis and urinary tract obstruction. The signs and symptoms of renal disease in the elderly are commonly nonspecific. The occurrence of symptoms of other disorders (heart failure, dementia) can mask the symptoms of renal disease and delay or prevent diagnosis and treatment. Patients often develop signs and symptoms of nephrotic syndrome, such as edema and proteinuria.

Hemodialysis and peritoneal dialysis have been used effectively in treating elderly patients (Levy, Morgan & Brown, 2004). Although there is no specific age limitation for renal transplantation, concomitant disorders (eg, coronary artery disease, peripheral vascular disease) have made it a less common treatment for the elderly. However, the outcome is comparable to that of younger patients. Some elderly patients elect not to undergo dialysis or transplantation. Conservative management, including nutritional therapy, fluid control, and medications such as phosphate binders, may be considered in patients who are not suitable for or elect not to have dialysis or transplantation.

Dialysis

Dialysis is used to remove fluid and uremic waste products from the body when the kidneys are unable to do so. It may also be used to treat patients with edema that does not respond to other treatment, hepatic coma, hyperkalemia, hypercalcemia, hypertension, and uremia. Methods of therapy include hemodialysis, CRRT, and peritoneal dialysis. The need for dialysis may be acute or chronic.

Acute dialysis is indicated when there is a high and increasing level of serum potassium, fluid overload, or impending pulmonary edema, increasing acidosis, pericarditis, and severe confusion. It may also be used to remove certain medications or other toxins (poisoning or medication overdose) from the blood.

Chronic or maintenance dialysis is indicated in ESRD in the following instances: the presence of uremic signs and symptoms affecting all body systems (nausea and vomiting, severe anorexia, increasing lethargy, mental confusion), hyperkalemia, fluid overload not responsive to diuretics and fluid restriction, and a general lack of well-being. An urgent indication for dialysis in patients with chronic renal failure is pericardial friction rub.

(text continues on page 1537)

CHART 44-5

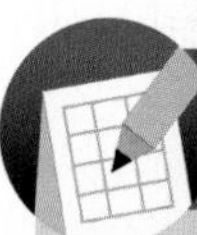

Plan of Nursing Care — The Patient With Chronic Renal Failure

Nursing Diagnosis: Excess fluid volume related to decreased urine output, dietary excesses, and retention of sodium and water
Goal: Maintenance of ideal body weight without excess fluid

NURSING INTERVENTIONS	RATIONALE	EXPECTED OUTCOMES
1. Assess fluid status: a. Daily weight b. Intake and output balance c. Skin turgor and presence of edema d. Distention of neck veins e. Blood pressure, pulse rate, and rhythm f. Respiratory rate and effort	1. Assessment provides baseline and ongoing database for monitoring changes and evaluating interventions.	• Demonstrates no rapid weight changes • Maintains dietary and fluid restrictions • Exhibits normal skin turgor without edema • Exhibits normal vital signs • Exhibits no neck vein distention • Reports no difficulty breathing or shortness of breath • Performs oral hygiene frequently • Reports decreased thirst • Reports decreased dryness of oral mucous membranes
2. Limit fluid intake to prescribed volume.	2. Fluid restriction will be determined on basis of weight, urine output, and response to therapy.	
3. Identify potential sources of fluid: a. Medications and fluids used to take or administer medications: oral and intravenous b. Foods	3. Unrecognized sources of excess fluids may be identified.	
4. Explain to patient and family rationale for fluid restriction.	4. Understanding promotes patient and family cooperation with fluid restriction.	
5. Assist patient to cope with the discomforts resulting from fluid restriction.	5. Increasing patient comfort promotes compliance with dietary restrictions.	
6. Provide or encourage frequent oral hygiene.	6. Oral hygiene minimizes dryness of oral mucous membranes.	

Nursing Diagnosis: Imbalanced nutrition; less than body requirements related to anorexia, nausea, vomiting, dietary restrictions, and altered oral mucous membranes
Goal: Maintenance of adequate nutritional intake

NURSING INTERVENTIONS	RATIONALE	EXPECTED OUTCOMES
1. Assess nutritional status: a. Weight changes b. Laboratory values (serum electrolyte, BUN, creatinine, protein, transferrin, and iron levels)	1. Baseline data allow for monitoring of changes and evaluating effectiveness of interventions.	• Consumes protein of high biologic value • Chooses foods within dietary restrictions that are appealing • Consumes high-calorie foods within dietary restrictions • Explains in own words rationale for dietary restrictions and relationship to urea and creatinine levels
2. Assess patient's nutritional dietary patterns: a. Diet history b. Food preferences c. Calorie counts	2. Past and present dietary patterns are considered in planning meals.	

Plan of Nursing Care — The Patient With Chronic Renal Failure (Continued)

NURSING INTERVENTIONS	RATIONALE	EXPECTED OUTCOMES
3. Assess for factors contributing to altered nutritional intake: a. Anorexia, nausea, or vomiting b. Diet unpalatable to patient c. Depression d. Lack of understanding of dietary restrictions e. Stomatitis	3. Information about other factors that may be altered or eliminated to promote adequate dietary intake is provided.	• Takes medications on schedule that does not produce anorexia or feeling of fullness • Consults written lists of acceptable foods • Reports increased appetite at meals • Exhibits no rapid increases or decreases in weight • Demonstrates normal skin turgor without edema; wound healing and acceptable plasma albumin levels
4. Provide patient's food preferences within dietary restrictions.	4. Increased dietary intake is encouraged.	
5. Promote intake of high biologic value protein foods: eggs, dairy products, meats.	5. Complete proteins are provided for positive nitrogen balance needed for growth and healing.	
6. Encourage high-calorie, low-protein, low-sodium, and low-potassium snacks between meals.	6. Reduces source of restricted foods and proteins and provides calories for energy, sparing protein for tissue growth and healing.	
7. Alter schedule of medications so that they are not given immediately before meals.	7. Ingestion of medications just before meals may produce anorexia and feeling of fullness.	
8. Explain rationale for dietary restrictions and relationship to kidney disease and increased urea and creatinine levels.	8. Promotes patient understanding of relationships between diet and urea and creatinine levels to renal disease.	
9. Provide written lists of foods allowed and suggestions for improving their taste without use of sodium or potassium.	9. Lists provide a positive approach to dietary restrictions and a reference for patient and family to use when at home.	
10. Provide pleasant surroundings at meal-times.	10. Unpleasant factors that contribute to patient's anorexia are eliminated.	
11. Weigh patient daily.	11. Allows monitoring of fluid and nutritional status.	
12. Assess for evidence of inadequate protein intake: a. Edema formation b. Delayed wound healing c. Decreased serum albumin levels	12. Inadequate protein intake can lead to decreased albumin and other proteins, edema formation, and delay in wound healing.	

Nursing Diagnosis: Deficient knowledge regarding condition and treatment
Goal: Increased knowledge about condition and related treatment

NURSING INTERVENTIONS	RATIONALE	EXPECTED OUTCOMES
1. Assess understanding of cause of renal failure, consequences of renal failure, and its treatment: a. Cause of patient's renal failure b. Meaning of renal failure	1. Provides baseline for further explanations and teaching.	• Verbalizes relationship of cause of renal failure to consequences • Explains fluid and dietary restrictions as they relate to failure of kidney's regulatory functions

continued >

CHART 44-5

Plan of Nursing Care — The Patient With Chronic Renal Failure (Continued)

NURSING INTERVENTIONS	RATIONALE	EXPECTED OUTCOMES
c. Understanding of renal function d. Relationship of fluid and dietary restrictions to renal failure e. Rationale for treatment (hemodialysis, peritoneal dialysis, transplantation)		• States in own words relationship of renal failure and need for treatment • Asks questions about treatment options, indicating readiness to learn • Verbalizes plans to continue as normal a life as possible • Uses written information and instructions to clarify questions and seek additional information
2. Provide explanation of renal function and consequences of renal failure at patient's level of understanding and guided by patient's readiness to learn.	2. Patient can learn about renal failure and treatment as he or she becomes ready to understand and accept the diagnosis and consequences.	
3. Assist patient to identify ways to incorporate changes related to illness and its treatment into lifestyle.	3. Patient can see that his or her life does not have to revolve around the disease.	
4. Provide oral and written information as appropriate about: a. Renal function and failure b. Fluid and dietary restrictions c. Medications d. Reportable problems, signs, and symptoms e. Follow-up schedule f. Community resources g. Treatment options	4. Provides patient with information that can be used for further clarification at home.	

Nursing Diagnosis: Activity intolerance related to fatigue, anemia, retention of waste products, and dialysis procedure
Goal: Participation in activity within tolerance

NURSING INTERVENTIONS	RATIONALE	EXPECTED OUTCOMES
1. Assess factors contributing to activity intolerance: a. Fatigue b. Anemia c. Fluid and electrolyte imbalances d. Retention of waste products e. Depression	1. Indicates factors contributing to severity of fatigue.	• Participates in increasing levels of activity and exercise • Reports increased sense of well-being • Alternates rest and activity • Participates in selected self-care activities
2. Promote independence in self-care activities as tolerated; assist if fatigued.	2. Promotes improved self-esteem	
3. Encourage alternating activity with rest.	3. Promotes activity and exercise within limits and adequate rest.	
4. Encourage patient to rest after dialysis treatments.	4. Adequate rest is encouraged after dialysis treatments, which are exhausting to many patients.	

CHART 44-5

Plan of Nursing Care **The Patient With Chronic Renal Failure (Continued)**

Nursing Diagnosis: Risk for situational low self-esteem related to dependency, role changes, change in body image, and change in sexual function
Goal: Improved self-esteem

NURSING INTERVENTIONS	RATIONALE	EXPECTED OUTCOMES
1. Assess patient's and family's responses and reactions to illness and treatment.	1. Provides data about problems encountered by patient and family in coping with changes in life.	• Identifies previously used coping styles that have been effective and those no longer possible due to disease and treatment (alcohol or drug use; extreme physical exertion)
2. Assess relationship of patient and significant family members.	2. Identifies strengths and supports of patient and family.	
3. Assess usual coping patterns of patient and family members.	3. Coping patterns that may have been effective in past may be harmful in view of restrictions imposed by disease and treatment.	• Patient and family identify and verbalize feelings and reactions to disease and necessary changes in their lives • Seeks professional counseling, if necessary, to cope with changes resulting from renal failure
4. Encourage open discussion of concerns about changes produced by disease and treatment: a. Role changes b. Changes in lifestyle c. Changes in occupation d. Sexual changes e. Dependence on health care team	4. Encourages patient to identify concerns and steps necessary to deal with them.	• Reports satisfaction with method of sexual expression
5. Explore alternate ways of sexual expression other than sexual intercourse.	5. Alternative forms of sexual expression may be acceptable.	
6. Discuss role of giving and receiving love, warmth, and affection.	6. Sexuality means different things to different people, depending on stage of maturity.	

Collaborative Problems: Hyperkalemia; pericarditis, pericardial effusion, and pericardial tamponade; hypertension; anemia; bone disease and metastatic calcifications
Goal: Absence of complications

NURSING INTERVENTIONS	RATIONALE	EXPECTED OUTCOMES
Hyperkalemia		
1. Monitor serum potassium levels. Notify physician if level greater than 5.5 mEq/L, and prepare to treat hyperkalemia.	1. Hyperkalemia causes potentially life-threatening changes in the body.	• Patient has normal potassium level • Experiences no muscle weakness or diarrhea.
2. Assess patient for muscle weakness, diarrhea, ECG changes (tall-tented T waves and widened QRS).	2. Cardiovascular signs and symptoms are characteristic of hyperkalemia.	• Exhibits normal ECG pattern • Vital signs are within normal limits
Pericarditis, Pericardial Effusion, and Pericardial Tamponade		
1. Assess patient for fever, chest pain, and a pericardial friction rub (signs of pericarditis) and, if present, notify physician.	1. About 30%–50% of chronic renal failure patients develop pericarditis due to uremia; fever, chest pain, and a pericardial friction rub are classic signs.	• Has strong and equal peripheral pulses • Absence of a paradoxical pulse

continued >

CHART 44-5

Plan of Nursing Care The Patient With Chronic Renal Failure (Continued)

NURSING INTERVENTIONS	RATIONALE	EXPECTED OUTCOMES
2. If patient has pericarditis, assess for the following every 4 hours: a. Paradoxical pulse > 10 mm Hg b. Extreme hypotension c. Weak or absent peripheral pulses d. Altered level of consciousness e. Bulging neck veins	2. Pericardial effusion is a common fatal sequela of pericarditis. Signs of an effusion include a paradoxical pulse (> 10 mm Hg drop in blood pressure during inspiration) and signs of shock due to compression of the heart by a large effusion. Cardiac tamponade exists when the patient is severely compromised hemodynamically.	• Absence of pericardial effusion or tamponade on cardiac ultrasound • Patient has normal heart sounds
3. Prepare patient for cardiac ultrasound to aid in diagnosis of pericardial effusion and cardiac tamponade.	3. Cardiac ultrasound is useful in visualizing pericardial effusions and cardiac tamponade.	
4. If cardiac tamponade develops, prepare patient for emergency pericardiocentesis.	4. Cardiac tamponade is a life-threatening condition, with a high mortality rate. Immediate aspiration of fluid from the pericardial space is essential.	
Hypertension		
1. Monitor and record blood pressure as indicated.	1. Provides objective data for monitoring. Elevated levels may indicate non-adherence to the treatment regimen.	• Blood pressure within normal limits • Reports no headaches, visual problems, or seizures • Edema is absent • Demonstrates compliance with dietary and fluid restrictions
2. Administer antihypertensive medications as prescribed.	2. Antihypertensive medications play a key role in treatment of hypertension associated with chronic renal failure.	
3. Encourage compliance with dietary and fluid restriction therapy.	3. Adherence to diet and fluid restrictions and dialysis schedule prevents excess fluid and sodium accumulation.	
4. Teach patient to report signs of fluid overload, vision changes, headaches, edema, or seizures.	4. These are indications of inadequate control of hypertension and the need to alter therapy.	
Anemia		
1. Monitor RBC count, hemoglobin, and hematocrit levels as indicated.	1. Provides assessment of degree of anemia.	• Patient has a normal skin color without pallor • Exhibits hematology values within acceptable limits • Experiences no bleeding from any site
2. Administer medications as prescribed, including iron and folic acid supplements, Epogen, and multivitamins.	2. RBCs need iron, folic acid, and vitamins to be produced. Epogen stimulates the bone marrow to produce RBC.	
3. Avoid drawing unnecessary blood specimens.	3. Anemia is worsened by drawing numerous specimens.	

CHART 44-5

Plan of Nursing Care The Patient With Chronic Renal Failure (Continued)

NURSING INTERVENTIONS	RATIONALE	EXPECTED OUTCOMES
4. Teach patient to prevent bleeding: avoid vigorous nose blowing and contact sports, and use a soft toothbrush.	4. Bleeding from anywhere in the body worsens anemia.	
5. Administer blood component therapy as indicated.	5. Blood component therapy may be needed if the patient has symptoms.	
Bone Disease and Metastatic Calcifications		
1. Administer the following medications as prescribed: phosphate binders, calcium supplements, vitamin D supplements.	1. Chronic renal failure causes numerous physiologic changes affecting calcium, phosphorus, and vitamin D metabolism.	• Exhibits serum calcium, phosphorus, and aluminum levels within acceptable ranges
2. Monitor serum lab values as indicated (calcium, phosphorus, aluminum levels) and report abnormal findings to physician.	2. Hyperphosphatemia, hypocalcemia, and excess aluminum accumulation are common in chronic renal failure.	• Exhibits no symptoms of hypocalcemia • Has no bone demineralization on bone scan
3. Assist patient with an exercise program.	3. Bone demineralization increases with immobility.	• Discusses importance of maintaining activity level and exercise program

Patients with no renal function can be maintained by dialysis for years; a patient beginning dialysis between 15 and 19 years of age has a greater than 80% chance of a 10-year survival (Levy et al., 2004). Although the costs of dialysis are usually reimbursable, limitations on the patient's ability to work resulting from illness and dialysis usually impose a great financial burden on the patient and family.

The decision to initiate dialysis should be reached only after thoughtful discussion among the patient, family, physician, and others as appropriate. Many potentially life-threatening issues are associated with the need for dialysis. The nurse can assist the patient and family by answering their questions, clarifying the information provided, and supporting their decision. The lifestyle changes that patients requiring hemodialysis eventually need to make are often overwhelming. Sometimes the news that a donor kidney is available for transplantation can be so disruptive to the changes in lifestyle made to accommodate hemodialysis that the patient may stall the process required for transplantation or refuse the kidney when it becomes available, choosing instead to continue with hemodialysis.

Successful kidney transplantation eliminates the need for dialysis. Not only is the quality of life much improved in patients with ESRD who undergo transplantation, but physiologic function is improved as well. Patients who undergo renal transplantation from living donors before dialysis is initiated generally have longer survival of the transplanted kidney than patients who receive transplantation after dialysis treatment is initiated (Danovitch, 2005).

Hemodialysis

Hemodialysis is the most common method of dialysis. More than 280,000 Americans currently receive chronic hemodialysis (USRDS, 2004). Hemodialysis is used for patients who are acutely ill and require short-term dialysis (days to weeks) and for patients with ESRD who require long-term or permanent therapy. A **dialyzer** (also referred to as an artificial kidney) serves as a synthetic semipermeable membrane, replacing the renal glomeruli and tubules as the filter for the impaired kidneys.

For patients with chronic renal failure, hemodialysis prevents death, although it does not cure renal disease and does not compensate for the loss of endocrine or metabolic activities of the kidneys. Treatments usually occur three times a week for 3 to 4 hours per treatment. Patients receive chronic or maintenance dialysis when they require dialysis therapy for survival and control of uremic symptoms. The trend in managing ESRD is to initiate treatment before the signs and symptoms associated with uremia become severe.

The objectives of hemodialysis are to extract toxic nitrogenous substances from the blood and to remove excess water. In hemodialysis, the blood, laden with toxins and nitrogenous wastes, is diverted from the patient to a machine, a dialyzer, where toxins are removed and the blood is returned to the patient.

Diffusion, osmosis, and ultrafiltration are the principles on which hemodialysis is based. The toxins and wastes in the blood are removed by **diffusion**—that is, they move from an area of higher concentration in the blood to an area of lower concentration in the **dialysate**. The dialysate is a solution made up of all the important electrolytes in their ideal extracellular concentrations. The electrolyte level in the patient's blood can be brought under control by properly adjusting the dialysate bath. The semipermeable membrane impedes the diffusion of large molecules, such as RBCs and proteins.

Excess water is removed from the blood by **osmosis**, in which water moves from an area of higher solute concentration (the blood) to an area of lower solute concentration (the dialysate bath). In **ultrafiltration**, water moves under high pressure to an area of lower pressure. This process is much more efficient than osmosis at water removal and is accomplished by applying negative pressure or a suctioning force to the dialysis membrane. Because patients with renal disease usually cannot excrete water, this force is necessary to remove fluid to achieve fluid balance.

The body's buffer system is maintained using a dialysate bath made up of bicarbonate (most common) or acetate, which is metabolized to form bicarbonate. The anticoagulant heparin is administered to keep blood from clotting in the dialysis circuit. Cleansed blood is returned to the body. By the end of the dialysis treatment, many waste products have been removed, the electrolyte balance has been restored to normal, and the buffer system has been replenished.

Dialyzers

Dialyzers are hollow-fiber devices containing thousands of tiny cellophane tubules that act as semipermeable membranes. The blood flows through the tubules while a solution (the dialysate) circulates around the tubules. The exchange of wastes from the blood to the dialysate occurs through the semipermeable membrane of the tubules (Fig. 44-3).

Dialyzers have undergone many technological changes in performance and biocompatibility. Biocompatibility refers to the ability of the dialyzer to accomplish its objectives without causing hypersensitive, allergic, or adverse reactions. Some dialyzers remove middle-weight molecules at a faster rate and ultrafiltrate at higher rates, which is thought to reduce neuropathy of the lower extremities, a complication of long-term hemodialysis. In general, the more efficient the dialyzer, the higher the cost.

Another technological advance is high-flux dialysis, which uses highly permeable membranes that increase the clearance of low- and mid-molecular-weight molecules. These special membranes are used with higher-than-traditional rates of flow for the blood entering and exiting the dialyzer (500 to 550 mL/min). High-flux dialysis requires the use of precise volumetric ultrafiltration control systems, and not every dialysis unit can perform this type of

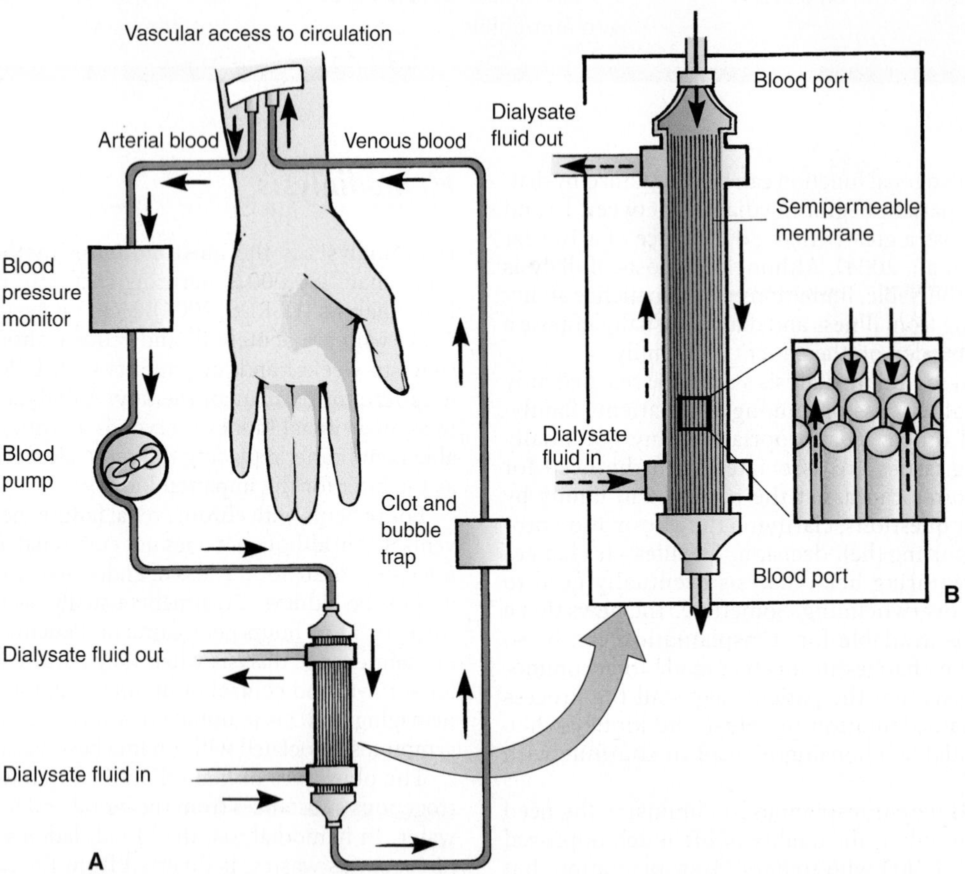

FIGURE 44-3. Hemodialysis system. (**A**) Blood from an artery is pumped into (**B**) a dialyzer where it flows through the cellophane tubes, which act as the semipermeable membrane (*inset*). The dialysate, which has the same chemical composition as the blood except for urea and waste products, flows in around the tubules. The waste products in the blood diffuse through the semipermeable membrane into the dialysate.

dialysis. High-flux dialysis increases the efficiency of treatments while shortening their duration and reducing the need for heparin.

Because of the high cost associated with hemodialysis, dialyzers can be reused in centers in the United States. Strict regulations apply to the reuse of dialyzers. Careful staff training and continuous monitoring of the program are essential (Levy et al., 2004).

Vascular Access

Access to the patient's vascular system must be established to allow blood to be removed, cleansed, and returned to the patient's vascular system at rates between 300 and 550 mL/minute. Several types of access are available.

Vascular Access Devices

Immediate access to the patient's circulation for acute hemodialysis is achieved by inserting a double-lumen large-bore catheter into the subclavian, internal jugular, or femoral vein (Fig. 44-4). This method of vascular access involves some risk (eg, hematoma, pneumothorax, infection, thrombosis of the subclavian vein, inadequate flow) and can be used for no longer than 3 weeks (Levy et al., 2004). The catheter is removed when no longer needed (eg, because the patient's condition has improved or another type of access has been established). Double-lumen, cuffed catheters may also be inserted into the internal jugular vein of patients requiring a central venous catheter for dialysis. These catheters can be used for long-term access.

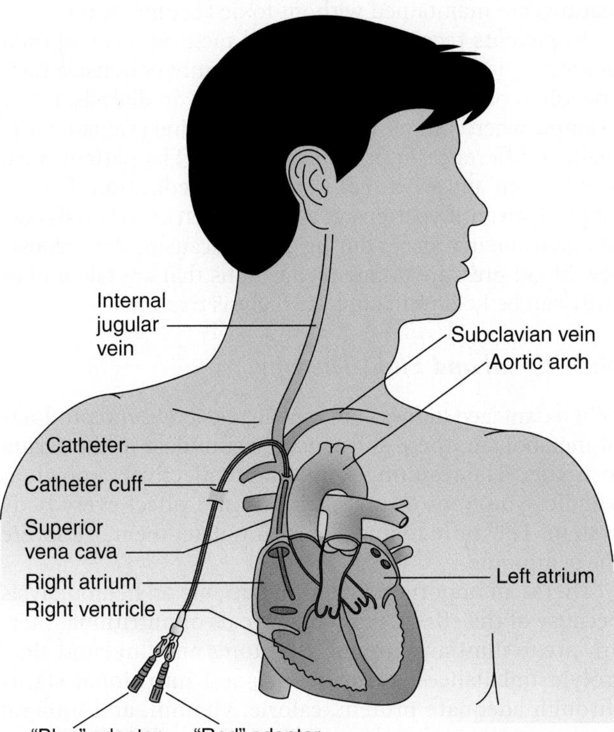

FIGURE 44-4. Double-lumen, cuffed hemodialysis catheter used in acute hemodialysis. The red adapter is attached to a blood line through which blood is pumped from the patient to the dialyzer. After the blood passes through the dialyzer (artificial kidney), it returns to the patient through the blue adapter.

Arteriovenous Fistula

The preferred method of permanent access is an **arteriovenous fistula** that is created surgically (usually in the forearm) by joining (anastomosing) an artery to a vein, either side-to-side or end-to-side (Fig. 44-5). Needles are inserted into the vessel to obtain blood flow adequate to pass through the dialyzer. The arterial segment of the fistula is used for arterial flow to the dialyzer and the venous segment for reinfusion of the dialyzed blood. The fistula should be allowed at least 14 days to mature (Rayner, Pisoni, Gillespie et al., 2003). This gives time for healing and for the venous segment of the fistula to dilate to accommodate two large-bore (14-, 15-, or 16-gauge) needles. The patient is encouraged to perform exercises to increase the size of these vessels (ie, squeezing a rubber ball for forearm fistulas) to accommodate the large-bore needles used in hemodialysis.

Arteriovenous Graft

An **arteriovenous graft** can be created by subcutaneously interposing a biologic, semibiologic, or synthetic graft material between an artery and vein (see Fig. 44-5). The most commonly used synthetic graft material is expanded polytetrafluoroethylene. Other synthetic materials are being used for the creation of these grafts. The Impra Vectra graft, for example, is made of Thoralon (polyetherurethaneurea and siloxane) and can be used in 24 hours. Access can be achieved in 10 days with Artegraft, another material that is a natural collagen vascular graft. Usually, a graft is created when the patient's vessels are not suitable for creation of a fistula. Patients with compromised vascular systems (eg, from diabetes) often need to have a graft to undergo hemodialysis. Grafts are usually placed in the arm but may be placed in the thigh or chest area (Leydig, 2005). Infection and thrombosis are the most common complications of arteriovenous grafts.

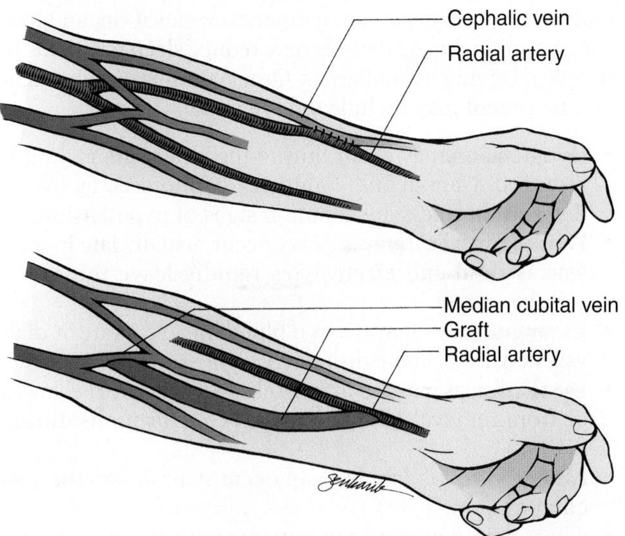

FIGURE 44-5. An internal arteriovenous fistula (*top*) is created by a side-to-side anastomosis of the artery and vein. A graft (*bottom*) can also be established between the artery and vein.

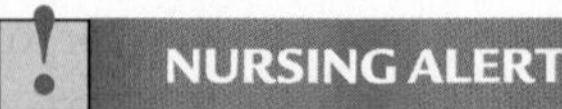

Failure of the permanent dialysis access (fistula or graft) accounts for most hospital admissions of patients undergoing chronic hemodialysis. Thus, protection of the access is of high priority.

Complications

Although hemodialysis can prolong life indefinitely, it does not alter the natural course of the underlying kidney disease, nor does it completely replace kidney function. The patient is subject to a number of problems and complications. A leading cause of death among patients undergoing maintenance hemodialysis is atherosclerotic cardiovascular disease (USRDS, 2004). Disturbances of lipid metabolism (hypertriglyceridemia) appear to be accentuated by hemodialysis. Heart failure, coronary heart disease and anginal pain, stroke, and peripheral vascular insufficiency may occur and may incapacitate the patient (Levy et al., 2004). Anemia and fatigue contribute to diminished physical and emotional well-being, lack of energy and drive, and apathy, although the use of erythropoietin (Epogen) before the start of dialysis has been shown to have a significant effect on hematocrit levels for the first 19 months after starting dialysis. Dialyzer clotting can be prevented by adjusting heparin doses.

Gastric ulcers and other GI problems result from the physiologic stress of chronic illness, medication, and related problems. Disturbed calcium metabolism leads to renal osteodystrophy that produces bone pain and fractures. Other problems include fluid overload associated with heart failure, malnutrition, infection, neuropathy, and pruritus.

Up to 85% of people undergoing hemodialysis experience major sleep problems that further complicate their overall health status. Early-morning or late-afternoon dialysis may be a risk factor for developing sleep disturbances. Interventions such as changing the temperature of the dialysate bath may prevent temperature elevation, and limiting napping during dialysis may reduce sleep problems in people receiving hemodialysis. Other complications of dialysis treatment may include the following:

- Hypotension may occur during the treatment as fluid is removed. Nausea and vomiting, diaphoresis, tachycardia, and dizziness are common signs of hypotension.
- Painful muscle cramping may occur, usually late in dialysis as fluid and electrolytes rapidly leave the extracellular space.
- Exsanguination may occur if blood lines separate or dialysis needles become dislodged.
- Dysrhythmias may result from electrolyte and pH changes or from removal of antiarrhythmic medications during dialysis.
- Air embolism is rare but can occur if air enters the vascular system.
- Chest pain may occur in patients with anemia or arteriosclerotic heart disease.
- Dialysis disequilibrium results from cerebral fluid shifts. Signs and symptoms include headache, nausea and vomiting, restlessness, decreased level of consciousness, and seizures. It is more likely to occur in acute renal failure or when blood urea nitrogen levels are very high (exceeding 150 mg/dL).

Nursing Management

During dialysis, the patient, the dialyzer, and the dialysate bath require constant monitoring because numerous complications are possible, including clotting of the circuit, air embolism, inadequate or excessive ultrafiltration (hypotension, cramping, vomiting), blood leaks, contamination, and access complications. The nurse in the dialysis unit has an important role in monitoring, supporting, assessing, and educating the patient. Nursing care of the patient and maintenance of the vascular access device are discussed later in this chapter in the section titled "Special Considerations: Care of the Hospitalized Patient on Dialysis."

Pharmacologic Therapy

Just as many medications are excreted wholly or in part by the kidneys, many medications are removed from the blood during hemodialysis; therefore, the physician may need to adjust the dosage. Metabolites of drugs that are bound to protein are not removed during dialysis. Removal of other drug metabolites depends on the weight and size of the molecule.

Patients undergoing hemodialysis who require medications (eg, cardiac glycosides, antibiotic agents, antiarrhythmic medications, antihypertensive agents) are monitored closely to ensure that blood and tissue levels of these medications are maintained without toxic accumulation.

In patients receiving dialysis, all medications and their dosages must be carefully evaluated. Antihypertensive therapy, often part of the regimen of patients on dialysis, is one example when communication, teaching, and evaluation can make a difference in patient outcomes. The patient must know when and when not to take the medication. For example, if an antihypertensive agent is taken on a dialysis day, hypotension may occur during dialysis, causing dangerously low blood pressure. Many medications that are taken once daily can be held until after the dialysis treatment.

Nutritional and Fluid Therapy

When damaged kidneys are unable to excrete end products of metabolism, these substances accumulate in the serum as toxins. The resulting symptoms, collectively known as uremic symptoms or uremic syndrome, affect every body system. The more toxins that accumulate, the more severe the symptoms.

Diet is an important factor for patients on hemodialysis because of the effects of uremia. Goals of nutritional therapy are to minimize uremic symptoms and fluid and electrolyte imbalances; to maintain good nutritional status through adequate protein, calorie, vitamin, and mineral intake; and to enable the patient to eat a palatable and enjoyable diet. Restricting dietary protein decreases the accumulation of nitrogenous wastes, reduces uremic symptoms, and may even postpone the initiation of dialysis for a few months. Restriction of fluid is also part of the dietary prescription because fluid accumulation may occur, leading to weight gain, heart failure, and pulmonary edema (Leydig, 2005).

With the initiation of hemodialysis, the patient usually requires some restriction of dietary protein, sodium, potassium, and fluid intake. Protein intake is restricted to about 1.2 to 1.3 g/kg/day ideal body weight per day; therefore, protein must be of high biologic quality and consist of the essential amino acids to prevent poor protein use and to maintain a positive nitrogen balance. Examples of foods high in biologic protein content include eggs, meat, milk, poultry, and fish. Sodium is usually restricted to 2 to 3 g/day; fluids are restricted to an amount equal to the daily urine output plus 500 mL/day. The goal for patients on hemodialysis is to keep their interdialytic (between dialysis treatments) weight gain under 1.5 kg. Potassium restriction depends on the amount of residual renal function and the frequency of dialysis (Levy et al., 2004).

Dietary restriction is an unwelcome change in lifestyle for many patients with chronic renal failure. Patients often feel stigmatized in social situations because there may be few food choices available for their diet. If the restrictions are ignored, life-threatening complications, such as hyperkalemia and pulmonary edema, may result. Thus, the patient may feel punished for responding to basic human drives to eat and drink. The nurse who cares for a patient with symptoms or complications resulting from dietary indiscretion must avoid harsh, judgmental, or punitive tones when communicating with him or her.

Meeting Psychosocial Needs

Patients requiring long-term hemodialysis are often concerned about the unpredictability of the illness and the disruption of their lives. They often have financial problems, difficulty holding a job, waning sexual desire and impotence, depression from being chronically ill, and fear of dying. Younger patients worry about marriage, having children, and the burden that they bring to their families. The regimented lifestyle that frequent dialysis treatments and restrictions in food and fluid intake impose is often demoralizing to the patient and family.

Dialysis alters the lifestyle of the patient and family. The amount of time required for dialysis and physician visits and being chronically ill can create conflict, frustration, guilt, and depression. It may be difficult for the patient, spouse, and family to express anger and negative feelings.

The nurse needs to give the patient and family the opportunity to express feelings of anger and concern about the limitations that the disease and treatment impose, possible financial problems, and job insecurity. If anger is not expressed, it may be directed inward and lead to depression, despair, and attempts at suicide (suicide is more prevalent in patients on dialysis); however, if anger is projected outward to other people, it may destroy already threatened family relationships.

Although these feelings are normal in this situation, they are often profound and overwhelming. Counseling and psychotherapy may be necessary. Depression may require treatment with antidepressant agents. Referring the patient and family to a mental health provider with expertise in the care of patients receiving dialysis may also be helpful. Clinical nurse specialists, psychologists, and social workers may be helpful in assisting the patient and family to cope with the changes brought about by renal failure and its treatment.

The sense of loss that the patient experiences cannot be underestimated because every aspect of a "normal life" is disrupted. Some patients use denial to deal with the overwhelming array of medical problems (eg, infections, hypertension, anemia, neuropathy). Staff who are tempted to label the patient as noncompliant must consider the impact of renal failure and its treatment on the patient and family and the coping strategies that they may use.

Patients and their families should be encouraged to discuss end-of-life options. Only between 21% and 25% of patients on hemodialysis have an advanced directive or living will. One researcher reported that among 20 patients encouraged to discuss and think about end-of-life issues, most patients chose to focus on living rather than dying (Calvin, 2004).

Promoting Home and Community-Based Care

TEACHING PATIENTS SELF-CARE

Preparing a patient for hemodialysis is challenging. Often the patient does not fully comprehend the impact of dialysis, and learning needs may go unrecognized. Good communication between dialysis staff and home care nurses is essential.

Assessment helps identify the learning needs of the patient and family members. In many cases, the patient is discharged home before learning needs and readiness to learn can be thoroughly evaluated; therefore, hospital-based nurses, dialysis staff, and home care nurses must work together to provide appropriate teaching that meets the patient's and family's changing needs and readiness to learn.

The diagnosis of chronic renal failure and the need for dialysis often overwhelm the patient and family. In addition, many patients with ESRD have depressed mentation, a shortened attention span, a decreased level of concentration, and altered perception. Therefore, teaching must occur in brief, 10- to 15-minute sessions, with time added for clarification, repetition, reinforcement, and questions from the patient and family. The nurse needs to convey a nonjudgmental attitude to enable the patient and family to discuss options and their feelings about those options. Team conferences are helpful for sharing information and providing every team member the opportunity to discuss the needs of the patient and family.

HOME HEMODIALYSIS

Although most patients who require hemodialysis undergo the procedure in an outpatient setting, home hemodialysis is an option for some. Home hemodialysis requires a highly motivated patient who is willing to take responsibility for the procedure and is able to adjust each treatment to meet the body's changing needs. It also requires the commitment and cooperation of a family member to assist the patient. However, many patients are not comfortable imposing on others this way and do not wish to subject family members to the feeling that their home is being turned into a clinic. The health care team never forces a patient to use home hemodialysis, because this treatment requires significant changes in the home and family. Home hemodialysis must be the patient's and family's decision.

NURSING RESEARCH PROFILE

Hemodialysis and End-of-Life Treatment

Calvin, A. O. (2004). Haemodialysis patients and end-of-life decisions: A theory of personal preservation. *Journal of Advanced Nursing, 46*(5), 558–566.

Purpose

There is a lack of knowledge about end-of-life treatment preferences of patients receiving hemodialysis in the acute care setting. Patients may be unable to express their treatment wishes and many have not documented their desires in advanced directives. The purpose of this study was to explore decisions about end-of-life treatment preferences (eg, cardiopulmonary resuscitation and mechanical ventilation) in patients receiving hemodialysis.

Design

In this qualitative study, 20 subjects (11 men and 9 women) were interviewed using an interview guide containing questions about end-of-life treatment plans and the use of advanced directives. All interviews were audiotaped and transcribed verbatim. The mean age of subjects was 56 years. Data collection and analysis spanned a 3-year period of time.

Findings

When prompted to think about and discuss end-of-life issues, patients receiving hemodialysis chose to focus on living rather than on dying. A substantive theory of personal preservation was developed. The theory postulated that patients use a decision process consisting of three phases: knowing the odds for survival, defining individuality ("beating the odds"), and personal preservation (being responsible and taking chances).

Nursing Implications

The theory of personal preservation furthers understanding of illness behavior and the process by which patients make decisions about end-of-life treatments. It can be used to increase the sensitivity of health care professionals to patient desires (choosing to focus on life) and to enhance communication between patients receiving hemodialysis and health care professionals.

The patient undergoing home hemodialysis and the caregiver assisting that patient must be trained to prepare, operate, and disassemble the dialysis machine; maintain and clean the equipment; administer medications (eg, heparin) into the machine lines; and handle emergency problems (hemodialysis dialyzer rupture, electrical or mechanical problems, hypotension, shock, and seizures). Because home hemodialysis places primary responsibility for the treatment on the patient and the family member, they must understand and be capable of performing all aspects of the hemodialysis procedure (Chart 44-6).

Before home hemodialysis is initiated, the home environment, household and community resources, and ability and willingness of the patient and family to carry out this treatment are assessed. The home is surveyed to see if electrical outlets, plumbing facilities, and storage space are adequate. Modifications may be needed to enable the patient and assistant to perform dialysis safely and to deal with emergencies.

Once home dialysis is initiated, the home care nurse must visit periodically to evaluate compliance with the recommended techniques, to assess the patient for complications, to reinforce previous teaching, and to provide reassurance.

CONTINUING CARE

The health care team's goal in treating patients with chronic renal failure is to maximize their vocational potential, functional status, and quality of life. To facilitate renal rehabilitation, appropriate follow-up and monitoring by members of the health care team (physicians, dialysis nurses, social worker, psychologist, home care nurses, and others as appropriate) are essential to identify and resolve problems early on. Many patients with chronic renal failure can resume relatively normal lives, doing the things that are important to them: traveling, exercising, working, or actively participating in family activities. If appropriate interventions are available early in the course of dialysis, the potential for better health improves, and the patient can remain active in family and community life. Outcome goals for renal rehabilitation include employment for those able to work, improved physical functioning of all patients, improved understanding about adaptation and options for living well, increased control over the effects of kidney disease and dialysis, and resumption of activities enjoyed before dialysis.

Continuous Renal Replacement Therapies

Several types of continuous renal replacement therapies (CRRT) are available and widely used in critical care units (Fig. 44-6). CRRT may be indicated for patients with acute or chronic renal failure who are too clinically unstable for traditional hemodialysis, for patients with fluid overload secondary to oliguric (low urine output) renal failure, and for patients whose kidneys cannot handle their acutely high metabolic or nutritional needs. CRRT does not produce rapid fluid shifts, does not require dialysis machines or dialysis personnel to carry out the procedures, and can be initiated quickly in hospitals without dialysis facilities.

All CRRT methods are similar in that they require access to the circulation and blood to pass through an artificial filter. A hemofilter (an extremely porous blood filter con-

CHART 44-6

HOME CARE CHECKLIST • Hemodialysis

At the completion of the home care instruction, the patient or caregiver will be able to:	Patient	Caregiver
• Discuss renal failure and its effects on the body.	✔	✔
• Describe the cause of renal failure and why hemodialysis is necessary.	✔	✔
• Describe the basic principles of hemodialysis.	✔	✔
• Discuss common problems that may occur during hemodialysis and their prevention and management.	✔	✔
• Demonstrate knowledge about prescribed medications and the reason for their use, potential side effects, guidelines on when to notify physician, and the schedule of medications on dialysis and nondialysis days.	✔	✔
• Acknowledge dietary and fluid restrictions, rationale, and consequences of noncompliance.	✔	✔
• Describe commonly measured laboratory values, results, and implications.	✔	✔
• List guidelines for prevention and detection of fluid overload, meaning of "dry" weight, and how to weigh self.	✔	✔
• Demonstrate vascular access care, how to check patency, signs and symptoms of infection, prevention of complications.	✔	✔
• Discuss strategies for detection, management, and relief of pruritus, neuropathy, and other complications of renal failure.	✔	✔
• Develop strategies to manage or reduce anxiety and maintain independence.	✔	✔
• Coordinate financial arrangements for dialysis and strategies to identify and obtain resources.	✔	✔

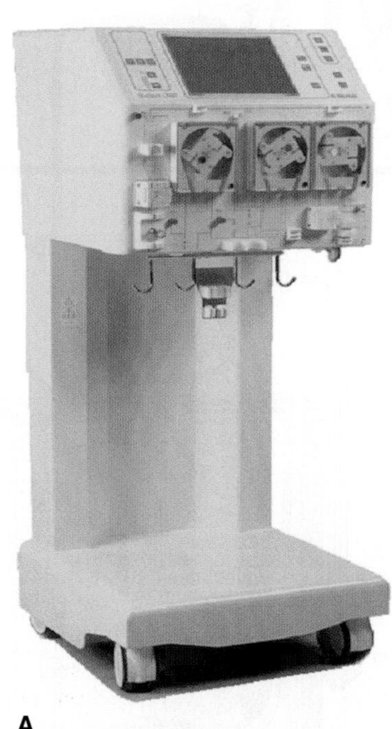

A

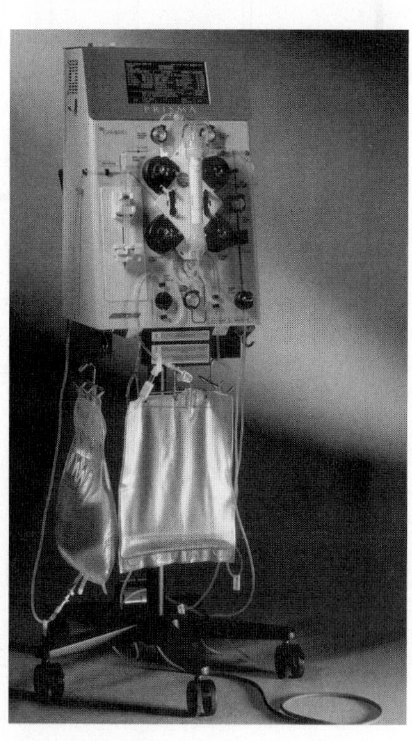

B

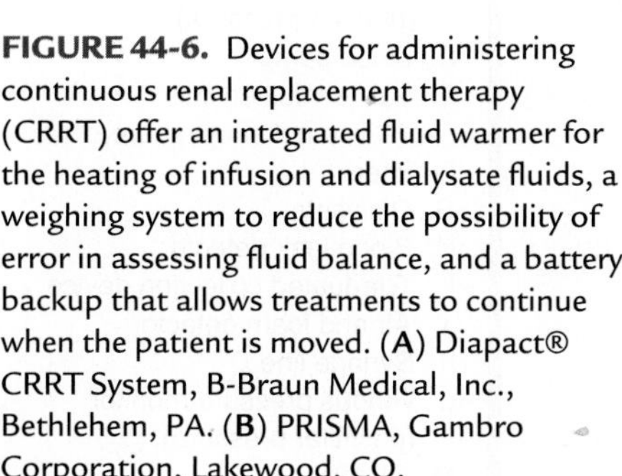

FIGURE 44-6. Devices for administering continuous renal replacement therapy (CRRT) offer an integrated fluid warmer for the heating of infusion and dialysate fluids, a weighing system to reduce the possibility of error in assessing fluid balance, and a battery backup that allows treatments to continue when the patient is moved. (**A**) Diapact® CRRT System, B-Braun Medical, Inc., Bethlehem, PA. (**B**) PRISMA, Gambro Corporation, Lakewood, CO.

taining a semipermeable membrane) is used in all methods (Kaplow & Barry, 2002).

Continuous arteriovenous hemofiltration (CAVH) and continuous arteriovenous hemodialysis (CAVHD) are techniques that are no longer commonly used (Morton et al., 2005).

Continuous Venovenous Hemofiltration

Continuous venovenous hemofiltration (CVVH) is used to manage acute renal failure. Blood from a double-lumen venous catheter is pumped (using a small blood pump) through a hemofilter and then returned to the patient through the same catheter. CVVH provides continuous slow fluid removal (ultrafiltration); therefore, hemodynamic effects are mild and better tolerated by patients with unstable conditions. CVVH does not require arterial access, and critical care nurses can set up, initiate, maintain, and terminate the system.

Continuous Venovenous Hemodialysis

Continuous venovenous hemodialysis (CVVHD) is similar to CVVH (Fig. 44-7). Blood is pumped from a double-

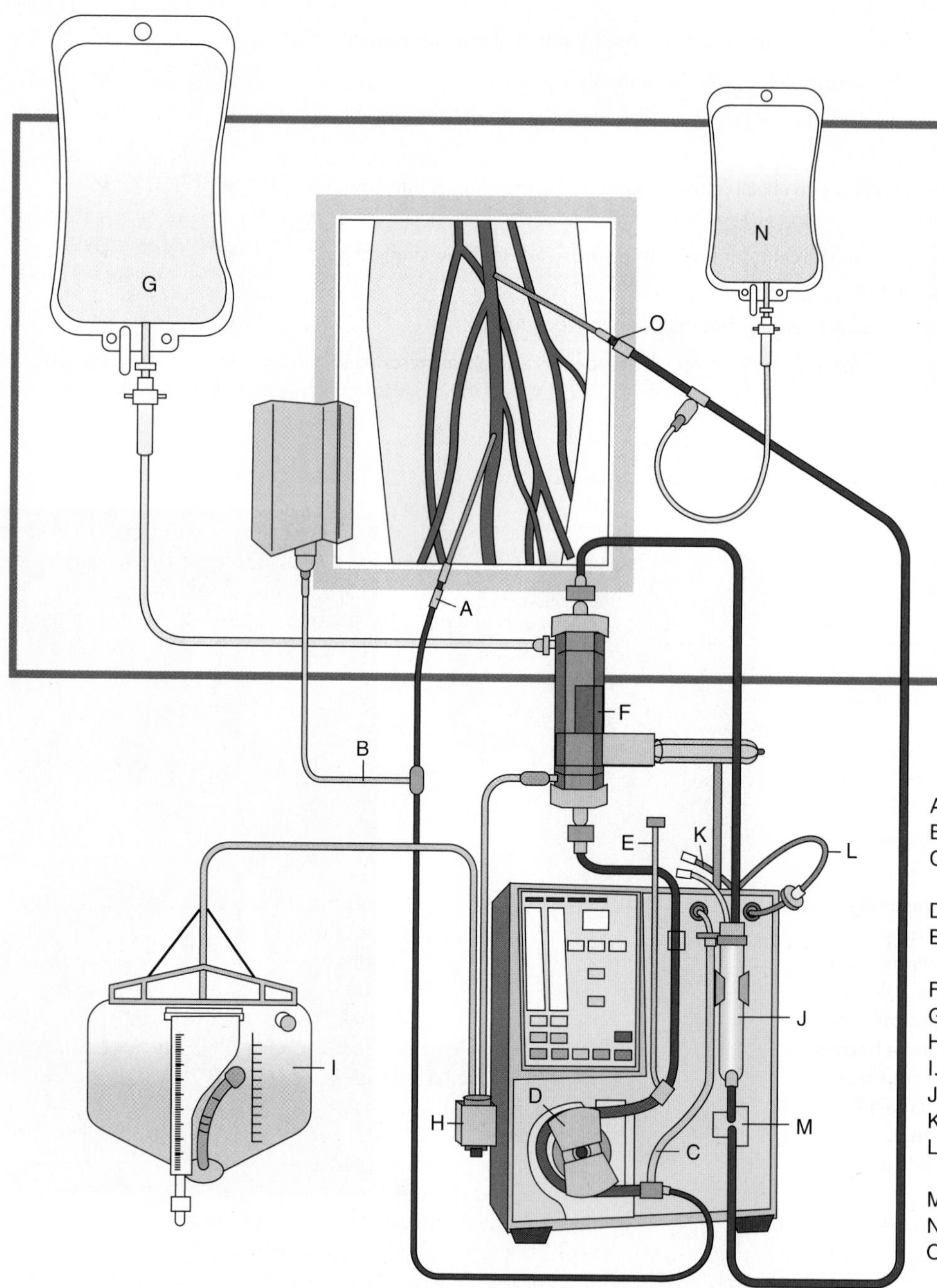

FIGURE 44-7. Continuous venovenous hemofiltration (CVVH) removes fluid (ultrafiltrate) slowly from the blood.

lumen venous catheter through a hemofilter and returned to the patient through the same catheter. In addition to the benefits of ultrafiltration, CVVHD uses a concentration gradient to facilitate the removal of uremic toxins and fluid. Therefore, no arterial access is required, hemodynamic effects are usually mild, and critical care nurses can set up, initiate, maintain, and terminate the system (Kaplow & Barry, 2002).

Peritoneal Dialysis

The goals of peritoneal dialysis are to remove toxic substances and metabolic wastes and to re-establish normal fluid and electrolyte balance. Peritoneal dialysis may be the treatment of choice for patients with renal failure who are unable or unwilling to undergo hemodialysis or renal transplantation. Patients who are susceptible to the rapid fluid, electrolyte, and metabolic changes that occur during hemodialysis experience fewer of these problems with the slower rate of peritoneal dialysis. Therefore, patients with diabetes or cardiovascular disease, many older patients, and those who may be at risk for adverse effects of systemic heparin are likely candidates for peritoneal dialysis. Additionally, severe hypertension, heart failure, and pulmonary edema not responsive to usual treatment regimens have been successfully treated with peritoneal dialysis.

In peritoneal dialysis, the peritoneal membrane that covers the abdominal organs and lines the abdominal wall serves as the semipermeable membrane (Kelley, 2004). The surface of the peritoneum constitutes a body surface area of about 22,000 cm^2. Sterile dialysate fluid is introduced into the peritoneal cavity through an abdominal catheter at intervals (Fig. 44-8). Urea and creatinine, metabolic end products normally excreted by the kidneys, are cleared from the blood by diffusion and osmosis as waste products move from an area of higher concentration (the peritoneal blood supply) to an area of lower concentration (the lining of the peritoneal cavity) across a semipermeable membrane (the peritoneal membrane). Urea is cleared at a rate of 15 to 20 mL/min, whereas creatinine is removed at a slower rate. With peritoneal dialysis, it usually takes 36 to 48 hours to achieve what hemodialysis accomplishes in 6 to 8 hours. Ultrafiltration (water removal) occurs in peritoneal dialysis through an osmotic gradient created by using a dialysate fluid with a higher glucose concentration.

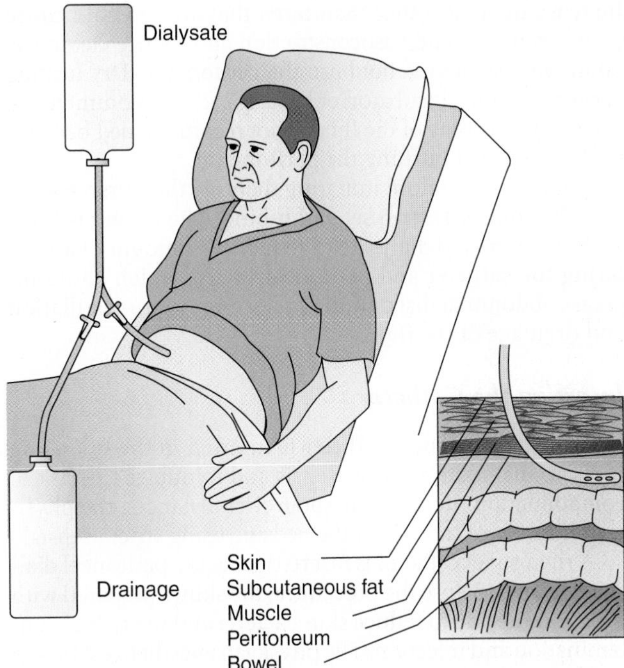

FIGURE 44-8. In peritoneal dialysis and in acute intermittent peritoneal dialysis, dialysate is infused into the peritoneal cavity by gravity, after which the clamp on the infusion line is closed. After a dwell time (when the dialysate is in the peritoneal cavity), the drainage tube is unclamped and the fluid drains from the peritoneal cavity, again by gravity. A new container of dialysate is infused as soon as drainage is complete. The duration of the dwell time depends on the type of peritoneal dialysis.

Procedure

As with other forms of treatment, the decision to begin peritoneal dialysis is made by the patient and family in consultation with the physician. The patient undergoing peritoneal dialysis may be acutely ill, thus requiring short-term treatment to correct severe disturbances in fluid and electrolyte status, or may have chronic renal failure and need to receive ongoing treatments.

Preparing the Patient

The nurse's preparation of the patient and family for peritoneal dialysis depends on the patient's physical and psychological status, level of alertness, previous experience with dialysis, and understanding of and familiarity with the procedure.

The nurse explains the procedure to the patient and obtains signed consent for it. Baseline vital signs, weight, and serum electrolyte levels are recorded. The patient is encouraged to empty the bladder and bowel to reduce the risk of puncturing internal organs. The nurse also assesses the patient's anxiety about the procedure and provides support and instruction. Broad-spectrum antibiotic agents may be administered to prevent infection. If the peritoneal catheter is to be inserted in the operating room, this is explained to the patient and family.

Preparing the Equipment

In addition to assembling the equipment for peritoneal dialysis, the nurse consults with the physician to determine the concentration of dialysate to be used and the medications to be added to it. Heparin may be added to prevent fibrin formation and resultant occlusion of the peritoneal catheter. Potassium chloride may be prescribed to prevent hypokalemia. Antibiotics may be added to treat **peritonitis** (inflammation of the peritoneal membrane). Regular insulin may be added for patients with diabetes; however, a larger-than-normal dose may be needed, because about 10% of the insulin binds to the wall of the dialysate container. All medications are added immediately before the solution is instilled. Aseptic technique is imperative.

Before medications are added, the dialysate is warmed to body temperature to prevent patient discomfort and abdominal pain and to dilate the vessels of the peritoneum to increase urea clearance. Solutions that are too cold cause pain, cramping, and vasoconstriction and reduce clearance. Solutions that are too hot burn the peritoneum. Dry heating (heating cabinet, incubator, or heating pad) is recommended. Microwave heating of the fluid is not recommended because of the danger of burning the peritoneum.

Immediately before initiating dialysis, the nurse assembles the administration set and tubing. The tubing is filled with the prepared dialysate to reduce the amount of air entering the catheter and peritoneal cavity, which could increase abdominal discomfort and interfere with instillation and drainage of the fluid.

Inserting the Catheter

Ideally, the peritoneal catheter is inserted in the operating room to maintain surgical asepsis and minimize the risk of contamination. However, in some circumstances, the physician inserts the catheter at the bedside using strict asepsis.

A rigid stylet catheter is inserted for acute peritoneal dialysis use only. Before the procedure, the skin is prepared with a local antiseptic to reduce skin bacteria and the risk of contamination and infection. The physician anesthetizes the site with a local anesthetic agent before making a small incision or stab wound in the lower abdomen, 3 to 5 cm below the umbilicus. Because this area is relatively free from large blood vessels, little bleeding occurs. A trocar is used to puncture the peritoneum as the patient tightens the abdominal muscles by raising the head. The catheter is threaded through the trocar and positioned. Previously prepared dialysate is infused into the peritoneal cavity, pushing the omentum (peritoneal lining extending from the abdominal organs) away from the catheter. The physician may then secure the catheter with a purse-string suture and apply antibacterial ointment and a sterile dressing over the site.

Catheters for long-term use (Tenckhoff, Swan, Cruz) are usually made of silicone and are radiopaque to permit visualization on x-ray. These catheters have three sections: (1) an intraperitoneal section, with numerous openings and an open tip to let dialysate flow freely; (2) a subcutaneous section that passes from the peritoneal membrane and tunnels through muscle and subcutaneous fat to the skin; and (3) an external section for connection to the dialysate system. Most of these catheters have two cuffs, which are made of Dacron polyester. The cuffs stabilize the catheter, limit movement, prevent leaks, and provide a barrier against microorganisms. One cuff is placed just distal to the peritoneum, and the other cuff is placed subcutaneously. The subcutaneous tunnel (5 to 10 cm long) further protects against bacterial infection (Fig. 44-9).

Performing the Exchange

Peritoneal dialysis involves a series of exchanges or cycles. An exchange is defined as the infusion, dwell, and drainage of the dialysate. This cycle is repeated throughout the course

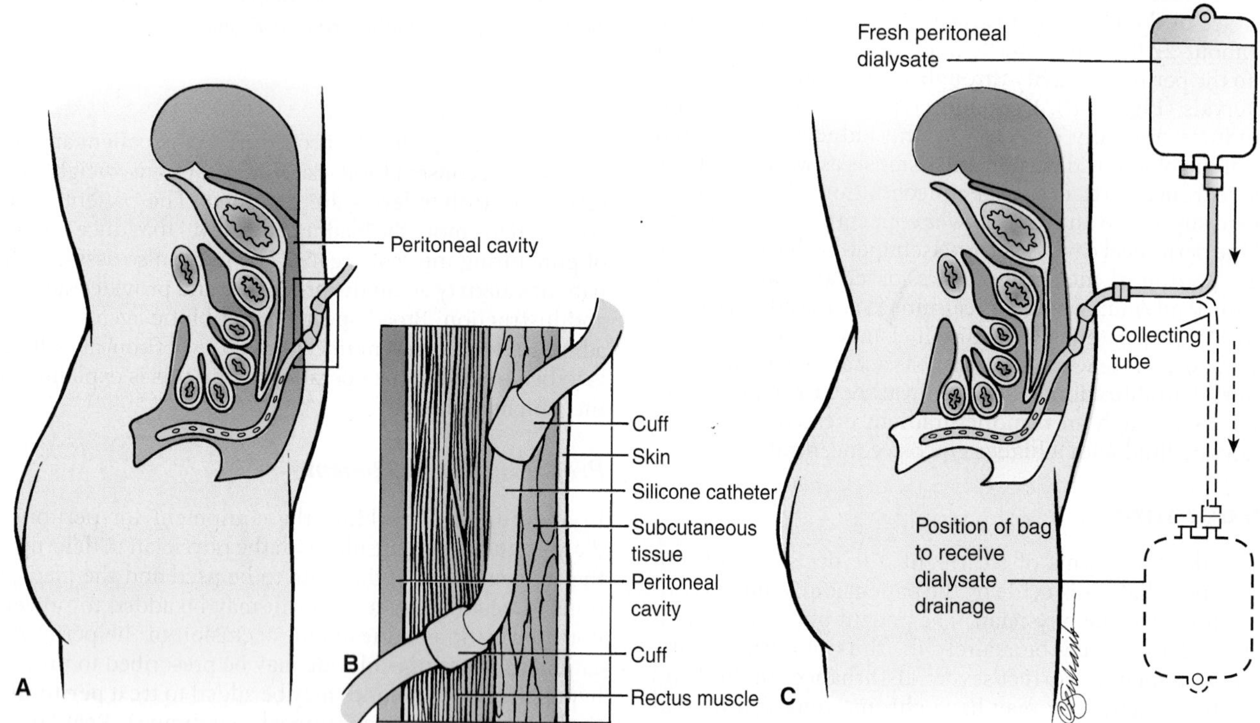

FIGURE 44-9. Continuous ambulatory peritoneal dialysis. (**A**) The peritoneal catheter is implanted through the abdominal wall. (**B**) Dacron cuffs and a subcutaneous tunnel provide protection against bacterial infection. (**C**) Dialysate flows by gravity through the peritoneal catheter into the peritoneal cavity. After a prescribed period of time, the fluid is drained by gravity and discarded. New solution is then infused into the peritoneal cavity until the next drainage period. Dialysis thus continues on a 24-hour-a-day basis during which the patient is free to move around and engage in his or her usual activities.

of the dialysis. The dialysate is infused by gravity into the peritoneal cavity. A period of about 5 to 10 minutes is usually required to infuse 2 to 3 L of fluid. The prescribed dwell, or equilibration, time allows diffusion and osmosis to occur. Diffusion of small molecules, such as urea and creatinine, peaks in the first 5 to 10 minutes of the dwell time. At the end of the dwell time, the drainage portion of the exchange begins. The tube is unclamped and the solution drains from the peritoneal cavity by gravity through a closed system. Drainage is usually completed in 10 to 30 minutes. The drainage fluid is normally colorless or straw-colored and should not be cloudy. Bloody drainage may be seen in the first few exchanges after insertion of a new catheter but should not occur after that time. The entire exchange (infusion, dwell time, and drainage) takes 30 to 45 minutes. The number of cycles or exchanges and their frequency are prescribed based on the patient's physical status and acuity of illness.

The removal of excess water during peritoneal dialysis is achieved by using a hypertonic dialysate with a high dextrose concentration that creates an osmotic gradient. Dextrose solutions of 1.5%, 2.5%, and 4.25% are available in several volumes, from 1000 mL to 3000 mL, allowing the dialysate selection to fit the patient's tolerance, size, and physiologic needs. The higher the dextrose concentration, the greater the osmotic gradient and the more water will be removed. Selection of the appropriate solution is based on the patient's fluid status.

Complications

Peritoneal dialysis is not without complications. Most are minor, but several, if unattended, can have serious consequences.

Acute Complications

PERITONITIS

Peritonitis is the most common and serious complication of peritoneal dialysis, although there has been a recent decrease in the rate of cases of peritonitis. It has been reported that the rate of peritonitis is 0.24 episodes per patient-year, and mortality rates are now between 2.3% and 3.4% (Bernardini, 2004). The organism responsible for peritoneal dialysis-related peritonitis is an important factor in clinical outcome and the basis of treatment guidelines. *Staphylococcus aureus* and *S. epidermidis* remain the most common gram-positive organisms responsible for peritonitis, although the rates of each have decreased. *Pseudomonas aeruginosa, Escherichia coli,* and *Klebsiella* species are the most common causes of gram-negative peritonitis.

Peritonitis is characterized by cloudy dialysate drainage, diffuse abdominal pain, and rebound tenderness. Hypotension and other signs of shock may occur if *S. aureus* is the responsible organism. The patient with peritonitis may be treated as an inpatient or outpatient (most common), depending on the severity of the infection and the patient's clinical status. Initially, one to three rapid exchanges with a 1.5% dextrose solution without added medications are completed to wash out causes of inflammation and to reduce abdominal pain. Drainage fluid is examined for cell count, and Gram's stain and culture are used to identify the organism and guide treatment. Antibiotic agents (aminoglycosides or cephalosporins) are usually added to subsequent exchanges until Gram stain or culture results are available for appropriate antibiotic determination. Intraperitoneal administration of antibiotics is as effective as IV administration. Antibiotic therapy continues for 10 to 14 days. Careful calculation of the antibiotic dosage helps prevent nephrotoxicity and further compromise of renal function.

Peritonitis that is unresolved after 2 to 3 days of appropriate therapy may necessitate catheter removal. The patient is maintained on hemodialysis and systemic antibiotics for about 1 month before a new catheter is inserted (Levy et al., 2004).

Regardless of which organism causes peritonitis, the patient with peritonitis loses large amounts of protein through the peritoneum. Acute malnutrition and delayed healing may result. Therefore, attention must be given to detecting and promptly treating peritonitis.

LEAKAGE

Leakage of dialysate through the catheter site may occur immediately after the catheter is inserted. Usually, the leak stops spontaneously if dialysis is withheld for several days to give the incision and exit site time to heal. During this time, it is important to reduce factors that might delay healing, such as undue abdominal muscle activity and straining during bowel movement. Leakage through the exit site or into the abdominal wall can occur for months or years after catheter placement. In many cases, leakage can be avoided by using small volumes (500 mL) of dialysate, gradually increasing the volume up to 2000 to 3000 mL.

BLEEDING

A bloody effluent (drainage) may be observed occasionally, especially in young, menstruating women. (The hypertonic fluid pulls blood from the uterus, through the opening in the fallopian tubes, and into the peritoneal cavity.) Bleeding is common during the first few exchanges after a new catheter insertion because some blood enters the abdominal cavity following insertion. In many cases, no cause can be found for the bleeding, although catheter displacement from the pelvis has occasionally been associated with bleeding. Some patients have had bloody effluent after an enema or from minor trauma. Invariably, bleeding stops in 1 to 2 days and requires no specific intervention. More frequent exchanges during this time may be necessary to prevent blood clots from obstructing the catheter.

Long-Term Complications

Hypertriglyceridemia is common in patients undergoing long-term peritoneal dialysis, suggesting that the therapy may accelerate atherogenesis. Despite this, the use of cardioprotective medications is relatively low, and many patients have suboptimal blood pressure control. Given the high burden of disease in these patients, beta-blockers and ACE inhibitors should be used to control hypertension or protect the heart, and the use of aspirin and statins should be considered.

Increases in blood pressure and fluid volume leading to left ventricular hypertrophy and dyslipidemias are the major causes of morbidity and mortality in patients undergoing peritoneal dialysis with comorbidities such as diabetes and vascular disease (Danovitch, 2005). Because cardiovascular disease is the cause of death in half of all patients with ESRD, the adequacy of dialysis is determined by its effects on risk for cardiovascular disease.

Other complications that may occur with long-term peritoneal dialysis include abdominal hernias (incisional, inguinal, diaphragmatic, and umbilical), probably resulting from continuously increased intra-abdominal pressure. The persistently elevated intra-abdominal pressure also aggravates symptoms of hiatal hernia and hemorrhoids. Low back pain and anorexia from fluid in the abdomen and a constant sweet taste related to glucose absorption may also occur.

Mechanical problems occasionally occur and may interfere with instillation or drainage of the dialysate. Formation of clots in the peritoneal catheter and constipation are factors that may contribute to these problems.

Approaches

Peritoneal dialysis can be performed using several different approaches: acute intermittent peritoneal dialysis; **continuous ambulatory peritoneal dialysis (CAPD)**; and **continuous cyclic peritoneal dialysis (CCPD)**.

Acute Intermittent Peritoneal Dialysis

Indications for acute intermittent peritoneal dialysis, a variation of peritoneal dialysis, include uremic signs and symptoms (nausea, vomiting, fatigue, altered mental status), fluid overload, acidosis, and hyperkalemia. Although peritoneal dialysis is not as efficient as hemodialysis in removing solute and fluid, it permits a more gradual change in the patient's fluid volume status and in waste product removal. Therefore, it may be the treatment of choice for the hemodynamically unstable patient. It can be carried out manually (the nurse warms, spikes, and hangs each container of dialysate) or by a cycler machine. Exchange times range from 30 minutes to 2 hours. A common routine is hourly exchanges consisting of a 10-minute infusion, a 30-minute dwell time, and a 20-minute drain time.

Maintaining the peritoneal dialysis cycle is a nursing responsibility. Strict aseptic technique is maintained when changing solution containers and emptying drainage containers. Vital signs, weight, intake and output, laboratory values, and patient status are frequently monitored. The nurse uses a flow sheet to document each exchange and records vital signs, dialysate concentration, medications added, exchange volume, dwell time, dialysate fluid balance for the exchange (fluid lost or gained), and cumulative fluid balance. The nurse also carefully assesses skin turgor and mucous membranes to evaluate fluid status and monitor the patient for edema.

If the peritoneal fluid does not drain properly, the nurse can facilitate drainage by turning the patient from side to side or raising the head of the bed. The catheter should never be pushed further into the peritoneal cavity. Other measures to promote drainage include checking the patency of the catheter by inspecting for kinks, closed clamps, or an air lock. The nurse monitors for complications, including peritonitis, bleeding, respiratory difficulty, and leakage of peritoneal fluid. Abdominal girth may be measured periodically to determine if the patient is retaining large amounts of dialysis solution. Additionally, the nurse must ensure that the peritoneal dialysis catheter remains secure and that the dressing remains dry. Physical comfort measures, frequent turning, and skin care are provided. The patient and family are educated about the procedure and are kept informed about progress (fluid loss, weight loss, laboratory values). Emotional support and encouragement are given to the patient and family during this stressful and uncertain time.

Continuous Ambulatory Peritoneal Dialysis

CAPD is a form of dialysis used for many patients with ESRD (Kelley, 2004). CAPD is performed at home by the patient or a trained caregiver who is usually a family member; the procedure allows the patient reasonable freedom and control of daily activities (Chart 44-7).

CAPD works on the same principles as other forms of peritoneal dialysis: diffusion and osmosis. Less extreme fluctuations in the patient's laboratory values occur with CAPD than with intermittent peritoneal dialysis or hemodialysis because the dialysis is constantly in progress. The serum electrolyte levels usually remain in the normal range.

PROCEDURE

The patient performs exchanges four or five times a day, 24 hours a day, 7 days a week, at intervals scheduled throughout the day (before meals and bedtime). Different manufacturers supply different equipment. A Y-shaped system, in which a bag containing dialysate solution comes already attached to one end of the "Y" and a sterile empty bag is attached to another arm of the "Y," is most commonly used. The patient washes his or her hands and dons a mask, and the patient or caregiver then removes the cap from the transfer set, which is an adaptor that provides a connection between the catheter and the tubing set. The set is attached to the end of the transfer set (the patient then can remove the mask), and the patient drains the fluid (effluent) from the peritoneal cavity through the catheter (over about 20 to 30 minutes) into the empty bag. The patient then instills the dialysate solution into the peritoneal cavity. Once the dialysate is infused, the patient dons a mask again, clamps off the transfer set and the tubing set, disconnects the tubing set, and applies a cap to maintain a closed system. This provides the patient with freedom and reduces the number of connections and disconnections necessary at the catheter end of the tubing, thereby reducing the risk for contamination and peritonitis (Levy et al., 2004).

The longer the dwell time, the better the clearance of middle-sized molecules. It is thought that these molecules may be significant uremic toxins. If dwell time is excessive, the patient absorbs some of the effluent back into the body.

COMPLICATIONS

To reduce the risk of peritonitis, the patient must use meticulous care to avoid contaminating the catheter, fluid, or tubing and to avoid accidentally disconnecting the catheter from the tubing. Excess manipulation is avoided and meticulous care of the catheter entry site is provided using a standardized protocol.

CHART 44-7

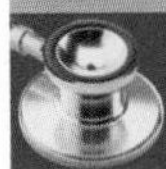

Assessing for Suitability for CAPD

Although CAPD is not suitable for all patients with end-stage renal disease (ESRD), it is a viable therapy for those who can perform self-care and exchanges and who can fit therapy into their own routines. Often, patients report having more energy and feeling healthier once they begin CAPD. Nurses can be instrumental in helping patients with ESRD find the dialysis therapy that best suits their lifestyle. Those considering CAPD need to investigate the advantages and disadvantages along with the indications and contraindications for this form of therapy.

ADVANTAGES

- Freedom from a dialysis machine
- Control over daily activities
- Opportunities to avoid dietary restrictions, increase fluid intake, raise serum hematocrit values, improve blood pressure control, avoid venipuncture, and gain a sense of well-being

DISADVANTAGES

- Continuous dialysis 24 hours a day, 7 days a week

INDICATIONS

- Patient's willingness, motivation, and ability to perform dialysis at home
- Strong family or community support system (essential for success), particularly if the patient is an older adult
- Special problems with long-term hemodialysis, such as dysfunctional or failing vascular access devices, excessive thirst, severe hypertension, postdialysis headaches, and severe anemia requiring frequent transfusion
- Interim therapy while awaiting kidney transplantation
- ESRD secondary to diabetes because hypertension, uremia, and hyperglycemia are easier to manage with CAPD than with hemodialysis

CONTRAINDICATIONS

- Adhesions from previous surgery (adhesions reduce clearance of solutes) or systemic inflammatory disease
- Chronic backache and preexisting disk disease, which could be aggravated by the continuous pressure of dialysis fluid in the abdomen
- Risk of complications, for example, in patients receiving immunosuppressive medications, which impede healing of the catheter site, and in patients with a colostomy, ileostomy, nephrostomy, or ileal conduit because of the risk of peritonitis. The risk for complications is not an absolute contraindication for CAPD therapy.
- Diverticulitis because CAPD has been associated with rupture of the diverticulum
- Severe arthritis or poor hand strength necessitating assistance in performing the exchange. However, blind or partially blind patients and those with other physical limitations can learn to perform CAPD.

NURSING MANAGEMENT

Meeting Psychosocial Needs. In addition to the complications of peritoneal dialysis previously described, patients who elect to use CAPD may experience altered body image because of the abdominal catheter and the bag and tubing. Waist size increases from 1 to 2 inches (or more) with fluid in the abdomen. This affects clothing selection and may make the patient feel "fat." Body image may be so altered that patients do not want to look at or care for the catheter for days or weeks. The nurse may arrange for the patient to talk with other patients who have adapted well to CAPD. Although some patients have no psychological problems with the catheter—they think of it as their lifeline and as a life-sustaining device—other patients feel they are doing exchanges all day long and have no free time, particularly in the beginning. They may experience depression because they feel overwhelmed with the responsibility of self-care.

Patients undergoing CAPD may also experience altered sexuality patterns and sexual dysfunction. The patient and partner may be reluctant to engage in sexual activities, partly because of the catheter being psychologically "in the way" of sexual performance. The peritoneal catheter, drainage bag, and about 2 L of dialysate may interfere with the patient's sexual function and body image as well. Although these problems may resolve with time, some problems may warrant special counseling. Questions by the nurse about concerns related to sexuality and sexual function often provide the patient with a welcome opportunity to discuss these issues and a first step toward their resolution.

Promoting Home and Community-Based Care

Teaching Patients Self-Care. Patients are taught as inpatients or outpatients to perform CAPD once their condition is medically stable. Training usually takes 5 days to 2 weeks. Patients are taught according to their own learning ability and knowledge level and only as much at one time as they can handle without feeling uncomfortable or becoming overwhelmed. Education topics for the patient and family who will be performing peritoneal dialysis at home are described in Chart 44-8. The use of an adult learning theory–based curriculum has been shown to improve patient outcomes such as peritonitis and exit site infection rates (Hall, Bogan, Dreis, et al., 2004).

CHART 44-8

HOME CARE CHECKLIST • Peritoneal Dialysis (CAPD or CCPD)

At the completion of the home care instruction, the patient or caregiver will be able to:	Patient	Caregiver
• Discuss basic information about normal kidney function.	✔	✔
• Discuss basic information about the disease process.	✔	✔
• Discuss the basic principles of peritoneal dialysis.	✔	✔
• Demonstrate catheter and exit site care.	✔	✔
• Demonstrate measurement of vital signs and weight measurement.	✔	✔
• Discuss monitoring and management of fluid balance.	✔	✔
• Discuss basic principles of aseptic technique.	✔	✔
• Demonstrate the CAPD exchange procedure using aseptic technique (CCPD patients should also demonstrate exchange procedure in case of failure or unavailability of cycling machine).	✔	✔
• Demonstrate cycler set-up procedure and maintenance if on CCPD.	✔	✔
• Discuss complications of peritoneal dialysis; prevention, recognition, and management of complications.	✔	✔
• Demonstrate procedure for adding medications to the dialysis solution.	✔	✔
• Demonstrate procedure for obtaining sterile dialysis fluid samples.	✔	✔
• Discuss routine laboratory tests needed and implications of results.	✔	✔
• Discuss dietary restrictions.	✔	✔
• Discuss medications: name of medications, their actions, potential side effects, and when to contact physician.	✔	✔
• Discuss ordering, storage, and inventory of dialysis supplies.	✔	✔
• Describe plan for follow-up care.	✔	✔
• Demonstrate maintenance of home dialysis records.	✔	✔
• Describe actions in case of emergency.	✔	✔

Because of protein loss with continuous peritoneal dialysis, the patient is instructed to eat a high-protein, well-balanced diet. The patient is also encouraged to increase his or her daily fiber intake to help prevent constipation, which can impede the flow of dialysate into or out of the peritoneal cavity. Many patients gain 3 to 5 lb within a month of initiating CAPD, so they may be asked to limit their carbohydrate intake to avoid excessive weight gain. Potassium, sodium, and fluid restrictions are not usually needed. Patients commonly lose about 2 to 3 L of fluid over and above the volume of dialysate infused into the abdomen during a 24-hour period, permitting a normal fluid intake even in an anephric patient (a patient without kidneys).

Continuing Care. Follow-up care through phone calls, visits to the outpatient department, and continuing home care assists patients in the transition to home and promotes their active participation in their own health care. Patients often depend on checking with the nurse to see if they are making the correct choices about dialysate or control of blood pressure, or simply to discuss a problem.

Patients may be seen by the CAPD team as outpatients once a month or more often if needed. The exchange procedure is evaluated at that time to see that strict aseptic technique is being used. The CAPD nurse changes the transfer set every 6 months (Levy et al., 2004). Infrequent tubing changes decrease the risk of contamination. Blood chemistry values are followed closely to make certain the therapy is adequate for the patient.

If a referral is made for home care, the home care nurse assesses the home environment and suggests modifications to accommodate the equipment and facilities needed to carry out CAPD. In addition, the nurse assesses the patient's and family's understanding of CAPD and their use of safe technique in performing CAPD. Additional assessments include checking for changes related to renal disease, complications such as peritonitis, and treatment-related problems such as heart failure, inadequate drainage, and weight gain or loss. The nurse continues to reinforce and clarify teaching about CAPD and renal disease and assesses the patient's and family's progress in coping with the procedure. In addition, the patient is reminded about the need to participate in appropriate health promotion activities and health screening (eg, gynecological examinations, colonoscopy).

Because of the projected high numbers of elderly patients who will develop ESRD, the nursing home or extended care facility is likely to become an increasingly important site for both rehabilitation and long-term management of patients with renal failure.

Continuous Cyclic Peritoneal Dialysis

CCPD combines overnight intermittent peritoneal dialysis with a prolonged dwell time during the day. The peritoneal catheter is connected to a cycler machine every evening, and the patient receives three to five 2- to 3-L exchanges during the night. In the morning, the patient caps off the catheter after infusing 2 to 3 L of fresh dialysate. This dialysate remains in the abdominal cavity until the tubing is reattached to the cycler machine at bedtime. Because the machine is very quiet, the patient can sleep. Moreover, the extra-long tubing allows the patient to move and turn normally during sleep (Kelley, 2004).

CCPD has a lower infection rate than other forms of peritoneal dialysis because there are fewer opportunities for contamination with bag changes and tubing disconnections. It also allows the patient to be free from exchanges throughout the day, making it possible to engage in work and activities of daily living more freely.

Special Considerations: Care of the Hospitalized Patient on Dialysis

Whether undergoing hemodialysis or peritoneal dialysis, the patient may be hospitalized for treatment of complications related to the dialysis treatment, the underlying renal disorder, or health problems not related to renal dysfunction or its treatment.

Nursing Management

Protecting Vascular Access

When the patient undergoing hemodialysis is hospitalized for any reason, care must be taken to protect the vascular access from damage. The nurse assesses the vascular access for patency and takes precautions to ensure that the extremity with the vascular access is not used for measuring blood pressure or for obtaining blood specimens; tight dressings, restraints, or jewelry over the vascular access must be avoided as well.

The bruit, or "thrill," over the venous access site must be evaluated at least every 8 hours. Absence of a palpable thrill or audible bruit may indicate blockage or clotting in the vascular access. Clotting can occur if the patient has an infection anywhere in the body (serum viscosity increases) or if the blood pressure has dropped. When blood flow is reduced through the access for any reason (hypotension, application of blood pressure cuff or tourniquet), the access can clot. If a patient has a hemodialysis catheter or implanted hemodialysis access device, the nurse must observe for signs and symptoms of infection such as redness, swelling, drainage from the exit site, fever, and chills. The nurse must assess the integrity of the dressing and change it as needed. Patients with renal disease are more prone to infection; therefore, infection control measures must be used for all procedures.

Taking Precautions During Intravenous Therapy

When the patient needs IV therapy, the rate of administration must be as slow as possible and should be strictly controlled by a volumetric infusion pump. Because patients on dialysis cannot excrete water, rapid or excessive administration of IV fluid can result in pulmonary edema. Accurate intake and output records are essential.

Monitoring Symptoms of Uremia

As metabolic end products accumulate, symptoms of uremia worsen. Patients whose metabolic rate accelerates (those receiving corticosteroid medications or parenteral nutrition, those with infections or bleeding disorders, those undergoing surgery) accumulate waste products more quickly and may require daily dialysis. These same patients are more likely than other patients receiving dialysis to experience complications.

Detecting Cardiac and Respiratory Complications

Cardiac and respiratory assessment must be conducted frequently. As fluid builds up, fluid overload, heart failure, and pulmonary edema develop. Crackles in the bases of the lungs may indicate pulmonary edema.

Pericarditis may result from the accumulation of uremic toxins. If not detected and treated promptly, this serious complication may progress to pericardial effusion and cardiac tamponade. Pericarditis is detected by the patient's report of substernal chest pain (if the patient can communicate), low-grade fever (often overlooked), and pericardial friction rub. A pulsus paradoxus (a decrease in blood pressure of more than 10 mm Hg during inspiration) is often present. When pericarditis progresses to effusion, the friction rub disappears, heart sounds become distant and muffled, ECG waves show very low voltage, and the pulsus paradoxus worsens.

The effusion may progress to life-threatening cardiac tamponade, noted by narrowing of the pulse pressure in addition to muffled or inaudible heart sounds, crushing chest pain, dyspnea, and hypotension. Although pericarditis, pericardial effusion, and cardiac tamponade can be detected by chest x-ray, they should also be detected through astute nursing assessment. Because of their clinical significance, assessment of the patient for cardiac complications is a priority.

Controlling Electrolyte Levels and Diet

Electrolyte alterations are common, and potassium changes can be life threatening. All IV solutions and medications to be administered are evaluated for their electrolyte content. Serum laboratory values are assessed daily. If blood transfusions are required, they may be administered during hemodialysis, if possible, so that excess potassium can be removed. Dietary intake must also be monitored. The patient's frustrations related to dietary restrictions typically increase if the hospital food is unappetizing. The nurse needs to recognize that this may lead to dietary indiscretion and hyperkalemia.

Hypoalbuminemia is an indicator of malnutrition in patients undergoing long-term or maintenance dialysis. Although some patients can be treated with adequate nutrition alone, some patients remain hypoalbuminemic for reasons that are poorly understood.

Managing Discomfort and Pain

Complications such as pruritus and pain secondary to neuropathy must be managed. Antihistamine agents, such as diphenhydramine hydrochloride (Benadryl), are commonly used, and analgesic medications may be prescribed. However, because elimination of the metabolites of medications occurs through dialysis rather than through renal excretion, medication dosages may need to be adjusted. Keeping the skin clean and well moisturized using bath oils, superfatted soap, and creams or lotions helps promote comfort and reduce itching. Teaching the patient to keep the nails trimmed to avoid scratching and excoriation and to apply lotion to the skin instead of scratching also promotes comfort.

Monitoring Blood Pressure

Hypertension in renal failure is common. It is usually the result of fluid overload and, in part, oversecretion of renin. Many patients undergoing dialysis receive some form of antihypertensive therapy and require intense teaching about its purpose and adverse effects. The trial-and-error approach that may be necessary to identify the most effective antihypertensive agent and dosage may confuse or alarm the patient if no explanation is provided. Antihypertensive agents must be withheld before dialysis to avoid hypotension due to the combined effect of the dialysis and the medication.

Typically these patients require single or multiple antihypertensive agents to achieve normal blood pressure, thus adding to the total number of medications needed on an ongoing basis.

Preventing Infection

Patients with ESRD commonly have low WBC counts (and decreased phagocytic ability), low RBC counts (anemia), and impaired platelet function. Together, these pose a high risk for infection and potential for bleeding after even minor trauma. Preventing and controlling infection are essential because the incidence of infection is high. Infection of the vascular access site and pneumonia are common.

Caring for the Catheter Site

Patients receiving CAPD usually know how to care for the catheter site; however, the hospital stay should be an opportunity to assess catheter care technique and correct misperceptions or deviations from recommended technique. Recommended daily or three-or-four-times-weekly routine catheter site care is typically performed during showering or bathing. The exit site should not be submerged in bath water. The most common cleaning method is soap and water; liquid soap is recommended. During care, the nurse and patient need to make sure that the catheter remains secure to avoid tension and trauma. The patient may wear a gauze or semitransparent dressing over the exit site.

Administering Medications

All medications and the dosage prescribed for any patient on dialysis must be closely monitored to avoid those that are toxic to the kidneys and may threaten remaining renal function. Medications are also scrutinized for potassium and magnesium content, because medications containing potassium or magnesium must be avoided. Care must be taken to evaluate all problems and symptoms that the patient reports without automatically attributing them to renal failure or to dialysis therapy.

Providing Psychological Support

Patients undergoing dialysis for a while may begin to reevaluate their status, the treatment modality, their satisfaction with life, and the impact of these factors on their families and support systems. Nurses must provide opportunities for these patients to express their feelings and reactions and to explore options. The decision to begin dialysis does not require that dialysis be continued indefinitely, and it is not uncommon for patients to consider discontinuing treatment. These feelings and reactions must be taken seriously, and the patient should have the opportunity to discuss them with the dialysis team as well as with a psychologist, psychiatrist, psychiatric nurse, trusted friend, or spiritual advisor. The patient's informed decision about discontinuing treatment, after thoughtful deliberation, should be respected.

Kidney Surgery

A patient may undergo surgery to remove obstructions that affect the kidney (tumors or calculi), to insert a tube for draining the kidney (nephrostomy, ureterostomy), or to remove the kidney involved in unilateral kidney disease, renal carcinoma, or kidney transplantation.

Preoperative Considerations

Surgery is performed only after a thorough evaluation of renal function. Patient preparation to ensure that optimal renal function is maintained is essential. Fluids are encouraged to promote increased excretion of waste products before surgery unless contraindicated because of preexisting renal or cardiac dysfunction. If kidney infection is present preoperatively, broad-spectrum antimicrobial agents may be prescribed to prevent bacteremia. Antibiotic agents must be given with extreme care because many are toxic to the kidneys. Coagulation studies (prothrombin time, partial thromboplastin time, platelet count) may be indicated if the patient has a history of bruising and bleeding. The preoperative preparation is similar to that described in Chapter 18.

Because many patients facing kidney surgery are apprehensive, the nurse encourages the patient to recognize and verbalize concerns. Confidence is reinforced by establishing a relationship of trust and by providing expert care. Patients faced with the prospect of losing a kidney may think that they will be dependent on dialysis for the rest of their lives. It is important to teach the patient and family that normal function may be maintained by a single healthy kidney.

Perioperative Concerns

Renal surgery requires various patient positions to expose the surgical site adequately. Three surgical approaches are common: flank, lumbar, and thoracoabdominal (Fig. 44-10). During surgery, plans are carried out for managing altered urinary drainage. These may include inserting a nephrostomy or other drainage tube.

Postoperative Management

Because the kidney is a highly vascular organ, hemorrhage and shock are the chief complications of renal surgery. Fluid and blood component replacement is frequently necessary in the immediate postoperative period to treat intraoperative blood loss.

Abdominal distention and paralytic ileus are fairly common after renal and ureter surgery and are thought to be due to a reflex paralysis of intestinal peristalsis and manipulation of the colon or duodenum during surgery. Abdominal distention is relieved by decompression through a nasogastric tube (see Chapter 38 for treatment of paralytic ileus). Oral fluids are permitted when the passage of flatus is noted.

If infection occurs, antibiotic agents are prescribed after a culture reveals the causative organism. The toxic effects that antibiotic agents have on the kidneys (nephrotoxicity) must be kept in mind when assessing the patient. Low-dose heparin therapy may be initiated postoperatively to prevent thromboembolism in patients who had any type of urologic surgery.

Nursing Process

The Patient Undergoing Kidney Surgery

Assessment

Immediate care of the patient who has undergone surgery of the kidney includes assessment of all body systems. Respiratory and circulatory status, pain level, fluid and electrolyte status, and patency and adequacy of urinary drainage systems are assessed.

Respiratory Status

As with any surgery, the use of anesthesia increases the risk for respiratory complications. Noting the location of the surgical incision assists the nurse in anticipating respiratory problems and pain. Respiratory status is assessed by monitoring the rate, depth, and pattern of respirations. The location of the incision frequently causes pain on inspiration and coughing; therefore, the patient tends to splint the chest wall and take shallow respirations. Auscultation is performed to assess normal and adventitious breath sounds.

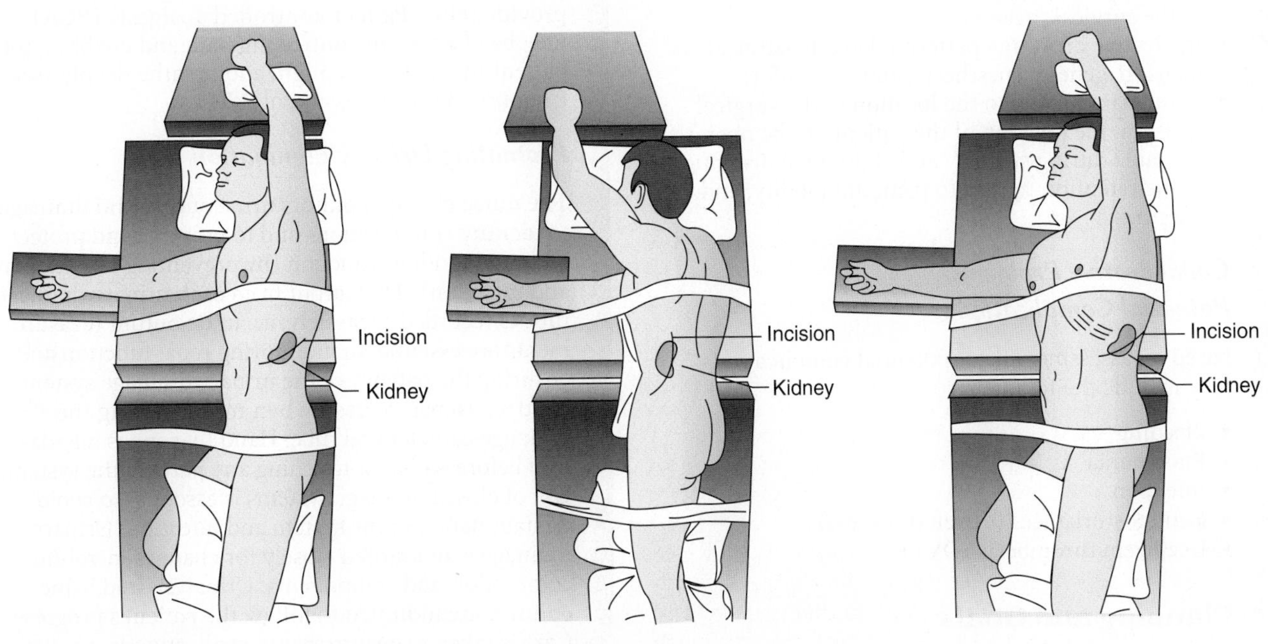

FIGURE 44-10. Patient positioning and incisional approaches (**A**, flank; **B**, lumbar; **C**, thoracoabdominal) for kidney surgery are associated with significant postoperative discomfort.

Circulatory Status and Blood Loss

The patient's vital signs and arterial or central venous pressure are monitored. Skin color and temperature and urine output provide information about circulatory status. The surgical incision and drainage tubes are observed frequently to help detect unexpected blood loss and hemorrhage.

Pain

Postoperative pain is a major problem for the patient because of the location of the surgical incision and patient's position on the operating table to permit access to the kidney. The location and severity of pain are assessed before and after analgesic medications are administered. Abdominal distention, which increases discomfort, is also noted.

Urinary Drainage

Urine output and drainage from tubes inserted during surgery are monitored for amount, color, and type or characteristics. Decreased or absent drainage is promptly reported to the physician because it may indicate obstruction that could cause pain, infection, and disruption of the suture lines.

Diagnosis

Nursing Diagnoses

Based on the history and assessment data and the type of surgical procedure performed, major nursing diagnoses for the patient include the following (additional diagnoses and interventions appear in the plan of nursing care in Chart 44-9).

- Ineffective airway clearance related to the location of the surgical incision
- Ineffective breathing pattern related to surgical incision, general anesthesia, and discomfort
- Acute pain related to the location of the surgical incision, the position of the patient on the operating table during surgery, and abdominal distention
- Urine retention related to pain, immobility, and anesthesia

Collaborative Problems/ Potential Complications

Based on assessment data, potential complications may include the following:

- Bleeding
- Pneumonia
- Infection
- Fluid disturbances (deficit or excess)
- Deep vein thrombosis (DVT)

Planning and Goals

The major goals for the patient include maintenance of effective airway clearance and breathing pattern, relief of pain and discomfort, maintenance of urinary elimination, and absence of complications.

Nursing Interventions

Maintaining Airway Clearance and Breathing Patterns

The surgical approaches to the kidney predispose the patient to respiratory complications and paralytic ileus. If the pleural cavity has been entered during surgery, a pneumothorax may occur, necessitating insertion of a chest tube. The incision is generally close to the diaphragm, and with a substernal incision, the nerves may be stretched and bruised. These factors can lead to pain and limited chest movement during inspiration; breathing patterns are altered or ineffective when the chest cannot fully expand. If the patient cannot generate an effective cough, either because of pain at the incision site and restricted movement or because of anesthesia, ineffective airway clearance may result.

Adequate use of analgesic medications is necessary to relieve pain so that the patient can take deep breaths and cough. When the analgesia is administered at regular, frequent intervals, the patient can perform deep-breathing and coughing exercises more effectively. The incentive spirometer (see Chapter 25) may be used to help maximize lung inflation. The patient is encouraged to cough after each deep breath to loosen secretions.

Relieving Pain

The patient may experience pain at the incision site as well as pain and discomfort from distention of the renal capsule (by tumor or blood clot), ischemia (from occlusion of blood vessels), and stretching of the intrarenal blood vessels. Muscle aches and pain stemming from the position of the patient on the operating table, which places anatomic and physiologic stresses on the body, are also common. Massage, moist heat, and analgesic medications as prescribed provide relief. Patient-controlled analgesia (PCA) may be effective in controlling pain and enabling the patient to ambulate, cough, and breathe deeply (see Chapter 13 for discussion of PCA).

Promoting Urinary Elimination

The nurse closely monitors urine output and drainage to identify complications and to preserve and protect remaining kidney function (by preventing obstruction and infection). The output from each urinary drainage tube is recorded separately; accurate output measurements are essential in monitoring renal function and ensuring the patency of the urinary drainage system.

Strict asepsis is used when manipulating the drainage catheter and tube. Hand hygiene is mandatory before and after touching any parts of the system. Use of closed drainage systems is essential to avoid contamination of the system and infection. Urinary drainage is monitored closely for changes in volume, color, odor, and components. Urinalysis and urine cultures are indicated to follow the patient's progress. Care is taken to ensure that the collection bag is suspended below the bladder to prevent reflux of urine into the urinary tract. The bag must be kept off the floor to prevent contamination.

(text continues on page 1558)

CHART 44-9

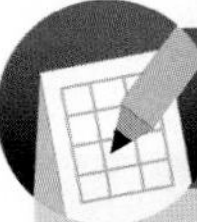

Plan of Nursing Care — Care of Patient Undergoing Kidney Surgery

Nursing Diagnosis: Ineffective airway clearance related to pain of high abdominal or flank incision, abdominal discomfort, and immobility; risk for ineffective breathing pattern related to high abdominal incision
Goal: Improved airway clearance

NURSING INTERVENTIONS	RATIONALE	EXPECTED OUTCOMES
1. Administer analgesics as prescribed.	1. Enables patient to take deep breaths and cough	• Takes deep breaths and coughs adequately when encouraged and assisted
2. Splint incision with hands or pillow to assist patient in coughing.	2. Splints incision and promotes adequate cough and prevention of atelectasis	• Exhibits respiratory rate of 12–18 breaths/min • Exhibits normal breath sounds without adventitious sounds
3. Assist patient to change positions frequently.	3. Promotes drainage and inflation of all lobes of the lungs	• Exhibits full thoracic excursion without shallow respirations
4. Encourage use of incentive spirometer if indicated or prescribed.	4. Encourages adequate deep breaths	• Uses incentive spirometer with encouragement
5. Assist with and encourage early ambulation.	5. Mobilizes pulmonary secretions	• Splints incision while taking deep breaths and coughing • Reports progressively less pain and discomfort with coughing and deep breaths • Exhibits normal blood gas levels and chest x-ray • Exhibits normal body temperature with no signs of atelectasis or pneumonia on assessment

Nursing Diagnosis: Acute pain and discomfort related to surgical incision, positioning, and stretching of muscles during kidney surgery
Goal: Relief of pain and discomfort

NURSING INTERVENTIONS	RATIONALE	EXPECTED OUTCOMES
1. Assess level of pain.	1. Provides baseline for later evaluation of pain relief strategies	• Reports relief of severe pain and discomfort
2. Administer analgesics as prescribed.	2. Promotes pain relief	• Takes analgesia as prescribed • States rationale for use of moist heat and massage
3. Apply moist heat and massage to areas with muscular aches and discomfort.	3. Promotes relaxation and relief of muscle pain and discomfort	• Exercises aching muscles within recommendations
4. Splint incision with hands or pillow during movement or deep breathing and coughing exercises.	4. Minimizes sensation of pulling or tension on incision and provides sense of support to the patient	• Gradually increases physical activity and exercise • Uses distraction, relaxation exercises, and imagery to relieve pain
5. Assist and encourage early ambulation.	5. Promotes resumption of muscle activity exercise	• Exhibits no behavioral manifestations of pain and discomfort (eg, restlessness, perspiration, verbal expressions of pain) • Participates in deep-breathing and coughing exercises

continued >

CHART 44-9

Plan of Nursing Care — Care of Patient Undergoing Kidney Surgery (Continued)

Nursing Diagnosis: Fear and anxiety related to diagnosis, outcome of surgery, and alteration in urinary function
Goal: Reduction of fear and anxiety

NURSING INTERVENTIONS	RATIONALE	EXPECTED OUTCOMES
1. Assess patient's anxiety and fear before surgery if possible.	1. Provides a baseline for postoperative assessment	• Verbalizes reactions and feelings to staff • Shares reactions and feelings with family or partner • Grieves appropriately for self and for changes in role and function • Identifies information needed to promote own adaptation and coping • Participates in activities and events in immediate environment • Accepts visit from ostomy group if indicated • Identifies support person or support group
2. Assess patient's knowledge about procedure and expected surgical outcome preoperatively.	2. Provides a basis for further teaching	
3. Evaluate the meaning of alterations resulting from surgical procedure for the patient and family or partner.	3. Enables understanding of patient's reactions and responses to expected and unexpected results of surgery	
4. Encourage patient to verbalize reactions, feelings, and fears.	4. Affirms patient's understanding of and ultimate resolution of feelings and fears	
5. Encourage patient to share feelings with spouse or partner.	5. Enables patient and partner to receive mutual support and reduces sense of isolation from each other	
6. Offer and arrange for visit from member of support group (eg, ostomy group, if indicated).	6. Provides support from another person who has encountered the same or a similar surgical procedure and an example of how others have coped with the alteration	

Nursing Diagnosis: Impaired urinary elimination related to urinary drainage; risk for infection related to altered urinary drainage
Goal: Maintenance of urinary elimination; infection-free urinary tract

NURSING INTERVENTIONS	RATIONALE	EXPECTED OUTCOMES
1. Assess urinary drainage system immediately.	1. Provides basis for further assessment and action	• Exhibits adequate urinary output and patent drainage system • Exhibits urinary output consistent with fluid intake • Demonstrates normal laboratory values: BUN, serum creatinine levels, urine specific gravity, and osmolality • Exhibits sterile urine on urine culture • Exhibits clear, dilute urine without debris or encrustation in the drainage system • States rationale for avoiding manipulation of catheter, drainage, or irrigation system
2. Assess adequacy of urinary output and patency of drainage system.	2. Provides baseline	
3. Use asepsis and hand hygiene when providing care and manipulating drainage system.	3. Prevents or reduces risk of contamination of urinary drainage system	
4. Maintain closed urinary drainage system.	4. Reduces risk of bacterial contamination and infection	
5. If irrigation of the drainage system is necessary, use sterile gloves and sterile irrigating solution and a closed drainage and irrigation system.	5. Permits irrigation when necessary while maintaining closed drainage system, minimizing risk of infection	

CHART 44-9

Plan of Nursing Care — Care of Patient Undergoing Kidney Surgery (Continued)

NURSING INTERVENTIONS

6. If irrigation is necessary and prescribed, perform it gently with sterile saline and the prescribed amount of irrigating fluid.
7. Assist patient in turning and moving in bed and when ambulating to prevent displacement or inadvertent removal of urinary stent or ureteral catheters if in place.
8. Observe urine color, volume, odor, and components.
9. Minimize trauma and manipulation of catheter, drainage system, and urethra.
10. Clean catheter gently with soap during bath, avoiding any to-and-fro movement of catheter.
11. Anchor drainage tube.
12. Maintain adequate fluid intake.
13. Assist with and encourage early ambulation while ensuring placement of urinary drainage system.
14. If patient is to be discharged with urinary drainage system (catheter) in place or a urinary diversion, instruct patient and family member in care.

RATIONALE

6. Maintains patency of the catheter or drainage system and prevents sudden increases in pressure in the urinary tract that may cause trauma, pressure on sutures or urinary tract structures, and pain
7. Prevents trauma from accidental displacement of urinary stent or ureteral catheter necessitating repeated instrumentation of the urinary tract (eg, cystoscopy) to replace them
8. Provides information about adequacy of urine output, condition and patency of drainage system, and debris in urine
9. Reduces risk of contamination of drainage system and eliminates site of bacterial invasion
10. Removes debris and encrustations without causing trauma to or contamination of urethra
11. Prevents movement or slipping of drainage tube, minimizing trauma to and contamination of urethra or catheter
12. Promotes adequate urine output and prevents urinary stasis
13. Minimizes cardiovascular and pulmonary complications while preventing loss, dislodging, or disruption of drainage system
14. Knowledge and understanding of the drainage system or urinary diversion are essential to prevent infection and other complications

EXPECTED OUTCOMES

- Exhibits normal placement of urinary stent or ureteral catheters until removed by physician
- Maintains closed urinary drainage system
- Exhibits normal body temperature without signs or symptoms of urinary tract infection
- Cleans catheter with soap and water
- Consumes adequate fluid intake (6 to 8 glasses of water or more per day, unless contraindicated)
- Urinary drainage system remains in place until physician removes or discontinues it
- Maintains urinary drainage system without infection or obstruction
- Maintains urinary diversion as instructed
- Maintains self-care so that environment is odor-free
- States rationale for close follow-up and maintains recommended schedule of appointments with health care providers

Nursing Diagnosis: Risk for imbalanced fluid volume related to surgical fluid loss, altered urinary output, parenteral fluid administration
Goal: Normal fluid balance will be maintained.

NURSING INTERVENTIONS

1. Weigh patient daily.
2. Take accurate intake and output measurements.

RATIONALE

1. Daily weight is the most sensitive indicator of fluid loss or gain
2. Detects fluid retention due to poor cardiac or renal output

EXPECTED OUTCOMES

- Patient's weight will be within 2–3 lb of patient's baseline.
- Intake that exceeds output will be detected early.

continued >

CHART 44-9

Plan of Nursing Care — Care of Patient Undergoing Kidney Surgery (Continued)

NURSING INTERVENTIONS	RATIONALE	EXPECTED OUTCOMES
3. Place all parenteral therapy on an infusion pump.	3. Ensures that the patient does not receive excess or insufficient intravenous fluids	• The exact amount of solution is infused with no adverse effects resulting from overinfusion or underinfusion.
4. Monitor amount and characteristics of urine.	4. Assists in early detection of possible complications of surgery or tube insertion	• Urine is clear and absent of blood, pus, or any foreign substances.
5. Monitor vital signs: temperature, pulse, respirations, and blood pressure.	5. When fluid volume or cardiac output is altered, vital signs are affected	• Temperature, pulse, respiration, and blood pressure are normal.
6. Auscultate heart and lungs every shift.	6. When fluid volume is increased because of poor cardiac or renal output, fluid accumulates in the lungs. Also, heart sounds change as heart failure develops; frequent auscultation ensures early detection.	• Normal heart and lung sounds are present.

Most urinary drainage systems do not require routine irrigation. However, if irrigation is necessary and prescribed, it should be performed carefully, with the use of sterile solution; with minimal pressure, consistent with the physician's instructions; and with strict asepsis without interruption of the closed drainage system.

Monitoring and Managing Potential Complications

Bleeding is a major complication of kidney surgery. If undetected and untreated, bleeding can result in hypovolemia and hemorrhagic shock. The nurse's role is to observe for these complications, to report their signs and symptoms, and to administer prescribed parenteral fluids and blood and blood components if complications occur. Monitoring of vital signs, skin condition, the urinary drainage system, the surgical incision, and the level of consciousness is necessary to detect evidence of bleeding, decreased circulating blood, and fluid volume and cardiac output. Frequent monitoring of vital signs (initially monitored at least at hourly intervals) and urinary output is necessary for early detection of these complications.

If bleeding goes undetected or is not detected promptly, the patient may lose significant amounts of blood and may experience hypoxemia. In addition to hypovolemic shock due to hemorrhage, this type of blood loss may precipitate a myocardial infarction or transient ischemic attack. Bleeding may be suspected when the patient experiences fatigue and when urine output is less than 30 mL per hour. As bleeding persists, late signs of hypovolemia occur, such as cool skin, flat neck veins, and change in level of consciousness or responsiveness. Transfusions of blood components are indicated, along with surgical repair of the bleeding vessel.

Pneumonia may be prevented through use of an incentive spirometer, adequate pain control, and early ambulation. Early signs of pneumonia include fever, increased heart and respiratory rates, and adventitious breath sounds.

Preventing infection is the rationale for using asepsis when changing dressings and handling and preparing catheters, other drainage tubes, central venous catheters, and IV catheters for administration of fluids. Insertion sites are monitored closely for signs and symptoms of inflammation: redness, drainage, heat, and pain. Special care must be taken to prevent urinary tract infection, which is associated with the use of indwelling urinary catheters. Catheters and other invasive tubes are removed as soon they are no longer needed.

Antibiotic agents are commonly administered postoperatively to prevent infection. If antibiotic agents are prescribed, serum creatinine and BUN values must be monitored closely because many antibiotic agents are toxic to the kidney or can accumulate to toxic levels if renal function is decreased.

Preventing fluid imbalance is critical when caring for a patient undergoing kidney surgery, because both fluid loss and fluid excess are possible adverse effects of the surgery. Fluid loss may occur during surgery as a result of excessive urinary drainage when the obstruction is removed, or it may occur if diuretic agents are used. Such loss may also occur with GI losses, with diarrhea resulting from antibiotic use, or with nasogastric drainage. When postoperative IV therapy is inadequate to match the output or fluids lost, a fluid deficit results. Fluid excess, or overload, may result from cardiac effects of anesthesia, administration of excessive amounts of fluids, or the patient's inability to excrete fluid because of changes in renal function. Decreased urine output may be an indication of fluid excess.

Astute assessment skills are needed to detect early signs of fluid excess (such as weight gain, pedal edema, urine output below 30 mL/h, and slightly elevated pulmonary wedge pressure, if available) before they become severe (appearance of adventitious breath sounds, shortness of breath).

Fluid excess may be treated with fluid restriction and administration of furosemide (Lasix) or other diuretic agents. If renal insufficiency is present, these medications may prove ineffective; therefore, dialysis may be necessary to prevent heart failure and pulmonary edema.

DVT may occur postoperatively because of surgical manipulation of the iliac vessels during surgery or prolonged immobility. Elastic compression stockings are applied, and the patient is monitored closely for signs and symptoms of thrombosis and encouraged to exercise the legs. Heparin may be administered postoperatively to reduce the risk of thrombosis. Specific nursing interventions for the patient undergoing kidney surgery are presented in the Plan of Nursing Care (Chart 44-9).

Promoting Home and Community-Based Care

TEACHING PATIENTS SELF-CARE

If the patient has a drainage system in place, measures are taken to ensure that both patient and family understand the importance of maintaining the system correctly at home and preventing infection. Verbal and written instructions and guidelines are provided to the patient and family at the time of hospital discharge. The patient may be asked to demonstrate management of the drainage system to ensure understanding. The importance of strategies to prevent postoperative complications (urinary tract infection and obstruction, DVT, atelectasis, and pneumonia) is stressed to the patient and family. Those signs, symptoms, problems, and questions that should be referred to the physician or other primary health care provider are reviewed by the nurse with the patient and family.

CONTINUING CARE

The need for postoperative assessment and care after renal surgery continues regardless of the setting: the home, subacute care unit, outpatient clinic or office, or rehabilitation facility. Referral for home care is indicated for the patient going home with a urinary drainage system in place. During the home visit, the home care nurse reviews the instructions and guidelines given to the patient at hospital discharge. The nurse assesses the patient's ability to carry out the instructions in the home and answers questions that the patient or family has about management of the drainage system and the surgical incision.

Additionally, the home care nurse obtains vital signs and assesses the patient for signs and symptoms of urinary tract infection and obstruction. The nurse also ensures that pain is adequately controlled and that the patient is complying with recommendations. The home care nurse encourages adequate fluid intake and increased levels of activity. Together the nurse, patient, and family review the signs, symptoms, problems, and questions that should be referred to the physician or other primary health care provider. If the patient has a drainage tube in place, the nurse assesses the site and the patency of the system and monitors the patient for complications, such as DVT, bleeding, or pneumonia.

Because it is easy for the patient, family, and health care team to focus on the patient's immediate disorder to the exclusion of other health issues, reminding the patient and family about the importance of participating in health promotion activities, including health screening, is key.

Evaluation

Expected Patient Outcomes

Expected patient outcomes may include:

1. Achieves effective airway clearance
    a. Exhibits clear and normal breath sounds, normal respiratory rate, and unrestricted thoracic excursion
    b. Performs deep-breathing exercises, coughs every 2 hours, and uses the incentive spirometer as directed
    c. Demonstrates normal temperature and vital signs
2. Reports progressive decrease in pain
    a. Requires analgesic medications at less frequent intervals
    b. Turns, coughs, and takes deep breaths as recommended
    c. Ambulates progressively
3. Maintains urinary elimination
    a. Demonstrates unobstructed urine flow from drainage tubes
    b. Exhibits normal fluid and electrolyte balance (normal skin turgor, serum electrolyte levels within normal range, absence of symptoms of imbalances)
    c. Reports no increase in pain, tenderness, or pressure at drainage site
    d. Exhibits cautious handling of drainage system
    e. Uses hand hygiene before and after handling drainage system, and handles it only when necessary
    f. States rationale for use and maintenance of a closed drainage system
4. Participates in self-care activities
5. Experiences no complications
    a. Demonstrates normal vital signs and arterial and central venous pressures, normal skin turgor, temperature, and color
    b. Exhibits no signs or symptoms of bleeding, shock, or hypovolemia (eg, decreased urine output, restlessness, rapid pulse)

c. Exhibits no signs or symptoms of infection (eg, fever or pain) or evidence of DVT (tenderness, redness, warmth or edema of calves)
d. Maintains normal fluid balance, without rapid weight gain or loss
e. Has clear breath sounds and no shortness of breath
f. Excretes urine at a rate of at least 30 mL per hour

Kidney Transplantation

Kidney transplantation has become the treatment of choice for most patients with ESRD. During the past 40 years, more than 400,000 kidney transplantations have been performed worldwide, and approximately 9000 are performed in the United States each year. In the United States, there are many more patients on the waiting list for kidney transplantation than there are organ donors (Danovitch, 2005). Patients choose kidney transplantation for various reasons, such as the desire to avoid dialysis or to improve their sense of well-being and the wish to lead a more normal life. Additionally, the cost of maintaining a successful transplantation is one-third the cost of dialysis treatment.

Kidney transplantation involves transplanting a kidney from a living donor or deceased donor to a recipient who has ESRD (Chart 44-10). Kidney transplants from well-matched living donors who are related to the patient (those with compatible ABO and HLA antigens) are slightly more successful than those from cadaver donors (Holechek, Hiller, Paredes, et al., 2003). The success rate increases if kidney transplantation from a living donor is performed before dialysis is initiated (Danovitch, 2005). The half-life of a renal graft is longer if from a living related donor than a deceased donor (Ponticelli, Villa, Cesana, et al., 2002). The mean ages of donor and recipient affect long-term graft survival (Dantal & Souillou, 2005).

Depending on the cause and symptoms of renal failure, a nephrectomy of the patient's own native kidneys may be performed before transplantation. The transplanted kidney is placed in the patient's iliac fossa anterior to the iliac crest. The ureter of the newly transplanted kidney is transplanted into the bladder or anastomosed to the ureter of the recipient (Fig. 44-11).

CHART 44-10

Kidney Donation

An inadequate number of available kidneys remains the greatest limitation to treating patients with end-stage renal disease successfully. For those interested in donating a kidney, the National Kidney Foundation provides written information describing the organ donation program and a card specifying the organs to be donated in the event of death.

The organ donation card is signed by the donor and two witnesses and should be carried by the donor at all times. Procurement of an adequate number of kidneys for potential recipients is still a major problem, despite national legislation that requires relatives of deceased patients or patients declared brain-dead to be asked if they would consider organ donation.

In some states in the United States, drivers can indicate their desire to be organ donors on their driver's license application or renewal.

Preoperative Management

Preoperative management goals include bringing the patient's metabolic state to a level as close to normal as possible, making sure that the patient is free of infection, and preparing the patient for surgery and the postoperative course.

Medical Management

A complete physical examination is performed to detect and treat any conditions that could cause complications after transplantation. Tissue typing, blood typing, and antibody screening are performed to determine compatibility of the tissues and cells of the donor and recipient. Other diagnostic tests must be completed to identify conditions requiring treatment before transplantation. The lower urinary tract is studied to assess bladder neck function and to detect ureteral reflux.

The patient must be free of infection at the time of renal transplantation because after surgery medications to prevent transplant rejection will be prescribed. These medications suppress the immune response, leaving the patient immunosuppressed and at risk of infection. Therefore, the patient is evaluated and treated for any infections, including gingival (gum) disease and dental caries.

A psychosocial evaluation is conducted to assess the patient's ability to adjust to the transplant, coping styles, social history, social support available, and financial resources. A history of psychiatric illness is important to obtain because psychiatric conditions are often aggravated by the corticosteroids needed for immunosuppression after transplantation. If a dialysis routine has been established, hemodialysis is often performed the day before the scheduled transplantation procedure to optimize the patient's physical status. However, it is preferable to avoid initiation of dialysis before transplantation when a donor kidney is available (Ponticelli et al., 2002).

Nursing Management

The nursing aspects of preoperative care for the patient undergoing renal transplant are similar to those for patients undergoing other types of elective abdominal surgery. Preoperative teaching can be conducted in a variety of settings, including the outpatient preadmission area, the hospital, or the transplantation clinic during the preliminary workup phase. Patient teaching addresses postoperative pulmonary hygiene, pain management options, dietary

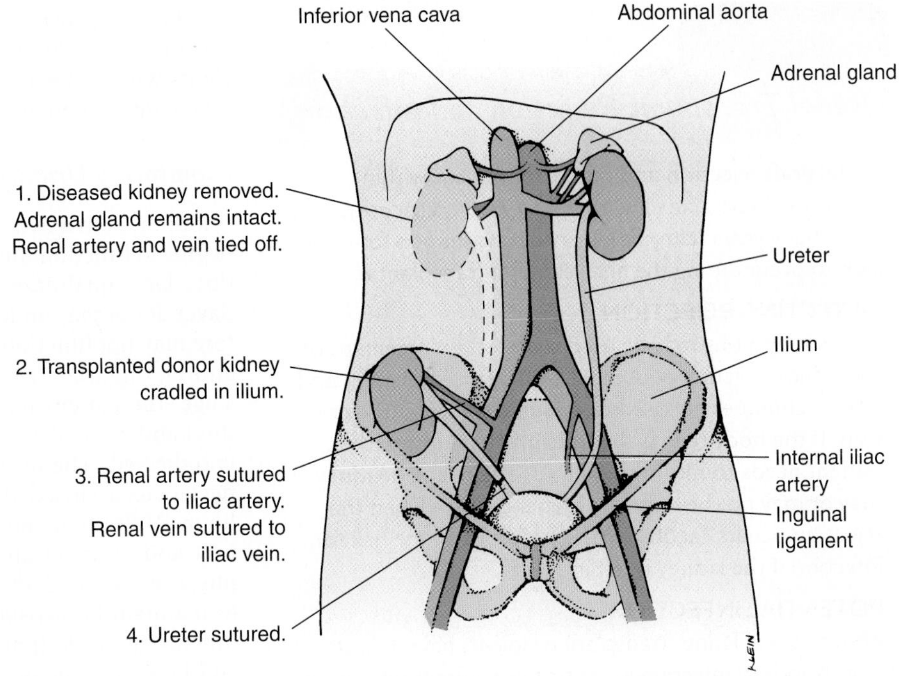
Inferior vena cava
Abdominal aorta
Adrenal gland
1. Diseased kidney removed. Adrenal gland remains intact. Renal artery and vein tied off.
Ureter
2. Transplanted donor kidney cradled in ilium.
Ilium
3. Renal artery sutured to iliac artery. Renal vein sutured to iliac vein.
Internal iliac artery
Inguinal ligament
4. Ureter sutured.

FIGURE 44-11. Renal transplantation: (1) The diseased kidney may be removed and the renal artery and vein tied off. (2) The transplanted kidney is placed in the iliac fossa. (3) The renal artery of the donated kidney is sutured to the iliac artery, and the renal vein is sutured to the iliac vein. (4) The ureter of the donated kidney is sutured to the bladder or to the patient's ureter.

restrictions, IV and arterial lines, tubes (indwelling catheter and possibly a nasogastric tube), and early ambulation. The patient who receives a kidney from a living related donor may be concerned about the donor and how the donor will tolerate the surgical procedure.

Most patients have been on dialysis for months or years before transplantation. Many have waited months to years for a kidney transplant and are anxious about the surgery, possible rejection, and the need to return to dialysis. Helping the patient to deal with these concerns is part of the nurse's role in preoperative management, as is teaching the patient about what to expect after surgery.

Postoperative Management

The goal of care is to maintain homeostasis until the transplanted kidney is functioning well. The patient whose kidney functions immediately has a more favorable prognosis than the patient whose kidney does not.

Medical Management

The survival of a transplanted kidney depends on the ability to block the body's immune response to the transplanted kidney. To overcome or minimize the body's defense mechanism, immunosuppressive agents are administered. The use of corticosteroid agents is limited because of long-term side effects (Woodle, Vincento, Lorber, et al., 2005). Cyclosporine is available in a microemulsion form (Neoral) that delivers the medication reliably, thus producing a steady-state serum concentration. Tacrolimus (Prograf) is similar to cyclosporine and about 100 times more potent. Mycophenolate mofetil (CellCept), sirolimus (Rapamune), and antithymocyte globulin (Thymoglobulin), as well as tacrolimus, are used in various combinations to prevent transplant rejection. Treatment with combinations of these new agents has dramatically improved survival rates. Immunosuppressive therapy after kidney transplantation continues to evolve (Halloran, 2004).

Doses of immunosuppressive agents are gradually reduced (tapered) over a period of several weeks, depending on the patient's immunologic response to the transplant. However, the patient is required to take some form of immunosuppressive therapy for the entire time that he or she has the transplanted kidney (Chart 44-11).

The risks associated with these medications include nephrotoxicity, hypertension, hyperlipidemia, hirsutism, tremor, and several types of cancers (Halloran, 2004). Sirolimus may have antineoplastic effects compared with cyclosporine (Stallone, Schena, Infante, et al., 2005); mycophenolate may increase the risk for cytomegalovirus disease.

Nursing Management

Assessing the Patient for Transplant Rejection

After kidney transplantation, the nurse assesses the patient for signs and symptoms of transplant rejection: oliguria, edema, fever, increasing blood pressure, weight gain, and swelling or tenderness over the transplanted kidney or graft. Patients receiving cyclosporine may not exhibit the usual signs and symptoms of acute rejection. In these patients, the only sign may be an asymptomatic rise in the serum creatinine level (more than a 20% rise is considered acute rejection).

Preventing Infection

The results of blood chemistry tests and leukocyte and platelet counts are monitored closely, because immuno-

CHART 44-11

Renal Transplant Rejection and Infection

Renal graft rejection and failure may occur within 24 hours (hyperacute), within 3 to 14 days (acute), or after many years (chronic). It is not uncommon for rejection to occur during the first year after transplantation.

DETECTING REJECTION

Ultrasonography may be used to detect enlargement of the kidney; percutaneous renal biopsy (most reliable) and x-ray techniques are used to evaluate transplant rejection. If the body rejects the transplanted kidney, the patient needs to return to dialysis. The rejected kidney may or may not be removed, depending on when the rejection occurs (acute versus chronic) and the risk for infection if the kidney is left in place.

POTENTIAL INFECTION

About 75% of kidney transplant recipients have at least one episode of infection in the first year after transplantation because of immunosuppressant therapy. Immunosuppressants of the past made the transplant recipient more vulnerable to opportunistic infections (candidiasis, cytomegalovirus, *Pneumocystis* pneumonia) and infection with other relatively nonpathogenic viruses, fungi, and protozoa, which can be a major hazard. Cyclosporine therapy has reduced the incidence of opportunistic infections because it selectively exerts its effect, sparing T cells that protect the patient from life-threatening infections. In addition, combination immunosuppressant therapy and improved clinical care have produced 1-year patient survival rates approaching 100% and graft survival exceeding 90%. Infections, however, remain a major cause of death at all points in time for kidney transplant recipients (Danovitch, 2005).

suppression depresses the formation of leukocytes and platelets. The patient is closely monitored for infection because of susceptibility to impaired healing and infection related to immunosuppressive therapy and complications of renal failure. Clinical manifestations of infection include shaking chills, fever, rapid heartbeat (tachycardia), and respirations (tachypnea), as well as either an increase or a decrease in WBCs (leukocytosis or leukopenia).

Infection may be introduced through the urinary tract, the respiratory tract, the surgical site, or other sources. Urine cultures are performed frequently because of the high incidence of bacteriuria during early and late stages of transplantation. Any type of wound drainage should be viewed as a potential source of infection because drainage is an excellent culture medium for bacteria. Catheter and drain tips may be cultured when removed by cutting off the tip of the catheter or drain (using aseptic technique) and placing the tip in a sterile container to be taken to the laboratory for culture.

The nurse ensures that the patient is protected from exposure to infection by hospital staff, visitors, and other patients with active infections. Careful hand hygiene by all who come in contact with the patient is imperative.

Monitoring Urinary Function

A kidney from a living donor related to the patient usually begins to function immediately after surgery and may produce large quantities of dilute urine. A kidney from a cadaver donor may undergo acute tubular necrosis and therefore may not function for 2 or 3 weeks, during which time anuria, oliguria, or polyuria may be present. During this stage, the patient may experience significant changes in fluid and electrolyte status. Therefore, careful monitoring is indicated. The output from the urinary catheter (connected to a closed drainage system) is measured every hour. IV fluids are administered on the basis of urine volume and serum electrolyte levels and as prescribed by the physician. Hemodialysis may be necessary postoperatively to maintain homeostasis until the transplanted kidney is functioning well. It also may be required if fluid overload and hyperkalemia occur (Perico, Cattaneo, Sayegh, et al., 2004). After successful renal transplantation, the vascular access device may clot, possibly from improved coagulation with the return of renal function. The vascular access for hemodialysis is monitored to ensure patency and to evaluate for evidence of infection.

Addressing Psychological Concerns

The rejection of a transplanted kidney remains a matter of great concern to the patient, the family, and the health care team for many months. The fears of kidney rejection and the complications of immunosuppressive therapy (Cushing's syndrome, diabetes, capillary fragility, osteoporosis, glaucoma, cataracts, acne, nephrotoxicity) place tremendous psychological stresses on the patient. Anxiety and uncertainty about the future and difficult posttransplantation adjustment are often sources of stress for the patient and family.

An important nursing function is the assessment of the patient's stress and coping. The nurse uses each visit with the patient to determine if the patient and family are coping effectively and the patient is adhering to the prescribed medication regimen. If indicated or requested, the nurse refers the patient for counseling.

Monitoring and Managing Potential Complications

The patient undergoing kidney transplantation is at risk for the postoperative complications that are associated with any surgical procedure. In addition, the patient's physical condition may be compromised because of the complications associated with long-standing renal failure and its treatment. Therefore, careful assessment for the complications related to renal failure and those associated with a major surgical procedure are important aspects of nursing care. Strategies that promote surgical recovery (breathing exercises, early ambulation, care of the surgical incision) are important aspects of postoperative care.

GI ulceration and corticosteroid-induced bleeding may occur. Fungal colonization of the GI tract (especially the mouth) and urinary bladder may occur secondary to corticosteroid and antibiotic therapy. Closely monitoring the patient and notifying the physician about the occurrence of these complications are important nursing interventions. In addition, the patient is monitored closely for signs and symptoms of adrenal insufficiency if the treatment has included use of corticosteroids.

Promoting Home and Community-Based Care

TEACHING PATIENTS SELF-CARE

The nurse works closely with the patient and family to be sure that they understand the need for continuing immunosuppressive therapy as prescribed. Additionally, the patient and family are instructed to assess for and report signs and symptoms of transplant rejection, infection, or significant adverse effects of the immunosuppressive regimen. These include decreased urine output; weight gain; malaise; fever; respiratory distress; tenderness over the transplanted kidney; anxiety; depression; changes in eating, drinking, or other habits; and changes in blood pressure. The patient is instructed to inform other health care providers (eg, dentist) about the kidney transplant and the use of immunosuppressive agents.

CONTINUING CARE

The patient needs to know that follow-up care after transplantation is a lifelong necessity. Individual verbal and written instructions are provided concerning diet, medication, fluids, daily weight, daily measurement of urine, management of intake and output, prevention of infection, resumption of activity, and avoidance of contact sports in which the transplanted kidney may be injured. Because of the risk for other potential complications, the patient is followed closely. Cardiovascular disease is now the major cause of morbidity and mortality after transplantation, due in part to the increasing age of patients with transplants. An additional problem is possible malignancy; patients receiving long-term immunosuppressive therapy have been found to develop cancers more frequently than the general population. The incidence rate of Kaposi's sarcoma in patients following organ transplant, for example, is 500 times the rate found in the general population (Stallone et al., 2005). Because of the usual need for health promotion along with the increased risks of malignancy because of immunosuppressive therapy, the patient is reminded of the importance of health promotion and health screening.

The American Association of Kidney Patients (listed at the end of this chapter) is a nonprofit organization that serves the needs of those with kidney disease. It can provide many helpful suggestions for patients and family members learning to cope with dialysis and transplantation.

Renal Cancer

Renal cancer accounts for about 3% of all cancers in adults in the United States and is the sixth leading cause of cancer deaths (Curti, 2004). It affects almost twice as many men as women. In the United States, the incidence of renal cancer at all stages has increased in the past 2 decades. The incidence of renal cell carcinoma is higher in both men and women with an increased body mass index (Bjorge, Trettli & Engeland, 2004). Tobacco use continues to be a significant risk factor for renal carcinoma (Chart 44-12).

The most common type of renal carcinoma comes from the renal epithelium and accounts for more than 85% of all kidney tumors. These tumors may metastasize early to the lungs, bone, liver, brain, and contralateral kidney. One quarter of patients have metastatic disease at the time of diagnosis. Although enhanced imaging techniques account for improved detection of early-stage kidney cancer, it is unknown why the rate of late-stage kidney cancers is higher (Cohen & McGovern, 2005).

Clinical Manifestations

Many renal tumors produce no symptoms and are discovered on a routine physical examination as a palpable abdominal mass. The classic triad of signs and symptoms, which occurs in only 10% of patients, are hematuria, pain, and a mass in the flank (Cohen & McGovern, 2005). The usual sign that first calls attention to the tumor is painless hematuria, which may be either intermittent and microscopic or continuous and gross. There may be a dull pain in the back from the pressure produced by compression of the ureter, extension of the tumor into the perirenal area, or hemorrhage into the kidney tissue. Colicky pains occur if a clot or mass of tumor cells passes down the ureter. Symptoms from metastasis may be the first manifestations of renal tumor and may include unexplained weight loss, increasing weakness, and anemia.

Assessment and Diagnostic Findings

The diagnosis of a renal tumor may require IV urography, cystoscopic examination, nephrotomograms, renal angiograms, ultrasonography, or a CT scan. These tests may be exhausting for patients already debilitated by the systemic effects of a tumor as well as for elderly patients and those who are anxious about the diagnosis and outcome. The nurse assists the patient to prepare physically and psychologically for these procedures and monitors carefully for signs and symptoms of dehydration and exhaustion.

CHART 44-12

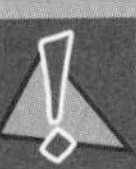

Risk Factors for Renal Cancer

- Gender: Affects men more than women
- Tobacco use
- Occupational exposure to industrial chemicals, such as petroleum products, heavy metals, and asbestos
- Obesity
- Unopposed estrogen therapy
- Polycystic kidney disease

Medical Management

The goal of management is to eradicate the tumor before metastasis occurs (Kirkali, Tuzel & Munga, 2002).

Surgical Management

A radical nephrectomy is the preferred treatment if the tumor can be removed. This includes removal of the kidney (and tumor), adrenal gland, surrounding perinephric fat and Gerota's fascia, and lymph nodes. Laparoscopic nephrectomy can be performed for removal of the kidney with a small tumor. This procedure incurs less morbidity and a shorter recovery time (Curti, 2004). Radiation therapy, hormonal therapy, or chemotherapy may be used along with surgery. Immunotherapy may also be helpful. For patients with bilateral tumors or cancer of a functional single kidney, nephron-sparing surgery (partial nephrectomy) may be considered. Favorable results have been achieved in patients with small local tumors and a normal contralateral kidney (Cohen & McGovern, 2005; Saranchuk, Tourijer, Hakimian et al., 2004).

Nephron-sparing surgery is increasingly being used to treat patients with solid renal lesions. The technical success rate of nephron-sparing surgery is excellent, and operative morbidity and mortality are low.

Patients with upper tract transitional cell carcinoma may benefit from laparoscopic nephroureterectomy. Although it is a lengthier surgical procedure, it has the same efficacy and is better tolerated by patients than open nephroureterectomy.

RENAL ARTERY EMBOLIZATION

In patients with metastatic renal carcinoma, the renal artery may be occluded to impede the blood supply to the tumor and thus kill the tumor cells. After angiographic studies are completed, a catheter is advanced into the renal artery, and embolizing materials (Gelfoam, autologous blood clot, steel coils) are injected into the artery and carried with the arterial blood flow to occlude the tumor vessels mechanically. This decreases the local blood supply, making removal of the kidney (nephrectomy) easier. It also stimulates an immune response because infarction of the renal cell carcinoma releases tumor-associated antigens that enhance the patient's response to metastatic lesions. The procedure may also reduce the number of tumor cells entering the venous circulation during surgical manipulation.

After renal artery embolization and tumor infarction, a characteristic symptom complex called postinfarction syndrome occurs, lasting 2 to 3 days. The patient has pain localized to the flank and abdomen, elevated temperature, and GI symptoms. Pain is treated with parenteral analgesic agents, and acetaminophen is administered to control fever. Antiemetic medications, restriction of oral intake, and IV fluids are used to treat the GI symptoms.

Pharmacologic Therapy

Currently, no pharmacologic agents are in widespread use for treatment of renal cell carcinoma, which is refractory to most chemotherapeutic agents (Curti, 2004). However, depending on the stage of the tumor, percutaneous partial or radical nephrectomy may be followed by treatment with chemotherapeutic agents. Radiation therapy may be used for palliation in patients who are not eligible for surgery.

Treatment with biologic response modifiers such as interleukin-2 (IL-2) is effective. IL-2, a protein that regulates cell growth, is used alone or in combination with lymphokine-activated killer cells (WBCs that have been stimulated by IL-2 to increase their ability to kill cancer cells). Interferon, another biologic response modifier, appears to have a direct antiproliferative effect on renal tumors. The study of these biologic agents and new biologic response modifiers has become a priority.

Another promising experimental approach to renal cell carcinoma is a vaccination to stimulate immune response. Those studied include autologous tumor cell–, autologous tumor cells with IL-2–, granulocyte-macrophage stimulating factor–, and dendritic cell–type vaccines (Curti, 2004).

If patients with renal cancer do not respond to immunotherapy, allogeneic stem-cell transplantation is an evolving therapy (Cohen & McGovern, 2005).

Nursing Management

The patient with a renal tumor usually undergoes extensive diagnostic and therapeutic procedures. Treatment includes surgery, radiation therapy, and medication (or systemic) therapy. After surgery, the patient usually has catheters and drains in place to maintain a patent urinary tract, to remove drainage, and to permit accurate measurement of urine output. Because of the location of the surgical incision, the position of the patient during surgery, and the nature of the surgical procedure, pain and muscle soreness are common.

The patient requires frequent analgesia during the postoperative period and assistance with turning. Turning, coughing, use of incentive spirometry, and deep breathing are encouraged to prevent atelectasis and other pulmonary complications. The patient and family require assistance and support to cope with the diagnosis and uncertainties about the prognosis. (See this chapter for discussion of postoperative care of the patient undergoing kidney surgery and Chapter 16 for discussion of care of the patient with cancer.)

Promoting Home and Community-Based Care

TEACHING PATIENTS SELF-CARE

The patient is taught to inspect and care for the incision and perform other general postoperative care. Additionally, the patient learns about activity and lifting restrictions, driving, and pain management. Instructions are provided about follow-up care and when to notify the physician about problems (fever, breathing difficulty, wound drainage, blood in the urine, pain or swelling of the legs).

The patient is encouraged to eat a healthy diet and to drink adequate liquids to avoid constipation and to maintain an adequate urine volume. Education and emotional support are provided related to the disease process, treatment plan, and continuing care because many patients are concerned about the loss of the other kidney, the possible need for dialysis, or the recurrence of cancer.

CONTINUING CARE

Follow-up care is essential to detect signs of metastases and to reassure the patient and family about the patient's status and well-being. The patient who has had surgery for renal carcinoma should have a yearly physical examination and chest x-ray, because late metastases are not uncommon. All subsequent symptoms should be evaluated with possible metastases in mind.

If follow-up chemotherapy is necessary, the patient and family are informed about the entire treatment plan or chemotherapy protocol, what to expect with each visit, and how and when to notify the physician. Periodic evaluation of remaining renal function (creatinine clearance, BUN and serum creatinine levels) may also be carried out periodically. A home care nurse may monitor the patient's physical status and psychological well-being and coordinate other services and resources needed by the patient.

Renal Trauma

The kidneys are protected by the rib cage and musculature of the back posteriorly and by a cushion of abdominal wall and viscera anteriorly. They are highly mobile and are fixed only at the renal pedicle (stem of renal blood vessels and the ureter). With traumatic injury, the kidneys can be thrust against the lower ribs, resulting in contusion and rupture. Rib fractures or fractures of the transverse process of the upper lumbar vertebrae may be associated with renal contusion or laceration. Failure to wear seat belts contributes to the incidence of renal trauma in motor vehicle crashes. Up to 80% of patients with renal trauma have associated injuries of other internal organs.

Injuries may be blunt (automobile and motorcycle crashes, falls, athletic injuries, assaults) or penetrating (gunshot wounds, stabbings) (Itagaki & Knight, 2004). Blunt renal trauma accounts for 80% to 90% of all renal injuries; penetrating renal trauma accounts for the remaining 10% to 20% (Brenner, 2004). Blunt renal trauma is classified into one of four groups, as follows:

- Contusion: bruises or hemorrhages under the renal capsule; capsule and collecting system intact
- Minor laceration: superficial disruption of the cortex; renal medulla and collecting system are not involved
- Major laceration: parenchymal disruption extending into cortex and medulla, possibly involving the collecting system
- Vascular injury: tears of renal artery or vein

The most common renal injuries are contusions, lacerations, ruptures, and renal pedicle injuries or small internal lacerations of the kidney (Fig. 44-12). The kidneys receive half of the blood flow from the abdominal aorta; therefore, even a fairly small renal laceration can produce massive bleeding. About 70% of patients are in shock when admitted to the hospital. In some cases, there is an isolated renal artery thrombosis (Kau, Patel, & Shah, 2004).

Clinical manifestations include pain, renal colic (due to blood clots or fragments obstructing the collecting system), hematuria, mass or swelling in the flank, ecchymoses, and lacerations or wounds of the lateral abdomen and flank. Hematuria is the most common manifestation of renal trauma; its presence after trauma suggests renal injury. There is no relationship between the degree of hematuria and the degree of injury. Hematuria may not occur, or it may be detectable only on microscopic examination. Signs and symptoms of hypovolemia and shock are likely with significant hemorrhage.

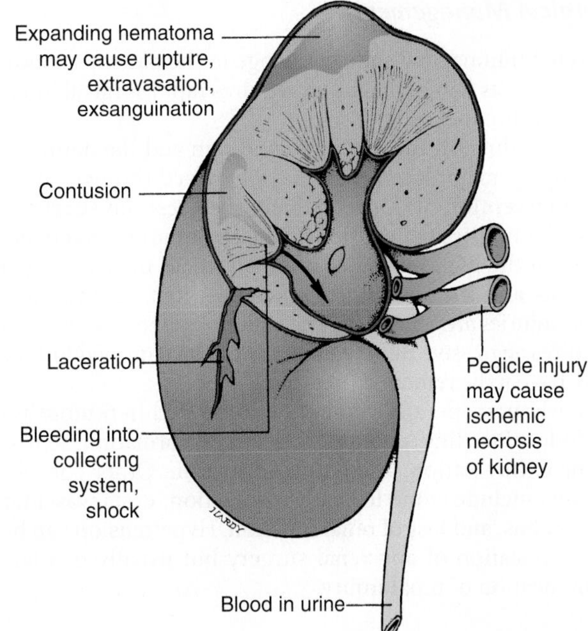

FIGURE 44-12. Types and pathophysiologic effects of renal injuries: contusions, lacerations, rupture, and pedicle injury.

Medical Management

The goals of management in patients with renal trauma are to control hemorrhage, pain, and infection as well as to preserve and restore renal function. All urine is saved and sent to the laboratory for analysis to detect RBCs and to evaluate the course of bleeding. Hematocrit and hemoglobin levels are monitored closely; decreasing values indicate hemorrhage.

The patient is monitored for oliguria and signs of hemorrhagic shock, because a pedicle injury or shattered kidney can lead to rapid exsanguination (lethal blood loss). An expanding hematoma may cause rupture of the kidney capsule. To detect hematoma, the area around the lower ribs, upper lumbar vertebrae, flank, and abdomen is palpated for tenderness. A palpable flank or abdominal mass with local tenderness, swelling, and ecchymosis suggests renal hemorrhage. The area of the original mass can be outlined with a marking pen so that the examiner can evaluate the area for change.

Renal trauma is often associated with other injuries to the abdominal organs (liver, colon, small intestines); therefore, the patient is assessed for skin abrasions, lacerations, and entry and exit wounds of the upper abdomen and lower thorax because these may be associated with renal injury.

With a contusion of the kidney, healing may take place with conservative measures. If the patient has microscopic hematuria and a normal IV urogram, outpatient management is possible. If gross hematuria or a minor laceration is present, the patient is hospitalized and kept on bed rest until the hematuria clears. Antimicrobial medications may be prescribed to prevent infection from perirenal hematoma or urinoma (a cyst containing urine). Patients with retroperitoneal hematomas may develop low-grade fever as absorption of the clot takes place.

Surgical Management

In renal trauma, any sudden change in the patient's condition suggests hemorrhage and requires rapid surgical intervention (Brenner, 2004).

Depending on the patient's condition and the nature of the injury, major lacerations may be treated through surgical intervention or conservatively (bed rest, no surgery). Vascular injuries require immediate exploratory surgery because of the high incidence of involvement of other organ systems and the serious complications that may result if these injuries are untreated. The patient is often in shock and requires aggressive fluid resuscitation. The damaged kidney may have to be removed (nephrectomy).

Early postoperative complications (within 6 months) include rebleeding, perinephritic abscess formation, sepsis, urine extravasation, and fistula formation. Other complications include stone formation, infection, cysts, vascular aneurysms, and loss of renal function. Hypertension can be a complication of any renal surgery but usually is a late complication of renal injury.

Nursing Management

The patient with renal trauma must be assessed frequently during the first few days after injury to detect flank and abdominal pain, muscle spasm, and swelling over the flank. During this time, the patient who has undergone surgery is instructed about care of the incision and the importance of an adequate fluid intake. In addition, instructions about changes that should be reported to the physician, such as fever, hematuria, flank pain, or any signs and symptoms of decreasing kidney function, are provided. Guidelines for gradually increasing activity, lifting, and driving are also provided in accordance with the physician's prescription.

Follow-up nursing care includes monitoring the blood pressure to detect hypertension and advising the patient to restrict activities for about 1 month after trauma to minimize the incidence of delayed or secondary bleeding. The patient should be advised to schedule periodic follow-up assessments of renal function (creatinine clearance, BUN and serum creatinine analyses). If a nephrectomy was necessary, the patient is advised to wear medical identification.

Critical Thinking Exercises

1 You are a staff nurse in an outpatient dialysis facility. A 50-year-old man with renal failure secondary to poorly controlled diabetes is scheduled to be seen in the clinic; it is anticipated that he will need dialysis in the near future. The patient and his wife require teaching about the dialysis options. Develop a teaching plan to explain the different types of dialysis, goals, and level of involvement on the part of the patient and family. How would you modify the approach if the patient is distraught and does not seem to hear what you are saying?

2 ebp A 45-year-old married woman with three teenage children visits the nephrology department to discuss options for dealing with her ESRD. Her healthy twin sister has begun the workup to donate one of her kidneys to her sister, and the preliminary reports show that a match is possible. The patient states that she does not want her sister to go through the process of kidney donation if dialysis is possible. Identify the evidence for and the criteria used to evaluate the strength of the evidence for dialysis compared to kidney transplantation.

3 You are treating a 35-year-old woman who is in the emergency department following a motor vehicle crash complaining of severe left-sided flank pain. Identify possible causes of her pain and laboratory tests that would be indicated. What nursing assessment and interventions should you make at this time? What explanations would you give the patient while awaiting the results of laboratory tests?

4 A 55-year-old man who is deaf has just had a catheter placed for peritoneal dialysis. His wife, his primary caretaker, is also deaf. Develop a teaching plan to explain peritoneal dialysis, goals, and level of involvement to the patient and family.

REFERENCES AND SELECTED READINGS

BOOKS

Bickley, L. S. & Szilagyi, P. G. (2003). *Bates' guide to physical examination and history taking* (8th ed.). Philadelphia: Lippincott Williams & Wilkins.

Brady, H. R. & Wilcox, C. S. (2003). *Therapy in nephrology and hypertension* (2nd ed.). St Louis: Elsevier Saunders.

Brenner, B. M (2004). *Brenner & Rector's the kidney* (7th ed.). Philadelphia: Saunders.

Danovitch, G. M. (Ed.) (2005). *Handbook of kidney transplantation.* Philadelphia: Lippincott Williams & Wilkins.

Goshorn, J. (2005). Acute renal failure. In M. L. Sole, D. G. Klein, & M. J. Moseley (Eds.). *Introduction to critical care nursing.* St Louis: Elsevier Saunders.

Hricik, D., Miller, R. T. & Sedor, J. R. (2003). *Nephrology secrets* (2nd ed.). Philadelphia: Hanley and Belfus.

Levy, J., Morgan, J. & Brown, E. (2004). *Oxford handbook of dialysis* (2nd ed.). Oxford: Oxford University Press.

Morton, P. G., Fontaine, D. K., Hudak, C. M., et al. (2005). *Critical care nursing: A holistic approach* (8th ed.). Philadelphia: Lippincott Williams & Wilkins.

Mulzahn, A., & Butera, E. (2006). *Contemporary nephrology nursing: Principles and practice* (2nd ed.). Pitman, NJ: American Nephrology Nurses' Association.

Porth, C. M. (2005). *Pathophysiology: Concepts of altered health states* (7th ed.). Philadelphia: Lippincott Williams & Wilkins.

Schrier, R. W. (Ed.) (2005). *Manual of nephrology* (6th ed.). Philadelphia: Lippincott Williams & Wilkins.

Stanley, M., Blair, K. A., & Beare, P. G. (2005). *Gerontological nursing: Promoting successful aging with older adults* (3rd ed.). Philadelphia: F. A. Davis.

Zonderman, J. & Doyle, R. (2006). *Springhouse nurse's drug guide 2006.* Philadelphia: Lippincott Williams & Wilkins.

JOURNALS

**Asterisks indicate nursing research articles.*

General

*Bengtson, A. & Drevenhorn, E. (2003). The nurse's role and skills in hypertension care. *Clinical Nurse Specialist, 17*(5), 260–268.

Brenner, Z. R. & Myer, S. (2003). Acetylcysteine and nephropathy. *American Journal of Nursing, 103*(3), 64AA-64DD.

Burrows-Hudson, S. (2005). Chronic kidney disease: An overview: Early and aggressive treatment is vital. *American Journal of Nursing, 105*(2), 40–50.

*Calvin, A. O. (2004). Haemodialysis patients and end-of-life decisions: A theory of personal preservation. *Journal of Advanced Nursing, 46*(5), 558–566.

Futterman, L. G. & Lemberg, L. (2002). Focus: hypertension for the aged population. *American Journal of Critical Care, 11*(1), 80–86.

Gersch, M. S. (2004). Treatment of dialysis catheter infections. *Journal of Vascular Access, 5*(11), 99–108.

Go, A. S., Chertow, G. M., Fan, D., et al. (2004). Chronic kidney disease and risks of death, cardiovascular events, and hospitalization. *New England Journal of Medicine, 351*(13), 1296–305.

Goodman, E. D. & Ballou, M. B. (2004). Perceived barriers and motivators to exercise in hemodialysis patients. *Nephrology Nursing Journal: Journal of the American Nephrology Nurses Association, 31*(1), 23–29.

Hinds, A. C. (2004). Obstructive uropathy: Considerations for nephrology nurses. *Nephrology Nursing Journal: Journal of the American Nephrology Nurses Association, 31*(2), 166–181.

Hyjariri, N., Afzali, B. & Goldsmith, D. J. (2004). Cardiac calcification in renal patients: What we do and don't know. *American Journal of Kidney Disease, 43*(2), 234–243.

Johnson, C. A., Levey, A. S, Coresh, J., et al. (2004). Clinical practice guidelines for chronic kidney disease in adults: Part II. Glomerular filtrations rate, proteinuria, and other markers. *American Family Physician, 70*(6), 869–876.

*Kugler, C., Vlaminck, H., Haverich A., et al. (2005) Nonadherance with diet and fluid restrictions among adults having hemodialysis. *Journal of Nursing Scholarship, 37*(1), 25–29.

Leydig, E. J. (2005). Are you endangering your patients? *RN, 68*(2), 29–31.

Mikrut, M. & Brockmiller-Sell, H. (2004). Sodium polystyrene sulfonate dosing guidelines for the treatment of adult hyperkalemia. *Hospital Pharmacy, 39*, 765–771.

Nguyen, T. V. & Dikun, M. (2004). Establishing an alteplase dosing protocol for hemodialysis-catheter thrombosis. *American Journal of Health-System Pharmacy, 61*(18), 1922–1924.

Painter, P., Carlson, L., Carey, S., et al. (2004). Determinants of exercise encouragement practices in hemodialysis staff. *Nephrology Nursing Journal: Journal of the American Nephrology Nurses Association, 31*(1), 67–74.

Pile, C. (2004). Hemodialysis vascular access: How do practice patterns affect outcomes? *Nephrology Nursing Journal: Journal of the American Nephrology Nurses Association, 31*(3), 305–308.

Sturm, B., Laggner, H., Ternes N., et al. (2005). Intravenous iron preparations and ascorbic acid: Effects on chelatable and bioavailable iron. *Kidney International, 67*(3), 1161–1176.

Szromba, C., Thies, M. A. & Ossman, S. S. (2002). Advancing chronic kidney disease care: New imperatives for recognition and intervention. *Nephrology Nursing Journal: Journal of the American Nephrology Nurses Association, 29*(6), 547–560.

*Thomas, S. A., Liehr, P., De Keyser, F., et al. (2002). A review of nursing research on blood pressure. *Journal of Nursing Scholarship, 34*(4), 313–321.

Thomas-Hawkins, C. & Zazworsky, D. (2005). Self-management of chronic kidney disease. *American Journal of Nursing, 105*(10), 40–49.

Thompson, E. J. & King, S. T. (2003). Acetylcysteine and Fenoldopam promising new approaches for preventing effects of contrast nephrotoxicity. *Critical Care Nurse, 23*(3), 39–46.

Tilley, B. (2004). Red blood cell physiology, Epogen alfa and iron. *Nephrology Nursing Journal: Journal of the American Nephrology Nurses Association, 31*(1), 75–78.

van Onna, M., Houben, A. J, Kroon, A. A., et al. (2003). Asymmetry of renal blood flow in patients with moderate to severe hypertension. *Hypertension, 41*(1), 108–120.

Wells, C. (2003). Optimizing nutrition in patients with chronic kidney disease. *Nephrology Nursing Journal: Journal of the American Nephrology Nurses Association, 30*(6), 637–648.

Acute Renal Failure

Bagshaw, S. M., Peets, A. D., Hameed, M., et al. (2004). Dialysis disequilibrium syndrome: Brain death following hemodialysis for metabolic acidosis and acute renal failure report. *BMC Nephrology, 5*(1), 9.

Bonventre, J. V. & Weinberg, J. M. (2003). Recent advances in the pathophysiology of ischemic acute renal failure. *Journal of the American Society of Nephrology, 14*(8), 2199–2210.

Campbell, D (2003). How acute renal failure puts the breaks on kidney function. *Nursing 2003, 33*(1), 59–64.

Criddle, L. M. (2003). Rhabdomyolysis pathophysiology, recognition, and management. *Critical Care Nurse, 23*(6), 14–32.

Delanaye, P., Bovy, C., de Leval, L., et al. (2004). Back pain and renal failure. *Lancet, 364*(9449), 1992.

D'Intini, V, Ronco, C, Bonello, M., et al. (2004). Renal replacement therapy in acute renal failure. *Best Practice & Research. Clinical Anesthesiology, 18*(1), 145–157.

Mehta, R. L. & Chertow, G. M. (2003). Acute renal failure definitions and classifications: Time for change. *Journal of the American Society of Nephrology, 14*(8), 2178–2187.

Singri, N., Ahya, S. N. & Levin, M. L. (2003). Acute renal failure. *Journal of the American Medical Association, 289*(6), 747–751.

Swartz, R., Perry, E. & Daley, J. (2004). The frequency of withdrawal from acute care is impacted by severe acute renal failure. *Journal of Palliative Medicine, 7*(5), 676–682.

Chronic Renal Failure

*Boulware, L. E., Jaar, B. B., Traver-Carr, M. E., et al. (2003). Screening for proteinuria in U.S. Adults: A cost-effectiveness analysis. *Journal of the American Medical Association, 290*(2), 3101–3114.

Fox, C. S., Larson, M. G., Leip, E. P., et al. (2004). Predictors of new-onset kidney disease in a community–based population. *Journal of American Medical Association, 291*(7), 844–850.

Holley, J. L. (2003). Advance care planning in the elderly chronic dialysis patient. *International Urology Nursing, 35*(4), 565–568.

Ikizier, T. A. (2004). Poor nutritional status and inflammation protein and energy: Recommended intake and nutritional supplementation in chronic dialysis patients. *Seminars in Dialysis, 17*(6), 471–478.

Qunibi, W. Y., Hootkins, R. E., McDowell, L. L., et al. (2004). Treatment of hyperphosphatemia in hemodialysis patients: The calcium acetate Renagel evaluation (CARE study). *Kidney International, 65*(5), 1914–1926.

Roy-Chaudhury, P. Kelly, B. S., Melhem, T., et al. (2005). Novel therapies for hemodialysis vascular access dysfunction: fact or fiction! *Blood Purification, 23*(1), 29–35.

Tangalos, E. G., Hoggard, J. G., Murray, A. M., et al. (2004). Treatment of kidney disease and anemia in elderly, long-term care residents. *Journal of the American Medical Directors Association, 5*(4), H1-H6.

U.S. Renal Data System (2004). *USRDS 2004 annual data report: Atlas of end-stage renal disease in the United States*. Bethesda, MD: National Institutes of Health, National Institute of Diabetes and Digestive and Kidney Diseases. Available at: http://www.usrds.org/adr.htm. Accessed July 10, 2006.

Disorders of the Kidney

Cashion, A. K. & Driscoll, C. J. (2004). Genetics and kidney dysfunction. *Nephrology Nursing Journal: Journal of the American Nephrology Nurses Association, 31*(1), 14–18.

Weening, J. J., D'Ageti, V. D, Schwartz, M. M., et al. (2004). The classification of glomerulonephritis in systemic lupus erythematosus revisited. *Kidney International, 65*(2), 521–530.

Dialysis

*Gordon, E. J., Leon, J. & Sehgal, A. (2003). Why are hemodialysis treatments shortened or skipped? Development of a taxonomy and relationship to patient subgroups. *Nephrology Nursing Journal: Journal of the American Nephrology Nurses Association, 30*(2), 209–217.

Bernardini, J. (2004). Peritoneal dialysis: Myths, barriers, and achieving optimum outcomes. *Nephrology Nursing Journal: Journal of the American Nephrology Nurses Association, 31*(5), 494–498.

*Hall, G., Bogan, A., Dreis, S., et al. (2004). New directions in dialysis patient training. *Nephrology Nursing Journal: Journal of the American Nephrology Nurses Association, 31*(2), 149–163.

Kaplow, R. & Barry, R. (2002). Continuous renal replacement therapies. *American Journal of Nursing: Journal of the American Nephrology Nurses Association, 102*(11), 26–33.

Kelley, K. T. (2004). How peritoneal dialysis works. *Nephrology Nursing Journal, 31*(5), 481–490.

Polaschek, N. (2003). The experience of living on dialysis: A literature review. *Nephrology Nursing Journal: Journal of the American Nephrology Nurses Association, 30*(3), 303–309.

Prowant, B. F. (2004). Peritoneal dialysis nursing: We've come a long way. *Nephrology Nursing Journal: Journal of the American Nephrology Nurses Association, 31*(5), 479–480.

Rayner, H. C., Pisoni, R. L., Gillespie, B. W., et al. (2003). Creation, cannulation and survival of arteriovenous fistulae: Data from the Dialysis Outcomes and Practice Patterns Study. *Kidney International, 63*(1), 323–30.

Kidney Transplantation

Dantal, J. & Souillou, J. P. (2005). Immunosuppressive drugs and risk of cancer after organ transplantation. *New England Journal of Medicine, 352*(13), 1371–1373.

Gonzalez, M. & Alonso, M. (2005). Pancreas islet cell transplantation in patients with type 1 diabetes mellitus after kidney transplant. *Transplant Procedure, 37*(3), 1443–1445.

Halloran, P. F. (2004). Immunosuppressive drugs for kidney transplantation. *New England Journal of Medicine, 351*(26), 2715–2729.

Heeger, P. S. & Hricik, D. (2002). Immune monitoring in kidney transplant recipients revisited. *Journal of American Society of Nephrology, 13*(1), 288–290.

Holechek, E. J., Hiller, J., Paredes, M., et al. (2003). Expanding the living organ donor pool: Positive crossmatch and ABO incompatible renal transplantation. *Nephrology Nursing Journal: Journal of the American Nephrology Nurses Association, 30*(2), 195–204.

Land, W. G. (2004). Aging and immunosuppression in kidney transplantation. *Experimental Clinical Transplant, 2*(2), 229–237.

Molzahn, A. E., & McCormick Starzomski, R. J. (2003). The supply of organs for transplantation: Issues and challenges. *Nephrology Nursing Journal: Journal of the American Nephrology Nurses Association, 30*(1), 17–28.

Najafian, N., Salama, A. D., Fedoseyeva, E. V., et al. (2002). Enzyme-linked immunosorbent spot assay analysis of peripheral blood lymphocyte reactivity to donor HLA-DR peptides: Potential novel assay for prediction of outcomes for renal transplant recipients. *Journal of American Society of Nephrology, 13*(1), 252–259.

Perico, N., Cattaneo, D., Sayegh, M. H., et al. (2004). Delayed graft function in kidney transplantation. *Lancet, 364*(9447), 1814–1827.

Ponticelli, C., Villa, A, Cesana, B., et al. (2002). Risk factors for late kidney allograft failure. *Kidney International, 62*(5), 1848–1854.

Transplant Patient DataSource. United Network for Organ Sharing. http://www.unos.org. Accessed July 10, 2006.

Woodle, E. S., Vincento, F., Lorber, M., et al. (2005). A multicenter pilot study of early (4-day) steroid cessation in renal transplant recipients under simulect, tacrolimus and sirolimus. *American Journal of Transplantation, 5*(1), 157–166.

Wolters, HH., Hendenreich, S., Dame, C., et al. (2005). Living donor kidney transplantation: Impact of differentiated immunosuppressive regime. *Transplant Procedures, 37*(3), 1616–1617.

Yakupogulu, Y. K. & Kahan, B. D. (2003). Sirolimus: a current perspective. *Experimental Clinical Transplant, 1*(1), 8–18.

Renal Carcinoma

Bjorge, T., Trettli, S. & Engeland A. (2004). Relation of height and body mass index to renal cell carcinoma in two million Norwegian men and women. *American Journal of Epidemiology, 160*(12), 1168–1176.

Cohen, H. T. & McGovern, F. J. (2005). Renal-cell carcinoma. *New England Journal of Medicine, 353*(23), 2477–2490.

Curti, B. D. (2004). Renal cell cancer. *Journal of the American Medical Association, 292*(1), 1684–1692.

Kirkali, Z., Tuzel, E., & Munga, U. (2002). Recent advances in kidney cancer and metastatic disease. *British Journal of Urology International, 88*(8), 818–824.

Ruppert-Kohlmayr A. J., Uggowitzer, M., Meissnitzer T., et al. (2004). Differentiation of renal clear cell carcinoma and renal papillary carcinoma using quantitative CT enhancement parameters. *American Journal of Roentgenology, 183*(5), 1387–1391.

Saranchuk, J. W., Tourijer, A. K., Hakimian P., et al. (2004). Partial nephrectomy for patients with solitary kidney: The Memorial Sloan-Kettering experience. *BJU International, 94*(9), 1323–1330.

Schips, L., Lipsky, K., Zigeuner R., et al. (2004). Does overweight impact on the prognosis of patients with renal cell carcinoma? A single center experience of 683 patients. *Journal of Surgical Oncology, 88*(2), 57–61.

Renal Trauma

Itagaki, M. W. & Knight, N. B. (2004). Kidney trauma in martial arts: A case report of kidney contusion in jujitsu. *American Journal of Sports Medicine, 32*(2), 522–524.

Kau, E., Patel, R. & Shah, O. (2004). Isolated renal vein thrombosis after blunt trauma. *Urology. 64*(4), 807–808.

RESOURCES

American Association of Kidney Patients, 3505 E. Frontage Road, Suite 315, Tampa, FL 33607; (800) 749–2257; http://www.aakp.org. Accessed July 10, 2006.

American Association of Nephrology Nurses, East Holly Avenue, Box 56, Pitman, NJ 08071; (888) 600-ANNA; http://www.annanurse.org. Accessed July 10, 2006.

American Foundation for Urologic Disease, 1128 N. Charles Street, Baltimore, MD 21201; (800) 242-2383; http://www.afud.org. Accessed July 10, 2006.

American Kidney Fund, 6110 Executive Blvd., Suite 1010, Rockville, MD 20852; (800) 638-8299; http://www.arbon.com/kidney. Accessed July 10, 2006.

National Institute of Diabetes and Digestive and Kidney Diseases, National Institutes of Health, Office of Communications and Public Liaison, NIDDK, NIH, Building 31, room 9A04 Center Drive, MSC 2560, Bethesda, MD 20892-2560; http://www.niddk.nih.gov. Accessed July 10, 2006.

National Kidney and Urologic Diseases Information Clearinghouse, Box NKUDIC, 9000 Rockville Pike, Bethesda, MD 20892; (301) 654-4415; http://www.niddk.nih.gov. Accessed July 10, 2006.

National Kidney Foundation, 20 East 33rd Street, New York, 10016; (800) 622-9010; http://www.kidney.org. Accessed July 10, 2006.

North American Society for Dialysis and Transplantation, c/o Wadi N. Suki, MD, 6550 Fannin, Suite 1273, Houston, TX 77030; (713) 790-3275.

United Network for Organ Sharing, Post Office Box 2484 Richmond, Virginia 23218; (888) 894-6361; http://www.unos.org. Accessed July 10, 2006.

CHAPTER 45

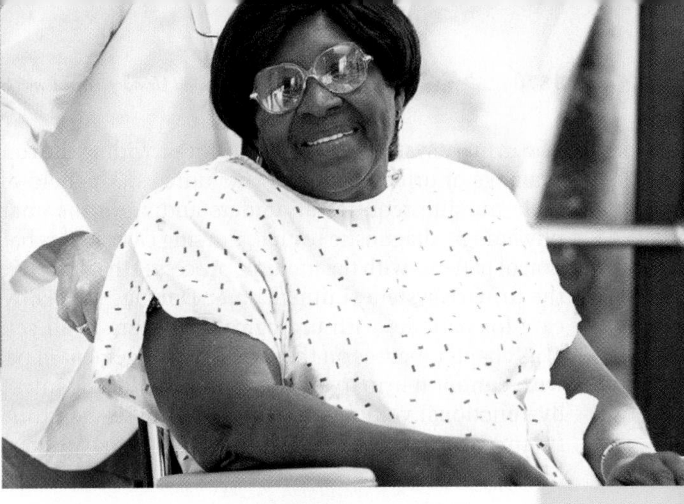

Management of Patients With Urinary Disorders

Learning Objectives

On completion of this chapter, the learner will be able to:

1. Identify factors contributing to upper and lower urinary tract infections (UTIs).
2. Use the nursing process as a framework for care of the patient with a UTI.
3. Differentiate between the various adult dysfunctional voiding patterns.
4. Develop a patient education plan for a patient who has mixed (stress and urge) urinary incontinence.
5. Identify potential causes of an obstruction of the urinary tract, and management of the patient with this condition.
6. Develop a teaching plan for the patient undergoing treatment for renal calculi (kidney stones).
7. Formulate preoperative and postoperative nursing diagnoses for the patient undergoing surgery for urinary diversion.

The urinary system is responsible for providing the route for drainage of urine formed by the kidneys. The field of urologic nursing requires an understanding of the anatomy, physiology, diagnostic testing, nursing care, and rehabilitation of patients with the multiple processes that interfere with the urinary system (Fillingham & Douglas, 2004). Nurses care for patients with urological disorders in all settings. This chapter focuses on the nursing management of patients with common urinary dysfunctions, including infections, dysfunctional voiding patterns, urolithiasis, genitourinary trauma, cancer of the urinary tract, and urinary diversions.

Infections of the Urinary Tract

Urinary tract infections (UTIs) are caused by pathogenic microorganisms in the urinary tract (the normal urinary tract is sterile above the urethra). UTIs are generally classified as infections involving the upper or lower urinary tract and further classified as uncomplicated or complicated, depending on other patient-related conditions (Chart 45-1).

Lower UTIs include bacterial **cystitis** (inflammation of the urinary bladder), bacterial **prostatitis** (inflammation of the prostate gland), and bacterial **urethritis** (inflammation of the urethra). There can be acute or chronic nonbacterial causes of inflammation in any of these areas that can be misdiagnosed as bacterial infections. Upper UTIs are much

CHART 45-1

Classifying Urinary Tract Infections

Urinary tract infections (UTIs) are classified by location: the lower urinary tract (which includes the bladder and structures below the bladder) or the upper urinary tract (which includes the kidneys and ureters). They can also be classified as uncomplicated or complicated UTIs.

LOWER UTIs

Cystitis, prostatitis, urethritis

UPPER UTIs

Acute pyelonephritis, chronic pyelonephritis, renal abscess, interstitial nephritis, perirenal abscess

UNCOMPLICATED LOWER OR UPPER UTIs

Community-acquired infection; common in young women and not usually recurrent

COMPLICATED LOWER OR UPPER UTIs

Often nosocomial (acquired in the hospital) and related to catheterization; occur in patients with urologic abnormalities, pregnancy, immunosuppression, diabetes mellitus, and obstructions and are often recurrent

Glossary

bacteriuria: more than 10^5 colonies of bacteria per milliliter of urine

continent urinary diversion (Kock or Charleston pouch): transplantation of the ureters to a segment of bowel with construction of an effective continence mechanism or valve

cystectomy: removal of the urinary bladder

cystitis: inflammation of the urinary bladder

dysuria: painful or difficult urination

frequency: voiding more often than every 3 hours

functional incontinence: physical impairments make it difficult or impossible for the patient to reach the toilet in time for voiding

iatrogenic incontinence: the involuntary loss of urine due to extrinsic medical factors, predominantly medications

ileal conduit: transplantation of the ureters to an isolated section of the terminal ileum, with one end of the ureters brought to the abdominal wall

interstitial cystitis: inflammation of the bladder wall that eventually causes disintegration of the lining and loss of bladder elasticity

micturition: voiding or urination

neurogenic bladder: bladder dysfunction that results from a disorder or dysfunction of the nervous system; may result in either urinary retention or bladder overactivity, resulting in urinary urgency and urge incontinence

nocturia: awakening at night to urinate

overflow incontinence: involuntary urine loss associated with overdistention of the bladder due to mechanical or anatomic bladder outlet obstruction

prostatitis: inflammation of the prostate gland

pyelonephritis: inflammation of the renal pelvis

pyuria: white blood cells in the urine

reflex incontinence: involuntary loss of urine due to hyperreflexia or involuntary urethral relaxation in the absence of normal sensations; usually associated with micturition (voiding)

residual urine: urine that remains in the bladder after voiding

stress incontinence: involuntary loss of urine through an intact urethra as a result of a sudden increase in intra-abdominal pressure

suprapubic catheter: a urinary catheter that is inserted through a suprapubic incision into the bladder

urge incontinence: involuntary loss of urine associated with urinary urgency due to hypersensory disorders of the bladder, motor instability, or both

urinary incontinence: involuntary or uncontrolled loss of urine from the bladder sufficient to cause a social or hygienic problem

urethritis: inflammation of the urethra

ureterosigmoidostomy: transplantation of the ureters into the sigmoid colon, allowing urine to flow through the colon and out the rectum

ureterovesical or **vesicoureteral reflux:** backward flow of urine from the bladder into one or both ureters

urethrovesical reflux: backward flow of urine from the urethra into the bladder

urosepsis: sepsis resulting from infected urine, most often a UTI

wound care specialist: a nurse specially educated in appropriate skin, wound, ostomy, and continence care; often referred to as an enterostomal therapist or a wound-ostomy-continence nurse (WOCN)

less common and include acute or chronic **pyelonephritis** (inflammation of the renal pelvis), interstitial nephritis (inflammation of the kidney), and renal abscesses. Upper and lower UTIs are further classified as uncomplicated or complicated, depending on other patient-related conditions (eg, whether the UTI is recurrent and the duration of the infection). Most uncomplicated UTIs are community-acquired. Complicated UTIs usually occur in people with urologic abnormalities or recent catheterization and are often acquired during hospitalization.

A UTI is the second most common reason patients seek health care (Porth, 2005). Most cases occur in women; one out of every five women in the United States will develop a UTI sometime during her lifetime. The urinary tract is the most common site of nosocomial infection, accounting for greater than 40% of the total number reported by hospitals and affecting about 600,000 patients each year. In most of these hospital-acquired UTIs, instrumentation of the urinary tract or catheterization is the precipitating cause. More than 250,000 cases of acute pyelonephritis occur in the United States each year, with 100,000 patients requiring hospitalization. Approximately 11.3 million women are diagnosed with UTIs in the United States annually, representing an expenditure of about $1.6 billion in direct heath care costs. This amount does not include the indirect costs associated with time lost from work and the negative impact on the person's lifestyle.

CHART 45-2

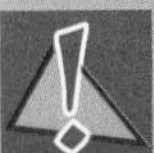

Risk Factors for Urinary Tract Infection

- Inability or failure to empty the bladder completely
- Obstructed urinary flow
  - Congenital abnormalities
  - Urethral strictures
  - Contracture of the bladder neck
  - Bladder tumors
  - Calculi (stones) in the ureters or kidneys
  - Compression of the ureters
  - Neurologic abnormalities
- Decreased natural host defenses or immunosuppression
- Instrumentation of the urinary tract (eg, catheterization, cystoscopic procedures)
- Inflammation or abrasion of the urethral mucosa
- Contributing conditions
  - Diabetes mellitus (increased urinary glucose levels create an infection-prone environment in the urinary tract)
  - Pregnancy
  - Neurologic disorders
  - Gout
  - Altered states caused by incomplete emptying of the bladder and urinary stasis

Lower Urinary Tract Infections

Several mechanisms maintain the sterility of the bladder: the physical barrier of the urethra, urine flow, ureterovesical junction competence, various antibacterial enzymes and antibodies, and antiadherent effects mediated by the mucosal cells of the bladder. Abnormalities or dysfunctions of these mechanisms are contributing risk factors for lower UTIs (Chart 45-2).

Pathophysiology

For infection to occur, bacteria must gain access to the bladder, attach to and colonize the epithelium of the urinary tract to avoid being washed out with voiding, evade host defense mechanisms, and initiate inflammation. Many UTIs result from fecal organisms that ascend from the perineum to the urethra and the bladder and then adhere to the mucosal surfaces.

Bacterial Invasion of the Urinary Tract

By increasing the normal slow shedding of bladder epithelial cells (resulting in bacteria removal), the bladder can clear even large numbers of bacteria. Glycosaminoglycan (GAG), a hydrophilic protein, normally exerts a nonadherent protective effect against various bacteria. The GAG molecule attracts water molecules, forming a water barrier that serves as a defensive layer between the bladder and the urine. GAG may be impaired by certain agents (cyclamate, saccharin, aspartame, and tryptophan metabolites). The normal bacterial flora of the vagina and urethral area also interfere with adherence of *Escherichia coli*. Urinary immunoglobulin A (IgA) in the urethra may also provide a barrier to bacteria.

Reflux

An obstruction to free-flowing urine is a problem known as **urethrovesical reflux**, which is the reflux (backward flow) of urine from the urethra into the bladder (Fig. 45-1). With coughing, sneezing, or straining, the bladder pressure increases, which may force urine from the bladder into the urethra. When the pressure returns to normal, the urine flows back into the bladder, bringing into the bladder bacteria from the anterior portions of the urethra. Urethrovesical reflux is also caused by dysfunction of the bladder neck or urethra. The urethrovesical angle and urethral closure pressure may be altered with menopause, increasing the incidence of infection in postmenopausal women. Reflux is most often noted in young children, and treatment is based on its severity.

Ureterovesical or **vesicoureteral reflux** refers to the backward flow of urine from the bladder into one or both ureters (see Fig. 45-1). Normally, the ureterovesical junction prevents urine from traveling back into the ureter. The ureters tunnel into the bladder wall so that the bladder musculature compresses a small portion of the ureter during normal voiding. When the ureterovesical valve is impaired by congenital causes or ureteral abnormalities, the bacteria may reach the kidneys and eventually destroy them (Porth, 2005).

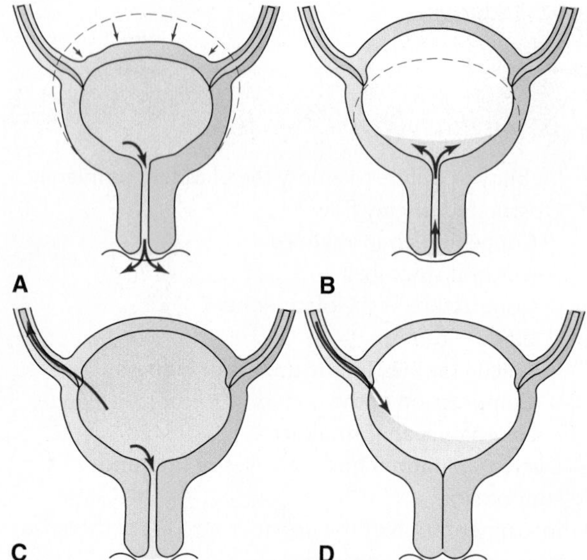

FIGURE 45-1. Mechanisms of urethrovesical and ureterovesical reflux may cause urinary tract infection. **Urethrovesical reflux:** With coughing and straining, bladder pressure rises, which may force urine from the bladder into the urethra. (**A**) When bladder pressure returns to normal, the urine flows back to the bladder (**B**), which introduces bacteria from the urethra to the bladder. **Ureterovesical reflux:** With failure of the ureterovesical valve, urine moves up the ureters during voiding (**C**) and flows into the bladder when voiding stops (**D**). This prevents complete emptying of the bladder. It also leads to urinary stasis and contamination of the ureters with bacteria-laden urine.

Uropathogenic Bacteria

Bacteriuria is generally defined as more than 10^5 colonies of bacteria per milliliter of urine. Because urine samples (especially in women) are commonly contaminated by the bacteria normally present in the urethral area, a bacterial count exceeding 10^5 colonies/mL of clean-catch midstream urine is the measure that distinguishes true bacteriuria from contamination. In men, contamination of the collected urine sample occurs less frequently; hence, bacteriuria can be defined as 10^4 colonies/mL urine. Community-acquired UTIs are among the most common bacterial infections in women (Porth, 2005).

The organisms most frequently responsible for UTIs are those normally found in the lower gastrointestinal (GI) tract. In a large-scale study of the types and prevalence of organisms of patients with UTIs in both the community and hospital, *E. coli* was responsible for 54.7% of UTIs. Isolation of *E. coli* is decreasing in comparison to previous observations, especially in males and in patients with indwelling bladder catheters, who instead had higher rates of *Pseudomonas* and *Enterococcus* organisms than females and noncatheterized patients (Porth, 2005).

Routes of Infection

Bacteria enter the urinary tract in three well-recognized ways: by the transurethral route (ascending infection), through the bloodstream (hematogenous spread), or by means of a fistula from the intestine (direct extension).

The most common route of infection is transurethral, in which bacteria (often from fecal contamination) colonize the periurethral area and subsequently enter the bladder by means of the urethra. In women, the short urethra offers little resistance to the movement of uropathogenic bacteria (Porth, 2005). Sexual intercourse or massage of the urethra forces the bacteria up into the bladder. This accounts for the increased incidence of UTIs in sexually active women. Bacteria may also enter the urinary tract by means of the blood (hematogenous spread) from a distant site of infection or through direct extension by way of a fistula from the intestinal tract.

Clinical Manifestations

A variety of signs and symptoms are associated with UTI. About half of all patients with bacteriuria have no symptoms. Signs and symptoms of an uncomplicated lower UTI (cystitis) include **dysuria** (painful or difficult urination), burning on urination, **frequency** (voiding more than every 3 hours), urgency, **nocturia** (awakening at night to urinate), incontinence, and suprapubic or pelvic pain. Hematuria and back pain may also be present (Bickley & Szilagyi, 2003). In older people, these symptoms are less common (see Gerontologic Considerations, below).

In patients with complicated UTIs, such as those with indwelling catheters, manifestations can range from asymptomatic bacteriuria to gram-negative sepsis with shock. Complicated UTIs often are due to a broader spectrum of organisms, have a lower response rate to treatment, and tend to recur. Many patients with catheter-associated UTIs are asymptomatic; however, any patient with a catheter who suddenly develops signs and symptoms of septic shock should be evaluated for **urosepsis** (sepsis resulting from infected urine).

Gerontologic Considerations

The incidence of bacteriuria in the elderly differs from that in younger adults. Bacteriuria increases with age and disability, and women are affected more frequently than men. UTI is the most common cause of acute bacterial sepsis in patients older than 65 years, in whom gram-negative sepsis carries a mortality rate exceeding 50%. Urologists see many asymptomatic older patients with bacteriuria, and 20% are women older than 65 years. In long-term care facilities, up to 50% of females have asymptomatic bacteriuria (Goldrick, 2005).

In the elderly population at large, structural abnormalities secondary to decreased bladder tone and neurogenic bladder (dysfunctional bladder) secondary to stroke or autonomic neuropathy of diabetes may prevent complete emptying of the bladder and increase the risk for UTI (Morton, Fontaine, Hudak, et al., 2005). When indwelling catheters are used, the risk for UTI increases dramatically. Elderly women often have incomplete emptying of the bladder and urinary stasis. In the absence of estrogen, postmenopausal women are susceptible to colonization and increased adherence of bacteria to the vagina and urethra. Oral or topical estrogen has been used to restore the glycogen content of vaginal epithelial cells and an acidic pH for some postmenopausal women with recurrent cystitis.

The antibacterial activity of prostatic secretions that protect men from bacterial colonization of the urethra and bladder decreases with aging. Although UTIs are rare in men, the prevalence of infection in men older than 50 years approaches that of women in the same age group. The increase of UTIs in men as they age is due largely to prostatic hyperplasia or carcinoma, strictures of the urethra, and neuropathic bladder. The use of catheterization or cystoscopy in evaluation or treatment may also contribute to the higher incidence of UTI in this group. The incidence of bacteriuria increases in men with confusion, dementia, or bowel or bladder incontinence. The most common cause of recurrent UTIs in elderly males is chronic bacterial prostatitis. Resection of the prostate gland may help reduce its incidence (see Chapter 49).

In institutionalized elderly patients, such as those in long-term care facilities, infecting pathogens are often resistant to many antibiotics. Factors that may contribute to UTI in elderly long-term care facility patients include high incidence of chronic illness, frequent use of antimicrobial agents, infected pressure ulcers, immobility and incomplete emptying of the bladder, and use of a bedpan rather than a commode or toilet (Chart 45-3).

Diligent hand hygiene, careful perineal care, and frequent toileting may decrease the incidence of UTIs seen in patients in long-term care facilities. The organisms responsible for UTIs in the institutionalized elderly may differ from those found in patients residing in the community; this is thought to be due in part to the frequent use of antibiotic agents by patients in long-term care facilities. *E. coli* is the most common organism seen in elderly patients in the community or hospital. However, patients with indwelling catheters are more likely to be infected with *Proteus*, *Klebsiella*, *Pseudomonas*, or *Staphylococcus* species. Patients who have been previously treated with antibiotics may be infected with *Enterococcus* species. Frequent reinfections are common in older adults.

The most common subjective presenting symptom of UTI in older adults is generalized fatigue. The most common objective finding is a change in cognitive functioning, especially in those with dementia, because these patients usually exhibit even more profound cognitive changes with the onset of a UTI (Midthum, 2004).

Controversy continues about the need for treatment of asymptomatic bacteriuria in institutionalized elderly patients, because resulting antibiotic-resistant organisms and sepsis may be greater threats to patients. Most experts now recommend withholding antibiotics unless symptoms develop. However, treatment regimens are generally the same as those for younger adults, although age-related changes in the intestinal absorption of medications and decreased renal function and hepatic flow may necessitate alterations in the antimicrobial regimen. Renal function must be monitored, and medication dosages should be altered accordingly.

CHART 45-3

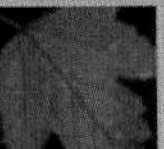

Gerontologic Considerations

Factors That Contribute to Urinary Tract Infection in Older Adults

- High incidence of chronic illness
- Frequent use of antimicrobial agents
- Presence of infected pressure ulcers
- Immunocompromise
- Cognitive impairment
- Immobility and incomplete emptying of bladder
- Use of a bedpan rather than a commode or toilet

NURSING ALERT

Elderly patients often lack the typical symptoms of UTI and sepsis. Although frequency, urgency, and dysuria may occur, nonspecific symptoms, such as altered sensorium, lethargy, anorexia, new incontinence, hyperventilation, and low-grade fever, may be the only clues.

Assessment and Diagnostic Findings

Results of various tests, such as bacterial colony counts, cellular studies, and urine cultures, help confirm the diagnosis of UTI. The American College of Obstetricians and Gynecologists (ACOG) recommends that all pregnant women be screened for asymptomatic bacteriuria, because pregnancy itself is a risk factor for UTIs; the bladder does not empty as well as it normally does. In an uncomplicated UTI, the strain of bacteria determines the antibiotic of choice.

Urine Cultures

Urine cultures are useful for documenting a UTI and can identify the specific organism present. UTI is diagnosed by bacteria in the urine culture. A colony count of at least 10^5 colony-forming units (CFU) per milliliter of urine on a clean-catch midstream or catheterized specimen is a major criterion for infection (Porth, 2005). However, UTI and subsequent sepsis have occurred with lower bacterial colony counts. About one third of women with symptoms of acute infections have negative midstream urine culture results and may go untreated if 10^5 CFU/mL is used as the criterion for infection. The presence of any bacteria in specimens obtained by suprapubic needle aspiration of the urinary bladder or catheterization (insertion of a tube into the urinary bladder) is considered indicative of infection.

The following groups of patients should have urine cultures obtained when bacteriuria is present:

- All men (because of the likelihood of structural or functional abnormalities)
- All children
- Women with a history of compromised immune function or renal problems
- Patients with diabetes mellitus
- Patients who have undergone recent instrumentation (including catheterization) of the urinary tract
- Patients who have been recently hospitalized or who live in long-term care facilities

- Patients with prolonged or persistent symptoms
- Patients with three or more UTIs in the past year
- Pregnant women
- Postmenopausal women
- Women who are sexually active or have new partners

Cellular Studies

Microscopic hematuria is present in about half of patients with an acute UTI (see Chapter 43). **Pyuria** (greater than 4 white blood cells [WBCs] per high-power field) occurs in all patients with UTI; however, it is not specific for bacterial infection. Pyuria can also be seen with kidney stones, interstitial nephritis, and renal tuberculosis.

Other Studies

A multiple-test dipstick often includes testing for WBCs, known as the leukocyte esterase test, and nitrite testing (Griess nitrate reduction test). If the leukocyte esterase test is positive, it is assumed that the patient has pyuria and should be treated. The Griess nitrate reduction test is considered positive if bacteria that reduce normal urinary nitrates to nitrites are present.

Tests for sexually transmitted diseases (STDs), also referred to as sexually transmitted infections (STIs), may be performed because acute urethritis caused by sexually transmitted organisms (ie, *Chlamydia trachomatis, Neisseria gonorrhoeae,* herpes simplex) or acute vaginitis infections (caused by *Trichomonas* or *Candida* species) may be responsible for symptoms similar to those of UTIs. Therefore, evaluation for STDs may be performed (see Chapter 70).

Diagnostic studies such as computed tomography (CT) and ultrasonography are useful diagnostic tools. A CT scan may detect pyelonephritis or abscesses, and ultrasonography is extremely sensitive for detecting obstruction, abscesses, tumors, and cysts. Transrectal ultrasonography (to assess the prostate and bladder) is the procedure of choice for men with recurrent or complicated UTIs. An intravenous (IV) urogram may be indicated to visualize the ureters or to detect strictures or stones, and it is necessary for an accurate diagnosis of reflux nephropathy (Fillingham & Douglas, 2004).

Medical Management

Management of UTIs typically involves pharmacologic therapy and patient education. The nurse teaches the patient about medication regimens and infection prevention measures.

Acute Pharmacologic Therapy

The ideal medication for treatment of UTI is an antibacterial agent that eradicates bacteria from the urinary tract with minimal effects on fecal and vaginal flora, thereby minimizing the incidence of vaginal yeast infections. (Yeast vaginitis occurs in as many as 25% of patients treated with antimicrobial agents that affect vaginal flora. Yeast vaginitis often causes more symptoms and is more difficult and costly to treat than the original UTI.) Additionally, the antibacterial agent should be affordable and should have few adverse effects and low resistance. Because the organism in initial, uncomplicated UTIs in women is most likely *E. coli* or other fecal flora, the agent should be effective against these organisms (Mehnert-Kay, 2005). Various treatment regimens have been successful in treating uncomplicated lower UTIs in women: single-dose administration, short-course (3 to 4 days) regimens, or 7- to 10-day regimens. The trend is toward a shortened course of antibiotic therapy for uncomplicated UTIs, because most cases are cured after 3 days of treatment (Zonderman & Doyle, 2006).

In a complicated UTI (ie, pyelonephritis), the general treatment of choice is usually a cephalosporin or an ampicillin/aminoglycoside combination. Patients in institutional settings may require 7 to 10 days of medication for the treatment to be effective. Other commonly used medications include trimethoprim-sulfamethoxazole (TMP-SMZ, Bactrim, Septra) and nitrofurantoin (Macrodantin, Furadantin). Occasionally, medications such as ampicillin or amoxicillin are used, but *E. coli* has developed resistance to these agents. Because of the problem of resistance, the fluoroquinolone ciprofloxacin (Cipro) is often used as a first-line agent (Mehnert-Kay, 2005).

Levofloxacin (Levaquin), another fluoroquinolone, is a good choice for short-course therapy of uncomplicated, mild to moderate UTIs. There is high patient adherence (95.6%) to the 3-day regimen and a high eradication rate (96.4%) for all pathogens. Before using levofloxacin in patients with complicated UTIs, the causative pathogen should be identified. Levofloxacin is used only when generic and less costly antibiotics are likely to be ineffective (Zonderman & Doyle, 2006).

Nitrofurantoin should not be used in patients with renal insufficiency because it is ineffective at glomerular filtration rates of less than 50 mL/min and may cause peripheral neuropathy. Phenazopyridine (Pyridium), a urinary analgesic, may be prescribed to relieve the discomfort associated with the infection (Zonderman & Doyle, 2006).

Regardless of the regimen prescribed, the patient is instructed to take all the doses prescribed, even if relief of symptoms occurs promptly. Longer medication courses are indicated for men, pregnant women, and women with pyelonephritis and other types of complicated UTIs. Hospitalization and IV antibiotics are occasionally needed.

Long-Term Pharmacologic Therapy

Although brief pharmacologic treatment of UTIs for 3 days is usually adequate in women, infection recurs in about 20% of women treated for uncomplicated UTIs. Infections that recur within 2 weeks of therapy do so because organisms of the original offending strain remain in the vagina. Relapses suggest that the source of bacteriuria may be the upper urinary tract or that initial treatment was inadequate or administered for too short a time. Recurrent infections in men are usually due to persistence of the same organism; further evaluation and treatment are indicated.

Reinfection with new bacteria is the reason for more than 90% of recurrent UTIs in women. If the diagnostic evaluation reveals no structural abnormalities in the urinary tract, the woman with recurrent UTIs may be instructed to begin treatment on her own whenever symptoms occur and to contact her health care provider only when symptoms persist, fever occurs, or the number of treatment episodes exceeds four in a 6-month period. The patient may be taught to use dip-slide culture devices to detect bacteria.

If infection recurs after completing antimicrobial therapy, another short course (3 to 4 days) of full-dose antimicrobial therapy followed by a regular bedtime dose of an antimicrobial agent may be prescribed. If there is no recurrence, medication is taken every other night for 6 to 7 months. Long-term use of antimicrobial agents decreases the risk of reinfection and may be indicated in patients with recurrent infections.

If recurrence is caused by persistent bacteria from preceding infections, the cause (ie, kidney stone, abscess), if known, must be treated. After treatment and sterilization of the urine, low-dose preventive therapy (trimethoprim with or without sulfamethoxazole) each night at bedtime is often prescribed.

Current evidence about the effectiveness of daily intake of cranberry juice to prevent UTIs is inconclusive (McMurdo, Bissett, Price, et al., 2005). Patients who like cranberry juice can be encouraged to include it in their increased fluid intake that will assist to flush bacteria (Dudek, 2006).

Nursing Process

The Patient With a Lower Urinary Tract Infection

Nursing care of the patient with a lower UTI focuses on treating the underlying infection and preventing its recurrence.

Assessment

A history of signs and symptoms related to UTI is obtained from the patient with a suspected UTI. The presence of pain, frequency, urgency, and hesitancy and changes in urine are assessed, documented, and reported. The patient's usual pattern of voiding is assessed to detect factors that may predispose him or her to UTI. Infrequent emptying of the bladder, the association of symptoms of UTI with sexual intercourse, contraceptive practices, and personal hygiene are assessed. The patient's knowledge about prescribed antimicrobial medications and preventive health care measures is also assessed. Additionally, the urine is assessed for volume, color, concentration, cloudiness, and odor, all of which are altered by bacteria in the urinary tract.

Diagnosis

Nursing Diagnoses

Based on the assessment data, the nursing diagnoses may include the following:

- Acute pain related to infection within the urinary tract
- Deficient knowledge about factors predisposing the patient to infection and recurrence, detection and prevention of recurrence, and pharmacologic therapy

Collaborative Problems/ Potential Complications

Based on assessment data, the following complications may develop:

- Sepsis (urosepsis)
- Renal failure, which may occur as the long-term result of either an extensive infective or inflammatory process

Planning and Goals

Major goals for the patient may include relief of pain and discomfort, increased knowledge of preventive measures and treatment modalities, and absence of complications.

Nursing Interventions

Relieving Pain

The pain associated with UTI is quickly relieved once effective antimicrobial therapy is initiated. Antispasmodic agents may also be useful in relieving bladder irritability and pain. Analgesic agents and the application of heat to the perineum help relieve pain and spasm. The patient is encouraged to drink liberal amounts of fluids (water is the best choice) to promote renal blood flow and to flush the bacteria from the urinary tract. Urinary tract irritants (eg, coffee, tea, citrus, spices, colas, alcohol) are avoided. Frequent voiding (every 2 to 3 hours) is encouraged to empty the bladder completely because this can significantly lower urine bacterial counts, reduce urinary stasis, and prevent reinfection.

Monitoring and Managing Potential Complications

Early recognition of UTI and prompt treatment are essential to prevent recurrent infection and the possibility of complications, such as renal failure, sepsis (urosepsis), strictures, and obstructions. The goal of treatment is to prevent infection from progressing and causing permanent renal damage and renal failure. Thus, the patient must be taught to recognize early signs and symptoms, to test for bacteriuria, and to initiate treatment as prescribed. Appropriate antimicrobial therapy, liberal fluid intake, frequent voiding, and hygienic measures are commonly prescribed for managing UTIs. The patient is instructed to notify the health care provider if fatigue, nausea, vomiting, or pruritus occurs. Periodic monitoring of renal function and evaluation for strictures, obstructions, or stones may be indicated for patients with recurrent UTIs.

Patients with UTIs, especially catheter-associated infection, are at increased risk for Gram-negative sepsis. Indwelling catheters should be avoided if possible and removed at the earliest opportunity. However, if an indwelling catheter is necessary, specific nursing interventions are initiated to prevent infection and urosepsis. These include the following:

- Using strict aseptic technique during insertion of the smallest catheter possible
- Securing the catheter with tape to prevent movement
- Frequently inspecting urine color, odor, and consistency
- Performing meticulous daily perineal care with soap and water
- Maintaining a closed system
- Following the manufacturer's instructions when using the catheter port to obtain urine specimens

Careful assessment of vital signs and level of consciousness may alert the nurse to kidney involvement or impending sepsis. Blood cultures that are positive for infection and elevated WBC counts must be reported immediately. At the same time, appropriate antibiotic therapy and increased fluid intake are prescribed (IV antibiotic therapy and fluids may be required). Aggressive early treatment is the key to reducing the mortality rate associated with Gram-negative sepsis, especially in elderly patients.

Promoting Home and Community-Based Care

TEACHING PATIENTS SELF-CARE

In helping patients learn about and prevent or manage a recurrent UTI, the nurse implements teaching that meets the patient's needs. Health-related behaviors that help prevent recurrent UTIs include practicing careful personal hygiene, increasing fluid intake to promote voiding and dilution of urine, urinating regularly and more frequently, and adhering to the therapeutic regimen. For a detailed discussion of patient teaching interventions, see Chart 45-4.

Evaluation

Expected Patient Outcomes

Expected patient outcomes may include:

1. Experiences relief of pain
   a. Reports absence of pain, urgency, dysuria, frequency, nocturia, or hesitancy on voiding
   b. Takes analgesic, antispasmodic, and antibiotic agents as prescribed

NURSING RESEARCH PROFILE

The Experience of Living With a Urinary Catheter

Wilde, M. H. (2003) Life with an indwelling urinary catheter: The dialectic of stigma and acceptance. *Qualitative Health Research, 13*(9), 1189–1204.

Purpose

Although many people live at home and in long-term care facilities with indwelling urinary catheters, there is little research about what life is like for these patients. The purpose of this study was to describe and interpret the experience of living with an indwelling urinary catheter among long-term (longer than 4 months) users of catheters.

Design

This study used a phenomenologic qualitative design, with a purposive sample of 14 community-dwelling adults, 10 of whom were recruited from a home care agency and another 4 from a urology practice. The participants, who ranged from 35 to 95 years of age and included 9 women and 5 men, were interviewed in their homes. The length of time they had had indwelling catheters ranged from 6 months to 18 years. The catheters were used because of urinary retention due to multiple sclerosis, cerebrovascular accident, enlarged prostate, or spinal cord injury. Interviews lasted 1 to 1½ hours; all interviews were audiotaped, then transcribed and analyzed using van Maren's qualitative methodology.

Findings

Analysis of the transcriptions generated three themes: adjustment by perceiving the catheter as a "part of me," shame and use of normalizing to respond to the shame, and embarrassment and use of humor to cope with the embarrassment. The study participants reported that the catheter was a constant, visible, and tangible reminder of chronic illness and of participants' vulnerability.

Living with an indwelling urinary catheter involved a constant pendulum swing between accepting it as a part of one's self and viewing it as a stigma. All participants reported that viewing the catheter as a stigma engendered feelings of alienation and vulnerability.

Nursing Implications

With increased insight into the experience of living with an indwelling urinary catheter, nurses who generally insert and change the urinary catheters can help guide patients' adjustment and minimize the stigma. Specific suggested strategies include coaching patients about ways of managing outside the home with a minimum number of events of urinary spillage and helping them develop ways of concealing the urine collection bag.

CHART 45-4

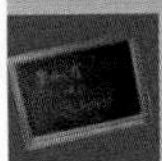

Patient Education

Preventing Recurrent Urinary Tract Infections

HYGIENE
- Shower rather than bathe in tub because bacteria in the bath water may enter the urethra.
- After each bowel movement, clean the perineum and urethral meatus from front to back. This will help reduce concentrations of pathogens at the urethral opening and, in women, the vaginal opening.

FLUID INTAKE
- Drink liberal amounts of fluids daily to flush out bacteria.
- Avoid coffee, tea, colas, alcohol, and other fluids that are urinary tract irritants.

VOIDING HABITS
- Void every 2 to 3 hours during the day and completely empty the bladder. This prevents overdistention of the bladder and compromised blood supply to the bladder wall. Both predispose the patient to UTI. Precautions expressly for women include voiding immediately after sexual intercourse.

THERAPY
- Take medication *exactly* as prescribed.
- If bacteria continue to appear in the urine, long-term antimicrobial therapy may be required to prevent colonization of the periurethral area and recurrence of infection.
- Special timing of administration may be required.
- For recurrent infection, consider acidification of the urine through ascorbic acid (vitamin C), 1,000 mg daily, or cranberry juice.
- If prescribed, test urine for presence of bacteria following manufacturer's and health care provider's instructions.
- Notify the primary health care provider if fever occurs or if signs and symptoms persist.
- Consult the primary health care provider regularly for follow-up.

2. Explains UTIs and their treatment
   a. Demonstrates knowledge of preventive measures and prescribed treatments
   b. Drinks 8 to 10 glasses of fluids daily
   c. Voids every 2 to 3 hours
   d. Voids urine that is clear and odorless
3. Experiences no complications
   a. Reports no symptoms of infection (fever, dysuria, frequency)
   b. Has normal renal function, negative urine and blood cultures
   c. Exhibits normal vital signs and temperature; no signs or symptoms of sepsis (urosepsis)
   d. Maintains adequate urine output more than 30 mL per hour

Upper Urinary Tract Infections

Pyelonephritis is a bacterial infection of the renal pelvis, tubules, and interstitial tissue of one or both kidneys. Causes involve either the upward spread of bacteria from the bladder or spread from systemic sources reaching the kidney via the bloodstream. It is not uncommon for bacteria that are causing a bladder infection to ascend into the kidney, causing pyelonephritis. An incompetent ureterovesical valve or obstruction occurring in the urinary tract increases the susceptibility of the kidneys to infection (see Fig. 45-1), because static urine provides a good medium for bacterial growth. Bladder tumors, strictures, benign prostatic hyperplasia, and urinary stones are some potential causes of obstruction that can lead to infections. Systemic infections (such as tuberculosis) can spread to the kidneys and result in abscesses.

Pyelonephritis may be acute or chronic. Acute pyelonephritis is usually manifested by enlarged kidneys with interstitial infiltrations of inflammatory cells. Abscesses may be noted on the renal capsule and at the corticomedullary junction. Eventually, atrophy and destruction of tubules and the glomeruli may result. When pyelonephritis becomes chronic, the kidneys become scarred, contracted, and nonfunctioning. Chronic pyelonephritis is a cause of chronic kidney disease that can result in the need for permanent renal replacement therapies such as transplantation or dialysis (Burrows-Hudson, 2005).

Acute Pyelonephritis

Clinical Manifestations

The patient with acute pyelonephritis is acutely ill with chills, fever, leukocytosis, bacteriuria and pyuria. Low back pain, flank pain, nausea and vomiting, headache, malaise, and painful urination are common findings. Physical examination reveals pain and tenderness in the area of the costovertebral angle (see Chapter 43, Fig. 43-6). In addition, symptoms of lower urinary tract involvement, such as dysuria and frequency, are common.

Assessment and Diagnostic Findings

An ultrasound study or a CT scan may be performed to locate any obstruction in the urinary tract. Relief of obstruction is essential to prevent the complications and eventual kidney damage. An IV pyelogram is rarely indicated during acute pyelonephritis because findings are normal in up to 75% of patients. Radionuclide imaging with gallium citrate and indium-111 (In^{111})–labeled WBCs may be useful to identify sites of infection that may not be visualized on CT scan or ultrasound. Urine culture and sensitivity tests are performed to determine the causative organism so that appropriate antimicrobial agents can be prescribed.

Medical Management

Patients with acute uncomplicated pyelonephritis are most often treated on an outpatient basis if they are not exhibiting dehydration, nausea or vomiting, or symptoms of sepsis. In addition, they must be responsible and reliable to ensure that all medications will be taken as prescribed. For outpatients, a 2-week course of antibiotics is recommended because renal parenchymal disease is more difficult to eradicate than mucosal bladder infections. Commonly prescribed agents include TMP-SMZ, ciprofloxacin, gentamicin with or without ampicillin, or a third-generation cephalosporin (Zonderman & Doyle, 2006). These medications must be used with great caution if the patient has renal or liver dysfunction.

Pregnant women may be hospitalized for 2 or 3 days of parenteral antibiotic therapy. Oral antibiotic agents may be prescribed once the patient is afebrile and showing clinical improvement.

A possible issue in acute pyelonephritis treatment is a chronic or recurring symptomless infection persisting for months or years. After the initial antibiotic regimen, the patient may need antibiotic therapy for up to 6 weeks if evidence of a relapse is seen. A follow-up urine culture is obtained 2 weeks after completion of antibiotic therapy to document clearing of the infection.

Hydration with oral or parenteral fluids is essential in all patients with UTIs when there is adequate kidney function. Hydration helps facilitate "flushing" of the urinary tract and reduces pain and discomfort.

Chronic Pyelonephritis

Repeated bouts of acute pyelonephritis may lead to chronic pyelonephritis.

Clinical Manifestations

The patient with chronic pyelonephritis usually has no symptoms of infection unless an acute exacerbation occurs. Noticeable signs and symptoms may include fatigue, headache, poor appetite, polyuria, excessive thirst, and weight loss. Persistent and recurring infection may produce progressive scarring of the kidney resulting in renal failure (see Chapter 44).

Assessment and Diagnostic Findings

The extent of the disease is assessed by an IV urogram and measurements of creatinine clearance, blood urea nitrogen, and creatinine levels. Bacteria, if detected in the urine, are eradicated if possible.

Complications

Complications of chronic pyelonephritis include end-stage renal disease (ESRD) (from progressive loss of nephrons secondary to chronic inflammation and scarring), hypertension, and formation of kidney stones (from chronic infection with urea-splitting organisms).

Medical Management

Long-term use of prophylactic antimicrobial therapy may help limit recurrence of infections and renal scarring (Tanagho & McAninch, 2004). Impaired renal function alters the excretion of antimicrobial agents and necessitates careful monitoring of renal function, especially if the medications are potentially toxic to the kidneys.

Nursing Management

The patient may require hospitalization or may be treated as an outpatient. When the patient requires hospitalization, fluid intake and output are carefully measured and recorded. Unless contraindicated, 3 to 4 L of fluids per day are encouraged to dilute the urine, decrease burning on urination, and prevent dehydration. The nurse assesses the patient's temperature every 4 hours and administers antipyretic and antibiotic agents as prescribed. Symptomatic patients are often more comfortable on bed rest.

Patient teaching focuses on prevention of further infection by consuming adequate fluids, emptying the bladder regularly, and performing recommended perineal hygiene. The importance of taking antimicrobial medications exactly as prescribed is stressed, as is the need for keeping follow-up appointments.

Adult Voiding Dysfunction

Both neurogenic and non-neurogenic disorders can cause adult voiding dysfunction (Table 45-1). The **micturition** (voiding or urination) process involves several highly coordinated neurologic responses that mediate bladder function. A functional urinary system allows for appropriate bladder filling and complete bladder emptying (see Chapter 43). If voiding dysfunction goes undetected and untreated, the upper urinary system may be compromised. Chronic incomplete bladder emptying from poor detrusor pressure results in recurrent bladder infection. Incomplete bladder emptying due to bladder outlet obstruction (such as benign prostatic hyperplasia), causing high-pressure detrusor contractions, can result in hydronephrosis from the high detrusor pressure that radiates up the ureters to the renal pelvis.

Urinary Incontinence

More than 17 million adults in the United States are estimated to have **urinary incontinence** (involuntary loss of urine from the bladder), with most of them experiencing overactive bladder syndrome, making this disorder more prevalent than diabetes or ulcer disease. Despite widespread media coverage, urinary incontinence remains underdiagnosed and underreported. Patients may be too embarrassed to seek help, causing them to ignore or conceal symptoms. Many patients resort to using absorbent pads or other devices without having their condition properly diagnosed and treated. Health care providers must be alert to subtle cues of urinary incontinence and stay informed about current management strategies (Newman, 2003).

The costs of care for patients with urinary incontinence include cost of absorbent products, medications, and surgical or nonsurgical treatment modalities as well as the psychosocial costs of urinary incontinence. These include embarrassment, loss of self-esteem, and social isolation.

Urinary incontinence affects people of all ages but is particularly common among the elderly; it can decrease an elderly person's ability to maintain an independent lifestyle. This increases dependence on caregivers and may lead to institutionalization. More than half of all nursing home resi-

TABLE 45-1 Conditions Causing Adult Voiding Dysfunction

Condition	Voiding Dysfunction	Treatment
Neurogenic Disorders		
Cerebellar ataxia	Incontinence or dyssynergia	Timed voiding; anticholinergics
Cerebrovascular accident	Retention or incontinence	Anticholinergics; bladder retraining
Dementia	Incontinence	Prompted voiding; anticholinergics
Diabetes mellitus	Incontinence and/or incomplete bladder emptying	Timed voiding; EMG/biofeedback; pelvic floor nerve stimulation; anticholinergics/antispasmodics; well-controlled blood glucose levels
Multiple sclerosis	Incontinence or incomplete bladder emptying	Timed voiding; EMG/biofeedback to learn pelvic muscle exercises and urge inhibition; pelvic floor nerve stimulation; antispasmodics
Parkinson's disease	Incontinence	Anticholinergics/antispasmodics
Spinal Cord Dysfunction		
Acute injury	Urinary retention	Indwelling catheter
Degenerative disease	Incontinence and/or incomplete bladder emptying	EMG/biofeedback; pelvic floor nerve stimulation; anticholinergics
Non-neurogenic Disorders		
"Bashful bladder"	Inability to initiate voiding in public bathrooms	Relaxation therapy; EMG/biofeedback
Overactive bladder	Urgency, frequency, and/or urge incontinence	EMG/biofeedback; pelvic floor nerve stimulation; bladder drill (see Chart 45-7); anticholinergics
Post general surgery	Acute urine retention	Catheterization
Post-prostatectomy	Incontinence	*Mild:* biofeedback; bladder drill (see Chart 45-7); pelvic floor nerve stimulation *Moderate/severe:* surgery—artificial sphincter
Stress incontinence	Incontinence with cough, laugh, sneeze, position change	*Mild:* biofeedback: bladder drill (see Chart 45-7); periurethral bulking with collagen *Moderate/severe:* surgery

dents have urinary incontinence. Although urinary incontinence is not a normal consequence of aging, age-related changes in the urinary tract predispose the older person to incontinence.

Although urinary incontinence is commonly regarded as a condition that occurs in older multiparous women, it is also common in young nulliparous women, especially during vigorous high-impact activity. Age, gender, and number of vaginal deliveries are established risk factors (Chart 45-5); they explain, in part, the increased incidence in women. Urinary incontinence is a symptom of many possible disorders.

Types of Incontinence

Stress incontinence is the involuntary loss of urine through an intact urethra as a result of sneezing, coughing, or changing position (Muller, 2005). It predominantly affects women who have had vaginal deliveries and is thought to be the result of decreasing ligament and pelvic floor support of the urethra and decreasing or absent estrogen levels within the urethral walls and bladder base. In men, stress incontinence is often experienced after a radical prostatectomy for prostate cancer because of the loss of urethral compression that the prostate had supplied before the surgery, and possibly bladder wall irritability.

Urge incontinence is the involuntary loss of urine associated with a strong urge to void that cannot be suppressed. The patient is aware of the need to void but is unable to reach a toilet in time (Muller, 2005). An uninhibited detrusor contraction is the precipitating factor. This can occur in a patient with neurologic dysfunction that impairs inhibition of bladder contraction or in a patient without overt neurologic dysfunction.

Reflex incontinence is the involuntary loss of urine due to hyperreflexia in the absence of normal sensations usually associated with voiding. This commonly occurs in patients with spinal cord injury because they have neither neurologically mediated motor control of the detrusor nor sensory awareness of the need to void (see Chapter 63).

Overflow incontinence is the involuntary loss of urine associated with overdistention of the bladder. Such overdistention results from the bladder's inability to empty normally, despite frequent urine loss. Both neurologic abnormalities (eg, spinal cord lesions) and factors that obstruct the outflow of urine (eg, tumors, strictures, and prostatic hyperplasia) can cause overflow incontinence (Muller, 2005).

Functional incontinence refers to those instances in which lower urinary tract function is intact but other factors, such as severe cognitive impairment (eg, Alzheimer's dementia), make it difficult for the patient to identify the need to void or physical impairments make it difficult or impos-

CHART 45-5

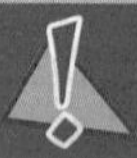

Risk Factors for Urinary Incontinence

- Pregnancy: vaginal delivery, episiotomy
- Menopause
- Genitourinary surgery
- Pelvic muscle weakness
- Incompetent urethra due to trauma or sphincter relaxation
- Immobility
- High-impact exercise
- Diabetes mellitus
- Stroke
- Age-related changes in the urinary tract
- Morbid obesity
- Cognitive disturbances: dementia, Parkinson's disease
- Medications: diuretics, sedatives, hypnotics, opioids
- Caregiver or toilet unavailable

sible for the patient to reach the toilet in time for voiding (Palmer, 2004).

Iatrogenic incontinence refers to the involuntary loss of urine due to extrinsic medical factors, predominantly medications. One such example is the use of alpha-adrenergic agents to decrease blood pressure. In some people with an intact urinary system, these agents adversely affect the alpha receptors responsible for bladder neck closing pressure; the bladder neck relaxes to the point of incontinence with a minimal increase in intra-abdominal pressure, thus mimicking stress incontinence. As soon as the medication is discontinued, the apparent incontinence resolves (Palmer, 2004).

Some patients have several types of urinary incontinence. This **mixed incontinence** is usually a combination of stress and urge incontinence (Muller, 2005).

Only with appropriate recognition of the problem, assessment, and referral for diagnostic evaluation and treatment can the outcome of incontinence be determined. All people with incontinence should be considered for evaluation and treatment.

Gerontologic Considerations

If nurses and other health care providers accept incontinence as an inevitable part of illness or aging or consider it irreversible and untreatable, it cannot be treated successfully. Collaborative, interdisciplinary efforts are essential in assessing and effectively treating urinary incontinence (Specht, 2005).

Many older people experience transient episodes of incontinence that tend to be abrupt in onset. When this occurs, the nurse should question the patient, as well as the family if possible, about the onset of symptoms and any signs or symptoms of a change in other organ systems. Acute UTI, infection elsewhere in the body, constipation, decreased fluid intake, a change in a chronic disease pattern, such as elevated blood glucose levels in patients with diabetes or decreased estrogen levels in menopausal women, can provoke the onset of urinary incontinence. If the cause is identified and modified or eliminated early at the onset of incontinence, the incontinence itself may be eliminated. Although the bladder of the older person is more vulnerable to altered detrusor activity, age alone is not a risk factor for urinary incontinence (Palmer, 2004).

Decreased bladder muscle tone is a normal age-related change found in the elderly. This leads to decreased bladder capacity, increased residual urine, and an increase in urgency (Morton et al., 2005).

Many medications affect urinary continence in addition to causing other unwanted or unexpected effects. Any medication administered needs to be assessed for potential interactions (Palmer, 2004; Fick, Cooper, Waller, et al., 2003).

Assessment and Diagnostic Findings

Once incontinence is recognized, a thorough history is necessary. This includes a detailed description of the problem and a history of medication use. The patient's voiding history, a diary of fluid intake and output, and bedside tests (eg, residual urine, stress maneuvers) may be used to help determine the type of urinary incontinence involved. Extensive urodynamic tests may be performed (see Chapter 43). Urinalysis and urine culture are performed to identify infection.

Urinary incontinence may be transient or reversible if the underlying cause is successfully treated and the voiding pattern reverts to normal (Chart 45-6).

Medical Management

Management depends on the type of urinary incontinence and its causes. Management of urinary incontinence may be behavioral, pharmacologic, or surgical in nature (Newman, 2003).

CHART 45-6

Causes of Transient Incontinence: DIAPPERS

Delirium
Infection of urinary tract
Atrophic vaginitis, urethritis
Pharmacologic agents (anticholinergics, sedatives, alcohol, analgesics, diuretics, muscle relaxants, adrenergic agents)
Psychological factors (depression, regression)
Excessive urine production (increased intake, diabetes insipidus, diabetic ketoacidosis)
Restricted activity
Stool impaction

Behavioral Therapy

Behavioral therapies are the first choice to decrease or eliminate urinary incontinence (Chart 45-7). In using these techniques, health care professionals help patients avoid potential adverse effects of pharmacologic or surgical interventions. Pelvic floor muscle exercises (sometimes called Kegel exercises) represent the cornerstone of behavioral intervention for addressing symptoms of stress, urge, and mixed incontinence (Muller, 2005). Other behavioral treatments include a voiding diary (Sampselle, 2003), biofeedback, verbal instruction (prompted voiding), and physical therapy (Melnyk & Fineout-Overholt, 2005).

Pharmacologic Therapy

Pharmacologic therapy works best when used as an adjunct to behavioral interventions. Anticholinergic agents inhibit bladder contraction and are considered first-line medications for urge incontinence. Several tricyclic antidepressant medications (eg, amitriptyline [Endep], amoxapine [Asendin]) can also decrease bladder contractions as well as increase bladder neck resistance (Karch, 2005). Stress incontinence may be treated with pseudoephedrine sulfate (Sudafed), which acts on alpha-adrenergic receptors, causing urinary retention; it needs to be used with caution in men with prostatic hyperplasia. Hormone therapy (eg, estrogen) taken orally, transdermally, or topically was once the treatment of choice for urinary incontinence in postmenopausal women. Estrogen is believed to decrease obstruction to urine flow by restoring the mucosal, vascular, and muscular integrity of the urethra. However, the results of the Women's Health Initiative showed that after 1 year of therapy, incontinence had increased, especially in women taking estrogen alone compared to placebo (Mennick, 2005). More controlled trials are needed in this area.

Surgical Management

Surgical correction may be indicated in patients who have not achieved continence using behavioral and pharmacologic therapy. Surgical options vary according to the underlying anatomy and the physiologic problem. Most procedures involve lifting and stabilizing the bladder or urethra to restore the normal urethrovesical angle or to lengthen the urethra (Tanagho & McAninch, 2004).

Women with stress incontinence may undergo an anterior vaginal repair, retropubic suspension, or needle suspension to reposition the urethra. Procedures to compress the urethra and increase resistance to urine flow include sling procedures and placement of periurethral bulking agents such as artificial collagen.

Periurethral bulking is a semipermanent procedure in which small amounts of artificial collagen are placed within the walls of the urethra to enhance the closing pressure of the urethra. This procedure takes only 10 to 20 minutes and may be performed under local anesthesia or moderate sedation. A cystoscope is inserted into the urethra. An instrument is inserted through the cystoscope to deliver a small amount of collagen into the urethral wall at locations selected by the urologist. The patient is usually discharged home after voiding. There are no restrictions following the procedure, although occasionally more than one collagen bulking session may be necessary if the initial procedure did not halt the stress urinary incontinence. Collagen placement anywhere in the body is considered semipermanent because its durability averages between 12 and 24 months, until the body absorbs the material. Periurethral bulking with collagen offers an alternative to surgery, as in a frail, elderly person. It is also an option for people who are seeking help with stress urinary incontinence who prefer to avoid surgery and who do not have access to behavioral therapies.

An artificial urinary sphincter can be used to close the urethra and promote continence. Two types of artificial sphincters are a periurethral cuff and a cuff inflation pump (Fillingham & Douglas, 2004).

Men with overflow and stress incontinence may undergo a transurethral resection to relieve symptoms of prostatic enlargement. An artificial sphincter can be used after prostatic surgery for sphincter incompetence (Fig. 45-2). After surgery, periurethral bulking agents can be injected into the periurethral area to increase compression of the urethra.

Nursing Management

Nursing management is based on the premise that incontinence is not inevitable with illness or aging and that it is often reversible and treatable. The nursing interventions are determined in part by the type of treatment that is undertaken. For behavioral therapy to be effective, the nurse must provide support and encouragement, because it is easy for the patient to become discouraged if therapy does not quickly improve the level of continence. Patient teaching is important and should be provided verbally and in writing (Chart 45-8). The patient should be taught to develop and use a log or diary to record timing of pelvic floor muscle exercises, frequency of voiding, any changes in bladder function, and any episodes of incontinence (Sampselle, 2003).

If pharmacologic treatment is used, its purpose is explained to the patient and family. It is important to educate patients who have mixed incontinence (both stress and urge incontinence) that anticholinergic and antispasmodic agents can help decrease urinary urgency and frequency and urge incontinence, but they do not decrease the urinary incontinence related to stress incontinence. If surgical correction is undertaken, the procedure and its desired outcomes are described to the patient and family. Follow-up contact with the patient enables the nurse to answer the patient's questions and to provide reinforcement and encouragement.

Urinary Retention

Urinary retention is the inability to empty the bladder completely during attempts to void. Chronic urine retention often leads to overflow incontinence (from the pressure of the retained urine in the bladder). **Residual urine** is urine that remains in the bladder after voiding. In a healthy adult younger than 60 years, complete bladder emptying should occur with each voiding. In adults older than 60 years, 50 to 100 mL of residual urine may remain after each voiding because of the decreased contractility of the detrusor muscle.

CHART 45-7

Behavioral Interventions for Urinary Incontinence

Behavioral strategies are largely carried out, coordinated, and monitored by the nurse. These interventions may or may not be augmented by the use of medications.

FLUID MANAGEMENT

One of the most common approaches is fluid management because adequate daily fluid intake of approximately 50 to 60 ounces (1,500 to 1,600 mL), taken as small increments between breakfast and the evening meal, helps to reduce urinary urgency related to concentrated urine production, decreases the risk of urinary tract infection, and maintains bowel functioning. (Constipation, resulting from inadequate daily fluid intake, can increase urinary urgency and/or urine retention.) The best fluid is water. Fluids containing caffeine, carbonation, alcohol, or artificial sweetener should be avoided because they irritate the bladder wall, thus resulting in urinary urgency. Some patients who have coexisting medical diagnoses, such as heart failure or end-stage renal disease, need to discuss their daily fluid limit with their primary health care provider.

STANDARDIZED VOIDING FREQUENCY

After establishing a patient's natural voiding and urinary incontinence tendencies, voiding on a schedule can be very effective in those with and without cognitive impairment, although patients with cognitive impairment may require assistance with this technique from nursing personnel or family members. The object is to purposely empty the bladder before the bladder reaches the critical volume that would cause an urge or stress incontinence episode. This approach involves the following:

- **Timed voiding** involves establishing a set voiding frequency (such as every 2 hours if incontinent episodes tend to occur 2 or more hours after voiding). The individual chooses to "void by the clock" at the given interval while awake, rather than wait until a voiding urge occurs.
- **Prompted voiding** is timed voiding that is carried out by staff or family members when the individual has cognitive difficulties that make it difficult to remember to void at set intervals. The caregiver checks the patient to assess if he or she has remained dry and, if so, assists the patient to use the bathroom while providing positive reinforcement for remaining dry.
- **Habit retraining** is timed voiding at an interval that is more frequent than the individual would usually choose. This technique helps to restore the sensation of the need to void in individuals who are experiencing diminished sensation of bladder filling due to various medical conditions such as a mild cerebrovascular accident (CVA).
- **Bladder retraining**, also known as "bladder drill," incorporates a timed voiding schedule and urinary urge inhibition exercises to inhibit voiding, or leaking urine, in an attempt to remain dry for a set time. When the first timing interval is easily reached on a consistent basis without urinary urgency or incontinence, a new voiding interval, usually 10 to 15 minutes beyond the last, is established. Again, the individual practices urge inhibition exercises to delay voiding or avoid incontinence until the next preset interval arrives. When an acceptable voiding interval is reached, the patient continues that timed voiding sequence throughout the day.

PELVIC MUSCLE EXERCISE (PME)

Also known as Kegel exercises, PME aims to strengthen the voluntary muscles that assist in bladder and bowel continence in both men and women. Research shows that written and/or verbal instruction alone is usually inadequate to teach an individual how to identify and strengthen the pelvic floor for sufficient bladder and bowel control. Biofeedback-assisted PME uses either electromyography or manometry to help the individual identify the pelvic muscles as he or she attempts to learn which muscle group is involved when performing PME. The biofeedback method also allows assessment of the strength of this muscle area.

PME involves gently tightening the same muscles used to stop flatus or the stream of urine for 5- to 10-second increments, followed by 10-second resting phases. To be effective, these exercises need to be performed 2 or 3 times a day for at least 6 weeks. Depending on the strength of the pelvic musculature when initially evaluated, anywhere from 10 to 30 repetitions of PME are prescribed at each session. Elderly patients may need to exercise for an even longer time to strengthen the pelvic floor muscles. Pelvic muscle exercises are helpful for women with stress, urge, or mixed incontinence and for men who have undergone prostate surgery.

VAGINAL CONE RETENTION EXERCISES

Vaginal cone retention exercises are an adjunct to the Kegel exercises. Vaginal cones of varying weight are inserted intravaginally twice a day. The patient tries to retain the cone for 15 minutes by contracting the pelvic muscles.

CHART 45-7 Behavioral Interventions for Urinary Incontinence, continued

TRANSVAGINAL OR TRANSRECTAL ELECTRICAL STIMULATION

Commonly used to treat urinary incontinence, electrical stimulation is known to elicit a passive contraction of the pelvic floor musculature, thus re-educating these muscles to provide enhanced levels of continence. This modality is often used with biofeedback-assisted pelvic muscle exercise training and voiding schedules. At high frequencies, it is effective for stress incontinence. At low frequencies, electrical stimulation can also relieve symptoms of urinary urgency, frequency, and urge incontinence. Intermediate ranges are used for mixed incontinence.

NEUROMODULATION

Neuromodulation via transvaginal or transrectal nerve stimulation of the pelvic floor inhibits detrusor overactivity and hypersensory bladder signals and strengthens weak sphincter muscles.

Urinary retention can occur postoperatively in any patient, particularly if the surgery affected the perineal or anal regions and resulted in reflex spasm of the sphincters. General anesthesia reduces bladder muscle innervation and suppresses the urge to void, impeding bladder emptying (Fillingham & Douglas, 2004).

Pathophysiology

Urinary retention may result from diabetes, prostatic enlargement, urethral pathology (infection, tumor, calculus), trauma (pelvic injuries), pregnancy, or neurologic disorders such as stroke, spinal cord injury, multiple sclerosis, or Parkinson's disease.

Some medications cause urinary retention, either by inhibiting bladder contractility or by increasing bladder outlet resistance. Medications that cause retention by inhibiting bladder contractility include anticholinergic agents (atropine sulfate, dicyclomine hydrochloride [Antispas, Bentyl]), antispasmodic agents (oxybutynin chloride [Ditropan], belladonna, and opioid suppositories), and tricyclic antidepressant medications (imipramine [Tofranil], doxepin [Sinequan]). Medications that cause urine retention by increasing bladder outlet resistance include alpha-adrenergic agents (ephedrine sulfate, pseudoephedrine), beta-adrenergic blockers (propranolol), and estrogens.

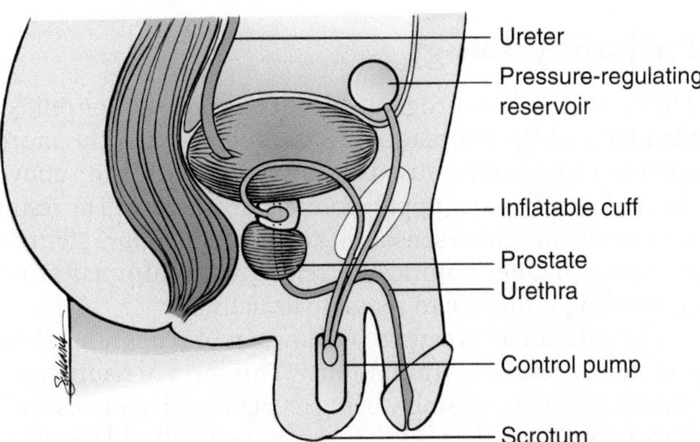

FIGURE 45-2. Male artificial urinary sphincter. An inflatable cuff is inserted surgically around the urethra or neck of the bladder. To empty the bladder, the cuff is deflated by squeezing the control pump located in the scrotum.

Assessment and Diagnostic Findings

The assessment of a patient for urinary retention is multifaceted because the signs and symptoms may be easily overlooked. The following questions serve as a guide in assessment:

- What was the time of the last voiding, and how much urine was voided?
- Is the patient voiding small amounts of urine frequently?
- Is the patient dribbling urine?

CHART 45-8

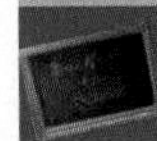

Patient Education

Strategies for Promoting Urinary Continence

- Increase your awareness of the amount and timing of all fluid intake.
- Avoid taking diuretics after 4 pm.
- Avoid bladder irritants, such as caffeine, alcohol, and aspartame (NutraSweet).
- Take steps to avoid constipation: drink adequate fluids, eat a well-balanced diet high in fiber, exercise regularly, and take stool softeners if recommended.
- Void regularly, 5 to 8 times a day (about every 2 to 3 hours):
  - First thing in the morning
  - Before each meal
  - Before retiring to bed
  - Once during night if necessary
- Perform all pelvic floor muscle exercises as prescribed, every day.
- Stop smoking (smokers usually cough frequently, which increases incontinence).

- Does the patient complain of pain or discomfort in the lower abdomen? (Discomfort may be relatively mild if the bladder distends slowly.)
- Is the pelvic area rounded and swollen (could indicate urine retention and a distended bladder)?
- Does percussion of the suprapubic region elicit dullness (possibly indicating urine retention and a distended bladder)?
- Are other indicators of urinary retention present, such as restlessness and agitation?
- Does a postvoid bladder ultrasound test reveal residual urine?

The patient may verbalize an awareness of bladder fullness and a sensation of incomplete bladder emptying. Signs and symptoms of UTI (hematuria, urgency, frequency, nocturia, and dysuria) may be present. A series of urodynamic studies, described in Chapter 43, may be performed to identify the type of bladder dysfunction and to aid in determining appropriate treatment. The patient may complete a voiding diary to provide a written record of the amount of urine voided and the frequency of voiding (Sampselle, 2003). Postvoid residual urine may be assessed either using straight catheterization or an ultrasound bladder scanner and is considered diagnostic of urinary retention if there is more than 100 mL of residual urine.

Complications

Urine retention can lead to chronic infection. Infections that are unresolved predispose the patient to renal calculi (urolithiasis or nephrolithiasis), pyelonephritis, and sepsis. The kidney may also eventually deteriorate if large volumes of urine are retained, causing hydronephrosis. In addition, urine leakage can lead to perineal skin breakdown, especially if regular hygiene measures are neglected.

Nursing Management

Management strategies are instituted to prevent overdistention of the bladder and to treat infection or correct obstruction. However, many problems can be prevented with careful assessment and appropriate nursing interventions. The nurse explains why normal voiding is not occurring and monitors urine output closely. The nurse also provides reassurance about the temporary nature of retention and successful management strategies.

Promoting Urinary Elimination

Nursing measures to encourage normal voiding patterns include providing privacy, ensuring an environment and a position conducive to voiding, and assisting the patient with the use of the bathroom or bedside commode, rather than a bedpan, to provide a more natural setting for voiding. The male patient may stand beside the bed while using the urinal; most men find this position more comfortable and natural.

Additional measures include applying warmth to relax the sphincters (ie, sitz baths, warm compresses to the perineum, showers), giving the patient hot tea, and offering encouragement and reassurance. Simple trigger techniques, such as turning on the water faucet while the patient is trying to void, may also be used. Other examples of trigger techniques are stroking the abdomen or inner thighs, tapping above the pubic area, and dipping the patient's hands in warm water. A combination of techniques may be necessary to initiate voiding.

After surgery or childbirth, prescribed analgesics should be administered because pain in the perineal area can make voiding difficult.

When the patient cannot void, catheterization is used to prevent overdistention of the bladder (see later discussion of neurogenic bladder and catheterization). In the case of prostatic obstruction, attempts at catheterization (by the urologist) may not be successful, requiring insertion of a **suprapubic catheter** (catheter inserted through a small abdominal incision into the bladder). After urinary drainage is restored, bladder retraining is initiated for the patient who cannot void spontaneously.

Promoting Home and Community-Based Care

In addition to the strategies listed for promoting urinary continence found in Chart 45-8, modifications to the home environment can provide simple and effective ways to assist in treating urinary incontinence and retention. For example, the patient may need to remove obstacles, such as throw rugs or other objects, to provide easy, safe access to the bathroom. Other modifications that the nurse may recommend include installing support bars in the bathroom; placing a bedside commode, bedpan, or urinal within easy reach; leaving lights on in the bedroom and bathroom; and wearing clothing that is easy to remove quickly.

Neurogenic Bladder

Neurogenic bladder is a dysfunction that results from a lesion of the nervous system and leads to urinary incontinence. It may be caused by spinal cord injury, spinal tumor, herniated vertebral disk, multiple sclerosis, congenital disorders (spina bifida or myelomeningocele), infection, or diabetes mellitus (see Chapters 41, 63, and 64).

Pathophysiology

The two types of neurogenic bladder are spastic (or reflex) bladder and flaccid bladder. Spastic bladder is the more common type and is caused by any spinal cord lesion above the voiding reflex arc (upper motor neuron lesion). The result is a loss of conscious sensation and cerebral motor control. A spastic bladder empties on reflex, with minimal or no controlling influence to regulate its activity.

Flaccid bladder is caused by a lower motor neuron lesion, commonly resulting from trauma. This form of neurogenic bladder is also increasingly being recognized in patients with diabetes mellitus. The bladder continues to fill and becomes greatly distended, and overflow incontinence occurs. The bladder muscle does not contract forcefully at any time. Because sensory loss may accompany a flaccid bladder, the patient feels no discomfort.

Assessment and Diagnostic Findings

Evaluation for neurogenic bladder involves measurement of fluid intake, urine output, and residual urine volume; urinalysis; and assessment of sensory awareness of bladder fullness and degree of motor control. Comprehensive urodynamic studies are also performed.

Complications

The most common complication of neurogenic bladder is infection resulting from urinary stasis and catheterization. Long-term complications include urolithiasis (stones in the urinary tract), vesicoureteral reflux, and hydronephrosis, all of which can lead to destruction of the kidney.

Medical Management

The problems resulting from neurogenic bladder disorders vary considerably from patient to patient and are a major challenge to the health care team. There are several long-term objectives appropriate for all types of neurogenic bladders:

- Preventing overdistention of the bladder
- Emptying the bladder regularly and completely
- Maintaining urine sterility with no stone formation
- Maintaining adequate bladder capacity with no reflux

Specific interventions include continuous, intermittent, or self-catheterization (discussed later in this chapter), use of an external condom-type catheter, a diet low in calcium (to prevent calculi), and encouragement of mobility and ambulation. A liberal fluid intake is encouraged to reduce the urinary bacterial count, reduce stasis, decrease the concentration of calcium in the urine, and minimize the precipitation of urinary crystals and subsequent stone formation.

A bladder retraining program may be effective in treating a spastic bladder or urine retention. Use of a timed, or habit, voiding schedule may be established. To further enhance emptying of a flaccid bladder, the patient may be taught to "double void." After each voiding, the patient is instructed to remain on the toilet, relax for 1 to 2 minutes, and then attempt to void again in an effort to further empty the bladder.

Pharmacologic Therapy

Parasympathomimetic medications, such as bethanechol (Urecholine), may help to increase the contraction of the detrusor muscle.

Surgical Management

In some cases, surgery may be carried out to correct bladder neck contractures or vesicoureteral reflux or to perform some type of urinary diversion procedure.

Catheterization

In patients with a urologic disorder or with marginal kidney function, care must be taken to ensure that urinary drainage is adequate and that kidney function is preserved. When urine cannot be eliminated naturally and must be drained artificially, catheters may be inserted directly into the bladder, the ureter, or the renal pelvis. Catheters vary in size, shape, length, material, and configuration. The type of catheter used depends on its purpose.

Catheterization is performed to achieve the following:

- Relieve urinary tract obstruction
- Assist with postoperative drainage in urologic and other surgeries
- Provide a means to monitor accurate urine output in critically ill patients
- Promote urinary drainage in patients with neurogenic bladder dysfunction or urine retention
- Prevent urinary leakage in patients with stage III to IV pressure ulcers (see Chapter 11)

A patient should be catheterized only if necessary, because catheterization commonly leads to UTI. Catheters impede most of the natural defenses of the lower urinary tract by obstructing the periurethral ducts, irritating the bladder mucosa, and providing an artificial route for organisms to enter the bladder. Organisms may be introduced from the urethra into the bladder during catheterization, or they may migrate along the epithelial surface of the urethra or external surface of the catheter. In addition, urinary catheters have been associated with other complications, such as bladder spasms, urethral strictures, and pressure necrosis.

INDWELLING CATHETERS

When an indwelling catheter cannot be avoided, a closed drainage system is essential. This drainage system is designed to prevent any disconnections, thereby reducing the risk of contamination. Triple-lumen catheters are commonly used after transurethral prostate surgery (see Chapter 49). This system has a triple-lumen indwelling urethral catheter attached to a closed sterile drainage system. With the triple-lumen catheter, urinary drainage occurs through one channel. The retention balloon of the catheter is inflated with water or air through the second channel, and the bladder is continuously irrigated with sterile irrigating solution through the third channel.

The spout (or drainage port) of any urinary drainage bag can become contaminated when opened to drain the bag. Bacteria enter the urinary drainage bag, multiply rapidly, and then migrate to the drainage tubing, catheter, and bladder. By keeping the drainage bag lower than the patient's bladder and not allowing urine to flow back into the bladder, this risk is minimized.

SUPRAPUBIC CATHETERS

Suprapubic catheterization allows bladder drainage by inserting a catheter or tube into the bladder through a suprapubic (above the pubis) incision or puncture (Fig. 45-3). The catheter or suprapubic drainage tube is then threaded into the bladder and secured with sutures or tape, and the area around the catheter is covered with a sterile dressing. The catheter is connected to a sterile closed drainage system, and the tubing is secured to prevent tension on the catheter. This may be a temporary measure to divert the flow of urine from the urethra when the urethral route is impassable (because of injuries, strictures, prostatic obstruction), after gynecologic or other abdominal surgery when bladder dysfunction is likely to occur, and occasionally after pelvic fractures.

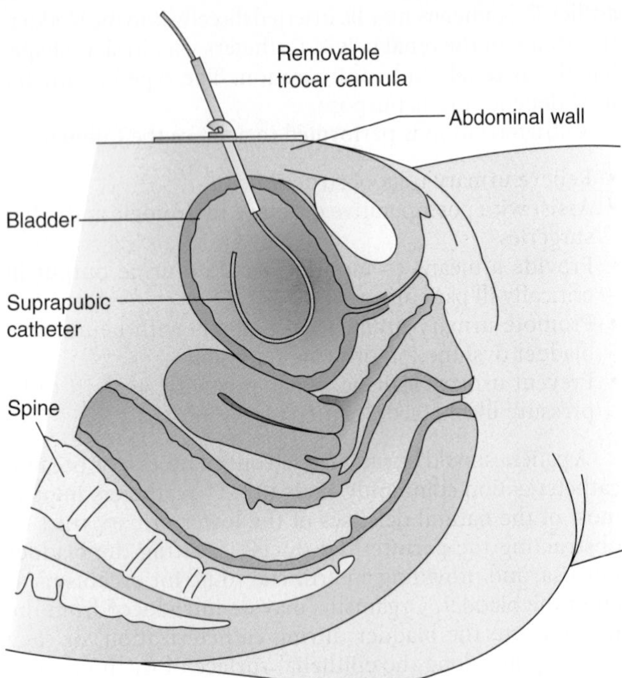

FIGURE 45-3. Suprapubic bladder drainage. A trocar cannula is used to puncture the abdominal and bladder walls. The catheter is threaded through the trocar cannula, which is then removed, leaving the catheter in place. The catheter is secured by tape or sutures to prevent unintentional removal.

Suprapubic bladder drainage may be maintained continuously for several weeks. When the patient's ability to void is to be tested, the catheter is clamped for 4 hours, during which time the patient attempts to void. After the patient voids, the catheter is unclamped, and the residual urine is measured. If the amount of residual urine is less than 100 mL on two separate occasions (morning and evening), the catheter is usually removed. However, if the patient complains of pain or discomfort, the suprapubic catheter is usually left in place until the patient can void successfully.

Suprapubic drainage offers certain advantages. Patients can usually void sooner after surgery than those with urethral catheters, and they may be more comfortable. The catheter allows greater mobility, permits measurement of residual urine without urethral instrumentation, and presents less risk of bladder infection. The suprapubic catheter is removed when it is no longer required, and a sterile dressing is placed over the site.

The patient requires liberal amounts of fluid to prevent encrustation around the catheter. Other potential problems include the formation of bladder stones, acute and chronic infections, and problems collecting urine. A **wound care specialist**/enterostomal therapist, also referred to as a wound-ostomy-continence nurse, may be consulted to assist the patient and family in selecting the most suitable urine collection system and to teach them about its use and care.

NURSING MANAGEMENT DURING CATHETERIZATION

Assessing the Patient and the System. For patients with indwelling catheters, the nurse assesses the drainage system to ensure that it provides adequate urinary drainage. The color, odor, and volume of urine are also monitored. An accurate record of fluid intake and urine output provides essential information about the adequacy of renal function and urinary drainage.

The nurse observes the catheter to make sure that it is properly anchored, to prevent pressure on the urethra at the penoscrotal junction in male patients, and to prevent tension and traction on the bladder in both male and female patients.

Patients at high risk for UTI from catheterization need to be identified and monitored carefully. These include women; older adults; and patients who are debilitated, malnourished, chronically ill, immunosuppressed, or have diabetes. They are observed for signs and symptoms of UTI: cloudy malodorous urine, hematuria, fever, chills, anorexia, and malaise. The area around the urethral orifice is observed for drainage and excoriation. Urine cultures provide the most accurate means of assessing a patient for infection.

Gerontologic Considerations. The elderly patient with an indwelling catheter may not exhibit the typical signs and symptoms of infection. Therefore, any subtle change in physical condition or mental status must be considered a possible indication of infection and promptly investigated because sepsis may occur before the infection is diagnosed. Figure 45-4 summarizes the sequence of events leading to infection and leakage of urine that often follow long-term use of an indwelling catheter in an elderly patient.

Preventing Infection. Certain principles of care are essential to prevent infection in patients with a closed urinary drainage system (Chart 45-9). The catheter is a foreign body in the urethra and produces a reaction in the urethral mucosa with some urethral discharge. Vigorous cleansing of the meatus while the catheter is in place is discouraged because the cleansing action can move the catheter back and forth, increasing the risk of infection. To remove obvious encrustations from the external catheter surface, the area can be washed gently with soap during the daily bath. The catheter is anchored as securely as possible to prevent it from moving in the urethra. Encrustations arising from urinary salts may serve as a nucleus for stone formation; however, using silicone catheters results in significantly less crust formation.

A liberal fluid intake, within the limits of the patient's cardiac and renal reserve, and an increased urine output must be ensured to flush the catheter and to dilute urinary substances that might form encrustations.

Urine cultures are obtained as prescribed or indicated when monitoring the patient for infection; many catheters have an aspiration (puncture) port from which a specimen can be obtained.

Bacteriuria is considered inevitable in patients with indwelling catheters; therefore, controversy remains about the usefulness of taking cultures and treating asymptomatic bacteriuria, because overtreatment may lead to resistant strains of bacteria. Continual observation for fever, chills and other signs and symptoms of systemic infection is necessary; these symptoms are generally treated aggressively.

Minimizing Trauma. Trauma to the urethra can be minimized by:

- Using an appropriate-sized catheter
- Lubricating the catheter adequately with a water-soluble lubricant during insertion

Physiology/Pathophysiology

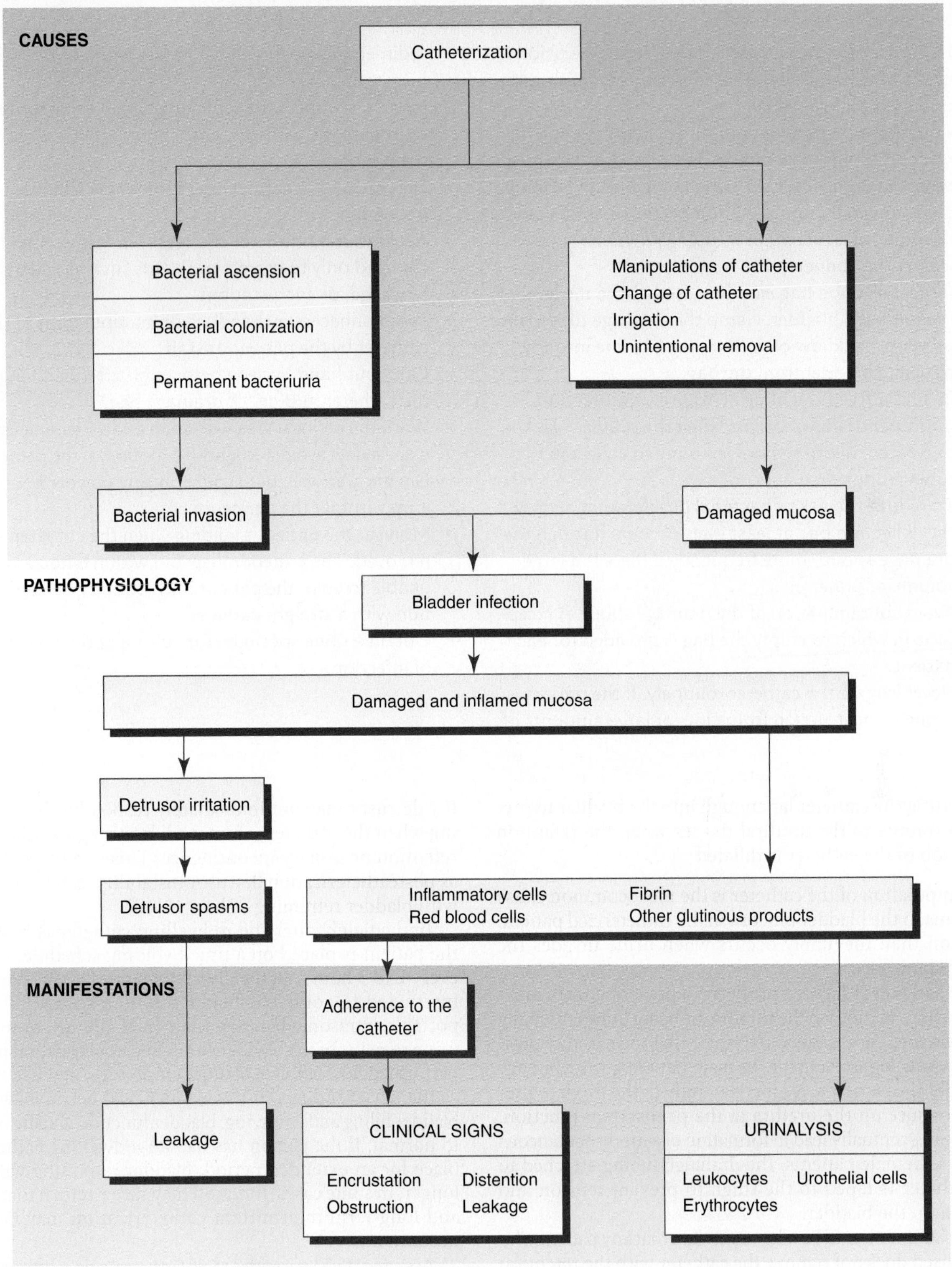

CAUSES

Catheterization

Bacterial ascension

Bacterial colonization

Permanent bacteriuria

Manipulations of catheter
Change of catheter
Irrigation
Unintentional removal

Bacterial invasion

Damaged mucosa

PATHOPHYSIOLOGY

Bladder infection

Damaged and inflamed mucosa

Detrusor irritation

Detrusor spasms

Inflammatory cells
Red blood cells
Fibrin
Other glutinous products

MANIFESTATIONS

Adherence to the catheter

Leakage

CLINICAL SIGNS
Encrustation
Obstruction
Distention
Leakage

URINALYSIS
Leukocytes
Erythrocytes
Urothelial cells

FIGURE 45-4. Pathophysiology and manifestations of bladder infection in long-term catheterized patients.

CHART 45-9

Preventing Infection in the Catheterized Patient

- Use scrupulous aseptic technique during insertion of the catheter. Use a preassembled, sterile, closed urinary drainage system.
- To prevent contamination of the closed system, *never* disconnect the tubing. The drainage bag must *never* touch the floor. The bag and collecting tubing are changed if contamination occurs, if urine flow becomes obstructed, or if tubing junctions start to leak at the connections.
- If the collection bag *must* be raised above the level of the patient's bladder, clamp the drainage tube. This prevents backflow of contaminated urine into the patient's bladder from the bag.
- Ensure a free flow of urine to prevent infection. Improper drainage occurs when the tubing is kinked or twisted, allowing pools of urine to collect in the tubing loops.
- To reduce the risk of bacterial proliferation, empty the collection bag at least every 8 hours through the drainage spout—more frequently if there is a large volume of urine.
- Avoid contamination of the drainage spout. A receptacle in which to empty the bag is provided for each patient.
- Never irrigate the catheter routinely. If the patient is prone to obstruction from clots or large amounts of sediment, use a three-way system with continuous irrigation.
- Never disconnect the tubing to obtain urine samples, to irrigate the catheter, or to ambulate or transport the patient.
- Never leave the catheter in place longer than is necessary.
- Avoid routine catheter changes. The catheter is changed only to correct problems such as leakage, blockage, or encrustations.
- Avoid unnecessary handling or manipulation of the catheter by the patient or staff.
- Carry out hand hygiene before and after handling the catheter, tubing, or drainage bag.
- Wash the perineal area with soap and water at least twice a day; avoid a to-and-fro motion of the catheter. Dry the area well, but avoid applying powder because it may irritate the perineum.
- Monitor the patient's voiding when the catheter is removed. The patient must void within 8 hours; if unable to void, the patient may require catheterization with a straight catheter.
- Obtain a urine specimen for culture at the first sign of infection.

- Inserting the catheter far enough into the bladder to prevent trauma to the urethral tissues when the retention balloon of the catheter is inflated

Manipulation of the catheter is the most common cause of trauma to the bladder mucosa in the catheterized patient. Infection then inevitably occurs when urine invades the damaged mucosa.

The catheter is secured properly to prevent it from moving, causing traction on the urethra, or being unintentionally removed, and care is taken to ensure that the catheter position permits leg movement. In male patients, the drainage tube (not the catheter) is taped laterally to the thigh to prevent pressure on the urethra at the penoscrotal junction, which can eventually lead to formation of a urethrocutaneous fistula. In female patients, the drainage tubing attached to the catheter is taped to the thigh to prevent tension and traction on the bladder.

Special care should be taken to ensure that any patient who is confused does not remove the catheter with the retention balloon still inflated, because this could cause bleeding and considerable injury to the urethra.

Retraining the Bladder. When an indwelling urinary catheter is in place, the detrusor muscle does not actively contract the bladder wall to stimulate emptying, because urine is continuously draining from the bladder. As a result, the detrusor may not immediately respond to bladder filling when the catheter is removed, resulting in either urine retention or urinary incontinence. This condition, known as postcatheterization detrusor instability, can be managed with bladder retraining (Chart 45-10).

Immediately after the indwelling catheter is removed, the patient is placed on a timed voiding schedule, usually every 2 to 3 hours. At the given time interval, the patient is instructed to void. The bladder is then scanned using a portable ultrasonic bladder scanner. If 100 mL or more of urine remains in the bladder, straight catheterization may be performed for complete bladder emptying. After a few days, as the nerve endings in the bladder wall become aware of bladder filling and emptying, bladder function usually returns to normal. If the person has had an indwelling catheter in place for an extended period, bladder retraining will take longer; in some cases, function may never return to normal and long-term intermittent catheterization may become necessary.

Assisting With Intermittent Self-Catheterization. Intermittent self-catheterization provides periodic drainage of urine from the bladder. By promoting drainage and eliminating excessive residual urine, intermittent catheterization protects the kidneys, reduces the incidence of UTIs, and improves continence. It is the treatment of choice in patients with spinal cord injury and other neurologic disorders, such

CHART 45-10

Bladder Retraining After Indwelling Catheterization

- Instruct the patient to drink a measured amount of fluid from 8 AM to 10 PM to avoid bladder overdistention. Offer no fluids (except sips) after 10 PM.
- At specific times, ask the patient to void by applying pressure over the bladder, tapping the abdomen, or stretching the anal sphincter with a finger to trigger the bladder.
- Immediately after the voiding attempt, catheterize the patient to determine the amount of residual urine.
- Measure the volumes of urine voided and obtained by catheterization.
- Palpate the bladder at repeated intervals to assess for distention.
- Instruct the patient who has no voiding sensation to be alert for any signs that indicate a full bladder, such as perspiration, cold hands or feet, or feelings of anxiety.
- Lengthen the intervals between catheterizations as the volume of residual urine decreases. Catheterization is usually discontinued when the volume of residual urine is less than 100 mL.

as multiple sclerosis, when the ability to empty the bladder is impaired. Self-catheterization promotes independence, results in few complications, and enhances self-esteem and quality of life.

When teaching the patient how to perform self-catheterization, the nurse must use aseptic technique to minimize the risk of cross-contamination. However, the patient may use a "clean" (nonsterile) technique at home, where the risk of cross-contamination is reduced. Either antibacterial liquid soap or povidone-iodine (Betadine) solution is recommended for cleaning urinary catheters at home. The catheter is thoroughly rinsed with tap water after soaking in the cleaning solution. It must dry before reuse. It should be kept in its own container, such as a plastic food-storage bag.

In teaching the patient, the nurse emphasizes the importance of frequent catheterization and emptying the bladder at the prescribed time. The average daytime clean intermittent catheterization schedule is every 4 to 6 hours and just before bedtime. If the patient is awakened at night with an urge to void, catheterization may be performed after an attempt is made to void normally.

The female patient assumes a Fowler's position and uses a mirror to help locate the urinary meatus. She inserts the lubricated catheter 7.5 cm (3 in) into the urethra, in a downward and backward direction. The male patient assumes a Fowler's or sitting position, lubricates the catheter, retracts the foreskin of the penis with one hand while grasping the penis and holding it at a right angle to the body. (This maneuver straightens the urethra and makes it easier to insert the catheter.) He inserts the catheter 15 to 25 cm (6 to 10 in) until urine begins to flow. After removal, the catheter is cleaned, rinsed, and wrapped in a paper towel or placed in a plastic bag or case. Patients who follow this routine should consult a primary health care provider at regular intervals to assess urinary function and to detect complications.

If the patient cannot perform intermittent self-catheterization, a family member may be taught to carry out the procedure at regular intervals during the day.

An alternative to self-catheterization that requires an extensive surgical procedure is creation of the Mitrofanoff umbilical appendicovesicostomy, which provides easy access to the bladder. In this procedure, the bladder neck is closed and the appendix is used to create access to the bladder from the skin surface through a submucosal tunnel created with the appendix. One end of the appendix is brought to the skin surface and used as a stoma and the other end is tunneled into the bladder. The appendix serves as an artificial urinary sphincter when an alternative is necessary to empty the bladder. A surgically prepared continent urine reservoir with a sphincter mechanism is required in cases of bladder cancer and severe **interstitial cystitis** (inflammation of the bladder wall). In males, various types of urological stomas may be used when a radical **cystectomy** (surgical removal of the bladder) is necessary (Fillingham & Douglas, 2004).

Urolithiasis and Nephrolithiasis

Urolithiasis and nephrolithiasis refer to stones (calculi) in the urinary tract and kidney, respectively. Urinary stones account for more than 320,000 hospital admissions each year. The occurrence of urinary stones occurs predominantly in the third to fifth decades of life and affects men more than women. About half of patients with a single renal stone have another episode within 5 years.

Pathophysiology

Stones are formed in the urinary tract when urinary concentrations of substances such as calcium oxalate, calcium phosphate, and uric acid increase. Referred to as supersaturation, this is dependent on the amount of the substance, ionic strength, and pH of the urine. Stones may be found anywhere from the kidney to the bladder and may vary in size from minute granular deposits, called sand or gravel, to bladder stones as large as an orange. The different sites of calculi formation in the urinary tract are shown in Figure 45-5.

Stone formation is not clearly understood, and there are a number of theories about their causes. One theory is that there is a deficiency of substances that normally prevent crystallization in the urine, such as citrate, magnesium, nephrocalcin, and uropontin (Porth, 2005). Another theory relates to fluid volume status of the patient (stones tend to occur more often in dehydrated patients). Certain factors favor the formation of stones, including infection, urinary stasis, and periods of immobility, all of which slow renal drainage and alter calcium metabolism. In addition, increased calcium concentrations in the blood and urine promote precipitation of calcium and formation of stones (about 75% of all renal stones are calcium-based). Causes of hyper-

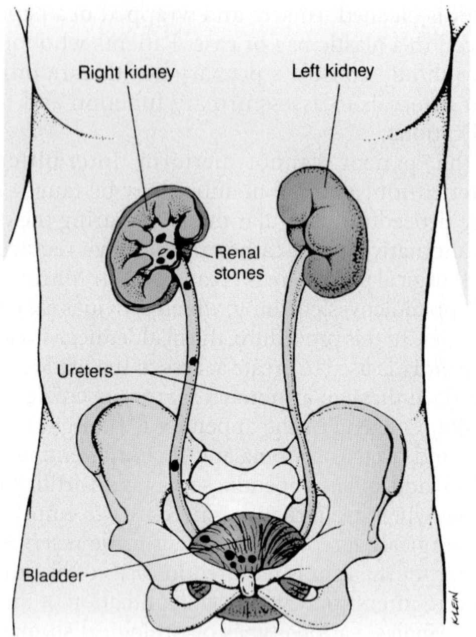

FIGURE 45-5. Examples of potential sites of calculi formation (urolithiasis) in the urinary tract.

calcemia (high serum calcium) and hypercalciuria (high urine calcium) include the following:

- Hyperparathyroidism
- Renal tubular acidosis
- Cancers
- Granulomatous diseases (eg, sarcoidosis, tuberculosis), which may cause increased vitamin D production by the granulomatous tissue
- Excessive intake of vitamin D
- Excessive intake of milk and alkali
- Myeloproliferative diseases (leukemia, polycythemia vera, multiple myeloma), which produce an unusual proliferation of blood cells from the bone marrow

For patients with stones containing uric acid, struvite, or cystine, a thorough physical examination and metabolic workup are indicated because of associated disturbances contributing to the stone formation. Uric acid stones (5% to 10% of all stones) may be seen in patients with gout or myeloproliferative disorders. Struvite stones account for 15% of urinary calculi and form in persistently alkaline, ammonia-rich urine caused by the presence of urease-splitting bacteria such as *Proteus, Pseudomonas, Klebsiella, Staphylococcus,* or *Mycoplasma* species. Predisposing factors for struvite stones include neurogenic bladder, foreign bodies, and recurrent UTIs. Cystine stones (1% to 2% of all stones) occur exclusively in patients with a rare inherited defect in renal absorption of cystine (an amino acid) (Porth, 2005).

Several conditions as well as certain metabolic risk factors predispose patients to stone formation. These include anatomic derangements such as polycystic kidney disease, horseshoe kidneys, chronic strictures, and medullary sponge disease. Urinary stone formation can occur in patients with inflammatory bowel disease and in those with an ileostomy or bowel resection because these patients absorb more oxalate. Medications known to cause stones in some patients include antacids, acetazolamide (Diamox), vitamin D, laxatives, and high doses of aspirin (Karch, 2005). However, in many patients, no cause may be found.

Clinical Manifestations

Signs and symptoms of stones in the urinary system depend on the presence of obstruction, infection, and edema. When stones block the flow of urine, obstruction develops, producing an increase in hydrostatic pressure and distending the renal pelvis and proximal ureter. Infection (pyelonephritis and UTI with chills, fever, and dysuria) can be a contributing factor with struvite stones (Porth, 2005). Some stones cause few, if any, symptoms while slowly destroying the functional units (nephrons) of the kidney; others cause excruciating pain and discomfort.

Stones in the renal pelvis may be associated with an intense, deep ache in the costovertebral region. Hematuria is often present; pyuria may also be noted. Pain originating in the renal area radiates anteriorly and downward toward the bladder in the female and toward the testis in the male. If the pain suddenly becomes acute, with tenderness over the costovertebral area, and nausea and vomiting appear, the patient is having an episode of renal colic. Diarrhea and abdominal discomfort may occur. These GI symptoms are due to renointestinal reflexes and the anatomic proximity of the kidneys to the stomach, pancreas, and large intestine.

Stones lodged in the ureter (ureteral obstruction) cause acute, excruciating, colicky, wavelike pain, radiating down the thigh and to the genitalia. Often, the patient has a desire to void, but little urine is passed, and it usually contains blood because of the abrasive action of the stone. This group of symptoms is called ureteral colic. Colic is mediated by prostaglandin E, a substance that increases ureteral contractility and renal blood flow and that leads to increased intraureteral pressure and pain. In general, the patient spontaneously passes stones 0.5 to 1 cm in diameter. Stones larger than 1 cm in diameter usually must be removed or fragmented (broken up by lithotripsy) so that they can be removed or passed spontaneously.

Stones lodged in the bladder usually produce symptoms of irritation and may be associated with UTI and hematuria. If the stone obstructs the bladder neck, urinary retention occurs. If infection is associated with a stone, the condition is far more serious, with urosepsis threatening the patient's life.

Assessment and Diagnostic Findings

The diagnosis is confirmed by x-rays of the kidneys, ureters, and bladder (KUB) or by ultrasonography, IV urography, or retrograde pyelography. Blood chemistries and a 24-hour urine test for measurement of calcium, uric acid, creatinine, sodium, pH, and total volume are part of the diagnostic workup. Dietary and medication histories and family history of renal stones are obtained to identify factors predisposing the patient to the formation of stones.

When stones are recovered (stones may be freely passed by the patient or removed through special procedures), chemical analysis is carried out to determine their composition. Stone analysis can provide a clear indication of the underlying disorder. For example, calcium oxalate or calcium phosphate stones usually indicate disorders of oxalate or calcium metabolism, whereas urate stones suggest a disturbance in uric acid metabolism (Porth, 2005).

Medical Management

The goals of management are to eradicate the stone, determine the stone type, prevent nephron destruction, control infection, and relieve any obstruction that may be present. The immediate objective of treatment of renal or ureteral colic is to relieve the pain until its cause can be eliminated. Opioid analgesics are administered to prevent shock and syncope that may result from the excruciating pain. Nonsteroidal anti-inflammatory drugs (NSAIDs) are effective in treating renal stone pain because they provide specific pain relief. They also inhibit the synthesis of prostaglandin E, reducing swelling and facilitating passage of the stone. Generally once the stone has passed, the pain is relieved. Hot baths or moist heat to the flank areas may also be useful. Unless the patient is vomiting or has heart failure or any other condition requiring fluid restriction, fluids are encouraged. This increases the hydrostatic pressure behind the stone, assisting it in its downward passage. A high, around-the-clock fluid intake reduces the concentration of urinary crystalloids, dilutes the urine, and ensures a high urine output.

Nutritional Therapy

Nutritional therapy plays an important role in preventing renal stones (Dudek, 2006) (Chart 45-11). Fluid intake is the mainstay of most medical therapy for renal stones. Unless fluids are contraindicated, patients with renal stones should drink eight to ten 8-ounce glasses of water daily or have IV fluids prescribed to keep the urine dilute. A urine output exceeding 2 L a day is advisable.

CALCIUM STONES. Historically, patients with calcium-based renal stones were advised to restrict calcium in their diet. However, recent evidence has questioned the advisability of this practice, except for patients with type II absorptive hypercalciuria (half of all patients with calcium stones), in whom stones are clearly due to excess dietary calcium. Liberal fluid intake is encouraged along with dietary restriction of protein and sodium. It is thought that a high-protein diet is associated with increased urinary excretion of calcium and uric acid, thereby causing a supersaturation of these substances in the urine. Similarly, a high sodium intake has been shown in some studies to increase the amount of calcium in the urine. Medications such as ammonium chloride may be used, and if increased parathormone production (resulting in increased serum calcium levels in blood and urine) is a factor in the formation of stones, therapy with thiazide diuretics may be beneficial in reducing the calcium loss in the urine and lowering the elevated parathormone levels (Porth 2005).

URIC ACID STONES. For uric acid stones, the patient is placed on a low-purine diet to reduce the excretion of uric acid in the urine. Foods high in purine (shellfish, anchovies, asparagus, mushrooms, and organ meats) are avoided, and other proteins may be limited. Allopurinol (Zyloprim) may be prescribed to reduce serum uric acid levels and urinary uric acid excretion.

CHART 45-11

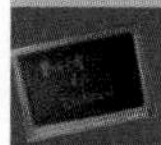

Patient Education

Preventing Kidney Stones

- Avoid protein intake; usually protein is restricted to 60 g/day to decrease urinary excretion of calcium and uric acid.
- A sodium intake of 3–4 g/day is recommended. Table salt and high-sodium foods should be reduced, because sodium competes with calcium for reabsorption in the kidneys.
- Low-calcium diets are not generally recommended, except for true absorptive hypercalciuria. Evidence shows that limiting calcium, especially in women, can lead to osteoporosis and does not prevent renal stones.
- Avoid intake of oxalate-containing foods (eg, spinach, strawberries, rhubarb, tea, peanuts, wheat bran).
- During the day, drink fluids (ideally water) every 1–2 hours.
- Drink two glasses of water at bedtime and an additional glass at each nighttime awakening to prevent urine from becoming too concentrated during the night.
- Avoid activities leading to sudden increases in environmental temperatures that may cause excessive sweating and dehydration.
- Contact your primary health care provider at the first sign of a urinary tract infection.

CYSTINE STONES. A low-protein diet is prescribed, the urine is alkalinized, and fluid intake is increased.

OXALATE STONES. A dilute urine is maintained and the intake of oxalate is limited. Many foods contain oxalate; however, only certain foods increase the urinary excretion of oxalate. These include spinach, strawberries, rhubarb, chocolate, tea, peanuts, and wheat bran.

Interventional Procedures

If the stone does not pass spontaneously or if complications occur, common interventions include endoscopic or other procedures—for example, ureteroscopy, extracorporeal shock wave lithotripsy (ESWL), or endourologic (percutaneous) stone removal.

Ureteroscopy (Fig. 45-6A) involves first visualizing the stone and then destroying it. Access to the stone is accomplished by inserting a ureteroscope into the ureter and then inserting a laser, electrohydraulic lithotriptor, or ultrasound device through the ureteroscope to fragment and remove the stones. A stent may be inserted and left in place for 48 hours or more after the procedure to keep the ureter patent. Hospital stays are generally brief, and some patients can be treated as outpatients.

ESWL is a noninvasive procedure used to break up stones in the calyx of the kidney (see Fig. 45-6B). After the stones

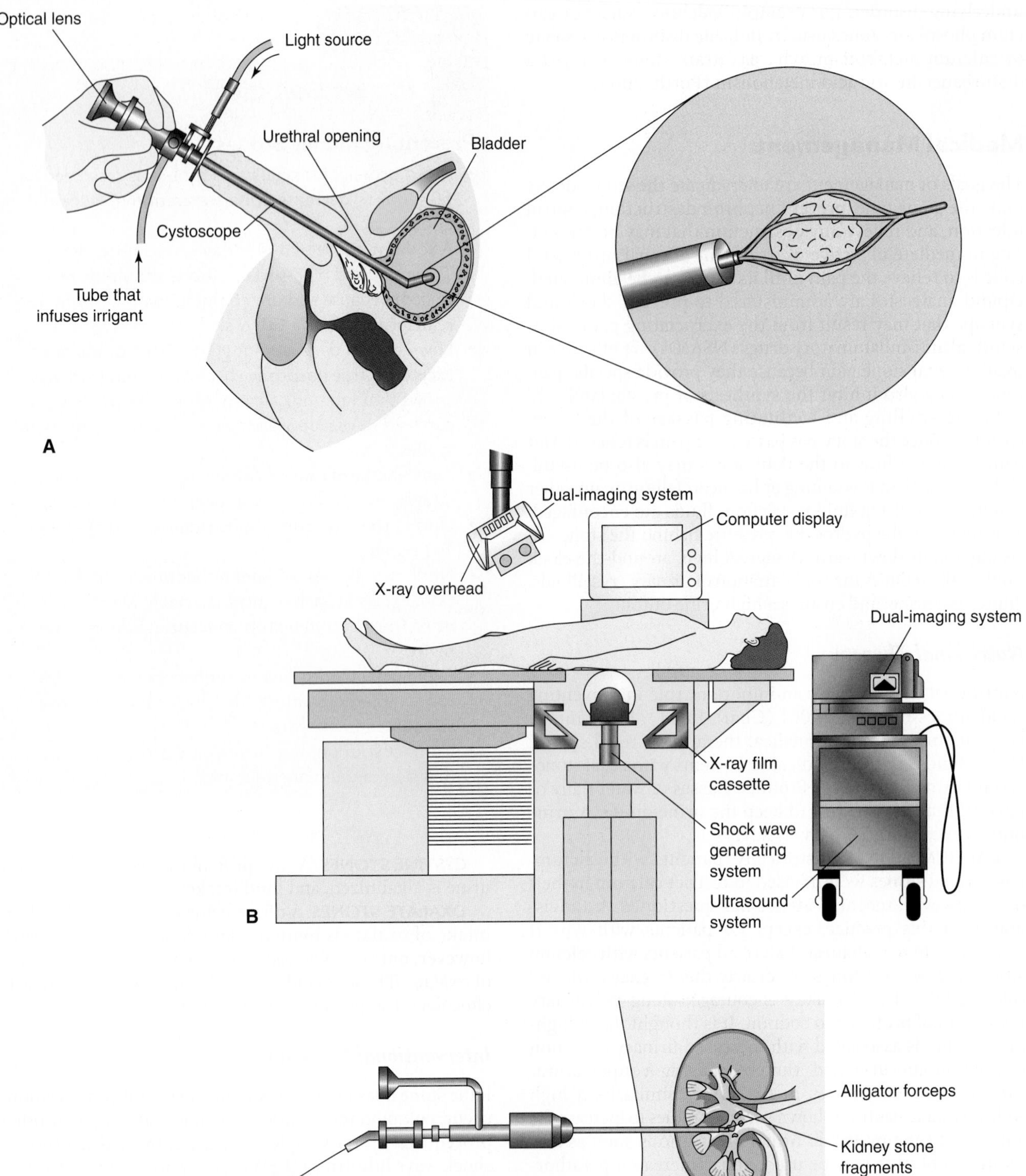

FIGURE 45-6. Methods of treating renal stones. (**A**) During a cystoscopy, which is used for removing small stones located in the ureter close to the bladder, a ureteroscope is inserted into the ureter to visualize the stone. The stone is then fragmented or captured and removed. (**B**) Extracorporeal shock wave lithotripsy (ESWL) is used for most symptomatic, nonpassable upper urinary tract stones. Electromagnetically generated shock waves are focused over the area of the renal stone. The high-energy dry shock waves pass through the skin and fragment the stone. (**C**) Percutaneous nephrolithotomy is used to treat larger stones. A percutaneous tract is formed and a nephroscope is inserted through it. Then the stone is extracted or pulverized.

are fragmented to the size of grains of sand, the remnants of the stones are spontaneously voided. In ESWL, a high-energy amplitude of pressure, or shock wave, is generated by the abrupt release of energy and transmitted through water and soft tissues. When the shock wave encounters a substance of different intensity (a renal stone), a compression wave causes the surface of the stone to fragment. Repeated shock waves focused on the stone eventually reduce it to many small pieces that are excreted in the urine.

Discomfort from the multiple shocks may occur, although the shock waves usually do not cause damage to other tissue. The patient is observed for obstruction and infection resulting from blockage of the urinary tract by stone fragments. All urine is strained after the procedure; voided gravel or sand is sent to the laboratory for chemical analysis. Several treatments may be necessary to ensure disintegration of stones. Although lithotripsy is a costly treatment, its cost is offset by a decrease in the length of hospital stay and avoidance of a surgical procedure.

Endourologic methods of stone removal (see Fig. 45-6C) may be used to extract renal calculi that cannot be removed by other procedures. A percutaneous nephrostomy or a percutaneous nephrolithotomy (which are similar procedures) may be performed. A nephroscope is introduced through a percutaneous route into the renal parenchyma. Depending on its size, the stone may be extracted with forceps or by a stone retrieval basket. If the stone is too large to initially be removed, an ultrasound probe inserted through a nephrostomy tube is used to pulverize the stone. Small stone fragments and stone dust are then removed from the collecting system.

Electrohydraulic lithotripsy is a similar method in which an electrical discharge is used to create a hydraulic shock wave to break up the stone. A probe is passed through the cystoscope, and the tip of the lithotriptor is placed near the stone. The strength of the discharge and pulse frequency can be varied. This procedure is performed under topical anesthesia. After the stone is extracted, the percutaneous nephrostomy tube is left in place for a time to ensure that the ureter is not obstructed by edema or blood clots. The most common complications are hemorrhage, infection, and urinary extravasation. After the tube is removed, the nephrostomy tract closes spontaneously.

Chemolysis, stone dissolution using infusions of chemical solutions (eg, alkylating agents, acidifying agents) for the purpose of dissolving the stone, is an alternative treatment sometimes used in patients who are at risk of complications of other types of therapy, who refuse to undergo other methods, or who have stones (struvite) that dissolve easily. A percutaneous nephrostomy is performed, and the warm chemical solution is allowed to flow continuously onto the stone. The solution exits the renal collecting system by means of the ureter or the nephrostomy tube. The pressure inside the renal pelvis is monitored during the procedure.

Several of these treatment modalities may be used in combination to ensure removal of the stones.

Surgical Management

Surgical removal was the major mode of therapy before the advent of lithotripsy. However, today, surgery is performed in only 1% to 2% of patients. Surgical intervention is indicated if the stone does not respond to other forms of treatment. It may also be performed to correct anatomic abnormalities within the kidney to improve urinary drainage. If the stone is in the kidney, the surgery performed may be a nephrolithotomy (incision into the kidney with removal of the stone) or a nephrectomy, if the kidney is nonfunctional secondary to infection or hydronephrosis. Stones in the kidney pelvis are removed by a pyelolithotomy, those in the ureter by ureterolithotomy, and those in the bladder by cystotomy. If the stone is in the bladder, an instrument may be inserted through the urethra into the bladder, and the stone is crushed in the jaws of this instrument. Such a procedure is called a cystolitholapaxy. Nursing management following kidney surgery is discussed in Chapter 44.

Nursing Process

The Patient With Kidney Stones

Assessment

The patient with suspected renal stones is assessed for pain and discomfort as well as associated symptoms, such as nausea, vomiting, diarrhea, and abdominal distention. The severity and location of pain are determined, along with any radiation of the pain. Nursing assessment also includes observing for signs and symptoms of UTI (chills, fever, dysuria, frequency, and hesitancy) and obstruction (frequent urination of small amounts, oliguria, or anuria). The urine is inspected for blood and is strained for stones or gravel.

The history focuses on factors that predispose the patient to urinary tract stones or that may have precipitated the current episode of renal or ureteral colic. The patient's knowledge about renal stones and measures to prevent their occurrence or recurrence is also assessed.

Diagnosis

Nursing Diagnoses

Based on the assessment data, the nursing diagnoses in the patient with renal stones may include the following:

- Acute pain related to inflammation, obstruction, and abrasion of the urinary tract
- Deficient knowledge regarding prevention of recurrence of renal stones

Collaborative Problems/Potential Complications

Based on assessment data, potential complications that may develop include the following:

- Infection and urosepsis (from UTI and pyelonephritis)
- Obstruction of the urinary tract by a stone or edema with subsequent acute renal failure

Planning and Goals

The major goals for the patient may include relief of pain and discomfort, prevention of recurrence of renal stones, and absence of complications.

Nursing Interventions

Relieving Pain

Severe and acute pain is often the presenting symptom of a patient with renal and urinary calculi and requires immediate attention. Opioid analgesic agents (IV or intramuscular) may be prescribed and administered to provide rapid relief along with an IV NSAID. The patient is encouraged and assisted to assume a position of comfort. If activity brings pain relief, the patient is assisted to ambulate. The pain level is monitored closely, and an increase in severity is reported promptly to the physician so that relief can be provided and additional treatment initiated.

Monitoring and Managing Potential Complications

Increased fluid intake is encouraged to prevent dehydration and increase hydrostatic pressure within the urinary tract to promote passage of the stone. If the patient cannot take adequate fluids orally, IV fluids are prescribed. The total urine output and patterns of voiding are monitored. Ambulation is encouraged as a means of moving the stone through the urinary tract.

All urine is strained through gauze because uric acid stones may crumble. Any blood clots passed in the urine should be crushed and the sides of the urinal and bedpan inspected for clinging stones. Because renal stones increase the risk of infection, sepsis, and obstruction of the urinary tract, the patient is instructed to report decreased urine volume and bloody or cloudy urine.

Patients with calculi require frequent nursing observation to detect the spontaneous passage of a stone. The patient is instructed to immediately report any sudden increases in pain intensity because of the possibility of a stone fragment obstructing a ureter. Vital signs, including temperature, are monitored closely to detect early signs of infection. UTIs may be associated with renal stones due to an obstruction from the stone or from the stone itself. All infections should be treated with the appropriate antibiotic agent before efforts are made to dissolve the stone.

Promoting Home and Community-Based Care

TEACHING PATIENTS SELF-CARE

Because the risk of recurring renal stones is high, the nurse provides education about the causes of kidney stones and recommendations to prevent their recurrence (see Chart 45-11). The patient is encouraged to follow a regimen to avoid further stone formation, including maintaining a high fluid intake because stones form more readily in concentrated urine. A patient who has shown a tendency to form stones should drink enough fluid to excrete greater than 2000 mL (preferably 3000 to 4000 mL) of urine every 24 hours.

Urine cultures may be performed every 1 to 2 months the first year and periodically thereafter. Recurrent UTI is treated vigorously. Because prolonged immobilization slows renal drainage and alters calcium metabolism, increased mobility is encouraged whenever possible. In addition, excessive ingestion of vitamins (especially vitamin D) and minerals is discouraged.

If lithotripsy, percutaneous stone removal, ureteroscopy, or other surgical procedures for stone removal have been performed, the nurse instructs the patient about the signs and symptoms of complications that need to be reported to the physician. The importance of follow-up to assess kidney function and to ensure the eradication or removal of all kidney stones is emphasized to the patient and family.

If ESWL has been performed, the nurse must provide instructions for home care and necessary follow-up. The patient is encouraged to increase fluid intake to assist in the passage of stone fragments, which may occur for 6 weeks to several months after the procedure. The patient and family are instructed about signs and symptoms that indicate complications, such as fever, decreasing urine output, and pain. It is also important to inform the patient to expect hematuria (it is anticipated in all patients), but it should disappear within 4 to 5 days. If the patient has a stent in the ureter, hematuria may be expected until the stent is removed. The patient is instructed to check his or her temperature daily and notify the physician if the temperature is greater than 38°C (about 101°F), or the pain is unrelieved by the prescribed medication. The patient is also informed that a bruise may be observed on the treated side of the back.

CONTINUING CARE

The patient is monitored closely in follow-up care to ensure that treatment has been effective and that no complications, such as obstruction, infection, renal hematoma, or hypertension, have developed. During the patient's visits to the clinic or physician's office, the nurse has the opportunity to assess the patient's understanding of ESWL and possible complications. Additionally, the nurse has the opportunity to assess the patient's understanding of factors that increase the risk of recurrence of renal calculi and strategies to reduce those risks.

The patient's ability to monitor urinary pH and interpret the results is assessed during follow-up visits to the clinic or physician's office. Because of the high risk of recurrence, the patient with renal stones needs to understand the signs and symptoms of stone formation, obstruction, and infection and the importance of reporting these signs promptly. If medications are prescribed for the prevention of stone formation, the actions and importance of the medications are explained to the patient.

Evaluation

Expected Patient Outcomes

Expected patient outcomes may include:

1. Reports relief of pain
2. States increased knowledge of health-seeking behaviors to prevent recurrence
   a. Consumes increased fluid intake (at least eight 8-ounce glasses of fluid per day)
   b. Participates in appropriate activity
   c. Consumes diet prescribed to reduce dietary factors predisposing to stone formation
   d. Recognizes symptoms (fever, chills, flank pain, hematuria) to be reported to health care provider
   e. Monitors urinary pH as directed
   f. Takes prescribed medication as directed to reduce stone formation
3. Experiences no complications
   a. Reports no signs or symptoms of infection or urosepsis
   b. Voids 200 to 400 mL per voiding of clear urine without evidence of bleeding
   c. Experiences absence of dysuria, frequency, and hesitancy
   d. Maintains normal body temperature

Genitourinary Trauma

Various types of injuries of the flank, back, or upper abdomen may result in trauma to the ureters, bladder, or urethra. Approximately 10% of all injuries seen in the emergency department involve the genitourinary system (Tanagho & McAninch, 2004). (Renal trauma is discussed in Chapter 44.)

Specific Injuries

Ureteral Trauma

Penetrating trauma and unintentional injury during surgery are the major causes of trauma to the ureters. Gunshot wounds account for 95% of ureteral injuries, which may range from contusions to complete transection. Unintentional injury to the ureter may occur during gynecologic or urologic surgery. There are no specific signs or symptoms of ureteral injury; many traumatic injuries are discovered during exploratory surgery. If the ureteral trauma is not detected and urine leakage continues, fistulas can develop.

IV urography detects 90% of ureteral injuries and can be performed on the operating table in patients undergoing emergent surgery. Surgical repair with placement of stents (to divert urine away from an anastomosis) is usually necessary.

Bladder Trauma

Injury to the bladder may occur with pelvic fractures and multiple trauma or from a blow to the lower abdomen when the bladder is full. Blunt trauma may result in contusion evident as an ecchymosis—a large, discolored bruise resulting from escape of blood into the tissues and involving a segment of the bladder wall—or in rupture of the bladder extraperitoneally, intraperitoneally, or both. Complications from these injuries include hemorrhage, shock, sepsis, and extravasation of blood into the tissues, which must be treated promptly.

Urethral Trauma

Urethral injuries usually occur with blunt trauma to the lower abdomen or pelvic region. Many patients also have associated pelvic fractures. The classic triad of symptoms comprises blood at the urinary meatus, inability to void, and a distended bladder.

Medical Management

The goals of management in patients with genitourinary trauma are to control hemorrhage, pain, and infection and to maintain urinary drainage. Genitourinary trauma is frequently associated with renal trauma (see Chapter 44). Hematocrit and hemoglobin levels are monitored closely; decreasing values indicate hemorrhage within the genitourinary system. The patient is also monitored for oliguria, signs of hemorrhagic shock, and signs and symptoms of acute peritonitis (Tanagho & McAninch, 2004).

Surgical Management

In urethral trauma, unstable patients who need monitoring of urine output may need a suprapubic catheter inserted. The patient is catheterized after urethrography is performed to minimize the risk of urethral disruption and extensive, long-term complications, such as stricture, incontinence, and impotence. Surgical repair may be performed immediately or at a later time. Delayed surgical repair tends to be the favored procedure because it is associated with fewer long-term complications, such as impotence, strictures, and incontinence. After surgery, an indwelling urinary catheter may remain in place for up to 1 month.

Nursing Management

The patient with genitourinary trauma should be assessed frequently during the first few days after injury to detect flank and abdominal pain, muscle spasm, and swelling over the flank.

During this time, patients can be instructed about care of the incision and the importance of an adequate fluid intake. In addition, instructions about changes that should be reported to the physician, such as fever, hematuria, flank pain, or any signs and symptoms of decreasing kidney function, are provided. The patient with a ruptured bladder may have gross bleeding for several days after repair. Guidelines for increasing activity gradually, lifting, and driving are also provided in accordance with the physician's prescription.

Follow-up nursing care includes monitoring the blood pressure to detect hypertension and advising the patient to restrict activities for about 1 month after trauma to minimize the incidence of delayed or secondary bleeding.

Urinary Tract Cancers

In 2005, the American Cancer Society (ACS) estimated that there were more than 100,000 new cases of urinary cancer, and more than 26,000 deaths. Urinary tract cancers include those of the urinary bladder; kidney and renal pelvis; ureters; and other urinary structures, such as the prostate. (Renal cancer is discussed in Chapter 44, and prostate cancer is discussed in Chapter 49.) Malignant tumors include transitional cell carcinomas (90%), squamous cell carcinomas (5% to 8%), adenocarcinomas (1% to 2%), sarcomas (less than 1%) and other types of cancers (Fillingham & Douglas, 2004).

Cancer of the Bladder

Cancer of the urinary bladder is more common in people between the ages of 50 and 70 years. It affects more men than women (4:1) and is more common in Caucasians than in African Americans. Bladder cancer is the fourth leading cause of cancer in American men, accounting for more than 13,000 deaths in the United States annually (ACS, 2006). Bladder cancer has a high worldwide incidence (Fillingham & Douglas, 2004).

Bladder cancer, combined with prostatic cancer, is the most common urologic malignancy, accounting for 90% of all tumors seen. Cancers arising from the prostate, colon, and rectum in males and from the lower gynecologic tract in females may metastasize to the bladder (Chart 45-12).

Tobacco use continues to be a leading risk factor for all urinary tract cancers. People who smoke get bladder cancer twice as often as those who do not smoke (ACS, 2006).

Clinical Manifestations

Bladder tumors usually arise at the base of the bladder and involve the ureteral orifices and bladder neck. Visible, painless hematuria is the most common symptom of bladder cancer. Infection of the urinary tract is a common complication, producing frequency, urgency, and dysuria. However, any alteration in voiding or change in the urine may indicate cancer of the bladder. Pelvic or back pain may occur with metastasis.

CHART 45-12

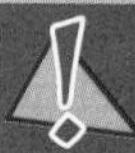

Risk Factors for Bladder Cancer

- Cigarette smoking: risk proportional to number of packs smoked daily and number of years of smoking
- Exposure to environmental carcinogens: dyes, rubber, leather, ink, or paint
- Recurrent or chronic bacterial infection of the urinary tract
- Bladder stones
- High urinary pH
- High cholesterol intake
- Pelvic radiation therapy
- Cancers arising from the prostate, colon, and rectum in males

Assessment and Diagnostic Findings

The diagnostic evaluation includes cystoscopy (the mainstay of diagnosis), excretory urography, CT, ultrasonography, and bimanual examination with the patient anesthetized. Biopsies of the tumor and adjacent mucosa are the definitive diagnostic procedures. Transitional cell carcinomas and carcinomas in situ shed recognizable cancer cells. Cytologic examination of fresh urine and saline bladder washings provide information about the prognosis and staging, especially for patients at high risk for recurrence of primary bladder tumors (Fillingham & Douglas, 2004).

Although the mainstay diagnostic tools such as cytology and CT have a high detection rate, they are costly. Newer diagnostic tools such as bladder tumor antigens, nuclear matrix proteins, adhesion molecules, cytoskeletal proteins, and growth factors are being studied to support the early detection and diagnosis of bladder cancer (ACS, 2006).

Medical Management

Treatment of bladder cancer depends on the grade of the tumor (the degree of cellular differentiation), the stage of tumor growth (the degree of local invasion and the presence or absence of metastasis), and the multicentricity (having many centers) of the tumor. The patient's age and physical, mental, and emotional status are considered when determining treatment modalities.

Surgical Management

Transurethral resection or fulguration (cauterization) may be performed for simple papillomas (benign epithelial tumors). These procedures, described in more detail in Chapter 49, eradicate the tumors through surgical incision or electrical current with the use of instruments inserted through the urethra. After this bladder-sparing surgery, intravesical administration of bacille Calmette-Guérin (BCG) is the treatment of choice. BCG is an attenuated live strain of *Mycobacterium bovis*, the causative agent for tuberculosis. The exact action of BCG is unknown, but it is thought to produce a local inflammatory as well as a systemic immunologic response (Sanger, Busche, Bentien et al., 2004).

Management of superficial bladder cancers presents a challenge because there are usually widespread abnormalities in the bladder mucosa. The entire lining of the urinary tract, or urothelium, is at risk because carcinomatous changes can occur in the mucosa of the bladder, renal pelvis, ureter, and urethra. About 25% to 40% of superficial tumors recur after transurethral resection or fulguration. Patients with benign papillomas should undergo cytology and cystoscopy periodically for the rest of their lives because aggressive malignancies may develop from these tumors.

A simple cystectomy or a radical cystectomy is performed for invasive or multifocal bladder cancer. Radical cystectomy in men involves removal of the bladder, prostate, and seminal vesicles and immediate adjacent perivesical tissues. In women, radical cystectomy involves removal of the bladder, lower ureter, uterus, fallopian tubes, ovaries, anterior vagina, and urethra. It may include removal of pelvic lymph nodes. Removal of the bladder requires a urinary diversion procedure. This is described later in this chapter.

Although radical cystectomy remains the standard of care for invasive bladder cancer in the United States, researchers are exploring trimodality therapy—transurethral resection of the bladder tumor, radiation, and chemotherapy—in an effort to spare patients the need for cystectomy. This approach to transitional cell bladder cancer mandates lifelong surveillance with periodic cystoscopy. Although most patients respond completely and their bladders remain free from invasive relapse, one fourth develop a relapse of noninvasive disease. This may be managed with transurethral resection of the bladder tumor and intravesical therapies but carries an additional risk that a late cystectomy may be required (Tanagho & McAninch, 2004).

Pharmacologic Therapy

Chemotherapy with a combination of methotrexate, 5-fluorouracil, vinblastine, doxorubicin (Adriamycin), and cisplatin has been effective in producing partial remission of transitional cell carcinoma of the bladder in some patients. IV chemotherapy may be accompanied by radiation therapy. Topical chemotherapy (intravesical chemotherapy or instillation of antineoplastic agents into the bladder, resulting in contact of the agent with the bladder wall) is considered when there is a high risk of recurrence, when cancer in situ is present, or when tumor resection has been incomplete. Topical chemotherapy delivers a high concentration of medication (thiotepa, doxorubicin, mitomycin, ethoglucid, and BCG) to the tumor to promote tumor destruction. Bladder cancer may also be treated by direct infusion of the cytotoxic agent through the bladder's arterial blood supply to achieve a higher concentration of the chemotherapeutic agent with fewer systemic toxic effects (Tanagho & McAninch, 2004).

BCG is now considered the most effective intravesical agent for recurrent bladder cancer, especially superficial transitional cell carcinoma, because it is an immunotherapeutic agent that enhances the body's immune response to cancer. BCG has a 43% advantage in preventing tumor recurrence, a significantly better rate than the 16% to 21% advantage of intravesical chemotherapy. In addition, BCG is particularly effective in the treatment of carcinoma in situ, eradicating it in more than 80% of cases. In contrast to intravesical chemotherapy, BCG has also been shown to decrease the risk of tumor progression.

The optimal course of BCG appears to be a 6-week course of weekly instillations, followed by a 3-week course at 3 months for tumors that do not respond. In high-risk cancers, maintenance BCG administered in a 3-week course at 6,12, 18, and 24 months may limit recurrence and prevent progression (Sanger, Busche, Bentien et al., 2004). However, the adverse effects associated with this prolonged therapy may limit its widespread applicability.

The patient is allowed to eat and drink before the instillation procedure. Once the bladder is full, the patient must retain the intravesical solution for 2 hours before voiding. At the end of the procedure, the patient is encouraged to void and to drink liberal amounts of fluid to flush the medication from the bladder.

Radiation Therapy

Radiation of the tumor may be performed preoperatively to reduce microextension of the neoplasm and viability of tumor cells, thus reducing the chances that the cancer may recur in the immediate area or spread through the circulatory or lymphatic systems. Radiation therapy is also used in combination with surgery or to control the disease in patients with inoperable tumors.

For more advanced bladder cancer or for patients with intractable hematuria (especially after radiation therapy), a large, water-filled balloon placed in the bladder produces tumor necrosis by reducing the blood supply of the bladder wall (hydrostatic therapy). The instillation of formalin, phenol, or silver nitrate relieves hematuria and strangury (slow and painful discharge of urine) in some patients.

Investigational Therapy

The use of photodynamic techniques in treating superficial bladder cancer is under investigation. This procedure involves systemic injection of a photosensitizing material (hematoporphyrin), which the cancer cell picks up. A laser-generated light then changes the hematoporphyrin in the cancer cell into a toxic medication. This process has received renewed interest with regulatory approval of several photosensitizing drugs and light applicators as potential palliative and curative treatments (Huang, 2005).

Urinary Diversions

Urinary diversion procedures are performed to divert urine from the bladder to a new exit site, usually through a surgically created opening (stoma) in the skin. These procedures are primarily performed when a bladder tumor necessitates cystectomy. Urinary diversion has also been used in managing pelvic malignancy, birth defects, strictures, trauma to the ureters and urethra, neurogenic bladder, chronic infection causing severe ureteral and renal damage, and intractable interstitial cystitis. It may also be used as a last resort in managing incontinence.

Controversy exists about the best method of establishing permanent diversion of the urinary tract. New techniques are frequently introduced in an effort to improve patient outcomes and quality of life. The age of the patient, condition of the bladder, body build, degree of obesity, degree of ureteral dilation, status of renal function, and the patient's learning ability and willingness to participate in postoperative care are all taken into consideration when determining the appropriate surgical procedure (Quallich & Ohl, 2003a).

The extent to which the patient accepts urinary diversion depends to a large degree on the location or position of the stoma, whether the drainage device (pouch or bag) establishes a watertight seal to the skin, and the patient's ability to manage the pouch and drainage apparatus (Quallich & Ohl, 2003b).

There are two types of urinary diversion. In a cutaneous urinary diversion, urine drains through an opening created in the abdominal wall and skin (Fig. 45-7). In a **continent urinary diversion**, a portion of the intestine is used to create a new reservoir for urine (Fig. 45-8).

Cutaneous Urinary Diversions

Ileal Conduit

The **ileal conduit** (ileal loop) is the oldest and most common of the urinary diversion procedures in use because of the low number of complications and surgeons' familiarity with the procedure. In an ileal conduit, the urine is diverted by implanting the ureter into a 12-cm loop of ileum that is led out through the abdominal wall. This loop of ileum is a simple conduit (passageway) for urine from the ureters to the surface. A loop of the sigmoid colon may also be used. An ileostomy bag is used to collect the urine. The resected (cut) ends of the remaining intestine are anastomosed (connected) to provide an intact bowel (Diepenbrock, 2004).

Stents, usually made of thin, pliable tubing, are placed in the ureters to prevent occlusion secondary to postsurgical edema. The bilateral ureteral stents allow urine to drain from the kidney to the stoma and provide a method

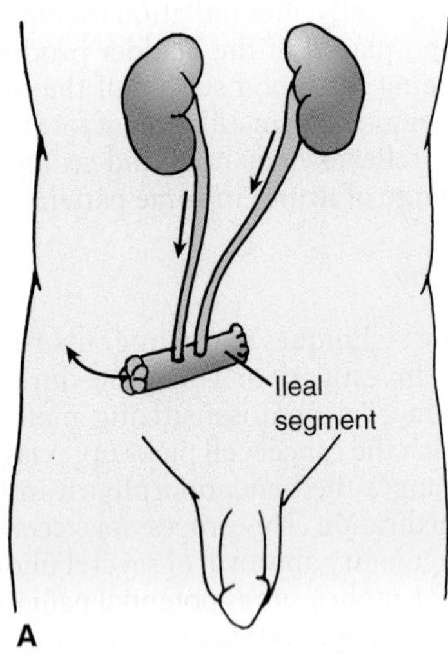

A

Conventional ileal conduit. The surgeon transplants the ureters to an isolated section of the terminal ileum (ileal conduit), bringing one end to the abdominal wall. The ureter may also be transplanted into the transverse sigmoid colon (colon conduit) or proximal jejunum (jejunal conduit).

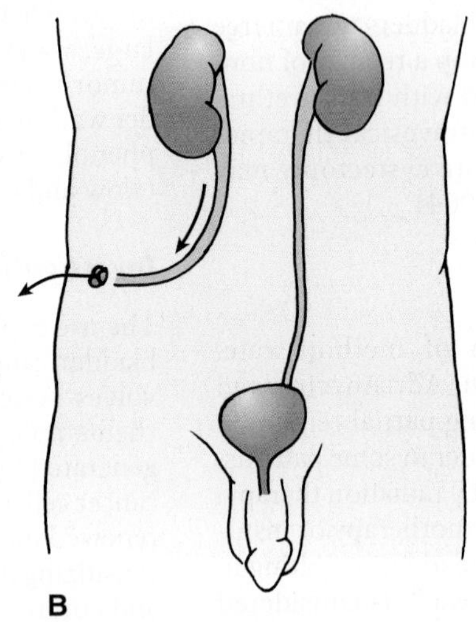

B

Cutaneous ureterostomy. The surgeon brings the detached ureter through the abdominal wall and attaches it to an opening in the skin.

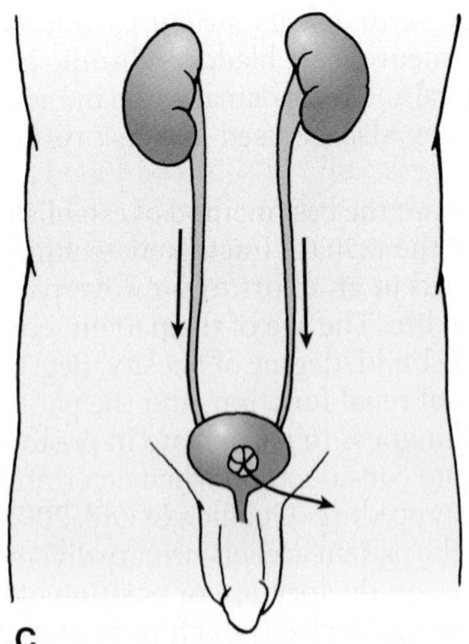

C

Vesicostomy. The surgeon sutures the bladder to the abdominal wall and creates an opening (stoma) through the abdominal and bladder walls for urinary drainage.

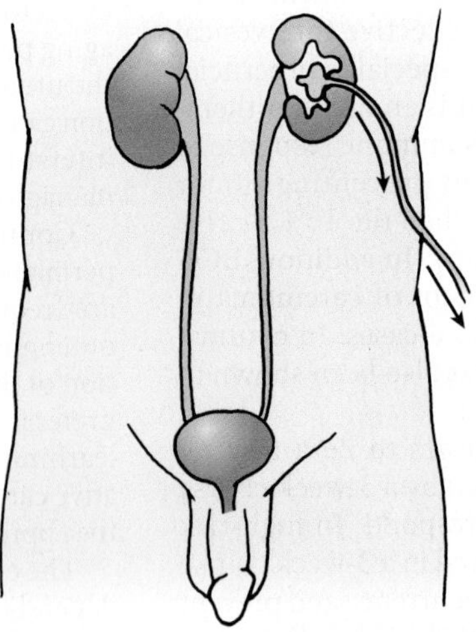

D

Nephrostomy. The surgeon inserts a catheter into the renal pelvis via an incision into the flank or, by percutaneous catheter placement, into the kidney.

FIGURE 45-7. Types of cutaneous diversions include (**A**) the conventional ileal conduit, (**B**) cutaneous ureterostomy, (**C**) vesicostomy, and (**D**) nephrostomy.

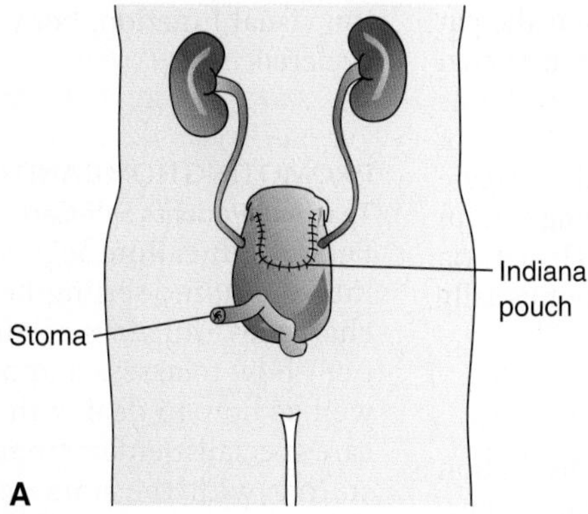

Indiana pouch. The surgeon introduces the ureters into a segment of ileum and cecum. Urine is drained periodically by inserting a catheter into the stoma.

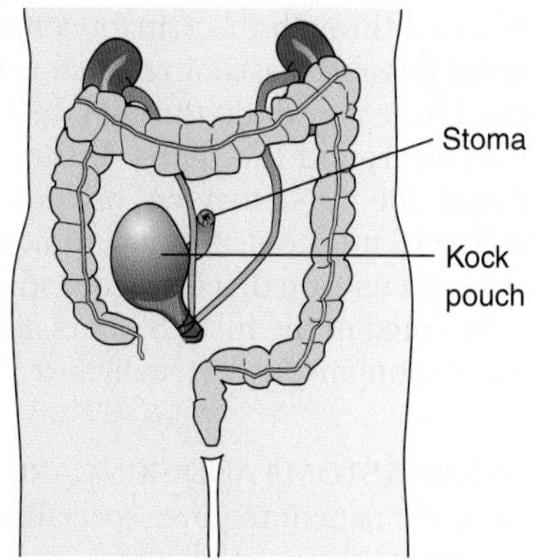

Continent ileal urinary diversions (Kock pouch). The surgeon transplants the ureters to an isolated segment of small bowel, ascending colon, or ileocolonic segment and develops an effective continence mechanism or valve. Urine is drained by inserting a catheter into the stoma.

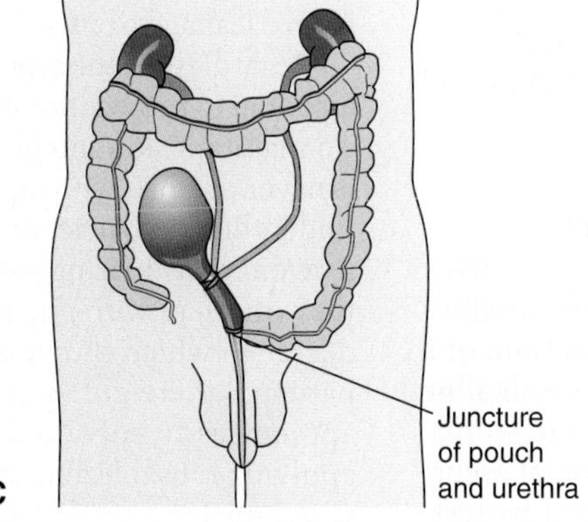

In male patients, the *Kock pouch* can be modified by attaching one end of the pouch to the urethra, allowing more normal voiding. The female urethra is too short for this modification.

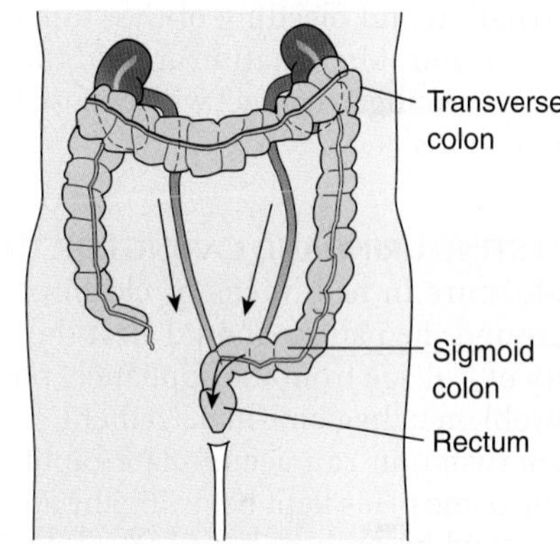

Ureterosigmoidostomy. The surgeon introduces the ureters into the sigmoid colon, thereby allowing urine to flow through the colon and out of the rectum.

FIGURE 45-8. Types of continent urinary diversions include (A) the Indiana pouch, (B and C) the Kock pouch, also called a continent ileal diversion, and (D) a ureterosigmoidostomy.

for accurate measurement of urine output. They may be left in place 10 to 21 days postoperatively. Jackson-Pratt tubes or other types of drains are inserted to prevent the accumulation of fluid in the space created by removal of the bladder.

After surgery, a skin barrier and a transparent, disposable urinary drainage bag are applied around the conduit and connected to drainage. A custom-cut appliance is used until the edema subsides and the stoma shrinks to normal size. The clear bag allows the stoma to be inspected and the patency of the stent and the urine output to be monitored. The ileal bag drains urine (not feces) continuously. The appliance (bag) usually remains in place as long as it is watertight; it is changed when necessary to prevent leakage of urine.

Complications

Complications that may follow placement of an ileal conduit include wound infection or wound dehiscence, urinary leakage, ureteral obstruction, hyperchloremic acidosis, small bowel obstruction, ileus, and gangrene of the stoma. Delayed complications include ureteral obstruction, contraction or narrowing of the stoma (stenosis), renal deterioration due to chronic reflux, pyelonephritis, and renal calculi.

Nursing Management

In the immediate postoperative period, urine volumes are monitored hourly. Throughout the patient's hospitalization, the nurse monitors closely for complications, reports signs and symptoms of them promptly, and intervenes quickly to prevent their progression.

A urine output below 30 mL/h may indicate dehydration or an obstruction in the ileal conduit, with possible backflow or leakage from the ureteroileal anastomosis. After the physician's order is obtained, a catheter may be inserted through the urinary conduit to monitor the patient for possible stasis or residual urine from a constricted stoma. Urine may drain through the bilateral ureteral stents as well as around the stents. If the ureteral stents are not draining, the nurse may be instructed to carefully irrigate with 5 to 10 mL sterile normal saline solution, being careful not to exert tension that could dislodge the stent. Hematuria may be noted in the first 48 hours after surgery but usually resolves spontaneously (Quallich & Ohl, 2003c).

PROVIDING STOMA AND SKIN CARE

Because the patient requires specialized care, a consultation is initiated with a wound care specialist/enterostomal therapist. The stoma is inspected frequently for color and viability. A healthy stoma is beefy red. A change from this normal color to a dark purplish color suggests that the vascular supply may be compromised. If cyanosis and a compromised blood supply persist, surgical intervention may be necessary. The stoma is not sensitive to touch, but the skin around the stoma becomes sensitive if urine or the appliance irritates it. The skin is inspected for (1) signs of irritation and bleeding of the stoma mucosa, (2) encrustation and skin irritation around the stoma (from alkaline urine coming in contact with exposed skin), and (3) wound infections.

TESTING URINE AND CARING FOR THE OSTOMY

Moisture in bed linens or clothing or the odor of urine around the patient should alert the nurse to the possibility of leakage from the appliance, potential infection, or a problem in hygienic management. Because severe alkaline encrustation can accumulate rapidly around the stoma, the urine pH is kept below 6.5 by administration of ascorbic acid by mouth. Urine pH can be determined by testing the urine draining from the stoma, not from the collecting appliance. A properly fitted appliance is essential to prevent exposure of the skin around the stoma to urine. If the urine is foul-smelling, the stoma is catheterized, if prescribed, to obtain a urine specimen for culture and sensitivity testing.

ENCOURAGING FLUIDS AND RELIEVING ANXIETY

Because mucous membrane is used in forming the conduit, the patient may excrete a large amount of mucus mixed with urine. This causes anxiety in many patients. To help relieve this anxiety, the nurse reassures the patient that this is a normal occurrence after an ileal conduit procedure. The nurse encourages adequate fluid intake to flush the ileal conduit and decrease the accumulation of mucus.

SELECTING THE OSTOMY APPLIANCE

Various urine collection appliances are available, and the nurse is instrumental in selecting an appropriate one. The urinary appliance may consist of one or two pieces and may be disposable (usually used once and discarded) or reusable. The choice of appliance is determined by the location of the stoma and by the patient's normal activity, manual dexterity, visual function, body build, economic resources, and preference.

PROMOTING HOME AND COMMUNITY-BASED CARE

Teaching Patients Self-Care

Patient education begins in the hospital but continues into the home setting because patients are usually discharged within days of surgery. The nurse teaches the patient how to assess and manage the urinary diversion as well as how to deal with body image changes. A wound care specialist/enterostomal therapist is invaluable in consulting with the nurse on various aspects of care and patient education.

Changing the Appliance. The patient and family are taught to apply and change the appliance so that they are comfortable carrying out the procedure and can do so proficiently. Ideally, the appliance system is changed before the system leaks and at a time that is convenient for the patient. Many patients find early morning most convenient because the urine output is reduced. A variety of appliances are available; an average collecting appliance lasts 3 to 7 days before leakage occurs.

Regardless of the type of appliance used, a skin barrier is essential to protect the skin from irritation and excoriation. To maintain skin integrity, a skin barrier or leaking pouch is never patched with tape to prevent accumulation of urine under the skin barrier or faceplate. The patient is instructed to avoid moisturizing soaps when cleaning the area because they interfere with the adhesion of the pouch. Because the degree to which the stoma protrudes is not the same in all patients, there are various accessories and custom-made appliances to solve individual problems. Guidelines for applying reusable and disposable systems are presented in Chart 45-13.

Controlling Odor. The patient is instructed to avoid foods that give the urine a strong odor (eg, asparagus, cheese, eggs). Today, most appliances contain odor barriers, but a few drops of liquid deodorizer or diluted white vinegar may be introduced through the drain spout into the bottom of the pouch with a syringe or eyedropper to reduce odors. Ascorbic acid by mouth helps acidify the urine and suppress urine odor. Patients should be cautioned not to put aspirin tablets in the pouch to control odor because they may ulcerate the stoma. Also, the patient is reminded that odor will develop if the pouch is worn longer than recommended and not cared for properly.

Managing the Ostomy Appliance. The patient is instructed to empty the pouch by means of a drain valve when it is one-third full because the weight of more urine will cause the pouch to separate from the skin. Some patients prefer wearing a leg bag attached with an adapter to the drainage apparatus. To promote uninterrupted sleep, a collecting bottle and tubing (one unit) are snapped onto an adapter that connects to the ileal appliance. A small amount of urine is left in the bag when the adapter is attached to prevent the bag from collapsing against itself. The tubing may be threaded down the pajama or pants leg to prevent kinking. The collecting bottle and tubing are rinsed daily

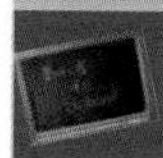

CHART 45-13

Patient Education

Using Urinary Diversion Collection Appliances

APPLYING A REUSABLE POUCH SYSTEM

1. Gather all necessary supplies.
2. Prepare new appliance according to the manufacturer's directions.
   - Apply double-faced adhesive disk that has been properly sized to fit the reusable pouch faceplate. Remove paper backing and set pouch aside, or apply thin layer of contact cement to one side of the reusable pouch faceplate. Set pouch aside.
3. Remove soiled pouch gently. Lay aside to clean later.
4. Clean peristomal skin (skin around stoma) with small amount of soap and water. Rinse thoroughly and dry. If a film of soap remains on the skin and the site does not dry, the appliance will not adhere adequately.
5. Use a wick (rolled gauze pad or tampon) over the stoma to absorb urine and keep the skin dry throughout the appliance change.
6. Inspect peristomal skin for irritation.
7. A skin protector wipe or barrier ring may be applied before centering the faceplate opening directly over the stoma.
8. Position appliance over stoma and press gently into place.
9. If desired, use a pouch cover or apply cornstarch under the pouch to prevent perspiration and skin irritation.
10. Clean soiled pouch and prepare for reuse.

APPLYING A DISPOSABLE POUCH SYSTEM

1. Gather all necessary supplies.
2. Measure stoma and prepare an opening in the skin barrier about an ⅛-inch larger than the stoma and the same shape as the stoma.
3. Remove paper backing from skin barrier and set aside.
4. Gently remove old appliance and set aside.
5. Clean peristomal skin with warm water and dry thoroughly.
6. Inspect peristomal skin (skin around stoma) for irritation.
7. Use a wick (rolled gauze pad or tampon) over the stoma to absorb urine and keep the skin dry during the appliance change.
8. Center opening of skin barrier over stoma and apply with firm, gentle pressure to attain a watertight seal.
9. If using a two-piece system, snap pouch onto the flanged wafer that adheres to skin.
10. Close drainage tap or spout at bottom of pouch.
11. A pouch cover can be used or cornstarch applied under pouch to prevent perspiration and skin irritation.
12. Apply hypoallergenic tape around the skin barrier in a picture-frame manner.
13. Dispose of soiled appliance.

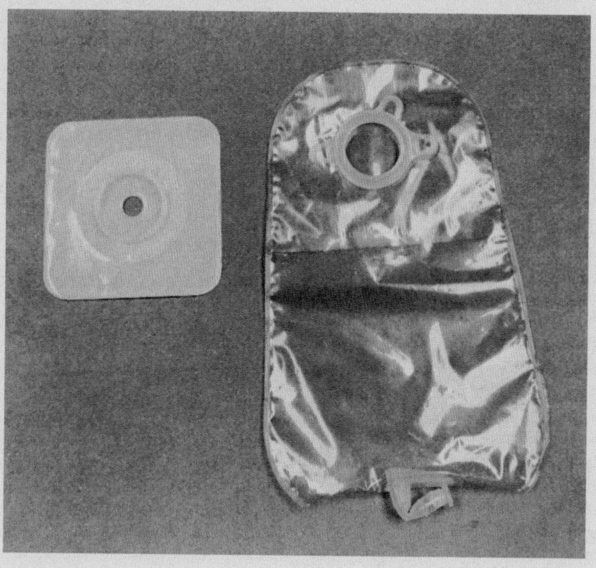

with cool water and once a week with a 3:1 solution of water and white vinegar.

Cleaning and Deodorizing the Appliance. Usually, the reusable appliance is rinsed in warm water and soaked in a 3:1 solution of water and white vinegar or a commercial deodorizing solution for 30 minutes. It is rinsed with tepid water and air-dried away from direct sunlight. (Hot water and exposure to direct sunlight dry the pouch and increase the incidence of cracking.) After drying, the appliance may be powdered with cornstarch and stored. Two appliances are necessary—one to be worn while the other is air-drying.

Continuing Care

Follow-up care is essential to determine how the patient has adapted to the body image changes and lifestyle changes. Referral for home care is indicated to determine how well the patient and family are coping with the changes necessitated by altered urinary drainage. The home care nurse assesses the patient's physical status and emotional response to urinary diversion. Additionally, the nurse assesses the ability of the patient and family to manage the urinary diversion and appliance, reinforces previous teaching, and provides additional information (eg, community resources, sources of ostomy supplies, insurance coverage for supplies).

As the postoperative edema subsides, the home care nurse assists in determining the appropriate changes needed in the ostomy appliance. The size of the stoma is measured every 3 to 6 weeks for the first few months postoperatively. The correct appliance size is determined by measuring the widest part of the stoma with a ruler. The permanent appliance should be no more than 1.6 mm (⅙ inch) larger than the diameter of the stoma and the same shape as the stoma to prevent contact of the skin with drainage.

The nurse teaches the patient and family about resources (see the list of resources at end of this chapter). Local chapters of the American Cancer Society (ACS) can provide medical equipment and supplies and other resources for the patient who has undergone ostomy surgery for cancer.

The home care nurse assesses the patient for potential long-term complications such as ureteral obstruction, stenosis, hernias, or deterioration of renal function, and reinforces previous teaching about these complications.

Cutaneous Ureterostomy

A cutaneous ureterostomy (see Fig. 45-7), in which the ureters are directed through the abdominal wall and attached to an opening in the skin, is used for selected patients with ureteral obstruction (ie, advanced pelvic cancer) because it requires less extensive surgery than other urinary diversion procedures. It is also an appropriate procedure for patients who have had previous abdominal irradiation.

A urinary appliance is fitted immediately after surgery. The management of the patient with a cutaneous ureterostomy is similar to the care of the patient with an ileal conduit, although the stomas are usually flush with the skin or retracted.

Continent Urinary Diversions

Continent Ileal Urinary Reservoir (Indiana Pouch)

The most common continent urinary diversion is the Indiana pouch, created for the patient whose bladder is removed or no longer functions. The Indiana pouch uses a segment of the ileum and cecum to form the reservoir for urine (see Fig. 45-8A). The ureters are tunneled through the muscular bands of the intestinal pouch and anastomosed. The reservoir is made continent by narrowing the efferent portion of the ileum and sewing the terminal ileum to the subcutaneous tissue, forming a continent stoma flush with the skin. The pouch is sewn to the anterior abdominal wall around a cecostomy tube. Urine collects in the pouch until a catheter is inserted and the urine is drained (Diepenbrock, 2004).

The pouch must be drained at regular intervals by a catheter to prevent absorption of metabolic waste products from the urine, reflux of urine to the ureters, and UTI. Postoperative nursing care of the patient with a continent ileal urinary pouch is similar to nursing care of the patient with an ileal conduit. However, these patients usually have additional drainage tubes (cecostomy catheter from the pouch, stoma catheter exiting from the stoma, ureteral stents, Penrose drain, as well as a urethral catheter). All drainage tubes must be carefully monitored for patency and amount and type of drainage. In the immediate postoperative period, the cecostomy tube is irrigated two or three times daily to remove mucus and prevent blockage.

Other variations of continent urinary reservoirs include the **Kock pouch** (U-shaped pouch constructed of ileum, with a nipple-like one-way valve; see Fig. 45-8B, C) and the **Charleston pouch** (uses the ileum and ascending colon as the pouch, with the appendix and colon junction serving as the one-way valve mechanism). With both of these methods, the pouch must be drained at regular intervals by a catheter.

Ureterosigmoidostomy

Ureterosigmoidostomy, another form of continent urinary diversion, is an implantation of the ureters into the sigmoid colon (see Fig. 45-8D). It is usually performed in patients who have had extensive pelvic irradiation, previous small bowel resection, or coexisting small bowel disease.

After surgery, voiding occurs from the rectum (for life), and an adjustment in lifestyle will be necessary because of urinary frequency. Drainage has a consistency equivalent to watery diarrhea, and the patient has some degree of nocturia. Patients usually need to plan activities around the frequent need to urinate, which in turn may affect the patient's social life. However, patients have the advantage of urinary control without having to wear an external appliance.

Nursing Management

In addition to the usual preoperative regimen, the patient may be placed on a liquid diet for several days preoperatively to reduce residue in the colon. Antibiotic agents (neomycin, kanamycin) are administered to disinfect the bowel. Ureterosigmoidostomy requires a competent anal sphincter, adequate renal function, and active renal peristalsis. The degree of anal sphincter control may be determined by assessing the patient's ability to retain enemas.

The postoperative regimen initially includes placing a catheter in the rectum to drain the urine and prevent reflux of urine into the ureters and kidneys. The tube is taped to the buttocks, and special skin care is given around the anus to prevent excoriation. Irrigations of the rectal tube may be prescribed, but force is never used because of the danger of introducing bacteria into the newly implanted ureters.

MONITORING FLUID AND ELECTROLYTES

In ureterosigmoidostomy, larger areas of the bowel mucosa are exposed to urine and electrolyte reabsorption. As a result, electrolyte imbalance and acidosis may occur. Potassium and magnesium in the urine may cause diarrhea. Fluid and electrolyte balance is maintained in the immediate postoperative period by closely monitoring the serum electrolyte levels and administering appropriate IV fluids. Acidosis may be prevented by placing the patient on a low-chloride diet supplemented with sodium potassium citrate.

The patient should be instructed never to wait longer than 2 to 3 hours before emptying urine from the intestine. This keeps rectal pressure low and minimizes the absorption of urinary constituents from the colon. It is essential to teach the patient about the symptoms of UTI: fever, flank pain, and dysuria.

RETRAINING THE ANAL SPHINCTER

After the rectal catheter is removed, the patient learns to control the anal sphincter through special sphincter exercises. At first, urination is frequent. With reassurance and encouragement and the passage of time, the patient gains greater control and learns to differentiate between the need to void and the need to defecate.

PROMOTING DIETARY MEASURES

Specific dietary instructions include avoidance of gas-forming foods (flatus can cause stress incontinence and offensive odors). Other ways to avoid gas are to avoid chewing gum, smoking, and any other activity that involves swallowing air. Salt intake may be restricted to prevent hyperchloremic acidosis. Potassium intake is increased through foods and medication because potassium may be lost in acidosis.

MONITORING AND MANAGING POTENTIAL COMPLICATIONS

Pyelonephritis (upper UTI) due to reflux of bacteria from the colon is fairly common. Long-term antibiotic therapy may be prescribed to prevent infection. A late complication is adenocarcinoma of the sigmoid colon, possibly from cellular changes due to exposure of the colonic mucosa to urine. Urinary carcinogens promote late malignant transformation of the colon after a ureterosigmoidostomy, warranting life-long medical follow-up.

Other Urinary Diversion Procedures

Variations on urinary diversion surgical procedures are devised frequently in an effort to identify and perfect procedures that will improve patient outcomes and reduce the incidence of postoperative problems. These include cecal, patched cecal, and Mainz reservoirs. These techniques involve isolating a part of the large intestine to form a reservoir for urine and creating an abdominal stoma. Another surgical procedure, the Camey procedure, uses a portion of the ileum as a bladder substitute. In this procedure, the isolated ileum serves as the reservoir for urine; it is anastomosed directly to the portion of the remaining urethra after cystectomy. This procedure permits emptying of the bladder through the urethra. However, the Camey procedure applies only to men because the entire urethra is removed when a cystectomy is performed in women.

Nursing Process

The Patient Undergoing Urinary Diversion Surgery

Preoperative Assessment

The following are key preoperative nursing assessment concerns:

- Cardiopulmonary function assessments are performed because patients undergoing cystectomy are often older people who may be at greater risk for cardiac and respiratory complications.
- A nutritional status assessment is important because of possible poor nutritional intake related to underlying health problems.
- Learning needs are assessed to evaluate the patient's and the family's understanding of the procedure and the changes in physical structure and function that result from the surgery. The patient's self-concept and self-esteem are assessed, in addition to methods for coping with stress and loss. The patient's mental status, manual dexterity and coordination, and preferred method of learning are noted because they will affect postoperative self-care.

Preoperative Nursing Diagnoses

Based on the assessment data, the preoperative nursing diagnoses for the patient undergoing urinary diversion surgery may include the following:

- Anxiety related to anticipated losses associated with the surgical procedure
- Imbalanced nutrition, less than body requirements related to inadequate nutritional intake
- Deficient knowledge about the surgical procedure and postoperative care

Preoperative Planning and Goals

The major goals for the patient may include relief of anxiety, improved preoperative nutritional status, and increased knowledge about the surgical procedure, expected outcomes, and postoperative care.

Preoperative Nursing Interventions

Relieving Anxiety

The threat of cancer and removal of the bladder create anxiety related to changes in body image. Patients may face problems adapting to an external appliance, a stoma, a surgical incision, and altered toileting habits. Men must also adapt to sexual impotency; a penile implant is considered if the patient is a candidate for the procedure. Women also have anxiety related to altered appearance, body image, and self-esteem. A supportive approach, both physical and psychosocial, is needed and includes assessing the patient's self-concept and manner of coping with stress and loss; helping the patient to identify ways to maintain his or her lifestyle and independence with as few changes as possible; and encouraging the patient to express fears and anxieties about the ramifications of the upcoming surgery. A visitor from the Ostomy Visitation Program of the ACS can provide emotional support and make adaptation easier both before and after surgery.

Ensuring Adequate Nutrition

In addition to cleansing the bowel to minimize fecal stasis, decompress the bowel, and minimize postoperative ileus, a low-residue diet is prescribed. In addition, antibiotic medications are administered to reduce pathogenic flora in the bowel and to reduce the risk of infection. Because the patient undergoing a urinary diversion procedure for cancer may be severely malnourished due to the tumor, radiation enteritis, and anorexia, enteral or parenteral nutrition may be prescribed to promote healing. Adequate preoperative hydration is imperative to ensure urine flow during surgery and to prevent hypovolemia during the prolonged surgical procedure.

Explaining Surgery and its Effects

Participation of a wound care specialist/enterostomal therapist is invaluable for informed preoperative teaching and postoperative care planning. Explanations of the surgical procedure, the appearance of the stoma, the rationale for preoperative bowel preparation, the reasons for wearing a collection device, and the anticipated effects of the surgery on sexual functioning are part of patient teaching. The placement of the stoma site is planned preoperatively with the patient standing, sitting, and lying down to locate the stoma away from bony prominences, skin creases, and folds. The stoma should also be placed away from old scars, the umbilicus, and the belt line.

For ease of self-care, the patient must be able to see and reach the site comfortably. The site is marked with indelible ink so that it can be located easily during surgery. The patient is assessed for allergies or sensitivity to tape or adhesives. Patch testing of certain appliances may be necessary before the ostomy equipment is selected. This is particularly important if the patient is or may be allergic to latex (see Chapter 18).

Preoperative Evaluation

To measure the effectiveness of care, the nurse evaluates the patient's preoperative anxiety level and nutritional status as well as pre-existing knowledge and expectations of surgery.

Expected Patient Outcomes

Expected patient outcomes may include:

1. Exhibits reduced anxiety about surgery and expected losses
   a. Verbalizes fears with health care team and family
   b. Expresses positive attitude about outcome of surgery
2. Exhibits adequate nutritional status
   a. Maintains adequate intake before surgery
   b. Maintains body weight
   c. States rationale for enteral or parenteral nutrition if needed
   d. Exhibits normal skin turgor, moist mucous membranes, adequate urine output, and absence of excessive thirst
3. Demonstrates knowledge about the surgical procedure and postoperative course
   a. Identifies limitations expected after surgery
   b. Discusses expected immediate postoperative environment (tubes, equipment, nursing surveillance)
   c. Practices deep breathing, coughing, and foot exercises

Postoperative Assessment

The role of the nurse in the immediate postoperative period is to prevent complications and to assess the patient carefully for any signs and symptoms of complications. The catheters and any drainage devices are monitored closely. Urine volume, patency of the drainage system, and color of the drainage are assessed. A sudden decrease in urine volume or increase in drainage is reported promptly to the physician because these may indicate obstruction of the urinary tract, inadequate blood volume, or bleeding. In addition, the patient's need for pain control is assessed regularly as with all postoperative patients.

Postoperative Diagnosis

Nursing Diagnoses

Based on the assessment data, the major postoperative nursing diagnoses for the patient following urinary diversion surgery may include the following:

- Risk for impaired skin integrity related to problems in managing the urine collection appliance
- Acute pain related to surgical incision
- Disturbed body image related to urinary diversion
- Potential for sexual dysfunction related to structural and physiologic alterations
- Deficient knowledge about management of urinary function

Collaborative Problems/ Potential Complications

Potential complications may include the following:

- Peritonitis due to disruption of anastomosis
- Stoma ischemia and necrosis due to compromised blood supply to stoma
- Stoma retraction and separation of mucocutaneous border due to tension or trauma

Postoperative Planning and Goals

The major goals for the patient may include maintaining skin integrity, relieving pain, increasing self-esteem, developing appropriate coping mechanisms to accept and deal with altered urinary function and sexuality, increasing knowledge about management of urinary function, and preventing potential complications.

Postoperative Nursing Interventions

Postoperative management focuses on monitoring urinary function, preventing postoperative complications (infection and sepsis, respiratory complications, fluid and electrolyte imbalances, fistula formation, and urine leakage), and promoting patient comfort. Catheters or drainage systems are monitored, and urine output is monitored carefully. A nasogastric tube is inserted during surgery to decompress the GI tract and to relieve pressure on the intestinal anastomosis. It is usually kept in place for several days after surgery. As soon as bowel function resumes, as indicated by bowel sounds, the passage of flatus, and a soft abdomen, oral fluids are permitted. Until that time, IV fluids and electrolytes are administered. The patient is assisted to ambulate as soon as possible to prevent complications of immobility.

Maintaining Skin Integrity

Strategies to promote skin integrity begin with reducing and controlling those factors that increase the patient's risk of poor nutrition and poor healing. As indicated previously, meticulous skin care and management of the drainage system are provided by the nurse until the patient can manage them and is comfortable doing so. Care is taken to keep the drainage system intact to protect the skin from exposure to drainage. Supplies must be readily available to manage the drainage in the immediate postoperative period. Consistency in implementing the skin care program throughout the postoperative period results in maintenance of skin integrity and patient comfort. Additionally, maintenance of skin integrity around the stoma enables the patient and family to adjust more easily to the alterations in urinary function and helps them learn skin care techniques.

Relieving Pain

Analgesic medications are administered liberally postoperatively to relieve pain and promote comfort, thereby allowing the patient to turn, cough, and perform deep-breathing exercises. Patient-controlled analgesia (PCA) and administration of analgesic agents regularly around the clock are two options that may be used to ensure adequate pain relief. A pain intensity scale is used to evaluate the adequacy of the medication and the approach to pain management.

Improving Body Image

The patient's ability to cope with the changes associated with the surgery depends to some degree on his or her body image and self-esteem before the surgery and the support and reaction of others. Allowing the patient to express concerns and anxious feelings can help, especially in adjusting to the changes in toileting habits. The nurse can also help improve the patient's self-concept by teaching the skills needed to be independent in managing the urinary drainage devices. Education about ostomy care is conducted in a private setting to encourage the patient to ask questions without fear of embarrassment. Explaining why the nurse must wear gloves when performing ostomy care can prevent the patient from misinterpreting the use of gloves as a sign of aversion to the stoma.

Exploring Sexuality Issues

Patients who experience altered sexual function as a result of the surgical procedure may mourn this loss. Encouraging the patient and partner to share their feelings about this loss with each other and acknowledging the importance of sexual function and expression may encourage the patient and partner to seek sexual counseling and to explore alternative ways of expressing sexuality. A visit from another "ostomate" who is functioning fully in society and family life may also assist the patient and family in recognizing that full recovery is possible.

Monitoring and Managing Potential Complications

Complications are not unusual because of the complexity of the surgery, the underlying reason (cancer, trauma) for the urinary diversion procedure, and the patient's frequently less-than-optimal nutritional status. Complications may include respiratory complications (eg., atelectasis, pneumonia), fluid and electrolyte imbalances, breakdown of any anastomosis, sepsis, fistula formation, fecal or urine leakage, and skin irritation. If these occur, the patient will remain hospitalized for an extended length of time and will probably require parenteral nutrition, GI decompression by means of nasogastric suction, and further surgery. The goals of management are to establish drainage, provide adequate nutrition for healing to occur, and prevent sepsis.

PERITONITIS

Peritonitis can occur postoperatively if urine leaks at the anastomosis. Signs and symptoms include abdominal pain and distention, muscle rigidity with guarding, nausea and vomiting, paralytic ileus (absence of bowel sounds), fever, and leukocytosis.

Urine output must be monitored closely, because a sudden decrease in output with a corresponding increase in drainage from the incision or drains may indicate urine leakage. In addition, the urine drainage device is observed for leakage. The pouch is changed if a leak is observed. Small leaks in the anastomosis may seal themselves, but surgery may be needed for larger leaks.

Vital signs (blood pressure, pulse and respiratory rates, temperature) are monitored. Changes in vital signs, as well as increasing pain, nausea and vomiting, and abdominal distention, are reported to the physician and may indicate peritonitis.

STOMA ISCHEMIA AND NECROSIS

The stoma is monitored because ischemia and necrosis of the stoma can result from tension on the mesentery blood vessels, twisting of the bowel segment (conduit) during surgery, or arterial insufficiency. The new stoma must be inspected at least every 4 hours to assess the adequacy of its blood supply. The stoma should be red or pink. If the blood supply to the stoma is compromised, the color changes to purple, brown, or black. These changes are reported immediately to the physician. The physician or wound care specialist/enterostomal therapist may insert a small, lubricated tube into the stoma and shine a flashlight into the lumen of the tube to assess for superficial ischemia or necrosis. A necrotic stoma requires surgical intervention. If the ischemia is superficial, the dusky stoma is observed and may slough its outer layer in several days.

STOMA RETRACTION AND SEPARATION

Stoma retraction and separation of the mucocutaneous border can occur as a result of trauma or tension on the internal bowel segment used for creation of the stoma. In addition, mucocutaneous separation can occur if the stoma does not heal as a result of accumulation of urine on the stoma and mucocutaneous border. Using a collection drainage pouch with an antireflux valve is helpful because the valve prevents urine from pooling on the stoma and mucocutaneous border. Meticulous skin care to keep the area around the stoma clean and dry promotes healing. If a separation of the mucocutaneous border occurs, surgery is not usually needed. The separated area is protected by applying karaya powder, stoma adhesive paste, and a properly fitted skin barrier and pouch. By protecting the separation, healing is promoted. If the stoma retracts into the peritoneum, surgical intervention is mandatory.

If surgery is needed to manage these complications, the nurse provides explanations to the patient and family. The need for additional surgery is usually perceived as a setback by the patient and family. Emotional support of the patient and family is provided along with physical preparation of the patient for surgery.

Promoting Home and Community-Based Care

TEACHING PATIENTS SELF-CARE

A major postoperative objective is to assist the patient to achieve the highest level of independence and self-care possible. The nurse and wound care specialist/enterostomal therapist work closely with the patient and family to instruct and assist them in all phases of managing the ostomy. Adequate supplies and complete instruction are necessary to enable the patient and a family member to develop competence and confidence in their skills. Written and verbal instructions are provided, and the patient is encouraged to contact the nurse or physician with follow-up questions. Follow-up telephone calls from the nurse to the patient and family after discharge may provide added support and provide another opportunity to answer their questions. Follow-up visits and reinforcement of correct skin care and appliance management techniques also promote skin integrity. Specific techniques for managing the appliance are described in Chart 45-13.

The patient is encouraged to participate in decisions regarding the type of collecting appliance and the time of day to change the appliance. The patient is assisted and encouraged to look at and touch the stoma early to overcome any fears. The patient and family need to know the characteristics of a normal stoma:

- Pink and moist, like the inside of the mouth
- Insensitive to pain because it has no nerve endings
- Vascular and may bleed when cleaned

Additionally, if a segment of the GI tract was used to create the urinary diversion, mucus may be visible in the urine. By learning what is normal, the patient and family become familiar with what signs and symptoms they should report to the physician or nurse and what problems they can handle themselves.

Information provided to the patient and the extent of involvement in self-care are determined by the patient's physical recovery and ability to accept and acquire the knowledge and skill needed for independence. Verbal and written instructions are provided, and the patient is given the opportunity to practice and demonstrate the knowledge and skills needed to manage urinary drainage.

CONTINUING CARE

Follow-up care is essential to determine how the patient has adapted to the body image changes and lifestyle adjustments. Visits from a home care nurse are important to assess the patient's adaptation to the home setting and management of the ostomy. Teaching and reinforcement may assist the patient and family to cope with altered urinary function. It is also necessary to assess for long-term complications that may occur, such as pouch leakage or rupture, stone formation, stenosis of the stoma, deterioration in renal function, or incontinence.

Long-term monitoring for anemia is performed to identify vitamin B deficiency, which may occur when a significant portion of the terminal ileum is removed. This may take several years to develop and can be treated with vitamin B injections. The patient and family are informed of the United Ostomy Association and any local ostomy support groups to provide ongoing support, assistance, and education.

Postoperative Evaluation

Expected Patient Outcomes

Expected patient outcomes may include:

1. Maintains skin integrity
   a. Maintains intact skin and demonstrates skill in managing drainage system and appliance
   b. States actions to take if skin excoriation occurs
2. Reports relief of pain
3. Exhibits improved body image as evidenced by the following:
   a. Voices acceptance of urinary diversion, stoma, and appliance
   b. Demonstrates increasingly independent self-care, including hygiene and grooming
   c. States acceptance of support and assistance from family members, health care providers, and other ostomates
4. Copes with sexuality issues
   a. Verbalizes concern about possible alterations in sexuality and sexual function
   b. Reports discussion of sexual concerns with partner and appropriate counselor
5. Demonstrates knowledge needed for self-care
   a. Performs self-care and proficient management of urinary diversion and appliance
   b. Asks questions relevant to self-management and prevention of complications
   c. Identifies signs and symptoms needing care from physician, nurse, or other health care providers
6. Absence of complications as evidenced by the following:
   a. Reports absence of pain or tenderness in abdomen
   b. Has temperature within normal range
   c. Reports no urine leakage from incision or drains
   d. Has urine output within desired volume limits
   e. Maintains stoma that is red or pink, moist, and appropriate in size without edema
   f. Has intact and healed border of the stoma

Critical Thinking Exercises

1 ebp As the head nurse in a long-term care facility, you are approached by the daughter of one of the residents. She requests that her mother, who can ambulate with assistance, have an indwelling urinary catheter inserted "for convenience sake." What is the evidence base that supports your response? Identify the criteria used to evaluate the strength of the evidence.

2 As one of the nurses in a busy urology practice, you are performing telephone triage. A 62-year-old man who was seen 2 days ago for increasing urinary frequency, including several awakenings at night, phones to report increasing abdominal pain. He states that he has not voided for more than 12 hours, although he has made several unsuccessful attempts. Explain the instructions you would provide. What medical and nursing interventions would you anticipate?

3 ebp A 50-year-old woman comes for her annual pelvic check-up with complaints of occasional urinary urgency, sometimes with "near incontinences" just as she reaches the toilet. She denies the intake of any potentially bladder-irritating substances, such as beverages containing caffeine or synthetic sweeteners. She also mentions that she is having difficulty with decreased lubrication during intercourse and her menses are irregular. On physical examination, thinning of the vaginal mucosa is noted. Identify the evidence for and the criteria used to evaluate the strength of the evidence for and against the use of estrogen in maintaining continence.

4 A 55-year-old man returns to your unit following a Camey procedure after cystectomy for bladder cancer. What immediate nursing assessment and interventions should you take at this time? Describe the nursing diagnoses and plan of care in the postoperative period. How will you modify the plan if the patient is a 75-year-old?

REFERENCES AND SELECTED READINGS

BOOKS

Bickley, L. S. & Szilagyi, P. G. (2003). *Bates' guide to physical examination and history taking* (8th ed.). Philadelphia: Lippincott Williams & Wilkins.

Diepenbrock, N. H. (2004). *Quick reference to critical care* (2nd ed.). Philadelphia: Lippincott Williams & Wilkins.

Dudek, S. G. (2006). *Nutrition essentials for nursing practice* (5th ed.). Philadelphia: Lippincott Williams & Wilkins.

Fillingham, S. & Douglas, J. (2004). *Urological nursing* (3rd ed). London: Elsevier.

Karch, A. (2005). *Lippincott's nursing drug guide.* Philadelphia: Lippincott Williams & Wilkins.

Melnyk, B. M. & Fineout-Overholt, E. (2005). *Evidence-based practice in nursing and healthcare: A guide to best practices.* Philadelphia: Lippincott, Williams & Wilkins.

Morton, P. G., Fontaine, D. K., Hudak, C. M., et al. (2005). *Critical care nursing: A holistic approach* (8th ed.). Philadelphia: Lippincott Williams & Wilkins.

Porth, C. M. (2005). *Pathophysiology: Concepts of altered health states* (7th ed.). Philadelphia: Lippincott Williams & Wilkins.

Schnell, Z., Leeuwen, A., & Kranpitz, T. (2003). *Davis's comprehensive handbook of laboratory and diagnostic tests with nursing implications.* Philadelphia: F. A. Davis Co.

Stanley, M., Blair, K. A., & Beare, P. G. (2005). *Gerontological nursing: Promoting successful aging with older adults* (3rd ed.). Philadelphia: F. A. Davis.

Tanagho, E. & McAninch, J. (Eds.) (2004). *Smith's general urology* (16th ed.). New York: McGraw-Hill.

Zonderman, J. & Doyle, R. (2006). *Springhouse nurse's drug guide 2006.* Philadelphia: Lippincott Williams & Wilkins.

JOURNALS

**Asterisks indicate nursing research articles.*

General

Albaugh, J. (2003). Urinary dysfunction and urodynamics in the elderly. *Urologic Nursing, 23*(2), 136–140.

Burrows-Hudson, S. (2005). Chronic kidney disease: An overview: Early and aggressive treatment is vital. *American Journal of Nursing, 105*(2), 40–50.

Hanson, K. (2003). Laboratory studies in the evaluation of urological disease: Part I. *Urologic Nursing, 23*(6), 400–404.

Hanson, K. (2003). Laboratory studies in the evaluation of urological disease: Part II. *Urologic Nursing 23*(6), 405–414.

Toughill, E. (2005). Indwelling catheters: Common mechanical and pathogenic problems. *American Journal of Nursing, 105*(5), 35–37.

Infections of the Urinary Tract

Goldrick, B. (2005). Infection in the older adult. Long term care poses particular risk. *American Journal of Nursing, 105*(6), 31–34.

Jackson, S. L., Boyko, E. J., Scholes, D. et al. (2004). Predictors of urinary tract infection after menopause: A prospective study. *American Journal of Medicine, 117*(12), 903–911.

McMurdo, M. E., Bissett, L. Y., Price, R. J., et al. (2005). Does ingestion of cranberry juice reduce symptomatic urinary tract infections in older people in hospital? *Age and Ageing, 34*(3), 256–261.

Mehnert-Kay, S. A. (2005). Diagnosis and management of uncomplicated urinary tract infections. *American Family Physician, 72*(3), 451–456.

Midthum, S. (2004) Criteria for urinary tract infection in the elderly: Variables that affect nursing assessment. *Urologic Nursing, 24*(3), 157–169.

Adult Voiding Dysfunction

Diokno, A. C., Sampselle, C. M., Herzog, A. R., et. al. (2004). Prevention of urinary incontinence by behavioral modification program: A randomized, controlled trial among older women in the community. *Journal of Urology, 171*(3), 1165–1171.

Fick, D. M., Cooper, J., Waller, J., et al. (2003). Updating criteria for potentially inappropriate medication use in older adults. *Archives of Internal Medicine, 163*(22), 2716–2724.

Gokula, R. (2004). Inappropriate use of urinary catheters in elderly patients at a midwestern community teaching hospital. *American Journal of Infection Control, 4*(32), 196–199.

*Klay, M. & Marfyak, K. (2005). Use of a continence nurse specialist in an extended care facility. *Urologic Nursing, 25*(2), 101–108.

Lekan-Rutledge, D. (2004). Urinary incontinence strategies for frail elderly women. *Urologic Nursing, 24*(4), 281–301.

Lekan-Rutledge, D., Doughty, D., Moore, K., et al. (2003). Promoting social continence: Products and devices in the management of urinary incontinence. *Urologic Nursing, 23*(6), 416–458.

Mennick, F. (2005). Urinary incontinence worsens with menopausal hormone therapy. *American Journal of Nursing, 105*(7), 22.

*Muller, N. (2005). What Americans understand and how they are affected by bladder control problems: Highlights of recent nationwide consumer research. *Urologic Nursing, 25*(2), 109–115.

Newman, D. (2003). Stress urinary incontinence in women. *American Journal of Nursing, 103*(8), 46–56.

Newman, D. (2004). Incontinence products and devices for the elderly. *Urologic Nursing, 24*(4), 317–333.

Palmer, M. (2004). Physiologic and psychologic age-related changes that affect urologic clients. *Urologic Nursing, 24*(4), 247–252.

Sampselle, C. (2003). Teaching women to use a voiding diary. *American Journal of Nursing, 103*(11), 62–64.

Specht, J. (2005). Nine myths of incontinence in older adults. *American Journal of Nursing, 105*(6), 58–70.

Wilde, M. H. (2004). Urinary catheter management for the older adult patient. *Clinical Geriatrics, 12*(4), 26–32.

Wilde, M. H. (2003). Life with an indwelling urinary catheter: The dialectic of stigma and acceptance. *Qualitative Health Research, 13*(9), 1189–1204.

Urolithiasis and Nephrolithiasis

*Schnelle, J. (2003). Translating clinical research into practice: A randomized controlled trial of exercise and incontinence care with nursing home patients. *Journal of American Geriatric Society, 50*(9), 1476–1483.

Urinary Tract Cancers

American Cancer Society Inc. (2006) Cancer facts and figures 2006. http://www.cancer.org/docroot/STT/stt_0.asp. Accessed July 14, 2006.

Huang, Z. (2005). A review of progress in clinical photodynamic therapy. *Technology in Cancer Research and Treatment, 4*(3), 283–293.

Sanger, C., Busche, A., Bentien, G. et al. (2004). Immunodominant PstS1 antigen of mycobacterium tuberculosis is a potent biological response modifier for the treatment of bladder cancer. *BioMedCentral Cancer, 86*(4), 1471–2407. http://www.biomedcentral.com/1471-2407/4/86. Accessed July 14, 2006.

Genitourinary Trauma

Armenakas, N. A., Pareek, G. & Fracchia, J. A. (2004). Iatrogenic bladder perforations: Long-term follow-up of 65 patients. *Journal of the American College of Surgeons, 198*(1), 78–82.

Ziran, B., Chamberlin, E., Shuler, F. D. et al. (2005). Delays and difficulty in the diagnosis of lower urologic injuries in the context of pelvic fractures. *Journal of Trauma-Injury and Critical Care, 58*(3), 533–537.

Urinary Diversions

Quallich, S. A. & Ohl, D. (2003a). Artificial urinary sphincter. Part I: Overview. *Urologic Nursing, 23*(4), 259–268.

Quallich, S. A. & Ohl, D. (2003b). Artificial urinary sphincter. Part II: Patient teaching and perioperative care. *Urologic Nursing, 23*(4), 269–273.

Quallich, S. A. & Ohl, D. (2003c). Artificial urinary sphincter case study. *Urologic Nursing, 23*(4), 274–275.

RESOURCES

American Cancer Society Inc., 1599 Clifton RD, NE Atlanta GA 30329, (404) 320-3333; http://www.cancer.org. Accessed July 14, 2006.

American Foundation for Urologic Disease, 1000 Corporate Boulevard, Linthicum, MD 21090, 1-800-828-7866 or 410-689-3990; http://www.afud.org. Accessed July 14, 2006.

American Urological Association, 1000 Corporate Boulevard Linthicum, MD 21090, 1-866-746-4282; http://www.auanet.org. Accessed July 14, 2006.

National Association for Continence, P.O. Box 1019 Charleston, NC 29402, 1-800-BLADDER (252-3337); http://www.nafac.org. Accessed July 14, 2006.

National Institute of Diabetes & Digestive and Kidney Diseases (NIDDK), National Institutes of Health, Building 31, Bethesda, MD 20892; http://www.niddk.nih.gov. Accessed July 14, 2006.

National Kidney Foundation, 30 East 33rd St., New York, NY 10016; (212) 889-2210; http://www.kidney.org. Accessed July 14, 2006.

UNIT 10

Reproductive Function

Case Study

Applying Concepts from NANDA, NIC, and NOC

A Patient With a Difficult Health Care Choice Involving Losses

Mrs. Cole is a 49-year-old woman who has been undergoing cancer staging after positive breast biopsy results. The surgeon has informed her that she has stage IIB infiltrating ductal carcinoma. The surgeon has discussed with her two different surgical approaches—breast conserving or modified radical mastectomy (MRM). If she chooses MRM, Mrs. Cole must decide whether she will undergo breast reconstruction or use a breast prosthesis. The nurse notes that Mrs. Cole is trembling and near tears. Mrs. Cole tells the nurse that she is uncertain about how her husband will respond if she chooses MRM. She is also concerned that she will not feel feminine after MRM but states she is very frightened about anything less since a friend died of metastatic breast cancer.

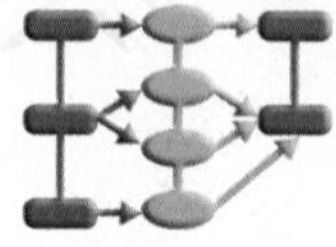

Turn to Appendix C to see a concept map that illustrates the relationships that exist between the nursing diagnoses, interventions, and outcomes for the patient's clinical problems.

Nursing Classifications and Languages

NANDA Nursing Diagnoses	NIC Nursing Interventions	NOC Nursing Outcomes Return to functional baseline status, stabilization of, or improvement in:
Decisional Conflict—Uncertainty about course of action to be taken when choice among competing actions involves risk, loss, or challenge to personal life values	**Active Listening**—Attending closely to and attaching significance to a patient's verbal and nonverbal messages	**Decision Making**—Ability to make judgments and choose between two or more alternatives
Anticipatory Grieving—Intellectual and emotional responses and behaviors by which individuals, families, and communities work through the process of modifying self-concept based on the perception of potential loss	**Decision-Making Support**—Providing information and support for a patient who is making a decision regarding health care	**Grief Resolution**—Adjustment to actual or impending loss
	Anticipatory Guidance—Preparation of a patient for an anticipated developmental and/or situational crisis **Grief Work Facilitation**—Assistance with the resolution of a significant loss **Emotional Support**—Provision of reassurance, acceptance and encouragement during times of stress	**Psychosocial Adjustment: Life Change**—Adaptive psychosocial response of an individual to a significant life change

NANDA International. (2005). *Nursing diagnoses: Definitions & classification 2005–2006.* Philadelphia: North American Nursing Diagnosis Association.

Dochterman, J. M. & Bulechek, G. M. (2004). *Nursing interventions classification (NIC)* (4th ed.). St. Louis: Mosby.

Iowa Outcomes Project. (2004). In Moorhead, S., Johnson, M. & Maas, M. (2004). *Nursing outcomes classification (NOC)* (3rd ed.). St. Louis: Mosby.

Dochterman, J. M. & Jones, D. A. (2003). *Unifying nursing languages: The harmonization of NANDA, NIC, and NOC.* Washington, D.C.: American Nurses Association.

CHAPTER 46

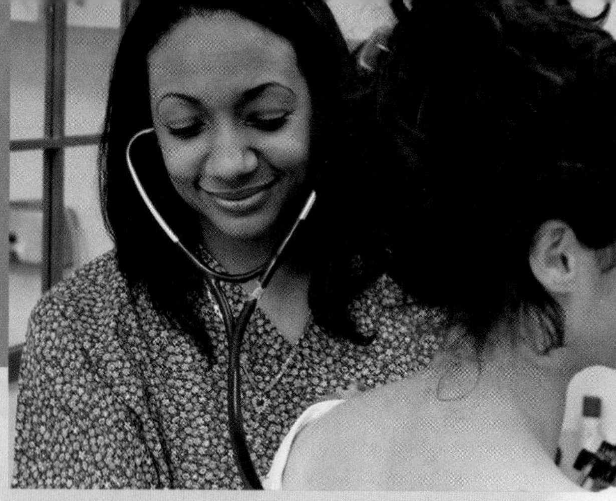

Assessment and Management of Female Physiologic Processes

Learning Objectives

On completion of this chapter, the learner will be able to:

1. Describe female reproductive function.
2. Describe approaches to effective sexual assessment.
3. Describe indicators of domestic violence and abuse of women and methods of identifying and treating women who are survivors of abuse.
4. Identify the diagnostic examinations and tests used to determine alteration in female reproductive function and describe the nurse's role before, during, and after these examinations and procedures.
5. Identify factors that cause menstrual disorders and related nursing implications.
6. Describe nursing care for patients with premenstrual syndrome.
7. Develop a teaching plan for women experiencing menopause.
8. Describe methods of contraception and implications for health care and education.
9. Describe the nursing management of the patient having an abortion.
10. Describe the causes and management of infertility.
11. Use the nursing process to plan for the care of the patient with ectopic pregnancies.
12. Discuss the healthy older woman and health teaching related to aging.

Women's health is evolving as more information about their health is being discovered. Nurses who work with women need to understand normal female anatomy and physiology and the physical, developmental, psychological, and social-cultural influences on women's health, health practices, and use of health care. Health assessment, maintenance, and promotion across the life span must consider women's growth and development, sexuality, contraception, preconception care, conception, prenatal care, effects of pregnancy on health, perimenopause, menopause, and aging. It is also necessary to consider how medications and diseases affect women. In addition, women's sexuality is complex and often affected by many factors, and related issues need careful evaluation and treatment. Because women use the health care system more often than men and make up the majority of health care workers, addressing women's health needs and concerns improves quality and access for women and their families.

Role of Nurses in Women's Health

As their presence in the labor market continues to increase, women face challenges in their roles, lifestyles, and family patterns. Furthermore, they encounter environmental hazards and stress, prompting some to focus greater attention on health and health-promoting practices. As a result, many women are taking a greater interest in and responsibility for their own health and health care, although not all women have the time, finances, or other resources to do so.

In recent years, many women have delayed pregnancy and childbearing until well after they have established careers. This is due in part to the wide variety of contraceptive methods that are available. Advances in the treatment of infertility have enabled many women previously unable to have children to become pregnant and have allowed couples well into their 40s to have children. Women who have many roles and multiple responsibilities (eg, workers, wives, mothers, parental caretakers) have to meet competing demands; many women have little time for themselves and may put the needs of others before their own health needs. Nurses must be sensitive to these needs and knowledgeable about preventive health care for women. Nurses are in an ideal position to encourage women to determine their own health goals and behaviors, teach about heath promotion and illness prevention, offer intervention strategies, and provide support, counseling, and ongoing monitoring. Areas of special interest in health promotion include the following:

- Personal hygiene
- Strategies for detecting and preventing disease, especially sexually transmitted diseases (STDs), also referred to as sexually transmitted infections (STIs), including human

Glossary

adnexa: the fallopian tubes and ovaries

amenorrhea: absence of menstrual flow

androgens: hormones produced by the ovaries and adrenals that affect many aspects of female health, including follicle development, libido, oiliness of hair and skin, and hair growth

cervix: bottom (inferior) part of the uterus that is located in the vagina

chandelier sign: pain on gentle movement of the cervix; associated with pelvic infection

corpus luteum: site of a follicle that changes after ovulation to produce progesterone

cystocele: weakness of the anterior vaginal wall that allows the bladder to protrude into the vagina

dysmenorrhea: painful menstruation

dyspareunia: difficult or painful sexual intercourse

endometrial ablation: procedure performed through a hysteroscope in which the lining of the uterus is burned away or ablated to treat abnormal uterine bleeding

endometriosis: condition in which endometrial tissue implants in other areas of the pelvis; may produce dysmenorrhea or infertility

endometrium: lining of the uterus

estrogen: hormone that develops and maintains the female reproductive system

follicle-stimulating hormone (FSH): hormone released by the pituitary gland to stimulate estrogen production and ovulation

fornix: upper part of the vagina

fundus: body of the uterus

graafian follicle: cystic structure that develops on the ovary as ovulation begins

hymen: tissue that covers the vaginal opening partially or completely before vaginal penetration

hysteroscopy: a procedure performed using a long telescope-like instrument inserted through the cervix to diagnose uterine problems

introitus: perineal opening to the vagina

luteal phase: stage in the menstrual cycle in which the endometrium becomes thicker and more vascular

luteinizing hormone (LH): hormone released by the pituitary gland that stimulates progesterone production

menarche: beginning of menstrual function

menopause: permanent cessation of menstruation resulting from the loss of ovarian follicular activity

menstruation: sloughing and discharge of the lining of the uterus if conception does not take place

osteoporosis: a disorder in which bones lose density and become porous and fragile

ovaries: almond-shaped reproductive organs that produce eggs at ovulation and play a major role in hormone production

ovulation: discharge of a mature ovum from the ovary

perimenopause: the period immediately prior to menopause and the first year after menopause

polyp (cervical or endometrial): growth of tissue on the cervix or endometrial lining; usually benign

progesterone: hormone produced by the corpus luteum

proliferative phase: stage in the menstrual cycle before ovulation when the endometrium proliferates

rectocele: weakness of the posterior vaginal wall that allows the rectal cavity to protrude into the submucosa of the vagina

secretory phase: stage of the menstrual cycle in which the endometrium becomes thickened, more vascular, and edematous

uterine prolapse: relaxation of pelvic tone that allows the cervix and uterus to descend into the lower vagina

immunodeficiency virus (HIV) infection and acquired immunodeficiency syndrome (AIDS)
- Issues related to sexuality and sexual function, such as contraception; preconception, prenatal, and postnatal care; sexual satisfaction; and menopause
- Diet, exercise, and health-promoting practices that maintain and enhance health
- Appropriate stress management to reduce the detrimental effects of stress on health and well-being
- Maintaining a normal weight for height and avoiding substance abuse and smoking
- Avoidance of unhealthy lifestyle and risk behaviors

Nurses who promote healthy ways of living also need to model that lifestyle for their patients. It is important that nurses promote positive practices and behaviors related to the reproductive and sexual health of all patients. Necessary strategies include the following:

- Recommending regular examinations to promote health, detect health problems at an early stage, assess problems related to gynecologic and reproductive function, and discuss questions or concerns related to sexual function and sexuality
- Providing an open, nonjudgmental environment (crucial in providing nursing and health care, and especially when patients are discussing personal issues). Nurses must convey understanding and sensitivity when discussing sensitive issues and must be alert to cues about unspoken patient concerns.
- Recognizing signs and symptoms of abuse and screening all patients in a private and safe environment
- Recognizing cultural differences and beliefs and respecting sexual orientation and concerns related to both

Anatomic and Physiologic Overview

Anatomy of the Female Reproductive System

The female reproductive system consists of external and internal structures. Other anatomic structures that affect the female reproductive system include the hypothalamus and pituitary gland of the endocrine system.

External Genitalia

The external genitalia (the vulva) include two thick folds of tissue called the labia majora and two smaller lips of delicate tissue called the labia minora, which lie within the labia majora. The upper portions of the labia minora unite, forming a partial covering for the clitoris, a highly sensitive organ composed of erectile tissue. Between the labia minora, below and posterior to the clitoris, is the urinary meatus, the external opening of the female urethra, which is about 3 cm (<1.5 inches) long. Below this orifice is a larger opening, the vaginal orifice or **introitus** (Fig. 46-1). On each side of the vaginal orifice is a vestibular (Bartholin's) gland, a bean-sized structure that empties its mucous secretion through a small duct. The opening of the duct lies within the labia minora, external to the hymen. The area between the vagina and rectum is called the perineum.

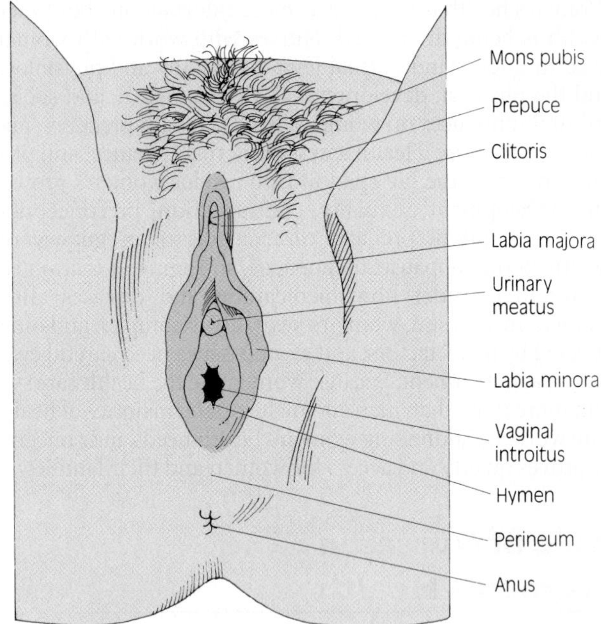

FIGURE 46-1. External female genitalia.

Internal Reproductive Structures

The internal structures consist of the vagina, uterus, ovaries, and fallopian or uterine tubes (Fig. 46-2).

VAGINA

The vagina, a canal lined with mucous membrane, is 7.5 to 10 cm (3 to 4 inches) long and extends upward and backward from the vulva to the cervix. Anterior to it are the bladder and the urethra, and posterior to it lies the rectum. The anterior and posterior walls of the vagina normally touch each other. The upper part of the vagina, the **fornix**, surrounds the **cervix** (the inferior part of the uterus).

UTERUS

The uterus, a pear-shaped, muscular organ, is about 7.5 cm (3 inches) long and 5 cm (2 inches) wide at its upper part. Its walls are about 1.25 cm (0.5 inch) thick. The size of the uterus varies, depending on parity (number of viable births) and uterine abnormalities (eg, fibroids, which are a type of tumor that may distort the uterus). A nulliparous woman (one who has not completed a pregnancy to the stage of fetal viability) usually has a smaller uterus than a multiparous woman (one who has completed two or more pregnancies to the stage of fetal viability). The uterus lies posterior to the bladder and is held in position by several ligaments. The round ligaments extend anteriorly and laterally to the internal inguinal ring and down the inguinal canal, where they blend with the tissues of the labia majora. The broad ligaments are folds of peritoneum extending from the lateral pelvic walls and enveloping the fallopian tubes. The uterosacral ligaments extend posteriorly to the sacrum. The uterus has two parts: the cervix, which projects into the vagina, and a larger upper part, the **fundus** or body, which

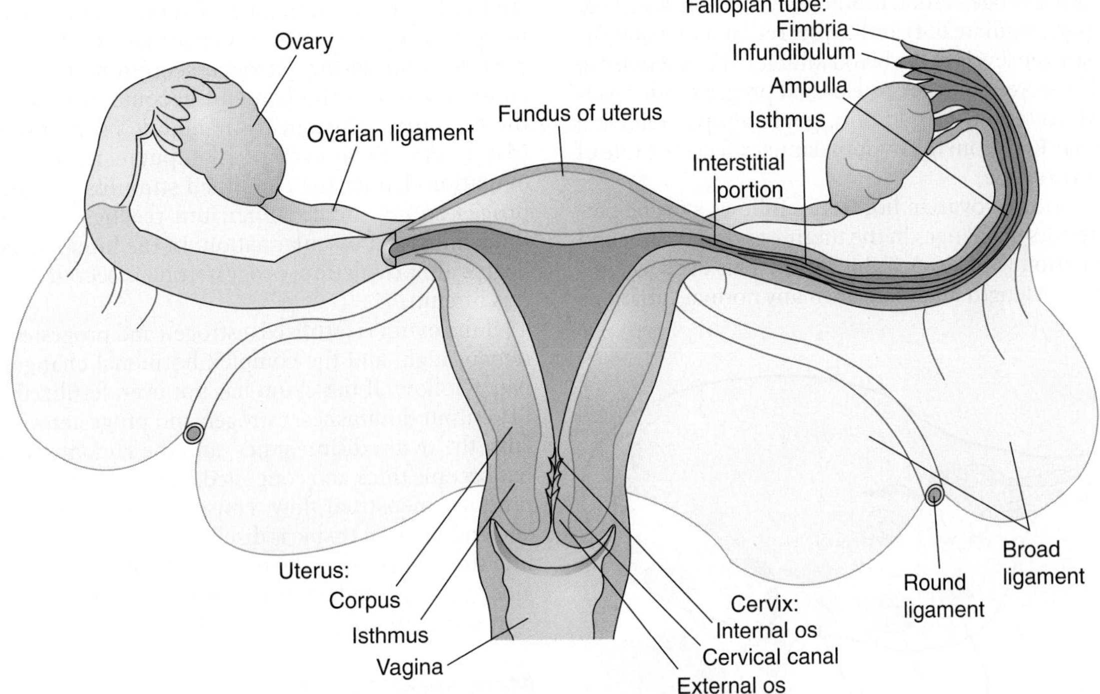

FIGURE 46-2. Internal female reproductive structures.

is covered posteriorly and partly anteriorly by peritoneum. The triangular inner portion of the fundus narrows to a small canal in the cervix that has constrictions at each end, referred to as the external os and internal os. The upper lateral parts of the uterus are called the cornua. From here, the oviducts or fallopian (or uterine) tubes extend outward, and their lumina are internally continuous with the uterine cavity (Porth, 2005).

OVARIES

The **ovaries** lie behind the broad ligaments, behind and below the fallopian tubes. They are oval bodies about 3 cm (1.2 inches) long. At birth, they contain thousands of tiny egg cells, or ova. The ovaries and the fallopian tubes together are referred to as the **adnexa.**

Function of the Female Reproductive System

Ovulation

At puberty (usually between 12 and 14 years of age, but earlier for some; 10 or 11 years of age is not uncommon), the ova begin to mature. During a period known as the follicular phase, an ovum enlarges as a type of cyst called a **graafian follicle** until it reaches the surface of the ovary, where transport occurs. The ovum (or oocyte) is discharged into the peritoneal cavity. This periodic discharge of matured ovum is referred to as **ovulation.** The ovum usually finds its way into the fallopian tube, where it is carried to the uterus. If it is penetrated by a spermatozoon, the male reproductive cell, a union occurs and conception takes place. After the discharge of the ovum, the cells of the graafian follicle undergo a rapid change. Gradually, they become yellow (**corpus luteum**) and produce **progesterone,** a hormone that prepares the uterus for receiving the fertilized ovum. Ovulation usually occurs 2 weeks prior to the next menstrual period.

Menstrual Cycle

The menstrual cycle is a complex process involving the reproductive and endocrine systems. The ovaries produce steroid hormones, predominantly estrogens and progesterone. Several different **estrogens** are produced by the ovarian follicle, which consists of the developing ovum and its surrounding cells. The most potent of the ovarian estrogens is estradiol. Estrogens are responsible for developing and maintaining the female reproductive organs and the secondary sex characteristics associated with the adult female. Estrogens play an important role in breast development and in monthly cyclic changes in the uterus (Porth, 2005).

Progesterone is also important in regulating the changes that occur in the uterus during the menstrual cycle. It is secreted by the corpus luteum, which is the ovarian follicle after the ovum has been released. Progesterone is the most important hormone for conditioning the **endometrium** (the mucous membrane lining the uterus) in preparation for implantation of a fertilized ovum. If pregnancy occurs, the progesterone secretion becomes largely a function of the placenta and is essential for maintaining a normal pregnancy. In addition, progesterone, working with estrogen, prepares the breast for producing and secreting milk. **Androgens** are also produced by the ovaries, but only in small amounts. These hormones are involved in the early development of the follicle and also affect the female libido (Porth, 2005).

Two gonadotropic hormones are released by the pituitary gland: **follicle-stimulating hormone** (FSH) and **luteinizing hormone** (LH). FSH is primarily responsible for stimulating the ovaries to secrete estrogen. LH is primarily responsible for stimulating progesterone production. Feedback mechanisms, in part, regulate FSH and LH secretion. For example, elevated estrogen levels in the blood inhibit FSH secretion but promote LH secretion, whereas elevated progesterone levels inhibit LH secretion. In addition, gonadotropin-releasing hormone (GnRH) from the hypothalamus affects the rate of FSH and LH release.

The secretion of ovarian hormones follows a cyclic pattern that results in changes in the uterine endometrium and in **menstruation** (Fig. 46-3; Table 46-1). This cycle is typically 28 days in length, but there are many normal variations (from 21 to 42 days). In the **proliferative phase** at the beginning of the cycle (just after menstruation), FSH output increases, stimulating estrogen secretion. This causes the endometrium to thicken and become more vascular. In the **secretory phase** near the middle portion of the cycle (day 14 in a 28-day cycle), LH output increases, stimulating ovulation. Under the combined stimulus of estrogen and progesterone, the endometrium reaches the peak of its thickening and vascularization. In the **luteal phase**, which begins after ovulation, progesterone is secreted by the corpus luteum.

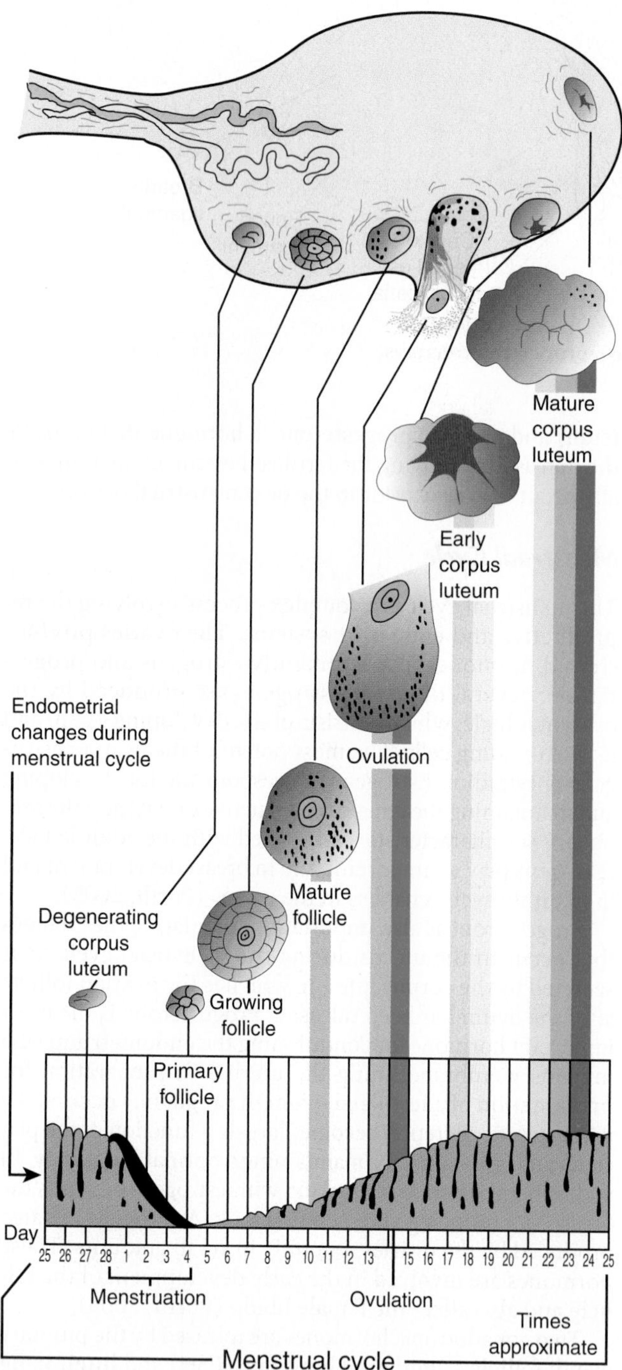

FIGURE 46-3. One menstrual cycle and the corresponding changes in the endometrium.

If the ovum is fertilized, estrogen and progesterone levels remain high, and the complex hormonal changes of pregnancy follow. If the ovum has not been fertilized, FSH and LH output diminishes, estrogen and progesterone secretion falls, the ovum disintegrates, and the endometrium, which has become thick and congested, becomes hemorrhagic. The product, menstrual flow, consisting of old blood, mucus, and endometrial tissue, is discharged through the cervix and into the vagina. After the menstrual flow stops, the cycle begins again; the endometrium proliferates and thickens from estrogenic stimulation, and ovulation recurs (Porth, 2005).

Menopausal Period

The menopausal period marks the end of a woman's reproductive capacity. It usually occurs between 45 and 52 years of age but may occur as early as 42 or as late as 55; the median age is 51 years. Perimenopause precedes this and can begin as early as 35 years of age. Physical, emotional, and menstrual changes may occur, and this transition offers an opportunity for health promotion and disease prevention teaching and counseling (Lyndaker & Hulton, 2004). **Menopause** is not a pathologic phenomenon but a normal part of aging and maturation. Menstruation ceases, and because the ovaries are no longer active, the reproductive organs become smaller. No more ova mature; therefore, no ovarian hormones are produced. (An earlier menopause may occur if the ovaries are surgically removed, or are destroyed by radiation or chemotherapy or because of an unknown etiology.) Besides changes in the reproductive system that reduce estrogen levels, multifaceted changes occur throughout the woman's body. These changes are neuroendocrinologic, biochemical, and metabolic and are related to normal maturation or aging (Table 46-2).

Assessment

A nurse who is obtaining information from a patient for the health history and performing physical assessment is in an ideal position to discuss the woman's general health issues, health promotion, and health-related concerns. Relevant topics include fitness, nutrition, cardiovascular risks, health screening, sexuality, menopause, abuse, health risk behaviors, and immunizations. Recommendations for health screening are summarized in Chart 46-1.

Health History

In addition to obtaining a general health history, the nurse asks about past illnesses and experiences that are specific

TABLE 46-1 Hormonal Changes During the Menstrual Cycle

(Times approximate)

Phase	Menstrual	Follicular	Ovulation	Luteal	Premenstrual
Days	1 2 3 4 5	6 7 8 9 10 11 12 13	14 15 16	17 18 19 20 21 22 23 24 25	26 27 28 1 2
Ovary	Degenerating corpus luteum; beginning follicular development	Growth and maturation of follicle	Ovulation	Active corpus luteum	Degenerating corpus luteum
Estrogen Production	Low	Increasing	High	Declining, then a secondary rise	Decreasing
Progesterone Production	None	Low	Low	Increasing	Decreasing
FSH Production	Increasing	High, then declining	Low	Low	Increasing
LH Production	Low	Low, then increasing	High	High	Decreasing
Endometrium	Degeneration and shedding of superficial layer. Coiled arteries dilate, then constrict again.	Reorganization and proliferation of superficial layer	Continued growth	Active secretion and glandular dilation; highly vascular; edematous	Vasoconstriction of coiled arteries; beginning degeneration

to a woman's health. Data should be collected about the following:

- Menstrual history (including **menarche**, length of cycles, length and amount of flow, presence of cramps or pain, bleeding between periods or after intercourse, bleeding after menopause)
- History of pregnancies (number of pregnancies, outcomes of pregnancies)
- History of exposure to medications (diethylstilbestrol [DES], immunosuppressive agents, others)
- Pain with menses (**dysmenorrhea**), pain with intercourse (**dyspareunia**), pelvic pain
- History of vaginal discharge and odor or itching
- History of problems with urinary function, including frequency, urgency, and incontinence
- History of bowel problems
- Sexual history

TABLE 46-2 Age-Related Changes in the Female Reproductive System

	Physiologic Changes	Signs and Symptoms
Cessation of ovarian function and decreased estrogen production	Decreased ovulation	Decreased/loss of ability to conceive; increased infertility
	Onset of menopause	Irregular menses with eventual cessation of menses
	Vasomotor instability and hormonal fluctuations	Hot flashes or flushing; night sweats, sleep disturbances; mood swings; fatigue
	Decreased bone formation	Bone loss and increased risk for osteoporosis and osteoporotic fractures; loss of height
	Decreased vaginal lubrication	Dyspareunia, resulting in lack of interest in sex
	Thinning of urinary and genital tracts	Increased risk for urinary tract infection
	Increased pH of vagina Thinning of pubic hair and shrinking of labia	Increased incidence of inflammation (atrophic vaginitis) with discharge, itching, and vulvar burning
Relaxation of pelvic musculature	Prolapse of uterus, cystocele, rectocele	Dyspareunia, incontinence, feelings of perineal pressure

CHART 46-1

Summary of Health Screening and Counseling Issues for Women

Ages 19–39

SEXUALITY AND REPRODUCTIVE ISSUES

Annual pelvic examination
Annual clinical breast exam
Contraceptive options
High-risk sexual behaviors

HEALTH AND RISK BEHAVIORS

Hygiene
Injury prevention
Nutrition
Exercise patterns
Risk for domestic abuse
Use of tobacco, drugs, and alcohol
Life stresses
Immunizations

DIAGNOSTIC TESTING*

Pap smear
STD screening as indicated

Ages 40–64

SEXUALITY AND REPRODUCTIVE ISSUES

Annual pelvic examination
Annual clinical breast exam
Contraceptive options
High-risk sexual behaviors
Menopausal concerns

HEALTH AND RISK BEHAVIORS

Hygiene
Bone loss and injury prevention
Nutrition
Exercise patterns
Risk for domestic abuse
Use of tobacco, drugs, and alcohol
Life stresses
Immunizations

DIAGNOSTIC TESTING*

Pap smear
Mammography
Cholesterol and lipid profile
Colorectal cancer screening
Bone mineral density testing
Thyroid-stimulating hormone testing
Hearing and eye examinations

Ages 65 and Over

SEXUALITY AND REPRODUCTIVE ISSUES

Annual pelvic examination
Annual clinical breast exam
High-risk sexual behaviors

HEALTH AND RISK BEHAVIORS

Hygiene
Injury prevention
Nutrition
Exercise patterns
Risk for domestic abuse
Use of tobacco, drugs, and alcohol
Life stresses
Immunizations

DIAGNOSTIC TESTING*

Pap smear
Mammography
Cholesterol and lipid profile
Colorectal cancer screening
Bone mineral density testing
Thyroid-stimulating hormone testing
Hearing and eye examinations

*Each individual's risks (family history, personal history) influence the need for specific assessments and their frequency.

- History of STDs and methods of treatment
- History of sexual abuse or physical abuse
- History of surgery or other procedures on reproductive tract structures (including female genital mutilation or female circumcision)
- History of chronic illness or disability that may affect health status, reproductive health, need for health screening, or access to health care
- History or family history of a genetic disorder

In collecting data related to reproductive health, the nurse is in a unique position to teach the patient about normal physiologic processes, such as menstruation and menopause, and to assess possible abnormalities. Many problems experienced by young or middle-aged women can be corrected easily. However, if they are allowed to go untreated, they may result in anxiety and health problems. Issues related to sexuality and sexual function are typically brought more often to the attention of the gynecologic or women's health care provider than other health care providers; however, any nurse caring for women should consider these issues part of routine health assessment.

Sexual History

A sexual assessment includes both subjective and objective data. Health and sexual histories, physical examination findings, and laboratory results are all part of the database. The purpose of a sexual history is to obtain information that provides a picture of a woman's sexuality and sexual prac-

GENETICS IN NURSING PRACTICE

Reproductive Disorders

Various reproductive disorders are influenced by genetic factors. Some examples are:

- Hereditary breast or ovarian cancer syndromes
- Hereditary nonpolyposis colon cancer syndrome (risk for uterine cancer)
- Müllerian aplasia
- 21-Hydroxylase deficiency (female masculinization)
- Turner syndrome (45,XO)
- Klinefelter syndrome (47,XXY)

NURSING ASSESSMENTS

Family History Assessment

- Assess family history for other family members with similar reproductive problems/abnormalities.
  - Inquire about ethnic background (eg, Ashkenazi Jewish populations and hereditary breast/ovarian cancer mutations).
  - Inquire about relatives with other cancers, including early-onset ovarian, uterine, renal, prostate cancers.

Patient Assessment

- In females with delayed puberty or primary amenorrhea, assess for clinical features of Turner syndrome (short stature, webbing of the neck, widely spaced nipples).
- In males with delayed puberty or infertility, assess for clinical features of Klinefelter syndrome (tall stature, gynecomastia, learning disabilities).
- Assess for other congenital anomalies in females with Müllerian defect, including renal and vertebral anomalies.

MANAGEMENT ISSUES SPECIFIC TO GENETICS

- Inquire whether genetics testing (DNA chromosomal, metabolic) has been carried out on affected family member(s).
  - If indicated, refer for further genetics counseling and evaluation so that family members can discuss inheritance, risk to other family members, availability of genetics testing, and gene-based interventions.
- Offer appropriate genetics information and resources.
- Assess patient's understanding of genetics information.
- Provide support to families with newly diagnosed gene-related reproductive disorders.
- Participate in management and coordination of care of patients with genetic conditions, individuals predisposed to develop or pass on a genetic condition.

GENETICS RESOURCES FOR NURSES AND THEIR PATIENTS ON THE WEB

Genetic Alliance: http://www.geneticalliance.org—a directory of support groups for patients and families with genetic conditions

American Cancer Society: http://www.cancer.org—offers general information about cancer and support resources for families

Gene Clinics: http://www.geneclinics.org—a listing of common genetic disorders with up-to-date clinical summaries, genetic counseling and testing information

National Organization of Rare Disorders: http://www.rarediseases.org—a directory of support groups and information for patients and families with rare genetic disorders

National Cancer Institute: http://www.nci.nih.gov—current information about cancer research, treatment, resources for health care providers, individuals and families

OMIM: Online Mendelian Inheritance in Man: http://www.ncbi.nlm.nih.gov/omim/stats/html—a complete listing of inherited genetic conditions

tices and to promote sexual health. The sexual history may enable a patient to discuss sexual matters openly and to discuss sexual concerns with an informed health professional. This information can be obtained with the health history after the gynecologic-obstetric or genitourinary history is completed. By incorporating the sexual history into the general health history, the nurse can move from areas of lesser sensitivity to areas of greater sensitivity after establishing initial rapport.

Taking the sexual history becomes a dynamic process reflecting an exchange of information between the patient and the nurse and provides the opportunity to clarify myths and explore areas of concern that the patient may not have felt comfortable discussing in the past. In obtaining a sexual history, the nurse must not assume the patient's sexual preference until clarified. When asking about sexual health, the nurse also cannot assume that the patient is married or unmarried. Asking a patient to label herself as single, married, widowed, or divorced may be interpreted as an inappropriate inquiry. Asking about a partner or about current meaningful relationships may be a less offensive way to initiate a sexual history.

The PLISSIT (Permission, Limited Information, Specific Suggestions, Intensive Therapy) model of sexual assessment and intervention may be used to provide a framework for nursing interventions (Annon, 1976). The assessment begins by introducing the topic and asking the woman for permission to discuss issues of sexual functioning with her.

The nurse can begin by explaining the purpose of obtaining a sexual history (eg, "I ask all my patients about their sexual health. May I ask you some questions about this?"). History taking continues by inquiring about present sexual activity and sexual orientation (eg, "Are you currently having sex with a man, a woman, or both?"). Inquiries about possible sexual dysfunction may include, "Are you having any problems related to your current sexual activity?" Such problems may be related to medication, life changes, disability, or the onset of physical or emotional illness. A patient can be asked about her thoughts on what is causing the current problem.

Information about sexual function can be introduced during the health history. As the discussion progresses, the nurse may offer specific suggestions for interventions. A professional who specializes in sex therapy may provide more intensive therapy if necessary. By initiating an assessment about sexual concerns, the nurse communicates to the patient that issues about changes or problems in sexual functioning are valid health topics for discussion and provides a safe environment for discussing these sensitive topics. Young women may be apprehensive about having irregular periods, may be concerned about STDs, or may need contraception. They may want information about using tampons, emergency contraception, or issues related to pregnancy. Perimenopausal women may have concerns about irregular menses. Menopausal women may be concerned about vaginal dryness and discomfort with intercourse. Women of any age may have concerns about relationships, sexual satisfaction, orgasm, or masturbation.

Risk of STDs can be assessed by asking about number of partners in the past year or in the patient's lifetime. An open-ended question related to the patient's need for further information should be included (eg, "Do you have any questions or concerns about your sexual health?"). The nurse should be aware that some women and men are using the Internet to seek partners and that obtaining sexual partners this way has been associated with an increased risk of STDs (McFarlane, Bull & Rietmeijer, 2000; U.S. Department of Health and Human Services [USDHHS], 2001).

Female Genital Mutilation

Female genital mutilation (FGM), or cutting, refers to the partial or total removal of the external female genitalia or other injury to female organs. People in some cultures view FGM as a rite of passage to womanhood and believe it promotes hygiene, protects virginity and family honor, prevents promiscuity, improves female attractiveness and male sexual pleasure, and enhances fertility. FGM is considered an acceptable practice in many cultures, mostly in Africa and the Middle East. However, FGM is a criminal act in the United States. Although more than 130 million girls and women worldwide have undergone FGM, many organizations (eg, World Health Organization, Amnesty International) consider it a health and human rights issue and are working to end it. An increasing number of women entering the United States health care system underwent FGM before coming to the United States (Nour, 2004), and others have undergone FGM since their arrival in this country.

Four types of FGM are known:

1. Type 1, or Sunna, FGM involves excision of the clitoral prepuce; total excision of the clitoral prepuce and glans. It is performed in Eritrea, Ethiopia, and Nigeria.
2. Type II FGM involves clitoridectomy with partial or total excision of the labia minora. It is performed in Sierra Leone, Gambia, and Guinea.
3. Type III, or pharaonic, FGM involves clitoridectomy, excision of the labia, and stitching or narrowing of the vaginal opening (referred to as infibulation). It is more likely to result in infertility than other types of FGM. It is performed in Somalia and northern Sudan.
4. Type IV, or unclassified, FGM includes pricking, piercing, or incision of the clitoris, the labia, or both, stretching of the clitoris or surrounding tissues, and introduction of corrosive substances into the vagina (Nour, 2004).

FGM is usually performed when a girl is between 4 and 10 years of age. Short-term complications of FGM include hemorrhage, cellulitis, lacerations, urinary dysfunction, and infection. Long-term complications include urinary dysfunction, chronic vaginitis and pelvic infections, inability to undergo pelvic examination, painful intercourse, impaired sexual response, anemia, increased risk of human immunodeficiency virus (HIV) infection due to tearing of scar tissue, and psychological and psychosexual sequelae. Because FGM can affect sexual function, menstrual hygiene, and bladder function, the possibility of FGM must be considered in the sexual history, particularly in women from cultures and countries where the practice is common.

Nurses who care for patients who have undergone FGM need to be sensitive, empathetic, knowledgeable, culturally competent, and nonjudgmental. Respect for others' health beliefs, practices, and behaviors, and recognition of the complexity of issues involved is crucial. Women who have undergone FGM may not think of themselves as mutilated, and the nurse should use the woman's terminology. Speculums are not used in some developing countries; the function of this instrument should be explained and an appropriate size speculum used to examine women who have experienced FGM (Nour, 2004).

Domestic Violence

Domestic violence is a broad term that includes child abuse, elder abuse, and abuse of women and men. Abuse can be emotional, physical, sexual, or economic. Abuse involves fear of one partner by another and control by threats, intimidation, and physical abuse. Abuse is related to the need to maintain control of a partner and is rooted in sex role inequality.

More than 6 million women experience domestic violence each year, and battered women are encountered daily in nursing practice. Battering involves repeated physical or sexual assault in a context of coercive control and, more broadly, emotional degradation, threats, and intimidation. Violence is rarely a one-time occurrence in a relationship; it usually continues and escalates in severity. This is an important point to emphasize when a woman states that her partner has hurt her but has promised to change. Batterers can change their behavior but not without extensive counseling and motivation. If a woman states that she is being hurt, sensitive care is required (Chart 46-2).

CHART 46-2 Guidelines for Managing Reported Domestic Abuse

ACTIONS	RATIONALE
1. Reassure the woman that she is not alone.	Women often believe that they are alone in experiencing abuse at the hands of their partners.
2. Express your belief that no one should be hurt, that abuse is the fault of the batterer and is against the law.	Lets the woman know that no one deserves to be abused and that she has not caused the abuse.
3. Assure the woman that her information is confidential, although it does become part of her medical record. **If children are suspected of being abused or are being abused, the law requires that this be reported to the authorities.** Some states require reporting of spousal or partner abuse. Domestic violence agencies and medical and nursing groups disagree with this policy and are trying to have it changed. Serious opposition is based on the fact that reporting does not and cannot currently guarantee a woman's safety and may place her in more danger. It may also interfere with a patient's willingness to discuss her personal life and concerns with care providers. This places a serious barrier in the way of comprehensive nursing care. If nurses are in doubt about laws on reporting abuse, they need to check with their local or state domestic violence agency.	Women are often afraid that their information will be reported to the police or protective services and their children may be taken away.
4. Document the woman's statement of abuse and take photographs of any visible injuries if written formal consent has been obtained. (Emergency departments usually have a camera available if one is not on the nursing unit.)	Provides documentation of injuries that may be needed for later legal or criminal proceedings.
5. Provide teaching: • Inform the woman that shelters are available to ensure safety for her and her children. (Lengths of stay in shelters vary by state but are often up to 2 months. Staff often assist with housing, jobs, and the emotional distress that accompanies the break-up of the family.) Provide list of shelters. • Inform the woman that violence gets worse, not better. • If the woman chooses to go to a shelter, let her make the call. • If the woman chooses to return to the abuser, remain nonjudgmental and provide information that will make her safer than she was before disclosing her situation. • Make sure that the woman has a 24-hour hotline telephone number that provides information and support (Spanish translation and a device for the deaf are also available), police number, and 911. • Assist her to set up a safety plan in case she decides to return home. (A safety plan is an organized plan for departure with packed bags and important papers hidden in a safe spot.)	These options may be life-saving for the woman and her children.

By knowing about this major public health problem, being alert to abuse-related problems, and learning how to elicit information from women about abuse in their lives, nurses can offer intervention for a problem that might otherwise go undetected and can save lives by making women safer through education and support. Asking each woman about violence in her life in a safe environment (ie, a private room with the door closed) is part of a comprehensive assessment and universal screening. Asking about abuse directly is effective in identifying the presence of abuse and should be included in the health history of all women (Chart 46-3). The third and fourth questions of the screening questionnaire are specifically directed at abuse in women with disabilities.

No specific signs or symptoms are diagnostic of battering; however, nurses may see an injury that does not fit the account of how it happened (eg, a bruise on the side of the upper arm after "I walked into a door"). Manifestations of abuse may involve suicide attempts, drug and alcohol abuse, frequent emergency department visits, vague pelvic pain, somatic complaints, and depression. However, there may be no obvious signs or symptoms. Women in abusive situations often report that they do not feel well, possibly due to the stress of fear and anticipation of impending abuse. Nurses need to be knowledgeable about abuse, ask every female patient about abuse in her life, provide resources and referral, and follow written protocols of their institution or agency to ensure comprehensive care (Nelson, Nygren, McInerny et al., 2004).

Incest and Childhood Sexual Abuse

More than one in five women has experienced incest or childhood sexual abuse, and nurses frequently encounter women who have been sexually traumatized. It has been reported that female survivors of sexual abuse have more health problems and undergo more surgery than women who were not victims of abuse. Victims of childhood sexual abuse are reported to experience more chronic depression, posttraumatic stress disorder, morbid obesity, marital instability, gastrointestinal problems, and headaches, as well as greater use of health care services, than people who were not victims. Chronic pelvic pain in women is often associated with physical violence, emotional neglect, and sexual abuse in childhood (McFarlane, Malecha, Watson, et al., 2005). Women who have experienced rape or sexual abuse may be very anxious about pelvic examinations, labor, pelvic or breast irradiation, or any treatment or examination that involves hands-on treatment or requires removal of clothing. Nurses should be prepared to offer support and referral to psychologists, community resources, and self-help groups.

CHART 46-3

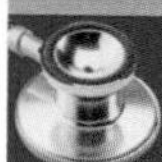

Screening for Abuse

Abuse Assessment Screen-Disability (AAS-D)

- Within the last year, have you been hit, slapped, kicked, pushed, shoved or otherwise physically hurt by someone?
- Within the last year, has anyone forced you to have sexual activities?
- Within the last year, has anyone prevented you from using a wheelchair, cane, respiratory, or other assistive devices?
- Within the last year, has anyone you depend on refused to help you with an important personal need, such as taking your medicine, getting to the bathroom, getting out of bed, bathing, getting dressed, or getting food or drink?

Center for Research on Women with Disabilities. Abuse Assessment Screen-Disability. http://www.bcm.edu/crowd/?PMID=1325m. Accessed July 9, 2006.

Rape and Sexual Assault

Sexual assault occurs every 6 minutes in the United States. Men, women, and children may be victims. Many rapes occur on dates. Sexual assault nurse examiners, emergency department staff, and gynecologists perform the painstaking collection of forensic evidence that is needed for criminal prosecution. Oral, anal, and genital tissue is examined for evidence of trauma, semen, or infection. Saliva, hair, and fingernail evidence is also collected. Cultures are obtained for STDs, and prophylactic antibiotics are prescribed. (The postexposure prophylaxis recommended by the Centers for Disease Control and Prevention consists of ceftriaxone, metronidazole, and azithromycin [CDC, 2002].) First injection of hepatitis B vaccine may also be given if the patient is not already immune, with subsequent doses given at 1 to 2 months and 4 to 6 months (CDC, 2004). HIV testing is offered and is repeated in 3 to 6 months. HIV prophylaxis is not universally recommended but is considered when mucosal exposure to contamination has occurred. Prophylaxis against chlamydia and gonorrhea are provided. Emergency contraception is explained and provided if requested and appropriate. Emotional counseling is provided, and follow-up treatment visits are arranged. Rape trauma syndrome is the emotional reaction to a sexual assault and may consist of shock, sleep disturbances, nightmares, flashbacks, anxiety, anger, mood swings, and depression. It is important and helpful for survivors to discuss the experience and to obtain professional counseling.

Screening for abuse, rape, and violence should be part of routine assessment, because women often do not report or seek treatment for assault. Often, the assailant is a partner, husband, or date. Nurses may encounter women with infections or pregnancies related to sexual assault who require support, understanding, and comprehensive care.

Health Issues in Women With Disabilities

Approximately 20% of women have disabilities and encounter physical, architectural, and attitudinal barriers that may limit their full participation in society. Women with disabilities may experience stereotyping and increased risk for abuse. They have reported that others, including health care providers, often equate them with their disability. Studies have shown that women with disabilities receive less primary health care and preventive health screening than other women, often because of access problems and health care providers who focus on the causes of disability rather than on health issues that are of concern to all women

(Smeltzer & Sharts-Hopko, 2005). To address these issues, the health history must include questions about barriers to health care encountered by women with disabilities and the effect of their disability on their health status and health care. Other issues to be addressed are identified in Chart 46-4. If a patient has hearing loss, vision loss, or another disability that affects communication, it may be necessary to obtain the assistance of an interpreter or to establish another method of communication. Nurses assessing women with disabilities may require additional time and the assistance of others to be certain that accurate information is obtained. Extra time may be needed to conduct the assessment in a sensitive and unhurried manner (Welner & Haseltine, 2002; Smeltzer & Sharts-Hopko, 2005). Women with disabilities may have had previous negative experiences with health care providers (Nosek, Hughes, Howland, et al., 2004), and it is important that nurses provide them with knowledgeable and sensitive care. See Chapter 10 for further discussion of health care of patients with disabilities.

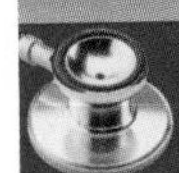

Gerontologic Considerations

Care of older women with gynecologic concerns requires knowledge and understanding. Many older women are functioning at various levels across the health spectrum; some function at a high level in their jobs or families, whereas others may be very ill. Nurses need to be prepared to care for older women who may be bright, energetic, and ambitious or who are coping with multiple family crises, including their own health as well as for those who are experiencing a life-altering or life-threatening health problem. Knowledge related to heart disease prevention, pharmacology, diet, signs of dementia or cognitive decline, osteoporosis prevention, gynecologic and breast cancers, and sexuality are important for providing high-level nursing care to older women. Health disparities, cultural competency, and end-of-life issues also need to be considered (Amin, Kuhle & Fitzpatrick, 2003).

Physical Assessment

Periodic examinations and routine cancer screening are important for all women. Annual breast and pelvic examinations are important for all women 18 years of age or older and for those who are sexually active, regardless of age. Patients deserve understanding and support because of the emotional and physical considerations associated with gynecologic examinations. Women may be embarrassed by the usual questions asked by a gynecologist or

CHART 46-4

Assessing a Woman With a Disability

HEALTH HISTORY

Address questions directly to the woman herself rather than to people accompanying her. Ask about:

- Self-care limitations resulting from her disability (ability to feed and dress self, use of assistive devices, transportation requirements, other assistance needed)
- Sensory limitations (lack of sensation, low vision, deaf or hard of hearing)
- Accessibility issues (ability to get to health care provider, transfer to examination table, accessibility of office/clinic of health care provider, previous experiences with health care providers, health screening practices; her understanding of physical examination)
- Cognitive or developmental changes that affect understanding
- Limitations secondary to disability that affect general health issues and reproductive health and health care
- Sexual function and concerns (those of all women and those that may be affected by the presence of a disabling condition)
- Menstrual history and menstrual hygiene practices
- Physical, sexual, or psychological abuse (including abuse by care providers; abuse by neglect, withholding or withdrawing assistive devices or personal or health care)
- Presence of secondary disabilities (ie, those resulting from the patient's primary disability: pressure ulcers, spasticity, osteoporosis, etc.)
- Health concerns related to aging with a disability

PHYSICAL ASSESSMENT

Provide instructions directly to the woman herself rather than to people accompanying her; provide written or audiotaped instructions.

Ask the woman what assistance she needs for the physical examination and provide assistance if needed:
—Undressing and dressing
—Providing a urine specimen
—Standing on scale to be weighed (provide alternative means of obtaining weight if she is unable to stand on scale)
—Moving on and off the examination table
—Assuming, changing, and maintaining positions

Consider the fatigue experienced by the woman during a lengthy exam and allow rest.

Provide assistive devices and other aids/methods needed to allow adequate communication with the patient (interpreters, signers, large-print written materials).

Complete examination that would be indicated for any other woman; having a disability is *never* justification for omitting parts of the physical examination, including the pelvic examination.

women's health care provider. Because gynecologic conditions are of a personal and private nature to most women, such information is shared only with those directly involved in patient care (as is true with all patient information).

Throughout the examination, the nurse explains the procedures to be performed. This not only encourages the woman to relax but also provides an opportunity for her to ask questions and minimizes the negative feelings that many women associate with gynecologic examinations.

The first pelvic examination is often anxiety-producing; the nurse can alleviate many of these feelings with explanations and teaching (Chart 46-5). It may be necessary to emphasize that a pelvic examination should not be painful except in the presence of a pelvic infection. Before the examination begins, the patient is asked to empty her bladder and to provide a urine specimen if urine tests are part of the total assessment. Voiding ensures patient comfort and eases the examination because a full bladder can make palpation of pelvic organs uncomfortable for the patient and difficult for the examiner.

Positioning

Although several positions may be used for the pelvic examination, the supine lithotomy position is used most commonly, although the upright lithotomy position (in which the woman assumes a semi-sitting posture) may also be used. This position offers several advantages:

- It is more comfortable for some women.
- It allows better eye contact between patient and examiner.
- It may provide an easier means for the examiner to carry out the bimanual examination.
- It enables the woman to use a mirror to see her anatomy (if she chooses) to visualize any conditions that require treatment or to learn about using certain types of contraceptive methods.

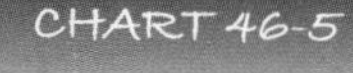

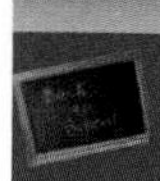

Patient Education

The Pelvic Examination

A pelvic examination includes assessment of the appearance of the vulva, vagina, and cervix and the size and shape of the uterus and ovaries to ensure reproductive health and absence of illness. The following should make the examination proceed more smoothly:

- You may have a feeling of fullness or pressure during the examination, but you should not feel pain. It is important to relax, because if you are very tense, you may feel discomfort.
- It is normal to feel uncomfortable and apprehensive.
- A narrow, warmed speculum will be inserted to visualize the cervix.
- A Papanicolaou (Pap) smear will be obtained and should not be uncomfortable.
- You may watch the examination with a mirror if you choose.
- The examination usually takes no longer than 5 minutes.
- Draping will be used to minimize exposure and reduce embarrassment.

In the supine lithotomy position, the patient lies on the table with her feet on foot rests or stirrups. She is encouraged to relax so that her buttocks are positioned at the edge of the examination table, and she is asked to relax and spread her thighs as widely apart as possible. If the patient is unable to lie safely on the examination table or unable to maintain the supine lithotomy position because of acute illness or disability, the Sims' position (or alternate positions) may be used. In Sims' position, the patient lies on her left side with her right leg bent at a 90-degree angle. The right labia may be retracted to gain adequate access to the vagina. The presence of a disability does not justify skipping any parts of the physical assessment, including the pelvic examination.

The following equipment is obtained and readily available: a good light source; a vaginal speculum; clean examination gloves; lubricant, spatula, cytobrush, glass slides, fixative solution or spray; and diagnostic testing supplies for screening for occult rectal blood if the woman is older than 40 years. Latex-free gloves should be available if the patient or clinician is allergic to latex. This allergy is becoming more prevalent in nurses and other health care providers and patients and is potentially life-threatening. Patients should be questioned about previous reactions to latex. (See Chapter 18 for a latex screening form and Chapter 53 for more information on latex allergy.)

Inspection

After the patient is prepared, the examiner inspects the labia majora and minora, noting the epidermal tissue of the labia majora; the skin fades to the pink mucous membrane of the vaginal introitus. Lesions of any type (eg, venereal warts, pigmented lesions [melanoma]) are evaluated. In the nulliparous woman, the labia minora come together at the opening of the vagina. In a woman who has delivered children vaginally, the labia minora may gape and vaginal tissue may protrude.

Trauma to the anterior vaginal wall during childbirth may have resulted in incompetency of the musculature, and a bulge caused by the bladder protruding into the submucosa of the anterior vaginal wall (**cystocele**) may be seen. Childbirth trauma may also have affected the posterior vaginal wall, producing a bulge caused by rectal cavity protrusion (**rectocele**). The cervix may descend under pressure through the vaginal canal and be seen at the introitus (**uterine prolapse**). See Chapter 47 for a discussion of these structural changes. To identify such protrusions, the examiner asks the patient to "bear down."

The introitus should be free of superficial mucosal lesions. The labia minora may be separated by the fingers of the gloved hand and the lower part of the vagina palpated. In women who have not had vaginal intercourse, a **hymen** of variable thickness may be felt circumferentially within the vaginal opening. The hymenal ring usually permits the insertion of one finger. Rarely, the hymen totally occludes the vaginal entrance (imperforate hymen).

In women who have had intercourse, a rim of scar tissue representing the remnants of the hymenal ring may be palpated circumferentially around the vagina near its opening. The greater vestibular glands (Bartholin's glands) lie between the labia minora and the remnants of the hymenal ring. An abscess of the Bartholin's gland can cause discomfort and requires incision and drainage.

Speculum Examination

The bivalved speculum, either metal or plastic, is available in many sizes. Metal specula are soaked, scrubbed, and sterilized between patients. Some clinicians and some patients prefer plastic specula, which permit one-time use. The speculum can be warmed with a heating pad or warm water to make insertion more comfortable for the patient. The speculum is not usually lubricated because commercial lubricants may interfere with cervical cytology (Papanicolaou [Pap] smear) findings.

The speculum is grasped in the dominant hand, with the thumb against the back of the thumb rest to keep the tips of the valves closed. The speculum is rotated slightly counterclockwise, and the vaginal orifice is held open by the thumb and the forefinger of the gloved nondominant hand by some examiners. Other examiners find that straight insertion of a speculum with downward pressure on the vagina is more comfortable for the patient. The speculum is gently inserted into the posterior portion of the introitus and slowly advanced to the top of the vagina; this should not be painful or uncomfortable for the woman. The tip of the speculum may then be elevated and the speculum rotated to a transverse position. The speculum is then slowly opened and the set-screw of the thumb rest is tightened to hold the speculum open (Fig. 46-4). The plastic speculum is operated in a similar manner.

INSPECTION OF THE CERVIX

The cervix is inspected. In nulliparous women, the cervix usually is 2 to 3 cm wide and smooth. In women who have borne children, the cervix may have a laceration, usually transverse, giving the cervical os a "fishmouth" appearance. Epithelium from the endocervical canal may have grown onto the surface of the cervix, appearing as beefy-red surface epithelium circumferentially around the os. Occasionally, the cervix of a woman whose mother took DES has a hooded appearance (a peaked aspect superiorly or a ridge of tissue surrounding it); this is evaluated by colposcopy when identified.

Malignant changes may not be obviously differentiated from the rest of the cervical mucosa. Small, benign cysts may appear on the cervical surface. These are usually bluish or white and are called nabothian cysts. A **polyp** of endocervical mucosa may protrude through the os and usually is dark red. Polyps can cause irregular bleeding; they are rarely malignant and usually are removed easily in an office or clinic setting. A carcinoma may appear as a cauliflower-like growth that bleeds easily when touched. Bluish coloration of the cervix is a sign of early pregnancy (Chadwick's sign).

PAP SMEAR

During the gynecologic examination, a Pap smear is obtained by rotating a small spatula at the os, followed by a cervical brush rotated in the os. The tissue obtained is spread on a glass slide and sprayed or fixed immediately, or inserted into liquid. A small broom-like device can also be used to obtain specimens for the Pap smear.

A specimen of any purulent material appearing at the cervical os is obtained for culture. A sterile applicator is used to obtain the specimen, which is immediately placed in an appropriate medium for transfer to a laboratory. In a patient who has a high risk of infection, routine cultures for gonococcal and chlamydial organisms are recommended

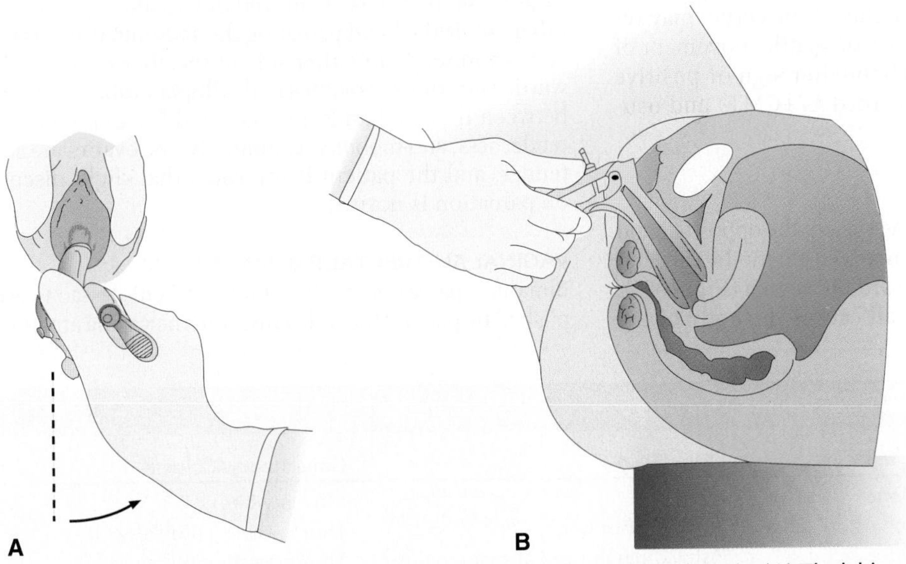

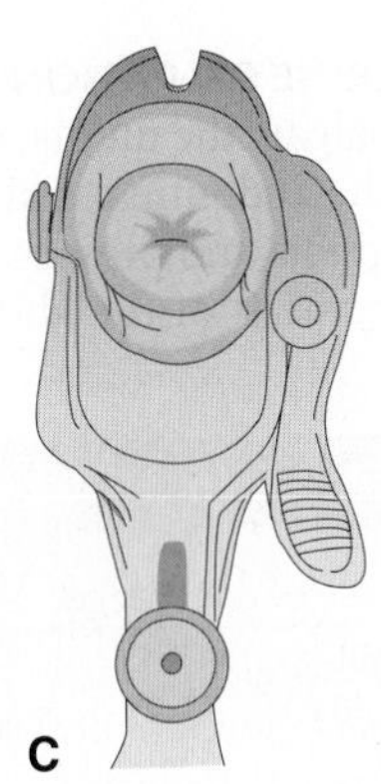

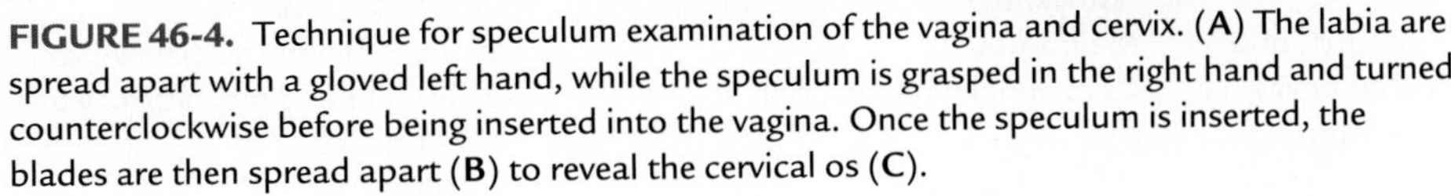

FIGURE 46-4. Technique for speculum examination of the vagina and cervix. (**A**) The labia are spread apart with a gloved left hand, while the speculum is grasped in the right hand and turned counterclockwise before being inserted into the vagina. Once the speculum is inserted, the blades are then spread apart (**B**) to reveal the cervical os (**C**).

because of the high incidence of both diseases and the complications of pelvic infection, fallopian tube damage, and subsequent infertility.

Vaginal discharge, which may be normal or may result from vaginitis, may be present. Discharge caused by bacteria (bacterial vaginosis) usually appears gray and purulent. Discharge caused by *Trichomonas* species infection is usually frothy, copious, and malodorous. Discharge caused by *Candida* species infection is usually thick and white-yellow and has a cottage-cheese appearance. Table 46-3 summarizes the characteristics of vaginal discharge found in different conditions.

The vagina is inspected as the examiner withdraws the speculum. It is smooth in young girls and thickens after puberty, with many rugae (folds) and redundancy in the epithelium. In menopausal women, the vagina thins and has fewer rugae because of decreased estrogen.

Some clinicians use PapSure to assist in the visual detection of cervical lesions. PapSure is a special light that is used following application of acetic acid. The effectiveness of this device is being evaluated.

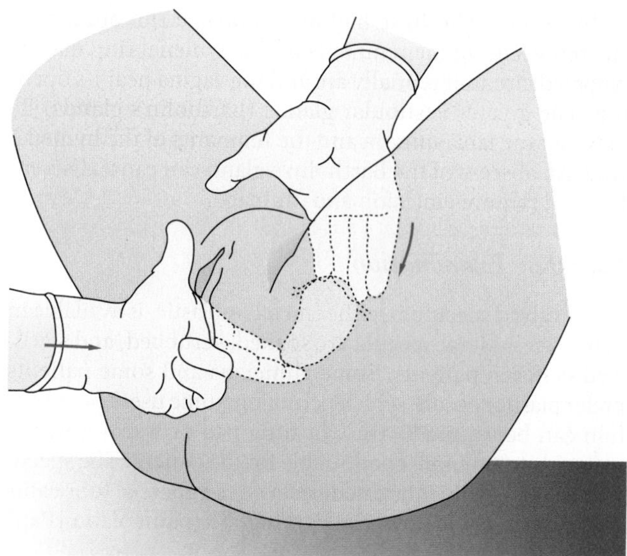

FIGURE 46-5. Technique for the bimanual examination of the pelvis.

Bimanual Palpation

To complete the pelvic examination, the examiner performs a bimanual examination, usually from a standing position. The examination is performed with the forefinger and middle finger of the gloved and lubricated hand. These fingers are placed in the vaginal orifice, while the other fingers are held tightly out of the way, with the thumb completely adducted. The fingers are advanced vertically along the vaginal canal, and the vaginal wall is palpated. Any firm part of the vaginal wall may represent old scar tissue from childbirth trauma but may also require further evaluation.

CERVICAL PALPATION

The cervix is palpated and assessed for its consistency, mobility, size, and position. The normal cervix is uniformly firm but not hard. Softening of the cervix is a finding in early pregnancy. Hardness and immobility of the cervix may reflect invasion by a neoplasm. Pain on gentle movement of the cervix is called a positive **chandelier sign** or positive cervical motion tenderness (recorded as +CMT) and usually indicates a pelvic infection.

UTERINE PALPATION

To palpate the uterus, the examiner places the opposite hand on the abdominal wall halfway between the umbilicus and the pubis and presses firmly toward the vagina (Fig. 46-5). Movement of the abdominal wall causes the body of the uterus to descend, and the organ becomes freely movable between the hand used to examine the abdomen and the fingers of the hand used to examine the pelvis. Uterine size, mobility, and contour can be estimated through palpation. Fixation of the uterus in the pelvis may be a sign of **endometriosis** or malignancy.

The body of the uterus is normally twice the diameter and twice the length of the cervix, curving anteriorly toward the abdominal wall. Some women have a retroverted or retroflexed uterus, which tips posteriorly toward the sacrum, whereas others have a uterus that is neither anterior nor posterior and is described as midline.

ADNEXAL PALPATION

Next, the right and left adnexal areas are palpated to evaluate the fallopian tubes and ovaries. The fingers of the hand examining the pelvis are moved first to one side, then to the other, while the hand palpating the abdominal area is moved correspondingly to either side of the abdomen and downward. The adnexa (ovaries and fallopian tubes) are trapped between the two hands and palpated for an obvious mass, tenderness, and mobility. Commonly, the ovaries are slightly tender, and the patient is informed that slight discomfort on palpation is normal.

VAGINAL AND RECTAL PALPATION

Bimanual palpation of the vagina and cul-de-sac is accomplished by placing the index finger in the vagina and the mid-

TABLE 46-3 Characteristics of Vaginal Discharge

Cause of Discharge	Symptoms	Odor	Consistency/Color
Physiologic	None	None	Mucus/white
Candida species infection	Itching, irritation	Yeast odor or none	Thin to thick, curdlike/white
Bacterial vaginosis	Odor	Fishy, often noticed after intercourse	Thin/grayish or yellow
Trichomonas species infection	Irritation, odor	Malodorous	Copious, often frothy/yellow-green
Atrophic	Vulvar or vaginal dryness	Occasional mild malodor	Usually scant and mucoid/may be blood-tinged

dle finger in the rectum. To prevent cross-contamination between the vaginal and rectal orifices, the examiner puts on new gloves. A gentle movement of these fingers toward each other compresses the posterior vaginal wall and the anterior rectal wall and assists the examiner in identifying the integrity of these structures. During this procedure, the patient may sense an urge to defecate. The nurse assures the patient that this is unlikely to occur. Ongoing explanations are provided to reassure and educate the patient about the procedure.

Gerontologic Considerations

Yearly examinations are important; they identify problems of the reproductive tract in aging women early. Some older women do not have regular gynecologic examinations. For example, a woman who delivered her children at home may never have had a pelvic examination. Some women regard it as an embarrassing and unpleasant procedure. Nurses play an important role; they can encourage all women to have an annual gynecologic examination. Nurses can make the examination a time for education and reassurance rather than a time of embarrassment.

Perineal pruritus is abnormal in elderly women and should be evaluated because it may indicate a disease process (diabetes or malignancy). Vulvar dystrophy, a thickened or whitish discoloration of tissue, may be visible, and biopsy is needed to rule out abnormal cells. Topical cortisone and hormone creams may be prescribed for symptomatic relief.

With relaxing pelvic musculature, uterine prolapse and relaxation of the vaginal walls can occur. Appropriate evaluation and surgical repair can provide relief if the patient is a candidate for surgery. After surgery, the patient should know that tissue repair and healing may require more time with aging. Pessaries (latex devices that provide support) are often used if surgery is contraindicated or before surgery to see if surgery can be avoided. They are fitted by a health care provider and may reduce discomfort and pressure. Use of a pessary requires the patient to have routine gynecologic examinations to monitor for irritation or infection. The patient must be assessed for allergy prior to insertion of a latex pessary (see Chapter 47 for details about pessaries).

Diagnostic Testing and Evaluation

Cytologic Test for Cancer (Pap Smear)

The Pap smear is used to detect cervical cancer. Before the introduction of the Pap smear by Papanicolaou in the 1930s, cervical cancer was the most common cause of cancer death in women. Because of the effectiveness of the Pap smear as a screening method, cervical cancer is now less common than breast or ovarian cancer.

Cervical secretions are gently removed from the cervical os and may be transferred to a glass slide and fixed immediately by spraying with a fixative or immersing in solution (Fig. 46-6). If the Pap smear reveals atypical cells, the liquid method allows for human papillomavirus (HPV) testing (see Chapter 47 for further discussion of HPV, a commonly transmitted STD that can cause venereal warts or cervical cancer). HPV DNA testing is helpful in some populations. HPV infection may be temporary, and further studies concerning the use of this testing modality to determine the best use of this assessment method are ongoing (Goldie, Kim & Wright, 2004).

The proper technique for obtaining a cervical specimen for cytologic study is described in Chart 46-6. A Pap smear should be performed when a patient is not menstruating, because blood usually interferes with interpretation. To avoid washing away cellular material, the patient should be instructed not to douche before having a Pap smear taken.

Both false-positive and false-negative results may be obtained. The Bethesda Classification system has been developed to promote consistency in reporting Pap smear results and to assist in standardizing management guidelines (Solomon, Davey, Kurman et al., 2001). Terminology includes the following categories:

- Low-grade squamous intraepithelial lesion (LSIL), which is equivalent to cervical intraepithelial neoplasia (CIN grade 1) and to mild changes related to exposure to HPV
- High-grade squamous intraepithelial lesion (HSIL), which equates to moderate and severe dysplasia, carcinoma in situ (CIS), and CIN grade 2 and CIN grade 3

These terms used on Pap smear findings are precursors to invasive carcinoma of the cervix.

The patient may incorrectly assume that an abnormal Pap smear signifies cancer. If the Pap smear (liquid immersion method) shows atypical cells and no high-risk HPV types are found, the next Pap smear is performed in 1 year. If a specific infection is causing inflammation, it is treated appropriately, and the Pap smear is repeated. If the repeat Pap smear reveals atypical squamous cells with high-risk HPV types, colposcopy is indicated. Pap smears that indicate LSIL should be repeated in 4 to 6 months and colposcopy performed if the LSIL has not resolved. Patients with Pap smears that indicate HGSIL and CIS require prompt colposcopy.

If the Pap smear results are abnormal, prompt notification, evaluation, and treatment are crucial. Notification of patients is often the responsibility of nurses in a women's health care practice or clinic. Pap smear follow-up is essential because appropriate follow-up can prevent cervical cancer. Many women do not adhere to recommendations—particularly those women who are young, those of low socioeconomic status, those who have difficulty coping with the diagnosis, and those without social support. Fear, lack of understanding, and childcare responsibilities have all been identified by women as reasons for poor follow-up. Women with a history of abuse, obese women, and women who had a negative gynecologic experience may also find returning for follow-up difficult. Interventions are tailored to meet the needs of the particular patient. Intensive telephone counseling, tracking systems, brochures, videos, and financial incentives have all been used to encourage follow-up. The nurse provides clear explanations and emotional support along with a carefully designed follow-up protocol designed to meet the needs of the specific patient (Abercrombie, 2001).

In 2006, the Committee on Adolescent Health Care of the American College of Obstetricians and Gynecologists (ACOG) issued a set of guidelines for the evaluation and management of abnormal cervical cytology and histology in

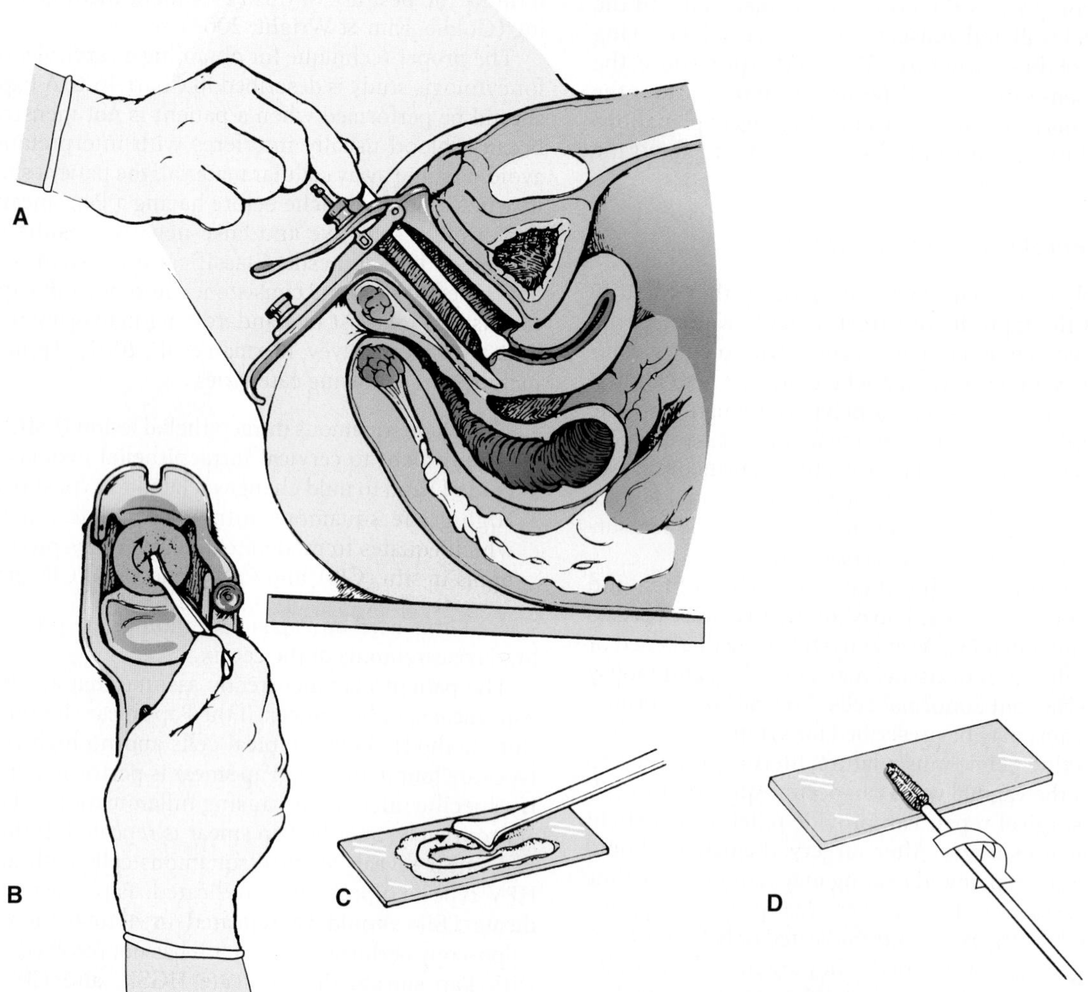

FIGURE 46-6. Method of using an Ayre spatula to obtain cervical secretions for cytology. (**A**) Speculum in place and the Ayre spatula in position at the cervical os. (**B**) The tip of the spatula is placed in the cervical os and the spatula rotated 360 degrees, firmly but nontraumatically. (**C**) Cellular material clinging to the spatula is then smeared smoothly on a glass slide. (**D**) Cytobrush is rotated in the cervical os and rolled onto a glass slide. Smear is then sprayed with fixative. *Note:* Liquid-based Pap smears are collected in the same way with a spatula and a brush, but then both are swirled separately in a bottle of solution and sent to the laboratory.

adolescent females. The committee stressed the need for a complete and accurate sexual history in making decisions about initiation of cervical cytology screening in adolescents. Because most CIN grades 1 and 2 regress in adolescents, surgical excision or destruction of cervical tissues is usually unnecessary. Specific screening and treatment recommendations were identified for adolescents with abnormalities detected on Pap tests and are available from ACOG (ACOG Committee on Adolescent Health Care, 2006).

Colposcopy and Cervical Biopsy

All suspicious Pap smears should be evaluated by colposcopy. The colposcope is a portable microscope (magnification from 10× to 25×) that allows the examiner to visualize the cervix and obtain a sample of abnormal tissue for analysis. Nurse practitioners and gynecologists require special training in this diagnostic technique.

After inserting a speculum and visualizing the cervix and vaginal walls, the examiner applies acetic acid to the cervix. Subsequent abnormal findings that indicate the need for biopsy include leukoplakia (white plaque visible before applying acetic acid), acetowhite tissue (white epithelium after applying acetic acid), punctation (dilated capillaries occurring in a dotted or stippled pattern), mosaicism (a tile-like pattern), and atypical vascular patterns.

An endocervical curettage may be performed during colposcopy. This analysis of tissue from the cervical canal is used to determine whether abnormal changes have occurred. If these biopsy specimens show premalignant cells or CIN, the

CHART 46-6 Guidelines for Obtaining an Optimal Pap Smear

ACTIONS	RATIONALE
1. Do not obtain a Pap smear if the woman is menstruating or has other frank bleeding (exception: high suspicion of neoplasia).	Blood obscures a proper reading of cells.
2. If performing more than one test (eg, Pap and GC), obtain the Pap smear first.	By performing the Pap smear first, the chance of a bloody smear is avoided.
3. Label the frosted end of the slide with the patient's name in pencil or label Thin-prep Pap bottle.	Ink may rub off or blur. Labeling with a pencil prevents improper identification.
4. Put on gloves before gently inserting the unlubricated speculum. (Speculum may be moistened with warm water.)	Gloves provide protection and warm water prevents discomfort. Lubricants may obscure cells on Pap smear.
5. Place the longer end of the Ayre spatula in the cervical canal and rotate it in a full circle to obtain a sample from the exocervix. Spread the material obtained onto the Pap smear slide.	This technique obtains a sampling of the exocervix and squamocolumnar junction.
6. Insert a cytobrush 2 cm into the cervical canal and rotate 180 degrees. Roll the brush onto the Pap smear slide. (With Thin-prep Pap smears, the brushings are not spread onto a slide. The spatula and brush are placed in a bottle of fixative and swirled.)	This technique obtains a sampling of the endocervical cells and may sample cells from the squamocolumnar junction if it is high in the canal.
7. In women who have had a hysterectomy for a gynecologic cancer, use a cotton applicator moistened with saline solution to obtain a sampling of cells from the vaginal cuff or posterior vagina. Women who have had a hysterectomy for benign conditions do not require frequent Pap smears.	Saline solution prevents drying, which makes interpretation difficult for the cytologist and prevents absorption of cells into the cotton, increasing the yield on the slide.
8. Immediately spray the slide or, if a Thin-prep, swirl the brush and spatula in the solution.	Exposure to air or light causes distortion of cells.

patient usually requires cryotherapy, laser therapy, or a cone biopsy (excision of an inverted tissue cone from the cervix).

Cryotherapy and Laser Therapy

Cryotherapy (freezing cervical tissue with nitrous oxide) and laser treatment are used in the outpatient setting. Cryotherapy may result in cramping and occasional feelings of faintness (vasovagal response). A watery discharge is normal for a few weeks after the procedure as the cervix heals.

Cone Biopsy and Loop Electrosurgical Excision Procedure

If endocervical curettage findings indicate abnormal changes or if the lesion extends into the canal, the patient may undergo a cone biopsy. This can be performed surgically or with a procedure called loop electrosurgical excision procedure (LEEP), which uses a laser beam.

Usually performed in the outpatient setting, LEEP is associated with a high success rate in removal of abnormal cervical tissue. The gynecologist excises a small amount of cervical tissue, and the pathologist examines the borders of the specimen to determine if disease is present. A patient who has received anesthesia for a surgical cone biopsy is advised to rest for 24 hours after the procedure and to leave any vaginal packing in place until it is removed (usually the next day). The patient is instructed to report any excessive bleeding.

The nurse or physician provides guidelines regarding postoperative sexual activity, bathing, and other activities. Because open tissue may be potentially exposed to HIV and other pathogens, the patient is cautioned to avoid intercourse until healing is complete and verified at follow-up. LEEP has a low incidence of complications but there is a slight future increase in the risk of cervical stenosis or premature deliveries (Crane, 2003).

Endometrial (Aspiration) Biopsy

Endometrial biopsy, a method of obtaining endometrial tissue, is performed when indicated as an outpatient procedure. A tissue sample obtained through biopsy permits diagnosis of cellular changes in the endometrium. Endometrial biopsy is usually indicated in cases of midlife irregular bleeding, postmenopausal bleeding, and irregular bleeding while taking hormone therapy or tamoxifen.

Women who undergo endometrial biopsy may experience slight discomfort. Usually, the procedure is performed without anesthesia. The examiner may apply a tenaculum (a clamp-like instrument that stabilizes the uterus) after the pelvic examination and then inserts a thin, hollow, flexible suction tube (Pipelle or sampler) through the cervix into the uterus.

Findings on aspiration may include normal endometrial tissue, hyperplasia, or endometrial cancer. Simple hyperplasia is an overgrowth of the uterine lining and is usually treated with progesterone. Complex hyperplasia, which refers to overgrowth of cells with abnormal features, is a risk factor for uterine cancer and is treated with progesterone and careful follow-up. Women who are overweight, who are older than 45 years, who have a history of nulliparity and infertility, or who have a family history of colon cancer seem to be at higher risk for hyperplasia. Endometrial cancer is discussed in Chapter 47.

Dilation and Curettage

Dilation and curettage (D & C) may be diagnostic (identifies the cause of irregular bleeding) or therapeutic (often temporarily stops irregular bleeding). The cervical canal is widened with a dilator, and the uterine endometrium is scraped with a curette. The purpose of the procedure is to secure endometrial or endocervical tissue for cytologic examination, to control abnormal uterine bleeding, and as a therapeutic measure for incomplete abortion.

Because D & C is usually carried out under anesthesia and requires surgical asepsis, it is usually performed in the operating room. However, it may take place in the outpatient setting with the patient receiving a local anesthetic supplemented with diazepam (Valium), midazolam (Versed), or meperidine (Demerol). The patient who receives these medications is carefully monitored until she has fully recovered.

The nurse explains the procedure, the physical and psychological preparation required, and expectations regarding postoperative discomfort and bleeding. The perineum is not shaved. The patient is instructed to void before the procedure. The patient is placed in the lithotomy position, the cervix is dilated with a dilating instrument, and endometrial scrapings are obtained by a curette. A perineal pad is placed over the perineum after the procedure, and excessive bleeding is reported. No restrictions are placed on dietary intake. If pelvic discomfort or low back pain occurs, mild analgesics usually provide relief. The physician indicates when sexual intercourse may be safely resumed. To reduce the risk of infection and bleeding, most physicians advise no vaginal penetration or use of tampons for 2 weeks.

Endoscopic Examinations

Laparoscopy (Pelvic Peritoneoscopy)

A laparoscopy involves inserting a laparoscope (a tube about 10 mm wide and similar to a small periscope) into the peritoneal cavity through a 2-cm (0.75-inch) incision below the umbilicus to allow visualization of the pelvic structures (Fig. 46-7). Laparoscopy may be used for diagnostic purposes (eg, in cases of pelvic pain when no cause can be found) or treatment. Laparoscopy facilitates many surgical procedures, such as tubal ligation, ovarian biopsy, myomectomy, hysterectomy, and lysis of adhesions (scar tissue that can cause pelvic discomfort). A surgical instrument (intrauterine sound or cannula) may be positioned inside the uterus to permit manipulation or movement during laparoscopy, affording better visualization. The pelvic organs can be visualized after the injection of a prescribed amount of carbon dioxide intraperitoneally into the cavity. Called insufflation, this technique separates the intestines from the pelvic organs. If a patient is undergoing sterilization, the fallopian or uterine tubes may be electrocoagulated, sutured, or ligated and a segment removed for histologic verification (clips are an alternative device for occluding the tubes).

After the laparoscopy is completed, the laparoscope is withdrawn, carbon dioxide is allowed to escape through the outer cannula, the small skin incision is closed with sutures or a clip, and the incision is covered with an adhesive bandage. The patient is carefully monitored for several

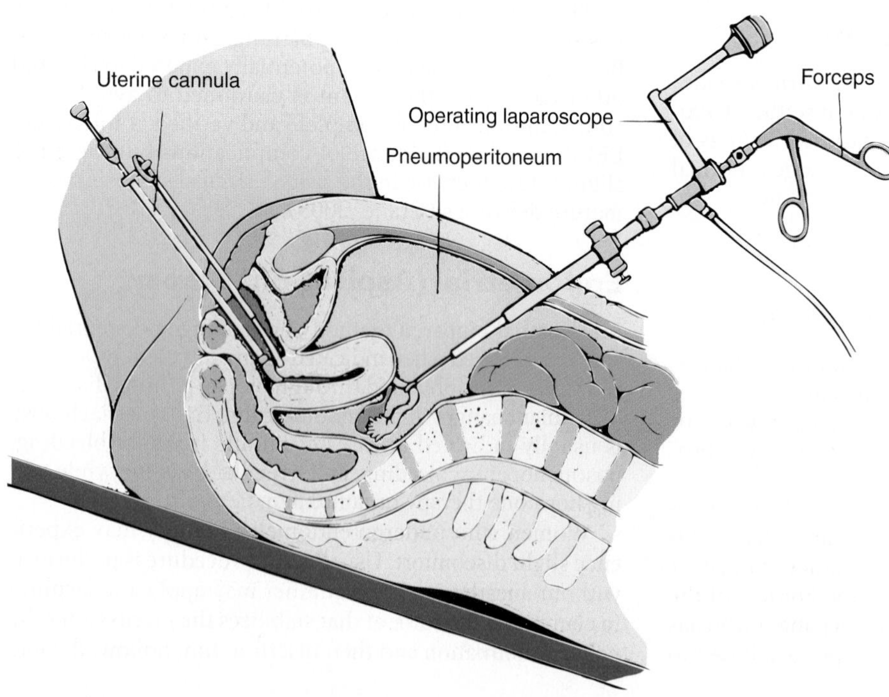

FIGURE 46-7. Laparoscopy. The laparoscope (*right*) is inserted through a small incision in the abdomen. A forceps is inserted through the scope to grasp the fallopian tube. To improve the view, a uterine cannula (*left*) is inserted into the vagina to push the uterus upward. Insufflation of gas creates an air pocket (pneumoperitoneum), and the pelvis is elevated (note the angle), which forces the intestines higher in the abdomen.

hours to detect any untoward signs indicating bleeding (most commonly from vascular injury to the hypogastric vessels), bowel or bladder injury, or burns from the coagulator. These complications are rare, making laparoscopy a cost-effective and safe short-stay procedure. The patient may experience abdominal or shoulder pain related to the use of carbon dioxide gas.

Hysteroscopy

Hysteroscopy (transcervical intrauterine endoscopy) allows direct visualization of all parts of the uterine cavity by means of a lighted optical instrument. The procedure is best performed about 5 days after menstruation ceases, in the estrogenic phase of the menstrual cycle. The vagina and vulva are cleansed, and a paracervical anesthetic block is performed or lidocaine spray is used. The instrument used for the procedure, a hysteroscope, is passed into the cervical canal and advanced 1 or 2 cm under direct vision. Uterine-distending fluid (normal saline solution or 5% dextrose in water) is infused through the instrument to dilate the uterine cavity and enhance visibility. Hysteroscopy, a safe procedure with few complications, is useful for evaluating endometrial pathology.

Hysteroscopy may be indicated as an adjunct to a D & C and laparoscopy in cases of infertility, unexplained bleeding, retained intrauterine device (IUD), and recurrent early pregnancy loss. Treatment for some conditions (eg, fibroid tumors) can be accomplished during this procedure, and sterilization may also be performed. Hysteroscopy is contraindicated in patients with cervical or endometrial carcinoma or acute pelvic inflammation.

Endometrial ablation (destruction of the uterine lining) is performed with a hysteroscope and resector (cutting loop), roller ball (a barrel-shaped electrode) or laser beam in cases of severe bleeding not responsive to other therapies. Performed in an outpatient setting under general, regional, or local anesthesia, this rapid procedure is an alternative to hysterectomy for some patients. Following uterine distension with fluid infusion, the lining of the uterus is destroyed. Hemorrhage, perforation, and burns can occur.

Other Diagnostic Procedures

Many diagnostic procedures are helpful in evaluating pelvic conditions. These may include x-rays, barium enemas, gastrointestinal x-ray series, intravenous urography, and cystography studies. In addition, because the uterus, ovaries, and fallopian tubes are near the structures of the urinary tract, urologic diagnostic studies, such as x-ray study of the kidney, ureters, and bladder (KUB) and pyelography are used, as are angiography and radioisotope scanning, if needed. Other diagnostic procedures include hysterosalpingography and computed tomography (CT) scanning.

Hysterosalpingography or Uterotubography

Hysterosalpingography (HSG) is an x-ray study of the uterus and the fallopian tubes after injection of a contrast agent. The diagnostic procedure is performed to evaluate infertility or tubal patency and to detect any abnormal condition in the uterine cavity. Sometimes the procedure is therapeutic because the flowing contrast agent flushes debris or loosens adhesions.

Prior to hysterosalpingography, laxatives and an enema may be administered to evacuate the intestinal tract so that gas shadows do not distort the x-ray findings. An analgesic agent may be prescribed. The patient is placed in the lithotomy position and the cervix is exposed with a bivalved speculum. A cannula is inserted into the cervix and the contrast agent is injected into the uterine cavity and the fallopian tubes. X-rays are taken to show the path and the distribution of the contrast agent.

Some patients experience nausea, vomiting, cramps, and faintness. After the test, the patient is advised to wear a perineal pad for several hours, because the radiopaque contrast agent may stain clothing.

Computed Tomography

CT has several advantages over ultrasonography (described below), even though it involves radiation exposure and is more costly. It is more effective than ultrasonography for obese patients or for patients with a distended bowel. CT can also demonstrate a tumor and any extension into the retroperitoneal lymph nodes and skeletal tissue, although it has limited value in diagnosing other gynecologic abnormalities.

Ultrasonography

Ultrasonography (or ultrasound) is a useful adjunct to the physical examination, particularly in obstetric patients or in patients with abnormal pelvic examination findings. It may be used to evaluate endometrial polyps, a frequent and usually benign cause of bleeding in older women Ultrasonography is a simple procedure based on sound wave transmission that uses pulsed ultrasonic waves at frequencies exceeding 20,000 Hz (formerly cycles per second) by way of a transducer placed in contact with the abdomen (abdominal scan) or a vaginal probe (vaginal ultrasound). Mechanical energy is converted into electrical impulses, which in turn are amplified and recorded on an oscilloscope screen while a photograph or video recording of the patterns is taken. The entire procedure takes usually less than 10 minutes and involves no ionizing radiation and no discomfort other than a full bladder, which is necessary for good visualization during an abdominal scan. (A vaginal ultrasound or sonogram does not require a full bladder.) Saline may be instilled into the uterus (saline infusion sonogram) to help delineate endometrial polyps or fibroids.

Magnetic Resonance Imaging

Magnetic resonance imaging (MRI) produces patterns that are finer and more definitive than other imaging procedures, and it does not expose patients to radiation. However, MRI is more costly.

NURSING ALERT

All metal devices, including medication skin patches with foil backing, must be removed before MRI is performed to avoid burns.

Management of Female Physiologic Processes

Many health concerns of women are related to normal changes or abnormalities of the menstrual cycle and may result from women's lack of understanding of the menstrual cycle, developmental changes, and factors that may affect the pattern of the menstrual cycle. Educating women about the menstrual cycle and changes over time is an important aspect of the nurse's role in providing quality care to women. Teaching should begin early, so that menstruation and the lifelong changes in the menstrual cycle can be anticipated and accepted as a normal part of life.

Menstruation

Menstruation, a cyclic vaginal flow of tissue that lines the uterus, occurs about every 28 days during the reproductive years, although normal cycles can vary from 21 to 42 days. The flow usually lasts 4 to 5 days, during which time 50 to 60 mL (4 to 12 teaspoons) of blood are lost.

A perineal pad is generally used to absorb menstrual discharge. Deodorant-treated pads are available, but some women are allergic or sensitive to the deodorants. Tampons are also used extensively; there is no significant evidence of untoward effects from their use, provided that there is no difficulty in inserting them. However, no tampons should be used for more than 4 to 6 hours, and superabsorbent tampons should not be used because of their association with toxic shock syndrome. If a tampon is difficult to remove, the vagina feels dry, or the tampon shreds when removed, less absorbent tampons should be used. If the string breaks or retracts, a woman should squat in a comfortable position, insert one finger into the vagina, try to locate the tampon, and remove it. If the woman feels uncomfortable attempting this maneuver or if she cannot remove the tampon, she should consult a gynecologic health care provider promptly.

Psychosocial Considerations

Girls who are approaching menarche (the onset of menstruation) should be instructed about the normal process of the menstrual cycle before it occurs. Psychologically, it is much healthier and appropriate to refer to this event as a "period" rather than as "being sick." With adequate nutrition, rest, and exercise, most women feel little discomfort, although some report breast tenderness and a feeling of fullness 1 or 2 days before menstruation begins. Others report fatigue and some discomfort in the lower back, legs, and pelvis on the first day and temperament or mood changes. Slight deviations from a usual pattern of daily living are considered normal, but excessive deviation may require evaluation. Regular exercise and a healthy diet have been found to decrease discomfort for some women. Heating pads may be very effective for cramps, as may nonsteroidal anti-inflammatory drugs (NSAIDs). Women with excessive cramping or dysmenorrhea are referred to a women's health care provider; oral contraceptives may be prescribed following evaluation.

Cultural Considerations

Culture refers to knowledge, beliefs, customs, and values acquired as members of a racial, ethnic, religious, or social group. The United States is becoming more culturally diverse. Various aspects of culture affect many health care encounters, and these encounters can be positive if nurses understand the various cultures of their patients.

Cultural views and beliefs about menstruation differ. Some women believe that it is detrimental to change a pad or tampon too frequently; they think that allowing the discharge to accumulate increases the flow, which is considered desirable. Some women believe they are vulnerable to illness during menstruation. Others believe it is harmful to swim, shower, have their hair permed, have their teeth filled, or eat certain foods during menstruation. They may also avoid using contraception during menstruation.

In such situations, nurses are in a position to provide women with facts in an accepting and culturally sensitive manner. The objective is to be mindful of these unexpressed, deep-rooted beliefs and to provide the facts with care. Aspects of gynecologic problems cannot always be expressed easily. The nurse needs to convey confidence and openness and to offer facts to facilitate communication. Suggestions to improve care include overcoming language barriers, providing appropriate materials in the patient's language, asking about traditional beliefs and dietary practices, and asking about their fears regarding care (Mattson, 2000). Patience, sensitivity, and a desire to learn about other cultures and groups will enhance the nursing care of all women (Chart 46-7).

Perimenopause

Perimenopause is the period extending from the first signs of menopause—usually hot flashes, vaginal dryness, or irregular menses—to beyond the complete cessation of menses. It has also been defined as the period around menopause, lasting to 1 year after the last menstrual period. Women often have varied beliefs about aging, and these must be considered by nurses caring for or educating perimenopausal patients.

Nursing Management

Perimenopausal women often benefit from information about the subtle physiologic changes they are experiencing. Perimenopause has been described as an opportune time for teaching women about health promotion and disease prevention strategies. When discussing health-related concerns with midlife women, nurses should consider the following issues:

- Sexuality, fertility, contraception, and STDs
- Unintended pregnancy (if contraception is not used correctly and consistently)
- Oral contraceptive use. Oral contraceptives provide perimenopausal women with protection against uterine cancer, ovarian cancer, anemia, pregnancy, and fibrocystic breast changes as well as relief from perimenopausal symptoms. This option should be discussed

CHART 46-7

Health Care for Women Who Are Lesbians

Lesbians can generally be defined as women who have sex with or primary emotional partnerships with women, but there is no universally accepted definition; variability exists in relationships and sexual preferences. Lesbians are found in every ethnic group and socioeconomic class. They can be single, celibate, divorced, teens, and seniors. Most experts believe that sexual orientation is not a conscious choice.

Lesbians have often encountered insensitivity in health care encounters. When they are asked if they are sexually active and respond affirmatively, contraception is immediately urged as health care providers may assume incorrectly that they practice heterosexual intercourse. Similar to many other marginalized groups of women, they often underuse health care. Some health care providers are homophobic, and discrimination against lesbians has been found in health care (Blackwell & Blackwell, 1999). Whether heterosexual or homosexual, nurses need to consider lesbianism within the continuum of human sexual behavior and need to use gender-neutral questions and terms that are nonjudgmental and accepting. Lesbian teens are at risk for suicide and STDs. Many lesbians do participate in heterosexual activity and often consider themselves at low risk for STDs. Because HPV, herpes infections, and other organisms implicated in STDs are transmitted by secretions and contact, they may need information on STDs and contraception. If sex toys are used and not cleaned, pelvic infections can occur.

Lesbians may smoke and drink more alcohol, may have a higher body mass index, may bear fewer or no children, and often have fewer health preventive screenings than heterosexual women (Carroll, 1999). These factors may predispose them to colon, lung, endometrial, ovarian, and breast cancer, as well as cardiovascular disease and diabetes. Nurses need to understand the unique needs of this population and provide appropriate and sensitive care.

with perimenopausal women. (Women who smoke and are 35 years of age or older should not take oral contraceptives because of an increased risk for cardiovascular disease.) Contraception is discussed in detail later in this chapter.

- Breast health. About 16% of cases of breast cancer occur in perimenopausal women, so breast self-examination, routine physical examinations, and mammograms are essential. (Although the effectiveness of breast self-examination is currently being questioned, women should be encouraged to report changes.) Women need to be aware that diet and exercise are crucial to their health.

Menopause

Menopause is the permanent physiologic cessation of menses associated with declining ovarian function; during this time, reproductive function diminishes and ends. Postmenopause is the period beginning from about 1 year after menses cease. Menopause is associated with some atrophy of breast tissue and genital organs, loss in bone density, and vascular changes.

Menopause starts gradually and is usually signaled by changes in menstruation. The monthly flow may increase, decrease, become irregular, and finally cease. Often, the interval between periods is longer; a lapse of several months between periods is not uncommon. Changes signaling menopause begin to occur as early as the late 30s, when ovulation occurs less frequently, estrogen levels fluctuate, and FSH levels increase in an attempt to stimulate estrogen production.

Clinical Manifestations

Because of these hormonal changes, some women notice irregular menses, breast tenderness, and mood changes long before menopause occurs. The hot or warm flashes and night sweats reported by some women are thought to be due to hormonal changes and denote vasomotor instability. They may vary in intensity from a barely perceptible warm feeling to a sensation of extreme warmth accompanied by profuse sweating, causing discomfort, sleep disturbances and subsequent fatigue, and occasionally, embarrassment. Other physical changes may include bone loss (discussed later in this chapter).

The entire genitourinary system is affected by the reduced estrogen level. Changes in the vulvovaginal area may include a gradual thinning of pubic hair and a gradual shrinkage of the labia. Vaginal secretions decrease, and women may report dyspareunia (discomfort during intercourse). The vaginal pH increases during menopause, predisposing women to bacterial infections and atrophic vaginitis. Discharge, itching, and vulvar burning may result.

Some women report fatigue, forgetfulness, weight gain, irritability, trouble sleeping, feeling "blue," and feelings of panic. Menopausal complaints need to be evaluated carefully, because they may indicate other disorders. Most women have few problems and are relieved to be free from menstrual periods.

Psychological Considerations

Women's reactions and feelings related to loss of reproductive capacity may vary. Some women may experience role confusion, whereas others experience a sense of sexual and personal freedom. Women may be relieved that the childbearing phase of their lives is over. Each woman's personality and circumstances affect her response and must be considered on an individual basis. Nurses need to be sensitive to all possibilities and take their cues from the patient.

Medical Management

Women approaching menopause often have many concerns about their health. Some have concerns based on a family

NURSING RESEARCH PROFILE

Perimenopausal Health Information

Lyndaker, C. & Hulton, L. (2004). The influence of age on symptoms of perimenopause. *Journal of Obstetric, Gynecologic and Neonatal Nursing, 33*(3), 340–347.

Purpose

Women in perimenopause have questions about this transitional period that can span 15 to 25 years. Researchers do not agree about the length of perimenopause and its associated symptoms. This study was designed to determine symptoms and association with age, explore the severity of symptoms, and identify which symptoms women discuss with their health care provider. This study used a descriptive exploratory research design with a structured questionnaire to identify symptoms of perimenopause and their severity, women's recognition that these symptoms were evidence of perimenopause, and women's discussion of these symptoms with a health care provider. Data were analyzed in terms of differences between age groups and symptomatology.

Design

More than 1600 prospective participants were chosen from two universities and a community hospital, because they were likely to have insurance and see health care providers regularly. After Institutional Review Board (IRB) approval, the Menopause Symptom List (MSL) questionnaire was distributed. The 418 women who returned completed questionnaires (30% response rate) were subjects. One-way analysis of variance was used to test differences between age groups and frequency of symptoms.

Findings

The frequency and severity of perimenopausal symptoms increased as age increased. The authors reported significant differences ($p < .05$) by age groups in number of episodes of sleeplessness, moodiness, and depression, and poor concentration ($p < .005$). Significant differences were also found in age groups for severity of depression ($p < .05$) and poor concentration ($p < .005$). Women reported that they discussed feelings of depression, headaches, moodiness, and palpitations with their health care providers more often than other symptoms. Many women did not attribute these problems to perimenopause.

Nursing Implications

Education and anticipatory guidance for perimenopausal women should begin when women are in their 30s, because many symptoms occurred as early as 35 years of age. Being knowledgeable about the cause of symptoms may reduce a woman's discomfort associated with the onset of symptoms as well as her concerns and fears. The importance of health promotion behaviors, including the proposed changes in treatment of menopausal symptoms based on the findings of the Women's Health Initiative study, should be stressed to women who are approaching perimenopause and menopause.

history of heart disease, osteoporosis, or cancer. Each woman needs to be as knowledgeable as possible about her options and should be encouraged to discuss her concerns with her primary health care provider so that she can make an informed decision about managing menopausal symptoms and maintaining her health. Decisions about management have become more difficult because of the findings of the Women's Health Initiative study. In a controlled trial of hormone therapy (HT) in more than 16,600 women, the WHI demonstrated that the risks of HT outweigh its benefits (WHI, 2002). The WHI study, which was supposed to last for 8.5 years, was halted after 5.2 years because women receiving HT had a higher risk for invasive breast cancer than women receiving placebo. Although the absolute risk of breast cancer is low for an individual woman taking HT, the risk was contrary to the intended effects of HT, that is, to preserve health and prevent disease.

Hormone Therapy

Until recently, HT was prescribed to prevent hot flashes, reduce the risk for osteoporotic fractures, and decrease the risk for cardiovascular disease. Contrary to long-held beliefs, HT or menopausal hormonal therapy (National Institutes of Health, 2005) (previously referred to as hormone replacement therapy or HRT) has been found to increase some health problems and to be less effective in preventing others than previously believed. Although HT decreases hot flashes and reduces the risk for osteoporotic fractures as well as colorectal cancer, it was found to increase the risk for breast cancer, heart attack, stroke, and blood clots (WHI, 2002). Thus, the benefits of HT were determined to be inadequate given the increased risk of breast cancer and these other disorders. Because of these findings, many women discontinued HT or are reluctant to begin HT. Some women have elected to use HT in low doses on the advice of their health care providers; however, the effect of these low doses has not been studied. The current recommendation for treatment of hot flashes with HT is to use the lowest dose possible for the shortest time possible (AHA, 2002). Nurses need to be knowledgeable about these issues to be able to respond to women's questions about HT use.

METHODS OF ADMINISTRATION

There are several different approaches for use of HT for those women who elect to take it. Both estrogen and progestin are prescribed for women who have not had a hysterectomy; progestin prevents proliferation of the uterine lining and hyperplasia. Women who no longer have a uterus because of hysterectomy can take estrogen without progestin (ie, unopposed estrogen) because there is no longer a risk for estrogen-induced hyperplasia of the uterine lining. There is a slight increase of risk of stroke in women taking estrogen alone following hysterectomy, but their risk for breast cancer is unchanged (WHI, 2002).

Some women take both estrogen and progestin daily; others take estrogen for 25 consecutive days each month, with progestin taken in cycles (eg, 10 to 14 days of the month). Women who take HT for 25 days often experience bleeding after completing the progestin. Other women take estrogen and progesterone every day and usually experience no bleeding. They occasionally have irregular spotting, which should be evaluated by their health care provider.

Estrogen patches, which are replaced once or twice weekly, are another option but require a progestin along with them if the woman still has a uterus. Another type of patch provides estrogen and progestin treatment. Vaginal treatment with an estrogen cream, suppository, or an estradiol vaginal ring (Estring) may be used for vaginal dryness or atrophic vaginitis. Estring is a small, flexible vaginal ring that slowly releases estrogen in small doses over 3 months.

RISKS AND BENEFITS

The changes that occur during menopause increase women's risks for atherosclerosis, angina, and coronary artery disease. Because of the findings of the WHI, the American Heart Association (AHA) has recommended against initiating HT for primary and secondary prevention of cardiovascular disease or stroke (AHA, 2002). HT is contraindicated in women with a history of breast cancer, vascular thrombosis, impaired liver function, some cases of uterine cancer, and undiagnosed abnormal vaginal bleeding. Because the risk for thromboembolic phenomena is increased, women who elect to take HT should be taught the signs and symptoms of deep vein thrombosis and pulmonary embolism and instructed to report these signs and symptoms immediately. Women taking HT should be assessed for leg redness, tenderness, chest pain, and shortness of breath. Further, they need to be informed about the importance of regular follow-up care, including a yearly physical examination and mammogram. An endometrial biopsy is indicated for women with any irregular bleeding. Because the risk for complications increases the longer HT is used, HT should be used for the shortest time possible (AHA, 2002). Estrogen alone or in combination with a progestin does not reduce risk for dementia or cognitive impairment (Shumaker, Legault, Kuller et al., 2004).

MAKING A DECISION ABOUT HORMONE THERAPY

Although the results of the WHI study may make the decision about use of HT easy for some women, it remains a difficult decision for those who could benefit from it because of disruptive symptoms of menopause and evidence of bone loss. Women often seek information about alternatives to HT use; therefore, nurses must be knowledgeable about other approaches women can use to promote their health in the perimenopausal and postmenopausal period. The decisions women make related to HT use must be individualized, based on their current health, risk factors, family history, and severity of symptoms.

Alternative Therapy for Hot Flashes

Problematic hot flashes have been treated with venlafaxine (Effexor), paroxetine (Paxil), gabapentin (Neurontin), and clonidine (Catapres). These medications have been found to reduce hot flashes and are alternatives for women who elect not to use HT. Similarly, vitamin B_6 (in doses of less than 200 mg) and vitamin E may be effective in decreasing hot flashes. Some women are interested in other alternative treatments (eg, natural estrogens and progestins, black cohosh, ginseng, dong quai, soy products, and several other herbal preparations); however, few scientific data exist about the safety or effectiveness of these remedies. Therefore, assessment of menopausal patients should address their use of complementary and alternative therapies and supplements. The North American Menopause Society (listed at the end of this chapter) provides additional suggestions.

Maintaining Bone Health

Osteoporosis, a disease characterized by low bone mass and microarchitectural deterioration of bone tissue, occurs with menopause and leads to enhanced bone fragility and increased risk for fracture. Other factors that increase a woman's risk for osteoporosis include a thin body frame, race (Caucasian or Asian), family history of osteoporosis, nulliparity, early menopause, moderate to heavy alcohol ingestion, smoking, caffeine use, sedentary lifestyle, and a diet low in calcium. Approximately 13% to 18% of women in the United States 50 years of age and older have osteoporosis and another 37% to 50% have osteopenia (Amin, Kuhle & Fitzpatrick, 2003). Women are advised to remain active and to begin a regular exercise program of weight-bearing activity, such as walking; to take a calcium supplement; to decrease or stop smoking; and to discuss with their health care provider the use of pharmacologic agents (bisphosphonates, calcitonin, parathyroid hormone, HT) to reduce bone loss if indicated (NIH Consensus Statement, 2001; USDHHS, 2004). Osteoporosis and its treatment are described in detail in Chapter 68.

Maintaining Cardiovascular Health

The American Heart Association (2002) recommends a variety of strategies to lower risk for heart disease in women. These include lifestyle changes and behavioral strategies. Diet, exercise, stress reduction, and a healthy lifestyle all contribute to older women's cardiac health and are an essential part of health promotion. Regular physical exercise increases the heart rate and high-density lipoprotein (HDL) levels. Weight-bearing exercise (eg, walking, jogging) at least four times a week is recommended. Pharmacologic therapy (eg, aspirin, beta-blockers, "statins," angiostatin-converting enzyme [ACE] inhibitors) may be indicated in women who have cardiovascular disease or are at high risk for it. Prevention and treatment of cardiovascular disease are discussed in detail in Chapter 26.

Behavioral Strategies

Regular physical exercise, including weight-bearing exercise, raises the heart rate, increases high-density lipoprotein (HDL) levels, and helps maintain bone mass. It may also reduce stress, enhance well-being, and improve self-image. Loss of muscle tissue is mediated by exercise; weight-bearing exercise (eg, walking, jogging) at least four times a week is recommended.

Women are also encouraged to participate in other health-promoting activities. These include regular health screening recommended for women at the time of menopause: gynecologic examinations, mammograms, colonoscopy, fecal occult blood testing, and bone mineral density testing if risk factors for osteoporosis are present.

Nutritional Therapy

Women are encouraged to decrease their fat and caloric intake and increase their intake of whole grains, fiber, fruit, and vegetables. Women of all ages tend to ingest less than the recommended amount of calcium; therefore, they should be encouraged to increase their intake of foods high in calcium (eg, nonfat yogurt, green leafy vegetables, seafood, and calcium-fortified foods). Calcium and vitamin D supplementation may be helpful in reducing bone loss and preventing the morbidity associated with fractures secondary to osteoporosis.

Nursing Management

Nurses can encourage women to view menopause as a natural change resulting in freedom from symptoms related to menses. No relationship exists between menopause and mental health problems; however, social circumstances (eg, adolescent children, ill partners, and dependent or ill parents) that may coincide with menopause can be very stressful.

Measures should be taken to promote general health. The nurse explains to the patient that cessation of menses is a normal occurrence that is rarely accompanied by nervous symptoms or illness. The current expected life span after menopause for the average woman is 30 to 35 years, which may encompass as many years as the childbearing phase of her life. Normal sexual urges continue, and women retain their usual response to sex long after menopause. Many women enjoy better health after menopause than before, especially those who have experienced dysmenorrhea. The individual woman's evaluation of herself and her worth, now and in the future, is likely to affect her emotional reaction to menopause. Patient teaching and counseling regarding healthy lifestyles, health promotion, and health screening are of paramount importance (Chart 46-8).

Menstrual Disorders

Menstrual disorders may include premenstrual syndrome (PMS); dysmenorrhea; amenorrhea; and excessive bleeding, irregular bleeding, or bleeding between cycles or unrelated to cycles. These disorders need to be discussed with a health care provider and managed individually. Dysmenorrhea may be due to endometriosis or anatomic abnormalities, or it can be a normal variation. Amenorrhea may be related to pregnancy, thyroid disorders, anatomic abnormalities, and eating disorders. Excessive bleeding may be due to fibroids, clotting disorders, thyroid disorders, and miscarriage. Irregular bleeding may be secondary to hormonal changes in adolescence or perimenopause or due to ectopic pregnancy, threatened abortion, or a variety of other factors.

Premenstrual Syndrome

Premenstrual syndrome (PMS) is a combination of symptoms that occur before the menses and subside with the onset of menstrual flow (Chart 46-9). The cause is unknown, but serotonin regulation is currently the most plausible theory. Other hormones may also be involved. Dietary factors may play a role because carbohydrates may affect serotonin. PMS is diagnosed if symptoms occur during the five days prior to onset of menses, disappear within four days of the onset of menses and have occurred through several cycles. Severe symptoms have been labeled as premenstrual dysphoric disorder (DiCarlo, Palomba, Tommaselli et al., 2001). This severe form of PMS, which interferes with the woman's schoolwork, job, or social or family life, is uncommon. PMS tends to become less symptomatic with menopause, but may be predictive of menopausal difficulties with depression, decreased libido, and insomnia (Freeman, Sammel, Rinaudo et al., 2004).

Clinical Manifestations

Major symptoms of PMS include physical symptoms such as headache, fatigue, low back pain, painful breasts, and a feeling of abdominal fullness. Behavioral and emotional symptoms may include general irritability, mood swings, fear of losing control, binge eating, and crying spells. Symptoms vary widely from one woman to another and from one cycle to the next in the same woman. Great variability is found in the degree of symptoms. Many women are affected to some degree, but some are severely affected.

A generally stressful life and problematic relationships may be related to the intensity of physical symptoms. Some women report moderate to severe life disruption secondary to PMS that negatively affects their interpersonal relationships. PMS may also be a factor in reduced productivity, work-related injuries, and absenteeism.

Medical Management

Because there is no single treatment or known cure for PMS, women should chart their symptoms so they can anticipate and therefore cope with them. Exercise is encouraged for all women, because it may be helpful and is part of general health promotion. Although women have been advised to avoid caffeine, high-fat foods, and refined sugars, little research demonstrates the efficacy of dietary changes. Alternative therapies that have been used include vitamins B and E, magnesium, and oil of evening primrose capsules. No studies have evaluated the effectiveness of these therapies.

CHART 46-8

HOME CARE CHECKLIST • The Woman Approaching Menopause

At the completion of the home care instruction, the patient or caregiver will be able to:	Patient	Caregiver
• Describe menopause as a normal period in a woman's life.	✔	✔
• State that fatigue and stress may worsen hot flashes.	✔	✔
• State that a nutritious diet and weight control will enhance physical and emotional well-being.	✔	✔
• State the importance of exercising for 30 minutes three or four times a week to maintain good health.	✔	✔
• Describe involvement in outside activities as beneficial in reducing anxiety and tension.	✔	✔
• Identify the following as changes that often occur in midlife: departure of children, aging, dependence of parents, possible loss of loved ones.	✔	✔
• Describe this phase of life as having the potential for intellectual growth, personal accomplishment, and initiation of new activities.	✔	✔
• State the following points about sexual activity:		
Frequent sexual activity helps to maintain the elasticity of the vagina.	✔	
Contraception is advised until 1 year passes without menses.	✔	
Safer sex is important at any age.	✔	
Sexual functioning may be enhanced at midlife.	✔	
• Identify the importance of an annual physical examination to screen for problems and to promote general health.	✔	
• Identify strategies and methods to prevent or manage the following problems:		
Itching or burning of vulvar areas: see primary health care provider to rule out dermatologic abnormalities and, if appropriate, to obtain a prescription for a lubricating or hormonal cream.	✔	
Dyspareunia (painful intercourse) due to vaginal dryness; use a water-soluble lubricant, such as K-Y Jelly, Astro-Glide, Replens, hormone cream, or contraceptive foam.	✔	
Decreased perineal muscle tone and bladder control: practice Kegel exercises daily (contract the perineal muscles as though stopping urination; hold for 5–10 seconds and release; repeat frequently during the day).	✔	
Dry skin: use mild emollient skin cream and lotions to prevent dry skin.	✔	
Weight control: join a weight-reduction support group such as Weight Watchers or a similar group if appropriate, or consult a registered dietitian for guidance about the tendency to gain weight, particularly around the hips, thighs, and abdomen.	✔	
Osteoporosis: observe recommended calcium and vitamin D intake, including calcium supplements, if indicated, to slow the process of osteoporosis; avoid smoking, alcohol, and excessive caffeine, all of which increase bone loss. Perform weight-bearing exercises. Undergo bone density testing when appropriate.	✔	
Risk for urinary tract infection (UTI): drink 6 to 8 glasses of water daily and take vitamin C (500 mg) as a possible way to reduce the incidence of UTI related to atrophic changes of the urethra.	✔	
Vaginal bleeding: report any bleeding after 1 year of no menses to a primary health care provider *immediately, no matter how minimal.*	✔	

Pharmacologic remedies include selective serotonin reuptake inhibitors (eg, fluoxetine [Prozac, Sarafem]), gonadotropin-releasing hormone (GnRH) agonists, prostaglandin inhibitors (eg, ibuprofen and naproxen [Anaprox]), diuretics, antianxiety agents, and calcium supplements.

Nursing Management

The nurse establishes rapport with the patient and obtains a health history, noting the time when symptoms began and their nature and intensity. The nurse then determines whether the onset of symptoms occurs before or shortly after the menstrual flow begins. In addition, the nurse can show the patient how to record the timing and intensity of symptoms. A nutritional history is also elicited to determine if the diet is high in salt, caffeine, or alcohol or low in essential nutrients.

The patient's goals may include reduction of anxiety, mood swings, crying, binge eating, fear of losing control, improved coping with day-to-day stressors, improved

CHART 46-9

Causes, Manifestations, and Treatment of Premenstrual Syndrome

CAUSE

- Unknown; may be related to hormonal changes combined with other factors (diet, stress, and lack of exercise)
- Many women have some symptoms related to menses, but PMS affects 2% to 5% of women and is a complex of symptoms that result in dysfunction.

PHYSICAL SYMPTOMS

- Fluid retention (eg, bloating, breast tenderness)
- Headache
- Swelling

AFFECTIVE SYMPTOMS

- Depression
- Anger
- Irritability
- Anxiety
- Confusion
- Withdrawal
- Symptoms begin in the 5 days preceding menses and relief occurs within 4 days of onset of menses. Dysfunction usually occurs in relationships, parenting, work, or school.

TREATMENT

- Use of social support and family resources
- Nutritious diet consisting of whole grains, fruits, and vegetables; increased water intake may help
- Serotonin reuptake inhibitors
- Alprazolam (Xanax) has been effective but risk of physical and psychological dependence is high.
- Spironolactone, a diuretic, may be effective in treating fluid retention.
- Initiation/maintenance of exercise program
- Stress reduction techniques

relationships with family and coworkers, and increased knowledge about PMS. Positive coping measures are facilitated. This may involve encouraging the woman's partner to offer support and assistance with childcare. The patient can try to plan her working time to accommodate the days she is less productive because of PMS. The nurse encourages the patient to use exercise, meditation, imagery, and creative activities to reduce stress. The nurse also encourages the patient to take medications as prescribed and provides instructions about the desired effects of the medications. Enrolling in a PMS group that meets to discuss problems may help the patient learn to recognize and understand what she is experiencing.

If the patient has severe symptoms of PMS or premenstrual dysphoric disorder, the nurse assesses her for suicidal, uncontrollable, and violent behavior. Any suggestions of suicidal tendencies must be evaluated by psychiatric consultation immediately. In rare cases, uncontrollable behavior may lead to violence toward family members. If abuse of children or other members of a patient's family is suspected, reporting protocols are implemented and followed. Referral is made for immediate psychiatric or psychological care and counseling.

Dysmenorrhea

Primary dysmenorrhea is painful menstruation, with no identifiable pelvic pathology. It occurs at the time of menarche or shortly thereafter. It is characterized by crampy pain that begins before or shortly after the onset of menstrual flow and continues for 48 to 72 hours. Pelvic examination findings are normal. Dysmenorrhea is thought to result from excessive production of prostaglandins, which causes painful contraction of the uterus and arteriolar vasospasm. Psychological factors, such as anxiety and tension, may also contribute to dysmenorrhea. As women become older, dysmenorrhea often decreases and frequently completely resolves after childbirth.

In secondary dysmenorrhea, pelvic pathology such as endometriosis, tumor, or pelvic inflammatory disease (PID) contributes to symptoms. Patients with secondary dysmenorrhea frequently have pain that occurs several days before menses, with ovulation, and occasionally with intercourse.

Assessment and Diagnostic Findings

A complete pelvic examination is performed to rule out possible disorders, such as endometriosis, PID, adenomyosis, and fibroid uterus. A laparoscopy is usually required to identify organic causes.

Management

In primary dysmenorrhea, the reason for the discomfort is explained, and the patient is assured that menstruation is a normal function of the reproductive system. If the patient is young and accompanied by her mother, the mother may also need reassurance. Many young women expect to have painful periods if their mothers did. The discomfort of cramps can be treated once anxiety and concern over its cause are dispelled by adequate explanation. Symptoms usually subside with appropriate medication. Aspirin, a mild prostaglandin inhibitor, may be taken at recommended doses every 4 hours. Other useful prostaglandin antagonists include NSAIDs such as ibuprofen (Motrin), naproxen (Aleve, Anaprox, Naprosyn), and mefenamic acid (Ponstel). If one medication does not provide relief, another may be recommended. Usually these medications are well tolerated, but some women experience gastrointestinal side effects. Contraindications include allergy, peptic ulcer history, sensitivity to aspirin-like medications, asthma, and pregnancy. Low-dose oral contraceptives provide relief in more than 90% of patients and are indicated in women with dysmenorrhea who are sexually active but do not desire pregnancy.

Continuous low-level local heat may also be effective in relieving primary dysmenorrhea. The mechanism is not clearly known; the heat may counteract the activity of hormones that cause the uterus to contract. Heat is a vasodilator that increases blood flow and may counteract constriction and muscle contraction. Heat therapy and medication have been found to work well in combination.

The patient is encouraged to continue her usual activities and to increase physical exercise if possible, because this relieves discomfort for some women. Taking analgesic agents before cramps start, in anticipation of discomfort, is advised.

Management of secondary dysmenorrhea is directed at diagnosis and treatment of the underlying cause (eg, endometriosis or PID). The same analgesic agents used for primary dysmenorrhea may be part of the management of secondary dysmenorrhea due to endometriosis.

Amenorrhea

Amenorrhea (absence of menstrual flow) is a symptom of a variety of disorders and dysfunctions. Primary amenorrhea (delayed menarche) refers to the situation in which young women older than 16 years of age have not begun to menstruate but otherwise show evidence of sexual maturation, or in which young women have not begun to menstruate and have not begun to show development of secondary sex characteristics by 14 years of age. Amenorrhea may be of considerable concern but is often due to minor variations in body build, heredity, environment, and physical, mental, and emotional development.

The nurse encourages the patient to express her concerns and anxiety about this problem, because the patient may feel that she is different from her peers. A complete physical examination, careful health history, and simple laboratory tests help rule out possible causes, such as physiologic disorders, metabolic or endocrine difficulties, and systemic diseases. Treatment is directed toward correcting any abnormalities.

Secondary amenorrhea (an absence of menses for three cycles or 6 months after a normal menarche) may be caused by pregnancy, tension, emotional upset, eating disorders, exercise, or stress. In adolescents, secondary amenorrhea is usually caused by minor emotional upset related to being away from home, attending college, tension due to schoolwork, or interpersonal problems. However, the second most common cause is pregnancy, so a pregnancy test is almost always indicated.

Secondary nutritional disturbances may also be factors. Obesity can result in anovulation and subsequent amenorrhea. Eating disorders, such as anorexia and bulimia, are characterized by lack of menses because the decrease in body fat and caloric intake affects hormonal function. Intense exercise can induce menstrual disturbances. Competitive female athletes often experience amenorrhea. If they do, they may be placed on HT to prevent bone loss related to low estrogen levels. On occasion, a pituitary or thyroid dysfunction may cause amenorrhea. These dysfunctions can be treated successfully by treatment of the underlying endocrine disorder. Infrequent periods (oligomenorrhea) may be related to thyroid disorders, polycystic ovarian syndrome, or premature ovarian failure. Again, evaluation by a primary health care provider is necessary.

Abnormal Uterine Bleeding

Dysfunctional uterine bleeding is abnormal bleeding that has no known organic cause. The bleeding is defined as irregular, painless bleeding of endometrial origin that may be excessive, prolonged, or without pattern. Dysfunctional uterine bleeding can occur at any age but is most common at opposite ends of the reproductive life span. It is usually secondary to anovulation (lack of ovulation) and is common in adolescents and women approaching menopause.

Adolescents account for many cases of abnormal uterine bleeding, because they often do not ovulate as their pituitary-ovarian axis matures. Perimenopausal women also experience this condition due to irregular ovulation because of their decreasing ovarian hormone production. The remaining causes are often related to fibroids, obesity, or hypothalamic dysfunction.

Abnormal or unusual vaginal bleeding that is atypical in time or amount must be evaluated, because it may be a manifestation of a major, life-threatening disorder. A physical examination is performed, and the patient is evaluated for conditions such as pregnancy, neoplasm, infection, anatomic abnormalities, endocrine disorders, trauma, blood dyscrasias, platelet dysfunction, and hypothalamic disorders. Women of any age require evaluation to identify a specific cause of abnormal uterine bleeding. Pregnancy testing and hormonal evaluation are usually part of the initial assessment. Treatment often consists of hormones or oral contraceptives.

Menorrhagia

Menorrhagia is prolonged or excessive bleeding at the time of the regular menstrual flow. In early life the cause is usually related to endocrine disturbance, whereas in later life it usually results from inflammatory disturbances, tumors of the uterus, or hormonal imbalance. Emotional disturbances may also affect bleeding.

Women with menorrhagia are urged to see a primary health care provider and to describe the amount of bleeding by pad count and saturation (ie, absorbency of perineal pad or tampon and number saturated hourly). Persistent heavy bleeding can result in anemia (Sharts-Hopko, 2001).

Metrorrhagia

Metrorrhagia (vaginal bleeding between regular menstrual periods) is probably the most significant form of menstrual dysfunction because it may signal cancer, benign tumors of the uterus, or other gynecologic problems. This condition warrants early diagnosis and treatment. Although bleeding between menstrual periods by women taking oral contraceptives is usually not serious, irregular bleeding by women taking HT should be evaluated.

Menometrorrhagia is heavy vaginal bleeding between and during periods. It, too, requires evaluation.

Postmenopausal Bleeding

Bleeding 1 year after menses cease at menopause must be investigated, and a malignant condition must be considered until proved otherwise. An endometrial biopsy or a D & C is indicated. A vaginal ultrasound can also be used in postmenopausal bleeding to measure the thickness of the endometrial lining. The uterine lining in postmenopausal women should be thin because of low estrogen levels. A lining thicker than 5 mm usually warrants evaluation by endometrial biopsy or saline sonogram.

Dyspareunia

Dyspareunia (difficult or painful intercourse) can be superficial, deep, primary, or secondary and may occur at the beginning of, during, or after intercourse. This problem can be embarrassing for women to discuss because they may believe that it is their problem if their partner is not experiencing discomfort. Dyspareunia may be related to many factors, including injury during childbirth; lack of vaginal lubrication; a history of incest, sexual abuse, or assault; endometriosis; pelvic infection; vaginal atrophy with menopause; gastrointestinal disorders; fibroids; urinary tract infection; STDs; or vulvodynia (vulvar pain that affects women of all ages without any discernible physical cause). Depending on the cause of dyspareunia, counseling, extra lubrication, or antidepressants may be prescribed, and surgery to expand or repair the vaginal opening is occasionally needed. Women's health issues related to sexuality may be affected by many factors. Thus, these issues need to be taken seriously, carefully assessed, and treated.

Contraception

Each year, more than half of the pregnancies in the United States are unintended. Although unintended pregnancies occur in women of all ages, incomes, and racial and ethnic groups, the highest rates occur among adolescents, lower-income women, and African-American women. Adolescents are more likely to experience pregnancy complications and are more prone to have low-birthweight babies. In addition, adolescent mothers are less likely to obtain a high school diploma and are more likely to live in poverty.

Women often fail to use effective methods of contraception consistently or at all. Of the women who undergo abortions, many were not using contraception when they became pregnant, and others have never used any method of contraception. Fewer unwanted pregnancies may reduce the number of abortions, abused children, stressed families, and infant mortality and morbidity.

Nurses can assist with information and support. Women can be asked directly when they plan to have their next pregnancy and about their need for contraception. Many women who are sexually active or who are considering becoming sexually active can benefit from learning about contraception. Nurses who are involved in helping patients make contraceptive choices need to listen, educate, take time to answer questions, and assist patients in choosing the method they prefer. It is important for women to receive unbiased and nonjudgmental information, understand the benefits and risks of each method, learn about alternatives and how to use them, and receive positive reinforcement and acceptance of their choice. Some women fear that contraception will cause cancer or weight gain.

Although contraception is available in developing countries, it is not used as much as it is in more developed countries. Family planning has been identified as a high priority in Asia, Latin America, the Middle East, and Africa (Cleland & Ali, 2004).

Abstinence

Abstinence, or celibacy, is the only completely effective means of preventing pregnancy. Abstinence may not be a desired or available option for many women because of cultural expectations and their own and their partner's values and sexual needs.

Sterilization

After abstinence, sterilization by bilateral tubal occlusion or vasectomy is the most effective means of contraception. Both procedures must be considered permanent, because neither is easily reversible. Women and men who choose these methods should be certain that they no longer wish to have children, no matter how the circumstances in their life may change. Often, decisions are made that may be regretted later. Some gynecologists suggest a waiting period to ensure that patients are certain about a potentially irreversible decision.

Tubal Ligation

Sterilization by tubal ligation is one of the most common surgical procedures performed on women. Tubal ligation is usually performed as a same-day surgical procedure and is carried out by laparoscopy, with the patient receiving a general or local anesthetic. The laparoscope, a small periscope-like optical instrument, is inserted through a small umbilical incision. Carbon dioxide is introduced to lift other abdominal organs away from the tubal area. The fallopian tubes are visualized and may be coagulated, sutured (Pomeroy procedure), or ligated with silicone bands or a spring clip, thereby disrupting their patency. The use of spring clips is associated with the highest rate of pregnancy following sterilization. Another procedure, transcervical tubal occlusion procedure, uses a 0.6-inch metal coil or spring that is inserted into the fallopian tubes through the cervix, thus avoiding the need for laparoscopy or a surgical incision. This method, referred to as the Essure procedure, is performed via hysteroscopy and obstructs the tubes by inducing scar tissue. Women who have had this procedure should abstain from unprotected intercourse for 3 months to avoid pregnancy until the scar tissue develops and the effectiveness of the procedure is verified by hysterosalpingography (HSG).

Despite a very high rate of effectiveness, all women who have undergone tubal ligation but miss a period should be tested for pregnancy, because ectopic and intrauterine pregnancies, although rare, may occur. Ovulation and menstruation are not affected by sterilization, although some women report heavier menstrual bleeding and more cramping after tubal ligation.

Before undergoing tubal ligation, the patient should be informed that an IUD, if present, will be removed. If the patient is taking oral contraceptives, she usually continues them up to the time of the procedure. If a laparoscopic procedure is performed, the patient may experience postoperative abdominal or shoulder discomfort for a few days, related to the carbon dioxide gas and the manipulation of organs. The patient is instructed to report heavy bleeding, fever, or pain that persists or increases. She should avoid intercourse, strenuous exercise, and lifting for 2 weeks. Risks associated with tubal ligation are minimal and are more often related to anesthesia than to the surgery itself. Risk is increased in women with diabetes, previous abdominal or pelvic surgery, or obesity.

Vasectomy

Vasectomy (male sterilization) and hysteroscopic/laparoscopic tubal ligation are compared in Chart 46-10. See Chapter 49 for a discussion of vasectomy.

Hormonal Contraception

Estrogens and progestins are currently used by many women to prevent pregnancy. Oral contraceptives block ovarian stimulation by preventing the release of FSH from the anterior pituitary gland. In the absence of FSH, a follicle does not ripen, and ovulation does not occur. Progestins (synthetic forms of progesterone) suppress the LH surge, prevent ovulation, and also render the cervical mucus impenetrable to sperm. Synthetic estrogens and progestin, found in many hormonal contraceptive agents, differ in androgenic activity. Hormonal contraceptive agents may be oral, transdermal, vaginal, or injectable.

Benefits and Risks

Benefits of hormonal contraceptive use include a reduction in the incidence of benign breast disease; improvement in acne; and reduced risk of uterine and ovarian cancers, anemia, and pelvic infection. In general, prolonged hormonal contraceptive use has resulted in no definite long-term undesirable effects, although there is an increased risk of gallbladder problems (eg, cholestasis). Resumption of normal menses is delayed 2 to 3 months or longer in about 20% of hormonal contraceptive users. Risks include venous thromboembolism, although the incidence of venous thromboembolism has decreased, because the estrogen concentrations used today are less than early preparations. Venous thromboembolism is less than half as likely with hormonal contraceptives than with pregnancy. Fetal anomalies do not appear to be a concern, and normal reproductive tract function and fertility resume after hormonal contraceptive use is discontinued. However, most health care providers recommend that women who wish to become pregnant use a barrier contraceptive method for 1 to 2 months after stopping hormonal contraceptives before attempting to become

CHART 46-10

Comparison of Sterilization Methods

Vasectomy

ADVANTAGES
- Highly effective
- Relieves the female of the contraceptive burden
- Inexpensive in the long run
- Permanent
- Highly acceptable procedure to most clients
- Very safe
- Quickly performed

DISADVANTAGES
- Expensive in the short term
- Serious long-term effects suggested (although currently unproved)
- Permanent (although reversal is possible, it is expensive and requires a highly technical and major surgery, and its results cannot be guaranteed)
- Regret in 5%–10% of patients
- No protection against STDs, including HIV
- Not effective until sperm remaining in the reproductive system are ejaculated

Hysteroscopic and Laparoscopic Tubal Sterilization

ADVANTAGES
- Low incidence of complications
- Short recovery
- Leaves small or no scar
- Quickly performed

DISADVANTAGES
- Permanent
- Reversal difficult and expensive
- Sterilization procedures technically difficult
- Requires surgeon, operating room (aseptic conditions), trained assistants, medications, surgical equipment (Essure [insertion of a coil or spring in the fallopian tubes] requires hysteroscopy rather than surgery)
- Expensive at the time performed
- If failure, high probability of ectopic pregnancy
- No protection against STDs, including HIV

pregnant to permit a normal period for accurate dating of the pregnancy.

A few patients experience adverse reactions when using hormonal contraceptives. These include nausea, depression, headache, leg cramps, and breast soreness. Usually, these symptoms subside after 3 or 4 months. Because such symptoms are sometimes related to sodium and water retention caused by estrogen, a smaller dose of the hormone or a different hormonal combination may alleviate the problem. Many patients experience spotting in the first month of use of hormonal contraceptive or if they use it irregularly, so they need to be reassured and advised to use the contraceptive agent as prescribed. Chart 46-11 compares different oral contraceptive regimens, and Chart 46-12 describes the benefits and risks of oral contraceptive use.

Clinical trials have shown no evidence of weight gain with hormone contraceptive use. However, many young women are reluctant to use hormonal contraceptive agents because of fear of weight gain (Gallo, Grimes, Schulz, et al., 2004).

Contraindications

Absolute contraindications to hormonal contraceptives include current or past thromboembolic disorder, cerebrovascular disease, or artery disease; migraine headaches with visual auras; known or suspected breast cancer; known or suspected current or past estrogen-dependent neoplasia; pregnancy; current or past benign or malignant liver tumor; liver dysfunction; clotting disorders, congenital hyperlipidemia and abnormal vaginal bleeding (Kaunitz & Mestman, 2004).

Relative contraindications include hypertension, bile-induced jaundice, acute phase of mononucleosis, and sickle cell disease. Controlled hypertension in otherwise healthy young nonsmokers is generally not a contraindication to use of combination agents but does require a low dose and careful blood pressure monitoring. Women older than 35 years who smoke are at risk for cardiac problems and should not use hormonal contraceptives. Occasionally, neuro-ocular complications arise, but a cause-and-effect relationship has not been established. If visual disturbances occur, hormonal contraceptives should be discontinued. Chart 46-13 summarizes patient education guidelines that are important for women using combination hormonal contraceptives.

Some medical conditions require special precautions. Women with seizure disorders taking antiseizure medications that can increase hepatic enzyme levels may experience decreased contraception efficacy. Progestin-only pills should not be used with these antiseizure medications for the same reason. Because antiseizure medications may be used to treat bipolar disorder, migraine headaches, and chronic pain syndromes, a complete list of medications taken by the patient should be obtained. Hormonal contraception use is contraindicated with any disorder of arterial narrowing or clotting disorders. Injectable hormonal contraceptives (eg, Depo-Provera) are effective in patients who are taking antiseizure medications.

Some diabetes specialists allow their patients to use hormonal contraceptives with careful glucose monitoring. Women with diabetes who are older than 35 years should not use combination oral contraceptives because they may increase risk for vascular disease.

Patients with leiomyomas (fibroid tumors) are monitored carefully if they use hormonal contraceptives. If fibroids enlarge, they are advised to discontinue combined contraceptive agents and choose another contraceptive method.

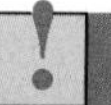

NURSING ALERT

Patients need to be aware that hormonal contraceptives protect them from pregnancy but not from STDs or HIV infection. In addition, sex with multiple partners or sex without a condom may also result in chlamydial and other infections, including HIV infection.

CHART 46-11

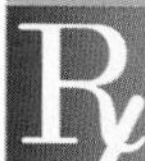

PHARMACOLOGY • Comparison of Oral Contraceptive Regimens

There are two kinds of oral contraceptives: combined and progestin only. Combined methods consist of an estrogen and a progestin, usually leading to a lighter-than-normal menstrual flow, which results from withdrawal.

COMBINED PREPARATIONS (pills, transdermal patches, vaginal rings)

- Each dose contains estrogen and progestin.
- Monophasic preparations supply the same dose of estrogen and progestin for 21 days.
- Biphasic preparations and triphasic pills vary the amount of hormonal components during the cycle.

PROGESTIN-ONLY "MINI" PREPARATIONS

- Each dose contains progestin only (estrogen is not contained in a progestin-only preparation).
- Preparations provide less protection against conception than combined preparations.
- About 40% of women taking progestin only have ovulatory cycles.
- Progestin-only preparations are useful for women who have had estrogen-related side effects on combination pills (eg, headaches, hypertension, leg pain, chloasma or skin discoloration, weight gain, or nausea).
- Progestin-only preparations are useful for lactating women who need a hormonal contraceptive method.
- Depo-Provera, a progestin-only injection, lasts for 3 months.

CHART 46-12

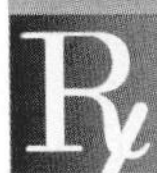

PHARMACOLOGY · Benefits and Risks of Combination Hormonal Contraceptives

BENEFITS

- Decreased cramps and bleeding
- Regular bleeding cycle
- Decreased incidence of anemia
- Decrease in acne with some formulations
- Protection from uterine and ovarian cancer
- Decreased incidence of ectopic pregnancy
- Protection from benign breast disease
- Decreased incidence of pelvic infection

RISKS

- Rare in healthy women
- Bothersome side effects (eg, breakthrough bleeding, breast tenderness)
- Nausea, weight gain, mood changes
- Small increased risk of developing blood clots, stroke, or heart attack, related more to smoking than to oral contraceptive use alone
- Possible increased incidence of benign liver tumors and gallbladder disorders
- No protection from STDs (possible increased risk with unsafe sex)

Methods of Hormonal Contraception

Chart 46-14 lists hormonal methods of birth control approved by the Food and Drug Administration (FDA).

ORAL CONTRACEPTIVES

Many women currently use oral contraceptive preparations of synthetic estrogens and progestins. A variety of formulations are available. Newer options include extended regimens of oral hormonal contraceptive agents. Extended regimens are an option for women who have heavy or uncomfortable menstrual bleeding or who wish to have fewer periods. With the use of these regimens, women may have an increased occurrence of breakthrough bleeding; the blood may be dark brown rather than red. It may be more difficult to tell if a pregnancy occurs with this method, although pregnancy is unlikely if pills are taken as prescribed. Studies are ongoing to assess the risks of exposure to increased estrogen resulting from this method. One extended-regimen option is Seasonale, an FDA-approved combination of ethinyl estradiol and levonorgestrel. Pills are taken for 84 days and then a placebo is taken for seven days, resulting in four withdrawal bleeding episodes per year instead of 12 to 14 with other oral contraceptives. The safety profile of Seasonale is comparable to that of other oral contraceptives and continues to be studied (Burkman & Miller, 2004).

TRANSDERMAL CONTRACEPTIVES

Ortho Evra is a thin, beige, matchbook-sized skin patch that releases an estrogen and a progestin continuously. It is changed every week for 3 weeks, and no patch is used during the fourth week, resulting in withdrawal bleeding. The effectiveness of Ortho Evra is comparable to that of oral contraceptives. Its risks are similar to those of oral contraceptives and include an increased risk of blood clots. The patch may be applied to the torso, chest, arms, or thighs; it should not be applied to the breasts. The patch is convenient and more easily remembered than a daily pill but is not as effective for women who weigh more than 198 pounds. In addition, it may also irritate skin conditions (eg, psoriasis) in some women.

CHART 46-13

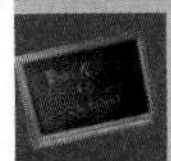

Patient Education

Using Combination Contraceptives

- Use condoms to protect against sexually transmitted diseases.
- Take pill at exactly the same time every day *or* put the patch on once a week *or* remove the vaginal ring after 3 weeks.
- Stop smoking or cut down on smoking.
- Report the following symptoms immediately:
  A —abdominal pains
  C —chest pains
  H —headaches
  E —eye problems (blurred vision or spots)
  S —severe leg pains

CHART 46-14

Examples of FDA-Approved Hormonal Contraceptive Methods

COMBINATION

Combination oral contraceptive pills
Vaginal ring (NuvaRing)
Transdermal patch (Ortho Evra)

PROGESTIN-ONLY METHODS

Progestin-only pills or minipills (Norgestrel)
Progestin-only emergency contraception (Plan B)
Once-every-3-months injection (DepoProvera)
Levonorgestrel-releasing intrauterine system (Mirena)

VAGINAL CONTRACEPTIVES

NuvaRing is a vaginal ring that releases estrogen and progestin. It is inserted in the vagina for 3 weeks and then removed, resulting in withdrawal bleeding. It is as effective as oral contraceptives. NuvaRing is flexible, does not require sizing or fitting, and is effective when placed anywhere in the vagina. Patients are occasionally reluctant to consider vaginal methods of contraception unless discussed openly and as a convenient alternative to other routes of administration. Some women are uncomfortable with this method and may fear that the ring may migrate upwards or be uncomfortable or be noticed by a partner. The nurse can be helpful in dispelling misconceptions. The patient can be informed that while some women notice a slight increase in vaginal discharge, this effective method of contraception has been found to increase the vaginal health-promoting lactobacillus (Veres, Miller & Burrington, 2004).

INJECTABLE CONTRACEPTIVES

An intramuscular injection of Depo-Provera (a long-acting progestin) every 3 months inhibits ovulation and provides a reliable, private, and convenient contraceptive method. It can be used by lactating women and those with hypertension, liver disease, migraine headaches, heart disease, and hemoglobinopathies. Women who use this method must be prepared for irregular or no bleeding. With continued use, irregular bleeding episodes and spotting decrease, and amenorrhea usually occurs.

Advantages of Depo-Provera include reduction of menorrhagia, dysmenorrhea, and anemia due to heavy menstrual bleeding. It may reduce the risk of pelvic infection, has been associated with improvement in hematologic status in women with sickle cell disease, and does not interfere with the efficacy of antiseizure agents.

Possible side effects of Depo-Provera include irregular menstrual bleeding, bloating, headaches, hair loss, decreased sex drive, bone loss, and weight loss or weight gain. The contraceptive does not protect against STDs. Fertility may be delayed when women discontinue this method; therefore, other methods of contraception may be more appropriate for the woman who wishes to conceive within a year of discontinuing contraception. While Depo-Provera is used, bone density is decreased and may be a risk for future osteoporosis. Severe allergic response is rare but possible following injection (Selo-Ojeme, Tillisi & Welch, 2004).

Depo-Provera is contraindicated in women who are pregnant and those who have abnormal vaginal bleeding of unknown cause, breast or pelvic cancer, or sensitivity to synthetic progestin. The long-term effects on infants of nursing mothers who use Depo-Provera are unknown but are thought to be negligible.

Intrauterine Device

An IUD is a small plastic device, usually T-shaped, that is inserted into the uterine cavity to prevent pregnancy. A string attached to the IUD is visible and palpable at the cervical os. An IUD prevents conception by causing a local inflammatory reaction that is toxic to spermatozoa and blastocysts, thus preventing fertilization. The IUD does not work by causing abortion.

Advantages include effectiveness over a long period of time, few if any systemic effects, and reduction of patient error. This reversible method of birth control is as effective as sterilization and more effective than barrier methods.

Disadvantages include possible excessive bleeding, cramps, and backaches; a slight risk of tubal pregnancy; slight risk of pelvic infection on insertion; displacement of the device; and, rarely, perforation of the cervix and uterus. If a pregnancy occurs with an IUD in place, the device is removed immediately to avoid infection. Spontaneous abortion (miscarriage) may occur on removal. An IUD is not usually used in women who have not had children, because a small nulliparous uterus may not tolerate it. Women with multiple partners, women with heavy or crampy periods, or those with a history of ectopic pregnancy or pelvic infection should be encouraged to use other methods of contraception. Some clinicians test for chlamydia and gonorrhea prior to insertion to prevent PID.

The Copper T 380A (ParaGard), an IUD that has been available for 15 years, is effective for at least 10 years. Copper has an antispermatic effect. The Levonorgestrel Intrauterine System (LNG-IUS; Mirena), another IUD, releases levonorgestrel, a synthetic progestin used in oral contraceptives, and is effective for at least 5 years. It has also been used therapeutically as it was found to reduce heavy bleeding and may prevent the need for hysterectomy in some women with heavy vaginal bleeding.

Mechanical Barriers

Diaphragm

The diaphragm is an effective contraceptive device that consists of a round, flexible spring (50 to 90 mm wide) covered with a dome-like latex rubber cup. A spermicidal (contraceptive) jelly or cream is used to coat the concave side of the diaphragm before it is inserted deep into the vagina, covering the cervix. The diaphragm is a spermicide holder; the spermicide inhibits spermatozoa from entering the cervical canal. The diaphragm is not felt by the user or her partner when properly fitted and inserted. Because women vary in size, the diaphragm must be sized and fitted by an experienced clinician. The woman is instructed in using and caring for the device. A return demonstration ensures that the woman can insert the diaphragm correctly and that it covers the cervix.

Each time that the woman uses the diaphragm, she should examine it carefully. By holding it up to a bright light, she should ensure that it has no pinpoint holes, cracks, or tears. She then applies spermicidal jelly or cream and positions the diaphragm to cover the cervix completely. The diaphragm should remain in place at least 6 hours after coitus (no more than 12 hours). Additional spermicide is necessary if more than 6 hours have passed before intercourse occurs and before each act of repeated intercourse. On removal, the diaphragm should be cleansed thoroughly with mild soap and water, rinsed, and dried before being stored in its original container.

Disadvantages include allergic reactions in those who are sensitive to latex and an increased incidence of urinary tract infections. Toxic shock syndrome has been reported in some diaphragm users but is rare.

NURSING ALERT

The nurse must assess the woman for possible latex allergy because use of latex barrier methods (eg, diaphragm, cervical cap, male condoms) may cause severe allergic reactions, including anaphylaxis, in patients with latex allergy.

Cervical Cap

The cervical cap is much smaller (22 to 35 mm) than the diaphragm and covers only the cervix. If a woman can feel her cervix, she can usually learn to use a cervical cap. The chief advantage is that the cap may be left in place for 2 days after coitus. Although convenient to use, the cervical cap may cause cervical irritation; therefore, before fitting a cap, most clinicians obtain a Pap smear and repeat the smear after 3 months. The cap is used with a spermicide and does not require additional spermicide for repeated exposure.

Contraceptive Sponge

The sponge is another barrier method of contraception. It is a made of soft, disposable polyurethane foam that is moistened with water and inserted into the vagina before intercourse. It contains and releases a spermicide (eg, nonoxynol-9) that is continuously released into the vagina in small amounts through a 24-hour wear time. The sponge is left in place in the vagina for at least 6 hours after intercourse and can be kept in place for up to 24 additional hours without the need to replace it with repeated acts of intercourse during that period of time. The sponge is sold over-the-counter and does not require a prescription or special fitting by a health care provider. The sponge should not be used by women with allergy to polyurethrane. It should not be used during menstruation. Women who have a history of toxic shock syndrome should not use the contraceptive sponge.

Female Condom

The female condom was developed to give control of barrier protection to women—to provide them with protection from STDs and HIV as well as pregnancy. The female condom (Reality) consists of a cylinder of polyurethane enclosed at one end by a closed ring that covers the cervix and at the other end by an open ring that covers the perineum (Fig. 46-8). Advantages include some degree of protection from STDs (HPV, herpes simplex virus, and HIV). Disadvantages include the inability to use the female condom with some coital positions (ie, standing).

Spermicides

Spermicides are made from nonoxynol-9 or octoxynol and are available over the counter as foams, gels, films, and suppositories and also on condoms. Nonoxynol-9 has been found to be associated with minute tears in vaginal tissue with frequent use, possibly increasing the possibility of contracting HIV from an infected partner (Stephenson, 2000). This substance also may increase the risk of latex allergy when used with a condom by leaching out a natural rubber protein from the latex (Greydanus, Patel & Rimsza, 2001).

Spermicides are effective, relatively inexpensive chemical contraceptives when used with condoms. Products with

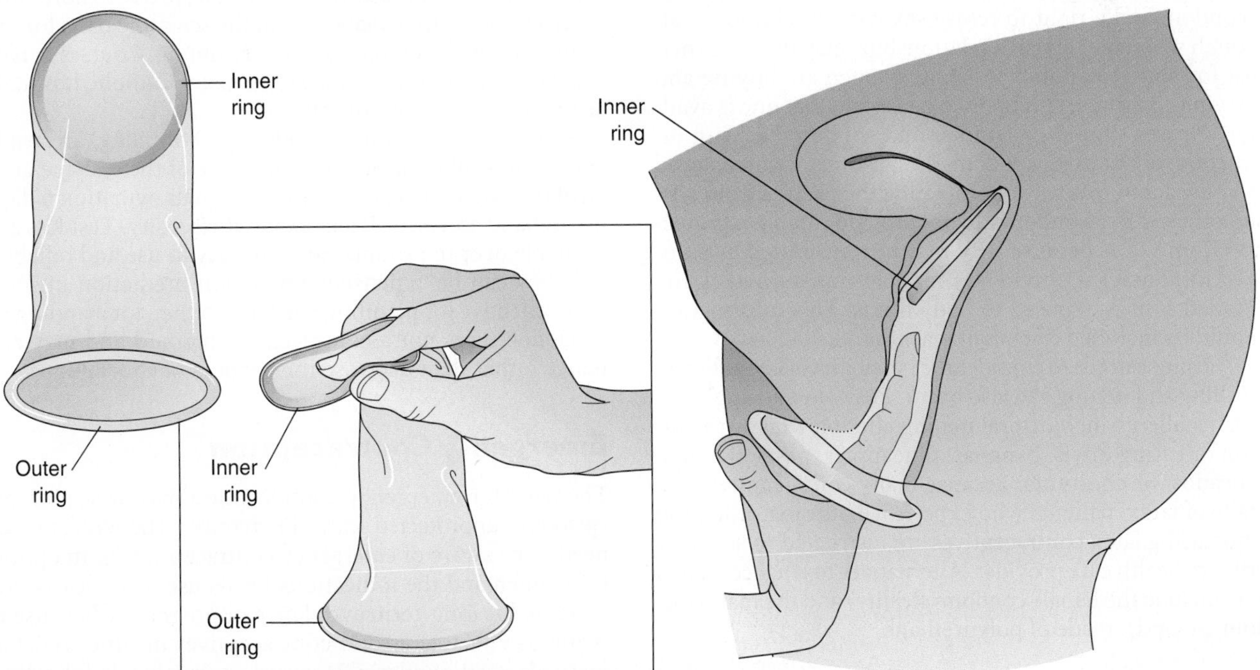

FIGURE 46-8. Female condom. To insert the female condom, hold the inner ring between the thumb and middle finger. Put the index finger on the pouch between the thumb and other fingers and squeeze the ring. Slide the condom into the vagina as far as it will go. The inner ring keeps the condom in place.

the highest doses of nonoxynol-9 have been found to be more effective; gels with less than 100 mg are less effective than those containing 100 mg or more (Raymond, Lien Chen, & Luoto, 2004). When spermicides are used alone, they are better than no contraception at all, they can be used without a partner's cooperation, and they may provide some protection from gonorrhea and chlamydia. Spermicides may cause burning, rash, or irritation in either partner; this condition is usually temporary. The problem is often alleviated by changing to another brand of spermicide.

Nonoxynol-9 (N-9), which is the spermicide that is released from the contraceptive sponge and is the major component of other spermicides, provides little if any protection against bacterial STDs or HIV. If used frequently, nonoxynol-9 may actually increase the risk for HIV because it may cause small disruptions in the wall of the vagina.

Male Condom

The male condom is an impermeable, snug-fitting cover applied to the erect penis before it enters the vaginal canal. The tip of the condom is pinched while being applied to leave space for ejaculate. If no space is left, ejaculation may cause a tear or hole in the condom and reduce its effectiveness. The penis, with the condom held in place, is removed from the vagina while still erect to prevent the ejaculate from leaking. Condoms are now available in large and small sizes.

The condom is an effective method when used with contraceptive foam. The latex condom also creates a barrier against transmission of STDs that are transmitted by fluids (gonorrhea, chlamydial infection, and HIV) and may reduce the risk of herpes virus transmission. However, natural condoms (those made from animal tissue) do not protect against HIV infection. Nurses need to reassure women that they have a right to insist on their male partners using a condom and a right to refuse sex without condoms, although women in abusive relationships may increase their risk for abuse by doing so. Some women are buying and carrying condoms with them to be certain that one is available. Nurses should be familiar and comfortable with instructions about using condoms, because many women need to know about this way of protecting themselves from HIV and other STDs. Condoms do not provide complete protection from STDs, because HPV may be transmitted by skin-to-skin contact. Other STDs may be transmitted if any abraded skin is exposed to body fluids. This information should be included in patient teaching.

The nurse needs to consider the possibility of latex allergy. Swelling and itching can also occur. Possible warning signs of latex allergy include oral itching after blowing up a balloon or eating kiwis, bananas, pineapples, passion fruits, avocados, or chestnuts. Because many contraceptives are made of latex, patients who experience burning or itching while using latex contraceptives are instructed to see their primary health care provider. Alternatives to latex condoms may include the female condom (Reality) and the male condom (Avanti), made of polyurethane.

Coitus Interruptus or Withdrawal

Coitus interruptus (removing the penis from the vagina before ejaculation) requires careful control by the male partner. Although it is a frequently used method of preventing pregnancy and better than no method, it is considered an unreliable method of contraception.

Rhythm and Natural Methods

Natural family planning is any method of conception regulation that is based on awareness of signs and symptoms of fertility during a menstrual cycle. The advantages of natural contraceptive methods include the following: (1) they are not hazardous to health, (2) they are inexpensive, and (3) they are approved by some religions that do not approve of other methods of contraception. The disadvantage is that they require discipline by the couple, who must monitor the menstrual cycle and abstain from sex during the fertile phase.

There are four general methods of natural family planning: (1) the calendar method, (2) the basal body temperature method, (3), the ovulation method, and (4) the symptothermal method. The calendar and basal body temperature methods are older than the ovulation method and the symptothermal method. Combinations of these methods are often used (Fehring, 2004). The fertile phase (in which sexual abstinence is required) is estimated to occur about 14 days before menstruation, although it may occur between the 10th and 17th days. Spermatozoa can fertilize an ovum up to 72 hours after intercourse, and the ovum can be fertilized for 24 hours after leaving the ovary. The pregnancy rate with the rhythm (ie, calendar) method is about 40% yearly.

Women who carefully determine their "safe period," based on a precise recording of menstrual dates for at least 1 year, and who follow a carefully worked-out formula may achieve very effective protection. A long abstinence period during each cycle is required. These prerequisites require more time and control than many couples have. Changes in cervical mucus and basal body temperature due to hormonal changes related to ovulation form the scientific basis for the symptothermal method of ovulatory timing. Courses in natural family planning are offered at many Catholic hospitals and some family planning clinics.

Ovulation detection methods (eg, Ovulindex) are available in most pharmacies. The presence of the enzyme guaiacol peroxidase in cervical mucus signals ovulation 6 days beforehand and also affects mucosal viscosity. Test kits are available over the counter and are easy to use and reliable, but they can be expensive. Ovulation prediction kits are more effective for planning conception than for avoiding it.

Douching is not a contraceptive method and may enhance rather than decrease the chances of conception.

Emergency Contraception

The need for emergency contraception may arise after an episode of unprotected sexual intercourse. Therefore, nurses need to be aware of emergency contraception as an option for women and the indications for its use. It is clearly not suitable for long-term avoidance of pregnancy because it is not as effective as oral contraceptives or other reliable methods used regularly. However, it is valuable following intercourse, when a pregnancy is not intended and in emergency situations such as rape, a defective or torn condom or diaphragm, or other situations that may result in unwanted conception. All women need to be made aware of emergency contraception and how to obtain it.

Methods of Emergency Contraception

HORMONAL METHODS

A properly timed, adequate dose of estrogen and a progestin or progestin-only medication after intercourse without effective contraception, or when a method has failed, can prevent pregnancy by inhibiting or delaying ovulation. This method does not interrupt an established pregnancy and does not cause an abortion.

Emergency contraception is currently available only with prescription and is not available over the counter. Emergency contraceptives may also be dispensed by pharmacists without a prescription in some states. The sooner emergency contraception is taken, the more effective it is. It is considered safe and effective by the FDA and can be prescribed or purchased as Plan B (progestin only) packages of emergency contraception with patient literature. It can also be prescribed as a specific number of contraceptive pills, depending on the medication and dose used.

Alternatively, a dose of oral contraceptives (ie, levonorgestrel and ethinyl estradiol) is given and repeated in 12 hours. This method must be used not more than 5 days following intercourse. Nausea, a common side effect, can be minimized by taking the medication with meals and with an antiemetic agent. Other side effects, such as breast soreness and irregular bleeding, may occur but are transient. Patients who use this method should be advised of the potential failure rate and also counseled about other contraceptive methods. There are no known contraindications to the use of this method except an established pregnancy in which case it will not work (Trussell, Ellertson, Stewart, et al., 2004).

The nurse reviews with the patient instructions for emergency contraception based on the medication regimen prescribed. If the woman is breastfeeding, a progestin-only formulation is prescribed. To avoid exposing infants to synthetic hormones through breast milk, the patient can manually express milk and bottle-feed for 24 hours after treatment. The patient should be informed that her next menstrual period may begin a few days earlier or a few days later than expected. She is instructed to return for a pregnancy test if she has not had a menstrual period in 3 weeks and should be offered another visit to provide a regular method of contraception if she does not have one currently.

POSTCOITAL IUD INSERTION

Postcoital IUD insertion, another form of emergency contraception, involves insertion of a copper-bearing IUD within 5 days of coitus in women who want this method of contraception; however, it may be inappropriate for some women or if other contraindications exist. The mechanism of action is unknown, but it is thought that the IUD interferes with fertilization (Trussell et al., 2004). The patient may experience discomfort on insertion and heavier menstrual periods and increased cramping. Contraindications include a confirmed or suspected pregnancy or any contraindication to regular copper IUD use. The patient must be informed that there is a risk that insertion of an IUD may disrupt a pregnancy that is already present.

Nursing Management

Patients who use emergency contraception may be anxious, embarrassed, and lacking information about birth control. The nurse must be supportive and nonjudgmental and provide facts and appropriate patient teaching. If the patient repeatedly uses this method of birth control, she should be informed that the failure rate with this method is higher than with a regularly used method. A toll-free telephone information service (1-888-Not-2-Late) operates 24 hours a day in English and Spanish and provides information and referrals to health care providers. Nurses can educate and inform women about emergency contraception options to reduce unwanted pregnancies and abortions. See the list of resources at the end of this chapter for more information.

Abortion

Interruption of pregnancy or expulsion of the product of conception before the fetus is viable is called abortion. The fetus is generally considered to be viable any time after the fifth to sixth month of gestation.

Spontaneous Abortion

It is estimated that 1 of every 5 to 10 conceptions ends in spontaneous abortion. Most of these occur because an abnormality in the fetus makes survival impossible. Other causes may include systemic diseases, hormonal imbalance, or anatomic abnormalities. If a pregnant woman experiences bleeding and cramping, a threatened abortion is diagnosed because an actual abortion is usually imminent. Spontaneous abortion occurs most commonly in the second or third month of gestation.

There are various types of spontaneous abortion, depending on the nature of the process (threatened, inevitable, incomplete, or complete). In a threatened abortion, the cervix does not dilate. With bed rest and conservative treatment, the abortion may be prevented. If not, an abortion is imminent. If only some of the tissue is passed, the abortion is referred to as incomplete. An emptying or evacuation procedure (D & C, or dilation and evacuation [D & E]) or administration of oral misoprostol (Cytotec) is usually required to remove the remaining tissue (Blanchard, 2004). If the fetus and all related tissue are spontaneously evacuated, the abortion is termed complete, and no further treatment is required.

Habitual Abortion

Habitual or recurrent abortion is defined as successive, repeated, spontaneous abortions of unknown cause. As many as 60% of abortions may result from chromosomal anomalies. After two consecutive abortions, the patient is referred for genetic counseling and testing, and other possible causes are explored.

If bleeding occurs in a patient with a history of habitual abortion, conservative measures, such as bed rest and administration of progesterone to support the endometrium, are attempted to save the pregnancy. Supportive counseling is crucial in this stressful condition. Bed rest, sexual abstinence, a light diet, and no straining on defecation may be recommended in an effort to prevent spontaneous abortion. If infection is suspected, antibiotics may be prescribed.

In the condition known as incompetent or dysfunctional cervix, the cervix dilates painlessly in the second trimester of pregnancy, often resulting in a spontaneous abortion. In such cases, a surgical procedure called cervical cerclage may be used to prevent the cervix from dilating prematurely although its effectiveness is unclear. It involves placing a purse-string suture around the cervix at the level of the internal os. Bed rest is usually advised to keep the weight of the uterus off the cervix. The patient and her health care providers must be informed that such a suture is in place in this high-risk pregnancy. About 2 to 3 weeks before term or the onset of labor, the suture is cut. Delivery is usually by cesarean section.

Medical Management

After a spontaneous abortion, all tissue passed vaginally is saved for examination if possible. The patient and all personnel who care for her are alerted to save any discharged material. In the rare case of heavy bleeding, the patient may require blood component transfusions and fluid replacement. An estimate of the bleeding volume can be determined by recording the number of perineal pads and the degree of saturation over 24 hours. When an incomplete abortion occurs, oxytocin may be prescribed to cause uterine contractions before D & E or uterine suctioning.

Nursing Management

Because patients experience loss and anxiety, emotional support and understanding are important aspects of nursing care. The responses of women who desperately want to become pregnant are very different from those of women who do not want to be pregnant but may be frightened by the possible consequences of an abortion (ie, miscarriage).

The nurse must be aware that a woman who has had a spontaneous abortion often experiences grief. However, the grief reaction may be delayed and may cause other problems until resolved. There may be many reasons for a delayed grief reaction. The woman's friends may not have known that she was pregnant; the woman may not have seen her lost fetus and can only imagine the gender, size, and characteristics of the child who never developed; there is usually no burial service; and people who know about the loss (family, friends, caregivers) may encourage denial by rarely talking about the loss or by discouraging the woman from crying.

Providing opportunities for the patient to talk and express her emotions helps and also provides clues for the nurse in planning more specific care. Those closest to the patient are encouraged to give emotional support and to allow the patient to talk and freely express her grief. Unresolved grief may manifest itself in persistent vivid memories of the events surrounding the loss, persistent sadness or anger, and episodes of overwhelming emotion when recalling the loss. Dysfunctional grief may require the assistance of a skilled therapist.

Elective Abortion

A voluntary induced termination of pregnancy is called an elective abortion and is usually performed by skilled health care providers. In 1973, the United States Supreme Court in Roe v. Wade ruled that decisions about abortion reside with a woman and her physician in the first trimester. During the second trimester, the state may regulate practice in the interest of a woman's health and during the final weeks of pregnancy may choose to protect the life of the fetus, except when necessary to preserve the life or health of the woman. Legislation has been passed to increase access to abortion clinics and to prevent violence toward those who work in such facilities.

The rate of abortion, which remained unchanged from 1980 to 1990, decreased 15% from 1990 to 1995. Rates since 2000 have decreased from those in 1999, and the decline has been steady for a decade (Whitcomb, 2004; Stubblefield, Carr-Ellis, & Borgatta, 2004). However, the rate has increased among unmarried Caucasian girls younger than 15 years of age, unmarried non-Caucasian girls 15 to 19 years of age, and married non-Caucasian women 20 to 24 years of age. The United States' rates of abortion are among the highest in the industrialized Western world. These numbers indicate the need for effective contraceptive education, information about emergency contraception, and counseling.

Medical Management

Before the abortion procedure is performed (Chart 46-15), a nurse or counselor trained in pregnancy counseling should talk with the patient and explore her fears, feelings, and options. The nurse then identifies the patient's choice (ie, continuing pregnancy and parenthood; continuing pregnancy followed by adoption; or terminating pregnancy by abortion). If abortion is chosen, the patient has a pelvic examination to determine uterine size. Laboratory studies before an abortion must include a pregnancy test to confirm the pregnancy, hematocrit to rule out anemia, and Rh determination. Patients with anemia may need an iron supplement, and patients who are Rh-negative may require RhoGAM to prevent isoimmunization. Before the procedure, all patients should be screened for STDs to prevent introducing pathogens upward through the cervix during the procedure.

NURSING ALERT

Women who have resorted to unskilled attempts to end a pregnancy are often critically ill because of infection, hemorrhage, or uterine rupture. If a woman has undergone such efforts to end a pregnancy, prompt medical attention, broad-spectrum antibiotics and replacement of fluids and blood components may be required before careful attempts are made to evacuate the uterus.

Patients may opt for a type of abortion that ends a pregnancy by using medication rather than surgery. Mifepristone (RU-486, Mifeprex) is used only in early pregnancy (up to 49 days from the last menstrual period). It works by blocking progesterone. Cramping and bleeding similar to a heavy menstrual period will occur. After counseling and consent and often a sonogram to confirm the pregnancy, mifepristone

CHART 46-15

Types of Elective Abortions

VACUUM ASPIRATION

- The cervix is dilated manually with instrumentation or by laminaria (small suppositories made of seaweed that swells as it absorbs water).
- A uterine aspirator is introduced.
- Suction is applied, and tissue is removed from the uterus.

This is the most common type of termination procedure and is used early in pregnancy, up to 14 weeks. Laminaria may be used to soften and dilate the cervix prior to the procedure.

DILATION AND EVACUATION

Cervical dilation with laminaria followed by vacuum aspiration

LABOR INDUCTION

These procedures account for less than 1% of all terminations and generally take place in an inpatient setting.

1. Installation of saline or urea results in uterine contractions.
   - Although rare, serious complications can occur, including cardiovascular collapse, cerebral edema, pulmonary edema, renal failure, and disseminated intravascular coagulopathy (DIC).
2. Prostaglandins
   - Prostaglandins are introduced into the amniotic fluid or by vaginal suppository or intramuscular injection in later pregnancy.
   - Strong uterine contractions begin within 4 hours and usually result in abortion.
   - Gastrointestinal side effects (eg, nausea, vomiting, diarrhea, and abdominal cramping) and fever can occur.
3. Intravenous oxytocin
   Used for later abortions for genetic indications.
   Requires patient to go through labor.

MEDICAL ABORTION

Mifepristone

- Mifepristone (formerly known as RU-486) is a progesterone antagonist that prevents implantation of the ovum.
- Administered orally within 10 days of an expected menstrual period, mifepristone produces a medical abortion in most patients.
- Combined with a prostaglandin suppository, mifepristone causes abortion in up to 95% of patients.
- Prolonged bleeding may occur. Other side effects may include abdominal pain, nausea, vomiting, and diarrhea. This method may not be used in women with adrenal failure, asthma, long-term corticosteroid therapy, an IUD in place, porphyria, or a history of allergy to mifepristone or other prostaglandins. It is less effective when used in pregnancies more than 49 days from the beginning of the last menstrual period.

Methotrexate

- Methotrexate has also been used to terminate pregnancy because it is a teratogen that is lethal to the fetus. It has been found to have minimal risk and few side effects in the woman. Its low cost may provide an alternative for some women.

Misoprostol

- Misoprostol is a synthetic prostaglandin analog that produces cervical effacement and uterine contractions.
- Inserted vaginally, misoprostol is effective in terminating a pregnancy in about 75% of cases.
- When combined with methotrexate or mifepristone, misoprostol's effectiveness rate is high.

is administered. This is followed by a dose of misoprostol orally or vaginally. If the pregnancy persists, a suction aspiration is performed (Creinin, Fox, Teal, et al., 2004). Contraindications include ectopic pregnancy, adrenal failure, allergy to the medications, bleeding disorder, irritable bowel syndrome, or uncontrolled seizure disorders (Stubblefield et al., 2004). Several deaths from sepsis have been reported following medical abortion; the morbidity and mortality associated with medical abortion are being monitored closely by researchers and the U.S. Food and Drug Administration (Fisher, Reagan & Zaki, 2006).

Nursing Management

Patient teaching is an important aspect of care for women who elect to terminate a pregnancy. A patient undergoing elective abortion is informed about what the procedure entails and the expected course after the procedure. The patient is scheduled for a follow-up appointment 2 weeks after the procedure and is instructed in recognizing and reporting signs and symptoms of complications (ie, fever, heavy bleeding, or pain).

Available contraceptive methods are reviewed with the patient at this time. Effectiveness depends on the method used and the extent to which the woman and her partner follow the instructions for use. A woman who has used any method of birth control should be assessed for her understanding of the method and its potential side effects and her satisfaction with the method. If the woman has not been using contraception, the nurse explains all methods and their benefits and risks and helps the patient make a contraceptive choice for use after abortion. Increasingly important related teaching issues are the need to use barrier contraceptive devices (ie, condoms) for protection against transmission of STDs and HIV infection, and the availability of emergency contraception.

Psychological support is another important aspect of nursing care. The nurse needs to be aware that women terminate pregnancies for many reasons. Some women terminate pregnancies because of severe genetic defects. Women who have been raped or impregnated in incestuous relationships or by an abusive partner may elect to terminate their pregnancies. Patients with infertility may elect to undergo selective termination if they become pregnant with multiple fetuses. In pregnancies with multiple gestation, adverse outcomes are directly proportional to the number of fetuses in the uterus. Such multifetal reductions are specialized procedures that are stressful and difficult for the parents; therefore, psychological support and understanding are required. The care of a woman undergoing termination of pregnancy is stressful, and assistance needs to be provided in a safe and nonjudgmental way. Nurses have the right to refuse to participate in a procedure that is against their religious beliefs but are professionally obligated not to impose their beliefs or judgments on their patients.

Infertility

Infertility is defined as a couple's inability to achieve pregnancy after 1 year of unprotected intercourse. Primary infertility refers to a couple who has never had a child. Secondary infertility means that at least one conception has occurred, but currently the couple cannot achieve a pregnancy. In the United States, infertility affects 6 million couples. It is a complex physical problem, and its causes are usually related to azoospermia, anovulation, or tubal obstruction. For infertile women who wish to bear children, infertility can be stressful and difficult (Hart, 2002).

Pathophysiology

Ovarian and Ovulation Factors

Diagnostic studies performed to determine if ovulation is regular and whether the progestational endometrium is adequate for implantation may include a serum progesterone level and an ovulation index. The ovulation index involves a urine-stick test to determine whether the surge in LH that precedes follicular rupture has occurred. Ovulatory dysfunction is complex, but many women with ovulation disorders have polycystic ovary syndrome, described in Chapter 47, and may be treated with clomiphene to induce ovulation or insulin sensitizing agents. Once insulin levels are normalized, ovulation often occurs. Some women have high prolactin levels, which inhibit ovulation, and they are treated with dopaminergic drugs after a pituitary adenoma is ruled out by MRI. If a woman has premature ovarian failure, oocyte donation may be considered (Smith, Pfeifer & Collins, 2003).

Tubal Factors

Hysterosalpingography (HSG) is used to rule out uterine or tubal abnormalities. Water- or oil-based dye injected into the uterus through the cervix produces an outline of the shape of the uterine cavity and the patency of the tubes. This process sometimes removes mucus or tissue that is lodged in the tubes. Laparoscopy permits direct visualization of the tubes and other pelvic structures and can assist in identifying conditions that may interfere with fertility (eg, endometriosis).

Uterine Factors

Fibroids, polyps, and congenital malformations are possible conditions in this category. Their presence may be determined by pelvic examination, hysteroscopy, saline sonogram (a variation of a sonogram), and HSG. Endometriosis is associated with reduced fertility and is found in 10% of infertile women (Smith, Pfeifer & Collins, 2003). Even mild endometriosis can inhibit fertility, although no causal relationship has been shown.

Semen Factors

An analysis of semen provides information about the number of sperm (density), percentage of moving forms, quality of forward movement (forward progression), and morphology (shape and form). From 2 to 6 mL of watery alkaline semen is normal. A normal count has 60 to 100 million sperm/mL. However, the incidence of impregnation is lessened only when the count decreases to less than 20 million sperm/mL.

Other Male Factors

Men may also be affected by varicoceles, varicose veins around the testicle, which decrease semen quality by increasing testicular temperature. Retrograde ejaculation or ejaculation into the bladder is assessed by urinalysis after ejaculation. Blood tests for male partners may include measuring testosterone; FSH and LH (both of which are involved in maintaining testicular function); and prolactin levels.

Medical Management

The treatment of infertility is complex and often requires advanced technology. The specific type of treatment depends on the cause of the problem, if it can be identified. As many as one third of all infertile couples have normal test results for ovulation, sperm production, and fallopian tube patency. Pharmacologic treatment may be used to stimulate ovulation. Other techniques may be necessary. The health outcomes of children conceived with assisted reproductive technology are being studied (Schieve, Rasmussen, Buch, et al., 2004).

Pharmacologic Therapy

Pharmacologically induced ovulation is undertaken when women do not ovulate on their own or ovulate irregularly. Women older than 37 years are less likely to be fertile. These couples are often treated with clomiphene (Clomid) to stimulate ovulation. Gonadotropin treatment may also be used if conception does not occur. Various other medications are used, depending on the primary cause of infertility (Chart 46-16). These medications have not been shown

CHART 46-16

PHARMACOLOGY • Medications That Induce Ovulation

- Clomiphene citrate (Clomid, Serophene) is an estrogen antagonist that increases gonadotropin release, resulting in follicular rupture or ovulation. Clomiphene is used when the hypothalamus is not stimulating the pituitary gland to release follicle-stimulating hormone (FSH) and luteinizing hormone (LH). This medication stimulates follicles in the ovary. It is usually taken for 5 days beginning on the fifth day of the menstrual cycle. Ovulation should occur 4 to 8 days after the last dose. Patients receive instructions about timing intercourse to facilitate fertilization.
- Menotropin (Repronex, Pergonal), a combination of FSH and LH, may be used to stimulate the ovaries to produce eggs. These agents are used for women with deficiencies in FSH and LH. When followed by administration of human chorionic gonadotropin, menotropin stimulates the ovaries, so monitoring by ultrasound and hormone levels is essential because overstimulation may occur.
- Follitropin alpha (Gonal-F), follitropin beta (Follistim), and urofollitropin (Bravelle) may be used to treat ovulation disorders or to stimulate a follicle and egg production for intrauterine insemination or in vitro fertilization or other assisted reproductive technologies.
- Gonadotropin-releasing hormone agonists (leuprolide [Lupron, Synarel]) suppress FSH, prevent premature egg release, and shrink fibroids.
- Bromocriptine (Parlodel) may be used in treatment of infertility due to elevated prolactin levels.
- Progesterone (Prometrium Crinone, progesterone in oil) vaginal suppositories help improve the uterine lining after ovulation.
- Urofollitropin (Metrodin, Bravelle), which contains FSH with a small amount of LH, is used in some disorders (eg, polycystic ovarian syndrome) to stimulate follicle growth. Clomiphene is then used to stimulate ovulation.
- Chorionic gonadotropin (Ovidrel, Novarel, Pregnyl), which mimics LH, releases an egg after hyperstimulation and supports the corpus luteum.
- Metformin may be used in polycystic ovarian syndrome to induce regular ovulation.
- Aspirin and heparin may be used to prevent recurrent pregnancy loss in patients with elevated antiphospholipid antibodies.

to increase the risk of ovarian or breast cancer (Kashyap, Moher, Fung et al., 2004).

Blood tests and ultrasounds are used to monitor ovulation. Multiple pregnancies (ie, twins, triplets or more) may occur with use of these medications. Ovarian hyperstimulation syndrome (OHSS) may also occur. This condition is characterized by enlarged multicystic ovaries and is complicated by a shift of fluid from the intravascular space into the abdominal cavity. The fluid shift can result in ascites, pleural effusion, and edema; hypovolemia may also result. Risk factors include younger age, history of polycystic ovarian syndrome, high serum estradiol levels, a larger number of follicles, and pregnancy. If the woman is pregnant, she is producing human chorionic gonadotropin, which can worsen OHSS. Symptoms include abdominal discomfort, distention, weight gain, and ovarian enlargement. This condition may be moderate, severe, or critical. OHSS is prevented by careful monitoring and adjustment of medication dosage.

Management in mild and moderate cases of OHSS consists of activity restrictions, monitoring of urine output, and frequent office visits as designated by the reproductive endocrinologist. Patients with severe OHSS are hospitalized for monitoring and treatment. Severe OHSS is characterized by clinical ascites, hypovolemia, oliguria, hemoconcentration, electrolyte imbalance, and ovarian size greater than 10 cm. Treatment of severe OHSS includes use of an indwelling catheter for strict monitoring of fluid intake and output and daily measurements of weight and abdominal circumference. Intravenous fluids and heparin are administered as prescribed. Patients are permitted to ambulate as tolerated. Critical OHSS is life-threatening and is characterized by tense ascites that may be accompanied by hydrothorax, renal failure, and ARDS. Volume expanders, diuretic agents, hemodialysis, and intubation may be required (Copeland, 2000).

Artificial Insemination

Artificial insemination is the deposit of semen into the female genital tract by artificial means. If the sperm cannot penetrate the cervical canal normally, artificial insemination using a partner's or husband's semen or that of a donor may be considered. When the sperm of the woman's partner is defective or absent (azoospermia) or when there is a risk of transmitting a genetic disease, donor sperm may be used. Safeguards are put in place to address legal, ethical, emotional, and religious issues. Written consent is obtained to protect all parties involved, including the woman, the donor, and the resulting child. The donor's semen is frozen, and the donor is evaluated to ensure that he is free of genetic disorders and STDs, including HIV infection.

Indications for artificial insemination include: (1) the male partner's inability to deposit semen in the vagina, which may be due to premature ejaculation, pronounced hypospadias (a displaced male urethra), or dyspareunia (painful intercourse experienced by the woman), (2) inability of semen to be transported from the vagina to the uterine cavity (this is usually due to faulty chemical conditions and may occur with an abnormal cervical discharge), and (3) a single or lesbian woman's desire to have a child. Methods of insemination include intracervical insemination (ICI) and intrauterine insemination (IUI).

Certain conditions must be met before semen is transferred to the vagina or uterus. The woman must have no abnormalities of the genital system, the fallopian tubes must be patent, and ova must be available. In the male, sperm need to be normal in shape, amount, motility, and endurance. The time of ovulation should be determined as accurately as possible so that the 2 or 3 days during which fertilization is possible each month can be targeted for treatment.

Ultrasonography and blood studies of varying hormone levels are used to pinpoint the best time for insemination and to monitor for OHSS. Fertilization seldom occurs from a single insemination. Usually, insemination is attempted between days 10 and 17 of the cycle; three different attempts may be made during one cycle. The woman may have received clomiphene or other medications to stimulate ovulation before insemination. The recipient is placed in the lithotomy position on the examination table, a speculum is inserted, and the vagina and cervix are swabbed with a cotton-tipped applicator to remove any excess secretions. The sperm are washed before insertion to remove biochemicals and to select the most active sperm. Semen is drawn into a sterile syringe, and a cannula is attached. The semen is then directed to the external os. In IUI, semen is placed into the uterine cavity.

In Vitro Fertilization

In vitro fertilization (IVF) involves ovarian stimulation, egg retrieval, fertilization, and embryo transfer. This procedure is accomplished by first stimulating the ovary to produce multiple eggs or ova, usually with medications, because success rates are greater with more than one embryo. Many different protocols exist for inducing ovulation with one or more agents. Patients are carefully selected and evaluated, and cycles are carefully monitored using ultrasound and hormone levels. At the appropriate time, the ova are recovered by transvaginal ultrasound retrieval. Sperm and eggs are coincubated for up to 36 hours, and the embryos are transferred about 48 hours after retrieval. Implantation should occur in 3 to 5 days.

Gamete intrafallopian transfer (GIFT), a variation of IVF, is the treatment of choice for patients with ovarian failure. GIFT is considered in unexplained infertility and when there is religion-based discomfort with IVF. The most common indications for IVF and GIFT are irreparable tubal damage, endometriosis, unexplained infertility, inadequate sperm, and exposure to DES. Success rates for GIFT vary from 20% to 30%. The ovaries are stimulated with gonadotropin derivatives, and follicles are observed with vaginal ultrasound. Once the oocyte is mature, it is retrieved by laparoscopy or transvaginally with ultrasound guidance. The oocyte (unfertilized egg) is removed and drawn into a catheter, where it is mixed with sperm that was obtained shortly before the oocyte retrieval. The most motile fraction of sperm is selected by a washing process. The oocyte and sperm are then inserted into the fallopian tube, where fertilization occurs. The latter method avoids anesthesia.

Other Assisted Reproductive Technologies

In intracytoplasmic sperm injection (ICSI), an ovum is retrieved as described previously, and a single sperm is injected through the zona pellucida, through the egg membrane, and into the cytoplasm of the oocyte. The fertilized egg is then transferred back to the donor. ICSI is the treatment of choice in severe male factor infertility.

Women who cannot produce their own eggs (ie, premature ovarian failure) have the option of using the eggs of a donor after stimulation of the donor's ovaries. The recipient also receives hormones in preparation for these procedures. Couples may also choose this modality if the female partner has a genetic disorder that may be passed on to children.

Nursing Management

Nursing interventions appropriate when working with couples during infertility evaluations include the following: assisting in reducing stress in the relationship, encouraging cooperation, protecting privacy, fostering understanding, and referring the couple to appropriate resources when necessary. Because infertility evaluations and treatments are expensive, time-consuming, invasive, stressful, and not always successful, couples need support in working together to deal with this process.

Resolve, Inc., a nonprofit self-help group that provides information and support for infertile patients, was founded by a nurse who experienced difficulty conceiving. The literature on infertility that is produced by this group is an important resource for patients and professionals. Most areas of the country have local support groups. More information can be obtained by visiting the Resolve web site or writing to Resolve, Inc. (see address at the end of this chapter).

Smoking is strongly discouraged because it has an adverse effect on the success of assisted reproduction. Diet, exercise, stress reduction techniques, folic acid supplementation, health maintenance, and disease prevention are emphasized in many infertility programs. Couples may also consider adoption, child-free living, and gestational carriers (use of surrogate to carry the fetus for the infertile couple). Nurses can be helpful listeners and information resources in these deliberations.

Preconception/Periconception Health Care

Nurses can be instrumental in encouraging all women of childbearing age, including those with chronic illness or disabilities, to consider issues that may affect health during pregnancy. Women who plan their pregnancies and are healthy and well informed tend to have better outcomes (Moos, 2004). This is an important issue because half of all pregnancies in the United States are unintended.

Nurses can make a difference through education and counseling; preconception counseling can decrease the incidence of birth defects. Women who smoke should be encouraged to stop smoking, and it may help to offer smoking cessation classes. Women should take folic acid supplements to prevent neural tube defects. Women with diabetes should have good glycemic control prior to conception. It is necessary to assess rubella immunity and other immunizations as well as a family history of genetic defects; genetic counseling may be appropriate. Women taking teratogenic medications and women concerned about genetic disorders should be encouraged to discuss effective contraception and childbearing plans with their health care provider.

Ectopic Pregnancy

The incidence of ectopic pregnancy may be decreasing, and the risk of death due to ectopic pregnancy is decreasing, although there are no standard reporting guidelines. However, ectopic pregnancy remains the leading cause of pregnancy-related death in the first trimester. Ectopic pregnancy occurs when a fertilized ovum (a blastocyst) becomes implanted on any tissue other than the uterine lining (eg, the fallopian tube, ovary, abdomen, cervix or scar tissue from previous caesarean section). The most common site of ectopic implantation is the fallopian tube (Fig. 46-9).

Possible causes of ectopic pregnancy include salpingitis, peritubal adhesions (after pelvic infection, endometriosis, appendicitis), structural abnormalities of the fallopian tube (rare and usually related to DES exposure), previous ectopic pregnancy (after one ectopic pregnancy the risk of recurrence is 7% to 15%; Lemus, 2000), previous tubal surgery, multiple previous induced abortions (particularly if followed by infection), tumors that distort the tube, and IUD and progestin-only contraceptives. PID appears to be the major risk factor. Improved antibiotic therapy for PID usually prevents total tubal closure but may leave a stricture or narrowing, predisposing to ectopic implantation. The odds of recurrent ectopic pregnancy are three times higher if an infectious pathology caused the first ectopic pregnancy. After a second ectopic pregnancy occurs, assisted reproduction is considered.

Risk factors are important, but all women need to be educated about early treatment and have a high index of suspicion in the case of a period that does not seem normal, the presence of pain, or pain with a suspected pregnancy. Women often wait until after a missed period to begin prenatal care but should be evaluated as early as possible, especially if they are experiencing discomfort. Women may have fatal hemorrhage with ruptured ectopic pregnancies if they delay seeking attention or if their health care providers are not alert to the possibility of this diagnosis.

Clinical Manifestations

Signs and symptoms vary depending on whether tubal rupture has occurred. Delay in menstruation from 1 to 2 weeks followed by slight bleeding (spotting) or a report of a slightly abnormal period suggests the possibility of an ectopic pregnancy. Symptoms may begin late, with vague soreness on the affected side (probably due to uterine contractions and distention of the tube), and may proceed to sharp, colicky pain. Most patients experience some pelvic or abdominal pain and some spotting or bleeding. Gastrointestinal symptoms, dizziness, or lightheadedness may occur. Patients frequently think the abnormal bleeding is a menstrual period, especially if a recent period occurred and was normal.

If implantation occurs in the fallopian tube, the tube becomes more and more distended and can rupture if the ectopic pregnancy remains undetected for 4 to 6 weeks or longer after conception. When the tube ruptures, the ovum is discharged into the abdominal cavity, and the woman experiences agonizing pain, dizziness, faintness,

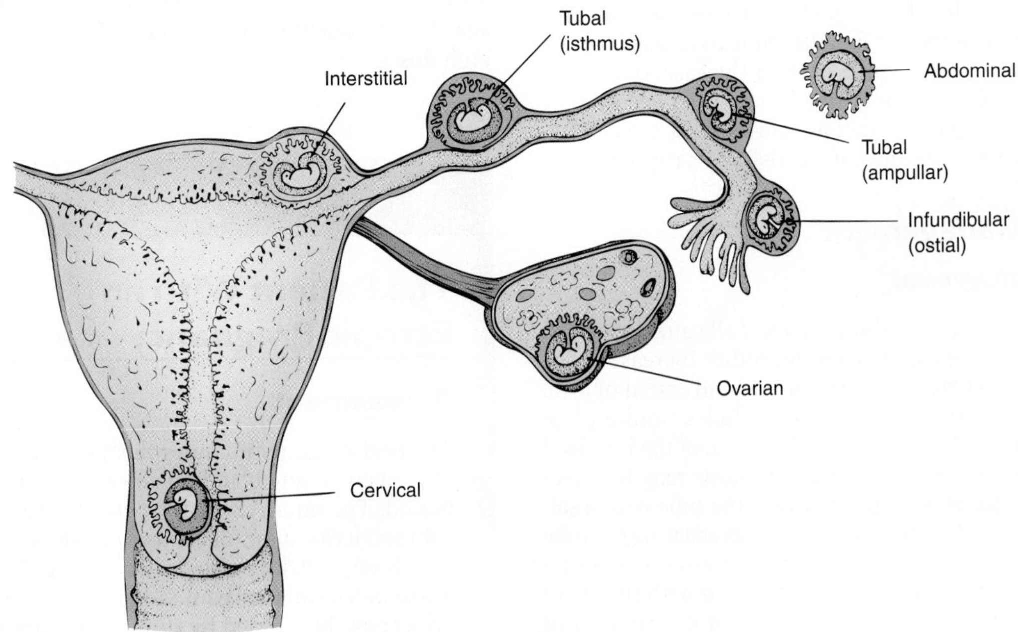

FIGURE 46-9. Sites of ectopic pregnancy.

and nausea and vomiting. These symptoms are related to the peritoneal reaction to blood escaping from the tube. Air hunger and symptoms of shock may occur, and the signs of hemorrhage—rapid and thready pulse, decreased blood pressure, subnormal temperature, restlessness, pallor, and sweating—are evident. Later, the pain becomes generalized in the abdomen and radiates to the shoulder and neck because of accumulating intraperitoneal blood that irritates the diaphragm.

Assessment and Diagnostic Findings

Ectopic pregnancies must be diagnosed promptly to prevent life-threatening hemorrhage, the major complication of rupture. During vaginal examination, a large mass of clotted blood that has collected in the pelvis behind the uterus or a tender adnexal mass may be palpable, although no abnormal findings are sometimes detectable. If an ectopic pregnancy is suspected, the patient is evaluated by sonography and the beta subunit of human chorionic gonadotropin (hCG) levels. If the ultrasound results are inconclusive, the beta-hCG test is repeated to evaluate the rate of rise in the level. The levels of hCG (the diagnostic hormone of pregnancy) double in early normal pregnancies every 3 days but are reduced in abnormal or ectopic pregnancies. A less-than-normal increase is cause for suspicion. Serum progesterone levels are also measured. Levels less than 5 ng/mL are considered abnormal; levels greater than 25 ng/mL are associated with a normally developing pregnancy.

Ultrasound, the usual method of diagnosis, can detect a pregnancy between 5 and 6 weeks from the time of the last menstrual period. Detectable fetal heart movement outside the uterus on ultrasound is firm evidence of an ectopic pregnancy. On occasion, an ultrasound study is not definitive and the diagnosis must be made with combined diagnostic aids (beta-hCG and progesterone levels, ultrasound, pelvic examination, and clinical judgment). Studies using ultrasound with Doppler flow, in which color indicates perfusion, may be useful.

Occasionally, the clinical picture makes the diagnosis relatively easy. However, when the clinical signs and symptoms are inconclusive, which is often the case, other procedures have value. Laparoscopy can be used because the physician can visually detect an unruptured tubal pregnancy and thereby circumvent the risk of its rupture.

Medical Management

Surgical Management

When surgery is performed early, almost all patients recover rapidly; if tubal rupture occurs, mortality increases. The type of surgery is determined by the size and extent of local tubal damage. Conservative surgery includes "milking" an ectopic pregnancy from the tube. Resection of the involved fallopian tube with end-to-end anastomosis may be effective. Some surgeons attempt to salvage the tube with a salpingotomy, which involves opening and evacuating the tube and controlling bleeding. More extensive surgery includes removing the tube alone (salpingectomy) or with the ovary (salpingo-oophorectomy). Depending on the amount of blood lost, blood component therapy and treatment of hemorrhagic shock may be necessary before and during surgery. Surgery may also be indicated in women unlikely to comply with close monitoring or those who live too far away from a health care facility to obtain the monitoring needed with nonsurgical management.

Methotrexate, a chemotherapeutic agent and folic acid antagonist, may be used after surgery to treat any remaining embryonic or early pregnancy tissue, as indicated by a persistent or increasing beta-hCG level. The beta-hCG test is repeated 2 weeks after surgery to ensure that the level is decreasing.

Pharmacologic Therapy

Another option is the use of methotrexate without surgery. Because methotrexate stops the pregnancy from progressing by interfering with DNA synthesis and the multiplication of cells, it interrupts early, small, unruptured ectopic pregnancies. The patient must be hemodynamically stable, have no active renal or hepatic disease, have no evidence of thrombocytopenia or leukopenia, and have a very small, unruptured ectopic pregnancy on ultrasound. Other indications may include no fetal cardiac activity, no active bleeding, and a beta-hCG level of <2000 mIU/mL. The medication is administered intramuscularly or orally. Some patients may be treated with intratubal injection of methotrexate. Complete blood count and tests of liver and renal function are conducted to monitor the patient; blood typing is performed in anticipation of the need for transfusions.

Until the pregnancy is resolved, the patient is advised to refrain from alcohol, intercourse, and vitamins containing folic acid, because these may exacerbate the adverse effects of methotrexate. Abdominal pain may occur within 5 to 10 days and may indicate termination of the pregnancy. This requires careful assessment by the health care provider. Serum levels of beta-hCG are monitored carefully, and these levels should gradually decrease. Ultrasound may also be used for monitoring. Side effects of methotrexate include abdominal cramping, mucositis, and renal and hepatic damage. Allergic reactions have occurred in patients receiving high doses.

Nursing Process

The Patient With an Ectopic Pregnancy

Assessment

The health history includes the menstrual pattern and any (even slight) bleeding since the last menstrual period. The nurse elicits the patient's description of pain and its location. The nurse asks the patient whether any sharp, colicky pains have occurred. Then the nurse notes whether pain radiates to the shoulder and neck (possibly caused by rupture and pressure on the diaphragm).

In addition, the nurse monitors vital signs, level of consciousness, and the nature and amount of vaginal bleeding. If possible, the nurse assesses how the patient is coping with the abnormal pregnancy and likely loss.

Diagnosis

Nursing Diagnoses

Based on the assessment data, major nursing diagnoses may include the following:

- Acute pain related to the progression of the tubal pregnancy
- Anticipatory grieving related to the loss of pregnancy and effect on future pregnancies
- Deficient knowledge related to the treatment and effect on future pregnancies

Collaborative Problems/ Potential Complications

Based on the assessment data, major complications may include the following:

- Hemorrhage
- Hemorrhagic shock

Planning and Goals

The major goals may include relief of pain; acceptance and resolution of grief and pregnancy loss; increased knowledge about ectopic pregnancy, its treatment, and its outcome; and absence of complications.

Nursing Interventions

Relieving Pain

The abdominal pain associated with ectopic pregnancy may be described as cramping or severe continuous pain. If the patient is to have surgery, preanesthetic medications may provide pain relief. Postoperatively, analgesic agents are administered liberally; this promotes early ambulation and enables the patient to cough and take deep breaths.

Supporting the Grieving Process

Patients' distress levels vary. If the pregnancy was desired, loss may or may not be expressed verbally by the patient and her partner. The impact may not be fully realized until much later. The nurse should be available to listen and provide support. The patient's partner, if appropriate, should participate in this process. Even if the pregnancy was unplanned, a loss has been experienced, and a grief reaction may follow. Severe and persistent psychological distress may require referral for psychological counseling.

Monitoring and Managing Potential Complications

Potential complications of ectopic pregnancy are hemorrhage and shock. Careful assessment is essential to detect the development of these complications. Continuous monitoring of vital signs, level of consciousness, amount of bleeding, and intake and output provides information about the possibility of hemorrhage and the need to prepare for IV therapy. Bed rest is indicated. Hematocrit, hemoglobin, and blood gas levels are monitored to assess hematologic status and adequacy of tissue perfusion. Significant deviations in these laboratory values are reported immediately, and the patient is prepared for possible surgery. Blood component therapy may be required if blood loss has been rapid and extensive. If hypovolemic shock occurs, the treatment is directed toward reestablishing tissue perfusion and adequate blood volume. See Chapter 15 for a discussion of the IV fluids and medications used in treating shock.

The nurse has an important role in prevention by being alert to patients with abnormal bleeding who may be at risk for an ectopic pregnancy and referring them immediately for care. It is necessary to keep a high index of suspicion in daily practice when a woman of child-bearing age, particularly one who is not using an effective method of contraception consistently, reports abdominal discomfort or abnormal bleeding.

Promoting Home and Community-Based Care

TEACHING PATIENTS SELF-CARE

If the patient has experienced life-threatening hemorrhage and shock, these complications are addressed and treated before any in-depth teaching can begin. At this time, the patient's and the nurse's attention is focused on the crisis, not on learning. At a later time, the patient begins to ask questions about what happened and why certain procedures were performed. Procedures are explained in terms that the distressed and apprehensive patient can understand. The patient's partner is included in teaching and explanations when possible. After the patient recovers from postoperative discomfort, it may be more appropriate to address any questions and concerns that she and her partner have, including the effect of this pregnancy or its treatment on future pregnancies. The patient should be advised that ectopic pregnancies may recur. The patient is informed about possible complications and instructed to report early signs and symptoms. It is important to review signs and symptoms with the patient and instruct her to report an abnormal menstrual period promptly. Patient teaching is based on the needs of the patient and partner and must take into consideration their distress and grief.

CONTINUING CARE

Because of the risk of subsequent ectopic pregnancies, the patient is advised to seek preconception counseling before considering future pregnancies and to seek early prenatal care. Psychological support and counseling may be advisable for the patient and her partner to help them deal with the loss of the pregnancy. Follow-up contact allows the nurse to answer questions and clarify information for the patient and her partner. In addition, it provides an opportunity to assess the ability of the patient and her partner to cope with the loss of the pregnancy.

Evaluation

Expected Patient Outcomes

Expected patient outcomes may include:

1. Experiences relief of pain
   a. Reports a decrease in pain and discomfort
   b. Ambulates as prescribed; performs coughing and deep breathing
2. Begins to accept loss of pregnancy and expresses grief by verbalizing feelings and reactions to loss
3. Verbalizes an understanding of the causes of ectopic pregnancy
4. Experiences no complications
   a. Exhibits no signs of bleeding, hemorrhage, or shock
   b. Has decreased amounts of discharge (on perineal pad)
   c. Has normal skin color and turgor
   d. Exhibits stable vital signs and adequate urine output
   e. Levels of beta-hCG return to normal

Critical Thinking Exercises

1 ebp A 57-year-old woman has recently been diagnosed with osteoporosis. She is considering beginning hormone therapy (HT) to prevent further bone loss but is concerned about its risks. What information would you give to her? What is the evidence base for that information? What criteria would you use to assess the strength of the evidence? What resources would you recommend to her?

2 A 20-year-old college student comes to the student health clinic for a gynecologic examination because she anticipates having sex with her new boyfriend. She asks you for advice about hormonal contraceptives versus barrier methods of contraception. What advice would you give her? How would you teach her about using a barrier method of contraception if that is what she chooses? How would you modify your teaching if she informed you that her new boyfriend has other partners? What other teaching would you provide to her?

3 ebp You are working in a women's health practice and are responsible for educating women about menopause and health promotion. Your patient is overweight and has a family history of heart disease. She has no time for exercise and eats mostly fast food. During your initial conversation, you learn that she has a high level of stress and a high-pressure job. How would you proceed? What is the evidence base for the strategies that you would suggest to her to reduce stress and lose weight? What criteria would you use to assess the strength of that evidence? How would you use that evidence to develop a teaching plan for her?

4 During a checkup, a 23-year-old woman tells you that she has a new boyfriend and is not concerned about sexual risks of STDs because she only plans on having oral sex. How would you address the educational needs of this patient? How would your teaching differ if her new partner is a woman?

5 At a health clinic, you meet a 45-year-old woman with multiple sclerosis (MS) who uses a wheelchair most of the time. She is approaching menopause and is concerned about how her physical limitations secondary to MS might affect her health related to menopause. Describe what health promotion issues would be relevant and the actions, including patient teaching, that are warranted.

REFERENCES AND SELECTED READINGS

BOOKS

Advisory Committee on Immunization Practices. (2003). *Adult immunization schedule by age group and medical conditions. United States, 2003–2004.* Atlanta, GA: Centers for Disease Control and Prevention.

American Cancer Society. (2005). *Cancer facts and figures 2005.* Atlanta, GA: Author.

American College of Obstetricians and Gynecologists (ACOG). *2004 compendium of selected publications.* Washington, DC: Author.

Andrews, M. & Boyle, J. (Eds.). (2003). *Transcultural concepts in nursing care* (4th ed.). Philadelphia: Lippincott William & Wilkins.

Association of Reproductive Health Professionals. (2004a). *Communicating with patients: A quick reference guide for clinicians.* Washington, DC.: Author.

Association of Reproductive Health Professionals. (2004b). *Administration of hormonal contraceptive drugs: A quick reference guide for clinicians.* Washington, DC.: Author.

Association of Reproductive Health Professionals. (2004c). *Manual vacuum aspiration (MVA): A quick reference guide for clinicians.* Washington, DC.: Author.

Hawkins, J., Roberto-Nichols, D., & Stanley-Haney, J. (2004). *Protocols for nurse practitioners in gynecologic settings* (7th ed.). New York: Tiresias Press.

National Osteoporosis Foundation. (2003). *Physician's guide to prevention and treatment of osteoporosis.* Washington, DC: Author.

North American Menopause Society. (2004). *Menopause core curriculum study guide.* Cleveland: Author. Available at http://www.menopause.org. Accessed July 9, 2006.

Sherwin, B., & Parish, B. (2002). *Women, medicine, ethics and the law.* Burlington, VT: Ashgate.

Smeltzer, S. C. & Sharts-Hopko. (2005). *A providers' guide for the care of women with physical disabilities and chronic health conditions.* Chapel Hill, NC: North Carolina Office on Disability & Health.

U.S. Department of Health and Human Services. (2001). *Surgeon general's call to action to promote sexual health and responsible sexual behavior.* Washington, DC: U.S. Government Printing Office.

U.S. Department of Health and Human Services. (2004). *Bone health and osteoporosis: A report of the Surgeon General.* Rockville, MD: U.S. Department of Health and Human Services. Washington, D.C.

U.S. Department of Health and Human Services (2005). *The Surgeon General's call to action to improve the health and wellness of persons with disabilities.* Rochville, MD: U.S. Department of Health and Human Services.

Welner, S. & Haseltine, F. (2002). *Welner's guide to the care of women with disabilities.* Philadelphia: Lippincott Williams & Wilkins, 2004.

Youngkin, E. & Davis, M. (2004). *Women's health.* Upper Saddle, NJ: Pearson Education Inc.

JOURNALS

**Asterisks indicate nursing research articles.*

General

Amin, S., Kuhle, C., & Fitzpatrick, L. (2003). Comprehensive evaluation of the older woman. *Mayo Clinic Proceedings, 78*(9), 1157–1185.

Centers for Disease Control and Prevention (CDC). (2002). Sexually transmitted diseases treatment guidelines, 2002. *MMWR-Morbidity and Mortality Weekly Report, 51*(RR-6), 1–85.

Cleves, M., Hobbs, C., Collins, H., et al. (2004). Folic acid use by women receiving routine gynecologic care. *Obstetrics and Gynecology, 103*(4), 746–753.

Drumright, L., Gorbach, P., & Homes, K. (2004). Do people really know their sex partners? Concurrency, knowledge of partner behavior and sexually transmitted infections within partnerships. *Sexually Transmitted Diseases, 31*(7), 437–442.

Kass-Wolf, J. (2004). Calcium in women: Healthy bones and much more. *Journal of Obstetric, Gynecologic, and Neonatal Nursing, 33*(1), 21–33.

McFarlane, M., Bull, S. S., & Rietmeijer, C. A. (2000). The Internet as a newly emerging risk environment for sexually transmitted diseases. *Journal of the American Medical Association, 284*(4), 443–446.

Moos, M. (2004). Preconceptional health promotion: Progress in changing a prevention paradigm. *Journal of Perinatal and Neonatal Nursing, 18*(1), 2–13.

Nosek, M., Hughes, R., Howland, C., et al. (2004). The meaning of health for women with physical disabilities: A qualitative analysis. *Family and Community Health, 27*(1), 6–21.

Peck, S. A. (2001). The importance of the sexual health history in the primary care setting. *Journal of Obstetric, Gynecologic and Neonatal Nursing, 30*(3), 269–274.

Salonia, A., Munarriz, R., Naspro, R., et al. (2004). Women's sexual dysfunction: A pathophysiological review. *BJU International, 93*(8), 1156–1164.

Sandelowski, M. (2000). "This most dangerous instrument": Propriety, power and the vaginal speculum. *Journal of Obstetric, Gynecologic, and Neonatal Nursing, 29*(1), 73–82.

Smeltzer, S. C. (2000). Double jeopardy: Women with disabilities. *American Journal of Nursing, 100*(8), 11.

Abortion

Bartlett, L., Berg, C., Shulman, H., Zane, S., Green, C., Whitehead, S., et al. (2004). Risk factors for legal induced abortion-related mortality in the US. *Obstetrics and Gynecology, 103*(4), 729–744.

Blanchard, K. (2004). Two regimens of misoprostol for treatment of incomplete abortion. *Obstetrics and Gynecology, 103*(5), 860–870.

Creinin, M., Fox, J., Teal, S., Chen, A., Schaff, E., & Meyn, L. (2004). A randomized comparison of misoprostol 6 to 8 hours versus 24 hours after mifepristone for abortion. *Obstetrics and Gynecology, 103*(5) Part 1, 851–865.

Doyle, N., Flores, D., & Ramin, S. (2004). Medical vs surgical management of missed abortion: An economic analysis. *Obstetrics and Gynecology,* 103(4) S-6S.

Fisher, M., Reagan, S. & Zaki, S. R. (2006). Deaths from *Clostridium sordellii* after medical abortion. *New England Journal of Medicine, 354*(15), 1645–1647.

Grimes, D. (2004). Emergency contraception: Politics trumps science at the FDA. *Obstetrics and Gynecology,* (2), 220–221.

Grimes, D., & Creinin, M. (2004). Induced abortion: An overview for internists. *Annals of Internal Medicine, 140*(8), 620–626.

Grossman, D., Ellertson, C., Grimes, D., & Walker, D. (2004). Routine follow-up visits after first-trimester induced abortion. *Obstetrics and Gynecology, 103*(4), 738–745.

Stubblefield, P., Carr-Ellis, S., Borgatta, L. (2004) Methods for induced abortion. *Obstetrics and Gynecology, 104*(1), 174–185.

Taylor, D. & Hwang, A. (2003–2004). Mifepristone for medical abortion. *AWHONN Lifelines, 7*(6), 524–529.

Whitcomb, D. (2004). Abortion surveillance. *AWHONN Lifelines, 8*(2), 112–114.

Conception Control

Alan Guttmacher Institue. (2004). *Contraceptive use: Facts in brief.* Available at http://www.guttmacher.org. Accessed July 9, 2006.

Barron, M., & Daly, K. (2001). Expert in fertility appreciation: The Creighton model practitioner. *Journal of Obstetric, Gynecologic and Neonatal Nursing, 30*(4), 386–391.

Burkman, R., & Miller, C. (2004). Extended and continuous use of hormonal contraceptives. *Dialogues in Contraception, 8*(4), 1–4.

Burkman, R., & Collins, J. (2004). Hormonal contraception and cancer: Protective effects and risks. *Dialogues in Contraception, 8*(6), 5–7.

Cleland, J., & Ali, M. (2004). Reproductive consequences of contraceptive failure in 19 developing countries. *Obstetrics and Gynecology, 104*(2), 314–318.

Fehring, R. (2004). The future of professional education in natural family planning. *Journal of Obstetric, Gynecologic and Neonatal Nursing, 33*(1), 34–43.

Gallo, M., Grimes, D., Schulz, K., et al. (2004). Combination estrogen progestin contraceptives and body weight: Systematic review of randomized controlled trials. *Obstetrics and Gynecology, 103*(2), 359–373.

Grimes, D. (2002). Switching emergency contraception to over-the-counter status. *New England Journal of Medicine, 347*(11), 846–849.

Greydanus, D., Patel, D., & Rimsza, M. (2001). Contraception in the adolescent: An update. *Pediatrics, 107*(3), 562–573.

Jamieson, D., Costello, C., Trussell, J., et al (2004). Risk of pregnancy after vasectomy. *Obstetrics and Gynecology, 103*(5), Part 1, 848–850.

Kartoz, C. (2004). New options for teen pregnancy prevention. *Maternal Child Nursing, 29*(1), 30–35.

Kaunitz, A., & Mestman, J. (2004). Hormonal contraception in women with common medical conditions: Benefits and risks of use. *Dialogues in Contraception, 8*(6), 1–4.

Kerin, J., Cooper, J., Price, T., et al. (2003). Hysteroscopic sterilization using a micro-insert device: Results of a multicentre phase II study. *Human Reproduction, 18*(6), 1223–1230.

Muchowski, K. & Paladine, H. (2004) An ounce of prevention: The evidence supporting periconception health care. *Journal of Family Practice, 53*(2), 126–133.

Raymond, E., Lien Chen, P., & Luoto, J. (2004). Contraceptive effectiveness and safety of five nonoxynol-9 spermicides: A randomized trial. *Obstetrics and Gynecology, 103*(3), 430–439.

Ross, B., Potter, L., Armstrong, K. (2004). Improving patient educational literature: An understandable patient package insert for "the Pill." *Journal of Obstetric, Gynecologic and Neonatal Nursing, 31*(2), 198–207.

Trussell, J., Ellertson, C., Stewart, F., et al. (2004). The role of emergency contraception. *American Journal of Obstetrics and Gynecology, 190*(4), Supplement 4, S30–38.

Veres, S., Miller, L., & Burrington, B. (2004). A comparison between the vaginal ring and oral contraceptives. *Obstetrics and Gynecology, 104*(3), 555–563.

Westhof, C. (2003). Emergency contraception. *New England Journal of Medicine, 349*(19), 1830–1835.

Cultural Differences in Health Care of Women

Carroll, N. (1999). Optimal gynecologic and obstetric care for lesbians. *Obstetrics & Gynecology, 93*(4), 611–613.

Cesario, S. (2001). Care of the native American woman: Strategies for practice education and research. *Journal of Obstetric, Gynecologic and Neonatal Nursing, 30*(1), 13–18.

Cochran, S. D., Mays, V. M., Bowen, D., et al. (2001). Cancer-related risk indicators and preventive screening behaviors among lesbians and bisexual women. *American Journal of Public Health, 91*(4), 591–597.

Green-Hernandez, C., Quinn, A., Denman, S., et al. (2004). Making primary care culturally competent. *Nurse Practitioner, 29*(6), 49–55.

Marazzo, J. & Stine, K. (2004). Reproductive health history of lesbians: implications of care. *American Journal of Obstetrics and Gynecology, 190*(5), 1298–1304.

Varney, J. (2004). Health needs of women who have sex with women: Maybe new subspecialty is needed. *BMJ, 328*(7), 437–463.

Ectopic Pregnancy

Anderson, F., Hogan, J., & Ansbacher, R. (2004). Sudden death: Ectopic pregnancy mortality. *Obstetrics and Gynecology, 103*(6), 1218–1223.

Leke, R., Goyaux, N., Matsuda, T., et al. (2004) Ectopic pregnancy in Africa: A population based study. *Obstetrics and Gynecology, 103*(4), 692–697.

Sowter, M. & Farquhar, C. (2004). Ectopic pregnancy: An update. *Current Opinion in Obstetrics and Gynecology, 16*(4), 289–293.

Staka, M. Zeringue, E., & Goldman, J. (2004) A rare drug reaction to methotrexate after treatment for ectopic pregnancy. *Obstetrics and Gynecology, 105*(5 Part 2), 1047–1048.

Infertility

Brinton, L., Lamb, E., Moghissi, K., et al. (2004). Ovarian cancer risk after the use of ovulation stimulating drugs. *Obstetrics and Gynecology, 103*(6), 1194–99.

Hart, V. A. (2002). Infertility and the role of psychotherapy. *Issues in Mental Health Nursing, 23*(1), 31–41.

Kashyap, S., Moher, D., Fung, M. & Rosenwaks, Z. (2004) Assisted reproductive technology and the incidence of ovarian cancer: a meta-analysis. *Obstetrics and Gynecology, 103*(4), 785–794.

Schieve, L., Rasmussen, S., Buch, G., Schendel, D., Reynolds, M., & Wright, V. (2004). Are children born after assisted reproductive technology at increased risk for adverse health outcomes? *Obstetrics and Gynecology, 103*(6), 1154–1163.

Smith, S., Pfeifer, S., & Collins, J. (2003) Diagnosis and management of female infertility. *Journal of the American Medical Association, 290*(13), 1767–1770.

Templeton, A. (2004) The multiple gestation epidemic: The role of assisted reproductive technologies. *American Journal of Obstetrics and Gynecology, 190*(4), 894–898.

Menstruation, Irregular Bleeding, Perimenopause, PMS, and Menopause

American Heart Association. Questions and answers about HRT. http://www.americanheart.org. Accessed July 9, 2006.

Aschenbrenner, D. HRT (2004). Reconsidered: What should you tell patients about it now? *American Journal of Nursing, 104*(6), 51–53.

Barron, M. (2004). Proactive management of menstrual cycle abnormalities in young women. *Journal of Perinatal and Neonatal Nursing, 18*(2), 81–92.

Dell, D., Moskowitz, D., & Sondheimer, S. (2001). PMS and PMDD: Identification and treatment. *Contemporary Obstetrics & Gynecology, 46*(4), 15–24.

Fitzpatrick, L. (2004). Menopause and hot flashes: No easy answers to a complex problem. *Mayo Clinic Proceedings, 79*(6), 735–737.

Freeman, E., Sammel, P., Rinaudo, J., et al. (2004) Premenstrual syndrome as a predictor of menopausal symptoms. *Obstetrics and Gynecology, 103*(5), 960–966.

Garry, R. (1995). Good practice with endometrial ablation. *Obstetrics and Gynecology, 86*(1), 144–151.

Hendrix, S. (2003). Menopausal hormone therapy informed consent. *American Journal of Obstetrics and Gynecology, 189*(4, Suppl.), S31–S36.

*Lyndaker, C., & Hulton, L. (2004). The influence of age on symptoms of perimenopause. *Journal of Obstetric, Gynecologic and Neonatal Nursing, 33*(3), 340–347.

Manson, J., & Martin, K. (2003) Estrogen plus progestin and coronary heart disease. *New England Journal of Medicine, 349*(1), 523–534.

McEvoy, M., Chang, J., & Coupey, S. (2004). Common menstrual disorders in adolescence: nursing interventions. *Maternal Child Nursing, 29*(1), 41–49.

National Institutes of Health. (2005). National Institutes of Health State-of-the Science Conference Statement: Management of menopause-related symptoms. *Annals of Internal Medicine, 142*(12, Part 1), 1003–1013.

National Institutes of Health Consensus Development Panel on Osteoporosis, Prevention, Diagnosis and Therapy. (2001). Osteoporosis prevention, diagnosis, and therapy. *Journal of the American Medical Association, 285*(6), 785–795.

Selo-Ojeme, D., Tillisi, A., & Welch, C. (2004). Anaphylaxis from medroxyprogesterone acetate. *Obstetrics and Gynecology, 103*(5, Part 2), 1045–46.

Sharts-Hopko, N. C. (2001). Hysterectomy for nonmalignant conditions. *American Journal of Nursing, 101*(9), 32–40.

Shumaker, S. A., Legault, C., Kuller, L., et al. (2004). Conjugated equine estrogens and incidence of probable dementia and mild cognitive impairment in postmenopausal women. *Journal of the American Medical Association, 291*(24), 2947–2958.

Taylor, M. (2001). Psychological consequences of surgical menopause. *Journal of Reproductive Medicine, 46*(3 Suppl.), 317–324, 333–336.

Tice, J., Ettinger, B., Ensrud, K., et al. (2003) Phytoestrogen supplements for the treatment of hot flashes: The Isoflavone Clover Extract (ICE) Study, a randomized controlled trial. *Obstetrics and Gynecology Survey, 58*(11), 732–733.

Vandenakker, C. B., & Glass, D. D. (2001). Menopause and aging with disability. *Physical and Medical Rehabilitation Clinics of North America, 12*(1), 133–151.

Writing Group for Women's Health Initiative Investigators. (2002). Risks and benefits of estrogen plus progestin in healthy postmenopausal women: Principal results from the Women's Health Initiative randomized controlled trial. *Journal of the American Medical Association, 288*(3), 321–333.

Mutilation, Domestic Violence, Physical and Sexual Assault

Dunn, L., & Oths, K. (2004) Prenatal predictors of intimate partner abuse. *Journal of Obstetric, Gynecologic, and Neonatal Nursing, 31*(1), 54–53.

*Harner, H. (2004). Domestic violence and trauma care in teenage pregnancy: Does paternal age make a difference? *Journal of Obstetric, Gynecologic and Neonatal Nursing, 33*(3), 312–319.

Kaplan, D. W., Feinstein, R. A., Fisher, M. M., et al. (2001). Care of the adolescent sexual assault victim. *Pediatrics, 107*(6), 1476–1479.

*McFarlane, J. Malecha, A., Watson, K., et al. (2005). Intimate partner sexual assault against women: Frequency, health consequences, and treatment outcomes. *Obstetrics and Gynecology, 105*(1), 99–108.

*McFarlane, J., Hughes, R. B., Nosek, M. A., et al. (2001). Abuse Assessment Screen-Disability (AAS-D), measuring frequency, type, and perpetrator of abuse toward women with physical disabilities. *Journal of Women's Health & Gender-Based Medicine, 10*(9), 861–866.

Medrano, M., Brzyski, R., Bernstein, D., et al. (2004) Childhood abuse and neglect histories in low-income women: prevalence in a menopausal population. *Menopause, 11*(2), 208–213.

Nelson, H. D., Nygren, P., McInerney, Y., et al. (2004). Screening women and elderly adults for family and intimate partner violence. A review of the evidence for the U.S. Preventive Services Task Force. *Annals of Internal Medicine, 140*(5), 387–396.

Nour, N. (2004 April). Female genital cutting: Clinical and cultural guidelines. *Obstetrics and Gynecology Survey, 59*(4), 272–279.

Rickert, V., Vaughan, R., & Wiemann, C. (2003) Violence against young women: Implications for clinicians. *Contemporary Obstetrics/Gynecology*, 48, 30–35.

Sugar, N., Fine, D., & Eckert, L. (2004) Physical injury after sexual assault: Findings of a large case series. *American Journal of Obstetrics and Gynecology, 190*(1), 71–6.

Pap Smears and Follow-Up Treatment

Abercrombie, P. D. (2001). Improving adherence to abnormal Pap smear follow-up. *Journal of Obstetric, Gynecologic and Neonatal Nursing, 30*(1), 80–88.

Choma, K. (2003). ASC-US HPV testing. *American Journal of Nursing, 103*(2), 42–50.

Committee on Adolescent Health Care of the American College of Obstetricians and Gynecologists. (2006). Evaluation and management of abnormal cervical cytology and histology in the adolescent. ACOG Committee Opinion, 330. *Obstetrics & Gynecology, 107*(4), 963–968.

Crane, J. (2003) Pregnancy outcome after loop electrosurgical excision procedure: a systemic review. *Obstetrics and Gynecology, 102,* 1058–62.

Franco, E., Duarte-Franco, E., & Ferenczy, A. (2001). Cervical cancer: Epidemiology, prevention and the role of human papillomavirus infection. *Canadian Medical Association Journal, 164*(7), 1017–1025.

Goldie, S., Kim, J., & Wright, T. (2004). Cost-effectiveness of HPV DNA testing for cervical cancer screening in women aged 30 or more. *Obstetrics and Gynecology, 103*(4), 619–638.

Huntington, J., Oliver, L., Anna, L., et al. (2004). What is the best approach for patients with ASCUS detected on Pap smear? *Journal of Family Practice, 53*(3), 240–241.

Koutsky, L., Ault, K., & Wheeler, C. (2002). A controlled trial of a human papillomavirus type 16 vaccine. *New England Journal of Medicine, 347*(21), 645–651.

McNeely, S. (2003). New cervical cancer screening techniques. *American Journal of Obstetrics and Gynecology, 189*(4), S40–41.

Moore, D. H. (2006). Cervical cancer. *Obstetrics and Gynecology, 107*(5), 1152–1161.

Padilla-Paz, L., Carlson, J., Twiggs, L., et al. (2004). Evidence supporting the current management guidelines for high grade squamous intraepithelial lesion cytology. *Journal of Lower Genital Tract Disease, 8*(2), 139–146.

Schiffman, M. (2004). Evidence-based screening and management guidelines address the realistic concerns of practicing clinicians and pathologists. *Journal of Lower Genital Tract Disease, 8*(2), 150–154.

Skinner, E., Gehrig, P., & Van Le, L. (2004). High-grade squamous intraepithelial lesions: abbreviating posttreatment surveillance. *Obstetrics and Gynecology, 103*(3), 488–492.

U.S. Preventive Services Task Force. (2003). Screening for cervical cancer: Recommendations and Rationale. *American Journal of Nursing, 103*(11), 101–109.

Wee, C., McCarthy, E., Davis, R., et al. (2000). Screening for cervical and breast cancer: Is obesity an unrecognized barrier to preventive care? *Annals of Internal Medicine, 132*(9), 697–704.

Wright, T. C., Jr., Cox, J. T., Massad, L. S., et al. (2002). ASCCP-Sponsored Consensus Conference. 2001 Consensus Guidelines for the management of women with cervical cytological abnormalities. *Journal of the American Medical Association, 287*(16), 2120–2129.

RESOURCES

American College of Obstetricians and Gynecologists (ACOG), 409 12th St. SW, P.O. Box 96920, Washington, DC 20090-6920; http://www.acog.org. Accessed July 9, 2006.

American Public Health Association and the Maternal Child Health Community Leadership Institute. Understanding the health culture of recent immigrants to the United States: a cross-cultural maternal health information catalog. 800 I Street, NW, Washington, DC 20001; (202) 777-2742; http://www.apha.org/ppp/maternal. Accessed July 9, 2006.

American Society for Reproductive Medicine (ASRM), 209 Montgomery Highway, Birmingham, AL 35216; (205) 978-5000; http://www.asrm.org. Accessed July 9, 2006.

Amnesty International, 322 Eighth Ave., New York, NY 10001 (212) 807-8400; http://www.amnesty.org (resource for activists to end female genital mutilation). Accessed July 9, 2006.

Association of Reproductive Health Professionals, 2401 Pennsylvania Ave NW, Suite 350, Washington, DC 20037; (202) 466-3826; http://www.arhp.org. Accessed July 9, 2006.

Association of Women's Health, Obstetrical and Neonatal Nurses (AWHONN), 2000 L Street NW, Suite 740, Washington, DC 20036; (800) 673-8499; http://www.awhonn.org. Accessed July 9, 2006.

Department of Adolescent Health, American Medical Association, 515 North State St., Chicago, IL 60610; Adolescent Health on Line at http://www.ama-assn.org/ama/pub/category/1947.html. Accessed July 9, 2006.

D.E.S. Action USA, 610 16th Street, Suite 301, Oakland, CA 94612; (510) 465-4011; http://www.desaction.org. Accessed July 9, 2006.

Emergency Contraception; Office of Population Research, Princeton University, Princeton, NJ 08540; (888) Not-2-Late; http://opr.princeton.edu/ec. Accessed July 9, 2006.

Family Violence Prevention Fund, 383 Rhode Island St., Suite 304, San Francisco, CA 94103; (415) 252-8900; http://www.endabuse.org. Accessed July 9, 2006.

Female Genital Mutilation Education and Networking Project, http://www.fgmnetwork.org; e-mail: fgm@fgmnetwork.org. Accessed July 9, 2006.

Health Promotion for Women with Disabilities Project, Villanova University College of Nursing, 800 Lancaster Ave., Villanova, PA 19085; (610) 519-6828; http://www.nursing.villanova.edu/WomenWithDisabilities. Accessed July 9, 2006.

Healthy People 2010, http://www.healthy people.gov (lists goals for health in 2010 and progress toward those goals). Accessed July 9, 2006.

Jacob's Institute of Women's Health, 409 12th St SW, Washington, DC; (202) 863-4990; http://www.jiwh.org. Accessed July 9, 2006.

National Association of Nurse Practitioners in Women's Health (NPWH); (202) 543-9693; e-mail: info@npwh.org; http://www.npwh.org/index.html. Accessed July 9, 2006.

National Coalition Against Domestic Violence, 503 Capitol Court, NE, Suite 300, Washington, DC 20002; http://www.ncadv.org. Accessed July 9, 2006.

National Osteoporosis Foundation, 1150 17th St. NW, Suite 500, Washington, DC 20036; (800) 223-9994; http://www.nof.org. Accessed July 9, 2006.

North American Menopause Society, P.O. Box 94527, Cleveland, OH 44101; (800) 772-5342; http://www.menopause.org. Accessed July 9, 2006.

Nursing Network on Violence Against Women International, 1801 H Street, Suite B5-165, Modesto, CA 95354; (888) 909-9993. http://www.nnvawi.org. Accessed July 9, 2006.

Planned Parenthood Federation of America, 810 Seventh Ave., New York, NY 10019; (212) 541-7800; http://www.plannedparenthood.org. Accessed July 9, 2006.

Research, Action and Information Network for the Bodily Integrity of Women (RAINBO), 915 Broadway, Suite 1109, New York, NY 10010-7108; (212) 477-3318; e-mail: Info@rainbow.org; http://www.rainbo.org. Accessed July 9, 2006.

Resolve National Headquarters, 1310 Broadway, Somerville, MA 02144; (617) 623-0744; e-mail: resolveinc@aol.com. http://www.resolve.org. Accessed July 9, 2006.

Sexuality Information and Education Council of the United States, 130 W. 42nd St., Suite 350, New York, NY 10036; (212) 819-9770; http://www.siecus.org. Accessed July 9, 2006.

World Health Organization Department of Women's Health; 525 23 St. NW, Washington, DC 20037; (202) 974-3000; http://www.who.int/frh-whd/fgm/index.htm. Accessed July 9, 2006.

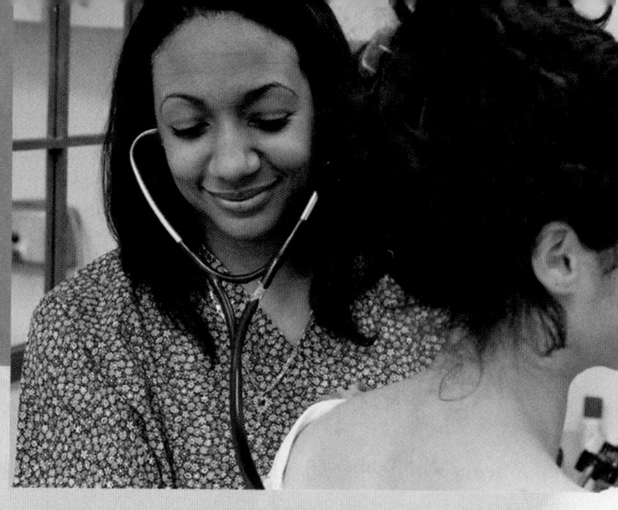

CHAPTER 47

Management of Patients With Female Reproductive Disorders

Learning Objectives

On completion of this chapter, the learner will be able to:

1. Compare the various types of vaginal infections and the signs, symptoms, and treatments of each.
2. Develop a teaching plan for the patient with a vaginal infection.
3. Use the nursing process as a framework for care of the patient with a vulvovaginal infection.
4. Use the nursing process as a framework for care of the patient with genital herpes.
5. Discuss the signs and symptoms, management, and nursing care implications of malignant disorders of the female reproductive tract.
6. Use the nursing process as a framework for care of the patient undergoing a hysterectomy.
7. Describe indications for a wide excision of the vulva, or vulvectomy, and the preoperative and postoperative nursing interventions.
8. Compare nursing interventions indicated for the patient undergoing radiation therapy and chemotherapy for cancer of the female reproductive tract.

Disorders of the female reproductive system can be minor or serious but are usually anxiety-producing and often distressing. Some disorders are self-limited and cause only minor inconvenience to the woman; others are life-threatening and require immediate attention and long-term therapy. Many disorders are managed by the patient at home, whereas others require hospitalization and surgical intervention. All disorders require that nurses have knowledge, understanding, and skill in patient teaching. Nurses must also be sensitive to the woman's concerns and possible discomfort in discussing and dealing with these disorders.

Vulvovaginal Infections

Vulvovaginal infections are common problems, and nurses have an important role in providing information that may prevent their occurrence. To prevent these infections, women need to understand their own anatomy and vulvovaginal health.

The vagina is protected against infection by its normally low pH (3.5 to 4.5), which is maintained in part by the actions of *Lactobacillus acidophilus*, the dominant bacteria in a healthy vaginal ecosystem. These bacteria suppress the

Glossary

abscess: a collection of purulent material

acquired immunodeficiency syndrome (AIDS): a disease transmitted by body fluids that results in impaired immune response

Bartholin's cyst: a cyst in a paired vestibular gland in the vulva

brachytherapy: radiation delivered by an internal device placed close to the tumor

candidiasis: infection caused by *Candida* species or yeast; also referred to as monilial vaginitis or yeast infection

chancre: painless lesion caused by syphilis

choriocarcinoma: a type of gestational neoplasm

colporrhaphy: repair of the vagina

condylomata: warty growths indicative of the human papillomavirus (HPV)

conization: procedure in which a cone-shaped piece of cervical tissue is removed as a result of detection of abnormal cells; also called cone biopsy

cryotherapy: destruction of tissue by freezing (eg, with liquid nitrogen)

cystocele: bulging of the bladder downward into the vagina

dermoid cyst: ovarian tumor of undefined origin that consists of undifferentiated embryonal cells

douche: rinsing the vaginal canal with fluid

dysplasia: term related to abnormal cell changes found on Pap smear and cervical biopsy reports

endocervicitis: inflammation of the mucosa and the glands of the cervix

endometriosis: endometrial tissue in abnormal locations; causes pain with menstruation, scarring, and possible infertility

fibroid tumor: usually benign tumor of the uterus that may cause irregular bleeding; also called myoma or leiomyoma

fistula: abnormal opening between two organs or sites (eg, vesicovaginal, between bladder and vagina; rectovaginal, between rectum and vagina)

hydatidiform mole: a type of gestational trophoblastic neoplasm

hyphae: microscopic findings that indicate monilia

hysterectomy: surgical removal of the uterus

lactobacilli: vaginal bacteria that limit the growth of other bacteria by producing hydrogen peroxide

laparoscope: surgical device inserted through a periumbilical incision to facilitate visualization and surgical procedures

lichen sclerosus: benign disorder of the vulva that usually occurs when estrogen levels are low; characterized by itching

liposomal therapy: chemotherapy delivered in a liposome, a nontoxic drug carrier

loop electrocautery excision procedure (LEEP): procedure in which laser energy is used to remove a portion of cervical tissue after abnormal biopsy findings

mucopurulent cervicitis (MCP): inflammation of the cervix with exudate; almost always related to a chlamydial infection

myomectomy: removal of uterine fibroids though an abdominal incision

oophorectomy: surgical removal of an ovary

pelvic exenteration: major surgical procedure in which the pelvic organs are removed

pelvic inflammatory disease (PID): infection of uterus and fallopian tubes, usually from a sexually transmitted disease

perineorrhaphy: surgical repair of perineal lacerations

rectocele: bulging of the rectum into the vagina

salpingo-oophorectomy: removal of the ovary and its fallopian tube (removal of the fallopian tube alone is a salpingectomy)

salpingitis: inflammation of the fallopian tube

toxic shock syndrome (TSS): a rare but potentially life-threatening infection caused by a toxin produced by *Staphylococcus aureus;* commonly associated with, but not exclusive to, use of super-absorbent tampons

vaginal vault: term used to describe the vagina following a hysterectomy, which involves removal of the uterus including the cervix

vaginitis: inflammation of the vagina, usually secondary to infection

vestibulitis: inflammation of the vulvar vestibule, or tissue around the opening of the vagina, that often causes pain with intercourse (dyspareunia)

vulvar dystrophy: thickening or lesions of the vulva; usually causes itching and may require biopsy to exclude malignancy

vulvectomy: removal of the tissue of the vulva

vulvitis: inflammation of the vulva, usually secondary to infection or irritation

vulvodynia: painful condition that affects the vulva

growth of anaerobes and produce lactic acid, which maintains normal pH. They also produce hydrogen peroxide, which is toxic to anaerobes. The risk of infection increases if a woman's resistance is reduced by stress or illness, if the pH is altered, or if a pathogen is introduced. Continued research into causes and treatments is needed, along with better ways to encourage growth of **lactobacilli.**

The epithelium of the vagina is highly responsive to estrogen, which induces glycogen formation. The subsequent breakdown of glycogen into lactic acid assists in producing a low vaginal pH. When estrogen decreases during lactation and menopause, glycogen also decreases. With reduced glycogen formation, infections may occur. In addition, as estrogen production ceases during the perimenopausal and postmenopausal periods, the vagina and labia may atrophy (thin), making the vaginal area more susceptible to infection. When patients are treated with antibiotics, the normal vaginal flora are reduced. This results in altered pH and growth of fungal organisms. Other factors that may initiate or predispose to infections include contact with an infected partner and wearing tight, nonabsorbent, and heat- and moisture-retaining clothing (Chart 47-1).

Vaginitis (inflammation of the vagina) occurs when *Candida* or *Trichomonas* species or other bacteria invade the vagina (Table 47-1). The normal vaginal discharge, which may occur in slight amounts during ovulation or just before the onset of menstruation, becomes more profuse when vaginitis occurs. Urethritis may accompany vaginitis because of the proximity of the urethra to the vagina. Discharge that occurs with vaginitis may produce itching, odor, redness, burning, or edema, which may be aggravated by voiding and defecation. After the causative organism has been identified, appropriate treatment (discussed later) is prescribed. This may include an oral medication or a local medication that may be inserted into the vagina using an applicator.

CHART 47-1

Risk Factors for Vulvovaginal Infections

- Premenarche
- Pregnancy
- Perimenopause/Menopause
- Poor personal hygiene
- Tight undergarments
- Synthetic clothing
- Frequent douching
- Allergies
- Use of oral contraceptives
- Use of broad-spectrum antibiotics
- Diabetes mellitus
- Low estrogen levels
- Intercourse with infected partner
- Oral-genital contact (yeast can inhabit the mouth and intestinal tract)
- HIV infection

Candidiasis

Vulvovaginal **candidiasis** is a fungal or yeast infection caused by strains of Candida (see Table 47-1). *Candida albicans* accounts for most cases, but other strains, such as *Candida glabrata,* may also be implicated. Many women with a healthy vaginal ecosystem harbor *Candida* but are asymptomatic. Certain conditions favor the change from an asymptomatic state to colonization with symptoms. For example, use of antibiotics decreases bacteria, thereby altering the natural protective organisms usually present in the vagina. Although infections can occur at any time, they may occur more commonly in pregnancy or with a systemic condition such as diabetes mellitus or human immunodeficiency virus (HIV) infection, or when patients are taking medications such as corticosteroids or oral contraceptives.

Clinical Manifestations

Clinical manifestations include a vaginal discharge that causes pruritus (itching) and subsequent irritation. The discharge may be watery or thick but has a white, cottage cheese-like appearance. Symptoms are usually more severe just before menstruation and may be less responsive to treatment during pregnancy. Diagnosis is made by microscopic identification of spores and **hyphae** on a glass slide prepared from a discharge specimen mixed with potassium hydroxide. With candidiasis, the pH is 4.5 or less.

Medical Management

The goal of management is to eliminate symptoms. Treatments include antifungal agents such as miconazole (Monistat), nystatin (Mycostatin), clotrimazole (Gyne-Lotrimin), and terconazole (Terazol) cream. These agents are inserted into the vagina with an applicator at bedtime. There are 1-night, 3-night, and 7-night treatment courses available. Oral medication (fluconazole [Diflucan]) is also available. Fluconazole is given in a one-pill dose; relief should be noted within 3 days.

Some vaginal creams are available without a prescription; however, patients are cautioned to use these creams only if they are certain that they have a yeast or monilial infection. Many patients use these remedies for problems other than yeast infections. If a woman is uncertain about the cause of her symptoms or if relief has not been obtained after using these creams, she should be instructed to seek health care promptly. Yeast infections can become recurrent and may be related to cell-mediated immunity. Women with recurrent yeast infections benefit from a comprehensive gynecologic assessment.

Bacterial Vaginosis

Bacterial vaginosis is caused by an overgrowth of anaerobic bacteria and *Gardnerella vaginalis* normally found in the vagina and an absence of lactobacilli (see Table 47-1). It is characterized by a fish-like odor that is particularly noticeable after sexual intercourse or during menstruation as a result of an increase in vaginal pH. It is usually accompanied by

TABLE 47-1 Vaginal Infections and Vaginitis

Infection	Cause	Clinical Manifestations	Management Strategies
Candidiasis	*Candida albicans,glabrata,* or *tropicalis*	Inflammation of vaginal epithelium, producing itching, reddish irritation White, cheeselike discharge clinging to epithelium	Eradicate the fungus by administering an antifungal agent. Frequently used brand names of vaginal creams and suppositories are Monistat, Femstat, Terazol, and Gyne-Lotrimin. Review other causative factors (eg, antibiotic therapy, nylon underwear, tight clothing, pregnancy, oral contraceptives). Assess for diabetes and HIV infection in patients with recurrent monilia.
Gardnerella-associated bacterial vaginosis	*Gardnerella vaginalis* and vaginal anaerobes	Usually no edema or erythema of vulva or vagina Gray-white to yellow-white discharge clinging to external vulva and vaginal walls	Administer metronidazole (Flagyl), with instructions about avoiding alcohol while taking this medication. If infection is recurrent may treat partner.
Trichomonas vaginalis vaginitis (STD)	*Trichomonas vaginalis*	Inflammation of vaginal epithelium, producing burning and itching Frothy yellow-white or yellow-green vaginal discharge	Relieve inflammation, restore acidity, and reestablish normal bacterial flora; provide oral metronidazole for patient and partner.
Bartholinitis (infection of greater vestibular gland)	*Escherichia coli* *Trichomonas vaginalis* Staphylococcus Streptococcus Gonococcus	Erythema around vestibular gland Swelling and edema Abscessed vestibular gland	Drain the abscess; provide antibiotic therapy; excise gland of patients with chronic bartholinitis.
Cervicitis: acute and chronic	Chlamydia Gonococcus Streptococcus Many pathogenic bacteria	Profuse purulent discharge Backache Urinary frequency and urgency	Determine the cause: perform cytologic examination of cervical smear and appropriate cultures. Eradicate the gonococcal organism, if present: penicillin (as directed) or spectinomycin or tetracycline, if patient is allergic to penicillin. Tetracycline, doxycycline (Vibramycin) to eradicate chlamydia. Eradicate other causes.
Atrophic vaginitis	Lack of estrogen; glycogen deficiency	Discharge and irritation from alkaline pH of vaginal secretions	Provide topical vaginal estrogen therapy; improve nutrition if necessary; relieve dryness through use of moisturizing medications.

a heavier-than-normal discharge. Risk factors include douching after menses, smoking, multiple sex partners, other sexually transmitted diseases (STDs) (also referred to as sexually transmitted infections [STIs]), and increased sexual activity.

Clinical Manifestations

Bacterial vaginosis can occur throughout the menstrual cycle and does not produce local discomfort or pain. More than half of patients with bacterial vaginosis do not notice any symptoms. Discharge, if noticed, is gray to yellowish white. The fish-like odor can be detected readily by adding a drop of potassium hydroxide to a glass slide with a sample of vaginal discharge, which releases amines. Under the microscope, vaginal cells are coated with bacteria and are described as "clue cells." The pH of the discharge is usually greater than 4.7 because of the amines that result from enzymes from anaerobes. Lactobacilli, which serve as a natural host defense, are usually absent. Bacterial vaginosis is not considered a serious condition; however, it has been associated with premature labor, endometritis, and recurrent urinary tract infection.

Medical Management

Metronidazole (Flagyl), administered orally twice a day for 1 week, is effective; a vaginal gel is also available. Clindamycin

(Cleocin) vaginal cream or ovules (oval suppositories) are also effective. Treatment of patients' partners does not seem to be effective, but use of condoms may be helpful. Patients with recurrent bacterial vaginosis should be tested for other STDs and assessed for use of sex toys or other intravaginal devices that may harbor bacteria (Hillier, 2004).

Trichomoniasis

Trichomonas vaginalis is a flagellated protozoan that causes a common, usually sexually transmitted vaginitis that is often called "trich." It is the second most common sexually transmitted infection in the United States (Soper, 2004), where about 5 million cases occur each year (U.S. Surgeon General's Report, 2001). It may be transmitted by an asymptomatic carrier who harbors the organism in the urogenital tract (see Table 47-1). It may increase the risk of contracting HIV from an infected partner and may play a role in development of cervical neoplasia, postoperative infections, adverse pregnancy outcomes, pelvic inflammatory disease (PID), and infertility.

Clinical Manifestations

Clinical manifestations include a vaginal discharge that is thin (sometimes frothy), yellow to yellow-green, malodorous, and very irritating. An accompanying vulvitis may result, with vulvovaginal burning and itching. Diagnosis is made most often by microscopic detection of the causative organisms or less frequently by culture. Inspection with a speculum often reveals vaginal and cervical erythema (redness) with multiple small petechiae ("strawberry spots"). Testing of a trichomonal discharge demonstrates a pH greater than 4.5.

Medical Management

The most effective treatment for trichomoniasis is metronidazole (Flagyl). Both partners receive a one-time loading dose or a smaller dose three times a day for 1 week. The one-time dose is more convenient; consequently, compliance tends to be greater. The week-long treatment has occasionally been noted to be more effective. Some patients complain of an unpleasant but transient metallic taste when taking metronidazole. Nausea and vomiting, as well as a hot, flushed feeling (disulfiram-like reaction), occur when this medication is taken with an alcoholic beverage. In view of these side effects, patients taking metronidazole are strongly advised to abstain from alcohol.

Metronidazole is not prescribed without examination. It is contraindicated in patients with some blood dyscrasias or central nervous system diseases, in the first trimester of pregnancy, and in women who are breastfeeding.

Gerontologic Considerations

After menopause, the vaginal mucosa becomes thinner and may atrophy. This condition can be complicated by infection from pyogenic bacteria, resulting in atrophic vaginitis (see Table 47-1). Leukorrhea (vaginal discharge) may cause itching and burning. Management is similar to that for bacterial vaginosis if bacteria are present. Estrogenic hormones, either taken orally or inserted into the vagina in a cream form, can also be effective in restoring the epithelium.

Nursing Process

The Patient With a Vulvovaginal Infection

Assessment

The woman with vulvovaginal symptoms should be examined as soon as possible after the onset of symptoms. She should be instructed not to **douche** because doing so removes the vaginal discharge needed to make the diagnosis. The area is observed for erythema, edema, excoriation, and discharge. Each of the infection-producing organisms produces its own characteristic discharge and effect (see Table 47-1). The patient is asked to describe any discharge and other symptoms, such as odor, itching, or burning. Dysuria often occurs as a result of local irritation of the urinary meatus. A urinary tract infection may need to be ruled out by obtaining a urine specimen for culture and sensitivity testing.

The patient is asked about the occurrence of factors that may contribute to vulvovaginal infection:

- Physical and chemical factors, such as constant moisture from tight or synthetic clothing, perfumes and powders, soaps, bubble bath, poor hygiene, and use of feminine hygiene products
- Psychogenic factors (eg, stress, fear of STDs, abuse)
- Medical conditions or endocrine factors, such as a predisposition to *Monilia* in a patient who has diabetes
- Use of medications such as antibiotics, which may alter the vaginal flora and allow an overgrowth of monilial organisms
- New sex partner, multiple sex partners, previous vaginal infection

The patient is also asked about factors that could contribute to infection, including hygiene practices (douching), and use or nonuse of condoms and other barrier methods of birth control.

The nurse may prepare a vaginal smear (wet mount) to assist in diagnosing the infection. A common method for preparing the smear is to collect vaginal secretions with an applicator and place the secretions on two separate glass slides. A drop of saline solution is added to one slide and a drop of 10% potassium hydroxide is added to another slide for examination under a microscope. If bacterial vaginosis is present, the slide with normal saline solution added shows epithelial cells dotted with bacteria (clue cells). If *Trichomonas* species is present, small motile cells are seen. In the presence of yeast, the potassium hydroxide slide reveals typical characteristics. Discharge associated with bacterial vaginosis produces a strong odor when mixed with potassium hydroxide. This is called a positive "whiff test." Testing the pH of the discharge with Nitrazine paper assists in proper diagnosis.

Diagnosis

Nursing Diagnoses

Based on the nursing assessment and other data, major nursing diagnoses may include the following:

- Discomfort related to burning, odor, or itching from the infectious process
- Anxiety related to stressful symptoms
- Risk for infection or spread of infection
- Deficient knowledge about proper hygiene and preventive measures

Planning and Goals

Major goals may include relief of discomfort, reduction of anxiety related to symptoms, prevention of reinfection or infection of sexual partner, and acquisition of knowledge about methods for preventing vulvovaginal infections and managing self-care.

Nursing Interventions

Relieving Discomfort

Treatment with the appropriate medication usually relieves discomfort. Sitz baths may be occasionally recommended and may provide temporary relief of symptoms.

Reducing Anxiety

Vulvovaginal infections are upsetting and require treatment. The patient who experiences such an infection may be very anxious about the significance of the symptoms and possible causes. Explaining the cause of symptoms may reduce anxiety related to fear of a more serious illness. Discussing ways to help prevent vulvovaginal infections may help patients adopt specific strategies to decrease infection and the related symptoms.

Preventing Reinfection or Spread of Infection

The patient needs to be informed about the importance of adequate treatment of herself and her partner, if indicated. Other strategies to prevent persistence or spread of infection include abstaining from sexual intercourse when infected, treatment of sexual partners, and minimizing irritation of the affected area. When medications such as antibiotic agents are prescribed for any infection, the nurse instructs the patient about the usual precautions related to using these agents. If vaginal itching occurs several days after use, the patient can be reassured that this is usually not an allergic reaction but may be a yeast or monilial infection resulting from altered vaginal bacteria. Treatment for monilial infection is prescribed.

Another goal of treatment is to reduce tissue irritation caused by scratching or wearing tight clothing. The area needs to be kept clean by daily bathing and adequate hygiene after voiding and defecation. The use of a hairdryer on a cool setting will dry the area and application of topical corticosteroids may decrease irritation.

When teaching the patient about medications such as suppositories and devices such as applicators to dispense cream or ointment, the nurse may demonstrate the procedure by using a plastic model of the pelvis and vagina. The nurse should also stress the importance of hand washing before and after each administration of medication. To prevent the medication from escaping from the vagina, the patient should recline for 30 minutes after it is inserted, if possible. The patient is informed that seepage of medication may occur, and the use of a perineal pad may be helpful.

Promoting Home and Community-Based Care

TEACHING PATIENTS SELF-CARE

Vulvovaginal conditions are treated on an outpatient basis, unless a patient has other medical problems. Patient teaching, tact, and reassurance are important aspects of nursing care. Women may express embarrassment, guilt, or anger and may be concerned that the infection may be serious or that it may have been acquired from a sex partner. (In some instances, treatment plans include the partner.)

In addition to reviewing ways of relieving discomfort and preventing reinfection, the nurse assesses each patient's learning needs relative to the immediate problem. The patient needs to know the characteristics of normal as opposed to abnormal discharge. Questions often arise about douching. Normally, douching and use of feminine hygiene sprays are unnecessary because daily baths or showers and proper hygiene after voiding and defecating keep the perineal area clean. Douching tends to eliminate normal flora, reducing the body's ability to ward off infection. In addition, repeated douching may result in vaginal epithelial breakdown and chemical irritation and has been associated with other pelvic disorders.

However, therapeutic douching may be recommended and prescribed to reduce unpleasant, abnormal odors; to remove excessive discharge; to change the pH (eg, vinegar douches); and to serve as an antiseptic irrigating solution. The procedure is reviewed with the patient, as is the care and cleaning of equipment so that it is properly disinfected.

In the case of recurrent yeast infections, the perineum should be kept as dry as possible. Loose-fitting cotton instead of tight-fitting synthetic, nonabsorbent, heat-retaining underwear is recommended. Use of talcum powder should be discouraged.

Vulvar self examination is a good health practice for all women. Becoming familiar with one's own anatomy and reporting anything that seems new or different may result in early detection and treatment of any new disorders. Nurses can also play a role in teaching women about the risks of unprotected intercourse, particularly with partners who have sex with other men or women.

Evaluation

Expected Patient Outcomes

Expected patient outcomes may include:

1. Experiences reduced discomfort
   a. Cleans the perineum as instructed
   b. Reports that itching is relieved
   c. Maintains urine output within normal limits and without dysuria
2. Experiences relief of anxiety
3. Remains free from infection
   a. Has no signs of inflammation, pruritus, odor, or dysuria
   b. Notes that vaginal discharge appears normal (thin, clear, not frothy)
4. Participates in self-care
   a. Takes medication as prescribed
   b. Wears absorbent underwear
   c. Avoids unprotected sexual intercourse
   d. Douches only as prescribed
   e. Performs vulvar self examination regularly and reports any new findings to care provider

Human Papillomavirus

Human papillomavirus (HPV) infection is sexually transmitted and is the most common sexually transmitted disease (STD) among young, sexually active people. An estimated 5.5 million people become infected with HPV each year in the United States (U.S. Surgeon General's Report, 2001). More than 80 strains exist, some of which are associated with cervical abnormalities, including dysplasia and cancer. Infections can be latent (asymptomatic and detected only by DNA hybridization tests for HPV), subclinical (visualized only after application of acetic acid followed by inspection under magnification), or clinical (visible condylomata acuminata).

Pathophysiology

The most common strains of HPV, 6 and 11, usually cause **condylomata** (warty growths) on the vulva. These are often visible or may be palpable by patients. Condylomata are rarely premalignant but are an outward manifestation of the virus. Strains 6 and 11 are associated with a low risk for cervical cancer. Some HPV strains (16, 18, 31, 33 and 45) may not cause condylomata but do affect the cervix, resulting in abnormal Papanicolaou (Pap) smears. The effects of these strains are usually invisible on examination but may be seen on colposcopy. They may cause cervical changes that may appear as koilocytosis on Pap smear. These strains are associated with a higher risk of cervical cancer (U.S. Surgeon General's Report, 2001); half of all cervical cancers are caused by HPV 16 and 18. However, most women with HPV infection do not develop cervical cancer.

The incidence of HPV in young, sexually active women is high. The infection often disappears due to an effective immune system response. It is thought that two proteins produced by high-risk types of HPV interfere with tumor suppression by normal cells. Risk factors include being sexually active, having multiple sex partners, and having sex with a partner who has or has had multiple partners. Alcohol consumption and drug use are risk factors, because both impair careful decision making, judgment, and self-care (Association of Reproductive Health Practitioners, 2001).

In October, 2005, the results of a multinational clinical drug study of a vaccine for HPV were announced, indicating that the vaccine is very effective in preventing transmission of two HPV strains, which together cause about 70% of cervical cancer cases.

In 2006, the Advisory Committee on Immunization Practices (ACIP) of the CDC recommended that the newly licensed vaccine against HPV be routinely administered to girls 11 to 12 years of age, that is, before they become sexually active. Although the vaccine is considered an important medical breakthrough, it is controversial because of fears that it will increase the likelihood of adolescents becoming sexually active. Immunization will not replace other strategies important in prevention of HPV or the need for cervical cancer screening.

Medical Management

Treatment of external genital warts includes topical application of trichloroacetic acid, podophyllin (Podofin, Podocon), and chemotherapeutic agents, and injections of interferon administered by a health care provider. Topical agents that can be applied by patients to external lesions include podofilox (Condylox) and imiquimod (Aldara). Because the safety of podophyllin, imiquimod, and podofilox during pregnancy has not been determined, these agents should not be used during pregnancy. Electrocautery and laser therapy are alternative therapies that may be indicated for patients with a large number or area of genital warts (Centers for Disease Control and Prevention [CDC], 2002).

Treatment usually eradicates perineal warts or condylomata. However, they may resolve spontaneously without treatment and may also recur even with treatment.

If the treatment includes application of a topical agent by the patient, she needs to be carefully instructed in the use of the agent prescribed and must be able to identify the warts and be able to apply the medication to them. The patient is instructed to anticipate mild pain or local irritation with the use of these agents (CDC, 2002).

Women with HPV should have annual Pap smears because of the potential of HPV to cause **dysplasia** (changes in cervical cells). Much remains unknown about subclinical and latent HPV disease. Women are often exposed to HPV by partners who are unknowing carriers. Use of condoms can reduce the likelihood of transmission, but transmission can also occur during skin-to-skin contact in areas not covered by condoms. In many cases, patients are angry about having warts or HPV and do not know who infected them because the incubation period can be long and partners may have no symptoms. Acknowledging the emotional distress that occurs when an STD is diagnosed and providing support and facts are important nursing actions.

Herpesvirus Type 2 Infection (Herpes Genitalis, Herpes Simplex Virus)

Herpes genitalis is a recurrent, life-long viral infection that causes herpetic lesions (blisters) on the external genitalia and occasionally the vagina and cervix. It is an STD but may also be transmitted asexually from wet surfaces or by self-transmission (ie, touching a cold sore and then touching the genital area). The initial infection is usually very painful and lasts about 1 week, but it can also be asymptomatic. Recurrences are less painful and usually produce minor itching and burning. Some patients have few or no recurrences, whereas others have frequent bouts. Recurrences are often associated with stress, sunburn, dental work, or inadequate rest or nutrition—all situations that may tax the immune system.

Since the late 1970s, the incidence of herpes infection has increased fivefold among Caucasian adolescents and young adults. At least 50 million people in the United States have genital herpes infection, and most have not been diagnosed (CDC, 2002). The prevalence of other STDs has decreased slightly, possibly because of increased condom use, but herpes can be transmitted by contact with skin not covered by a condom. Transmission is possible even when a carrier does not have symptoms (subclinical shedding). Lesions increase vulnerability to HIV infection and other STDs. Vaccines for herpes genitalis are in clinical trials.

Pathophysiology

Of the known herpesviruses, six affect humans: (1) herpes simplex type 1 (HSV-1), which usually causes cold sores of the lips; (2) herpes simplex type 2 (HSV-2), or genital herpes; (3) varicella zoster, or shingles; (4) Epstein-Barr virus; (5) cytomegalovirus (CMV); and (6) human B-lymphotrophic virus. HSV-2 appears to be the cause of about 80% of genital and perineal lesions; HSV-1 may cause about 20%.

There is considerable overlap between HSV-1 and HSV-2, which are clinically indistinguishable. Close human contact by the mouth, oropharynx, mucosal surface, vagina, or cervix appears necessary to acquire the infection. Other susceptible sites are skin lacerations and conjunctivae. Usually, the virus is killed at room temperature by drying. When viral replication diminishes, the virus ascends the peripheral sensory nerves and remains inactive in the nerve ganglia. Another outbreak may occur when the host is subjected to stress. In pregnant women with active herpes, infants delivered vaginally may become infected with the virus. There is a risk of fetal morbidity and mortality if this occurs; therefore, a cesarean delivery may be performed if the virus recurs near the time of delivery.

Clinical Manifestations

Itching and pain accompany the process as the infected area becomes red and edematous. Primary infection may begin with macules and papules and progress to vesicles and ulcers. The vesicular state often appears as a blister, which later coalesces, ulcerates, and encrusts. In women, the labia are the usual primary site, although the cervix, vagina, and perianal skin may be affected. In men, the glans penis, foreskin, or penile shaft is typically affected. Influenza-like symptoms may occur 3 or 4 days after the lesions appear. Inguinal lymphadenopathy (enlarged lymph nodes in the groin), minor temperature elevation, malaise, headache, myalgia (aching muscles), and dysuria (pain on urination) are often noted. Pain is evident during the first week and then decreases. The lesions subside in about 2 weeks unless secondary infection occurs.

Rarely, complications may arise from extragenital spread, such as to the buttocks, upper thighs, or even the eyes as a result of touching lesions and then touching other areas. Patients should be advised to wash their hands after contact with lesions. Other potential problems are aseptic meningitis, neonatal transmission, and severe emotional stress related to the diagnosis.

Medical Management

There is currently no cure for HSV-2 infection, but treatment is aimed at relieving the symptoms. Management goals are preventing the spread of infection, making patients comfortable, decreasing potential health risks, and initiating a counseling and education program. The antiviral agents acyclovir (Zovirax), valacyclovir (Valtrex), and famciclovir (Famvir) can suppress symptoms and shorten the course of the infection. Other antiviral agents are also available. All of them are effective at reducing the duration of lesions and preventing recurrences. Resistance and long-term side effects do not appear to be major problems. Recurrent episodes are much milder than the initial episode.

Nursing Process

The Patient With a Genital Herpesvirus Infection

Assessment

The health history and a physical and pelvic examination are important in establishing the nature of the infectious condition. In addition, patients are assessed for risk of STDs. The perineum is inspected for painful lesions. Inguinal nodes are assessed and are often enlarged and tender during an occurrence of HSV.

Diagnosis

Nursing Diagnoses

Based on the assessment data, major nursing diagnoses may include the following:

- Acute pain related to the genital lesions
- Risk for infection or spread of infection
- Anxiety related to the diagnosis
- Deficient knowledge about the disease and its management

Planning and Goals

Major goals may include relief of pain and discomfort, control of infection and its spread, relief of anxiety, knowledge of and adherence to the treatment regimen and self-care, and knowledge about implications for the future.

Nursing Interventions

Relieving Pain

The lesions should be kept clean, and proper hygiene practices are advocated. Sitz baths ease discomfort. Clothing should be clean, loose, soft, and absorbent. Aspirin and other analgesics are usually effective in controlling pain. Occlusive ointments and powders are avoided because they prevent the lesions from drying.

If there is considerable pain and malaise, bed rest may be required. The patient is encouraged to increase fluid intake, to be alert for possible bladder distention, and to contact her primary health care provider immediately if she cannot void because of discomfort. Painful voiding may occur if urine comes in contact with the herpes lesions. Discomfort with urination can be reduced by pouring warm water over the vulva during voiding or by sitz baths. When oral acyclovir or other antiviral agents are prescribed, the patient is instructed about when to take the medication and what side effects to note, such as rash and headache. Rest, fluids, and a nutritious diet are recommended to promote recovery.

Preventing Infection and Its Spread

The risk of reinfection and spread of infection to others or to other structures of the body can be reduced by hand washing, use of barrier methods with sexual contact, and adherence to prescribed medication regimens. Avoidance of contact when obvious lesions are present does not eliminate the risk because the virus can be shed in the absence of symptoms, and lesions may not be visible to women. Avoiding stress, sunburn, and other stress-producing situations may decrease the episodes of recurrence.

Relieving Anxiety

Concern about the presence of herpes infection, future occurrences of lesions, and the impact of the infection on future relationships and childbearing may cause considerable patient anxiety. Nurses can be an important support, listening to patients' concerns and providing information and instruction. The patient may be angry with her partner if the partner is the probable source of the infection. The patient may need assistance and support in discussing the infection and its implications with her current sexual partners and in future sexual relationships. The nurse can refer the patient to a support group to assist in coping with the diagnosis (see Resources at the end of the chapter).

Increasing Knowledge About the Disease and Its Treatment

Patient teaching is an essential part of nursing care of the patient with a genital herpes infection. This includes an adequate explanation about the infection and how it is transmitted, management and treatment strategies, strategies to minimize spread of infection, the importance of adherence to the treatment regimen, and self-care strategies. Because of the increased risk of HIV and other STDs in the presence of skin lesions, an important part of patient education involves instructing the patient to protect herself from exposure to HIV and other STDs. Further details are included in Chart 47-2.

Promoting Home and Community-Based Care

TEACHING PATIENTS SELF-CARE

Genital herpes causes physical pain and emotional distress. Usually, the patient is upset on learning the diagnosis. Therefore, when counseling the patient, the nurse should explain the causes of the condition and the manner in which it can be managed. Questions are encouraged because they may indicate that the patient is receptive to learning.

The nurse can provide reassurance that the lesions will heal and that recurrences can be minimized by adopting a healthful lifestyle and by taking prescribed medications. Self-care measures for people with genital herpes appear in Chart 47-2.

Evaluation

Expected Patient Outcomes

Expected patient outcomes may include:

1. Experiences a reduction in pain and discomfort
2. Keeps infection under control
   a. Demonstrates proper hygiene techniques
   b. Takes medication as prescribed
   c. Consumes adequate fluids
   d. Assesses own current lifestyle (diet, adequate fluid intake, safer sex practices, stress management)
3. Uses strategies to reduce anxiety
   a. Verbalizes issues and concerns related to genital herpes infection
   b. Discusses strategies to deal with issues and concerns with current and future sexual partners
   c. Initiates contact with support group if indicated
4. Demonstrates knowledge about genital herpes and strategies to control and minimize recurrences
   a. Identifies methods of transmission of herpes infection and strategies to prevent transmission to others
   b. Discusses strategies to reduce recurrence of lesions
   c. Takes medications as prescribed
   d. Reports no recurrence of lesions

CHART 47-2

HOME CARE CHECKLIST • The Patient With Genital Herpes

At the completion of the home care instruction, the patient or caregiver will be able to:	Patient	Caregiver
• State that herpes is transmitted mainly by direct contact.	✔	✔
• State that abstinence from sex is required for a brief period (intercourse is avoided during treatment, but other options such as hand-holding and kissing are acceptable).	✔	✔
• State that intercourse during a herpes outbreak not only increases the risk of transmission but also increases the likelihood of contracting HIV and other STDs.	✔	✔
• State that transmission is possible even in the absence of active lesions.	✔	✔
• State that condoms may provide some protection against viral transmission.	✔	✔
• Explain that obstetric care provider should be informed about the history of herpes. In cases of recurrence at time of delivery, cesarean section may be considered.	✔	✔
• Describe appropriate hygiene practices (hand washing, perineal cleanliness, gentle washing of lesions with mild soap and running water and lightly drying lesions) and importance of avoiding occlusive ointments, strong perfumed soaps, or bubble bath.	✔	✔
• State that control of the condition may require changes in sexual behavior and use of medications.	✔	✔
• Describe strategies to avoid self-infection (eg, avoid touching lesions during an outbreak).	✔	✔
• Explain rationale for avoiding self-infection (ie, lesions can become infected from germs on the hand, and the virus from the lesion can be transmitted from the hand to another area of the body or another person).	✔	✔
• Describe health promotion strategies: wear loose, comfortable clothing; eat a balanced diet; get adequate rest and relaxation.	✔	✔
• State rationale for avoiding exposure to the sun as it can cause recurrences (and skin cancer).	✔	✔
• Identify importance of taking medications as prescribed, keeping follow-up appointments with health care provider, and reporting repeated recurrences (may not be as severe as the initial episode).	✔	✔
• Describe possible benefits of joining a group to share solutions and experiences and hear about newer treatments, such as HELP (Herpetics Engaged in Living Productively).	✔	✔

Endocervicitis and Cervicitis

Endocervicitis is an inflammation of the mucosa and the glands of the cervix that may occur when organisms gain access to the cervical glands after intercourse and, less often, after procedures such as abortion, intrauterine manipulation, or vaginal delivery. If untreated, the infection may extend into the uterus, fallopian tubes, and pelvic cavity. Inflammation can irritate the cervical tissue, resulting in spotting or bleeding and **mucopurulent cervicitis.**

Chlamydia and Gonorrhea

Chlamydia and gonorrhea are the most common causes of endocervicitis, although *Mycoplasma* may also be involved. Chlamydia causes about 3 million infections every year in the United States; it is most commonly found in young, sexually active people with more than one partner and is transmitted through sexual intercourse (Miller, Ford, Morris et al., 2004; U.S. Surgeon General's Report, 2001). It can result in serious complications, including pelvic infection, an increased risk for ectopic pregnancy, and infertility. As many as 40% of untreated women develop PID. One in 20 women of reproductive age in the United States is infected. Chlamydial infections of the cervix often produce no symptoms, but cervical discharge, dyspareunia, dysuria, and bleeding may occur. Other complications include conjunctivitis and perihepatitis. If pregnant women are infected, stillbirth, neonatal death, and premature labor may occur. Infants born to infected mothers may experience prematurity, conjunctivitis, and pneumonia.

Chlamydial infection and gonorrhea often coexist. As many as 25% of females who have chlamydial infections also have gonorrhea. The inflamed cervix that results from this infection may leave a woman more vulnerable to HIV transmission from an infected partner. Gonorrhea is also a major cause of PID, tubal infertility, ectopic pregnancy, and chronic pelvic pain. Fifty percent of women with gonorrhea have no symptoms, but without treatment, 40% may develop PID. In males, urethritis and epididymitis may occur. Diagnosis can be confirmed by culture, smear, or other methods, using a swab to obtain a sample of cervical discharge or penile discharge from the patient's partner. Some studies have implicated chlamydial infection as a factor in increased risk of cervical cancer, but more studies are needed to confirm this finding (American Cancer Society [ACS], 2002).

Medical Management

The Centers for Disease Control and Prevention (CDC) recommends treating chlamydia with doxycycline for 1 week or with a single dose of azithromycin (Zithromax). Because of the high incidence of coinfection with chlamydia and gonorrhea, treatment for gonorrhea should include treatment for chlamydia as well (CDC, 2002). Partners must also be treated. Pregnant women are cautioned not to take tetracycline because of potential adverse effects on the fetus. In these cases, erythromycin may be prescribed. Results are usually good if treatment begins early. Possible complications from delayed treatment are tubal disease, ectopic pregnancy, PID, and infertility.

Cultures for chlamydia and other STDs should be obtained from all patients who have been sexually assaulted when they first seek medical attention; patients are treated prophylactically. Cultures should then be repeated in 2 weeks. Annual screening for chlamydia is recommended for all sexually active young women and older women with new sex partners or multiple partners (CDC, 2002).

Nursing Management

All sexually active women may be at risk for chlamydia, gonorrhea, and other STDs, including HIV. Nurses can assist patients in assessing their own risk. Recognition of risk is a first step before changes in behavior occur. Patients should be discouraged from assuming that a partner is "safe" without open, honest discussion. Nonjudgmental attitudes, educational counseling, and role playing may be helpful.

Because chlamydia, gonorrhea, and other STDs may have a serious effect on future health and fertility and because many of these disorders can be prevented by the use of condoms and spermicides and careful choice of partners, nurses can play a major role in counseling patients about safer sex practices. Exploring options with patients, addressing knowledge deficits, and correcting misinformation may reduce morbidity and mortality.

Promoting Home and Community-Based Care

TEACHING PATIENTS SELF-CARE

Nurses can educate women and help them develop communication skills and initiate discussions about sex with their partners. Communicating with partners about sex, risk, postponing intercourse, and using safer sex behaviors, including use of condoms, may be lifesaving. Some young women report having sex but not being comfortable enough to discuss sexual risk issues. Nurses can pose the question, "If you are uncomfortable talking about sex with this person, how do you feel about having a sexual relationship with this person?"

Reinforcing the need for annual screening for chlamydia and other STDs is an important part of patient teaching. Instructions also include the need for the patient to abstain from sexual intercourse until all of her sex partners are treated (CDC, 2002). The CDC has revised its guidelines in an effort to protect young women from infertility; it recommends rescreening of all women with chlamydial infections 3 to 4 months after treatment is completed.

Pelvic Infection (Pelvic Inflammatory Disease)

Pelvic inflammatory disease (PID) is an inflammatory condition of the pelvic cavity that may begin with cervicitis and may involve the uterus (endometritis), fallopian tubes (**salpingitis**), ovaries (oophoritis), pelvic peritoneum, or pelvic vascular system. Infection, which may be acute, subacute, recurrent, or chronic and localized or widespread, is usually caused by bacteria but may be attributed to a virus, fungus, or parasite. Gonorrheal and chlamydial organisms are the most likely causes. CMV has also been implicated. This condition can result in the fallopian tubes becoming narrowed and scarred, which increases the risk of ectopic pregnancy (fertilized eggs become trapped in the tube), infertility, recurrent pelvic pain, tubo-ovarian **abscess**, and recurrent disease. Rupture of a tubo-ovarian abscess has a 5% to 10% mortality rate and usually necessitates a complete hysterectomy. PID is a common gynecologic cause of hospital admissions in the United States. The true incidence of PID is unknown because some cases are asymptomatic.

Pathophysiology

The exact pathogenesis of PID has not been determined, but it is presumed that organisms usually enter the body through the vagina, pass through the cervical canal, colonize the endocervix, and move upward into the uterus. Under various conditions, the organisms may proceed to one or both fallopian tubes and ovaries and into the pelvis. In bacterial infections that occur after childbirth or abortion, pathogens are disseminated directly through the tissues that support the uterus by way of the lymphatics and blood vessels (Fig. 47-1). In pregnancy, the increased blood supply required by the placenta provides more pathways for infection. These postpartum and postabortion infections tend to be unilateral. Infections can cause perihepatic inflammation when the organism invades the peritoneum.

In gonorrheal infections, the gonococci pass through the cervical canal and into the uterus, where the environment, especially during menstruation, allows them to multiply rapidly and spread to the fallopian tubes and into the pelvis (see Fig. 47-1). The infection is usually bilateral. In rare instances, organisms (eg, tuberculosis) gain access to the reproductive organs by way of the bloodstream from the lungs (see Fig. 47-1). One of the most common causes of salpingitis (inflammation of the fallopian tube) is chlamydia, possibly accompanied by gonorrhea.

Pelvic infection is most commonly caused by sexual transmission but can also occur with invasive procedures such as endometrial biopsy, surgical abortion, hysteroscopy, or

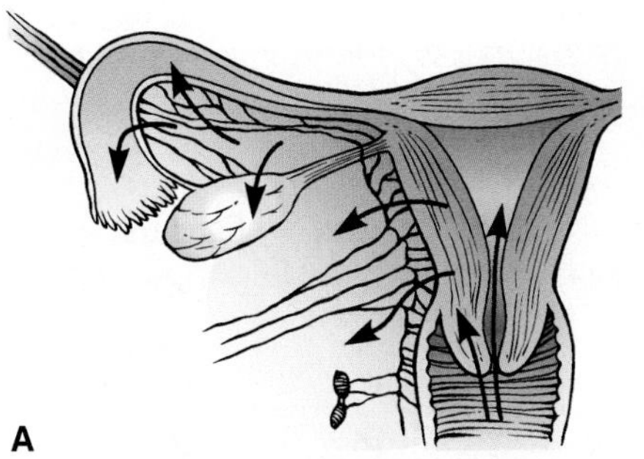

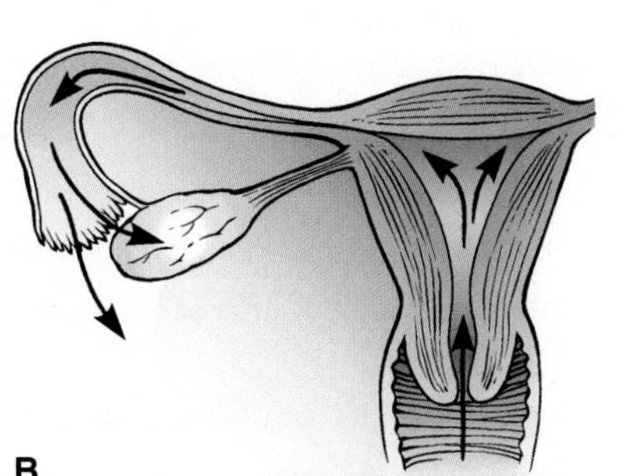

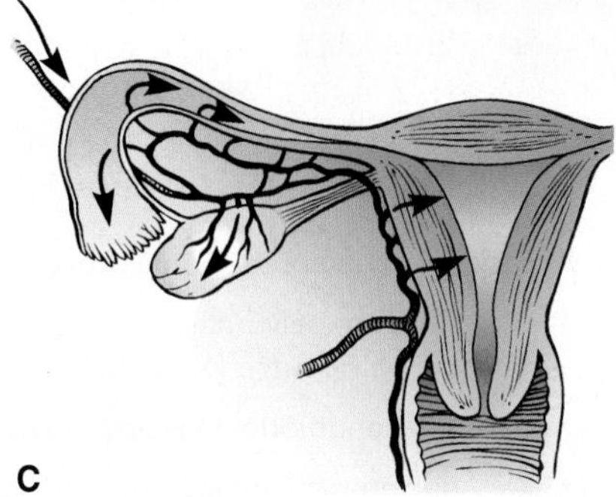

FIGURE 47-1. Pathway by which microorganisms spread in pelvic infections. (**A**) Bacterial infection spreads up the vagina into the uterus and through the lymphatics. (**B**) Gonorrhea spreads up the vagina into the uterus and then to the tubes and ovaries. (**C**) Bacterial infection can reach the reproductive organs through the bloodstream (hematogenous spread).

insertion of an intrauterine device. Bacterial vaginosis, a vaginal infection, may predispose women to pelvic infection. Risk factors include early age at first intercourse, multiple sexual partners, frequent intercourse, intercourse without condoms, sex with a partner with an STD, and a history of STDs or previous pelvic infection.

Clinical Manifestations

Symptoms of pelvic infection usually begin with vaginal discharge, dyspareunia, lower abdominal pelvic pain, and tenderness that occurs after menses. Pain may increase with voiding or with defecation. Other symptoms include fever, general malaise, anorexia, nausea, headache, and possibly vomiting. On pelvic examination, intense tenderness may be noted on palpation of the uterus or movement of the cervix (cervical motion tenderness). Symptoms may be acute and severe or low-grade and subtle.

Complications

Pelvic or generalized peritonitis, abscesses, strictures, and fallopian tube obstruction may develop. Obstruction may cause an ectopic pregnancy in the future if a fertilized egg cannot pass a tubal stricture, or scar tissue may occlude the tubes, resulting in sterility. Adhesions are common and often result in chronic pelvic pain; they eventually may require removal of the uterus, fallopian tubes, and ovaries. Other complications include bacteremia with septic shock and thrombophlebitis with possible embolization.

Medical Management

Broad-spectrum antibiotic therapy is prescribed. Women with mild infections may be treated as outpatients, but hospitalization may be necessary. Intensive therapy includes bed rest, intravenous (IV) fluids, and IV antibiotic therapy. If the patient has abdominal distention or ileus, nasogastric intubation and suction are initiated. Careful monitoring of vital signs and symptoms assists in evaluating the status of the infection. Treatment of sexual partners is necessary to prevent reinfection.

Nursing Management

Infection takes a toll, both physically and emotionally. The patient may feel well one day and experience vague symptoms and discomfort the next. She may also suffer from constipation and menstrual difficulties.

A hospitalized patient is maintained on bed rest and is usually placed in the semi-Fowler's position to facilitate dependent drainage. Accurate recording of vital signs and the characteristics and amount of vaginal discharge is necessary as a guide to therapy.

The nurse administers analgesic agents as prescribed for pain relief. Heat applied safely to the abdomen may also provide some pain relief and comfort. In addition, the nurse minimizes the transmission of infection to others by carefully handling perineal pads with gloves, discarding the soiled pad according to hospital guidelines for disposal of biohazardous material, and performing meticulous hand hygiene.

Promoting Home and Community-Based Care

TEACHING PATIENTS SELF-CARE

The patient must be informed of the need for precautions and must be encouraged to take part in procedures to prevent infecting others and protect herself from reinfection. If a partner is not well known or has had other sexual partners recently, use of condoms may prevent life-threatening infection and its sequelae. If reinfection occurs or if the infection spreads, symptoms may include abdominal pain, nausea and vomiting, fever, malaise, malodorous purulent vaginal discharge, and leukocytosis. Patient teaching consists of explaining how pelvic infections occur, how they can be controlled and avoided, and their signs and symptoms. Guidelines and instructions provided to the patient are summarized in Chart 47-3.

All patients who have had PID need to be informed of the signs and symptoms of ectopic pregnancy (pain, abnormal bleeding, delayed menses, faintness, dizziness, and shoulder pain) because they are prone to this complication. (See Chapter 46 for a discussion of ectopic pregnancy.)

CHART 47-3

HOME CARE CHECKLIST • The Patient With Pelvic Inflammatory Disease

At the completion of the home care instruction, the patient or caregiver will be able to:	Patient	Caregiver
• State that any pelvic pain or abnormal discharge, particularly after sexual exposure, childbirth, or pelvic surgery, should be evaluated as soon as possible.	✔	✔
• State that antibiotics may be prescribed after insertion of intrauterine devices (IUDs).	✔	✔
• Describe proper perineal care procedures (wiping from front to back after defecation or urination).	✔	✔
• State that douching reduces the natural flora that combat infecting organisms and may introduce bacteria upward.	✔	✔
• Identify the importance of consulting a health care provider if unusual vaginal discharge or odor is noted.	✔	✔
• Discuss the importance of following health practices (ie, proper nutrition, exercise, and weight control), and safer sex practices (ie, using condoms, avoiding multiple sexual partners).	✔	✔
• Explain the importance of consistent use of condoms before intercourse or any penile–vaginal contact if there is any chance of transmitting infection.	✔	✔
• State that a gynecologic examination should be performed at least once a year.	✔	✔

Human Immunodeficiency Virus Infection and Acquired Immunodeficiency Syndrome

Any discussion of vulvovaginal infections and STDs must include the topic of HIV and **acquired immunodeficiency syndrome (AIDS)**, which is described in Chapter 52.

The incidence of HIV infection and AIDS in women is increasing. Females represent the fastest-growing segment of the AIDS epidemic. Most are in the reproductive age group, and more than 70% are African American or Hispanic. More than 50% have been exposed through sexual contact with HIV-infected partners. Women who exchange sex for drugs are at high risk, just as are women who engage in anal intercourse. Heterosexual transmission is the leading cause of new HIV infection in women, surpassing IV/injection drug use as the most common mode of transmission. Younger women are disproportionally at higher risk; 25% to 50% of all women who acquire HIV heterosexually do so in adolescence or in their early 20s. Women are nine times more likely to contract HIV from men than men are from women. Factors that may account for this difference include a higher quantity of HIV in semen as compared with vaginal secretions, a larger inoculum on ejaculation, retention of HIV-infected semen in the vagina, and traumatic microscopic mucosal injury during intercourse. The presence of genital ulcers or a friable cervix increases risk. Intercourse during menses may also increase risk. In addition, any break in skin integrity increases the possibility of infection (eg, a herpetic lesion or syphilitic **chancre** could provide a portal of entry). Women need to be informed about the dangers of unprotected sex.

Syphilis appears to accelerate in HIV-positive patients and proceeds directly from primary to tertiary disease in some patients. Chlamydia is associated with a high risk of HIV (which may be related to inflammatory changes of the cervix, providing entry sites). HIV-positive women have a higher rate of HPV, and this risk increases as their CD4 cell count decreases. Infections with HPV and HIV together increase the risk of malignant transformation and cervical cancer. This risk also increases as the CD4 cell count decreases. Thus, women with HIV infection should have frequent Pap smears. HIV-positive women also have larger and more painful herpes lesions with more recurrences, probably related to immunosuppression from their disease. Treatment with acyclovir or other antiviral agents is appropriate for such patients. Pneumonitis, esophagitis, and disseminated skin involvement are common; candidiasis also occurs frequently in this population; oral candidiasis may signal rapidly advancing disease. Gynecologic infections and malignancies are gender-specific manifestations of HIV; many HIV-infected women have gynecologic disorders, including candidiasis, PID, anogenital warts, and cervical dysplasia (United States Public Health Services, 2000).

Women with HIV and women with partners who have HIV must be counseled about safer sex. Consistent use of condoms with an HIV-infected partner can keep seroconversion rates to about 1%, but inconsistent use results in an annual 7.2% seroconversion rate. Because there is a risk of perinatal transmission, decisions to conceive or to use contraception must be based on teaching, accurate information and care. The use of antiretroviral agents by pregnant women significantly decreases perinatal transmission of HIV infection. Therefore, the use of these agents during pregnancy is critical and must also be discussed. For women who choose to avoid conception, use of condoms alone and with oral contraceptives are possible choices.

After informed consent is obtained, women who are at risk for HIV are offered testing by a specially trained nurse or counselor. Because patients may be reluctant to discuss risk-taking behavior, routine screening should be offered to all women. Early detection permits early treatment to delay progression of the disease. The nurse plays a crucial role in educating patients about HIV and prevention of HIV infection and AIDS.

Use of antiretroviral therapy has been improving, but barriers to use of health services by disadvantaged women include lack of insurance, current drug use, and difficulty keeping appointments. Depression and abuse are issues that the nurse needs to assess in this population. Prevention of cervical neoplasia and PID need to be part of the teaching for women at risk. The nurse also needs to remember that many women do not see themselves as at risk for acquiring HIV infection.

Other issues that nurses need to be aware of in women who are at risk of HIV include the following:

- Frequent use of spermicides containing nonoxynol-9 may increase the risk of HIV transmission due to irritation.
- Some protease inhibitors lessen the effectiveness of oral contraceptives, particularly those containing ethinyl estradiol; therefore, condoms should be used because of reduced effectiveness of oral contraceptives.
- Plan B is an effective method of emergency contraception when needed (described in Chapter 46).
- Pregnancy does not seem to accelerate the course of HIV infection.
- Perinatal transmission risk is low with use of antiretroviral treatments and caesarean section. Breastfeeding is not recommended.
- Some advanced reproductive technologies can be used to reduce risk of transmission, including artificial insemination and sperm washing.
- Bacterial vaginosis, trichomoniasis, PID, and genital ulcers are common disorders among women who are HIV positive.

Structural Disorders

Fistulas of the Vagina

A **fistula** is an abnormal, tortuous opening between two internal hollow organs or between an internal hollow organ and the exterior of the body. The name of the fistula indicates the two areas that are connected abnormally: a vesicovaginal fistula is an opening between the bladder and the vagina, and a rectovaginal fistula is an opening between the rectum and the vagina (Fig. 47-2). Fistulas may be congenital in origin. However, in adults, breakdown usually occurs because of tissue damage resulting from injury sustained during surgery, vaginal delivery, radiation therapy, or disease processes such as carcinoma.

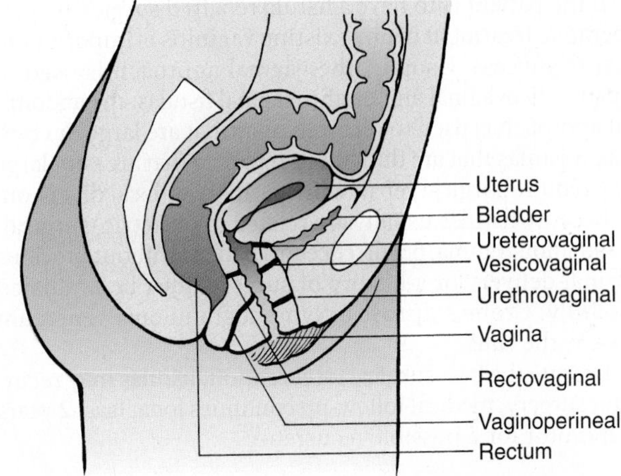

FIGURE 47-2. Common sites for vaginal fistulas: *Vesicovaginal*—bladder and vagina. *Urethrovaginal*—urethra and vagina. *Vaginoperineal*—vagina and perineal area. *Ureterovaginal*—ureter and vagina. *Rectovaginal*—rectum and vagina.

Clinical Manifestations

Symptoms depend on the specific defect. For example, in a patient with a vesicovaginal fistula, urine escapes continuously into the vagina. With a rectovaginal fistula, there is fecal incontinence, and flatus is discharged through the vagina. The combination of fecal discharge with leukorrhea results in malodor that is difficult to control.

Assessment and Diagnostic Findings

A history of the symptoms experienced by the patient is important to identify the structural alterations and to assess the impact of the symptoms on the patient's quality of life. In addition, the use of methylene blue dye helps delineate the course of the fistula. In vesicovaginal fistula, the dye is instilled into the bladder and appears in the vagina. After a negative methylene blue test result, indigo carmine is injected IV; the appearance of the dye in the vagina indicates a ureterovaginal fistula. Cystoscopy or IV pyelography may then be used to determine the exact location.

Medical Management

The goal is to eliminate the fistula and to treat infection and excoriation. A fistula may heal without surgical intervention, but surgery is often required. If the primary care provider determines that a fistula will heal without surgical intervention, care is planned to relieve discomfort, prevent infection, and improve the patient's self-concept and self-care abilities. Measures to promote healing include proper nutrition, cleansing douches and enemas, rest, and administration of prescribed intestinal antibiotics. A rectovaginal fistula heals faster when the patient eats a low-residue diet and when the affected tissue drains properly. Warm perineal irrigations promote healing.

Sometimes a fistula does not heal on its own and cannot be surgically repaired. In this situation, care must be planned and implemented on an individual basis. Cleanliness, frequent sitz baths, and deodorizing douches are required, as are perineal pads and protective undergarments. Meticulous skin care is necessary to prevent excoriation. Applying bland creams or lightly dusting with cornstarch may be soothing. In addition, attending to the patient's social and psychological needs is an essential aspect of care.

If the patient is to have a fistula repaired surgically, preoperative treatment of any existing vaginitis is important to ensure success. Usually, the vaginal approach is used to repair vesicovaginal and urethrovaginal fistulas; the abdominal approach is used to repair fistulas that are large or complex. Fistulas that are difficult to repair or that are very large may require surgical repair with a urinary or fecal diversion.

Because fistulas usually are related to obstetric, surgical, or radiation trauma, occurrence in a patient without previous vaginal delivery or a history of surgery must be evaluated carefully. Crohn's disease or lymphogranuloma venereum may be the cause.

Despite the best surgical intervention, fistulas may recur. After surgery, medical follow-up continues for at least 2 years to monitor for a possible recurrence.

Pelvic Organ Prolapse: Cystocele, Rectocele, Enterocele

Age and parity can put strain on the ligaments and structures that make up the female pelvis. Childbirth can result in tears of the levator sling musculature, resulting in structural weakness. Hormone deficiency also may play a role. Some degree of prolapse (weakening of the vaginal walls allowing the pelvic organs to descend and protrude into the vaginal canal) may be found in many older women. Risk factors include age, parity, and delivery of large babies (Nygaard, Bradley & Brandt, 2004).

Cystocele is a downward displacement of the bladder toward the vaginal orifice (Fig. 47-3) resulting from damage to the anterior vaginal support structures. It usually results from injury and strain during childbirth. The condition usually appears some years later when genital atrophy associated with aging occurs, but younger, multiparous, premenopausal women may also be affected.

Rectocele and perineal lacerations may affect the muscles and tissues of the pelvic floor and may occur during childbirth. Because of muscle tears below the vagina, the rectum may pouch upward, thereby pushing the posterior wall of the vagina forward. This structural abnormality is called a **rectocele.** Sometimes the lacerations may completely sever the fibers of the anal sphincter (complete tear). An enterocele is a protrusion of the intestinal wall into the vagina. Prolapse (if complete prolapse occurs, it may also be referred to as procidentia) results from a weakening of the support structures of the uterus itself; the cervix drops and may protrude from the vagina.

Clinical Manifestations

Because a cystocele causes the anterior vaginal wall to bulge downward, the patient may report a sense of pelvic pressure, fatigue, and urinary problems such as incontinence, frequency, and urgency. Back pain and pelvic pain may occur as well. The symptoms of rectocele resemble those of cystocele, with one exception: instead of urinary symptoms, patients may experience rectal pressure. Constipation, uncontrollable gas, and fecal incontinence may occur in patients with complete tears. Prolapse can result in feelings of pressure and ulcerations and bleeding. Dyspareunia may occur with these disorders.

Medical Management

Kegel exercises, which involve contracting or tightening the vaginal muscles, are prescribed to help strengthen these weakened muscles. The exercises are more effective in the early stages of a cystocele. Kegel exercises are easy to perform and are recommended for all women, including those with strong pelvic floor muscles (Chart 47-4).

Pessaries can be used to avoid surgery. This device is inserted into the vagina and positioned to keep an organ, such as the bladder, uterus, or intestine, properly aligned when a cystocele, rectocele, or prolapse has occurred. Pessaries are usually ring-shaped or doughnut-shaped and are made of various materials, such as rubber or plastic (Fig. 47-4). Rubber pessaries must be avoided in women with latex allergy. The size and type of pessary are selected and fitted by a gynecologic health care provider. The patient should have the pessary removed, examined, and cleaned by her health care provider at prescribed intervals. At these checkups, vaginal

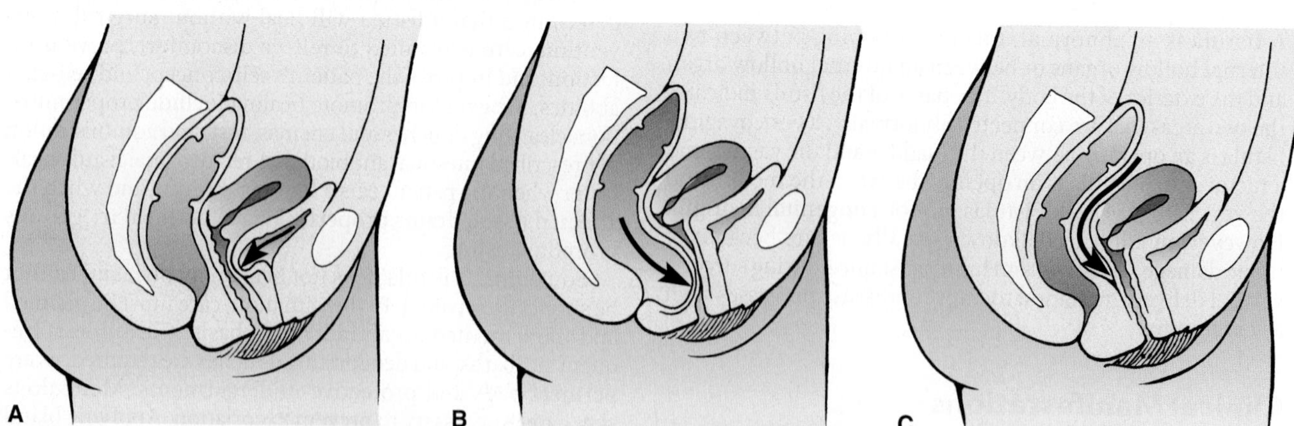

FIGURE 47-3. Diagrammatic representation of the three most common types of pelvic floor relaxation: (**A**) cystocele, (**B**) rectocele, and (**C**) enterocele. *Arrows* depict sites of maximum protrusion.

CHART 47-4

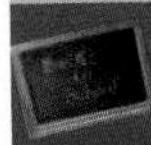

Patient Education

Performing Kegel (Pelvic Muscle) Exercises

Purposes: To strengthen and maintain the tone of the pubococcygeal muscle, which supports the pelvic organs; reduce or prevent stress incontinence and uterine prolapse; enhance sensation during sexual intercourse; and hasten postpartum healing

1. Become aware of pelvic muscle function by "drawing in" the perivaginal muscles and anal sphincter as if to control urine or defecation, but not contracting the abdominal, buttock, or inner thigh muscles.
2. Sustain contraction of the muscles for up to 10 seconds, followed by at least 10 seconds of relaxation.
3. Perform these exercises 30–80 times a day.

walls should be examined for pressure points or signs of irritation. Normally, the patient experiences no pain, discomfort, or discharge with a pessary, but if chronic irritation occurs, alternative measures may be needed.

Surgical Management

In many cases, surgery helps correct structural abnormalities. The procedure to repair the anterior vaginal wall is called anterior **colporrhaphy**, repair of a rectocele is called a posterior colporrhaphy, and repair of perineal lacerations is called a **perineorrhaphy**. These repairs are frequently performed laparoscopically, resulting in short hospital stays and good outcomes. A **laparoscope** is inserted through a small abdominal incision, the pelvis is visualized, and surgical repairs are performed.

Uterine Prolapse

Usually, the uterus and the cervix lie at right angles to the long axis of the vagina and with the body of the uterus inclined slightly forward. The uterus is normally freely movable on examination. Individual variations may result in an anterior, middle, or posterior uterine position. A backward positioning of the uterus, known as retroversion and retroflexion, is not uncommon (Fig. 47-5).

If the structures that support the uterus weaken (typically from childbirth), the uterus may work its way down the vaginal canal (prolapse) and even appear outside the vaginal orifice (procidentia) (Fig. 47-6). As the uterus descends, it may pull the vaginal walls and even the bladder and rectum with it. Symptoms include pressure and urinary problems (incontinence or retention) from displacement of the bladder. The problems are aggravated when a woman coughs, lifts a heavy object, or stands for a long time. Normal activities, even walking up stairs, may aggravate the problem.

Medical Management

Pessaries and surgery are two options for treatment. If surgery is the method of treatment used, the uterus is sutured back into place and repaired to strengthen and tighten the muscle bands. In postmenopausal women, the uterus may be removed (**hysterectomy**) or repaired by colpopexy. For elderly women or those who are too ill to tolerate surgery, pessaries may be the treatment of choice.

Nursing Management

Implementing Preventive Measures

Some problems related to "relaxed" pelvic muscles (cystocele, rectocele, and uterine prolapse) may be prevented. During pregnancy, early visits to the health care provider permit

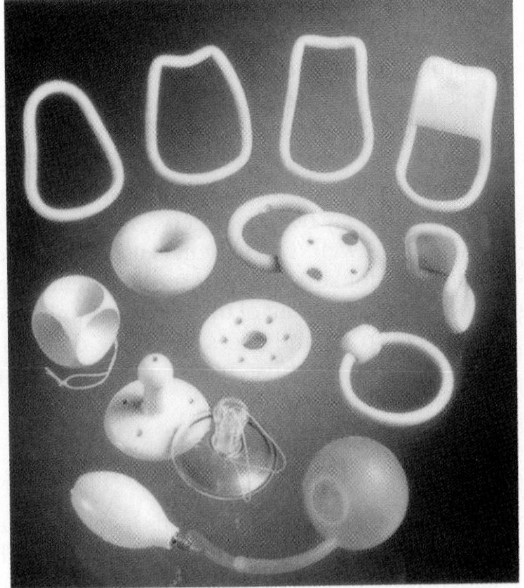

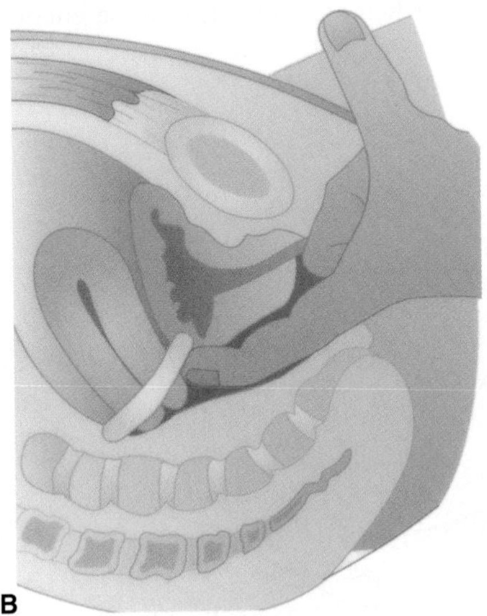

FIGURE 47-4. Examples of pessaries. (**A**) Various shapes and sizes of pessaries available. (**B**) Insertion of one type of pessary.

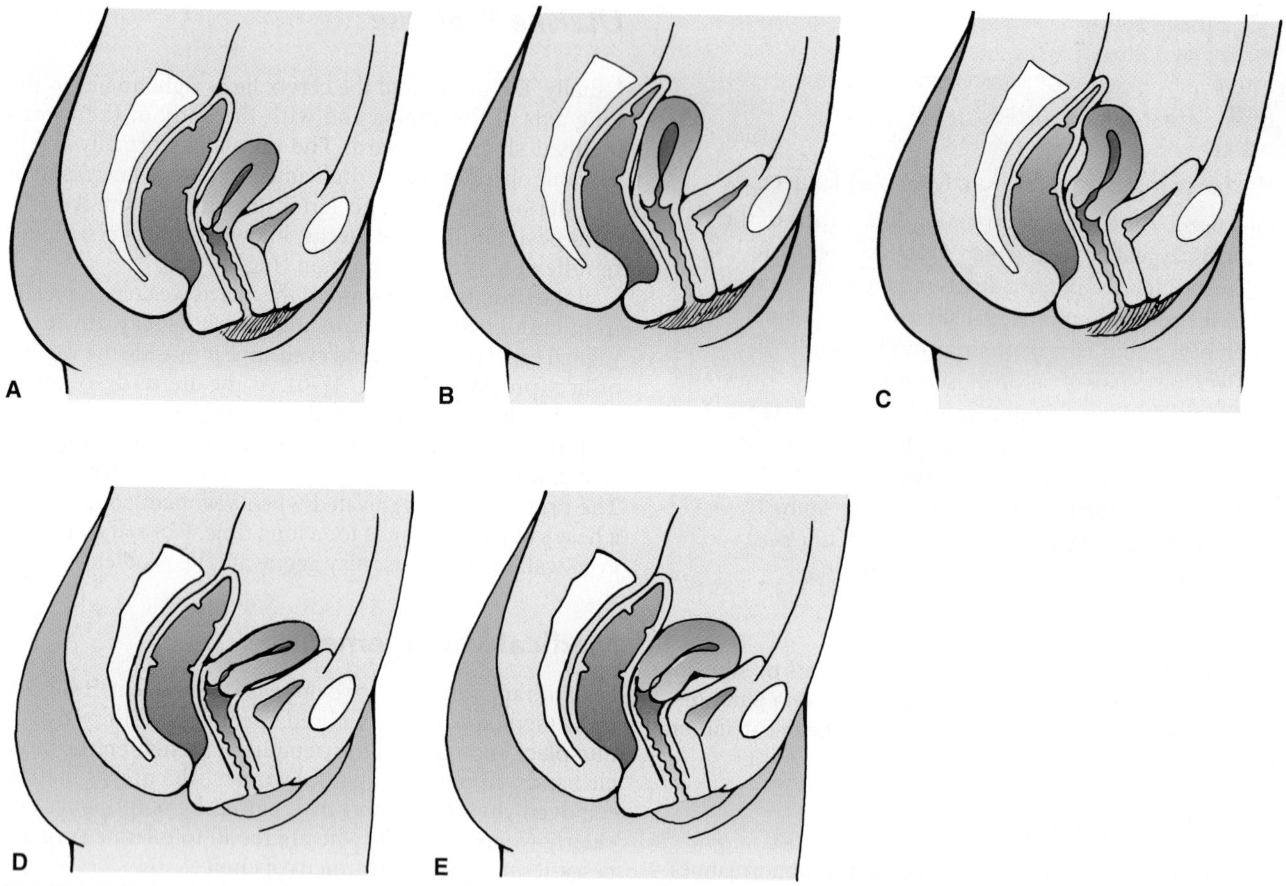

FIGURE 47-5. Positions of the uterus. (**A**) The most common position of the uterus detected on palpation. (**B**) In *retroversion* the uterus turns posteriorly as a whole unit. (**C**) In *retroflexion* the fundus bends posteriorly. (**D**) In *anteversion* the uterus tilts forward as a whole unit. (**E**) In *anteflexion* the uterus bends anteriorly.

early detection of problems. During the postpartum period, the woman can be taught to perform Kegel exercises to strengthen the muscles that support the uterus.

Delays in obtaining evaluation and treatment may result in complications such as infection, cervical ulceration, cystitis, and hemorrhoids. The nurse encourages the patient to obtain prompt treatment for these structural disorders.

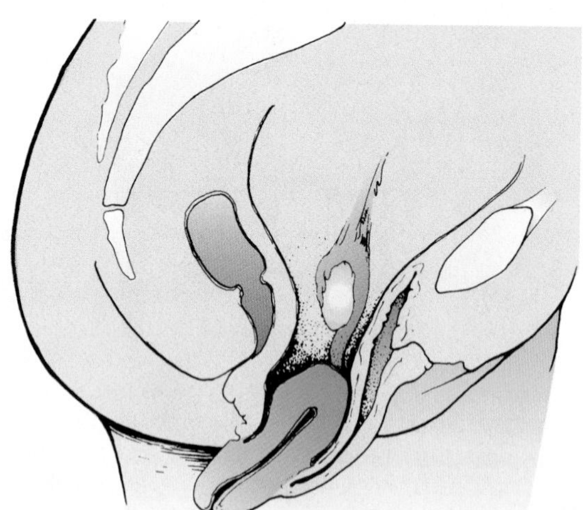

FIGURE 47-6. Complete prolapse of the uterus through the introitus.

Implementing Preoperative Nursing Care

Before surgery, the patient needs to know the extent of the proposed surgery, the expectations for the postoperative period, and the effect of surgery on future sexual function. In addition, the patient having a rectocele repair needs to know that before surgery, a laxative and a cleansing enema may be prescribed. She may be asked to administer these at home the day before surgery. A perineal shave may be prescribed as well. The patient is usually placed in a lithotomy position for surgery, with special attention given to moving both legs in and out of the stirrups simultaneously to prevent muscle strain and excess pressure on the legs and thighs. Other preoperative interventions are similar to those described in Chapter 18.

Initiating Postoperative Nursing Care

Immediate postoperative goals include preventing infection and pressure on any existing suture line. This may require perineal care and may preclude using dressings. The patient is encouraged to void within a few hours after surgery for cystocele and complete tear. If the patient does not void within this period and reports discomfort or pain in the bladder region after 6 hours, she will need to be catheterized. Some physicians prefer to leave an indwelling catheter in place for 2 to 4 days, so some women may return home with a catheter in place. Various other bladder care methods are described in Chapter 44. After each voiding or bowel movement, the perineum is cleansed with warm, sterile saline solution and dried with sterile absorbent material if a perineal incision has been made.

After an external perineal repair, several methods are used in caring for the sutures. In one method, the sutures are left alone until healing occurs (in 5 to 10 days). Thereafter, daily vaginal douches with sterile saline solution may be administered during recovery. In another method—the wet method—small, sterile saline douches are administered twice daily, beginning on the day after surgery and continuing throughout recovery. A heat lamp or hair dryer may be used to help dry the area and promote healing. Commercially available sprays containing combined antiseptic and anesthetic solutions are soothing and effective, and an ice pack applied locally may relieve discomfort. However, the weight of the ice bag must rest on the bed, not on the patient.

Routine postoperative care is similar to that given after abdominal surgery. The patient is positioned in bed with her head and knees elevated slightly. The patient may go home the day of or the day after surgery; the duration of the hospital stay depends on the surgical approach used.

After surgery for a complete perineal laceration (through the rectal sphincter), special care and attention are required. The bladder is drained through the catheter to prevent strain on the sutures. Throughout recovery, stool-softening agents are administered nightly after the patient begins a soft diet.

Promoting Home and Community-Based Care

TEACHING PATIENTS SELF-CARE

Predischarge instructions include information pertaining to the gynecologist's postoperative instructions related to douching, using mild laxatives, performing exercise as recommended, and avoiding lifting heavy objects or standing for prolonged periods. The patient is instructed to report any pelvic pain, unusual discharge, inability to carry out personal hygiene, and vaginal bleeding.

CONTINUING CARE

The patient is advised to continue with perineal exercises, which are recommended to improve muscle strength and tone. She is reminded to return to the gynecologist for a follow-up visit and to consult with the physician about when it is safe to resume sexual intercourse.

Benign Disorders

Vulvitis, an inflammation of the vulva, may occur with other disorders, such as diabetes, dermatologic problems, or poor hygiene, or it may be secondary to irritation from a vaginal discharge related to a specific vaginitis.

Vulvodynia is a chronic syndrome of vulvar discomfort. Symptoms may include burning, stinging, irritation, or excoriation. It has been described as primary, with onset at first tampon insertion or sexual experience, or secondary, beginning months or years after first tampon insertion or sexual experience. It may be classified as organic if it has a known cause (infection, trauma, or irritants) or idiopathic if no cause is known. It seems to be similar to a peripheral neuralgia and may respond to treatment with tricyclic antidepressants. Etiology is unknown.

Cyclic vulvitis is a subset of vulvodynia and is characterized by episodes of vulvar discomfort. Typical complaints are recurrent itching and burning, often worsening with menses and after sexual intercourse. Erythema and swelling may occur. It is often related to candidal infection, and fungal cultures are often positive. There are two types of vulvodynia: vulvar vestibulitis and dysesthetic vulvodynia (Edwards, 2003). Vulvar **vestibulitis** syndrome is a chronic persistence of severe pain on touch to the vestibular area or attempted vaginal entry, and physical findings of vestibular erythema. Treatment methods vary. Research is ongoing to identify treatment for vulvar vestibulitis, but topical treatments (ie, estrogens, corticosteroids, trichloroacetic acid), surgery, and interferon have been used. Biofeedback has also been used. The pain of dysesthetic vulvodynia is not limited to the vestibule and can occur without touch or pressure.

Vulvar Cysts

Bartholin's cyst results from the obstruction of a duct in one of the paired vestibular glands located in the posterior third of the vulva, near the vestibule. This cyst is the most common of vulvar tumors. A simple cyst may be asymptomatic, but an infected cyst or abscess may cause discomfort. Infection may be due to a gonococcal organism, *Escherichia coli,* or *Staphylococcus aureus* and can cause an abscess with or without involving the inguinal lymph nodes. Skene's duct cysts may result in pressure, dyspareunia, altered urinary stream, and pain, especially if infection is present. Vestibular cysts, located inferior to the hymen, may also occur. Cysts can be treated by resection or with laser, ablation with silver nitrate and puncture (Marzano & Haefner, 2004). Asymptomatic cysts do not require treatment. Malignancy can occur, usually in women older than 50 years of age, so drainage and biopsy may be considered.

Medical Management

The usual treatment for a Bartholin's cyst is incision and drainage followed by antibiotic therapy. If a cyst is asymptomatic, treatment is unnecessary. Moist heat or sitz baths may promote drainage and resolution. If surgery is necessary, a Word Bartholin gland catheter is usually used. This catheter, a short latex stem with an inflatable bulb at the distal end, creates a tract that preserves the gland and allows for drainage. A nonopioid analgesic agent may be administered before this outpatient procedure. A local anesthetic agent is injected, and the cyst is incised or lanced and irrigated with normal saline; the catheter is inserted and inflated with 2 to 3 mL of water. The catheter stem is then tucked into the vagina to allow freedom of movement. The catheter is left in place for 4 to 6 weeks until the tract reepithelializes. The patient is informed that discharge should be expected, as the catheter allows drainage of the cyst. She is instructed to contact her primary health care provider if pain occurs because the bulb may be too large for the cavity and fluid may need to be removed. Routine hygiene is encouraged.

Skene's duct cysts can be excised or drained with a Word catheter. Vestibular cysts are excised if symptomatic.

Vulvar Dystrophy

Vulvar dystrophy is a condition found in older women that causes dry, thickened skin on the vulva or slightly raised, whitish papules, fissures, or macules. Symptoms usually consist of varying degrees of itching, but some patients have no symptoms. A few patients with vulvar cancer have associated dystrophy (vulvar cancer is discussed later in this chapter). Biopsy with careful follow-up is the standard intervention. Benign dystrophies include lichen planus, simplex chronicus, **lichen sclerosus**, squamous cell hyperplasia, vulvar vestibulitis, and other dermatoses.

Medical Management

Topical corticosteroids (ie, hydrocortisone creams) are the usual treatment. Petrolatum jelly may relieve pruritus. Use is decreased as symptoms resolve. Topical corticosteroids are effective in treating squamous cell hyperplasia. Treatment is often complete in 2 to 3 weeks; this condition is not likely to recur after treatment is complete.

If malignant cells are detected on biopsy, local excision, laser therapy, local chemotherapy, and immunologic treatment are used. Vulvectomy is avoided, if possible, to spare the patient from the stress of disfigurement and possible sexual dysfunction.

Nursing Management

Key nursing responsibilities for patients with vulvar dystrophies focus on teaching. Important topics include hygiene and self-monitoring for signs and symptoms of complications.

Promoting Home and Community-Based Care

TEACHING PATIENTS SELF-CARE

Instructions for patients with benign vulvar dystrophies include the importance of maintaining good personal hygiene and keeping the vulva dry. Lanolin or hydrogenated vegetable oil is recommended for relief of dryness. Sitz baths may help but should not be overused because dryness may result or increase. The patient is instructed to notify her primary health care provider about any change or ulceration, because biopsy may be necessary to rule out squamous cell carcinoma.

By encouraging all patients to perform genital self-examinations regularly and have any itching, lesions, or unusual symptoms assessed by a health care provider, nurses can help prevent complications and progression of vulvar lesions.

Ovarian Cysts

The ovary is a common site for cysts, which may be simple enlargements of normal ovarian constituents, the graafian follicle, or the corpus luteum, or they may arise from abnormal growth of the ovarian epithelium. About 98% of cysts that occur in women 29 years of age and younger are benign. In women older than 50 years of age, only 50% of these cysts are benign.

Dermoid cysts are tumors that are thought to arise from parts of the ovum that normally disappear with ripening (maturation). Their origin is undefined, and they consist of undifferentiated embryonal cells. They grow slowly and are found during surgery to contain a thick, yellow, sebaceous material arising from the skin lining. Hair, teeth, bone, and many other tissues are found in a rudimentary state within these cysts. Dermoid cysts are only one type of lesion that may develop. Many other types can occur, and treatment usually depends on the type.

The patient may or may not report acute or chronic abdominal pain. Symptoms of a ruptured cyst mimic various acute abdominal emergencies, such as appendicitis or ectopic pregnancy. Larger cysts may produce abdominal swelling and exert pressure on adjacent abdominal organs.

Polycystic ovary syndrome (PCOS) is a complex endocrine condition involving a disorder in the hypothalamic–pituitary and ovarian network or axis resulting in chronic anovulation and androgen excess. It occurs in approximately 4% of women of childbearing age (Guzick, 2004). Characteristics include insulin resistance, hyperandrogenism, and altered gonadotropin dynamics. Symptoms are related to androgen excess. Irregular periods resulting from lack of regular ovulation, infertility, obesity, and hirsutism may be presenting complaints. Cysts form in the ovaries because the hormonal milieu cannot cause ovulation on a regular basis. Onset may occur at menarche or later. When pregnancy is desired, medications to stimulate ovulation are often effective. Women with PCOS may develop insulin resistance and metabolic syndrome and may be at higher risk for diabetes and cardiac disorders in later life. Clomid (Clomiphene) is often used to induce ovulation when pregnancy is desired. Metformin (Glucophage) is also used to decrease the hyperinsulinemia that occurs with PCOS.

Medical Management

The treatment of large ovarian cysts is usually surgical removal. However, oral contraceptives may be used in young, healthy patients to suppress ovarian activity and resolve small cysts that appear to be fluid-filled or physiologic. Oral contraceptives are also usually prescribed to treat PCOS. Weight management is often part of the treatment plan.

Postoperative nursing care after surgery to remove an ovarian cyst is similar to that after abdominal surgery, with one exception. The marked decrease in intra-abdominal pressure resulting from removal of a large cyst usually leads to considerable abdominal distention. This complication may be prevented to some extent by applying a snug-fitting abdominal binder.

Some surgeons discuss the option of a hysterectomy when a woman is undergoing bilateral ovary removal because of a suspicious mass; it may increase life expectancy, avoid a later second surgery, and save on health care costs. It is preventive in that future cancer is avoided, as is benign disease that might require hysterectomy. Patient preference is a priority in determining its appropriateness.

Benign Tumors of the Uterus: Fibroids (Leiomyomas, Myomas)

Myomatous or **fibroid tumors** of the uterus are estimated to occur in 20% to 40% of women during their reproductive years. It is thought that women are genetically predisposed to develop this condition, which is almost always benign. Fibroids arise from the muscle tissue of the uterus and can be solitary or multiple, in the lining (intracavitary), muscle wall (intramural), and outside surface (serosal) of the uterus. They develop slowly in women between 25 and 40 years of age and may become large. A growth spurt with enlargement of the fibroid tumor may occur in the decade before menopause, possibly related to anovulatory cycles and high levels of unopposed estrogen. Fibroids are a common reason for hysterectomy, because they often result in menorrhagia that can be difficult to control.

Clinical Manifestations

Fibroids may cause no symptoms, or they may produce abnormal vaginal bleeding. Other symptoms are due to pressure on the surrounding organs and include pain, backache, pressure, bloating, constipation, and urinary problems. Menorrhagia (excessive bleeding) and metrorrhagia (irregular bleeding) may occur because fibroids may distort the uterine lining (Fig. 47-7). Fibroids may interfere with fertility.

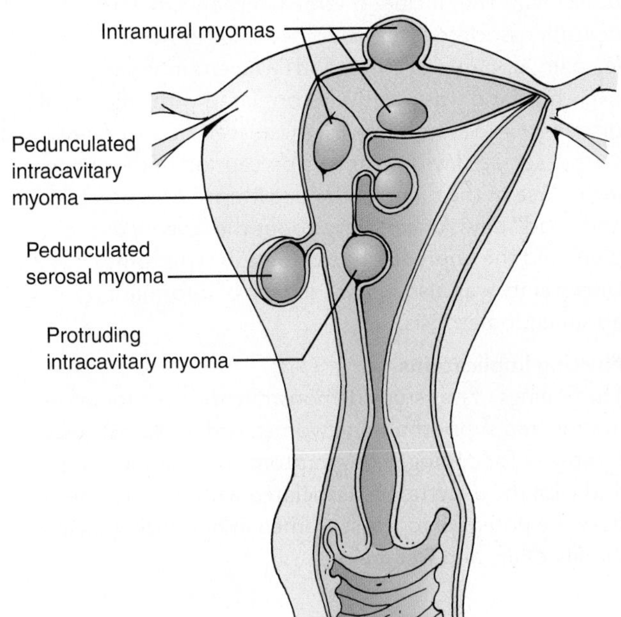

FIGURE 47-7. Myomas (fibroids). Those that impinge on the uterine cavity are called intracavitary myomas.

Medical Management

Treatment of uterine fibroids may include medical or surgical intervention and depends to a large extent on the size, symptoms, and location, as well as the woman's age and her reproductive plans. Fibroids usually shrink and disappear during menopause, when estrogen is no longer produced. Simple observation and follow-up may be all the management that is necessary. The patient with minor symptoms is closely monitored. If she plans to have children, treatment is as conservative as possible. As a rule, large tumors that produce pressure symptoms should be removed (**myomectomy**). The uterus may be removed (hysterectomy) if symptoms are bothersome and childbearing is completed (see later discussion of nursing care for a patient having a hysterectomy).

Several other alternatives to hysterectomy have been developed for the treatment of excessive bleeding due to fibroids. These include the following:

- Hysteroscopic resection of myomas: a laser is used through a hysteroscope passed through the cervix; no incision or overnight stay is needed
- Laparoscopic myomectomy: removal of a fibroid through a laparoscope inserted through a small abdominal incision
- Laparoscopic myolysis: a laser or electrical needles are used to cauterize and shrink the fibroid
- Laparoscopic cryomyolysis: electric current is used to coagulate the fibroid
- Uterine artery embolization (UAE), polyvinyl alcohol or gelatin particles are injected into the blood vessels that supply the fibroid via the femoral artery, resulting in infarction and resultant shrinkage. This percutaneous image–guided therapy offers an alternative to hormone therapy or surgery. UAE may result in infrequent but serious complications such as pain, infection, amenorrhea, necrosis and bleeding. Although rare, deaths and ovarian failure have been reported (Wallach & Vlahos, 2004). UAE is normally used in women who have completed childbearing. Women need to consider this procedure and its possible complications carefully, especially if they have not completed childbearing (American College of Obstetricians and Gynecologists [ACOG], 2004).

Medications (eg, leuprolide [Lupron]) or other GnRH analogs, which induce a temporary menopause-like environment, may be prescribed to shrink the fibroids. This treatment consists of monthly injections, which may cause hot flashes and vaginal dryness. Treatment is usually short term (ie, before surgery) to shrink the fibroids, allowing easier surgery, and to alleviate anemia, which may occur due to heavy menstrual flow. This treatment is short term because it leads to vasomotor symptoms and loss of bone density.

Antifibrotic agents are under investigation for long-term treatment of fibroids. Mifepristone (RU-486, Mifeprex), a progesterone antagonist, has also been prescribed; it appears to be effective but can result in endometrial hyperplasia. Progestins have been reported to be effective. Norethindrone (Aygestin) and medroxyprogesterone acetate (Provera) are used (Wallach & Vlahos, 2004).

Endometriosis

Endometriosis is a chronic disease that affects between 5% to 15% of women of reproductive age. It is a benign lesion or lesions with cells similar to those lining the uterus growing aberrantly in the pelvic cavity outside the uterus. Often, extensive endometriosis causes few symptoms, whereas an isolated lesion may produce severe symptoms. It is a major cause of chronic pelvic pain and infertility. In order of frequency, pelvic endometriosis involves the ovary, uterosacral ligaments, cul-de-sac, rectovaginal septum, uterovesical peritoneum, cervix, outer surface of the uterus, umbilicus, laparotomy scar tissue, hernial sacs, and appendix.

Endometriosis has been diagnosed more frequently as a result of the increased use of laparoscopy, but diagnosis can be delayed, and women with this problem often feel as if their complaints are being dismissed. Before laparoscopy became widely available, major surgery was necessary before a diagnosis could be made. There is a high incidence among patients who bear children late and among those who have fewer children. In countries where tradition favors early marriage and early childbearing, endometriosis is rare. There also appears to be a familial predisposition to endometriosis; it is more common in women whose close female relatives are affected. Other factors that may suggest increased risk include a shorter menstrual cycle (less than every 27 days), flow longer than 7 days, outflow obstruction, and younger age at menarche. Characteristically, endometriosis is found in young, nulliparous women between 25 and 35 years of age. It is also found in adolescents, particularly those with dysmenorrhea that does not respond to nonsteroidal anti-inflammatory drugs (NSAIDs) or oral contraceptives.

Pathophysiology

Misplaced endometrial tissue responds to and depends on ovarian hormonal stimulation. During menstruation, this ectopic tissue bleeds, mostly into areas having no outlet, which causes pain and adhesions. The lesions are typically small and puckered, with a blue/brown/gray powder-burn appearance and brown or blue-black appearance, indicating concealed bleeding. They may also have an atypical appearance as red, white, petechial, and reddish-brown implants.

Endometrial tissue contained within an ovarian cyst has no outlet for the bleeding; this formation is referred to as a pseudocyst or chocolate cyst. Adhesions, cysts, and scar tissue may result, causing pain and infertility. Endometriosis has been found in many body organs (Lemaire, 2004), and its etiology is unclear.

NURSING RESEARCH PROFILE

Women's Views of Endometriosis

Lemaire, G. S. (2004). More than just menstrual cramps: Symptoms and uncertainty among women with endometriosis. *Journal of Obstetric, Gynecologic and Neonatal Nursing, 33*(1), 71–79.

Purpose

Although endometriosis is a fairly common disorder of the female reproductive tract, its effects on women's lives are not well known. The purpose of this study was to examine women's reported symptoms of endometriosis and to explore the relationships among these symptoms and the women's emotional distress, uncertainty, and preferences for information about the disease.

Design

A cross-sectional, descriptive correlational design was used to investigate the relationships among symptoms, distress, uncertainty, and preferences for information. The convenience sample consisted of 298 women who had received a diagnosis of endometriosis. Investigator-developed instruments included an endometriosis symptom checklist, adequacy of information survey, and a 15-item Feelings and Reactions (FAR) scale. In addition, the Mishel Uncertainty in Illness Scale-Community form and a modification of the Krantz Health Opinion Survey Information Subscale were completed by the women.

Findings

Women reported multiple symptoms; the most common were fatigue, menstrual cramping, and nonmenstrual pelvic pain. They included some symptoms that are not typically associated with endometriosis (eg, joint pain, leg pain, urinary tract infection). Uncertainty was relatively high and was positively correlated with emotional distress ($r = .37$, $p < .001$). Highest levels of uncertainty were associated with women's perception of the changing course of their illness, the occurrence of "good" and "bad" days, uncertainty about the severity of the pain, and the unpredictable change in symptoms. Uncertainty was also related to lack of information about endometriosis.

Nursing Implications

The findings of this study demonstrate the need for information and support among women with endometriosis. Strategies for coping with symptoms of endometriosis and with the uncertainty associated with this disorder have the potential to assist women in optimizing their quality of life and well-being.

Currently the best-accepted theory regarding the origin of endometrial lesions is the transplantation theory, which suggests that a backflow of menses (retrograde menstruation) transports endometrial tissue to ectopic sites through the fallopian tubes. Transplantation of tissue can also occur during surgery if endometrial tissue is transferred inadvertently by way of surgical instruments. Retrograde menstruation has been found to occur in many women, not just those with endometriosis. Why some women develop this condition and others do not is unknown. Endometrial tissue can also be spread by lymphatic or venous channels.

Clinical Manifestations

Symptoms vary but include dysmenorrhea, dyspareunia, and pelvic discomfort or pain. Dyschezia (pain with bowel movements) and radiation of pain to the back or leg may occur. Depression, loss of work due to pain, and relationship difficulties may result. Infertility may occur because of fibrosis and adhesions or because of a variety of substances (prostaglandins, cytokines, other factors) produced by the implants.

Assessment and Diagnostic Findings

A health history, including an account of the menstrual pattern, is necessary to elicit specific symptoms. On bimanual pelvic examination, fixed tender nodules are sometimes palpated, and uterine mobility may be limited, indicating adhesions. Laparoscopic examination confirms the diagnosis and helps stage the disease. In stage 1, patients have superficial or minimal lesions; stage 2, mild involvement; stage 3, moderate involvement; and stage 4, extensive involvement and dense adhesions, with obliteration of the cul-de-sac.

Medical Management

Treatment depends on the symptoms, the patient's desire for pregnancy, and the extent of the disease. If the woman does not have symptoms, routine examination may be all that is required. Other therapy for varying degrees of symptoms may be NSAIDs, oral contraceptives, GnRH agonists, or surgery. Pregnancy often alleviates symptoms because neither ovulation nor menstruation occurs.

Pharmacologic Therapy

Palliative measures include use of medications, such as analgesic agents and prostaglandin inhibitors, for pain. Hormonal therapy is effective in suppressing endometriosis and relieving dysmenorrhea (menstrual pain). Oral contraceptives are used frequently. Side effects that may occur with oral contraceptives include fluid retention, weight gain, or nausea. These can usually be managed by changing brands or formulations. Depo-Provera, an injectable contraceptive agent, may also be used.

Several types of hormonal therapy are also available in addition to oral contraceptives. A synthetic androgen, danazol (Danocrine), causes atrophy of the endometrium and subsequent amenorrhea. The medication inhibits the release of gonadotropin with minimal overt sex hormone stimulation. The drawbacks of this medication are that it is expensive and may cause troublesome side effects such as fatigue, depression, weight gain, oily skin, decreased breast size, mild acne, hot flashes, and vaginal atrophy. GnRH agonists decrease estrogen production and cause subsequent amenorrhea. Side effects are related to low estrogen levels (eg, hot flashes and vaginal dryness). Loss of bone density is often offset by concurrent use of estrogen. Leuprolide (Lupron), an GnRH agonist, is injected monthly to suppress hormones, induce an artificial menopause, and thereby avoid menstrual effects and relieve endometriosis. Some clinicians prescribe a combination of therapies. Most women continue treatment despite side effects, and symptoms diminish for 80% to 90% of women with mild to moderate endometriosis. Hormonal medications are not used in patients with a history of abnormal vaginal bleeding or liver, heart, or kidney disease. Bone density is followed carefully because of the risk of bone loss; hormone therapy is usually short-term.

Assisted reproductive techniques may be warranted and effective in women with infertility secondary to endometriosis (Olive & Pritts, 2002).

Surgical Management

If conservative measures are not helpful, surgery may be necessary to relieve pain and enhance the possibility of pregnancy. Surgery may be combined with use of medical therapy. The procedure selected depends on the patient. Laparoscopy may be used to fulgurate (cut with high-frequency current) endometrial implants and to release adhesions. Laser surgery is another option made possible by laparoscopy. Laser therapy vaporizes or coagulates the endometrial implants, thereby destroying this tissue. Other surgical options include endocoagulation and electrocoagulation, laparotomy, abdominal hysterectomy, **oophorectomy**, bilateral **salpingo-oophorectomy**, and appendectomy. For women older than 35 years of age or those willing to sacrifice reproductive capability, total hysterectomy is an option. Endometriosis recurs in many women.

Nursing Management

The health history and physical examination focus on specific symptoms (eg, pain) and when and how long they have been bothersome, the effect of prescribed medications, and the woman's reproductive plans. This information helps in determining the treatment plan. Explaining the various diagnostic procedures may help to alleviate the patient's anxiety. Patient goals include relief of pain, dysmenorrhea, dyspareunia, and avoidance of infertility.

As the treatment progresses, the woman with endometriosis and her partner may find that pregnancy is not easily possible, and the psychosocial impact of this realization must be recognized and addressed. Alternatives, such as in vitro fertilization or adoption, may be discussed at an appropriate time and referrals offered.

The nurse's role in patient education is to dispel myths and encourage the patient to seek care if dysmenorrhea or dyspareunia occurs. The Endometriosis Association (listed at the end of this chapter) is a helpful resource for patients seeking further information and support for this condition, which can cause disabling pain and severe emotional distress.

Chronic Pelvic Pain

Chronic pelvic pain is a common disorder of women that may be related to several of the previously discussed gynecologic disorders. Fifteen to 20% of women have chronic pelvic pain—that is, pelvic pain that persists for more than 6 months. It may be cyclic or intermittent and noncyclic. Causes may be reproductive, genitourinary, or gastrointestinal. A history of abuse, PID, endometriosis, interstitial cystitis, musculoskeletal disorders, irritable bowel syndrome, and previous surgery resulting in abdominal adhesions may be associated with chronic pelvic pain.

Chronic pelvic pain is often difficult to treat. Treatment depends on physical and diagnostic test results and may include antidepressants, analgesics, oral contraceptives, GnRH agonists, exercise, and surgery.

Adenomyosis

In adenomyosis, the tissue that lines the endometrium invades the uterine wall. The incidence is highest in women 40 to 50 years of age. Symptoms include hypermenorrhea (excessive and prolonged bleeding), acquired dysmenorrhea, polymenorrhea (abnormally frequent bleeding), and premenstrual staining. Physical examination findings on palpation include an enlarged, firm, and tender uterus. Treatment depends on the severity of bleeding and pain. Hysterectomy may offer greater relief than more conservative therapies.

Endometrial Hyperplasia

This condition, a build-up of endometrial tissue, is a precursor to endometrial cancer and often results from unopposed estrogen from any source. Estrogen alone without progesterone in a woman with a uterus can cause this condition. Women with anovulatory cycles, PCOS, or obesity may all have high circulating levels of estrogen. Tamoxifen may also be a causative factor. Diagnosis is by biopsy or ultrasound findings of thickness of the endometrium. Hyperplasia with atypia on a pathology or biopsy report indicates risk for progression. Progestin treatment may be effective but hysterectomy may be advised if a woman has atypia on Pap smear and is postmenopausal. Abnormal bleeding is the most common symptom.

Malignant Conditions

The estimated incidence and estimated mortality for female reproductive cancers in the United States are (American Cancer Society, 2006),

- Cervical cancer: about 9,710 new cases and 3,700 deaths
- Uterine cancer: about 41,200 new cases and 7,350 deaths
- Ovarian cancer: about 20,180 new cases and 15,310 deaths
- Vaginal cancer: about 2,420 new cases and 820 deaths
- Vulvar cancer: about 3,740 new cases and 880 deaths

Cervical cancer is the second most prevalent cancer in women worldwide and the fifth leading cause of cancer deaths. Worldwide, the incidence is declining. Pap smears in developed countries have resulted in increased detection of preinvasive lesions and decreased cancer death rates. Eighty percent of all cases of cervical cancer are found in developing countries, where early detection methods are often not available.

Although death rates for cancer are decreasing in the United States and other developed countries, cancer in developing countries is increasing. Many of these cases affect women. Although infectious diseases and HIV are often high priorities in these countries, the toll of increasing malignancies needs to be considered where 80% of cervical cancer deaths occur. HPV vaccine may be helpful in reducing the incidence of HPV and cervical cancer.

Although some cancers are difficult to detect or prevent, annual pelvic examination with a Pap smear is a painless and relatively inexpensive method of early detection. Health care providers can encourage women to follow this health practice by providing non-stressful examinations that are educational and supportive and offering an opportunity for patients to ask questions and clarify misinformation. If more women understood that the gynecologic examination and Pap smear do not have to be uncomfortable or embarrassing, early detection rates would likely improve, and lives would be saved.

Many women diagnosed with gynecologic malignancy experience depression and anxiety. The occurrence of physical symptoms has been shown to increase psychological distress (Fowler, Carpenter, Gupta, et al., 2004). Intervention directed toward physical and psychological symptoms requires a multidisciplinary approach.

Nurses should be aware of ongoing clinical trials that are being conducted to identify effective treatments for many conditions. They are often in a position to answer questions about clinical trials and to encourage patients to consider participation if appropriate. Participation in cancer research varies but enrollment is low for all patient groups. This may be due in part to women being unaware of ongoing relevant research and the potential for improved health status (Murthy, Krumholz, & Gross, 2004).

Cancer of the Cervix

Carcinoma of the cervix is predominantly squamous cell cancer. Cervical cancer is less common than it once was because of early detection of cell changes by Pap smear. However, it is still the third most common female reproductive cancer and affects more than 10,000 women in the United States every year (American Cancer Society, 2005). Risk factors are presented in Chart 47-5.

Pap screening can identify preinvasive lesions and prevent cancer (Benard et al., 2004). Preventive measures include

CHART 47-5

Risk Factors for Cervical Cancer

- Sexual activity:
  Multiple sex partners
  Early age (younger than 20) at first coitus (exposes the vulnerable young cervix to potential viruses from a partner)
- Sex with uncircumcised males
- Sexual contact with males whose partners have had cervical cancer
- Early childbearing
- Exposure to human papillomavirus
- HIV infection and other causes of immunodeficiency
- Smoking and exposure to secondhand smoke
- Exposure to diethylstilbestrol (DES) in utero
- Family history of cervical cancer
- Low socioeconomic status (may be related to early marriage and early childbearing)
- Nutritional deficiencies (folate, beta-carotene, and vitamin C levels are lower in women with cervical cancer than in women without it)
- Chronic cervical infection
- Overweight status

regular pelvic examinations and Pap tests for all women, especially older women past childbearing age (decreases the chance of dying from cervical cancer from 1 in 250 to 1 in 2,000). In developing countries with limited resources, the American College of Obstetrics and Gynecology (ACOG) advocates visible inspection with acetic acid followed by cryotherapy (ACOG, Cervical Cancer Prevention, 2004). Preventive counseling should include delaying first intercourse, avoiding HPV infection, education about reproductive health and safer sex, smoking cessation, and considering HPV immunization.

Clinical Manifestations

There are several different types of cervical cancer. Most cancers originate in squamous cells, while the remainder are adenocarcinomas or mixed adenosquamous carcinomas. Adenocarcinomas begin in mucus-producing glands and are often due to HPV infection. Most cervical cancers, if not detected and treated, spread to regional pelvic lymph nodes, and local recurrence is not uncommon. Early cervical cancer rarely produces symptoms. If symptoms are present, they may go unnoticed as a thin watery vaginal discharge often noticed after intercourse or douching. When symptoms such as discharge, irregular bleeding, or pain or bleeding after sexual intercourse occur, the disease may be advanced. Advanced disease should not occur if all women have access to gynecologic care and avail themselves of it. The nurse's role in access and utilization is crucial and may prevent the delay of detection of cervical cancer until the advanced stage.

In advanced cervical cancer, the vaginal discharge gradually increases and becomes watery and, finally, dark and foul-smelling from necrosis and infection of the tumor. The bleeding, which occurs at irregular intervals between periods (metrorrhagia) or after menopause, may be slight (just enough to spot the undergarments) and occurs usually after mild trauma or pressure (eg, intercourse, douching, or bearing down during defecation). As the disease continues, the bleeding may persist and increase. Leg pain, dysuria, rectal bleeding, and edema of the extremities signal advanced disease.

As the cancer advances, it may invade the tissues outside the cervix, including the lymph glands anterior to the sacrum. In one-third of patients with invasive cervical cancer, the disease involves the fundus. The nerves in this region may be affected, producing excruciating pain in the back and the legs that is relieved only by large doses of opioid analgesic agents. If the disease progresses, it often produces extreme emaciation and anemia, usually accompanied by fever due to secondary infection and abscesses in the ulcerating mass, and by fistula formation. Because the survival rate for in situ cancer is 100% and the rate for women with more advanced stages of cervical cancer decreases dramatically, early detection is essential.

Assessment and Diagnostic Findings

Diagnosis may be made on the basis of abnormal Pap smear results, followed by biopsy results identifying severe dysplasia (cervical intraepithelial neoplasia type III [CIN III], high-grade squamous intraepithelial lesions [HGSIL] [also referred to as HSIL], or carcinoma in situ; see below). HPV infections are usually implicated in these conditions. Biopsy results may indicate carcinoma in situ. Carcinoma in situ is technically classified as severe dysplasia and is defined as cancer that has extended through the full thickness of the epithelium of the cervix, but not beyond. This is often referred to as preinvasive cancer.

In its very early stages, invasive cervical cancer is found microscopically by Pap smear. In later stages, pelvic examination may reveal a large, reddish growth or a deep, ulcerating lesion. The patient may report spotting or bloody discharge.

When the patient has been diagnosed with invasive cervical cancer, clinical staging estimates the extent of the disease so that treatment can be planned more specifically and prognosis reasonably predicted. Adopted by the International Federation of Gynecology and Obstetrics and included in the NIH Consensus Conference on Cervical Cancer (1996), the TNM (tumor, nodes, and metastases) system is the most widely used staging system. The TNM classification is also used in describing cancer stages. In this system, T refers to the extent of the primary tumor, N to lymph node involvement, and M to metastasis, or spread of the disease.

Signs and symptoms are evaluated, and x-rays, laboratory tests, and special examinations, such as punch biopsy and colposcopy, are performed. Depending on the stage of the cancer, other tests and procedures may be performed to determine the extent of disease and appropriate treatment. These tests include dilation and curettage (D & C), computed tomography (CT), MRI, IV urography, cystography, and barium x-ray studies.

Medical Management

Precursor or Preinvasive Lesions

When precursor lesions, such as low-grade squamous intraepithelial lesion (LGSIL), which is also referred to as LSIL (CIN I and II or mild to moderate dysplasia), are found by colposcopy and biopsy, careful monitoring by frequent Pap smears or conservative treatment is possible. Conservative treatment may consist of monitoring, **cryotherapy** (freezing with nitrous oxide), or laser therapy. A **loop electrocautery excision procedure (LEEP)** may also be used to remove abnormal cells. In this procedure, a thin wire loop with laser is used to cut away a thin layer of cervical tissue. LEEP is an outpatient procedure usually performed in a gynecologist's office; it takes only a few minutes. Analgesia is given before the procedure, and a local anesthetic agent is injected into the area. This procedure allows the pathologist to examine the removed tissue sample to determine if the borders of the tissue are disease-free. Another procedure called a cone biopsy or **conization** (removing a cone-shaped portion of the cervix) is performed when biopsy findings demonstrate CIN III or HGSIL, equivalent to severe dysplasia and carcinoma in situ.

If preinvasive cervical cancer (carcinoma in situ) occurs when a woman has completed childbearing, a simple hysterectomy (removal of the uterus only) is usually recommended. If a woman has not completed childbearing and invasion is less than 1 mm, conization may be sufficient. Frequent reexaminations are necessary to monitor for recurrence.

Patients who have precursor or premalignant lesions need reassurance that they do not have invasive cancer. However, the importance of close follow-up is emphasized because the condition, if untreated for a long time, may progress to cancer. Patients with cervical cancer in situ also need to know that this is usually a slow-growing and nonaggressive type of cancer that is not expected to recur after appropriate treatment.

Invasive Cancer

Treatment of invasive cervical cancer depends on the stage of the lesion, the patient's age and general health, and the judgment and experience of the physician. Surgery and radiation treatment (intracavitary and external) are most often used. Surgical procedures that may be used to treat cervical cancer are summarized in Chart 47-6. When tumor invasion is less than 3 mm, a hysterectomy is often sufficient. Invasion exceeding 3 mm usually requires a radical hysterectomy with pelvic node dissection and aortic node assessment. Stage 1B1 tumors are treated with radical hysterectomy and radiation. Stage 1B2 tumors are treated individually because no single correct course of treatment has been identified, and many variable options may be considered.

A procedure called a radical trachelectomy is an alternative to hysterectomy in women with invasive cervical cancer who are young and want to have children (Dargent, Martin, Sacchetoni, et al., 2000). In this procedure, the cervix is gripped with retractors and pulled down into the vagina until it is visible. The affected tissue is excised while the rest of the cervix and uterus remain intact. A drawstring suture is used to close the cervix.

CHART 47-6

Surgical Procedures for Cervical Cancer

- Total hysterectomy—removal of the uterus, cervix, and ovaries
- Radical hysterectomy—removal of the uterus, ovaries, fallopian tubes, proximal vagina, and bilateral lymph nodes through an abdominal incision (*Note:* "radical" indicates that an extensive area of the paravaginal, paracervical, parametrial, and uterosacral tissues is removed with the uterus.)
- Radical vaginal hysterectomy—vaginal removal of the uterus, ovaries, fallopian tubes, and proximal vagina
- Bilateral pelvic lymphadenectomy—removal of the common iliac, external iliac, hypogastric, and obturator lymphatic vessels and nodes
- Pelvic exenteration—removal of the pelvic organs, including the bladder or rectum and pelvic lymph nodes, and construction of diversional conduit, colostomy, and vagina
- Radical trachelectomy—removal of the cervix and selected nodes to preserve childbearing capacity in a woman of reproductive age with cervical cancer

Frequent follow-up after surgery by a gynecologic oncologist is imperative because the risk of recurrence is 35% after treatment for invasive cervical cancer. Recurrence usually occurs within the first 2 years. Recurrences are often in the upper quarter of the vagina, and ureteral obstruction may be a sign. Weight loss, leg edema, and pelvic pain may be signs of lymphatic obstruction and metastasis. Micrometastases have been found in patients with negative lymph nodes, and further research is necessary to determine whether this has an impact on recurrence or prognosis (Lentz, Muderspach, Felix, et al., 2004).

Radiation, which is often part of treatment to reduce recurrent disease, may be delivered by an external beam or by **brachytherapy** (method by which the radiation source is placed near the tumor) or both. The field to be irradiated and dose of radiation are determined by stage, volume of tumor, and lymph node involvement. Treatment can be administered daily for 4 to 6 weeks followed by one or two treatments of intracavitary radiation. Interstitial therapy may be used when vaginal placement has become impossible due to tumor or stricture.

Platinum-based agents are being used to treat advanced cervical cancer. They are often used in combination with radiation therapy, surgery, or both. Studies are ongoing to find the best approach to treat advanced cervical cancer. Vaginal stenosis is a frequent side effect of radiation. Sexual activity, with lubrication, is preventive, as is use of a vaginal dilator to avoid severe permanent vaginal stenosis.

Some patients with recurrences of cervical cancer are considered for **pelvic exenteration**, in which a large portion of the pelvic contents is removed. This is a complex, extensive surgical procedure that is reserved for those with a high likelihood of cure. Unilateral leg edema, sciatica, and ureteral obstruction indicate likely disease progression. Patients with these symptoms have advanced disease and are not considered candidates for this major surgical procedure. Surgery is often complex because it is performed close to the bowel, bladder, ureters, and great vessels. Complications can be considerable and include pulmonary emboli, pulmonary edema, myocardial infarction, cerebrovascular accident, hemorrhage, sepsis, small bowel obstruction, fistula formation, obstruction of the ileal conduit, bladder dysfunction, and pyelonephritis, most often in the first 18 months. Vein constriction must be avoided postoperatively. Patients with varicose veins or a history of thromboembolic disease may be treated prophylactically with heparin. Pneumatic compression stockings are prescribed to reduce the risk of deep vein thrombosis (DVT). Nursing care of these patients is complex and requires coordination and care by experienced health care professionals. Pelvic exenteration is discussed in further detail later in this chapter.

Cancer of the Uterus (Endometrium)

Cancer of the uterine endometrium (fundus or corpus) has increased in incidence, partly because women are living longer and because reporting is more accurate; however, its incidence seems to be leveling off. Most uterine cancers are endometrioid (that is, originating in the lining of the uterus). After breast, colorectal, and lung cancer, endometrial cancer is the fourth most common cancer in women and the most common pelvic neoplasm. Cumulative exposure to estrogen is considered the major risk factor (Chart 47-7). This exposure occurs with the use of estrogen replacement therapy without the use of progestin, early menarche, late menopause, nulliparity, and anovulation. Other risk factors include infertility, diabetes, hypertension, gallbladder disease, and obesity (ACS, 2004). Tamoxifen may also cause proliferation of the uterine lining, and women receiving this medication for treatment or prevention of breast cancer are monitored by their oncologists and gynecologic health care providers.

CHART 47-7

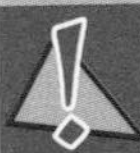

Risk Factors for Uterine Cancer

- Age: at least 55 years; median age, 61 years
- Postmenopausal bleeding
- Obesity that results in increased estrone levels (related to excess weight) resulting from conversion of androstenedione to estrone in body fat, which exposes the uterus to unopposed estrogen
- Unopposed estrogen therapy (estrogen used without progesterone, which offsets the risk of unopposed estrogen)
- Other: nulliparity, truncal obesity, late menopause (after 52 years of age) and, possibly, use of tamoxifen

Assessment and Diagnostic Findings

All women should be encouraged to have annual checkups, including a gynecologic examination. Any woman who is experiencing irregular bleeding should be evaluated promptly. If a menopausal woman experiences bleeding, an endometrial aspiration or biopsy is performed to rule out hyperplasia, a possible precursor of endometrial cancer. The procedure is quick and painless. Ultrasonography can also be used to measure the thickness of the endometrium. (Postmenopausal women should have a very thin endometrium due to low levels of estrogen; a thicker lining warrants further investigation.) A biopsy or aspiration is diagnostic.

Medical Management

Treatment of endometrial cancer consists of total hysterectomy (discussed later in this chapter) and bilateral salpingo-oophorectomy and node sampling. Depending on the stage, the therapeutic approach is individualized and is based on stage, type, differentiation, degree of invasion, and node involvement. Adjuvant radiation may be used in a patient who is considered high risk. The effects of adjuvant therapy and node sampling on survival are inconclusive (Randall & Armstrong, 2003). Whole pelvis radiotherapy is used if there is any spread beyond the uterus. Preoperative and postoperative treatments for stage II and beyond may include pelvic, abdominal, and vaginal intracavitary radiation. Recurrent cancer usually occurs inside the **vaginal vault** or in the upper vagina, and metastasis usually occurs in lymph nodes or the ovary. Recurrent lesions in the vagina are treated with surgery and radiation. Recurrent lesions beyond the vagina are treated with hormonal therapy or chemotherapy. Progestin therapy is used frequently. Patients should be prepared for such side effects as nausea, depression, rash, or mild fluid retention with this therapy.

Cancer of the Vulva

Primary cancer of the vulva represents 4% of all gynecologic malignancies and is seen mostly in postmenopausal women, although its incidence in younger women is increasing. The median age for cancer limited to the vulva is 50 years, whereas the median age for invasive vulvar cancer is 70 years (ACS, 2005). Possible risk factors include smoking, HPV infection, HIV infection, and immunosuppression. Squamous cell carcinoma accounts for most primary vulvar tumors. Less common are Bartholin's gland cancer, vulvar sarcoma, and malignant melanoma. Little is known about what causes this disease; however, increased risk may be related to chronic vulvar irritation. In younger women, HPV infection may be implicated, especially types 16, 18, and 31. Prevention includes delaying onset of sexual activity to avoid early exposure to HPV and avoidance of smoking. Regular pelvic examinations, Pap smears, and vulvar self-examination are helpful in early detection.

Clinical Manifestations

Long-standing pruritus and soreness are the most common symptoms of vulvar cancer. Itching occurs in half of all patients with vulvar malignancy. Bleeding, foul-smelling discharge, and pain may also be present and are usually signs of advanced disease. Cancerous lesions of the vulva are visible and accessible and grow relatively slowly. Early lesions appear as a chronic dermatitis; later, patients may note a lump that continues to grow and becomes a hard, ulcerated, cauliflower-like growth. Biopsy should be performed on any vulvar lesion that persists, ulcerates, or fails to heal quickly with proper therapy. Vulvar malignancies may appear as a lump or mass, redness, or a lesion that fails to heal.

Nurses are in an ideal position to encourage women to perform vulvar self-examinations regularly. Using a mirror, patients can see what constitutes normal female anatomy and learn about changes that should be reported (eg, lesions, ulcers, masses, and persistent itching). Nurses must urge women to seek health care if they notice anything abnormal, because vulvar cancer is one of the most curable of all malignant conditions.

Medical Management

Vulvar intraepithelial lesions are preinvasive and are also called vulvar carcinoma in situ. They may be treated by local excision, laser ablation, chemotherapeutic creams (ie, 5-fluorouracil), or cryosurgery.

When invasive vulvar carcinoma exists, primary treatment may include wide excision or removal of the vulva (**vulvectomy**). An effort is made to individualize treatment, depending on the extent of the disease. A wide excision is performed only if lymph nodes are normal. More pervasive lesions require vulvectomy with deep pelvic node dissection. Vulvectomy is very effective at prolonging life but is frequently followed by complications (ie, scarring, wound breakdown, leg swelling, vaginal stenosis, or rectocele). To reduce complications, only necessary tissue is removed. External beam radiation may be used, resulting in sunburn-like irritation that resolves in 6 to 12 months.

If a widespread area is involved or the disease is advanced, a radical vulvectomy with bilateral groin dissection may be performed. Antibiotic and heparin prophylaxis may be prescribed preoperatively and continued postoperatively to prevent infection, DVT, and pulmonary emboli. Elastic compression stockings are applied to reduce the risk of DVT.

Although the role of systemic chemotherapy in the treatment of vulvar cancer remains to be determined, chemotherapy may be useful when used in combination with radiation therapy for the treatment of advanced disease. The combination of radiation and chemotherapy may reduce the size of the cancer, resulting in less extensive subsequent surgery (ACS, 2005).

Clinical trials to determine the most effective treatment are difficult to conduct, because there are few patients with this condition. Morbidity with recurrence of the disease is high, and patterns of recurrence vary. Reconstruction after vulvectomy is being studied and initial patient responses are positive (Hockel & Dornhofer, 2004).

Nursing Process

The Patient Undergoing Vulvar Surgery

Assessment

The health history is a valuable tool for establishing rapport with the patient. The reason the patient is seeking health care is apparent. What the nurse can tactfully elicit is the reason why a delay, if any, occurred, in seeking health care—for example, because of modesty, economics, denial, neglect, or fear (abusive partners sometimes prevent women from seeking health care). Factors involved in any delay in seeking health care and treatment may also affect recovery. The patient's health habits and lifestyle are assessed, and her receptivity to teaching is evaluated. Psychosocial factors are also assessed. Preoperative preparation and psychological support begin at this time.

Diagnosis

Nursing Diagnoses

Based on all the assessment data, the major nursing diagnoses may include the following:

- Anxiety related to the diagnosis and surgery
- Acute pain related to the surgical incision and subsequent wound care
- Impaired skin integrity related to the wound and drainage
- Sexual dysfunction related to change in body image
- Self-care deficit related to lack of understanding of perineal care and general health status

Collaborative Problems/ Potential Complications

Based on assessment data, potential complications may include the following:

- Wound infection and sepsis
- DVT
- Hemorrhage

Planning and Goals

Major goals may include acceptance of and preparation for surgical intervention, relief of pain, maintenance of skin integrity, return to optimal sexual function, ability to perform adequate and appropriate self-care, and absence of complications.

Preoperative Nursing Interventions

Relieving Anxiety

The patient must be allowed time to talk and ask questions. Fear often decreases when a woman of childbearing age who is to undergo wide excision of the vulva or vulvectomy learns that the possibility for subsequent sexual relations is good and that pregnancy is possible after a wide excision. The nurse must know what information the physician has given the patient about the surgery to reinforce that information and address the patient's questions and concerns.

Preparing Skin for Surgery

Skin preparation may include cleansing the lower abdomen, inguinal areas, upper thighs, and vulva with a detergent germicide for several days before the surgical procedure. The patient may be instructed to do this at home.

Postoperative Nursing Interventions

Relieving Pain

Because of the wide excision, the patient may experience severe pain and discomfort even with minimal movement. Inadequate pain relief inhibits the patient's mobility and increases the likelihood of complications. Therefore, analgesic agents are administered preventively (ie, around the clock at designated times) to relieve pain and increase the patient's comfort level. Patient-controlled analgesia may be used to provide pain relief and promote patient comfort. Careful positioning using pillows usually increases comfort, as do soothing back rubs. A low Fowler's position or, occasionally, a pillow placed under the knees reduces pain by relieving tension on the incision; however, efforts must be made to avoid pressure behind the knees, which increases the risk of DVT. Positioning the patient on her side, with pillows between her legs and against the lumbar region, provides comfort and reduces tension on the surgical wound.

Improving Skin Integrity

A pressure-reducing mattress may be used to prevent pressure ulcers. Moving from one position to another requires time and effort; use of an overbed trapeze bar may help the patient to move herself more easily. Ambulation may be attempted on the second day.

The extent of the surgical incision and the type of dressing are considered when choosing strategies to promote skin integrity. Intact skin needs to be protected from drainage and moisture, and dressings must be changed as needed to ensure patient comfort, to perform wound care and irrigation (if prescribed), and to permit observation of the surgical site. When the patient returns from the operating room, perineal dressings are more likely to remain in place and be comfortable if a T-binder is used.

The wound is cleansed daily with warm, normal saline irrigations or other antiseptic solutions as prescribed. A transparent dressing or Xeroform gauze may be in place over the wound to minimize exposure to the air and subsequent pain. The appearance of the surgical site and the characteristics of drainage are assessed and documented. After the dressings are removed, a bed cradle may be used to keep the bed linens away from the surgical site. The nurse must protect the patient from exposure when visitors arrive or someone else enters the room.

Supporting Positive Sexuality and Sexual Function

The patient who undergoes vulvar surgery usually experiences concerns about the effects of the surgery on her body image, sexual attractiveness, and functioning. Establishing a trusting nurse–patient relationship is important for the patient to feel comfortable expressing her concerns and fears. The patient is encouraged to share and discuss her concerns with her sexual partner.

Because alterations in sexual sensation and functioning depend on the extent of surgery, the nurse needs to know about any structural and functional changes resulting from the surgery. Consulting with the surgeon will clarify which changes to expect, and referring the patient and her partner to a sex counselor may help them address these changes and resume satisfying sexual activity.

Monitoring and Managing Potential Complications

INFECTION

The location, extent, and exposure of the surgical site and incision put the patient at risk for contamination of the site and infection and sepsis. The patient is monitored closely for local and systemic signs and symptoms of infection: purulent drainage, redness, increased pain, fever, and an increased white blood cell count. The nurse assists in obtaining tissue specimens for culture if infection is suspected and administers antibiotic agents as prescribed. Hand hygiene, always a crucial infection-preventing measure, is of particular importance whenever there is an extensive area of exposed tissue. Catheters, drains, and dressings are handled carefully and with gloves to avoid cross-contamination. A low-residue diet prevents straining on defecation and wound contamination. Sitz baths are discouraged after a wide excision because of the risk for infection.

DEEP VEIN THROMBOSIS

The patient is at risk for DVT because of the positioning required during surgery, postoperative edema, and the usually prolonged immobility needed to promote healing. Elastic compression stockings are applied, and the patient is encouraged and reminded to perform ankle exercises to minimize venous pooling, which leads to DVT. The patient is encouraged and assisted in changing positions by using the overhead trapeze. Pressure behind the knees is avoided when positioning the patient, because this may increase venous pooling. The patient is assessed for signs and symptoms of DVT (leg pain, redness, warmth, edema) and pulmonary embolism (chest pain, tachycardia, dyspnea). Fluid intake is encouraged to prevent dehydration, which also increases the risk for DVT.

HEMORRHAGE

The extent of the surgical incision and possibly wide excision of tissue increase the risk of postoperative bleeding and hemorrhage. Although the pressure dressings that are applied after surgery minimize the risk, the patient must be monitored closely for signs of hemorrhage and resulting hypovolemic shock. These signs may include decreased blood pressure, increased pulse rate, decreased urine output, decreased mental status, and cold, clammy skin.

If hemorrhage and shock occur, interventions include fluid replacement, blood component therapy, and vasopressor medications. Laboratory results (eg, hematocrit and hemoglobin levels) and hemodynamic monitoring are used to assess the patient's response to treatment. Depending on the specific cause of hemorrhage, the patient may be returned to the operating room. The patient who experiences hemorrhage is anxious and apprehensive. Providing brief explanations of the procedures being performed and offering reassurance that the problem has been identified and is being taken care of may reduce the anxiety and fears of the patient and her family.

Promoting Home and Community-Based Care

TEACHING PATIENTS SELF-CARE

Preparing the patient for hospital discharge begins before hospital admission. The patient and family are informed about what to expect during the immediate postoperative and recovery periods. Posthospital care requires giving complete instructions to a family member or significant other who will help care for the patient at home and to the home care nurse who will provide follow-up care. Depending on the changes resulting from the surgery, the patient and her family may need instruction about wound care, urinary catheterization, and possible complications. The patient is encouraged to share her concerns and to assume increasing responsibility for her own care. She is encouraged and assisted in learning to care for the surgical wound.

CONTINUING CARE

Shortened hospital stays may result in the patient's discharge during the early postoperative recovery stage. Thus, home care referral or discharge to a subacute facility may be indicated. During this phase, the patient's physical status and psychological responses to the surgery are assessed. In addition, the patient is assessed for complications and healing of the surgical site. During home visits, the patient's environment is assessed to determine if modifications are needed to facilitate patient care. The home care nurse uses the home visit to reinforce previous teaching and to assess the patient's and the family's understanding of and adherence to the prescribed treatment strategies. Follow-up phone calls by the nurse to the patient between home visits are usually reassuring to the patient and family, who may be responsible for performing complex care procedures. Attention to the patient's psychological responses is important, because the patient may become discouraged and depressed because of alterations in body image and a slow recovery. Communication between the nurse involved in the patient's immediate postoperative care and the home care nurse is essential to ensure continuity of care.

Evaluation

Expected Patient Outcomes

Expected patient outcomes may include:

1. Adjusts to the trauma of the surgical experience
   a. Uses available resources in coping with and alleviating emotional stress
   b. Asks questions related to postoperative expectations
   c. Demonstrates willingness to discuss alternative approaches to sexual expression
2. Obtains pain relief
   a. Reports progressive decrease in pain and discomfort
   b. Assumes position of comfort
3. Maintains skin integrity
   a. States rationale for use of a special mattress or other device
   b. Uses overhead trapeze to change position frequently
   c. Exhibits healing of surgical site without excoriated skin
   d. Cares for incision and surgical site as instructed
4. Exhibits positive outlook about sexuality and sexual functioning
   a. Verbalizes concerns and anxieties about sexual functioning
   b. Discusses options and alternative approaches to sexual intercourse
   c. Follows up with sexual counselor or therapist, if indicated
5. Increases participation in self-care activities
   a. Demonstrates self-care activities as instructed
   b. Identifies signs and symptoms of complications that should be reported to the nurse or physician
   c. Properly cleans the surgical site after voiding and defecation
6. Absence of complications
   a. Is free of any signs and symptoms of infection: has normal vital signs (temperature, blood pressure, pulse rate); has no purulent discharge
   b. Identifies activities to prevent DVT: avoids crossing legs or sitting with pressure against knees; exercises ankles and legs
   c. Exhibits no signs or symptoms of DVT (leg pain, redness, warmth, edema)
   d. Demonstrates no signs or symptoms of hemorrhage

Cancer of the Vagina

Cancer of the vagina is rare and usually takes years to develop. Primary cancer of the vagina is usually squamous in origin. Malignant melanoma and sarcomas can occur. Risk factors include previous cervical cancer, in utero exposure to diethylstilbestrol (DES), previous vaginal or vulvar cancer, previous radiation therapy, history of HPV, or pessary use. Any patient with previous cervical cancer should be examined regularly for vaginal lesions.

Before 1970, vaginal cancer occurred primarily in postmenopausal women. In the 1970s, it was shown that maternal ingestion of DES, prescribed from 1938 to 1971 to enhance pregnancy outcomes, affected female offspring who were exposed in utero. DES was prescribed under many brand names, and it is unclear how many pregnant women received it. It is estimated that 5 to 10 million women in the United States and their fetuses were exposed to DES (Blunt, 2004). All patients should be asked about DES exposure if they were born or were pregnant between 1938 and 1971. Benign genital tract abnormalities, such as vaginal adenosis (abnormal tissue growth), cervical irregularities (collars, hoods, septae, cockscombs), and uterine abnormalities, have occurred in approximately one-third of exposed women. Clear cell carcinoma of the vagina or cervix may also occur as a result of DES exposure; the risk is 0.14 to 1.4 in 1000 women. However, most female offspring of mothers who took DES are now between 30 and 60 years of age, and diagnosis of this condition has been decreasing. Vigilance is still necessary, because it is unknown how long women remain at risk (ACS, 2005). Colposcopy is indicated for all women exposed to DES in utero. If colposcopic examination discloses adenosis or a significant cervical lesion, follow-up is essential. The risk of breast cancer related to DES exposure is also higher. In addition, women whose sons were exposed to DES in utero may have more epididymal cysts.

Vaginal pessaries, used to support prolapsed tissues, can be a source of chronic irritation. As such, they have been associated with vaginal cancer, but only when the devices were not cared for properly (ie, the device was not cleaned regularly or the patient did not return to the health care provider regularly for vaginal examinations).

Patients often do not have symptoms but may report slight bleeding after intercourse, spontaneous bleeding, vaginal discharge, pain, and urinary or rectal symptoms (or both). Diagnosis is often by Pap smear of the vagina. Encouraging close follow-up by health care providers is the primary focus of nursing interventions with women who were exposed to DES in utero. Emotional support for mothers and their daughters is essential.

Medical Management

Treatment of early lesions may be by local excision, topical chemotherapy, or laser. Laser therapy is a common treatment option in early vaginal and vulvar cancer. Surgery for more advanced lesions depends on the size and the stage of the cancer. If radical vaginectomy is required, a vagina can be reconstructed with tissue from the intestine, muscle, or skin grafts. After vaginal reconstructive surgery and radiation, regular intercourse may be helpful in preventing vaginal stenosis. Water-soluble lubricants are helpful in reducing painful intercourse (dyspareunia).

Following surgery, radiation therapy may be administered by a variety of methods, including external beam radiation, which is usually an outpatient procedure, or brachytherapy, which is internal radiation therapy. Internal radiation may be given with intracavitary-radioactive material contained in a seed, wire, needle, or tube, which is placed into a cavity such as the uterus or vagina. Interstitial radiation is another type of internal radiation treatment in which the radioactive material is placed in or near the cancer but not into a body cavity and is used in cervical and ovarian malignancies. These treatments may be high dose for a short period or low dose, which may take longer. Treatment during hospitalization or during outpatient therapy depends on several factors, including the status of the patient and the mode of delivery.

Cancer of the Fallopian Tubes

Malignancies of the fallopian tube are rare and are the least common type of genital cancer. This type of cancer can occur at any age; the average age at diagnosis is 55 years. Symptoms include abdominal pain, abnormal bleeding, and vaginal discharge. An enlarged fallopian tube may be found on sonogram if dilated and fluid filled or it may appear or be palpated as a mass. Surgery followed by radiation therapy is the usual treatment.

Cancer of the Ovary

Ovarian cancer causes more deaths than any other cancer of the female reproductive system. Despite careful physical examination, ovarian tumors are often difficult to detect because they are usually deep in the pelvis. No early screening mechanism exists at present, although tumor markers are being explored. Transvaginal ultrasound and CA-125 antigen testing may be reassuring for women who have a high risk for this condition, and clinical trials are underway to evaluate the effect of screening on mortality from ovarian cancer. Studies are also examining target populations most likely to benefit from this screening, as well as compliance, costs, and the physical and psychological effects of screening (Luce, Dow, & Holcomb, 2003). Tumor-associated antigens are helpful in determining follow-up care after diagnosis and treatment but not in early general screening.

Epidemiology

The risk of ovarian cancer increases with age and peaks in women in their late 70s. Its incidence is highest in industrialized countries, except for Japan, where the incidence is low. A woman with ovarian cancer has a threefold to fourfold increased risk for breast cancer, and a woman with breast cancer has an increased risk for ovarian cancer. However, most women who develop ovarian cancer have no known risk factors, and no definitive causative factors have been determined. Oral contraceptives appear to have a protective effect. Risk factors include nulliparity; infertility; use of talcum powder in the genital area, which has been debated as a potential risk factor due to asbestos contamination in the past (ACS, 2005); and heredity. Many health care providers advocate pelvic examinations every 6 months for women who have one or two relatives with ovarian cancer.

Advances in knowledge of genetics are changing the approaches to detecting and treating breast and ovarian cancer. Some families have specific genes that predispose them to various cancers. BRCA-1 is a genetic mutation that results in an increased risk for breast and ovarian cancer. BRCA-2 is another genetic mutation that may result in an increased risk for both female and male breast cancers as well as of ovarian cancer. Other mutations are also under study.

Genetic testing is indicated when three or more cases of closely related family members have premenopausal breast cancer or ovarian cancer. One member with cancer is tested, and if the results are positive, other members without cancer may undergo testing. This testing is available at centers with genetics counselors or nurses with expertise in genetics counseling.

Much more needs to be learned about the risks associated with some mutations, the reliability of testing, and the efficacy of follow-up. Confidentiality and insurance risks are ethical issues that need clarification. Because there are no primary methods of preventing breast or ovarian cancer, emotional distress is also an issue. Patients with concerns about their family history should be referred to a cancer genetics center to obtain information and testing, if indicated. Women with inherited types of ovarian cancer tend to be younger when the diagnosis is made than the average age at the time of diagnosis of 59 years. Prophylactic oophorectomy in women with genetic mutations has been found to be associated with a decrease in the risk of ovarian and other gynecologic cancers as well as breast cancer and is an option for women who have completed childbearing (ACS, 2004; Rebbeck et al., 2002). Hereditary nonpolyposis colon cancer increases the risk of uterine cancer and slightly increases the risk for ovarian cancer (ACS, 2004). Oral contraceptives, hysterectomy, pregnancy, and lactation may be preventive.

Pathophysiology

Types of tumors include germ cell tumors, which arise from the cells that produce eggs; stromal cell tumors, which arise in connective tissue cells that produce hormones; and epithelial tumors, which originate from the outer surface of the ovary. Most ovarian cancers are epithelial in origin. Of the many different cell types in ovarian cancer, epithelial tumors constitute 90%. Germ cell tumors and stromal tumors make up the other 10%.

Primary peritoneal carcinoma is closely related to ovarian cancer. Extraovarian primary peritoneal carcinoma (EOPPC) resembles ovarian cancer histologically and can occur in women with and without ovaries. Symptoms and treatment are similar. Because of the possibility of EOPPC, oophorectomy does not guarantee that the patient will not develop carcinoma following hysterectomy.

Clinical Manifestations

Symptoms of ovarian cancer are nonspecific and include increased abdominal girth, pelvic pressure, bloating, back pain, constipation, abdominal pain, urinary urgency, indigestion, flatulence, increased waist size, leg pain, and pelvic pain (Mandel, Melancon, & Muntz, 2004). Symptoms are often vague, and many women ignore them. Ovarian cancer is often silent, but enlargement of the abdomen from an accumulation of fluid is the most common sign. All woman with gastrointestinal symptoms and without a known diagnosis must be evaluated with ovarian cancer in mind. Vague, undiagnosed, persistent gastrointestinal symptoms should alert the nurse to the possibility of an early ovarian malignancy. A palpable ovary in a woman who has gone through menopause is investigated, because ovaries normally become smaller and less palpable after menopause.

Assessment and Diagnostic Findings

Any enlarged ovary must be investigated. Pelvic examination often does not detect early ovarian cancer, and pelvic imaging techniques are not always definitive. Ovarian tumors are classified as benign if there is no proliferation or invasion, borderline if there is proliferation but no invasion, and malignant if there is invasion. Fifteen percent of all new cases of ovarian tumors are classified as borderline and have low malignancy potential. However, by the time of diagnosis, about 75% of ovarian cancers have metastasized, and about 60% have spread beyond the pelvis.

Medical Management

Surgical Management

Surgical staging, exploration, and reduction of tumor mass are the basics of treatment. Surgical removal is the treatment of choice; the preoperative workup usually includes a barium enema or colonoscopy, upper gastrointestinal series, MRI, ultrasound, chest x-rays, and IV urography. CT may be used preoperatively to rule out intra-abdominal metastasis. Staging the tumor by the TNM system is performed to guide treatment (Chart 47-8). Likely treatment involves a total ab-

CHART 47-8

Stages of Ovarian Cancer

I Cancer is contained within the ovary (or ovaries).

II Cancer is in one or both ovaries and has involved other organs (ie, uterus, fallopian tubes, bladder, the sigmoid colon, or the rectum) within the pelvis.

III Cancer involves one or both ovaries, and one or both of the following are present: (1) cancer has spread beyond the pelvis to the lining of the abdomen; (2) cancer has spread to lymph nodes.

IV The most advanced stage of ovarian cancer. Cancer is in one or both ovaries. There is distant metastasis to the liver, lungs, or other organs outside the peritoneal cavity; ovarian cancer cells in the pleural cavity are evidence of stage IV disease.

dominal hysterectomy with removal of the fallopian tubes and ovaries and possibly, the omentum (bilateral salpingo-oophorectomy and omentectomy); tumor debulking; para-aortic and pelvic lymph node sampling; diaphragmatic biopsies; random peritoneal biopsies; and cytologic washings. Postoperative management may include radiation or chemotherapy.

Borderline tumors resemble ovarian cancer but have much more favorable outcomes. Women diagnosed with this type of cancer tend to be younger (early 40s). A conservative surgical approach is now used. The affected ovary is removed, but the uterus and the contralateral ovary may remain in place. Adjuvant therapy may not be warranted.

Pharmacologic Therapy

Chemotherapy is usually administered intravenously on an outpatient basis using a combination of platinum and taxane agents. Paclitaxel plus carboplatin are most often used because of their excellent clinical benefits and manageable toxicity. Leukopenia, neurotoxicity, and fever may occur.

Paclitaxel (Taxol) causes microtubules within the cells to gather and prevents the breakdown of these threadlike structures. In general, cells cannot function when they are clogged with microtubules and cannot divide. Because this medication often causes leukopenia, patients may need to take granulocyte colony-stimulating factor as well. Paclitaxel is contraindicated in patients with hypersensitivity to medications formulated in polyoxyethylated castor oil and in patients with baseline neutropenia. Because of possible adverse cardiac effects, paclitaxel is not used in patients with cardiac disorders. Hypotension, dyspnea, angioedema, and urticaria indicate severe reactions that usually occur soon after the first and second doses are administered. The nurse must be prepared to assist in treating anaphylaxis. Patients should be prepared for inevitable hair loss.

Carboplatin (Paraplatin) may be used in the initial treatment and in patients with recurrence. It should be used with caution in patients with renal impairment. Usually, six cycles are given. A positive clinical response is normalization of the tumor marker, CA-125, negative CT results, and a normal physical and gynecologic examination.

Liposomal therapy, delivery of chemotherapy in a liposome, allows the highest possible dose of chemotherapy to the tumor target with a reduction in adverse effects. Liposomes are used as drug carriers because they are nontoxic, biodegradable, easily available, and relatively inexpensive. This encapsulated chemotherapy allows increased duration of action and better targeting. The encapsulation of doxorubicin lessens the incidence of nausea, vomiting, and alopecia. Patients must be monitored for bone marrow suppression. Gastrointestinal and cardiac effects may also occur. These medications are administered as a slow IV infusion over 60 to 90 minutes by oncology nurses.

Genetics engineering and identification of cancer genes may make gene therapy a future possibility; gene therapy is under investigation. Radiation may be helpful and is more useful in some types of ovarian cancer than others. It may be delivered by external beam.

Chemotherapy is the most common form of treatment in advanced ovarian cancer.

Emerging proteomic technologies (tissue-based protein analysis) look promising; they may allow earlier diagnosis and treatment decision making. New biomarkers need further validation, but protein signature patterns are now being evaluated in clinical trials. These technologies may help in development of individualized treatment strategies for epithelial ovarian cancer. Osteopontin, a naturally occurring protein found in all body fluids, may be useful as a marker for ovarian cancer. Research is underway to evaluate its clinical usefulness in identification of early ovarian cancer (Kim, Skates, Uede et al., 2002).

Recurrence of ovarian cancer is common, and many patients may require treatment with multiple agents. Therefore, ovarian cancer may be considered a chronic disease, with treatment directed toward control of the cancer, maintenance of quality of life, and palliation. Liposomal preparations, intraperitoneal drug administration, anti-cancer vaccines, monoclonal antibodies directed against cancer antigens, gene therapy, and antiangiogenic treatments (to prevent formation of new blood vessels in an effort to halt growth of ovarian cancer) are often used in the treatment of recurrence. Specific modalities may include gemcitabine, liposomal doxorubicin, and topotecan. Specific strategies may be used to treat neutropenia and thrombocytopenia and to prevent nephrotoxicity and neurotoxicity (Almadrones, 2003).

Nursing Management

Nursing measures include those related to the patient's treatment plan, which may include surgery, chemotherapy, radiation, palliation, or a combination of these. Emotional support, comfort measures, and information, plus attentiveness and caring, are important components of nursing care for the patient and her family.

Nursing interventions after pelvic surgery to remove the tumor are similar to those after other abdominal surgeries. If ovarian cancer occurs in a young woman and the tumor is unilateral, it is removed. Childbearing, if desired, is encouraged in the near future. After childbirth, surgical reexploration may be performed, and the remaining ovary may be removed. If both ovaries are involved, surgery is performed and chemotherapy follows.

Patients with advanced ovarian cancer may develop ascites and pleural effusion. Nursing care may include administering IV fluids prescribed to alleviate fluid and electrolyte imbalances, administering parenteral nutrition to provide adequate nutrition, providing postoperative care after intestinal bypass to alleviate an obstruction, controlling pain, and managing drainage tubes. Comfort measures for women with ascites may include providing small frequent meals, decreasing fluid intake, administering diuretic agents, and providing rest. Patients with pleural effusion may experience shortness of breath, hypoxia, pleuritic chest pain, and cough. Thoracentesis is usually performed to relieve these symptoms. The patient with ovarian cancer often has complex needs and benefits from the assistance and support of an oncology nurse specialist.

Hysterectomy

Hysterectomy is the surgical removal of the uterus to treat cancer, dysfunctional uterine bleeding, endometriosis, nonmalignant growths, persistent pain, pelvic relaxation and prolapse, and previous injury to the uterus. The number of hysterectomies in the United States per year has stabilized at 600,000, despite an increase in the number of women who have reached the age at which this procedure is likely to be performed. The number is thought to be stabilizing because women often seek second opinions, and the number of other therapeutic options (ie, laser therapy, endometrial ablation, and medications to shrink fibroid tumors) has increased.

Hysterectomy can be performed using a variety of surgical approaches. A total hysterectomy involves removal of the uterus and the cervix. Hysterectomy can be supracervical or subtotal, in which the uterus is removed but the cervix is spared. Malignant conditions usually require a total abdominal hysterectomy and bilateral salpingo-oophorectomy (removal of fallopian tubes and ovaries). In radical hysterectomy, the uterus and surrounding tissue are removed, including the upper third of the vagina and pelvic lymph nodes. Hysterectomy can be performed through the vagina, through an abdominal incision, or laparoscopically (in which the uterus is removed in sections through small incisions using a laparoscope).

A laparoscopically assisted approach can also be used for vaginal hysterectomy, with excellent results and rapid recovery. This procedure is performed as a short-stay procedure or ambulatory surgery in carefully selected patients. It also can be used effectively in patients who are obese (Heinberg, Crawford, Weitzen, et al., 2004).

Preoperative Management

The physical preparation of a patient undergoing a hysterectomy is similar to that of a patient undergoing a laparotomy. The lower half of the abdomen and the pubic and perineal regions may be shaved, and these areas are cleaned with soap and water (some surgeons do not require that patients be shaved). To prevent contamination and injury to the bladder or intestinal tract, the intestinal tract and the bladder need to be empty before the patient is taken to the operating room. An enema and antiseptic douche may be prescribed the evening before surgery, and the patient may be instructed to administer these treatments at home. Preoperative medications may be administered before surgery to help the patient relax.

Postoperative Management

The principles of general postoperative care for abdominal surgery apply, with particular attention given to peripheral circulation to prevent thrombophlebitis and DVT (noting varicosities, promoting circulation with leg exercises, and using elastic compression stockings). Major risks are infection and hemorrhage. In addition, because the surgical site is close to the bladder, voiding problems may occur, particularly after a vaginal hysterectomy.

Edema or nerve trauma may cause temporary loss of bladder tone (bladder atony), and an indwelling catheter may be inserted. During surgery, the handling of the bowel may cause paralytic ileus and interfere with bowel functioning.

Nursing Process

The Patient Undergoing a Hysterectomy

Assessment

The health history and the physical and pelvic examination are completed, and laboratory tests are performed. Additional assessment data include the patient's psychosocial responses, because the need for a hysterectomy may elicit strong emotional reactions. If the hysterectomy is performed to remove a malignant tumor, anxiety related to fear of cancer and its consequences adds to the stress of the patient and her family. Women who have had a hysterectomy may be at greater risk for psychological symptoms, physical symptoms, postmenopausal syndrome, and increased use of health care postoperatively. Alternatively, women may note improved physical and mental health after hysterectomy.

Diagnosis

Nursing Diagnoses

Based on all the assessment data, the major nursing diagnoses may include the following:

- Anxiety related to the diagnosis of cancer, fear of pain, possible perception of loss of femininity or childbearing potential
- Disturbed body image related to altered fertility and fears about sexuality and relationships with partner and family
- Acute pain related to surgery and other adjuvant therapy
- Deficient knowledge of the perioperative aspects of hysterectomy and postoperative self-care

Collaborative Problems/ Potential Complications

Based on assessment data, potential complications may include the following:

- Hemorrhage
- DVT
- Bladder dysfunction

Planning and Goals

The major goals may include relief of anxiety, acceptance of loss of the uterus, absence of pain or discomfort, increased knowledge of self-care requirements, and absence of complications.

Nursing Interventions

Relieving Anxiety

Anxiety stems from several factors: unfamiliar environment, the effects of surgery on body image and reproductive ability, fear of pain and other discomfort, and, possibly, feelings of embarrassment about exposure of the genital area in the perioperative period. The nurse needs to determine what the experience means to the patient and how to assist her in expressing her feelings. Throughout the pre- and postoperative and recovery periods, explanations are given about physical preparations and procedures that are performed.

Patient education addresses the outcomes of surgery, possible feelings of loss, and options for management of symptoms of menopause. Women vary in their preferences; many want a choice of treatment options, a part in decision making, accurate and useful information at the appropriate time, support from their health care providers, and access to professional and lay support systems.

Improving Body Image

The patient may have strong emotional reactions to having a hysterectomy and strong personal feelings related to the diagnosis, views of significant others who may be involved (family, partner), religious beliefs, and fears about prognosis. Concerns such as the inability to have children and the effect on femininity may surface, as may questions about the effects of surgery on sexual relationships, function, and satisfaction. The patient needs reassurance that she will still have a vagina and that she can experience sexual intercourse after temporary postoperative abstinence while tissues heal. Information that sexual satisfaction and orgasm arise from clitoral stimulation rather than from the uterus reassures many women. Most women note some change in sexual feelings after hysterectomy, but they vary in intensity. In some cases, the vagina is shortened by surgery, and this may affect sensitivity or comfort.

When hormonal balance is upset, as usually occurs in reproductive system disturbances, the patient may experience depression and heightened emotional sensitivity to people and situations. The nurse needs to approach and evaluate each patient individually in light of these factors. A nurse who exhibits interest, concern, and willingness to listen to the patient's fears will help the patient progress through the surgical experience.

Relieving Pain

Postoperative pain and discomfort are common. Therefore, the nurse assesses the intensity of the patient's pain and administers analgesia as prescribed. In some circumstances, a nasogastric tube may be inserted before the patient leaves the operating room to prevent discomfort from abdominal distention, especially if excessive handling of the viscera was required or if a large tumor was removed. Excision of a large tumor could cause edema because of the sudden release of pressure. In the postoperative period, fluids and food may be restricted for 1 or 2 days. If the patient has abdominal distention or flatus, a rectal tube and application of heat to the abdomen may be prescribed. When abdominal auscultation reveals return of bowel sounds and peristalsis, additional fluids and a soft diet are permitted. Early ambulation facilitates the return of normal peristalsis.

Monitoring and Managing Potential Complications

HEMORRHAGE

Vaginal bleeding and hemorrhage may occur after hysterectomy. To detect these complications early, the nurse counts the perineal pads used, assesses the extent of saturation with blood, and monitors vital signs. Abdominal dressings are monitored for drainage if an abdominal surgical approach was used. In preparation for hospital discharge, the nurse gives prescribed guidelines for activity restrictions to promote healing and to prevent postoperative bleeding. Because many women may go home the day of surgery or within a day or two, they are instructed to contact the nurse or surgeon if bleeding is excessive.

DEEP VEIN THROMBOSIS

Because of positioning during surgery, postoperative edema, and decreased activity postoperatively, the patient is at risk for DVT and pulmonary embolism (PE). To minimize the risk, elastic compression stockings are applied. In addition, the patient is encouraged and assisted to change positions frequently, although pressure under the knees is avoided, and to exercise her legs and feet while in bed. The nurse helps the patient ambulate early in the postoperative period. In addition, the nurse assesses for DVT or phlebitis (leg pain, redness, warmth, edema) and PE (chest pain, tachycardia, dyspnea). If the patient is being discharged home soon after surgery, she is instructed to avoid prolonged sitting in a chair with pressure at the knees, sitting with crossed legs, and inactivity. Furthermore, she is instructed to contact her health care provider if symptoms of DVT or PE occur.

BLADDER DYSFUNCTION

Because of possible difficulty in voiding postoperatively, occasionally an indwelling catheter may be inserted before or during surgery and is left in place in the immediate postoperative period. If a catheter is in place, it is usually removed shortly after the patient begins to ambulate. After the catheter is removed, urinary output is monitored; additionally, the abdomen is assessed for distention. If the patient does not void within a prescribed time, measures are initiated to encourage voiding (eg, assisting the patient to the bathroom, pouring warm water over the perineum). If the patient cannot void, catheterization may be necessary. Occasionally, the patient may be discharged home with the catheter in place and needs to be instructed in its management.

Promoting Home and Community-Based Care

TEACHING PATIENTS SELF-CARE

The information provided to the patient is tailored to her needs. She must know what limitations or restrictions, if any, to expect. She is instructed to check the surgical incision daily and to contact her primary health care provider if redness or purulent drainage or discharge occurs. She is informed that her periods are now over but that she may have a slightly bloody discharge for a few days; if bleeding recurs after this time, it should be reported immediately. The patient is instructed about the importance of an adequate oral intake and of maintaining bowel and urinary tract function. The patient is informed that she is likely to recover quickly; however, postoperative fatigue, which may occur following any surgical procedure, is not unusual.

The patient should resume activities gradually. This does not mean sitting for long periods, because doing so may cause blood to pool in the pelvis, increasing the risk of thromboembolism. The nurse explains that showers are preferable to tub baths to reduce the possibility of infection and to avoid the dangers of injury that may occur when getting in and out of the bathtub. The patient is instructed to avoid straining, lifting, having sexual intercourse, or driving until her surgeon permits her to resume these activities. Vaginal discharge, foul odor, excessive bleeding, any leg redness or pain, or an elevated temperature should be reported to the primary health care provider promptly. The nurse should be familiar with information given to patients by their surgeons regarding all activities and restrictions to reinforce them and prevent confusion.

CONTINUING CARE

Follow-up telephone contact provides the nurse with the opportunity to determine whether the patient is recovering without problems and to answer any questions that may have arisen. The patient is reminded about postoperative follow-up appointments. If the patient's ovaries were removed, hormone therapy (HT, previously referred to as hormone replacement therapy or HRT) may be considered. Providing information about the findings of the Women's Health Initiative (2002) study about the benefits and risks of HT promotes informed decision making about its use. The patient is reminded to discuss HT and alternative therapies with her primary care provider.

Evaluation

Expected Patient Outcomes

Expected patient outcomes may include:

1. Experiences decreased anxiety
2. Has improved body image
   a. Discusses changes resulting from surgery with her partner
   b. Verbalizes understanding of her disorder and the treatment plan
   c. Displays minimal depression or anxiety
3. Experiences minimal pain and discomfort
   a. Reports relief of abdominal pain and discomfort
   b. Ambulates without pain
4. Verbalizes knowledge and understanding of self-care
   a. Practices deep-breathing, turning, and leg exercises as instructed
   b. Increases activity and ambulation daily
   c. Reports adequate fluid intake and adequate urinary output
   d. Identifies reportable symptoms
   e. Schedules and keeps follow-up appointments
5. Absence of complications
   a. Has minimal vaginal bleeding and exhibits normal vital signs
   b. Ambulates early
   c. Notes no chest or calf pain and no redness, tenderness, or swelling in the extremities
   d. Reports no urinary problems or abdominal distention

Radiation Therapy

Radiation may be used in the treatment of cervical, uterine and ovarian cancers either alone or in combination with surgery and chemotherapy. Several approaches are used to deliver radiation to the female reproductive system: external radiation, intraoperative radiation therapy (IORT), and internal (intracavitary) irradiation or brachytherapy. The cervix and uterus can serve as a receptacle for radioactive sources for internal radiation therapy.

Methods of Radiation Therapy

External Radiation Therapy

This method of delivering radiation destroys cancerous cells at the skin surface or deeper in the body. Other methods of delivering radiation therapy are more commonly used to treat cancer of the female reproductive system than this method.

Intraoperative Radiation Therapy

Intraoperative radiation therapy (IORT) allows radiation to be applied directly to the affected area during surgery. An electron beam is directed at the disease site. This direct-view irradiation may be used when para-aortic nodes are involved or for unresectable (inoperable) or partially resectable neoplasms. Benefits include accurate beam direction (which precisely limits the radiation to the tumor) and the ability during treatment to block sensitive organs from radiation. IORT is usually combined with external beam irradiation preoperatively or postoperatively.

Internal (Intracavitary) Irradiation

After the patient receives an anesthetic agent and an examination, specially prepared applicators are inserted into the endometrial cavity and vagina. These devices are not loaded with radioactive material until the patient returns to her room. X-rays are obtained to verify the precise relationship of the applicator to the normal pelvic anatomy and to the tumor. When this step is completed, the radiation oncologist loads the applicators with predetermined amounts of radioactive material. This procedure, called afterloading, allows for precise control of the radiation exposure received by the patient, with minimal exposure of physicians, nurses, and other health care personnel. A patient undergoing internal radiation treatment remains isolated in private rooms until the application is completed. Adjacent rooms may need to be evacuated and a lead shield placed at the doorway to the patient's room.

Of the various applicators developed for intracavitary treatment, some are inserted into the endometrial cavity and endocervical canal as multiple small irradiators (eg, Heyman capsules). Others consist of a central tube (a tandem or intrauterine "stem") placed through the dilated endocervical canal into the uterine cavity, which remains in a fixed relationship with the irradiators placed in the upper vagina on each side of the cervix (vaginal ovoids) (Fig. 47-8).

When the applicator is inserted, an indwelling urinary catheter is also inserted. Vaginal packing is inserted to keep the applicator in place and to keep other organs, such as the bladder and rectum, as far from the radioactive source as possible. The objective of the internal treatment is to maintain the distribution of internal radiation at a fixed dosage throughout the application, which may last 24 to 72 hours, depending on dose calculations made by the radiation physicist.

Automated high-dose rate (HDR) intracavitary brachytherapy systems have been developed that allow outpatient radiation therapy. Treatment time is shorter, thereby decreasing patient discomfort. Staff exposure to radiation is also avoided. Isotopes of radium and cesium are used for intracavitary irradiation.

NURSING CONSIDERATIONS FOR RADIATION SAFETY

Various radioactive elements are used in intracavitary therapy. Regardless of the specific agent used, diligent nursing care must be provided. The patient is carefully monitored and care is provided. However, the nursing staff must minimize radiation exposure to themselves as much as possible by:

- Minimizing the amount of time near a radioactive source
- Maximizing the distance from the radioactive source
- Using required shielding to minimize exposure

Nurses who are or may be pregnant should not be involved in the immediate care of such patients. Nursing visits to patients should be planned to minimize the amount of time the nurse is in contact with the patient. In addition, to minimize radiation exposure, the nurse remains as far away (ie, at the entrance to the room) from the radiation source as possible but makes special efforts to provide some time to discuss the patient's anxieties and fears.

The Radiation Safety Department will give specific safety precautions to those people who will be in contact with the patient, including health care providers and family. Nurses caring for the patient will receive instructions about safe times and distances related to care provision to ensure that their occupational exposure is *a*s *l*ow *a*s *r*easonably *a*chievable (ALARA). Other instructions vary but may include the following:

- Wear film badges or pocket ion chambers to monitor exposure.
- Wear rubber gloves to dispose of any soiled matter that may be contaminated. (However, these gloves do not provide protection from sealed radiation sources.)
- Follow specific laundry and housekeeping directions.
- Keep the patient restricted to her room and allow no visitors who are or may be pregnant or who are younger than 18 years of age.
- Explain that a discharge survey is usually performed by Radiation Safety Department personnel before the patient leaves the room to ensure that all sources of radiation have been removed.

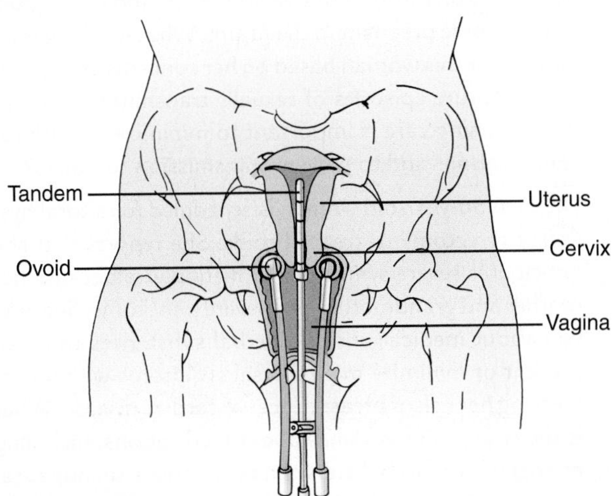

FIGURE 47-8. Placement of tandem and ovoids for internal radiation therapy.

NURSING PRIORITIES FOR PATIENT CARE

Of the many nursing concerns, primary concerns include providing the patient with emotional support and physical comfort and not dislodging the applicator. Although the radiation oncologist takes steps to secure the internal applicator in place and nursing personnel need not be preoccupied with the fear that the applicator will be prematurely extruded, they should monitor to see that the applicator or the radioactive sources have not been dislodged. Should this happen, the nurse should avoid touching the radioactive object and notify the Radiation Safety Department at once.

The nurse needs to explain that during the treatment, the patient must stay on absolute bed rest. She may move from side to side with her back supported by a pillow, and the head of the bed may be raised to 15 degrees. She should be encouraged to practice deep-breathing and coughing exercises and to flex and extend the feet to stretch the calf muscles, promoting circulation and venous return. Elastic compression stockings are worn to prevent venous pooling. Back care, though appreciated by the patient, needs to be performed within the minimal time allowed at the bedside.

Usually, the patient receives a low-residue diet to prevent frequent bowel movements. In addition, a urinary catheter is in place and must be inspected frequently to ensure that it drains properly. The chief hazard of improper drainage is that the bladder may become distended and its walls exposed to radiation. Although perineal care is not performed at this time, any profuse discharge should be reported immediately to the radiation oncologist or gynecologic surgeon.

Additional nursing interventions include observing the patient for temperature elevation, nausea, and vomiting. These symptoms should be reported because they may indicate such complications as infection or perforation.

Patient teaching includes informing the patient that abdominal fullness, cramping, backache, and the urge to void are normal feelings during therapy. Severe pain should not occur. Administering mild opioid agents, muscle relaxants, or sedative medications may be helpful.

APPLICATOR REMOVAL

The radiation oncologist calculates precisely the radiation dose. At the end of the prescribed period, the nurse may be requested to assist a physician in removing the applicator. Because the sources are afterloaded, they can be removed by the physician in the same manner as they were inserted. This does not require local or general anesthesia and is performed in the patient's room. However, it may be necessary to medicate the patient with a mild sedative agent before the applicator is removed.

POST-TREATMENT CARE

Progressive ambulation is recommended after any period of enforced bed rest. Diet may be offered as tolerated. The patient may shower as soon as she wishes but should be instructed not to douche after removal of the applicator. Because the cervix may have been dilated, any chance of bacterial contamination should be minimized.

Both before and after treatment, nurses caring for patients undergoing radiation therapy need to assess any misconceptions about this mode of treatment that the patient and family may have. The oncology clinical nurse specialist may be a valuable resource for information and problem solving, if necessary. Resources for further clinical and patient information are listed at the end of Chapter 16.

Side Effects of Radiation Therapy

Radiation side effects are cumulative and tend to appear when the total dose exceeds the body's natural capacity to repair the damage caused by radiation. Radiation enteritis, resulting in diarrhea and abdominal cramping, and radiation cystitis, manifested by urinary frequency, urgency, and dysuria, may occur. These effects are manifestations of the normal tissues' response to radiation therapy. Occasionally, severe reactions require interrupting treatment until normal tissue repair occurs. Fatigue is one of the most bothersome side effects and is often not relieved by rest.

The radiation oncologist and nurse must carefully inform the patient in advance about possible side effects and implement management strategies if they occur. Such measures include dietary control (restricting the amount of fiber, roughage, and lactose) and the use of antispasmodic medications. The purpose of a low-residue diet is to prevent frequent bowel movements and to prevent exposure of the intestines to radiation. An oncology dietitian may be consulted.

Evaluating the patient's and family's physical, emotional, and learning needs is part of the nursing assessment before and during treatment. Information overload, along with anxiety that impairs learning, must be anticipated.

Any method of therapy requires adequate preparation, education, and emotional support. The patient who has been adequately prepared, supported, and educated before treatment through expert nursing care finds it easier to cope with the rigors and stress of cancer and its treatment.

Critical Thinking Exercises

1 When visiting the employee health center to obtain her annual influenza vaccine, a 48-year-old woman with a history of breast cancer and previous mastectomy reports that she has been experiencing vague abdominal discomfort, bloating, flatulence, and increased waist size over the last six months. Her next annual physical examination is 6 months from now. What additional information is it important to obtain from her? What recommendations for further follow-up and health care would you provide?

2 A 75-year-old woman with a history of angina and osteoarthritis is scheduled to undergo radical vulvectomy. She reports that she is very anxious because she has never been hospitalized before and is unsure of what to expect. Describe the preoperative teaching for her and the postoperative care that can be anticipated. How will her history of angina and osteoarthritis affect her care? What modifications in care, postoperative teaching and discharge planning may be necessary because of these health issues?

3 A 25-year-old woman with a diagnosis of severe pelvic inflammatory disease (PID) has been admitted to the hospital for intravenous (IV) antibiotics. When you discuss the disorder with her, she expresses concern about the effect of PID on future sexual relationships and on her ability to become pregnant in the future. What teaching is indicated for this woman based on her concerns and on her risk for future episodes of sexually transmitted disease? What nursing care is important to minimize the risk for complications and to prevent transmission to others?

4 ebp A 50-year-old woman is scheduled for a total hysterectomy to treat fibroids. She reports that she anticipates severe symptoms of menopause because her mother and grandmother had severe symptoms. She asks you about medications and herbal substances that can prevent or minimize menopausal symptoms without increasing her risk of breast cancer or cardiac disease. What is the strength of evidence about medications, including estrogen, and herbal substances to reduce menopausal symptoms? What criteria would you use to determine the strength of that evidence?

5 A 49-year-old woman is scheduled for surgery to repair a rectovaginal fistula. She has multiple sclerosis (MS) and has used a wheelchair for 15 years because of limited mobility. How would you modify her pre- and postoperative nursing care in view of her MS and limited mobility? What discharge planning will be important for her?

REFERENCES AND SELECTED READINGS

BOOKS

American Cancer Society. (2006). *Cancer facts and figures*. Atlanta, GA: Author.

American College of Obstetricians and Gynecologists. (2003). *Compendium of selected publications*. Washington, DC: Author.

American College of Obstetricians and Gynecologists. (2002). *Guidelines for women's health care*. Washington, DC: Author.

American Cancer Society. (2004). *Cancer facts and figures*. Atlanta, GA: Author.

American Cancer Society. (2005). *Cancer facts and figures*. Atlanta, GA: Author.

Emans, J., Laufer, M., & Goldstein, D. (2004). *Pediatric and adolescent gynecology* (4th ed.). Philadelphia: Lippincott Williams & Wilkins.

Holmes, K. K., Sparling, P. F., Mardh, P. C., et al. (2000). *Sexually transmitted diseases*. New York: McGraw-Hill.

ACOG Committee on Practice Bulletin—Gynecology. (2004). ACOG Chronic pelvic pain. Practice Bulletin No. 51. *Obstetrics & Gynecology, 103*(3), 589–605.

U.S. Public Health Service. (2000). *Healthy people 2010*. Washington, DC: U.S. Department of Health and Human Services.

U.S. Surgeon General. (2001). *The Surgeon General's call to action to promote sexual health and responsible sexual behavior*. Washington, DC: U.S. Department of Health and Human Services.

Youngkin, E. & Davis, M. (2004). *Women's health: A primary care clinical guide*. Upper Saddle River, NJ: Pearson Prentice Hall.

JOURNALS

**Asterisks indicate nursing research articles.*

General

Centers for Disease Control and Prevention. (2002). Sexually transmitted diseases treatment guidelines, 2002. *MMWR: Morbidity and Mortality Weekly Report, 51*(RR06), 1–80.

McCrink, A. (2004). Evaluating the female pelvic floor. *AWHONN Lifelines, 7*(6), 514–522.

Nelson, H. D., Humphrey, L. L., Nygren, P., et al. (2002). Postmenopausal hormone replacement therapy: Scientific review. *Journal of the American Medical Association, 288*(7), 872–881.

Women's Health Initiative. (2002). Risks and benefits of estrogen plus progestin in healthy postmenopausal women: Principal results from the Women's Health Initiative randomized controlled trial. *Journal of the American Medical Association, 288*(3), 321–333.

Benign Vulvar Disorders

Edwards, L. (2003). New concepts in vulvodynia. *American Journal of Obstetrics & Gynecology, 189*(3) Supplement, S24–S30.

Marzano, D., & Haefner, H. (2004). The Bartholin gland cyst: Past, present and future. *Journal of Lower Genital Tract Disease, 8*(3), 1195–2004.

Benign Ovarian Disorders

Guzick, D. (2004). Polycystic ovary syndrome. *Obstetrics and Gynecology, 103*(1), 181–193.

Rotterdam ESHRE/ASRM-sponsored PCOS consensus workshop group. (2004). Revised 2003 consensus on diagnostic criteria and long-term health risks related to polycystic ovary syndrome (PCOS). *Human Reproduction, 19*(1), 41–47.

Tsilchorozidou, T., & Prelevic, G. (2003). The role of metformin in the management of polycystic ovary syndrome. *Current Opinion in Obstetrics and Gynecology, 15*(6), 483–488.

Benign Uterine Disorders

ACOG Committee Opinion. (2004). Uterine artery embolization. *Obstetrics and Gynecology, 103*(2), 403–404.

Andrews, R. T., Spies, J. B., Sacks, D., et al. (2004). Patient care and uterine artery embolization for leiomyomata. *Journal of Vascular & Interventional Radiology, 15*(2, Part 1), 115–120.

Freeman, S. (2002). Dysfunctional uterine bleeding. *Advance for Nurse Practitioners, 10*(12), 20–28.

Hovsepian, D., Siskin, G., Bonn, J., et al. (2004). Quality improvement guidelines for uterine artery embolization for symptomatic leiomyomata. *Journal of Vascular & Interventional Radiology, 15*(6), 535–541.

Maher, C. F., Qatawneh, A. M., Dwyer, P. L., et al. (2004). Abdominal sacral colpopexy or vaginal sacrospinous colpopexy for vaginal vault prolapse: A prospective randomized study. *American Journal of Obstetrics and Gynecology, 190*(1), 20–26.

Montgomery, B., Daum, G., & Dunton, C. (2004). Endometrial hyperplasia: A review. *Obstetrics and Gynecoly Survey, 59*(5), 368–378.

Nygaard, I., Bradley, C., & Berandt, D. (2004). Pelvic organ prolapse in older women: Prevalence and risk factors. *Obstetrics & Gynecology, 104*(3), 489–497.

Steinauer, J., Pritts, E. A., Jackson, R., et al. (2004). Systematic review of mifepristone for the treatment of uterine leiomyomata. *Obstetrics & Gynecology, 103*(6), 1331–1336.

Wallach, E., & Vlahos, N. (2004). Uterine myomas: An overview of development, clinical features and management. *Obstetrics & Gynecology, 104*(2), 393–406.

Endometriosis

*Denny, E. (2004). Women's experiences of endometriosis. *Journal of Advances in Nursing*. 46(6), 641–648.

*Lemaire, G. S. (2004). More than just menstrual cramps: Symptoms and uncertainty among women with endometriosis. *Journal of Obstetrical, Gynecologic, and Neonatal Nurses, 33*(1), 71–79.

Human Papillomavirus

Choma, K. K. (2003). ASC-US and HPV testing. *American Journal of Nursing, 103*(2), 42–50.

Koutsky, L. A., Ault, K. A., Wheeler, C. M., et al. (2002). A controlled trial of human papillomavirus type 16 vaccine. *New England Journal of Medicine, 347*(21), 1645–1651.

Hysterectomy

DeCherney, A., Bachmann, G., Isaacson, K., et al. (2002). Postoperative fatigue negatively impacts the daily lives of patients recovering from hysterectomy. *Obstetrics and Gynecology, 99*(1), 51–57.

Garry, R., Fountain, J., Mason, S., et al. (2004). The eVALuate study: Two parallel randomised trials, one comparing laparoscopic with abdominal hysterectomy, the other comparing laparoscopic with vaginal hysterectomy. *British Medical Journal, 328*(7432), 129.

Heinberg, E., Crawford, B., Weitzen, S., et al. (2004). Total laparoscopic hysterectomy in obese versus nonobese patients. *Obstetrics and Gynecology, 103*(4), 674–680.

Katz, A. (2003). Sexuality after hysterectomy: A review of the literature and discussion of the nurses' role. *Journal of Advanced Nursing, 42*(3), 297–303.

Kovac, S. (2004). Transvaginal hysterectomy: Rationale and surgical approach. *Obstetrics and Gynecology, 103*(6), 1321–1325.

Torpy, J., & Lynm, C. (2004). Hysterectomy. *Journal of the American Medical Association, 291*(12), 1526.

Reproductive Malignancy

ACOG Statement of Policy (2004). Cervical cancer prevention in low resource settings. *Obstetrics and Gynecology, 103*(3), 607–609.

*Ahlberg, K., Ekman, T., Wallgreen, A., et al. (2004). Fatigue, psychological distress, coping and quality of life in patients with uterine cancer. *Journal of Advanced Nursing, 45*(2), 205–213.

Almadrones, L. A., (2003). Treatment advances in ovarian cancer. *Cancer Nursing, 26*(Supplement 6S), 16S-20S.

Benard, V., Eheman, C., Lawson, H., et al. (2004). Cervical screening in the national breast and cervical cancer early detection program. *Obstetrics and Gynecology, 103*(3), 564–571.

Blunt, E. (2004). Diethylstilbestrol exposure: It's still an issue. *Holistic Nursing Practice, 18*(4), 187–191.

Bowcock, S., Shee, C., Rassam, S., et al. (2004). Chemotherapy for cancer patients who present late. *British Medical Journal, 328*(7453), 1430–1432.

Cannistra, S. A. (2004). Cancer of the ovary. *New England Journal of Medicine, 351*(24), 2519–2529.

Daly, M. B. & Ozols, R. F. (2004). Symptoms of ovarian cancer-where to set the bar. *Journal of the American Medical Association, 291*(22), 2755–2756

Ekman, I., Bergbom, I., Ekman, T., et al. (2004). Maintaining normality and support are central issues when receiving chemotherapy for ovarian cancer. *Cancer Nursing, 27*(3), 177–182.

Eltabbakh, G. H., Yildiram, Z., & Adamowicz, R. (2004). Paclitaxel and carboplatin as second-line therapy in women with platinum-sensitive ovarian carcinoma treated with platinum and paclitaxel as first-line therapy. *American Journal of Clinical Oncology, 27*(1), 46–50.

Fowler, J., Carpenter, K., Gupta, P., et al. (2004). The gynecologic oncology consult: Symptom presentation and concurrent symptoms of depression and anxiety. *Obstetrics and Gynecology, 103*(6), 1211–1216.

Goff, B., Mandel, L., Melancon, C., et al. (2004). Frequency of symptoms of ovarian cancer in women presenting to primary care clinics. *Journal of the American Medical Association, 291*(22), 2705–2712.

Harris, L. L. (2002). Ovarian cancer: Screening for early detection. *American Journal of Nursing, 102*(10), 46–52.

Hockel, M., & Dornhofer, N. (2004). Anatomical reconstruction after vulvectomy. *Obstetrics and Gynecology, 103*(5,Part 2), 1125–28.

Kim, J-H., Skates, S. J., Uede, T., et al. (2002). Osteopontin as a potential diagnostic biomarker for ovarian cancer. *Journal of the American Medical Association, 287*(13), 1671–75.

Lentz, S., Muderspach, L., Felix, J., et al. (2004). Identification of micrometastases in histologically negative lymph nodes of early stage cervical cancer patients. *Obstetrics and Gynecology, 103*(6), 1204–1210.

Luce, T., Dow, K. H., & Holcomb, L. (2003). Early diagnosis key to epithelial ovarian cancer detection. *Nurse Practitioner, 28*(12), 41–47.

Murthy, V. H., Krumholz, H. M., & Gross, C. P. (2004). Participation in cancer clinical trials: Race-, sex-, and age-based disparities. *Journal of the American Medical Association, 291*(22), 2720–2726.

Pasacreta, J., Jacobs, L., & Cataldo, J. (2002). Genetic testing for breast and ovarian cancer risk: The psychosocial issues. *American Journal of Nursing, 102*(12), 40–49.

Patlas, J., Rosen, B., Chapman, W., et al. (2004). Sonographic diagnosis of primary malignant tumors of the fallopian tube. *Ultrasound Quarterly, 20*(2), 59–64.

Posadas, E. M., Davidson, B., & Kohn, E. C. (2004). Proteomics and ovarian cancer: Implications for diagnosis and treatment: A critical review of the recent literature. *Current Opinion in Oncology, 16*(5), 478–484.

Randall, T., & Armstrong, K. (2003). Differences in treatment and outcome between African American and white women with endometrial cancer. *Journal of Clinical Oncology, 21*(22), 4200–4206.

Rebbeck, T. R, Lynch, H. T, Neuhausen, S. L., et al. (2002). Prophylactic oophorectomy in carriers of BRCA1 or BRCA2 mutations. *New England Journal of Medicine, 346*(21), 1616–1622.

Rose, P. G., Nerenstone, S., Brady, M. F. (2004). Secondary surgical cytoreduction for advanced ovarian carcinoma. *New England Journal of Medicine, 351*(24), 2489–2497.

Shinn, S. (2004). Taking a stand against cervical cancer. *Nursing 2004, 34*(5), 36–41.

Wilson, C., Tobin, S., & Young, R. (2004). The exploding worldwide cancer burden: The impact of cancer on women. *International Journal of Gynecologic Cancer, 14*(1), 1–11.

STDs, Vaginitis, and Vulvovaginal Infections and Pelvic Infections

Adams, A., Southwick, K., Jui, J., et al. (2004). Electronic reporting of pelvic inflammatory disease from an emergency department. *Sexually Transmitted Diseases, 31*(6), 327–330.

Allen-Davis, J., Beck, A., Parker, R., et al. (2002). Assessment of vulvovaginal complaints: Accuracy of telephone triage and in-office diagnosis. *Obstetrics and Gynecology, 99*(1), 18–22.

Clark, R., & Dumestre, J. (2004). Women and human immunodeficiency virus: Unique management issues. *American Journal of Medical Sciences, 328*(1), 17–25.

Feroli, K. L. & Burstein, G. R. (2003). Adolescent sexually transmitted diseases: New recommendations for diagnosis, treatment and prevention. *MCN: American Journal of Maternal Child Nursing, 28*(2), 113–118.

Hader, S., Smith, D., Moore, J., et al. (2001). HIV infection in women in the US: Status at the millennium. *Journal of the American Medical Association, 285*(9), 1186–1192.

Hillier, S. (2004). Treatment of recurrent bacterial vaginosis. *Clinician Reviews, 14*(6), 98–101.

Kimberlin, D., & Rouse, D. (2004). Genital herpes. *New England Journal of Medicine, 350*(19), 1970–1977.

Klebanoff, J., Schwebke, J., Zhang, J., et al. (2004). Vulvovaginal symptoms in women with bacterial vaginosis. *Obstetrics and Gynecology, 104*(2), 267–272.

Ledger, W., & Monif, G. (2004). A growing concern: Inability to diagnose vulvovaginal infections correctly. *Obstetrics and Gynecology, 103*(4), 782–784.

Miller, W., Ford, C., Morris, M., et al. (2004). Prevalence of chlamydia and gonococcal infections among young adults in the US. *Journal of the American Medical Association, 291*(18), 2161–2276.

Mitchell, H. (2004). Vaginal discharge—causes, diagnosis and treatment. *British Medical Journal, 328*(7451), 1306–1308.

Schwebke, J., Desmond, R., & Kim, O. (2004) Predictors of bacterial vaginosis in adolescent women who douche. *Sexually Transmitted Diseases, 31*(7), 433–436.

Shah, A., & Panjabi, C. (2004). Human seminal plasma allergy: A review of a rare phenomenon. *Clinical & Experimental Allergy, 34*(6), 827–838.

Soper, D. (2004). Trichomoniasis: Under control or undercontrolled. *American Journal of Obstetrics and Gynecology, 190*(1), 281–290.

RESOURCES

American Cancer Society, 1599 Clifton Road NE, Atlanta, GA 30329; (800) ACS-2345; http://www.cancer.org. Accessed July 10, 2006.

American Social Health Association, P.O. Box 13827, Research Triangle Park, NC 27709; (800) 227-8922; http://www.ashastd.org/std/std.html; teen website: http://www.iwannaknow.org. Accessed July 11, 2006.

Association of Reproductive Health Professionals, 2401 Pennsylvania Avenue, Suite 350, Washington, DC 20037-1718; (202) 466-3825; http://www.arhp.org. Accessed July 11, 2006.

AWHONN: Association of Women's Health, Obstetrical and Neonatal Nurses, 2000 L St., NW, Suite 7400, Washington, DC 20036; http://www.awhonn.org. Accessed July 11, 2006.

Cancer Journey: Issues for Survivors. A leader's guide and videotape available from the National Cancer Institute (1-800-4-CANCER)

Centers for Disease Control and Prevention, Office of Women's Health, 1600 Clifton Road, MS: D-51, Atlanta, GA 30033; (404) 639-7230; http://www.cdc.gov/od/owh/whstd.htm. Accessed July 11, 2006.

Endometriosis Association, 8585 N. 76th Place, Milwaukee, WI 53223; (800) 992-3636; http://www.endometriosisassn.org. Accessed July 11, 2006.

Gay and Lesbian Medical Association, 459 Fulton St., Suite 107, San Francisco, CA 94102; (415) 225-4547; http://www.glma.org/home.html.

Herpes Hotline: (919) 361-8488.

Herpetics Engaged in Living Productively (HELP), 260 Sheridan Avenue, Palo Alto, CA 94306.

National AIDS Hotline: (800) 342-AIDS; http://www.ashastd.org/nah.

National Ovarian Cancer Coalition, 500 NE Spanish River Boulevard, Suite 8, Boca Raton, FL 33432, (561) 393-0005; (888)-ovarian; http://www.ovarian.org. Accessed July 11, 2006.

National STD Hotline: (800) 227-8922 or (800) 342-2437; http://www.ashastd.org/nah. Accessed July 11, 2006.

Ovarian Cancer National Alliance, 910 17thStreet, Suite 1190, Washington, DC, 20006; (202)331-1332; http://www.ovariancancer.org. Accessed July 11, 2006.

Planned Parenthood Federation of America, 810 Seventh Avenue, New York, NY 10019; (800) 829-PPFA; http://www.plannedparenthood.org/sti/.

Resolve: The National Infertility Association, 1310 Broadway, Somerville, MA 02144; (888) 623-0744; http://www.resolve.org.

Women's Cancer Network, Gynecologic Cancer Foundation, 230 W. Monroe, Suite 2528, Chicago, IL 60606, 312-578-1439, FAX: 312-578-9769 http://www.wcn.org. Accessed July 11, 2006.

CHAPTER 48

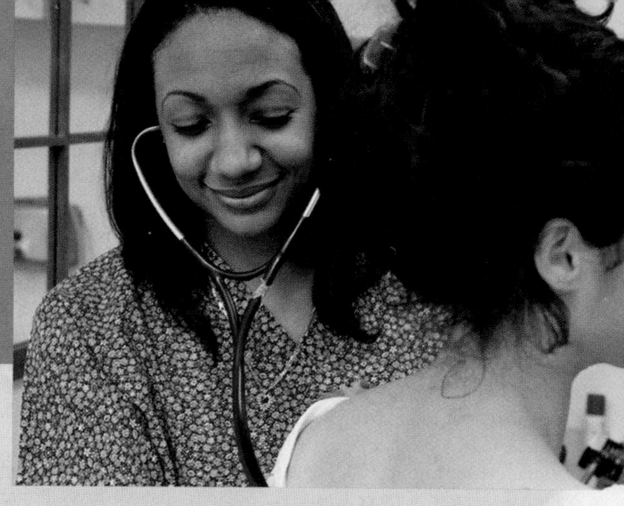

Assessment and Management of Patients With Breast Disorders

Learning Objectives

On completion of this chapter, the learner will be able to:

1. Summarize the guidelines for the early detection of breast cancer.
2. Develop a teaching plan for breast self-examination for patients and consumer groups.
3. Identify the diagnostic tests used to detect breast disorders.
4. Describe the different modalities used to treat breast cancer.
5. Use the nursing process as a framework for care of the patient undergoing breast cancer surgery.
6. Describe the physical, psychosocial, and rehabilitative needs of the patient who has had breast surgery for the treatment of breast cancer.

In many cultures, the breast plays a significant role in a woman's sexuality and self-identity. A breast disorder, whether benign or malignant, can cause great anxiety and fear of potential disfigurement, loss of sexual attractiveness, and even death. Nurses, therefore, must have expertise in the assessment and management of not only the physical symptoms but also the psychosocial symptoms of breast disorders.

Anatomic and Physiologic Overview

Male and female breasts mature comparably until puberty, when in females estrogen and other hormones initiate breast development. This development usually occurs from 10 to 16 years of age, although the range can vary from 9 to 18 years. Stages of breast development are described as Tanner stages 1 through 5.

- Stage 1 describes a prepubertal breast.
- Stage 2 is breast budding, the first sign of puberty in a female.
- Stage 3 involves further enlargement of breast tissue and the areola (a darker tissue ring around the nipple).
- Stage 4 occurs when the nipple and areola form a secondary mound on top of the breast tissue.
- Stage 5 is the continued development of a larger breast with a single contour.

The breasts are located between the second and sixth ribs over the pectoralis muscle from the sternum to the midaxillary line. An area of breast tissue, called the tail of Spence,

Glossary

adjuvant chemotherapy: use of anticancer medications in addition to other treatments (i.e., surgery, radiation) to delay or prevent a recurrence of the disease

aromatase inhibitors: medications that block the production of estrogens by the adrenal glands

atypical hyperplasia: abnormal increase in the number of cells in a specific area within the ductal or lobular areas of the breast; this abnormal proliferation increases the risk for cancer

benign proliferative breast disease: various types of atypical, yet noncancerous, breast tissue that increase the risk for breast cancer

brachytherapy: form of partial breast radiation in which a radioactive source is placed within the lumpectomy site

BRCA-1 and **BRCA-2:** genes on chromosome 17 that, when damaged or mutated, place a woman at greater risk for breast cancer and/or ovarian cancer compared with women who do not have the mutation

breast conservation treatment: surgery to remove a breast tumor and a margin of tissue around the tumor without removing any other part of the breast; may or may not include lymph node removal and radiation therapy

dose-dense chemotherapy: administration of chemotherapeutic agents at standard doses with shorter time intervals between each cycle of treatment

ductal carcinoma in situ (DCIS): cancer cells that start in the ductal system of the breast but have not penetrated the surrounding tissue

estrogen and progesterone receptor assay: test to determine whether the breast tumor is nourished by hormones; this information helps in determining prognosis and treatment

fibrocystic breast changes: term used to describe certain benign changes in the breast, typically associated with palpable nodularity, lumpiness, swelling, or pain

fine-needle aspiration (FNA): removal of fluid for diagnostic analysis from a cyst or cells from a mass using a needle and syringe

galactography: use of mammography after an injection of radiopaque dye to diagnose problems in the ductal system of the breast

gynecomastia: overdeveloped breast tissue typically seen in adolescent boys

lobular carcinoma in situ (LCIS): atypical change and proliferation of the lobular cells of the breast; previously considered a premalignant condition but now considered a marker of increased risk for invasive breast cancer

lymphedema: chronic swelling of an extremity due to interrupted lymphatic circulation, typically from an axillary lymph node dissection

mammoplasty: surgical procedure to reconstruct or change the size or shape of the breast; can be performed for reduction or augmentation

mastalgia: breast pain, usually related to hormonal fluctuations or irritation of a nerve

mastitis: inflammation or infection of the breast

modified radical mastectomy: removal of the breast tissue, nipple–areola complex, and a portion of the axillary lymph nodes

neoadjuvant chemotherapy: preoperative chemotherapy; it is administered preoperatively to shrink a large tumor

Paget disease: form of breast cancer that begins in the ductal system and involves the nipple, areola, and surrounding skin

prophylactic mastectomy: removal of the breast to reduce the risk of breast cancer in women considered to be at high risk for development of the disease

sentinel lymph node: first lymph node(s) in the lymphatic basin that receives drainage from the primary tumor in the breast; identified by a radioisotope and/or blue dye

stereotactic biopsy: computer-guided method of core needle biopsy that is useful when masses in the breast cannot be felt but can be visualized using mammography

surgical biopsy: procedure in which an entire mass or a portion of it is surgically removed for examination under a microscope by a pathologist

tissue expander followed by permanent implant: series of surgical procedures used to reconstruct the breast after a mastectomy; involves stretching the skin and muscle before inserting the permanent implant

total mastectomy: removal of the breast tissue and nipple–areola complex

transverse rectus abdominis myocutaneous (TRAM) flap: method of breast reconstruction in which a flap of skin, fat, and muscle from the lower abdomen, with its attached blood supply, is rotated to the mastectomy site

ultrasonography: imaging method using high-frequency sound waves to diagnose whether masses are solid or fluid-filled

extends into the axilla. Fascial bands, called Cooper's ligaments, support the breast on the chest wall. The inframammary fold (or crease) is a ridge of fat at the bottom of the breast.

Each breast contains 12 to 20 cone-shaped lobes, which are made up of glandular elements (lobules and ducts) and separated by fat and fibrous tissue that binds the lobes together. Milk is produced in the lobules and then carried through the ducts to the nipple. Figure 48-1 shows the anatomy of the fully developed breast.

Assessment

Health History

When a patient presents with a breast problem, the nurse conducts a general health assessment, including history of medical disorders and previous surgery; family history of cancer; gynecologic and obstetric history; present medications (including prescriptions, vitamins, and herbal); past and present use of hormonal contraceptives, hormone therapy (HT), or fertility treatments; and social habits (eg, smoking, drinking alcohol). Psychosocial information, such as the patient's marital status, occupation, and availability of resources and support people, is obtained. Any recent x-rays or other diagnostic tests are noted. Focused questions pertaining to the breast disorder are asked concerning the onset of the disorder and the length of time it has been present. In addition, the patient is asked if any masses are palpable and if there is any associated pain, swelling, redness, nipple discharge, or skin changes. Knowledge and comfort in practicing breast self-examination (BSE) should also be ascertained from the patient.

Physical Assessment: Female Breast

A female breast examination can be conducted during any general physical or gynecologic examination or whenever the patient reports an abnormality. The American Cancer Society (ACS) recommends that women at average risk for breast cancer undergo a clinical breast examination at least every 3 years while in their 20s and 30s and then annually thereafter (Chart 48-1). A thorough breast examination, including instruction in BSE, takes at least 10 minutes.

Inspection

Examination begins with inspection. The patient is asked to disrobe to the waist and sit in a comfortable position facing the examiner. The breasts are inspected for size and symmetry. A slight variation in the size of each breast is common and generally normal. The skin is inspected for color, venous pattern, thickening, or edema. Erythema (redness) may indicate benign local inflammation or superficial lymphatic invasion by a neoplasm. A prominent venous pattern can signal increased blood supply required by a tumor. Edema and pitting of the skin may result from a neoplasm blocking

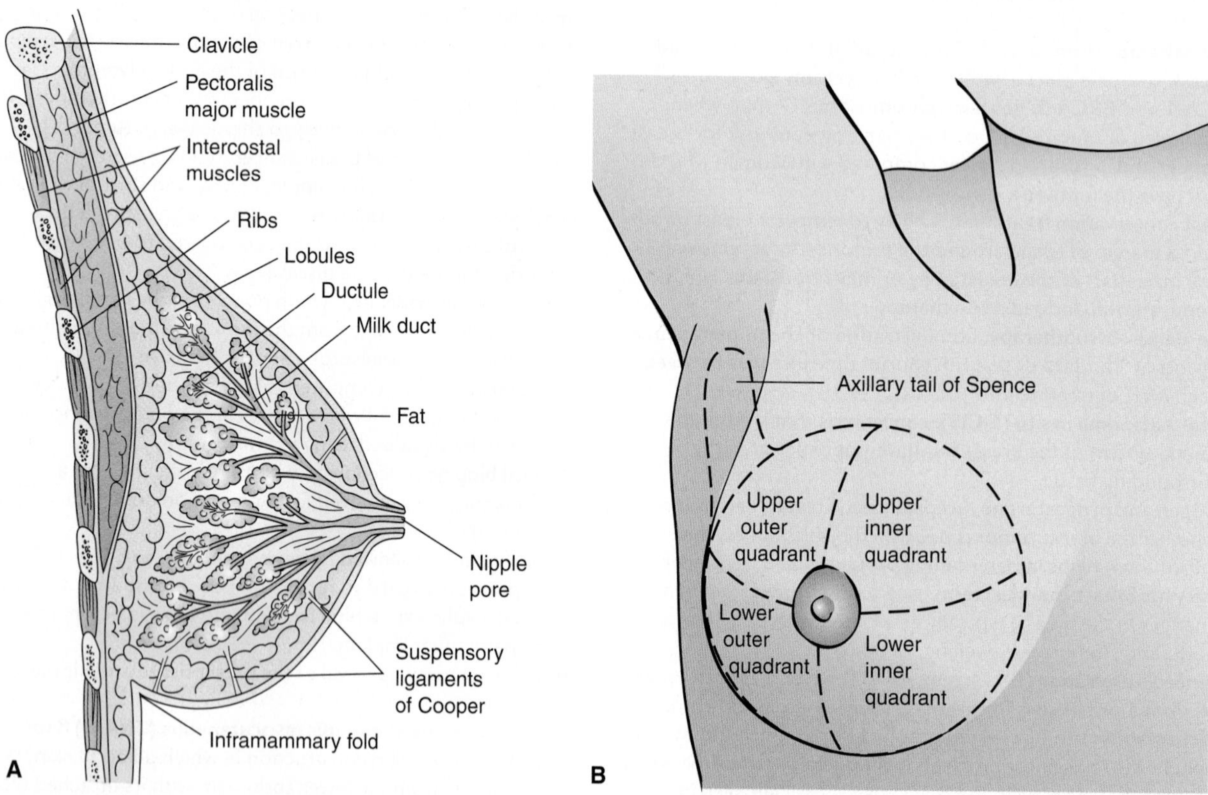

FIGURE 48-1. (A) Anatomy of the breast. (B) Areas of breast, including the tail of Spence. Adapted from Weber, J., & Kelley, J. (2003). *Health assessment in nursing* (2nd ed.). Philadelphia: Lippincott Williams & Wilkins.

CHART 48-1

American Cancer Society Guidelines for Early Detection of Breast Cancer

WOMEN AT AVERAGE RISK

- Begin mammography at 40 years of age.
- For women in their 20s and 30s, it is recommended that clinical breast examination be part of a periodic health examination, preferably at least every 3 years. Asymptomatic women 40 years of age and older should continue to receive a clinical breast examination as part of a periodic health examination, preferably annually.
- Beginning in their 20s, women should be told about the benefits and limitations of breast self-examination (BSE). The importance of prompt reporting of any new breast symptoms to a health care professional should be emphasized. Women who choose to do BSE should receive instruction and have their technique reviewed on the occasion of a periodic health examination. It is acceptable for women to choose not to do BSE or to do BSE irregularly.
- Women should have an opportunity to become informed about the benefits, limitations, and potential harms associated with regular screening.

OLDER WOMEN

- Screening decisions in older women should be individualized by considering the potential benefits and risks of mammography in the context of current health status and estimated life expectancy. As long as a woman is in reasonably good health and would be a candidate for treatment, she should continue to be screened with mammography.

WOMEN AT INCREASED RISK

- Women at increased risk for breast cancer might benefit from additional screening strategies beyond those offered to women of average risk, such as earlier initiation of screening, shorter screening intervals, or the addition of screening modalities other than mammography and physical examination, such as ultrasound or magnetic resonance imaging. However, the currently available evidence is insufficient to justify recommendations for any of these screening approaches.

Smith, R. A., Saslow, D., Sawyer, K. A. et al. (2003). American Cancer Society guidelines for breast cancer screening: Update 2003. *CA: A Cancer Journal for Clinicians, 53*(3), 141–169.

lymphatic drainage, giving the skin an orange-peel appearance (peau d'orange), a classic sign of advanced breast cancer. Nipple inversion of one or both breasts is not uncommon and is significant only when of recent origin. Ulceration, rashes, or spontaneous nipple discharge requires evaluation. Examples of abnormal breast findings can be found in Chart 48-2.

To elicit skin dimpling or retraction that may otherwise go undetected, the examiner instructs the patient to raise both arms overhead. This maneuver normally elevates both breasts equally. The patient is then instructed to place her hands on her waist and push in. These movements, which cause contraction of the pectoral muscles, do not normally alter the breast contour or nipple direction. Any dimpling or retraction during these position changes suggests an underlying mass. The clavicular and axillary regions are inspected for swelling, discoloration, lesions, or enlarged lymph nodes.

Palpation

The breasts are palpated with the patient sitting up (upright) and lying down (supine). In the supine position the patient's shoulder is first elevated with a small pillow to help balance the breast on the chest wall. Failure to do this allows the breast tissue to slip laterally, and a breast mass may be missed. The entire surface of the breast and the axillary tail is systematically palpated using the flat part (pads) of the 2nd, 3rd, and 4th fingertips, held together, making dime-sized circles. The examiner may choose to proceed in a clockwise direction, following imaginary concentric circles from the outer limits of the breast toward the nipple. Other acceptable methods are to palpate from each number on the face of the clock toward the nipple in a clockwise fashion or along imaginary vertical lines on the breast (Fig. 48-2).

Palpation of the axillary and clavicular areas is easily performed with the patient seated (Fig. 48-3). To examine the axillary lymph nodes, the examiner gently abducts the patient's arm from the thorax. With the left hand, the patient's left forearm is grasped and supported. The right hand is then free to palpate the axillae. Any lymph nodes that may be lying against the thoracic wall are noted. Normally, these lymph nodes are not palpable, but if they are enlarged, their location, size, mobility, and consistency are noted. During palpation, the examiner notes any patient-reported tenderness or masses. If a mass is detected, it is described by its location (e.g., left breast, 2 cm from the nipple at 2 o'clock position). Size, shape, consistency, border delineation, and mobility are included in the description.

The breast tissue of the adolescent is usually firm and lobular, whereas that of the postmenopausal woman is more likely to feel thinner and fattier. During pregnancy and lactation, the breasts are firmer and larger with lobules that are more distinct. Hormonal changes cause the areola to darken. Cysts are commonly found in menstruating women and are usually well defined and freely movable. Premenstrually, cysts may be larger and more tender. Malignant tumors, on the other hand, tend to be hard, poorly defined, and nontender. A physician should further evaluate any abnormalities detected during inspection and palpation.

Physical Assessment: Male Breast

Breast cancer can occur in men. Examination of the male breast and axillae should be included in a physical examination. The nipple and areola are inspected for masses and nipple discharge. The same procedure for palpating the female axillae is used when assessing the male axillae.

Gynecomastia is the firm enlargement of glandular tissue beneath and immediately surrounding the areola of the

CHART 48-2

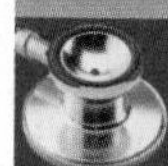

Assessing the Breasts

Abnormal Breast Findings

RETRACTION SIGNS

- Signs include skin dimpling, creasing, or changes in the contour of the breast or nipple
- Secondary to fibrosis or scar tissue formation in the breast
- Retraction signs may appear only with position changes or with breast palpation.

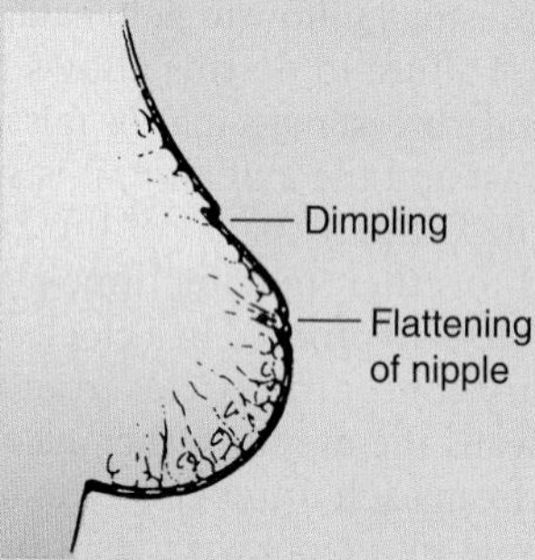

Retraction signs

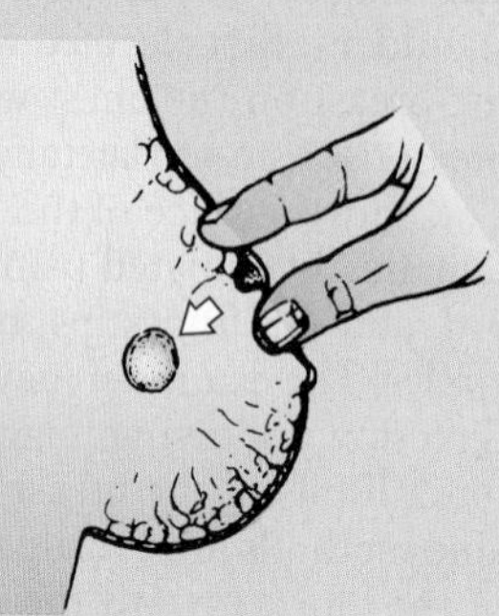

Retraction with compression

BREAST CANCER MASS (MALIGNANT TUMOR)

- Usually occurs as a single mass (lump) in one breast
- Usually nontender
- Irregular shape
- Firm, hard, embedded in surrounding tissue
- Referral and biopsy indicated for definitive diagnosis

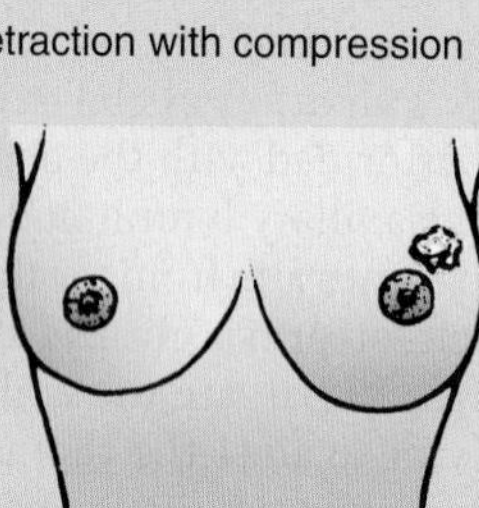

Breast cancer mass

BREAST CYST (BENIGN MASS)

- Occur as single or multiple lumps in one or both breasts
- Usually tender (omitting caffeine reduces tenderness); tenderness increases during premenstrual period
- Round shape
- Soft or firm, mobile
- Referral and biopsy indicated for definitive diagnosis, especially for first mass; later masses may be evaluated over time by a specialist

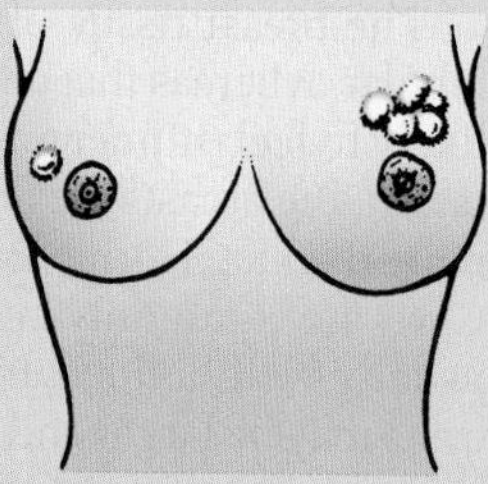

Breast cysts

FIBROADENOMA (BENIGN BREAST LUMP)

- Usually occurs as a single mass in women aged 15–35 years
- Usually nontender
- May be round or lobular
- Firm, mobile, and not fixed to breast tissue or chest wall
- No premenstrual changes
- Referral and biopsy indicated for definitive diagnosis

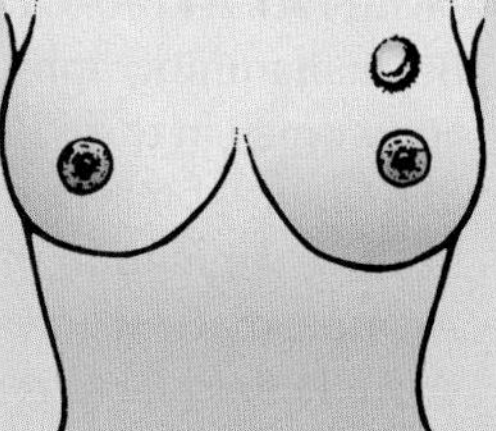

Fibroadenoma

INCREASED VENOUS PROMINENCE

- Associated with breast cancer if unilateral
- Unilateral localized increase in venous pattern associated with malignant tumors
- Normal with breast enlargement associated with pregnancy and lactation if bilateral and bilateral symmetry

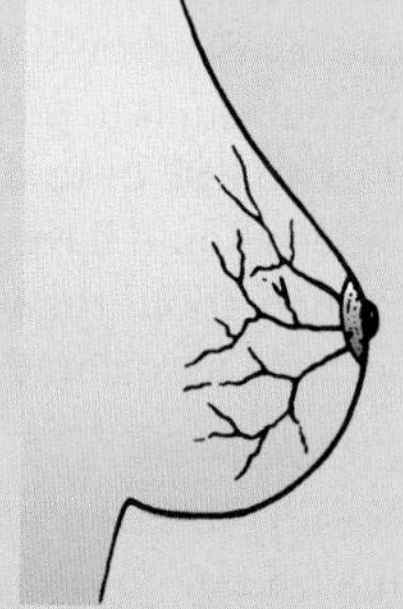

Increased venous prominence

PEAU D'ORANGE (EDEMA)

- Associated with breast cancer
- Caused by interference with lymphatic drainage
- Breast skin has orange peel appearance
- Skin pores enlarge
- May be noted on the areola
- Skin becomes thick, hard, immobile
- Skin discoloration may occur

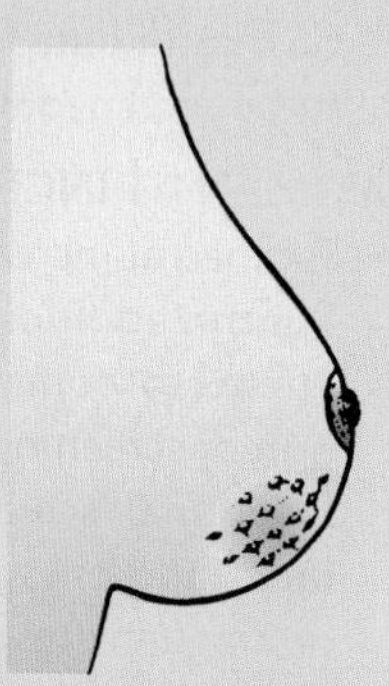

Peau d'orange

NIPPLE INVERSION

- Considered normal if long-standing
- Associated with fibrosis and malignancy if recent development

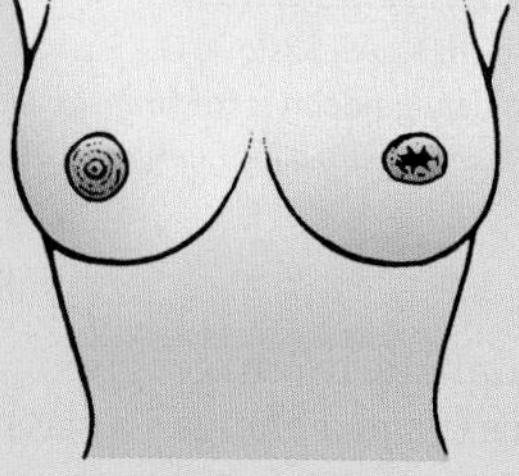

Nipple inversion

CHART 48-2

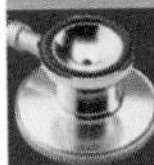

Assessing the Breasts, continued

ACUTE MASTITIS (INFLAMMATION OF THE BREASTS)

- Associated with lactation but may occur at any age
- Nipple cracks or abrasions noted
- Breast skin reddened and warm to touch
- Tenderness
- Systemic signs include fever and increased pulse

PAGET DISEASE (MALIGNANCY OF MAMMARY DUCTS)

- Early signs: erythema of nipple and areola
- Late signs: thickening, scaling, and erosion of the nipple and areola

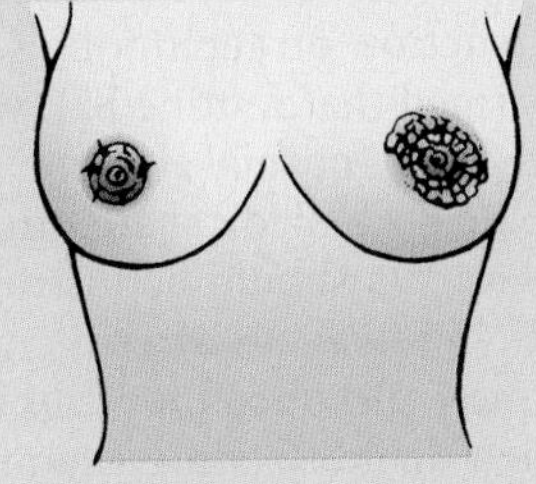

Paget disease

male. This is different from the enlargement of soft, fatty tissue, which is caused by obesity.

Diagnostic Evaluation

Breast Self-Examination

The nurse plays an important role in BSE education, a modality used for the early detection of breast cancer. BSE can be taught in a variety of settings—either on a one-to-one basis or in a group. It can also be initiated by a health care practitioner during a patient's routine physical examination.

Variations in breast tissue occur during the menstrual cycle, pregnancy, and the onset of menopause. Women on hormone therapy (HT, formerly referred to as hormone replacement therapy or HRT) can also experience fluctuations. Normal changes must be distinguished from those that may signal disease. Most women notice increased tenderness and lumpiness before their menstrual periods; therefore, BSE is best performed after menses (day 5 to day 7, counting the first day of menses as day 1). Also, many women have grainy-textured breast tissue, but these areas are usually less nodular after menses. Younger women may find BSE particularly difficult because of the density of their breast tissue. As women age, their breasts become fattier and may be easier to examine.

It is estimated that only 25% to 30% of women perform BSE proficiently and regularly each month. Some find BSE to be anxiety-producing; others find it too difficult to differentiate between normal changes and worrisome findings. Even women who perform BSE and detect a change may delay seeking medical attention because of fear, economic factors, lack of education, and modesty. Despite these factors, many women discover their own breast cancers. For this reason, BSE should be taught and encouraged but not overemphasized. Recent changes in the early detection guidelines of the ACS now recommend that women, beginning in their early 20s, should be told about the benefits and limitations of

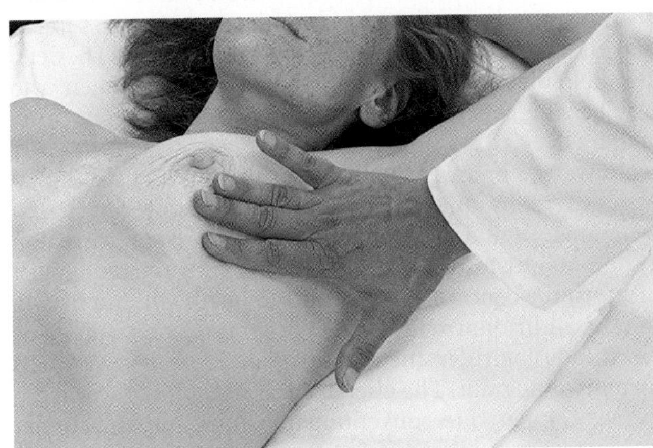

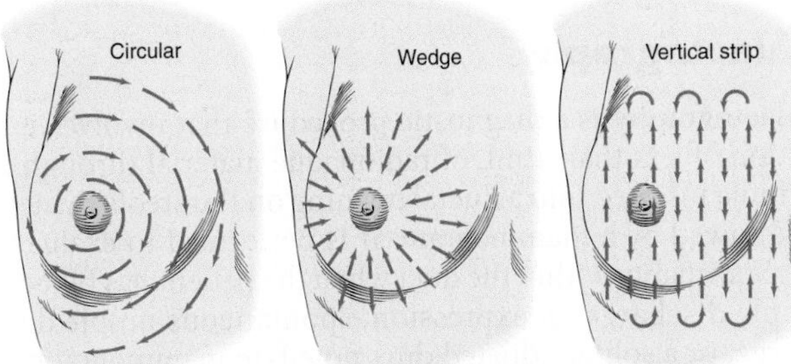

FIGURE 48-2. Breast examination with the woman in a supine position (above). The entire surface of the breast is palpated from the outer edge of the breast to the nipple. Alternative palpation patterns are circular or clockwise, wedge, and vertical strip (below). From Weber, J. & Kelley, J. (2003). *Health assessment in nursing* (2nd ed.). Philadelphia: Lippincott Williams & Wilkins.

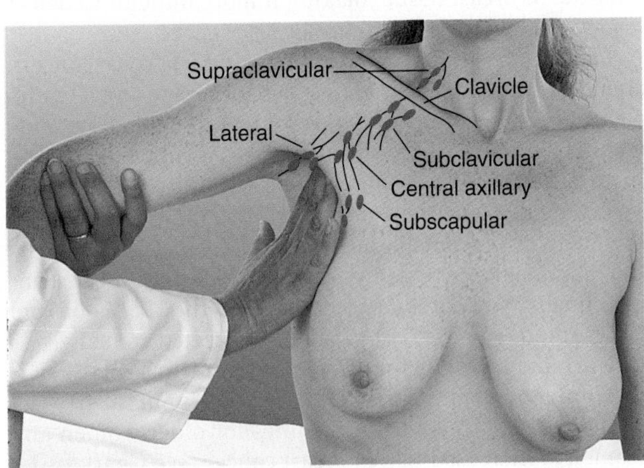

FIGURE 48-3. Palpating axillary nodes in breast examination.

BSE. It is then up to the individual woman whether to perform BSE regularly, irregularly, or not at all (see Chart 48-1).

Instructions about BSE should also be provided to men if they have a family history of breast cancer, because they may have an increased risk for male breast cancer.

Patients who elect to perform BSE should receive proper instruction on technique (Chart 48-3). They should be informed that routine BSE will help them become familiar with their "normal abnormalities." If a change occurs, they should seek medical attention.

Patients should be instructed about optimal timing for BSE (5 to 7 days after menses begin for premenopausal women and once monthly for postmenopausal women). When demonstrating examination techniques, the feel of normal breast tissue should be reviewed and ways to identify breast changes discussed. Patients should then perform a BSE demonstration on themselves or on a breast model. Patients who have had breast cancer surgery should be instructed to examine their breast or chest wall for any new changes or nodules that may indicate a recurrence of the disease.

BSE videos, shower cards, and pamphlets can be obtained from local chapters of the ACS. The National Cancer Institute in Bethesda, MD, offers a program for nurses on BSE instruction, and it also provides teaching aids.

Mammography

Mammography is a breast-imaging technique that has been shown to reduce breast cancer mortality rates. It can detect nonpalpable lesions and assist in diagnosing palpable masses. The procedure takes about 15 minutes and can be performed in a hospital radiology department or independent imaging center. Two views are taken of each breast. The breast is mechanically compressed from top to bottom (craniocaudal view) and side to side (mediolateral oblique view) (Fig. 48-4). Women may experience some fleeting discomfort because maximum compression is necessary for proper visualization. The new mammogram is compared with previous mammograms, and any changes may indicate a need for further investigation. Mammography may detect a breast tumor before it is clinically palpable (ie, smaller than 1 cm); however, it has limitations. The false-negative rate ranges between 5% and 10%. Younger women, or those taking HT, may have dense breast tissue, making it more difficult to detect lesions with mammography.

Patients scheduled for a mammogram may voice concern about exposure to radiation. The radiation exposure is equivalent to about 1 hour of exposure to sunlight, so patients would have to have many mammograms in a year to increase their cancer risk. The benefits of this test outweigh the risks. To ensure that a mammogram is reliable, it is important that a woman find a reputable facility. A facility that is certified by the Mammography Quality Standards Act must meet stringent quality standards, be accredited by the U.S. Food and Drug Administration (FDA), and be inspected annually.

Current mammographic screening guidelines of the ACS recommend a mammogram every year beginning at 40 years of age. The ACS also has guidelines for older women and women at increased risk of breast cancer (see Chart 48-1). Women who are at increased risk due to a strong family history should seek the opinion of a breast specialist regarding the optimal age to begin screening mammography. A general guideline is to begin screening ten years earlier than the age at which the youngest family member developed breast cancer but not before 25 years of age. In families with a history of breast cancer, a downward shift in age of diagnosis of about 10 years is seen (eg, grandmother diagnosed with breast cancer at 48 years of age, mother diagnosed with breast cancer at 38 years of age, then daughter should begin screening at age 28 years of age).

Despite the decreased mortality rates associated with mammographic screening, many women are not undergoing this simple procedure. Only 56.9% of non-Hispanic white women older than 40 years of age reported having mammography within the past year (Ward, Jemal, Cokkinides et al., 2004). The percentage was even lower for women in racial and ethnic minority groups, particularly those who immigrated to the United States in the past 10 years. Low rates of screening were also seen in women with less education and no health insurance coverage. The implementation of screening programs such as the National Breast and Cervical Cancer Early Detection Program of the Centers for Disease Control and Prevention (CDC) helps low-income, uninsured, and underserved women gain access not only to mammograms but to clinical breast examinations, Papanicolaou (Pap) tests, diagnostic testing for abnormal screening tests, and surgical consultation (CDC, 2004). The program was established in 1991 and has currently provided more than 4 million screening examinations and diagnosed more than 17,000 patients with breast cancer. Nurses are in key positions to educate women about the current ACS screening guidelines and the benefits of mammography. They can also help identify and provide information to women who may benefit from such screening programs as the one operated by the CDC.

Newer techniques for breast screening include digital mammography and computer-assisted detection (CAD) programs. Digital mammography records x-ray images on a computer instead of on film, thus allowing the radiologist to adjust the contrast and focus on an image without having to take additional x-rays. CAD programs are designed to assist radiologists in the identification of suspicious areas on a mammogram. The effectiveness of both of these techniques compared to conventional mammography is under investigation.

Galactography

Galactography is a diagnostic procedure that involves injection of less than 1 mL of radiopaque material through a cannula inserted into a ductal opening on the areola, which is followed by a mammogram. It is performed to evaluate an abnormality within the duct when the patient has bloody nipple discharge on expression, spontaneous nipple discharge, or a solitary dilated duct noted on mammography.

Ultrasonography

Ultrasonography (ultrasound) is used as a diagnostic adjunct to mammography to help distinguish fluid-filled cysts from other lesions. A thin coating of lubricating jelly is spread

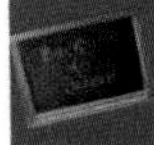

Patient Education

Breast Self-Examination (BSE)

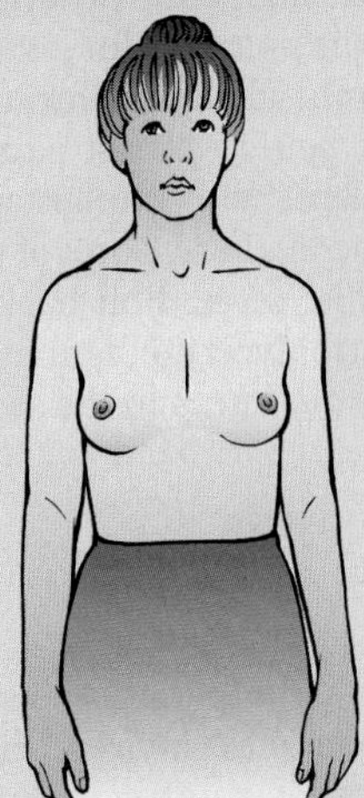

STEP 1

1. Stand in front of a mirror.
2. Check both breasts for anything unusual.
3. Look for discharge from the nipple, puckering, dimpling, or scaling of the skin.

The next two steps are done to check for any changes in the contour of your breasts. As you do them, you should be able to feel your muscles tighten.

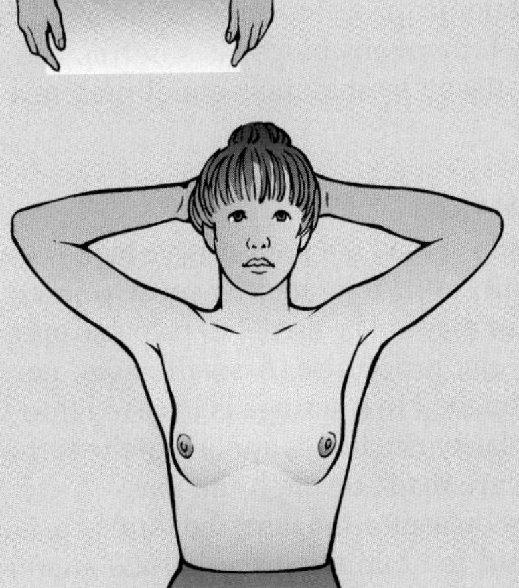

STEP 2

1. Watch closely in the mirror as you clasp your hands behind your head and press your hands forward.
2. Note any change in the contour of your breasts.

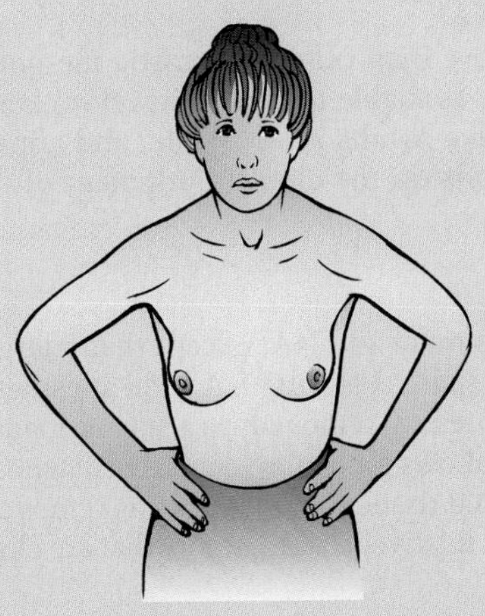

STEP 3

1. Next, press your hands firmly on your hips and bow slightly toward the mirror as you pull your shoulders and elbows forward.
2. Note any change in the contour of your breasts.

Some women do the next part of the examination in the shower. Your fingers will glide easily over soapy skin, so you can concentrate on feeling for changes inside the breast.

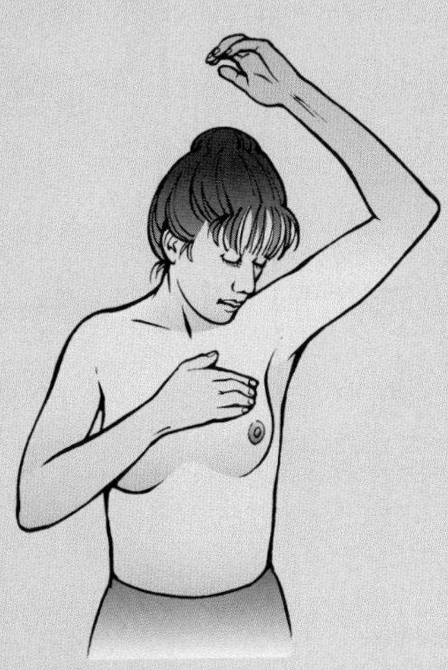

STEP 4

1. Raise your left arm.
2. Use 3 or 4 fingers of your right hand to feel your left breast firmly, carefully, and thoroughly.
3. Beginning at the outer edge, press the flat part of your fingers in small circles, moving the circles slowly around the breast.
4. Gradually work toward the nipple.
5. Be sure to cover the whole breast.
6. Pay special attention to the area between the breast and the underarm, including the underarm itself.
7. Feel for any unusual lumps or masses under the skin.
8. If you have any spontaneous discharge during the month—whether or not it is during your BSE—see your doctor.
9. Repeat the examination on your right breast.

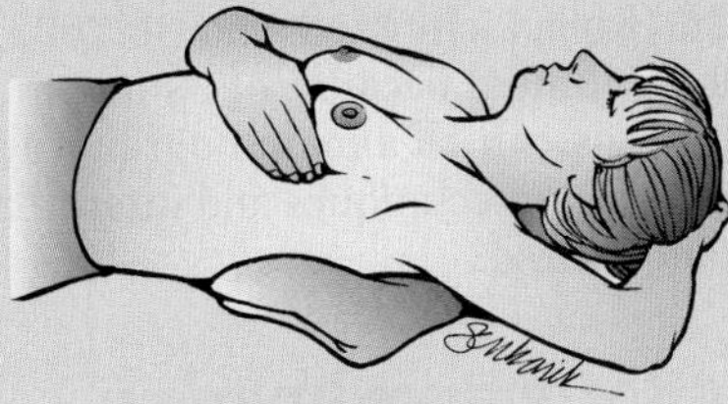

STEP 5

1. Step 4 should be repeated lying down.
2. Lie flat on your back with your left arm over your head and a pillow or folded towel under your left shoulder. (This position flattens your breast and makes it easier to check.)
3. Use the same circular motion described above.
4. Repeat on your right breast.

Adapted from U.S. Department of Health and Human Services, Public Health Service, *What you need to know about breast cancer*. Bethesda, MD: National Institutes of Health.

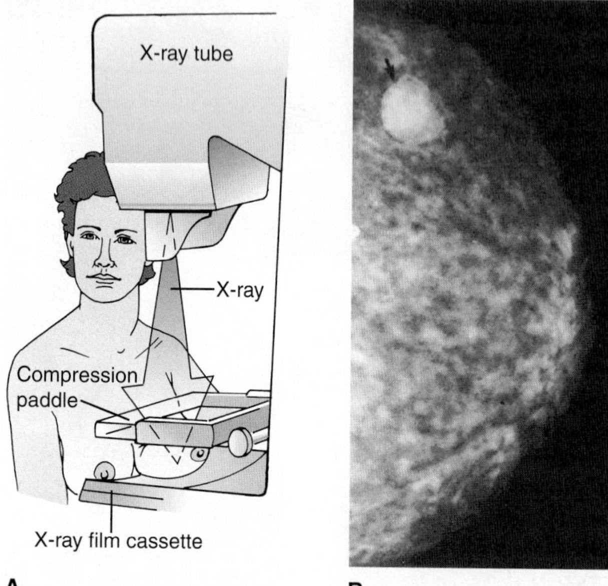

FIGURE 48-4. The mammography procedure (**A**) relies on x-ray imaging to produce the mammogram (**B**), which in this case reveals a breast lump.

over the area to be imaged. A transducer is then placed on the breast. The transducer transmits high-frequency sound waves through the skin toward the area of concern. The sound waves that are reflected back form a two-dimensional image, which is then displayed on a computer screen. No radiation is emitted during the procedure. The technique diagnoses cysts with great accuracy but cannot definitively rule out malignant lesions.

Ultrasonography is also being used with increasing frequency to screen women with dense breasts. In a study of more than 11,000 women, screening ultrasound increased the number of women diagnosed with nonpalpable invasive cancers by 42% (Kolb, Lichy & Newhouse, 2002). However, the procedure is limited because of its inability to detect microcalcifications, which a mammogram can detect. In addition, examination techniques and interpretation criteria are not standardized.

Magnetic Resonance Imaging

Magnetic resonance imaging (MRI) of the breast is an emerging technology that is highly sensitive and has become a useful diagnostic adjunct to mammography. A magnet is linked to a computer that creates detailed images of the breast without exposure to radiation. An intravenous (IV) injection of gadolinium, a contrast dye, is given to improve visibility. The patient lies face down and the breast is placed through a depression in the table. A coil is placed around the breast, and the patient is placed inside the MRI machine. The entire procedure takes about 30 to 40 minutes.

MRI is most useful in patients with proven breast cancer when assessing for multifocal (more than one tumor in the same quadrant of the breast) or multicentric (more than one tumor in different quadrants of the breast) disease, chest wall involvement, tumor recurrence, or response to chemotherapy. The procedure can also identify occult (undetectable) breast cancer and determine the integrity of saline or silicone breast implants. Recent studies have shown that MRI may be used as a screening tool to identify breast cancer in women at high risk for the disease (Kriege, Brekelmans, Boetes, et al., 2004).

Some disadvantages of MRI include high cost, variations in technique and interpretation, and the potential for patient claustrophobia. The procedure cannot always accurately distinguish between malignant and benign breast conditions. MRI is contraindicated in patients with implantable metal devices (eg, aneurysm clips, pacemakers, ports of tissue expanders) because of the metallic force. Foil-backed medication patches (eg, nicotine, nitroglycerine, fentanyl) should be removed prior to MRI to avoid burns to the skin.

Procedures for Tissue Analysis

Percutaneous Biopsy

Percutaneous biopsy is performed on an outpatient basis to sample palpable and nonpalpable lesions. Less invasive than a surgical biopsy, percutaneous biopsy is a needle or core biopsy that obtains tissue by making a small puncture in the skin.

FINE-NEEDLE ASPIRATION

Fine-needle aspiration (FNA) is a noninvasive biopsy technique that is generally well tolerated by most women. A local anesthetic may or may not be used. For palpable masses, a surgeon performs the procedure. A small gauge needle (25- or 22-gauge) attached to a syringe is inserted into the mass or area of nodularity. Suction is applied to the syringe, and multiple passes are made through the mass. A simple cyst often disappears on aspiration, and the fluid is usually discarded. If no fluid is obtained, any cellular material obtained in the hub of the needle is spread on a glass slide or placed in a preservative and sent to the laboratory for analysis. For nonpalpable masses, the same procedure can be performed by a radiologist using ultrasound guidance (ultrasound-guided FNA).

FNA is less expensive than other diagnostic methods, and results are usually available quickly. However, false-negative or false-positive results are possible, and appropriate follow-up depends on the clinical judgment of the treating physician.

CORE NEEDLE BIOPSY

Core needle biopsy is similar to FNA, except that a larger gauge needle is used (usually 14-gauge). A local anesthetic is applied, and tissue cores are removed via a spring-loaded device. This procedure allows for a more definitive diagnosis than FNA, because actual tissue, not just cells, is removed. It is often performed for relatively large tumors that are close to the skin surface.

STEREOTACTIC CORE BIOPSY

Stereotactic core biopsy is performed on nonpalpable lesions detected by mammography. The patient lies prone on the stereotactic table. The breast is suspended through an opening in the table and compressed between two x-ray plates. Images are then obtained using digital mammography. The exact coordinates of the lesion to be sampled are located with the aid of a computer. Next, a local anesthetic is injected into the entry site on the breast. A small nick is made in the skin, a core needle is inserted, and samples of the tissue are taken for pathologic examination. Often, several passes are taken to ensure that the lesion is well-sampled. Post biopsy films are then taken to check that sampling has been adequate A small titanium clip is often placed at the biopsy site so that the site can easily be located if further treatment is indicated.

Stereotactic biopsy is quite accurate and often allows the patient to avoid a surgical biopsy. However, there is a small false-negative rate. Appropriate follow-up depends on the final pathologic diagnosis and the clinical judgment of the treating physician. Use of a titanium clip does not preclude subsequent MRIs.

ULTRASOUND-GUIDED CORE BIOPSY

This procedure is performed on nonpalpable lesions found by ultrasound. The principles are similar to those of stereotactic core biopsy, but the computer coordination and mammographic compression are not necessary. Ultrasound-guided core biopsy does not use radiation and is also faster and less expensive than stereotactic core biopsy.

MRI-GUIDED CORE BIOPSY

Recently, the technology has become available to perform core biopsies under MRI guidance. This procedure is currently available at a small number of facilities.

Surgical Biopsy

Surgical biopsy is usually performed using local anesthesia and IV sedation. After an incision is made, the lesion is excised and sent to a laboratory for pathologic examination.

TYPES OF SURGICAL BREAST BIOPSY

Excisional Biopsy. Excisional biopsy is the standard procedure for complete pathological assessment of a palpable breast mass. The entire mass, plus a margin of surrounding tissue, is removed. This type of biopsy may also be referred to as a lumpectomy. Depending on the clinical situation, a frozen section analysis of the specimen may be performed at the time of the biopsy by the pathologist who does an immediate reading intraoperatively and provides a provisional diagnosis. This can help confirm a diagnosis in a patient who had no previous tissue analysis performed.

Incisional Biopsy. Incisional biopsy surgically removes a portion of a mass. This is performed to confirm a diagnosis and to conduct special studies (eg, ER/PR, Her-2/neu) that will aid in determining treatment and are discussed later in this chapter. Complete excision of the area may not be possible or immediately beneficial to the patient, depending on the clinical situation. This procedure is often performed on women with locally advanced breast cancer or on women with suspected cancer recurrence, whose treatment may depend on the results of these special studies. However, pathological information may be easily obtained from core needle biopsy, and incisional biopsy is becoming less common.

Wire Needle Localization. Wire needle localization is a technique used to locate nonpalpable masses or suspicious calcium deposits detected on a mammogram, ultrasound, or MRI that require an excisional biopsy. The radiologist inserts a long, thin wire through a needle, which is then inserted into the area of abnormality using x-ray or ultrasound guidance (whichever imaging technique originally identified the abnormality). The wire remains in place after the needle is withdrawn to ensure the precise location. The patient is then taken to the operating room, where the surgeon follows the wire to the tip and excises the area.

NURSING MANAGEMENT

During the preoperative visit, the nurse assesses the patient for any specific educational, physical, or psychosocial needs that she may have. This can be accomplished by reviewing her medical and psychosocial history and encouraging her to verbalize her fears, concerns, and questions. Patients are often worried not only about the procedure but also about the potential implications of the pathology results. Providing a thorough explanation about what to expect in a supportive manner can help alleviate anxiety. Patients often have difficulty absorbing all the information given to them; therefore, written materials should be provided to reinforce teaching.

The nurse instructs the patient to discontinue any agents that can increase the risk of bleeding, including products containing aspirin, nonsteroidal anti-inflammatory drugs, vitamin E supplements, herbal substances (such as gingko biloba and garlic supplements), and warfarin. The patient may be instructed not to eat or drink for several hours or after midnight the night before the procedure, depending on the type of biopsy planned. Most breast biopsy procedures today are performed with the use of moderate sedation and local anesthesia.

Immediate postoperative assessment includes monitoring the effects of the anesthesia and inspecting the surgical dressing for any signs of bleeding. Once the sedation has worn off, the nurse reviews the care of the biopsy site, pain management, and activity restrictions with the patient. Prior to discharge from the ambulatory surgical center or the office, the patient must be able to tolerate fluids, ambulate, and void. The patient must have somebody to accompany her home. The dressing covering the incision is usually removed after 48 hours, but the Steri-Strips, which are applied directly over the incision, should remain in place for approximately 7 to 10 days. The use of a supportive bra following surgery is encouraged to limit movement of the breast and reduce discomfort. A follow-up telephone call from the nurse 24 to 48 hours after the procedure can provide the patient with the opportunity to ask any questions and can be a source of great comfort and reassurance.

Most women return to their usual activities the day after the procedure but are encouraged to avoid jarring or high-impact activities for 1 week to promote healing of the biopsy site. Discomfort is usually minimal, and most women find acetaminophen sufficient for pain relief, although a mild opioid may be prescribed if needed.

Follow-up after the biopsy includes a return visit to the surgeon for discussion of the final pathology report and assessment of the healing of the biopsy site. Depending on the results of the biopsy, the nurse's role varies. If the pathology report is benign, the nurse reviews incision care and explains what the patient should expect as the biopsy site heals (ie, changes in sensation may occur weeks or months after the biopsy due to nerve injury within the breast tissue). If a diagnosis of cancer is made, the nurse's role changes dramatically. This is discussed in depth later in this chapter.

Conditions Affecting the Nipple

Nipple Discharge

Nipple discharge in a woman who is not lactating may be related to many causes, such as carcinoma, papilloma, pituitary adenoma, cystic breasts, and various medications. Oral contraceptives, pregnancy, HT, chlorpromazine-type medications, and frequent breast stimulation may be contributing factors. In some athletic women, nipple discharge may occur during running or aerobic exercises. Nipple discharge should be evaluated by a health care provider, but it is not often a cause for alarm. One in three women has clear discharge on expression, which is usually normal. A green discharge could indicate an infection. Any discharge that is spontaneous, persistent, or unilateral is of more concern. Although bloody discharge can indicate a malignancy, it is often caused by a benign wartlike growth on the lining of the duct called an intraductal papilloma.

Nipple discharge should be evaluated for the presence of occult (hidden) blood by performing a guaiac test. A galactogram can also be performed to detect abnormalities within the duct that may be causing the discharge. If there is a high level of suspicion, a surgical biopsy called a duct excision may be indicated.

Fissure

A fissure is a longitudinal ulcer that may develop in breastfeeding women. If the nipple becomes irritated, a painful, raw area may form and become a site of infection. Daily washing with water, massage with breast milk or lanolin, and exposure to air are helpful. Breastfeeding can be continued with the use of a nipple shield if necessary. If the fissure is severe or extremely painful, the woman is advised to stop breastfeeding. A breast pump can be used until breastfeeding can be resumed. Persistent ulceration requires further diagnosis and therapy. Guidance from a nurse or lactation consultant may be helpful because nipple irritation can result from improper positioning (ie, the infant has not grasped the areola fully) during breastfeeding.

Breast Infections

Mastitis

Mastitis, an inflammation or infection of breast tissue, occurs most commonly in breastfeeding women, although it may also occur in nonlactating women. The infection may result from a transfer of microorganisms to the breast by the patient's hands or from a breastfed infant with an oral, eye, or skin infection. Mastitis may also be caused by blood-borne organisms. As inflammation progresses, the breast texture becomes tough or doughy, and the patient complains of dull to severe pain in the infected region. A nipple that is discharging purulent material, serum, or blood should be investigated.

Treatment consists of antibiotics and local application of cold compresses to relieve discomfort. A broad-spectrum antibiotic agent may be prescribed for 7 to 10 days. The patient should wear a snug bra and perform personal hygiene carefully. Adequate rest and hydration are important aspects of management.

Lactational Abscess

A breast abscess may develop as a consequence of acute mastitis. The area affected becomes tender and red. Purulent matter can usually be aspirated with a needle, but incision and drainage may be required. Specimens of the aspirated material are obtained for culture so that an organism-specific antibiotic can be prescribed.

Benign Conditions of the Breast

Breast Pain

Breast pain (**mastalgia**) may be cyclical or noncyclical. Cyclical pain is usually related to hormonal fluctuations and accounts for nearly 75% of all complaints. Noncyclical pain is far less common and does not vary with the menstrual cycle. Women who experience injury or trauma to the breast or those who had a breast biopsy may experience noncyclical pain. Patients should be reassured that breast pain is rarely indicative of cancer. However, if the pain persists after menses begin, the patient should see her primary health care provider.

Medical Management

If pain and tenderness are severe, danazol (Danocrine) may be prescribed. This agent has an antiestrogenic effect, thereby decreasing breast pain and nodularity. Danazol is used only in severe cases because of its potential side effects, which include weight gain, irregular menstrual periods, and androgenic changes (virilization).

Nursing Management

The nurse may recommend that the patient wear a supportive bra both day and night for a week, decrease her salt and caffeine intake, and take ibuprofen as needed for its anti-inflammatory actions. Vitamin E supplements or oil of evening primrose (an over-the-counter herbal preparation) may also be helpful.

Cysts

Cysts are fluid-filled sacs that develop as breast ducts dilate. Cysts occur most commonly in women 30 to 55 years of age and may be exacerbated during perimenopause. Although their cause is unknown, cysts usually disappear after menopause, suggesting that estrogen is a factor. Cystic areas often fluctuate in size and are usually larger premenstrually. They may be painless or may become very tender premenstrually. Occasionally, a patient may report an intermittent shooting sensation or a dull ache. Various breast masses are compared in Table 48-1. Cysts that are confirmed on an ultrasound and are not bothersome can often be left alone. To confirm a diagnosis or to relieve pain, FNA can be performed. Cysts do not increase the risk of breast cancer.

"**Fibrocystic breast changes,**" which is often called "fibrocystic breast disease," is a nonspecific term used to describe an array of benign findings. The changes do not necessarily indicate a cystic process.

Fibroadenomas

Fibroadenomas are firm, round, movable, benign tumors. They can occur from puberty to menopause with a peak incidence at 30 years of age. These masses are nontender and are sometimes removed for definitive diagnosis.

Benign Proliferative Breast Disease

The two most common diagnoses of **benign proliferative breast disease** found on biopsy are atypical hyperplasia and lobular carcinoma in situ. These diagnoses increase a woman's risk of breast cancer.

Atypical Hyperplasia

Atypical hyperplasia is an abnormal increase in the ductal (atypical ductal hyperplasia) or lobular (atypical lobular hyperplasia) cells in the breast and is usually found incidentally in mammographic abnormalities. Atypical hyperplasia increases a woman's risk for breast cancer about 4 to 5 times compared with that of the general population. This risk can be 10 times greater if the patient has a first-degree relative with breast cancer (Pinder & Ellis, 2003).

Lobular Carcinoma in Situ

Lobular carcinoma in situ (LCIS) is characterized by a proliferation of cells within the breast lobules. LCIS is usually found incidentally on pathologic diagnosis, because it cannot be seen on mammography and does not form a palpable lump. The term LCIS is misleading as it is not a carcinoma. Historically, LCIS was considered a premalignant condition but is now considered a marker of increased risk for invasive carcinoma. The invasive carcinoma can be either ductal or lobular in origin and can develop in either breast. LCIS increases a woman's risk of breast cancer about 8 to 10 times compared with that of the general population (Simpson, Gale, Fulford, et al., 2003).

Other Benign Conditions

Cystosarcoma phyllodes is a rare fibroepithelial lesion that tends to grow rapidly. It is rarely malignant and is treated with surgical excision. If it is malignant, mastectomy may follow. Lymph node removal is usually not performed, because metastasis is rare.

TABLE 48-1 Comparison of Various Breast Masses

The most common breast masses are due to cysts, fibroadenomas, or malignancy. Biopsy is usually needed for confirmation, but the following characteristics are diagnostic clues:

Characteristics	Cysts	Fibroadenomas	Malignancy
Age	30–55 years, regress after menopause except with use of estrogen therapy	Puberty to menopause	30–90 years; most common, 40–80 years
Number	Single or multiple	Usually single	Usually single
Shape	Round	Round, disk, or lobular	Irregular or stellate
Consistency	Soft to firm, usually elastic	Usually firm	Firm or hard
Mobility	Mobile	Mobile	May be fixed to skin or underlying tissues
Tenderness	Usually tender	Usually nontender	Usually nontender
Retraction signs	Absent	Absent	May be present

Fat necrosis is a condition of the breast that is often associated with a history of trauma. Surgical procedures such as a breast biopsy can cause fat necrosis. It may be indistinguishable from carcinoma, and the entire mass is usually excised.

Gigantomastia or macromastia (overly large breasts) is a problem for some women. Weight loss and various medications rarely help. Reduction mammoplasty (discussed later in this chapter) is an elective procedure for the patient who is physically or emotionally distressed by this condition.

Superficial thrombophlebitis of the breast (Mondor disease) is an uncommon condition that is usually associated with pregnancy, trauma, or breast surgery. Pain and redness occur as a result of a superficial thrombophlebitis in the vein that drains the outer part of the breast. The mass is usually linear, tender, and erythematous. Treatment consists of analgesics and heat.

Malignant Conditions of the Breast

Breast cancer is a major health problem in the United States. At present, there is no cure. It is estimated that more than 212,000 women and 1700 men develop the disease and more than 41,000 die of it annually (Jemal, Siegel, Ward, et al., 2006). Incidence rates have steadily increased from 1980 to 2000 although the rate of increase slowed in the 1990s. Between 1990 and 2002, the mortality for breast cancer decreased by 2.3%, suggesting that the combination of early detection and improved treatment modalities is having an effect on overall survival.

Current statistics indicate that over an entire lifetime (birth to death), a woman's risk for developing breast cancer is 1 in 8. When broken down by age, the risk by age 39 years is 1 in 209, and it increases to 1 in 24 by age 59 years. Approximately 80% of breast cancers are diagnosed after 50 years of age (Jemal et al., 2006).

Types of Breast Cancer

Ductal Carcinoma in Situ

The increased use of mammography as a screening tool has contributed to the dramatic increase in the diagnosis of **ductal carcinoma in situ (DCIS)**. An estimated 62,000 new cases are diagnosed annually (Jemal et al., 2006). DCIS is characterized by the proliferation of malignant cells inside the milk ducts without invasion into the surrounding tissue. Therefore, it is a noninvasive form of cancer (also called intraductal carcinoma). DCIS is frequently manifested on a mammogram with the appearance of calcifications, and it is considered breast cancer stage 0.

If DCIS is left untreated, there is an increased likelihood that it will progress to invasive cancer. Deciding on the best surgical treatment option can be very complex. DCIS can be categorized in terms of its aggressiveness depending on a variety of factors, including histological subtype (comedo is more aggressive than noncomedo), size of tumor, and whether it is multicentric (present in different quadrants of the breast). These factors, together with patient preference, are important determinants in making treatment decisions. The most traditional treatment is total or simple mastectomy (removal of the breast only), with a cure rate of 98% to 99% (Burstein, Polyak, Wong et al., 2004). The trend today is toward less aggressive surgery; **breast conservation treatment** (limited surgery followed by radiation) is being performed with increasing frequency. In rare cases, lumpectomy alone is an option. The National Surgical Adjuvant Breast and Bowel Project B-24 study demonstrated that the addition of tamoxifen (Nolvadex) significantly reduced local recurrence rates after surgery and radiation (Vogel, Costantino, Wickerham et al., 2003). The medication is usually prescribed for 5 years.

Invasive Cancer

The American Cancer Society (ACS, 2005a) maintains records and disseminates estimates for various types of cancer.

INFILTRATING DUCTAL CARCINOMA

Infiltrating ductal carcinoma, the most common histologic type of breast cancer, accounts for 75% of all cases. The tumors arise from the duct system and invade the surrounding tissues. They often form a solid irregular mass in the breast.

INFILTRATING LOBULAR CARCINOMA

Infiltrating lobular carcinoma accounts for 5% to 10% of breast cancers. The tumors arise from the lobular epithelium and typically occur as an area of ill-defined thickening in the breast. They are often multicentric and can be bilateral.

MEDULLARY CARCINOMA

Medullary carcinoma accounts for about 5% of breast cancers, and it tends to be diagnosed more often in women younger than 50 years. The tumors grow in a capsule inside a duct. They can become large and may be mistaken for a fibroadenoma. The prognosis is often favorable.

MUCINOUS CARCINOMA

Mucinous carcinoma accounts for about 3% of breast cancers and often presents in postmenopausal women 75 years and older. A mucin producer, the tumor is also slow-growing and thus the prognosis is more favorable than in many other types.

TUBULAR DUCTAL CARCINOMA

Tubular ductal carcinoma accounts for about 2% of breast cancers. Because axillary metastases are uncommon with this histology, prognosis is usually excellent.

INFLAMMATORY CARCINOMA

Inflammatory carcinoma is a rare (1% to 2%) and aggressive type of breast cancer that has unique symptoms. The cancer is characterized by diffuse edema and brawny erythema of the skin, often referred to as peau d'orange (resembling an orange peel). This is due to malignant cells blocking the lymph channels in the skin. An associated mass may or may not be present; if there is, it is often a large area of indiscrete thickening. Inflammatory carcinoma can be confused with an infection because of its presentation. The disease can spread to other parts of the body rapidly. Chemotherapy often plays an initial role in controlling disease progression, but radiation and surgery may also be useful.

PAGET DISEASE

Paget disease of the breast accounts for 1% of diagnosed breast cancer cases. Symptoms typically include a scaly, erythematous, pruritic lesion of the nipple. Paget disease often represents ductal carcinoma in situ of the nipple but may have an invasive component. Mammography should be performed followed by a biopsy of the involved skin area.

Risk Factors

There is no single, specific cause of breast cancer. A combination of hormonal, genetic, and possibly environmental factors may lead to an increased risk for its development (Chart 48-4).

Nongenetic Risk Factors

GENDER AND AGE

Gender is the most obvious risk factor for breast cancer; 99% of the cases occur in women. Increasing age is also associated with an increasing risk of breast cancer, the risk is greatest after 50 years of age (ACS, 2004b).

PERSONAL HISTORY

Once a woman has been treated for breast cancer, her risk of developing cancer in the same or opposite breast is significantly increased.

CHART 48-4

Risk Factors for Breast Cancer

- Female gender
- Increasing age
- Personal history of breast cancer
- Family history of breast cancer
- Genetic mutations (BRCA-1 and BRCA-2 mutations are responsible for majority of inherited breast cancer cases)
- Hormonal factors
  - Early menarche
  - Late menopause
  - Nulliparity
  - First child after 30 years of age
  - Hormone therapy (HT)
- Exposure to ionizing radiation during adolescence and early adulthood
- History of benign proliferative breast disease
- Obesity
- High-fat diet (controversial)
- Alcohol intake

HORMONAL FACTORS

The role of hormones and their relationship to breast cancer remains controversial. However, the relationship between estrogen exposure and breast cancer is widely accepted. Endogenous factors, including early menarche (before 12 years of age), nulliparity, first child after 30 years of age, and late menopause (after age 55 years of age), are minor risk factors. The mechanism by which these factors influence risk appears to involve repeated exposure to estrogen during the menstrual cycles (ACS, 2004b).

The role of exogenous hormones has been a source of debate. In the Women's Health Initiative (WHI) trial, women were assigned to receive an estrogen plus progestin or a placebo. A 5.6-year follow-up showed a 24% increase in the risk of breast cancer in women taking hormone therapy (Chlebowksi, Hendrix, Langer, et al, 2003). Another arm of the WHI trial compared women taking estrogen alone to those taking a placebo and demonstrated that estrogen may lead to a possible reduction in the risk for breast cancer. However, these findings require further study (Women's Health Initiative Steering Committee, 2004). There is no evidence that use of oral contraceptives increases the risk of breast cancer.

RADIATION EXPOSURE

Women who receive radiation during adolescence and early adulthood are at an increased risk of breast cancer, which suggests that exposure to radiation causes potential aberrations while the breast tissue is still developing. Women at particularly high risk are those who received mantle radiation (to the chest area) for treatment of Hodgkin disease in their younger years.

BENIGN PROLIFERATIVE BREAST DISEASE

The risk of breast cancer more than quadruples in women with atypical ductal hyperplasia, atypical lobar hyperplasia, or LCIS.

FAT INTAKE AND OBESITY

Studies of dietary fat intake and the risk of breast cancer have been conflicting. Past epidemiologic studies found that there is a lower incidence of breast cancer in countries in which the diet is low in fat. In contrast, studies in the United States have not shown that the risk of breast cancer is related to fat intake. A recent Swedish study examined 11,726 postmenopausal women and did find a significantly increased risk for breast cancer with increased fat intake (Mattisson, Wirfalt, Wallstrom et al., 2004). More research is needed to confirm these findings. Obesity has been shown to increase the risk of breast cancer in postmenopausal women. Studies have shown that maintaining a healthy weight in early life has a protective effect against breast cancer after menopause; therefore, it is prudent to modify dietary fat intake (King, Marks, Mandell et al., 2003).

ALCOHOL USE

Research has shown that use of alcohol increases the risk of breast cancer slightly (Mattisson et al., 2004). Women who consume one drink a day have a small increase in risk. With increasing alcohol intake (2 to 5 drinks a day), the risk may double. Women who consumed more than approximately 1.5 glasses of wine a day are twice as likely to develop breast cancer when compared with women who drink little or no alcohol. Women who reportedly consumed large amounts of alcohol, including beer and spirits, had a nonsignificantly elevated risk for breast cancer.

OTHER POSSIBLE RISK FACTORS

The role of smoking in breast cancer remains unclear. There is currently no conclusive link between cigarette smoking and the risk of breast cancer. However, some studies suggest that cigarette smoking may play a role—the earlier a woman begins smoking, the greater the risk. There is also no evidence that silicone breast implants, use of antiperspirants, underwire bras, and induced or spontaneous abortion increase risk for breast cancer.

Genetic Risk Factors

More than 80% of all breast cancer cases are sporadic, meaning that patients have no known family history of the disease. The remaining cases are either familial (there is a family history of breast cancer but it is not passed on genetically) or genetically acquired. In familial cases, the risk is determined by which family member has the disease. Having a first-degree relative (mother, sister, daughter) increases the risk twofold. This risk is higher if the relative was premenopausal at the time of the diagnosis of breast cancer. Having two first-degree relatives increases the risk of breast cancer fivefold. Having a father or brother with the disease poses a similar risk.

Breast cancer can be genetically inherited, resulting in significant risk. Approximately 5% to 10% of breast cancer cases develop as a result of genetic mutations. Factors that may indicate a genetic link include multiple first-degree relatives with early-onset breast cancer, breast and ovarian cancer in the same family, male breast cancer, and Ashkenazi Jewish background. **BRCA-1** and **BRCA-2** are tumor suppressor genes that normally function to identify damaged DNA and thereby restrain abnormal cell growth. Mutations in these genes are responsible for the majority of hereditary breast cancer in the United States. BRCA mutations are associated with a 55% to 85% estimated lifetime risk for the disease. Carriers also have a significantly increased risk for ovarian cancer—approaching 30% (Antoniou, Pharoah, Narod et al., 2003; King et al., 2003). Male BRCA mutation carriers are also at increased risk for breast cancer, particularly if they carry the BRCA-2 germline mutation. Mutations in BRCA genes may also cause an increased risk for melanoma and cancer of the colon, prostate, and pancreas.

Protective Factors

Certain factors may be protective in relation to the development of breast cancer. Regular exercise has been shown to decrease the risk for breast cancer. In the WHI study, 35-year-old women who performed strenuous physical activity that produced sweating and increased heart rate (eg, aerobics, tennis, or jogging) at least 3 times a week decreased their risk of breast cancer by 14%. Those who did 1.25 to 2.5 hours/week of brisk walking or equivalent exercise reduced their risk by 18% (McTiernan, Kooperberg, White et al., 2003).

Breastfeeding is also thought to decrease risk because it prevents the return of menstruation, thereby decreasing exposure to endogenous estrogen. Having completed a full-term pregnancy before 30 years of age is also thought to be protective.

Breast Cancer Prevention Strategies in the High-Risk Patient

Patients often overestimate or underestimate their risk for developing breast cancer. A consultation with a breast specialist is of paramount importance prior to embarking on any of the prevention strategies that follow. Once patients have an accurate assessment of their risk along with the knowledge of the pros and cons of each prevention strategy, they can make a decision that is most appropriate for their situation.

Long-Term Surveillance

Long-term surveillance is a form of secondary prevention that focuses on early detection of the disease. As recommended by the ACS, women at high risk may benefit from additional screening (see Chart 48-1). Clinical breast examinations may be performed twice a year starting as early as 25 years of age. Mammograms may also be performed as early as 25 years of age (see Chart 48-1 for a discussion of mammogram recommendations for women at high risk). Data concerning the effectiveness of BSE are limited. In addition to yearly mammography, other screening tests, including MRI and ultrasound of the breast, may be useful. Although there is growing evidence that MRI is more sensitive than mammography in BRCA-1 and BRCA-2 carriers (Warner, Plewes, Hill et al., 2004), currently, there are no specific guidelines regarding its performance. Due to the insufficient evidence about optimal screening guidelines in women at increased risk for breast cancer, the ACS recommends that patients and their physicians both participate in the decision-making process concerning what follow-up is most appropriate (Smith, Saslow, Sawyer, et al., 2003).

Chemoprevention

Chemoprevention is a primary prevention modality that aims at preventing the disease before it starts. In April 1998, the results of the Breast Cancer Prevention Trial were released to the general public. This national, randomized, double-blind clinical trial evaluated tamoxifen (Nolvadex) (20 mg daily for 5 years) versus a placebo in more than 13,000 women considered to be at high risk for breast cancer. The women who received tamoxifen had a 49% reduction in the incidence of breast cancer (Fisher, Constantino, Wickerham et al., 1998), suggesting that tamoxifen was an effective chemopreventive agent. Subsequently, the FDA approved its use in high-risk women. Nurses can help women who are considering this option by providing them with information about the benefits, risks, and possible side effects of tamoxifen.

Raloxifene (Evista) is another medication that shows promise as a chemopreventive agent. Raloxifene is now approved by the FDA for the prevention and treatment of osteoporosis. The Multiple Outcomes of Raloxifene Evaluation trial in postmenopausal women with osteoporosis found that women who received raloxifene instead of placebo had a 76% reduction in invasive breast cancer (Cummings, Eckert, Krueger et al., 1999).

A subsequent national, randomized clinical trial, the Study of Tamoxifen and Raloxifene (STAR), compared these two agents in postmenopausal women for the prevention of breast cancer (Vogel, Costantino, Wickerham et al., 2006). Initial results showed that raloxifene is as effective as tamoxifen in reducing breast cancer risk with fewer side effects.

Prophylactic Mastectomy

Prophylactic mastectomy is another primary prevention modality. This procedure can reduce the risk of cancer by 90% (Rebbeck, Friebel, Lynch et al., 2004) and is sometimes referred to as a "risk-reducing" mastectomy. The procedure consists of a total mastectomy (removal of breast tissue only) and is usually accompanied by immediate breast reconstruction. Possible candidates include women with a strong family history of breast cancer, a diagnosis of LCIS or atypical hyperplasia, a BRCA gene mutation, an extreme fear of cancer ("cancer phobia"), or previous cancer in one breast.

A patient who is considering prophylactic mastectomy is often faced with a very controversial and emotional decision. A multidisciplinary approach should be used to help the patient arrive at a decision that is best for her. Consultation with a genetics counselor, plastic surgeon, medical oncologist, and psychiatrist can be invaluable. The patient needs to understand that this surgery is elective and not emergent. The nurse can play a valuable role in providing the patient with information, clarification, and support during the decision-making process.

Clinical Manifestations

Breast cancers can occur anywhere in the breast but are usually found in the upper outer quadrant, where the most breast tissue is located. Generally, the lesions are nontender, fixed rather than mobile, and hard with irregular borders. Complaints of diffuse breast pain and tenderness with menstruation are usually associated with benign breast disease.

With the increased use of mammography, more women are seeking treatment at earlier stages of the disease. These women often have no signs or symptoms other than a mammographic abnormality. Unfortunately, some women with advanced disease seek initial treatment after ignoring symptoms. Advanced signs may include skin dimpling, nipple retraction, or skin ulceration.

Assessment and Diagnostic Findings

Techniques to determine the diagnosis of breast cancer include various types of biopsy, which have been described previously. Tumor staging and analysis of additional prognostic factors are used to determine the prognosis and optimal treatment regimen (see below).

Staging

Staging involves classifying the cancer by the extent of disease. Clinical staging involves the physician's estimate of the size of the breast tumor and the extent of axillary lymph node involvement. Such staging is determined by physical examination and imaging studies.

The staging of breast cancer has become complex. Classification of tumors that are stage 0 (DCIS, LCIS, or Paget disease of the nipple with no invasion), stage I (tumors that are 2 cm or less with no involvement of axillary lymph nodes), and stage IV (tumors of any size, with distant metastases) is fairly straightforward. However, classification of tumors that are stage II and stage III, which represent a wide spectrum of breast cancers, is more difficult. Factors that play a role in determining stages II and III include the number and characteristics of axillary lymph nodes, the status of other regional lymph nodes such as internal mammary nodes or supraclavicular nodes, and the presence or absence of involvement of the skin or underlying muscle. Based on these factors, stage II and stage III breast cancers are further subdivided into stage IIA, IIB, IIIA, IIIB, and IIIC. For a detailed explanation of the staging system, the reader is referred to the American Joint Committee on Cancer Staging Manual or to the ACS web site at http://www.cancer.org (Greene, Page, Fleming et al., 2002). Other diagnostic tests may be performed before or after the surgery to help in the staging of the disease. The extent of testing often depends on the clinical presentation of the disease and may include chest x-rays, CT, MRI, bone scans, and blood work (complete blood count, comprehensive metabolic panel, tumor markers (ie, carcinoembryonic antigen, CA15-3).

Prognosis

Several different factors must be taken into consideration when determining the prognosis of a patient with breast cancer. The two most important factors are tumor size and whether the tumor has spread to the lymph nodes under the arm (axilla).

Generally, the smaller the tumor, the better the prognosis. Carcinoma of the breast is not a pathologic entity that develops overnight. It starts with a genetic alteration in a single cell and takes time to divide and double in size. A carcinoma may double in size 30 times to become 1 cm or larger, at which point it becomes clinically apparent. Doubling time varies, but breast tumors are often present for several years before they become palpable. Nurses can reassure patients that once breast cancer is diagnosed, they have a safe period of several weeks to make decisions regarding treatment.

Prognosis also depends on the extent of spread of the breast cancer. Table 48-2 shows the 5-year survival rate by stage of disease. The most common route of regional spread is to the axillary lymph nodes. Other sites of lymphatic spread include the internal mammary and supraclavicular nodes (Fig. 48-5). Distant metastasis can affect any organ, but the most common sites are bone, lung, liver, pleura, adrenals, skin, and brain.

In addition to the type of breast cancer and the stage, other factors may help determine prognosis (Chart 48-5). Excessive number of copies of certain genes (amplification) or excessive amounts of their protein product (overexpression)

TABLE 48-2 Breast Cancer Survival by Stage

Stage	Five-Year Survival Rate (%)*
0	100
I	98
IIA	88
IIB	76
IIIA	56
IIIB	49
IIIC	**
IV	16

*The 5-year survival rate refers to the percentage of patients who live *at least* 5 years after their cancer is diagnosed. Five-year rates are used to produce a standard way of discussing prognosis. Of course, many people live much longer than 5 years. Five-year relative survival rates exclude patients dying of other diseases. This means that anyone who died of another cause, such as heart disease, is not counted.

**Survival rates are not yet available for patients with stage IIIC breast cancer because this stage was defined only a few years ago.

Source: American Cancer Society's website http://www.cancer.org (accessed July 3, 2006). Reprinted with permission.

may represent a poorer prognosis. The Her-2/neu oncogene is the classic example; approximately 25% to 30% of invasive breast cancers, which typically involve the more aggressive tumors, have amplification or overexpression of the Her-2/neu gene (Emens & Davidson, 2004). Research concerning the prognostic usefulness of the proliferative rate (S-phase fraction) and DNA content (ploidy) of a tumor is ongoing.

Surgical Management

The main goal of surgery is to obtain local control of the disease. With breast cancer being diagnosed today at earlier

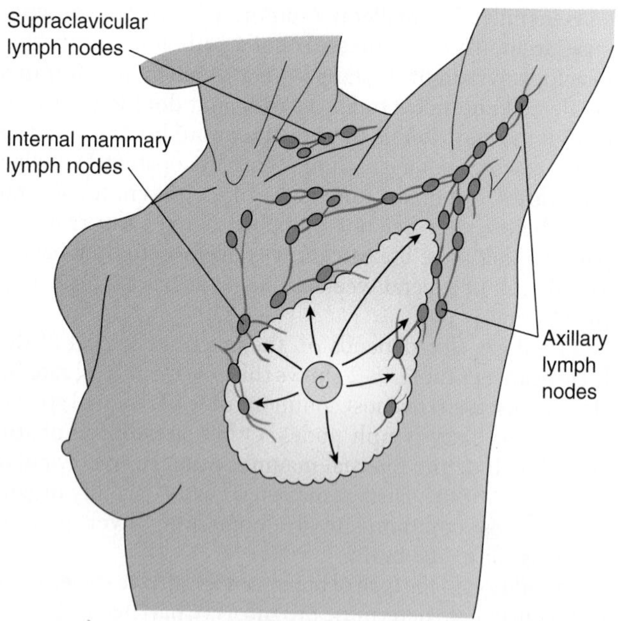

FIGURE 48-5. Lymphatic drainage of the breast.

CHART 48-5

Pathologic Factors Associated With Favorable Prognosis for Breast Cancer

- Noninvasive tumors or invasive tumors <1 cm
- Negative axillary lymph nodes
- Estrogen receptor (ER) and progesterone receptor (PR) proteins
- Well-differentiated tumors
- Low expression of HER-2/neu oncogene
- No vascular or lymphatic invasion
- Diploid tumors with low S-phase fraction

stages, options for less invasive surgical procedures are available. Surgical treatment options for noninvasive and invasive breast cancer are summarized in Table 48-3.

Modified Radical Mastectomy

Modified radical mastectomy is performed to treat invasive breast cancer. The procedure involves removal of the entire breast tissue, including the nipple-areola complex. In addition, a portion of the axillary lymph nodes are also removed in axillary lymph node dissection (ALND). If immediate breast reconstruction is desired, the patient is referred to a plastic surgeon prior to the mastectomy so that she has the opportunity to explore all available options. In modified radical mastectomy, the pectoralis major and pectoralis minor muscles are left intact, unlike in radical mastectomy, in which the muscles are removed. Radical mastectomy is rarely performed today.

Total Mastectomy

Like modified radical mastectomy, **total mastectomy** (i.e., simple mastectomy) also involves removal of the breast

TABLE 48-3 Surgical Treatment Options for Noninvasive and Invasive Breast Cancer

Noninvasive Breast Cancer	Invasive Breast Cancer
Breast conservation* alone	Breast conservation* with one of the following: Sentinel lymph node biopsy Axillary lymph node dissection
Total mastectomy alone	Total mastectomy with sentinel lymph node biopsy or Modified radical mastectomy

*Breast conservation treatment includes lumpectomy, wide excision, partial or segmental mastectomy, and quadrantectomy. These are relatively synonymous terms that describe removal of varying amounts of breast tissue.

and nipple-areola complex but does not include ALND. Total mastectomy may be performed for patients with noninvasive breast cancer (eg, DCIS), which does not have a tendency to spread to the lymph nodes. It may also be performed prophylactically for patients who are at high risk for breast cancer (eg, LCIS, BRCA mutation). A total mastectomy may also be performed in conjunction with sentinel lymph node biopsy (SLNB) for patients with invasive breast cancer.

Breast Conservation Treatment

The goal of breast conservation treatment (ie, lumpectomy, wide excision, partial or segmental mastectomy, quadrantectomy) is to excise the tumor in the breast completely and obtain clear margins while achieving an acceptable cosmetic result. If the procedure is being performed to treat a noninvasive breast cancer, lymph node removal is not necessary. For an invasive breast cancer, lymph node removal (SLNB or ALND) is indicated. The lymph nodes are removed through a separate semicircular incision in the axilla. In 1990, the National Institutes of Health (NIH) issued a consensus statement that breast conservation along with radiation therapy in stage I and stage II breast cancer resulted in a survival rate equal to that of modified radical mastectomy.

Sentinel Lymph Node Biopsy (SLNB)

As previously discussed, the status of the lymph nodes is the most important prognostic factor in breast cancer. Approximately two-thirds of women with early-stage breast cancer who have an ALND have negative nodes. In the mid-1990s, SLNB emerged as a less invasive alternative to ALND and is now considered a standard of care for the treatment of early-stage breast cancer. ALND is associated with potential morbidity, including lymphedema, cellulitis, decreased arm mobility, and sensory changes. Studies have shown that SLNB is highly accurate and is associated with a local recurrence rate similar to that of ALND (Naik, Fey, Gemignani et al., 2004; Veronesi, Pagnelli, Viale et al., 2003). Table 48-4 compares sentinel lymph node biopsy and axillary lymph node dissection.

The **sentinel lymph node**, which is the first node (or nodes) in the lymphatic basin that receives drainage from the primary tumor in the breast, is identified by injecting a radioisotope and/or blue dye into the breast; the radioisotope and/or dye then travels via the lymphatic pathways to the node. In SLNB, the surgeon uses a hand-held probe to locate the sentinel lymph node, excises it, and sends it for pathologic analysis, which is often performed immediately during the surgery using frozen section analysis. If the sentinel lymph node is positive, the surgeon can proceed with an immediate ALND, thus sparing the patient a return trip to the operating room and additional anesthesia. (The patient could also opt to return for additional surgery at a later time.) If the sentinel lymph node is negative, a standard ALND is not needed, thus sparing the patient the sequelae of the procedure. After the operation is complete, all the specimens are sent to pathology for more thorough analysis.

NURSING MANAGEMENT

Patients who undergo SLNB in conjunction with breast conservation are generally discharged the same day. Patients who undergo SLNB with total mastectomy usually stay in the hospital overnight, possibly longer if breast reconstruction is being performed. The patient must be informed that although frozen section analysis is highly accurate, false-negative results can occur. A negative sentinel lymph node on frozen section analysis may show metastatic disease on subsequent analysis, indicating that ALND is still necessary. The patient should also be reassured that the radioisotope and blue dye are generally safe. The patient may notice a blue-green discoloration in the urine or stool for the first 24 hours as the blue dye is excreted. The incidence of lymphedema, decreased arm mobility, and seroma formation (collection of serous fluid) in the axilla is generally low, but the patient should be prepared for this possibility. A recent study demonstrated that women who have SLNB alone have neuropathic sensations similar to those who undergo ALND, although the prevalence and severity of these sensations and the resulting distress are lower with SLNB (Baron, Fey, Borgen & Van Zee, 2004).

The nurse must not overlook the psychosocial needs of the patient who has undergone SLNB. Although SLNB is a less invasive procedure than ALND and results in a shorter

TABLE 48-4 Comparison of Sentinel Lymph Node Biopsy and Axillary Lymph Node Dissection

Sentinel Lymph Node Biopsy (SLNB)	Axillary Lymph Node Dissection (ALND)
Shorter operating room time (approximately 15 to 30 minutes)	Longer operating room time (approximately 60 to 90 minutes)
No surgical drain	Surgical drain
Local anesthesia with IV moderate sedation as outpatient surgery (unless being performed in conjunction with total mastectomy)	General anesthesia; usually overnight admission
Lymphedema incidence approximately 0% to 7%	Lymphedema incidence approximately 10% to 30%
Presence of neuropathic sensations postoperatively (prevalence lower than after axillary lymph node dissection)	Presence of neuropathic sensations postoperatively
Decreased range of motion in affected arm unlikely postoperatively but may occur	Decreased range of motion likely postoperatively
Seroma (collection of serous fluid in the axilla) may occur postoperatively	Seroma may occur postoperatively

recovery period, a patient who has undergone SLNB also has many difficult issues surrounding her breast cancer diagnosis and treatment. The nurse must listen, provide emotional support, and refer the patient to appropriate specialists when indicated.

Nursing Process

The Patient Undergoing Surgery for Breast Cancer

Assessment

The health history is a valuable tool to assess the patient's reaction to the diagnosis and her ability to cope with it. Pertinent questions include the following:

- How is the patient responding to the diagnosis?
- What coping mechanisms does she find most helpful?
- What psychological or emotional supports does she have and use?
- Is there a partner, family member, or friend available to assist her in making treatment choices?
- What are her educational needs?
- Is she experiencing any discomfort?

Diagnosis

Preoperative Nursing Diagnoses

Based on the health history and other assessment data, major preoperative nursing diagnoses may include the following:

- Deficient knowledge about the planned surgical treatments
- Anxiety related to the diagnosis of cancer
- Fear related to specific treatments and body image changes
- Risk for ineffective coping (individual or family) related to the diagnosis of breast cancer and related treatment options
- Decisional conflict related to treatment options

Postoperative Nursing Diagnoses

Based on the health history and other assessment data, major postoperative nursing diagnoses may include the following:

- Pain and discomfort related to surgical procedure
- Disturbed sensory perception related to nerve irritation in affected arm, breast, or chest wall
- Disturbed body image related to loss or alteration of the breast
- Risk for impaired adjustment related to the diagnosis of cancer and surgical treatment
- Self-care deficit related to partial immobility of upper extremity on operative side
- Risk for sexual dysfunction related to loss of body part, change in self-image, and fear of partner's responses
- Deficient knowledge: drain management after breast surgery
- Deficient knowledge: arm exercises to regain mobility of affected extremity
- Deficient knowledge: hand and arm care after an axillary lymph node dissection (ALND)

Collaborative Problems/ Potential Complications

Based on the assessment data, potential complications may include the following:

- Lymphedema
- Hematoma/seroma formation
- Infection

Planning and Goals

The major goals may include increased knowledge about the disease and its treatment; reduction of preoperative and postoperative fear, anxiety, and emotional stress; improvement of decision-making ability; pain management; improvement in coping abilities; improvement in sexual function; and the absence of complications.

Preoperative Nursing Interventions

Providing Education and Preparation About Surgical Treatments

Patients with newly diagnosed breast cancer are expected to absorb an abundance of new information during a very emotionally difficult time. The nurse plays a key role in reviewing treatment options by reinforcing information provided to the patient and answering any questions. The nurse fully prepares the patient for what to expect before, during, and after surgery. Patients undergoing breast conservation with ALND, or a total or modified radical mastectomy, generally remain in the hospital overnight (or longer if they have immediate reconstruction). Surgical drains will be inserted in the mastectomy incision and in the axilla if the patient undergoes an ALND. A surgical drain is generally not needed after a SLNB. The patient should be informed that she will go home with the drain(s) and that complete instructions about drain care will be provided prior to discharge. In addition, the patient should be informed that she will often have decreased arm and shoulder mobility after an ALND and that she will be shown range-of-motion exercises prior to discharge. The patient should also be reassured that appropriate analgesia and comfort measures will be provided to alleviate any postoperative discomfort.

Reducing Fear and Anxiety and Improving Coping Ability

The nurse must help the patient cope with the physical as well as the emotional effects of surgery. Many fears may emerge during the preoperative phase. These can include fear of pain, mutilation (after mastectomy), and loss of sexual attractiveness; concern about inability to care for oneself and one's family; concern about taking time off from work; and coping with an uncertain future. Providing the patient with realistic expectations about the healing process and expected recovery can help alleviate fears. Maintaining open communication and assuring the patient that she can contact the nurse at any time with questions or concerns can be a source of comfort. The patient should also be made aware of available resources at the treatment facility as well as in the breast cancer community such as social workers, psychiatrists, and support groups. Some women find it helpful and reassuring to talk to a breast cancer survivor who has undergone similar treatments.

Promoting Decision-Making Ability

The patient may be eligible for more than one therapeutic approach; she may be presented with treatment options and then asked to make a choice. This can be very frightening for some patients, and they may prefer to have someone else make the decision for them (e.g., surgeon, family member). The nurse can be instrumental in ensuring that the patient and family members truly understand their options. The nurse can then help the patient weigh the risks and benefits of each option. The patient may be presented with the option of having breast conservation treatment followed by radiation or a mastectomy. The nurse can explore the issues with the individual patient by asking questions such as the following:

- How would you feel about losing your breast?
- Are you considering breast reconstruction?
- If you choose to retain your breast, would you consider undergoing radiation treatments 5 days a week for 5 to 6 weeks?

Questions such as these can help the patient focus. Once the patient's decision is made, it is very important to support it.

Postoperative Nursing Interventions

Relieving Pain and Discomfort

Many patients tolerate the breast surgery quite well and have minimal pain during the postoperative period. This is particularly true of the less invasive procedures such as breast conservation treatment with SLNB. However, all patients must be carefully assessed, because individual patients can have varying degrees of pain. Patients who have had more invasive procedures such as a modified radical mastectomy with immediate reconstruction may have considerably more pain. All patients are discharged home with analgesic medication (e.g., oxycodone and acetaminophen [Percocet] or propoxyphene and acetaminophen [Darvocet]) and are encouraged to take it if needed. An over-the-counter analgesic such as acetaminophen may provide sufficient relief. Sometimes patients complain of a slight increase in pain after the first few days of surgery; this may occur as patients regain sensation around the surgical site and become more active. However, patients who report excruciating pain must be evaluated to rule out any potential complications such as infection or a hematoma. Alternative methods of pain management such as taking warm showers and using distraction methods (eg, guided imagery) may also be helpful.

Managing Postoperative Sensations

Because nerves in the skin and axilla are often cut or injured during breast surgery, patients experience a variety of sensations. Common sensations include tenderness, soreness, numbness, tightness, pulling, and twinges. These sensations may occur along the chest wall, in the axilla, and along the inside aspect of the upper arm. After mastectomy, some patients experience phantom sensations and report a feeling that the breast and/or nipple are still present. Overall, patients do not find these sensations severe or distressing (Baron et al., 2004). Sensations usually persist for several months and then begin to diminish, although some may persist for as long as 2 years and possibly longer. Patients should be reassured that this is a normal part of healing and that these sensations are not indicative of a problem.

Promoting Positive Body Image

Patients who have undergone mastectomy often find it very difficult to view the surgical site for the first time. No matter how prepared the patient may think she is, the appearance of an absent breast can be very emotionally distressing. Some patients who have undergone breast conservation treatment may find it difficult to view their surgical incisions, although this is rare. Ideally, the patient sees the incision for the first time when she is with the nurse or another health care provider who is available for support.

The nurse first assesses the patient's readiness and provides gentle encouragement. It is important to maintain a patient's privacy while assisting her as she views the incision; this allows her to express feelings safely to the nurse. Asking the patient what she perceives, acknowledging her feelings, and allowing her to express her emotions are important nursing actions. Reassuring the patient that her feelings are a normal response to breast cancer surgery may be comforting. If the patient has not had immediate reconstruction, providing her with a temporary breast form to place

NURSING RESEARCH PROFILE

Sensory Morbidity After Breast Cancer Surgery

Baron, R. H., Fey, J. V., Borgen, P. I., et al. (2004). Eighteen sensations after breast cancer surgery: A two-year comparison of sentinel lymph node biopsy and axillary lymph node dissection. *Oncology Nursing Forum, 31*(4), 691–698.

Purpose

Although women with breast cancer often report distressing sensations following surgery, these sensations have not been well described. The purpose of this study was to compare the prevalence, severity, and level of distress associated with sensations after sentinel lymph node biopsy (SLNB) and axillary lymph node dissection (ALND) at 3 to 15 days (baseline) and 24 months after breast cancer surgery. Differences in sensations after SLNB and ALND have rarely been addressed by researchers, making it difficult for clinicians to provide effective symptom management.

Design

This descriptive study prospectively evaluated sensations in 197 women who had SLNB and in 97 women who had more extensive ALND. Eighteen sensations were measured using the Breast Sensation Assessment Scale; women completed the scale five times over a 24-month period, beginning 3 to 15 days after surgery during their initial postoperative visit and by mail at 3, 6, 12, and 24 months after surgery.

Findings

The prevalence and severity of sensations and the resulting level of distress were lower in those women who had SLNB compared to those who had ALND. Tenderness and soreness were prevalent at baseline in both groups and remained so over 2 years in women who had SLNB. Numbness and tightness were prevalent in women who had ALND and continued over 2 years; however, they decreased in prevalence over time. The majority of sensations were generally not reported to be severe or distressing.

Nursing Implications

Nurses can use the results of this study to provide women undergoing ALND and SLNB with accurate education about postoperative sensations. It is necessary to provide this information to women undergoing these procedures to help them anticipate these sensations, thus reducing anxiety and distress.

in her bra on discharge can help alleviate feelings of embarrassment or self-consciousness.

Promoting Positive Adjustment and Coping

Providing ongoing assessment of how the patient is coping with her diagnosis of breast cancer and her surgical treatment is important in determining her overall adjustment. Assisting the patient in identifying and mobilizing her support systems can be beneficial to her well-being. The patient's spouse or partner may need guidance, support, and education as well. The patient and partner may benefit from a wide network of available community resources, including the Reach to Recovery program of the ACS, advocacy groups, or a spiritual advisor. Encouraging the patient to discuss issues and concerns with other patients who have had breast cancer may help her to understand that her feelings are normal and that other women who have had breast cancer can provide invaluable support and understanding.

The patient may also have considerable anxiety about the treatments that will follow surgery (i.e., chemotherapy and radiation) and their implications. Providing her with information about the plan of care and referring her to the appropriate members of the health care team also promote coping during recovery. Some women require additional support to adjust to their diagnosis and the changes that it brings. If a woman displays ineffective coping, consultation with a mental health practitioner may be indicated.

Table 48-5 summarizes the needs and nursing interventions for patients and their partners at various stages of the breast cancer experience. Chart 48-6 provides strategies for initiating conversations with patients and their partners during different phases of therapy.

Improving Sexual Function

Once discharged from the hospital, most patients are physically allowed to engage in sexual activity. However, any change in the patient's body image, self-esteem, or the response of her partner may increase her anxiety level and affect sexual function. Some partners may have difficulty looking at the incision, whereas others may be completely unaffected. Encouraging the patient to openly discuss how she feels about herself and about possible reasons for a decrease in libido (e.g., fatigue, anxiety, self-consciousness) may help clarify issues for her. Helpful suggestions for the patient may include varying the time of day for sexual activity (when the patient is less tired), assuming positions that are more comfortable, and expressing affection using alternative measures (e.g., hugging, kissing, manual stimulation).

TABLE 48-5 Needs and Nursing Interventions for Patients and Partners According to Phase of the Breast Cancer Experience

Diagnostic Phase	Postsurgical Phase	Adjuvant Therapy Phase	Ongoing Recovery Phase
Needs and Interventions Related to the Health Care System			
Minimize uncertainty: • correct misinformation • discuss surgical options • explore resources • explain health care system logistics	Establish confidence in health care: • encourage questions • provide information on postoperative care • promote a sense of control	Develop a supportive network: • clarify information • discuss side effects and management • assist in decision making	Maintain association with professionals: • encourage regular follow-up exams, changes in diet and exercise • teach early detection skills • provide realistic reassurance
Needs and Interventions Related to Physical Well-Being			
Prevent disease advancement: • expedite early treatment • reduce anxiety through timely care	Promote physical well-being: • provide information on the healing process • discuss self-care	Minimize adverse physical outcomes: • promote recovery from surgery • teach side effects management	Maintain a positive outlook: • assess perception of physical change • encourage healthful behaviors
Needs and Interventions Related to Psychological Well-Being			
Protect emotional well-being: • alter perceptions of the illness • foster active participation in health care • identify ways to reduce anxiety	Develop a framework of expectations: • describe the treatment process • discuss potential emotional sequelae • support a positive self-image • help to accept altered roles	Manage stress: • identify feelings of vulnerability • provide information on adjuvant therapies and potential side effects • encourage communication of needs	Redefine self and partner: • normalize activities of daily living • reprioritize values, needs, and expectations • incorporate health-promoting behaviors
Needs and Interventions Related to Social Support			
Establish trusting communication: • explore the meaning of the diagnosis • examine treatment options • foster the ability to ask for help	Establish a supportive network: • consider sources of emotional support	Understand family members' responses: • interpret others' reactions	Cultivate ongoing support: • promote an understanding of how to live as a cancer survivor

Reproduced with permission from Hoskins, C. N., & Haber, J. (2000). Adjusting to breast cancer. *American Journal of Nursing, 100*(4), 26–32.

Most patients and their partners adjust with minimal difficulty if they openly discuss their concerns. However, if issues cannot be resolved, a referral for counseling (e.g., psychologist, psychiatrist, psychiatric clinical nurse specialist, social worker, sex therapist) may be helpful. The ambulatory care nurse in the outpatient clinic or hospital should inquire whether the patient is having difficulty with sexuality issues, because many patients are reluctant or embarrassed to bring it up themselves.

Monitoring and Managing Potential Complications

LYMPHEDEMA

Lymphedema occurs in about 10% to 30% of patients who undergo ALND and in about 0% to 7% of patients who have SLNB (Leidenius, Leivonen, Vironen, et al., 2005; Wilke, McCall, Posther, et al., 2006). Risk factors for lymphedema include increasing age, obesity, presence of extensive axillary disease, radiation treatment, and injury or infection to the extremity (Golshan, Martin & Dowlatshahi, 2003). Lymphedema results if functioning lymphatic channels are inadequate to ensure a return flow of lymph fluid to the general circulation. After axillary lymph nodes are removed, collateral circulation must assume this function. Transient edema in the postoperative period occurs until collateral circulation has completely taken over this function, which generally occurs within a month. Performing prescribed exercises, elevating the arm above the heart several times a day, and gentle muscle pumping (making a fist and releasing) can help reduce the transient edema. The patient

CHART 48-6

Talking With Patients and Partners

For patients in the diagnostic phase: We've talked about your recent breast cancer diagnosis. It's natural for you to be full of feelings, concerns, and fears about yourself and your family. Sometimes it's hard to find someone to speak freely with. Would you share what you've been thinking, feeling, and worrying about recently?

For partners in the diagnostic phase: We've talked about your partner's recent breast cancer diagnosis. It's natural for you to have a lot of feelings, concerns, and fears about your partner, yourself, and your family. Partners often feel that they have to be strong for the patient or for others and that they aren't entitled to express their own concerns. Would you share what you've been thinking about, feeling, or worrying about recently?

For patients in the postsurgical phase: Many women who have had breast surgery, especially mastectomy or extensive lumpectomy are concerned not only with their own loss, but with how their partner will accept it. How have you felt about losing [part of] your breast? How has it changed your body image? Your sense of your sexuality? Your desire for intimacy?

For partners in the postsurgical phase: Many partners of women who have had breast surgery are concerned, as are the women themselves, about how they'll respond to the loss. How have you felt about your partner's losing [part of] her breast? How has it changed her attractiveness for you? Your sexual feelings toward her? Your desire for intimacy?

For patients in the adjuvant therapy phase: Given the type of therapy (radiation, chemotherapy, hormone therapy) you're going to have, what side effects do you anticipate? What do you know about them? Let's talk about ways to reduce and handle potential side effects.

For partners in the adjuvant therapy phase: Given the type of therapy (radiation, chemotherapy, hormone therapy) your partner is going to have, what side effects do you anticipate? What do you know about them? Let's talk about ways to reduce and handle potential side effects, and how it might help you to be familiar with them.

For patients in the ongoing recovery phase: As you plan your return to a full work schedule, what measures—setting priorities, delegating responsibility, managing stress—might help you make the necessary physical and emotional adjustments? What have you learned about balancing work, family, and play in your life?

For partners in the ongoing recovery phase: As your partner plans her return to a full work-schedule, what strategies have you thought about using to make your own physical and emotional adjustments, so that you don't continue to be overburdened at work and at home?

Reproduced with permission from Hoskins, C. N., & Haber, J. (2000). Adjusting to breast cancer. *American Journal of Nursing, 100*(4), 26-32.

needs reassurance that this transient swelling is not lymphedema.

Once lymphedema develops, it tends to be chronic, so preventive strategies are vital. After ALND, the patient is taught hand and arm care to prevent injury or trauma to the affected extremity, thus decreasing the likelihood for lymphedema development (Chart 48-7). The patient is instructed to follow these guidelines for the rest of her life. She is also instructed to contact the physician or a nurse immediately if she suspects that she has lymphedema, because early intervention provides the best chance for control. If allowed to progress without treatment, the swelling can become more difficult to manage. Treatment may consist of a course of antibiotics if an infection is present. A referral to a rehabilitation specialist (e.g., occupational or physical therapist) may be necessary for a compression sleeve and/or glove, exercises, manual lymph drainage, and a discussion of ways to modify daily activities to avoid worsening lymphedema.

HEMATOMA OR SEROMA FORMATION

Hematoma formation (collection of blood inside the cavity) may occur after either mastectomy or breast conservation and usually develops within the first 12 hours after surgery. The nurse assesses for signs and symptoms of a hematoma at the surgical site, which may include swelling, tightness, pain, and bruising of the skin. The surgeon should be notified immediately for gross swelling or increased bloody output from the drain. Depending on the surgeon's assessment, a compression wrap may be applied to the incision for approximately 12 hours, or the patient may be returned to the operating room so that the incision may

CHART 48-7

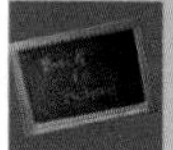

Patient Education

Hand and Arm Care After Axillary Lymph Node Dissection

- Avoid blood pressures, injections, and blood draws in affected extremity.
- Use sunscreen (higher than 15 SPF) for extended exposure to sun.
- Apply insect repellent to avoid insect bites.
- Wear gloves for gardening.
- Use cooking mitt for removing objects from oven.
- Avoid cutting cuticles; push them back during manicures.
- Use electric razor for shaving armpit.
- Avoid lifting objects greater than 5–10 pounds.
- If a trauma or break in the skin occurs, wash the area with soap and water, and apply an over-the-counter antibacterial ointment (Bacitracin or Neosporin).
- Observe the area and extremity for 24 hours; if redness, swelling, or a fever occurs, call the surgeon or nurse.

be reopened to identify the source of bleeding. Some hematomas are small, and the body absorbs the blood naturally. The patient may take warm showers or apply warm compresses to help increase the absorption. A hematoma usually resolves in 4 to 5 weeks.

A seroma, a collection of serous fluid, may accumulate under the breast incision after mastectomy or breast conservation or in the axilla. Signs and symptoms may include swelling, heaviness, discomfort, and a sloshing of fluid. Seromas may develop temporarily after the drain is removed or if the drain is in place and becomes obstructed. Seromas rarely pose a threat and may be treated by unclogging the drain or manually aspirating the fluid with a needle and syringe. Large, long-standing seromas that have not been aspirated could lead to infection. Small seromas that are not bothersome to the patient usually resolve on their own.

INFECTION

Although infection is rare, it is a risk after any surgical procedure. This risk may be higher in patients with accompanying conditions such as diabetes, immune disorders, and advanced age, as well as in those with poor hygiene. Patients are taught to monitor for signs and symptoms of infection (redness, warmth around incision, tenderness, foul-smelling drainage, temperature greater than 100.4°F, chills) and to contact the surgeon or nurse for evaluation. Treatment consists of oral or IV antibiotics (for more severe infections) for 1 or 2 weeks. Cultures are taken of any foul-smelling discharge.

Promoting Home and Community-Based Care

TEACHING PATIENTS SELF-CARE

Patients who undergo breast cancer surgery receive a tremendous amount of information preoperatively and postoperatively. It is often difficult for the patient to absorb all of the information, partly because of the emotional distress that often accompanies the diagnosis and treatment. Prior to discharge, the nurse must assess the patient's readiness to assume self-care responsibilities, and any gaps in knowledge must be identified. Teaching may need to be reviewed and reinforced to ensure that the patient and family are prepared to manage the necessary home care. The nurse reiterates symptoms the patient should report, such as infection, seroma, hematoma, or arm swelling. All teaching should be reinforced during office visits and by telephone.

Most patients are discharged 1 or 2 days after ALND and/or mastectomy (possibly later if they have had immediate reconstruction) with surgical drains in place. Initially, the drainage fluid appears bloody, but it gradually changes to a serosanguineous and then a serous fluid over the next several days. The patient is given instructions about drainage management at home (Chart 48-8). If the patient lives alone and drainage management is difficult for her, a referral for a home care nurse should be made. The drains are usually removed when the output is less than 30 mL in a 24-hour period (approximately 7 to 10 days). The home care nurse also reviews pain management and incision care.

Generally, the patient may shower on the second postoperative day and wash the incision and drain site with soap and water to prevent infection. If immediate reconstruction has been performed, showering may be contraindicated until the drain is removed. A dry dressing may be applied to the incision each day for 7 days. The patient should know that sensation may be decreased in the operative area because the nerves were disrupted during surgery, and gentle care is needed to avoid injury. After the incision has completely healed (usually after 4 to 6 weeks), lotions or creams may be applied to the area to increase skin elasticity. The patient can begin to use deodorant on the affected side, although many women note that they no longer perspire as much as before the surgery.

After ALND, patients are taught arm exercises on the affected side to restore range of motion (Chart 48-9). After SLNB, patients may also benefit from these exercises, although they are less likely to have decreased range of motion than those who have undergone ALND. Range of motion exercises are initiated on the second postoperative day, although instruction often occurs on the first postoperative day. The goals of the

CHART 48-8

HOME CARE CHECKLIST • Surgical Breast Cancer Patient With a Drainage Device

At the completion of the home care instruction, the patient or caregiver will be able to:	Patient	Caregiver
• Demonstrate how to empty and measure fluid from the drainage device	✔	✔
• Demonstrate how to milk clots through the tubing of the drainage device	✔	✔
• State observations that require contacting the physician or nurse (eg, sudden change in color of drainage, sudden cessation of drainage, signs or symptoms of an infection)	✔	✔
• Care for the drain site as per surgeon's recommendation	✔	✔
• Identify when the drain is ready for removal (usually when draining less than 30 mL for a 24-hour period)	✔	✔

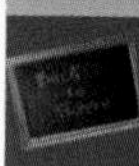

CHART 48-9

Patient Education

Exercise After Breast Surgery

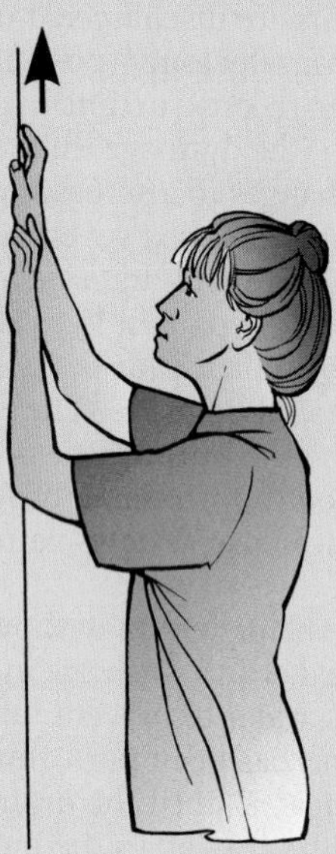

1. *Wall handclimbing.* Stand facing the wall with feet apart and toes as close to the wall as possible. With elbows slightly bent, place the palms of the hand on the wall at shoulder level. By flexing the fingers, work the hands up the wall until arms are fully extended. Then reverse the process, working the hands down to the starting point.

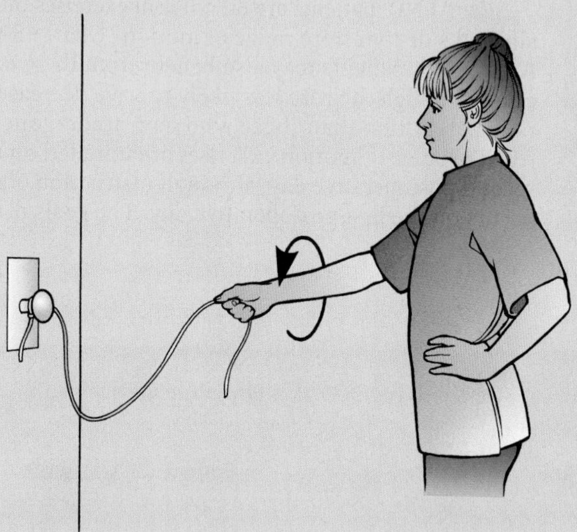

2. *Rope turning.* Tie a light rope to a doorknob. Stand facing the door. Take the free end of the rope in the hand on the side of surgery. Place the other hand on the hip. With the rope-holding arm extended and held away from the body (nearly parallel with the floor), turn the rope, making as wide swings as possible. Begin slowly at first; speed up later.

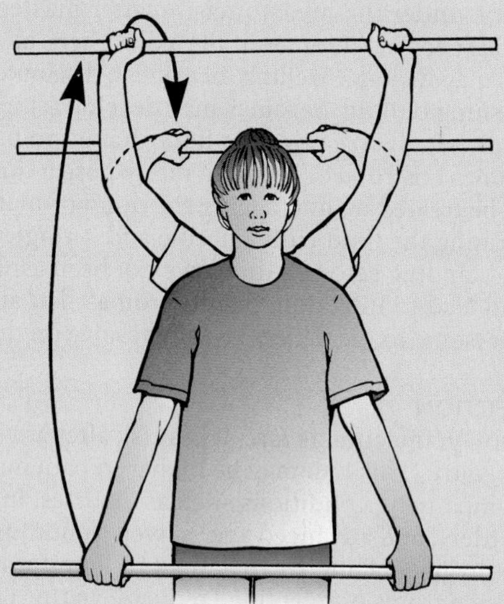

3. *Rod or broomstick lifting.* Grasp a rod with both hands, held about 2 feet apart. Keeping the arms straight, raise the rod over the head. Bend elbows to lower the rod behind the head. Reverse maneuver, raising the rod above the head, then return to the starting position.

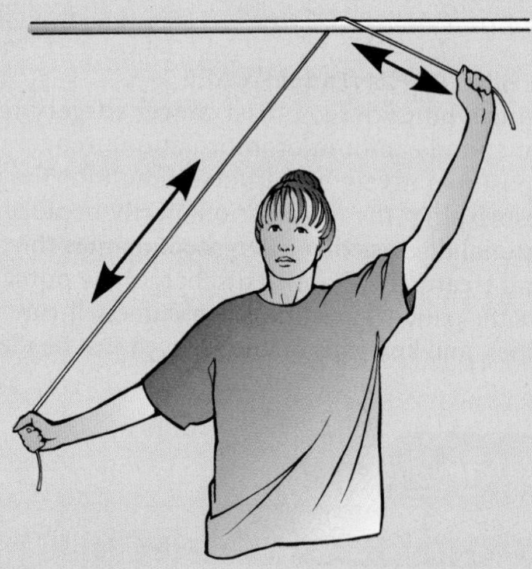

4. *Pulley tugging.* Toss a light rope over a shower curtain rod or doorway curtain rod. Stand as nearly under the rope as possible. Grasp an end in each hand. Extend the arms straight and away from the body. Pull the left arm up by tugging down with the right arm, then the right arm up and the left down in a see-sawing motion.

exercise regimen are to increase circulation and muscle strength, prevent joint stiffness and contractures, and restore full range of motion. The patient is instructed to perform range of motion exercises at home 3 times a day for 20 minutes at a time until full range of motion is restored (generally 4 to 6 weeks). Most patients find that after the drain is removed, range of motion returns quickly if they have adhered to their exercise program.

If the patient is having any discomfort, taking an analgesic 30 minutes before beginning the exercises can be helpful. Taking a warm shower before exercising can also loosen stiff muscles and provide comfort. When exercising, the patient is encouraged to use the muscles in both arms and to maintain proper posture. Specific exercises may need to be prescribed and introduced gradually if the patient has had skin grafts; has a tense, tight surgical incision; or has had immediate reconstruction. Self-care activities, such as brushing the teeth, washing the face, and brushing the hair, are physically and emotionally therapeutic because they aid in restoring arm function and provide a sense of normalcy for the patient.

The patient is instructed about postoperative activity limitation. Generally, heavy lifting (more than 5 to 10 lbs) is avoided for about 4 to 6 weeks, although normal household and work-related activities are promoted to maintain muscle tone. Brisk walking, use of stationary bikes and stepping machines, and stretching exercises may begin as soon as the patient feels comfortable. Once the drain is removed, the patient may begin to drive if she has full arm range of motion and is no longer taking opioid analgesics. General guidelines for activity focus on the gradual introduction of previous activities (e.g., bowling, weight-training) once fully healed, although checking with the physician or nurse beforehand is recommended.

CONTINUING CARE

Patients who have difficulty managing their postoperative care at home may benefit from a home health care referral. The home care nurse assesses the patient's incision and surgical drain(s), adequacy of pain management, adherence to the exercise plan, and overall physical and psychological functioning. In addition, the home care nurse reinforces previous teaching and communicates important physiologic findings and psychosocial issues to the patient's primary care provider, nurse, or surgeon.

The frequency of follow-up visits after surgery may vary but generally should occur every 3 to 6 months for the first several years. The patient may alternate visits with the surgeon, medical oncologist, or radiation oncologist, depending on the treatment regimen. The ambulatory care nurse can also be a great source of comfort and security for the patient and family and should encourage them to telephone if they have any questions or concerns. It is common for people to ignore routine health care when a major health issue arises, so women who have been treated for breast cancer should be reminded of the importance of participating in routine health screening.

Evaluation

EXPECTED PREOPERATIVE PATIENT OUTCOMES

Expected preoperative patient outcomes may include:

1. Exhibits knowledge about diagnosis and surgical treatment options
   a. Asks relevant questions about diagnosis and available surgical treatments
   b. States rationale for surgery
   c. Describes advantages and disadvantages of treatment options
2. Verbalizes willingness to deal with anxiety and fears related to the diagnosis and the effects of surgery on self-image and sexual functioning
3. Demonstrates ability to cope with diagnosis and treatment
   a. Verbalizes feelings appropriately and recognizes normalcy of mood lability
   b. Proceeds with treatment in timely fashion
   c. Discusses impact of diagnosis and treatment on family and work
4. Demonstrates ability to make decisions regarding treatment options in timely fashion

EXPECTED POSTOPERATIVE PATIENT OUTCOMES

Expected postoperative patient outcomes may include:

1. Reports that pain has decreased and states pain and discomfort management strategies are effective
2. Identifies postoperative sensations and recognizes that they are a normal part of healing
3. Exhibits clean, dry, and intact surgical incisions without signs of inflammation or infection
4. Lists the signs and symptoms of infection to be reported to the nurse or surgeon
5. Verbalizes feelings regarding change in body image
6. Discusses meaning of the diagnosis, surgical treatment, and fears appropriately
7. Participates actively in self-care activities
   a. Performs exercises as prescribed
   b. Participates in self-care activities as prescribed
8. Discusses issues of sexuality and resumption of sexual relations
9. Demonstrates knowledge of postdischarge recommendations and restrictions
   a. Describes follow-up care and activities
   b. Demonstrates appropriate care of incisions and drainage system
   c. Demonstrates arm exercises and describes exercise regimen and activity limitations during postoperative period
   d. Describes care of affected arm and hand and lists indications to contact the surgeon or nurse
10. Experiences no complications
    a. Identifies signs and symptoms of reportable complications (eg, redness, heat, pain, edema)
    b. Explains how to contact appropriate health care providers in case of complications

Radiation Therapy

Radiation therapy is used to decrease the chance of a local recurrence in the breast by eradicating residual microscopic cancer cells. Breast conservation treatment followed by radiation therapy for stage I and II breast cancer results in a survival rate equal to that of a modified radical mastectomy (Fisher, Anderson, Brant et al., 2002). If radiation therapy, which is part of breast conservation treatment (Chart 48-10), is contraindicated, a mastectomy would then be indicated.

External-beam radiation (the most common type) typically begins about 6 weeks after breast conservation to allow the surgical site to heal. If systemic chemotherapy is indicated, radiation therapy usually begins after its completion. Before radiation begins, the patient undergoes a planning session called a simulation where the anatomic areas to be treated are mapped out and then identified with small permanent ink markings. External beam radiation, which delivers high-energy photons from a linear accelerator, is administered to the entire breast region. Each treatment lasts only a few minutes and is generally given 5 days a week for 5 to 6 weeks. After completion of radiation to the entire breast, many patients receive a "boost," a dose of radiation to the lumpectomy site where the cancer cells were located. The boost consists of the same dose of radiation but is less penetrating and directed to a smaller area. The treatments are not painful.

Because most breast cancer recurrences appear at or near the lumpectomy site, the need for whole breast radiation is now being questioned. Partial breast radiation (radiation to the lumpectomy site alone) is now being evaluated at some institutions in carefully selected patients. One approach is **brachytherapy**, which delivers partial breast radiation by placing a radioactive source within the lumpectomy site. This technique can lead to an improved quality of life, because the treatments are administered over 4 to 5 days instead of 5 to 6 weeks. Another approach is intraoperative radiation therapy (IORT), in which a single intense dose of radiation is delivered to the surgical site in the operating room immediately following the lumpectomy. Short-term results comparing IORT to the standard treatment are similar in terms of local recurrence and survival (Cuncins-Hearn, Saunders, Walsh et al., 2004). Many questions remain unanswered, and longer follow-up with larger studies is needed to document the efficacy of IORT and to evaluate the cosmetic results. Although not widely used today after mastectomy, postoperative radiation is indicated for women at high risk for cancer recurrence (ie, chest wall involvement, four or more positive nodes, tumors larger than 5 cm, positive surgical margins).

Side Effects

Generally, radiation therapy is well tolerated. Acute side effects consist of mild to moderate erythema, breast edema, and fatigue. Occasionally, skin breakdown may occur in the inframammary fold or near the axilla toward the end of treatment. Fatigue can be depressing, as can the frequent trips to the radiation oncology unit for treatment. The patient needs to be reassured that the fatigue is normal and not a sign of recurrence. Side effects usually resolve within a few weeks to a few months after treatment is completed. Rare long-term effects of radiation therapy include pneumonitis, rib fracture, and breast fibrosis.

Nursing Management

Self-care instructions for patients receiving radiation are provided to assist in the maintenance of skin integrity during the treatments and for several weeks after completion. They pertain only to the area being treated and not to the rest of the body.

- Use mild soap with minimal rubbing.
- Avoid perfumed soaps or deodorants.
- Use hydrophilic lotions (Lubriderm, Eucerin, Aquaphor) for dryness.
- Use a nondrying, antipruritic soap (Aveeno) if pruritus occurs.
- Avoid tight clothes, underwire bras, excessive temperatures, and ultraviolet light.

Follow-up care includes teaching the patient to minimize sun exposure to the treated area (i.e., using sunblock with an SPF of 15 or above) and reassuring the patient that minor twinges and shooting pain in the breast are normal after radiation treatment.

CHART 48-10

Contraindications to Breast-Conservation Treatment

Note: Breast-conservation treatment includes both surgery and radiation.

ABSOLUTE CONTRAINDICATIONS

- First or second trimester of pregnancy
- Presence of multicentric disease in the breast
- Prior radiation to the breast or chest region

RELATIVE CONTRAINDICATIONS

- History of collagen vascular disease
- Large tumor-to-breast ratio
- Tumor beneath nipple

Systemic Treatments

Chemotherapy

Adjuvant chemotherapy involves the use of anticancer agents in addition to other treatments (i.e., surgery, radiation) to delay or prevent a recurrence of breast cancer. It is considered for patients who have positive lymph nodes or who have invasive tumors greater than or equal to 1 cm, regardless of nodal status (NIH, 2000). Table 48-6 outlines general indications for adjuvant treatment. A survival benefit has been shown in premenopausal and postmenopausal women who received chemotherapy, although data are limited in women older than 70 years. Chemotherapy is most commonly initiated after breast surgery and before radiation.

Chemotherapy regimens for breast cancer combine several agents (polychemotherapy), generally administered over a period of 3 to 6 months. Decisions regarding the optimal

TABLE 48-6 General Indications for Adjuvant Chemotherapy and Hormonal Therapy for Breast Cancer

Nodal Status, Tumor Size	Hormone Receptor Status	Adjuvant Treatment
Node negative, <1 cm	Positive	Tamoxifen or aromatase inhibitor*
Node negative, <1 cm	Negative	None
Node negative, ≥1 cm	Positive	Chemotherapy followed by tamoxifen or aromatase inhibitor*
Node negative, ≥1 cm	Negative	Chemotherapy
Node positive, any tumor size	Positive	Chemotherapy followed by tamoxifen or aromatase inhibitor*
Node positive, any tumor size	Negative	Chemotherapy

*Only postmenopausal women have the option of receiving an aromatase inhibitor. They may receive an aromatase inhibitor alone, or they may receive tamoxifen first followed by an aromatase inhibitor.

Note: These are only general guidelines. Recommendations may vary depending on factors such as prognostic variables, patient age, and comorbid conditions.

regimen are based on a variety of factors, including tumor characteristics (i.e., tumor size, lymph node status, hormone receptor status, Her-2/neu status) and the patient's age, physical status, and existing comorbid conditions. A regimen of cyclophosphamide, methotrexate, and fluorouracil (CMF), which historically has been the most widely used adjuvant therapy, is usually well tolerated and may be considered for patients who are at a low risk of recurrence. CMF also may be considered for use in patients who have a high risk for cardiac toxicity (a potential side effect of anthracycline-based regimens) or who have other limiting comorbidities. Anthracycline-based regimens (e.g., doxorubicin, epirubicin) have been shown to result in a small improvement in survival compared to non–anthracycline-based regimens (NIH, 2000). Cyclophosphamide, doxorubicin (Adriamycin), and fluorouracil (CAF), and doxorubicin and cyclophosphamide (AC) are examples of combination regimens often administered to higher risk patients.

The taxanes (paclitaxel, docetaxel), a newer category of chemotherapeutic agents, are being incorporated into treatment regimens for patients with larger, node-negative cancers and for those with positive axillary lymph nodes. The addition of four cycles of paclitaxel (Taxol; T) after a standard course of AC (regimen known as ACT) has been found to increase the disease-free period and improve overall survival in patients with operable breast cancer and positive lymph nodes (Henderson, Berry, Denetri, et al., 2003).

Much attention has been focused on **dose-dense chemotherapy**, the administration of chemotherapeutic agents at standard doses with shorter time intervals between each cycle of treatment. Patients who received ACT every 2 weeks compared to those who received it on the conventional schedule of every 3 weeks had an improved disease-free and overall survival (Citron, Berry, Cirrincione et al., 2003). Long-term follow-up of this study as well as other clinical trials are ongoing to determine optimal treatment regimens, doses, and timing.

SIDE EFFECTS

Today, many of the side effects of adjuvant chemotherapy can be managed well, allowing patients to maintain their daily routines and work schedules. This has been due in a large part to the meticulous educational and psychological preparation provided to patients and their families by oncology nurses, oncologists, social workers, and other members of the health care team. In addition, strides have been made in the effectiveness of antiemetic agents used to alleviate nausea and vomiting and the use of hematopoietic growth factors to treat neutropenia and anemia.

Common physical side effects of chemotherapy for breast cancer may include nausea, vomiting, bone marrow suppression, taste changes, alopecia (hair loss), mucositis, skin changes, and fatigue. A weight gain of more than 10 pounds occurs in about half of all patients; the cause is unknown. Premenopausal women may also experience temporary or permanent amenorrhea leading to sterility.

Specific side effects vary with the type of chemotherapeutic agent used. In general, CMF and the taxanes are better tolerated than the anthracyclines. However, the taxanes can cause peripheral neuropathy, arthralgias, and myalgias, particularly at high doses. During taxane administration, hypersensitivity reactions may occur; therefore, the patient must be premedicated. Alopecia is also common. The side effects of the anthracyclines may be more severe and include cardiotoxicity in addition to nausea and vomiting, bone marrow suppression, and alopecia. Their vesicant properties can lead to tissue necrosis if infiltration of the medication infusion occurs.

NURSING MANAGEMENT

Nurses play an important role in helping patients manage the physical and psychosocial sequelae of chemotherapy. (Chapter 16 provides an in-depth discussion of side effect management.) Instructing the patient about the use of antiemetics and reviewing the optimal dosage schedule can help minimize nausea and vomiting. The different classes of antiemetic agents include serotonin (5HT-3) receptor antagonists (palonosetron [Aloxi], granisetron [Kytril], ondansetron [Zofran]); neurokinin-1 receptor antagonists (aprepitant [Emend]); dopamine receptor antagonists (prochlorperazine [Compazine], metoclopramide [Reglan]); benzodiazepines (lorazepam [Ativan]); and corticosteroids (dexamethasone [Decadron]). Measures to ease the symptoms of mucositis may include rinsing with normal saline or sodium bicarbonate solution, avoiding hot and spicy foods, and using a soft toothbrush.

Some patients may require hematopoietic growth factors to minimize the effects of chemotherapy-induced neutropenia and anemia. Granulocyte colony-stimulating

NURSING RESEARCH PROFILE

Vomiting During Chemotherapy Treatment for Breast Cancer

Dibble, S. L., Casey, K., Nussey, B., et al. (2004). Chemotherapy-induced vomiting in women treated for breast cancer. *Oncology Nursing Forum, 31*(1), E1–E8.

Purpose

Nausea and vomiting are side effects of chemotherapy that have caused some women to delay or even discontinue their treatments. Research has shown that 5-HT3 receptor antagonists are effective in treating vomiting during the acute phase (within the first 24 hours) of vomiting. This study examined the acute and delayed (after 24 hours) incidence and intensity of chemotherapy-induced vomiting since the advent of the 5-HT3 antagonists.

Design

This descriptive study longitudinally evaluated 303 women from 40 urban and rural outpatient facilities. Researchers obtained demographic data about the study participants as well as information about their diagnosis and treatment regimen, including chemotherapy dosages and antiemetics prescribed. Participants also completed a daily log of their vomiting experience through two consecutive cycles of chemotherapy; the log consisted of a three-item vomiting experience subscale from the Rhodes Index of Nausea, Vomiting, and Retching. Women also completed an exit survey about strategies they used to alleviate chemotherapy-induced vomiting.

Findings

Eighty-two percent of women experienced no acute vomiting, and 48% experienced no delayed vomiting. However, women who did experience vomiting found it to be severe, with the worst vomiting occurring on the day of chemotherapy administration and the following 3 days. Risk factors associated with significant vomiting included younger age, higher body mass index, history of car sickness, and minority status.

Nursing Implications

Despite the availability of effective antiemetic medications, vomiting remains a significant problem for some women receiving chemotherapy for treatment of breast cancer. Nurses should understand that some patients are more likely than others to experience chemotherapy-induced vomiting. This allows nurses to teach patients about appropriate management strategies and to ensure that available antiemetic medications are used effectively.

factors (G-CSFs) boost the white blood cell count, helping reduce the incidence of neutropenic fever and infection. The short-acting form, filgrastim (Neupogen), is injected subcutaneously for 7 to 10 days after chemotherapy administration. The long-acting form, pegfilgrastim (Neulasta), is injected once, 24 hours after chemotherapy. Erythropoietin growth factor increases the production of red blood cells, thus decreasing the symptoms of anemia. The short-acting form, epoetin alfa (Epogen) is usually administered weekly. The long-acting form, darbepoetin alfa (Aranesp), is administered every 2 weeks. The nurse instructs the patient and family on proper injection technique of hematopoietic growth

CHART 48-11

HOME CARE CHECKLIST • Self-Administration of Hematopoietic Growth Factors

At the completion of the home care instruction, the patient or caregiver will be able to:	Patient	Caregiver
• State the purpose for the injections	✔	✔
• Identify the equipment necessary for self-injection	✔	✔
• Identify appropriate body sites for self-injection	✔	✔
• Demonstrate how to draw up the solution in a syringe if indicated (note: darbepoetin and pegfilgrastim come in prefilled syringes)	✔	✔
• Demonstrate how to give an injection properly	✔	✔
• State possible side effects of medication	✔	✔
• Demonstrate correct disposal of sharps	✔	✔
• Describe proper storage of supplies	✔	✔
• State reasons for contacting the physician or nurse (eg, excessive pain, fever)	✔	✔

factors and about symptoms that require follow-up with a physician (Chart 48-11).

To prevent some of the emotional trauma associated with alopecia, it often helps to have a patient obtain a wig before hair loss begins to occur. The nurse may provide a list of wig suppliers in the patient's geographic region. Familiarity with creative ways to use scarves and turbans may also help minimize the patient's distress. The patient needs reassurance that new hair will grow back when treatment is completed, although the color and texture may be different. The ACS offers a program called "Look Good, Feel Better" that provides useful tips for applying cosmetics during chemotherapy.

Chemotherapy may negatively affect the patient's self-esteem, sexuality, and sense of well-being. This, combined with the stress of a potentially life-threatening disease, can be overwhelming. Providing support and promoting open communication are important aspects of nursing care. Referring the patient to the dietitian, social worker, psychiatrist, or spiritual advisor can provide additional support. Numerous community support and advocacy groups are available for patients and their families. Complementary therapies, such as guided imagery, meditation, and relaxation exercises, can also be used in conjunction with conventional treatments.

Hormonal Therapy

The use of **adjuvant hormonal therapy**, with or without the addition of chemotherapy, is considered in women who have hormone receptor–positive tumors (see Table 48-6). Its use can be determined by the results of an **estrogen and progesterone receptor assay**. About two-thirds of breast cancers are dependent on estrogen for growth and express a nuclear receptor that binds to the estrogen; thus, they are estrogen receptor–positive (ER+). Similarly, tumors that express the progesterone receptor are progesterone receptor–positive (PR+). Hormonal therapy involves the use of medications that compete with estrogen by binding to the receptor sites (selective estrogen receptor modulators [SERMs]), or by blocking estrogen production (**aromatase inhibitors**). Generally, tumors that are ER+/PR+ have the greatest likelihood of responding to hormonal therapy and have a more favorable prognosis than those that are ER–/PR–. Premenopausal and perimenopausal women are more likely to have non–hormone-dependent lesions, whereas postmenopausal women are more likely to have hormone-dependent lesions.

Traditionally, the SERM tamoxifen has been the primary hormonal agent used in treatment of premenopausal and postmenopausal breast cancer and remains the mainstay in premenopausal women. As a SERM, tamoxifen has estrogen antagonistic (estrogen-blocking) and agonistic (estrogen-like) effects on certain tissues. Its antagonistic effects in the breast prevent estrogen from binding to the receptor sites, thus preventing tumor growth. Tamoxifen has positive agonistic effects on blood lipid profiles and bone mineral density in postmenopausal women. It also has agonistic effects on endometrial tissue and blood coagulation processes, leading to an increased incidence of endometrial cancer and thromboembolic events (e.g., deep vein thrombosis, superficial phlebitis, pulmonary embolism). Nevertheless, the benefits of tamoxifen in women with breast cancer outweigh the risks.

The aromatase inhibitors anastrazole (Arimidex), letrozole (Femara), and exemestane (Aromasin) are now becoming important components in the hormonal management of postmenopausal women. Most of the circulating estrogens in postmenopausal women are derived from the conversion of the adrenal androgen androstenedione to estrone and the conversion of testosterone to estradiol. Aromatase inhibitors work by blocking the enzyme aromatase from performing the conversion, thereby decreasing the level of circulating estrogen in peripheral tissues. The Arimidex and Tamoxifen: Alone or in Combination (ATAC) trial, which compared anastrozole to tamoxifen either alone or in combination, demonstrated that anastrozole was superior to tamoxifen in terms of disease-free survival (Baum, Buzdar, Cuzick, et al., 2003). Another study found a significant disease-free survival in patients who received 5 years of letrozole following the completion of 5 years of tamoxifen (Goss, Ingle, Martino et al., 2003). Patients who took tamoxifen for 2 to 3 years and then took exemestane experienced benefits similar to patients who took tamoxifen alone for 5 years (Coombes, Hall, Gibson et al., 2004). These data ensure that aromatase inhibitors will play an increasingly central role in the long-term management and follow up of early-stage breast cancer. Table 48-7 outlines the adverse effects of adjuvant hormonal therapy. Chart 48-12 outlines appropriate patient education to manage the adverse effects.

Targeted Therapy

One of the most exciting areas of research in the systemic treatment of breast cancer involves the use of targeted therapies. Trastuzumab (Herceptin) is a monoclonal antibody that binds specifically to the HER-2/neu protein. This protein, which regulates cell growth, is present in small amounts on the surface of normal breast cells and in most breast cancers. Approximately 25% to 30% of tumors overexpress (overproduce) the HER-2/neu protein and are associated

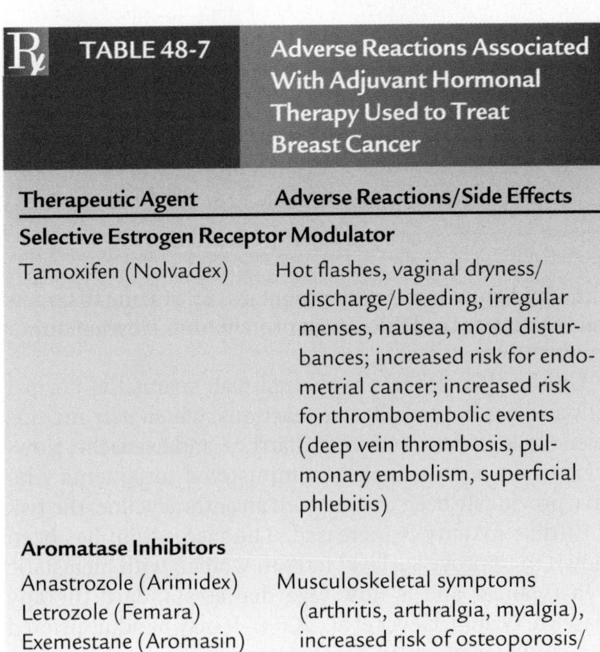

TABLE 48-7 Adverse Reactions Associated With Adjuvant Hormonal Therapy Used to Treat Breast Cancer

Therapeutic Agent	Adverse Reactions/Side Effects
Selective Estrogen Receptor Modulator	
Tamoxifen (Nolvadex)	Hot flashes, vaginal dryness/discharge/bleeding, irregular menses, nausea, mood disturbances; increased risk for endometrial cancer; increased risk for thromboembolic events (deep vein thrombosis, pulmonary embolism, superficial phlebitis)
Aromatase Inhibitors	
Anastrozole (Arimidex) Letrozole (Femara) Exemestane (Aromasin)	Musculoskeletal symptoms (arthritis, arthralgia, myalgia), increased risk of osteoporosis/fractures, nausea/vomiting, hot flashes, fatigue, mood disturbances

CHART 48-12

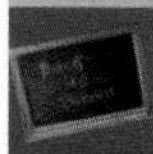

Patient Education

Managing Side Effects of Adjuvant Hormonal Therapy in Breast Cancer

HOT FLASHES
- Wear breathable, layered clothing.
- Avoid caffeine and spicy foods.
- Perform breathing exercises (paced respirations).
- Consider medications (vitamin E, antidepressants) or acupuncture.

VAGINAL DRYNESS
- Use vaginal moisturizers for everyday dryness (eg, Replens, Vitamin E suppository).
- Apply vaginal lubrication during intercourse (eg, Astroglide, K-Y jelly).

NAUSEA AND VOMITING
- Consume a bland diet.
- Try to take medication in the evening.

MUSCULOSKELETAL SYMPTOMS
- Take nonsteroidal analgesics as recommended.
- Take warm baths.

RISK OF ENDOMETRIAL CANCER
- Report any irregular bleeding to a gynecologist for evaluation.

RISK FOR THROMBOEMBOLIC EVENTS
- Report any redness, swelling, or tenderness in the lower extremities, or any unexplained shortness of breath.

RISK FOR OSTEOPOROSIS OR FRACTURES
- Undergo a baseline bone density scan.
- Perform regular weight-bearing exercises.
- Take calcium supplements with vitamin D.
- Take bisphosphonates (eg, alendronate) or calcitonin as prescribed.

with rapid growth and poor prognosis. Trastuzumab targets and inactivates the HER-2/neu protein, thus slowing tumor growth.

Unlike chemotherapy, trastuzumab spares the normal cells and has limited adverse reactions, which may include fever, chills, nausea, vomiting, diarrhea, and headache. However, when trastuzumab is administered to patients who have previously been treated with an anthracycline, the risk of cardiac toxicity is increased. The medication has been shown to improve survival rates in women with metastatic breast cancer and is now regarded as standard therapy (Baselga, Gianni, Geyer et al., 2004). It may be administered as a single agent or in combination with chemotherapy. Research to evaluate its efficacy in the adjuvant setting is currently ongoing.

Treatment of Recurrent and Metastatic Breast Cancer

Despite the advances made in the treatment of breast cancer, recurrences occur in some women. The disease may recur locally (on the chest wall or in the conserved breast), regionally (in the remaining lymph nodes), or systemically (in distant organs). In metastatic disease, the bone, usually the hips, spine, ribs, or pelvis, is the most common site of spread. Other sites of metastasis include the lungs, liver, pleura, and brain.

The overall prognosis and optimal treatment are determined by a variety of factors such as the site and extent of recurrence, the time to recurrence from the original diagnosis, history of prior treatments, the patient's performance status, and any existing comorbid conditions. Patients with bone metastases generally have a longer overall survival compared with metastases in visceral organs.

Local recurrence in the absence of systemic disease is treated aggressively with surgery, radiation, and hormonal therapy. Chemotherapy may also be used for tumors that are not hormonally sensitive. Local recurrence may be an indicator that systemic disease will develop in the future, particularly if it occurs within 2 years of the original diagnosis.

Metastatic breast cancer involves control of the disease rather than cure. Treatment includes hormonal therapy, chemotherapy, and targeted therapy. Surgery or radiation may be indicated in select situations. Premenopausal women who have hormonally dependent tumors may eliminate the production of estrogen by the ovaries through oophorectomy (removal of the ovaries) or suppression of estrogen production by medications such as leuprolide (Lupron) or goserelin (Zoladex).

Patients with advanced breast cancer are monitored closely for signs of disease progression. Baseline studies are obtained at the time of recurrence. These may include complete blood count; comprehensive metabolic panel; tumor markers (ie, carcinoembryonic antigen, CA 15-3); bone scan; CT of the chest, abdomen, and pelvis; and MRI of symptomatic areas. Additional x-rays may be performed to evaluate areas of pain or abnormal areas seen on bone scan (eg, long bones, pelvis). These studies are repeated at regular intervals to assess for effectiveness of treatment and to monitor progression of disease.

Nursing Management

Nurses play an important role in not only educating patients and managing their symptoms but in providing emotional support. Many patients find that recurrence of the disease is more distressing than the initial cancer diagnosis. They not only have to contend with another round of treatments but are faced with a greater uncertainty about their future and long-term survival. The nurse can help the patient identify coping strategies and set priorities to optimize quality of life. Family members and significant others should be included in the treatment plan and follow-up care. Referrals to support groups, psychiatry, social work, and complementary medicine programs (eg, guided imagery, meditation, yoga) should be made as indicated.

Nurses also play important roles in providing palliative care, if indicated. The highest priorities should include alleviating pain and providing comfort measures. A frank discussion with the patient and family regarding their preferences for end-of-life care should occur before the need arises, to ensure a smooth transition without disruption of care. Referrals to hospice and home health care should be initiated as necessary. Chapter 16 provides more information on the general care of the patient with advanced cancer. Chapter 17 discusses end-of-life care.

Reconstructive Breast Surgery

Breast reconstruction is elective surgery that can enhance a woman's self-image and sense of well-being. Women desire reconstruction for a variety of physical and psychological reasons. Therefore, it is important that the health care team conduct a thorough assessment prior to reconstructive surgery to evaluate the woman's underlying desire, motivation, and expectations. Preparing a woman realistically could help her to avoid potential disappointment. A variety of reconstructive options are available today for women who desire a correction in the size or the shape of the breast, including reduction **mammoplasty** (breast reduction), augmentation mammoplasty (breast enlargement), and mastopexy (breast lift). Several options are also available to reconstruct the breast after a mastectomy.

Reduction Mammoplasty

Reduction mammoplasty is usually performed on women who have breast hypertrophy (excessively large breasts). The weight of the enlarged breasts can cause discomfort, fatigue, embarrassment, and poor posture.

Reduction mammoplasty is an outpatient procedure that is performed under general anesthesia. Most commonly, an anchor-shaped incision that circles the areola is made, extending downward and following the natural curve of the crease beneath the breast (inframammary fold). Depending on the size of the breast, the nipple may be moved up to a higher position while still attached to the breast tissue or it may be separated and transplanted to a new location. Drains are placed in the incision and remain for 2 to 5 days.

During the preoperative consultation, the patient should be informed that there is a possibility that sensory changes of the nipple (such as numbness) may occur. These sensations are normal and usually resolve after several months but can sometimes persist. The procedure may also make breastfeeding impossible, although some women have breastfed successfully. The patient must also be aware that if she gains weight (usually more than 10 pounds), her breasts may also enlarge.

After reduction mammoplasty, many women verbalize feelings of extreme satisfaction, possibly because of the relief they experience. The patient is instructed to wear a supportive bra 24 hours a day for 2 weeks to prevent tension on the swollen breast and incision line. Vigorous exercise (eg, jumping, jogging) should be avoided for about 6 weeks after surgery.

Augmentation Mammoplasty

Augmentation mammoplasty is requested by women who desire larger or fuller breasts. The procedure is performed by placing a breast implant either under the pectoralis muscle (subpectoral) or under the breast tissue (subglandular). The subpectoral approach is preferred because it interferes less with clinical breast examinations and mammograms. The incision line can be placed in the inframammary fold, in the axilla, or around the areola. The procedure is performed as an outpatient procedure under general anesthesia. A drain is not necessary. Postoperative instructions are the same as for reduction mammoplasty.

Saline implants are typically used for augmentation mammoplasty. In the past, silicone implants were used; however, after concerns about the risk of their causing autoimmune diseases, they were removed from the market. Today, women who choose to have silicone implants must enroll in an FDA-approved study, in which information about implant safety is collected prospectively for 5 years. Women with breast implants should be aware that mammograms may be more difficult to read, and they should seek experienced breast radiologists.

Mastopexy

Mastopexy is performed when the patient is happy with the size of her breasts but wishes to have the shape improved and a lift performed. The procedure is also an outpatient surgery, and postoperative instructions are the same as for reduction mammoplasty.

Reconstructive Procedures After Mastectomy

Breast reconstruction can provide a significant psychological benefit for women who are already struggling with the emotional distress of losing a breast. A consultation with a plastic surgeon can help the patient understand procedures for which she is a candidate and the pros and cons of each. Factors to consider include body size and shape, comorbid conditions (eg, hypertension, diabetes mellitus, obesity), personal habits such as smoking, and patient preference. The patient must be informed that although breast reconstruction can provide a good cosmetic result, it will never precisely duplicate the natural breast. Realistic preparation can help the patient avoid unrealistic expectations. Once reconstruction is complete, the opposite breast may require augmentation, reduction, or mastopexy, to achieve symmetry on both sides. The patient must also be informed that breast reconstruction will not interfere with breast cancer treatments nor will it affect the risk for cancer recurrence. Reconstruction is considered an integral component in the surgical treatment of breast cancer and is usually covered by insurance companies.

Many women elect immediate reconstruction at the time of the mastectomy operation. This can be a benefit in that it saves the woman from undergoing general anesthesia a second time, and it saves the cost and stress of future hospitalizations. However, it does increase the length of the surgical procedure. Delayed reconstruction is preferable in women who are having a difficult time deciding on the type of reconstruction they desire. It may also be preferable in patients with advanced disease such as inflammatory breast cancer where the breast cancer treatments should be given without delay. Any delays in healing after immediate reconstruction may interfere with the initiation of treatment.

TISSUE EXPANDER FOLLOWED BY PERMANENT IMPLANT

Breast reconstruction using a **tissue expander followed by a permanent implant** is the simplest and most common method used today (Fig. 48-6). To accommodate an implant, the skin remaining after a mastectomy and the underlying muscle must gradually be stretched by a process called tissue expansion. The surgeon places a balloon-like device called a tissue expander through the mastectomy incision underneath the pectoralis muscle. A small amount of saline is injected through a metal port intraoperatively to partially inflate the expander. Then, for about 6 to 8 weeks, at weekly intervals, the patient receives additional saline injections through the port until the expander is fully inflated. It remains fully expanded for about 6 weeks to allow the skin to loosen. The expander is then exchanged for a permanent implant. This is usually performed as outpatient surgery.

Advantages of this expansion procedure are a shorter operating time and a shorter recuperation period than for autologous reconstruction (see Tissue Transfer Procedures, below). A disadvantage is a tendency for the implant to feel firm and round, with little natural ptosis (sag). Women with a small to medium opposite breast with little ptosis are good candidates for this procedure. Women who have had radiation or who have connective tissue disease are not good candidates because of the decreased elasticity of the skin.

The patient must be instructed not to have an MRI while the tissue expander is in place, because the port contains metal. This is not an issue once the permanent implant is in place. The patient should also be informed that for the rest of her life she should not engage in any exercises that will develop the pectoralis muscle, because this can result in distortion of the reconstructed breast.

TISSUE TRANSFER PROCEDURES

Autologous reconstruction is the use of the patient's own tissue to create a breast mound. A flap of skin, fat, and muscle with its attached blood supply is rotated to the mastectomy site to create a mound that simulates the breast. Donor sites may include the **transverse rectus abdominis myocutaneous (TRAM) flap** (abdominal muscle) (Fig. 48-7), gluteal flap (buttock muscle), or the latissimus dorsi flap (back muscle) (Fig. 48-8). The results more closely resemble a real breast, because the skin and fat from the donor sites are similar in consistency to a natural breast. These procedures avoid the use of synthetic material. However, they are far more complex and involve longer operative time (ranging from about 5 to 10 hours total time for the mastectomy and reconstruction) and longer recuperation than a tissue expander procedure. The risk for potential complications (eg, infection, bleeding, flap necrosis) is also greater. Therefore, patients must be in relatively good health, and those with medical conditions (eg, atherosclerosis, pulmonary disease, heart failure) that affect circulation or compromise oxygen delivery are not good candidates. Other poor candidates include those with uncontrolled type 1 diabetes mellitus or morbid obesity, and heavy smokers.

The TRAM flap is the most commonly performed tissue transfer procedure. A free TRAM procedure may also be performed; in this case, the skin, fat, muscle, and blood supply are completely detached from the body and then transplanted to the mastectomy site using microvascular surgery (use of a microscope to reconnect the vessels). Postoperatively, patients who have undergone TRAM procedures often face a lengthy recovery (often 6 to 8 weeks) and have incisions both at the mastectomy site and at the donor site in the abdomen. The nurse must assess the newly constructed breast site for changes in color, circulation, and temperature, because flap loss is a potential complication. Mottling or an obvious decrease in skin temperature is reported to the surgeon immediately. Breathing and leg exercises are essential, because the patient is more limited in her activity and is at greater risk for respiratory complications and deep vein thrombosis. Measures to help the patient reduce tension on

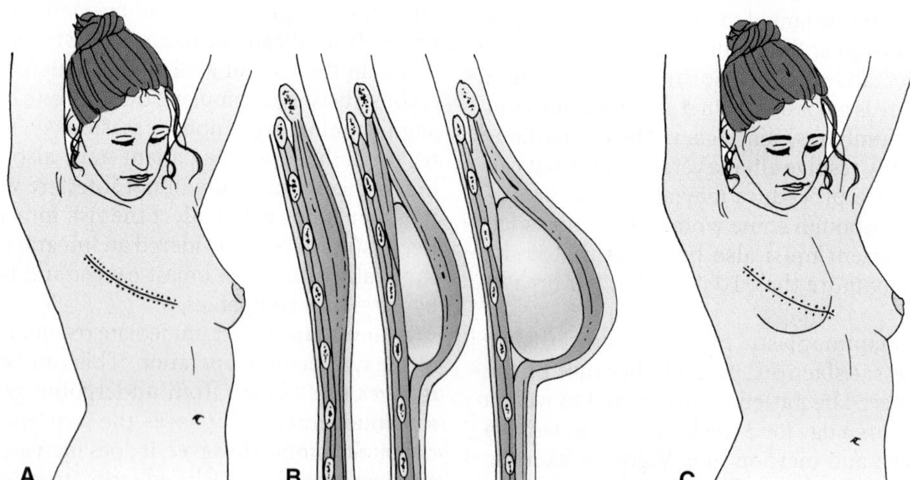

FIGURE 48-6. Breast reconstruction with tissue expander. (**A**) Mastectomy incision line prior to tissue expansion. (**B**) The expander is placed under the pectoralis muscle and is gradually filled with saline solution through a port to stretch the skin enough to accept a permanent implant. (**C**) The breast mound is restored. Although permanent, scars will fade with time. The nipple and areola are reconstructed later. Adapted from "Breast Reconstruction," American Society of Plastic and Reconstructive Surgeons, Arlington Heights, IL.

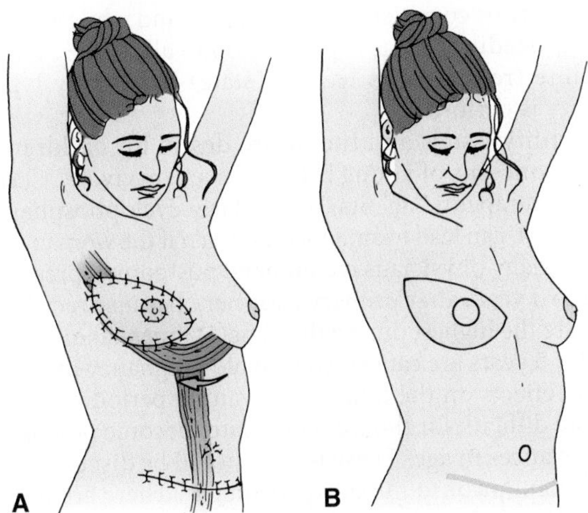

FIGURE 48-7. Breast reconstruction: transverse rectus abdominis myocutaneous (TRAM) flap. (**A**) A breast mound is created by tunneling abdominal skin, fat, and muscle to the mastectomy site. (**B**) Final location of scars. Adapted from "Breast Reconstruction," American Society of Plastic and Reconstructive Surgeons, Arlington Heights, IL.

the abdominal incision during the first postoperative week include elevating the head of the bed 45 degrees and flexing the patient's knees.

Once the patient is able to ambulate, she can protect the surgical incision by splinting it and will gradually achieve a more upright position. The patient is instructed to avoid high impact activities and lifting (more than 5 to 10 pounds for 6 to 8 weeks after surgery) to prevent stress on the incision.

NIPPLE–AREOLA RECONSTRUCTION

After the breast mound has been created and the site has healed, some women choose to have nipple–areola reconstruction. This is a minor surgical procedure carried out either in the physician's office or at an outpatient surgical facility. The most common method of creating a nipple is with the use of local flaps (skin and fat from the center of the new breast mound), which are wrapped around each other to create a projecting nipple. The areola is created using a skin graft. The most common donor site is the upper inner thigh, because this skin has darker pigmentation than the skin on the reconstructed breast. After the nipple graft has healed, micropigmentation (tattooing) can be performed to achieve a more natural color. The surgeon can usually match the reconstructed nipple–areola complex with that of the contralateral breast for an acceptable cosmetic result.

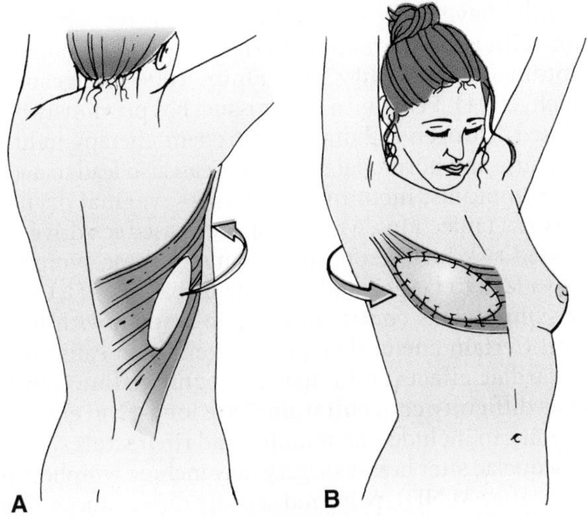

FIGURE 48-8. Breast reconstruction: latissimus dorsi flap. (**A**) The latissimus muscle with an ellipse of skin is rotated from the back to the mastectomy site. (**B**) Because the flap is usually not bulky enough to provide an adequate breast mound, an implant is often also required. Adapted from "Breast Reconstruction," American Society of Plastic and Reconstructive Surgeons, Arlington Heights, IL.

Prosthetics

Not all patients desire or are candidates for reconstructive surgery. A breast prosthesis, an external form which simulates the breast, is another option. Prostheses are available in different shapes, sizes, colors, and materials, although they are most often made of silicone. They can be placed inside a pocket in a bra or can adhere directly to the chest wall. The nurse can provide the patient with the names of shops where she can be fitted for a prosthesis, or the patient can call the Reach to Recovery program of the ACS for appropriate referrals. The patient should be encouraged to find a shop that has a comfortable, supportive atmosphere and employs a certified prosthetics consultant. Generally, medical supply shops are not recommended, because often they do not have the appropriate resources to ensure the proper fitting of a prosthesis.

Prior to discharge from the hospital, the nurse usually provides the patient with a temporary, lightweight, cotton-filled form that can be worn until the surgical incision is well healed (4 to 6 weeks). After that, the patient can be fitted for a prosthesis. Insurance companies generally cover the cost of the prosthesis and the special bras that hold it in place. A breast prosthesis can provide a psychological benefit and assist the woman in resuming proper posture, because it helps balance the weight of the remaining breast.

Special Issues in Breast Cancer Management

Implications of Genetics Testing

The rapid advancement in genetics has brought new knowledge about genetically inherited breast cancer, but it has also raised potential ethical and psychosocial issues. Although the actual testing for the BRCA-1 and BRCA-2 genes involves a simple blood test, it is these issues that must be addressed. Before undergoing genetics testing, a person should meet either with a clinician who has expertise in this area or with a certified genetics counselor to discuss risk factors as well as the benefits, sequelae, and limitations of testing.

How people react when they receive their actual test results is not always easy to predict. A negative test in a person who comes from a family with a known mutation may lead to enormous relief. However, a negative test in a family with no known mutation may be a source of undue reassurance; the possibility of existing genes that cannot yet be detected remains. A negative test may also lead to feelings of guilt in a person whose family members did not receive favorable test results; this is known as "survivor's guilt." A positive test could act as a motivator in a person to pursue appropriate screening and/or treatment, or it could cause tremendous anxiety, depression, and worry.

In addition, test results may be ambiguous, leading to feelings of confusion and uncertainty. People must be informed that not all gene carriers develop breast cancer (incomplete penetrance) and that not all noncarriers are protected.

Other issues include those of cost: Who should pay for genetics testing and the services that relate to it? Difficult ethical questions arise concerning whether the person who is tested should disclose the test results. Is it ethical to withhold results from family members who may be at risk? If they are told, what effect will it have on them? People considering testing must be informed that there is no guarantee that test results will remain confidential. Once confidentiality is breached, it could unleash potential discrimination in employment and insurability. Genetics testing should be performed as part of a research protocol to protect the patient (research data are kept separate from the patient's medical record).

People must be well informed of all of the issues and potential implications prior to undergoing genetics testing. Nurses play a role in educating and counseling patients and their family members about the implications of genetics testing. Nurses provide support and clarification and make referrals to appropriate specialists when indicated.

Pregnancy and Breast Cancer

Breast cancer during pregnancy is defined as breast cancer diagnosed during gestation or within 1 year of childbirth and occurs in 1 in 3000 women (Middleton, Amin, Gwyn et al., 2003). Due to increased levels of hormones produced during pregnancy and subsequent lactation, the breast tissue becomes tender and swollen, making it more difficult to detect a mass. A breast mass could potentially be missed, leading to a delay in diagnosis. Practicing monthly BSEs and undergoing clinical breast examinations during prenatal visits could help avoid a delay.

If a mass is found during pregnancy, ultrasound is the preferred diagnostic method, because it involves no exposure to radiation. If indicated, mammography with appropriate shielding, FNA, and biopsy can be performed. Modified radical mastectomy remains the most common form of surgical treatment. SLNB is typically not performed because of the unknown effects of the radioisotope and the blue dye on the fetus. Breast conservation treatment may be considered if the breast cancer is diagnosed during the third trimester. Radiation can then be delayed until after delivery, because it is contraindicated during pregnancy. Chemotherapy should be avoided during the first trimester; the fetal organs are still developing, and it poses a great risk for fetal malformations. However, chemotherapy has been administered during the second and third trimesters with few reported abnormalities. Long-term effects on the fetus are still being studied. If a woman is close to term, a cesarean section may be performed as soon as maturation of the fetus allows, and then treatment is initiated. If aggressive disease is detected early in pregnancy and chemotherapy is advised, termination of the pregnancy may be considered. If a mass is found while a woman is breastfeeding, she is urged to stop to allow the breast to involute (return to its baseline state) before any type of surgery is performed.

Fertility issues and the future desire for children are major concerns of young breast cancer survivors. Certain chemotherapeutic agents, particularly cyclophosphamide (Cytoxan), can lead to amenorrhea. Even if the woman is still fertile, many physicians recommend postponing pregnancy for 2 to 3 years after primary treatment because recurrence rates are the highest during this time. Women taking tamoxifen for 5 years are cautioned to avoid pregnancy due to potential effects on the fetus. This waiting period may make it more difficult for the woman to later become pregnant as she advances in age. These issues should be discussed with the patient prior to initiating treatment. There are options today that may help to preserve a woman's fertility, and prior to the onset of chemotherapy she should seek the opinion of a reproductive specialist (Hassey-Dow & Kuhn, 2004). Fertile Hope, a national nonprofit organization, can also provide updated information on reproduction (Fertile Hope, 2004).

Quality of Life and Survivorship

With increased early detection and improved treatment modalities, women with breast cancer have become the largest group of cancer survivors. However, the treatment or simply the diagnosis of breast cancer may have long-term effects that negatively affect the patient and her family. It is important that nurses learn about these effects so that appropriate interventions can be provided to optimize quality of life. The nurse can be pivotal in providing education and support to the patient as she makes very difficult and emotional decisions. The patient should be prepared early for the potential long-term effects of the disease and its treatments so she has realistic expectations and can make informed decisions.

Studies have shown that long-term survivors have difficulty with issues pertaining to sexuality and menopausal symptoms (Casso, Buist, & Talpin, 2004; Helgeson & Tomich, 2004). Fertility, a major issue, has previously been discussed. Estrogen withdrawal from chemotherapy-induced menopause and hormonal treatments can also lead to a variety of symptoms, including hot flashes, vaginal dryness, urinary tract infections, weight gain, decreased sex drive, and increased risk for osteoporosis. Some of these symptoms can also lead to fatigue and sleep disturbances. HT to alleviate symptoms is contraindicated in women with breast cancer. Certain chemotherapeutic agents can cause long-term cardiac effects and impaired cognitive functioning, such as difficulty concentrating. Rare long-term effects of radiation can include pneumonitis and rib fractures. Long-term sequelae after breast surgery may include lymphedema (mainly after ALND), pain, and sensory disturbances. Once lymphedema develops, it tends to be a chronic problem, so prevention strategies (discussed earlier) are vital. Patients have also reported sensations such as tenderness and soreness 2 years after their surgical procedure (Baron et al., 2004).

Long-term psychosocial sequelae may include anxiety, depression, uncertainty about the future, and fear of recurrence. Many of these sequelae may affect the patient's partner and children (Loerzel, 2004). In the workplace, the patient may suffer from fear of discrimination, concern over coworkers' reactions, fear of losing benefits, and lack of physical stamina.

Gerontologic Considerations

When deciding on the optimal treatment modality for an elderly patient—whether it be surgery, radiation, chemotherapy, hormonal therapy, or any combination—age alone should not be the single determining factor. Many older women, regardless of their advancing chronological age, remain in excellent health. Therefore, the woman's treatment preferences should play a strong role in the decision-making process. For example, a woman's desire to have breast reconstruction following mastectomy or breast conservation treatment followed by radiation rather than mastectomy should be respected.

It should not be assumed that elderly women are less concerned about their appearance than their younger counterparts. In a study of 563 women who were 67 years of age or older, 31% reported that body image was an important factor in making decisions about treatment for breast cancer. Women who underwent mastectomy but preferred breast conservation had the poorest body image (Figueiredo, Cullen, Hwang et al., 2004). Research studies in women older than 70 years are lacking, and nurses can play important roles in conducting research about these patients.

A thorough assessment must be performed before any treatment is initiated, and careful monitoring must occur throughout the course of treatment to avoid complications. The physical and psychosocial assessment of the older woman should include general health, currently existing comorbidities, performance status, cognitive status, current medications, available resources, and support systems.

Breast Health of Women With Disabilities

Women with a variety of disabilities may be unable to detect changes in their own breasts. Those with decreased sensation in their fingers may be unable to palpate even large breast masses and those with vision loss may be unable to detect changes in the appearance of their breasts. Women with disabilities tend to undergo mammography less often than recommended and less often than other women (Shootman & Jeffe, 2003). They may lack transportation to the imaging facility, and they may be unable to undress without assistance, stand, or maintain positioning for a mammogram. Many imaging facilities do not have accessible mammography equipment and staff members may be unfamiliar with modifications in positioning needed to obtain acceptable scans in women with disabilities (Smeltzer & Sharts-Hopko, 2005). Further, health care providers often neglect to recommend health screening, including mammograms, for women with disabilities despite the fact that they have the same risks for breast cancer as other women and generally have a normal or near-normal life expectancy (U.S. Department of Human Services, 2005). The more severe the disability, the less likely it is for a woman to undergo mammography. For those women with disabilities who cannot be adequately positioned for a mammogram, ultrasound may be used as an alternative; however, these women may need more frequent clinical breast examinations.

Women who have had repeated x-ray exposure because of disability-related health issues may be concerned about exposure to additional x-rays for mammograms. However, the benefits of mammography are generally thought to outweigh the risks.

Women with disabilities who are diagnosed and treated for breast cancer tend to be offered breast conservation surgery less often than other women, although women with disabilities have the same concerns for body image as other women and should be provided health care that is the same as that provided for all women.

An essential role of the nurse is to assist women with disabilities to identify accessible health screening and to advocate for greater accessibility of imaging centers and other health care facilities. Reminding women of the need for recommended clinical breast examinations and mammograms is an important part of nursing care.

Diseases of the Male Breast

Gynecomastia

Gynecomastia, or overdeveloped breast tissue, is the most common breast condition in the male. Adolescent boys can be affected by this condition because of hormones secreted by the testes. This type of gynecomastia is virtually always benign and resolves spontaneously in 1 to 2 years. Gynecomastia can also occur in older men and usually presents as a firm, tender mass underneath the areola. In these patients, gynecomastia may be diffuse and related to use of certain medications (eg, digitalis, ranitidine). It may also be associated with certain conditions, including feminizing testicular tumors, infection in the testes, and liver disease resulting from factors such as alcohol abuse or a parasitic infection.

Patients in their late teens to late forties presenting with idiopathic (unknown cause) gynecomastia should have a testicular examination and possibly a testicular ultrasound. Treatment of the enlarged breast tissue is based on patient preference and is usually reserved for those men who cannot tolerate the cosmetic appearance of the breast or who have severe pain associated with the condition. Observation is acceptable in most cases, because gynecomastia may resolve on its own. Surgical removal of the tissue through a small incision around the areola is the best treatment option. Liposuction performed by a plastic surgeon is another possibility, although this does not allow for pathologic examination of the tissue.

Male Breast Cancer

Cancer of the male breast accounts for less than 1% of all cases of breast cancer. The average age at the time of diagnosis is 67 years (Giordano, Cohen, Buzdar et al., 2004), but the disease may occur in younger men, especially if there is a genetic link. There is a well-documented link to mutations in the BRCA-2 gene in men with breast cancer; men with a BRCA-2 mutation have a 7% lifetime risk of breast cancer

(ACS, 2004c; Liede, Karlan & Narod, 2004). In sporadic cases of male breast cancer (no known family history), risk factors may include a history of mumps orchitis, radiation exposure, and Klinefelter's syndrome (a chromosomal condition reflecting decreased testosterone levels). Liver disease due to factors such as alcohol abuse or a parasitic infection, which compromises estrogen metabolism, may also lead to an increase in rates of male breast cancer. Symptoms include a painless lump beneath the areola, nipple retraction, bloody nipple discharge, or skin ulceration. Diagnostic tests and treatment modalities are similar to those used for women.

Early detection is uncommon in male breast cancer because of the rare nature of the disease. Neither patient nor physician suspects male breast cancer early in its development. Treatment generally consists of a total mastectomy with either SLNB or ALND. If the pectoralis muscle is involved, **neoadjuvant** (preoperative) **chemotherapy** and radical mastectomy may be indicated. Radiation therapy may be used postoperatively. As in women with breast cancer, prognosis depends on the stage of disease at presentation. Involvement of the axillary lymph nodes is the most important prognostic indicator.

Male breast cancers are very likely to be estrogen receptor positive, and tamoxifen, although it has several side effects, is a mainstay of treatment. Overall, survival rates by stage of disease are similar for males and females with breast cancer (Giordano et al., 2004).

Critical Thinking Exercises

1 A 49-year-old woman has a high risk of breast cancer because she has a strong family history. For the past 10 years, she has been having yearly mammograms. She is concerned about the amount of radiation exposure she has received and asks if she should have yearly breast ultrasounds instead. What would you advise?

2 A 34-year-old woman, who is pregnant for the first time, is in the middle of her first trimester. She has just been diagnosed with a 3-cm malignant mass in her breast. What treatment options are available for this patient? What resources would be appropriate to provide to her?

3 ebp A 40-year-old woman with breast cancer has been taking tamoxifen for a year. She is having terrible hot flashes and wants to know if she could take hormone therapy (HT). She also asks if her risk of osteoporosis is increased and asks what she can do to reduce the risk. How would you respond to her question and concerns? What advice can you give her to manage her hot flashes and to reduce her risk for osteoporosis? What is the evidence base for your responses to her questions? How will you evaluate the strength of the evidence?

4 A 60-year-old woman has had several benign breast biopsies in the past. She has heard about a blood test to check for the breast cancer gene and she would like to go have this test promptly. How would you address this request? What are the implications of genetics testing?

5 A 72-year-old frail woman who lives alone is scheduled for a modified radical mastectomy. Describe the postoperative care of this patient, including discharge planning. How would you modify your care if she has a severe hearing impairment?

REFERENCES AND SELECTED READINGS

BOOKS

American Cancer Society. (2005a). *Cancer facts and figures.* Atlanta, GA: Author.

American Cancer Society. (2005b). *Detailed guide: Breast cancer.* Atlanta, GA: Author.

American Cancer Society. (2005c). *Breast cancer in men, 2005.* Atlanta, GA: Author.

American Cancer Society. (2005d). *Cancer prevention and early detection facts and figures, 2005.* Atlanta, GA: Author.

American Cancer Society. (2005e). *Breast cancer facts and figures, 2005–2006.* Atlanta, GA: Author.

American Cancer Society. (2005f). *Breast cancer treatment guidelines for patients.* Atlanta, GA: Author.

Bickley, L. S., & Szilagyi, P. G. (2003). *Bates' guide to physical examination and history taking* (8th ed.). Philadelphia: Lippincott Williams & Wilkins.

Bland, K. I., & Copeland, E. M. III (Eds.). (2004). *The breast: Comprehensive management of benign and malignant disorders* (3rd ed.). Philadelphia: W. B. Saunders.

Dow, K. H. (2002). *Pocket guide to breast cancer* (2nd ed.). Boston: Jones & Bartlett.

Dow, K. H. (Ed.) (2004). *Contemporary issues in breast cancer* (2nd ed.). Boston: Jones & Bartlett.

Greene, F. L., Page, D. L., Fleming, I. D., et al. (2002). *AJCC cancer staging manual* (6th ed.). New York: Springer-Verlag.

Harris, J. R., Lippman, M. E., Morrow, M., & Osborne, C. K. (Eds.) (2004). *Diseases of the breast* (3rd ed.). Philadelphia: Lippincott Williams & Wilkins.

Loerzel, V. (2004). Support and survivorship issues. In K. Hassey-Dow (Ed.), *Contemporary issues in breast cancer* (pp. 313–322). Sudbury, MA: Jones and Bartlett.

Love, S. M. (2000). *Dr. Susan Love's breast book.* Reading, MA: Addison-Wesley.

Smeltzer, S. C. & Sharts-Hopko, N. C. (2005). *A provider's guide for the care of women with physical disabilities and chronic health conditions.* Chapel Hill, NC: North Carolina Office on Disability & Health.

U.S. Department of Health and Human Services. (2005). *The Surgeon General's call to action to improve the health and wellness of persons with disabilities.* Washington, DC: U.S. Department of Health and Human Services, Office of the Surgeon General.

Weber, J., & Kelley, J. (2003). *Health assessment in nursing* (2nd ed.). Philadelphia: Lippincott Williams & Wilkins.

Yarbro, C. H., Frogge, M. H. & Goodman, M. (Eds.) (2005). *Cancer nursing: Principles and practices* (6th ed.). Sudbury, MA: Jones & Bartlett.

JOURNALS

**Asterisks indicate nursing research articles.*

Breast Cancer Risk and Prevention

Antoniou, A., Pharoah, P., Narod, S. et al. (2003). Average risks of breast and ovarian cancer associated with BRCA1 or BRCA2 mutations detected in case series unselected for family history: A combined analysis of 22 studies. *American Journal of Human Genetics, 72*(5), 1117–1130.

Chlebowksi, R. T., Hendrix, S. L., Langer, R. D. et al. (2003). Influence of estrogen plus progestin on breast cancer and mammography in healthy postmenopausal women. *Journal of the American Medical Association, 289*(24), 3243–3253.

Cummings, S. R., Eckert, S., Krueger, K. A., et al. (1999). The effect of raloxifene on risk of breast cancer in postmenopausal women: Results from the MORE randomized trial. *Journal of the American Medical Association, 281*(23), 2189–2197.

Fisher, B., Costantino, J. P., Wickerham, D. L., et al. (1998). Tamoxifen for prevention of breast cancer. Report of the National Surgical Adjuvant Breast and Bowel Project P-1 Study. *Journal of the National Cancer Institute, 90*(18), 1371–1388.

Jemal, A., Siegel, R., Ward, E., et al. (2006). Cancer statistics, 2006. *CA: A Cancer Journal for Clinicians, 56*(2), 106–130.

King, M. C., Marks, J. H., Mandell, J. B. et al. (2003). Breast and ovarian cancer risks due to inherited mutations in BRCA1 and BRCA2. *Science, 302*(5645), 643–646.

Mattisson, I., Wirfalt, E., Wallstrom, P. et al. (2004). High fat and alcohol intakes are risk factors of postmenopausal breast cancer: A prospective study from the Malmo diet and cancer cohort. *International Journal of Cancer, 110*(4), 589–597.

McTiernan, A., Kooperberg, C., White, E., et al. (2003). Recreational physical activity and the risk of breast cancer in postmenopausal women. *Journal of the American Medical Association, 290*(10), 1331–1336.

Pinder, S. E. & Ellis, I. O. (2003). Ductal carcinoma in situ (DCIS) and atypical ductal hyperplasia (ADH)-current definitions and classification. *Breast Cancer Research, 5*(5), 254–257.

Rebbeck, T. R., Friebel, T., Lynch, H. T. et al. (2004). Bilateral prophylactic mastectomy reduces breast cancer risk in BRCA1 and BRCA2 mutation carriers: The PROSE study group. *Journal of Clinical Oncology, 22*(6), 1055–1062.

Simpson, P. T., Gale, T., Fulford, L. G. et al. (2003). Pathology of atypical lobular hyperplasia and lobular carcinoma in situ. *Breast Cancer Research, 5*(5), 258–262.

Smith, R. A., Saslow, D., Sawyer, K. et al. (2003). American Cancer Society guidelines for breast cancer screening: Update 2003. *CA: A Cancer Journal for Clinicians, 53*(3), 141–169.

Warner, E., Plewes, D. B., Hill, K. A. et al. (2004). Surveillance of BRCA1 and BRCA2 mutation carriers with magnetic resonance imaging, ultrasound, mammography, and clinical breast examination. *Journal of the American Medical Association, 292*(11), 1317–1325.

Women's Health Initiative Steering Committee. (2004). Effects of conjugated equine estrogen in postmenopausal women with hysterectomy. *Journal of the American Medical Association, 291*(14), 1701–1712.

Cancer

Burstein, H. J., Polyak, K., Wong, J. S. et al. (2004). Ductal carcinoma in situ of the breast. *New England Journal of Medicine, 350*(14), 1430–1441.

Emens, L. A. & Davidson, N. E. (2004). Trastuzumab in breast cancer. *Oncology*. 18(9), 1117–1128.

Figueiredo, M. I., Cullen, J., Hwang, Y. T. et al. (2004). Breast cancer treatment in older women: does getting what you want improve your long-term body image and mental health? *Journal of Clinical Oncology, 22*(19), 4002–4009.

Giordano, S. H., Cohen, D. S., Buzdar, A. U. et al. (2004). Breast carcinoma in men: A population based study. *Cancer, 101*(1), 51–57.

Liede, A., Karlan, B. Y. & Narod, S. A. (2004). Cancer risks for male carriers of germline mutations in BRCA1 or BRCA2: A review of the literature. *Journal of Clinical Oncology, 22*(4), 735–742.

Vogel, V. G., Costantino, J. P., Wickerham, D. L. et al., (2003). National surgical adjuvant breast and bowel project update: prevention trials and endocrine therapy of ductal carcinoma in situ. *Clinical Cancer Research, 9*(Suppl.), 495S–501S.

Chemotherapy

Baselga, J., Gianni, L., Geyer, C. et al. (2004). Future options with trastuzumab for primary systemic and adjuvant therapy. *Seminars in Oncology, 31*,(5 Suppl. 10), 51–57.

Citron, M. L., Berry, D. A., Cirrincione, C. et al. (2003). Randomized trial of dose-dense versus conventionally scheduled and sequential versus concurrent combination chemotherapy as postoperative adjuvant treatment of node-positive primary breast cancer: First report of intergroup trial C9741/cancer and leukemia group B trial 9741. *Journal of Clinical Oncology, 21*(8), 1431–1439.

*Dibble, S. L., Casey, K., Nussey, B. et al. (2004). Chemotherapy-induced vomiting in women treated for breast cancer. *Oncology Nursing Forum, 31*(1), E1–E8.

Henderson, I. C., Berry, D. A., Demetri, G. D. et al. (2003). Improved outcomes from adding sequential paclitaxel but not from escalating doxorubicin dose in an adjuvant chemotherapy regimen for patients with node-postive primary breast cancer. *Journal of Clinical Oncology, 21*(6), 976–983.

National Institutes of Health. (2000). Adjuvant therapy for breast cancer. *NIH Consensus Statement Online, 17*(4), 1–23. Accessed July 3, 2006.

Vogel, V. G., Costantino, J. P., Wickerham, D. L., et al. (2006). Effects of tamoxifen vs. raloxifene on the risk of developing invasive breast cancer and other disease outcomes. *Journal of the American Medical Association, 295*(5), 2727–2741.

Hormonal Therapy

Baum, M., Buzdar, A., Cuzick, J., et al. (2003). Anastrozole alone or in combination with tamoxifen versus tamoxifen alone for adjuvant treatment of postmenopausal women with early-stage breast cancer: results of the ATAC trial efficacy and safety update analysis. *Cancer, 98*(9), 1802–1810.

Coombes, R. C., Hall, E., Gibson L. J., et al. (2004). A randomized trial of exemestane after two to three years of tamoxifen therapy in postmenopausal women with primary breast cancer. *New England Journal of Medicine, 350*(11), 1081–1092.

Goss, P. E., Ingle, J. N., Martino, S. et al. (2003). A randomized trial of letrozole in postmenopausal women after five years of tamoxifen therapy for early-stage breast cancer. *New England Journal of Medicine, 349*(19), 1793–1802.

Pregnancy and Breast Cancer

Dow, K. H. & Kuhn, D. (2004). Fertility options in young breast cancer survivors: A review of the literature. *Oncology Nursing Forum, 31*, E46–E53.

Middleton, L. P., Amin, M., Gwyn, K. et al. (2003) Breast carcinoma in pregnant women. *Cancer*. 98(5), 1055–1060.

Psychological Aspects of Breast Cancer

Casso, D., Buist, D., & Taplin, S. (2004). Quality of life of 5–10 year breast cancer survivors diagnosed between age 40 and 49. *Health and Quality of Life Outcomes, 2*(1), 25.

Helgeson, V. S. & Tomich, P. L. (2005). Surviving cancer: A comparison of 5-year disease-free breast cancer survivors with healthy women. *Psycho-Oncology, 14*(4), 307–317.

Hoskins, C. N., & Haber, J. (2000). Adjusting to breast cancer. *American Journal of Nursing, 100*(4), 26–32.

*Overcash, J. A. (2004). Using narrative research to understand the quality of life of older women with breast cancer. *Oncology Nursing Forum, 31*(6), 1153–1159.

Radiation

Cuncins-Hearn, A., Saunders, C., Walsh, D. et al. (2004). A systematic review of intraoperative radiotherapy in early breast cancer. *Breast Cancer Research and Treatment, 85*(3), 271–280.

Screening, BSE, and Mammography

Centers for Disease Control and Prevention. (2004). The National Breast and Cervical Cancer Early Detection Program, 2004/2005 Fact Sheet. Available at: http://www.cdc.gov/cancer/nbccedp/about2004.htm. Accessed July 3, 2006.

Kolb, T. M., Lichy, J., & Newhouse, J. H. (2002). Comparison of the performance of screening mammography, physical examination, and breast US and evaluation of factors that influence them: an analysis of 27,825 patient evaluations. *Radiology, 225*(1), 165–175.

Kriege, M., Brekelmans, C. T., Boetes, C. et al. (2004). Efficacy of MRI and mammography for breast-cancer screening in women with a familial or genetic predisposition. *New England Journal of Medicine, 351*(5), 427–437.

Shootman, M. & Jeffe, D. B. (2003). Identifying factors associated with disability-related differences in breast cancer screening (United States). *Cancer Causes and Control, 14*(2), 97–107.

Ward, E., Jemal, A., Cokkinides, V. et al. (2004). Cancer disparities by race/ethnicity and socioeconomic status. *CA: A Cancer Journal for Clinicians, 54*(2), 78–93.

Surgical Treatment of Breast Cancer

*Baron, R. H., Fey, J. V., Borgen, P. I., et al. (2004). Eighteen sensations after breast cancer surgery: A two-year comparison of sentinel lymph node biopsy and axillary lymph node dissection. *Oncology Nursing Forum, 31*(4), 691–698.

Fisher, B., Anderson, S., Bryant, J., et al. (2002). Twenty-year follow-up of a randomized trial comparing total mastectomy, lumpectomy, and lumpectomy plus irradiation for the treatment of invasive breast cancer. *New England Journal of Medicine.* 347(16), 1233–1241.

Golshan, M., Martin, W. J., & Dowlatshahi, K (2003). Sentinel lymph node biopsy lowers the rate of lymphedema when compared with standard axillary lymph node dissection. *American Surgeon, 69*(3), 209–211.

Leidenius, M., Leivonen, M., Vironen, J., et al. (2005). The consequences of long-time arm morbidity in node-negative breast cancer patients with sentinel node biopsy or axillary clearance. *Journal of Surgical Oncology, 92*(1), 23–31.

Naik, A. M., Fey, J, Gemignani, M. et al. (2004). The risk of axillary relapse after sentinel lymph node biopsy for breast cancer is comparable with that of axillary lymph node dissection: a follow-up study of 4008 procedures. *Annals of Surgery, 240*(3). 462–468.

Veronesi, U., Pagnelli, G., Viale, G. et al. (2003). A randomized comparison of sentinel-node biopsy with routine axillary dissection in breast cancer. *New England Journal of Medicine, 349*(6), 546–553.

Wilke, L. G., McCall, L. M., Posther, K. E., et al. (2006). Surgical complications associated with sentinel lymph node biopsy: results from a prospective international cooperative group trial. *Annals of Surgical Oncology, 13*(4), 491–500.

RESOURCES

AGENCIES

American Cancer Society, 1599 Clifton Road, NE, Atlanta, GA 30329-4251; (800) ACS-2345; http://www.cancer.org (extensive professional and patient literature is available, including booklets on reconstruction, radiation, and chemotherapy). Accessed July 3, 2006.

American Cancer Society Breast Health Department, 19 West 56th Street, New York, NY 10019; (212) 586-8700; http://www.cancer.org. Accessed July 3, 2006.

American Society of Plastic and Reconstructive Surgeons, 444 East Algonquin Road, Arlington Heights, IL 60005; (800) 635-0635; http://www.plastic surgery.org. Accessed July 3, 2006.

National Breast Cancer Coalition, 1101 17 Street NW, Suite 1300, Washington, DC 20036; (800) 622-2838; http://www.natlbcc.org. (This activist group has raised funds and consciousness levels regarding breast cancer and was instrumental in obtaining funds for research on prevention.) Accessed July 3, 2006.

National Cancer Institute, Public Inquiry Section, Office of Cancer Communications, National Cancer Institute, Building 31, Room 10 A 24, Bethesda, MD 20892; (800) 422-6237; http://www.cancernet.nci.nih.gov. (Patient materials can be ordered on the following topics: biopsies, treatment options, mastectomy, radiation, chemotherapy, reconstruction, diet, and clinical trials.) Accessed July 3, 2006.

National Lymphedema Network, 1611 Telegraph Avenue, Suite 1111, Oakland, CA 94612; (800) 541-3259; http://lymphnet.org. Accessed July 3, 2006.

Oncology Nursing Society, 125 Enterprise Drive, Pittsburgh, PA 15275; (866) 257-4ONS; http://www.ons.org. Accessed July 3, 2006.

Reach to Recovery Program—I Can Cope Program. (Information available through local American Cancer Society chapters).

Susan G. Komen Breast Cancer Foundation, 5005 LBJ Freeway, Suite 250, Dallas, TX 75244; (800) I'M AWARE (800-462-9273); http://www.komen.org. Accessed July 3, 2006.

Y-ME Breast Cancer Support Program, 212 West Van Buren, Suite 1000, Chicago, IL 60607; (800) 221-2141; http://www.y-me.org. Accessed July 3, 2006.

Young Survival Coalition, 155 6th Avenue, New York, NY 10013; (212) 206-6610; http://www.youngsurvival.org. Accessed July 3, 2006.

WEBSITES

Abramson Cancer Center of the University of Pennsylvania, 3400 Spruce Street-2 Donner, Philadelphia, PA 19101-4283; fax: 215-349-5445 (educational resource for patients with cancer); http:www.oncolink.upenn.edu. Accessed July 3, 2006.

Cancer Care, Inc., 275 Seventh Avenue, New York, NY 10001; 212-712-8400 or 1-800-813-HOPE (4673). Produced by Cancer Care, Inc. Provides telephone services and free teleconference seminars; http://www.cancercare.org. Accessed July 3, 2006.

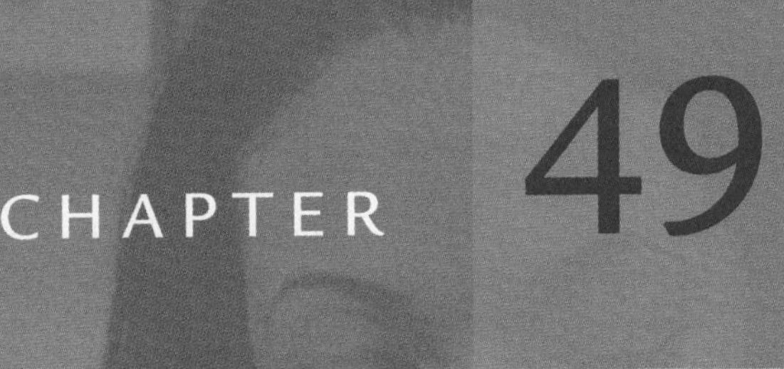

CHAPTER 49

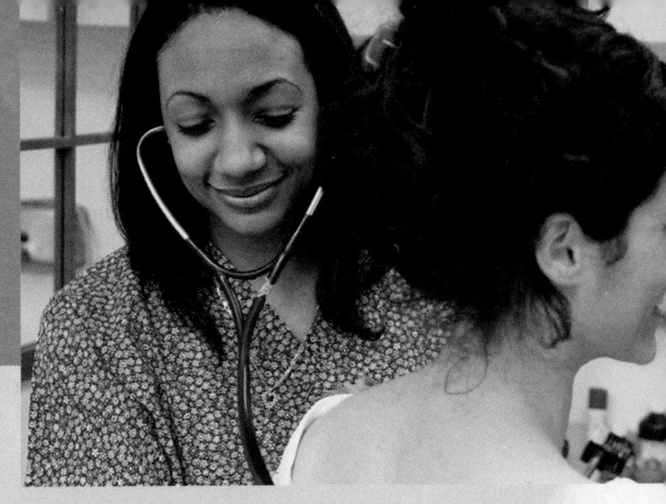

Assessment and Management of Problems Related to Male Reproductive Processes

Learning Objectives

On completion of this chapter, the learner will be able to:

1. Describe structures and function of the male reproductive system.
2. Discuss nursing assessment of the male reproductive system and identify diagnostic tests that complement assessment.
3. Discuss the causes and management of male sexual dysfunction.
4. Compare the types of prostatectomy with regard to advantages and disadvantages.
5. Use the nursing process as a framework for care of the patient undergoing prostatectomy.
6. Describe the nursing management of patients with testicular cancer.
7. Describe the various conditions affecting the penis, including pathophysiology, clinical manifestations, and management.

Disorders of the male reproductive system include a wide variety of conditions that usually affect both urinary and reproductive systems. Because these disorders focus on the genitalia, and in some instances on sexuality, the patient may experience anxiety and embarrassment. The nurse must recognize the patient's need for privacy as well as his need for education. This requires an openness to discuss critical and sensitive issues with the patient as well as effective assessment, management, and communication on the part of the nurse.

Anatomic and Physiologic Overview

In the male, several organs serve as parts of both the urinary tract and the reproductive system. Disorders in the male reproductive organs may interfere with the functions of one or both of these systems. As a result, diseases of the male reproductive system are usually treated by a urologist. The structures in the male reproductive system include the

Glossary

benign prostatic hyperplasia (BPH): noncancerous enlargement or hypertrophy of the prostate. BPH is the most common pathologic condition in older men and the second most common cause of surgical intervention in men older than 60 years of age.

Bowen's disease: form of squamous cell carcinoma in situ of the penile shaft

circumcision: excision of the foreskin, or prepuce, of the glans penis

cryosurgery of the prostate: localized treatment of the prostate by application of freezing temperatures

cryptorchidism: most common congenital defect, characterized by failure of one or both of the testes to descend into the scrotum

epididymitis: infection of the epididymis that usually descends from an infected prostate or urinary tract; also may develop as a complication of gonorrhea

erectile dysfunction: also called impotence; the inability to either achieve or maintain an erection sufficient to accomplish sexual intercourse

hydrocele: a collection of fluid, generally in the tunica vaginalis of the testis, although it also may collect within the spermatic cord

nocturia: urination during the night

orchiectomy: surgical removal of one or both of the testes

orchitis: inflammation of the testes (testicular congestion) caused by pyogenic, viral, spirochetal, parasitic, traumatic, chemical, or unknown factors

penile cancer: represents about 0.5% of malignancies in men in the United States; can involve the glans, the body of the penis, the urethra, and regional or distant lymph nodes

penis: male organ for copulation and urination; consists of glans penis, body, and root

Peyronie's disease: buildup of fibrous plaques in the sheath of the corpus cavernosum, causing curvature of the penis when it is erect

phimosis: condition in which the foreskin is constricted so that it cannot be retracted over the glans; can occur congenitally or from inflammation and edema

priapism: an uncontrolled, persistent erection of the penis from either neural or vascular causes, including medications, sickle cell thrombosis, leukemic cell infiltration, spinal cord tumors, and tumor invasion of the penis or its vessels

prostate cancer: the most common cancer in men; risk factors include increasing age, African American race, and possibly a high-fat diet; the genetic association of prostate cancer and the increased incidence within certain families are being investigated

prostate gland: gland that lies just below the neck of the bladder, surrounds the urethra, and is traversed by the ejaculatory duct, a continuation of the vas deferens; produces a secretion that is chemically and physiologically suitable to the needs of the spermatozoa in their passage from the testes

prostate-specific antigen (PSA): substance that is produced by the prostate gland and measured in a blood specimen; PSA levels are increased with prostate cancer; the PSA test is used in combination with digital rectal examination to detect prostate cancer

prostatism: obstructive and irritative symptom complex that includes increased frequency and hesitancy in starting urination, a decrease in the volume and force of the urinary stream, acute urinary retention, and recurrent urinary tract infections

prostatitis: inflammation of the prostate gland caused by infectious agents (bacteria, fungi, mycoplasma) or various other problems (eg, urethral stricture, prostatic hyperplasia)

spermatogenesis: production of sperm in the testes

testes: the ovoid sex glands encased in the scrotum; the testes produce sperm

testicular cancer: the most common cancer in men 15 to 35 years of age and the second most common malignancy in those 35 to 39 years of age; its cause is unknown

testosterone: male sex hormone secreted by the testes; induces and preserves the male sex characteristics

transurethral resection of the prostate (TUR or TURP): resection of the prostate through endoscopy; the surgical and optical instrument is introduced directly through the urethra to the prostate, and the gland is then removed in small chips with an electrical cutting loop

varicocele: an abnormal dilation of the veins of the pampiniform venous plexus in the scrotum (the network of veins from the testis and the epididymis, which constitute part of the spermatic cord)

vasectomy: also called male sterilization; ligation and transection of part of the vas deferens, with or without removal of a segment of the vas to prevent the passage of the sperm from the testes

testes, the vas deferens (ductus deferens) and seminal vesicles, the penis, and certain accessory glands, such as the prostate gland and Cowper's gland (bulbourethral gland) (Fig. 49-1).

The **testes** have a dual function: **spermatogenesis** (production of sperm) and secretion of the male sex hormone **testosterone**, which induces and preserves the male sex characteristics. The testes are formed in the embryo, within the abdominal cavity, near the kidney. During the last month of fetal life, they descend posterior to the peritoneum and pierce the abdominal wall in the groin. Later, they progress along the inguinal canal into the scrotum. In this descent, they are accompanied by blood vessels, lymphatics, nerves, and ducts, which support the tissue and make up the spermatic cord. This cord extends from the internal inguinal ring through the abdominal wall and the inguinal canal to the scrotum. As the testes descend into the scrotum, a tubular extension of peritoneum accompanies them. Normally, this tissue is obliterated during fetal development; the only remaining portion is that which covers the testes, the tunica vaginalis. (If this peritoneal process is not obliterated but remains open into the abdominal cavity, a potential sac remains into which abdominal contents may enter to form an indirect inguinal hernia.)

The testes are encased in the scrotum, which keeps them at a slightly lower temperature than the rest of the body to facilitate spermatogenesis. The testes consist of numerous seminiferous tubules in which the spermatozoa form. Collecting tubules transmit the spermatozoa into the epididymis, a hoodlike structure lying on the testes and containing winding ducts that lead into the vas deferens. This firm, tubular structure passes upward through the inguinal canal to enter the abdominal cavity behind the peritoneum. It then extends downward toward the base of the bladder. An outpouching from this structure is the seminal vesicle, which acts as a reservoir for testicular secretions. The tract is continued as the ejaculatory duct, which passes through the prostate gland to enter the urethra. Testicular secretions take this pathway when they exit the penis during ejaculation.

The **penis** has a dual function: it is the organ for copulation and for urination. Anatomically, it consists of the glans penis, the body, and the root. The glans penis is the soft, rounded portion at the distal end of the penis. The urethra, the tube that carries urine, opens at the tip of the glans. The glans is naturally covered or protected by elongated penile skin—the foreskin—which may be retracted to expose the glans. However, many men have had the foreskin removed (circumcision) as newborns. The body of the penis is composed of erectile tissues containing numerous blood vessels that become distended, leading to an erection during sexual excitement. The urethra, which passes through the penis, extends from the bladder through the prostate to the distal end of the penis.

The **prostate gland** lies just below the neck of the bladder. It surrounds the urethra and is traversed by the ejaculatory duct, a continuation of the vas deferens. This gland produces a secretion that is chemically and physiologically suitable to the needs of the spermatozoa in their passage from the testes. Cowper's gland lies below the prostate, within the posterior aspect of the urethra. This gland empties its secretions into the urethra during ejaculation, providing lubrication.

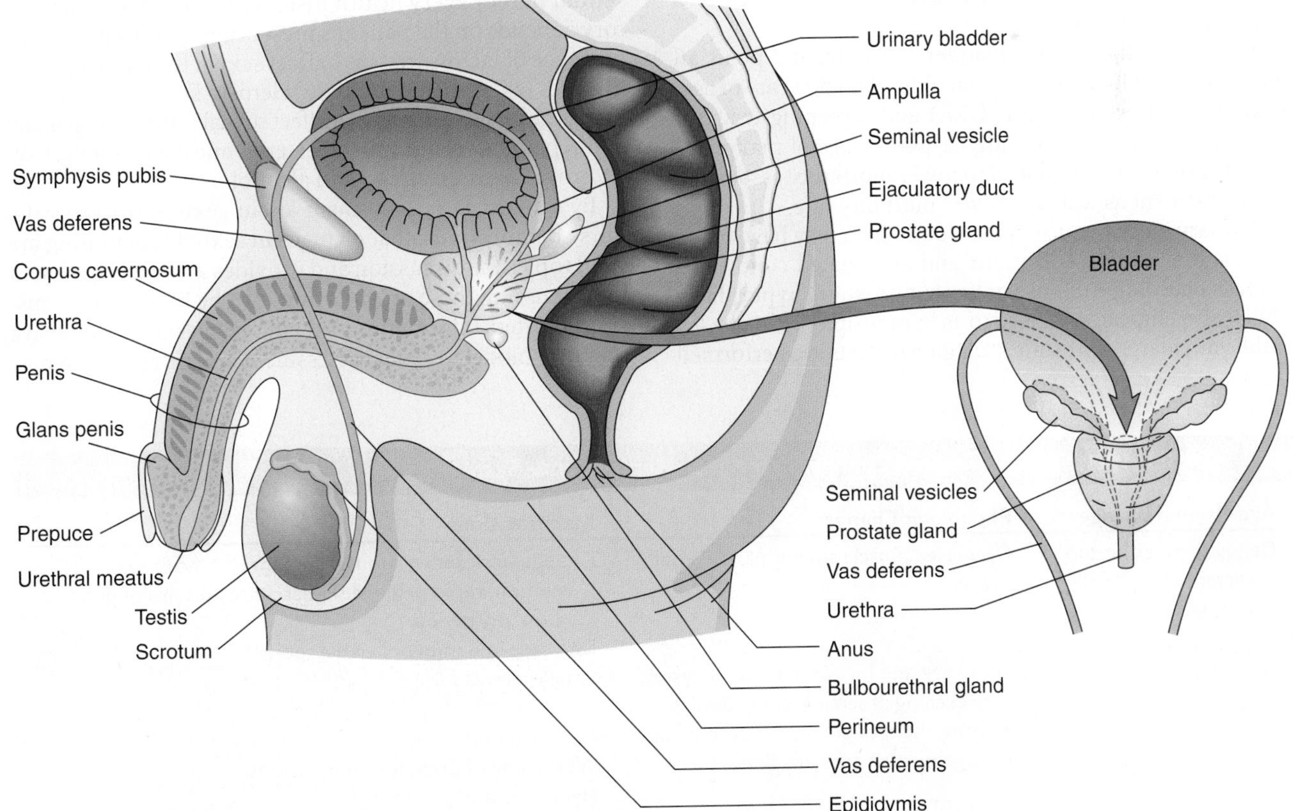

FIGURE 49-1. Structures of the male reproductive system.

Gerontologic Considerations

As men age, the prostate gland enlarges, prostate secretion decreases, the scrotum hangs lower, the testes become smaller and more firm, and pubic hair becomes sparser and stiffer. Changes in gonadal function include a decline in plasma testosterone levels and reduced production of progesterone (Table 49-1). Other changes include decreasing sexual function, slower sexual responses, an increased incidence of genitourinary tract cancer, and urinary incontinence.

Male reproductive capability is maintained with advancing age. Although degenerative changes occur in the seminiferous tubules, spermatogenesis continues. However, libido (sexual desire) and potency decrease (Araujo, Mohr, & McKinlay, 2004). Vascular problems cause about half of the cases of impotence in men older than 50 years of age (Shabsigh & Anastasiadis, 2003).

Hypogonadism occurs in up to one fourth of older men. The relationship of hypogonadism to impotence is uncertain. This decline is more evident in men older than 60 years of age (Foresta, Caretta, Garolla, et al., 2003). In older men, the sexual response slows. Erection takes longer, and full erections may not be attained until orgasm. Sexual function is affected by several factors, such as psychological problems, illnesses, and medications. In general, the entire sexual act takes longer. In older men, ejaculatory control increases; however, if the erection is partially lost, there may be difficulty in attaining a full erection again, and resolution may occur without orgasm. Sexual activity is closely correlated with the man's sexual activity in his earlier years; if he was more active than average as a young man, he will most likely continue to be more active than average in his later years (Jones, 2003).

Cancers of the kidney, bladder, prostate, and penis all have increased incidence in men older than 50 years of age. Digital rectal examination (DRE) and screening tests for hematuria may uncover a higher percentage of malignancies at earlier stages and lead to lower morbidity associated with treatment as well as a lower mortality rate.

Urinary incontinence in the elderly man may have many causes, including medications and age-related conditions such as neurologic disease or **benign prostatic hyperplasia** (BPH; also clinically referred to as hypertrophy or by the lay public as enlarged prostate). Diagnostic tests are performed to exclude reversible causes of urinary incontinence. For some patients with severe incontinence, augmentation cystoplasty (repair of the bladder) with placement of an artificial urinary sphincter may help alleviate this problem.

Assessment

Health History and Clinical Manifestations

Male sexuality is a complex phenomenon that is strongly influenced by personal, cultural, and social factors. Sexuality and male reproductive function become concerns in the presence of illness (Kelly, 2004). The nurse is challenged to bridge the gap between theoretical views about male sexuality and its importance to human beings. Assessment of male reproductive function begins with an evaluation of urinary function and symptoms. This assessment also includes a focus on sexual function as well as manifestations of sexual dysfunction. The patient is asked about his usual state of health and any recent change in general physical and sexual activity. Any symptoms or changes in function are explored fully and described in detail. These symptoms, collectively referred to as prostatism, may include those associated with an obstruction caused by an enlarged prostate gland: increased urinary frequency, decreased force of urine stream, "double" or "triple" voiding (the patient needs to urinate two or three times over a period of several minutes to completely empty his bladder). The patient is also assessed for **dysuria**, **hematuria**, and hematospermia (blood in the ejaculate).

Assessment of sexual function and dysfunction is an essential part of every health history. The extent of the history depends on the patient's presenting symptoms and the presence of factors that may affect sexual function: chronic illnesses (eg, diabetes, multiple sclerosis, stroke, cardiac disease), use of medications that affect sexual function (eg, many antihypertensive and anticholesterolemic medications, psychotropic agents), stress, and alcohol use.

By initiating an assessment about sexual concerns, the nurse demonstrates that changes in sexual functioning are valid topics for discussion and provides a safe environment for discussing these sensitive topics. The PLISSIT (*p*ermission, *l*imited *i*nformation, *s*pecific *s*uggestions, *i*ntensive *t*herapy) model of sexual assessment and intervention may

TABLE 49-1 Age-Related Changes in the Male Reproductive System

Age-Related Changes	Physiologic Changes	Manifestations
Decrease in sex hormone secretion, especially testosterone	Decreased muscle strength and sexual energy	Changes in sexual response: prolonged time to reach full erection, rapid penile detumescence and prolonged refractory period Decrease in number of viable sperm
	Shrinkage and loss of firmness of testes; thickening of seminiferous tubules	Smaller testes
	Fibrotic changes of corpora cavernosa	Erectile dysfunction
	Enlargement of prostate gland	Weakening of prostatic contractions Hyperplasia of prostate gland Signs and symptoms of obstruction of lower urinary tract (urgency, frequency, nocturia)

NURSING RESEARCH PROFILE

Older Men's Perceptions of Health Care Needs

Loeb, S. J. (2004). Older men's health: Motivation, self-ratings, and behaviors. *Nursing Research, 53*(3), 198–206.

Purpose

Because elderly men participate in fewer health screenings, experience poorer health, have shorter life expectancies, and delay longer in seeking health care than women, data about the health and well-being of older men are limited. Older men are often ignored by researchers because of the misperception that they experience a better quality of life than older women do. The purpose of this study was to examine the relationships among health motivation, self-rated health status, and health behaviors in community-residing older men.

Design

A convenience sample of 135 men who were 55 years of age and older participated in this descriptive, correlational study. They completed several questionnaires, including a demographic data tool, the Older Men's Health Promotion and Screening Inventory, the Health-Promotion Activities of Older Adults Measure, and the Health Determinism Index. Sites of data collection, both rural and urban, included senior centers, exercise classes, safe driving classes, and a fast food restaurant.

Findings

Men who participated in the study ranged from 55 to 91 years of age, and the majority (78.5%) were Caucasian. Data analysis revealed that men with greater intrinsic motivation rated their health as better ($p \leq .001$) and assessed their lifestyles as healthier ($p \leq .001$) than those who were extrinsically motivated. Health motivation was not related significantly to participation in health-promoting activities, health screenings, or health promotion programs. Men who participated in health-promoting activities attended more health promotion programs. Men who believed that they would benefit more from health promotion behaviors participated in more health screenings than those who did not anticipate much benefit. Men from urban areas anticipated significantly more benefits from health promotion activities and participated in a greater number of health screenings than those from rural areas.

Nursing Implications

The nurse has a valuable role in promoting healthy behaviors among all groups of people, including elderly men. Education programs are key strategies to enhance awareness of health needs in older men and to develop positive perceptions of the potential benefits of health-promoting activities and behaviors. When developing and implementing health education strategies designed to target health promotion in elderly men, it is necessary to consider differences in perceptions of men about benefits of health-promoting activities.

be used to provide a framework for nursing interventions (Annon, 1976). It is designed to provide a graded counseling approach that allows health care professionals to deal with sexual issues with a level of comfort and expertise (McInnes, 2003). The model begins by asking the patient's permission (P) to discuss sexual functioning. Limited information (LI) about sexual function may then be provided to the patient. As the discussion progresses, the nurse may offer specific suggestions (SS) for interventions. A professional who specializes in sex therapy may provide more intensive therapy (IT) as needed.

Patients may find it difficult to express their feelings and concerns regarding their sexuality, especially after a body image change. Discussing sexuality with patients who have an illness or disability can be uncomfortable for nurses and other health care providers; this, in turn, makes discussion of these issues more difficult and uncomfortable for patients. Health care professionals may unconsciously have stereotypes about the sexuality of people who are ill or have a disability (eg, the belief that people with disabilities are asexual or should be sexually inactive). In addition, patients are often embarrassed to initiate a discussion about sexual issues with their health care providers (Black, 2004).

Physical Assessment

In addition to the customary aspects of the physical examination, two essential components address disorders of the male genital or reproductive system: the digital rectal exam (DRE) and the testicular examination.

Digital Rectal Examination

The DRE is recommended as part of the regular health checkup for every man older than 40 years of age; it is invaluable in screening for cancer of the prostate gland. The DRE enables the examiner to assess the size, shape, and consistency of the prostate gland (Fig. 49-2). Tenderness of the prostate gland on palpation and the presence and consistency of any nodules are noted. Although this examination may be embarrassing for the patient, it is an important screening tool.

Testicular Examination

The male genitalia are inspected for abnormalities and palpated for masses. The scrotum is palpated carefully for nodules, masses, or inflammation. Examination of the scrotum can reveal such disorders as **hydrocele**, hernia, or tumor

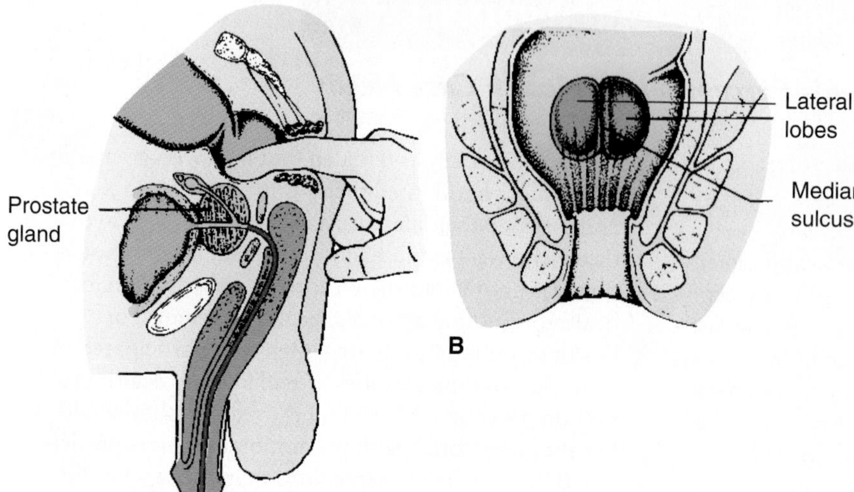

FIGURE 49-2. (**A**) Palpation of the prostate gland during digital rectal examination (DRE) enables the examiner to assess the size, shape, and texture of the gland. (**B**) The prostate is round, with a palpable median sulcus or groove separating the two lobes. It should feel rubbery and free of nodules and masses.

of the testis. The penis is inspected and palpated for ulcerations, nodules, inflammation, and discharge. The testicular examination provides an excellent opportunity to instruct the patient about techniques for testicular self-examination (TSE) and its importance in early detection of testicular cancer (see later discussion). TSE should begin during adolescence.

Diagnostic Evaluation

Prostate-Specific Antigen Test

The prostate gland produces a substance known as **prostate-specific antigen (PSA).** It can be measured in a blood specimen, and levels increase with prostate cancer. A number of other conditions (eg, BPH, transurethral resection of the prostate, acute urinary retention, acute prostatitis) can cause an elevated PSA level in the absence of prostate cancer. PSA levels are measured in nanograms per milliliter (ng/mL). In most laboratories, the range of values generally considered normal is 0.2 to 4.0 ng/mL. Values greater than 4.0 are considered elevated. The use of age-specific reference ranges for populations with a low incidence of prostate cancers (eg, Chinese) helps minimize unnecessary biopsies (Wu & Huang, 2004).

Prostate cancer screening with serum PSA testing has become common practice (Antenor, Han, Roehl, et al., 2004). An annual PSA test, along with DRE, is recommended by the American Cancer Society (ACS) (2005) for men at high risk, including those with a family history of prostate cancer and African American men. PSA is also useful to monitor patients for recurrence after treatment for cancer of the prostate, based on evidence-based algorithms (Liao & Datta, 2004).

Ultrasonography

Transrectal ultrasound (TRUS) may be performed in patients with abnormalities detected by DRE and in those with elevated PSA levels. After DRE has been completed, a lubricated, condom-covered, rectal probe transducer is inserted into the rectum, along the anterior wall. Water may be introduced into the condom to help transmit sound waves to the prostate. TRUS may be used in detecting nonpalpable prostate cancers and in staging localized prostate cancer. Needle biopsies of the prostate are commonly guided by TRUS.

Prostate Fluid or Tissue Analysis

Specimens of prostate fluid or tissue may be obtained for culture if disease or inflammation of the prostate gland is suspected. A biopsy of the prostate gland may be necessary to obtain tissue for histologic examination. This may be performed at the time of prostatectomy or by means of a perineal or transrectal needle biopsy.

Tests of Male Sexual Function

If the patient cannot engage in sexual intercourse to his satisfaction, a detailed history is obtained. Nocturnal penile tumescence tests may be conducted in a sleep laboratory to monitor changes in penile circumference during sleep (using a mercury strain gauge placed around the penis); the results help identify the cause of erectile dysfunction. Additional tests, including psychological evaluations, are also part of the diagnostic workup and are usually conducted by a specialized team of health care providers.

Disorders of Male Sexual Function

Erectile Dysfunction

Erectile dysfunction, also called impotence, is the inability to achieve or maintain an erection sufficient to accomplish intercourse. The man may report decreased frequency of erections, inability to achieve a firm erection, or rapid detumescence (subsiding of erection). Incidence ranges from 25% to 50% in men older than 65 years of age. The physiology of erection and ejaculation is complex and involves sympathetic and parasympathetic components. Erection involves the release of nitric oxide into the corpus cavernosum during sexual stimulation. Its release in turn activates cyclic guanosine monophosphate (cGMP), causing smooth muscle relaxation. This allows flow of blood into the corpus cavernosum, resulting in erection (Porth, 2005).

Erectile dysfunction has both psychogenic and organic causes. Psychogenic causes include anxiety, fatigue, depression, and pressure to perform sexually. However, organic impotence may account for more impotence than has been previously realized. Organic causes include occlusive vascular disease, endocrine disease (diabetes, pituitary tumors, hypogonadism with testosterone deficiency, hyperthyroidism, and hypothyroidism), cirrhosis, chronic renal failure, genitourinary conditions (radical pelvic surgery), hematologic conditions (Hodgkin disease, leukemia), neurologic disorders (neuropathies, parkinsonism, spinal cord injury, multiple sclerosis), trauma to the pelvic or genital area, alcohol, medications (Chart 49-1), and drug abuse.

Assessment and Diagnostic Findings

The diagnosis of erectile dysfunction requires a sexual and medical history; an analysis of presenting symptoms; a physical examination, including a neurologic examination; a detailed assessment of all medications, alcohol, and drugs used; and various laboratory studies. Nocturnal penile tumescence tests are conducted in sleep laboratories to monitor changes in penile circumference. The nocturnal penile tumescence test can help to determine whether erectile impotence has an organic or a psychological cause. In healthy men, nocturnal penile erections closely parallel rapid eye movement (REM) sleep in occurrence and duration. Organically impotent men show inadequate sleep-related erections that correspond to their waking performance. Arterial blood flow to the penis is measured using a Doppler probe. In addition, nerve conduction tests and extensive psychological evaluations are carried out. Figure 49-3 describes the evaluation and treatment of erectile dysfunction.

CHART 49-1

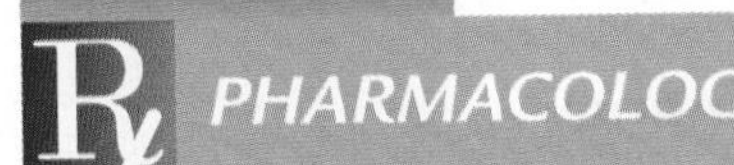

PHARMACOLOGY

Classes of Medications Associated With Erectile Dysfunction

- Antiadrenergics and antihypertensives: guanethidine (Ismelin), clonidine (Catapres), hydralazine (Apresoline), metoprolol (Lopressor)
- Anticholinergics and phenothiazines: prochlorperazine (Compazine), trihexyphenidyl (Artane)
- Anti-seizure agents: carbamazepine (Tegretol)
- Antifungals: ketoconazole (Nizoral)
- Antihormone (prostate cancer treatment): flutamide (Eulexin), leuprolide (Lupron)
- Antipsychotics: haloperidol (Haldol), chlorpromazine (Thorazine)
- Antispasmodics: oxybutynin (Ditropan)
- Anxiolytics, sedative-hypnotics, tranquilizers: lorazepam (Ativan), triazolam (Halcion)
- Beta-blockers: nadolol (Corgard)
- Calcium channel blockers: nifedipine (Adalat, Procardia)
- Carbonic anhydrase inhibitors: acetazolamide (Diamox)
- H_2 antagonists: nizatidine (Axid)
- Nonsteroidal anti-inflammatory drugs: naproxen (Naprosyn)
- Thiazide diuretics: hydrochlorothiazide (HydroDIURIL)
- Tricyclic antidepressants: amitriptyline (Elavil), desipramine (Norpramin)

Medical Management

Treatment can be medical, surgical, or both, depending on the cause (Table 49-2). Nonsurgical therapy includes treating associated conditions, such as alcoholism, and readjusting antihypertensive agents or other medications. Endocrine therapy may be instituted for erectile dysfunction secondary to hypothalamic-pituitary-gonadal dysfunction and may reverse the condition. Insufficient penile blood flow may be treated with vascular surgery. Patients with erectile dysfunction from psychogenic causes are referred to a health care provider or therapist who specializes in sexual dysfunction. Patients with erectile dysfunction secondary to organic causes may be candidates for penile implants.

Pharmacologic Therapy

Phosphodiesterase-5 (PDE-5) inhibitors are oral medications that are used to treat erectile dysfunction. Sildenafil (Viagra), the first of these agents, was introduced in 1998 in the United States. Other PDE-5 inhibitors include vardenafil (Levitra) and tadalafil (Cialis). PDE-5 is an enzyme found in trabecular smooth muscle that inactivates cGMP, the nucleotide that causes the cavernosal relaxation necessary for erection to occur. By blocking the inhibition of PDE-5, these pharmacologic agents facilitate corporeal smooth muscle relaxation in response to sexual stimulation (Porth, 2005).

When these PDE-5 inhibitors are taken about 1 hour before sexual activity, they are effective in producing an erection with stimulation; the erection can last about 60 to 120 minutes (Fazio & Brock, 2004). These medications have side effects, including headache, flushing, and dyspepsia. PDE-5 inhibitors are contraindicated in men who take organic nitrates, because together these drugs can cause side effects such as severe hypotension (Porth, 2005). PDE-5 inhibitors should be used with caution in patients with retinopathy, especially in those with diabetic retinopathy. Patient teaching related to the use of these medications is summarized in Chart 49-2.

Other pharmacologic measures to induce erections include injecting vasoactive agents, such as alprostadil, papaverine, and phentolamine, directly into the penis. Complications include **priapism** (a persistent abnormal erection) and development of fibrotic plaques at the injection sites. Alprostadil is also formulated in a gel pellet that can be inserted into the urethra to create an erection.

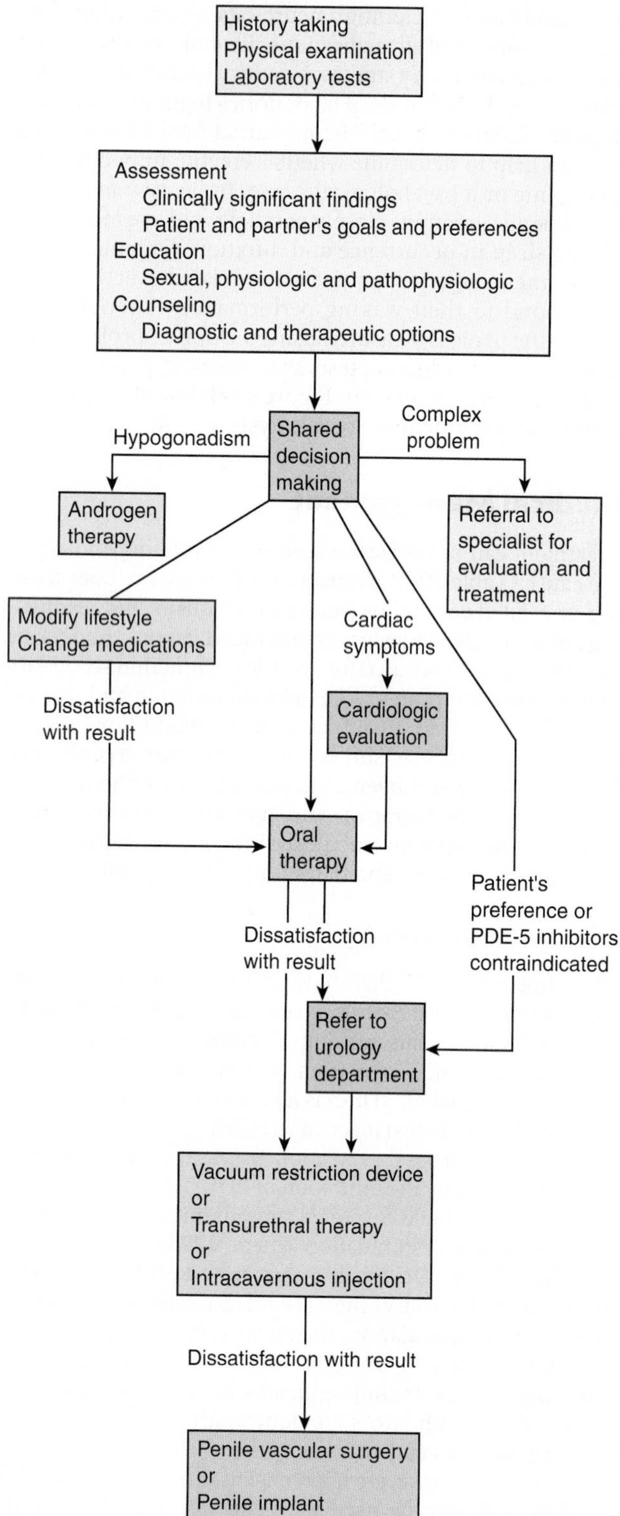

FIGURE 49-3. Evaluation and treatment of men with erectile dysfunction. From Lue, T. F. (2000). Erectile dysfunction. *New England Journal of Medicine, 342*(24), 1807. © 2000 Massachusetts Medical Society. All rights reserved. Used with permission.

Penile Implants

Penile implants are available in two types: the semirigid rod and the inflatable prosthesis. The semirigid rod (eg, the Small-Carrion prosthesis) results in a permanent semi-erection. The inflatable prosthesis simulates natural erections and natural flaccidity. Complications after implantation include infection, erosion of the prosthesis through the skin (more common with the semirigid rod than with the inflatable prosthesis), and persistent pain, which may require removal of the implant. Subsequent cystoscopic surgery, such as **transurethral resection of the prostate** (**TUR** or **TURP**), is more difficult with a semirigid rod than with the inflatable prosthesis. Factors to consider in choosing a prosthesis are the patient's activities of daily living and social activities and the expectations of the patient and his partner. Ongoing counseling for the patient and his partner is usually necessary to help them adapt to the prosthesis.

Negative-Pressure Devices

Negative-pressure (vacuum) devices may also be used to induce an erection. A plastic cylinder is placed over the flaccid penis, and negative pressure is applied. When an erection is attained, a constriction band is placed around the base of the penis to maintain the erection. Although many men find this method satisfactory, others experience premature loss of penile rigidity or pain when applying suction or during intercourse.

Nursing Management

Personal satisfaction and the ability to sexually satisfy a partner are common concerns of patients. Men with illnesses and disabilities may need the assistance of a sex therapist to find, implement, and integrate their sexual beliefs and behaviors into a healthy and satisfying lifestyle. The nurse can inform patients about support groups for men with erectile dysfunction and their partners. Information about Impotence Anonymous for patients and I-Anon for their partners can be found at the end of this chapter.

Disorders of Ejaculation

Premature ejaculation occurs when a man cannot control the ejaculatory reflex and, once aroused, reaches orgasm before or shortly after intromission. It is the most common type of ejaculatory dysfunction in men. Inhibited or retarded ejaculation is the involuntary inhibition of the ejaculatory reflex. The spectrum of responses ranges from occasional ejaculation through intercourse or self-stimulation to complete inability to ejaculate under any circumstances. Retrograde ejaculation occurs when semen travels toward the bladder instead of exiting the body.

Treatment modalities depend on the nature and severity of the ejaculation problem. Behavioral therapies may be indicated for treatment of premature ejaculation; these therapies often involve both the man and his sexual partner. "Homework" assignments are often given to the couple to encourage them to identify their sexual needs and to

(text continues on page 1750)

TABLE 49-2 Treatments for Erectile Dysfunction

Method	Description	Advantages and Disadvantages	Duration
Pharmacologic therapy • Oral medication (sildenafil [Viagra]; vardenafil [Levitra]; tadalafil [Cialis]) 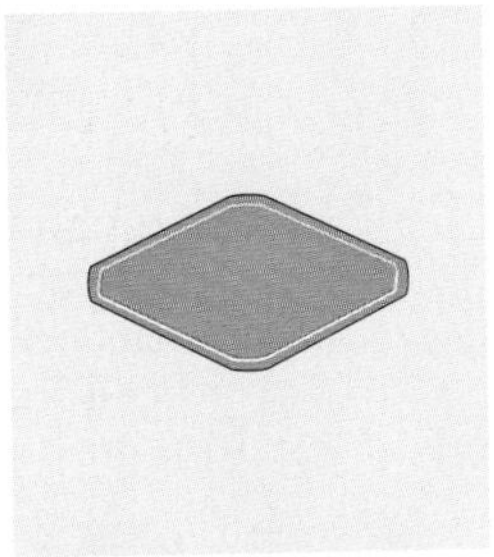 Oral medication	Smooth muscle relaxant causing blood to flow into penis	Can cause headache and diarrhea Contraindicated for men taking nitrate medications Used with caution in patients with retinopathy, especially diabetic retinopathy	Taken orally 1 hour before intercourse Stimulation is required to achieve erection Erection can last 1 hour
• Injection (alprostadil, papaverine, phentolamine) 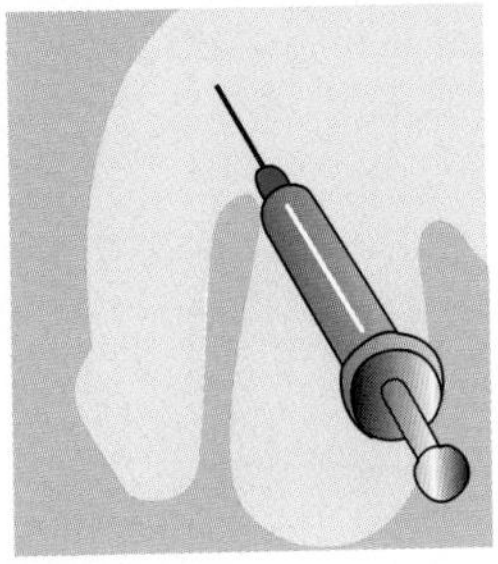 Penile injection	Smooth muscle relaxant causing blood to flow into penis	Firm erections are achievable in more than 50% of cases Pain at injection site; plaque formation, risk of priapism	Injection 20 minutes before intercourse Erection can last up to 1 hour
• Urethral suppository (alprostadil) 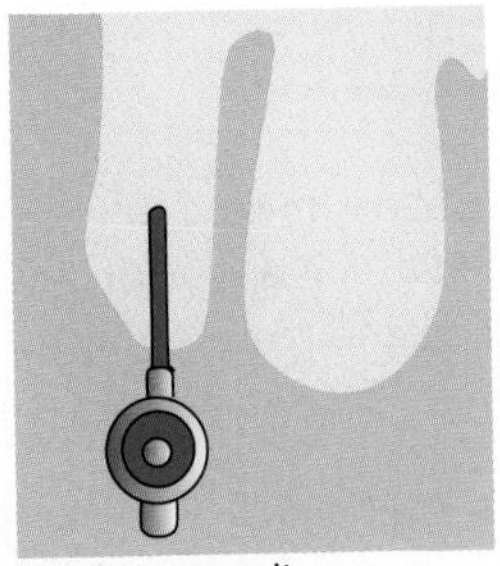 Penile suppository	Smooth muscle relaxant causing blood to flow into penis	May be used twice a day Not recommended with pregnant partners	Inserted 10 minutes before intercourse Erection can last up to 1 hour

continued >

TABLE 49-2 Treatments for Erectile Dysfunction (Continued)

Method	Description	Advantages and Disadvantages	Duration
Penile implants • Semirigid rod • Inflatable Penile implant	Surgically implanted into corpus cavernosum	Reliable Requires surgery Healing takes up to 3 weeks Subsequent cystoscopic surgery is difficult Semirigid rod results in permanent semierection	Indefinite Inflatable prosthesis: saline returns from penile receptacle to reservoir
Negative-pressure (vacuum) devices Penile vacuum pump	Induction of erection with vacuum; maintained with constriction band around base of penis	Few side effects Cumbersome to use before intercourse Vasocongestion of penis can cause pain or numbness	To prevent penile injury, constriction band must not be left in place for longer than 1 hour

CHART 49-2

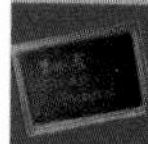

Patient Education

The medications sildenafil (Viagra), vardenafil (Levitra), and tadalafil (Cialis) have been approved for the treatment of erectile dysfunction. These agents are known as phosphodiesterase-5 (PDE-5) inhibitors. PDE-5 is a type of enzyme found almost exclusively in the penis. The PDE-5 inhibitors slow the release of nitric oxide and temporarily restore the body's natural sexual response by increasing the capability of blood flow to the penis. They work only when a man is sexually stimulated.

Pharmacologic Treatment of Erectile Dysfunction

	SILDENAFIL (VIAGRA)	VARDENAFIL (LEVITRA)	TADALAFIL (CIALIS)
Recommended dose	Initial dose is 25 mg. Usual dose is 50 mg. Maximal dose is 100 mg/24 hours.	Usual dose is 10 mg. Maximum dose is 20 mg/24 hours. If you are 65 years of age or older, the starting dose is 5 mg.	Dosage range is 5–20 mg, based on individual response. Maximum dose is 20 mg/24 hours. For patients with decreased liver or kidney function, the maximum dose is 10 mg every 48 hours.

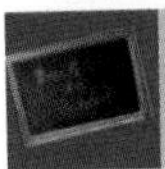

CHART 49-2 ***Patient Education, continued***

Pharmacologic Treatment of Erectile Dysfunction

	SILDENAFIL (VIAGRA)	VARDENAFIL (LEVITRA)	TADALAFIL (CIALIS)
When to take	Take the medication 30 minutes to 4 hours before intercourse. *There must be sexual stimulation to produce an erection.* If you fall asleep or need to go out in public, you will have no erection if there is no stimulation.	Follow the same directions as with sildenafil; take the medication 1 hour before intercourse. The peak action occurs in 30 to 120 minutes. *There must be sexual stimulation to produce an erection.* If you fall asleep or need to go out in public, you will have no erection if there is no stimulation.	Take the medication before sexual activity. Effect peaks at 30 minutes to 6 hours; effect may last up to 36 hours. *There must be sexual stimulation to produce an erection.*
Frequency of use	If you take this medication more than once a day, it will not have an increased effect. You may take it 7 days per week if you wish, but only once in 24 hours. It does not build up in your bloodstream. Remember to take it only when you want to have intercourse.	The recommended frequency for this medication is 10 mg in 24 hours.	The effects of this medication may last up to 36 hours. This allows for increased spontaneity in the sexual experience.
Side effects	Side effects include headache, flushing, indigestion, nasal congestion, abnormal vision, diarrhea, dizziness, and rash. You may also have low blood sugar and abnormal liver function tests; your physician can determine this.	Side effects include headache, flushing, runny nose, indigestion, sinusitis, flulike syndrome, dizziness, nausea, back pain, and joint pain. Tell your physician if you experience any of these effects. You may also have abnormally elevated liver enzymes; your physician can determine this.	Side effects are similar to those of sildenafil and vardenafil. Tadalafil may also cause back pain and muscle aches. Tell your physician if you experience any of these side effects.
Contraindications	Do not take if you are taking nitrate medications such as nitroglycerine (eg, Nitrobid) or isosorbide mononitrate (eg, Imdur). Do not take if you have high uncontrolled blood pressure, coronary artery disease, or have had a heart attack within the past 6 months. Do not take if you have been diagnosed with a cardiac dysrhythmia or kidney or liver dysfunction.		
Drug interactions	This medication can react with other medications that you may be taking. Provide your physician and pharmacist with a complete list of all prescribed as well as over-the-counter medications that you are using.		
Use of PDE-5 inhibitors with penile injections or urethral suppositories	The use of PDE-5 inhibitors with other forms of therapy for erectile dysfunction has not been tested and should be avoided.		

communicate those needs to each other. In some cases, pharmacologic and behavioral therapy together may be effective.

Neurologic disorders (eg, spinal cord injury, multiple sclerosis, neuropathy secondary to diabetes), surgery (prostatectomy), and medications are the most common causes of inhibited ejaculation. Chemical, vibratory, and electrical methods of stimulation have been used with some success. Treatment is usually multidisciplinary and addresses the physical and psychological factors that are often involved in inhibited ejaculation (Jones, 2003).

For men with retrograde ejaculation, the urine may be collected after ejaculation; sperm are then collected from the urine for use in artificial insemination (Aust & Lewis-Jones, 2004). In men with spinal cord injury, electroejaculation may be used to obtain sperm for artificial insemination (Giulini, Pesce, Madgar, et al., 2004). This procedure is performed with the use of an electroejaculator, which has a specially designed probe that is inserted into the rectum next to the prostate. The device generates a current that stimulates the nerves and produces contraction of the pelvic muscles, resulting in what is known as mechanical ejaculation (Shieh, Chen, Wang, et al., 2003).

The effects of trauma, chronic illness, and physical disability on sexual function can be profound. In addition to psychogenic factors, the physical changes associated with illness and injury can impair sexual function, resulting in disorders of ejaculation.

Infections of the Male Genitourinary Tract

Acute uncomplicated cystitis in adult men is uncommon but occasionally occurs in men whose sexual partners have vaginal infections with *Escherichia coli*. Asymptomatic bacteriuria may also result from genitourinary manipulation, catheterization, or instrumentation. Urinary tract infections in the male are discussed in Chapter 45.

More than 15 million people develop sexually transmitted diseases (STDs; also referred to as sexually transmitted infections, or STIs) (Chorba, Tao, & Irwin, 2004). The incidence of STDs has declined over the past several years, except in specific populations, including men who have sex with men. STDs affect people from all walks of life—from all social, educational, economic, and racial backgrounds. The single greatest risk factor for contracting an STD is the number of sexual partners. As the number of partners increases, so does the risk for exposure to a person infected with an STD.

Several diseases are classified as STDs: urethritis (gonococcal and nongonococcal), genital ulcers (genital herpes infections, primary syphilis, chancroid, granuloma inguinale, and lymphogranuloma venereum), genital warts (human papillomavirus [HPV]), scabies, pediculosis pubis, molluscum contagiosum, hepatitis and enteric infections, proctitis, and acquired immunodeficiency syndrome (AIDS). Trichomoniasis and STDs characterized by genital ulcers are thought to increase susceptibility to human immunodeficiency virus (HIV) infection. Trichomoniasis is associated with nonchlamydial, nongonococcal urethritis.

Treatment of STDs must be targeted at the patient as well as his sexual partners and sometimes an unborn child. A thorough history that includes a sexual history is crucial to identify patients at risk and to direct care and teaching. Partners of men with STDs must also be examined, treated, and counseled to prevent reinfection and complications in both partners and to limit the spread of the disease. Sexual abstinence during treatment and recovery is advised to prevent the transmission of STDs. Use of synthetic condoms for at least 6 months after completion of treatment is recommended to decrease transmission of HPV infection as well as other STDs. It is important to examine and test for other STDs, because patients who have one STD may also have another. Use of spermicides with nonoxynol 9 (known as "N-9") is discouraged; these agents do not protect against HIV infection and may increase the risk for transmission of the virus (Shlay, McClung, Patnaik, et al., 2004). See Chapters 52 and 70 for more detailed discussions of HIV infection and AIDS and other STDs.

Conditions of the Prostate

Prostatitis

Prostatitis is an inflammation of the prostate gland that is caused by infectious agents (bacteria, fungi, mycoplasma) or other conditions (eg, urethral stricture, prostatic hyperplasia). *E. coli* is the most commonly isolated organism. Microorganisms are usually carried to the prostate from the urethra. Prostatitis syndromes are classified as acute bacterial (type I), chronic bacterial (type II), chronic prostatitis/chronic pelvic pain syndrome (CP/CPPS) (type III), and asymptomatic inflammatory prostatitis (type IV) (Wolfgang, 2004).

Clinical Manifestations

Symptoms of prostatitis may include perineal discomfort, burning, urgency, frequency, and pain with or after ejaculation. Prostatodynia (pain in the prostate) is manifested by pain on voiding or perineal pain without evidence of inflammation or bacterial growth in the prostate fluid.

Acute bacterial prostatitis may produce sudden fever and chills and perineal, rectal, or low back pain. Urinary symptoms, such as dysuria, frequency, urgency, and **nocturia** (urination during the night), may occur. Some patients do not have symptoms. Chronic bacterial prostatitis is a major cause of relapsing urinary tract infection in men. Symptoms are usually mild, consisting of frequency, dysuria, and occasionally urethral discharge. High temperature and chills are uncommon.

Complications of prostatitis include swelling of the prostate gland and urinary retention. Other complications include epididymitis, bacteremia, and pyelonephritis.

Assessment and Diagnostic Findings

The diagnosis of prostatitis requires a careful history, culture of prostate fluid or tissue, and occasionally a histologic examination of the tissue. To locate the source of a lower genitourinary infection (bladder neck, urethra, prostate), it is necessary to collect a divided urinary specimen for segmental urine culture. After cleaning the glans penis and retracting the foreskin (if present), the patient voids 10 to 15 mL of urine into a container. This represents urethral urine. Without interrupting the urinary stream, he collects 50 to 75 mL of urine in a second container; this represents bladder urine.

If the patient does not have acute prostatitis, the physician immediately performs a prostatic massage and collects any prostatic fluid that is expressed into a third container. If it is not possible to collect prostatic fluid, the patient voids a small quantity of urine. The specimen may contain the bacteria present in the prostatic fluid. Urinalysis after prostate examination commonly reveals many white blood cells.

Medical Management

The goal of therapy for acute bacterial prostatitis is to avoid the complications of abscess formation and septicemia. A broad-spectrum antibiotic agent (to which the causative organism is sensitive) is administered for 10 to 14 days. Intravenous (IV) administration of the agent may be necessary to achieve high serum and tissue levels; the agent may be administered at home. The patient is encouraged to remain on bed rest to alleviate symptoms quickly. Comfort is promoted with analgesic agents (to relieve pain), antispasmodic medications and bladder sedatives (to relieve bladder irritability), sitz baths (to relieve pain and spasm), and stool softeners (to prevent pain from straining).

Chronic bacterial prostatitis is difficult to treat because most antibiotics diffuse poorly from the plasma into the prostatic fluid. Treatment includes alpha-adrenergic blockers (eg, tamsulosin [Flomax]) as well as antibiotics. Alpha-adrenergic blockers are used to promote relaxation of the bladder and prostate. Antibiotics, including trimethoprim-sulfamethoxazole (TMP-SMZ) or a fluoroquinolone, may be prescribed, and continuous therapy with low-dose antibiotics to suppress the infection may also be indicated. The patient is advised that the urinary tract infection may recur and is taught to recognize its symptoms.

Other treatment modalities for chronic prostatitis include reducing the retention of prostatic fluid by ejaculation through sexual intercourse or masturbation, antispasmodics, sitz baths, stool softeners, and evaluation of sexual partners to reduce the possibility of cross-infection. The treatment of nonbacterial prostatitis is directed toward relief of symptoms.

Nursing Management

If the patient experiences symptoms of acute prostatitis (fever, severe pain and discomfort, inability to urinate, malaise), he may be hospitalized for IV antibiotic therapy. Nursing management includes administration of prescribed antibiotics and provision of comfort measures, including prescribed analgesic agents and sitz baths.

The patient with chronic prostatitis is usually treated on an outpatient basis and needs to be instructed about the importance of continuing antibiotic therapy.

Promoting Home and Community-Based Care

TEACHING PATIENTS SELF-CARE

The nurse instructs the patient to complete the prescribed course of antibiotics. If IV antibiotics are to be administered at home, the nurse instructs the patient and family about correct and safe administration. Arrangements for a home care nurse to oversee administration may be needed. Hot sitz baths (10 to 20 minutes) may be taken several times daily. Fluids are encouraged to satisfy thirst but are not "forced," because an effective medication level must be maintained in the urine. Foods and liquids that have diuretic action or that increase prostatic secretions, such as alcohol, coffee, tea, chocolate, cola, and spices, should be avoided. A suprapubic catheter may be necessary for severe urinary retention. During periods of acute inflammation, sexual arousal and intercourse should be avoided.

To minimize discomfort, the patient should avoid sitting for long periods. Medical follow-up is necessary for at least 6 months to 1 year, because prostatitis caused by the same or different organisms can recur.

Benign Prostatic Hyperplasia (Enlarged Prostate)

In approximately one half of men 50 years and older, the prostate gland enlarges, extending upward into the bladder and obstructing the outflow of urine by encroaching on the vesical orifice. This condition, known as BPH, is evident in 80% of men 80 years of age and older. In the United States, BPH is responsible for 375,000 hospital stays each year (Gilchrist, 2004).

Pathophysiology

The cause of BPH is uncertain, but studies suggest that estradiol levels may have a relationship to prostate size among men with testosterone levels above the median (Roberts, Jacobson, Rhodes, et al., 2004). Many African American men develop BPH at a much younger age (40 years) than Caucasian men do, whereas Asian men are unlikely to develop BPH (Gilchrist, 2004). Recent studies have identified smoking (both current and former smoking), heavy alcohol consumption, hypertension, heart disease, and diabetes as risk factors associated with BPH in African American men (Joseph, Harlow, Wei, et al., 2003). Other studies suggest that dietary factors may affect prostate growth and BPH (Denmark-Wahnefried, Robertson, Polascik, et al., 2004).

The hypertrophied lobes of the prostate may obstruct the vesical neck or prostatic urethra, causing incomplete emptying of the bladder and urinary retention. As a result, a gradual dilation of the ureters (hydroureter) and kidneys (hydronephrosis) can occur. Urinary tract infections may result from urinary stasis. Urine remaining in the urinary tract serves as a medium for infective organisms.

Clinical Manifestations

The obstructive and irritative symptoms associated with BPH include increased frequency of urination, nocturia, urgency, hesitancy in starting urination, abdominal straining with urination, a decrease in the volume and force of the urinary stream, interruption of the urinary stream, dribbling (urine dribbles out after urination), a sensation that the bladder has not been completely emptied, acute urinary retention (more than 60 mL of urine remaining in the bladder after urination), and recurrent urinary tract infections. Ultimately, azotemia (accumulation of nitrogenous waste products) and renal failure can occur with chronic urinary retention and large residual volumes. Generalized symptoms may also be noted, including fatigue, anorexia, nausea, vomiting, and epigastric discomfort. Other disorders producing similar symptoms include urethral stricture, prostate cancer, neurogenic bladder, and urinary bladder stones.

Assessment and Diagnostic Findings

DRE reveals a large, rubbery, and nontender prostate gland. Diagnostic studies may be indicated to determine the degree to which the prostate is enlarged, the presence of any changes in the bladder wall, and the efficiency of renal function. These tests may include urinalysis and urodynamic studies to assess urine flow. Renal function tests, including serum creatinine levels, may be performed to determine whether there is renal impairment from prostatic back-pressure and to evaluate renal reserve. Complete blood studies are performed. Because hemorrhage is a major complication of prostate surgery, all clotting defects must be corrected. A high percentage of patients with BPH have cardiac or respiratory complications, or both, because of their age; therefore, cardiac and respiratory function is also assessed.

Medical Management

The treatment plan depends on the cause of BPH, the severity of the obstruction, and the patient's condition. If the patient is admitted on an emergency basis because he cannot void, he is immediately catheterized. The ordinary catheter may be too soft and pliable to advance through the urethra into the bladder. In such cases, a thin wire called a stylet is introduced (by a urologist) into the catheter to prevent the catheter from collapsing when it encounters resistance. In severe cases, metal catheters with a pronounced prostatic curve may be used. Sometimes an incision is made into the bladder (a suprapubic cystostomy) to provide drainage.

Pharmacologic Therapy

Pharmacologic treatment for BPH includes use of alpha-adrenergic blockers and 5-alpha-reductase inhibitors (Kirby, 2004). Alpha-adrenergic blockers (eg, terazosin [Hytrin], doxazosin [Cardura], tamsulosin [Flomax]) relax the smooth muscle of the bladder neck and prostate. Alfuzosin (Uroxatral) is an extended-release alpha-adrenergic antagonist that exerts its effects on the prostate, bladder neck, and posterior urethra. The smooth muscle blockade improves urine flow and relieves BPH symptoms (Laustsen & Wimett, 2003).

Because a hormonal component of BPH has been identified, one method of treatment involves hormonal manipulation with antiandrogen agents (eg, finasteride [Proscar], dutasteride [Avodart]). In clinical studies, 5-alpha-reductase inhibitors such as finasteride have been effective in preventing the conversion of testosterone to dihydrotestosterone (DHT). Decreased levels of DHT lead to decreased glandular cell activity and prostate size. Side effects include gynecomastia (breast enlargement), erectile dysfunction, and flushing.

Other Therapies

Other treatment options for BPH include transurethral incision of the prostate (TUIP), balloon dilation, transurethral laser resection, transurethral needle ablation, and microwave thermotherapy (National Institutes of Health, 2004).

TUIP may be an option for men with only slightly enlarged prostate glands. An electric current or laser beam is used to make incisions in the prostate to decrease resistance to flow of urine out of the bladder. No tissue is removed.

Resection of the prostate can be performed with ultrasound guidance. The treated tissue either vaporizes or becomes necrotic and sloughs. The procedure is performed in the outpatient setting and usually results in less postoperative bleeding than in a traditional surgical prostatectomy.

Transurethral needle ablation uses low-level radiofrequencies to produce localized heat that destroys prostate tissue while sparing the urethra, nerves, muscles, and membranes. The radiofrequencies are delivered by thin needles placed in the prostate gland through use of a catheter. The body then resorbs the dead tissue.

Microwave thermotherapy involves the application of heat to the prostatic tissue. A transurethral probe is inserted into the urethra, and microwaves are carefully directed to the prostate tissue. A water-cooling system helps minimize damage to the urethra and decreases the discomfort from the procedure. The tissue becomes necrotic and sloughs.

Saw palmetto is a herbal product used to treat the symptoms associated with BPH. The active element comes from the fruit of the American dwarf palm tree. Research has shown that the efficacy of saw palmetto is similar to that of medications such as finasteride, and the herbal product may be better tolerated and less expensive (Gordon & Shaughnessy, 2003). In theory, it functions by interfering with the conversion of testosterone to DHT. In addition, saw palmetto may directly block the ability of DHT to stimulate prostate cell growth. It should not be used with finasteride, dutasteride, or medications containing estrogen.

Finally, "watchful waiting," in which patients are monitored periodically for severity of symptoms, physical findings, laboratory tests, and diagnostic urologic tests, is the appropriate treatment for many patients, because the likelihood of progression of the disease or the development of complications is unknown.

Cancer of the Prostate

Prostate cancer is the most common cancer in men other than nonmelanoma skin cancer. It is the second most common cause of cancer death in American men, exceeded only by lung cancer, and is responsible for 10% of cancer-related deaths in men. Among men diagnosed with prostate cancer, 98% survive at least 5 years, 84% survive at least 10 years, and 56% survive 15 years (ACS, 2005).

Prostate cancer is common in the United States and northwestern Europe but is rare in Asia, Africa, Central America, and South America. The worldwide incidence of prostate cancer is highest in African American men, and they are more likely to die of prostate cancer than men in any other racial or ethnic group. Possible factors that may explain the increased mortality rate in African American men include their lower level of engagement in the health care system, disparities in health care, and cultural and structural constraints. The African-American Hereditary Prostate Cancer Study examined characteristics of African American men with hereditary prostate cancer. Its findings suggest a strong genetic link that increases the risk of early onset of the disease (Ahaghotu, Baffoe-Bonnie, Kittles, et al., 2004). These results support the need for education about prostate cancer and diagnostic screening for African American men. Efforts are underway to reduce the incidence and mortality of prostate cancer in this population. Researchers are currently examining the effect of a model of independent decision making related to prostate screening in African American men to determine whether it has an effect on screening behavior, early diagnosis, and intervention for prostate cancer (Sellers & Ross, 2003). Culturally sensitive promotional campaigns, teaching and counseling about prostate cancer, screening, and treatment are important in increasing awareness of the high incidence of prostate cancer and mortality rates in African American men (Wilkinson, List, Sinner, et al., 2003).

Other risk factors for prostate cancer include increasing age; the incidence of prostate cancer increases rapidly after the age of 50 years, and more than 70% of cases occur in men older than 65 years of age. A familial predisposition may occur in men who have a father or brother previously diagnosed with prostate cancer, especially if their relatives were diagnosed at a young age. A number of studies have identified an association of *BRCA2* mutation with an increased risk of prostate cancer (Kirchhoff, Kauff, Mitra, et al., 2004). The risk of prostate cancer is also greater in men who consume a diet containing excessive amounts of red meat or dairy products that are high in fat (ACS, 2005). Efforts are underway to identify additional risk factors for prostate cancer.

Large-scale studies are in progress to determine whether prostate cancer can be prevented by use of selected supplements or finasteride (Proscar). Additional studies suggest a weak protective effect of carotene, especially beta-carotene, against prostate cancer (Bosetti, Talamini, Montella, et al., 2004). Research has suggested that beta-blockers and long-term use of alpha-blockers to treat hypertension may prevent prostate cancer (Perron, Bairati, Harel, et al., 2004).

Clinical Manifestations

Cancer of the prostate in its early stages rarely produces symptoms. The symptoms that develop from urinary obstruction occur late in the disease. This cancer tends to vary in its course. If the neoplasm is large enough to encroach on the bladder neck, signs and symptoms of urinary obstruction occur (difficulty and frequency of urination, urinary retention, and decreased size and force of the urinary stream). Other symptoms may include blood in the urine or semen and painful ejaculation. Hematuria may result if the cancer invades the urethra or bladder, or both.

Prostate cancer can metastasize to bone and lymph nodes. Symptoms related to metastases include backache, hip pain, perineal and rectal discomfort, anemia, weight loss, weakness, nausea, and oliguria (decreased urine output). These symptoms may be the first indications of prostate cancer.

Assessment and Diagnostic Findings

If prostate cancer is detected early, the likelihood of cure is high. It can be diagnosed through an abnormal finding with the DRE, serum PSA, or TRUS with biopsy. Higher rates of detection are documented with the use of combined diagnostic modalities. Routine repeated rectal palpation of the gland (preferably by the same examiner) is important, because early cancer may be detected as a nodule within the substance of the gland or as an extensive hardening in the posterior lobe. The more advanced lesion is "stony hard" and fixed. DRE also provides useful clinical information about the rectum, anal sphincter, and quality of stool.

The diagnosis of prostate cancer is confirmed by a histologic examination of tissue removed surgically by TUR, open prostatectomy, or transrectal needle biopsy. Fine-needle aspiration is a quick, painless method of obtaining prostate cells for cytologic examination and determining the stage of disease.

Most prostate cancers are detected when a man seeks medical attention for symptoms of urinary obstruction or are found by DRE. Cancer detected when TURP is performed for clinically benign disease and lower urinary tract symptoms occurs in about 1 out of 10 cases (National Institutes of Health, 2004). Rarely do patients have other signs and symptoms, such as azotemia (nitrogen compounds in the blood), weakness, anemia, or bone pain.

PSA is a neutral serine protease (protein) produced by both normal and neoplastic ductal epithelium of the prostate. By measuring the amount of this antigen in the blood, it is possible to detect prostate cancer. Therefore, PSA is referred to as a biologic marker or tumor marker. (Tumor markers are substances that are synthesized by the tumor cells and released into the circulation in abnormal amounts.)

The PSA level indicates the presence of prostate tissue. The level of PSA in the blood is proportional to the total prostatic mass and does not necessarily indicate malignancy. There are limitations in the relationship of serum PSA to prostate cancer volume and higher stages of prostate cancer as measured by the Gleason score, which is the system used most often to grade prostate cancer and to guide the physician in determining the most appropriate treatment (Stamey, Caldwell, McNeal, et al., 2004). Debates about acceptable PSA thresholds persist among clinicians. Recent advances in PSA testing have allowed more effective detection of prostate cancer even if PSA levels are not high (Otto & de Koning, 2004). The combination of DRE and PSA testing appears to be a cost-effective method of detecting prostate cancer.

The ACS (2005) recommends that every man older than 50 years of age have an annual DRE and PSA test as part of his regular health checkup. These tests are recommended for younger men (40 to 45 years of age) if they are at high risk for prostate cancer.

A variety of diagnostic tests may also be necessary. TRUS is indicated for men who have elevated PSA levels and abnormal DRE findings. TRUS helps detect nonpalpable prostate cancers and assists with staging of localized prostate cancer. Needle biopsies of the prostate are commonly guided by TRUS. Other tests include bone scans to detect metastatic bone disease, skeletal x-ray studies to identify bone metastases, excretory urography to detect changes caused by ureteral obstruction, renal function tests, and computed tomography (CT) or lymphangiography to identify metastases in the pelvic lymph nodes.

The radiolabeled monoclonal antibody capromab pendetide with indium 111 (ProstaScint) is an antibody that is attracted to the prostate-specific membrane antigen found on prostate cancer cells. It is capable of detecting recurrent prostate cancer at low PSA levels (Wilkinson & Chodak, 2004). The radioactive element attached to the antibody is visible with scanning, allowing assessment of spread of disease. ProstaScint is approved by the U.S. Food and Drug Administration for evaluation of metastatic disease and for postprostatectomy assessment of recurrent disease in patients with an increasing PSA (Ellis, Kim, & Foor, 2004).

Complications

Men with prostate cancer commonly experience sexual dysfunction before the diagnosis is made. Each treatment for prostate cancer (see later discussion) further increases the incidence of sexual problems. With nerve-sparing radical prostatectomy, the likelihood of recovering the ability to have erections is better for men who are younger and in whom both neurovascular bundles are spared. Hormonal therapy also affects the central nervous system mechanisms that mediate sexual desire and arousability.

PDE-5 inhibitors (discussed earlier; see Chart 49-02) may be effective for treatment of erectile dysfunction in younger men after radical retropubic prostatectomy, especially if the neurovascular bundles were preserved (Ogura, Ichioka, Terada, et al., 2004). They may improve erectile function in men with partial or moderate erectile dysfunction after radiation therapy for localized prostate cancer (Incrocci, Hop & Slob, 2004).

Medical Management

Treatment is based on the stage of the disease and the patient's age and symptoms. Treatment is often guided by the use of a nomogram. Nomograms are instruments based on multiple variables that are used to calculate the predicted probability that a patient will have a specified outcome (Di Blasio, Rhee, Cho, et al., 2003). Incorporation of data from clinical assessment, laboratory tests, and TRUS into a prebiopsy nomogram significantly improves the prediction of prostate carcinoma, reduces the number of unnecessary prostate biopsies, and assists in the treatment decision process. Nursing care of the patient with cancer of the prostate is summarized in the plan of nursing care in Chart 49-3.

Surgical Management

Radical prostatectomy is the complete surgical removal of the prostate, seminal vesicles, tips of the vas deferens, and often the surrounding fat, nerves, and blood vessels. It is considered the standard first-line treatment for prostate cancer. Laparoscopic radical prostatectomy is a new approach to surgical treatment of localized cancer of the prostate; however, because the technique has been performed for only a few years, data regarding long-term cancer control and functional results are not available. Although sexual impotence follows radical prostatectomy, laparoscopic radical prostatectomy offers advantages of low morbidity and favorable postoperative outcomes, including quality of life (Touijer & Guillonneau, 2004). Surgical approaches are discussed in detail later in this chapter.

Radiation Therapy

If prostate cancer is detected in its early stage, the treatment may be curative radiation therapy. Two major forms of radiation therapy are used to treat cancer of the prostate: teletherapy (external) and brachytherapy (internal).

Teletherapy (external-beam radiation therapy) involves 6 to 7 weeks of daily (5 days/week) radiation treatments. Intensity-modulated radiation therapy (IMRT) has revolutionized the delivery of external-beam radiation therapy. IMRT sets a dose for the target volume and restricts the dose to adjacent structures. It is thought to be accurate within 1 to 3 millimeters.

Brachytherapy involves the implantation of interstitial radioactive seeds under anesthesia. The surgeon uses ultrasound guidance to place 80 to 100 seeds, and the patient returns home after the procedure. Exposure of others to radiation is minimal, but the patient should avoid close contact with pregnant women and infants for up to 2 months. Radiation safety guidelines include straining urine for seeds and using a condom during sexual intercourse for 2 weeks after implantation, to catch any seeds that pass through the urethra.

Side effects of teletherapy and brachytherapy, which usually are transitory, include inflammation of the rectum, bowel, and bladder (proctitis, enteritis, and cystitis) due to their proximity to the prostate and the radiation doses (Abel, Dafoe-Lambie, Butler, et al., 2003). Irritation of the bladder and urethra from radiation therapy can cause pain with urination and during ejaculation until the irritation subsides. However, there is a greater preservation of sexual potency with radiation therapy than with surgery. For patients with clinically localized but high-risk prostate cancer, multimodal treatment may result in improved cancer control. In patients with larger tumors, combination therapy (radiation therapy followed by hormonal therapy) may improve overall survival (Eastham, 2003).

Hormonal Therapy

In the early 1940s, it was determined that most prostate cancers were androgen-dependent and could be controlled by androgen withdrawal. Hormonal therapy for advanced prostate cancer suppresses androgenic stimuli to the prostate by decreasing the level of circulating plasma testosterone or interrupting the conversion to or binding of DHT. As a result, the prostatic epithelium atrophies (decreases in size). This effect is accomplished either by surgical castration (**orchiectomy**, removal of the testes), which has traditionally been the mainstay of hormonal treatment, or by the administration of medications. Orchiectomy decreases plasma testosterone levels, because about 93% of circulating testosterone is of testicular origin (7% is from the adrenal glands).

(text continues on page 1760)

CHART 49-3

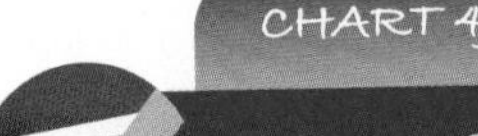

Plan of Nursing Care The Patient With Prostate Cancer

Nursing Diagnosis: Anxiety related to concern and lack of knowledge about the diagnosis, treatment plan, and prognosis
Goal: Reduced stress and improved ability to cope

NURSING INTERVENTIONS	RATIONALE	EXPECTED OUTCOMES
1. Obtain health history to determine the following: a. Patient's concerns b. His level of understanding of his health problem c. His past experience with cancer d. Whether he knows his diagnosis of malignancy and its prognosis e. His support systems and coping methods	1. Nurse clarifies information and facilitates patient's understanding and coping.	• Appears relaxed • States that anxiety has been reduced or relieved • Demonstrates understanding of illness, diagnostic tests, and treatment when questioned • Engages in open communication with others
2. Provide education about diagnosis and treatment plan: a. Explain in simple terms what diagnostic tests to expect, how long they will take, and what will be experienced during each test. b. Review treatment plan and allow patient to ask questions.	2. Helping the patient to understand the diagnostic tests and treatment plan will help decrease his anxiety and promote cooperation.	
3. Assess his psychological reaction to his diagnosis/prognosis and how he has coped with past stresses.	3. This information provides clues in determining appropriate measures to facilitate coping.	
4. Provide information about institutional and community resources for coping with prostate cancer: social services, support groups, community agencies.	4. Institutional and community resources can help the patient and family cope with the illness and treatment on an ongoing basis.	

Nursing Diagnosis: Urinary retention related to urethral obstruction secondary to prostatic enlargement or tumor and loss of bladder tone due to prolonged distention/retention
Goal: Improved pattern of urinary elimination

NURSING INTERVENTIONS	RATIONALE	EXPECTED OUTCOMES
1. Determine patient's usual pattern of urinary function.	1. Provides a baseline for comparison and goal to work toward	• Voids at normal intervals • Reports absence of frequency, urgency, or bladder fullness • Displays no palpable suprapubic distention after voiding • Maintains balanced intake and output
2. Assess for signs and symptoms of urinary retention: amount and frequency of urination, suprapubic distention, complaints of urgency and discomfort.	2. Voiding 20 to 30 mL frequently and output less than intake suggest retention.	

continued >

CHART 49-3

Plan of Nursing Care — The Patient With Prostate Cancer (Continued)

NURSING INTERVENTIONS	RATIONALE	EXPECTED OUTCOMES
3. Catheterize patient to determine amount of residual urine.	3. Determines amount of urine remaining in bladder after voiding	
4. Initiate measures to treat retention:	4. Promotes voiding	
a. Encourage assuming normal position for voiding.	a. Usual position provides relaxed conditions conducive to voiding.	
b. Recommend using Valsalva maneuver preoperatively, if not contraindicated.	b. Valsalva maneuver exerts pressure to force urine out of bladder.	
c. Administer prescribed cholinergic agent.	c. Stimulates bladder contraction	
d. Monitor effects of medication.	d. If unsuccessful, another measure may be required.	
5. Consult with physician regarding intermittent or indwelling catheterization; assist with procedure as required.	5. Catheterization will relieve urinary retention until the specific cause is determined; it may be an obstruction that can be corrected only surgically.	
6. Monitor catheter function; maintain sterility of closed system; irrigate as required.	6. Adequate functioning of catheter is to be ensured to empty bladder and to prevent infection.	
7. Prepare patient for surgery if indicated.	7. Surgical removal of obstruction may be necessary.	

Nursing Diagnosis: Deficient knowledge related to the diagnosis of: cancer, urinary difficulties, and treatment modalities
Goal: Understanding of the diagnosis and ability to care for self

NURSING INTERVENTIONS	RATIONALE	EXPECTED OUTCOMES
1. Encourage communication with the patient.	1. This is designed to establish rapport and trust.	• Discusses his concerns and problems freely • Asks questions and shows interest in his disorder • Describes activities that help or hinder recovery • Identifies ways of attaining/maintaining bladder control • Demonstrates satisfactory technique and understanding of catheter care • Lists signs and symptoms that must be reported should they occur
2. Review the anatomy of the involved area.	2. Orientation to one's anatomy is basic to understanding its function.	
3. Be specific in selecting information that is relevant to the patient's particular treatment plan.	3. This is based on the treatment plan; as it varies with each patient, individualization is desirable.	
4. Identify ways to reduce pressure on the operative area after prostatectomy: a. Avoid prolonged sitting (in a chair, long automobile rides), standing, walking. b. Avoid straining, such as during exercises, bowel movement, lifting, and sexual intercourse.	4. This is to prevent bleeding; such precautions are in order for 6 to 8 weeks postoperatively.	

CHART 49-3

Plan of Nursing Care — The Patient With Prostate Cancer (Continued)

NURSING INTERVENTIONS	RATIONALE	EXPECTED OUTCOMES
5. Familiarize patient with ways of attaining/maintaining bladder control.	5. These measures will help control frequency and dribbling and aid in preventing retention.	
a. Encourage urination every 2 to 3 hours; discourage voiding when supine.	a. By sitting or standing, patient is more likely to empty his bladder.	
b. Avoid drinking cola and caffeine beverages; urge a cutoff time in the evening for drinking fluids to minimize frequent voiding during the night.	b. Spacing the kind and amount of liquid intake will help to prevent frequency.	
c. Describe perineal exercises to be performed every hour.	c. Exercises will assist him in starting and stopping the urinary stream.	
d. Develop a schedule with patient that will fit into his routine.	d. A schedule will assist in developing a workable pattern of normal activities.	
6. Demonstrate catheter care; encourage his questions; stress the importance of position of urinary receptacle.	6. By requiring a return demonstration of care, collection, and emptying of the device, he will become more independent and also can prevent backflow of urine, which can lead to infection.	

Nursing Diagnosis: Imbalanced nutrition: less than body requirements related to decreased oral intake because of anorexia, nausea, and vomiting caused by cancer or its treatment
Goal: Maintain optimal nutritional status

NURSING INTERVENTIONS	RATIONALE	EXPECTED OUTCOMES
1. Assess the amount of food eaten.	1. This assessment will help determine nutrient intake.	• Responds positively to his favorite foods
2. Routinely weigh patient.	2. Weighing the patient on the same scale under similar conditions can help monitor changes in weight.	• Assumes responsibility for his oral hygiene
3. Elicit patient's explanation of why he is unable to eat more.	3. His explanation may present easily corrected practices.	• Reports absence of nausea and vomiting.
4. Cater to his individual food preferences (eg, avoiding foods that are too spicy or too cold).	4. He will be more likely to consume larger servings if food is palatable and appealing.	• Notes increase in weight after improved appetite
5. Recognize effect of medication or radiation therapy on appetite.	5. Many chemotherapeutic agents and radiation therapy promote anorexia.	
6. Inform patient that alterations in taste can occur.	6. Aging and the disease process can reduce taste sensitivity. In addition, smell and taste can be altered as a result of the body's absorption of byproducts of cellular destruction (brought on by malignancy and its treatment).	

continued >

CHART 49-3

Plan of Nursing Care The Patient With Prostate Cancer (Continued)

NURSING INTERVENTIONS	RATIONALE	EXPECTED OUTCOMES
7. Use measures to control nausea and vomiting: a. Administer prescribed antiemetics, around the clock if necessary. b. Provide oral hygiene after vomiting episodes. c. Provide rest periods after meals.	7. Prevention of nausea and vomiting can stimulate appetite.	
8. Provide frequent small meals and a comfortable and pleasant environment.	8. Smaller portions of food are less overwhelming to the patient.	
9. Assess patient's ability to obtain and prepare foods.	9. Disability or lack of social support can hinder the patient's ability to obtain and prepare foods.	

Nursing Diagnosis: Sexual dysfunction related to effects of therapy: chemotherapy, hormonal therapy, radiation therapy, surgery
Goal: Ability to resume/enjoy modified sexual functioning

NURSING INTERVENTIONS	RATIONALE	EXPECTED OUTCOMES
1. Determine from nursing history what effect patient's medical condition is having on his sexual functioning.	1. Usually decreased libido and, later, impotence may be experienced.	• Describes the reasons for changes in sexual functioning • Discusses with appropriate health care personnel alternative approaches and methods of sexual expression • Includes partner in discussions related to changes in sexual function
2. Inform patient of the effects of prostate surgery, orchiectomy (when applicable), chemotherapy, irradiation, and hormonal therapy on sexual function.	2. Treatment modalities may alter sexual function, but each is evaluated separately with regard to its effect on a particular patient.	
3. Include his partner in developing understanding and in discovering alternative, satisfying close relations with each other.	3. The bonds between a couple may be strengthened with new appreciation and support that had not been evident before the current illness.	

Nursing Diagnosis: Pain related to progression of disease and treatment modalities
Goal: Relief of pain

NURSING INTERVENTIONS	RATIONALE	EXPECTED OUTCOMES
1. Evaluate nature of patient's pain, its location and intensity using pain rating scale.	1. Determining nature and causes of pain and its intensity helps to select proper pain-relief modality and provide baseline for later comparison.	• Reports relief of pain • Expects exacerbations, reports their quality and intensity, and obtains relief • Uses pain relief strategies appropriately and effectively • Identifies strategies to avoid complications of analgesic use (eg, constipation)
2. Avoid activities that aggravate or worsen pain.	2. Bumping the bed is an example of an action that can intensify the patient's pain.	

CHART 49-3

Plan of Nursing Care — The Patient With Prostate Cancer (Continued)

NURSING INTERVENTIONS	RATIONALE	EXPECTED OUTCOMES
3. Because pain is usually related to bone metastasis, ensure that patient's bed has a bed board on a firm mattress. Also, protect the patient from falls/injuries.	3. This will provide added support and is more comfortable. Protecting the patient from injury protects him from additional pain.	
4. Provide support for affected extremities.	4. More support, coupled with reduced movement of the part, helps in pain control.	
5. Prepare patient for radiation therapy if prescribed.	5. Radiation therapy may be effective in controlling pain.	
6. Administer analgesics or opioids at regularly scheduled intervals as prescribed.	6. Analgesics alter perception of pain and provide comfort. Regularly scheduled analgesics around the clock rather than PRN provide more consistent pain relief.	
7. Initiate bowel program to prevent constipation.	7. Opioid analgesics and inactivity contribute to constipation.	

Nursing Diagnosis: Impaired physical mobility and activity intolerance related to tissue hypoxia, malnutrition, and exhaustion and to spinal cord or nerve compression from metastases
Goal: Improved physical mobility

NURSING INTERVENTIONS	RATIONALE	EXPECTED OUTCOMES
1. Assess for factors causing limited mobility (eg, pain, hypercalcemia, limited exercise tolerance).	1. This information offers clues to the cause; if possible, cause is treated.	• Achieves improved physical mobility • Relates that short-term goals are encouraging him because they are attainable
2. Provide pain relief by administering prescribed medications.	2. Analgesics/opioids allow the patient to increase his activity more comfortably.	
3. Encourage use of assistive devices: cane, walker.	3. Support may offer the security needed to become mobile.	
4. Involve significant others in helping patient with range-of-motion exercises, positioning, and walking.	4. Assistance from partner or others encourages patient to repeat activities and achieve goals.	
5. Provide positive reinforcement for achievement of small gains.	5. Encouragement stimulates improvement of performance.	
6. Assess nutritional status.	6. See Nursing Diagnosis: Imbalanced nutrition: less than body requirements.	

continued >

CHART 49-3

Plan of Nursing Care **The Patient With Prostate Cancer (Continued)**

Collaborative Problems: Hemorrhage, infection, bladder neck obstruction
Goal: Absence of complications

NURSING INTERVENTIONS	RATIONALE	EXPECTED OUTCOMES
1. Alert the patient to changes that may occur (after discharge) and that need to be reported:	1. Certain changes signal beginning complications, which call for nursing and medical interventions.	• Experiences no bleeding or passage of blood clots • Reports no pain around the catheter • Experiences normal frequency or urination • Reports normal urinary output • Maintains bladder control
a. Continued bloody urine; passing blood clots	a. Hematuria with or without blood clot formation may occur postoperatively.	
b. Pain; burning around the catheter	b. Indwelling urinary catheters may be a source of infections.	
c. Frequency of urination	c. Urinary frequency may be caused by urinary tract infections or by bladder neck obstruction, resulting in incomplete voiding.	
d. Diminished urinary output	d. Bladder neck obstruction decreases the amount of urine that is voided.	
e. Increasing loss of bladder control	e. Urinary incontinence may be a result of urinary retention.	

As a result, the testicular stimulus required for continued prostatic growth is removed, resulting in prostatic atrophy.

However, orchiectomy often results in significant morbidity. Although the procedure does not cause the side effects associated with other hormonal therapies (described later), it is associated with considerable emotional impact. Because patients who have prostate cancer are living longer with the disease, health care providers have now begun to focus their attention on effective therapeutic modalities that promote an acceptable quality of life. Hormonal therapy, which is used to control rather than cure prostate cancer, is a viable therapeutic option for men with advanced prostate cancer. Research indicates that the most appropriate choice, timing, and actual benefits of hormonal therapy are uncertain (Miyamoto & Messing, 2004).

Effective hormonal alternatives to orchiectomy include the nonsteroidal antiandrogen bicalutamide (Casodex) (Fradet, 2004). Estrogen therapy, usually in the form of diethylstilbestrol (DES), has long been used to inhibit the gonadotropins responsible for testicular androgenic activity, thereby removing the androgenic hormone that promotes the growth of the malignancy. DES relieves symptoms of advanced prostate cancer, reduces tumor size, decreases pain from metastatic nodules, and promotes well-being. However, DES significantly increases the risk of thromboembolism, pulmonary embolism, myocardial infarction, and stroke. Other side effects of estrogen therapy include impotence, decreased libido, difficulty in achieving orgasm, decreased sperm production, and gynecomastia (enlargement of breasts in men).

Newer hormonal therapies include luteinizing hormone–releasing hormone (LHRH) agonists (leuprolide [Lupron] and goserelin [Zoladex]) and antiandrogen agents, such as flutamide (Eulexin). LHRH suppresses testicular androgen, whereas flutamide causes adrenal androgen suppression. The most common uses of LHRH agonists are the following: (1) in the adjuvant and neoadjuvant setting (i.e., before use of hormonal suppressive agents), in combination with radiation therapy; (2) in combination with radical prostatectomy; and (3) in the treatment of recurrence indicated by an elevation in the PSA but without clinical or x-ray evidence (Moul & Fowler, 2003). Cyproterone acetate is a synthetic progesterone derivative that provides effective, competitive inhibition of androgens at the target cells. In contrast to estrogen, the newer hormonal agents are associated with a lower incidence of cardiovascular side effects, gynecomastia, and decreased sexual function. Hot flushing can occur with orchiectomy or LHRH agonist therapy, because these treatment modalities increase hypothalamic activity, which stimulates the thermoregulatory centers of the body.

Chemotherapy

The management of hormone-refractory cancer of the prostate remains somewhat controversial. Administration of second-line hormonal therapy using ketoconazole is an option. High-dose ketoconazole (HDK) lowers testosterone through its abilities to decrease both testicular and endocrine production of androgen. Use of HDK is considered a form of androgen deprivation therapy. The agent is also classified as a cytochrome P450 enzyme inhibitor; thus, it allows chemotherapy agents to have a direct effect on cancer cells, causing cell death (Lam, 2004).

Recent studies have shown clear benefits in terms of survival with chemotherapy treatment that includes paclitaxel (Taxol) and docetaxel (Taxotere) for non–androgen-dependent prostate cancer (Beer, Garzotto, Henner, et al., 2004). Other studies are underway to determine the importance of the vascular endothelial growth factor system. Tumor angiogenesis is essential for tumor growth, including growth of prostate carcinomas and other high-grade cancers. Therefore, antiangiogenic treatment in combination with conventional therapies may play a future role in treatment (Steranou, Batistatou, Kamina, et al., 2004). Gene-based therapy in prostate cancer is an emerging and promising adjuvant to conventional treatment strategies.

Other Therapies

Cryosurgery of the prostate is used to ablate prostate cancer in patients who cannot tolerate surgery and in those with recurrent prostate cancer. Transperineal probes are inserted into the prostate under ultrasound guidance to freeze the tissue directly. Chemotherapy agents, such as doxorubicin, cisplatin, and cyclophosphamide, may also be used.

Keeping the urethral passage patent may require repeated TURs. If this is impractical, catheter drainage is instituted by way of the suprapubic or transurethral route. For men with advanced prostate cancer, palliative measures are indicated. Although cure is unlikely with advanced prostate cancer, many men survive for a long period apparently free of metastatic disease.

Bone lesions resulting from metastasis of prostate cancer can be very painful. Opioid and nonopioid medications are used to control the pain. External-beam radiation therapy can be delivered to skeletal lesions to relieve pain. Radiopharmaceuticals, such as strontium 89, can be injected IV to treat multiple sites of bone metastasis (Gunawardana, Lichtenstein, Better, et al., 2004). Antiandrogen therapies are used in an effort to reduce the circulating androgens. If antiandrogen therapies are not effective, medications such as prednisone and mitoxantrone have been effective in reducing pain and improving quality of life. In advanced prostate cancer, blood transfusions are administered to maintain adequate hemoglobin levels when bone marrow is replaced by tumor.

More than one third of men with a diagnosis of prostate cancer elect to use some form of complementary and alternative medicine (CAM). Because of lack of research on many forms of CAM, patients often rely on anecdotal information to make decisions about its use. Nurses play a vital role in assisting patients to locate and evaluate available information about CAM to ensure that harmful forms are avoided (Eng, Ramsum, Verhoef, et al., 2003).

The Patient Undergoing Prostate Surgery

Prostate surgery may be indicated for the patient with BPH or prostate cancer. The objectives before prostate surgery are to assess the patient's general health status and to establish optimal renal function. Prostate surgery should be performed before acute urinary retention develops and damages the upper urinary tract and collecting system or, in the case of prostate cancer, before cancer progresses.

Surgical Procedures

Several approaches can be used to remove the hypertrophied portion of the prostate gland: TURP, suprapubic prostatectomy, perineal prostatectomy, retropubic prostatectomy, TUIP, and laparoscopic radical prostatectomy (Table 49-3). In these approaches, the surgeon removes all hyperplastic tissue, leaving behind only the capsule of the prostate. The transurethral approaches (TURP, TUIP) are closed procedures; the other three are open procedures (ie, a surgical incision is required). The procedure chosen depends on the underlying disorder, the patient's age and physical status, and patient preference.

Transurethral Resection of the Prostate

TURP, the most common procedure used, can be carried out through endoscopy. The surgical and optical instrument is introduced directly through the urethra to the prostate, which can then be viewed directly. The gland is removed in small chips with an electrical cutting loop (Fig. 49-4A). This procedure, which requires no incision, may be used for glands of varying size and is ideal for patients who have small glands and for those who are considered poor surgical risks. Newer technology uses bipolar electrosurgery and reduces the risk of electrical shock (Bishop, 2003). It also eliminates the risk of TUR syndrome (hyponatremia, hypovolemia). TUR syndrome is a potential but rare complication of TURP that occurs in approximately 2% of men who undergo the procedure (Chart 49-4).

TURP usually requires an overnight hospital stay. Urethral strictures are more frequent than with non-transurethral procedures, and repeated procedures may be necessary because the residual prostatic tissue grows back. TURP rarely causes erectile dysfunction but may trigger retrograde ejaculation, because removal of prostatic tissue at the bladder neck can cause the seminal fluid to flow backward into the bladder rather than forward through the urethra during ejaculation.

Suprapubic Prostatectomy

Suprapubic prostatectomy is one method of removing the gland through an abdominal incision. An incision is made into the bladder, and the prostate gland is removed from above (see Fig. 49-4B). Such an approach can be used for a gland of any size, and few complications occur, although blood loss may be greater than with the other methods. Another disadvantage is the need for an abdominal incision, with the concomitant hazards of any major abdominal surgical procedure.

Perineal Prostatectomy

Perineal prostatectomy involves removal of the gland through an incision in the perineum (see Fig. 49-4C). This approach is practical when other approaches are not possible and is useful for an open biopsy. Postoperatively, the wound may easily become contaminated because the incision is near

TABLE 49-3 Comparing Surgical Approaches for Treatment of Prostate Disorders

The surgical approach of choice depends on (1) the size of the gland, (2) the severity of the obstruction, (3) the age of the patient, (4) the condition of patient, and (5) the presence of associated diseases.

Surgical Approach	Advantages	Disadvantages	Nursing Implications
Transurethral Resection (TUR or TURP) (removal of prostatic tissue by instrument introduced through urethra)	Avoids abdominal incision Safer for surgical-risk patient Shorter hospitalization and recovery periods Lower morbidity rate Causes less pain	Requires highly skilled surgeon Recurrent obstruction, urethral trauma, and stricture may develop. Delayed bleeding may occur.	Monitor for hemorrhage. Observe for symptoms of urethral stricture (dysuria, straining, weak urinary stream).
Open Surgical Removal			
Suprapubic approach	Technically simple Offers wide area of exploration Permits exploration for cancerous lymph nodes Allows more complete removal of obstructing gland Permits treatment of associated bladder lesions	Requires surgical approach through the bladder Control of hemorrhage difficult Urine may leak around the suprapubic tube. Recovery may be prolonged and uncomfortable.	Monitor for indications of hemorrhage and shock. Provide meticulous aseptic care to the area around suprapubic tube.
Perineal approach	Offers direct anatomic approach Permits gravity drainage Particularly effective for radical cancer therapy Allows hemostasis under direct vision Low mortality rate Low incidence of shock Ideal for very old, frail, and poor-surgical-risk patients with large prostate	Higher postoperative incidence of impotence and urinary incontinence Possible damage to rectum and external sphincter Restricted operative field Greater potential for infection	Avoid using rectal tubes or thermometers and enemas after perineal surgery. Use drainage pads to absorb excess urinary drainage. Provide foam rubber ring for patient comfort in sitting. Anticipate urinary leakage around the wound for several days after the catheter is removed.
Retropubic approach	Avoids incision into the bladder Permits surgeon to see and control bleeding Shorter recovery period Less bladder sphincter damage	Cannot treat associated bladder disease Increased incidence of hemorrhage from prostatic venous plexus; pubic osteitis	Monitor for hemorrhage. Anticipate posturinary leakage for several days after removing the catheter.
Transurethral Incision (TUIP)	Results comparable to TURP Low incidence of erectile dysfunction and retrograde ejaculation No bladder neck contracture	Requires highly skilled surgeon Recurrent obstruction and urethral trauma Delayed bleeding	Monitor for hemorrhage.
Laparoscopic Radical Prostatectomy (LPR)	Minimally invasive technique Improved patient satisfaction and quality of life Short convalescense More rapid return to normal activity Short indwelling catheter duration Decreased blood loss Improved magnification of operative field	Lack of tactile sensation available with open prostatectomy Inability to palpably assess for induration and palpable nodules Inability to delineate the proximity of involvement of the neurovascular bundles due to lack of palpation Technically demanding	Observe for symptoms of urethral stricture (dysuria, straining, weak urinary stream. Monitor for hemorrhage and shock. Provide meticulous aseptic care to the area around suprapubic tube. Monitor for changes in bowel function. Avoid using rectal tubes or thermometers and enemas after perineal surgery. Use drainage pads to absorb excess urinary drainage. Provide foam rubber ring for patient comfort in sitting. Anticipate urinary leakage around the wound for several days after the catheter is removed.

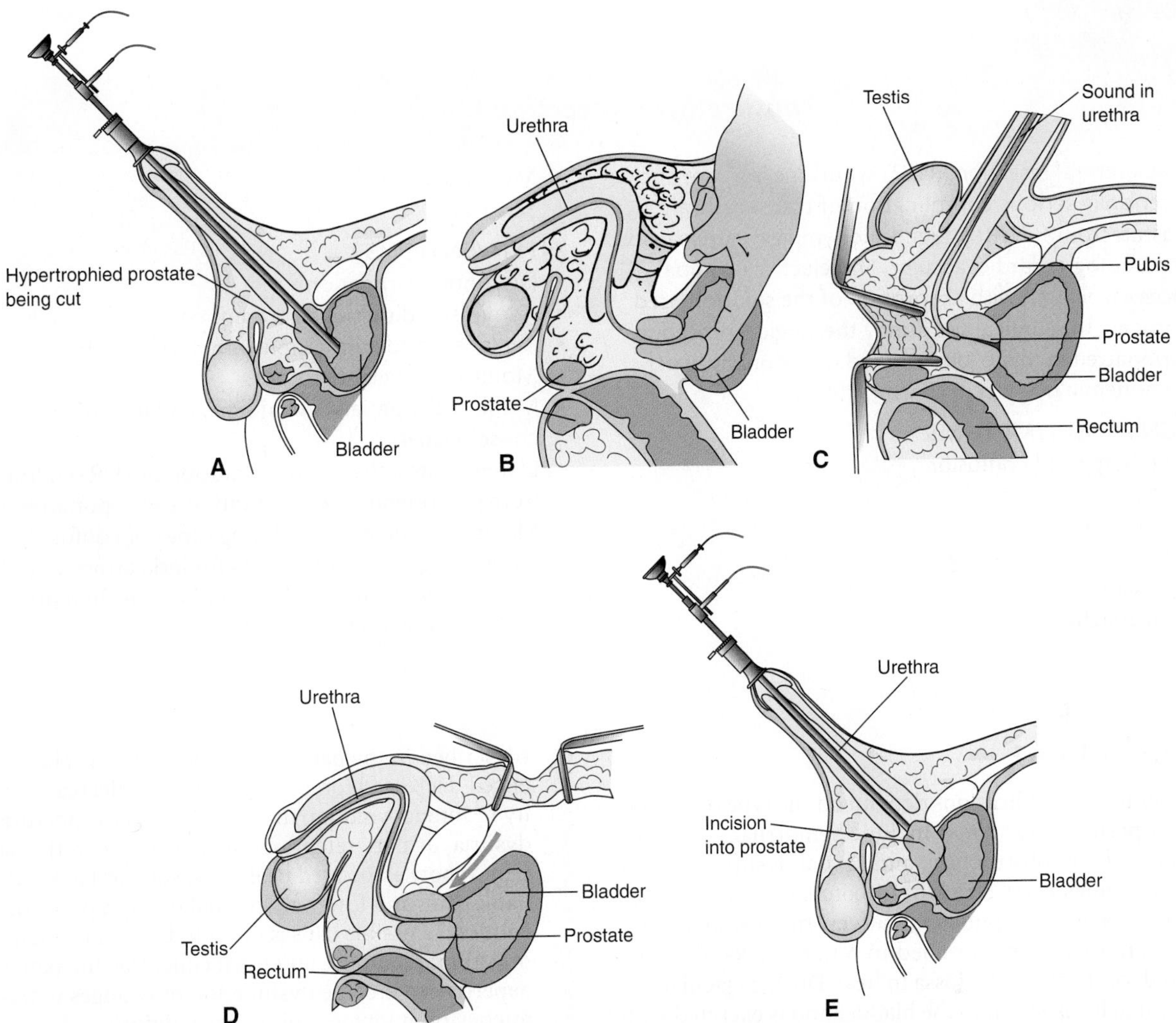

FIGURE 49-4. Prostate surgery procedures. (**A**) Transurethral resection (TUR). A loop of wire connected with a cutting current is rotated in the cystoscope to remove shavings of prostate at the bladder orifice. (**B**) Suprapubic prostatectomy. With an abdominal approach, the prostate is shelled out of its bed. (**C**) Perineal prostatectomy. Two retractors on the left spread the perineal incision to provide a view of the prostate. (**D**) Retropubic prostatectomy is performed through a low abdominal incision. Note two abdominal retractors and *arrow* pointing to the prostate gland. (**E**) Transurethral incision of prostate (TUIP) involves one or two incisions into the prostate to reduce pressure on the urethra.

the rectum. Incontinence, impotence, and rectal injury are more likely with this approach.

Retropubic Prostatectomy

Retropubic prostatectomy is more common than the suprapubic approach. The surgeon makes a low abdominal incision and approaches the prostate gland between the pubic arch and the bladder without entering the bladder (see Fig. 49-4D). This procedure is suitable for large glands located high in the pelvis. Although blood loss can be better controlled and the surgical site is easier to visualize, infections can readily start in the retropubic space.

Transurethral Incision of the Prostate

TUIP is another procedure used to treat BPH. An instrument is passed through the urethra (see Fig. 49-4E). One or two incisions are made in the prostate and prostate capsule to reduce the prostate's pressure on the urethra and to reduce urethral constriction. TUIP is indicated when the prostate gland is small (30 g or less), and it is an effective treatment for many cases of BPH. TUIP can be performed on an outpatient basis and has a lower complication rate than other invasive prostate procedures.

Laparoscopic Radical Prostatectomy

Laparoscopic radical prostatectomy provides better visualization of the surgical site and surrounding areas than other surgical procedures. In addition, patients who undergo this procedure have been shown to experience less bleeding and reduced need for blood transfusion, shorter hospital stays, less postoperative pain, and more rapid return to normal activity compared to those who undergo open radical prostatectomy (Touijer & Guillonneau, 2004). Further research is needed to assess long-term outcomes.

CHART 49-4

Transurethral Resection Syndrome

Transurethral resection (TUR) syndrome is a rare but potentially serious complication of transurethral prostatectomy (TURP). Signs and symptoms are caused by neurologic, cardiovascular, and electrolyte imbalances associated with absorption of the solution used to irrigate the surgical site during the surgical procedure. Hyponatremia, hypovolemia, and occasionally hyperammonemia may occur (Eaton, 2003).

SIGNS AND SYMPTOMS

- Lethargy and confusion
- Hypotension
- Tachycardia
- Nausea and vomiting
- Collapse
- Headache
- Muscle spasms
- Seizures

INTERVENTIONS

- Discontinue irrigation.
- Administer diuretics as prescribed.
- Replace bladder irrigation with normal saline.
- Monitor intake and output.
- Monitor the patient's vital signs and level of consciousness.
- Differentiate lethargy and confusion of TUR syndrome from postoperative disorientation and hyponatremia.
- Maintain patient safety during times of confusion.
- Assess lung and heart sounds for indications of pulmonary edema, heart failure, or both as fluid moves back into the intravascular space.

Complications

Postoperative complications depend on the type of prostatectomy performed and may include hemorrhage, clot formation, catheter obstruction, and sexual dysfunction. All prostatectomies carry a risk of impotence because of potential damage to the pudendal nerves. In most instances, sexual activity may be resumed in 6 to 8 weeks, the time required for the prostatic fossa to heal. During ejaculation, the seminal fluid goes into the bladder and is excreted with the urine. The anatomic changes in the posterior urethra lead to retrograde ejaculation. A vasectomy may be performed during surgery to prevent infection from spreading from the prostatic urethra through the vas and into the epididymis.

After total prostatectomy (usually for cancer), impotence almost always results. For the patient for whom this is unacceptable, options are available to produce erections sufficient for sexual intercourse: prosthetic penile implants, negative-pressure (vacuum) devices, and pharmacologic interventions (see earlier discussion and Table 49-2).

Nursing Process

The Patient Undergoing Prostatectomy

Assessment

The nurse assesses how the underlying disorder (BPH or prostate cancer) has affected the patient's lifestyle. Questions to ask during assessment include the following: Has the patient's activity level or activity tolerance changed? What is his presenting urinary problem (described in the patient's own words)? Has he experienced decreased force of urinary flow, decreased ability to initiate voiding, urgency, frequency, nocturia, dysuria, urinary retention, hematuria? Does the patient report associated problems, such as back pain, flank pain, and lower abdominal or suprapubic discomfort? Possible causes of such discomfort include infection, retention, and renal colic. Has the patient experienced erectile dysfunction or changes in frequency or enjoyment of sexual activity?

The nurse obtains further information about the patient's family history of cancer and heart or kidney disease, including hypertension. Has he lost weight? Does he appear pale? Can he raise himself out of bed and return to bed without assistance? Can he perform usual activities of daily living? This information helps determine how soon the patient will be able to return to normal activities after prostatectomy.

Diagnosis

Based on the assessment data, the patient's major nursing diagnoses may include the following.

Preoperative Nursing Diagnoses

- Anxiety about surgery and its outcome
- Acute pain related to bladder distention
- Deficient knowledge about factors related to the disorder and the treatment protocol

Postoperative Nursing Diagnoses

- Acute pain related to the surgical incision, catheter placement, and bladder spasms
- Deficient knowledge about postoperative care and management

Collaborative Problems/ Potential Complications

Based on the assessment data, the potential complications may include the following:

- Hemorrhage and shock
- Infection
- Deep vein thrombosis
- Catheter obstruction
- Sexual dysfunction

Planning and Goals

The major preoperative goals for the patient may include reduced anxiety and learning about his prostate disorder and the perioperative experience. The major postoperative goals may include maintenance of fluid volume balance, relief of pain and discomfort, ability to perform self-care activities, and absence of complications.

Preoperative Nursing Interventions

Reducing Anxiety

The patient is frequently admitted to the hospital on the morning of surgery. Because contact with the patient may be limited before surgery, the nurse must establish communication with the patient to assess his understanding of the diagnosis and of the planned surgical procedure. The nurse clarifies the nature of the surgery and expected postoperative outcomes. In addition, the nurse familiarizes the patient with the preoperative and postoperative routines and initiates measures to reduce anxiety. Because the patient may be sensitive and embarrassed discussing problems related to the genitalia and sexuality, the nurse provides privacy and establishes a trusting and professional relationship. Guilt feelings often surface if the patient falsely assumes a cause-and-effect relationship between sexual practices and his current problems. He is encouraged to verbalize his feelings and concerns.

Relieving Discomfort

If the patient experiences discomfort before surgery, he is prescribed bed rest, analgesic agents are administered, and measures are initiated to relieve anxiety. If he is hospitalized, the nurse monitors his voiding patterns, watches for bladder distention, and assists with catheterization if indicated. An indwelling catheter is inserted if the patient has continuing urinary retention or if laboratory test results indicate azotemia (accumulation of nitrogenous waste products in the blood). The catheter can help decompress the bladder gradually over several days, especially if the patient is elderly and hypertensive and has diminished renal function or urinary retention that has existed for many weeks. For a few days after the bladder begins draining, the blood pressure may fluctuate and renal function may decline. If the patient cannot tolerate a urinary catheter, he is prepared for a cystostomy (see Chapters 44 and 45).

Providing Instruction

Before surgery, the nurse reviews with the patient the anatomy of the affected structures and their function in relation to the urinary and reproductive systems, using diagrams and other teaching aids if indicated. This instruction often takes place during the preadmission testing visit or in the urologist's office. The nurse explains what will take place as the patient is prepared for diagnostic tests and then for surgery (depending on the type of prostatectomy planned). The nurse also describes the type of incision, which varies with the surgical approach (directly over the bladder, low on the abdomen, or in the perineal area; in the case of a transurethral procedure, no incision will be made), and informs the patient about the likely type of urinary drainage system, the type of anesthesia, and the recovery room procedure. The amount of information given is based on the patient's needs and questions. The nurse explains procedures expected to occur during the immediate perioperative period, answers questions the patient or family may have, and provides emotional support. In addition, the nurse provides the patient with information about postoperative pain management.

Preparing the Patient

If the patient is scheduled for a prostatectomy, the preoperative preparation described in Chapter 18 is provided. Elastic compression stockings are applied before surgery and are particularly important for prevention of deep vein thrombosis (DVT) if the patient is placed in a lithotomy position during surgery. An enema is usually administered at home on the evening before surgery or on the morning of surgery to prevent postoperative straining, which can induce bleeding.

Postoperative Nursing Interventions

Maintaining Fluid Balance

During the postoperative period, the patient is at risk for imbalanced fluid volume because of the irrigation of the surgical site during and after surgery. With irrigation of the urinary catheter to prevent its obstruction by blood clots, fluid may be absorbed through the open surgical site and retained, increasing the risk of excessive fluid retention, fluid imbalance, and water intoxication. The urine output and the amount of fluid used for irrigation must be closely monitored to determine whether irrigation fluid is being retained and to ensure an adequate urine output. An intake and output record, including the amount of fluid used for irrigation, must be maintained. The patient also is monitored for electrolyte imbalances (eg, hyponatremia), increasing blood pressure, confusion, and respiratory distress. These signs and symptoms are documented and reported to the surgeon. The risk of fluid and electrolyte imbalance is greater in elderly patients with preexisting cardiovascular or respiratory disease.

Relieving Pain

After a prostatectomy, the patient is assisted to sit and dangle his legs over the side of the bed on the day of surgery. The next morning, he is assisted to ambulate. If pain is present, the cause and location are determined and the severity of pain and discomfort is assessed. The pain may be related to the incision or may be the result of excoriation of the skin at the catheter site. It may be in the flank area, indicating a kidney problem, or it may be caused by bladder spasms. Bladder irritability can initiate bleeding and result in clot formation, leading to urinary retention.

Patients experiencing bladder spasms may note an urgency to void, a feeling of pressure or fullness in the bladder, and bleeding from the urethra around the catheter. Medications that relax the smooth muscles can help ease the spasms, which can be intermittent and severe; these medications include flavoxate (Urispas) and oxybutynin (Ditropan). Warm compresses to the pubis or sitz baths may also relieve the spasms.

The nurse monitors the drainage tubing and irrigates the system as prescribed to relieve any obstruction that may cause discomfort. Usually, the catheter is irrigated with 50 mL of irrigating fluid at a time. It is important to make sure that the same amount is recovered in the drainage receptacle. Securing the catheter drainage tubing to the leg or abdomen can help decrease tension on the catheter and prevent bladder irritation. Discomfort may be caused by dressings that are too snug, saturated with drainage, or improperly placed. Analgesic agents are administered as prescribed.

After the patient is ambulatory, he is encouraged to walk but not to sit for prolonged periods, because this increases intra-abdominal pressure and the possibility of discomfort and bleeding. Prune juice and stool softeners are provided to ease bowel movements and to prevent excessive straining. An enema, if prescribed, is administered with caution to avoid rectal perforation.

Monitoring and Managing Potential Complications

After prostatectomy, the patient is monitored for major complications such as hemorrhage, infection, DVT, catheter obstruction, and sexual dysfunction.

HEMORRHAGE

The immediate dangers after a prostatectomy are bleeding and hemorrhagic shock. This risk is increased with BPH, because a hyperplastic prostate gland is very vascular. Bleeding may occur from the prostatic bed. Bleeding may also result in the formation of clots, which then obstruct urine flow. The drainage normally begins as reddish-pink and then clears to a light pink within 24 hours after surgery. Bright red bleeding with increased viscosity and numerous clots usually indicates arterial bleeding. Venous blood appears darker and less viscous. Arterial hemorrhage usually requires surgical intervention (eg, suturing or transurethral coagulation of bleeding vessels), whereas venous bleeding may be controlled by applying prescribed traction to the catheter so that the balloon holding the catheter in place applies pressure to the prostatic fossa. The surgeon applies traction by securely taping the catheter to the patient's thigh if hemorrhage occurs.

Nursing management includes assistance in implementing strategies to stop the bleeding and to prevent or reverse hemorrhagic shock. If blood loss is extensive, fluids and blood component therapy may be administered. If hemorrhagic shock occurs, treatments described in Chapter 15 are initiated.

Nursing interventions include closely monitoring vital signs; administering medications, IV fluids, and blood component therapy as prescribed; maintaining an accurate record of intake and output; and carefully monitoring drainage to ensure adequate urine flow and patency of the drainage system. The patient who experiences hemorrhage and his family are often anxious and benefit from explanations and reassurance about the event and the procedures that are performed.

INFECTION

After perineal prostatectomy, the surgeon usually changes the dressing on the first postoperative day. Further dressing changes may become the responsibility of the nurse or home care nurse. Careful aseptic technique is used, because the potential for infection is great. Dressings can be held in place by a double-tailed, T-binder bandage or a padded athletic supporter. The tails cross over the incision to give double thickness, and then each tail is drawn up on either side of the scrotum to the waistline and fastened.

Rectal thermometers, rectal tubes, and enemas are avoided because of the risk of injury and bleeding in the prostatic fossa. After the perineal sutures are removed, the perineum is cleansed as indicated. A heat lamp may be directed to the perineal area to promote healing. The scrotum is protected with a towel while the heat lamp is in use. Sitz baths are also used to promote healing.

Urinary tract infections and epididymitis are possible complications after prostatectomy. The patient is assessed for their occurrence; if they occur, the nurse administers antibiotics as prescribed.

Because the risk for infection continues after discharge from the hospital, the patient and family need to be instructed to monitor for signs and symptoms of infection (fever, chills, sweating, myalgia, dysuria, urinary frequency, and urgency). The patient and family are instructed to contact the urologist if these symptoms occur.

DEEP VEIN THROMBOSIS

Because patients undergoing prostatectomy have a high incidence of DVT and pulmonary embolism, the physician may prescribe prophylactic (preventive) low-dose heparin therapy. The nurse assesses the patient frequently after surgery for manifestations of DVT and applies elastic compression stockings to reduce the risk for DVT and pulmonary embolism. Nursing and medical management of DVT and pulmonary embolism are described in Chapters 31 and 23, respectively. The patient who is receiving heparin must be closely monitored for excessive bleeding.

OBSTRUCTED CATHETER

After a TUR, the catheter must drain well; an obstructed catheter produces distention of the prostatic capsule and resultant hemorrhage. Furosemide (Lasix) may be prescribed to promote urination and initiate postoperative diuresis, thereby helping to keep the catheter patent.

The nurse observes the lower abdomen to ensure that the catheter has not become blocked. An overdistended bladder manifests a distinct, rounded swelling above the pubis.

The drainage bag, dressings, and incisional site are examined for bleeding. The color of the urine is noted and documented; a change in color from pink to amber indicates reduced bleeding. Blood pressure, pulse, and respirations are monitored and compared with baseline preoperative vital signs to detect hypotension. The nurse also observes the patient for restlessness, diaphoresis, pallor, any drop in blood pressure, and an increasing pulse rate.

Drainage of the bladder may be accomplished by gravity through a closed sterile drainage system. A three-way drainage system is useful in irrigating the bladder and preventing clot formation (Fig. 49-5). Continuous irrigation may be used with TUR. Some urologists leave an indwelling catheter attached to a dependent drainage system. Gentle irrigation of the catheter may be prescribed to remove any obstructing clots.

If the patient complains of pain, the tubing is examined. The drainage system is irrigated, if indicated and prescribed, to clear any obstruction. Usually, the catheter is irrigated with 50 mL of irrigating fluid at a time. The amount of fluid recovered in the drainage bag must equal the amount of fluid injected. Overdistention of the bladder is avoided, because it can induce secondary hemorrhage by stretching the coagulated blood vessels in the prostatic capsule.

To prevent traction on the bladder, the drainage tube (not the catheter) is taped to the shaved inner thigh. If a cystostomy catheter is in place, it is taped to the abdomen. The nurse explains the purpose of the catheter to the patient and assures him that the urge to void results from the presence of the catheter and from bladder spasms. He is cautioned not to pull on the catheter, because this causes bleeding and subsequent catheter blockage, which leads to urinary retention.

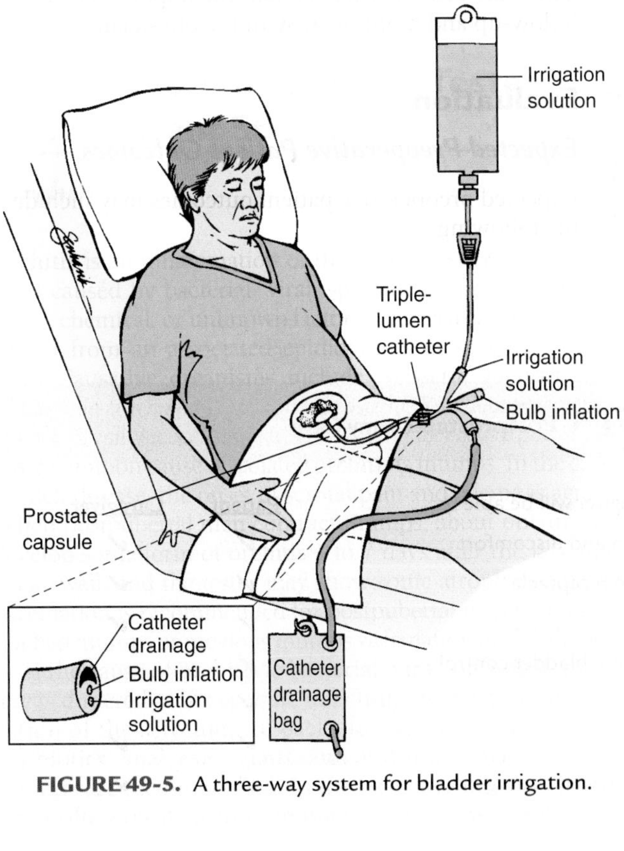

FIGURE 49-5. A three-way system for bladder irrigation.

COMPLICATIONS WITH CATHETER REMOVAL

After the catheter is removed (usually when the urine appears clear), urine may leak around the wound for several days in the patient who has undergone perineal, suprapubic, or retropubic surgery. The cystostomy tube may be removed before or after the urethral catheter is removed. Some urinary incontinence may occur after catheter removal, and the patient is informed that this is likely to subside over time.

SEXUAL DYSFUNCTION

Depending on the type of surgery, the patient may experience sexual dysfunction related to erectile dysfunction, decreased libido, and fatigue. These issues may become a concern to the patient soon after surgery or in the weeks to months of rehabilitation. Several options to restore erectile function are discussed with the patient by the surgeon or urologist. These options may include medications, surgically placed implants, or negative-pressure devices. A decrease in libido is usually related to the impact of the surgery on the man's body. Reassurance that the usual level of libido will return after recuperation from surgery is often helpful for the patient and his partner. The patient should be aware that he may experience fatigue during rehabilitation from surgery. This fatigue may also decrease his libido and alter his enjoyment of usual activities.

Nursing interventions include assessing for the presence of sexual dysfunction after surgery. Providing a private and confidential environment to discuss issues of sexuality is important. The emotional challenges of prostate surgery and its consequences need to be carefully explored with the patient and his partner. Providing the opportunity to discuss these issues can be very beneficial to the patient. For patients who demonstrate significant problems adjusting to their sexual dysfunction, a referral to a sex therapist may be indicated.

Promoting Home and Community-Based Care

TEACHING PATIENTS SELF-CARE

The patient undergoing prostatectomy may be discharged within several days. The length of the hospital

Testicular Cancer

Testicular cancer is the most common cancer in men between the ages of 15 and 40 years, although it can occur in males of any age. It is estimated that there are almost 9000 new cases of testicular cancer and almost 400 deaths in the United States annually. It is a highly treatable and usually curable form of cancer. The cure rate is greater than 90% for all stages of the disease (ACS, 2005).

Classification of Testicular Tumors

The testicles contain several types of cells, each of which may develop into one or more types of cancer. The type of cancer determines the appropriate treatment and affects the prognosis. Testicular cancers are classified as germinal or nongerminal (stromal). Secondary testicular cancers may also occur.

Germinal Tumors

More than 90% of all cancers of the testicle are germinal; germinal tumors may be further classified as seminomas or nonseminomas. About half of all germinal tumors are seminomas, or tumors that develop from the sperm-producing cells of the testes. Seminomas tend to remain localized, whereas nonseminomatous tumors grow quickly. In addition, nonseminomas tend to develop earlier in life than seminomas, usually occurring in men in their 20s. Examples of nonseminomas include teratocarcinomas, choriocarcinomas, yolk sac carcinomas, and embryonal carcinomas. Most tumors are mixtures of at least two different tumor types.

Nongerminal Tumors

Testicular cancer may also develop in the supportive and hormone-producing tissues, or stroma, of the testicles. The two main types of stromal tumors are Leydig cell tumors and Sertoli cell tumors. Although these tumors infrequently spread beyond the testicle, a small number metastasize and tend to be resistant to chemotherapy and radiation therapy.

Secondary Testicular Tumors

Secondary testicular tumors are those that have metastasized to the testicle from other organs. Lymphoma is the most common cause of secondary testicular cancer. Cancers may also spread to the testicles from the prostate gland, lung, skin (melanoma), kidney, and other organs. The prognosis with these cancers is usually poor, because they typically also spread to other organs. Treatment depends on the specific type of cancer (ACS, 2005).

Risk Factors

Risk factors for testicular cancer include undescended testicles (**cryptorchidism**), a family history of testicular cancer, and cancer of one testicle, which increases the risk in the other testicle. Other risk factors include race and ethnicity: Caucasian American men have a five times greater risk than that of African American men and more than double the risk of Asian American men. Occupational hazards, including exposure to chemicals encountered in mining, oil and gas production, and leather processing, have been suggested as possible risk factors. An association of prenatal exposure to DES with testicular cancer has been suggested, but scientific evidence is lacking. Recent studies have demonstrated that vasectomy does not pose a greater risk of testicular cancer (ACS, 2005).

Clinical Manifestations

The symptoms appear gradually, with a mass or lump on the testicle and usually painless enlargement of the testis. The patient may report heaviness in the scrotum, inguinal area, or lower abdomen. Backache (from retroperitoneal node extension), abdominal pain, weight loss, and general weakness may result from metastasis. Enlargement of the testis without pain is a significant diagnostic finding. Testicular tumors tend to metastasize early, spreading from the testis to the lymph nodes in the retroperitoneum and to the lungs.

Assessment and Diagnostic Findings

Monthly TSEs are effective in detecting testicular cancer (Chart 49-6). Accurate monthly self-assessment by the patient and annual testicular examinations can reveal signs and lead to early diagnosis and treatment of this disease. Teaching men of all ages to perform TSE is an important health promotion intervention for early detection of testicular cancer. Because testicular cancer occurs most often in young adults, TSE should begin during adolescence.

Human chorionic gonadotropin and alpha-fetoprotein are tumor markers that may be elevated in patients with testicular cancer. Tumor marker levels in the blood are used for diagnosis, staging, and monitoring the response to treatment. Other diagnostic tests include IV urography to detect any ureteral deviation caused by a tumor mass, lymphangiography to assess the extent of tumor spread to the lymphatic system, and ultrasound examination to determine the presence and size of the testicular mass.

A CT of the abdomen and pelvis is performed to determine the extent of the disease in the retroperitoneum and pelvis. A chest x-ray is commonly performed to assess for metastasis in the lungs. Depending on the patient's signs and symptoms and results of the chest x-ray, CT of the chest may be performed. Magnetic resonance imaging (MRI) may be performed to assess the brain and spinal cord for metastasis. Positron emission tomography (PET) is used to evaluate enlarged lymph nodes for active tumor. Microscopic analysis of tissue is the only definitive way to determine whether cancer is present, but it is usually performed at the time of surgery rather than as a part of the diagnostic workup, to reduce the risk of promoting spread of the cancer (ACS, 2005).

Medical Management

Testicular cancer, one of the most curable solid tumors, is highly responsive to treatment. The goals of management are to eradicate the disease and achieve a cure. Treatment selection is based on the cell type and the anatomic extent

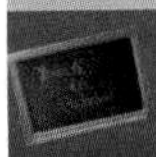

CHART 49-6

Patient Education

Testicular Self-Examination

Testicular self-examination (TSE) is to be performed once a month. The test is neither difficult nor time-consuming. A convenient time is usually after a warm bath or shower when the scrotum is more relaxed.

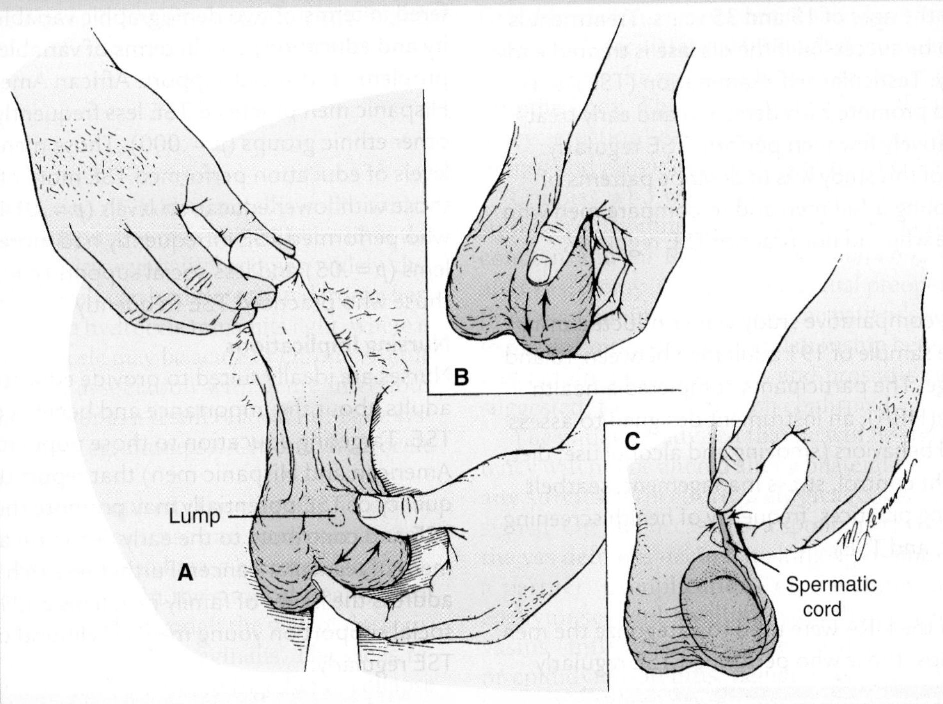

1. Use both hands to palpate the testis. The normal testicle is smooth and uniform in consistency.
2. With the index and middle fingers under the testis and the thumb on top, roll the testis gently in a horizontal plane between the thumb and fingers (**A**).
3. Feel for any evidence of a small lump or abnormality.
4. Follow the same procedure and palpate upward along the testis (**B**).
5. Locate and palpate the epididymis (**C**), a cord-like structure on the top and back of the testicle that stores and transports sperm. Also locate and palpate the spermatic cord.
6. Repeat the examination for the other testis, epididymis, and spermatic cord. It is normal to find that one testis is larger than the other.
7. If you find any evidence of a small, pea-like lump or if the testis is swollen (possibly from an infection or tumor), consult your physician.

of the disease. The testis is removed by orchiectomy through an inguinal incision with a high ligation of the spermatic cord. A gel-filled prosthesis can be implanted. After unilateral orchiectomy for testicular cancer, most patients experience no impairment of endocrine function. However, some patients have decreased hormonal levels, suggesting that the unaffected testis is not functioning at normal levels. Retroperitoneal lymph node dissection (RPLND) may be performed after orchiectomy to prevent lymphatic spread of the cancer. More recently, laparoscopic RPLND has become a preferred alterative to the more invasive open RPLND for early-stage nonseminomatous germ cell testicular cancer (Bhayani, Allaf & Kavoussi, 2004). Although libido and orgasm are usually unimpaired after RPLND, the patient may develop ejaculatory dysfunction with resultant infertility. Because sperm quality is reduced in men with testicular cancer, banking of sperm before treatment may be considered (Ragni, Somigliana, Restelli, et al., 2003).

As previously stated, testicular cancers are classified as either seminomas or nonseminomas for determining treatment; seminomatous types are more sensitive to radiation therapy. Research has demonstrated that for stage IIA/B seminomas, radiation therapy alone provides excellent results for the majority of patients. Postoperative irradiation

Nursing Management

Ice bags are applied intermittently to the scrotum for several hours after surgery to reduce swelling and to relieve discomfort. The nurse advises the patient to wear cotton, Jockey-type briefs for added comfort and support. He may become greatly concerned about the discoloration of the scrotal skin and superficial swelling. These are temporary conditions that occur frequently after vasectomy and may be relieved by sitz baths.

Sexual intercourse may be resumed as desired, although fertility remains for a varying time after vasectomy, until the spermatozoa stored distal to the severed vas deferens have been evacuated. Other methods of contraception should be used until infertility is confirmed by an examination of ejaculate. To determine sterility, some physicians examine a specimen 4 weeks after the vasectomy, and others examine two consecutive specimens 1 month apart. Still others consider a patient sterile after 36 ejaculations.

Vasovasostomy (Sterilization Reversal)

Microsurgical techniques are used to reverse a vasectomy (vasovasostomy) and restore patency to the vas deferens. Many men have sperm in their ejaculate after a reversal, and 40% to 75% can impregnate a partner.

Banking Sperm

Storing fertile semen in a sperm bank before a vasectomy is an option for men who face an unforeseen life event and may want to father a child at a later time. In addition, if a man is about to undergo a procedure or treatment (eg, radiation therapy to the pelvis, chemotherapy) that may affect his fertility, sperm banking may be considered. This procedure usually requires several visits to the facility where the sperm is stored under hypothermic conditions. The semen is produced by masturbation and collected in a sterile container for storage.

Conditions Affecting the Penis

Hypospadias and Epispadias

Hypospadias and epispadias are congenital anomalies of the urethral opening. In hypospadias, the urethral opening is a groove on the underside of the penis. In epispadias, the urethral opening is on the dorsum. These anatomic abnormalities may be repaired by various types of plastic surgery, usually when the boy is very young.

Phimosis

Phimosis, a condition in which the foreskin is constricted so that it cannot be retracted over the glans, can occur congenitally or as a result of inflammation and edema. With the trend away from routine circumcision of newborns, early instruction should be given about cleansing the prepuce. If the preputial area is not cleaned, normal secretions accumulate, causing inflammation (balanitis), which can lead to adhesions and fibrosis. The thickened secretions become encrusted with urinary salts and calcify, forming calculi in the prepuce. In elderly men, penile carcinoma may develop. Phimosis is corrected by circumcision (see later discussion).

Paraphimosis is a condition in which the foreskin is retracted behind the glans and, because of narrowness and subsequent edema, cannot be returned to its usual position (covering the glans). Paraphimosis is treated by firmly compressing the glans to reduce its size and then pushing the glans back while simultaneously moving the prepuce forward (manual reduction). Circumcision is usually indicated after the inflammation and edema subside.

Cancer of the Penis

Cancer of the penis appears on the skin of the penis as a painless, wartlike growth or ulcer. Cancer of the penis can involve the glans, the coronal sulcus under the prepuce, the corporal bodies, the urethra, and regional or distant lymph nodes. **Bowen's disease** is a form of squamous cell carcinoma in situ of the penile shaft. Typically, a man delays seeking treatment for more than a year, probably because of guilt, embarrassment, or ignorance.

Cancer of the penis can develop in each of the various types of cells of the penis. The type of cancer determines the seriousness of the disease. About 95% of **penile cancers** develop from the flat skin cells called squamous cells. This particular type of cancer of the penis can develop anywhere on the penis; however, it is most common on the foreskin. Melanomas and basal cell carcinomas each account for 2% of all diagnosed penile cancers. Unlike basal cell cancer, melanoma is more serious and can spread rapidly. Sarcomas of the penis account for 1% of penile cancers. They develop from blood vessels, smooth muscle, or other connective tissue cells. Verrucous carcinoma is an uncommon form of squamous cell carcinoma that can occur on the penis. It resembles a benign and precancerous condition such as a genital wart. It is considered low-grade and can spread deeply into the tissue, but rarely to distant parts of the body (ACS, 2005).

Known risk factors for penile cancer include HPV infection, smoking, smegma (oily secretions from the skin, dead skin cells, and bacteria under the foreskin), phimosis (constricted foreskin), previous treatment of psoriasis, age (55 years and older), and AIDS. It is also suggested that circumcision leads to improved hygiene and thus decreases the risk of penile cancer (ACS, 2005).

Prevention

According to the ACS (2005), the best way to reduce the risk of penile cancer is to avoid known risk factors whenever possible. In the past, circumcision has been suggested as a major step toward prevention. This suggestion was based on studies that reported much lower penile cancer rates among circumcised men than among uncircumcised men. Avoiding sexual practices that are likely to result in HPV infection may reduce the risk of penile cancer.

Medical Management

Surgery is the most common treatment of all forms of penile cancer. Surgical procedures include simple excision, electrodesiccation and curettage, cryosurgery, Mohs' surgery (microscopically controlled surgery), laser surgery, wide local excision, circumcision, and surgical removal of part of the penis or the entire penis (penectomy). Partial penectomy is preferred to total penectomy if possible, because patients can then participate in sexual intercourse and stand for urination. The shaft of the penis can still respond to sexual arousal with an erection and has the sensory capacity for orgasm and ejaculation. Total penectomy is indicated if the tumor is not amenable to conservative treatment. After a total penectomy, the patient may still experience orgasm with stimulation of the perineum and scrotal area.

Topical chemotherapy with 5-fluorouracil cream is an option in selected patients. Radiation therapy is used to treat small squamous cell carcinomas of the penis and for palliation in advanced tumors or cases of lymph node metastasis.

Priapism

Priapism is an uncontrolled, persistent erection of the penis that causes the penis to become large, hard, and painful. It results from either neural or vascular causes, including sickle cell thrombosis, leukemic cell infiltration, spinal cord tumors or injury, and tumor invasion of the penis or its vessels. It may also occur with use of medications that affect the central nervous system, antihypertensive agents, antidepressant medications, and substances injected into the penis to treat erectile dysfunction. This condition can cause gangrene and often results in impotence, whether or not it is treated.

Priapism is a urologic emergency. The goal of therapy is to improve venous drainage of the corpora cavernosa to prevent ischemia, fibrosis, and impotence. The initial treatment is directed at relieving the erection and includes bed rest and sedation. The corpora may be irrigated with an anticoagulant, which allows stagnant blood to be aspirated. Shunting procedures to divert the blood from the turgid corpora cavernosa to the venous system (corpora cavernosa–saphenous vein shunt) or into the corpus spongiosum–glans penis compartment may be attempted.

Peyronie's Disease

Peyronie's disease involves the buildup of fibrous plaques in the sheath of the corpus cavernosum. These plaques are not visible when the penis is relaxed. However, when the penis is erect, curvature occurs that can be painful and can make sexual intercourse difficult or impossible. Peyronie's disease occurs primarily in middle-aged and older men. Although the plaques may shrink over time, surgical removal may be necessary.

Urethral Stricture

Urethral stricture is a condition in which a section of the urethra is narrowed. It can occur congenitally or from a scar along the urethra. Traumatic injury to the urethra (eg, from instrumentation or infections) can result in strictures. Treatment involves dilation of the urethra or, in severe cases, urethrotomy (surgical removal of the stricture).

Circumcision

Circumcision is the excision of the foreskin, or prepuce, of the glans penis. It is usually performed in infancy. In adults, it is part of the treatment for phimosis, paraphimosis, and recurrent infections of the glans and foreskin and also may be performed at the personal desire of the patient.

Postoperatively, a petrolatum (Vaseline) gauze dressing is applied and changed as indicated. The patient is observed for bleeding. Because considerable pain may occur after circumcision, analgesic agents are administered as needed.

Critical Thinking Exercises

1 A 54-year-old electrical engineer who has just been diagnosed with prostate cancer is now admitted to undergo a laparoscopic radical prostatectomy. As you are preparing him for surgery, he asks you if the surgery will cause him to be impotent and if this is the best procedure for treatment of his prostate cancer. Describe your immediate response to this patient and the rationale behind your response. Briefly explain resources that you could make immediately available to this patient.

2 A 78-year-old man with type 2 diabetes has undergone TURP. What immediate postoperative assessment is indicated when he arrives from the postanesthetic care unit and for the first 24 hours after surgery? Later during his hospital stay, your patient develops urosepsis and is eventually discharged with an indwelling urinary catheter. What discharge teaching and preparation are indicated for this patient? How would your discharge teaching and preparation differ if the patient lived alone? If he had significant visual impairment caused by diabetic retinopathy?

3 A 28-year-old man is seeking treatment for urinary frequency. He informs you that he believes that he has a urinary tract infection. When you are obtaining the health history, he reports that he has multiple sexual partners outside his marriage. He has undergone treatment for gonorrhea within the past 6 months. Briefly discuss the incidence of acute uncomplicated cystitis in males. What are your major concerns regarding the patient's complaint of urinary frequency? Describe important aspects

that must be addressed when teaching this patient about safer sex. What community resources should you make available to this patient and his wife?

4 One of your patients, a 32-year-old man with a spinal cord injury, tells you that he has seen an advertisement on television for vardenafil (Levitra). He asks you if it would help him to have an erection. How would you respond, and what information would you give him about Levitra? How would your approach differ if your patient were a 46-year-old man with sexual dysfunction caused by long-standing diabetes? If he were a 58-year-old man who experiences angina with exertion?

5 ebp A college athlete who describes his health as excellent comes to the student health clinic because he noticed a walnut-size mass in his testicle when showering. Describe the specific components of the history and physical examination that would be appropriate. What would be your concerns, and what referrals would be warranted for him? What is the evidence base for the effectiveness of testicular self-examination in detection of testicular cancer? How strong is that evidence, and what criteria did you use to determine the strength of the evidence?

6 During a community health fair, you are approached by a 49-year-old African American man who asks you about his risk of prostate cancer. He informs you that his father has been recently diagnosed with prostate cancer and is scheduled to begin treatment within the next week. He wants you to explain his risk of developing prostate cancer. Develop a plan to address this issue with him at the health fair and provide the rationale for your plan. How would your responses differ if you saw the patient during an office visit to follow-up an elevated PSA test result?

REFERENCES AND SELECTED READINGS

BOOKS

Abel, P. & Lalani, E. (Eds.). (2003). *Prostate cancer: Clinical and scientific aspects—Bridging the gap.* London: Imperial College Press.

Abeloff, M., Armitage, J., Niederhuber, M., et al. (Eds.) (2004). *Clinical oncology* (2nd ed.). Philadelphia: Churchill Livingstone.

American Cancer Society. (2005). *Cancer facts and figures 2005.* Atlanta: Author.

Annon, J. S. (1976). *Behavioral treatment of sexual problems: Brief therapy.* Hagerstown, MD: Harper & Row.

Broderick, G. (2005). *Oral pharmacotherapy for sexual dysfunction: A guide to clinical management.* Totowa, NJ: Humana Press.

Campbell, M. F., Retik, A. B. & Walsh, P. C. (Eds.). (2002). *Campbell's urology* (8th ed.). Philadelphia: W. B. Saunders.

Chorba, T., Tao, G., & Irwin, K. L. (2004). Sexually transmitted diseases. In Litwin, M. S. & Saigal, C. S. (Eds.). *Urologic diseases in America.* NIH Pub. No. 04-5512. U.S. Department of Health and Human Services, Public Health Service, National Institutes of Health, National Institute of Diabetes and Digestive and Kidney Diseases. Washington, DC: US Government Publishing Office.

DeVita, V., Hellman, S. & Rosenberg, S. (Eds.) (2005). *Cancer: Principles and practice of oncology* (7th ed.). Philadelphia: Lippincott Williams & Wilkins.

Fabrizio, M. D., Soderdahl, D., & Schellhammer, P. F. (2003). Laparoscopic radical prostatectomy. In Cadeddu, J. A. (Ed.). *Laparoscopic urologic oncology.* Totowa, NJ: Humana Press.

Jones, S. J. (2003). *Overcoming impotence: A leading urologist tells you everything you need to know.* Amherst, NY: Prometheus Books.

Kantoff, P. W., Carroll, A. V. & D'Amico, A. V. (Eds.) (2002). *Prostate cancer: Principles and practice.* Philadelphia: Lippincott Williams & Wilkins.

Klein, E. A. (Ed.) (2004). *Management of prostate cancer* (Current Clinical Oncology). Totowa, NJ: Humana Press.

Kufe, D., Pollock, R., Weicheslbaum, R., et al. (2003). *Holland-Frei cancer medicine.* Philadelphia: B. C. Decker.

National Institutes of Health. (2004). *Prostate enlargement: Benign prostatic hyperplasia.* NIH Publication No. 04-3012. Bethesda, MD: U.S. Department of Health and Human Services.

Otto, S. (Ed). (2003). *Oncology nursing clinical reference.* St. Louis: Mosby.

Perez, C. A., Brady, L. W., Halperin, E. C., et al. (Eds.). (2004). *Principles and practices of radiation oncology* (3rd ed.). Philadelphia: Lippincott Williams & Wilkins.

Plaut, S., Graziottin, A. & Heaton, J. (2004). *Sexual dysfunction fast facts series.* London: Health Press.

Porth, C. M. (2005). *Pathophysiology: Concepts of altered health states* (7th ed.). Philadelphia: Lippincott Williams & Wilkins.

Richie, J. & D'Amico, A. (Eds.). (2004). *Urologic oncology.* Philadelphia: Elsevier/Saunders.

Segraves, B., (2005). *Handbook of sexual dysfunction.* New York: Marcel Dekker.

U.S. Surgeon General. (2001). *U.S. Surgeon General's call to action to promote sexual health and responsible sexual behavior.* Washington, DC: United States Public Health Service.

Yarbro, C. H., Frogge, M. H. & Goodman, M. (2004). *Cancer symptom management* (3rd ed.). Sudbury, MA: Jones & Bartlett.

JOURNALS

**Asterisks indicate nursing research articles.*

General

Kelly, D. (2004). Male sexuality in theory and practice. *Nursing Clinics of North America, 39*(2), 341–356.

*Loeb, S. J. (2004). Older men's health: Motivation, self-ratings, and behaviors. *Nursing Research, 53*(3), 198–206.

McInnes, R. A. (2003). Chronic illness and sexuality. *Medical Journal of Australia, 179*(5), 263–266.

O'Donnell, A. B., Araujo, A. B. & McKinlay, J. B. (2004). The health of normally aging men: The Massachusetts male aging study (1987–2004). *Experimental Gerontology, 39*(7), 975–984.

Sussman, D. O. (2004). Pharmacokinetics, pharmacodynamics, and efficacy of phosphodiesterase type 5 inhibitors. *Journal of the American Osteopathic Association, 104*(3 Suppl 4), S11–S15.

Wren, T. (2004). Penile and testicular disorders. *Nursing Clinics of North America, 39*(2), 319–326.

*Wynd, C. A. (2002). Testicular self-examination in young adult men. *Nursing Research, 34*(3), 251–255.

Youngkin, E. Q. (2004). The myths and truths of mature intimacy: Mature guidance for nurse practitioners. *Advance for Nurse Practitioners, 12*(9), 45–48.

Epididymitis

Cole, F. L. & Vogler, R. (2004). The acute, nontraumatic scrotum: Assessment, diagnosis, and management. *Journal of the American Academy of Nurse Practitioners, 16*(2), 50–56.

De Backer, A. I., Mortele, K. J., De Roeck, J., et al. (2004). Tuberculous epididymitis associated with abdominal lymphadenopathy. *European Radiology, 14*(4), 748–751.

Kodner, C. (2003). Sexually transmitted infections in men. *Primary Care: Clinics in Office Practice, 30*(1), 173–191.

Benign Prostatic Hyperplasia

Denmark-Wahnefried, W., Robertson, P. J., Polascik, T. J., et al. (2004). Pilot study to explore effects of low-fat, flaxseed-supplement diet on proliferation of benign prostatic epithelium and prostate-specific antigen. *Urology, 63*(5), 900–904.

Gilchrist, K. (2004). Benign prostatic hyperplasia: Is it a precursor to prostatic cancer? *Nurse Practitioner, 29*(6), 30–37.

Gordon, A. E. & Shaughnessy, A. D. (2003). Saw palmetto for prostate disorders. *American Family Physician, 67*(6), 1281–1283.

Joseph, M. A., Harlow, S. D., Wei, J. T., et al. (2003). Risk factors for lower urinary tract symptoms in a population-based sample of African-American men. *American Journal of Epidemiology, 157*(10), 906–914.

Kirby, R. S. (2004). Selecting long-term medical therapy for BPH. *Contemporary Urology, 16*(1), 12,15–16,18.

Laustsen, G. & Wimett, L. (2004). Drug approval highlights for 2003. *Nurse Practitioner, 29*(2), 8–21.

Roberts, R. O., Jacobson, D. J., Rhodes, T., et al. (2004). Serum sex hormones and measures of benign prostatic hyperplasia. *Prostate, 61*(2), 124–131.

Sexual Dysfunction

Araujo, A. B., Mohr, B. A. & McKinlay, J. B. (2004). Changes in sexual function in middle-aged and older men: Longitudinal data from the Massachusetts Male Aging Study. *Journal of the American Geriatrics Society, 52*(9), 1502–1509.

Aust, T. R. & Lewis-Jones, D. I. (2004). Retrograde ejaculation and male infertility. *Hospital Medicine, 65*(6), 361–364.

Black, P. K. (2004). Psychological, sexual and cultural issues for patients with a stoma. *British Journal of Nursing, 13*(12), 692–697.

Fazio, L. & Brock, G. (2004). Erectile dysfunction: Management update. *Canadian Medical Association Journal, 170*(9), 1429–1437.

Foresta, C., Caretta, N., Garolla, A., et al. (2003). Erectile function in elderly: Role of androgens. *Journal of Endocrinological Investigation, 26* (3 Suppl), 77–81.

Giulini, S., Pesce, F., Madgar, I., et al. (2004). Influence of multiple transrectal electroejaculations on semen parameters and intracytoplasmic sperm injection outcome. *Fertility and Sterility, 82*(1), 200–204.

Shabsigh, R. (2003). Hypogonadism and erectile dysfunction: The role for testosterone therapy. *International Journal of Impotence Research, 15*(4), S9–S13.

Shell, J. A. (2002). Evidence-based practice for symptom management in adults with cancer: Sexual dysfunction. *Oncology Nursing Forum, 29*(1), 53–69.

Shieh, J. Y., Chen, S. U., Wang, Y. H., et al. (2003). A protocol of electro-ejaculation and systematic assisted reproductive technology achieved high efficiency and efficacy for pregnancy for anejaculatory men with spinal cord injury. *Archives of Physical Medicine and Rehabilitation, 84*(4), 535–540.

Stipetich, R. L., Abel, L. J., Blatt, H. J., et al. (2002). Nursing assessment of sexual function following permanent prostate brachytherapy for patients with early-stage prostate cancer. *Clinical Journal of Oncology Nursing, 6*(5), 271–274.

Sexually Transmitted Diseases

Shlay, J. C., McClung, M. W., Patnaik, J. L., et al. (2004). Comparison of sexually transmitted disease prevalence by reported condom use: Errors among consistent condom users seen at an urban sexually transmitted disease clinic. *Sexually Transmitted Diseases, 31*(9), 526–532.

Sternberg, P. & Hubley, J. (2004). Evaluating men's involvement as a strategy in sexual and reproductive health promotion. *Health Promotion International, 19*(3), 389–396.

Vazquez, F., Otero, L., Ordas, J., et al. (2004). Up to date in sexually transmitted infections: Epidemiology, diagnostic approaches and treatments. *Enfermedades Infecciosas y Microbiologia Clinica, 22*(7), 392–411.

Erectile Dysfunction

Ahmed-Jushuf, I. H., Griffiths, V., Hall, J., et al. (2004). Treatment of erectile dysfunction. *International Journal of STD and AIDS, 15*(9), 639.

Derouet, H., Osterhage, J. & Sittinger, H. (2004). Erectile dysfunction: Epidemiology, physiology, etiology, diagnosis, and therapy. *Urologue, 43*(2), 197–207.

Dinsmore, W. (2004). Treatment of erectile dysfunction. *International Journal of STD and AIDS, 15*(4), 215–221.

Heaton, J. P. & Adams, M. A. (2004). Causes of erectile dysfunction. *Endocrine, 23*(2–3), 119–123.

Lewis, J. H., Rosen, R., Goldstein, I., et al. (2003). Erectile dysfunction: A panel's recommendations for management. *American Journal of Nursing, 103*(10), 48–57.

Milbank, A. J. & Montague, D. K. (2004). Surgical management of erectile dysfunction. *Endocrine, 23*(2–3), 161–165.

Shabsigh, R. & Anastasiadis, A. G. (2003). Erectile dysfunction. *Annual Review of Medicine, 54*, 153–168.

Wijesinha, S. (2003). Male reproductive health. *Australian Family Physician, 32*(6), 408–411.

Cancer of the Penis

Singh, I. & Khaitan, A. (2003). Current trends in the management of carcinoma of the penis: A review. *International Urology and Nephrology, 35*(2), 215–225.

Stancik, I. & Holtl, W. (2003). Penile cancer: Review of the recent literature. *Current Opinion in Urology, 13*(6), 467–472.

Syed, S., Eng, T. Y., Thomas, C. R., et al. (2003). Current issues in the management of advanced squamous cell carcinoma of the penis. *Urologic Oncology, 21*(6), 431–438.

Windahl, T., Skeppner, E., Andersson, S. O., et al. (2004). Sexual function and satisfaction in men after laser treatment for penile carcinoma. *Journal of Urology, 172*(2), 648–651.

Prostate Cancer

Abel, L., Dafoe-Lambie, J., Butler, W. M., et al. (2003). Treatment outcomes and quality-of-life issues for patients treated with prostate brachytherapy. *Clinical Journal of Oncology Nursing, 7*(1), 48–54.

Ahaghotu, C., Baffoe-Bonnie, A., Kittles, R., et al. (2004). Clinical characteristics of African-American men with hereditary prostate cancer: The AAHPC Study. *Prostate Cancer and Prostatic Disease, 7*(2), 165–169.

Antenor, J. A., Han, M., Roehl, K., et al. (2004). Relationship between initial prostate specific antigen level and subsequent prostate cancer detection in a longitudinal screening study. *Journal of Urology, 172*(1), 90–93.

Beer, T. M., Garzotto, M., Henner, W. D., et al. (2004). Multiple cycles of intermittent chemotherapy in metastatic androgen-independent prostate cancer. *British Journal of Cancer, 91*(8), 1425–1427.

Bosetti, C., Talamini, R., Montella, M., et al. (2004). Retinol, carotenoids and the risk of prostate cancer: A case-control study from Italy. *International Journal of Cancer, 112*(4), 689–692.

Calabrese, D. A. (2004). Prostate cancer in older men. *Urologic Nursing, 24*(4), 258–264.

Di Blasio, C. J., Rhee, A. C., Cho, D., et al. (2003). Predicting clinical end points: Treatment nomograms in prostate cancer. *Seminars in Oncology, 30*(5), 567–586.

Eastham, J. A. (2003). High-risk localized prostate cancer: Multimodal treatment strategies combining neoadjuvant hormonal therapy and/or chemotherapy with radical prostatectomy. *Expert Opinion on Emerging Drugs, 8*(2), 291–295.

Ellis, R. J., Kim, E., & Foor, R. (2004). Role of ProstaScint for brachytherapy in localized prostate adenocarcinoma. *Expert Review of Molecular Diagnostics, 4*(4), 435–441.

Eng, J., Ramsum, D., Verhoef, M., et al. (2003). A population-based survey of complementary and alternative medicine use in men recently diagnosed with prostate cancer. *Integrative Cancer Therapies, 2*(3), 212–216.

Fradet, Y. (2004). Bicalutamide (Casodex) in the treatment of prostate cancer. *Expert Review of Anticancer Therapy, 4*(1), 37–48.

Gunawardana, D., Lichtenstein, M., Better, N., et al. (2004). Results of strontium-89 therapy in patients with prostate cancer resistant to chemotherapy. *Clinical Nuclear Medicine, 29*(2), 81–85.

Incrocci, L., Hop, W. C., & Slob, A. K. (2003). Efficacy of sildenafil in an open label study as a continuation of a double-blind study in the treatment of erectile dysfunction after radiotherapy for prostate cancer. *Urology, 62*(1), 116–120.

Kirchhoff, T., Kauff, N. D., Mitra, N., et al. (2004). BRCA mutations and risk of prostate in Ashkenazi Jews. *Clinical Cancer Research, 10*(9), 2918–2921.

Lam, R. (2004). High dose ketoconazole plus hydrocortisone (HDK + HC). *Prostate Cancer Research Institute, 7*(2). Available at http://www.prostate-cancer.org/education/anderprv/Lam_HDK.html. Accessed July 30, 2006.

Liao, Z. & Datta, M. W. (2004). A simple computer program for calculating PSA recurrence in prostate cancer patients. *BMC Urology, 19*(4), 8.

Miyamoto, H. & Messing, E. M. (2004). Early versus late hormonal therapy for prostate cancer. *Current Urology Reports, 5*(3), 188–196.

Moul, J. W. & Fowler, J. E. Jr. (2003). Evolution of therapeutic approaches with luteinizing hormone-releasing hormone agonists in 2003. *Urology, 62*(6 Suppl. 1), 20–28.

Ogura, K., Ichioka, K., Terada, N., et al. (2004). Role of sildenafil citrate in treatment of erectile dysfunction after radical retropubic. *International Journal of Urology, 11*(3), 159–163.

Otto, S. J. & de Koning, H. G. (2004). Update on screening and early detection of prostate cancer. *Current Opinion in Urology, 14*(3), 151–156.

Perron, L., Bairati, I., Harel, F., et al. (2004). Antihypertensive drug use and the risk of prostate cancer (Canada). *Cancer Causes Control, 15*(6), 535–541.

Rocco, B., Matei, D. & deCobelli, O. (2004). Prostate cancer with low PSA levels. *New England Journal of Medicine, 35*(17), 1802–1803.

Sellers, D. B. & Ross, L. E. (2003). African American men, prostate cancer screening and informed decision making. *Journal of the National Medical Association, 95*(7), 618–625.

Sharifi, N., Gulley, J. L., & Dahut, W. L. (2005). Androgen deprivation therapy for prostate cancer. *Journal of the American Medical Association, 292*(2), 238–244.

Stamey, T. A., Caldwell, M., McNeal, J. E., et al. (2004). The prostate specific antigen era in the United States is over for prostate cancer: What happened in the last 20 years? *Journal of Urology, 172*(4, Part 1), 1297–1301.

Steranou, D., Batistatou, A., Kamina, S., et al. (2004). Expression of vascular endothelial growth factor (VEGF) and association with microvessel density in benign prostatic hyperplasia and prostate cancer. *In Vivo, 18*(2), 155–160.

Wilkinson, S. & Chodak, G. (2004). An evaluation of intermediate-dose ketoconazole in hormone refractory prostate cancer. *European Urology, 45*(5), 581–584.

Wilkinson, S., List, M., Sinner, M., et al. (2003). Educating African-Americans about prostate cancer: Impact on awareness and knowledge. *Urology, 61*(2), 308–313.

Woods, V., Montgomery, S. & Herring, R. P. (2004). Recruiting black/African American men for research on prostate cancer prevention. *Cancer, 100*(5), 1017–1025.

Wu, T. T. & Huang, J. K. (2004). The clinical usefulness of prostate-specific antigen (PSA) level and age-specific PSA reference ranges for detecting prostate cancer in Chinese. *Urology International, 72*(3), 208–211.

Prostate Surgery

Bishop, P. (2003). Bipolar transurethral resection of the prostate: A new approach. *AORN Journal, 77*(5), 979–983.

Chambers A. (2002). Transurethral resection syndrome: It does not have to be a mystery. *AORN Journal, 75*(1), 156–164,166,168–170.

Eaton, J. (2003). Detection of hyponatremia in the PACU. *Journal of PeriAnesthesia Nursing, 18*(6), 392–397.

Touijer, A. K. & Guillonneau, B. (2004). Laparoscopic radical prostatectomy. *Urological Oncology, 22*(2), 133–138.

Trabulski, E. J. & Guillonneau, B. (2005). Laparoscopic radical prostatectomy. *Journal of Urology, 173*(4), 1072–1079.

Testicular Cancer

Bhayani, S. B., Allaf, M. E. & Kavoussi, L. R. (2004). Laparoscopic RPLND for clinical stage I nonseminomatous germ cell testicular cancer: Current status. *Urologic Oncology, 22*(2), 145–148.

Brown, C. G. (2003). Testicular cancer: An overview. *MedSurg Nursing, 12*(1), 37–43.

Chung, P. W., Gospodarowicz, M. K., Panzarella, T., et al. (2004). Stage II testicular seminoma: Patterns of recurrence and outcome of treatment. *European Urology, 45*(6), 754–759.

Lipphardt, M. E. & Albers, P. (2004). Late relapse of testicular cancer. *World Journal of Urology, 22*(1), 47–54.

Raghavan, D. (2003). Testicular cancer: Maintaining the high cure rate. *Oncology, 17*(2), 218–229,234–237,293–294.

Ragni, G., Somigliana, E., Restelli, L., et al. (2003). Sperm banking and rate of assisted reproduction treatment: Insights form a 15-year cryopreservation program for male cancer patients. *Cancer, 97*(7), 1624–1629.

Taylor, J. S., Dube, C. E., Pipas, C. F., et al. (2004). Teaching the testicular exam: A model curriculum from "A" to "Zack." *Family Medicine, 36*(3), 209–213.

Prostatitis

Hua, V. N. & Schaeffer, A. J. (2004). Acute and chronic prostatitis. *Medical Clinics of North America, 88*(2), 483–494.

Kravchick, S., Cytron, S., Agulansky, L., et al. (2004). Acute prostatitis in middle-aged men: A prospective study. *BJU International, 93*(1), 93–96.

Pontari, M. A. & Ruggieri, M. R. (2004). Mechanisms in prostatitis/chronic pelvic pain syndrome. *Journal of Urology, 172*(3), 839–845.

Wolfgang, W. (2004). Treating chronic prostatitis: Antibiotics no, alpha-blockers maybe. *Annals of Internal Medicine, 141*(8), 639–640.

RESOURCES

Agencies

American Cancer Society, 1599 Clifton Road NE, Atlanta, GA 30326; 800-ACS-2345; Man-to-Man Support Group; http://www.cancer.org. Accessed June 2, 2006.

American Foundation for Urologic Disease, Prostate Cancer Support Network, 300 West Pratt, Suite 401, Baltimore, MD 21201-2463; 800-828-7866; http://www.afud.org. Accessed June 2, 2006.

CancerCare, 275 Seventh Avenue, New York, NY 10001; 800-813-HOPE (ext. 4673); http://www.cancercare.org. Accessed June 2, 2006.

Centers for Disease Control and Prevention, 1600 Clifton Road, Atlanta, GA 30333; 404-634-3311; http://www.cdc.gov/cancer/prostate/. Accessed June 2, 2006.

Impotence Anonymous and I-Anon, Impotence World Association, P.O. Box 410, Bowie, MD 20718-0410; 800-669-1603.

National Cancer Institute, Office of Cancer Communications, Building 31, Room 10A24, Bethesda, MD 20892; 800-4-CANCER; http://www.nci.nih.gov. Accessed June 2, 2006.

National Prostate Cancer Coalition, 1158 Fifteenth Street, NW, Washington, DC 20005; 888-245-9455; http://www.4npcc.org. Accessed June 2, 2006.

Us TOO International Prostate Cancer Survivor Support Group, 930 North York Road, Suite 50, Hinsdale, IL 60521-2993; 800-80-US-TOO; http://www.ustoo.com. Accessed June 2, 2006.

Printed Materials

Alterowitz, R. & Alterowitz, B. (2004). *Intimacy with impotence: The couple's guide to better sex after prostate disease.* Cambridge, MA: Da Capo.

Centeno, A. & Onik, G., (2004). *Prostate cancer: A patient's guide to treatment.* Omaha: Addicus Books.

Douglass, W. C. (2003). *Prostate problems: Safe, simple, effective relief.* Miami: Rhino Publishing.

Grimm, P., Blasko, J., & Sylvester, J., (2004). *The prostate cancer treatment book.* Hauppauge, NY: McGraw-Hill.

Kirby, R., Chapple, C., Barclay, C., Kassianos, G. (Eds.) (2005). *BPH best medicine.* Oxford: CSF Medical Communications Ltd.

Klein, E., Jamnicky, L., & Nam, R. (2004). *So you're having prostate surgery.* New York: John Wiley & Sons.

Marks, S., (2003). *Prostate and cancer: A family guide to diagnosis, treatment and survival* (3rd ed.). Philadelphia: Perseus.

Rosario, D. & MacDiarmid., S. (2005). *Rapid reference to BPH.* Rapid Reference Series. St. Louis: Mosby.

Rous, S. (2002). *The prostate book* (2nd ed.). New York: W. W. Norton.

Scardino, P. (2005). *Dr. Peter Scardino's prostate book: A comprehensive guide to overcoming and understanding prostate cancer, prostatitis, and prostate enlargement.* New York: Avery.

Simone, C. (2004). *The truth about prostate health: Prostate cancer, prevention, cancer life extension.* Princeton: Princeton Institute.

Schultz, R. E., & Oliver, A. W. (2000). *Humanizing prostate cancer: A physician-patient perspective.* White Stone, VA: Brandylane Publishers.

Wainrib, B. R., Haber, S. & Maguire, J. (2000). *Men, women and prostate cancer* (2nd ed.). Oakland, CA: New Harbinger Publications.

Walsh, P. C. & Worthington, J. F. (1997). *The prostate: A guide for men and the women who love them.* New York: Warner Books.

Walsh, P. C. & Worthington, J. F. (2002). *Dr. Patrick Walsh's guide to surviving prostate cancer.* New York: Warner Books.

UNIT 11

Immunologic Function

Case Study

Applying Concepts from NANDA, NIC, and NOC

An Immunosuppressed Patient With a History of Oral Infections

Mrs. Baker is a 52-year-old mother of three with severe rheumatoid arthritis. She has been taking prednisone, 10 mg daily for 6 months, as part of a treatment plan that will also include nonsteroidal anti-inflammatory drugs (NSAIDs) and disease-modifying antirheumatic drugs (DMARDs). Although her physician has tried to taper the prednisone, each time the dose is reduced Mrs. Baker experiences a painful flare-up of her rheumatoid arthritis and symptoms of steroid withdrawal. Mrs. Baker states that when her symptoms flare, she takes an extra dose of prednisone. She has had oral candidal disease twice in the preceding 3 months and has had frequent upper respiratory tract infections.

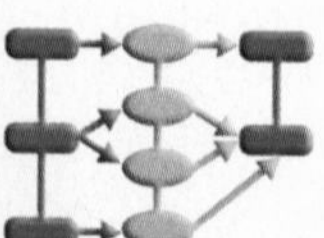

Turn to Appendix C to see a concept map that illustrates the relationships that exist between the nursing diagnoses, interventions, and outcomes for the patient's clinical problems.

Nursing Classifications and Languages

NANDA Nursing Diagnoses	NIC Nursing Interventions	NOC Nursing Outcomes Return to functional baseline status, stabilization of, or improvement in:
Risk for Infection—At risk for being invaded by pathogenic organisms	**Infection Protection**—Prevention and early detection of infection in a patient at risk	**Infection Severity**—Severity of infection and associated symptoms
Impaired Oral Mucous Membrane—Disruption of the lips and soft tissues of the oral cavity	**Infection Control**—Minimizing the acquisition and transmission of infectious agents	**Tissue Integrity: Skin and Mucous Membranes**—Structural intactness and normal physiologic function of skin and mucous membranes
Risk for Ineffective Therapeutic Regimen Management—Having the potential for developing a pattern of regulating and integrating into daily living a program for treatment of illness and the sequelae of illness that is unsatisfactory for meeting specific health goals	**Oral Health Maintenance**—Maintenance and promotion of oral hygiene and dental health for the patient at risk for developing oral or dental lesions	**Knowledge: Treatment Regimen**—Extent of understanding conveyed about the safe use of medication
	Teaching: Prescribed Medication—Preparing a patient to safely take prescribed medications and monitor their effects	

NANDA International (2005). *Nursing diagnoses: Definitions and classification 2005–2006.* Philadelphia: North American Nursing Diagnosis Association.
Dochterman, J. C. M. & Bulechek, G. M. (2004). *Nursing interventions classification (NIC)* (4th ed.). St. Louis: Mosby.
Iowa Outcomes Project © 2004. In Moorhead, S., Johnston, M. & Maas, M. (2004). *Nursing outcomes classification (NOC)* (3rd ed.). St. Louis: Mosby.
Dochterman, J. M. & Jones, D. A. (2003). *Unifying nursing languages: The harmonization of NANDA, NIC, and NOC.* Washington, D.C.: American Nurses Association.

CHAPTER 50

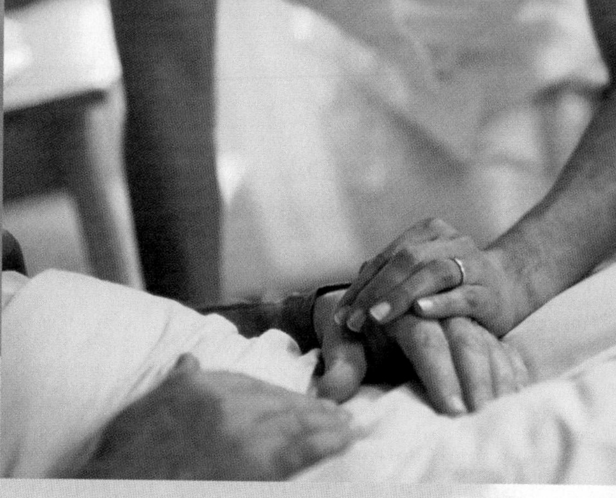

Assessment of Immune Function

Learning Objectives

On completion of this chapter, the learner will be able to:

1. Describe the body's general immune responses.
2. Discuss the stages of the immune response.
3. Differentiate between cellular and humoral immune responses.
4. Describe the effects of selected variables on function of the immune system.
5. Use assessment parameters for determining the patient's status of immune function.

The term **immunity** refers to the body's specific protective response to an invading foreign agent or organism. The immune system functions as the body's defense mechanism against invasion and allows a rapid response to foreign substances in a specific manner. Responses occur at the genetic and cellular levels. Any qualitative or quantitative change in the components of the immune system can produce profound effects on the integrity of the human organism. Immune function is affected by a variety of factors, such as central nervous system integrity, emotional status, medications, and the stress of illness, trauma, or surgery. Dysfunctions involving the immune system occur across the life span. Many are genetically based; others are acquired. Immune memory is a property of the immune system that provides protection against harmful microbial agents despite the timing of re-exposure to the agent. Tolerance is the process by which the immune system is programmed to eliminate foreign substances such as microbes, toxins, and cellular mutations but maintains the ability to accept self-antigens. Some credence is given to the concept of surveillance, in which the immune system is in a perpetual state of vigilance, screening and rejecting any invader that is recognized as foreign to the host. The term **immunopathology** refers to the study of diseases that result from dysfunctions within the immune system. Disorders of the immune system may stem from excesses or deficiencies of immunocompetent cells, alterations in the function of these cells, immunologic attack on self-antigens, or inappropriate or exaggerated responses to specific antigens (Table 50-1).

TABLE 50-1 Immune System Disorders

Disorder	Description
Autoimmunity	Normal protective immune response paradoxically turns against or attacks the body, leading to tissue damage
Hypersensitivity	Body produces inappropriate or exaggerated responses to specific antigens
Gammopathies	Immunoglobulins are overproduced
Immune deficiencies	
Primary	Deficiency results from improper development of immune cells or tissues; usually congenital or inherited
Secondary	Deficiency results from some interference with an already developed immune system; usually acquired later in life

To gain insight into immunopathology and the growing number of immunologic disorders, and to assess and care

Glossary

agglutination: clumping effect occurring when an antibody acts as a cross-link between two antigens

antibody: a protein substance developed by the body in response to and interacting with a specific antigen

antigen: substance that induces the production of antibodies

antigenetic determinant: the specific area of an antigen that binds with an antibody combining site and determines the specificity of the antigen-antibody reaction.

apoptosis: programmed cell death that results from the digestion of DNA by endonucleases

B-cells: cells that are important for producing a humoral immune response

cellular immune response: the immune system's third line of defense, involving the attack of pathogens by T-cells

complement: series of enzymatic proteins in the serum that, when activated, destroy bacteria and other cells

cytokines: generic term for non-antibody proteins that act as intercellular mediators, as in the generation of immune response

cytotoxic T-cells: lymphocytes that lyse cells infected with virus; also play a role in graft rejection

epitope: any component of an antigen molecule that functions as an antigenetic determinant by permitting the attachment of certain antibodies

genetics engineering: emerging technology designed to enable replacement of missing or defective genes

helper T-cells: lymphocytes that attack foreign invaders (antigens) directly

humoral immune response: the immune system's second line of defense; often termed the antibody response

immunity: the body's specific protective response to an invading foreign agent or organism

immunopathology: study of diseases resulting in dysfunctions within the immune system

immunoregulation: complex system of checks and balances that regulates or controls immune responses

interferons: proteins formed when cells are exposed to viral or foreign agents; capable of activating other components of the immune system

lymphokines: substances released by sensitized lymphocytes when they come in contact with specific antigens

memory cells: cells that are responsible for recognizing antigens from previous exposure and mounting an immune response

natural killer cells (NK cells): lymphocytes that defend against microorganisms and malignant cells

null lymphocytes: lymphocytes that destroy antigens already coated with the antibody

opsonization: the coating of antigen–antibody molecules with a sticky substance to facilitate phagocytosis

phagocytic cells: cells that engulf, ingest, and destroy foreign bodies or toxins

phagocytic immune response: the immune system's first line of defense, involving white blood cells that have the ability to ingest foreign particles

stem cells: precursors of all blood cells; reside primarily in bone marrow

suppressor T-cells: lymphocytes that decrease B-cell activity to a level at which the immune system is compatible with life

T-cells: cells that are important for producing a cellular immune response

for people with immunologic disorders, the nurse needs to understand the immune system and how it functions; to recognize its importance in understanding disease processes; and to apply this knowledge in making appropriate patient care decisions.

Anatomic and Physiologic Overview

Anatomy of the Immune System

The immune system is composed of an integrated collection of various cell types, each with a designated functional role in defending against infection and invasion by other organisms. Supporting this system are molecules that are responsible for the interactions, modulations, and regulation of the system. These molecules and cells participate in specific interactions with immunogenic **epitopes** (antigenic determinants) present on foreign materials and initiate a series of actions in a host, including the inflammatory response, the lysis of microbial agents, and the disposal of foreign toxins. The major components of the immune system include the bone marrow, the white blood cells (WBCs) produced by the bone marrow, and the lymphoid tissues, including the thymus gland, the spleen, the lymph nodes, the tonsils and adenoids, and similar tissues in the gastrointestinal, respiratory, and reproductive systems (Fig. 50-1).

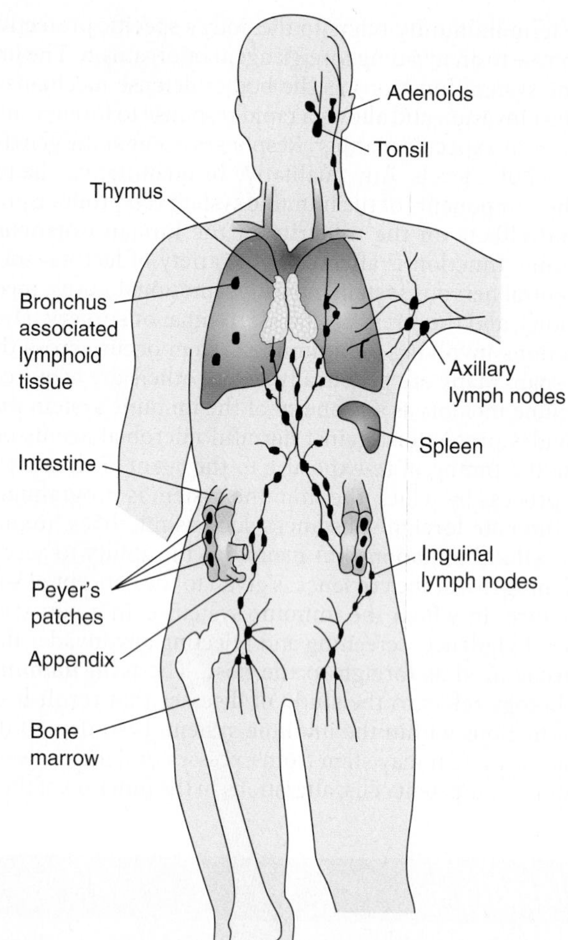

FIGURE 50-1. Central and peripheral lymphoid organs and tissues. From Porth, C. M. (2005). *Pathophysiology: Concepts of altered health states* (7th ed.). Philadelphia: Lippincott Williams & Wilkins.

Bone Marrow

The WBCs involved in immunity are produced in the bone marrow (Fig. 50-2). Like other blood cells, lymphocytes are generated from stem cells, which are undifferentiated cells. Descendants of **stem cells** become lymphocytes—the B-lymphocytes (**B-cells**), and the T-lymphocytes (**T-cells**) (Fig. 50-3). B-lymphocytes mature in the bone marrow and then enter the circulation. T-lymphocytes move from the bone marrow to the thymus, where they mature into several kinds of cells with different functions.

Lymphoid Tissues

The spleen, composed of red and white pulp, acts somewhat like a filter. The red pulp is the site where old and injured red blood cells (RBCs) are destroyed. The white pulp contains concentrations of lymphocytes. The lymph nodes are distributed throughout the body. They are connected by lymph channels and capillaries, which remove foreign material from the lymph system before it enters the bloodstream. The lymph nodes also serve as centers for immune cell proliferation. The remaining lymphoid tissues contain immune cells that defend the body's mucosal surfaces against microorganisms.

Immune Function

CONCEPTS in action ANIMATION There are two general types of immunity: natural (innate) and acquired (adaptive). Natural immunity is a nonspecific immunity that is present at birth. Acquired or specific immunity develops after birth. Natural immune responses to a foreign invader are very similar from one encounter to the next, regardless of the number of times the invader is encountered; in contrast, acquired responses increase in intensity with repeated exposure to the invading agent (Porth, 2005). Although each type of immunity has a distinct role in defending the body against harmful invaders, the various components usually act in an interdependent manner.

Natural Immunity

The natural (innate) immune system provides rapid nonspecific immunity and is present at birth. Because of its nonspecificity, it has a broad spectrum of defense against and resistance to infection. Natural (innate) immunity provides a nonspecific response to any foreign invader, regardless of the invader's composition. The basis of this defense mechanism is the ability to distinguish between friend and foe or "self" and "non-self." Natural (innate) immunity co-coordinates the initial response to pathogens through the production of cytokines and other effector molecules, which either activate cells for control of the pathogen (by elimination) or promote the development of the acquired immune

Physiology/Pathophysiology

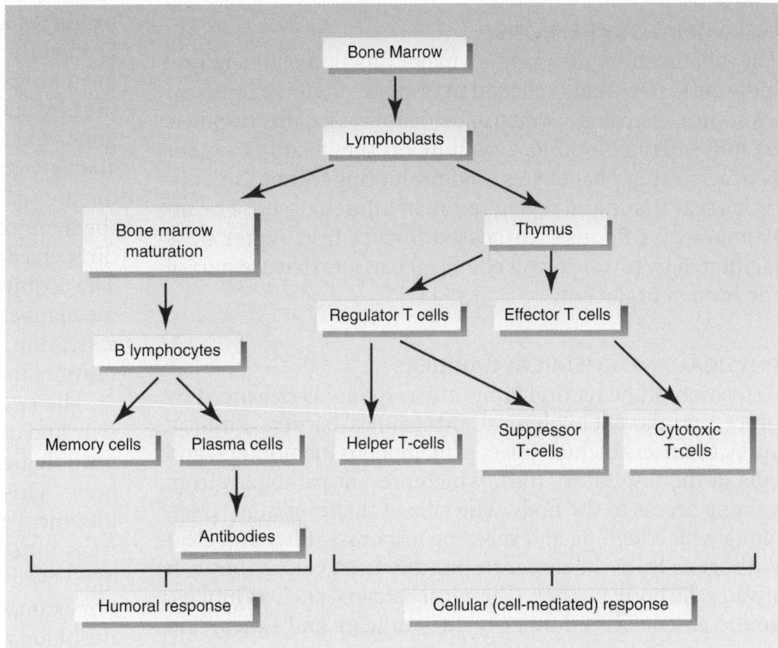

FIGURE 50-2. Development of cells of the immune system.

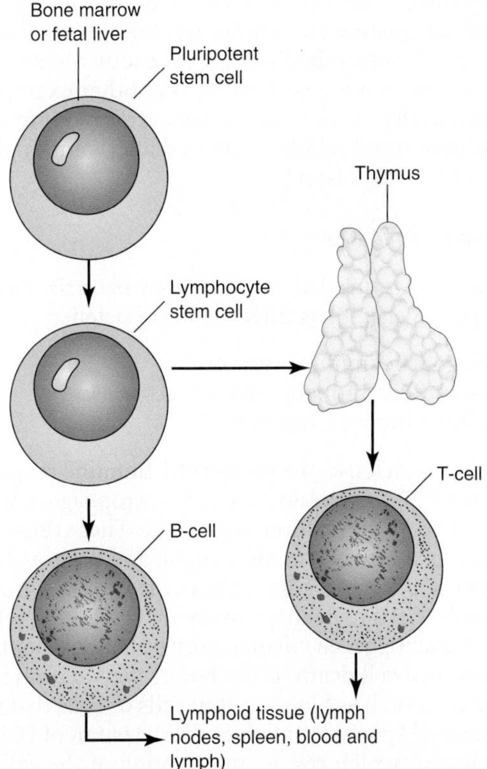

FIGURE 50-3. Lymphocytes originate from stem cells in the bone marrow. B-lymphocytes mature in the bone marrow before entering the bloodstream, whereas T-lymphocytes mature in the thymus, where they also differentiate into cells with various functions. From Porth, C. M. (2002). *Pathophysiology: Concepts of altered health states* (7th ed.). Philadelphia: Lippincott Williams & Wilkins.

response. The cells involved in this response include macrophages, dendritic cells, and natural killer (NK) cells, which have the ability to recognize and respond to a wide variety of pathogens long before the development of antigen-specific acquired immunity. The early events in this immune response are critical in determining the nature of the adaptive immune response. Innate immune mechanisms can be divided into two stages: immediate (generally occurring within 4 hours) and delayed (occurring between 4 and 96 hours after exposure).

WHITE BLOOD CELL ACTION

Cellular response is key to the effective initiation of the immune response. WBCs, or leukocytes, participate in both the natural and the acquired immune responses. Granular leukocytes, or granulocytes (so called because of granules in their cytoplasm), fight invasion by foreign bodies or toxins by releasing cell mediators, such as histamine, bradykinin, and prostaglandins, and engulfing the foreign bodies or toxins. Granulocytes include neutrophils, eosinophils, and basophils.

Neutrophils (also called polymorphonuclear leukocytes, or PMNs, because their nuclei have multiple lobes) are the first cells to arrive at the site where inflammation occurs. Eosinophils and basophils, other types of granulocytes, increase in number during allergic reactions and stress responses. Nongranular leukocytes include monocytes or macrophages (referred to as histiocytes when they enter tissue spaces) and lymphocytes. Monocytes also function as **phagocytic cells**, engulfing, ingesting, and destroying greater numbers and quantities of foreign bodies or toxins than granulocytes do. Lymphocytes, consisting of B-cells and T-cells, play major roles in humoral and cell-mediated immune responses. About 60% to 70% of lymphocytes in the blood are T-cells, and about 10% to 20% are B-cells (Porth, 2005).

INFLAMMATORY RESPONSE

The inflammatory response is a major function of the natural immune system that is elicited in response to tissue injury or invading organisms. Chemical mediators assist this response by minimizing blood loss, walling off the invading organism, activating phagocytes, and promoting formation of fibrous scar tissue and regeneration of injured tissue. The inflammatory response (discussed further in Chapter 6) is facilitated by physical and chemical barriers that are part of the human organism.

PHYSICAL AND CHEMICAL BARRIERS

Activation of the natural immunity response is enhanced by processes inherent in physical and chemical barriers. Physical surface barriers include intact skin, mucous membranes, and cilia of the respiratory tract, which prevent pathogens from gaining access to the body. The cilia of the respiratory tract, along with coughing and sneezing responses, filter and clear pathogens from the upper respiratory tract before they can invade the body further. Chemical barriers, such as mucus, acidic gastric secretions, enzymes in tears and saliva, and substances in sebaceous and sweat secretions, act in a nonspecific way to destroy invading bacteria and fungi. Viruses are countered by other means, such as interferon. **Interferon**, one type of biologic response modifier, is a nonspecific viricidal protein that is naturally produced by the body and is capable of activating other components of the immune system.

IMMUNE REGULATION

Regulation of the immune response involves balance and counterbalance. Dysfunction of the natural immune system can occur when the immune components are inactivated or when they remain active long after their effects are beneficial. A successful immune response eliminates the responsible antigen. Immunodeficiencies are characterized by inactivation or impairment of immune components, and disorders with an inflammatory component (eg, asthma, allergy, arthritis) are characterized by persistent inflammatory responses. The immune system's recognition of one's own tissues as "foreign" rather than as self is the basis for many autoimmune disorders. Despite the fact that the immune response is critical to the prevention of disease, it must be well controlled to curtail immunopathology. Most microbial infections induce an inflammatory response mediated by T-cells and cytokines, which, in excess, can cause tissue damage. Therefore, regulatory mechanisms must be in place to suppress or halt the immune response. This is mainly achieved by the production of cytokines and transformation of growth factor that inhibits macrophage activation. In some cases, T-cell activation is so overwhelming that these mechanisms fail and pathology results. Research on **immunoregulation** holds the promise of preventing graft rejection and aiding the body in eliminating cancerous or infected cells (Schwartz, 2003).

Acquired Immunity

Acquired (adaptive) immunity—immunologic responses acquired during life but not present at birth—usually develops as a result of prior exposure to an antigen through immunization (vaccination) or by contracting a disease, both of which generate a protective immune response. Weeks or months after exposure to the disease or vaccine, the body produces an immune response that is sufficient to defend against the disease on re-exposure. In contrast to the rapid but nonspecific innate immune response, this form of immunity relies on the recognition of specific foreign antigens. The two components of the immune response are strongly interrelated. Events occurring early in infection dictate the direction of the adaptive response and activate the acquired immune effector mechanisms, which have a direct feedback on the cells of the innate (natural) system. The acquired immune response is broadly divided into two mechanisms: the cell-mediated response, involving T-cell activation, and effector mechanisms, involving B-cell maturation and production of antibodies.

The two types of acquired immunity are known as active and passive. In active acquired immunity, the immunologic defenses are developed by the person's own body. This immunity typically lasts many years or even a lifetime. Passive acquired immunity is temporary immunity transmitted from a source outside the body that has developed immunity through previous disease or immunization. For example, immune globulin or antiserum, obtained from the blood plasma of people with acquired immunity, is used in emergencies to provide immunity to diseases when the risk for contracting a specific disease is great (eg, after exposure to hepatitis) and there is not enough time for a person to develop adequate active immunity. Immunity resulting from the transfer of antibodies from the mother to an infant in utero or through breast-feeding is another example of passive immunity. Active and passive acquired immunity involve humoral and cellular (cell-mediated) immunologic responses (described later).

Response to Invasion

When the body is invaded or attacked by bacteria, viruses, or other pathogens, it has three means of defense:

- The phagocytic immune response
- The humoral or antibody immune response
- The cellular immune response

The first line of defense, the **phagocytic immune response**, involves the WBCs (granulocytes and macrophages), which have the ability to ingest foreign particles. These cells move to the point of attack, where they engulf and destroy the invading agents. Phagocytes also remove the body's own dying or dead cells. Cells in necrotic tissue that are dying release substances that trigger an inflammatory response. **Apoptosis**, or programmed cell death, is the body's way of destroying worn-out cells such as blood or skin cells or cells that need to be renewed. Apoptosis involves the digestion of DNA by endonucleases, which results in targeting of the cells for phagocytosis (Jegathesan, Liebenthat, Arnett, et al., 2004).

Unlike macrophages, eosinophils are only weakly phagocytic. On activation, eosinophils probably kill parasites by releasing specific chemical mediators into the extracellular fluid. Additionally, eosinophils secrete leukotrienes, prostaglandins, and various cytokines (Abbas & Lichtman, 2005).

A second protective response, the **humoral immune response** (sometimes called the **antibody** response), begins with the B-lymphocytes, which can transform themselves into plasma cells that manufacture antibodies. These antibodies are highly specific proteins that are transported in the bloodstream and attempt to disable invaders. The third mechanism of defense, the **cellular immune response**, also involves the T-lymphocytes, which can turn into special cytotoxic (or killer) T-cells that can attack the pathogens.

The structural part of the invading or attacking organism that is responsible for stimulating antibody production is called an **antigen** (or an immunogen). For example, an antigen can be a small patch of proteins on the outer surface of a microorganism. Not all antigens are naturally immunogenic; some must be coupled to other molecules to stimulate the immune response. A single bacterium or large molecule, such as a diphtheria or tetanus toxin, may have several antigens, or markers, on its surface, thus inducing the body to produce a number of different antibodies. Once produced, an antibody is released into the bloodstream and carried to the attacking organism. There, it combines with the antigen, binding with it like an interlocking piece of a jigsaw puzzle (Fig. 50-4). There are four well-defined stages in an immune response: recognition, proliferation, response, and effector.

RECOGNITION STAGE

Recognition of antigens as foreign, or non-self, by the immune system is the initiating event in any immune response. The body must first recognize invaders as foreign before it can react to them. The body accomplishes recognition using lymph nodes and lymphocytes for surveillance. Lymph nodes are widely distributed internally throughout the body and in the circulating blood, as well as externally near the body's surfaces. They continuously discharge small lymphocytes into the bloodstream. These lymphocytes patrol the tissues and vessels that drain the areas served by that node.

Lymphocytes recirculate from the blood to lymph nodes and from the lymph nodes back into the bloodstream, in a never-ending series of patrols. Some circulating lymphocytes can survive for decades. Some of these small, hardy cells maintain their solitary circuits for a person's entire lifetime.

The exact way in which circulating lymphocytes recognize antigens on foreign surfaces is not known; however, recognition is thought to depend on specific receptor sites on the surface of the lymphocytes. Macrophages play an important role in helping the circulating lymphocytes process the antigens. Both macrophages and neutrophils have receptors for antibodies and complement; as a result, they coat microorganisms with antibodies, complement, or both, enhancing phagocytosis. The engulfed microorganisms are then subjected to a wide range of toxic intracellular molecules. When foreign materials enter the body, circulating lymphocytes come into physical contact with the surfaces of these materials. Upon contact with the foreign material, lymphocytes, with the help of macrophages, either remove the antigen from the surface or obtain an imprint of its structure, which becomes important in subsequent re-exposure to the antigen.

In a streptococcal throat infection, for example, the streptococcal organism gains access to the mucous membranes of the throat. A circulating lymphocyte moving through the tissues of the throat comes in contact with the organism. The lymphocyte, familiar with the surface markers on the cells of its own body, recognizes the antigens on the microbe as different (non-self) and the streptococcal organism as antigenic (foreign). This triggers the second stage of the immune response—proliferation.

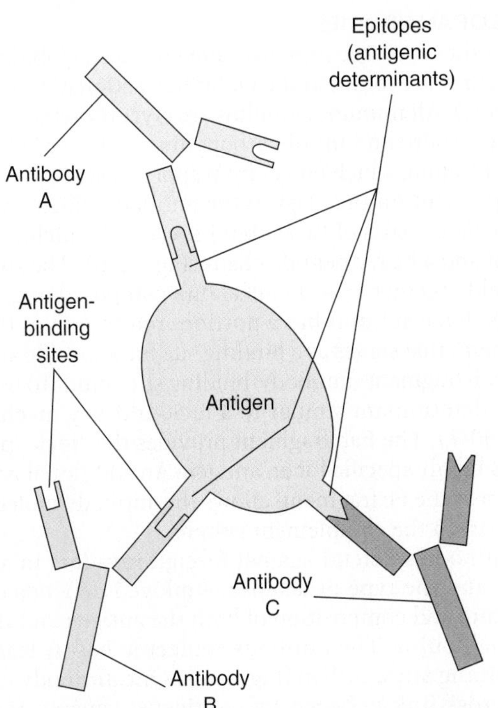

FIGURE 50-4. Complement-mediated immune responses. From Porth, C. M. (2005). *Pathophysiology: Concepts of altered health states* (7th ed.). Philadelphia: Lippincott Williams & Wilkins.

PROLIFERATION STAGE

The circulating lymphocyte containing the antigenic message returns to the nearest lymph node. Once in the node, the sensitized lymphocyte stimulates some of the resident dormant T- and B-lymphocytes to enlarge, divide, and proliferate. T-lymphocytes differentiate into cytotoxic (or killer) T-cells, whereas B-lymphocytes produce and release antibodies. Enlargement of the lymph nodes in the neck in conjunction with a sore throat is one example of the immune response.

RESPONSE STAGE

In the response stage, the differentiated lymphocytes function in either a humoral or a cellular capacity. The production of antibodies by the B-lymphocytes in response to a specific antigen begins the humoral response. Humoral refers to the fact that the antibodies are released into the bloodstream and therefore reside in the plasma (fluid fraction of the blood).

With the initial cellular response, the returning sensitized lymphocytes migrate to areas of the lymph node other than those areas containing lymphocytes programmed to become plasma cells. Here, they stimulate the residing lymphocytes to become cells that will attack microbes directly rather than through the action of antibodies. These transformed lymphocytes are known as cytotoxic (killer) T-cells.

The T stands for thymus, signifying that during embryologic development of the immune system, these T-lymphocytes spent time in the thymus of the developing fetus, where they were genetically programmed to become T-lymphocytes rather than the antibody-producing B-lymphocytes. Viral rather than bacterial antigens induce a cellular response. This response is manifested by the increasing number of T-lymphocytes (lymphocytosis) seen in the blood tests of people with viral illnesses such as infectious mononucleosis. (Cellular immunity is discussed in further detail later in this chapter.)

Most immune responses to antigens involve both humoral and cellular responses, although one usually predominates. For example, during transplant rejection, the cellular response predominates, whereas in the bacterial pneumonias and sepsis, the humoral response plays the dominant protective role (Chart 50-1).

EFFECTOR STAGE

In the effector stage, either the antibody of the humoral response or the cytotoxic (killer) T-cell of the cellular response reaches and connects with the antigen on the surface of the foreign invader. The connection initiates a series of events that in most instances results in the total destruction of the invading microbes or the complete neutralization of the toxin. The events involve interplay of antibodies (humoral immunity), complement, and action by the cytotoxic T-cells (cellular immunity). Figure 50-5 summarizes the stages of the immune response.

Humoral Immune Response

The humoral response is characterized by the production of antibodies by B-lymphocytes in response to a specific antigen. Although the B-lymphocyte is ultimately responsible for the production of antibodies, both the macrophages of natural immunity and the special T-cell lymphocytes of cellular immunity are involved in recognizing the foreign substance and in producing antibodies.

ANTIGEN RECOGNITION

Several theories explain the mechanisms by which B-lymphocytes recognize the invading antigen and respond by producing antibodies. It is known that B-lymphocytes recognize and respond to invading antigens in more than one way.

The B-lymphocytes appear to respond to some antigens by directly triggering antibody formation; however, in response to other antigens, they need the assistance of T-cells to trigger antibody formation. The T-lymphocytes are part of a surveillance system that is dispersed throughout the body and recycles through the general circulation, tissues, and lymphatic system. With the assistance of macrophages, the T-lymphocytes are believed to recognize the antigen of a foreign invader. The T-lymphocyte picks up the antigenic message, or "blueprint," of the antigen and returns to the nearest lymph node with that message.

B-lymphocytes stored in the lymph nodes are subdivided into thousands of clones, each responsive to a single group of antigens having almost identical characteristics. When the antigenic message is carried back to the lymph node, specific clones of the B-lymphocyte are stimulated to enlarge, divide, proliferate, and differentiate into plasma cells capable of producing specific antibodies to the antigen. Other B-lymphocytes differentiate into B-lymphocyte clones with a memory for the antigen. These memory cells are responsible for the more exaggerated and rapid immune response in a person who is repeatedly exposed to the same antigen (Clancy, McVicar & Baird, 2002).

ROLE OF ANTIBODIES

Antibodies are large proteins called immunoglobulins (because they are found in the globulin fraction of the plasma proteins). All immunoglobulins are glycoproteins and contain a certain amount of carbohydrate. The carbohydrate concentration, which ranges from approximately 3% to 13%, is dependent on the class of the antibody. Each antibody molecule consists of two subunits, each of which contains a light and a heavy peptide chain (Fig. 50-6). The subunits are held together by a chemical link composed of disulfide bonds. Each subunit has a portion, referred to as the Fab fragment, that serves as a binding site for a specific antigen. The Fab fragment (antibody-binding site) binds to the antigenic determinant similar to a lock-and-key mechanism (Fig. 50-7). The Fab fragment provides the "lock" portion that is highly specific for an antigen. An additional portion, known as the Fc fragment, allows the antibody molecule to take part in the complement system.

Antibodies defend against foreign invaders in several ways, and the type of defense employed depends on the structure and composition of both the antigen and the immunoglobulin. The antibody molecule has at least two combining sites, or Fab fragments. One antibody can act as a cross-link between two antigens, causing them to bind or clump together. This clumping effect, referred to as **agglutination**, helps clear the body of the invading

CHART 50-1

Differences in Cellular and Humoral Immune Responses

HUMORAL RESPONSES (B-CELLS)
- Bacterial phagocytosis and lysis
- Anaphylaxis
- Allergic hay fever and asthma
- Immune complex disease
- Bacterial and some viral infections

CELLULAR RESPONSES (T-CELLS)
- Transplant rejection
- Delayed hypersensitivity (tuberculin reaction)
- Graft-versus-host disease
- Tumor surveillance or destruction
- Intracellular infections
- Viral, fungal, and parasitic infections

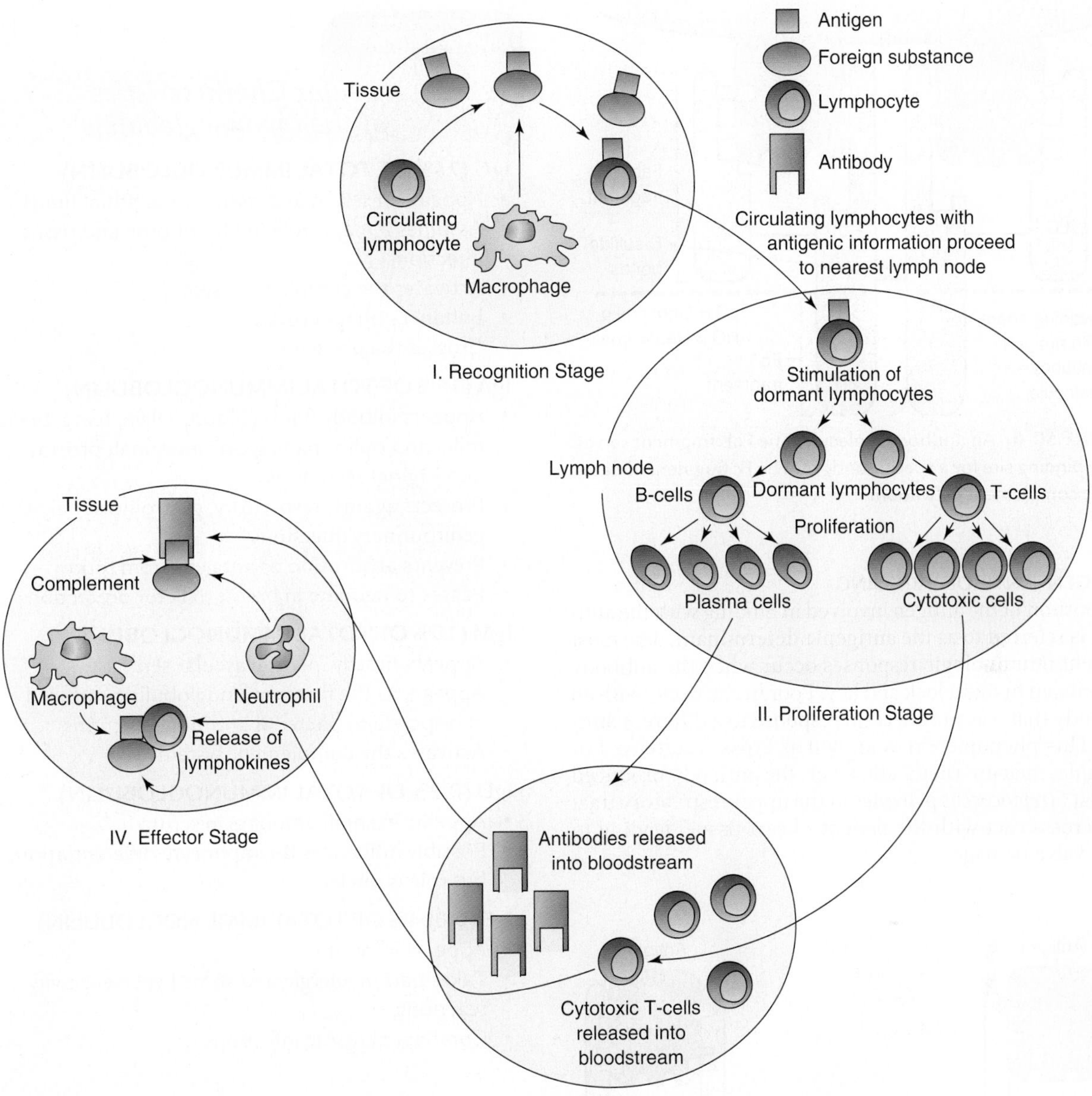

FIGURE 50-5. Stages of the immune response. (**I**) In the *recognition stage,* antigens are recognized by circulating lymphocytes and macrophages. (**II**) In the *proliferation stage,* the dormant lymphocytes proliferate and differentiate into cytotoxic (killer) T-cells or B-cells responsible for formation and release of antibodies. (**III**) In the *response stage,* the cytotoxic T-cells and the B-cells perform cellular and humoral functions, respectively. (**IV**) In the *effector stage,* antigens are destroyed or neutralized through the action of antibodies, complement, macrophages, and cytotoxic T-cells.

organism by facilitating phagocytosis. Some antibodies assist in removal of offending organisms through **opsonization.** In this process, the antigen–antibody molecule is coated with a sticky substance that also facilitates phagocytosis.

Antibodies also promote the release of vasoactive substances, such as histamine and slow-reacting substance, two of the chemical mediators of the inflammatory response. Antibodies do not function in isolation; rather, they mobilize other components of the immune system to defend against the invader. The typical role of antibodies is to focus components of the natural immune system on the invader. This includes activation of the complement system and activation of phagocytosis (Abbas & Lichtman, 2005).

The body can produce five different types of immunoglobulins (Ig). Each of the five types, or classes, is identified by a specific letter of the alphabet: IgA, IgD, IgE, IgG, and IgM. Classification is based on the chemical structure and biologic role of the individual immunoglobulin. Major characteristics of the immunoglobulins are summarized in Chart 50-2.

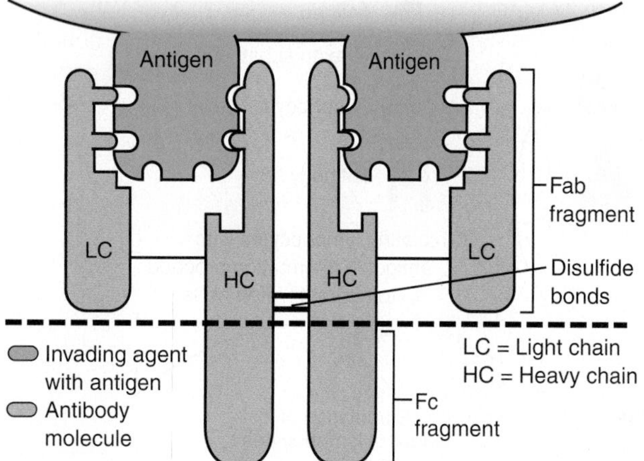

FIGURE 50-6. An antibody molecule. The Fab fragment serves as the binding site for a specific antigen. The Fc fragment initiates classic complement activation.

ANTIGEN–ANTIBODY BINDING

The portion of the antigen involved in binding with the antibody is referred to as the **antigenic determinant.** The most efficient immunologic responses occur when the antibody and antigen fit like a lock and key. Poor fit can occur with an antibody that was produced in response to a different antigen. This phenomenon is known as cross-reactivity. For example, in acute rheumatic fever, the antibody produced against *Streptococcus pyogenes* in the upper respiratory tract may cross-react with the patient's heart tissue, leading to heart valve damage.

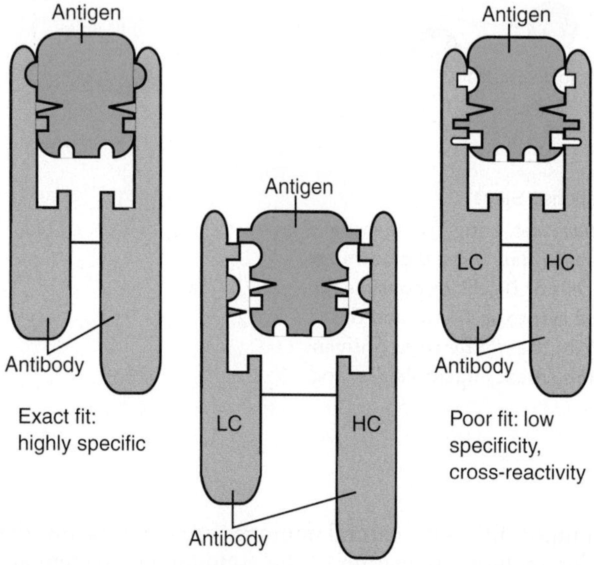

FIGURE 50-7. Antigen–antibody binding. (*Left*) A highly specific antigen–antibody complex. (*Middle*) No match and therefore, no immune response. (*Right*) Poor fit or match with low specificity; antibody reacts to antigen with similar characteristics, producing cross-reactivity.

CHART 50-2

Major Characteristics of the Immunoglobulins

IgG (75% OF TOTAL IMMUNOGLOBULIN)
- Appears in serum and tissues (interstitial fluid)
- Assumes a major role in bloodborne and tissue infections
- Activates the complement system
- Enhances phagocytosis
- Crosses the placenta

IgA (15% OF TOTAL IMMUNOGLOBULIN)
- Appears in body fluids (blood, saliva, tears, breast milk, and pulmonary, gastrointestinal, prostatic, and vaginal secretions)
- Protects against respiratory, gastrointestinal, and genitourinary infections
- Prevents absorption of antigens from food
- Passes to neonate in breast milk for protection

IgM (10% OF TOTAL IMMUNOGLOBULIN)
- Appears mostly in intravascular serum
- Appears as the first immunoglobulin produced in response to bacterial and viral infections
- Activates the complement system

IgD (0.2% OF TOTAL IMMUNOGLOBULIN)
- Appears in small amounts in serum
- Possibly influences B-lymphocyte differentiation, but role is unclear

IgE (0.004% OF TOTAL IMMUNOGLOBULIN)
- Appears in serum
- Takes part in allergic and some hypersensitivity reactions
- Combats parasitic infections

Cellular Immune Response

The B-lymphocytes are responsible for humoral immunity, and the T-lymphocytes are primarily responsible for cellular immunity. Stem cells continuously migrate from the bone marrow to the thymus gland, where they develop into T-cells. T-cells continue to develop in the thymus gland, despite the partial degeneration of the gland that occurs at puberty. By spending time in the thymus, these cells are programmed to become T-cells rather than antibody-producing B-lymphocytes. Several types of T-cells exist, each with designated roles in the defense against bacteria, viruses, fungi, parasites, and malignant cells. T-cells attack foreign invaders directly rather than by producing antibodies.

Cellular reactions are initiated by the binding of an antigen to an antigen receptor located on the surface of a T-cell. This may occur with or without the assistance of macrophages. The T-cells then carry the antigenic message, or blueprint, to the lymph nodes, where the production of other T-cells is stimulated. Some T-cells remain in the lymph nodes and retain a memory for the antigen. Other T-cells migrate from the lymph nodes into the general circulatory system and ultimately to the tissues, where they remain until they either come in contact with their respective antigens or die.

ROLE OF T-LYMPHOCYTES

T-cells include effector T-cells, suppressor T-cells, and memory T-cells. Two major categories of effector T-cells exist: helper T-cells and cytotoxic T-cells. These effector T-cells participate in the destruction of foreign organisms. T-cells interact closely with B-cells, indicating that humoral and cellular immune responses are not separate, unrelated processes, but rather, branches of the immune response that interact.

Helper T-cells are activated on recognition of antigens and stimulate the rest of the immune system. When activated, helper T-cells secrete **cytokines,** which attract and activate B-cells, cytotoxic T-cells, NK cells, macrophages, and other cells of the immune system. Separate subpopulations of helper T-cells produce different types of cytokines and determine whether the immune response will be the production of antibodies or a cell-mediated immune response. Helper T-cells produce **lymphokines,** one category of cytokines. These lymphokines activate other T-cells (eg, interleukin-2 [IL-2]), natural and cytotoxic T-cells (eg, interferon-γ), and other inflammatory cells (eg, tumor necrosis factor). Helper T-cells produce IL-4 and IL-5, lymphokines that activate B-cells to grow and differentiate (Table 50-2).

Cytotoxic T-cells (killer T-cells) attack the antigen directly by altering the cell membrane and causing cell lysis (disintegration) and by releasing cytolytic enzymes and cytokines. Lymphokines can recruit, activate, and regulate other lymphocytes and WBCs. These cells then assist in destroying the invading organism. Delayed-type hypersensitivity is an example of an immune reaction that protects the body from antigens through the production and release of lymphokines (see later discussion).

Another type of cell, the **suppressor T-cell,** has the ability to decrease B-cell production, thereby keeping the immune response at a level that is compatible with health (eg, sufficient to fight infection adequately without attacking the body's healthy tissues). **Memory cells** are responsible for recognizing antigens from previous exposure and mounting an immune response (Table 50-3).

TABLE 50-2 Cytokines and Their Biologic Activity

Cytokine*	Biologic Activity
Interleukin-1 (α and β)	Promotes differentiation of T- and B-lymphocytes, natural killer (NK) cells, and null cells
Interleukin-2	Stimulates growth of T-lymphocytes and special activated killer lymphocytes (known as lymphocyte-activated killer cells [LAK cells])
Interleukin-3	Stimulates growth of mast cells and other blood cells
Interleukin-4	Stimulates growth of T- and B-lymphocytes, mast cells, and macrophages
Interleukin-5	Stimulates antibody responses
Interleukin-6	Stimulates growth and function of B-lymphocytes and antibodies
Interleukin-7	Stimulates growth of pre-B, CD4+ and CD8+ T-lymphocytes and activates mature T-lymphocytes
Interleukin-8	Promotes chemotaxis and activation of neutrophils
Interleukin-9	Stimulates growth and proliferation of T-lymphocytes
Interleukin-10	Inhibits interferon-gamma and mononuclear cell inflammation
Interleukin-11	Promotes induction of acute phase proteins
Interleukin-12	Introduces helper T-lymphocytes
Interleukin-13	Inhibits mononuclear phagocyte inflammation and promotes differentiation of B-cells
Interleukin-16	Promotes chemotaxis CD4+ T-lymphocytes and eosinophils
Permeability factor	Increases vascular permeability, allowing white cells into area
Interferon-γ	Activates macrophages; increases expression of class I and II MHC antigen processing and presentation
Interferon (type 1α and type β)	Exerts antiviral activity in body cells; induces class I antigen expression; activates NK cells
Migration inhibitory factor	Suppresses movement of macrophages, keeping macrophages in area of foreign cells
Skin reactive factor	Induces inflammatory response
Cytotoxic factor (lymphotoxin)	Kills certain antigenic cells
Macrophage chemotactic factor	Attracts macrophages into the area
Lymphocyte blastogenic factor	Stimulates more lymphocytes, recruiting additional lymphocytes into the area
Macrophage aggregation factor	Causes clumping of macrophages and lymphocytes
Macrophage activation factor	Allows macrophages to adhere to surfaces more readily
Proliferation inhibitor factor	Inhibits growth of certain antigenic cells
Cytophilic antibody	Binds to an Fc receptor on macrophages, thereby permitting macrophages to bind to antigens
Tumor necrosis factor-alpha	Stimulates inflammation, wound healing, and tissue remodeling
Tumor necrosis factor-beta	Mediates inflammation and graft rejection

*Cytokines are biologically active substances that are released by cells to regulate growth and function of other cells within the immune system. Lymphocytes produce lymphokines, and monocytes and macrophages produce monokines. This table lists some of the cytokines that play a role in immune system functioning. MHC = major histocompatibility complex.

TABLE 50-3 Lymphocytes Involved in Immune Responses

Type of Immune Response	Cell Type	Function
Humoral	B-lymphocyte	Produces antibodies or immunoglobulins (IgA, IgD, IgE, IgG, IgM)
Cellular	T-lymphocyte	
	Helper T	Attacks foreign invaders (antigens) directly Initiates and augments inflammatory response
	Helper T_1	Increases activated cytotoxic T-cells
	Helper T_2	Increases B-cell antibody production
	Suppressor T	Suppresses the immune response
	Memory T	Remembers contact with an antigen and on subsequent exposures mounts an immune response
	Cytotoxic T (killer T)	Lyses cells infected with virus; plays a role in graft rejection
Nonspecific	Non-T or non-B lymphocyte	
	Null cell	Destroys antigens already coated with antibody
	Natural killer (NK) cell (granular lymphocyte)	Defends against microorganisms and some types of malignant cells; produces cytokines

ROLES OF NULL LYMPHOCYTES AND NATURAL KILLER CELLS

Null lymphocytes and NK cells are other lymphocytes that assist in combating organisms. These cells are distinct from B-cells and T-cells and lack the usual characteristics of those cells. **Null lymphocytes**, a subpopulation of lymphocytes, destroy antigens already coated with antibody. These cells have special Fc receptor sites on their surface that allow them to connect with the Fc end of antibodies; this is known as antibody-dependent, cell-mediated cytotoxicity.

Natural killer cells, another subpopulation of lymphocytes, defend against microorganisms and some types of malignant cells (Goodfellow, 2003). NK cells are capable of directly killing invading organisms and producing cytokines. The helper T-cells contribute to the differentiation of null and NK cells.

Complement System

Circulating plasma proteins, known as **complement**, are made in the liver and activated when an antibody connects with its antigen. Complement plays an important role in the immune response. Destruction of an invading or attacking organism or toxin is not achieved merely by the binding of the antibody and antigens; it also requires activation of complement, the arrival of killer T-cells, or the attraction of macrophages. Complement has three major physiologic functions: defending the body against bacterial infection, bridging natural and acquired immunity, and disposing of immune complexes and the byproducts associated with inflammation. Complement-mediated immune responses are summarized in Table 50-4.

The proteins that comprise complement interact sequentially with one another in a cascading or "falling domino" effect. The complement cascade is important to modifying the effector arm of the immune system. Activation of complement allows important events, such as removal of infectious agents and initiation of the inflammatory response, to take place. These events involve active parts of the pathway that enhance chemotaxis of macrophages and granulocytes, alter blood vessel permeability, change blood vessel diameters, cause cells to lyse, alter blood clotting, and cause other points of modification. These macrophages and granulocytes continue the body's defense by devouring the antibody-coated microbes and by releasing bacterial products.

There are several ways to activate the complement system: the classic pathway, the alternative pathway, and the lectin pathway (Abbas & Lichtman, 2005).

CLASSIC PATHWAY OF COMPLEMENT ACTIVATION

The classic pathway (the first method discovered) is activated by antigen–antibody complexes; it begins when antibody binds to a cell surface and ends with lysis of the cell. This involves the reaction of the first of the circulating complement proteins (C1) with the receptor site of the Fc portion of an antibody molecule after formation of an antigen–antibody complex. The activation of the first complement component then activates all the other components, in the following sequence: C4, C2, C3, C5, C6, C7, C8, and C9. (The components are named in the sequence in which they were discovered.)

ALTERNATIVE AND LECTIN PATHWAYS

The alternative and lectin pathways of complement are activated without the formation of antigen–antibody complexes. These pathways can be initiated by the release of bacterial products, such as endotoxins. When complement is activated without the formation of antigen–antibody complexes, the process bypasses the first three components (C1, C4, and C2) and begins with C3. Regardless of the method, once activated, the complement system destroys cells by altering or damaging the cell membrane of the antigen, by chemically attracting phagocytes to the antigen (chemotaxis), and by rendering the antigen more vulnerable to phagocytosis (opsonization). The complement system enhances the inflammatory response by releasing vasoactive substances.

Complement components, prostaglandins, leukotrienes, and other inflammatory mediators all contribute to the

TABLE 50-4 Complement-Mediated Immune Responses

Response	Complement Products	Effects
Cytolysis	C5b–C9	Lysis and destruction of cell membranes of body's cells or of pathogens
Opsonization	C3b, C5b	Targeting of the antigen so that it can be easily engulfed and digested by macrophages and other phagocytic cells
Chemotaxis	C3a, C5a	Chemical attraction of neutrophils and phagocytic cells to the antigen
Anaphylaxis	C3a, C5a	Activation of mast cells and basophils with release of inflammatory mediators that produce smooth muscle contraction and increased vascular permeability

From Porth, C. M. (2005). *Pathophysiology: Concepts of altered health states* (7th ed.). Philadelphia: Lippincott Williams and Wilkins.

recruitment of inflammatory cells, as do chemokines, a group of cytokines. The activated neutrophils pass through the vessel walls to accumulate at the site of infection, where they phagocytose complement-coated microbes (Abbas & Lichtman, 2005). This response is usually therapeutic and can be lifesaving if the cell attacked by the complement system is a true foreign invader, such as a streptococcal or staphylococcal organism. However, if that cell is actually part of the person—for example, a cell of the brain or liver, the tissue lining the blood vessels, or the cells of a transplanted organ or skin graft—the result can be devastating disease and even death. This vigorous and deadly attack on the material identified as foreign is underscored by the resulting purulent material (the remains of microbes, granulocytes, macrophages, T-cells, plasma proteins, complement, and antibodies) that accumulates in wound infections and abscesses. In addition, many autoimmune diseases (eg, systemic lupus erythematosus) and disorders characterized by chronic infection (eg, hepatitis C, bacterial endocarditis) and necrosis (eg, myocardial infarction, stroke) are thought to be caused in part by continued or chronic activation of complement, which in turn results in chronic inflammation (Perl, 2004).

The RBCs (erythrocytes) and platelets (thrombocytes) also have a role in the immune response. RBCs and platelets have complement receptors and, as a result, play an important role in the clearance of immune complexes that consist of antigen, antibody, and components of the complement system (Abbas & Lichtman, 2005).

Role of Interferons

Biologic response modifiers, such as the interferons, continue to be investigated to determine their roles in the immune system and their potential therapeutic effects in disorders characterized by disturbed immune responses (Korholz & Kiess, 2003). Interferons have antiviral and antitumor properties. In addition to responding to viral infection, interferons are produced by T-lymphocytes, B-lymphocytes, and macrophages in response to antigens. They are thought to modify the immune response by suppressing antibody production and cellular immunity. They also facilitate the cytolytic role of macrophages and NK cells. Interferons are undergoing extensive testing to evaluate their effectiveness in treating tumors and acquired immunodeficiency syndrome (AIDS). Some interferons are already used to treat immune-related disorders (eg, multiple sclerosis) and chronic inflammatory conditions (eg, chronic hepatitis).

Advances in Immunology

Genetics Engineering

One of the more remarkable evolving technologies is **genetics engineering**, which uses recombinant DNA technology. Two facets exist with this technology. The first permits scientists to combine genes from one type of organism with genes of a second organism. This type of technology allows cells and microorganisms to manufacture proteins, monokines, and lymphokines, which can alter and enhance immune system function. The second facet of recombinant DNA technology involves gene therapy (Moreland, 2004). If a particular gene is abnormal or missing, experimental recombinant DNA technology may be capable of restoring normal gene function. For example, a recombinant gene is inserted onto a virus particle. When the virus particle splices its genes, the virus automatically inserts the missing gene, and theoretically corrects the genetic anomaly. Extensive research into recombinant DNA technology and gene therapy is ongoing (Perl, 2004).

Stem Cells

Stem cells are potentially immortal cells that are capable of self-renewal and differentiation; they continually replenish the body's entire supply of both RBCs and WBCs. Some stem cells, described as totipotent cells, have tremendous capacity to self-renew and differentiate. Embryonic stem cells, described as pluripotent, give rise to numerous cell types that are able to form tissues (Porth, 2005). Research has shown that stem cells can restore an immune system that has been destroyed. Stem cell transplantation has been carried out in humans with certain types of immune dysfunction, such as severe combined immunodeficiency (SCID); clinical trials using stem cells are underway in patients with a variety of disorders having an autoimmune component, including systemic lupus erythematosus, rheumatoid arthritis, scleroderma, and multiple sclerosis. Research with embryonic stem cells has enabled investigators to make substantial gains in developmental biology, gene therapy, therapeutic tissue engineering, and the treatment of a variety of diseases. However, along with these remarkable opportunities, many ethical challenges arise, which are largely based on concerns about safety, efficacy, resource allocation, and human cloning (Cogle, Guthrie, Sanders, et al., 2003).

Assessment

An assessment of immune function begins during the health history and physical examination. Areas to be assessed include nutritional status; infections and immunizations; allergies; disorders and disease states, such as autoimmune disorders, cancer, and chronic illnesses; surgeries; medications; and blood transfusions. In addition to inspection of general characteristics, palpation of the lymph nodes and examinations of the skin, mucous membranes, and respiratory, gastrointestinal, musculoskeletal, genitourinary, cardiovascular, and neurosensory systems are performed (Moorhead, Johnson & Maas, 2004) (Chart 50-3).

CHART 50-3

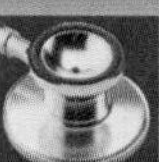

Assessing for Immune Dysfunction

Be on the alert for the following signs and symptoms:

RESPIRATORY SYSTEM
- Changes in respiratory rate
- Cough (dry or productive)
- Abnormal lung sounds (wheezing, crackles, rhonchi)
- Rhinitis
- Hyperventilation
- Bronchospasm

CARDIOVASCULAR SYSTEM
- Hypotension
- Tachycardia
- Dysrhythmia
- Vasculitis
- Anemia

GASTROINTESTINAL SYSTEM
- Hepatosplenomegaly
- Colitis
- Vomiting
- Diarrhea

GENITOURINARY SYSTEM
- Frequency and burning on urination
- Hematuria
- Discharge

MUSCULOSKELETAL SYSTEM
- Joint mobility, edema, and pain

SKIN
- Rashes
- Lesions
- Dermatitis
- Hematomas or purpura
- Edema or urticaria
- Inflammation
- Discharge

NEUROSENSORY SYSTEM
- Cognitive dysfunction
- Hearing loss
- Visual changes
- Headaches and migraines
- Ataxia
- Tetany

Health History

The history should note the patient's age along with information about past and present conditions and events that may provide clues to the status of the patient's immune system.

Gender

There are differences in the immune system functions of men and women. For example, many autoimmune diseases have a higher incidence in females than in males (Abbas & Lichtman, 2005). During the reproductive years, women have a stronger immune response than men do, a phenomenon generally believed to be a result of hormonal differences.

Gerontologic Considerations

Age is an important factor, because people at the extremes of the life span are more likely to develop problems related to immune system functioning than are middle-aged adults (Table 50-5). The greatest impact of aging on the immune system is on cell-mediated immunity; age has a lesser but substantial impact on humoral immunity. The frequency and severity of infections are increased in elderly people, possibly due to a decreased ability to respond adequately to invading organisms. Both the production and the function of T- and B-lymphocytes may be impaired. Responses to antigen stimulation may be altered, with increasing proportions of lymphocytes becoming unresponsive with age (Porth, 2005). The data regarding the effects of aging on immunity and infection are inconclusive and sometimes conflicting. However, aging has an impact on the immune system that can best be summarized as immunosenescence, a condition thought to be a result of involution of the thymus (Rosenthal & Kavic, 2004).

Declining function of various organ systems associated with increasing age also contributes to impaired immunity. Decreased gastric secretions and motility allow normal intestinal flora to proliferate and produce infection, causing gastroenteritis and diarrhea. Decreased renal circulation, filtration, absorption, and excretion contribute to the risk for urinary tract infections. Moreover, prostatic enlargement or a neurogenic bladder can impede urine passage and impair bacterial clearance through the urinary system. Urinary stasis, common in elderly people, permits the growth of microorganisms. Exposure to tobacco and environmental toxins impairs pulmonary function. Prolonged exposure to these agents decreases the elasticity of lung tissue, the effectiveness of cilia, and the ability to cough effectively. These impairments hinder the removal of infectious organisms and toxins, increasing the elderly person's susceptibility to pulmonary infections and cancers. The skin becomes thinner and less elastic. The increased incidence of peripheral neuropathy and the accompanying decreased sensation and circulation may lead to stasis ulcers, pressure

TABLE 50-5 Age-Related Changes in Immunologic Function

Body System	Changes	Consequences
Immune	Impaired function of B- and T-lymphocytes Failure of lymphocytes to recognize mutant or abnormal cells Decreased antibody production Failure of immune system to differentiate "self" from "non-self" Suppressed phagocytic immune response	Suppressed responses to pathogenic organisms with increased risk for infection Increased incidence of cancers Anergy (lack of response to antigens applied to the skin [PPD, allergens]) Increased incidence of autoimmune diseases Absence of typical signs and symptoms of infection and inflammation Dissemination of organisms usually destroyed or suppressed by phagocytes (eg, reactivation or spread of tuberculosis)
Gastrointestinal	Decreased gastric secretions and motility Decreased phagocytosis by the liver's Kupffer cells Altered nutritional intake with inadequate protein intake	Proliferation of intestinal organisms resulting in gastroenteritis and diarrhea Increased incidence and severity of hepatitis B; increased incidence of liver abscesses Suppressed immune response
Urinary	Decreased kidney function and changes in lower urinary tract function (enlargement of prostate gland, neurogenic bladder). Altered genitourinary tract flora.	Urinary stasis and increased incidence of urinary tract infections
Pulmonary	Impaired ciliary action due to exposure to smoke and environmental toxins	Impaired clearance of pulmonary secretions; increased incidence of respiratory infections
Integumentary	Thinning of skin with less elasticity; loss of adipose tissue	Increased risk of skin injury, breakdown and infection
Circulatory	Impaired microcirculation	Stasis and pressure ulcers
Neurologic function	Decreased sensation and slowing of reflexes	Increased risk of injury, skin ulcers, abrasions, and burns

ulcers, abrasions, and burns. Impaired skin integrity predisposes elderly people to infection from organisms that are part of normal skin flora.

The incidence of autoimmune diseases also increases with aging, possibly from a decreased ability of antibodies to differentiate between self and non-self. Failure of the surveillance system to recognize mutant or abnormal cells also may be responsible, in part, for the high incidence of cancer associated with increasing age.

Nutrition

The importance of optimal nutrition in enhancing immunity is gaining greater recognition. Inadequate intake of vitamins that are essential for DNA and protein synthesis may lead to protein–calorie deficiency and subsequently to impaired immune function. Vitamins also help in the regulation of cell proliferation and maturation of immune cells. Excess or deficiency of trace elements (ie, copper, iron, manganese, selenium, or zinc) in the diet generally suppresses immune function.

Fatty acids are the building blocks that make up the structural components of cell membranes. Lipids are precursors of vitamins A, D, E, and K as well as cholesterol. Both excess and deficiency of fatty acids have been found to suppress immune function.

Depletion of protein reserves results in atrophy of lymphoid tissues, depression of antibody response, reduction in the number of circulating T-cells, and impaired phagocytic function. As a result, susceptibility to infection is greatly increased. During periods of infection or serious illness, nutritional requirements may be further altered, potentially contributing to depletion of protein, fatty acid, vitamin, and trace elements and causing even greater risk of impaired immune response and sepsis. Nutritional intake that supports a competent immune response plays an important role in reducing the incidence of infections; patients whose nutritional status is compromised have a delayed postoperative recovery and often experience more severe infections and delayed wound healing. The nurse must assess the patient's nutritional status and caloric intake. The nurse is responsible for assuming a proactive role in ensuring the best possible nutritional intake for all patients as a vital step in preventing untoward treatment outcomes.

Infection and Immunization

The patient is asked about childhood and adult immunizations and the usual childhood diseases. Known past or present exposure to tuberculosis is assessed, and the dates and results of any tuberculin tests (purified protein derivative [PPD] or tine test) and chest x-rays are obtained. Recent exposure to any infections and the exposure dates are elicited. It is important for the nurse to assess whether the patient has been exposed to any sexually transmitted diseases (STDs) or bloodborne pathogens such as hepatitis A, B, C, D, and E viruses and HIV virus. A history of STDs such as gonorrhea, syphilis, HPV infection, and chlamydia can alert the nurse that the patient may have been exposed to HIV infection or to hepatitis. A history of past and present infections and the dates and types of treatments, along with a history of any multiple persistent infections, fevers of unknown origin, lesions or sores, or any type of drainage, are obtained.

Allergy

The patient is asked about any allergies, including types of allergens (eg, pollens, dust, plants, cosmetics, food, medications, vaccines, latex), the symptoms experienced, and seasonal variations in occurrence or severity in the symptoms. A history of testing and treatments, including prescribed and over-the-counter medications, that the patient has taken or is currently taking for these allergies and the effectiveness of the treatments is obtained. All medication and food allergies are listed on an allergy alert sticker and placed on the front of the patient's health record or chart to alert others. Continued assessment for potential allergic reactions in the patient is vital.

Disorders and Diseases

AUTOIMMUNE DISORDERS

Autoimmune disorders affect people of both genders of all ages, ethnicities, and social classes. The patient is asked about any autoimmune disorders, such as lupus erythematosus, rheumatoid arthritis, or psoriasis. The onset, severity, remissions and exacerbations, functional limitations, treatments that the patient has received or is currently receiving, and the effectiveness of the treatments are described. Although most specific autoimmune disorders are rare, together they affect approximately 5% of the United States population. The occurrence of different autoimmune diseases within a family strongly suggests a genetic predisposition to more than one autoimmune disease (Moser, Gaffney, Peterson, et al., 2004).

In general, autoimmune disorders are more common in females than in males. This is believed to result from the activity of the sex hormones. The ability of sex hormones to modulate immunity has been well established. There is evidence that estrogen modulates the activity of T-lymphocytes (especially suppressor cells), whereas androgens act to preserve IL-2 production and suppressor cell activity. The effects of sex hormones on B-cells are less pronounced. Estrogen activates the autoimmune-associated B-cell population that expresses the CD5 marker (an antigenic marker on the B-cell). Estrogen tends to enhance immunity, whereas androgen tends to be immunosuppressive.

NEOPLASTIC DISEASE

If there is a history of cancer in the family, the type of cancer, age at onset, and relationship (maternal or paternal) of the patient to the affected family members is noted. Dates and results of any cancer screening tests for the patient are obtained. A history of cancer in the patient is also obtained, along with the type of cancer, date of diagnosis, and treatment modalities used. Immunosuppression contributes to the development of cancers; however, cancer itself is immunosuppressive. Large tumors can release antigens into the blood, and these antigens combine with circulating antibodies and prevent them from attacking the tumor cells. Furthermore, tumor cells may possess special blocking factors that coat tumor cells and prevent their destruction by killer T-lymphocytes. During the early development of tumors, the body may fail to recognize the tumor antigens as foreign and subsequently fail to initiate destruction of the malignant cells. Hematologic cancers, such as leukemia and lymphoma, are associated with altered production and function of WBCs and lymphocytes (Chiorazzi, Rai & Ferrarini, 2005).

All treatments that the patient has received or is currently receiving, such as radiation or chemotherapy, are recorded in the health history. Radiation destroys lymphocytes and decreases the ability to mount an effective immune response. The size and extent of the irradiated area determine the extent of immunosuppression. Whole-body irradiation may leave the patient totally immunosuppressed. Chemotherapy also affects bone marrow function, destroying cells that contribute to an effective immune response and resulting in immunosuppression.

CHRONIC ILLNESS AND SURGERY

The health assessment includes a history of chronic illness, such as diabetes mellitus, renal disease, chronic obstructive pulmonary disease (COPD), or fibromyalgia (Karper & Stasik, 2003). The onset and severity of illnesses, as well as treatment that the patient is receiving for the illness, are obtained. Chronic illness may contribute to immune system impairments in various ways. Renal failure is associated with a deficiency in circulating lymphocytes. In addition, immune defenses may be altered by acidosis and uremic toxins. In diabetes, an increased incidence of infection has been associated with vascular insufficiency, neuropathy, and poor control of serum glucose levels. Recurrent respiratory tract infections are associated with COPD as a result of altered inspiratory and expiratory function and ineffective airway clearance. Additionally, a history of organ transplantation or surgical removal of the spleen, lymph nodes, or thymus is noted, because these conditions may place the patient at risk for impaired immune function (Clancy et al., 2002).

SPECIAL PROBLEMS

Conditions such as burns and other forms of injury and infection may contribute to altered immune system function. Major burns cause impaired skin integrity and compromise the body's first line of defense. Loss of large amounts of serum occurs with burn injuries and depletes the body of essential proteins, including immunoglobulins. The physiologic and psychological stressors associated with surgery or injury stimulate cortisol release from the adrenal cortex; increased serum cortisol also contributes to suppression of normal immune responses.

Medications and Blood Transfusions

A list of past and present medications is obtained. In large doses, antibiotics, corticosteroids, cytotoxic agents, salicylates, nonsteroidal anti-inflammatory drugs (NSAIDs), and anesthetics can cause immune suppression (Table 50-6).

A history of blood transfusions is obtained, because previous exposure to foreign antigens through transfusion may be associated with abnormal immune function. Additionally,

℞ TABLE 50-6 Selected Medications and Effects on the Immune System

Drug Classification (and Examples)	Effects on the Immune System
Antibiotics (in large doses)	**Bone marrow suppression**
ceftriaxone (Rocefin)	Eosinophilia, hemolytic anemia, hypoprothrombinemia, neutropenia, thrombocytopenia
cefuroxime sodium (Ceftin)	Eosinophilia, hemolytic anemia, hypoprothrombinemia, neutropenia, thrombocytopenia
chloramphenicol (Chloromycetin)	Leukopenia, aplastic anemia
dactinomycin (Cosmogen)	Agranulocytosis, neutropenia
fluoroquinolones (Cipro, Levaquin, Tequin)	Hemolytic anemia, methemoglobinemia, eosinophilia, leukopenia, pancytopenia
gentamicin sulfate (Garamycin)	Agranulocytosis, granulocytosis
macriolides (erythromycin, Zithromax, Biaxin)	Neutropenia, leukopenia
penicillins	Agranulocytosis
streptomycin	Leukopenia, neutropenia, pancytopenia
vancomycin (Vancocin, Vancoled)	Transient leukopenia
Antithyroid drugs	
propylthiouracil (PTU)	Agranulocytosis, leukopenia
Nonsteroidal anti-inflammatory drugs (NSAIDs) (in large doses)	**Inhibit Prostaglandin Synthesis or Release**
aspirin	Agranulocytosis
cox-2 inhibitors	Anemia, allergy, no major other adverse affects to the immune system
ibuprofen (Advil, Motrin)	Leukopenia, neutropenia
indomethacin (Indocid, Indocin)	Agranulocytosis, leukopenia
phenylbutazone	Pancytopenia, agranulocytosis, aplastic anemia
Adrenal corticosteroids	**Immunosuppression**
prednisone	
Antineoplastic agents (cytotoxic agents)	**Immunosuppression**
alkylating agents	Leukopenia, bone marrow suppression
cyclophosphamide (Cytoxan)	Leukopenia, neutropenia
mechlorethamine HCl (Mustargen)	Agranulocytosis, neutropenia
cyclosporine	Leukopenia, inhibits T-lymphocyte function
Antimetabolites	**Immunosuppression**
fluorouracil (pyrimidine antagonist)	Leukopenia, eosinophilia
methotrexate (folic acid antagonist)	Leukopenia, aplastic bone marrow
mercaptopurine (6-MP) (purine antagonist)	Leukopenia, pancytopenia

although the risk of HIV transmission through blood transfusion is extremely low in patients who received a transfusion after 1985 (the year that testing of blood for HIV was initiated in the United States), a small risk remains.

The patient is also asked about use of herbal agents and over-the-counter medications. Because many of these products have not been subjected to rigorous testing, their effects have not been fully identified. It is important, therefore, to ask patients about their use of these substances, to document their use, and to educate patients about untoward effects that may alter immune responsiveness.

Lifestyle Factors

Like any other body system, the functions of the immune system depend on other body systems. Poor nutritional status, smoking, excessive consumption of alcohol, illicit drug use, STDs, and occupational or residential exposure to environmental radiation and pollutants have been associated with impaired immune function and are assessed in a detailed patient history. Although factors that are not consistent with a healthy lifestyle are predominately responsible for ineffective immune function, positive lifestyle factors can also negatively affect immune function and require assessment. For example, rigorous exercise or competitive exercise—usually considered a positive lifestyle factor—can be a physiologic stressor and cause negative effects on immune response (Buyukyazi, Kutukculer, Kutlu, et al., 2004). This outcome is compounded if the athlete also faces the stressful environmental conditions while undergoing exercise. This phenomenon has been investigated in studies, for example, of marathon runners. Given the cumulative impact of various environmental stressors on the immune system, every effort should be made to minimize the athlete's exposure to stressors other than the exercise performed (Malm, 2004).

Psychoneuroimmunologic Factors

The patient assessment also addresses psychoneuroimmunologic factors. The bidirectional pathway between the brain and immune system is referred to as psychoneuroimmunology, a field that has been the focus of research and discussion over the last several decades (Starkweather, Witek-Janusek & Mathews, 2005; Vines, Gupta, Whiteside, et al., 2003). It is thought that the immune response is regulated and modulated in part by neuroendocrine influences. Lymphocytes and macrophages have receptors that are capable of responding to neurotransmitters and endocrine hormones. Lymphocytes can produce and secrete adrenocorticotropic hormone and endorphin-like compounds. Cells in the brain, especially in the hypothalamus, can recognize prostaglandins, interferons, and interleukins as well as histamine and serotonin, which are released during the inflammatory process. Like all other biologic systems functioning in the interest of homeostasis, the immune system is integrated with other psychophysiologic processes and is subject to regulation and modulation by the brain.

Conversely, the immune processes can affect neural and endocrine function, including behavior. Growing evidence indicates that a measurable immune system response can be positively influenced by biobehavioral strategies such as relaxation and imagery techniques, biofeedback, humor, hypnosis, and conditioning. Therefore, the assessment should address the patient's general psychological status and the patient's use of and response to these strategies.

Physical Examination

On physical examination (see Chart 50-3), the skin and mucous membranes are assessed for lesions, dermatitis, purpura (subcutaneous bleeding), urticaria, inflammation, or any discharge. Any signs of infection are noted. The patient's temperature is recorded, and the patient is observed for chills and sweating. The anterior and posterior cervical, axillary, and inguinal lymph nodes are palpated for enlargement; if palpable nodes are detected, their location, size, consistency, and reports of tenderness on palpation are noted. Joints are assessed for tenderness, swelling, increased warmth, and limited range of motion. The patient's respiratory, cardiovascular, genitourinary, and neurosensory status is evaluated for signs and symptoms indicative of immune dysfunction. Any functional limitations or disabilities the patient may have are also assessed.

NURSING RESEARCH PROFILE

Therapeutic Back Massage and Immune Function in Spouses of Cancer Patients

Goodfellow, L. (2003). The effects of therapeutic back massage on psychophysiologic variables and immune function in spouses of patients with cancer. *Nursing Research, 52*(5), 318–328.

Purpose

The diagnosis, treatment, and continuing management of cancer are major stressors, not only for the patient but also for the patient's spouse, who is often the primary caregiver in the home and supporter. Research suggests that a high stress level may have prolonged effects on the health and well-being of the spouse of an ill partner. Therapeutic back massage (TBM) has been shown to enhance relaxation and, because relaxation reduces stress levels, it may have a positive correlation with optimal immune function. This study was undertaken to determine whether TBM influences psychosocial, physiologic, and immune function variables in spouses of patients with cancer.

Design

An experimental design was used with random assignment of 42 spouses to either the experimental (TBM) group or the control group. The effects of a 20-minute TBM were measured at three points: before intervention, immediately after intervention, and 20 minutes after intervention. Variables measured included natural killer cell activity (NKCA), heart rate, systolic and diastolic blood pressure, mood, and perceived stress. Data were collected about mood using the Profile of Mood States (POMS) and about perceived stress using the Visual Analogue Scale (VAS). Descriptive statistics and two-way repeated-measures analysis of variance (RANOVA) tests were used to analyze the data.

Findings

The RANOVA determined the effects of TBM and showed significant interactions, including a positive change in mood measured on the POMS ($p = .0005$), a decrease in stress measured on the VAS ($p = .001$), as well as a decrease in heart rate and blood pressure, at the two postintervention time points in the TBM group, compared with the control group. Inverse relationships between mood and NKCA ($r = -41$, $p = .009$), and between perceived stress and NKCA ($r = -37$, $p = .017$) were found, providing evidence that TBM may help elevate mood and decrease perceived stress in spouses of patients with cancer.

Nursing Implications

Nurses may find these results particularly useful in clinical practice. TBM can be easily taught to family members, and this study suggests it may help spouses face the challenge of living with and caring for an ill partner. The effect of TBM on NKCA is an area that needs further investigation.

CHART 50-4

Selected Tests for Evaluating Immunologic Status

Various laboratory tests may be performed to assess immune system activity or dysfunction. The studies assess leukocytes and lymphocytes, humoral immunity, cellular immunity, phagocytic cell function, complement activity, hypersensitivity reactions, specific antigen–antibodies, or HIV infection.

LEUKOCYTE AND LYMPHOCYTE TESTS
- White blood cell count and differential
- Bone marrow biopsy

HUMORAL (ANTIBODY-MEDIATED) IMMUNITY TESTS
- B-cell quantification with monoclonal antibody
- In vivo immunoglobulin synthesis with T-cell subsets
- Specific antibody response
- Total serum globulins and individual immunoglobulins (by electrophoresis, immunoelectrophoresis, single radial immunodiffusion, nephelometry, isohemagglutinin techniques)

CELLULAR (CELL-MEDIATED) IMMUNITY TESTS
- Total lymphocyte count
- T-cell and T-cell subset quantification with monoclonal antibody
- Delayed hypersensitivity skin test
- Cytokine production
- Lymphocyte response to mitogens, antigens, and allogenic cells
- Helper and suppressor T-cell functions

PHAGOCYTIC CELL FUNCTION TESTS
- Nitroblue tetrazolium reductase assay

COMPLEMENT COMPONENT TESTS
- Total serum hemolytic complement
- Individual complement component titrations
- Radial immunodiffusion
- Electroimmunoassay
- Radioimmunoassay
- Immunonephelometric assay
- Immunoelectrophoresis

HYPERSENSITIVITY TESTS
- Scratch test
- Patch test
- Intradermal test
- Radioallergosorbent test (RAST)

SPECIFIC ANTIGEN-ANTIBODY TESTS
- Radioimmunoassay
- Immunofluorescence
- Agglutination
- Complement fixation test

HIV INFECTION TESTS
- Enzyme-linked immunosorbent assay (ELISA)
- Western blot
- CD4 and CD8 cell counts
- P24 antigen test
- Polymerase chain reaction (PCR)

Diagnostic Evaluation

A series of blood tests and skin tests and a bone marrow biopsy may be performed to evaluate the patient's immune competence. Specific laboratory and diagnostic tests are discussed in greater detail along with individual disease processes in subsequent chapters in this unit. Selected laboratory and diagnostic tests used to evaluate immune competence are summarized in Chart 50-4.

Nursing Management

The nurse needs to be aware that patients undergoing evaluation for possible immune system disorders experience not only physical pain and discomfort with certain types of diagnostic procedures, but many psychological reactions as well. For example, patients may fear test results that demonstrate decreased immune function, because the diminished immune system can make them more prone to certain infections, cancers, and other disorders. It is the nurse's role to counsel, educate, and support patients throughout the diagnostic process. Further, many patients may be extremely anxious about the results of diagnostic tests and the possible implications of those results for their employment, insurance, and personal relationships. This is an ideal time for the nurse to provide counseling and education, should these interventions be warranted.

Critical Thinking Exercises

1 A 36-year-old man was camping and hiking with his partner when he began to run a high temperature and developed a non-productive cough. He is diagnosed with *Pneumocystis* pneumonia (PCP) and started on antibiotic therapy. He asks why he has developed this problem. How would you respond? What diagnostic tests would you expect to be ordered? Why?

2 ebp A 68-year-old woman is hospitalized for a kidney transplantation, and immunosuppressant medications are prescribed. Describe the parameters you

would use to assess her immune function. How would altered immune function affect the care that you provide? Develop an evidence-based teaching plan for the patient and her family before hospital discharge. Discuss the criteria used to assess the strength of that evidence.

3 A 24-year-old woman presents to her physician's office for a chief complaint of a "facial rash." She is diagnosed with systemic lupus erythematosus (SLE). She asks for information about the disease, why it occurs, what the laboratory tests showed, and what effect it will have on her health status and lifestyle. What nursing observations and assessments are indicated? Identify patient teaching that is appropriate.

REFERENCES AND SELECTED READINGS

BOOKS

Abbas, A. K. & Lichtman, A. H. (2004). *Basic immunology: Functions and disorders of the immune system* (2nd ed.). Philadelphia: W. B. Saunders.

Abbas, A. K. & Lichtman, A. H. (2005). *Cellular and molecular immunology* (5th ed.). Philadelphia: Elsevier Saunders.

Brashers, V. (2002). *Clinical applications of pathophysiology: Assessment, diagnostic reasoning, and management* (2nd ed.). St. Louis: Mosby.

Clancy, J., McVicar, A. J. & Baird, N. (2002). *Perioperative practice: Fundamentals of homeostasis*. New York: Routledge.

Dains, J., Bauman, L. & Scheibel, P. (2003). *Advanced health assessment and clinical diagnosis* (2nd ed.). St. Louis: Mosby.

Goroll, A. H. & Mulley, A. G. Jr. (2002). *Primary care medicine recommendations* (4th ed.). Philadelphia: Lippincott Williams & Wilkins.

Katzung, B. (2004). *Basic and clinical pharmacology* (9th ed.). New York: McGraw-Hill.

Korholz, D. & Kiess, W. (2003). *Methods in molecular biology: Cytokines and colony stimulating factors*. Totowa, NJ: Humana Press.

Lehne, R. (2004). *Pharmacology for nursing care*. St. Louis: Mosby.

Moorhead, S., Johnson, M. & Maas, M. (2004). *Nursing outcomes classification (NOC)* (3rd ed.). St. Louis: Mosby.

Moreland, L. W. (2004). *Rheumatology and immunology therapy: A to Z essentials*. New York: Springer.

Perl, A. (2004). *Autoimmunity: Methods and protocols*. Totowa, NJ: Humana Press.

Porth, C. M. (2005). *Pathophysiology: Concepts of altered health states* (7th ed.). Philadelphia: Lippincott Williams & Wilkins.

JOURNALS

**Asterisks indicate nursing research articles.*

Buyukyazi, G., Kutukculer, N., Kutlu, N., et al. (2004). Differences in the cellular and humoral immune system between middle-aged men with different intensity and duration of physically training. *Journal of Sports Medicine and Physical Fitness, 44*(2), 207–214.

Chiorazzi, N., Rai, K. R. & Ferrarini, M. (2005). Chronic lymphocytic leukemia. *New England Journal of Medicine, 352*(8), 804–815.

Cogle, C., Guthrie, S., Sanders, R., et al. (2003). An overview of stem cell research and regulatory issues. *Mayo Clinic Proceedings, 78*(8), 993–1003.

*Farran, C., Loukissa, D., Lindeman, D., et al. (2004). Caring for self while caring for others: The two-track life of coping with Alzheimer's disease. *Journal of Gerontological Nursing, 30*(5), 38–45.

Fehder, W. P. & Douglas, S. D. (2001). Interactions between the nervous and immune systems. *Seminars in Clinical Neuropsychiatry, 6*(4), 229–240.

*Garand, L., Buckwalter, K., Lubaroff, D., et al. (2002). A pilot study of immune and mood outcomes of a community-based intervention for dementia caregivers: The PLST intervention. *Archives of Psychiatric Nursing, 16*(4), 156–167.

*Goodfellow, L. (2003). The effects of therapeutic back massage on psychophysiologic variables and immune function in spouses of patients with cancer. *Nursing Research, 52*(5), 318–328.

Jegathesan, J., Liebenthat, J. A., Arnett, M. G., et al. (2004). Apoptosis: Understanding the new molecular pathway. *MedSurg Nursing, 13*(6), 371–377.

*Karper, W. & Stasik, S. (2003). A successful long-term exercise program for women with fibromyalgia syndrome and chronic fatigue and immune dysfunction syndrome. *Clinical Nurse Specialist, 17*(5), 243–248.

King, S. E. (2004). Therapeutic cancer vaccines: An emerging treatment option. *Clinical Journal of Oncology Nursing, 8*(3), 271–278.

Lentz, A. K. & Feezor, R. J. (2003). Principles of immunology. *Nutrition in Clinical Practice, 18*(6), 451–460.

Malm, C. (2004). Exercise immunology: The current state of man and mouse. *Sports Medicine, 34*(9), 555–566.

McCowen, K. C. & Bistrian, R. (2003). Immunonutrition: Problematic or problem solving? *American Journal of Clinical Nutrition, 77*(4), 764–770.

Moser, K., Gaffney, P., Peterson, E., et al. (2004). Keys to unlocking the mysteries of rheumatic autoimmune disease. *Minnesota Medicine, 87*(5), 46–51.

*Motzer, S., Jarrett, M., Heitkemper, M. & Tsuju, J. (2002). Natural killer cell function and psychological distress in women with and without irritable bowel syndrome. *Biological Research for Nursing, 4*(1), 31–42.

Rose, N. (2004). Autoimmune disease 2002: An overview. *Journal of Investigative Dermatology, 9*(Suppl 1), 1–4.

Rosenthal, R. A. & Kavic, S. M. (2004). Assessment and management of the geriatric patient. *Critical Care Medicine, 32*(4), S92–S105.

Schwartz, R. S. (2003). Shattuck lecture: Diversity of the immune repertoire and immunoregulation. *New England Journal of Medicine, 348*(11), 1017–1026.

Starkweather, A., Witek-Janusek, L. & Mathews, H. L. (2005) Applying the psychoneuroimmunology framework to nursing research. *Journal of Neuroscience Nursing, 37*(1), 56–62.

*Vines, S., Gupta, S., Whiteside, T., et al. (2003). The relationship between chronic pain, immune function, depression, and health behaviors. *Biological Research for Nursing, 5*(1), 18–29.

RESOURCES

Centers for Disease Control and Prevention, 1600 Clifton Road, Atlanta, GA 30333-3311; http://www.cdc.gov. Accessed June 2, 2006.

National Institute of Allergy and Infectious Disease, Office of Communication and Public Liaison, 6610 Rockville Pike, MSC 6612, Bethesda, MD 20892-6612; http://www.niaid.nih.gov/. Accessed June 2, 2006.

National Institutes of Health, 9000 Rockville Pike, Bethesda, MD 20892; http://www.nih.gov; for toll-free information line for NIH departments: http://www.nih.gov/health/infoline.htm. Accessed June 2, 2006.

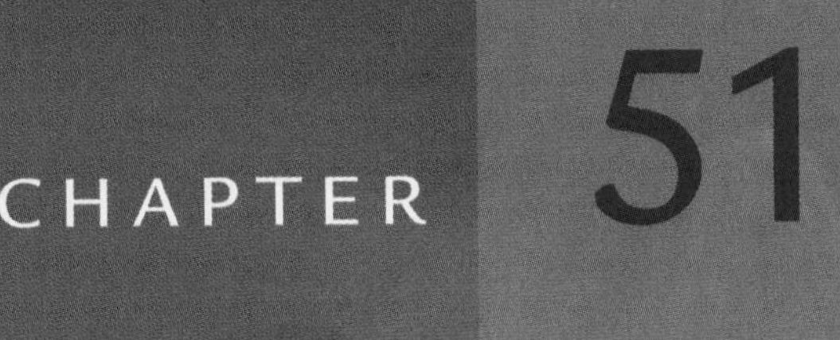

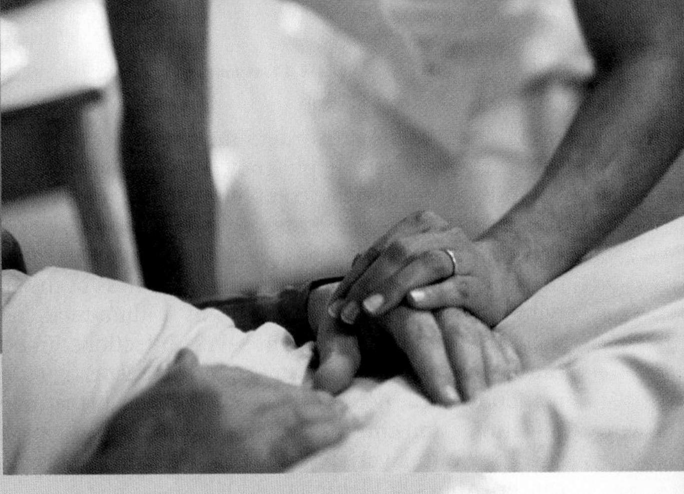

CHAPTER 51

Management of Patients With Immunodeficiency

Learning Objectives

On completion of this chapter, the learner will be able to:

1. Compare the different types of primary immunodeficiency disorders and their causes, clinical manifestations, management, potential complications, and common treatment modalities.
2. Discuss treatment plans for patients with immunodeficiency disorders.
3. Describe the nursing management of the patient with an immunodeficiency.
4. Identify the essential teaching needs for a patient with an immunodeficiency.

Immunodeficiency disorders may be caused by a defect in or a deficiency of phagocytic cells, B-lymphocytes, T-lymphocytes, or the complement system. The specific symptoms and their severity, age at onset, and prognosis depend on the immune system components affected and their degree of functional impairment. Regardless of the underlying cause, the cardinal symptoms of immunodeficiency include chronic or recurrent severe infections, infections caused by unusual organisms or by organisms that are normal body flora, poor response to standard treatment for infections, and chronic diarrhea. In addition, the patient is susceptible to a variety of secondary disorders, including cancer (Abbas & Lichtman, 2004).

Immunodeficiencies can be classified as either primary or secondary and by the affected components of the immune system. Primary immunodeficiency diseases are genetic in origin and are caused by intrinsic defects in the cells of the immune system. In contrast, secondary immunodeficiencies, such as acquired immunodeficiency syndrome (AIDS), are caused by triggers such as infection with human immunodeficiency virus (HIV). Essential elements of effective nursing care include knowledge of the immune system and potential secondary disorders, skillful assessment, symptom management, and sensitivity and responsiveness to the learning needs of the patient and caregiver.

Primary Immunodeficiencies

Primary immunodeficiencies represent inborn errors of immune function and include a variety of syndromes that render patients more susceptible to infections. Primary immunodeficiencies can be fatal if not treated. They are seen primarily in infants and young children. Occasionally, adults present with clinical episodes of infectious diseases that are beyond the scope of normal immunocompetence. Examples include infections that are unusually persistent, recurrent, or resistant to treatment and those involving unexpected dissemination of disease or atypical pathogens. Although some immunodeficiencies have mild presentations and good outcomes, others result in severe infection and significant morbidity and mortality. To date, more than 100 immunodeficiencies of genetic origin have been identified (Riminton & Limaye, 2004). Common primary immunodeficiencies include disorders of humoral immunity (affecting B-cell differentiation or antibody production), T-cell defects, and combined B- and T-cell defects, phagocytic disorders, and complement deficiencies. These disorders may involve one or more components of the immune system. Symptoms of immune deficiency disorders are related to the deficient component (Table 51-1). Major signs and symptoms include multiple infections despite aggressive treatment, infections with unusual or opportunistic organisms, failure to thrive or poor growth, and a positive family history (Cooper, Pommering & Koranyi, 2003).

Phagocytic Dysfunction

Pathophysiology

A variety of primary defects of phagocytes may occur; almost all of them are genetic in origin and affect the innate immune system. In some types of phagocytic disorders, the neutrophils are impaired so that they cannot exit the circulation and travel to sites of infection. As a result, the patient cannot initiate a normal inflammatory response against pathogenic organisms. In some disorders, the neutrophil count may be very low; in others, it may be very high because the neutrophils remain in the vascular system. A clinically important feature of phagocytic cell disorders is the relatively narrow spectrum of disease-specific infections found, such as chronic granulomatous disease (Abbas & Lichtman, 2005; Rosenzweig & Holland, 2004).

Clinical Manifestations

In phagocytic cell disorders, there is an increased incidence of bacterial and fungal infections caused by organisms that are normally nonpathogenic. People with these disorders may also develop fungal infections from *Candida* organisms and viral infections from herpes simplex or herpes zoster

Glossary

agammaglobulinemia: disorder marked by an almost complete lack of immunoglobulins or antibodies

angioneurotic edema: condition marked by development of urticaria and an edematous area of skin, mucous membranes, or viscera

ataxia: loss of muscle coordination

ataxia-telangiectasia: autosomal recessive disorder affecting T- and B-cell immunity primarily seen in children and resulting in a degenerative brain disease

hypogammaglobulinemia: lack of one or more of the five immunoglobulins; caused by B-cell deficiency

immunocompromised host: person with a secondary immunodeficiency and associated immunosuppression

panhypoglobulinemia: general lack of immunoglobulins in the blood

severe combined immunodeficiency disease (SCID): disorder involving a complete absence of humoral and cellular immunity resulting from an X-linked or autosomal genetic abnormality

telangiectasia: vascular lesions caused by dilated blood vessels

thymic hypoplasia: T-cell deficiency that occurs when the thymus gland fails to develop normally during embryogenesis; also known as DiGeorge syndrome

Wiskott-Aldrich syndrome (WAS): immunodeficiency characterized by thrombocytopenia and the absence of T- and B-cells

TABLE 51-1 Selected Primary Immunodeficiency Disorders

Immune Component	Disorder	Major Symptoms	Treatment
Phagocytic cells	Hyperimmunoglobulinemia E (HIE) syndrome	Bacterial, fungal, and viral infections; deep-seated cold abscesses	Antibiotic therapy and treatment for viral and fungal infections Granulocyte-macrophage colony-stimulating factor (GM-CSF); granulocyte colony-stimulating factor (G-CSF)
B-lymphocytes	Sex-linked agammaglobulinemia (Bruton's disease)	Severe infections soon after birth	Passive pooled plasma or gammaglobulin
	Common variable immunodeficiency (CVID)	Bacterial infections, infection with *Giardia lamblia*	Intravenous immunoglobulin (IVIG) Metronidazole (Flagyl) Quinacrine HCl (Atabrine)
		Pernicious anemia	Vitamin B_{12}
		Chronic respiratory infections	Antimicrobial therapy
	Immunoglobulin A (IgA) deficiency	Predisposition to recurrent infections, adverse reactions to blood transfusions or immunoglobulin, autoimmune diseases, hypothyroidism	None
	IgC_2 deficiency	Heightened incidence of infectious diseases	Pooled immunoglobulin
T-lymphocytes	Thymic hypoplasia (DiGeorge syndrome)	Recurrent infections; hypoparathyroidism, hypocalcemia, tetany, convulsions, congenital heart disease, possible renal abnormalities; abnormal facies	Thymus graft
	Chronic mucocutaneous candidiasis	*Candida albicans* infections of mucous membrane, skin, and nails; endocrine abnormalities (hypoparathyroidism, Addison's disease)	Antifungal agents: Topical: miconazole Oral: clotrimazole, ketoconazole IV: amphotericin B
B- and T-lymphocytes	Ataxia-telangiectasia	Ataxia with progressive neurologic deterioration, telangiectasia (vascular lesions), recurrent infections; malignancies	Antimicrobial therapy; management of presenting symptoms; fetal thymus transplant, IV immunoglobulin
	Nezelof's syndrome	Severe infections, malignancies	Antimicrobial therapy; IV immunoglobulin, bone marrow transplantation; thymus transplantation; thymus factors
	Wiskott-Aldrich syndrome	Thrombocytopenia, resulting in bleeding, infections; malignancies	Antimicrobial therapy; splenectomy with continuous antibiotic prophylaxis; IV immunoglobulin and bone marrow transplantation
	Severe combined immunodeficiency disease (SCID)	Overwhelming severe fatal infections soon after birth (also includes opportunistic infections)	Antimicrobial therapy; IV immunoglobulin and bone marrow transplantation
Complement system	Angioneurotic edema	Episodes of edema in various parts of the body, including respiratory tract and bowels	Pooled plasma, androgen therapy
	Paroxysmal nocturnal hemoglobinuria (PNH)	Lysis of erythrocytes due to lack of decay-accelerating factor (DAF) on erythrocytes	None

virus. These patients experience recurrent cutaneous abscesses, chronic eczema, bronchitis, pneumonia, chronic otitis media, and sinusitis. In one type of phagocytic disorder, hyperimmunoglobulinemia E syndrome (formerly known as Job syndrome), white blood cells cannot initiate an inflammatory response to infectious organisms. This results in recurrent skin and pulmonary abscesses; abnormalities of connective tissue, skeleton, and dentition; and extremely elevated levels of immunoglobulin (IgE) (Cohen & Powderly, 2004).

Although patients with phagocytic cell disorders may be asymptomatic, severe neutropenia may be accompanied by deep and painful mouth ulcers, gingivitis, stomatitis, and cellulitis. Death from overwhelming infection occurs in about 10% of patients with severe neutropenia. Chronic granulomatous disease, another type of primary phagocytic disorder, produces recurrent or persistent infections of the soft tissues, lungs, and other organs; these are resistant to aggressive treatment with antibiotics (Canbakan, Ozyilmaz, Capan, et al., 2003; Cohen & Powderly, 2004).

Assessment and Diagnostic Findings

Diagnosis is based on the history, signs and symptoms, and laboratory analysis by the nitroblue tetrazolium reductase test (see Chart 50-3 in Chapter 50), which indicates the cytocidal (causing death of cells) activity of the phagocytic cells. A history of recurrent infection and fever in a child, and occasionally in an adult, is an important key to the diagnosis. Failure of an infection to resolve with usual treatment is also an important indicator. Warning signs of primary immunodeficiency disorders are summarized in Chart 51-1.

Medical Management

Neutropenic patients continue to be at increased risk for development of severe infections despite substantial advances in supportive care. Epidemiologic shifts occur periodically and need to be detected early, because they influence prophylactic, empiric, and specific strategies for medical management. Although it is effective in preventing some bacte-

CHART 51-1

The 10 Warning Signs of Primary Immune Deficiency

Primary immune deficiency causes children and adults to have infections that come back frequently or are unusually hard to cure. In America alone, up to 1/2 million people suffer from one or more of the 70 known primary immune deficiency diseases.

If you or your child is affected by more than one of the following conditions, speak to your doctor about the possible presence of primary immune deficiency.

1. Eight or more new ear infections within 1 year.
2. Two or more serious sinus infections within 1 year.
3. Two or more months on antibiotics with little effect.
4. Two or more pneumonias within 1 year.
5. Failure of an infant to gain weight or grow normally.
6. Recurrent, deep skin or organ abscesses.
7. Persistent thrush in mouth or elsewhere on skin, after age 1.
8. Need for intravenous antibiotics to clear infections.
9. Two or more deep-seated infections such as meningitis, osteomyelitis, cellulitis, or sepsis.
10. A family history of primary immune deficiency.

Though the primary immune deficiency diseases can be serious, they are rarely fatal and can generally be controlled. Primary immune deficiency should not be confused with AIDS. Primary immune deficiency can be diagnosed through blood tests and should be detected as soon as possible to prevent avoidable permanent damage. As with all disease, only direct examination by a physician should be used to determine the presence of primary immune deficiency.

Educational materials developed by the Jeffrey Modell Foundation Medical Advisory Board, New York, NY. Used with permission.

rial and some fungal infections, prophylaxis must be used with caution, because it is associated with the emergence of resistance. The choices for empiric therapy include combination regimens and monotherapy. Specific choices depend on local factors (epidemiology, susceptibility/resistance patterns, availability). Home and inpatient settings are also available, and the selection of setting depends on the patient's risk category. Early diagnosis and appropriate treatment of many fungal and viral infections remains suboptimal in many cases. Attention to infection control and prevention are important strategies, especially with the emergence of multidrug-resistant organisms (Rolston, 2004). Although granulocyte transfusions are sometimes used, they are seldom successful because of the short half-life of these cells. Treatment with granulocyte-macrophage colony-stimulating factor (GM-CSF) or granulocyte colony-stimulating factor (G-CSF) may prove successful, because these proteins draw nonlymphoid stem cells from the bone marrow and hasten their maturation. Hematopoietic stem cell transplantation (HSCT) may also be used to treat primary immunodeficiencies (Antoine, Muller, Cant, et al, 2003). After HSCT the deficient cell types in the blood regenerate (Moreland, 2004).

B-Cell Deficiencies

Pathophysiology

Two types of inherited B-cell deficiencies exist. The first type results from lack of differentiation of B-cell precursors into mature B-cells. As a result, plasma cells are absent, and the germinal centers from all lymphatic tissues disappear, leading to a complete absence of antibody production against invading bacteria, viruses, and other pathogens. This syndrome is called sex-linked **agammaglobulinemia** (Bruton's disease), because all antibodies disappear from the patient's plasma. B-cells in the peripheral blood and the immunoglobulins IgG, IgM, IgA, IgD, and IgE are low or absent. Infants born with this disorder suffer from severe infections starting soon after birth. Males are at a high risk for having X-linked agammaglobulinemia if they have an affected male relative. Early detection and prompt initiation of treatment with gamma-globulin is essential. More than 10% of patients with X-linked agammaglobulinemia are hospitalized for infection at less than 6 months of age; the prognosis of this condition depends on prompt recognition and treatment (Porth, 2005).

The second type of B-cell deficiency results from a lack of differentiation of B-cells into plasma cells. Only diminished antibody production occurs with this disorder. Although plasma cells are the most vigorous producers of antibodies, affected patients have normal lymph follicles and many B-lymphocytes that produce some antibodies. This syndrome, called **hypogammaglobulinemia**, is a frequently occurring immunodeficiency. It is also called common variable immunodeficiency (CVID), a term that encompasses a variety of defects ranging from immunoglobulin A (IgA) deficiency, in which only the plasma cells that produce IgA are absent, to the other extreme, in which there is severe **panhypoglobulinemia** (general lack of immunoglobulins in the blood).

CVID is the most common primary immunodeficiency seen in adults; it can occur in either gender. Most patients are diagnosed as adults, and delay in recognition of the disease is common. CVID is characterized by recurrent bacterial infections, especially of the upper and lower respiratory airways, and is also associated with an increased incidence of autoimmune and neoplastic disorders. Several T- and B-cell defects have been described, although the underlying cause is still unknown. The etiology of this disorder is believed to be multifactorial (DiRenzo, Pasqui & Auteri, 2004).

Clinical Manifestations

Infants with sex-linked agammaglobulinemia usually become symptomatic after the natural loss of maternally transmitted immunoglobulins, which occurs at about 5 to 6 months of age. Symptoms of recurrent pyogenic infections usually occur by that time.

More than half of patients with CVID develop pernicious anemia. Lymphoid hyperplasia of the small intestine and spleen and gastric atrophy detected by biopsy of the stomach are common findings. Other autoimmune diseases, such as arthritis and hypothyroidism, frequently develop in patients with CVID. Young adults who develop the disease also have an increased incidence of chronic lung disease, hepatitis, gastric cancer, and malabsorption that results in chronic diarrhea (Sewell, Buckland & Jolles, 2003). CVID must be distinguished from secondary immunodeficiency diseases caused by protein-losing enteropathy, nephrotic syndrome, or burns.

Patients with CVID are susceptible to infections with encapsulated bacteria, such as *Haemophilus influenzae, Streptococcus pneumoniae,* and *Staphylococcus aureus.* Frequent respiratory tract infections typically lead to chronic progressive bronchiectasis and pulmonary failure. Commonly, infection with *Giardia lamblia* occurs. Opportunistic infections with *Pneumocystis* pneumonia (PCP), however, are seen only in patients who have a concomitant deficiency in T-cell immunity.

Assessment and Diagnostic Findings

Sex-linked agammaglobulinemia may be diagnosed by the marked deficiency or complete absence of all serum immunoglobulins. The diagnosis of CVID is based on the history of bacterial infections, quantification of B-cell activity, and reported signs and symptoms. The number of B-lymphocytes and the total and specific immunoglobulin levels are measured. Measuring only the total serum globulin level is inadequate, because a compensatory overproduction of one globulin may mask the loss of another globulin or the deficiency of a globulin that is present in very low amounts. Antibody titers to confirm successful childhood vaccination are determined by specific serologic tests. Previous successful childhood immunization indicates that B-cells were functioning adequately earlier in life. If the patient exhibits signs and symptoms suggestive of pernicious anemia, hemoglobin and hematocrit levels are also obtained. Biopsies of the small intestine, spleen, and stomach may also be conducted to assess for lymphoid hyperplasia.

Medical Management

Patients with primary phagocytic disorders may be treated with intravenous immunoglobulin (IVIG). Other interventions aimed at overcoming the immunologic defects in CVID, such as interleukin-2 therapy, are being studied, but there is as yet insufficient evidence to support their routine use (Perl, 2004). Those who are receiving adequate treatment with IVIG usually do not require prophylactic antibiotics unless they also have chronic respiratory disease. Antimicrobial therapy is prescribed for respiratory infections to prevent complications such as pneumonia, sinusitis, and otitis media. Intestinal infestation with *G. lamblia* is treated with a 10-day course of metronidazole (Flagyl) or a 7-day course of quinacrine hydrochloride (Atabrine). Patients with pernicious anemia receive parenteral injections of vitamin B_{12} at monthly intervals. Management may also include physical therapy with postural drainage for patients with chronic lung disease or bronchiectasis (Sewell et al., 2003).

T-Cell Deficiencies

Pathophysiology

Defects in T-cells lead to opportunistic infections. Most primary T-cell immunodeficiencies are genetic in origin. Although an increased susceptibility to infection is common, symptoms can vary considerably depending on the type of T-cell defect. Because the T-cells play a regulatory role in immune system function, the loss of T-cell function is usually accompanied by some loss of B-cell activity.

DiGeorge syndrome, or **thymic hypoplasia**, is one example of a primary T-cell immunodeficiency. This rare, complex, multisystem genetic abnormality is caused by the absence of several genes on chromosome 22 (Markert, Alexieff, Li, et al., 2004). The variation in symptoms is a result of differences in the amount of genetic material affected. T-cell deficiency occurs when the thymus gland fails to develop normally during embryogenesis. It often manifests in the neonatal period as a cardiac anomaly. DiGeorge syndrome is one of the few immunodeficiency disorders with symptoms that manifest almost immediately after birth (Walker, 2002).

Chronic mucocutaneous candidiasis, with or without endocrinopathy, is another T-cell disorder associated with a selective defect in T-cell immunity; it is thought to be caused by an autosomal recessive inheritance that affects both males and females. It is considered an autoimmune disorder involving the thymus and other endocrine glands. The disease causes extensive morbidity resulting from endocrine dysfunction.

Clinical Manifestations

Infants born with DiGeorge syndrome have hypoparathyroidism with resultant hypocalcemia resistant to standard therapy, congenital heart disease, cleft palate and lip, dysmorphic facial features, and possibly renal abnormalities (Moreland, 2004). These infants are susceptible to yeast, fungal, protozoan, and viral infections and are particularly susceptible to childhood diseases (chickenpox, measles, rubella), which are usually severe and may be fatal. Many of these infants are also born with congenital heart defects, which can result in heart failure. The most frequent presenting sign in patients with DiGeorge syndrome is hypocalcemia that is resistant to standard therapy. It usually occurs within the first 24 hours of life (Walker, 2002).

The initial presentation of chronic mucocutaneous candidiasis may be a result of either chronic candidal infection or idiopathic endocrinopathy. Patients may survive to the second or third decade of life. Problems may include hypocalcemia and tetany secondary to hypofunction of the parathyroid glands. Hypofunction of the adrenal cortex (Addison's disease) is the major cause of death in these patients; it may develop suddenly and without any history of previous symptoms.

Assessment and Diagnostic Findings

Prompt diagnosis is necessary for appropriate management. Markert and colleagues (2004) reported on an analysis of five infants presenting with infections, skin rashes, and lymphadenopathy after the newborn period. T-cell count and function varied greatly in each patient, and initial laboratory testing did not suggest athymia. Consequently, the authors suggest that diagnostic protocols include a comprehensive immunologic analysis.

Medical Management

Patients with T-cell deficiency should receive prophylaxis for PCP. General care includes management of hypocalcemia and correction of cardiac abnormalities. Hypocalcemia is controlled by oral calcium supplementation in conjunction with administration of vitamin D or parathyroid hormone. Congenital heart disease frequently results in heart failure, and these patients may require immediate surgical intervention in a tertiary care center. Transplantation of fetal thymus, postnatal thymus, or human leukocyte antigen (HLA)-matched bone marrow has been used for permanent reconstitution of T-cell immunity. In patients with DiGeorge syndrome, T-cell function improves with age and often is normal by 5 years of age (Abbas & Lichtman, 2005). IVIG therapy may be used if an antibody deficiency exists. This therapy may also be used to control recurrent infections. Prolonged survival has been reported after successful transplantation of thymus gland or spontaneous remission of immunodeficiency, which occurs in some patients (Markert et al., 2004).

Combined B-Cell and T-Cell Deficiencies

Pathophysiology

T-cell and B-cell immune deficiencies comprise a heterogeneous group of disorders, all characterized by profound impairment in the development or function of the cellular, the humoral, or both parts of the immune system. A variety of inherited (autosomal recessive and X-linked) conditions fit this description. These conditions are typified by disruption of the normal communication system of B-cells and T-cells and impairment of the immune response, and they appear early in life (Cohen & Powderly, 2004).

Ataxia-telangiectasia is an autosomal recessive neurodegenerative disorder that arises because of a defect on chromosome 11; the ataxia-telangiectasia mutation that affects both T- and B-cell immunity (Moreland, 2004). In 40% of patients with this disease, a selective IgA deficiency exists. IgA and IgG subclass deficiencies, along with IgE deficiencies, have been identified. Variable degrees of T-cell deficiencies are observed and become more severe with advancing age. The disease is associated with neurologic, vascular, endocrine, hepatic, and cutaneous abnormalities. It is accompanied by progressive cerebellar ataxia, telangiectasias, recurrent bacterial infection of the sinuses and lungs, and an increased incidence of cancer.

Both B-cells and T-cells are missing in **severe combined immunodeficiency disease (SCID)**. SCID is a phenotypic term that is used for a wide variety of congenital and hereditary immunologic defects characterized by early onset of infections, defects in both B-cell and T-cell systems, lymphoid aplasia, and thymic dysplasia. It is one of the most common causes of primary immunodeficiencies. Inheritance of this disorder can be X-linked, autosomal recessive, or sporadic. The exact incidence of SCID is unknown; it is recognized as a rare disease in most population groups, with an incidence of about 1 case in 1,000,000. This illness occurs in all racial groups and both genders (Fischer, 2003).

Wiskott-Aldrich syndrome (WAS), a variation of SCID, is an inherited immunodeficiency caused by a variety of mutations in the gene encoding the WAS protein. It is characterized by frequent infections, thrombocytopenia with small platelets, eczema, and increased risk for autoimmune disorders and malignancies. Vasculitides and autoimmune hemolytic anemia are the two most common autoimmune manifestations and often cause considerable morbidity and mortality. Many patients require bone marrow transplantation. The prognosis is poor, because most affected infants develop overwhelming fatal infections (Schurman & Candotti, 2003).

Clinical Manifestations

The onset of **ataxia** (loss of muscle coordination) and **telangiectasia** (vascular lesions caused by dilated blood vessels) occurs in the first 4 years of life. Many patients, however, remain symptom-free for 10 years or longer. As the patient approaches the second decade of life, chronic lung disease, cognitive impairment, neurologic symptoms, and physical disability become severe. Long-term survivors develop progressive deterioration of immunologic and neurologic functions. Some affected patients have lived until the fifth decade of life. The primary causes of death in these patients are overwhelming infection and lymphoreticular or epithelial cancer.

The onset of symptoms occurs within the first 3 months of life in most patients with SCID. Symptoms include respiratory infections and pneumonia (often secondary to PCP infection), thrush, diarrhea, and failure to thrive. Many of these infections are resistant to treatment. Shedding of viruses such as respiratory syncytial virus or cytomegalovirus from the respiratory and gastrointestinal tracts is persistent. Maculopapular and erythematous skin rashes may occur. Vomiting, fever, and a persistent rash are also common manifestations (Schurman & Candotti, 2003).

Medical Management

Treatment of ataxia-telangiectasia includes early management of infections with antimicrobial therapy, management of chronic lung disease with postural drainage and physical therapy, and management of other presenting symptoms. Other treatments include transplantation of fetal thymus tissue and IVIG administration (Chart 51-2).

Treatment options for SCID include stem cell and bone marrow transplantation. HSCT has been the definitive therapy for SCID since the first successful transplant in 1968. The ideal donor is an HLA-identical sibling. Improvements continue in the use of HSCT to treat patients with SCID, as well as other primary immunodeficiencies. Evidence demonstrates that transplantation of allogeneic hematopoietic stem cells can cause an enhanced improvement over time (Antoine et al., 2003). Other treatment regimens include administration of IVIG or thymus-derived factors and thymus gland transplantation. Gene therapy has been used, but the results have thus far been disappointing. As treatment improves, an increasing number of patients who previously would have died in infancy are living to adulthood.

Nursing Management

Many patients require immunosuppression to ensure engraftment of depleted bone marrow during certain transplantation procedures. For this reason, nursing care must be meticulous, with attention to preventing infection. Use of appropriate infection control precautions and thorough hand hygiene are essential. It is also essential that the nurse protect the patient through reverse isolation procedures, by donning protective clothing, and by using other precautions to insure a safe environment. Recent evidence suggests that rigorous protective measures do not necessarily contribute to the reduction of infection in neutropenic patients (Mank & van der Lelie, 2002); however, institutional policies related to protective care must be followed scrupulously until definitive evidence demonstrates that precautions are unnecessary (Larson & Nirenberg, 2004). The patient's condition must be monitored at all times, because some patients experience complications that can be fatal.

Deficiencies of the Complement System

The complement system is an integral part of the immune system, and alterations in normal components of complement can result in increased susceptibility to infectious diseases and immune-mediated disorders. Improved techniques to identify the individual components of the complement system have led to a steady increase in the number of deficiencies identified. Disorders of the complement system can be primary or secondary. C2 and C3 component deficiencies result in diminished resistance to bacterial infections.

CHART 51-2

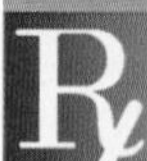

PHARMACOLOGY · Managing an Intravenous Immunoglobulin (IVIG) Infusion

Previously available only for intramuscular injection, immunoglobulin can now be administered for replacement therapy as an IV infusion in greater, more effective doses without painful side effects. Variables affecting the risk and intensity of adverse events associated with the administration of IVIG include patient age, underlying condition, history of migraine, cardiovascular and/or renal disease, dose, concentration, rate of infusion, as well as specific data related to the precise lot of the product being used. The nurse must assess all of these variables before starting the IVIG infusion and continue to assess to anticipate adverse effects if any of these variables are present in the patient being treated (Pierce & Jain, 2003).

HOW SUPPLIED

Immunoglobulin is supplied in a 5% solution or a lyophilized powder with a reconstituting diluent prepared from Cohn fraction II obtained from pools of 1,000 to 10,000 donors. Currently, a number of different IV preparations are approved for use and have been shown to be effective and safe by the U.S. Food and Drug Administration.

DOSAGE

The optimal dose is that determined by the patient's response. In most instances, an IV dose of 100 to 400 mg/kg of body weight is administered monthly or more frequently to ensure adequate serum levels of immunoglobulin G.

ADVERSE EFFECTS

- Complaints of flank pain, shaking chills, and tightness in the chest, terminating with a slight rise in body temperature
- Hypotension (possible with severe reactions)
- Anaphylactic reactions

GUIDELINES FOR NURSING MANAGEMENT

- Weigh the patient before treatment.
- Obtain vital signs before, during, and after treatment.
- Administer the prescribed pretreatment prophylactic aspirin or IV antihistamine, such as diphenhydramine (Benadryl).
- Understand that long-term tolerance of an older IVIG product does not necessarily imply tolerance to a newer product, even if it is technically superior. Caution should be exercised when changing IVIG products as they are not biologically equivalent.
- Be aware that corticosteroids may be used to prevent possible severe reactions.
- Administer the IV infusion at a slow rate, not to exceed 3 mL/min.
- Assess the patient for adverse reactions, including the early signs of anaphylactic shock; prepare to slow the infusion rate if necessary.
- Be aware that patients with low gammaglobulin levels have more severe reactions than those with normal levels (eg, patients who receive gammaglobulin for thrombocytopenia or Kawasaki disease).
- Keep in mind that patients who have an immunoglobulin A (IgA) deficiency have IgE antibodies to IgA, which requires administration of plasma or immunoglobulin replacement from IgA-deficient patients. Because all IV immunoglobulin preparations contain some IgA, they may cause an anaphylactic reaction in patients with IgE anti-IgA antibodies.
- Remember that the risk for transmission of hepatitis, HIV, or other known viruses is extremely low.
- Be cognizant that the pharmacokinetics of IgG differ when smaller doses are given more frequently, as is commonly done with subcutaneous regimens. Differences include lower peaks and higher troughs, which may be preferable for some patients.

Hereditary **angioneurotic edema** results from the deficiency of C1-esterase inhibitor, which opposes the release of inflammatory mediators. The clinical picture of this autosomal dominant disorder includes recurrent attacks of edema formation in the subcutaneous tissue, gastrointestinal tract, and upper airway (Moreland, 2004). Although the disease is mild in childhood and becomes more severe after puberty, first episodes have been reported later in life. Food allergy has often been linked to this disorder, although recent evidence has implicated a C1-esterase inhibitor deficiency. The fluctuations in hormone levels at the beginning of adolescence, in the perimenopausal period, during pregnancy, and during the use of oral contraceptives can precipitate edematous attacks that usually disappear after the onset of menopause (Andre, Veysseyre-Balter, Rousset, et al., 2003; Visy, Fust, Varga, et al., 2004).

Paroxysmal nocturnal hemoglobinuria is an acquired clonal stem cell disorder resulting from a somatic mutation in the hematopoietic stem cell. It is characterized by intravascular hemolysis, cytopenia, frequent infections, bone marrow hyperplasia, and a high incidence of life-threatening venous thrombosis. An absent glycosylphosphatidylinositol (GPI)-anchored receptor prevents several proteins from binding to the erythrocyte membrane. These include the complement-regulatory proteins, CD55 and CD59, the absence of which results in enhanced complement-mediated lysis. Patients with this disorder present with anemia and hemoglobinuria. Laboratory diagnosis can include specialized

NURSING RESEARCH PROFILE

Preventing Infection in Hospitalized Neutropenic Patients with Cancer

Larson, E. & Nirenberg, A. (2004). Evidence-based nursing practice to prevent infection in hospitalized neutropenic patients with cancer. *Oncology Nursing Forum, 31*(4), 717–723.

Purpose

Hospitalized patients with cancer and neutropenia are at high risk for infection. The purpose of this study was to review research that has assessed the effectiveness of selected nursing interventions used in hospitals to prevent health care–associated infections in patients with cancer and neutropenia.

Design

A search of the literature used the key words "low microbial diets," "protective clothing and environments," "personal hygiene," and "oral care" to search English-language articles from PubMed; the *Cumulative Index of Nursing and Allied Health Literature;* the National Guideline Clearing House, 1980–June, 2003; and Cochrane Database of Systematic Reviews. The identified articles were then reviewed and classified into levels of evidence.

Findings

Few studies demonstrated the effectiveness of low microbial food and water or protective environments and clothing in reducing infections in patients with cancer and neutropenia, and hospitals vary in these practices. Skin asepsis reduces microbial counts, but data regarding its effect on infections are lacking. Many studies were characterized by insufficient sample sizes or use of multiple interventions, yet many consensus guidelines were identified. At the highest level of evidence, support was found for the clinical practice of using ice chips to prevent mucositis.

Implications for Nursing

Nurses practicing in areas with patients who are neutropenic should know that, although the evidence base for clinical practices such as a low microbial diet, protective environments and clothing, and special skin asepsis regimens is weak, the authors have identified some of these practices as prudent and reasonable. Evidence supports the clinical practice of using ice chips to prevent mucositis. More studies with sufficient sample sizes addressing nursing practices such as the role of protective environments, room placement, antiseptic bathing, and prevention and treatment of oral complications are clearly needed.

tests, such as the sucrose hemolysis test, Ham acid hemolysis test, and fluorescent-activated cell analysis. Treatment is mainly supportive, consisting of transfusion therapy, anticoagulation therapy, and antibiotic therapy. HSCT may be curative (Schwartz, 2004; Smith, 2004).

Secondary Immunodeficiencies

Secondary immunodeficiencies are more common than primary immunodeficiencies and frequently occur as a result of underlying disease processes or the treatment of these diseases. Common causes of secondary immunodeficiencies include malnutrition, chronic stress, burns, uremia, diabetes mellitus, certain autoimmune disorders, certain viruses, exposure to immunotoxic medications and chemicals, and self-administration of recreational drugs and alcohol. AIDS, the most common secondary immunodeficiency disorder, is discussed in detail in Chapter 52. Patients with secondary immunodeficiencies have immunosuppression and are often referred to as **immunocompromised hosts.**

Medical management of secondary immunodeficiencies includes diagnosis and treatment of the underlying disease process. Interventions include teaching the patient to control or avoid factors that contribute to immunosuppression, treating the underlying condition, and using sound principles of infection control.

Nursing Management for Patients With Immunodeficiencies

Nursing management includes assessment, patient teaching, selected interventions, and supportive care. Assessment of the patient for infection and timely initiation of treatment are essential. Nursing care of patients with primary and secondary immunodeficiencies depends on the underlying cause of the immunodeficiency, the type of immunodeficiency, and its severity. Because immunodeficiencies result in a compromised immune system and a high risk for infection, careful assessment of the patient's immune status is essential. The assessment focuses on the history of past infections, particularly the type and frequency of infection; methods of and response to past treatments; signs and symptoms of any current skin, respiratory, oral, gastrointestinal, or genitourinary infection; and measures taken by the patient to prevent infection. The nurse assesses and monitors the patient for signs and symptoms of infection (Chart 51-3). Advances in science have had the effect of expanding the spectrum of dysfunctional immune responses, leading to larger numbers of patients diagnosed with immunodeficiencies. Many patients develop oral manifestations and need education about their role in promoting good dental hygiene.

CHART 51-3

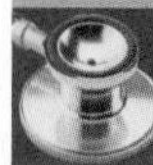

Assessing for Infection

Be on the alert for the following signs and symptoms:
- Fever with or without chills
- Cough with or without sputum
- Shortness of breath
- Difficulty breathing
- Difficulty swallowing
- White patches in the oral cavity
- Swollen lymph nodes
- Nausea with or without vomiting
- Persistent diarrhea
- Frequency, urgency, or pain on urination
- Change in the character of the urine
- Lesions on the face, lips, or perianal area
- Redness, swelling, or drainage from skin lesions
- Persistent vaginal discharge with or without perianal itching
- Persistent abdominal pain

Because the inflammatory response may be blunted, the patient is observed for subtle and unusual signs and changes in physical status. Vital signs and the development of pain, neurologic signs, cough, and skin and oral lesions are monitored and reported immediately. Pulse rate and respiratory rate should be counted for a full minute, because even subtle changes can signal deterioration in the patient's clinical status. Thorough auscultation and assessment of the breath sounds are also important in detecting changes in respiratory status that would signal an existing or impending infection. Any unusual response to treatment or a significant change in the patient's clinical condition must be promptly reported to the physician.

The nurse continuously monitors laboratory values (ie, white blood cell count and differential cell count) for changes indicative of infection. Culture and sensitivity reports from wound drainage, lesions, sputum, stool, urine, and blood are monitored to identify pathogenic organisms and appropriate antimicrobial therapy. Changes in laboratory results and subtle changes in clinical status must be reported to the physician, because the immunocompromised patient may fail to develop typical signs and symptoms of infection.

Assessment also focuses on nutritional status; stress level and coping skills; use of alcohol, drugs, or tobacco; and general hygiene practices, all of which may affect immune function. Strategies the patient has used to reduce the risk of infection are identified and evaluated for their appropriateness and effectiveness (Dudek, 2006). Other aspects of nursing care are directed toward reducing the patient's risk for infection, assisting with medical measures aimed at improving immune status and treating infection, achieving optimal nutritional status, and maintaining respiratory, bowel, and bladder function. The patient's ability to demonstrate acceptable hand hygiene must be assessed, and the patient must be encouraged to cough and perform deep-breathing exercises at regular intervals. Teaching good dental hygiene measures reduces the potential for oral lesions, as do instructions on measures to protect the integrity of the skin. Attention to strict aseptic technique when performing invasive procedures, such as dressing changes, venipunctures, and bladder catheterizations, is essential. Other aspects of nursing care include assisting the patient to manage stress, to incorporate lifelong patterns of physiologic safety, and to adopt behaviors that strengthen immune system function.

If the patient is a candidate for any of the newer or experimental therapies (gene therapy, bone marrow transplantation, immunomodulators such as interferon-γ), the patient and family must be informed about the potential risks and benefits of the treatment regimen. A major role of the nurse is to develop and maintain a knowledge base in these evolving treatment modalities, in order to help the patient and family understand the treatment options and cope with the uncertainties of treatment outcomes.

Promoting Home and Community-Based Care

Teaching Patients Self-Care

The patient and caregivers require instruction about the signs and symptoms that indicate infection and about the potential for atypical symptoms secondary to underlying immunosuppression. They need to be informed of the necessity of continuous monitoring for subtle changes in the patient's physical health status and of the importance of seeking immediate health care if changes are detected. Patients should be advised that they know themselves best; therefore, whenever they experience a symptom that is not typical for them, they should contact their health care provider, who will determine and initiate appropriate therapy. Instruction needs to be provided about prophylactic medication regimens, including dosage, indications, times, actions, potential interactions, and side effects. Patients and their families are also instructed about the importance of continuing treatment regimens without interruption and incorporating these routines into their daily living patterns. The patient is instructed about the importance of avoiding others with infections and avoiding crowds, and about other ways to prevent infection (Chart 51-4).

The patient who is to receive IVIG at home will need information about the expected benefits and outcomes of the treatment as well as expected adverse reactions and their management (Chart 51-5). Patients who can perform self-infusion at home must be instructed in sterile technique, medication dosages, administration rate, and detection and management of adverse reactions (Berger, 2004).

Continuing Care

Encouraging the patient and family to be active partners in the management of the immunodeficiency is the key to successful outcomes and a favorable prognosis. The patient must be made aware that all health-related instructions are lifelong, that follow-up with all scheduled appointments is essential, and that it is the patient's responsibility to notify the primary care provider of any early signs or symptoms

CHART 51-4

HOME CARE CHECKLIST • Infection Prevention for the Patient With Immunodeficiency

At the completion of the home care instruction, the patient or caregiver will be able to:	Patient	Caregiver
• Identify signs and symptoms of infection to report to the health care provider, such as fever, chills; wet or dry cough; breathing problems; white patches in the mouth; swollen glands; nausea; vomiting; persistent abdominal pain; persistent diarrhea; problems with urination; red, swollen, or draining wounds; sores or lesions on the body; and persistent vaginal discharge with or without itching.	✔	✔
• Demonstrate correct handwashing procedure.	✔	✔
• State rationale for thorough handwashing before eating, after using the bathroom, and before and after performing health care procedures.	✔	✔
• State rationale for use of cream and emollients to prevent or manage dry, chaffed, or cracked skin.	✔	✔
• Demonstrate recommended personal hygiene in bathing and foot care to prevent bacterial and fungal diseases.	✔	✔
• State rationale for avoiding contact with people who have known illness or who have recently been vaccinated.	✔	✔
• Verbalize understanding of ways to maintain a well-balanced diet and adequate calories.	✔	✔
• State the reason for avoiding the eating of raw fruits and vegetables, cooking all foods thoroughly, and immediately refrigerating all leftover food.	✔	✔
• Identify the rationale for frequent cleaning of kitchen and bathroom surfaces with disinfectant.	✔	✔
• Identify rationale and benefits of avoiding alcohol, tobacco, and unprescribed medications.	✔	✔
• State rationale for taking prescribed medications as directed.	✔	✔
• Verbalize ways to cope with stress successfully, plans for regular exercise, and rationale for obtaining adequate rest.	✔	✔

CHART 51-5

HOME CARE CHECKLIST • Home Infusion of Intravenous Immunoglobulin (IVIG)

At the completion of the home care instruction, the patient or caregiver will be able to:	Patient	Caregiver
• Identify the benefits and expected outcome of IVIG.	✔	✔
• Demonstrate how to check for patency of IV access device.	✔	✔
• Demonstrate how to prepare IVIG.	✔	✔
• Demonstrate how to infuse IVIG.	✔	✔
• Demonstrate how to clean and maintain IV equipment.	✔	✔
• Identify side effects and adverse effects of IVIG.	✔	✔
• State rationale for prophylactic use of aspirin and an antihistamine before treatment begins.	✔	✔
• Verbalize understanding of emergency measures for anaphylactic shock.	✔	✔

of infection, however subtle they may be. If the patient's treatment includes IVIG and the patient or family cannot administer treatment, a referral for home care or an infusion service may be warranted.

Critical Thinking Exercises

1 A 70-year-old woman with an extensive past medical history, including chronic obstructive pulmonary disease, angina, hypercholesterolemia, hypothyroidism, gastroesophageal reflux disease (GERD), osteoporosis and arthritis, is referred to the allergy and immunology clinic for evaluation of her immune status. In addition to the 21 medications she routinely takes, she has received several courses of antibiotics in the previous months for recurrent infections. What diagnostic tests would you expect to be ordered? Why? What further assessment data would you want to obtain from this patient?

2 The mother of your 17-year-old nephew contacts you to discuss his frequent illnesses. She asks whether there may be something serious underlying his frequent bouts of colds, viruses and sinus infections. She describes them as "seeming to run into one another; he has lost so much time from school." Identify the 10 warning signs of primary immune deficiency that you would consider when responding to this mother's dilemma.

3 ebp You are the charge nurse on a general medical unit to which most of the patients with depressed immune competence are admitted. A nurse approaches you for advice on the best infection control practices to use with a patient who has just been admitted with a WBC of 1,000. Identify the infection control measures that are indicated. Describe the evidence base for the infection control measures you identified and the criteria used to evaluate the strength of that evidence.

REFERENCES AND SELECTED READINGS

BOOKS

Abbas, A. K., & Lichtman, A. H. (2004). *Basic immunology*. Philadelphia: W. B. Saunders.

Abbas, A. K. & Lichtman, A. H. (2005). *Cellular and molecular immunology* (5th ed.). Philadelphia: Elsevier Saunders.

Cohen, J. & Powderly, W. G. (2004). *Infectious diseases* (2nd ed.). St. Louis: Mosby.

Dudek, S. G. (2006). *Nutrition essentials for nursing practice* (5th ed.). Philadelphia: Lippincott Williams & Wilkins.

Jarvis, C. (2003). *Physical examination and health assessment*. Philadelphia: W. B. Saunders.

Moorhead, S., Johnson, M. & Maas, M. (2004). *Nursing outcomes classification (NOC)* (3rd ed.). St. Louis: Mosby.

Moreland, L. W. (2004). *Rheumatology and immunology therapy: A to Z essentials*. New York: Springer.

Nairn, R. & Helbert, M. (2004). *Immunology for medical students*. St. Louis: Mosby.

Perl, A. (2004). *Autoimmunity: Methods and protocols*. Totowa, NJ: Humana Press.

Porth, C. M. (2005). *Pathophysiology: Concepts of altered health states* (7th ed.). Philadelphia: Lippincott Williams & Wilkins.

Rabson, A., Roitt, I. & Delves, P. (2004). *Really essential medical immunology*. Malden, MA: Blackwell Science.

Rosen, F. & Ceha, R. (2004). *Case studies in immunology: A clinical companion* (4th ed.). New York: Garland Publishing.

Tierney, L. M., McPhee, S. J. & Papadakis, M. A. (2004). *Current medical diagnosis and treatment* (44th ed.). Stamford, CT: Appleton & Lange.

JOURNALS

Asterisks indicate nursing research articles.

Andre, F., Veysseyre-Balter, C., Rousset, H., et al. (2003). Exogenous estrogen as an alternative to food allergy in the etiology of angioneurotic edema. *Toxicology, 185*(1–2), 155–160.

Antoine, C., Muller, S., Cant, A., et al. (2003). Long-term survival and transplantation of hematopoietic stem cells for immunodeficiencies: Report of the European experience. *Lancet, 361*(9357), 553–560.

Berger, M. (2004). Subcutaneous immunoglobulin replacement in primary immunodeficiencies. *Clinical Immunology, 112*(1), 1–7.

Buckley, R. H. (2002). Primary immunodeficiency diseases: Dissectors of the immune system. *Immunological Reviews, 185*(7), 206–219.

Canbakan, S., Ozyilmaz, E., Capan, N., et al. (2003). Hyper IgE syndrome in an adult. *ACI International, 15*(2), 82–84.

Cooper, M., Pommering, T. & Koranyi, K. (2003). Primary immunodeficiencies. *American Family Physician, 68*(10), 2001–2008.

DiRenzo, M., Pasqui, A. & Auteri, A. (2004). Common variable immunodeficiency: A review. *Clinical and Experimental Medicine, 3*(4), 211–217.

Fischer, A. (2003). Have we seen the last variant of severe combined immunodeficiency? *New England Journal of Medicine, 349*(10), 1789–1792.

*Hansen, S., Gardulf, A., Andersson, E., et al. (2004). Women with primary antibody deficiencies requiring IgG replacement therapy: Their perception of prenatal care during pregnancy. *Journal of Obstetric, Gynecologic, and Neonatal Nursing, 33*(5), 604–609.

*Larson, E. & Nirenberg, A. (2004). Evidence-based nursing practice to prevent infection in hospitalized neutropenic patients with cancer. *Oncology Nursing Forum, 31*(4), 717–723.

*Mank, A. & van der Lelie, H. (2002). Is there still an indication for nursing patients with prolonged neutropenia in protective isolation? *European Journal of Oncology Nursing, 7*(1), 17–23.

Markert, M., Alexieff, M., Li, J., et al. (2004). Complete DiGeorge syndrome: Development of rash, lymphadenopathy, and oligoclonal T cells in 5 cases. *Journal of Allergy and Clinical Immunology, 113*(4), 734–741.

Pierce, L. & Jain, N. (2003). Risks associated with the use of intravenous immunoglobulin. *Transfusion Medicine Reviews, 17*(4), 241–251.

Riminton, D. & Limaye, S. (2004). Primary immunodeficiency diseases in adulthood. *Internal Medicine Journal, 34*(6), 348–354.

Rolston, K. (2004). Management of infections in the neutropenic patient. *Annual Review of Medicine, 55*(6), 519–526.

Rosenzweig, S. & Holland, S. (2004). Phagocyte immunodeficiencies and their infections. *Journal of Allergy and Clinical Immunology, 113*(4), 620–626.

*Saleh, U. & Brockopp, D. (2001). Hope among patients with cancer hospitalized for bone marrow transplantation. *Cancer Nursing, 24*(4), 308–314.

*Saleh, U. & Brockopp, D. (2001). Quality of life one year following bone marrow transplantation: Psychometric evaluation of the quality of life in bone marrow transplant survivors tool. *Oncology Nursing Forum, 28*(9), 1457–1464.

Schurman, S. & Candotti, F. (2003). Autoimmunity in Wiskott-Aldrich syndrome. *Current Opinion in Rheumatology, 15*(4), 446–453.

Schwartz, R. (2004). Black mornings, yellow sunsets: A day with paroxysmal nocturnal hemoglobinuria. *New England Journal of Medicine, 350*(6), 537–538.

Sewell, W. A., Buckland, M. & Jolles, S. R. (2003). Therapeutic strategies in common variable immunodeficiency. *Drugs, 63*(13), 1359–1371.

Smith, L. (2004). Paroxysmal nocturnal hemoglobinuria. *Clinical Laboratory Science, 17*(3), 172–177.

*So, W., Dodgson, J. & Tai, J. (2003). Fatigue and quality of life among Chinese patients with hematologic malignancy after bone marrow transplantation. *Cancer Nursing, 26*(3), 211–219.

Visy, B., Fust, G., Varga, L., et al. (2004). Sex hormones in hereditary angioneurotic edema. *Clinical Endocrinology, 60*(4), 508–515.

Walker, S. (2002). DiGeorge syndrome in the neonate: Helping parents understand its implications. *Journal of Neonatal Nursing, 8*(6), 191–194.

*Young, L., Polzin, J., Todd, S. et al. (2002). Validation of the nursing diagnosis anxiety in adult patients undergoing bone marrow transplant. *International Journal of Nursing Terminologies and Classifications, 13*(3), 88–100.

RESOURCES

Centers for Disease Control and Prevention, 1600 Clifton Road, Atlanta, GA 30333; 404-639-3311 or 800-311-3435; http://www.cdc.gov. Accessed June 2, 2006.

The Immune Deficiency Foundation (IDF), 40 W. Chesapeake Avenue, Suite 308, Towson, MD 21204; 800-296-4433; http://www.primaryimmune.org. Accessed June 2, 2006.

National Institute of Allergy and Infectious Disease, NIAID Office of Communications and Public Liaison, NIH, 6610 Rockledge Drive, Bethesda, MD 20892-6612; 301-496-5717; http://www.niaid.nih.gov. Accessed June 2, 2006.

National Institutes of Health, 9000 Rockville Pike, Bethesda, MD 20892; 301-496-4000; http://www.nih.gov. Accessed June 2, 2006.

National Library of Medicine, 8600 Rockville Pike, Bethesda, MD 20894; 888-FIND-NLM, 888-346-3656, 301-594-5983; http://www.nlm.nih.gov. Accessed June 2, 2006.

National Primary Immunodeficiency Resource Center/Jeffrey Modell Foundation; 1-866-INFO-4-PI; http://www.info4pi.org. Accessed June 2, 2006.

CHAPTER 52

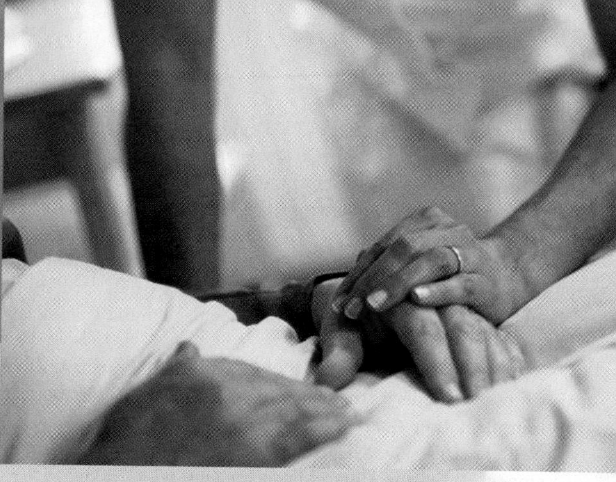

Management of Patients With HIV Infection and AIDS

Learning Objectives

On completion of this chapter, the learner will be able to:

1. Describe the modes of transmission of HIV infection.
2. Describe the pathophysiology of HIV infection.
3. Explain the physiology underlying the clinical manifestations of HIV infection.
4. Describe the management of patients with HIV infection.
5. Discuss the nursing interventions appropriate for patients with HIV infection and AIDS.
6. Use the nursing process as a framework for care of the patient with AIDS.

Although progress has been made in treating human immunodeficiency virus (HIV) infection and acquired immunodeficiency syndrome (AIDS), the epidemic remains a critical public health issue in all communities across the country and around the world. Prevention, early detection, and ongoing treatment remain important aspects of care for people with HIV infection and AIDS. Nurses in all settings encounter people with this disease; therefore, nurses need an understanding of the disorder, knowledge of the physical and psychological consequences associated with the diagnosis, and expert assessment and clinical management skills to provide optimal care for people with HIV infection and AIDS.

In 1987, just 6 years after the first cases of AIDS were reported, the U.S. Food and Drug Administration (FDA) approved the first antiretroviral agent; in 1988, the first randomized controlled trial of primary prophylaxis of *Pneumocystis jiroveci* pneumonia (PCP; formerly called *P. carinii* pneumonia) appeared in the literature; and in 1995, protease inhibitors joined the growing number of antiretroviral agents. Improved treatment of HIV and AIDS has resulted in increased survival times; the estimated number of deaths among people with AIDS in 2002 represented a 14% decline since 1998 (Centers for Disease Control and Prevention [CDC], 2005).

HIV Infection and AIDS

Since acquired immunodeficiency syndrome (AIDS) was first recognized more than 20 years ago, remarkable progress has been made in improving the quality and duration of life

Glossary

alpha-interferon: protein substance that the body produces in response to infection

anergy: loss or weakening of the body's immunity to an irritating agent or antigen

B-cell lymphoma: common malignancy in patients with HIV/AIDS

candidiasis: yeast infection of skin or mucous membrane

CCR5: cell surface molecule that is needed along with the CD4 molecule to fuse with the membranes of the host's immune system cells

cytomegalovirus (CMV): a species-specific herpes virus that may cause retinitis in people with AIDS

EIA (enzyme immunoassay): a blood test that can determine the presence of antibodies to HIV in the blood or saliva; also referred to as **enzyme-linked immunosorbent assay (ELISA)**. Positive results must be validated, usually with Western blot test.

HIV-1: retrovirus isolated and recognized as the etiologic agent of AIDS

HIV-2: virus closely related to HIV-1 that has also been found to cause AIDS

HIV encephalopathy: degenerative neurologic condition characterized by a group of clinical presentations including loss of coordination, mood swings, loss of inhibitions, and widespread cognitive dysfunctions; formerly referred to as AIDS dementia complex (ADC)

human papillomavirus (HPV): virus that causes venereal warts

Kaposi's sarcoma: malignancy that involves the epithelial layer of blood and lymphatic vessels

macrophage: large immune cell that devours invading pathogens and other intruders. Can harbor large quantities of HIV without being killed, acting as a reservoir of the virus.

monocyte: large white blood cell that ingests microbes or other cells and foreign particles. When a monocyte enters tissues, it develops into a macrophage.

***Mycobacterium avium* complex (MAC):** opportunistic infection caused by mycobacterial organisms that commonly causes a respiratory illness but can also infect other body systems

opportunistic infection: illness caused by various organisms, some of which usually do not cause disease in persons with normal immune systems

p24 antigen: blood test that measures viral core protein; accuracy of test is limited because the p24 antibody binds with the antigen and makes it undetectable

peripheral neuropathy: disorder characterized by sensory loss, pain, muscle weakness, and wasting of muscles in the hands or legs and feet

***Pneumocystis jiroveci* pneumonia (PCP):** common opportunistic lung infection caused by an organism, initially thought to be a protozoan but now believed to be a fungus based on its structure

polymerase chain reaction (PCR): a sensitive laboratory technique that can detect and quantify HIV in a person's blood or lymph nodes

primary infection: 4- to 7-week period of rapid viral replication immediately following infection; also known as acute HIV infection

progressive multifocal leukoencephalopathy (PML): opportunistic infection that infects brain tissue and causes damage to the brain and spinal cord

protease inhibitor: medication that inhibits the function of protease, an enzyme needed for HIV replication

provirus: viral genetic material in the form of DNA that has been integrated into the host genome. When it is dormant in human cells, HIV is in a proviral form.

retrovirus: a virus that carries genetic material in RNA instead of DNA and contains reverse transcriptase

reverse transcriptase: enzyme that transforms single-stranded RNA into a double-stranded DNA

viral load test: measures the quantity of HIV RNA in the blood

viral set point: amount of virus present in the blood after the initial burst of viremia and the immune response that follows

wasting syndrome: involuntary weight loss of 10% of baseline body weight with chronic diarrhea or chronic weakness and documented fever.

Western blot assay: a blood test that identifies antibodies to HIV and is used to confirm the results of an EIA (ELISA) test

window period: time from infection with HIV until seroconversion detected on HIV antibody test

for people with HIV infection. During the first decade, this progress was associated with the recognition of opportunistic disease processes, more effective therapy for complications, and introduction of prophylaxis against common **opportunistic infections.** The second decade witnessed progress in the development of highly active antiretroviral therapies (HAART) as well as continuing progress in the treatment of opportunistic infections. The third decade has focused on issues of adherence to therapy, development of second-generation medications to treat HIV disease, and continued pressure to develop a vaccine. The HIV serologic test, an enzyme immunoassay (EIA; formerly enzyme-linked immunosorbent assay [ELISA]), became available in 1984, allowing early diagnosis of the infection before onset of symptoms. Since then, HIV infection has been best managed as a chronic disease and most appropriately managed in an outpatient care setting.

Epidemiology

In the fall of 1982, the CDC issued a case definition of AIDS after the first 100 cases were reported. Since then, the CDC has revised the case definition a number of times (1985, 1987, and 1993). All 50 states, the District of Columbia, United States dependencies and possessions, and independent nations in free association with the United States report AIDS cases to the CDC using a uniform surveillance case definition and case report form (CDC, 2005). Starting in the late 1990s, many more states began to implement HIV case reporting in response to the changing epidemic and the need for information on the numbers and characteristics of people with HIV infection who had not yet developed AIDS.

Thirty-three areas report integrated HIV and AIDS surveillance data, but these areas represent only about 43% of the epidemic in the United States (CDC, 2005). From 2000 through 2003, the estimated number of HIV/AIDS cases in the 33 areas with confidential name-based HIV infection reporting remained relatively stable. African Americans accounted for 50% of all HIV/AIDS cases diagnosed in 2003, and males accounted for 72% of the cases. During that same period, the estimated number of cases in the reporting areas increased each year among men who have sex with men and among heterosexual adults and adolescents and decreased among intravenous (IV)/injection drug users. These patterns were also found in numbers of AIDS cases reported during the period 1999 to 2003. Three states (California, Florida, and New York) reported 43% of the cumulative AIDS cases and 41% of the AIDS cases reported to the CDC in 2004 (CDC, 2005). Through 2004, a total of about 920,000 people had been reported as having AIDS in the United States, dependencies, possessions, and associated nations.

Worldwide, AIDS kills more than 8,000 people every day, 1 person every 10 seconds (UNAIDS, 2006). Since the beginning of the epidemic, AIDS has claimed almost 39 million lives; the gender distribution of newly HIV-infected adults in 2005 was approximately 50% men and 50% women; unsafe sex was the predominant mode of transmission. The earliest confirmed case of HIV infection was found in blood drawn from an African man in 1959 (Stephenson, 1998). Although factors associated with the spread of HIV in Africa remain unknown, possibilities include the reuse of unsterilized needles in large-scale vaccination campaigns that began in Africa in the 1960s; however, social changes such as easier access to transportation, increasing population density, and more frequent sexual contacts may have been more important (Stephenson, 1998).

HIV Transmission

HIV-1 is transmitted in body fluids containing HIV or infected CD4+ T lymphocytes. These fluids include blood, seminal fluid, vaginal secretions, amniotic fluid, and breast milk. Mother-to-child transmission of HIV-1 may occur in utero, at the time of delivery, or through breast-feeding, but most perinatal infections are thought to occur after exposure during delivery (Ferrigno & DeHovitz, 2004). Inflammation and breaks in the skin or mucosa result in the increased probability of exposure to HIV. HIV is not transmitted through casual contact (Chart 52-1). Because HIV is harbored within lymphocytes, a type of white blood cell, any exposure to infected blood results in a significant risk of infection. The amount of virus and infected cells in the body fluid is associated with the risk of new infection after exposure to that fluid.

Blood and blood products can transmit HIV to recipients. However, the risk associated with transfusions has been virtually eliminated as a result of voluntary self-deferral, completion of a detailed health history, extensive testing, heat treatment of clotting factor concentrates, and more effective virus inactivation methods. Donated blood is tested for antibodies to HIV-1, **HIV-2**, and **p24 antigen**; in addition, since 1999, nucleic acid amplification testing (NAT) has been performed (CDC, 2003). However, blood donated during the **window period** after infection is infectious even though it tests negative for HIV antibodies. The window period is the period of time between initial infection with HIV and development of a positive antibody test for HIV. Although antibodies usually are detected within 3 to 6 months, the window period can last up to 1 year.

Gerontologic Considerations

The number of people between the ages of 55 and 64 years living with AIDS more than doubled between the years 1998 and 2003 (from 19,258 to 38,997) (CDC, 2005). HIV infection in middle-aged and older populations

CHART 52-1

Risk Behaviors Associated With HIV Infection and AIDS

- Sharing infected injection drug use equipment
- Having sexual relations with infected individuals (both male and female)

Also at risk are people who received HIV-infected blood or blood products (especially before blood screening was instituted in 1985) and infants born to mothers with HIV infection.

may be underreported and underdiagnosed because health care professionals erroneously believe that older adults are not at risk for HIV infection. Also, HIV-related dementia in the older adult may mimic Alzheimer's disease and may be misdiagnosed.

In fact, several factors put older adults at risk for HIV infection:

- Many older adults are sexually active but do not use condoms, viewing them only as a means of unneeded birth control.
- Many older adults do not consider themselves at risk for HIV infection.
- Older gay men, who grew up and lived in an era when disclosure of their sexual orientation was not acceptable and who have lost long-time partners, may begin new relationships with younger men.
- Older adults may be IV/injection drug users.
- Older adults may have received HIV-infected blood through transfusions before 1985.
- Normal age-related changes include a reduction in immune system function, which puts the older adult at greater risk for infections, cancers, and autoimmune disorders. Many older adults also experience the loss of loved ones, resulting in depression and bereavement (Heckman, Kochman & Sikkema, 2004), factors that are associated with depressed immune function.

Physical strain and the number of comorbidities were significant predictors of the adequacy of social support in older adults with HIV (Shippy & Karpiak, 2005).

CHART 52-2

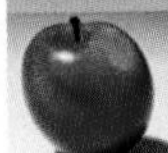

Health Promotion

Safer Sexual Behaviors

- Advise patients to abstain from sharing sexual fluids.
- Advise patients to reduce the number of sexual partners to one.
- Advise patients to always use latex condoms. If the patient is allergic to latex, nonlatex condoms should be used.
- Advise patients to avoid reusing condoms.
- Advise patients to avoid using cervical caps or diaphragms without using a condom as well.
- Advise patients to always use dental dams for oral-genital or anal stimulation.
- Advise patients to avoid anal intercourse because this practice may injure tissues.
- Advise patients to avoid manual-anal intercourse ("fisting").
- Advise patients not to ingest urine or semen.
- Educate patients about nonpenetrative sexual activities, such as body massage, social kissing (dry), mutual masturbation, fantasy, and sex films.
- Advise patients to avoid sharing needles, razors, toothbrushes, sex toys, or blood-contaminated articles.
- Advise HIV-seropositive patients to inform previous, present, and prospective sexual and drug-using partners of their HIV-positive status. If the patient is concerned for his or her safety, advise the patient that many states have established mechanisms through the public health department in which professionals are available to notify exposed people.
- Advise HIV-seropositive patients to avoid having unprotected sex with another HIV-seropositive person. Cross-infection with that person's HIV can increase the severity of infection.
- Advise HIV-seropositive patients to avoid donating blood, plasma, body organs, or sperm.

Prevention of HIV Infection

Until an effective vaccine is developed, preventing HIV by eliminating or reducing risky behaviors is essential. Primary prevention efforts through effective educational programs are vital for control and prevention. HIV is not transmitted by casual contact.

Preventive Education

Effective educational programs have been initiated to educate the public regarding safer sexual practices to decrease the risk of transmitting HIV-1 infection to sexual partners (Chart 52-2). Other than abstinence, consistent and correct use of condoms (Chart 52-3) is the only method proven to decrease the risk for sexual transmission of HIV infection. Latex condoms should be used during vaginal or anal intercourse. Nonlatex condoms made of natural materials such as lambskin are available for people with latex allergy but will not protect against HIV infection. A condom should be used for oral contact with the penis, and a dental dam (a piece of latex used by dentists to isolate a tooth for treatment) should be used for oral contact with the vagina or rectum.

The use of a **microbicide**, nonoxynol-9 (N-9), was widely advocated to reduce the risk of HIV infection until a clinical trial conducted in almost 1000 female commercial sex workers in African countries revealed that those who used N-9 intravaginally along with condoms were 50% more likely to be infected with HIV than those who did not use the N-9 gel. Based on these results, it is now recommended that intravaginal application of N-9 not be used as a means of HIV prevention. Further research throughout the world continues to investigate the use of other microbicides, especially since these methods are often controlled by the female sex partner.

Other topics important in preventive education include the importance of avoiding sexual practices that might cut or tear the lining of the rectum, penis, or vagina and avoiding sexual contact with multiple partners or people who are known to be HIV positive or IV/injection drug users. In addition, people who are HIV positive or who use injection drugs should be instructed not to donate blood or share drug equipment with others.

The Harm Reduction model (Goodroad, 2003) recognizes that abstinence from addicting drugs might not be a

CHART 52-3

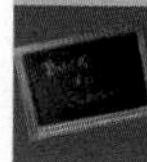

Patient Education

The Right Way to Use a Male Condom

1. Put on a new condom before any kind of sex.
2. Hold the condom by the tip to squeeze out the air.

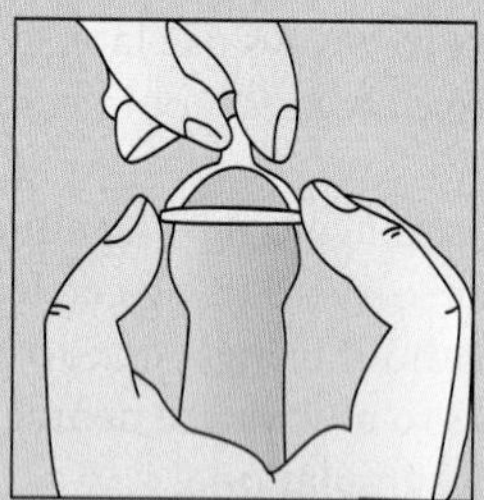

3. Unroll the condom all the way over the erect penis.

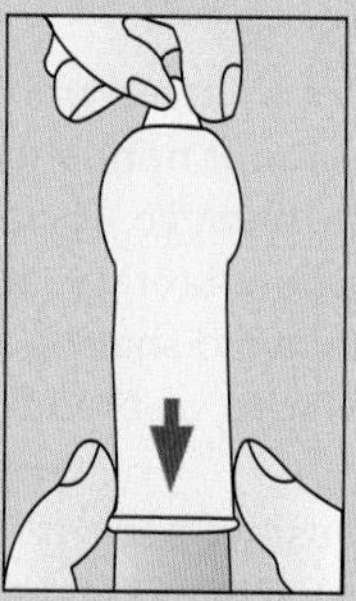

4. Have sex.
5. Hold the condom so it cannot come off the penis.
6. Pull out.
7. Use a new condom if you want to have sex again or if you want to have sex in a different place (eg, in the anus and then in the vagina).

   Keep condoms cool and dry. Never use skin lotions, baby oil, petroleum jelly, or cold cream with condoms. The oil in these products will cause the condom to break. Products made with water (such as K-Y jelly or glycerin) are safer to use.

realistic short-term goal. This model recommends working with drug users to assist them to increase their healthy behaviors. Increasingly, needle exchange programs are available so that IV/injection drug users can obtain sterile drug equipment at no cost. Extensive research has demonstrated that needle exchange programs do not promote increased drug use; on the contrary, they have been found to decrease the incidence of bloodborne infections in people who use IV/injection drugs (Taliaferro & Williams, 2003). In the absence of needle exchange programs, IV/injection drug users should be instructed on methods to clean their syringes and advised to avoid sharing cotton and other drug use equipment. Drug users interested in treatment programs should be referred to those programs.

Related Reproductive Education

Because HIV infection in women often occurs during the childbearing years, family planning issues need to be addressed. Attempts to achieve pregnancy by couples in which only one partner has HIV expose the unaffected partner to the virus. Efforts at artificial insemination using processed semen from an HIV-infected partner are underway. Studies are needed, because HIV has been found in the spermatozoa of patients with AIDS, and it is possible that HIV can replicate in the male germ cell. Women considering pregnancy need to have adequate information about the risks for transmitting HIV infection to themselves, their partner, and their future children, and about the benefits of taking antiretroviral agents to reduce perinatal HIV transmission. The desire of women who are HIV-positive to bear children is strong despite health risks to these women, their children, and society in general (Wesley, 2003). Women who are HIV-positive should be instructed not to breast feed their infants, because HIV is transmitted through breast milk (Riley & Yawetz, 2005).

Certain contraceptive methods may pose additional health risks for women. Estrogen in oral contraceptives may increase a woman's risk for HIV infection. In addition, women infected with HIV who use estrogen oral contraceptives have shown increased shedding of HIV in vaginal and cervical secretions. The intrauterine contraceptive device (IUD) may also increase the risk for HIV transmission, because the device's string may serve as a means to transmit the virus. The female condom is as effective in preventing pregnancy as other barrier methods, such as the diaphragm and the male condom. Unlike the diaphragm, the female condom is also effective in preventing the transmission of HIV infection and sexually transmitted diseases (STDs). The female condom has the distinction of being the first barrier method that can be controlled by the woman (see Chapter 46).

Transmission to Health Care Providers

Standard Precautions

In 1996, efforts were made by the CDC and its Hospital Infection Control Practices Advisory Committee (HICPAC) to reduce the risk for exposure of health care workers to HIV through the development of Standard Precautions. Standard Precautions incorporate the major features of Universal Precautions (designed to reduce the risk of transmission of bloodborne pathogens) and Body Substance Isolation (designed to reduce the risk of transmission of pathogens from moist body substances); they are applied to all patients receiving care in health care facilities, regardless of their diagnosis or presumed infectious status (Chart 52-4). Standard Precautions apply to blood; all body fluids, secretions, and excretions (except sweat), regardless of whether they contain visible blood; nonintact skin; and mucous membranes (Chiarello, Panlilio, & Cardo, 2004). The primary purpose of Standard Precautions is to prevent the transmission of nosocomial infection. The first tier, referred to as Standard Precautions, was developed to reduce the risk for exposure from all recognized or unrecognized sources of infections in hospitals.

NURSING RESEARCH PROFILE

Childbearing Among Black Women With and Without HIV Infection

Wesley, Y. (2003). Desire for children among Black women with and without HIV infection. *Journal of Nursing Scholarship, 35*(1), 37–43.

Purpose

Childbearing is often seen as a woman's obligation and is still valued by women even after being diagnosed with HIV infection. This study asked three research questions: (1) Is there a relationship between self-esteem, self-efficacy, and desire for children? (2) Does desire for children vary in relation to HIV status? (3) Are demographic factors better predictors of desire for children than self-esteem and self-efficacy?

Design

This study was based on a general proposition from the symbolic interaction model. Black women, who were either HIV-positive or HIV-negative, were recruited from an inner-city community health center. Usable responses were obtained from 58 HIV-positive and 50 HIV-negative women. Participants completed the Modified Index of Parenthood Motivation, the General Self-Efficacy subscale of the Self-Efficacy Scale, the Rosenberg Self-Esteem Scale, and a demographic survey.

Findings

Independent group *t* tests showed a significant difference between HIV-positive and HIV-negative women in age ($t = -1.99$, $p = .05$), education ($t = 2.2$, $p = .03$), employment ($t = 4.30$, $p = .00$), income ($t = 2.73$, $p = .01$), and number of elective abortions ($t = 2.05$, $p = .04$). HIV-negative women were significantly younger, more educated, reported fewer abortions, and were more likely to be employed than HIV-positive women. Data analysis revealed no significant difference between the two groups of women on their motivation to have children as measured by the Modified Index of Parenthood Motivation. HIV-negative women had significantly greater general self-efficacy ($t = 2.57$, $p = .01$) and self-esteem ($t = 2.50$, $p = .01$) than the HIV-positive women. Women who were HIV-positive and who already had children had significantly greater ($p = .03$) self-esteem than did those without children.

Nursing Implications

Desire for children did not vary as a function of HIV status. Increased desire for children was related to increased general self-efficacy in women with HIV infection. Nurses need to examine their personal beliefs about pregnancy in women with HIV infection to determine how their personal beliefs and values affect their professional practice. In order to establish and maintain a trusting relationship, nurses must acknowledge that some HIV-infected women may make childbearing choices that seem risky. Nurses need to explore how they can best support these women in their choices and present strategies that will minimize risk and maximize positive outcomes.

Large-scale studies of exposed health care workers continue to be conducted by the CDC and other groups. In November 2000, the Needlestick Safety and Prevention Act became law, mandating that health care facilities use devices to protect against sharps injuries.

Postexposure Prophylaxis for Health Care Providers

Postexposure prophylaxis in response to the exposure of health care personnel to blood or other body fluids has been proven to reduce the risk for HIV infection. The CDC recommends that all health care providers who have sustained a significant exposure to HIV be counseled and offered anti-HIV postexposure prophylaxis, if appropriate (Chart 52-5). Some clinicians are considering the use of postexposure prophylaxis for patients exposed to HIV as a result of high-risk sexual behavior or possible contact through IV/injection drug use. This use of postexposure prophylaxis is controversial because of concern that it may be substituted for safer sex practices and safer IV/injection drug use. Postexposure prophylaxis should not be considered an acceptable method of preventing HIV infection.

The medications recommended for postexposure prophylaxis are those used to treat established HIV infection. Ideally, prophylaxis needs to start immediately after exposure; therapy started more than 72 hours after exposure is thought to offer no benefit.

The recommended course of therapy involves taking the prescribed medications for 4 weeks. Those who choose postexposure prophylaxis must be prepared for the side effects of the medications and must be willing to face the unknown long-term risks, because HIV often becomes resistant to the medications used to treat it. If the person becomes infected despite prophylaxis, viral drug resistance may reduce future treatment options. The cost is also of concern; the cost of a medication regimen ranges from $500 to more than $1,000, in addition to the costs of testing and counseling. Health insurance may not cover the costs of medications, laboratory tests, and counseling.

Pathophysiology

Because HIV infection is an infectious disease, it is important to understand how HIV integrates itself into a person's immune system and how immunity plays a role in the course

CHART 52-4

Standard Precautions

The following guidelines prevent the transmission of infection during patient care for all patients, regardless of known or unknown infectious status. **Barrier protection** should be used at all times to prevent skin and mucous membrane contamination with blood, body fluids containing visible blood, or other body fluids (cerebrospinal, synovial, pleural, peritoneal, pericardial, and amniotic fluids, semen and vaginal secretions). Barrier protection should be used with ALL tissues. The type of barrier protection used should be appropriate for the type of procedures being performed and the type of exposure anticipated. Examples of barrier protection include disposable lab coats, gloves, and eye and face protection. Private rooms and rooms specially equipped with ventilation systems should be used as indicated.

1. Gloves are to be worn when there is a potential for hand or skin contact with blood, other potentially infectious material, or items and surfaces contaminated with these materials.
   - Clean, nonsterile gloves can be used to protect the nurse's hands.
   - Change gloves after contact with materials that may contain a high concentration of microorganisms even when working with the same patient.
   - Remove gloves promptly after use, before touching noncontaminated items and environmental surfaces, and before going to another patient.
2. **Face protection** (face shield, mask, eye protection) should be worn during procedures that are likely to generate droplets of blood or body fluid to prevent exposure to mucous membranes of the mouth, nose, and eyes.
3. **Environmental Control**
   - Ensure that the hospital has adequate procedures for the routine care, cleaning, and disinfection of environmental surfaces, beds, bed rails, bedside equipment, and other frequently touched surfaces.
   - Ensure that procedures are being followed.
   - Advocate for the purchase and correct use of the safest equipment
4. **Patient Care Equipment**
   - Handle used patient care equipment soiled with blood, body fluids, secretions, and excretions in a manner that prevents skin and mucous membrane exposures, contamination of clothing, and transfer of microorganisms to other patients and environment.
   - Ensure that reusable equipment is not used for the care of another patient until it has been cleaned and reprocessed appropriately.
   - Ensure that single-use items are discarded properly.
   - Use mouthpieces, resuscitation bags, or other ventilation devices as an alternative to mouth-to-mouth resuscitation methods.
   - Handle, transport, and process used linen soiled with blood, body fluids, secretions, and excretions in a manner that prevents skin and mucous membrane exposures and contamination of clothing and that avoids transfer of microorganisms to other patients and environments.
5. **Protective body clothing** such as disposable laboratory coats should be worn whenever there is a potential for splashing of blood or body fluids.
   - Wear a clean, nonsterile gown to protect skin and prevent soiling of clothing during procedures and patient care activities that are likely to generate splashes or sprays of blood, body fluids, secretions, or excretions.
   - Remove a soiled gown promptly, avoiding contact with clean clothes, and wash hands/perform hand hygiene to prevent the transfer of microorganisms to other patients or environments.
6. **Wash hands** thoroughly and immediately if contaminated with blood, body fluids containing visible blood, or other body fluids to which universal precautions apply.
   - Use soap and water or antimicrobial agent or waterless antiseptic agent.
   - Wash hands during procedures for the same patient to prevent cross-contamination of different body sites.
   - Wash hands immediately and other skin surfaces after gloves are removed.
7. **Avoid accidental injuries** that can be caused by needles, scalpel blades, laboratory instruments, and so on when performing procedures, cleaning instruments, handling sharp instruments, disposing of used needles or pipettes, and similar activities. Used needles, disposable syringes, scalpel blades, pipettes, and other sharp items are to be placed in puncture-resistant containers marked with a biohazard symbol for disposal.
   - Use "needleless" systems correctly whenever possible.
   - Never recap used needles or otherwise manipulate them by using both hands or use any technique that involves directing the point of the needle toward any part of the body.
   - Use either a one-handed scoop technique or a mechanical device designed for holding the needle sheath.

CHART 52-4 Standard Precautions, continued

- Do not remove used needles from disposable syringes by hand and do not bend, break, or otherwise manipulate used needles by hand.
- Place used disposable syringes and needles, scalpel blades, and other sharp items in appropriate puncture-resistant containers as close as practical to the area in which the items were used.
- Place reusable syringes and needles in a puncture-resistant container for transport to the reprocessing area.

Adapted from Garner, J. S. (1996). Guidelines for isolation precautions in hospitals. *Infection Control and Hospital Epidemiology, 17*(1), 53–80; Boyce, J. M. & Pittet, D. Healthcare Infection Control Practices Advisory Committee; HICPAC/SHEA/APIC/IDSA Hand Hygiene Task Force. (2002). Guideline for hand hygiene in health-care settings. *Morbidity and Mortality Weekly Report, 51*(RR-16),1–45. Further information is available at: http://www.niehs.nih.gov/odhsb/biosafe/univers.htm. Accessed June 2, 2006.

of infection. This knowledge is also essential for understanding medication therapy and vaccine development.

Viruses are intracellular parasites. HIV belongs to a group of viruses known as **retroviruses.** These viruses carry their genetic material in the form of ribonucleic acid (RNA) rather than deoxyribonucleic acid (DNA). As shown in Figure 52-1A, HIV consists of a viral core containing the viral RNA, surrounded by an envelope consisting of protruding glycoproteins (GP). For HIV to enter the targeted cell, the membrane of the viral envelope must be fused with the plasma membrane of the cell, a process mediated by the envelope glycoproteins of HIV (Goff, 2004).

The HIV life cycle is complex (see Fig. 52-1B) and consists of eight steps (Porth, 2005):

1. The HIV GP120 and GP41 attach to the uninfected CD4 cell surface (receptor) and fuse with the cell membrane.
2. The viral core contents are emptied into the host cell, a process known as "uncoating."
3. HIV enzyme **reverse transcriptase** copies the viral genetic material from RNA into double-stranded DNA.
4. Double-stranded DNA is spliced into the cellular DNA by the action of integrase, another HIV enzyme.
5. Using the integrated DNA or **provirus** as a blueprint, the cell makes new viral proteins and viral RNA.
6. HIV protease cleaves the new proteins (polyproteins).
7. The new proteins join the viral RNA into new viral particles.
8. New viral particles bud from the cell and start the process all over.

Perhaps the least understood aspects of the HIV life cycle are the events that occur immediately after entry of the viral core into the host CD4+ cell. The process of viral assembly

CHART 52-5 Postexposure Prophylaxis for Health Care Providers

If you sustain a puncture injury, such as a needlestick, take the following actions immediately:

- Wash the area with soap and water.
- Alert your supervisor/nursing faculty and initiate the injury-reporting system used in the setting.
- Identify the source patient, who may need to be tested for HIV, hepatitis B, and hepatitis C. State laws will determine whether written informed consent must be obtained from the source patient before his or her testing. OraQuick rapid testing should be used if possible if the HIV status of the source patient is unknown, because results can be available within 20 minutes.
- Report as quickly as possible to the employee health services, the emergency department, or other designated treatment facility. This visit should be documented in the health care worker's confidential medical record.
- Give consent for baseline testing for HIV, hepatitis B, and hepatitis C. Confidential HIV testing can be performed up to 72 hours after the exposure but should be performed as soon as the health care worker can give informed consent for baseline testing.
- Get postexposure prophylaxis for HIV in accordance with CDC guidelines (http://www.hivguidelines.org. Accessed June 2, 2006). Start the prophylaxis medications within 2 hours after exposure. Make sure that you are being monitored for symptoms of toxicity. Practice safer sex until follow-up testing is complete. Continue the HIV medications for 4 weeks.
- Follow up with postexposure testing at 1 month, 3 months, and 6 months, and perhaps 1 year.
- Document the exposure in detail for your own records as well as for the employer.

Worthington, K. (2001). You've been stuck: What do you do? *American Journal of Nursing, 101*(3), 104; Agins, B. (2003). *HIV prophylaxis following occupational exposure.* New York: AIDS Institute, New York State Department of Health.

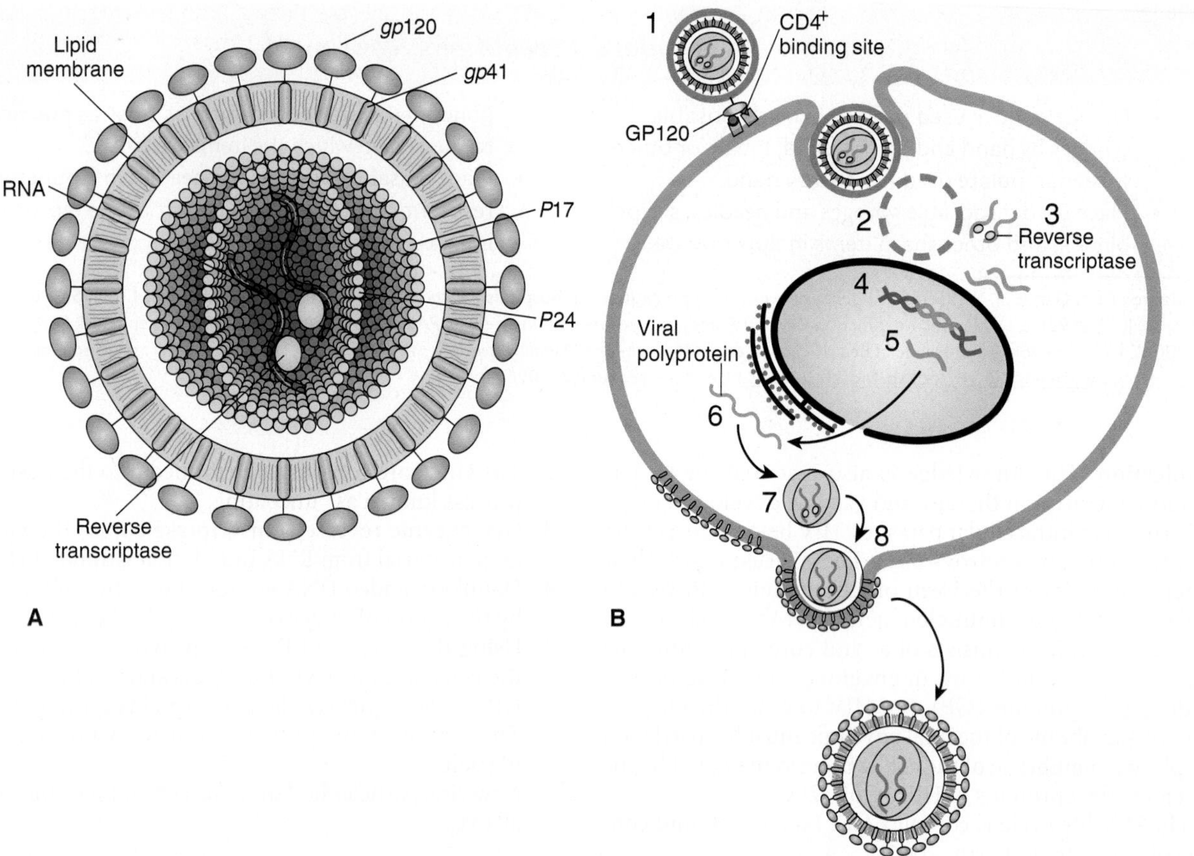

FIGURE 52-1. (**A**) Structure of HIV-1. A glycoprotein envelope surrounds the virus, which carries its genetic material in RNA. Knobs, consisting of proteins GP120 and GP41, protrude from the envelope. These proteins are essential for binding the virus to the CD4+ T lymphocyte. (**B**) Life cycle of HIV-1: (1) Attachment of the HIV virus to a CD4+ receptor; (2) internalization and uncoating of the virus with viral RNA and reverse transcriptase; (3) reverse transcription, which produces a mirror image of the viral RNA and double-stranded DNA molecule; (4) integration of viral DNA into host DNA using the integrase enzyme; (5) transcription of the inserted viral DNA to produce viral messenger RNA; (6) translation of viral messenger RNA to create viral polyprotein; (7) cleavage of viral polyprotein into individual viral proteins that make up the new virus; and (8) assembly and release of the new virus from the host cell. From Porth, C. (2005). *Pathophysiology: Concepts of altered health states* (7th ed.). Philadelphia: Lippincott Williams & Wilkins.

is intimately linked to its subsequent reversal (disassembly). Interactions occur between viral proteins and cellular factors in the cells that produce virus and frequently influence events at the next round of infection (Sedaghat & Siliciano, 2004). In resting (nondividing) cells, HIV can apparently survive in a latent state as an integrated provirus that produces few or no viral particles. These resting CD4+ T cells can be stimulated to produce new particles if something reactivates them. When a T cell that harbors this integrated DNA (also known as provirus) becomes activated against HIV or other microbes, the cell replicates and begins to produce new copies of both RNA and viral proteins. Activation of the infected cell may be achieved by antigens, mitogens, certain cytokines (tumor necrosis factor-α [TNF] or interleukin-1 [IL-1]), or virus gene products of such viruses as **cytomegalovirus** (CMV), Epstein-Barr virus, herpes simplex virus, and hepatitis viruses. Consequently, whenever the infected T cell is activated, HIV replication and budding occur, which often destroys the host cell. Newly formed HIV is then released into the blood plasma and infects other CD4+ cells (see Fig. 52-1B).

HIV-1 mutates quickly, at a relatively constant rate, with about 1% of the virus's genetic material changing annually. Over the years, subtypes A, B, C, D, F, G, H, J, and K constitute the major group of HIV-1 or group M, along with two additional groups of viruses (O and N). The pandemic of HIV/AIDS reflects many subepidemics coexisting in different regions of the world and in different populations (Hu, Pieniazek, & Mastro, 2004).

All viruses target specific cells. Lymphocytes consist of three major populations: T cells, B cells, and natural killer cells. Mature T cells are phenotypically composed of two major subpopulations, defined by cell surface reciprocal expression of CD4 or CD8. Approximately two thirds of peripheral blood T cells are CD4+ and approximately one third are CD8+. Most people have about 700 to 1000 CD4+ cells/mm^3, but as low as 500 cells/mm^3 can be considered "normal." HIV targets cells with the CD4 glycoprotein, which is expressed on the surface of T lymphocytes, **monocytes**, dendritic cells, and brain microglia. A major function of CD4 binding is to induce conformational changes in the GP120 glycoprotein of the HIV envelope that contribute to the formation or exposure of the binding site for the chemokine receptors. Most primary clinical isolates of HIV use the chemokine receptor **CCR5** for entry. HIV-1 isolates that appear later in the course of infection often use other chemokine receptors, such as CXCR4, in addition to CCR5 (Goff, 2004). HIV must attach to both the CD4 and the CCR5 binding sites in order to infect CD4+ cells. CD4 fits into a recessed pocket in the viral envelope GP120 that may simply be too inaccessible to be easily reached by antibodies.

A mutation of CCR5 that is common among Caucasians, but not other ethnic groups, has been identified. About 1% of Caucasians lack functional CCR5 and are highly protected against HIV infection even if exposed (although protection is not absolute); about 18% are not markedly protected against infection but, if infected, demonstrate significantly slower rates of disease progression (Kaslow, Tang & Dorak, 2004).

Stages of HIV Disease

The stage of HIV disease is based on clinical history, physical examination, laboratory evidence of immune dysfunction, signs and symptoms, and infections and malignancies. The CDC standard case definition of AIDS categorizes HIV infection and AIDS in adults and adolescents on the basis of clinical conditions associated with HIV infection and CD4+ T-cell counts. The classification system (Table 52-1)

TABLE 52-1 Classification System for HIV Infection and Expanded AIDS Surveillance Case Definition for Adolescents and Adults

Diagnostic Categories	Clinical Categories		
CD4+ T-Cell Category	*A* *Asymptomatic, Acute (Primary) HIV or PGL*	*B* *Symptomatic, Not (A) or (C) Conditions*	*C* *AIDS-Indicator Conditions*
(1) ≥500/μL	A1	B1	C1
(2) 200–499/μL	A2	B2	C2
(3) <200/μL AIDS-indicator T-cell count	A3	B3	C3

People with AIDS-indicator conditions (clinical category C) and those in categories A3 or B3 are considered to have AIDS.

Clinical Category A

Includes one or more of the following in an adult or adolescent with confirmed HIV infection and without conditions in clinical categories B and C:

- Asymptomatic HIV infection
- Persistent generalized lymphadenopathy (PGL)
- Acute (primary) HIV infection with accompanying illness or history of acute HIV infection

Clinical Category B

Examples of conditions in clinical category B include, but are not limited to, the following:

- Bacillary angiomatosis
- Candidiasis, oropharyngeal (thrush) or vulvovaginal (persistent, frequent, or poorly responsive to therapy)
- Cervical dysplasia (moderate or severe)/cervical carcinoma in situ
- Constitutional symptoms, such as fever (38.5°C) or diarrhea exceeding 1 month in duration
- Hairy leukoplakia, oral
- Herpes zoster (shingles), involving at least two distinct episodes or more than one dermatome
- Idiopathic thrombocytopenic purpura
- Listeriosis
- Pelvic inflammatory disease, particularly if complicated by tuboovarian abscess
- Peripheral neuropathy

Clinical Category C

Examples of conditions in adults and adolescents include the following:

- Candidiasis of bronchi, trachea, or lungs; esophagus
- Cervical cancer, invasive
- Coccidioidomycosis, disseminated or extrapulmonary
- Cryptococcosis, extrapulmonary
- Cryptosporidiosis, chronic intestinal (exceeding 1 month's duration)
- Cytomegalovirus disease (other than liver, spleen, or lymph nodes)
- Cytomegalovirus retinitis (with loss of vision)
- Encephalopathy, HIV-related
- Herpes simplex: chronic ulcer(s) (exceeding 1 month's duration); or bronchitis, pneumonitis, or esophagitis
- Histoplasmosis, disseminated or extrapulmonary
- Isosporiasis, chronic intestinal (exceeding 1 month's duration)
- Kaposi's sarcoma
- Lymphoma, Burkitt's (or equivalent term); immunoblastic (or equivalent term); primary, of brain
- *Mycobacterium avium* complex or *M. kansasii*, disseminated or extrapulmonary
- *Mycobacterium tuberculosis*, any site (pulmonary or extrapulmonary)
- *Mycobacterium*, other species or unidentified species, disseminated or extrapulmonary
- *Pneumocystis jiroveci* pneumonia
- Pneumonia, recurrent
- Progressive multifocal leukoencephalopathy
- *Salmonella* septicemia, recurrent
- Toxoplasmosis of brain
- Wasting syndrome due to HIV

Adapted from Centers for Disease Control, U.S. Department of Health and Human Services. (1992). 1993 revised classification system for HIV infection and expanded surveillance case definition for AIDS among adolescents and adults. *MMWR CDC Recommendations and Reports, 41* (RR-17), 1–19.

groups clinical conditions into one of three categories, denoted A, B, and C.

Primary Infection (Acute HIV Infection, Acute HIV Syndrome)

The period from infection with HIV to the development of antibodies to HIV is known as **primary infection.** This period is characterized by intense viral replication and widespread dissemination of HIV throughout the body. Symptoms associated with the viremia range from none to severe flu-like symptoms. During primary infection, a window period occurs, during which a person with HIV infection tests negative on the HIV antibody blood test. Although antibodies to the HIV envelope glycoproteins typically can be detected in the sera of HIV-infected individuals by 2 to 3 weeks after infection, most of these antibodies lack the ability to inhibit virus infection. By the time neutralizing antibodies can be detected, HIV-1 is firmly established in the host. During this period, there are high levels of viral replication and destruction of CD4+ T cells, resulting in high levels of HIV in the blood and a dramatic drop in CD4+ T-cell counts from the normal level of 500 to 1500 cells/mm^3 of blood. About 3 weeks into this acute phase, the person may display symptoms reminiscent of mononucleosis, such as fever, enlarged lymph nodes, rash, muscle aches, and headaches. These symptoms resolve within another 1 to 3 weeks as the immune system begins to gain some control over the virus. That is, the CD4+ T-cell population responds in ways that cause other immune cells, such as CD8+ lymphocytes, to increase their killing of infected, virus-producing cells. The body produces antibody molecules in an effort to contain the virus; they bind to free HIV particles (outside cells) and assist in their removal. This balance between the amount of HIV in the body and the immune response is referred to as the **viral set point**; it results in a steady state of infection that can last for years.

Primary HIV infection (Sedaghat & Siliciano, 2004), the time during which the viral burden set point is achieved, includes the acute symptomatic and early infection phases. During this initial stage, viral replication is associated with dissemination in lymphoid tissue and a distinct immunologic response. The final level of the viral set point is inversely correlated with disease prognosis; that is, the higher the viral set point, the poorer the prognosis. The primary infection stage is part of CDC category A.

HIV Asymptomatic (CDC Category A: More Than 500 CD4+ T Lymphocytes/mm^3)

When a viral set point is reached, a chronic, clinically asymptomatic state begins. Despite its best efforts, the immune system rarely if ever fully eliminates the virus. By about 6 months, the rate of viral replication reaches a lower but relatively steady state that is reflected in the maintenance of viral levels at a kind of "set point." This set point varies greatly from patient to patient and dictates the subsequent rate of disease progression; on average, 8 to 10 years pass before a major HIV-related complication develops. In this prolonged, chronic stage, patients feel well and have few if any symptoms. Apparent good health continues because CD4+ T-cell levels remain high enough to preserve defensive responses to other pathogens.

HIV Symptomatic (CDC Category B: 200 to 499 CD4+ T Lymphocytes/mm^3)

Over time, the number of CD4+ T cells gradually falls. Category B consists of symptomatic conditions in HIV-infected patients that are not included in the conditions listed in category C. These conditions must also meet one of the following criteria: (1) the condition is due to HIV infection or a defect in cellular immunity, or (2) the condition is considered to have a clinical course or to require management that is complicated by HIV infection. If a person was once treated for a category B condition and has not developed a category C disease but is now symptom-free, that person's illness is considered category B.

AIDS (CDC Category C: Fewer Than 200 CD4+ T Lymphocytes/mm^3)

When the CD4+ T-cell level drops below 200 cells/mm^3 of blood, the person is said to have AIDS. As levels decrease to fewer than 100 cells/mm^3, the immune system is significantly impaired. Once a patient has had a category C condition, he or she remains in category C. This classification has implications for entitlements (ie, disability benefits, housing, and food stamps), because these programs are often linked to an AIDS diagnosis. Although the revised classification emphasizes CD4+ T-cell counts, it allows for CD4+ percentages (percentage of CD4+ T cells compared with total lymphocytes). The CD4+ percentage is less subject to variation on repeated measurements than is the absolute CD4+ T-cell count. A CD4+ percentage of less than 14% of the total lymphocytes is consistent with an AIDS diagnosis. The percentage, as compared with the absolute number of CD4+ T cells, becomes particularly important when the patient has a heightened immune response to infections in addition to HIV. One complication of advanced HIV infection is anemia, which may be caused by HIV, opportunistic diseases, or medications (Orlando, 2003).

Assessment and Diagnostic Findings

During the first stage of HIV infection, the patient may be asymptomatic or may exhibit various signs and symptoms. The patient's health history should alert the health care provider about the need for HIV screening based on the patient's sexual practices, IV/injection drug use, and receipt of blood transfusions. Additionally, exposure to body fluids containing infected blood while providing care to others with HIV infection, such as through needlesticks, should alert health care providers to possible HIV infection. Patients who are in later stages of HIV infection may have a variety of symptoms related to their immunosuppressed state. Several screening tests are used to diagnose HIV infection. Others are used to assess the stage and severity of the infection. Table 52-2 identifies common blood tests.

HIV Antibody Tests

Before an HIV antibody test is performed, the meaning of the test and possible test results are explained, and informed consent for the test is obtained from the patient. State laws should be consulted about specific requirements

TABLE 52-2 Selected Laboratory Tests for Diagnosing and Tracking HIV and Assessing Immune Status

Test	Findings in HIV Infection
EIA (enzyme immunoassay)	Antibodies are detected, resulting in positive results and marking the end of the window period
Western blot	Also detects antibodies to HIV; used to confirm EIA
Viral load	Measures HIV RNA in the plasma
CD4/CD8 ratio	These are markers found on lymphocytes. HIV kills CD4+ cells, which results in a significantly impaired immune system.

related to testing for HIV. When the result of the HIV antibody test is received, it is carefully explained to the patient in private (Chart 52-6). All test results are kept confidential. Education and counseling about the test result and about preventing transmission are essential. The patient's psychological response to a seropositive test result may include feelings of panic, depression, and hopelessness. The social and interpersonal consequences of a positive test result can be devastating. The patient may lose his or her sexual partner and health insurance because of disclosure. The patient may experience discrimination in employment and housing, as well as social ostracism. For these reasons and others, a patient who tests positive may need ongoing counseling as well as referrals for social, financial, medical, and psychological support services. Patients whose test results are seronegative may develop a false sense of security, possibly resulting in continued high-risk behaviors or feelings that they are immune to the virus. These patients may need ongoing counseling to help modify high-risk behaviors and to encourage returns for repeated testing. Other patients may experience anxiety regarding the uncertainty of their status.

When a person is infected with HIV, the immune system responds by producing antibodies against the virus, usually within 3 to 12 weeks after infection. In 1985, the FDA licensed an HIV-1 antibody assay that used approximately 5 to 7 mL of blood. Samples are tested using two different laboratory techniques to determine the presence of antibodies to HIV. The **EIA (enzyme immunoassay)** test, formerly referred to as the **ELISA (enzyme-linked immunosorbent assay)** test, identifies antibodies directed specifically against HIV. The **Western blot assay** is used to confirm seropositivity when the EIA result is positive. Adults whose blood contains antibodies for HIV are seropositive.

In addition to this HIV-1 antibody assay, two additional techniques are now available. The OraSure test uses saliva to perform an EIA antibody test. Using less than a drop of blood, the **OraQuick Rapid HIV-1 Antibody Test** quickly (approximately 20 minutes) and reliably (99.6% accuracy) detects antibodies to HIV-1 (Hemmila, 2004). The OraQuick test is becoming the standard method of testing in settings where a delay would seriously affect treatment, such as in labor and delivery rooms or in emergency departments when the HIV status of a sexual abuser is unknown. Home-based testing for HIV antibodies using a small amount of blood was first proposed in 1985 but was not approved by the FDA until 1995. Although home testing kits are commercially available, they raise concerns because of the lack of counseling and the possibility of inaccurate results, including both false-positive and false-negative results.

CHART 52-6

HIV Test Results: Implications for Patients

INTERPRETATION OF POSITIVE TEST RESULTS

- Antibodies to HIV are present in the blood (the patient has been infected with the virus, and the body has produced antibodies).
- HIV is active in the body, and the patient can transmit the virus to others.
- Despite HIV infection, the patient does not necessarily have AIDS.
- The patient is not immune to HIV (the antibodies do not indicate immunity).

INTERPRETATION OF NEGATIVE TEST RESULTS

- Antibodies to HIV are not present in the blood at this time, which can mean that the patient has not been infected with HIV or, if infected, the body has not yet produced antibodies (window period—usually 3 weeks to 6 months).
- The patient should continue taking precautions. The test result does not mean that the patient is immune to the virus, nor does it mean the patient is not infected; it just means that the body may not have produced antibodies yet.

Viral Load Tests

Target amplification methods quantify HIV RNA or DNA levels in the plasma and have replaced p24 antigen capture assays. Target amplification methods include reverse transcriptase–**polymerase chain reaction** (RT-PCR) and nucleic acid sequence–based amplification (NASBA). A widely used **viral load test** measures plasma HIV RNA levels. Currently, these tests are used to track viral load and response to treatment of HIV infection. RT-PCR is also used to detect HIV in high-risk seronegative people before antibodies are measurable, to confirm a positive EIA result, and to screen neonates. HIV culture or quantitative plasma culture and plasma viremia are additional tests that measure viral burden, but they are used infrequently. Viral load is a better predictor of the risk for HIV disease progression than the CD4+ count. The lower the viral load, the longer the time to AIDS diagnosis and the longer the survival time.

Treatment of HIV Infection

Protocols on treatment of HIV disease change relatively often. The U.S. Department of Health and Human Services (DHHS) convenes a team of HIV specialists from across the country to evaluate the latest evidence and make recommendations that are widely disseminated (Department of Health and Human Services Panel on Antiretroviral Guidelines for Adults and Adolescents [DHHS Panel], 2006). Treatment decisions are individualized based on a number of factors, including CD4+ T-cell count, HIV RNA (viral load), severe symptoms of HIV disease or AIDS, and willingness of the patient to adhere to a lifelong treatment regimen. The CD4+ count is usually the most important consideration in decisions to initiate antiretroviral therapy (DHHS Panel; 2006). Treatment should be offered to all patients with primary infection (acute HIV syndrome, as previously described). In general, antiretroviral medications should be offered to individuals with a T-cell count of less than 350 cells/mm^3 or plasma HIV RNA levels exceeding 100,000 copies/mL (Hammer, 2005; DHHS Panel, 2006). Some clinicians and patients, however, are choosing not to start medications until the CD4+ cell count decreases to approximately 200 cells/mm^3. Monitoring the DHHS web site for updates of the recommendations is essential before caring for patients with HIV/AIDS (DHHS Panel, 2006).

The increasing number of antiretroviral agents (Table 52-3) and the rapid evolution of new information have introduced extraordinary complexity into the treatment of HIV infection (DHHS Panel, 2006). Adherence to long-term treatment is required to manage many chronic illnesses, such as hypertension, diabetes, and asthma, yet overall adherence rates remain unacceptably low (30% to 50%) (Chesney, 2004). Antiretroviral regimens are complex, have major side effects, pose difficulties with regard to adherence, and carry serious potential consequences; these include viral resistance resulting from nonadherence to the medication regimen or suboptimal levels of antiretroviral agents. The goals of treatment include maximal and sustained suppression of viral load, restoration or preservation of immunologic function, improved quality of life, and reduction of HIV-related morbidity and mortality. The DHHS Guidelines recommend viral load testing at the time of diagnosis of HIV disease and every 3 to 4 months thereafter in the untreated person; T-cell counts should be measured at diagnosis and usually every 3 to 6 months thereafter (DHHS Panel, 2006).

It is difficult to predict which patients will adhere to medication regimens (Holzemer, Corless, Nokes, et al., 2004). Perceived engagement with the health care provider has been associated with greater adherence to HIV medication regimens (Bakken, Holzemer, Brown, et al., 2000). Individualized plans of care that take into consideration housing and social support issues, in addition to health indicators, are essential. Adherence to the antiretroviral treatment plan involves very complex behavior that can change over the duration of the medication regimen (Reynolds, 2004). Self-reported adherence measures can distinguish clinically meaningful patterns of medication-taking behaviors; therefore, nurses should ask patients if they are taking their medications as prescribed (Nieuwkerk & Oort, 2005). Factors associated with nonadherence include active substance abuse, depression, and lack of social support. Gender, race, pregnancy, and history of past substance use have not been associated with nonadherence (DHHS Panel, 2006). Chart 52-7 summarizes various strategies that health care providers can encourage to promote treatment regimen adherence. Every health care encounter should be used as an opportunity to briefly review the treatment regimen and identify any new issues.

Results of therapy are evaluated with viral load tests (DHHS Panel, 2006). Viral load levels should be measured immediately before initiation of antiretroviral therapy and again after 2 to 8 weeks, because in most patients adherence to a regimen of potent antiretroviral agents should result in a large decrease in the viral load by 2 to 8 weeks. The viral load should continue to decline over the following weeks, and in most individuals it will drop below detectable levels (currently defined as less than 50 RNA copies/mL) by 16 to 20 weeks. The rate of viral load decline toward undetectable levels is affected by the baseline T-cell count, the initial viral load, the potency of the medication, adherence to the medication regimen, prior exposure to antiretroviral agents, and the presence of any opportunistic infections. The confirmed absence of a viral load response should prompt the health care team to reevaluate the regimen. The CD4+ count should increase by 100 to 150 cells/mm^3 per year, with an accelerated response in the first 3 months (DHHS Panel, 2006).

All medications have adverse effects (see Table 52-3). Many of the antiretroviral agents that prolong life may simultaneously cause lipodystrophy syndrome and place the person at risk for early-onset hypercholesterolemia, heart disease, and diabetes (Norris & Dreher, 2004). Fat redistribution syndrome, which consists of lipoatrophy, lipohypertrophy, or both in localized areas (Sanchez & Friedman-Kien, 2004), is also known as lipodystrophy syndrome or pseudo-Cushing's syndrome. This syndrome is one of the most frequent systemic side effects associated with the use of antiretroviral medications, especially protease inhibitors (Sanchez & Friedman-Kien, 2004). Many people who have lipodystrophy experience an increase in fat loss in the legs, arms, and face or a buildup of fat around the abdomen and at the base of the neck, or both. Patients may also experience an increase in breast size. These changes in body image can be very disturbing to people living with HIV/AIDS, and they have been reported to occur in 6% to 80% of patients receiving HAART (see later discussion).

Facial wasting, characterized as a sinking of the cheeks, eyes, and temples caused by the loss of fat tissue under the skin, may be treated by injectable fillers such as poly-L-lactic acid (Sculptra) (FDA News, 2004) (Fig. 52-2). Hepatotoxicity associated with certain protease inhibitors may limit the use of these agents, especially in patients with underlying liver dysfunction (DHHS Panel, 2006).

There are more than 20 approved antiretroviral agents, belonging to four classes, with which to design combination regimens containing at least three medications. The four classes are the nucleoside/nucleotide reverse transcriptase inhibitors (NRTI), non-nucleoside reverse transcriptase inhibitors (NNRTI), protease inhibitors, and fusion inhibitors (DHHS Panel, 2006). Fusion and entry inhibitors (such as enfuvirtide [T-20]) act by targeting GP120 during

TABLE 52-3 Antiretroviral Agents*

*Regimens should be individualized based on the advantages and disadvantages of each combination such as pill burden, dosing frequency, toxicities, drug-drug interaction potential, co-morbid conditions, and level of plasma HIV-RNA. There are four classes of medications.

Generic Name (Abbreviation) and Trade Names	Food Effect	Adverse Events
Nucleoside Reverse Transcriptase Inhibitors (NRTIs)		
Abacavir (ABC) Ziagen Trizivir (ABC + ZDV, + 3TC) Epzicom (ABC + 3TC)	Can be taken without regard to meals. Alcohol increases abacavir levels 41%. Abacavir has no effect on alcohol.	Hypersensitivity reaction which can be fatal; symptoms may include fever, rash, nausea, vomiting, malaise or fatigue, loss of appetite, respiratory symptoms such as sore throat, cough, shortness of breath.
Didanosine (ddL) Videx Videx EC	Levels decrease 55%; take ½ hour before or 2 hours after meals.	Pancreatitis; peripheral neuropathy; nausea; diarrhea. Lactic acidosis with fatty degeneration of the liver (rare but potentially life-threatening toxicity associated with use of NRTIs).
Emtricitabine (FTC) Emtriva Truvada (FTC + TDF)	Can be taken without regard to meals.	Minimal toxicity; lactic acidosis with hepatic steatosis (rare but potentially life-threatening toxicity with use of NRTIs).
Lamivudine (3TC) Epivir Combivir (3TC + ZDV) Epizicom (3TC + ABC) Trizivir (3TC + ZDV, + ABC)	Can be taken without regard to meals.	Minimal toxicity; lactic acidosis with hepatic steatosis (rare but potentially life-threatening toxicity with use of NRTIs).
Stavudine (d4T) Zerit	Can be taken without regard to meals.	Peripheral neuropathy; lipodystrophy; rapidly progressive ascending neuromuscular weakness (rare); pancreatitis; lactic acidosis with hepatic steatosis (higher incidence with d4T than with other NRTIs), hyperlipidemia.
Tenofovir disoproxil fumarate (TDF) Viread Truvada (TDF + FTC)	Can be taken without regard to meals.	Asthenia, headache, diarrhea, nausea, vomiting, and flatulence; renal insufficiency; lactic acidosis with hepatic steatosis (rare but potentially life-threatening toxicity with use of NRTIs)
Zalcitabine (ddC) Hivid	Can be taken without regard to meals.	Peripheral neuropathy; stomatitis; lactic acidosis with hepatic steatosis (rare but potentially life-threatening toxicity with use of NRTIs); pancreatitis.
Zidovudine (AZT or ZDV) Retrovir Combivir (AZT + 3TC) Trizivir (AZT + 3TC, + ABC)	Can be taken without regard to meals.	Bone marrow suppression; macrocytic anemia or neutropenia; gastrointestinal intolerance, headache, insomnia, asthenia; lactic acidosis with hepatic steatosis (rare but potentially life-threatening toxicity with use of NRTIs)
Non-nucleoside Reverse Transcriptase Inhibitors (NNRTIs)		
Delavirdine (DLV) Rescriptor	Can be taken without regard to meals.	Rash (rare cases of Stevens-Johnson syndrome have been reported); increased transaminase levels; headaches.
Efavirenz (EFV) Sustiva	High-fat/high caloric meals increase peak plasma concentrations of capsules by 39% and tablets by 79%; take on an empty stomach.	Rash (rare cases of Stevens-Johnson syndrome have been reported); central nervous system symptoms (dizziness, somnolence, insomnia, abnormal dreams, confusion, abnormal thinking, impaired concentration, amnesia, agitation, depersonalization, hallucinations, and euphoria); increased transaminase levels; false-positive cannabinoid test; teratogenic in monkeys.
Nevirapine (NVP) Viramune	Take without regard to meals.	Rash including Stevens-Johnson syndrome, symptomatic hepatitis including fatal hepatic necrosis has been reported.
Protease Inhibitors (PIs)		
Amprenavir (APV) Agenerase	High-fat meal decreases blood concentration 21%; can be taken with or without food, but high-fat meal should be avoided.	GI intolerance; nausea; vomiting; diarrhea; rash; oral paresthesias; hyperlipidemia; transaminase elevation; hyperglycemia; fat maldistribution; possible increased bleeding episodes in patients with hemophilia (Note: oral solution contains propylene glycol).

continued >

TABLE 52-3 Antiretroviral Agents* (Continued)

Generic Name (Abbreviation) and Trade Names	Food Effect	Adverse Events
Atazanavir (ATV) Reyataz	Administration with food increases bioavailability. Should be taken with food; avoid taking with antacids.	Indirect hyperbilirubinemia; prolonged PR interval—some patients experienced asymptomatic first-degree AV block; use with caution in patients with underlying conduction defects or on concomitant medications that can cause PR prolongation; hyperglycemia; fat maldistribution, possible increased bleeding episodes in patients with hemophilia.
Fosamprenavir (f-APV) Lexiva	Can be taken without regard to meals.	Skin rash (19%); diarrhea; nausea; vomiting; headache; hyperlipidemia; transaminase elevation; hyperglycemia; fat maldistribution; possible increased bleeding episodes in patients with hemophilia.
Indinavir (IDV) Crixivan	For unboosted IDV: Should be taken 1 hour before or 2 hours after meals; may take with skim or low-fat meal. For RTV-boosted IDV: Can be taken with or without food.	Nephrolithiasis; GI intolerance; nausea; indirect hyperbilirubinemia; hyperlipidemia; headache, asthenia; blurred vision; dizziness; rash; metallic taste; thrombocytopenia; alopecia; and hemolytic anemia; hyperglycemia; fat maldistribution; possible increased bleeding episodes in patients with hemophilia.
Lopinavir + ritonavir (LPV/r) Kaletra	Should be taken with food.	GI intolerance; nausea; vomiting; diarrhea; asthenia; hyperlipidemia (especially hypertriglyceridemia) elevated serum transaminase; hyperglycemia; fat maldistribution; possible increased bleeding episodes in patients with hemophilia
Nelfinavir (NFV) Viracept	Should be taken with a meal or snack.	Diarrhea; hyperlipidemia; hyperglycemia; fat maldistribution; possible increased bleeding episodes in patients with hemophilia; serum transaminase elevation.
Ritonavir (RTV) Norvir	Should be taken with food if possible; may improve tolerability.	GI intolerance; nausea; vomiting; diarrhea; paresthesias—circumoral and extremities; hyperlipidemia, especially hypertriglyceridemia; hepatitis; asthenia; taste perversion; hyperglycemia; fat maldistribution; possible increased bleeding in patients with hemophilia.
Saquinavir hard gel capsule (SQV-hgc) Invirase Saquinavir soft gel capsule (SQV-sgc) Fortovase	Hard gel: Should be taken within 2 hours of a meal when taken with RTV. Soft gel: Should be taken with or up to 2 hours after a meal.	GI intolerance; nausea; diarrhea; abdominal pain and dyspepsia; headache; hyperlipidemia; elevated transaminase enzymes; hyperglycemia; fat maldistribution; possible increased bleeding episodes in patients with hemophilia.
Fusion Inhibitors		
Enfuvirtide (T-20) Fuzeon	Injected subcutaneously, so meals are not an issue.	Local injection site reactions—almost 100% of patients (pain, erythema, induration, nodules and cysts, pruritus, ecchymosis); increased rate of bacterial pneumonia; hypersensitivity reaction—symptoms may include rash, fever, nausea, vomiting, chills, rigors, hypotension, or elevated serum transaminases; may recur on challenge.

Department of Health and Human Services Panel on Antiretroviral Guidelines for Adults and Adolescents—A Working Group of the Office of AIDS Research Advisory Council. (2006.) *Guidelines for the use of antiretroviral agents in HIV-1-infected adults and adolescents, May 4, 2006.* Available at http://AIDSinfor.nih.gov. Accessed July 28, 2006.

the attachment stage of the HIV life cycle (see Fig. 52-2). Unlike the other three classes of medications, which are administered orally, T-20 is administered by subcutaneous injection twice a day (DHHS Panel, 2006).

In order to achieve sustained viral suppression, patients must take more than one antiretroviral medication. Combination therapy is defined as a regimen containing at least two antiretroviral agents; HAART was defined originally as a regimen that includes at least one **protease inhibitor** (Agins, 2003), but this definition has evolved. As new medications are developed and research is completed, the number and types of recommended drug combinations continue to change (DHHS Panel, 2006). In addition, some pharmaceutical companies have combined two to three agents into one tablet or capsule (such as Kaletra, which is a combination of lopinavir and ritonavir), so a patient may

CHART 52-7

HOME CARE CHECKLIST • Adhering to Medication Therapy for HIV

At the completion of the home care instruction, the patient or caregiver will be able to:	Patient	Caregiver
• Verbalize knowledge of each medication name.	✔	✔
• State the action of each medication.	✔	✔
• State the correct times that medications are to be taken.	✔	✔
• Identify special guidelines to follow when taking medications (eg, with meals, on an empty stomach, medications that are not to be taken together).	✔	✔
• Demonstrate methods of keeping track of the medication regimen and storage of the prescribed medications and use reminders such as beepers and/or pill boxes.	✔	✔
• Identify specific laboratory tests such as viral load that are necessary to monitor the effectiveness of the prescribed medication regimen.	✔	✔
• List expected side effects of each medication.	✔	✔
• Identify side effects that should be reported to health care providers.	✔	✔
• Explain the importance of and necessity for adherence with prescribed medication regimen.	✔	✔
• Demonstrate correct administration of IM, SC, or IV medications.	✔	✔
• Demonstrate correct use and safe disposal of needles, syringes, and other IV equipment.	✔	✔
• Discuss with health care providers any problems that he or she is having with side effects and adherence.	✔	✔
• Discuss episodes of nonadherence to the medication regimen.	✔	✔

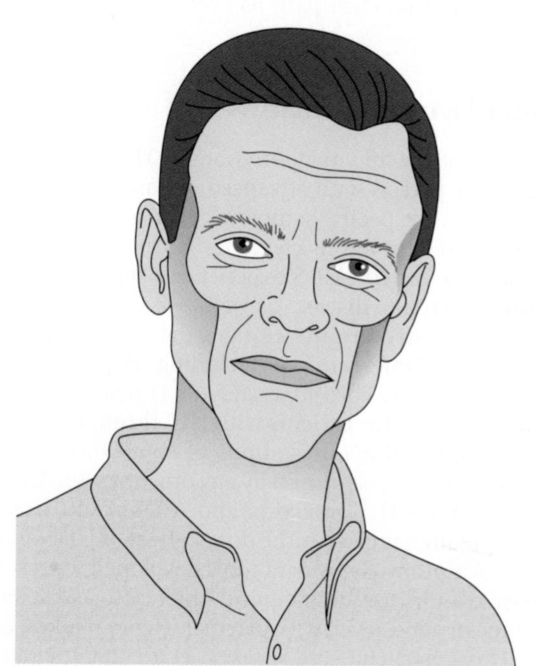

FIGURE 52-2. Facial lipoatrophy.

be taking one tablet or capsule that contains two different medications. With a decrease in the number of tablets or capsules that the patient must take ("pill burden"), the patient is more likely to adhere to prescribed regimens and achieve sustained viral suppression. Efforts are underway to develop additional combinations of antiretroviral medications. One medication made available in 2006, Atripla, combines Sustiva (efavirenz), Emtriva (emtricitabine), and Viread (tenofovir disoproxil fumarate) in a single tablet for once-a-day use. It is anticipated that simplifying treatment regimens and decreasing the number of medications that must be taken each day may increase patients' adherence to therapy (U.S. Food and Drug Administration, 2006).

Drug Resistance

Drug resistance can be broadly defined as the ability of pathogens to withstand the effects of medications that are intended to be toxic to them. Resistance develops as a result of spontaneous genetic mutation of the pathogens or in response to exposure to the medication. Factors associated with the development of drug resistance include serial monotherapy (taking one medication at a time), inadequate suppression of virus replication with suboptimal treatment regimens, difficulty with adherence to complex and toxic regimens, and initiation of therapy late in the course of HIV infection. HIV-1 may find refuge in organ sanctuaries, such as behind the blood–brain barrier, where diminished drug concentrations in the central nervous system (CNS) might induce the development of drug-resistant mutants. HIV-1 persists in lymphoid tissue even in people who appear to have responded well to antiviral therapy (Horowitz & Wormser, 2004).

Resistance testing has a number of limitations and is more helpful in determining which antiretroviral agents should be eliminated rather than which ones should be used. Deciding whether a medication regimen is effective or ineffective is a complex phenomenon. Some patients demonstrate inconsistent results on virologic, immunologic, and clinical parameters. In general, virologic failure occurs first, followed by immunologic failure, and finally by clinical progression. These events may be separated by months to years (DHHS Panel, 2006). Genotypic testing determines the sequence of viral RNA encoding relevant genes, which allows detection of amino acid mutations that are either proven or suspected to be associated with phenotypic resistance. Phenotypic testing determines the drug concentration needed to inhibit replication of a recombinant virus by 50% of a patient's isolate, when compared with a susceptible reference. This generates a prediction of the likely susceptibility of that virus to the available HAART medications (Daar, Gallant, Markowitz, et al., 2004).

In addition to resistance testing, several factors must be considered in choosing medications for a new regimen, once the prior regimen has failed. These factors include the patient's past treatment history, viral load, and medication tolerance; the likelihood of the patient's adhering to the medication regimen; and concomitant medical conditions or medications. Resistance testing is of greatest value when it is performed before drugs are discontinued or immediately afterward (within 4 weeks). Drug resistance testing is not advised for patients with a viral load of less than 1000 copies/mL, because amplification of the virus is unreliable (DHHS Panel, 2006).

Treatment Interruption and Reinstitution Based on CD4+ Cell Count

It may be safe and appropriate to temporarily discontinue antiretroviral therapy after immune competence has been reestablished and is stable. Although the evidence is not definitive, a sustained CD4+ count of between 500 and 800 cells/mm^3 may indicate that antiretroviral medications can be discontinued. If the CD4+ counts fall to between 350 and 400 cells/mm^3, antiretroviral therapy should be restarted (DHHS Panel, 2006).

Patients who elect to interrupt therapy should be counseled that the HIV viral load will increase, usually to pretreatment levels, which results in an increased risk for transmission to others during risky behaviors such as unsafe sex and sharing IV/injection drug use equipment. Because of drug toxicities, drug resistance, quality of life issues, and the high cost of medications, the complex medication regimen is often difficult for patients to follow, and some patients may choose to take a "drug holiday." Through an open, honest partnership between the health care provider and the patient, these options can be explored and their effectiveness maximized. Structured intermittent therapy, characterized by alternating short periods (eg, 7 days) on and off medication, appears to be ineffective.

Immunomodulator Therapy

Combating HIV infection requires not only agents that will inhibit viral growth but also those that will restore or bolster the damaged immune system. New therapies are needed to restore immune function, and immunologic markers need to be identified to predict the success of therapy. Current clinical research is testing the effectiveness of IL-2, IL-12, and other cytokines and lymphokines, but results thus far are mixed (Allende & Lane, 2004).

Vaccines

Vaccine research for HIV has two potential areas of application: prevention of new infections, and therapy for those already infected with HIV (therapeutic vaccine) (Allende & Lane, 2004). HIV-1 is a uniquely difficult target for the development of vaccines. Since HIV-1 was discovered, researchers have been working to develop a vaccine. A vaccine is a substance that triggers the production of antibodies to destroy the offending organism. Most vaccines activate the humoral arm of the immune system, which stimulates the production of protective antibodies. In addition to antibodies, B lymphocytes take the form of memory B cells. These cells do not produce antibodies immediately, but they respond vigorously to subsequent exposure. Vaccines that stimulate the cellular arm of the immune system are being developed. Since 1995, a variety of vaccines have been under study that use different strategies to prevent HIV infection in animals and humans. Some researchers are exploring whether variations in immunization schedules, including boosters, or use of a combination of several vaccines will result in stronger or more durable responses. Creation of an HIV vaccine is feasible, and a worldwide research network has been created. Cooperation among all nations is growing, and resources are being allocated by resource-rich countries to develop a worldwide vaccine and to create and support the infrastructure needed to facilitate testing of vaccine immunogens. Many different strategies are being attempted, but no clear path has yet emerged (Allende & Lane, 2004).

Clinical Manifestations

Treatment of specific manifestations of HIV infection and AIDS in the person with advanced disease focuses on the management of specific symptoms (Kirton, 2003). These are discussed later in this chapter.

Patients with HIV/AIDS experience a number of symptoms related to the disease, as well as side effects of treatment. Nurses need to understand the causes, signs and symptoms, and interventions, including self-care strategies (Chou, Holzemer, Portillo, et al., 2004) that can enhance the quality of life for patients with HIV throughout the illness. The clinical manifestations of HIV/AIDS are widespread and may involve virtually any organ system. Diseases associated with HIV infection and AIDS result from infections, malignancies, or the direct effect of HIV on body tissues. Symptom assessment tools developed for research purposes can be useful in clinical practice to assess symptom intensity and severity (Holzemer, Henry, Nokes, et al., 1999; Holzemer, Hudson, Kirksey, et al., 2001; Nokes & Bakken, 2002). Fatigue is frequently cited by people living with HIV/AIDS as one of the most bothersome symptoms.

Fatigue has a multifactorial etiology (Sullivan & Dworkin, 2003). People with HIV/AIDS use a variety of self-care strategies to minimize common symptoms, which can arise from HIV disease, comorbidities, or the effects of medications used to treat HIV and opportunistic infections (Chou et al., 2004).

Immune reconstitution syndromes have been described for mycobacterial infections, including disease caused by *Mycobacterium avium* complex (MAC) and *Mycobacterium tuberculosis;* PCP; toxoplasmosis; hepatitis B and hepatitis C; CMV infection; varicella-zoster virus infection; cryptococcal infection; and progressive multifocal leukoencephalopathy. Immune reconstitution syndromes are characterized by fever and worsening of the clinical manifestations of the opportunistic infection, or the appearance of new manifestations, developing weeks after the initiation of antiretroviral therapy. It is important to determine the absence or reappearance of the underlying opportunistic infection, new drug toxicity, or a new opportunistic infection. If the syndrome represents an immune reactivation syndrome, adding nonsteroidal anti-inflammatory agents (NSAIDs) or corticosteroids to alleviate the inflammatory reaction is appropriate. The inflammation might take weeks to months to subside (Benson, Kaplan, Masur, et al., 2004). The nurse should be alert to signs of immune reconstitution syndrome and advise the patient to seek health care if he or she is feeling sicker with no clear explanation.

Respiratory Manifestations

Shortness of breath, dyspnea (labored breathing), cough, chest pain, and fever are associated with various opportunistic infections, such as those caused by *P. jiroveci, Mycobacterium avium-intracellulare,* CMV, and *Legionella* species.

PNEUMOCYSTIS PNEUMONIA (PCP)

The most common infection in people with AIDS is ***Pneumocystis* pneumonia.** The current guidelines on treatment of opportunistic infections (Benson et al., 2004) refer to the causative organism as *P. jiroveci* instead of *P. carinii,* although the infection is still abbreviated as PCP. PCP was one of the first opportunistic infections described in association with AIDS, and it is the most common opportunistic infection resulting in the diagnosis of AIDS. Without prophylactic therapy (discussed later), 80% of all people infected with HIV will develop PCP.

The clinical presentation of PCP in HIV infection is generally less acute than in people who are immunosuppressed as a result of other conditions. The time between the onset of symptoms and the actual documentation of disease may be weeks to months. Patients with AIDS initially develop nonspecific signs and symptoms, such as nonproductive cough, fever, chills, shortness of breath, dyspnea, and occasionally chest pain. PCP may be present despite the absence of crackles. Arterial oxygen concentrations in patients who are breathing room air may be mildly decreased, indicating minimal hypoxemia.

If left untreated, PCP eventually progresses and causes significant pulmonary impairment and, ultimately, respiratory failure. A few patients have a dramatic onset and a fulminating course involving severe hypoxemia, cyanosis, tachypnea, and altered mental status. Respiratory failure can develop within 2 to 3 days after the initial appearance of symptoms.

PCP can be diagnosed definitively by identifying the organism in lung tissue or bronchial secretions. This is accomplished by such procedures as sputum induction, bronchial-alveolar lavage, and transbronchial biopsy (by fiberoptic bronchoscopy).

MYCOBACTERIUM AVIUM COMPLEX

***Mycobacterium avium* complex** (MAC) disease is a common opportunistic infection in people with AIDS. MAC comprises a group of acid-fast bacilli (mycobacteria) that includes *M. avium, M. intracellulare,* and *M. scrofulaceum.* MAC usually causes respiratory infection but is also commonly found in the gastrointestinal tract, lymph nodes, and bone marrow. Most patients with AIDS who have T-cell counts lower than 100 cells/mm^3 have widespread disease at diagnosis and are debilitated. MAC infections are associated with rising mortality rates.

TUBERCULOSIS

M. tuberculosis tends to occur in IV/injection drug users and other groups with a preexisting high prevalence of tuberculosis (TB) infection. TB that occurs late in HIV infection is characterized by absence of an immune response to the tuberculin skin test. This is known as **anergy**, and it occurs because the compromised immune system can no longer respond to the TB antigen. In the later stages of HIV infection, TB may be associated with dissemination to extrapulmonary sites such as the CNS, bone, pericardium, stomach, peritoneum, and scrotum. Multidrug-resistant strains of the bacillus have emerged and are often associated with lack of adherence to antituberculosis medication regimens.

Immune reconstitution syndrome (also known as paradoxical reactions) seem to occur more often among patients with TB. Patients can experience high fevers, worsening lymphadenopathy or transient to severe worsening of pulmonary infiltrates, and expanding CNS lesions. Such "paradoxical reactions" may be more common among HIV-1–infected patients with TB disease who were started on potent antiretroviral agents, compared to those who were not started on these agents or to patients with TB disease who are not HIV-1–infected. Reduction of HIV-1 RNA levels and marked increases in CD4+ T-lymphocyte counts have been associated with the occurrence of paradoxical reactions in patients with TB disease or MAC. Although the majority of reactions occur within the first few weeks after initiation of ART, some have occurred up to several months after the initiation of TB therapy or ART (Benson et al., 2004).

Gastrointestinal Manifestations

The gastrointestinal manifestations of AIDS include loss of appetite, nausea, vomiting, oral and esophageal candidiasis, and chronic diarrhea. Diarrhea is a problem in 50% to 90% of all AIDS patients. Gastrointestinal symptoms may be related to the direct effect of HIV on the cells lining the intestines. Some of the enteric pathogens that occur most frequently, identified by stool cultures or intestinal biopsy, are *Cryptosporidium muris, Salmonella* species, *Isospora belli, Giardia lamblia,* CMV, *Clostridium difficile,* and *M. avium-intracellulare.* In patients with AIDS, the effects of diarrhea can be devastating in terms of profound weight loss (more than 10% of body weight), fluid and electrolyte imbalances, perianal skin excoriation, weakness, and inability to perform the usual activities of daily living.

ORAL CANDIDIASIS

Candidiasis, a fungal infection, occurs in almost all patients with AIDS and AIDS-related conditions. Commonly preceding other life-threatening infections, it is characterized by creamy-white patches in the oral cavity. If left untreated, oral candidiasis progresses to involve the esophagus and stomach. Associated signs and symptoms include difficult and painful swallowing and retrosternal pain. Some patients also develop ulcerating oral lesions and are particularly susceptible to dissemination of candidiasis to other body systems.

WASTING SYNDROME

Wasting syndrome is part of the category C case definition for AIDS. Diagnostic criteria include profound involuntary weight loss exceeding 10% of baseline body weight and either chronic diarrhea for more than 30 days or chronic weakness and documented intermittent or constant fever in the absence of any concurrent illness that could explain these findings. This protein–energy malnutrition is multifactorial. In some AIDS-associated illnesses, patients experience a hypermetabolic state in which excessive calories are burned and lean body mass is lost. This state is similar to that seen in sepsis or trauma and can lead to organ failure. The distinction between cachexia (wasting) and malnutrition, or between cachexia and simple weight loss, is important, because the metabolic derangement seen in wasting syndrome may not be modified by nutritional support alone.

Anorexia, diarrhea, gastrointestinal malabsorption, and lack of nutrition in chronic disease all contribute to wasting syndrome. Progressive tissue wasting, however, may occur with only modest gastrointestinal involvement and without diarrhea. TNF and IL-1 are cytokines that play important roles in AIDS-related wasting syndrome. Both act directly on the hypothalamus to cause anorexia. Cytokine-induced fever accelerates the body's metabolism by 14% for every 1°F increase in temperature. TNF causes inefficient use of lipids by reducing enzymes that are needed for fat metabolism, whereas IL-1 triggers the release of amino acids from muscle tissue. People with AIDS generally experience increased protein metabolism in relation to fat metabolism, which results in significant decreases in lean body mass due to muscle and protein breakdown.

Hypertriglyceridemia, seen in people with AIDS and attributed to chronically elevated cytokine levels, can persist for months without tissue wasting and loss of lean body mass. It is believed that infections and sepsis lead to transient increases in TNF, IL-1, and other cell mediators above the chronically elevated levels that are often seen with AIDS. These transient increases in TNF and IL-1 trigger muscle wasting.

Oncologic Manifestations

Patients with AIDS have a higher than usual incidence of cancer, possibly related to HIV stimulation of developing cancer cells or to the immune deficiency that allows cancer-causing substances, such as viruses, to transform susceptible cells into malignant cells. Kaposi's sarcoma, certain types of B-cell lymphomas, and invasive cervical carcinoma are included in the CDC classification of AIDS-related malignancies. Carcinomas of the skin, stomach, pancreas, rectum, and bladder also occur more frequently than expected in people with AIDS.

KAPOSI'S SARCOMA

Kaposi's sarcoma (KS), the most common HIV-related malignancy, is a disease that involves the endothelial layer of blood and lymphatic vessels. It is associated with human herpes virus 8 (HHV-8) transmission. When first noted in 1872 by Dr. Moritz Kaposi, KS characteristically manifested as lower-extremity skin lesions in elderly men of Eastern European ancestry. This form, referred to as classic KS, is slow to progress and is easily treated. An endemic form of KS, found in children and young men in equatorial Africa, is more virulent than the classic form. Acquired KS occurs in patients who are treated with immunosuppressive agents and commonly in patients who have undergone organ transplantation. In such patients, KS usually resolves once the dose of the immunosuppressive medication is decreased or discontinued. In people with AIDS, epidemic KS is most often seen among male homosexuals and bisexuals.

Although the histopathology of all forms of KS is virtually identical, the clinical manifestations differ: AIDS-related KS exhibits a more variable and aggressive course, ranging from localized cutaneous lesions to disseminated disease involving multiple organ systems. Cutaneous signs may be the first manifestation of HIV, appearing in more than 90% of HIV-infected patients as the immune functions deteriorate. These skin signs correlate to low CD4+ counts. Cutaneous lesions can appear anywhere on the body and are usually brownish pink to deep purple. They may be flat or raised and surrounded by ecchymoses (hemorrhagic patches) and edema (Fig. 52-3). Rapid development of lesions involving large areas of skin is associated with extensive disfigurement. The location and size of some lesions

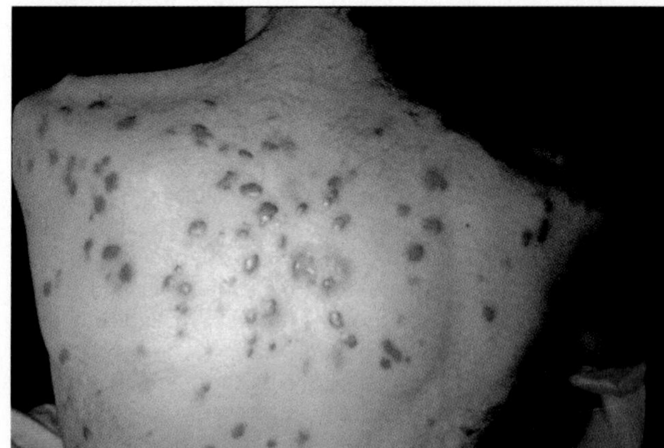

FIGURE 52-3. Lesions of the AIDS-related Kaposi's sarcoma. Whereas some patients may have lesions that remain flat, others experience extensively disseminated, raised lesions with edema. From DeVita, V. T. Jr., Hellman, S., & Rosenberg, S. (Eds.). *AIDS: Etiology, diagnosis, treatment, and prevention* (4th ed.). Philadelphia: Lippincott Williams & Wilkins.

can lead to venous stasis, lymphedema, and pain. Ulcerative lesions disrupt skin integrity and increase discomfort and susceptibility to infection. The most common sites of visceral involvement are the lymph nodes, gastrointestinal tract, and lungs. Involvement of internal organs may eventually lead to organ failure, hemorrhage, infection, and death.

Diagnosis of KS is confirmed by biopsy of suspected lesions. Prognosis depends on the extent of the tumor, the presence of other symptoms of HIV infection, and the CD4+ count. Death may result from tumor progression. More often, however, it results from other complications of HIV infection.

B-CELL LYMPHOMAS

B-cell lymphomas are the second most common malignancy occurring in people with AIDS. Lymphomas associated with AIDS usually differ from those occurring in the general population. Patients with AIDS are typically much younger than the usual population affected by non-Hodgkin lymphoma. In addition, AIDS-related lymphomas tend to develop outside the lymph nodes, most commonly in the brain, bone marrow, and gastrointestinal tract. These types of lymphomas are characteristically of a higher grade, indicating aggressive growth and resistance to treatment. The course of AIDS-related lymphomas includes multiple sites of organ involvement and complications related to opportunistic infections. Although aggressive combination chemotherapy is frequently successful in the treatment of non-Hodgkin lymphoma that is not associated with HIV infection, treatment is less successful in people with AIDS because of severe hematologic toxicity and complications of opportunistic infections that can occur from treatment.

Neurologic Manifestations

An estimated 80% of all patients with AIDS experience some form of neurologic involvement during the course of HIV infection. Many neuropathologic disorders are underreported, because patients may have neurologic involvement without overt signs or symptoms. Neurologic complications involve central, peripheral, and autonomic functions. Neurologic dysfunction results from direct effects of HIV on nervous system tissue, opportunistic infections, primary or metastatic neoplasms, cerebrovascular changes, metabolic encephalopathies, or complications secondary to therapy. Immune system response to HIV infection in the CNS includes inflammation, atrophy, demyelination, degeneration, and necrosis.

HIV ENCEPHALOPATHY

HIV encephalopathy was formerly referred to as AIDS dementia complex (Chart 52-8). It is a clinical syndrome that is characterized by a progressive decline in cognitive, behavioral, and motor functions. Substantial evidence exists that HIV encephalopathy is a direct result of HIV infection. HIV has been found in the brain and cerebrospinal fluid (CSF) of patients with HIV encephalopathy. The brain cells infected by HIV are predominantly the CD4+ cells of monocyte-**macrophage** lineage. HIV infection is thought to trigger the release of toxins or lymphokines that result in cellular dysfunction or interference with neurotransmitter function rather than cellular damage.

Signs and symptoms may be subtle and difficult to distinguish from fatigue, depression, or the adverse effects of treatment for infections and malignancies. Early manifestations include memory deficits, headache, difficulty concentrating, progressive confusion, psychomotor slowing, apathy, and ataxia. Later stages include global cognitive impairments, delay in verbal responses, a vacant stare, spastic paraparesis, hyperreflexia, psychosis, hallucinations, tremor, incontinence, seizures, mutism, and death.

Confirming the diagnosis of HIV encephalopathy can be difficult. Extensive neurologic evaluation includes a computed tomography scan, which may indicate diffuse cerebral atrophy and ventricular enlargement. Other tests that may detect abnormalities include magnetic resonance imaging, analysis of CSF through lumbar puncture, and brain biopsy.

CRYPTOCOCCUS NEOFORMANS

A fungal infection, *C. neoformans* is another common opportunistic infection among patients with AIDS, and it causes neurologic disease. Cryptococcal meningitis is characterized by symptoms such as fever, headache, malaise, stiff neck, nausea, vomiting, mental status changes, and seizures. Diagnosis is confirmed by CSF analysis.

PROGRESSIVE MULTIFOCAL LEUKOENCEPHALOPATHY

Progressive multifocal leukoencephalopathy (PML) is a demyelinating CNS disorder that affects the oligodendroglia. It occurs in about 3% of AIDS patients. Clinical manifestations often begin with mental confusion and rapidly progress to include blindness, aphasia, muscle weakness, paresis (partial or complete paralysis), and death. Treatments have greatly reduced the threat of mortality associated with this disorder.

OTHER NEUROLOGIC DISORDERS

Other common infections involving the nervous system include *T. gondii*, CMV, and *M. tuberculosis* infections. Additional neurologic manifestations include both central and peripheral neuropathies. Vascular myelopathy is a degenerative disorder that affects the lateral and posterior columns of the spinal cord, resulting in progressive spastic paraparesis, ataxia, and incontinence. HIV-related **peripheral neuropathy** is thought to be a demyelinating disorder; it is associated with pain and numbness in the extremities, weakness, diminished deep tendon reflexes, orthostatic hypotension, and impotence.

Depressive Manifestations

The prevalence of depression among people with HIV infection is unknown. The causes of depression are multifactorial and may include a history of preexisting mental illness, neuropsychiatric disturbances, and psychosocial factors. Depression also occurs in people with HIV infection in response to the physical symptoms, including pain and weight loss, and the lack of someone to talk with about their concerns. People with HIV/AIDS who are depressed may experience irrational guilt and shame, loss of self-esteem, feelings of helplessness and worthlessness, and suicidal ideation.

CHART 52-8

Care of the Patient With HIV Encephalopathy

DISTURBED THOUGHT PROCESSES
- Assess mental status and neurologic functioning.
- Monitor for medication interactions, infections, electrolyte imbalance, and depression.
- Frequently orient the patient to time, place, person, reality, and the environment.
- Use simple explanations.
- Teach the patient to perform tasks in incremental steps.
- Provide memory aids (clocks and calendars).
- Provide memory aids for medication administration.
- Post activity schedule.
- Give positive feedback for appropriate behavior.
- Teach caretakers how to orient patient to time, place, person, reality, and the environment.
- Encourage the patient to designate a responsible person to assume power of attorney.

DISTURBED SENSORY PERCEPTION
- Assess sensory impairment.
- Decrease amount of stimuli in the patient's environment.
- Correct inaccurate perceptions.
- Provide reassurance and safety if the patient displays fear.
- Provide a secure and stable environment.
- Teach caregivers how to recognize inaccurate sensory perceptions.
- Teach caregivers techniques to correct inaccurate perceptions.
- Teach the patient and caregivers to report any changes in the patient's vision to the patient's health care provider.

RISK FOR INJURY
- Assess the patient's level of anxiety, confusion, or disorientation.
- Assess the patient for delusions or hallucinations.
- Remove potentially dangerous objects from the patient's environment.
- Structure the environment for safety (ensure adequate lighting, avoid clutter, provide bed rails if needed).
- Supervise smoking.
- Do not let the patient drive a car if confusion is present.
- Instruct the patient and caregiver in home safety.
- Provide assistance as needed for ambulation and in getting in and out of bed.
- Pad headboard and side rails if the patient has seizures.

SELF-CARE DEFICITS
- Encourage activities of daily living within the patient's level of ability.
- Encourage independence but assist if the patient cannot perform an activity.
- Demonstrate any activity that the patient is having difficulty accomplishing.
- Monitor food and fluid intake.
- Weigh patient weekly.
- Encourage the patient to eat, and offer nutritious meals, snacks, and adequate fluids.
- If patient is incontinent, establish a routine toileting schedule.
- Teach caregivers how to meet the patient's self-care needs.

Integumentary Manifestations

Cutaneous manifestations are associated with HIV infection and the accompanying opportunistic infections and malignancies. KS (described earlier) and opportunistic infections such as herpes zoster and herpes simplex are associated with painful vesicles that disrupt skin integrity. Molluscum contagiosum is a viral infection characterized by deforming plaque formation. Seborrheic dermatitis is associated with an indurated, diffuse, scaly rash involving the scalp and face. Patients with AIDS may also exhibit a generalized folliculitis associated with dry, flaking skin or atopic dermatitis, such as eczema or psoriasis. Up to 60% of patients treated with trimethoprim-sulfamethoxazole (TMP-SMZ) develop a drug-related rash that is pruritic with pinkish-red macules and papules. Regardless of the origin of these rashes, patients experience discomfort and are at increased risk for additional infection from disrupted skin integrity.

Endocrine Manifestations

The endocrine manifestations of HIV infection are not completely understood. At autopsy, endocrine glands show infiltration and destruction from opportunistic infections or neoplasms. Endocrine function may also be affected by therapeutic agents.

Gynecologic Manifestations

Persistent, recurrent vaginal candidiasis may be the first sign of HIV infection in women. Past or present genital ulcer disease is a risk factor for the transmission of HIV infection. Women with HIV infection are more susceptible to and have increased rates of incidence and recurrence of genital ulcer disease and venereal warts. Ulcerative STDs such as chancroid, syphilis, and herpes are more severe in women with HIV infection. **Human papillomavirus (HPV)** causes venereal warts and is a risk factor for cervical intraepithelial neoplasia, a cellular change that is frequently a precursor to cervical cancer. Women with HIV are 10 times more likely to develop cervical intraepithelial neoplasia than those not infected with HIV. There is a strong association between abnormal Pap smears and HIV seropositivity. HIV-seropositive women with cervical carcinoma present at a more advanced stage of disease and have more persistent and recurrent disease and a shorter interval to recurrence and death than women without HIV infection.

A significant percentage of women who require hospitalization for pelvic inflammatory disease have HIV infection. Women with HIV are at increased risk for pelvic inflammatory disease, and the associated inflammation may potentiate the transmission of HIV infection. Moreover, women with HIV infection appear to have a higher incidence of menstrual abnormalities, including amenorrhea or bleeding between periods, than do women without HIV infection. The failure of health care providers to consider HIV infection in women may lead to a later diagnosis, thereby denying these patients appropriate treatment.

Medical Management

Treatment of Infections

GENERAL INFECTIONS

TMP-SMZ (Bactrim, Septra) is an antibacterial agent used to treat various organisms causing infection. People with HIV infection who have a T-cell count of less than 200 cells/mm^3 should receive chemoprophylaxis against PCP with TMP-SMZ. PCP prophylaxis can be safely discontinued in patients who are responding to HAART with a sustained increase in T lymphocytes. TMP-SMZ also confers cross-protection against toxoplasmosis and some common respiratory bacterial infections. Patients with AIDS who are treated with TMP-SMZ experience a high incidence of adverse effects, such as fever, rashes, leukopenia, thrombocytopenia, and renal dysfunction. Reintroduction of TMP-SMZ using a gradually increasing dose (desensitization) may be successful in up to 70% of patients.

PNEUMOCYSTIS PNEUMONIA

In the past several years, there have been many advances in the treatment of PCP. TMP-SMZ, the treatment of choice for PCP in patients with AIDS and in immunocompromised patients without HIV infection, is available in both IV and oral preparations. Pentamidine (Pentacarinat, Pentam 300, NebuPent), an antiprotozoal medication, is used as an alternative agent for combating PCP. If adverse effects develop or if the patient does not improve clinically when treated with TMP-SMZ, the health care provider may recommend pentamidine. Intramuscular administration is avoided because of the potential for painful sterile abscess formation. In addition, IV pentamidine can cause severe hypotension if it is administered too rapidly. Other adverse effects include impaired glucose metabolism leading to the development of diabetes mellitus from damage to the pancreas, renal damage, hepatic dysfunction, and neutropenia. Initially, the success of aerosolized pentamidine led to its use as a treatment for mild to moderate PCP. However, it has proved to be less effective and more costly than TMP-SMZ, and early relapses are common. Because of these limitations, aerosolized pentamidine should not be used (Benson et al., 2004). The combination of TMP-SMZ and pentamidine has shown no additional benefit and is avoided because of the cumulative toxic effects that may result.

MYCOBACTERIUM AVIUM COMPLEX

Chemoprophylaxis against disseminated MAC disease is indicated for HIV-infected people with T-cell counts lower than 50 cells/mm^3. Treatment for MAC infections involves use of either clarithromycin (Biaxin) or azithromycin (Zithromax). The combination of azithromycin with rifabutin (Mycobutin) is more effective, but the additional cost, increased occurrence of adverse effects, potential for drug interactions, and lack of demonstrated difference in survival do not warrant the recommendation of both medications. Secondary prophylaxis for disseminated MAC may be discontinued in patients who have sustained increases (eg, longer than 6 months) in CD4 counts (greater than 100 cells/mm^3) in response to HAART, have completed 12 months of MAC therapy, and have no signs or symptoms attributable to MAC. Primary prophylaxis for disseminated MAC may be discontinued in patients who have responded to HAART with CD4 counts of 100 cells/mm^3 or higher for at least 3 months and may be reintroduced if counts decrease to 50 to 100 cells/mm^3 (Horowitz & Wormser, 2004).

MENINGITIS

Current primary therapy for cryptococcal meningitis is IV amphotericin B with or without oral flucytosine (5-FC, Ancobon) or fluconazole (Diflucan). Serious potential adverse effects of amphotericin B include anaphylaxis, renal and hepatic impairment, electrolyte imbalances, anemia, fever, and severe chills. Intrathecal administration of amphotericin B has been used in place of or in combination with IV administration in patients who have failed to respond to IV administration. Until fluconazole, an antifungal agent, was approved and used for lifelong suppressive therapy, frequent relapses and high mortality rates often necessitated prolonged therapy with amphotericin B. In some instances, the patient continues to receive IV amphotericin in the home setting. Oral fluconazole is used as suppressive therapy when the CSF tests negative for the organism. This medication is less toxic and better tolerated than amphotericin B.

CYTOMEGALOVIRUS RETINITIS

Retinitis caused by CMV is a leading cause of blindness in patients with AIDS. Prophylaxis with oral ganciclovir may be considered for HIV-infected people who have CD4+ T-cell counts of less than 50 cells/mm^3. Two antiviral agents, ganciclovir (DHPG, Cytovene, Vitrasert) and foscarnet (Foscavir), offer effective treatment but not a cure for CMV retinitis. Because ganciclovir and foscarnet do not kill the virus but rather control its growth, they must be taken for life. Relapse rates associated with the two agents are similar. Discontinuation of the medication is associated with the relapse of retinitis within 1 month.

A common adverse reaction to ganciclovir is severe neutropenia, which limits the concomitant use of zidovudine (AZT, Compound S, Retrovir). Intravitreal injections of ganciclovir have been effective for patients who cannot tolerate systemic ganciclovir because of severe neutropenia, infection at the venous access site, or the need to take zidovudine. Zidovudine may be given with foscarnet (Foscavir). Common adverse reactions to foscarnet are nephrotoxicity, including acute renal failure, and electrolyte imbalances, including hypocalcemia, hyperphosphatemia, and hypomagnesemia, which can be life-threatening. Other common adverse effects include seizures, gastrointestinal disturbances, anemia, phlebitis at the infusion site, and low back pain. Possible bone marrow suppression (producing a decrease in white blood cell and platelet counts), oral candidiasis, and liver and renal impairments require close patient monitoring.

OTHER INFECTIONS

Oral acyclovir, famciclovir, or valacyclovir may be used to treat infections caused by herpes simplex or herpes zoster. Esophageal or oral candidiasis is treated topically with clotrimazole (Mycelex) oral troches or nystatin suspension. Chronic refractory infection with candidiasis (thrush) or esophageal involvement is treated with ketoconazole (Nizoral) or fluconazole (Diflucan).

Antidiarrheal Therapy

Although many forms of diarrhea respond to treatment, it is not unusual for this condition to recur and become a chronic problem for the HIV patient. Therapy with octreotide acetate (Sandostatin), a synthetic analogue of somatostatin, has been shown to be effective in managing chronic severe diarrhea. High concentrations of somatostatin receptors have been found in the gastrointestinal tract and in other tissues. Somatostatin inhibits many physiologic functions, including gastrointestinal motility and intestinal secretion of water and electrolytes.

Chemotherapy

KAPOSI'S SARCOMA

Management of KS is usually difficult because of the variability of symptoms and the organ systems involved. KS is rarely life-threatening except when there is pulmonary or gastrointestinal involvement. The treatment goals are to reduce symptoms by decreasing the size of the skin lesions, to reduce discomfort associated with edema and ulcerations, and to control symptoms associated with mucosal or visceral involvement. No one treatment has been shown to increase survival. Localized treatment includes surgical excision of the lesions or application of liquid nitrogen to local skin lesions and injections of intraoral lesions with dilute vinblastine. Injection of intraoral lesions has been associated with local pain and skin irritation. Radiation therapy is effective as a palliative measure to relieve localized pain due to tumor mass (especially in the legs) and for KS lesions that are in sites such as the oral mucosa, conjunctiva, face, and soles of the feet.

Interferon is known for its antiviral and antitumor effects. Patients with cutaneous KS treated with **alpha-interferon** have experienced tumor regression and improved immune system function. Positive responses have been observed in 30% to 50% of patients, with the best responses seen in those with limited disease and no opportunistic infections. Alpha-interferon is administered by the IV, intramuscular, or subcutaneous route. Patients may self-administer interferon at home or receive interferon in an outpatient setting.

LYMPHOMA

Successful treatment of AIDS-related lymphomas has been limited because of the rapid progression of these malignancies. Combination chemotherapy and radiation therapy regimens may produce an initial response, but it is usually short-lived. Because standard regimens for non-AIDS lymphomas have been ineffective, many clinicians suggest that AIDS-related lymphomas should be studied as a separate group in clinical trials.

Antidepressant Therapy

Treatment for depression in people with HIV infection involves psychotherapy integrated with pharmacotherapy. If depressive symptoms are severe and of sufficient duration, treatment with antidepressants may be initiated. Antidepressants such as imipramine (Tofranil), desipramine (Norpramin), and fluoxetine (Prozac) may be used, because these medications also alleviate the fatigue and lethargy that are associated with depression. A psychostimulant such as methylphenidate (Ritalin) may be used in low doses in patients with neuropsychiatric impairment. Electroconvulsive therapy may be an option for patients with severe depression who have not responded to pharmacologic interventions.

Nutrition Therapy

Malnutrition increases the risk for infection and may also increase the incidence of opportunistic infections. Nutrition therapy should be integrated into the overall management plan and should be tailored to meet the nutritional needs of the patient, whether by oral diet, enteral tube feedings, or parenteral nutritional support, if needed. As with all patients, a healthy diet is essential for the patient with HIV infection. For all patients with AIDS who experience unexplained weight loss, calorie counts should be obtained to evaluate nutritional status and initiate appropriate therapy. The goal is to maintain the ideal weight and, when necessary, to increase weight.

Appetite stimulants have been successfully used in patients with AIDS-related anorexia. Megestrol acetate (Megace), a synthetic oral progesterone preparation used to treat breast cancer, promotes significant weight gain and inhibits cytokine IL-1 synthesis. In patients with HIV infection, it increases body weight primarily by increasing body fat stores. Dronabinol (Marinol), which is a synthetic tetrahydrocannabinol (THC), the active ingredient in marijuana, has been used to relieve nausea and vomiting associated with cancer chemotherapy. Preliminary results show that after beginning dronabinol therapy, almost all patients with HIV infection experience a modest weight gain. The effects on body composition are unknown.

Oral supplements may be used to supplement diets that are deficient in calories and protein. Ideally, oral supplements should be lactose-free (many people with HIV infection are intolerant to lactose), high in calories and easily digestible protein, low in fat with the fat easily digestible, palatable, inexpensive, and tolerated without causing diarrhea. Advera is a nutritional supplement that has been developed specifically for people with HIV infection and AIDS. Parenteral nutrition is the final option because of its prohibitive cost and associated risks, including risk of infections.

Complementary and Alternative Modalities

Traditional Western medicine focuses on the treatment of disease. These treatments or interventions are taught in medical schools and are used by physicians in the care of patients. Complementary and alternative medicine (CAM) is often viewed as consisting of unconventional and unorthodox treatments or interventions that are not traditionally taught in medical schools. These modalities and therapies stress the need to treat the whole person, recognizing the interaction of the body, mind, and spirit. What is considered to be CAM in one culture may actually be a traditional therapy in another. People with HIV infection report substantial use of CAM for symptom management. The use of CAM in HIV infection and AIDS often results because of disillusionment with standard medical treatment, which to date has provided no cure. Combined with traditional therapies, CAM may improve the patient's overall well-being. However, there can be adverse drug–drug interactions between certain CAM therapies (eg, St. John's wort) and some antiretroviral medications (Panel on Clinical Practices, 2004).

CAM can be divided into four categories:

- Spiritual or psychological therapies may include humor, hypnosis, faith healing, guided imagery, and positive affirmations.
- Nutritional therapies may include vegetarian or macrobiotic diets, vitamin C or beta-carotene supplements, and turmeric, which contains curcumin, a food spice supplement. Chinese herbs, such as traditional herbal mixtures, are also used, in addition to compound Q (a Chinese cucumber extract) and *Momordica charantia* (bitter melon), which is given as an enema.
- Drug and biologic therapies include medications and other substances not approved by the FDA. Examples are *N*-acetylcysteine, pentoxifylline (Trental), and 1-chloro-2, 4-dinitrobenzene. Also included in this category are oxygen therapy, ozone therapy, and urine therapy.
- Treatment with physical forces and devices may include acupuncture, acupressure, massage therapy, reflexology, therapeutic touch, yoga, and crystals.

Although there is insufficient research on the effects of CAM, there is a growing body of literature reporting benefits for modalities involving nutrition, exercise, psychosocial treatment, and Chinese medicine.

Many patients who use these therapies do not report use of CAM to their health care providers. To obtain a complete health history, the nurse should ask about the patient's use of alternative therapies. Patients may need to be encouraged to report their use of CAM to their primary health care provider. Problems may arise, for example, when patients are using CAM while participating in clinical drug trials; alternative therapies can have significant adverse side effects, making it difficult to assess the effects of the medications in the clinical trial. The nurse needs to become familiar with the potential adverse side effects of these therapies. The nurse who suspects that CAM is causing a side effect needs to discuss this with the patient, the alternative therapy provider, and the primary health care provider. It is important for the nurse to view CAM with an open mind and to try to understand the importance of this treatment to the patient. This approach will improve communication with the patient and reduce conflict.

Supportive Care

Patients who are weak and debilitated as a result of chronic illness associated with HIV infection typically require many kinds of supportive care. Nutritional support may be as simple as providing assistance in obtaining or preparing meals. For patients with more advanced nutritional impairment resulting from decreased intake, wasting syndrome, or gastrointestinal malabsorption associated with diarrhea, parenteral feedings may be required. Imbalances that result from nausea, vomiting, and profuse diarrhea often necessitate IV fluid and electrolyte replacement.

Skin breakdown associated with KS, perianal skin excoriation, or immobility is managed with thorough and meticulous skin care involving regular turning, cleansing, and applications of medicated ointments and dressings.

Pain associated with skin breakdown, abdominal cramping, peripheral neuropathy, or KS is managed by administering analgesics at regular intervals around the clock. Relaxation and guided imagery may be helpful in reducing pain and anxiety.

Pulmonary symptoms, such as dyspnea and shortness of breath, may be related to infection, KS, or fatigue. For patients with these symptoms, oxygen therapy, relaxation training, and energy conservation techniques may be helpful. Patients with severe respiratory dysfunction may require mechanical ventilation. Before mechanical ventilation is instituted, the procedure is explained to the patient and the caregiver. If the patient elects to not be placed on mechanical ventilation, his or her wishes should be followed. Ideally, the patient has prepared an advance directive identifying preferences for treatments and end-of-life care, including hospice care. If the patient has not identified preferences in advance, treatment options are described so that the patient can make informed decisions and have those wishes respected.

Nursing Process

The Patient With AIDS

The nursing care of patients with AIDS is challenging because of the potential for any organ system to be the target of infections or cancer. In addition, this disease is complicated by many emotional, social, and ethical issues. The plan of care for the patient with AIDS (Chart 52-9) is individualized to meet the needs of the patient. Care includes many of the

(text continues on page 1844)

CHART 52-9

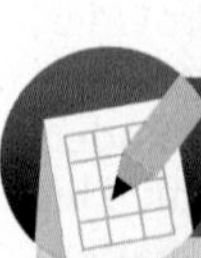

Plan of Nursing Care Care of the Patient With AIDS

Nursing Diagnosis: Diarrhea related to enteric pathogens or HIV infection
Goal: Resumption of usual bowel habits

NURSING INTERVENTIONS	RATIONALE	EXPECTED OUTCOMES
1. Assess patient's normal bowel habits.	1. Provides baseline for evaluation	• Exhibits return to normal bowel patterns • Reports decreasing episodes of diarrhea and abdominal cramping • Identifies and avoids foods that irritate the gastrointestinal tract • Appropriate therapy is initiated as prescribed. • Exhibits normal stool cultures • Maintains adequate fluid intake • Maintains body weight and reports no additional weight loss • States rationale for avoiding smoking • Enrolls in program to stop smoking • Uses medication as prescribed • Maintains adequate fluid status • Exhibits normal skin turgor, moist mucous membranes, adequate urine output, and absence of excessive thirst
2. Assess for diarrhea: frequent, loose stools; abdominal pain or cramping, volume of liquid stools, and exacerbating and alleviating factors.	2. Detects changes in status, quantifies loss of fluid, and provides basis for nursing measures	
3. Obtain stool cultures and administer antimicrobial therapy as prescribed.	3. Identifies pathogenic organism; therapy targets specific organism	
4. Initiate measures to reduce hyperactivity of bowel:	4. Promotes bowel rest, which may decrease acute episodes	
a. Maintain food and fluid restrictions as prescribed. Suggest BRAT diet (*b*ananas, *r*ice, *a*pplesauce, *t*ea and *t*oast).	a. Reduces stimulation of bowel	
b. Discourage smoking.	b. Eliminates nicotine, which acts as bowel stimulant	
c. Avoid bowel irritants such as fatty or fried foods, raw vegetables, and nuts. Offer small, frequent meals.	c. Prevents stimulation of bowel and abdominal distention and promotes adequate nutrition	
5. Administer anticholinergic antispasmodics and opioids or other medications as prescribed.	5. Decreases intestinal spasms and motility	
6. Maintain fluid intake of at least 3 L unless contraindicated.	6. Prevents hypovolemia	

Nursing Diagnosis: Risk for infection related to immunodeficiency
Goal: Absence of infection

NURSING INTERVENTIONS	RATIONALE	EXPECTED OUTCOMES
1. Monitor for infection: fever, chills, and diaphoresis; cough; shortness of breath; oral pain or painful swallowing; creamy-white patches in oral cavity; urinary frequency, urgency, or dysuria; redness, swelling, or drainage from wounds; vesicular lesions on face, lips, or perianal area.	1. Allows for early detection of infection, essential for prompt initiation of treatment. Repeated and prolonged infections contribute to patient's debilitation.	• Identifies reportable signs and symptoms of infection • Reports signs and symptoms of infection if present • Exhibits and reports absence of fever, chills, and diaphoresis • Exhibits normal (clear) breath sounds without adventitious breath sounds • Maintains weight • Reports adequate energy level without excessive fatigue
2. Teach patient or caregiver about need to report possible infection.	2. Allows early detection of infection	

CHART 52-9

Plan of Nursing Care Care of the Patient With AIDS (Continued)

NURSING INTERVENTIONS	RATIONALE	EXPECTED OUTCOMES
3. Monitor white blood cell count and differential.	3. Identifies elevated WBC possibly associated with infection	• Reports absence of shortness of breath and cough • Exhibits pink, moist oral mucous membranes without fissures or lesions • Takes appropriate therapy as prescribed • Experiences no infection • States rationale for strategies to avoid infection • Modifies activities to reduce exposure to infection or infectious persons • Practices "safer sex" • Avoids sharing eating utensils and toothbrush • Exhibits normal body temperature • Uses recommended techniques to maintain cleanliness of skin, skin lesions, and perianal area • Has others handle pet excreta and cleanup • Uses recommended cooking techniques
4. Obtain cultures of wound drainage, skin lesions, urine, stool, sputum, mouth, and blood as prescribed. Administer antimicrobial therapy as prescribed.	4. Assists in determining offending organism to initiate appropriate treatment	
5. Instruct patient in ways to prevent infection: a. Clean kitchen and bathroom surfaces with disinfectants. b. Clean hands thoroughly after exposure to body fluids. c. Avoid exposure to others' body fluids or sharing eating utensils. d. Turn, cough, and deep breathe, especially when activity is decreased. e. Maintain cleanliness of perianal area. f. Avoid handling pet excreta or cleaning litter boxes, bird cages, or aquariums. g. Cook meat and eggs thoroughly.	5. Minimizes exposure to infection and transmission of HIV infection to others	
6. Maintain aseptic technique when performing invasive procedures such as venipunctures, bladder catheterizations, and injections.	6. Prevents hospital-acquired infections	

Nursing Diagnosis: Ineffective airway clearance related to *Pneumocystis* pneumonia, increased bronchial secretions, and decreased ability to cough related to weakness and fatigue
Goal: Improved airway clearance

NURSING INTERVENTIONS	RATIONALE	EXPECTED OUTCOMES
1. Assess and report signs and symptoms of altered respiratory status, tachypnea, use of accessory muscles, cough, color and amount of sputum, abnormal breath sounds, dusky or cyanotic skin color, restlessness, confusion, or somnolence.	1. Indicates abnormal respiratory function	• Maintains normal airway clearance: Respiratory rate <20 breaths/min Unlabored breathing without use of accessory muscles and flaring nares (nostrils) Skin color pink (without cyanosis) Alert and aware of surroundings Arterial blood gas values normal Normal breath sounds without adventitious breath sounds
2. Obtain sputum sample for culture prescribed. Administer antimicrobial therapy as prescribed.	2. Aids in identification of pathogenic organisms	

continued >

CHART 52-9

Plan of Nursing Care — Care of the Patient With AIDS (Continued)

NURSING INTERVENTIONS	RATIONALE	EXPECTED OUTCOMES
3. Provide pulmonary care (cough, deep breathing, postural drainage, and vibration) every 2 to 4 hours.	3. Prevents stasis of secretions and promotes airway clearance	• Begins appropriate therapy • Takes medication as prescribed • Reports improved breathing • Maintains clear airway
4. Assist patient in attaining semi- or high Fowler's position.	4. Facilities breathing and airway clearance	• Coughs and takes deep breaths every 2–4 hours as recommended
5. Encourage adequate rest periods.	5. Maximizes energy expenditure and prevents excessive fatigue	• Demonstrates appropriate positions and practices postural drainage every 2–4 hours
6. Initiate measures to decrease viscosity of secretions: a. Maintain fluid intake of at least 3 L per day unless contraindicated. b. Humidify inspired air as prescribed. c. Consult with physician concerning use of mucolytic agents delivered through nebulizer or IPPB treatment.	6. Facilitates expectoration of secretions; prevents stasis of secretions	• Reports reduced breathing difficulty when in semi- or high Fowler's position • Practices energy-conserving strategies and alternates rest with activity • Demonstrates reduction in thickness (viscosity) of pulmonary secretions • Reports increased ease in coughing up sputum
7. Perform tracheal suctioning as needed.	7. Removes secretions if patient is unable to do so	• Uses humidified air or oxygen as prescribed and indicated
8. Administer oxygen therapy as prescribed.	8. Increases availability of oxygen	• Indicates need for assistance with removal of pulmonary secretions
9. Assist with endotracheal intubation; maintain ventilator settings as prescribed.	9. Maintains ventilation	• Understands need for and cooperates with endotracheal intubation and use of a mechanical ventilator • Verbalizes concerns about respiratory difficulty, intubation, and mechanical ventilation

Nursing Diagnosis: Imbalanced nutrition, less than body requirements, related to decreased oral intake
Goal: Improvement of nutritional status

NURSING INTERVENTIONS	RATIONALE	EXPECTED OUTCOMES
1. Assess for malnutrition with height, weight, age, BUN, serum protein, and albumin, transferrin levels, hemoglobin, hematocrit, and cutaneous anergy.	1. Provides objective measurement of nutritional status	• Identifies factors limiting oral intake and uses resources to promote adequate dietary intake • Reports increased appetite • States understanding of nutritional needs
2. Obtain dietary history, including likes and dislikes and food intolerances.	2. Defines need for nutritional education; helps individualize interventions	• Identifies ways to reduce factors that limit oral intake
3. Assess factors that interfere with oral intake.	3. Provides basis and directions for interventions	• Rests before meals • Eats in pleasant, odor-free environment

CHART 52-9

Plan of Nursing Care — Care of the Patient With AIDS (Continued)

NURSING INTERVENTIONS	RATIONALE	EXPECTED OUTCOMES
4. Consult with dietitian to determine patient's nutritional needs.	4. Facilitates meal planning	• Arranges meals to coincide with visitors' visits
5. Reduce factors limiting oral intake:	5. Addresses factors limiting intake:	• Reports increased dietary intake • Uses oral hygiene before meals
a. Encourage patient to rest before meals.	a. Minimizes fatigue, which can decrease appetite	• Takes analgesics before meals as prescribed
b. Plan meals so that they do not occur immediately after painful or unpleasant procedures.	b. Decreases noxious stimuli	• Identifies ways to increase protein and caloric intake • Identifies foods high in protein and calories
c. Encourage patient to eat meals with visitors or others when possible.	c. Limits social isolation	• Consumes foods high in protein and calories • Reports decreased rate of weight loss.
d. Encourage patient to prepare simple meals or to obtain assistance with meal preparation if possible.	d. Limits energy expenditure	• Maintains adequate intake • States rationale for enteral or parenteral nutrition if needed
e. Serve small, frequent meals: 6 per day.	e. Prevents overwhelming patient	• Demonstrates skill in preparing alternate sources of nutrition
f. Limit fluids 1 hour before meals and with meals.	f. Reduces satiety	
6. Instruct patient in ways to supplement nutrition: consume protein-rich foods (meat, poultry, fish) and carbohydrates (pasta, fruit, breads).	6. Provides additional proteins and calories	
7. Consult with physician and dietitian about alternative feeding (enteral or parenteral nutrition).	7. Provides nutritional support if patient is unable to take sufficient amounts by mouth	
8. Consult with social worker or community liaison about financial assistance if patient cannot afford food.	8. Increases availability of resources and nutrition	

Nursing Diagnosis: Deficient knowledge related to means of preventing HIV transmission
Goal: Increased knowledge concerning means of preventing disease transmission

NURSING INTERVENTIONS	RATIONALE	EXPECTED OUTCOMES
1. Instruct patient, family, and friends about routes of transmission of HIV.	1. Knowledge about disease transmission can help prevent spread of disease; may also alleviate fears.	• Patient, family, and friends state means of transmission.
2. Instruct patient, family, and friends about means of preventing transmission of HIV:	2. Reduces transmission risk	• Reports and demonstrates practices to reduce exposure of others to HIV
a. Avoid sexual contact with multiple partners, and use precautions if sexual partner's HIV status is not certain.	a. The risk of infection increases with the number of sexual partners, male or female, and sexual contact with those who engage in high-risk behaviors.	• Demonstrates knowledge of safer sexual practices • Identifies means of preventing disease transmission

continued >

CHART 52-9

Plan of Nursing Care — Care of the Patient With AIDS (Continued)

NURSING INTERVENTIONS	RATIONALE	EXPECTED OUTCOMES
b. Use condoms during sexual intercourse (vaginal, anal, oral–genital); avoid mouth contact with the penis, vagina, or rectum; avoid sexual practices that can cause cuts or tears in the lining of the rectum, vagina, or penis.	b. Risk of HIV transmission is reduced.	• States that sexual partners are informed about patient's positive HIV status in blood • Avoids IV/injection drug use and sharing of drug equipment with others
c. Avoid sex with prostitutes and others at high risk.	c. Many prostitutes are infected with HIV through sexual contact with multiple partners or IV/injection drug use.	
d. Do not use IV/injection drugs; if addicted and unable or unwilling to change behavior, use clean needles and syringes.	d. Clean needles and syringes are the only way to prevent HIV transmission for those who continue to use drugs. Taking precautions is important for those who are antibody positive to prevent transmitting HIV.	
e. Women who may have been exposed to HIV through sexual or drug practices should consult with a physician before becoming pregnant; consider use of antiretroviral agents if pregnant.	e. HIV can be transmitted from mother to child in utero; use of antiretroviral agents during pregnancy significantly reduces perinatal transmission of HIV.	

Nursing Diagnosis: Social isolation related to stigma of the disease, withdrawal of support systems, isolation procedures, and fear of infecting others
Goal: Decreased sense of social isolation

NURSING INTERVENTIONS	RATIONALE	EXPECTED OUTCOMES
1. Assess patient's usual patterns of social interaction.	1. Establishes basis for individualized interventions	• Shares with others the need for valued social interaction • Demonstrates interest in events, activities, and communication • Verbalizes feelings and reactions to diagnosis, prognosis, and life changes • Identifies modes of transmission of HIV • States ways of preventing transmission of AIDS virus to others while maintaining contact with valued friends and relatives • Reveals AIDS diagnosis to others when appropriate
2. Observe for behaviors indicative of social isolation, such as decreased interaction with others, hostility, noncompliance, sad affect, and stated feelings of rejection or loneliness.	2. Promotes early detection of social isolation, which may be manifested in several ways	
3. Provide instruction concerning modes of transmission of HIV.	3. Provides accurate information, corrects misconceptions, and alleviates anxiety	
4. Assist patient to identify and explore resources for support and positive mechanisms for coping (eg, contact with family, friends, AIDS task force).	4. Enables mobilization of resources and supports	

CHART 52-9

Plan of Nursing Care — Care of the Patient With AIDS (Continued)

NURSING INTERVENTIONS	RATIONALE	EXPECTED OUTCOMES
5. Allow time to be with patient other than for medications and procedures.	5. Promotes feelings of self-worth and provides social interaction	• Identifies resources (ie, family, friends, and support groups) • Uses resources when appropriate • Accepts offers of assistance and support • Reports decreased sense of isolation • Maintains contacts with those of importance to him or her • Develops or continues hobbies that effectively serve as diversion or distraction
6. Encourage participation in diversional activities such as reading, television, or hand crafts.	6. Provides distraction	

Collaborative Problems: Opportunistic infections; impaired breathing; wasting syndrome and fluid and electrolyte imbalances; adverse reaction to medications
Goal: Absence of complications

NURSING INTERVENTIONS	RATIONALE	EXPECTED OUTCOMES
Opportunistic Infections		
1. Monitor vital signs.	1. Changes in vital signs such as increases in pulse rate, respirations, blood pressure, and temperature may indicate infection.	• Exhibits stable vital signs • Experiences control of infection • Identifies signs and symptoms correctly and experiences no complications • Identifies signs and symptoms that are reportable to the physician • Takes medications as prescribed
2. Obtain laboratory specimens and monitor test results.	2. Smears and cultures can identify causative agents such as bacteria, fungi, and protozoa, and sensitivity studies can identify antibiotics or other medications effective against the causative agent.	
3. Instruct the patient and caregiver about signs and symptoms of infection and the need to report them early.	3. Early recognition of symptoms facilitates prompt treatment and avoids extra complications.	
Impaired Breathing		
1. Monitor respiratory rate and pattern.	1. Rapid shallow breathing, diminished breath sounds, and shortness of breath may indicate respiratory failure resulting in hypoxia.	• Maintains stable respiratory rate and pattern within the normal limits • Exhibits no adventitious lung sounds; normal breath sounds • Has stable pulse rate and blood pressure within normal limits, and exhibits no evidence of hypoxia • Oxygen saturation levels within acceptable range
2. Auscultate the chest for breath sounds and abnormal lung sounds.	2. Crackles and wheezes may indicate fluid in the lungs, which disrupts respiratory function and alters the blood's oxygen-carrying capacity.	
3. Monitor pulse rate, blood pressure, and oxygen saturation levels.	3. Changes in pulse rate, blood pressure, and oxygen levels may indicate the development of respiratory or cardiac failure.	

continued >

CHART 52-9

Plan of Nursing Care — Care of the Patient With AIDS (Continued)

NURSING INTERVENTIONS	RATIONALE	EXPECTED OUTCOMES
Wasting Syndrome and Fluid and Electrolyte Disturbances		
1. Monitor weight and laboratory values for nutritional status.	1. Weight loss, malnutrition, and anemia are common in HIV infection and increase risk for superinfection.	• Maintains stable weight • Eats a nutritious diet • Attains and maintains hemoglobin, hematocrit, and ferritin levels within normal limits • Sustains fluid and electrolyte balance within normal limits • Exhibits no signs and symptoms of dehydration
2. Monitor intake and output and laboratory values for fluid and electrolyte imbalance (potassium, sodium, calcium, phosphorus, magnesium, and zinc).	2. Chronic diarrhea, inadequate oral intake, vomiting, and profuse sweating deplete electrolytes. Small intestine inflammation may impair the absorption of fluids and electrolytes.	
3. Monitor for and report signs and symptoms of dehydration.	3. Fluid loss results in decreased circulating volume leading to tachycardia, dry skin and mucous membranes, poor skin turgor, elevated urine specific gravity, and thirst. Early detection allows early treatment.	
Reactions to Medications		
1. Monitor for medication interactions.	1. People with HIV infection receive many medications for HIV and for disease complications. Early detection of medication interactions is necessary to prevent complications.	• Experiences no serious side effects or complications from medications • Correctly describes medication regimen and complies with therapy, including adaptations in eating routines and type of food used with prescribed medications
2. Monitor for and promptly report side effects from antiretroviral agents.	2. Side effects from antiretroviral agents can be life-threatening. Serious side effects include anemia, pancreatitis, peripheral neuropathy, mental confusion, and persistent nausea and vomiting. Corrective measures need to be instituted.	
3. Instruct the patient and caregiver in the medication regimen.	3. Knowledge of the medication purpose, correct administration, side effects, and strategies to manage or prevent side effects promote safety and greater compliance with treatment.	

interventions and concerns cited in the section on supportive care.

Assessment

Nursing assessment includes identification of potential risk factors, including a history of risky sexual practices or IV/injection drug use. The patient's physical status and psychological status are assessed. All factors affecting immune system functioning are thoroughly explored.

Nutritional Status

Nutritional status is assessed by obtaining a dietary history and identifying factors that may interfere with oral intake, such as anorexia, nausea, vomiting, oral pain, or difficulty swallowing. In addition, the patient's ability to purchase and prepare food is assessed. Weight history (ie, changes over time); anthropometric measurements; and blood urea nitrogen (BUN), serum protein, albumin, and transferrin levels provide objective measurements of nutritional status.

Skin Integrity

The skin and mucous membranes are inspected daily for evidence of breakdown, ulceration, or infection. The oral cavity is monitored for redness, ulcerations, and the presence of creamy-white patches indicative of candidiasis. Assessment of the perianal area for excoriation and infection in patients with profuse diarrhea is important. Wounds are cultured to identify infectious organisms.

Respiratory Status

Respiratory status is assessed by monitoring the patient for cough, sputum production (ie, amount and color), shortness of breath, orthopnea, tachypnea, and chest pain. The presence and quality of breath sounds are investigated. Other measures of pulmonary function include chest x-ray results, arterial blood gas values, pulse oximetry, and pulmonary function test results.

Neurologic Status

Neurologic status is determined by assessing level of consciousness; orientation to person, place, and time; and memory lapses. Mental status is assessed as early as possible to provide a baseline. The patient is also assessed for sensory deficits (visual changes, headache, or numbness and tingling in the extremities), motor involvement (altered gait, paresis, or paralysis), and seizure activity.

Fluid and Electrolyte Balance

Fluid and electrolyte status is assessed by examining the skin and mucous membranes for turgor and dryness. Dehydration may be indicated by increased thirst, decreased urine output, postural hypotension, weak and rapid pulse, and urine specific gravity of 1.025 or more. Electrolyte imbalances, such as decreased serum sodium, potassium, calcium, magnesium, and chloride, typically result from profuse diarrhea. The patient is assessed for signs and symptoms of electrolyte deficits, including decreased mental status, muscle twitching, muscle cramps, irregular pulse, nausea and vomiting, and shallow respirations.

Knowledge Level

The patient's level of knowledge about the disease and the modes of disease transmission is evaluated. In addition, the level of knowledge of family and friends is assessed. The patient's psychological reaction to the diagnosis of HIV infection or AIDS is important to explore. Reactions vary among patients and may include denial, anger, fear, shame, withdrawal from social interactions, and depression. It is often helpful to gain an understanding of how the patient has dealt with illness and major life stresses in the past. The patient's resources for support are also identified.

Diagnosis

Nursing Diagnoses

The list of potential nursing diagnoses is extensive because of the complex nature of this disease. However, based on assessment data, major nursing diagnoses for the patient may include the following:

- Impaired skin integrity related to cutaneous manifestations of HIV infection, excoriation, and diarrhea
- Diarrhea related to enteric pathogens or HIV infection
- Risk for infection related to immunodeficiency
- Activity intolerance related to weakness, fatigue, malnutrition, impaired fluid and electrolyte balance, and hypoxia associated with pulmonary infections
- Disturbed thought processes related to shortened attention span, impaired memory, confusion, and disorientation associated with HIV encephalopathy
- Ineffective airway clearance related to PCP, increased bronchial secretions, and decreased ability to cough related to weakness and fatigue
- Pain related to impaired perianal skin integrity secondary to diarrhea, KS, and peripheral neuropathy
- Imbalanced nutrition, less than body requirements, related to decreased oral intake
- Social isolation related to stigma of the disease, withdrawal of support systems, isolation procedures, and fear of infecting others
- Anticipatory grieving related to changes in lifestyle and roles and unfavorable prognosis
- Deficient knowledge related to HIV infection, means of preventing HIV transmission, and self-care

Collaborative Problems/ Potential Complications

Based on the assessment data, possible complications may include the following:

- Opportunistic infections
- Impaired breathing or respiratory failure
- Wasting syndrome and fluid and electrolyte imbalance
- Adverse reaction to medications

Planning and Goals

Goals for the patient may include achievement and maintenance of skin integrity, resumption of usual bowel patterns, absence of infection, improved activity tolerance, improved thought processes, improved airway clearance, increased comfort, improved nutritional status, increased socialization, expression of grief, increased knowledge regarding disease prevention and self-care, and absence of complications.

Nursing Interventions

Promoting Skin Integrity

The skin and oral mucosa are assessed routinely for changes in appearance, location and size of lesions, and evidence of infection and breakdown. The patient is encouraged to maintain a balance between rest and mobility whenever possible. Patients who are immobile are assisted to change position every 2 hours. Devices such as alternating-pressure mattresses and low-air-loss beds are used to prevent skin breakdown. Patients are encouraged to avoid scratching; to use nonabrasive, nondrying soaps; and to apply nonperfumed skin moisturizers to dry skin surfaces. Regular oral care is also encouraged.

Medicated lotions, ointments, and dressings are applied to affected skin surfaces as prescribed. Adhesive tape is avoided. Skin surfaces are protected from friction and rubbing by keeping bed linens free of wrinkles and avoiding tight or restrictive clothing. Patients with foot lesions are advised to wear cotton socks and shoes that do not cause the feet to perspire. Antipruritic, antibiotic, and analgesic agents are administered as prescribed.

The perianal region is assessed frequently for impairment of skin integrity and infection. The patient is instructed to keep the area as clean as possible. The perianal area is cleaned after each bowel movement with nonabrasive soap and water to prevent further excoriation and breakdown of the skin and infection. If the area is very painful, soft cloths or cotton sponges may be less irritating than washcloths. In addition, sitz baths or gentle irrigation may facilitate cleaning and promote comfort. The area is dried thoroughly after cleaning. Topical lotions or ointments may be prescribed to promote healing. Wounds are cultured if infection is suspected, so that the appropriate antimicrobial treatment can be initiated. Debilitated patients may require assistance in maintaining hygienic practices.

Promoting Usual Bowel Patterns

Bowel patterns are assessed for diarrhea. The nurse monitors the frequency and consistency of stools and the patient's reports of abdominal pain or cramping associated with bowel movements. Factors that exacerbate frequent diarrhea are also assessed. The quantity and volume of liquid stools are measured to document fluid volume losses. Stool cultures are obtained to identify pathogenic organisms.

The patient is counseled about ways to decrease diarrhea. The physician may recommend restriction of oral intake to rest the bowel during periods of acute inflammation associated with severe enteric infections. As the patient's dietary intake is increased, foods that act as bowel irritants, such as raw fruits and vegetables, popcorn, carbonated beverages, spicy foods, and foods of extreme temperatures, should be avoided. Small, frequent meals help to prevent abdominal distention. The physician may prescribe medications such as anticholinergic antispasmodics or opioids, which decrease diarrhea by decreasing intestinal spasms and motility. Administering antidiarrheal agents on a regular schedule may be more beneficial than administering them on an as-needed basis. Antibiotics and antifungal agents may also be prescribed to combat pathogens identified by stool cultures. The nurse also assesses the self-care strategies being used by the patient to control diarrhea (Orlando, 2003).

Preventing Infection

The patient and caregivers are instructed to monitor for signs and symptoms of infection: fever; chills; night sweats; cough with or without sputum production; shortness of breath; difficulty breathing; oral pain or difficulty swallowing; creamy-white patches in the oral cavity; unexplained weight loss; swollen lymph nodes; nausea; vomiting; persistent diarrhea; frequency, urgency, or pain on urination; headache; visual changes or memory lapses; redness, swelling, or drainage from skin wounds; and vesicular lesions on the face, lips, or perianal area. The nurse also monitors laboratory test results that indicate infection, such as the white blood cell count and differential. The physician may decide to culture specimens of wound drainage, skin lesions, urine, stool, sputum, mouth, and blood to identify pathogenic organisms and the most appropriate antimicrobial therapy. The patient is instructed to avoid others with active infections such as upper respiratory infections.

Improving Activity Tolerance

Activity tolerance is assessed by monitoring the patient's ability to ambulate and perform activities of daily living. Patients may be unable to maintain their usual levels of activity because of weakness, fatigue, shortness of breath, dizziness, and neurologic involvement. Assistance in planning daily routines that maintain a balance between activity and rest may be necessary. In addition, patients benefit from instructions about energy conservation techniques, such as sitting while washing or while preparing meals. Personal items that are frequently used should be kept within the patient's reach. Measures such as relaxation and guided imagery may be beneficial because they decrease anxiety, which contributes to weakness and fatigue.

Collaboration with other members of the health care team may uncover other factors associated with increasing fatigue and strategies to address them. For example, if fatigue is related to anemia, administering epoetin alfa (Epogen) as prescribed may relieve fatigue and increase activity tolerance.

Maintaining Thought Processes

The patient is assessed for alterations in mental status that may be related to neurologic involvement, metabolic abnormalities, infection, side effects of treatment, and coping mechanisms. Manifestations of neurologic impairment may be difficult to distinguish from psy-

NURSING RESEARCH PROFILE

Exercise As a Self-Care Activity

Ramirez-Marrero, F., Smith, B. & Melendez-Brau, N. (2004). Physical and leisure activity, body composition, and life satisfaction in HIV-positive Hispanics in Puerto Rico. *Journal of the Association of Nurses in AIDS Care, 15*(4), 68–77.

Purpose

Decreases in lean body mass and increases in abdominal fat observed in HIV-positive people receiving highly active antiretroviral therapy (HAART) increase their risk for developing chronic conditions such as cardiovascular disease or diabetes. The purposes of this research were to (1) describe physical and leisure-time activity, body composition, life satisfaction, and depression in HIV-positive Hispanics living in Puerto Rico; and (2) compare body composition, leisure time, CD4 counts, life satisfaction, and depression in those individuals classified as physically active or inactive.

Design

A descriptive survey design was used to examine psychological (life satisfaction, depression), behavioral (physical and leisure-time activity), and biophysical (body composition, CD4 counts) characteristics in HIV-positive men ($n = 43$) and women ($n = 25$) who were receiving ambulatory health care. The study participants in the convenience sample, all of whom were taking HAART medications, completed an instrument packet consisting of four separate questionnaires: Life Satisfaction Index, Beck Depression Inventory, Leisure Activity Inventory, and Seven-Day Physical Activity Recall. Biophysical parameters included measurements of body composition and CD4 counts; the outcomes of the study were based on the objectives identified in *Healthy People 2010*.

Findings

A criterion of 300 kcal/day of physical activity was used to categorize participants into the physically active group or the inactive group. Independent two-tailed *t* tests were used to examine differences in the variables of interest by gender. No differences in physical activity were found between males and females. The physically active group had lower body weight, lower body mass index (BMI), lower limb and trunk skin folds, and lower trunk circumference; they spent less time watching television and had higher life satisfaction scores.

Nursing Implications

Exercise was defined as physical activity that was planned, structured, and repetitive. Many of the participants, particularly women, were overweight and had a BMI indicative of obesity. With the advent of HAART, HIV has evolved into a chronic illness, and as people grow older they often develop chronic illnesses that are exacerbated by excess weight. Nurses need to integrate counseling about weight management in their care, assist patients to differentiate between exercise and usual physical activity, and teach patients that the recommendation for a healthy lifestyle is 30 minutes daily of at least moderate-intensity physical activity. The results of this research suggest that exercise is helpful in physical and psychological well-being for men and women who are HIV-positive.

chological reactions to HIV infection, such as anger and depression.

If the patient experiences altered mental or cognitive status, family members are instructed to speak to the patient in simple, clear language and give the patient sufficient time to respond to questions. Family members are instructed to orient the patient to the daily routine by talking about what is taking place during daily activities. They are encouraged to provide the patient with a regular daily schedule for medication administration, grooming, meal times, bedtimes, and awakening times. Posting the schedule in a prominent area (eg, on the refrigerator), providing nightlights for the bedroom and bathroom, and planning safe leisure activities allow the patient to maintain a regular routine in a safe manner. Activities that the patient previously enjoyed are encouraged. These should be easy to accomplish and fairly short in duration. The nurse encourages the family to remain calm and not to argue with the patient while protecting the patient from injury. Around-the-clock supervision may be necessary, and strategies can be implemented to prevent the patient from engaging in potentially dangerous activities, such as driving, using the stove, or mowing the lawn. Strategies for improving or maintaining functional abilities and for providing a safe environment are used for patients with HIV encephalopathy (see Chart 52-8).

Improving Airway Clearance

Respiratory status, including rate, rhythm, use of accessory muscles, and breath sounds; mental status; and skin color must be assessed at least daily. Any cough and the quantity and characteristics of sputum are documented. Sputum specimens are analyzed for infectious organisms. Pulmonary therapy (coughing, deep breathing, postural drainage, percussion, and vibration) is provided as often as every 2 hours to prevent stasis of secretions and to promote airway clearance. Because of weakness and fatigue, many patients require assistance in attaining a position (such as a high Fowler's or semi-Fowler's position) that facilitates breathing and airway clearance. Adequate rest is essential to minimize energy expenditure and prevent excessive fatigue. The fluid volume status is evaluated so that adequate hydration can be maintained. Unless contraindicated because of renal or cardiac disease, daily intake of 3 L of fluid is encouraged. Humidified oxygen may be prescribed, and nasopharyngeal or tracheal suctioning, intubation, and mechanical ventilation may be necessary to maintain adequate ventilation.

Relieving Pain and Discomfort

The patient is assessed for the quality and severity of pain associated with impaired perianal skin integrity, the lesions of KS, and peripheral neuropathy. In addition, the effects of pain on elimination, nutrition, sleep, affect, and communication are explored, along with exacerbating and relieving factors. Cleaning the perianal area, as previously described, can promote comfort. Topical anesthetics or ointments may be prescribed. Use of soft cushions or foam pads may increase comfort while sitting. The patient is instructed to avoid foods that act as bowel irritants. Antispasmodics and antidiarrheal medications may be prescribed to reduce the discomfort and frequency of bowel movements. If necessary, systemic analgesic agents may also be prescribed. Pain from KS is frequently described as a sharp, throbbing pressure, and heaviness, if lymphedema is present. Pain management may include use of NSAIDs and opioids plus nonpharmacologic approaches such as relaxation techniques. When NSAIDs are administered to patients who are receiving zidovudine, hepatic and hematologic status must be monitored.

The patient with pain related to peripheral neuropathy frequently describes it as burning, numbness, and "pins and needles." Pain management approaches may include opioids, tricyclic antidepressants, and elastic compression stockings to equalize pressure. Tricyclic antidepressants have been found to be helpful in controlling the symptoms of neuropathic pain. They also potentiate the actions of opioids and can be used to relieve pain without increasing the dose of the opioid.

Improving Nutritional Status

Nutritional status is assessed by monitoring weight, dietary intake, and serum albumin, BUN, protein, and transferrin levels. The patient is also assessed for factors that interfere with oral intake, such as anorexia, oral and esophageal candidal infection, nausea, pain, weakness, fatigue, and lactose intolerance (Dudek, 2006). Based on the results of assessment, the nurse can implement specific measures to facilitate oral intake. The dietitian is consulted to determine the patient's nutritional requirements.

Control of nausea and vomiting with antiemetic medications administered on a regular basis may increase the patient's dietary intake. Inadequate food intake resulting from pain caused by oral lesions or a sore throat may be managed by administering prescribed opioids and viscous lidocaine (the patient is instructed to rinse the mouth and swallow). Additionally, the patient is encouraged to eat foods that are easy to swallow and to avoid rough, spicy, or sticky food items and foods that are excessively hot or cold. Oral hygiene before and after meals is encouraged. If fatigue and weakness interfere with intake, the nurse encourages the patient to rest before meals. If the patient is hospitalized, meals should be scheduled so that they do not occur immediately after painful or unpleasant procedures. The patient with diarrhea and abdominal cramping is encouraged to avoid foods that stimulate intestinal motility and abdominal distention, such as fiber-rich foods or lactose, if the patient is intolerant to lactose. The patient is instructed about ways to enhance the nutritional value of meals. Adding eggs, butter, or fortified milk (milk to which powdered skim milk has been added to increase the caloric content) to gravies, soups, or milkshakes can provide additional calories and protein. Supplements such as puddings, powders, milkshakes, and Advera (a nutritional product specifically designed for people with HIV infection or AIDS) may also be useful (Dudek, 2006). Patients who cannot maintain their nutritional status through oral intake may require enteral feedings or parenteral nutrition.

Decreasing the Sense of Isolation

People with AIDS are at risk for double stigmatization. They have what society refers to as a "dreaded disease," and they may have a lifestyle that differs from what is considered acceptable by many people. Many people with AIDS are young adults at a developmental stage that is usually associated with establishing intimate relationships, personal goals and career goals, as well as having and raising children. Their focus changes as they are faced with a disease that threatens their life expectancy with no cure. In addition, they may be forced to reveal hidden lifestyles or behaviors to family, friends, coworkers, and health care providers. As a result, people with HIV infection may be overwhelmed with emotions such as anxiety, guilt, shame, and fear. They also may be faced with multiple losses, such as loss of financial security; normal roles and functions; self-esteem; privacy; ability to control bodily functions; ability to interact meaningfully with the environment; and sexual functioning, as well as rejection by sexual partners, family, and friends. Some patients may harbor feelings of guilt because of their lifestyle or because they may have infected others in current or previous relationships. Other patients may feel anger toward sexual partners who transmitted the virus to them. Infection control measures used in the hospital or at home may further contribute to the patient's emotional isolation. Any or all of these stressors may cause the patient with AIDS to withdraw both physically and emotionally from social contact.

Nurses are in a key position to provide an atmosphere of acceptance and understanding for people with AIDS and their families and partners. The patient's usual level of social interaction is assessed as early as possible to provide a baseline for monitoring changes in behaviors that suggest social isolation (eg, decreased interaction with staff or family, hostility, noncompliance). Patients are encouraged to express feelings of isolation and loneliness, with the assurance that these feelings are not unique or abnormal.

Providing information about how to protect themselves and others may help patients avoid social isolation. Patients, family, and friends must be reassured that AIDS is not spread through casual contact. Education of ancillary personnel, nurses, and physicians will help to reduce factors that might contribute to patients' feelings of isolation. Patient care conferences that address the psychosocial issues associated with AIDS may help sensitize the health care team to patients' needs.

Coping With Grief

The nurse can help the patient verbalize feelings and explore and identify resources for support and mechanisms for coping, especially when the patient is grieving anticipated losses. The patient is encouraged to maintain contact with family, friends, and coworkers and to use local or national AIDS support groups and hotlines. If possible, losses are identified and addressed. The patient is encouraged to continue usual activities whenever possible. Consultations with mental health counselors are useful for many patients.

Monitoring and Managing Potential Complications

OPPORTUNISTIC INFECTIONS

Patients who are immunosuppressed are at risk for opportunistic infections. Therefore, anti-infective agents may be prescribed and laboratory tests obtained to monitor their effect. Signs and symptoms of opportunistic infections, including fever, malaise, difficulty breathing, nausea or vomiting, diarrhea, difficulty swallowing, and any occurrences of swelling or discharge, should be reported.

RESPIRATORY FAILURE

Impaired breathing is a major complication that increases the patient's discomfort and anxiety and may lead to respiratory and cardiac failure. The respiratory rate and pattern are monitored, and the lungs are auscultated for abnormal breath sounds. The patient is instructed to report shortness of breath and increasing difficulty in carrying out usual activities. Pulse rate and rhythm, blood pressure, and oxygen saturation are monitored. Suctioning and oxygen therapy may be prescribed to ensure an adequate airway and to prevent hypoxia. Mechanical ventilation may be necessary for the patient who cannot maintain adequate ventilation as a result of pulmonary infection, fluid and electrolyte imbalance, or respiratory muscle weakness. Arterial blood gas values are used to guide ventilator settings. If the patient is intubated, methods must be established to allow communication with the nurse and others. Attention must be given to assisting the patient receiving mechanical ventilation to cope with the stress associated with intubation and ventilator assistance. The possible need for mechanical ventilation in the future should be discussed early in the course of the disease, when the patient is able to make known his or her preferences about treatment. The use of mechanical ventilation should be consistent with the patient's decisions about end-of-life treatment. (Further discussion of end-of-life care can be found in Chapter 17.)

CACHEXIA AND WASTING

Wasting syndrome and fluid and electrolyte disturbances, including dehydration, are common complications of HIV infection and AIDS. The patient's nutritional and electrolyte status is evaluated by monitoring weight gains or losses, skin turgor, ferritin levels, hemoglobin and hematocrit values, and electrolyte levels. Fluid and electrolyte status is monitored on an ongoing basis; fluid intake and output and urine specific gravity may be monitored daily if the patient is hospitalized with complications. The skin is assessed for dryness and adequate turgor. Vital signs are monitored for decreased systolic blood pressure or increased pulse rate on sitting or standing. Signs and symptoms of electrolyte disturbances, such as muscle cramping, weakness, irregular pulse, decreased mental status, nausea, and vomiting, are documented and reported to the physician. Serum electrolyte values are monitored, and abnormalities are reported.

The nurse helps the patient select foods that will replenish electrolytes, such as oranges and bananas (potassium) and cheese and soups (sodium) (Dudek, 2006). A fluid intake of 3 L or more per day, unless contraindicated, is encouraged to replace fluid lost with diarrhea, and measures to control diarrhea are initiated. If fluid and electrolyte imbalances persist, the nurse administers IV fluids and electrolytes as prescribed. Effects of parenteral therapy are monitored.

SIDE EFFECTS OF MEDICATIONS

Adverse reactions are of concern in patients who receive many medications to treat HIV infection or its complications. Many medications can cause severe toxic effects. Information about the purpose of the medications, their correct administration, side effects, and strategies to manage or prevent side effects is provided. Patients and their caregivers need to know which signs and symptoms of side effects should be reported immediately to their primary health care provider (see Table 52-3).

In addition to medications used to treat HIV infection, other medications that may be required include opioids, tricyclic antidepressants, and NSAIDs for pain relief; medications for treatment of opportunistic infections; antihistamines (diphenhydramine) for relief of pruritus; acetaminophen or aspirin for management of fever; and antiemetic agents for control of nausea and vomiting. Concurrent use of these medications can cause many drug interactions, resulting in hepatic and hematologic abnormalities. Therefore, careful monitoring of laboratory test results is essential.

During each contact with the patient, it is important for the nurse to ask not only about side effects but also about how well the patient is managing the medication regimen. The nurse may be able to assist the patient in organizing and planning the medication schedule to promote adherence to the medication regimen.

Promoting Home and Community-Based Care

TEACHING PATIENTS SELF-CARE

Patients, families, and friends are instructed about the routes of transmission of HIV. As discussed earlier, the nurse discusses precautions the patient can use to avoid transmitting HIV sexually (see Charts 52-2 and 52-3) or through sharing of blood. Patients and their families or caregivers must receive instructions about how to prevent disease transmission, including handwashing techniques and methods for safely handling and disposing of items soiled with body fluids. Clear guidelines about avoiding and controlling infection, regular health care appointments, symptom management, nutrition, rest, and exercise are necessary. The importance of personal and environmental hygiene is emphasized. Caregivers are taught many of the guidelines (Standard Precautions) described in Chart 52-4. Kitchen and bathroom surfaces should be cleaned regularly with disinfectants to prevent growth of fungi and bacteria. Patients with pets are encouraged to have another person clean areas soiled by animals, such as bird cages and litter boxes. If this is not possible, patients should use gloves and should wash their hands after they clean the area. Patients are advised to avoid exposure to others who are sick or who have been recently vaccinated. The importance of avoiding smoking, excessive alcohol, and over-the-counter and street drugs is emphasized. Patients who are HIV positive or who inject drugs are instructed not to donate blood. IV/injection drug users who are unwilling to stop using drugs are advised to avoid sharing drug equipment with others.

Caregivers in the home are taught how to administer medications, including IV preparations. The medication regimens used for patients with HIV infection and AIDS are often complex and expensive. Patients receiving combination therapies for treatment of HIV infection and its complications require careful teaching about the importance of taking medications as prescribed and explanations and assistance in fitting the medication regimen into their lives (see Chart 52-7). If the patient requires enteral or parenteral nutrition, instruction is provided to the patient and family about how to administer nutritional therapies at home. Home care nurses provide ongoing teaching and support for the patient and family.

CONTINUING CARE

Many people with AIDS remain in their community and continue their usual daily activities, whereas others can no longer work or maintain their independence. Families or caregivers may need assistance in providing supportive care. There are many community-based organizations that provide a variety of services for people living with HIV infection and AIDS; nurses can help identify these services.

Community health nurses, home care nurses, and hospice nurses are in an excellent position to provide the support and guidance so often needed in the home setting. As hospital costs continue to rise and insurance coverage continues to decline, the complexity of home care increases. Home care nurses are key to the safe and effective administration of parenteral antibiotics, chemotherapy, and nutrition in the home.

During home visits, the nurse assesses the patient's physical and emotional status and home environment. The patient's adherence to the therapeutic regimen is assessed, and strategies are suggested to assist with adherence. The patient is assessed for progression of disease and for adverse side effects of medications. Previous teaching is reinforced, and the importance of keeping follow-up appointments is stressed.

Complex wound care or respiratory care may be required in the home. Patients and families are often unable to meet these skilled care needs without assistance. Nurses may refer patients to community programs that offer a range of services for patients, friends, and families, including help with housekeeping, hygiene, and meals; transportation and shopping; individual and group therapy; support for caregivers; telephone networks for the homebound; and legal and financial assistance. These services are typically provided by both professionals and nonprofessional volunteers. A social worker may be consulted to identify sources of financial support, if needed.

Home care and hospice nurses are increasingly called on to provide physical and emotional support to patients and families as patients with AIDS enter the terminal stages of disease. This support takes on special meaning when people with AIDS lose friends and when family members fear the disease or feel anger concerning the patient's lifestyle. The nurse encourages the patient and family to discuss end-of-life decisions and to ensure that care is consistent with those decisions, all comfort measures are employed, and the patient is treated with dignity at all times.

Evaluation

Expected Patient Outcomes

Expected patient outcomes may include:

1. Maintains skin integrity
2. Resumes usual bowel habits
3. Experiences no infections
4. Maintains adequate level of activity tolerance
5. Maintains usual level of thought processes
6. Maintains effective airway clearance
7. Experiences increased sense of comfort and less pain
8. Maintains adequate nutritional status

9. Experiences decreased sense of social isolation
10. Progresses through grieving process
11. Reports increased understanding of AIDS and participates in self-care activities as possible
12. Remains free of complications

Detailed outcomes are included in the plan of nursing care for a patient with AIDS (see Chart 52-9).

Emotional and Ethical Concerns

Nurses in all settings are called on to provide care for patients with HIV infection. In doing so, they encounter not only the physical challenges of this epidemic but also emotional and ethical concerns. The concerns raised by health care professionals involve issues such as fear of infection, responsibility for giving care, values clarification, confidentiality, developmental stages of patients and caregivers, and poor prognostic outcomes.

Many patients with HIV infection have engaged in "stigmatized" behaviors. Because these behaviors challenge some traditional religious and moral values, nurses may feel reluctant to care for these patients. In addition, health care providers may still have fear and anxiety about disease transmission despite education concerning infection control and the low incidence of transmission to health care providers (see Chart 52-5). Nurses are encouraged to examine their personal beliefs and to use the process of values clarification to approach controversial issues. The American Nurses Association's Code for Nurses can also be used to help resolve ethical dilemmas that might affect the quality of care given to patients with HIV infection and AIDS.

Nurses are responsible for protecting the patient's right to privacy by safeguarding confidential information. Inadvertent disclosure of confidential patient information may result in personal, financial, and emotional hardships for the patient. The controversy surrounding confidentiality concerns the circumstances in which information may be disclosed to others. Health care team members need accurate patient information to conduct assessment, planning, implementation, and evaluation of patient care. Failure to disclose HIV status could compromise the quality of patient care. Sexual partners of HIV-infected patients should know about the potential for infection and the need to engage in safer sex practices, as well as the possible need for testing and health care. Nurses are advised to discuss concerns about confidentiality with nurse administrators and to consult professional nursing organizations such as the Association of Nurses in AIDS Care and legal experts in their state to identify the most appropriate course of action. Chart 52-10 explores issues related to revealing one's HIV status.

CHART 52-10

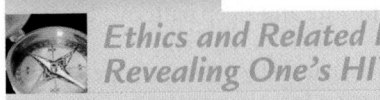

Ethics and Related Issues: Revealing One's HIV Status

Should All People Who Are Infected With HIV Be Required to Reveal This Status to All Their Sexual and Drug-Sharing Contacts?

SITUATION

The human immunodeficiency virus (HIV) causes HIV infection, which progresses to AIDS, a disease that is currently incurable and ultimately fatal. Many HIV-positive people are aware that they carry the virus but refuse to share this information with others, especially their sexual partners or IV/injection drug contacts. Because sexual contacts and needle-sharing partners are at risk for developing the disease, would a policy that requires notification of contacts infringe on the liberty and privacy of the known HIV-infected person?

DILEMMA

The person's right to privacy conflicts with notifying all people who are contacts either through sexual or needle-sharing behavior (autonomy versus justice). The person's right to privacy conflicts with society's need to contain the deadly virus and stem a deadly epidemic (autonomy versus justice).

DISCUSSION

1. What arguments would you offer in favor of notifying all the person's contacts?
2. What arguments would you offer against notifying all or some of the person's contacts?
3. Each state has various laws that pertain to whether contacts can be notified and who is responsible for notifying contacts. Is there a law for contact notification in the state in which you live? If there is such a law in your state, who is responsible for contact notification?
4. What would you do if the person responsible for contact notification refuses to do so based on his own beliefs for confidentiality of HIV infection status?
5. How would you respond if the HIV-positive person said that he or she is afraid to notify his or her contact because of fear of a violent response?

AIDS has had a high mortality rate, but advances in antiretroviral and multidrug therapy have demonstrated promise in slowing or controlling disease progression. It is not known whether current treatment regimens will remain effective, because viral drug resistance has developed with most previous medications. Most nurses in the United States have never faced an epidemic in which many young and middle-aged adults experience serious illness and may die during the usual course of the disease process. Nurses may struggle with the value and meaning of their professional roles as they witness repeated instances of deterioration. Exposure to so many deaths among patients at the same developmental stage as many nurses can create feelings of stress. Contributing to this stress are personal fears of contagion or disapproval of the patient's lifestyle and behaviors. Unlike cancer or other diseases, AIDS is associated with controversies challenging our legal and political systems as well as religious and personal beliefs.

Nurses who feel stressed and overburdened may experience physical and mental distress in the form of fatigue, headache, changes in appetite and sleep patterns, helplessness, irritability, apathy, negativity, and anger.

Many strategies have been used by nurses to cope with the stress associated with caring for AIDS patients. Education and provision of up-to-date information help to alleviate apprehension and prepare nurses to deliver safe, high-quality patient care. Interdisciplinary meetings allow participants to support one another and provide comprehensive patient care. Staff support groups give nurses an opportunity to solve problems and explore values and feelings about caring for AIDS patients and their families; they also provide a forum for grieving. Other sources of support include nursing administrators, peers, and spiritual advisors.

Critical Thinking Exercises

1 A 43-year-old man who has been using IV/injection drugs for 20 years says that he is not going to stop his use of drugs but wants to reduce his risk for HIV infection. What would you teach him? What types of community agencies could provide resources to this patient?

2 During a code response in the intensive care unit, a nursing student was inadvertently stuck with a needle used on a homeless patient who has AIDS. The student states that he is not concerned about contracting any diseases as a result. As his clinical instructor or the nurse manager of the ICU, what actions should you take? What reporting and documentation are needed? What testing, treatment, and counseling are indicated for the student?

3 ebp During a home visit to a family in which two adolescents are HIV positive, you are instructing the adolescents, their siblings, and their parents about strategies to protect the adolescents from other infections and to protect other family members from HIV transmission. What is the evidence for strategies that you plan to discuss with the adolescents and their family members? What is the strength of that evidence, and what criteria would you use to evaluate the strength of the evidence?

4 A 48-year-old man presents to the emergency department intoxicated and combative. He is bleeding from several stab wounds. An OraQuick Rapid HIV-1 Antibody Test is performed because of the likely exposure to health care personnel to body fluids. What are the implications of a positive OraQuick Rapid HIV-1 Antibody Test? How would care in the emergency department be modified because of a positive test result? What are the legal ramifications of obtaining this test if the patient's ability to consent to testing is questioned?

5 You are making a home visit to a patient with AIDS who is exhibiting early signs of dementia and encephalopathy. Describe the aspects of the home environment that you would assess to ensure safety and adequate care. How would you modify your assessment if the patient lived alone in a third-floor apartment without an elevator? If the patient lived in a rural setting? If the patient had a physical disability that limited his ability to leave his apartment?

REFERENCES AND SELECTED READINGS

BOOKS

Agins, B. (2003). *HIV prophylaxis following occupational exposure.* New York: AIDS Institute, New York State Department of Health.

Allende, M. & Lane, H. C. (2004). Immune-based therapies for HIV infection. In Wormser, G. (Ed.). *AIDS and other manifestations of HIV infection.* San Diego: Elsevier Academic Press.

Chesney, M. (2004). Review: Adherence to HAART regimens. In Laurence, J. (Ed.). *Medication adherence in HIV/AIDS.* Larchmont, NY: Mary Ann Liebert.

Chiarello, L., Panlilio, A., & Cardo, D. (2004). Infection control considerations to prevent HIV transmission in healthcare settings. In Wormser, G. (Ed). *AIDS and other manifestations of HIV infection.* San Diego: Elsevier Academic Press.

Daar, E., Gallant, J., Markowitz, M., et al. (2004). *Consensus Development Panel for the Resistance Testing clinical guide.* New York: World Health, CME.

Department of Health and Human Services Panel (DHHS Panel) on Antiretroviral Guidelines for Adults and Adolescents—A Working Group of the Office of AIDS Research Advisory Council. (2006). *Guidelines for the use of antiretroviral agents in HIV-1-infected adults and adolescents, May 4, 2006.* Available at http://AIDSinfor.nih.gov. Accessed July 28, 2006.

Dudek, S. G. (2006). *Nutrition essentials for nursing practice* (5th ed.). Philadelphia: Lippincott Williams & Wilkins.

Ferrigno, L. & DeHovitz, J. (2004). HIV disease in women. In Wormser, G. (Ed.). *AIDS and other manifestations of HIV infection.* San Diego: Elsevier Academic Press.

Goff, S. (2004). Introduction to retroviruses. In Wormser, G. (Ed.). *AIDS and other manifestations of HIV infection.* San Diego: Elsevier Academic Press.

Goodroad, B. (2003). Managing antiretroviral therapy. In Kirton, C. (Ed.). *ANAC's core curriculum for HIV/AIDS nursing.* Thousand Oaks, CA: Sage Publishers.

Heckman, T., Kochman, A. & Sikkema, K. (2004). Depressive symptoms in older adults living with HIV disease: Application of the Chronic Illness Quality of Life model. In Emlet, C. (Ed.). *HIV/AIDS and older adults: Challenges for individuals, families, and communities.* New York: Springer.

*Holzemer, W., Corless, I., Nokes, K., et al. (2004). Predictors of self-reported adherence in persons living with HIV disease. In Laurence, J. (Ed.). *Medication adherence in HIV/AIDS.* Larchmont, NY: Mary Ann Liebert.

Horowitz, H. & Wormser, G. (2004). Care of the adult patient with HIV infection. In Wormser, G. (Ed.). *AIDS and other manifestations of HIV infection.* San Diego: Elsevier Academic Press.

Hu, D., Pieniazek, D., & Mastro, T. (2004). The genetic diversity and global molecular epidemiology of HIV. In Wormser, G. (Ed.). *AIDS and other manifestations of HIV infection.* San Diego: Elsevier Academic Press.

Kaslow, R., Tang, J. & Dorak, T. (2004). The role of host genetic variation in HIV infection and its manifestations. In Wormser, G. (Ed.). *AIDS and other manifestations of HIV infection.* San Diego: Elsevier Academic Press.

Kirton, C. (2003). *ANAC's core curriculum for HIV/AIDS nursing.* Thousand Oaks, CA: Sage Publishers.

Orlando, D. (2003). Anemia. In Kirton, C. (Ed.). *ANAC's core curriculum for HIV/AIDS nursing*. Thousand Oaks, CA: Sage Publishers.

Orlando, D. (2003). Diarrhea, recurrent or chronic. In Kirton, C. (Ed.). *ANAC's core curriculum for HIV/AIDS nursing*. Thousand Oaks, CA: Sage Publishers.

Porth, C. (2005). *Pathophysiology: Concepts of altered health states* (7th ed.). Philadelphia: Lippincott Williams & Wilkins.

Sanchez, M. & Friedman-Kien, A. (2004). Skin manifestations of HIV infection. In Wormser, G. (Ed.). *AIDS and other manifestations of HIV infection*. San Diego: Elsevier Academic Press.

Sedaghat, A. & Siliciano, R. (2004). Immunodeficiency in HIV-1 infection. In Wormser, G. (Ed.). *AIDS and other manifestations of HIV infection*. San Diego: Elsevier Academic Press.

Taliaferro, D. & Williams, G. (2003). Substance users. In Kirton, C. (Ed). *ANAC's core curriculum for HIV/AIDS nursing*. Thousand Oaks, CA: Sage Publishers.

JOURNALS

**Asterisks indicate nursing research articles.*

American Red Cross. (2001). This month's HIV/AIDS facts. Available at: http://www.redcross.org. Accessed June 2, 2006.

*Bakken, S., Holzemer, W., Brown, M. A., et al. (2000). Relationships between perception of engagement with health care provider and demographic characteristics, health status, and adherence to therapeutic regimen in persons with HIV/AIDS. *AIDS Patient Care and STDs, 14*(4), 189–197.

Benson, C., Kaplan, J., Masur, H., et al. (2004). Treating opportunistic infections among HIV infected adults and adolescents. *MMWR, 53*(RR-15), 1–112. Available at: http://www.cdc.gov/mmwr/preview/mmwrhtml/rr5315a1.htm. Accessed June 2, 2006.

Capili, B. & Annastasi, J. K. (2006). HIV and hyperlipidemia: Current recommendations and treatment. *MedSurg Nursing, 15*(1), 14–19, 35.

Centers for Disease Control and Prevention. (2002). Guideline for hand hygiene in healthcare settings. *MMWR CDC Recommendations and Reports, 51*(RR-16), 1–45.

Centers for Disease Control and Prevention. (2003). How safe is the blood supply in the United States? December 15. Available at: http://www.cdc.gov/hiv/pubs/faq/faq15.htm. Accessed June 2, 2006.

Centers for Disease Control and Prevention. (2005). *HIV/AIDS Surveillance Report, 2003, 15*(1), 1–46. Atlanta: Author. Available at: http://www.cdc.gov/hiv/topics/surveillance/resources/reports/2003report/default.htm. Accessed June 2, 2006.

Centers for Disease Control and Prevention. (2005). Cases of HIV infection and AIDS in the United States, 2004. *HIV/AIDS Surveillance Report, 2004, 16*(1), 1–46. Available at http://www.cdc.gov/hiv/stats/hasrlink.htm. Accessed July 28, 2006.

Centers for Disease Control and Prevention. (2005). AIDS cases by state and metropolitan area provided for the Ryan White CARE Act, June 2005. *HIV/AIDS Surveillance Supplemental Report, 22*(1), 1–9. Available at http://www.cdc.gov/hiv/stats/hasrlink.htm. Accessed July 28, 2006.

Centers for Disease Control and Prevention. (2006). Rapid HIV test distribution—United States, 2003–2005. *MMWR, Morbidity and Mortality Weekly Report, 55*(24), 673–676.

Centers for Disease Control and Prevention. (2006). Reported CD4+ T-lymphocyte results for adults and adolescents with HIV/AIDS—33 states. *HIV/AIDS Surveillance Report, Supplemental Report, 11*(2), 1–31. Atlanta: Author. Available at http://www.cdc.gov/hiv/stats/hasrlink.htm. Accessed July 28, 2006.

Centers for Disease Control and Prevention, U.S. Department of Health and Human Services. (1992). 1993 revised classification system for HIV infection and expanded surveillance case definition for AIDS among adolescents and adults. *MMWR CDC Recommendations and Reports, 41*(RR-17), 1–19.

*Chou, F., Holzemer, W., Portillo, C., et al. (2004). Self-care strategies and sources of information for HIV/AIDS symptom management. *Nursing Research, 53*(5), 332–339.

Coyne, P. J., Lyne, M. E. & Watson, A. C. (2002). Symptom management in people with AIDS. *American Journal of Nursing, 102*(9), 48–56.

Daughtry, L., Bankston, J., & Deshotels, J. (2002). HIV meds: Keeping trouble at bay. *RN, 65*(2), 31–35.

FDA News. (2004). FDA Approves Sculptra for HIV patients. August 3. Available at: http://www.fda.gov/bbs/topics/news/2004/NEW01100.html. Accessed June 2, 2006.

Hammer, S. M. (2005). Management of newly diagnosed HIV infection. *New England Journal of Medicine, 353*(16), 1702–1710.

Hemmila, D. (2004). The wait is over: New rapid-results tests for HIV could encourage more patients to be screened and help halt the spread of the virus. August 25. Available at: http://www.NurseWeek.com/news/Features/04-08/HIVRapidResultsTest.asp. Accessed June 2, 2006.

*Holzemer, W., Henry, S., Nokes, K., et al. (1999). Validation of the Sign and Symptom Checklist for Persons with HIV Disease. *Journal of Advanced Nursing, 30*(5), 1041–1049.

*Holzemer, W., Hudson, A., Kirksey, K., et al. (2001). The Revised Sign and Symptom Check-List for HIV (SSC-HIVrev). *Journal of the Association of Nurses in AIDS Care, 12*(5), 60–70.

Huang, L., Quartin, A., Jones, D., et al. (2006). Intensive care of patients with HIV infection. *New England Journal of Medicine, 355*(2), 173–181.

*Kirksey, K., Goodroad, B., Kemppainen, J., et al. (2002). Complementary therapy use in persons with HIV/AIDS. *Journal of Holistic Nursing, 20*(3), 264–278.

Merson, M. H. (2006). The HIV-AIDS pandemic at 25: The global response. *New England Journal of Medicine, 354*(23), 2414–2417.

Nieuwkerk, P. & Oort, F. (2005). Self-reported adherence to antiretroviral therapy for HIV infection and virologic treatment response: A meta-analysis. *Journal of Acquired Immune Deficiency Syndrome, 38*(4), 445–448.

*Nokes, K. & Bakken, S. (2002). Issues associated with measuring symptoms status: HIV/AIDS case illustration. *Journal of the New York State Nurses Association, 33*(2), 17–21.

*Nokes, K., Wheeler, K. & Kendrew, J. (1994). Development of an HIV assessment tool. *Image: Journal of Nursing Scholarship, 26*(2), 133–138.

Norris, A. & Dreher, H. M. (2004). Lipodystrophy syndrome: The morphologic and metabolic effects of antiretroviral therapy in HIV infection. *Journal of the Association of Nurses in AIDS Care, 15*(6), 46–64.

*Ramirez-Marrero, F., Smith, B., Melendez-Brau, N., et al. (2004). Physical and leisure activity, body composition, and life satisfaction in HIV-positive Hispanics in Puerto Rico. *Journal of the Association of Nurses in AIDS Care, 15*(4), 68–77.

Reynolds, N. (2004). Adherence to antiretroviral therapies: State of the science. *Current HIV Research, 2*(3), 207–214.

Riley, L. E. & Yawetz, S. (2005). Case 32-2005: A 34-year-old HIV-positive woman who desired to become pregnant. *New England Journal of Medicine, 353*(16), 1725–1732.

Shippy, A. & Karpiak, S. (2005). Perceptions of support among older adults with HIV. *Research on Aging, 27*(3), 290–306.

Stephenson, J. (1998). Studies reveal early impact of HIV infection, effects of treatment. *Journal of American Medical Association, 279*(9), 641–642.

Sullivan, P. & Dworkin, M. (2003). Prevalence and correlates of fatigue among persons with HIV infection. *Journal of Pain and Symptom Management, 25*(4), 329–333.

UNAIDS. (2006). *2006 report on the global AIDS epidemic: A UNAIDS 10th anniversary special edition. Executive summary*. Geneva: World Health Organization.

Universal Precautions: Biological Safety. Available at: http://www.niehs.nih.gov/odhsb/biosafe/univers.htm. Accessed June 2, 2006.

U.S. Food and Drug Administration. (2002). FDA approves new rapid HIV test kit. [News release]. Available at: http://www.fda.gov/bbs/topics/NEWS/2002/NEW00852.html. Accessed June 2, 2006.

U.S. Food and Drug Administration. (2006). FDA approves the first once-a-day three-drug combination tablet for treatment of HIV-1. Available at http://www.fda.gov/bbs/topics/NEWS/2006/NEW01408.html. Accessed July 31, 2006.

*Wesley, Y. (2003). Desire for children among Black women with and without HIV infection. *Journal of Nursing Scholarship, 35*(1), 37–43.

World Health Organization. (2005). HIV/AIDS facts and figures. Available at: http://w3.whosea.org/EN/Section10/Section18/Section348.htm. Accessed June 2, 2006.

Worthington, K. (2001). You've been stuck: What do you do? *American Journal of Nursing, 101*(3), 104.

RESOURCES

AIDS Action Council, 875 Connecticut NW, Suite 700, Washington, DC 20003; 202-986-1300; fax 202-986-1345; http://www.aidsaction.org. Accessed June 2, 2006.

AIDS Community Research Initiative of America, 230 W. 38th St., 17th floor, New York, NY 10018; 212-924-3934; fax 212-924-3936; http://www.acria.org/acria.html. Accessed June 2, 2006.

AIDS Education and Training Centers (ETCs) Program, 5600 Fishers Lane, Room 9A-39, Rockville, MD 20857; 301-443-6364; fax 301-433-9887.

AIDS Information Service, 800-448-0440 (Spanish available); fax 800-519-3739; e-mail: ContactUs@aidsinfo.nih/gov.

All About Blood; http://www.aabb.org/Content/About_Blood/. Accessed June 2, 2006.

American Red Cross; http://www.redcross.org. Accessed June 2, 2006.

Antiretroviral medication information Web sites: http://www.AIDSmeds.com; http://www.projectinform.org; http://www.sfaf.org; http://www.HIVInSite.com; http://www.amfAR.org; http://www.natap.org; http://www.thebody.com (many of these sites are coordinated by persons living with HIV/AIDS). Accessed June 2, 2006.

Centers for Disease Control and Prevention, 1600 Clifton Rd., Atlanta, GA 30333; 404-639-3311; AIDS hotline: 800-342-2437; Spanish: 800-344-7432; http://www.cdc.gov. Accessed June 2, 2006.

Gay Men's Health Crisis Network, 119 W. 24th St., New York, NY 10011; 800-AIDS-NYC, 800-243-7692; http://www.gmhc.org. Accessed June 2, 2006.

Hemophilia and AIDS/HIV Network for the Dissemination of Information, The National Hemophilia Foundation, 116 W. 32nd St., 11th Floor, New York, NY 10001; 212-328-3700; 800-42-HANDI; fax 212-328-3777; http://www.hemophilia.org. Accessed June 2, 2006.

HRSA National Clinician's Post-exposure Prophylaxis hotline (health care providers only): 888-HIV-4911.

HRSA National HIV Telephone Consultation Service: 800-933-3413.

Living with HIV/AIDS; http://www.cdc.gov/hiv/pubs/brochure/livingwithhiv.htm. Accessed June 2, 2006.

National Association of People With AIDS, 1413 K Street, NW, 7th Floor, Washington, DC 20005; 202-898-0414; fax 202-898-0435; http://www.napwa. org. Accessed June 2, 2006.

National Pediatric and Family HIV Resource Center, University of Medicine and Dentistry, 30 Bergen St., ADMC #4, Newark, NJ 07103; 973-972-0410; http://www.womenchildrenhiv.org. Accessed June 2, 2006.

Office of Minority Health Resource Center, P.O. Box 37337, Washington, DC 20013; 800-444-6472; TDD: 301-230-7199; public inquiries: 404-639-3534; 800-311-3435; http://www.omhrc.gov. Accessed June 2, 2006.

National Pediatric HIV Resource Center; 800-362-0071.

Pharmaceutical Research and Manufacturers of America, 1100 Fifteenth St., NW, Washington, DC 20005; 202-835-3400; http://www.phrma.org. Accessed June 2, 2006.

Treatment Information Service: Glossary of HIV/AIDS-related terms (2002); 800-448-0440.

CHAPTER 53

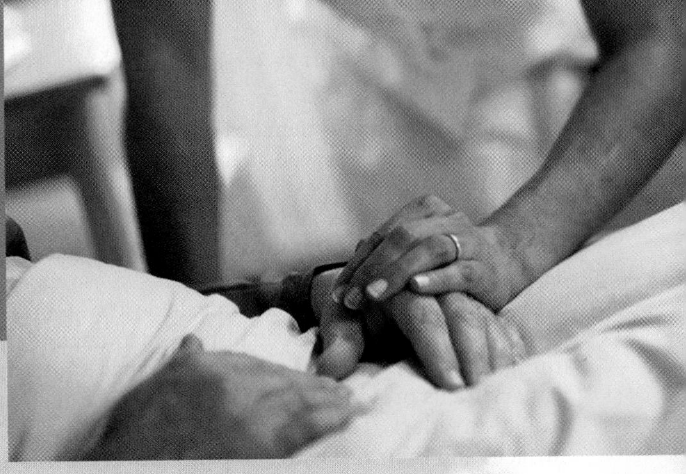

Assessment and Management of Patients With Allergic Disorders

Learning Objectives

On completion of this chapter, the learner will be able to:

1. Explain the physiologic events involved with allergic reactions.
2. Describe the types of hypersensitivity.
3. Describe the management of patients with allergic disorders.
4. Describe measures to prevent and manage anaphylaxis.
5. Use the nursing process as a framework for care of the patient with allergic rhinitis.
6. Discuss the different allergic disorders according to type.

The human body is menaced by a host of potential invaders—allergens as well as microbial organisms—that constantly threaten its defenses. After penetrating those defenses, these allergens and organisms, if allowed to continue unimpeded, disrupt the body's enzyme systems and destroy its vital tissues. To protect against these agents, the body is equipped with an elaborate defense system.

The epithelial cells that coat the skin and make up the lining of the respiratory, gastrointestinal, and genitourinary tracts provide the first line of defense against microbial invaders. The structure and continuity of these surfaces and their resistance to penetration are initial deterrents to invaders.

One of the most effective defense mechanisms is the body's capacity to equip itself rapidly with weapons (antibodies) individually designed to meet each new invader, namely specific protein antigens. Antibodies react with antigens in a variety of ways: (1) by coating the antigens' surfaces if they are particular substances, (2) by neutralizing the antigens if they are toxins, and (3) by precipitating the antigens out of solution if they are dissolved.

The antibodies prepare the antigens so that the phagocytic cells of the blood and the tissues can dispose of them. However, although this system is normally protective, in some cases the body produces inappropriate or exaggerated responses to specific antigens, and the result is an allergic or hypersensitivity disorder.

Allergic Reaction: Physiologic Overview

An allergic reaction is a manifestation of tissue injury resulting from interaction between an antigen and an antibody. **Allergy** is an inappropriate and often harmful response of the immune system to normally harmless substances. In this case, the substance is termed an **allergen.** Allergy is a hypersensitive reaction to a specific allergen that is initiated by immunological mechanisms and is usually mediated by immunoglobulin E (IgE) antibodies, which are produced in response to the allergen. **Atopy** refers to allergic reactions that are characterized by the action of IgE antibodies and a genetic predisposition to allergic reactions. It refers to a predisposition to produce IgE antibodies in response to low-dose allergens and consequently to develop typical symptoms such as rhinitis, asthma, wheezing, or eczema. Atopy is diagnosed through personal and family history and is confirmed by the presence of high levels of allergen-specific IgE in serum or by positive skin prick tests (Holgate & Lack, 2005).

When the body encounters an **antigen,** usually a protein that the body's defenses recognize as foreign, a series of events occurs in an attempt to render the invader harmless, destroy it, and remove it from the body. When lymphocytes respond to the antigen, **antibodies** (protein substances that

Glossary

allergen: substance that causes manifestations of allergy

allergy: inappropriate and often harmful immune system response to substances that are normally harmless

anaphylaxis: clinical response to an immediate immunologic reaction between a specific antigen and antibody

angioneurotic edema: condition characterized by urticaria and diffuse swelling of the deeper layers of the skin

antibody: protein substance developed by the body in response to and interacting with a specific antigen

antigen: substance that induces the production of antibodies

antihistamine: medication that opposes the action of histamine

atopic dermatitis: type I hypersensitivity involving inflammation of the skin evidenced by itching, redness, and a variety of skin lesions

atopy: term often used to describe immunoglobulin E-mediated diseases (ie, atopic dermatitis, asthma, and allergic rhinitis) with a genetic component

B lymphocyte: cells that are important in producing circulating antibodies

bradykinin: polypeptide that stimulates nerve fibers and causes pain

eosinophil: granular leukocyte

epitope: an immunologically active site on an antigen; a single antigen can have several different epitopes that elicit responses from different antibodies

erythema: diffuse redness of the skin

hapten: incomplete antigen

histamine: substance in the body that causes increased gastric secretion, dilation of capillaries, and constriction of the bronchial smooth muscle

hypersensitivity: abnormal heightened reaction to a stimulus of any kind

immunoglobulins: a family of closely related proteins capable of acting as antibodies

leukotrienes: a group of chemical mediators that initiate the inflammatory response

lymphokines: substances released by sensitized lymphocytes when they contact specific antigens

mast cells: connective tissue cells that contain heparin and histamine in their granules

prostaglandins: unsaturated fatty acids that have a wide assortment of biologic activity

rhinitis: inflammation of the nasal mucosa

serotonin: chemical mediator that acts as a potent vasoconstrictor and bronchoconstrictor

T lymphocytes: cells that can cause graft rejection, kill foreign cells, or suppress production of antibodies

urticaria: hives

protect against antigens) are produced. Common allergic reactions occur when the immune system of a susceptible person responds aggressively to a substance that is normally harmless (eg, dust, weeds, pollen, dander). Chemical mediators released in allergic reactions may produce symptoms ranging from mild to life-threatening.

The many cells and organs of the immune system secrete various substances that are important in the immune response. These parts of the immune system must work together to ensure adequate defense against antigens without destroying the body's own tissues through an overly aggressive reaction.

Function of Immunoglobulins

Antibodies that are formed by lymphocytes and plasma cells in response to an immunogenic stimulus constitute a group of serum proteins called **immunoglobulins.** Grouped into five classes (IgE, IgD, IgG, IgM, and IgA), antibodies can be found in the lymph nodes, tonsils, appendix, and Peyer's patches of the intestinal tract or circulating in the blood and lymph. Each antibody molecule is composed of two identical heavy (H) chains and two identical light (L) chains. Each chain contains one variable region and one or more constant regions. The constant regions determine the class (eg, IgE, IgD) of each antibody and allow each class of antibody to interact with specific effector cells and molecules. The variable regions contain antigen-binding sites (Porth, 2005). Antibodies are capable of binding with a wide variety of antigens, which include macromolecules and small chemicals (Abbas & Lichtman, 2004). Antibodies of the IgM, IgG, and IgA classes have definite and well-established protective functions. These include neutralization of toxins and viruses and precipitation, agglutination, and lysis of bacteria and other foreign cellular material. (See Chapter 50 for further discussion of these functions.)

Immunoglobulins of the IgE class are involved in allergic disorders and some parasitic infections, evidenced by elevation of IgE concentrations. IgE-producing cells are located in the respiratory and intestinal mucosa. Two or more IgE molecules bind together to an allergen and trigger **mast cells** or basophils to release chemical mediators, such as histamine, serotonin, kinins, slow-reacting substance of anaphylaxis (SRS-A), and the neutrophil factor, which produces allergic skin reactions, asthma, and hay fever.

Antibodies combine with antigens in a special way, likened to keys fitting into a lock. Antigens (the keys) fit only certain antibodies (the locks). Hence, the term "specificity" refers to the specific reaction of an antibody to an antigen. There are many variations and complexities in these patterns. The strength with which one antigen-binding surface of an antibody binds to one **epitope**, an immunologically active site on an antigen, is known as the affinity of the interaction (Abbas & Lichtman, 2004).

Antibody molecules are bivalent; that is, they have two combining sites. Therefore, the antibody easily becomes a cross-link between two antigen groups, causing them to clump together (agglutination). By this action, foreign invaders are cleared from the bloodstream. Agglutination is the means for determining blood group in laboratory tests.

Role of B Cells

B cells, or **B lymphocytes**, are programmed to produce one specific antibody. On encountering a specific antigen, B cells stimulate production of plasma cells, the site of antibody production. The result is the outpouring of antibodies for the purpose of destroying and removing the antigen.

Role of T Cells

T cells, or **T lymphocytes**, assist the B cells in producing antibodies. T cells secrete substances known as **lymphokines** that encourage cell growth, promote cell activation, direct the flow of cell activity, destroy target cells, and stimulate the macrophages. Macrophages present the antigen to the T cells and initiate the immune response. They also digest antigens and assist in removing cells and other debris. The antigen-binding site of a T cell has a structure much like that of an immunoglobulin. It recognizes epitopes through complementary interactions. Unlike a specific antibody, a T cell does not bind free antigens.

Function of Antigens

Antigens are divided into two groups: complete protein antigens and low-molecular-weight substances. Complete protein antigens, such as animal dander, pollen, and horse serum, stimulate a complete humoral response. (See Chapter 50 for a discussion of humoral immunity.) Low-molecular-weight substances, such as medications, function as **haptens** (incomplete antigens), binding to tissue or serum proteins to produce a carrier complex that initiates an antibody response. The term "hapten" is derived from the Greek word *haptien* ("to fasten"). The proteins or other immunogens that haptens are fastened to are known as carriers.

In an allergic reaction, the production of antigen-specific IgE antibodies requires active communication between macrophages, T cells, and B cells. When the allergen is absorbed through the respiratory tract, gastrointestinal tract, or skin, allergen sensitization occurs. The macrophage processes the antigen and presents it to the appropriate T cell. B cells that are influenced by the T cell mature into allergen-specific IgE-secreting plasma cells that synthesize and secrete antigen-specific IgE antibody.

Function of Chemical Mediators

Mast cells, which play a major role in IgE-mediated immediate hypersensitivity, are located in the skin and mucous membranes. When mast cells are stimulated by antigens, powerful chemical mediators are released that cause a sequence of physiologic events resulting in symptoms of immediate hypersensitivity (Fig. 53-1). There are two types of chemical mediators: primary and secondary. Primary mediators are preformed and are found in mast cells or basophils. Secondary mediators are inactive precursors that are formed or released in response to primary mediators. The most prevalent known primary and secondary mediators are described in the following sections. Table 53-1 summarizes the actions of primary and secondary chemical mediators.

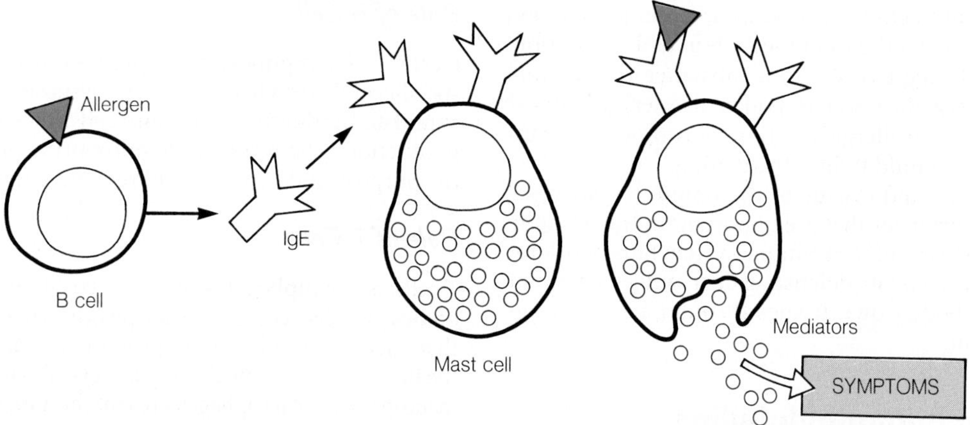

FIGURE 53-1. Allergen triggers B cell to make IgE antibody, which attaches to mast cell. When that allergen reappears, it binds to the IgE and triggers the mast cell to release its chemicals. Courtesy of U.S. Dept. of Health and Human Services, National Institutes of Health.

Primary Mediators

IgE-mediated inflammation occurs when an antigen binds to the IgE antibodies that occupy certain receptors on mast cells. Within minutes, this binding causes the mast cell to degranulate, releasing certain preformed mediators. A two-phase response results. There is an initial immediate effect on blood vessels, smooth muscles, and glandular secretions. This is followed a few hours later by cellular infiltration of the involved site. This type of response is commonly known as an immediate hypersensitivity response.

HISTAMINE

Histamine plays an important role in the immune response. Histamine is released from mast cell granules where it is stored. Maximal intensity is reached within about 15 minutes after antigen contact. The effects of histamine release include erythema; localized edema in the form of wheals; pruritus; contraction of bronchial smooth muscle, resulting in wheezing and bronchospasm; dilation of small venules and constriction of larger vessels; and increased secretion of gastric and mucosal cells, resulting in diarrhea. Histamine action results from stimulation of histamine 1 (H_1)

TABLE 53-1 Chemical Mediators of Hypersensitivity

Mediators	Action
Primary Mediators	
Preformed and found in mast cells or basophils	
Histamine (preformed in mast cells)	Vasodilation Smooth muscle contraction, increased vascular permeability, increased mucus secretions
Eosinophil chemotactic factor of anaphylaxis (ECF-A) (preformed in mast cells)	Attracts eosinophils
Platelet-activating factor (PAF) (requires synthesis by mast cells, neutrophils, and macrophages)	Smooth muscle contraction Incites platelets to aggregate and release serotonin and histamine
Prostaglandins (chemically derived from arachidonic acid; require synthesis by cells)	D and F series → bronchoconstriction E series → bronchodilation D, E, and F series → vasodilation
Basophil kallikrein (preformed in mast cells)	Frees bradykinin, which causes bronchoconstriction, vasodilation, and nerve stimulation
Secondary Mediators	
Inactive precursors formed or released in response to primary mediators	
Bradykinin (derived from precursor kininogen)	Smooth muscle contraction, increased vascular permeability, stimulates pain receptors, increased mucus production
Serotonin (preformed in platelets)	Smooth muscle contraction, increased vascular permeability
Heparin (preformed in mast cells)	Anticoagulant
Leukotrienes (derived from arachidonic acid and activated by mast cell degranulation) C, D, and E or slow-reacting substance of anaphylaxis (SRS-A)	Smooth muscle contraction, increased vascular permeability

and histamine 2 (H_2) receptors found on different types of lymphocytes, particularly T-lymphocyte suppressor cells and basophils. H_1 receptors are found predominantly on bronchiolar and vascular smooth muscle cells; H_2 receptors are found on gastric parietal cells.

Certain medications are categorized by their action at these receptors. Diphenhydramine (Benadryl) is an example of an **antihistamine**, a medication that displays an affinity for H_1 receptors. Cimetidine (Tagamet) and ranitidine (Zantac) target H_2 receptors to inhibit gastric secretions in peptic ulcer disease.

EOSINOPHIL CHEMOTACTIC FACTOR OF ANAPHYLAXIS

Eosinophil chemotactic factor of anaphylaxis (ECF-A) is preformed in the mast cells and affects movement of **eosinophils** (granular leukocytes) to the site of allergens. It is released from disrupted mast cells.

PLATELET-ACTIVATING FACTOR

Platelet-activating factor (PAF) is responsible for initiating platelet aggregation and leukocyte infiltration at sites of immediate hypersensitivity reactions. It also causes bronchoconstriction and increased vascular permeability (Porth, 2005).

PROSTAGLANDINS

Prostaglandins, composed of unsaturated fatty acids, produce smooth muscle contraction as well as vasodilation and increased capillary permeability (Hepner & Castells, 2003a). The fever and pain that occur with inflammation in allergic responses are due in part to the prostaglandins.

Secondary Mediators

LEUKOTRIENES

Leukotrienes are chemical mediators that initiate the inflammatory response. They are metabolites released by mucosal mast cells and collectively make up what was once termed SRS-A. Leukotrienes cause smooth muscle contraction, bronchial constriction, mucus secretion in the airways, and the typical wheal-and-flare reaction of the skin. Compared with histamine, leukotrienes are 100 to 1000 times more potent in causing bronchospasm. Many manifestations of inflammation can be attributed in part to leukotrienes. Medications categorized as leukotriene antagonists or modifiers, such as zileuton (Zyflo), zafirlukast (Accolate), and montelukast (Singulair), block the synthesis or action of leukotrienes and prevent the signs and symptoms associated with asthma.

BRADYKININ

Bradykinin is a polypeptide with the ability to cause increased vascular permeability, vasodilation, hypotension, and contraction of many types of smooth muscle, such as the bronchi. Increased permeability of the capillaries results in edema. Bradykinin stimulates nerve cell fibers and produces pain.

SEROTONIN

Serotonin acts as a potent vasoconstrictor and causes contraction of bronchial smooth muscle.

Hypersensitivity

Although the immune system defends the host against infections and foreign antigens, immune responses can themselves cause tissue injury and disease. An immune response to an antigen may result in sensitivity when challenged with that antigen; **hypersensitivity** is a reflection of excessive or aberrant immune responses (Abbas & Lichtman, 2004).

A hypersensitivity reaction is an abnormal, heightened reaction to any type of stimulus. It usually does not occur with the first exposure to an allergen. Rather, the reaction follows a re-exposure after sensitization in a predisposed person. Sensitization initiates the humoral response or buildup of antibodies. To promote understanding of the immunopathogenesis of disease, hypersensitivity reactions have been classified into four specific types of reactions (Fig. 53-2). Most allergies are identified as either type I or type IV hypersensitivity reactions.

Anaphylactic (Type I) Hypersensitivity

The most severe form of hypersensitivity reaction, the most severe immune-mediated reaction, is **anaphylaxis.** An unanticipated severe allergic reaction that is often explosive in onset, anaphylaxis is characterized by edema in many tissues, including the larynx, and is often accompanied by hypotension, bronchospasm, and cardiovascular collapse in severe cases. Type I or anaphylactic hypersensitivity is an immediate reaction beginning within minutes of exposure to an antigen. This reaction is mediated by IgE antibodies rather than IgG or IgM antibodies. It typically occurs on re-exposure to a specific antigen and requires the release of proinflammatory mediators. In turn, the plasma cells produce IgE antibodies in the lymph nodes, where helper T cells aid in promoting this reaction. The IgE antibodies bind to membrane receptors on mast cells found in connective tissue and basophils. During re-exposure, the antigen binds to adjacent IgE antibodies, activating a cellular reaction that triggers degranulation and the release of chemical mediators (histamine, leukotrienes, and ECF-A) (Hepner & Castells, 2003a).

Primary chemical mediators are responsible for the symptoms of type I hypersensitivity because of their effects on the skin, lungs, and gastrointestinal tract. If chemical mediators continue to be released, a delayed reaction may occur and may last for up to 24 hours. Clinical symptoms are determined by the amount of the allergen, the amount of mediator released, the sensitivity of the target organ, and the route of allergen entry. Type I hypersensitivity reactions may include both local and systemic anaphylaxis.

Cytotoxic (Type II) Hypersensitivity

Type II, or cytotoxic, hypersensitivity occurs when the system mistakenly identifies a normal constituent of the body as foreign. This reaction may be the result of a cross-reacting antibody, possibly leading to cell and tissue damage. Type II hypersensitivity involves the binding of either IgG or IgM antibody to the cell-bound antigen. The result of antigen–antibody binding is activation of the complement cascade (see Chapter 50) and destruction of the cell to which the antigen is bound.

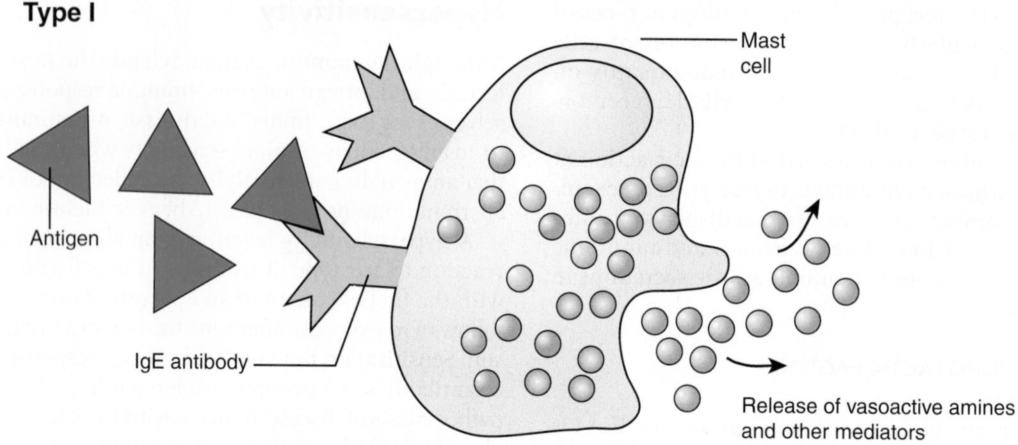

Type I. An anaphylactic reaction is characterized by vasodilation, increased capillary permeability, smooth muscle contraction, and eosinophilia. Systemic reactions may involve laryngeal stridor, angioedema, hypotension, and bronchial, GI, or uterine spasm; local reactions are characterized by hives. Examples of type I reactions include extrinsic asthma, allergic rhinitis, systemic anaphylaxis, and reactions to insect stings.

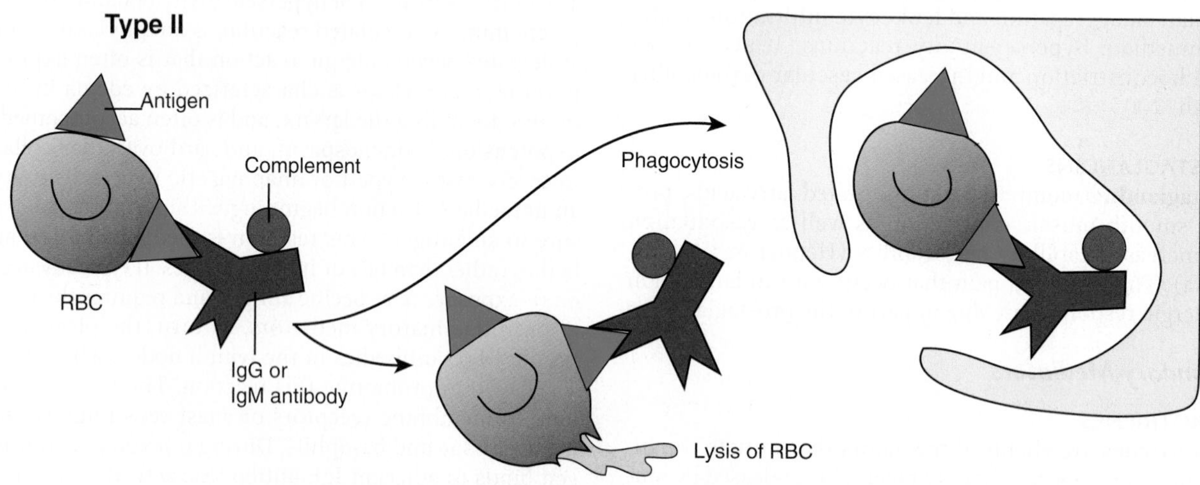

Type II. A cytotoxic reaction, which involves the binding of either the IgG or IgM antibody to a cell-bound antigen, may lead to eventual cell and tissue damage. The reaction is the result of mistaken identity when the system identifies a normal constituent of the body as foreign and activates the complement cascade. Examples of type II reactions are myasthenia gravis, Goodpasture's syndrome, pernicious anemia, hemolytic disease of the newborn, transfusion reaction, and thrombocytopenia.

FIGURE 53-2. Four types of hypersensitivity reactions.

Type II hypersensitivity reactions are associated with several disorders. For example, in myasthenia gravis, the body mistakenly generates antibodies against normal nerve ending receptors. In Goodpasture syndrome, it generates antibodies against lung and renal tissue, producing lung damage and renal failure. A type II hypersensitivity reaction resulting in red blood cell destruction is associated with drug-induced immune hemolytic anemia, Rh-hemolytic disease of the newborn, and incompatibility reactions in blood transfusions (see Chapter 33).

Immune Complex (Type III) Hypersensitivity

Type III, or immune complex, hypersensitivity involves immune complexes that are formed when antigens bind to antibodies. These complexes are cleared from the circulation by phagocytic action. If these type III complexes are deposited in tissues or vascular endothelium, two factors contribute to injury: the increased amount of circulating complexes and the presence of vasoactive amines. As a result, there is an increase in vascular permeability and tissue injury. The joints and kidneys are particularly susceptible to this type of injury. Type III hypersensitivity is associated with systemic lupus erythematosus, rheumatoid arthritis, certain types of nephritis, and some types of bacterial endocarditis. These are discussed elsewhere in this text.

Delayed-Type (Type IV) Hypersensitivity

Type IV, or delayed-type hypersensitivity, also known as cellular hypersensitivity, occurs 24 to 72 hours after exposure to an allergen. It is mediated by sensitized T cells and macrophages. An example of this reaction is the effect of an intradermal injection of tuberculin antigen or purified

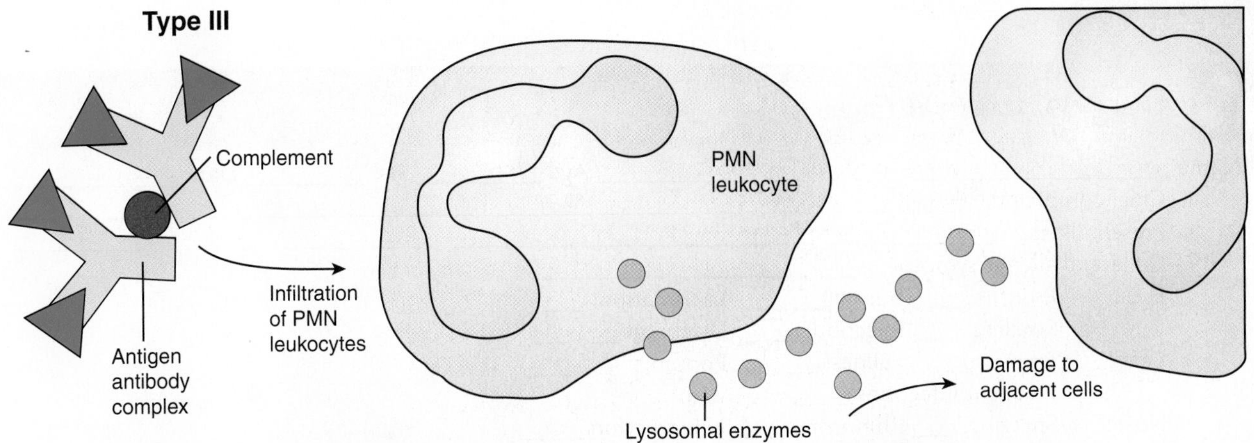

Type III. An immune complex reaction is marked by acute inflammation resulting from formation and deposition of immune complexes. The joints and kidneys are particularly susceptible to this kind of reaction, which is associated with systemic lupus erythematosus, serum sickness, nephritis and rheumatoid arthritis. Some signs and symptoms include urticaria, joint pain, fever, rash, and adenopathy (swollen glands).

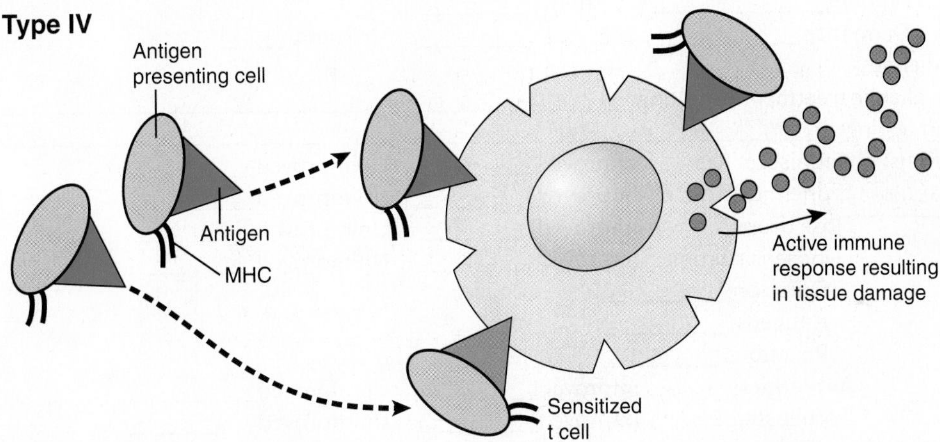

Type IV. A delayed, or cellular, reaction occurs 1 to 3 days after exposure to an antigen. The reaction, which results in tissue damage, involves activity by lymphokines, macrophages, and lysozymes. Erythema and itching are common; a few examples include contact dermatitis, graft-versus-host disease, Hashimoto's thyroiditis, and sarcoidosis.

FIGURE 53-2. Continued

protein derivative (PPD). Sensitized T cells react with the antigen at or near the injection site. Lymphokines are released and attract, activate, and retain macrophages at the site. These macrophages then release lysozymes, causing tissue damage. Edema and fibrin are responsible for the positive tuberculin reaction.

An example of a type IV hypersensitivity reaction is contact dermatitis resulting from exposure to allergens such as cosmetics, adhesive tape, topical agents (eg, povidone-iodine), medication additives, and plant toxins. The most common immune-mediated reaction to local anesthetics is a type IV hypersensitivity reaction (Hepner & Castells, 2003a). The primary exposure results in sensitization. Re-exposure causes a hypersensitivity reaction composed of low-molecular-weight molecules (haptens) that bind with proteins or carriers and are then processed by Langerhans cells in the skin. The symptoms that occur include itching, erythema, and raised lesions.

Assessment and Diagnostic Evaluation

Health History and Clinical Manifestations

A comprehensive allergy history and a thorough physical examination provide useful data for the diagnosis and management of allergic disorders. An assessment form is useful for obtaining and organizing this information (Chart 53-1).

CHART 53-1

Allergy Assessment Form

Name ______ Age ______ Sex ______ Date ______

I. Chief complaint: ______

II. Present illness: ______

III. Collateral allergic symptoms: ______

Eyes: Pruritus ____ Burning ____ Lacrimation ____
Swelling ____ Injection ____ Discharge ____

Ears: Pruritus ____ Fullness ____ Popping ____
Frequent infections ____

Nose: Sneezing ____ Rhinorrhea ____ Obstruction ____
Pruritus ____ Mouth-breathing ____
Purulent discharge ____

Throat: Soreness ____ Postnasal discharge ____
Palatal pruritus ____ Mucus in the morning ____

Chest: Cough ____ Pain ____ Wheezing ____
Sputum ____ Dyspnea ____
Color ____ Rest ____
Amount ____ Exertion ____

Skin: Dermatitis ____ Eczema ____ Urticaria ____

IV. Family allergies

V. Previous allergic treatment or testing: ______

Prior skin testing: ______

Medications:

Antihistamines Improved ____ Unimproved ____
Bronchodilators Improved ____ Unimproved ____
Nose drops Improved ____ Unimproved ____
Hyposensitization Improved ____ Unimproved ____
Duration ____
Antigens ____
Reactions ____
Antibiotics Improved ____ Unimproved ____
Corticosteroids Improved ____ Unimproved ____

VI. Physical agents and habits: ______

Tobacco for ____ years
Cigarettes ____ packs/day
Cigars ____ per day
Pipes ____ per day
Never smoked ____
Bothered by smoke ____

Bothered by:

Alcohol ____ Air cond. ____
Heat ____ Muggy weather ____
Cold ____ Weather changes ____
Perfumes ____ Chemicals ____
Paints ____ Hair spray ____
Insecticides ____ Newspapers ____
Cosmetics ____ Latex ____

VII. When symptoms occur: ______

Time and circumstances of 1st episode: ______

Prior health: ______

Course of illness over decades: progressing ____ regressing ____

Time of year: ______ Exact dates: ______

Perennial ____
Seasonal ____
Seasonally exacerbated ____

Monthly variations (menses, occupation): ______

Time of week (weekends vs. weekdays): ______

Time of day or night: ______

After insect stings: ______

CHART 53-1 *Allergy Assessment Form, continued*

VIII. Where symptoms occur: ______

Living where at onset: ______

Living where since onset: ______

Effect of vacation or major geographic change: ______

Symptoms better indoors or outdoors: ______

Effect of school or work: ______

Effect of staying elsewhere nearby: ______

Effect of hospitalization: ______

Effect of specific environments: ______

Do symptoms occur around: ______

old leaves ____ hay ____ lakeside ____ barns ____

summer homes ____ damp basement ____ dry attic ____

lawnmowing ____ animals ____ other ____

Do symptoms occur after eating:

cheese ____ mushrooms ____ beer ____ melons ____

bananas ____ fish ____ nuts ____ citrus fruits ____

other foods (list) ______

Home: city ____ rural ____

house ____ age ____

apartment ____ basement ____ damp ____ dry ____

heating system ____

pets (how long) ____ dog ____ cat ____ other ____

Bedroom:	Type	Age	*Living room:*	Type	Age
Pillow	____	____	Rug	____	____
Mattress	____	____	Matting	____	____
Blankets	____	____	Furniture	____	____
Quilts	____	____			
Furniture	____	____			

Anywhere in home symptoms are worse: ______

IX. What does patient think makes symptoms worse? ______

X. Under what circumstances is patient free of symptoms? ______

XI. Summary and additional comments: ______

The degree of difficulty and discomfort experienced by the patient because of allergic symptoms and the degree of improvement in those symptoms with and without treatment are assessed and documented. The relationship of symptoms to exposure to possible allergens is noted.

Diagnostic Evaluation

Diagnostic evaluation of the patient with allergic disorders commonly includes blood tests, smears of body secretions, skin tests, and the radioallergosorbent test (RAST). Results of laboratory blood studies provide supportive data for various diagnostic possibilities; however, they are not the major criteria for the diagnosis of allergic disease.

Complete Blood Count With Differential

The white blood cell (WBC) count is usually normal except with infection. Eosinophils, which are granular leukocytes, normally make up 1% to 3% of the total number of WBCs. A level between 5% and 15% is nonspecific but does suggest allergic reaction. Higher percentages of eosinophils are considered to represent moderate to severe eosinophilia. Moderate eosinophilia is defined as 15% to 40% eosinophils and is found in patients with allergic disorders; in patients with malignancy, immunodeficiencies, parasitic infections, or congenital heart disease; and in patients receiving peritoneal dialysis. Severe eosinophilia is defined as 50% to 90% eosinophils and is found in the idiopathic hypereosinophilic syndrome.

Eosinophil Count

An actual count of eosinophils can be obtained from blood samples or smears of secretions. A total eosinophil count can be obtained from a blood sample with the use of special diluting fluids that hemolyze erythrocytes and stain the eosinophils. During symptomatic episodes, smears obtained from nasal secretions, conjunctival secretions, and sputum of allergic patients usually reveal eosinophils, indicating an active allergic response.

Total Serum Immunoglobulin E Levels

High total serum IgE levels support the diagnosis of allergic disease. However, a normal IgE level does not exclude the diagnosis of an allergic disorder. IgE levels are not as sensitive as the paper radioimmunosorbent test (PRIST) or the enzyme-linked immunosorbent assay (ELISA). Indications for determining IgE levels include the following:

- Evaluation of immunodeficiency
- Evaluation of drug reactions
- Initial laboratory screening for allergic bronchopulmonary aspergillosis
- Evaluation of allergy among children with bronchiolitis
- Differentiation of allergic and nonallergic dermatitis
- Differentiation of allergic and nonallergic asthma and rhinitis

Skin Tests

Skin testing entails the intradermal injection or superficial application (epicutaneous) of solutions at several sites. Depending on the suspected cause of allergic signs and symptoms, several different solutions may be applied at separate sites. These solutions contain individual antigens representing an assortment of allergens most likely to be implicated in the patient's disease. Positive reactions (wheal-and-flare) are clinically significant when correlated with the history, physical findings, and results of other laboratory tests.

The results of skin tests complement the data obtained from the history. They indicate which of several antigens are most likely to provoke symptoms and provide some clue to the intensity of the patient's sensitization. The dosage of the antigen (allergen) injected is also important. Most patients are hypersensitive to more than one allergen. Under testing conditions, they may not react (although they usually do) to the specific allergens that induce their attacks.

In cases of doubt about the validity of the skin tests, a RAST or a provocative challenge test may be performed. If a skin test is indicated, there is a reasonable suspicion that a specific allergen is producing symptoms in an allergic patient. However, several precautionary steps must be observed before skin testing with allergens is performed:

- Testing is not performed during periods of bronchospasm.
- Epicutaneous tests (scratch or prick tests) are performed before other testing methods, in an effort to minimize the risk of systemic reaction.
- Emergency equipment must be readily available to treat anaphylaxis.

TYPES OF SKIN TESTS

The methods of skin testing include prick skin tests, scratch tests, and intradermal skin testing (Fig. 53-3). After negative prick or scratch tests, intradermal skin testing is performed with allergens that are suggested by the patient's history to be problematic. The back is the most suitable area of the body for skin testing, because it permits the performance of many tests. The multitest applicator is a commercially available device with multiple test heads that allows simultaneous administration of antigens by multiple punctures at different sites. A negative response on a skin test cannot be interpreted as an absence of sensitivity to an allergen. Such a response may occur with insufficient sensitivity of the test or with use of an inappropriate allergen in testing. Therefore, it is essential to observe the patient undergoing skin testing for an allergic reaction even if the previous response was negative.

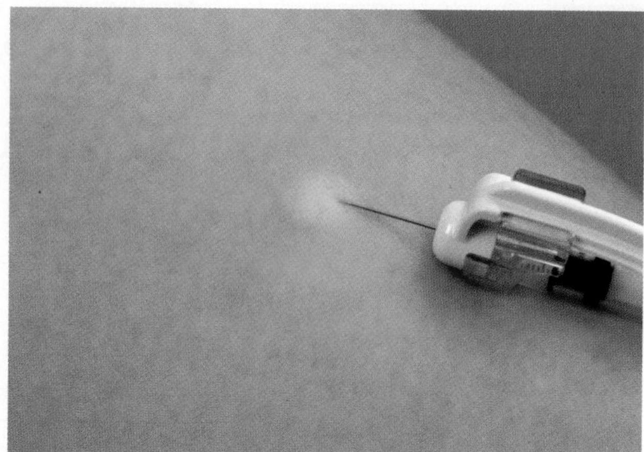

FIGURE 53-3. Intradermal testing. A 0.5-mL or 1-mL sterile syringe with a 26/27 gauge intradermal needle is used to inject 0.02 to 0.03 mL of intradermal allergen. The needle is inserted with the bevel facing upward and the syringe parallel to the skin. The skin is penetrated superficially, and a small amount of the allergen solution is injected to create a bleb (raised area) approximately 5 mm in diameter. A separate sterile syringe and needle are used for each injection. From Taylor, C., Lillis C., & LeMone, P. (2005). *Fundamentals of nursing: The art and science of nursing care* (5th ed.). Philadelphia: Lippincott Williams & Wilkins.

INTERPRETATION OF SKIN TEST RESULTS

Familiarity with and consistent use of a grading system are essential. The grading system used should be identified on a skin test sheet for later interpretation. A positive reaction, evidenced by the appearance of an urticarial wheal (round, reddened skin elevation) (Fig. 53-4), localized **erythema** (diffuse redness) in the area of inoculation or contact, or pseudopodia (irregular projection at the end of a wheal) with associated erythema is considered indicative of sensitivity to the corresponding antigen.

False-negative results may occur because of improper technique, outdated allergen solutions, or prior use of medications that suppress skin reactivity. Corticosteroids and antihistamines, including over-the-counter allergy medications, suppress skin test reactivity and are usually withheld for 48 to 96 hours before testing, depending on the duration of their activity. False-positive results may occur because of improper preparation or administration of allergen solutions.

Interpretation of positive or negative skin tests must be based on the history, physical examination, and other laboratory test results. The following guidelines are used for the interpretation of skin test results:

- Skin tests are more reliable for diagnosing atopic sensitivity in patients with allergic rhinoconjunctivitis than in patients with asthma.
- Positive skin tests correlate highly with food allergy.
- The use of skin tests to diagnose immediate hypersensitivity to medications is limited, because metabolites of medications, not the medications themselves, are usually responsible for causing hypersensitivity.

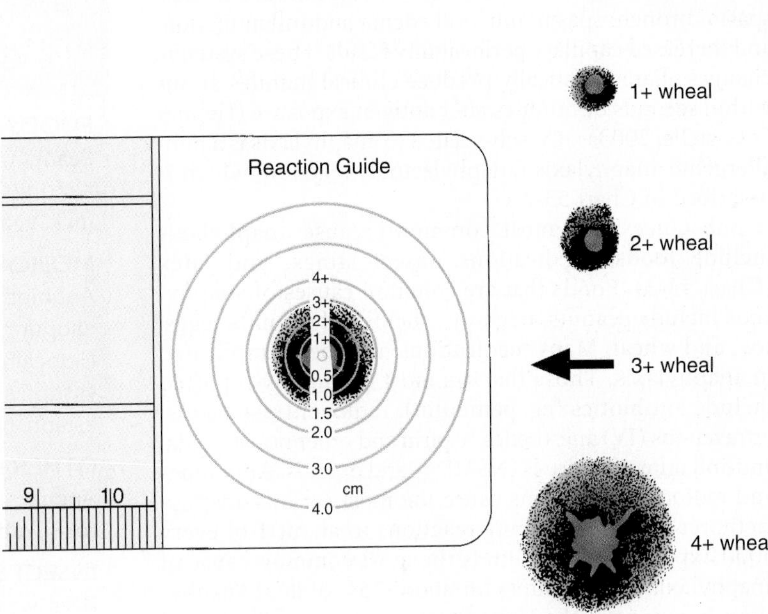

FIGURE 53-4. Interpretation of reactions: Negative = wheal soft with minimal erythema. 1+ = wheal present (5–8 mm) with associated erythema. 2+ = wheal (7–10 mm) with associated erythema. 3+ = wheal (9–15 mm), slight pseudopodia possible with associated erythema. 4+ = wheal (12 mm+) with pseudopodia and diffuse erythema.

Provocative Testing

Provocative testing involves the direct administration of the suspected allergen to the sensitive tissue, such as the conjunctiva, nasal or bronchial mucosa, or gastrointestinal tract (by ingestion of the allergen), with observation of target organ response. This type of testing is helpful in identifying clinically significant allergens in patients who have a large number of positive tests. Major disadvantages of this type of testing are the limitation of one antigen per session and the risk of producing severe symptoms, particularly bronchospasm, in patients with asthma.

Radioallergosorbent Test (RAST)

RAST is a radioimmunoassay that measures allergen-specific IgE. A sample of the patient's serum is exposed to a variety of suspected allergen particle complexes. If antibodies are present, they will combine with radiolabeled allergens. After the serum is centrifuged, radioimmunoassay detects the allergen-specific IgE antibody. Test results are then compared with control values. In addition to detecting an allergen, RAST indicates the quantity of allergen necessary to evoke an allergic reaction. Values are reported on a scale from 0 to 5. Values of 2 or greater are considered significant. The major advantages of RAST over other tests include decreased risk of systemic reaction, stability of antigens, and lack of dependence on skin reactivity modified by medications. The major disadvantages include limited allergen selection and reduced sensitivity compared with intradermal skin tests, lack of immediate results, and higher cost.

Allergic Disorders

There are two types of IgE-mediated allergic reactions: atopic and nonatopic disorders. Although the underlying immunologic reactions of the two types of disorders are the same, the predisposing factors and manifestations are different. The atopic disorders are characterized by a hereditary predisposition and production of a local reaction to IgE antibodies, which manifests in one or more of the following three atopic disorders: allergic rhinitis, asthma, and atopic dermatitis/eczema. The nonatopic disorders lack the genetic component and organ specificity of the atopic disorders (Porth, 2005). Latex allergy (see later discussion) may be a type I or type IV hypersensitivity reaction, although true latex allergy is considered to be a type I hypersensitivity reaction (Hepner & Castells, 2003b). Contact dermatitis is considered to be a type IV hypersensitivity reaction.

Anaphylaxis

Anaphylaxis is a clinical response to an immediate (type I hypersensitivity) immunologic reaction between a specific antigen and an antibody. The reaction results from a rapid release of IgE-mediated chemicals, which can induce a severe, life-threatening allergic reaction. It is estimated that between 3.3 and 43 million people in the United States (1.24% to 16.8% of the population) are at risk for anaphylaxis (Hepner & Castells, 2003a).

Pathophysiology

Anaphylaxis is caused by the interaction of a foreign antigen with specific IgE antibodies found on the surface membrane of mast cells and peripheral blood basophils. The subsequent release of histamine and other bioactive mediators causes activation of platelets, eosinophils, and neutrophils. Histamine, prostaglandins, and inflammatory leukotrienes are potent vasoactive mediators that are implicated in the vascular permeability changes, flushing, urticaria, angioedema, hypotension, and bronchoconstriction that characterize anaphylaxis (Hepner & Castells, 2003a). Smooth muscle spasm, bronchospasm, mucosal edema and inflammation, and increased capillary permeability result. These systemic changes characteristically produce clinical manifestations within seconds or minutes after antigen exposure (Hepner & Castells, 2003a). Closely related to anaphylaxis is a nonallergenic anaphylaxis (anaphylactoid) reaction, which is described in Chart 53-2.

Substances that most commonly cause anaphylaxis include foods, medications, insect stings, and latex (Chart 53-3). Foods that are common causes of anaphylaxis include peanuts, tree nuts, shellfish, fish, milk, eggs, soy, and wheat. Many medications have been implicated in anaphylaxis. Those that are most frequently reported include antibiotics (eg, penicillin), radiocontrast agents, intravenous (IV) anesthetics, aspirin and other nonsteroidal anti-inflammatory drugs (NSAIDs), and opioids. Antibiotics and radiocontrast agents cause the most serious anaphylactic reactions, producing reactions in about 1 of every 5000 exposures. Penicillin is the most common cause of anaphylaxis and accounts for about 75% of fatal anaphylactic reactions in the United States each year. The actual prevalence of penicillin allergy in the general population is unknown; however, the incidence of self-reported penicillin allergy ranges from 1% to 10%. It has been reported that 80% to 90% of those patients with self-reported penicillin allergy have no evidence of IgE antibodies to penicillin on skin testing (Park & Li, 2005).

The diagnosis of risk of anaphylaxis is determined by prick and intradermal skin testing. Skin testing of patients who have clinical symptoms consistent with a type I, IgE-mediated reaction has been recommended (Hepner & Castells, 2003a).

CHART 53-2

Nonallergenic Anaphylaxis (Anaphylactoid Reaction)

Closely resembling anaphylaxis is an anaphylaxis-like reaction that is caused by the release of mast cell and basophil mediators triggered by non–IgE-mediated events. A nonallergenic anaphylaxis reaction may occur with medications, food, exercise, or cytotoxic antibody transfusions. The reaction may be local or systemic. Local reactions usually involve urticaria and angioedema at the site of the antigen exposure. Although possibly severe, nonallergenic anaphylaxis reactions are rarely fatal. Systemic reactions occur within about 30 minutes after exposure and involve cardiovascular, respiratory, gastrointestinal, and integumentary organ systems. For the most part, the treatment of nonallergenic anaphylaxis reaction is identical to that of anaphylaxis (Hepner & Castells, 2003a; Johansson, Hourihane, Bousquet, et al., 2005).

CHART 53-3

Common Causes of Anaphylaxis

FOODS

Peanuts, tree nuts (eg, walnuts, pecans, cashews, almonds), shellfish (eg, shrimp, lobster, crab), fish, milk, eggs, soy, wheat

MEDICATIONS

Antibiotics, especially penicillin and sulfa antibiotics, allopurinol, radiocontrast agents, anesthetic agents (lidocaine, procaine), vaccines, hormones (insulin, vasopressin, adrenocorticotropic hormone [ACTH], aspirin, nonsteroidal anti-inflammatory drugs [NSAIDs]).

OTHER PHARMACEUTICAL/BIOLOGIC AGENTS

Animal serums (tetanus antitoxin, snake venom antitoxin, rabies antitoxin), antigens used in skin testing

INSECT STINGS

Bees, wasps, hornets, yellow jackets, ants, including fire ants

LATEX

Medical and nonmedical products containing latex

Clinical Manifestations

Anaphylactic reactions produce a clinical syndrome that affects multiple organ systems due to the acute release of mediators from tissue mast cells and basophils by cross-linking of IgE antibodies (Hepner & Castells, 2003a). Reactions may be categorized as mild, moderate, or severe. The time from exposure to the antigen to onset of symptoms is a good indicator of the severity of the reaction: the faster the onset, the more severe the reaction. The severity of previous reactions does not determine the severity of subsequent reactions, which could be the same, more, or less severe. The severity depends on the degree of allergy and the dose of allergen (McLean-Tooke, Bethune, Fay, et al., 2003).

Mild systemic reactions consist of peripheral tingling and a sensation of warmth, possibly accompanied by a sensation of fullness in the mouth and throat. Nasal congestion, periorbital swelling, pruritus, sneezing, and tearing of the eyes can also be expected. Onset of symptoms begins within the first 2 hours after exposure.

Moderate systemic reactions may include flushing, warmth, anxiety, and itching in addition to any of the milder symptoms. More serious reactions include bronchospasm and edema of the airways or larynx with dyspnea, cough, and wheezing. The onset of symptoms is the same as for a mild reaction.

Severe systemic reactions have an abrupt onset with the same signs and symptoms described previously. These symptoms progress rapidly to bronchospasm, laryngeal edema, severe dyspnea, cyanosis, and hypotension. Dysphagia (difficulty swallowing), abdominal cramping, vomiting, diarrhea,

NURSING RESEARCH PROFILE

Emergency Epinephrine for Home IV Antibiotic Therapy

Dobson, P., Boyle, M., & Loewenthal, M. (2004). Home intravenous antibiotic therapy and allergic drug reactions: Is there a case for routine supply of anaphylaxis kits? *Journal of Infusion Nursing, 27*(6), 425–430.

Purpose

The administration of parenteral antibiotic therapy in the home has become a convenient, cost-effective alternative to its administration in the hospital or outpatient facility. Because of the risk of allergic reactions with IV antibiotic therapy, it has been suggested that epinephrine be available in case of anaphylaxis; however, few data exist about the implications of providing epinephrine to all patients receiving antibiotic therapy in the home. This study was conducted to estimate the risk of allergic reactions among patients receiving IV antibiotics in the home and to identify the potential advantages and disadvantages of providing injectable epinephrine for use by these patients if an allergic reaction occurs.

Design

A prospective descriptive study was conducted to assess the severity and nature of allergic reactions associated with home IV antibiotic therapy. The sample consisted of more than 700 patients consecutively admitted to a program for IV administration of antibiotics at home. Data were collected from 770 patients who received 1000 courses of therapy with 25 different antibiotics for 37 conditions, for a total of more than 21,000 patient-days of antibiotic therapy. All patients received the first dose of the IV antibiotic under medical supervision, and all had ready access to a telephone and transport in case of emergency. Patients who reported a history of reaction to a specific medication did not receive that compound.

Findings

Prospective data collected included the medication administered, its dose, mode of administration of home IV therapy care, and complications, including adverse drug reactions. A drug reaction was defined as allergic in nature by an immunologist, was not attributable to any other patient-related factors, and required cessation of the antibiotic thought to be responsible for the reaction. The patients in the study experienced 28 allergic reactions, most commonly nonexfoliative or nonbullous skin rash, with the mean time to allergic reaction being 19.6 days (range, 1 to 39 days). Allergic reactions occurred in 2% of the penicillin courses, 3.2% of the cephalosporin courses, and 5.8% of the vancomycin courses. Reactions to vancomycin occurred 2.5 times more often ($p = .0374$) than reactions to other antibiotics. Penicillin, cephalosporin, and vancomycin were administered by 24-hour infusion, which may have affected the rate of sensitivity. Delayed oral angioedema occurred in 3 patients (0.4%) and resolved with discontinuation of the antibiotic. No episodes of anaphylaxis were observed.

Nursing Implications

Although it has been suggested that patients receiving IV antibiotic therapy at home should have epinephrine available for emergency administration, the results of this study and the potential disadvantages of issuing epinephrine to these patients suggest that this strategy may not provide a net benefit. These disadvantages are the adverse effects of epinephrine, which range from anxiety, pallor, and palpitations to more severe events, including myocardial infarction and death in vulnerable patients. The researchers suggest that issuing epinephrine may be dangerous if factors such as patient age, cardiac history, concurrent medications, pregnancy, allergy history, and whether the person is receiving a first or subsequent dose of antibiotic are not considered. Although patients with a history of anaphylaxis may be appropriate candidates for a supply of epinephrine autoinjectors, careful screening of recipients of home IV antibiotic therapy and administration of the first dose under supervision may be more effective. The potential for progression of oral angioedema to laryngeal edema is of particular concern and highlights the need for provision of support services to people receiving home IV therapy.

and seizures can also occur. Cardiac arrest and coma may follow.

Prevention

Strict avoidance of potential allergens is an important preventive measure for the patient at risk for anaphylaxis. Patients at risk for anaphylaxis from insect stings should avoid areas populated by insects and should use appropriate clothing, insect repellent, and caution to avoid further stings.

If avoidance of exposure to allergens is impossible, the patient should be instructed to carry and administer epinephrine to prevent an anaphylactic reaction in the event of exposure to the allergen. People who are sensitive to insect bites and stings, those who have experienced food or medication reactions, and those who have experienced idiopathic or exercise-induced anaphylactic reactions should always carry an emergency kit that contains epinephrine. The EpiPen from Dey Pharmaceuticals (Napa, CA) is a commercially available first-aid device that delivers premeasured doses of 0.3 mg (EpiPen) or 0.15 mg (EpiPen Jr.) of epinephrine (Fig. 53-5). The autoinjection system requires no preparation, and the self-administration technique is uncomplicated. The patient must be given an opportunity to demonstrate the correct technique for use; an EpiPen training device can be used for teaching correct technique. Verbal and written information about the emergency kit, as well as strategies to avoid exposure to threatening allergens, must also be provided.

Screening for allergies before a medication is prescribed or first administered is an important preventive measure. A careful history of any sensitivity to suspected antigens must be obtained before administering any medication, particularly in parenteral form, because this route is associated with the most severe anaphylaxis. Nurses caring for patients in any setting (hospital, home, outpatient diagnostic testing sites, long-term care facilities) must assess patients' risks for anaphylactic reactions. Patients are asked about previous exposure to contrast agents used for diagnostic tests and any allergic reactions, as well as reactions to any medications, foods, insect stings, and latex. People who are predisposed to anaphylaxis should wear some form of identification, such as a medical alert bracelet, which names allergies to medications, food, and other substances.

People who are allergic to insect venom may require venom immunotherapy, which is used as a control measure and not a cure. Immunotherapy administered after an insect sting is very effective in reducing the risk of anaphylaxis from future stings (Gruchalla, 2004). Insulin-allergic patients with diabetes and those who are allergic to penicillin may require desensitization. Desensitization is based on controlled anaphylaxis, with a gradual release of mediators. Patients who undergo desensitization are cautioned that there should be no lapses in therapy, because this may lead to the reappearance of the allergic reaction when the use of the medication is resumed.

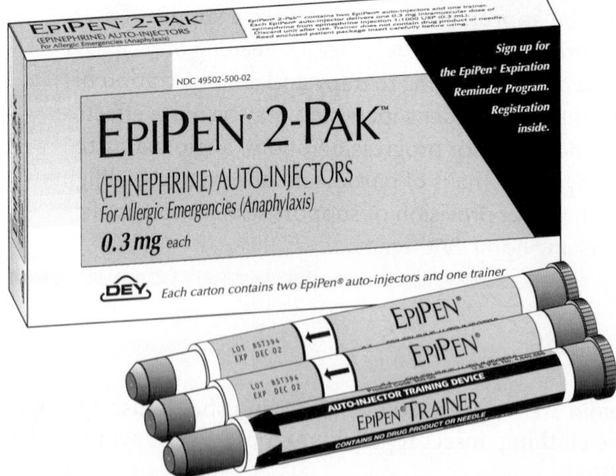

FIGURE 53-5. The EpiPen and EpiPen Jr. Autoinjectors are commercially available first-aid devices that administer premeasured doses of epinephrine. An EpiPen training device is available for patients to practice correct self-injection technique. Courtesy of Dey Pharmaceuticals, Napa, CA.

Medical Management

Management depends on the severity of the reaction. Initially, respiratory and cardiovascular functions are evaluated. If the patient is in cardiac arrest, cardiopulmonary resuscitation is instituted. Oxygen is provided in high concentrations during cardiopulmonary resuscitation or if the patient is cyanotic, dyspneic, or wheezing. Epinephrine, in a 1:1000 dilution, is administered subcutaneously in the upper extremity or thigh and may be followed by a continuous IV infusion. Most adverse events associated with administration of epinephrine (ie, adrenaline) occur when the dose is excessive or it is given intravenously. Patients at risk for adverse effects include elderly patients and those with hypertension, arteriopathies, or known ischemic heart disease (McLean-Tooke et al., 2003).

Antihistamines and corticosteroids may also be administered to prevent recurrences of the reaction (Timoney, Eagan, & Sklarin, 2003) and to treat urticaria and angioedema. IV fluids (eg, normal saline solution), volume expanders, and vasopressor agents are administered to maintain blood pressure and normal hemodynamic status. In patients with episodes of bronchospasm or a history of bronchial asthma or chronic obstructive pulmonary disease, aminophylline and corticosteroids may also be administered to improve airway patency and function. If hypotension is unresponsive to vasopressors, glucagon may be administered intravenously for its acute inotropic and chronotropic effects.

Patients who have experienced anaphylactic reactions and received epinephrine should be transported to the local emergency department for observation and monitoring because of the risk for a "rebound" reaction 4 to 10 hours after the initial allergic reaction. Patients with severe reactions are monitored closely for 12 to 14 hours in a facility that can provide emergency care, if needed. Because of the potential for recurrence, patients with even mild reactions must be informed about this risk (Al-Muhsen, Clarke & Kagan, 2003).

Nursing Management

If a patient is experiencing an allergic response, the nurse's initial action is to assess the patient for signs and symptoms of anaphylaxis. The nurse assesses the airway, breathing pattern, and other vital signs. The patient is observed for signs of increasing edema and respiratory distress. Prompt notification of the physician and preparation for initiation of emergency measures (intubation, administration of emergency medications, insertion of IV lines, fluid administration, oxygen administration) are important to reduce the severity of the reaction and to restore cardiovascular function. The nurse documents the interventions used and the patient's vital signs and response to treatment.

The patient who has recovered from anaphylaxis needs an explanation of what occurred and instruction about avoiding future exposure to antigens and how to administer emergency medications to treat anaphylaxis. The patient must be instructed about antigens that should be avoided and about other strategies to prevent recurrence of anaphylaxis. All patients who have experienced an anaphylactic reaction should receive a prescription for preloaded syringes of epinephrine. The nurse instructs the patient and family in their use and has the patient and family demonstrate correct administration (Chart 53-4).

Allergic Rhinitis

Allergic **rhinitis** (hay fever, seasonal allergic rhinitis) is the most common form of respiratory allergy presumed to be mediated by an immediate (type I hypersensitivity) immunologic reaction, and it is among the top 10 reasons for visits to primary care physicians (Wang, Chan & Smith, 2004). It affects about 10% to 25% of the United States population (Gendo & Larson, 2004). The symptoms are similar to those of viral rhinitis but are usually more persistent and demonstrate seasonal variation; rhinitis is considered to be the allergic form if the symptoms are caused by an allergen-specific IgE-mediated immunologic response. However, a sizable proportion of patients with rhinitis have mixed rhinitis, or coexisting allergic and nonallergic rhinitis (Holgate & Lack, 2005). The proportion of patients with the allergic form of rhinitis increases with age. It often occurs with other conditions, such as allergic conjunctivitis, sinusitis, and asthma. If symptoms are severe, allergic rhinitis may interfere with sleep, leisure, and school or work activities (Plaut & Valentine, 2005). If left untreated, many complications may result, such as allergic asthma, chronic nasal obstruction, chronic otitis media with hearing loss, anosmia (absence of the sense of smell), and, in children, orofacial dental deformities. Early diagnosis and adequate treatment are essential to reduce complications and relieve symptoms.

Because allergic rhinitis is induced by airborne pollens or molds, it is characterized by the following seasonal occurrences:

- Early spring—tree pollen (oak, elm, poplar)
- Early summer—rose pollen (rose fever), grass pollen (Timothy, red-top)
- Early fall—weed pollen (ragweed)

Each year attacks begin and end at about the same time. Airborne mold spores require warm, damp weather. Although there is no rigid seasonal pattern, these spores appear in early spring, are rampant during the summer, then taper off and disappear by the first frost.

Pathophysiology

Sensitization begins by ingestion or inhalation of an antigen. On re-exposure, the nasal mucosa reacts by the slowing of ciliary action, edema formation, and leukocyte (primarily eosinophil) infiltration. Histamine is the major mediator of allergic reactions in the nasal mucosa. Tissue edema results from vasodilation and increased capillary permeability.

CHART 53-4

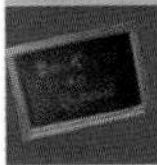

Patient Education

Self-Administration of Epinephrine

Practice this technique using a training device.

1. Carefully uncap the Epipen device, holding it so that the injecting end is upright.

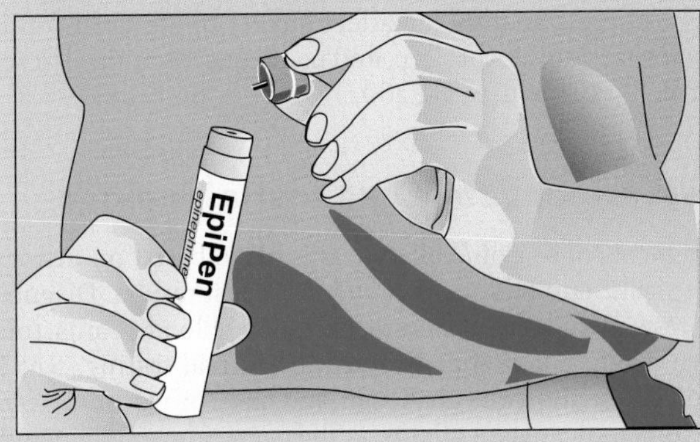

2. Position the device at the middle portion of the thigh.

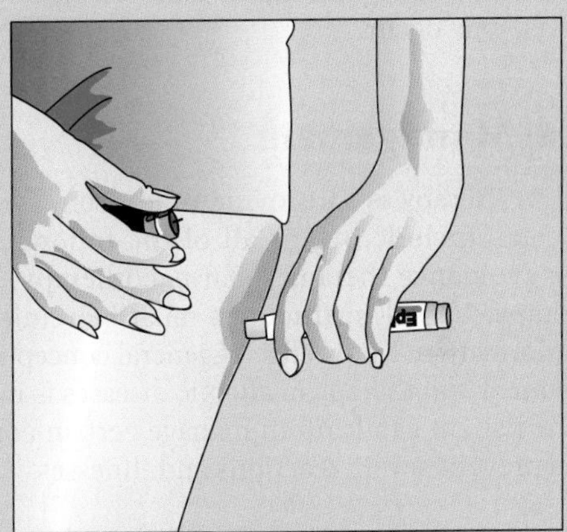

3. Push the device into the thigh as far as possible. The Epipen device will autoinject a premeasured dose of epinephrine into the subcutaneous tissue.

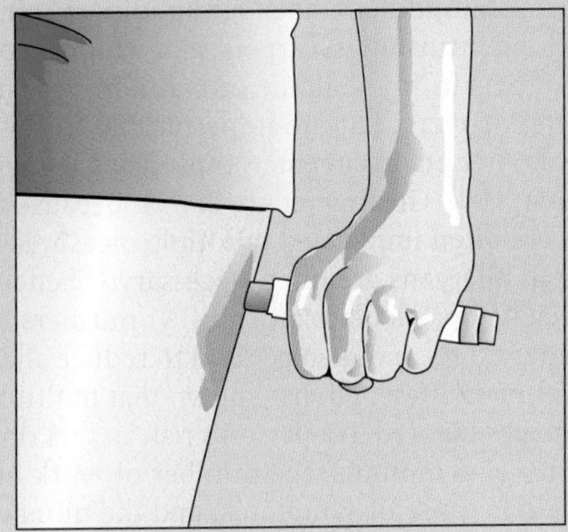

Clinical Manifestations

Typical signs and symptoms of allergic rhinitis include sneezing and nasal congestion; clear, watery nasal discharge; and nasal itching. Itching of the throat and soft palate is common. Drainage of nasal mucus into the pharynx results in multiple attempts to clear the throat and results in a dry cough or hoarseness. Headache, pain over the paranasal sinuses, and epistaxis can accompany allergic rhinitis. The symptoms of this chronic condition depend on environmental exposure and intrinsic host responsiveness. Allergic rhinitis can affect quality of life by also producing fatigue, loss of sleep, and poor concentration (Ratner, Ehrlich, Fineman, et al., 2002).

Assessment and Diagnostic Findings

Diagnosis of seasonal allergic rhinitis is based on history, physical examination, and diagnostic test results. Diagnostic tests include nasal smears, peripheral blood counts, total serum IgE, epicutaneous and intradermal testing, RAST, food elimination and challenge, and nasal provocation tests. Results indicative of allergy as the cause of rhinitis include increased IgE and eosinophil levels and positive reactions on allergen testing. False-positive and false-negative responses to these tests, particularly skin testing and provocation tests, may occur.

Medical Management

The goal of therapy is to provide relief from symptoms. Therapy may include one or all of the following interventions: avoidance therapy, pharmacotherapy, and immunotherapy. Verbal instructions must be reinforced by written information. Knowledge of general concepts regarding assessment and therapy in allergic diseases is important so that the patient can learn to manage certain conditions as well as prevent severe reactions and illnesses.

Avoidance Therapy

In avoidance therapy, every attempt is made to remove the allergens that act as precipitating factors. Simple measures and environmental controls are often effective in decreasing symptoms. Examples include use of air conditioners, air cleaners, humidifiers, and dehumidifiers; removal of dust-catching furnishings, carpets, and window coverings; removal of pets from the home or bedroom; use of pillow and mattress covers that are impermeable to dust mites; and a smoke-free environment (Simpson & Custovic, 2003; Terreehorst, Hak, Oosting, et al., 2003). Because multiple allergens are often implicated, multiple measures to avoid exposure to allergens are often necessary (Sheffer, 2004). High-efficiency particulate air (HEPA) purifiers and vacuum cleaner filters may also be used to reduce allergens in the environment. Research has shown that multiple avoidance strategies tailored to a person's risk factors can reduce the severity of symptoms, the number of work or school days missed because of symptoms, and the number of unscheduled health care visits for treatment (Morgan, Crain, Gruchalla, et al., 2004). In many cases, it is impossible to avoid exposure to all environmental allergens, so pharmacologic therapy or immunotherapy is needed.

Pharmacologic Therapy

ANTIHISTAMINES

Antihistamines, now classified as H_1-receptor antagonists (or H_1-blockers), are used in the management of mild allergic disorders. H_1-blockers bind selectively to H_1 receptors, preventing the actions of histamines at these sites. They do not prevent the release of histamine from mast cells or basophils. The H_1-antagonists have no effect on H_2 receptors, but they do have the ability to bind to nonhistaminic receptors. The ability of certain antihistamines to bind to and block muscarinic receptors underlies several of the prominent anticholinergic side effects of these medications.

Oral antihistamines, which are readily absorbed, are most effective when given at the first occurrence of symptoms, because they prevent the development of new symptoms. The effectiveness of these medications is limited to certain patients with hay fever, vasomotor rhinitis, **urticaria** (hives), and mild asthma. They are rarely effective in other conditions or in any severe conditions.

Antihistamines are the major class of medications prescribed for the symptomatic relief of allergic rhinitis. The major side effect is sedation, although H_1-antagonists are less sedating than earlier antihistamines (Simons, 2004). Additional side effects include nervousness, tremors, dizziness, dry mouth, palpitations, anorexia, nausea, and vomiting. Antihistamines are contraindicated during the third trimester of pregnancy; in nursing mothers and newborns; in children and elderly people; and in patients whose conditions may be aggravated by muscarinic blockade (eg, asthma, urinary retention, open-angle glaucoma, hypertension, prostatic hyperplasia).

Newer antihistamines are called second-generation or nonsedating H_1-receptor antagonists. Unlike first-generation H_1-receptor antagonists, they do not cross the blood–brain barrier and do not bind to cholinergic, serotoninergic, or alpha-adrenergic receptors (Simons, 2004). They bind to peripheral rather than central nervous system H_1 receptors, causing less sedation. Examples of these medications are loratadine (Claritin), cetirizine (Zyrtec), and fexofenadine (Allegra). These are summarized in Table 53-2.

ADRENERGIC AGENTS

Adrenergic agents, vasoconstrictors of mucosal vessels, are used topically (nasal and ophthalmic formulations) in addition to the oral route. The topical route (drops and sprays) causes fewer side effects than oral administration; however, the use of drops and sprays should be limited to a few days to avoid rebound congestion. Adrenergic nasal decongestants are applied topically to the nasal mucosa for the relief of nasal congestion. They activate the alpha-adrenergic receptor sites on the smooth muscle of the nasal mucosal blood vessels, reducing local blood flow, fluid exudation, and mucosal edema. Topical ophthalmic drops are used for symptomatic relief of eye irritations caused by allergies. Potential side effects include hypertension, dysrhythmias, palpitations, central nervous system stimulation, irritability, tremor, and tachyphylaxis (acceleration of hemodynamic

TABLE 53-2 Selected H_1-Antihistamines

H_1-Antihistamine	Contraindications	Major Side Effects	Nursing Implications and Patient Teaching
First-Generation H_1-Antihistamines (Sedating)			
Diphenhydramine (Benadryl)	Allergy to any antihistamines Third trimester of pregnancy Lactation Use cautiously with narrow-angle glaucoma, asthma, stenosing peptic ulcer, BPH or bladder neck obstruction, pregnancy, elderly patients	Drowsiness, confusion, dizziness, dry mouth, nausea, vomiting, photosensitivity, urinary retention	Administer with food if gastrointestinal upset occurs. Caution patients to avoid alcohol, driving, or engaging in any hazardous activities until CNS response to medication is stabilized. Suggest sucking on sugarless lozenges or ice chips for relief of dry mouth. Encourage use of sunscreen and hat while outdoors. Assess for urinary retention; monitor urinary output.
Chlorpheniramine (Chlor-Trimeton)	Allergy to any antihistamines Third trimester of pregnancy Lactation Use cautiously with narrow-angle glaucoma, asthma, stenosing peptic ulcer, BPH or bladder neck obstruction, pregnancy, elderly patients	Drowsiness, sedation, and dizziness, although less than other sedating agents; confusion, dry mouth, nausea, vomiting, urinary retention, epigastric distress, thickening of bronchial secretions	Caution patients to avoid alcohol, driving, or engaging in any hazardous activities until CNS response to medication is stabilized. Suggest sucking on sugarless lozenges or ice chips for relief of dry mouth. Recommend use of humidifier.
Hydroxyzine (Atarax)	Allergy to hydroxyzine or cetirizine (Zyrtec), pregnancy, lactation	Drowsiness, dry mouth, involuntary motor activity, including tremor and seizures	Caution patients to avoid alcohol, driving, or engaging in any hazardous activities until CNS response to medication is stabilized. Suggest sucking on sugarless lozenges or ice chips for relief of dry mouth. Instruct patients to report tremors.
Second-Generation H_1-Antihistamines (Nonsedating)			
Cetirizine (Zyrtec)	Allergy to any antihistamines Narrow-angle glaucoma Asthma Stenosing peptic ulcer BPH or bladder neck obstruction Lactation	Dry nasal mucosa, thickening of bronchial secretions	Can be taken without regard to meals. Instruct patients to use caution if driving or performing tasks that require alertness. Recommend use of humidifier.
Desloratadine (Clarinex)	Allergy to loratadine (Alavert, Claritin) Lactation Use cautiously with renal or hepatic impairment or with pregnancy	Somnolence, nervousness, dizziness, fatigue, dry mouth	Can be taken without regard to meals. Suggest sucking on sugarless lozenges or ice chips for relief of dry mouth. Recommend use of humidifier.
Loratadine (Alavert, Claritin)	Allergy to any antihistamines Narrow-angle glaucoma Asthma Stenosing peptic ulcer BPH or bladder neck obstruction	Headache, nervousness, dizziness, depression, edema, increased appetite	Instruct patients to take on empty stomach (1 h before or 2 h after meals or food). Instruct patients to avoid alcohol and to use caution if driving or performing tasks that require alertness. Suggest sucking on sugarless lozenges or ice chips for relief of dry mouth. Recommend use of humidifier.
Fexofenadine (Allegra)	Allergy to any antihistamines Pregnancy Lactation Use with caution with hepatic or renal impairment and in elderly patients	Fatigue, drowsiness, GI upset	Should not be administered within 15 min of ingestion of antacids. Instruct patients to use caution if driving or performing tasks that require alertness. Recommend use of humidifier.

BPH = benign prostatic hyperplasia, CNS = central nervous system.

and tingling sensations. In addition to these symptoms, hoarseness, wheezing, hives, rash, erythema, and edema are noted. Any relationship between emotional problems or stress and the triggering of allergy symptoms is assessed.

Diagnosis

Nursing Diagnoses

Based on the assessment data, the patient's major nursing diagnoses may include the following:

- Ineffective breathing pattern related to allergic reaction
- Deficient knowledge about allergy and the recommended modifications in lifestyle and self-care practices
- Ineffective individual coping with chronicity of condition and need for environmental modifications

Collaborative Problems/ Potential Complications

Based on assessment data, potential complications may include the following:

- Anaphylaxis
- Impaired breathing
- Nonadherence to the therapeutic regimen

Planning and Goals

The goals for the patient may include restoration of normal breathing pattern, increased knowledge about the causes and control of allergic symptoms, improved coping with alterations and modifications, and absence of complications.

Nursing Interventions

Improving Breathing Pattern

The patient is instructed and assisted to modify the environment to reduce the severity of allergic symptoms or to prevent their occurrence. The patient is instructed to reduce exposure to people with upper respiratory tract infections. If an upper respiratory infection occurs, the patient is encouraged to take deep breaths and to cough frequently to ensure adequate gas exchange and prevent atelectasis. The patient is instructed to seek medical attention, because the presence of allergy symptoms along with an upper respiratory tract infection may compromise adequate lung function. Adherence to medication schedules and other treatment regimens is encouraged and reinforced.

Promoting Understanding of Allergy and Allergy Control

Instruction includes strategies to minimize exposure to allergens and explanation about desensitization procedures and correct use of medications. The nurse informs and reminds the patient of the importance of keeping appointments for desensitization procedures, because dosages are usually adjusted on a weekly basis, and missed appointments may interfere with the dosage adjustment.

Patients also need to understand that medications for allergy control should be used only when the allergy is apparent. This is usually on a seasonal basis. Continued use of medications when not required can cause an increased tolerance to the medication, with the result that the medication will not be effective when needed.

Coping With a Chronic Disorder

Although allergic reactions are infrequently life-threatening, they require constant vigilance to avoid allergens and modification of the lifestyle or environment to prevent recurrence of symptoms. Allergic symptoms are often present year-round and create discomfort and inconvenience for the patient. Although patients may not feel ill during allergy seasons, they often do not feel well either. The need to be alert for possible allergens in the environment may be tiresome, placing a burden on the patient's ability to lead a normal life. Stress related to these difficulties may in turn increase the frequency or severity of symptoms.

To assist the patient in adjusting to these modifications, the nurse must have an appreciation of the difficulties encountered by the patient. The patient is encouraged to verbalize feelings and concerns in a supportive environment and to identify strategies to deal with them effectively.

Monitoring and Managing Potential Complications

ANAPHYLAXIS AND IMPAIRED BREATHING

Respiratory and cardiovascular functioning can be significantly altered during allergic reactions by the reaction itself or by the medications used to treat reactions. The respiratory status is evaluated by monitoring the respiratory rate and pattern and by assessing for breathing difficulties or abnormal lung sounds. The pulse rate and rhythm and blood pressure are monitored to assess cardiovascular status regularly or any time the patient reports symptoms such as itching or difficulty breathing. In the event of signs and symptoms suggestive of anaphylaxis, emergency medications and equipment must be available for immediate use.

NONADHERENCE TO THE THERAPEUTIC REGIMEN

Knowing about the treatment regimen does not ensure adherence. Having the patient identify potential barriers and explore acceptable solutions for effective management of the condition (eg, installing tile floors rather than carpet, not gardening in the spring) can increase adherence to the treatment regimen.

Promoting Home and Community-Based Care

TEACHING PATIENTS SELF-CARE

The patient is instructed about strategies to minimize exposure to allergens, the actions and adverse effects of medications, and the correct use of medications. The patient should know the name, dose, frequency, actions, and side effects of all medications taken.

Instruction about strategies to control allergic symptoms is based on the needs of the patient as determined by the results of tests, the severity of symptoms, and the motivation of the patient and family to deal with the condition. Suggestions for patients who are sensitive to dust and mold in the home are given in Chart 53-6. Additional nursing interventions for allergy management are presented in Chart 53-7.

If the patient is to undergo immunotherapy, the nurse reinforces the physician's explanation regarding the purpose and procedure. Instructions are given regarding the series of injections, which usually are administered initially every week and then at 2- to 4-week intervals. These instructions include remaining in the physician's office or the clinic for at least 30 minutes after the injection so that emergency treatment may be given if the patient has a reaction; avoiding rubbing or scratching the injection site; and continuing with the series for the period of time required. In addition, the patient and family are instructed about emergency treatment of severe allergic symptoms.

Because antihistamines may produce drowsiness, the patient is cautioned about this and other side effects of the particular medication. Operating machinery, driving a car, and performing activities that require intense concentration should be postponed. The patient is also informed about the dangers of drinking alcohol when taking these medications, because they tend to exaggerate the effects of alcohol.

The patient must be aware of the effects caused by overuse of the sympathomimetic agents in nose drops or sprays. A condition referred to as rhinitis medicamentosa may result (Fig. 53-6). After topical application of the medication, a rebound period occurs in which the nasal mucous membranes become more edematous and congested than they were before the medication was used. Such a reaction encourages the

CHART 53-6

HOME CARE CHECKLIST • Allergy Management

At the completion of the home care instruction, the patient or caregiver will be able to:	Patient	Caregiver
• Verbalize how to maintain a dust-free environment by removing drapes, curtains, and venetian blinds and replacing them with pull shades; covering the mattress with a hypo-allergenic cover that can be zipped; and removing rugs and replacing them with wood flooring or linoleum.	✔	✔
• Identify rationale for washing the floor and dusting and vacuuming daily.	✔	✔
• Identify rationale for replacing stuffed furniture with wood pieces that can easily be dusted.	✔	✔
• State rationale for wearing a mask whenever cleaning is being done.	✔	✔
• Identify rationale for avoiding use of tufted bedspreads, stuffed toys, and feather pillows and replacing them with washable cotton material.	✔	✔
• State rationale for avoiding the use of any clothing that causes itching.	✔	✔
• Verbalize ways to reduce dust in the house as a whole by using steam or hot water for heating rather than air and using air filters or air conditioning.	✔	✔
• Verbalize ways to reduce exposure to pollens or molds by identifying seasons of the year when pollen counts are high; wearing a mask at times of increased exposure (windy days and when grass is being cut); and avoiding contact with weeds, dry leaves, and freshly cut grass.	✔	✔
• State rationale for seeking air-conditioned areas at the height of the allergy season.	✔	✔
• State rationale for avoiding sprays and perfumes.	✔	✔
• State rationale for use of hypoallergenic cosmetics.	✔	✔
• State rationale for taking prescribed medications as ordered.	✔	✔
• Identify specific foods that may cause allergic symptoms. (Examples of foods that can cause allergic reactions are fish, nuts, eggs, and chocolate.)	✔	✔
• Develop a list of foods to avoid.	✔	✔

CHART 53-7

Selected Nursing Strategies for Allergy Management

- Identify the patient's known allergens (eg, medications, foods, insects, environmental allergens).
- Describe the patient's typical allergic reaction and its severity.
- Document the patient's allergies (eg, medications, foods, insects, environmental allergens) in the patient's medical record.
- Post allergy alerts appropriately.
- Encourage the patient to wear a medical alert band and to carry information about allergies at all times.
- Monitor the patient closely after administration of new medications and exposure to new foods, contrast agents, latex, and other allergens.
- Investigate potential for allergic reactions with all new medications through consultation with the pharmacist.
- Instruct the patient to question all medications and new foods.
- Identify early manifestations of allergic reactions.
- Administer emergency treatment for allergic reactions.
- Monitor the patient's response and status for 24 hours after a severe allergic reaction.
- Instruct the patient and family about emergency home management of allergic reaction.
- Instruct the patient and family about avoidance measures to reduce risk of exposure to allergens.

use of more medication, and a cyclic pattern results. The topical agent must be discontinued immediately and completely to correct this problem.

CONTINUING CARE

Follow-up telephone calls to the patient are often reassuring to the patient and family and provide an opportunity for the nurse to answer any questions. The patient is reminded to keep follow-up appointments and is informed about the importance of continuing with treatment. The importance of participating in health promotion activities and health screening is also emphasized.

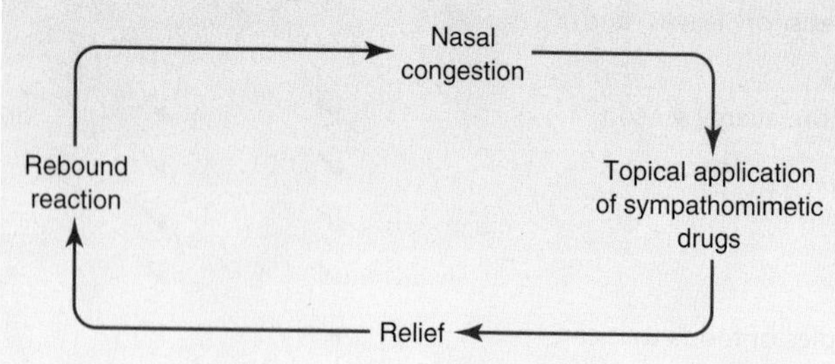

FIGURE 53-6. Rhinitis medicamentosa. This cyclic pattern results from overuse of sympathomimetic nose drops or sprays.

Evaluation

Expected Patient Outcomes

Expected patient outcomes may include the following:

1. Exhibits normal breathing patterns
   a. Demonstrates lungs clear on auscultation
   b. Exhibits absence of adventitious breath sounds (crackles, rhonchi, wheezing)
   c. Has a normal respiratory rate and pattern
   d. Reports no complaints of respiratory distress (shortness of breath, difficulty on inspiration or expiration)
2. Demonstrates knowledge about allergy and strategies to control symptoms
   a. Identifies causative allergens, if known
   b. States methods of avoiding allergens and controlling indoor and outdoor precipitating factors
   c. Removes from the environment items that retain dust
   d. Wears a dampened mask if dust or mold may be a problem
   e. Avoids smoke-filled rooms and dust-filled or freshly sprayed areas
   f. Uses air conditioning for a major part of the day
   g. Takes antihistamines as prescribed; participates in hyposensitization program, if applicable
   h. Describes name, purpose, side effects, and method of administration of prescribed medications
   i. Identifies when to seek immediate medical attention for severe allergic responses
   j. Describes activities that are possible, including ways to participate in activities without activating the allergies
3. Experiences relief of discomfort while adapting to the inconveniences of an allergy
   a. Relates the emotional aspects of the allergic response
   b. Demonstrates use of measures to cope positively with allergy
4. Demonstrates absence of complications
   a. Exhibits vital signs within normal limits
   b. Reports no symptoms or episodes of anaphylaxis (urticaria, itching, peripheral tingling, fullness in the mouth and throat, flushing, difficulty swallowing) or coughing, wheezing, or difficulty breathing
   c. Demonstrates correct procedure to self-administer emergency medications to treat severe allergic reaction
   d. Correctly states medication names, dose and frequency of administration, and medication actions
   e. Correctly identifies side effects and untoward signs and symptoms to report to physician
   f. Discusses acceptable lifestyle changes and solutions for identified potential barriers to adherence to treatment and medication regimen

Contact Dermatitis

Contact dermatitis, a type IV delayed hypersensitivity reaction, is an acute or chronic skin inflammation that results from direct skin contact with chemicals or allergens. There are four basic types: allergic, irritant, phototoxic, and photoallergic (Table 53-4). Eighty percent of cases are caused by excessive exposure to or additive effects of irritants (eg, soaps, detergents, organic solvents). Skin sensitivity may develop after brief or prolonged periods of exposure, and the clinical picture may appear hours or weeks after the sensitized skin has been exposed.

Clinical Manifestations

Symptoms include itching, burning, erythema, skin lesions (vesicles), and edema, followed by weeping, crusting, and finally drying and peeling of the skin. In severe responses, hemorrhagic bullae may develop. Repeated reactions may be accompanied by thickening of the skin and pigmentary changes. Secondary invasion by bacteria may develop in skin that is abraded by rubbing or scratching. Usually, there are no systemic symptoms unless the eruption is widespread.

Assessment and Diagnostic Findings

The location of the skin eruption and the history of exposure aid in determining the condition. However, in cases of obscure irritants or an unobservant patient, the diagnosis can be extremely difficult, often involving many trial-and-error procedures before the cause is determined. Patch tests on the skin with suspected offending agents may clarify the diagnosis.

Atopic Dermatitis

Atopic dermatitis is a type I immediate hypersensitivity disorder characterized by inflammation and hyperreactivity of the skin. Other terms used to describe this skin disorder include atopic eczema, atopic dermatitis/eczema, and atopic dermatitis/eczema syndrome (AEDS). In a revised classification system developed to clarify terminology, AEDS includes both allergic and nonallergic disorders. Allergic AEDS can be further classified as IgE-associated AEDS or non-IgE–associated AEDS (Johansson & Bieber, 2002). The term atopic dermatitis is currently the most commonly used of these terms and is used in the following discussion.

TABLE 53-4 Types, Testing, and Treatment of Contact Dermatitis

Type	Etiology	Clinical Presentation	Diagnostic Testing	Treatment
Allergic	Results from contact of skin and allergenic substance. Has a sensitization period of 10–14 days.	Vasodilation and perivascular infiltrates on the dermis Intracellular edema Usually seen on dorsal aspects of hand	Patch testing (contraindicated in acute, widespread dermatitis)	Avoidance of offending material Burow's solution or cool water compress Systemic corticosteroids (prednisone) for 7–10 days Topical corticosteroids for mild cases Oral antihistamines to relieve pruritus
Irritant	Results from contact with a substance that chemically or physically damages the skin on a nonimmunologic basis. Occurs after first exposure to irritant or repeated exposures to milder irritants over an extended time.	Dryness lasting days to months Vesiculation, fissures, cracks Hands and lower arms most common areas	Clinical picture Appropriate negative patch tests	Identification and removal of source of irritation Application of hydrophilic cream or petrolatum to soothe and protect Topical corticosteroids and compresses for weeping lesions Antibiotics for infection and oral antihistamines for pruritus
Phototoxic	Resembles the irritant type but requires sun and a chemical in combination to damage the epidermis.	Similar to irritant dermatitis	Photopatch test	Same as for allergic and irritant dermatitis
Photoallergic	Resembles allergic dermatitis but requires light exposure in addition to allergen contact to produce immunologic reactivity.	Similar to allergic dermatitis	Photopatch test	Same as for allergic and irritant dermatitis

Atopic dermatitis affects 15% to 20% of children and 1% to 3% of adults in developed countries (Ashcroft, Dimmock, Garside, et al., 2005). Most patients have significant elevations of serum IgE and peripheral eosinophilia. Pruritus and hyperirritability of the skin are the most consistent features of atopic dermatitis and are related to large amounts of histamine in the skin. Excessive dryness of the skin with resultant itching is related to changes in lipid content, sebaceous gland activity, and sweating. In response to stroking of the skin, immediate redness appears on the skin and is followed in 15 to 30 seconds by pallor, which persists for 1 to 3 minutes. Lesions develop secondary to the trauma of scratching and appear in areas of increased sweating and hypervascularity. Atopic dermatitis is chronic, with remissions and exacerbations. This condition has a tendency to recur, with remission from adolescence to age 20.

It is important to note that atopic dermatitis is often the first step in a process that leads to asthma and allergic rhinitis. It is the result of interactions between susceptibility genes, the environment, defective function of the skin barrier, and immunologic responses.

Medical Management

Treatment of patients with atopic dermatitis must be individualized. Guidelines for treatment include decreasing itching and scratching by wearing cotton fabrics, washing with a mild detergent, humidifying dry heat in winter, maintaining room temperature at 20°C to 22.2°C (68°F to 72°F), using antihistamines such as diphenhydramine (Benadryl), and avoiding animals, dust, sprays, and perfumes. Keeping the skin moisturized with daily baths to hydrate the skin and the use of topical skin moisturizers is encouraged. Topical corticosteroids are used to prevent inflammation, and any infection is treated with antibiotics to eliminate *Staphylococcus aureus* when indicated. Use of immunosuppressive agents, such as cyclosporine (Neoral, Sandimmune), tacrolimus (Prograf, Protopic), and pimecrolimus (Elidel), may be effective in inhibiting T cells and mast cells involved in atopic dermatitis (Leung, Boguniewicz & Howell, 2004). Research is needed to assess the effectiveness and the adverse side effects of medications used to treat atopic dermatitis (Ashcroft et al., 2005).

Nursing Management

Patients who experience atopic dermatitis and their families require assistance and support from the nurse to cope with the disorder. The symptoms are often disturbing to the patient and disruptive to the family. The appearance of the skin may affect the patient's self-esteem and his or her willingness to interact with others. Instructions and counseling about strategies to incorporate preventive measures and treatments into the lifestyle of the family may be helpful.

The patient and family need to be aware of signs of secondary infection and of the need to seek treatment if infection occurs. The nurse also teaches the patient and family about the side effects of medications used in treatment.

To avoid the risk of developing eczema vaccinatum, patients and close contacts of patients with atopic dermatitis should be cautioned to avoid vaccination with smallpox or contact with someone who has recently received smallpox vaccination. Eczema vaccinatum is a localized or generalized cutaneous dissemination of vaccinia virus. Although this illness is usually mild and self-limited, it can be severe or fatal (Naleway, Belongia, Greenless, et al., 2003).

Dermatitis Medicamentosa (Drug Reactions)

Dermatitis medicamentosa, a type I hypersensitivity disorder, is the term applied to skin rashes associated with certain medications. Although people react differently to each medication, certain medications tend to induce eruptions of similar types. Rashes are among the most common adverse reactions to medications and occur in approximately 2% to 3% of hospitalized patients.

In general, drug reactions appear suddenly, have a particularly vivid color, manifest with characteristics that are more intense than the somewhat similar eruptions of infectious origin, and, with the exception of bromide and the iodide rashes, disappear rapidly after the medication is withdrawn. Rashes may be accompanied by systemic or generalized symptoms. On discovery of a medication allergy, patients are warned that they have a hypersensitivity to a particular medication and are advised not to take it again. Patients should carry information identifying the hypersensitivity with them at all times.

Skin eruptions related to medication therapy suggest more serious hypersensitivities. Frequent assessment and prompt reporting of the appearance of any eruptions are important so that early treatment can be initiated. Some cutaneous drug reactions may be associated with a clinical complex that involves other organs. These are known as complex drug reactions.

Urticaria and Angioneurotic Edema

Urticaria (hives) is a type I hypersensitive allergic reaction of the skin characterized by the sudden appearance of pinkish, edematous elevations that vary in size and shape, itch, and cause local discomfort. They may involve any part of the body, including the mucous membranes (especially those of the mouth), the larynx (occasionally with serious respiratory complications), and the gastrointestinal tract.

Each hive remains for a few minutes to several hours before disappearing. For hours or days, clusters of these lesions may come, go, and return episodically. If this sequence continues for longer than 6 weeks, the condition is called chronic urticaria.

Angioneurotic edema involves the deeper layers of the skin, resulting in more diffuse swelling rather than the discrete lesions characteristic of hives. On occasion, this reaction covers the entire back. The skin over the reaction may appear normal but often has a reddish hue. The skin does not pit on pressure, as ordinary edema does. The regions most often involved are the lips, eyelids, cheeks, hands, feet, genitalia, and tongue; the mucous membranes of the larynx, the bronchi, and the gastrointestinal canal may also be affected, particularly in the hereditary type (see discussion in the following section). Swellings may appear suddenly, in a few seconds or minutes, or slowly, in 1 or 2 hours. In the latter case, their appearance is often preceded by itching or burning sensations. Seldom does more than a single swelling appear at one time, although one may develop while another is disappearing. Infrequently, swelling recurs in the same region. Individual lesions usually last 24 to 36 hours. On rare occasions, swelling may recur with remarkable regularity at intervals of 3 to 4 weeks.

Hereditary Angioedema

Hereditary angioedema, although not an immunologic disorder in the usual sense, is included because of its resemblance to allergic angioedema and because of the potential seriousness of the condition. Symptoms are caused by edema of the skin, the respiratory tract, or the digestive tract. Attacks may be precipitated by trauma, or they may seem to occur spontaneously.

Clinical Manifestations

When skin is involved, the swelling usually is diffuse, does not itch, and usually is not accompanied by urticaria. Gastrointestinal edema may cause abdominal pain severe enough to suggest the need for surgery. Typically, attacks last 1 to 4 days and are harmless; however, attacks can occasionally affect the subcutaneous and submucosal tissues in the region of the upper airway and can be associated with respiratory obstruction and asphyxiation. This disorder is inherited as an autosomal dominant trait. Approximately 85% of patients with this disorder have one nonproductive gene, and the remaining 15% have a gene mutation (Parslow, Stites, Terr, et al., 2001).

Medical Management

Attacks usually subside within 3 to 4 days, but during this time the patient should be observed carefully for signs of laryngeal obstruction, which may necessitate tracheostomy as a life-saving measure. Epinephrine, antihistamines, and corticosteroids are usually used in treatment, but their success is limited.

Food Allergy

IgE-mediated food allergy, a type I hypersensitivity reaction, occurs in 6% to 8% of children and about 2% of the adult population (Beyer & Teuber, 2004); it is thought to occur in people who have a genetic predisposition combined with exposure to allergens early in life through the gastrointestinal or respiratory tract or nasal mucosa (Long, 2002). Researchers have also identified a second type of food allergy, a non-IgE–mediated food allergy syndrome in which T cells play a major role (Eigenmann & Frossard, 2003).

Almost any food can cause allergic symptoms. Any food can contain an allergen that results in anaphylaxis. The most common offenders are seafood (lobster, shrimp, crab, clams, fish), legumes (peanuts, peas, beans, licorice), seeds (sesame, cottonseed, caraway, mustard, flaxseed, sunflower seeds), tree nuts, berries, egg white, buckwheat, milk, and chocolate. Peanut and tree nut (eg, cashew, walnut) allergies are responsible for most severe food allergy reactions. In more than 70% of children with peanut allergy, symptoms develop at their first known exposure, suggesting unknown exposure through breast milk or another source (Al-Muhsen et al., 2003). Pregnant and breast-feeding women who are aware of a family history of allergy (mother, father, or a sibling of the unborn infant with asthma, eczema, hay fever, or other allergy) should avoid peanuts and peanut-containing foods during pregnancy as a precaution (Sheetz & McIntyre, 2005).

One of the dangers of food allergens is that they may be hidden in other foods and not apparent to people who are susceptible to the allergen. For example, peanuts and peanut butter are often used in salad dressings and Asian, African, and Mexican cooking and may result in severe allergic reactions, including anaphylaxis. Previous contamination of equipment with allergens (eg, peanuts) during preparation of another food product (eg, chocolate cake) is enough to produce anaphylaxis in people with severe allergy.

Clinical Manifestations

The clinical symptoms are classic allergic symptoms (urticaria, dermatitis, wheezing, cough, laryngeal edema, angioedema) and gastrointestinal symptoms (itching; swelling of lips, tongue, and palate; abdominal pain; nausea; cramps; vomiting; and diarrhea).

Assessment and Diagnostic Findings

A careful diagnostic workup is required in any patient with a suspected food hypersensitivity. Included are a detailed allergy history, a physical examination, and pertinent diagnostic tests. Skin testing is used to identify the source of symptoms and is useful in identifying specific foods as causative agents.

Medical Management

Therapy for food hypersensitivity includes elimination of the food responsible for the hypersensitivity (Chart 53-8). Pharmacologic therapy is necessary for patients who cannot avoid exposure to offending foods and for patients with multiple food sensitivities not responsive to avoidance measures. Medication therapy involves the use of H_1-blockers, antihistamines, adrenergic agents, corticosteroids, and cromolyn sodium. Another essential aspect of management is teaching patients and family members how to recognize and manage the early stages of an acute anaphylactic reaction. Many food allergies disappear with time, particularly in children. About one third of proven allergies disappear in 1 to 2 years if the patient carefully avoids the offending food. However, peanut allergy has been reported to persist throughout adulthood in some people (Beyer & Teuber, 2004).

CHART 53-8

HOME CARE CHECKLIST • Managing Food Allergies

At the completion of the home care instruction, the patient or caregiver will be able to:	Patient	Caregiver
• Verbalize understanding of the need to maintain an allergen-free diet.	✔	✔
• Demonstrate reading of food labels to identify hidden allergens in food.	✔	✔
• Identify ways to manage an allergen-free diet when eating away from home.	✔	✔
• State the need to wear a medical alert medallion or bracelet.	✔	✔
• List symptoms of food allergy.	✔	✔
• Demonstrate emergency administration of epinephrine.	✔	✔
• State the importance of replacing epinephrine when outdated.	✔	✔
• State the importance of prompt treatment of allergic reactions and health care follow-up.	✔	✔

Nursing Management

In addition to participating in management of the allergic reaction, the nurse focuses on preventing future exposure of the patient to the food allergen. If a severe allergic or anaphylactic reaction to food allergens has occurred, the nurse must instruct the patient and family about strategies to prevent its recurrence. The patient is instructed about the importance of carefully assessing foods prepared by others for obvious as well as hidden sources of food allergens and of avoiding locations and facilities where those allergens are likely to be present. This includes careful reading of food labels and monitoring the preparation of food by others to be sure that exposure to even minute amounts of allergenic foods is avoided. The patient and family must be knowledgeable about early signs and symptoms of allergic reactions and must be proficient in emergency administration of epinephrine if a reaction occurs. The nurse also advises the patient to wear a medical alert bracelet or to carry identification and emergency equipment at all times. Patients' food allergies should be noted on their medical records, because there may be risk of allergic reactions not only to food but also to some medications containing similar substances (Karch & Karch, 2003). Pregnant women and those who are breastfeeding are instructed to avoid eating peanuts or food containing peanuts to minimize the risk of peanut allergy in their children (Sheetz & McIntyre, 2005).

Serum Sickness

Serum sickness is an immune-complex type III hypersensitivity. It has traditionally resulted from the administration of therapeutic antisera of animal sources for the treatment or prevention of infectious diseases such as tetanus, pneumonia, rabies, diphtheria, botulism, and venomous snake and black widow spider bites. With the advent of human antitetanus serum and antibiotics, classic serum sickness is much less common now. However, various medications (primarily penicillin) may cause a serum sickness–like reaction similar to that caused by foreign sera.

The introduction of monoclonal and polyclonal antibody therapy to treat a variety of immunologic disorders necessitates increased surveillance for serum sickness with their use.

Clinical Manifestations

Symptoms are caused by a reaction and immunologic attack on the serum or medication. Antibodies appear to be of the IgE and IgM classes. Early manifestations, beginning 6 to 10 days after administration of the medication, include an inflammatory reaction at the site of injection of the medication, followed by regional and generalized lymphadenopathy and fever. There is usually a skin rash, which may be urticarial or purpuric. Joints are frequently tender and swollen. Vasculitis may occur in any organ but is most commonly observed in the kidney, resulting in proteinuria and, occasionally, casts in the urine and renal dysfunction (Tanriover, Chuang, Fishbach, et al., 2005). There may be mild to severe cardiac involvement. Peripheral neuritis may cause temporary paralysis of the upper extremities or may be widespread, causing Guillain-Barré syndrome.

Medical Management

The usual course lasts for several days to a few weeks if untreated, but the patient responds promptly and completely if treated with antihistamines and corticosteroids. Aggressive therapy, including ventilator support, may be necessary if peripheral neuritis and Guillain-Barré syndrome occur. Use of therapeutic plasma exchange to treat patients with serum sickness in the renal transplant population has been reported (Tanriover et al., 2005).

Nursing Management

See Chapter 64 for nursing management of Guillain-Barré syndrome.

Latex Allergy

Latex allergy, the allergic reaction to natural rubber proteins, has been implicated in rhinitis, conjunctivitis, contact dermatitis, urticaria, asthma, and anaphylaxis. Latex allergy and hypersensitivity were first reported in 1927. The current prevalence of latex allergy is unknown. However, from 1989 until the mid-1990s the number of cases steadily increased (Ranta & Ownby, 2004), and since that time, the prevalence has been steadily declining, possibly because of the use of nonpowdered latex and latex-free gloves. Although it is widely held that the increase in latex allergy among health care professionals was caused by the implementation of universal or standard precautions, a recent study did not support this idea (McCall, Horwitz & Kammeyer-Mueller, 2003).

Natural rubber latex is derived from the sap of the rubber tree (*Hevea brasiliensis*). The conversion of the liquid rubber latex into a finished product entails the addition of more than 200 chemicals. The proteins in the natural rubber latex (Hevea proteins) or the various chemicals that are used in the manufacturing process are thought to be the source of the allergic reactions. Not all objects composed of latex have the same ability to stimulate an allergic response. For example, the antigenicity of latex gloves can vary widely depending on the manufacturing method used.

Populations at risk include health care workers, patients with atopic allergies or multiple surgeries, people working in factories that manufacture latex products, females, and patients with spina bifida. Because more food handlers, hairdressers, auto mechanics, and police are now wearing latex gloves, they may also be at risk for latex allergy. It is estimated that 1% to 3% of the general population have an allergy to latex and that about 3% to 12% of health care workers are sensitized (Ranta & Ownby, 2004). Patients are at risk for anaphylactic reactions due to contact with latex during medical treatments, especially surgical procedures. Latex is the second most common cause of anaphylactic reactions during the intraoperative period, preceded only by muscle relaxants (Hebl, Hall & Sprung, 2004).

Food that has been handled by people wearing latex gloves may stimulate an allergic response. Cross-reactions have been reported in people who are allergic to certain food products, such as kiwis, bananas, pineapples, mangos, passion fruit, avocados, and chestnuts (Hepner & Castells, 2003a).

Routes of exposure to latex products can be cutaneous, percutaneous, mucosal, parenteral, or aerosol. Allergic reactions are more likely with parenteral or mucous membrane exposure but can also occur with cutaneous contact or inhalation (Hepner & Castells, 2003a). The most frequent source of exposure is cutaneous, which usually involves the wearing of natural latex gloves. The powder used to facilitate putting on latex gloves can become a carrier of latex proteins from the gloves; when the gloves are put on or removed, the particles become airborne and can be inhaled or settle on skin, mucous membranes, or clothing. Mucosal exposure can occur from the use of latex condoms, catheters, airways, and nipples. Parenteral exposure can occur from IV lines or hemodialysis equipment. In addition to latex-derived medical devices, many household items also contain latex. Examples of medical and household items containing latex and a list of alternative products are found in Table 53-5. It is estimated that more than 40,000 medical devices and nonmedical products contain latex. Although non-latex gloves and other items have a low potential to stimulate an allergic response, chemical additives used in their manufacture have been associated with allergic symptoms (Yip & Roman, 2003).

Clinical Manifestations

Several different types of reactions to latex are possible (Table 53-6). Irritant contact dermatitis, a nonimmunologic response, may be caused by mechanical skin irritation or an alkaline pH associated with latex gloves. Common symptoms of irritant dermatitis include erythema and pruritus. These symptoms can be eliminated by changing glove brands or by using powder-free gloves. Use of hand lotion before donning latex gloves can worsen the symptoms, because lotions may leach latex proteins from the gloves, increasing skin exposure and the risk of developing true allergic reactions (Yip & Roman, 2003).

Delayed hypersensitivity to latex, a type IV reaction mediated by T cells in the immune system, is localized to the area of exposure and is characterized by symptoms of contact dermatitis, including vesicular skin lesions, papules, pruritus, edema, erythema, and crusting and thickening of the skin. These symptoms usually appear on the back of the hands. This reaction is thought to be caused by chemicals that are used in the manufacturing of latex products. It is the most common allergic reaction to latex. Although not usually life-threatening, delayed hypersensitivity reactions often require major changes in the patient's home and work environment to avoid further exposure. People who are sensitized to latex are at increased risk for development of type I allergic reactions (Hepner & Castells, 2000b).

Immediate hypersensitivity, a type I allergic reaction, is mediated by the IgE mast cell system. Symptoms can include rhinitis, conjunctivitis, asthma, and anaphylaxis. The term "latex allergy" is usually used to describe the type I reaction. Clinical manifestations have a rapid onset and can include urticaria, wheezing, dyspnea, laryngeal edema, bronchospasm, tachycardia, angioedema, hypotension, and cardiac arrest.

Localized itching, erythema, or local urticaria within minutes after exposure to latex are often the initial symptoms. Symptoms of subsequent reactions can include generalized urticaria, angioedema, rhinitis, conjunctivitis, asthma, and anaphylactic shock minutes after dermal or mucosal exposure to latex. An increasing number of people who are allergic to latex experience severe reactions characterized by generalized urticaria, bronchospasm, and hypotension (Association of Perioperative Registered Nurses, 2004).

Assessment and Diagnostic Findings

The diagnosis of latex allergy is based on the history and diagnostic test results (Hepner & Castells, 2000b). Sensitization is detected by skin testing, RAST, or ELISA. Skin tests have been unreliable because of variability in the techniques used; however, a new standardized skin testing reagent is expected to be available in the near future. Skin

TABLE 53-5 Selected Products Containing Natural Rubber Latex and Latex-Free Alternatives

Products Containing Latex	Examples of Latex-Safe Alternatives*
Hospital Environment	
Ace bandage (brown)	Ace bandage, white all cotton
Adhesive bandages, Band-Aid dressing, Telfa	Cotton pads and plastic or silk tape, Active Strip (3M), Duoderm
Anesthesia equipment	Neoprene anesthesia kit (King)
Blood pressure cuff, tubing, and bladder	Clean Cuff, single-use nylon or vinyl blood pressure cuffs or wrap with stockinette or apply over clothing
Catheters	All-silicone or vinyl catheters
Catheter leg bag straps	Velcro straps
Crutch axillary pads and hand grips, tips	Cover with cloth, tape
ECG pads	Baxter, Red Dot 3M ECG pads
Elastic compression stockings	Kendall SCD stockings with stockinette
Gloves	Dermaprene, Neoprene, polymer, or vinyl gloves
IV catheters	Jelko, Deseret IV catheters
IV rubber injection ports	Cover Y-sites and ports; do not puncture. Use three-way stopcocks on plastic tubing.
Levin tube	Salem sump tube
Medication vials	Remove rubber stopper.
Penrose drains	Jackson-Pratt, Zimmer hemovac drains
Prepackaged enema kits	Theravac, Fleet Ready-to-use
Pulse oximeters	Nonin oximeters
Resuscitation bags	Laerdal, Puritan Bennett, *certain* Ambu
Stethoscope tubing	PVC tubing; cover with latex-free stockinette
Syringes—single use (Monoject, B & D)	Terumo syringes, Abbott PCA Abboject
Suction tubing	PVC (Davol, Laerdal)
Tapes	Dermicel, Micropore
Thermometer probes	Diatec probe covers
Tourniquets	X-Tourn straps (Avcor)
Theraband	New Thera-band Exercisers, plastic tubing
Home Environment	
Balloons	Mylar balloons
Diapers, incontinence pads	Huggies, Always, *some* Attends
Condoms, diaphragms	Polyurethane products, Durex/Avanti and Reality products (female condom)
Feminine hygiene pad	Kimberly-Clark products
Wheelchair cushions	ROHO cushions, Sof Care bed/chair cushions

*Confirmation is essential to verify that all items are latex-free before using, especially if risk of latex allergy is present.

tests should be performed only by clinicians who have expertise in their administration and interpretation and who have the necessary equipment available to treat local or systemic allergic reactions to the reagent. Nasal challenge and dipstick tests may be useful in the future as screening tests for latex allergy.

Medical Management

The best treatment available for latex allergy is the avoidance of latex-based products, but this is often difficult because of their widespread use. Patients who have experienced an anaphylactic reaction to latex should be instructed to wear medical identification. Antihistamines and an emergency kit containing epinephrine should be provided to these patients, along with instructions about emergency management of latex allergy symptoms. Patients should be counseled to notify all health care workers as well as local paramedic and ambulance companies about their allergy. Warning labels can be attached to car windows to alert police and paramedics about the driver's or passenger's latex allergy in case of a motor vehicle crash. People with latex allergy should be provided with a list of alternative products and referred to local support groups; they are also urged to carry their own supply of nonlatex gloves.

People with type I latex sensitivity may be unable to continue to work if a latex-free work environment is not possible. This may occur with surgeons, dentists, operating room personnel, or intensive care nurses. Occupational implications for employees with type IV latex sensitivity are usually easier to manage by changing to nonlatex gloves and avoiding direct contact with latex-based medical equipment. Although latex-specific immunotherapy has been attempted, this method of treatment remains experimental.

Nursing Management

The nurse can assume a pivotal role in the management of latex allergies in both patients and staff. All patients should be asked about latex allergy, although special attention should be given to those at particularly high risk (eg, patients with spina bifida, patients who have undergone multiple

TABLE 53-6 Types of Reactions to Latex

Type of Reaction	Cause	Signs/Symptoms	Treatment
Irritant contact dermatitis	Damage to skin because of irritation and loss of epidermoid skin layer; not an allergic reaction. Can be caused by excessive use of soaps and cleansers, multiple handwashings, inadequate hand drying, mechanical irritation (eg, sweating, rubbing inside powdered gloves), exposure to chemicals added during the manufacturing of gloves, and alkaline pH of powdered gloves. Reaction may occur with first exposure, is usually benign, and is not life-threatening.	Acute: redness, edema, burning, discomfort, itching Chronic: dry, thickened, cracked skin	Referral for diagnostic testing Avoidance of exposure to irritant Thorough washing and drying of hands Use of powder-free gloves with more frequent changes of gloves Changing glove types Use of water- or silicone-based moisturizing creams, lotions, or topical barrier agents Avoidance of oil- or petroleum-based skin agents with latex products, because they cause breakdown of the latex product
Allergic contact dermatitis	Delayed hypersensitivity (type IV) reaction. Usually affects only area in contact with latex; reaction is usually to chemical additives used in the manufacturing process rather than to latex itself. Cause of reaction is T cell–mediated sensitization to additives of latex. Reaction is not life-threatening and is far more common than a type I reaction. Slow onset; occurs 18 to 24 hours after exposure. Resolves within 3 to 4 days after exposure. More severe reactions may occur with subsequent exposures.	Pruritus, erythema, swelling, crusty thickened skin, blisters, other skin lesions	Referral for diagnosis (patch tests) and treatment Thorough washing and drying of hands Use of water- or silicone-based moisturizing creams, lotions, or topical barrier agents Avoidance of oil- or petroleum-based products unless they are latex compatible Avoidance of identified causative agent, because continued exposure to latex products in presence of breaks in skin may contribute to latex protein sensitization
Latex allergy	Type I IgE-mediated immediate hypersensitivity to plant proteins in natural rubber latex. In sensitized people, anti-latex IgE antibody stimulates mast cell proliferation and basophil histamine release. Exposure can be through contact with the skin, mucous membranes, or internal tissues, or through inhalation of traces of powder from latex gloves. Severe reactions usually occur shortly after parenteral or mucous membrane exposure. People with any type I reaction to latex are at high risk of anaphylaxis. Local swelling, redness, edema, itching, and systemic reactions, including anaphylaxis, occur within minutes after exposure.	Rhinitis, flushing, conjunctivitis, urticaria, laryngeal edema, bronchospasm, asthma, severe vasodilation angioedema, anaphylaxis, cardiovascular collapse, death	Immediate treatment of reaction with epinephrine, fluids, vasopressors, and corticosteroids, and airway and ventilator support, with close monitoring for recurrence for next 12 to 14 hours Prompt referral for diagnostic evaluation Treatment and diagnostic evaluation in latex-free environment Strict avoidance of allergy testing and management Assessment of all patients for symptoms of latex allergy Teaching of patients and family members about the disorder and about the importance of preventing future reactions by avoiding latex Encouraging wearing of a medical alert bracelet that identifies latex allergy for emergency situations and carrying an EpiPen at all times and being prepared and able to use it

surgical procedures). Every time an invasive procedure must be performed, the nurse should consider the possibility of latex allergies. Nurses working in operating rooms, intensive care units, short procedure units, and emergency departments need to pay particular attention to latex allergy. See Chapter 18 for a latex allergy screening form.

Although the type I reaction is the most significant of the reactions to latex, care must be taken in the presence of irritant contact dermatitis and delayed hypersensitivity reaction to avoid further exposure of the person to latex. Patients with latex allergy are advised to notify their health care providers and to wear a medical information bracelet.

Patients must become knowledgeable about what products contain latex and what products are safe, nonlatex alternatives. They must also become knowledgeable about signs and symptoms of latex allergy and emergency treatment and self-injection of epinephrine in case of allergic reaction.

Nurses can be instrumental in establishing and participating in multidisciplinary committees to address latex allergy and to promote a latex-free environment. Latex allergy protocols and education of staff about latex allergy and precautions are important strategies to reduce this growing problem and to ensure assessment and prompt treatment of affected people.

Critical Thinking Exercises

1 ebp A 17-year-old woman has developed symptoms of asthma thought to be an allergic response to allergens in her environment. Develop an evidence-based plan for avoidance strategies for her while she is living at home and for her move next year to a college dormitory. Describe the strength of the evidence and criteria used to assess its strength. What instructional strategies and outcome measures will you use to educate her about avoidance strategies and to assess the effectiveness of their use?

2 A 35-year-old home health aide has developed symptoms of severe latex allergy. She is to receive instructions about self-administration of epinephrine if she experiences anaphylaxis. Develop a teaching plan for her and identify outcomes to measure the effectiveness of your teaching. Given her allergy to latex and the nature of her occupation, what other teaching or counseling is needed for her?

3 A 72-year-old man is admitted for emergency surgery to treat a strangulated hernia. He reports that he has severe allergies but is unable to be specific about the nature of his allergies or the allergic reactions that he has experienced in the past. He reports that he has had to use emergency epinephrine on several occasions in the past because of severe allergic reactions. What precautions are needed preoperatively, intraoperatively, and postoperatively for this patient to prevent the occurrence of severe allergic reactions? What interventions and nursing management would be indicated if he developed a severe allergic reaction?

REFERENCES AND SELECTED READINGS

BOOKS

Abbas, A. K. & Lichtman, A. H. (2004). *Basic immunology: Functions and disorders of the immune system*. Philadelphia: W. B. Saunders.

Adkinson, N. F., Yunginger, J. W., Busse, W., et al. (Eds.). (2003). *Middleton's allergy: Principles and practice*. St. Louis: C. V. Mosby.

Buttaro, T. M., Trybulski, J., Bailey, P. P. & Sandberg-Cook, J. (2003). *Primary care: A collaborative practice*. St. Louis: Mosby.

Dochterman, J. M. & Bulechek, G. M. (2004). *Nursing interventions and classification (NIC)*. St. Louis: Mosby.

Gershwin, M. E. & Naguwa, S. M. (2005). *Allergy and immunology secrets*. Philadelphia: Elsevier-Mosby.

Karch, A. M. (2005). *Lippincott's nursing drug guide*. Philadelphia: Lippincott Williams & Wilkins.

Parslow, T. G., Stites, D. P., Terr, A. I., & Imboden, J. B. (2001). *Medical immunology*. New York: McGraw-Hill.

Porth, C. M. (2005). *Pathophysiology: Concepts of altered health states* (7th ed.). Philadelphia: Lippincott Williams & Wilkins.

Rabson, A., Roitt, I. M. & Delves, P. J. (2005). *Really essential medical immunology*. Malden, MA; Blackwell.

U.S. Department of Health and Human Services. (2003). *Airborne allergens: Something in the air*. NIH Publication No. 03-7045. Bethesda, MD: U.S. Department of Health and Human Services.

U.S. Department of Health and Human Services. (2004). *Food allergy: An overview*. NIH Publication No. 04-5518. Bethesda, MD: U.S. Department of Health and Human Services.

JOURNALS

Asterisks indicate nursing research articles.

Al-Muhsen, S., Clarke, A. E. & Kagan, R. S. (2003). Peanut allergy: An overview. *CMAJ: Canadian Medical Association Journal, 168*(10), 1279–1285.

Ashcroft, D. M., Dimmock, P., Garside, R., et al. (2005). Efficacy and tolerability of topical pimecrolimus and tacrolimus in the treatment of atopic dermatitis: Meta-analysis of randomised controlled trials. *British Medical Journal, 330*(7490), 516.

Association of Perioperative Registered Nurses. (2004). AORN latex guideline. *AORN Journal, 79*(3), 653–672.

Beltrani, V. S. (2005). Suggestions regarding a more appropriate understanding of atopic dermatitis. *Current Opinion in Allergy and Clinical Immunology, 5*(5), 413–418.

Beyer, K. & Teuber, S. (2004). The mechanism of food allergy: What do we know today? *Current Opinion in Allergy and Clinical Immunology, 4*(3), 197–199.

Chatzi, L., Prokopakis, E., Tzanakis, N., et al. (2005). Allergic rhinitis, asthma, and atopy among grape farmers in a rural population in Crete, Greece. *Chest, 127*(1), 372–378.

Clinton, G. J. (2005). Multiple-chemical sensitivity. *MedSurg Nursing, 14*(6), 365–369.

*Dobson, P., Boyle, M. & Loewenthal, M. (2004). Home intravenous antibiotic therapy and allergic drug reactions: Is there a case for routine supply of anaphylaxis kits? *Journal of Infusion Nursing, 27*(6), 425–430.

Eigenmann, P. A. & Frossard, C. P. (2003). The T lymphocyte in food-allergy disorders. *Current Opinion in Allergy and Clinical Immunology, 3*(3), 199–203.

Finegold, I. (2002). Is immunotherapy effective in allergic disease? *Current Opinion in Allergy and Clinical Immunology, 2*(6), 537–540.

Gendo, K. & Larson, E. B. (2004). Evidence-based diagnostic strategies for evaluating suspected allergic rhinitis. *Annals of Internal Medicine, 140*(4), 278–289.

Gibson, L. E. (2005). Atopic dermatitis. *Mayo Clinical Proceedings, 80*(1), 107.

Gruchalla, R. S. (2004). Immunotherapy in allergy to insect stings in children. *New England Journal of Medicine, 351*(7), 707–709.

Gruchalla, R. S. & Pirmohamed, M. (2006). Clinical practice: Antibiotic allergy. *New England Journal of Medicine, 354*(6), 601–609.

Hebl, J. R., Hall, B. A. & Sprung, J. (2004). Prolonged cardiovascular collapse due to unrecognized latex anaphylaxis. *Anesthesia and Analgesia, 98*(4), 1124–1126.

Hepner, D. L. & Castells, M. C. (2003a). Anaphylaxis during the perioperative period. *Anesthesia and Analgesia, 97*(5), 1381–1395.

Hepner, D. L. & Castells, M. C. (2003b). Latex allergy: An update. *Anesthesia and Analgesia, 96*(4), 1219–1229.

Holgate, S. T. & Lack, G. (2005). Improving the management of atopic disease. *Archives of Disease in Childhood, 90*(8), 826–831.

Hu, W., Kemp, A. & Kerridge, I. (2004). Making clinical decisions when the stakes are high and the evidence unclear. *British Medical Journal, 329*(7470), 852–854.

Huggins, J. L. & Looney, R. J. (2004). Allergen immunotherapy. *American Family Physician, 70*(4), 689–696, 703–704.

Johansson, S. G. O. & Bieber, T. B. (2002). New diagnostic classification of allergic skin disorders. *Current Opinion in Allergy and Immunology, 2*(5), 403–406.

Johansson, S. G. O., Hourihane, J. O'B., Bousquet, J., et al. (2005). Revised nomenclature for allergy for global use. Report of the Nomenclature Review Committee of the World Allergy Organization, October 2003. *Allergy and Clinical Immunology International—Journal of the World Allergy Organization, 17*(1), 4–8.

Karch, A. M. & Karch, F. E. (2003). It was a shock: Food allergies and some drugs don't mix well. *American Journal of Nursing, 103*(6), 27.

Leung, D. Y. M., Boguniewicz, M., Howell, M. D., et al. (2004). New insights into atopic dermatitis. *Journal of Clinical Investigation, 113*(5), 651–657.

Leynaert, B. & Sousson, D. (2003). Monitoring the quality of life in allergic disorders. *Current Opinion in Asthma and Immunology, 3*(3), 177–183.

Long, A. (2002). The nuts and bolts of peanut allergy. *New England Journal of Medicine, 346*(17), 1320–1322.

McCall, B. P., Horwitz, I. B., & Kammeyer-Mueller, J. D. (2003). Have health conditions associated with latex increased since the issuance of universal precautions? *American Journal of Public Health, 93*(4), 599–604.

McKevith, B. & Theobald, H. (2005). Common food allergies. *Nursing Standard, 19*(29), 39–42.

McLean-Tooke, A., Bethune, C. A., Fay, A. C., et al. (2003). Adrenaline in the treatment of anaphylaxis: What is the evidence? *British Medical Journal, 327*(7427), 1332–1335.

Milgrom, H., Tran, Z. V., & Demoly, P. (2003). Towards evidence-based practice of allergy and clinical immunology: Applying an evidence-based medicine approach to allergen avoidance. *Current Opinion in Allergy and Clinical Immunology, 3*(3), 155–157.

Morgan, W. J., Crain, E. F., Gruchalla, R S., et al. (2004). Results of a home-based environmental intervention among urban children with asthma. *New England Journal of Medicine, 351*(11), 1068–1080.

Naleway, A. L., Belongia, E. A., Greenless, R. T., et al. (2003). Eczematous skin disease and recall of past diagnoses: Implications for smallpox vaccination. *Annals of Internal Medicine, 139*(1), 1–7.

Park, M. A. & Li, J. T. (2005). Diagnosis and management of penicillin allergy. *Mayo Clinic Proceedings, 80*(3), 405–410.

Platts-Mills, T. A. (2003). Allergen avoidance in the treatment of asthma and rhinitis. *New England Journal of Medicine, 349*(3), 207–208.

Plaut, M. & Valentine, M. D. (2005). Allergic rhinitis. *New England Journal of Medicine, 353*(18), 1934–1944.

Ranta, P. & Ownby, D. (2004). A review of natural-rubber latex allergy in health care workers. *Clinical Infectious Diseases, 38*(2), 252–256.

Ratner, P. H., Ehrlich, P. M., Fineman, S. M., et al. (2002). Use of intranasal cromolyn sodium for allergic rhinitis. *Mayo Clinic Proceedings, 77*(4), 350–354.

Schmidt-Weber, C. B. & Blaser, K. (2005). New insights into the mechanisms of allergen-specific immunotherapy. *Current Opinion in Allergy and Clinical Immunology, 5*(5), 425–428.

Sheetz, A. H. & McIntyre, C. L. (2005). Anaphylaxis experienced by school children offers opportunities for ED nurse, school nurse collaboration. *Journal of Emergency Nursing, 31*(1), 102–104.

Sheffer, A. L. (2004). Allergen avoidance to reduce asthma-related morbidity. *New England Journal of Medicine, 351*(11), 1134–1136.

Simons, F. E. R. (2004). Advances in H_1-antihistamines. *New England Journal of Medicine, 351*(21), 2203–2217.

Simpson, A. & Custovic, A. (2003). Early pet exposure: Friend or foe? *Current Opinion in Allergy and Clinical Immunology, 3*(3), 7–14.

Simpson, A. & Custovic, A. (2005). Pets and the development of allergic sensitization. *Current Allergy and Asthma Reports, 5*(3), 212–220.

Tanriover, B., Chuang, P. Fishbach, B., et al. (2005). Polyclonal antibody-induced serum sickness in renal transplant recipients: Treatment with therapeutic plasma exchange. *Transplantation, 80*(2), 279–281.

Terreehorst, I., Hak, E., Oosting, A. J., et al. (2003). Evaluation of impermeable covers for bedding in patients with allergic rhinitis. *New England Journal of Medicine, 349*(3), 237–246.

Teuber, S. S. & Beyer, K. (2004). Peanut, tree nut and seed allergies. *Current Opinion in Allergy and Clinical Immunology, 4*(3), 201–203.

Timoney, J. P., Eagan, M. M. & Sklarin, N. T. (2003). Establishing clinical guidelines for the management of acute hypersensitivity reactions secondary to the administration of chemotherapy/biologic therapy. *Journal of Nursing Care Quality, 18*(1), 80–86.

Turjanmaa, K. (2005). The role of atopy patch tests in the diagnosis of allergy in atopic dermatitis. *Current Opinion in Allergy and Clinical Immunology, 5*(5), 429–436.

Uter, W., Johansen, J. D., Orton, D. I., et al. (2005). Clinical update on contact allergy. *Current Opinion in Allergy and Clinical Immunology, 5*(5), 429–436.

Von Bubnoff, D., Novak, N., Kraft, S., et al. (2003). The central role of FCεRI in allergy. *Clinical and Experimental Dermatology, 28*(2), 184–187.

Wang, D. Y., Chan, A. & Smith, J. D. (2004). Management of allergic rhinitis: A common part of practice in primary care clinics. *Allergy, 59*(3), 315–319.

William, H. C. (2005). Clinical practice: Atopic dermatitis. *New England Journal of Medicine, 353*(22), 2314–2324.

Yip, E. (2004). Consideration of barrier protection and latex protein allergy in the evaluation of medical gloves. *Journal of Infusion Nursing, 27*(4), 227–231.

Yip, E. & Roman, M. (2003). Latex protein allergy and your choice of gloves: A balanced consideration. *MedSurg Nursing, 12*(1), 20–26.

RESOURCES

American Academy of Allergy, Asthma and Immunology, 555 East Wells Street, Suite 1100, Milwaukee, WI 53202; 800-822-2762; http://www.aaaai.org. Accessed June 2, 2006.

American College of Allergy, Asthma and Immunology, 85 W. Algonquin Road, Suite 550, Arlington Heights, IL 60005; 800-842-7777; http://allergy.mcg. edu. Accessed June 2, 2006.

Asthma and Allergy Foundation of America, 1233 20th Street, NW, Suite 402, Washington, DC 20036; 800-727-8462 or 202-466-7643; http://www. aafa.org. Accessed June 2, 2006.

Centers for Disease Control and Prevention, 1600 Clifton Road, Atlanta, GA 30333; 404-639-3311 or 800-311-3435; http://www.cdc.gov. Accessed June 2, 2006.

Food Allergy and Anaphylaxis Network, 11781 Lee Jackson Highway, Suite 160; Fairfax, VA 22033; 800-929-4040; e-mail: faan@foodallergy.org; http://www.foodallergy.org. Accessed June 2, 2006.

National Institute of Allergy and Infectious Disease, NIAID Office of Communications and Public Liaison, NIH, Bldg. 31, Room 7A50, 31 Center Drive, MSC 2520, Bethesda, MD 20893; 301-496-5717; http://www3. niaid.nih.gov/. Accessed June 2, 2006.

Spina Bifida Association of America, 4590 MacArthur Blvd., NW, Suite 250, Washington, DC 20007; 800-621-3141; http://www.sbaa.org. Accessed June 2, 2006.

CHAPTER

54

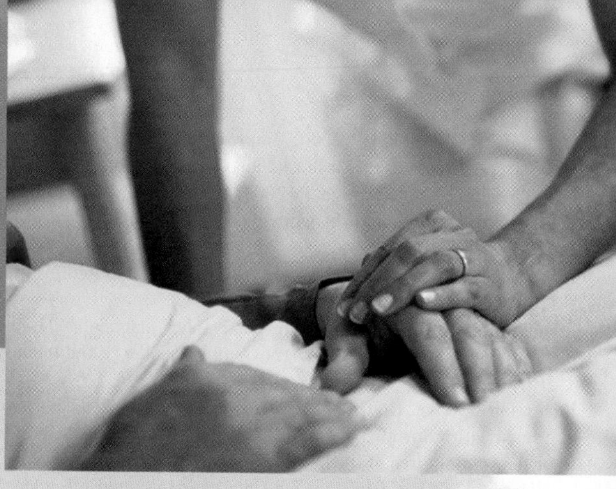

Assessment and Management of Patients With Rheumatic Disorders

Learning Objectives

On completion of this chapter, the learner will be able to:

1. Explain the processes of inflammation and degradation in the development of rheumatic diseases.
2. Describe the assessment and diagnostic findings that may be evidenced by patients with a suspected diagnosis of rheumatic disease.
3. Discuss appropriate nursing interventions based on nursing diagnoses and collaborative problems that commonly occur with rheumatic disorders.
4. Apply the nursing process as a framework for the care of the patient with a rheumatic disease, such as connective tissue disease or osteoarthritis.
5. Describe the systemic effects of a connective tissue disease.
6. Devise a teaching plan for the patient with newly diagnosed rheumatic disease.
7. Identify modifications in interventions to accommodate changes in patients' functional ability that may occur with disease progression.

Rheumatic diseases include common disorders such as osteoarthritis and less common conditions such as systemic lupus erythematosus (SLE) and scleroderma. These conditions can be life-threatening, or they can be minor illnesses. The problems caused by the rheumatic diseases include not only the obvious limitations in mobility and activities of daily living but also the more subtle systemic effects that can lead to organ failure and death or result in problems such as pain, fatigue, altered self-image, and sleep disturbances. The rheumatic disease may be the patient's primary health problem or a secondary diagnosis. Thorough understanding of rheumatic diseases and their effects on a patient's function and well-being is the key to developing an appropriate plan of nursing care.

Rheumatic Diseases

Commonly called arthritis (inflammation of a joint) and thought of as one condition, the rheumatic diseases are actually more than 100 different types of disorders that primarily affect skeletal muscles, bones, cartilage, ligaments, tendons, and joints in males and females of all ages. Some disorders are more likely to occur at a particular time of life or to affect one gender more than the other. The onset of these conditions may be acute or insidious, with a course possibly marked by periods of remission (a period when disease symptoms are reduced or absent) and exacerbation (a period when symptoms occur or increase). Treatment can be simple, aimed at localized relief, or it can be complex, directed toward relief of systemic effects. Permanent changes and disability may result from these disorders.

There are several approaches to the classification of rheumatic diseases. One basic system is to classify disease as either monoarticular (affecting a single joint) or polyarticular (affecting multiple joints), and then to further classify it as either inflammatory or noninflammatory. Conditions that may secondarily affect the musculoskeletal structure are also included, emphasizing the diversity of the rheumatic diseases.

Pathophysiology

Understanding the normal anatomy and physiology of the **diarthrodial** or **synovial** joints is key to understanding the pathophysiology of the rheumatic diseases. The function of the synovial joints is movement. Each synovial joint has a given range of motion, although range of motion of movable joints varies among people.

In a normal synovial joint, a smooth, almost friction-free, resilient surface for movement is provided by articular cartilage, which covers the bone end of the joint. Lining the inner surface of the fibrous capsule is the synovial membrane, which secretes fluid into the space between the bone ends. The synovial fluid functions as a shock absorber and a lubricant, allowing the joint to move freely.

The joint is the area most commonly affected by the inflammation and degeneration seen in rheumatic diseases. Despite the diversity of rheumatic diseases, from localized involvement of one joint to systemic, multisystem disorders, they all involve some degree of inflammation and degeneration, which may occur simultaneously. Inflammation is manifested in the joints as synovitis. In inflammatory rheumatic diseases, the primary process is inflammation caused by the immune response. Degeneration occurs as a secondary process, resulting from the effect of **pannus** (proliferation of newly formed synovial tissue infiltrated with inflammatory cells). The inflammation is a result of altered immune function. Conversely, in degenerative rheumatic diseases, inflammation occurs as a secondary process. This synovitis is usually milder, is more likely to be seen in advanced disease, and represents a reactive process. The synovitis is thought to result from mechanical irritation due to cartilage **matrix** products.

Inflammation

Inflammation involves a series of related steps. In response to the triggering event, the **antigen** stimulus activates monocytes and T lymphocytes (also called T cells). Next, the immunoglobulin antibodies form immune complexes with antigens. Phagocytosis of the immune complexes is initiated,

Glossary

ankylosis: fixation or immobility of a joint

antibody: a protein substance developed by the body in response to and interacting with a specific antigen

antigen: a substance that induces production of antibodies

arthroplasty: replacement of a joint

complement: a plasma protein associated with immunologic reactions

cytokines: generic term for nonantibody proteins that act as intercellular mediators, as in the generation of immune response

diarthrodial: a joint with two freely moveable parts

hemarthrosis: bleeding into the joint

joint effusion: the escape of fluid from the blood vessels or lymphatics into the joint space

leukotrienes: chemical mediators formed from constituents (ie, arachidonic acid) of cell membranes; they initiate and mediate the inflammatory response

matrix: noncellular component of tissue

osteophyte: a bony outgrowth or protuberance; spur

pannus: newly formed synovial tissue infiltrated with inflammatory cells

prostaglandins: lipid-soluble molecules synthesized from constituents (ie, arachidonic acid) from cell membranes; they mediate the inflammatory process

subchondral bone: bony plate that supports the articular cartilage

synovial: pertaining to the joint-lubricating fluid

tophi: accumulation of crystalline deposits in articular surfaces, bones, soft tissue, and cartilage generating an inflammatory reaction (joint effusion, pain, and edema) (Fig. 54-1).

During the next step, the immune response deviates from normal. Phagocytosis produces chemicals such as leukotrienes and prostaglandins. **Leukotrienes** contribute to the inflammatory process by attracting other white blood cells to the area. **Prostaglandins** act as modifiers to inflammation. In some cases, they increase inflammation; in other cases, they decrease it. Leukotrienes and prostaglandins produce enzymes such as collagenase that break down collagen, a vital part of a normal joint. The release of these enzymes in the joint causes edema, proliferation of synovial membrane and pannus formation, destruction of cartilage, and erosion of bone.

The immunologic inflammatory process begins when antigens are presented to T lymphocytes, leading to a proliferation of T and B cells. B cells are a source of **antibody**-forming cells, or plasma cells. In response to specific antigens, plasma cells produce and release antibodies. Antibodies combine with corresponding antigens to form pairs, or immune complexes. The immune complexes build up and are deposited in synovial tissue or other organs in the body, triggering the inflammatory reaction that can ultimately damage the involved tissue.

The systemic nature of the rheumatic diseases known as diffuse connective tissue diseases is reflected in the resultant widespread inflammatory process. Although focused in the joints, inflammation also involves other areas. The blood vessels (vasculitis and arteritis), lungs, heart, and kidneys may also be affected by the inflammation. In the joints, this inflammatory response is manifested as pannus extending throughout the joint space and, if persistent, eroding the articular cartilage, causing secondary degenerative changes to the joint.

Degeneration

Although the cause of degeneration of the articular cartilage is poorly understood, the process is known to be metabolically active and therefore is more accurately called "degradation." One theory of degradation is that genetic or hormonal influences, mechanical factors, or prior joint damage causes cartilage failure. Degradation of cartilage ensues, and increased mechanical stress on bone ends causes stiffening of bone tissue. Another theory is that bone stiffening occurs and results in increased mechanical stress on cartilage, which in turn initiates the processes of degradation.

Articular cartilage plays two essential mechanical roles in joint physiology. First, the articular cartilage provides a remarkably smooth weight-bearing surface and, with synovial fluid, results in extremely low friction during movement. Second, the cartilage transmits load or pressure to the bone, dissipating the mechanical stress. Specific factors have been implicated in association with degenerative joint changes.

MECHANICAL STRESS

Articular cartilage is highly resistant to wear under conditions of repeated movement. However, repetitive impact loading (velocity at which the force is applied) rapidly leads to joint failure at the cartilage level. When a person walks, three to four times the body weight is transmitted through the knee. A deep knee bend transmits up to nine times the body weight through the patellofemoral joint. As a joint undergoes repeated mechanical stress, the elasticity of the joint capsule, articular cartilage, and ligaments is reduced. The articular plate (**subchondral bone**) thins, and its ability to absorb shock decreases. The joint space narrows, accompanied by a loss of stability. When the articular plate disappears, bony spurs (**osteophytes**) form at the edges of the joint surfaces, and the capsule and synovial membranes thicken. The joint cartilage degenerates and atrophies (shrinks), the bones harden and hypertrophy (thicken) at their articular surfaces, and the ligaments calcify. As a result, sterile **joint effusions** (fluid escaping from the blood vessels or lymphatics into the joint cavity) and secondary synovitis may be present (Fig. 54-2).

ALTERED LUBRICATION

In addition to the changes in the articular cartilage and subchondral bone, lubrication of the joint is also a factor in joint degeneration. With joint loading (forces carried through the joint), lubrication depends on a film of interstitial fluid that is squeezed out of the cartilage on compression of the opposing surfaces of the joint. The mechanisms that normally operate under high weight loads to produce this lubricating film may be affected.

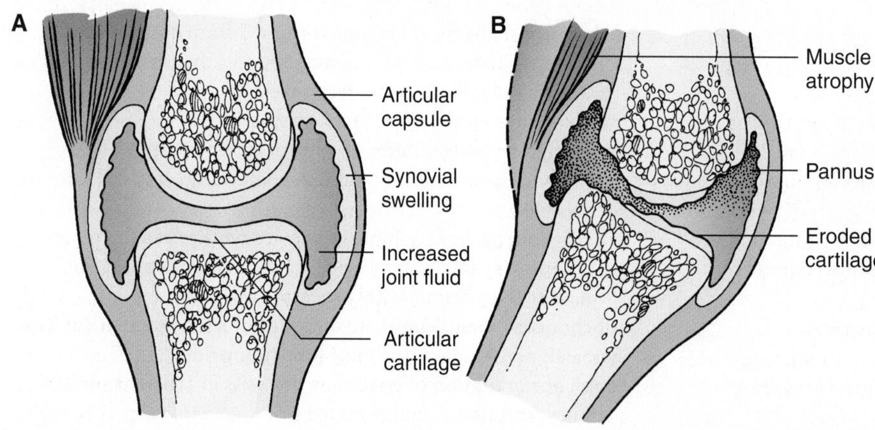

FIGURE 54-1. (**A**) Synovial swelling and fluid accumulation. (**B**) Pannus (a proliferation of synovial tissue), eroded articular cartilage, and joint space narrowing—all of which contribute to muscle atrophy and ankylosis (joint rigidity and immobility).

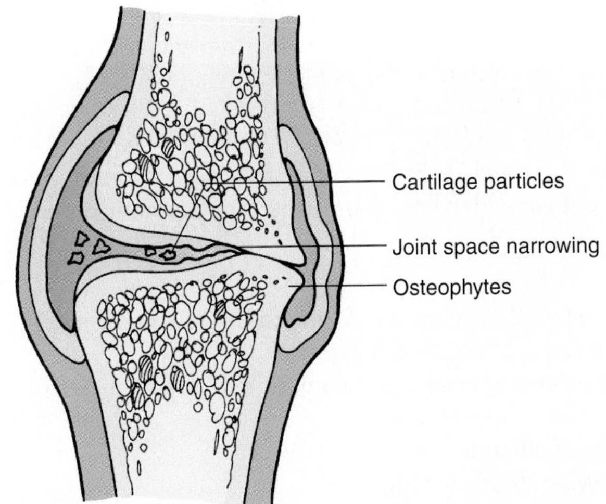

FIGURE 54-2. Joint space narrowing and osteophytes (bone spurs) are characteristic of degenerative changes in joints.

IMMOBILITY

Immobilization of a joint is another factor that can produce degenerative changes in articular cartilage. Although these changes are more marked and appear earlier in areas of contact, they also occur in areas not subject to mechanical compression. Cartilage degeneration due to joint immobility may result from loss of the pumping action of lubrication that occurs with joint movement. Approximately three weeks after remobilization of the joint, the cartilage abnormalities are reversed. However, impact exercising (eg, running) prevents reversal of the atrophy. Instead, slow, gradual range of motion is thought to be very important in preventing cartilage injury.

Clinical Manifestations

The symptom of a rheumatic disease that most commonly causes a person to seek medical attention is pain. Other common symptoms include joint swelling, limited movement, stiffness, weakness, and fatigue.

Assessment and Diagnostic Findings

Assessment begins with a general health history, which includes the onset of symptoms and how they evolved, family history, past health history, and any other contributing factors. Because many of the rheumatic diseases are chronic conditions, the health history should also include information about the patient's perception of the problem, previous treatments and their effectiveness, the patient's support systems, and the patient's current knowledge base and the source of that information. A complete health history is followed by a complete physical assessment.

Assessment for rheumatic diseases combines the physical examination with a functional assessment. Inspection of the patient's general appearance occurs during initial contact. Gait, posture, and general musculoskeletal size and structure are observed. Gross deformities and abnormalities in movement are noted. The symmetry, size, and contour of other connective tissues, such as the skin and adipose tissue, are also noted and recorded. Chart 54-1 outlines the important areas for consideration during the physical assessment. The functional assessment is a combination of history (what the patient reports that he or she can and cannot do) and examination (observation of activities: the patient demonstrates what he or she can and cannot do, such as dressing and getting in and out of a chair). Observation also includes the adaptations and adjustments the patient may have made (sometimes without awareness); for example, with shoulder or elbow involvement, the person may bend over to reach a fork, rather than raising the fork to the mouth.

The history and physical assessment data are supplemented by supportive or confirming diagnostic test findings. In some instances, tests are used to monitor the course of the disease. For example, the erythrocyte sedimentation rate (ESR) reflects inflammatory activity and, indirectly, the progression or remission of disease.

Diagnosis of a specific rheumatic disease may or may not be relatively simple and clear-cut. Commonly, observation of clinical signs and symptoms over time is needed to make the diagnosis. The combination of history, assessment, testing, and evolving manifestations of the disease may require explanation and interpretation to the patient with early disease. This is especially true for patients with multisystem rheumatic disease, such as one of the connective tissue diseases.

Many forms of rheumatic disease can be accurately diagnosed by the primary health care provider, but patients with more complicated signs and symptoms may need referral to a rheumatologist (a physician who specializes in diagnosing and treating rheumatic disease). Patients should know which type of rheumatic disease they have, not just that they have "arthritis" or "arthritis of the knee."

The following tests are commonly used for patients with rheumatic diseases.

Arthrocentesis

Arthrocentesis (needle aspiration of synovial fluid) may be performed not only to obtain a sample of synovial fluid for analysis but also to relieve pain caused by pressure of increased fluid volume, usually in the knee or shoulder. Synovial fluid is usually analyzed in cases such as suspected joint infection to determine the presence of inflammatory cells and to identify crystals in suspected gout or the presence of blood after trauma. The synovial fluid may provide a specific diagnosis. The presence of crystals is indicative of gout, and the presence of bacteria is indicative of infectious arthritis.

After the joint is anesthetized locally, a large-bore needle is inserted into the joint space to obtain a fluid specimen. Because this procedure has the potential for introducing bacteria into the joint, aseptic technique is essential. After the procedure, the patient is observed for signs of infection and **hemarthrosis** (bleeding into the joint).

Normally, synovial fluid is clear, viscous, straw-colored, and scanty in volume, with few cells. However, in inflammatory joint disease, the fluid may become cloudy, milky, or dark yellow and may contain numerous inflammatory cells, such as leukocytes (white blood cells), and **complement**

CHART 54-1

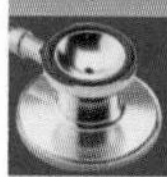

Assessing for Rheumatic Diseases

In addition to the head-to-toe assessment or systems review, the following are important areas of consideration to be noted when performing the complete physical assessment of a patient with a known or suspected rheumatic disease.

MANIFESTATION	SIGNIFICANCE
Skin (inquire and inspect)	
Rash, lesions	Associated with lupus erythematosus (LE), vasculitis, adverse effect of medication
Increased bruising	Associated with several rheumatic diseases and adverse effect of medication
Erythema	Sign of inflammation
Thinning	Adverse effect of medication
Warmth	Sign of inflammation
Photosensitivity	Associated with systemic lupus erythematosus (SLE), dermatomyositis, adverse effect of medication
Hair (inquire and inspect)	
Alopecia or thinning	Associated with rheumatic diseases or adverse effect of medication
Eye (inquire and inspect)	
Dryness, grittiness	Associated with Sjögren's syndrome (commonly occurring with rheumatoid arthritis [RA] and LE)
Decreased acuity or blindness	Associated with temporal arteritis, medication complications
Cataracts	Adverse effect of medication
Decreased peripheral vision	Adverse effect of medication
Conjunctivitis, uveitis	Associated with ankylosing spondylitis and Reiter's syndrome
Ear (inquire)	
Tinnitus	Adverse effect of medication
Decreased acuity	Adverse effect of medication
Mouth (inquire and inspect)	
Buccal, sublingual lesions	Associated with vasculitis, dermatomyositis, adverse effect of medication
Altered sense of taste	Adverse effect of medication
Dryness	Associated with Sjögren's syndrome
Dysphagia	Associated with myositis
Difficulty chewing	Associated with decreased range of motion of jaw
Chest (inspect and inquire)	
Pleuritic pain	Associated with RA and SLE
Decreased chest expansion	Associated with ankylosing spondylitis
Activity intolerance (dyspnea)	Associated with pulmonary hypertension in scleroderma
Cardiovascular system (inquire, inspect, palpate)	
Blanching of fingers on exposure to cold	Associated with Raynaud's phenomenon
Peripheral pulses	Deficit may indicate vascular involvement or edema associated with medication effect or rheumatic diseases, especially SLE or scleroderma
Abdomen (inquire and palpate)	
Altered bowel habits	Associated with scleroderma, spondylosis, ulcerative colitis, decreased physical mobility, medication effect
Nausea, vomiting, bloating, and pain	Adverse effect of medication
Weight change (measure)	Associated with RA (decreased), adverse effect of medication (increased or decreased)

CHART 54-1 Assessing for Rheumatic Diseases, continued

MANIFESTATION	SIGNIFICANCE
Genitalia (inquire and inspect)	
Dryness, itching	Associated with Sjögren's syndrome
Abnormal menses	Adverse effect of medication
Altered sexual performance	Fear of pain (or of pain caused by partner) and limitation of motion may affect sexual mobility.
Hygiene	Poor hygiene may be related to limitations in activities of daily living.
Urethritis, dysuria	Associated with ankylosing spondylitis and Reiter's syndrome
Lesions	Associated with vasculitis
Neurologic (inquire and inspect)	
Paresthesias of extremities; abnormal reflex pattern	Nerve compressions associated with carpal tunnel syndrome, spinal stenosis, etc.
Headaches	Associated with temporal arteritis, adverse effect of medication
Musculoskeletal (inspect and palpate)	
Joint redness, warmth, swelling, tenderness, deformity—location of first joint involved, pattern of progression, symmetry, acute vs chronic nature	Signs of inflammation
Joint range of motion	Decreased range of motion may indicate severity or progression of disease.
Surrounding tissue findings	
Muscle atrophy, subcutaneous nodules, popliteal cyst	Extra-articular manifestations
Muscle strength (grip)	Muscle strength decreases with increased disease activity.

(a plasma protein associated with immunologic reactions). The viscosity is reduced in inflammatory disease, and copious amounts of fluid may be present. Arthrocentesis is diagnostically valuable, but arthrocentesis of small joints (ie, fingers or wrist) may be difficult.

X-Ray Studies

X-rays are often used in evaluating patients with rheumatic disease. The timing of the studies influences their usefulness: it is unlikely that a patient with a 2-month history of joint inflammation will have demonstrable changes on an x-ray study, but someone with long-standing disease may show severe joint degeneration. X-rays can also be used to monitor disease activity and progression, demonstrating the loss of cartilage and narrowing of the joint space over time. In addition, x-rays can demonstrate cartilage abnormalities, joint erosions, abnormal bony growth, and osteopenia (decreased bone mineralization).

Bone Scans, Computed Tomography, and Magnetic Resonance Imaging

Bone scans reflect the degree to which the crystal lattice of bone takes up or absorbs a bone-seeking radioactive isotope. An area demonstrating increased uptake, such as a joint, is considered abnormal and indicative of inflammation due to infection or nondisplaced fractures. Computed tomography (CT) and magnetic resonance imaging (MRI) are techniques used to better visualize soft tissues. Bone scans, CT, and MRI are not the most cost-effective methods for detection of early disease, and they are not performed routinely at the time of diagnosis.

Tissue Biopsies

A muscle biopsy, carried out to examine skeletal muscle, is useful in diagnosing myositis. After administration of local anesthesia under sterile conditions in an outpatient setting or in an operating room, a surgical incision is made to obtain the desired specimen, which is sent to the laboratory for microscopic analysis. A pressure dressing is applied, and the affected extremity is immobilized for 12 to 24 hours.

An arterial biopsy may be performed to examine a specimen of an arterial wall using a procedure similar to that for a muscle biopsy. Most frequently the temporal artery is selected, but other arteries may be used as indicated. Arterial biopsy most often confirms inflammation of the vessel wall, or arteritis, a type of vasculitis.

A skin biopsy may be performed to confirm inflammatory connective tissue diseases such as scleroderma or lupus erythematosus (LE; a non-systemic form of lupus that is limited to skin symptoms). A specimen may be lightly scraped from the skin without causing discomfort. Deeper skin biopsies may be needed if scraping is insufficient.

Blood Tests

In general, laboratory studies in rheumatology are based on the assumption that most rheumatic diseases are autoimmune disorders. Although many of the tests are highly complex and technical, no single test used in isolation sufficiently supports a diagnosis of a rheumatic disease. Some of the most common blood studies are listed with their corresponding normal ranges and primary indications in Table 54-1. Because many of the tests require special laboratory techniques, they may not be performed in every health care facility. The physician determines which tests are necessary based on the symptoms, stage of disease, cost, and likely benefit of the test.

Gerontologic Considerations

Although people of all ages, from infancy through childhood, adolescence, and adulthood, may be affected, rheumatic disease is commonly thought of by the patient, family, and society as a whole as an inevitable consequence of aging. Many older people expect and accept the immobility and self-care problems related to the rheumatic diseases and do not seek help, thinking that nothing can be done. Careful diagnosis and appropriate treatment can improve the quality of life for older people. However, the rheumatic diseases do have some special implications for the older adult.

In elderly patients, other medical conditions may take precedence over the rheumatic disease, which commonly becomes a secondary diagnosis and concern. Identifying the effects of the rheumatic disease on the patient's lifestyle, independence, and other chronic or acute conditions is important.

The frequency, pattern of onset, clinical features, severity, and effects on function of the rheumatic disease in elderly patients may be different in very old patients. One disease, polymyalgia rheumatica, affects primarily people older than 50 years of age (Paget, 2001), whereas some disorders are less severe in elderly people than in younger patients. Another disease, osteoarthritis (OA), is the leading cause of disability and pain in the elderly (Porth, 2005). OA may account for more total disability among elderly patients than many diseases, such as stroke or cancer, that are considered more serious.

In some instances, the age of the patient and coexisting health problems make diagnosis difficult. A missed diagnosis is not unusual, because it is assumed that most older people with joint problems have OA. In addition, it may be difficult to differentiate problems associated with aging from those caused by a rheumatic disease. For example, rheumatoid arthritis (RA) that begins in the later years has been shown to differ prognostically and therapeutically from RA that begins in childhood or early adulthood. In the elderly patient with early RA, the onset is more likely to be abrupt, but the clinical course does not appear to differ from that of RA with an insidious onset.

For the elderly person who has had a diffuse connective tissue disease, the risk of osteoporosis is increased. Pain, loss of mobility, diminished self-image, and increasing morbidity can result from progressive osteoporosis. Therefore, diagnosis and treatment for osteoporosis should not be overlooked in this population. Pharmacologic therapy including analgesic agents, exercise, postural assistance, modification of activities of daily living, and psychological support can be useful.

Other conditions (eg, soft tissue problems such as bursitis) usually are not problematic by themselves. However, when combined with other health problems and the normal physiologic processes of aging, these conditions may significantly affect the patient's quality of life. In fact, the effects of most forms of rheumatic disease may lead to considerable changes in the patient's lifestyle, possibly threatening his or her independence. Decreased vision and altered balance, often present in elderly people, may be problematic if rheumatic disease in the lower extremities affects locomotion. Also, the combination of decreased hearing and visual acuity, memory loss, and depression contributes to failure to follow the treatment regimen in elderly patients. Special techniques for promoting patient safety, self-management, and strategies such as memory aids for medications may be necessary.

Partly because of the more frequent contact of the elderly with health care providers for a variety of health issues, overtreatment or inappropriate treatment is possible. Complaints of pain may be met with a prescription for an opioid analgesic rather than instructions for rest, use of an assistive device, and local comfort measures such as heat or cold. Acetaminophen may be appropriate and worth trying before other medications that pose a greater chance of side effects. Intra-articular corticosteroid injections, with their usually rapid relief of symptoms, may be requested by the patient who is unaware of the consequences of too-frequent use of this treatment. In addition, exercise programs may not be instituted or may be ineffective because the patient expects results to occur quickly or fails to appreciate the effectiveness of a program of exercise.

Pharmacologic treatment of rheumatic disease in older patients is more difficult than it is in younger patients. If therapeutic medications have an effect on the senses (hearing, cognition), this effect is intensified in the elderly. The cumulative effect of these medications is accentuated because of the physiologic changes of aging. For example, decreased renal function in the elderly alters the metabolism of certain medications, such as nonsteroidal anti-inflammatory drugs (NSAIDs). Elderly patients are more prone to side effects associated with the use of multiple-drug therapy for various disorders (Lehne, 2004).

Elderly patients with rheumatic disease may unnecessarily accept or endure pain, loss of ambulation, and difficulty with activities of daily living. The need to view oneself as capable of managing life independently despite increasing age may take considerable energy. The body image and self-esteem of the elderly person with rheumatic disease, combined with underlying depression, may interfere with the use of assistive devices such as canes. Use of adaptive equipment such as long-handled reachers or tongs may be viewed as evidence of aging rather than as a means of increasing independence.

The elderly person usually has a lifelong pattern of dealing with the stresses of daily life. Depending on the success of that pattern, the elderly person can often maintain a positive attitude and self-esteem when faced with a rheumatic disease, especially if support is available. Previous stress management strategies are assessed. If these strategies have been effective, the patient is encouraged and supported in their use. If they were ineffective, the nurse assists the patient in identifying alternative strategies, encourages use of new strategies, and assesses their effectiveness.

TABLE 54-1 Common Blood Studies for Rheumatic Diseases

Test	Normal Value	Significance
Serum		
Creatinine Metabolic waste excreted through the kidneys	0.6–1.2 mg/dL (50–110 μmol/L)	Increase may indicate renal damage in SLE, scleroderma, and polyarteritis.
Erythrocyte Sedimentation Rate (ESR) Measures the rate at which red blood cells settle out of unclotted blood in 1 hour	Westergren = *Men,* 0–15 mm/h, *Women,* 0–25 mm/h Wintrobe = *Men,* 0–9 mm/h, *Women* 0–15 mm/h	Increase is usually seen in inflammatory connective tissue diseases. An increase indicates rising inflammation, resulting in clustering of RBCs, which makes them heavier than normal. The higher the ESR, the greater the inflammatory activity.
Hematocrit Measures the size, capacity, and number of cells present in blood	*Men:* 42–52% *Women:* 35–47%	Decrease can be seen in chronic inflammation (anemia of chronic disease); also, blood loss through bowel due to medication.
Red Blood Cell Count Measures circulating erythrocytes	*Men:* Average 4.8 million/μL *Women:* Average 4.3 million/μL	Decrease can be seen in RA, SLE.
White Blood Cell Count Measures circulating leukocytes	5,000–10,000 cells/mm^3	Decrease may be seen in SLE.
VDRL (Venereal Disease Research Laboratory) Measures antibody to syphilis	Nonreactive	False-positive results are sometimes found with SLE.
Uric Acid Measures level of uric acid in serum	2.5–8 mg/dL (0.15–0.5 mmol/L)	Increase is seen with gout.
Serum Immunology		
Antinuclear Antibody (ANA) Measures antibodies that react with a variety of nuclear antigens If antibodies are present, further testing determines the type of ANA circulating in the blood (anti-DNA, anti-RNP).	Negative A few healthy adults have a positive ANA.	Positive test is associated with SLE, RA, scleroderma, Raynaud's disease, Sjögren's syndrome, necrotizing arteritis. The higher the titer, the greater the inflammation. The pattern of immunofluorescence (speckled, homogeneous, or nucleolar) helps determine the diagnosis.
Anti-DNA, DNA binding Titer measurement of antibody to double-stranded DNA	Negative	High titer is seen in SLE; increases in titer may indicate increase in disease activity.
Complement levels—C3, C4 Complement is a protein substance that binds with antigen–antibody complexes for the purpose of lysis. When the number of complexes increases markedly, complement is used for lysis, thus depleting the amount available in the blood.	C3: 55–120 mg/dL (550–1,200 mg/L) C4: 11–40 mg/dL (110–400 mg/L)	Decrease may be seen in RA and SLE. Decrease indicates autoimmune and inflammatory activity.
C-Reactive Protein Test (CRP) Shows presence of abnormal glycoprotein due to inflammatory process	<1 mg/dL (<10 mg/L)	A positive reading indicates active inflammation. Often is positive for RA and SLE
Immunoglobulin Electrophoresis Measures the values of immunoglobulins	IgA 50–300 mg/dL (0.5–3 g/L) IgG 635–1,400 mg/dL (6.35–14 g/L) IgM 40–280 mg/dL (0.4–238 g/L)	Increased levels are found in people who have autoimmune disorders.

continued >

TABLE 54-1 Common Blood Studies for Rheumatic Diseases (Continued)

Test	Normal Value	Significance
Rheumatoid Factor (RF)		
Determines the presence of abnormal antibodies seen in connective tissue disease	Negative	Positive titer > 1:80 Present in 80% of those with RA Positive RF may also suggest SLE, Sjögren's syndrome, or mixed connective tissue disease. The higher the titer (number at right of colon), the greater the inflammation.
Tissue Typing		
HLA-B27 Antigen		
Measures presence of HLA antigens, which are used for tissue recognition	Negative	Found in 80%–90% of those with ankylosing spondylitis and Reiter's syndrome.

Medical Management

A treatment program involving an interdisciplinary team, including the patient, is the basis for managing the rheumatic diseases. The chronic nature of most of these diseases mandates that the patient understand the disease, have the information necessary to make good self-management decisions, and be presented with a therapeutic program that is compatible with his or her lifestyle. Table 54-2 outlines the goals and strategies of basic rheumatic disease management.

Pharmacologic Therapy

Medications are used with the rheumatic diseases to manage symptoms, to control inflammation, and, in some instances, to modify the disease. Useful medications include the salicylates, NSAIDs, and disease-modifying antirheumatic drugs (DMARDs). Table 54-3 reviews the medications commonly used.

Controlling the inflammation related to the disease process helps manage pain, but this is often a delayed response. Nonopioid medications are often used for pain management, especially early in the treatment program, until other measures can be instituted (Burckhardt, 2001a). Short-term use of low-dose antidepressant medications, such as amitriptyline (Elavil), may be prescribed to reestablish adequate sleep patterns and improve pain management (Wegener, 2001).

TABLE 54-2 Goals and Strategies for Rheumatic Diseases

Major Goals	Management Strategy
Suppress inflammation and the autoimmune response	Optimize pharmacologic therapy (anti-inflammatory and disease-modifying agents)
Control pain	Protect joints; ease pain with splints, thermal modalities, relaxation techniques
Maintain or improve joint mobility	Implement exercise programs for joint motion and muscle strengthening and overall health
Maintain or improve functional status	Make use of adaptive devices and techniques
Increase patient's knowledge of disease process	Provide and reinforce patient teaching
Promote self-management by patient compliance with the therapeutic regimen	Emphasize compatibility of therapeutic regimen and lifestyle

Nonpharmacologic Pain Management

Nonpharmacologic methods of pain management are important. Methods used include therapeutic heat or cold and devices such as a cane or a wrist splint to protect and support the joint. A combination of methods may be required, because different methods often work better at different times.

Exercise and Activity

The ongoing nature of most rheumatic diseases makes it important to maintain and, when possible, improve joint mobility and overall functional status. An individualized exercise program is crucial to movement. Table 54-4 summarizes the exercises appropriate for patients with rheumatic diseases. Appropriate programs of exercise have been shown to decrease pain and improve function (Lorig, 2005). A mild analgesic may be suggested before exercise for a patient starting a program of exercise. Acute or prolonged pain associated with exercise should be reported to a health care provider for evaluation.

The major challenge for the patient and the health care provider is the need to adjust all aspects of treatment according to the activity of the disease. Especially for the patient with an active diffuse connective tissue disease, such as RA or SLE, activity levels may vary from day to day and even within a single day.

TABLE 54-3 Medications Used in Rheumatic Diseases

Medication	Action, Use, and Indication	Nursing Considerations
Salicylates *Acetylated* aspirin *Nonacetylated* choline salicylate (Arthropan, Trilisate) salsalate (Disalcid) sodium salicylate	*Action:* anti-inflammatory, analgesic, antipyretic Acetylated salicylates are platelet aggregation inhibitors. Anti-inflammatory doses will produce blood salicylate levels of 20–30 mg/dL.	Administer with meals to prevent gastric irritation. Assess for tinnitus, gastric intolerance, GI bleeding, and purpura. Monitor for possible confusion in the elderly.
Nonsteroidal Anti-inflammatory Drugs (NSAIDs) diclofenac (Voltaren) diflunisal (Dolobid) etodolac (Lodine) flurbiprofen (Ansaid) ibuprofen (Motrin) indomethacin (Indocin) ketoprofen (Orudis, Oruvail) meclofenamate (Meclomen) meloxicam (Mobic) nabumetone (Relafen) naproxen (Naprosyn) oxaprozin (DayPro) piroxicam (Feldene) sulindac (Clinoril) tolmetin sodium (Tolectin)	*Action:* anti-inflammatory, analgesic, antipyretic, platelet aggregation inhibitor Anti-inflammatory effect occurs 2–4 weeks after initiation. All NSAIDs are useful for short-term treatment of acute gout attack. NSAIDs are alternative to salicylates for first-line therapy in several rheumatic diseases.	Administer NSAIDs with food. Monitor for GI, CNS, cardiovascular, renal, hematologic, and dermatologic adverse effects. Avoid salicylates; use acetaminophen for additional analgesia. Watch for possible confusion in the elderly.
COX-2 inhibitors celecoxib (Celebrex)	*Action:* Inhibit only cyclooxygenase-2 (COX-2) enzymes, which are produced during inflammation, and spare COX-1 enzymes, which can be protective to the stomach	Monitoring the same as for other NSAIDs Increased risk of cardiovascular events, including myocardial infarction and stroke Appropriate for the elderly and patients who are at high risk for gastric ulcers
Disease-Modifying Antirheumatic Drugs (DMARDs)		
Antimalarials hydroxychloroquine (Plaquenil) chloroquine (Aralen)	*Action:* Anti-inflammatory, inhibits lysosomal enzymes Slow-acting, onset may take 2–4 months Useful in RA and SLE	Administer concurrently with NSAIDs. Assess for visual changes, GI upset, skin rash, headaches, photosensitivity, bleaching of hair. Emphasize need for ophthalmologic examinations (every 6–12 mo).
Gold-containing compounds aurothioglucose (Solganol) gold sodium thiomalate (Myochrysine) auranofin (Ridaura)	*Action:* Inhibits T- and B-cell activity, suppresses synovitis during active stage of rheumatoid disease Slow-acting, onset may take 3–6 months IM preparations are given weekly for about 6 months, then every 2–4 weeks	Administer concurrently with NSAIDs. Assess for stomatitis, diarrhea, dermatitis, proteinuria, hematuria, bone marrow suppression (decreased WBCs and/or platelets), CBC and urinalysis with every other injection
sulfasalazine (Azulfidine)	*Action:* Anti-inflammatory, reduces lymphocyte response, inhibits angiogenesis Useful in RA, seronegative spondyloarthropathies	Administer concurrently with NSAIDs. Do not use in patients with allergy to sulfa medications or salicylates. Emphasize adequate fluid intake. Assess for GI upset, skin rash, headache, liver abnormalities, anemia.
penicillamine (Cuprimine, Depen)	*Action:* Anti-inflammatory, inhibits T-cell function, impairs antigen presentation Slow-acting, onset may take 2–3 months Useful in RA and systemic sclerosis	Administer concurrently with NSAIDs. Assess for GI irritation, decreased taste, skin rash or itching, bone marrow suppression, proteinuria with CBC, and urinalysis every 2–4 wk.

continued >

TABLE 54-3 Medications Used in Rheumatic Diseases (Continued)

Medication	Action, Use, and Indication	Nursing Considerations
Immunosuppressives methotrexate (Rheumatrex) azathioprine (Imuran) cyclophosphamide (Cytoxan)	*Action:* Immune suppression, affects DNA synthesis and other cellular effects Have teratogenic potential; azathioprine and cyclophosphamide reserved for more aggressive or unresponsive disease Methotrexate is "gold standard" for RA treatment; also useful in SLE.	Assess for bone marrow suppression, GI ulcerations, skin rashes, alopecia, bladder toxicity, increased infections. Monitor CBC, liver enzymes, creatinine every 2–4 wk. Advise patient of contraceptive measures because of teratogenicity.
cyclosporine (Neoral)	*Action:* Immune suppression by inhibiting T lymphocytes Used for severe, progressive RA, unresponsive to other DMARDs Used in combination with methotrexate	Assess slow dose titration upward until response noted or toxicity occurs. Assess for toxic effects: bleeding gums, fluid retention, hair growth, tremors. Monitor blood pressure and creatinine every 2 wk until stable.
Immunomodulators		
Pyrimidine synthesis inhibitor leflunomide (Arava)	*Action:* Has antiproliferative and anti-inflammatory effects. Used in moderate to severe RA. May be used alone or in combination with other DMARDs (except methotrexate).	Long half-life; requires loading dose followed by daily administration. Assess for diarrhea, hair loss, skin rash, mouth sores. Monitor liver function tests. Contraindicated in pregnancy and breastfeeding. Administered orally.
Tumor necrosis factor blocking agents adalimumab (Humira) etanercept (Enbrel) infliximab (Remicade)	*Action:* Biologic response modifier that binds to tumor necrosis factor (TNF), a cytokine involved in inflammatory and immune responses. Used in moderate to severe RA unresponsive to methotrexate. Can be used alone or with methotrexate or other DMARDs. Humira is administered every 1–2 wk, and Enbrel is administered twice a wk.	Patient should be tested for tuberculosis before beginning this medication. Teach patient subcutaneous self-injection of adalimumab (Humira) or etanercept (Enbrel). Infliximab (Remicade) is administered by IV over 2 h or more. Medication must be refrigerated. Monitor for injection site reactions. Educate patient about increased risk for infection and to withhold medication if fever occurs.
Interleukin-1 receptor antagonist anakinra (Kineret)	*Action:* Human interleukin-1 (IL-1) receptor antagonist; blocks IL-1 receptors, decreasing inflammatory and immunologic responses. Used in moderate to severe RA unresponsive to methotrexate. Can be used alone or with methotrexate or DMARDs other than TNF blocking agents	Administered daily by subcutaneous injection. Teach patient subcutaneous self-injection to be administered daily. Medication must be refrigerated. Monitor for injection site reactions. Educate patient about increased risk for infection and to withhold medication if fever occurs.
Corticosteroids prednisone prednisolone hydrocortisone	*Action:* Anti-inflammatory Used for shortest duration and at lowest dose possible to minimize adverse effects Useful for unremitting RA, SLE, polymyalgia rheumatica, myositis, arteritis Fast-acting; onset in days Intra-articular injections useful for joints unresponsive to NSAIDs	Assess for toxicity: cataracts, GI irritation, hyperglycemia, hypertension, fractures, avascular necrosis, hirsutism, psychosis. Joints most amenable to injections include ankles, knees, hips, shoulders, and hands. Repeated injections can cause joint damage.
Topical Analgesics capsaicin (Zostrix)	*Action:* analgesic	Teach patient to apply sparingly, avoid areas of open skin, avoid contact with eyes and mucous membranes. Wash hands carefully after application. Assess for local skin irritation.

CBC, complete blood count; CNS, central nervous system; GI, gastrointestinal; RA, rheumatoid arthritis; SLE, systemic lupus erythematosus; WBCs, white blood cells.

TABLE 54-4 Exercises to Promote Mobility

Type of Exercise	Purpose	Recommended Performance	Precautions
Range of motion	Maintain flexibility and joint motion	Active or active/self-assisted at least daily	Reduce number of repetitions when inflammation is present
Isometric exercise	Improve muscle tone, static endurance, and strength; prepares for dynamic and weight-bearing exercises	Perform at 70% of maximal voluntary contraction daily	Monitor blood pressure, because isometric exercises may increase blood pressure and decrease blood flow to muscles
Dynamic exercise	Maintain or increase dynamic strength and endurance; increase muscle power; enhance synovial blood flow; promote strength of bone and cartilage	Start with repetitions against gravity and add progressive resistance; perform 2–3 days per week	May increase biomechanical stress on unstable or misaligned joints
Aerobic exercise	Improve cardiovascular fitness and endurance	Perform 3–5 days per week for 20–30 minutes of moderate-intensity exercise	Progress slowly as activity tolerance and fitness improve
Aquatic exercise	Water supports or resists movement; warm water may provide muscle relaxation	Provides buoyant medium for performance of dynamic or aerobic exercise	Warm water (84–92°F or 29–33°C); deep water to minimize joint compression; nonslip footwear for safety and comfort; receive appropriate instruction in a program designed for people with arthritis

Adapted from Minor, M. A. & Westby, M. D. (2001). Rest and exercise. In Robbins, L., Burckhardt, C. S., Hannan, M. T. (Eds.). *Clinical care in the rheumatic diseases.* Atlanta: Association of Rheumatology Health Professionals.

Nursing Process

The Patient With a Rheumatic Disease

Assessment

The depth and focus of the nursing assessment depend on several factors: the health care setting (clinic or office, home, extended care facility, or hospital), the role of the nurse (home care nurse; nurse practitioner; hospital, clinic, or office nurse), and the needs of the patient. The nurse is often the first health care team member to come in contact with the patient. This enables the nurse to assess the patient's perceptions of the disorder and situation, actions taken to relieve symptoms, plans for treatment, and expectations. The nurse's assessment may lead to identifying issues and concerns that can be addressed by nursing interventions and, through collaboration with other team members, to achieving the expected patient outcomes.

The health history and physical assessment focus on current and past symptoms, such as fatigue, weakness, pain, stiffness, fever, or anorexia, and the effects of these symptoms on the patient's lifestyle and self-image. Because the rheumatic diseases affect many body systems, the history and physical assessment include a review and examination of all systems, with particular attention given to those areas most commonly affected, including the musculoskeletal system (see Chart 54-1).

The patient's psychological and mental status and social support systems are also assessed, as well as his or her ability to participate in daily activities, comply with the treatment regimen, and manage self-care. The information obtained can give insight into the patient's understanding of the medication regimen and may reveal misuse of medications, failure to follow the treatment regimen, or use of potentially harmful unproven remedies. Additional areas assessed include the patient's understanding, motivation, knowledge, coping abilities, past experiences, preconceptions, and fears. The effects of the disease on the patient's self-concept and coping abilities are also assessed. The patient's perception of the condition and its impact influences the decisions, choices, and actions associated with treatment recommendations.

In addition, the patient's response to having a chronic disorder or a disability is assessed. Patients' and families' responses to illness are discussed in detail in Chapter 7, and chronic illness and disability are addressed in detail in Chapter 10.

Diagnosis

Nursing Diagnoses

Although many nursing diagnoses are appropriate for the patient with a rheumatic disease, the following are a few of the most common ones:

- Acute and chronic pain related to inflammation and increased disease activity, tissue damage, fatigue, or lowered tolerance level

- Fatigue related to increased disease activity, pain, inadequate sleep/rest, deconditioning, inadequate nutrition, and emotional stress/depression
- Disturbed sleep pattern related to pain, depression, and medications
- Impaired physical mobility related to decreased range of motion, muscle weakness, pain on movement, limited endurance, lack of or improper use of ambulatory devices
- Self-care deficits related to contractures, fatigue, or loss of motion
- Disturbed body image related to physical and psychological changes and dependency imposed by chronic illness
- Ineffective coping related to actual or perceived lifestyle or role changes

Collaborative Problems/ Potential Complications

Based on assessment data, potential complications may include the following:

- Adverse effects of medications

Planning and Goals

The major goals for the patient may include relief of pain and discomfort, relief of fatigue, promotion of restorative sleep, increased mobility, maintenance of self-care, improved body image, effective coping, and absence of complications.

Nursing Interventions

An understanding of the underlying disease process (ie, degeneration or inflammation, including degeneration resulting from inflammation or vice versa) guides the nurse's critical thinking processes. In addition, knowledge about whether the condition is localized or more widely systemic influences the scope of the nursing activity.

Some rheumatic diseases (eg, OA) are more localized alterations in which control of symptoms such as pain or stiffness is possible. Others (eg, gout) have a known cause and specific treatment to control the symptoms. The diseases that usually present the greatest challenge are those with systemic manifestations, such as the diffuse connective tissue diseases. The plan of nursing care in Chart 54-2 details the nursing interventions to be considered for each nursing diagnosis.

Relieving Pain and Discomfort

Medications are used on a short-term basis to relieve acute pain. Because the pain may be persistent, nonopioid analgesics such as acetaminophen are often used. After administering medications, the nurse needs to reassess pain levels at intervals. With persistent pain, assessment findings should be compared with baseline measurements and evaluations. Additional measures include exploring coping skills and strategies that have worked in the past.

The patient needs to understand the importance of taking medications, such as NSAIDs and DMARDs, exactly as prescribed to achieve maximum benefits. These benefits include relief of pain and anti-inflammatory action as the disease is brought under control. Because disease control and pain relief are delayed, the patient may mistakenly believe the medication is ineffective or may think of the medication as merely "pain pills," taking them only sporadically and failing to achieve control over the disease activity. Alternatively, the patient may not understand the need to continue the medication for its anti-inflammatory actions once pain control has been achieved.

A weight reduction program may be recommended to relieve stress on painful joints. Heat applications are also helpful in relieving pain, stiffness, and muscle spasm. Superficial heat may be applied in the form of warm tub baths or showers and warm moist compresses. Paraffin baths (dips), which offer concentrated heat, are helpful to patients with wrist and small-joint involvement. Maximum benefit is achieved within 20 minutes after application. More frequent use for shorter lengths of time is most beneficial. Therapeutic exercises can be carried out more comfortably and effectively after heat has been applied.

However, in some patients, heat may actually increase pain, muscle spasm, and synovial fluid volume. If the inflammatory process is acute, cold applications in the form of moist packs or an ice bag may be tried. Both heat and cold are analgesic to nerve pain receptors and can relax muscle spasms (Robinson, Brosseau, Casimiro, et al., 2006). Safe use of heat and cold must be evaluated and taught, particularly to patients with impaired sensation. Further study of the effectiveness of these modalities is needed.

The use of braces, splints, and assistive devices for ambulation, such as canes, crutches, and walkers, eases pain by limiting movement or stress from weight bearing on painful joints. Acutely inflamed joints can be rested by applying splints to limit motion. Splints also support the joint to relieve spasm. Canes and crutches can relieve stress from inflamed and painful weight-bearing joints while promoting safe ambulation. Cervical collars may be used to support the weight of the head and limit cervical motion. A metatarsal bar or special pads may be put into the patient's shoes if foot pain or deformity is present (Egan, Brosseau, Farmer, et al., 2006).

Other strategies for decreasing pain include muscle relaxation techniques, imagery, self-hypnosis, and distraction.

Decreasing Fatigue

Fatigue related to rheumatic disease can be both acute (brief and relieved by rest or sleep) and chronic. Chronic fatigue, related to the disease process, is persistent, cumulative, and not eliminated by rest but is

(text continues on page 1903)

CHART 54-2

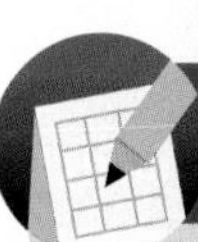

Plan of Nursing Care — Care of the Patient With a Rheumatic Disease

Nursing Diagnosis: Acute and chronic pain related to inflammation and increased disease activity, tissue damage, fatigue, or lowered tolerance level
Goal: Improvement in comfort level; incorporation of pain management techniques into daily life

NURSING INTERVENTIONS	RATIONALE	EXPECTED OUTCOMES
1. Provide variety of comfort measures a. Application of heat or cold b. Massage, position changes, rest c. Foam mattress, supportive pillow, splints d. Relaxation techniques, diversional activities	1. Pain may respond to nonpharmacologic interventions such as joint protection, exercise, relaxation, and thermal modalities.	• Identifies factors that exacerbate or influence pain response • Identifies and uses pain management strategies • Verbalizes decrease in pain • Reports signs and symptoms of side effects in timely manner to prevent additional problems • Verbalizes that pain is characteristic of rheumatic disease • Establishes realistic pain-relief goals • Verbalizes that pain often leads to the use of nontraditional and unproven self-treatment methods • Identifies changes in quality or intensity of pain
2. Administer anti-inflammatory, analgesic, and slow-acting antirheumatic medications as prescribed.	2. Pain of rheumatic disease responds to individual or combination medication regimens.	
3. Individualize medication schedule to meet patient's need for pain management.	3. Previous pain experiences and management strategies may be different from those needed for persistent pain.	
4. Encourage verbalization of feelings about pain and chronicity of disease.	4. Verbalization promotes coping.	
5. Teach pathophysiology of pain and rheumatic disease, and assist patient to recognize that pain often leads to unproven treatment methods.	5. Knowledge of rheumatic pain and appropriate treatment may help patient avoid unsafe, ineffective therapies.	
6. Assist in identification of pain that leads to use of unproven methods of treatment.	6. The impact of pain on an individual's life often leads to misconceptions about pain and pain management techniques.	
7. Assess for subjective changes in pain.	7. The individual's description of pain is a more reliable indicator than objective measurements such as change in vital signs, body movement, and facial expression.	

Nursing Diagnosis: Fatigue related to increased disease activity, pain, inadequate sleep/rest, deconditioning, inadequate nutrition, and emotional stress/depression
Goal: Incorporates as part of daily activities strategies necessary to modify fatigue

NURSING INTERVENTIONS	RATIONALE	EXPECTED OUTCOMES
1. Provide instruction about fatigue a. Describe relationship of disease activity to fatigue.	1. The patient's understanding of fatigue will affect his or her actions. a. The amount of fatigue is directly related to the activity of the disease.	• Self-evaluates and monitors fatigue pattern • Verbalizes the relationship of fatigue to disease activity

continued >

CHART 54-2

Plan of Nursing Care Care of the Patient With a Rheumatic Disease (Continued)

NURSING INTERVENTIONS	RATIONALE	EXPECTED OUTCOMES
b. Describe comfort measures while providing them.	b. Relief of discomfort can relieve fatigue.	• Uses comfort measures as appropriate
c. Develop and encourage a sleep routine (warm bath and relaxation techniques that promote sleep).	c. Effective bedtime routine promotes restorative sleep.	• Practices effective sleep hygiene and routine • Makes use of various assistive devices (splints, canes) and strategies (bed rest, relaxation techniques) to ease different kinds of fatigue
d. Explain importance of rest for relieving systematic, articular, and emotional stress.	d. Different kinds of rest are needed to relieve fatigue and are based on patient need and response.	• Incorporates time management strategies in daily activities
e. Explain how to use energy conservation techniques (pacing, delegating, setting priorities).	e. A variety of measures can be used to conserve energy.	• Uses appropriate measures to prevent physical and emotional fatigue
f. Identify physical and emotional factors that can cause fatigue.	f. Awareness of the various causes of fatigue provides the basis for measures to modify the fatigue.	• Has an established plan to ensure well-paced, therapeutic activity schedule • Adheres to therapeutic program
2. Facilitate development of appropriate activity/rest schedule.	2. Alternating rest and activity conserves energy while allowing most productivity.	• Follows a planned conditioning program
3. Encourage adherence to the treatment program.	3. Overall control of disease activity can decrease the amount of fatigue.	• Consumes a nutritious diet consisting of appropriate food groups and recommended daily allowance of vitamins and minerals
4. Refer to and encourage a conditioning program.	4. Deconditioning resulting from lack of mobility, understanding, and disease activity contributes to fatigue.	
5. Encourage adequate nutrition, including source of iron from food and supplements.	5. A nutritious diet can help counteract fatigue.	

Nursing Diagnosis: Impaired physical mobility related to decreased range of motion, muscle weakness, pain on movement, limited endurance, lack of or improper use of ambulatory devices
Goal: Attains and maintains optimal functional mobility

NURSING INTERVENTIONS	RATIONALE	EXPECTED OUTCOMES
1. Encourage verbalization regarding limitations in mobility.	1. Mobility is not necessarily related to deformity. Pain, stiffness, and fatigue may temporarily limit mobility. The degree of mobility is not synonymous with the degree of independence. Decreased mobility may influence a person's self-concept and lead to social isolation.	• Identifies factors that interfere with mobility • Describes and uses measures to prevent loss of motion • Identifies environmental (home, school, work, community) barriers to optimal mobility • Uses appropriate techniques and/or assistive equipment to aid mobility

CHART 54-2

Plan of Nursing Care — Care of the Patient With a Rheumatic Disease (Continued)

NURSING INTERVENTIONS	RATIONALE	EXPECTED OUTCOMES
2. Assess need for occupational or physical therapy consultation: a. Emphasize range of motion of affected joints. b. Promote use of assistive ambulatory devices. c. Explain use of safe footwear. d. Use individual appropriate positioning/posture.	2. Therapeutic exercises, proper footwear, and/or assistive equipment may improve mobility. Correct posture and positioning are necessary for maintaining optimal mobility.	• Identifies community resources available to assist in managing decreased mobility
3. Assist to identify environmental barriers.	3. Furniture and architectural adaptations may enhance mobility.	
4. Encourage independence in mobility and assist as needed. a. Allow ample time for activity b. Provide rest period after activity. c. Reinforce principles of joint protection and work simplification.	4. Changes in mobility may lead to a decrease in personal safety.	
5. Initiate referral to community health agency.	5. The degree of mobility may be slow to improve or may not improve with intervention.	

Nursing Diagnosis: Self-care deficits related to contractures, fatigue, or loss of motion
Goal: Achieves self-care independently or with the use of resources

NURSING INTERVENTIONS	RATIONALE	EXPECTED OUTCOMES
1. Assist patient to identify self-care deficits and factors that interfere with ability to perform self-care activities.	1. The ability to perform self-care activities is influenced by the disease activity and the accompanying pain, stiffness, fatigue, muscle weakness, loss of motion, and depression.	• Identifies factors that interfere with the ability to perform self-care activities • Identifies alternative methods for meeting self-care needs • Uses alternative methods for meeting self-care needs • Identifies and uses other health care resources for meeting self-care needs
2. Develop a plan based on the patient's perceptions and priorities on how to establish and achieve goals to meet self-care needs, incorporating joint protection, energy conservation, and work simplification concepts. a. Provide appropriate assistive devices. b. Reinforce correct and safe use of assistive devices. c. Allow patient to control timing of self-care activities.	2. Assistive devices may enhance self-care abilities. Effective planning for changes must include the patient who must accept and adopt the plan.	

continued >

CHART 54-2

Plan of Nursing Care — Care of the Patient With a Rheumatic Disease (Continued)

NURSING INTERVENTIONS	RATIONALE	EXPECTED OUTCOMES
d. Explore with the patient different ways to perform difficult tasks or ways to enlist the help of someone else.		
3. Consult with community health care agencies when individuals have attained a maximum level of self-care yet still have some deficits, especially regarding safety.	3. Individuals differ in ability and willingness to perform self-care activities. Changes in ability to care for self may lead to a decrease in personal safety.	

Nursing Diagnosis: Disturbed body image related to physical and psychological changes and dependency imposed by chronic illness
Goal: Adapts to physical and psychological changes imposed by the rheumatic disease

NURSING INTERVENTIONS	RATIONALE	EXPECTED OUTCOMES
1. Help patient identify elements of control over disease symptoms and treatment. 2. Encourage patient's verbalization of feelings, perceptions, and fears. a. Help to assess present situation and identify problems. b. Assist to identify past coping mechanisms. c. Assist to identify effective coping mechanisms.	1. The individual's self-concept may be altered by the disease or its treatment. 2. The individual's coping strategies reflect the strength of his or her self-concept.	• Verbalizes an awareness that changes taking place in self-concept are normal responses to rheumatic disease and other chronic illnesses • Identifies strategies to cope with altered self-concept

Nursing Diagnosis: Ineffective coping related to actual or perceived lifestyle or role changes
Goal: Use of effective coping behaviors for dealing with actual or perceived limitations and role changes

NURSING INTERVENTIONS	RATIONALE	EXPECTED OUTCOMES
1. Identify areas of life affected by disease. Answer questions and dispel possible myths. 2. Develop plan for managing symptoms and enlisting support of family and friends to promote daily function.	1. The effects of disease may be more or less manageable once identified and explored reasonably. 2. By taking action and involving others appropriately, patient develops or draws on coping skills and community support.	• Names functions and roles affected and not affected by disease process • Describes therapeutic regimen and states actions to take to improve, change, or accept a particular situation, function, or role

CHART 54-2

Plan of Nursing Care — Care of the Patient With a Rheumatic Disease (Continued)

Collaborative Problems: Complications secondary to effects of medications
Goal: Absence or resolution of complications

NURSING INTERVENTIONS	RATIONALE	EXPECTED OUTCOMES
1. Perform periodic clinical assessment and laboratory evaluation.	1. Skillful assessment helps detect early symptoms of side effects of medications.	• Complies with monitoring procedures and experiences minimal side effects
2. Instruct in correct self-administration, potential side effects, and importance of monitoring.	2. The patient needs accurate information about medications and potential side effects to avoid or manage them.	• Takes medication as prescribed and lists potential side effects • Identifies strategies to reduce or manage side effects
3. Counsel regarding methods to reduce side effects and manage symptoms.	3. Appropriate identification and early intervention may minimize complications.	• Reports that side effects or complications have subsided
4. Administer medications in modified doses as prescribed if complications occur.	4. Modifications may help minimize side effects or other complications.	

influenced by biologic, psychological, social, and personal factors.

Disease-related factors that may influence the amount and severity of fatigue include persistent pain, sleep disturbance, impaired physical activity, and disease duration. Pain increases fatigue because additional physical and emotional energy is required to deal with it. It may also cause the patient to expend more energy to do tasks in a way that causes less pain.

Efforts are aimed at modifying and reducing the fatigue. Energy may be regained by the use of rest periods. The patient's needs determine the type and amount of rest needed. Naps or nighttime sleep can provide systemic rest. Splints can provide articular rest by limiting motion and stress on the joints. Relaxation techniques can provide emotional rest. Inactivity may lead to deconditioning and fatigue, so measures to build endurance should be instituted. Conditioning exercise, such as walking, swimming, or biking, requires gradual progression of activity and monitoring of disease activity.

Psychosocial factors with an effect on fatigue include depression, learned helplessness, and perceived social support (Lorig, 2005). These factors affect the patient's perception and evaluation of the fatigue. Improvement of functional status can improve mood. The patient is taught strategies to conserve energy, such as planning and grouping activities to minimize the number of times needed to climb the stairs each day and sitting down to prepare meals.

Promoting Restorative Sleep

Restful sleep is important in helping the patient to cope with pain, minimize physical fatigue, and deal with the changes necessitated by a chronic disease. In patients with acute disease, sleep time is frequently reduced and fragmented by prolonged awakenings. Stiffness, depression, and medications may also compromise the quality of sleep and increase daytime fatigue. A sleep-inducing routine, medication, and comfort measures may help improve the quality of sleep.

Teaching sleep hygiene strategies may be helpful in promoting restorative sleep. These strategies include establishing a set time to sleep and a regular wake-up time, creating a quiet sleep environment with a comfortable room temperature, avoiding factors that interfere with sleep (eg, use of alcohol and caffeine), using relaxation exercises, and getting out of bed and engaging in another activity (eg, reading) if unable to sleep (Dochterman & Bulechek, 2004).

Increasing Mobility

Proper body positioning is essential to minimize stress on inflamed joints and prevent deformities that limit mobility. All joints should be supported in a position of optimal function. When in bed, the patient should lie flat on a firm mattress, with feet positioned against a footboard and with only one pillow under the head because of the risk of dorsal kyphosis. A pillow should not be placed under the knees, because this promotes flexion contracture. The patient should lie prone several times daily to prevent hip flexion contracture.

Active and active/self-assisted range-of-motion exercises are encouraged because they prevent joint stiffness and increase mobility (Steultjens, Bouter, Dekker, et al., 2006). Active/self-assisted exercises involve the use of overhead pulleys or wand exercises (shoulder exercises using a wand, stick, or cane). Measures to reinforce proper body posture and increase mobility include walking erect and using chairs with straight backs. When seated, the patient should rest the feet flat on the floor and the shoulders and hips against the back of the chair.

Care must be taken so that splinting for comfort does not restrict mobility later. The knee is splinted at full extension and the wrist at slight dorsiflexion. Because of the predominant strength of flexor muscles, the joints should not be permitted to "freeze" in positions of flexion. This can be prevented by regularly removing the splint and exercising the joint through a range of motion. Splint modification may be needed when changes occur in joint structure.

In addition, assistive devices may be necessary for mobility. They should be properly fitted, and the patient should be instructed in their correct and safe use. A cane, long enough to allow for only a slight bend of the elbow, should be held in the hand opposite the affected side. Forearm-trough style crutches (platform crutches) may be needed to protect the upper extremities if the disease also involves the hands and wrists. This is especially important for the patient undergoing rehabilitation after lower extremity joint reconstructive surgery. Assistive devices can mean the difference between dependence and independence in mobility; however, they may also alter the patient's body image, which can become a barrier to adherence to the treatment regimen.

Facilitating Self-Care

Adaptive equipment may increase the patient's independence. However, when introducing adaptive equipment, the nurse must be sensitive to the patient's feelings by demonstrating acceptance and positive attitudes about using these devices. The nurse needs to keep in mind that a patient's deformity does not necessarily equate with the severity of limitations or disability. For example, swollen (edematous) hands may be more limiting than deformed hands. The nurse in a hospital or extended care facility can help preserve the patient's independence by making available adaptive equipment for eating, toileting, bathing, and dressing. In the home, the nurse can encourage use of these devices. Again, by relieving pain, stiffness, and fatigue, the nurse may increase the patient's ability to perform self-care (Lorig, 2005).

Improving Body Image and Coping

All aspects of the patient's life, including perception of self, work role, social life, sexual function, and financial status, may be altered because of the unpredictability and uncertainty of the course of a rheumatic disease. Body image changes can cause social isolation and depression. The nurse and the family need to understand and be sensitive to the patient's emotional reactions to the disease and provide support and assistance when appropriate. Communication should be encouraged so that the patient and family verbalize feelings, perceptions, and fears related to the disease. The nurse helps the patient and family identify areas in which they have some control over disease symptoms and treatment. The nurse also encourages commitment to the treatment program, which is a key to positive outcomes, as well as use of effective coping strategies.

Monitoring and Managing Potential Complications

Medications used for treating rheumatic diseases have the potential for serious and adverse effects. Therefore, an important aspect of care is avoiding medication-induced complications. The clinician bases the prescribed medication regimen on clinical findings and past medical history, then monitors for side effects with periodic clinical assessments and laboratory testing. The nurse has a major role in working with the primary care provider and pharmacist to help the patient recognize and deal with side effects from medications. These side effects may include gastrointestinal bleeding or irritation, bone marrow suppression, kidney or liver toxicity, infection, oral ulcers, rashes, and changes in vision. Other signs and symptoms include bruising, breathing problems, dizziness, jaundice, dark urine, black or bloody stools, diarrhea, nausea and vomiting, and headaches. Systemic and local infections, which can often be masked by high doses of corticosteroids, need close monitoring (see Table 54-3 for more information about administration considerations).

Patient instruction also includes teaching correct techniques for self-administration of medications, methods of reducing side effects, and measures to ensure regular monitoring. The nurse can be available for consultation between physician visits. If side effects occur, the medication may need to be stopped or the dose reduced. The patient may experience an increase in symptoms while the complication is being resolved or a new medication is being initiated. In such cases, the nurse's counseling regarding symptom management may relieve potential anxiety and distress.

Promoting Home and Community-Based Care

TEACHING PATIENTS SELF-CARE

Patient teaching is an essential aspect of nursing care of the patient with rheumatic disease to enable the patient to maintain as much independence as possible, to take medications accurately and safely, and to use adaptive devices correctly. Patient teaching focuses on the disorder itself, the possible changes related to the disorder, the therapeutic regimen prescribed to treat it, the potential side effects of medications, strategies to maintain independence and function, and patient safety in the home (Chart 54-3).

The patient and family are encouraged to verbalize their concerns and ask questions. Pain, fatigue, and depression can interfere with the patient's ability to learn and should be addressed before teaching is initi-

CHART 54-3

HOME CARE CHECKLIST • The Patient with Rheumatic Disease

At the completion of the home care instruction, the patient or caregiver will be able to:	Patient	Caregiver
• Explain the nature of the disease and principles of disease management.	✔	✔
• Describe the medication regimen (name of medications, dosage, schedule of administration, precautions, potential side effects, and desired effects).	✔	✔
• Identify monitoring procedures and strategies that should be implemented.	✔	✔
• Identify sources of additional information, if necessary.	✔	✔
• Demonstrate accurate and safe self-administration of medications.	✔	✔
• Describe and demonstrate use of pain management techniques.	✔	✔
• Demonstrate use of joint protection techniques in activities of daily living (ADLs).	✔	✔
• Demonstrate ability to perform self-care activities independently or with assistive devices.	✔	
• Demonstrate a safe exercise program.	✔	
• Demonstrate a relaxation technique.	✔	

ated. Various educational strategies may then be used, depending on the patient's previous knowledge base, interest level, degree of comfort, social or cultural influences, and readiness to learn. The nurse instructs the patient about basic disease management and necessary adaptations in lifestyle. Because suppression of inflammation and autoimmune responses requires the use of anti-inflammatory, disease-modifying antirheumatic and immunosuppressive agents, the patient is taught about prescribed medications, including type, dosage, rationale, potential side effects, self-administration, and required monitoring procedures. If hospitalized, the patient is encouraged to practice new self-management skills with support from caregivers and significant others. The nurse then reinforces disease management skills during each patient contact. Barriers to compliance are assessed, and measures are taken to promote adherence to medications and the treatment program.

CONTINUING CARE

Depending on the severity of the disorder and the patient's resources and supports, referral for home care may or may not be warranted. However, the patient who is elderly or frail, has a rheumatic disorder that limits function significantly, and lives alone may need a referral for home care.

The impact of rheumatic disease on everyday life is not always evident when the patient is seen in the hospital or in an ambulatory care setting. The increased frequency with which nurses see patients in the home provides opportunities for recognizing problems and implementing interventions aimed at improving the quality of life of patients with rheumatic disorders. The patient encountered in the home setting often has a rheumatic disease that is secondary to the primary reason for the visit. In such cases, the problems caused by the rheumatic disease may interfere with the treatment of the primary condition. For example, a patient who is recovering from coronary artery surgery may have been instructed to exercise but is unable or only partially able to do so because of the rheumatic disease. Conversely, treatment of the primary condition can cause or increase problems related to the rheumatic disease. For example, the cardiac patient who has been instructed to walk long distances every day may find that doing so increases the symptoms of OA in the knees.

During home visits, the nurse has the opportunity to assess the home environment and its adequacy for patient safety and management of the disorder. Adherence to the treatment program can be more easily monitored in the home setting, where physical and social barriers to adherence are more readily identified. For example, a patient with diabetes who requires insulin may be unable to fill the syringe accurately or unable to administer the insulin because of impaired joint mobility. Appropriate adaptive equipment needed for increased independence is often identified more readily when the nurse sees how the patient functions in the home. Any barriers to adherence are identified, and appropriate referrals are made.

For patients at risk for impaired skin integrity, the home care nurse can closely monitor skin status and also instruct, provide, or supervise the patient and family in preventive skin care measures. The nurse also assesses the patient's need for assistance in the home and supervises home health aides, who may meet many of the needs of the patient with a rheumatic disease. Referrals to physical and occupational therapists may be made as problems are identified and limitations increase. A home care nurse may visit the home to make sure the patient can function as independently as possible despite mobility problems and can safely manage treatments and pharmacotherapy. The patient and family should be informed about support services such as Meals on Wheels and local Arthritis Foundation chapters.

Because many of the medications used to suppress inflammation are injectable, the nurse may administer the medication to the patient or teach self-injection. These frequent contacts allow the nurse to reinforce other disease management techniques.

The nurse also assesses the patient's physical and psychological status, adequacy of symptom management, and adherence to the management plan. Previous teaching is reinforced with emphasis on potential side effects of medications and changes in physical status that indicate disease progression and the need to contact the health care provider for reevaluation; otherwise, patients may wait until their next appointment. The importance of follow-up appointments is emphasized to the patient and family.

Patients with chronic disorders often focus on the chronic disease and neglect general health issues; therefore, the patient and family should be reminded about the importance of participating in other health promotion activities and health screening (eg, immunizations, cholesterol screening, bone density testing, gynecologic examinations, mammography, colonoscopy).

Evaluation

Expected Patient Outcomes

Expected patient outcomes may include the following:

1. Experiences relief of pain or improved comfort level
   a. Identifies factors that cause or increase pain
   b. Identifies realistic goals for pain relief
   c. Uses pain management strategies safely and effectively
   d. Reports decreased pain and increased comfort level
2. Experiences reduction in level of fatigue
   a. Identifies factors that contribute to fatigue
   b. Verbalizes the relationship of fatigue to disease activity
   c. Schedules periodic rest periods and identifies and uses other measures to prevent or modify fatigue
   d. Reports decreased level of fatigue
   e. Practices energy conservation strategies
3. Improves sleep patterns
   a. Reports fewer nighttime awakenings
   b. Adheres to sleep-inducing routine
   c. Reports feeling rested on awakening
4. Increases or maintains level of mobility
   a. Identifies factors that impede mobility
   b. Participates in activities and exercises that promote or maintain mobility
   c. Uses assistive devices appropriately and safely
   d. Demonstrates normal or acceptable body alignment and posture
5. Maintains self-care activities
   a. Participates in self-care activities within capabilities
   b. Uses adaptive equipment and alternative methods to increase participation in self-care activities
   c. Maintains self-care at highest possible level
6. Experiences improved body image and coping
   a. Verbalizes concerns about the impact of rheumatic disease on appearance and function
   b. Sets and achieves meaningful goals
   c. States acceptance of self-worth
   d. Adapts to body image changes caused by disease
   e. Identifies and uses effective coping strategies
7. Experiences absence of complications
   a. Takes medications as prescribed
   b. States potential side effects of medications and names reportable side effects
   c. Verbalizes understanding of rationale for monitoring
   d. Complies with recommendations for monitoring
   e. Identifies strategies to reduce risks of side effects

Diffuse Connective Tissue Diseases

Diffuse connective tissue disease refers to a group of disorders that are chronic in nature and are characterized by diffuse inflammation and degeneration in the connective tissues. These disorders share similar clinical features and may affect some of the same organs. The characteristic clinical course is one of exacerbations and remissions. Although the diffuse connective tissue diseases have unknown causes, they are thought to be the result of immunologic abnormalities. They include RA, SLE, scleroderma, polymyositis, and polymyalgia rheumatica.

Rheumatoid Arthritis

RA is commonly used as the prototype for inflammatory arthritis. RA affects 0.5% to 1% of the general population worldwide, with a female-to-male ratio between 2:1 and 4:1 (Firestein, 2005).

Pathophysiology

In RA, the autoimmune reaction (Fig. 54-3) primarily occurs in the synovial tissue. Phagocytosis produces enzymes within the joint. The enzymes break down collagen, causing edema, proliferation of the synovial membrane, and ultimately pannus formation. Pannus destroys cartilage and erodes the bone. The consequence is loss of articular surfaces and joint motion. Muscle fibers undergo degenerative changes. Tendon and ligament elasticity and contractile power are lost.

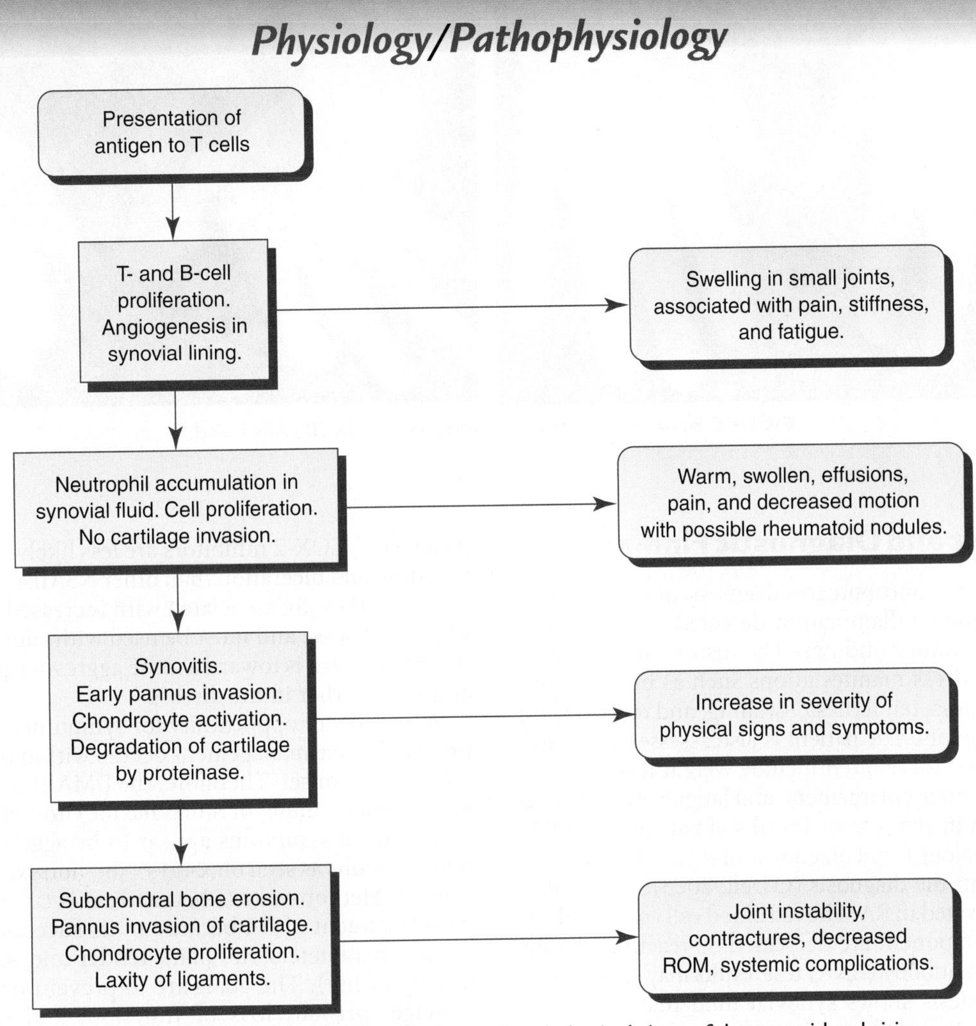

FIGURE 54-3. Pathophysiology and associated physical signs of rheumatoid arthritis.

Clinical Manifestations

Clinical manifestations of RA vary, usually reflecting the stage and severity of the disease. Joint pain, swelling, warmth, erythema, and lack of function are classic symptoms. Palpation of the joints reveals spongy or boggy tissue. Often fluid can be aspirated from the inflamed joint. Characteristically, the pattern of joint involvement begins in the small joints of the hands, wrists, and feet. As the disease progresses, the knees, shoulders, hips, elbows, ankles, cervical spine, and temporomandibular joints are affected. The onset of symptoms is usually acute. Symptoms are usually bilateral and symmetric. In addition to joint pain and swelling, another classic sign of RA is joint stiffness, especially in the morning, lasting at least 30 to 45 minutes (Harris, 2005).

In the early stages of disease, even before bony changes occur, limitation in function can occur when there is active inflammation in the joints. Joints that are hot, swollen, and painful are not easily moved. The patient tends to guard or protect these joints by immobilizing them. Immobilization for extended periods can lead to contractures, creating soft tissue deformity.

Deformities of the hands and feet are common in RA (Fig. 54-4). The deformity may be caused by misalignment resulting from swelling, progressive joint destruction, or the subluxation (partial dislocation) that occurs when one bone slips over another and eliminates the joint space.

RA is a systemic disease with multiple extra-articular features. Most common are fever, weight loss, fatigue, anemia, lymph node enlargement, and Raynaud's phenomenon (cold- and stress-induced vasospasm causing episodes of digital blanching or cyanosis). Rheumatoid nodules may be noted in patients with more advanced RA, and they develop at some time in the course of the disease in about 25% of patients (O'Dell, 2005). These nodules are usually nontender and movable in the subcutaneous tissue. They usually appear over bony prominences such as the elbow, are varied in size, and can disappear spontaneously. Nodules occur only in people who have rheumatoid factor. The nodules often are associated with rapidly progressive and destructive disease. Other extra-articular features include arteritis, neuropathy, scleritis, pericarditis, splenomegaly, and Sjögren's syndrome (dry eyes and dry mucous membranes).

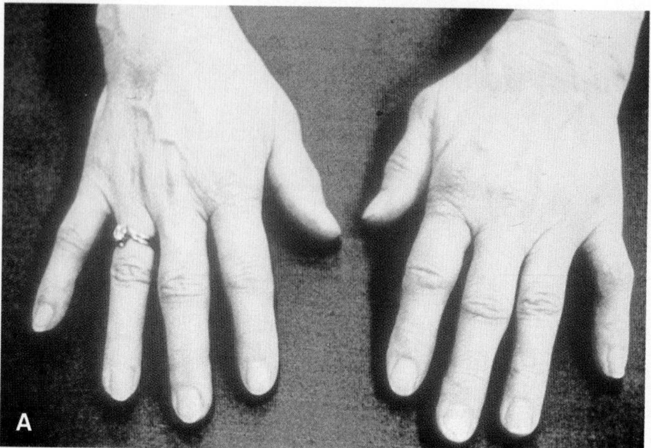

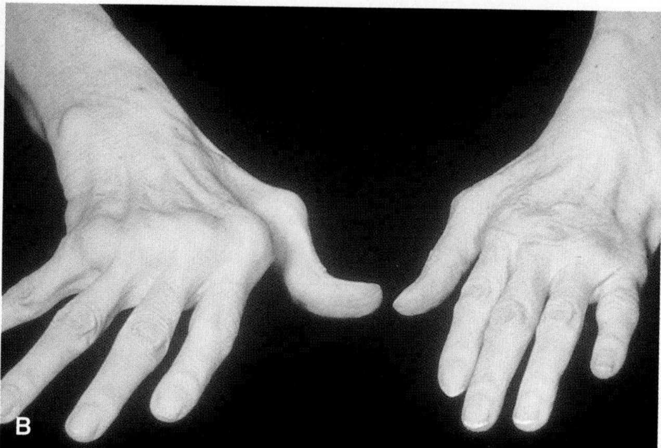

FIGURE 54-4. Rheumatoid arthritis. (**A**) Early. (**B**) Advanced.

Assessment and Diagnostic Findings

Several factors can contribute to a diagnosis of RA: rheumatoid nodules, joint inflammation detected on palpation, and certain laboratory findings. The history and physical examination address manifestations such as bilateral and symmetric stiffness, tenderness, swelling, and temperature changes in the joints. The patient is also assessed for extra-articular changes; these often include weight loss, sensory changes, lymph node enlargement, and fatigue. Rheumatoid factor is present in about three fourths of patients with RA, but its presence alone is not diagnostic of RA, and its absence does not rule out the diagnosis (O'Dell, 2005). The ESR is significantly elevated in RA. The red blood cell count and C4 complement component are decreased. C-reactive protein and antinuclear antibody (ANA) test results may also be positive. Arthrocentesis shows synovial fluid that is cloudy, milky, or dark yellow and contains numerous inflammatory components, such as leukocytes and complement.

X-ray studies, performed to help diagnose and monitor the progression of disease, show characteristic bony erosions and narrowed joint spaces occurring later in the disease.

Medical Management

Early Rheumatoid Arthritis

In patients with early RA, treatment begins with education, a balance of rest and exercise, and referral to appropriate community agencies (such as the Arthritis Foundation) for support. Medical management begins with therapeutic doses of salicylates or NSAIDs. When used in full therapeutic dosages, these medications provide both anti-inflammatory and analgesic effects. Taking medications as prescribed to maintain a consistent blood level is necessary to optimize the effectiveness of the anti-inflammatory medication.

Several cyclo-oxygenase 2 (COX-2) inhibitors, another class of NSAIDs, have been approved for treatment of RA. Cyclo-oxygenase is an enzyme that is involved in the inflammatory process. COX-2 inhibitors block the enzyme involved in inflammation (COX-2) while leaving intact the enzyme involved in protecting the stomach lining (COX-1). As a result, COX-2 inhibitors are less likely to cause gastric irritation and ulceration than other NSAIDs (Lehne, 2004); however, they are associated with increased risk of cardiovascular disease and must be used with caution. The trend in management is toward a more aggressive pharmacologic approach earlier in the disease.

A window of opportunity for symptom control and improved disease management occurs within the first 2 years after disease onset. Therefore, the DMARDs (antimalarials, gold, penicillamine, or sulfasalazine) are initiated early in treatment. If symptoms appear to be aggressive (ie, early bony erosions as seen on x-rays), methotrexate may be considered. Methotrexate (Rheumatrex) is currently the standard treatment of RA because of its success in improving disease parameters (ie, pain, tender and swollen joints, quality of life). The goals are to prevent or control joint damage, prevent loss of function, and decrease pain (American College of Rheumatology, 2002).

An alternative treatment approach for RA has emerged in the area of biologic therapies. Biologic response modifiers are a group of agents that consist of molecules produced by cells of the immune system or by cells that participate in the inflammatory reactions (Toussirot & Wendling, 2004). Recent studies (St. Clair, van der Heijde, Smolen, et al., 2004; Voulgari, Alamanos, Nikas, et al., 2005) using tumor necrosis factor-alpha (TNF-α) inhibitors in combination with other medications, have shown that patients demonstrate significant improvement based on American College of Rheumatology criteria (Felson et al., 1995). Four examples of biologic response modifiers that are currently available are etanercept (Enbrel), infliximab (Remicade), adalimumab (Humira) and anakinra (Kineret). Etanercept, infliximab, and adalimumab inhibit the function of TNF-α, a key **cytokine** known to play a role in the disease process in RA (Porth, 2005), whereas anakinra inhibits the function of interleukin-1, another cytokine that contributes to the destruction of the joint (Furst, 2004). Research in this area is ongoing.

Additional analgesia may be prescribed for periods of extreme pain. Opioid analgesics are avoided because of the potential for continuing need for pain relief. Nonpharmacologic pain management techniques (eg, relaxation techniques, heat and cold applications) are taught.

Moderate, Erosive Rheumatoid Arthritis

For moderate, erosive RA, a formal program with occupational and physical therapy is prescribed to educate the patient about principles of joint protection, pacing activities, work simplification, range of motion, and muscle-strengthening exercises. The patient is encouraged to participate actively in the management program. The medication program is reevaluated periodically, and appropriate changes are made if indicated. Cyclosporine (Neoral), an immunosuppressant, may be added to enhance the disease-modifying effect of methotrexate.

Persistent, Erosive Rheumatoid Arthritis

For persistent, erosive RA, reconstructive surgery and corticosteroids are often used. Reconstructive surgery is indicated when pain cannot be relieved by conservative measures and the threat of loss of independence is eminent. Surgical procedures include synovectomy (excision of the synovial membrane), tenorrhaphy (suturing of a tendon), arthrodesis (surgical fusion of the joint), and **arthroplasty** (surgical repair and replacement of the joint). Surgery is not performed during disease flares.

Systemic corticosteroids are used when the patient has unremitting inflammation and pain or needs a "bridging" medication while waiting for the slower DMARDs (eg, methotrexate) to begin taking effect. Low-dose corticosteroid therapy is prescribed for the shortest time necessary to minimize side effects. Single large joints that are severely inflamed and fail to respond promptly to the measures outlined previously may be treated by local injection of a corticosteroid (Zvaifler & Corr, 2005).

Advanced, Unremitting Rheumatoid Arthritis

For advanced, unremitting RA, immunosuppressive agents are prescribed because of their ability to affect the production of antibodies at the cellular level. These include high-dose methotrexate (Rheumatrex), cyclophosphamide (Cytoxan), azathioprine (Imuran), and leflunomide (Arava). However, these medications are highly toxic and can produce bone marrow suppression, anemia, gastrointestinal disturbances, and rashes.

Through all stages of RA, depression and sleep deprivation may require the short-term use of low-dose antidepressant medications, such as amitriptyline (Elavil), paroxetine (Paxil), or sertraline (Zoloft), to reestablish an adequate sleep pattern and to manage chronic pain.

The U.S. Food and Drug Administration has approved a medical device for use in treating patients with more severe and long-standing RA who have had no response to or are intolerant of DMARDs. The device, a protein A immunoadsorption column (Prosorba Column), is used in 12 weekly 2-hour apheresis treatments to bind immunoglobulin G (IgG) (ie, circulating immune complex). In this unique population of patients, a significant improvement using the American College of Rheumatology criteria for improvement has been demonstrated (Roth, 2004).

Nutrition Therapy

Patients with RA frequently experience anorexia, weight loss, and anemia. A dietary history identifies usual eating habits and food preferences. Food selection should include the daily requirements from the basic food groups, with emphasis on foods high in vitamins, protein, and iron for tissue building and repair. For the patient who is extremely anorexic, small, frequent feedings with increased protein supplements may be prescribed. Some medications (ie, oral corticosteroids) used in RA treatment stimulate the appetite and, when combined with decreased activity, may lead to weight gain. Therefore, patients may need to be counseled about eating a healthy, calorie-restricted diet.

Nursing Management

Nursing care of the patient with RA follows the basic plan of care presented earlier (see Chart 54-2). The most common issues for the patient with RA include pain, sleep disturbance, fatigue, altered mood, and limited mobility. The patient with newly diagnosed RA needs information about the disease to make daily self-management decisions and to cope with having a chronic disease.

Because of repeated contact with the patient, the nurse has the opportunity to assess and intervene in patient concerns and issues that occur with the diagnosis of a chronic illness such as RA and the resulting disability. Because the disease commonly affects young women, major concerns may be related to the effects of the disease on childbearing potential, caring for family, or work responsibilities. The patient with a chronic illness may seek a "cure" or have questions about alternative therapies.

Systemic Lupus Erythematosus

The overall prevalence of SLE is estimated to be 1 per 1000 or 2000 persons. It occurs 10 times more frequently in women than in men and approximately three times more frequently in African Americans than in Caucasians (Edworthy, 2005).

Pathophysiology

SLE is a result of disturbed immune regulation that causes an exaggerated production of autoantibodies. This immunoregulatory disturbance is brought about by some combination of genetic factors, hormonal factors (as evidenced by the usual onset during the childbearing years), and environmental factors (eg, sunlight, thermal burns). Certain medications, such as hydralazine (Apresoline), procainamide (Pronestyl), isoniazid (INH), chlorpromazine (Thorazine), and some antiseizure medications, have been implicated in chemical or drug-induced SLE.

In SLE, the increase in autoantibody production is thought to result from abnormal suppressor T-cell function, which leads to immune complex deposition and tissue damage. Inflammation stimulates antigens, which in turn stimulate additional antibodies, and the cycle repeats.

Clinical Manifestations

The onset of SLE may be insidious or acute. For this reason, SLE may remain undiagnosed for many years. SLE is an

NURSING RESEARCH PROFILE

Living With Rheumatoid Arthritis

Iaquinta, M. L. & Larrabee, J. H. (2004). Phenomenological lived experience of patients with rheumatoid arthritis. *Journal of Nursing Care Quality, 19*(3), 280–289.

Purpose

Rheumatoid arthritis (RA) is a chronic, progressive, inflammatory disease of unknown etiology that causes disability as well as morbidity and mortality. RA affects the physiologic, psychological, social, spiritual, and economic aspects of life of people with the disease. A greater understanding of patient experiences is necessary to improve quality of care. The purpose of this study was to explore patients' verbal descriptions of their experiences with RA, investigate their views of the nurse's role in care, and consider the patient's role as a comanager of the disease.

Design

A qualitative research design with a phenomenological approach was used. Purposive sampling was used to recruit six Caucasian women, who ranged from 43 to 67 years of age and who had had RA from 7 to 38 years. Informed written consent was obtained from eligible participants, and audiotaped interviews lasting 1 to 2 hours were conducted. Demographic data, transcripts of the interviews, and the investigator's impressions and insights were analyzed. To evaluate the overall meaning of the patient's comments, transcripts were read and reread. Meanings and themes were identified from significant statements.

Findings

Six clusters of themes emerged from the analysis and descriptions of RA phenomena considered by the study participants. These six topics were grieving while growing, persuading self and others of RA's authenticity, cultivating resilience, confronting negative feelings, navigating the health care system, and masterminding new lifeways.

- Grieving allowed personal growth by assisting the person to rise above circumstances and bear suffering.
- Persuading self and others of RA's authenticity involved validation of the disease as well as being understood by family.
- Cultivating resilience referred to the sense of determination expressed by the participants.
- Confronting negative feelings of anger, fear, frustration, self-consciousness, and depression was identified as an important activity.
- Navigating the health care system addressed interactions between the participants and physicians and nurses.
- Masterminding new lifeways involved methods of management, adaptation to change, development of new skills, and reconciliation of lost abilities.

Nursing Implications

The findings of this study demonstrate the need for nurses to understand patients' views of RA, to provide support during difficult times, to encourage patients to verbalize their concerns, and to demonstrate compassion. Nurses also need to acknowledge patients as comanagers of RA, because the person lives with the unpredictability of the disease on a daily basis. Including the patient in disease management can result in favorable outcomes and improve the quality of patient care.

autoimmune systemic disease that can affect any body system. Involvement of the musculoskeletal system, with arthralgias and arthritis (synovitis), is a common presenting feature of SLE. Joint swelling, tenderness, and pain on movement are also common. Frequently, these are accompanied by morning stiffness.

Several different types of skin manifestations may occur in patients with SLE, including subacute cutaneous lupus erythematosus, which involves papulosquamous or annular polycyclic lesions, and discoid lupus erythematosus, which is a chronic rash that has erythematous papules or plaques and scaling and can cause scarring and pigmentation changes. The most familiar skin manifestation (occurring in more than 50% of patients with SLE) is an acute cutaneous lesion consisting of a butterfly-shaped rash across the bridge of the nose and cheeks (Petri, 2005) (Fig. 54-5). In some cases of discoid lupus erythematosus, only skin involvement occurs. In some patients with SLE, the initial skin involvement is the precursor to more systemic involvement. The lesions often worsen during exacerbations (flares) of the systemic disease and possibly are provoked by sunlight or artificial ultraviolet light. Oral ulcers, which may accompany skin lesions, may involve the buccal mucosa or the hard palate. The ulcers occur in crops and are often associated with exacerbations.

Pericarditis is the most common cardiac manifestation. Women who have SLE are also at risk for early atherosclerosis.

Serum creatinine levels and urinalysis are used in screening for renal involvement. Early detection allows for prompt treatment so that renal damage can be prevented. Renal involvement may lead to hypertension, which also requires careful monitoring and management.

Central nervous system involvement is widespread, encompassing the entire range of neurologic disease. The varied and frequent neuropsychiatric presentations of SLE are now widely recognized. These are generally demonstrated by subtle changes in behavior patterns or cognitive ability.

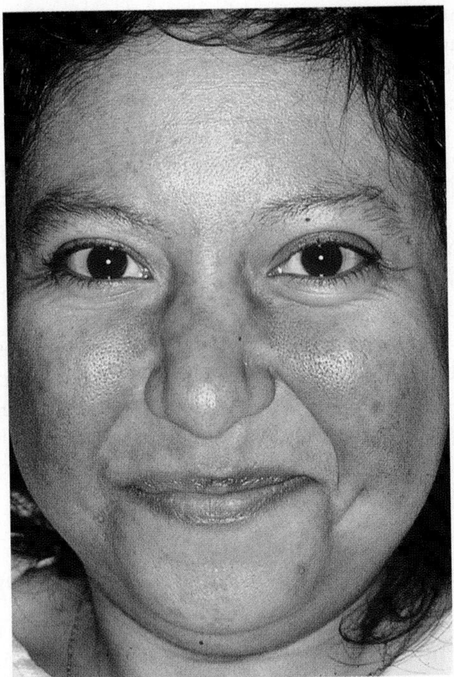

FIGURE 54-5. The characteristic butterfly rash of systemic lupus erythematosus.

Depression and psychosis are common (Edworthy, 2005; Petri, 2005).

Assessment and Diagnostic Findings

Diagnosis of SLE is based on a complete history, physical examination, and blood tests. Typically, assessment reveals classic symptoms, including fever, fatigue, weight loss, and possibly arthritis, pleurisy, and pericarditis. Interactions with the patient and family may provide further evidence of systemic involvement.

In addition to the general assessment performed for any patient with a rheumatic disease, assessment for known or suspected SLE has special features. The skin is inspected for erythematous rashes. Cutaneous erythematous plaques with an adherent scale may be observed on the scalp, face, or neck. Areas of hyperpigmentation or depigmentation may be noted, depending on the phase and type of the disease. The patient should be questioned about skin changes (because these may be transitory) and specifically about sensitivity to sunlight or artificial ultraviolet light. The scalp should be inspected for alopecia and the mouth and throat for ulcerations reflecting gastrointestinal involvement.

Cardiovascular assessment includes auscultation for pericardial friction rub, possibly associated with myocarditis and accompanying pleural effusions. The pleural effusions and infiltrations, which reflect respiratory insufficiency, are demonstrated by abnormal lung sounds. Papular, erythematous, and purpuric lesions developing on the fingertips, elbows, toes, and extensor surfaces of the forearms or lateral sides of the hand that may become necrotic suggest vascular involvement.

Joint swelling, tenderness, warmth, pain on movement, stiffness, and edema may be detected on physical examination. The joint involvement is often symmetric and similar to that found in RA.

The neurologic assessment is directed at identifying and describing any central nervous system changes. The patient and family members are asked about any behavioral changes, including manifestations of neurosis or psychosis. Signs of depression are noted, as are reports of seizures, chorea, or other central nervous system manifestations.

No single laboratory test confirms SLE; rather, blood testing reveals moderate to severe anemia, thrombocytopenia, leukocytosis, or leukopenia and positive ANAs. Other diagnostic immunologic tests support but do not confirm the diagnosis. Hematuria may be found on urinalysis.

Medical Management

Treatment of SLE includes management of acute and chronic disease. Although SLE can be life-threatening, advances in its treatment have led to improved survival and reduced morbidity. Acute disease requires interventions directed at controlling increased disease activity or exacerbations that can involve any organ system. Disease activity is a composite of clinical and laboratory features that reflect active inflammation secondary to SLE. Management of the more chronic condition involves periodic monitoring and recognition of meaningful clinical changes requiring adjustments in therapy (Hahn, 2005).

The goals of treatment include preventing progressive loss of organ function, reducing the likelihood of acute disease, minimizing disease-related disabilities, and preventing complications from therapy. Management of SLE involves regular monitoring to assess disease activity and therapeutic effectiveness.

Pharmacologic Therapy

Medication therapy for SLE is based on the concept that local tissue inflammation is mediated by exaggerated or heightened immune responses, which can vary widely in intensity and require different therapies at different times. Corticosteroids are the single most important medication available for treatment. They are used topically for cutaneous manifestations, in low oral doses for minor disease activity, and in high doses for major disease activity. Intravenous (IV) administration of corticosteroids is an alternative to traditional high-dose oral use. Antimalarial medications are effective for managing cutaneous, musculoskeletal, and mild systemic features of SLE. The NSAIDs used for minor clinical manifestations are often used along with corticosteroids in an effort to minimize corticosteroid requirements.

Immunosuppressive agents (alkylating agents and purine analogues) are used because of their effect on immune function. These medications are generally reserved for patients who have serious forms of SLE that have not responded to conservative therapies (Hahn, 2005; National Institutes of Health, 2001; Wofsy, 2005).

Nursing Management

Nursing care of the patient with SLE is based on the fundamental plan presented earlier in the chapter (see Chart 54-2).

The most common nursing diagnoses include fatigue, impaired skin integrity, body image disturbance, and lack of knowledge for self-management decisions. The disease or its treatment may produce dramatic changes in appearance and considerable distress for the patient. The changes and the unpredictable course of SLE necessitate expert assessment skills and nursing care and sensitivity to the psychological reactions of the patient. The patient may benefit from participation in support groups, which can provide disease information, daily management tips, and social support. Because sun and ultraviolet light exposure can increase disease activity or cause an exacerbation, patients should be taught to avoid exposure or to protect themselves with sunscreen and clothing.

Because of the increased risk of involvement of multiple organ systems, patients should understand the need for routine periodic screenings as well as health promotion activities. A dietary consultation may be indicated to ensure that the patient is knowledgeable about dietary recommendations, given the increased risk of cardiovascular disease, including hypertension and atherosclerosis. The nurse instructs the patient about the importance of continuing prescribed medications and addresses the changes and potential side effects that are likely to occur with their use. The patient is reminded of the importance of monitoring because of the increased risk of systemic involvement, including renal and cardiovascular effects.

Scleroderma

Scleroderma ("hard skin") is a relatively rare disease that is poorly understood; the cause is unknown. Its incidence is 18 to 20 people per million per year (Seibold, 2005).

Pathophysiology

Like other diffuse connective tissue diseases, scleroderma (also known as systemic sclerosis) has a variable course with remissions and exacerbations. Its prognosis is not as optimistic as that of SLE. The disease commonly begins with skin involvement. Mononuclear cells cluster on the skin and stimulate lymphokines to stimulate procollagen. Insoluble collagen is formed and accumulates excessively in the tissues. Initially, the inflammatory response causes edema formation, with a resulting taut, smooth, and shiny skin appearance. The skin then undergoes fibrotic changes, leading to loss of elasticity and movement. Eventually, the tissue degenerates and becomes nonfunctional. This chain of events, from inflammation to degeneration, also occurs in blood vessels, major organs, and body systems (Korn, 2005).

Clinical Manifestations

Scleroderma starts insidiously with Raynaud's phenomenon and swelling in the hands. The skin and the subcutaneous tissues become increasingly hard and rigid and cannot be pinched up from the underlying structures. Wrinkles and lines are obliterated. The skin is dry because sweat secretion over the involved region is suppressed. The extremities stiffen and lose mobility. The condition spreads slowly; for years, these changes may remain localized in the hands and the feet. The face appears masklike, immobile, and expressionless, and the mouth becomes rigid.

The changes within the body, although not visible directly, are vastly more important than the visible changes. The left ventricle of the heart is involved, resulting in heart failure. The esophagus hardens, interfering with swallowing. The lungs become scarred, impeding respiration. Digestive disturbances occur because of hardening (sclerosing) of the intestinal mucosa. Progressive renal failure may occur.

The patient may manifest a variety of symptoms referred to as the CREST syndrome. CREST stands for *c*alcinosis (calcium deposits in the tissues), *R*aynaud's phenomenon, *e*sophageal hardening and dysfunction, *s*clerodactyly (scleroderma of the digits), and *t*elangiectasia (capillary dilation that forms a vascular lesion).

Assessment and Diagnostic Findings

Assessment focuses on the sclerotic changes in the skin, contractures in the fingers, and color changes or lesions in the fingertips. Assessment of systemic involvement requires a systems review with special attention to gastrointestinal, pulmonary, renal, and cardiac symptoms. Limitations in mobility and self-care activities should be assessed, along with the impact the disease has had (or will have) on body image.

There is no one conclusive test to diagnose scleroderma. A skin biopsy is performed to identify cellular changes specific to scleroderma. Pulmonary studies show ventilation–perfusion abnormalities. Echocardiography identifies pericardial effusion (often present with cardiac involvement). Esophageal studies demonstrate decreased motility in most patients with scleroderma. Blood tests may detect ANAs, indicating a connective tissue disorder and possibly distinguishing the subgroup (diffuse or limited) of scleroderma. A positive ANA test result is common in patients with scleroderma.

Medical Management

Treatment of scleroderma depends on the clinical manifestations. All patients require counseling, during which realistic individual goals may be determined. Support measures include strategies to decrease pain and limit disability. A moderate exercise program is encouraged to prevent joint contractures. Patients are advised to avoid extreme temperatures and to use lotion to minimize skin dryness.

Pharmacologic Therapy

No medication regimen has proved effective in modifying the disease process in scleroderma, but various medications are used to treat organ system involvement. Calcium channel blockers and other antihypertensive agents may provide improvement in symptoms of Raynaud's phenomenon. Anti-inflammatory medications can be used to control arthralgia, stiffness, and general musculoskeletal discomfort (Seibold, 2005).

Nursing Management

The nursing care of the patient with scleroderma is based on the fundamental plan of nursing care presented earlier (see Chart 54-2). The most common nursing diagnoses of the patient with scleroderma are impaired skin integrity; self-care deficits; imbalanced nutrition, less than body requirements; and disturbed body image. The patient with advanced disease may also have impaired gas exchange, decreased cardiac output, impaired swallowing, and constipation.

Providing meticulous skin care and preventing the effects of Raynaud's phenomenon are major nursing challenges. Patient teaching must include the importance of avoiding cold and protecting the fingers with mittens in cold weather and when shopping in the frozen-food section of the grocery store. Warm socks and properly fitting shoes are helpful in preventing ulcers. Careful, frequent inspection for early ulcers is important. Smoking cessation is critical.

Polymyositis

Polymyositis is one of a group of diseases that are termed idiopathic inflammatory myopathies. It is a rare condition, with an incidence estimated at 5 to 10 cases per million adults per year (Miller, 2005).

Pathophysiology

Polymyositis is classified as autoimmune because autoantibodies are present. However, these antibodies do not cause damage to muscle cells, indicating only an indirect role in tissue damage. The pathogenesis is multifactorial, and a genetic predisposition is likely. Drug-induced disease is rare. Some evidence suggests a viral link.

Clinical Manifestations

The onset ranges from sudden with rapid progression to very slow and insidious. Proximal muscle weakness is typically a first symptom. Muscle weakness is usually symmetric and diffuse. Dermatomyositis, a related condition, is most commonly identified by an erythematous smooth or scaly lesion found over the joint surface.

Assessment and Diagnostic Findings

A complete history and physical examination help exclude other muscle-related disorders. As with other diffuse connective tissue disorders, no single test confirms polymyositis. An electromyogram is performed to rule out degenerative muscle disease. A muscle biopsy may reveal inflammatory infiltrate in the tissue. Serum studies indicate increased muscle enzyme activity.

Medical Management

Management involves high-dose corticosteroid therapy initially, followed by a gradual dosage reduction over several months as muscle enzyme activity decreases. Patients who do not respond to corticosteroids require the addition of an immunosuppressive agent. Plasmapheresis, lymphapheresis, and total-body irradiation have been used if there is no response to corticosteroids and immunosuppressive medications. The antimalarial agent hydroxychloroquine (Plaquenil) may be effective for skin rashes. Physical therapy is initiated slowly, with range-of-motion exercises to maintain joint mobility, followed by gradual strengthening exercises (Wortmann, 2005).

Nursing Management

Nursing care is based on the fundamental plan of nursing care presented earlier (see Chart 54-2). The most frequent nursing diagnoses for the patient with polymyositis are impaired physical mobility, fatigue, self-care deficit, and insufficient knowledge of self-management techniques.

Patients with polymyositis may have symptoms similar to those of other inflammatory diseases. However, proximal muscle weakness is characteristic, making activities such as combing the hair, reaching overhead, and using stairs difficult. Therefore, use of assistive devices may be recommended, and referral to occupational or physical therapy may be warranted.

Polymyalgia Rheumatica

Pathophysiology

The underlying mechanism involved with polymyalgia rheumatica is unknown. This disease occurs predominately in Caucasians and often in first-degree relatives. An association with the genetic marker HLA-DR4 suggests a familial predisposition. Immunoglobulin deposits in the walls of inflamed temporal arteries also suggest an autoimmune process.

Clinical Manifestations

Polymyalgia rheumatica is characterized by severe proximal muscle discomfort with mild joint swelling. Severe aching in the neck, shoulder, and pelvic muscles is common. Stiffness is noticeable most often in the morning and after periods of inactivity. Systemic features include low-grade fever, weight loss, malaise, anorexia, and depression. Because polymyalgia rheumatica usually occurs in people 50 years of age and older, it may be confused with, or disregarded as, an inevitable consequence of aging.

Giant cell arteritis, sometimes associated with polymyalgia rheumatica, may cause headaches, changes in vision, and jaw claudication. These symptoms should be evaluated immediately because of the potential for a sudden and permanent loss of vision if the condition is left untreated. Polymyalgia rheumatica and giant cell arteritis typically have a self-limited course, lasting several months to several years (Paget, 2001).

Assessment and Diagnostic Findings

Polymyalgia rheumatica and giant cell arteritis are found almost exclusively in people older than 50 years of age.

Polymyalgia rheumatica has an annual incidence rate of 52 cases per 100,000 people older than 50 years. Giant cell arteritis varies by geographic location and has a reported incidence of 7 to 19 cases per 100,000 people in the United States (Kremers & Gabriel, 2005).

Assessment focuses on musculoskeletal tenderness, weakness, and decreased function. Careful attention should be directed toward assessing the head (for changes in vision, headaches, and jaw claudication).

Often, diagnosis is difficult because of the lack of specificity of tests. A markedly high ESR is a screening test but is not definitive. Diagnosis is more likely to be made by eliminating other potential diagnoses, but this is highly dependent on the skills and experience of the diagnostician. The dramatic and immediate response to treatment with corticosteroids is considered by some to be diagnostic.

Medical Management

The treatment for patients with polymyalgia rheumatica (without giant cell arteritis) is moderate doses of corticosteroids. NSAIDs are sometimes used for mild disease. The treatment for patients with giant cell arteritis is rapid initiation of and strict adherence to a regimen of corticosteroids. This is essential to avoid the complication of blindness.

Nursing Management

Nursing care of the patient with polymyalgia rheumatica is based on the fundamental plan of nursing care presented earlier (see Chart 54-2). The most common nursing diagnoses are pain and insufficient knowledge of the medication regimen.

A management concern is that the patient will take the prescribed medication, frequently corticosteroids, until symptoms improve and then discontinue the medication. The decision to discontinue the medication should be based on clinical and laboratory findings and the physician's prescription. Nursing implications are related to helping the patient prevent and monitor side effects of medications (eg, infections, diabetes mellitus, gastrointestinal problems, and depression) and adjust to those side effects that cannot be prevented (eg, increased appetite and altered body image).

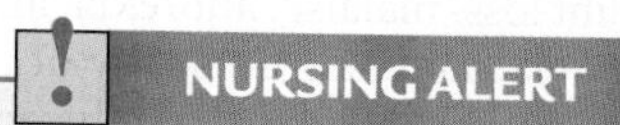

The nurse must emphasize to the patient the need for continued adherence to the prescribed medication regimen to avoid complications of giant cell arteritis, such as blindness.

The loss of bone mass with corticosteroid use increases the risk of osteoporosis in this already at-risk population. Interventions to promote bone health, such as adequate dietary calcium and vitamin D, measurement of bone mineral density, weight-bearing exercise, smoking cessation, and reduction of alcohol consumption if indicated, should be emphasized (Hellman & Hunder, 2005).

Degenerative Joint Disease (Osteoarthritis)

Osteoarthritis (OA), also known as degenerative joint disease or osteoarthrosis (even though inflammation may be present), is the most common and most frequently disabling of the joint disorders. OA is both overdiagnosed and trivialized; it is frequently overtreated or undertreated. The functional impact of OA on quality of life, especially for elderly patients, is often ignored.

OA has been classified as primary (idiopathic), with no prior event or disease related to the OA, and secondary, resulting from previous joint injury or inflammatory disease. The distinction between primary and secondary OA is not always clear.

Increasing age directly relates to the degenerative process in the joint, because the ability of the articular cartilage to resist microfracture with repetitive low loads diminishes with age. OA often begins in the third decade of life and peaks between the fifth and sixth decades. By 40 years of age, 90% of the population have degenerative joint changes in their weight-bearing joints, even though clinical symptoms are usually absent. Prevalence of OA is about 70% in people between the ages of 55 and 74 years (Hooper, Holderbaum, & Moskowitz, 2005).

Pathophysiology

OA may be thought of as the end result of many factors that, when combined, predispose the patient to the disease. OA affects the articular cartilage, subchondral bone (the bony plate that supports the articular cartilage), and synovium. A combination of cartilage degradation, bone stiffening, and reactive inflammation of the synovium occurs. The basic degenerative process in the joint exemplified in OA is presented in Figure 54-6. Understanding of OA has been greatly expanded beyond what previously was thought of as simply "wear and tear" related to aging. Risk factors for OA are summarized in Chart 54-4.

Congenital and developmental disorders of the hip are well known for predisposing a person to OA of the hip. These include congenital subluxation–dislocation of the hip, acetabular dysplasia, Legg-Calvé-Perthes disease, and slipped capital femoral epiphysis.

Obesity is now a well-recognized risk factor for the development of OA (DiCesare & Abramson, 2005; Hough, 2005). Being overweight or obese also increases symptoms associated with the disease (DiCesare & Abramson, 2005). Research has shown that a weight loss of 10% improved function by 28% in people with OA affecting the knee (Christensen, Astrup, & Bliddal, 2005).

Clinical Manifestations

The primary clinical manifestations of OA are pain, stiffness, and functional impairment. The pain is caused by an inflamed synovium, stretching of the joint capsule or ligaments, irritation of nerve endings in the periosteum over osteophytes, trabecular microfracture, intraosseous hypertension, bursitis, tendinitis, and muscle spasm. Stiffness,

Physiology/Pathophysiology

Genetic and hormonal factors
Mechanical injury
Previous joint damage
Other
Chondrocyte response
Release of cytokines
Stimulation, production, and release of proteolytic enzymes, metalloproteases, collagenase
Resulting damage predisposes to more....

FIGURE 54-6. Pathophysiology of osteoarthritis.

which is most commonly experienced in the morning or after awakening, usually lasts less than 30 minutes and decreases with movement. Functional impairment results from pain on movement and limited motion caused by structural changes in the joints.

Although OA occurs most often in weight-bearing joints (hips, knees, cervical and lumbar spine), the proximal and distal finger joints are also often involved. Characteristic bony nodes may be present; on inspection and palpation, these are usually painless, unless inflammation is present.

CHART 54-4

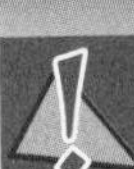

Risk Factors for Osteoarthritis

- Increased age
- Obesity
- Previous joint damage
- Repetitive use (occupational or recreational)
- Anatomic deformity
- Genetic susceptibility

Assessment and Diagnostic Findings

Diagnosis of OA is complicated because only 30% of patients with changes seen on x-ray report symptoms (Hooper et al., 2005). Physical assessment of the musculoskeletal system reveals tender and enlarged joints. Inflammation, when present, is not the destructive type seen in the connective tissue diseases such as RA. OA is characterized by a progressive loss of the joint cartilage, which appears on x-ray as a narrowing of the joint space. In addition, reactive changes occur at the joint margins and on the subchondral bone in the form of osteophytes (spurs) as the cartilage attempts to regenerate. Neither the presence of osteophytes nor joint space narrowing alone is specific for OA; however, when combined, these are sensitive and specific findings. In early or mild OA, there is only a weak correlation between joint pain and synovitis. Blood tests are not useful in the diagnosis of OA.

Medical Management

Although no treatment halts the degenerative process, certain preventive measures can slow the progress if undertaken early enough. These include weight reduction, prevention of injuries, perinatal screening for congenital hip disease, and ergonomic modifications.

Conservative treatment measures include patient education, the use of heat, weight reduction, joint rest and avoidance of joint overuse, orthotic devices (eg, splints, braces) to support inflamed joints, isometric and postural exercises, and aerobic exercise. Other miscellaneous physical modalities, such as massage, yoga, pulsed electromagnetic fields, transcutaneous electrical nerve stimulation (TENS), and music therapy, have unproven value in the treatment of OA. Occupational and physical therapy can help the patient adopt self-management strategies.

Patients with arthritis often use complementary and alternative therapies, many of which are not traditionally taught in American medical schools and are not traditionally available in American hospitals. These may include herbal and dietary supplements, other special diets, acupuncture, acupressure, wearing copper bracelets or magnets, and participation in tai chi. Currently, research is under way to determine the effectiveness of many of these treatments (Little, Parsons & Logan, 2006; Rao, Kroenke, Mihaliak, et al., 2003).

Pharmacologic Therapy

Pharmacologic management of OA is directed toward symptom management and pain control. Selection of medication is based on the patient's needs, the stage of disease, and the risk of side effects. Medications are used in conjunction with nonpharmacologic strategies. In most patients with OA, the initial analgesic therapy is acetaminophen. Some patients respond to the nonselective NSAIDs, and patients who are at increased risk for gastrointestinal complications, especially gastrointestinal bleeding, have been managed effectively with COX-2 inhibitors (Lozada, 2005; Stitik, Kaplan, Kamen, et al., 2005). However, COX-2 inhibitors must be used with caution because of the associated risk of cardiovascular disease. Other medications that may be

NURSING RESEARCH PROFILE

Pain and Mobility Management of Osteoarthritis

Baird, C. L. & Sands, L. (2004). A pilot study of the effectiveness of guided imagery with progressive muscle relaxation to reduce chronic pain and mobility difficulties of osteoarthritis. *Pain Management Nursing, 5*(3), 97–104.

Purpose

Osteoarthritis (OA), the most common rheumatic disorder in older adults, is associated with chronic pain that leads to limited mobility, disability, and difficulty in maintaining independence. Guided imagery (GI) and progressive muscle relaxation (PMR) have been shown to decrease pain and lessen mobility difficulties in other disease processes. The purpose of this pilot study was to test the effectiveness of GI with PMR to decrease chronic pain and mobility difficulties in patients with OA.

Design

This longitudinal, randomized, clinical trial pilot study included a sample of 28 women with OA who ranged in age from 65 to 93 years. Initially, they completed a questionnaire about their pain, mobility, and demographics. Then they were randomly assigned to either an intervention group or a control group. Intervention group participants ($n = 18$) received a personalized audiotape and instruction in using GI with PMR. In addition, they were asked to complete a journal three times a week describing their symptoms and how often they performed GI. Control group participants ($n = 10$) received standard care and also completed a journal three times a week describing their arthritis symptoms and what they were doing to manage them. Twelve weeks after enrollment, all subjects completed a questionnaire regarding their pain and mobility.

Findings

Subjects in the intervention group reported a significant decrease in pain ($p = .001$) and in mobility difficulty ($p = .005$); members of the control group reported no change in pain and an increase in mobility difficulty over the 12-week period. Journal recordings of the subjects in the intervention group revealed that they were using GI consistently; 89% used GI at least once a day, 49% used GI at least twice a day, and 11% used GI three to four times a day.

Nursing Implications

GI with PMR is an easy-to-teach, inexpensive, nonpharmacologic, and easy-to-use self-management technique for the treatment of OA and other chronic disorders. The findings of this study demonstrate that health care providers can provide instruction about this technique to patients with OA in the hope that it will lead to decreased pain and improved mobility. This approach seems useful, but further research is needed to determine its long-term effectiveness.

considered are the opioids and intra-articular corticosteroids. Topical analgesics such as capsaicin (Capsin, Zostrix) and methylsalicylate are also used (Lozada, 2005; Lozada & Altman, 2005).

Other therapeutic approaches include glucosamine and chondroitin. Although it has been suggested that these substances modify cartilage structure (Lozada & Altman, 2005; Zochling, Mardi, Lapsley, et al., 2004), studies have not shown them to be effective (Towheed, Maxwell, Anastassiades, et al., 2006). Viscosupplementation, the intra-articular injection of hyaluronic acid, is thought to provide a short-term lubricant and biomechanical benefit as well as an analgesic effect by buffering synovial nerve endings directly; it may also have some anti-inflammatory effects and stimulating effects on synovial lining cells to produce hyaluronic acid (Lozada, 2005; Lozada & Altman, 2005; Stitik et al., 2005).

Surgical Management

In moderate to severe OA, when pain is severe or because of loss of function, surgical intervention may be used. The procedures most commonly used are osteotomy (to alter the distribution of weight within the joint) and arthroplasty. In arthroplasty, diseased joint components are replaced with artificial products (see Chapter 67).

Tidal irrigation (lavage) of the knee involves the introduction of a large volume of saline into the joint through cannulas and then removal of this fluid. In some cases, this procedure provides pain relief for up to 6 months (Lozada & Altman, 2005).

Nursing Management

The nursing management of the patient with OA includes both pharmacologic and nonpharmacologic approaches. The nonpharmacologic interventions are used first and continued with the addition of pharmacologic agents. Pain management and optimal functional ability are major goals of nursing intervention. The patient's understanding of the disease process and symptom pattern is critical to a plan of care. Because patients with OA usually are older, they may have other health problems. Commonly they are overweight, and they may have a sedentary lifestyle. Weight loss and exercise are important approaches to pain and disability improvement (Christensen et al., 2005; Lozada, 2005). A referral for physical therapy or to an exercise program for people with similar problems can be very helpful. Canes or other assistive devices for ambulation should be considered. Exercises such as walking should be begun in moderation and increased gradually. Patients should plan their daily exercise for a time when the pain is least severe or plan to use an analgesic, if appropriate, before exercising. Adequate pain management is important for the success of an exercise program. Open discussion regarding the use of complementary and alternative therapies is important to maintain safe practices for patients looking for a "cure."

Spondyloarthropathies

The spondyloarthropathies are another category of systemic inflammatory disorders of the skeleton. The spondyloarthropathies include ankylosing spondylitis, reactive arthritis (Reiter's syndrome), and psoriatic arthritis. Spondyloarthritis is also associated with inflammatory bowel diseases such as regional enteritis (Crohn's disease) and ulcerative colitis.

These rheumatic diseases share several clinical features. The inflammation tends to occur peripherally at the sites of attachment—at tendons, joint capsules, and ligaments. Periosteal inflammation may be present. Many patients have arthritis of the sacroiliac joints. Onset tends to occur during young adulthood, with the disease affecting men more often than women. There is a strong tendency for these conditions to occur in families. Frequently, the HLA-B27 genetic marker is found.

Types of Spondyloarthropathies

Ankylosing Spondylitis

Ankylosing spondylitis affects the cartilaginous joints of the spine and surrounding tissues. Occasionally, the large synovial joints, such as the hips, knees, or shoulders, may be involved. Ankylosing spondylitis is more prevalent in males than in females and is usually diagnosed in the second or third decade of life. The disease is more severe in males, and significant systemic involvement is likely. Back pain is the characteristic feature. As the disease progresses, ankylosis of the entire spine may occur, leading to respiratory compromise and complications.

Reactive Arthritis (Reiter's Syndrome)

The disease process involved in Reiter's syndrome is called reactive because the arthritis occurs after an infection. It mostly affects young adult males and is characterized primarily by urethritis, arthritis, and conjunctivitis. Dermatitis and ulcerations of the mouth and penis may also be present. Low back pain is common.

Psoriatic Arthritis

Psoriatic arthritis is characterized by synovitis, polyarthritis, and spondylitis. Both psoriasis and arthritis are common conditions, and one theory suggests that the overlap of the two conditions is a chance occurrence. However, epidemiologic data suggest that the prevalence of arthritis in patients with psoriasis is 7% to 42%, exceeding the rate in the general population. Similarly, the prevalence of psoriasis in persons with arthritis is 2.6% to 7.0%, compared with 0.1% to 2.8% in the general population, supporting the theory that these two processes occur together in a unique disease process (Gladman, 2005).

Medical Management

Medical management of spondyloarthropathies focuses on treating pain and maintaining mobility by suppressing inflammation. For the patient with ankylosing spondylitis, good body positioning and posture are essential, so that if **ankylosis** (fixation) does occur, the patient is in the most functional position. Maintaining range of motion with a regular exercise and muscle-strengthening program is especially important.

Pharmacologic Management

NSAIDs and corticosteroids often produce marked improvement in back, skin, and joint symptoms. Sulfasalazine (Azulfidine) and methotrexate (Rheumatrex) may help with peripheral joint disease. Methotrexate is also used to control psoriasis. More recently, anti-TNF therapy is under investigation for treatment of the spondyloarthropathies (Stokes & Kremer, 2003).

Surgical Management

Surgical management may include total hip replacement (see Chapter 67).

Nursing Management

Major nursing interventions in the spondyloarthropathies are related to symptom management and maintenance of optimal functioning. Affected patients are primarily young men. Their major concerns are often related to prognosis and job modification, especially among those who perform physical work. Patients may also express concerns about leisure and recreational activities.

Metabolic and Endocrine Diseases Associated with Rheumatic Disorders

Metabolic and endocrine diseases may be associated with rheumatic disorders. These include biochemical abnormalities (amyloidosis and scurvy), endocrine diseases (diabetes mellitus and acromegaly), immunodeficiency diseases (human immunodeficiency virus [HIV] infection, acquired immunodeficiency syndrome [AIDS]), and some inherited disorders (hypermobility syndromes). However, the most common conditions are the crystal-induced arthropathies, in which crystals such as monosodium urate (gout) or calcium pyrophosphate (calcium pyrophosphate dihydrate disease [CPPD] or pseudogout) are deposited within joints and other tissues.

Gout

Gout is a heterogeneous group of conditions related to a genetic defect of purine metabolism that results in hyperuricemia. Oversecretion of uric acid or a renal defect resulting in decreased excretion of uric acid, or a combination of both, occurs. The prevalence of gout is reported to be less than 1% to 15.3%, and it appears to be on the rise. The incidence increases with age and body mass index. It occurs more commonly in males than in females (Wortmann & Kelley, 2005).

In primary hyperuricemia, elevated serum urate levels or manifestations of urate deposition appear to be consequences of faulty uric acid metabolism. Primary hyperuricemia may be caused by severe dieting or starvation, excessive intake of foods that are high in purines (shellfish, organ meats), or heredity. In secondary hyperuricemia, gout is a clinical feature secondary to any of a number of genetic or acquired processes, including conditions in which there is an increase in cell turnover (leukemia, multiple myeloma, some types of anemias, psoriasis) and an increase in cell breakdown. Altered renal tubular function, either as a major action or as an unintended side effect of certain pharmacologic agents (eg, diuretics such as thiazides and furosemide), low-dose salicylates, or ethanol, can contribute to uric acid underexcretion.

Pathophysiology

Hyperuricemia (serum concentration greater than 7 mg/dL) can but does not always cause monosodium urate crystal deposition (Becker & Jolly, 2005). However, as uric acid levels increase, the risk becomes greater. Attacks of gout appear to be related to sudden increases or decreases of serum uric acid levels. When the urate crystals precipitate within a joint, an inflammatory response occurs, and an attack of gout begins. With repeated attacks, accumulations of sodium urate crystals, called **tophi**, are deposited in peripheral areas of the body, such as the great toe, the hands, and the ear. Renal urate lithiasis (kidney stones), with chronic renal disease secondary to urate deposition, may develop.

The finding of urate crystals in the synovial fluid of asymptomatic joints suggests that factors other than crystals may be related to the inflammatory reaction. Recovered monosodium urate crystals are coated with immunoglobulins that are mainly IgG. IgG enhances crystal phagocytosis, thereby demonstrating immunologic activity.

Clinical Manifestations

Manifestations of the gout syndrome include acute gouty arthritis (recurrent attacks of severe articular and periarticular inflammation), tophi (crystalline deposits accumulating in articular tissue, osseous tissue, soft tissue, and cartilage), gouty nephropathy (renal impairment), and uric acid urinary calculi. Four stages of gout can be identified: asymptomatic hyperuricemia, acute gouty arthritis, intercritical gout, and chronic tophaceous gout. The subsequent development of gout is directly related to the duration and magnitude of the hyperuricemia. Therefore, the commitment to lifelong pharmacologic treatment of hyperuricemia is deferred until there is an initial attack of gout.

For hyperuricemic people who are going to develop gout, acute arthritis is the most common early clinical manifestation. The metatarsophalangeal joint of the big toe is the most commonly affected joint (90% of patients) (Porth, 2005). The tarsal area, ankle, or knee may also be affected. Less commonly, the wrists, fingers, and elbows may be affected. Trauma, alcohol ingestion, dieting, medications, surgical stress, or illness may trigger the acute attack. The abrupt onset often occurs at night, awakening the patient with severe pain, redness, swelling, and warmth of the affected joint. Early attacks tend to subside spontaneously over 3 to 10 days even without treatment. The attack is followed by a symptom-free period (the intercritical stage) until the next attack, which may not come for months or years. However, with time, attacks tend to occur more frequently, to involve more joints, and to last longer.

Tophi are generally associated with more frequent and severe inflammatory episodes. Higher serum concentrations of uric acid are also associated with more extensive tophus formation. Tophi most commonly occur in the synovium, olecranon bursa, subchondral bone, infrapatellar and Achilles tendons, and subcutaneous tissue on the extensor surface of the forearms and overlying joints. They have also been found in the aortic walls, heart valves, nasal and ear cartilage, eyelids, cornea, and sclerae. Joint enlargement may cause a loss of joint motion. Uric acid deposits may cause renal stones and kidney damage.

Medical Management

A definitive diagnosis of gouty arthritis is established by polarized light microscopy of the synovial fluid of the involved joint. Uric acid crystals are seen within the polymorphonuclear leukocytes in the fluid. Colchicine (oral or parenteral), an NSAID such as indomethacin, or a corticosteroid is prescribed to relieve an acute attack of gout. Management of hyperuricemia, tophi, joint destruction, and renal disorders is usually initiated after the acute inflammatory process has subsided. Uricosuric agents, such as probenecid (Benemid), correct hyperuricemia and dissolve deposited urate. When reduction of the serum urate level is indicated, uricosuric agents are the medications of choice. If the patient has, or is at risk for, renal insufficiency or renal calculi (kidney stones), allopurinol, a xanthine oxidase inhibitor, is also effective (Wortmann & Kelley, 2005). Corticosteroids may be used in patients who have no response to other therapy. If the patient experiences several acute episodes or there is evidence of tophi formation, prophylactic treatment is considered. Specific treatment is based on the serum uric acid level, 24-hour urinary uric acid excretion, and renal function (Table 54-5).

Nursing Management

Historically, gouty arthritis was thought to be a condition of royalty and the very rich, with the disease attributed to "high living." This has not been shown to be entirely true. Although severe dietary restriction is not necessary, the nurse should encourage the patient to restrict consumption

TABLE 54-5 Medications Used to Treat Gout

Medication	Actions and Use	Nursing Implications
colchicine	Lowers the deposition of uric acid and interferes with leukocyte infiltration, thus reducing inflammation; does not alter serum or urine levels of uric acid; used in acute and chronic management	*Acute management:* Administer when attack begins; dosage increased until pain is relieved or diarrhea develops *Chronic management:* Causes GI upset in most patients
probenecid (Benemid)	Uricosuric agent; inhibits renal reabsorption of urates and increases the urinary excretion of uric acid; prevents tophi formation	Be alert for nausea and rash.
allopurinol (Zyloprim)	Xanthine oxidase inhibitor; interrupts the breakdown of purines before uric acid is formed; inhibits xanthinoxidase because it blocks uric acid formation	Monitor for side effects, including bone marrow depression, vomiting, and abdominal pain.

of foods high in purines, especially organ meats, and to limit alcohol intake. Maintenance of normal body weight should be encouraged. In an acute episode of gouty arthritis, pain management with prescribed medications is essential, along with avoidance of factors that increase pain and inflammation, such as trauma, stress, and alcohol. During the intercritical period, the patient feels well and may abandon preventive behaviors, which may result in an acute attack. Acute attacks are most effectively treated if therapy is begun early in the course.

Fibromyalgia

Fibromyalgia is a common syndrome that involves chronic fatigue, generalized muscle aching, and stiffness. Two percent of the United States population is affected by this syndrome, with a prevalence rate of 3.4% in women and 0.5% in men (Bradley & Alarcón, 2005). Although criteria for the classification of fibromyalgia were identified in 1990 (Wolfe, Smythe, Yunus, et al., 1990), controversy exists as to whether this diagnosis represents a unique syndrome. The cause is unknown, and no specific pathologic characteristics have been identified.

Medical Management

Treatment consists of attention to the specific symptoms reported by the patient. NSAIDs may be used to treat the diffuse muscle aching and stiffness. Tricyclic antidepressants are used to improve or restore normal sleep patterns. In addition, selective serotonin reuptake inhibitors and anticonvulsants have been effective in preliminary reports (Goldenberg, 2004). Individualized programs of exercise are used to decrease muscle weakness and discomfort and to improve the general deconditioning that occurs in affected patients (Lash, Ehrlich-Jones & McCoy, 2003).

Nursing Management

Typically, patients with fibromyalgia have endured their symptoms for a long period of time. They may feel as if their symptoms have not been taken seriously. Nurses need to pay special attention to supporting these patients and providing encouragement as they begin their program of therapy. Patient support groups may be helpful. Careful listening to patients' descriptions of their concerns and symptoms is essential to help them make the changes that are necessary to improve their quality of life (Lash et al., 2003; Schaefer, 2005).

Arthritis Associated with Infectious Organisms

Arthritis, tenosynovitis, and bursitis can be associated with infectious organisms. Some inflammation of joints, tendons, and bursae is directly related to infection caused by bacterial, viral, fungal, or parasitic agents. Bacterial arthritis is the most rapidly destructive form of infectious arthritis. There are two major classes of bacterial arthritis: that caused by *Neisseria gonorrhoeae* and that caused by a nongonococcal bacterium. The most prevalent of the nongonococcal organisms include *Staphylococcus aureus* and the various streptococcal variants. Less common pathogens are related to syphilis, tuberculosis, leprosy, fungi (particularly coccidioidomycosis), mycoplasmas, and viral agents such as rubella, parvovirus, and hepatitis B.

Clinical Manifestations

The characteristic symptom is acute onset of a warm, swollen joint. Culture of the bacterium from the synovial fluid confirms the diagnosis. The patient often immobilizes the joint and elevates the affected extremity because of pain and swelling. Fever may be high, or it may be absent. Signs of systemic infection may be absent in elderly patients, in those with diabetes, and in those with suppressed immune systems. Diagnosis and treatment may be delayed by patients with preexisting arthritic conditions if they attribute the symptoms to a flare-up of arthritis.

Management

This condition is a medical emergency necessitating early diagnosis and appropriate treatment to eliminate the causative organism; otherwise, the joint may be destroyed relatively quickly. Treatment consists of parenteral antibiotics and drainage of the joint. The results of cultures are used to determine the appropriate antibiotic therapy. Immobilization of the joint and repeated joint aspirations may be necessary along with IV antibiotics. Nursing management focuses on providing pain relief, administering antibiotics, and assisting the patient with self-care activities. If the patient is sent home on IV antibiotic therapy, the nurse arranges for home care and instructs the patient and care providers in safe administration of the drug and changes that should be reported to a health care provider.

Neoplasms and Neurovascular, Bone, and Extra-Articular Disorders

Primary neoplasms of joints, tendon sheaths, and bursae are rare. Most neoplasms are benign, arising from the synovium. These benign tumors include lipoma, hemangioma, fibroma, and tumor-like lesions such as ganglion, bursitis, and synovial cyst. Malignant tumors include primary tumors, such as synovial and bone sarcomas, and secondary involvement as manifestations of joint invasion by leukemia, lymphoma, myeloma, or metastasis. Neoplasms may manifest as back or neck pain.

Neurovascular disorders include the compression syndromes, such as those with peripheral entrapment (eg, carpal tunnel syndrome), radiculopathy, and spinal stenosis. Raynaud's phenomenon and erythromelalgia (throbbing and burning pain often affecting the hands and feet) are also included in this category.

Bone and cartilage disorders include osteoporosis, osteomalacia, hypertrophic osteoarthropathy, diffuse idiopathic skeletal hyperostosis, Paget's disease, osteonecrosis, avascular necrosis, costochondritis, osteolysis or chondrolysis, and biomechanical or anatomic abnormalities. Notably, these conditions involve resorption, destruction, infection, or remodeling of bone.

Extra-articular rheumatism is a descriptive term for a group of conditions that affect structures other than the joints. Included are general and regional pain syndromes, low back pain and intervertebral disk disorders, tendonitis and bursitis, and ganglion cysts.

Miscellaneous Disorders

The last category in the classification of the rheumatic diseases is aptly labeled miscellaneous disorders because it contains a mix of disorders that are frequently associated with arthritis and other conditions. These include the direct consequences of trauma (including internal derangement and loose bodies of joints), pancreatic disease (related to avascular necrosis or osteonecrosis), sarcoidosis (a multisystem disorder particularly of the lymph nodes and lungs), and palindromic rheumatism (an uncommon variety of recurring and acute arthritis and periarthritis that in some may progress to RA but is characterized by symptom-free periods of days to months). Other conditions include villonodular synovitis, chronic active hepatitis, and drug-related rheumatic syndromes. The nursing interventions related to these varied conditions are specific to the multisystemic problems experienced by the patient. However, the musculoskeletal components should not be neglected or overlooked. Further information about these rare disorders can be found in specialty references.

Critical Thinking Exercises

1 A 29-year-old woman with RA recently gave birth to her first child. She states that during her pregnancy her arthritis symptoms seemed to decrease, but now she is having difficulty taking care of her infant because of joint pain, stiffness, and swelling, especially in her hands and wrists. What modifications can be made to help her to care for her child? What resources are available for her?

2 ebp A 79-year-old woman with a 10-year history of OA of the right knee complains of pain every day and difficulty walking. Currently she uses a walker to ambulate and needs to stop and rest every so often because of the pain. What treatment options are available? Develop an evidence-based plan of care for her.

3 A 20-year-old woman complains of alopecia, skin rash, joint pain, weight loss, and fatigue. Her family states that she does not "seem like herself" lately. A diagnosis of SLE is made. What can you explain to her about her diagnosis and her treatment options?

4 You are caring for a patient with a rheumatic disorder. NSAIDs, corticosteroids, and a biologic response modifier have been prescribed. How do the actions of these medications differ? What instructions and recommendations would you give to the patient to ensure their safe administration?

REFERENCES AND SELECTED READINGS

BOOKS

Becker, M. A. & Jolly, M. (2005). Clinical gout and the pathogenesis of hyperuricemia. In Koopman, W. J. & Moreland, L. W. (Eds.). *Arthritis and allied conditions: A textbook of rheumatology* (15th ed.). Philadelphia: Lippincott Williams & Wilkins.

Belza, B. (2001). Fatigue. In Robbins, L., Burckhardt, C. S., Hannan, M. T., et al. (Eds.). *Clinical care in the rheumatic diseases*. Atlanta: Association of Rheumatology Health Professionals.

Bradley, L. A. & Alarcón, G. S. (2005). Fibromyalgia. In Koopman, W. J. & Moreland, L. W. (Eds.). *Arthritis & allied conditions: A textbook of rheumatology* (15th ed.). Philadelphia: Lippincott Williams & Wilkins.

Burckhardt, C. (2001a). Pain management. In Robbins, L., Burckhardt, C. S., Hannan, M. T., et al. (Eds.). *Clinical care in the rheumatic diseases*. Atlanta: Association of Rheumatology Health Professionals.

Burckhardt, C. S. (2001b). Fibromyalgia. In Robbins, L., Burckhardt, C. S., Hannan, M. T., et al. (Eds.). *Clinical care in the rheumatic diseases.* Atlanta: Association of Rheumatology Health Professionals.

Dochterman, M. M. & Bulechek, G. M. (2004). *Nursing interventions classification (NIC)* (4th ed.). St. Louis: Mosby.

DiCesare, P. E. & Abramson, S. B. (2005). Pathogenesis of osteoarthritis. In Harris, E. D., Budd, R. C., Genovese, M. C., et al. (Eds.). *Kelley's textbook of rheumatology* (7th ed.). Philadelphia: Elsevier Saunders.

Edworthy, S. M. (2005). Clinical manifestations of systemic lupus erythematosus. In Harris, E. D., Budd, R. C., Genovese, M. C., et al. (Eds.). *Kelley's textbook of rheumatology* (7th ed.). Philadelphia: Elsevier Saunders.

Firestein, G. S. (2005). Etiology and pathogenesis of rheumatoid arthritis. In Harris, E. D., Budd, R. C., Genovese, M. C., et al. (Eds.). *Kelley's textbook of rheumatology* (7th ed.). Philadelphia: Elsevier Saunders.

Gladman, D. D. (2005). Psoriatic arthritis. In Harris, E. D., Budd, R. C., Genovese, M. C., et al. (Eds.). *Kelley's textbook of rheumatology* (7th ed.). Philadelphia: Elsevier Saunders.

Hahn, B. H. (2005). Management of systemic lupus erythematosus. In Harris, E. D., Budd, R. C., Genovese, M. C., et al. (Eds.). *Kelley's textbook of rheumatology* (7th ed.). Philadelphia: Elsevier Saunders.

Harris, E. D. (2005). Clinical features of rheumatoid arthritis. In Harris, E. D., Budd, R. C., Genovese, M. C., et al. (Eds.). *Kelley's textbook of rheumatology* (7th ed.). Philadelphia: Elsevier Saunders.

Hellman, D. B., & Hunder, G. G. (2005). Giant cell arteritis and polymyalgia rheumatica. In Harris, E. D., Budd, R. C., Genovese, M. C., et al. (Eds.). *Kelley's textbook of rheumatology* (7th ed.). Philadelphia: Elsevier Saunders.

Hooper, M. M., Holderbaum, D., & Moskowitz, R. W. (2005). Clinical and laboratory findings in osteoarthritis. In Koopman, W. J. & Moreland, L. W. (Eds.). *Arthritis and allied conditions: A textbook of rheumatology* (15th ed.). Philadelphia: Lippincott Williams & Wilkins.

Hough, A. J. Jr. (2005). Pathology of osteoarthritis. In Koopman, W. J. & Moreland, L. W. (Eds.). *Arthritis and allied conditions: A textbook of rheumatology* (15th ed.). Philadelphia: Lippincott Williams & Wilkins.

Korn, J. (2005). Pathogenesis of systemic sclerosis. In Koopman, W. J. & Moreland, L. W. (Eds.). *Arthritis and allied conditions: A textbook of rheumatology* (15th ed.). Philadelphia: Lippincott Williams & Wilkins.

Kremers, H. M. & Gabriel, S. E. (2005). Epidemiology of the rheumatic diseases. In Harris, E. D., Budd, R. C., Genovese, M. C., et al. (Eds.). *Kelley's textbook of rheumatology* (7th ed.). Philadelphia: Elsevier Saunders.

Lehne, R. A. (2004). *Pharmacology for nursing care* (5th ed.). St. Louis: W. B. Saunders.

Lorig, K. R. (2005). Education of patients. In Harris, E. D., Budd, R. C., Genovese, M. C., et al. (Eds.). *Kelley's textbook of rheumatology* (7th ed.). Philadelphia: Elsevier Saunders.

Lozada, C. J. (2005). Management of osteoarthritis. In Harris, E. D., Budd, R. C., Genovese, M. C., et al. (Eds.). *Kelley's textbook of rheumatology* (7th ed.). Philadelphia: Elsevier Saunders.

Lozada, C. J. & Altman, R. D. (2005). Management of osteoarthritis. In Koopman, W. J. & Moreland, L. W. (Eds.). *Arthritis and allied conditions: A textbook of rheumatology* (15th ed.). Philadelphia: Lippincott Williams & Wilkins.

Miller, F. W. (2005). Inflammatory myopathies: Polymyositis, dermatomyositis, and related conditions. In Koopman, W. J. & Moreland, L. W. (Eds.). *Arthritis and allied conditions: A textbook of rheumatology* (15th ed.). Philadelphia: Lippincott Williams & Wilkins.

Minor, M. A. & Westby, M. D. (2001). Rest and exercise. In Robbins, L., Burckhardt, C. S., Hannan, M. T., et al. (Eds.). *Clinical care in the rheumatic diseases.* Atlanta: Association of Rheumatology Health Professionals.

National Institutes of Health, National Institute of Arthritis and Musculoskeletal and Skin Diseases. (2001). *Lupus: A patient care guide for nurses and other health professionals.* Bethesda, MD: NIH.

O'Dell, J. R. (2005). Rheumatoid arthritis: The clinical picture. In Koopman, W. J. & Moreland, L. W. (Eds.). *Arthritis and allied conditions: A textbook of rheumatology* (15th ed.). Philadelphia: Lippincott Williams & Wilkins.

Paget, S. A. (2001). Polymyalgia rheumatica. In Robbins, L., Burckhardt, C. S., Hannan, M. T., et al. (Eds.). *Clinical care in the rheumatic diseases.* Atlanta: Association of Rheumatology Health Professionals.

Parker, J. C., Wright, G. E. & Smarr, K. L. (2001). Psychological assessment. In Robbins, L., Burckhardt, C. S., Hannan, M. T., et al. (Eds.). *Clinical care in the rheumatic diseases.* Atlanta: Association of Rheumatology Health Professionals.

Petri, M. A. (2005). Systemic lupus erythematosus: Clinical aspects. In Koopman, W. J. & Moreland, L. W. (Eds.). *Arthritis and allied conditions: A textbook of rheumatology* (15th ed.). Philadelphia: Lippincott Williams & Wilkins.

Porth, C. M. (2005). *Pathophysiology: Concepts of altered health status* (7th ed.). Philadelphia: Lippincott Williams & Wilkins.

Seibold, J. R. (2005). Scleroderma. In Harris, E. D., Budd, R. C., Genovese, M. C., et al. (Eds.). *Kelley's textbook of rheumatology* (7th ed.). Philadelphia: Elsevier Saunders.

Wegener, S. T. (2001). Sleep problems. In Robbins, L., Burckhardt, C. S., Hannan, M. T., et al. (Eds.). *Clinical care in the rheumatic diseases.* Atlanta: Association of Rheumatology Health Professionals.

Wofsy, D. (2005). Therapy of systemic lupus erythematosus. In Koopman, W. J. & Moreland, L. W. (Eds.). *Arthritis and allied conditions: A textbook of rheumatology* (15th ed.). Philadelphia: Lippincott Williams & Wilkins.

Wortmann, R. L. (2005). Inflammatory diseases of muscle and other myopathies. In Harris, E. D., Budd, R. C., Genovese, M. C., et al. (Eds.). *Kelley's textbook of rheumatology* (7th ed.). Philadelphia: Elsevier Saunders.

Wortmann, R. L., & Kelley, W. N. (2005). Gout and hyperuricemia. In Harris, E. D., Budd, R. C., Genovese, M. C., et al. (Eds.). *Kelley's textbook of rheumatology* (7th ed.). Philadelphia: Elsevier Saunders.

Zvaifler, N. J., & Corr, M. (2005). The evaluation and treatment of rheumatoid arthritis. In Koopman, W. J. & Moreland, L. W. (Eds.). *Arthritis and allied conditions: A textbook of rheumatology* (15th ed.). Philadelphia: Lippincott Williams & Wilkins.

JOURNALS

**Asterisks indicate nursing research articles.*

General

Centers for Disease Control and Prevention. (2002). Racial/ethnic differences in the prevalence and impact of doctor-diagnosed arthritis—United States, 2002. *MMWR, 54*(5), 119–123.

Centers for Disease Control and Prevention. (2004). Update: Direct and indirect costs of arthritis and other rheumatic conditions—United States, 1997. (2004). *MMWR, 53*(18), 388–389.

Fontaine, K. R., Bartlett, S. J. & Heo, M. (2005). Are health care professionals advising adults with arthritis to become more physically active? *Arthritis Care and Research, 53*(2), 279–283.

Fontaine, K. R., Heo, M. & Bathon, J. (2004). Are US adults with arthritis meeting public health recommendations for physical activity? *Arthritis and Rheumatism, 50*(2), 624–628.

Rao, J. K. & Hootman, J. M. (2004). Prevention research and rheumatic disease. *Current Opinion in Rheumatology, 16*(2), 119–124.

Rao, J. K., Kroenke, K., Mihaliak, K. A., et al. (2003). Rheumatology patients' use of complementary therapies: Results from a one-year longitudinal study. *Arthritis and Rheumatism, 49*(5), 619–625.

Soeken, K. L. (2004). Selected CAM therapies for arthritis-related pain: The evidence from systematic reviews. *Clinical Journal of Pain, 20*(1), 13–18.

Rheumatoid Arthritis

American College of Rheumatology, Subcommittee on Rheumatoid Arthritis Guidelines. (2002). Guidelines for the management of rheumatoid arthritis, 2002 update. *Arthritis and Rheumatism, 46*(2), 328–346.

Anderson, D. L. (2004). TNF inhibitors: A new age in rheumatoid arthritis treatment. *American Journal of Nursing, 104*(2), 60–68.

Bourguignon, C., Labyak, S. E., & Taibi, D. (2003). Investigating sleep disturbances in adults with rheumatoid arthritis. *Holistic Nursing Practice, 17*(5), 241–249.

Capriotti, T. (2004). The "alphabet" of rheumatoid arthritis treatment. *MedSurg Nursing, 13*(6), 420–428.

Egan, M., Brosseau, L., Farmer, M., et al. (2006). Splints and orthosis for treating rheumatoid arthritis. *The Cochrane Library,* 1: CD004018.

Fair, B. S. (2003). Contrasts in patients' and providers' explanations of rheumatoid arthritis. *Journal of Nursing Scholarship, 35*(4), 339–344.

Felson, D. T., Anderson, J. J., Boers, M., et al. (1995). American College of Rheumatology preliminary definition of improvement in rheumatoid arthritis. *Arthritis and Rheumatism, 38*(6), 727–735.

Furst, D. E. (2004). Anakinra: Review of recombinant human interleukin-1 receptor antagonist in the treatment of rheumatoid arthritis. *Clinical Therapeutics, 26*(12), 1960–1975.

*Iaquinta, M. L., & Larrabee, J. H. (2004). Phenomenological lived experience of patients with rheumatoid arthritis. *Journal of Nursing Care Quality, 19*(3), 280–289.

Little, C. V. & Parsons, T. (2006). Herbal therapy for treating rheumatoid arthritis. *The Cochrane Library,* 1: CD002948.

*Melanson, P. M. & Downe-Wamboldt, B. (2003). Confronting life with rheumatoid arthritis. *Journal of Advanced Nursing, 42*(2), 125–133.

Robinson, V. A., Brosseau, L., Casimiro, L., et al. (2006). Thermotherapy for treating rheumatoid arthritis. *The Cochrane Library,* 1: CD002826.

Roth, S. (2004). Effects of Prosorba Column apheresis in patients with chronic refractory rheumatoid arthritis. *Journal of Rheumatology, 31*(11), 2131–2135.

St. Clair, E. W., van der Heijde, D. M. F., Smolen, J. S., et al. (2004). Combination of infliximab and methotrexate therapy for early rheumatoid arthritis. *Arthritis and Rheumatism, 50*(11), 3432–3443.

Steultjens, E. E. M., Bouter, L. L. M., Dekker, J. J., et al. (2006). Occupational therapy for rheumatoid arthritis. *The Cochrane Library,* 1: CD003114.

Toussirot, E. & Wendling, D. (2004). The use of TNF-α blocking agents in rheumatoid arthritis: An overview. *Expert Opinion on Pharmacotherapy, 5*(3), 581–594.

Voulgari, P. V., Alamanos, Y., Nikas, S. N., et al. (2005). Infliximab therapy in established rheumatoid arthritis: An observational study. *American Journal of Medicine, 118*(5), 515–520.

Osteoarthritis

American College of Rheumatology. (2000). Recommendations for the medical management of osteoarthritis of the hip and knee. *Arthritis and Rheumatism, 43*(9), 1905–1915.

*Baird, C. L. & Sands, L. (2004). A pilot study of the effectiveness of guided imagery with progressive muscle relaxation to reduce chronic pain and mobility difficulties of osteoarthritis. *Pain Management Nursing, 5*(3), 97–104.

*Baird, C. L., Schmeiser, D., & Yehle, K. T. (2003). Self-caring of women with osteoarthritis living at different levels of independence. *Health Care for Women International, 24*(7), 617–634.

Blakeley, J. A. & Ribeiro, V. E. S. (2004). Gucosamine and osteoarthritis. *American Journal of Nursing, 104*(2), 54–59.

Christensen, R., Astrup, A., & Bliddal, H. (2005). Weight loss: The treatment of choice for knee osteoarthritis? *OsteoArthritis and Cartilage, 13*(1), 20–27.

*Gaines, J. M., Metter, E. J. & Talbot, L. A. (2004). The effect of neuromuscular electrical stimulation on arthritis knee pain in older adults with osteoarthritis of the knee. *Applied Nursing Research, 17*(3), 201–206.

Little, C. V., Parsons, T., & Logan, S. (2006). Herbal therapy for treating osteoarthritis. *The Cochrane Library,* 1: CD002947.

*McCaffrey, R. & Freeman, E. (2003). Effect of music on chronic osteoarthritis pain in older people. *Journal of Advanced Nursing, 44*(5), 517–524.

Stitik, T. P., Kaplan, R. J., Kamen, L. B., et al. (2005). Rehabilitation of orthopedic and rheumatologic disorders: 2. Osteoarthritis assessment, treatment, and rehabilitation. *Archives of Physical Medicine and Rehabilitation, 86*(3 Suppl. 1), S48–S55.

*Tak, S. H. & Laffrey, S. C. (2003). Life satisfaction and its correlates in older women with osteoarthritis. *Orthopaedic Nursing, 22*(3), 182–189.

Towheed, T. E., Maxwell, L., Anastassiades, T. P., et al. (2006). Glucosamine therapy for treating osteoarthritis. *The Cochrane Library,* 1: CD002946.

Tsai, P-F. & Tak, S. (2003). Disease-specific pain measures for osteoarthritis of the knee or hip. *Geriatric Nursing, 24*(2), 106–109.

Zochling, J., March, L., Lapsley, H., et al. (2004). Use of complementary medicines for osteoarthritis: A prospective study. *Annals of Rheumatic Disease, 63*(5), 549–554.

Systemic Lupus Erythematosus

Goodman, D., Morrissey, S., Graham, D., et al. (2005). Illness representations of systemic lupus erythematosus. *Qualitative Health Research, 15*(5), 606–619.

*Mendelson, C. (2003). Gentle hugs: Internet listservs as sources of support for women with lupus. *Advances in Nursing Science, 26*(4), 299–306.

Pullen, R. L., Cannon, J. D. & Rushing, J. D. (2003). Managing organ-threatening systemic lupus erythematosus. *MedSurg Nursing, 12*(6), 368–379.

*Sohng, K. Y. (2003). Effects of a self-management course for patients with systemic lupus erythematosus. *Journal of Advanced Nursing, 42*(5), 479–486.

Other Specific Rheumatic Diseases

Diep, J. T. & Gorevic, P. D. (2005). Geriatric autoimmune diseases: Systemic lupus erythematosus, Sjögren's syndrome, and myositis. *Geriatrics, 60*(5), 32–38.

Goldenberg, D. L. (2004). Update on the treatment of fibromyalgia. *Bulletin on the Rheumatic Diseases, 53*(1), 1–7.

Lash, A. A., Ehrlich-Jones, L. & McCoy, D. (2003). Fibromyalgia: Evolving concepts and management in primary care settings. *MedSurg Nursing, 12*(3), 145–159,190.

*Schaefer, K. M. (2005). The lived experience of fibromyalgia in African American women. *Holistic Nursing Practice, 19*(1), 17–25.

Stokes, D. G. & Kremer, J. M. (2003). Potential of tumor necrosis factor neutralization strategies in rheumatologic disorders other than rheumatoid arthritis. *Seminars in Arthritis and Rheumatism, 33*(1), 1–18.

Wolfe, F., Smythe, H. A., Yunus, M. B., et al. (1990). The American College of Rheumatology 1990 criteria for the classification of fibromyalgia: Report of the multicenter criteria committee. *Arthritis and Rheumatism, 33*(2), 160–172.

RESOURCES

American College of Rheumatology and Association of Rheumatology Health Professionals, 1800 Century Place, Suite 250, Atlanta, GA 30345; 404-633-3777; http://www.rheumatology.org. Accessed June 2, 2006.

American Fibromyalgia Syndrome Association, Inc., 6380 E. Tanque Verde Road, Suite D, Tucson, AZ 85615; 520-733-1570; http://www.afsafund.org. Accessed June 2, 2006.

Arthritis Foundation, P.O. Box 7669, Atlanta, GA 30357; 404-872-7100 or 800-568-4045 (information line); http://www.arthritis.org. Accessed June 2, 2006.

Centers for Disease Control & Prevention, 1600 Clifton Road, Atlanta, GA 30333; 404-639-3534 or 800-311-3435; http://www.cdc.gov. Accessed June 2, 2006.

Lupus Foundation of America, Inc., 2000 L Street, NW, Suite 710, Washington, DC 20036; 800-558-0121; http://www.lupus.org. Accessed June 2, 2006.

National Institute of Arthritis and Musculoskeletal and Skin Diseases, National Institutes of Health, Building 31, Room 4C02, 31 Center Drive—MSC 2350, Bethesda, MD 20892; 301-496-8190; http://www.niams.nih.gov. Accessed June 2, 2006.

Scleroderma Foundation, 12 Kent Way, Suite 101, Byfield, MA 01922; 978-463-5843 or 800-722-4673; http://www.scleroderma.org. Accessed June 2, 2006.

Sjögren's Syndrome Foundation, 8120 Woodmont Avenue, Suite 530, Bethesda, MD 20814; 301-718-0300; http://www.sjogrens.org. Accessed June 2, 2006.

Spondylitis Association of America, P.O. Box 5872, Sherman Oaks, CA 91413; 800-777-8189; http://www.spondylitis.org. Accessed June 2, 2006.

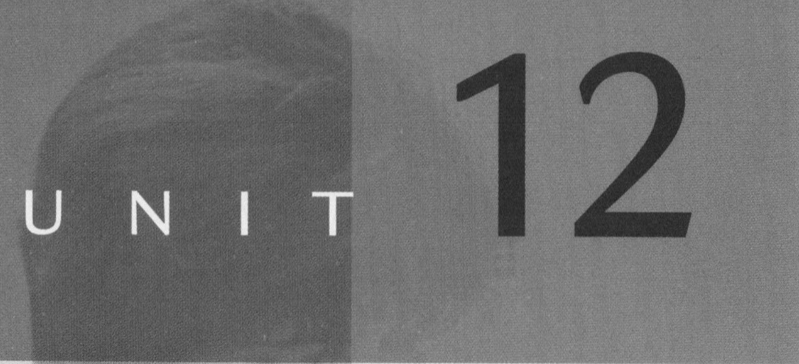

Integumentary Function

Case Study
Applying Concepts from NANDA, NIC, and NOC

A Patient With a Thermal Injury

An 87-year-old man who lives with his wife at an assisted living residence. He filled a basin of water to soak his feet and immersed his left foot in the basin before checking the water temperature. He sustained a deep partial-thickness burn on his foot and ankle and has been admitted to the residence's skilled nursing unit. The nurse notes that the skin of his left foot is bright red and there are three 2- to 4-cm blisters on the dorsum. The burn is quite painful and he cannot bear weight on his foot. His wife states that she is concerned because he is not eating his meals.

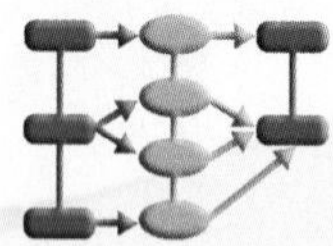

Turn to Appendix C to see a concept map that illustrates the relationships that exist between the nursing diagnoses, interventions, and outcomes for the patient's clinical problems.

Nursing Classifications and Languages

NANDA Nursing Diagnoses	NIC Nursing Interventions	NOC Nursing Outcomes Return to functional baseline status, stabilization of, or improvement in:
Impaired Skin Integrity—Altered epidermis and/or dermis	**Skin Care: Topical Treatments**—Application of topical substances or manipulation of devices to promote skin integrity and minimize skin breakdown	**Wound Healing: Secondary Intention**—Extent of regeneration of cells and tissues in an open wound
Acute Pain—Unpleasant sensory and emotional experience arising from actual or potential tissue damage or described in terms of such damage; sudden or slow onset of any intensity from mild to severe with an anticipated or predictable end and a duration of less than 6 months	**Wound Care**—Prevention of wound complications and promotion of wound healing	**Pain Control**—Personal actions to control pain
Risk for Infection—At increased risk for being invaded by pathogenic organisms	**Pain Management**—Alleviation of pain or reduction in pain to a level of comfort that is acceptable to the patient	**Infection Severity**—Severity of infection and associated symptoms
Risk for Imbalanced Nutrition: Less Than Body Requirements—At risk for intake of nutrients insufficient to meet metabolic needs	**Infection Protection**—Prevention and early detection of infection in a patient at risk	**Nutritional Status**—Extent to which nutrients are available to meet metabolic needs
	Nutrition Management—Assisting with or providing a balanced dietary intake of foods and fluids	

NANDA International (2005). *Nursing diagnoses: Definitions & classification 2005–2006.* Philadelphia: North American Nursing Diagnosis Association.

Dochterman, J. M., & Bulechek, G. M. (2004). *Nursing interventions classification (NIC)* (4th ed.). St. Louis: Mosby.

Iowa Outcomes Project (2004). In Moorhead, S., Johnson, M. & Maas, M. (2004). *Nursing outcomes classification (NOC)* (3rd ed.). St. Louis: Mosby.

Dochterman, J. M., & Jones, D. A. (2003). *Unifying nursing languages: The harmonization of NANDA, NIC, and NOC.* Washington, DC: American Nurses Association.

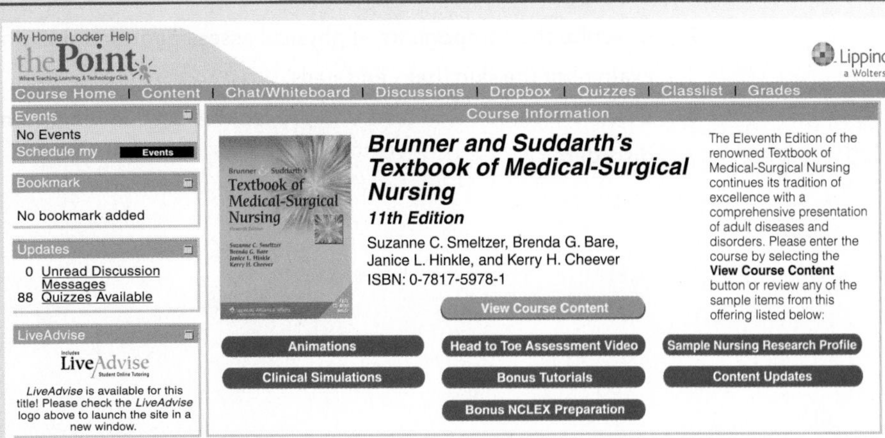

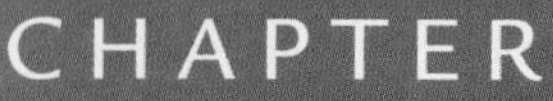

CHAPTER 55

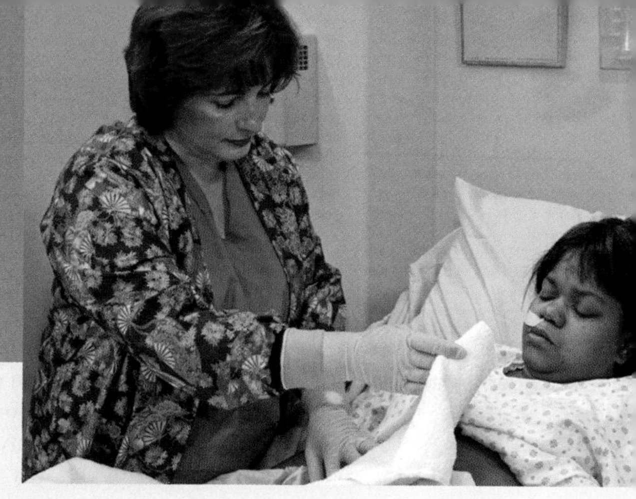

Assessment of Integumentary Function

Learning Objectives

On completion of this chapter, the learner will be able to:

1. Identify the structures and functions of the skin.
2. Differentiate the composition and function of each skin layer: epidermis, dermis, and subcutaneous tissue.
3. Identify and describe primary and secondary skin lesions and their pattern and distribution.
4. Recognize common skin eruptions and manifestations associated with systemic disease.
5. Describe the normal aging process of the skin and skin changes common in elderly patients.
6. List appropriate questions that help elicit information during an assessment of the skin.
7. Describe the components of physical assessment that are most useful when examining the skin, hair, and nails.
8. Discuss common skin tests and procedures used in diagnosing skin and related disorders.

Skin disorders are encountered frequently in nursing practice. Skin-related disorders account for up to 10% of all ambulatory patient visits in the United States (Fleischer, Feldman, & Rapp, 2000). Because the skin mirrors the general condition of the patient, many systemic conditions may be accompanied by dermatologic manifestations.

The psychological stress of illness or various personal and family problems is commonly exhibited outwardly as dermatologic problems. Any hospitalized patient may suddenly develop itching and a rash from the treatment regimen. In certain systemic conditions, such as hepatitis and some cancers, dermatologic manifestations may be the first sign of the disorder.

Anatomic and Physiologic Overview

The largest organ system of the body, the skin is indispensable for human life. Skin forms a barrier between the internal organs and the external environment and participates in many vital body functions. The skin is contiguous with the mucous membrane at the external openings of the digestive, respiratory, and urogenital systems. Because skin disorders are readily visible, dermatologic complaints are commonly the primary reason that a patient seeks health care.

Anatomy of the Skin, Hair, Nails, and Glands of the Skin

The skin is composed of three layers: epidermis, dermis, and subcutaneous tissue (Fig. 55-1). The epidermis is an outermost layer of stratified epithelial cells and composed predominantly of keratinocytes. It ranges in thickness from about 0.1 mm on the eyelids to about 1 mm on the palms of the hands and soles of the feet. Four distinct layers compose the epidermis; from innermost to outermost they are the stratum germinativum, stratum granulosum, stratum lucidum, and stratum corneum. Each layer becomes more differentiated (ie, mature and with more specific functions) as it rises from the basal stratum germinativum layer to the outermost stratum corneum layer.

Epidermis

The epidermis, which is contiguous with the mucous membranes and the lining of the ear canals, consists of live, continuously dividing cells covered on the surface by dead cells that were originally deeper in the dermis but were pushed upward by the newly developing, more differentiated cells underneath. This external layer is almost completely replaced every 3 to 4 weeks. The dead cells contain large amounts of **keratin**, an insoluble, fibrous protein that forms the outer barrier of the skin and has the capacity to repel pathogens and prevent excessive fluid loss from the body. Keratin is the principal hardening ingredient of the hair and nails.

Melanocytes are the special cells of the epidermis that are primarily involved in producing the pigment **melanin**, which colors the skin and hair. The more melanin in the tissue, the darker the color. Most of the skin of dark-skinned people and the darker areas of the skin on light-skinned people (eg, the nipple) contain larger amounts of this pigment. Normal skin color depends on race and varies from pale, almost ivory, to deep brown, almost pure black. Systemic disease affects skin color as well. For example, the skin appears bluish when there is insufficient oxygenation of the blood, yellow-green in people with jaundice, or red or flushed when there is inflammation or fever (Table 55-1).

Production of melanin is controlled by a hormone secreted from the hypothalamus of the brain called *melanocyte-*

Glossary

alopecia: loss of hair from any cause
anagen phase: active phase of hair growth
dermatosis: any abnormal skin condition
erythema: redness of the skin caused by congestion of the capillaries
hirsutism: the condition of having excessive hair growth
hyperpigmentation: increase in the melanin of the skin, resulting in an increase in pigmentation
hypopigmentation: decrease in the melanin of the skin, resulting in a loss of pigmentation
keratin: an insoluble, fibrous protein that forms the outer layer of skin
Langerhans cells: dendritic clear cells in the epidermis that carry surface receptors for immunoglobulin and complement and that are active participants in delayed hypersensitivity of the skin
lichenification: leathery thickening of the skin
Merkel cells: cells of the epidermis that play a role in transmission of sensory messages
melanin: the substance responsible for coloration of the skin
melanocytes: cells of the skin that produce melanin
petechiae: pinpoint red spots that appear on the skin as a result of blood leakage into the skin
rete ridges: undulations and furrows that appear at the dermis–epidermis junction and are responsible for cementing together the two layers
sebaceous glands: glands that exist within the epidermis and secrete sebum to keep the skin soft and pliable
sebum: fatty secretion of the sebaceous glands
telangiectases: red marks on the skin caused by distention of the superficial blood vessels
vitiligo: a localized or widespread condition characterized by destruction of the melanocytes in circumscribed areas of the skin, resulting in white patches
Wood's light: a blue light used for diagnosing skin conditions

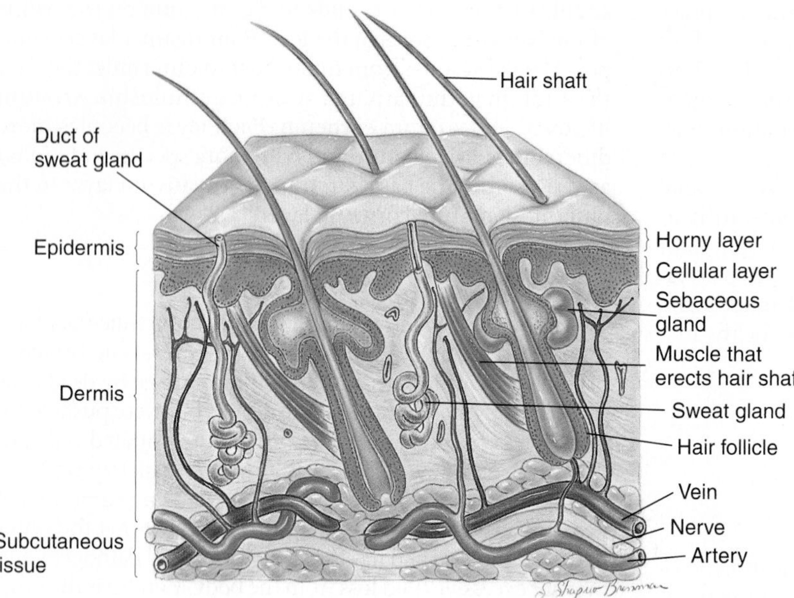

FIGURE 55-1. Anatomic structures of the skin. From Bickley, L. S. & Szilagyi, P. G. (2003). *Bates' guide to physical examination and history taking* (8th ed.). Philadelphia: Lippincott Williams & Wilkins.

stimulating hormone. It is believed that melanin can absorb ultraviolet light in sunlight.

Two other types of cells are common to the epidermis: Merkel and Langerhans cells. **Merkel cells** are receptors that transmit stimuli to the axon through a chemical synapse. **Langerhans cells** are believed to play a significant role in cutaneous immune system reactions. These accessory cells of the afferent immune system process invading antigens and transport the antigens to the lymph system to activate the T lymphocytes.

The characteristics of the epidermis vary in different areas of the body. It is thickest over the palms of the hands and soles of the feet and contains increased amounts of keratin. The thickness of the epidermis can increase with use and can result in calluses forming on the hands or corns forming on the feet.

The junction of the epidermis and dermis is an area of many undulations and furrows called **rete ridges.** This junction anchors the epidermis to the dermis and permits the free exchange of essential nutrients between the two layers. This interlocking between the dermis and epidermis produces ripples on the surface of the skin. On the fingertips, these ripples are called *fingerprints.* They are a person's most individual physical characteristic, and they rarely change.

Dermis

The dermis makes up the largest portion of the skin, providing strength and structure. It is composed of two layers: papillary and reticular. The papillary dermis lies directly beneath the epidermis and is composed primarily of fibroblast cells capable of producing one form of collagen, a component of connective tissue. The reticular layer lies beneath the papillary layer and also produces collagen and elastic bundles. The dermis is also made up of blood and lymph vessels, nerves, sweat and sebaceous glands, and hair roots. The dermis is often referred to as the "true skin."

Subcutaneous Tissue

The subcutaneous tissue, or hypodermis, is the innermost layer of the skin. It is primarily adipose tissue, which provides a cushion between the skin layers, muscles, and bones. It promotes skin mobility, molds body contours, and insulates the body. Fat is deposited and distributed according to the person's gender and in part accounts for the difference in body shape between men and women. Overeating results in increased deposition of fat beneath the skin. The subcutaneous tissues and the amount of fat deposited are important factors in body temperature regulation.

Hair

An outgrowth of the skin, hair is present over the entire body except for the palms and soles. The hair consists of a root formed in the dermis and a hair shaft that projects beyond the skin. It grows in a cavity called a *hair follicle.* Proliferation of cells in the bulb of the hair causes the hair to form (see Fig. 55-1).

Hair follicles undergo cycles of growth and rest. The rate of growth varies; beard growth is the most rapid, followed by hair on the scalp, axillae, thighs, and eyebrows. The growth or **anagen phase** may last up to 6 years for scalp hair, whereas the telogen or resting phase lasts approximately 4 months. During telogen, hair is shed from the body. The hair follicle recycles into the growing phase spontaneously, or it can be induced by plucking out hairs. Growing and resting hairs can be found side by side on all parts of the body. About 90% of the 100,000 hair follicles on a normal scalp are in the growing phase at any one time, and 50 to 100 scalp hairs are shed each day.

There is a small bulge on the side of the hair follicle that houses the stem cells that migrate down to the follicle root and begin the cycle of reproducing the hair shaft. These bulges also contain the stem cells that migrate upward to reproduce skin. The location of these cells on the side of the hair shaft rather than at the base is a factor in hair loss.

TABLE 55-1 Select Cutaneous Manifestations of Systemic Diseases

Common cutaneous manifestations of systemic diseases include *pruritus* (itching), which may result from chronic renal disease, scabies, pediculosis (lice), obstructive biliary disease with jaundice, Hodgkin's or non-Hodgkin's lymphoma, or medication reactions; *pallor*, which suggests anemia or a cardiopulmonary disorder; and *skin thickening and hardening*, such as that which occurs with scleroderma and dermatomyositis.

	Manifestation	Systemic Disease
Scale 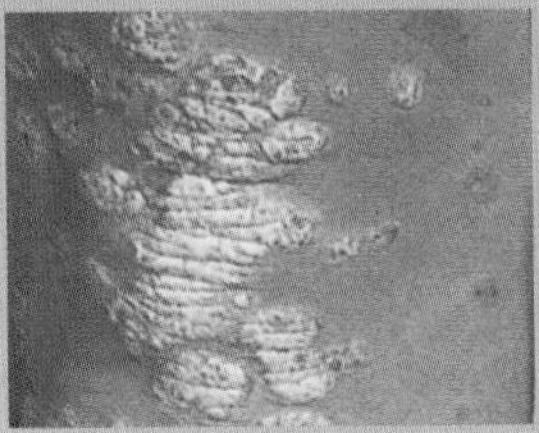	Plaques with scales (on the front of a knee)	Psoriasis
Ecchymosis 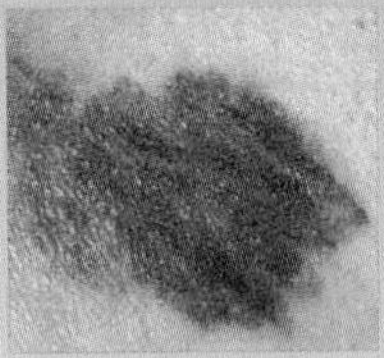 / Purpura 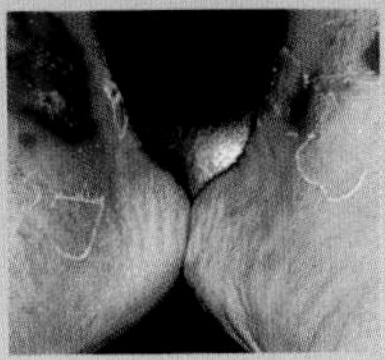	Ecchymosis (bruise) and purpura (bleeding into the skin)	Platelet disorder, vessel fragility
Urticaria 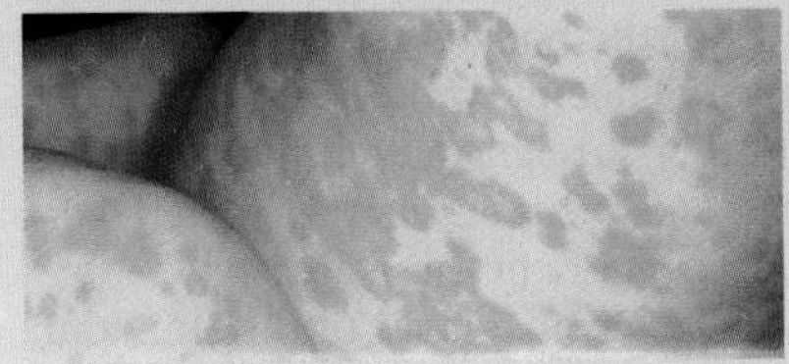	Urticaria (wheals or hives)	Infections, allergic reactions
Plaque 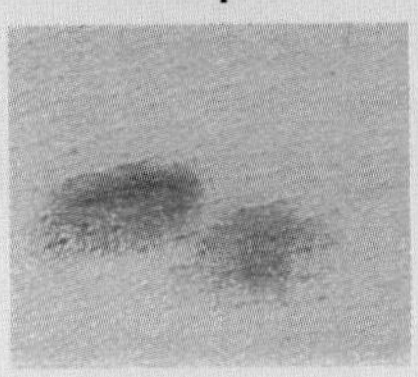 / Nodule 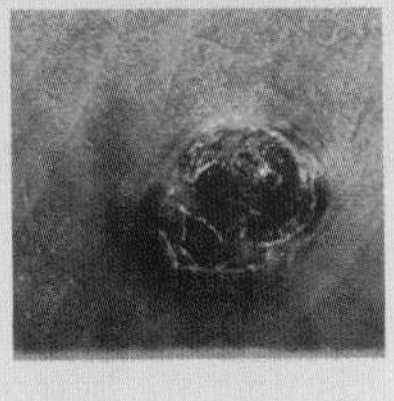	Cutaneous lesions: blue-red or dark brown plaques and nodules	Kaposi's sarcoma
Café-au-lait spot	Macular, tan *café-au-lait* spots	Neurocutaneous disorders, such as neurofibromatosis (von Recklinghausen's disease)
Ulcerated lesion 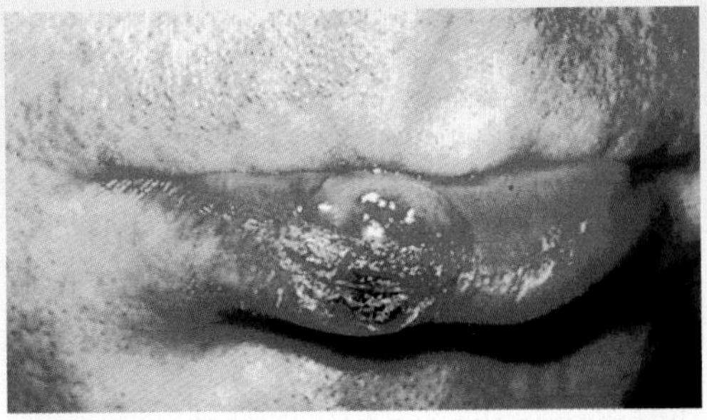	Painless chancre or ulcerated lesion	Syphilis

In conditions in which inflammation causes damage to the root of the hair, regrowth is possible. However, if inflammation causes damage to the side of the hair follicle, stem cells are destroyed and the hair does not grow.

In certain locations on the body, hair growth is controlled by sex hormones. The most vivid example is the growth of hair on the face (ie, beard and mustache), chest, and back, which is controlled by the male hormones known as androgens. Some women with higher levels of testosterone have hair in the areas generally thought of as masculine, such as the face, chest, and lower abdomen. This is often a normal genetic variation, but if it appears along with irregular menses and weight changes, it may indicate a hormonal imbalance.

Hair in different parts of the body serves different functions. The hairs of the eyes (ie, eyebrows and lashes), nose, and ears filter out dust, bugs, and airborne debris. The hair of the skin provides thermal insulation in lower animals. This function is enhanced during cold or fright by piloerection (ie, hairs standing on end), caused by contraction of the tiny erector muscles attached to the hair follicle. The piloerector response that occurs in humans is probably vestigial (ie, rudimentary).

Hair color is supplied by various amounts of melanin within the hair shaft. Gray or white hair reflects the loss of pigment. Hair quantity and distribution can be affected by endocrine conditions. For example, Cushing's syndrome causes **hirsutism**, especially in women, and hypothyroidism (ie, underactive thyroid) causes changes in hair texture. In many cases, chemotherapy and radiation therapy cause hair thinning or weakening of the hair shaft, resulting in partial or complete **alopecia** from the scalp and other parts of the body.

Nails

On the dorsal surface of the fingers and toes, a hard, transparent plate of keratin, called the *nail,* overlies the skin. The nail grows from its root, which lies under a thin fold of skin called the cuticle. The nail protects the fingers and toes by preserving their highly developed sensory functions, such as for picking up small objects.

Nail growth is continuous throughout life, with an average growth of 0.1 mm daily. Growth is faster in fingernails than toenails and tends to slow with aging. Complete renewal of a fingernail takes about 170 days, whereas toenail renewal takes 12 to 18 months.

Glands of the Skin

There are two types of skin glands: sebaceous glands and sweat glands (see Fig. 55-1). The **sebaceous glands** are associated with hair follicles. The ducts of the sebaceous glands empty **sebum** onto the space between the hair follicle and the hair shaft. For each hair there is a sebaceous gland, the secretions of which lubricate the hair and render the skin soft and pliable.

Sweat glands are found in the skin over most of the body surface, but they are heavily concentrated in the palms of the hands and soles of the feet. Only the glans penis, the margins of the lips, the external ear, and the nail bed are devoid of sweat glands. Sweat glands are subclassified into two categories: eccrine and apocrine.

The eccrine sweat glands are found in all areas of the skin. Their ducts open directly onto the skin surface. The thin, watery secretion called *sweat* is produced in the basal coiled portion of the eccrine gland and is released into its narrow duct. Sweat is composed of predominantly water and contains about one half of the salt content of the blood plasma. Sweat is released from eccrine glands in response to elevated ambient temperature and elevated body temperature. The rate of sweat secretion is under the control of the sympathetic nervous system. Excessive sweating of the palms and soles, axillae, forehead, and other areas may occur in response to pain and stress.

The apocrine sweat glands are larger than eccrine sweat glands and are located in the axillae, anal region, scrotum, and labia majora. Their ducts generally open onto hair follicles. The apocrine glands become active at puberty. In women, they enlarge and recede with each menstrual cycle. Apocrine glands produce a milky sweat that is sometimes broken down by bacteria to produce the characteristic underarm odor. Specialized apocrine glands called *ceruminous glands* are found in the external ear, where they produce cerumen (ie, wax).

Functions of the Skin

Protection

The skin covering most of the body is no more than 1 mm thick, but it provides very effective protection against invasion by bacteria and other foreign matter. The thickened skin of the palms and soles protects against the effects of the constant trauma that occurs in these areas.

The epidermis is the outermost layer of the skin and is composed of several layers of keratinocytes that change character as they migrate to the surface. The stratum corneum, the outer layer of the epidermis, provides the most effective barrier to epidermal water loss and penetration of environmental factors such as chemicals, microbes, and insect bites.

Various lipids are synthesized in the stratum corneum and are the basis for the barrier function of this layer. These are long-chain lipids that are better suited than phospholipids for water resistance. The presence of these lipids in the stratum corneum creates a relatively impermeable barrier for water egress and for the entry of toxins, microbes, and other substances that come in contact with the surface of the skin.

Some substances do penetrate the skin but meet resistance in trying to move through the channels between the cell layers of the stratum corneum. Microbes and fungi, which are part of the body's normal flora, cannot penetrate unless there is a break in the skin barrier.

The dermis–epidermis junction is the basal layer, which is composed of collagen. The basal layer serves four functions. It acts as a scaffold for tissue organization and a template for regeneration; it provides selective permeability for filtration of serum; it is a physical barrier between different types of cells; and it binds the epithelium to underlying cell layers.

Sensation

The receptor endings of nerves in the skin allow the body to constantly monitor the conditions of the immediate environment. The primary functions of the receptors in the skin are to sense temperature, pain, light touch, and pressure (or heavy touch). Different nerve endings respond to each of the different stimuli. Although the nerve endings are distributed over the entire body, they are more concentrated in some areas than in others. For example, the fingertips are more densely innervated than the skin on the back.

Fluid Balance

The stratum corneum, the outermost layer of the epidermis, has the capacity to absorb water, thereby preventing an excessive loss of water and electrolytes from the internal body and retaining moisture in the subcutaneous tissues. When skin is damaged, as occurs with a severe burn, large quantities of fluids and electrolytes may be lost rapidly, possibly leading to circulatory collapse, shock, and death.

The skin is not completely impermeable to water. Small amounts of water continuously evaporate from the skin surface. This evaporation, called *insensible perspiration*, amounts to approximately 600 mL daily in a normal adult. Insensible water loss varies with the body and ambient temperature. In a person with a fever, the loss can increase. During immersion in water, the skin can accumulate water up to three or four times its normal weight, such as the swelling of the skin that occurs after prolonged bathing.

Temperature Regulation

The body continuously produces heat as a result of the metabolism of food, which produces energy. This heat is dissipated primarily through the skin. Three major physical processes are involved in loss of heat from the body to the environment. The first process, radiation, is the transfer of heat to another object of lower temperature situated at a distance. The second process, conduction, is the transfer of heat from the body to a cooler object in contact with it. The third process, convection, which consists of movement of warm air molecules away from the body, is the transfer of heat by conduction to the air surrounding the body.

Evaporation from the skin aids heat loss by conduction. Heat is conducted through the skin into water molecules on its surface, causing the water to evaporate. The water on the skin surface may be from insensible perspiration, sweat, or the environment.

Normally, all of these mechanisms for heat loss are used. However, when the ambient temperature is very high, radiation and convection are ineffective, and evaporation becomes the only means of heat loss.

Under normal conditions, metabolic heat production is balanced by heat loss, and the internal temperature of the body is maintained constant at approximately 37°C (98.6°F). The rate of heat loss depends primarily on the surface temperature of the skin, which is a function of the skin blood flow. Under normal conditions, the total blood circulated through the skin is approximately 450 mL per minute, or 10 to 20 times the amount of blood required to provide necessary metabolites and oxygen. Blood flow through these skin vessels is controlled primarily by the sympathetic nervous system. Increased blood flow to the skin results in more heat delivered to the skin and a greater rate of heat loss from the body. In contrast, decreased skin blood flow decreases the skin temperature and helps conserve heat for the body. When the temperature of the body begins to fall, as occurs on a cold day, the blood vessels of the skin constrict, thereby reducing heat loss from the body.

Sweating is another process by which the body can regulate the rate of heat loss. Sweating does not occur until the core body temperature exceeds 37°C, regardless of skin temperature. In extremely hot environments, the rate of sweat production may be as high as 1 L per hour. Under some circumstances (eg, emotional stress), sweating may occur as a reflex and may be unrelated to the need to lose heat from the body.

Vitamin Production

Skin exposed to ultraviolet light can convert substances necessary for synthesizing vitamin D (cholecalciferol). Vitamin D is essential for preventing osteoporosis and rickets, a condition that causes bone deformities and results from a deficiency of vitamin D, calcium, and phosphorus.

Immune Response Function

Recent research has confirmed a definite action of **Langerhans cells** (specialized cells in the skin) in facilitating the uptake of IgE-associated allergens. This action plays a pivotal role in the pathogenesis of atopic dermatitis and other allergic diseases such as asthma and allergic rhinitis. These findings support the concept of a systemic regulatory mechanism as a trigger for allergic diseases and suggest that this trigger can be aggravated by local inflammation of atopic eczema (Semper, Heron, Woolard, et al., 2003).

Gerontologic Considerations

The skin undergoes many physiologic changes associated with normal aging. A lifetime of excessive sun exposure, systemic diseases, and poor nutrition can increase the range of skin problems and the rapidity with which they appear. In addition, certain medications (eg, antihistamines, antibiotics, diuretics) are photosensitizing and increase the damage that results from sun exposure. The outcome is an increasing vulnerability to injury and to certain diseases. Skin problems are common among older people.

Before conducting a skin assessment, the nurse needs to be aware of significant changes that occur with aging. The major changes in the skin of older people include dryness, wrinkling, uneven pigmentation, and various proliferative lesions. Cellular changes associated with aging include a thinning at the junction of the dermis and epidermis. This results in fewer anchoring sites between the two skin layers, which means that even minor injury or stress to the epidermis can cause it to shear away from the dermis. This phenomenon may account for the increased vulnerability of aged skin to trauma. With increasing age, the epidermis and dermis thin and flatten, causing wrinkles, sags, and overlapping skin folds (Fig. 55-2).

Loss of the subcutaneous tissue substances of elastin, collagen, and fat diminishes the protection and cushioning of underlying tissues and organs, decreases muscle

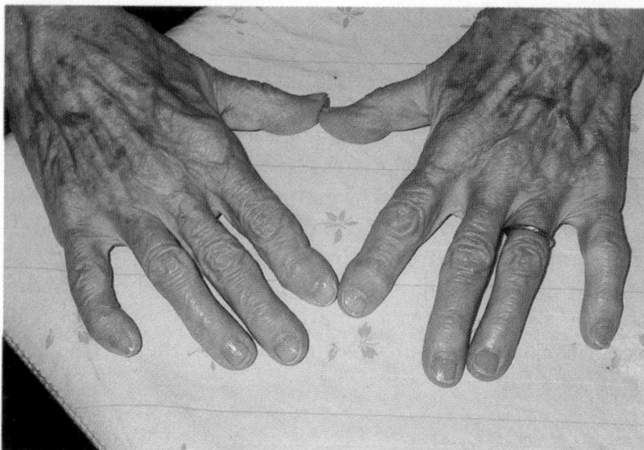

FIGURE 55-2. Hands with wrinkling and overlapping folds common to aging skin.

tone, and results in the loss of the insulating properties of fat.

Cellular replacement slows as a result of aging. As the dermal layers thin, the skin becomes fragile and transparent. The blood supply to the skin also changes with age. Vessels, especially the capillary loops, decrease in number and size. These vascular changes contribute to the delayed wound healing commonly seen in the elderly patient. Sweat and sebaceous glands decrease in number and functional capacity, leading to dry and scaly skin. Reduced hormonal levels of androgens are thought to contribute to declining sebaceous gland function.

Hair growth gradually diminishes, especially over the lower legs and dorsum of the feet. Thinning is common in the scalp, axilla, and pubic areas. Other functions affected by normal aging include the barrier function of skin, sensory perception, and thermoregulation.

Photoaging, or damage from excessive sun exposure, has detrimental effects on the normal aging of skin. A lifetime of outdoor work or outdoor activities (eg, construction work, lifeguarding, sunbathing) without prudent use of sunscreens can lead to profound wrinkling; increased loss of elasticity; mottled, pigmented areas; cutaneous atrophy; and benign or malignant lesions.

Many skin lesions are part of normal aging. Recognizing these lesions enables the examiner to assist the patient to feel less anxious about changes in skin. Chart 55-1 summarizes some skin lesions that are expected to appear as the skin ages. These are normal and require no special attention unless the skin becomes infected or irritated.

CHART 55-1

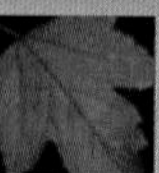

Benign Changes in Elderly Skin

- Cherry angiomas (bright red "moles")
- Diminished hair, especially on scalp and pubic area
- Dyschromias (color variations)
  - Solar lentigo (liver spots)
  - Melasma (dark discoloration of the skin)
  - Lentigines (freckles)
- Neurodermatitis (itchy spots)
- Seborrheic keratoses (crusty brown "stuck-on" patches)
- Spider angiomas
- Telangiectasias (red marks on skin caused by stretching of the superficial blood vessels)
- Wrinkles
- Xerosis (dryness)
- Xanthelasma (yellowish waxy deposits on upper and lower eyelids)

Assessment

Health History and Clinical Manifestations

When caring for patients with dermatologic disorders, the nurse obtains important information through the health history and direct observations. The nurse's skill in physical assessment and an understanding of the anatomy and function of the skin can ensure that deviations from normal are recognized, reported, and documented.

During the health history interview, the nurse asks about any family and personal history of skin allergies; allergic reactions to food, medications, and chemicals; previous skin problems; and skin cancer. The names of cosmetics, soaps, shampoos, and other personal hygiene products are obtained if there have been any recent skin problems noticed with the use of these products. The health history contains specific information about the onset, signs and symptoms, location, and duration of any pain, itching, rash, or other discomfort experienced by the patient. Chart 55-2 lists selected questions useful in obtaining appropriate information.

Physical Assessment

Assessment of the skin involves the entire skin area, including the mucous membranes, scalp, hair, and nails. The skin is a reflection of a person's overall health, and alterations commonly correspond to disease in other organ systems. Inspection and palpation are techniques commonly used in examining the skin. The room must be well lighted and warm. A penlight may be used to highlight lesions. The patient completely disrobes and is adequately draped. Gloves are worn during skin examination if a rash or lesions are to be palpated. However, it is important to avoid making the patient feel as if he or she cannot be touched. Touching skin lesions indicates a level of acceptance of the patient.

Assessing General Appearance

The general appearance of the skin is assessed by observing color, temperature, moisture or dryness, skin texture (rough or smooth), lesions, vascularity, mobility, and the condition of the hair and nails. Skin turgor, possible edema, and elasticity are assessed by palpation.

Skin color varies from person to person and ranges from ivory to deep brown to almost pure black. The skin of ex-

GENETICS IN NURSING PRACTICE

Integumentary Conditions

Integumentary conditions influenced by genetic factors include the following:

- Albinism
- Eczema
- Hypohidrotic ectodermal dysplasia
- Incontinentia pigmenti
- Neurofibromatosis type 1
- Pseudoxanthoma elasticum
- Psoriasis

NURSING ASSESSMENTS

Family History Assessment

- Assess for other closely related family members with integumentary impairment or abnormalities.
- Inquire about the nature and type of skin lesions and age at onset (eg, skin involvement with incontinentia pigmenti occurs in the first few weeks of life with blistering of the skin, whereas lesions of neurofibromatosis type 1 may appear in early childhood through adulthood).
- Note gender of affected individuals (eg, mostly females with incontinentia pigmenti, mostly males with hypohidrotic ectodermal dysplasia).
- Inquire about the presence of other clinical features, such as unusual hair, teeth, or nails; thrombocytopenia; recurrent infections.

Patient Assessment

- Assess for related clinical features, such as sparse eyebrows and eyelashes, abnormally shaped teeth, alopecia, nail abnormalities (eg, hypohidrotic ectodermal dysplasia).
- Assess for related alterations in vision, such as nystagmus or strabismus; albinism; retinal abnormalities (eg, pseudoxanthoma elasticum); Lisch nodules and/or optic glioma (neurofibromatosis type 1).

MANAGEMENT ISSUES SPECIFIC TO GENETICS

- Inquire whether DNA mutation or other genetics testing has been performed on affected family members.
- If indicated, refer for further genetics counseling and evaluation so that family members can discuss inheritance, risk to other family members, availability of genetics testing, and gene-based interventions.
- Offer appropriate genetics information and resources.
- Assess patient's understanding of genetics information.
- Provide support to families with newly diagnosed genetics-related integumentary conditions.
- Participate in management and coordination of care for patients with genetic conditions and for individuals predisposed to develop or pass on a genetic condition.

GENETICS RESOURCES

Genetic Alliance—a directory of support groups for patients and families with genetic conditions; http://www.geneticalliance.org

Gene Clinics—a listing of common genetic disorders with clinical summaries and genetic counseling and testing information; http://www.geneclinics.org

National Organization of Rare Disorders—a directory of support groups and information for patients and families with rare genetic disorders; http://www.rarediseases.org

Online Mendelian Inheritance in Man (OMIM)—a complete listing of inherited genetic conditions; http://www.ncbi.nlm.nih.gov/omim/stats/html

posed portions of the body, especially in sunny, warm climates, tends to be more pigmented than the rest of the body. The vasodilation that occurs with fever, sunburn, and inflammation produces a pink or reddish hue to the skin. Pallor is an absence of or a decrease in normal skin color and vascularity and is best observed in the conjunctivae or around the mouth.

The bluish hue of cyanosis indicates cellular hypoxia and is easily observed in the extremities, nail beds, lips, and mucous membranes. Jaundice, a yellowing of the skin, is directly related to elevations in serum bilirubin and is often first observed in the sclerae and mucous membranes (Fig. 55-3).

Erythema

Erythema is redness of the skin caused by the congestion of capillaries. In light-skinned people, it is easily observed at any location where it appears. To determine possible inflammation, the skin is palpated for increased warmth and for smoothness (ie, edema) or hardness (ie, intracellular infiltration). Because dark skin tends to assume a purple-gray cast when an inflammatory process is present, it may be difficult to detect erythema.

Rash

In instances of pruritus (ie, itching) the patient is asked to indicate which areas of the body are involved. The skin is then stretched gently to decrease the reddish tone and make the rash more visible. Pointing a penlight laterally across the skin may highlight the rash, making it easier to observe. The differences in skin texture are then assessed by running the tips of the fingers lightly over the skin. The borders of the rash may be palpable. The patient's mouth and ears are included in the examination (sometimes rubeola, or measles, causes a red cast to appear on the ears). The patient's temperature is assessed, and the lymph nodes are palpated.

CHART 55-2

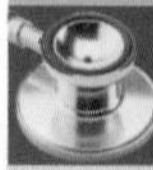

Assessing for Skin Disorders

Patient history relevant to skin disorders may be obtained by asking the following questions:

- When did you first notice this skin problem? (Also investigate duration and intensity.)
- Has it occurred previously?
- Are there any other symptoms?
- What site was first affected?
- What did the rash or lesion look like when it first appeared?
- Where and how fast did it spread?
- Do you have any itching, burning, tingling, or crawling sensations?
- Is there any loss of sensation?
- Is the problem worse at a particular time or season?
- How do you think it started?
- Do you have a history of hay fever, asthma, hives, eczema, or allergies?
- Who in your family has skin problems or rashes?
- Did the eruptions appear after certain foods were eaten? Which foods?
- When the problem occurred, had you recently consumed alcohol?
- What relation do you think there may be between a specific event and the outbreak of the rash or lesion?
- What medications are you taking?
- What topical medication (ointment, cream, salve) have you put on the lesion (including over-the-counter medications)?
- What skin products or cosmetics do you use?
- What is your occupation?
- What in your immediate environment (plants, animals, chemicals, infections) might be precipitating this disorder? Is there anything new, or are there any changes in the environment?
- Does anything touching your skin cause a rash?
- How has this affected you (or your life)?
- Is there anything else you wish to talk about in regard to this disorder?

Cyanosis

Cyanosis is the bluish discoloration that results from a lack of oxygen in the blood. It appears with shock or with respiratory or circulatory compromise. In people with light skin, cyanosis manifests as a bluish hue to the lips, fingertips, and nail beds. Other indications of decreased tissue perfusion include cold, clammy skin; a rapid, thready pulse; and rapid, shallow respirations. The conjunctivae of the eyelids are examined for pallor and **petechiae**.

In a person with dark skin, the skin usually assumes a grayish cast. To detect cyanosis, the areas around the mouth and lips and over the cheekbones and earlobes should be observed.

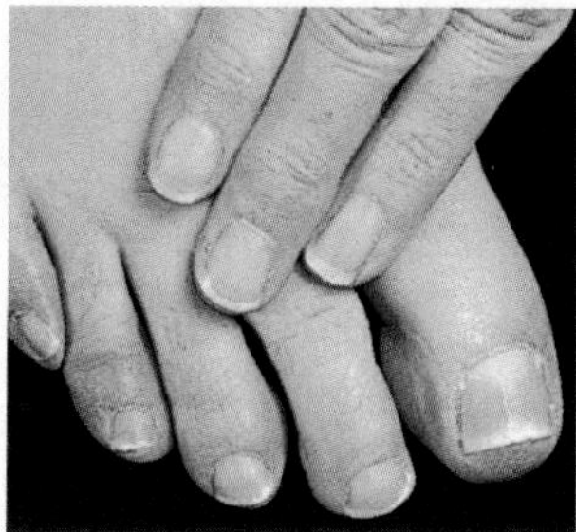

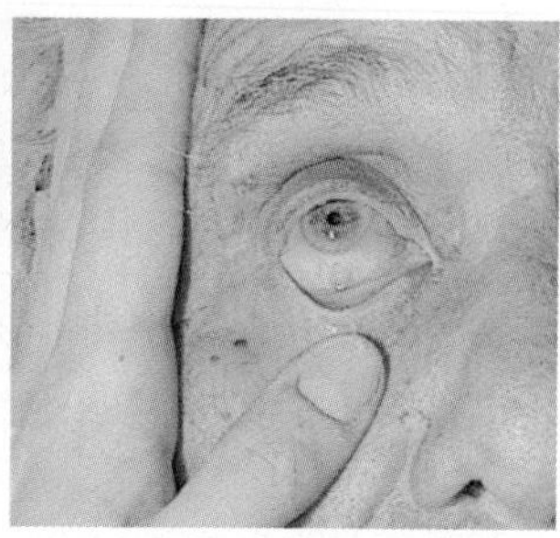

FIGURE 55-3. Examples of skin color changes: the bluish tint of cyanosis (*left*) and the yellow hue of jaundice (*right*).

Color Changes

Almost every process that occurs on the skin causes some color change. For example, **hypopigmentation** may be caused by a fungal infection, eczema, or **vitiligo**; **hyperpigmentation** can occur after sun injury, or as a result of aging.

Changes in skin color in people with dark skin are more noticeable and may cause more concern because the discoloration is more readily visible. Some variation in skin pigment levels is considered normal. Examples include the pigmented crease across the bridge of the nose, pigmented streaks in the nails, and pigmented spots on the sclera of the eye.

ASSESSING PATIENTS WITH DARK SKIN

The color gradations that occur in people with dark skin are largely determined by genetics; they may be described as light, medium, or dark. In people with dark skin, melanin is produced at a faster rate and in larger quantities than in people with light skin. Healthy dark skin has a reddish base or undertone. The buccal mucosa, tongue, lips, and nails normally are pink. The degree of pigmentation of the patient's skin may affect the appearance of a lesion. Lesions may be black, purple, or gray instead of the tan or red seen in patients with light skin. Dark pigment responds with discoloration after injury or inflammation, and patients with dark skin more often experience postinflammatory hyperpigmentation than those with lighter skin. The hyperpigmentation eventually fades but may require months to a year to do so.

In general, people with dark skin suffer the same skin conditions as those with light skin. They are less likely to have skin cancer but more likely to have keloid or scar formation and disorders resulting from occlusion or blockage of hair follicles.

Table 55-2 provides an overview of color changes in light-skinned and dark-skinned people, and the following section provides specific guidelines for assessing dark and light skin.

ASSESSING SKIN LESIONS

Skin lesions are the most prominent characteristics of dermatologic conditions. They vary in size, shape, and cause and are classified according to their appearance and origin. Skin lesions can be described as primary or secondary. Primary lesions are the initial lesions and are characteristic of the disease itself. Secondary lesions result from external

TABLE 55-2 Color Changes in Light and Dark Skin

Etiology	Light Skin	Dark Skin
Pallor		
Anemia—decreased hematocrit Shock—decreased perfusion, vasoconstriction	Generalized pallor	Brown skin appears yellow-brown, dull; black skin appears ashen gray, dull. (Observe areas with least pigmentation: conjunctivae, mucous membranes.)
Local arterial insufficiency	Marked localized pallor (lower extremities, especially when elevated)	Ashen gray, dull; cool to palpation
Albinism—total absence of pigment melanin	Whitish pink	Tan, cream, white
Vitiligo—a condition characterized by destruction of the melanocytes in circumscribed areas of the skin (may be localized or widespread)	Patchy, milky white spots, often symmetric bilaterally	Same
Cyanosis		
Increased amount of unoxygenated hemoglobin:	Dusky blue	Dark but dull, lifeless; only severe cyanosis is apparent in skin. (Observe conjunctivae, oral mucosa, nail beds.)
Central—chronic heart and lung diseases cause arterial desaturation Peripheral—exposure to cold, anxiety	Nail beds dusky	
Erythema		
Hyperemia—increased blood flow through engorged arterial vessels, as in inflammation, fever, alcohol intake, blushing	Red, bright pink	Purplish tinge, but difficult to see. (Palpate for increased warmth with inflammation, taut skin, and hardening of deep tissues.)
Polycythemia—increased red blood cells, capillary stasis	Ruddy blue in face, oral mucosa, conjunctivae, hands and feet	Well concealed by pigment. (Observe for redness in lips.)
Carbon monoxide poisoning	Bright, cherry red in face and upper torso	Cherry red nail beds, lips, and oral mucosa
Venous stasis—decreased blood flow from area, engorged venules	Dusky rubor of dependent extremities (a prelude to necrosis with pressure ulcer)	Easily masked. (Use palpation to identify warmth or edema.)
Jaundice		
Increased serum bilirubin concentration (>2–3 mg/100 mL) due to liver dysfunction or hemolysis, as after severe burns or some infections	Yellow first in sclerae, hard palate, and mucous membranes; then over skin	Check sclerae for yellow near limbus; do not mistake normal yellowish fatty deposits in the periphery under eyelids for jaundice. (Jaundice is best noted at junction of hard and soft palate, on palms.)
Carotenemia—increased level of serum carotene from ingestion of large amounts of carotene-rich foods	Yellow-orange tinge in forehead, palms and soles, and nasolabial folds, but no yellowing in sclerae or mucous membranes	Yellow-orange tinge in palms and soles
Uremia—renal failure causes retained urochrome pigments in the blood	Orange-green or gray overlying pallor of anemia; may also have ecchymoses and purpura	Easily masked. (Rely on laboratory and clinical findings.)
Brown-Tan		
Addison's disease—cortisol deficiency stimulates increased melanin production	Bronzed appearance, an "external tan"; most apparent around nipples, perineum, genitalia, and pressure points (inner thighs, buttocks, elbows, axillae)	Easily masked. (Rely on laboratory and clinical findings.)
Café-au-lait spots—caused by increased melanin pigment in basal cell layer	Tan to light brown, irregularly shaped, oval patch with well-defined borders often not visible in the very dark skinned person	

causes, such as scratching, trauma, infections, or changes caused by wound healing. Depending on the stage of development, skin lesions are further categorized according to type and appearance (Chart 55-3).

A preliminary assessment of the eruption or lesion helps identify the type of **dermatosis** and indicates whether the lesion is primary or secondary. At the same time, the anatomic distribution of the eruption should be observed, because certain diseases affect certain sites of the body and are distributed in characteristic patterns and shapes (Figs. 55-4 and 55-5). To determine the extent of the regional distribution, the left and right sides of the body should be compared while the color and shape of the lesions are assessed. After observation, the lesions are palpated to determine their texture, shape, and border and to see if they are soft and filled with fluid or hard and fixed to the surrounding tissue.

A metric ruler is used to measure the size of the lesions so that any further extension can be compared with this baseline measurement. Skin lesions are described clearly and in detail on the patient's health record, using precise terminology.

After the characteristic distribution of the lesions has been determined, the following information should be obtained and described clearly and in detail:

- Color of the lesion
- Any redness, heat, pain, or swelling
- Size and location of the involved area
- Pattern of eruption (eg, macular, papular, scaling, oozing, discrete, confluent)
- Distribution of the lesion (eg, bilateral, symmetric, linear, circular)

If acute open wounds or lesions are found on inspection of the skin, a comprehensive assessment should be made and documented. This assessment should address the following issues:

- Wound bed: Inspect for necrotic and granulation tissue, epithelium, exudate, color, and odor.
- Wound edges and margins: Observe for undermining (ie, extension of the wound under the surface skin), and evaluate for condition.
- Wound size: Measure in millimeters or centimeters, as appropriate, to determine diameter and depth of the wound and surrounding erythema.
- Surrounding skin: Assess for color, suppleness and moisture, irritation, and scaling.

Assessing Vascularity and Hydration

After the color of the skin has been evaluated and lesions have been inspected, an assessment of vascular changes in the skin is performed. A description of vascular changes includes location, distribution, color, size, and the presence of pulsations. Common vascular changes include petechiae, ecchymoses, **telangiectases**, angiomas, and venous stars.

Skin moisture, temperature, and texture are assessed primarily by palpation. The turgor (ie, elasticity) of the skin, which decreases in normal aging, may be a factor in assessing the hydration status of a patient.

Assessing the Nails and Hair

A brief inspection of the nails includes observation of configuration, color, and consistency. Many alterations in the nail or nail bed reflect local or systemic abnormalities in progress or resulting from past events (Fig. 55-6). Transverse depressions known as Beau's lines in the nails may reflect retarded growth of the nail matrix because of severe illness or, more commonly, local trauma. Ridging, hypertrophy, and other changes may also be visible with local trauma. Paronychia, an inflammation of the skin around the nail, is usually accompanied by tenderness and erythema. The angle between the normal nail and its base is 160 degrees. When palpated, the nail base is usually firm. Clubbing is manifested by a straightening of the normal angle (180 degrees or greater) and softening of the nail base. The softened area feels sponge-like when palpated.

The hair assessment is carried out by inspection and palpation. Gloves are worn by the examiner, and the examination room should be well lighted. Separating the hair so that the condition of the skin underneath can be easily seen, the nurse assesses color, texture, and distribution. The wooden end of a cotton swab can be used to make small parts in the hair so that the scalp can be inspected. Any abnormal lesions, evidence of itching, inflammation, scaling, or signs of infestation (ie, lice or mites) are documented.

COLOR AND TEXTURE

Natural hair color ranges from white to black. Hair begins to turn gray with age, initially during the third decade of life, when the loss of melanin begins to become apparent. However, it is not unusual for the hair of younger people to turn gray as a result of hereditary traits. The person with albinism (ie, partial or complete absence of pigmentation) has a genetic predisposition to white hair from birth. The natural state of the hair can be altered by using hair dyes, bleaches, and curling or relaxing products. The types of products used are identified in the assessment.

The texture of scalp hair ranges from fine to coarse, silky to brittle, oily to dry, and shiny to dull, and hair can be straight, curly, or kinky. Dry, brittle hair may result from overuse of hair dyes, hair dryers, and curling irons or from endocrine disorders, such as thyroid dysfunction. Oily hair is usually caused by increased secretion from the sebaceous glands close to the scalp. If the patient reports a recent change in hair texture, the underlying reason is pursued; the alteration may arise simply from the overuse of commercial hair products or from changing to a new shampoo.

DISTRIBUTION

Body hair distribution varies with location. Hair over most of the body is fine, except in the axillae and pubic areas, where it is coarse. Pubic hair, which develops at puberty, forms a diamond shape extending up to the umbilicus in boys and men. Female pubic hair resembles an inverted triangle. If the pattern found is more characteristic of the opposite gender, it may indicate an endocrine problem and further investigation is in order. Racial differences in hair are expected, such as straight hair in Asians and curly, coarser hair in people of African descent.

Men tend to have more body and facial hair than women. Loss of hair, or alopecia, can occur over the entire body or be confined to a specific area. Scalp hair loss may be localized to patchy areas or may range from generalized thinning to total baldness. When assessing scalp hair loss, it is im-

CHART 55-3

Primary and Secondary Skin Lesions

Primary Skin Lesions

Primary skin lesions are original lesions arising from previously normal skin. Secondary lesions can originate from primary lesions and are the progression of the primary disease to a different appearance.

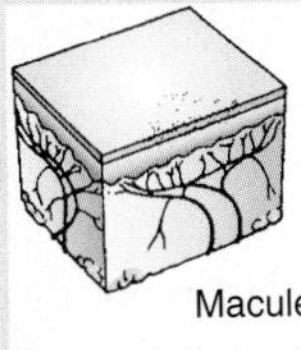
Macule

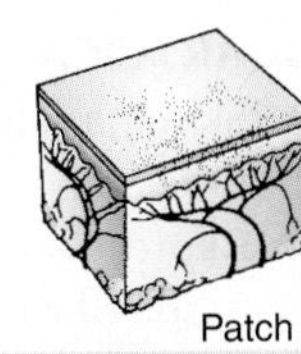
Patch

MACULE, PATCH

Flat, nonpalpable skin color change (color may be brown, white, tan, purple, red)

- *Macule:* <1 cm, circumscribed border
- *Patch:* >1 cm, may have irregular border

Examples:

Freckles, flat moles, petechia, rubella, vitiligo, port wine stains, ecchymosis

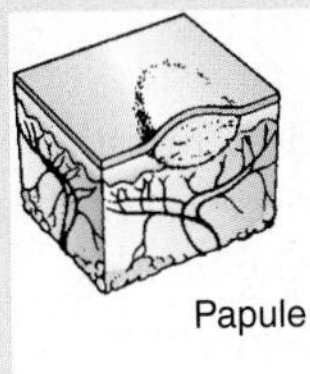
Papule

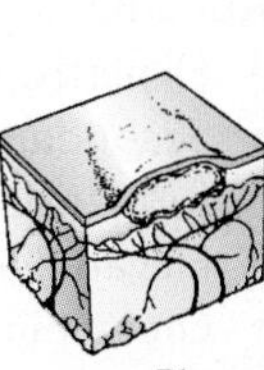
Plaque

PAPULE, PLAQUE

Elevated, palpable, solid mass

Circumscribed border

Plaque may be coalesced papules with flat top

- *Papule:* <0.5 cm
- *Plaque:* >0.5 cm

Examples:

Papules: Elevated nevi, warts, lichen planus

Plaques: Psoriasis, actinic keratosis

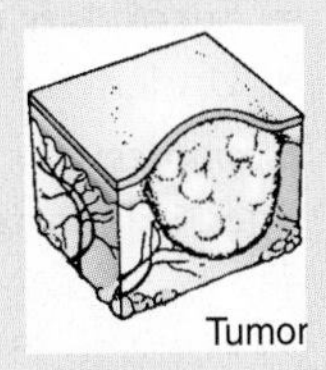
Tumor

NODULE, TUMOR

Elevated, palpable, solid mass

Extends deeper into the dermis than a papule

- *Nodule:* 0.5–2 cm; circumscribed
- *Tumor:* >1–2 cm; tumors do not always have sharp borders

Examples:

Nodules: Lipoma, squamous cell carcinoma, poorly absorbed injection, dermatofibroma

Tumors: Larger lipoma, carcinoma

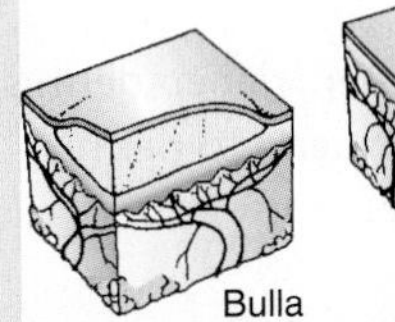
Bulla

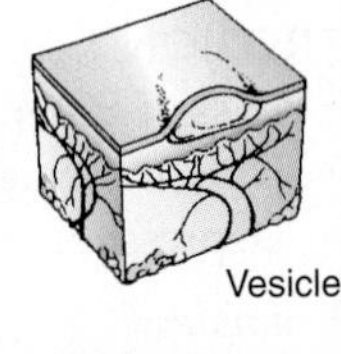
Vesicle

VESICLE, BULLA

Circumscribed, elevated, palpable mass containing serous fluid

- *Vesicle:* <0.5 cm
- *Bulla:* >0.5 cm

Examples:

Vesicles: Herpes simplex/zoster, chickenpox, poison ivy, second-degree burn (blister)

Bulla: Pemphigus, contact dermatitis, large burn blisters, poison ivy, bullous impetigo

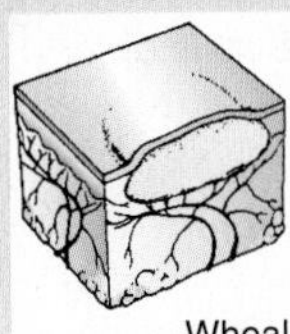
Wheal

WHEAL

- Elevated mass with transient borders
- Often irregular
- Size and color vary
- Caused by movement of serous fluid into the dermis
- Does not contain free fluid in a cavity (as, for example, a vesicle does)

Examples:

Urticaria (hives), insect bites

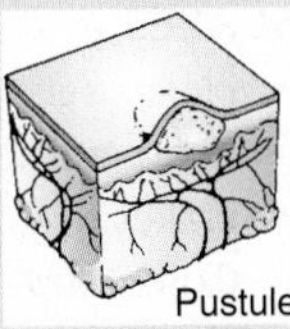
Pustule

PUSTULE

- Pus-filled vesicle or bulla

Examples:

Acne, impetigo, furuncles, carbuncles

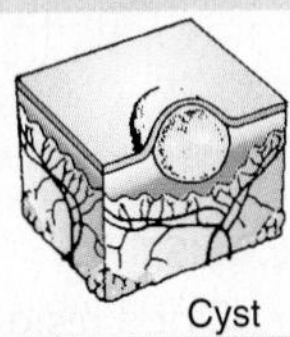
Cyst

CYST

- Encapsulated fluid-filled or semisolid mass
- In the subcutaneous tissue or dermis

Examples:

Sebaceous cyst, epidermoid cysts

continued >

CHART 55-3 *Primary and Secondary Skin Lesions, continued*

Secondary Skin Lesions

Secondary skin lesions result from changes in primary lesions.

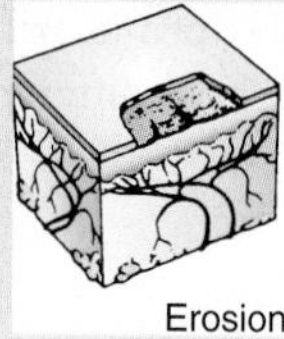
Erosion

EROSION
- Loss of superficial epidermis
- Does not extend to dermis
- Depressed, moist area

Examples:
Ruptured vesicles, scratch marks

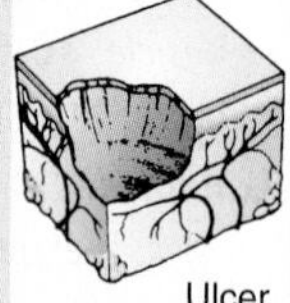
Ulcer

ULCER
- Skin loss extending past epidermis
- Necrotic tissue loss
- Bleeding and scarring possible

Examples:
Stasis ulcer of venous insufficiency, pressure ulcer

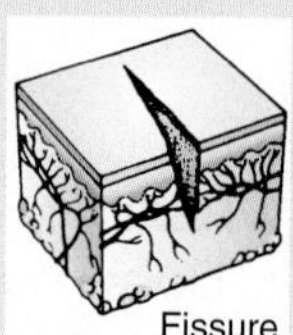
Fissure

FISSURE
- Linear crack in the skin
- May extend to dermis

Examples:
Chapped lips or hands, athlete's foot

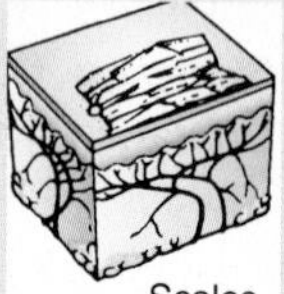
Scales

SCALES
- Flakes secondary to desquamated, dead epithelium
- Flakes may adhere to skin surface
- Color varies (silvery, white)
- Texture varies (thick, fine)

Examples:
Dandruff, psoriasis, dry skin, pityriasis rosea

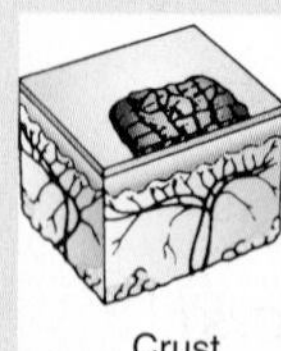
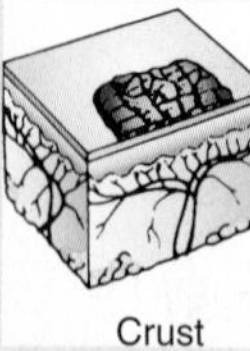
Crust

CRUST
- Dried residue of serum, blood, or pus on skin surface
- Large, adherent crust is a scab

Examples:
Residue left after vesicle rupture: impetigo, herpes, eczema

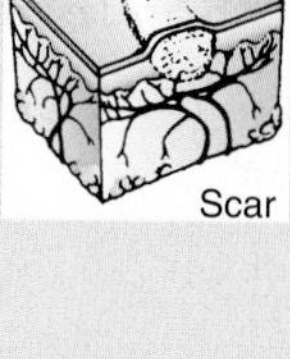
Scar

SCAR (CICATRIX)
- Skin mark left after healing of a wound or lesion
- Represents replacement by connective tissue of the injured tissue
- Young scars: red or purple
- Mature scars: white or glistening

Examples:
Healed wound or surgical incision

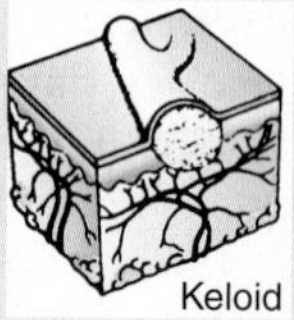

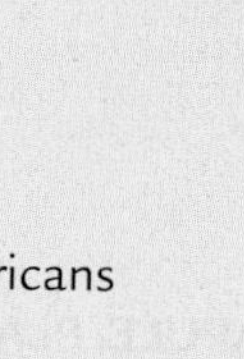
Keloid

KELOID
- Hypertrophied scar tissue
- Secondary to excessive collagen formation during healing
- Elevated, irregular, red
- Greater incidence among African Americans

Examples:
Keloid of ear piercing or surgical incision

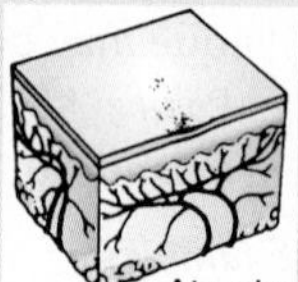

Atrophy

ATROPHY
- Thin, dry, transparent appearance of epidermis
- Loss of surface markings
- Secondary to loss of collagen and elastin
- Underlying vessels may be visible

Examples:
Aged skin, arterial insufficiency

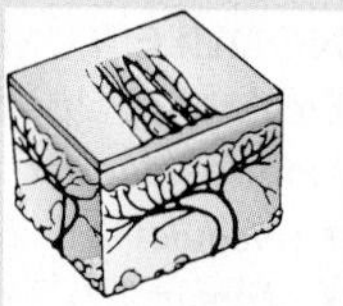

Lichenification

LICHENIFICATION
- Thickening and roughening of the skin
- Accentuated skin markings
- May be secondary to repeated rubbing, irritation, scratching

Examples:
Contact dermatitis

CHART 55-3 Primary and Secondary Skin Lesions, continued

Vascular Skin Lesions

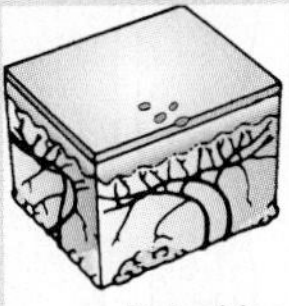
Petechiae

PETECHIA (*PL.* PETECHIAE)

- Round red or purple macule
- Small: 1–2 mm
- Secondary to blood extravasation
- Associated with bleeding tendencies or emboli to skin

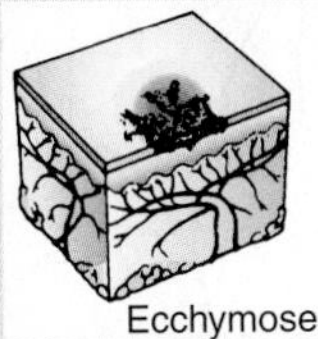
Ecchymoses

ECCHYMOSIS (*PL.* ECCHYMOSES)

- Round or irregular macular lesion
- Larger than petechia
- Color varies and changes: black, yellow, and green hues
- Secondary to blood extravasation
- Associated with trauma, bleeding tendencies

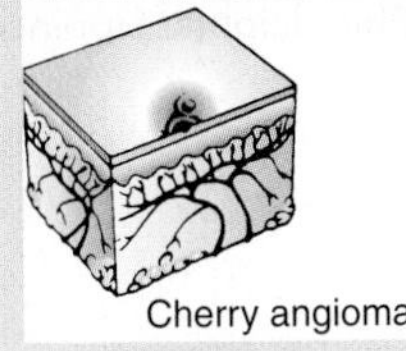
Cherry angioma

CHERRY ANGIOMA

- Papular and round
- Red or purple
- Noted on trunk, extremities
- May blanch with pressure
- Normal age-related skin alteration
- Usually not clinically significant

Spider angioma

SPIDER ANGIOMA

- Red, arteriole lesion
- Central body with radiating branches
- Noted on face, neck, arms, trunk
- Rare below the waist
- May blanch with pressure
- Associated with liver disease, pregnancy, vitamin B deficiency

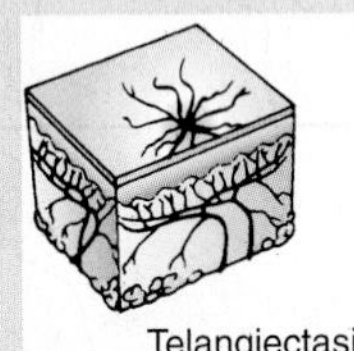
Telangiectasia

TELANGIECTASIA (VENOUS STAR)

- Shape varies: spider-like or linear
- Color bluish or red
- Does not blanch when pressure is applied
- Noted on legs, anterior chest
- Secondary to superficial dilation of venous vessels and capillaries
- Associated with increased venous pressure states (varicosities)

portant to investigate the underlying cause with the patient. Patchy hair loss may be from habitual hair pulling or twisting; excessive traction on the hair (eg, braiding too tightly); excessive use of dyes, straighteners, and oils; chemotherapeutic agents (eg, doxorubicin, cyclophosphamide); fungal infection; or moles or lesions on the scalp. Regrowth may be erratic, and distribution may never attain the previous thickness.

HAIR LOSS

The most common cause of hair loss is male pattern baldness, which affects more than one half of the male population and is believed to be related to heredity, aging, and androgen (male hormone) levels. Androgen is necessary for male pattern baldness to develop. The pattern of hair loss begins with receding of the hairline in the frontal-temporal area and progresses to gradual thinning and complete loss of hair over the top of the scalp and crown. Figure 55-7 illustrates the typical pattern of male hair loss.

OTHER CHANGES

Male pattern hair distribution may be seen in some women at the time of menopause, when the hormone estrogen is no longer produced by the ovaries. In women with hirsutism, excessive hair may grow on the face, chest, shoulders, and pubic area. When menopause is ruled out as the underlying cause, hormonal abnormalities related to pituitary or adrenal dysfunction must be investigated.

Because patients with skin conditions may be viewed negatively by others, these patients may become distraught

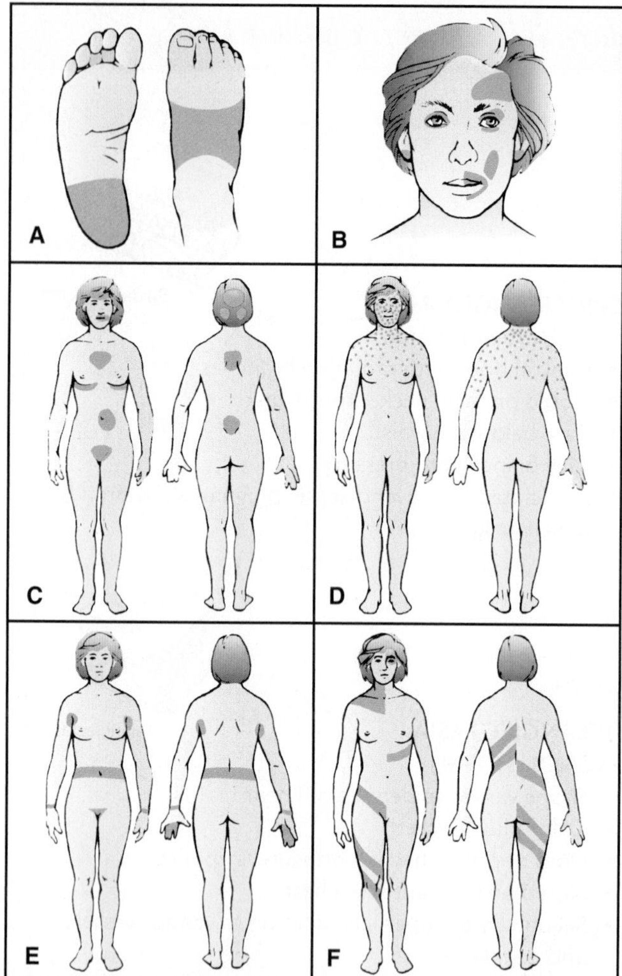

FIGURE 55-4. Anatomic distribution of common skin disorders. (**A**) Contact dermatitis (shoes). (**B**) Contact dermatitis (cosmetics, perfumes, earrings). (**C**) Seborrheic dermatitis. (**D**) Acne. (**E**) Scabies. (**F**) Herpes zoster (shingles).

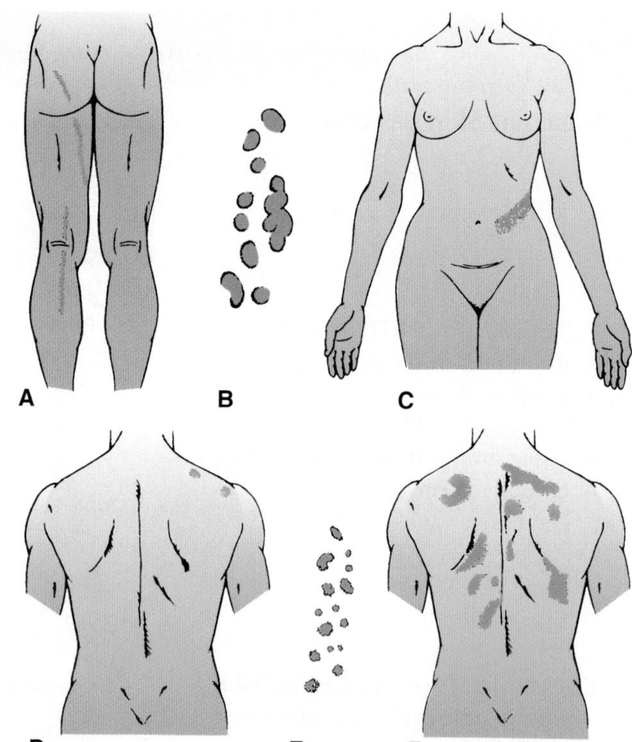

FIGURE 55-5. Skin lesion configurations. (**A**) Linear (in a line). (**B**) Annular and arciform (circular or arcing). (**C**) Zosteriform (linear along a nerve route). (**D**) Grouped (clustered). (**E**) Discrete (separate and distinct). (**F**) Confluent (merged). From Weber, J. W., & Kelley, J. (2003). *Health assessment in nursing* (2nd ed.). Philadelphia: Lippincott Williams & Wilkins.

and avoid interaction with people. Skin conditions can lead to disfigurement, isolation, job loss, and economic hardship.

Some conditions may subject the patient to a protracted illness, leading to feelings of depression, frustration, self-consciousness, poor self-image, and rejection. Itching and skin irritation, which are features of many skin diseases, may be a constant annoyance. These discomforts may result in loss of sleep, anxiety, and depression, all of which reinforce the general distress and fatigue that frequently accompany skin disorders.

For patients suffering such physical and psychological discomforts, the nurse needs to provide understanding, explanations of the problem, appropriate instructions related to treatment, nursing support, and encouragement. It is imperative to overcome any aversion that may be felt when caring for patients with unattractive skin disorders. The nurse should show no sign of hesitancy when approaching patients with skin disorders. Such hesitancy only reinforces the psychological trauma of the disorder.

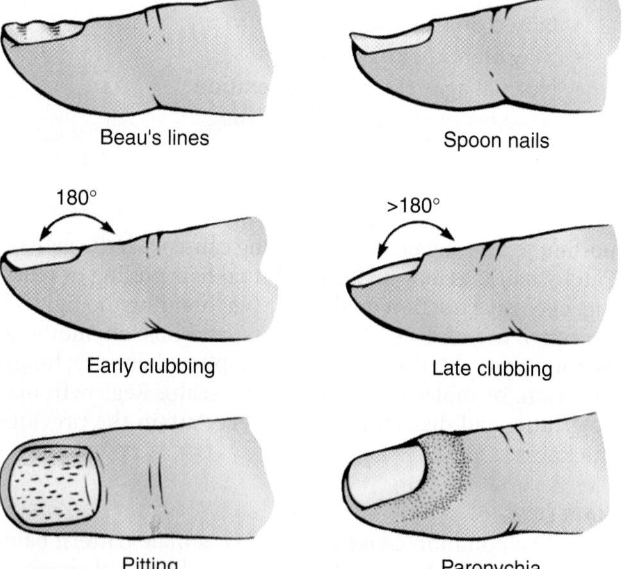

FIGURE 55-6. Common nail disorders. From Weber, J. W., & Kelley, J. (2003). *Health assessment in nursing* (2nd ed.). Philadelphia: Lippincott Williams & Wilkins.

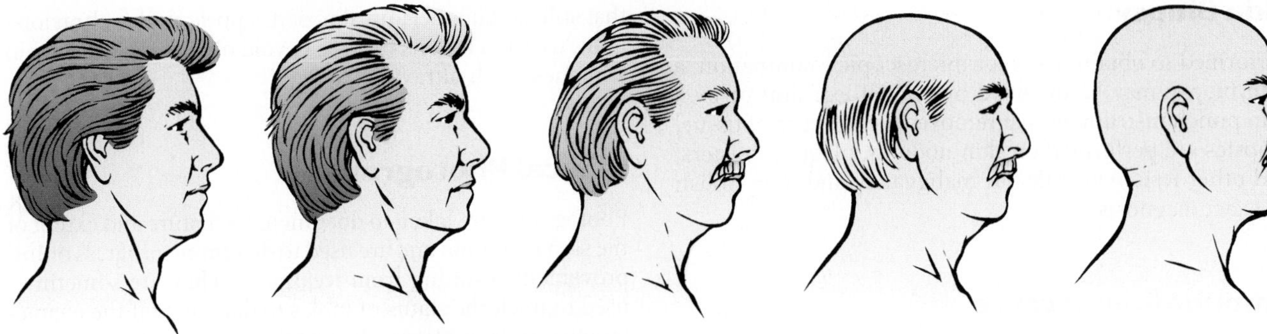

FIGURE 55-7. The progression of male pattern baldness.

Consequences of Selected Systemic Diseases

Skin Disorders in Diabetes Mellitus

Because diabetes causes changes in circulation and cell nutrition, it can have a great impact on skin status. Some of the more common skin problems encountered in diabetes are discussed in this section.

Diabetic Dermopathy

Diabetic dermopathy (shin spots) occurs in about 50% of patients with diabetes. These lesions are found on the lower anterior legs, forearms, and thighs and over other bony prominences. They are caused by breakdown of the small vessels that supply the skin. Each spot starts as a dull red bump, smaller than a pencil eraser. It slowly spreads to about one inch (the size of a quarter), becomes more scaly, and eventually leaves a brownish scar on the skin. The lesions are usually bilateral and occur in linear clusters.

Stasis Dermatitis

Stasis dermatitis is not unique to diabetes, but because of the blood vessel damage that results from diabetes, it is very common in patients with this disease. Large vessels are damaged, compromising circulation to the lower arms and legs. The skin suffers from lack of nutrients, becoming very dry and fragile. Minor injuries heal more slowly, and ulcers form easily. The skin takes on a thick leathery texture and a yellowish, waxy hue.

Skin Infections

The skin of patients with diabetes is prone to bacterial and fungal infections. Bacterial infections appear as small pimples around hair follicles. The most frequently affected sites include the lower legs, lower abdomen, and buttocks. Sometimes these lesions enlarge to become furuncles or carbuncles. If the blood glucose level is not well controlled, these infections may be very slow to heal.

Fungal infections are quite common in areas that remain moist all the time (under breasts, upper thighs, in axilla). *Candida* (ie, yeast) infections appear beefy red and have small pustules around the border of the area, with the skin appearing moist and raw.

Dermatophyte infections are dry and only minimally red, with more scale. Common sites are the toenails and feet.

Nurses must be alert to the signs of these common infections. If necessary, they should bring them to the attention of the physician and help the patient or family learn basic skin maintenance techniques.

Leg and Foot Ulcers

Because of changes in peripheral nerves, patients with diabetes do not always sense minor injuries to the lower legs and feet. Infections begin and if left untreated may lead to ulcerations. Ulcerations are often not noticed and become quite large before being treated. Ulcerations unresponsive to treatment are a leading cause of diabetic foot and leg amputations.

Cutaneous Signs of Human Immunodeficiency Virus Disease

Cutaneous signs may be the first manifestation of human immunodeficiency virus (HIV), appearing in more than 90% of HIV-infected people as immune function deteriorates. These skin signs correlate with low CD4 counts and may become very atypical in immunocompromised people. Some disorders such as Kaposi's sarcoma, oral hairy leukoplakia, facial molluscum contagiosum, and oral candidiasis may suggest that CD4 counts are less than 200 to 300 cell/μL. Being sensitive to these changes can alert the nurse so that early intervention can be initiated (Odom, James, & Berger, 2000).

Diagnostic Evaluation

As previously discussed, it is important to inspect the primary and secondary lesions and their configuration and distribution. Certain diagnostic procedures may also be used to help identify skin conditions.

Skin Biopsy

Performed to obtain tissue for microscopic examination, a skin biopsy may be obtained by scalpel excision or by a skin punch instrument that removes a small core of tissue. Biopsies are performed on skin nodules, plaques, blisters, and other lesions to rule out malignancy and to establish an exact diagnosis.

Immunofluorescence

Designed to identify the site of an immune reaction, immunofluorescence testing combines an antigen or antibody with a fluorochrome dye. Antibodies can be made fluorescent by attaching them to a dye. Direct immunofluorescence tests on skin are techniques to detect autoantibodies directed against portions of the skin. The indirect immunofluorescence test detects specific antibodies in the patient's serum.

Patch Testing

Performed to identify substances to which the patient has developed an allergy, patch testing involves applying the suspected allergens to normal skin under occlusive patches. The development of redness, fine elevations, or itching is considered a weak positive reaction; fine blisters, papules, and severe itching indicate a moderately positive reaction; and blisters, pain, and ulceration indicate a strong positive reaction (see Chapter 53).

Skin Scrapings

Tissue samples are scraped from suspected fungal lesions with a scalpel blade moistened with oil so that the scraped skin adheres to the blade. The scraped material is transferred to a glass slide, covered with a coverslip, and examined microscopically. The spores and hyphae of dermatophyte infections, as well as infestations such as scabies, can be visualized.

Tzanck Smear

The Tzanck smear is a test used to examine cells from blistering skin conditions, such as herpes zoster, varicella, herpes simplex, and all forms of pemphigus. The secretions from a suspected lesion are applied to a glass slide, stained, and examined.

Wood's Light Examination

Wood's light is a special lamp that produces long-wave ultraviolet rays, which result in a characteristic dark purple fluorescence. The color of the fluorescent light is best seen in a darkened room, where it is possible to differentiate epidermal from dermal lesions and hypopigmented and hyperpigmented lesions from normal skin. The patient is reassured that the light is not harmful to skin or eyes. Lesions that still contain melanin almost disappear under ultraviolet light, whereas lesions that are devoid of melanin increase in whiteness with ultraviolet light.

Clinical Photographs

Photographs are taken to document the nature and extent of the skin condition and are used to determine progress or improvement resulting from treatment. They are sometimes used to track the status of moles to document if the characteristics of the mole are changing.

Critical Thinking Exercises

1 You are caring for an elderly African-American woman who is hospitalized with a stroke. She has hemiparesis of her right arm and leg and is receiving physical therapy. Because of the patient's age and her limited mobility, what assessment parameters would you use to determine her risk of developing pressure ulcers? How will your assessment of the skin of this patient differ from the assessment of the skin of a Caucasian patient?

2 ebp You are volunteering at the skin cancer screening booth at a community health fair. A middle-aged man approaches you and asks about risk factors for skin cancer. He states that he is an avid golfer and plays golf year round. Identify the evidence to support the use of protection from the sun, including sunscreens, to prevent skin cancer. Discuss the strength of the evidence that supports the use of sunscreens. Identify the criteria used to evaluate the strength of the evidence for this practice.

REFERENCES AND SELECTED READINGS

BOOKS

Bickley, L. S., & Szilagyi, P. G. (2003). *Bates' guide to physical examination and history taking* (8th ed.). Philadelphia: Lippincott Williams & Williams.

Champion, R. H., Burton, J. L., Burns, D. A., et al. (1998). *Rook/Wilkinson/Ebling textbook of dermatology* (7th ed.). Boston: Blackwell Science.

Fitzpatrick, T. B., Johnson, R. A., Wolff, K., et al. (2001). *Color atlas & synopsis of clinical dermatology* (4th ed.). New York: McGraw-Hill.

Freedberg, I. M., Eisen, A. Z., Austen, K. F., et al. (2003). *Fitzpatrick's dermatology in general medicine* (5th ed.). New York: McGraw-Hill.

Odom, R. B., James, W. D., & Berger, T. G. (2000). *Andrews' diseases of the skin* (9th ed.). Philadelphia: W. B. Saunders.

Weber, J. W., & Kelley, J. (2003). *Health assessment in nursing* (2nd ed.). Philadelphia: Lippincott Williams & Wilkins.

JOURNALS

Draelos, Z. D. (1997). Understanding African-American hair. *Dermatology Nursing, 9*(4), 227–231.

Fleischer, A. B., Feldman, S. R., & Rapp, S. R. (2000). The magnitude of skin disease in the United States. *Dermatologic Clinics, 17*(2), 322–327.

Hayden, M. L. (2005). Did that medication cause this rash? *Nursing 2005, 35*(9), 62–64.

Jaworski, C., & Gilliam, A. C. (1999). Immunopathology of the hair follicle. *Dermatologic Clinics, 17*(3), 561–568.

Semper, A. E., Heron, K., Woolard, A. D., et al. (2003). Surface expression of Fc Epsilor Ri on Langerhans' cells. *Journal of Allergy and Clinical Immunology, 112*(2), 411–419.

Sun Safety Facts (2005). The Skin Cancer Foundation, April 10, 2005. Available at: www.skincancer.org.

Weinstock, M. A., & Rossi, J. S. (1998). The Rhode Island Sun Smart Project: A scientific approach to skin cancer prevention. *Clinical Dermatology, 16*(4), 411–413.

RESOURCES

American Academy of Dermatology, 930 N. Meacham Road, Schaumberg, IL 60168; 708-330-0230; www.aad.org. Accessed August 26, 2006.

Dermatology Online Atlas, a cooperation between the Department of Clinical Social Medicine (University of Heidelberg) and the Department of Dermatology (University of Erlangen); http://www.dermis.net. Accessed August 26, 2006.

Medscape online sources for medical information; http://www.medscape.com. Accessed August 26, 2006.

New Zealand Dermatology Society, 46 Kennedy Road, Auckland, New Zealand; http://www.dermnetnz.org. Accessed August 26, 2006.

Skin Cancer Foundation, 575 Park Ave. S., New York, NY 10016; 1-800-SKIN-490; http://www.skincancer.org. Accessed August 26, 2006.

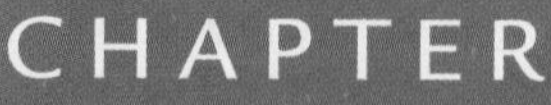

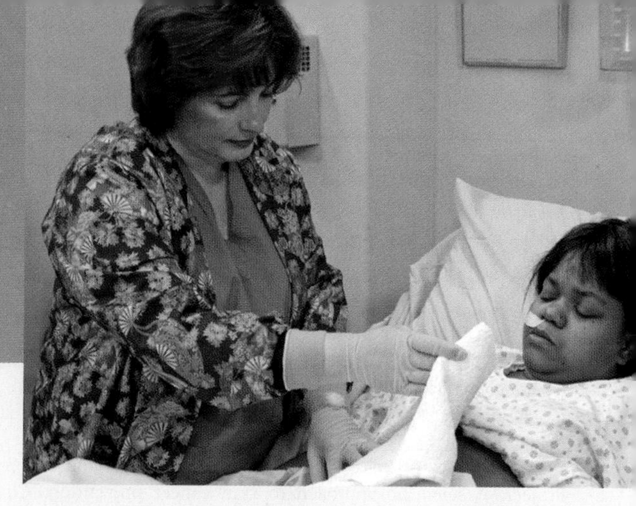

CHAPTER 56

Management of Patients With Dermatologic Problems

Learning Objectives

On completion of this chapter, the learner will be able to:

1. Describe the general management of the patient with an abnormal skin condition.
2. Use the nursing process as a framework for care of the patient with psoriasis.
3. Describe the health education needs of the patient with infections of the skin and parasitic skin diseases.
4. Use the nursing process as a framework for care of patients with noninfectious, inflammatory dermatoses.
5. Describe the management and nursing care of the patient with skin cancer.
6. Use the nursing process as a framework for care of the patient with malignant melanoma.
7. Describe characteristics of the various types of Kaposi's sarcoma.
8. Compare the various types of dermatologic and plastic reconstructive surgeries.
9. Use the nursing process as a framework for care of the patient undergoing facial reconstructive surgery.

Nursing care for patients with dermatologic problems includes administering topical and systemic medications, managing wet dressings and other special dressings, and providing therapeutic baths. The four major objectives of therapy are to prevent additional damage, prevent secondary infection, reverse the inflammatory process, and relieve the symptoms.

Skin Care for Patients With Skin Conditions

Some skin problems are markedly aggravated by soap and water, and bathing routines are modified according to the condition. Denuded skin, whether the area of desquamation is large or small, is excessively prone to damage by chemicals and trauma. The friction of a towel, if applied with vigor, is sufficient to produce a brisk inflammatory response that causes any existing lesion to flare up and extend.

Protecting the Skin

The essence of skin care in bathing a patient with skin problems is as follows:

- A mild, lipid-free soap or soap substitute is used.
- The area is rinsed completely and blotted dry with a soft cloth.
- Deodorant soaps are avoided.

Special care is necessary when changing dressings. Pledgets saturated with oil, sterile saline, or another prescribed solution help to loosen crusts, remove exudates, or free an adherent dry dressing.

Preventing Secondary Infection

Potentially infectious skin lesions should be regarded strictly as such, and proper precautions should be observed until the diagnosis is established. Most lesions with purulent drainage contain infectious material. The nurse and physician must adhere to standard precautions and wear gloves when inspecting the skin or changing a dressing. Proper disposal of any contaminated dressing is carried out according to Occupational Safety and Health Administration (OSHA) regulations.

Reversing the Inflammatory Process

The type of skin lesion (eg, oozing, infected, or dry) usually determines the type of local medication or treatment that is prescribed. As a rule, if the skin is acutely inflamed (ie, hot, red, and swollen) and oozing, it is best to apply wet dressings and soothing lotions. For chronic conditions in which the skin surface is dry and scaly, water-soluble emulsions, creams, ointments, and pastes are used. The therapy is modified as the responses of the skin indicate. The patient and the nurse should note whether the medication or dressings seem to irritate the skin. The success or failure of therapy usually depends on adequate instruction and motivation of the patient and family, and the support of health care personnel promotes adherence to instructions.

Wound Care for Skin Conditions

There are three types of wound dressings: passive, interactive, and active. Passive dressings have only a protective function and maintain a moist environment for natural healing. They include those that just cover the area (eg, DuoDERM, Tegaderm) and may remain in place for several days. Interactive dressings are capable of absorbing wound exudate while (1) maintaining a moist environment in the area of the wound and (2) allowing the surrounding skin to remain dry. They include hydrocolloids, alginates, and hydrogels. It is thought that interactive dressings are able to modify the physiology of the wound environment by modulating and stimulating cellular activity and by releasing growth

Glossary

acantholysis: separation of epidermal cells from each other due to damage or abnormality of the intracellular substance
balneotherapy: a bath with therapeutic additives
carbuncle: localized skin infection involving several hair follicles
cheilitis: dry, cracking, inflamed skin at the corners of the mouth
comedones: the primary lesions of acne, caused by sebum blockage in the hair follicle
cytotoxic: destructive of cells
débridement: removal of necrotic or dead tissue by mechanical, surgical, or autolytic means
dermatitis: any inflammation of the skin
dermatosis: any abnormal skin lesion
epidermopoiesis: development of epidermal cells
fibrinolytic: a substance that acts to break up fibrin, the fine filaments of blood clots
furuncle: localized skin infection of a single hair follicle
hydrophilic: a material that absorbs moisture
hydrophobic: a material that repels moisture
hygroscopic: a material that absorbs moisture from the air
lichenification: thickening of the horny layer of the skin
liniments: lotions with added oil for increased softening of the skin
mitogenic: a substance that stimulates mitosis or cell division and reproduction
plasmapheresis: removal of whole blood from the body, separation of its cellular elements by centrifugation, and reinfusion of them suspended in saline or some other plasma substitute, thereby depleting the body's own plasma without depleting its cells
pyodermas: bacterial skin infections
striae: bandlike streaks on the skin, distinguished by color, texture, depression, or elevation from the tissue in which they are found; usually purplish or white
suspensions: liquid preparations in which powder is suspended, requiring shaking before use
tinea: a superficial fungal infection on the skin or scalp
xerosis: overly dry skin

factor (Thanh, Pham, & Veves, 2002). Active dressings improve the healing process and decrease healing time. They include skin grafts and biologic skin substitutes. Both interactive and active dressings create a moist environment at the interface of the wound with the dressing.

Because so many wound care products are available, it is often difficult to select the most appropriate product for a specific wound (Chart 56-1). Selection of products should be made carefully because of their expense. Both clinical efficacy and health-related outcomes (eg, decreased pain, increased mobility) should be used to measure the success of a product for a wound. Even with the availability of a large variety of dressings, an appropriate selection can be made if certain principles are maintained. These principles are referred to as the five rules of wound care (Krasner, Rodehaver, & Sibbald, 2002):

- **Rule 1: Categorization.** The nurse learns about dressings by generic category and compares new products with those that already make up the category. The nurse becomes familiar with indications, contraindications, and side effects. The best dressing may be created by combining products in different categories to achieve several goals at the same time. These categories are discussed in subsequent sections.
- **Rule 2: Selection.** The nurse selects the safest and most effective, easy-to-use, and cost-effective dressing possible. In many cases, nurses carry out the physician's prescriptions for dressings, but they must be prepared to give the physician feedback about the dressing's effect on the wound, ease of use for the patient, and other considerations when applicable.
- **Rule 3: Change.** The nurse changes dressings based on patient, wound, and dressing assessments, not on standardized routines.

CHART 56-1

Wound Care Products

Adhesives	Foam dressings
Adhesive removers	Gauze dressings
Adhesive skin closures	Growth factors
Adhesive tapes	Hydrocolloid dressings
Alginate dressings	Hydrogel dressings
Antibiotics	Leg ulcer wraps, compression bandages or wraps
Antimicrobials	Lubricating, stimulating sprays
Antiseptics	Moisturizers
Bandages	Moisture barrier ointments
Biosynthetic dressings	Ointments
Cleansers	Perineal cleansers
Collagen dressings	Skin sealants
Composite dressings	Transparent film dressings
Contact layers	Wound fillers: pastes, powders, beads, etc.
Creams or skin protectant pastes	Wound pouches
Dressing covers	
Enzyme débriding agents	

NURSING ALERT

It is believed that the natural wound-healing process should not be disrupted. Unless the wound is infected or has a heavy discharge, it is common to leave chronic wounds covered for 48 to 72 hours and acute wounds for 24 hours.

- **Rule 4: Evolution.** As the wound progresses through the phases of wound healing, the dressing protocol is altered to optimize wound healing. It is rare, especially in cases of chronic wounds, that the same dressing material is appropriate throughout the healing process. It is assumed that the nurse and the patient or family have access to a wide variety of products and are knowledgeable about their use. The nurse teaches the patient or family caregiver about wound care and ensures that the family has access to appropriate dressing choices.
- **Rule 5: Practice.** Practice with dressing material is required for the nurse to learn the performance parameters of the particular dressing. Refining the skills of applying appropriate dressings correctly and learning about new dressing products are essential nursing responsibilities. Dressing changes should not be delegated to unlicensed personnel; these techniques require the knowledge base and assessment skills of professional nurses.

Autolytic Débridement

Autolytic **débridement** is a process that uses the body's own digestive enzymes to break down necrotic tissue. The wound is kept moist with occlusive dressings. Eschar and necrotic debris are softened, liquefied, and separated from the bed of the wound.

Several commercially available products contain the same enzymes that the body produces naturally. These are called enzymatic débriding agents; examples include Accu-Zyme, collagenase (Santyl), Granulex, and Zymase. Application of these products speeds the rate at which necrotic tissue is removed. This method is still slower and no more effective than surgical débridement. When enzymatic débridement is being used under an occlusive dressing, a foul odor is produced by the breakdown of cellular debris. This odor does not indicate that the wound is infected. The nurse should expect this reaction and help the patient and family understand the reason for the odor.

Categories of Dressings

Table 56-1 is a guide to wound dressing functions and categories.

Occlusive Dressings

Occlusive dressings may be commercially produced or made inexpensively from sterile or nonsterile gauze squares or wrap. Occlusive dressings cover topical medication that is applied to a skin lesion. The area is kept airtight by using plastic film (eg, plastic wrap). Plastic film is thin and read-

TABLE 56-1 Quick Guide to Wound Dressing Function and Categories

Function	Action	Example
Absorption	Absorbs exudate	Alginates, composite dressings, foams, gauze, hydrocolloids, hydrogels
Cleansing	Removes purulent drainage, foreign debris, and devitalized tissue	Wound cleansers
Débridement	*Autolytic;* covers a wound and allows enzymes to self-digest sloughed skin	Absorption beads, pastes, powders; alginates; composite dressings; foams; hydrate gauze; hydrogels; hydrocolloids; transparent films; wound care systems
	Chemical or enzymatic; applied topically to break down devitalized tissue	Enzymatic débridement agents
	Mechanical; removes devitalized tissue with mechanical force	Wound cleansers, gauze (wet to dry), whirlpool
Diathermy	Produces electrical current to promote warmth and new tissue growth	
Hydration	Adds moisture to a wound	Gauze (saturated with saline) solution, hydrogels, wound care systems
Maintain moist environment	Manages moisture levels in a wound and maintains a moist environment	Composites, contact layers, foams, gauze (impregnated or saturated), hydrogels, hydrocolloids, transparent films, wound care systems
Manage high-output wounds	Manages excessive quantities of exudate	Pouching systems
Pack or fill dead space	Prevents premature wound closure or fills shallow areas and provides absorption	Absorbent beads, powders, pastes; alginates, composites, foams, gauze (impregnated and non-impregnated)
Protect and cover wound	Provides protection from the external environment	Composites, compression bandages/wraps, foams, gauze dressings, hydrogels, hydrocolloids, transparent film dressings
Protect periwound skin	Prevents moisture and mechanical trauma from damaging delicate tissue around wound	Composites, foams, hydrocolloids, pouching systems, skin sealants, transparent film dressings
Provide therapeutic compression	Provides appropriate levels of support to the lower extremities in venous stasis disease	Compression bandages, wraps, support stockings

ily adapts to all sizes, body shapes, and skin surfaces. Plastic surgical tape containing a corticosteroid in the adhesive layer can be cut to size and applied to individual lesions. Generally, plastic wrap should be used no more than 12 hours each day.

Wet Dressings

Wet dressings (wet compresses applied to the skin) were traditionally used for acute, weeping, inflammatory lesions. They have become almost obsolete because of the many newer products available for wound care.

Moisture-Retentive Dressings

Commercially produced moisture-retentive dressings can perform the same functions as wet dressings but are more efficient at removing exudate because of their higher moisture-vapor transmission rate; some have reservoirs that can hold excessive exudate. A number of moisture-retentive dressings are already impregnated with saline solution, petrolatum, zinc-saline solution, hydrogel, or antimicrobial agents, thereby eliminating the need to coat the skin to avoid maceration. The main advantages of moisture-retentive dressings over wet dressings are improved fibrinolysis, accelerated epidermal resurfacing, reduced pain, fewer infections, less scar tissue, gentle autolytic débridement, and decreased frequency of dressing changes (Alvarez, Patel, Booker, et al., 2004). Depending on the product used and the type of dermatologic problem encountered, most moisture-retentive dressings may remain in place from 12 to 24 hours; some can remain in place as long as a week.

HYDROGELS

Hydrogels are polymers with 90% to 95% water content. They are available in impregnated sheets or as gel in a tube. Their high moisture content makes them ideal for autolytic débridement of wounds. They are semitransparent, allowing for wound inspection without dressing removal. They are comfortable and soothing for the painful wound. They require a secondary dressing to keep them in place. Hydrogels are appropriate for superficial wounds with high serous output, such as abrasions, skin graft sites, and draining venous ulcers.

HYDROCOLLOIDS

Hydrocolloids are composed of a water-impermeable, polyurethane outer covering separated from the wound by a hydrocolloid material. They are adherent and nonpermeable to water vapor and oxygen. As water evaporates over the wound, it is absorbed into the dressing, which softens and discolors with the increased water content. The dressing can be removed without damage to the wound. As the dressing absorbs water, it produces a foul-smelling, yellowish covering over the wound. This is a normal chemical interaction between the dressing and wound exudate and should not be confused with purulent drainage from the wound. Unfortunately, most of the hydrocolloid dressings are opaque, limiting inspection of the wound without removal of the dressing.

Available in sheets and in gels, hydrocolloids are a good choice for exudative wounds and for acute wounds. Easy to use and comfortable, hydrocolloid dressings promote débridement and formation of granulation tissue. They do not have to be removed for bathing. Most can be left in place for as long as 7 days.

FOAM DRESSINGS

Foam dressings consist of microporous polyurethane with an absorptive **hydrophilic** (water-absorbing) surface that covers the wound and a **hydrophobic** (water-resistant) backing to block leakage of exudate. They are nonadherent and require a secondary dressing to keep them in place. Moisture is absorbed into the foam layer, decreasing maceration of surrounding tissue. A moist environment is maintained, and removal of the dressing does not damage the wound. The foams are opaque and must be removed for wound inspection. Foams are a good choice for exudative wounds. They are especially helpful over bony prominences because they provide contoured cushioning.

CALCIUM ALGINATES

Calcium alginates are derived from seaweed and consist of very absorbent calcium alginate fibers. They are hemostatic and bioabsorbable and can be used as sheets or mats of absorbent material. As the exudate is absorbed, the fibers turn into a viscous hydrogel. They are useful in areas where the tissue is more irritated or macerated. The alginate dressing forms a moist pocket over the wound while the surrounding skin stays dry. The dressing also reacts with wound fluid and forms a foul-smelling coating. Alginates work well when packed into a deep cavity, wound, or sinus tract with heavy drainage (Krastner et al., 2002). They are nonadherent and require a secondary dressing.

Advances in Wound Treatment

Increasing understanding of how skin heals has led to several advances in therapy. Growth factors are cytokines or proteins that have potent **mitogenic** activity (Long, Falabella, Valencia, et al., 2001). Low levels of cytokines circulate in the blood continuously, but activated platelets release increased amounts of preformed growth factors into a wound. This increase in cytokines in the wound stimulates cellular growth and granulation of skin. Regranex gel contains becaplermin, a platelet-derived growth factor, which is applied to the wound to stimulate healing. Apligraf is a skin construct (ie, bioengineered skin substitute) imbedded in a dressing that also contains cytokines and fibroblasts. When applied to wounds, these agents stimulate platelet activity and potentially decrease wound healing time (Paquette & Falanga, 2002).

Bioengineered skin substitutes have emerged in the past 20 years as the most effective method for management of chronic wounds. Most of these skin substitutes are cultures of keratinocytes delivered on a petrolatum gauze. They work by maintaining wound moisture, providing a structure for regeneration of cells, and supplying beneficial cytokines. A partial list of these substitutes includes AlloDerm, Apligraf, Dermagraf, Epicel, and Laserskin.

Some oral medications are being investigated for their benefits in healing chronic venous ulcers of the lower legs. Pentoxifylline (Trental) increases peripheral blood flow by decreasing the viscosity of blood. It has some **fibrinolytic** action and decreases leukocyte adhesion to the wall of the blood vessels. Enteric-coated aspirin has also been shown to be of value, although its exact mechanism is still not clear (Long et al., 2001).

Medical Management

Therapeutic Baths (Balneotherapy)

Baths or soaks, known as **balneotherapy**, are useful when large areas of skin are affected. The baths remove crusts, scales, and old medications and relieve the inflammation and pruritus (itching) that accompany acute dermatoses. Additional information about therapeutic baths is given in Chart 56-2.

Pharmacologic Therapy

Because skin is easily accessible, topical medications are often used. High concentrations of some medications can be applied directly to the affected site with little systemic absorption and therefore with few systemic side effects. However, some medications are readily absorbed through the skin and can produce systemic effects. Because topical preparations may induce allergic contact **dermatitis** in sensitive patients, any untoward response should be reported immediately and the medication discontinued.

Medicated lotions, creams, ointments, and powders are frequently used to treat skin lesions. In general, moisture-retentive dressings, with or without medication, are used in the acute stage; lotions and creams are reserved for the subacute stage; and ointments are used when inflammation has become chronic and the skin is dry with scaling or **lichenification.**

With all types of topical medication, the patient is taught to apply the medication gently but thoroughly and, when necessary, to cover the medication with a dressing to protect clothing. Table 56-2 lists some commonly used topical preparations.

LOTIONS

Lotions are frequently used to replenish lost skin oils or to relieve pruritus. They are usually applied directly to the skin, but a dressing soaked in the lotion can be placed on the affected area. Lotions must be applied every 3 or 4 hours for sustained therapeutic effect. If left in place for a longer period, they may crust and cake on the skin.

CHART 56-2

Therapeutic Baths

Types of Therapeutic Baths

BATH SOLUTION	EFFECTS AND USES
Water	Same effect as wet dressings
Saline	Used for widely disseminated lesions
Colloidal (Aveeno, oatmeal)	Antipruritic, soothing
Sodium bicarbonate (baking soda)	Cooling
Starch	Soothing
Medicated tars	Psoriasis and chronic eczema
Bath oils	Antipruritic and emollient action; acute and subacute generalized eczematous eruptions

Nursing Interventions

- Fill the tub half full.
- Keep the water at a comfortable temperature.
- Do not allow the water to cool excessively.
- Use a bath mat, because *medications added to the bath can cause the tub to be slippery.*
- Apply an emollient cream to damp skin after the bath if lubrication is desired.
- Because tars are volatile, the bath area should be well ventilated.
- Maintain a constant room temperature without drafts.
- Encourage the patient to wear light, loose clothing after the bath.

Lotions are of two types: suspensions and liniments. **Suspensions** consist of a powder in water, requiring shaking before application, and clear solutions, containing completely dissolved active ingredients. A suspension such as calamine lotion provides a rapid cooling and drying effect as it evaporates, leaving a thin, medicinal layer of powder on the affected skin. **Liniments** are lotions with oil added to prevent crusting. Because lotions are easy to use, therapeutic compliance is generally high.

POWDERS

Powders usually have a talc, zinc oxide, bentonite, or cornstarch base and are dusted on the skin with a shaker or with cotton sponges. Although their therapeutic action is brief, powders act as **hygroscopic** agents that absorb and retain moisture from the air and reduce friction between skin surfaces and clothing or bedding.

CREAMS

Creams may be suspensions of oil in water or emulsions of water in oil, with additional ingredients to prevent bacterial and fungal growth. Both may cause an allergic reaction such as contact dermatitis. Oil-in-water creams are easily applied and usually are the most cosmetically acceptable to the patient. Although they can be used on the face, they tend to have a drying effect. Water-in-oil emulsions are greasier and are preferred for drying and flaking dermatoses. Creams usually are rubbed into the skin by hand. They are used for their moisturizing and emollient effects.

GELS

Gels are semisolid emulsions that become liquid when applied to the skin or scalp. They are cosmetically acceptable to the patient because they are not visible after application, and they are greaseless and nonstaining. The newer water-based gels appear to penetrate the skin more effectively and cause less stinging on application. They are especially useful for acute dermatitis in which there is weeping exudate (eg, poison ivy).

PASTES

Pastes are mixtures of powders and ointments and are used in inflammatory blistering conditions. They adhere to the skin and may be difficult to remove without using an oil (eg, olive oil, mineral oil). Pastes are applied with a wooden tongue depressor or gloved hand.

OINTMENTS

Ointments retard water loss and lubricate and protect the skin. They are the preferred vehicle for delivering medication to chronic or localized dry skin conditions, such as

℞ **TABLE 56-2 Common Topical Preparations and Medications**

Preparation	Product Name
Bath preparations	
With tar	Balnetar, Doak Oil, Lavatar
With colloidal oatmeal	Aveeno Oilated Bath Powder
With oatmeal and mineral oil	Aveeno Bath Oil, Nutra Soothe
With mineral oil	Nutraderm Bath Oil, Lubath, Alpha-Keri Bath Oil
Moisturizer creams	Acid Mantle Cream, Curel Cream, Dermasil, Eucerin, Lubriderm, Noxzema Skin Cream
Moisturizer ointments	Aquaphor Ointment, Eutra Swiss Skin Cream, Vaseline Ointment
Topical anesthetics	lidocaine (Xylocaine) of various strengths in the form of spray, ointment, gel; EMLA cream (lidocaine 2.5% and prilocaine 2.5%)
Topical antibiotics	bacitracin, Polysporin (bacitracin and polymixin B), Bactroban ointment or cream (mupirocin 2%), erythromycin 2% (Emgel, Eryderm Solution), clindamycin phosphate 1% (Cleocin cream, gel, solution), gentamicin sulfate 1% (Garamycin cream or ointment), 1% silver sulfadiazine cream (Silvadene)

eczema or psoriasis. Ointments are applied with a wooden tongue depressor or gloved hand.

SPRAYS AND AEROSOLS

Spray and aerosol preparations may be used on any widespread dermatologic condition. They evaporate on contact and are used infrequently.

CORTICOSTEROIDS

Corticosteroids are widely used in treating dermatologic conditions to provide anti-inflammatory, antipruritic, and vasoconstrictive effects. The patient is taught to apply this medication according to strict guidelines, using it sparingly but rubbing it into the prescribed area thoroughly. Absorption of topical corticosteroid is enhanced when the skin is hydrated or the affected area is covered by an occlusive or moisture-retentive dressing. Inappropriate use of topical corticosteroids can result in local and systemic side effects, especially when the medication is absorbed through inflamed and excoriated skin, is used under occlusive dressings, or is used for long periods on sensitive areas. Local side effects may include skin atrophy and thinning, **striae** (bandlike streaks), and telangiectasia. Thinning of the skin results from the ability of corticosteroids to inhibit skin collagen synthesis. The thinning process can be reversed by discontinuing the medication, but striae and telangiectasia are permanent. Systemic side effects may include hyperglycemia and symptoms of Cushing's syndrome. Caution is required when applying corticosteroids around the eyes for two reasons: (1) long-term use may cause glaucoma or cataracts, and (2) the anti-inflammatory effect of corticosteroids may mask existing viral or fungal infections.

Concentrated (fluorinated) corticosteroids are never applied on the face or intertriginous areas (ie, axilla and groin) because these areas have a thinner stratum corneum and absorb the medication much more quickly than areas such as the forearm or legs. Persistent use of concentrated topical corticosteroids in any location may produce acne-like dermatitis, known as steroid-induced acne, and hypertrichosis (excessive hair growth). Because some topical corticosteroid preparations are available without prescription, patients should be cautioned about prolonged and inappropriate use. Table 56-3 lists topical corticosteroid preparations according to potency.

Rx TABLE 56-3 Potency: Topical Corticosteroids

Potency	Topical Corticosteroid	Preparations
OTC	0.5–1.0% hydrocortisone	cr, lot, oint
Lowest	dexamethasone 0.1% (Decaderm)	cr, oint, aerosol, gel
	alclometasone 0.05% (Aclovate)	cr, oint
	hydrocortisone 2.5% (Hytone)	cr, lot, oint
Low–medium	desonide 0.05% (DesOwen, Tridesilon)	cr, lot, oint
	fluocinolone acetonide 0.025% (Synalar)	cr, solution
	hydrocortisone valerate 0.2% (Westcort)	cr, solution
	betamethasone valerate 0.1% (Valisone)	cr, oint
	fluticasonepropionate 0.05% (Cutivate)	cr, oint
Medium–high	triamcinolone acetonide 0.1–0.5% (Aristocort)	cr, oint, lot
	fluocinonide 0.05% (Lidex)	cr, oint, gel
	desoximetasone 0.05–0.25% (Topicort)	cr, oint, gel
	fluocinolone 0.2% (Synalar)	cr, oint
	diflorasone diacetate 0.05% (Psorcon)	cr, oint
Very high	clobetasol propionate 0.05% (Temovate)	cr, oint, gel
	betamethasone dipropionate 0.05% (Diprolene)	cr, oint, gel
	halobetasole propionate 0.05% (Ultravate)	cr, oint

cr, cream; lot, lotion; oint, ointment; OTC, over the counter

INTRALESIONAL THERAPY

Intralesional therapy consists of injecting a sterile suspension of medication (usually a corticosteroid) into or just below a lesion. Although this treatment may have an anti-inflammatory effect, local atrophy may result if the medication is injected into subcutaneous fat. Skin lesions treated with intralesional therapy include psoriasis, keloids, and cystic acne. Occasionally, immunotherapeutic and antifungal agents are administered as intralesional therapy.

SYSTEMIC MEDICATIONS

Systemic medications are also prescribed for skin conditions. These include corticosteroids for short-term therapy for contact dermatitis or for long-term treatment of a chronic dermatosis, such as pemphigus vulgaris. Other frequently used systemic medications include antibiotics, antifungals, antihistamines, sedatives, tranquilizers, analgesics, and **cytotoxic** (destructive of cells) agents.

Nursing Management

Management begins with a health history, direct observation, and a complete physical examination. Chapter 55 provides a description of integumentary assessment. Because of its visibility, a skin condition is usually difficult to ignore or conceal from others and may therefore cause the patient emotional distress. The major goals for the patient may include maintenance of skin integrity, relief of discomfort, promotion of restful sleep, self-acceptance, knowledge about skin care, and avoidance of complications.

Nursing management for patients who must perform self-care for skin problems, such as applying medications and dressings, focuses mainly on teaching the patient how to wash the affected area and pat it dry, apply medication to the lesion while the skin is moist, cover the area with plastic (eg, Telfa pads, plastic wrap, vinyl gloves, plastic bag) if recommended, and cover it with an elastic bandage, dressing, or paper tape to seal the edges. Dressings that contain or cover a topical corticosteroid should be removed for 12 of every 24 hours to prevent skin thinning, striae, and telangiectasias (small, red lesions caused by dilation of blood vessels).

Other forms of dressings, such as those used to cover topical medications, include soft cotton cloth and stretchable cotton dressings (eg, Surgitube, Tubegauz) that can be used for fingers, toes, hands, and feet. The hands can be covered with disposable polyethylene or vinyl gloves sealed at the wrists; the feet can be wrapped in plastic bags covered by cotton socks. Gloves and socks that are already impregnated with emollients, making application to the hands and feet more convenient, are also available. When large areas of the body must be covered, cotton cloth topped by an expandable stockinette can be used. Disposable diapers or cloths folded in diaper fashion are useful for dressing the groin and the perineal areas. Axillary dressings can be made of cotton cloth, or a commercially prepared dressing may be used and taped in place or held by dress shields. A turban or plastic shower cap is useful for holding dressings on the scalp. A face mask, made from gauze with holes cut out for the eyes, nose, and mouth, may be held in place with gauze ties looped through holes cut in the four corners of the mask.

CHART 56-3

Systemic Disorders Associated With Generalized Pruritus

Chronic renal disease
Obstructive biliary disease (primary biliary cirrhosis, extrahepatic biliary obstruction, drug-induced cholestasis)
Endocrine disease (thyrotoxicosis, hypothyroidism, diabetes mellitus)
Psychiatric disorders (emotional stress, anxiety, neurosis, phobias)
Malignancies (polycythemia vera, Hodgkin's disease, lymphoma, leukemia, multiple myeloma, mycosis fungoides, and cancers of the lung, breast, central nervous system, and gastrointestinal tract)
Neurologic disorders (multiple sclerosis, brain abscess, brain tumor)
Infestations (scabies, lice, other insects)
Pruritus of pregnancy (pruritic urticarial papules of pregnancy [PUPP], cholestasis of pregnancy, pemphigoid of pregnancy)
Folliculitis (bacterial, candidiasis, dermatophyte)
Skin conditions (seborrheic dermatitis, folliculitis, iron deficiency anemia, atopic dermatitis)

Pruritus

General Pruritus

Pruritus (itching) is one of the most common symptoms of patients with dermatologic disorders. Itch receptors are unmyelinated, penicillate (brush-like) nerve endings that are found exclusively in the skin, mucous membranes, and cornea. Although pruritus is usually caused by primary skin disease with resultant rash or lesions, it may occur without a rash or lesion. This is referred to as essential pruritus, which generally has a rapid onset, may be severe, and interferes with normal daily activities.

Pruritus may be the first indication of a systemic internal disease such as diabetes mellitus, blood disorders, or cancer (occult malignancy of the breast or colon; lymphoma). It may also accompany renal, hepatic, and thyroid diseases (Chart 56-3). Some common oral medications such as aspirin, antibiotics, hormones (ie, estrogens, testosterone, or oral contraceptives), and opioids (ie, morphine or cocaine) may cause pruritus directly or by increasing sensitivity to ultraviolet light. Certain soaps and chemicals, radiation therapy, prickly heat (miliaria), and contact with woolen garments are also associated with pruritus. Pruritus may also be caused by psychological factors, such as excessive stress in family or work situations.

Gerontologic Considerations

Pruritus occurs frequently in elderly people as a result of dry skin. Elderly people are also more likely to have a systemic illness that triggers pruritus, are at higher risk for occult malignancy, and are more likely to be taking multiple medications than younger people. All of these factors increase the incidence of pruritus in elderly people.

Pathophysiology

Scratching the pruritic area causes the inflamed cells and nerve endings to release histamine, which produces more pruritus, generating a vicious itch–scratch cycle. If the patient responds to an itch by scratching, the integrity of the skin may be altered, and excoriation, redness, raised areas (ie, wheals), infection, or changes in pigmentation may result. Pruritus usually is more severe at night and is less frequently reported during waking hours, probably because the person is distracted by daily activities. At night, when there are few distractions, the slightest pruritus cannot be easily ignored. Severe itching can be debilitating.

Medical Management

A thorough history and physical examination usually provide clues to the underlying cause of the pruritus, such as hay fever, allergy, recent administration of a new medication, or a change of cosmetics or soaps. After the cause has been identified, treatment of the condition should relieve the pruritus. Signs of infection and environmental clues, such as warm, dry air or irritating bed linens, should be identified. In general, washing with soap and hot water is avoided. Bath oils containing a surfactant that makes the oil mix with bath water (eg, Lubath, Alpha-Keri) may be sufficient for cleaning. However, an elderly patient or a patient with unsteady balance should avoid adding oil because it increases the danger of slipping in the bathtub. A warm bath with a mild soap followed by application of a bland emollient to moist skin can control **xerosis** (dry skin). Applying a cold compress, ice cube, or cool agents that contain menthol and camphor (which constrict blood vessels) may also help relieve pruritus.

Pharmacologic Therapy

Topical corticosteroids may be beneficial as anti-inflammatory agents to decrease itching. Oral antihistamines are even more effective because they can overcome the effects of histamine release from damaged mast cells. An antihistamine, such as diphenhydramine (Benadryl) or hydroxyzine (Atarax), prescribed in a sedative dose at bedtime is effective in producing a restful and comfortable sleep. Nonsedating antihistamine medications such as fexofenadine (Allegra) are more appropriate to relieve daytime pruritus. Tricyclic antidepressants, such as doxepin (Sinequan), may be prescribed for pruritus of neuropsychogenic origin. If pruritus continues, further investigation of a systemic problem is advised.

Nursing Management

The nurse reinforces the reasons for the prescribed therapeutic regimen and counsels the patient on specific points of care. If baths have been prescribed, the patient is reminded to use tepid (not hot) water and to shake off the excess water and blot between intertriginous areas (body folds) with a towel. Rubbing vigorously with the towel is avoided because this overstimulates the skin and causes more itching. It also removes water from the stratum corneum. Immediately after bathing, the skin should be lubricated with an emollient to trap moisture.

The patient is instructed to avoid situations that cause vasodilation. Examples include exposure to an overly warm environment and ingestion of alcohol or hot foods and liquids. All can induce or intensify pruritus. Using a humidifier is helpful if environmental air is dry. Activities that result in perspiration should be limited because perspiration may irritate and promote pruritus. If the patient is troubled at night with itching that interferes with sleep, the nurse can advise wearing cotton clothing next to the skin rather than synthetic materials. The room should be kept cool and humidified. Vigorous scratching should be avoided and nails kept trimmed to prevent skin damage and infection. When the underlying cause of pruritus is unknown and further testing is required, the nurse explains each test and the expected outcome.

Perineal and Perianal Pruritus

Pruritus of the genital and anal regions may be caused by small particles of fecal material lodged in the perianal crevices or attached to anal hairs. Alternatively, it may result from perianal skin damage caused by scratching, moisture, and decreased skin resistance as a result of corticosteroid or antibiotic therapy. Other possible causes of perianal itching include local irritants such as scabies and lice, local lesions such as hemorrhoids, fungal or yeast infections, and pinworm infestation. Conditions such as diabetes mellitus, anemia, hyperthyroidism, and pregnancy may also result in pruritus. Occasionally, no cause can be identified.

Management

The patient is instructed to follow proper hygiene measures and to discontinue home and over-the-counter remedies. The perineal or anal area should be rinsed with lukewarm water and blotted dry with cotton balls. Premoistened tissues may be used after defecation. Cornstarch can be applied in the skinfold areas to absorb perspiration.

As part of health teaching, the nurse instructs the patient to avoid bathing in water that is too hot and to avoid using bubble baths, sodium bicarbonate, and detergent soaps, all of which aggravate dryness. To keep the perineal or perianal skin as dry as possible, patients should avoid wearing underwear made of synthetic fabrics. Local anesthetic agents should not be used because of possible allergic effects. The patient should also avoid vasodilating agents or stimulants (eg, alcohol, caffeine) and mechanical irritants such as rough or woolen clothing. A diet that includes adequate fiber may help maintain soft stools and prevent minor trauma to the anal mucosa.

Secretory Disorders

The main secretory function of the skin is performed by the sweat glands, which help regulate body temperature. These glands excrete perspiration that evaporates, thereby cooling the body. The sweat glands are located in various parts of the body and respond to different stimuli. Those on the trunk generally respond to thermal stimulation; those on the palms and soles respond to nervous stimulation; and those in the axillae and on the forehead respond to both kinds of stimulation. Normal perspiration has no odor. Body odor is produced by the increase in bacteria on the skin and the interaction of bacterial waste products with the chemicals of perspiration. As a rule, moist skin is warm, and dry skin is cool, but this is not always true. It is not unusual to observe warm, dry skin in a dehydrated patient and very hot, dry skin in some febrile states.

Normally, sweat can be controlled with the use of antiperspirants and deodorants. Most antiperspirants are aluminum salts that block the opening to the sweat duct. Pure deodorants inhibit bacterial growth and block the metabolism of sweat; they have no antiperspirant effect. Fragrance-free deodorants are available for those with sensitive skin.

Hydradenitis Suppurativa

Hydradenitis suppurative is a chronic suppurative folliculitis of the perianal, axillary, and genital areas or under the breasts. It develops after puberty and can produce abscesses or sinuses with scarring. The cause is unknown, but it appears to have a genetic basis.

Pathophysiology

Abnormal blockage of the sweat glands causes recurring inflammation, nodules, and draining sinus tracts. Eventually, hypertrophic bands of scar tissue form in the area of the sweat glands.

Clinical Manifestations

The condition occurs more frequently in the axilla but also appears in inguinal folds, on the mons pubis, and around the buttocks. The patient can be extremely uncomfortable with multiple suppurative lesions within a small area.

Management

Management is often difficult. Hot compresses and oral antibiotics are used frequently. Isotretinoin (Accutane) or etretinate can be tried; careful monitoring for side effects is important. Incision and drainage of large suppurating areas with gauze packs inserted to facilitate drainage is often necessary. Rarely, the entire area is excised, removing the scar tissue and any infection. This surgery is drastic and attempted only as a last resort.

Seborrheic Dermatoses

Seborrhea is excessive production of sebum (secretion of sebaceous glands) in areas where sebaceous glands are normally found in large numbers, such as the face, scalp, eyebrows, eyelids, sides of the nose and upper lip, malar regions (cheeks), ears, axillae, under the breasts, groin, and gluteal crease of the buttocks. Seborrheic dermatitis is a chronic inflammatory disease of the skin with a predilection for areas that are well supplied with sebaceous glands or lie between skin folds, where the bacteria count is high.

Clinical Manifestations

Two forms of seborrheic dermatoses can occur, an oily form and a dry form. Either form may start in childhood and continue throughout life. The oily form appears moist or greasy. There may be patches of sallow, greasy skin, with or without scaling, and slight erythema, predominantly on the forehead, nasolabial fold, beard area, scalp, and between adjacent skin surfaces in the regions of the axillae, groin, and breasts. Small pustules or papulopustules resembling acne may appear on the trunk. The dry form, consisting of flaky desquamation of the scalp with a profuse amount of fine, powdery scales, is commonly called dandruff. The mild forms of the disease are asymptomatic. When scaling occurs, it is often accompanied by pruritus, which may lead to scratching and secondary infections and excoriation.

Seborrheic dermatitis has a genetic predisposition. Hormones, nutritional status, infection, and emotional stress influence its course. The remissions and exacerbations of this condition should be explained to the patient. If a person has not previously been diagnosed with this condition and suddenly appears with a severe outbreak, a complete history and physical examination should be considered.

Medical Management

Because there is no known cure for seborrhea, the objective of therapy is to control the disorder and allow the skin to repair itself. Seborrheic dermatitis of the body and face may respond to a topically applied corticosteroid cream, which allays the secondary inflammatory response. However, this medication should be used with caution near the eyelids, because it can induce glaucoma and cataracts in predisposed patients. Patients with seborrheic dermatitis may develop a secondary candidal (yeast) infection in body creases or folds. To avoid this, patients should be advised to ensure maximum aeration of the skin and to clean areas where there are creases or folds in the skin carefully. Patients with persistent candidiasis should be evaluated for diabetes.

The mainstay of dandruff treatment is proper, frequent shampooing (at least three times weekly) with medicated shampoos. Two or three different types of shampoo should be used in rotation to prevent the seborrhea from becoming resistant to a particular shampoo. The shampoo is left on at least 5 to 10 minutes. As the condition of the scalp improves, the treatment can be less frequent. Antiseborrheic shampoos include those containing selenium sulfide suspension, zinc pyrithione, salicylic acid or sulfur compounds, and tar shampoo that contains sulfur or salicylic acid.

Nursing Management

A person with seborrheic dermatitis is advised to avoid external irritants, excessive heat, and perspiration; rubbing and scratching prolong the disorder. To avoid secondary infection, the patient should air the skin and keep skin folds clean and dry.

Instructions for using medicated shampoos are reinforced for people with dandruff who require treatment. Frequent shampooing is contrary to some cultural practices; the nurse should be sensitive to these differences when teaching the patient about home care.

The patient is cautioned that seborrheic dermatitis is a chronic problem that tends to reappear. The goal is to keep it under control. Patients need to be encouraged to adhere to the treatment program. Those who become discouraged and disheartened by the effect on body image should be treated with sensitivity and encouraged to express their feelings.

Acne Vulgaris

Acne vulgaris is a common follicular disorder affecting susceptible hair follicles, most commonly found on the face, neck, and upper trunk. It is characterized by **comedones** (primary acne lesions), both closed and open, and by papules, pustules, nodules, and cysts.

Acne is the most commonly encountered skin condition in adolescents and young adults between the ages of 12 and 35 years. It accounts for approximately 15% of all dermatology visits (Torpy, 2004). Both males and females are affected equally, although onset is slightly earlier in females. This may be because females reach puberty at a younger age than males. Acne becomes more marked at puberty and during adolescence because the endocrine glands that influence the secretions of the sebaceous glands are functioning at peak activity. Acne appears to stem from an interplay of genetic, hormonal, and bacterial factors. In most cases, there is a family history of acne.

Pathophysiology

During childhood, the sebaceous glands are small and virtually nonfunctioning. These glands are under endocrine control, especially by the androgens. During puberty, androgens stimulate the sebaceous glands, causing them to enlarge and secrete a natural oil, sebum, which rises to the top of the hair follicle and flows out onto the skin surface. In adolescents who develop acne, androgenic stimulation produces a heightened response in the sebaceous glands so that acne occurs when accumulated sebum plugs the pilosebaceous ducts. This accumulated material forms comedones.

Clinical Manifestations

The primary lesions of acne are comedones. Closed comedones (whiteheads) are obstructive lesions formed from impacted lipids or oils and keratin that plug the dilated follicle. These small, whitish papules with minute follicular openings generally cannot be seen. Closed comedones may evolve into open comedones, in which the contents of the ducts are in open communication with the external environment. The color of open comedones (blackheads) results not from dirt but from an accumulation of lipid, bacterial, and epithelial debris.

Although the exact cause is unknown, some closed comedones may rupture, resulting in an inflammatory reaction caused by leakage of follicular contents (eg, sebum, keratin, bacteria) into the dermis. This inflammatory response may result from the action of certain skin bacteria, such as *Propionibacterium acnes,* that live in the hair follicles and break down the triglycerides of the sebum into free fatty acids and glycerin. The resultant inflammation is seen clinically as erythematous papules, inflammatory pustules, and inflammatory cysts. Mild papules and cysts drain and heal on their own without treatment. Deeper papules and cysts cause scarring of the skin. Acne is usually graded as mild, moderate, or severe based on the number and type of lesions (eg, comedones, papules, pustules, cysts).

Assessment and Diagnostic Findings

The diagnosis of acne is based on the history and physical examination, evidence of lesions characteristic of acne, and age. Acne does not occur until puberty. The presence of the typical comedones along with excessively oily skin is characteristic. Oiliness is more prominent in the midfacial area; other parts of the face may appear dry. When there are numerous lesions, some of which are open, the person may exude a distinct sebaceous odor. Women may report a history of flare-ups a few days before menses. Biopsy of lesions is seldom necessary for a definitive diagnosis.

Medical Management

The goals of management are to reduce bacterial colonies, decrease sebaceous gland activity, prevent the follicles from becoming plugged, reduce inflammation, combat secondary infection, minimize scarring, and eliminate factors that predispose the person to acne. The therapeutic regimen depends on the type of lesion (eg, comedone, papule, pustule, cyst). The duration of treatment depends on the extent and severity of the acne. In severe cases, treatment may extend over years.

There is no predictable cure for the disease, but combinations of therapies are available that can effectively control its activity. Table 56-4 summarizes the treatment modalities for acne vulgaris. Topical treatment may be all that is needed to treat mild to moderate lesions and superficial inflammatory lesions.

Nutrition and Hygiene Therapy

Although food restrictions have been recommended from time to time in treating acne, diet is not believed to play

℞ TABLE 56-4 Commonly Prescribed Treatments of Acne Vulgaris

Type of Therapy	Prescribed Treatment Agent
Topical	benzoyl peroxide wash, gel benzoyl peroxide and erythromycin (Benzamycin gel) benzoyl peroxide and sulfur (Benzulfoid cream) resorcinol (as ingredient in other preparations) salicylic acid (as ingredient in other preparations) sulfur (as ingredient in other preparations) tretinoin (Retin A, Avita) other comedogenics (adapalene [Differen], azelaic acid [Azelex], tazorotene [Tazorac]) topical antibiotics
Systemic	oral antibiotics (erythromycin, tetracycline, doxycycline, minocin, penicillins) isotretinoin (Accutane) hormones: corticosteroids high dose for anti-inflammatory action low dose to suppress androgenic action intralesional for anti-inflammatory action antiandrogens oral contraceptives (women only)
Surgical	extraction of comedo contents drainage of pustules and cysts excision of sinus tracts and cysts intralesional corticosteroids for anti-inflammatory action cryotherapy dermabrasion for scars laser resurfacing of scars

Treatments listed are common but do not include all available forms of therapy.

a major role in therapy. However, the elimination of a specific food or food product associated with a flare-up of acne, such as chocolate, cola, fried foods, or milk products, should be promoted. Maintenance of good nutrition equips the immune system for effective action against bacteria and infection.

For mild cases of acne, washing twice each day with a cleansing soap may be all that is required. These soaps can remove the excessive skin oil and the comedo in most cases. Oil-free cosmetics and creams should be chosen. These products are usually designated as useful for acne-prone skin.

Topical Pharmacologic Therapy

Over-the-counter acne medications contain either salicylic acid or benzoyl peroxide, both of which are very effective at removing the sebaceous follicular plugs. However, the skin of some people is sensitive to these products, which can cause irritation or excessive dryness, especially when used with some prescribed topical medications. The patient should be instructed to discontinue use of the product if severe irritation occurs.

BENZOYL PEROXIDE

Benzoyl peroxide preparations are widely used because they produce a rapid and sustained reduction of inflammatory lesions. They depress sebum production and promote breakdown of comedo plugs. They also produce an antibacterial effect by suppressing *P. acnes*. Initially, benzoyl peroxide causes redness and scaling, but the skin usually adjusts quickly to its use. Typically, the patient applies a gel of benzoyl peroxide once daily. In many instances, this is the only treatment needed. Benzoyl peroxide, benzoyl erythromycin (Benzamycin), and benzoyl sulfur (Sulfoxyl) are available over the counter and by prescription. Vitamin A acid (tretinoin) applied topically is used to clear the keratin plugs from the pilosebaceous ducts. Vitamin A acid speeds the cellular turnover, forces out the comedones, and prevents new comedones.

The patient should be informed that symptoms may worsen during early weeks of therapy because inflammation may occur during the process. Erythema and peeling also frequently result. Improvement may take 8 to 12 weeks. Some patients cannot tolerate this therapy. The patient is cautioned against sun exposure while using this topical medication because it may cause an exaggerated sunburn. Package insert directions should be followed carefully.

TOPICAL ANTIBIOTICS

Topical antibiotic treatment for acne is common. Topical antibiotics suppress the growth of *P. acnes;* reduce superficial free fatty acid levels; decrease comedones, papules, and pustules; and produce no systemic side effects. Common topical preparations include tetracycline, clindamycin, and erythromycin.

Systemic Pharmacologic Therapy

ORAL ANTIBIOTICS

Oral antibiotics, such as tetracycline, doxycycline, and minocycline, administered in small doses over a long period are very effective in treating moderate and severe acne, especially when the acne is inflammatory and results in pustules, abscesses, and scarring. Therapy may continue for months to years. The tetracycline family of antibiotics is contraindicated in children younger than 12 years and in pregnant women. Although tetracyclines are considered safe for long-term use in most cases, administration during pregnancy can affect the development of teeth, causing enamel hypoplasia and permanent discoloration of teeth in infants. Side effects of tetracyclines include photosensitivity, nausea, diarrhea, cutaneous infection in either gender, and vaginitis in women. In some women, broad-spectrum antibiotics may suppress normal vaginal bacteria and predispose the patient to candidiasis, a fungal infection.

ORAL RETINOIDS

Synthetic vitamin A compounds (ie, retinoids) are used with dramatic results in patients with nodular cystic acne unresponsive to conventional therapy. One compound is isotretinoin (Accutane, Sotret). Isotretinoin is also used for active inflammatory papular pustular acne that has a tendency to scar. Isotretinoin reduces sebaceous gland size and inhibits sebum production. It also causes the epidermis to shed (epidermal desquamation), thereby unseating and expelling existing comedones.

The most common side effect, experienced by almost all patients, is **cheilitis** (inflammation of the lips). Dry and chafed skin and mucous membranes are frequent side effects. These changes are reversible with the withdrawal of the medication. Most importantly, isotretinoin, like other vitamin A metabolites, is teratogenic in humans, meaning that it can have an adverse effect on a fetus, causing central nervous system and cardiovascular defects and structural abnormalities of the face. Effective contraceptive measures for women of childbearing age are mandatory during treatment and for about 4 to 8 weeks thereafter. To avoid additive toxic effects, patients are cautioned not to take vitamin A supplements while taking isotretinoin.

HORMONE THERAPY

Estrogen therapy (including progesterone–estrogen preparations) suppresses sebum production and reduces skin oiliness. It is usually reserved for young women when the acne begins somewhat later than usual and tends to flare up at certain times in the menstrual cycle. Estrogen in the form of estrogen-dominant oral contraceptive compounds may be administered on a prescribed cyclic regimen. Estrogen is not administered to male patients because of undesirable side effects such as enlargement of the breasts and decrease in body hair.

Surgical Management

Surgical treatment of acne consists of comedo extraction, injections of corticosteroids into the inflamed lesions, and incision and drainage of large, fluctuant (moving in palpable waves), nodular cystic lesions. Cryosurgery (freezing with liquid nitrogen) may be used for nodular and cystic forms of acne. Patients with deep scars may be treated with deep abrasive therapy (dermabrasion), in which the epidermis and some superficial dermis are removed down to the level of the scars.

Comedones may be removed with a comedo extractor. The site is first cleaned with alcohol. The opening of the extractor is then placed over the lesion, and direct pressure is applied to cause extrusion of the plug through the extractor. Removal of comedones leads to erythema, which may take several weeks to subside. Recurrence of comedones after extraction is common because of the continuing activity of the pilosebaceous glands.

Nursing Management

Nursing care of patients with acne consists largely of monitoring and managing potential complications of skin treatments. Major nursing activities include patient education, particularly in proper skin care techniques, and managing potential problems related to the skin disorder or therapy. Providing positive reassurance, listening attentively, and being sensitive to the feelings of the patient with acne are essential for the patient's psychological well-being and understanding of the disease and treatment plan.

Preventing Scarring

Prevention of scarring is the ultimate goal of therapy. The chance of scarring increases as the grade of acne increases. Grades III and IV (25 to more than 50 comedones, papules, or pustules) usually require longer-term therapy with systemic antibiotics or isotretinoin. Patients should be warned that discontinuing these medications can exacerbate acne, lead to more flare-ups, and increase the chance of deep scarring. Furthermore, manipulation of the comedones, papules, and pustules increases the potential for scarring.

When acne surgery is prescribed to extract deep-seated comedones or inflamed lesions or to incise and drain cystic lesions, the intervention itself may result in further scarring. Dermabrasion, which levels existing scar tissue, can also increase scar formation. Hyperpigmentation or hypopigmentation also may affect the tissue involved. The patient should be informed of these potential outcomes before choosing surgical intervention for acne.

Preventing Infection

Female patients receiving long-term antibiotic therapy with tetracycline should be advised to watch for and report signs and symptoms of oral or vaginal candidiasis, a yeast-like fungal infection.

Promoting Home and Community-Based Care

TEACHING PATIENTS SELF-CARE

In addition to instructions for taking prescribed medications, patients are instructed to wash the face and other affected areas with mild soap and water twice each day to remove surface oils and prevent obstruction of the oil glands. They are cautioned to avoid scrubbing the face; acne is not caused by dirt and cannot be washed away.

Mild abrasive soaps and drying agents are prescribed to eliminate the oily feeling that troubles many patients. At the same time, patients are cautioned to avoid excessive abrasion because it makes acne worse. Excessive abrasion causes minute scratches on the skin surface and increases possible bacterial contamination. Soap itself can irritate the skin.

All forms of friction and trauma are avoided, including propping the hands against the face, rubbing the face, and wearing tight collars and helmets. Patients are instructed to avoid manipulation of pimples or blackheads. Squeezing merely worsens the problem, because a portion of the blackhead is pushed down into the skin, which may cause the follicle to rupture. Because cosmetics, shaving creams, and lotions can aggravate acne, these substances are best avoided unless the patient is advised otherwise. There is no evidence that a particular food can cause or aggravate acne. In general, eating a nutritious diet helps the body maintain a strong immune system.

Infectious Dermatoses

Bacterial Skin Infections

Also called **pyodermas**, pus-forming bacterial infections of the skin may be primary or secondary. Primary skin infections originate in previously normal-appearing skin and are usually caused by a single organism. Secondary skin infections arise from a preexisting skin disorder or from disruption of the skin integrity from injury or surgery. In either case, several microorganisms may be implicated (eg, *Staphylococcus aureus*, group A streptococci). The most common primary bacterial skin infections are impetigo and folliculitis. Folliculitis may lead to furuncles or carbuncles.

Impetigo

Impetigo is a superficial infection of the skin caused by staphylococci, streptococci, or multiple bacteria. Bullous impetigo, a more deep-seated infection of the skin caused by *S. aureus*, is characterized by the formation of bullae (large, fluid-filled blisters) from original vesicles. The bullae rupture, leaving raw, red areas.

The exposed areas of the body, face, hands, neck, and extremities are most frequently involved. Impetigo is contagious and may spread to other parts of the patient's skin or to other members of the family who touch the patient or use towels or combs that are soiled with the exudate of the lesions.

Impetigo is seen in people of at all ages. It is particularly common in children living in poor hygienic conditions. It often follows pediculosis capitis (head lice), scabies (itch mites), herpes simplex, insect bites, poison ivy, or eczema. Chronic health problems, poor hygiene, and malnutrition may predispose an adult to impetigo. There is some indication that excessive use of antibacterial soaps may create resistant bacteria and contribute to the problem. Some people have been identified as asymptomatic carriers of *S. aureus*, usually in the nasal passages.

Clinical Manifestations

The lesions of impetigo begin as small, red macules, which quickly become discrete, thin-walled vesicles that rupture and become covered with a loosely adherent honey-yellow crust (Fig. 56-1). These crusts are easily removed to reveal smooth, red, moist surfaces on which new crusts soon develop. If the scalp is involved, the hair is matted, which distinguishes the condition from ringworm.

Medical Management

Systemic antibiotic therapy is the usual treatment. It reduces contagious spread, treats deep infection, and prevents acute glomerulonephritis (kidney infection), which may occur as a consequence of streptococcal skin diseases. In nonbullous impetigo, benzathine penicillin or oral penicillin may be prescribed. In bullous impetigo, a penicillinase-resistant penicillin (eg, cloxacillin [Cloxapen], dicloxacillin [Dycill]) may be used. In penicillin-allergic patients, erythromycin is an effective alternative.

Topical antibacterial therapy (eg, mupirocin [Bactroban]) may be prescribed when the disease is limited to a small area; the medication must be applied to the lesions several times daily for a week. The treatment regimen may be impossible for some patients or their caregivers to follow. Topical antibiotics generally are not as effective as systemic therapy in eradicating or preventing the spread of streptococci from the respiratory tract, thereby increasing the risk of developing glomerulonephritis.

When topical therapy is prescribed, lesions are soaked or washed with soap solution to remove the central site of bacterial growth, giving the topical antibiotic an opportunity to reach the infected site. After the crusts are removed, a topical antibiotic cream is applied. Gloves are worn when providing patient care. An antiseptic solution, such as povidone–iodine (Betadine), may be used to clean the skin, reduce bacterial content in the infected area, and prevent spread.

Nursing Management

The nurse instructs the patient and family members to bathe at least once daily with bactericidal soap. Cleanliness and good hygiene practices help prevent the spread of the lesions from one skin area to another and from one person to another. Each person should have a separate towel and washcloth. Because impetigo is a contagious disorder, infected people should avoid contact with other people until the lesions heal.

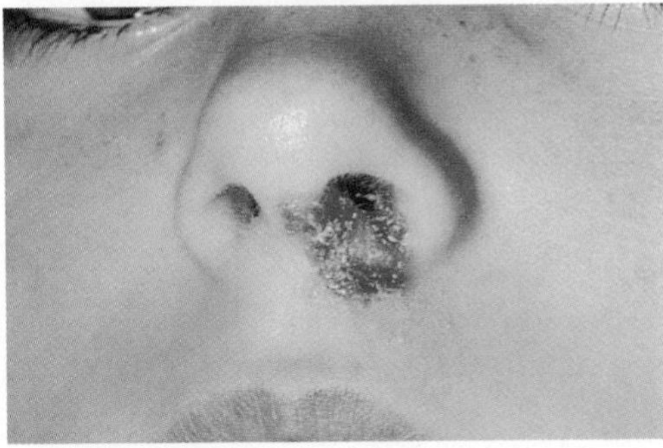

FIGURE 56-1. Impetigo of the nostril.

Folliculitis, Furuncles, and Carbuncles

Folliculitis is an infection of bacterial or fungal origin that arises within the hair follicles. Lesions may be superficial or deep. Single or multiple papules or pustules appear close to the hair follicles. Folliculitis commonly affects the beard area of men who shave and women's legs. Other areas include the axillae, trunk, and buttocks.

Pseudofolliculitis barbae (shaving bumps) are an inflammatory reaction that occurs predominately on the faces of African-American and other curly-haired men as a result of shaving. The sharp ingrowing hairs have a curved root that grows at a more acute angle and pierces the skin, provoking an irritative reaction. The only entirely effective treatment is to avoid shaving. Other treatments include using special lotions or antibiotics or using a hand brush to dislodge the hairs mechanically. If the patient must remove facial hair, a depilatory cream or electric razor may be used.

A **furuncle** (boil) is an acute inflammation arising deep in one or more hair follicles and spreading into the surrounding dermis. It is a deep form of folliculitis. Furunculosis refers to multiple or recurrent lesions. Furuncles may occur anywhere on the body but are more prevalent in areas subjected to irritation, pressure, friction, and excessive perspiration, such as the back of the neck, the axillae, and the buttocks.

A furuncle may start as a small, red, raised, painful pimple. Frequently, the infection progresses and involves the skin and subcutaneous fatty tissue, causing tenderness, pain, and surrounding cellulitis. The area of redness and induration represents an effort of the body to keep the infection localized. The bacteria (usually staphylococci) produce necrosis of the invaded tissue. The characteristic pointing of a boil follows in a few days. When this occurs, the center becomes yellow or black, and the boil is said to have "come to a head."

A **carbuncle** is an abscess of the skin and subcutaneous tissue that represents an extension of a furuncle that has invaded several follicles and is large and deep-seated. It is usually caused by a staphylococcal infection. Carbuncles appear most commonly in areas where the skin is thick and inelastic; the back of the neck and the buttocks are common sites. In carbuncles, the extensive inflammation frequently prevents a complete walling off of the infection; purulent material may be absorbed, resulting in high fever, pain, leukocytosis, and even extension of the infection to the bloodstream.

Furuncles and carbuncles are more likely to occur in patients with underlying systemic diseases, such as diabetes or hematologic malignancies, and in those receiving immunosuppressive therapy for other diseases. Both are more prevalent in hot climates, especially on skin beneath occlusive clothing.

Medical Management

In treating staphylococcal infections, it is important not to rupture or destroy the protective wall of induration that localizes the infection. The boil or pimple should never be squeezed.

Follicular disorders, including folliculitis, furuncles, and carbuncles, are usually caused by staphylococci, although if the immune system is impaired, the causative organisms may be gram-negative bacilli. Systemic antibiotic therapy, selected by culture and sensitivity study, is generally indicated. Oral cloxacillin, dicloxacillin, and flucloxacillin (Floxapen) are first-line medications. Cephalosporins and erythromycin are also effective. To promote comfort, bed rest is advised for patients who have boils on the perineum or in the anal region, and a course of systemic antibiotic therapy is indicated to prevent the spread of the infection.

When the pus has localized and is fluctuant, a small incision with a scalpel can speed resolution by relieving the tension and ensuring direct evacuation of the pus and slough. The patient is instructed to keep the draining lesion covered with a dressing.

Nursing Management

Intravenous (IV) fluids, fever reduction, and other supportive treatments are indicated for patients who are acutely ill from infection. Warm, moist compresses hasten resolution of the furuncle or carbuncle. The surrounding skin may be cleaned gently with antibacterial soap, and an antibacterial ointment may be applied. Soiled dressings are handled according to standard precautions. Nursing personnel should carefully follow isolation precautions to avoid becoming carriers of staphylococci. Disposable gloves are worn when caring for these patients.

NURSING ALERT

Nurses must take special precautions in caring for boils on the face, because the skin area drains directly into the cranial venous sinuses. Sinus thrombosis with fatal pyemia can develop after manipulating a boil in this location. The infection can travel through the sinus tract and penetrate the brain cavity, causing brain abscess.

PROMOTING HOME AND COMMUNITY-BASED CARE

Teaching Patients Self-Care. To prevent and control staphylococcal skin infections such as boils and carbuncles, the staphylococcal pathogen must be eliminated from the skin and environment. Efforts must be made to increase the patient's resistance and provide a hygienic environment. If lesions are actively draining, the mattress and pillow should be covered with plastic material and wiped off with disinfectant daily; the bed linens, towels, and clothing should be laundered after each use; and the patient should use an antibacterial soap and shampoo for an indefinite period, often several months.

Recurrent infection is prevented with the use of long-term antibiotic therapy (longer than about 3 months). The patient must take the full dose for the time prescribed. The purulent exudate is a source of reinfection or transmission of infection to caregivers. If the patient has a history of recurrent infections, a carrier state may exist, which should be investigated and treated with an antibacterial cream such as mupirocin.

Viral Skin Infections

Herpes Zoster

Herpes zoster, also called shingles, is an infection caused by the varicella-zoster virus, a member of a group of DNA viruses. The viruses causing chickenpox and herpes zoster are indistinguishable, hence the name varicella-zoster virus. The disease is characterized by a painful vesicular eruption along the area of distribution of the sensory nerves from one or more posterior ganglia. After a case of chickenpox runs its course, the varicella-zoster viruses responsible for the outbreak lie dormant inside nerve cells near the brain and spinal cord. Later, when these latent viruses are reactivated because of declining cellular immunity, they travel by way of the peripheral nerves to the skin, where the viruses multiply and create a red rash of small, fluid-filled blisters. About 10% of adults get shingles during their lifetimes, usually after 50 years of age. There is an increased frequency of herpes zoster infections among patients with weakened immune systems and cancers, especially leukemias and lymphomas.

Clinical Manifestations

The eruption is usually accompanied or preceded by pain, which may radiate over the entire region supplied by the affected nerves. The pain may be burning, lancinating (tearing or sharply cutting), stabbing, or aching. Some patients have no pain, but itching and tenderness may occur over the area. Sometimes, malaise and gastrointestinal disturbances precede the eruption. The patches of grouped vesicles appear on the red and swollen skin. The early vesicles, which contain serum, later may become purulent, rupture, and form crusts. The inflammation is usually unilateral, involving the thoracic, cervical, or cranial nerves in a bandlike configuration. The blisters are usually confined to a narrow region of the face or trunk (Fig. 56-2). The clinical course varies from 1 to 3 weeks. If an ophthalmic nerve is involved, the patient may have eye pain. Inflammation and

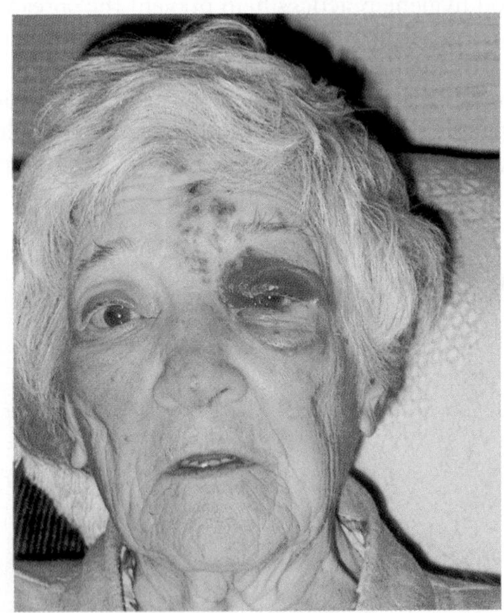

FIGURE 56-2. Herpes zoster (shingles).

a rash on the trunk may cause pain with the slightest touch. The healing time varies from 7 to 26 days.

Herpes zoster in healthy adults is usually localized and benign. However, in immunosuppressed patients, the disease may be severe and disabling.

Medical Management

There is evidence that infection is arrested if oral antiviral agents such as acyclovir (Zovirax), valacyclovir (Valtrex), or famciclovir (Famvir) are administered within 24 hours of the initial eruption. IV acyclovir, if started early, is effective in significantly reducing the pain and halting the progression of the disease. In older patients, the pain from herpes zoster may persist as postherpetic neuralgia for months after the skin lesions disappear.

The goals of herpes zoster management are to relieve the pain and to reduce or avoid complications, which include infection, scarring, and postherpetic neuralgia and eye complications. Pain is controlled with analgesics, because adequate pain control during the acute phase helps prevent persistent pain patterns. Systemic corticosteroids may be prescribed for patients older than 50 years of age to reduce the incidence and duration of postherpetic neuralgia (persistent pain of the affected nerve after healing). Healing usually occurs more quickly in those who have been treated with corticosteroids. Triamcinolone (Aristocort, Kenacort, Kenalog) injected subcutaneously under painful areas is effective as an anti-inflammatory agent.

Ophthalmic herpes zoster occurs when an eye is involved. This is considered an ophthalmic emergency, and the patient should be referred to an ophthalmologist immediately to prevent the possible sequelae of keratitis, uveitis, ulceration, and blindness.

People who have been exposed to varicella by primary infection or by vaccination are not at risk for infection after exposure to patients with herpes zoster.

Nursing Management

The patient and family members are instructed about the importance of taking antiviral agents as prescribed and in keeping follow-up appointments with the health care provider. The nurse assesses the patient's discomfort and response to medication and collaborates with the physician to make necessary adjustments to the treatment regimen. The patient is taught how to apply wet dressings or medication to the lesions and to follow proper hand hygiene techniques to avoid spreading the virus.

Diversionary activities and relaxation techniques are encouraged to ensure restful sleep and to alleviate discomfort. A caregiver may be required to assist with dressings, particularly if the patient is elderly and unable to apply them. Family members or a home care nurse may need to help with dressing changes. Food preparation for patients who cannot care for themselves or prepare nourishing meals must be arranged.

Herpes Simplex

Herpes simplex is a common skin infection. There are two types of the causative virus, which are identified by viral typing. Generally, herpes simplex type 1 occurs on the mouth and type 2 occurs in the genital area, but both viral types can be found in both locations. About 85% of adults worldwide are seropositive for herpes type 1. The prevalence of type 2 is lower; type 2 usually appears at the onset of sexual activity. Serologic testing shows that many more people are infected than have a history of clinical disease.

Herpes simplex is classified as a true primary infection, a nonprimary initial episode, or a recurrent episode. True primary infection is the initial exposure to the virus. A nonprimary initial episode is the initial episode of either type 1 or type 2 in a person previously infected with the other type. Recurrent episodes are subsequent episodes of the same viral type.

Types of Herpes Simplex

OROLABIAL HERPES

Orolabial herpes, also called fever blisters or cold sores, consists of erythematous-based clusters of grouped vesicles on the lips. A prodrome of tingling or burning with pain may precede the appearance of the vesicles by up to 24 hours. Certain triggers, such as sunlight exposure or increased stress, may cause recurrent episodes. Fewer than 1% of people with primary orolabial herpes infections develop herpetic gingivostomatitis. This complication occurs more often in children and young adults than in other age groups. The onset is often accompanied by high fever, regional lymphadenopathy, and generalized malaise. Another complication of orolabial herpes is the development of erythema multiforme, an acute inflammation of the skin and mucous membranes with characteristic lesions that have the appearance of targets (ie, concentric red rings with white bands between the red rings).

GENITAL HERPES

Genital herpes, or type 2 herpes simplex, manifests with a broad spectrum of clinical signs. Minor infections may produce no symptoms at all; severe primary infections with type 1 can cause systemic flulike illness. Lesions appear as grouped vesicles on an erythematous base initially involving the vagina, rectum, or penis. New lesions can continue to appear for 7 to 14 days. Lesions are symmetric and usually cause regional lymphadenopathy. Fever and flulike symptoms are common. Typical recurrences begin with a prodrome of burning, tingling, or itching about 24 hours before the vesicles appear. As the vesicles rupture, erosions and ulcerations begin to appear. Severe infections can cause extensive erosions of the vaginal or anal canal. For further information, see Chapter 47.

Assessment and Diagnostic Findings

Herpes simplex infections are confirmed in several ways. Generally, the appearance of the skin eruption is strongly suggestive. Viral cultures and rapid assays are available, and the type of test used depends on lesion morphology. Acute vesicular lesions are more likely to react positively to the rapid assay, whereas older, crusted patches are better diagnosed with viral culture. In all cases, it is imperative to obtain enough viral cells for testing, and careful collection methods are therefore important. All crusts should be gently removed or vesicles gently unroofed. A sterile cotton swab premoistened in viral culture preservative is used to swab the base of the vesicle to obtain a specimen for analysis.

Complications

Eczema herpeticum is a condition in which patients with eczema contract herpes that spreads throughout the eczematous areas. The same type of spread of herpes can occur in severe seborrhea, scabies, and other chronic skin conditions. Eczema herpeticum is managed with oral or IV acyclovir.

Herpetic whitlow is an infection of the pulp of a fingertip with herpes type 1 or 2. There is tenderness and erythema of the cuticle. Deep-seated vesicles appear within 24 hours.

Most cases of neonatal infection with herpes occur during delivery by contact of the infant with the mother's active ulcerations. Rarely, in mothers who have primary infections during pregnancy, intrauterine neonatal infections occur. Fetal anomalies include skin lesions, microcephaly, encephalitis, and intracerebral calcifications.

Medical Management

In many patients, recurrent orolabial herpes represents more of a nuisance than a disease. Because sun exposure is a common trigger, people with recurrent orolabial herpes should use a sunscreen liberally on the lips and face. Topical treatment with drying agents may accelerate healing. In more severe outbreaks or in patients with identified triggers, intermittent treatment with 200 mg acyclovir (Zovirax) administered five times each day for 5 days is often started as soon as the earliest symptoms occur.

Treatment of genital herpes depends on the severity, the frequency, and the psychological impact of recurrences and on the infectious status of the sexual partner. For people who have mild or rare outbreaks, no treatment may be required. For those who have more severe outbreaks, but for whom outbreaks are still infrequent, intermittent treatment as described for oral lesions can be used. Because intermittent treatment reduces the duration of the infection by only 24 to 36 hours, it should be initiated as early as possible.

Patients who have more than six recurrences per year may benefit from suppressive therapy. Use of acyclovir, valacyclovir (Valtrex), or famciclovir (Famvir) suppresses 85% of recurrences, and 20% of patients are free of recurrences during suppressive therapy. Suppressive therapy also reduces viral shedding by almost 95%, making the person less contagious. Treatment with suppressive doses of oral antiviral medications prevents recurrent erythema multiforme (acute eruption of macules, papules, and vesicles with a multiform appearance).

Management of genital herpes in pregnancy differs among clinicians. Routine prenatal cultures do not predict shedding at the time of delivery. The use of scalp electrodes during delivery should be avoided because they increase the risk for infection in the newborn. Because the risk for neonatal herpes is greater in women with their initial episode during pregnancy, suppression therapy should be started in these women to reduce outbreaks during the third trimester. All women with active lesions at the time of delivery undergo cesarean section.

In immunocompromised patients, suppression therapy should be considered. In severe infections of hospitalized patients, IV acyclovir is prescribed.

Fungal (Mycotic) Skin Infections

Fungi, tiny members of a subdivision of the plant kingdom that feed on organic matter, are responsible for various common skin infections. In some cases, they affect only the skin and its appendages (hair and nails). In other cases, internal organs are involved, and the diseases may be life-threatening. However, superficial infections rarely cause even temporary disability and respond readily to treatment. Secondary infection with bacteria, *Candida,* or both organisms may occur.

The most common fungal skin infection is **tinea**, which is also called ringworm because of its characteristic appearance of a ring or rounded tunnel under the skin. Tinea infections affect the head, body, groin, feet, and nails. Table 56-5 summarizes the tinea infections.

To obtain a specimen for diagnosis, the lesion is cleaned and a scalpel or glass slide is used to remove scales from the margin of the lesion. The scales are dropped onto a slide to which potassium hydroxide has been added. The diagnosis is made by examination of the infected scales microscopically for spores and hyphae or by isolating the organism in culture. Under Wood's light, a specimen of infected hair appears fluorescent; this may be helpful in diagnosing some cases of tinea capitis.

Tinea Pedis: Athlete's Foot

Tinea pedis (athlete's foot) is the most common fungal infection. It may be especially prevalent in people who use communal showers or swimming pools.

Clinical Manifestations

Tinea pedis may appear as an acute or chronic infection on the soles of the feet or between the toes. The toenail may also be involved. Lymphangitis and cellulitis occur occasionally when bacterial superinfection occurs. Sometimes, a mixed infection involving fungi, bacteria, and yeast occurs.

Medical Management

During the acute, vesicular phase, soaks of Burow's solution or potassium permanganate solutions are used to remove the crusts, scales, and debris and to reduce the inflammation. Topical antifungal agents (eg, miconazole [Lotrimin AF], clotrimazole [Lotrimin; Desenex]) are applied to the infected areas. Topical therapy is continued for several weeks because of the high rate of recurrence.

Nursing Management

Footwear provides a favorable environment for fungi, and the causative fungus may be in the shoes or socks. Because moisture encourages the growth of fungi, the patient is instructed to keep the feet as dry as possible, including the areas between the toes. Small pieces of cotton can be placed between the toes at night to absorb moisture. Socks should

TABLE 56-5 Tinea (Ringworm) Infections

Type and Location	Clinical Manifestations	Treatment
Tinea capitis (head) Contagious fungal infection of the hair shaft	• Common in children • Oval, scaling, erythematous patches • Small papules or pustules on the scalp • Brittle hair that breaks easily	• Griseofulvin for 6 weeks • Shampoo hair 2 or 3 times with Nizoral or selenium sulfide shampoo.
Tinea corporis (body)	• Begins with red macule, which spreads to a ring of papules or vesicles with central clearing • Lesions found in clusters • Many spread to the hair, scalp, or nails. • Very pruritic • An infected pet may be the source.	• Mild conditions: topical antifungal creams • Severe conditions: griseofulvin or terbinafine
Tinea cruris (groin area; "jock itch")	• Begins with small, red scaling patches, which spread to form circular elevated plaques • Very pruritic • Clusters of pustules may be seen around borders.	• Mild conditions: topical antifungal creams • Severe conditions: griseofulvin or terbinafine
Tinea pedis (foot; "athlete's foot")	• Soles of one or both feet have scaling and mild redness with maceration in the toe webs. • More acute infections may have clusters of clear vesicles on dusky base.	• Soak feet in vinegar and water solution. • Resistant infections: griseofulvin or terbinafine • Terbinafine (Lamisil) daily for 3 months
Tinea ungum (toenails; affects about 50% of adults)	• Nails thicken, crumble easily, and lack luster. • Whole nail may be destroyed.	• Itraconazole (Sporanox) in pulses of 1 week a month for 3 months in cases of terbinafine failure

be made of cotton, and hosiery should have cotton feet, because cotton is an effective absorber of moisture.

For people whose feet perspire excessively, perforated shoes allow aeration of the feet. Plastic- or rubber-soled footwear should be avoided. Talcum powder or antifungal powder applied twice daily helps keep the feet dry. Several pairs of shoes should be alternated so that they can dry completely before being worn again.

Tinea Corporis: Ringworm of the Body

In tinea corporis (ringworm of the body) the typical ringed lesion appears on the face, neck, trunk, and extremities (Fig. 56-3). Animal (nonhuman) varieties are known to cause an intense inflammatory reaction in humans. Humans make contact with animal varieties through contact with pets or objects that have been in contact with an animal.

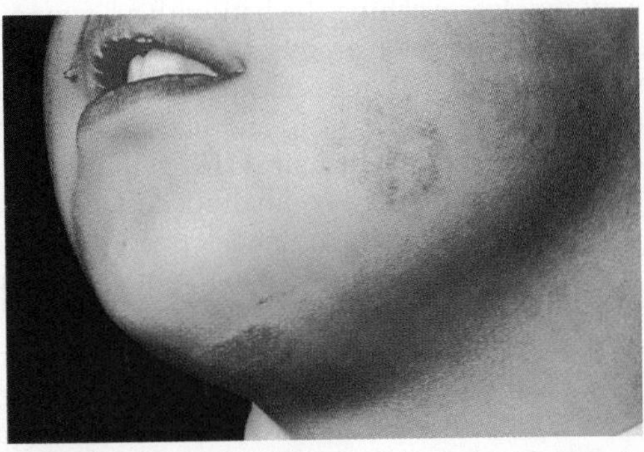

FIGURE 56-3. Tinea corporis (ringworm) of the face.

Medical Management

Topical antifungal medication may be applied to small areas. Oral antifungal agents are used only in extensive cases. Side effects of oral antifungal agents include photosensitivity, skin rashes, headache, and nausea. Newer antifungal agents, including itraconazole (Sporanox), fluconazole (Diflucan), and terbinafine (Lamisil), have been more effective with fewer systemic side effects than griseofulvin (Grifulvin V) in patients with chronic fungal (dermatophyte) infections.

Nursing Management

The patient is instructed to use a clean towel and washcloth daily. Because fungal infections thrive in heat and moisture, all skin areas and skin folds that retain moisture must be dried thoroughly. Clean cotton clothing should be worn next to the skin.

Tinea Capitis: Ringworm of the Scalp

Ringworm of the scalp is a contagious fungal infection of the hair shafts and a common cause of hair loss in children. Any child with scaling of the scalp should be considered to have tinea capitis until proven otherwise. Clinical examination reveals one or several round, red scaling patches. Small pustules or papules may be seen at the edges of such patches. As the hairs in the affected areas are invaded by the fungi, they become brittle and break off at or near the surface of the scalp, leaving bald patches with the classic sign of black dots, which are the broken ends of hairs. Because most cases of tinea capitis heal without scarring, the hair loss is only temporary.

Medical Management

Griseofulvin, an antifungal agent, is prescribed for patients with tinea capitis. Topical agents do not provide an effective cure because the infection occurs within the hair shaft and below the surface of the scalp. However, topical agents can be used to inactivate organisms already on the hair. This minimizes contagion and eliminates the need to clip the hair. Infected hairs break off anyway, and noninfected ones may remain in place. The hair should be shampooed two or three times weekly, and a topical antifungal preparation (eg, ketoconazole [Nizoral]) should be applied to reduce dissemination of the organisms.

Nursing Management

Because tinea capitis is contagious, the patient and family should be instructed to set up a hygiene regimen for home use. Each person should have a separate comb and brush and should avoid exchanging hats and other headgear. All infected members of the family must be examined, because familial infections are relatively common. Household pets should also be examined.

Tinea Cruris: Ringworm of the Groin

Tinea cruris (jock itch) is ringworm infection of the groin, which may extend to the inner thighs and buttock area. It occurs most frequently in young joggers, obese people, and those who wear tight underclothing. The incidence of tinea cruris is increased among people with diabetes.

Management

Mild infections may be treated with topical medication such as clotrimazole, miconazole, or terbinafine (Lamisil) for at least 3 to 4 weeks to ensure eradication of the infection. Oral antifungal agents (eg, ketoconazole [Nizoral]) may be required for more severe infections. Heat, friction, and maceration (from sweating) predispose the patient to the infection. The nurse instructs the patient to avoid excessive heat and humidity as much as possible and to avoid wearing synthetic (eg, nylon) underwear, tight-fitting clothing, and a wet bathing suit. The groin area should be cleaned, dried thoroughly, and dusted with a topical antifungal agent such as tolnaftate (Tinactin) as a preventive measure, because the infection is likely to recur.

Tinea Unguium: Ringworm of the Nails

Tinea unguium (onychomycosis) is a chronic fungal infection of the toenails or, less commonly, the fingernails. It is usually caused by *Trichophyton* species (*T. rubrum, T. mentagrophytes*) or *Candida albicans*. It is usually associated with long-standing fungal infection of the feet. The nails become thickened, friable (ie, easily crumbled), and lusterless. In time, debris accumulates under the free edge of the nail. Ultimately, the nail plate separates. Because of the chronicity of this infection, the entire nail may be destroyed.

Management

An oral antifungal agent is prescribed for 6 weeks when the fingernails are involved and 12 weeks when the toenails are involved. Selection of the antifungal agent depends on the causative fungus. Candidal infections are treated with fluconazole (Diflucan) or itraconazole (Sporanox). Griseofulvin is no longer considered effective therapy because of its long treatment course and poor cure rate. Response to oral antifungal agents in treating infections of the toenails is poor at best. Frequently, when the treatment stops, the infection returns.

Parasitic Skin Infestations

Pediculosis: Lice Infestation

Lice infestation affects people of all ages. Three varieties of lice infest humans: *Pediculus humanus capitis* (head louse), *Pediculus humanus corporis* (body louse), and *Phthirus pubis* (pubic louse or crab louse). Lice are called ectoparasites because they live on the outside of the host's body. They depend on the host for their nourishment, feeding on human blood approximately five times each day. They inject their digestive juices and excrement into the skin, which causes severe itching.

Pediculosis Capitis

Pediculosis capitis is an infestation of the scalp by the head louse. The female louse lays her eggs (nits) close to the scalp. The nits become firmly attached to the hair shafts with a tenacious substance. The young lice hatch in about 10 days and reach maturity in 2 weeks.

CLINICAL MANIFESTATIONS

Head lice are found most commonly along the back of the head and behind the ears. The eggs are visible to the naked eye as silvery, glistening oval bodies that are difficult to remove from the hair. The bite of the insect causes intense pruritus, and the resultant scratching often leads to secondary bacterial infection, such as impetigo or furunculosis. The infestation is more common in children and people with long hair. Head lice may be transmitted directly by physical contact or indirectly by infested combs, brushes, wigs, hats, and bedding.

MEDICAL MANAGEMENT

Treatment involves washing the hair with a shampoo containing lindane (Kwell) or pyrethrin compounds with piperonyl butoxide (RID or R&C Shampoo). The patient is instructed to shampoo the scalp and hair according to the product directions. After the hair is rinsed thoroughly, it is combed with a fine-toothed comb dipped in vinegar to remove any remaining nits or nit shells freed from the hair shafts. They are extremely difficult to remove and may have to be picked off one by one.

All articles, clothing, towels, and bedding that may have lice or nits should be washed in hot water—at least 54°C (130°F)—or dry-cleaned to prevent re-infestation. Upholstered furniture, rugs, and floors should be vacuumed frequently. Combs and brushes are also disinfected with the shampoo. All family members and close contacts are treated. Complications such as severe pruritus, pyoderma, and dermatitis are treated with antipruritics, systemic antibiotics, and topical corticosteroids.

NURSING MANAGEMENT

The nurse informs the patient that head lice may infest anyone and are not a sign of uncleanliness. Because the condition spreads rapidly, treatment must be started immediately. School epidemics may be managed by having all of the students shampoo their hair on the same night. Students should be warned not to share combs, brushes, and hats. Each family member should be inspected for head lice daily for at least 2 weeks. The patient should be instructed that lindane may be toxic to the central nervous system when used more frequently or for longer periods of time than specified in the package insert.

Pediculosis Corporis and Pubis

Pediculosis corporis is an infestation of the body by the body louse. This is a disease of unwashed people or those who live in close quarters and do not change their clothing (eg, survivors of natural disasters who must live with others in temporary housing without access to running water and clean clothes). Pediculosis pubis is extremely common. The infestation is generally localized in the genital region and is transmitted chiefly by sexual contact.

CLINICAL MANIFESTATIONS

Chiefly involved are those areas of the skin that come in closest contact with the underclothing (ie, neck, trunk, and thighs). The body louse lives primarily in the seams of underwear and clothing, to which it clings as it pierces the skin with its proboscis. Its bites cause characteristic minute hemorrhagic points. Widespread excoriation may appear as a result of intense pruritus and scratching, especially on the trunk and neck. Among the secondary lesions produced are parallel linear scratches and a slight degree of eczema. In long-standing cases, the skin may become thick, dry, and scaly, with dark pigmented areas.

Pruritus is the most common symptom of pediculosis pubis, particularly at night. Reddish-brown dust (ie, excretions of the insects) may be found in the patient's underclothing. The pubic area should be examined with a magnifying glass for lice crawling down a hair shaft or nits cemented to the hair or at the junction with the skin. Infestation by pubic lice may coexist with sexually transmitted diseases such as gonorrhea, herpes, or syphilis. There may also be infestation of the hairs of the chest, armpit, beard, and eyelashes. Gray-blue macules may sometimes be seen on the trunk, thighs, and axillae as a result of either the reaction of the insects' saliva with bilirubin (converting it to biliverdin) or an excretion produced by the salivary glands of the louse.

MEDICAL MANAGEMENT

The patient is instructed to bathe with soap and water, after which a prescription scabicide (lindane [Kwell] or 5% permethrin [Elimite]) is applied to affected areas of the skin and to hairy areas, according to the product directions. An alternative topical therapy is an over-the-counter strength of permethrin (1% Nix). If the eyelashes are involved, petrolatum may be thickly applied twice daily for 8 days, followed by mechanical removal of any remaining nits.

Complications, such as severe pruritus, pyoderma, and dermatitis, are treated with antipruritics, systemic antibiotics, and topical corticosteroids. Body lice can transmit epidemic rickettsial disease (eg, epidemic typhus, relapsing fever, and trench fever) to humans. The causative organism may be in the gastrointestinal tract of the insect and may be excreted on the skin surface of the infested person.

NURSING MANAGEMENT

All family members and sexual contacts must be treated and instructed about personal hygiene and methods to prevent or control infestation. The patient and partner must also be scheduled for a diagnostic workup for coexisting sexually transmitted disease. All clothing and bedding should be machine washed in hot water or dry-cleaned.

Scabies

Scabies is an infestation of the skin by the itch mite *Sarcoptes scabiei*. The disease may be found in people living in substandard hygienic conditions, but it can occur in anyone. Infestations may or may not be associated with sexual activity. The mites frequently involve the fingers, and hand contact may produce infection. In children, overnight stays with friends or the exchange of clothes may be a source of infection. Health care personnel who have prolonged hands-on physical contact with an infected patient may become infected.

Clinical Manifestations

It takes approximately 4 weeks from the time of contact for the patient's symptoms to appear. The patient complains of severe itching caused by a delayed type of immunologic reaction to the mite or its fecal pellets. During examination, the patient is asked where the pruritus is most severe. A magnifying glass and a penlight are held at an oblique angle to the skin while a search is made for the small, raised burrows created by the mites. The burrows may be multiple, straight or wavy, brown or black, threadlike lesions, most commonly observed between the fingers and on the wrists. Other sites are the extensor surfaces of the elbows, the knees, the edges of the feet, the points of the elbows, around the nipples, in the axillary folds, under pendulous breasts, and in or near the groin or gluteal fold, penis, or scrotum. Red, pruritic eruptions usually appear between adjacent skin areas. However, the burrow is not always visible. Any patient with a rash may have scabies.

One classic sign of scabies is the increased itching that occurs during the overnight hours, perhaps because the increased warmth of the skin has a stimulating effect on the parasite. Hypersensitivity to the organism and its products of excretion also may contribute to the pruritus. If the infection has spread, other members of the family and close friends also complain of pruritus about a month later.

Secondary lesions are quite common and include vesicles, papules, excoriations, and crusts. Bacterial superinfection may result from constant excoriation of the burrows and papules.

Gerontologic Considerations

Elderly patients living in long-term care facilities are susceptible to outbreaks of scabies because of close living quarters, poor hygiene due to limited physical ability, and the potential for incidental spread of the organisms by staff members. Although pruritus may be severe in the older patient, the vivid inflammatory reaction seen in younger people seldom occurs. Scabies may not be recognized in the elderly person; the pruritus may erroneously be attributed to the dry skin of old age or to anxiety.

Health care personnel in extended-care facilities should wear gloves when providing hands-on care for a patient suspected of having scabies until the diagnosis is confirmed and treatment completed. It is advisable to treat all residents, staff, and families of patients at the same time to prevent reinfection. Because geriatric patients may be more sensitive to side effects of the scabicides, they should be closely observed for reactions.

Assessment and Diagnostic Findings

The diagnosis is confirmed by recovering *S. scabiei* or the mites' byproducts from the skin. A sample of superficial epidermis is scraped from the top of the burrows or papules with a small scalpel blade. The scrapings are placed on a microscope slide and examined through a microscope at low power to demonstrate evidence of the mite.

Medical Management

The patient is instructed to take a warm, soapy bath or shower to remove the scaling debris from the crusts and then to dry thoroughly and allow the skin to cool. A prescription scabicide, such as lindane (Kwell), crotamiton (Eurax), or 5% permethrin (Elimite), is applied thinly to the entire skin from the neck down, sparing only the face and scalp (which are not affected in scabies). The medication is left on for 12 to 24 hours, after which the patient is instructed to wash thoroughly. One application may be curative, but it is advisable to repeat the treatment in 1 week.

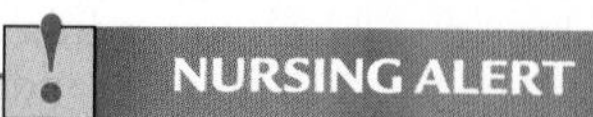

The patient must understand medication instructions, because application of a scabicide immediately after bathing and before the skin dries and cools increases percutaneous absorption of the scabicide and the potential for central nervous system abnormalities such as seizures.

Nursing Management

The patient should wear clean clothing and sleep between freshly laundered bed linens. All bedding and clothing should be washed in hot water and dried on the hot dryer cycle. If bed linens or clothing cannot be washed in hot water, dry-cleaning is advised.

After treatment is completed, the patient should apply an ointment, such as a topical corticosteroid, to skin lesions because the scabicide may irritate the skin. The patient's hypersensitivity does not cease on destruction of the mites. Pruritus may continue for several weeks as a manifestation of hypersensitivity, particularly in atopic (allergic) people. This is not a sign that the treatment has failed. The patient is instructed (1) not to apply more scabicide, because it will cause more irritation and increased itching, and (2) not to take frequent hot showers, because they can dry the skin and produce pruritus. Oral antihistamines such as diphenhydramine (Benadryl) or hydroxyzine (Atarax) can help control the pruritus.

All family members and close contacts should be treated simultaneously to eliminate the mites. Some scabicides are approved for use in infants and pregnant women. If scabies is sexually transmitted, the patient may require treatment for coexisting sexually transmitted disease. Scabies may also coexist with pediculosis.

Contact Dermatitis

Contact dermatitis is an inflammatory reaction of the skin to physical, chemical, or biologic agents. The epidermis is damaged by repeated physical and chemical irritations. Contact dermatitis may be of the primary irritant type, in which a nonallergic reaction results from exposure to an irritating substance, or it may be an allergic reaction resulting from exposure of sensitized people to contact allergens. Allergic dermatoses are discussed in Chapter 53. Common causes of irritant dermatitis are soaps, detergents, scouring compounds, and industrial chemicals. Predisposing factors include extremes of heat and cold, frequent contact with soap and water, and a preexisting skin disease (Chart 56-4).

Clinical Manifestations

The eruptions begin when the causative agent contacts the skin. The first reactions include pruritus, burning, and erythema, followed closely by edema, papules, vesicles, and oozing or weeping. In the subacute phase, these vesicular changes are less marked, and they alternate with crusting, drying, fissuring, and peeling. If repeated reactions occur or if the patient continually scratches the skin, lichenification and pigmentation occur. Secondary bacterial invasion may follow.

Medical Management

The objectives of management are to rest the involved skin and protect it from further damage. The distribution pattern of the reaction is identified to differentiate between allergic and irritant contact dermatitis. A detailed history is obtained. If possible, the offending irritant is removed. Local irritation should be avoided, and soap is not generally used until healing occurs.

Many preparations are advocated for relieving dermatitis. In general, a bland, unmedicated lotion is used for small patches of erythema. Cool, wet dressings also are applied

CHART 56-4

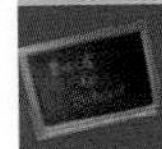

Patient Education

Strategies for Avoiding Contact Dermatitis

The following precautions may help prevent repeated cases of contact dermatitis. Follow these instructions for at least 4 months after your skin appears to be completely healed.

- Study the pattern and location of your dermatitis and think about which things have touched your skin and which things may have caused the problem.
- Try to avoid contact with these materials.
- Avoid heat, soap, and rubbing, all of which are external irritants.
- Choose bath soaps, laundry detergents, and cosmetics that do not contain fragrance.
- Avoid using a fabric softener dryer sheet (Bounce, Cling Free). Fabric softeners that are added to the washer may be used.
- Avoid topical medications, lotions, or ointments, except those specifically prescribed for your condition.
- Wash your skin thoroughly immediately after exposure to possible irritants.
- When wearing gloves (for example, for washing dishes or general cleaning), be sure they are cotton-lined. Do not wear them more than 15 or 20 minutes at a time.

over small areas of vesicular dermatitis. Finely cracked ice added to the water often enhances its antipruritic effect.

Wet dressings usually help clear the oozing eczematous lesions. A thin layer of cream or ointment containing a corticosteroid then may be used. Medicated baths at room temperature are prescribed for larger areas of dermatitis. For severe, widespread conditions, a short course of systemic corticosteroids may be prescribed.

Noninfectious Inflammatory Dermatoses

Psoriasis

Considered one of the most common skin diseases, psoriasis affects approximately 2% of the population, appearing more often in people of European ancestry. It is thought that this chronic, noninfectious, inflammatory disease stems from a hereditary defect that causes overproduction of keratin. Onset may occur at any age, but psoriasis is most common in people between 15 and 35 years of age. Psoriasis has a tendency to improve and then recur periodically throughout life (Porth, 2005).

Pathophysiology

Although the primary cause of psoriasis is unknown, a combination of specific genetic makeup and environmental stimuli may trigger the onset of disease. Current evidence supports an immunologic basis for the disease (Porth, 2005). Periods of emotional stress and anxiety aggravate the condition, and trauma, infections, and seasonal and hormonal changes also are trigger factors.

Epidermal cells are produced at a rate that is about six to nine times faster than normal. The cells in the basal layer of the skin divide too quickly, and the newly formed cells move so rapidly to the skin surface that they become evident as profuse scales or plaques of epidermal tissue. The psoriatic epidermal cell may travel from the basal cell layer of the epidermis to the stratum corneum and be cast off in 3 to 4 days, which is in sharp contrast to the normal 26 to 28 days. As a result of the increased number of basal cells and rapid cell passage, the normal events of cell maturation and growth cannot take place. This abnormal process does not allow the normal protective layers of the skin to form.

Clinical Manifestations

Lesions appear as red, raised patches of skin covered with silvery scales. The scaly patches are formed by the buildup of living and dead skin resulting from the vast increase in the rate of skin-cell growth and turnover (Fig. 56-4). If the scales are scraped away, the dark-red base of the lesion is exposed, producing multiple bleeding points. These patches are not moist and may be pruritic. One variation of this condition is called guttate (in the shape of a drop) psoriasis because the lesions remain about 1 cm wide and are scattered like raindrops over the body. This variation is believed to be associated with a recent streptococcal throat infection. Psoriasis may range in severity from a cosmetic source of annoyance to a physically disabling and disfiguring disorder.

Particular sites of the body tend to be affected most by this condition; they include the scalp, the extensor surface of the elbows and knees, the lower part of the back, and the geni-

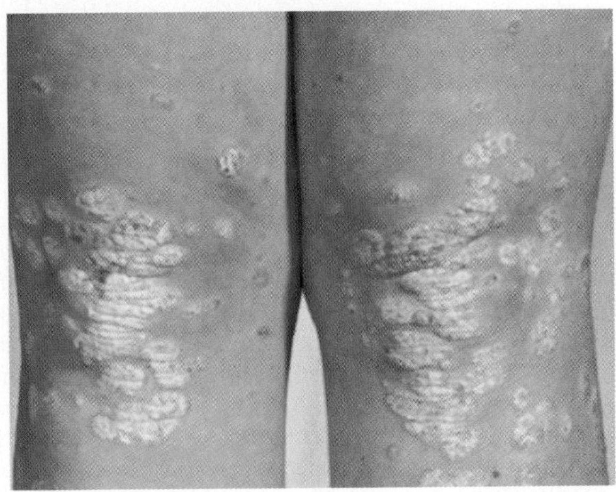

FIGURE 56-4. Psoriasis. Courtesy of Roche Laboratories.

talia. Bilateral symmetry is a feature of psoriasis. In approximately one fourth to one half of patients, the nails are involved, with pitting, discoloration, crumbling beneath the free edges, and separation of the nail plate. When psoriasis occurs on the palms and soles, it can cause pustular lesions called palmar pustular psoriasis.

Complications

Asymmetric rheumatoid factor–negative arthritis of multiple joints occurs in about 5% of people with psoriasis. The arthritic development can occur before or after the skin lesions appear. The relationship between arthritis and psoriasis is not understood, although recent studies suggest an interplay between genetics, environmental factors, and the immune system (Porth, 2005). Psoriatic arthritis is discussed in more detail later in this chapter.

Erythrodermic psoriasis, an exfoliative psoriatic state, involves disease progression that involves the total body surface. The patient is acutely ill, with fever, chills, and an electrolyte imbalance. Erythrodermic psoriasis often appears in people with chronic psoriasis after infections, after exposure to certain medications, or following withdrawal of systemic corticosteroids.

Assessment and Diagnostic Findings

The presence of the classic plaque-type lesions generally confirms the diagnosis of psoriasis. Because the lesions tend to change histologically as they progress from early to chronic plaques, biopsy of the skin is of little diagnostic value. There are no specific blood tests for diagnosing the condition. When in doubt, the health care provider should assess for signs of nail and scalp involvement and for a positive family history.

Medical Management

The goals of management are to slow the rapid turnover of epidermis, to promote resolution of the psoriatic lesions, and to control the natural cycles of the disease. There is no known cure.

The therapeutic approach should be one that the patient understands; it should be cosmetically acceptable and minimally disruptive of lifestyle. Treatment involves the commitment of time and effort by the patient and possibly the family. First, any precipitating or aggravating factors are addressed. An assessment is made of lifestyle, because psoriasis is significantly affected by stress. The patient is informed that treatment of severe psoriasis can be time-consuming, expensive, and aesthetically unappealing at times.

The most important principle of psoriasis treatment is gentle removal of scales. This can be accomplished with baths. Oils (eg, olive oil, mineral oil, Aveeno Oilated Oatmeal Bath) or coal tar preparations (eg, Balnetar) can be added to the bath water and a soft brush used to scrub the psoriatic plaques gently. After bathing, the application of emollient creams containing alpha-hydroxy acids (eg, Lac-Hydrin, Penederm) or salicylic acid continues to soften thick scales. The patient and family should be encouraged to establish a regular skin care routine that can be maintained even when the psoriasis is not in an acute stage.

Pharmacologic Therapy

With the recent addition of biologic medications, four types of therapy are now commonly used: topical, intralesional, oral, and injectable (Table 56-6).

TOPICAL AGENTS

Topically applied agents are used to slow the overactive epidermis without affecting other tissues. These agents

℞ TABLE 56-6 Current Pharmacologic Treatment for Psoriasis

Topical Agents	Use	Selected Agents
Biologicals	Moderate to severe lesions	Cyclosporine (Neoral), alefacept (Amevive), etanercept (Enbrel), infliximab (Remicade)
Topical corticosteroids	Mild to moderate lesions	Aristocort, Kenalog, Valisone
	Moderate to severe lesions	Lidex, Psorcon, Cutivate
	Severe lesions	Temovate, Diprolene, Ultravate
	Lesions on face and groin	Aclovate, DesOwen, Hytone 2.5%
Topical nonsteroidals	Mild to severe	Retinoids such as tazarotene (Tazorac) Vitamin D_3 derivative calcipotriene (Dovonex)
Coal tar products	Mild to moderate lesions	Coal tar and salicylic acid ointment (Aquatar, Estar gel, Fototar, Zetar); anthralin (AnthraDerm, Dritho-Cream); Neutrogena T-Derm, Psori Gel
Medicated shampoos	Scalp lesions	Neutrogena T-Gel, T-Sal, Zetar, Head & Shoulders, Desenex, Selsun Blue, Bakers P&S (emulsifying agent with phenol, saline solution, and mineral oil)
Intralesional therapy	Thick plaques and nails	Kenalog, Cordran-impregnated tape, Fluoroplex
Systemic therapy	Extensive lesions and nails	Methotrexate (Folex, Mexate); hydrourea (Hydrea); retinoic acid (Tegison) (not to be used in women of childbearing age)
	Psoriatic arthritis	Oral gold (auranofin), etrentinate, methotrexate
Photochemotherapy	Moderate to severe lesions	UVA or UVB light with or without topical medications PUVA (combines UVA light with oral psoralens, or topical tripsoralen)

include lotions, ointments, pastes, creams, and shampoos. Topical corticosteroids may be applied for their anti-inflammatory effect. Choosing the correct strength of corticosteroid for the involved site and choosing the most effective vehicle base are important aspects of topical treatment. In general, high-potency topical corticosteroids should not be used on the face and intertriginous areas, and their use on other areas should be limited to a 4-week course of twice-daily applications. A 2-week break should be taken before repeating treatment with the high-potency corticosteroids. For long-term therapy, moderate-potency corticosteroids are used. On the face and intertriginous areas, only low-potency corticosteroids are appropriate for long-term use (see Table 56-3).

Occlusive dressings may be applied to increase the effectiveness of the corticosteroid. Large plastic bags may be used—one for the upper body with openings cut for the head and arms and one for the lower body with openings for the legs. Large rolls of tubular plastic can be used to cover the arms and legs. Another option is a vinyl jogging suit. The medication is applied, and the suit is put on over it. The hands can be wrapped in gloves, the feet in plastic bags, and the head in a shower cap. Occlusive dressings should not remain in place longer than 8 hours. The skin should be inspected carefully for the appearance of atrophy, hypopigmentation, striae, and telangiectasias, all side effects of corticosteroids.

NURSING ALERT

When plastic substances are used, the nurse needs to check for flammability. Some thin plastic films burn slowly (if touched by a lighted cigarette), whereas others burst rapidly into flame. The patient should be cautioned not to smoke while wrapped in a plastic dressing.

When psoriasis involves large areas of the body, topical corticosteroid treatment can be expensive and involve some systemic risk. The more potent corticosteroids, when applied to large areas of the body, have the potential to cause adrenal suppression through percutaneous absorption of the medication. In this event, other treatment modalities (eg, nonsteroidal topical medications, ultraviolet light) may be used instead or in combination to decrease the need for corticosteroids.

Two topical nonsteroidal treatments introduced within the past few years are calcipotriene (Dovonex) and tazarotene (Tazorac). Treatment with these agents tends to suppress **epidermopoiesis** (ie, development of epidermal cells) and cause sloughing of the rapidly growing epidermal cells. Calcipotriene 0.05% is a derivative of vitamin D_2. It works by decreasing the mitotic turnover of the psoriatic plaques. Its most common side effect is local irritation. The intertriginous areas and face should be avoided when using this medication. The patient should be monitored for symptoms of hypercalcemia. Calcipotriene is available as a cream for use on the body and a solution for the scalp. It is not recommended for use by elderly patients because of their more fragile skin or by pregnant or lactating women.

Tazarotene, a retinoid, causes sloughing of the scales covering psoriatic plaques. As with other retinoids, it causes increased sensitivity to sunlight by loss of the outermost layer of skin, so the patient should be cautioned to use an effective sunscreen and avoid other photosensitizers (eg, tetracycline, antihistamines). Tazarotene is listed as a Category X drug in pregnancy; reports indicate evidence of fetal risk, and the risk of use in pregnant women clearly outweighs any possible benefits. A negative result on a pregnancy test should be obtained before initiating this medication in women of childbearing age, and an effective contraceptive should be continued during treatment. Side effects include burning, erythema, or irritation at the site of application and worsening of psoriasis.

INTRALESIONAL AGENTS

Intralesional injections of the corticosteroid triamcinolone acetonide (Aristocort, Kenalog-10, Trymex) can be administered directly into highly visible or isolated patches of psoriasis that are resistant to other forms of therapy. Care must be taken to ensure that the medication is not injected into normal skin.

SYSTEMIC AGENTS

Although systemic corticosteroids may cause rapid improvement of psoriasis, their usual risks and the possibility of triggering a severe flare-up on withdrawal limit their use. Systemic cytotoxic preparations, such as methotrexate, have been used in treating extensive psoriasis that fails to respond to other forms of therapy.

Methotrexate appears to inhibit DNA synthesis in epidermal cells, thereby reducing the turnover time of the psoriatic epidermis. However, the medication can be toxic, especially to the liver, kidneys, and bone marrow. Laboratory studies must be monitored to ensure that the hepatic, hematopoietic, and renal systems are functioning adequately. The patient should avoid drinking alcohol while taking methotrexate, because alcohol ingestion increases the possibility of liver damage. The medication is teratogenic (produces physical defects in the fetus) and thus should not be administered to pregnant women.

Hydroxyurea (Hydrea) also inhibits cell replication by affecting DNA synthesis. The patient is monitored for signs and symptoms of bone marrow depression.

Cyclosporine A, a cyclic peptide used to prevent rejection of transplanted organs, has shown some success in treating severe, therapy-resistant cases of psoriasis. However, its use is limited by side effects such as hypertension and nephrotoxicity.

Oral retinoids (ie, synthetic derivatives of vitamin A and its metabolite, vitamin A acid) modulate the growth and differentiation of epithelial tissue. Etretinate is especially useful for severe pustular or erythrodermic psoriasis. Etretinate is a teratogen with a very long half-life; it cannot be used in women with childbearing potential.

PHOTOCHEMOTHERAPY

One treatment for severely debilitating psoriasis is a psoralen (phototoxic) medication (eg, methoxsalen) combined with ultraviolet-A (PUVA) light therapy. Ultraviolet light is the portion of the electromagnetic spectrum containing wavelengths ranging from 180 to 400 nm. In this treatment, the patient takes a photosensitizing medication (usually 8-methoxypsoralen) in a standard dose and is subsequently exposed to long-wave ultraviolet light as the medication plasma levels peak. Although the mechanism of action is not completely understood, it is thought that when psoralen-treated skin is exposed to ultraviolet-A light, the psoralen binds with DNA and decreases cellular proliferation. PUVA is not without its hazards; it has been associated with long-term risks of skin cancer, cataracts, and premature aging of the skin (Porth, 2005).

The PUVA unit consists of a chamber that contains high-output black-light lamps and an external reflectance system. The exposure time is calibrated according to the specific unit in use and the anticipated tolerance of the patient's skin. The patient is usually treated two or three times each week until the psoriasis clears. An interim period of 48 hours between treatments is necessary; it takes this long for any burns resulting from PUVA therapy to become evident.

After the psoriasis clears, the patient begins a maintenance program. Once little or no disease is active, less potent therapies are used to keep minor flare-ups under control.

Ultraviolet-B (UVB) light therapy is also used to treat generalized plaques. UVB light ranges from 270 to 350 nm, although research has shown that a narrow range, 310 to 312 nm, is the action spectrum. It is used alone or combined with topical coal tar. Side effects are similar to those of PUVA therapy. Another development in light therapy is the narrow-band UVB, which ranges from 311 to 312 nm, decreasing exposure to harmful ultraviolet energy while providing more intense, specific therapy (Koo, Lowe, & Lew-Kaya, 2000).

If access to a light treatment unit is not feasible, the patient can expose himself or herself to sunlight. The risks of all light treatments are similar and include acute sunburn reaction; exacerbation of photosensitive disorders such as lupus, rosacea, and polymorphic light eruption; as well as other skin changes such as increased wrinkles, thickening, and an increased risk for skin cancer.

Excimer lasers have come into use in treating psoriasis. These lasers function at 308 nm. Studies show that medium-sized psoriatic plaques clear in four to six treatments and remain clear for up to 9 months. A laser can be more effective on the scalp or on other hard-to-treat areas, because it can be aimed very specifically on the plaque (Lask & Lowe, 2000). Table 56-6 summarizes the treatment options.

Nursing Process

Care of the Patient With Psoriasis

Assessment

The nursing assessment focuses on the appearance of the normal skin, the appearance of the skin lesions, and how the patient is coping with the psoriatic skin condition. The notable manifestations are red, scaling papules that coalesce to form oval, well-defined plaques. Silver-white scales may also be present. Adjacent skin areas show red, smooth plaques with a macerated surface. It is important to examine the areas especially prone to psoriasis: elbows, knees, scalp, gluteal cleft, and all nails (for small pits).

Psoriasis may cause despair and frustration for the patient; observers may stare, comment, ask embarrassing questions, or even avoid the person. The disease can eventually exhaust the patient's resources, interfere with his or her job, and negatively affect many aspects of life. Teenagers are especially vulnerable to the psychological effects of this disorder. The family, too, is affected, because time-consuming treatments and constant shedding of scales may disrupt home life and cause resentment. The patient's frustrations may be expressed through hostility directed at health care personnel and others.

The nurse assesses the impact of the disease on the patient and the coping strategies used for conducting normal activities and interactions with family and friends. Many patients need reassurance that the condition is not infectious, is not a reflection of poor personal hygiene, and is not skin cancer. The nurse can create an environment in which the patient feels comfortable discussing important quality-of-life issues related to his or her psychosocial and physical response to this chronic illness.

Diagnosis

Nursing Diagnoses

Based on the nursing assessment data, the patient's major nursing diagnoses may include the following:

- Deficient knowledge about the disease process and treatment
- Impaired skin integrity related to lesions and inflammatory response
- Disturbed body image related to embarrassment about appearance and self-perception of uncleanliness

Collaborative Problems/ Potential Complications

Based on the assessment data, potential complications include the following:

- Infection
- Psoriatic arthritis

Planning and Goals

Major goals for the patient may include increased understanding of psoriasis and the treatment regimen, achievement of smoother skin with control of lesions, development of self-acceptance, and absence of complications.

Nursing Interventions

Promoting Understanding

The nurse explains with sensitivity that although there is no cure for psoriasis and lifetime management is necessary, the condition can usually be controlled. The pathophysiology of psoriasis is reviewed, as are the factors that provoke it—irritation or injury to the skin (eg, cut, abrasion, sunburn), current illness (eg, pharyngeal streptococcal infection), and emotional stress. It is emphasized that repeated trauma to the skin and an unfavorable environment (eg, cold) or a specific medication (eg, lithium, beta-blockers, indomethacin) may exacerbate psoriasis. The patient is cautioned about taking any nonprescription medications because some may aggravate mild psoriasis.

Reviewing and explaining the treatment regimen are essential to ensure compliance. For example, if the patient has a mild condition confined to localized areas, such as the elbows or knees, application of an emollient to maintain softness and minimize scaling may be all that is required. Most patients need a comprehensive plan of care that ranges from using topical medications and shampoos to more complex and lengthy treatment with systemic medications and photochemotherapy, such as PUVA therapy. Patient education materials that include a description of the therapy and specific guidelines are helpful but cannot replace face-to-face discussions of the treatment plan.

Increasing Skin Integrity

To avoid injuring the skin, the patient is advised not to pick at or scratch the affected areas. Measures to prevent dry skin are encouraged because dry skin worsens psoriasis. Too-frequent washing produces more soreness and scaling. Water should be warm, not hot, and the skin should be dried by patting with a towel rather than by rubbing. Emollients have a moisturizing effect, providing an occlusive film on the skin surface so that normal water loss through the skin is halted and allowing the trapped water to hydrate the stratum corneum. A bath oil or emollient cleansing agent can comfort sore and scaling skin. Softening the skin can prevent fissures.

Improving Self-Concept and Body Image

A therapeutic relationship between health care professionals and the patient with psoriasis is one that includes education and support. After the treatment regimen is established, the patient should begin to feel more confident and empowered in carrying it out and in using coping strategies that help him or her deal with the altered self-concept and body image brought about by the disease. Introducing the patient to successful coping strategies used by others with psoriasis and making suggestions for reducing or coping with stressful situations at home, school, and work can facilitate a more positive outlook and acceptance of the chronicity of the disease.

Monitoring and Managing Potential Complications

PSORIATIC ARTHRITIS

The diagnosis of psoriasis, especially when it is accompanied by the complication of arthritis, is usually difficult to make. Psoriatic arthritis involving the sacroiliac and distal joints of the fingers may be overlooked, especially if the patient has the typical psoriatic lesions. However, patients who complain of mild joint discomfort and some pitting of the fingernails may not be diagnosed with psoriasis until the more obvious cutaneous lesions appear.

The complaint of joint discomfort in the patient with psoriasis should be noted and evaluated. The symptoms of psoriatic arthritis can mimic the symptoms of Reiter's disease and ankylosing spondylitis, and a definitive diagnosis must be made. Treatment of the condition usually involves joint rest, application of heat, and salicylates.

The patient requires education about the care and treatment of the involved joints and the need for compliance with therapy. The incidence of psoriatic arthropathy is unknown because the symptoms are so variable. However, it is believed that when the psoriasis is extensive and a family history of inflammatory arthritis is elicited, the chance that the patient will develop psoriatic arthritis increases substantially. It is recommended that a rheumatologist be consulted to assist in the diagnosis and treatment of the arthropathy.

Promoting Home and Community-Based Care

TEACHING PATIENTS SELF-CARE

Printed patient education materials may be provided to reinforce face-to-face discussions about treatment guidelines and other considerations. Patients using topical corticosteroid preparations repeatedly on the face and around the eyes should be aware that cataract development is possible. Strict guidelines for applying these medications should be emphasized because overuse can result in skin atrophy, striae, and medication resistance.

PUVA, which is reserved for moderate to severe psoriasis, produces photosensitization, which means that the skin is sensitive to the sun until methoxsalen has been excreted from the body in about 6 to 8 hours. Patients undergoing PUVA treatments should avoid exposure to the sun. If exposure is unavoidable, the skin must be protected with sunscreen and clothing. Gray- or green-tinted wraparound sunglasses should be worn to protect the eyes during and after treatment, and ophthalmologic examinations should be performed on a regular basis. Nausea associated with methoxsalen (a psoralen medication) is lessened when the medication is taken with food. Lubricants and bath oils may be used to help remove scales and prevent excessive dryness. No other creams or oils are to be used except on areas that have been shielded from ultraviolet light. Contraceptives should be used by sexually active women of reproductive age, because the teratogenic effect of PUVA has not been determined. The patient is kept under constant and careful supervision and is encouraged to recognize unusual changes in the skin.

If indicated, referral may be made to a mental health professional who can help to ease emotional strain and give support. Belonging to a support group may also help patients recognize that they are not alone in experiencing life adjustments in response to a visible, chronic disease. The National Psoriasis Foundation publishes periodic bulletins and reports about new and relevant developments in this condition.

Chart 56-5 is a Home Care Checklist for the patient with psoriasis.

Evaluation

Expected Patient Outcomes

Expected patient outcomes may include the following:

1. Demonstrates knowledge and understanding of disease process and its treatment
   a. Describes psoriasis and the prescribed therapy
   b. Verbalizes that trauma, infection, and emotional stress may be trigger factors
   c. Maintains control with appropriate therapy
   d. Demonstrates proper application of topical therapy
2. Achieves smoother skin and control of lesions
   a. Exhibits no new lesions
   b. Keeps skin lubricated and soft
3. Develops self-acceptance
   a. Identifies someone with whom to discuss feelings and concerns
   b. Expresses optimism about outcomes of treatment
4. Absence of complications
   a. Has no joint discomfort
   b. Reports control of cutaneous lesions with no extension of disease

Exfoliative Dermatitis

Exfoliative dermatitis is a serious condition characterized by progressive inflammation in which generalized erythema and scaling occur. It may be associated with chills, fever, prostration, severe toxicity, and a pruritic scaling of the skin. There is a profound loss of stratum corneum (ie, outermost layer of the skin), which causes capillary leakage, hypoproteinemia, and negative nitrogen balance. Because of widespread dilation of cutaneous vessels, large amounts of body heat are lost, and exfoliative dermatitis has a marked effect on the entire body.

Exfoliative dermatitis has a variety of causes. It is considered to be a secondary or reactive process to an underlying skin or systemic disease. It may appear as a part of the lymphoma group of diseases and may precede the clinical manifestations of lymphoma. Preexisting skin disorders that have been implicated as a cause include psoriasis, atopic dermatitis, and contact dermatitis. It also appears as a severe reaction to many medications, including penicillin and phenylbutazone. The cause is unknown in approximately 25% of cases (Odom, James, & Berger, 2000).

Clinical Manifestations

This condition starts acutely as a patchy or a generalized erythematous eruption accompanied by fever, malaise, and occasionally gastrointestinal symptoms. The skin color changes from pink to dark red. After a week, the characteristic exfoliation (ie, scaling) begins, usually in the form of thin flakes that leave the underlying skin smooth and red, with new scales forming as the older ones come off. Hair loss may accompany this disorder. Relapses are common. The systemic effects include high-output heart failure, intestinal disturbances, breast enlargement, elevated levels of uric acid in the blood (ie, hyperuricemia), and temperature disturbances.

Medical Management

The objectives of management are to maintain fluid and electrolyte balance and to prevent infection. The treatment is individualized and supportive and should be initiated as soon as the condition is diagnosed.

The patient may be hospitalized and placed on bed rest. All medications that may be implicated are discontinued. A

CHART 56-5

HOME CARE CHECKLIST • The Patient With Psoriasis

At the completion of the home care instruction, the patient or caregiver will be able to:	Patient	Caregiver
• Describe the etiology of psoriasis.	✔	✔
• Describe optimal skin maintenance practices to maintain moisture of skin and prevent infection.	✔	✔
• Demonstrate correct application of prescribed topical medications.	✔	✔
• Describe common side effects of oral medication, if prescribed.	✔	✔
• Demonstrate appropriate therapeutic bath technique, if prescribed.	✔	✔
• Verbalize optimism about condition.	✔	
• Identify a support person with whom to discuss feelings and concerns.	✔	

comfortable room temperature should be maintained because the patient does not have normal thermoregulatory control as a result of temperature fluctuations caused by vasodilation and evaporative water loss. Fluid and electrolyte balance must be maintained because there is considerable water and protein loss from the skin surface. Administration of plasma volume expanders may be indicated.

Nursing Management

Continual nursing assessment is carried out to detect infection. The disrupted, erythematous, moist skin is susceptible to infection and becomes colonized with pathogenic organisms, which produce more inflammation. Antibiotics, which are prescribed if infection is present, are selected on the basis of culture and sensitivity.

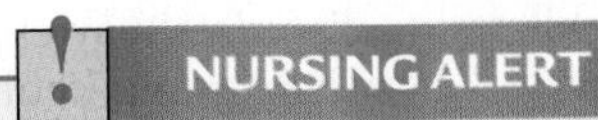

The nurse observes the patient for signs and symptoms of heart failure because hyperemia and increased cutaneous blood flow can produce high-output cardiac failure.

Hypothermia may occur because increased blood flow in the skin, coupled with increased water loss through the skin, leads to heat loss by radiation, conduction, and evaporation. Changes in vital signs are closely monitored and reported.

As in any acute dermatitis, topical therapy is used to provide symptomatic relief. Soothing baths, compresses, and lubrication with emollients are used to treat the extensive dermatitis. The patient is likely to be extremely irritable because of the severe pruritus. Oral or parenteral corticosteroids may be prescribed when the disease is not controlled by more conservative therapy. When a specific cause is known, more specific therapy may be used. The patient is advised to avoid all irritants in the future, particularly medications that are known to cause the disease.

Blistering Diseases

Blisters of the skin have many origins, including bacterial, fungal, or viral infections; allergic contact reactions; burns; metabolic disorders; and immunologically mediated reactions. Some of these have been discussed previously (eg, herpes simplex and zoster infections, contact dermatitis). Immunologically mediated diseases are autoimmune reactions and represent a defect of IgM, IgE, IgG, and C3. Some of these conditions are life-threatening; others become chronic.

The diagnosis is always made by histologic examination of a biopsy specimen, usually by a dermatopathologist. A specimen from the blister and surrounding skin demonstrates **acantholysis** (separation of epidermal cells from each other because of damage to or an abnormality of the intracellular substance). Circulating antibodies may be detected by immunofluorescent studies of the patient's serum.

Pemphigus

Pemphigus is a group of serious diseases of the skin characterized by the appearance of bullae (blisters) of various sizes on apparently normal skin (Fig. 56-5) and mucous membranes. Pemphigus is an autoimmune disease involving immunoglobulin G. It is thought that the pemphigus antibody is directed against a specific cell-surface antigen in epidermal cells. A blister forms from the antigen–antibody reaction. The level of serum antibody is predictive of disease severity. Genetic factors may also have a role in its development, with the highest incidence among those of Jewish or Mediterranean descent. This disorder usually occurs in men and women in middle and late adulthood. The condition may be associated with penicillins and captopril and with myasthenia gravis.

Clinical Manifestations

Most patients present with oral lesions appearing as irregularly shaped erosions that are painful, bleed easily, and heal slowly. The skin bullae enlarge, rupture, and leave large, painful eroded areas that are accompanied by crusting and oozing. A characteristic offensive odor emanates from the bullae and the exuding serum. There is blistering or sloughing of uninvolved skin when minimal pressure is applied (Nikolsky's sign). The eroded skin heals slowly, and large areas of the body eventually are involved. Bacterial superinfection is common.

Complications

The most common complications arise when the disease process is widespread. Before the advent of corticosteroid and immunosuppressive therapy, patients were very susceptible to secondary bacterial infection. Skin bacteria have relatively easy access to the bullae as they ooze, rupture, and leave denuded areas exposed to the environment. Fluid and electrolyte imbalance results from fluid and protein loss as the bullae rupture. Hypoalbuminemia is common when the disease process includes extensive areas of the body skin surface and mucous membranes.

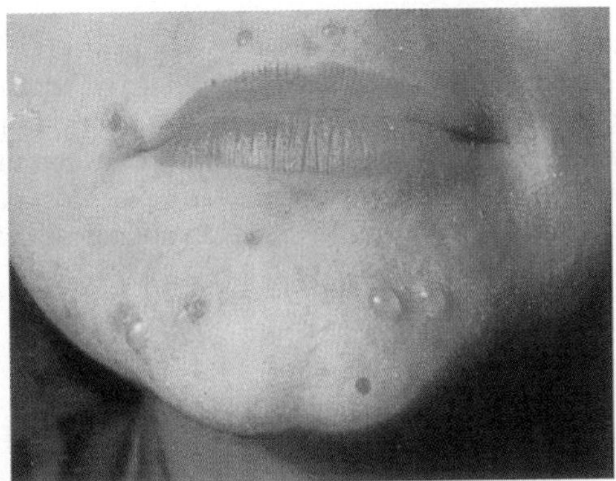

FIGURE 56-5. Vesicles on the chin (in pemphigus). From Hall, J. C. (1999). *Sauer's manual of skin diseases.* Philadelphia: Lippincott Williams & Wilkins.

Management

The goals of therapy are to bring the disease under control as rapidly as possible, to prevent loss of serum and the development of secondary infection, and to promote re-epithelization (ie, renewal of epithelial tissue).

Corticosteroids are administered in high doses to control the disease and keep the skin free of blisters. The high dosage level is maintained until remission is apparent. In some cases, corticosteroid therapy must be maintained for life. High-dose corticosteroid therapy has serious toxic effects (see Chapter 42).

Immunosuppressive agents (eg, azathioprine, cyclophosphamide, gold) may be prescribed to help control the disease and reduce the corticosteroid dose. **Plasmapheresis** temporarily decreases the serum antibody level and has been used with variable success, although it is generally reserved for life-threatening cases.

Bullous Pemphigoid

Bullous pemphigoid is an acquired disease of flaccid blisters appearing on normal or erythematous skin. It appears more often on the flexor surfaces of the arms, legs, axilla, and groin. Oral lesions, if present, are usually transient and minimal. When the blisters break, the skin has shallow erosions that heal fairly quickly. Pruritus can be intense, even before the appearance of the blisters. Bullous pemphigoid is common in the elderly, with a peak incidence at about 60 years of age. There is no gender or racial predilection, and the disease can be found throughout the world.

Management

Medical treatment includes topical corticosteroids for localized eruptions and systemic corticosteroids for widespread involvement. Systemic corticosteroids (eg, prednisone) may be continued for months, in alternate-day doses. The patient needs to understand the implications of long-term corticosteroid therapy (see Chapter 42).

Dermatitis Herpetiformis

Dermatitis herpetiformis is an intensely pruritic, chronic disease that manifests with small, tense blisters that are distributed symmetrically over the elbows, knees, buttocks, and nape of the neck. It is most common between the ages of 20 and 40 years but can appear at any age. Most patients with dermatitis herpetiformis have a subclinical defect in gluten metabolism.

Management

Most patients respond to dapsone (combination of tetracycline and nicotinamide) and to a gluten-free diet. All patients should be screened for glucose-6-phosphate dehydrogenase (G6PD) deficiency, because dapsone can induce severe hemolysis in those with this deficiency. Patients benefit from dietary counseling because the dietary restrictions are life-long, and a gluten-free diet is often difficult to follow. They need emotional support as they deal with the process of learning new habits and accepting major changes in their lives.

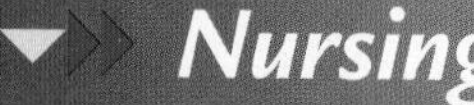

Nursing Process

Care of the Patient With Blistering Diseases

Assessment

Patients with blistering disorders may experience significant disability. There is constant itching and possible pain in the denuded areas of skin. There may be drainage from the denuded areas, which may be malodorous. Effective assessment and nursing management become a challenge.

Disease activity is monitored clinically by examining the skin for the appearance of new blisters. Areas where healing has occurred may show signs of hyperpigmentation. Particular attention is given to assessing for signs and symptoms of infection.

Diagnosis

Nursing Diagnoses

Based on nursing assessment data, the patient's major nursing diagnoses may include the following:

- Acute pain of skin and oral cavity related to blistering and erosions
- Impaired skin integrity related to ruptured bullae and denuded areas of the skin
- Anxiety and ineffective coping related to the appearance of the skin and no hope of a cure
- Deficient knowledge about medications and side effects

Collaborative Problems/ Potential Complications

Based on the assessment data, potential complications include the following:

- Infection and sepsis related to loss of protective barrier of skin and mucous membranes
- Fluid volume deficit and electrolyte imbalance related to loss of tissue fluids

Planning and Goals

The major goals for the patient may include relief of discomfort from lesions, skin healing, reduced anxiety and improved coping capacity, and absence of complications.

Nursing Interventions

Relieving Oral Discomfort

The patient's entire oral cavity may be affected with erosions and denuded surfaces. Necrotic tissue may develop over these areas, adding to the patient's discomfort and interfering with food intake. Weight loss and hypoproteinemia may result. Meticulous oral hygiene is important to keep the oral mucosa clean and allow the epithelium to regenerate. Frequent rinsing of the mouth is prescribed to rid the mouth of debris and to soothe ulcerated areas. Commercial mouthwashes are avoided. The lips are kept moist with lanolin, petrolatum, or lip balm. Cool mist therapy helps to humidify environmental air.

Enhancing Skin Integrity and Relieving Discomfort

Cool, wet dressings or baths are protective and soothing. The patient with painful and extensive lesions should be premedicated with analgesics before skin care is initiated. Patients with large areas of blistering have a characteristic odor that decreases when secondary infection is controlled. After the patient's skin is bathed, it is dried carefully and dusted liberally with nonirritating powder (eg, cornstarch), which enables the patient to move about freely in bed. Fairly large amounts are necessary to keep the patient's skin from adhering to the sheets. Tape should never be used, because it may produce more blisters. Hypothermia is common, and measures to keep the patient warm and comfortable are priority nursing activities. The nursing management of patients with bullous skin conditions is similar to that for patients with extensive burns (see Chapter 57).

Reducing Anxiety

Attention to the psychological needs of the patient requires listening to the patient, being available, providing expert nursing care, and educating the patient and the family. The patient is encouraged to express anxieties, discomfort, and feelings of hopelessness. Arranging for a family member or a close friend to spend more time with the patient can be supportive. When patients receive information about the disease and its treatment, uncertainty and anxiety often decrease, and the patient's capacity to act on his or her own behalf is enhanced. Psychological counseling may assist the patient in dealing with fears, anxiety, and depression.

Monitoring and Managing Potential Complications

INFECTION AND SEPSIS

The patient is susceptible to infection because the barrier function of the skin is compromised. Bullae are also susceptible to infection, and sepsis may follow. The skin is cleaned to remove debris and dead skin and to prevent infection.

Secondary infection may be accompanied by an unpleasant odor from skin or oral lesions. *C. albicans* of the mouth (ie, thrush) commonly affects patients receiving high-dose corticosteroid therapy. The oral cavity is inspected daily, and any changes are reported. Oral lesions are slow to heal.

Infection is the leading cause of death in patients with blistering diseases. Particular attention is given to assessment for signs and symptoms of local and systemic infection. Seemingly trivial complaints or minimal changes are investigated, because corticosteroids can mask or alter typical signs and symptoms of infection. The patient's vital signs are monitored, and temperature fluctuations are documented. The patient is observed for chills, and all secretions and excretions are monitored for changes suggesting infection. Results of culture and sensitivity tests are monitored. Antimicrobial agents are administered as prescribed, and response to treatment is assessed. Health care personnel must perform effective hand hygiene and wear gloves.

In hospitalized patients, environmental contamination is reduced as much as possible. Protective isolation measures and standard precautions are warranted.

FLUID AND ELECTROLYTE IMBALANCE

Extensive denudation of the skin leads to fluid and electrolyte imbalance because of significant loss of fluids and sodium chloride from the skin. This sodium chloride loss is responsible for many of the systemic symptoms associated with the disease and is treated by IV administration of saline solution.

A large amount of protein and blood is also lost from the denuded skin areas. Blood component therapy may be prescribed to maintain the blood volume, hemoglobin level, and plasma protein concentration. Serum albumin, protein, hemoglobin, and hematocrit values are monitored.

The patient is encouraged to maintain adequate oral fluid intake. Cool, nonirritating fluids are encouraged to maintain hydration. Small, frequent meals or snacks of high-protein, high-calorie foods (eg, oral nutritional supplements, eggnog, milkshakes) help maintain nutritional status. Parenteral nutrition is considered if the patient cannot eat an adequate diet.

Evaluation

Expected Patient Outcomes

Expected patient outcomes may include the following:

1. Reports relief from pain of oral lesions
   a. Identifies therapies that reduce pain
   b. Uses mouthwashes and anesthetic or antiseptic aerosol mouth spray
   c. Drinks chilled fluids at 2-hour intervals
2. Achieves skin healing
   a. States purpose of therapeutic regimen
   b. Cooperates with soaks and bath regimen
   c. Reminds caregivers to use liberal amounts of nonirritating powder on bed linens

3. Reports that anxiety and ability to cope with the condition have improved
   a. Verbalizes concerns about condition, self, and relationships with others
   b. Participates in self-care
4. Experiences no complications
   a. Has cultures from bullae, skin, and orifices that are negative for pathogenic organisms
   b. Has no purulent drainage
   c. Shows signs that skin is clearing
   d. Has normal body temperature
   e. Keeps intake record to ensure adequate fluid intake and normal fluid and electrolyte balance
   f. Verbalizes the rationale for IV infusion therapy
   g. Has urine output within normal limits
   h. Has serum chemistry and hemoglobin and hematocrit values within normal limits

Toxic Epidermal Necrolysis and Stevens-Johnson Syndrome

Toxic epidermal necrolysis (TEN) and Stevens-Johnson syndrome (SJS) are potentially fatal skin disorders and the most severe forms of erythema multiforme. These diseases are mucocutaneous reactions that constitute a spectrum of reactions, with TEN being the most severe. The mortality rate from TEN is 30% to 35%. TEN and SJS are triggered by a reaction to medications. Antibiotics, especially sulfonamides, antiseizure agents, NSAIDs, and sulfonamides are the most frequent medications implicated (Porth, 2005).

Clinical Manifestations

TEN and SJS are characterized initially by conjunctival burning or itching, cutaneous tenderness, fever, cough, sore throat, headache, extreme malaise, and myalgias (ie, aches and pains). These signs are followed by a rapid onset of erythema involving much of the skin surface and mucous membranes, including the oral mucosa, conjunctiva, and genitalia. In severe cases of mucosal involvement, there may be danger of damage to the larynx, bronchi, and esophagus from ulcerations. Large, flaccid bullae develop in some areas; in other areas, large sheets of epidermis are shed, exposing the underlying dermis. Fingernails, toenails, eyebrows, and eyelashes may be shed along with the surrounding epidermis. The skin is excruciatingly tender, and the loss of skin leaves a weeping surface similar to that of a total-body, partial-thickness burn; hence the condition is also referred to as "scalded skin syndrome."

These conditions occur in all ages and both genders. The incidence is increased in older people because of their use of many medications. People who are immunosuppressed, including those with human immunodeficiency virus (HIV) infection and acquired immunodeficiency syndrome (AIDS), have a high risk of SJS and TEN. Although the incidence of TEN and SJS in the general population is about 2 to 3 cases per 1 million people in the United States, the risk associated with sulfonamides in HIV-positive individuals may approach 1 case per 1000 (Porth, 2005). Most patients with TEN have an abnormal metabolism of the medication; the mechanism leading to TEN seems to be a cell-mediated cytotoxic reaction.

Complications

Sepsis and keratoconjunctivitis are complications of TEN and SJS. Unrecognized and untreated sepsis can be life-threatening. Keratoconjunctivitis can impair vision and result in conjunctival retraction, scarring, and corneal lesions.

Assessment and Diagnostic Findings

Histologic studies of frozen skin cells from a fresh lesion and cytodiagnosis of collections of cellular material from a freshly denuded area are conducted. A history of use of medications known to precipitate TEN or SJS may confirm medication reaction as the underlying cause.

Immunofluorescent studies may be performed to detect atypical epidermal autoantibodies. A genetic predisposition to erythema multiforme has been suggested but has not been confirmed in all cases.

Medical Management

The goals of treatment include control of fluid and electrolyte balance, prevention of sepsis, and prevention of ophthalmic complications. Supportive care is the mainstay of treatment.

All nonessential medications are discontinued immediately. If possible, the patient is treated in a regional burn center, because aggressive treatment similar to that for severe burns is required. Skin loss may approach 100% of the total body surface area. Surgical débridement or hydrotherapy in a Hubbard tank (large steel tub) may be performed to remove involved skin.

Tissue samples from the nasopharynx, eyes, ears, blood, urine, skin, and unruptured blisters are obtained for culture to identify pathogenic organisms. IV fluids are prescribed to maintain fluid and electrolyte balance, especially in the patient who has severe mucosal involvement and who cannot easily take oral nourishment. Because an indwelling IV catheter may be a site of infection, fluid replacement is carried out by nasogastric tube and then orally as soon as possible.

Initial treatment with systemic corticosteroids is controversial. Some experts argue for early high-dose corticosteroid treatment. However, in most cases, the risk of infection, the complication of fluid and electrolyte imbalance, the delay in the healing process, and the difficulty in initiating oral corticosteroids early in the course of the disease outweigh the perceived benefits. In patients with TEN thought to result from a medication reaction, corticosteroids may be administered; however, the patient should be closely monitored for adverse effects.

One report has shown that administration of IV immunoglobulin (IVIG) to 10 patients led to improvement within 48 hours and skin healing within 1 week. This response is dramatically better than that obtained with immunosuppressives, and IVIG may become the treatment of choice (Rutter & Luger, 2001).

Protecting the skin with topical agents is crucial. Various topical antibacterial and anesthetic agents are used to prevent wound sepsis and to assist with pain management. Systemic antibiotic therapy is used with extreme caution. Temporary biologic dressings (eg, pigskin, amniotic membrane) or plastic semipermeable dressings (eg, Vigilon) may be used to reduce pain, decrease evaporation, and prevent secondary infection until the epithelium regenerates. Meticulous oropharyngeal and eye care is essential when there is severe involvement of the mucous membranes and the eyes.

Nursing Process

Care of the Patient With Toxic Epidermal Necrolysis or Stevens-Johnson Syndrome

Assessment

A careful inspection of the skin is made, including its appearance and the extent of involvement. The normal skin is closely observed to determine if new areas of blisters are developing. Drainage from blisters is monitored for amount, color, and odor. The oral cavity is inspected daily for blistering and erosive lesions; the patient is assessed daily for itching, burning, and dryness of the eyes. The patient's ability to swallow and drink fluids, as well as speak normally, is determined.

The patient's vital signs are monitored, and special attention is given to the presence and character of fever and the respiratory rate, depth, rhythm, and cough. The characteristics and amount of respiratory secretions are observed. Assessment for high fever, tachycardia, and extreme weakness and fatigue is essential because these factors indicate the process of epidermal necrosis, increased metabolic needs, and possible gastrointestinal and respiratory mucosal sloughing. Urine volume, specific gravity, and color are monitored. The insertion sites of IV lines are inspected for signs of local infection. Body weight is recorded daily.

The patient is asked to describe fatigue and pain levels. An attempt is made to evaluate the patient's level of anxiety. The patient's basic coping mechanisms are assessed, and effective coping strategies are identified.

Diagnosis

Nursing Diagnoses

Based on the assessment data, the patient's major nursing diagnoses may include the following:

- Impaired tissue integrity (ie, oral, eye, and skin) related to epidermal shedding
- Deficient fluid volume and electrolyte losses related to loss of fluids from denuded skin
- Risk for imbalanced body temperature (ie, hypothermia) related to heat loss secondary to skin loss
- Acute pain related to denuded skin, oral lesions, and possible infection
- Anxiety related to the physical appearance of the skin and prognosis

Collaborative Problems/ Potential Complications

Based on the assessment data, potential complications include the following:

- Sepsis
- Conjunctival retraction, scars, and corneal lesions

Planning and Goals

The major goals for the patient may include skin and oral tissue healing, fluid balance, prevention of heat loss, relief of pain, reduced anxiety, and absence of complications.

Nursing Interventions

Maintaining Skin and Mucous Membrane Integrity

The local care of the skin is an important area of nursing management. The skin denudes easily, even when the patient is lifted and turned; thus, it may be necessary to place the patient on a circular turning frame. The nurse applies the prescribed topical agents that reduce the bacterial population of the wound surface. Warm compresses, if prescribed, should be applied gently to denuded areas. The topical antibacterial agent may be used in conjunction with hydrotherapy in a tank, bathtub, or shower. The nurse monitors the patient's condition during the treatment and encourages the patient to exercise the extremities during hydrotherapy.

The painful oral lesions make oral hygiene difficult. Careful oral hygiene is performed to keep the oral mucosa clean. Prescribed mouthwashes, anesthetics, or coating agents are used frequently to rid the mouth of debris, soothe ulcerative areas, and control foul mouth odor. The oral cavity is inspected several times each day, and any changes are documented and reported. Petrolatum or a prescribed ointment is applied to the lips.

Attaining Fluid Balance

The vital signs, urine output, and sensorium are observed for indications of hypovolemia. Mental changes from fluid and electrolyte imbalance, sensory overload, or sensory deprivation may occur. Laboratory test results are evaluated, and abnormal results are reported. The patient is weighed daily (with a bed scale if necessary).

Oral lesions may result in dysphagia, making tube feeding or parenteral nutrition necessary until oral ingestion can be tolerated. A daily calorie count and accurate recording of all intake and output are essential.

Preventing Hypothermia

The patient with TEN is prone to chilling. Dehydration may be made worse by exposing the denuded skin to a continuous current of warm air. The patient is usually sensitive to changes in room temperature. Measures similar to those implemented for a burn patient, such as cotton blankets, ceiling-mounted heat lamps, and heat shields, are useful in maintaining body temperature. To minimize shivering and heat loss, the nurse should work rapidly and efficiently when large wounds are exposed for wound care. The patient's temperature is monitored frequently.

Relieving Pain

The nurse assesses the patient's pain, its characteristics, factors that influence the pain, and the patient's behavioral responses. Prescribed analgesics are administered on a regular schedule, and the nurse documents pain relief and any side effects. Analgesics are administered before painful treatments are performed. Providing thorough explanations and speaking calmly to the patient during treatments can allay the anxiety that may intensify pain. Offering emotional support and reassurance and implementing measures that promote rest and sleep are basic in achieving pain control. As the pain diminishes and the patient has more physical and emotional energy, self-management techniques for pain relief, such as progressive muscle relaxation and imagery, may be taught.

Reducing Anxiety

Because the lifestyle of the patient with TEN has been abruptly changed to one of complete dependence, an assessment of his or her emotional state may reveal anxiety, depression, and fear of dying. The patient can be reassured that these reactions are normal. The patient also needs nursing support, honest communication, and hope that the situation can improve. The patient is encouraged to express his or her feelings. Listening to the patient's concerns and being readily available with skillful and compassionate care are important anxiety-relieving interventions. Emotional support by a psychiatric nurse, spiritual advisor, psychologist, or psychiatrist may be helpful to promote coping during the long recovery period.

Monitoring and Managing Potential Complications

SEPSIS

The major cause of death from TEN is infection, and the most common sites of infection are the skin and mucosal surfaces, lungs, and blood. The organisms most often involved are *S. aureus*, *Pseudomonas*, *Klebsiella*, *Escherichia coli*, *Serratia*, and *Candida*. Monitoring vital signs closely and noticing changes in respiratory, renal, and gastrointestinal function may quickly detect the beginning of an infection. Strict asepsis is always maintained during routine skin care measures. Hand hygiene and wearing sterile gloves when carrying out procedures are essential. When the condition involves a large portion of the body, the patient should be in a private room to prevent possible cross-infection from other patients. Visitors should wear protective garments and wash their hands before and after coming into contact with the patient. People with any infections or infectious disease should not visit the patient until they are no longer a danger to the patient.

CONJUNCTIVAL RETRACTION, SCARS, AND CORNEAL LESIONS

The eyes are inspected daily for signs of pruritus, burning, and dryness, which may indicate progression to keratoconjunctivitis, the principal eye complication. Applying a cool, damp cloth over the eyes may relieve burning sensations. The eyes are kept clean and observed for signs of discharge or discomfort, and the progression of symptoms is documented and reported. Administering an eye lubricant, when prescribed, may alleviate dryness and prevent corneal abrasion. Using eye patches or reminding the patient to blink periodically may also counteract dryness. The patient is instructed to avoid rubbing the eyes or putting any medication into the eyes that has not been prescribed or approved by the physician.

Promoting Home and Community-Based Care

TEACHING PATIENTS SELF-CARE

Patients with TEN or SJS with involvement of large areas of the skin require care that is similar to that of patients with thermal burns. As the patient completes the acute inpatient stage of illness, the focus is directed toward rehabilitation and outpatient care or care in a rehabilitation center. Throughout this care, the patient and family members are involved in the care and are instructed in the procedures, such as wound care and dressing changes, that will need to be continued at home. The patient and family members are assisted in acquiring dressing supplies that will be needed at home.

The patient and family members are also provided with instructions about pain management, nutrition, measures to increase mobility, and prevention of complications, including prevention of infection. They are taught the signs and symptoms of complications and instructed when to notify the health care provider. When appropriate, instructions are provided in writing to the patient and family so they can refer to these instructions when necessary at later times.

CONTINUING CARE

Interdisciplinary follow-up care is imperative to ensure that the patient's progress continues. Some patients will require care in a rehabilitation center before returning home. Others will require outpatient physical and occupational therapy for an extended period. When the patient returns home, the home care nurse coordinates the care provided by the various members of the health care team (eg, physician, physical therapist, occupational therapist, dietician). The nurse also monitors the patient's progress, provides ongoing assessment to identify complications, and monitors the patient's adherence to the plan of care. The patient's adaptation to the home care environment and the patient's and family's needs for support and assistance are also assessed. Referrals to community agencies are made as appropriate.

Evaluation

Expected Patient Outcomes

Expected patient outcomes may include the following:

1. Achieves increasing skin and oral tissue healing
   a. Demonstrates areas of healing skin
   b. Swallows fluids and speaks clearly
2. Attains fluid balance
   a. Demonstrates laboratory values within normal ranges
   b. Maintains urine volume and specific gravity within acceptable range
   c. Shows stable vital signs
   d. Increases intake of oral fluids without discomfort
   e. Gains weight, if appropriate
3. Attains thermoregulation
   a. Registers body temperature within normal range
   b. Reports no chills
4. Achieves pain relief
   a. Uses analgesics as prescribed
   b. Uses self-management techniques for relief of pain
5. Appears less anxious
   a. Discusses concerns freely
   b. Sleeps for progressively longer periods
6. Absence of complications, such as sepsis and impaired vision
   a. Body temperature within normal range
   b. Laboratory values within normal ranges
   c. Has no abnormal discharges or signs of infection
   d. Continues to see objects at baseline acuity level
   e. Shows no signs of keratoconjunctivitis

Ulcerations

Superficial loss of surface tissue as a result of death of cells is called an ulceration. A simple ulcer, such as the kind found in a small, superficial, partial-thickness burn, tends to heal by granulation if kept clean and protected from injury. If exposed to the air, the serum that escapes dries and forms a scab, under which the epithelial cells grow and cover the surface completely. Certain diseases cause characteristic ulcers (eg, tuberculous ulcers, syphilitic ulcers).

Ulcers related to problems with arterial circulation are seen in patients with peripheral vascular disease, arteriosclerosis, Raynaud's disease, and frostbite. In these patients, treatment of the ulcers is concurrent with treatment of the arterial disease (see Chapter 31). Nursing management includes the use of the dressings discussed at the beginning of this chapter. If nursing interventions are instituted early in the progression of an ulcer, the condition can often be effectively improved. Surgical amputation of an affected limb is a last resort.

Pressure ulcers involve breakdown of the skin due to prolonged pressure, friction and shear forces, and insufficient blood supply, usually at bony prominences. Information about these ulcers is presented in Chapter 11.

Skin Tumors

Benign Skin Tumors

Cysts

Cysts of the skin are epithelium-lined cavities that contain fluid or solid material. Epidermal cysts (epidermoid cysts) occur frequently and may be described as slow-growing, firm, elevated tumors found most frequently on the face, neck, upper chest, and back. Removal of the cysts provides a cure.

Pilar cysts (trichilemmal cysts), formerly called sebaceous cysts, are most frequently found on the scalp. They originate from the middle portion of the hair follicle and from the cells of the outer hair root sheath. Treatment is surgical removal.

Seborrheic and Actinic Keratoses

Seborrheic keratoses are benign, wartlike lesions of various sizes and colors, ranging from light tan to black. They are usually located on the face, shoulders, chest, and back and are the most common skin tumors seen in middle-aged and elderly people. They may be cosmetically unacceptable to the patient. A black keratosis may be erroneously diagnosed as malignant melanoma. Treatment is removal of the tumor tissue by excision, electrodesiccation (destruction of the skin lesions by monopolar high-frequency electric current) and curettage, or application of carbon dioxide or liquid nitrogen. However, there is no harm in allowing these growths to remain, because there is no medical significance to their presence.

Actinic keratoses are premalignant skin lesions that develop in chronically sun-exposed areas of the body. They appear as rough, scaly patches with underlying erythema. A small percentage of these lesions gradually transform into cutaneous squamous cell carcinoma; they are usually removed by cryotherapy or shave excision.

Verrucae: Warts

Warts are common, benign skin tumors caused by infection with the human papillomavirus, which belongs to the DNA virus group. People of all ages may be affected, but the warts occur most frequently between the ages of 12 and 16 years. There are many types of warts.

As a rule, warts are asymptomatic, except when they occur on weight-bearing areas, such as the soles of the feet. They may be treated with locally applied laser therapy, liquid nitrogen, salicylic acid plasters, or electrodesiccation.

Warts occurring on the genitalia and perianal areas are known as condylomata acuminata. They may be transmitted sexually and are treated with liquid nitrogen, cryosurgery, electrosurgery, topically applied trichloroacetic acid, and curettage. Condylomata that affect the uterine cervix predispose the patient to cervical cancer (see Chapter 47).

Angiomas

Angiomas are benign vascular tumors that involve the skin and the subcutaneous tissues. They are present at birth and may occur as flat, violet-red patches (port-wine angiomas) or as raised, bright-red, nodular lesions (strawberry angiomas). The latter tend to involute spontaneously within the first few years of life, but port-wine angiomas usually persist indefinitely. Most patients use masking cosmetics (ie, Covermark or Dermablend) to camouflage the lesions. The argon laser is being used on various angiomas with some success. Treatment of strawberry angiomas is more successful if undertaken as soon after birth as possible.

Pigmented Nevi: Moles

Moles are common skin tumors of various sizes and shades, ranging from yellowish brown to black. They may be flat, macular lesions or elevated papules or nodules that occasionally contain hair. Most pigmented nevi are harmless lesions. However, in rare cases, malignant changes occur, and a melanoma develops at the site of the nevus. Some authorities believe that all congenital moles should be removed, because they may have a higher incidence of malignant change. However, depending on the quantity and location, this may be impractical. Nevi that show a change in color or size, become symptomatic (eg, itch), or develop irregular borders should be removed to determine if malignant changes have occurred. Moles that occur in unusual places should be examined carefully for any irregularity and for notching of the border and variation in color. Early melanomas may display some redness and irritation and areas of bluish pigmentation where the pigment-containing cells have spread deeper into the skin. Late melanomas have areas of paler color, where pigment cells have stopped producing melanin. Nevi larger than 1 cm should be examined carefully. Excised nevi should be examined histologically.

Keloids

Keloids are benign overgrowths of fibrous tissue at the site of a scar or trauma. They appear to be more common among dark-skinned people. Keloids are asymptomatic but may cause disfigurement and cosmetic concern. The treatment, which is not always satisfactory, consists of surgical excision, intralesional corticosteroid therapy, and radiation.

Dermatofibroma

A dermatofibroma is a common, benign tumor of connective tissue that occurs predominantly on the extremities. It is a firm, dome-shaped papule or nodule that may be skin-colored or pinkish brown. Excisional biopsy is the recommended method of treatment.

Neurofibromatosis: Von Recklinghausen's Disease

Neurofibromatosis is a hereditary condition manifested by pigmented patches (café-au-lait macules), axillary freckling, and cutaneous neurofibromas that vary in size. Developmental changes may occur in the nervous system, muscles, and bone. Malignant degeneration of the neurofibromas occurs in some patients.

Malignant Skin Tumors

Skin cancer is the most common cancer in the United States. If the incidence continues at the present rate, an estimated one of eight fair-skinned Americans will eventually develop skin cancer, especially basal cell carcinoma (Chart 56-6). Because the skin is easily inspected, skin cancer is readily seen and detected and is the most successfully treated type of cancer.

Exposure to the sun is the leading cause of skin cancer; incidence is related to the total amount of exposure to the sun. Sun damage is cumulative, and harmful effects may be

CHART 56-6

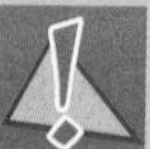

Risk Factors for Skin Cancer

Changes in the ozone layer from the effects of worldwide industrial air pollutants, such as chlorofluorocarbons, have prompted concern that the incidence of skin cancers, especially malignant melanoma, will increase. The ozone layer, a stratospheric blanket of bluish, explosive gas formed by the sun's ultraviolet radiation, varies in depth with the seasons and is thickest at the North and South Poles and thinnest at the equator. Scientists believe that it helps protect the earth from the effects of solar ultraviolet radiation. Proponents of this theory predict an increase in skin cancers as a consequence of changes in the ozone layer. Other skin cancer risk factors follow:

- Fair-skinned, fair-haired, blue-eyed people, particularly those of Celtic origin, with insufficient skin pigmentation to protect underlying tissues
- People who sustain sunburn and who do not tan
- Chronic sun exposure (certain occupations, such as farming, construction work)
- Exposure to chemical pollutants (industrial workers in arsenic, nitrates, coal, tar and pitch, oils and paraffins)
- Sun-damaged skin (elderly people)
- History of x-ray therapy for acne or benign lesions
- Scars from severe burns
- Chronic skin irritations
- Immunosuppression
- Genetic factors

severe by 20 years of age. The increase in skin cancer probably reflects changing lifestyles and the emphasis on sunbathing and related activities in light of changes in the environment, such as holes in the Earth's ozone layer. Protective measures should be used throughout life, and nurses should inform patients about risk factors associated with skin cancer.

Basal Cell and Squamous Cell Carcinoma

The most common types of skin cancer are basal cell carcinoma (BCC) and squamous cell (epidermoid) carcinoma (SCC). The third most common type, malignant melanoma, is discussed separately. Skin cancer is diagnosed by biopsy and histologic evaluation.

Clinical Manifestations

BCC is the most common type of skin cancer. It generally appears on sun-exposed areas of the body and is more prevalent in regions where the population is subjected to intense and extensive exposure to the sun. The incidence is proportional to the age of the patient (average: 60 years) and the total amount of sun exposure, and it is inversely proportional to the amount of melanin in the skin.

BCC usually begins as a small, waxy nodule with rolled, translucent, pearly borders; telangiectatic vessels may be present. As it grows, it undergoes central ulceration and sometimes crusting (Fig. 56-6). The tumors appear most frequently on the face. BCC is characterized by invasion and erosion of contiguous (adjoining) tissues. It rarely metastasizes, but recurrence is common. However, a neglected lesion can result in the loss of a nose, an ear, or a lip. Other variants of BCC may appear as shiny, flat, gray or yellowish plaques.

SCC is a malignant proliferation arising from the epidermis. Although it usually appears on sun-damaged skin, it may arise from normal skin or from preexisting skin lesions. It is of greater concern than BCC because it is a truly invasive carcinoma, metastasizing by the blood or lymphatic system.

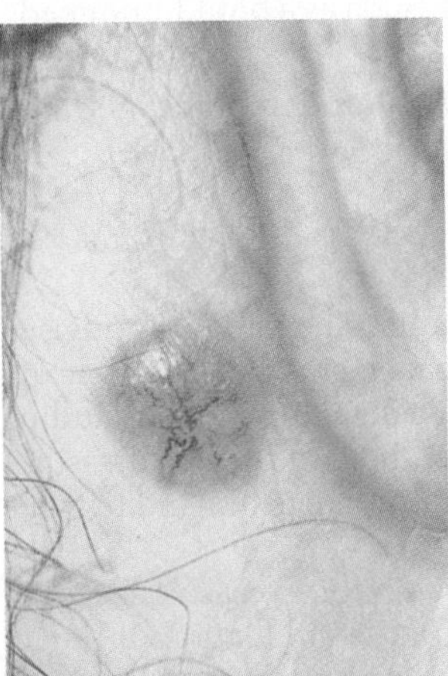
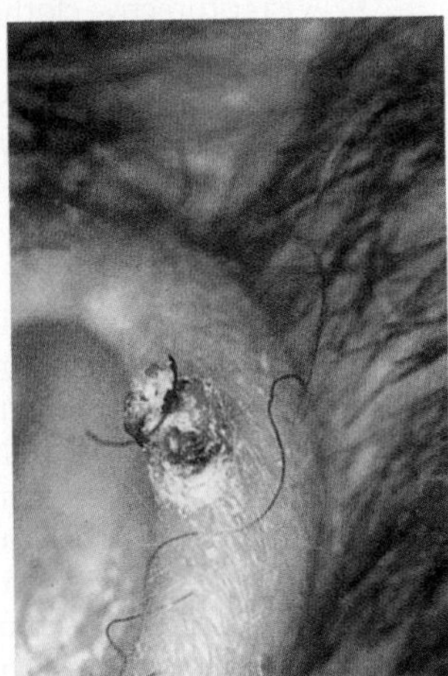

FIGURE 56-6. Basal cell carcinoma (*left*) and squamous cell carcinoma (*right*). Reprinted by permission from *New England Journal of Medicine, 326,* 169–170, 1992.

Metastases account for 75% of deaths from SCC. The lesions may be primary, arising on the skin and mucous membranes, or they may develop from a precancerous condition, such as actinic keratosis (lesions occurring in sun-exposed areas), leukoplakia (premalignant lesion of the mucous membrane), or scarred or ulcerated lesions. SCC appears as a rough, thickened, scaly tumor that may be asymptomatic or may involve bleeding (see Fig. 56-6). The border of an SCC lesion may be wider, more infiltrated, and more inflammatory than that of a BCC lesion. Secondary infection can occur. Exposed areas, especially of the upper extremities and of the face, lower lip, ears, nose, and forehead, are common sites.

The incidence of BCC and SCC is increased in all immunocompromised people, including those infected with HIV. Clinically, the tumors have the same appearance as in non–HIV-infected people; however, in HIV patients, the tumors may grow more rapidly and recur more frequently. These tumors are managed the same as those for the general population. Frequent follow-up (every 4 to 6 months) is recommended to monitor for recurrence.

Prognosis

The prognosis for BCC is usually good because tumors remain localized. Although some require wide excision with resultant disfigurement, the risk for death from BCC is low. The prognosis for SCC depends on the incidence of metastases, which is related to the histologic type and the level or depth of invasion. Usually, SCC arising in sun-damaged areas is less invasive and rarely causes death, whereas SCC that arises without a history of sun or arsenic exposure or scar formation appears to have a greater chance for spread. Regional lymph nodes should be evaluated for metastases.

Medical Management

The goal of treatment is to eradicate the tumor. The treatment method depends on the tumor location; the cell type, location, and depth; the cosmetic desires of the patient; the history of previous treatment; whether the tumor is invasive; and whether metastatic nodes are present. The management of BCC and SCC includes surgical excision, Mohs' micrographic surgery, electrosurgery, cryosurgery, and radiation therapy.

SURGICAL MANAGEMENT

The primary goal is to remove the tumor entirely. The best way to maintain cosmetic appearance is to place the incision properly along natural skin tension lines and natural anatomic body lines. In this way, scars are less noticeable. The size of the incision depends on the tumor size and location but usually involves a length-to-width ratio of 3:1.

The adequacy of the surgical excision is verified by microscopic evaluation of sections of the specimen. When the tumor is large, reconstructive surgery with use of a skin flap or skin grafting may be required. The incision is closed in layers to enhance cosmetic effect. A pressure dressing applied over the wound provides support. Infection after a simple excision is uncommon if proper surgical asepsis is maintained.

Mohs' Micrographic Surgery. Mohs' micrographic surgery is the technique that is most accurate and that best conserves normal tissue. The procedure removes the tumor layer by layer. The first layer excised includes all evident tumor and a small margin of normal-appearing tissue. The specimen is frozen and analyzed by section to determine if all the tumor has been removed. If not, additional layers of tissue are shaved and examined until all tissue margins are tumor-free. In this manner, only the tumor and a safe, normal-tissue margin are removed. Mohs' surgery is the recommended tissue-sparing procedure, with extremely high cure rates for BCC and SCC. It is the treatment of choice and the most effective for tumors around the eyes, nose, upper lip, and auricular and periauricular areas (Bowen, White, & Gerwels, 2005).

Electrosurgery. Electrosurgery is the destruction or removal of tissue by electrical energy. The current is converted to heat, which then passes to the tissue from a cold electrode. Electrosurgery may be preceded by curettage (excising the skin tumor by scraping its surface with a curette). Electrodesiccation is then implemented to achieve hemostasis and to destroy any viable malignant cells at the base of the wound or along its edges. Electrodesiccation is useful for lesions smaller than 1 to 2 cm (0.4 to 0.8 in) in diameter.

This method takes advantage of the fact that the tumor is softer than surrounding skin and therefore can be outlined by a curette, which "feels" the extent of the tumor. The tumor is removed and the base cauterized. The process is repeated twice. Usually, healing occurs within a month.

Cryosurgery. Cryosurgery destroys the tumor by deep-freezing the tissue. A thermocouple needle apparatus is inserted into the skin, and liquid nitrogen is directed to the center of the tumor until the tumor base is −40°C to −60°C. Liquid nitrogen has the lowest boiling point of all cryogens, is inexpensive, and is easy to obtain. The tumor tissue is frozen, allowed to thaw, and then refrozen. The site thaws naturally and then becomes gelatinous and heals spontaneously. Swelling and edema follow the freezing. The appearance of the lesion varies. Normal healing, which may take 4 to 6 weeks, occurs faster in areas with a good blood supply.

RADIATION THERAPY

Radiation therapy is frequently performed for cancer of the eyelid, the tip of the nose, and areas in or near vital structures (eg, facial nerve). It is reserved for older patients, because x-ray changes may be seen after 5 to 10 years, and malignant changes in scars may be induced by irradiation 15 to 30 years later.

The patient should be informed that the skin may become red and blistered. A bland skin ointment prescribed by the physician may be applied to relieve discomfort. The patient should also be cautioned to avoid exposure to the sun.

CHART 56-7

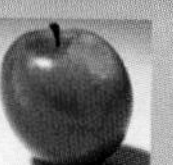

Health Promotion

Preventing Skin Cancer

- Teach patients that sunscreens are rated in strength from 4 (weakest) to 50 (strongest). The solar protection factor, or SPF, indicates how much longer a person can stay in the sun before the skin begins to redden. For example, if the person can normally stay in the sun for 10 minutes before reddening begins, an SPF of 4 will protect the person from reddening for about 40 minutes.
- Remind patients that up to 50% of ultraviolet rays can penetrate loosely woven clothing.
- Remind patients that ultraviolet light can penetrate cloud cover, and a sunburn can still occur.
- Teach children to avoid all but modest sun exposure and to use a sunscreen regularly for lifelong protection.
- Advise patients to:
  - Avoid tanning if their skin burns easily, never tans, or tans poorly.
  - Avoid unnecessary exposure to the sun, especially during the time of day when ultraviolet radiation (sunlight) is most intense (10 AM to 3 PM).
  - Avoid sunburns.
  - Apply a sunscreen daily to block harmful sun rays.
  - Use a sunscreen with an SPF of 15 or higher that protects against both ultraviolet-A (UVA) and ultraviolet-B (UVB) light.
  - Reapply water-resistant sunscreens after swimming, if heavily sweating, and every 2 to 3 hours during prolonged periods of sun exposure.
  - Avoid applying oils before or during sun exposure (oils do not protect against sunlight or sun damage).
  - Use a lip balm that contains a sunscreen with an SPF of 15 or higher.
  - Wear protective clothing, such as a broad-brimmed hat and long sleeves.
  - Avoid using sun lamps for indoor tanning, and avoid commercial tanning booths.

Nursing Management

Because many skin cancers are removed by excision, patients are usually treated in outpatient surgical units. The role of the nurse is to teach the patient about prevention of skin cancer and about self-care after treatment (Chart 56-7).

PROMOTING HOME AND COMMUNITY-BASED CARE

Teaching Patients Self-Care. The wound is usually covered with a dressing to protect the site from physical trauma, external irritants, and contaminants. The patient is advised when to report for a dressing change or is given written and verbal information on how to change dressings, including the type of dressing to purchase, how to remove dressings and apply fresh ones, and the importance of hand hygiene before and after the procedure.

The patient is advised to watch for excessive bleeding and tight dressings that compromise circulation. If the lesion is in the perioral area, the patient is instructed to drink liquids through a straw and limit talking and facial movement. Dental work should be avoided until the area is completely healed.

After the sutures are removed, an emollient cream may be used to help reduce dryness. Applying a sunscreen over the wound is advised to prevent postoperative hyperpigmentation if the patient spends time outdoors.

Follow-up examinations should be at regular intervals, usually every 3 months for a year, and should include palpation of the adjacent lymph nodes. The patient should also be instructed to seek treatment for any moles that are subject to repeated friction and irritation, and to watch for indications of potential malignancy in moles as described previously. The importance of lifelong follow-up evaluations is emphasized.

Teaching About Prevention. Studies show that regular daily use of a sunscreen with a solar protection factor (SPF) of at least 15 can reduce the recurrence of skin cancer by as much as 40%. The sunscreen should be applied to head, neck, arms, and hands every morning at least 30 minutes before leaving the house and reapplied every 4 hours if the skin perspires. Intermittent application of sunscreen only when exposure is anticipated has been shown to be less effective than daily use. Research (Darlington, Williams, Neale, et al., 2003) has shown that daily use of sunscreen on the hands and face reduces the total incidence of solar keratoses, which are precursors of SCC, but has no effect on the overall incidence of BCC. These data are inconsistent, but one theory is that people have a false sense of security when wearing sunscreen and tend to stay out in the sun for longer periods. This longer exposure is believed to contribute to the increasing incidence of melanoma. Although the evidence is insufficient, nurses should discuss the issues with patients who are at high risk of skin cancer.

Malignant Melanoma

A malignant melanoma is a cancerous neoplasm in which atypical melanocytes are present in the epidermis and the dermis (and sometimes the subcutaneous cells). It is the most lethal of all the skin cancers and is responsible for about 3% of all cancer deaths (Porth, 2005).

Malignant melanoma can occur in one of several forms: superficial spreading melanoma, lentigo-maligna melanoma, nodular melanoma, and acral-lentiginous melanoma. These types have specific clinical and histologic features as well as different biologic behaviors. Most melanomas arise from cutaneous epidermal melanocytes, but some appear in preexisting nevi (ie, moles) in the skin or develop in the uveal tract of the eye. Melanomas occasionally appear simultaneously with cancer of other organs.

The worldwide incidence of melanoma doubles every 10 years, an increase that is probably related to increased recreational sun exposure and changes in the ozone layer and improved methods of early detection. Peak incidence occurs between the ages of 20 and 45 years. The incidence of melanoma is increasing faster than that of almost any other cancer, and the mortality rate is increasing faster than that of any other cancer except lung cancer. Between 1973 and 1995, the age-adjusted incidence of melanoma increased more than 100%, from 5.7 per 100,000 people to 13.3 per 100,000 people. Men older than 65 years of age represent 22% of newly diagnosed cases, whereas women older than 65 years of age represent 14% of newly diagnosed cases (U.S. Preventive Services Task Force, 2004).

Risk Factors

The cause of malignant melanoma is unknown, but ultraviolet rays are strongly suspected, based on indirect evidence such as the increased incidence of melanoma in countries near the equator and in people younger than 30 years who have used a tanning bed more than 10 times per year. Ethnicity is a risk factor; in general, 1 in 100 Caucasians acquires melanoma each year. As many as 10% of patients with melanoma are members of melanoma-prone families who have multiple changing moles (dysplastic nevi) that are susceptible to malignant transformation. Patients with dysplastic nevus syndrome have been found to have unusual moles, larger and more numerous moles, lesions with irregular outlines, and pigmentation located all over the skin. Microscopic examination of dysplastic moles shows disordered, faulty growth. Chart 56-8 lists risk factors for malignant melanoma.

Research has identified a gene that resides on chromosome 9p, the absence of which increases the likelihood that potentially mutagenic DNA damage will escape repair before cell division. The absence of this gene can be identified in melanoma-prone families (Price, Herlyn, Dent, et al., 2005).

Clinical Manifestations

SUPERFICIAL SPREADING MELANOMA

Superficial spreading melanoma occurs anywhere on the body and is the most common form of melanoma. It usually affects middle-aged people and occurs most frequently on the trunk and lower extremities. The lesion tends to be circular, with irregular outer portions. The margins of the lesion may be flat or elevated and palpable (Fig. 56-7). This type of melanoma may appear in a combination of colors, with hues of tan, brown, and black mixed with gray, blue-black, or white. Sometimes a dull pink rose color can be seen in a small area within the lesion.

LENTIGO-MALIGNA MELANOMA

Lentigo-maligna melanoma is a slowly evolving, pigmented lesion that occurs on exposed skin areas, especially the dorsum of the hand, the head, and the neck in elderly people. Often, the lesion is present for many years before it is examined by a physician. It first appears as a tan, flat lesion, but in time it undergoes changes in size and color.

CHART 56-8

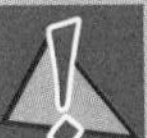

Risk Factors for Malignant Melanoma

- Fair-skinned or freckled, blue-eyed, light-haired people of Celtic or Scandinavian origin
- People who burn and do not tan or who have a significant history of severe sunburn
- Environmental exposure to intense sunlight (older Americans retiring to the southwestern United States appear to have a higher incidence)
- History of melanoma (personal or family)
- Skin with giant congenital nevi

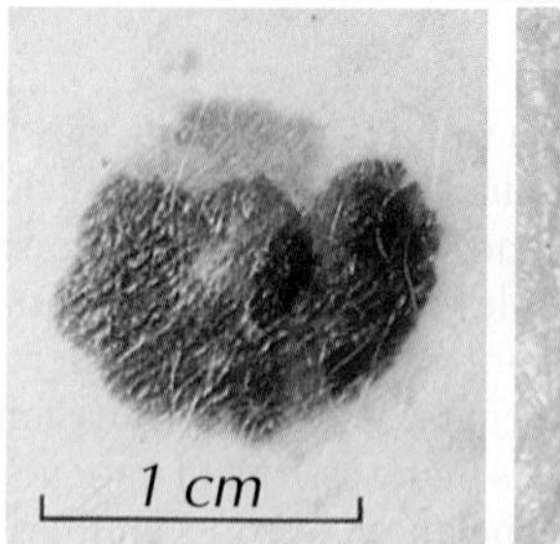

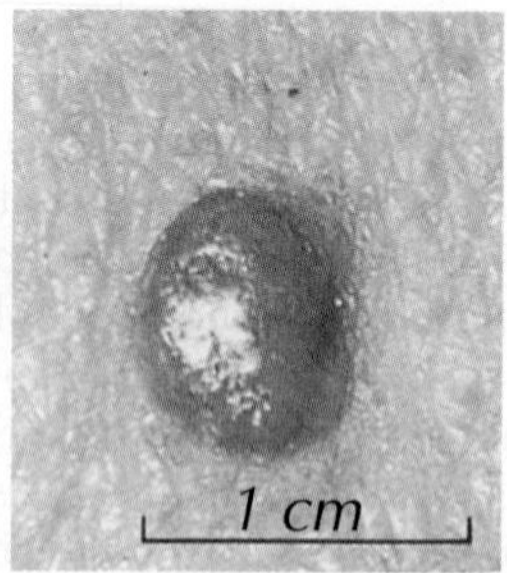

FIGURE 56-7. Two forms of malignant melanoma: superficial spreading (*left*) and nodular (*right*). From Bickley, L. S., & Szilagyi, P. (2003). *Bates' guide to physical examination and history taking* (8th ed.). Philadelphia: Lippincott Williams & Wilkins.

NODULAR MELANOMAS

Nodular melanoma is a spherical, blueberry-like nodule with a relatively smooth surface and a relatively uniform, blue-black color (see Fig. 56-7). It may be dome-shaped with a smooth surface. It may have other shadings of red, gray, or purple. Sometimes, nodular melanomas appear as irregularly shaped plaques. The patient may describe this as a blood blister that fails to resolve. A nodular melanoma invades directly into adjacent dermis (ie, vertical growth) and therefore has a poorer prognosis.

ACRAL-LENTIGINOUS MELANOMA

Acral-lentiginous melanoma occurs in areas not excessively exposed to sunlight and where hair follicles are absent. It is found on the palms of the hands, on the soles, in the nail beds, and in the mucous membranes in dark-skinned people. These melanomas appear as irregular, pigmented macules that develop nodules. They may become invasive early.

Assessment and Diagnostic Findings

Biopsy results confirm the diagnosis of melanoma. An excisional biopsy specimen provides information on the type, level of invasion, and thickness of the lesion. An excisional biopsy specimen that includes a 1-cm margin of normal tissue and a portion of underlying subcutaneous fatty tissue is sufficient for staging a melanoma in situ or an early, noninvasive melanoma. Incisional biopsy should be performed when the suspicious lesion is too large to be removed safely without extensive scarring. Biopsy specimens obtained by shaving, curettage, or needle aspiration are not considered reliable histologic proof of disease.

A thorough history and physical examination should include a meticulous skin examination and palpation of regional lymph nodes that drain the lesional area. Because melanoma occurs in families, a positive family history of melanoma is investigated so that first-degree relatives, who may be at high risk for melanoma, can be evaluated for atypical lesions. After the diagnosis of melanoma has been confirmed, a chest x-ray, complete blood cell count, liver function tests, and radionuclide or computed tomography scans are usually performed to stage the extent of disease.

Prognosis

The prognosis for long-term (5-year) survival is considered poor when the lesion is more than 1.5 mm thick or there is regional lymph node involvement. A person with a thin lesion and no lymph node involvement has a 3% chance of developing metastases and a 95% chance of surviving 5 years. If regional lymph nodes are involved, there is a 20% to 50% chance of surviving 5 years. Patients with melanoma on the hand, foot, or scalp have a better prognosis; those with lesions on the torso have an increased chance of metastases to the bone, liver, lungs, spleen, and central nervous system. Men and elderly patients also have poor prognoses.

Medical Management

Treatment depends on the level of invasion and the depth of the lesion. Surgical excision is the treatment of choice for small, superficial lesions. Deeper lesions require wide local excision, after which skin grafting may be necessary. Regional lymph node dissection is commonly performed to rule out metastasis, although new surgical approaches call for only sentinel node biopsy. This technique is used to sample the nodes nearest the tumor and to spare the patient the long-term sequelae of extensive removal of lymph nodes if the sample nodes are negative.

Immunotherapy for treatment of melanoma has had varied success. Immunotherapy modifies immune function and other biologic responses to cancer. Several forms of immunotherapy (eg, bacillus Calmette-Guérin vaccine, *Corynebacterium parvum,* levamisole) offer encouraging results. Some investigational therapies include biologic response modifiers (eg, interferon-alpha, interleukin-2), adaptive immunotherapy (ie, lymphokine-activated killer cells), and monoclonal antibodies directed at melanoma antigens. One of these, aldesleukin (Proleukin), shows promise in preventing recurrence of melanoma. Laboratory assay of tyrosinase, an enzyme believed to be produced only by melanoma cells, is under investigation. Several other studies are attempting to develop and test autologous immunization against specific tumor cells. These studies are in the experimental stage but show promise for future development of a vaccine against melanoma (Piepkorn, 2000).

Current treatments for metastatic melanoma rarely if ever produce a satisfactory outcome. Further surgical intervention may be performed to debulk the tumor or to remove part of the organ involved (eg, lung, liver, or colon). However, the rationale for more extensive surgery is for relief of symptoms, not for cure. Chemotherapy for metastatic melanoma may be used; however, only a few agents (eg, dacarbazine, nitrosoureas, cisplatin) have been effective in controlling the disease.

When the melanoma is located in an extremity, regional perfusion may be used; the chemotherapeutic agent is perfused directly into the area that contains the melanoma. This approach delivers a high concentration of cytotoxic agents while avoiding systemic, toxic side effects. The limb is perfused for 1 hour with high concentrations of the medication at temperatures of 39°C to 40°C (102.2°F to 104°F) with a perfusion pump. Inducing hyperthermia enhances the effect of the chemotherapy so that a smaller total dose can be used. The goal of regional perfusion is control of the metastasis, especially if it is used in combination with surgical excision of the primary lesion and with regional lymph node dissection.

Nursing Process

Care of the Patient With Malignant Melanoma

Assessment

Assessment of the patient with malignant melanoma is based on the patient's history and symptoms. The patient is asked specifically about pruritus, tenderness, and pain, which are not features of a benign nevus. The patient is also questioned about changes in preexisting moles or the development of new, pigmented lesions. People at risk are assessed carefully.

A magnifying lens and good lighting are needed for inspecting the skin for irregularity and changes in the mole. Signs that suggest malignant changes are referred to as the ABCDs of moles (Chart 56-9).

Common sites of melanomas are the skin of the back, the legs (especially in women), between the toes, and on the feet, face, scalp, fingernails, and backs of hands. In dark-skinned people, melanomas are most likely to occur in less pigmented sites: palms, soles, subungual areas, and mucous membranes. Satellite lesions (ie, those situated near the mole) are inspected.

Diagnosis

Nursing Diagnoses

Based on the nursing assessment data, the patient's major nursing diagnoses may include the following:

- Acute pain related to surgical excision and grafting
- Anxiety and depression related to possible life-threatening consequences of melanoma and disfigurement
- Deficient knowledge about early signs of melanoma

Collaborative Problems/ Potential Complications

Based on the assessment data, potential complications include the following:

- Metastasis
- Infection of the surgical site

Planning and Goals

The major goals for the patient may include relief of pain and discomfort, reduced anxiety and depression, increased knowledge of early signs of melanoma, and absence of complications.

Nursing Interventions

Relieving Pain and Discomfort

Surgical removal of melanoma in different locations presents different challenges, taking into consideration the removal of the primary melanoma, the intervening lymphatic vessels, and the lymph nodes to which metastases may spread. Nursing management of the patient having surgery in these regions is discussed in the appropriate chapters.

Nursing interventions after surgery for a malignant melanoma center on promoting comfort, because wide excision surgery may be necessary. A split-thickness or full-thickness skin graft may be necessary when large defects are created by surgical removal of a melanoma. Anticipating the need for and administering appropriate analgesic medications are important.

Reducing Anxiety and Depression

Psychological support is essential when disfiguring surgery is performed. Support includes allowing the patient to express feelings about the seriousness of

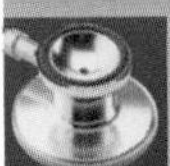

Assessing the ABCDs of Moles

A FOR ASYMMETRY

- The lesion does not appear balanced on both sides. If an imaginary line were drawn down the middle, the two halves would not look alike.
- The lesion has an irregular surface with uneven elevations (irregular topography) either palpable or visible. A change in the surface may be noted from smooth to scaly.
- Some nodular melanomas have a smooth surface.

B FOR IRREGULAR BORDER

- Angular indentations or multiple notches appear in the border.
- The border is fuzzy or indistinct, as if rubbed with an eraser.

C FOR VARIEGATED COLOR

- Normal moles are usually a uniform light to medium brown. Darker coloration indicates that the melanocytes have penetrated to a deeper layer of the dermis.
- Colors that may indicate malignancy if found together within a single lesion are shades of red, white, and blue; shades of blue are ominous.
- White areas within a pigmented lesion are suspicious.
- Some malignant melanomas, however, are not variegated but are uniformly colored (bluish-black, bluish-gray, bluish-red).

D FOR DIAMETER

- A diameter exceeding 6 mm (about the size of a pencil eraser) is considered more suspicious, although this finding without other signs is not significant. Many benign skin growths are larger than 6 mm, whereas some early melanomas may be smaller.

the cutaneous neoplasm, understanding the patient's anger and depression, and conveying understanding of these feelings. During the diagnostic workup and staging of the depth, type, and extent of the tumor, the nurse answers questions, clarifies information, and helps clarify misconceptions. Learning that he or she has a melanoma can cause the patient considerable fear and anguish. Pointing out the patient's resources, past effective coping mechanisms, and social support systems helps the patient cope with the diagnosis and need for treatment and continuing follow-up. Family members should be included in all discussions to enable them to clarify information, ask questions that the patient might be reluctant to ask, and provide emotional support to the patient.

Monitoring and Managing Potential Complications

METASTASIS

The prognosis for malignant melanoma is related to metastasis: the deeper and thicker (more than 4 mm) the melanoma, the greater is the likelihood of metastasis. If the melanoma is growing radially (ie, horizontally) and is characterized by peripheral growth with minimal or no dermal invasion, the prognosis is favorable. When the melanoma invades the dermal layer, the prognosis is poor. Lesions with ulceration have a poor prognosis. Melanomas of the trunk appear to have a poorer prognosis than those of other sites, perhaps because the network of lymphatics in the trunk permits metastasis to regional lymph nodes.

The role of the nurse in caring for the patient with metastatic disease is to provide holistic care. The nurse must be knowledgeable about the most effective current therapies and must deliver supportive care, provide and clarify information about the therapy and the rationale for its use, identify potential side effects of therapy and ways to manage them, and instruct the patient and family about the expected outcomes of treatment. The nurse monitors and documents symptoms that may indicate metastasis: lung (eg, difficulty breathing, shortness of breath, increasing cough), bone (eg, pain, decreased mobility and function, pathologic fractures), and liver (eg, change in liver enzyme levels, pain, jaundice). Nursing care is based on the patient's symptoms and emotional needs.

Although the chance of a cure for malignant melanoma that has metastasized is poor, the nurse encourages hope while maintaining a realistic perspective about the disease and ultimate outcome. Furthermore, the nurse provides time for the patient to express fears and concerns regarding future activities and relationships, offers information about support groups and contact people, and arranges palliative and hospice care if appropriate (see Chapter 17).

Promoting Home and Community-Based Care

TEACHING PATIENTS SELF-CARE

The best hope of decreasing the incidence of skin cancer lies in educating patients about the early signs. Patients at risk are taught to examine their skin and scalp monthly in a systematic manner and to seek prompt medical attention if changes are detected (Chart 56-10). The nurse also points out that a key factor in the development of melanoma is exposure to sunlight. Because melanoma is thought to be genetically linked, the family as well as the patient should be taught sun-avoiding measures and the importance of annual assessment by a health care provider.

Evaluation

Expected Patient Outcomes

Expected patient outcomes may include the following:

1. Experiences relief of pain and discomfort
   a. States pain is diminishing
   b. Exhibits healing of surgical scar without heat, redness, or swelling
2. Is less anxious
   a. Expresses fears and fantasies
   b. Asks questions about medical condition
   c. Requests facts about melanoma
   d. Identifies support and comfort provided by family member or significant other
3. Demonstrates understanding of the means for detecting and preventing melanoma
   a. Demonstrates how to conduct self-examination of skin on a monthly basis
   b. Verbalizes the following danger signals of melanoma: change in size, color, shape, or outline of mole, mole surface, or skin around mole
   c. Identifies measures to protect self from exposure to sunlight
4. Experiences absence of complications
   a. Recognizes abnormal signs and symptoms that should be reported to physician
   b. Complies with recommended follow-up procedures and prevention strategies

Metastatic Skin Tumors

The skin is an important, although not a common, site of metastatic cancer. All types of cancer may metastasize to the skin, but carcinoma of the breast is the primary source of cutaneous metastases in women. Other sources include cancer of the large intestine, ovaries, and lungs. In men, the most common primary sites are the lungs, large intestine, oral cavity, kidneys, or stomach. Skin metastases from melanomas are found in both genders. The clinical appearance of metastatic skin lesions is not distinctive, except perhaps in some cases of breast cancer in which diffuse, brawny hardening of the skin of the involved breast is seen. In most instances, metastatic lesions occur as multiple cutaneous or subcutaneous nodules of various sizes that may be skin-colored or different shades of red.

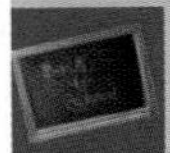

CHART 56-10

Patient Education

Periodic Self-Examination

Prevention of melanoma/skin cancer is the best weapon against these diseases, but if a melanoma should develop, it is almost always curable if caught in the early stages. Practice periodic self-examination to aid in early recognition of any new or developing lesion. The following is one way of self-examination that will ensure that no area of the body is neglected. To perform your self-examination, you will need a full-length mirror, a hand mirror, and a brightly lit room.

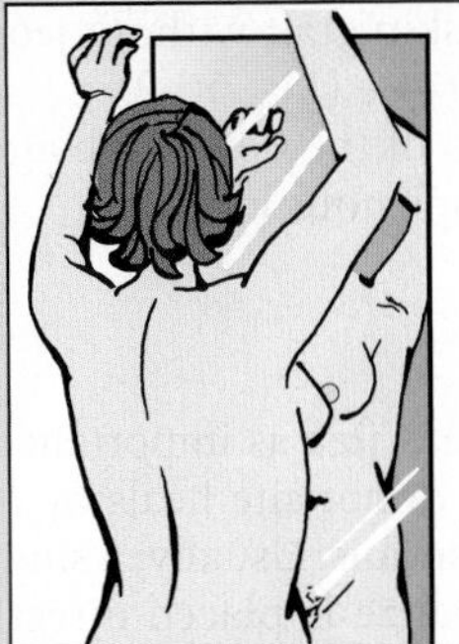	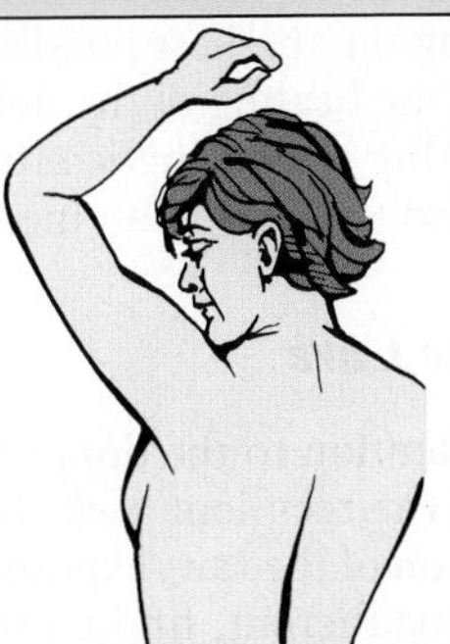	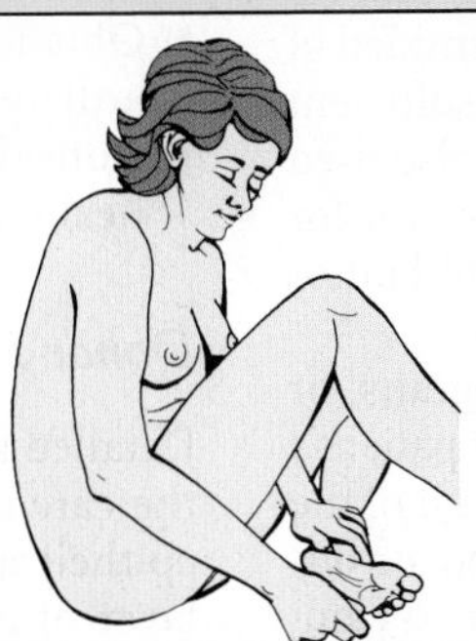	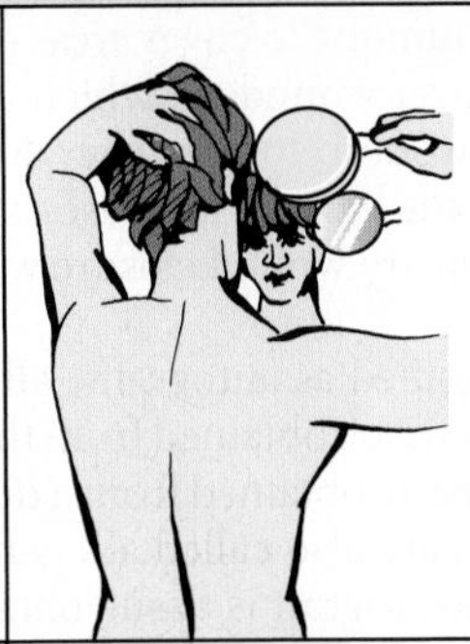	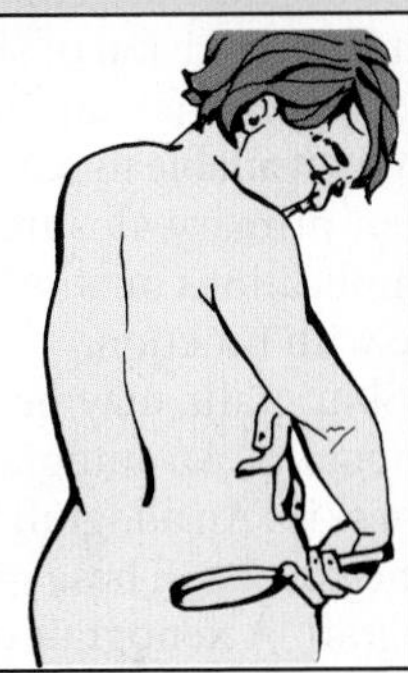
1 Examine the body front and back in the mirror, then the right and left sides, with the arms raised.	**2** Bend the elbows, looking carefully at the forearms, back of the upper arms, and palms.	**3** Next, look at the back of the legs and feet, the spaces between the toes, and the soles of the feet.	**4** Examine the back of the neck and the scalp with a hand mirror. Part the hair to lift.	**5** Finally, check the back and buttocks with a hand mirror.

Kaposi's Sarcoma

Kaposi's sarcoma (KS) is a malignancy of endothelial cells that line the small blood vessels. KS is manifested clinically by lesions of the skin, oral cavity, gastrointestinal tract, and lungs. The skin lesions consist of reddish-purple to dark-blue macules, plaques, or nodules. KS is subdivided into three categories:

- **Classic KS** occurs predominantly in men of Mediterranean or Jewish ancestry between 40 and 70 years of age. Most patients have nodules or plaques on the lower extremities that rarely metastasize beyond this area. Classic KS is chronic, relatively benign, and rarely fatal.
- **Endemic (African) KS** affects people predominantly in the eastern half of Africa near the equator. Men are affected more often than women, and children can be affected as well. The disease may resemble classic KS or it may infiltrate and progress to lymphadenopathic forms.
- **Immunosuppression-associated KS** occurs in transplant recipients and people with AIDS. This form of KS is characterized by local skin lesions and disseminated visceral and mucocutaneous diseases. The greater the degree of immunosuppression, the higher the incidence of KS. Immunosuppression-related KS that results from AIDS is an aggressive tumor that involves multiple body organs. Its presentation resembles that of KS associated with immunosuppressive therapy. Most patients are between the ages of 20 and 40 years. More information on AIDS-related KS can be found in Chapter 52.

Dermatologic and Plastic Reconstructive Surgery

The word *plastic* comes from a Greek word meaning *to form.* Plastic or reconstructive surgery is performed to reconstruct or alter congenital or acquired defects to restore or improve the body's form and function. Often, the terms "plastic" and "reconstructive" are used interchangeably. This type of surgery includes closure of wounds, removal of skin tumors, repair of soft tissue injuries or burns, correction of deformities, and repair of cosmetic defects. Plastic surgery can be used to repair many parts of the body and numerous structures, such as bone, cartilage, fat, fascia, mucous membrane, muscle, nerve, and cutaneous structures. Bone inlays and transplants for deformities and nonunion can be performed, muscle can be transferred, nerves can be reconstructed and spliced, and cartilage can be replaced. As important as any of these measures is the reconstruction of the cutaneous tissues around the neck and the face; this is usually referred to as aesthetic or cosmetic surgery.

Wound Coverage: Grafts and Flaps

Various surgical techniques, including skin grafts and flaps, are used to cover skin wounds.

Skin Grafts

Skin grafting is a technique in which a section of skin is detached from its own blood supply and transferred as free tissue to a distant (recipient) site. Skin grafting can be used to repair almost any type of wound and is the most common form of reconstructive surgery.

Skin grafts are commonly used to repair defects that result from excision of skin tumors, to cover areas denuded of skin (eg, burns), and to cover wounds in which insufficient skin is available to permit wound closure. They are also used when primary closure of the wound increases the risk for complications or when primary wound closure would interfere with function.

Skin grafts may be classified as autografts, allografts, or xenografts. An autograft is tissue obtained from the patient's own skin. An allograft is tissue obtained from a donor of the same species. These grafts are also called allogeneic or homograft. A xenograft or heterograft is tissue obtained from another species.

Grafts are also referred to by their thickness. A skin graft may be a split-thickness (ie, thin, intermediate, or thick) or a full-thickness graft, depending on the amount of dermis included in the specimen. A split-thickness graft can be cut at various thicknesses and is commonly used to cover large wounds or defects for which a full-thickness graft or flap is impractical (Fig. 56-8). A full-thickness graft consists of epidermis and the entire dermis without the underlying fat. It is used to cover wounds that are too large to be closed directly.

Donor Site Selection

The donor site is selected with several criteria in mind:

- Achieving the closest possible color match
- Matching the texture and hair-bearing qualities
- Obtaining the thickest possible skin graft without jeopardizing the healing of the donor site (Fig. 56-9)
- Considering the cosmetic effects of the donor site after healing, so that it is in an inconspicuous location

Donor Site Care

Detailed attention to the donor site is just as important as the care of the recipient area. The donor site heals by reepithelization of the raw, exposed dermis. Usually, a single layer of nonadherent, fine-mesh gauze is placed directly over the donor site. Absorbent gauze dressings are then placed on top to absorb blood or serum from the wound. A membrane dressing (eg, Op-Site) may be used and provides certain advantages. It is transparent and allows the wound

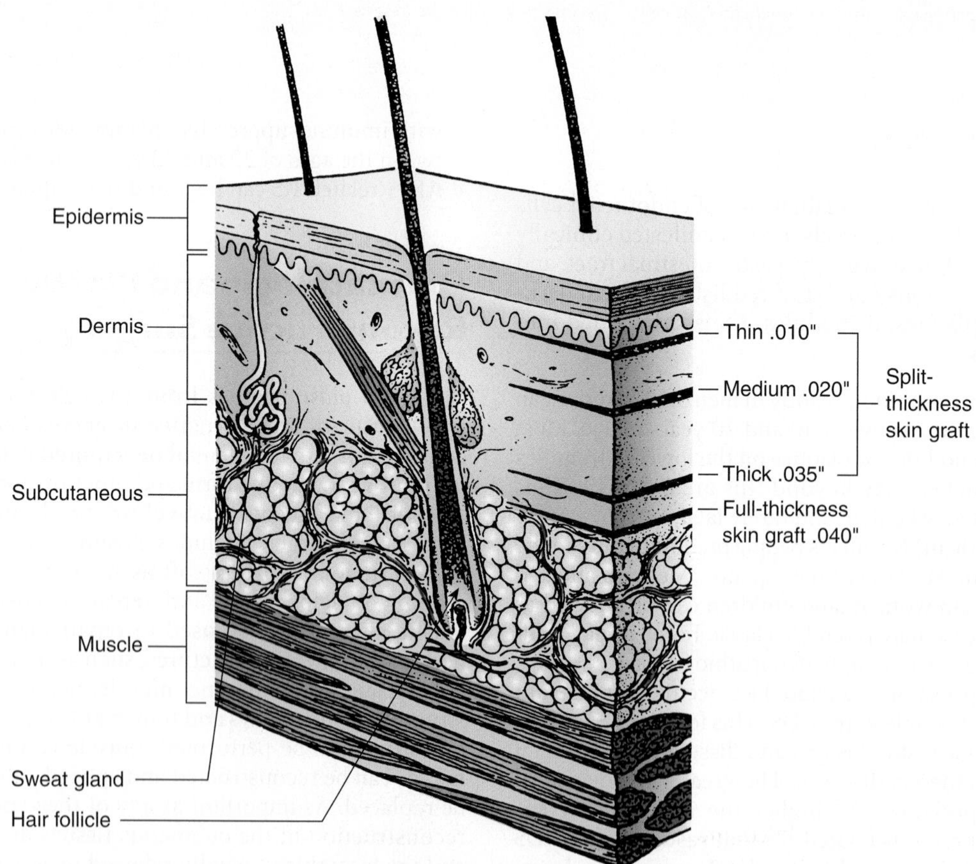

FIGURE 56-8. Layers of skin appropriate for split-thickness and full-thickness graft.

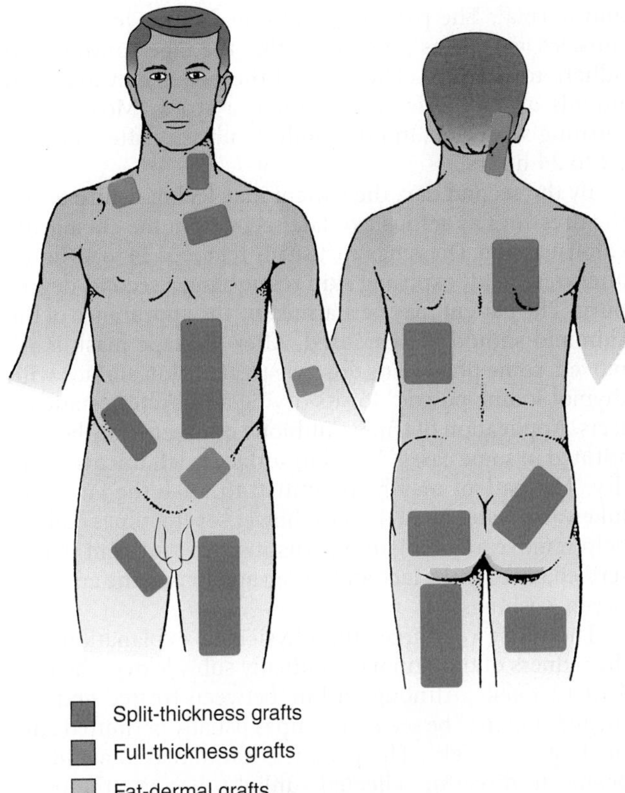

FIGURE 56-9. Common donor skin graft sites. Blue skin areas are appropriate for full-thickness grafts; green areas are used for split-thickness grafts; rose sites are used for fat-dermal grafts.

to be observed without disturbing the dressing, and it permits the patient to shower without fear of saturating the dressing with water.

After healing, the patient is instructed to keep the donor site soft and pliable with cream (eg, lanolin, olive oil). Both the donor site and the grafted area must be protected from exposure to extremes in temperature, external trauma, and sunlight because these areas are sensitive, especially to thermal injuries.

Graft Application

A graft is obtained by a variety of instruments: razor blades, skin-grafting knives, electric- or air-powered dermatomes, or drum dermatomes. The skin graft is taken from the donor or host site and applied to the desired site, called the recipient site or graft bed.

For a graft to survive and be effective, certain conditions must be met:

- The recipient site must have an adequate blood supply so that normal physiologic function can resume.
- The graft must be in close contact with its bed to avoid accumulation of blood or fluid between the graft and the recipient site.
- The graft must be fixed firmly (immobilized) so that it remains in place on the recipient site.
- The area must be free of infection.

The graft, when applied to the recipient site, may be sutured in place. It may be slit and spread apart to cover a greater area. The process of revascularization (establishing the blood supply) and reattachment of a skin graft to a recipient bed is referred to as a "take." After a skin graft is put in place, it may be left exposed (in areas that are impossible to immobilize) or covered with a light dressing or a pressure dressing, depending on the area of the body.

Nursing Interventions

The nurse instructs the patient to keep the affected part immobilized as much as possible. For a graft to the face, strenuous activity must be avoided. A graft on the hand or arm may be immobilized with a splint. When a graft is placed on a lower extremity, the part is kept elevated because the new capillary connections are fragile and excess venous pressure may cause rupture. When ambulation is permitted, the patient wears an elastic stocking to counterbalance venous pressure.

The nurse instructs the patient, family member, or other caregiver to inspect the dressing daily. Unusual drainage or an inflammatory reaction around the wound margin suggests infection and should be reported to the physician. Any fluid, purulent drainage, blood, or serum that has collected is gently evacuated by the surgeon, because accumulation of this material would cause the graft to separate from its bed.

When the graft appears pink, it is vascularized. After 2 to 3 weeks, the surgeon may prescribe that either mineral oil or a lanolin cream or one of the newer creams that are specific for scar prevention be massaged into the wound to moisten the graft. Because there may be loss of feeling or sensation in the grafted area for a prolonged period, the application of heating pads and exposure to sun are avoided to prevent burns and further skin trauma.

Flaps

Another form of wound coverage is provided by flaps. A flap is a segment of tissue that remains attached at one end (ie, a base or pedicle) while the other end is moved to a recipient area. Its survival depends on functioning arterial and venous blood supplies and lymphatic drainage in its pedicle or base. A flap differs from a graft in that a portion of the tissue is attached to its original site and retains its blood supply. An exception is the free flap, which is described below.

Flaps may consist of skin, mucosa, muscle, adipose tissue, omentum, and bone. They are used for wound coverage and provide bulk, especially when bone, tendon, blood vessels, or nerve tissue is exposed. Flaps are used to repair defects caused by congenital deformity, trauma, or tumor ablation (removal, usually by excision) in an adjacent part of the body.

Flaps offer an aesthetic solution because a flap retains the color and texture of the donor area, is more likely to survive than a graft, and can be used to cover nerves, tendons, and blood vessels. However, several surgical procedures are usually required to advance a flap. The major complication is necrosis of the pedicle or base as a result of failure of the blood supply.

Free Flaps

A striking advance in reconstructive surgery is the use of free flaps or free-tissue transfer achieved by microvascular techniques. A free flap is completely severed from the body and transferred to another site. A free flap receives early vascular supply from microvascular anastomosis with vessels at the recipient site. The procedure usually is completed in one step, eliminating the need for a series of surgical procedures to move the flap. Microvascular surgery allows surgeons to use a variety of donor sites for tissue reconstruction.

Chemical Face Peeling

Chemical face peeling, a technique that involves applying a chemical mixture to the face for superficial destruction of the epidermis and the upper layers of the dermis, treats fine wrinkles, keratoses, and pigment problems. It is especially useful for wrinkles at the upper and lower lip, forehead, and periorbital areas.

Pretreatment may consist of cleansing the face and hair for several days before the procedure with a hexachlorophene detergent. Pretreatment medication (ie, analgesic and tranquilizer for moderate sedation) may be prescribed to alleviate apprehension and control pain. This permits the patient to be sedated but conscious during the procedure, although some patients request general anesthesia.

The type of chemical used depends on the planned depth of the peel. A phenol-based chemical in an oil–water emulsion is commonly used because it produces a controlled, predictable chemical burn. The chemical is applied systematically to the face with cotton-tipped applicators. The conscious patient feels a burning sensation at this time. A mask of waterproof adhesive may then be applied directly to the skin and molded closely to the contours of the face, thereby acting as an occlusive dressing that increases the chemical penetration and action. Some surgeons believe that equally good results can be obtained with occlusive tape. After the tape mask is applied, the burning sensation continues, and the tape mask remains in place for 12 to 24 hours. Frequent small doses of analgesics and tranquilizers are prescribed to keep the patient comfortable.

Complications

Complications may arise when the chemically induced burn cannot be controlled. Complications include pigment changes, infection, milia (ie, small inclusion cysts that disappear after several months), scarring, atrophy, sensitivity changes, and long-term (4 to 5 months) erythema or pruritus.

Management

Because chemical face peeling is performed in the physician's office or in an outpatient surgical department, most care takes place in the home. After 6 to 8 hours, the face becomes edematous and the eyelids usually swell shut. The patient should be reassured that this reaction is expected and normal. The patient is cautioned to move the facial muscles as little as possible so that the tape continues to adhere to the skin. The head of the bed is elevated, and liquids are administered through a straw. Most of the burning sensation and discomfort subsides after the first 12 to 24 hours.

By the second day, the patient may feel moisture under the dressings as serous exudate seeps from the chemically exfoliated skin. Dressings are usually removed 24 to 48 hours after treatment, exposing skin resembling a second-degree burn. The patient may be alarmed by the appearance of the skin and should be reassured. After the tape mask is removed, some physicians dust the treated skin surface with thymol-iodine powder for its drying and bacteriostatic effects. Application of triple-antibiotic ointment may be substituted in some cases. The skin surface is left uncovered to dry. The patient may be permitted to wash the face with lukewarm water or advised to shower several times daily to help remove any remaining crusting. An ointment is prescribed to cover the face and soften and loosen the crust between washings.

The nurse reinforces the physician's explanation that the redness of the skin will gradually subside over the next 4 to 12 weeks. Although a line between treated and untreated skin may be seen, makeup is usually permitted after the first few weeks. The patient is cautioned to avoid exposure to direct or reflected sunlight, because the treatment reduces the natural protection of the skin from sun. The skin will probably never tan evenly again. Blotchy pigmentation can occur with exposure to the sun.

Dermabrasion

Dermabrasion is a form of skin abrasion used to correct acne scarring, aging, and sun-damaged skin. A special instrument (ie, motor-driven wire brush, diamond-impregnated disk, or serrated wheel) is used in the procedure. The epidermis and some superficial dermis are removed, while enough of the dermis is preserved to allow reepithelization of the treated areas. Results are best in the face because it is rich in intradermal epithelial elements.

Preparation and Procedure

The primary reason for undergoing dermabrasion is to improve appearance. The physician explains to the patient what can be expected from dermabrasion. The patient should also be informed about the nature of the postoperative dressing, what discomfort may be experienced, and how long it will be before the tissues look normal.

Dermabrasion may be performed in the physician's office, the operating room, or an outpatient setting. It is performed under local anesthesia or moderate sedation. During the procedure, some surgeons use refrigerant anesthetics to turn the skin into a numb, solid mass of rigid tissue and to provide a momentarily bloodless surgical field. During and after planing, the area is irrigated with copious amounts of saline solution to remove debris and allow the surgeon to see the area. A dressing impregnated with ointment is usually applied to the abraded surface.

Management

The nurse instructs the patient about postoperative effects. Edema occurs during the first 48 hours and may cause the eyelids to close. The head of the bed is elevated to hasten fluid drainage. Erythema occurs and can last for weeks or months. After 24 hours, the dressing may be removed if the physician allows. When the serum oozing from the skin begins to gel, the patient applies the prescribed ointment to the face several times each day to prevent hard crusting and to keep the abraded areas soft and flexible. Clear-water cleansing or soaking of the face to remove crusts from the healing skin is started when directed by the physician.

The patient is advised to avoid extreme cold and heat and excessive straining or lifting, which may bruise delicate new capillaries. Direct or reflected sunlight should be avoided for 3 to 6 months and a sunscreen used.

Facial Reconstructive Surgery

Reconstructive procedures on the face are individualized to the patient's needs and desired outcomes. They are performed to repair deformities or restore normal function as much as possible. They may vary from closure of small defects to complicated procedures involving implantation of prosthetic devices to conceal a large defect or reconstruct a lost part of the face (eg, nose, ear, jaw). Each surgical procedure is customized and involves a variety of incisions, flaps, and grafts.

In correcting a primary defect, the surgeon may have to create a secondary defect. Although the procedure may restore some function, such as eating or talking, the cosmetic or aesthetic results may be limited. The original appearance of a patient who has severe damage to soft tissue and bone structure can seldom be restored. Multiple surgical procedures may be required. The process of facial reconstruction is often slow and tedious.

Assessment

The face is a part of the body that every person desires to keep at its best or improve, because most human interactions involve the face. Anxiety and depression are common when the appearance and function of the face are affected by injury or disease. Patients with facial changes frequently mourn for the lost part, suffer a loss of self-esteem because of reactions or rejection by others, and withdraw and isolate themselves. Health care providers can acknowledge to the patient that anxiety and depression are appropriate for what the patient is experiencing.

The nurse assesses the patient's emotional responses and identifies strengths as well as usual coping mechanisms to determine how the patient will handle the surgical procedure. Areas in which the patient and family need extra support are identified.

The preoperative assessment determines the extent of disfigurement and improvement that can be anticipated, as well as the patient's understanding and acceptance of these limitations. The nurse reinforces facts and clarifies misconceptions after the surgeon has fully informed the patient about the procedure, the functional defects that may result, the possible need for a tracheostomy or other prosthesis, and the probability of additional surgery. The nurse instructs the patient about various postoperative measures: IV therapy, the use of a nasogastric tube to allow gastric decompression and prevent vomiting, and the frequent and lengthy periods that may be required to care for wounds, flaps, and skin grafts and to change dressings. Extra time is needed when presenting this information to anxious patients because they may not be able to concentrate or comprehend what is being said.

Nursing Management

Maintaining Airway and Pulmonary Function

The immediate concern after facial reconstruction is maintenance of an adequate airway. If the patient has regained consciousness, mental confusion with combative, anxious behavior may be a sign of hypoxia (reduced oxygen supply to tissues) or of unrelieved pain. Sedatives or opioids are not prescribed if the patient is hypoxic because they may impair oxygenation. However, if the patient's behavior is in response to pain, pain relief measures, including analgesics, are administered as prescribed. If the patient shows signs of restlessness, the airway is carefully inspected to detect laryngeal edema or accumulation of tracheobronchial mucus. Secretions are suctioned as necessary until the patient can manage the secretions without help. If the patient has a tracheostomy, suctioning is performed with sterile technique to prevent infection and cross-contamination. Chapter 25 provides information on care of the patient with a tracheostomy.

Relieving Pain and Achieving Comfort

Facial edema is an uncomfortable but natural consequence of facial reconstructive surgery. The patient's head and upper torso are kept slightly elevated (if the blood pressure is stable) to minimize facial edema. Catheters attached to closed drainage may be in place to keep the tissues in close apposition and to remove serous discharge. If extensive reconstruction has been performed, the patient's head should be properly aligned and supported so that minimal stress is placed on the suture line.

Analgesics are prescribed to relieve pain. If bone grafts have been used for reconstruction, there is usually considerable pain in the donor area. If the patient has head and neck cancer and increasing levels of pain, comprehensive nursing management is required (see Chapters 13 and 35).

Maintaining Adequate Nutrition

Fluids may be offered to the patient after oral and pharyngeal edema diminishes, the incisional areas and flaps heal, and the patient can swallow saliva. Gradually, soft foods are added as tolerated. If the patient cannot meet nutritional needs by the oral route, enteral nutrition is initiated. The formula strength and feeding rate are gradually increased until the desired daily caloric level is attained. See Chapter 36 for more information about nursing management of the patient who requires enteral feedings. Patients who have had radical surgery for large, encroaching neoplasms may have difficulty resuming eating. Positive nutrition is reflected in weight gain, and nutritional status is monitored by measuring body weight daily and assessing serum protein and electrolyte levels periodically.

Enhancing Communication

Communication problems may range from minimal difficulty to the loss of oral speech. Some tumors and injuries require extensive surgery involving the larynx, tongue, and mandible. Paper, pen or pencil, and a firm writing surface should be provided. If the patient cannot read and write, a pictograph board may be used. Referral to a speech therapist may be necessary for the patient who has undergone structural changes. The family may become frustrated by the patient's inability to communicate. The patient soon senses this, and both parties may withdraw. Allowing the family to vent their feelings and fears (away from the patient) is important.

Improving Self-Concept

Success in rehabilitating the patient undergoing reconstructive surgery depends on the relationships among the patient and the nurse, the physician, and other members of the health care team. Mutual trust, respect, and clear lines of communication are essential. Unhurried care provides emotional reassurance and support.

The kinds of dressings worn, the unusual positions to be maintained, and the temporary incapacity experienced can cause distress. Reinforcement of the patient's successful coping strategies improves self-esteem. If prosthetic devices are used, the patient is taught how to use and care for them to gain a sense of greater independence. Once involved in self-care activities, the patient may feel some control over what was previously an overwhelming situation.

Patients with severe disfigurement are encouraged to socialize to experience the reactions of others in a more protected environment. Gradually, they can widen their sphere of contact. Every effort is made to cover or mask defects. Patients may require support by members of the mental health team to accept their changed appearance.

Promoting Family Coping

The family is informed about the patient's appearance after surgery, the supportive equipment, and the ways that the equipment aids recovery. It is helpful to accompany the family during their first postoperative visit to help them cope with the changes they will see.

A major role of the nurse is to support the family in their decision to participate (or not to participate) in the patient's treatment. Nursing interventions also include helping the family members communicate by suggesting ways to reduce anxiety and stress and to promote problem solving and decision making. These activities encourage family members and promote growth.

Monitoring and Managing Potential Complications

Secondary infection is a primary concern after reconstructive surgery. The source of infection depends on the location and extent of the procedure, the suture line, and the pedicle flap.

The mouth is inspected to determine the location of sutures (when present) so that they are not disturbed during the cleaning process. The mouth is cleaned according to protocol several times daily. Loose blood clots may be removed with gentle swabbing. The patient is advised not to loosen clots with the tongue because this may cause bleeding. The patient is instructed not to use fingers to clean or remove blood clots because this may introduce organisms that cause infection.

The suture line remains under stress for several days after surgery because of edema, increased drainage, and hematoma formation. The nurse assesses the suture line carefully for signs of increased tension and infection (ie, elevated temperature, increasing edema, redness, bleeding, and increased pain) with each dressing change. Dressings may need to be changed many times each day until the drainage begins to decrease. Drainage and edema are expected after reconstructive surgery; however, both should decrease, and the process is hastened by using properly placed, functioning suction devices and elevating the head of the bed about 45 degrees. The nurse inspects the suction devices, empties them promptly, and documents the amount and consistency of drainage, as well as any unusual odor. When drainage is not removed or if saturated dressings are left unchanged for long periods, infection is likely. Strict asepsis must be maintained in wound care.

A pedicle flap used in reconstruction may become a source of infection if its circulation becomes compromised. Poor circulation may result from a hematoma forming beneath the flap and causing increased pressure on the underlying vasculature. The nurse inspects the flap for changes in color and temperature indicative of poor circulation. Signs of necrosis, increased drainage, or an odor may be a warning of an infection and should be reported promptly. Reinforcing preoperative teaching about wound healing, the need for strict sterile technique, good personal hygiene, and the need to restrict movement and stress on the operative site is an important part of the nurse's role in postoperative care and in the prevention of secondary infection.

Face Lift

Rhytidectomy (face lift) is a surgical procedure that removes soft tissue folds and minimizes cutaneous wrinkles on the face. It is performed to create a more youthful appearance.

Psychological preparation requires that the patient recognize the limitations of surgery and the fact that miraculous rejuvenation will not occur. The patient is informed that the face may appear bruised and swollen after the dressings are removed and that several weeks may pass before the edema subsides.

The procedure is performed under local anesthesia or moderate sedation, often in the outpatient setting. The incisions are concealed in natural skin folds and creases and areas hidden by hair. Loose skin, separated from underlying muscle, is pulled upward and backward. Excess skin that overlaps the incision line is removed. Liposuction-assisted rhytidectomy is being performed more frequently.

In this procedure, fat is suctioned from the body through a cannula inserted through a small incision.

Management

The nurse encourages the patient to rest quietly for the first 2 postoperative days until the dressings are removed. The head of the bed is elevated, and neck flexion is discouraged to avoid compromising the circulation and the suture line. The patient may feel some tightness of the face and neck from pressure created by the newly tightened muscles, fascia, and skin. Analgesics may be prescribed to relieve discomfort. A liquid diet may be given by means of straws, and a soft diet is permitted if chewing is not too uncomfortable.

When the dressings are removed, the skin is gently cleaned of crusting and oozing and coated with the prescribed topical ointment. Any hair matted with drainage may be combed with warm water and a wide-toothed comb.

The patient is advised not to lift or bend for 7 to 10 days because this activity may increase edema and provoke bleeding. Activities are gradually resumed. When all sutures are removed, the hair may be shampooed and blown dry with warm, not hot, air to avoid burning the ears, which may be numb for a while.

The patient needs to know that a face lift will not stop the aging process and that with time the tissues will resume the downward drift. Some patients have two or more face lifts.

Sudden pain indicates that blood is accumulating underneath the skin flaps; it should be reported to the surgeon immediately. Complications include sloughing of the skin, deformities of the face and neck, and partial facial paralysis. Cigarette smoking has been implicated as a cause of skin slough in some patients.

Laser Treatment of Cutaneous Lesions

Lasers are devices that amplify or generate highly specialized light energy. They can mobilize immense heat and power when focused at close range and are valuable tools in surgical procedures. The argon laser, carbon dioxide (CO_2) laser, and tunable pulse-dye laser are used in dermatologic surgery. Each type of laser emits its own wavelength within the color spectrum.

Argon Laser

The argon laser produces a visible blue-green light that is absorbed by vascular tissue and is therefore useful in treating vascular lesions: port-wine stains, telangiectases, vascular tumors, and pigmented lesions. The argon beam can penetrate approximately 1 mm of skin and reach the pigmented layer, causing protein coagulation in this area. An immediate effect is that tiny blood vessels under the skin coagulate, causing the area to turn a much lighter color. A crust forms within a few days.

During the procedure, the patient may require local anesthesia (lidocaine), but only if the lesion, such as a port-wine stain, is wider than 0.5 cm. Laser beams, regardless of type, are reflected and scattered in all directions during the treatment. Laser radiation is hazardous to the eye, and the eyes of the patient and all personnel involved in the surgical procedure and those who are within the immediate surgical environment must be protected with orange, argon light–absorbing safety goggles.

Management

Cold compresses are usually applied over the treatment area for approximately 6 hours to minimize edema, exudate, and loss of capillary permeability. The nurse advises the patient that swelling will subside in 1 to 2 days and will be followed by a crust that will last 7 to 10 days. The nurse instructs the patient to avoid picking at the crust, to apply an antibacterial ointment sparingly until the crust separates, to avoid applying makeup until the wound heals, and to avoid exposure to the sun. Sunscreen is to be used when exposure is unavoidable.

Carbon Dioxide Laser

The CO_2 laser emits invisible light in the infrared spectrum that is absorbed at the skin surface because of the high water content of the skin and the long wavelength of the CO_2 light. As the laser beam strikes tissue, it is absorbed by the intracellular and extracellular water, which vaporizes, destroying the tissue. The CO_2 laser is a precise surgical instrument that vaporizes and excises tissue with minimal damage. Because the beam can seal blood and lymphatic vessels, it creates a dry surgical field that makes many procedures easier and quicker. Therefore, it is safe to use on patients with bleeding disorders or those receiving anticoagulant therapy. It is useful for removing epidermal nevi, tattoos, certain warts, skin cancer, ingrown toenails, and keloids. Incisions made with the laser beam heal and scar much like those made by a scalpel.

In addition to wearing safety goggles, the patient and personnel wear laser-grade surgical masks to avoid inhaling the byproduct smoke, referred to as a plume.

Management

Immediately after undergoing CO_2 laser surgery, the treated area turns a charcoal color. The wound is covered with antibacterial ointment and a nonadhesive dressing. The patient is instructed to keep the wound dry except for gentle cleansing with mild soap several times each day. After the skin is cleaned, a prescribed ointment and light dressing are applied.

Because nerve endings and lymphatic vessels are sealed by the laser, less edema and pain follow the laser procedure than with conventional surgery. A mild analgesic is sufficient to maintain patient comfort. Wound healing occurs by secondary intention, with granulation tissue appearing within a week; complete healing occurs in several weeks. Sun exposure to the area should be avoided for approximately 6 months. Application of a sunscreen with an SPF of greater than 15 is recommended, especially for people at high risk for skin cancer from sun exposure, who need to block UVB and UVA light.

Pulse-Dye Laser

The tunable pulse-dye laser with various wavelengths is the latest laser available for dermatologic surgery. It is especially useful in treating cutaneous vascular lesions such as port-wine stains and telangiectasia. Eye protection used for the argon and CO_2 lasers is insufficient when the pulse-dye laser is in use. Special eyeglasses, such as those made of didymium glass, are required for the patient and all personnel. The procedure is generally painless. For procedures requiring anesthesia, lidocaine without epinephrine is sufficient because local vasoconstriction (which epinephrine induces) is unnecessary.

Management

The patient should be informed that there may be stinging in the treated area for several hours. Applying ice to the area and a light antibacterial ointment followed by a nonstick dressing (eg, Telfa) usually eases discomfort.

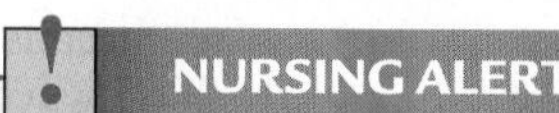

Telfa pads contain latex and should not be used on patients who are latex sensitive. Other dressings, such as petrolatum-impregnated gauze, should be used to prevent the dressing from adhering to the wound.

If crusting occurs, the patient is advised to wash the area gently with soap and water, reapply the antibacterial cream twice daily, and avoid wearing makeup until the crust disappears. Sun exposure should be avoided as well; sunscreens with an SPF of greater than 15 should be used for 3 to 4 months after the treatment. Complete removal of the lesion at one session, especially a port-wine stain, is rare. The patient should be informed that several treatments may be necessary.

Critical Thinking Exercises

1 ebp You are caring for an elderly woman in her home. She has a long history of peripheral vascular disease and now has developed a venous stasis ulcer on her lower leg just above the ankle. Her physician has prescribed a moisture-retentive dressing that is impregnated with hydrogel. The dressing is to be changed every 3 days, and the patient asks you why the dressing is not changed every day. How would you explain to the patient the purpose of the dressing? Identify the evidence that supports the use of moisture-retentive dressings for venous ulcers. Discuss the strength of the evidence regarding their effectiveness in the promotion of wound healing.

2 You are caring for a middle-aged woman who has recently been diagnosed with diabetes mellitus. On preparing for discharge, she tells you that she has had itchy, dry, flaky skin during the winter months for several years, and that she bathes every morning and night to try to get rid of the itching and dryness. She also states that it is difficult for her to avoid scratching her itchy skin. What teaching would you provide to this patient? What are this patient's risks of developing more serious skin conditions if the dryness and itching of her skin continue?

3 You are assigned to the emergency department and are caring for a young adult who is being treated for heatstroke following a golf game on a very hot day. As he is awaiting discharge he tells you that he is concerned about developing skin cancer because he spends so much time in the sun. After providing the patient with information about risk factors for, and prevention of, heatstroke, what other patient education would you provide? What are the risk factors for skin cancer? What health promotion strategies would be encouraged for this patient?

REFERENCES AND SELECTED READINGS

American Cancer Society. (2005). *Cancer facts and figures*. Atlanta, GA: Author.

Baran, R., & Maibach, H. I. (2004). *Textbook of cosmetic dermatology* (3rd ed.). New York: Taylor & Francis Group.

Barton, S. (Ed.). (2001). *Clinical evidence* (5th ed.). London: BJM Publishing.

Champion, R. H., Burton, J. L., Burns, D. A., et al. (2000). *Rook/Wilkinson/Ebling textbook of dermatology* (7th ed.). Boston: Blackwell Science.

Demis, D. J. (Ed.). (1998). *Clinical dermatology*. Philadelphia: Lippincott-Raven.

Fitzpatrick, T. B., Johnson, R. A., Wolff, K., et al. (2005). *Color atlas and synopsis of clinical dermatology* (7th ed.). New York: McGraw-Hill.

Freedberg, I. M., Eisen, A. Z., & Austen, K. F. (2003). *Fitzpatrick's dermatology in general medicine* (6th ed.). New York: McGraw-Hill.

Hall, J. C. (2006). *Sauer's manual of skin diseases* (9th ed.). Philadelphia: Lippincott Williams & Wilkins.

Krasner, D., Rodeheaver, G., & Sibbald, G. (2002). *Chronic wound care: A clinical source book for healthcare professionals*. Malvern, PA: HMP Communications.

Lask, G., & Lowe, N. (2000). *Lasers in cutaneous and cosmetic surgery*. Philadelphia: Elsevier.

Mallory, S. B., & Treadwell, P. A. (2004). *Handbook of pediatric dermatology* (2nd ed.). Boca Raton, FL: CRC Press.

Murphy, J. L. (2004). *Nurse practitioners' prescribing reference*. New York: Prescribing Reference.

Odom, R. B., James, W. D., & Berger, T. G. (Eds.). (2000). *Andrews' diseases of the skin* (9th ed.). Philadelphia: W. B. Saunders.

Porth, C. M. (2005). Pathophysiology. *Concepts of altered health states* (7th ed.). Philadelphia: Lippincott Williams & Wilkins.

age and in adults younger than 40 years of age. Inhalation injuries in combination with cutaneous burns worsen the prognosis. Outcome depends on the depth and extent of the burn as well as on the preinjury health status and age of the patient. Acute care of patients with burn injuries has improved to the point that survival is expected for most patients (Sheridan & Thompkins, 2004).

Classification of Burns

Burn injuries are described according to the depth of the injury and the extent of body surface area injured.

Burn Depth

[illegible]rns are classified according to the depth of tissue destruc[illegible]n as superficial partial-thickness injuries, deep partial-[illegible]hickness injuries, or full-thickness injuries (Table 57-1). These three categories are similar to, but not the same as, first-, second-, and third-degree burns, respectively. (See Chapter 55 for a review of the layers of the skin.)

- In a superficial partial-thickness burn, the **epidermis** is destroyed or injured and a portion of the **dermis** may be injured. The damaged skin may be painful and appear red and dry, as in sunburn, or it may blister.
- A deep partial-thickness burn involves destruction of the epidermis and upper layers of the dermis and injury to deeper portions of the dermis. The wound is painful, appears red, and exudes fluid. Capillary refill follows tissue blanching. Hair follicles remain intact. Deep partial-thickness burns take longer to heal and are more likely to result in hypertrophic scars.
- A full-thickness burn involves total destruction of epidermis and dermis and, in some cases, destruction of underlying tissue. Wound color ranges widely from white to red, brown, or black. The burned area is painless because nerve fibers are destroyed. The wound appears leathery; hair follicles and sweat glands are destroyed (Fig. 57-1).

Burn depth determines whether epithelialization will occur. Determining burn depth can be difficult even for the experienced burn care provider. The following factors are considered in determining the depth of a burn:

- How the injury occurred
- Causative agent, such as flame or scalding liquid
- Temperature of the burning agent
- Duration of contact with the agent
- Thickness of the skin

Extent of Body Surface Area Injured

Various methods are used to estimate the total body surface area (TBSA) affected by burns; among them are the rule of nines, the Lund and Browder method, and the palm method.

Rule of Nines

The **rule of nines** (Fig. 57-2) is a quick way to estimate the extent of burns. The system assigns percentages in multiples of nine to major body surfaces.

TABLE 57-1 Characteristics of Burns According to Depth

Depth of Burn and Causes	Skin Involvement	Symptoms	Wound Appearance	Recuperative Course
Superficial Partial-Thickness (Similar to First Degree)				
Sunburn Low-intensity flash	Epidermis; possibly a portion of dermis	Tingling Hyperesthesia (supersensitivity) Pain that is soothed by cooling	Reddened; blanches with pressure; dry Minimal or no edema Possible blisters	Complete recovery within a week; no scarring Peeling
Deep Partial-Thickness (Similar to Second Degree)				
Scalds Flash flame Contact	Epidermis, upper dermis, portion of deeper dermis	Pain Hyperesthesia Sensitive to cold air	Blistered, mottled red base; broken epidermis; weeping surface Edema	Recovery in 2 to 4 weeks Some scarring and depigmentation contractures Infection may convert it to full thickness
Full-Thickness (Similar to Third Degree)				
Flame Prolonged exposure to hot liquids Electric current Chemical Contact	Epidermis, entire dermis, and sometimes subcutaneous tissue; may involve connective tissue, muscle, and bone	Pain free Shock Hematuria (blood in the urine) and possibly hemolysis (blood cell destruction) Possible entrance and exit wounds (electrical burn)	Dry; pale white, leathery, or charred Broken skin with fat exposed Edema	Eschar sloughs Grafting necessary Scarring and loss of contour and function; contractures Loss of digits or extremity possible

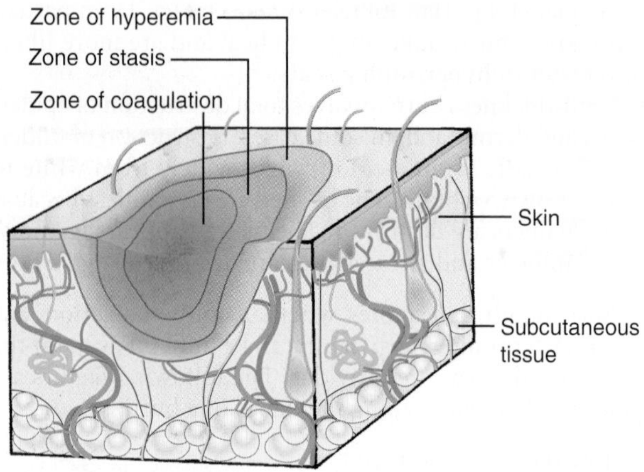

FIGURE 57-1. Zones of burn injury. Each burned area has three zones of injury. The inner zone (known as the area of coagulation, where cellular death occurs) sustains the most damage. The middle area, or zone of stasis, has a compromised blood supply, inflammation, and tissue injury. The outer zone—the zone of hyperemia—sustains the least damage.

Lund and Browder Method

A more precise method of estimating the extent of a burn is the Lund and Browder method, which recognizes that the percentage of surface area of various anatomic parts, especially the head and legs, changes with growth. Because of changes in body proportion with growth, the calculated TBSA changes with age as well. By dividing the body into very small areas and providing an estimate of the proportion of TBSA accounted for by each body part, one can obtain a reliable estimate of TBSA burned. The initial evaluation is made on arrival of the patient at the hospital and is revised on the second and third postburn days, because the demarcation usually is not clear until then.

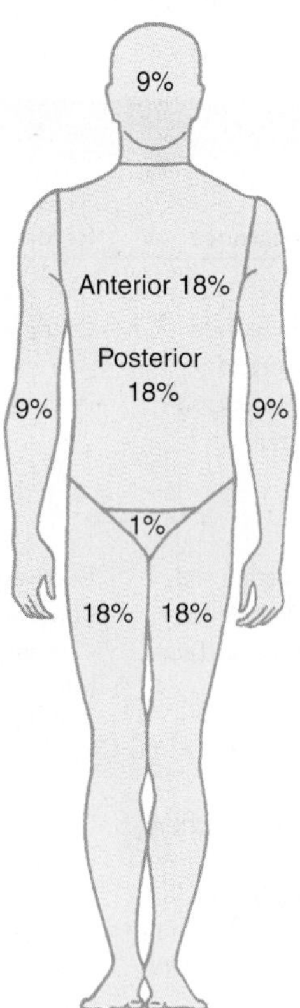

FIGURE 57-2. The rule of nines: Estimated percentage of total body surface area (TBSA) in the adult is arrived at by sectioning the body surface into areas with a numerical value related to nine. (Note: The anterior and posterior head total 9% of TBSA.)

Palm Method

In patients with scattered burns, the palm method may be used to estimate the extent of the burns. The size of the patient's palm is approximately 1% of the TBSA.

Electrical Burns

Electrical injury accounts for a small percentage of burn unit admissions each year, yet it is one of the worst types of burn injuries that can be sustained. The devastating effects of an electrical injury can cause lifelong neurovascular problems. High-voltage (more than 1000 volts) injury can cause tissue and bone destruction resulting in amputations and possible loss of life as the result of cardiac and respiratory abnormalities. A true electrical injury results when a current of electricity travels through the body and exits to the ground itself. With a true electrical injury, there is an entrance wound and an exit wound. An arc injury is the result of the electricity's traveling on the outside of the body or arcing around it. Often the clothes catch fire because of the high energy. The patient ends up with a flame burn and often small spider-like markings that make a path on the skin. The cutaneous injury from electrical sources is usually small compared with the damage under the surface of the skin. Electricity travels through areas of least resistance and destroys everything in its path—nerves and blood vessels first. The stronger the current and the longer the duration of contact, the more severe the injury.

For a patient with an electrical burn, once the patient is out of the path of the electricity, emergency care can safely be provided. The ABCs of emergency care are always followed. An electrical current immediately contracts muscles as it travels through the body, and cardiac dysrhythmias and spinal injuries often result from the muscular contraction. A cardiac monitor should be used for at least 24 hours after the injury or until the patient is stable. Until it is known that the patient has no fractures, it is imperative that a neck collar remain in place and that the patient be logrolled to eliminate the chance of further spinal cord injury. With high-voltage electrical injuries, cervical spine immobilization is a priority until cervical spine injury is ruled out.

For a patient with an electrical burn, prompt administration of intravenous (IV) fluids and monitoring of urine output are critical components of care. Patients with electrical burns are prone to acute renal failure because of the release of myoglobin from the destruction of muscle and tissue. Myoglobin can constrict renal arteries and block urine flow through the kidneys. Patients can have gross hematuria on admission to the hospital. Administration of high amounts of IV fluids helps maintain the flow of urine.

It is difficult to assess the amount of fluid a patient will require because the electrical injury creates so much damage inside the body. The nurse should expect 75 to 100 mL/hour of urine output for an adult patient who is receiving fluid resuscitation.

In patients with electrical injuries, neurovascular checks of affected extremities are very important. A person can have neurovascular complications for as long as 2 years after the incident occurred. Baseline neurologic and functional status must be assessed as soon as possible to rule out any abnormalities that might appear at a later date (DeBoer & O'Connor, 2004; O'Keefe Gatewood & Zane, 2004).

Pathophysiology

Burns are caused by transfer of energy from a heat source to the body. Heat may be transferred through conduction or electromagnetic radiation. Burns are categorized as thermal (including electrical burns), radiation, or chemical. Tissue destruction results from coagulation, protein denaturation, or ionization of cellular contents. The skin and the mucosa of the upper airways are the sites of tissue destruction. Deep tissues, including the viscera, can be damaged by electrical burns or by prolonged contact with a heat source. Disruption of the skin can lead to increased fluid loss, infection, hypothermia, scarring, compromised immunity, and changes in function, appearance, and body image.

The depth of the injury depends on the temperature of the burning agent and the duration of contact with the agent. For example, in the case of scald burns in adults, 1 second of contact with hot tap water at 68.9°C (156°F) may result in a burn that destroys both the epidermis and the dermis, causing a full-thickness (third-degree) injury. Fifteen seconds of exposure to hot water at 56.1°C (133°F) results in a similar full-thickness injury. Temperatures less than 111°F can be tolerated for long periods without injury.

Burns that do not exceed 25% TBSA produce a primarily local response. Burns that exceed 25% TBSA may produce both a local and a systemic response and are considered major burn injuries. The systemic response is caused by the release of cytokines and other mediators into the systemic circulation. The release of local mediators and changes in blood flow, tissue edema, and infection can cause progression of the burn injury.

Pathophysiologic changes resulting from major burns during the initial burn-shock period include tissue hypoperfusion and organ hypofunction secondary to decreased cardiac output, followed by a hyperdynamic and hypermetabolic phase. The incidence, magnitude, and duration of pathophysiologic changes in burns are proportional to the extent of burn injury, with a maximal response seen in burns covering 60% or more TBSA.

The initial systemic event after a major burn injury is hemodynamic instability, which results from loss of capillary integrity and a subsequent shift of fluid, sodium, and protein from the intravascular space into the interstitial spaces. Figure 57-3 illustrates the pathophysiologic processes in acute major burns. Hemodynamic instability involves cardiovascular, fluid and electrolyte, blood volume, pulmonary, and other mechanisms.

Cardiovascular Alterations

Hypovolemia is the immediate consequence of fluid loss and results in decreased perfusion and oxygen delivery. Cardiac output decreases before any significant change in blood volume is evident. As fluid loss continues and vascular volume decreases, cardiac output continues to decrease and the blood pressure drops. This is the onset of burn shock. In response, the sympathetic nervous system releases catecholamines, resulting in an increase in peripheral resistance (vasoconstriction) and an increase in pulse rate. Peripheral vasoconstriction further decreases cardiac output. Myocardial contractility may be suppressed by the release of inflammatory cytokine necrosis factor (Ahrns, 2004). Studies suggest that blocking endotoxin release prevents myocardial depression in the burn-shock phase (Saffle, 2003).

Prompt fluid resuscitation maintains the blood pressure in the low-normal range and improves cardiac output. Despite adequate fluid resuscitation, cardiac filling pressures (central venous pressure, pulmonary artery pressure, and pulmonary artery wedge pressure) remain low during the burn-shock period. If inadequate fluid resuscitation occurs, distributive shock occurs (see Chapter 15).

Generally, the greatest volume of fluid leak occurs in the first 24 to 36 hours after the burn, peaking by 6 to 8 hours. As the capillaries begin to regain their integrity, burn shock resolves and fluid returns to the vascular compartment. As fluid is reabsorbed from the interstitial tissue into the vascular compartment, blood volume increases. If renal and cardiac function is adequate, urinary output increases. Diuresis continues for several days to 2 weeks.

At the time of burn injury, some red blood cells may be destroyed and others damaged, resulting in anemia. Despite this, the hematocrit may be elevated due to plasma loss. Blood losses sustained during surgical procedures, wound care, and diagnostic studies and ongoing hemolysis further contribute to anemia. Blood transfusions are required periodically to maintain adequate hemoglobin levels for oxygen delivery. Abnormalities in coagulation, including a decrease in platelets (thrombocytopenia) and prolonged clotting and prothrombin times, also occur with burn injury.

Fluid and Electrolyte Alterations

Edema is defined as the presence of excessive fluid in the tissue spaces (Supple, 2004). Local edema caused by thermal injury is often extensive. As previously noted, in burns involving less than 25% TBSA, the loss of capillary integrity and shift of fluid are localized to the burn itself, resulting in blister formation and edema only in the area of injury. Patients with more severe burns develop massive systemic edema. Edema is usually maximal after 24 hours. It begins to resolve 1 to 2 days after the burn and usually is completely resolved within 7 to 10 days. Edema in burn wounds can be reduced by avoiding excessive fluid administration during the early postburn period. Unnecessary overresuscitation increases edema formation in both burned and nonburned tissue.

As the taut, burned tissue becomes unyielding to the edema underneath its surface, it begins to act like a tourniquet, especially if the burn is circumferential. As edema increases, pressure on small blood vessels and nerves in the

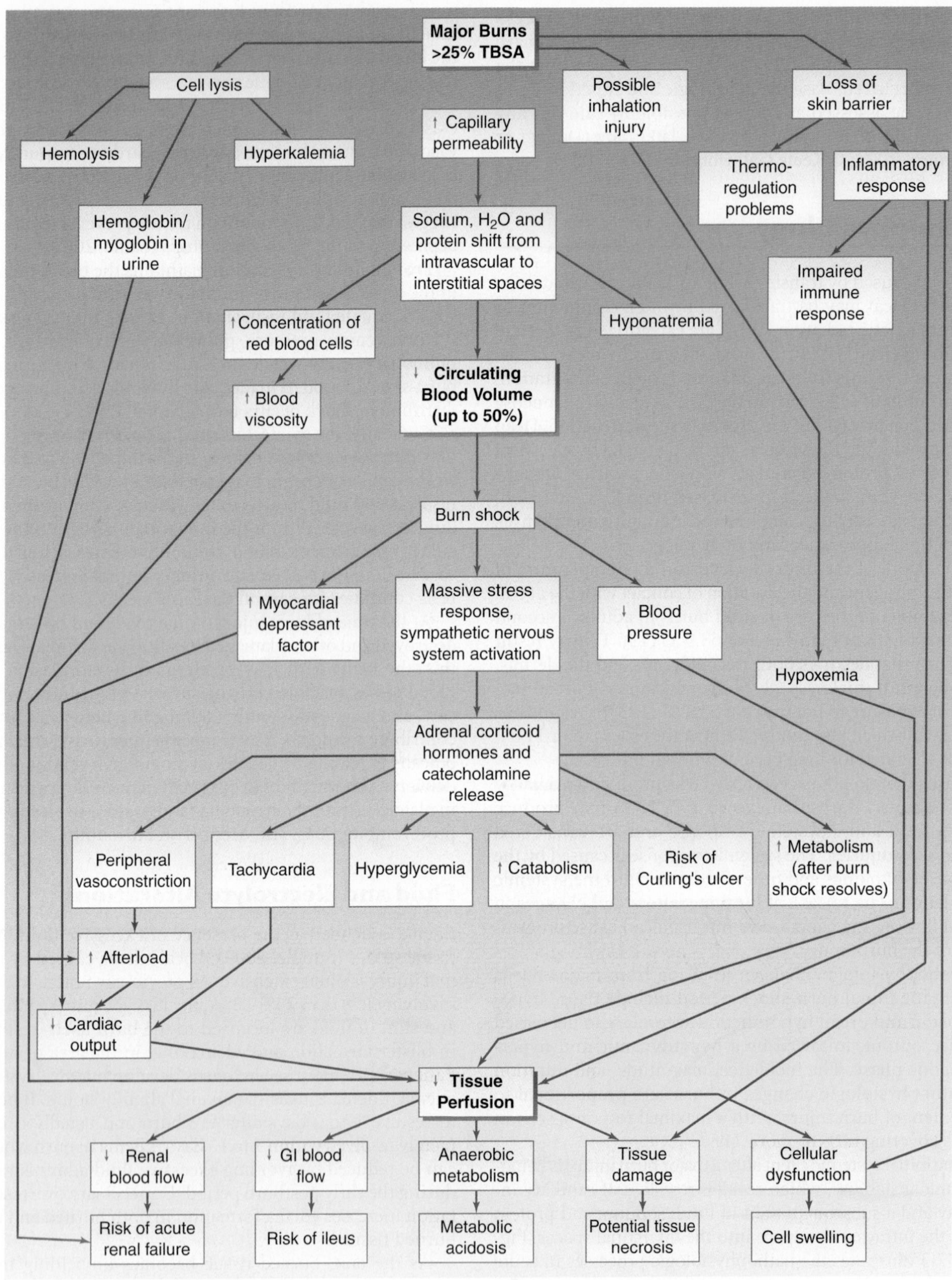

FIGURE 57-3. Overview of physiologic changes that occur after major burn.

distal extremities causes an obstruction of blood flow and consequent ischemia. This complication is similar to a compartment syndrome. The physician may need to perform an **escharotomy**, a surgical incision into the **eschar** (devitalized tissue resulting from a burn), to relieve the constricting effect of the burned tissue (Demling, 2005a).

Circulating blood volume decreases dramatically during burn shock. In addition, evaporative fluid loss through the burn wound may reach 3 to 5 L or more over a 24-hour period until the burn surfaces are covered.

During burn shock, serum sodium levels vary in response to fluid resuscitation. Usually, hyponatremia (sodium depletion) is present. Hyponatremia is also common during the first week of the acute phase, as water shifts from the interstitial space to the vascular space.

Immediately after burn injury, hyperkalemia (excessive potassium) results from massive cell destruction. Hypokalemia (potassium depletion) may occur later with fluid shifts and inadequate potassium replacement.

Pulmonary Alterations

Inhalation injury necessitates prolonged hospitalization and is a major cause of morbidity and mortality in patients with burn injuries. An inhalation injury can occur when a person is trapped inside a burning structure or involved in an explosion that leads to the inhalation of superheated air and noxious gas. Often, people escape from a burning home safely, but, once they are outside, realize that their loved ones, pets, or valuable items are still inside the burning home. They then re-enter the burning home and are overcome with toxic smoke and fumes and become disoriented or unconscious (McCall & Cahill, 2005; Sheridan & Thompkins, 2004).

Inhalation injury has a significant impact on a patient's ability to survive. Deterioration in severely burned patients can occur without obvious evidence of a smoke inhalation injury. Bronchoconstriction (caused by release of histamine, serotonin, and thromboxane, a powerful vasoconstrictor) and chest constriction secondary to circumferential full-thickness chest burns cause this deterioration. Even without pulmonary injury, hypoxia (oxygen starvation) may be present. Early in the postburn period, catecholamine release in response to the stress of the burn injury alters peripheral blood flow, thereby reducing oxygen delivery to the periphery. Later, hypermetabolism and continued catecholamine release lead to increased tissue oxygen consumption, which can lead to hypoxia. To ensure that adequate oxygen is available to the tissues, supplemental oxygen may be needed.

Pulmonary injuries fall into several categories: upper airway injury; inhalation injury below the glottis, including carbon monoxide poisoning; and restrictive defects. Upper airway injury results from direct heat or edema. It is manifested by mechanical obstruction of the upper airway, including the pharynx and larynx. Because of the cooling effect of rapid vaporization in the pulmonary tract, direct heat injury does not normally occur below the level of the bronchus. Upper airway injury is treated by early nasotracheal or endotracheal intubation.

Inhalation injury below the glottis results from inhaling the products of incomplete combustion or noxious gases. These products include carbon monoxide, sulfur oxides, nitrogen oxides, aldehydes, cyanide, ammonia, chlorine, phosgene, benzene, and halogens. The injury results directly from chemical irritation of the pulmonary tissues at the alveolar level. Inhalation injuries below the glottis cause loss of ciliary action, hypersecretion, severe mucosal edema, and possibly bronchospasm. The pulmonary surfactant is reduced, resulting in atelectasis (collapse of alveoli). Expectoration of carbon particles in the sputum is the cardinal sign of this injury.

Carbon monoxide is probably the most common cause of inhalation injury, because it is a byproduct of the combustion of organic materials and therefore is present in smoke. The pathophysiologic effects are caused by tissue hypoxia, a result of carbon monoxide combining with hemoglobin to form **carboxyhemoglobin**, which competes with oxygen for available hemoglobin-binding sites. The affinity of hemoglobin for carbon monoxide is 250 times greater than that for oxygen. Treatment usually consists of early intubation and mechanical ventilation with 100% oxygen. However, some patients require only oxygen therapy, depending on the extent of pulmonary injury and edema. Administering 100% oxygen is essential to accelerate the removal of carbon monoxide from the hemoglobin molecule (DeBoer & O'Connor, 2004).

Restrictive defects arise when edema develops under full-thickness burns encircling the neck and thorax. Chest excursion may be greatly restricted, resulting in decreased tidal volume. In such situations, escharotomy is necessary (Supple, 2004).

Pulmonary abnormalities are not always immediately apparent. More than half of all patients with burn injuries with pulmonary involvement do not initially demonstrate pulmonary signs and symptoms. Any patient with possible inhalation injury must be observed for at least 24 hours for respiratory complications. Airway obstruction may occur very rapidly or develop in hours. Decreased lung compliance, decreased arterial oxygen levels, and respiratory acidosis may occur gradually over the first 5 days after a burn.

Indicators of possible pulmonary damage include the following:

- History indicating that the burn occurred in an enclosed area
- Burns of the face or neck
- Singed nasal hair
- Hoarseness, voice change, dry cough, stridor, sooty sputum
- Sooty or bloody sputum
- Labored breathing or tachypnea (rapid breathing) and other signs of reduced oxygen levels (hypoxemia)
- Erythema and blistering of the oral or pharyngeal mucosa

Diagnosis of inhalation injury is an important priority for many patients with burn injuries. Serum carboxyhemoglobin levels and arterial blood gas levels are frequently used to assess for inhalation injuries. Fiberoptic bronchoscopy and xenon 133 (^{133}Xe) ventilation–perfusion scans can also be used to aid diagnosis in the early postburn period. Pulmonary function studies may be useful in diagnosing decreased lung compliance or obstructed airflow (Fitzpatrick & Cioffi, 2002; McCall & Cahill, 2005; Sheridan & Thompkins, 2004).

Pulmonary complications secondary to inhalation injuries include acute respiratory failure and acute respiratory distress syndrome (ARDS). Respiratory failure occurs when impairment of ventilation and gas exchange is life-threatening. The immediate intervention is intubation and mechanical ventilation. If ventilation is impaired by restricted chest excursion, immediate chest escharotomy is needed. ARDS may develop in the first few days after the burn injury, secondary to systemic and pulmonary responses to the burn and inhalation injury (Supple, 2004). Respiratory failure and ARDS are discussed in Chapter 23.

Renal Alterations

Renal function may be altered as a result of decreased blood volume. Destruction of red blood cells at the injury site results in free hemoglobin in the urine. If muscle damage occurs (eg, from electrical burns), myoglobin is released from the muscle cells and excreted by the kidney. Adequate fluid volume replacement restores renal blood flow, increasing the glomerular filtration rate and urine volume. If there is inadequate blood flow through the kidneys, the hemoglobin and myoglobin occlude the renal tubules, resulting in acute tubular necrosis and renal failure (see Chapter 44).

Immunologic Alterations

The immunologic defenses of the body are greatly altered by burn injury. Serious burn injury diminishes resistance to infection. As a result, sepsis continues to be the leading cause of morbidity and mortality in patients with thermal injuries (Bowler, Jones, Walker, et al., 2004; Neely, Fowler, Kagan, et al., 2004). The loss of skin integrity is compounded by the release of abnormal inflammatory factors, altered levels of immunoglobulins and serum complement, impaired neutrophil function, and a reduction in lymphocytes (lymphocytopenia). Research suggests that burn injury results in loss of T-helper lymphocytes (Saffle, 2003; Gosain & Gamelli, 2005a). There is a significant impairment of the production and release of granulocytes and macrophages from bone marrow after burn injury. The resulting immunosuppression places the patient with burn injury at high risk for sepsis.

Thermoregulatory Alterations

Loss of skin also results in an inability to regulate body temperature. Patients with burn injuries may therefore exhibit low body temperatures in the early hours after injury. Then, as hypermetabolism resets core temperatures, the patient becomes hyperthermic for much of the postburn period, even in the absence of infection.

Gastrointestinal Alterations

Two potential gastrointestinal complications may occur: paralytic ileus (absence of intestinal peristalsis) and Curling's ulcer. Decreased peristalsis and bowel sounds are manifestations of paralytic ileus resulting from burn trauma. Gastric distention and nausea may lead to vomiting unless gastric decompression is initiated. Gastric bleeding secondary to massive physiologic stress may be signaled by occult blood in the stool, regurgitation of "coffee ground" material from the stomach, or bloody vomitus. These signs suggest gastric or duodenal erosion (Curling's ulcer).

Patients with large burn wounds are at risk for abdominal compartment syndrome, especially if fluid resuscitation is delayed (Sheridan & Thompkins, 2004). Fluid shifts into the abdominal cavity cause increased abdominal distention, decreasing urine output and resulting in hypotension and difficulty with ventilation. Bladder pressures greater than 25 to 30 mm Hg over time are an indicator of increasing abdominal pressure. Drainage of fluid via an abdominal tap or laparotomy aids in reducing abdominal pressure.

Three components of the gastrointestinal tract are altered after burn injury: the mucosal barrier becomes permeable, the permeability allows for overgrowth of gastrointestinal bacteria, and the bacteria translocate to other organs, causing infection. Patients are unable to defend against their own bacteria due to immunosuppression in burn injury. In addition, alcohol ingestion is common in the burn population. Alcohol is known to affect intestinal integrity and immune response, leading to translocation of bacteria and possible bleeding complications (Gosain & Gamelli, 2005b).

Management of Burn Injury

Burn care must be based on burn depth and local response, the extent of the injury, and the presence of a systemic response. Burn care then proceeds through three phases: emergent/resuscitative phase, acute/intermediate phase, and rehabilitation phase. Although priorities exist for each of the phases, the phases overlap, and assessment and management of specific problems and complications are not limited to these phases but take place throughout burn care. The three phases and the priorities for care are summarized in Table 57-2.

Emergent/Resuscitative Phase

On-the-Scene Care

The first priority of on-the-scene care for a person who has been burned is to prevent injury to the rescuer. If needed, fire and emergency medical services should be requested at the first opportunity. Usually, rescue workers cool the wound, establish an airway, supply oxygen, and insert at least one large-bore IV line. Chart 57-3 describes additional emergency procedures that are carried out at the burn scene.

The burned person's appearance can be frightening at first. Although the local effects of a burn are the most evident, the systemic effects pose a greater threat to life. Therefore, it is important to remember the ABCs of all trauma care during the early postburn period:

- Airway
- Breathing
- Circulation; cervical spine immobilization for patients with high-voltage electrical injuries and if indicated for other injuries; cardiac monitoring for patients with all

TABLE 57-2 Phases of Burn Care

Phase	Duration	Priorities
Emergent/resuscitative	From onset of injury to completion of fluid resuscitation	• First aid • Prevention of shock • Prevention of respiratory distress • Detection and treatment of concomitant injuries • Wound assessment and initial care
Acute/intermediate	From beginning of diuresis to near completion of wound closure	• Wound care and closure • Prevention or treatment of complications, including infection • Nutritional support
Rehabilitation	From major wound closure to return to individual's optimal level of physical and psychosocial adjustment	• Prevention of scars and contractures • Physical, occupational, and vocational rehabilitation • Functional and cosmetic reconstruction • Psychosocial counseling

electrical injuries for at least 24 hours after cessation of dysrhythmia

The circulatory system must also be assessed quickly. Apical pulse and blood pressure are monitored frequently. Tachycardia (abnormally rapid heart rate) and slight hypotension are expected soon after the burn. The neurologic status is assessed quickly in the patient with extensive burns. Often the patient is awake and alert initially, and vital information can be obtained at that time. A secondary head-to-toe survey of the patient is carried out to identify other potentially life-threatening injuries. Prevention of shock in a patient with burns is imperative (DeBoer & O'Connor, 2004).

CHART 57-3

Emergency Procedures at the Burn Scene

- **Extinguish the flames.** When clothes catch fire, the flames can be extinguished if the person falls to the floor or ground and rolls ("drop and roll"); anything available to smother the flames, such as a blanket, rug, or coat, may be used. Standing still forces the person to breathe flames and smoke, and running fans the flames. If the burn source is electrical, the electrical source must be disconnected.
- **Cool the burn.** After the flames are extinguished, the burned area and adherent clothing are soaked with *cool* water, briefly, to cool the wound and halt the burning process. Once a burn has been sustained, the application of cool water is the best first-aid measure. Soaking the burn area intermittently in cool water or applying cool towels gives immediate and striking relief from pain and limits local tissue edema and damage. However, *never* apply ice directly to the burn, *never* wrap the person in ice, and *never* use cold soaks or dressings for longer than several minutes; such procedures may worsen the tissue damage and lead to hypothermia in people with large burns.
- **Remove restrictive objects.** If possible, remove clothing immediately. Adherent clothing may be left in place once cooled. Other clothing and all jewelry, including all piercings, should be removed to allow for assessment and to prevent constriction secondary to rapidly developing edema.
- **Cover the wound.** The burn should be covered as quickly as possible to minimize bacterial contamination and decrease pain by preventing air from coming into contact with the injured surface. Sterile dressings are best, but any clean, dry cloth can be used as an emergency dressing. Ointments and salves should *not* be used. Other than the dressing, no medication or material should be applied to the burn wound.
- **Irrigate chemical burns.** Chemical burns resulting from contact with a corrosive material are irrigated immediately. Most chemical laboratories have a high-pressure shower for such emergencies. If such an injury occurs at home, brush off the chemical agent, remove clothes immediately, and rinse all areas of the body that have come in contact with the chemical. Rinsing can occur in the shower or any other source of continuous running water. If a chemical gets in or near the eyes, the eyes should be flushed with cool, clean water immediately. Outcomes for the patient with chemical burns are significantly improved by rapid, sustained flushing of the injury at the scene.

NURSING ALERT

Breathing must be assessed and a patent airway established immediately during the initial minutes of emergency care. Immediate therapy is directed toward establishing an airway and administering humidified 100% oxygen. If such a high concentration of oxygen is not available under emergency conditions, oxygen by mask or nasal cannula is given initially. If qualified personnel and equipment are available and the victim has severe respiratory distress or airway edema, the rescuers can insert an endotracheal tube and initiate manual ventilation.

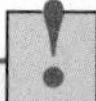

NURSING ALERT

No food or fluid is given by mouth, and the patient is placed in a position that will prevent aspiration of vomitus, because nausea and vomiting typically occur due to paralytic ileus resulting from the stress of injury.

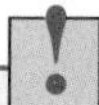

NURSING ALERT

If necessary, a blood pressure cuff can be placed around a patient's burned extremity. The cuff must be of the correct size with accommodations made for bulky dressings.

Medical Management

The patient is transported to the nearest emergency department. The hospital and physician are alerted that the patient is en route to the emergency department so that life-saving measures can be initiated immediately by a trained team.

Initial priorities in the emergency department remain airway, breathing, and circulation. For mild pulmonary injury, 100% humidified oxygen is administered and the patient is encouraged to cough so that secretions can be removed by suctioning. For more severe situations, it is necessary to remove secretions by bronchial suctioning and to administer bronchodilators and mucolytic agents. If edema of the airway develops, endotracheal intubation may be necessary. Continuous positive airway pressure and mechanical ventilation may also be required to achieve adequate oxygenation.

After adequate respiratory function and circulatory status have been established, the patient is assessed for cervical spinal injuries or head injury if he or she was involved in an explosion, a fall, a jump, or an electrical injury. Once the patient's condition is stable, attention is directed to the burn wound itself. All clothing and jewelry are removed. For chemical burns, flushing of the exposed areas is continued. The patient is checked for contact lenses. These are removed immediately if chemicals have contacted the eyes or if facial burns have occurred.

It is important to validate an account of the burn scenario provided by the patient, witnesses at the scene, and paramedics. Information needs to include the time of the burn injury, the source of the burn, the place where the burn occurred, how the burn was treated at the scene, and any history of falling with the injury. A history of preexisting diseases, allergies, medications, and the use of drugs, alcohol, and tobacco is obtained at this point to aid in plan the patient's care. A large-bore (16- or 18-gauge) IV catheter should be inserted in a nonburned area (if not inserted earlier). Most patients have a central venous catheter inserted so that large amounts of IV fluids can be administered quickly and central venous pressures can be monitored.

If the burn exceeds 20% to 25% TBSA, a nasogastric tube should be inserted and connected to low intermittent suction. Often, patients with large burns become nauseated as a result of the gastrointestinal effects of the burn injury, such as paralytic ileus (absence of peristalsis), and the effects of medication such as opioids. All patients who are intubated should have a nasogastric tube inserted to decompress the abdomen and prevent vomiting.

The physician evaluates the patient's general condition, assesses the burn, determines the priorities of care, and directs the individualized plan of treatment, which is divided into systemic management and local care of the burned area. Nonsterile gloves, caps, and gowns are worn by personnel while assessing the exposed burned areas. Clean technique is maintained while assessing burn wounds.

Assessment of both the TBSA burned and the depth of the burn is completed after soot and debris have been gently cleansed from the burn wound. Careful attention is paid to keeping the patient warm during wound assessment and cleansing. Assessment is repeated frequently throughout burn wound care. Photographs may be taken of the burn areas initially and periodically throughout treatment; in this way, the initial injury and burn wound can be documented. Such documentation is invaluable for insurance and legal claims.

Clean sheets are placed under and over the patient to protect the burn wound from contamination, maintain body temperature, and reduce pain caused by air currents passing over exposed nerve endings. An indwelling urinary catheter is inserted to permit more accurate monitoring of urine output and renal function for patients with moderate to severe burns. Baseline height, weight, arterial blood gases, hematocrit, electrolyte values, blood alcohol level, drug panel, urinalysis, and chest x-rays are obtained. If the patient is elderly or has an electrical burn, a baseline electrocardiogram (ECG) is obtained. Because burns are contaminated wounds, tetanus prophylaxis is administered if the patient's immunization status is not current or is unknown.

Although the major focus of care during the emergent phase is physical stabilization, the nurse must also attend to the patient's and family's psychological needs. Burn injury is a crisis, one that causes varying emotional responses. The patient's and family's coping abilities and available supports are assessed. Circumstances surrounding the burn injury should be considered when providing care. Individualized psychosocial support must be given to the patient and family. Because the patient is usually anxious and in pain, those in attendance should provide reassurance and support, explanations of procedures, and adequate pain relief. Because poor tissue perfusion accompanies burn injuries, only IV analgesia (usually morphine) is administered, titrated for the patient. If the patient wishes to see a spiritual advisor, one is notified.

Transfer to a Burn Center

The depth and extent of the burn are considered in determining whether the patient should be transferred to a burn center. Patients with major burns, those who are at the extremes of the age continuum, those with coexisting health problems that may affect recovery, and those with circumstances that increase their risk for acute and long-term complications are transferred to a burn center. Chart 57-4 lists the American Burn Association's criteria for burn center referral after initial assessment and management.

If the patient is to be transported to a burn center, the following measures, listed in order of importance, are instituted before transfer:

- A patent airway is ensured.
- Adequate peripheral circulation is established in any burned extremity.
- A secure IV catheter is inserted with lactated Ringer's solution infusing at the rate required to maintain a urine output of at least 30 mL per hour.
- An indwelling urinary catheter is inserted.
- Adequate pain relief is attained.
- Wounds are covered with a clean, dry sheet, and the patient is kept comfortably warm.

All assessments and treatments are documented, and this information is provided to the burn center personnel. The transferring facility must relay accurate intake and output totals to burn center personnel so that adequate fluid resuscitation measures will continue.

CHART 57-4

Classification of Extent of Burn Injury

MINOR BURN INJURY

- Second-degree burn of <15% total body surface area (TBSA) in adults or <10% TBSA in children
- Third-degree burn of <2% TBSA not involving special care areas (eyes, ears, face, hands, feet, perineum, joints)
- Excludes all patients with electrical injury, inhalation injury, or concurrent trauma and all poor-risk patients (eg, extremes of age, intercurrent disease)

MODERATE, UNCOMPLICATED BURN INJURY

- Second-degree burns of 15–25% TBSA in adults or 10–20% in children
- Third-degree burns of <10% TBSA not involving special care areas
- Excludes electrical injury, inhalation injury, or concurrent trauma and all poor-risk patients (eg, extremes of age, intercurrent disease)

MAJOR BURN INJURY

- Second-degree burns >25% TBSA in adults or >20% in children
- All third-degree burns >10% TBSA
- All burns involving eyes, ears, face, hands, feet, perineum, joints
- All inhalation injury, electrical injury, or concurrent trauma, and all poor-risk patients

From Morton, P. G., Fontaine, D. K., Hudak, C. M., et al. (2005). *Critical care nursing: A holistic approach* (8th ed.). Philadelphia: Lippincott Williams & Wilkins.

Management of Fluid Loss and Shock

Next to managing respiratory difficulties, the most urgent need is preventing irreversible shock by replacing lost fluids and electrolytes. As stated previously, survival of the patient with burn injury depends on adequate fluid resuscitation. Table 57-3 summarizes the fluid and electrolyte changes in the emergent phase of burn care. Baseline weight and laboratory test results are obtained as well. These parameters must be monitored closely in the immediate postburn (resuscitation) period. Controversy continues regarding the definition of adequate resuscitation and the optimal fluid type for resuscitation. Refinement of resuscitation techniques remains an active area of burn research (Atiyeh, Gunn & Hayek, 2005).

FLUID REPLACEMENT THERAPY

The total volume and rate of IV fluid replacement are gauged by the patient's response and guided by the resuscitation formula. The adequacy of fluid resuscitation is determined by monitoring urine output totals, an index of renal perfusion. Urine output totals of 30 to 50 mL/hour (0.5 to 1.0 mL/kg/hour) have been used as resuscitation goals. Other indicators of adequate fluid replacement are a systolic blood pressure exceeding 100 mm Hg, a pulse rate less than 110 beats/minute, or both.

NURSING ALERT

Clinical parameters are far more important in resuscitation than any formula. Indeed, the patient's individual response is the key to assessing the adequacy of fluid resuscitation.

Additional gauges of fluid requirements and response to fluid resuscitation include hematocrit and hemoglobin and serum sodium levels. Within the first 24 hours after injury, if the hematocrit and the hemoglobin levels decrease or if the urinary output exceeds 50 mL/hour, the rate of IV fluid administration may be decreased. One goal is to maintain serum sodium levels in the normal range during fluid replacement.

Appropriate resuscitation end points for patients with burn injuries remain unresolved, although some studies

TABLE 57-3 Fluid and Electrolyte Changes in the Emergent/Resuscitative Phase

Fluid accumulation phase (shock phase)
Plasma → interstitial fluid (edema at burn site)

Observation	Explanation
Generalized dehydration	Plasma leaks through damaged capillaries.
Reduction of blood volume	Secondary to plasma loss, fall of blood pressure, and diminished cardiac output
Decreased urinary output	Secondary to: Fluid loss Decreased renal blood flow Sodium and water retention caused by increased adrenocortical activity Hemolysis of red blood cells, causing hemoglobinuria and myonecrosis or myoglobinuria
Potassium (K^+) excess	Massive cellular trauma causes release of K^+ into extracellular fluid (ordinarily, most K^+ is intracellular).
Sodium (Na^+) deficit	Large amount of Na^+ is lost in trapped edema fluid and exudate and by shift into cells as K^+ is released from cells (ordinarily most Na^+ is extracellular).
Metabolic acidosis (base-bicarbonate deficit)	Loss of bicarbonate ions accompanies sodium loss.
Hemoconcentration (elevated hematocrit)	Liquid blood component is lost into extravascular space.

have examined hemodynamic and oxygen transport as resuscitation end points. Minute-to-minute base deficit sensors have been used to measure levels of PCO_2 in the tissues during fluid resuscitation to determine cellular perfusion, which is the major goal of fluid resuscitation in burn injury (Light, Jeng, Jain, et al., 2004). Successful resuscitation is associated with increased delivery of oxygen and consumption of oxygen with declining serum lactate levels (Demling, 2005a). Factors that are associated with the increased fluid requirements include delayed resuscitation, scald burn injuries, inhalation injuries, high-voltage electrical injuries, hyperglycemia, alcohol intoxication, and chronic diuretic therapy. Second 24-hour postburn fluid infusion rates incorporate both the maintenance amount of fluid and any additional fluid needs secondary to evaporative water loss through the burn wound.

FLUID REQUIREMENTS

The projected fluid requirements for the first 24 hours are calculated by the clinician based on the extent of the burn injury. Some combination of fluid categories may be used, including colloids (whole blood, plasma, and plasma expanders) and crystalloids/electrolytes (physiologic sodium chloride or lactated Ringer's solution). Adequate fluid resuscitation results in slightly decreased blood volume levels during the first 24 postburn hours and restoration of plasma levels to normal by the end of 48 hours. Oral and enteral resuscitation can be successful in adults with less than 20% TBSA and in children with less than 10% to 15% TBSA (Atiyeh et al., 2005).

Formulas have been developed for estimating fluid loss based on the estimated percentage of burned TBSA and the weight of the patient. The length of time since the burn injury occurred is also very important in calculating estimated fluid needs. Formulas must be adjusted so that initiation of fluid replacement reflects the time of injury. Resuscitation formulas are approximations only and are individualized to meet the requirements of each patient. The various formulas are discussed later and are summarized in Chart 57-5.

As early as 1978, the NIH Consensus Development Conference on Supportive Therapy in Burn Care established that salt and water are required in patients with burn injury, but that colloid may or may not be useful during the first 24 to 48 postburn hours. The consensus formula provides for the volume of an isotonic solution to be administered during the first 24 hours in a range of 2 to 4 mL/kg per percent of body surface burned. As with the other formulas, half of the calculated total should be given over the first 8 postburn hours, and the other half should be given over the next 16 hours. The rate and volume of the infusion must be regulated according to the patient's response by changing the hourly infusion rates. Fluid boluses are recommended only in the presence of marked hypotension, not low urine output. Although the consensus formula is commonly used today, there is still not complete agreement about which fluid resuscitation formula is best for burn injury. Again, practitioners should take note that the resuscitation formulas serve only as guidelines, and the patient's response to fluid therapy is the best parameter to use (Atiyeh et al., 2005).

With large burns, there is a failure of the sodium–potassium pump (a physiologic mechanism involved in fluid–electrolyte balance) at the cellular level. Therefore, patients with very large burns may need proportionately more milliliters of fluid per percent of burn than those with smaller burns. Also, patients with electrical injury, pulmonary injury, or delayed fluid resuscitation and those who were burned while intoxicated may need additional fluids.

The following example illustrates use of the consensus formula in a 70-kg (154-lb) patient with a 50% TBSA burn:

1. Consensus formula: 2 to 4 mL/kg/% TBSA
2. $2 \times 70 \times 50 = 7000$ mL/24 hours
3. Plan to administer: first 8 hours = 3500 mL, or 437 mL/hour; next 16 hours = 3500 mL, or 219 mL/hour

Most fluid replacement formulas use isotonic electrolyte solutions. Regardless of which standard replacement formula is used, the patient receives approximately the same fluid volume and sodium replacement during the first 48 hours.

CHART 57-5

Guidelines and Formulas for Fluid Replacement in Burn Patients

CONSENSUS FORMULA

Lactated Ringer's solution (or other balanced saline solution): 2–4 mL × kg body weight × % total body surface area (TBSA) burned. Half to be given in first 8 h; remaining half to be given over next 16 h.

EVANS FORMULA

1. Colloids: 1 mL × kg body weight × % TBSA burned
2. Electrolytes (saline): 1 mL × body weight × % TBSA burned
3. Glucose (5% in water): 2000 mL for insensible loss

Day 1: Half to be given in first 8 h; remaining half over next 16 h.

Day 2: Half of previous day's colloids and electrolytes; all of insensible fluid replacement.

Maximum of 10,000 mL over 24 h. Second- and third-degree (partial- and full-thickness) burns exceeding 50% TBSA are calculated on the basis of 50% TBSA.

BROOKE ARMY FORMULA

1. Colloids: 0.5 mL × kg body weight × % TBSA burned
2. Electrolytes (lactated Ringer's solution): 1.5 mL × kg body weight × % TBSA burned
3. Glucose (5% in water): 2000 mL for insensible loss

Day 1: Half to be given in first 8 h; remaining half over next 16 h

Day 2: Half of colloids; half of electrolytes; all of insensible fluid replacement.

Second- and third-degree (partial- and full-thickness) burns exceeding 50% TBSA are calculated on the basis of 50% TBSA.

PARKLAND/BAXTER FORMULA

Lactated Ringer's solution: 4 mL × kg body weight × % TBSA burned

Day 1: Half to be given in first 8 h; half to be given over next 16 h

Day 2: Varies. Colloid is added.

HYPERTONIC SALINE SOLUTION

Concentrated solutions of sodium chloride (NaCl) and lactate with concentration of 250–300 mEq of sodium per liter, administered at a rate sufficient to maintain a desired volume of urinary output. Do not increase the infusion rate during the first 8 postburn hours. Serum sodium levels must be monitored closely. Goal: Increase serum sodium level and osmolality to reduce edema and prevent pulmonary complications.

Another fluid replacement method requires hypertonic electrolyte solutions. This method uses concentrated solutions of sodium chloride and lactate (a balanced salt solution) so that the resulting fluid has a concentration of 250 to 300 mEq of sodium. The rationale for this replacement method is the increased serum osmolality will cause fluid to be pulled back into the vascular space from the interstitial space. Reduced systemic and pulmonary edema has been reported after administration of hypertonic solutions.

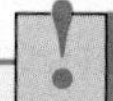

NURSING ALERT

Formulas are only a guide. The patient's response, evidenced by heart rate, blood pressure, and urine output, is the primary determinant of actual fluid therapy and must be assessed at least hourly. Patient outcomes are improved by optimal fluid resuscitation.

Nursing Management

Assessment data obtained by prehospital providers (rescuers such as emergency medical technicians) are shared with the physician and nurse in the emergency department. Nursing assessment in the emergent phase of burn injury focuses on the major priorities for any trauma patient; the burn wound is a secondary consideration. Aseptic management of the burn wounds and invasive lines continues.

The nurse monitors vital signs frequently. Respiratory status is monitored closely, and apical, carotid, and femoral pulses are evaluated. Cardiac monitoring is indicated if the patient has a history of cardiac disease, electrical injury, or respiratory conditions, or if the pulse is dysrhythmic or the rate is abnormally slow or rapid.

If all extremities are burned, determining blood pressure may be difficult. A sterile dressing applied under the blood pressure cuff protects the wound from contamination. Because increasing edema makes blood pressure difficult to auscultate, a Doppler (ultrasound) device or a noninvasive electronic blood pressure device may be helpful. In patients with severe burns, an arterial catheter is used for blood pressure measurement and for collecting blood specimens. Peripheral pulses of burned extremities are checked hourly; the Doppler device is useful for this. Elevation of burned extremities is crucial to decrease edema. Elevation of the lower extremities on pillows and of the upper extremities on pillows or by suspension using IV poles may be helpful.

Large-bore IV catheters and an indwelling urinary catheter are inserted, if not already in place, and the nurse's assessment includes monitoring of fluid intake and output. Urine output, an indicator of renal perfusion, is monitored carefully and measured hourly. The amount of urine first obtained when the urinary catheter was inserted is recorded. This may assist in determining the extent of preburn renal function and fluid status. Urine specific gravity, pH, and glucose, acetone, protein, and hemoglobin levels are assessed frequently.

Burgundy-colored urine suggests the presence of hemochromogen and myoglobin resulting from muscle damage. This is associated with deep burns caused by electrical injury or prolonged contact with flames. Glycosuria, a common finding in the early postburn hours, results from the release of stored glucose from the liver in response to stress.

Although not responsible for calculating the patient's fluid requirements, the nurse needs to know the maximum volume of fluid the patient should receive. Infusion pumps and rate controllers are used to deliver a complex regimen of IV fluids prescribed. Administering and monitoring IV therapy are major nursing responsibilities.

Body temperature, body weight, preburn weight, and history of allergies, tetanus immunization, past medical and surgical disorders, current illnesses, and use of medications are assessed. A head-to-toe assessment is performed, focusing on signs and symptoms of concomitant illness, injury, or developing complications. If the patient has facial burns, his or her eyes should be examined for injury to the corneas. An ophthalmologist is consulted for complete assessment via fluorescent staining.

Assessing the extent of the burn wound continues and is facilitated with anatomic diagrams (described previously). In addition, the nurse works with the physician to assess the depth of the wound and areas of full- and partial-thickness injury. Assessment of the circumstances surrounding the injury is important. Obtaining a history of the burn injury can help in planning the care for the patient. Assessment should include the time of injury, mechanism of burn, whether the burn occurred in a closed space, the possibility of inhalation of noxious chemicals, and any related trauma.

The neurologic assessment focuses on the patient's level of consciousness, psychological status, pain and anxiety levels, and behavior.

The patient's and family's understanding of the injury and treatment is assessed as well. Ethical dilemmas, such as those discussed in Chart 57-6, may also occur.

Nursing care of the patient during the emergent/resuscitative phase of burn injury is detailed in the plan of nursing care in Chart 57-7.

Gerontologic Considerations

Comorbid conditions coupled with the burn injury contribute to the high mortality rates of patients 65 years and older. Demling (2005b) reported that more than 60% of elderly patients with burn injuries admitted to the hospital had moderate to severe protein–energy malnutrition, which contributed to an increase in infection compared with well-nourished elderly burn patients. Decreased function of the

CHART 57-6

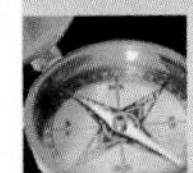

Ethics and Related Issues

When a Family's Request Conflicts With a Patient's Request for Information, What Should the Health Care Team Do?

SITUATION

A woman is brought to the burn center with second-degree and third-degree burns over 60% of her body as well an inhalation injury, which she received in a house fire. Although she is intubated and in critical condition, she is awake and responsive. Her children did not survive the fire. The burn team is not sure if the patient knows about her children. Family members have asked the burn team not to tell the patient until they arrive at the hospital. Despite the extent of the patient's injuries, she is able to use her dominant hand and writes a note to the nurse, "Kids?"

DILEMMA

The physician believes that the burn team should abide by the wishes of family members, so that they can support the patient when she receives the news about her children. On the other hand, the nurse believes that the burn team should answer the patient's questions, because the patient is alert and asking for the information. Soon, the patient will be heavily sedated and most likely be unable to respond.

DISCUSSION

Nurses are faced with this dilemma daily in a burn center. Some nurses believe that the wishes of the physician and the family should be honored, whereas others believe that the wishes of the patient should be respected. The nurse should relay news—whether good or bad—to the patient in a realistic and compassionate manner when asked. Family members will still be able to provide support to the patient and not be burdened by having to give bad news. The nurse can ask the patient what she knows about the situation. Although the patient cannot talk, she might be able to communicate in writing with the nurse. Many times patients do know what has happened but are not clear as to the details of the situation.

DISCUSSION

1. What arguments can be made to support the wishes of the physician?
2. What arguments can be made to support the wishes of the nurse?
3. Might communicating with the nurse in writing allow the patient to express what might have happened?
4. If it is decided that the patient should receive the news about her children, should it be the nurse who relays the news—whether good or bad?

NURSING RESEARCH PROFILE

Burns and Neurologic Conditions

Alden, N. E., Rabbitts, A., Rolls, J. A., et al. (2004). Burn injury in patients with early-onset neurological impairments. *Journal of Burn Care and Rehabilitation, 25*(1), 107–111.

Purpose

The purpose of this study was to obtain information about burn injury in people with early-onset neurologic impairment to better understand the circumstances of burn injury and to address burn care and burn prevention in this population.

Design

This retrospective study considered all patients admitted to a large urban burn center from August 1997 through July 2001. The study group included patients with burn injuries who had preexisting early-onset neurologic disorders, such as cerebral palsy, mental retardation, autism, spina bifida, and attention deficit hyperactivity disorder. A comparison group included patients with burn injuries but without early-onset neurologic impairment. Data obtained included type of impairment, age, gender, percent of total body surface area burned, length of hospital stay (LOS), admission to the intensive care unit (ICU), need for ventilator support and days on a ventilator, need for operative treatment, occurrence of aspiration, and patient's disposition. Information about the circumstances of the burn injury in the study group was also obtained.

Findings

Of the more than 3500 patients admitted to the burn center over a 4-year period, 51 patients met criteria for the study group. Sixty-two percent of patients in both groups were male. The average age of patients in the study group (18.4 ± 13.4 years) and in the comparison group (29.6 ± 24.6 years) were not significantly different. The percentages of patients in each group requiring ICU admission and ventilator support were not significantly different, but the LOS was significantly higher ($p < .001$) in the study group (22.3 ± 8.1 days) than in the comparison group (13.7 ± 17.4 days). Type, severity, and circumstances of burns in the study and comparison groups did not differ significantly.

Nursing Implications

The extended LOS of the study group may be due in part to the special needs of patients with early-onset neurologic impairments and the coordination of care and services, which is often difficult for their families and caregivers. Services already established may have been interrupted or suspended because of hospitalization. The need for special wound care after burn injury may also have contributed to the longer LOS, suggesting the need for nurses to teach wound care to caretakers and home care service providers. Early efforts to reestablish services before discharge are a priority. In addition, nurses can provide information to patients, caregivers, and home care service providers to promote safety, especially with cooking and bathing, common circumstances of burn in the study group. Nurses can also teach them to identify an injury when it occurs and to seek medical attention promptly. Advocating for monitoring and control of water temperature in group homes and facilities may prevent burns during bathing. Discharge planning should begin immediately on admission to the hospital, paying particular attention to the high-risk needs of the patient and ensuring adequate supervision on return home.

cardiovascular, renal, and pulmonary systems increases the need for close observation of elderly patients with even relatively minor burns during the emergent and acute phases. Acute renal failure is much more common in elderly patients than in those younger than 40 years of age. The margin of difference between hypovolemia and fluid overload is very small. Suppressed immunologic response, a high incidence of malnutrition, and an inability to withstand metabolic stressors (eg, a cold environment) further compromise the elderly person's ability to heal. As a result of these issues in elderly patients who sustain burn injury, close monitoring and prompt treatment of complications are mandatory.

Acute/Intermediate Phase

The acute or intermediate phase of burn care follows the emergent/resuscitative phase and begins 48 to 72 hours after the burn injury. During this phase, attention is directed toward continued assessment and maintenance of respiratory and circulatory status, fluid and electrolyte balance, and gastrointestinal function. Infection prevention, burn wound care (ie, wound cleaning, topical antibacterial therapy, wound dressing, dressing changes, wound débridement, and wound grafting), pain management, and nutritional support are priorities at this stage and are discussed in detail in the following sections.

Airway obstruction caused by upper airway edema can take as long as 48 hours to develop. Changes detected by x-ray and arterial blood gas analysis may occur as the effects of resuscitative fluid and the chemical reactions of smoke ingredients with lung tissues become apparent. Pulmonary complications are not unusual in burn injury. Those with ventilator-associated pneumonia (VAP) have a 40% mortality rate, increasing to 60% to 77% for VAP with an inhala-

(text continues on page 2015)

CHART 57-7

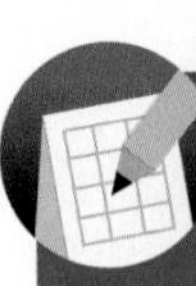

Plan of Nursing Care Care of the Patient During the Emergent/Resuscitative Phase of Burn Injury

Nursing Diagnosis: Impaired gas exchange related to carbon monoxide poisoning, smoke inhalation, and upper airway obstruction
Goal: Maintenance of adequate tissue oxygenation

NURSING INTERVENTIONS	RATIONALE	EXPECTED OUTCOMES
1. Provide humidified oxygen.	1. Humidified oxygen provides moisture to injured tissues; supplemental oxygen increases alveolar oxygenation.	• Absence of dyspnea • Respiratory rate between 12 and 20 breaths/min • Lungs clear on auscultation • Arterial oxygen saturation >96% by pulse oximetry • Arterial blood gas levels within normal limits
2. Assess breath sounds, and respiratory rate, rhythm, depth, and symmetry. Monitor patient for signs of hypoxia.	2. These factors provide baseline data for further assessment and evidence of increasing respiratory compromise.	
3. Observe for the following: a. Erythema or blistering of lips or buccal mucosa b. Singed nostrils c. Burns of face, neck, or chest d. Increasing hoarseness e. Soot in sputum or tracheal tissue in respiratory secretions	3. These signs indicate possible inhalation injury and risk of respiratory dysfunction.	
4. Monitor arterial blood gas values, pulse oximetry readings, and carboxyhemoglobin levels.	4. Increasing $PaCO_2$ and decreasing PaO_2 and O_2 saturation may indicate need for mechanical ventilation.	
5. Report labored respirations, decreased depth of respirations, or signs of hypoxia to physician immediately.	5. Immediate intervention is indicated for respiratory difficulty.	
6. Prepare to assist with intubation and escharotomies.	6. Intubation allows mechanical ventilation. Escharotomy enables chest excursion in circumferential chest burns.	
7. Monitor mechanically ventilated patient closely.	7. Monitoring allows early detection of decreasing respiratory status or complications of mechanical ventilation.	

Nursing Diagnosis: Ineffective airway clearance related to edema and effects of smoke inhalation
Goal: Maintain patent airway and adequate airway clearance

NURSING INTERVENTIONS	RATIONALE	EXPECTED OUTCOMES
1. Maintain patent airway through proper patient positioning, removal of secretions, and artificial airway if needed.	1. A patent airway is crucial to respiration.	• Patent airway • Respiratory secretions are minimal, colorless, and thin

CHART 57-7

Plan of Nursing Care — Care of the Patient During the Emergent/Resuscitative Phase of Burn Injury (Continued)

NURSING INTERVENTIONS	RATIONALE	EXPECTED OUTCOMES
2. Provide humidified oxygen.	2. Humidity liquefies secretions and facilitates expectoration.	• Respiratory rate, pattern, and breath sounds normal
3. Encourage patient to turn, cough, and deep breathe. Encourage patient to use incentive spirometry. Suction as needed.	3. These activities promote mobilization and removal of secretions.	

Nursing Diagnosis: Fluid volume deficit related to increased capillary permeability and evaporative losses from the burn wound
Goal: Restoration of optimal fluid and electrolyte balance and perfusion of vital organs

NURSING INTERVENTIONS	RATIONALE	EXPECTED OUTCOMES
1. Observe vital signs (including central venous pressure or pulmonary artery pressure, if indicated) and urine output, and be alert for signs of hypovolemia or fluid overload.	1. Hypovolemia is a major risk immediately after the burn injury. Overresuscitation might cause fluid overload.	• Serum electrolytes within normal limits • Urine output between 0.5 and 1.0 mL/kg/hr • Blood pressure higher than 90/60 mm Hg • Heart rate less than 120 beats/min • Exhibits clear sensorium • Voids clear yellow urine with specific gravity within normal limits
2. Monitor urine output at least hourly and weigh patient daily.	2. Output and weight provide information about renal perfusion, adequacy of fluid replacement, and fluid requirement and fluid status.	
3. Maintain IV lines and regulate fluids at appropriate rates, as prescribed.	3. Adequate fluids are necessary to maintain fluid and electrolyte balance and perfusion of vital organs.	
4. Observe for symptoms of deficiency or excess of serum sodium, potassium, calcium, phosphorus, and bicarbonate.	4. Rapid shifts in fluid and electrolyte status are possible in the postburn period.	
5. Elevate head of patient's bed and elevate burned extremities.	5. Elevation promotes venous return.	
6. Notify physician immediately of decreased urine output, blood pressure, central venous, pulmonary artery, or pulmonary artery wedge pressures, or increased pulse rate.	6. Because of the rapid fluid shifts in burn shock, fluid deficit must be detected early so that distributive shock does not occur.	

Nursing Diagnosis: Hypothermia related to loss of skin microcirculation and open wounds
Goal: Maintenance of adequate body temperature

NURSING INTERVENTIONS	RATIONALE	EXPECTED OUTCOMES
1. Provide a warm environment through use of heat shield, space blanket, heat lights, or blankets.	1. A stable environment minimizes evaporative heat loss.	• Body temperature remains 36.1° to 38.3°C (97° to 101°F) • Absence of chills or shivering

continued >

CHART 57-7

Plan of Nursing Care Care of the Patient During the Emergent/Resuscitative Phase of Burn Injury (Continued)

NURSING INTERVENTIONS	RATIONALE	EXPECTED OUTCOMES
2. Work quickly when wounds must be exposed.	2. Minimal exposure minimizes heat loss from wound.	
3. Assess core body temperature frequently.	3. Frequent temperature assessments help detect developing hypothermia.	

Nursing Diagnosis: Pain related to tissue and nerve injury and emotional impact of injury
Goal: Control of pain

NURSING INTERVENTIONS	RATIONALE	EXPECTED OUTCOMES
1. Use pain intensity scale to assess pain level (ie, 1 to 10). Differentiate restlessness due to pain from restlessness due to hypoxia.	1. Pain level provides baseline for evaluating effectiveness of pain relief measures. Hypoxia can cause similar signs and must be ruled out before analgesic medication is administered.	• States pain level is decreased • Absence of nonverbal cues of pain
2. Administer intravenous opioid analgesics as prescribed. Observe for respiratory depression in the patient who is not mechanically ventilated. Assess response to analgesic.	2. Intravenous administration is necessary because of altered tissue perfusion from burn injury.	
3. Provide emotional support and reassurance.	3. Emotional support is essential to reduce fear and anxiety resulting from burn injury. Fear and anxiety increase the perception of pain.	

Nursing Diagnosis: Anxiety related to fear and the emotional impact of burn injury
Goal: Minimization of patient's and family's anxiety

NURSING INTERVENTIONS	RATIONALE	EXPECTED OUTCOMES
1. Assess patient's and family's understanding of burn injury, coping skills, and family dynamics.	1. Previous successful coping strategies can be fostered for use in the present crisis. Assessment allows planning of individualized interventions.	• Patient and family verbalize understanding of emergent burn care • Able to answer simple questions
2. Individualize responses to the patient's and family's coping level.	2. Reactions to burn injury are extremely variable. Interventions must be appropriate to the patient's and family's present level of coping.	

CHART 57-7

Plan of Nursing Care — Care of the Patient During the Emergent/Resuscitative Phase of Burn Injury (Continued)

NURSING INTERVENTIONS	RATIONALE	EXPECTED OUTCOMES
3. Explain all procedures to the patient and the family in clear, simple terms.	3. Increased understanding alleviates fear of the unknown. High levels of anxiety may interfere with understanding of complex explanations.	
4. Maintain adequate pain relief.	4. Pain increases anxiety.	
5. Consider administering prescribed anti-anxiety medications if the patient remains extremely anxious despite nonpharmacologic interventions.	5. Anxiety levels during the emergent phase may exceed the patient's coping abilities. Medication decreases physiologic and psychological anxiety responses.	

Collaborative Problems: Acute respiratory failure, distributive shock, acute renal failure, compartment syndrome, paralytic ileus, Curling's ulcer
Goal: Absence of complications

NURSING INTERVENTIONS	RATIONALE	EXPECTED OUTCOMES
Acute Respiratory Failure		
1. Assess for increasing dyspnea, stridor, changes in respiratory patterns.	1. Such signs reflect deteriorating respiratory status.	• Arterial blood gas values within acceptable limits: PaO_2 >80 mm Hg, $PaCO_2$ <50 mm Hg • Breathes spontaneously with adequate tidal volume • Chest x-ray findings normal • Absence of cerebral signs of hypoxia
2. Monitor pulse oximetry, arterial blood gas values for decreasing PaO_2 and oxygen saturation, and increasing $PaCO_2$.	2. Such signs reflect decreased oxygenation status.	
3. Monitor chest x-ray results.	3. X-ray may disclose pulmonary injury.	
4. Assess for restlessness, confusion, difficulty attending to questions, or decreasing level of consciousness.	4. Such manifestations may indicate cerebral hypoxia.	
5. Report deteriorating respiratory status immediately to physician.	5. Acute respiratory failure is life-threatening, and immediate intervention is required.	
6. Prepare to assist with intubation or escharotomies as indicated.	6. Intubation allows mechanical ventilation. Escharotomies allow improved chest excursion with respirations.	
Distributive Shock		
1. Assess for decreasing urine output and blood pressure as well as increasing pulse rate. (If hemodynamic monitoring is used, assess for decreasing pulmonary artery and pulmonary artery wedge pressures and cardiac output.)	1. Such signs and symptoms may indicate distributive shock and inadequate intravascular volume.	• Urine output between 0.5 and 1.0 mL/kg/hr • Blood pressure within patient's normal range (usually >90/60 mm Hg) • Heart rate within patient's normal range (usually <110/min)

continued >

CHART 57-7

Plan of Nursing Care — Care of the Patient During the Emergent/Resuscitative Phase of Burn Injury (Continued)

NURSING INTERVENTIONS	RATIONALE	EXPECTED OUTCOMES
2. Assess for progressive edema as fluid shifts occur.	2. As fluid shifts into the interstitial spaces in burn shock, edema occurs and may compromise tissue perfusion.	• Pressures and cardiac output remain within normal limits
3. Adjust fluid resuscitation in collaboration with the physician in response to physiologic findings.	3. Optimal fluid resuscitation prevents distributive shock and improves patient outcomes.	
Acute Renal Failure		
1. Monitor urine output and blood urea nitrogen (BUN) and serum creatinine levels.	1. These values reflect renal function.	• Adequate urine output • BUN and serum creatinine values remain normal
2. Report decreased urine output or increased BUN and creatinine values to physician.	2. These laboratory values indicate possible renal failure.	
3. Assess urine for hemoglobin or myoglobin.	3. Hemoglobin or myoglobin in the urine points to an increased risk of renal failure.	
4. Administer increased fluids as prescribed.	4. Fluids help to flush hemoglobin and myoglobin from renal tubules, decreasing the potential for renal failure.	
Compartment Syndrome		
1. Assess peripheral pulses hourly with Doppler ultrasound device.	1. Assessment with Doppler device substitutes for auscultation and indicates characteristics of arterial blood flow.	• Absence of paresthesias or symptoms of ischemia of nerves and muscles • Peripheral pulses detectable by Doppler
2. Assess warmth, capillary refill, sensation, and movement of extremity hourly. Compare affected with unaffected extremity.	2. These assessments indicate characteristics of peripheral perfusion.	
3. Remove blood pressure cuff after each reading.	3. Cuff may act as a tourniquet as extremities swell.	
4. Elevate burned extremities.	4. Elevation reduces edema formation.	
5. Report loss of pulse or sensation or presence of pain to physician immediately.	5. These signs and symptoms may indicate inadequate tissue perfusion.	
6. Prepare to assist with escharotomies.	6. Escharotomies relieve the constriction caused by swelling under circumferential burns and improve tissue perfusion.	
Paralytic Ileus		
1. Maintain nasogastric tube on low intermittent suction until bowel sounds resume.	1. This measure relieves gastric and abdominal distention, also prevents vomiting.	• Absence of abdominal distention • Normal bowel sounds within 48 hours
2. Auscultate for bowel sounds, abdominal distention.	2. As bowel sounds resume, feeding may be slowly initiated. Abdominal distention reflects inadequate decompression.	

CHART 57-7

Plan of Nursing Care — Care of the Patient During the Emergent/Resuscitative Phase of Burn Injury (Continued)

NURSING INTERVENTIONS	RATIONALE	EXPECTED OUTCOMES
Curling's Ulcer		
1. Assess gastric aspirate for pH and blood.	1. Acidic pH indicates need for antacids or histamine blockers. Blood indicates possible gastric bleeding.	• Absence of abdominal distention • Normal bowel sounds within 48 hours • Gastric aspirate and stools do not contain blood
2. Assess stools for occult blood.	2. Blood in stools may indicate gastric or duodenal ulcer.	
3. Administer histamine blockers and antacids as prescribed.	3. Such medications reduce gastric acidity and risk of ulceration.	

tion injury. Bronchial washing or bronchioalveolar lavage can assist in the diagnosis and treatment of pneumonia (Wahl, Ahrns, Brandt, et al., 2005). Ideally, the best practice is to remove the endotracheal tube as soon as possible so that a route for pathogens is not accessible to the lungs. The arterial blood gas values and other parameters determine the need for intubation and mechanical ventilation.

As capillaries regain integrity, 48 or more hours after the burn, fluid moves from the interstitial to the intravascular compartment and diuresis begins (Table 57-4). If cardiac or renal function is inadequate, for instance in an elderly patient or in a patient with preexisting cardiac disease, fluid overload occurs and symptoms of congestive heart failure may result (see Chapter 30). Early detection allows for early intervention and carefully calculated fluid intake (Supple, 2004). Cautious administration of vasoactive medications, diuretics, and fluid restriction may be used to support circulatory function and prevent fluid overload, heart failure, and pulmonary edema.

TABLE 57-4 Fluid and Electrolyte Changes in the Acute Phase

Fluid remobilization phase (state of diuresis)
Interstitial fluid → plasma

Observation	Explanation
Hemodilution (decreased hematocrit)	Blood cell concentration is diluted as fluid enters the intravascular compartment; loss of red blood cells destroyed at burn site
Increased urinary output	Fluid shift into intravascular compartment increases renal blood flow and causes increased urine formation.
Sodium (Na^+) deficit	With diuresis, sodium is lost with water; existing serum sodium is diluted by water influx.
Potassium (K^+) deficit (occurs occasionally in this phase)	Beginning on the fourth or fifth postburn day, K^+ shifts from extracellular fluid into cells.
Metabolic acidosis	Loss of sodium depletes fixed base; relative carbon dioxide content increases.

Cautious administration of fluids and electrolytes continues during this phase of burn care because of the shifts in fluid from the interstitial to the intravascular compartment, losses of fluid from large burn wounds, and the patient's physiologic responses to the burn injury. Blood components are administered as needed to treat blood loss and anemia.

Fever is common in patients after burn shock resolves. A resetting of the core body temperature in severely burned patients results in a body temperature a few degrees higher than normal for several weeks after the burn. Bacteremia and septicemia also cause fever in many patients. Acetaminophen (Tylenol) and hypothermia blankets may be required to maintain body temperature in a range of 37.2° to 38.3°C (99° to 101°F) so as to reduce metabolic stress and tissue oxygen demand.

Central venous, peripheral arterial, or pulmonary artery thermodilution catheters may be required for monitoring venous and arterial pressures, pulmonary artery pressures, pulmonary capillary wedge pressures, or cardiac output. However, invasive vascular lines are generally avoided, unless deemed essential, because they provide an additional port for infection in an already greatly compromised patient.

Infection progressing to septic shock is the major cause of death in patients who have survived the first few days after a major burn. The immunosuppression that accompanies extensive burn injury places the patient at high risk of sepsis. The infection that begins within the burn site may spread to the bloodstream (Neely et al., 2004).

Infection Prevention

Despite aseptic precautions and the use of topical antimicrobial agents, the burn wound is an excellent medium for bacterial growth and proliferation. Bacteria such as *Staphylococcus, Proteus, Pseudomonas, Escherichia coli,* and *Klebsiella* find optimal conditions for growth within the burn wound. The burn eschar is a nonviable crust with no blood supply; therefore, neither polymorphonuclear leukocytes or antibodies nor systemic antibiotics can reach the area. Phenomenal numbers of bacteria—more than 1 billion per gram of tissue—may appear and subsequently spread to the bloodstream or release their toxins, which reach distant sites. Staphylococci and enterococci are the organisms responsible for more than 50% of nosocomial bloodstream infections in patients with burn injuries. Fungi such as *Candida albicans* also grow easily in burn wounds.

When the burn wound is healing through spontaneous reepithelialization or is being prepared for skin grafting, it must be protected from sepsis. Burn wound sepsis has these characteristics:

- 10^5 bacteria per gram of tissue
- Inflammation
- Sludging and thrombosis of dermal blood vessels

A primary source of bacterial infection appears to be the patient's intestinal tract, the source of most microbes. The intestinal mucosa normally serves as a barrier to keep the internal environment free from a variety of pathogens. After a severe burn injury, the intestinal mucosal barrier becomes markedly permeable (Gosain & Gamelli, 2005b). Because of this impaired barrier, the disturbed microbial flora and endotoxins found in the intestinal lumen pass freely into the systemic circulation, finally causing infection. If the intestinal mucosa receives some type of protection against permeability change, infection can be avoided. Early enteral feeding is one strategy to help avoid this increased intestinal permeability and prevent early endotoxin translocation (De-Souza & Greene, 2005).

Infection impedes burn wound healing by promoting excessive inflammation and damaging tissue. A major secondary source of pathogenic microbes is the environment. Infection control is a major role of the burn team in providing appropriate burn wound care. Cap, gown, mask, and gloves are worn while caring for the patient with open burn wounds. Clean technique is used when caring directly for burn wounds.

Tissue specimens are obtained for culture regularly to monitor colonization of the wound by microbial organisms. These may be swab, surface, or tissue biopsy cultures. Swab or surface cultures are noninvasive, simple, and painless. However, data obtained from such cultures apply only to the area sampled; therefore, invasive wound biopsy cultures may be required. Antibiotics are seldom prescribed prophylactically because of the risk of promoting resistant strains of bacteria. Systemic antibiotics are administered when there is documentation of burn wound sepsis or other positive cultures such as urine, sputum, or blood. By the time a patient demonstrates signs of sepsis, the infection has already affected large parts of the body (Ahrens & Vollman, 2003). Sensitivity of the organisms to the prescribed antibiotics should be determined before administration. Several parenteral antimicrobial agents may be administered together to treat the infection. Careful attention is paid to antibiotic use in the burn unit, because inappropriate use of antibiotics significantly affects the microbial flora present in the burn unit and increases the risk of drug resistance.

Wound Cleaning

Various measures are used to clean the burn wound. **Hydrotherapy** can be used to clean the wounds. If the patient is ambulatory, the wounds can be cleansed in a shower. The wounds of nonambulatory patients can be cleansed using shower carts—mobile stretchers made with removable sides, drainage holes, and positioning capabilities. Retractable shower hoses suspended from walls and ceilings provide the nurse with easy access to a water source for washing the wounds. Unstable patients have their wounds washed at the bedside. Total immersion hydrotherapy is performed in some settings. Because of the high risk for infection and sepsis, the use of plastic liners, water filters, and thorough decontamination of hydrotherapy equipment and wound care areas is required to prevent cross-contamination. The temperature of the water is maintained at 37.8°C (100°F), and the temperature of the room should be maintained between 26.6° and 29.4°C (80° to 85°F). Hydrotherapy, in whatever form, should be limited to a 20- to 30-minute period to prevent chilling of the patient and additional metabolic stress.

During the bath, the patient is encouraged to be as active as possible. Hydrotherapy provides an excellent opportunity for exercising the extremities and cleaning the entire body. When the patient is removed from the tub after the bath, any residue adhering to the body is washed away with a clear water spray or shower. Unburned areas, including the hair, must be washed regularly as well. At the time of wound cleaning, all skin is inspected for any hints of redness, breakdown, or local infection. Hair in and around the burn area, except the eyebrows, should be clipped short. Intact blisters should be left alone and débrided only if they rupture or break.

Conscientious management of the burn wound is essential. When nonviable loose skin is removed, aseptic conditions must be established. Wound cleaning is usually performed at least daily in wound areas that are not undergoing surgical intervention. When the eschar begins to separate from the viable tissue beneath (approximately 1.5 to 2 weeks after the burn), more frequent cleaning and débridement may be in order.

After the burn wounds are cleaned, they are gently patted with towels, and the prescribed method of wound care is performed. Physician preferences, the availability of skilled nursing staff, and resources in terms of number of personnel, supplies, and time must be considered in choosing the best method for a given patient. Whatever the method, the goal is to protect the wound from overwhelming proliferation of pathogenic organisms and invasion of deeper tissues until either spontaneous healing or skin grafting can be achieved.

Patient comfort and ability to participate in the prescribed treatment are also important considerations. Wound care procedures, particularly tub baths, are metabolically stressful. Therefore, the patient is assessed for signs of chilling, fatigue, changes in hemodynamic status, and pain unrelieved by analgesic medications or relaxation techniques.

Topical Antibacterial Therapy

There is general agreement that some form of antimicrobial therapy applied to the burn wound is the best method of local care in extensive burn injury. Topical antibacterial therapy does not sterilize the burn wound; it simply reduces the number of bacteria so that the overall microbial population can be controlled by the body's host defense mechanisms. Criteria for choice of topical agents include the following:

- They are effective against gram-negative organisms and even fungi.
- They are clinically effective.
- They penetrate the eschar but are not systemically toxic.
- They do not lose their effectiveness, allowing another infection to develop.
- They are cost-effective, available, and acceptable to the patient.
- They are easy to apply and remove, minimizing nursing care time.

For more than 50 years, it has been recognized that silver has bacteriostatic and bacteriocidal properties that make it an excellent treatment agent for burn injuries (Heggers, Goodheart, Washington, et al., 2005). Silver is effective against *Pseudomonas aeruginosa, Staphylococcus aureus, Enterococcus, Serratia marcescens,* and *C. albicans*. Methods of applying silver to burn wounds include liquid, cream, metallic foil, and hydrofiber sheeting (Caruso, Foster, Hermans, et al., 2004). Use of 0.5% liquid silver nitrate solution or cream-based topical agents such as silver sulfadiazine can have an immediate effect. Continuous silver application can be provided with the slow-release silver dressings such as Acticoat, Aquacel, Silversorb, or Silverlon. The advantages of the slow-release dressings are less discomfort and less need to change the wound dressing frequently (Bowler et al., 2004; Caruso et al., 2004; Heggers et al., 2005).

Table 57-5 describes three commonly used topical agents, silver sulfadiazine (Silvadene), silver nitrate, and mafenide acetate (Sulfamylon), two of which contain silver. Many other topical agents are available, including povidone–iodine ointment 10% (Betadine), gentamicin sulfate, nitrofurazone (Furacin), Dakin's solution, acetic acid, miconazole, and clotrimazole. Bacitracin or a triple antibiotic agent may be used for facial burns or on skin grafts initially.

No single topical medication is universally effective, and use of different agents at different times in the postburn period may be necessary. Bacteriologic cultures are required to monitor the effect of topical medications. Prudent use and alternation of antimicrobial agents result in less resistant strains of bacteria, greater effectiveness of the agents, and a decreased risk of sepsis.

Before any topical agent is reapplied, the previously applied topical agent must be thoroughly removed. The number of times the dressings are changed and soaked is planned to promote optimal therapeutic use of the topical agent.

Wound Dressing

When the wound is clean, the burned areas are patted dry and the prescribed topical agent is applied; the wound is then covered with several layers of dressings. A light dressing is used over joint areas to allow for motion (unless the particular area has a graft and motion is contraindicated). A light dressing is also applied over areas for which a splint has been designed to conform to the body contour for proper positioning. Circumferential dressings should be applied distally to proximally. If the hand or foot is burned, the fingers and toes should be wrapped individually to promote adequate healing.

Burns to the face may be left open to air once they have been cleaned and the topical agent has been applied. Careful attention must be given to ensure that the topical agent does not interfere with the eyes or mouth. A light dressing can be applied to the face to absorb excess exudates that might run into the eyes, causing irritation.

There is a role for occlusive dressings in treating specific wounds. An occlusive dressing is a thin gauze that is impregnated with a topical antimicrobial agent or is applied after application of a topical antimicrobial agent. Occlusive dressings are most often used over areas with new skin grafts. Their purpose is to protect the graft, promoting an optimal condition for its adherence to the recipient site. Ideally, these dressings remain in place for 3 to 5 days, at which time they are removed for examination of the graft.

When occlusive dressings are applied, precautions are taken to prevent two body surfaces from touching, such as fingers or toes, ear and scalp, the areas under the breasts, any point of flexion, or between the genital folds. Functional body alignment positions are maintained by using splints or by careful positioning of the patient.

Close communication and cooperation among the patient, surgeon, nurse, and other health care team members are essential for optimal burn wound care. Different wound areas on a given patient may require different wound care techniques. Diagrams posted at the bedside are useful to inform staff of the current prescription for wound care, splints to be applied over dressings, and the exercise regimen to be followed before dressings are reapplied.

NURSING ALERT

Dressings impede circulation if they are too tightly wrapped. The peripheral pulses must be checked frequently and burned extremities elevated on two pillows. If the patient's pulse is diminished, the dressings should be loosened.

Dressings are changed in the patient's unit, in the hydrotherapy room, or in the treatment area approximately 20 minutes after an analgesic agent is administered. They may also be changed in the operating room after the patient is anesthetized. A mask, goggles, hair cover, disposable plastic apron or cover gown, and gloves are worn by health care personnel when removing the dressings. The outer dressings are slit with blunt scissors, and the soiled dressings are removed and disposed of in accordance with established procedures for contaminated materials.

Dressings that adhere to the wound can be removed more comfortably if they are moistened with tap water or if the patient is allowed to soak for a few moments in the tub. The

TABLE 57-5 Overview of Selected Topical Antibacterial Agents Used for Burn Wounds

Agent	Indication	Application	Nursing Implications
Silver sulfadiazine 1% (Silvadene) water-soluble cream	• Most bactericidal agent • Minimal penetration of eschar	Apply 1/16-inch layer of cream with a sterile glove 1–3 times daily.	• Watch for leukopenia 2–3 days after initiation of therapy. (Leukopenia usually resolves within 2–3 days.) • Anticipate formation of pseudo-eschar (proteinaceous gel), which is removed easily after 72 hours.
Mafenide acetate 5% to 10% (Sulfamylon) hydrophilic-based cream	• Effective against gram-negative and gram-positive organisms • Diffuses rapidly through eschar • In 10% strength, it is the agent of choice for electrical burns because of its ability to penetrate thick eschar.	Apply thin layer with sterile glove twice a day and leave open as prescribed; if the wound is dressed, change the dressing every 6 hours as prescribed.	• Monitor arterial blood gas levels and discontinue as prescribed, if acidosis occurs. Mafenide acetate is a strong carbonic anhydrase inhibitor that may reduce renal buffering and cause metabolic acidosis. • Premedicate the patient with an analgesic before applying mafenide acetate because this agent causes severe burning pain for up to 20 minutes after application.
Silver nitrate 0.5% aqueous solution	• Bacteriostatic and fungicidal • Does *not* penetrate eschar	Apply solution to gauze dressing and place over wound. Keep the dressing wet but covered with dry gauze and dry blankets to decrease vaporization. Remoisten every 2 hours, and redress wound twice a day.	• Monitor serum sodium (Na^+) and potassium (K^+) levels and replace as prescribed. Silver nitrate solution is hypotonic and acts as wick for sodium and potassium. • Protect bed linen and clothing from contact with silver nitrate, which stains everything it touches black.
Acticoat	• Effective against gram-negative and gram-positive organisms and some yeasts and molds • Delivers a uniform, antimicrobial concentration of silver to the burn wound	Moisten with sterile water only (*never* use normal saline). Apply directly to wound. Cover with absorbent secondary dressing. Remoisten every 3–4 hours with sterile water.	• Do not use oil-based products or topical antimicrobials with Acticoat burn dressing. Keep Acticoat moist, not saturated. May produce a "pseudoeschar" from silver after application. • Can be left in place for 3–5 days. Also available in Acticoat 7, which can be left in place for up to 7 days without the need to change the dressing.

remaining dressings are carefully and gently removed. The patient may participate in removing the dressings, providing some degree of control over this painful procedure. The wounds are then cleaned and débrided to remove debris, any remaining topical agent, exudate, and dead skin. Sterile scissors and forceps may be used to trim loose eschar and encourage separation of devitalized skin. During this procedure, the wound and surrounding skin are carefully inspected. The color, odor, size, exudate, signs of reepithelialization, and other characteristics of the wound and the eschar and any changes from the previous dressing change are noted.

Wound Débridement

As debris accumulates on the wound surface, it can retard keratinocyte migration, thus delaying the epithelialization process. **Débridement**, another facet of burn wound care, has two goals:

- To remove tissue contaminated by bacteria and foreign bodies, thereby protecting the patient from invasion of bacteria
- To remove devitalized tissue or burn eschar in preparation for grafting and wound healing

There are three types of débridement—natural, mechanical, and surgical.

Natural Débridement

With natural débridement, the dead tissue separates from the underlying viable tissue spontaneously. After partial- and full-thickness burns, bacteria that are present at the interface of the burned tissue and the viable tissue underneath gradually liquefy the fibrils of **collagen** that hold the eschar in place for the first or second postburn week. Proteolytic and other natural enzymes cause this phenomenon. However, use of antibacterial topical agents tends to slow this natural process of eschar separation. It is advantageous to the patient to speed this process through other means, such as mechanical or surgical débridement, thereby reducing the time during which bacterial invasion and other iatrogenic problems may arise.

Mechanical Débridement

Mechanical débridement involves the use of surgical scissors, scalpels, and forceps to separate and remove the eschar. This technique can be performed by skilled physicians, nurses, or physical therapists and is usually done with daily dressing changes and wound cleaning procedures. Débridement by these means is carried out to the point of pain and bleeding. Hemostatic agents or pressure can be used to stop bleeding from small vessels. Wet-to-dry dressings are not advocated in burn care because of the chance of removing viable cells along with necrotic tissue. Dressing changes alone aid the removal of wound debris.

Topical enzymatic débridement agents are available to promote débridement of the burn wounds. Because such agents do not have antimicrobial properties, they should be used together with topical antibacterial therapy to protect the patient from bacterial invasion. Heavy metals such as silver deactivate the débriding agent; therefore, caution is necessary to ensure that the débriding agent does not interfere with the topical antimicrobial agent. Separate dressings are used to prevent this from occurring.

Surgical Débridement

Early surgical excision to remove devitalized tissue along with early burn wound closure is now recognized as one of the most important factors contributing to survival in a patient with a major burn injury. Aggressive surgical wound closure has reduced the incidence of burn wound sepsis, thus improving survival rates (Burke, 2005). Early excision is carried out before the natural separation of eschar is allowed to occur.

Surgical débridement is an operative procedure involving either primary **excision** (surgical removal of tissue) of the full thickness of the skin down to the fascia (tangential excision) or shaving of the burned skin layers gradually down to freely bleeding, viable tissue. Surgical excision is initiated early in burn wound management. This may be performed a few days after the burn or as soon as the patient is hemodynamically stable and edema has decreased. Ideally, the wound is then covered immediately with a skin graft, if needed, and an occlusive dressing. If the wound bed is not ready for a skin graft at the time of excision, a temporary biologic dressing may be used until a skin graft can be applied during subsequent surgery.

The use of surgical excision carries with it risks and complications, especially with large burns. The procedure creates a high risk of extensive blood loss (as much as 100 to 125 mL of blood per percent of body surface excised) and lengthy operating and anesthesia times. However, when conducted in a timely and efficient manner, surgical excision results in shorter hospital stays and possibly a decreased risk of complications from invasive burn wound sepsis.

Gerontologic Considerations

Eschar separation in full-thickness burns is typically delayed in elderly patients, and older patients are frequently poor risks for surgical excision. For these reasons, prolonged hospitalization, immobilization, and associated problems may be common. If the elderly patient can tolerate surgery, early excision with skin grafting is the treatment of choice, because it decreases the mortality rate in this population. Prevention of complications of prolonged hospitalization, immobility, and surgery is essential in the care of the elderly burn patient.

Wound Grafting

If wounds are deep (full-thickness) or extensive, spontaneous reepithelialization is not possible. Therefore, coverage of the burn wound is necessary until coverage with a graft of the patient's own skin (**autograft**) is possible. The purposes of wound coverage are to decrease the risk of infection; prevent further loss of protein, fluid, and electrolytes through the wound; and minimize heat loss through evaporation. Several methods of wound coverage are available; some are temporary until grafting with permanent coverage is possible. Wound coverage may consist of biologic, biosynthetic, synthetic, and autologous methods or a combination of these approaches, as described in Table 57-6.

The main areas for skin grafting include the face (for cosmetic and psychological reasons); functional areas, such as the hands and feet; and areas that involve joints. Grafting permits earlier functional ability and reduces wound **contractures.** When burns are very extensive, the chest and abdomen may be grafted first to reduce the burn surface.

Granulation tissue fills the space created by the wound, creates a barrier to bacteria, and serves as a bed for epithelial cell growth. Richly vascular granulation tissue is pink, firm, shiny, and free of exudate and debris. It should have a bacterial count of less than 100,000 per gram of tissue to optimize graft success. If the wound is not ready for skin grafting, the burn wound is excised and allowed to granulate. Once the wound is excised, a wound covering is applied to keep the wound bed moist and promote the granulation process.

Biologic Dressings (Homografts and Heterografts)

Biologic dressings have several uses. In extensive burns, they save lives by providing temporary wound coverage

TABLE 57-6 Temporary and Permanent Burn Wound Coverings

Name	Source	Type of Covering	Advantages	Disadvantages
Biobrane	Biosynthetic nylon on silastic membrane Collagen derivative	Temporary	Protects wound from fluid and protein loss Reduces pain Can remain in place for weeks Multiple uses over wide-meshed grants, donor sites, and partial-thickness burns Indefinite shelf life	Wound surface must be free of infection
Aquacel Ag	Sodium carboxymethyl-cellulose and ionic silver	Temporary	Ionic silver immediately kills pathogens Reduces pain Can remain in place up to 14 days Highly absorbent, creating moist wound environment	Difficult to cover joints Painful to remove if it needs to be removed prematurely Use on partial-thickness wounds only
BCG Matrix	Biosynthetic beta-glucan enmeshed with collagen	Temporary	Covers partial-thickness wounds and donor sites Can be left in place until wound heals	High cost Requires that wound be clean and free of infection
Allograft (homograft)	Human fresh or cryo-preserved	Temporary	Covers large areas Used until wound is ready for autografting Aids in revascularization of wound Protects granulation tissue Decreases evaporation of water and protein from wound	Availability and high cost Eventual rejection Questionable transmission of disease
Xenograft (heterograft)	Pig, rabbit, dog, lizard; fresh, frozen or freeze-dried	Temporary	Readily available Long shelf life Decreases pain of wound Protects granulation tissue Covers large areas Aids in wound débridement when removed	Eventual rejection Can be used only with noninfected partial-thickness wounds
Integra	Dermal replacement; dermal matrix covered by autograft	Permanent	Cryopreserved—easy to transport Multiple uses: burns, dermal ulcers Donor site smaller with less scarring Used for burn wound covering and reconstruction	Wound surface must be free of infection for "take" High cost Rigorous postoperative care Need to stage procedures
Alloderm	Nonimmunogenic dermal replacement Freeze-dried acellular allogenic dermis engrafted with a thick epithelial autograft	Permanent	Supports autograft Less scarring and contracture formation Multiple uses in dental, abdominal, burn, and reconstructive surgery High percentage of "take"	Wound surface must be free of infection for "take" High cost
Cultured epithelial autograft (CEA)	Patient's own cells autologous cultured epithelium	Permanent Permanent	Life-saving for very large full-thickness burns Covers large areas of wound from cells obtained from small biopsy of skin	Length of time to grow skin Tedious postoperative care with immobility Easily infected, fragile and affected by shear Difficult to handle graft High cost of grafts and process Increased scarring and contractures

TABLE 57-6 Temporary and Permanent Burn Wound Coverings (Continued)

Name	Source	Type of Covering	Advantages	Disadvantages
Apligraf CEA	Cultured keratinocytes with allodermis cultured fibroblast matrix		Bioengineered Better growth potential than CEA Good graft "take" with less chance of rejection Less scarring Multiple uses in different wounds	High cost New in wound care market; limited experience with use
		Permanent		
Autograft	Patient's own skin		Ideal and safest wound covering Reduced healing time and scarring Sheet-, meshed-, or postage stamp-size grafts possible No rejection by patient's immune system	Need to stage procedures Limited amount of skin available with large burns Creates donor site wound Healing of recipient areas with irregular pattern

and protecting the granulation tissue until autografting is possible. Biologic dressings are commonly used in patients with large areas of burn and little remaining normal skin donor sites. Biologic dressings may also be used to débride wounds after eschar separation. With each biologic dressing change, débridement occurs. Once the biologic dressing appears to be "taking," or adhering to the granulating surface with minimal underlying exudation, the patient is ready for an autologous skin graft.

Biologic dressings also provide temporary immediate coverage for clean, superficial burns and decrease the wound's evaporative water and protein loss. They decrease pain by protecting nerve endings and are an effective barrier against water loss and entry of bacteria. When applied to superficial partial-thickness wounds, they seem to speed healing. Biologic materials can be left open or covered. They stay in place for varying lengths of time but are removed in instances of infection or rejection.

Biologic dressings consist of **homografts** (or allografts) and **heterografts** (or xenografts). Homografts are skin obtained from living or recently deceased humans. The amniotic membrane (amnion) from the human placenta may also be used as a biologic dressing. Heterografts consist of skin taken from animals (usually pigs). Most biologic dressings are used as temporary coverings of burn wounds and are eventually rejected because of the body's immune reaction to them as foreign.

Homografts tend to be the most expensive biologic dressings. They are available from skin banks in fresh and cryopreserved (frozen) forms. Homografts are thought to provide the best infection control of all the biologic or biosynthetic dressings available. Revascularization occurs within 48 hours, and the graft may be left in place for several weeks.

Amnion is less expensive and is available in hospitals with burn centers and specialized tissue banks, which obtain and process it in cooperation with obstetric services. However, screening for viral disease is difficult.

Pigskin is available from commercial suppliers. It is available fresh, frozen, or lyophilized (freeze-dried) for longer shelf life. Pigskin is widely used for temporary covering of clean wounds such as superficial partial-thickness wounds and donor sites. Although pigskin does not vascularize, it does adhere to clean superficial wounds and provides excellent pain control while the underlying wound epithelializes (Atiyeh et al., 2005).

Biosynthetic and Synthetic Dressings

Problems with availability, sterility, and cost have prompted the search for biosynthetic and synthetic skin substitutes, which may eventually replace biologic dressings as temporary wound coverings. A widely used synthetic dressing is **Biobrane**, which is composed of a nylon, Silastic membrane combined with a collagen derivative. The material is semitransparent and sterile. It has an indefinite shelf life and is less costly than homograft or pigskin. Like biologic dressings, Biobrane protects the wound from fluid loss and bacterial invasion.

Biobrane adheres to the wound fibrin, which binds to the nylon–collagen material. Within 5 days, cells migrate into the nylon mesh. In general, adherence to the wound surface correlates directly with low bacterial counts. When the Biobrane dressing adheres to the wound, the wound remains stable and the Biobrane can remain in place for 3 to 4 weeks. Biobrane dressings (Fig. 57-4) readily adhere to donor sites and meticulously clean débrided partial-thickness wounds; they remain until spontaneous epithelialization and wound healing occur. Biobrane can be laid on top of a wide-meshed autograft to protect the wound until the autograft epithelium grows out to close the interstices. As the Biobrane gradually separates, it is trimmed, leaving a healed wound.

Biobrane is also useful for intermediate or long-term closure of a surgically excised wound until an autograft becomes available. Like biologic dressings, Biobrane should not be used over grossly contaminated or necrotic wounds. Removal of Biobrane after several weeks is similar to but easier than removal of a vascularized allograft and leaves a bleeding granulation bed that readily accepts an autograft.

Another temporary wound covering is BCG Matrix. This dressing combines beta-glucan, a complex carbohydrate, with collagen in a meshed reinforced wound dressing. Beta-glucan is known to stimulate macrophages, which are

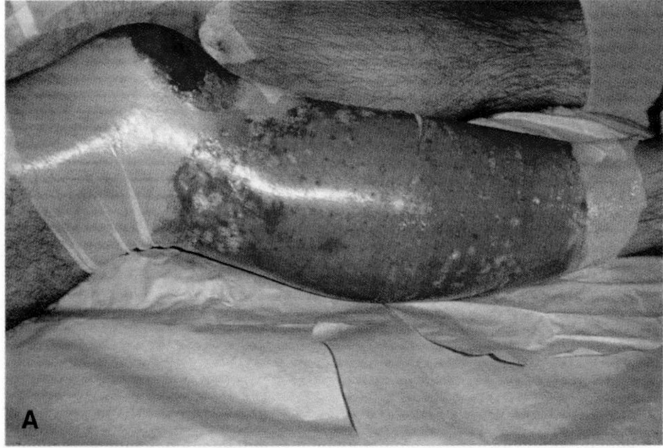

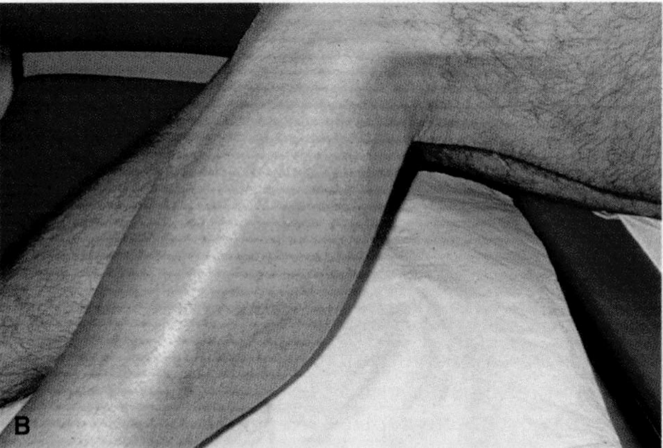

FIGURE 57-4. (**A**) Use of Biobrane dressing for full-thickness burn wound. Biobrane dressing applied to lower extremity partial-thickness burn. (**B**) Healed full-thickness burn wound after use of Biobrane. Used with permission. Bertek Pharmaceuticals, Research Triangle Park, NC.

vital in the inflammatory process of healing. BCG Matrix is a temporary wound covering intended for use with partial-thickness burns and donor sites. It is applied immediately after cleaning and débridement. If the burn wound surface remains free of infection, BCG Matrix can be left in place until healing is complete (Atiyeh et al., 2005).

Several other synthetic dressings are available for burn wound care. Op-Site, a thin, transparent, polyurethane elastic film, can be used to cover clean partial-thickness wounds and donor sites. This dressing is occlusive and waterproof but permeable to water vapor and air; this permeability not only provides protection from microbial contamination but also allows for the exchange of gases, which occurs much more quickly in a moist environment. Other synthetic dressings used for burn wounds include Tegaderm, N-Terface, and DuoDerm.

Burns that are between superficial and deep partial thickness in depth can be treated with a temporary biologic covering called TransCyte, a material composed of human newborn fibroblasts that are cultured on the nylon mesh of Biobrane. The thin silicone membrane bonded to the mesh provides a moisture vapor barrier for the wound. TransCyte is used to treat burns in which the depth is indeterminate. TransCyte delivers a variety of biologically active proteins, which may benefit the wound healing process. Research has shown that wounds treated with TransCyte healed more quickly and with less hypertrophic scarring than burns treated with the traditional silver sulfadiazine protocols (Cone, 2005).

Dermal Substitutes

In an attempt to develop the ideal burn wound covering product, dermal substitutes have been created. It is believed skin substitutes enhance the healing process of an open wound when autologous skin is unavailable or limited for use (Ehrlich, 2004). Two such products are Integra Artificial Skin and Alloderm.

Artificial skin (**Integra**) is the newest type of dermal substitute. A dermal analogue, Integra is composed of two main layers. The epidermal layer, consisting of silicone, acts as a bacterial barrier and prevents water loss from the dermis. The dermal layer is composed of animal collagen. It interfaces with the open wound surface and allows migration of fibroblasts and capillaries into the material. This "neodermis" becomes a permanent structure. The artificial dermis is biodegraded and reabsorbed. The outer silicone membrane is removed 2 weeks after application and is replaced with the patient's own skin in the form of a thin epidermal skin graft. When a thinner autologous donor graft is used, donor site healing is quicker. Long-term effects of Integra include minimal contracture formation. The graft site is very pliable, almost eliminating the need for repeated cosmetic surgery. Most importantly, Integra has resulted in less hypertrophic scarring (Fig. 57-5), thus reducing the need for compression devices once the burn wound has healed. Because Integra allows for earlier excision and coverage of the burn wound, metabolic demands of the patient are reduced. Integra allows for the increased survivability of patients with burn injuries and improves the functional and cosmetic qualities of the healed burns. The combination of Integra with cultured skin substitutes has demonstrated promise in burn management (Atiyeh et al., 2005; Heimbach, Warden, Luterman, et al., 2003, Sheridan & Thompkins, 2004).

Another promising dermal substitute is **Alloderm.** It is processed dermis from human cadaver skin, which can be used as the dermal layer for skin grafts. When a **donor site** (the area from which skin is taken to provide a skin graft for another part of the body) is harvested for an autologous skin graft, both the epidermal and the dermal layers of skin are removed from the donor site. Alloderm provides a permanent dermal layer replacement. Its use allows the burn surgeon to harvest a thinner skin graft, consisting of the epidermal layer only. The patient's epidermal layer is placed directly over the dermal base (Alloderm). The new graft is then treated according to the burn unit's protocol. Use of Alloderm has also resulted in less scarring and contractures with healed grafts; donor sites heal much more quickly than conventional donor sites, because only the epidermal layer has been harvested. This is important when donor sites are limited because of extensive burns (Sheridan & Thompkins, 2004).

Autografts

Autografts remain the preferred material for definitive burn wound closure after excision. Autografts are the ideal means

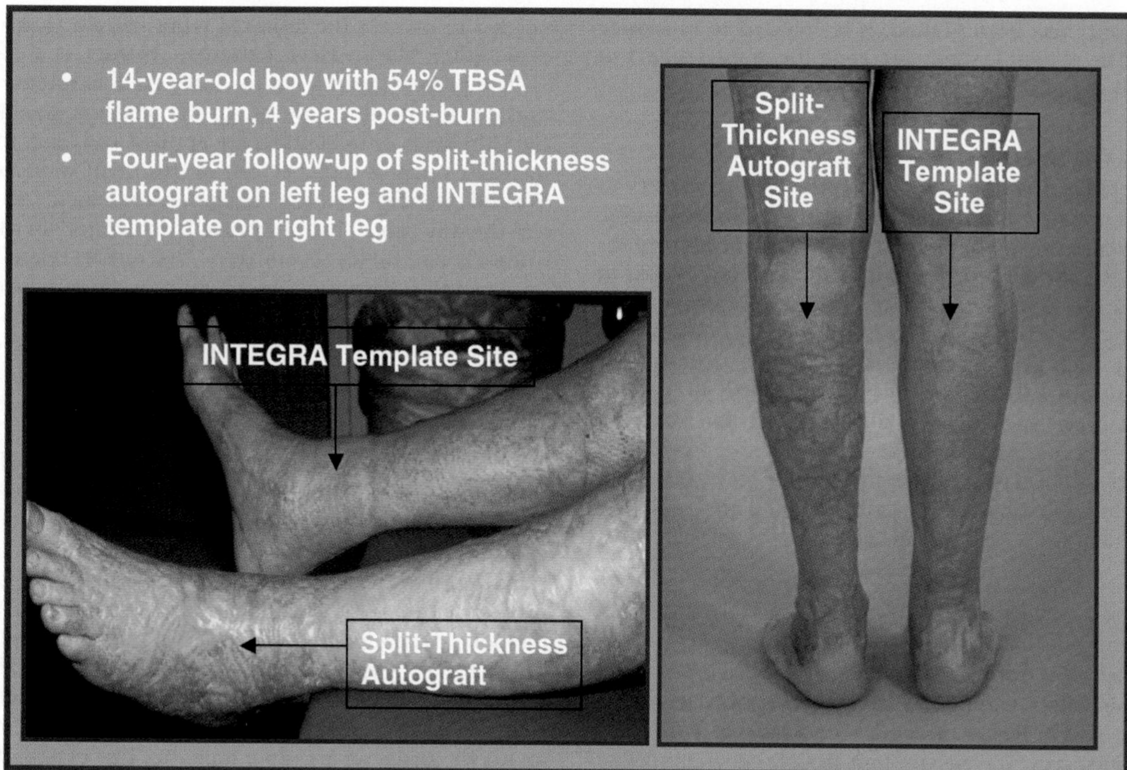

FIGURE 57-5. Comparison of Integra template site (right leg) to split thickness autograft site (left leg). Used with permission from Glenn Warden, MD.

of covering burn wounds, because the grafts are the patient's own skin and therefore are not rejected by the patient's immune system. They can be split-thickness, full-thickness, pedicle flaps, or epithelial grafts. Full-thickness autografts and pedicle flaps are commonly used for reconstructive surgery, which may take place months or years after the initial injury.

Split-thickness autografts can be applied in sheets or in postage stamp–like pieces, or they can be expanded by meshing so that they cover 1.5 to 9 times more than a given donor site area. Skin meshers enable the surgeon to cut tiny slits into a sheet of donor skin, making it possible to cover large areas with smaller amounts of donor skin. These expanded grafts adhere to the recipient site more easily than sheet grafts and prevent the accumulation of blood, serum, air, or purulent material under the graft. However, any kind of graft other than a sheet graft contributes to scar formation as it heals. Use of expanded grafts may be necessary in large wounds but should be viewed as a compromise in terms of cosmesis.

If blood, serum, air, fat, or necrotic tissue lies between the recipient site and the graft, there may be partial or total loss of the graft. Infection or mishandling of the graft and trauma during dressing changes account for most other instances of graft loss. Use of split-thickness grafts allows the remaining donor site to retain sweat glands and hair follicles and minimizes donor site healing time.

A **cultured epithelial autograft** (CEA) provides permanent coverage of large wounds when harvesting of skin for autografting is not an option. This involves a biopsy of the patient's skin in an unburned area. Keratinocytes are isolated, and epithelial cells are cultured in a laboratory. The original epithelial cell sample can multiply to 10,000 times its original size over 30 days. These cells are then attached to the burn wound. Varying degrees of success have been reported, and results are encouraging. However, the disadvantages of the CEA are that the grafts are thin and fragile and can shear easily. Research has shown that the outcomes with use of CEA are not as positive as once hoped (Supp, Karpinski & Boyce, 2004). Patients have longer hospital stays and higher hospital costs and require more surgical procedures than those treated by traditional methods. In addition, patients require more reconstructive procedures in the first 1 to 2 years after injury. Therefore, CEA use is very limited and is reserved for burn patients whose donor sites are limited (Sheridan & Thompkins, 2004).

CARE OF THE GRAFT SITE

Occlusive dressings are commonly used initially after grafting to immobilize the graft. Occupational therapists may be helpful in constructing splints to immobilize newly grafted areas to prevent dislodging of the graft. Homografts, heterografts, or synthetic dressings may also be used to protect grafts. The graft may be left open with skin staples to immobilize it, which allows close observation of progress.

The first dressing change is usually performed 2 to 5 days after surgery, or earlier in the case of purulent drainage or a foul odor. If the graft is dislodged, sterile saline compresses help prevent drying of the graft until the physician reapplies it.

The patient is positioned and turned carefully to avoid disturbing the graft or putting pressure on the graft site. If an extremity has been grafted, it is elevated to minimize edema. The patient begins exercising the grafted area 5 to 7 days after grafting.

CARE OF THE DONOR SITE

A moist gauze dressing is applied at the time of surgery to maintain pressure and to stop any oozing. A thrombostatic agent such as thrombin or epinephrine may be applied directly to the site as well. The donor site may be covered in several ways, from single-layer gauze impregnated with petrolatum, scarlet red, or bismuth to new biosynthetic dressings such as Biobrane or BCG Matrix. Acticoat can also be used as a dressing on donor sites. With all types of covering, donor sites must remain clean, dry, and free from pressure. Because a donor site is usually a partial-thickness wound, it will heal spontaneously within 7 to 14 days with proper care. Donor sites are painful, and additional pain management must be a part of the patient's care.

Pain Management

Pain is inevitable during recovery from any burn injury. Pain in patients with burn injuries has been described as one of the most severe forms of acute pain (Jaffe & Patterson, 2004). Burn pain travels through peripheral receptors to central detection via nociceptive tracts. The inflammatory response of the burn injury exacerbates the pain responses during dressing changes. Burn pain changes in time as the wound is covered with new skin, healing takes place, and scars form. Management of the often-severe pain is one of the most difficult challenges facing the burn team. Many factors contribute to the patient's pain experience. These factors include but are not limited to the severity of the pain, the adequacy of the health care provider's assessment of the pain, the appropriateness and adequacy of pharmacologic treatment of pain, the multiple procedures involved in burn care (eg, wound care, rehabilitative exercises), and appropriate evaluation of the effectiveness of pain relief measures. The outstanding features of burn pain are its intensity and long duration. Furthermore, necessary wound care carries with it the anticipation of pain and anxiety (Carrougher, Ptacek, Sharar, et al., 2003; Sheridan & Thompkins, 2004).

In partial-thickness burns, the nerve endings are exposed, resulting in excruciating pain with exposure to air currents. Although nerve endings are destroyed in full-thickness burns, the margins of the burn wound are hypersensitive to pain, and there is pain in adjacent structures. Healing of full-thickness burns creates significant discomfort as regenerating nerve endings become entrapped in scar formation. Most severe burns are a combination of partial-thickness and full-thickness burns.

Patients have reported three types of burn pain: background or resting pain, procedural pain, and breakthrough pain. Background pain is pain that exists on a 24-hour basis. Procedural pain is pain caused by manipulation of the wound bed during dressing changes or range-of-motion exercises. Breakthrough pain occurs when blood levels of analgesic agents decrease below the level required to control background pain. The patient's pain level must be assessed throughout the day, because each type of pain is different, and various pain management strategies may be needed to address the different types of pain (Carrougher et al., 2003; Martin-Herz, Patterson, Honari, et al., 2003).

The primary pain from the burn itself is intense in the initial acute postburn phase. In the next few weeks, until the skin heals or skin grafts are applied and heal, the pain intensity remains high because of treatment-induced pain. Wound cleaning, dressing changes, débridement, and physical therapy can all cause intense pain. Donor sites may be intensely painful for several days. Discomfort related to tissue healing, such as itching, tingling, and tightness of contracting skin and joints, adds to the duration, if not the intensity, of pain over weeks or months. Because pain cannot be eliminated short of complete anesthesia, the goal is to minimize the pain with analgesic agents to an acceptable goal set by the patient.

Opioid administration via the IV route, particularly in the emergent and acute phases of burn management, remains the mainstay for pharmacologic management of burn pain (DeBoer & O'Connor, 2004). Use of opioids is complicated by the fluctuation in the bioavailability of a drug, protein binding of the drug, and drug clearance related to the hemodynamic and fluid volume shifts that occur with a burn injury. Absorption of the opioid also may be affected. Titration of analgesic agents to obtain pain relief while minimizing side effects is crucial. The patient's requirements for analgesia are often high, but fear of addiction on the part of the patient and the health care provider hampers adequate opioid administration.

Morphine sulfate remains the analgesic of choice for treatment of acute burn pain. It is titrated to obtain pain relief based on the patient's self-report of pain using a standardized pain rating scale (see Chapter 13) (Carrougher et al., 2003; Martin-Herz et al., 2003).

Fentanyl is another useful opioid for burn pain, particularly procedural burn pain. It has been shown to be effective for management of intense pain of short duration. Fentanyl has a rapid onset, high potency, and short duration, all of which make it effective for use with burn wound procedures. However, its anticholinergic metabolite properties increase the risk of delirium. Appropriate cardiac and respiratory monitoring must be carried out during its administration.

Patient-controlled analgesia (PCA), in which a pump is used to administer a continuous infusion of an opioid, maintains a steady level of opioid for pain relief and enables the patient to administer intermittent doses of pain medication. Use of continuous infusion requires close monitoring of the patient's responses.

Sustained-release opioids, such as MS Contin or oxycodone (OxyContin), have also been used successfully in the treatment of burn pain. These medications can effectively treat the resting pain that is often associated with burn injury. Additional medications must be prescribed with these medications to cover breakthrough pain.

Some burn units use self-administered nitrous oxide during burn wound procedures. The need for proper ventilation and monitoring equipment and the availability of qualified personnel to monitor administration of nitrous oxide limit its use.

Anxiety and pain go hand in hand for burn patients. The entire burn experience can produce severe anxiety, which can, in turn, exacerbate pain. Therefore, the ideal pain management regimen must incorporate the treatment of pain and anxiety and must be individualized for each patient. Sedation with anxiolytic medications such as lorazepam (Ativan) and midazolam (Versed) may be indicated in addition to the administration of opioids.

Research has shown that sleep deprivation leads to increased reports of pain, and vice versa, in patients with burns. The problem arises with administration of opioids, which affect various sleep stages by decreasing rapid eye movement (REM) sleep, leading to hyperarousal. Many other agents used to treat burn injury, such as bronchodilators and antipruritics, interfere with sleep, which in turn can interfere with pain management (Jaffe & Patterson, 2004).

The use of nonpharmacologic measures aids in the management of burn pain. These measures include relaxation techniques, deep breathing exercises, distraction, guided imagery, hypnosis, therapeutic touch, humor, and information giving, as well as music therapy (Ferguson & Voll, 2004). Researchers have found that music affects both physiologic and psychological aspects of the pain experience. It diverts the patient's attention from the painful stimulus; provides reality orientation, distraction, and sensory stimulation; and allows for patient self-expression (Calne, 2004).

Nutritional Support

Burn injuries produce profound metabolic abnormalities fueled by the exaggerated stress response to the injury. The body's response has been classified as hyperdynamic, hypermetabolic, and hypercatabolic. Hypermetabolism can affect morbidity and mortality by increasing the risk for infection and slowing the healing rate. Patients' metabolic demands vary with the extent of the burn injury and age (Demling, 2005b). Hypermetabolism is evident immediately after a burn injury. The degree of the response depends on the size of the burn and the patient's age, body composition, size, and genetic response to insult (Dudek, 2006). Persistent hypermetabolism may last up to 1 year after burn injury.

Major metabolic abnormalities seen after a burn injury include increased catabolic hormones (cortisol and catechols); decreased anabolic hormones (human growth factor and testosterone); a marked increase in the metabolic rate; a sustained increase in body temperature; a marked increase in glucose demands; rapid skeletal muscle breakdown with amino acids serving as the energy source; lack of ketosis, indicating that fat is not a major source of calories; and catabolism that does not respond to nutrient intake (Pereira, Murphy & Herndon, 2005). Therefore, it is essential to control the stress response by increasing the anabolic process through adequate nutrition and increased muscle activity, decreasing heat loss from wounds, and maintaining a warm environment. Controlling secondary stress, such as pain and anxiety, also helps control the stress response.

The most important of these interventions is to provide adequate nutrition and calories to decrease catabolism (Supple, 2004). Healing of the burn wound consumes large quantities of energy. Patients with burns greater than 40% TBSA have resting metabolic rates twice that of normal (Pereira et al., 2005). Effective nutrition management depends on how well the energy expenditure due to the burn injury can be estimated and matched with appropriate amounts of micronutrients, carbohydrates, lipids, and protein. The goal of nutritional support is to promote a state of positive nitrogen balance by optimizing nutrition to match nutrient utilization (Flynn, 2004). The nutritional support required is based on the patient's preburn status and the TBSA burned.

Several formulas exist for estimating the daily metabolic expenditure and caloric requirements of patients with burn injuries. The most commonly used formulas are the Curreiri formula, which uses body weight and percent burn, and a variation of the Harris-Benedict equation, which determines basal energy requirements based on stress and burn size (Slone, 2004). Protein requirements may range from 1.5 to 4.0 g of protein per kilogram of body weight every 24 hours. Lipids are included in the nutritional support of every burn patient because of their importance for wound healing, cellular integrity, and absorption of fat-soluble vitamins. Carbohydrates are included to meet caloric requirements as high as 5000 calories per day and to spare protein, which is essential for wound healing. The patient also needs adequate vitamins and minerals. Existing formulas may underestimate the daily metabolic expenditures associated with burns. The formulas fail to account for added stressors such as pain, anxiety, daily dressing changes, and decreased activity levels. These must be considered when estimating appropriate nutritional support. Research findings have brought about changes in specific guidelines for estimating energy expenditure during the various phases of postburn recovery. Indirect calorimetry is the most effective method for predicting the nutritional requirements of the patient (Sheridan & Thompkins, 2004).

The enteral route of feeding is far superior to the parenteral route. Enteral feedings preserve the intestinal barrier function and absorption of peptides and amino acids, which leads to higher nitrogen retention. Feedings are started as soon as possible. Nasojejunal feeding tubes help prevent aspiration and allow for continuous, uninterrupted feedings during surgical procedures.

If the oral route is used, high-protein, high-calorie meals and supplements are given. Inhalation injury and prolonged intubation lead to dysphagia in patients with burn injuries. Speech therapists work closely with the burn team to help the patient preserve swallowing function. Their work enables the patient to eat with less risk of aspiration and less energy consumption (Dubose et al., 2005; Snyder & Ubben, 2003). Dietary consultations are useful in helping patients meet their nutritional needs. Daily calorie counts aid in assessing the adequacy of nutritional intake. Overfeeding must be avoided, because it increases metabolism, oxygen consumption, and carbon dioxide production (Saffle, 2003).

Patients lose a great deal of weight during recovery from severe burns. Reserve fat deposits are catabolized, fluids are lost, and caloric intake may be limited. Because a burn injury decreases the patient's resistance to infection and disease, the nutritional status must be improved and maintained even though the patient has a poor appetite and is weak. One goal of nutrition management is to decrease or stop the catabolic process and promote protein anabolism. Beta-blockers that alter the catabolic state in children with burn injuries are also being investigated (Supple, 2004). Supplemental vitamins and minerals, including the nonessential amino acid glutamine, are given to provide support when the patient is in the hypermetabolic, infection–prone state of acute burn injury (Sheridan & Thompkins, 2004). In addition, research is focused on aggressive alteration of the hyperglycemic response and administration of insulin therapy to promote wound healing. Other treatment modalities include early excision and skin grafting of the burn wound, aggressive prevention or treatment of infections, and adequate exercise with physical therapy to lessen muscle wasting and increase strength. Additional pharmacologic modalities used to alter the hypermetabolic state of burn injury include the use of oxandrolone (Oxandrin), an anabolic steroid; an adrenergic antagonist (propranolol [Indural]); and the anabolic protein, recombinant human growth hormone (Pereira et al., 2005).

Indications for parenteral nutrition include weight loss greater than 10% of normal body weight, inadequate intake of enteral nutrition due to clinical status, prolonged wound exposure, and malnutrition or debilitated condition before injury. The risk of infection at the site of the central venous catheter required for parenteral nutrition must be considered. Furthermore, the risk of Curling's ulcer continues in the acute phase.

Disorders of Wound Healing

Disorders of wound healing in patients with burn injuries result from excessive abnormal healing or inadequate new tissue formation. Hypertrophic scarring and keloid formation result from excessive abnormal healing.

Scars

One of the most devastating sequelae of a burn injury is the formation of **hypertrophic scars.** Hypertrophic scarring can cause severe contracture across involved joints. Therefore, prevention and management of this type of scarring is essential (see later discussion). However, these scars are limited to the area of injury and gradually regress over time.

Clinicians cannot reliably predict or prevent the formation of hypertrophic scars. Hypertrophic scars are more common in children, in people with dark skin, and in areas of stretch or motion. The pathophysiology of these scars is not completely understood, but they are characterized by an overabundant formation of matrix, especially collagen, in wounds that heal by granulation (Ehrlich, 2004).

Hypertrophic scars and wound contractures are more likely to occur if the initial burn injury extends below the level of the deep dermis. Healing of such deep wounds results in the replacement of normal integument with highly metabolically active tissues that lack the normal architecture of the skin. In the collagen layer beneath the epithelium, many fibroblasts proliferate gradually. Myofibroblasts, cells that have the ability to contract, are also present in immature wounds. As the myofibroblasts contract, the collagen fibers, which normally lie in flat bundles, tend to form a wavy pattern. Eventually the collagen bundles take on a supercoiled appearance, and collagen nodules develop. The scar becomes red (because of its hypervascular nature), raised, and hard.

Burn personnel must be proactive in the prevention and management of scar formation. Compression measures are instituted early in burn wound treatment. Ace wraps are used initially to help promote adequate circulation, but they can also be used as the first form of compression. Scar management occurs mainly in the rehabilitative phase, after the wounds are closed.

Keloids

A large, heaped-up mass of scar tissue, a keloid, may develop and extend beyond the wound surface. Keloids tend to be found in people with darkly pigmented skin, tend to grow outside of wound margins, and are likely to recur after surgical excision.

Failure to Heal

Failure of the wound to heal may result from many factors, including infection, an underlying disease process, shearing, pressure, or inadequate nutrition. A serum albumin level of less than 2 g/dL is usually a factor in impaired healing in the patient with burns.

Contractures

Contractures are another concern as wounds heal. The burn wound tissue shortens because of the force exerted by the fibroblasts and the flexion of muscles in natural wound healing. An opposing force provided by splints, traction, and purposeful movement and positioning is used to counteract deformity in burns affecting joints.

Nursing Process

Care of the Patient During the Acute Phase

Assessment

Continued assessment of the patient during the early weeks after the burn injury focuses on hemodynamic alterations, wound healing, pain and psychosocial responses, and early detection of complications. Assessment of respiratory and fluid status remains the highest priority for detection of potential complications.

The nurse assesses vital signs frequently. Continued assessment of peripheral pulses is essential for the first few postburn days while edema continues to increase, potentially damaging peripheral nerves and restricting blood flow. Observation of the electrocardiogram may give clues to cardiac dysrhythmias resulting from potassium imbalance, preexisting cardiac disease, or the effects of electrical injury or burn shock.

Assessment of residual gastric volumes and pH in the patient with a nasogastric tube is also important. Blood in the gastric fluid or in the stools must also be noted and reported.

Assessment of the burn wound requires an experienced eye, hand, and sense of smell. Important wound assessment features include size, color, odor, eschar, exudate, abscess formation under the eschar, epithelial buds (small pearl-like clusters of cells on the wound surface), bleeding, granulation tissue appearance, status of grafts and donor sites, and quality of surrounding skin. Any significant changes in the wound are reported to the physician, because they usually indicate burn wound or systemic sepsis and require immediate intervention.

Other significant and ongoing assessments focus on pain and psychosocial responses, daily body weights, caloric intake, general hydration, and serum electrolyte, hemoglobin, and hematocrit levels. Assessment for excessive bleeding from blood vessels adjacent to areas of surgical exploration and débridement is necessary as well.

Gerontologic Considerations

In elderly patients, a careful history of preburn medications and preexisting illnesses is essential. Nursing assessment of the elderly patient with burns should include particular attention to pulmonary function, response to fluid resuscitation, and signs of mental confusion or disorientation. Because of lowered resistance, burn wound sepsis and lethal systemic septicemia are more likely in elderly patients. Furthermore, fever may not be present in the elderly to signal such events. Therefore, surveillance for other signs of infection becomes even more important. Nursing care of the elderly patient with burn injuries promotes early mobilization, aggressive pulmonary care, and attention to preventing complications.

Diagnosis

Nursing Diagnoses

Based on the assessment data, priority nursing diagnoses in the acute phase of burn care may include the following:

- Excessive fluid volume related to resumption of capillary integrity and fluid shift from the interstitial to the intravascular compartment
- Risk for infection related to loss of skin barrier and impaired immune response
- Imbalanced nutrition, less than body requirements, related to hypermetabolism and wound healing needs
- Impaired skin integrity related to open burn wounds
- Acute pain related to exposed nerves, wound healing, and treatments
- Impaired physical mobility related to burn wound edema, pain, and joint contractures
- Ineffective coping related to fear and anxiety, grieving, and forced dependence on health care providers
- Interrupted family processes related to burn injury
- Deficient knowledge about the course of burn treatment

Collaborative Problems/ Potential Complications

Based on the assessment data, potential complications that may develop in the acute phase of burn care may include:

- Heart failure and pulmonary edema
- Sepsis
- Acute respiratory failure
- Acute respiratory distress syndrome
- Visceral damage (electrical burns)

Planning and Goals

The major goals for the patient may include restoration of normal fluid balance, absence of infection, attainment of anabolic state and normal weight, improved skin integrity, reduction of pain and discomfort, optimal physical mobility, adequate patient and family coping, adequate patient and family knowledge of burn treatment, and absence of complications. Achieving these goals requires a collaborative, interdisciplinary approach to patient management.

Nursing Interventions

Restoring Normal Fluid Balance

To reduce the risk of fluid overload and consequent heart failure and pulmonary edema, the nurse closely monitors IV and oral fluid intake, using IV infusion pumps to minimize the risk of rapid fluid infusion. To monitor changes in fluid status, careful intake and output and daily weights are obtained. Changes, including those of blood pressure and pulse rate, are reported to the physician (invasive hemodynamic monitoring is avoided because of the high risk of infection). Low-dose dopamine to increase renal perfusion and diuretics may be prescribed to promote increased urine output. The nurse's role is to administer these medications as prescribed and to monitor the patient's response.

Preventing Infection

A major part of the nurse's role during the acute phase of burn care is detecting and preventing infection. The nurse is responsible for providing a clean and safe environment and for closely scrutinizing the burn wound to detect early signs of infection. Culture results and white blood cell counts are monitored.

Clean technique is used for wound care procedures. Aseptic technique is used for any invasive procedures, such as insertion of IV lines and urinary catheters or tracheal suctioning. Meticulous hand hygiene before and after each patient contact is also an essential component of preventing infection, even though gloves are worn to provide care.

The nurse protects the patient from sources of contamination, including other patients, staff members, visitors, and equipment. Invasive lines and tubing must be routinely changed according to recommendations of the CDC. Tube feeding reservoirs, ventilator circuits, and drainage containers are replaced regularly. Fresh flowers, plants, and fresh fruit baskets are not permitted in the patient's room because of the risk of microorganism growth. Visitors are screened to avoid exposure of the immunocompromised patient to pathogens.

Patients can inadvertently promote migration of microorganisms from one burned area to another by touching their wounds or dressings. Bed linens also can spread infection through either colonization with wound microorganisms or fecal contamination. Regular bathing of unburned areas and changing of linens can help prevent infection.

Maintaining Adequate Nutrition

Oral fluids should be initiated slowly after bowel sounds resume. The patient's tolerance is recorded. If vomiting and distention do not occur, fluids may be increased gradually and the patient may be advanced to a normal diet or to tube feedings.

The nurse collaborates with the dietitian or nutrition support team to plan a protein- and calorie-rich diet that is acceptable to the patient. Family members may be encouraged to bring nutritious and favorite foods to the hospital. Milkshakes and sandwiches made with meat, peanut butter, and cheese may be offered as snacks between meals and late in the evening. High-calorie nutritional supplements such as Ensure and Resource may be provided. Caloric intake must be documented. Vitamin and mineral supplements may be prescribed.

If caloric goals cannot be met by oral feeding, a feeding tube is inserted and used for continuous or bolus feedings of specific formulas. The volume of residual gastric secretions should be checked to ensure absorption. Parenteral nutrition may also be required but should be used only if gastrointestinal function is compromised (see Chapter 36).

The patient should be weighed each day and his or her weights graphed. The patient can use this information to set goals for nutritional intake and to monitor weight loss and gain. Ideally, the patient will lose no more than 5% of preburn weight if aggressive nutritional management is implemented.

The patient with anorexia requires encouragement and support from the nurse to increase food intake. The patient's surroundings should be as pleasant as possible at mealtime. Catering to food preferences and offering high-protein, high-vitamin snacks are ways of encouraging the patient to increase intake.

Promoting Skin Integrity

Wound care is usually the single most time-consuming element of burn care after the emergent phase. The physician prescribes the desired topical antibacterial agents and specific biologic, biosynthetic, or synthetic wound coverings and plans for surgical excision and grafting. The nurse needs to make astute assessments of wound status, use creative approaches to wound dressing, and support the patient during the emotionally distressing and very painful experience of wound care.

The nurse serves as the coordinator of the complex aspects of wound care and dressing changes for the patient. The nurse must be aware of the rationale and nursing implications for the various wound management approaches. Nursing functions include assessing and recording any changes or progress in wound healing and keeping all members of the health care team informed of changes in the wound or in treatment. A diagram, updated daily by the nurse responsible for the patient's care, helps inform all those concerned about the latest wound care procedures in use for the patient.

The nurse also assists the patient and family by providing instruction, support, and encouragement to take an active part in dressing changes and wound care when appropriate. Discharge planning needs for wound care are anticipated early in the course of burn management, and the strengths of the patient and family are assessed and used in preparing for the patient's eventual discharge and home care.

Relieving Pain and Discomfort

Pain measures, discussed earlier, are continued during the acute phase of burn recovery. Analgesic agents and anxiolytic medications are administered as prescribed. Frequent assessment of pain and discomfort is essential. To increase its effectiveness, analgesic medication is provided before the pain becomes severe. Nursing interventions such as teaching the patient relaxation techniques, giving the patient some control over wound care and analgesia, and providing frequent reassurance are helpful. Guided imagery may be effective in altering the patient's perceptions of and responses to pain. Other pain-relieving approaches include distraction through video programs or video games, hypnosis, biofeedback, and behavioral modification.

The nurse assesses the patient's sleep patterns daily. Lack of sleep and rest interferes with healing, comfort, and restoration of energy. If necessary, sedatives are prescribed on a regular basis in addition to analgesics and anxiolytics.

The nurse works quickly to complete treatments and dressing changes to reduce pain and discomfort. The patient is encouraged to take analgesic medications before painful procedures. The patient's response to the medication and other interventions is assessed and documented.

Healing burn wounds are typically described by patients as itchy and tight. Oral antipruritic agents, a cool environment, frequent lubrication of the skin with water or a silica-based lotion, exercise and splinting to prevent skin contracture, and diversional activities all help promote comfort in this phase.

Promoting Physical Mobility

An early priority is to prevent complications of immobility. Deep breathing, turning, and proper positioning are essential nursing practices that prevent atelectasis and pneumonia, control edema, and prevent pressure ulcers and contractures. These interventions are modified to meet the patient's needs. Low-air-loss and rotation beds may be useful, and early sitting and ambulation are encouraged. If the lower extremities are burned, elastic pressure bandages should be applied before the patient is placed in an upright position. These bandages promote venous return and minimize edema formation.

The burn wound is in a dynamic state for at least 1 year after wound closure. During this time, aggressive efforts must be made to prevent contracture and hypertrophic scarring. Both passive and active range-of-motion exercises are initiated from the day of admission and are continued after grafting, within prescribed limitations. Splints or functional devices may be applied to extremities for contracture control. The nurse monitors the splinted areas for signs of vascular insufficiency and nerve compression.

Strengthening Coping Strategies

In the acute phase of burn care, the patient is facing the reality of the burn trauma and is grieving over obvious losses. Depression, regression, and manipulative behavior are common responses of patients who have burn injuries. Withdrawal from participation in required treatments and regression must be viewed with an understanding that such behavior may help the patient cope with an enormously stressful event. Although most patients recover emotionally from a burn injury, some have more difficult psychological reactions to the injury and its outcomes (Morton, Willebrand, Gerhard, et al. 2005).

Personality characteristics, rather than the size or severity of the injury, determine the ability of the patient to cope after burn injury (Kidal, Willebrand, Andersson, et al., 2004). Difficulty coping along with other psychological stressors often limits the patient's physical and psychological recovery (Fauerbach, Lezotte, & Hills, 2005). Patients who experience a burn injury tend to have high rates of involvement in risky behaviors (eg, alcohol and substance abuse, depression) before the injury (Morton et al., 2005). They may also have poor coping skills. Coping styles and perceived threat of death at the time of the burn injury are strong predictors of how well the patient recovers psychologically in the postburn period (Willebrand, Anderson & Ekselius, 2004). Intrusive thoughts of the burn event and reliving it over and over may also occur and can indicate posttraumatic stress disorder.

Much of the patient's energy goes into maintaining vital physical functions and wound healing in the early postburn weeks, leaving little emotional energy for coping in a more effective manner. The nurse can assist the patient to develop effective coping strategies by setting specific expectations for behavior, promoting truthful communication to build trust, helping the patient practice appropriate strategies, and giving positive reinforcement when appropriate. Most importantly, the nurse and all members of the health care team must demonstrate acceptance of the patient.

The patient frequently vents feelings of anger. At times the anger may be directed inward because of a sense of guilt, perhaps for causing the fire or even for surviving when loved ones perished. The anger may be directed outward toward those who escaped unharmed or toward those who are now providing care. One way to help the patient handle these emotions is to enlist someone to whom the patient can vent feelings without fear of retaliation. A nurse, social worker, psychiatric liaison nurse, or spiritual advisor who is not involved in direct care activities may fill this role successfully.

Patients with burn injuries are very dependent on health care team members during the long period of treatment and recovery. However, even when physically unable to contribute much to self-care, they should be included in decisions regarding care and encouraged to assert their individuality in terms of preferences and recognition of their unique identities. As the patient improves in mobility and strength, the nurse works with the patient to set realistic expectations for self-care, including self-feeding, assistance with wound care procedures, exercise, and planning for the future. Many patients respond positively to the use of contractual agreements and other strategies that recognize their independence and their specific role as part of the health care team moving toward the goal of self-care. Consultation with psychiatric/mental health care providers may be helpful to assist the patient in developing effective coping strategies.

Supporting Patient and Family Processes

Family functioning is disrupted with burn injury. One of the nurse's responsibilities is to support the patient and family and to address their spoken and unspoken concerns. Family members need to be instructed about ways that they can support the patient as adaptation to burn trauma occurs. The family also needs support from the health care team. The burn injury has tremendous psychological, economic, and practical impact on the patient and family. Referrals for social services or psychological counseling should be made as appropriate. This support continues into the rehabilitation phase.

Patients who experience major burns are commonly sent to burn centers far from home. Because burn injuries are sudden and unexpected, family roles are disrupted. Therefore, both the patient and the family need thorough information about the patient's burn care and expected course of treatment. Patient and family education begins at the initiation of burn management. Barriers to learning are assessed and considered in teaching. The preferred learning styles of both the patient and family are assessed. This information is used to tailor teaching activities. The nurse assesses the ability of the patient and family to grasp and cope with the information. Verbal information is supplemented by videos, models, or printed materials if available. Patient and family education is a priority in the acute and rehabilitation phases.

Nurses must remain sensitive to the possibility of changing family dynamics. It is not unusual for the provider in the family to be the one who is injured. Roles begin to change, which adds more stress to the family. In addition, families are often relocated due to loss of property from the fire. Social services play an integral part in providing support at this time.

Monitoring and Managing Potential Complications

HEART FAILURE AND PULMONARY EDEMA

The patient is assessed for fluid overload, which may occur as fluid is mobilized from the interstitial compartment back into the intravascular compartment. If the cardiac and renal systems cannot compensate for the excess vascular volume, heart failure and pulmonary edema may result. The patient is assessed for signs of heart failure, including decreased cardiac output, oliguria, jugular vein distention, edema, and the onset of an S_3 or S_4 heart sound. If invasive hemodynamic monitoring is used, increasing central venous, pulmonary artery, and wedge pressures indicate increased fluid volume.

Crackles in the lungs and increased difficulty with respiration may indicate a fluid buildup in the lungs, which is reported promptly to the physician. In the meantime, the patient is positioned comfortably, with the head of the bed raised (if not contraindicated because of other treatments or injuries) to promote lung expansion and gas exchange. Management of this complication includes providing supplemental oxygen, administering IV diuretic agents, carefully assessing the patient's response, and providing vasoactive medications, if indicated.

SEPSIS

The signs of early systemic sepsis are subtle and require a high index of suspicion and very close monitoring of changes in the patient's status. Early signs of sepsis may include increased temperature, increased pulse rate, widened pulse pressure, and flushed dry skin in unburned areas. As with many observations of the patient with a burn injury, one needs to look for patterns or trends in the data. (See Chapter 15 for a more detailed discussion of septic shock.)

Wound and blood cultures are performed as prescribed, and results are reported to the physician immediately. The nurse also observes for and reports early signs of sepsis and promptly intervenes, administering prescribed IV fluids and antibiotics to prevent septic shock, a complication with a high mortality rate. Antibiotics must be administered as scheduled to maintain proper blood concentrations. Serum antibiotic levels are monitored for evidence of maximal effectiveness, and the patient is monitored for toxic side effects.

ACUTE RESPIRATORY FAILURE AND ACUTE RESPIRATORY DISTRESS SYNDROME

The patient's respiratory status is monitored closely for increased difficulty in breathing, change in respiratory pattern, or onset of adventitious (abnormal) sounds. Typically at this stage, signs and symptoms of injury to the respiratory tract become apparent. Respiratory failure may follow. As described previously, signs of hypoxia (decreased oxygen to the tissues), decreased breath sounds, wheezing, tachypnea, stridor, and sputum tinged with soot (or in some cases containing sloughed tracheal tissue) are among the many possible findings. Patients receiving mechanical ventilation must be assessed for a decrease in tidal volume and lung compliance. The key sign of the onset of ARDS is hypoxemia while receiving 100% oxygen, with decreased lung compliance and significant shunting. The physician should be notified immediately of deteriorating respiratory status.

Medical management of the patient with acute respiratory failure requires intubation and mechanical ventilation (if not already in use). If ARDS has developed, higher oxygen levels, positive end-expiratory pressure, and pressure support are used with mechanical ventilation to promote gas exchange across the alveolar–capillary membrane (see Chapter 25).

VISCERAL DAMAGE

The nurse must be alert to signs of necrosis of visceral organs due to electrical injury. Tissues affected are usually located between the entrance and exit wounds of the electrical burn. All patients with electrical burns should undergo cardiac monitoring, with dysrhythmias being reported to the physician. Careful attention must also be paid to signs or reports of pain related to deep muscle ischemia. To minimize the severity of complications, visceral ischemia must be detected as early as possible. In the operating room, the physician may perform **fasciotomies** to relieve the swelling and ischemia in the muscles and fascia and to promote oxygenation of the injured tissues. Because of the deep incisions involved with fasciotomies, the patient must be monitored carefully for signs of excessive blood loss and hypovolemia.

Evaluation

Expected Patient Outcomes

Expected patient outcomes may include the following:

1. Achieves optimal fluid balance
   a. Maintains intake and output and body weight that correlate with expected pattern
   b. Exhibits vital signs and hemodynamic values within designated limits
   c. Demonstrates increased urine output in response to diuretic and vasoactive medications
   d. Has heart rate less than 110 beats/min in normal sinus rhythm
2. Has no localized or systemic infection
   a. Has wound culture results showing minimal bacteria
   b. Has normal urine and sputum culture results
3. Demonstrates anabolic nutritional status
   a. Gains weight daily after initial loss secondary to fluid diuresis and no oral intake of food or fluid

   b. Shows no signs of protein, vitamin, or mineral deficiencies
   c. Meets required nutritional needs entirely by oral intake
   d. Participates in selecting diet containing prescribed nutrients
   e. Exhibits normal serum protein levels
4. Demonstrates improved skin integrity
   a. Exhibits generally intact skin that remains free of infection, pressure, and injury
   b. Demonstrates remaining open wound areas that are pink, re-epithelializing, and free of infection
   c. Demonstrates donor graft sites that are clean and healing
   d. Has healed wounds that are soft and smooth
   e. Demonstrates skin that is lubricated and elastic
5. Has minimal pain
   a. Requests analgesic agents before specific wound care procedures or physical therapy activities
   b. Reports minimal pain
   c. Gives no physiologic, verbal, or nonverbal cues that pain is moderate or severe
   d. Uses pain control measures such as nitrous oxide, relaxation, imagery, and distraction techniques to cope with and alleviate pain and discomfort
   e. Can sleep without being disturbed by pain
   f. Reports that skin is comfortable, with no pruritus or tightness
6. Demonstrates optimal physical mobility and function
   a. Improves range of motion of joints daily
   b. Demonstrates preinjury range of motion of all joints
   c. Has no signs of calcification around the joints
   d. Participates in activities of daily living
7. Uses appropriate coping strategies to deal with postburn problems
   a. Verbalizes reactions to burns, therapeutic procedures, losses
   b. Identifies coping strategies used effectively in previous stressful situations
   c. Accepts dependency on health care providers during acute phase
   d. Verbalizes realistic view of problems resulting from burn injury and plans for future
   e. Cooperates with health care providers in required therapy
   f. Participates in decision making regarding care
   g. Begins to manage grief over losses resulting from burn injury and circumstances surrounding injury (eg, death of others, damage to home or other property)
   h. States realistic objectives for plastic surgery, further medical intervention, and results
   i. Verbalizes realistic abilities and goals
   j. Displays hopeful attitude toward future
8. Relates appropriately in patient/family processes
   a. Patient and family verbalize feelings regarding change in family interactions
   b. Family emotionally supports the patient during the hospitalization
   c. Family states that their own needs are being met
9. Patient and family verbalize understanding of the treatment course
   a. State rationales for the various aspects of treatment
   b. State realistic time period for recovery
10. Absence of complications
   a. Lungs clear on auscultation
   b. Exhibits no dyspnea or orthopnea and can breathe easily when standing, sitting, and lying down
   c. Exhibits no S_3 or S_4 heart sounds or jugular venous distention
   d. Exhibits adequate urine output
   e. Exhibits normal blood, sputum, and urine culture results
   f. Maintains arterial blood gas values or O_2 saturation within normal or acceptable limits
   g. Has normal lung compliance
   h. Has no visceral organ damage
   i. Has stable cardiac rhythm

Rehabilitation Phase

Although long-term aspects of burn care are discussed last in this chapter, rehabilitation begins immediately after the burn has occurred—as early as the emergent period—and often extends for years after injury. In the aftermath of the acute stages of burn injury, the patient increasingly focuses on the alterations in self-image and lifestyle that may occur. Wound healing, psychosocial support, and restoration of maximal functional activity remain priorities so that the patient can have the best quality of life both personally and socially (Civaia, Fedele, Gallino, et al., 2003; Sheridan & Thompkins, 2004). The body goes through many changes as it heals. As the burn wound becomes a burn scar, the burn survivor may be faced with new complications, as listed in Table 57-7 (Regojo & Wright, 2001). The focus on maintaining fluid and electrolyte balance and improving nutritional status continues. Reconstructive surgery to improve body appearance and function is often needed.

Burn injuries can have a major impact on quality of life. Changes in physical activity and social, psychological, and employment status may occur. Improving the social comfort of the patient who has survived a burn injury helps in the recovery of self-esteem (Lawrence & Fauerbach, 2004). Therefore, psychological and vocational counseling and referral to support groups may be helpful to promote recovery and quality of life. Family members also need support and guidance in assisting the patient to return to optimal health.

Prevention of Hypertrophic Scarring

Treatment modalities that are theoretically based on wound healing and scar formation are used to prevent scar contractures and excess hypertrophic tissue. These

TABLE 57-7 Complications in Rehabilitation Phase of Burn Care

Complications	Contributing Factors	Interventions
Neuropathies, peripheral neuropathies, mononeuropathies, multimono-neuropathies, nerve entrapment	Electrical injury, large deep burns, improper positioning, edema, scar tissue	Assess peripheral pulses and sensation (neurovascular checks). Prevent edema and pressure by elevation, positioning, and prevention of constricting dressings. Assess splints for proper fit and application. Consult occupational therapy (OT) and physical therapy (PT) for positioning.
Heterotopic ossification (abnormal formation of bone in response to soft tissue trauma)	Prolonged immobility	Perform gentle range-of-motion exercises.
Hypertrophic scarring	Partial- and full-thickness burns	Keep skin pliable and soft. Apply pressure garments as prescribed. Massage.
Contractures	Partial- and full-thickness burns	Maintain position of joints in alignment. Perform gentle range of motion exercises. Consult OT and PT for exercises and positioning recommendations.
Wound breakdown	Sheer, pressure, inadequate nutrition	Teach patient about importance of good nutrition. Protect wound from pressure and shearing forces.
Gait deviations	Pain, burn wound, donor site, scarring of joints, electrical injury of the brain	Provide adequate pain management. Consult OT and PT. Promote ambulation and mobility training.
Complex regional pain syndrome (previous reflex sympathetic dystrophy)	Trauma and burns	Provide adequate pain management. Consult OT and PT for exercises. Promote gentle motion of affected extremities.
Joint instability	Burn wound, burn scar and contractures	Maintain joint through appropriate application of splints. Monitor joint pinning if indicated. Consult OT and PT.

include the use of pressure garments, massage, lubrication, exercise, splints, manual lymphatic drainage and injectable steroids (Palmieri, Petuskey, Bagley, et al., 2003; Serghiou, Holmes & McCauley, 2004). The wound is in a dynamic state for 1.5 to 2 years after the burn occurs. If appropriate measures are instituted during this active period, the scar tissue loses its redness and softens. Healed areas that are prone to hypertrophic scarring require the patient to wear a pressure garment (Fig. 57-6). These devices are especially useful for partial-thickness wounds that needed more than 2 weeks to heal and for the edges of grafted skin. Application of elastic pressure garments loosens collagen bundles and encourages parallel orientation of the collagen to the skin surface, with the disappearance of the dermal nodules. As pressure continues over time, there is a restructuring of the collagen and a decrease in vascularity and cellularity. However, pressure needs to be continuous. Many areas of the body are difficult to compress due to the contours or the presence of cartilage. Silastic inserts are used under the pressure garments to enhance scar compression. Gentle superficial massage aids in softening the connective tissue (Civaia et al., 2003).

The physical therapist, occupational therapist, or a representative of the manufacturer of elastic pressure garments measures the patient for correct fit. While awaiting the arrival of the garment, soft, tubular, knitted elastic pressure bandages can be used to help desensitize the patient's skin, protect healing areas, apply pressure, and promote venous return. The patient must be instructed about the need for lubrication and protection of the healing skin and the need to use pressure garments for at least 1 year after the injury. A program including elastic pressure garments, splints, and exercise under the supervision of an experienced physical and occupational therapy team is recommended for optimal functional and cosmetic results.

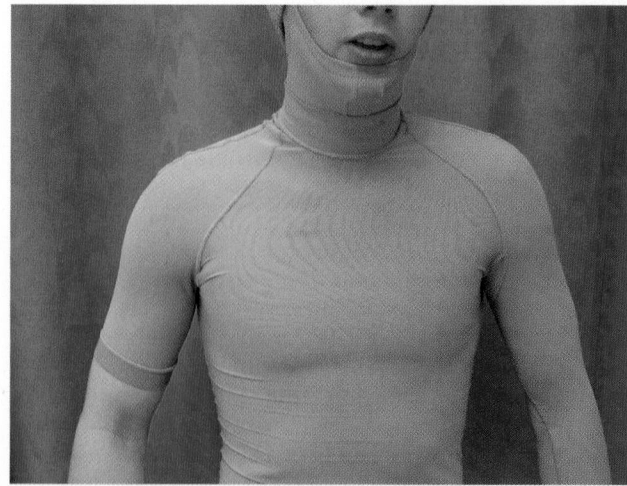

FIGURE 57-6. Elastic pressure garments. Application of pressure garments helps prevent hypertrophic burn scarring. Used with permission of Jobst Institute, Inc., Toledo, OH.

Nursing Process

Care of the Patient During the Rehabilitation Phase

Assessment

Information about the patient's educational level, occupation, leisure activities, cultural background, religion, and family interactions is obtained early. The patient's self-concept, mental status, emotional response to the injury and hospitalization, level of intellectual functioning, previous hospitalizations, response to pain and pain relief measures, and sleep pattern are also essential components of a comprehensive assessment. Information about the patient's general self-concept, self-esteem, and coping strategies in the past are valuable in addressing emotional needs.

Ongoing physical assessments related to rehabilitation goals include range of motion of affected joints, functional abilities in activities of daily living, early signs of skin breakdown from splints or positioning devices, evidence of neuropathies (neurologic damage), activity tolerance, and quality or condition of healing skin. The patient's participation in care and ability to demonstrate self-care in such areas as ambulation, eating, wound cleaning, and applying pressure wraps are documented on a regular basis. In addition to these assessment parameters, specific complications and treatments require additional specific assessments; for example, the patient undergoing primary excision requires postoperative assessment.

Recovery from burn injury involves every system of the body. Therefore, assessment of the patient with a burn injury must be comprehensive and continuous. Priorities vary at different points during the rehabilitation phase. Understanding the pathophysiologic responses to burn injury forms the framework for detecting early progress or signs and symptoms of complications. Early detection leads to early intervention and enhances the potential for successful rehabilitation.

Diagnosis

Nursing Diagnoses

Based on the assessment data, priority nursing diagnoses in the long-term rehabilitation phase of burn care may include the following:

- Activity intolerance related to pain on exercise, limited joint mobility, muscle wasting, and limited endurance
- Disturbed body image related to altered physical appearance and self-concept
- Deficient knowledge about postdischarge home care and follow-up needs

Collaborative Problems/ Potential Complications

Based on the assessment data, potential complications that may develop in the rehabilitation phase include:

- Contractures
- Inadequate psychological adaptation to burn injury

Planning and Goals

The major goals for the patient include increased participation in activities of daily living; increased understanding of the injury, treatment, and planned follow-up care; adaptation and adjustment to alterations in body image, self-concept, and lifestyle; and absence of complications.

Nursing Interventions

Promoting Activity Tolerance

Nursing interventions that must be carried out according to a strict regimen and the pain that accompanies movement take their toll on the patient. The patient may become confused and disoriented and lack the energy to participate optimally in care. The nurse must schedule care in such a way that the patient has periods of uninterrupted sleep. A good time for planned patient rest is after the stress of dressing changes and exercise, while pain interventions and sedatives are still effective. This plan must be communicated to family members and other care providers.

The patient may have insomnia related to frequent nightmares about the burn injury or to other fears and anxieties about the outcome of the injury. The nurse listens to and reassures the patient and administers hypnotic agents, as prescribed, to promote sleep.

Reducing metabolic stress by relieving pain, preventing chilling or fever, and promoting the physical integrity of all body systems help the patient conserve energy for therapeutic activities and wound healing.

The nurse incorporates physical therapy exercises in the patient's care to prevent muscle atrophy and to maintain the mobility required for daily activities. The patient's activity tolerance, strength, and endurance gradually increase if activity occurs over increasingly longer periods. Fatigue, fever, and pain tolerance are monitored and used to determine the amount of activity to be encouraged on a daily basis. Activities such as family visits and recreational or play therapy (eg, video games, radio, TV) can provide diversion, improve the patient's outlook, and increase tolerance for physical activity. In elderly patients and those with chronic illnesses and disabilities, rehabilitation must take into account preexisting functional abilities and limitations.

Improving Body Image and Self-Concept

Patients who have survived burn injuries frequently suffer profound losses. These include not only a loss of body image due to disfigurement but also losses of personal property, homes, loved ones, and ability to work. They lack the benefit of anticipatory grief often seen in a patient who is approaching surgery or dealing with the terminal illness of a loved one.

As care progresses, the patient who is recovering from burns becomes aware of daily improvement and begins to exhibit basic concerns: Will I be disfigured or be disabled? How long will I be in the hospital? What about my job and family? Will I ever be independent again? How can I pay for my care? Was my burn the result of my carelessness? As the patient expresses such concerns, the nurse must take time to listen and to provide realistic support. The nurse can refer the patient to a support group, such as those usually available at regional burn centers or through organizations such as the Phoenix Society. Through participation in such groups, the patient will meet others with similar experiences and learn coping strategies to help him or her deal with losses. Interaction with other burn survivors allows the patient to see that adaptation to the burn injury is possible. If a support group is not available, visits from other survivors of burn injuries can be helpful to the patient coping with such a traumatic injury.

A major responsibility of the nurse is to constantly assess the patient's psychosocial reactions. Questions to consider include the following: What are the patient's fears and concerns? Does the patient fear loss of control of care, independence, or sanity itself? Is the patient afraid of rejection by family and loved ones? Does he or she fear being unable to cope with pain or physical appearance? Does the patient have concerns about sexuality, including sexual function? Being aware of these anxieties and understanding the basis of the patient's fears enable the nurse to provide support and to cooperate with other members of the health care team in developing a plan to help the patient deal with these feelings.

When caring for a patient with a burn injury, the nurse needs to be aware that there are prejudices and misunderstandings in society about those who are viewed as different. Opportunities and accommodations available to others are often denied those who are disfigured. Such amenities include social participation, employment, prestige, various roles, and status. The health care team must actively promote a healthy body image and self-concept in patients with burn injuries so that they can accept or challenge others' perceptions of those who are disfigured or disabled. Survivors themselves must show others who they are, how they function, and how they want to be treated.

The nurse can help patients practice their responses to people who may stare or inquire about their injury once they are discharged from the hospital. The nurse can help patients build self-esteem by recognizing their uniqueness—for example, with small gestures such as providing a birthday cake, combing the patient's hair before visiting hours, giving information about the availability of a cosmetician to enhance appearance, and teaching the patient ways to direct attention away from a disfigured body to the self within. Consultants such as psychologists, social workers, vocational counselors, and teachers are valuable participants in assisting burn patients to regain their self-esteem.

Monitoring and Managing Potential Complications

CONTRACTURES

With early and aggressive physical and occupational therapy, contractures are rarely a long-term complication. However, surgical intervention is indicated if a full range of motion in the burn patient is not achieved. (See Chapter 11 for a discussion of prevention of contractures.)

IMPAIRED PSYCHOLOGICAL ADAPTATION TO THE BURN INJURY

Some patients, particularly those with limited coping skills or psychological function or a history of psychiatric problems before the burn injury, may not achieve adequate psychological adaptation to the burn injury. Psychological counseling or psychiatric referral may be made to assess the patient's emotional status, to help the patient develop coping skills, and to intervene if major psychological issues or ineffective coping is identified.

Promoting Home and Community-Based Care

TEACHING PATIENTS SELF-CARE

As the inpatient phase of recovery becomes shorter, the focus of rehabilitative interventions is directed toward outpatient care or care in a rehabilitation center. In the long term, much of the care of healing burns will be performed by the patient and others at home. Throughout the phases of burn care, efforts are made to prepare the patient and family for the care that will continue at home. They are instructed about the measures and procedures that they will need to perform. For example, patients commonly have small areas of clean, open wounds that are healing slowly. They are instructed to wash these areas daily with mild soap and water and to apply the prescribed topical agent or dressing.

In addition to instructions about wound care, patients and families require careful written and verbal instructions about pain management, nutrition, and prevention of complications. Information about specific exercises and use of pressure garments and splints is reviewed with both the patient and the family, and written instructions are provided for their use at home. The patient and family are taught to recognize abnormal signs and report them to the physician. This information helps the patient progress successfully through the rehabilitative phase of burn management. The patient and family are assisted in planning for the patient's continued care by identifying and acquiring supplies and equipment that are needed at home (Chart 57-8).

CONTINUING CARE

Follow-up care by an interdisciplinary burn care team is necessary. Preparations should begin during the early stages of care. Patients who receive care in a burn center usually return to the burn clinic or center periodically for evaluation by the burn team, modification of home care instructions, and planning for reconstructive surgery. Other patients receive ongoing care from the surgeon who cared for them during the acute phase of their management. Still other patients require the services of a rehabilitation center and may be transferred to such a center for aggressive rehabilitation before going home. Many patients require outpatient physical or occupational therapy, often several times weekly. It is often the nurse who is responsible for coordinating all aspects of care and ensuring that the patient's needs

CHART 57-8

HOME CARE CHECKLIST • The Patient with a Burn Injury

At the completion of the home care instruction, the patient or caregiver will be able to:	Patient	Caregiver
MENTAL HEALTH		
Identify strategies to promote own mental health; for example:		
• Remember that changes in lifestyle take time.	✔	✔
• Resume previous interests and activities gradually.	✔	
• Take one day at a time to regain physical and mental strength.	✔	
• Be aware of own feelings and fears and discuss them with selected others.	✔	✔
• Expect concerns, frustrations, and depression about changes in appearance.	✔	✔
• Be honest with self, family, and friends about needs, hopes, and fears.	✔	✔
• Realize that emotional adjustment to the burn injury will occur with time.	✔	✔
BURN SKIN PRECAUTIONS AND WOUND CARE		
Identify the following skin precautions and wound care:		
• Wear sun block with the highest SPF possible to protect burned skin from the sun.	✔	
• Avoid further trauma to burned skin; leave unbroken blisters that may form.	✔	✔
• Lubricate healed burned skin with mild lotion (as prescribed); avoid scratching.	✔	
• Wear wide-brimmed hats if face has been burned to protect the area from the sun.	✔	
• Use only mild soap and lotion (ie, products without perfume) on burned areas.	✔	✔
EXERCISE		
Describe the following guidelines for exercise:		
• Do as much for self as possible.	✔	
• Adhere to the exercise regimen given by the therapist.	✔	
• Participate in exercise every day, several times a day, even when "not feeling like it."	✔	
NUTRITION		
Identify the following guidelines for nutrition:		
• Eat a diet high in calories and protein.	✔	
• Drink adequate volume of fluids to prevent constipation associated with use of analgesic medications.	✔	
PAIN MANAGEMENT		
Describe the following steps for managing pain:		
• Avoid situations that require alertness (analgesic agents may produce drowsiness).	✔	
• Take analgesic medication as prescribed (30 minutes before painful procedures such as dressing changes).	✔	
• Use relaxation and distraction to relieve pain and discomfort.	✔	
THERMOREGULATION		
Identify strategies to compensate for inability to regulate body temperature:		
• Dress to accommodate cold and hot weather or environment.	✔	
• Avoid extremes of temperature.	✔	

continued >

CHART 57-8 HOME CARE CHECKLIST • The Patient with a Burn Injury

CLOTHING CONSIDERATIONS State the following strategies in selection of clothing to wear:	Patient	Caregiver
• Avoid tight clothing over burned areas.	✔	
• Select white cotton, loose-fitting clothing so that dyes in colored clothes do not irritate healing skin.	✔	
• Wear clothing and gloves to protect healing skin from unnecessary bruises, bumps, and scratches.	✔	
MANAGEMENT OF BURN SCAR Describe the following strategies to manage burn scar:		
• Massage and stretch skin to maintain/increase its elasticity.	✔	✔
• Use lotion for massage as recommended by therapist.	✔	✔
• Wear compression garments 23 hours a day.	✔	
RESUMPTION OF SEXUAL RELATIONS Identify the following guidelines regarding resumption of sexual relationships:		
• Realize that resumption of sexual relationships is the rule rather than the exception.	✔	✔
• Expect sensitivity of and around the genital area for several months if these areas were burned.	✔	
• Resume sexual activity slowly; endurance will increase with time.	✔	

Adapted with permission from Orlando Regional Medical Center Burn Unit's *Personal Guide to Burn Care.*

are met. Such coordination is an important aspect of assisting the patient to achieve independence.

Patients who return home after a severe burn injury, those who cannot manage their own burn care, and those with inadequate support systems need referral for home care. For example, elderly patients commonly lack family members who can provide home care; therefore, social services and community nursing services must be contacted to provide optimal care and supervision after hospital discharge. During visits to the patient at home, the home care nurse assesses the patient's physical and psychological status as well as the adequacy of the home setting for safe and adequate care. The nurse monitors the patient's progress and adherence to the plan of care and notes any problems that interfere with the patient's ability to carry out the care. During the visit, the nurse assists the patient and family with wound care and exercises. Patients with severe or persistent depression or difficulty adjusting to changes in their social or occupational roles are identified and referred to the burn team for possible referral to a psychologist, psychiatrist, or vocational counselor.

The burn team or home care nurse identifies community resources that may be helpful for the patient and family. Several burn patient support groups and other organizations throughout the United States offer services for burn survivors. They provide caring people (often people who have themselves recovered from burn injuries) who can visit the patient in the hospital or home or telephone the patient and family periodically to provide support and counseling about skin care, cosmetics, and problems related to psychosocial adjustment. Such organizations, and many regional burn centers, sponsor group meetings and social functions at which outpatients are welcome. Some also provide school-reentry programs and are active in burn prevention activities. If more information is needed regarding burn prevention, the American Burn Association can help locate the nearest burn center and offer current burn prevention tips (see Chart 57-2).

Because so much attention is given to the burn wound and the treatments that are necessary to treat the burn wound and prevent complications, the patient, family, and health care providers may inadvertently ignore the patient's ongoing needs for health promotion and screening. Therefore, the patient and family are reminded of the importance of periodic health screening and preventive care (eg, gynecologic examinations, dental care).

Evaluation

Expected Patient Outcomes

Expected patient outcomes may include the following:

1. Demonstrates activity tolerance required for desired daily activities
   a. Obtains adequate sleep daily

b. Reports absence of nightmares or sleep disturbances
c. Shows gradually increasing tolerance and endurance in physical activities
d. Can concentrate during conversations
e. Has energy available to sustain desired daily activities
2. Adapts to altered body image
a. Verbalizes accurate description of alterations in body image and accepts physical appearance
b. Demonstrates interest in resources that may improve body appearance and function
c. Uses cosmetics, wigs, and prostheses as desired to achieve acceptable appearance
d. Socializes with significant others, peers, and usual social group
e. Seeks and achieves return to role in family, school, and community as a contributing member
3. Demonstrates knowledge of required self-care and follow-up care
a. Describes surgical procedures and treatments accurately
b. Verbalizes detailed plan for follow-up care
c. Demonstrates ability to perform wound care and prescribed exercises
d. Returns for follow-up appointments as scheduled
e. Identifies resource people and agencies to contact for specific problems
4. Exhibits no complications
a. Demonstrates full range of motion
b. Shows no signs of withdrawal or depression
c. Displays no psychotic behaviors

Burn Care in the Home

More and more burns are being treated exclusively in outpatient settings, including wound clinics, physicians' offices, clinics, and emergency departments. The outpatient setting is appropriate for the care of minor burns and most moderate burns. However, a number of factors must be considered in determining the appropriate site of care. These factors include the age of the patient, the extent and depth of the burn, the availability of family support systems and community resources to assist the patient, the patient's adherence to the prescribed plan of care, and the distance from home to the outpatient setting.

Initially, looking at and touching the burn wound may be difficult and even frightening to some family members and patients. However, with encouragement and support, most can handle burn wound care with little need for daily professional care. Instructions, both verbal and written, are given to the patient about burn wound care, pain management strategies, the need for adequate nutrition, and the importance of exercise and rest. Instruction is also given about signs and symptoms of infection that should be reported to the physician. The importance of notifying the physician about complications early and of keeping follow-up appointments is emphasized to the patient and family.

Critical Thinking Exercises

1 A 75-year-old woman was scalded in the bathtub, where she sustained 25% full-thickness wounds to both lower legs before being found by her niece. It is not known how long the woman was in the tub. She has been independent and living alone for the past 15 years; however, her niece has offered to have her aunt come and live with her family. On admission to the emergency department, the woman's temperature is 94°F (35.5°C) and her weight is 111 lb (50 kg). She has diabetes as well as a history of heart failure and hypertension. What are the priorities in her medical and nursing care during the emergent phase of burn care? What assessment parameters would you monitor closely? What would be the best wound care for her? Is she a likely candidate for skin grafting? What type of discharge planning needs will she have?

2 A man with a history of chronic obstructive pulmonary disease who was smoking a cigarette while using his home oxygen sustained superficial partial-thickness burns to his face, including his nose, lips, and chin. This is his second admission for the same type of injury in less than 1 year. His pulse oximetry is 91% and his vital signs are stable. What emergency care and interventions should you provide to this patient? How should you treat the wounds on his face? Soon after admission to the hospital, he asks for a cigarette and states that he wants to be discharged. What resources do you use to address his immediate needs and long-term discharge needs?

3 An 18-year-old woman sustained second-degree burns from a tanning bed. Her burns cover her entire chest, abdomen, back, and legs. She has large blisters on her chest and the backs of her knees. Using the rule of nines, estimate the percent of TBSA burned; estimate her fluid resuscitation needs. Describe nursing care, including patient teaching, that is important for this patient. She is rating her pain level 10 out of 10. What comfort measures can you use to manage her pain?

4 A 38-year-old man suffered an electrical burn when he touched a high-voltage wire on the job. What are the priorities of on-the-scene rescuers in this situation? Compare the consequences of an electrical burn to those of other thermal burns along with specific assessment parameters and medical management and nursing care that can be anticipated during his hospital stay.

5 ebp A 50-year-old man who weighs 111 lb (50 kg) was transferred to the emergency department after his truck caught fire. He has circumferential burns on both of his legs, his anterior chest, and his entire right upper extremity. He was unable to extricate himself from the truck and suffered inhalation burns as well. Using the rule of nines chart, estimate the percent of TBSA burned. What are the emergency priorities for this patient? What are the fluid resuscitation requirements for this patient based on his percent of burn and his weight? What assessment parameters

would you monitor closely? What pain management strategies would be indicated for this patient? What is the evidence for use of pharmacologic and nonpharmacologic pain management strategies for this patient? How strong is that evidence, and what criteria would you use to evaluate the strength of that evidence? How would you use that evidence in providing care for this patient?

REFERENCES AND SELECTED READINGS

BOOKS

Appleby, T. (2005). Burns. In Morton, P. G., Fontaine, D. K., Hudak, C. M., et al. *Critical care nursing: A holistic approach*. Philadelphia: Lippincott Williams & Wilkins.

Calne, S. (2004). Minimising pain at wound dressing-related procedures: A consensus document. In Calne, S. (Ed.). *Principles of best practice: A World Union of Wound Healing Societies' initiative*. London: Medical Education Partnership/Viking Print Services.

Centers for Disease Control and Prevention, National Center for Injury Prevention and Control. (2003). *10 leading causes of death, United States 2003*. Atlanta: Author.

Dudek, S. G. (2006). *Nutrition essentials for nursing practice* (5th ed.). Philadelphia: Lippincott Williams and Wilkins.

Fitzpatrick, J. C. & Cioffi, W. G. (2002). Diagnosis and treatment of inhalation injury. In Herndon, D. N. (Ed.). *Total burn care* (2nd ed.). Philadelphia: W. B. Saunders.

Hall, J. R. (2005). *Children playing with fire*. Quincy, MA: National Fire Protection Association.

Herndon, D. N. (2002). *Total burn care*. Philadelphia: W. B. Saunders.

Karter, M. J. Jr. (2005). *Fire loss in the United States during 2004*. Quincy, MA: National Fire Protection Association.

Munster, A. M. (2002). The immunological response and strategies for intervention. In Herndon, D. N. (Ed.). *Total burn care* (2nd ed.). Philadelphia: W. B. Saunders.

Regojo, P. S. & Wright, S. (2001). A holistic approach to burn rehabilitation. In Derstine, J. B. & Hargrove, S. (Eds.). *Comprehensive rehabilitation nursing*. Philadelphia: W. B. Saunders.

Serghiou, M. A., Young, E. B., Ott, S., et al. (2002). Comprehensive rehabilitation of the burned patient. In Herndon, D. N. (Ed.). *Total burn care* (2nd ed.). Philadelphia: W. B. Saunders.

Wolf, S., Prough, D. S., & Herndon, D. N. (2002). Critical care in the severely burned: Organ support and management of complications. In Herndon, D. N. (Ed.). *Total burn care* (2nd ed.). Philadelphia: W. B. Saunders.

JOURNALS

**Asterisks indicate nursing research articles.*

Ahrens, T. & Vollman, K. (2003). Severe sepsis management: Are we doing enough? *Critical Care Nurse, 23*(5 Suppl), 2–15.

*Alden, N. E., Rabbits, A., Rolls, J. A., et al. (2004). Burn injury in patients with early-onset neurological impairments. *Journal of Burn Care and Rehabilitation, 25*(1), 107–111.

Ahrns, K. S. (2004). Trends in burn resuscitation: Shifting the focus from fluids to adequate endpoint monitoring, edema control, and adjuvant therapies. *Critical Care Nursing Clinics of North America, 16*(1), 75–98.

Atiyeh, B. S., Gunn, S. W. & Hayek, S. N. (2005). State of the art in burn treatment. *World Journal of Surgery, 29*(2), 131–148.

Bowler, P. G., Jones, S. A., Walker, M., et al. (2004). Microbicidal properties of a silver-containing hydrofiber dressing against a variety of burn wound pathogens. *Journal of Burn Care and Rehabilitation, 25*(2), 192–196.

Burke, J. F. (2005). Burn treatment's evolution in the 20th century. *Journal of the American College of Surgeons, 200*(2), 152–153.

Centers for Disease Control and Prevention, National Center for Injury Prevention and Control. (2004). *10 leading causes of unintentional injury deaths, United States 2001–2002, all races, both sexes*. Available at: http://www.cdc.gov/ncipc/pub-res/unintentional_activity/2004/01_overviewUI.htm. Accessed Aug. 1, 2006.

Carrougher, G. J., Ptacek, J. T., Sharar, S. R., et al. (2003). Comparison of patient satisfaction and self-reports of pain in adult burn-injured patients. *Journal of Burn Care and Rehabilitation, 24*(1), 1–8.

Caruso, D. M., Foster, K. N., Hermans, M. H., et al. (2004). Aquacel Ag in the management of partial thickness burns: Results of a clinical trial. *Journal of Burn Care and Rehabilitation, 25*(1), 89–96.

Cone, J. B. (2005). What's new in general surgery: Burns and metabolism. *Journal of the American College of Surgeons, 200*(4), 607–615.

Civaia, A., Fedele, C., Gallino, A., & Oliva, R. (2003). The rehabilitative management of burn patients in the post-acute phase. *Annals of Burns and Fire Disasters, 16*(1) 10–18.

DeBoer, S. & O'Connor, A. (2004). Prehospital and emergency department burn care. *Critical Care Nursing Clinics of North America, 16*(1), 61–74.

Demling, R. H. (2005a). The burn edema process: Current concepts. *Journal of Burn Care and Rehabilitation, 26*(3), 207–228.

Demling, R. H. (2005b). The incidence and impact of pre-existing protein energy malnutrition on outcomes in the elderly burn patient population. *Journal of Burn Care and Rehabilitation, 26*(1), 94–100.

De-Souza, D. A. & Greene, L. J. (2005). Intestinal permeability and systemic infection in critically ill patients: Effect of glutamine. *Critical Care Medicine, 33*(5), 1125–1135.

Dewar, D. J., Magson, C. L., Fraser, J. F., et al. (2004). Hot beverage scalds in Australian children. *Journal of Burn Care and Rehabilitation, 25*(3), 224–227.

Downs, C. E. & Sweet, D. (2003). Burn center reporting system. U.S. Consumer Product Safety Commission. *Consumer Product Safety Review, 8*(2), 1–2.

DuBose, C., Groher, M. G., Mann, G. C., Mozingo, D. W. (2005). Pattern of dysphagia recovery after thermal burn injury. *Journal of Burn Care and Rehabilitation, 26*(3), 233–237.

Ehrlich, H. P. (2004). Understanding experimental biology of skin equivalent: From laboratory to clinical use in patients with burns and chronic wounds. *American Journal of Surgery, 187*(5A), 29S–33S.

Fauerbach, J. A., Lezotte, D., Hills, R. A., et al. (2005). Burden of burn: A norm-based inquiry into the influence of burn size and distress on recovery of physical and psychosocial function. *Journal of Burn Care and Rehabilitation, 26*(1), 21–32.

Ferguson, S. L. & Voll, K. V. (2004). Burn pain and anxiety: The use of music relaxation during rehabilitation. *Journal of Burn Care and Rehabilitation, 25*(1), 8–14.

Flynn, M. B. (2004). Nutritional support for the burn-injured patient. *Critical Care Nursing Clinics of North America, 16*(1), 139–144.

Gosain, A. & Gamelli, R. (2005a). Role of the gastrointestinal tract in burn sepsis. *Journal of Burn Care and Rehabilitation, 26*(1), 85–91.

Gosain, A. & Gamelli, R. (2005b). A primer in cytokines. *Journal of Burn Care and Rehabilitation, 26*(1), 7–12.

Heggers, J., Goodheart, R., Washington, J., et al. (2005). Therapeutic efficacy of three silver dressings in an infected animal model. *Journal of Burn Care and Rehabilitation, 26*(1), 53–56.

Heimbach, D. M., Warden, G. D., Luterman, A., et al. (2003). Multicenter postapproval clinical trial of Integra dermal regeneration template for burn treatment. *Journal of Burn Care and Rehabilitation, 24*(1), 42–48.

Jaffe, S. E. & Patterson, D. R. (2004). Treating sleep problems in patients with burn injuries: Practical considerations. *Journal of Burn Care and Rehabilitation, 25*(3), 294–305.

Kidal, M., Willebrand, M., Andersson, G., et al. (2004). Personality characteristics and perceived health problems after burn injury. *Journal of Burn Care and Rehabilitation, 25*(3), 228–235.

LaBorde, P. (2004). Burn epidemiology: The patient, the nation, the statistics, and the data resources. *Critical Care Nursing Clinics of North America, 16*(1), 13–25.

Lawrence, J. & Fauerbach, J. (2003). Personality, coping, chronic stress, social support and PTSD symptoms among adult burn survivors. *Journal of Burn Care and Rehabilitation, 24*(1), 63–72.

Light, T. D., Jeng, J. C., Jain, A. K., et al. (2004). Real time monitors, ischemia reperfusion, titration endpoints, and ultra precise burn resuscitation. *Journal of Burn Care and Rehabilitation, 25*(1), 33–44.

Mancuso, M. G., Bishop, M. G., Blakeney, P., et al. (2003). Impact on the family: Psychosocial adjustment of siblings of children who survive serious burns. *Journal of Burn Care and Rehabilitation, 24*(2), 110–118.

Martin-Herz, S. P., Patterson, D. R., Honari, S., et al. (2003). Pediatric pain control practices of North American burn centers. *Journal of Burn Care and Rehabilitation, 24*(1), 26–36.

McCabe, C. J. (2003). Trauma: An annotated bibliography of recent trauma. *American Journal of Emergency Medicine, 22*(5), 405–424.

McCall, J. & Chaill, T. (2005). Respiratory care of the burn patient. *Journal of Burn Care and Rehabilitation, 26*(3), 200–206.

McGwin, G. Jr., Cross, J. M., Ford, J. W., et al. (2003). Long-term trends in mortality according to age among adult burn patients. *Journal of Burn Care and Rehabilitation, 24*(1), 21–25.

Meyer, W. J. 3rd., Blakeney, P. Russell, W., et al. (2004). Psychological problems reported by young adults who were burned as children. *Journal of Burn Care and Rehabilitation, 25*(1), 98–106.

Morton, K., Willebrand, M., Anderson, G., et al. (2004). Personality characteristics and perceived health problems after burn injury. *Journal of Burn Care and Rehabilitation, 25*(3), 228–235.

Neely, A., Fowler, L. A., Kagan, R. J., et al. (2004). Procalcitonin in pediatric burn patients: An early indicator of sepsis? *Journal of Burn Care and Rehabilitation, 25*(1), 76–80.

O'Keefe Gatewood, M. & Zane, R. (2004). Lightning injuries. *Emergency Medical Clinics of North America, 22*(2), 369–403.

Palmieri, T. L., Petuskey, K., Bagley, A., et al. (2003). Alterations in functional movement after axillary burn scar contracture: A motion analysis study. *Journal of Burn Care and Rehabilitation, 24*(2), 104–108.

Patterson, D. R., Finch, C. P., Wiechman, S. A., et al. (2003). Premorbid mental health status of adult burn patients: Comparison with a normative sample. *Journal of Burn Care and Rehabilitation, 24*(5), 347–350.

Pereira, C., Murphy, K. & Herndon, D. (2005). Altering metabolism. *Journal of Burn Care and Rehabilitation, 26*(3), 194–199.

Riordan, C. L., McDonough, M., Davidson, J. M., et al. (2003). Noncontact laser Doppler imaging in burn depth analysis of the extremities. *Journal of Burn Care and Rehabilitation, 24*(4), 177–186.

Saffle, J. R. (2003). What's new in general surgery: Burns and metabolism. *Journal of the American College of Surgeons, 196*(20), 267–289.

Santos, A. P., Wilson, A. K., Hornung, C. A., et al. (2005). Methamphetamine laboratory explosions: A new and emerging burn injury. *Journal of Burn Care and Rehabilitation, 26*(3), 228–232.

Serghiou, M. A., Holmes, C. L. & McCauley, R. L. (2004). A survey of current rehabilitation trends for burn injuries to the head and neck. *Journal of Burn Care and Rehabilitation, 25*(6), 514–518.

Sheridan, R. L. & Thompkins, R. G. (2004). What's new in burns and metabolism. *Journal of American College of Surgeons, 198*(2), 243–283.

Slone, D. S. (2004). Nutritional support of the critically ill and injured patients. *Critical Care Nursing Clinics of North America, 20*(1), 135–157.

Snyder, C. & Ubben, P. (2003). Use of speech pathology services in the burn unit. *Journal of Burn Care and Rehabilitation,* 24(4), 217–221.

Supp, A., Neely, A. N., Supp, D. M., et al. (2005). Evaluation of cytotoxicity and antimicrobial activity of Acticoat burn dressings for management of microbial contamination in cultured skin substitutes grafted to athymic mice. *Journal of Burn Care and Rehabilitation, 26*(3), 238–246.

Supp, D. M., Karpinski, A. & Boyce, S., (2004). Vascular endothelial growth factor overexpression increases vascularization by murine but not human endothelial cells in cultured skin substitutes grafted to athymic mice. *Journal of Burn Care and Rehabilitation, 25*(4), 337–345.

Supple, K. G. (2004). Physiologic response to burn injury. *Critical Care Nursing Clinics of North America, 16*(1), 119–126.

Thompkins, R. (2003). Outcomes measurement in pediatric burn care: An agenda for research. Executive summary and final report. *Journal of Burn Care and Rehabilitation, 24*(5), 269–274.

Tompkins, D. & Rossi, L. A. (2005). Care of outpatient burns. Available at: http://www.worldburn.org/documents/burncare/pdf. Accessed June 2, 2006.

Thompson, N. J., Waterman, M. B. & Sleet, D. A. (2004). Using behavioral science to improve fire escape behaviors in response to a smoke alarm. *Journal of Burn Care and Rehabilitation, 25*(2), 179–188.

U.S. Fire Administration/National Fire Data Center. (2004a). Kitchen fires. *Topical Fire Research Series, 4*(4), 1–5.

U.S. Fire Administration/National Fire Data Center. (2004b). Fire risk. *Topical Fire Research Series, 4*(7), 1–6.

U.S. Fire Administration/National Fire Data Center. (2005a). Fatal fires. *Topical Fire Research Series, 5*(1), 1–6.

U.S. Fire Administration/National Fire Data Center. (2005b). Structure cooking fires. *Topical Fire Research Series, 5*(6), 1–4.

U.S. Fire Administration/National Fire Data Center. (2005c). Residential smoking fires and casualties. *Topical Fire Research Series, 5*(5), 1–6.

Wahl, W. L., Ahrns, K. S., Brandt, M. M., et al. (2005). Bronchoalveolar lavage in diagnosis of ventilator-associated pneumonia in patients with burns. *Journal of Burn Care and Rehabilitation, 26*(1), 57–61.

Wibbenmeyer, L. A., Amelon, M. J., Torner, J. C., et al. (2003). Population-based assessment of burn injury in southern Iowa: Identification of children and young-adult at risk groups and behaviors. *Journal of Burn Care and Rehabilitation, 24*(4), 192–202.

Willebrand, M., Andersson, G. & Ekselius, L. (2004). Prediction of psychological health after an accidental burn. *Journal of Trauma, 57*(2), 367–374.

Also see issues of *The Journal of Burn Care and Rehabilitation* and *Burns—The Journal of the International Society for Burn Injuries.*

RESOURCES

Alisa Ann Ruch Burn Foundation, 20944 Sherman Way, Suite 115, Canoga Park, CA 91303; 818-883-7700; http://www.aarbf.org. Accessed June 2, 2006.

American Burn Association, 625 N. Michigan Ave., Suite 1530, Chicago, IL 60611; 800-548-BURN; http://www.ameriburn.org. Accessed June 2, 2006.

American Red Cross. P.O. Box 37243, Washington, DC 20013; 800-HELPNOW; http://www.redcross.org. Accessed June 2, 2006.

Association of Home Appliance Manufacturers, Suite 402, 111 19th Street, NW, Washington, DC 20036; 202-872-5955; http://www.aham.org. Accessed June 2, 2006.

Burn Children Recovery Foundation, P.O. Box 246, Arlington, VA 98223; 800-799-BURN; http://www.burnchildrenrecovery.org.

Burn Foundation, 1128 Walnut St., Philadelphia, PA 19107; 215-629-9200; e-mail: burnctrs@aol.com.

Burn Institute, 3702 Ruffin Rd. #101, San Diego, CA 92123; 858-541-2277; http://www.burninstitute.org. Accessed June 2, 2006.

Burn Prevention; 610-481-9810; http://www.burnprevention.org. Accessed June 2, 2006.

Chemical Educational Foundation, 1560 Wilson Boulevard, Suite 1250, Arlington, VA 22209; 703-527-6223; http://www.chemed.org. Accessed June 2, 2006.

Cool the Burn; http://www.regionshospital.com. Accessed June 2, 2006.

Firefighters Pacific Burn Institute, 3823 V Street #4, Sacramento, CA 95817; 916-739-8525; http://www.ffburn.org. Accessed June 2, 2006.

Integra Life Sciences Corporation 311 Enterprise Drive, Plainsboro, NJ 08536; 800-654-2873, fax 609-275-5363; http://www.integra-ls.com. Accessed June 2, 2006.

International Association of Fire Fighters Burn Foundation, 1750 New York Ave., NW, Washington, DC 20006; 202-737-8484; http://www.iaff.org. Accessed June 2, 2006.

International Medical Education Foundation; burnsurgery.org. Accessed June 2, 2006.

International Society for Burn Injuries; Dr. Ronald Tompkins, Massachusetts, General Hospital, GRB1302, 55 Fruit Street, Boston, MA 02114-2696; 617-726-3447, fax 617-367-8936; rtompkins@partners.org; Dr. Jacques Latarjet, M.D., 9 rue Grignard, 69365 Lyon, France; 478-http://www.worldburn.org. Accessed Aug. 3, 2006.

Lifecell Corporation, One Millennium Way, Branchburg, NJ 08876; 908-947-1100; http://www.lifecell.com. Accessed June 2, 2006.

National Burn Center Reporting System Report Form, U.S. Consumer Product Safety Commission; http://www.cpsc.gov/burnctr.html. Accessed June 2, 2006.

Phoenix Society for Burn Survivors, Inc., 1835 R. W. Berends Drive, SW, Grand Rapids, MI 49519; 800-888-2876; http://www.phoenix-society.org. Accessed June 2, 2006.

UNIT 13

Sensorineural Function

Case Study

Applying Concepts from NANDA, NIC, and NOC

A Patient With Impaired Vision and Decreased Attention to One Side of the Body

Mr. Martin is a 60-year-old man who has had several strokes. Ophthalmologic testing reveals that he has homonymous hemianopsia of the left visual field and visual spatial neglect; as a result he has limited vision in the left visual fields of both eyes. He has difficulty in many areas, such as bumping into objects and ignoring the left side of his body.

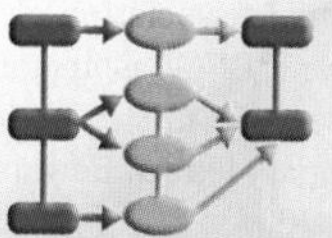

Turn to Appendix C to see a concept map that illustrates the relationships that exist between the nursing diagnoses, interventions, and outcomes for the patient's clinical problems.

Nursing Classifications and Languages

NANDA Nursing Diagnoses	NIC Nursing Interventions	NOC Nursing Outcomes Return to functional baseline status, stabilization of, or improvement in:
Disturbed Sensory Perception: Visual—Change in the amount or patterning of incoming stimuli accompanied by a diminished, exaggerated, distorted, or impaired response to such stimuli	**Communication Enhancement: Visual Deficit**—Assistance in accepting and learning alternative methods for living with diminished vision	**Vision Compensation Behavior**—Personal actions to compensate for visual impairment
Unilateral Neglect—Lack of awareness and attention to one side of the body	**Unilateral Neglect Management**—Protecting and safely reintegrating the affected part of the body while helping the patient adapt to disturbed perceptual abilities	**Safe Home Environment**—Physical arrangements to minimize environmental factors that might cause physical harm or injury in the home
Risk for Injury—At risk for injury as a result of environmental conditions interacting with the individual's adaptive and defensive resources	**Positioning**—Deliberative placement of the patient or a body part to promote physiological and/or psychological well-being	**Physical Injury Severity**—Severity of injuries from trauma

NANDA International (2005). *Nursing diagnoses: definitions & classification 2005–2006.* Philadelphia: North American Nursing Diagnosis Association.

Dochterman, J. M., & Bulechek, G. M. (2004). *Nursing interventions classification (NIC)* (4th ed.). St. Louis: Mosby.

Iowa Outcomes Project (2004). In Moorhead, S., Johnson, M., & Maas, M. (2004). *Nursing outcomes classification (NOC)* (3rd ed.). St. Louis: Mosby.

Dochterman, J. M., & Jones, D. A. (2003). *Unifying nursing languages: the harmonization of NANDA, NIC, and NOC.* Washington, DC: American Nurses Association.

CHAPTER 58

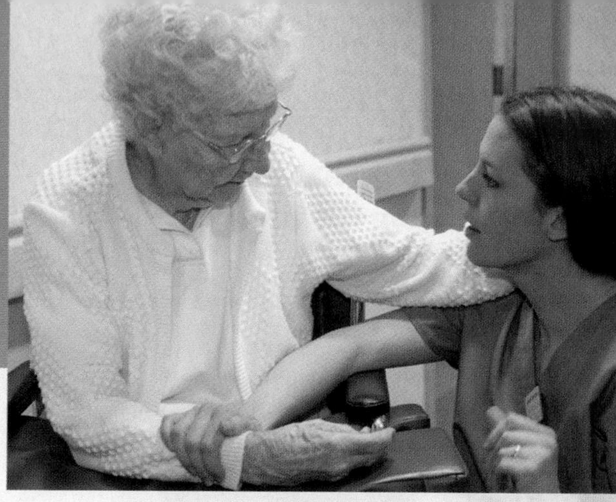

Assessment and Management of Patients With Eye and Vision Disorders

Learning Objectives

On completion of this chapter, the learner will be able to:

1. Identify significant eye structures and describe their functions.
2. Identify diagnostic tests for assessment of vision and evaluation of visual disabilities.
3. Discuss clinical features, diagnostic assessment and examinations, medical or surgical management, and nursing management of ocular disorders.
4. Describe therapeutic effects of ophthalmic medications.
5. Define low vision and blindness and differentiate between functional and visual impairment.
6. List and describe assessment and management strategies for low vision.
7. Demonstrate orientation and mobility techniques for patients with low vision in a hospital setting.
8. Demonstrate instillation of eye drops and ointment.
9. Discuss general discharge instructions for patients after ocular surgery.
10. Discuss strategies for patient safety in ophthalmology.

The ability to see the world clearly can easily be taken for granted. The eye is a sensitive, highly specialized sense organ subject to various disorders, many of which lead to impaired vision. Impaired vision may affect a person's independence in self-care, work and lifestyle choices, sense of self-esteem, safety, ability to interact with society and the environment, and overall quality of life. Many of the leading causes of visual impairment are associated with aging (eg, cataracts, glaucoma, macular degeneration), and two thirds of the population with impaired vision is older than 65 years of age. Younger people are also at risk for eye disorders, particularly traumatic injuries. The rapidly changing technological advances of ophthalmic surgery affect all age groups. These include refractive procedures, as well as implantation of intraocular lenses and telescopic devices.

Although most people with eye disorders are treated in an ambulatory care setting, many patients receiving health care have an eye disease as a comorbid condition. In addition to understanding the prevention, treatment, and consequences of eye disorders, nurses in all settings assess visual acuity in those at risk (eg, patients who are elderly, those with diabetes or acquired immunodeficiency syndrome [AIDS]), refer patients to eye care specialists as appropriate, implement measures to prevent further visual loss, and help patients adapt to impaired vision.

Anatomic and Physiologic Overview

Unlike most organs of the body, the eye is available for external examination, and its anatomy is more easily assessed than many other body parts (Fig. 58-1). The eyeball, or globe, sits in a protective bony structure known as the orbit. Lined with muscle and connective and adipose tissues, the orbit is about 4 cm high, wide, and deep, and it is shaped roughly like a four-sided pyramid, surrounded on three sides by the sinuses: ethmoid (medially), frontal (superiorly), and maxillary (inferiorly). The optic nerve and the ophthalmic artery

Glossary

accommodation: process by which the eye adjusts for near distance (eg, reading) by changing the curvature of the lens to focus a clear image on the retina

anterior chamber: space in the eye bordered anteriorly by the cornea and posteriorly by the iris and pupil

aphakia: absence of the natural lens

astigmatism: refractive error in which light rays are spread over a diffuse area rather than sharply focused on the retina, a condition caused by differences in the curvature of the cornea and lens

binocular vision: normal ability of both eyes to focus on one object and fuse the two images into one

blindness: inability to see, usually defined as corrected visual acuity of 20/400 or less, or a visual field of no more than 20 degrees in the better eye

chemosis: edema of the conjunctiva

cones: retinal photoreceptor cells essential for visual acuity and color discrimination

diplopia: seeing one object as two; double vision

emmetropia: absence of refractive error

enucleation: complete removal of the eyeball and part of the optic nerve

evisceration: removal of the intraocular contents through a corneal or scleral incision; the optic nerve, sclera, extraocular muscles, and sometimes, the cornea are left intact

exenteration: surgical removal of the entire contents of the orbit, including the eyeball and lids

hyperemia: "red eye" resulting from dilation of the vasculature of the conjunctiva

hyperopia: farsightedness; a refractive error in which the focus of light rays from a distant object is behind the retina

hyphema: blood in the anterior chamber

hypopyon: collection of inflammatory cells that has the appearance of a pale layer in the inferior anterior chamber of the eye

injection: congestion of blood vessels

keratoconus: cone-shaped deformity of the cornea

keratopathy, bullous: corneal edema with painful blisters in the epithelium due to excessive corneal hydration

limbus: junction of the cornea and sclera

miotics: medications that cause pupillary constriction

mydriatics: medications that cause pupillary dilation

myopia: nearsightedness; a refractive error in which the focus of light rays from a distant object is anterior to the retina

neovascularization: growth of abnormal new blood vessels

nystagmus: involuntary oscillation of the eyeball

papilledema: swelling of the optic disc due to increased intracranial pressure

photophobia: ocular pain on exposure to light

posterior chamber: space between the iris and vitreous

proptosis: downward displacement of the eyeball resulting from an inflammatory condition of the orbit or a mass within the orbital cavity

ptosis: drooping eyelid

refraction: determination of the refractive errors of the eye and correction by lenses

rods: retinal photoreceptor cells essential for bright and dim light

scotomas: blind or partially blind areas in the visual field

strabismus: a condition in which there is deviation from perfect ocular alignment

sympathetic ophthalmia: an inflammatory condition created in the fellow eye by the affected eye (without useful vision); the condition may become chronic and result in blindness (of the fellow eye)

trachoma: a bilateral chronic follicular conjunctivitis of childhood that leads to blindness during adulthood, if left untreated

vitreous humor: gelatinous material (transparent and colorless) that fills the eyeball behind the lens

Note: Common abbreviations related to vision and eye health are OD (oculus dexter, right eye), OS (oculus sinister, left eye), and OU (oculus uterque, both eyes).

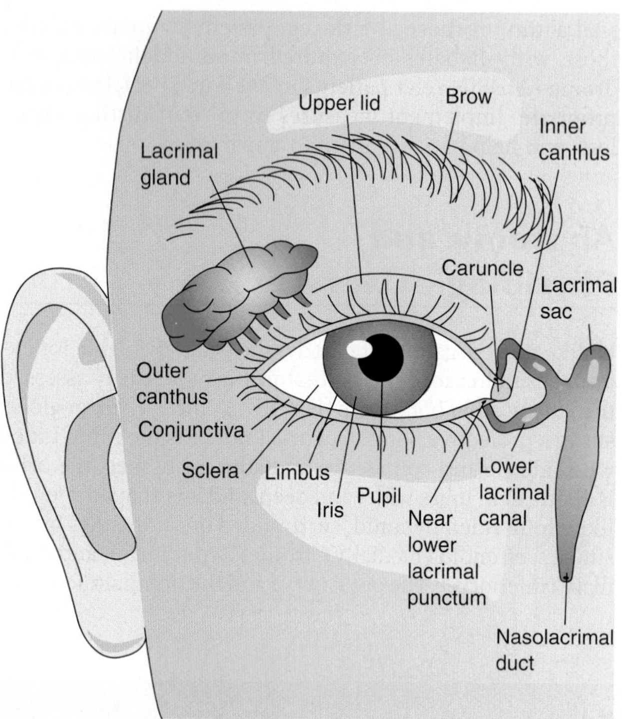

FIGURE 58-1. External structures of the eye and position of the lacrimal structures.

enter the orbit at its apex through the optic foramen. The eyeball is moved though all fields of gaze by the extraocular muscles. The four rectus muscles and two oblique muscles (Fig. 58-2) are innervated by cranial nerves (CN) III, IV, and VI. Normally, the movements of the two eyes are coordinated, and the brain perceives a single image.

The eyelids, composed of thin elastic skin that covers striated and smooth muscles, protect the anterior portion of the eye. The eyelids contain multiple glands, including sebaceous, sweat, and accessory lacrimal glands, and they are lined with conjunctival material. The upper lid normally covers the uppermost portion of the iris and is innervated by the oculomotor nerve (CN III). The lid margins contain meibomian glands, the inferior and superior puncta, and the eyelashes. The triangular spaces formed by the junction of the eyelids are known as the inner or medial canthus and the outer or lateral canthus. With every blink of the eyes, the lids wash the cornea and conjunctiva with tears.

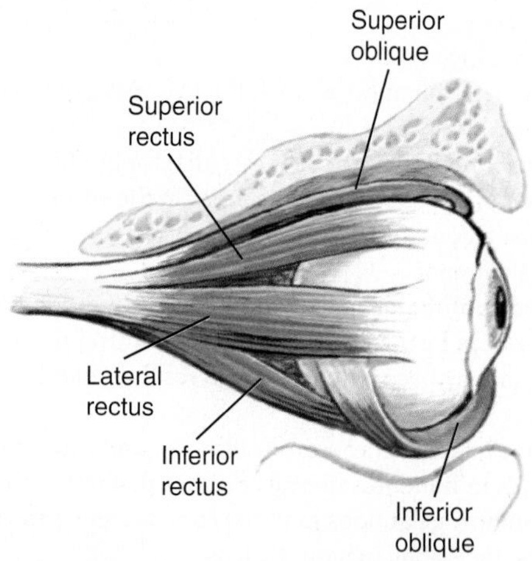

FIGURE 58-2. The extraocular muscles responsible for eye movement. The medial rectus muscle (not shown) is responsible for opposing the movement of the lateral rectus muscle.

Tears are vital to eye health. They are formed by the lacrimal gland and the accessory lacrimal glands. A healthy tear is composed of three layers: lipoid, aqueous, and mucoid. If there is a defect in the composition of any of these layers, the integrity of the cornea may be compromised. Tears are secreted in response to reflex or emotional stimuli.

The conjunctiva, a mucous membrane, provides a barrier to the external environment and nourishes the eye. The goblet cells of the conjunctiva secrete lubricating mucus. The bulbar conjunctiva covers the sclera, whereas the palpebral conjunctiva lines the inner surface of the upper and lower eyelids. The junction of the two portions is known as the fornix.

The sclera, commonly known as the white of the eye, is a dense, fibrous structure that makes up the posterior five sixths of the eye (Fig. 58-3). The sclera helps maintain the shape of the eyeball and protects the intraocular contents from trauma. The sclera may have a slightly bluish tinge in young children, a dull white color in adults, and a slightly yellowish color in the elderly. Externally, it is overlaid with conjunctiva, which is a thin, transparent, mucous membrane that contains fine blood vessels. The conjunctiva meets the cornea at the **limbus** on the outermost edge of the iris.

The cornea (Fig. 58-4), a transparent, avascular, domelike structure, forms the most anterior portion of the eyeball and is the main refracting surface of the eye. It is composed of five layers: epithelium, Bowman's membrane, stroma, Descemet's membrane, and endothelium. The epithelial cells are capable of rapid replication and are completely replaced every 7 days.

Behind the cornea lies the **anterior chamber**, filled with a continually replenished supply of clear aqueous humor, which nourishes the cornea. The aqueous humor is produced by the ciliary body, and its production is related to the intraocular pressure (IOP). Normal IOP is 10 to 21 mm Hg.

The uvea consists of the iris, the ciliary body, and the choroid. The iris, or colored part of the eye, is a highly vascularized, pigmented collection of fibers surrounding the pupil. The pupil is a space that dilates and constricts in response to light. Normal pupils are round and constrict symmetrically when a bright light shines on them. About 20% of the population have pupils that are slightly unequal in size but that respond equally to light. Dilation and constriction are controlled by the sphincter and dilator pupillae muscles. The dilator muscles are controlled by the sympathetic nervous system, whereas the sphincter muscles are controlled by the parasympathetic nervous system.

Directly behind the pupil and iris lies the lens, a colorless and almost completely transparent, biconvex structure held in position by zonular fibers. It is avascular and has no nerve or pain fibers. The lens enables focusing for near vision and refocusing for distance vision. The ability to focus and refocus is called **accommodation.** The lens is suspended behind the iris by the zonules and is connected to the ciliary body. The ciliary body controls accommodation

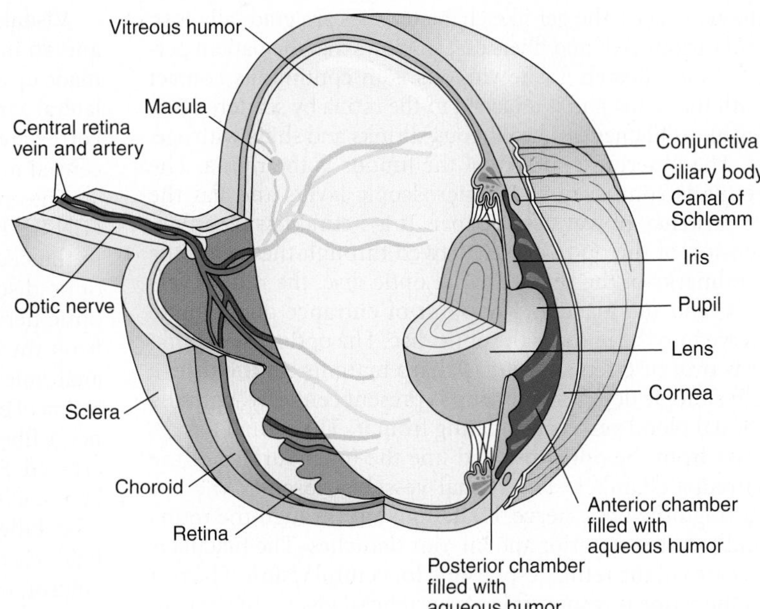

FIGURE 58-3. Three-dimensional cross-section of the eye.

through the zonular fibers and the ciliary muscles. The aqueous humor is anterior to the lens; posterior to the lens is the vitreous humor. All cells formed throughout life are retained by the lens, which makes the cell structure of the lens susceptible to the degenerative effects of aging. The lens continues to grow throughout life, laying down fibers in concentric rings. This gradual thickening becomes evident in the fifth decade of life and eventually results in an increasingly dense core or nucleus, which can limit accommodative powers.

The **posterior chamber** is a small space between the vitreous and the iris. Aqueous fluid is manufactured in the posterior chamber by the ciliary body. This aqueous fluid flows from the posterior chamber into the anterior chamber, from which it drains through the trabecular meshwork into the canal of Schlemm.

The choroid lies between the retina and the sclera. It is avascular tissue, supplying blood to the portion of the sensory retina closest to it.

The ocular fundus is the largest chamber of the eye and contains the **vitreous humor**, a clear, gelatinous substance, composed mostly of water and encapsulated by a hyaloid membrane. The vitreous humor occupies about two thirds of the eye's volume and helps maintain the shape of the eye. As

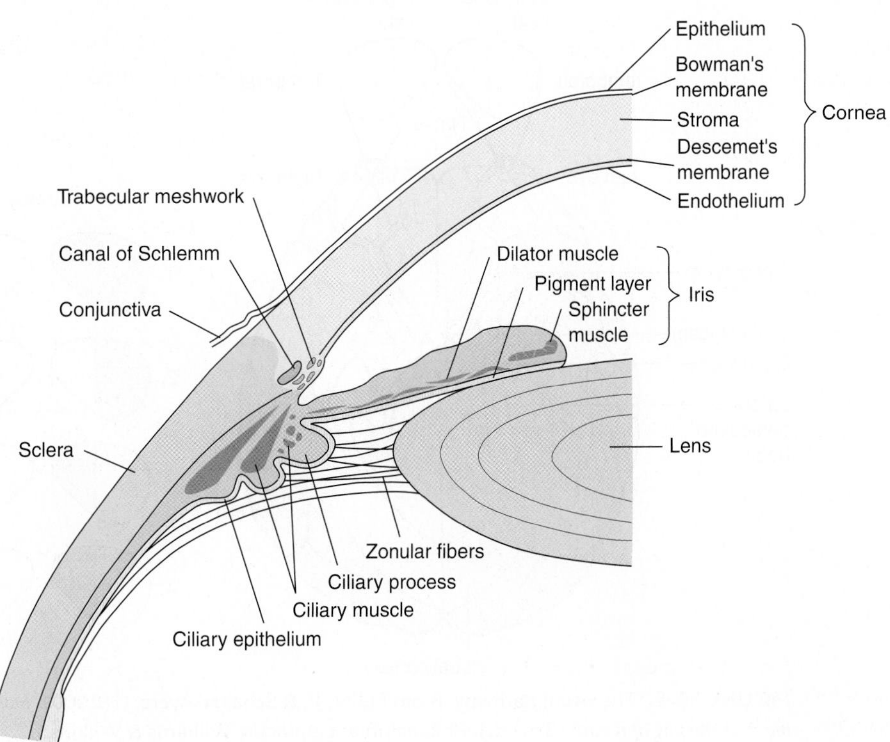

FIGURE 58-4. Internal structures of the eye. From Goldblum, K. (Ed.) (1997). *Core curriculum for ophthalmic nursing, American Society of Ophthalmic Registered Nurses.* Dubuque, IA: Kendall/Hall Publishing.

the body ages, the gel-like characteristics are gradually lost, and various cells and fibers cast shadows that the patient perceives as "floaters." The vitreous is in continuous contact with the retina and is attached to the retina by scattered collagenous filaments. The vitreous shrinks and shifts with age.

The innermost surface of the fundus is the retina. The retina is composed of 10 microscopic layers and has the consistency of wet tissue paper. It is neural tissue, an extension of the optic nerve. Viewed through the pupil, the landmarks of the retina are the optic disc, the retinal vessels, and the macula. The point of entrance of the optic nerve into the retina is the optic disc. The optic disc is pink; it is oval or circular and has sharp margins. In the disc, a physiologic depression or cup is present centrally, with the retinal blood vessels emanating from it. The retinal tissues arise from the optic disc and line the inner surface of the vitreous chamber. The retinal vessels also enter the eye through the optic nerve, branching out through the retina and forming superior and inferior branches. The macula is the area of the retina responsible for central vision. The rest of the retina is responsible for peripheral vision. In the center of the macula is the most sensitive area, the fovea, which is avascular and surrounded by the superior and inferior vascular arcades. Two important layers of the retina are the retinal pigment epithelium (RPE) and the sensory retina. A single layer of cells constitutes the RPE, and these cells have numerous functions, including the absorption of light. The sensory retina contains the photoreceptor cells: **rods** and **cones.** These are long, narrow cells shaped like rods or cones. The rods are mainly responsible for night vision or vision in low light, whereas the cones provide the best vision for bright light, color vision, and fine detail. Cones are distributed throughout the retina, with their greatest concentration in the fovea. Rods are absent in the fovea (Porth, 2005).

Visual acuity depends on a healthy, functioning eyeball and an intact visual pathway (Fig. 58-5). This pathway is made up of the retina, optic nerve, optic chiasm, optic tracks, lateral geniculate bodies, and optic radiations and the visual cortex area of the brain. The pathway is an extension of the central nervous system.

The optic nerve is also known as the second cranial nerve (CN II). Its purpose is to transmit impulses from the retina to the occipital lobe of the brain. The optic nerve head, or optic disc, is the physiologic blind spot in each eye. The optic nerve leaves the eye and then meets the optic nerve from the other eye at the optic chiasm. The chiasm is the anatomic point at which the nasal fibers from the nasal retina of each eye cross to the opposite side of the brain. The nerve fibers from the temporal retina of each eye remain uncrossed. Fibers from the right half of each eye, which would be the left visual field, carry impulses to the right occipital lobe. Fibers from the left half of each eye, or the right visual field, carry impulses to the left occipital lobe. Beyond the chiasm, these fibers are known as the optic tract. The optic tract continues on to the lateral geniculate body. The lateral geniculate body leads to the optic radiations and then to the cortex of the occipital lobe of the brain.

Assessment

Ocular History

The nurse, through careful questioning, elicits the necessary information that can lead to the diagnosis of an ophthalmic condition. Pertinent questions to ask during the interview can be found in Chart 58-1.

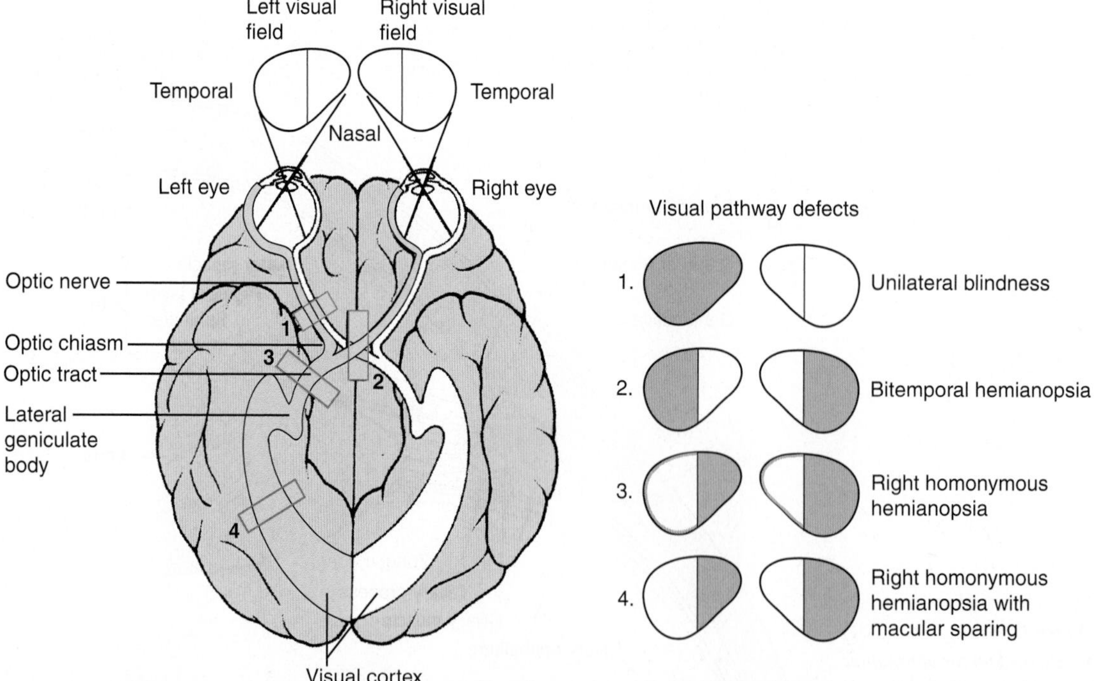

FIGURE 58-5. The visual pathway. From Fuller, J., & Schaller-Ayers, J. (2000). *Health assessment: A nursing approach* (3rd ed.). Philadelphia: Lippincott Williams & Wilkins.

GENETICS IN NURSING PRACTICE

Eye and Vision Disorders

Several eye and vision disorders are associated with genetic abnormalities. Some examples are:

- Albinism
- Aniridia
- Color blindness
- Glaucoma
- Homocystinuria
- Isolated familial congenital cataracts
- Leber hereditary optic neuropathy
- Leber congenital amaurosis
- Marfan syndrome
- Retinitis pigmentosa

NURSING ASSESSMENTS

Family History Assessment

- Assess history of family members with glaucoma, cataracts, night blindness (retinitis pigmentosa), color blindness, or other vision impairment.
- Inquire about the age of onset of symptoms (the onset of Leber congenital amaurosis is in childhood, while the onset of Leber hereditary optic neuropathy is in young adulthood).
- Inquire about family members with other disorders that may include visual impairment, such as cutaneous, metabolic, or connective tissue disorders and hearing loss.

Patient Assessment

- Assess for other systemic and/or clinical features such as cutaneous or skeletal conditions, or hearing loss.

MANAGEMENT ISSUES SPECIFIC TO GENETICS

- Inquire whether DNA gene mutation or other genetics testing has been performed on any affected family members.
- If indicated, refer for further genetics counseling and evaluation so that family members can discuss inheritance, risk to other family members, availability of genetics testing, and gene-based interventions.
- Offer appropriate genetics information and resources.
- Assess patient's understanding of genetics information.
- Provide support to families with newly diagnosed genetic-related sensorineural disorders.
- Participate in management and coordination of care of patients with genetic conditions and individuals predisposed to develop or pass on a genetic condition

GENETICS RESOURCES

Genetic Alliance—a directory of support groups for patients and families with genetic conditions, http://www.geneticalliance.org

Gene Clinics—a listing of common genetic disorders with up-to-date clinical summaries, genetic counseling and testing information, http://www.geneclinics.org

National Organization of Rare Disorders—a directory of support groups and information for patients and families with rare genetic disorders, http://www.rarediseases.org

OMIM: Online Mendelian Inheritance in Man—a complete listing of inherited genetic conditions, http://www.ncbi.nlm.nih.gov/omim/stats/html

Visual Acuity

Following the health history, the patient's visual acuity is assessed. This is an essential part of the eye examination and a measure against which all therapeutic outcomes are based.

Most people are familiar with the standard Snellen chart. It is composed of a series of progressively smaller rows of letters and is used to test distance vision. The fraction 20/20 is considered the standard of normal vision. Most people can see the letters on the line designated as 20/20 from a distance of 20 feet. A person whose vision is 20/200 can see an object from 20 feet away that a person with 20/20 vision can see from 200 feet away (Bickley & Szilagyi, 2003).

The patient is positioned at the prescribed distance, usually 20 feet, from the chart and is asked to read the smallest line that he or she can see. The patient should wear distance correction (eyeglasses or contact lenses) if required, and each eye should be tested separately. If the patient cannot read the 20/20 line, he or she is given a pinhole occluder and asked to read again using the eye in question. A makeshift occluder may be created by making a pinhole in an index card and asking the patient to look through the pinhole. Squinting produces the same effect. Patients should be encouraged to read more letters and to guess, if necessary. Often, patients avoid guessing and prefer not to try at all rather than to make a mistake. The patient should be encouraged to read every letter possible.

Visual acuity is then recorded. If the patient reads all five letters from the 20/20 line with the right eye (OD) and three of the five letters on the 20/15 line with the left eye (OS), the examiner writes OD 20/20, OS 20/15-2.

If the patient cannot read the largest letter on the chart (the 20/200 line), the patient should be moved toward the chart or the chart moved toward the patient until the patient can identify the largest letter on the chart. If the patient can recognize only the letter E on the top line at a distance of 10 feet, the visual acuity would be recorded as 10′/200. If the patient cannot see the letter E at any distance, the examiner should determine if the patient can

CHART 58-1

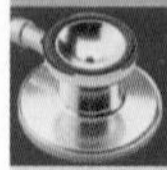

Assessment

Taking an Ocular History

- What does the patient perceive to be the problem?
- Is visual acuity diminished?
- Does the patient experience blurred, double, or distorted vision?
- Is there pain; is it sharp or dull; is it worse when blinking?
- Is the discomfort an itching sensation or more of a foreign body sensation?
- Are both eyes affected?
- Is there a history of discharge? If so, inquire about color, consistency, odor.
- What is the duration of the problem?
- Is this a recurrence of a previous condition?
- How has the patient self-treated?
- What makes the symptoms improve or worsen?
- Has the condition affected performance of activities of daily living (ADLs)?
- Are there any systemic diseases? What medications are used in their treatment?
- What concurrent ophthalmic conditions does the patient have?
- Is there an ophthalmic surgery history?
- Have other family members had the same symptoms or condition?

count fingers (CF). The examiner holds up a random number of fingers and asks the patient to count the number he or she sees. If the patient correctly identifies the number of fingers at 3 feet, the examiner would record CF/3′.

If the patient cannot count fingers, the examiner raises one hand up and down or moves it side to side and asks in which direction the hand is moving. This level of vision is known as hand motion (HM). A patient who can perceive only light is described as having light perception (LP). The vision of a patient who cannot perceive light is described as no light perception (NLP).

External Eye Examination

After the visual acuity has been recorded, an external eye examination is performed. The position of the eyelids is noted. Commonly, the upper 2 mm of the iris are covered by the upper lid. The patient is examined for **ptosis** (drooping eyelid) and for lid retraction (too much of the eye exposed). Sometimes, the upper or lower lid turns out, affecting closure. The lid margins and lashes should have no edema, erythema, or lesions. The examiner looks for scaling or crusting, and the sclera is inspected. A normal sclera is opaque and white. Lesions on the conjunctiva, discharge, and tearing or blinking are noted.

The room should be darkened so that the pupils can be examined. The pupillary response is checked with a penlight to determine if the pupils are equally reactive and regular. A normal pupil is black. An irregular pupil may result from trauma, previous surgery, or a disease process.

The patient's eyes are observed in primary or direct gaze, and any head tilt is noted. A tilt may indicate cranial nerve palsy. The patient is asked to stare at a target; each eye is covered and uncovered quickly while the examiner looks for any shift in gaze. The examiner observes for **nystagmus** (ie, oscillating movement of the eyeball). The extraocular movements of the eyes are tested by having the patient follow the examiner's finger, pencil, or a hand light through the six cardinal directions of gaze (ie, up, down, right, left, and both diagonals). This is especially important when screening patients for ocular trauma or for neurologic disorders.

Diagnostic Evaluation

Direct Ophthalmoscopy

A direct ophthalmoscope is a hand-held instrument with various plus and minus lenses. The lenses can be rotated into place, enabling the examiner to bring the cornea, lens, and retina into focus sequentially. The examiner holds the ophthalmoscope in the right hand and uses the right eye to examine the patient's right eye. The examiner switches to the left hand and left eye when examining the patient's left eye. During this examination, the room should be darkened, and the patient's eye should be on the same level as the examiner's eye. The patient and the examiner should be comfortable, and both should breathe normally. The patient is given a target to gaze at and is encouraged to keep both eyes open and steady.

When the fundus is examined, the vasculature comes into focus first. The veins are larger in diameter than the arteries. The examiner focuses on a large vessel and then follows it toward the midline of the body, which leads to the optic nerve. The central depression in the disc is known as the cup. The normal cup is about one-third the size of the disc. The size of the physiologic optic cup should be estimated and the disc margins described as sharp or blurred. A silvery or coppery appearance, which indicates arteriolosclerosis, should be noted. The periphery of the retina is examined by having the patient shift his or her gaze. The last area of the fundus to be examined is the macula, because this area is the most sensitive to light. The retina of a young person often has a glistening effect, sometimes referred to as a cellophane reflex.

The healthy fundus should be free of any lesions. The examiner looks for intraretinal hemorrhages, which may appear as red smudges or, if the patient has hypertension, may look somewhat flame-shaped. Lipid may be present in the retina of patients with hypercholesterolemia or diabetes. This lipid has a yellowish appearance. Soft exudates that have a fuzzy, white appearance (cotton-wool spots) should be noted. The examiner looks for microaneurysms, which look like little red dots, and nevi. Drusen (small, hyaline, globular growths), commonly found in macular degeneration, appear as yellowish areas with indistinct edges. Small drusen have a more distinct edge. The examiner should sketch the fundus and document any abnormalities.

Indirect Ophthalmoscopy

The indirect ophthalmoscope is an instrument commonly used by the ophthalmologist to see larger areas of the retina, although in an unmagnified state. It produces a bright and intense light. The light source is affixed with a pair of binocular lenses mounted on the examiner's head. The ophthalmoscope is used with a hand-held, 20-diopter lens.

Slit-Lamp Examination

The slit lamp is a binocular microscope mounted on a table. This instrument enables the user to examine the eye with magnification of 10 to 40 times the real image. The illumination can be varied from a broad to a narrow beam of light for different parts of the eye. For example, by varying the width and intensity of the light, the anterior chamber can be examined for signs of inflammation. Cataracts may be evaluated by changing the angle of the light. When a hand-held contact lens, such as a three-mirror lens, is used with the slit lamp, the angle of the anterior chamber may be examined, as may the ocular fundus.

Color Vision Testing

The ability to differentiate colors has a dramatic effect on the activities of daily living. For example, the inability to differentiate between red and green can compromise traffic safety. Some careers (eg, commercial art, color photography, airline pilot, electrician) may be closed to people with significant color deficiencies. The photoreceptor cells responsible for color vision are the cones, and the greatest area of color sensitivity is in the macula, the area of densest cone concentration.

A screening test, such as the polychromatic plates discussed in the next paragraph, can be used to establish whether a person's color vision is within normal range. Color vision deficits can be inherited. For example, red–green color deficiencies are inherited in an X-linked manner, affecting approximately 8% of men and 0.4% of women. Acquired color vision losses may be caused by medications (eg, digitalis) or pathology (eg, cataracts). A simple test, such as asking a patient if the red top on a bottle of eye drops appears redder to one eye than the other, can be an effective tool. A difference in the perception of the intensity of the color red between the two eyes can be a symptom of a neurologic problem and may provide information about the location of the lesion.

Because alteration in color vision sometimes indicates conditions of the optic nerve, color vision testing is often performed in a neuro-ophthalmologic workup. The most common color vision test is performed using Ishihara polychromatic plates. These plates are bound together in a booklet. On each plate of this booklet are dots of primary colors that are integrated into a background of secondary colors. The dots are arranged in simple patterns, such as numbers or geometric shapes. Patients with diminished color vision may be unable to identify the hidden shapes. Patients with central vision conditions (eg, macular degeneration) have more difficulty identifying colors than those with peripheral vision conditions (eg, glaucoma) because central vision identifies color.

Amsler Grid

The Amsler grid is a test often used for patients with macular problems, such as macular degeneration. It consists of a geometric grid of identical squares with a central fixation point. The grid should be viewed by the patient wearing normal reading glasses. Each eye is tested separately. The patient is instructed to stare at the central fixation spot on the grid and report any distortion in the squares of the grid itself. For patients with macular problems, some of the squares may look faded, or the lines may be wavy. Patients with age-related macular degeneration are commonly given these Amsler grids to take home. The patient is encouraged to check them frequently, as often as daily, to detect any early signs of distortion that may indicate the development of a neovascular choroidal membrane, an advanced stage of macular degeneration characterized by the growth of abnormal choroidal vessels.

Ultrasonography

Lesions in the globe or the orbit may not be directly visible and are evaluated by ultrasonography. Ultrasonography is a very valuable diagnostic technique, especially when the view of the retina is obscured by opaque media such as cataract or hemorrhage. Ultrasonography can be used to identify orbital tumors, retinal detachment, and changes in tissue composition.

Special techniques can also be used to calculate the power for an intraocular lens implant and to obtain more anatomic information, showing cross-sectional images. Vitreous hemorrhage, retinal detachment, and tumors can be evaluated with minimal discomfort for the patient. Three-dimensional images can be created and the entire ultrasound examination can be recorded for later use.

Optical Coherence Tomography

Optical coherence tomography is an emerging technology that involves low coherence interferometry. Light is used to evaluate retinal and macular diseases as well as anterior segment conditions. This method is noninvasive and involves no physical contact with the eye.

Color Fundus Photography

Fundus photography is used to detect and document retinal lesions. The patient's pupils are widely dilated during the procedure, and visual acuity is diminished for about 30 minutes due to retinal "bleaching" by the intense flashing lights. The resulting fundus photographs can be viewed stereoscopically so that elevations such as macular edema can be identified.

Fluorescein Angiography

Fluorescein angiography evaluates clinically significant macular edema, documents macular capillary nonperfusion, and identifies retinal and choroidal **neovascularization** (growth of abnormal new blood vessels) in age-related macular degeneration. It is an invasive procedure in which fluorescein dye is injected, usually into an antecubital vein. Within 10 to 15 seconds, this dye can be seen coursing through the retinal vessels. Over a 10-minute period, serial black-and-white photographs are taken of the retinal vasculature. The dye may impart a gold tone to the skin of some patients, and urine may turn deep yellow or orange. This discoloration usually disappears in 24 hours.

Indocyanine Green Angiography

Indocyanine green angiography is used to evaluate abnormalities in the choroidal vasculature, conditions often seen in macular degeneration. Indocyanine green dye is injected intravenously (IV), and multiple images are captured using digital videoangiography over a period of 30 seconds to 20 minutes. The dye is generally well tolerated, but some patients experience nausea and vomiting. Allergic reactions are rare; however, indocyanine green angiography is contraindicated in patients with a history of iodide reactions.

Tonometry

Tonometry measures IOP by determining the amount of force or pressure necessary to indent or flatten (applanate) a small anterior area of the globe of the eye. The principle involved is that a soft eye is dented more easily than a hard eye. Pressure is measured in millimeters of mercury (mm Hg). High readings indicate high pressure; low readings indicate low pressure. The procedure is noninvasive and usually painless. A topical anesthetic eye drop is instilled in the lower conjunctival sac, and the tonometer is then used to measure the IOP.

Two of the most commonly used tonometers are the applanation tonometer and the Tono-Pen. The applanation tonometer is generally used by the more skilled examiner. A drop of fluorescein dye and an anesthetic drop are instilled in the eye. The applanation tip is pressed against the cornea and the examiner, looking through the slit lamp, obtains the IOP reading. The Tono-Pen is a portable, battery-operated, handheld tonometer that is commonly used in many clinical settings. A disposable cover is placed over the tip of the instrument, and it is held against the anesthetized cornea for a few seconds. The tension reading is displayed in a liquid crystal display window.

Perimetry Testing

Perimetry testing evaluates the field of vision. A visual field is the area or extent of physical space visible to an eye in a given position. Its average extent is 65 degrees upward, 75 degrees downward, 60 degrees inward, and 95 degrees outward when the eye is in the primary gaze (ie, looking directly forward). It has a three-dimensional contour representing areas of relative retinal sensitivity: visual acuity is sharpest at the very top of the field and declines progressively toward the periphery. Visual field testing (ie, perimetry) helps identify which parts of the patient's central and peripheral visual fields have useful vision. It is most helpful in detecting central **scotomas** (blind areas in the visual field) in macular degeneration and the peripheral field defects in glaucoma and retinitis pigmentosa.

The two methods of perimetric testing are manual and automated perimetry. Manual perimetry involves the use of moving (kinetic) or stationary (static) stimuli or targets. An example of kinetic manual perimetry is the tangent screen. A tangent screen is a black felt material mounted on a wall that has a series of concentric circles bisected by straight lines emanating from the center. It tests the central 30 degrees of the visual field. Automated perimetry uses stationary targets, which are more difficult to detect than moving targets. In this test, a computer projects light randomly in different areas of a hollow dome while the patient looks through a telescopic opening and depresses a button whenever he or she detects the light stimulus. Automated perimetry is more accurate than manual perimetry.

Impaired Vision

Refractive Errors

In refractive errors, vision is impaired because a shortened or elongated eyeball prevents light rays from focusing sharply on the retina. Blurred vision from refractive error can be corrected with eyeglasses or contact lenses. The appropriate eyeglass or contact lens is determined by **refraction.** Ophthalmic refraction consists of placing various types of lenses in front of the patient's eyes to determine which lens best improves the patient's vision.

The depth of the eyeball is important in determining refractive error (Fig. 58-6). Patients for whom the visual image focuses precisely on the macula and who do not need eyeglasses or contact lenses are said to have **emmetropia** (nor-

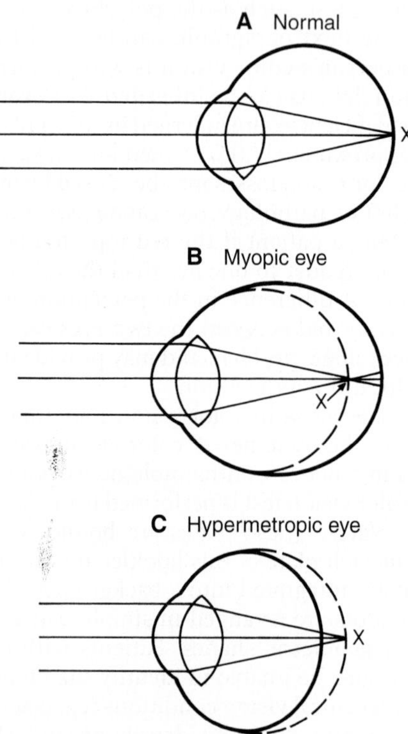

FIGURE 58-6. Eyeball shape determines visual acuity in refractive errors. (**A**) Normal eye. (**B**) Myopic eye. (**C**) Hypermetropic eye.

mal vision). People who have **myopia** are said to be nearsighted. They have deeper eyeballs; thus, the distant visual image focuses in front of, or short of, the retina. Myopic people experience blurred distance vision. When people have a shorter depth to their eyes, the visual image focuses beyond the retina; the eyes are shallower and are called hyperopic. People with **hyperopia** are farsighted. These patients experience near vision blurriness, whereas their distance vision is excellent.

Another important cause of refractive error is **astigmatism**, an irregularity in the curve of the cornea. Because astigmatism causes a distortion of the visual image, acuity of distance and near vision can be decreased. Hard contact lenses, which by means of their tear film correct astigmatic errors, or soft toric contact lenses with a cylinder correction may be used in place of eyeglasses for patients with astigmatism.

Ophthalmology has entered the era of customized vision correction in its desire to achieve "super-normal vision." A new method of measuring refractive error that includes sphere, cylinder, and higher-order aberrations is called wavefront technology. The most promising application for this technology is wavefront-guided refractive surgery. A customized laser ablation pattern is generated to reshape the cornea (Yeh & Azar, 2004).

Low Vision and Blindness

Low vision is a general term describing visual impairment that requires patients to use devices and strategies in addition to corrective lenses to perform visual tasks. Low vision is defined as a best corrected visual acuity (BCVA) of 20/70 to 20/200.

Blindness is defined as a BCVA that can range from 20/400 to no light perception (NLP). The clinical definition of absolute blindness is the absence of light perception. Legal blindness is a condition of impaired vision in which a person has a BCVA that does not exceed 20/200 in the better eye or whose widest visual field diameter is 20 degrees or less. This definition neither equates with functional ability nor classifies the degrees of visual impairment. Legal blindness ranges from an inability to perceive light to having some vision remaining. A person who meets the criteria for legal blindness may be eligible for government financial assistance.

Impaired vision is often accompanied by difficulty in performing functional activities. People with visual acuity of 20/80 to 20/100 with a visual field restriction of 60 degrees to greater than 20 degrees can read at a nearly normal level with optical aids. Their visual orientation is near normal but requires increased scanning of the environment (ie, systematic use of head and eye movements). In a visual acuity range of 20/200 to 20/400 with a 20-degree to greater than 10-degree visual field restriction, the person can read slowly with optical aids. His or her visual orientation is slow, with constant scanning of the environment. People in this category may have the ability to negotiate their environment without auxiliary aids. This ability is termed "travel vision." People with hand motion (HM) vision or no vision may benefit from the use of mobility devices (eg, cane, guide dog) and should be encouraged to learn Braille and to use computer aids.

The most common causes of blindness and visual impairment among adults 40 years of age or older are diabetic retinopathy, macular degeneration, glaucoma, and cataracts (Prevent Blindness America, 2002). Macular degeneration is more prevalent among Caucasians, whereas glaucoma is more prevalent among African Americans. Age-related changes in the eye are summarized in Table 58-1.

TABLE 58-1 Age-Related Changes in the Eye

The External Eye	Structural Change	Functional Change	History & Physical Findings
Eyelids and lacrimal structures	Loss of skin elasticity and orbital fat, decreased muscle tone; wrinkles develop	Lid margins turn in, causing lashes to irritate cornea and conjunctiva (entropian); or lid margins may turn out, resulting in increased corneal exposure (ectropian).	Reports of burning, foreign body sensation, increased tearing (epiphoria); injection, inflammation, and ulceration may occur
Refractive changes; presbyopia	Loss of accommodative power in the lens with age	Reading materials must be held at increasing distance in order to focus.	Patient reports, "Arms are too short!"; need for increased light; reading glasses or bifocals needed
Cataract	Opacities in the normally crystalline lens	Interference with the focus of a sharp image on the retina	Patients report increased glare, decreased vision, changes in color values (blue and yellow especially affected)
Posterior vitreous detachment	Liquefaction and shrinkage of vitreous body	May lead to retinal tears and detachment	Reports light flashes, cobwebs, floaters
Age-related macular degeneration (AMD)	Drusen (yellowish aging spots in the retina) appear and coalesce in the macula. Abnormal choroidal blood vessels may lead to formation of fibrotic disciform scars in the macula.	Central vision is affected; onset is more gradual in dry AMD, more rapid in wet AMD; distortion and loss of central vision may occur.	Reading vision is affected; words may be missing letters, faded areas appear on the page, straight lines may appear wavy; drusen, pigmentary changes in retina; abnormal submacular choroidal vessels

Assessment and Diagnostic Testing

The assessment of low vision includes a thorough history and the examination of distance and near visual acuity, visual field, contrast sensitivity, glare, color perception, and refraction. Specially designed, low-vision visual acuity charts are used to evaluate patients.

Patient Interview

During history taking, the cause and duration of the patient's visual impairment are identified. Patients with retinitis pigmentosa, for example, have a genetic abnormality. Patients with diabetic macular edema typically have fluctuating visual acuity. Patients with macular degeneration have central acuity problems. Central acuity problems cause difficulty in performing activities that require finer vision, such as reading. People with peripheral field defects have more difficulties with mobility. The patient's customary activities of daily living (ADLs), medication regimen, habits (eg, smoking), acceptance of the physical limitations brought about by the visual impairment, and realistic expectations of low-vision aids must be identified and included in the plan of care, including provision of guidelines for safety and referrals to social services.

Contrast-Sensitivity Testing and Glare Testing

Contrast-sensitivity testing measures visual acuity in different degrees of contrast. The initial test may take the form of simply turning on the lights while testing the distance acuity. If the patient can read better with the lights on, the patient can benefit from magnification. Glare testing enables the examiner to obtain a more realistic evaluation of the patient's ability to function in his or her environment. Glare can reduce a person's ability to see, especially in patients with cataracts. Devices that test glare, such as the Brightness Acuity Tester, produce three degrees of bright light to create a dazzle effect while the patient is viewing a target, such as Snellen letters on the wall. The lights have been calibrated to imitate certain objects that create glare, such as a car's headlights at night.

Medical Management

Managing low vision involves magnification and image enhancement through the use of low-vision aids and strategies and referrals to social services and community agencies serving those with visual impairment. The goals are to optimize the patient's remaining vision, whether central or peripheral, and assist the patient to perform customary activities. Low-vision aids include optical and nonoptical devices (Table 58-2). The optical devices include convex lens aids, such as magnifiers and spectacles; telescopic devices; antireflective lenses that diminish glare; and electronic reading systems, such as closed-circuit television and computers with large print. Continuing advances in computer software provide very useful products for patients with low vision. Scanners and the appropriate software enable the user to scan printed material and have it read by computer voice or enlarge the print for reading. Magnifiers can be hand-held or attached to a stand with or without illumination. Telescopic devices can be spectacle telescopes or clip-on or hand-held loupes.

The Internet continues to expand, and a telephone system has been developed that allows access to the Internet and e-mail using voice commands (Chart 58-2).

Referrals to community agencies may be necessary for patients with low vision who live alone and cannot self-administer their medications. Community agencies, such as the Lighthouse National Center for Vision and Aging, offer services to patients with low vision that include training in independent living skills and the provision of occupational

TABLE 58-2 Activities Affected by Visual Impairment and Visual Aids

Activity	Optical Aids	Nonoptical Aids
Shopping	Hand magnifier	Lighting, color cues
Fixing a snack	Bifocals	Color cues, consistent storage plan
Eating out	Hand magnifier	Flashlight, portable lamp
Identifying money	Bifocals, hand magnifier	Arrange paper money in wallet compartments
Reading print	High-power spectacle, bifocals, hand magnifier, stand magnifier, closed-circuit television	Lighting, high-contrast print, large print, reading slit
Writing	Hand magnifier, focusable telescope, closed-circuit television	Lighting, bold-tip pen, black ink
Using a telephone	Hand magnifier	Large print dial or touch tone buttons, hand-printed directory
Crossing streets	Telescope	Cane, ask directions
Finding taxis and bus signs	Telescope	Ask for assistance
Reading medication labels	Hand magnifier	Color codes, large print
Reading stove dials	Hand magnifier	Color codes, raised dots
Adjusting the thermostat	Hand magnifier	Enlarged print model
Using a computer	Spectacles	High-contrast color, large-print program
Reading signs	Spectacles	Move closer
Watching sporting event	Telescope	Sit in front rows

Adapted from Vaughn, D. G., Asbury, T., & Riorda-Eva, P. (Eds.). (1999). *General ophthalmology*. Stamford, CT: Appleton & Lange.

CHART 58-2

Web Access for the Visually Impaired

People with impaired vision need not be left behind in the computer age. Various technologies are available. A list of general equipment needs follows:

- Computer: software specifically developed for people with visual impairment.
- Internet service provider (eg, AOL, Netscape, Earthlink, Comcast)
- Screen-reader program: converts text on the computer screen to synthesized speech (eg, JAWS for Windows, Windows Eyes, Slimware Window Bridge, ProTalk 32, Hal Screen Reader, WinVision, WYNN, outSPOKEN for Windows)
- Browser program to navigate the World Wide Web (eg, Microsoft Internet Explorer, IBM Home Page Reader)

and recreational activities and a wide variety of assistive devices for vision enhancement and orientation and mobility.

Ophthalmologists have worked for years toward visual restoration for people who are blind, and computer technology now provides opportunities for restoring sight. Research is ongoing all over the world. Retinal implants for those whose optic nerves are functional as well as cortical implants for those whose optic nerves are diseased are being developed. For example, an experimental artificial silicon retina microchip is being developed for the treatment of patients with retinitis pigmentosa (Chow, Chow, Packo, et al., 2004). The rapid changes in technology and miniaturization of computer chips may enable dramatic advances in synthetic vision in the future.

Nursing Management

Coping with blindness involves three types of adaptation: emotional, physical, and social. The emotional adjustment to blindness or severe visual impairment determines the success of the physical and social adjustments of the patient. Successful emotional adjustment means acceptance of blindness or severe visual impairment.

Promoting Coping Efforts

Effective coping may not occur until the patient recognizes the permanence of the blindness. Clinging to false hopes of regaining vision hampers effective adaptation to blindness. A newly blind patient and his or her family members (especially those who live with the patient) undergo the various steps of grieving: denial and shock, anger and protest, restitution, loss resolution, and acceptance. The ability to accept the changes that must come with visual loss and willingness to adapt to those changes influence the successful rehabilitation of the patient who is blind. Additional aspects to consider are value changes, independence–dependence conflicts, coping with stigma, and learning to function in social settings without visual cues and landmarks.

Promoting Spatial Orientation and Mobility

A person who is blind or severely visually impaired requires strategies for adapting to the environment. ADLs, such as walking to a chair from a bed, require spatial concepts. The person needs to know where he or she is in relation to the rest of the room, to understand the changes that may occur, and to know how to approach the desired location safely. This requires a collaborative effort between the patient and the responsible adult who serves as the sighted guide.

A patient whose visual impairment results from a chronic progressive eye disorder, such as glaucoma, has better cognitive mapping skills than the patient who becomes blind suddenly. Patients with progressive eye disorders develop the use of spatial and topographic concepts early and gradually; hence, remembering a room layout is easier for them. Patients who become blind suddenly have more difficulty in adjusting, and emotional and behavioral issues of coping with blindness may hinder their learning. These patients require intensive emotional support. The nurse must assess the degree of physical assistance the person with vision loss requires and communicate this to other health care personnel.

In the hospital, the bedside table and the call button must always be within reach. The parts of the call button are explained, and the patient is taught to touch and press the buttons or dials until the activity is mastered. The patient must be familiarized with the location of the telephone, water pitcher, and other objects on the bedside table. The food tray's composition is likened to the face of a clock; for example, the main plate may be described as being at 12 o'clock or the coffee cup at 3 o'clock. All articles and furniture must remain in the same positions throughout the patient's hospitalization. The nurse should introduce herself upon entering a patient's room and alert the patient to his or her departure. Such habits are always polite and help in the care of a patient with vision loss.

The nurse should be aware of the importance of techniques in providing physical assistance, encouraging independence, and ensuring safety. Specific guidelines for interacting with the patient with vision loss are presented in Chart 58-3. The readiness of the patient and his or her family to learn must be assessed before initiating orientation and mobility training.

Promoting Home and Community-Based Care

The nurse, social worker, family, and others collaborate to assess the patient's home condition and support system. If available, a low-vision specialist or occupational therapist should be consulted, particularly for patients for whom identifying and administering medications pose problems. The level of visual acuity and patient preference help determine appropriate interventions. Some private and nonprofit services are identified in the Resources section at the end of this chapter.

Other interventions that are appropriate for some people with low vision or blindness include Braille and guide dogs. Recent rapid advances in technology have led to the

CHART 58-3

Guidelines for Interacting With People Who Are Blind Or Have Low Vision

- Remember that the only difference between you and people who are blind or have low vision is that they are not able to see through their eyes what you are able to see through yours.
- Do not be uncomfortable when in the company of a person who is blind or has low vision. Talk with the person as you would talk with any other individual, honestly and without pity; do not be concerned about using words like "see" and "look." There is no need to raise your voice unless the person asks you to do so.
- Identify yourself as you approach the person and before you make physical contact. Tell the person your name and your role. If another person approaches, introduce him or her. When you leave the room, be sure to tell the person that you are leaving and if anyone else remains in the room.
- It is often appropriate to touch the person's hand or arm lightly to indicate that you are about to speak.
- When talking, face the person and speak directly to him or her using a normal tone of voice.
- Be specific when communicating direction. Mention a specific distance or use clock cues when possible (eg, walk left about 2 yards; walk about 20 feet to the right; the telephone is at 2 o'clock). Avoid using phrases such as "over there."
- When you offer to assist someone, allow the person to hold onto your arm just above the elbow and to walk a half-step behind you.
- When offering the person a seat, place the person's hand on the back or the arm of the seat.
- When you are about to go up or down a flight of stairs, tell the person and place his or her hand on the banister.
- Make sure that the environment is free of obstacles; close doors and cabinets so they are not in the path.
- Offer to read written information, such as a menu.
- If you serve food to the person, use clock cues to specify where everything is on the plate.
- When the person who is blind or who has low vision is a patient in a health care facility:
  - Make sure all objects the person will need are close at hand.
  - Identify the location of objects that the person may need (eg, "The call light is near your right hand"; "The telephone is on the table on the left side of your bed.")
  - Remove obstacles that may be in the person's pathway and could cause a fall.
  - Place all assistive devices the person uses close at hand; let the person feel the devices so that he or she knows their location.
- Do not distract the service animal unless the owner has given permission.
- Ask the person, "How can I help you?" At some times the person needs help, but at other times help may not be needed.

This material is adapted from and based in part on *Achieving Physical and Communication Accessibility,* a publication of the National Center for Access Unlimited; *Community Access Facts,* an Adaptive Environments Center publication; and *The Ten Commandments of Interacting with People with Mental Health Disabilities,* a publication of The Ability Center of Greater Toledo.

erroneous conclusion by some that Braille is an outmoded communication tool. There has been an ever-increasing reliance on print magnification technology as well as computer-assisted speech output. However, although the use of Braille may be less important for adults who have already learned language and grammar skills, educators and low-vision specialists have continued to advocate that children who are legally blind be given the opportunity to learn Braille. One study (Ryles, 1996) has found that future employment success is increased when Braille is used as the original medium for children learning to read.

Guide dogs, also known as Seeing-Eye dogs, are dogs that are specially bred, raised, and rigorously trained to assist people who are blind. The guide dog is a constant companion to the person who is blind (also referred to as the animal's handler) and is allowed on airplanes and in restaurants, stores, hotels, and other public places. With the assistance of the guide dog, the person who is blind can be extremely mobile and accomplish normal activities both within and outside of the home and workplace. A dog in harness is a working dog, not a pet. The dog should not be distracted from his job by well-intentioned strangers who want to pet, feed, or play with him. The dog's handler should always be consulted before approaching the working guide dog. Most health care facilities have a service animal policy that outlines the responsibilities of the handler with regard to the care of the animal.

Glaucoma

Glaucoma is a group of ocular conditions characterized by optic nerve damage. The optic nerve damage is related to the IOP caused by congestion of aqueous humor in the eye. There is a range of pressures that have been considered "normal" but that may be associated with vision loss in some patients. Glaucoma is one of the leading causes of irreversible blindness in the world and is the leading cause of blindness among adults in the United States. It is estimated that at least 3 million Americans have glaucoma and that 5 to 10 million more are at risk (Schachat, Quigley, Schein, et al., 2004). Glaucoma is more prevalent among people older than 40 years of age, and the incidence increases with age. It is also more prevalent among men than women and in African-American and Asian populations (Chart 58-4). There is no cure for glaucoma, but research continues.

Physiology

Aqueous humor flows between the iris and the lens, nourishing the cornea and lens. Most (90%) of the fluid then flows out of the anterior chamber, draining through the spongy trabecular meshwork into the canal of Schlemm and the episcleral veins (Fig. 58-7). About 10% of the aqueous fluid exits through the ciliary body into the suprachoroidal space and then drains into the venous circulation of the ciliary body, choroid, and sclera. Unimpeded outflow of aqueous fluid depends on an intact drainage system and an open angle (about 45 degrees) between the iris and the cornea. A narrower angle places the iris closer to the trabecular meshwork, diminishing the angle. The amount of aqueous humor produced tends to decrease with age, in systemic diseases such as diabetes, and in ocular inflammatory conditions.

IOP is determined by the rate of aqueous production, the resistance encountered by the aqueous humor as it flows out of the passages, and the venous pressure of the episcleral veins that drain into the anterior ciliary vein. When aqueous fluid production and drainage are in balance, the IOP is between 10 and 21 mm Hg. When aqueous fluid is inhibited from flowing out, pressure builds up within the eye. Fluctuations in IOP occur with time of day, exertion, diet, and medications. IOP tends to increase with blinking, tight lid squeezing, and upward gazing. Systemic conditions such as hypertension and intraocular conditions such as uveitis and retinal detachment have been associated with elevated IOP.

CHART 58-4

Risk Factors for Glaucoma

- Family history of glaucoma
- African-American race
- Older age
- Diabetes mellitus
- Cardiovascular disease
- Migraine syndromes
- Nearsightedness (myopia)
- Eye trauma
- Prolonged use of topical or systemic corticosteroids

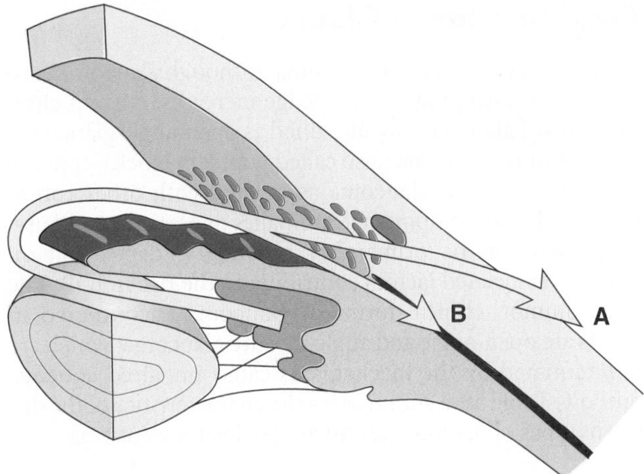

FIGURE 58-7. Normal outflow of aqueous humor. (**A**) Trabecular meshwork. (**B**) Uveoscleral route. From Kanski, J. J. (2003). *Clinical ophthalmology*. Oxford: Butterworth-Heinemann Ltd.

Pathophysiology

There are two accepted theories regarding how increased IOP damages the optic nerve in glaucoma. The direct mechanical theory suggests that high IOP damages the retinal layer as it passes through the optic nerve head. The indirect ischemic theory suggests that high IOP compresses the microcirculation in the optic nerve head, resulting in cell injury and death. Some glaucomas appear as exclusively mechanical, and some are exclusively ischemic types. Typically, most cases are a combination of both. Regardless of the cause of damage, glaucomatous changes typically evolve through clearly discernible stages (Chart 58-5).

CHART 58-5

Stages of Glaucoma

1. **Initiating events.** Precipitating factors include illness, emotional stress, congenital narrow angles, long-term use of corticosteroids, and use of mydriatics (ie, medications causing pupillary dilation). These events lead to the second stage.
2. **Structural alterations in the aqueous outflow system.** Tissue and cellular changes caused by factors that affect aqueous humor dynamics lead to structural alterations and to the third stage.
3. **Functional alterations.** Conditions such as increased intraocular pressure or impaired blood flow create functional changes that lead to the fourth stage.
4. **Optic nerve damage.** Atrophy of the optic nerve is characterized by loss of nerve fibers and blood supply. This fourth stage inevitably progresses to the fifth stage.
5. **Visual loss.** Progressive loss of vision is characterized by visual field defects.

Classification of Glaucoma

There are several types of glaucoma. Although glaucoma classification is changing as knowledge increases, current clinical forms of glaucoma are identified as open-angle glaucoma, angle-closure glaucoma (also called pupillary block), congenital glaucoma, and glaucoma associated with other conditions, such as developmental anomalies or corticosteroid use. Glaucoma can be primary or secondary, depending on whether associated factors contribute to the rise in IOP. The two common clinical forms of glaucoma encountered in adults are open-angle and angle-closure glaucoma, which are differentiated by the mechanisms cause impaired aqueous outflow. Table 58-3 summarizes the characteristics of the different types of open-angle and angle-closure glaucoma.

Clinical Manifestations

Glaucoma is often called the "silent thief of sight" because most patients are unaware that they have the disease until they have experienced visual changes and vision loss. The patient may not seek health care until he or she experiences blurred vision or "halos" around lights, difficulty focusing, difficulty adjusting eyes in low lighting, loss of peripheral vision, aching or discomfort around the eyes, and headache.

Assessment and Diagnostic Findings

The purpose of a glaucoma workup is to establish the diagnostic category, assess the optic nerve damage, and formulate a treatment plan. The patient's ocular and medical history must be detailed to investigate the history of predisposing factors. Four major types of examinations are used in glaucoma evaluation, diagnosis, and management: tonometry to measure the IOP, ophthalmoscopy to inspect the optic nerve, gonioscopy to examine the filtration angle of the anterior chamber, and perimetry to assess the visual fields.

The changes in the optic nerve related to glaucoma are pallor and cupping of the optic nerve disc. The pallor of the optic nerve is caused by a lack of blood supply that results

TABLE 58-3 Glaucoma Types, Clinical Manifestation, and Treatment

Types of Glaucoma	Clinical Manifestations	Treatment
Open-Angle Glaucoma		
Usually bilateral, but one eye may be more severely affected than the other. In all three types of open-angle glaucoma, the anterior chamber angle is open and appears normal.		
Chronic open-angle glaucoma (COAG)	Optic nerve damage, visual field defects, IOP >21 mm Hg. May have fluctuating IOPs. Usually no symptoms but possible ocular pain, headache, and halos.	Decrease IOP 20% to 50%. Additional topical and oral agents added as necessary. If medical treatment is unsuccessful, laser trabeculoplasty (LT) can decrease intraocular pressure by 20%. Glaucoma filtering surgery if continued optic nerve damage despite medication therapy and LT.
Normal tension glaucoma	IOP ≤ 21 mm Hg. Optic nerve damage, visual field defects.	Treatment similar to COAG, however, the best management for normal tension glaucoma management is yet to be established. Goal is to lower the IOP by at least 30%.
Ocular hypertension	Elevated IOP. Possible ocular pain or headache.	Decrease IOP by at least 20%.
Angle-Closure (Pupillary Block) Glaucoma		
Obstruction in aqueous humor outflow due to the complete or partial closure of the angle from the forward shift of the peripheral iris to the trabecula. The obstruction results in an increased IOP.		
Acute angle-closure glaucoma (AACG)	Rapidly progressive visual impairment, periocular pain, conjunctival hyperemia, and congestion. Pain may be associated with nausea, vomiting, bradycardia, and profuse sweating. Reduced central visual acuity, severely elevated IOP, corneal edema. Pupil is vertically oval, fixed in a semi-dilated position, and unreactive to light and accommodation.	Ocular emergency; administration of hyperosmotics, azetazolamide, and topical ocular hypotensive agents, such as pilocarpine and beta-blockers (betaxolol). Possible laser incision in the iris (iridotomy) to release blocked aqueous and reduce IOP. Other eye is also treated with pilocarpine eye drops and/or surgical management to avoid a similar spontaneous attack.
Subacute angle-closure glaucoma	Transient blurring of vision, halos around lights; temporal headaches and/or ocular pain; pupil may be semi-dilated.	Prophylactic peripheral laser iridotomy. Can lead to acute or chronic angle-closure glaucoma if untreated.
Chronic angle-closure glaucoma	Progression of glaucomatous cupping and significant visual field loss; IOP may be normal or elevated; ocular pain and headache.	Management similar to that for COAG: includes laser iridotomy and medications.

IOP, intraocular pressure.

from cellular destruction. Cupping is characterized by exaggerated bending of the blood vessels as they cross the optic disc, resulting in an enlarged optic cup that appears more basin-like compared with a normal cup. The progression of cupping in glaucoma is caused by the gradual loss of retinal nerve fibers accompanied by the loss of blood supply, resulting in increased pallor of the optic disc.

As the optic nerve damage increases, visual perception in the area is lost. The localized areas of visual loss (ie, scotomas) represent loss of retinal sensitivity and are measured and mapped by perimetry. The results are mapped on a graph. In patients with glaucoma, the graph has a distinct pattern that is different from other ocular diseases and is useful in establishing the diagnosis. Figure 58-8 shows the progression of visual field defects caused by glaucoma.

Medical Management

The aim of all glaucoma treatment is prevention of optic nerve damage. Lifelong therapy is almost always necessary because glaucoma cannot be cured. Treatment focuses on pharmacologic therapy, laser procedures, surgery, or a combination of these approaches, all of which have potential complications and side effects. The object is to achieve the greatest benefit at the least risk, cost, and inconvenience to the patient. Although treatment cannot reverse optic nerve damage, further damage can be controlled. The goal is to maintain an IOP within a range unlikely to cause further damage.

The initial target for IOP among patients with elevated IOP and those with low-tension glaucoma with progressive visual field loss is typically set at 30% lower than the current pressure. The patient is monitored for changes in the appearance of the optic nerve. If there is evidence of progressive damage, the target IOP is again lowered until the optic nerve shows stability.

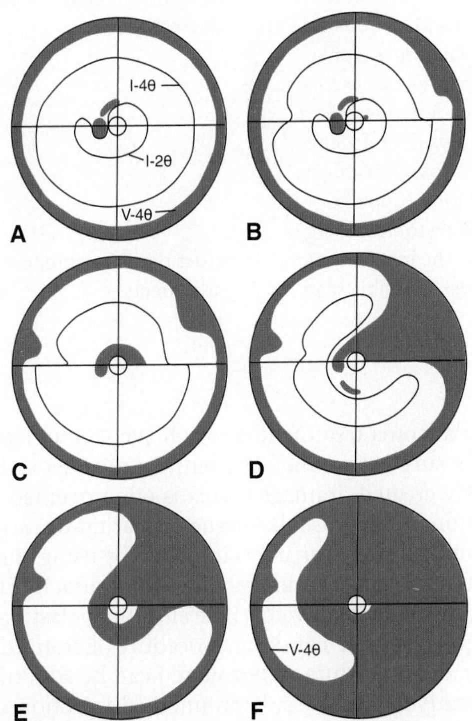

FIGURE 58-8. Progression of glaucomatous visual field defects. A central scotoma at 10 to 20 degrees of fixation near the blind spot is the initial significant finding (**A, B**). As the glaucoma progresses, the scotomas enlarge and deepen, resulting in peripheral vision loss. (**C**) Defect within 5 degrees of fixation point nasally. (**D**) Peripheral involvement enlarges. (**E**) Ringlike scotoma. (**F**) Eventually, vision is lost. The resulting "island of vision" becomes the characteristic visual field appearance of glaucoma and correlates with the "tunnel vision," in which peripheral vision is lost. From Kanski, J. J. (2003). *Clinical ophthalmology*. Oxford: Butterworth-Heinemann Ltd.

Pharmacologic Therapy

Medical management of glaucoma relies on systemic and topical ocular medications that lower IOP. Periodic follow-up examinations are essential to monitor IOP, the appearance of the optic nerve, the visual fields, and side effects of medications. Therapy takes into account the patient's health and stage of glaucoma. Comfort, affordability, convenience, lifestyle, and personality are factors to consider in the patient's adherence to the medical regimen.

The patient is usually started on the lowest dose of topical medication and then advanced to increased concentrations until the desired IOP level is reached and maintained. Because of their efficacy, minimal dosing (can be used once each day), and low cost, beta-blockers are the preferred initial topical medications. One eye is treated first, with the other eye used as a control in determining the efficacy of the medication; once efficacy has been established, treatment of the other eye is started. If the IOP is elevated in both eyes, both are treated. When results are not satisfactory, a new medication is substituted. The main markers of the efficacy of the medication in glaucoma control are lowering of the IOP to the target pressure, appearance of the optic nerve head, and the visual field.

Several types of ocular medications are used to treat glaucoma (Table 58-4), including **miotics** (medications that cause pupillary constriction), adrenergic agonists (ie, sympathomimetic agents), beta-blockers, alpha$_2$-agonists (ie, adrenergic agents), carbonic anhydrase inhibitors, and prostaglandins. Cholinergics (ie, miotics) increase the outflow of the aqueous humor by affecting ciliary muscle contraction and pupil constriction, allowing flow through a larger opening between the iris and the trabecular meshwork. Adrenergic agonists increase aqueous outflow but primarily decrease aqueous production with an action similar to beta-blockers and carbonic anhydrase inhibitors.

Surgical Management

In *laser trabeculoplasty* for glaucoma, laser burns are applied to the inner surface of the trabecular meshwork to open the intratrabecular spaces and widen the canal of Schlemm, thereby promoting outflow of aqueous humor and decreasing IOP. The procedure is indicated when IOP is inadequately controlled by medications; it is contraindicated when the trabecular meshwork cannot be fully visualized because of narrow angles. A serious complication of this procedure is a transient increase in IOP (usually 2 hours after surgery) that may become persistent. IOP assessment in the immediate postoperative period is essential.

TABLE 58-4 Medications Used in the Management of Glaucoma

Medication	Action	Side Effects	Nursing Implications
Cholinergics (miotics) (pilocarpine, carbachol)	Increases aqueous fluid outflow by contracting the ciliary muscle and causing miosis (constriction of the pupil) and opening of trabecular meshwork	Periorbital pain, blurry vision, difficulty seeing in the dark	Caution patients about diminished vision in dimly lit areas.
Adrenergic agonists (dipivefrin, epinephrine)	Reduces production of aqueous humor and increases outflow	Eye redness and burning; can have systemic effects, including palpitations, elevated blood pressure, tremor, headaches, and anxiety	Teach patients punctal occlusion to limit systemic effects (described in Chart 58-13).
Beta-blockers (betaxolol, timolol)	Decreases aqueous humor production	Can have systemic effects, including bradycardia, exacerbation of pulmonary disease, and hypotension	Contraindicated in patients with asthma, chronic obstructive pulmonary disease, second- or third-degree heart block, bradycardia, or cardiac failure; teach patients punctal occlusion to limit systemic effects
Alpha-adrenergic agonists (apraclonidine, brimonidine)	Decreases aqueous humor production	Eye redness, dry mouth and nasal passages	Teach patients punctal occlusion to limit systemic effects.
Carbonic anhydrase inhibitors (acetazolamide, methazolamide, dorzolamide)	Decreases aqueous humor production	Oral medications (acetazolamide and methazolamide) associated with serious side effects, including anaphylactic reactions, electrolyte loss, depression, lethargy, gastrointestinal upset, impotence, and weight loss; side effects of topical form (dorzolamide) include topical allergy	Do not administer to patients with sulfa allergies; monitor electrolyte levels.
Prostaglandin analogs (latanoprost)	Increases uveoscleral outflow	Darkening of the iris, conjunctival redness, possible rash	Instruct patients to report any side effects.

In *laser iridotomy* for pupillary block glaucoma, an opening is made in the iris to eliminate the pupillary block. Laser iridotomy is contraindicated in patients with corneal edema, which interferes with laser targeting and strength. Potential complications are burns to the cornea, lens, or retina; transient elevated IOP; closure of the iridotomy; uveitis; and blurring. Pilocarpine is usually prescribed to prevent closure of the iridotomy.

Filtering procedures for chronic glaucoma are used to create an opening or fistula in the trabecular meshwork to drain aqueous humor from the anterior chamber to the subconjunctival space into a bleb, thereby bypassing the usual drainage structures. This allows the aqueous humor to flow and exit by different routes (ie, absorption by the conjunctival vessels or mixing with tears). *Trabeculectomy* is the standard filtering technique used to remove part of the trabecular meshwork. Complications include hemorrhage, an extremely low (hypotony) or elevated IOP, uveitis, cataracts, bleb failure, bleb leak, and endophthalmitis. Unlike other surgical procedures, the filtering procedure's goal in glaucoma treatment is to achieve incomplete healing of the surgical wound. The outflow of aqueous humor in a newly created drainage fistula is circumvented by the granulation of fibrovascular tissue or scar tissue formation on the surgical site. Scarring is inhibited by using antifibrosis agents such as the antimetabolites fluorouracil (Efudex) and mitomycin (Mutamycin). Like all antineoplastic agents, they require special handling procedures before, during, and after the procedure. Fluorouracil can be administered intraoperatively and by subconjunctival injection during follow-up; mitomycin is much more potent and is administered only intraoperatively.

Drainage implants or *shunts* are open tubes implanted in the anterior chamber to shunt aqueous humor to an attached plate in the conjunctival space. These implants are used when failure has occurred with one or more trabeculectomies in which antifibrotic agents were used. A fibrous capsule develops around the episcleral plate and filters the aqueous humor, thereby regulating the outflow and controlling IOP.

Nursing Management

Promoting Home and Community-Based Care

TEACHING PATIENTS SELF-CARE

The medical and surgical management of glaucoma slows the progression of glaucoma but does not cure it. The lifelong therapeutic regimen mandates patient education. The nature of the disease and the importance of strict adherence to the medication regimen must be included in a teaching plan to help ensure compliance. A thorough patient interview is essential to determine systemic conditions, current systemic and ocular medications, family history, and problems with compliance to glaucoma medications. Then the medication program can be discussed, particularly the interactions of glaucoma-control medications with other medications. For example, the diuretic effect of acetazolamide has an additive effect on the diuretic effects of other antihypertensive medications and can result in hypokalemia. The effects of glaucoma-control medications on vision must also be explained. Miotics and sympathomimetics result in altered focus; therefore, patients need to be cautious in navigating their surroundings. Information about instilling ocular medication and preventing systemic absorption with punctal occlusion is given in the section on ophthalmic medications.

Nurses in all settings encounter patients with glaucoma. Even patients with longstanding disease and those with glaucoma as a secondary diagnosis should be assessed for knowledge level and compliance with the therapeutic regimen. Chart 58-6 contains points to review with patients with glaucoma.

CONTINUING CARE

For the patient with severe glaucoma and impaired function, referral to services that assist the patient in performing ADLs may be needed. The loss of peripheral vision impairs mobility the most. These patients need to be referred for low vision and rehabilitation services. Patients who meet the criteria for legal blindness should be offered referrals to agencies that can assist them in obtaining federal assistance.

Reassurance and emotional support are important aspects of care. A lifelong disease involving possible loss of sight has psychological, physical, social, and vocational ramifications. The family must be integrated into the plan of care, and because the disease has a familial tendency, family members should be encouraged to undergo examinations at least once every 2 years to detect glaucoma early.

CHART 58-6

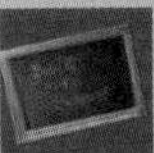

Patient Education

Managing Glaucoma

- Know your intraocular pressure (IOP) measurement and the desired range.
- Be informed about the extent of your vision loss and optic nerve damage.
- Keep a record of your eye pressure measurements and visual field test results to monitor your own progress.
- Review all your medications (including over-the-counter and herbal medications) with your ophthalmologist, and mention any side effects each time you visit.
- Ask about potential side effects and drug interactions of your eye medications.
- Ask whether generic or less costly forms of your eye medications are available.
- Review the dosing schedule with your ophthalmologist and inform him or her if you have trouble following the schedule.
- Participate in the decision-making process. Let your doctor know what dosing schedule works for you and other preferences regarding your eye care.
- Have the nurse observe you instilling eye medication to determine whether you are administering it properly.
- Be aware that glaucoma medications can cause adverse effects if used inappropriately. Eye drops are to be administered as prescribed, not when eyes feel irritated.
- Ask your ophthalmologist to send a report to your doctor after each appointment.
- Keep all follow-up appointments.

Cataracts

A cataract is a lens opacity or cloudiness (Fig. 58-9). Cataracts rank behind only arthritis and heart disease as a leading cause of disability in older adults. Cataracts affect nearly 20.5 million Americans who are 40 years of age or older, or about one in every six people in this age range. By 80 years of age, more than half of all Americans have cataracts. According to the World Health Organization, cataract is the leading cause of blindness in the world (Prevent Blindness America, 2002).

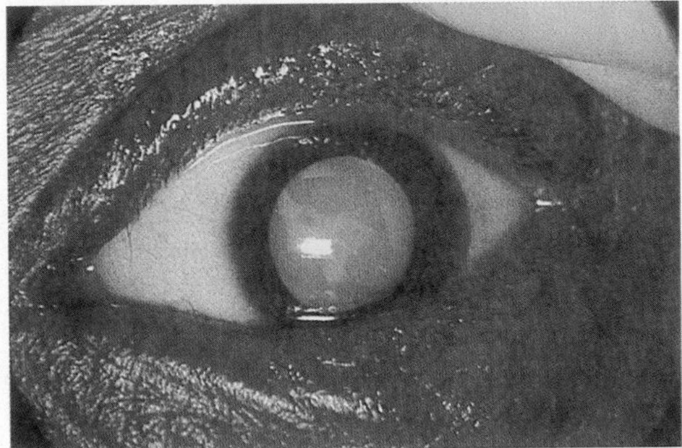

FIGURE 58-9. A cataract is a cloudy or opaque lens. On visual inspection, the lens appears gray or milky. From Rubin, E., Gorstein, F., Rubin, R., et al. (2005). *Pathology* (4th ed.). Philadelphia: Lippincott Williams & Wilkins.

Pathophysiology

Cataracts can develop in one or both eyes at any age for a variety of causes (Chart 58-7). Recent studies have linked cataract risk to lower income and educational level, smoking history for 35 or more pack-years, and high triglyceride levels in men (Klein, Klein, Lee, et al, 2003). Visual impairment normally progresses at the same rate in both eyes over many years or in a matter of months. The three most common types of senile (age-related) cataracts are defined by their location in the lens: nuclear, cortical, and posterior subcapsular. The extent of visual impairment depends on their size, density, and location in the lens. More than one type can be present in one eye.

A nuclear cataract is caused by central opacity in the lens and has a substantial genetic component. It is associated with myopia (ie, nearsightedness), which worsens when the cataract progresses. If dense, the cataract severely blurs vision. Periodic changes in prescription eyeglasses help manage this condition.

A cortical cataract involves the anterior, posterior, or equatorial cortex of the lens. A cataract in the equator or periphery of the cortex does not interfere with the passage of light through the center of the lens and has little effect on vision. Cortical cataracts progress at a highly variable rate. Vision is worse in very bright light. Studies show that people with the highest levels of sunlight exposure have twice the risk of developing cortical cataracts as those with low-level sunlight exposure (West, Muñoz, Schein, et al., 1998).

Posterior subcapsular cataracts occur in front of the posterior capsule. This type typically develops in younger people and, in some cases, is associated with prolonged corticosteroid use, diabetes, or ocular trauma. Near vision is diminished, and the eye is increasingly sensitive to glare from bright light (eg, sunlight, headlights). Studies in the United States have shown that Caucasians are more likely to develop nuclear and posterior subcapsular cataracts, whereas cortical cataracts are more prevalent among African Americans (West et al., 1998). Some studies have found that occupational sun exposure in people between 20 and 29 years of age is associated with nuclear cataract formation (Neale, Purdie, Hirst, et al., 2003).

CHART 58-7

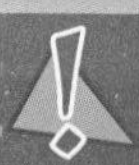

Risk Factors for Cataract Formation

Aging

- Loss of lens transparency
- Clumping or aggregation of lens protein (which leads to light scattering)
- Accumulation of a yellow-brown pigment due to the breakdown of lens protein
- Decreased oxygen uptake
- Increase in sodium and calcium
- Decrease in levels of vitamin C, protein, and glutathione (an antioxidant)

Associated Ocular Conditions

- Retinitis pigmentosa
- Myopia
- Retinal detachment and retinal surgery
- Infection (eg, herpes zoster, uveitis)

Toxic Factors

- Corticosteroids, especially at high doses and in long-term use
- Alkaline chemical eye burns, poisoning
- Cigarette smoking
- Calcium, copper, iron, gold, silver, and mercury, which tend to deposit in the pupillary area of the lens

Nutritional Factors

- Reduced levels of antioxidants
- Poor nutrition
- Obesity

Physical Factors

- Dehydration associated with chronic diarrhea, use of purgatives in anorexia nervosa, and use of hyperbaric oxygenation
- Blunt trauma, perforation of the lens with a sharp object or foreign body, electric shock
- Ultraviolet radiation in sunlight and x-ray

Systemic Diseases and Syndromes

- Diabetes mellitus
- Down syndrome
- Disorders related to lipid metabolism
- Renal disorders
- Musculoskeletal disorders

Clinical Manifestations

Painless, blurry vision is characteristic of cataracts. The person perceives that surroundings are dimmer, as if his or her glasses need cleaning. Light scattering is common, and the person experiences reduced contrast sensitivity, sensitivity to glare, and reduced visual acuity. Other effects include myopic shift, astigmatism, monocular **diplopia** (double vision), color shift (the aging lens becomes progressively more absorbent at the blue end of the spectrum), brunescens (color values shift to yellow-brown), and reduced light transmission.

Assessment and Diagnostic Findings

Decreased visual acuity is directly proportionate to cataract density. The Snellen visual acuity test, ophthalmoscopy, and slit-lamp biomicroscopic examination are used to establish the degree of cataract formation. The degree of lens opacity does not always correlate with the patient's functional status. Some patients can perform normal activities despite clinically significant cataracts. Others with less lens opacification have a disproportionate decrease in visual acuity; hence, visual acuity is an imperfect measure of visual impairment.

Medical Management

No nonsurgical (medications, eyedrops, eyeglasses) treatment cures cataracts or prevents age-related cataracts. Results from the Age-Related Eye Disease Research Study (2001), a randomized, placebo-controlled trial, found no benefit from antioxidant supplements, vitamins C and E, beta-carotene, and selenium. However, cigarette smoking, long-term use of corticosteroids, especially at high doses, sunlight and ionizing radiation, diabetes, obesity, and eye injuries can increase the risk for cataracts. In the early stages of cataract development, glasses, contact lenses, strong bifocals, or magnifying lenses may improve vision.

Surgical Management

In general, if reduced vision from cataract does not interfere with normal activities, surgery may not be needed. In deciding when cataract surgery is to be performed, the patient's functional and visual status should be a primary consideration. Surgery is performed on an outpatient basis and usually takes less than 1 hour, with the patient being discharged in 30 minutes or less afterward. Although complications from cataract surgery are uncommon, they can have significant effects on vision (Table 58-5). Restoration of visual function through a safe and minimally invasive procedure is the surgical goal, which is achieved with advances in topical anesthesia, smaller wound incision (ie, clear cornea incision), and lens design (ie, foldable and more accurate intraocular lens measurements).

Injection-free topical and intraocular anesthesia, such as 1% lidocaine gel applied to the surface of the eye, eliminates the hazards of regional (retrobulbar and peribulbar) anesthesia, such as ocular perforation, retrobulbar hemorrhage, optic injuries, diplopia, and ptosis, and is ideal for patients receiving anticoagulants. Furthermore, patients can communicate and cooperate during surgery. Intravenous (IV) moderate sedation may used to minimize anxiety and discomfort.

When both eyes have cataracts, one eye is treated first, with at least several weeks, preferably months, separating the two procedures. Because cataract surgery is performed to improve visual functioning, the delay for the other eye gives time for the patient and the surgeon to evaluate whether the results from the first surgery are adequate to preclude the need for a second operation. The delay also provides time for the first eye to recover; if there are any complications, the surgeon may decide to perform the second procedure differently.

INTRACAPSULAR CATARACT EXTRACTION

In intracapsular cataract extraction, the entire lens (ie, nucleus, cortex, and capsule) is removed and fine sutures are used to close the incision. From the late 1800s until the 1970s, it was the technique of choice for cataract extraction. It is infrequently performed today but is still indicated when there is a need to remove the entire lens, such as with a subluxated cataract (ie, partially or completely dislocated lens).

EXTRACAPSULAR CATARACT EXTRACTION

The extracapsular cataract extraction technique involves smaller incisional wounds (less trauma to the eye) and maintains the posterior capsule of the lens, reducing postoperative complications, particularly aphakic retinal detachment and cystoid macular edema. A portion of the anterior capsule is removed, allowing extraction of the lens nucleus and cortex. The posterior capsule and zonular support are left intact. An intact zonular–capsular diaphragm provides the needed safe anchor for the posterior chamber intraocular lens (IOL). After the pupil has been dilated and the surgeon has made a small incision on the upper edge of the cornea, a viscoelastic substance (clear gel) is injected into the space between the cornea and the lens. This prevents the space from collapsing and facilitates insertion of the IOL.

PHACOEMULSIFICATION

This method of extracapsular surgery uses an ultrasonic device that liquefies the nucleus and cortex, which are then suctioned out through a tube. The posterior capsule is left intact. Because the incision is even smaller than the standard extracapsular cataract extraction, the wound heals more rapidly, and there is early stabilization of refractive error and less astigmatism. Hardware and software advances in ultrasonic technology—including new phaco needles that are used to cut and aspirate the cataract—permit safe and efficient removal of nearly all cataracts through a clear cornea incision. With increasing frequency, self-sealing (sutureless) clear corneal incisions (temporal part of the cornea) are performed with phacoemulsification, minimizing postoperative astigmatism and thus decreasing bleeding and subconjunctival hemorrhage and speeding recovery of visual acuity.

However, studies have revealed an increased incidence of postoperative endophthalmitis, or inflammation of ocular tissue (Taban, Behrens, Newcomb, et al., 2005). An in vitro study concluded that the transient reduction of IOP might result in poor wound apposition with the potential fluid flow across the cornea and into the anterior chamber increasing the risk of endophthalmitis. Innovations are underway for laser phacoemulsification with low heat generation and smaller incision size, minimizing induced astigmatism, improving wound integrity, and promoting the use of injectable IOLs (Hoffman, Fine, & Packer, 2005).

LENS REPLACEMENT

After removal of the crystalline lens, the patient is referred to as *aphakic* (ie, without lens). The lens, which focuses light on the retina, must be replaced for the patient to see clearly. There are three lens replacement options: aphakic eyeglasses, contact lenses, and IOL implants.

Aphakic glasses, although effective, are rarely used. Objects are magnified by 25%, making them appear closer than they actually are. This magnification creates distortion. Peripheral vision is also limited, and **binocular vision** (ie, ability of both eyes to focus on one object and fuse the two images into one) is impossible if the other eye is phakic (normal).

Contact lenses provide patients with almost normal vision, but because contact lenses need to be removed occasionally, the patient also needs a pair of aphakic glasses. Contact lenses are not advised for patients who have difficulty inserting, removing, and cleaning them. Frequent handling and improper disinfection increase the risk for infection.

TABLE 58-5 Potential Complications of Cataract Surgery

Complication	Effects	Management and Outcome
Immediate Preoperative		
Retrobulbar hemorrhage: can result from retrobulbar infiltration of anesthetic agents if the short ciliary artery is located by the injectia	Increased IOP, proptosis, lid tightness, and subconjunctival hemorrhage with or without edema	Emergent lateral canthotomy (slitting of the canthus) is performed to stop central retinal perfusion when the IOP is dangerously elevated. If this procedure fails to reduce IOP, a puncture of the anterior chamber with removal of fluid is considered. The patient must be closely monitored for at least a few hours. Postponement of cataract surgery for 2 to 4 weeks is advised. Complications such as iris prolapse, vitreous loss, and choroidal hemorrhage could result in a catastrophic visual outcome.
Intraoperative Complications		
Rupture of the posterior capsule	May result in loss of vitreous	Anterior vitrectomy is required if vitreous loss occurs.
Suprachoroidal (expulsive) hemorrhage: profuse bleeding into the suprachoroidal space	Extrusion of intraocular contents from the eye or opposition of retinal surfaces	Closure of the incision and administration of a hyperosmotic agent to reduce IOP or corticosteroids to reduce intraocular inflammation. Vitrectomy is performed 1 to 2 weeks later. Visual prognosis is poor; some useful vision may be salvaged on rare occasions.
Early Postoperative Complications		
Acute bacterial endophthalmitis: devastating complication that occurs in about 1 in 1000 cases; the most common causative organisms are *Staphylococcus epidermidis, S. aureus, Pseudomonas* and *Proteus* species	Characterized by marked visual loss, pain, lid edema, hypopyon, corneal haze, and chemosis	Managed by aggressive antibiotic therapy. Broad-spectrum antibiotics are administered while awaiting culture and sensitivity results. Once results are obtained, the appropriate antibiotics are administered via intravitreal injection. Corticosteroid therapy is also administered.
Toxic anterior segment syndrome: noninfectious inflammation that is a complication of anterior chamber surgery; caused by a toxic agent such as an agent used to sterilize surgical instruments	Corneal edema occurs less than 24 hours after surgery; symptoms include reduced visual acuity and pain.	If there is no growth of microorganisms, the treatment is topical steroids alone.
Late Postoperative Complications		
Suture-related problems	Toxic reactions or mechanical injury from broken or loose sutures	Suture removal relieves the symptoms. Topical corticosteroids are used when the incision is not healed and sutures cannot be removed.
Malposition of the IOL	Results in astigmatism, sensitivity to glare, or appearance of halos	Miotics are used for mild cases, whereas IOL removal and replacement is necessary for severe cases.
Chronic endophthalmitis	Persistent, low-grade inflammation and granuloma	Corticosteroids and antibiotics are administered systemically. If the condition persists, removal of the IOL and capsular bag, vitrectomy, and intravitreal injection of antibiotics are required.
Opacification of the posterior capsule (most common late complication of extracapsular cataract extraction)	Visual acuity is diminished.	YAG laser is used to create a hole in the posterior capsule. Blurred vision is cleared immediately.

IOL, intraocular lens; IOP, intraocular pressure.

Insertion of IOLs during cataract surgery is the usual approach to lens replacement. After cataract extraction, or phacoemulsification, the surgeon implants an IOL. Extracapsular cataract extraction and posterior chamber IOLs are associated with a relatively low incidence of complications (eg, hyphema, macular edema, secondary glaucoma, damage to the corneal endothelium). IOL implantation is contraindicated in patients with recurrent uveitis, proliferative diabetic retinopathy, neovascular glaucoma, or rubeosis iridis.

The most common IOL is the single-focus lens. Eyeglasses are still needed for distant or close vision, because the single-focus lens, unlike the natural lens of the eye, cannot alter its shape to bring objects at different distances into focus. Multifocal IOLs reduce the need for eyeglasses but patients can experience halos and glare. In the future, aging patients may benefit from a combined surgical approach using customized IOLs and refractive surgery for a customized vision correction.

TOXIC ANTERIOR SEGMENT SYNDROME

Also known as toxic endothelial cell destruction or sterile endophthalmitis, toxic anterior segment syndrome is a noninfectious inflammation caused by a toxic agent after an uncomplicated and uneventful surgery. This relatively newly recognized disorder is a complication of anterior chamber surgery. Investigations have shown that it may be caused by toxins from improperly rinsed surgical instruments soaked in enzymatic detergents, residue from instruments sterilized with plasma gas, abnormalities in the pH or ionic composition of irrigation solutions, ophthalmic viscoelastic devices, intraocular medications, or even the finish of the IOL (Parikh & Edelhauser, 2003).

Toxic anterior segment syndrome is characterized by corneal edema less than 24 hours after surgery, compared to the classic endophthalmitis, which appears 48 to 72 hours after surgery and is bacterial in nature. Like the classic endophthalmitis, the symptoms include reduction in visual acuity and pain. In the absence of microorganism growth, improvement has occurred with topical steroid treatment alone.

Nursing Management

The patient with cataracts should receive the usual preoperative care for ambulatory surgical patients undergoing eye surgery. According to the study on Medical Testing for Cataract Surgery, routine preoperative testing before cataract surgery does not improve health or clinical outcomes. Hence, the standard battery of preoperative tests (eg, complete blood count, electrocardiogram, urinalysis) should be prescribed only if they are indicated by the patient's medical history (Smith, Khoury, Shields, et al., 2000).

Providing Preoperative Care

It has been common practice to withhold any anticoagulant therapy (eg, aspirin, warfarin [Coumadin]) to reduce the risk for retrobulbar hemorrhage (after retrobulbar injection) for 5 to 7 days before surgery. However, a recent study showed that the risk of adverse events for patients who continued anticoagulant therapy before cataract surgery was very low (0.1% to 0.8%). The researchers speculated that regular users of aspirin or warfarin are already at higher risk for transient ischemic attacks or angina and suggest that patients may not need to discontinue these medications prior to surgery (Katz, Feldman, Bass et al., 2003).

Dilating drops are administered every 10 minutes for four doses at least 1 hour before surgery. Additional dilating drops may be administered in the operating room (immediately before surgery) if the affected eye is not fully dilated. Antibiotic, corticosteroid, and anti-inflammatory drops may be administered prophylactically to prevent postoperative infection and inflammation.

Providing Postoperative Care

After recovery from anesthesia, the patient receives verbal and written instructions about how to protect the eye, administer medications, recognize signs of complications, and obtain emergency care. Activities to be avoided are identified in Chart 58-8. The nurse also explains that there should be minimal discomfort after surgery and instructs the patient to take a mild analgesic agent, such as acetaminophen, as needed. Antibiotic, anti-inflammatory, and corticosteroid eye drops or ointments are prescribed postoperatively. A clinical pathway for the care of patients undergoing ambulatory cataract surgery is presented in Appendix B at the end of this textbook.

Promoting Home and Community-Based Care

TEACHING PATIENTS SELF-CARE

To prevent accidental rubbing or poking of the eye, the patient wears a protective eye patch for 24 hours after surgery, followed by eyeglasses worn during the day and a metal shield worn at night for 1 to 4 weeks. The nurse instructs the patient and family in applying and caring for the eye shield. Sunglasses should be worn while outdoors during the day because the eye is sensitive to light.

Slight morning discharge, some redness, and a scratchy feeling may be expected for a few days. A clean, damp washcloth may be used to remove slight morning eye discharge. Because cataract surgery increases the risk for retinal detachment, the patient must know to notify the surgeon if new floaters (dots) in vision, flashing lights, decrease in vision, pain, or increase in redness occurs.

CONTINUING CARE

The eye patch is removed after the first follow-up appointment. The patient may experience blurring of vision for several days to weeks. Sutures, if used, are left in the eye but alter the curvature of the cornea, resulting in temporary blurring and some astigmatism. Vision gradually improves as the eye heals. Patients with IOL implants have functional vision on the first day after surgery. Vision is stabilized when the eye is completely healed, usually within 6 to 12 weeks, when final corrective prescription is completed. Visual correction is needed for any remaining nearsightedness or farsightedness (even in patients with IOL implants).

CHART 58-8

HOME CARE CHECKLIST • Intraocular Lens Implant

At the completion of the home care instruction, the patient or caregiver will be able to:	Patient	Caregiver
• Wear glasses or metal eye shield at all times following surgery as instructed by the physician.	✔	
• Always wash hands before touching or cleaning the postoperative eye.	✔	✔
• Clean postoperative eye with a clean tissue; wipe the closed eye with a single gesture from the inner canthus outward.	✔	✔
• Bathe or shower; shampoo hair cautiously or seek assistance.	✔	
• Avoid lying on the side of the affected eye the night after surgery.	✔	
• Keep activity light (eg, walking, reading, watching television). Resume the following activities only as directed by the physician: driving, sexual activity, unusually strenuous activity.	✔	
• Remember not to lift, push, or pull objects heavier than 15 lb.	✔	
• Avoid bending or stooping for an extended period.	✔	
• Be careful when climbing or descending stairs.	✔	
• Know when to contact the physician.*	✔	✔

*Contact the physician immediately if any of the following problems occur before the next physician's appointment: (1) vision changes; (2) continuous flashing lights appear to the affected eye; (3) redness, swelling, or pain increase in the eye; (4) the amount or type of eye drainage changes; (5) the eye is injured in any way; (6) significant pain is not relieved by acetaminophen.

Corneal Disorders

Corneal Dystrophies

Corneal dystrophies are inherited as autosomal dominant traits and manifest when the person is about 20 years of age. They are characterized by deposits in the corneal layers. Decreased vision is caused by the irregular corneal surface and corneal deposits. Corneal endothelial decompensation leads to corneal edema and blurring of vision. Persistent edema leads to **bullous keratopathy** (formation of blisters that cause pain and discomfort on rupturing). This condition is usually associated with primary open-angle glaucoma.

A bandage contact lens is used to flatten the bullae, protect the exposed corneal nerve endings, and relieve discomfort. Symptomatic treatments, such as hypertonic drops or ointment (5% sodium chloride), may reduce epithelial edema; lowering the IOP also reduces stromal edema.

Keratoconus

Keratoconus is a condition characterized by a conical protuberance of the cornea with progressive thinning on protrusion and irregular astigmatism. This hereditary condition has a higher incidence among women. Onset occurs at puberty; the condition may progress for more than 20 years and is bilateral. Corneal scarring occurs in severe cases. Blurred vision is a prominent symptom. Rigid, gas-permeable contact lenses correct irregular astigmatism and improve vision. Advances in contact lens design have reduced the need for surgery. Penetrating keratoplasty is indicated when contact lens correction is no longer effective.

Corneal Surgeries

Among the surgical procedures used to treat diseased corneal tissue are phototherapeutic keratectomy (PTK) and keratoplasty. The success rate of ocular surface transplantation using autologous oral mucosal epithelium or amniotic membrane recipient-derived bone stem cells is now reasonable. Tissue rejection remains a major cause of failure (Nishida, Yamato, Hayashida, et al., 2004).

Phototherapeutic Keratectomy

PTK is a laser procedure that is used to treat diseased corneal tissue by removing or reducing corneal opacities and smoothing the anterior corneal surface to improve functional vision. PTK is a safer, more effective (when indicated) alternative than penetrating or lamellar keratoplasty. PTK is contraindicated in patients with active herpetic keratitis because the ultraviolet rays may reactivate latent virus. Common side effects are induced hyperopia and stromal haze. Complications are delayed reepithelization (particularly in patients with diabetes) and bacterial keratitis. Postoperative management consists of oral analgesics for eye pain. Reepithelization is promoted with a pressure patch or therapeutic soft contact lens. Antibiotic and corticosteroid ointments and nonsteroidal anti-inflammatory agents (NSAIDs) are prescribed postoperatively. Follow-up examinations are required for up to 2 years.

Keratoplasty

Keratoplasty (corneal transplantation or corneal grafting) involves replacing abnormal host tissue with healthy donor (cadaver) corneal tissue. Common indications are keratoconus, corneal dystrophy, corneal scarring from herpes simplex keratitis, and chemical burns.

Several factors affect the success of the graft: the condition of the ocular structures (eg, lids, conjunctiva), tear film function, adequacy of blinking, and viability of the donor endothelium. Tissue that is typically not used for grafting (Chart 58-9) includes tissue that may be the source of disease transmission from donor to recipient; corneas with functionally compromised endothelium; and corneas from donors who have undergone laser-assisted in situ keratomileusis (LASIK), because the cornea is no longer intact. Conditions such as glaucoma, retinal disease, and **strabismus** (deviation in ocular alignment) can negatively influence the outcome. The surgeon determines the graft size before the procedure, and the appropriate size is marked on the surface of the cornea. The surgeon prepares the donor cornea and the recipient bed, removes the diseased cornea, places the donor cornea on the recipient bed, and sutures it in place. Sutures remain in place for 12 to 18 months. Potential complications include early graft failure due to poor quality of donor tissue, surgical trauma, acute infection, and persistently increased IOP and late graft failure due to rejection.

CHART 58-9

Contraindications to the Use of Donor Tissue for Corneal Transplantation: Donor Characteristics

Systemic Disorders

- Death from unknown cause
- Creutzfeldt-Jacob disease
- AIDS or high risk for HIV infection
- Hepatitis
- Eye infection, systemic infection

Intrinsic Eye Disease

- Retinoblastoma
- Ocular inflammation
- Malignant tumors of anterior segment
- Disorders of the conjunctiva or corneal surface involving the optical zone of the cornea

Other

- History of eye trauma
- Corneal scars
- Previous surgical procedure
- Corneal graft
- LASIK eye surgery

Postoperatively, the patient receives **mydriatics** (medications causing pupillary dilation) for 2 weeks and topical corticosteroids for 12 months (daily doses for 6 months and tapered doses thereafter). These mydriatics and corticosteroid drops should be preservative-free to prevent a reactive inflammation (Kanski, 2003). Patients typically describe a sensation of postoperative eye discomfort rather than acute pain.

Nursing Management

The nurse reinforces the surgeon's recommendations and instructions regarding visual rehabilitation and visual improvement by explaining why a technically successful graft may initially produce disappointing results because the procedure has produced a new optical surface, and only after several months do patients start seeing the natural and true colors of their environment. Correction of a resultant refractive error with eyeglasses or contact lenses determines the final visual outcome. The nurse assesses the patient's support system and his or her ability to comply with long-term follow-up, which includes frequent clinic visits for several months for tapering of topical corticosteroid therapy, selective suture removal, and ongoing evaluation of the graft site and visual acuity. The nurse also initiates appropriate referrals to community services when indicated.

Because graft failure is an ophthalmic emergency that can occur at any time, the primary goal of nursing care is to teach the patient to identify signs and symptoms of graft failure. The early symptoms are blurred vision, discomfort, tearing, or redness of the eye. Decreased vision results after graft destruction. The patient must contact the ophthalmologist as soon as symptoms occur. Treatment of graft rejection involves prompt administration of hourly topical corticosteroids and periocular corticosteroid injections. Systemic immunosuppressive agents may be necessary for severe, resistant cases.

Refractive Surgeries

Refractive surgeries are cosmetic, elective procedures performed to recontour corneal tissue and correct refractive errors so that eyeglasses or contact lenses are no longer needed. Both photorefractive keratectomy (PRK) and LASIK use an excimer laser (193-nm-wavelength argon fluoride laser), which can evaporate corneal tissue very cleanly with almost no damage to the epithelial cells. Newer excimer lasers have a smaller spot size, a robust tracking system for eye movements, and wavefront custom ablation technology. These advances have minimized or eliminated aberrations induced by conventional laser vision correction as well as preexisting aberrations; they have improved treatment accuracy and therefore have provided for better vision. Postoperative night vision problems also have been reduced (Mrochen, Bueeler, Iseli, et al., 2004).

Laser vision correction alters the major optical function of the eye and thereby carries certain surgical risks. The patient must fully understand the benefits, potential risks and complications, common side effects, and limitations of the procedure. Refractive surgery does not alter the normal aging process of the eye. If the reason for the procedure is to meet vision requirements for the patient's occupation, the results must satisfy both the patient and the employer. Precise visual outcome cannot be guaranteed. Typically, patients must be at least 18 years of age.

The corneal structure must be normal and the refractive error must be stable. The patient is required to discontinue using contact lenses for a period before the procedure (2 to 3 weeks for soft lenses and 4 weeks for hard lenses). Patients with conditions that are likely to adversely affect corneal wound healing (eg, corticosteroid use, immunosuppression, elevated IOP) are not good candidates for the procedure. Any superficial eye disease must be diagnosed and fully treated before a refractive procedure.

Patient satisfaction is the ultimate goal; therefore, patient education and counseling about potential risks, complications, and postoperative follow-up are critical. Minimal postoperative care includes topical corticosteroid or NSAID and antibiotic drops.

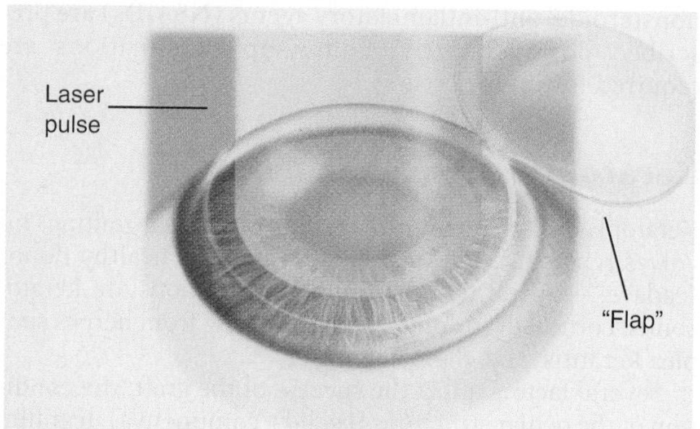

FIGURE 58-10. LASIK combines delicate surgical procedures and laser treatment. A flap is surgically created and lifted to one side. A laser is then applied to the cornea to reshape it. With permission from The Wilmer Laser Vision Center, Lutherville, MD.

Laser Vision Correction Photorefractive Keratectomy (PRK)

PRK is used to treat myopia and hyperopia with or without astigmatism. The excimer laser is applied directly to the cornea according to carefully calculated measurements. For myopia, the relative curvature is decreased; for hyperopia, the relative curvature is increased. A bandage contact lens is placed over the cornea to promote epithelial healing and reduce pain, which is similar to that of a severe corneal abrasion. The major limitations of this procedure are postoperative pain, subepithelial haze, and prolonged recovery of vision.

Laser-Assisted In Situ Keratomileusis (LASIK)

An improvement over PRK, particularly for correcting high (severe) myopia, LASIK involves flattening the anterior curvature of the cornea by removing a stromal lamella or layer. The surgeon creates a corneal flap with a microkeratome, which is an automatic corneal shaper similar to a carpenter's plane. The surgeon retracts a flap of corneal tissue less than one third of the thickness of a human hair to access the corneal stroma and then uses the excimer laser on the stromal bed to reshape the cornea according to calculated measurements (Fig. 58-10). LASIK causes less postoperative discomfort, has fewer side effects, and is safer than PRK. The patient has no corneal haze and requires less postoperative care. However, with LASIK, the cornea has been invaded at a deeper level, and any complications are more significant than those that can occur with PRK. With the increasing success and popularity of LASIK, PRK is now reserved for patients who are unsuitable for LASIK, such as people with very thin corneas.

Perioperative Complications

SURGICALLY INDUCED ABNORMALITIES

Corneal surface irregularities can occur after LASIK treatment. These include central islands (central areas of stiffness or elevation), decentered ablations due to misalignment of the laser treatment or from involuntary eye movement during laser treatment, and forms of irregular astigmatism. Symptoms of central islands and decentered ablations include monocular diplopia or ghost images, halos, glare, decreased visual acuity, and contrast sensitivity in low light.

DIFFUSE LAMELLAR KERATITIS

As LASIK increases in popularity and is performed more often, the vision-threatening complication known as diffuse lamellar keratitis (DLK) is reported more often. DLK is a peculiar, noninfectious, inflammatory reaction in the lamellar interface after LASIK. DLK is characterized by a white, granular, diffuse, culture-negative lamellar keratitis occurring in the first week after surgery. No single agent appears to be the sole cause of DLK; rather, the cause is multifactorial. DLK is diagnosed by identifying cells in the lamellar interface by slit-lamp examination from postoperative day 1. Depending on the severity of the condition, treatment methods range from administering corticosteroid drops to intervening surgically.

Phakic Intraocular Lenses

Because the results of refractive surgery on high (severe) myopia, hyperopia, and astigmatism are less predictable, there has been increasing interest in the use of phakic IOL implantation in patients who retain their natural lens. These phakic IOLs may be used in either the anterior or posterior chamber, and design improvements continue to be made. The implantation of such devices is reversible because the natural lens is left in place and the normal architecture of the cornea is preserved. This procedure may provide more predictable refractive results than procedures that alter the corneal curvature. Potential complications include cataract, iritis or uveitis, endothelial cell loss, and increased IOP.

Although phakic IOL implantation provides a more predictable alternative to corneal refractive surgery, more controlled, longitudinal multicenter trials are needed to evaluate its long-term safety.

Conductive Keratoplasty

A recent innovation in refractive surgery for the correction of low to mild hyperopia uses the principles of thermal keratoplasty by applying radiofrequency current to the peripheral cornea using a thin, hand-held probe. It does not involve the removal of cornea tissue. Clinical trials have shown that postprocedure visual acuity, predictability, and stability are as good as, if not better than, with other refractive procedures (McDonald, Durrie, Asbell, et al., 2004).

Retinal Disorders

Although the retina is composed of multiple microscopic layers, the two innermost layers, the sensory retina and the retinal pigment epithelium (RPE), are the most relevant to common retinal disorders. Just as the film in a camera captures an image, so does the retina, the neural tissue of the eye. The rods and cones, the photoreceptor cells, are found in the sensory layer of the retina. Beneath the sensory layer lies the RPE, the pigmented layer. When the rods and cones are stimulated by light, an electrical impulse is generated, and the image is transmitted to the brain.

Retinal Detachment

Retinal detachment refers to the separation of the RPE from the sensory layer. The four types of retinal detachment are rhegmatogenous, traction, a combination of rhegmatogenous and traction, and exudative. *Rhegmatogenous detachment* is the most common form. In this condition, a hole or tear develops in the sensory retina, allowing some of the liquid vitreous to seep through the sensory retina and detach it from the RPE (Fig. 58-11). People at risk for this type of detachment include those with high myopia or **aphakia** after cataract surgery. Trauma may also play a role in rhegmatogenous retinal detachment. Between 5% and 10% of all rhegmatogenous retinal detachments are associated with proliferative retinopathy, a retinopathy associated with diabetic neovascularization (see Chapter 41).

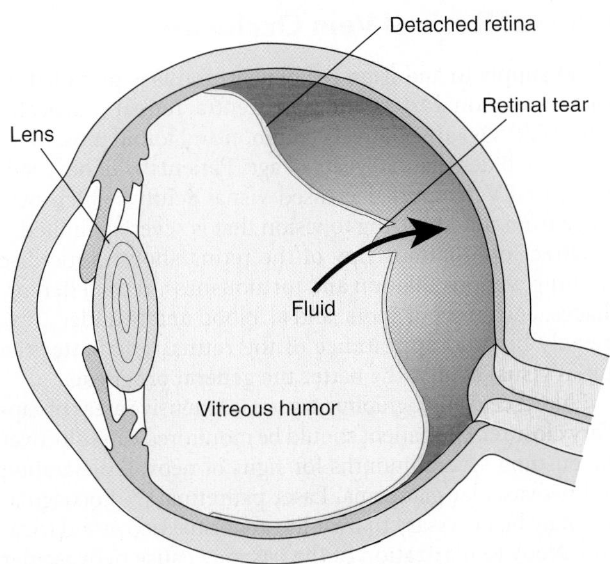

FIGURE 58-11. Retinal detachment.

Tension, or a pulling force, is responsible for *traction retinal detachment*. An ophthalmologist must ascertain all of the areas of retinal break and identify and release the scars or bands of fibrous material providing traction on the retina. Generally, patients with this condition have developed fibrous scar tissue from conditions such as diabetic retinopathy, vitreous hemorrhage, or the retinopathy of prematurity. The hemorrhages and fibrous proliferation associated with these conditions exert a pulling force on the delicate retina.

Patients can have both rhegmatogenous and traction retinal detachment. *Exudative retinal detachments* are the result of the production of a serous fluid under the retina from the choroid. Conditions such as uveitis and macular degeneration may cause the production of this serous fluid.

Clinical Manifestations

Patients may report the sensation of a shade or curtain coming across the vision of one eye, cobwebs, bright flashing lights, or the sudden onset of a great number of floaters. Patients do not complain of pain.

Assessment and Diagnostic Findings

After visual acuity is determined, the patient must have a dilated fundus examination using an indirect ophthalmoscope as well as slit-lamp biomicroscopy. Stereo fundus photography and fluorescein angiography are commonly used during the evaluation.

Increasingly, optical coherence tomography and ultrasound are used for the complete retinal assessment, especially if the view is obscured by a dense cataract or vitreal hemorrhage. All retinal breaks, all fibrous bands that may be causing traction on the retina, and all degenerative changes must be identified.

Surgical Management

In rhegmatogenous detachment, an attempt is made to surgically reattach the sensory retina to the RPE. In traction detachment, the source of traction must be removed and the sensory retina reattached. New surgical techniques as well as advances in instrumentation have led to an increased rate of success of surgical reattachment and better visual outcomes. The most commonly used surgical interventions are the scleral buckle, the pars plana vitrectomy, and pneumatic retinopexy.

Scleral Buckle

The retinal surgeon compresses the sclera (often with a scleral buckle or a silicone band; Fig. 58-12) to indent the scleral wall from the outside of the eye and bring the two retinal layers in contact with each other. This type of surgery has a high success rate in the hands of experienced retinal surgeons. It causes less damage to the lens of the eye in phakic patients, and there is a low risk of endophthalmitis.

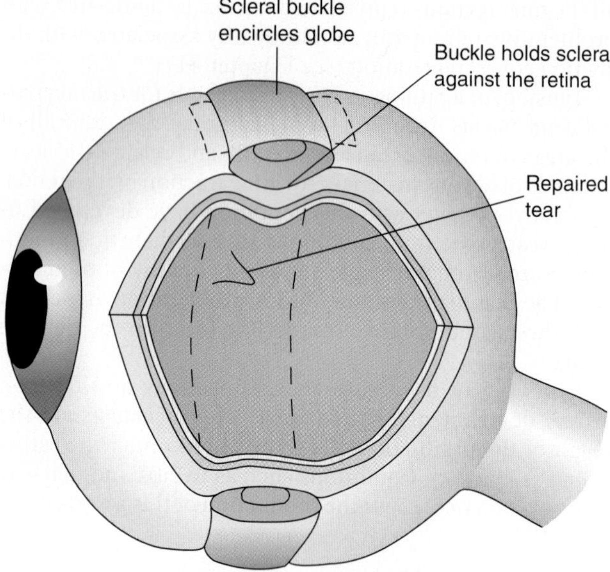

FIGURE 58-12. Scleral buckle.

However, there is an increased incidence of diplopia and other complications, such as induced myopia and increased postoperative pain.

Pars Plana Vitrectomy

A vitrectomy is an intraocular procedure in which 1- to 4-mm incisions are made at the pars plana. One incision allows the introduction of a light source, and another incision serves as the portal for the vitrectomy instrument. The surgeon dissects preretinal membranes under direct visualization while the retina is stabilized by an intraoperative vitreous substitute.

This surgical technique was originally introduced as a treatment for eyes with conditions that were previously inoperable (eg, vitreous hemorrhage, proliferative diabetic retinopathy). Technologic improvements, including the use of operating microscopes, microinstrumentation, and instruments that combine vitreous cutting, aspiration, and illumination capabilities in one device, have advanced vitreoretinal surgery. The techniques of vitreoretinal surgery can be used in various procedures, including the removal of foreign bodies, vitreous opacities such as blood, and dislocated lenses. Traction on the retina may be relieved through vitrectomy and may be combined with scleral buckling to repair retinal breaks. Treatment of macular holes includes vitrectomy, laser photocoagulation, air-fluid-gas exchanges, and the use of growth factor.

Pneumatic Retinopexy

This technique is used for the repair of a rhegmatogenous retinal detachment. It is the least invasive of the three procedures described. A gas bubble, silicone oil, or perfluorocarbon and liquids may be injected into the vitreous cavity to help push the sensory retina up against the RPE. Postoperative positioning of the patient is critical, because the injected bubble must float into a position overlying the area of detachment, providing consistent pressure to reattach the sensory retina. Argon laser photocoagulation or cryotherapy is also used to "spot-weld" small holes (Chang, Pelzek, Nguyen, et al., 2003).

Nursing Management

For the most part, nursing interventions consist of educating the patient and providing supportive care.

Promoting Comfort

If a gas tamponade is used to flatten the retina, the patient may have to be specially positioned to make the gas bubble float into the best position. Some patients must lie face down or on their side for days. Patients and family members should be made aware of these special needs beforehand so that the patient can be made as comfortable as possible.

Teaching About Complications

In many cases, vitreoretinal procedures are performed on an outpatient basis, and the patient is seen the next day for a follow-up examination and closely monitored thereafter as required. Postoperative complications may include increased IOP, endophthalmitis, development of other retinal detachments, development of cataracts, and loss of turgor of the eye. Patients must be taught the signs and symptoms of complications, particularly of increasing IOP and postoperative infection.

Retinal Vascular Disorders

Loss of vision can occur from occlusion of a retinal artery or vein. Such occlusions may result from atherosclerosis, cardiac valvular disease, venous stasis, hypertension, or increased blood viscosity. Associated risk factors include diabetes mellitus, glaucoma, and aging.

Central Retinal Vein Occlusion

Blood supply to and from the ocular fundus is provided by the central retinal artery and vein. Central retinal vein occlusions (CRVOs) are relatively common and found most often in people older than 50 years of age. Patients who have suffered a CRVO report decreased visual acuity, which may range from mild blurring to vision that is severely limited.

Direct ophthalmoscopy of the retina shows optic disc swelling, venous dilation and tortuousness, retinal hemorrhages, cotton-wool spots, and a "blood and thunder" (extremely bloody) appearance of the retina. The better the initial visual acuity, the better the general prognosis.

Fluorescein angiography may show extensive areas of capillary closure. The patient should be monitored carefully over the ensuing several months for signs of neovascularization and neovascular glaucoma. Laser panretinal photocoagulation may be necessary to treat the abnormal neovascularization. Neovascularization of the iris may cause neovascular glaucoma, which may be difficult to control. Macular edema, macular nonperfusion, and vitreous hemorrhage from the neovascularization are among the potential complications of CRVO.

Branch Retinal Vein Occlusion

Some patients with branch retinal vein occlusion (BRVO) are symptom-free, whereas others complain of a sudden loss of vision if the macular area is involved. A more gradual loss of vision may occur if macular edema associated with BRVO develops. Studies have found that a grid-like pattern of laser burns helps reduce macular edema and improves visual acuity by two or more lines on the Snellen chart (Esrick, Subramanian, Heier, et al., 2005).

On examination, the ocular fundus appears similar to that found in CRVO; however, only those portions of the retina affected by the obstructive veins have what is known as a "blood and thunder" appearance. The occlusions generally occur at the arteriovenous crossings. The diagnostic evaluation and follow-up assessments are the same as for CRVO. Potential complications are similar. Associated conditions include glaucoma, systemic hypertension, diabetes mellitus, hyperlipidemia, and hyperviscosity syndrome.

Central Retinal Artery Occlusion

Patients with central retinal artery occlusion, a relatively rare disorder that accounts for approximately 1 in 10,000 ophthalmologic visits, present with a sudden loss of vision. Visual acuity is reduced to being able to count the examiner's fingers, or the field of vision is tremendously restricted. A relative afferent pupillary defect is present. Examination of the ocular fundus reveals a pale retina with a cherry-red spot at the fovea. The retinal arteries are thin, and emboli are occasionally seen in the central retinal artery or its branches. Central retinal artery occlusion is a true ocular emergency. Various treatments are used; the ophthalmologist may perform ocular massage, anterior chamber paracentesis, IV administration of hyperosmotic agents such as acetazolamide, and high concentrations of oxygen. Most visual loss associated with central retinal artery occlusion is severe and permanent.

Macular Degeneration

Macular degeneration is the most common cause of visual loss in people older than age 60 (Schachat et al., 2004). Commonly called age-related macular degeneration (AMD), it is characterized by tiny, yellowish spots called drusen (Fig. 58-13) beneath the retina. Most people older than 60 years of age have at least a few small drusen. There is a wide range of visual loss in patients with macular degeneration, but most patients do not experience total blindness. Central vision is generally the most affected, with most patients retaining peripheral vision (Fig. 58-14). There are two types of AMD, commonly known as the dry type and wet type.

Between 85% and 90% of people with AMD have the dry or nonexudative type, in which the outer layers of the retina slowly break down (Fig. 58-15). With this breakdown comes the appearance of drusen. When the drusen occur outside of the macular area, patients generally have no symptoms. When the drusen occur within the macula, however, there is a gradual blurring of vision that patients may notice when

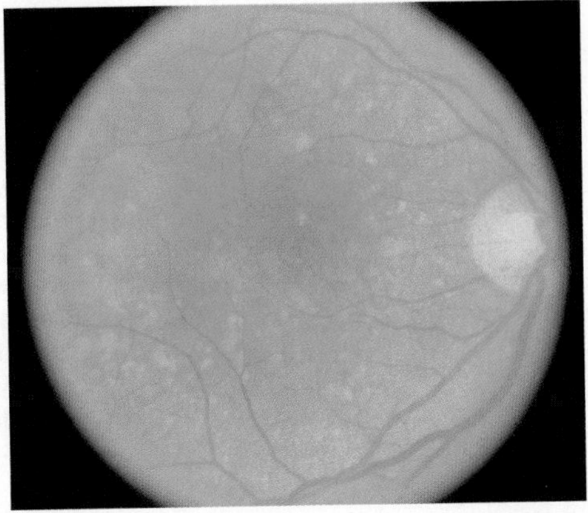

FIGURE 58-13. Retina showing drusen and age-related macular degeneration (AMD).

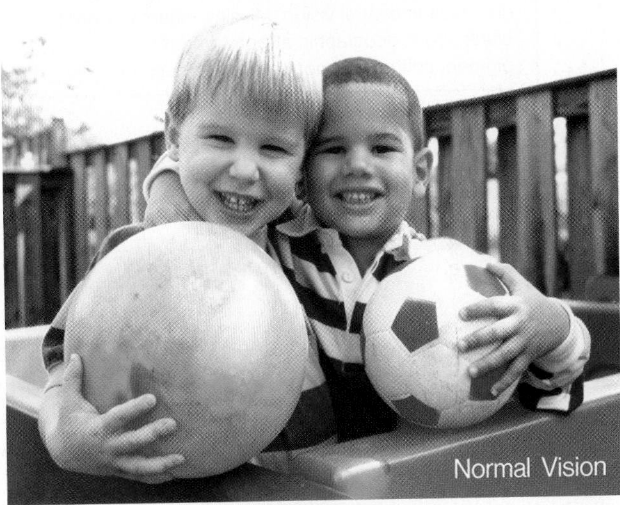

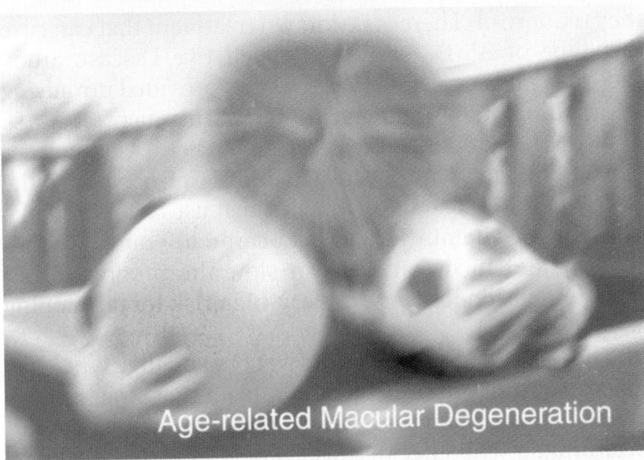

FIGURE 58-14. Visual loss associated with macular degeneration. Photos courtesy of the National Eye Institute/National Institutes of Health.

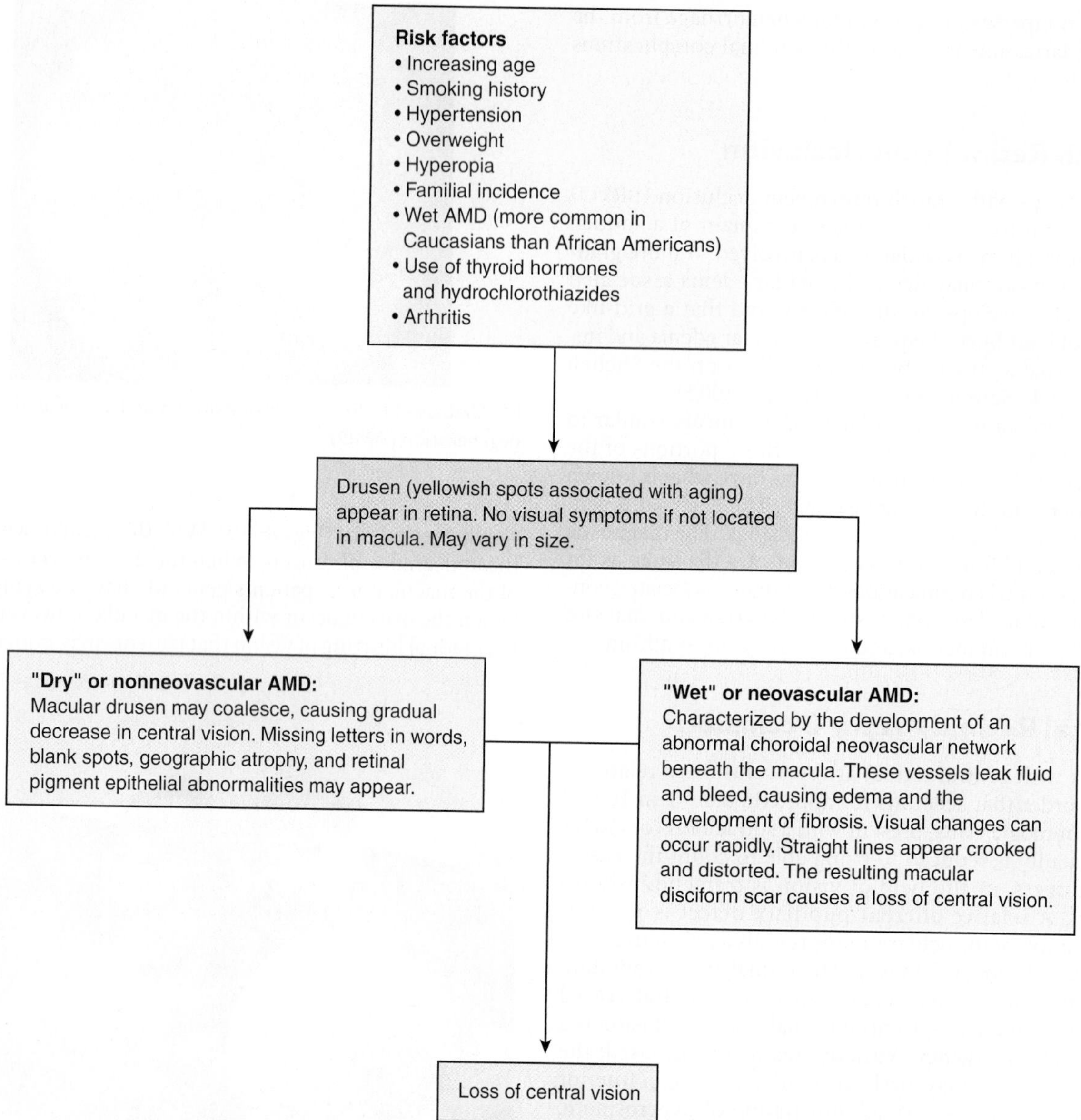

Risk factors
• Increasing age
• Smoking history
• Hypertension
• Overweight
• Hyperopia
• Familial incidence
• Wet AMD (more common in Caucasians than African Americans)
• Use of thyroid hormones and hydrochlorothiazides
• Arthritis
Drusen (yellowish spots associated with aging) appear in retina. No visual symptoms if not located in macula. May vary in size.
"Dry" or nonneovascular AMD:
Macular drusen may coalesce, causing gradual decrease in central vision. Missing letters in words, blank spots, geographic atrophy, and retinal pigment epithelial abnormalities may appear.
"Wet" or neovascular AMD:
Characterized by the development of an abnormal choroidal neovascular network beneath the macula. These vessels leak fluid and bleed, causing edema and the development of fibrosis. Visual changes can occur rapidly. Straight lines appear crooked and distorted. The resulting macular disciform scar causes a loss of central vision.
Loss of central vision

FIGURE 58-15. Progression of age-related macular degeneration (AMD): pathways to vision loss.

they try to read. There is no known treatment that can cure this type of AMD. The Age-Related Eye Disease Study (2001), a multicenter clinical trial, has provided promising information about the prevention and treatment of AMD. The study was designed to determine whether large doses of macronutrients are effective in preventing or slowing the course of AMD. The study revealed that use of antioxidants (vitamin C, vitamin E, and beta-carotene) and minerals (zinc oxide) in megadoses can slow the progression of AMD and vision loss for people at high risk for developing advanced AMD.

The second type of AMD, the wet or exudative type, may have an abrupt onset. Patients complain that straight lines appear crooked and distorted or that letters in words appear broken. This effect results from proliferation of abnormal blood vessels growing under the retina, within the choroid layer of the eye, a condition known as choroidal neovascularization. The affected vessels can leak fluid and blood, elevating the retina. Some patients can be treated with the argon laser to stop the leakage from these vessels. However, this treatment is not ideal because vision may be affected by the laser treatment and abnormal vessels often grow back after treatment.

Medical Management

Photodynamic Therapy

Visual loss from choroidal neovascularization lesions in AMD is a growing problem. With the growth of these new vessels from the choriocapillary layer, fibrous tissue develops that can, over months, destroy central vision. Laser treatment has been used to close these abnormal vessels, but the very process of photocoagulation carries with it some level of retinal destruction, albeit less than the natural scarring that would occur in the untreated eye.

Photodynamic therapy (PDT) has been developed in an attempt to ameliorate the choroidal neovascularization while causing minimal damage to the retina. Studies have shown that PDT can reduce the risk of visual loss for certain groups of patients who have classic subfoveal choroidal neovascularization due to macular degeneration. PDT is a two-step process (Fig. 58-16). Verteporfin, a photosensitive dye, is infused IV over 10 minutes. Fifteen minutes after the start of the infusion, a diode laser is used to treat the abnormal network of vessels. The dye within the vessels takes up the energy of the diode laser but the surrounding retina does not, avoiding damage to adjacent areas. Multiple treatments may be necessary over time. Overall, some patients may experience an improvement in vision, but most often the result has been to stabilize or slow visual loss (Azab, Benchaboune, Blinder, et al., 2004).

Verteporfin is a light-activated dye, so patient education is important preoperatively. The dye within the blood vessels near the surface of the skin could become activated with exposure to strong light. This would include bright sunlight, tanning booths, halogen lights, and the bright lights used in dental offices and operating rooms; ordinary indoor light is not a problem. The patient should be instructed to bring dark sunglasses, gloves, a wide-brimmed hat, long-sleeved shirt, and slacks to the setting where PDT will be performed. The patient must be cautioned to avoid exposure to direct sunlight or bright light for 5 days after treatment. If the patient must go outdoors within the first 5 days after treatment, he or she should wear a long-sleeved shirt and slacks made of tightly woven fabrics. Gloves, shoes, socks, sunglasses, and a wide-brimmed hat should also be worn if the patient has to go outdoors during daylight hours during this period. Inadvertent sunlight exposure can lead to severe blistering of the skin and sunburn that may require plastic surgery.

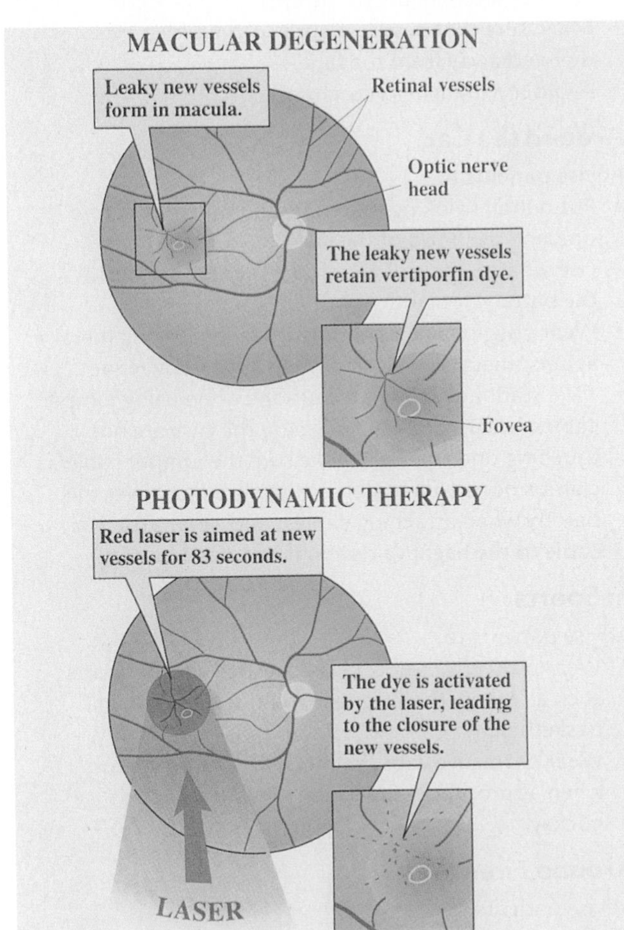

FIGURE 58-16. Photodynamic therapy (PDT) for slowing the progression of age-related macular degeneration. Light-sensitive verteporfin dye is injected into defective vessels. A special laser activates the dye, which releases singlet oxygen that is toxic to endothelial cells, shutting down the vessels without damaging the retina. With permission from Valenz, K. D. (2001). Laser surgery shines as ray of hope. *Helix, 18*(3), 12–13.

Nursing Management

Nursing management is primarily educational. Most patients benefit from the use of bright lighting and magnification devices and from referral to a low vision center. Some low vision centers send representatives to the patient's home or place of employment to evaluate the living and working conditions and make recommendations to improve lighting, thereby improving vision and promoting safety. The home care nurse can make the same assessment and recommendations.

Amsler grids are given to patients to use in their home to monitor for a sudden onset or distortion of vision. These may provide the earliest sign that macular degeneration is getting worse. Patients should be encouraged to use these grids and to look at them, one eye at a time, several times each week with glasses on. If there is a change in the grid (eg, if the lines or squares appear distorted or faded), the patient should notify the ophthalmologist immediately and should arrange to be seen promptly.

Ongoing Research

Angiogenesis

An important component of the effort against neovascular AMD is research into the development and progression of angiogenesis (abnormal blood vessel formation). Studies continue toward identification of agents that can be used to inhibit angiogenesis. This has implications for ocular neovascularization and the treatment of other disorders, such as solid tumors (Hera, Keramidas, Peoc'h, et al., 2005).

Vasoproliferation in exudative AMD is believed to be caused by an underlying angiogenic stimulus known as vascular endothelial growth factor (VEGF). Research is ongoing in phase III trials on two intravitreal agents designed to inhibit angiogenesis. Macugen (pegaptanib sodium) is designed to inhibit the ability of VEGF to bind to cellular receptors. Thus far Macugen has been shown to be safe and more effective than placebo (Eyetech Study Group, 2003). Lucentis (ranibizumab) is designed to bind and inactivate all isoforms of VEGF. The results of animal studies and a small study of 64 patients have been promising. A larger phase III trial is underway.

Macular Translocation

Wet macular degeneration is characterized by the development of an abnormal choroidal neovascularization membrane, to the detriment of central vision. One approach to this problem is the surgical procedure known as macular translocation, in which a 360-degree retinal detachment is surgically created and the retina is gently lifted and resettled, placing the macular area a slight distance away from the area of choroidal neovascularization. Laser treatment can then be applied to the abnormal neovascular network, with minimal damage to the macula. This surgical technique is being refined.

Orbital and Ocular Trauma

Whether affecting the eye or the orbit, trauma to the eye and surrounding structures may have devastating consequences for vision. It is preferable to prevent injury rather than treat it. Chart 58-10 details safety measures to prevent orbital and ocular trauma.

Orbital Trauma

Injury to the orbit is usually associated with a head injury; hence, the patient's general medical condition must first be

CHART 58-10

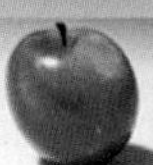

Preventing Eye Injuries

In and Around the House

Advise patients to:

- Make sure that all spray nozzles are directed away from themselves before pressing down on the handle.
- Read instructions carefully before using cleaning fluids, detergents, ammonia, or harsh chemicals, and to wash hands thoroughly after use.
- Use grease shields on frying pans to decrease spattering.
- Wear special goggles to shield their eyes from fumes and splashes when using powerful chemicals.
- Use opaque goggles to avoid burns from sunlamps.

In the Workshop

Advise patients to:

- Protect their eyes from flying fragments, fumes, dust particles, sparks, and splashed chemicals by wearing safety glasses.
- Read instructions thoroughly before using tools and chemicals, and follow precautions for their use.

Around Children

Advise patients to:

- Pay attention to age and maturity level of a child when selecting toys and games, and to avoid projectile toys, such as darts and pellet guns.
- Supervise children when they are playing with toys or games that can be dangerous.
- Teach children the correct way to handle potentially dangerous items, such as scissors and pencils.

In the Garden

Advise patients to:

- Avoid letting anyone stand at the side of or in front of a moving lawn mower.
- Pick up rocks and stones before going over them with the lawn mower (stones can be hurled out of the rotary blades and rebound off curbs or walls, causing severe injury to the eye).
- Make sure that pesticide spray can nozzles are directed away from the face.
- Avoid low-hanging branches.

Around the Car

Advise patients to:

- Put out all smoking materials and matches before opening the hood of the car.
- Use a flashlight, not a match or lighter, to look at the battery at night.
- Wear goggles when grinding metal or striking metal against metal while performing auto body repair.
- Take standard safety precautions when using jumper cables (wear goggles; make sure the cars are not touching one another; make sure the jumper cable clamps never touch each other; never lean over the battery when attaching cables; and never attach a cable to the negative terminal of a dead battery).

In Sports

Advise patients to:

- Wear protective safety glasses, especially for sports such as racquetball, squash, tennis, baseball, and basketball.
- Wear protective caps, helmets, or face protectors when appropriate, especially for sports such as ice hockey.

Around Fireworks

Advise patients to:

- Wear eye glasses or safety goggles.
- Avoid using explosive fireworks.
- Never allow children to ignite fireworks.
- Avoid standing near others when lighting fireworks.
- Douse duds in water instead of attempting to relight them.

stabilized before conducting an ocular examination. Only then is the globe assessed for soft tissue injury. During inspection, the face is meticulously assessed for underlying fractures, which should always be suspected in cases of blunt trauma. To establish the extent of ocular injury, visual acuity is assessed as soon as possible, even if it is only a rough estimate. Soft tissue orbital injuries often result in damage to the optic nerve. Major ocular injuries indicated by a soft globe, prolapsing tissue, ruptured globe, and hemorrhage, require immediate surgical attention.

Soft Tissue Injury and Hemorrhage

The signs and symptoms of soft tissue injury from blunt or penetrating trauma include tenderness, ecchymosis, lid swelling, **proptosis** (ie, downward displacement of the eyeball), and hemorrhage. Closed injuries lead to contusions with subconjunctival hemorrhage, commonly known as a *black eye*. Blood accumulates in the tissues of the conjunctiva. Hemorrhage may be caused by a soft tissue injury to the eyelid or by an underlying fracture.

Management of soft tissue hemorrhage that does not threaten vision is usually conservative and consists of thorough inspection, cleansing, and repair of wounds. Cold compresses are used in the early phase, followed by warm compresses. Hematomas that appear as swollen, fluctuating areas may be surgically drained or aspirated; if they are causing significant orbital pressure, they may be surgically evacuated.

Penetrating injuries or a severe blow to the head can result in severe optic nerve damage. Visual loss can be sudden or delayed and progressive. Immediate loss of vision after an ocular injury is usually irreversible. Delayed visual loss has a better prognosis. Corticosteroid therapy is indicated to reduce optic nerve swelling. Surgery, such as optic nerve decompression, may be performed.

Orbital Fractures

Orbital fractures are detected by facial x-rays. Depending on the orbital structures involved, orbital fractures can be classified as blowout, zygomatic or tripod, maxillary, midfacial, orbital apex, and orbital roof fractures. Blowout fractures result from compression of soft tissue and the sudden increase in orbital pressure when the force is transmitted to the orbital floor, the area of least resistance.

The inferior rectus and inferior oblique muscles, with their fat and fascial attachments, or the nerve that courses along the inferior oblique muscle may become entrapped, and the globe may be displaced inward (ie, enophthalmos). Computed tomography (CT) can identify the muscle and its auxiliary structures that are entrapped. These fractures are usually caused by blunt small objects, such as a fist, knee, elbow, or tennis or golf ball.

Orbital roof fractures are dangerous because of potential complications to the brain. Surgical management of these fractures requires a neurosurgeon and an ophthalmologist. The most common indications for surgical intervention are displacement of bone fragments disfiguring the normal facial contours, interference with normal binocular vision caused by extraocular muscle entrapment, interference with mastication in zygomatic fracture, and obstruction of the nasolacrimal duct. Surgery is usually nonemergent, and a period of 10 to 14 days gives the ophthalmologist time to assess ocular function, especially the extraocular muscles and the nasolacrimal duct. Emergency surgical repair is usually not performed unless the globe is displaced to the maxillary sinus. Surgical repair is primarily directed at freeing the entrapped ocular structures and restoring the integrity of the orbital floor.

Foreign Bodies

Foreign bodies that enter the orbit are usually tolerated, except for copper, iron, and vegetable materials such as those from plants or trees, which may cause purulent infection. X-rays and CT scans are used to identify the foreign body. A careful history is important, especially if the foreign body has been in the orbit for a period of time and the incident forgotten. It is important to identify metallic foreign bodies because they prohibit the use of magnetic resonance imaging (MRI) as a diagnostic tool.

After the extent of the orbital damage is assessed, the decision to use conservative treatment or surgical removal is made. In general, orbital foreign bodies are removed if they are superficial and anterior in location; have sharp edges that may affect adjacent orbital structures; or are composed of copper, iron, or vegetable material. Surgical intervention is directed at preventing further ocular injury and maintaining the integrity of the affected areas. Cultures are usually obtained, and the patient is placed on prophylactic IV antibiotics that are later changed to oral antibiotics.

Ocular Trauma

Ocular trauma is the leading cause of blindness among children and young adults, especially male trauma victims. The most common circumstances of ocular trauma are occupational injuries (eg, construction industry), sports (eg, baseball, basketball, racquet sports, boxing), weapons (eg, air guns, BB guns), assault, motor vehicle crashes (eg, broken windshields), and explosions (eg, blast fragments).

There are two types of ocular trauma in which the first response is critical: chemical burn and foreign object in the eye. With a chemical burn, the eye should be immediately irrigated with tap water or normal saline. With a foreign body, no attempt should be made to remove the foreign object. The object should be protected from jarring or movement to prevent further ocular damage. No pressure or patch should be applied to the affected eye. All traumatic eye injuries should be protected using a metal shield if available or a stiff paper cup until medical treatment can be obtained (Fig. 58-17).

Assessment and Diagnostic Findings

A thorough history is obtained, particularly assessing the patient's ocular history, such as preinjury vision in the affected

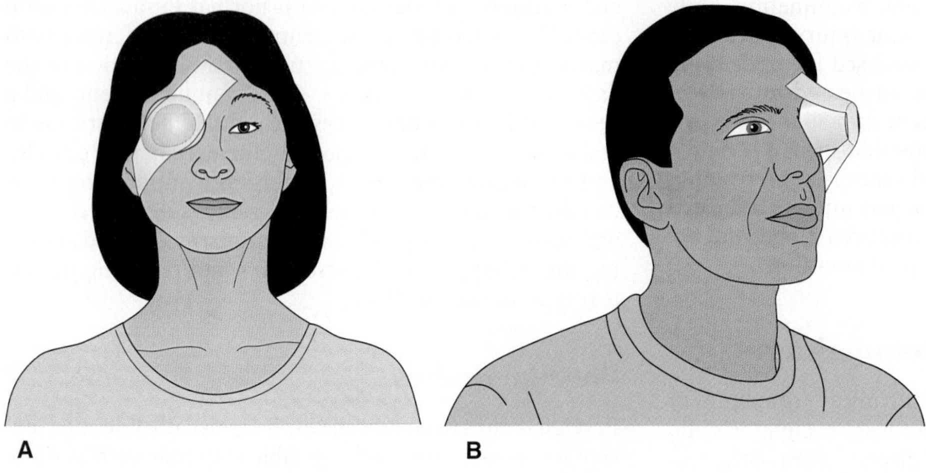

FIGURE 58-17. Two kinds of eye patches. (**A**) Aluminum shield. (**B**) Stiff paper cup shield (innovative substitute when aluminum shield is unavailable).

eye or past ocular surgery. Details related to the injury that help in the diagnosis and assessment of need for further tests include the nature of the ocular injury (ie, blunt or penetrating trauma); the type of activity that caused the injury to determine the nature of the force striking the eye; and whether onset of vision loss was sudden, slow, or progressive. For chemical eye burns, the chemical agent must be identified and tested for pH if the agent is available. The corneal surface is examined for foreign bodies, wounds, and abrasions, after which the other external structures of the eye are examined. Pupillary size, shape, and light reaction of the pupil of the affected eye are compared with the other eye. Ocular motility (ability of the eyes to move synchronously up, down, right, and left) is also assessed.

Medical Management

Splash Injuries

Splash injuries are irrigated with normal saline solution before further evaluation occurs. In cases of a ruptured globe, cycloplegic agents (agents that paralyze the ciliary muscle) or topical antibiotics must be deferred because of potential toxicity to exposed intraocular tissues. Further manipulation of the eye must be avoided until the patient is under general anesthesia. Parenteral, broad-spectrum antibiotics are initiated. Tetanus antitoxin is administered, if indicated, as well as analgesics. (Tetanus prophylaxis is recommended for full-thickness ocular and skin wounds.) Any topical ophthalmic medication (eg, anesthetic, dyes) must be sterile.

Foreign Bodies and Corneal Abrasions

After removal of a foreign body from the surface of the eye, an antibiotic ointment is applied and the eye is patched. The eye is examined daily for evidence of infection until the wound is completely healed.

Contact lens wear is a common cause of corneal abrasion. The patient experiences severe pain and **photophobia** (ocular pain on exposure to light). Corneal epithelial defects are treated with antibiotic ointment and a pressure patch to immobilize the eyelids. Topical anesthetic eye drops must not be given to the patient to take home for repeated use after corneal injury because their effects mask further damage, delay healing, and can lead to permanent corneal scarring. Corticosteroids are avoided while the epithelial defect exists.

Penetrating Injuries and Contusions of the Eyeball

Sharp penetrating injury or blunt contusion force can rupture the eyeball. When the eye wall, cornea, and sclera rupture, rapid decompression or herniation of the orbital contents into adjacent sinuses can occur. In general, blunt traumatic injuries (with an increased incidence of retinal detachment, intraocular tissue avulsion, and herniation) have a worse prognosis than penetrating injuries. Most penetrating injuries result in marked loss of vision with the following signs: hemorrhagic **chemosis** (edema of the conjunctiva), conjunctival laceration, shallow anterior chamber with or without an eccentrically placed pupil, **hyphema** (hemorrhage within the chamber), or vitreous hemorrhage.

Hyphema is caused by contusion forces that tear the vessels of the iris and damage the anterior chamber angle. Preventing rebleeding and prolonged increased IOP are the goals of treatment for hyphema. In severe cases, the patient is hospitalized with moderate activity restriction. An eye shield is applied. Topical corticosteroids are prescribed to reduce inflammation. An antifibrinolytic agent, aminocaproic acid (Amicar), stabilizes clot formation at the site of hemorrhage. Aspirin is contraindicated.

A ruptured globe and severe injuries with intraocular hemorrhage require surgical intervention. Vitrectomy is performed for traumatic retinal detachments. Primary **enucleation** (complete removal of the eyeball and part of the optic nerve) is considered only if the globe is irreparable and has no light perception. It is a general rule that enucleation is performed within 2 weeks of the initial injury (in an eye that has no useful vision after sustaining penetrating injury) to prevent the risk of **sympathetic ophthalmia** (an inflammation created in the uninjured eye by the affected eye that can result in blindness of the uninjured eye).

Intraocular Foreign Bodies

A patient who complains of blurred vision and discomfort should be questioned carefully about recent injuries and exposures. Patients may be injured in a number of different situations and experience an intraocular foreign body (IOFB). Precipitating circumstances can include working in construction; striking metal against metal; being involved in a motor vehicle crash with facial injury; a gunshot wound; grinding-wheel work; and an explosion.

IOFB is diagnosed and localized by slit-lamp biomicroscopy and indirect ophthalmoscopy, as well as CT or ultrasonography. MRI is contraindicated because most foreign bodies are metallic and magnetic. It is important to determine the composition, size, and location of the IOFB and affected eye structures. Every effort should be made to identify the type of IOFB and whether it is magnetic. Iron, steel, copper, and vegetable matter cause intense inflammatory reactions. The incidence of endophthalmitis is also high. If the cornea is perforated, tetanus prophylaxis and IV antibiotics are administered. The extraction route (ie, surgical incision) of the foreign body depends on its location and composition and associated ocular injuries. Specially designed IOFB forceps and magnets are used to grasp and remove the foreign body. Any damaged area of the retina is treated to prevent retinal detachment.

Ocular Burns

Alkali, acid, and other chemically active organic substances, such as Mace and tear gas, cause chemical burns. Alkali burns (eg, lye, ammonia) result in the most severe injury because they penetrate the ocular tissues rapidly and continue to cause damage long after the initial injury is sustained. They also cause an immediate rise in IOP. Acids (eg, bleach, car batteries, refrigerant) generally cause less damage because the precipitated necrotic tissue proteins form a barrier to further penetration and damage. Chemical burns may appear as superficial punctate keratopathy (ie, spotty damage to the cornea), subconjunctival hemorrhage, or complete marbleizing of the cornea.

In treating chemical burns, every minute counts. Immediate tap-water irrigation should be started on site before transport of the patient to an emergency department. Only a brief history and examination are performed. The corneal surfaces and conjunctival fornices are immediately and copiously irrigated with normal saline or any neutral solution. A local anesthetic is instilled, and a lid speculum is applied to overcome blepharospasm (ie, spasms of the eyelid muscles that result in closure of the lids). Particulate matter must be removed from the fornices using moistened, cotton-tipped applicators and minimal pressure on the globe. Irrigation continues until the conjunctival pH normalizes (between 7.3 and 7.6). The pH of the corneal surface is checked by placing a pH paper strip in the fornix. Antibiotics are instilled, and the eye is patched.

The goal of intermediate treatment is to prevent tissue ulceration and promote reepithelization. Intense lubrication using nonpreserved (ie, without preservatives to avoid allergic reactions) artificial tears is essential. Reepithelization is promoted with patching or therapeutic soft lenses. The patient is usually monitored daily for several days. Prognosis depends on the type of injury and adequacy of the irrigation immediately after exposure. Long-term treatment consists of two phases: restoration of the ocular surface through grafting procedures and surgical restoration of corneal integrity and optical clarity.

Thermal injury is caused by exposure to a hot object (eg, curling iron, tobacco, ash), whereas photochemical injury results from ultraviolet irradiation or infrared exposure (eg, exposure to the reflections from snow, sun gazing, viewing an eclipse of the sun without an adequate filter). These injuries can cause corneal epithelial defect, corneal opacity, conjunctival chemosis and **injection** (congestion of blood vessels), and burns of the eyelids and periocular region. Antibiotics and a pressure patch for 24 hours constitute the treatment of mild injuries. Scarring of the eyelids may require oculoplastic surgery, whereas corneal scarring may require corneal surgery.

Infectious and Inflammatory Conditions

Inflammation and infections of eye structures are common. Eye infection is a leading cause of blindness worldwide. Table 58-6 summarizes selected common infections and their treatment.

Dry Eye Syndrome

Dry eye syndrome, or keratoconjunctivitis sicca, is a deficiency in the production of any of the aqueous, mucin, or lipid tear film components; lid surface abnormalities; or epithelial abnormalities related to systemic diseases (eg, thyroid disorders, Parkinson's disease), infection, injury, or complications of medications (eg, antihistamines, oral contraceptives, phenothiazines).

Clinical Manifestations

The most common complaint in dry eye syndrome is a scratchy or foreign body sensation. Other symptoms include itching, excessive mucus secretion, inability to produce tears, a burning sensation, redness, pain, and difficulty moving the lids.

Assessment and Diagnostic Findings

Slit-lamp examination shows an absent or interrupted tear meniscus at the lower lid margin, and the conjunctiva is thickened, edematous, and hyperemic and has lost its luster. A tear meniscus is the crescent-shaped edge of the tear film in the lower lid margin. Chronic dry eyes may result in chronic conjunctival and corneal irritation that can lead to corneal erosion, scarring, ulceration, thinning, or perforation that can seriously threaten vision. Secondary bacterial infection can occur.

Management

Management of dry eye syndrome requires the complete cooperation of the patient with a regimen that needs to be followed at home for a long period; otherwise, complete relief of symptoms is unlikely. Instillation of artificial tears

TABLE 58-6 Common Infections and Inflammatory Disorders of Eye Structures

Disorder	Description	Management
Hordeolum (stye)	Acute suppurative infection of the glands of the eyelids caused by *Staphylococcus aureus*. The lid is red and edematous with a small collection of pus in the form of an abscess. There is considerable discomfort.	Warm compresses are applied directly to the affected lid area three to four times a day for 10–15 minutes. If the condition is not improved after 48 hours, incision and drainage may be indicated. Application of topical antibiotics may be prescribed thereafter.
Chalazion	Sterile inflammatory process involving chronic granulomatous inflammation of the meibomian glands; can appear as a single granuloma or multiple granulomas in the upper or lower eyelids.	Warm compresses applied three to four times a day for 10–15 minutes may resolve the inflammation in the early stages. Most often, however, surgical excision is indicated. Corticosteroid injection to the chalazion lesion may be used for smaller lesions.
Blepharitis	Chronic bilateral inflammation of the eyelid margins. There are two types: staphylococcal and seborrheic. Staphylococcal blepharitis is usually ulcerative and is more serious due to the involvement of the base of hair follicles. Permanent scarring can result.	The seborrheic type is chronic and is usually resistant to treatment, but the milder cases may respond to lid hygiene. Staphylococcal blepharitis requires topical antibiotic treatment. Instructions on lid hygiene (to keep the lid margins clean and free of exudates) are given to the patient.
Bacterial keratitis	Infection of the cornea by *Staphylococcus aureus, Streptococcus pneumoniae,* and *Pseudomonas aeruginosa*	Fortified (high-concentration) antibiotic eyedrops are administered every 30 minutes around the clock for the first few days, then every 1–2 hours. Systemic antibiotics may be administered. Cycloplegics are administered to reduce pain caused by ciliary spasm. Corticosteroid therapy and subconjunctival injections of antibiotics are controversial.
Herpes simplex keratitis	Leading cause of corneal blindness in the United States. Symptoms are severe pain, tearing, and photophobia. The dendritic ulcer has a branching, linear pattern with feathery edges and terminal bulbs at its ends. Herpes simplex keratitis can lead to recurrent stromal keratitis and persist to 12 months with residual corneal scarring.	Many lesions heal without treatment and residual effects. The treatment goal is to minimize the damaging effect of the inflammatory response and eliminate viral replication within the cornea. Penetrating keratoplasty is indicated for corneal scarring and must be performed when the herpetic disease has been inactive for many months.

during the day and an ointment at night is the usual regimen to hydrate and lubricate the eye and preserve a moist ocular surface. Anti-inflammatory medications are also used, and moisture chambers (eg, moisture chamber spectacles, swim goggles) may provide additional relief.

Patients may become hypersensitive to chemical preservatives such as benzalkonium chloride and thimerosal. For these patients, preservative-free ophthalmic solutions are used. Management of the dry eye syndrome also includes the concurrent treatment of infections, such as chronic blepharitis and acne rosacea, and treating the underlying systemic disease, such as Sjögren's syndrome (an autoimmune disease).

In advanced cases of dry eye syndrome, surgical treatment that includes punctal occlusion, grafting procedures, and lateral tarsorrhaphy (uniting the edges of the lids) are options. Punctal plugs are made of silicone material for the temporary or permanent occlusion of the puncta. This helps preserve the natural tears and prolongs the effects of artificial tears. Short-term occlusion is performed by inserting punctal or silicone rods in all four puncta. If tearing is induced, the upper plugs are removed, and the remaining lower plugs are removed in another week. Permanent occlusion is performed only in severe cases among adults who do not develop tearing after partial occlusion and who have results on a repeated Schirmer's test of 2 mm or less (filter paper is used to measure tear production).

Conjunctivitis

Conjunctivitis (inflammation of the conjunctiva) is the most common ocular disease worldwide. It is characterized by a pink appearance (hence the common term *pink eye*) because of subconjunctival blood vessel congestion.

Clinical Manifestations

General symptoms include foreign body sensation, scratching or burning sensation, itching, and photophobia. Conjunctivitis may be unilateral or bilateral, but the infection usually starts in one eye and then spreads to the other eye by hand contact.

Assessment and Diagnostic Findings

The four main clinical features important to evaluate are the type of discharge (watery, mucoid, purulent, or mucopurulent), type of conjunctival reaction (follicular or papillary), presence of pseudomembranes or true membranes, and presence or absence of lymphadenopathy (enlargement of the preauricular and submandibular lymph nodes where the eyelids drain). Pseudomembranes consist of coagulated exudate that adheres to the surface of the inflamed conjunctiva. True membranes form when the exudate adheres to the superficial layer of the conjunctiva, and removal results in bleeding. Follicles are multiple, slightly elevated lesions encircled by tiny blood vessels; they look like grains of rice. Papillae are hyperplastic conjunctival epithelium in numerous projections that are usually seen as a fine mosaic pattern under slit-lamp examination. Diagnosis is based on the distinctive characteristics of ocular signs, acute or chronic presentation, and identification of any precipitating events. Positive results of swab smear preparations and cultures confirm the diagnosis.

Types of Conjunctivitis

Conjunctivitis is classified according to its cause. The major causes are microbial infection, allergy, and irritating toxic stimuli. A wide spectrum of organisms can cause conjunctivitis, including bacteria (eg, *Chlamydia*), viruses, fungus, and parasites. Conjunctivitis can also result from an existing ocular infection or can be a manifestation of a systemic disease.

Microbial Conjunctivitis

BACTERIAL CONJUNCTIVITIS

Bacterial conjunctivitis can be acute or chronic. The acute type can develop into a chronic condition. Signs and symptoms can vary from mild to severe. Chronic bacterial conjunctivitis is usually seen in patients with lacrimal duct obstruction, chronic dacryocystitis, and chronic blepharitis. The most common causative microorganisms are *Streptococcus pneumoniae, Haemophilus influenzae,* and *Staphylococcus aureus.*

Bacterial conjunctivitis manifests with an acute onset of redness, burning, and discharge. There is papillary formation, conjunctival irritation, and injection in the fornices. The exudates are variable but are usually present on waking in the morning. The eyes may be difficult to open because of adhesions caused by the exudate. Purulent discharge occurs in severe acute bacterial infections, whereas mucopurulent discharge appears in mild cases. In gonococcal conjunctivitis, the symptoms are more acute. The exudate is profuse and purulent, and there is lymphadenopathy. Pseudomembranes may be present.

Chlamydial conjunctivitis includes **trachoma** (a bilateral chronic follicular conjunctivitis of childhood that leads to blindness during adulthood if left untreated) and inclusion conjunctivitis. Trachoma is an ancient disease and is the leading cause of preventable blindness in the world. It is prevalent in areas with hot, dry, and dusty climates and in areas with poor living conditions. It is spread by direct contact or fomites, and the vectors can be insects such as flies and gnats. The onset of trachoma in children is usually insidious, but it can be acute or subacute in adults. The initial symptoms include red inflamed eyes, tearing, photophobia, ocular pain, purulent exudates, preauricular lymphadenopathy, and lid edema. Initial ocular signs include follicular and papillary formations. At the middle stage of the disease, there is an acute inflammation with papillary hypertrophy and follicular necrosis, after which trichiasis (turning inward of hair follicles) and entropion begin to develop. The lashes that are turned in rub against the cornea and, after prolonged irritation, cause corneal erosion and ulceration. The late stage of the disease is characterized by scarred conjunctiva, subepithelial keratitis, abnormal vascularization of the cornea (pannus), and residual scars from the follicles that look like depressions in the conjunctiva (Herbert's pits). Severe corneal ulceration can lead to perforation and blindness.

Inclusion conjunctivitis affects sexually active people who have genital chlamydial infection. Transmission is by oral–genital sex or hand-to-eye transmission. Indirect transmission can occur in inadequately chlorinated swimming pools. The eye lesions usually appear a week after exposure and may be associated with a nonspecific urethritis or cervicitis. The discharge is mucopurulent, follicles are present, and there is lymphadenopathy.

VIRAL CONJUNCTIVITIS

Viral conjunctivitis can be acute and chronic. The discharge is watery, and follicles are prominent. Severe cases include pseudomembranes. The common causative organisms are adenovirus and herpes simplex virus. Conjunctivitis caused by adenovirus is highly contagious. The condition is usually preceded by symptoms of upper respiratory infection. Corneal involvement causes extreme photophobia. Symptoms include extreme tearing, redness, and foreign body sensation that can involve one or both eyes. There is lid edema, ptosis, and conjunctival **hyperemia** (dilation of the conjunctival blood vessels) (Fig. 58-18). These signs and symptoms vary from mild to severe and may last for 2 weeks. Viral conjunctivitis, although self-limited, tends to last longer than bacterial conjunctivitis.

Epidemic keratoconjunctivitis (EKC) is a highly contagious viral conjunctivitis that is easily transmitted from one

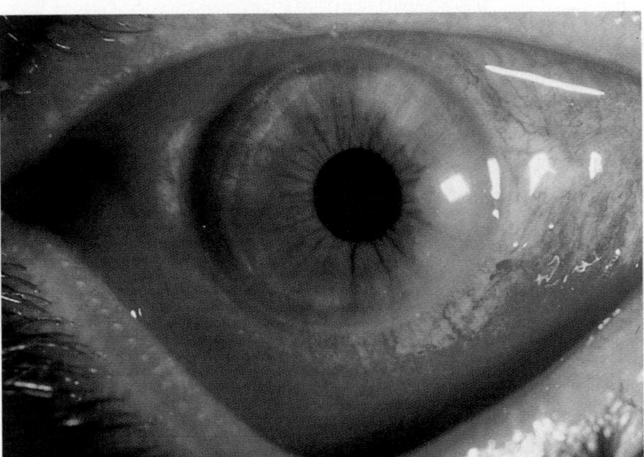

FIGURE 58-18. Conjunctival hyperemia in viral conjunctivitis.

person to another among household members, schoolchildren, and health care workers. The outbreak of epidemics is seasonal, especially during the summer when people use swimming pools. Epidemic keratoconjunctivitis is most often accompanied by preauricular lymphadenopathy and occasionally periorbital pain. There are marked follicular and papillary formations. Epidemic keratoconjunctivitis can lead to keratopathy.

Allergic Conjunctivitis

Immunologic or allergic conjunctivitis is a hypersensitivity reaction that occurs as part of allergic rhinitis (hay fever), or it can be an independent allergic reaction. The patient usually has a history of an allergy to pollens and other environmental allergens. There is extreme pruritus, epiphora (ie, excessive secretion of tears), injection, and usually severe photophobia. The stringlike mucoid discharge is usually associated with rubbing the eyes because of severe pruritus. Vernal conjunctivitis is also known as seasonal conjunctivitis because it appears mostly during warm weather. There may be large formations of papillae that have a cobblestone appearance. It is more common in children and young adults. Most affected people have a history of asthma or eczema.

Toxic Conjunctivitis

Chemical conjunctivitis can be the result of medications; chlorine from swimming pools; exposure to toxic fumes among industrial workers; or exposure to other irritants such as smoke, hair sprays, acids, and alkalis.

Management

The management of conjunctivitis depends on the type. Most types of mild and viral conjunctivitis are self-limiting, benign conditions that may not require treatment and laboratory procedures. For more severe cases, topical antibiotics, eye drops, or ointments are prescribed. Patients with gonococcal conjunctivitis require urgent antibiotic therapy. If left untreated, this ocular disease can lead to corneal perforation and blindness. The systemic complications can include meningitis and generalized septicemia.

Bacterial Conjunctivitis

Acute bacterial conjunctivitis is almost always self-limiting, lasting 2 weeks if left untreated. If treated with antibiotics, it may last a few days, except for gonococcal and staphylococcal conjunctivitis.

For trachoma, usually broad-spectrum antibiotics are administered topically and systemically. Surgical management includes the correction of trichiasis (eyelashes growing inward toward the conjuctiva and cornea) to prevent conjunctival scarring.

Adult inclusion conjunctivitis requires 1 week of antibiotics. Prevention of reinfection is important, and affected individuals and their sexual partners must seek treatment for sexually transmitted disease, if indicated.

Viral Conjunctivitis

Viral conjunctivitis is not responsive to any treatment. Cold compresses may alleviate some symptoms. It is extremely important to remember that viral conjunctivitis, especially epidemic keratoconjunctivitis, is highly contagious. Patients must be made aware of the contagious nature of the disease, and adequate instructions must be given (Chart 58-11). These instructions should include an emphasis on hand hygiene and avoiding sharing of hand towels, face cloths,

CHART 58-11

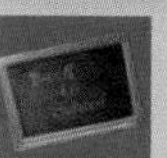

Patient Education

Instructions for Patients With Viral Conjunctivitis

Viral conjunctivitis is a highly contagious eye infection. It can easily spread from one person to another. The symptoms can be alarming, but they are not serious. The following information will help you understand this eye condition and how to take care of yourself and/or your family member at home.

- Your eyes will look red and will have watery discharge, and your lids will be swollen for about a week.
- You will experience eye pain, a sandy sensation in your eye, and sensitivity to light.
- Symptoms will resolve after about 1 week.
- You may use light cold compresses over your eyes for about 10 minutes four to five times a day to soothe the pain.
- You may use artificial tears for the sandy sensation in your eye and mild pain medications such as acetaminophen (Tylenol).
- You need to stay at home. Children must not play outside. You may return to work or school after 7 days when the redness and discharge have cleared. You may obtain a doctor's note to return to work or school.
- Do not share towels, linens, makeup, or toys.
- Wash your hands thoroughly with soap and water frequently, including and before and after you apply artificial tears or cold compresses.
- Use a new tissue every time you wipe the discharge from your eye. You may dampen the tissue with clean water to clean the outside of the eye.
- You may wash your face and take a shower as you normally do.
- Discard all of your makeup articles. You must not apply makeup until the disease is over.
- You may wear dark glasses if bright lights bother you.
- If the discharge from your eye turns yellowish and puslike or you experience changes in your vision, you need to return to the health care provider for an examination.

and eye drops. Tissues should be directly discarded into a covered trash can.

Proper steps must be taken to avoid nosocomial infections. Frequent hand hygiene and procedures for environmental cleaning and disinfection of equipment used for eye examination must be strictly followed at all times. To prevent spread during outbreaks of conjunctivitis caused by adenovirus, health care facilities must set aside specified areas for treating patients with or suspected of having conjunctivitis caused by adenovirus to prevent spread. All forms of tonometry must be avoided unless medically indicated. All multidose medications must be discarded at the end of each day or when contaminated. Infected employees and others must not be allowed to work or attend school until symptoms have resolved, which can take 3 to 7 days.

Allergic Conjunctivitis

Patients with allergic conjunctivitis, especially recurrent vernal or seasonal conjunctivitis, are usually given corticosteroids in ophthalmic preparations. Depending on the severity of the disease, they may be given oral preparations. Use of vasoconstrictors, such as topical epinephrine solution, cold compresses, ice packs, and cool ventilation usually provide comfort by decreasing swelling.

Toxic Conjunctivitis

For conjunctivitis caused by chemical irritants, the eye must be irrigated immediately and profusely with saline or sterile water.

Uveitis

Inflammation of the uveal tract (uveitis) can affect the iris, the ciliary body, or the choroid. There are two types of uveitis: nongranulomatous and granulomatous.

The more common type of uveitis is the nongranulomatous type, which manifests as an acute condition with pain, photophobia, and a pattern of conjunctival injection, especially around the cornea. The pupil is small or irregular, and vision is blurred. There may be small, fine precipitates on the posterior corneal surface and cells in the aqueous humor (ie, cell and flare). If the uveitis is severe, a **hypopyon** (accumulation of pus in the anterior chamber) may occur. The condition may be unilateral or bilateral and may be recurrent. Repeated attacks of nongranulomatous anterior uveitis can cause anterior synechiae (peripheral iris adheres to the cornea and impedes outflow of aqueous humor). Posterior synechiae (adherence of the iris and lens) block aqueous outflow from the posterior chamber. Secondary glaucoma can result from either anterior or posterior synechiae. Cataracts may also occur as a sequela to uveitis.

Granulomatous uveitis can have a more insidious onset and can involve any portion of the uveal tract. It tends to be chronic. Symptoms such as photophobia and pain may be minimal. Vision is markedly and adversely affected. Conjunctival injection is diffuse, and there may be vitreous clouding. In a severe posterior uveitis, such as chorioretinitis, there may be retinal and choroidal hemorrhages.

Management

Because photophobia is a common symptom, patients should wear dark glasses outdoors. Ciliary spasm and synechia are best avoided through mydriasis; cyclopentolate (Cyclogyl) and atropine are commonly used. Local corticosteroid drops, such as Pred Forte 1% and Flarex 0.1%, instilled four to six times a day are also used to decrease inflammation. In very severe cases, systemic corticosteroids, as well as intravitreal corticosteroids, may be used. The National Eye Institute of the National Institutes of Health is conducting a clinical trial to examine the safety and effectiveness of treating uveitis with daclizumab, a monoclonal antibody. Daclizumab (Zenapax) is designed to prevent a specific chemical interaction needed by immune cells, such as lymphocytes, to produce inflammation.

If the uveitis is recurrent, a careful history prior to a medical workup should be initiated to discover any underlying causes. This evaluation should include a complete history, physical examination, and diagnostic tests, including a complete blood cell count, erythrocyte sedimentation rate, antinuclear antibodies, and Venereal Disease Research Laboratory (VDRL) and Lyme disease titers. Underlying causes include autoimmune disorders such as ankylosing spondylitis and sarcoidosis as well as toxoplasmosis, herpes zoster virus, ocular candidiasis, histoplasmosis, herpes simplex virus, tuberculosis, and syphilis.

Orbital Cellulitis

Orbital cellulitis is inflammation of the tissues surrounding the eye and may result from bacterial, fungal, or viral inflammatory conditions of contiguous structures, such as the face, oropharynx, dental structures, or intracranial structures. It can also result from foreign bodies and from a preexisting ocular infection, such as dacryocystitis and panophthalmitis, or from generalized septicemia. Infection of the sinuses is the most frequent cause. Infection originating in the sinuses can spread easily to the orbit through the thin bony walls and foramina or by means of the interconnecting venous system of the orbit and sinuses. The most common causative organisms are staphylococci and streptococci in adults and *H. influenzae* in children. The symptoms include pain, lid swelling, conjunctival edema, **proptosis**, and decreased ocular motility. With such edema, optic nerve compression can occur and IOP may increase.

The severe intraorbital tension caused by abscess formation and the impairment of optic nerve function in orbital cellulitis can result in permanent visual loss. Because of the orbit's proximity to the brain, orbital cellulitis can lead to life-threatening complications, such as intracranial abscess and cavernous sinus thrombosis.

Management

Immediate administration of high-dose, broad-spectrum, systemic antibiotics is indicated. Cultures and Gram-stained smears are obtained. Monitoring changes in visual acuity, degree of proptosis, central nervous system function (eg, nausea, vomiting, fever, cognitive changes), displacement of the globe, extraocular movements, pupillary signs, and the fundus is extremely important. Consultation with an otolaryngologist is necessary, especially when sinusitis is suspected. In the event of abscess formation or progressive loss of vision, surgical drainage of the abscess or sinus is performed. Sinusotomy and antibiotic irrigation are also performed.

Orbital and Ocular Tumors

Benign Tumors of the Orbit

Benign tumors can develop from infancy and grow rapidly or slowly and present in later life. Some benign tumors are superficial and are easily identifiable by external presentation, palpation, and x-rays, but some are deep and may require a CT scan for a more thorough and precise diagnosis. There can be a significant proptosis, and visual function may be jeopardized. Benign tumors are masses characterized by the lack of infiltration in the surrounding tissues. Examples are cystic dermoid cysts and mucocele, hemangiomas, lymphangiomas, lacrimal tumors, and neurofibromas.

To prevent recurrence, benign masses are excised completely when possible. Sometimes, excision is difficult because of the involvement of some portions of the orbital bones, such as deep dermoid cysts, in which dissection of the bone is required. Subtotal resection may be indicated in deep benign tumors that intertwine with other orbital structures, such as optic nerve meningiomas. Complete removal of the tumor may endanger visual function.

Benign Tumors of the Eyelids

Benign tumors include a wide variety of neoplasms and increase in frequency with age. Nevi may be unpigmented at birth and may enlarge and darken in adolescence or may never acquire any pigment at all. Hemangiomas are vascular capillary tumors that may be bright, superficial, strawberry-red lesions (ie, strawberry nevus) or bluish and purplish deeper lesions. Milia are small, white, slightly elevated cysts of the eyelid that may occur in multiples. Xanthelasma are yellowish, lipoid deposits on both lids near the inner angle of the eye that commonly appear as a result of the aging of the skin or a lipid disorder. Molluscum contagiosum lesions are flat, symmetric growths along the lid margin caused by a virus that can result in conjunctivitis and keratitis if debris gets into the conjunctival sac.

Treatment of benign congenital lid lesions is rarely indicated, except when visual function is affected. Corticosteroid injection to the hemangioma lesion is usually effective, but surgical excision may be performed. Benign lid lesions usually present aesthetic problems rather than visual function problems. Surgical excision, or electrocautery, is primarily performed for cosmetic reasons, except for cases of molluscum contagiosum, for which surgical intervention is performed to prevent an infectious process that may ensue.

Benign Tumors of the Conjunctiva

Conjunctival nevus, a congenital, benign neoplasm, is a flat, slightly elevated, brown spot that becomes pigmented during late childhood or adolescence. This should be differentiated from the pigmented lesion melanosis acquired at middle age, which tends to wax and wane and become malignant melanoma. Keratin- and sebum-containing dermoid cysts are congenital and can be found in the conjunctiva. Dermolipoma is a congenital tumor that manifests as a smooth, rounded growth in the conjunctiva near the lateral canthus. Papillomas are usually soft with irregular surfaces and appear on the lid margins. Treatment consists of surgical excision.

Malignant Tumors of the Orbit

Rhabdomyosarcoma is the most common malignant primary orbital tumor in childhood, but it can also develop in elderly people. The symptoms of rhabdomyosarcoma include sudden painless proptosis of one eye followed by lid swelling, conjunctival chemosis, and impairment of ocular motility. Imaging of these tumors establishes the size, configuration, location, and stage of the disease; delineates the degree of bone destruction; and is useful in estimating the field for radiation therapy, if needed. The most common site of metastasis is the lung.

Management of these primary malignant orbital tumors involves three major therapeutic modalities: surgery, radiation therapy, and adjuvant chemotherapy. The degree of orbital destruction is important in planning the surgical approach. Resection often involves removal of the eyeball. The psychological needs of the patient and family are paramount in planning the management approach.

Malignant Tumors of the Eyelid

Basal cell carcinoma is the most common malignant tumor of the eyelid. Squamous cell carcinoma occurs less frequently but is considered the second most common malignant tumor. Malignant melanoma is rare. Malignant eyelid tumors occur more frequently among people with a fair complexion who have a history of chronic exposure to the sun.

Basal cell carcinoma appears as a painless nodule that may ulcerate. The lesion is invasive, spreads to the surrounding tissues, and grows slowly but does not metastasize. It usually appears on the lower lid margin near the inner canthus with a pearly white margin. Squamous cell carcinoma of the eyelids may resemble basal cell carcinoma initially because it also grows slowly and painlessly. It tends to ulcerate and invade the surrounding tissues, but it can metastasize to the regional lymph nodes. Malignant melanoma may not be pigmented and can arise from nevi. It spreads to the surrounding tissues and metastasizes to other organs.

Complete excision of these carcinomas is followed by reconstruction with skin grafting if the surgical excision is extensive. The ocular postoperative site and the graft donor site are monitored for bleeding. Donor graft sites may include the buccal mucosa, the thigh, or the abdomen. The patient is referred to an oncologist for evaluation of the need for radiation therapy treatment and monitoring for metastasis. Early diagnosis and surgical management are the basis of a good prognosis. These conditions have life-threatening consequences, and surgical excisions may result in facial disfigurement. Emotional support is an extremely important aspect of nursing management.

Malignant Tumors of the Conjunctiva

Conjunctival carcinoma most often grows in the exposed areas of the conjunctiva. The typical lesions are usually gelatinous and whitish due to keratin formation. They grow gradually, and deep invasion and metastasis are rare. Malignant melanoma is rare but may arise from a preexisting nevus or acquired melanosis during middle age. Squamous cell carcinoma is also rare but invasive.

The management is surgical incision. Some benign tumors and most malignant tumors recur. To avoid recurrences, patients usually undergo radiation therapy and cryotherapy after the excision of malignant tumors. Cosmetic disfigurement may result from extensive excision when deep invasion by the malignant tumor is involved.

Malignant Tumors of the Globe

Retinoblastoma, a malignant tumor of the retina, occurs in childhood, is hereditary, and requires complete enucleation if there is to be a chance for successful outcome (Chart 58-12). Ocular melanoma, another cancer, primarily occurs in adults. This rare, malignant choroidal tumor is often discovered on a retinal examination. In its early stages, it could be mistaken for a nevus. Many ophthalmologists may practice for decades and never encounter this lesion. For this reason, any patient who is suspected of having ocular melanoma should be immediately referred to an ocular oncologist with experience in this disease.

Although many patients do not have symptoms in the early stages, some patients complain of blurred vision or a change in eye color. A number of such tumors have been found in people with blindness who have painful eyes. In addition to a complete physical examination to discover any evidence of metastasis (to the liver, lung, and breast), retinal fundus photography, fluorescein angiography, and ultrasonography are performed. The diagnosis is confirmed at biopsy after enucleation.

Tumors are classified according to boundary lines (apical height and basal diameter) as small, medium, or large. Small tumors are generally monitored, whereas medium and large tumors require treatment. Treatment consists of radiation, enucleation, or both. Radiation therapy may be achieved by external beam performed in repeated episodes over several days or through the implantation of a small plaque that contains radioactive iodine pellets (I-125) over the tumor.

CHART 58-12

Ocular Effects of Selected Genetic Conditions

The mapping of the human genome has enhanced the opportunity to understand the genetic component of ophthalmic disorders and to develop new methods of prevention and treatment. Apparently more than one gene is involved in any particular condition, making genetic counseling an important part of the care and prevention of inherited diseases. Ocular effects of some genetic conditions follow.

Retinoblastoma

A malignant retinal tumor occurring in 1 of every 15,000 live births, it is hereditary in 30% to 40% of cases. All bilateral cases are hereditary. The retinoblastoma gene is found on chromosome 13, region q14. If this gene is inhibited, the growth in retinal cells is unchecked and the retinoblastoma results. Signs and symptoms include an initial leukocoria or "white" pupil with a peculiar light reflection and possibly strabismus as well. Less frequent signs are uveitis, glaucoma, hyphema, nystagmus, and periorbital cellulitis. Treatment for this life-threatening tumor is enucleation, if the tumor is large and unilateral. If the eye is removed before cancer spreads to the optic nerve, the cure rate is greater than 90%.

Marfan Syndrome

Ophthalmic consequences may include amblyopia and dislocation of the lens. Patients are often myopic and may be at increased risk for retinal detachment.

Leber Congenital Amaurosis

To date, four genes have been implicated in this disorder, which is characterized by decreased vision and onset in childhood, generally before 7 years of age. It accounts for 10% to 18% of cases of congenital blindness (some infants may be blind from birth). Other signs and symptoms include strabismus, nystagmus, photophobia, cataracts, and keratoconus.

Surgical Procedures and Enucleation

Orbital Surgeries

Orbital surgeries may be performed to repair fractures, remove a foreign body, or remove benign or malignant growths. Surgical procedures involving the orbit and lids affect facial appearance (cosmesis). The goals are to recover and preserve visual function and to maintain the anatomic relationship of the ocular structures to achieve cosmesis. During the repair of orbital fractures, the orbital bones are realigned to follow the anatomic positions of facial structures.

Orbital surgical procedures involve working around delicate structures of the eye, such as the optic nerve, retinal blood vessels, and ocular muscles. Complications of orbital surgical procedures may include blindness as a result of damage to the optic nerve and its blood supply. Sudden pain and loss of vision may indicate intraorbital hemorrhage or compression of the optic nerve. Ptosis and diplopia may result from trauma to the extraocular muscles during the surgical procedure, but these conditions typically resolve after a few weeks.

Prophylaxis with IV antibiotics is the usual postoperative regimen after orbital surgery, especially with repair of orbital fractures and intraorbital foreign body removal. IV corticosteroids are used if there is a concern about optic nerve swelling. Topical ocular antibiotics are typically instilled, and antibiotic ointments are applied externally to the skin suture sites.

For the first 24 to 48 hours postoperatively, ice compresses are applied over the periocular area to decrease periorbital swelling, facial swelling, and hematoma. The head of the patient's bed should be elevated to a comfortable position (30 to 45 degrees).

Discharge teaching should include medication instructions for oral antibiotics, instillation of ophthalmic medications, and application of ocular compresses.

Enucleation

Enucleation is the removal of the entire eye and part of the optic nerve. It may be performed for the following conditions:

- Severe injury resulting in prolapse of uveal tissue or loss of light projection (the ability to identify the direction of the light source) or perception
- An irritated, blind, painful, deformed, or disfigured eye, usually caused by glaucoma, retinal detachment, or chronic inflammation
- An eye without useful vision that is producing or has produced sympathetic ophthalmia in the other eye
- Intraocular tumors that are untreatable by other means

The procedure for enucleation involves the separation and cutting of each of the ocular muscles, dissection of the Tenon's capsule (fibrous membrane covering the sclera), and cutting of the optic nerve from the eyeball. The insertion of an orbital implant typically follows, and the conjunctiva is closed. A large pressure dressing is applied over the area.

Evisceration involves the surgical removal of the intraocular contents through an incision or opening in the cornea or sclera. Evisceration may be performed to treat severe ocular trauma with ruptured globe, severe ocular inflammation, or severe ocular infection. The optic nerve, sclera, extraocular muscles, and sometimes the cornea are left intact. The main advantage of evisceration over enucleation is that the final cosmetic result and motility after fitting the ocular prosthesis are enhanced. This procedure would be more acceptable to a patient whose body image is severely threatened. The main disadvantage is the high risk of sympathetic ophthalmia.

Exenteration is the removal of the eyelids, the eye, and various amounts of orbital contents. It is indicated in malignancies in the orbit that are life-threatening or when more conservative modalities of treatment have failed or are inappropriate. An example is squamous cell carcinoma of the paranasal sinuses, skin, and conjunctiva with deep orbital involvement. In its most extensive form, exenteration may include the removal of all orbital tissues and resection of the orbital bones.

Ocular Prostheses

Orbital implants and conformers (ocular prostheses usually made of silicone rubber) maintain the shape of the eye after enucleation or evisceration to prevent a contracted, sunken appearance. The temporary conformer is placed over the conjunctival closure after the implantation of an orbital implant. A conformer is placed after the enucleation or evisceration procedure to protect the suture line, maintain the fornices, prevent contracture of the socket in preparation for the ocular prosthesis, and promote the integrity of the eyelids.

All ocular prosthetics have limitations in their motility. There are two designs of eye prostheses. The anophthalmic ocular prostheses are used in the absence of the globe. Scleral shells look just like the anophthalmic prosthesis (Fig. 58-19) but are thinner and fit over a globe with intact corneal sensation. An eye prosthesis usually lasts about 6 years, depending on the quality of fit, comfort, and cosmetic appearance. When the anophthalmic socket is completely healed, conformers are replaced with prosthetic eyes.

An ocularist is a specially trained and skilled professional who makes prosthetic eyes. After the ophthalmologist is satisfied that the anophthalmic socket is completely healed and is ready for prosthetic fitting, the patient is referred to an ocularist. The healing period is usually 6 to 8 weeks. It is advisable for the patient to have a consultation with the ocularist before the fitting. Obtaining accurate information and verbalizing concerns can lessen anxiety about wearing an ocular prosthesis.

Medical Management

Removal of an eye has physical, social, and psychological ramifications for any person. The significance of loss of the eye and vision must be addressed in the plan of care. The patient's preparation should include information about the surgical procedure and placement of orbital implants and conformers and the availability of ocular prosthetics to en-

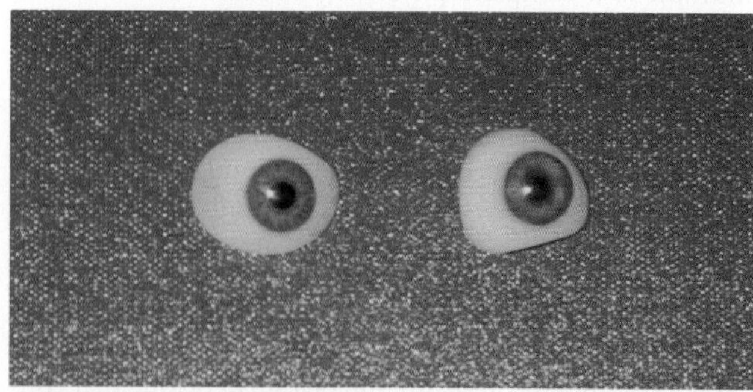

FIGURE 58-19. Eye prostheses. (*Left*) Anophthalmic ocular prosthesis. (*Right*) Scleral shell.

hance cosmetic appearance. In some cases, patients may choose to see an ocularist before the surgery to discuss ocular prosthetics.

Nursing Management

Teaching About Postsurgical and Prosthetic Care

Patients who undergo eye removal need to know that they will usually have a large ocular pressure dressing, which is typically removed after a week, and that an ophthalmic topical antibiotic ointment is applied in the socket three times daily.

After the removal of an eye, there is a loss of depth perception. Patients must be advised to take extra caution in their ambulation and movement to avoid miscalculations that may result in injury. It may take some time to adjust to monocular vision.

The patient must be advised that conformers may accidentally fall out of the socket. If this happens, the conformer must be washed, wiped dry, and placed back in the socket.

When surgical eye removal is unexpected, such as in severe ocular trauma, leaving no time for the patient and family to prepare for the loss, the nurse's role in providing emotional support is crucial.

Promoting Home and Community-Based Care

TEACHING PATIENTS SELF-CARE

Patients need to be taught how to insert, remove, and care for the prosthetic eye. Proper hand hygiene must be observed before inserting and removing an ocular prosthesis. A suction cup may be used if there are problems with manual dexterity. Precautions, such as draping a towel over the sink and closing the sink drain, must be taken to avoid loss of the prosthesis. When instructing patients or family members, a return demonstration is important to assess the level of understanding and ability to perform the procedure.

Before insertion, the inner punctal or outer lateral aspects and the superior and inferior aspects of the prosthesis must be identified by locating the identifying marks, such as a reddish color in the inner punctal area. For people with low vision, other forms of identifying markers, such as dots or notches, are used. The upper lid is raised high enough to create a space; then the patient learns to slide the prosthesis up, underneath, and behind the upper eyelid. Meanwhile, the patient pulls the lower eyelid down to help put the prosthesis in place and to have its inferior edge fall back gradually to the lower eyelid. The lower eyelid is checked for correct positioning.

To remove the prosthesis, the patient cups one hand on the cheek to catch the prosthesis, places the forefinger of the free hand against the midportion of the lower eyelid, and gazes upward. Gazing upward brings the inferior edge of the prosthesis nearer the inferior eyelid margin. With the finger pushing inward, downward, and laterally against the lower eyelid, the prosthesis slides out, and the cupped hand acts as the receptacle.

CONTINUING CARE

An eye prosthesis can be worn and left in place for several months. Hygiene and comfort are usually maintained with daily irrigation of the prosthesis in place with normal saline solution, hard contact lens solution, or artificial tears. In the case of dry eye symptoms, the use of ophthalmic ointment lubricants or oil-based drops, such as vitamin E and mineral oil, can be helpful. Removing crusting and mucous discharge that accumulate overnight is performed with the prosthesis in place. Malpositions may occur when wiping or rubbing the prosthesis in the socket. The prosthesis can be repositioned with the use of clean fingers. Proper wiping of the prosthesis should be a gentle temporal-to-nasal motion to avoid malpositions.

The prosthesis needs to be removed and cleaned when it becomes uncomfortable and when there is increased mucous discharge. The socket should also be rendered free of mucus and inspected for any signs of infection. Any unusual discomfort, irritation, or redness of the globe or eyelids may indicate excessive wear, debris under the shell, or lack of proper hygiene. Any infection or irritation that does not resolve needs medical attention.

Ocular Consequences of Systemic Disease

Diabetic Retinopathy

Of all of the medical disorders that the nurse encounters, diabetes mellitus is one of the most common, and it can have devastating effects on the patient. In the United States today, diabetes is the leading cause of new cases of blindness in people between 20 and 74 years of age (Prevent Blindness America, 2002). Before the discovery of insulin in the 1920s, diabetic retinopathy was relatively rare because most people with diabetes did not survive for more than 1 or 2 years. However, with the many advancements in the treatment of diabetes, more and more patients are able to survive and enjoy relatively normal lifespans, but they are also confronted with the complications of long-term diabetes. One of the most serious complications is retinopathy. Chapter 41 provides a detailed discussion of diabetic retinopathy.

Cytomegalovirus Retinitis

Many ophthalmic complications have been associated with AIDS. Cytomegalovirus (CMV) is the most common cause of retinal inflammation in patients with AIDS. Early symptoms of CMV retinitis vary from patient to patient. Some patients complain of floaters or a decrease in peripheral vision. Some have a paracentral or central scotoma, whereas others have fluctuations in vision from macular edema. The retina often becomes thin and atrophic and susceptible to retinal tears and breaks.

CMV retinitis generally takes one of three forms: hemorrhagic, brushfire, or granular. In the hemorrhagic type, large areas of white, necrotic retina may be associated with retinal hemorrhage. In the brushfire type, a yellow-white margin begins at the edge of burned-out atrophic retina. This retinitis expands and, if untreated, involves the entire retina. In the granular type, white granular lesions in the periphery of the retina gradually expand. The white, feathery infiltration of the retina destroys sensory retina and leads to necrosis, optic atrophy, and retinal detachment.

Medical Management

Pharmacologic Therapy

Pharmacologic agents available for treatment of CMV retinitis include ganciclovir (Cytovene), foscarnet (Foscavir), and cidofovir (Vistide).

Ganciclovir is administered intravenously, orally, or intravitreously in the acute stage of CMV retinitis. In a relatively new mode of ganciclovir administration, a 4-mm intraocular implant, or insert, containing ganciclovir embedded in a polymer-based system slowly releases the medication. The insert is surgically placed in the posterior segment of the eye, and the medication diffuses locally to the site of the infection over a period of 5 to 8 months before the insert must be replaced. This method of administration is effective; a study that combined the use of the intravitreous implant with oral ganciclovir demonstrated a reduction in the risk of new CMV disease as well as a delay in the progression of the retinitis (Martin, Kuppermann, Wolitz, et al., 1999). When administered systemically, ganciclovir is a very potent medication; it can cause neutropenia, thrombocytopenia, anemia, and elevated serum creatinine levels. The surgically implanted sustained-release insert enables higher concentrations of ganciclovir to reach the CMV retinitis, but there are risks and complications associated with the inserts, including endophthalmitis, retinal detachment, and hypotony.

Foscarnet inhibits viral DNA replication. It may be the medication of choice when ganciclovir is ineffective. It may be administered by IV or intravitreal injections. The combination of foscarnet and ganciclovir has been more effective than either medication alone. Nephrotoxicity may occur with systemic foscarnet, and renal function must be monitored carefully.

Cidofovir impedes CMV replication and is administered IV. Cidofovir has been shown to delay the progression of CMV retinitis significantly. Nephrotoxicity, proteinuria, and increased serum creatinine levels are significant side effects.

In the late 1990s, the routine management of patients with AIDS, including those with CMV retinitis, changed with the introduction of highly active antiretroviral therapy (HAART). HAART is a combination of two or three medications of different categories. For example, a nucleoside analog such as zidovudine administered in combination with one or more protease inhibitors such as ritonavir has led to a suppression of human immunodeficiency virus (HIV) replication for sustained periods. The immune system can then recover to a functional level. Several patients who had been treated for CMV retinitis have been able to discontinue treatment for CMV retinitis as their immune systems rebounded. However, some patients develop immune recovery uveitis, characterized by intraocular inflammation, cystoid macular edema, and the formation of epiretinal membranes. Immune recovery uveitis is managed by corticosteroids or by injection of corticosteroids into the sub-Tenon's area of the eye.

Hypertension-Related Eye Changes

Hypertension can shorten the lifespan by as many as 20 years and affects the eye as well as the heart, brain, and kidneys. Hypertension of longstanding duration goes hand in hand with atherosclerosis, and the associated retinal changes are evidenced by the development of retinal arteriolar changes, such as tortuousness, narrowing, and a change in light reflex. Funduscopic examination reveals a copper or silver coloration of the arterioles and venous compression (arteriovenous nicking) at the arteriolar and venous crossings. Intraretinal hemorrhages from hypertension appear flame-shaped because they occur in the nerve fiber layer of the retina.

Hypertension can also occur as an acute consequence of conditions such as pheochromocytoma, acute renal failure, and pregnancy-induced hypertension. The retinopathy associated with these crisis states is extensive, and the manifestations include cotton-wool spots, retinal hemorrhages, retinal edema, and retinal exudates, often clustered around the macula.

The choroid is also affected by the profound and abrupt rise in blood pressure and resulting vasoconstriction, and ischemia may result in serous retinal detachments and infarction of the RPE. Ischemic optic neuropathy and **papilledema** (swelling of the optic disc due to increased IOP) may also result. Blood pressure in these more severe stages should be lowered in a controlled gradual fashion to avoid ischemia of the optic nerve and brain secondary to a too-rapid fall in blood pressure. For further information about hypertension, see Chapter 32.

Concepts in Ocular Medication Administration

The main objective of ocular medication delivery is to maximize the amount of medication that reaches the ocular site of action in sufficient concentration to produce a beneficial therapeutic effect. This is determined by the dynamics of ocular pharmacokinetics: absorption, distribution, metabolism, and excretion.

Topical administration of ocular medications results in only a 1% to 7% absorption rate by the ocular tissues. Ocular absorption involves the entry of a medication into the aqueous humor through the different routes of ocular medication administration. The rate and extent of aqueous humor absorption are determined by the characteristics of the medication and the anatomy and physiology of the eye. Natural barriers of absorption that diminish the efficacy of ocular medications include the following:

- *Limited size of the conjunctival sac.* The conjunctival sac can hold only 50 μL, and any excess is wasted. The volume of one eye drop from commercial topical ocular solutions typically ranges from 20 to 35 μL.
- *Corneal membrane barriers.* The epithelial, stromal, and endothelial layers are barriers to absorption.
- *Blood–ocular barriers.* Blood–ocular barriers prevent high ocular tissue concentration of most ophthalmic medica-

tions because they separate the bloodstream from the ocular tissues and keep foreign substances from entering the eye, thereby limiting a medication's efficacy.
- *Tearing, blinking, and drainage.* Increased tear production and drainage due to ocular irritation or an ocular condition may dilute or wash out an instilled eye drop; blinking expels an instilled eye drop from the conjunctival sac.

Distribution of an ocular medication into the various ocular tissues varies by tissue type; the various tissues (eg, conjunctiva, cornea, lens, iris, ciliary body, choroids) absorb medications to varying degrees. Medications penetrate the corneal epithelium by diffusion by passing through the cells (intracellular) or by passing between the cells (intercellular). Water-soluble (hydrophilic) medications diffuse through the intracellular route, and fat-soluble (lipophilic) medications diffuse through the intercellular route. Topical administration usually does not reach the retina in significant concentrations. Because the space between the ciliary process and the lens is small, medication diffusion in the vitreous is slow. When high concentrations of medication in the vitreous are required, intraocular injection is often chosen to bypass the natural ocular anatomic and physiologic barriers.

Aqueous solutions are most commonly used for the eye. They are the least expensive medications and interfere least with vision. However, corneal contact time is brief because tears dilute the medication. Ophthalmic ointments have extended retention time in the conjunctival sac and provide a higher concentration than eye drops. The major disadvantage of ointments is the blurred vision that results after application. In general, eyelids and eyelid margins are best treated with ointments. The conjunctiva, limbus, cornea, and anterior chamber are treated most effectively with instilled solutions or suspensions. Subconjunctival injection may be necessary for better absorption in the anterior chamber. If high medication concentrations are required in the posterior chamber, intravitreal injections or systemically absorbed medications are considered. Contact lenses and collagen shields soaked in antibiotics are alternative delivery methods for treating corneal infections.

Of all these delivery methods, the topical route of administration—instilled eye drops and applied ointments—remains the most common. Topical instillation, which is the least invasive method, permits self-administration of medication and produces fewer side effects.

Preservatives are commonly used in ocular medications. Benzalkonium chloride, for example, prevents the growth of organisms and enhances the corneal permeability of most medications; however, some patients are allergic to this preservative. This may be suspected even if the patient had never before experienced an allergic reaction to systemic use of the medication in question. Eye drops without preservatives can be prepared by pharmacists.

Commonly Used Ocular Medications

Common ocular medications include topical anesthetic, mydriatic, and cycloplegic agents that reduce IOP; anti-infective medications, corticosteroids, NSAIDs, antiallergy medications, eye irrigants, and lubricants.

Topical Anesthetics

One or two drops of proparacaine hydrochloride (Ophthaine 0.5%) and tetracaine hydrochloride (Pontocaine 0.5%) are instilled before diagnostic procedures such as tonometry and gonioscopy and in minor ocular procedures such as removal of sutures or conjunctival or corneal scrapings. Topical anesthetics are also used for severe eye pain to allow the patient to open his or her eyes for examination or treatment (eg, eye irrigation for chemical burns). Anesthesia occurs within 20 seconds to 1 minute and lasts 10 to 20 minutes. The nurse must instruct the patient not to rub his or her eyes while anesthetized because this may result in corneal damage.

Most patients are not allowed to take topical anesthetics home because of the risk of overuse. Patients with corneal abrasions and erosions experience severe pain and are often tempted to overuse topical anesthetic eye drops. Overuse of these drops results in softening of the cornea. Prolonged use of anesthetic drops can delay wound healing and can lead to permanent corneal opacification and scarring, resulting in visual loss.

Mydriatics and Cycloplegics

Mydriasis, or pupil dilation, is the main objective of the administration of mydriatic and cycloplegic agents (Table 58-7). These two types of medications function differently and are used in combination to achieve the maximal dilation that is needed during surgery and fundus examinations to give the ophthalmologist a better view of the internal eye structures. **Mydriatics** potentiate alpha-adrenergic sympathetic effects that result in the relaxation of the ciliary muscle. This causes the pupil to dilate. However, this sympathetic action alone is not enough to sustain mydriasis because of its short duration of action. The strong light used during an eye examination also stimulates miosis (ie, pupillary contraction). Cycloplegic medications are administered to paralyze the iris sphincter.

The patient is instructed about the temporary effects of mydriasis on vision, such as glare and the inability to focus properly. The patient may have difficulty reading. The effects of the various mydriatics and cycloplegics can last 3 hours to several days. The patient is advised to wear sunglasses (most eye clinics provide protective sunglasses). The ability to drive is dependent on the person's age, vision, and comfort level. Some patients can drive safely with the use of sunglasses, whereas others may need to be driven home.

Mydriatic and cycloplegic agents affect the central nervous system. Their effects are most prominent in children and elderly patients; these patients must be assessed closely for symptoms, such as increased blood pressure, tachycardia, dizziness, ataxia, confusion, disorientation, incoherent speech, and hallucination. These medications are contraindicated in patients with narrow angles or shallow anterior chambers and in patients taking monoamine oxidase inhibitors or tricyclic antidepressants.

Medications Used to Treat Glaucoma

Therapeutic medications for glaucoma are used to lower IOP by decreasing aqueous production or increasing aqueous outflow. Because glaucoma calls for lifetime therapy, the

TABLE 58-7 Mydriatics and Cycloplegics

Medication	Available Preparation/ Concentration	Indication/Dosage	Peak		Recovery Time	
			Mydriasis	Cycloplegia	Mydriasis	Cycloplegia
phenylephrine (Neo-Synephrine)	Solutions (2.5%, 10%)	Administered with cycloplegics in pupillary dilation for ophthalmoscopy and surgical procedures every 5–10 min × 3 or until the pupils are fully dilated	10–60 min	—	3–6 h	—
atropine (Atropine Ophthalmic)	Ointment (0.5%–2%) Solutions (0.5%–3%)	In glaucoma, uveitis, or after surgery, 2× to 4× daily	30–40 min	60–180 min	7–10 d	6–12 d
scopolamine (Isopto Hyoscine Ophthalmic)	Solution (0.25%)	Same as atropine	20–30 min	30–60 min	3–7 d	3–7 d
homatropine (Homatropine HBR)	Solution (5%–2.5%)	Same as atropine and scopolamine	40–60 min	30–60 min	1–3 d	1–3 d
cyclopentolate (AK-Pentolate)	Solution (0.5%–2%)	Administered with mydriatics q 5–10 min × 3 or until the pupils are fully dilated for ophthalmoscopy and surgical procedures	30–60 min	25–75 min	1 d	6–24 h
tropicamide (Mydriacyl)	Solution (0.25%–1%)		20–40 min	20–35 min	6 h	<6 h

Data on peak and recovery time from *Ophthalmic Drug Facts by Facts and Comparisons* (1998), pp. 45 and 49. Copyright 1998 by Facts and Comparisons, a Wolters Kluwer Company. Adapted with permission.

patient must be instructed regarding both the ocular and systemic side effects of the medications.

Most antiglaucoma medications affect the accommodation of the lens and limit light entry through a constricted pupil. Visual acuity and the ability to focus may be affected. Factors to consider in selecting glaucoma medications are efficacy, systemic and ocular side effects, convenience, and cost.

Anti-infective Medications

Anti-infective medications include antibiotic, antifungal, and antiviral agents. Most are available as drops, ointments, or subconjunctival or intravitreal injections. Antibiotics include penicillin, cephalosporins, aminoglycosides, and fluoroquinolones. The main antifungal agent is amphotericin B. Side effects of amphotericin are serious and include severe pain, conjunctival necrosis, iritis, and retinal toxicity. Antiviral medications include acyclovir and ganciclovir. They are used to treat ocular infections associated with herpesvirus and CMV. Patients receiving ocular anti-infective agents are subject to the same side effects and adverse reactions as those receiving oral or parenteral medications.

Corticosteroids and Nonsteroidal Anti-Inflammatory Drugs

The topical preparations of corticosteroids are commonly used in inflammatory conditions of the eyelids, conjunctiva, cornea, anterior chamber, lens, and uvea. In posterior segment diseases that involve the posterior sclera, retina, and optic nerve, the topical agents are less effective, and parenteral and oral routes are preferred. Because these topical eye drop preparations are suspensions, the patient is instructed to shake the bottle several times to promote mixture of the medication and maximize its therapeutic effect. The most common ocular side effects of long-term topical corticosteroid administration are glaucoma, cataracts, susceptibility to infection, impaired wound healing, mydriasis, and ptosis. High IOP may develop, which is reversible after corticosteroid use is discontinued. To avoid the side effects of corticosteroids, NSAIDs are used as an alternative in controlling inflammatory eye conditions and postoperatively to reduce inflammation. NSAID therapy in combination with topical and oral preparations is an important adjunct therapy in managing uveitis.

Antiallergy Medications

Ocular hypersensitivity reactions, such as allergic conjunctivitis, are extremely common. These conditions result primarily from responses to environmental allergens. Most allergens are airborne or carried to the eye by the hand or by other means, although allergic reactions may also be drug-induced. Corticosteroids are commonly used as anti-inflammatory and immunosuppressive agents to control ocular hypersensitivity reactions.

Ocular Irrigants and Lubricants

Most irrigating solutions are used to cleanse the external lids to maintain lid hygiene, to irrigate the external corneal surface to regain normal pH (eg, in chemical burns), to irrigate the corneal surface to eliminate debris, or to inflate the globe intraoperatively. These solutions have various compositions that include sodium, potassium, magnesium, calcium, bicarbonate, glucose, and glutathione (ie, substance found in the aqueous humor). Sterile irrigating solutions, such as Dacriose, for lid hygiene are available. Irrigating solutions are safe to use with an intact corneal surface; however, the corneal surface should not be irrigated in cases of threatened corneal perforation. For patients with severe corneal ulcer, specific orders must be obtained regarding whether it is safe to irrigate the corneal surface or just to cleanse the external lids. Although it is good practice to promote hygiene, prevention of complications must be the primary concern. Normal saline solutions are commonly used to irrigate the corneal surface when chemical burns occur.

Lubricants, such as artificial tears, help alleviate corneal irritation, such as dry eye syndrome. Artificial tears are topical preparations of methyl or hydroxypropyl cellulose that are prepared as eye drop solutions, ointments, or ocular inserts (inserted at the lower conjunctival cul-de-sac once each day). The eye drops can be instilled as often as every hour, depending on the severity of symptoms.

Nursing Management

The objectives in administering ocular medications are to ensure proper administration to maximize the therapeutic effects and to ensure the safety of the patient by monitoring for systemic and local side effects. Absorption of eye drops by the nasolacrimal duct is undesirable because of the potential systemic side effects of ocular medications. To diminish systemic absorption and minimize the side effects, it is important to occlude the puncta (Chart 58-13). This is especially important for patients who are most vulnerable to medication overdose, including elderly people, children, infants, women who are lactating or are pregnant, and patients with cardiac, pulmonary, hepatic, or renal disease. A 1-minute interval between instillation of different types of ocular drops is recommended.

Before the administration of ocular medications, the nurse warns the patient that blurred vision, stinging, and a burning sensation are symptoms that ordinarily occur after instillation and are temporary. Risk for interactions of the ocular medication with other ocular and systemic medications must be emphasized; therefore, a careful patient interview regarding the medications being taken must be obtained.

Emphasis must be placed on hand hygiene techniques before and after medication instillation. The tip of the eye drop bottle or the ointment tube must never touch any part of the eye. The medication must be recapped immediately after each use. If a patient who instills his or her own medications cannot feel the eye drops when they are instilled, the eye medication may be refrigerated, because a cold drop is easier to detect. A 5-minute interval between successive administrations allows adequate drug retention and absorption. The patient or the caregiver at home should be asked to demonstrate actual eye drop or ointment instillation and punctal occlusion.

Issues in Ophthalmology

Issues that arise in any area of health care usually pose more questions than answers. In ophthalmology, the well-being of the patient physically, emotionally, financially, socially, and spiritually can be at risk when vision is threatened. Patients with a deteriorating eye condition often worry about the impact that visual loss will have on their lives. As they experience visual distortions, scotomas, or gradual visual loss, what was a vague worry can become a consuming preoccupation. The patient may equate a decrease in visual acuity with a loss of independence. The loss of a driver's license may force a patient to relocate or give up or change careers.

Major goals should include the preservation of vision and the prevention of further visual loss in patients who have already experienced some degree of loss. Effective communication is essential to promote rehabilitation of the distressed patient. The nurse together with the patient should establish goals. The nurse listens to the patient, tries to determine his or her level of health care need, and makes suggestions and recommendations. Lines of communication must be kept open so that the patient is comfortable exploring all treatment options.

Patient Safety

With the advent of the report from the Institute of Medicine (2000) on medical errors, the nurse must be aware of patient safety practices unique to ophthalmology and must be an active participant in the development of a culture of safety. High-volume, efficient, fast-paced procedures characterize ophthalmic practice. This means that patient identification is critical. Active identification (asking the patient his or her name versus asking, "Are you Ms. Smith?") and a second identifier (birth date, history, hospital number) must be verified before any procedure. As with other organs involving laterality, the correct eye must be verified before medication administration and surgery. Verification of the correct eye before surgery with the involvement of the patient or caregiver (for pediatric patients and adults with cognitive impairment) must be done before initiating any procedure or transferring the patient to another unit. Marking of the operative eye by the surgeon and a final verification of the correct eye by the surgeon, anesthesiologist, and nurse immediately before incision must be performed in all cases.

Cataract surgery with an IOL implant is one of the most frequently performed surgeries. Each facility must have a policy for multiple checks and verification of the IOL type, power, and diopter, as well as the operative eye. The surgeon, scrub nurse or technician, and circulating nurse should each verify the correct IOL measurements, the correct patient, and the patient's chart.

CHART 58-13

Instilling Eye Medications

- Shake suspensions or "milky" solutions to obtain the desired medication level.
- Wash hands thoroughly before and after the procedure.
- Ensure adequate lighting.
- Read the label of the eye medication to make sure it is the correct medication.
- Assume a comfortable position.
- Do not touch the tip of the medication container to any part of the eye or face.
- Hold the lower lid down; do not press on the eyeball. Apply gentle pressure to the cheek bone to anchor the finger holding the lid.

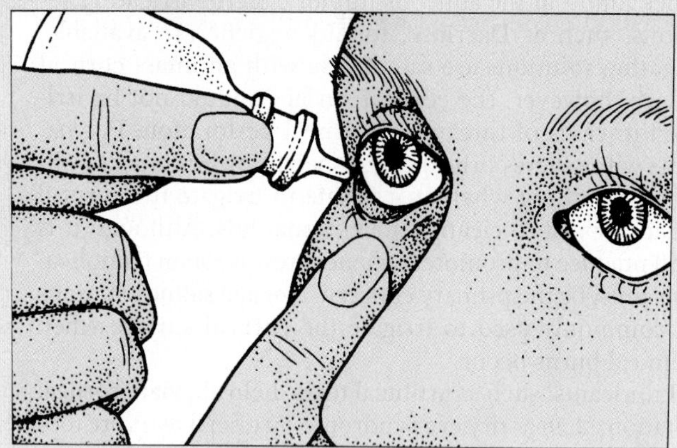

- Instill eye drops before applying ointments.
- Apply a ½-inch ribbon of ointment to the lower conjunctival sac.

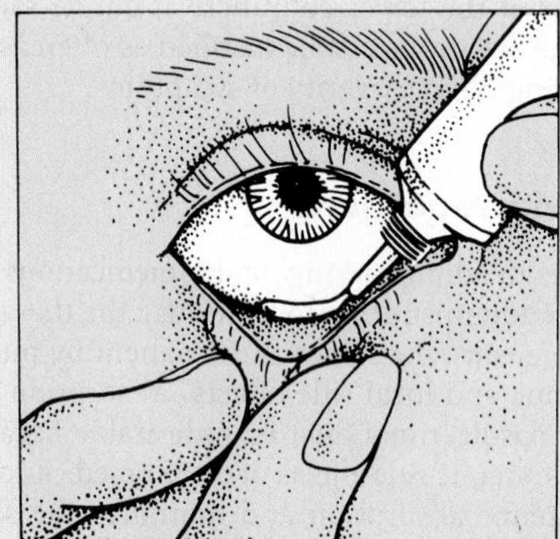

- Keep the eyelids closed, and apply gentle pressure on the inner canthus (punctal occlusion) near the bridge of the nose for 1 or 2 minutes immediately after instilling eyedrops.
- Using a clean tissue, gently pat skin to absorb excess eyedrops that run onto the cheeks.
- Wait 5 to 10 minutes before instilling another eye medication.

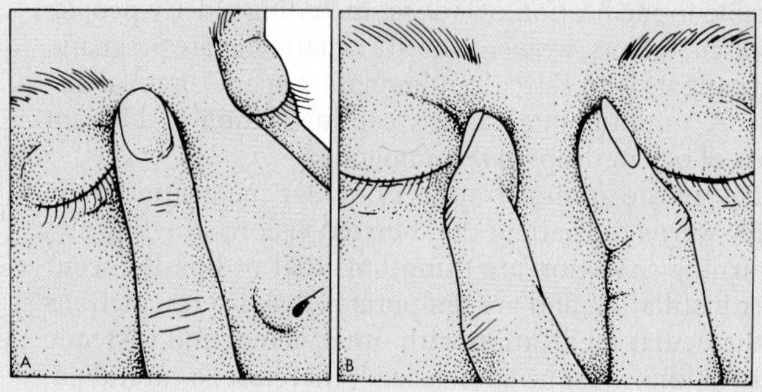

Critical Thinking Exercises

1 You are working in the health center of an assisted living facility for senior citizens. An 86-year-old resident who has previously been diagnosed with "dry" age-related macular degeneration has noted some changes in her vision. On checking her vision with her glasses on, you are relieved to find that her vision is close to 20/20 in each eye. However, the patient complains that some of the letters seem to be missing on some of the lines, especially with her right eye. In addition, she seems to have some visual distortion: she cannot tell the letter *D* from the letter *O*. The patient has a follow-up appointment scheduled with her retinologist in 4 months. Should she be seen

sooner? What additional tests could you perform in the office? What could be the etiology of her complaints?

2 ebp You are employed in an eye clinic in which the majority of patients are elderly and the majority of medications that are prescribed for these patients are topical agents. Develop an evidence-based teaching plan for patients and caregivers that provides instructions in the proper administration of ocular drops and ointments. What evidence supports the medication administration techniques and associated safety precautions that you have included in the teaching plan? What evidence supports the principles of learning that you considered regarding the elderly population that the clinic serves? What is the strength of the evidence? What criteria would you use to determine the strength of the evidence?

3 In the emergency department, you are caring for a man who has been involved in a motor vehicle crash in which there was a broken windshield. He states that he has a headache and a stiff neck, that his vision is "blurry," and that he has a "scratching pain" in his right eye. He requests a cold compress for his eyes. How would you respond to this patient's request? What diagnostic tests do you anticipate would be used to determine the cause for the patient's symptoms of blurred vision and pain in the eye? What information would you communicate to the physician?

REFERENCES AND SELECTED READINGS

BOOKS

Allen, D. (2004). The mechanical and hydrodynamic aspects of phacoemulsification. In M. Yanoff & J. S. Duker (Eds.), *Ophthalmology*. St. Louis: Mosby.

Azar, D. T., Yoo, S. H., Malecaze, F., et al. (2004). Phakic intraocular lenses. In M. Yanoff & J. S. Duker (Eds.), *Ophthalmology*. St. Louis: Mosby.

Bartlett, J. D., Bennett, E. S., & Fiscella, R. G. (Eds.). (2004). *Ophthalmic drug facts, 2005*. St. Louis: Facts & Comparisons.

Barouch, F. C., & Miller, J. W. (2004). Anti-vascular endothelial growth factor strategies for the treatment of choroidal neovascularization from age-related macular degeneration. In *Ocular pharmacology and drug delivery*. Philadelphia: Lippincott Williams & Wilkins.

Bearelly, S., & Fekrat, S. (2004). Controversy in the management of retinal venous occlusive disease. In *Controversies and advancements in the treatment of retinal disease*. Philadelphia: Lippincott Williams & Wilkins.

Bhatia, L. S., & Chen, T. C. (2004). New Ahmed valve designs. In *Surgical innovations in ophthalmology*. Philadelphia: Lippincott Williams & Wilkins.

Bickley, L. S., & Szilagyi, P. G. (2003). *Bates' guide to physical examination and history taking* (8th ed.). Philadelphia: Lippincott Williams & Wilkins.

Comer, G. M., & Ciulla, T. A. (2004). Diagnostic imaging of retinal disease. In *Controversies and advancements in the treatment of retinal disease*. Philadelphia: Lippincott Williams & Wilkins.

Fernandez-Suntay, J. P., Pineda II, R., & Azar, D. T. (2004). Conductive keratoplasty. In *Surgical innovations in ophthalmology*. Philadelphia: Lippincott Williams & Wilkins.

Fine, I. H., Packer, M., & Hoffman, R. S. (2004). Small incision cataract surgery. In M. Yanoff & J. S. Duker (Eds.), *Ophthalmology*. St. Louis: Mosby.

Freedman, J. (2004). Drainage implants. In M. Yanoff & J. S. Duker (Eds.), *Ophthalmology*. St. Louis: Mosby.

Fynn-Thompson, N., & Pineda, R., II (2004). Antibiotic advances in ophthalmology. In *Ocular pharmacology and drug delivery*. Philadelphia: Lippincott Williams & Wilkins.

Gardiner, M. F., Pineda, R., & Dana, M. R. (2004). Laser cataract surgery: past, present, and evolving technologies. In *Surgical innovations in ophthalmology*. Philadelphia: Lippincott Williams & Wilkins.

Kanski, J. J. (2003). *Clinical ophthalmology: A systematic approach* (5th ed.). Boston: Butterworth-Heinemann.

Kim, R. W., & Heier, J. S. (2004). Innovative treatments for exudative age-related macular degeneration. In *Controversies and advancements in the treatment of retinal disease*. Philadelphia: Lippincott Williams & Wilkins.

Park, R. I. (2004). The bionic eye: retinal prostheses. In *Controversies and advancements in the treatment of retinal disease*. Philadelphia: Lippincott Williams & Wilkins.

Porth, C. M. (2005). *Pathophysiology. Concepts of altered health states* (7th ed.). Philadelphia: Lippincott Williams & Wilkins.

Prevent Blindness America. (2002). *Vision problems in the US*. Schaumberg, IL: Prevent Blindness America/National Eye Institute.

Rhee, D. J., Pyfer, M. F., & Rhee, D. M. (2004). *The Wills eye manual: office of emergency room diagnosis and treatment of eye disease* (4th ed.). Philadelphia: Lippincott Williams & Wilkins.

Salmon, J., & Kanski, J. (2004). *Glaucoma: A colour manual of diagnosis and treatment* (3rd ed.). Oxford, UK: Butterworth-Heinemann

Schachat, A. P., Quigley, H. A., Schein, O. D., et al. (2004). *Vision: The Johns Hopkins White Papers*. New York: Medletter Associates.

Shields, M. B. (2005). *Textbook of glaucoma* (5th ed.). Philadelphia: Lippincott Williams & Wilkins.

Subramanian, M. L., & Topping, T. M. (2004). Controversies in the management of primary retinal detachments. In *Controversies and advancements in the treatment of retinal disease*. Philadelphia: Lippincott Williams & Wilkins.

Tipperman, R. (2004). Cataract surgery 2003. In C. J. Rapuano (Ed.), *Yearbook of ophthalmology 2004*. Philadelphia: Mosby.

Vaughn, D. G., Asbury, T., & Riorda-Eva, P. (Eds.). (2003). *General ophthalmology* (16th ed.). Stamford, CT: Appleton & Lange.

Vavvas, D., & Foster, C. S. (2004). Immunomodulatory medications in uveitis. In *Ocular pharmacology and drug delivery*. Philadelphia: Lippincott Williams & Wilkins.

Viola, R. S. (2004). Conjunctivitis. In R. Rakel & E. T. Bope (Eds.), *Conn's current therapy* (56th ed.). Philadelphia: W. B. Saunders.

Whitcher, J. (2004). Blindness. In D. G. Vaughn, T. Asbury, & P. Riorda-Eva (Eds.), *General ophthalmology* (16th ed.). Stamford, CT: Appleton & Lange.

JOURNALS

Age-Related Eye Disease Study Research Group. (2000). Risk factors associated with age-related macular degeneration. *Ophthalmology, 107*(12), 2224–2232.

Age-Related Eye Disease Study Research Group. (2001). A randomized, placebo-controlled clinical trial of high-dose supplementation with vitamins C and E, beta-carotene, and zinc for age-related macular degeneration and vision loss. *Archives of Ophthalmology, 119*(10), 1439–1452.

Azab, M., Benchaboune, M., Blinder, K. J., et al. (2004). Treatment of age-related macular degeneration with photodynamic therapy and verteporfin. *Retina, 24*(1), 1–12.

Brown, M. M., Brown, G. C., Sharma, S., et al. (2003). Quality of life associated with visual loss. *Ophthalmology, 110*(6), 1076–1081.

Chang, T. S., Pelzek, C. D., Nguyen, R. L., et al. (2003). Inverted pneumatic retinopexy: A method of treating retinal detachments associated with inferior retinal breaks. *Ophthalmology, 110*(3), 589–594.

Cho, E., Seddon, J., Rosner, B., et al. (2004). Prospective study of intake of fruits, vegetables, vitamins, and carotenoids and risk of age-related maculopathy. *Archives of Ophthalmology, 122*(6), 883–892.

Chow, A. Y., Chow, V. Y., Packo, K. H., et al. (2004). The artificial silicon retina microchip for the treatment of vision loss from retinitis pigmentosa. *Archives of Ophthalmology, 122*(4), 460–469.

Clouser, S. (2004). Toxic anterior segment syndrome: How one surgery center recognized and solved its problem. *Insight, 29*(1), 4–7.

Congdon, N. G., Friedman, D. S., & Lietman, T. (2003). Important causes of visual impairment in the world today. *Journal of the American Medical Association, 290*(15), 2057–2060.

Esrick, E., Subramanian, M. L., Heier, J. S., et al. (2005). Multiple laser treatments for macular edema attributable to branch retinal vein occlusion. *American Journal of Ophthalmology, 139*(4), 653–657.

Eyetech Study Group (2003). Anti-vascular endothelial growth factor therapy for subfoveal choroidal neovascularization secondard to age-related macular degeneration: Phase II study results. *Ophthalmology, 110*(5), 979–986.

Grehn, F. (2001). World health problem of glaucoma. *Journal of Glaucoma, 10*(Suppl.1), 82–84.

Hera, R., Keramidas, M., Peoc'h, M., et al. (2005). Expression of VEGF and angiopoietins in subfoveal membranes from patients with age-related macular degeneration. *American Journal of Ophthalmology, 139*(4), 589–596.

Hiller, R., Sperduto, R. D., Reed, G. F., et al. (2003). Serum lipids and age-related lens opacities: A longitudinal investigation. *Ophthalmology, 110*(3), 578–583.

Hoffman, R., Fine, I. H., & Packer, M. (2005). New phacoemulsification technology. *Current Opinion in Ophthalmology, 16*(1), 38–43.

Holland, E. J., & Schwartz, G. S. (2004). The Paton lecture ocular surface transplantation: 10 years' experience. *Cornea, 23*(5), 425–431.

Huang, D., Li, Y., & Radhakrishnan, S. (2004). Optical coherence tomography of the anterior segment of the eye. *Ophthalmology Clinics of North America, 17*(1), 1–6.

Hwang, D. G. (2004) Fluoroquinolone resistance in ophthalmology and the potential for newer ophthalmic fluoroquinolones. *Survey of Ophthalmology, 49*(Suppl. 2), 79–83.

Jabs, D. (2004.) AIDS and ophthalmology in 2004. *Archives of Ophthalmology, 122*(7), 1040–1042.

Katz, J., Feldman, M. A., Bass, E. B., et al. & Study of Medical Testing for Cataract Surgery Team. (2003). Risks and benefits of anticoagulant and antiplatelet medication use before cataract surgery. *Ophthalmology, 110*(9), 1784–1788.

Klein, B. E. K., Klein, R., Lee, K. E., et al. (2003). Socioeconomic and lifestyle factors and the 10-year incidence of age-related cataracts. *American Journal of Ophthalmology, 136*(3), 506–512.

Leslie, T., Aitken, D. A., Barrie, T., et al. (2003). Residual debris as a potential cause of postphaco-emulsification endophthalmitis. *Eye, 17*(4), 506–512.

Liu, H., Routley, I., & Teichmann, K. D. (2001). Toxic endothelial cell destruction from intraocular benzalkonium chloride. *Journal of Cataract and Refractive Surgery, 27,* 1746–1750.

Lois, N. (2004). Neovascular age-related macular degeneration. *Comprehensive Ophthalmology Update, 5*(3), 141–161.

Luo, B. P., & Brown, G. C. (2004) Update on the ocular manifestations of systemic arterial hypertension. *Current Opinion in Ophthalmology, 15*(3), 203–210.

Martin, D. F., Kuppermann, B. D., Wolitz, R. A., et al. (1999). Oral ganciclovir for patients with cytomegalovirus retinitis treated with a ganciclovir implant. Roche Ganciclovir Study Group. *New England Journal of Medicine, 340*(14), 1063–1070.

McDonald, M. B., Durrie, D., Asbell, P., et al. (2004). Treatment of presbyopia with conductive keratoplasty: Six-month results of the 1-year United States FDA clinical trial. *Cornea, 23*(7), 661–668.

McDonnell, P. J., Taban, M., Sarayba, M., et al. (2003). Dynamic morphology of clear corneal cataract incisions. *Ophthalmology, 110*(12), 2342–2348.

Mendoza, J. F., & Ferretti, Y. (2003). Immune recovery uveitis in AIDS patients with cytomegalovirus retinitis treated with highly active retroviral therapy in Venezuela. *Retina, 23*(4), 495–502.

Mrochen, M., Bueeler, M., Iseli, H. P., et al. (2004). Transferring wavefront measurements into corneal ablations: An overview of related topics. *Journal of Refractive Surgery, 20*(5), S550–554.

Neale, R. E., Purdie, J. L., Hirst, L. W., et al. (2003). Sun exposure as a risk factor for nuclear cataract. *Epidemiology, 14*(6), 707–712.

Nishida, K., Yamato, M., Hayashida, Y., et al. (2004). Corneal reconstruction with tissue-engineered cell sheets composed of autologous oral mucosal epithelium. *New England Journal of Medicine, 351*(12), 1187–1196.

Parikh, C. H., & Edelhauser, H. F. (2003). Ocular surgical pharmacology: Corneal endothelial safety and toxicity. *Current Opinion in Ophthalmology, 14*(4), 178–185.

Parikh, C., Sippy, B. D., Martin, D. F., et al. (2002). Effects of enzymatic sterilization detergents on the corneal endothelium. *Archives of Ophthalmology, 120,* 165–172.

Preshel, N., Hardten, D., & Lindstrom, R. L. (2000). LASIK after penetrating keratoplasty. *International Ophthalmology Clinic, 40*(3), 111–123.

Ryles, R. (1996). The impact of Braille reading skills on employment, income, education, and reading habits. *Journal of Visual Impairment and Blindness, 90*(3), 219–226.

Smiddy, W. E. (2004). Optical coherence tomography comes of age. *American Journal of Ophthalmology, 138*(5), 845–846.

Smith, C. A., Khoury, J. M., Shields, S. M., et al. (2000). Unexpected corneal endothelial cell decompensation after intraocular surgery with instruments sterilized by plasma gas. *Ophthalmology, 107*(8), 1561–1566.

Sommer, A. (2004). Global health, global vision [editorial]. *Archives of Ophthalmology, 122*(6), 911–912.

Spelsberg, H., Reinhard, T., Henke, L., et al. (2004). Penetrating limbokeratoplasty and lattice corneal dystrophy. *Ophthalmology, 111*(8), 1528–1533.

Taban, M., Behrens, A., Newcomb, R. I., et al. (2005). Acute endophthalmitis following cataract surgery: a systematic review of the literature. *Archives of Ophthalmology, 123*(5), 613–620.

Tomany, S. C., Cruikshanks, K., Klein, R., et al. (2004). Sunlight and the 10-year incidence of age-related maculopathy. *Archives of Ophthalmology, 122*(3), 750–757.

Voo, I., Mavrofrides, E., & Puliafito, C. A. (2004). Clinical applications of optical coherence tomography for the diagnosis and management of macular diseases. *Ophthalmology Clinics of North America, 17*(1), 21–31.

West, S. K., Muñoz, B., Schein, O. D., et al. (1998). Racial differences in lens opacities: the Salisbury Eye Evaluation (SEE) project. *American Journal of Epidemiology, 148*(11), 1033–1039.

Wong, T. Y., & Mitchell, P. (2004). Hypertensive retinopathy. *New England Journal of Medicine, 351*(22), 2310–2317.

Yeh, I., & Azar, D. T. (2004). The future of wavefront sensing and customization. *Ophthalmology Clinics of North America, 17*(2), 247–260.

RESOURCES

American Academy of Ophthalmology, P.O. Box 7424, San Francisco, CA 94120-7424; http://www.aao.org/news/eyenet. Accessed July 21, 2006.

American Council of the Blind, 1155 15th St. N.W., Suite 720, Washington, DC 20005; http://www.acb.org. Accesssed July 21, 2006.

American Society of Ophthalmic Registered Nurses, P.O. Box 193030, San Francisco, CA 94119-3030; http://webeye.ophth.uiowa.edu/asorn. Accessed July 21, 2006.

Association for Macular Diseases, Inc., 210 East 64th St., New York, NY 10021; http://www.macular.org. Accessed July 21, 2006.

Foundation Fighting Blindness, Executive Plaza I, Suite 800, 11350 McCormick Road, Hunt Valley, MD 21031-1014; http://www.blindness.org. Accessed July 21, 2006.

Glaucoma Research Foundation, 490 Post St., Suite 830, San Francisco, CA 94102; http://www.glaucoma.org. Accessed July 21, 2006.

Lighthouse National Center for Vision and Aging, 111 E. 59th St., New York, NY 10022; http://www.lighthouse.org. Accessed July 21, 2006.

Macular Degeneration Foundation, P.O. Box 9752, San Jose, CA 95157; http://www.eyesight.org. Accessed July 21, 2006.

National Association for Visually Handicapped, 22 W. 21st St., 6th Floor, New York, NY 10010; http://www.navh.org. Accessed July 21, 2006.

National Eye Institute Information Office, Bldg. 31, Rm. 6A-32, 31 Center Drive MSC2510, Bethesda, MD 20892-2510; http://www.nei.nih.gov. Accessed July 21, 2006.

Prevent Blindness America, 500 E. Remington Road, Schaumburg, IL 60173; http://www.prevent-blindness.org. Accessed July 21, 2006.

Research to Prevent Blindness, 645 Madison Ave., New York, NY 10022-1010; http://www.rpbusa.org. Accessed July 21, 2006.

VISION Community Services, 818 Mt. Auburn St., Watertown, MA 02172; 617-926-4232, 1-800-852-3029; http://www.mablind.org/VCSHomePage.htm. Accessed July 21, 2006.

Vision World Wide, Inc., 5707 Brockton Dr., Suite 302, Indianapolis, IN 46220-5481; http://www.visionww.org. Accessed July 21, 2006.

CHAPTER 59

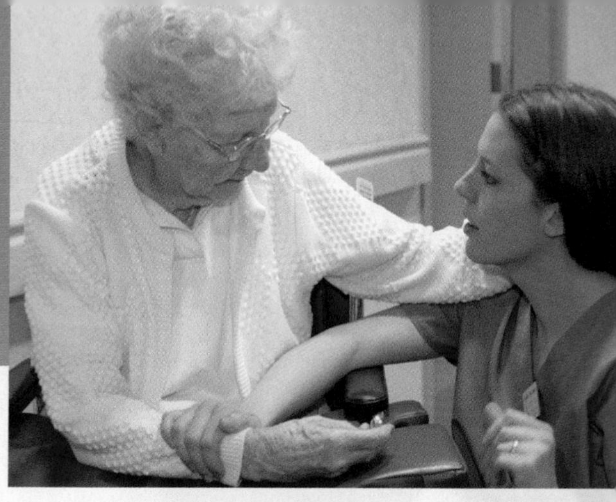

Assessment and Management of Patients With Hearing and Balance Disorders

Learning Objectives

On completion of this chapter, the learner will be able to:

1. Describe methods used to assess hearing and diagnose hearing and balance disorders.
2. List the manifestations that may be exhibited by a person with a hearing disorder.
3. Identify ways to communicate effectively with a person with a hearing disorder.
4. Differentiate problems of the external ear from those of the middle ear and inner ear.
5. Compare the various types of surgical procedures used for managing middle ear disorders and appropriate nursing care.
6. Describe the teaching topics that need to be addressed for patients undergoing middle ear and mastoid surgery.
7. Describe the different types of inner ear disorders, including the clinical manifestations, diagnosis, and management.

The ear is a sensory organ with dual functions—hearing and balance. The sense of hearing is essential for normal development and maintenance of speech as well as the ability to communicate with others. Balance, or equilibrium, is essential for maintaining body movement, position, and coordination.

The delicate structure and function of the ear make early detection and accurate diagnosis of disorders necessary for preservation of normal hearing and balance. Among the professionals involved in the diagnosis and treatment of these disorders are otolaryngologists, pediatricians, internists, and nurses. Nurses involved in the specialty of otolaryngology can become certified through the Society of Otorhinolaryngology and Head and Neck Nurses, Inc.

This chapter addresses the assessment and management of hearing and balance disorders common to the adult population. The pediatric otolaryngology literature provides information on otologic disorders pertaining to that population.

Anatomic and Physiologic Overview

The cranium encloses and protects the brain and surrounding structures, providing attachment for various muscles that control head and jaw movements. Eight bones form the cranium: the occipital bone, the frontal bone, two parietal bones, two temporal bones, the sphenoid bone, and the ethmoid bone. Some of these bones contain sinuses, which are cavities lined with mucous membranes and connected to the nasal cavity. The ears are located on either side of the cranium at approximately eye level.

Anatomy of the External Ear

The external ear includes the auricle (pinna) and the external auditory canal (Fig. 59-1). The external ear is separated from the middle ear by a disk-like structure called the tympanic membrane (eardrum).

Auricle

The auricle, attached to the side of the head by skin, is composed mainly of cartilage, except for the fat and subcutaneous tissue in the earlobe. The auricle collects the sound waves and directs vibrations into the external auditory canal.

External Auditory Canal

The external auditory canal is approximately 2.5 cm long. The lateral third is an elastic cartilaginous and dense fibrous framework to which thin skin is attached. The medial two thirds is bone lined with thin skin. The external auditory canal ends at the tympanic membrane (Chart 59-1).

The skin of the canal contains hair, sebaceous glands, and ceruminous glands, which secrete a brown, waxlike substance called cerumen (ear wax). The ear's self-cleaning mechanism moves old skin cells and cerumen to the outer part of the ear.

Just anterior to the external auditory canal is the temporomandibular joint. The head of the mandible can be felt by placing a fingertip in the external auditory canal while the patient opens and closes the mouth.

Glossary

acute otitis media: inflammation in the middle ear lasting less than 6 weeks

cholesteatoma: tumor of the middle ear or mastoid, or both, that can destroy structures of the temporal bone

chronic otitis media: repeated episodes of acute otitis media causing irreversible tissue damage and persistent tympanic membrane perforation

conductive hearing loss: loss of hearing in which efficient sound transmission to the inner ear is interrupted by some obstruction or disease process

deafness: partial or complete loss of the ability to hear

dizziness: altered sensation of orientation in space

endolymphatic hydrops: dilation of the endolymphatic space of the inner ear; the pathologic correlate of Ménière's disease

exostoses: small, hard, bony protrusions in the lower posterior bony portion of the ear canal

hearing loss: dysfunction of any component of the auditory system (conductive hearing loss; sensorineural hearing loss; mixed hearing loss)

labyrinthitis: inflammation of the labyrinth of the inner ear

Ménière's disease: condition of the inner ear characterized by a triad of symptoms: episodic vertigo, tinnitus, and fluctuating sensorineural hearing loss

middle ear effusion: fluid in the middle ear without evidence of infection

myringotomy (ie, tympanotomy): incision in the tympanic membrane

nystagmus: involuntary rhythmic eye movement

ossiculoplasty: surgical reconstruction of the middle ear bones to restore hearing

otalgia: sensation of fullness or pain in the ear

otitis externa (ie, external otitis): inflammation of the external auditory canal

otorrhea: drainage from the ear

otosclerosis: a condition characterized by abnormal spongy bone formation around the stapes

presbycusis: progressive hearing loss associated with aging

rhinorrhea: drainage from the nose

sensorineural hearing loss: loss of hearing related to damage of the end organ for hearing or cranial nerve VIII, or both

tinnitus: subjective perception of sound with internal origin; unwanted noises in the head or ear

tympanoplasty: surgical repair of the tympanic membrane

vertigo: illusion of movement in which the individual or the surroundings are sensed as moving

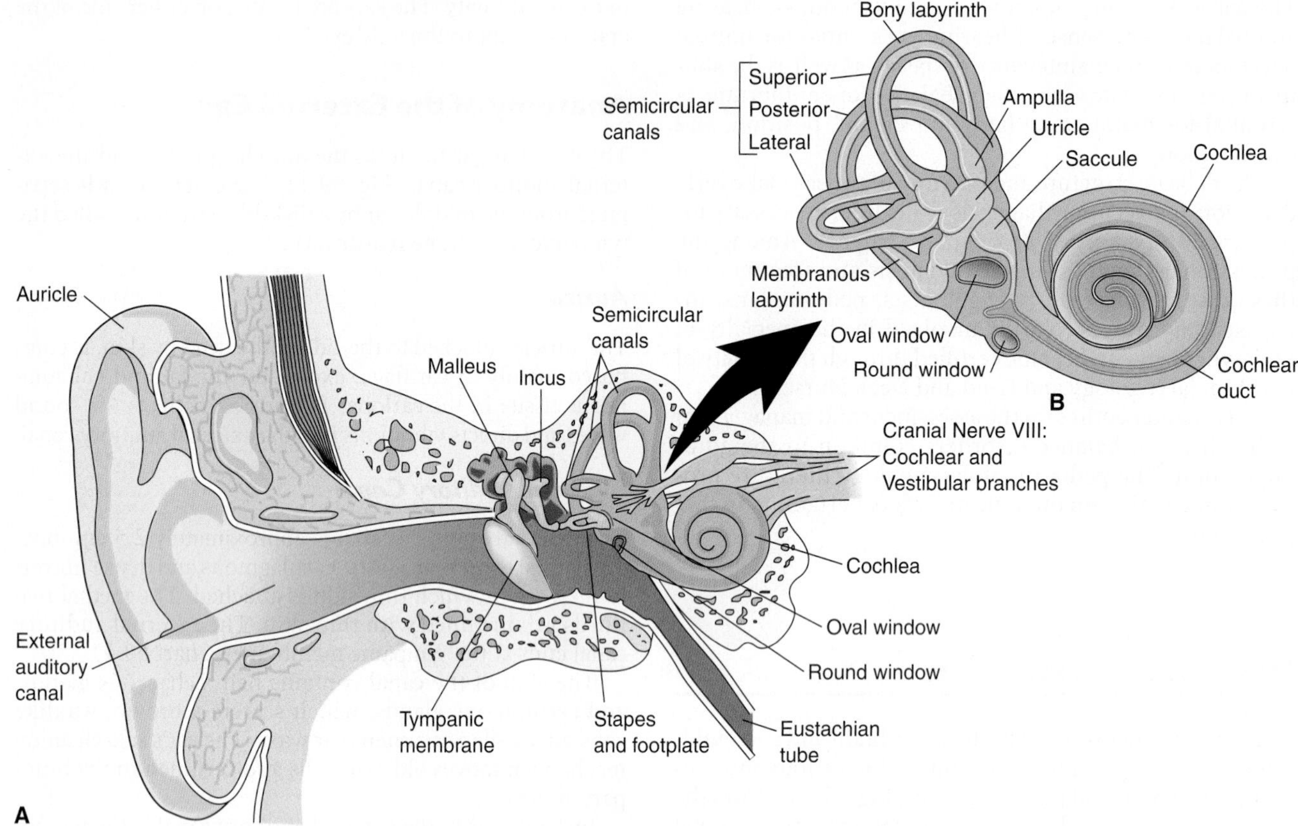

FIGURE 59-1. (A) Anatomy of the ear. (B) The inner ear.

Anatomy of the Middle Ear

The middle ear, an air-filled cavity, includes the tympanic membrane laterally and the otic capsule medially. The middle ear cleft lies between the two. The middle ear is connected by the eustachian tube to the nasopharynx and is continuous with air-filled cells in the adjacent mastoid portion of the temporal bone.

The eustachian tube, which is approximately 1 mm wide and 35 mm long, connects the middle ear to the nasopharynx. Normally, the eustachian tube is closed, but it opens by action of the tensor veli palatini muscle when the person performs a Valsalva maneuver, yawns, or swallows. It drains normal and abnormal secretions of the middle ear and equalizes pressure in the middle ear with that of the atmosphere.

Tympanic Membrane

The tympanic membrane (eardrum), about 1 cm in diameter and very thin, is normally pearly gray and translucent. It consists of three layers of tissue: an outer layer, continuous with the skin of the ear canal; a fibrous middle layer; and an inner mucosal layer, continuous with the lining of the middle ear cavity. Approximately 80% of the tympanic membrane is composed of all three layers and is called the pars tensa. The remaining 20% lacks the middle layer and is called the pars flaccida. The absence of this fibrous middle layer makes the pars flaccida more vulnerable to pathologic disorders than the pars tensa. Distinguishing landmarks of the tympanic membrane include the annulus, the fibrous border that attaches the eardrum to the temporal bone; the short process of the malleus; the long process of the malleus; the umbo of the malleus, which attaches to the tympanic membrane in the center; the pars flaccida; and the pars tensa (Fig. 59-2).

The tympanic membrane protects the middle ear and conducts sound vibrations from the external canal to the ossicles. The sound pressure is magnified 22 times as a result of transmission from a larger area to a smaller one.

Ossicles

The middle ear contains the three smallest bones (the ossicles) of the body: the malleus, the incus, and the stapes. The ossicles, which are held in place by joints, muscles, and ligaments, assist in the transmission of sound. Two small fenestrae (oval and round windows), located in the medial wall of the middle ear, separate the middle ear from the inner ear. The footplate of the stapes sits in the oval window, secured by a fibrous annulus (ring-shaped structure). The footplate transmits sound to the inner ear. The round window, covered by a thin membrane, provides an exit for sound vibrations (see Fig. 59-1).

Anatomy of the Inner Ear

The inner ear is housed deep within the temporal bone. The organs for hearing (cochlea) and balance (semicircular canals), as well as cranial nerves VII (facial nerve) and

CHART 59-1

Definition of Terms: Ear Anatomy

Acoustic: pertaining to sound or the sense of hearing

Cerumen: yellow or brown, waxlike secretion found in the external auditory canal

Cochlea: the winding, snail-shaped bony tube that forms a portion of the inner ear and contains the organ of Corti, the transducer for hearing

Cochlear (acoustic) nerve: the division of the eighth cranial (vestibulocochlear) nerve, which goes to the cochlea

Eustachian tube: the 3- to 4-cm tube that extends from the middle ear to the nasopharynx

External auditory canal: the canal leading from the external auditory meatus to the tympanic membrane; about 2.5 cm in length

External ear: the portion of the ear that consists of the auricle and external auditory canal; it is separated from the middle ear by the tympanic membrane

Incus: the second of the three ossicles in the middle ear; it articulates with the malleus and stapes; the anvil

Inner ear: the portion of the ear that consists of the cochlea, vestibule, and semicircular canals

Internal auditory canal: a canal in the petrous portion of the temporal bone, which houses the facial and vestibulocochlear nerves (cranial nerves VII and VIII)

Malleus: the first (most lateral) and largest of the three ossicles in the middle ear; it is connected to the tympanic membrane laterally and articulates with the incus; the hammer

Middle ear: the small, air-filled cavity in the temporal bone that contains the three ossicles

Organ of Corti: the end organ of hearing, located in the cochlea

Ossicle: a small bone; there are three in the middle ear: malleus, incus, and stapes

Oval window: a fenestra (aperture) between the vestibule of the inner ear and the middle ear, occupied by the base of the stapes

Pinna: the outer part of the external ear, which collects and directs sound waves into the external auditory canal; the auricle

Round window: a fenestra between the middle ear and the inner ear at the base of the cochlea, occupied by the round window membrane

Semicircular canals: the superior, posterior, and lateral bony tubes that form part of the inner ear; contain the receptor organs for balance

Stapes: the third (most medial) ossicle of the middle ear; it articulates with the incus, and its footplate fits into the oval window; the stirrup

Temporal bone: a bone on both sides of the skull at its base; composed of the squamous, mastoid, and petrous portions

Tympanic membrane: the membrane that separates the middle ear from the external auditory canal; also referred to as the eardrum

Vestibulocochlear nerve: cranial nerve VIII; contains the cochlear (acoustic) portion and the vestibular portion

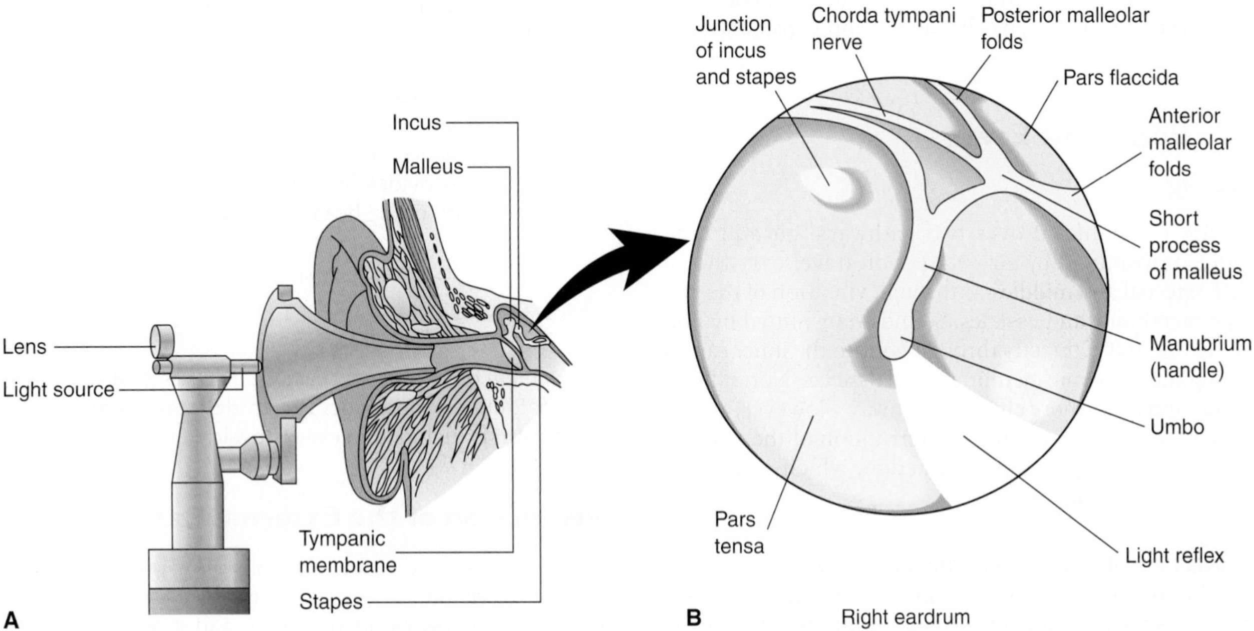

FIGURE 59-2. (A) Technique for using the otoscope to see (B) the tympanic membrane.

VIII (vestibulocochlear nerve), are all part of this complex anatomy (see Fig. 59-1). The cochlea and semicircular canals are housed in the bony labyrinth. The bony labyrinth surrounds and protects the membranous labyrinth, which is bathed in a fluid called perilymph.

Membranous Labyrinth

The membranous labyrinth is composed of the utricle, the saccule, the cochlear duct, the semicircular canals, and the organ of Corti. The membranous labyrinth contains a fluid called endolymph. The three semicircular canals—posterior, superior, and lateral, which lie at 90-degree angles to one another—contain sensory receptor organs, arranged to detect rotational movement. These receptor end organs are stimulated by changes in the rate or direction of a person's movement. The utricle and saccule are involved with linear movements.

Organ of Corti

The organ of Corti is located in the cochlea, a snail-shaped, bony tube about 3.5 cm long with two and a half spiral turns. Membranes separate the cochlear duct (scala media) from the scala vestibuli, and the scala tympani from the basilar membrane. The organ of Corti is located on the basilar membrane stretching from the base to the apex of the cochlea. As sound vibrations enter the perilymph at the oval window and travel along the scala vestibuli, they pass through the scala tympani, enter the cochlear duct, and cause movement of the basilar membrane. The organ of Corti, also called the end organ for hearing, transforms mechanical energy into neural activity and separates sounds into different frequencies. This electrochemical impulse travels through the acoustic nerve to the temporal cortex of the brain to be interpreted as meaningful sound. In the internal auditory canal, the cochlear (acoustic) nerve, arising from the cochlea, joins the vestibular nerve, arising from the semicircular canals, utricle, and saccule, to become the vestibulocochlear nerve (cranial nerve VIII). This canal also houses the facial nerve and the blood supply from the ear to the brain.

Function of the Ears

Hearing

Hearing is conducted over two pathways: air and bone. Sounds transmitted by air conduction travel over the air-filled external and middle ear through vibration of the tympanic membrane and ossicles. Sounds transmitted by bone conduction travel directly through bone to the inner ear, bypassing the tympanic membrane and ossicles. Normally, air conduction is the more efficient pathway. However, a defect in the tympanic membrane or interruption of the ossicular chain disrupts normal air conduction, which results in a conductive **hearing loss**.

SOUND CONDUCTION AND TRANSMISSION

Sound enters the ear through the external auditory canal and causes the tympanic membrane to vibrate. These vibrations transmit sound through the lever action of the ossicles to the oval window as mechanical energy. This mechanical energy is then transmitted through the inner ear fluids to the cochlea, stimulating the hair cells, and is subsequently converted to electrical energy. The electrical energy travels through the vestibulocochlear nerve to the central nervous system, where it is interpreted in its final form as sound.

Vibrations transmitted by the tympanic membrane to the ossicles of the middle ear are transmitted to the cochlea, located in the labyrinth of the inner ear. The stapes rocks, causing vibrations (waves) in fluids contained in the inner ear. These fluid waves cause movement of the basilar membrane, stimulating the hair cells of the organ of Corti in the cochlea to move in a wavelike manner. The movements of the tympanic membrane set up electrical currents that stimulate the various areas of the cochlea. The hair cells set up neural impulses that are encoded and then transferred to the auditory cortex in the brain, where they are decoded into a sound message.

The footplate of the stapes receives impulses transmitted by the incus and the malleus from the tympanic membrane. The round window, which opens on the opposite side of the cochlear duct, is protected from sound waves by the intact tympanic membrane, permitting motion of the inner ear fluids by sound wave stimulation. For example, in the normally intact tympanic membrane, sound waves stimulate the oval window first, and a lag occurs before the terminal effect of the stimulus reaches the round window. However, this lag phase is changed when a perforation of the tympanic membrane allows sound waves to impinge on the oval and round windows simultaneously. This effect cancels the lag and prevents the maximal effect of inner ear fluid motility and its subsequent effect in stimulating the hair cells in the organ of Corti. The result is a reduction in hearing ability (Fig. 59-3).

Balance and Equilibrium

Body balance is maintained by the cooperation of the muscles and joints of the body (proprioceptive system), the eyes (visual system), and the labyrinth (vestibular system). These areas send their information about equilibrium, or balance, to the brain (cerebellar system) for coordination and perception in the cerebral cortex. The brain obtains its blood supply from the heart and arterial system. A problem in any of these areas, such as arteriosclerosis or impaired vision, can cause a disturbance of balance. The vestibular apparatus of the inner ear provides feedback regarding the movements and the position of the head and body in space.

Assessment

Assessment of hearing and balance involves inspection of the external, middle, and inner ear. Evaluation of gross hearing acuity also is included in every physical examination.

Inspection of the External Ear

Inspection of the external ear is a simple procedure, but it is often overlooked. The external ear is examined by inspection and direct palpation; the auricle and surrounding tissues should be inspected for deformities, lesions, and discharge,

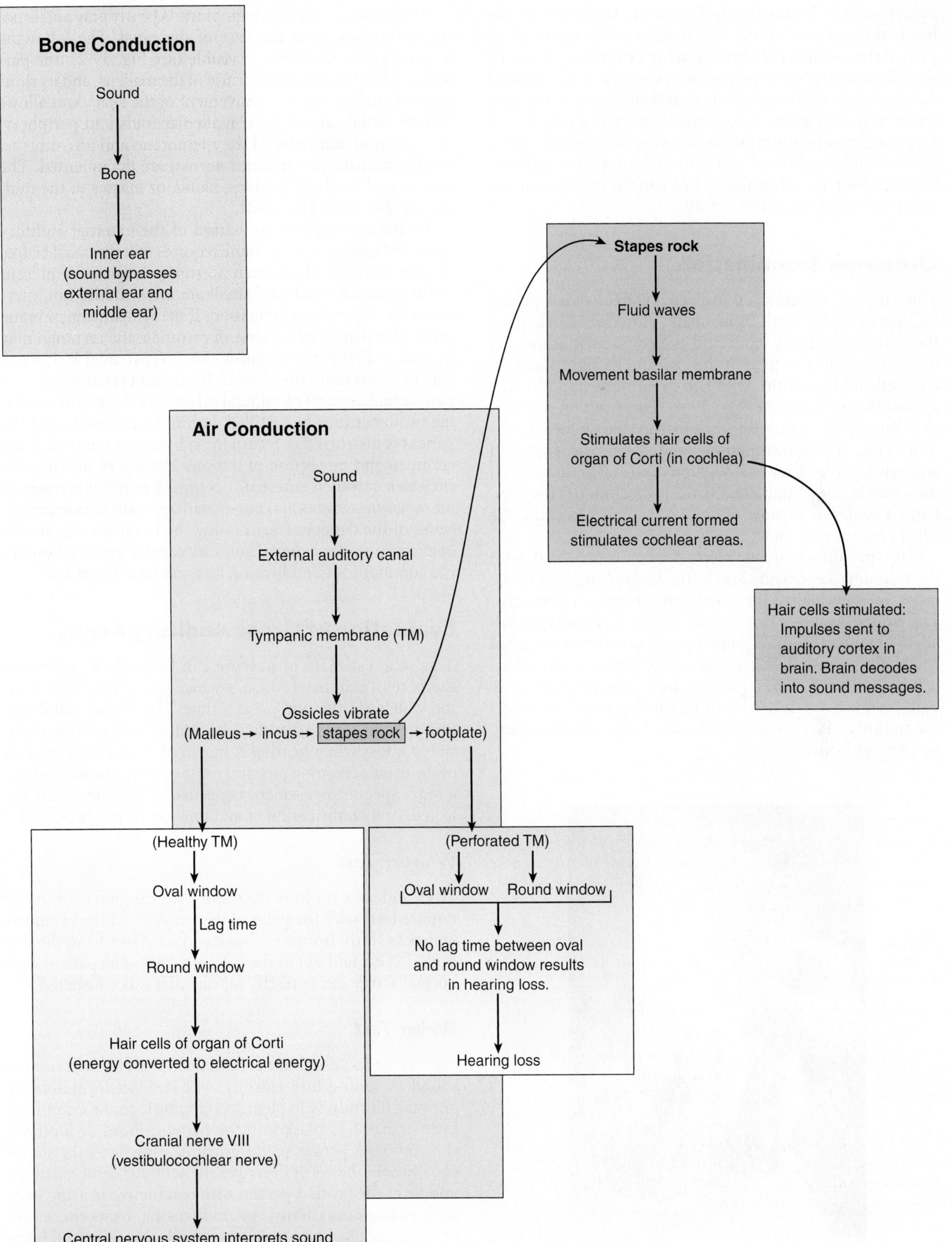

FIGURE 59-3. Bone conduction compared to air conduction.

as well as size, symmetry, and angle of attachment to the head. Manipulation of the auricle does not normally elicit pain. If this maneuver is painful, acute external otitis is suspected. Tenderness on palpation in the area of the mastoid may indicate acute mastoiditis or inflammation of the posterior auricular node. Occasionally, sebaceous cysts and tophi (subcutaneous mineral deposits) are present on the pinna. A flaky scaliness on or behind the auricle usually indicates seborrheic dermatitis and can be present on the scalp and facial structures as well.

Otoscopic Examination

The tympanic membrane is inspected with an otoscope and indirect palpation with a pneumatic otoscope. To examine the external auditory canal and tympanic membrane, the otoscope should be held in the examiner's right hand, in a pencil-hold position, with the examiner's hand braced against the patient's face (Fig. 59-4). This position prevents the examiner from inserting the otoscope too far into the external canal. Using the opposite hand, the auricle is grasped and gently pulled back to straighten the canal in the adult. If the canal is not straightened with this technique, the tympanic membrane is more difficult to visualize because the canal obstructs the view.

The speculum is slowly inserted into the ear canal, with the examiner's eye held close to the magnifying lens of the otoscope to visualize the canal and tympanic membrane. The largest speculum that the canal can accommodate (usually 5 mm in an adult) is guided gently down into the canal and slightly forward. Because the distal portion of the canal is bony and covered by a sensitive layer of epithelium, only light pressure can be used without causing pain. The external auditory canal is examined for discharge, inflammation, or a foreign body.

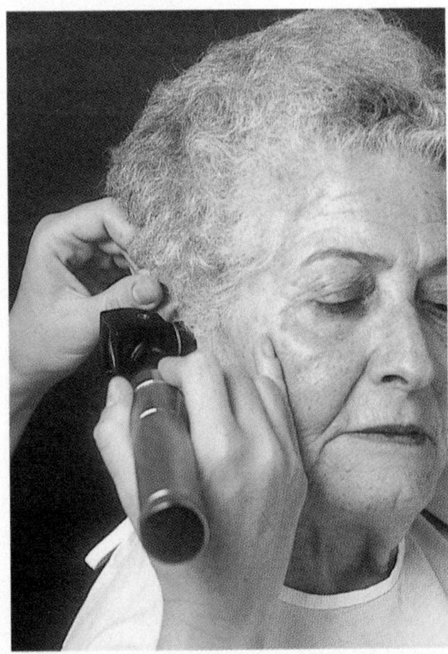

FIGURE 59-4. Proper technique for examining the ear. Hold the otoscope in the right or left hand, in a "pencil-hold" position. Steady the hand against the patient's head to avoid inserting the otoscope too far into the external canal.

The healthy tympanic membrane is pearly gray and is positioned obliquely at the base of the canal. The following landmarks are identified, if visible (see Fig. 59-2): the pars tensa, the umbo, the manubrium of the malleus, and its short process. A slow, circular movement of the speculum allows further visualization of the malleolar folds and periphery. The position and color of the membrane and any unusual markings or deviations from normal are documented. The presence of fluid, air bubbles, blood, or masses in the middle ear also should be noted.

Proper otoscopic examination of the external auditory canal and tympanic membrane requires that the canal be free of large amounts of cerumen. Cerumen is normally present in the external canal, and small amounts should not interfere with otoscopic examination. If the tympanic membrane cannot be visualized because of cerumen, the cerumen may be removed by gently irrigating the external canal with warm water (unless contraindicated). If adherent cerumen is present, a small amount of mineral oil or over-the-counter cerumen softener may be instilled within the ear canal, and the patient is instructed to return for subsequent removal of the cerumen and inspection of the ear. The use of instruments such as a cerumen curette for cerumen removal is reserved for otolaryngologists and nurses with specialized training because of the danger of perforating the tympanic membrane or excoriating the external auditory canal. Cerumen buildup is a common cause of hearing loss and local irritation.

Evaluation of Gross Auditory Acuity

A general estimate of hearing can be made by assessing the patient's ability to hear a whispered phrase or a ticking watch, testing one ear at a time. The Weber and Rinne tests may be used to distinguish conductive loss from sensorineural loss when hearing is impaired. These tests are part of the usual screening physical examination and are useful if a more specific assessment is needed, if hearing loss is detected, or if confirmation of audiometric results is desired.

Whisper Test

To exclude one ear from the testing, the examiner covers the untested ear with the palm of the hand. Then the examiner whispers softly from a distance of 1 or 2 feet from the unoccluded ear and out of the patient's sight. The patient with normal acuity can correctly repeat what was whispered.

Weber Test

The Weber test uses bone conduction to test lateralization of sound. A tuning fork (ideally, 512 Hz), set in motion by grasping it firmly by its stem and tapping it on the examiner's knee or hand, is placed on the patient's head or forehead (Fig. 59-5). A person with normal hearing hears the sound equally in both ears or describes the sound as centered in the middle of the head. A person with **conductive hearing loss**, such as from otosclerosis or otitis media, hears the sound better in the affected ear. A person with **sensorineural hearing loss**, resulting from damage to the cochlear or vestibulocochlear nerve, hears the sound in the better-hearing ear. The Weber test is useful for detecting unilateral hearing loss (Table 59-1).

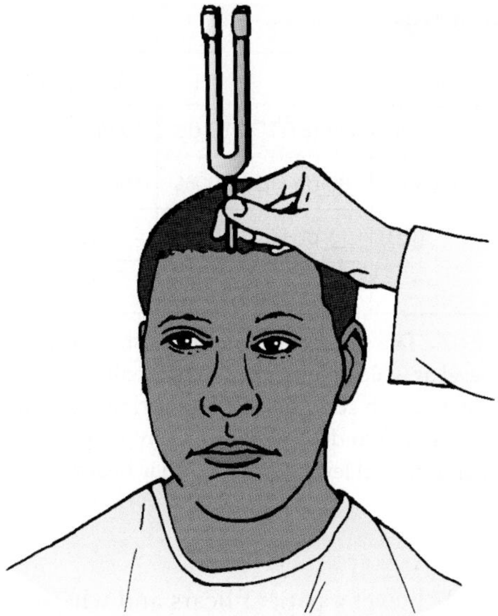

FIGURE 59-5. The Weber test assesses bone conduction of sound. From Weber, J. W., & Kelley, J. (2003). *Health assessment in nursing* (2nd ed.). Philadelphia: Lippincott Williams & Wilkins.

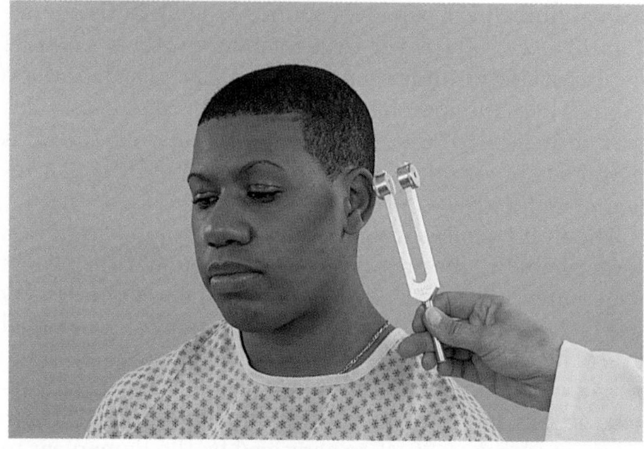

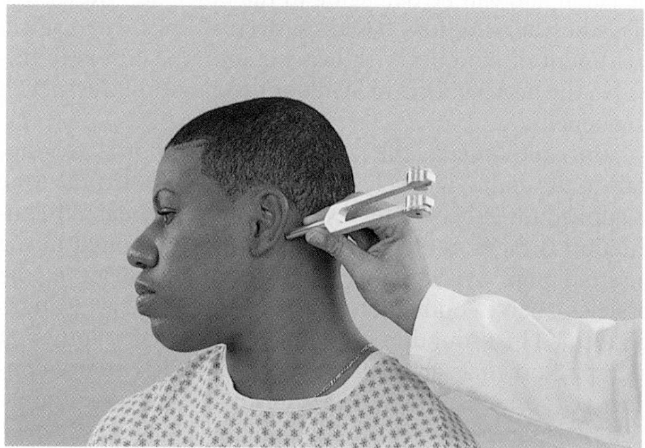

FIGURE 59-6. The Rinne test assesses both air and bone conduction of sound. From Weber, J., & Kelley, J. (2003). *Health assessment in nursing* (2nd ed., p. 218). Philadelphia: Lippincott Williams & Wilkins. © B. Proud.

Rinne Test

In the Rinne test (pronounced *rin-ay*), the examiner shifts the stem of a vibrating tuning fork between two positions: 2 inches from the opening of the ear canal (for air conduction) and against the mastoid bone (for bone conduction) (Fig. 59-6). As the position changes, the patient is asked to indicate which tone is louder or when the tone is no longer audible.

The Rinne test is useful for distinguishing between conductive and sensorineural hearing loss. A person with normal hearing reports that air-conducted sound is louder than bone-conducted sound. A person with a conductive hearing loss hears bone-conducted sound as long as or longer than air-conducted sound. A person with a sensorineural hearing loss hears air-conducted sound longer than bone-conducted sound.

Diagnostic Evaluation

Many diagnostic procedures are available to measure the auditory and vestibular systems indirectly. These tests are usually performed by an audiologist whose clinical competence is certified by the American Speech-Language-Hearing Association.

Audiometry

In detecting hearing loss, audiometry is the single most important diagnostic instrument. Audiometric testing is of two kinds: pure-tone audiometry, in which the sound stimulus consists of a pure or musical tone (the louder the tone before the patient perceives it, the greater the hearing loss), and speech audiometry, in which the spoken word is used to determine the ability to hear and discriminate sounds and words.

When evaluating hearing, three characteristics are important: frequency, pitch, and intensity. *Frequency* refers to the number of sound waves emanating from a source per second, measured as cycles per second, or Hertz (Hz). The

TABLE 59-1 Comparison of Weber and Rinne Tests

Hearing Status	Weber	Rinne
Normal hearing	Sound is heard equally in both ears.	Air conduction is audible longer than bone conduction.
Conductive hearing loss	Sound heard best in affected ear (hearing loss).	Sound heard as long or longer in affected ear (hearing loss).
Sensorineural hearing loss	Sound heard best in normal hearing ear.	Air conduction is audible longer than bone conduction in affected ear.

normal human ear perceives sounds ranging in frequency from 20 to 20,000 Hz. The frequencies from 500 to 2,000 Hz are important in understanding everyday speech and are referred to as the speech range or speech frequencies. *Pitch* is the term used to describe frequency; a tone with 100 Hz is considered of low pitch, and a tone of 10,000 Hz is considered of high pitch.

The unit for measuring loudness (*intensity* of sound) is the decibel (dB), the pressure exerted by sound. Hearing loss is measured in decibels, a logarithmic function of intensity that is not easily converted into a percentage. The critical level of loudness is approximately 30 dB. The shuffling of papers in quiet surroundings is about 15 dB; a low conversation, 40 dB; and a jet plane 100 feet away, about 150 dB. Sound louder than 80 dB is perceived by the human ear to be harsh and can be damaging to the inner ear. Table 59-2 classifies hearing loss based on decibel level. In surgical treatment of patients with hearing loss, the aim is to improve the hearing level to 30 dB or better within the speech frequencies.

With audiometry, the patient wears earphones and signals to the audiologist when a tone is heard. When the tone is applied directly over the external auditory canal, air conduction is measured. When the stimulus is applied to the mastoid bone, bypassing the conductive mechanism (ie, the ossicles), nerve conduction is tested. For accuracy, testing is performed in a soundproof room. Responses are plotted on a graph known as an audiogram, which differentiates conductive from sensorineural hearing loss. Speech discrimination is also measured (Fig. 59-7).

SPEECH HEARING TESTS						
TEST		R	L	BIN	SF
Sp. Reception Threshold (SRT)		10 db	10 db	db	db
Sp. Discrim. Scores	80 db HL	100%	100%	%	%
(PB)	___db HL	%	%	%	%
	___db HL	%	%	%	%

FIGURE 59-7. The speech reception threshold is the sound intensity level at which a patient is just capable of correctly identifying simple speech stimuli. Speech discrimination determines the patient's ability to distinguish different sounds, in the form of words, at a decibel level where sound is heard.

Tympanogram

A tympanogram, or impedance audiometry, measures middle ear muscle reflex to sound stimulation and compliance of the tympanic membrane by changing the air pressure in a sealed ear canal. Compliance is impaired with middle ear disease.

Auditory Brain Stem Response

The auditory brain stem response is a detectable electrical potential from cranial nerve VIII and the ascending auditory pathways of the brain stem in response to sound stimulation. Electrodes are placed on the patient's forehead. Acoustic stimuli (eg, clicks) are made in the ear. The resulting electrophysiologic measurements can determine at which decibel level a patient hears and whether there are any impairments along the nerve pathways (eg, tumor on cranial nerve VIII).

TABLE 59-2 Severity of Hearing Loss

Loss in Decibels	Interpretation
0–15	Normal hearing
>15–25	Slight hearing loss
>25–40	Mild hearing loss
>40–55	Moderate hearing loss
>55–70	Moderate to severe hearing loss
>70–90	Severe hearing loss
>90	Profound hearing loss

Electronystagmography

Electronystagmography is the measurement and graphic recording of the changes in electrical potentials created by eye movements during spontaneous, positional, or calorically evoked nystagmus. It is also used to assess the oculomotor and vestibular systems and their corresponding interaction. It helps diagnose conditions such as **Ménière's disease** and tumors of the internal auditory canal or posterior fossa. Any vestibular suppressants, such as sedatives, tranquilizers, antihistamines, and alcohol, are withheld for 24 hours before testing. Prior to the test, the procedure is explained to the patient.

Platform Posturography

Platform posturography is used to investigate postural control capabilities such as vertigo. It can be used to evaluate if a person's vertigo is becoming worse or to evaluate the person's response to treatment. The integration of visual, vestibular, and proprioceptive cues (ie, sensory integration) with motor response output and coordination of the lower limbs is tested. The patient stands on a platform, surrounded by a screen, and different conditions such as a moving platform with a moving screen or a stationary platform with a moving screen are presented. The responses from the patient on six different conditions are measured and indicate which of the anatomic systems may be impaired. Preparation for the testing is the same as for electronystagmography.

Sinusoidal Harmonic Acceleration

Sinusoidal harmonic acceleration, or a rotary chair, is used to assess the vestibulo-ocular system by analyzing compensatory eye movements in response to the clockwise and counterclockwise rotation of the chair. Although such testing cannot identify the side of the lesion in unilateral disease, it helps identify disease (eg, Ménière's disease and tumors of the auditory canal) and evaluate the course of recovery. The same patient preparation is required as for electronystagmography.

Middle Ear Endoscopy

With endoscopes with very small diameters and acute angles, the ear can be examined by an endoscopist specializing in otolaryngology. Middle ear endoscopy is performed safely and effectively as an office procedure to evaluate suspected perilymphatic fistula and new-onset conductive hearing loss, the anatomy of the round window before transtympanic treatment of Ménière's disease, and the tympanic cavity before ear surgery to treat chronic middle ear and mastoid infections.

The tympanic membrane is anesthetized topically for about 10 minutes before the procedure. Then, the external auditory canal is irrigated with sterile normal saline solution. With the aid of a microscope, a tympanotomy is created with a laser beam or a myringotomy knife, so that the endoscope can be inserted into the middle ear cavity. Video and photo documentation can be accomplished through the scope.

Hearing Loss

More than 28 million people in the United States have some form of hearing impairment (Isaacson & Vora, 2003). Hearing loss is greater in men than in women. By the year 2050, about one of every five people in the United States, or almost 58 million people, will be 55 years of age or older. Of this population, almost half can expect to have a hearing impairment (U.S. Public Health Service, 2000).

Approximately 10 million people in the United States have irreversible hearing loss (Isaacson & Vora, 2003). It is estimated that more than 30 million people are exposed on a daily basis to noise levels that produce hearing loss. Occupations such as carpentry, plumbing, and coal mining have the highest risk of noise-induced hearing loss. Hearing loss is an important health issue, and studies indicate that as people age, hearing screening and treatment are indicated (Cruickshanks, Tweed, Wiley, et al., 2003).

Conductive hearing loss usually results from an external ear disorder, such as impacted cerumen, or a middle ear disorder, such as otitis media or otosclerosis. In such instances,

GENETICS IN NURSING PRACTICE

Hearing Disorders

SELECTED HEARING DISORDERS INFLUENCED BY GENETIC FACTORS

- Autosomal dominant hearing loss
- Autosomal recessive hearing loss (eg, connexin 26 gene)
- Otosclerosis
- Pendred syndrome
- Usher syndrome
- Waardenburg syndrome

NURSING ASSESSMENTS

Family History Assessment

- Assess for other family members in several generations with hearing loss (autosomal dominant hearing loss)
- Inquire about genetic relatedness (eg, individuals who are related, such as first cousins, have a higher chance to share the same recessive genes—autosomal recessive hearing loss)
- Inquire about age at onset of hearing loss

Patient Assessment

- Assess for related genetic conditions, such as vision impairment (eg, retinitis pigmentosa in Usher syndrome; thyroid disorder in Pendred syndrome)
- Assess for iris, pigment, and hair alterations (white forelock) seen in Waardenburg syndrome

MANAGEMENT ISSUES SPECIFIC TO GENETICS

- Inquire whether DNA gene mutation or other genetics testing has been performed on affected family members.
- If indicated, refer for further genetics counseling and evaluation so that family members can discuss inheritance, risk to other family members, availability of genetics testing, and gene-based interventions.
- Offer appropriate genetics information and resources.
- Assess patient's understanding of genetics information.
- Provide support to families with newly diagnosed genetic-related sensorineural disorders.
- Participate in management and coordination of care of patients with genetic conditions, and individuals predisposed to develop or pass on a genetic condition.

GENETICS RESOURCES

Genetic Alliance—a directory of support groups for patients and families with genetic conditions; http://www.geneticalliance.org

Gene Clinics—a listing of common genetic disorders with up-to-date clinical summaries, genetic counseling and testing information; http://www.geneclinics.org

National Organization of Rare Disorders—a directory of support groups and information for patients and families with rare genetic disorders; http://www.rarediseases.org

OMIM: Online Mendelian Inheritance in Man—a complete listing of inherited genetic conditions; http://www.ncbi.nlm.nih.gov/omim/stats/html

the efficient transmission of sound by air to the inner ear is interrupted. A sensorineural loss involves damage to the cochlea or vestibulocochlear nerve.

Mixed hearing loss and functional hearing loss also may occur. Patients with mixed hearing loss have conductive loss and sensorineural loss, resulting from dysfunction of air and bone conduction. A functional (or psychogenic) hearing loss is nonorganic and unrelated to detectable structural changes in the hearing mechanisms; it is usually a manifestation of an emotional disturbance.

Clinical Manifestations

Early manifestations of hearing impairment and loss may include tinnitus, increasing inability to hear when in a group, and a need to turn up the volume of the television. Hearing impairment can also trigger changes in attitude, the ability to communicate, the awareness of surroundings, and even the ability to protect oneself, affecting a person's quality of life. In a classroom, a student with impaired hearing may be uninterested and inattentive and have failing grades. A person at home may feel isolated because of an inability to hear the clock chime, the refrigerator hum, the birds sing, or the traffic pass. A pedestrian who is hearing-impaired may attempt to cross the street and fail to hear an approaching car. People with impaired hearing may miss parts of a conversation. Many people are unaware of their gradual hearing impairment. Often, it is not the person with the hearing loss but the people with whom he or she is communicating who recognize the impairment first (Chart 59-2).

For various reasons, some people with hearing loss refuse to seek medical attention or wear a hearing aid. Others feel self-conscious wearing a hearing aid. Insightful people generally ask those with whom they are trying to communicate to let them know whether difficulties in communication exist. These attitudes and behaviors should be taken into account when counseling patients who need hearing assistance. The decision to wear a hearing aid is a personal one that is affected by these attitudes and behaviors.

Prevention

Many environmental factors have an adverse effect on the auditory system and, with time, result in permanent sensorineural hearing loss. The most common is noise. Noise (unwanted and unavoidable sound) has been identified as one of today's environmental hazards. The volume of noise that surrounds us daily has increased into a potentially dangerous source of physical and psychological damage.

Loud, persistent noise has been found to cause constriction of peripheral blood vessels, increased blood pressure and heart rate (because of increased secretion of adrenalin), and increased gastrointestinal activity. Although research is needed to address the overall effects of noise on the human body, a quiet environment is more conducive to peace of mind. A person who is ill feels more at ease when noise is kept to a minimum.

Numerous factors contribute to hearing loss (Chart 59-3). *Noise-induced hearing loss* refers to hearing loss that follows a long period of exposure to loud noise (eg, heavy machinery, engines, artillery). *Acoustic trauma* refers to hearing loss caused by a single exposure to an extremely intense noise, such as an explosion. Usually, noise-induced hearing loss occurs at a high frequency (about 4000 Hz). However, with continued noise exposure, the hearing loss can become more severe and include adjacent frequencies. The minimum noise level known to cause noise-induced hearing loss, regardless of duration, is about 85 to 90 dB.

Noise exposure is inherent in many jobs (eg, mechanics, printers, pilots, musicians) and in hobbies such as wood-

CHART 59-2

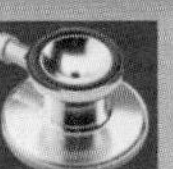

Assessing for Hearing Loss

Be on the alert for the following signs and symptoms:

Speech deterioration: The person who slurs words or drops word endings, or produces flat-sounding speech, may not be hearing correctly. The ears guide the voice, both in loudness and in pronunciation.

Fatigue: If a person tires easily when listening to conversation or to a speech, fatigue may be the result of straining to hear. Under these circumstances, the person may become irritable very easily.

Indifference: It is easy for the person who cannot hear what others say to become depressed and disinterested in life in general.

Social withdrawal: Not being able to hear what is going on causes the hearing-impaired person to withdraw from situations that might prove embarrassing.

Insecurity: Lack of self-confidence and fear of mistakes create a feeling of insecurity in many hearing-impaired people. No one likes to say the wrong thing or do anything that might appear foolish.

Indecision and procrastination: Loss of self-confidence makes it increasingly difficult for a hearing-impaired person to make decisions.

Suspiciousness: The hearing-impaired person, who often hears only part of what is being said, may suspect that others are talking about him or her, or that portions of the conversation are deliberately spoken softly so that he or she will not hear them.

False pride: The hearing-impaired person wants to conceal the hearing loss and thus often pretends to be hearing when he or she actually is not.

Loneliness and unhappiness: Although everyone wishes for quiet now and then, *enforced* silence can be boring and even somewhat frightening. People with a hearing loss often feel isolated.

Tendency to dominate the conversation: Many hearing-impaired people tend to dominate the conversation, knowing that as long as it is centered on them and they can control it, they are not so likely to be embarrassed by some mistake.

CHART 59-3

Risk Factors for Hearing Loss

- Family history of sensorineural impairment
- Congenital malformations of the cranial structure (ear)
- Low birth weight (<1500 g)
- Use of ototoxic medications (eg, gentamicin, loop diuretics)
- Recurrent ear infections
- Bacterial meningitis
- Chronic exposure to loud noises
- Perforation of the tympanic membrane

working and hunting. The Occupational Safety and Health Administration requires that workers wear ear protection to prevent noise-induced hearing loss when exposed to noise above the legal limits. Ear protection against noise is the most effective preventive measure available. There are no medications that protect against noise-induced hearing loss; hearing loss is permanent because the hair cells in the organ of Corti are destroyed.

Gerontologic Considerations

About 30% of people 65 years of age and older and 50% of people 75 years and older have hearing difficulties. The cause is unknown; linkages to diet, metabolism, arteriosclerosis, stress, and heredity have been inconsistent (Cruickshanks et al., 2003).

With aging, changes occur in the ear that may eventually lead to hearing deficits. Although few changes occur in the external ear, cerumen tends to become harder and drier, posing a greater chance of impaction. In the middle ear, the tympanic membrane may atrophy or become sclerotic. In the inner ear, cells at the base of the cochlea degenerate. A familial predisposition to sensorineural hearing loss is also seen, manifested by inability to hear high-frequency sounds, followed in time by the loss of middle and lower frequencies. The term **presbycusis** is used to describe this progressive hearing loss.

In addition to age-related changes, other factors can affect hearing in the elderly population, such as lifelong exposure to loud noises (eg, jets, guns, heavy machinery, circular saws). Certain medications, such as aminoglycosides and aspirin, have ototoxic effects when renal changes (eg, in the older person) result in delayed medication excretion and increased levels of the medications in the blood. Many older people take quinine for treatment of leg cramps, and quinine can cause a hearing loss. Psychogenic factors and other disease processes (eg, diabetes) also may be partially responsible for sensorineural hearing loss.

When hearing loss occurs, proper evaluation and treatment are warranted. *Healthy People 2010* identifies eight objectives for decreasing the problems caused by hearing loss. One of these objectives is for people diagnosed with hearing loss or **deafness** to use rehabilitation services and supplemental devices to improve communication with other people. Resources are available in workplaces and in schools. The Individuals with Disabilities Education Act (IDEA) was developed to ensure that children and adults, including elderly adults, receive the same opportunities in the educational system as those without hearing impairment (U.S. Public Health Service, 2000).

Even with the best medical care, people with hearing loss must learn to adjust to it. Care of elderly patients includes recognizing emotional reactions related to hearing loss, such as suspicion of others because of an inability to hear adequately; frustration and anger, with repeated statements such as, "I didn't hear what you said"; and feelings of insecurity because of the inability to hear the telephone or alarms. The Americans with Disabilities Act (ADA) of 1990 requires that all emergency services are accessible to people who have text message telephones (TTYs). In addition, in 1998, the Department of Justice mandated that all 911 centers in the United States be accessible to people with TTYs.

Medical Management

If a hearing loss is permanent or untreatable or if the patient elects not to be treated, aural rehabilitation (discussed at the end of the chapter) may be beneficial.

Nursing Management

Nurses who understand the different types of hearing loss are more successful in adopting a communication style to fit the needs and preferences of every patient. Trying to speak in a loud voice to a person who cannot hear high-frequency sounds only makes understanding more difficult. However, strategies such as talking into the less-impaired ear and using gestures and facial expressions can help (Chart 59-4).

A major issue for many people who are deaf or hearing-impaired is that they have other health problems that often do not receive attention, in large part because of communication barriers with their health care practitioners. To meet the health care needs of these patients, practitioners are legally obligated to make accommodations for a patient's inability to hear. Providing interpreters for those who can communicate through sign language is essential in many situations so that the practitioner can effectively communicate with the patient.

During health care and screening procedures, the practitioner (eg, dentist, physician, nurse) must be aware that patients who are deaf or hearing-impaired are unable to read lips, see a signer, or read written materials in the dark rooms required during some diagnostic tests. The same situation exists if the practitioner is wearing a mask or not in sight (eg, x-ray studies, magnetic resonance imaging [MRI], colonoscopy).

Nurses and other health care practitioners must work with patients who are deaf or hearing-impaired and their families to identify practical and effective means of communication. Nurses can serve as catalysts throughout the health care system to ensure that accommodations are made to meet the communication needs of these patients.

CHART 59-4

Communicating With People Who Are Hearing-Impaired

For the person who is hearing-impaired whose speech is difficult to understand:

- Consider how the person prefers to communicate with others. Do not assume that writing, gestures, or other means are the best or preferred technique.
- Consider if the person uses sign language. Interpreters are available from the American Sign Language Inc., Interpreting Service (ASLI). These specialists provide the best means of communication, providing accurate, professional services.
- Devote full attention to what the person is saying. Look and listen—do not try to attend to another task while listening.
- Engage the speaker in conversation when it is possible for you to anticipate the replies. This enables you to become accustomed to any peculiarities in speech patterns.
- Try to determine the essential context of what is being said; you can often fill in the details from context.
- Do not try to appear as if you understand if you do not.
- If you cannot understand at all or have serious doubt about your ability to understand what is being said, have the person write the message rather than risk misunderstanding. Having the person repeat the message in speech, after you know its content, also aids you in becoming accustomed to the person's pattern of speech.
- Written communication is an excellent resource. Written material should be written at a third-grade level so that the majority of people can understand it.

For the person who is hearing-impaired who speech reads:

- When speaking, always face the person as directly as possible.
- Make sure your face is as clearly visible as possible. Locate yourself so that your face is well lighted; avoid being silhouetted against strong light. Do not obscure the person's view of your mouth in any way; avoid talking with any object held in your mouth.
- Be sure that the patient knows the topic or subject before going ahead with what you plan to say. This enables the person to use contextual clues in speech reading.
- Speak slowly and distinctly, pausing more frequently than you would normally.
- If you question whether some important direction or instruction has been understood, check to be certain that the patient has the full meaning of your message.
- If for any reason your mouth must be covered (as with a mask) and you must direct or instruct the patient, write the message.

Conditions of the External Ear

Cerumen Impaction

Cerumen normally accumulates in the external canal in various amounts and colors. Although wax does not usually need to be removed, impaction occasionally occurs, causing **otalgia**, a sensation of fullness or pain in the ear, with or without a hearing loss. Accumulation of cerumen as a cause of hearing loss is especially significant in the elderly population. Attempts to clear the external auditory canal with matches, hairpins, and other implements are dangerous because trauma to the skin, infection, and damage to the tympanic membrane can occur.

Management

Cerumen can be removed by irrigation, suction, or instrumentation. Unless the patient has a perforated eardrum or an inflamed external ear (ie, otitis externa), gentle irrigation usually helps remove impacted cerumen, particularly if it is not tightly packed in the external auditory canal. For successful removal, the water stream must flow behind the obstructing cerumen to move it first laterally and then out of the canal. To prevent injury, the lowest effective pressure should be used. However, if the eardrum behind the impaction is perforated, water can enter the middle ear, producing acute vertigo and infection. If irrigation is unsuccessful, direct visual, mechanical removal can be performed on a cooperative patient by a trained health care provider.

Instilling a few drops of warmed glycerin, mineral oil, or half-strength hydrogen peroxide into the ear canal for 30 minutes can soften cerumen before its removal. Ceruminolytic agents, such as peroxide in glyceryl (Debrox), are available; however, these compounds may cause an allergic dermatitis reaction. Using any softening solution two or three times a day for several days is generally sufficient. If the cerumen cannot be dislodged by these methods, instruments, such as a cerumen curette, aural suction, and a binocular microscope for magnification, can be used.

Foreign Bodies

Some objects are inserted intentionally into the ear by adults who may have been trying to clean the external canal or relieve itching or by children who introduce peas, beans, pebbles, toys, and beads. Insects may also enter the ear canal. In either case, the effects may range from no symptoms to profound pain and decreased hearing.

Management

Removing a foreign body from the external auditory canal can be quite challenging. The three standard methods for removing foreign bodies are the same as those for removing cerumen: irrigation, suction, and instrumentation. The contraindications for irrigation are also the same. Foreign vegetable bodies and insects tend to swell; thus, irrigation is contraindicated. Usually, an insect can be dislodged by instilling mineral oil, which will kill the insect and allow it to be removed.

Attempts to remove a foreign body from the external canal may be dangerous in unskilled hands. The object may be pushed completely into the bony portion of the canal, lacerating the skin and perforating the tympanic membrane. In some circumstances, the foreign body may have to be extracted in the operating room with the patient under general anesthesia.

External Otitis (Otitis Externa)

External otitis, or **otitis externa**, refers to an inflammation of the external auditory canal. Causes include water in the ear canal (swimmer's ear); trauma to the skin of the ear canal, permitting entrance of organisms into the tissues; and systemic conditions, such as vitamin deficiency and endocrine disorders. Bacterial or fungal infections are most frequently encountered. The most common bacterial pathogens associated with external otitis are *Staphylococcus aureus* and *Pseudomonas* species. The most common fungus isolated in both normal and infected ears is *Aspergillus*. External otitis is often caused by a dermatosis such as psoriasis, eczema, or seborrheic dermatitis. Even allergic reactions to hair spray, hair dye, and permanent wave lotions can cause dermatitis, which clears when the offending agent is removed.

Clinical Manifestations

Patients usually report pain, discharge from the external auditory canal, aural tenderness (usually not present in middle ear infections), and occasionally fever, cellulitis, and lymphadenopathy. Other symptoms may include pruritus and hearing loss or a feeling of fullness. On otoscopic examination, the ear canal is erythematous and edematous. Discharge may be yellow or green and foul-smelling. In fungal infections, hairlike black spores may even be visible.

Medical Management

The principles of therapy are aimed at relieving the discomfort, reducing the swelling of the ear canal, and eradicating the infection. Patients may require analgesics for the first 48 to 92 hours. If the tissues of the external canal are edematous, a wick should be inserted to keep the canal open so that liquid medications (eg, Burow's solution, antibiotic otic preparations) can be introduced. These medications may be administered by dropper at room temperature. Such medications usually combine antibiotic and corticosteroid agents to soothe the inflamed tissues. For cellulitis or fever, systemic antibiotics may be prescribed. For fungal disorders, antifungal agents are prescribed.

Nursing Management

Nurses should instruct patients not to clean the external auditory canal with cotton-tipped applicators and to avoid events that traumatize the external canal such as scratching the canal with the fingernail or other objects. Trauma may lead to infection of the canal. Patients should also avoid getting the canal wet when swimming or shampooing the hair. A cotton ball can be covered in a water-insoluble gel such as petroleum jelly and placed in the ear as a barrier to water contamination. Infection can be prevented by using antiseptic otic preparations after swimming (eg, Swim Ear, Ear Dry), unless there is a history of tympanic membrane perforation or a current ear infection (Chart 59-5).

Malignant External Otitis

A more serious, although rare, external ear infection is malignant external otitis (temporal bone osteomyelitis). This is a progressive, debilitating, and occasionally fatal infection of the external auditory canal, the surrounding tissue, and the base of the skull. *Pseudomonas aeruginosa* is usually the infecting organism in patients with low resistance to infection (eg, patients with diabetes). Successful treatment includes control of the diabetes, administration of antibiotics (usually intravenously), and aggressive local wound care. Standard parenteral antibiotic treatment includes the combination of an antipseudomonal agent and an aminoglycoside, both of which have potentially serious side effects. Because aminoglycosides are nephrotoxic and ototoxic, serum aminoglycoside levels and renal and auditory function must be monitored during therapy. Local wound care includes limited débridement of the infected tissue, including bone and cartilage, depending on the extent of the infection.

Masses of the External Ear

Exostoses are small, hard, bony protrusions found in the lower posterior bony portion of the ear canal; they usually

CHART 59-5

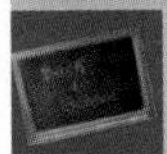

Patient Education

Prevention of Otitis Externa

- Protect the external canal when swimming, showering, or washing hair. Ear plugs or a swim cap should be worn. Drying the external canal afterward with a hair dryer on low heat may be suggested.
- Alcohol drops may be placed in the external canal to act as an astringent to help prevent infection after water exposure.
- Prevent trauma to the external canal. Procedures, foreign objects (eg, bobby pin), scratching, or any other trauma to the canal that breaks the skin integrity may cause infection.
- If otitis externa is diagnosed, refrain from any water sport activity for approximately 7 to 10 days to allow the canal to heal completely. Recurrence is highly likely unless you allow the external canal to heal completely.

occur bilaterally. The skin covering the exostosis is normal. It is believed that exostoses are caused by an exposure to cold water, as in scuba diving or surfing. The usual treatment, if any, is surgical excision.

Malignant tumors also may be found in the external ear. Most common are basal cell carcinomas on the pinna and squamous cell carcinomas in the ear canal. If untreated, squamous cell carcinoma may spread through the temporal bone, causing facial nerve paralysis and hearing loss. Carcinomas must be treated surgically.

Gapping Earring Puncture

Gapping earring puncture results from wearing heavy pierced earrings for a long time or after an infection, or as a reaction from the earring or other impurities in the earring. This deformity can only be corrected surgically. The edges of the perforations are excised on the lateral and medial surfaces of the earlobe. The entire tract is removed, joining the above two incisions and resulting in a much larger defect that is closed separately on each surface.

Conditions of the Middle Ear

Tympanic Membrane Perforation

Perforation of the tympanic membrane is usually caused by infection or trauma. Sources of trauma include skull fracture, explosive injury, or a severe blow to the ear. Less frequently, perforation is caused by foreign objects (eg, cotton-tipped applicators, bobby pins, keys) that have been pushed too far into the external auditory canal. In addition to tympanic membrane perforation, injury to the ossicles and even the inner ear may result from this type of action. Attempts by patients to clear the external auditory canal should be discouraged. During infection, the tympanic membrane can rupture if the pressure in the middle ear exceeds the atmospheric pressure in the external auditory canal.

Medical Management

Although most tympanic membrane perforations heal spontaneously within weeks after rupture, some may take several months to heal. Some perforations persist because scar tissue grows over the edges of the perforation, preventing extension of the epithelial cells across the margins and final healing. In the case of a head injury or temporal bone fracture, a patient is observed for evidence of cerebrospinal fluid **otorrhea** or **rhinorrhea**—a clear, watery drainage from the ear or nose, respectively. While healing, the ear must be protected from water.

Surgical Management

Perforations that do not heal on their own may require surgery. The decision to perform a **tympanoplasty** (surgical repair of the tympanic membrane) is usually based on the need to prevent potential infection from water entering the ear or the desire to improve the patient's hearing. Performed on an outpatient basis, tympanoplasty may involve a variety of surgical techniques. In all techniques, tissue (commonly from the temporalis fascia) is placed across the perforation to allow healing. Surgery is usually successful in closing the perforation permanently and improving hearing.

Acute Otitis Media

Ear infections can occur at any age; however, they are most commonly seen in children. Approximately three out of four children experience an ear infection by the time they are 3 years of age. **Acute otitis media** (AOM) is an acute infection of the middle ear, usually lasting less than 6 weeks. The pathogens that cause acute otitis media are usually *Streptococcus pneumoniae, Haemophilus influenzae,* and *Moraxella catarrhalis,* which enter the middle ear after eustachian tube dysfunction caused by obstruction related to upper respiratory infections, inflammation of surrounding structures (eg, sinusitis, adenoid hypertrophy), or allergic reactions (eg, allergic rhinitis). Bacteria can enter the eustachian tube from contaminated secretions in the nasopharynx and the middle ear from a tympanic membrane perforation. A purulent exudate is usually present in the middle ear, resulting in a conductive hearing loss.

Clinical Manifestations

The symptoms of otitis media vary with the severity of the infection. The condition, usually unilateral in adults, may be accompanied by otalgia. The pain is relieved after spontaneous perforation or therapeutic incision of the tympanic membrane. Other symptoms may include drainage from the ear, fever, and hearing loss. On otoscopic examination, the external auditory canal appears normal. The tympanic membrane is erythematous and often bulging. Patients report no pain with movement of the auricle. Table 59-3 differentiates acute external otitis from AOM. Risk factors for AOM include age (younger than 12 months), chronic upper respiratory infections, medical conditions that predispose to ear infections (Down syndrome, cystic fibrosis, cleft palate), and chronic exposure to secondhand cigarette smoke.

Medical Management

The outcome of AOM depends on the efficacy of therapy (the prescribed dose of an oral antibiotic and the duration of therapy), the virulence of the bacteria, and the physical status of the patient. With early and appropriate broad-spectrum antibiotic therapy, otitis media may resolve with no serious sequelae. If drainage occurs, an antibiotic otic preparation is usually prescribed. The condition may become subacute (lasting 3 weeks to 3 months), with persistent purulent discharge from the ear. Rarely does permanent hearing loss occur. Secondary complications involving the mastoid and other serious intracranial complications, such as meningitis or brain abscess, although rare, can occur.

Surgical Management

An incision in the tympanic membrane is known as **myringotomy** or **tympanotomy.** The tympanic membrane is numbed with a local anesthetic such as phenol or by ion-

TABLE 59-3 Clinical Features of Otitis

Feature	Acute Otitis Externa	Acute Otitis Media
Otorrhea	May or may not be present	Present if tympanic membrane perforates; discharge is profuse
Otalgia	Persistent, may awaken patient at night	Relieved if tympanic membrane ruptures
Aural tenderness	Present on palpation of auricle	Usually absent
Systemic symptoms	Absent	Fever, upper respiratory infection, rhinitis
Edema of external auditory canal	Present	Absent
Tympanic membrane	May appear normal	Erythema, bulging, may be perforated
Hearing loss	Conductive type	Conductive type

tophoresis (ie, electrical current flows through a lidocaine-and-epinephrine solution to numb the ear canal and tympanic membrane). The procedure is painless and takes less than 15 minutes. Under microscopic guidance, an incision is made through the tympanic membrane to relieve pressure and to drain serous or purulent fluid from the middle ear.

Normally, this procedure is unnecessary for treating AOM, but it may be performed if pain persists. Myringotomy also allows the drainage to be analyzed (by culture and sensitivity testing) so that the infecting organism can be identified and appropriate antibiotic therapy prescribed. The incision heals within 24 to 72 hours.

If AOM recurs and there is no contraindication, a ventilating, or pressure-equalizing, tube may be inserted. The ventilating tube, which temporarily takes the place of the eustachian tube in equalizing pressure, is retained for 6 to 18 months. The ventilating tube is then extruded with normal skin migration of the tympanic membrane, with the hole healing in nearly every case. Ventilating tubes are used to treat recurrent episodes of AOM.

Serous Otitis Media

Serous otitis media (**middle ear effusion**) involves fluid, without evidence of active infection, in the middle ear. In theory, this fluid results from a negative pressure in the middle ear caused by eustachian tube obstruction. When this condition occurs in adults, an underlying cause for the eustachian tube dysfunction must be sought. Middle ear effusion is frequently seen in patients after radiation therapy or barotrauma and in patients with eustachian tube dysfunction from a concurrent upper respiratory infection or allergy. Barotrauma results from sudden pressure changes in the middle ear caused by changes in barometric pressure, as in scuba diving or airplane descent. A carcinoma (eg, nasopharyngeal cancer) obstructing the eustachian tube should be ruled out in adults with persistent unilateral serous otitis media.

Clinical Manifestations

Patients may complain of hearing loss, fullness in the ear or a sensation of congestion, or popping and crackling noises, which occur as the eustachian tube attempts to open. The tympanic membrane appears dull on otoscopy, and air bubbles may be visualized in the middle ear. Usually, the audiogram shows a conductive hearing loss.

Management

Serous otitis media need not be treated medically unless infection (ie, AOM) occurs. If the hearing loss associated with middle ear effusion is significant, a myringotomy can be performed, and a tube may be placed to keep the middle ear ventilated. Corticosteroids in small doses may decrease the edema of the eustachian tube in cases of barotrauma. Decongestants have not proved effective. A Valsalva maneuver, which forcibly opens the eustachian tube by increasing nasopharyngeal pressure, may be cautiously performed; this maneuver may cause worsening pain or perforation of the tympanic membrane.

Chronic Otitis Media

Chronic otitis media is the result of recurrent AOM causing irreversible tissue pathology and persistent perforation of the tympanic membrane. Chronic infections of the middle ear damage the tympanic membrane, destroy the ossicles, and involve the mastoid. Before the discovery of antibiotics, infections of the mastoid were life-threatening. Today, acute mastoiditis is rare in developed countries.

Clinical Manifestations

Symptoms may be minimal, with varying degrees of hearing loss and a persistent or intermittent, foul-smelling otorrhea. Pain is not usually experienced, except in cases of acute mastoiditis, when the postauricular area is tender and may be erythematous and edematous. Otoscopic examination may show a perforation, and cholesteatoma can be identified as a white mass behind the tympanic membrane or coming through to the external canal from a perforation.

Cholesteatoma is an ingrowth of the skin of the external layer of the eardrum into the middle ear. It is generally caused by a chronic retraction pocket of the tympanic membrane, creating a persistently high negative pressure of the middle ear. The skin forms a sac that fills with degenerated skin and sebaceous materials. The sac can attach to the structures of the middle ear or mastoid, or both.

Chronic otitis media can cause chronic mastoiditis and lead to the formation of cholesteatoma. It can occur in the middle ear, mastoid cavity, or both, often dictating the type of surgery to be performed. If untreated, cholesteatoma will continue to enlarge, possibly causing damage to the facial nerve and horizontal canal and destruction of other surrounding structures.

Cholesteatomas are the third most common benign tumor of the inner ear, seen in approximately 9.2 people per 100,000 people annually (Rash, 2004). Cholesteatomas usually do not cause pain; however, if treatment or surgery is delayed, they may destroy structures of the temporal bone. These fast-growing tumors may cause severe sequelae such as hearing loss or neurologic disorders. Congenital cholesteatomas are usually found in children and may cause severe bone loss of the incus. Cholesteatomas found in elderly patients generally develop in the external canal.

Cholesteatomas may be asymptomatic or they may cause hearing loss, facial pain and paralysis, tinnitus, or vertigo. Audiometric tests often show a conductive or mixed hearing loss. Based on presenting symptoms, diagnosis may be made by visual examination or by computed tomography (CT) or MRI. Therapy includes treatment of the acute infection and surgical removal of the mass to restore hearing.

Medical Management

Local treatment of chronic otitis media consists of careful suctioning of the ear under otoscopic guidance. Instillation of antibiotic drops or application of antibiotic powder is used to treat purulent discharge. Systemic antibiotics are prescribed only in cases of acute infection.

Surgical Management

Surgical procedures, including tympanoplasty, ossiculoplasty, and mastoidectomy, are used if medical treatments are ineffective.

TYMPANOPLASTY

The most common surgical procedure for chronic otitis media is a tympanoplasty, or surgical reconstruction of the tympanic membrane. Reconstruction of the ossicles may also be required. The purposes of a tympanoplasty are to reestablish middle ear function, close the perforation, prevent recurrent infection, and improve hearing.

There are five types of tympanoplasties. The simplest surgical procedure, type I (myringoplasty), is designed to close a perforation in the tympanic membrane. The other procedures, types II through V, involve more extensive repair of middle ear structures. The structures and the degree of involvement can differ, but all tympanoplasty procedures include restoring the continuity of the sound conduction mechanism.

Tympanoplasty is performed through the external auditory canal with a transcanal approach or through a postauricular incision. The contents of the middle ear are carefully inspected, and the ossicular chain (malleus and incus unit) is evaluated. Ossicular interruption is most frequent in chronic otitis media, but problems of reconstruction can also occur with malformations of the middle ear and ossicular dislocations due to head injuries. Dramatic improvement in hearing can result from closure of a perforation and reestablishment of the ossicles. Surgery is usually performed in an outpatient facility under moderate sedation or general anesthesia.

OSSICULOPLASTY

Ossiculoplasty is the surgical reconstruction of the middle ear bones to restore hearing. Prostheses made of materials such as Teflon, stainless steel, and hydroxyapatite are used to reconnect the ossicles, thereby reestablishing the sound conduction mechanism. However, the greater the damage, the lower the success rate for restoring normal hearing.

MASTOIDECTOMY

The objectives of mastoid surgery are to remove the cholesteatoma, gain access to diseased structures, and create a dry (noninfected) and healthy ear. If possible, the ossicles are reconstructed during the initial surgical procedure. Occasionally, extensive disease or damage dictates that this be performed as part of a second-stage operation.

A mastoidectomy is usually performed through a postauricular incision. Infection is eliminated by removing the mastoid air cells. A second mastoidectomy may be necessary to check for recurrent or residual cholesteatoma. The hearing mechanism may be reconstructed at this time. The success rate for correcting this conductive hearing loss is approximately 75%. Surgery is usually performed in an outpatient setting. The patient has a mastoid pressure dressing, which can be removed 24 to 48 hours after surgery. Although infrequently injured, the facial nerve, which runs through the middle ear and mastoid, is at some risk for injury during mastoid surgery. As the patient awakens from anesthesia, any evidence of facial paresis should be reported to the physician.

Nursing Process

The Patient Undergoing Mastoid Surgery

Although several otologic surgical procedures are performed under moderate sedation, mastoid surgery is performed using general anesthesia.

Assessment

The health history includes a complete description of the ear disorder, including infection, otalgia, otorrhea, hearing loss, and vertigo. Data are collected about the duration and intensity of the disorder, its causes, and previous treatments. Information is obtained about other health problems and all medications that the patient is taking. Medication allergies and family history of ear disease also should be obtained.

Physical assessment addresses erythema, edema, otorrhea, lesions, and characteristics such as odor and color of discharge. The results of the audiogram are reviewed.

Nursing Diagnoses

Based on the assessment data, the major nursing diagnoses may include the following:

- Anxiety related to surgical procedure, potential loss of hearing, potential taste disturbance, and potential loss of facial movement

- Acute pain related to mastoid surgery
- Risk for infection related to mastoidectomy; placement of grafts, prostheses, and electrodes; and surgical trauma to surrounding tissues and structures
- Disturbed auditory sensory perception related to ear disorder, surgery, or packing
- Risk for trauma related to impaired balance or vertigo during the immediate postoperative period
- Disturbed sensory perception related to potential damage to facial nerve (cranial nerve VII) and chorda tympani nerve
- Impaired skin integrity related to ear surgery, incisions, and graft sites
- Deficient knowledge about mastoid disease, surgical procedure, and postoperative care and expectations

Planning and Goals

The major goals of caring for a patient undergoing mastoidectomy include reduction of anxiety; freedom from pain and discomfort; prevention of infection; stable or improved hearing and communication; absence of vertigo and related injury; absence of or adjustment to sensory or perceptual alterations; return of skin integrity; and increased knowledge regarding the disease, surgical procedure, and postoperative care.

Nursing Interventions

Reducing Anxiety

The nurse reinforces the information discussed by the otologic surgeon with the patient, including anesthesia, the location of the incision (postauricular), and expected surgical results (eg, hearing, balance, taste, facial movement). The patient also is encouraged to discuss any anxieties and concerns about the surgery.

Relieving Pain

Although most patients complain very little about incisional pain after mastoid surgery, they do have some ear discomfort. Aural fullness or pressure after surgery is caused by residual blood or fluid in the middle ear. The prescribed analgesic may be taken for the first 24 hours after surgery and then only as needed.

A wick or external auditory canal packing is used if a tympanoplasty was performed at the time of the mastoidectomy. For the next 2 to 3 weeks after surgery, the patient may experience sharp, shooting pains intermittently as the eustachian tube opens and allows air to enter the middle ear. Constant, throbbing pain accompanied by fever may indicate infection and should be reported to the physician.

Preventing Infection

Measures are initiated to prevent infection in the operated ear. The external auditory canal wick, or packing, may be impregnated with an antibiotic solution before instillation. Prophylactic antibiotics are administered as prescribed, and the patient is instructed to prevent water from entering the external auditory canal for 6 weeks. A cotton ball or lamb's wool covered with a water-insoluble substance (eg, petroleum jelly) and placed loosely in the ear canal usually prevents water contamination and should be used when the patient showers or washes his or her hair, or in any situations in which water may enter the ear. The postauricular incision should be kept dry for 2 days. Signs of infection such as an elevated temperature and purulent drainage should be reported. Some serosanguineous drainage from the external auditory canal is normal after surgery.

Improving Hearing and Communication

Hearing in the operated ear may be reduced for several weeks because of edema, accumulation of blood and tissue fluid in the middle ear, and dressings or packing. Measures are initiated to improve hearing and communication, such as reducing environmental noise, facing the patient when speaking, speaking clearly and distinctly without shouting, providing good lighting if the patient relies on speech reading, and using nonverbal clues (eg, facial expression, pointing, gestures) and other forms of communication. Family members or significant others are instructed about effective ways to communicate with the patient. If the patient uses assistive hearing devices, one can be used in the unaffected ear.

Preventing Injury

Vertigo may occur after mastoid surgery if the semicircular canals or other areas of the inner ear are traumatized. Antiemetics or antivertiginous medications (eg, antihistamines) can be prescribed if a balance disturbance or vertigo occurs. Safety measures such as assisted ambulation are implemented to prevent falls and injury.

Preventing Altered Sensory Perception

Facial nerve injury is a potential, although rare, complication of mastoid surgery. The patient is instructed to report immediately any evidence of facial nerve (cranial nerve VII) weakness, such as drooping of the mouth on the operated side, slurred speech, decreased sensation, and difficulty swallowing. A more frequent occurrence is a temporary disturbance in the chorda tympani nerve, a small branch of the facial nerve that runs through the middle ear. Patients experience a taste disturbance and dry mouth on the side of surgery for several months until the nerve regenerates.

Promoting Wound Healing

The patient is instructed to avoid heavy lifting, straining, exertion, and nose blowing for 2 to 3 weeks after surgery to prevent dislodging the tympanic membrane graft or ossicular prosthesis.

Promoting Home and Community-Based Care

TEACHING PATIENTS SELF-CARE

Patients require instruction about prescribed medication therapy, such as analgesics and antivertiginous agents (eg, antihistamines) prescribed for balance disturbance. Teaching includes information about the expected effects and potential side effects of the medication. Patients also need instruction about any activity restrictions. Possible complications such as infection, facial nerve weakness, or taste disturbances, including the signs and symptoms to report immediately, should be addressed (Chart 59-6).

CONTINUING CARE

Some patients, particularly elderly patients, who have had mastoid surgery may require the services of a home care nurse for a few days after returning home. However, most people find that assistance from a family member or a friend is sufficient. The caregiver and patient are cautioned that the patient may experience some vertigo and will therefore require help with ambulation to avoid falling. Any symptoms of complications are to be reported promptly to the surgeon. The importance of scheduling and keeping follow-up appointments is also stressed.

CHART 59-6

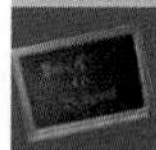

Patient Education

Self-Care After Middle Ear or Mastoid Surgery

Postoperative instructions for patients who have had middle ear and mastoid surgery may vary among otolaryngologists. General teaching guidelines for the patient may include:

- Take antibiotics and other medications as prescribed.
- Blow nose gently one side at a time for 1 week after surgery.
- Sneeze and cough with the mouth open for a few weeks after surgery.
- Avoid heavy lifting (>10 lb), straining, and bending over for a few weeks after surgery.
- Popping and crackling sensations in the operative ear are normal for approximately 3 to 5 weeks after surgery.
- Temporary hearing loss is normal in the operative ear due to fluid, blood, or packing in the ear.
- Report excessive or purulent ear drainage to the physician. Some slightly bloody or serosanguineous drainage from the ear is normal after surgery.
- Change the cotton ball in the ear as needed.
- Avoid getting water in the operative ear for 2 weeks after surgery. You may shampoo the hair 2 to 3 days postoperatively if the ear is protected from water by saturating a cotton ball with petroleum jelly (or some other water-insoluble substance) and loosely placing it in the ear. If the postauricular suture line becomes wet, pat (not rub) the area and cover it with a thin layer of antibiotic ointment.

Evaluation

Expected Patient Outcomes

Expected patient outcomes may include:

1. Demonstrates reduced anxiety about surgical procedure
   a. Verbalizes and exhibits less stress, tension, and irritability
   b. Verbalizes acceptance of the results of surgery and adjustment to possible hearing impairment
2. Remains free of discomfort or pain
   a. Exhibits no facial grimacing, moaning, or crying, and reports absence of pain
   b. Uses analgesics appropriately
3. Demonstrates no signs or symptoms of infection
   a. Has normal vital signs, including temperature
   b. Demonstrates absence of purulent drainage from the external auditory canal
   c. Describes method for preventing water from contaminating packing
4. Exhibits signs that hearing has stabilized or improved
   a. Describes surgical goal for hearing and judges whether the goal has been met
   b. Verbalizes that hearing has improved
5. Remains free of injury and trauma because of vertigo
   a. Reports absence of vertigo or balance disturbance
   b. Experiences no injury or fall
   c. Modifies environment to prevent falls and injuries (eg, night light, no clutter on stairs)
6. Adjusts to or remains free from altered sensory perception
   a. Reports no taste disturbance, mouth dryness, or facial weakness
7. Demonstrates no skin breakdown
   a. Lists ways to prevent dislodging graft or prosthesis
8. Verbalizes the reasons for and methods of care and treatment
   a. Shares knowledge with family about treatment protocol
   b. Discusses the discharge plan formulated with the nurse with regard to rest periods, medication, and activities permitted and restricted
   c. Lists symptoms that should be reported to health care personnel
   d. Keeps follow-up appointments

Otosclerosis

Otosclerosis involves the stapes and is thought to result from the formation of new, abnormal spongy bone, especially around the oval window, with resulting fixation of the stapes. The efficient transmission of sound is prevented because the stapes cannot vibrate and carry the sound as conducted from the malleus and incus to the inner ear. Otosclerosis is more common in women and frequently hereditary, and pregnancy may worsen it.

Clinical Manifestations

Otosclerosis may involve one or both ears and manifests as a progressive conductive or mixed hearing loss. The patient may or may not complain of tinnitus. Otoscopic examination usually reveals a normal tympanic membrane. Bone conduction is better than air conduction on Rinne testing. The audiogram confirms conductive hearing loss or mixed loss, especially in the low frequencies.

Medical Management

There is no known nonsurgical treatment for otosclerosis. However, some physicians believe the use of sodium fluoride can mature the abnormal spongy bone growth and prevent the breakdown of the bone tissue. Amplification with a hearing aid also may help (Porth, 2005).

Surgical Management

One of two surgical procedures may be performed, the stapedectomy or the stapedotomy. A stapedectomy involves removing the stapes superstructure and part of the footplate and inserting a tissue graft and a suitable prosthesis (Fig. 59-8). The surgeon drills a small hole into the footplate to hold a prosthesis. The prosthesis bridges the gap between the incus and the inner ear, providing better sound conduction. Stapes surgery is very successful; approximately 95% of patients experience resolution of conductive hearing loss. Balance disturbance or true vertigo, which rarely occurs in other middle ear surgical procedures, may occur during the postoperative period for several days. Long-term balance disorders are rare (Roland, 2004).

Middle Ear Masses

Other than cholesteatoma, masses in the middle ear are rare. Glomus jugulare tumor is a tumor that arises from the jugular vein. A histologically identical tumor that arises from Jacobson's nerve (in the temporal bone of the skull) and remains limited to the middle ear is known as a glomus tympanicum. On otoscopy, a red blemish on or behind the tympanic membrane is indicative of a glomus tumor. Glomus jugulare tumors are rarely malignant; however, due to their location, treatment may be necessary to relieve symptoms. The treatment for glomus tumors is surgical excision, except in poor surgical candidates, in whom radiation therapy is used.

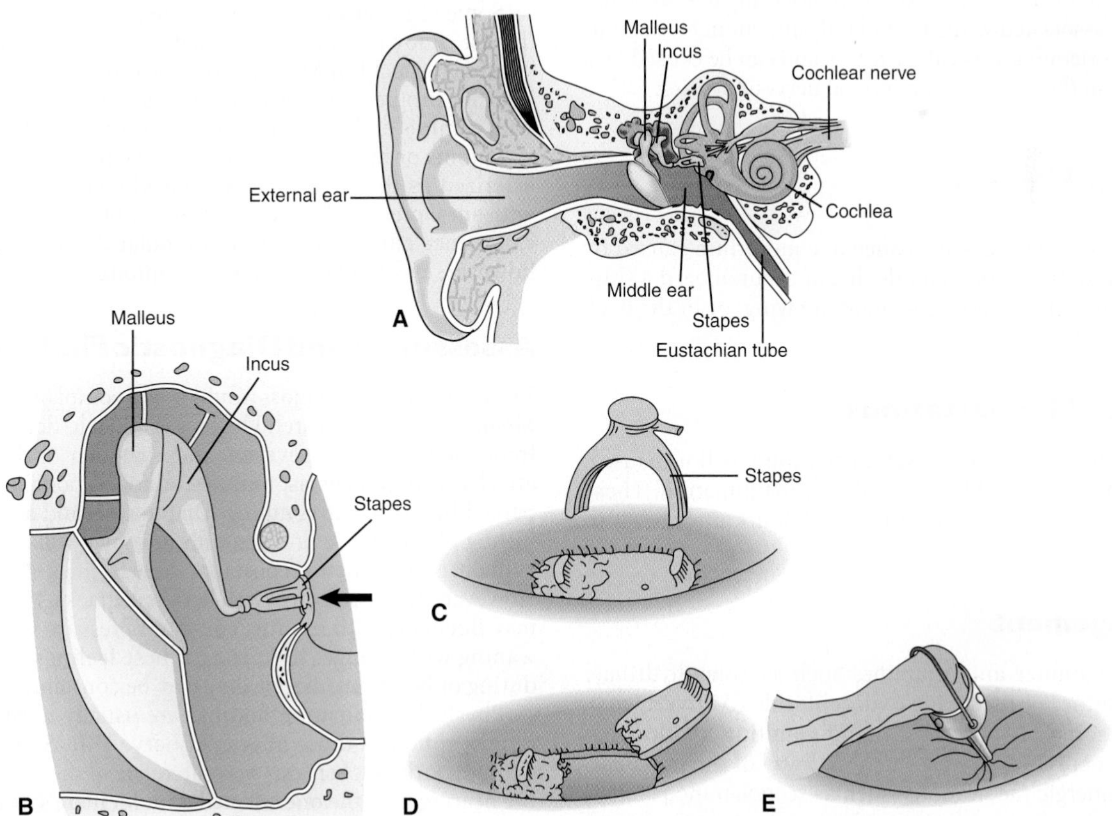

FIGURE 59-8. Stapedectomy for otosclerosis. (**A**) Normal anatomy. (**B**) Arrow points to sclerotic process at the foot of the stapes. (**C**) Stapes broken away surgically from its diseased base. The hole in the footplate provides an area where an instrument can grasp the plate. (**D**) The footplate is removed from its base. Some otosclerotic tissue may remain, and tissue is placed over it. (**E**) Robinson stainless-steel prosthesis in position.

A facial nerve neuroma is a tumor on cranial nerve VII, the facial nerve. These types of tumors are usually not visible on otoscopic examination but are suspected when a patient presents with a facial nerve paresis. X-ray evaluation is used to identify the site of the tumor along the facial nerve. The treatment is surgical removal.

Conditions of the Inner Ear

Almost 8 million American adults are affected by a chronic problem with balance and an additional 2.4 million are affected by dizziness alone. Disorders of balance are a major cause of falls of elderly people (NIDCD, 2005).

The term **dizziness** is used frequently by patients and health care providers to describe any altered sensation of orientation in space. **Vertigo** is defined as the misperception or illusion of motion of the person or the surroundings. Most people with vertigo describe a spinning sensation or say they feel as though objects are moving around them. Ataxia is a failure of muscular coordination and may be present in patients with vestibular disease. Syncope, fainting, and loss of consciousness are not forms of vertigo and usually indicate disease in the cardiovascular system.

Nystagmus is an involuntary rhythmic movement of the eyes. Nystagmus occurs normally when a person watches a rapidly moving object (eg, through the side window of a moving car or train). However, pathologically it is an ocular disorder associated with vestibular dysfunction. Nystagmus can be horizontal, vertical, or rotary and can be caused by a disorder in the central or peripheral nervous system.

Motion Sickness

Motion sickness is a disturbance of equilibrium caused by constant motion. For example, it can occur aboard a ship, while riding on a merry-go-round or swing, or in the back seat of a car.

Clinical Manifestations

The syndrome manifests itself in sweating, pallor, nausea, and vomiting caused by vestibular overstimulation. These manifestations may persist for several hours after the stimulation stops.

Management

Over-the-counter antihistamines such as dimenhydrinate (Dramamine) or meclizine hydrochloride (Antivert) may provide some relief of nausea and vomiting by blocking the conduction of the vestibular pathway of the inner ear. Anticholinergic medications, such as scopolamine patches, may also be effective because they antagonize the histamine response. These must be replaced every few days. Side effects such as dry mouth and drowsiness may occur. Potentially hazardous activities such as driving a car or operating heavy machinery should be avoided if drowsiness occurs.

Ménière's Disease

Ménière's disease is an abnormal inner ear fluid balance caused by a malabsorption in the endolymphatic sac or a blockage in the endolymphatic duct. **Endolymphatic hydrops**, a dilation in the endolymphatic space, develops, and either increased pressure in the system or rupture of the inner ear membrane occurs, producing symptoms of Ménière's disease.

Ménière's disease affects more than 2.4 million people in the United States. More common in adults, it has an average age of onset in the 40s, with symptoms usually beginning between the ages of 20 and 60 years. Ménière's disease appears to be equally common in both genders and occurs bilaterally in about 20% of patients. About 50% of the patients who have Ménière's disease have a positive family history of the disease.

Clinical Manifestations

Symptoms of Ménière's disease include fluctuating, progressive sensorineural hearing loss; **tinnitus** or a roaring sound; a feeling of pressure or fullness in the ear; and episodic, incapacitating vertigo, often accompanied by nausea and vomiting. These symptoms range in severity from a minor nuisance to extreme disability, especially if the attacks of vertigo are severe. At the onset of the disease, perhaps only one or two of the symptoms are manifested.

Some clinicians believe that there are two subsets of the disease, known as atypical Ménière's disease: cochlear and vestibular. Cochlear Ménière's disease is recognized as a fluctuating, progressive sensorineural hearing loss associated with tinnitus and aural pressure in the absence of vestibular symptoms or findings. Vestibular Ménière's disease is characterized as the occurrence of episodic vertigo associated with aural pressure but no cochlear symptoms. Patients may experience either cochlear or vestibular disease symptoms; however, eventually all of these symptoms develop.

Assessment and Diagnostic Findings

Vertigo is usually the most troublesome complaint related to Ménière's disease. A careful history is taken to determine the frequency, duration, severity, and character of the vertigo attacks. Vertigo may last minutes to hours, possibly accompanied by nausea or vomiting. Diaphoresis and a persistent feeling of imbalance or disequilibrium may waken patients at night. Some patients report that these feelings last for days. However, they usually feel well between attacks. Hearing loss may fluctuate, with tinnitus and aural pressure waxing and waning with changes in hearing. These feelings may occur during or before attacks, or they may be constant.

Physical examination findings are usually normal, with the exception of those of cranial nerve VIII. Sounds from a tuning fork (Weber test) may lateralize to the ear opposite the hearing loss, the one affected with Ménière's disease. An audiogram typically reveals a sensorineural hearing loss in the affected ear. This can be in the form of a "Pike's Peak" pattern, which looks like a hill or mountain. A sensorineural loss in the low frequencies occurs as the disease progresses. The electronystagmogram may be normal or may show reduced vestibular response.

Medical Management

Most patients with Ménière's disease can be successfully treated with diet and medication. Many patients can control their symptoms by adhering to a low-sodium (2000 mg/day) diet. Chart 59-7 describes dietary guidelines that may be useful in Ménière's disease. The amount of sodium is one of many factors that regulate the balance of fluid within the body. Sodium and fluid retention disrupts the delicate balance between endolymph and perilymph in the inner ear. Psychological evaluation may be indicated if a patient is anxious, uncertain, fearful, or depressed.

Pharmacologic Therapy

Pharmacologic therapy for Ménière's disease consists of antihistamines such as meclizine (Antivert), which suppress the vestibular system. Tranquilizers such as diazepam (Valium) may be used in acute instances to help control vertigo. Antiemetics such as promethazine (Phenergan) suppositories help control the nausea and vomiting and the vertigo because of their antihistamine effect. Diuretic therapy (eg, hydrochlorothiazide) may relieve symptoms by lowering the pressure in the endolymphatic system. Intake of foods containing potassium (eg, bananas, tomatoes, oranges) is necessary if the patient takes a diuretic that causes potassium loss. There is no scientific basis for the use of vasodilators, such as nicotinic acid, papaverine hydrochloride (Pavabid), and methantheline bromide (Banthine), to alleviate the symptoms, but they are often used in conjunction with other therapies.

CHART 59-7

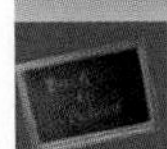

Patient Education

Dietary Guidelines for Patients with Ménière's Disease

- Limit foods high in salt or sugar. Be aware of foods with hidden salts and sugars.
- Eat meals and snacks at regular intervals to stay hydrated. Missing meals or snacks may alter the fluid level in the inner ear.
- Eat fresh fruits, vegetables, and whole grains. Limit the amount of canned, frozen, or processed foods with high sodium content.
- Drink plenty of fluids daily. Water, milk, and low-sugar fruit juices are recommended. Limit intake of coffee, tea, and soft drinks. Avoid caffeine because of its diuretic effect.
- Limit alcohol intake. Alcohol may change the volume and concentration of the inner ear fluid and may worsen symptoms.
- Avoid monosodium glutamate (MSG), which may increase symptoms.
- Avoid aspirin and aspirin-containing medications. Aspirin may increase tinnitus and dizziness.

Surgical Management

Although most patients respond well to conservative therapy, some continue to have disabling attacks of vertigo. If these attacks reduce their quality of life, patients may elect to undergo surgery for relief. However, hearing loss, tinnitus, and aural fullness may continue, because the surgical treatment of Ménière's disease is aimed at eliminating the attacks of vertigo (Silverstein, Lewis, & Jackson, 2003).

ENDOLYMPHATIC SAC DECOMPRESSION

Endolymphatic sac decompression, or shunting, theoretically equalizes the pressure in the endolymphatic space. A shunt or drain is inserted in the endolymphatic sac through a postauricular incision. This procedure is favored by many otolaryngologists as a first-line surgical approach to treat the vertigo of Ménière's disease because it is relatively simple and safe and can be performed on an outpatient basis.

MIDDLE AND INNER EAR PERFUSION

Ototoxic medications, such as streptomycin or gentamicin, can be administered to patients by infusion into the middle and inner ear. These medications are used to destroy vestibular function and decrease vertigo. The success rate for eliminating vertigo is about 85%, but the risk of significant hearing loss is high. After the procedure, many patients have a period of imbalance that lasts several weeks.

INTRAOTOLOGIC CATHETERS

In an attempt to deliver medication directly to the inner ear, catheters are being developed to provide a conduit from the outer ear to the inner ear. The route of the catheter is from the external ear canal through or around the tympanic membrane and to the round window niche or membrane. Medicinal fluids can be placed against the round window for a direct route to the inner ear fluids.

Potential uses of these catheters include treatment for sudden hearing loss and various disorders causing intractable vertigo. Future applications may include tinnitus and slowly progressing sensorineural hearing loss. Intratympanic injections of ototoxic medications for round window membrane diffusion can be used to decrease vestibular function. Established surgical techniques can be used for the patient with vertigo who has not responded to medical or physical therapeutic modalities.

VESTIBULAR NERVE SECTIONING

Vestibular nerve sectioning provides the greatest success rate (approximately 98%) in eliminating the attacks of vertigo. It can be performed by a translabyrinthine approach (ie, through the hearing mechanism) or in a manner that can conserve hearing (ie, suboccipital or middle cranial fossa), depending on the degree of hearing loss. Most patients with incapacitating Ménière's disease have little or no effective hearing. Cutting the nerve prevents the brain from receiving input from the semicircular canals. This procedure requires a brief hospital stay. A plan of nursing care for the patient with vertigo is presented in Chart 59-8.

(text continues on page 2118)

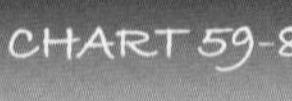

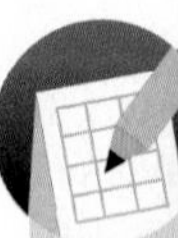

Plan of Nursing Care Care of the Patient With Vertigo

Nursing Diagnosis: Risk for injury related to altered mobility because of gait disturbance and vertigo
Goal: Remains free of any injuries associated with imbalance and/or falls

NURSING INTERVENTIONS	RATIONALE	EXPECTED OUTCOMES
1. Assess for vertigo, including history, onset, description of attacks, duration, frequency, and any associated ear symptoms (hearing loss, tinnitus, aural fullness).	1. History provides basis for interventions.	• Experiences no falls due to balance disturbance • Fear and anxiety are reduced • Performs exercises as prescribed • Takes prescribed medications appropriately • Assumes safe position when vertigo is present • Keeps head still when vertigo is present • Identifies a characteristic fullness or sense of pressure in the ear as occurring before a full-blown attack • Reports measures that help reduce vertigo
2. Assess extent of disability in relation to activities of daily living.	2. Extent of disability indicates risk of falling.	
3. Teach or reinforce vestibular/balance therapy as prescribed.	3. Exercises hasten labyrinthine compensation, which may decrease vertigo and gait disturbance.	
4. Administer, or teach administration of, antivertiginous medications and/or vestibular sedation medication; instruct patient about side effects.	4. Alleviates acute symptoms of vertigo	
5. Encourage patient to sit down when dizzy.	5. Decreases possibility of falling and injury	
6. Place pillow on each side of head to restrict movement.	6. Movement aggravates vertigo.	
7. Assist patient in identifying aura that suggests an impending attack.	7. Recognition of aura may trigger the need to take medication before an attack occurs, thereby minimizing the severity of effects.	
8. Recommend that the patient keep eyes open and stare straight ahead when lying down and experiencing vertigo.	8. Sensation of vertigo decreases and motion decelerates if eyes are kept in a fixed position.	

Nursing Diagnosis: Impaired adjustment related to disability requiring change in lifestyle due to unpredictability of vertigo
Goal: Modifies lifestyle to decrease disability and exert maximum control and independence within limits posed by chronic vertigo

NURSING INTERVENTIONS	RATIONALE	EXPECTED OUTCOMES
1. Encourage patient to identify personal strengths and roles that can still be fulfilled.	1. Maximizes sense of regaining control and independence	• Exerts maximum control of environment and independence within limits imposed by vertigo • Is informed about condition • Family and significant others are included in rehabilitation process • Uses strengths and potentials to engage in the most independent and constructive lifestyle
2. Provide information about vertigo and what to expect.	2. Reduces fear and anxiety	
3. Include family and significant others in rehabilitative process.	3. Perceived beliefs of significant others are important for patient's adherence to medical regimen.	

CHART 59-8

Plan of Nursing Care — Care of the Patient With Vertigo (Continued)

NURSING INTERVENTIONS	RATIONALE	EXPECTED OUTCOMES
4. Encourage patient to maintain sense of control by making decisions and assuming more responsibility for care.	4. Reinforces positive psychological and social outcomes	

Nursing Diagnosis: Risk for deficient fluid volume related to increased fluid output, altered intake, and medications
Goal: Maintains normal fluid and electrolyte balance

NURSING INTERVENTIONS	RATIONALE	EXPECTED OUTCOMES
1. Assess, or have patient assess, intake and output (including emesis, liquid stools, urine, and diaphoresis). Monitor laboratory values.	1. Accurate records provide basis for fluid replacement.	• Laboratory values within normal limits • Alert and oriented; vital signs within normal limits, skin turgor normal; electrolytes normal • Mucous membranes are moist • Vomiting or diarrhea has stopped; usual oral intake resumed
2. Assess indicators of dehydration, including blood pressure (orthostasis), pulse, skin turgor, mucous membranes, and level of consciousness.	2. Prompt recognition of dehydration allows early intervention.	
3. Encourage oral fluids as tolerated; discourage beverages containing caffeine (a vestibular stimulant).	3. Oral replacement is begun as soon as possible to replace losses. Caffeine may increase diarrhea.	
4. Administer, or teach administration of, antiemetics and antidiarrheal medication as prescribed and needed. Instruct patient in side effects.	4. Antiemetics reduce nausea and vomiting, reducing fluid losses and improving oral intake. Antidiarrheal medication reduces intestinal motility and fluid losses.	

Nursing Diagnosis: Anxiety related to threat of, or change in, health status and disability effects of vertigo
Goal: Experiences less or no anxiety

NURSING INTERVENTIONS	RATIONALE	EXPECTED OUTCOMES
1. Assess level of anxiety. Help patient identify coping skills used successfully in the past.	1. Guides therapeutic interventions and participation in self-care. Past coping skills can relieve anxiety.	• Fear and anxiety about attacks of vertigo reduced or eliminated • Acquires knowledge and skills to deal with vertigo • Feels less tension, apprehension, and uncertainty • Uses stress management techniques when needed • Avoids upsetting encounters • Repeats instructions given and verbalizes understanding of treatments
2. Provide information about vertigo and its treatment.	2. Increased knowledge helps to decrease anxiety.	
3. Encourage patient to discuss anxieties and explore concerns about vertigo attacks.	3. Promotes awareness and understanding of relationship between anxiety level and behavior	
4. Teach patient stress management techniques or make appropriate referral.	4. Improved stress management can reduce the frequency and severity of some vertiginous attacks.	

continued >

CHART 59-8

Plan of Nursing Care — Care of the Patient With Vertigo (Continued)

NURSING INTERVENTIONS	RATIONALE	EXPECTED OUTCOMES
5. Provide comfort measures and avoid stress-producing activities.	5. Stressful situations may exacerbate symptoms of the condition.	
6. Instruct patient in aspects of treatment regimen.	6. Patient knowledge helps to decrease anxiety.	

Nursing Diagnosis: Risk for trauma related to impaired balance
Goal: Reduces the risk of trauma by adapting the home environment and by using assistive devices as necessary

NURSING INTERVENTIONS	RATIONALE	EXPECTED OUTCOMES
1. Assess for balance disturbance and/or vertigo by taking history and by examination for nystagmus, positive Romberg, and inability to perform tandem Romberg.	1. Peripheral vestibular disorders cause these signs and symptoms.	• Has adapted home environment or uses rehabilitative devices to reduce risk of falling • Ambulates with needed assistance • Visual and proprioceptive risks identified • Activity level increased • Home environment free of hazards
2. Assist with ambulation when indicated.	2. Abnormal gait can predispose patient to unsteadiness and falls.	
3. Assess for visual acuity and proprioceptive deficits.	3. Balance depends on visual, vestibular, and proprioceptive systems.	
4. Encourage increased activity level with or without use of assistive devices.	4. Increased activity may help retrain balance system.	
5. Help identify hazards in home environment.	5. Adaptation of home environment can reduce risk of falls during rehabilitative process.	

Nursing Diagnosis: Ineffective coping related to personal vulnerability and effects of vertigo
Goal: Develops coping skills necessary to decrease vulnerability and unmet needs and demonstrates effective coping

NURSING INTERVENTIONS	RATIONALE	EXPECTED OUTCOMES
1. Assess cognitive appraisal of illness and factors that may be contributing to inability to cope.	1. To improve patient's self-image and to enhance coping process	• Copes effectively with vertigo • Has acquired knowledge and skills to cope with vertigo • Verbalizes less threatening appraisal of situation • Is involved in outside activities • Identifies specific strategies for coping • Uses support groups or counseling as appropriate
2. Provide factual information about treatment and future health status.	2. Clarifies any misinformation or confusion	
3. Encourage and help patient to participate in decision making about adjustments in lifestyle.	3. Helps patient regain sense of power and control in self-care with activities of daily living	
4. Encourage patient to maintain diversional or recreational activities, exercise, and social events.	4. Social isolation and avoiding pleasant activities intensify isolation and reduce ability to cope with vertigo.	

CHART 59-8

Plan of Nursing Care — Care of the Patient With Vertigo (Continued)

NURSING INTERVENTIONS	RATIONALE	EXPECTED OUTCOMES
5. Help patient identify personal strengths and develop coping strategies based on previous positive experiences in dealing with stress, and situational supports.	5. Enhances patient's strengths that help maintain hope	
6. Refer patient to support groups or counseling as indicated.	6. May help patient feel less alone and isolated	

Nursing Diagnosis: Deficient diversional activity related to environmental lack of such activity
Goal: Engages in diversional activities

NURSING INTERVENTIONS	RATIONALE	EXPECTED OUTCOMES
1. Assess level and type of diversional activity to plan appropriate activities.	1. Boredom may be exhibited as well as depression; helps determine tolerances as well as preferences.	• Verbalizes decreased feelings of boredom and appears alert and animated • Seeks realistic opportunities for involvement in diversional activities.
2. Discuss usual pattern of diversional activities with patient. Suggest opportunities to continue meaningful diversional activities.	2. To provide information about perceived and actual stressors that influence activity level; to support patient's sense of self-worth and productivity.	

Nursing Diagnosis: Self-care deficit: feeding, bathing/hygiene, dressing/grooming, toileting, related to labyrinth dysfunction and episodes of vertigo
Goal: Able to care for self

NURSING INTERVENTIONS	RATIONALE	EXPECTED OUTCOMES
1. Administer, or teach administration of, antiemetics and other prescribed medications to relieve nausea and vomiting associated with vertigo.	1. Antiemetics and sedative-type medications depress stimuli in the cerebellum.	• Carries out necessary functions during symptom-free periods. Takes medications to relieve nausea, vomiting, or vertigo. • Carries out daily activities • Accepts dietary plan and reports its effectiveness. • Drinks fluids in sufficient amounts
2. Encourage patient to perform self-care when free of vertigo.	2. Spacing activities is important because episodes of vertigo vary in occurrence.	
3. Review diet with patient and caregivers. Offer fluids as necessary.	3. Sodium restriction helps improve an inner ear fluid imbalance in some patients, thereby decreasing vertigo. Fluids help prevent dehydration.	

continued >

CHART 59-8

Plan of Nursing Care — Care of the Patient With Vertigo (Continued)

Nursing Diagnosis: Powerlessness related to illness regimen and being helpless in certain situations due to vertigo/balance disturbance
Goal: Experiences increased sense of control over life and activities despite vertigo/balance disturbance

NURSING INTERVENTIONS	RATIONALE	EXPECTED OUTCOMES
1. Assess patient's needs, values, attitudes, and readiness to initiate activities. 2. Provide opportunities for patient to express feelings about self and illness. 3. Help patient identify previous coping behaviors that were successful.	1. Involving patient in planning activities and care enhances potential for mastery. 2. Expressing feelings increases understanding of individual coping styles and defense mechanisms. 3. Awareness increases understanding of stressors that trigger feeling of powerlessness. Awareness of past successes enhances self-confidence.	• Does not restrict activities unnecessarily due to vertigo • Verbalizes positive feelings about own ability to achieve a sense of power and control • Identifies previous successful coping behaviors

Tinnitus

Tinnitus is a symptom of an underlying disorder of the ear that is associated with hearing loss. This condition affects approximately 10% of the U.S. population between 40 and 70 years of age. The severity of tinnitus may range from mild to severe. Patients describe tinnitus as a roaring, buzzing, or hissing sound in one or both ears. Numerous factors may contribute to the development of tinnitus, including several ototoxic substances (Chart 59-9). Underlying disorders that contribute to tinnitus may include thyroid disease, hyperlipidemia, vitamin B_{12} deficiency, psychological disorders (eg, depression, anxiety), fibromyalgia, otologic disorders (Ménière's disease, acoustic neuroma), and neurologic disorders (head injury, multiple sclerosis).

A physical examination should be performed to determine the cause of tinnitus. Diagnostic testing determines if hearing loss is present. An audiograph speech discrimination test or a tympanogram may be used to help determine the cause. Some forms of tinnitus are irreversible; therefore, patients may need teaching and counseling about ways of adjusting to their treatment and dealing with tinnitus in the future.

CHART 59-9

Rx PHARMACOLOGY

Selected Ototoxic Substances

- **Diuretics:** ethacrynic acid, furosemide, acetazolamide
- **Chemotherapeutic agents:** cisplatin, nitrogen mustard
- **Antimalarial agents:** quinine, chloroquine
- **Anti-inflammatory agents:** salicylates (aspirin), indomethacin
- **Chemicals:** alcohol, arsenic
- **Aminoglycoside antibiotics:** amikacin, gentamicin, kanamycin, netilmicin, neomycin, streptomycin, tobramycin
- **Other antibiotics:** erythromycin, minocycline, polymyxin B, vancomycin
- **Metals:** gold, mercury, lead

Labyrinthitis

Labyrinthitis, an inflammation of the inner ear, can be bacterial or viral in origin. Bacterial labyrinthitis is rare because of antibiotic therapy, but it sometimes occurs as a complication of otitis media. The infection can spread to the inner ear by penetrating the membranes of the oval or round windows. Viral labyrinthitis is a common diagnosis, but little is known about this disorder, which affects hearing and balance. The most common viral causes are mumps, rubella, rubeola, and influenza. Viral illnesses of the upper respiratory tract and herpetiform disorders of the facial and acoustic nerves (ie, Ramsay Hunt syndrome) also cause labyrinthitis.

Clinical Manifestations

Labyrinthitis is characterized by a sudden onset of incapacitating vertigo, usually with nausea and vomiting, various degrees of hearing loss, and possibly tinnitus. The first episode is usually the worst; subsequent attacks, which usually occur over a period of several weeks to months, are less severe.

Management

Treatment of bacterial labyrinthitis includes IV antibiotic therapy, fluid replacement, and administration of an antihistamine (eg, meclizine) and antiemetic medications. Treatment of viral labyrinthitis is based on the patient's symptoms.

Benign Paroxysmal Positional Vertigo

Benign paroxysmal positional vertigo is a brief period of incapacitating vertigo that occurs when the position of the patient's head is changed with respect to gravity, typically by placing the head back with the affected ear turned down. The onset is sudden and followed by a predisposition for positional vertigo, usually for hours to weeks but occasionally for months or years.

Benign paroxysmal positional vertigo is thought to be due to the disruption of debris within the semicircular canal. This debris is formed from small crystals of calcium carbonate from the inner ear structure, the utricle. This is frequently stimulated by head trauma, infection, or other events. In severe cases, vertigo may easily be induced by any head movement. The vertigo is usually accompanied by nausea and vomiting; however, hearing impairment does not generally occur (Hain, 2002).

Bed rest is recommended for patients with acute symptoms. There are repositioning techniques that can be used to treat vertigo. The canalith repositioning procedure is commonly used. This noninvasive procedure, which involves quick movements of the body, rearranges the debris in the canal. The procedure is performed by placing the patient in a sitting position, turning the head to a 45-degree angle on the affected side, and then quickly moving the patient to the supine position. The procedure is safe, inexpensive, and easy to perform.

Patients with acute vertigo may be treated with meclizine for 1 to 2 weeks. After this time, the meclizine is stopped, and the patient is reassessed. Patients who continue to have severe positional vertigo may be premedicated with prochlorperazine (Compazine) 1 hour before the canalith repositioning procedure is performed.

Vestibular rehabilitation can be used in the management of vestibular disorders. This strategy promotes active use of the vestibular system through an interdisciplinary team approach, including medical and nursing care, stress management, biofeedback, vocational rehabilitation, and physical therapy. A physical therapist prescribes balance exercises that help the brain compensate for the impairment to the balance system (see Chart 59-8).

Ototoxicity

A variety of medications may have adverse effects on the cochlea, vestibular apparatus, or cranial nerve VIII. All but a few, such as aspirin and quinine, cause irreversible hearing loss. At high doses, aspirin toxicity can produce bilateral tinnitus. IV medications, especially the aminoglycosides, are the most common cause of ototoxicity, and they destroy the hair cells in the organ of Corti (see Chart 59-9).

To prevent loss of hearing or balance, patients receiving potentially ototoxic medications should be counseled about the side effects of these medications. These medications should be used with caution in patients who are at high risk for complications, such as children, the elderly, pregnant patients, patients with kidney or liver problems, and patients with current hearing disorders. Blood levels of the medications should be monitored, and patients receiving long-term IV antibiotics should be monitored with an audiogram twice each week during therapy.

Acoustic Neuroma

Acoustic neuromas are slow-growing, benign tumors of cranial nerve VIII, usually arising from the Schwann cells of the vestibular portion of the nerve. Most acoustic tumors arise within the internal auditory canal and extend into the cerebellopontine angle to press on the brain stem, possibly destroying the vestibular nerve. Most acoustic neuromas are unilateral, except in von Recklinghausen's disease (neurofibromatosis type 2), in which bilateral tumors occur (Roland, 2003).

Acoustic neuromas develop in one of every 10,000 people per year. These neuromas account for 5% to 10% of all intracranial tumors and seem to occur with equal frequency in men and women at any age, although most occur during middle age.

Assessment and Diagnostic Findings

The most common assessment findings of patients with acoustic neuromas are unilateral tinnitus and hearing loss with or without vertigo or balance disturbance. It is important to identify asymmetry in audiovestibular test results so that further workup can be performed to rule out an acoustic neuroma. MRI with a paramagnetic contrast agent (ie, gadolinium or Magnevist) is the imaging study of choice. If the patient is claustrophobic or cannot undergo an MRI for other reasons or if the scan is unavailable, a CT scan with contrast dye is performed. However, MRI is more sensitive than CT in delineating a small tumor.

Management

Surgical removal of acoustic tumors is the treatment of choice because these tumors do not respond well to radiation or chemotherapy. Because treatment of acoustic tumors crosses several specialties, the interdisciplinary treatment approach involves a neurologist and a neurosurgeon. The objective of the surgery is to remove the tumor while preserving facial nerve function. Most acoustic tumors have damaged the cochlear portion of cranial nerve VIII, and hearing is impaired. In these patients, the surgery is performed using a translabyrinthine approach, and the hearing mechanism is destroyed. If hearing is still good before surgery, a suboccipital or middle cranial fossa approach to removing the tumor may be used. This procedure exposes the lateral third of the internal auditory canal and preserves hearing.

Complications of surgery include facial nerve paralysis, cerebrospinal fluid leakage, meningitis, and cerebral edema. Death from acoustic neuroma surgery is rare.

Aural Rehabilitation

If hearing loss is permanent or cannot be treated by medical or surgical means or if the patient elects not to undergo surgery, aural rehabilitation may be beneficial. The purpose of aural rehabilitation is to maximize the communication skills of the person with hearing impairment. Aural rehabilitation includes auditory training, speech reading, speech training, and the use of hearing aids and hearing guide dogs.

Auditory training emphasizes listening skills, so the person who is hearing-impaired concentrates on the speaker. Speech reading (formerly known as lip reading) can help fill the gaps left by missed or misheard words. The goals of speech training are to conserve, develop, and prevent deterioration of current communication skills.

It is important to identify the type of hearing impairment a person has so that rehabilitative efforts can be directed at his or her particular need. Surgical correction may be all that is necessary to treat and improve a conductive hearing loss by eliminating the cause of the hearing loss (Fig. 59-9). With advances in hearing aid technology, amplification for patients with sensorineural hearing loss is more helpful than ever.

Hearing Aids

A hearing aid is a device through which speech and environmental sounds are received by a microphone, converted to electrical signals, amplified, and reconverted to acoustic signals. Many aids available for sensorineural hearing loss depress the low frequencies, or tones, and enhance hearing for the high frequencies. A general guideline for assessing the patient's need for a hearing aid is a hearing loss ex-

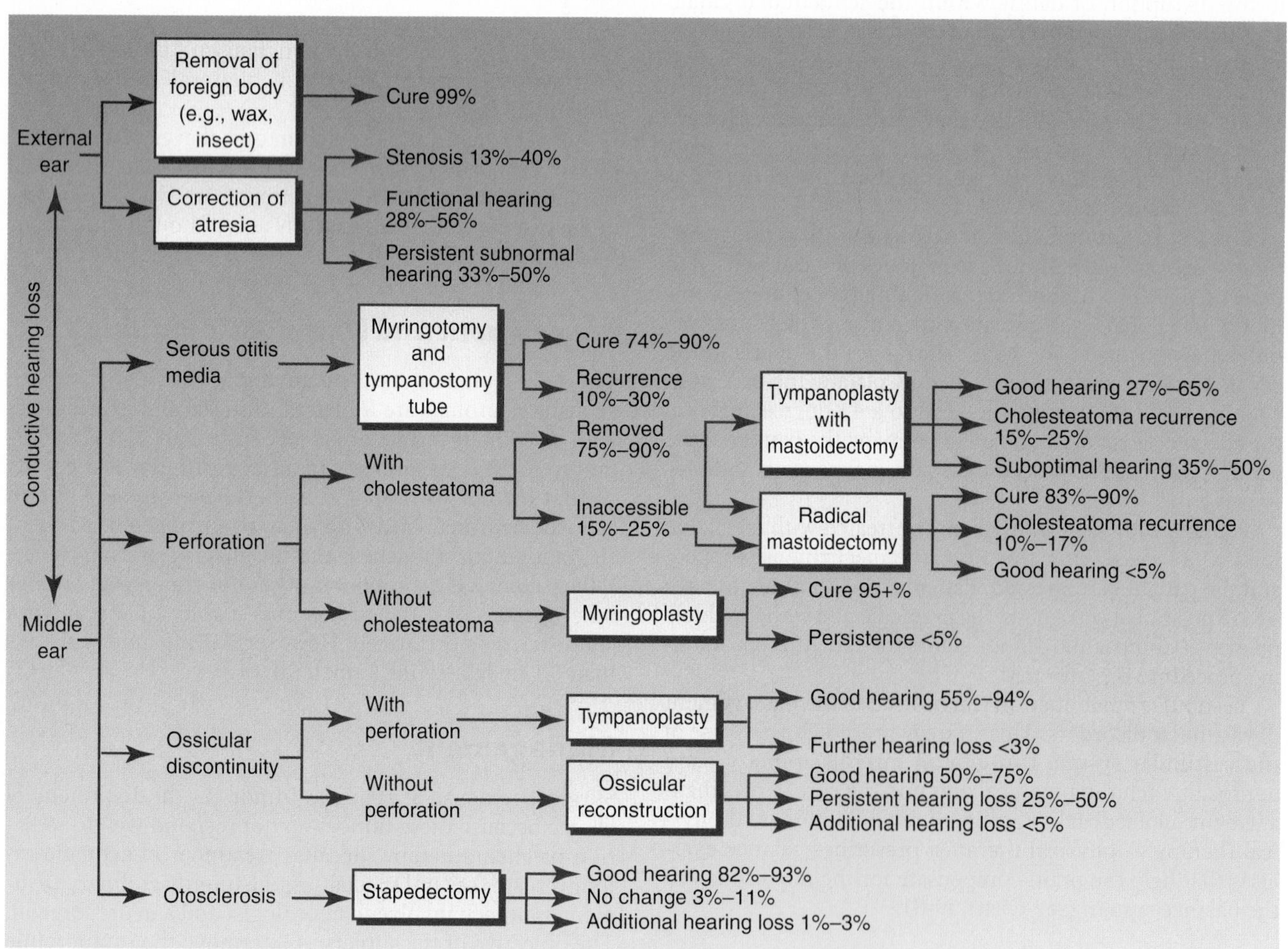

FIGURE 59-9. Management flow chart for conductive hearing loss. The flow chart indicates how the diagnosis determines the management of the patient and predicts the outcome. From Jafek, B. W., & Balkany, T. J. Conductive hearing loss. In B. Eiseman (Ed.). *Prognosis of surgical disease.* Philadelphia: W. B. Saunders.

ceeding 30 dB in the range of 500 to 2000 Hz in the better-hearing ear.

The evolution in technology has led to the availability of many smaller and more effective hearing aids. It is estimated that 98% of all hearing aids sold today are behind-the-ear, in-the-ear, or in-the-canal types (Table 59-4).

A hearing aid should be fitted according to the patient's needs (eg, type of hearing loss, manual dexterity, and preferences), rather than the brand name, by a certified audiologist licensed to dispense hearing aids. Many states have consumer protection laws that allow the hearing aid to be returned after a trial use if the patient is not completely satisfied.

A hearing aid makes sounds louder, but it does not improve a patient's ability to discriminate words or understand speech. People who have low discrimination scores (ie, 20%) on audiograms may derive little benefit from a hearing aid. Hearing aids amplify all sounds, including background noise, which may be disturbing to the wearer. Chart 59-10 identifies additional problems associated with hearing aid use. Computerized hearing aids are available to compensate for background noise or allow amplification at certain programmed frequencies rather than at all frequencies. Occasionally, depending on the type of hearing loss, binaural aids (ie, one for each ear) may be indicated. Chart 59-11 provides tips for hearing aid care.

To protect the health and safety of people with hearing impairments, the U.S. Food and Drug Administration (FDA) has established certain regulations. A medical evaluation of the impairment by a physician must be obtained within 6 months before the purchase of a hearing aid. However, the written statement from a physician may be waived if the patient (a fully informed adult 18 years of age or older) signs a document to this effect. Health care professionals who dispense hearing aids are required to refer prospective users to a physician if any of the following otologic conditions are evident:

- Visible congenital or traumatic deformity of the ear
- Active drainage from the ear within the previous 90 days

CHART 59-10

Hearing Aid Problems

Whistling Noise

Loose ear mold
Improperly made
Improperly worn
Worn out

Improper Aid Selection

Too much power required in aid, with inadequate separation between microphone and receiver
Open mold used inappropriately

Inadequate Amplification

Dead batteries
Cerumen in ear
Cerumen or other material in mold
Wires or tubing disconnected from aid
Aid turned off or volume too low
Improper mold
Improper aid for degree of loss

Pain from Mold

Improperly fitted mold
Ear skin or cartilage infection
Middle ear infection
Ear tumor
Unrelated conditions of the temporomandibular joint, throat, or larynx

TABLE 59-4 Hearing Aids

Site (and Range of Hearing Loss)	Advantages	Disadvantages
Body, usually on the trunk (mild–profound)	Separation of receiver and microphone prevents acoustic feedback, allowing high amplification. Generally used in a school setting.	Bulky; requires long wire, which may be cosmetically displeasing; some loss of high-frequency response
Behind the ear (mild–profound)	Economical; powerful, with no long wires; easily used by children—adapts easily as the child grows, with only the ear mold needing replacement.	Large size
In the ear (mild–moderately severe)	One-piece custom fit to contour of ear; no tubes or cords; miniature microphone is located in the ear, which is a more natural placement; more cosmetically appealing due to easy concealment	Smaller size limits output; patients who have arthritis or cannot perform tasks requiring good manual dexterity may have difficulty with the small size of aid and/or battery; can require more repair than the behind-the-ear aid
In the canal (mild–moderately severe)	Same as in-the-ear aids; less visible, so more cosmetically pleasing	Even smaller than in-the-ear aids; requires good manual dexterity

CHART 59-11

Patient Education

Tips for Hearing Aid Care

CLEANING

- The ear mold is the only part of the hearing aid that may be washed frequently.
- Wash ear mold daily with soap and water.
- Allow the ear mold to dry completely before it is snapped into the receiver.
- Clean the cannula with a small pipe cleaner-like device.
- Proper care of the ear device and keeping the ear canal clean and dry can prevent complications.

MALFUNCTIONING

- Inadequate amplification, a whistling noise, or pain from the mold can occur when a hearing aid is not functioning properly.
- Check for malfunctions:
  - Is the switch on properly?
  - Are the batteries charged and positioned correctly?
- If the hearing aid is still not working properly, notify the hearing aid dealer.
- If the unit requires extended time for repair, the dealer may lend you a hearing aid until the repair can be accomplished.

RECOGNIZING COMPLICATIONS

- Common medical complications include external otitis media and pressure ulcers in the external auditory canal. Signs and symptoms of these infections include painful ear, especially when the external ear is touched, canal swelling, redness, difficulty hearing, pain radiating to the jaw area, and fever.
- If any of these symptoms are present, notify your health care provider for evaluation. You may need medication to treat infection, pain, or both.

- Sudden or rapidly progressive hearing loss within the previous 90 days
- Complaints of dizziness or tinnitus
- Unilateral hearing loss that occurred suddenly or within the previous 90 days
- Audiometric air–bone gap of 15 dB or more at 500, 1000, and 2000 Hz
- Significant accumulation of cerumen or a foreign body in the external auditory canal
- Pain or discomfort in the ear

A user instruction brochure is provided with every hearing aid device. In this brochure, the following information is presented:

- Notification that good health practice requires a medical evaluation before purchasing a hearing aid
- Notification that any of the eight otologic conditions previously listed should be investigated by a physician before purchase of a hearing aid
- Instructions for proper use, maintenance, and care of the hearing aid, as well as instructions for replacing or recharging the batteries
- Repair service information
- Description of avoidable conditions that could damage the hearing aid
- List of any known side effects that may warrant physician consultation (eg, skin irritation, accelerated cerumen accumulation)

Implanted Hearing Devices

Three types of implanted hearing devices are commercially available or in the investigational stage: the cochlear implant, the bone conduction device, and the semi-implantable hearing device. Cochlear implants are for patients with little or no hearing. Bone conduction devices, which transmit sound through the skull to the inner ear, are used in patients with a conductive hearing loss if a hearing aid is contraindicated (eg, those with chronic infection). The device is implanted postauricularly under the skin into the skull, and an external device—worn above the ear, not in the canal—transmits the sound through the skin. Currently there are two types of implantable hearing aids. The bone anchored hearing aid (BAHA) is implanted behind the ear in the mastoid area. The middle ear implantation (MEI) is implanted in the middle ear cavity. The BAHA is used for conductive or mixed hearing loss while the MEI is used for sensorineural hearing loss.

Cochlear Implant

A cochlear implant is an auditory prosthesis used for people with profound sensorineural hearing loss bilaterally who do not benefit from conventional hearing aids. The hearing loss may be congenital or acquired. An implant does not restore normal hearing; rather, it helps the person detect medium to loud environmental sounds and conversation. The implant provides stimulation directly to the auditory nerve, bypassing the nonfunctioning hair cells of the inner ear. The microphone and signal processor, worn outside the body, transmit electrical stimuli to the implanted electrodes. The electrical signals stimulate the auditory nerve fibers and then the brain, where they are interpreted.

Worldwide, more than 59,000 people have received a cochlear implant. In the United States, more than 13,000 adults and 10,000 children have cochlear implants (Garber et al., 2002).

Candidates for a cochlear implant, who are usually at least 1 year of age, are selected after careful screening by otologic history, physical examination, audiologic testing, x-rays, and psychological testing. Criteria for choosing adults who may benefit from a cochlear implant include the following:

- Profound sensorineural hearing loss in both ears
- Inability to hear and recognize speech well with hearing aids

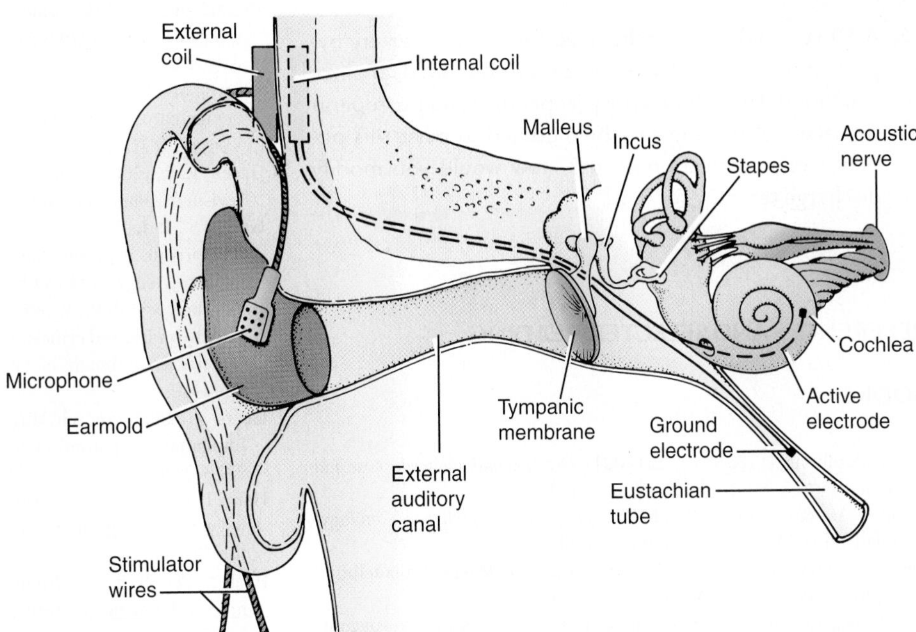

FIGURE 59-10. The cochlear implant. The internal coil has a stranded electrode lead. The electrode is inserted through the round window into the scala tympani of the cochlea. The external coil (the transmitter) is held in alignment with the internal coil (the receiver) by a magnet. The microphone receives the sound. The stimulator wire receives the signal after it has been filtered, adjusted, and modified so that the sound is at a comfortable level for the patient. Sound is passed by the external transmitter to the inner coil receiver by magnetic conduction and is then carried by the electrode to the cochlea.

- No medical contraindication to a cochlear implant or general anesthesia
- Indications that being able to hear would enhance the patient's life

The surgery involves implanting a small receiver in the temporal bone through a postauricular incision and placing electrodes into the inner ear (Fig. 59-10). The microphone and transmitter are worn on an external unit. The patient undergoes extensive cochlear rehabilitation with the multidisciplinary team, which includes an audiologist and speech pathologist. Several months may be needed to learn to interpret the sounds heard. Children and adults who lost their hearing before they learned to speak take much longer to acquire speech. There are wide variations of success with cochlear implants, and there is also controversy about their use, especially among the Deaf community. Patients who have had a cochlear implant are cautioned that an MRI will inactivate the implant; MRI is to be used only when there is no other diagnostic option.

Hearing Guide Dogs

Specially trained dogs (service dogs) are available to assist the person with a hearing loss. People who live alone are eligible to apply for a dog trained by International Hearing Dog, Inc. The dog reacts to the sound of a telephone, a doorbell, an alarm clock, a baby's cry, a knock at the door, a smoke alarm, or an intruder. The dog alerts its master by physical contact; the dog then runs to the source of the noise. In public, the dog positions itself between the person with hearing impairment and any potential hazard that the person cannot hear, such as an oncoming vehicle or a loud, hostile person. In many states, a certified hearing guide dog is legally permitted access to public transportation, public eating places, and stores, including food markets.

Critical Thinking Exercises

1 You are visiting an elderly man for a postoperative home visit following a cholecystectomy. He tells you that he has had severe leg cramps at nighttime and has started taking quinine daily. He has noticed a significant improvement in the leg cramps. During your assessment, you also learn that he has a significant hearing loss, and his wife tells you that she thinks that his hearing has worsened over the past several months; however, she attributes his hearing loss to old age and to anxiety regarding his recent surgery. Devise a teaching plan for this patient and his wife. Provide a rationale for each part of the plan.

2 A 20-year-old man, a member of a college swim team, has recurrent external otitis—his third episode in the past 6 weeks. He is being treated at an ear-nose-throat clinic. Devise an evidence-based practice teaching plan for this patient.

3 An elderly man comes to the outpatient dialysis clinic. He tells you that he has started becoming dizzy in the morning after breakfast and has noticed a continuous roaring sound in his right ear. How would you assess this patient? Explain your rationale for the assessment questions. List potential causes of the patient's problems and provide patient education to prevent further complications.

4 A young man has recently been diagnosed with Ménière's disease. Develop a teaching plan that focuses on control of the patient's symptoms. Provide a rationale for each component of the teaching plan.

5 A 50-year-old man is scheduled for coronary artery bypass graft surgery. He has been profoundly deaf since childhood. How should the preoperative and postoperative plans of nursing care be modified to meet this patient's communication needs? How would you modify discharge teaching for him?

REFERENCES AND SELECTED READING

BOOKS

Alper, C., Eibling, D., & Myers, E. (2001). *Decision making in ear, nose and throat disorders.* Philadelphia: W. B. Saunders.

Canalis, A., & Lambert, P. (2000). *The ear: comprehensive otology.* Philadelphia: Lippincott Williams & Wilkins.

Cash, J., & Glass, C. (2000). *Family practice guidelines.* Philadelphia: Lippincott Williams & Wilkins.

Cooley, D., Grossan, M., & Hoffman, D. (2002). The ins and outs of common ear problems. In *Patient care for the nurse practitioner: 6.* Montvale, NJ: Medical Economics Company.

Goroll, A., Mulley, A. G., Jr., & May, L. A. (Eds.). (2000). *Primary care medicine: Office evaluation and management of the adult patient.* Philadelphia: Lippincott Williams & Wilkins.

Harris, L. L., & Huntoon, M. B. (1998). *Core curriculum for otorhinolaryngology and head/neck nursing.* New Smyrna Beach, FL: Society of Otorhinolaryngology and Head & Neck Nurses.

National Institute on Deafness and Other Communication Disorders (NIDCD). (2005). Strategic Plan. FY 2006-2008. www.nidcd.nih.gov/Stategic.Resources/about/plans/strategic/strategic06-08.pdf. Accessed July 20, 2006.

Noble, J., Greene, H. L., & Levinson, W. (2001). *Textbook of primary care medicine.* St. Louis: C. V. Mosby.

Patton, K., & Thibodeau, G. (2000). *Mosby's handbook of anatomy & physiology.* St. Louis: C. V. Mosby.

Porth, C. M. (2005). Pathophysiology. Concepts of altered health status. Philadelphia: Lippincott Williams & Wilkins.

Society of Otorhinolaryngology and Head & Neck Nurses, Inc. (1996). *Nursing practice guidelines for care of the otorhinolaryngology head and neck patient.* New Smyrna Beach, FL: Author.

Woodson, G. (2001). *Ear, nose and throat disorders in primary care.* Philadelphia: Harcourt Health Sciences.

U.S. Public Health Service. (2000). *Healthy People 2010.* Washington, DC: Author.

JOURNALS

Battista, R., & Esquivel, C. (2003). *Middle ear, ossiculoplasty.* Feb. 7, 2003. Available at http://www.emedicine.com/ent/topic219.htm. Accessed August 26, 2006.

Cavenish, R. (1998). Adult hearing loss. *American Journal of Nursing, 98*(8), 50–51.

Christianson, J., & Leigh, I. (2004). Children with cochlear implants: changing parent and deaf community perspectives. *Archives of Otolaryngology and Head & Neck Surgery, 130*(7), 673–677.

Cruickshanks, K., Tweed, T., Wiley, T., et al. (2003). The 5-year incidence and progression of hearing loss. *Archives of Otolaryngology and Head & Neck Surgery, 129*(3), 1041–1046.

Densert, B., & Sass, K. (2001). Control of symptoms in patients with Meniere's disease using middle ear pressure applications: Two-year follow-up. *Acta Otolaryngologica, 121*(5), 616–621.

Donaldson, J. (2004). *Middle ear, acute otitis media. Surgical treatment.* Available at: http://www.emedicine.com/ent/topic211.htm. Accessed August 26, 2006.

Epley, J. M. (1992). The canalith repositioning procedure: For treatment of benign paroxysmal positional vertigo. *Otolaryngology and Head & Neck Surgery, 107*(3), 399–404.

Gacek, R. R. (2003). Pathology of benign paroxysmal positional vertigo revisited. *Annals of Otology, Rhinology & Laryngology, 112*(7), 574–582.

Garber S., Ridgely, S., Bradley, M., et al. (2002). Payment under public and private insurance and access to cochlear implants. *Archives of Otolaryngology and Head & Neck Surgery, 128*(3), 1145–1152.

Garcia-Berrocal, J. R., Ramirez-Camacho, R., Trinidad, A., et al. (2004). Controversies and criticisms on designs for experimental autoimmune labyrinthitis. *Annals of Otology, Rhinology & Laryngology, 113*(5), 404–410.

Geers, A. (2004). Speech, language, and reading skills after early cochlear implantation. *Journal of the American Medical Association, 291*(12), 2378–2380.

Hain, T. (2002). *Benign paroxysmal positional vertigo.* Available at http://www.tchain.com/otoneurology/disorders/bppv/bppv.html. Accessed July 20, 2006.

Healthy People 2010. *Healthy Hearing 2010.* Available at: http://www.nidcd.nih.gov/health/healthyhearing/what_hh/objectives.asp. Accessed July 20, 2006.

Isaacson, J., & Vora, N. (2003). Differential diagnosis and treatment of hearing loss. *American Family Physician, 15*(3), 1125–1132.

Kaplan, S. L., Mason, E. O., Wald, E. R., et al. (2000). Pneumococcal mastoiditis in children. *Pediatrics, 106*(5), 695–699.

Kitahara, T., Kondoh, K., & Morihana, T. (2004). Surgical management of special cases of intractable Meniere's disease: Unilateral cases with intact canals and bilateral cases. *Annals of Otorhinolaryngology, 113*(5), 339–403.

Korres, S., Babatsouras, D., & Ferekidis, E. (2004). Electronystagmographic findings in benign paroxymal positional vertigo. *Annals of Otology, Rhinology & Laryngology, 113*(4), 313.

Rabinowitz, P. (2000). Noise-induced hearing loss. *American Family Physician, 6*(5), 2749–2760.

Rash, E. (2004). Recognize cholesteatomas early. *Nurse Practitioner, 29*(2), 24–29.

Rizer, F. (2004). *Inner ear, tinnitus.* Available at: http://www.emedicine.com/ent/topic235.htm. Accessed August 26, 2006.

Roland, P. S. (2003). *Skull base, acoustic neuroma (vestibular schwannoma).* Available at: www.emedicine.com/ent/topic239.htm. Accessed August 26, 2006.

Roland, P. S. (2004). *Otosclerosis.* Available at: http://www.emedicine.com/ped/topic1692.htm. Accessed August 26, 2006.

Rovers, M., Schilder, A., Zielhuis, G., et al. (2004). Otitis media. *Lancet, 363*(9407), 465–473.

Silverstein, H., Lewis, W., & Jackson, L. E. (2003). Changing trends in the surgical treatment of Meniere's disease: Results of a 10-year survey. *Ear, Nose, and Throat Journal, 82*(3), 185–194.

Vibert, D., Kompis, M., & Hausler, R. (2003). Benign paroxysmal positional vertigo in older females may be related to osteoporosis and osteopenia. *Annals of Otology, Rhinology, & Laryngology, 112*(10), 885–889.

RESOURCES

Acoustic Neuroma Association, P.O. Box 12402, Atlanta, GA 30355; 770-205-8211; http://ANAusa.org. Accessed July 19, 2006.

Alexander Graham Bell Association for the Deaf, Inc., 3417 Volta Place, NW, Washington, DC 20007; 202-337-5220; http://www.agbell.org. Accessed July 19, 2006.

American Academy of Audiology, 8201 Greensboro Dr., Suite 300, McLean, VA 22102; 703-790-8466; http://www.audiology.com. Accessed July 19, 2006.

American Academy of Facial Plastic and Reconstructive Surgery, 1101 Vermont Ave., NW, Suite 220, Washington, DC 20005; 703-299-9291; http://www.aafprs.org. Accessed July 19, 2006.

American Academy of Otolaryngology and Head & Neck Surgery, One Prince Street, Alexandria, VA 22314; 703-836-4444; http://www.entnet.org. Accessed July 19, 2006.

American Board of Facial Plastic & Reconstructive Surgery, One Prince Street, Suite 310, Alexandria, VA 22314; 703-549-3223; http://www.abfprs.org. Accessed July 19, 2006.

American Speech-Language-Hearing Association, 10801 Rockville Pike, Rockville, MD 20852; 1-800-638-8255; http://www.asha.org. Accessed July 19, 2006.

American Tinnitus Association, P.O. Box 5, Portland, OR 97207; http://www.ata.org; http://www.surgeon.org. Accessed July 19, 2006.

International Hearing Dog, Inc., 5901 E. 89th Ave., Henderson, CO 80640; 303-287-3277; www.ihdi.org. Accessed July 19, 2006.

National Institute on Deafness and Other Communication Disorders, National Institutes of Health, Building 31, Room 3c35 9000, Rockville Pike, Bethesda, MD 20892; http://www.nidcd.nih.gov. Accessed July 19, 2006.

Self-Help for Hard of Hearing People, Inc., 7910 Woodmont Ave., Suite 1200, Bethesda, MD 20814; 301-657-2248; http://www.shhh.org. Accessed July 19, 2006.

Society of Otorhinolaryngology and Head & Neck Nurses, Inc., 116 Canal Street, Suite A, New Smyrna Beach, FL 32168; 904-428-1695; http://www.sohnnurse.com. Accessed July 19, 2006.

Vestibular Disorders Association, P.O. Box 4467, Portland, OR 97208; 503-229-7705; http://www.vestibular.org. Accessed July 19, 2006.

UNIT 14

Neurologic Function

Case Study

Applying Concepts from NANDA, NIC, and NOC

A Patient With Brain Injury And A History of Alcohol Abuse

Mr. Williams is a 56-year-old man with a history of alcohol abuse. On the evening before his admission to the hospital, Mr. Williams fell down a flight of stairs while intoxicated, hitting the front and left side of his head. He was admitted to the neurologic intensive care unit (NICU) and diagnosed with a traumatic brain injury. After several days in the NICU, Mr. Williams developed increased intracranial pressure (ICP) and is being treated for alcohol withdrawal. When family members come to visit, they admit to a significant history of alcoholism in the family.

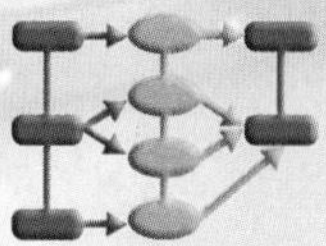

Turn to Appendix C to see a concept map that illustrates the relationships that exist between the nursing diagnoses, interventions, and outcomes for the patient's clinical problems.

Nursing Classifications and Languages

NANDA Nursing Diagnoses	NIC Nursing Interventions	NOC Nursing Outcomes Return to functional baseline status, stabilization of, or improvement in:
Decreased Intracranial Adaptive Capacity—Intracranial fluid dynamic mechanisms that normally compensate for increases in intracranial volumes are compromised, resulting in repeated disproportionate increases in increased intracranial pressure (ICP) in response to a variety of noxious stimuli	**Neurologic Monitoring**—Collection and analysis of patient data to prevent or minimize neurologic complications	**Neurological Status**—Ability of the peripheral and central nervous system to receive, process, and respond to internal and external stimuli
Risk for Injury—At risk of injury as a result of environmental conditions interacting with the individual's adaptive and defensive resources	**Cerebral Edema Management**—Limitation of secondary cerebral injury resulting from swelling of brain tissue	**Seizure Control**—Personal actions to reduce or minimize the occurrence of seizure episodes
Dysfunctional Family Processes: Alcoholism—Psychosocial, spiritual, and physiological functions of the family unit are chronically disorganized, which leads to conflict, denial of problems, resistance to change, ineffective problem solving, and a series of self-perpetuating crises	**Medication Administration**—Preparing, giving, and evaluating the effectiveness of prescription and nonprescription drugs	**Physical Injury Severity**—Severity of injuries from trauma
	Surveillance: Safety—Purposeful and ongoing collection and analysis of information about the patient and the environment for use in promoting and maintaining patient safety	**Family Coping**—Family actions to manage stressors that tax family resources
	Family support—Promotion of family values, interests and goals	

NANDA International (2005). *Nursing diagnoses: Definitions and classification 2005–2006.* Philadelphia: North American Nursing Diagnosis Association.
Dochterman, J. M. & Bulechek, G. M. (2004). *Nursing interventions classification (NIC)* (4th ed.). St. Louis: Mosby.
Iowa Outcomes Project (2004). In Moorhead, S., Johnson, M. & Maas, M. (2004). *Nursing outcomes classification (NOC)* (3rd ed.). St. Louis: Mosby.
Dochterman, J. M. & Jones, D. A. (2003). *Unifying nursing languages: The harmonization of NANDA, NIC, and NOC.* Washington, D.C.: American Nurses Association.

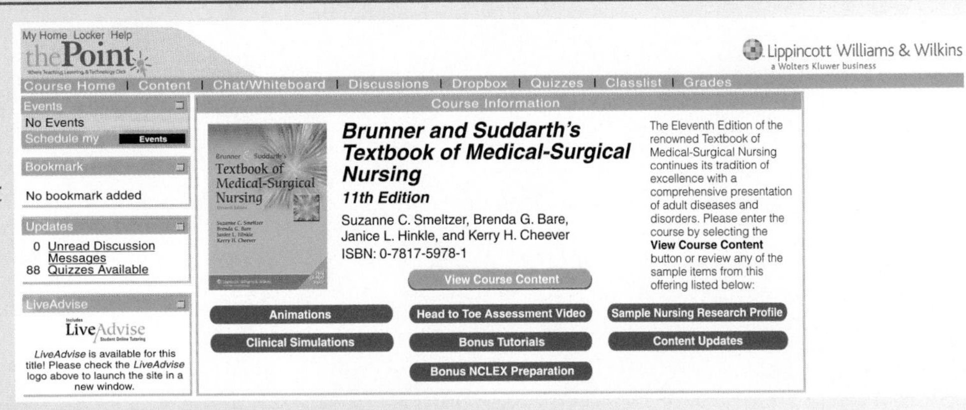

CHAPTER 60

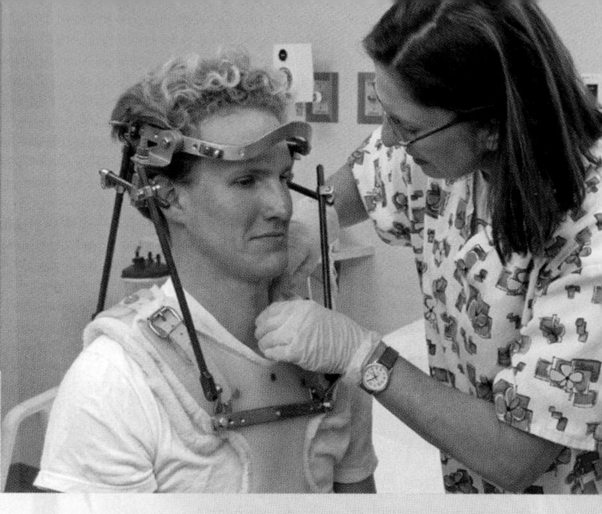

Assessment of Neurologic Function

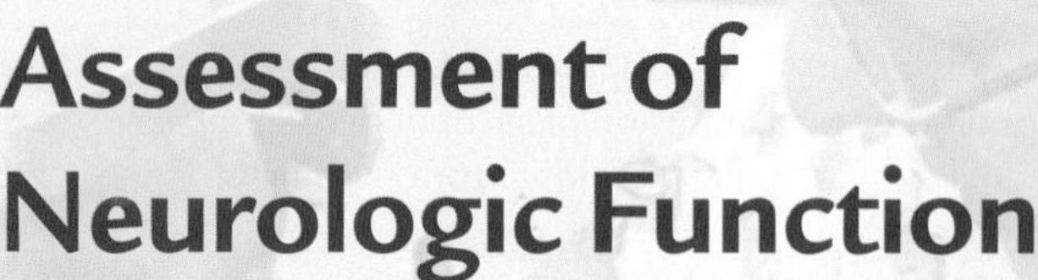

Learning Objectives

On completion of this chapter, the learner will be able to:

1. Describe the structures and functions of the central and peripheral nervous systems.
2. Differentiate between pathologic changes that affect motor control and those that affect sensory pathways.
3. Compare the functioning of the sympathetic and parasympathetic nervous systems.
4. Describe the significance of physical assessment to the diagnosis of neurologic dysfunction.
5. Describe changes in neurologic function associated with aging and their impact on neurologic assessment findings.
6. Describe diagnostic tests used for assessment of suspected neurologic disorders and the related nursing implications.

Nurses in many practice settings encounter patients with altered neurologic function. Disorders of the nervous system can occur at any time during the life span and can vary from mild, self-limiting symptoms to devastating, life-threatening disorders. Nurses must be skilled in the assessment of the neurologic system, whether the assessment is generalized or focused on specific areas of function. In either case, assessment requires knowledge of the anatomy and physiology of the nervous system and an understanding of the array of tests and procedures used to diagnose neurologic disorders. Knowledge about the nursing implications and interventions related to assessment and diagnostic testing is also essential.

Anatomic and Physiologic Overview

The nervous system consists of two divisions: the central nervous system (CNS), including the brain and spinal cord, and the peripheral nervous system, which includes cranial and spinal nerves. The peripheral nervous system can be further divided into the somatic, or voluntary, nervous system, and the autonomic, or involuntary, nervous system. The function of the nervous system is control of all motor, sensory, autonomic, cognitive, and behavioral activities. The nervous system has approximately 10 million sensory neurons that send information about the internal and external environment to the brain and 500,000 motor neurons that control the muscles and glands. The brain itself contains more than 100 billion cells that link the motor and sensory pathways, monitor the body's processes, respond to the internal and external environment, maintain homeostasis, and direct all psychological, biologic, and physical activity through complex chemical and electrical messages (Roscigno, 2004; Bader & Littlejohns, 2004).

Anatomy of the Nervous System

Cells of the Nervous System

The basic functional unit of the brain is the neuron (Fig. 60-1). It is composed of a cell body, a dendrite, and an axon. The **dendrite** is a branch-type structure with synapses for receiving electrochemical messages. The **axon** is a long projection that carries impulses away from the cell body. Nerve cell bodies occurring in clusters are called ganglia or nuclei. A cluster of cell bodies with the same function is called a center (eg, the respiratory center). Neuroglial cells, smaller types of nerve cells, support, protect, and nourish neurons (Bader & Littlejohns, 2004).

Neurotransmitters

Neurotransmitters communicate messages from one neuron to another or from a neuron to a specific target tissue. Neurotransmitters are manufactured and stored in synaptic vesicles. They enable conduction of impulses across the synaptic cleft. Each neurotransmitter has an affinity for specific receptors in the postsynaptic bulb. When released, the neurotransmitter crosses the synaptic cleft and binds to receptors in the postsynaptic cell membrane. The action of a neurotransmitter is to potentiate, terminate, or modulate a specific action, and it can either excite or inhibit the activity of the target cell. Usually, multiple neurotransmitters are at work in the neural synapse. Various substances serve as neurotransmitters (Bader & Littlejohns, 2004; Hickey, 2003); major neurotransmitters are described in Table 60-1.

Glossary

agnosia: loss of ability to recognize objects through a particular sensory system; may be visual, auditory, or tactile

ataxia: inability to coordinate muscle movements, resulting in difficulty in walking, talking, and performing self-care activities

autonomic nervous system: division of the nervous system that regulates the involuntary body functions

axon: portion of the neuron that conducts impulses away from the cell body

Babinski reflex (sign): a reflex action of the toes, indicative of abnormalities in the motor control pathways leading from the cerebral cortex

clonus: abnormal movement marked by alternating contraction and relaxation of a muscle occurring in rapid succession

delirium: transient loss of intellectual function, usually due to systemic problems

dendrite: portion of the neuron that conducts impulses toward the cell body

dysphagia: difficulty swallowing

flaccid: displaying lack of muscle tone; limp, floppy

parasympathetic nervous system: division of the autonomic nervous system active primarily during nonstressful conditions, controlling mostly visceral functions

photophobia: inability to tolerate light

position (postural) sense: awareness of position of parts of the body without looking at them; also referred to as proprioception

reflex: an automatic response to stimuli

rigidity: increase in muscle tone at rest characterized by increased resistance to passive stretch

Romberg test: test for cerebellar dysfunction requiring the patient to stand with feet together, eyes closed and arms extended; inability to maintain the position, with either significant stagger or sway, is a positive test

spasticity: sustained increase in tension of a muscle when it is passively lengthened or stretched

sympathetic nervous system: division of the autonomic nervous system with predominantly excitatory responses, the "fight-or-flight" system

tone: tension present in a muscle at rest

vertigo: an illusion of movement, usually rotation

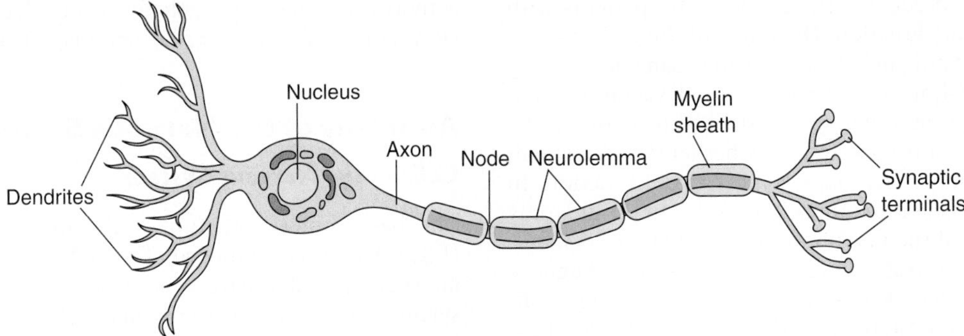

FIGURE 60-1. Neuron.

Many neurologic disorders are due, at least in part, to an imbalance in neurotransmitters—that is, an increase in gamma-aminobutyric acid (GABA) in alcohol withdrawal seizures (Prendergast, 2004), a decrease in dopamine in Parkinson's disease (Dawson & Dawson, 2003), and a decrease in acetylcholine in myasthenia gravis (Porth, 2005). In fact, probably all brain functions are modulated through neurotransmitter receptor site activity, including memory and other cognitive processes (Hickey, 2003).

There are two types of receptors: direct and indirect. Direct receptors are also known as inotropic because they are linked to ion channels and allow passage of ions when opened. They can be excitatory or inhibitory and are rapid-acting (measured in milliseconds). Indirect receptors affect metabolic processes in the cell, which can take from seconds to hours to occur. Receptor sites are an expanding area of research because they are often the target for the action and development of new medications. These medications either block or stimulate neurotransmitters at receptor sites and thus provide relief from symptoms (Dawson & Dawson, 2003; Prendergast, 2004). Receptor sites are also sites for the action of addictive drugs.

Another important area of ongoing research is diagnostic testing that can detect abnormal levels of neurotransmitters in the brain. Positron emission tomography (PET), for example, can detect dopamine, serotonin, and acetylcholine (DeKosky & Marek, 2003). Single photon emission computed tomography (SPECT), similar to PET, can detect changes in some neurotransmitters such as dopamine in Parkinson's disease (DeKosky & Marek, 2003). Both PET and SPECT are discussed in more detail later in this chapter.

The Central Nervous System

ANATOMY OF THE BRAIN

The brain is divided into three major areas: the cerebrum, the brain stem, and the cerebellum. The cerebrum is composed of two hemispheres, the thalamus, the hypothalamus, and the basal ganglia. In addition, connections for the olfactory (cranial nerve I) and optic (cranial nerve III) nerves are found in the cerebrum. The brain stem includes the midbrain, pons, medulla, and connections for cranial nerves II and IV through XII. The cerebellum is located under the cerebrum and behind the brain stem (Fig. 60-2). The brain accounts for approximately 2% of the total body weight; in an average young adult, the brain weighs approximately 1,400 g whereas in an average elderly person, the brain weighs approximately 1,200 g (Hickey, 2003).

Cerebrum. The cerebrum consists of two hemispheres that are incompletely separated by the great longitudinal

TABLE 60-1 Major Neurotransmitters

Neurotransmitter	Source	Action
Acetylcholine (major transmitter of the parasympathetic nervous system)	Many areas of the brain; autonomic nervous system	Usually excitatory; parasympathetic effects sometimes inhibitory (stimulation of heart by vagal nerve)
Serotonin	Brain stem, hypothalamus, dorsal horn of the spinal cord	Inhibitory, helps control mood and sleep, inhibits pain pathways
Dopamine	Substantia nigra and basal ganglia	Usually inhibits, affects behavior (attention, emotions) and fine movement
Norepinephrine (major transmitter of the sympathetic nervous system)	Brain stem, hypothalamus, post-ganglionic neurons of the sympathetic nervous system	Usually excitatory; affects mood and overall activity
Gamma-aminobutyric acid (GABA)	Spinal cord, cerebellum, basal ganglia, some cortical areas	Excitatory
Enkephalin, endorphin	Nerve terminals in the spine, brain stem, thalamus and hypothalamus, pituitary gland	Excitatory; pleasurable sensation, inhibits pain transmission

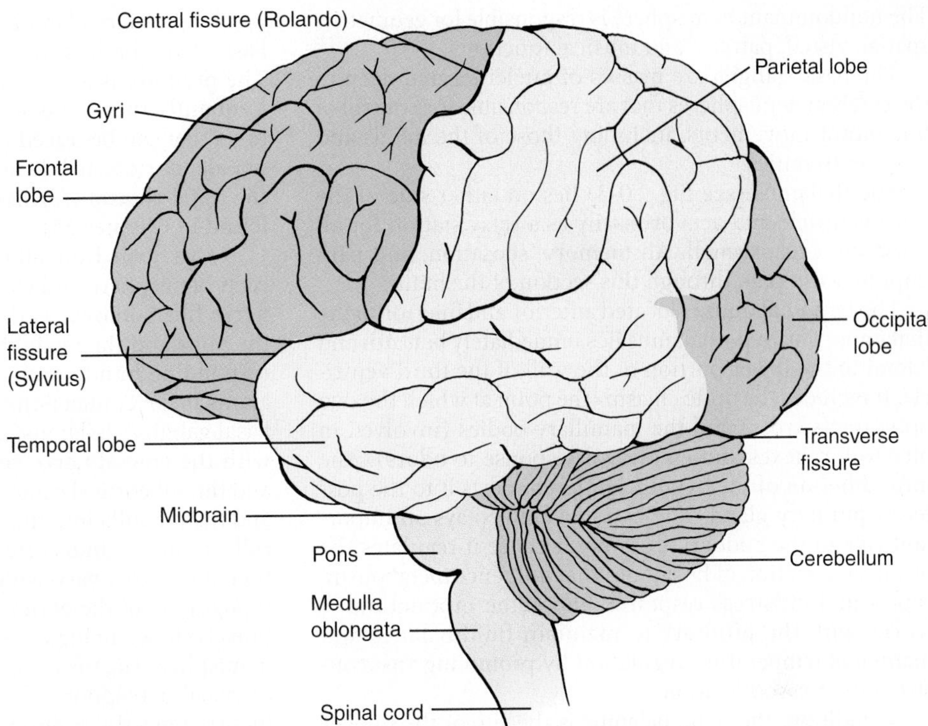

FIGURE 60-2. View of the external surface of the brain showing lobes, cerebellum, and brain stem.

fissure. This sulcus separates the cerebrum into the right and left hemispheres. The two hemispheres are joined at the lower portion of the fissure by the corpus callosum. The outside surface of the hemispheres has a wrinkled appearance that is the result of many folded layers or convolutions called gyri, which increase the surface area of the brain, accounting for the high level of activity carried out by such a small-appearing organ. The external or outer portion of the cerebrum (the cerebral cortex) is made up of gray matter approximately 2 to 5 mm in depth; it contains billions of neurons/cell bodies, giving it a gray appearance. White matter makes up the innermost layer and is composed of nerve fibers and neuroglia (support tissue) that form tracts or pathways connecting various parts of the brain with one another (transverse and association pathways) and the cortex to lower portions of the brain and spinal cord (projection fibers). The cerebral hemispheres are divided into pairs of frontal, parietal, temporal, and occipital lobes. The four lobes are as follows (see Fig. 60-2):

- Frontal—the largest lobe, located in the front of the skull. The major functions of this lobe are concentration, abstract thought, information storage or memory, and motor function. It also contains Broca's area, critical for motor control of speech. The frontal lobe is also responsible in large part for a person's affect, judgment, personality, and inhibitions (Diepenbrock, 2004).
- Parietal—a predominantly sensory lobe located near the crown of the head. This lobe analyzes sensory information and relays the interpretation of this information to the thalamus and other cortical areas. It is also essential to a person's awareness of the body in space, as well as orientation in space and spatial relations (Diepenbrock, 2004).
- Temporal—contains the auditory receptive areas located around the temples. The temporal lobe contains a vital area called the interpretive area that provides integration of somatization, visual, and auditory areas and plays the most dominant role of any area of the cortex in thinking (Diepenbrock, 2004).
- Occipital—the posterior lobe of the cerebral hemisphere located at the lower back of the head, is responsible for visual interpretation (Diepenbrock, 2004).

The corpus callosum (Fig. 60-3) is a thick collection of nerve fibers that connects the two hemispheres of the brain and is responsible for the transmission of information from one side of the brain to the other. Information transferred includes sensation, memory, and learned discrimination. Right-handed people and some left-handed people have cerebral dominance on the left side of the brain for verbal, linguistic, arithmetical, calculating, and analytic functions.

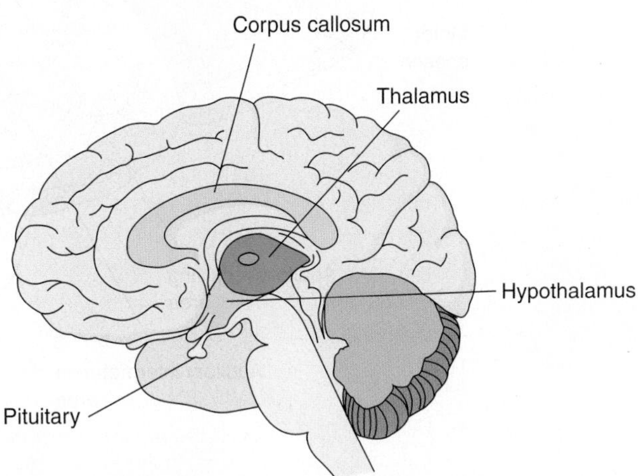

FIGURE 60-3. Medial view of the brain.

The nondominant hemisphere is responsible for geometric, spatial, visual, pattern, and musical functions.

The basal ganglia are masses of nuclei located deep in the cerebral hemispheres that are responsible for control of fine motor movements, including those of the hands and lower extremities.

The thalamus (see Fig. 60-3) lies on either side of the third ventricle and acts primarily as a relay station for all sensation except smell. All memory, sensation, and pain impulses also pass through this section of the brain.

The hypothalamus is located anterior and inferior to the thalamus. The hypothalamus lies immediately beneath and lateral to the lower portion of the wall of the third ventricle. It includes the optic chiasm (the point at which the two optic tracts cross) and the mamillary bodies (involved in olfactory reflexes and emotional response to odors). The infundibulum of the hypothalamus connects it to the posterior pituitary gland. The hypothalamus plays an important role in the endocrine system because it regulates the pituitary secretion of hormones that influence metabolism, reproduction, stress response, and urine production. It works with the pituitary to maintain fluid balance and maintains temperature regulation by promoting vasoconstriction or vasodilatation.

In addition, the hypothalamus is the site of the hunger center and is involved in appetite control. It contains centers that regulate the sleep–wake cycle, blood pressure, aggressive and sexual behavior, and emotional responses (ie, blushing, rage, depression, panic, and fear). The hypothalamus also controls and regulates the autonomic nervous system.

The pituitary gland is located in the sella turcica at the base of the brain and is connected to the hypothalamus. The pituitary is a common site of brain tumors in adults; frequently they are detected by physical signs and symptoms that can be traced to the pituitary, such as hormonal imbalance or visual disturbances secondary to pressure on the optic chiasm (further information on brain tumors is found in Chapter 65).

Nerve fibers from all portions of the cortex converge in each hemisphere and exit in the form of a tight bundle of nerve fibers known as the internal capsule. After entering the pons and the medulla, each bundle crosses to the corresponding bundle from the opposite side. Some of these axons make connections with axons from the cerebellum, basal ganglia, thalamus, and hypothalamus; some connect with the cranial nerve cells. Other fibers from the cortex and the subcortical centers are channeled through the pons and the medulla into the spinal cord. Although the various cells in the cerebral cortex are quite similar in appearance, their functions vary widely, depending on location. The topography of the cortex in relation to certain of its functions is shown in Figure 60-4. The posterior portion of each hemisphere (ie, the occipital lobe) is devoted to all aspects of visual perception. The lateral region, or temporal lobe, incorporates the auditory center. The midcentral zone, or parietal zone, posterior to the fissure of Rolando, is concerned with sensation; the anterior portion is concerned with voluntary muscle movements. The large area behind the forehead (ie, the frontal lobes) contains the association pathways that determine emotions, attitudes, and responses

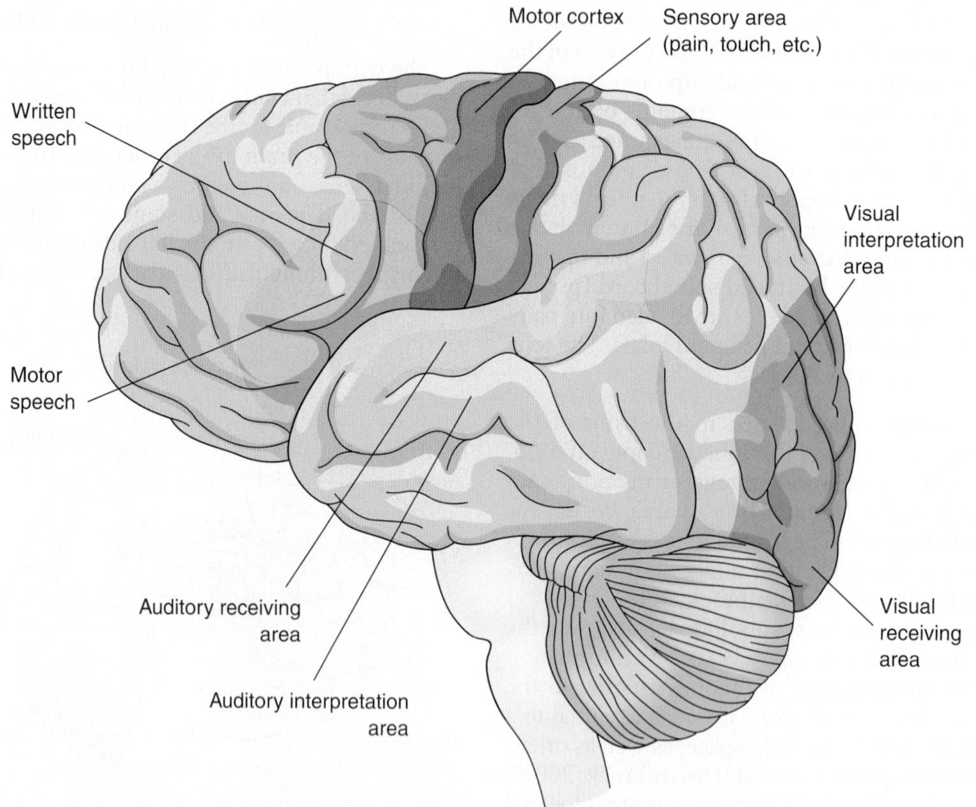

FIGURE 60-4. Topography of the cortex as it relates to function.

and contributes to the formation of thought processes. Damage to the frontal lobes as a result of trauma or disease is by no means incapacitating from the standpoint of muscular control or coordination, but it can affect a person's personality, as reflected by basic attitudes, sense of humor and propriety, self-restraint, and motivations. (Neurologic trauma and disease states that may result in frontal lobe damage are discussed in later chapters in this unit.)

Brain Stem. The brain stem consists of the midbrain, pons, and medulla oblongata (see Fig. 60-2). The midbrain connects the pons and the cerebellum with the cerebral hemispheres; it contains sensory and motor pathways and serves as the center for auditory and visual reflexes. Cranial nerves III and IV originate in the midbrain. The pons is situated in front of the cerebellum between the midbrain and the medulla and is a bridge between the two halves of the cerebellum, and between the medulla and the cerebrum. Cranial nerves V through VIII connect to the brain in the pons. The pons contains motor and sensory pathways. Portions of the pons also control the heart, respiration, and blood pressure.

The medulla oblongata contains motor fibers from the brain to the spinal cord and sensory fibers from the spinal cord to the brain. Most of these fibers cross, or decussate, at this level. Cranial nerves IX through XII connect to the brain in the medulla.

Cerebellum. The cerebellum is separated from the cerebral hemispheres by a fold of dura mater, the *tentorium cerebelli*. The cerebellum has both excitatory and inhibitory actions and is largely responsible for coordination of movement. It also controls fine movement, balance, **position (postural) sense** or proprioception (awareness of where each part of the body is), and integration of sensory input.

STRUCTURES PROTECTING THE BRAIN

The brain is contained in the rigid skull, which protects it from injury. The major bones of the skull are the frontal, temporal, parietal, and occipital bones. These bones join at the suture lines (Fig. 60-5).

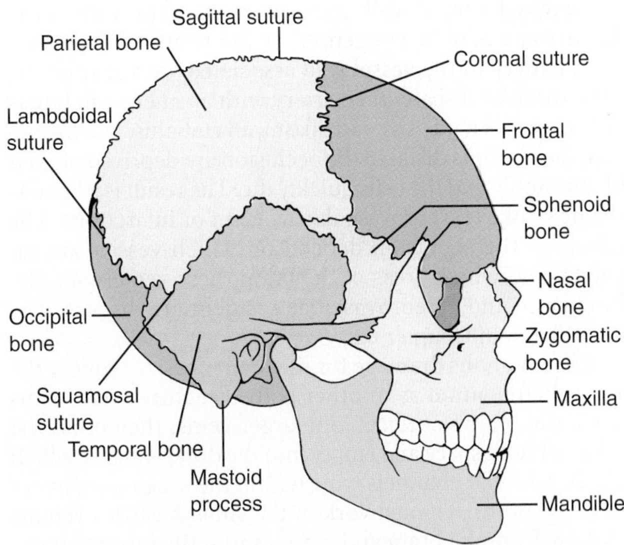

FIGURE 60-5. Bones and sutures of the skull.

The meninges (fibrous connective tissues that cover the brain and spinal cord) provide protection, support, and nourishment to the brain and spinal cord. The layers of the meninges are the dura, arachnoid, and pia mater (Fig. 60-6).

- Dura mater—the outermost layer; covers the brain and the spinal cord. It is tough, thick, inelastic, fibrous, and gray. There are four extensions of the dura: the falx cerebri, which separates the two hemispheres in a longitudinal plane; the tentorium, which is an infolding of the dura that forms a tough, membranous shelf; the falx cerebelli, which is between the two lateral lobes of the cerebellum; and the diaphragm sellae, which provides a "roof" for the sella turcica. The tentorium supports the hemispheres and separates them from the lower part of the brain. When excess pressure occurs in the cranial cavity, brain tissue may be compressed against the tentorium or displaced downward, a process called herniation. Between the dura mater and the skull in the cranium, and between the periosteum and the dura in the vertebral column, is the epidural space, a potential space.
- Arachnoid—the middle membrane; an extremely thin, delicate membrane that closely resembles a spider web (hence the name arachnoid). It appears white because it has no blood supply. The arachnoid layer contains the choroid plexus, which is responsible for the production of cerebrospinal fluid (CSF). This membrane also has unique finger-like projections, arachnoid villi, that absorb CSF. In the normal adult, approximately 500 mL of CSF is produced each day; all but 125 to 150 mL is absorbed by the villi (Hickey, 2003). When blood enters the system (from trauma or hemorrhagic stroke), the villi become obstructed and hydrocephalus (increased size of ventricles) may result. The subdural space is between the dura and the arachnoid layer, and the subarachnoid space is between the arachnoid and pia layers and contains the CSF.
- Pia mater—the innermost membrane; a thin, transparent layer that hugs the brain closely and extends into every fold of the brain's surface.

CEREBROSPINAL FLUID

CSF, a clear and colorless fluid with a specific gravity of 1.007, is produced in the ventricles and is circulated around the brain and the spinal cord through the ventricular system. There are four ventricles: the right and left lateral and the third and fourth ventricles. The two lateral ventricles open into the third ventricle at the interventricular foramen or the foramen of Monro. The third and fourth ventricles connect via the aqueduct of Sylvius. The fourth ventricle supplies CSF to the subarachnoid space and down the spinal cord on the dorsal surface. CSF is returned to the brain and is then circulated around the brain, where it is absorbed by the arachnoid villi.

CSF is produced in the choroid plexus of the lateral, third, and fourth ventricles. The ventricular and subarachnoid system contains approximately 150 mL of fluid; each lateral ventricle normally contains 25 mL of CSF (Bader & Littlejohns, 2004).

The composition of CSF is similar to other extracellular fluids (such as blood plasma), but the concentrations of the various constituents are different. The laboratory report of CSF analysis usually contains information on color, specific

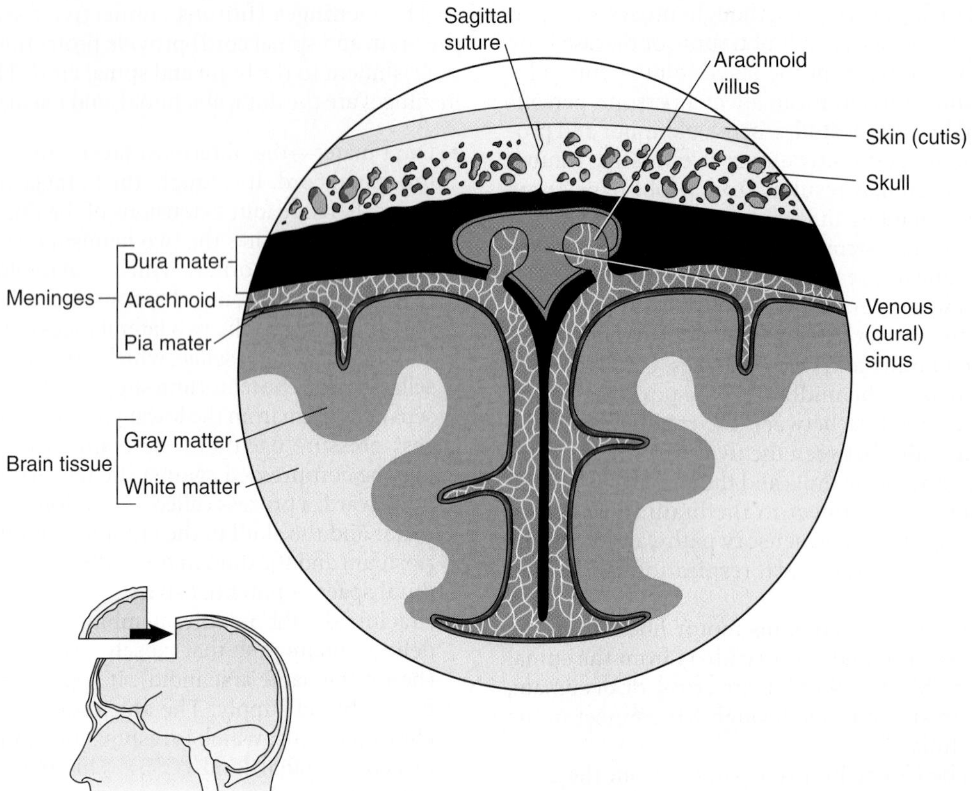

FIGURE 60-6. Meninges and related structures.

gravity, protein count, white blood cell count, glucose, and other electrolyte levels (see Appendix B, Table B-5). The CSF may also be tested for immunoglobulins or lactate (Hickey, 2003). Normal CSF contains a minimal number of white blood cells and no red blood cells.

CEREBRAL CIRCULATION

The cerebral circulation receives approximately 15% of the cardiac output, or 750 mL per minute. The brain does not store nutrients and has a high metabolic demand that requires the high blood flow. The brain's blood pathway is unique because it flows against gravity; its arteries fill from below, and the veins drain from above. In contrast to other organs that may tolerate decreases in blood flow because of their good collateral circulation, the brain has poor collateral blood flow, which may result in irreversible tissue damage when blood flow is occluded for even short time periods.

Arteries. Two internal carotid arteries and two vertebral arteries and their extensive system of branches provide the blood supply to the brain. The internal carotids arise from the bifurcation of the common carotid and supply much of the anterior circulation of the brain. The vertebral arteries branch from the subclavian arteries, flow back and upward on either side of the cervical vertebrae, and enter the cranium through the foramen magnum. The vertebral arteries join to become the basilar artery at the level of the brain stem; the basilar artery divides to form the two branches of the posterior cerebral arteries. The vertebrobasilar arteries supply most of the posterior circulation of the brain.

At the base of the brain surrounding the pituitary gland, a ring of arteries is formed between the vertebral and internal carotid arterial chains. This ring is called the circle of Willis and is formed from the branches of the internal carotid arteries, anterior and middle cerebral arteries, and anterior and posterior communicating arteries (Fig. 60-7). Functionally, the posterior portion of the circulation and the anterior or carotid circulation usually remain separate. The arteries of the circle of Willis can provide collateral circulation if one or more of the four vessels supplying it become occluded or are ligated.

The arterial anastomoses along the circle of Willis are frequent sites of aneurysms that can form when the pressure at a weakened arterial wall causes an outward protuberance. Aneurysms may be congenital or the result of degenerative changes in the vessel wall associated with arteriosclerotic vascular disease. If an artery with an aneurysm bursts or becomes occluded by vasospasm, an embolus, or a thrombus, the neurons distal to the occlusion are deprived of their blood supply and the cells quickly die. The result is a hemorrhagic stroke (cerebrovascular accident or infarction). The effects of the occlusion depend on which vessels are involved and which areas of the brain these vessels supply. Aneurysm and cerebrovascular accident are discussed in more detail in Chapter 62.

Veins. Venous drainage for the brain does not follow the arterial circulation as in other body structures. The veins reach the brain's surface, join larger veins, then cross the subarachnoid space and empty into the dural sinuses, which are the vascular channels lying within the tough dura mater (see Fig. 60-6). The network of the sinuses carries venous outflow from the brain and empties into the internal jugular vein, returning the blood to the heart. Cerebral veins and sinuses are unique because, unlike other veins in the body,

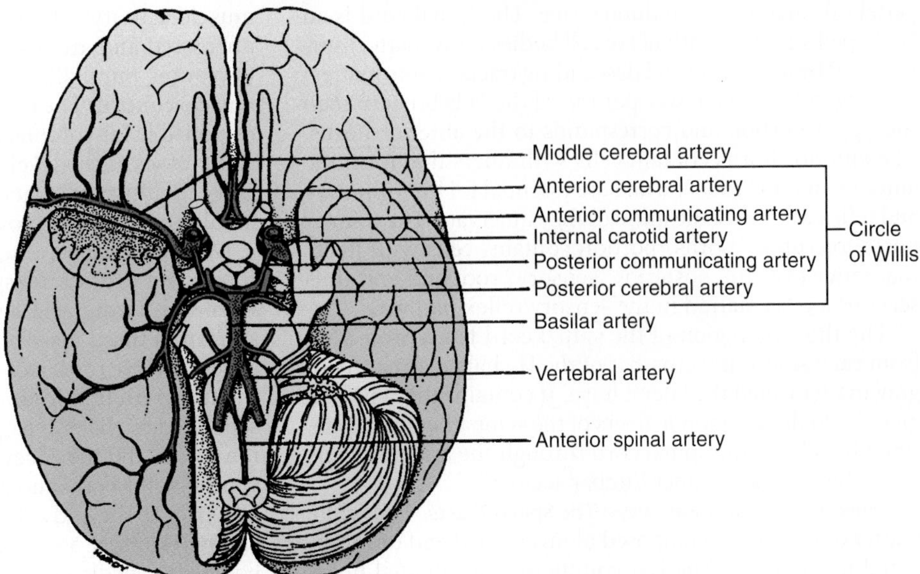

FIGURE 60-7. Arterial blood supply of the brain, including the circle of Willis, as viewed from the ventral surface.

they do not have valves to prevent blood from flowing backward and depend on both gravity and blood pressure.

BLOOD–BRAIN BARRIER

The CNS is inaccessible to many substances that circulate in the blood plasma (eg, dyes, medications, and antibiotics). After entering the blood, many substances cannot reach the neurons of the CNS because of the blood–brain barrier. This barrier is formed by the endothelial cells of the brain's capillaries, which form continuous tight junctions, creating a barrier to macromolecules and many compounds. All substances entering the CSF must filter through the capillary endothelial cells and astrocytes (Hickey, 2003). The blood–brain barrier has a protective function but can be altered by trauma, cerebral edema, and cerebral hypoxemia; this has implications in the treatment and selection of medication for CNS disorders.

ANATOMY OF THE SPINAL CORD

The spinal cord and medulla form a continuous structure extending from the cerebral hemispheres and serving as the connection between the brain and the periphery. Approximately 45 cm (18 in) long and about the thickness of a finger, it extends from the foramen magnum at the base of the skull to the lower border of the first lumbar vertebra, where it tapers to a fibrous band called the *conus medullaris.* Continuing below the second lumbar space are the nerve roots that extend beyond the conus, which are called the *cauda equina* because they resemble a horse's tail. Similar to the brain, the spinal cord consists of gray and white matter. Gray matter in the brain is external and white matter is internal; in the spinal cord, gray matter is in the center and is surrounded on all sides by white matter (Fig. 60-8).

The spinal cord is surrounded by the meninges, dura, arachnoid, and pia layers. Between the dura mater and the

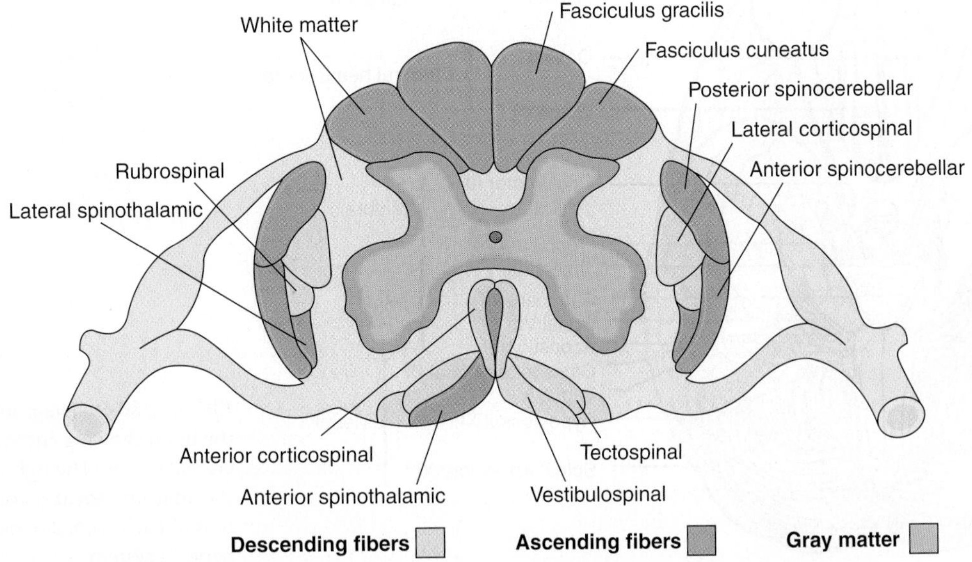

FIGURE 60-8. Cross-sectional diagram of the spinal cord showing major spinal tracts.

vertebral canal is the epidural space. The spinal cord is an H-shaped structure with nerve cell bodies (gray matter) surrounded by ascending and descending tracts (white matter) (see Fig. 60-8). The lower portion of the H is broader than the upper portion and corresponds to the anterior horns. The anterior horns contain cells with fibers that form the anterior (motor) root end and are essential for the voluntary and reflex activity of the muscles they innervate. The thinner posterior (upper horns) portion contains cells with fibers that enter over the posterior (sensory) root end and thus serve as a relay station in the sensory/reflex pathway.

The thoracic region of the spinal cord has a projection from each side at the crossbar of the H-shaped structure of gray matter called the lateral horn. It contains the cells that give rise to the autonomic fibers of the sympathetic division. The fibers leave the spinal cord through the anterior roots in the thoracic and upper lumbar segments.

Sensory and Motor Pathways: The Spinal Tracts. The white matter of the cord is composed of myelinated and unmyelinated nerve fibers. The fast-conducting myelinated fibers form bundles that also contain glial cells. Fiber bundles with a common function are called tracts.

There are six ascending tracts. Two conduct sensation, principally the perception of touch, pressure, vibration, position, and passive motion from the same side of the body. Before reaching the cerebral cortex, these fibers cross to the opposite side in the medulla. The two spinocerebellar tracts conduct sensory impulses from muscle spindles, providing necessary input for coordinated muscle contraction. They ascend essentially uncrossed and terminate in the cerebellum. The last two spinothalamic tracts are responsible for conduction of pain, temperature, proprioception, fine touch, and vibratory sense from the upper body to the brain. They ascend, cross to the opposite side of the brain, and terminate in the thalamus (Hickey, 2003).

There are eight descending tracts. The two corticospinal tracts conduct motor impulses to the anterior horn cells from the opposite side of the brain and control voluntary muscle activity. The three vestibulospinal tracts descend uncrossed and are involved in some autonomic functions (sweating, pupil dilation, and circulation) and involuntary muscle control. The corticobulbar tract conducts impulses responsible for voluntary head and facial muscle movement and crosses at the level of the brain stem. The rubrospinal and reticulospinal tracts conduct impulses involved with involuntary muscle movement.

Vertebral Column. The bones of the vertebral column surround and protect the spinal cord and normally consist of 7 cervical, 12 thoracic, and 5 lumber vertebrae, as well as the sacrum (a fused mass of 5 vertebrae), and terminate in the coccyx. Nerve roots exit from the vertebral column through the intervertebral foramina (openings). The vertebrae are separated by disks, except for the first and second cervical, the sacral, and the coccygeal vertebrae. Each vertebra has a ventral solid body and a dorsal segment or arch, which is posterior to the body. The arch is composed of two pedicles and two laminae supporting seven processes. The vertebral body, arch, pedicles, and laminae all encase and protect the spinal cord.

The Peripheral Nervous System

The peripheral nervous system includes the cranial nerves, the spinal nerves, and the autonomic nervous system.

CRANIAL NERVES

Twelve pairs of cranial nerves emerge from the lower surface of the brain and pass through the foramina in the skull. Three are entirely sensory (I, II, VIII), five are motor (III, IV, VI, XI, and XII), and four are mixed (V, VII, IX, and X), because they have both sensory and motor functions (Diepenbrock, 2004; Hickey, 2003). The cranial nerves are numbered in the order in which they arise from the brain. For example, cranial nerves I and II attach in the cerebral hemispheres, whereas cranial nerves IX, X, XI, and XII attach at the medulla (Fig. 60-9). Most cranial nerves innervate the head, neck,

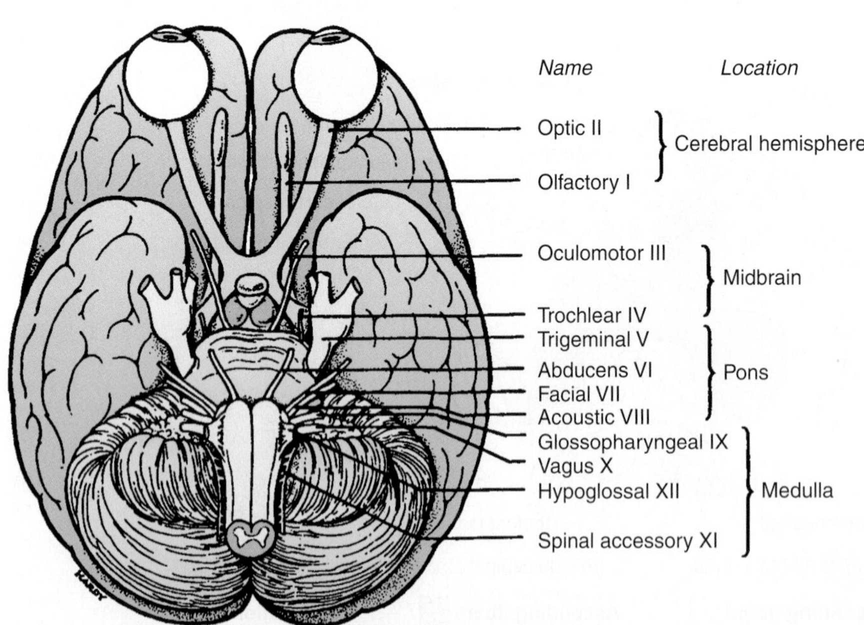

FIGURE 60-9. Diagram of the base of the brain showing entrance or exit of the cranial nerves. The right column shows the anatomic location of the connection of each cranial nerve to the central nervous system.

and special sense structures. Table 60-2 lists the names and primary functions of the cranial nerves.

SPINAL NERVES

The spinal cord is composed of 31 pairs of spinal nerves: 8 cervical, 12 thoracic, 5 lumbar, 5 sacral, and 1 coccygeal. Each spinal nerve has a ventral root and a dorsal root (Fig. 60-10).

The dorsal roots are sensory and transmit sensory impulses from specific areas of the body known as dermatomes (Fig. 60-11) to the dorsal ganglia. The sensory fiber may be somatic, carrying information about pain, temperature, touch, and position sense (proprioception) from the tendons, joints, and body surfaces; or visceral, carrying information from the internal organs.

The ventral roots are motor and transmit impulses from the spinal cord to the body, and these fibers are also either somatic or visceral. The visceral fibers include autonomic fibers that control the cardiac muscles and glandular secretions.

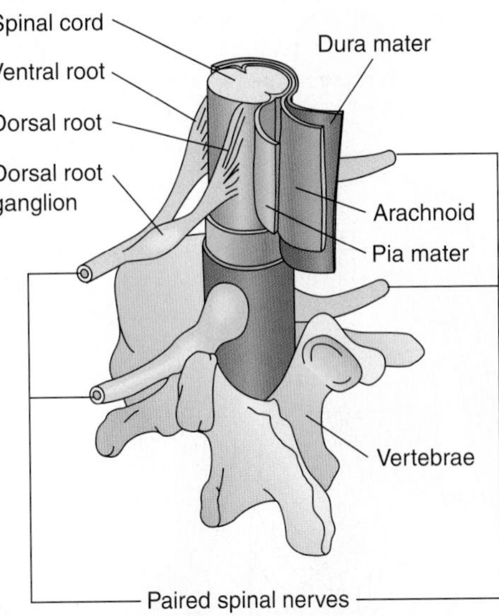

FIGURE 60-10. Spinal cord and meninges. Reproduced from Porth, C. M. (2005). *Pathology: Concepts of altered health states* (7th ed.). Philadelphia: Lippincott Williams & Wilkins.

AUTONOMIC NERVOUS SYSTEM

The **autonomic nervous system** regulates the activities of internal organs such as the heart, lungs, blood vessels, digestive organs, and glands. Maintenance and restoration of internal homeostasis is largely the responsibility of the autonomic nervous system. There are two major divisions: the **sympathetic nervous system,** with predominantly excitatory responses, most notably the "fight or flight" response, and the **parasympathetic nervous system,** which controls mostly visceral functions.

The autonomic nervous system innervates most body organs. Although usually considered part of the peripheral nervous system, this system is regulated by centers in the spinal cord, brain stem, and hypothalamus. The autonomic nervous system has two neurons in a series extending between the centers in the CNS and the organs innervated. The first neuron, the preganglionic neuron, is located in the brain or spinal cord, and its axon extends to the autonomic ganglia. There, it synapses with the second neuron, the postganglionic neuron, located in the autonomic ganglia, and its axon synapses with the target tissue and innervates the effector organ. Its regulatory effects are exerted not on individual cells but on large expanses of tissue and on entire organs. The responses elicited do not occur instantaneously but after a lag period. These responses are sustained far longer than other neurogenic responses to ensure maximal functional efficiency on the part of receptor organs, such as blood vessels.

The autonomic nervous system transmits its impulses by way of nerve pathways, enhanced by chemical mediators, resembling the endocrine system in this respect. This accounts for the quality of these responses. Electrical impulses, conducted through nerve fibers, stimulate the formation of specific chemical agents at strategic locations within the muscle mass; the diffusion of these chemicals within the muscle is responsible for the contraction.

The hypothalamus is the major subcortical center for the regulation of visceral and somatic activities, serving an inhibitory–excitatory role in the autonomic nervous system. The hypothalamus has connections that link the autonomic system with the thalamus, the cortex, the olfactory apparatus, and the pituitary gland. Located here are the mechanisms for the control of visceral and somatic reactions

TABLE 60-2 Cranial Nerves

Cranial Nerve	Type	Function
I (olfactory)	Sensory	Sense of smell
II (optic)	Sensory	Visual acuity and visual fields
III (oculomotor)	Motor	Muscles that move the eye and lid, pupillary constriction, lens accommodation
IV (trochlear)	Motor	Muscles that move the eye
V (trigeminal)	Mixed	Facial sensation, corneal reflex, mastication
VI (abducens)	Motor	Muscles that move the eye
VII (facial)	Mixed	Facial expression and muscle movement, salivation and tearing, taste, sensation in the ear
VIII (acoustic)	Sensory	Hearing and equilibrium
IX (glossopharyngeal)	Mixed	Taste, sensation in pharynx and tongue, pharyngeal muscles, swallowing
X (vagus)	Mixed	Muscles of pharynx, larynx, and soft palate; sensation in external ear, pharynx, larynx, thoracic and abdominal viscera; parasympathetic innervation of thoracic and abdominal organs
XI (spinal accessory)	Motor	Sternocleidomastoid and trapezius muscles
XII (hypoglossal)	Motor	Movement of the tongue

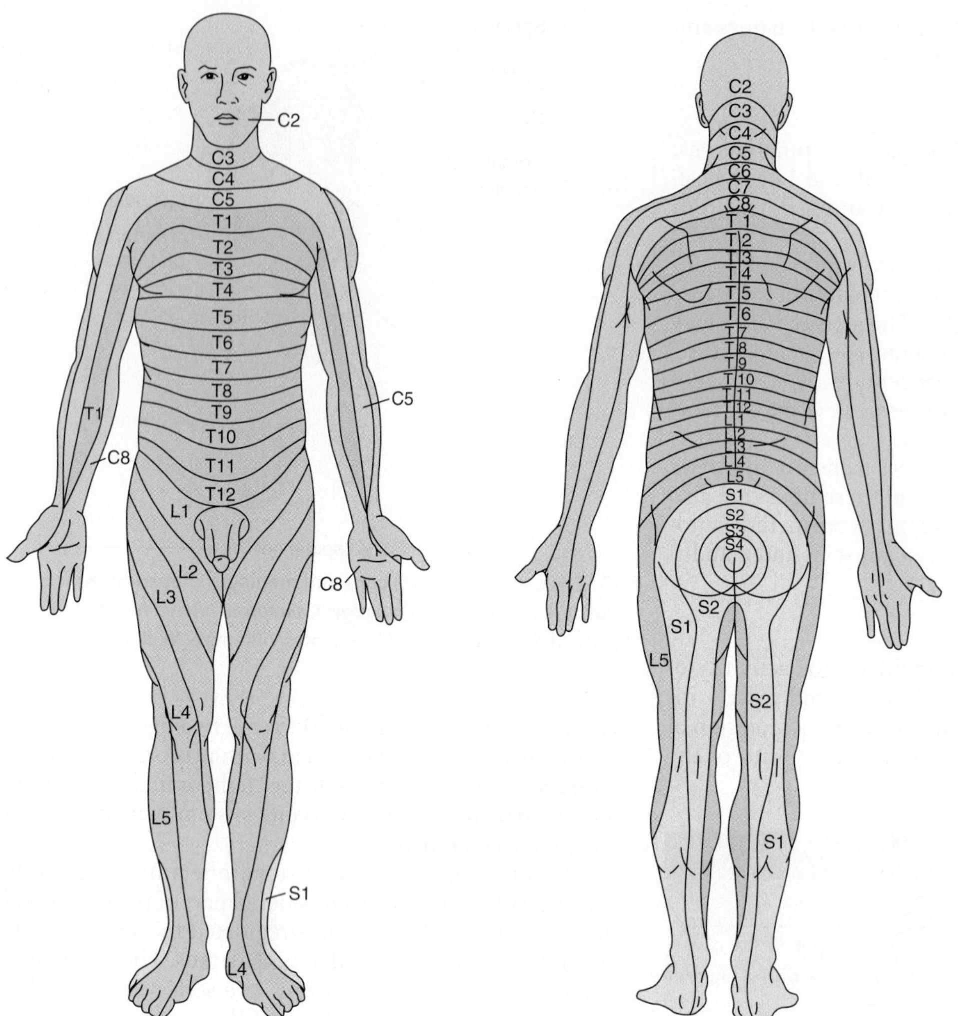

FIGURE 60-11. Dermatome distribution.

that were originally important for defense or attack and are associated with emotional states (eg, fear, anger, anxiety); for the control of metabolic processes, including fat, carbohydrate, and water metabolism; for the regulation of body temperature, arterial pressure, and all muscular and glandular activities of the gastrointestinal tract; for control of genital functions; and for the sleep cycle.

The autonomic nervous system is separated into the anatomically and functionally distinct sympathetic and parasympathetic divisions. Most of the tissues and the organs under autonomic control are innervated by both systems. Sympathetic stimuli are mediated by norepinephrine and parasympathetic impulses are mediated by acetylcholine. These chemicals produce opposing and mutually antagonistic effects. Both divisions produce stimulatory and inhibitory effects. For example, the parasympathetic division causes contraction (stimulation) of the urinary bladder muscles and a decrease (inhibition) in heart rate, whereas the sympathetic division produces relaxation (inhibition) of the urinary bladder and an increase (stimulation) in the rate and force of the heartbeat. Table 60-3 compares the sympathetic and the parasympathetic effects on the different systems of the body.

Sympathetic Nervous System. The sympathetic division of the autonomic nervous system is best known for its role in the body's "fight-or-flight" response. Under stress from either physical or emotional causes, sympathetic impulses increase greatly. As a result, the bronchioles dilate for easier gas exchange; the heart's contractions are stronger and faster; the arteries to the heart and voluntary muscles dilate, carrying more blood to these organs; peripheral blood vessels constrict, making the skin feel cool but shunting blood to essential organs; the pupils dilate; the liver releases glucose for quick energy; peristalsis slows; hair stands on end; and perspiration increases. The main sympathetic neurotransmitter is norepinephrine (noradrenaline), and this increase in sympathetic discharge is the same as if the body has been given an injection of adrenalin—hence, the term adrenergic is often used to refer to this division.

Sympathetic neurons are located primarily in the thoracic and the lumbar segments of the spinal cord, and their axons, or the preganglionic fibers, emerge by way of anterior nerve roots from the eighth cervical or first thoracic segment to the second or third lumbar segment. A short distance from the cord, these fibers diverge to join a chain, composed of 22 linked ganglia, that extends the entire length of the spinal column, adjacent to the vertebral bodies on both sides. Some form multiple synapses with nerve cells within the chain. Others traverse the chain without making connections or losing continuity to join large "pre-

TABLE 60-3 Autonomic Effects of the Nervous System

Structure or Activity	Parasympathetic Effects	Sympathetic Effects
Pupil of the Eye	Constricted	Dilated
Circulatory System		
Rate and force of heartbeat	Decreased	Increased
Blood vessels		
In heart muscle	Constricted	Dilated
In skeletal muscle	*	Dilated
In abdominal viscera and the skin	*	Constricted
Blood pressure	Decreased	Increased
Respiratory System		
Bronchioles	Constricted	Dilated
Rate of breathing	Decreased	Increased
Digestive System		
Peristaltic movements of digestive tube	Increased	Decreased
Muscular sphincters of digestive tube	Relaxed	Contracted
Secretion of salivary glands	Thin, watery saliva	Thick, viscid saliva
Secretions of stomach, intestine, and pancreas	Increased	*
Conversion of liver glycogen to glucose	*	Increased
Genitourinary System		
Urinary bladder		
Muscle walls	Contracted	Relaxed
Sphincters	Relaxed	Contracted
Muscles of the uterus	Relaxed; variable	Contracted under some conditions; varies with menstrual cycle and pregnancy
Blood vessels of external genitalia	Dilated	*
Integumentary System		
Secretion of sweat	*	Increased
Pilomotor muscles	*	Contracted (goose-flesh)
Adrenal Medulla	*	Secretion of epinephrine and norepinephrine

* No direct effect.
From Hickey, J. (2003). *Clinical practice of neurological and neurosurgical nursing* (5th ed.). Philadelphia: Lippincott Williams & Wilkins.

vertebral" ganglia in the thorax, the abdomen, or the pelvis or one of the "terminal" ganglia in the vicinity of an organ, such as the bladder or the rectum (Fig. 60-12). Postganglionic nerve fibers originating in the sympathetic chain rejoin the spinal nerves that supply the extremities and are distributed to blood vessels, sweat glands, and smooth muscle tissue in the skin. Postganglionic fibers from the prevertebral plexuses (eg, the cardiac, pulmonary, splanchnic, and pelvic plexuses) supply structures in the head and neck, thorax, abdomen, and pelvis, respectively, having been joined in these plexuses by fibers from the parasympathetic division.

The adrenal glands, kidneys, liver, spleen, stomach, and duodenum are under the control of the giant celiac plexus, commonly known as the solar plexus. This receives its sympathetic nerve components by way of the three splanchnic nerves, composed of preganglionic fibers from nine segments of the spinal cord (T4 to L1), and is joined by the vagus nerve, representing the parasympathetic division. From the celiac plexus, fibers of both divisions travel along the course of blood vessels to their target organs.

Sympathetic Syndromes. Certain syndromes are distinctive to diseases of the sympathetic nerve trunks. Among these are dilation of the pupil of the eye on the same side as a penetrating wound of the neck (evidence of disturbance of the cervical sympathetic cord); temporary paralysis of the bowel (indicated by the absence of peristaltic waves and the distention of the intestine by gas) after fracture of any one of the lower dorsal or upper lumbar vertebrae with hemorrhage into the base of the mesentery; and the marked variations in pulse rate and rhythm that often follow compression fractures of the upper six thoracic vertebrae. Sympathetic storming, a syndrome that is associated with changes in level of consciousness, altered vital signs, diaphoresis, and agitation, may result from hypothalamic stimulation of the sympathetic nervous system following traumatic brain injury (Lempe, 2004).

Parasympathetic Nervous System. The parasympathetic nervous system functions as the dominant controller for most visceral effectors. During quiet, nonstressful conditions, impulses from parasympathetic fibers (cholinergic) predominate. The fibers of the parasympathetic system are located in two sections, one in the brain stem and the other from spinal segments below L2. Because of the location of these fibers, the parasympathetic system is referred to as the craniosacral division, as distinct from the thoracolumbar (sympathetic) division of the autonomic nervous system.

The parasympathetic nerves arise from the midbrain and the medulla oblongata. Fibers from cells in the midbrain travel with the third oculomotor nerve to the ciliary ganglia, where postganglionic fibers of this division are joined by those of the sympathetic system, creating controlled opposition, with a delicate balance maintained between the two at all times.

Motor and Sensory Functions of the Nervous System

MOTOR SYSTEM FUNCTION

The motor cortex, a vertical band within each cerebral hemisphere, controls the voluntary movements of the body. The exact locations within the brain at which the voluntary

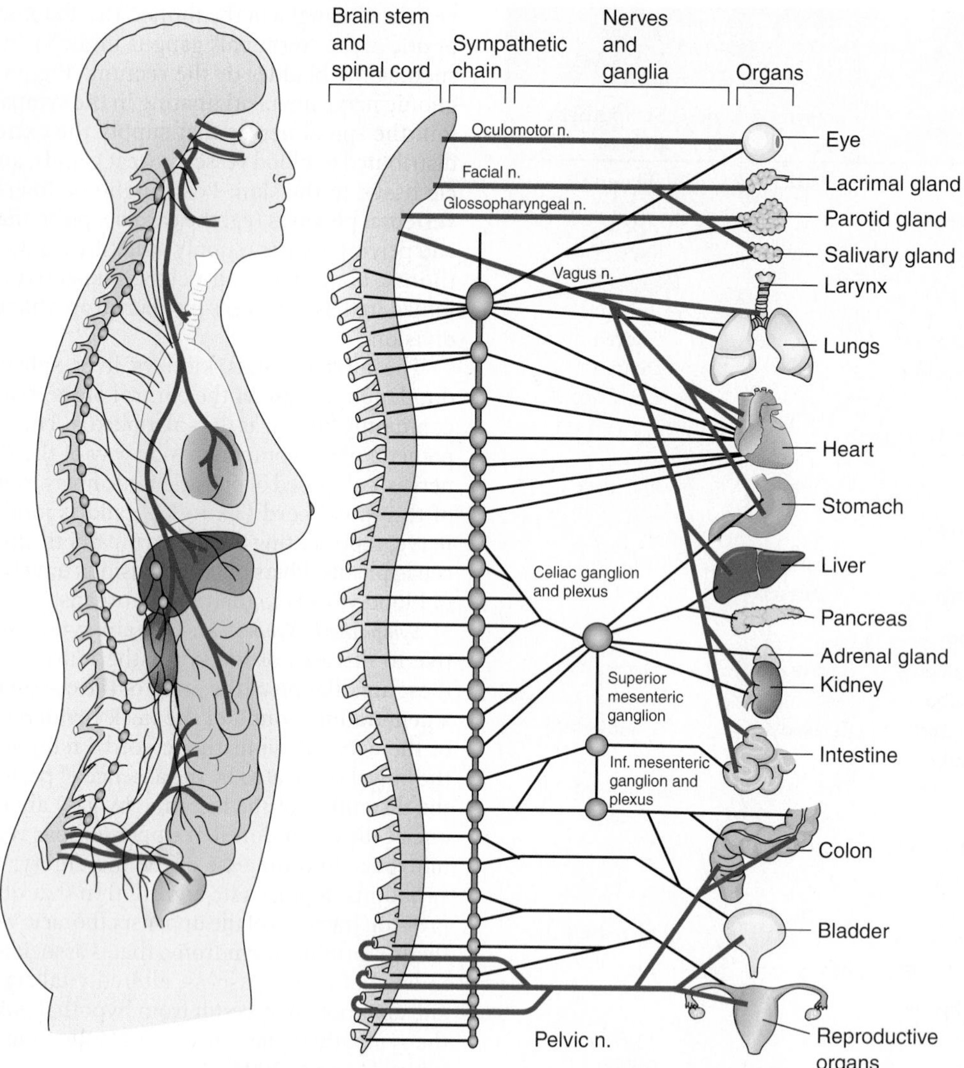

FIGURE 60-12. Anatomy of the autonomic nervous system.

movements of the muscles of the face, thumb, hand, arm, trunk, and leg originate are known (Fig. 60-13). To initiate muscle movement, these particular cells must send the stimulus along their fibers. Stimulation of these cells with an electric current also results in muscle contraction. En route to the pons, the motor fibers converge into a tight bundle known as the internal capsule. A comparatively small injury to the capsule results in paralysis in more muscles than does a much larger injury to the cortex itself.

Within the medulla, the motor axons from the cortex form the motor pathways or tracts, notably the corticospinal or pyramidal tracts. Here, most of the fibers cross (or decussate) to the opposite side, continuing as a crossed pyramidal tract. The remaining fibers enter the spinal cord on the same side as the direct pyramidal tract. Each fiber in this tract finally crosses to the opposite side of the cord and terminates within the gray matter of the anterior horn on that side, in proximity to a motor nerve cell. Fibers of the crossed pyramidal tract terminate within the anterior horn and make connections with anterior horn cells on the same side. All of the motor fibers of the spinal nerves represent extensions of these anterior horn cells, with each of these fibers communicating with only one particular muscle fiber.

The motor system is complex, and motor function depends on the integrity of the corticospinal tracts, the extrapyramidal system, and cerebellar function. A motor impulse consists of a two-neuron pathway (described below). The motor nerve pathways are contained in the spinal cord. Some represent the pathways of the so-called extrapyramidal system, establishing connections between the anterior horn cells and the automatic control centers located in the basal ganglia and the cerebellum. Others are components of reflex arcs, forming synaptic connections between anterior horn cells and sensory fibers that have entered adjacent or neighboring segments of the spinal cord.

Upper and Lower Motor Neurons. The voluntary motor system consists of two groups of neurons: upper motor neurons and lower motor neurons. Upper motor neurons originate in the cerebral cortex, the cerebellum, and the brain stem. Their fibers make up the descending motor pathways, are located entirely within the CNS, and modulate the activity of the lower motor neurons. Lower motor neurons are located either in the anterior horn of the spinal cord gray matter or within cranial nerve nuclei in the brain stem. Axons of lower motor neurons in both sites extend through peripheral nerves and terminate in skeletal mus-

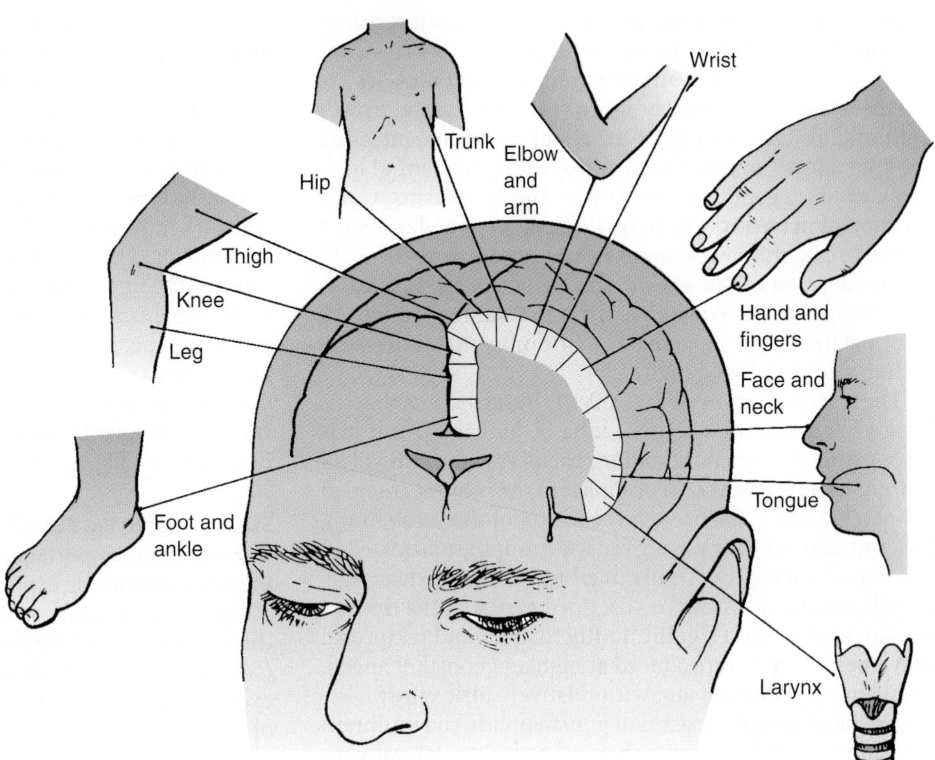

FIGURE 60-13. Diagrammatic representation of the cerebrum showing locations for control of motor movement of various parts of the body.

cle. Lower motor neurons are located in both the CNS and the peripheral nervous system.

The motor pathways from the brain to the spinal cord, as well as from the cerebrum to the brain stem, are formed by upper motor neurons. They begin in the cortex of one side of the brain, descend through the internal capsule, cross to the opposite side in the brain stem, descend through the corticospinal tract, and synapse with the lower motor neurons in the cord. The lower motor neurons receive the impulse in the posterior part of the cord and run to the myoneural junction located in the peripheral muscle. The clinical features of lesions of upper and lower motor neurons are discussed in the following sections and in Table 60-4.

Upper Motor Neuron Lesions. Upper motor neuron lesions can involve the motor cortex, the internal capsule, the spinal cord, and other structures of the brain through which the corticospinal tract descends. If the upper motor neurons are damaged or destroyed, as frequently occurs with stroke or spinal cord injury, paralysis (loss of voluntary movement) results. However, because the inhibitory influences of intact upper motor neurons are now impaired, **reflex** (involuntary) movements are uninhibited, and hence hyperactive deep tendon reflexes, diminished or absent superficial reflexes, and pathologic reflexes such as a Babinski response occur. Severe leg spasms can occur as the result of an upper motor neuron lesion; the spasms result from the preserved reflex arc, which lacks inhibition along the spinal cord below the level of injury. There is little or no muscle atrophy, and muscles remain permanently tense, exhibiting spastic paralysis or paresis (weakness).

TABLE 60-4 Comparison of Upper Motor Neuron and Lower Motor Neuron Lesions

Upper Motor Neuron Lesions	Lower Motor Neuron Lesions
Loss of voluntary control	Loss of voluntary control
Increased muscle tone	Decreased muscle tone
Muscle spasticity	Flaccid muscle paralysis
No muscle atrophy	Muscle atrophy
Hyperactive and abnormal reflexes	Absent or decreased reflexes

Paralysis associated with upper motor neuron lesions can affect a whole extremity, both extremities, or an entire half of the body. Hemiplegia (paralysis of an arm and leg on the same side of the body) can be the result of an upper motor neuron lesion. If hemorrhage, an embolus, or a thrombus destroys the fibers from the motor area in the internal capsule, the arm and the leg of the opposite side become stiff, weak, or paralyzed, and the reflexes are hyperactive (further discussion of hemiplegia is found in Chapter 62). If both legs are paralyzed, the condition is called paraplegia. If all four extremities are paralyzed, the condition is called quadriplegia or tetraplegia. (Additional discussion of these disorders appears in Chapter 63.)

Lower Motor Neuron Lesions. A patient is considered to have lower motor neuron damage if a motor nerve is damaged between the muscle and the spinal cord. The result of lower motor neuron damage is muscle paralysis. Reflexes are lost, and the muscle becomes **flaccid** (limp) and atrophied from disuse. If the patient has injured the spinal trunk and it can heal, use of the muscles connected to that section of the spinal cord may be regained. However, if the anterior horn motor cells are destroyed, the nerves cannot regenerate and the muscles are never useful again.

Flaccid paralysis and atrophy of the affected muscles are the principal signs of lower motor neuron disease. Lower motor neuron lesions can be the result of trauma, infection (poliomyelitis), toxins, vascular disorders, congenital malformations, degenerative processes, and neoplasms. Compression of nerve roots by herniated intervertebral disks is a common cause of lower motor neuron dysfunction.

Coordination of Movement. The smoothness, accuracy, and strength that characterize the muscular movements of a normal person are attributable to the influence of the cerebellum and the basal ganglia.

The cerebellum (see Fig. 60-2), described earlier, is located beneath the occipital lobe of the cerebrum; it is responsible for the coordination, balance, and timing of all muscular movements that originate in the motor centers of the cerebral cortex. Through the action of the cerebellum, the contractions of opposing muscle groups are adjusted in relation to each other to maximal mechanical advantage; muscle contractions can be sustained evenly at the desired tension and without significant fluctuation, and reciprocal movements can be reproduced at high and constant speed, in stereotyped fashion and with relatively little effort.

The basal ganglia, masses of gray matter in the midbrain beneath the cerebral hemispheres, border the lateral ventricles and lie in proximity to the internal capsule. The basal ganglia play an important role in planning and coordinating motor movements and posture. Complex neural connections link the basal ganglia with the cerebral cortex. The major effect of these structures is to inhibit unwanted muscular activity; disorders of the basal ganglia result in exaggerated, uncontrolled movements.

Impaired cerebellar function, which may occur as a result of an intracranial injury or some type of an expanding mass (eg, a hemorrhage, abscess, or tumor), results in loss of muscle tone, weakness, and fatigue. Depending on the area of the brain affected, the patient has different motor symptoms or responses. The patient may demonstrate decorticate, decerebrate, or flaccid posturing, usually as a result of cerebral trauma (Diepenbrock, 2004). For further explanation of this, see Figure 61-1 in Chapter 61. Decortication (decorticate posturing) is the result of lesions of the internal capsule or cerebral hemispheres; the patient has flexion and internal rotation of the arms and wrists and extension, internal rotation, and plantar flexion of the feet. Decerebration (decerebrate posturing), the result of lesions at the midbrain, is more ominous than decortication. The patient has extension and external rotation of the arms and wrists and extension, plantar flexion, and internal rotation of the feet. Flaccid posturing is usually the result of lower brain stem dysfunction; the patient has no motor function, is limp, and lacks motor tone.

Flaccidity preceded by decerebration in a patient with cerebral injury indicates severe neurologic impairment, which may herald brain death. However, before brain death is declared, spinal cord injury must be ruled out, the effects of all neuromuscular paralyzing agents must have worn off, and any other possible treatable causes of neurologic impairment must be investigated.

Tumors, infection, or abscess and increased intracranial pressure can all affect the cerebellum. Cerebellar signs, such as ataxia, incoordination, and seizures, as well as CSF obstruction and compression of the brain stem may be seen. Signs of increased intracranial pressure, including vomiting, headache, and changes in vital signs and level of consciousness, are especially common when CSF flow is obstructed.

Destruction or dysfunction of the basal ganglia leads not to paralysis but to muscle rigidity, with disturbances of posture and movement. The patient tends to have involuntary movements. These may take the form of coarse tremors, most often in the upper extremities, particularly in the distal portions; athetosis, movement of a slow, squirming, writhing, twisting type; or chorea, marked by spasmodic, purposeless, irregular, uncoordinated motions of the trunk and the extremities, and facial grimacing. Disorders due to lesions of the basal ganglia include Parkinson's disease, Huntington's disease (see Chapter 65), and spasmodic torticollis.

SENSORY SYSTEM FUNCTION

Integrating Sensory Impulses. The thalamus, a major receiving and transmitting center for the afferent sensory nerves, is a large structure connected to the midbrain. It lies next to the third ventricle and forms the floor of the lateral ventricle (see Fig. 60-3). The thalamus integrates all sensory impulses except olfaction. It plays a role in the conscious awareness of pain and the recognition of variation in temperature and touch. The thalamus is responsible for the sense of movement and position and the ability to recognize the size, shape, and quality of objects.

Receiving Sensory Impulses. Afferent impulses travel from their points of origin to their destinations in the cerebral cortex via the ascending pathways directly, or they may cross at the level of the spinal cord or in the medulla, depending on the type of sensation that is registered. Sensory information may be integrated at the level of the spinal cord or may be relayed to the brain. Knowledge of these pathways is important for neurologic assessment and for understanding symptoms and their relationship to various lesions.

Sensory impulses convey sensations of heat, cold, and pain. The axons enter the spinal cord by way of the posterior root, specifically in the posterior gray column of the spinal cord, where they make connections with the cells of secondary neurons. Pain and temperature fibers cross immediately to the opposite side of the cord and course upward to the thalamus. Fibers carrying sensations of touch, light pressure, and localization do not connect immediately with the second neuron but ascend the cord for a variable distance before entering the gray matter and completing this connection. The axon of the secondary neuron crosses the cord and proceeds upward to the thalamus.

Position and vibratory sensations are produced by stimuli arising from muscles, joints, and bones. These stimuli are conveyed, uncrossed, all the way to the brain stem by the axon of the primary neuron. In the medulla, synaptic connections are made with cells of the secondary neurons, whose axons cross to the opposite side and then proceed to the thalamus.

Sensory Losses. Destruction of a sensory nerve results in total loss of sensation in its area of distribution. Transection of the spinal cord yields complete anesthesia below the level of injury. Selective destruction or degeneration of the posterior columns of the spinal cord is responsible for a loss of position and vibratory sense in segments distal to the lesion, without loss of touch, pain, or temperature perception. A lesion, such as a cyst, in the center of the spinal cord causes dissociation of sensation—loss of pain at the level of the lesion. This occurs because the fibers carrying pain and temperature cross within the cord immediately on entering; thus, any lesion that divides the cord longitudinally divides these fibers. Other sensory fibers ascend the cord for variable distances, some even to the medulla, before crossing, thereby bypassing the lesion and avoiding destruction.

Lesions affecting the posterior spinal nerve roots may cause impairment of tactile sensation, including intermittent severe pain that is referred to their areas of distribution. Tingling of the fingers and the toes can be a prominent symptom of spinal cord disease, presumably due to degenerative changes in the sensory fibers that extend to the thalamus (ie, belonging to the spinothalamic tract).

Assessment: The Neurologic Examination

Health History

An important aspect of the neurologic assessment is the history of the present illness. The initial interview provides an excellent opportunity to systematically explore the patient's current condition and related events while simultaneously observing overall appearance, mental status, posture, movement, and affect. Depending on the patient's condition, the nurse may need to rely on yes-or-no answers to questions, on a review of the medical record, or input from the family or a combination of these.

Neurologic disease may be stable or progressive, characterized by symptom-free periods as well as fluctuations in symptoms. The health history therefore includes details about the onset, character, severity, location, duration, and frequency of symptoms and signs; associated complaints; precipitating, aggravating, and relieving factors; progression, remission, and exacerbation; and the presence or absence of similar symptoms among family members. The nurse may also use the interview to inquire about any family history of genetic diseases.

A review of the medical history, including a system-by-system evaluation, is part of the health history. The nurse should be aware of any history of trauma or falls that may have involved the head or spinal cord. Questions regarding the use of alcohol, medications, and illicit drugs are also relevant. The history-taking portion of the neurologic assessment is critical and, in many cases of neurologic disease, leads to an accurate diagnosis.

Clinical Manifestations

The clinical manifestations of neurologic disease are as varied as the disease processes themselves. Symptoms may be subtle or intense, fluctuating or permanent, inconvenient or devastating. An introduction to some of the most common symptoms associated with neurologic disease is given in this chapter. Detailed discussions regarding how specific symptoms relate to a particular disorder are covered in later chapters in this unit.

Pain

Pain is considered an unpleasant sensory perception and emotional experience associated with actual or potential tissue damage or described in terms of such damage. Pain is therefore considered multidimensional and entirely subjective. Pain can be acute or chronic. In general, acute pain lasts for a relatively short period of time and remits as the pathology resolves. In neurologic disease, this type of pain is often associated with spinal disk disease (Coles, 2004), trigeminal neuralgia, or other neuropathic pathology (eg, postherpetic neuralgia or painful neuropathies). In contrast, chronic or persistent pain extends for long periods of time and may represent a low level of pathology. This type of pain can occur with many degenerative and chronic neurologic conditions (eg, cerebral palsy) (McKearnan, Kieckhefer, Engel, et al, 2004). See Chapter 13 for a more detailed discussion of pain.

Seizures

Seizures are the result of abnormal paroxysmal discharges in the cerebral cortex, which then manifest as an alteration in sensation, behavior, movement, perception, or consciousness (Hickey, 2003). The alteration may be short, such as in a blank stare that lasts only a second, or of longer duration, such as a tonic-clonic grand mal seizure that can last several minutes. The type of seizure activity is a direct result of the area of the brain affected. Seizures can occur as isolated events, such as when induced by a high fever, alcohol or drug withdrawal, or hypoglycemia. A seizure may also be the first obvious sign of a brain lesion.

Dizziness and Vertigo

Dizziness is an abnormal sensation of imbalance or movement. It is fairly common in the elderly and one of the most common complaints encountered by health professionals (Traccis, Zoroddu, Zecca, et al, 2004). Dizziness can have a variety of causes, including viral syndromes, hot weather, roller coaster rides, and middle ear infections, to name a few. One difficulty confronting health care providers when assessing dizziness is the vague and varied terms patients use to describe the sensation.

About 50% of all patients with dizziness have **vertigo**, which is defined as an illusion of movement, usually rotation (Traccis, et al., 2004). Vertigo is usually a manifestation of vestibular dysfunction. It can be so severe as to result in spatial disorientation, light-headedness, loss of equilibrium (staggering), and nausea and vomiting.

Visual Disturbances

Visual defects that cause people to seek health care can range from the decreased visual acuity associated with aging to sudden blindness caused by glaucoma. Normal vision depends on functioning visual pathways through the retina and optic chiasm and the radiations into the visual cortex in the occipital lobes. Lesions of the eye itself (eg, cataract), lesions along the pathway (eg, tumor), or lesions in the visual cortex (from stroke) interfere with normal visual acuity. Abnormalities of eye movement (as in the nystagmus associated with multiple sclerosis) can also compromise vision by causing diplopia or double vision.

GENETICS IN NURSING PRACTICE

Neurologic Disorders

DISEASES AND CONDITIONS INFLUENCED BY GENETIC FACTORS

- Alzheimer disease
- Amyotrophic lateral sclerosis (ALS)
- Duchenne muscular dystrophy
- Epilepsy
- Friedrich ataxia
- Huntington disease
- Myotonic dystrophy
- Neurofibromatosis type I
- Parkinson's disease
- Spina bifida
- Tourette syndrome

NURSING ASSESSMENTS

Family History Assessment

- Assess for other similarly affected relatives with neurologic impairment.
- Inquire about age of onset (eg, present at birth—spina bifida; developed in childhood—Duchenne muscular dystrophy; developed in adulthood—Huntington disease, Alzheimer disease, amyotrophic lateral sclerosis)
- Inquire about the presence of related conditions such as mental retardation and/or learning disabilities (neurofibromatosis type I).

Patient Assessment

- Assess for the presence of other physical features suggestive of an underlying genetic condition, such as skin lesions seen in neurofibromatosis type 1 (café-au-lait spots).
- Assess for other congenital abnormalities (eg, cardiac, ocular).

MANAGEMENT SPECIFIC TO GENETICS

- Inquire whether DNA mutation or other genetic testing has been performed on affected family members.
- If indicated, refer for further genetic counseling and evaluation so that family members can discuss inheritance, risk to other family members, availability of genetics testing and gene-based interventions.
- Offer appropriate genetics information and resources.
- Assess patient's understanding of genetics information.
- Provide support to families with newly diagnosed genetic-related neurologic disorders.
- Participate in management and coordination of care of patients with genetic conditions and individuals predisposed to develop or pass on a genetic condition.

GENETICS RESOURCES FOR NURSES AND THEIR PATIENTS ON THE WEB

Genetic Alliance: http://www.geneticalliance.org—a directory of support groups for patients and families with genetic conditions

Gene Clinics: http://www.geneclinics.org—a listing of common genetic disorders with up-to-date clinical summaries, genetic counseling and testing information

National Organization of Rare Disorders: http://www.rarediseases.org—a directory of support groups and information for patients and families with rare genetic disorders

OMIM: Online Mendelian Inheritance in Man: http://www.nchi.nlm.nih.gov/omim/stats/html—a complete listing of inherited genetic conditions

Weakness

Weakness, specifically muscle weakness, is a common manifestation of neurologic disease. Weakness frequently coexists with other symptoms of disease and can affect a variety of muscles, causing a wide range of disability. Weakness can be sudden and permanent, as in stroke, or progressive, as in many neuromuscular diseases such as amyotrophic lateral sclerosis. Any muscle group can be affected.

Abnormal Sensation

Numbness, abnormal sensation, or loss of sensation is a neurologic manifestation of both central and peripheral nervous system disease. Altered sensation can affect small or large areas of the body. It is frequently associated with weakness or pain and is potentially disabling. Both numbness and weakness can significantly affect balance and coordination.

Physical Examination

The neurologic examination is a systematic process that includes a variety of clinical tests, observations, and assessments designed to evaluate the neurologic status of a complex system. Although the neurologic examination is often limited to a simple screening, the examiner must be able to conduct a thorough neurologic assessment when the patient's history or other physical findings warrant it. An example of such a situation that is becoming more common is the need to assess comatose survivors of cardiac arrest (Johkura, Komiyama & Kuroiwa, 2004; Freeman and Hedges, 2003). Many neurologic rating scales exist; some of the more common ones are discussed in this chapter, but an in-depth discussion of all rating scales is beyond the scope of this chapter. Two recent review articles describe many neurologic rating scales: Booth, Boone, Tomlinson, et al., 2004, and Lindeboom, Vermeulen, Holman, et al., 2003.

The brain and spinal cord cannot be examined as directly as other systems of the body. Thus, much of the neurologic examination is an indirect evaluation that assesses the function of the specific body part or parts controlled or innervated by the nervous system. A neurologic assessment is divided into five components: cerebral function, cranial nerves, motor system, sensory system, and reflexes. As in other parts of the physical assessment, the neurologic examination follows a logical sequence and progresses from higher levels of cortical function, such as abstract thinking, to lower levels of function, such as the determination of the integrity of peripheral nerves.

Assessing Cerebral Function

Cerebral abnormalities may cause disturbances in mental status, intellectual functioning, and thought content and in patterns of emotional behavior. There may also be alterations in perception, motor and language abilities, as well as lifestyle.

Interpretation and documentation of neurologic abnormalities, particularly mental status abnormalities, should be specific and nonjudgmental. Lengthy descriptions and the use of terms such as "inappropriate" or "demented" should be avoided. Terms such as these often mean different things to different people and are therefore not useful when describing behavior. The examiner records and reports specific observations regarding orientation, level of consciousness, emotional state, or thought content, all of which permit comparison by others over time. Analysis and the conclusions that may be drawn from these findings usually depend on the examiner's knowledge of neuroanatomy, neurophysiology, and neuropathology.

MENTAL STATUS

An assessment of mental status begins by observing the patient's appearance and behavior, noting dress, grooming, and personal hygiene. Posture, gestures, movements, facial expressions, and motor activity often provide important information about the patient. The patient's manner of speech and level of consciousness are also assessed (Munro, 2004). Is the patient's speech clear and coherent? Is the patient alert and responsive or drowsy and stuporous?

Assessing orientation to time, place, and person assists in evaluating mental status. Does the patient know what day it is, what year it is, and the name of the president of the United States? Is the patient aware of where he or she is? Is the patient aware of who the examiner is and of his or her purpose for being in the room? Is the capacity for immediate memory intact? (See Chapter 12, Chart 12-1.)

INTELLECTUAL FUNCTION

A person with an average IQ can repeat seven digits without faltering and can recite five digits backward. The examiner might ask the patient to count backward from 100 or to subtract 7 from 100, then 7 from that, and so forth (called serial 7s). The capacity to interpret well-known proverbs tests abstract reasoning, which is a higher intellectual function; for example, does the patient know what is meant by "a stitch in time saves nine"? Patients with damage to the frontal cortex appear superficially normal until one or more tests of integrative capacity are performed. Questions designed to assess this capacity might include the ability to recognize similarities: how are a mouse and dog or pen and pencil alike? Can the patient make judgments about situations: for example, if the patient arrived home without a house key, what alternatives are there?

THOUGHT CONTENT

During the interview, it is important to assess the patient's thought content. Are the patient's thoughts spontaneous, natural, clear, relevant, and coherent? Does the patient have any fixed ideas, illusions, or preoccupations? What are his or her insights into these thoughts? Preoccupation with death or morbid events, hallucinations, and paranoid ideation are examples of unusual thoughts or perceptions that require further evaluation.

EMOTIONAL STATUS

An assessment of cerebral functioning also includes the patient's emotional status. Is the patient's affect (external manifestation of mood) natural and even, or irritable and angry, anxious, apathetic or flat, or euphoric? Does his or her mood fluctuate normally, or does the patient unpredictably swing from joy to sadness during the interview? Is affect appropriate to words and thought content? Are verbal communications consistent with nonverbal cues?

PERCEPTION

The examiner may now consider more specific areas of higher cortical function. **Agnosia** is the inability to interpret or recognize objects seen through the special senses. The patient may see a pencil but not know what it is called or what to do with it. The patient may even be able to describe it but not to interpret its function. The patient may experience auditory or tactile agnosia as well as visual agnosia. Each of the dysfunctions implicates a different part of the cortex (Table 60-5).

Screening for visual and tactile agnosia provides insight into the patient's cortical interpretation ability. The patient is shown a familiar object and asked to identify it by name. Placing a familiar object (eg, key, coin) in the patient's hand and having him or her identify it with both eyes closed is an easy way to assess tactile interpretation.

MOTOR ABILITY

Assessment of cortical motor integration is carried out by asking the patient to perform a skilled act (throw a ball, move a chair). Successful performance requires the ability to

TABLE 60-5 Types of Agnosia and Corresponding Sites of Lesions

Type of Agnosia	Affected Cerebral Area
Visual	Occipital lobe
Auditory	Temporal lobe (lateral and superior portions)
Tactile	Parietal lobe
Body parts and relationships	Parietal lobe (posteroinferior regions)

understand the activity desired and normal motor strength. Failure signals cerebral dysfunction.

LANGUAGE ABILITY

The person with normal neurologic function can understand and communicate in spoken and written language. Does the patient answer questions appropriately? Can he or she read a sentence from a newspaper and explain its meaning? Can the patient write his or her name or copy a simple figure that the examiner has drawn? A deficiency in language function is called aphasia. Different types of aphasia result from injury to different parts of the brain (Table 60-6). Aphasia is discussed in detail in Chapter 62.

IMPACT ON LIFESTYLE

The nurse assesses the impact the neurologic impairment has on the patient's lifestyle. Issues to consider include the limitations imposed on the patient by any deficit and the patient's role in society, including family and community roles. The plan of care that the nurse develops needs to address and support adaptation to the neurologic deficit and continued function to the extent possible within the patient's support system.

Examining the Cranial Nerves

Chart 60-1 describes how to assess the cranial nerves. Opposite sides of the face and neck are compared throughout the examination (Diepenbrock, 2004; Rasmor & Brown, 2003).

Examining the Motor System

A thorough examination of the motor system includes an assessment of muscle size, tone, and strength, coordination, and balance. The patient is instructed to walk across the room while the examiner observes posture and gait. The muscles are inspected, and palpated if necessary, for their size and symmetry. Any evidence of atrophy or involuntary movements (tremors, tics) is noted. Muscle **tone** (the tension present in a muscle at rest) is evaluated by palpating various muscle groups at rest and during passive movement. Resistance to these movements is assessed and documented. Abnormalities in tone include **spasticity** (increased muscle tone), **rigidity** (resistance to passive stretch), and flaccidity.

MUSCLE STRENGTH

Assessing the patient's ability to flex or extend the extremities against resistance tests muscle strength. The function of an individual muscle or group of muscles is evaluated by placing the muscle at a disadvantage. The quadriceps, for example, is a powerful muscle responsible for straightening the leg. Once the leg is straightened, it is exceedingly difficult for the examiner to flex the knee. Conversely, if the knee is flexed and the patient is asked to straighten the leg against resistance, a more subtle disability can be elicited. The evaluation of muscle strength compares the sides of the body to each other. For example, the right upper extremity is compared to the left upper extremity. In this way, subtle differences in muscle strength can be more easily detected and accurately described.

Clinicians use a five-point scale to rate muscle strength. A 5 indicates full power of contraction against gravity and resistance or normal muscle strength; 4 indicates fair but not full strength against gravity and a moderate amount of resistance or slight weakness; 3 indicates just sufficient strength to overcome the force of gravity or moderate weakness; 2 indicates the ability to move but not to overcome the force of gravity or severe weakness; 1 indicates minimal contractile power (weak muscle contraction can be palpated but no movement is noted) or very severe weakness; and 0 indicates no movement (Lehman, Hayes, LaCroix, et al., 2003). A stick figure may be used to record muscle strength and is a precise form of documenting findings. Distal and proximal strength in both upper and lower extremities is recorded using the five-point scale (Fig. 60-14).

Assessment of muscle strength may be as detailed as necessary. One may quickly test the strength of the proximal muscles of the upper and lower extremities, always comparing both sides. The strength of the finer muscles that control the function of the hand (hand grasp) and the foot (dorsiflexion and plantar flexion) can then be assessed.

BALANCE AND COORDINATION

Cerebellar influence on the motor system is reflected in balance control and coordination. Coordination in the hands and upper extremities is tested by having the patient perform rapid, alternating movements and point-to-point testing. First, the patient is instructed to pat his or her thigh as fast as possible with each hand separately. Then the patient is instructed to alternately pronate and supinate the hand as rapidly as possible. Lastly, the patient is asked to touch each of the fingers with the thumb in a consecutive motion. Speed, symmetry, and degree of difficulty are noted.

Point-to-point testing is accomplished by having the patient touch the examiner's extended finger and then his or her own nose. This is repeated several times. This assessment is then carried out with the patient's eyes closed.

Coordination in the lower extremities is tested by having the patient run the heel down the anterior surface of the tibia of the other leg. Each leg is tested in turn. **Ataxia** is defined as incoordination of voluntary muscle action, particularly of the muscle groups used in activities such as walking or reaching for objects. The presence of ataxia or tremors (rhythmic, involuntary movements) during these movements suggests cerebellar disease.

It is not necessary to carry out each of these assessments for coordination. During a routine examination, it is advisable to perform a simple screening of the upper and lower extremities by having the patient perform either rapid, alternating movements or point-to-point testing. When abnormalities are observed, a more thorough examination is indicated.

TABLE 60-6 Types of Aphasia and Region of Brain Involved

Type of Aphasia	Brain Area Involved
Auditory-receptive	Temporal lobe
Visual-receptive	Parietal-occipital area
Expressive speaking	Inferior posterior frontal areas
Expressive writing	Posterior frontal area

CHART 60-1

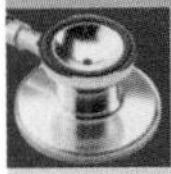

Assessing Cranial Nerve Function

CRANIAL NERVE	CLINICAL EXAMINATION
I (olfactory)	With eyes closed, the patient is asked to identify familiar odors (coffee, tobacco). Each nostril is tested separately.
II (optic)	Snellen eye chart; visual fields; ophthalmoscopic examination
III (oculomotor) IV (trochlear)	For cranial nerves III, IV, and VI: test for ocular rotations, conjugate movements, nystagmus. Test for pupillary reflexes, and inspect eyelids for ptosis.
V (trigeminal)	Have patient close the eyes. Touch cotton to forehead, cheeks, and jaw. Sensitivity to superficial pain is tested in these same three areas by using the sharp and dull ends of a broken tongue blade. Alternate between the sharp point and the dull end. Patient reports "sharp" or "dull" with each movement. If responses are incorrect, test for temperature sensation. Test tubes of cold and hot water are used alternately. While the patient looks up, *lightly* touch a wisp of cotton against the temporal surface of each cornea. A blink and tearing are normal responses. Have the patient clench and move the jaw from side to side. Palpate the masseter and temporal muscles, noting strength and equality.
VI (abducens)	
VII (facial)	Observe for symmetry while the patient performs facial movements: smiles, whistles, elevates eyebrows, frowns, tightly closes eyelids against resistance (examiner attempts to open them). Observe face for flaccid paralysis (shallow nasolabial folds). Patient extends tongue. Ability to discriminate between sugar and salt is tested.
VIII (acoustic)	Whisper or watch-tick test Test for lateralization (Weber test) Test for air and bone conduction (Rinne test)
IX (glossopharyngeal)	Assess patient's ability to swallow and discriminate between sugar and salt on posterior third of the tongue.
X (vagus)	Depress a tongue blade on posterior tongue, or stimulate posterior pharynx to elicit gag reflex. Note any hoarseness in voice. Check ability to swallow. Have patient say "ah." Observe for symmetric rise of uvula and soft palate.
XI (spinal accessory)	Palpate and note strength of trapezius muscles while patient shrugs shoulders against resistance. Palpate and note strength of each sternocleidomastoid muscle as patient turns head against opposing pressure of the examiner's hand.
XII (hypoglossal)	While the patient protrudes the tongue, any deviation or tremors are noted. The strength of the tongue is tested by having the patient move the protruded tongue from side to side against a tongue depressor.

The **Romberg test** is a screening test for balance. The patient stands with feet together and arms at the side, first with eyes open and then with both eyes closed for 20 to 30 seconds. The examiner stands close to reassure the patient of support if he or she begins to fall. Slight swaying is normal, but a loss of balance is abnormal and is considered a positive Romberg test. Additional cerebellar tests for balance in the ambulatory patient include hopping in place, alternating knee bends, and heel-to-toe walking (both forward and backward).

Examining the Reflexes

The motor reflexes are involuntary contractions of muscles or muscle groups in response to abrupt stretching near the site of the muscle's insertion. The tendon is struck directly with a reflex hammer or indirectly by striking the examiner's thumb, which is placed firmly against the tendon. Testing these reflexes enables the examiner to assess involuntary reflex arcs that depend on the presence of afferent stretch receptors, spinal synapses, efferent motor fibers, and a variety of modifying influences from higher levels. Common reflexes that may be tested include the deep tendon reflexes (biceps, brachioradialis, triceps, patellar, and ankle reflexes) and superficial or cutaneous reflexes (abdominal reflexes and plantar or Babinski response) (Fig. 60-15).

TECHNIQUE

A reflex hammer is used to elicit a deep tendon reflex. The handle of the hammer is held loosely between the thumb and index finger, allowing a full swinging motion. The wrist motion is similar to that used during percussion. The extremity

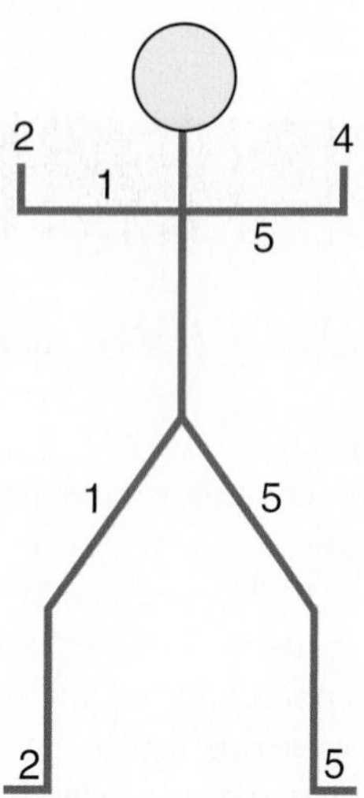

FIGURE 60-14. A stick figure may be used to record muscle strength as follows: 5, full range of motion against gravity and resistance; 4, full range of motion against gravity and a moderate amount of resistance; 3, full range of motion against gravity only; 2, full range of motion when gravity is eliminated; 1, a weak muscle contraction when muscle is palpated, but no movement; and 0, complete paralysis.

is positioned so that the tendon is slightly stretched. This requires a sound knowledge of the location of muscles and their tendon attachments. The tendon is then struck briskly, and the response is compared with that on the opposite side of the body. A wide variation in reflex response may be considered normal; however, it is more important that the reflexes be symmetrically equivalent. When the comparison is made, both sides should be equivalently relaxed and each tendon struck with equal force.

Valid findings depend on several factors: proper use of the reflex hammer, proper positioning of the extremity, and a relaxed patient (Bickley & Szilagyi, 2003). If the reflexes are symmetrically diminished or absent, the examiner may use isometric contraction of other muscle groups to increase reflex activity. For example, if lower extremity reflexes are diminished or absent, the patient is instructed to lock the fingers together and pull in opposite directions. Having the patient clench the jaw or press the heels against the floor or examining table may similarly elicit more reliable biceps, triceps, and brachioradialis reflexes.

GRADING THE REFLEXES

The absence of reflexes is significant, although ankle jerks (Achilles reflex) may be normally absent in older people. Deep tendon reflex responses are often graded on a scale of 0 to 4+ (Rasmor & Brown, 2003). A 4+ indicates a hyperactive reflex, often indicating pathology; 3+ indicates a response that is more brisk than average but may be normal or indicative of disease; 2+ indicates an average or normal response; 1+ indicates a hypoactive or diminished response; and 0 indicates no response. As stated previously, scale ratings are highly subjective. Findings can be recorded as a fraction, indicating the scale range (eg, 2/4). Some examiners prefer to use the terms present, absent, and diminished when describing reflexes. As with muscle strength recording, a stick figure such as the one shown in Chart 60-2 may also be used to record numerical findings.

BICEPS REFLEX

The biceps reflex is elicited by striking the biceps tendon of the flexed elbow. The examiner supports the forearm with one arm while placing the thumb against the tendon and striking the thumb with the reflex hammer. The normal response is flexion at the elbow and contraction of the biceps (see Fig. 60-15*A*).

TRICEPS REFLEX

To elicit a triceps reflex, the patient's arm is flexed at the elbow and positioned in front of the chest. The examiner supports the patient's arm and identifies the triceps tendon by palpating 2.5 to 5 cm (1 to 2 in) above the elbow. A direct blow on the tendon normally produces contraction of the triceps muscle and extension of the elbow (see Fig. 60-15*B*).

BRACHIORADIALIS REFLEX

With the patient's forearm resting on the lap or across the abdomen, the brachioradialis reflex is assessed. A gentle strike of the hammer 2.5 to 5 cm (1 to 2 in) above the wrist results in flexion and supination of the forearm (Bickley & Szilagyi, 2003).

PATELLAR REFLEX

The patellar reflex is elicited by striking the patellar tendon just below the patella. The patient may be in a sitting or a lying position. If the patient is supine, the examiner supports the legs to facilitate relaxation of the muscles. Contractions of the quadriceps and knee extension are normal responses (see Fig. 60-15*C*).

ANKLE REFLEX

To elicit an ankle (Achilles) reflex, the foot is dorsiflexed at the ankle and the hammer strikes the stretched Achilles tendon (see Fig. 60-15*D*). This reflex normally produces plantar flexion. If the examiner cannot elicit the ankle reflex and suspects that the patient cannot relax, the patient is instructed to kneel on a chair or similar elevated, flat surface. This position places the ankles in dorsiflexion and reduces any muscle tension in the gastrocnemius. The Achilles tendons are struck in turn, and plantar flexion is usually demonstrated (Bickley & Szilagyi, 2003).

CLONUS

When reflexes are very hyperactive, a phenomenon called **clonus** may be elicited. If the foot is abruptly dorsiflexed, it may continue to "beat" two or three times before it settles into a position of rest. Occasionally with central nervous system disease this activity persists, and the foot does not come to rest while the tendon is being stretched but persists in repetitive activity. The unsustained clonus associated with normal but hyperactive reflexes is not considered pathologic. Sustained clonus always indicates the presence of central nervous system disease and requires further evaluation.

SUPERFICIAL REFLEXES

The major superficial reflexes include corneal, gag or swallowing, upper/lower abdominal, cremasteric (men only), plantar, and perianal. These reflexes are graded differently than the motor reflexes and are noted to be present (+) or absent (−). Of these, only the corneal, gag, and plantar reflexes are tested commonly.

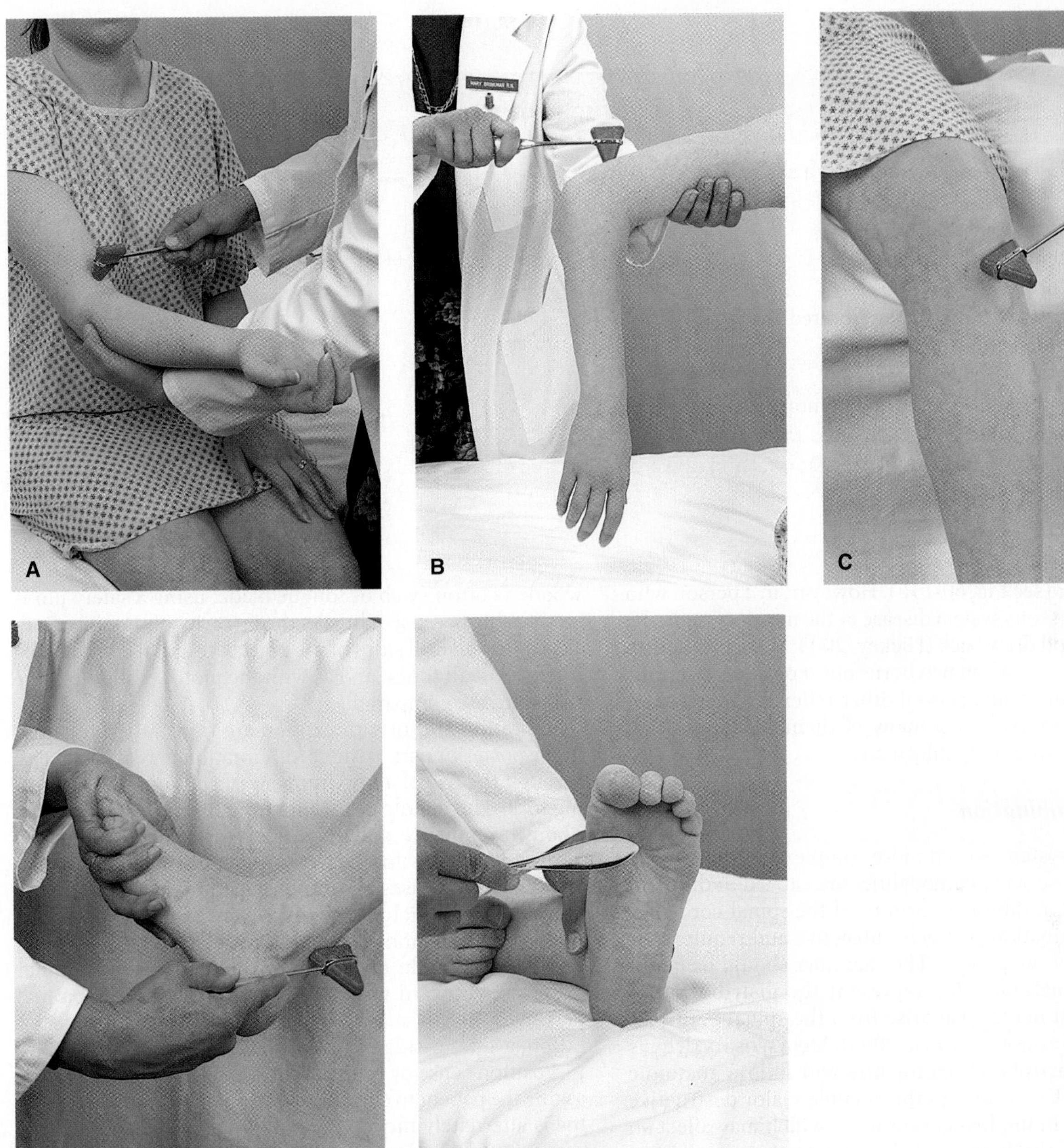

FIGURE 60-15. Techniques for eliciting major reflexes. (**A**) Biceps reflex. (**B**) Triceps reflex. (**C**) Patellar reflex. (**D**) Ankle or Achilles reflex. (**E**) Babinski response. From Weber, J. & Kelley, J. (2003). *Health assessment in nursing* (2nd ed.). Philadelphia: Lippincott Williams & Wilkins. © B. Proud.

The corneal reflex is tested carefully using a clean wisp of cotton and lightly touching the outer corner of each eye on the sclera. The reflex is present if the action elicits a blink. Conditions such as a cerebrovascular accident or coma might result in loss of this reflex, either unilaterally or bilaterally. Loss of this reflex indicates the need for eye protection and possible lubrication to prevent corneal damage.

The gag reflex is elicited by gently touching the back of the pharynx with a cotton-tipped applicator; first on one side of the uvula and then the other. Positive response is an equal elevation of the uvula and "gag" with stimulation. Absent response on one or both sides can be seen following a cerebrovascular accident and requires careful evaluation and treatment of the resultant swallowing dysfunction to prevent aspiration of food and fluids.

The plantar reflex is elicited by stroking the lateral side of the foot with a tongue blade or the handle of a reflex hammer. Stimulation normally causes toe flexion. Toe fanning (positive Babinski) is an abnormal response and is discussed below (Weber & Kelley, 2003).

BABINSKI RESPONSE

A well-known reflex indicative of central nervous system disease affecting the corticospinal tract is the **Babinski reflex.** In a person with an intact central nervous system, if the lateral aspect of the sole of the foot is stroked, the toes contract and

CHART 60-2

Documenting Reflexes

Deep tendon reflexes are graded on a scale of 0 to 4:

0	No response
1+	Diminished (hypoactive)
2+	Normal
3+	Increased (may be interpreted as normal)
4+	Hyperactive (hyperreflexia)

The deep tendon responses and plantar reflexes are commonly recorded on stick figures. The arrow points downward if the plantar response is normal and upward if the response is abnormal.

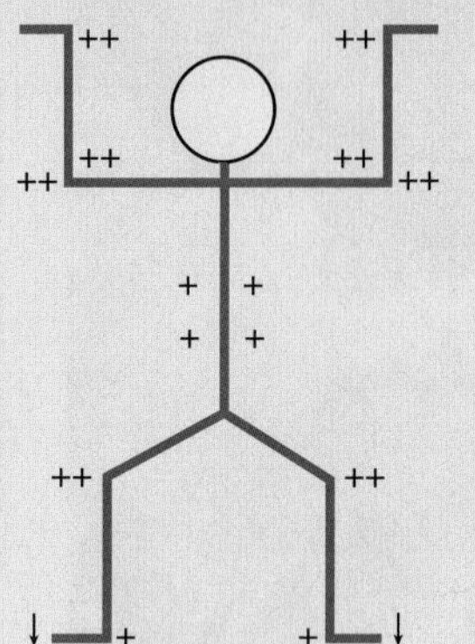

draw together (see Fig. 60-15*E*). However, in a person who has central nervous system disease of the motor system, the toes fan out and draw back (Hickey, 2003; Weber & Kelley, 2003). This is normal in newborns but represents a serious abnormality in adults. Several other reflexes convey similar information. Although many of them are interesting, they are not particularly informative.

Sensory Examination

The sensory system is even more complex than the motor system, because sensory modalities are carried in different tracts located in different portions of the spinal cord. The sensory examination is largely subjective and requires the cooperation of the patient. The examiner should be familiar with dermatomes that represent the distribution of the peripheral nerves that arise from the spinal cord (see Fig. 60-11) (Rasmor & Brown, 2003). Most sensory deficits result from peripheral neuropathy and follow anatomic dermatomes. Exceptions to this include major destructive lesions of the brain; loss of sensation, which may affect an entire side of the body; and the neuropathies associated with alcoholism, which occur in a glove-and-stocking distribution (ie, over the entire hand or foot in areas traditionally covered by a glove or sock).

Assessment of the sensory system involves tests for tactile sensation, superficial pain, vibration, and position sense (proprioception). During the sensory assessment, the patient's eyes are closed. Simple directions and reassurance that the examiner will not hurt or startle the patient encourage the cooperation of the patient.

Tactile sensation is assessed by lightly touching a cotton wisp to corresponding areas on each side of the body. The sensitivity of proximal parts of the extremities is compared with that of distal parts.

Pain and temperature sensations are transmitted together in the lateral part of the spinal cord, so it is unnecessary to test for temperature sense in most circumstances. Determining the patient's sensitivity to a sharp object can assess superficial pain perception. The patient is asked to differentiate between the sharp and dull ends of a broken wooden cotton swab or tongue blade; using a safety pin is inadvisable because it breaks the integrity of the skin. Both the sharp and dull sides of the object are applied with equal intensity at all times, and as with the motor evaluation, the two sides are compared.

Vibration and proprioception are transmitted together in the posterior part of the cord. Vibration may be evaluated through the use of a low-frequency (128- or 256-Hz) tuning fork. The handle of the vibrating fork is placed against a bony prominence, and the patient is asked if he or she feels a sensation and is instructed to signal the examiner when the sensation ceases. Common locations used to test for vibratory sense include the distal joint of the great toe and the proximal thumb joint. If the patient does not perceive the vibrations at the distal bony prominences, the examiner progresses upward with the tuning fork until the patient perceives the vibrations. As with all measurements of sensation, a side-to-side comparison is made.

Position sense or proprioception may be determined by asking the patient to close both eyes and indicate, as the great toe is alternately moved up and down, in which direction movement has taken place. Vibration and position sense are often lost together, frequently in circumstances in which all others remain intact.

Integration of sensation in the brain is evaluated next. This may be performed by testing two-point discrimination—when the patient is touched with two sharp objects simultaneously, are they perceived as two or as one? If touched simultaneously on opposite sides of the body, the patient should normally report being touched in two places. If only one site is reported, the one not being recognized is said to demonstrate extinction. Another test of higher cortical sensory ability is stereognosis. The patient is instructed to close both eyes and identify a variety of objects (eg, keys, coins) that are placed in one hand by the examiner.

Gerontologic Considerations

During the normal aging process, the nervous system undergoes many changes, and it is extremely vulnerable to general systemic illness. Changes throughout the nervous system that occur with age vary in degree. Nerve fibers that connect directly to muscles show little decline in function with age, as do simple neurologic functions that involve a number of connections in the spinal cord. Disease in the elderly often makes it difficult to distinguish normal from abnormal changes. It is important for clinicians not to attribute abnormality or dysfunction to aging without appropriate investigation (Stotts & Deitrich, 2004). Pain in the absence of disease, for example, is not a normal part of aging and should be assessed, diagnosed, and treated (Hanks-Bell, Halvey & Paice, 2004).

Structural Changes

A number of alterations occur with increasing age. Brain weight decreases, as does the number of synapses. A loss of neurons occurs in select regions of the brain. Cerebral blood flow and metabolism are reduced. Temperature regulation becomes less efficient. In the peripheral nervous system, myelin is lost, resulting in a decrease in conduction velocity in some nerves. There is an overall reduction in muscle bulk and the electrical activity within muscles. Taste buds atrophy and nerve cell fibers in the olfactory bulb degenerate (Heckman, Heckman, Lang, et al., 2003). Nerve cells in the vestibular system of the inner ear, cerebellum, and proprioceptive pathways also degenerate. Deep tendon reflexes can be decreased or in some cases absent. Hypothalamic function is modified such that stage IV sleep is reduced. There is an overall slowing of autonomic nervous system responses. Pupillary responses are reduced or may not appear at all in the presence of cataracts.

Motor Alterations

There is an overall reduction in muscle bulk, with atrophy most easily noted in the hands. Changes in motor function often result in a flexed posture, shuffling gait, and rigidity of movement. These changes can create difficulties for the older person in maintaining or recovering balance. Strength and agility are diminished, and reaction time and movement time are decreased. Repetitive movements and mild tremors may be noted during an examination and may be of concern to the person. Observation of gait may reveal a wide-based gait with balance difficulties.

Sensory Alterations

Sensory isolation due to visual and hearing loss can cause confusion, anxiety, disorientation, misinterpretation of the environment, and feelings of inadequacy. Sensory alterations may require modification of the home environment, such as large-print reading materials or sound enhancement for the telephone, as well as extra orientation to new surroundings. Simple explanations of routines, the location of the bathroom, and how to operate the call bell or light are just a few examples of information the elderly patient may need when hospitalized.

Temperature Regulation and Pain Perception

Other manifestations of neurologic changes are related to temperature regulation and pain. The elderly patient may feel cold more readily than heat and may require extra covering when in bed; a room temperature somewhat higher than usual may be desirable. Reaction to painful stimuli may be decreased with age. Because pain is an important warning signal, caution must be used when hot or cold packs are used. The older patient may be burned or suffer frostbite before being aware of any discomfort. Complaints of pain, such as abdominal discomfort or chest pain, may be more serious than the patient's perception might indicate and thus require careful evaluation (Hanks-Bell et al., 2004). Two pain syndromes that are common in the neurological system in older adults are diabetic neuropathies and postherpetic neuropathies (Hanks-Bell et al., 2004).

Taste and Smell Alterations

The acuity of the taste buds decreases with age; along with an altered olfactory sense, this may cause a decreased appetite and subsequent weight loss. Extra seasoning often increases food intake as long as it does not cause gastric irritation. A decreased sense of smell due to atrophy of olfactory organs may present a safety hazard, because elderly people living alone may be unable to detect household gas leaks or fires. Smoke and carbon monoxide detectors, important for all, are critical for the elderly.

Tactile and Visual Alterations

Another neurologic alteration in the elderly patient is the dulling of tactile sensation due to a decrease in the number of areas of the body responding to all stimuli and in the number and sensitivity of sensory receptors. There may be difficulty in identifying objects by touch, and because fewer tactile cues are received from the bottom of the feet, the person may become confused about body position and location.

These factors, combined with sensitivity to glare, decreased peripheral vision, and a constricted visual field, may result in disorientation, especially at night when there is little or no light in the room. Because the elderly person takes longer to recover visual sensitivity when moving from a light to dark area, night-lights and a safe and familiar arrangement of furniture are essential.

Mental Status

Mental status is evaluated when obtaining the history. Areas of judgment, intelligence, memory, affect, mood, orientation, speech, and grooming are assessed. Family members who bring the patient to the attention of the health care provider may have noticed changes in the patient's mental status. Drug toxicity should always be suspected as a causative factor when the patient has a change in mental status. **Delirium** (mental confusion, usually with delusions and hallucinations) is seen in elderly patients who have underlying central nervous system damage or are experiencing an acute condition such as infection, adverse medication reaction, or dehydration. Many elderly patients admitted to the hospital have delirium, and the cause is often reversible and treatable (eg, drug toxicity, vitamin B deficiency, thyroid disease). Depression may produce impairment of attention and memory. In elderly patients, delirium, which is an acute change in mental status attributable to a treatable medical problem, must be differentiated from dementia, which is a chronic and irreversible deterioration of cognitive status.

Nursing Implications

Nursing care for patients with age-related changes to the nervous system and for patients with long-term neurologic disability who are aging should include the previously described modifications. In addition, the consequences of any neurologic deficit and its impact on overall function such as activities of daily living, use of assistive devices, and individual coping should be assessed and considered in planning patient care.

Patient teaching is also affected, because the nurse must understand the altered responses and the changing needs of the elderly patient before beginning to teach. When caring for the elderly patient, the nurse adapts activities such as preoperative teaching, diet therapy, and instruction about new medications, their timing, and doses to the patient's needs and capabilities. The nurse considers the presence of decline in fine motor movement and failing vision. When using visual materials for teaching or menu selection, adequate lighting without glare, contrasting colors, and large print are used to offset visual difficulties caused by rigidity and opacity of the lens in the eye and slower pupillary reaction.

Procedures and preparations needed for diagnostic tests are explained, taking into account the possibility of impaired hearing and slowed responses in the elderly. Even with hearing loss, the elderly patient often hears adequately if the speaker uses a low-pitched, clear voice; shouting only makes it harder for the patient to understand the speaker. Providing auditory and visual cues aids understanding; if the patient has a significant hearing or visual loss, assistive devices, a signer, or a translator may be needed.

Teaching at an unrushed pace and using reinforcement enhance learning and retention. Material should be short, concise, and concrete. Vocabulary is matched to the patient's ability, and terms are clearly defined. The elderly patient requires adequate time to receive and respond to stimuli, to learn, and to react. These measures allow comprehension, memory, and formation of association and concepts.

Diagnostic Evaluation

Computed Tomography Scanning

Computed tomography (CT) scanning makes use of a narrow x-ray beam to scan the body part in successive layers. The images provide cross-sectional views of the brain, with distinguishing differences in tissue densities of the skull, cortex, subcortical structures, and ventricles. The brightness of each slice of the brain in the final image is proportional to the degree to which it absorbs x-rays. The image is displayed on an oscilloscope or TV monitor and is photographed and stored digitally (Grey & Ailinani, 2003).

Lesions in the brain are seen as variations in tissue density differing from the surrounding normal brain tissue. Abnormalities of tissue indicate possible tumor masses, brain infarction, displacement of the ventricles, and cortical atrophy (Som & Curtin, 2003). Whole-body CT scanners allow sections of the spinal cord to be visualized. The injection of a water-soluble iodinated contrast agent into the subarachnoid space through lumbar puncture improves the visualization of the spinal and intracranial contents on these images. The CT scan, along with magnetic resonance imaging (MRI), has largely replaced myelography as a diagnostic procedure for the diagnosis of herniated lumbar disks.

CT scanning is usually performed first without contrast material and then with intravenous (IV) contrast enhancement. The patient lies on an adjustable table with the head held in a fixed position while the scanning system rotates around the head and produces cross-sectional images. The patient must lie with the head held perfectly still without talking or moving the face, because head motion distorts the image.

CT scanning is noninvasive and painless and has a high degree of sensitivity for detecting lesions. With advances in CT scanning, the number of disorders and injuries that can be diagnosed is increasing (Selman, 2004).

Nursing Interventions

Essential nursing interventions include preparation for the procedure and patient monitoring. Preparation includes teaching the patient about the need to lie quietly throughout the procedure. A review of relaxation techniques may be helpful for patients with claustrophobia.

Sedation can be used if agitation, restlessness, or confusion will interfere with a successful study. Ongoing patient monitoring during sedation is necessary. If a contrast agent is used, the patient must be assessed before the CT scan for an iodine/shellfish allergy, because the contrast agent is iodine-based. An IV line for injection of the contrast agent and a period of fasting (usually 4 hours) are required prior to the study. Patients who receive an IV or inhalation contrast agent are monitored during and after the procedure for allergic reactions and other side effects, including flushing, nausea, and vomiting.

Positron Emission Tomography

Positron emission tomography (PET) is a computer-based nuclear imaging technique that produces images of actual organ functioning. The patient either inhales a radioactive gas or is injected with a radioactive substance that emits positively charged particles. When these positrons combine with negatively charged electrons (normally found in the body's cells), the resultant gamma rays can be detected by a scanning device that produces a series of two-dimensional views at various levels of the brain. This information is integrated by a computer and gives a composite picture of the brain at work.

PET permits the measurement of blood flow, tissue composition, and brain metabolism and thus indirectly evaluates brain function. The brain is one of the most metabolically active organs, consuming 80% of the glucose the body uses. PET measures this activity in specific areas of the brain and can detect changes in glucose use.

In addition, PET is useful in showing metabolic changes in the brain (Alzheimer disease), locating lesions (brain tumor, epileptogenic lesions), identifying blood flow and oxygen metabolism in patients with strokes, evaluating new therapies for brain tumors (Henze, Mohammed, Schlemmer, et al., 2004), and revealing biochemical abnormalities associated with mental illness. The isotopes used have a very short half-life and are expensive to produce, requiring specialized equipment for production. PET scanning has been useful in research settings for the last 20 years and is now becoming more available in clinical settings. Improvements in scanning itself and the production of isotopes, as well as the advent of reimbursement by third-party payers, has increased the availability of PET studies.

Nursing Interventions

Key nursing interventions include patient preparation, which involves explaining the test and teaching the patient about inhalation techniques and the sensations (eg, dizziness, lightheadedness, and headache) that may occur. The IV injection of the radioactive substance produces similar side effects. Relaxation exercises may reduce anxiety during the test.

Single Photon Emission Computed Tomography

Single photon emission computed tomography (SPECT) is a three-dimensional imaging technique that uses radionuclides and instruments to detect single photons. It is a perfusion study that captures a moment of cerebral blood flow at the time of injection of a radionuclide. Gamma photons are emitted from a radiopharmaceutical agent administered to the patient and are detected by a rotating gamma camera or cameras; the image is sent to a minicomputer. This approach allows areas behind overlying structures or background to be viewed, greatly increasing the contrast between normal and abnormal tissue. It is relatively inexpensive, and the duration is similar to that of a CT scan.

SPECT is useful in detecting the extent and location of abnormally perfused areas of the brain, thus allowing detection, localization, and sizing of stroke (before it is visible by CT scan), localization of seizure foci in epilepsy, detecting tumor progression (Henze et al., 2004), and evaluation of perfusion before and after neurosurgical procedures. Pregnancy and breastfeeding are contraindications to SPECT.

Nursing Interventions

The nursing interventions for SPECT primarily include patient preparation and patient monitoring. Teaching about what to expect before the test can allay anxiety and ensure patient cooperation during the test. Premenopausal women are advised to practice effective contraception before and for several days after testing, and the woman who is breastfeeding is instructed to stop nursing for the time period recommended by the nuclear medicine department (Hinkle, 2002).

The nurse may need to accompany and monitor the patient during transport to the nuclear medicine department for the scan. Patients are monitored during and after the procedure for allergic reactions to the radiopharmaceutical agent. In a few institutions, nurses with special education and training inject the contrast agent before a SPECT scan (Fischbach, 2002).

Magnetic Resonance Imaging

Magnetic resonance imaging (MRI) uses a powerful magnetic field to obtain images of different areas of the body (Fig. 60-16). This diagnostic test involves altering hydrogen ions in the body. Placing the patient into a powerful magnetic field causes the hydrogen nuclei (protons) within the body to align like small magnets in a magnetic field. In combination with radiofrequency pulses, the protons emit signals, which are converted to images. An MRI scan can be performed with or without a contrast agent and can identify a cerebral abnormality earlier and more clearly than other diagnostic tests (Selman, 2004). It can provide information about the chemical changes within cells, allowing the clinician to monitor a tumor's response to treatment. It is particularly useful in the diagnosis of multiple sclerosis and can describe the activity and extent of disease in the brain and spinal cord. MRI does not involve ionizing radiation. At present, MRI is most valuable in the diagnosis of nonacute conditions, because the test takes up to an hour to complete (Grey & Ailinani, 2003).

Several newer MRI scanning techniques, including magnetic resonance angiography (MRA), diffusion-weighted imaging (DWI), perfusion-weighted imaging (PWI), and fluid attenuation inversion recovery (FLAIR), are becoming more widely used. The use of MRA allows visualization of the cerebral vasculature without the administration of an arterial contrast agent. Research shows the promise of DWI, PWI, FLAIR, and other new techniques for clearer visualization and the early diagnosis of ischemic stroke (Tanenbaum, 2005).

Nursing Interventions

Patient preparation should include teaching relaxation techniques and informing the patient that he or she will be able to talk to the staff by means of a microphone located inside the scanner. Many MRI suites provide headphones so patients can listen to the music of their choice during the procedure.

Before the patient enters the room where the MRI is to be performed, all metal objects and credit cards (the magnetic field can erase them) are removed. This includes medication patches that have a metal backing; these can cause burns if not removed (Karch, 2004). No metal objects may be brought into the room where the MRI is located; this includes oxygen tanks, traditional ventilators, or even stethoscopes. The magnetic field generated by the unit is so strong that any metal-containing items will be strongly attracted and literally can be pulled away with such force that they fly like projectiles toward the magnet. There is a risk of severe

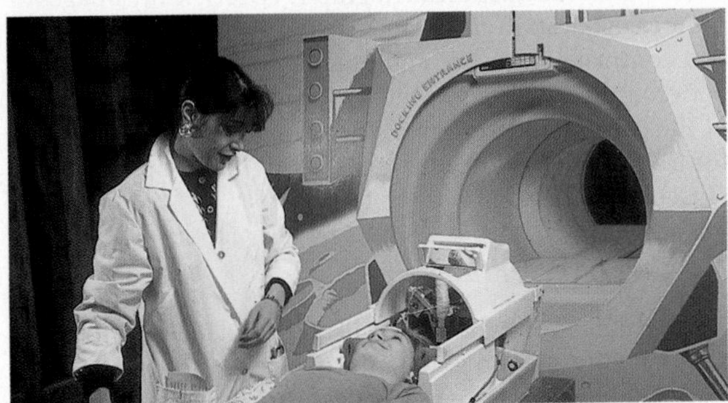

FIGURE 60-16. Technician explains what to expect during an MRI.

injury and death; furthermore, damage to a very expensive piece of equipment may occur. A patient history is obtained to determine the presence of any metal objects (eg, aneurysm clips, orthopedic hardware, pacemakers, artificial heart valves, intrauterine devices). These objects could malfunction, be dislodged, or heat up as they absorb energy. Cochlear implants will be inactivated by MRI; therefore, other imaging procedures are considered.

The patient lies on a flat platform that is moved into a tube housing the magnet. The scanning process is painless, but the patient hears loud thumping of the magnetic coils as the magnetic field is being pulsed. Because the MRI scanner is a narrow tube, patients may experience claustrophobia; sedation may be prescribed in these circumstances. Newer versions of MRI machines (open MRI) are less claustrophobic than the earlier devices and are available in some locations. However, the images produced on these machines are not optimal, and traditional devices are preferable for accurate diagnosis.

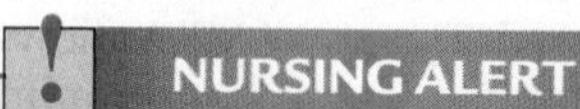

For patient safety, the nurse must make sure no patient care equipment (eg, portable oxygen tanks) that contains metal or metal parts enters the room where the MRI is located. The patient must be assessed for the presence of medication patches with foil backing (such as nicotine) that may cause a burn.

Cerebral Angiography

Cerebral angiography is an x-ray study of the cerebral circulation with a contrast agent injected into a selected artery. Cerebral angiography is a valuable tool to investigate vascular disease, aneurysms, and arteriovenous malformations. It is frequently performed before craniotomy to assess the patency and adequacy of the cerebral circulation and to determine the site, size, and nature of the pathologic processes (Fischbach, 2002).

Most cerebral angiograms are performed by threading a catheter through the femoral artery in the groin and up to the desired vessel. Alternatively, direct puncture of the carotid or vertebral artery or retrograde injection of a contrast agent into the brachial artery may be performed.

In digital subtraction angiography (DSA), x-ray images of the area in question are obtained before and after the injection of a contrast agent. The computer analyzes the differences between the two images and produces an enhanced image of the carotid and vertebral arterial systems. The injection for a DSA can be administered through a peripheral vein (Fischbach, 2002).

Nursing Interventions

The patient should be well hydrated, and clear liquids are usually permitted up to the time of a regular arteriogram or DSA. Before going to the x-ray department, the patient is instructed to void. The locations of the appropriate peripheral pulses are marked with a felt-tip pen. The patient is instructed to remain immobile during the angiogram process and is told to expect a brief feeling of warmth in the face, behind the eyes, or in the jaw, teeth, tongue, and lips, and a metallic taste when the contrast agent is injected.

After the groin is shaved and prepared, a local anesthetic is administered to prevent pain at the insertion site and to reduce arterial spasm. A catheter is introduced into the femoral artery, flushed with heparinized saline, and filled with contrast agent. Fluoroscopy is used to guide the catheter to the appropriate vessels. During injection of the contrast agent, images are made of the arterial and venous phases of circulation through the brain.

Nursing care after cerebral angiography includes observation for signs and symptoms of altered cerebral blood flow. In some instances, patients may experience major or minor arterial blockage due to embolism, thrombosis, or hemorrhage, producing a neurologic deficit. Signs of such an occurrence include alterations in the level of responsiveness and consciousness, weakness on one side of the body, motor or sensory deficits, and speech disturbances. Therefore, it is necessary to observe the patient frequently for these signs and to report them immediately if they occur.

The injection site is observed for hematoma formation (a localized collection of blood), and an ice bag may be applied intermittently to the puncture site to relieve swelling and discomfort. Because a hematoma at the puncture site or embolization to a distant artery affects the peripheral pulses, these pulses are monitored frequently. The color and temperature of the involved extremity are assessed to detect possible embolism.

Myelography

A myelogram is an x-ray of the spinal subarachnoid space taken after the injection of a contrast agent into the spinal subarachnoid space through a lumbar puncture. It outlines the spinal subarachnoid space and shows any distortion of the spinal cord or spinal dural sac caused by tumors, cysts, herniated vertebral disks, or other lesions. Water-based agents have replaced oil-based agents, and their use has reduced side effects and complications; these agents disperse upward through the CSF. Myelography is performed less frequently today because of the sensitivity of CT and MRI scanning (Hickey, 2003).

Nursing Interventions

Because many patients have misconceptions about myelography, the nurse clarifies the explanation given by the physician and answers questions. The patient is informed about what to expect during the procedure and should be aware that changes in position may be made during the procedure. The meal that normally would be eaten before the procedure is omitted. A sedative may be prescribed to help the patient cope with this rather lengthy test. Patient preparation for lumbar puncture is discussed later in this chapter.

After myelography, the patient lies in bed with the head of the bed elevated 30 to 45 degrees. The patient is advised to remain in bed in the recommended position for 3 hours or as prescribed by the physician. The patient is encouraged to drink liberal amounts of fluid for rehydration and replacement of CSF and to decrease the incidence of post–lumbar puncture headache. The blood pressure, pulse, respiratory rate, and temperature are monitored, as well as the patient's ability to void. Untoward signs include headache, fever, stiff neck, **photophobia** (sensitivity to light), seizures, and signs of chemical or bacterial meningitis (Pullen, 2004).

Noninvasive Carotid Flow Studies

Noninvasive carotid flow studies use ultrasound imagery and Doppler measurements of arterial blood flow to evaluate carotid and deep orbital circulation. The graph produced indicates blood velocity. Increased blood velocity can indicate stenosis or partial obstruction. These tests are often obtained before arteriography, which carries a higher risk of stroke or death (Hickey, 2003). Carotid Doppler, carotid ultrasonography, oculoplethysmography, and ophthalmodynamometry are four common noninvasive vascular techniques that permit evaluation of arterial blood flow and detection of arterial stenosis, occlusion, and plaques. These vascular studies allow noninvasive imaging of extracranial and intracranial circulation (Selman, 2004).

Transcranial Doppler

Transcranial Doppler uses the same noninvasive techniques as carotid flow studies except that it records the blood flow velocities of the intracranial vessels (Selman, 2004). Flow velocities of the basal artery can be measured through thin areas of the temporal and occipital bones of the skull. A hand-held Doppler probe emits a pulsed beam; the signal is reflected by the moving red blood cells within the blood vessels. Transcranial Doppler sonography is a noninvasive technique that is helpful in assessing vasospasm (a complication following subarachnoid hemorrhage), altered cerebral blood flow found in occlusive vascular disease or stroke, and other cerebral pathology.

Nursing Interventions

When a carotid flow study or transcranial Doppler is scheduled, the procedure is described to the patient. The patient is informed that this is a noninvasive test, that a hand-held transducer will be placed over the neck and the orbits of the eyes, and that some type of water-soluble jelly is used on the transducer. Either one of these low-risk tests can be performed at the patient's bedside.

Electroencephalography

An electroencephalogram (EEG) represents a record of the electrical activity generated in the brain (Selman, 2004). It is obtained through electrodes applied on the scalp or through microelectrodes placed within the brain tissue. It provides a physiologic assessment of cerebral activity.

The EEG is a useful test for diagnosing and evaluating seizure disorders, coma, or organic brain syndrome. Tumors, brain abscesses, blood clots, and infection may cause abnormal patterns in electrical activity. The EEG is also used in making a determination of brain death.

Electrodes are applied to the scalp to record the electrical activity in various regions of the brain. The amplified activity of the neurons between any two of these electrodes is recorded on continuously moving paper; this record is called the encephalogram.

For a baseline recording, the patient lies quietly with both eyes closed. The patient may be asked to hyperventilate for 3 to 4 minutes and then look at a bright, flashing light for photic stimulation. These activation procedures are performed to evoke abnormal electrical discharges, such as seizure potentials. A sleep EEG may be recorded after sedation because some abnormal brain waves are seen only when the patient is asleep. If the epileptogenic area is inaccessible to conventional scalp electrodes, nasopharyngeal electrodes may be used.

Depth recording of EEG is performed by introducing electrodes stereotactically (radiologically placed using instrumentation) into a target area of the brain, as indicated by the patient's seizure pattern and scalp EEG. It is used to identify patients who may benefit from surgical excision of epileptogenic foci.

Special transsphenoidal, mandibular, and nasopharyngeal electrodes can be used, and video recording combined with EEG monitoring and telemetry is used in hospital settings to capture epileptiform abnormalities and their sequelae. Some epilepsy centers provide long-term ambulatory EEG monitoring with portable recording devices.

Nursing Interventions

To increase the chances of recording seizure activity, it is sometimes recommended that the patient be deprived of sleep on the night before the EEG. Antiseizure agents, tranquilizers, stimulants, and depressants should be withheld 24 to 48 hours before an EEG because these medications can alter the EEG wave patterns or mask the abnormal wave patterns of seizure disorders (Hickey, 2003). Coffee, tea, chocolate, and cola drinks are omitted in the meal before the test because of their stimulating effect. However, the meal is not omitted, because an altered blood glucose level can also cause changes in the brain wave patterns.

The patient is informed that the standard EEG takes 45 to 60 minutes, 12 hours for a sleep EEG. The patient is assured that the procedure does not cause an electric shock and that the EEG is a diagnostic test, not a form of treatment. An EEG requires patient cooperation and ability to lie quietly during the test. Sedation is not advisable, because it may lower the seizure threshold in patients with a seizure disorder and it alters brain wave activity in all patients. The nurse needs to check the physician's prescription regarding the administration of antiseizure medication prior to testing.

Routine EEGs use a water-soluble lubricant for electrode contact, which at the conclusion of the study can be wiped off and removed by shampooing. Sleep EEGs involve the use of collodion glue for electrode contact, which requires acetone for removal.

Electromyography

An electromyogram (EMG) is obtained by inserting needle electrodes into the skeletal muscles to measure changes in the electrical potential of the muscles and the nerves leading to them (Selman, 2004). The electrical potentials are shown on an oscilloscope and amplified so that both the sound and appearance of the waves can be analyzed and compared simultaneously.

An EMG is useful in determining the presence of neuromuscular disorders and myopathies. It helps distinguish weakness due to neuropathy (functional or pathologic changes in the peripheral nervous system) from weakness resulting from other causes.

Nursing Interventions

The procedure is explained, and the patient is warned to expect a sensation similar to that of an intramuscular injection as the needle is inserted into the muscle. The muscles examined may ache for a short time after the procedure.

Nerve Conduction Studies

Nerve conduction studies are performed by stimulating a peripheral nerve at several points along its course and recording the muscle action potential or the sensory action potential that results. Surface or needle electrodes are placed on the skin over the nerve to stimulate the nerve fibers. This test is useful in the study of peripheral neuropathies.

Evoked Potential Studies

Evoked potential studies are extensions of nerve conduction tests (Selman, 2004). Electrodes are applied to the scalp, and an external stimulus is applied to peripheral sensory receptors to elicit changes in the brain waves. Evoked changes are detected with the aid of computerized devices that extract the signal, display it on an oscilloscope, and store the data on magnetic tape or disk. These studies are based on the concept that any insult or dysfunction that can alter neuronal metabolism or disturb membrane function may change evoked responses in brain waves. In neurologic diagnosis, they reflect nerve conduction times in the peripheral nervous system. In clinical practice, the visual, auditory, and somatosensory systems are most often tested.

In visual evoked responses, the patient looks at a visual stimulus (flashing lights, a checkerboard pattern on a screen). The average of several hundred stimuli is recorded by EEG leads placed over the occipital lobe. The transit time from the retina to the occipital area is measured using computer-averaging methods.

Auditory evoked responses or brain stem–evoked responses are measured by applying an auditory stimulus (repetitive auditory click) and measuring the transit time via the brain stem into the cortex. Specific lesions in the auditory pathway modify or delay the response.

In somatosensory evoked responses, the peripheral nerves are stimulated (electrical stimulation through skin electrodes) and the transit time along the spinal cord to the cortex is measured and recorded from scalp electrodes.

These tests are used to detect a deficit in spinal cord conduction and to monitor spinal cord function during surgical procedures. Because myelinated fibers conduct impulses at a higher rate of speed, nerves with an intact myelin sheath record the highest velocity. Demyelination of nerve fibers leads to a decrease in speed of conduction, as found in Guillain-Barré syndrome, multiple sclerosis, and polyneuropathies.

Nursing Interventions

There is no specific patient preparation other than to explain the procedure and to reassure the patient and encourage him or her to relax. The patient is advised to remain perfectly still throughout the recording to prevent artifacts (signals not generated by the brain) that interfere with the recording and interpretation of the test.

Lumbar Puncture and Examination of Cerebrospinal Fluid

A lumbar puncture (spinal tap) is carried out by inserting a needle into the lumbar subarachnoid space to withdraw CSF. The test may be performed to obtain CSF for examination, to measure and reduce CSF pressure, to determine the presence or absence of blood in the CSF, to detect spinal subarachnoid block, and to administer antibiotics intrathecally (into the spinal canal) in certain cases of infection.

The needle is usually inserted into the subarachnoid space between the third and fourth or fourth and fifth lumbar vertebrae. Because the spinal cord divides into a sheaf of nerves at the first lumbar vertebra, insertion of the needle below the level of the third lumbar vertebra prevents puncture of the spinal cord.

A successful lumbar puncture requires that the patient be relaxed; an anxious patient is tense, and this may increase the pressure reading. CSF pressure with the patient in a lateral recumbent position is normally 70 to 200 mm H_2O. Pressures of more than 200 mm H_2O are considered abnormal.

A lumbar puncture may be risky in the presence of an intracranial mass lesion because intracranial pressure is decreased by the removal of CSF, and the brain may herniate downward through the tentorium and the foramen magnum.

Queckenstedt's Test

A lumbar manometric test (Queckenstedt's test) may be performed by compressing the jugular veins on each side of the neck during the lumbar puncture. The increase in pressure caused by the compression is noted; then the pressure is released and pressure readings are made at 10-second intervals. Normally, CSF pressure rises rapidly in response to compression of the jugular veins and returns quickly to normal when the compression is released. A slow rise and fall in pressure indicates a partial block due to a lesion compressing the spinal subarachnoid pathways. If there is no pressure change, a complete block is indicated. This test is not performed if an intracranial lesion is suspected.

See Chart 60-3 for nursing guidelines for assisting with a lumbar puncture.

Cerebrospinal Fluid Analysis

The CSF should be clear and colorless. Pink, blood-tinged, or grossly bloody CSF may indicate a cerebral contusion, laceration, or subarachnoid hemorrhage. Sometimes with a difficult lumbar puncture, the CSF initially is bloody because of local trauma but then becomes clearer. Usually, specimens are obtained for cell count, culture, and glucose

CHART 60-3

Guidelines for Assisting With a Lumbar Puncture

A needle is inserted into the subarachnoid space through the third and fourth or fourth and fifth lumbar interface to withdraw spinal fluid.

PREPROCEDURE

1. Determine whether written consent for the procedure has been obtained.
2. Explain the procedure to the patient and describe sensations that are likely during the procedure (ie, a sensation of cold as the site is cleansed with solution, a needle prick when local anesthetic is injected).
3. Determine whether the patient has any questions or misconceptions about the procedure; reassure the patient that the needle will not enter the spinal cord or cause paralysis.
4. Instruct the patient to void before the procedure.

PROCEDURE

1. The patient is positioned on one side at the edge of the bed or examining table with back toward the physician; the thighs and legs are flexed as much as possible to increase the space between the spinous processes of the vertebrae, for easier entry into the subarachnoid space.

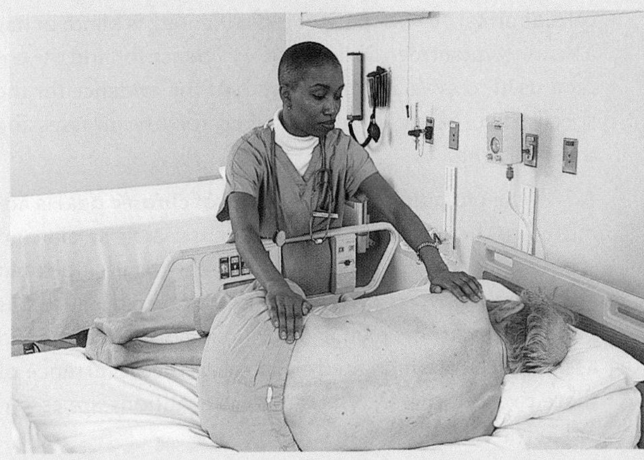

© B. Proud.

2. A small pillow may be placed under the patient's head to maintain the spine in a horizontal position; a pillow may be placed between the legs to prevent the upper leg from rolling forward.
3. The nurse assists the patient to maintain the position to avoid sudden movement, which can produce a traumatic (bloody) tap.
4. The patient is encouraged to relax and is instructed to breathe normally, because hyperventilation may lower an elevated pressure.
5. The nurse describes the procedure step by step to the patient as it proceeds.
6. The physician cleanses the puncture site with an antiseptic solution and drapes the site.
7. The physician injects local anesthetic to numb the puncture site, and then inserts a spinal needle into the subarachnoid space through the third and fourth or fourth and fifth lumbar interspace.
8. A specimen of CSF is removed and usually collected in three test tubes, labeled in order of collection. A pressure reading may be obtained. The needle is withdrawn.
9. The physician applies a small dressing to the puncture site.
10. The tubes of CSF are sent to the laboratory immediately.

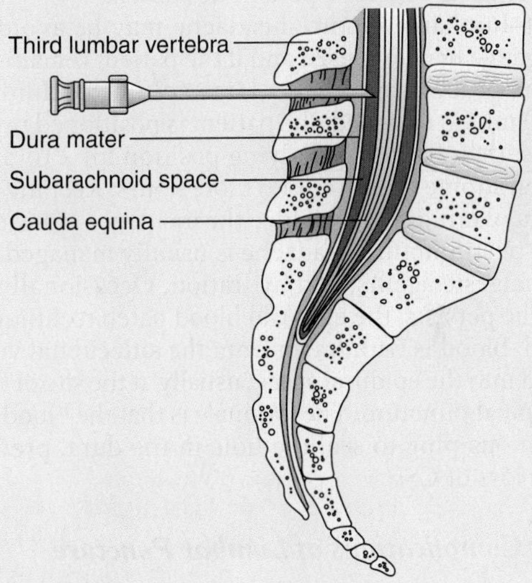

POSTPROCEDURE

1. Instruct the patient to lie prone for 2 to 3 hours to separate the alignment of the dural and arachnoid needle punctures in the meninges, to reduce leakage of CSF.
2. Monitor the patient for complications of lumbar puncture; notify physician if complications occur.
3. Encourage increased fluid intake to reduce the risk of post-procedure headache.

and protein testing. The specimens should be sent to the laboratory immediately because changes will take place and alter the result if the specimens are allowed to stand. (See Table B-5 in Appendix B for the normal values of CSF.)

Post–Lumbar Puncture Headache

A post–lumbar puncture headache, ranging from mild to severe, may occur a few hours to several days after the procedure. This is the most common complication, occurring in 15% to 30% of patients. It is a throbbing bifrontal or occipital headache, dull and deep in character. It is particularly severe on sitting or standing but lessens or disappears when the patient lies down.

The headache is caused by CSF leakage at the puncture site. The fluid continues to escape into the tissues by way of the needle track from the spinal canal. It is then absorbed promptly by the lymphatics. As a result of this leak, the supply of CSF in the cranium is depleted to a point at which it is insufficient to maintain proper mechanical stabilization of the brain. This leakage of CSF allows settling of the brain when the patient assumes an upright position, producing tension and stretching the venous sinuses and pain-sensitive structures. Both traction and pain are lessened and the leakage is reduced when the patient lies down.

Post–lumbar puncture headache may be avoided if a small-gauge needle is used and if the patient remains prone after the procedure. When a large volume of fluid (more than 20 mL) is removed, the patient is positioned prone for 2 hours, then flat in a side-lying position for 2 to 3 hours, and then supine or prone for 6 more hours. Keeping the patient flat overnight may reduce the incidence of headaches.

The postpuncture headache is usually managed by bed rest, analgesic agents, and hydration. Occasionally, if the headache persists, the epidural blood patch technique may be used. Blood is withdrawn from the antecubital vein and injected into the epidural space, usually at the site of the previous spinal puncture. The rationale is that the blood acts as a gelatinous plug to seal the hole in the dura, preventing further loss of CSF.

Other Complications of Lumbar Puncture

Herniation of the intracranial contents, spinal epidural abscess, spinal epidural hematoma, and meningitis are rare but serious complications of lumbar puncture. Other complications include temporary voiding problems, slight elevation of temperature, backache or spasms, and stiffness of the neck.

Promoting Home and Community-Based Care

Teaching Patients Self-Care

Many diagnostic tests that were once performed as part of a hospital stay are now carried out in short-procedure units or outpatient testing settings or units. As a result, family members often provide the postprocedure care. Therefore, the patient and family must receive clear verbal and written instructions about precautions to take after the procedure, complications to watch for, and steps to take if complications occur. Because many patients undergoing neurologic diagnostic studies are elderly or have neurologic deficits, provisions must be made to ensure that transportation and postprocedure care and monitoring are available.

Continuing Care

Contacting the patient and family after diagnostic testing enables the nurse to determine whether they have any questions about the procedure or whether the patient had any untoward results. During these phone calls, teaching is reinforced and the patient and family are reminded to make and keep follow-up appointments. Patients, family members, and health care providers are focused on the immediate needs, issues, or deficits that necessitated the diagnostic testing. This is also a good time to remind them of the need for and importance of continuing health promotion and screening practices and to make referrals to appropriate health care providers.

Critical Thinking Exercises

1. ebp Identify the approach and techniques you would use to perform a neurologic screening examination on a 58-year-old woman. How would your approach and technique differ if your patient is recovering from a cardiac arrest? If your patient is disoriented, is blind, or has a hearing impairment? Identify the evidence for and the criteria used to evaluate the strength of the evidence for the specific neurologic scales identified for use in assessing these patients.
2. A 78-year-old patient with a history of chronic pain is admitted to the hospital to rule out an ischemic stroke and is scheduled for an MRI. Explain why the MRI is indicated and what, if any, precautions must be taken because this patient has chronic pain. What nursing observations and assessments are indicated because of the occurrence of these two disorders? What safety precautions are essential in the MRI suite, and why?
3. You are caring for a patient who is scheduled to undergo a lumbar puncture. How can you best assist and support the patient during the procedure? What laboratory studies would you expect to be ordered on the CSF sample? What postprocedure restrictions can you expect and prepare the patient for?

REFERENCES AND SELECTED READINGS

BOOKS

Bader, M. K. & Littlejohns, J. R. (2004) *AANN core curriculum for neuroscience nursing* (4th ed.). St Louis: Elsevier Inc.

Bickley, L. S., & Szilagyi, P. G. (2003). *Bates' guide to physical examination and history taking* (8th ed.). Philadelphia: Lippincott Williams & Wilkins.

Diepenbrock, N. H. (2004). *Quick reference to critical care* (2nd ed.). Philadelphia: Lippincott Williams & Wilkins.

Dochterman, J. C., & Bulechek, G. M. (2004). *Nursing interventions classification (NIC)* (4th ed.). St. Louis: Mosby.

Fischbach, F. (2002). *Common laboratory and diagnostic tests* (3rd ed.). Philadelphia: Lippincott Williams & Wilkins.

Grey, M. & Ailinani, J. M. (2003). *CT and MRI pathology: A pocket atlas.* New York: McGraw-Hill Company.

Hickey, J. (2003). *Clinical practice of neurologic and neurosurgical nursing* (5th ed.). Philadelphia: Lippincott Williams & Wilkins.

Moorhead, S., Johnson, M. & Maas, M. (2004). *Nursing outcomes classification (NOC)* (3rd ed.). St. Louis: Mosby.

NANDA International. (2003). *Nursing diagnoses; Definitions and classification 2003–2004.* Philadelphia: North American Nursing Diagnosis Association.

Orient, J. (2005). *Sapira's art and science of bedside diagnosis* (3rd ed.). Philadelphia: Lippincott Williams & Wilkins.

Porth, C. M. (2005). *Pathophysiology: Concepts of altered health states* (7th ed.). Philadelphia: Lippincott Williams & Wilkins.

Rice, J. N., Robichaux, C. & Leonard, A. (2005). Nervous system alterations. In M. L. Sole, D. G. Klein, & M. J. Moseley (Eds.). *Introduction to critical care nursing.* St. Louis: Elsevier Saunders.

Som, P. & Curtin, H. D. (2003). *Head and neck imaging* (4th ed.). St. Louis: Mosby.

Somjen, G. (2004). *Ions in the brain: Normal function, seizures and stroke.* Oxford, UK: Oxford University Press.

Weber, J. & Kelley, J. (2003). *Health assessment in nursing* (2nd ed.). Philadelphia: Lippincott Williams & Wilkins.

Winn, H. R. (2003). *Youman's neurological surgery* (5th ed., Vols. 1–4). Philadelphia: W. B. Saunders.

JOURNALS

Booth, C. M., Boone, R. H., Tomlinson, G., et al. (2004). Is this patient dead, vegetative, or severely neurologically impaired? *Journal of the American Medical Association, 291*(7), 870–879.

Coles, M. C. (2004). S1 radiculopathy due to adenocarcinoma: A case study. *Journal of Neuroscience Nursing, 36*(1), 40–41.

Cunning, S. (1999). Preventing secondary brain injuries. *Dimensions in Critical Care Nursing, 18*(5), 20–22.

Dawson, T. M. & Dawson, V. L. (2003). Molecular pathways of neurodegeneration in Parkinson's disease. *Science, 302*(5646), 819–822.

DeKosky, S. T. & Marek, K. (2003). Looking backward to move forward: Early detection of neurodegenerative disorders. *Science, 302*(5646), 830–834.

Freeman, J. J., & Hedges, C. (2003). Cardiac arrest: The effect on the brain. *American Journal of Nursing, 103*(6), 50–54.

Hanks-Bell, M., Halvey, K. & Paice, J. A. (2004). Pain assessment and management in aging. *Online Journal of Issues in Nursing, 9*(3), 1–10.

Haymore, J. (2004). A neuron in a haystack: Advanced neurological assessment. *AACN Clinical Issues, 15*(4), 568–581.

Heckman, J. G., Heckman, S. M., Lang, C. J. G., et al. (2003). Neurological aspects of taste disorders. *Archives of Neurology, 60*(5), 667–671.

Henze, M., Mohammed, A., Schlemmer, H. P., et al. (2004). PET and SPECT for detection of tumor progression in irradiated low-grad astrocytoma: A receiver-operating characteristic analysis. *Journal of Nuclear Medicine, 45*(4), 579–586.

Hinkle, J. L. (2002). SPECT: A powerful imaging tool. *American Journal of Nursing, 102*(3), 24A–24G.

Johkura, K., Komiyama, A., and Kuroiwa, Y (2004). Vertical conjugate eye deviation in post resuscitation coma. *Annals of Neurology, 56*(6), 878–881.

Karch, A. M. (2004). Don't get burnt by the MRI. *American Journal of Nursing, 104*(8), 31.

Lehman, C. A., Hayes, J. M., LaCroix, M., et al. (2003). Development and implementation of a problem-focused neurologic assessment system. *Journal of Neuroscience Nursing, 35*(4), 185–192.

Lempe, D. M. (2004). Riding out the storm: Sympathetic storming after traumatic brain injury. *Journal of Neuroscience Nursing, 36*(1), 4–9.

Lindeboom, R., Vermeulen, M., Holman, M. M., et al. (2003). Activities of daily living instruments: Optimizing scales for neurologic assessments. *Neurology, 60*(5), 738–742.

McKearnan, K. A., Kieckhefer, G. M., Engel, J. M., et al. (2004). Pain in children with cerebral palsy: A review. *Journal of Neuroscience Nursing, 36*(5), 252–259.

Munro, N. (2004). Evidence-based assessment: No more pride or prejudice. *AACN Clinical Issues, 15*(4), 501–505.

Prendergast, M. A. (2004). Do women possess a unique susceptibility to the neurotoxic effects of alcohol? *Journal of the American Medical Women's Association, 59*(3), 225–227.

Pullen, R. (2004). Assessing for signs of meningitis. *Nursing, 34*(5), 18.

Rasmor, M., & Brown, C. M. (2003). Physical examination for the occupational health nurse. *AAOHN Journal, 51*(9), 390–401.

Roscigno, C. I. (2004). Neuronal pathway finding: From neurons to initial neural networks. *Journal of Neuroscience Nursing, 36*(5), 263–272.

Selman, J. E. (2004). How to choose the proper imaging test. *Clinical Advisor, 7*(2), 56–62.

Stotts, N. A., & Deitrich, C. E. (2004). The challenge to come: The care of older adults. *American Journal of Nursing, 104*(8), 40–47.

Tanenbaum, L. N. (2005). 3T MRI in clinical practice. *Applied Radiology, 35*(1), 8–17.

Traccis, S., Zoroddu, G. F., Zecca, M. T., et al. (2004). Evaluating patients with vertigo: Bedside examination. *Neurological Sciences, 24*(Suppl. 1), S16-S19.

CHAPTER 61

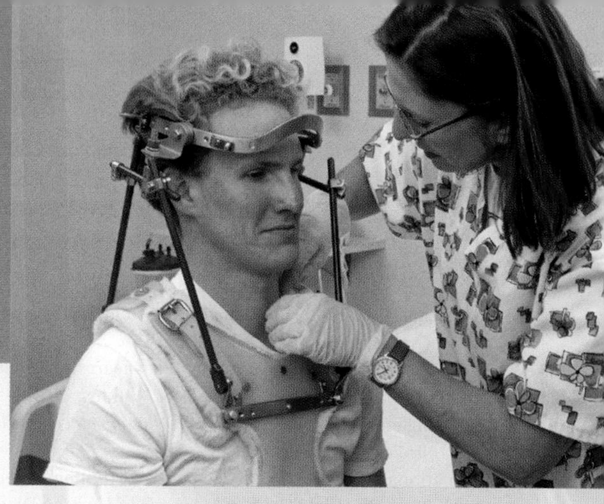

Management of Patients With Neurologic Dysfunction

Learning Objectives

On completion of this chapter, the learner will be able to:

1. Describe the nursing needs of patients with various neurologic dysfunctions.
2. Describe the multiple needs of the patient with altered level of consciousness.
3. Use the nursing process as a framework for care of the patient with altered level of consciousness.
4. Identify the early and late clinical manifestations of increased intracranial pressure.
5. Use the nursing process as a framework for care of the patient with increased intracranial pressure.
6. Describe the needs of the patient undergoing intracranial or transsphenoidal surgery.
7. Use the nursing process as a framework for care of the patient undergoing intracranial or transsphenoidal surgery.
8. Identify the various types and causes of seizures.
9. Use the nursing process to develop a plan of care for the patient experiencing seizures.
10. Identify the needs of the patient experiencing headaches.

This chapter presents care of the patient with an altered level of consciousness, the patient with increased **intracranial pressure** (ICP), and the patient who is undergoing neurosurgical procedures, experiencing seizures, or experiencing headaches. Some of the disorders in this chapter, such as headaches and seizures, may be symptoms of dysfunction in another body system. Alternatively, headaches and seizures can be symptoms of a severe disruption of the neurologic system. These disorders can also be diagnosed at times as "idiopathic," or without an identifiable cause. The commonalities of these disorders are often the behaviors and needs of the patient and the approaches nurses use to support the patient.

The central nervous system (CNS) contains a vast network of neurons that control the body's vital functions. Yet this system is vulnerable, and its optimal function depends on several key factors. First, the neurologic system relies on its structural integrity for support and homeostasis, but this integrity may be disrupted. Examples of structural disruption include head injury, brain tumor, intracranial hemorrhage, infection, and stroke. As brain tissue expands in the inflexible cranium, ICP rises and cerebral perfusion is impaired. Further expansion places pressure on vital centers, which can cause permanent neurologic deficits or lead to brain death.

Second, the neurologic system relies on the body's ability to maintain a homeostatic environment. It requires the delivery of the essential elements of oxygen and glucose, as well as filtration of substrates that are toxic to the neurons. The functions of the neurologic system may be decreased or absent due to the effect of toxic substrates or the body's inability to provide essential substrates. Sepsis, hypovolemia, myocardial infarction, respiratory arrest, hypoglycemia, electrolyte imbalance, drug and/or alcohol overdose, encephalopathy, and ketoacidosis are all examples of such circumstances. Some conditions can be treated and reversed; others result in permanent neurologic deficits and disabilities.

Although the specialty of neuroscience nursing requires an understanding of neuroanatomy, neurophysiology, neurodiagnostic testing, critical care nursing, and rehabilitation nursing, nurses in all settings care for patients with neurologic disorders. Ongoing assessment of the patient's

Glossary

akinetic mutism: unresponsiveness to the environment; the patient makes no movement or sound but sometimes opens the eyes

altered level of consciousness: condition of being less responsive to and aware of environmental stimuli

autoregulation: ability of cerebral blood vessels to dilate or constrict to maintain stable cerebral blood flow despite changes in systemic arterial blood pressure

brain death: irreversible loss of all functions of the entire brain, including the brain stem

coma: prolonged state of unconsciousness

craniotomy: a surgical procedure that involves entry into the cranial vault

craniectomy: a surgical procedure that involves removal of a portion of the skull

Cushing's response: brain's attempt to restore blood flow by increasing arterial pressure to overcome the increased intracranial pressure

Cushing's triad: three classic signs—bradycardia, hypertension, and bradypnea—seen with pressure on the medulla as a result of brain stem herniation

decerebration: an abnormal body posture associated with a severe brain injury, characterized by extreme extension of the upper and lower extremities

decortication: an abnormal posture associated with severe brain injury, characterized by abnormal flexion of the upper extremities and extension of the lower extremities

epidural monitor: a sensor placed between the skull and the dura to monitor intracranial pressure

epilepsy: a group of syndromes characterized by paroxysmal transient disturbances of brain function.

fiberoptic monitor: a system that uses light refraction to determine intracranial pressure

herniation: abnormal protrusion of tissue through a defect or natural opening

intracranial pressure: pressure exerted by the volume of the intracranial contents within the cranial vault

locked-in syndrome: condition resulting from a lesion in the pons in which the patient lacks all distal motor activity (tetraplegia) but cognition is intact

microdialysis: procedure in which an intracranial catheter is inserted near an injured area of brain to measure lactate, pyruvate, glutamate, and glucose levels

migraine headache: a severe, unrelenting headache often accompanied by symptoms such as nausea, vomiting, and visual disturbances

Monro-Kellie hypothesis: theory that states that due to limited space for expansion within the skull, an increase in any one of the cranial contents—brain tissue, blood, or CSF—causes a change in the volume of the others

persistent vegetative state: condition in which the patient is wakeful but devoid of conscious content, without cognitive or affective mental function

primary headache: a headache for which no specific organic cause can be found

seizures: paroxysmal transient disturbance of the brain resulting from a discharge of abnormal electrical activity

status epilepticus: episode in which the patient experiences multiple seizure bursts with no recovery time in between

secondary headache: headache identified as a symptom of another organic disorder (eg, brain tumor, hypertension)

subarachnoid screw or bolt: device placed into the subarachnoid space to measure intracranial pressure

transsphenoidal: surgical approach to the pituitary via the sphenoid sinuses

ventriculostomy: a catheter placed in one of the lateral ventricles of the brain to measure intracranial pressure and allow for drainage of fluid

neurologic function and health needs, identification of problems, mutual goal setting, development and implementation of care plans (including teaching, counseling, and coordinating activities), and evaluation of the outcomes of care are nursing actions integral to the recovery of the patient. The nurse also collaborates with other members of the health care team to provide essential care, offer a variety of solutions to problems, help the patient and family gain control of their lives, and explore the educational and supportive resources available in the community. The goals are to achieve as high a level of function as possible and to enhance the quality of life for the patient with neurologic impairment and his or her family.

Altered Level of Consciousness

An **altered level of consciousness** (LOC) is apparent in the patient who is not oriented, does not follow commands, or needs persistent stimuli to achieve a state of alertness. LOC is gauged on a continuum with a normal state of alertness and full cognition (consciousness) on one end and coma on the other end. **Coma** is a clinical state of unarousable unresponsiveness in which there are no purposeful responses to internal or external stimuli, although nonpurposeful responses to painful stimuli and brain stem reflexes may be present (Hickey, 2003). The duration of coma is usually limited to 2 to 4 weeks. **Akinetic mutism** is a state of unresponsiveness to the environment in which the patient makes no voluntary movement. **Persistent vegetative state** is a condition in which the unresponsive patient resumes sleep-wake cycles after coma but is devoid of cognitive or affective mental function. **Locked-in syndrome** results from a lesion affecting the pons and results in tetraplegia (formerly called quadriplegia) and inability to speak, but vertical eye movements and lid elevation remain intact and are used to indicate responsiveness (Ropper, Gress, Diringer, et al., 2004). The level of responsiveness and consciousness is the most important indicator of the patient's condition.

Pathophysiology

Altered LOC is not a disorder itself; rather, it is a result of multiple pathophysiologic phenomena. The cause may be neurologic (head injury, stroke), toxicologic (drug overdose, alcohol intoxication), or metabolic (hepatic or renal failure, diabetic ketoacidosis).

The underlying cause of neurologic dysfunction is disruption in the cells of the nervous system, neurotransmitters, or brain anatomy (see Chapter 60). A disruption in the basic functional units (neurons) or neurotransmitters results in faulty impulse transmission, impeding communication within the brain or from the brain to other parts of the body. These disruptions are caused by cellular edema or other mechanisms, such as disruption of chemical transmission at receptor sites by antibodies.

Intact anatomic structures of the brain are needed for normal function. The two hemispheres of the cerebrum must communicate, via an intact corpus callosum, and the lobes of the brain (frontal, parietal, temporal, and occipital) must communicate and coordinate their specific functions (see Chapter 60). Additional anatomic structures of importance are the cerebellum and the brain stem. The cerebellum has both excitatory and inhibitory actions and is largely responsible for coordination of movement. The brain stem contains areas that control the heart, respiration, and blood pressure. Disruptions in the anatomic structures are caused by trauma, edema, pressure from tumors, or other mechanisms, such as an increase or decrease in the circulation of blood or cerebrospinal fluid (CSF).

Clinical Manifestations

Alterations in LOC occur along a continuum, and the clinical manifestations depend on where the patient is on this continuum. As the patient's state of alertness and consciousness decreases, changes will ultimately occur in the pupillary response, eye opening response, verbal response, and motor response. However, initial alterations in LOC may be reflected by subtle behavioral changes, such as restlessness or increased anxiety. The pupils, normally round and quickly reactive to light, become sluggish (response is slower); as the patient becomes comatose, the pupils become fixed (no response to light). The patient in a coma does not open the eyes, respond verbally, or move the extremities in response to a request to do so.

Assessment and Diagnostic Findings

The patient with an altered LOC is at risk for alterations in every body system. A complete assessment is performed, with particular attention to the neurologic system. The neurologic examination should be as complete as the LOC allows (American Association of Neuroscience Nurses [AANN], 2005). It includes an evaluation of mental status, cranial nerve function, cerebellar function (balance and coordination), reflexes, and motor and sensory function. LOC, a sensitive indicator of neurologic function, is assessed based on the criteria in the Glasgow Coma Scale: eye opening, verbal response, and motor response (Rice, Robichaux & Leonard, 2005). The patient's responses are rated on a scale from 3 to 15. A score of 3 indicates severe impairment of neurologic function, brain death, or pharmacologic inhibition of the neurologic response. A score of 15 indicates that the patient is fully responsive (see Chapter 63).

If the patient is comatose and has localized signs such as abnormal pupillary and motor responses, it is assumed that neurologic disease is present until proven otherwise. If the patient is comatose but pupillary light reflexes are preserved, a toxic or metabolic disorder is suspected. Common diagnostic procedures used to identify the cause of unconsciousness include computed tomography (CT) scanning, magnetic resonance imaging (MRI), and electroencephalography. Less common procedures include positron emission tomography (PET) and single photon emission computed tomography (SPECT; see Chapter 60). Laboratory tests include analysis of blood glucose, electrolytes, serum ammonia, and liver function tests; blood urea nitrogen levels; serum osmolality; calcium level; and partial thromboplastin and prothrombin times. Other studies may be used to evaluate serum ketones, alcohol and drug concentrations, and arterial blood gases.

NURSING RESEARCH PROFILE

Testing a Device for Measuring Pupil Size and Reactivity

Meeker, M., Du, R., Bacchetti, P., et al. (2005). Pupil examination: Validity and clinical utility of an automated pupillometer. *Journal of Neuroscience Nursing, 37*(1), 34–40.

Purpose

The size and reactivity of the pupil is a critical component of the examination of many patients with neurologic disorders and provides important information. The purpose of this study was to test the accuracy and reliability of an automated pupillometer compared with the standard manual examination with a penlight or similar light source.

Design

The design of the study was a descriptive comparison with the 20 subjects serving as their own controls. Each patient was examined by two groups of three examiners using both manual examination with a penlight or similar light source and a portable automated pupillometer. The pupillometer is a portable, battery-operated automated device with a screen and digital video camera that measures pupil size and reactivity. Measurements were made before and after the examination with a static pupillometer to determine the mean "true" size of the pupil. All of the subjects were in an intensive care unit; 10 had acute intracranial processes including hemorrhagic stroke or traumatic brain injury, and 10 had medical diagnoses of acute pancreatitis, necrotizing fascitis, or pneumonia.

Findings

The degree of error in pupil size measurement was greater for manual examination than for the automated pupillometer. The automated pupillometer was consistent in all but one patient in determining pupillary reactivity.

Nursing Implications

Nurses in intensive care units may see pupillometers used more frequently to augment manual examinations. This study found that an automated device is more accurate and reliable in measuring pupil size and reactivity. The device may be a beneficial addition to the clinical assessment of the neurologically impaired patient.

Complications

Potential complications for the patient with altered LOC include respiratory failure, pneumonia, pressure ulcers, and aspiration. Respiratory failure may develop shortly after the patient becomes unconscious. If the patient cannot maintain effective respirations, care (insertion of an airway, mechanical ventilation) is initiated to provide adequate ventilation and protect the airway. Pneumonia is common in patients receiving mechanical ventilation or in those who cannot maintain and clear the airway. The patient with altered LOC is subject to all the complications associated with immobility, such as pressure ulcers, venous stasis, musculoskeletal deterioration, and disturbed gastrointestinal functioning. Pressure ulcers may become infected and serve as a source of sepsis. Aspiration of gastric contents or feedings may occur, precipitating the development of aspiration pneumonia or airway occlusion.

Medical Management

The first priority of treatment for the patient with altered LOC is to obtain and maintain a patent airway. The patient may be orally or nasally intubated, or a tracheostomy may be performed. Until the ability of the patient to breathe on his or her own is determined, a mechanical ventilator is used to maintain adequate oxygenation and ventilation. The circulatory status (blood pressure, heart rate) is monitored to ensure adequate perfusion to the body and brain. An intravenous (IV) catheter is inserted to provide access for IV fluids and medications. Neurologic care focuses on the specific neurologic pathology, if known. Nutritional support, via a feeding tube or a gastrostomy tube, is initiated as soon as possible. In addition to measures designed to determine and treat the underlying causes of altered LOC, other medical interventions are aimed at pharmacologic management and prevention of complications.

Nursing Process

The Patient With an Altered Level of Consciousness

Assessment

Assessment of the patient with an altered LOC depends on the patient's circumstances, but clinicians often start by assessing the verbal response. Determining the patient's orientation to time, person, and place assesses verbal response. The patient is asked to identify the day, date, or season of the year and to identify where he or she is or to identify the clinicians, family members, or visitors present. Other questions such as, "Who is the president?" or "What is the next holiday?" may be helpful in determining the patient's processing of information in the environment. (Verbal response cannot be evaluated if the patient is intubated or has a tracheostomy, and this should be clearly documented.)

Alertness is measured by the patient's ability to open the eyes spontaneously or in response to a vocal or noxious stimulus (pressure or pain). Patients with severe neurologic dysfunction cannot do this. The nurse assesses for periorbital edema (swelling around the eyes) or trauma, which may prevent the patient from opening the eyes, and documents any such condition that interferes with eye opening.

Motor response includes spontaneous, purposeful movement (eg, the awake patient can move all four extremities with equal strength on command), movement only in response to painful stimuli, or abnormal posturing (Hickey, 2003; Seidel, Ball, Dains, et al., 2003). If the patient is not responding to commands, the motor response is tested by applying a painful stimulus (firm but gentle pressure) to the nailbed or by squeezing a muscle. If the patient attempts to push away or withdraw, the response is recorded as purposeful or appropriate ("patient withdraws to painful stimuli"). This response is considered purposeful if the patient can cross the midline from one side of the body to the other in response to painful stimuli. An inappropriate or nonpurposeful response is random and aimless. Posturing may be decorticate or decerebrate (Fig. 61-1; see also Chapter 60). The most severe neurologic impairment results in flaccidity. The motor response cannot be elicited if the patient has been administered pharmacologic paralyzing agents.

In addition to LOC, the nurse monitors parameters such as respiratory status, eye signs, and reflexes on an ongoing basis. Table 61-1 summarizes the assessment and the clinical significance of the findings. Body functions (circulation, respiration, elimination, fluid and electrolyte balance) are examined in a systematic and ongoing manner.

Diagnosis

Nursing Diagnoses

Based on the assessment data, the major nursing diagnoses may include the following:

- Ineffective airway clearance related to altered LOC
- Risk of injury related to decreased LOC
- Deficient fluid volume related to inability to take fluids by mouth
- Impaired oral mucous membrane related to mouth-breathing, absence of pharyngeal reflex, and altered fluid intake
- Risk for impaired skin integrity related to immobility
- Impaired tissue integrity of cornea related to diminished or absent corneal reflex
- Ineffective thermoregulation related to damage to hypothalamic center
- Impaired urinary elimination (incontinence or retention) related to impairment in neurologic sensing and control
- Bowel incontinence related to impairment in neurologic sensing and control and also related to changes in nutritional delivery methods
- Disturbed sensory perception related to neurologic impairment
- Interrupted family processes related to health crisis

Collaborative Problems/ Potential Complications

Based on the assessment data, potential complications may include:

- Respiratory distress or failure
- Pneumonia
- Aspiration
- Pressure ulcer
- Deep vein thrombosis (DVT)
- Contractures

Planning and Goals

The goals of care for the patient with altered LOC include maintenance of a clear airway, protection from injury, attainment of fluid volume balance, achievement of intact oral mucous membranes, maintenance of normal skin integrity, absence of corneal irritation, attainment of effective thermoregulation, and effective urinary elimination. Additional goals include bowel continence, accurate perception of environmental stimuli, maintenance of intact family or support system, and absence of complications (Rice et al., 2005).

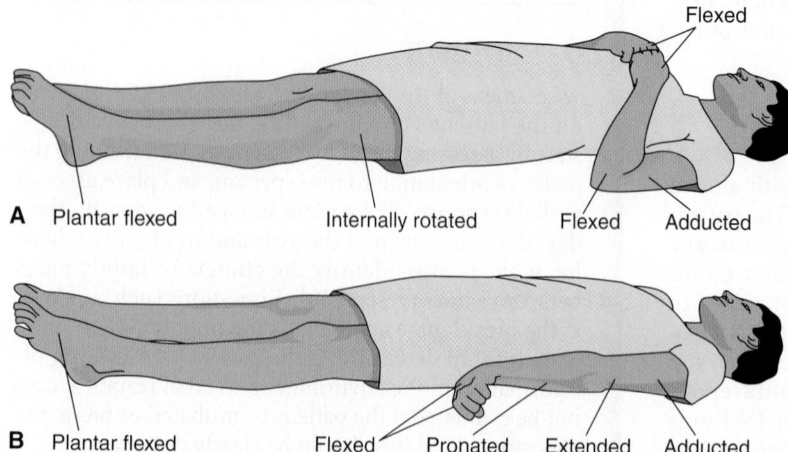

FIGURE 61-1. Abnormal posture response to stimuli. **(A)** Decorticate posturing, involving adduction and flexion of the upper extremities, internal rotation of the lower extremities, and plantar flexion of the feet. **(B)** Decerebrate posturing, involving extension and outward rotation of upper extremities and plantar flexion of the feet.

TABLE 61-1 Nursing Assessment of the Unconscious Patient

Examination	Clinical Assessment	Clinical Significance
Level of responsiveness or consciousness	Eye opening; verbal and motor responses; pupils (size, equality, reaction to light)	Obeying commands is a favorable response and demonstrates a return to consciousness.
Pattern of respiration	Respiratory pattern	Disturbances of respiratory center of brain may result in various respiratory patterns.
	Cheyne-Stokes respiration	Suggests lesions deep in both hemispheres; area of basal ganglia and upper brain stem
	Hyperventilation	Suggests onset of metabolic problem or brain stem damage
	Ataxic respiration with irregularity in depth/rate	Ominous sign of damage to medullary center
Eyes		
Pupils (size, equality, reaction to light)	Equal, normally reactive pupils	Suggests that coma is toxic or metabolic in origin
	Equal or unequal diameter	Helps determine location of lesion
	Progressive dilation	Indicates increasing intracranial pressure
	Fixed dilated pupils	Indicates injury at level of midbrain
Eye movements	Normally, eyes should move from side to side.	Functional and structural integrity of brain stem is assessed by inspection of extraocular movements; usually absent in deep coma.
Corneal reflex	When cornea is touched with a wisp of clean cotton, blink response is normal.	Tests cranial nerves V and VII; helps determine location of lesion if unilateral; absent in deep coma
Facial symmetry	Asymmetry (sagging, decrease in wrinkles)	Sign of paralysis
Swallowing reflex	Drooling versus spontaneous swallowing	Absent in coma Paralysis of cranial nerves X and XII
Neck	Stiff neck	Subarachnoid hemorrhage, meningitis
	Absence of spontaneous neck movement	Fracture or dislocation of cervical spine
Response of extremity to noxious stimuli	Firm pressure on a joint of the upper and lower extremity	Asymmetric response in paralysis
	Observe spontaneous movements.	Absent in deep coma
Deep tendon reflexes	Tap patellar and biceps tendons.	Brisk response may have localizing value Asymmetric response in paralysis Absent in deep coma
Pathologic reflexes	Firm pressure with blunt object on sole of foot, moving along lateral margin and crossing to the ball of foot	Flexion of the toes, especially the great toe, is normal except in newborn Dorsiflexion of toes (especially great toe) indicates contralateral pathology of corticospinal tract (Babinski reflex) Helps determine location of lesion in brain

continued >

TABLE 61-1 Nursing Assessment of the Unconscious Patient (Continued)

Examination	Clinical Assessment	Clinical Significance
Abnormal posture	Observation for posturing (spontaneous or in response to noxious stimuli) Flaccidity with absence of motor response Decorticate posture (flexion and internal rotation of forearms and hands) Decerebrate posture (extension and external rotation)	Deep extensive brain lesion Seen with cerebral hemisphere pathology and in metabolic depression of brain function Decerebrate posturing indicates deeper and more severe dysfunction than does decorticate posturing; implies brain pathology; poor prognostic sign.

Because the unconscious patient's protective reflexes are impaired, the quality of nursing care provided literally may mean the difference between life and death. The nurse must assume responsibility for the patient until the basic reflexes (coughing, blinking, and swallowing) return and the patient becomes conscious and oriented. Therefore, the major nursing goal is to compensate for the absence of these protective reflexes.

Nursing Interventions

Maintaining the Airway

The most important consideration in managing the patient with altered LOC is to establish an adequate airway and ensure ventilation. Obstruction of the airway is a risk because the epiglottis and tongue may relax, occluding the oropharynx, or the patient may aspirate vomitus or nasopharyngeal secretions.

The accumulation of secretions in the pharynx presents a serious problem. Because the patient cannot swallow and lacks pharyngeal reflexes, these secretions must be removed to eliminate the danger of aspiration. Elevating the head of the bed to 30 degrees helps prevent aspiration. Positioning the patient in a lateral or semiprone position also helps, because it permits the jaw and tongue to fall forward, thus promoting drainage of secretions.

Positioning alone is not always adequate, however. Suctioning and oral hygiene may be required. Suctioning is performed to remove secretions from the posterior pharynx and upper trachea. Before and after suctioning, the patient is hyperoxygenated and adequately ventilated to prevent hypoxia (Hickey, 2003). In addition to these interventions, chest physiotherapy and postural drainage may be initiated to promote pulmonary hygiene, unless contraindicated by the patient's underlying condition. The chest should be auscultated at least every 8 hours to detect adventitious breath sounds or absence of breath sounds.

Despite these measures, or because of the severity of impairment, the patient with altered LOC often requires intubation and mechanical ventilation. Nursing actions for the mechanically ventilated patient include maintaining the patency of the endotracheal tube or tracheostomy, providing frequent oral care, monitoring arterial blood gas measurements, and maintaining ventilator settings (see Chapter 25).

NURSING ALERT

If the patient begins to emerge from unconsciousness, every measure that is available and appropriate for calming and quieting the patient should be used. Any form of restraint is likely to be countered with resistance, leading to self-injury or to a dangerous increase in ICP. Therefore, physical restraints should be avoided if possible; a written prescription must be obtained if their use is essential for the patient's well-being.

Protecting the Patient

For the protection of the patient, side rails are padded. Two rails are kept in the raised position during the day and three at night; however, raising all four side rails is considered a restraint by the Joint Commission on Accreditation of Healthcare Organizations. Care should be taken to prevent injury from invasive lines and equipment, and other potential sources of injury should be identified, such as restraints, tight dressings, environmental irritants, damp bedding or dressings, and tubes and drains.

Protection also includes protecting the patient's dignity during altered LOC. Simple measures such as providing privacy and speaking to the patient during nursing care activities preserve the patient's dignity. Not speaking negatively about the patient's condition or prognosis is also important, because patients in a light coma may be able to hear. The comatose patient has an increased need for advocacy, and the nurse is responsible for seeing that these advocacy needs are met (Hickey, 2003).

Maintaining Fluid Balance and Managing Nutritional Needs

Hydration status is assessed by examining tissue turgor and mucous membranes, assessing intake and output trends, and analyzing laboratory data. Fluid needs are met initially by administering the required IV fluids. However, IV solutions (and blood component therapy) for patients with intracranial conditions must be administered slowly. If they are administered too rapidly, they can increase ICP. The quantity of fluids administered may be restricted to minimize the possibility of cerebral edema.

If the patient does not recover quickly and sufficiently enough to take adequate fluids and calories by mouth, a feeding or gastrostomy tube will be inserted for the administration of fluids and enteral feedings (Dudek, 2006; Worthington, 2004).

Providing Mouth Care

The mouth is inspected for dryness, inflammation, and crusting. The unconscious patient requires conscientious oral care, because there is a risk of parotitis if the mouth is not kept scrupulously clean. The mouth is cleansed and rinsed carefully to remove secretions and crusts and to keep the mucous membranes moist. A thin coating of petrolatum on the lips prevents drying, cracking, and encrustations. If the patient has an endotracheal tube, the tube should be moved to the opposite side of the mouth daily to prevent ulceration of the mouth and lips.

Maintaining Skin and Joint Integrity

Preventing skin breakdown requires continuing nursing assessment and intervention. Special attention is given to unconscious patients, because they cannot respond to external stimuli. Assessment includes a regular schedule of turning to avoid pressure, which can cause breakdown and necrosis of the skin. Turning also provides kinesthetic (sensation of movement), proprioceptive (awareness of position), and vestibular (equilibrium) stimulation. After turning, the patient is carefully repositioned to prevent ischemic necrosis over pressure areas. Dragging or pulling the patient up in bed must be avoided, because this creates a shearing force and friction on the skin surface (see Chapter 11).

Maintaining correct body position is important; equally important is passive exercise of the extremities to prevent contractures. The use of splints or foam boots aids in the prevention of foot drop and eliminates the pressure of bedding on the toes. The use of trochanter rolls to support the hip joints keeps the legs in proper alignment. The arms are in abduction, the fingers lightly flexed, and the hands in slight supination. The heels of the feet are assessed for pressure areas. Specialty beds, such as fluidized or low-air-loss beds, may be used to decrease pressure on bony prominences (Hickey, 2003).

Preserving Corneal Integrity

Some unconscious patients have their eyes open and have inadequate or absent corneal reflexes. The cornea may become irritated, dried out, or scratched, leading to ulceration. The eyes may be cleansed with cotton balls moistened with sterile normal saline to remove debris and discharge (Hickey, 2003). If artificial tears are prescribed, they may be instilled every 2 hours. Periorbital edema (swelling around the eyes) often occurs after cranial surgery. Cold compresses may be prescribed, and care must be exerted to avoid contact with the cornea. Eye patches should be used cautiously because of the potential for corneal abrasion from contact with the patch.

Maintaining Body Temperature

High fever in the unconscious patient may be caused by infection of the respiratory or urinary tract, drug reactions, or damage to the hypothalamic temperature-regulating center. A slight elevation of temperature may be caused by dehydration. The environment can be adjusted, depending on the patient's condition, to promote a normal body temperature. If body temperature is elevated, a minimum amount of bedding—a sheet, small drape, or towel—is used. The room may be cooled to 18.3°C (65°F). However, if the patient is elderly and does not have an elevated temperature, a warmer environment is needed.

Because of damage to the temperature center in the brain or severe intracranial infection, unconscious patients often develop very high temperatures. Such temperature elevations must be controlled, because the increased metabolic demands of the brain can exceed cerebral circulation and oxygenation, resulting in cerebral deterioration (Diringer, 2004; Hickey, 2003). Persistent hyperthermia with no identified clinical source of infection indicates brain stem damage and a poor prognosis.

NURSING ALERT

The body temperature of an unconscious patient is never taken by mouth. Rectal or tympanic (if not contraindicated) temperature measurement is preferred to the less accurate axillary temperature.

Strategies for reducing fever include:

- Removing all bedding over the patient (with the possible exception of a light sheet or small drape)
- Administering acetaminophen as prescribed
- Giving cool sponge baths and allowing an electric fan to blow over the patient to increase surface cooling
- Using a hypothermia blanket
- Frequent temperature monitoring is indicated to assess the patient's response to the therapy and to prevent an excessive decrease in temperature and shivering.

Preventing Urinary Retention

The patient with an altered LOC is often incontinent or has urinary retention. The bladder is palpated or scanned at intervals to determine whether urinary retention is present, because a full bladder may be an overlooked cause of overflow incontinence. A portable bladder ultrasound instrument is a useful tool in bladder management and retraining programs (O'Farrell, Vandervoort, Bisnaire, et al., 2001).

If the patient is not voiding, an indwelling urinary catheter is inserted and connected to a closed drainage system. A catheter may also be inserted during the acute phase of illness to monitor urinary output. Because catheters are a major factor in causing urinary tract infection, the patient is observed for fever and cloudy urine. The area around the urethral orifice is inspected for drainage. The urinary catheter is usually removed if the patient has a stable cardiovascular system and if no diuresis, sepsis, or voiding dysfunction existed before the onset of coma. Although many unconscious patients urinate spontaneously after catheter removal, the bladder should be palpated or scanned with a portable ultrasound device periodically for urinary retention (O'Farrell et al., 2001). An intermittent catheterization program may be initiated to ensure complete emptying of the bladder at intervals, if indicated.

An external catheter (condom catheter) for the male patient and absorbent pads for the female patient can be used for unconscious patients who can urinate spontaneously although involuntarily. As soon as consciousness is regained, a bladder-training program is initiated (Hickey, 2003). The incontinent patient is monitored frequently for skin irritation and skin breakdown. Appropriate skin care is implemented to prevent these complications.

Promoting Bowel Function

The abdomen is assessed for distention by listening for bowel sounds and measuring the girth of the abdomen with a tape measure. There is a risk for diarrhea from infection, antibiotics, and hyperosmolar fluids. Frequent loose stools may also occur with fecal impaction. Commercial fecal collection bags are available for patients with fecal incontinence.

Immobility and lack of dietary fiber can cause constipation. The nurse monitors the number and consistency of bowel movements and performs a rectal examination for signs of fecal impaction. Stool softeners may be prescribed and can be administered with tube feedings. To facilitate bowel emptying, a glycerin suppository may be indicated. The patient may require an enema every other day to empty the lower colon.

Providing Sensory Stimulation

Once increased ICP is not a problem, sensory stimulation can help overcome the profound sensory deprivation of the unconscious patient. Efforts are made to restore the sense of daily rhythm by maintaining usual day and night patterns for activity and sleep. The nurse touches and talks to the patient and encourages family members and friends to do so. Communication is extremely important and includes touching the patient and spending enough time with the patient to become sensitive to his or her needs. It is also important to avoid making any negative comments about the patient's status or prognosis in the patient's presence.

The nurse orients the patient to time and place at least once every 8 hours. Sounds from the patient's usual environment may be introduced using a tape recorder. Family members can read to the patient from a favorite book and may suggest radio and television programs that the patient previously enjoyed as a means of enriching the environment and providing familiar input (Hickey, 2003).

When arousing from coma, many patients experience a period of agitation, indicating that they are becoming more aware of their surroundings but still cannot react or communicate in an appropriate fashion. Although this is disturbing for many family members, it is actually a positive clinical sign. At this time, it is necessary to minimize stimulation by limiting background noises, having only one person speak to the patient at a time, giving the patient a longer period of time to respond, and allowing for frequent rest or quiet times. After the patient has regained consciousness, videotaped family or social events may assist the patient in recognizing family and friends and allow him or her to experience missed events.

Various programs of structured sensory stimulation for patients with brain injury have been developed to improve outcomes. Although these are controversial programs with inconsistent results, some research supports the concept of providing structured stimulation (Davis & Gimenez, 2003).

Meeting the Family's Needs

The family of the patient with altered LOC may be thrown into a sudden state of crisis and go through the process of severe anxiety, denial, anger, remorse, grief, and reconciliation. Depending on the disorder that caused the altered LOC and the extent of the patient's recovery, the family may be unprepared for the changes in the cognitive and physical status of their loved one. If the patient has significant residual deficits, the family may require considerable time, assistance, and support to come to terms with these changes. To help family members mobilize resources and coping skills, the nurse reinforces and clarifies information about the patient's condition, permits the family to be involved in care, and listens to and encourages ventilation of feelings and concerns while supporting decision making about posthospitalization management and placement (Bond, Draeger, Mandleco, et al., 2003). Families may benefit from participation in support groups offered through the hospital, rehabilitation facility, or community organizations.

In some circumstances, the family may need to face the death of their loved one. The patient with a neurologic disorder is often pronounced brain dead before the heart stops beating. The term **brain death** describes irreversible loss of all functions of the entire brain, including the brain stem (Booth, Boone, Tomlinson, et al., 2004). The term may be misleading to the family because, although brain function has ceased, the patient appears to be alive, with the heart rate and blood pressure sustained by vasoactive medications and breathing continued by mechanical ventilation. When discussing a patient who is brain dead with family members, it is important to provide accurate, timely, understandable, and consistent information (Henneman & Karras, 2004). End-of-life care is discussed in Chapter 17.

Monitoring and Managing Potential Complications

Pneumonia, aspiration, and respiratory failure are potential complications in any patient who has a depressed LOC and who cannot protect the airway or turn, cough, and take deep breaths. The longer the period of unconsciousness, the greater the risk for pulmonary complications.

Vital signs and respiratory function are monitored closely to detect any signs of respiratory failure or distress. Total blood count and arterial blood gas measurements are assessed to determine whether there are adequate red blood cells to carry oxygen and whether ventilation is effective. Chest physiotherapy and suctioning are initiated to prevent respiratory complications such as pneumonia. If pneumonia develops, cultures are obtained to identify the organism so that appropriate antibiotics can be administered.

The patient with altered LOC is monitored closely for evidence of impaired skin integrity, and strategies to prevent skin breakdown and pressure ulcers are continued through all phases of care, including hospitalization, rehabilitation, and home care. Factors that contribute to impaired skin integrity (eg, incontinence, inadequate dietary intake, pressure on bony prominences, edema) are addressed. If pressure ulcers develop, strategies to promote healing are undertaken. Care is taken to prevent bacterial contamination of pressure ulcers, which may lead to sepsis and septic shock. Assessment and management of pressure ulcers are discussed in Chapter 11.

The patient should also be monitored for signs and symptoms of deep vein thrombosis (DVT). Patients who develop DVT are at risk for pulmonary embolism. Prophylaxis such as subcutaneous heparin or low-molecular-weight heparin (Fragmin, Orgaran) should be prescribed if not contraindicated (Kurtoglu, Yanar, Bilsel, et al., 2004). Thigh-high elastic compression stockings or pneumatic compression devices should also be prescribed to reduce the risk for clot formation. The nurse observes for signs and symptoms of DVT.

Evaluation

Expected Patient Outcomes

Expected patient outcomes may include the following:

1. Maintains clear airway and demonstrates appropriate breath sounds
2. Experiences no injuries
3. Attains or maintains adequate fluid balance
   a. Has no clinical signs or symptoms of dehydration
   b. Demonstrates normal range of serum electrolytes
   c. Has no clinical signs or symptoms of overhydration
4. Achieves healthy oral mucous membranes
5. Maintains normal skin integrity
6. Has no corneal irritation
7. Attains or maintains thermoregulation
8. Has no urinary retention
9. Has no diarrhea or fecal impaction
10. Receives appropriate sensory stimulation
11. Family members cope with crisis
    a. Verbalize fears and concerns
    b. Participate in patient's care and provide sensory stimulation by talking and touching
12. Patient is free of complications
    a. Has arterial blood gas values or O_2 saturation levels within normal range
    b. Displays no signs or symptoms of pneumonia
    c. Exhibits intact skin over pressure areas
    d. Does not develop DVT or pulmonary embolism (PE)

Increased Intracranial Pressure

The rigid cranial vault contains brain tissue (1400 g), blood (75 mL), and CSF (75 mL). The volume and pressure of these three components are usually in a state of equilibrium and produce the ICP. ICP is usually measured in the lateral ventricles, with the normal pressure being 10 to 20 mm Hg (Hickey, 2003).

The **Monro-Kellie hypothesis** states that, because of the limited space for expansion within the skull, an increase in any one of the components causes a change in the volume of the others. Because brain tissue has limited space to expand, compensation typically is accomplished by displacing or shifting CSF, increasing the absorption or diminishing the production of CSF, or decreasing cerebral blood volume. Without such changes, ICP will begin to rise. Under normal circumstances, minor changes in blood volume and CSF volume occur constantly due to alterations in intrathoracic pressure (coughing, sneezing, straining), posture, blood pressure, and systemic oxygen and carbon dioxide levels (Bader & Littlejohns, 2004; Hickey, 2003).

Pathophysiology

Increased ICP affects many patients with acute neurologic conditions. This is because pathologic conditions alter the relationship between intracranial volume and ICP. Although elevated ICP is most commonly associated with head injury, it also may be seen as a secondary effect in other conditions, such as brain tumors, subarachnoid hemorrhage, and toxic and viral encephalopathies. Increased ICP from any cause decreases cerebral perfusion, stimulates further swelling (edema), and may shift brain tissue through openings in the rigid dura, resulting in **herniation**, a dire and frequently fatal event.

Decreased Cerebral Blood Flow

Increased ICP may significantly reduce cerebral blood flow, resulting in ischemia and cell death. In the early stages of cerebral ischemia, the vasomotor centers are stimulated and the systemic pressure rises to maintain cerebral blood flow.

Usually, this is accompanied by a slow bounding pulse and respiratory irregularities. These changes in blood pressure, pulse, and respiration are important clinically because they suggest increased ICP.

The concentration of carbon dioxide in the blood and in the brain tissue also plays a role in the regulation of cerebral blood flow. An increase in carbon dioxide partial pressure ($PaCO_2$) causes cerebral vasodilation, leading to increased cerebral blood flow and increased ICP. A decrease in $PaCO_2$ has a vasoconstrictive effect, limiting blood flow to the brain (Rice et al., 2005). Decreased venous outflow may also increase cerebral blood volume, thus raising ICP.

Cerebral Edema

Cerebral edema or swelling is defined as an abnormal accumulation of water or fluid in the intracellular space, extracellular space, or both, associated with an increase in the volume of brain tissue. Edema can occur in the gray, white, or interstitial matter. As brain tissue swells within the rigid skull, several mechanisms attempt to compensate for the increasing ICP. These compensatory mechanisms include autoregulation and decreased production and flow of CSF. **Autoregulation** refers to the brain's ability to change the diameter of its blood vessels automatically to maintain a constant cerebral blood flow during alterations in systemic blood pressure. This mechanism can be impaired in patients who are experiencing a pathologic and sustained increase in ICP.

Cerebral Response to Increased Intracranial Pressure

As ICP rises, compensatory mechanisms in the brain work to maintain blood flow and prevent tissue damage. The brain can maintain a steady perfusion pressure if the arterial systolic blood pressure is 50 to 150 mm Hg and the ICP is less than 40 mm Hg. Changes in ICP are closely linked with cerebral perfusion pressure (CPP). The CPP is calculated by subtracting the ICP from the mean arterial pressure. For example, if the mean arterial pressure is 100 mm Hg and the ICP is 15 mm Hg, then the CPP is 85 mm Hg. The normal CPP is 70 to 100 mm Hg (Hickey, 2003). As ICP rises and the autoregulatory mechanism of the brain is overwhelmed, the CPP can increase to greater than 100 mm Hg or decrease to less than 50 mm Hg. Patients with a CPP of less than 50 mm Hg experience irreversible neurologic damage. Therefore, the CPP must be maintained at 70 to 80 mm Hg to ensure adequate blood flow to the brain. If ICP is equal to mean arterial pressure, cerebral circulation ceases (Rice et al., 2005).

A clinical phenomenon known as the **Cushing's response** (or Cushing's reflex) is seen when cerebral blood flow decreases significantly. When ischemic, the vasomotor center triggers an increase in arterial pressure in an effort to overcome the increased ICP. A sympathetically mediated response causes an increase in the systolic blood pressure with a widening of the pulse pressure and cardiac slowing. This response is seen clinically as an increase in systolic blood pressure, widening of the pulse pressure, and reflex slowing of the heart rate. It is a late sign requiring immediate intervention; however, perfusion may be recoverable if the Cushing's response is treated rapidly.

At a certain point, the brain's ability to autoregulate becomes ineffective and decompensation (ischemia and infarction) begins. When this occurs, the patient exhibits significant changes in mental status and vital signs. The bradycardia, hypertension, and bradypnea associated with this deterioration are known as **Cushing's triad**, a grave sign. At this point, herniation of the brain stem and occlusion of the cerebral blood flow occur if therapeutic intervention is not initiated. Herniation refers to the shifting of brain tissue from an area of high pressure to an area of lower pressure (Fig. 61-2). The herniated tissue exerts pressure on the brain area into which it has shifted, which interferes with the blood supply in that area. Cessation of cerebral blood flow results in cerebral ischemia, infarction, and brain death.

Clinical Manifestations

If ICP increases to the point at which the brain's ability to adjust has reached its limits, neural function is impaired; this may be manifested at first by clinical changes in LOC and later by abnormal respiratory and vasomotor responses.

NURSING ALERT

The earliest sign of increasing ICP is a change in LOC. Slowing of speech and delay in response to verbal suggestions are other early indicators.

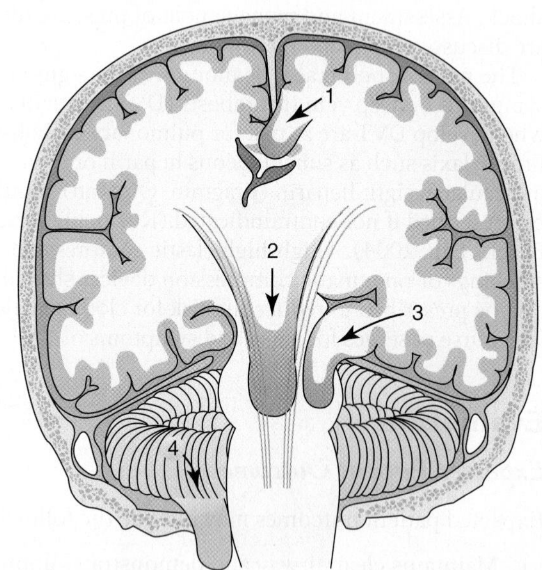

FIGURE 61-2. Brain with intracranial shifts from supratentorial lesions. (1) Herniation of the cingulate gyrus under the falx cerebri. (2) Central transtentorial herniation. (3) Uncal herniation of the temporal lobe into the tentorial notch. (4) Infratentorial herniation of the cerebral tonsils. Courtesy of Carole Hilmer, C.M.I. Reprinted from Porth, C.M. (2005). *Pathophysiology: Concepts of altered health states* (7th ed.). Philadelphia: Lippincott Williams & Wilkins.

Any sudden change in the patient's condition, such as restlessness (without apparent cause), confusion, or increasing drowsiness, has neurologic significance. These signs may result from compression of the brain due to swelling from hemorrhage or edema, an expanding intracranial lesion (hematoma or tumor), or a combination of both.

As ICP increases, the patient becomes stuporous, reacting only to loud or painful stimuli. At this stage, serious impairment of brain circulation is probably taking place, and immediate intervention is required. As neurologic function deteriorates further, the patient becomes comatose and exhibits abnormal motor responses in the form of **decortication** (abnormal flexion of the upper extremities and extension of the lower extremities), **decerebration** (extreme extension of the upper and lower extremities), or flaccidity (see Fig. 61-1). If the coma is profound, with the pupils dilated and fixed and respirations impaired or absent, death is usually inevitable.

Assessment and Diagnostic Findings

The diagnostic studies used to determine the underlying cause of increased ICP are discussed in detail in Chapter 60. The most common diagnostic tests are CT scanning and MRI. The patient may also undergo cerebral angiography, PET, or SPECT. Transcranial Doppler studies provide information about cerebral blood flow. The patient with increased ICP may also undergo electrophysiologic monitoring to observe cerebral blood flow indirectly. Evoked potential monitoring measures the electrical potentials produced by nerve tissue in response to external stimulation (auditory, visual, or sensory). Lumbar puncture is avoided in patients with increased ICP, because the sudden release of pressure in the lumbar area can cause the brain to herniate (Bader & Littlejohns, 2004). (See Chapter 60 for further discussion of lumbar puncture and other diagnostic tests.)

Complications

Complications of increased ICP include brain stem herniation, diabetes insipidus, and syndrome of inappropriate antidiuretic hormone (SIADH).

Brain stem herniation results from an excessive increase in ICP in which the pressure builds in the cranial vault and the brain tissue presses down on the brain stem. This increasing pressure on the brain stem results in cessation of blood flow to the brain, leading to irreversible brain anoxia and brain death.

Diabetes insipidus is the result of decreased secretion of antidiuretic hormone (ADH). The patient has excessive urine output, decreased urine osmolality, and serum hyperosmolarity (Suarez, 2004). Therapy consists of administration of fluids, electrolyte replacement, and vasopressin (desmopressin, DDAVP) therapy. Diabetes insipidus is discussed in Chapters 14 and 42.

SIADH is the result of increased secretion of ADH. The patient becomes volume-overloaded, urine output diminishes, and serum sodium concentration becomes dilute. Treatment of SIADH includes fluid restriction (less than 800 mL/day with no free water), which is usually sufficient to correct the hyponatremia. Severe cases call for judicious administration of a 3% hypertonic saline solution (Ropper et al., 2004). The change in serum sodium concentration should not exceed a correction rate of approximately 1.3 mEq/L/hour. Rapid correction of sodium predisposes the patient to central pontine myelinolysis, a disorder in which the pontine white matter becomes demyelinated; this results in tetraplegia with cranial nerve deficits (Suarez, 2004). Patients with chronic SIADH may respond to lithium carbonate or demeclocycline, both of which act on the renal collecting tubule to block the action of ADH and increase free water excretion (Bader & Littlejohns, 2004). Further discussion of SIADH is presented in Chapters 14 and 42.

Medical Management

Increased ICP is a true emergency and must be treated promptly. Invasive monitoring of ICP is an important component of management. Immediate management to relieve increased ICP requires decreasing cerebral edema, lowering the volume of CSF, or decreasing cerebral blood volume while maintaining cerebral perfusion (Rice et al., 2005). These goals are accomplished by administering osmotic diuretics, restricting fluids, draining CSF, controlling fever, maintaining systemic blood pressure and oxygenation, and reducing cellular metabolic demands. Corticosteroids are not recommended in cases of increased ICP resulting from traumatic brain injury. Judicious use of hyperventilation is recommended only if the ICP is refractory to other measures and only for a short duration (Brain Trauma Foundation, 2003).

Monitoring Intracranial Pressure and Cerebral Oxygenation

The purposes of ICP monitoring are to identify increased pressure early in its course (before cerebral damage occurs), to quantify the degree of elevation, to initiate appropriate treatment, to provide access to CSF for sampling and drainage, and to evaluate the effectiveness of treatment. ICP can be monitored with the use of an intraventricular catheter (ventriculostomy), a subarachnoid bolt, an epidural or subdural catheter, or a fiberoptic transducer-tipped catheter placed in the subdural space or in the ventricle (Fig. 61-3).

When a **ventriculostomy** or ventricular catheter monitoring device is used for monitoring ICP, a fine-bore catheter is inserted into a lateral ventricle, preferably in the nondominant hemisphere of the brain (Hickey, 2003). The catheter is connected by a fluid-filled system to a transducer, which records the pressure in the form of an electrical impulse. In addition to obtaining continuous ICP recordings, the ventricular catheter allows CSF to drain, particularly during acute increases in pressure. The ventriculostomy can also be used to drain blood from the ventricle. Continuous drainage of CSF under pressure control is an effective method of treating intracranial hypertension.

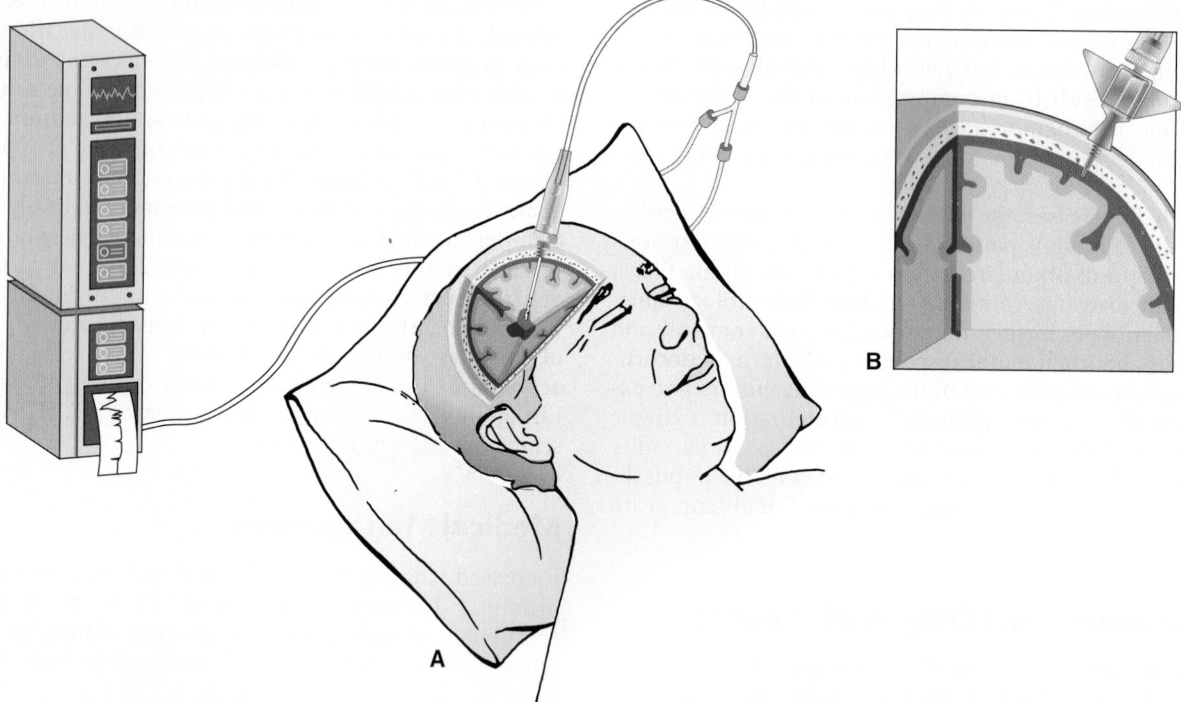

FIGURE 61-3. ICP monitoring. A fiberoptic, transducer-tipped device placed in (**A**) the ventricle or (**B**) the subarachnoid space. These devices connect to a pressure transducer and a display system.

Another advantage of a ventricular catheter is access for the intraventricular administration of medications and the occasional instillation of air or a contrast agent for ventriculography. Complications associated with its use include infection, meningitis, ventricular collapse, occlusion of the catheter by brain tissue or blood, and problems with the monitoring system (Fukunaga, Naritaka, Fukaya, et al., 2004; Rice et al., 2005).

The **subarachnoid screw or bolt** is a hollow device that is inserted through the skull and dura mater into the cranial subarachnoid space (Hickey, 2003). It has the advantage of not requiring a ventricular puncture. The subarachnoid screw is attached to a pressure transducer, and the output is recorded on an oscilloscope. The hollow screw technique also has the advantage of avoiding complications from brain shift and small ventricle size. Complications include infection and blockage of the screw by clot or brain tissue, which leads to a loss of pressure tracing and a decrease in accuracy at high ICP readings.

An **epidural monitor** uses a pneumatic flow sensor and functions without electricity. The epidural ICP monitoring system has a low incidence of infection and complications and appears to read pressures accurately. Calibration of the system is maintained automatically, and abnormal pressure waves trigger an alarm system. One disadvantage of the epidural catheter is the inability to withdraw CSF for analysis.

A **fiberoptic monitor**, or transducer-tipped catheter, is an alternative to standard intraventricular, subarachnoid, and subdural systems (Hickey, 2003; Rice et al., 2005). The miniature transducer reflects pressure changes, which are converted to electrical signals in an amplifier and displayed on a digital monitor. The catheter can be inserted into the ventricle, subarachnoid space, subdural space, or brain parenchyma or under a bone flap. If inserted into the ventricle, it can also be used in conjunction with a CSF drainage device.

INTERPRETING INTRACRANIAL PRESSURE WAVEFORMS

Waves of high pressure and troughs of relatively normal pressure indicate changes in ICP. Waveforms are captured and recorded on an oscilloscope. These waves have been classified as A waves (plateau waves), B waves, and C waves (Fig. 61-4). The plateau waves (A waves) are transient, paroxysmal, recurring elevations of ICP that may last 5 to 20 minutes and range in amplitude from 50 to 100 mm Hg (AANN, 2005; Hickey, 2003). Plateau waves have clinical significance and indicate changes in vascular volume within the intracranial compartment that are beginning to compromise cerebral perfusion. The A waves may increase in amplitude and frequency, reflecting cerebral ischemia and brain damage that can occur before overt signs and symptoms of raised ICP are seen clinically. B waves are shorter (30 seconds to 2 minutes) and have smaller amplitude (up to 50 mm Hg). They have less clinical significance, but if seen in a series in a patient with depressed consciousness, they may precede the appearance of A waves. B waves may be seen in patients with intracranial hypertension and decreased intracranial compliance. C waves are small, rhythmic oscillations with frequencies of approximately six per minute. They appear to be related to rhythmic variations of the systemic arterial blood pres-

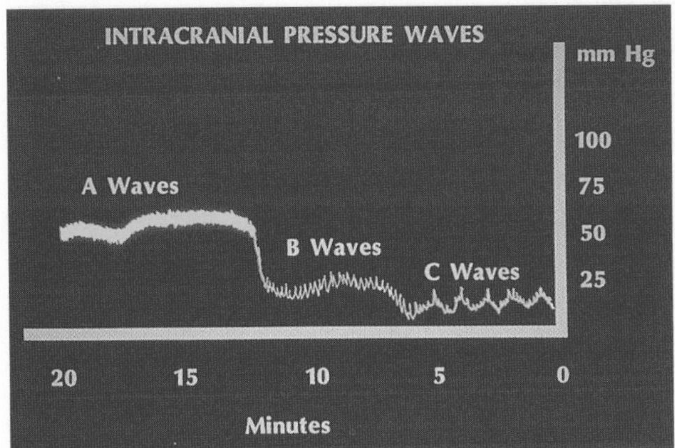

FIGURE 61-4. Intracranial pressure waves. Composite diagram of A (plateau) waves, which indicate cerebral ischemia; B waves, which indicate intracranial hypertension and variations in the respiratory cycle; and C waves, which relate to variations in systemic arterial pressure and respirations.

sure and respirations. The clinical significance of C waves is unknown (Hickey, 2003).

NEW TRENDS IN NEUROLOGIC MONITORING

New trends in neurologic monitoring include **microdialysis** of the patient with a brain injury (Nelson, Bellander, MacCallum, et al., 2004). Cortical probes are placed near the injured area and are used to measure levels of glutamate, lactate, pyruvate, and glucose, substances that reflect the metabolic function of the brain. Some researchers theorize that direct measurements of glucose and energy byproducts in the brain will lead to better management of these patients and, ultimately, to improved outcomes.

An additional new trend is monitoring of cerebral oxygenation through monitoring of the oxygen saturation in the jugular venous bulb ($SjvO_2$) or via a catheter in the brain. Cerebral oxygenation is thought to be important, because changes in cerebral perfusion may reflect an increase in ICP (Bader, Littlejohns & March, 2003). Readings taken from a catheter residing in the jugular outflow tract allow for a comparison of arterial and venous oxygen saturation, and the balance of cerebral oxygen supply and demand is demonstrated. Venous jugular desaturations can reflect early cerebral ischemia, alerting the clinician before an increase in ICP occurs. Minimizing cerebral desaturations can potentially improve outcomes (Bader et al., 2003; Stevens, 2004; Stocchetti, Canavesi, Magnoni, et al., 2004). This type of monitoring is now widely available and has been successfully used to identify secondary brain insults. A limiting factor is that this saturation reflects overall perfusion of the brain rather than that of a specific injured area (Suarez, 2004).

Another method of measuring cerebral oxygenation and temperature is by inserting a catheter in brain white matter (Bader et al., 2003). The most common system is LICOX (manufactured by Integra NeuroSciences, Plainsboro, NJ; Fig. 61-5). The system includes a monitor with a screen for the display of oxygen and temperature values and cables that connect to the monitoring probes in the brain (Bader et al., 2003).

Decreasing Cerebral Edema

Osmotic diuretics such as mannitol may be administered to dehydrate the brain tissue and reduce cerebral edema. They act by drawing water across intact membranes, thereby reducing the volume of the brain and extracellular fluid. An indwelling urinary catheter is usually inserted to monitor urinary output and to manage the resulting diuresis. If the patient is receiving osmotic diuretics, serum osmolality should be determined to assess hydration status. If a brain tumor is the cause of the increased ICP, corticosteroids (eg, dexamethasone) help reduce the edema surrounding the tumor.

Another method for decreasing cerebral edema is fluid restriction (Hickey, 2003). Limiting overall fluid intake leads to dehydration and hemoconcentration, which draws fluid across the osmotic gradient and decreases cerebral edema. Conversely, overhydration of the patient with increased ICP is avoided, because it increases cerebral edema.

Researchers have long hypothesized that lowering body temperature would decrease cerebral edema by reducing the oxygen and metabolic requirements of the brain, thus protecting the brain from continued ischemia. If body metabolism can be reduced by lowering the body temperature, the collateral circulation in the brain may be able to provide an adequate blood supply to the brain (Polderman, 2004). The effect of hypothermia on ICP requires more study; thus far, induced hypothermia has not consistently been shown to be beneficial for patients with brain injury. Inducing and maintaining hypothermia is a major clinical treatment and requires knowledge and skilled nursing observation and management (Alderson, Gadkary & Signorini, 2004).

Maintaining Cerebral Perfusion

Cardiac output may be manipulated to provide adequate perfusion to the brain. Improvements in cardiac output are made using fluid volume and inotropic agents such as dobutamine hydrochloride (Dobutrex) and norepinephrine bitartrate (Levophed). The effectiveness of the cardiac output is reflected in the CPP, which is maintained at greater than 70 mm Hg (Johnston, Steiner, Coles, et al., 2005). A lower CPP indicates that the cardiac output is insufficient to maintain adequate cerebral perfusion. $SjvO_2$ and LICOX, described earlier, assist in monitoring cerebral perfusion.

Reducing Cerebrospinal Fluid and Intracranial Blood Volume

CSF drainage is frequently performed, because the removal of CSF with a ventriculostomy drain can dramatically reduce ICP and restore CPP. Caution should be used in draining CSF, however, because excessive drainage may result in collapse of the ventricles and herniation.

Hyperventilation, which results in vasoconstriction, was previously used in patients with increased ICP. Recent research has demonstrated that hyperventilation may not be as beneficial as once thought (Brain Trauma Foundation, 2003). The reduction in the $PaCO_2$ may result in hypoxia, ischemia,

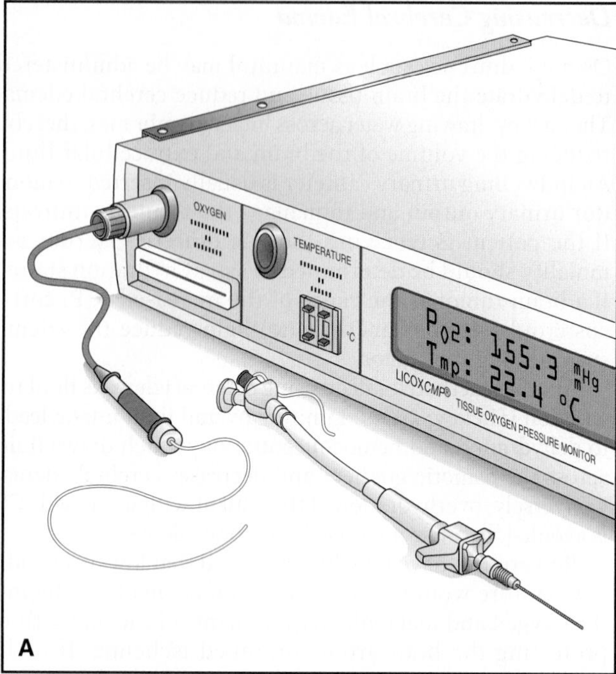

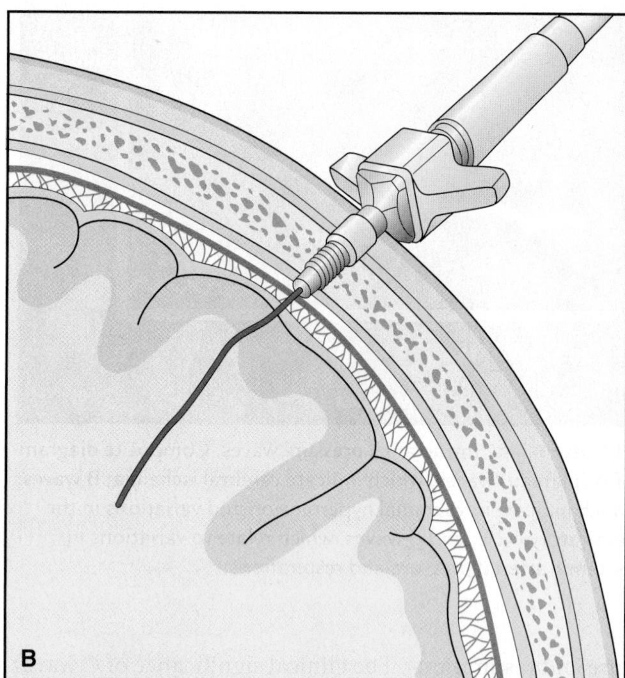

FIGURE 61-5. LICOX catheter system. (**A**) The brain tissue oxygen catheter and monitor. (**B**) Placement of the catheter in brain white matter. Redrawn with permission of Integra NeuroSciences, Plainsboro, NJ.

and an increase in cerebral lactate levels. Maintaining the $PaCO_2$ at 30 to 35 mm Hg may prove beneficial (Hickey, 2003). Hyperventilation is an option for patients whose ICP is unresponsive to conventional therapies, but it should be used judiciously.

Controlling Fever

Preventing a temperature elevation is critical, because fever increases cerebral metabolism and the rate at which cerebral edema forms. Strategies to reduce body temperature include administration of antipyretic medications, as prescribed, and use of a hypothermia blanket. Additional strategies for reducing fever were previously discussed in the Nursing Process section on altered LOC. The patient's temperature is monitored closely, and the patient is observed for shivering, which should be avoided because it is associated with increased oxygen consumption, increased levels of circulating catecholamines, and increased vasoconstriction (Diringer, 2004).

Maintaining Oxygenation

Arterial blood gases and pulse oximetry are monitored to ensure that systemic oxygenation remains optimal. Hemoglobin saturation can also be optimized to provide oxygen more efficiently at the cellular level.

Reducing Metabolic Demands

Cellular metabolic demands may be reduced through the administration of high doses of barbiturates if the patient is unresponsive to conventional treatment. The mechanism by which barbiturates decrease ICP and protect the brain is uncertain, but the resultant comatose state is thought to reduce the metabolic requirements of the brain, thus providing some cerebral protection (Censullo & Sebastian, 2003).

Another method of reducing cellular metabolic demand and improving oxygenation is the administration of pharmacologic paralyzing agents such as propofol (Diprivan). The patient who receives these agents cannot move; this decreases the metabolic demands and results in a decrease in cerebral oxygen demand. Because the patient cannot respond or report pain, sedation and analgesia must be provided, because the paralyzing agents do not provide either.

Patients receiving high doses of barbiturates or pharmacologic paralyzing agents require continuous cardiac monitoring, endotracheal intubation, mechanical ventilation, ICP monitoring, and arterial pressure monitoring. Pentobarbital (Nembutal), thiopental (Pentothal), and propofol (Diprivan) are the most common agents used for barbiturate or paralytic therapy (Bader & Littlejohns, 2004). Serum barbiturate levels must be routinely monitored (Hickey, 2003).

The ability to perform serial neurologic assessments is lost with the use of barbiturates or paralyzing agents. Therefore, other monitoring tools are needed to assess the patient's status and response to therapy. Important parameters that must be assessed include ICP, blood pressure, heart rate, respiratory rate, and response to ventilator therapy (eg, bucking the ventilator). The level of pharmacologic paralysis is adjusted based on serum levels of the medications administered and the assessed parameters. Potential complications include hypotension due to decreased sympathetic tone and myocardial depression (Bader & Littlejohns, 2004).

Nursing Process

The Patient With Increased Intracranial Pressure

Assessment

Initial assessment of the patient with increased ICP includes obtaining a history of events leading to the present illness and the pertinent past medical history. It is usually necessary to obtain this information from family or friends. The neurologic examination should be as complete as the patient's condition allows. It includes an evaluation of mental status, LOC, cranial nerve function, cerebellar function (balance and coordination), reflexes, and motor and sensory function. Because the patient is critically ill, ongoing assessment is more focused, including pupil checks, assessment of selected cranial nerves, frequent measurements of vital signs and ICP, and use of the Glasgow Coma Scale. Assessment of the patient with altered LOC is summarized in Table 61-1.

Diagnosis

Nursing Diagnoses

Based on the assessment data, the major nursing diagnoses for patients with increased ICP include the following:

- Ineffective airway clearance related to diminished protective reflexes (cough, gag)
- Ineffective breathing patterns related to neurologic dysfunction (brain stem compression, structural displacement)
- Ineffective cerebral tissue perfusion related to the effects of increased ICP
- Deficient fluid volume related to fluid restriction
- Risk for infection related to ICP monitoring system (fiberoptic or intraventricular catheter)

Other relevant nursing diagnoses are included in the section on altered LOC.

Collaborative Problems/ Potential Complications

Based on the assessment data, potential complications include:

- Brain stem herniation
- Diabetes insipidus
- SIADH

Planning and Goals

The goals for the patient include maintenance of a patent airway, normalization of respiration, adequate cerebral tissue perfusion through reduction in ICP, restoration of fluid balance, absence of infection, and absence of complications.

Nursing Interventions

Maintaining a Patent Airway

The patency of the airway is assessed. Secretions that are obstructing the airway must be suctioned with care, because transient elevations of ICP occur with suctioning (Hickey, 2003). The patient is hyperoxygenated before and after suctioning to maintain adequate oxygenation. Hypoxia caused by poor oxygenation leads to cerebral ischemia and edema. Coughing is discouraged, because coughing and straining increase ICP. The lung fields are auscultated at least every 8 hours to determine the presence of adventitious sounds or any areas of congestion. Elevating the head of the bed may aid in clearing secretions and improve venous drainage of the brain.

Achieving an Adequate Breathing Pattern

The patient must be monitored constantly for respiratory irregularities. Increased pressure on the frontal lobes or deep midline structures may result in Cheyne-Stokes respirations, whereas pressure in the midbrain can cause hyperventilation. If the lower portion of the brain stem (the pons and medulla) is involved, respirations become irregular and eventually cease.

If hyperventilation therapy is deemed appropriate to reduce ICP (by causing cerebral vasoconstriction and a decrease in cerebral blood volume), the nurse collaborates with the respiratory therapist in monitoring the $PaCO_2$, which is usually maintained at 30 to 35 mm Hg (Hickey, 2003).

A neurologic observation record (Fig. 61-6) is maintained, and all observations are made in relation to the patient's baseline condition. Repeated assessments of the patient are made (sometimes minute by minute) so that improvement or deterioration may be noted immediately. If the patient's condition deteriorates, preparations are made for surgical intervention.

Optimizing Cerebral Tissue Perfusion

In addition to ongoing nursing assessment, strategies are initiated to reduce factors contributing to the elevation of ICP (Table 61-2).

Proper positioning helps to reduce ICP. The head is kept in a neutral (midline) position, maintained with the use of a cervical collar if necessary, to promote venous drainage. Elevation of the head is maintained at 0 to 60 degrees to aid in venous drainage unless otherwise prescribed (Fan, 2004). Extreme rotation of the neck and flexion of the neck are avoided, because compression or distortion of the jugular veins increases ICP. Extreme hip flexion is also avoided, because this position causes an increase in intra-abdominal and intrathoracic pressures, which can produce an increase in ICP. Relatively minor changes in position can significantly affect ICP (Fan, 2004). If monitoring reveals that

(text continues on page 2178)

NURSING NEUROLOGICAL CRITICAL CARE FLOWSHEET

ADDRESSOGRAPH

	Date												
	Time												
	Initials												
Level of orientation (✓)	Person												
	Place												
	Date and time												
	No orientation												
Awakens to (✓)	Voice												
	Touch												
	Noxious stimuli												
	Painful stimuli												
	No response												
Best verbal response (✓)	Clear and appropriate												
	Clear and inappropriate												
	Difficulty speaking*												
	Perseveration												
	Aphasic expressive (non-fluent)												
	Aphasic receptive (fluent)												
	Sounds no speech												
	No verbal response												
	ETT/TRACH												
Best motor response (✓)	Moves all extremities purposefully												
	Withdraws and lifts to painful stimuli												
	Moves to painful stimuli												
	Decorticates (spinal reflex)												
	Decerebrates (spinal reflex)												
	No motor response												
Best motor strength upper extremities (✓)	No drifts (R/L)	R L	R L	R L	R L	R L	R L	R L	R L	R L	R L	R L	R L
	Drift (R/L)	R L	R L	R L	R L	R L	R L	R L	R L	R L	R L	R L	R L
	Can only lift forearm (R/L)	R L	R L	R L	R L	R L	R L	R L	R L	R L	R L	R L	R L
	Trace movement of hand or arm (R/L)	R L	R L	R L	R L	R L	R L	R L	R L	R L	R L	R L	R L
	Trace movement of fingers only (R/L)	R L	R L	R L	R L	R L	R L	R L	R L	R L	R L	R L	R L
	No motor response (R/L)	R L	R L	R L	R L	R L	R L	R L	R L	R L	R L	R L	R L
Best strength lower extremities (✓)	Raises leg off bed (R/L)	R L	R L	R L	R L	R L	R L	R L	R L	R L	R L	R L	R L
	Drags heel on bed and lifts knee (R/L)	R L	R L	R L	R L	R L	R L	R L	R L	R L	R L	R L	R L
	Trace movement of foot or leg (R/L)	R L	R L	R L	R L	R L	R L	R L	R L	R L	R L	R L	R L
	Trace movement of toes only (R/L)	R L	R L	R L	R L	R L	R L	R L	R L	R L	R L	R L	R L
	No response (R/L)	R L	R L	R L	R L	R L	R L	R L	R L	R L	R L	R L	R L
Seizure activity (✓)	No seizure activity												
	With loss of consciousness*												
	Without loss of consciousness*												
Ataxia (✓)	Gross ataxia												
	Fine motor ataxia												
	Does not apply												
ICP monitoring	Ventriculostomy mL												
	ICP mm Hg												
	Not applicable												

***= FURTHER DOCUMENTATION IS REQUIRED TO VALIDATE ASSESSMENT**

FIGURE 61-6. A neurologic assessment flow sheet.

PUPIL GAUGE (mm)

2 3 4 5 6

7 8 9

B=Brisk, S=Sluggish, F=Fixed

ADDRESSOGRAPH

	Date												
	Time												
	Initials												
Incision +/–	Dry and intact												
	Drainage												
Pupils: refer to above gauge (✓) (+)=Present (–)=Absent	Size (R/L)	R L	R L	R L	R L	R L	R L	R L	R L	R L	R L	R L	R L
	Regular (R/L)	R L	R L	R L	R L	R L	R L	R L	R L	R L	R L	R L	R L
	Irregular* (R/L)	R L	R L	R L	R L	R L	R L	R L	R L	R L	R L	R L	R L
	Reaction (R/L) (B) - (S) - (F)	R L	R L	R L	R L	R L	R L	R L	R L	R L	R L	R L	R L
	Ptosis (R/L) (+) (–)	R L	R L	R L	R L	R L	R L	R L	R L	R L	R L	R L	R L
	Gaze preference (R/L) (+)* (–)	R L	R L	R L	R L	R L	R L	R L	R L	R L	R L	R L	R L
Meningeal signs (+)=Present (–)=Absent	Headache												
	Nuchal rigidity												
	Photophobia												
Visual fields (+)=Present (–)=Absent* NA=Not applicable	Right upper outer												
	Right lower outer												
	Left upper outer												
	Left lower outer												
Nystagmus (+)=Present (–)=Absent	Lateral (R/L)	R L	R L	R L	R L	R L	R L	R L	R L	R L	R L	R L	R L
	Vertical (R/L)	R L	R L	R L	R L	R L	R L	R L	R L	R L	R L	R L	R L
Cranial nerves (+)=Present (–)=Absent	III, IV, VI, Extraocular movements												
	VII – Peripheral facial droop (R/L)	R L	R L	R L	R L	R L	R L	R L	R L	R L	R L	R L	R L
	XII – Tongue deviation (R/L)	R L	R L	R L	R L	R L	R L	R L	R L	R L	R L	R L	R L
	IX – Gag reflex												
	V, VII – Corneal reflex (R/L)	R L	R L	R L	R L	R L	R L	R L	R L	R L	R L	R L	R L
	X, IX – Cough reflex												
	Doll's eyes if appropriate												
Follows commands	Two step verbal command												
	One step verbal command												
	Unable to follow command												

***= FURTHER DOCUMENTATION IS REQUIRED TO VALIDATE ASSESSMENT**

Initials	Signature	Title	Initials	Signature	Title

FIGURE 61-6. Continued

TABLE 61-2 Increased Intracranial Pressure and Interventions

Factor	Physiology	Interventions	Rationale
Cerebral edema	Can be caused by contusion, tumor, or abscess; water intoxication (hypo-osmolality); alteration in the blood–brain barrier (protein leaks into the tissue, causing water to follow)	Administer osmotic diuretics as prescribed (monitor serum osmolality)	Promotes venous return
		Maintain head of bed elevated 30 degrees Maintain alignment of the head	Prevents impairment of venous return through the jugular veins
Hypoxia	A decrease in the PaO_2 causes cerebral vasodilation at <60 mm Hg.	Maintain PaO_2 greater than 60 mm Hg Maintain oxygen therapy Monitor arterial blood gas values Suction when needed Maintain a patent airway	Prevents hypoxia and vasodilation
Hypercapnia (elevated $PaCO_2$)	Causes vasodilation	Maintain $PaCO_2$ (normally 35–45 mm Hg) by establishing ventilation	Normalizing $PaCO_2$ minimizes vasodilation and thus reduces the cerebral blood volume
Impaired venous return	Increases the cerebral blood volume	Maintain head alignment Elevate head of bed 30 degrees	Hyperextension, rotation, or hyperflexion of the neck causes decreased venous return
Increase in intrathoracic or abdominal pressure	Increase in these pressures due to coughing, PEEP, Valsalva maneuver causes a decrease in venous return	Monitor arterial blood gas values and keep PEEP as low as possible Provide humidified oxygen	To keep secretions loose and easy to suction or expectorate
		Administer stool softeners as prescribed	Soft bowel movements will prevent straining or Valsalva maneuver

turning the patient raises ICP, rotating beds, turning sheets, and holding the patient's head during turning may minimize the stimuli that increase ICP.

The Valsalva maneuver, which can be produced by straining at defecation or even moving in bed, raises ICP and is to be avoided. Stool softeners may be prescribed. If the patient is alert and able to eat, a diet high in fiber may be indicated. Abdominal distention, which increases intra-abdominal and intrathoracic pressure and ICP, should be noted. Enemas and cathartics are avoided if possible. When moving or being turned in bed, the patient can be instructed to exhale (which opens the glottis) to avoid the Valsalva maneuver.

Mechanical ventilation presents unique problems for the patient with increased ICP. Before suctioning, the patient should be preoxygenated and briefly hyperventilated using 100% oxygen on the ventilator (Hickey, 2003). Suctioning should not last longer than 15 seconds. High levels of positive end-expiratory pressure (PEEP) are avoided, because they may decrease venous return to the heart and decrease venous drainage from the brain through increased intrathoracic pressure (Hickey, 2003).

Activities that increase ICP, as indicated by changes in waveforms, should be avoided if possible. Spacing of nursing interventions may prevent transient increases in ICP. During nursing interventions, the ICP should not increase more than 25 mm Hg, and it should return to baseline levels within 5 minutes. Patients with increased ICP should not demonstrate a significant increase in pressure or change in the ICP waveform. Patients with the potential for a significant increase in ICP may need sedation and a paralytic agent before initiation of nursing activities (Hickey, 2003).

Emotional stress and frequent arousal from sleep are avoided. A calm atmosphere is maintained. Environmental stimuli (eg, noise, conversation) should be minimal.

Maintaining Negative Fluid Balance

The administration of various osmotic and loop diuretics is part of the treatment protocol to reduce ICP. Corticosteroids may be used to reduce cerebral edema (except when it results from trauma), and fluids may be restricted (Brain Trauma Foundation, 2003). All of these treatment modalities promote dehydration.

Skin turgor, mucous membranes, urine output, and serum and urine osmolality are monitored to assess fluid status. If IV fluids are prescribed, the nurse ensures that they are administered at a slow to moderate rate with an IV infusion pump, to prevent too-rapid administration and avoid overhydration. For the patient receiving mannitol, the nurse observes for the possible development of heart failure and pulmonary edema, because the intent of treatment is to promote a shift of fluid from the intracellular compartment to the intravascular system, thus controlling cerebral edema.

For patients undergoing dehydrating procedures, vital signs, including blood pressure, must be monitored to assess fluid volume status. An indwelling urinary catheter is inserted to permit assessment of renal function and fluid status. During the acute phase, urine output is monitored hourly. An output greater than 250 mL/hour for 2 consecutive hours may indicate the onset of diabetes insipidus (Suarez, 2004). These patients also need careful oral hygiene, because mouth dryness occurs with dehydration. Frequently rinsing the mouth with nondrying solutions, lubricating the lips, and removing encrustations relieve dryness and promote comfort.

Preventing Infection

Risk for infection is greatest when ICP is monitored with an intraventricular catheter, and the risk of infection increases with the duration of the monitoring (Park, Garton, Kocan, et al., 2004). Most health care facilities have written protocols for managing these systems and maintaining their sterility; strict adherence to the protocols is essential.

Aseptic technique must be used when managing the system and changing the ventricular drainage bag. The drainage system is also checked for loose connections, because they can cause leakage and contamination of the CSF as well as inaccurate readings of ICP. The nurse observes the character of the CSF drainage and reports observations of increasing cloudiness or blood. The patient is monitored for signs and symptoms of meningitis: fever, chills, nuchal (neck) rigidity, and increasing or persistent headache. (See Chapter 64 for a discussion of meningitis.)

Monitoring and Managing Potential Complications

The primary complication of increased ICP is brain herniation resulting in death (see Fig. 61-2). Nursing management focuses on detecting early signs of increasing ICP, because medical interventions are usually ineffective once later signs develop. Frequent neurologic assessments and documentation and analysis of trends will reveal the subtle changes that may indicate increasing ICP.

DETECTING EARLY INDICATIONS OF INCREASING INTRACRANIAL PRESSURE

The nurse assesses for and immediately reports any of the following early signs or symptoms of increasing ICP:

- Disorientation, restlessness, increased respiratory effort, purposeless movements, and mental confusion; these are early clinical indications of increasing ICP because the brain cells responsible for cognition are extremely sensitive to decreased oxygenation
- Pupillary changes and impaired extraocular movements; these occur as the increasing pressure displaces the brain against the oculomotor and optic nerves (cranial nerves II, III, IV, and VI), which arise from the midbrain and brain stem (see Chapter 60)
- Weakness in one extremity or on one side of the body; this occurs as increasing ICP compresses the pyramidal tracts
- Headache that is constant, increasing in intensity, and aggravated by movement or straining; this occurs as increasing ICP causes pressure and stretching of venous and arterial vessels in the base of the brain

DETECTING LATER INDICATIONS OF INCREASING ICP

As ICP increases, the patient's condition worsens, as manifested by the following signs and symptoms:

- The LOC continues to deteriorate until the patient is comatose.
- The pulse rate and respiratory rate decrease or become erratic, and the blood pressure and temperature increase. The pulse pressure (the difference between the systolic and the diastolic pressures) widens. The pulse fluctuates rapidly, varying from bradycardia to tachycardia.
- Altered respiratory patterns develop, including Cheyne-Stokes breathing (rhythmic waxing and waning of rate and depth of respirations alternating with brief periods of apnea) and ataxic breathing (irregular breathing with a random sequence of deep and shallow breaths).
- Projectile vomiting may occur with increased pressure on the reflex center in the medulla.
- Hemiplegia or decorticate or decerebrate posturing may develop as pressure on the brain stem increases; bilateral flaccidity occurs before death.
- Loss of brain stem reflexes, including pupillary, corneal, gag, and swallowing reflexes, is an ominous sign of approaching death.

MONITORING INTRACRANIAL PRESSURE

Because clinical assessment is not always a reliable guide in recognizing increased ICP, especially in comatose patients, monitoring of ICP and cerebral oxygenation is an essential part of management (Hickey, 2003). ICP is monitored closely for continuous elevation or significant increase over baseline. The trend of ICP measurements over time is an important indication of the patient's underlying status. Vital signs are assessed when an increase in ICP is noted.

Strict aseptic technique is used when handling any part of the monitoring system. The insertion site is inspected for signs of infection. Temperature, pulse, and respirations are closely monitored for systemic signs of infection. All connections and stopcocks are checked for leaks, because even small leaks can distort pressure readings and lead to infection.

When ICP is monitored with a fluid system, the transducer is calibrated at a particular reference point, usually 2.5 cm (1 inch) above the ear with the patient in the supine position; this point corresponds to the level of the foramen of Monro (Fig. 61-7). CSF pressure readings depend on the patient's position. For subsequent pressure readings, the head should be in the same position relative to the transducer. Fiberoptic catheters are

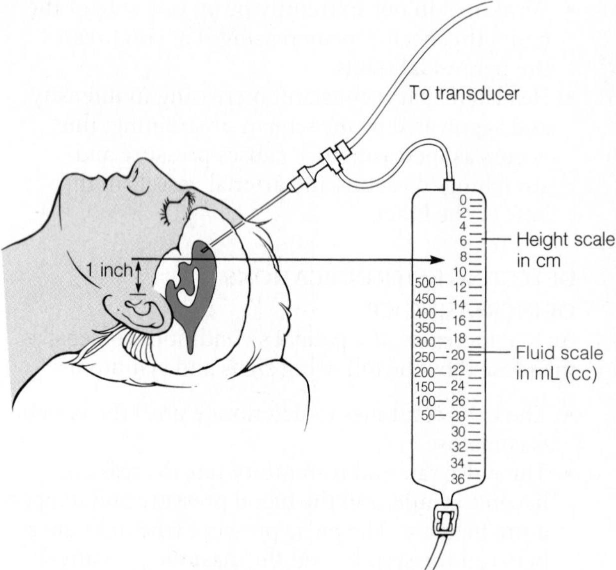

FIGURE 61-7. Location of the foramen of Monro for calibration of intracranial pressure monitoring system.

calibrated before insertion and do not require further referencing; they do not require the head of the bed to be at a specific position to obtain an accurate reading.

Whenever technology is associated with patient management, the nurse must be certain that the technological equipment is functioning properly. The most important concern, however, must be the patient who is attached to the equipment. The patient and family must be informed about the technology and the goals of its use. The patient's response is monitored, and appropriate comfort measures are implemented to ensure that the patient's stress is minimized.

ICP measurement is only one parameter; repeated neurologic checks and clinical examinations remain important measures. Astute observation, comparison of findings with previous observations, and interventions can assist in preventing life-threatening ICP elevations.

MONITORING FOR SECONDARY COMPLICATIONS

The nurse also assesses for complications of increased ICP, including diabetes insipidus and SIADH (see Chapters 14 and 42). Urine output should be monitored closely. Diabetes insipidus requires fluid and electrolyte replacement, along with the administration of vasopressin, to replace and slow the urine output. Serum electrolyte levels are monitored for imbalances. SIADH requires fluid restriction and monitoring of serum electrolyte levels.

Evaluation

Expected Patient Outcomes

Expected patient outcomes may include the following:

1. Maintains patent airway
2. Attains optimal breathing pattern
   a. Breathes in a regular pattern
   b. Attains or maintains arterial blood gas values within acceptable range
3. Demonstrates optimal cerebral tissue perfusion
   a. Increasingly oriented to time, place, and person
   b. Follows verbal commands; answers questions correctly
4. Attains desired fluid balance
   a. Maintains fluid restriction
   b. Demonstrates serum and urine osmolality values within acceptable range
5. Has no signs or symptoms of infection
   a. Has no fever
   b. Shows no signs of infection at arterial, IV, and urinary catheter sites
   c. Has no redness, swelling, or purulent drainage from invasive intracranial monitoring device
6. Absence of complications
   a. Has ICP values that remain within normal limits
   b. Demonstrates urine output and serum electrolyte levels within acceptable limits

Intracranial Surgery

A **craniotomy** involves opening the skull surgically to gain access to intracranial structures. This procedure is performed to remove a tumor, relieve elevated ICP, evacuate a blood clot, or control hemorrhage. The surgeon cuts the skull to create a bony flap, which can be repositioned after surgery and held in place by periosteal or wire sutures. One of two approaches through the skull is used: (1) above the tentorium (supratentorial craniotomy) into the supratentorial compartment, or (2) below the tentorium into the infratentorial (posterior fossa) compartment. A third approach, the **transsphenoidal** approach (through the mouth and nasal sinuses) is often used to gain access to the pituitary gland (Pertrovich, Jozsef, Yu, et al. 2003). Table 61-3 compares the three different surgical approaches: supratentorial, infratentorial, and transsphenoidal.

Alternatively, intracranial structures may be approached through burr holes (Fig. 61-8), which are circular openings made in the skull by either a hand drill or an automatic craniotome (which has a self-controlled system to stop the drill when the bone is penetrated). Burr holes are made as part of surgical treatment. They may be used to determine the presence of cerebral swelling and injury and the size and position of the ventricles. They are also a means of evacuating an intracranial hematoma or abscess and for making a bone flap in the skull that allows access to the ventricles for decompression, ventriculography, or shunting procedures. Other cranial procedures include **craniectomy** (excision of a portion of the skull) and cranioplasty (repair of a cranial defect using a plastic or metal plate).

Supratentorial and Infratentorial Approaches

Preoperative Management

Medical Management

Preoperative diagnostic procedures may include a CT scan to demonstrate the lesion and show the degree of surround-

TABLE 61-3 Comparison of Cranial Surgical Approaches

	Supratentorial	Infratentorial	Transsphenoidal
Site of Surgery	Above the tentorium	Below the tentorium, brain stem	Sella turcica
Incision Location	Incision is made above the area to be operated on; usually located behind the hairline.	Incision is made at the nape of the neck, around the occipital lobe.	Incision is made beneath the upper lip to gain access into the nasal cavity.
Selected Nursing Interventions	Maintain head of bed elevated 30–45 degrees, with neck in neutral alignment.	Maintain neck in straight alignment. Avoid flexion of the neck to prevent possible tearing of the suture line.	Maintain nasal packing in place and reinforce as needed. Instruct patient to avoid blowing the nose. Provide frequent oral care.
	Position patient on either side or back. (Avoid positioning patient on operative side if a large tumor has been removed.)	Position the patient on either side. (Check surgeon's preference for positioning of patient.)	Keep head of bed elevated to promote venous drainage and drainage from the surgical site.

ing brain edema, the ventricular size, and the displacement. An MRI scan provides information similar to that of a CT scan with improved tissue contrast, resolution, and anatomic definition and examines the lesion in multiple planes (Suarez, 2004). Cerebral angiography may be used to study a tumor's blood supply or obtain information about vascular lesions. Transcranial Doppler flow studies are used to evaluate the blood flow within intracranial blood vessels.

Most patients are prescribed an antiseizure medication such as phenytoin (Dilantin) or a phenytoin metabolite (Cerebyx) before surgery to reduce the risk of postoperative **seizures** (paroxysmal transient disturbances of the brain resulting from a discharge of abnormal electrical activity) (Hickey, 2003; Karch, 2005). Before surgery, corticosteroids such as dexamethasone (Decadron) may be administered to reduce cerebral edema if the patient has a brain tumor. Fluids may be restricted. A hyperosmotic agent (mannitol) and a diuretic agent such as furosemide (Lasix) may be administered IV immediately before and sometimes during surgery if the patient tends to retain fluid, as do many who have intracranial dysfunction. Antibiotics may be administered if there is a chance of cerebral contamination; diazepam (Valium) may be prescribed before surgery to allay anxiety.

Nursing Management

The preoperative assessment serves as a baseline against which postoperative status and recovery are compared. This assessment includes evaluating the LOC and responsiveness to stimuli and identifying any neurologic deficits, such as paralysis, visual dysfunction, alterations in personality or speech, and bladder and bowel disorders. Distal and proximal motor strength in both upper and lower extremities is recorded on a 5-point scale. Testing of motor function is discussed in Chapter 60 (see Fig. 60-14).

The patient's and family's understanding of and reactions to the anticipated surgical procedure and its possible

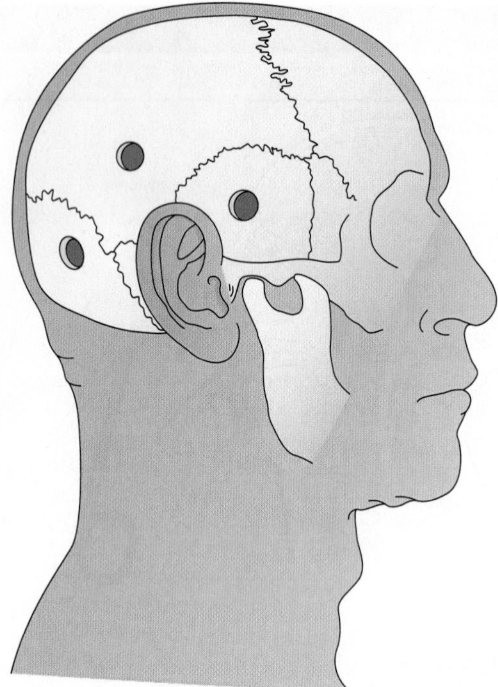

FIGURE 61-8. Burr holes may be used in neurosurgical procedures to make a bone flap in the skull, to aspirate a brain abscess, or to evacuate a hematoma.

CHART 61-1

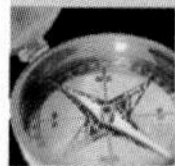

Ethics and Related Issues

What Ethical Principles Are Involved With Surrogate Consent?

SITUATION

A 35-year-old woman has had a brain injury, is in and out of a comatose state, and needs a craniotomy for removal of an epidural hematoma. The health care provider determines that the patient is unable to give informed consent for the procedure, so consent is obtained from the next of kin.

DILEMMA

The principle of autonomy for the patient conflicts with the principle of paternalism for the health care providers.

DISCUSSION

1. What are the essential elements of informed consent pertinent to this situation?
2. What mechanisms can the nursing staff use to assist them in resolving any dilemma they have regarding the patient's right to autonomy?

sequelae are assessed, as is the availability of support systems for the patient and family. Adequate preparation for surgery, with attention to the patient's physical and emotional status, can reduce the risk for anxiety, fear, and postoperative complications. The patient is assessed for neurologic deficits and their potential impact after surgery. For motor deficits or weakness or paralysis of the arms or legs, trochanter rolls are applied to the extremities, and the feet are positioned against a footboard. A patient who can ambulate is encouraged to do so. If the patient is aphasic, writing materials or picture and word cards showing the bedpan, glass of water, blanket, and other frequently used items may help improve communication.

Preparation of the patient and family includes providing information about what to expect during and after surgery. The surgical site is shaved and prepared immediately before surgery (usually in the operating room), so that any resultant superficial abrasions do not have time to become infected. An indwelling urinary catheter is inserted in the operating room to drain the bladder during the administration of diuretics and to permit urinary output to be monitored. The patient may have a central and arterial line placed for fluid administration and monitoring of pressures after surgery. The large head dressing applied after surgery may impair hearing temporarily. Vision may be limited if the eyes are swollen shut. If a tracheostomy or endotracheal tube is in place, the patient will be unable to speak until the tube is removed, so an alternative method of communication must be established.

An altered cognitive state may make the patient unaware of the impending surgery (Chart 61-1). Even so, encouragement and attention to the patient's needs are necessary. Whatever the state of awareness of the patient, the family needs reassurance and support, because they usually recognize the seriousness of brain surgery.

Postoperative Management

Postoperatively, an arterial line and a central venous pressure line may be in place to monitor and manage blood pressure and central venous pressure. The patient may be intubated and may receive supplemental oxygen therapy. Ongoing postoperative management is aimed at detecting and reducing cerebral edema, relieving pain and preventing seizures, and monitoring ICP and neurologic status.

Reducing Cerebral Edema

Medications to reduce cerebral edema include mannitol, which increases serum osmolality and draws free water from areas of the brain (with an intact blood–brain barrier). The fluid is then excreted by osmotic diuresis. Dexamethasone (Decadron) may be administered IV every 6 hours for 24 to 72 hours; the route is changed to oral as soon as possible, and the dosage is tapered over 5 to 7 days (Karch, 2005).

Relieving Pain and Preventing Seizures

Acetaminophen is usually prescribed for temperature exceeding 99.6°F (37.5°C) and for pain. The patient usually has a headache after a craniotomy as a result of stretching and irritation of nerves in the scalp during surgery. Codeine, administered IV, is often sufficient to relieve headache. Morphine sulfate may also be used in the management of postoperative pain in patients who have undergone a craniotomy (Roberts, 2004).

Antiseizure medication (phenytoin, diazepam) is prescribed for patients who have undergone supratentorial craniotomy because of the high risk for seizures after supratentorial neurosurgical procedures (Suarez, 2004). Serum levels are monitored to keep the medications within the therapeutic range.

Monitoring Intracranial Pressure

A patient undergoing intracranial surgery may have an ICP or cerebral oxygenation monitor inserted during surgery. Strict adherence to the written protocols for managing these systems is essential, as discussed earlier, for preventing infection and managing ICP. The system is removed after the ICP or cerebral oxygenation is normal and stable. The neurosurgeon must be notified immediately if the system is not functioning.

Nursing Process

The Patient Undergoing Intracranial Surgery

Assessment

After surgery, the frequency of postoperative monitoring is based on the patient's clinical status. Assessing respiratory function is essential, because even a small degree of hypoxia can increase cerebral ischemia. The respiratory rate and pattern are monitored, and arterial blood gas values are assessed frequently. Fluctuations in vital signs are carefully monitored and documented, because they may indicate increased ICP. The patient's temperature is measured to assess for hyperthermia secondary to infection or damage to the hypothalamus. Neurologic checks are made frequently to detect increased ICP resulting from cerebral edema or bleeding. A change in LOC or response to stimuli may be the first sign of increasing ICP.

The surgical dressing is inspected for evidence of bleeding and CSF drainage. The nurse must be alert to the development of complications; all assessments are carried out with these problems in mind. Chart 61-2 provides an overview of the nursing management of the patient who has undergone intracranial surgery. Seizures are a potential complication, and any seizure activity is carefully recorded and reported. Restlessness may occur as the patient becomes more responsive, or restlessness may be caused by pain, confusion, hypoxia, or other stimuli.

Diagnosis

Nursing Diagnoses

Based on the assessment data, the patient's major nursing diagnoses after intracranial surgery may include the following:

- Ineffective cerebral tissue perfusion related to cerebral edema
- Risk for imbalanced body temperature related to damage to the hypothalamus, dehydration, and infection
- Potential for impaired gas exchange related to hypoventilation, aspiration, and immobility
- Disturbed sensory perception related to periorbital edema, head dressing, endotracheal tube, and effects of ICP
- Body image disturbance related to change in appearance or physical disabilities

Other nursing diagnoses may include impaired communication (aphasia) related to insult to brain tissue and high risk for impaired skin integrity related to immobility, pressure, and incontinence; impaired physical mobility related to a neurologic deficit secondary to the neurosurgical procedure or to the underlying disorder may also occur.

Collaborative Problems/ Potential Complications

Potential complications include the following:

- Increased ICP
- Bleeding and hypovolemic shock
- Fluid and electrolyte disturbances
- Infection
- Seizures

Planning and Goals

The major goals for the patient include neurologic homeostasis to improve cerebral tissue perfusion, adequate thermoregulation, normal ventilation and gas exchange, ability to cope with sensory deprivation, adaptation to changes in body image, and absence of complications.

Nursing Interventions

Maintaining Cerebral Tissue Perfusion

Attention to the patient's respiratory status is essential, because even slight decreases in the oxygen level (hypoxia) or slight increases in the carbon dioxide level (hypercarbia) can affect cerebral perfusion, the clinical course, and the patient's outcome. The endotracheal tube is left in place until the patient shows signs of awakening and has adequate spontaneous ventilation, as evaluated clinically and by arterial blood gas analysis. Secondary brain damage can result from impaired cerebral oxygenation.

Some degree of cerebral edema occurs after brain surgery; it tends to peak 24 to 36 hours after surgery, producing decreased responsiveness on the second postoperative day. The control of cerebral edema was discussed earlier. Nursing strategies used to control factors that may raise ICP were presented in the previous Nursing Process section on increased ICP.

(text continues on page 2186)

CHART 61-2

Overview of Nursing Management for the Patient After Intracranial Surgery

POSTOPERATIVE INTERVENTIONS

Nursing Diagnosis: Risk for ineffective breathing pattern related to postoperative cerebral edema

Goal: Achievement of adequate respiratory function

1. Establish proper respiratory exchange to eliminate systemic hypercapnia and hypoxia, which increase cerebral edema.
   a. Unless contraindicated, place the patient in a lateral or a semiprone position to facilitate respiratory gas exchange until consciousness returns.
   b. Suction trachea and pharynx *cautiously* to remove secretions; suctioning can raise ICP.
   c. Maintain patient on controlled ventilation if prescribed to maintain normal ventilatory status; monitor arterial blood gas results to determine respiratory status.
   d. Elevate the head of the bed as prescribed.
   e. Administer nothing by mouth until active coughing and swallowing reflexes are demonstrated, to prevent aspiration.

Nursing Diagnosis: Risk for imbalanced fluid volume related to intracranial pressure or diuretics

Goal: Attainment of fluid and electrolyte balance

1. Monitor for polyuria, especially during first postoperative week; diabetes insipidus may develop in patients with lesions around the pituitary or hypothalamus.
   a. Monitor urinary specific gravity.
   b. Monitor serum and urinary electrolyte levels.
2. Evaluate patient's electrolyte status; patients may retain water and sodium.
   a. Early postoperative weight gain indicates fluid retention; a greater-than-estimated weight loss indicates negative water balance.
   b. Loss of sodium and chloride can produce weakness, lethargy, and coma.
   c. Low potassium levels can cause confusion, decreased level of responsiveness, and cardiac dysrhythmias.
3. Weigh patient daily; keep intake and output record.
4. Administer prescribed IV fluids cautiously—rate and composition depend on fluid deficit, urine output, and blood loss. Fluid intake and fluid losses should remain relatively equal.

Nursing Diagnosis: Disturbed sensory perception (visual/auditory) related to periorbital edema and head dressings

Goal: Compensate for sensory deprivation; prevent injury

1. Perform supportive measures until the patient can care for self.
   a. Change position as indicated; position changes can increase ICP.
   b. Administer prescribed analgesics (eg, codeine) that do not mask the level of responsiveness.
2. Use measures prescribed to relieve signs of periocular edema.
   a. Lubricate eyelids and around eyes with petrolatum.
   b. Apply light, cold compresses over eyes at specified intervals.
   c. Observe for signs of keratitis if cornea has no sensation.
3. Put extremities through range-of-motion exercises.
4. Evaluate and support patient during episodes of restlessness.
   a. Evaluate for airway obstruction, distended bladder, meningeal irritation from bloody CSF.
   b. Pad patient's hands and bed rails to prevent injury.
5. Reinforce blood-stained dressings with sterile dressing; blood-soaked dressings act as a culture medium for bacteria.
6. Orient patient frequently to time, place, and person.

MONITOR AND MANAGE COMPLICATIONS

1. Cerebral edema
   a. Assess patient's level of responsiveness/consciousness; decreased level of consciousness may be the first sign of increased ICP.
      (1) Eye opening (spontaneous, to sound, to pain); pupillary reactions to light
      (2) Response to commands
      (3) Assessment of spinal motor reflexes (pinch Achilles tendon, arm, or other body site)
      (4) Observation of patient's spontaneous activity
   b. Maintain a neurologic flow sheet to assess and document neurologic status, fluid administration, laboratory data, medications, and treatments.
   c. Evaluate for signs and symptoms of increasing ICP, which can lead to ischemia and further impairment of brain function.
      (1) Assess patient minute by minute, hour by hour, for
         - Diminished response to stimuli
         - Fluctuations of vital signs
         - Restlessness
         - Weakness and paralysis of extremities
         - Increasing headache
         - Changes or disturbances of vision; pupillary changes
      (2) Modify nursing management to prevent further increases in ICP.

CHART 61-2 Overview of Nursing Management for the Patient After Intracranial Surgery, continued

d. Control postoperative cerebral edema as prescribed.
   (1) Administer corticosteroids and osmotic diuretics as prescribed to reduce brain swelling.
   (2) Monitor fluid intake; avoid overhydration.
   (3) Maintain a normal temperature. Temperature control may be impaired in certain neurologic states, and fever increases the metabolic demands of the brain.
      - Monitor rectal temperature at specified intervals. Assess temperature of extremities, which may be cold and dry due to impaired heat-losing mechanisms (vasodilation and sweating).
      - Employ measures as prescribed to reduce fever: ice bags to axillae and groin; hypothermia blanket. Use ECG monitoring to detect dysrhythmias during hypothermia procedures.
   (4) Employ hyperventilation when prescribed and indicated (results in respiratory alkalosis, which causes cerebral vasoconstriction and reduces intracranial pressure).
   (5) Elevate head of bed to reduce ICP and facilitate respirations.
   (6) Avoid excessive stimuli.
   (7) Use ICP monitoring if patient is at risk for intracranial hypertension.

2. Intracranial hemorrhage
   a. Postoperative bleeding may be intraventricular, intracerebellar, subdural, or extradural.
   b. Observe for progressive impairment of state of consciousness and other signs of increasing ICP.
   c. Prepare deteriorating patient for return to surgery for evacuation of hematoma.
3. Seizures (greater risk with supratentorial operations)
   a. Administer prescribed antiseizure agents; monitor antiseizure medication blood levels.
   b. Observe for status epilepticus, which may occur after any intracranial surgery.
4. Infections
   a. Urinary tract infections
   b. Pulmonary infections related to aspiration secondary to depressed level of responsiveness; may result in atelectasis and aspiration pneumonia
   c. CNS infections (postoperative meningitis, CSF shunt infection)
   d. Surgical site infections/septicemia
5. Venous thrombosis
   a. Assess for pain, redness, warmth, and edema.
   b. Apply sequential compression device.
   c. Administer anticoagulant therapy as prescribed.
6. Leakage of CSF
   a. Differentiate between CSF and mucus.
      (1) Collect fluid on Dextrostix; if CSF is present, the indicator will have a positive reaction, as CSF contains glucose.
      (2) Assess for moderate elevation of temperature and mild neck rigidity.
   b. Caution patient against nose blowing or sniffing.
   c. Elevate head of bed as prescribed.
   d. Assist with insertion of lumbar CSF drainage system if inserted to reduce CSF pressure.
      (1) Ventricular catheters may be inserted in the patient undergoing surgery of the posterior fossa (ventriculostomy); the catheter is connected to a closed drainage system.
      (2) Administer antibiotics as prescribed.
7. Gastrointestinal ulceration (probably caused by stress response); monitor for signs and symptoms of hemorrhage, perforation, or both.

EVALUATION

Expected patient outcomes

1. Demonstrates normal breathing pattern
   a. Absence of crackles
   b. Demonstrates active swallowing and coughing reflexes
2. Attains/maintains fluid balance
   a. Takes fluids orally
   b. Maintains weight within expected range
3. Compensates for sensory deprivation
   a. Makes needs known
   b. Demonstrates improvement of vision
4. Exhibits absence of complications
   a. No evidence of increased ICP
   b. Opens eyes on request
   c. Obeys commands
   d. Has appropriate motor responses
   e. Shows increasing alertness
   f. No evidence of rhinorrhea, otorrhea, or CSF leakage
   g. Absence of fever
   h. No evidence of inflammation or infection at surgical site
   i. Absence of seizures
   j. No evidence of DVT or GI bleeding

Intraventricular drainage is carefully monitored, using strict asepsis when any part of the system is handled.

Vital signs and neurologic status (LOC and responsiveness, pupillary and motor responses) are assessed every 15 to 60 minutes. Extreme head rotation is avoided, because this raises ICP. After supratentorial surgery, the patient is placed on his or her back or side (on the unoperated side if a large lesion was removed) with one pillow under the head. The head of the bed may be elevated 30 degrees, depending on the level of the ICP and the neurosurgeon's preference. After posterior fossa (infratentorial) surgery, the patient is kept flat on one side (off the back) with the head on a small, firm pillow. The patient may be turned on either side, keeping the neck in a neutral position. When the patient is being turned, the body should be turned as a unit to prevent placing strain on the incision and possibly tearing the sutures. The head of the bed may be elevated slowly as tolerated by the patient.

The patient's position is changed every 2 hours, and skin care is given frequently. During position changes, care is taken to prevent disruption of the ICP monitoring system. A turning sheet placed under the patient's head to midthigh makes it easier to move and turn the patient safely.

Regulating Temperature

Moderate temperature elevation can be expected after intracranial surgery because of the reaction to blood at the operative site or in the subarachnoid space. Injury to the hypothalamic centers that regulate body temperature can occur during surgery. High fever is treated vigorously to combat the effect of an elevated temperature on brain metabolism and function.

Nursing interventions include monitoring the patient's temperature and using the following measures to reduce body temperature: removing blankets, applying ice bags to axilla and groin areas, using a hypothermia blanket as prescribed, and administering prescribed medications to reduce fever.

Conversely, hypothermia may be seen after lengthy neurosurgical procedures. Therefore, frequent measurements of rectal temperature are necessary. Rewarming should occur slowly to prevent shivering, which increases cellular oxygen demands.

Improving Gas Exchange

The patient undergoing neurosurgery is at risk for impaired gas exchange and pulmonary infections because of immobility, immunosuppression, decreased LOC, and fluid restriction. Immobility compromises the respiratory system by causing pooling and stasis of secretions in dependent areas and the development of atelectasis. The patient whose fluid intake is restricted may be more vulnerable to atelectasis as a result of inability to expectorate thickened secretions. Pneumonia can develop in neurosurgical patients related to aspiration and restricted mobility.

The nurse assesses the patient for signs of respiratory infection, which include temperature elevation, increased pulse rate, and changes in respiration, and auscultates the lungs for decreased breath sounds and adventitious sounds.

Repositioning the patient every 2 hours helps to mobilize pulmonary secretions and prevent stasis. After the patient regains consciousness, additional measures to expand collapsed alveoli can be instituted, such as yawning, sighing, deep breathing, incentive spirometry, and coughing (unless contraindicated). If necessary, the oropharynx and trachea are suctioned to remove secretions that cannot be raised by coughing; however, coughing and suctioning increase ICP. Therefore, suctioning should be used cautiously. Increasing the humidity in the oxygen delivery system may help to loosen secretions. The nurse and the respiratory therapist work together to monitor the effects of chest physical therapy.

Managing Sensory Deprivation

Periorbital edema is a common consequence of intracranial surgery, because fluid drains into the dependent periorbital areas when the patient has been positioned in a prone position during surgery. A hematoma may form under the scalp and spread down to the orbit, producing an area of ecchymosis (black eye).

Before surgery, the patient and family should be informed that one or both eyes may be edematous temporarily after surgery. After surgery, elevating the head of the bed (if not contraindicated) and applying cold compresses over the eyes will help reduce the edema. If periorbital edema increases significantly, the surgeon is notified, because this may indicate that a postoperative clot is developing or that there is increasing ICP and poor venous drainage. Health care personnel should announce their presence when entering the room to avoid startling the patient whose vision is impaired due to periorbital edema or neurologic deficits.

Additional factors that can affect sensation include a bulky head dressing, the presence of an endotracheal tube, and effects of increased ICP. The first postoperative dressing change is usually performed by the neurosurgeon. In the absence of bleeding or a CSF leak, every effort is made to minimize the size of the head dressing. If the patient requires an endotracheal tube for mechanical ventilation, every effort is made to extubate the patient as soon as clinical signs indicate it is possible. The patient is monitored closely for the effects of elevated ICP.

Enhancing Self-Image

The patient is encouraged to verbalize feelings and frustrations about any change in appearance. Nursing support is based on the patient's reactions and feelings. Factual information may need to be provided if the patient has misconceptions about puffiness about the face, periorbital bruising, and hair loss. Attention to grooming, the use of the patient's own clothing, and covering the head with a turban (and later a wig until hair growth occurs) are encouraged. Social interaction with close friends, family, and hospital personnel may increase the patient's sense of self-worth.

The family and social support system can be of assistance while the patient recovers from surgery.

Monitoring and Managing Potential Complications

Complications that may develop within hours after surgery include increased ICP, bleeding and hypovolemic shock, altered fluid and electrolyte balance (including water intoxication), infection, and seizures. These complications require close collaboration between the nurse and the surgeon.

MONITORING FOR INCREASED INTRACRANIAL PRESSURE AND BLEEDING

Increased ICP and bleeding are life-threatening to the patient who has undergone intracranial surgery. The following points must be kept in mind when caring for any patient who has undergone such surgery:

- An increase in blood pressure and decrease in pulse with respiratory failure may indicate increased ICP.
- An accumulation of blood under the bone flap (extradural, subdural, or intracerebral hematoma) may pose a threat to life. A clot must be suspected in any patient who does not awaken as expected or whose condition deteriorates. An intracranial hematoma is suspected if the patient has any new postoperative neurologic deficits (especially a dilated pupil on the operative side). In these circumstances, the patient is returned to the operating room immediately for evacuation of the clot if indicated.
- Cerebral edema, infarction, metabolic disturbances, and hydrocephalus are conditions that may mimic the clinical manifestations of a clot.

The patient is monitored closely for indicators of complications, and early signs and trends in clinical status are reported to the surgeon. Treatments are initiated promptly, and the nurse assists in evaluating the patient's response to treatment. The nurse also provides support to the patient and family.

Should signs and symptoms of increased ICP occur, efforts to decrease the ICP are initiated: alignment of the head in a neutral position without flexion to promote venous drainage, elevation of the head of the bed to 30 degrees (when prescribed), administration of mannitol (an osmotic diuretic), and possible administration of pharmacologic paralyzing agents.

MANAGING FLUID AND ELECTROLYTE DISTURBANCES

Fluid and electrolyte imbalances may occur because of the patient's underlying condition and its management or as complications of surgery. Fluid and electrolyte disturbances can contribute to the development of cerebral edema.

The postoperative fluid regimen depends on the type of neurosurgical procedure and is determined on an individual basis. The volume and composition of fluids are adjusted based on daily serum electrolyte values, along with fluid intake and output.

Sodium retention may occur in the immediate postoperative period. Serum and urine electrolytes, BUN, blood glucose, weight, and clinical status are monitored. Intake and output are measured in view of losses associated with fever, respiration, and CSF drainage. Fluids may have to be restricted in patients with cerebral edema.

Oral fluids are usually resumed after the first 24 hours (Hickey, 2003). The presence of gag and swallowing reflexes must be checked before initiation of oral fluids. Some patients with posterior fossa tumors have impaired swallowing, so fluids may need to be administered by alternative routes. The patient should be observed for signs and symptoms of nausea and vomiting as the diet is progressed (Hickey, 2003).

Patients undergoing surgery for brain tumor often receive large doses of corticosteroids and therefore tend to develop hyperglycemia. Serum glucose levels are measured every 4 to 6 hours. These patients are prone to gastric ulcers, so histamine-2 receptor antagonists (H_2 blockers) are prescribed to suppress the secretion of gastric acid. The patient also is monitored for bleeding and assessed for gastric pain.

If the surgical site is near to (or causes edema to) the pituitary gland and hypothalamus, the patient may develop symptoms of diabetes insipidus, which is characterized by excessive urinary output, elevated serum osmolality, decreased urine osmolality, hypernatremia, and a low urine specific gravity (Holcomb, 2002). The urine specific gravity is measured hourly, and fluid intake and output are monitored. Fluid replacement must compensate for urine output, and serum potassium levels must be monitored.

SIADH, which results in water retention with hyponatremia and serum hypo-osmolality, occurs in a wide variety of central nervous system disorders (brain tumor, head trauma) causing fluid disturbances. Nursing management includes careful intake and output measurements, specific gravity determinations of urine, and monitoring of serum and urine electrolyte levels while following directives for fluid restriction. SIADH is usually self-limited.

PREVENTING INFECTION

The patient undergoing neurosurgery is at risk for infection related to the neurosurgical procedure (brain exposure, bone exposure, wound hematomas) and the presence of IV and arterial lines for fluid administration and monitoring. Risk for infection is increased in patients who undergo lengthy intracranial operations and in those who have external ventricular drains in place longer than 48 to 72 hours (Park et al., 2004).

The incision site is monitored for redness, tenderness, bulging, separation, or foul odor. The dressing is often stained with blood in the immediate postoperative period. Because blood is an excellent culture medium for bacteria, the dressing is reinforced with sterile pads so that contamination and infection are avoided. A heavily stained or displaced dressing should be reported immediately. A drain is sometimes placed in the craniotomy incision to facilitate drainage.

After suboccipital surgical procedures, CSF may leak through the incision. This complication is dangerous because of the possibility of meningitis. Any sudden discharge of fluid from a cranial incision is reported at once, because a massive leak requires surgical repair. Attention should be paid to the patient who complains of a salty taste or "post-nasal drip," because this can be caused by CSF trickling down the throat. After a craniotomy, the patient is instructed to avoid coughing, sneezing, or nose blowing, which can cause CSF leakage by creating pressure on the operative site.

Aseptic technique is used when handling dressings, drainage systems, and IV and arterial lines. The patient is monitored carefully for signs and symptoms of infection, and cultures are obtained if infection is suspected. Appropriate antibiotics are administered as prescribed. Other causes of infection in the patient undergoing intracranial surgery, such as pneumonia and urinary tract infections, are similar to those in other postoperative patients.

MONITORING FOR SEIZURE ACTIVITY

Seizures and epilepsy may occur as complications after any intracranial neurosurgical procedure. Preventing seizures is essential to avoid further cerebral edema. Administering the prescribed antiseizure medication before and after surgery may prevent the development of seizures in subsequent months and years (Ropper et al., 2004). **Status epilepticus** (prolonged seizures without recovery of consciousness in the intervals between seizures) may occur after craniotomy and also may be related to the development of complications (hematoma, ischemia). The management of status epilepticus is described later in this chapter.

MONITORING AND MANAGING LATER COMPLICATIONS

Other complications may occur during the first 2 weeks or later and may compromise the patient's recovery. The most important of these are thromboembolic complications (DVT, pulmonary embolism), pulmonary and urinary tract infection, and pressure ulcers. Most of these complications may be avoided with frequent changes of position, adequate suctioning of secretions, thrombosis prophylaxis, early ambulation, and skin care.

Promoting Home and Community-Based Care

TEACHING PATIENTS SELF-CARE

The recovery of a neurosurgical patient at home depends on the extent of the surgical procedure and its success. The patient's strengths as well as limitations are assessed and explained to the family, along with the family's part in promoting recovery. Because administration of antiseizure medication is a priority, the patient and family are taught to use a check-off system, pill boxes, and alarms to ensure that the medication is taken as prescribed.

The patient and family are taught what to expect after surgery. Dietary restrictions usually are not required unless another health problem necessitates a special diet. Although shower or tub bathing is permitted, the scalp should be kept dry until all the sutures have been removed. A clean scarf or cap may be worn until a wig or hairpiece is purchased. If skull bone has been removed, the neurosurgeon may prescribe a protective helmet. After a craniotomy, the patient may require rehabilitation, depending on the postoperative level of function. The patient may require physical therapy for residual weakness and mobility issues. An occupational therapist is consulted to assist with self-care issues. If the patient is aphasic, speech therapy may be necessary.

CONTINUING CARE

Barring complications, patients are discharged from the hospital as soon as possible. Patients with severe motor deficits require extensive physical therapy and rehabilitation. Those with postoperative cognitive and speech impairments require psychological evaluation, speech therapy, and rehabilitation. The nurse collaborates with the physician and other health care professionals during hospitalization and home care to achieve as complete a rehabilitation as possible and to assist the patient in living with residual disability.

If tumor, injury, or disease makes the prognosis poor, care is directed toward making the patient as comfortable as possible. With return of the tumor or cerebral compression, the patient becomes less alert and aware. Other possible consequences include paralysis, blindness, and seizures. The home care nurse, hospice nurse, and social worker collaborate with the family to plan for additional home health care or hospice services or placement of the patient in an extended-care facility (see also the section on cerebral metastases in Chapter 65). The patient and family are encouraged to discuss end-of-life preferences for care; the patient's end-of-life preferences must be respected (see Chapter 17). The nurse involved in home and continuing care of patients after cranial surgery also needs to remind patients and family members of the need for health promotion and recommended health screening.

Evaluation

Expected Patient Outcomes

Expected patient outcomes may include the following:

1. Achieves optimal cerebral tissue perfusion
   a. Opens eyes on request; uses recognizable words, progressing to normal speech
   b. Obeys commands with appropriate motor responses
2. Maintains normal body temperature
   a. Registers normal body temperature

3. Has normal gas exchange
   a. Has arterial blood gas values within normal ranges
   b. Breathes easily; lung sounds are clear without adventitious sounds
   c. Takes deep breaths and changes position as directed
4. Copes with sensory deprivation
5. Demonstrates improving self-concept
   a. Pays attention to grooming
   b. Visits and interacts with others
6. Exhibits absence of complications
   a. Exhibits ICP within normal range
   b. Has minimal bleeding at surgical site; surgical incision is healing without evidence of infection
   c. Shows fluid balance and electrolyte levels within desired ranges
   d. Exhibits no evidence of seizures

An overview of care of the patient undergoing intracranial surgery is presented in Chart 61-2.

Transsphenoidal Approach

Tumors within the sella turcica and small adenomas of the pituitary can be removed through a transsphenoidal approach: an incision is made beneath the upper lip, and entry is then gained successively into the nasal cavity, sphenoidal sinus, and sella turcica (see Table 61-3). Although an otorhinolaryngologist may make the initial opening, the neurosurgeon completes the opening into the sphenoidal sinus and exposes the floor of the sella. Microsurgical techniques provide improved illumination, magnification, and visualization so that nearby vital structures can be avoided.

The transsphenoidal approach offers direct access to the sella turcica with minimal risk of trauma and hemorrhage (Pertrovich et al., 2003; Pickett, 2003). It avoids many of the risks of craniotomy, and the postoperative discomfort is similar to that of other transnasal surgical procedures. It may also be used for pituitary ablation (destruction) in patients with disseminated breast or prostatic cancer.

Complications

Manipulation of the posterior pituitary gland during surgery may produce transient diabetes insipidus of several days' duration (Bader & Littlejohns, 2004). It is treated with vasopressin but occasionally persists. Other complications include CSF leakage, visual disturbances, postoperative meningitis, pneumocephalus (air in the intracranial cavity), and SIADH (see Chapter 42).

Preoperative Management

Medical Management

The preoperative workup includes a series of endocrine tests (Pickett, 2003), rhinologic evaluation (to assess the status of the sinuses and nasal cavity), and neuroradiologic studies. Funduscopic examination and visual field determinations are performed, because the most serious effect of pituitary tumor is localized pressure on the optic nerve or chiasm. In addition, the nasopharyngeal secretions are cultured, because a sinus infection is a contraindication to an intracranial procedure through this approach. Corticosteroids may be administered before and after surgery, because the surgery involves removal of the pituitary, the source of adrenocorticotropic hormone (ACTH). Antibiotics may or may not be administered prophylactically (Bader & Littlejohns, 2004).

Nursing Management

Deep breathing is taught before surgery. The patient is instructed that after the surgery he or she will need to avoid vigorous coughing, blowing the nose, sucking through a straw, or sneezing, because these actions may place increased pressure at the surgical site and cause a CSF leak (Hickey, 2003).

Postoperative Management

Medical Management

Because the procedure disrupts the oral and nasal mucous membranes, management focuses on preventing infection and promoting healing. Medications include antimicrobial agents (which are continued until the nasal packing inserted at the time of surgery is removed), corticosteroids, analgesic agents for discomfort, and agents for the control of diabetes insipidus if necessary (Bader & Littlejohns, 2004).

Nursing Management

Vital signs are measured to monitor hemodynamic, cardiac, and ventilatory status. Because of the anatomic proximity of the pituitary gland to the optic chiasm, visual acuity and visual fields are assessed at regular intervals. One method is to ask the patient to count the number of fingers held up by the nurse. Evidence of decreasing visual acuity suggests an expanding hematoma.

The head of the bed is raised to decrease pressure on the sella turcica and to promote normal drainage. The patient is cautioned against blowing the nose or engaging in any activity that raises ICP, such as bending over or straining during urination or defecation.

Intake and output are measured as a guide to fluid and electrolyte replacement and to assess for diabetes insipidus. The urine specific gravity is measured after each voiding. Daily weight is monitored. Fluids are usually given after nausea ceases, and the patient then progresses to a regular diet.

The nasal packing inserted during surgery is checked frequently for blood or CSF drainage. The major discomfort is related to the nasal packing and to mouth dryness and thirst caused by mouth-breathing. Oral care is provided every 4 hours or more frequently. Usually, the teeth are not brushed until the incision above the teeth has healed. Warm saline mouth rinses and the use of a cool mist vaporizer are helpful. Petrolatum is soothing when applied to the lips. A room humidifier assists in keeping the mucous membranes moist. The packing is removed in 3 to 4 days, and only then can the area around the nares be cleaned with the prescribed solution to remove crusted blood and moisten the mucous membranes (Hickey, 2003).

Home care considerations include advising the patient to use a room humidifier to keep the mucous membranes moist and to soothe irritation. The head of the bed is elevated for at least 2 weeks after surgery.

Seizure Disorders

Seizures

Seizures are episodes of abnormal motor, sensory, autonomic, or psychic activity (or a combination of these) that result from sudden excessive discharge from cerebral neurons (Hickey, 2003). A part or all of the brain may be involved. The international classification of seizures differentiates between two main types: partial seizures that begin in one part of the brain, and generalized seizures that involve electrical discharges in the whole brain (Chart 61-3). In a simple partial seizure, consciousness remains intact, whereas in a complex partial seizure, consciousness is impaired. Unclassified seizures are so termed because of incomplete data.

CHART 61-3

International Classification of Seizures

PARTIAL SEIZURES (SEIZURES BEGINNING LOCALLY)

Simple partial seizures (with elementary symptoms, generally without impairment of consciousness)

- With motor symptoms
- With special sensory or somatosensory symptoms
- With autonomic symptoms
- Compound forms

Complex partial seizures (with complex symptoms, generally with impairment of consciousness)

- With impairment of consciousness only
- With cognitive symptoms
- With affective symptoms
- With psychosensory symptoms
- With psychomotor symptoms (automatisms)
- Compound forms

Partial seizures secondarily generalized

GENERALIZED SEIZURES (CONVULSIVE OR NONCONVULSIVE, BILATERALLY SYMMETRIC, WITHOUT LOCAL ONSET)

Tonic-clonic seizures
Tonic seizures
Clonic seizures
Absence (petit mal) seizures
Atonic seizures
Myoclonic seizures (bilaterally massive epileptic)
Unclassified seizures

The underlying cause is an electrical disturbance (dysrhythmia) in the nerve cells in one section of the brain; these cells emit abnormal, recurring, uncontrolled electrical discharges. The characteristic seizure is a manifestation of this excessive neuronal discharge. Associated loss of consciousness, excess movement or loss of muscle tone or movement, and disturbances of behavior, mood, sensation, and perception may also occur.

The specific causes of seizures are varied and can be categorized as idiopathic (genetic, developmental defects) and acquired. Causes of acquired seizures include:

- Cerebrovascular disease
- Hypoxemia of any cause, including vascular insufficiency
- Fever (childhood)
- Head injury
- Hypertension
- Central nervous system infections
- Metabolic and toxic conditions (eg, renal failure, hyponatremia, hypocalcemia, hypoglycemia, pesticides)
- Brain tumor
- Drug and alcohol withdrawal
- Allergies

Nursing Management

During a Seizure

A major responsibility of the nurse is to observe and record the sequence of signs. The nature of the seizure usually indicates the type of treatment that is required (Rho, Sankar & Cavazos, 2004). Before and during a seizure, the patient is assessed and the following items are documented:

- The circumstances before the seizure (visual, auditory, or olfactory stimuli, tactile stimuli, emotional or psychological disturbances, sleep, hyperventilation)
- The occurrence of an aura (a premonitory or warning sensation that can be visual, auditory, or olfactory)
- The first thing the patient does in the seizure—where the movements or the stiffness begins, conjugate gaze position, and the position of the head at the beginning of the seizure. This information gives clues to the location of the seizure origin in the brain. (In recording, it is important to state whether the beginning of the seizure was observed.)
- The type of movements in the part of the body involved
- The areas of the body involved (turn back bedding to expose patient)
- The size of both pupils and whether the eyes are open
- Whether the eyes or head turned to one side
- The presence or absence of automatisms (involuntary motor activity, such as lip smacking or repeated swallowing)
- Incontinence of urine or stool
- Duration of each phase of the seizure
- Unconsciousness, if present, and its duration
- Any obvious paralysis or weakness of arms or legs after the seizure
- Inability to speak after the seizure
- Movements at the end of the seizure
- Whether or not the patient sleeps afterward
- Cognitive status (confused or not confused) after the seizure

In addition to providing data about the seizure, nursing care is directed at preventing injury and supporting the patient, not only physically but also psychologically. Consequences such as anxiety, embarrassment, fatigue, and depression can be devastating to the patient (Rho et al., 2004). Steps to prevent or minimize injury are presented in Chart 61-4.

After a Seizure

After a patient has a seizure, the nurse's role is to document the events leading to and occurring during and after the seizure and to prevent complications (eg, aspiration, injury). The patient is at risk for hypoxia, vomiting, and pulmonary aspiration. To prevent complications, the patient is placed in the side-lying position to facilitate drainage of oral secretions, and suctioning is performed, if needed, to maintain a patent airway and prevent aspiration (see Chart 61-4). Seizure precautions are maintained, including having available functioning suction equipment with a suction catheter and oral airway. The bed is placed in a low position with two to three side rails up and padded, if necessary, to prevent injury to the patient. The patient may be drowsy and may wish to sleep after the seizure; he or she may not remember events leading up to the seizure and for a short time thereafter.

The Epilepsies

Epilepsy is a group of syndromes characterized by unprovoked, recurring seizures (Stafstrom & Rho, 2004). Epileptic syndromes are classified by specific patterns of clinical features, including age at onset, family history, and seizure type. Types of epilepsies are differentiated by how the seizure activity manifests (see Chart 61-3), the most common syndromes being those with generalized seizures and those with partial-onset seizures (Rho et al., 2004). Epilepsy can be primary (idiopathic) or secondary (when the cause is known and the epilepsy is a symptom of another underlying condition, such as a brain tumor).

Epilepsy affects an estimated 3% of people during their lifetime, and most forms of epilepsy occur in childhood (Chang & Lowenstein, 2003). The improved treatment of cerebrovascular disorders, head injuries, brain tumors, meningitis, and encephalitis has increased the number of patients at risk for seizures after recovery from these conditions. Also, advances in electroencephalography have aided in the diagnosis of epilepsy. The general public has been educated about epilepsy, which has reduced the stigma associated with it; as a result, more people are willing to acknowledge that they have epilepsy.

Although some evidence suggests that susceptibility to some types of epilepsy may be inherited, the cause of seizures in many people is unknown. Epilepsy can follow birth trauma, asphyxia neonatorum, head injuries, some infectious diseases (bacterial, viral, parasitic), toxicity (carbon monoxide and lead poisoning), circulatory problems, fever, metabolic and nutritional disorders, or drug or alcohol intoxication (Bader & Littlejohns, 2004). It is also associated with brain tumors, abscesses, and congenital malformations. Most cases of epilepsy are idiopathic (ie, the cause is unknown).

Pathophysiology

Messages from the body are carried by the neurons (nerve cells) of the brain by means of discharges of electrochemical energy that sweep along them. These impulses occur in bursts whenever a nerve cell has a task to perform. Sometimes, these cells or groups of cells continue firing after a task is finished. During the period of unwanted discharges, parts of the body controlled by the errant cells may perform erratically. Resultant dysfunction ranges from mild to incapacitating and often causes loss of consciousness (Hickey, 2003). If these uncontrolled, abnormal discharges occur repeatedly, a person is said to have an epileptic syndrome (Stafstrom & Rho, 2004). Epilepsy is not associated with intellectual level. People who have epilepsy without other brain or nervous system disabilities fall within the same intelligence ranges as the overall population. Epilepsy is not synonymous with mental retardation or illness. However, many people who have developmental disabilities because of serious neurologic damage also have epilepsy.

Clinical Manifestations

Depending on the location of the discharging neurons, seizures may range from a simple staring episode (absence seizure) to prolonged convulsive movements with loss of consciousness.

The initial pattern of the seizures indicates the region of the brain in which the seizure originates (see Chart 61-3). In simple partial seizures, only a finger or hand may shake, or the mouth may jerk uncontrollably. The person may talk unintelligibly, may be dizzy, and may experience unusual or unpleasant sights, sounds, odors, or tastes, but without loss of consciousness (Hickey, 2003).

In complex partial seizures, the person either remains motionless or moves automatically but inappropriately for time and place, or he or she may experience excessive emotions of fear, anger, elation, or irritability. Whatever the manifestations, the person does not remember the episode when it is over.

Generalized seizures, previously referred to as grand mal seizures, involve both hemispheres of the brain, causing both sides of the body to react (Hickey, 2003). Intense rigidity of the entire body may occur, followed by alternating muscle relaxation and contraction (generalized tonic–clonic contraction). The simultaneous contractions of the diaphragm and chest muscles may produce a characteristic epileptic cry. The tongue is often chewed, and the patient is incontinent of urine and feces. After 1 or 2 minutes, the convulsive movements begin to subside; the patient relaxes and lies in deep coma, breathing noisily. The respirations at this point are chiefly abdominal. In the postictal state (after the seizure), the patient is often confused and hard to arouse and may sleep for hours. Many patients report headache, sore muscles, fatigue, and depression (Rho et al., 2004).

Assessment and Diagnostic Findings

The diagnostic assessment is aimed at determining the type of seizures, their frequency and severity, and the factors that precipitate them (Rho et al., 2004; Stafstrom & Rho, 2004). A developmental history is taken, including events of pregnancy and childbirth, to seek evidence of

CHART 61-4 Guidelines for Seizure Care

Nursing Care During a Seizure

- Provide privacy and protect the patient from curious onlookers. (The patient who has an *aura* [warning of an impending seizure] may have time to seek a safe, private place.)
- Ease the patient to the floor, if possible.
- Protect the head with a pad to prevent injury (from striking a hard surface).
- Loosen constrictive clothing.
- Push aside any furniture that may injure the patient during the seizure.
- If the patient is in bed, remove pillows and raise side rails.
- If an aura precedes the seizure, insert an oral airway to reduce the possibility of the patient's biting the tongue or cheek.
- *Do not attempt to pry open jaws that are clenched in a spasm or to insert anything.* Broken teeth and injury to the lips and tongue may result from such an action.
- No attempt should be made to restrain the patient during the seizure, because muscular contractions are strong and restraint can produce injury.
- If possible, place the patient on one side with head flexed forward, which allows the tongue to fall forward and facilitates drainage of saliva and mucus. If suction is available, use it if necessary to clear secretions.

Nursing Care After the Seizure

- Keep the patient on one side to prevent aspiration. Make sure the airway is patent.
- There is usually a period of confusion after a grand mal seizure.
- A short apneic period may occur during or immediately after a generalized seizure.
- The patient, on awakening, should be reoriented to the environment.
- If the patient becomes agitated after a seizure (postictal), use calm persuasion and gentle restraint.

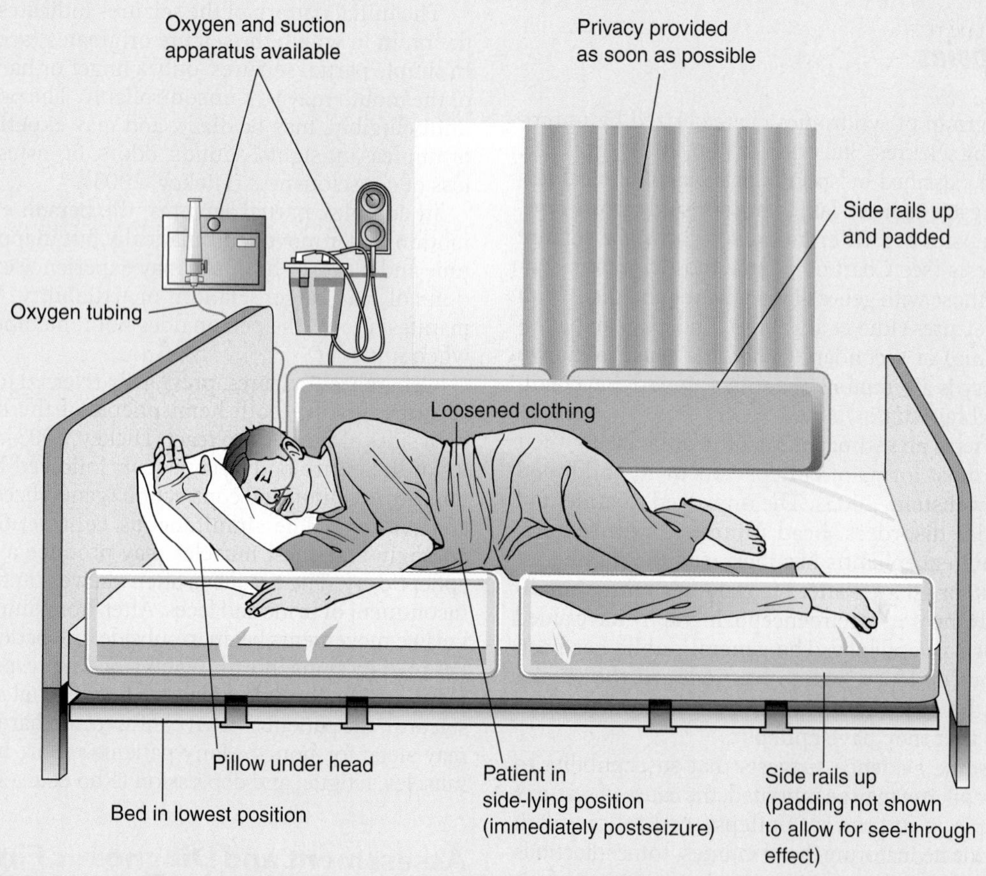

preexisting injury. The patient is also questioned about illnesses or head injuries that may have affected the brain. In addition to physical and neurologic evaluations, diagnostic examinations include biochemical, hematologic, and serologic studies. MRI is used to detect structural lesions such as focal abnormalities, cerebrovascular abnormalities, and cerebral degenerative changes (Bader & Littlejohns, 2004).

The electroencephalogram (EEG) furnishes diagnostic evidence for a substantial proportion of patients with epilepsy and assists in classifying the type of seizure (Rho et al., 2004). Abnormalities in the EEG usually continue between seizures or, if not apparent, may be elicited by hyperventilation or during sleep. Microelectrodes (depth electrodes) can be inserted deep in the brain to probe the action of single brain cells. Some people with clinical seizures have normal EEGs, whereas others who have never had seizures have abnormal EEGs. Telemetry and computerized equipment are used to monitor electrical brain activity while the patient pursues his or her normal activities and to store the readings on computer tapes for analysis. Video recording of seizures taken simultaneously with EEG telemetry is useful in determining the type of seizure as well as its duration and magnitude. This type of intensive monitoring is changing the treatment of severe epilepsy.

SPECT is an additional tool that is sometimes used in the diagnostic workup. It is useful for identifying the epileptogenic zone so that the area in the brain giving rise to seizures can be removed surgically (Cascino, Buchhalter & Mullan, 2004).

Epilepsy in Women

More than 1 million American women have epilepsy, and they face particular needs associated with the syndrome. Women with epilepsy often note an increase in seizure frequency during menses; this has been linked to the increase in sex hormones that alter the excitability of neurons in the cerebral cortex. The effectiveness of contraceptives is decreased by antiseizure medications. Therefore, patients should be encouraged to discuss family planning with their primary health care provider and to obtain preconception counseling if they are considering childbearing (Rho et al., 2004).

Women of childbearing age who have epilepsy require special care and guidance before, during, and after pregnancy. Many women note a change in the pattern of seizure activity during pregnancy. The risk for congenital fetal anomaly is two to three times higher in mothers with epilepsy. The effects of maternal seizures, antiseizure medications, and genetic predisposition are all mechanisms that contribute to possible malformation. Because the unborn infants of mothers who take certain antiseizure medications for epilepsy are at risk, these women need careful monitoring, including blood studies to detect the level of antiseizure medications taken throughout pregnancy (Karch, 2005). High-risk mothers (teenagers, women with histories of difficult deliveries, women who use illicit drugs (eg, crack, cocaine), and women with diabetes or hypertension) should be identified and monitored closely during pregnancy, because damage to the fetus during pregnancy and delivery can increase the risk for epilepsy. All of these issues need further study (Rho et al., 2004).

Because of bone loss associated with the long-term use of antiseizure medications, patients receiving antiseizure agents should be assessed for low bone mass and osteoporosis. They should be instructed about other strategies to reduce their risks for osteoporosis (Gross, Gidal & Pack, 2004).

Gerontologic Considerations

Elderly people have a high incidence of new-onset epilepsy (Bader & Littlejohns, 2004). Cerebrovascular disease is the leading cause of seizures in the elderly (Somjen, 2004). The increased incidence is also associated with stroke, head injury, dementia, infection, alcoholism, and aging. Treatment depends on the underlying cause. Because many elderly people have chronic health problems, they may be taking other medications that can interact with medications prescribed for seizure control. In addition, the absorption, distribution, metabolism, and excretion of medications are altered in the elderly as a result of age-related changes in renal and liver function. Therefore, elderly patients must be monitored closely for adverse and toxic effects of antiseizure medications and for osteoporosis. The cost of antiseizure medications can lead to poor adherence to the prescribed regimen in elderly patients on fixed incomes.

Prevention

Society-wide efforts are the key to prevention of epilepsy. Head injury is one of the main causes of epilepsy that can be prevented. Through highway safety programs and occupational safety precautions, lives can be saved and epilepsy due to head injury prevented; these programs are discussed in Chapter 63.

Medical Management

The management of epilepsy is individualized to meet the needs of each patient and not just to manage and prevent seizures. Management differs from patient to patient, because some forms of epilepsy arise from brain damage and others are caused by altered brain chemistry.

Pharmacologic Therapy

Many medications are available to control seizures, although the mechanisms of their actions are still unknown (French, Kanner, Bautista, et al., 2004). The objective is to achieve seizure control with minimal side effects. Medication therapy controls rather than cures seizures. Medications are selected on the basis of the type of seizure being treated and the effectiveness and safety of the medications. If properly prescribed and taken, medications control seizures in 70% to 80% of patients with seizures. The condition is not improved by any available medication in 20% of patients with generalized seizures, and in 30% of those with partial seizures, due to the nature of the seizure or the patient's inability to tolerate the side effects of medication (French et al., 2004).

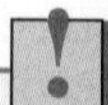

NURSING ALERT

Nurses must take care when administering lamotrigine (Lamictal), an antiseizure medication. The drug packaging was recently changed in an attempt to reduce medication errors, because this medication has been confused with terbinafine (Lamisil), labetalol hydrochloride (Trandate), lamivudine (Epivir), maprotiline (Ludiomil), and the combination of diphenoxylate and atropine (Lomotil). Patients with epilepsy are at risk for status epilepticus from having their medication regimen interrupted.

Treatment usually starts with a single medication. The starting dose and the rate at which the dosage is increased depend on the occurrence of side effects. The medication levels in the blood are monitored, because the rate of drug absorption varies among patients. Changing to another medication may be necessary if seizure control is not achieved or if toxicity makes it impossible to increase the dosage. The medication may need to be adjusted because of concurrent illness, weight changes, or increases in stress. Sudden withdrawal of these medications can cause seizures to occur with greater frequency or can precipitate the development of status epilepticus (Hickey, 2003).

Side effects of antiseizure agents may be divided into three groups: (1) idiosyncratic or allergic disorders, which manifest primarily as skin reactions; (2) acute toxicity, which may occur when the medication is initially prescribed; and (3) chronic toxicity, which occurs late in the course of therapy.

The manifestations of drug toxicity are variable, and any organ system may be involved. Gingival hyperplasia (swollen and tender gums) can be associated with long-term use of phenytoin (Dilantin), for example (Karch, 2005). Periodic physical and dental examinations and laboratory tests are performed for patients receiving medications that are known to have hematopoietic, genitourinary, or hepatic effects. Table 61-4 lists the medications in current use.

Surgical Management

Surgery is indicated for patients whose epilepsy results from intracranial tumors, abscesses, cysts, or vascular anomalies. Some patients have intractable seizure disorders that do not respond to medication. A focal atrophic process may occur secondary to trauma, inflammation, stroke, or anoxia. If the seizures originate in a reasonably well-circumscribed area

℞ TABLE 61-4 Major Antiseizure Medications

Medication	Dose-Related Side Effects	Toxic Effects
carbamazepine (Tegretol)	Dizziness, drowsiness, unsteadiness, nausea and vomiting, diplopia, mild leukopenia	Severe skin rash, blood dyscrasias, hepatitis
clonazepam (Klonopin)	Drowsiness, behavior changes, headache, hirsutism, alopecia, palpitations	Hepatotoxicity, thrombocytopenia, bone marrow failure, ataxia
ethosuximide (Zarontin)	Nausea and vomiting, headache, gastric distress	Skin rash, blood dyscrasias, hepatitis, systemic lupus erythematosus
felbamate (Felbatol)	Cognitive impairments, insomnia, nausea, headache, fatigue	Aplastic anemia, hepatotoxicity
gabapentin (Neurotonin)	Dizziness, drowsiness, somnolence, fatigue, ataxia, weight gain, nausea	Leukopenia, hepatotoxicity
lamotrigine (Lamictal)	Drowsiness, tremor, nausea, ataxia, dizziness, headache, weight gain	Severe rash (Stevens-Johnson syndrome)
levetiracetam (Keppra)	Somnolence, dizziness, fatigue	Unknown
oxacarbazepine (Trileptal)	Dizziness, somnolence, double vision, fatigue, nausea, vomiting, loss of coordination, abnormal vision, abdominal pain, tremor, abnormal gait	Hepatotoxicity
phenobarbital (Luminal)	Sedation, irritability, diplopia, ataxia	Skin rash, anemia
phenytoin (Dilantin)	Visual problems, hirsutism, gingival hyperplasia, dysrhythmias, dysarthria, nystagmus	Severe skin reaction, peripheral neuropathy, ataxia, drowsiness, blood dyscrasias
primidone (Mysoline)	Lethargy, irritability, diplopia, ataxia, impotence	Skin rash
tiagabine (Gabitril)	Dizziness, fatigue, nervousness, tremor, difficulty concentrating, dysarthria, weak or buckling knees, abdominal pain	Unknown
topiramate (Topamax)	Fatigue, somnolence, confusion, ataxia, anorexia, depression, weight loss	Nephrolithiasis
valproate (Depakote, Depakene)	Nausea and vomiting, weight gain, hair loss, tremor, menstrual irregularities	Hepatotoxicity, skin rash, blood dyscrasias, nephritis
zonisamide (Zonegran, Excegran)	Somnolence, dizziness, anorexia, headache, nausea, agitation, rash	Leukopenia, hepatotoxicity

of the brain that can be excised without producing significant neurologic deficits, the removal of the area generating the seizures may produce long-term control and improvement (Elisevich & Smith, 2002).

This type of neurosurgery has been aided by several advances, including microsurgical techniques, EEGs with depth electrodes, improved illumination and hemostasis, and the introduction of neuroleptanalgesic agents (droperidol and fentanyl). These techniques, combined with use of local anesthetic agents, enable the neurosurgeon to perform surgery on an alert and cooperative patient. Using special testing devices, electrocortical mapping, and the patient's responses to stimulation, the boundaries of the epileptogenic focus (ie, abnormal area of the brain) are determined. Any abnormal epileptogenic focus is then excised (Elisevich & Smith, 2002).

As an adjunct to medication and surgery in adolescents and adults with partial seizures, a generator may be implanted under the clavicle. The device is connected to the vagus nerve in the cervical area, where it delivers electrical signals to the brain to control and reduce seizure activity (Luders, 2004; Parmet, Lynm & Glass, 2004). An external programming system is used by the physician to change stimulator settings. Patients can turn the stimulator on and off with a magnet. Resection surgery significantly reduces the incidence of seizures in patients with refractory epilepsy; however, more research is needed to determine the effect of surgery on quality of life, anxiety, and depression, all issues for these patients (Spencer, Berg, Vickrey, et al., 2003).

Nursing Process

The Patient With Epilepsy

Assessment

The nurse elicits information about the patient's seizure history. The patient is asked about the factors or events that may precipitate the seizures. Alcohol intake is documented. The nurse determines whether the patient has an aura before an epileptic seizure, which may indicate the origin of the seizure (eg, seeing a flashing light may indicate that the seizure originated in the occipital lobe). Observation and assessment during and after a seizure assist in identifying the type of seizure and its management.

The effects of epilepsy on the patient's lifestyle are assessed (Stafstrom & Rho, 2004). What limitations are imposed by the seizure disorder? Does the patient have a recreational program? Social contacts? Is the patient working, and is it a positive or stressful experience? What coping mechanisms are used?

Diagnosis

Nursing Diagnoses

Based on the assessment data, the patient's major nursing diagnoses may include the following:

- Risk for injury related to seizure activity
- Fear related to the possibility of seizures
- Ineffective individual coping related to stresses imposed by epilepsy
- Deficient knowledge related to epilepsy and its control

Collaborative Problems/ Potential Complications

The major potential complications for patients with epilepsy are status epilepticus and medication side effects (toxicity).

Planning and Goals

The major goals for the patient may include prevention of injury, control of seizures, achievement of a satisfactory psychosocial adjustment, acquisition of knowledge and understanding about the condition, and absence of complications.

Nursing Interventions

Preventing Injury

Injury prevention for the patient with seizures is a priority. If the type of seizure the patient is having places him or her at risk for injury, the patient should be lowered gently to the floor (if not in bed), and any potentially harmful items nearby (eg, furniture) should be removed. The patient should never be restrained or forced into a position, nor should anyone attempt to insert anything into the patient's mouth once a seizure has begun. Patients for whom seizure precautions are instituted should have pads applied to the side rails while in bed.

Reducing Fear of Seizures

Fear that a seizure may occur unexpectedly can be reduced by the patient's adherence to the prescribed treatment regimen. Cooperation of the patient and family and their trust in the prescribed regimen are essential for control of seizures. The nurse emphasizes that the prescribed antiseizure medication must be taken on a continuing basis and that drug dependence or addiction does not occur. Periodic monitoring is necessary to ensure the adequacy of the treatment regimen, to prevent side effects, and to monitor for drug resistance (Rho et al., 2004).

In an effort to control seizures, factors that may precipitate them are identified, such as emotional disturbances, new environmental stressors, onset of menstruation in female patients, or fever (Rho et al., 2004). The patient is encouraged to follow a regular and moderate routine in lifestyle, diet (avoiding excessive stimulants), exercise, and rest (sleep deprivation may lower the seizure threshold). Moderate activity is therapeutic, but excessive exercise should be avoided. An additional dietary intervention, referred to as the ketogenic diet, may be helpful for control of seizures in some patients (Stafstrom & Rho, 2004). This high-protein, low-carbohydrate diet is most effective in children whose seizures have not been controlled with two antiepileptic medications, but it is sometimes used for adults who have had poor seizure control (Stafstrom & Rho, 2004).

Photic stimulation (bright flickering lights, television viewing) may precipitate seizures; wearing dark glasses or covering one eye may be preventive. Tension states (anxiety, frustration) induce seizures in some patients. Classes in stress management may be of value. Because seizures are known to occur with alcohol intake, alcoholic beverages should be avoided.

Improving Coping Mechanisms

The social, psychological, and behavioral problems that frequently accompany epilepsy can be more of a disability than the actual seizures. Epilepsy may be accompanied by feelings of stigmatization, alienation, depression, and uncertainty. The patient must cope with the constant fear of a seizure and the psychological consequences (Rho et al., 2004). Children with epilepsy may be ostracized and excluded from school and peer activities. These problems are compounded during adolescence and add to the challenges of dating, not being able to drive, and feeling different from other people. Adults face these problems in addition to the burden of finding employment, concerns about relationships and childbearing, insurance problems, and legal barriers. Alcohol abuse may complicate matters. Family reactions may vary from outright rejection of the person with epilepsy to overprotection. As a result, many people with epilepsy have psychological and behavioral problems.

Counseling assists the patient and family to understand the condition and the limitations it imposes. Social and recreational opportunities are necessary for good mental health. Nurses can improve the quality of life for patients with epilepsy by teaching them and their families about symptoms and their management (Bader & Littlejohns, 2004).

Providing Patient and Family Education

Perhaps the most valuable facets of care contributed by the nurse to the person with epilepsy are education and efforts to modify the attitudes of the patient and family toward the disorder. The person who experiences seizures may consider every seizure a potential source of humiliation and shame. This may result in anxiety, depression, hostility, and secrecy on the part of the patient and family. Ongoing education and encouragement should be given to patients to enable them to overcome these reactions. The patient with epilepsy should carry an emergency medical identification card or wear a medical information bracelet. The patient and family need to be educated about medications as well as care during a seizure.

Monitoring and Managing Potential Complications

Status epilepticus, the major complication, is described later in this chapter. Another complication is the toxicity of medications. The patient and family are instructed about side effects and are given specific guidelines to assess and report signs and symptoms that indicate medication overdose. Many antiseizure medications require careful monitoring for therapeutic levels. The patient should plan to have serum drug levels assessed at regular intervals. Many known drug interactions occur with antiseizure medications. A complete pharmacologic profile should be reviewed with the patient to avoid interactions that either potentiate or inhibit the effectiveness of the medications.

Promoting Home and Community-Based Care

TEACHING PATIENTS SELF-CARE

Thorough oral hygiene after each meal, gum massage, daily flossing, and regular dental care are essential to prevent or control gingival hyperplasia in patients receiving phenytoin (Dilantin). The patient is also instructed to inform all health care providers of the medication being taken, because of the possibility of drug interactions. An individualized comprehensive teaching plan is needed to assist the patient and family to adjust to this chronic disorder. Written patient education materials must be appropriate for the patient's reading level and must be provided in alternative formats if warranted (Murphy, Chesson, Berman et al., 2001). See Chart 61-5 for home care instruction points.

CONTINUING CARE

Because epilepsy is a long-term disorder, the use of costly medications can create a significant financial burden. The Epilepsy Foundation of America (EFA) offers a mail-order program to provide medications at minimal cost and access to life insurance. This organization also serves as a referral source for special services for people with epilepsy.

For many, overcoming employment problems is a challenge. State vocational rehabilitation agencies can provide information about job training. The EFA has a training and placement service. If seizures are not well controlled, information about sheltered workshops or home employment programs may be obtained. Federal and state agencies and federal legislation may be of assistance to people with epilepsy who experience job discrimination. As a result of the Americans with Disabilities Act, the number of employers who knowingly hire people with epilepsy is increasing, but barriers to employment still exist (Bader & Littlejohns, 2004).

People who have uncontrollable seizures accompanied by psychological and social difficulties can be referred to comprehensive epilepsy centers where continuous audio-video and EEG monitoring, specialized treatment, and rehabilitation services are available (Bader & Littlejohns, 2004). Patients and their families need to be reminded of the importance of following the prescribed treatment regimen and of keeping follow-up appointments. In addition, they are reminded of the importance of participating in health promotion activities and recommended health screenings to promote a

CHART 61-5

HOME CARE CHECKLIST • The Patient With Epilepsy

At the completion of the home instruction, the patient and caregiver will be able to:	Patient	Caregiver
• Take medications daily as prescribed to keep the drug level constant to prevent seizures. The patient should never discontinue medications, even if there is no seizure activity.	✔	
• Keep a medication and seizure chart, noting when medications are taken and any seizure activity.	✔	✔
• Notify the patient's physician if patient cannot take medications due to illness.	✔	✔
• Have antiseizure medication serum levels checked regularly. When testing is prescribed, the patient should report to the laboratory for blood sampling before taking morning medication.	✔	
• Avoid activities that require alertness and coordination (driving, operating machinery) until after the effects of the medication have been evaluated.	✔	
• Report signs of toxicity so dosage can be adjusted. Common signs include drowsiness, lethargy, dizziness, difficulty walking, hyperactivity, confusion, inappropriate sleep, and visual disturbances.	✔	✔
• Avoid over-the-counter medications unless approved by the patient's physician.	✔	
• Carry a medical alert bracelet or identification card specifying the name of the patient's antiseizure medication and physician.	✔	
• Avoid seizure triggers, such as alcoholic beverages, electrical shocks, stress, caffeine, constipation, fever, hyperventilation, hypoglycemia.	✔	
• Take showers rather than tub baths to avoid drowning if seizure occurs; never swim alone.	✔	
• Exercise in moderation in a temperature-controlled environment to avoid excessive heat.	✔	
• Develop regular sleep patterns to minimize fatigue and insomnia.	✔	✔
• Use the Epilepsy Foundation of America's special services, including help in obtaining medications, vocational rehabilitation, and coping with epilepsy.	✔	✔

healthy lifestyle. Genetic and preconception counseling is advised.

Evaluation

Expected Patient Outcomes

Expected patient outcomes may include the following:

1. Sustains no injury during seizure activity
   a. Complies with treatment regimen and identifies the hazards of stopping the medication
   b. Patient and family can identify appropriate care during seizure
2. Indicates a decrease in fear
3. Displays effective individual coping
4. Exhibits knowledge and understanding of epilepsy
   a. Identifies the side effects of medications
   b. Avoids factors or situations that may precipitate seizures (eg, flickering lights, hyperventilation, alcohol)
   c. Follows a healthy lifestyle by getting adequate sleep and eating meals at regular times to avoid hypoglycemia
5. Absence of complications

Status Epilepticus

Status epilepticus (acute prolonged seizure activity) is a series of generalized seizures that occur without full recovery of consciousness between attacks (Rice et al., 2005). The term has been broadened to include continuous clinical or electrical seizures (on EEG) lasting at least 30 minutes, even without impairment of consciousness. It is considered a medical emergency. Status epilepticus produces cumulative effects. Vigorous muscular contractions impose a heavy metabolic demand and can interfere with respirations. Some respiratory arrest at the height of each seizure produces venous congestion and hypoxia of the brain. Repeated episodes of cerebral anoxia and edema may lead to irreversible and fatal brain damage. Factors that precipitate status epilepticus include withdrawal of antiseizure medication, fever, and concurrent infection.

Medical Management

The goals of treatment are to stop the seizures as quickly as possible, to ensure adequate cerebral oxygenation, and to maintain the patient in a seizure-free state. An airway and adequate oxygenation are established. If the patient remains unconscious and unresponsive, a cuffed endotracheal tube is inserted. Intravenous diazepam (Valium), lorazepam (Ativan), or fosphenytoin (Cerebyx) is administered slowly in an attempt to halt seizures immediately. Other medications (phenytoin, phenobarbital) are administered later to maintain a seizure-free state.

An IV line is established, and blood samples are obtained to monitor serum electrolytes, glucose, and phenytoin levels (Rice et al., 2005). EEG monitoring may be useful in determining the nature of the seizure activity. Vital signs and neurologic signs are monitored on a continuing basis. An IV infusion of dextrose is administered if the seizure is caused by hypoglycemia. If initial treatment is unsuccessful, general anesthesia with a short-acting barbiturate may be used. The serum concentration of the antiseizure medication is measured, because a low level suggests that the patient was not taking the medication or that the dosage was too low. Cardiac involvement or respiratory depression may be life-threatening. The potential for postictal cerebral edema also exists.

Nursing Management

The nurse initiates ongoing assessment and monitoring of respiratory and cardiac function because of the risk for delayed depression of respiration and blood pressure secondary to administration of antiseizure medications and sedatives to halt the seizures. Nursing assessment also includes monitoring and documenting the seizure activity and the patient's responsiveness.

The patient is turned to a side-lying position, if possible, to assist in draining pharyngeal secretions. Suction equipment must be available because of the risk for aspiration. The IV line is closely monitored, because it may become dislodged during seizures.

A person who has received long-term antiseizure therapy has a significant risk for fractures resulting from bone disease (osteoporosis, osteomalacia, and hyperparathyroidism), a side effect of therapy. Therefore, during seizures, the patient is protected from injury with the use of seizure precautions and is monitored closely. No effort should be made to restrain movements. The patient having seizures can inadvertently injure nearby people, so nurses should protect themselves. Other nursing interventions for the person having seizures are presented in Chart 61-4.

Headache

Headache, or cephalgia, is one of the most common of all human physical complaints. Headache is a symptom rather than a disease entity; it may indicate organic disease (neurologic or other disease), a stress response, vasodilation (migraine), skeletal muscle tension (tension headache), or a combination of factors. A **primary headache** is one for which no organic cause can be identified. These types of headache include migraine, tension-type, and cluster headaches (Lipton, Bigal, Steiner, et al., 2004). Cranial arteritis is another common cause of headache. A classification of headaches was issued first by the Headache Classification Committee of the International Headache Society in 1988. The International Headache Society revised the headache classification in 2004; an abbreviated list is shown in Chart 61-6.

Migraine is a symptom complex characterized by periodic and recurrent attacks of severe headache lasting from 4 to 72 hours in adults. The cause of migraine has not been clearly demonstrated, but it is primarily a vascular disturbance that occurs more commonly in women and has a strong familial tendency. The typical time of onset is at puberty, and the incidence is highest in adults 20 to 35 years of age. There are six subtypes of **migraine headache**, including migraine with and without aura. Most patients have migraine without an aura.

Tension-type headaches tend to be chronic and less severe and are probably the most common type of headache. *Cluster headaches* are a severe form of vascular headache. They are seen five times more frequently in men than in women. Types of headaches not subsumed under these categories fall into the *Other Primary Headache* group and include headaches triggered by cough, exertion, and sexual activity (Lipton et al., 2004).

Cranial arteritis is a cause of headache in the older population, reaching its greatest incidence in those older than 70 years of age. Inflammation of the cranial arteries is characterized by a severe headache localized in the region of the temporal arteries. The inflammation may be generalized (in which case cranial arteritis is part of a vascular disease) or focal (in which case only the cranial arteries are involved).

A **secondary headache** is a symptom associated with an organic cause, such as a brain tumor or an aneurysm.

CHART 61-6

International Headache Society Classification of Headache

1. Migraine
2. Tension-type headache
3. Cluster headache and other trigeminal-autonomic cephalalgias
4. Other primary headaches
5. Headache attributed to head and/or neck trauma
6. Headache attributed to cranial or cervical vascular disorder
7. Headache attributed to nonvascular intracranial disorder
8. Headache attributed to a substance or its withdrawal
9. Headache attributed to infection
10. Headache attributed to disorder of homeostasis
11. Headache or facial pain attributed to disorder of cranium, neck, eyes, ears, nose, sinuses, teeth, mouth, or other facial or cranial structures
12. Headache attributed to psychiatric disorder
13. Cranial neuralgias and central causes of facial pain
14. Other headache

From Headache Classification Subcommittee of the International Headache Society. (2004). International classification of headache disorders (2nd ed.). *Cephalalgia, 24*(Suppl 1), 1–150.

Although most headaches do not indicate serious disease, persistent headaches require further investigation. Serious disorders related to headache include brain tumors, subarachnoid hemorrhage, stroke, severe hypertension, meningitis, and head injuries.

Assessment and Diagnostic Evaluation

The diagnostic evaluation includes a detailed history, a physical assessment of the head and neck, and a complete neurologic examination. Headaches may manifest differently in the same person over the course of a lifetime, and the same type of headache may manifest differently from patient to patient. The health history focuses on assessing the headache itself, with emphasis on the factors that precipitate or provoke it. The patient is asked to describe the headache in his or her own words.

Because headache is often the presenting symptom of various physiologic and psychological disturbances, a general health history is an essential component of the patient database. Headache may be a symptom of endocrine, hematologic, gastrointestinal, infectious, renal, cardiovascular, or psychiatric disease. Therefore, questions addressed in the health history should cover major medical and surgical illness as well as a body systems review.

The medication history can provide insight into the patient's overall health status. Antihypertensive agents, diuretic medications, anti-inflammatory agents, and monoamine oxidase (MAO) inhibitors are a few of the categories of medications that can provoke headaches. Although sometimes exaggerated in importance, emotional factors can play a role in precipitating headaches. Stress is thought to be a major initiating factor in migraine headaches; therefore, sleep patterns, level of stress, recreational interests, appetite, emotional problems, and family stressors are relevant. There is a strong familial tendency for headache disorders, and a positive family history may help in making a diagnosis.

A direct relationship may exist between exposure to toxic substances and headache. Careful questioning may uncover chemicals to which a worker has been exposed. Under the Right to Know law, employees have access to the material safety data sheets (commonly referred to as MSDSs) for all the substances with which they come in contact in the workplace. The occupational history also includes assessment of the workplace as a possible source of stress and for a possible ergonomic basis of muscle strain and headache.

A complete description of the headache itself is crucial. The nurse reviews the age at onset of headache; the headache's frequency, location, and duration; the type of pain; factors that relieve and precipitate the event; and associated symptoms. The data obtained should include the patient's own words about the headache in response to the following questions:

- What is the location? Is it unilateral or bilateral? Does it radiate?
- What is the quality—dull, aching, steady, boring, burning, intermittent, continuous, paroxysmal?
- How many headaches occur during a given period of time?
- What are the precipitating factors, if any—environmental (eg, sunlight, weather change), foods, exertion, other?
- What makes the headache worse (eg, coughing, straining)?
- What time (day or night) does it occur?
- How long does a typical headache last?
- Are there any associated symptoms, such as facial pain, lacrimation (excessive tearing), or scotomas (blind spots in the field of vision)?
- What usually relieves the headache (aspirin, nonsteroidal anti-inflammatory drugs, ergot preparation, food, heat, rest, neck massage)?
- Does nausea, vomiting, weakness, or numbness in the extremities accompany the headache?
- Does the headache interfere with daily activities?
- Do you have any allergies?
- Do you have insomnia, poor appetite, loss of energy?
- Is there a family history of headache?
- What is the relationship of the headache to your lifestyle or physical or emotional stress?
- What medications are you taking?

Diagnostic testing often is not helpful in the investigation of headache, because often there are few objective findings. In patients who demonstrate abnormalities on the neurologic examination, CT, cerebral angiography, or MRI may be used to detect underlying causes, such as tumor or aneurysm. Electromyography (EMG) may reveal a sustained contraction of the neck, scalp, or facial muscles. Laboratory tests may include complete blood count, erythrocyte sedimentation rate, electrolytes, glucose, creatinine, and thyroid hormone levels.

Pathophysiology

The cerebral signs and symptoms of *migraine* result from dysfunction of the brain stem pathways that normally modulate sensory input (Goadsby, Lipton & Ferrari, 2002). Abnormal metabolism of serotonin, a vasoactive neurotransmitter found in platelets and cells of the brain, plays a major role. The headache is preceded by a rise in plasma serotonin, which dilates the cerebral vessels, but migraines are more than just vascular headaches. The exact mechanism of pain in migraine is not completely understood but is thought to be related to the cranial blood vessels, the innervation of the vessels, and the reflex connections in the brain stem.

Migraines can be triggered by menstrual cycles, bright lights, stress, depression, sleep deprivation, fatigue, overuse of certain medications, and certain foods containing tyramine, monosodium glutamate, nitrites, or milk products. Foods in these categories include aged cheese and many processed foods. Use of oral contraceptives may be associated with increased frequency and severity of attacks in some women.

Emotional or physical stress may cause contraction of the muscles in the neck and scalp, resulting in *tension* headache. The pathophysiology of *cluster* headache is not fully understood. One theory is that it is caused by dilation of orbital and nearby extracranial arteries. *Cranial arteritis* is thought to represent an immune vasculitis in which immune complexes are deposited within the walls of affected blood vessels, producing vascular injury and inflammation. A biopsy may be performed on the involved artery to make the diagnosis.

Clinical Manifestations

Migraine

The migraine with aura can be divided into four phases: prodrome, aura, the headache, and recovery (headache termination and postdrome).

PRODROME

The prodrome phase is experienced by 60% of patients, with symptoms that occur hours to days before a migraine headache. Symptoms may include depression, irritability, feeling cold, food cravings, anorexia, change in activity level, increased urination, diarrhea, or constipation. Patients usually experience the same prodrome with each migraine headache.

Aura Phase

Aura occurs in up to 31% of patients who have migraines (Goadsby et al., 2002). The aura usually lasts less than 1 hour and may provide enough time for the patient to take the prescribed medication to avert a full-blown attack (see later discussion). This period is characterized by focal neurologic symptoms. Visual disturbances (ie, light flashes and bright spots) are common and may be hemianopic (affecting only half of the visual field). Other symptoms that may follow include numbness and tingling of the lips, face, or hands; mild confusion; slight weakness of an extremity; drowsiness; and dizziness.

This period of aura corresponds to the painless vasoconstriction that is the initial physiologic change characteristic of classic migraine. Cerebral blood flow studies performed during migraine headaches demonstrate that during all phases of the attack, cerebral blood flow is reduced throughout the brain, with subsequent loss of autoregulation and impaired carbon dioxide responsiveness.

Headache Phase

As vasodilation and a decline in serotonin levels occur, a throbbing headache (unilateral in 60% of patients) intensifies over several hours. This headache is severe and incapacitating and is often associated with photophobia, nausea, and vomiting. Its duration varies, ranging from 4 to 72 hours (Goadsby et al., 2002).

Recovery Phase

In the recovery phase (termination and postdrome), the pain gradually subsides. Muscle contraction in the neck and scalp is common, with associated muscle ache and localized tenderness, exhaustion, and mood changes. Any physical exertion exacerbates the headache pain. During this postheadache phase, patients may sleep for extended periods.

Other Headache Types

The *tension-type headache* is characterized by a steady, constant feeling of pressure that usually begins in the forehead, temple, or back of the neck. It is often band-like or may be described as "a weight on top of my head."

Cluster headaches are unilateral and come in clusters of one to eight daily, with excruciating pain localized to the eye and orbit and radiating to the facial and temporal regions. The pain is accompanied by watering of the eye and nasal congestion. Each attack lasts 15 minutes to 3 hours and may have a crescendo–decrescendo pattern (Hickey, 2003). The headache is often described as penetrating.

Cranial arteritis often begins with general manifestations, such as fatigue, malaise, weight loss, and fever. Clinical manifestations associated with inflammation (heat, redness, swelling, tenderness, or pain over the involved artery) usually are present. Sometimes a tender, swollen, or nodular temporal artery is visible. Visual problems are caused by ischemia of the involved structures.

Prevention

Prevention begins by having the patient avoid specific triggers that are known to initiate the headache syndrome. Preventive medical management of migraine involves the daily use of one or more agents that are thought to block the physiologic events leading to an attack. Medication therapy should be considered for migraine if attacks occur as often as 3 to 4 days per month (Goadsby et al., 2002). Treatment regimens vary greatly, as do patient responses; therefore, close monitoring is indicated.

Several proven or widely used medications for the prevention of migraine are available. Two beta-blocking agents, propranolol (Inderal) and metoprolol (Lopressor), inhibit the action of beta-receptors—cells in the heart and brain that control the dilation of blood vessels. This is thought to be a major reason for their antimigraine action. Other medications that are prescribed for migraine prevention include amitriptyline hydrochloride (Elavil), divalproex (Valproate), flunarizine, and serotonin antagonists (Pizotyline) (Goadsby et al., 2002).

Calcium antagonists (eg, verapamil) are widely used but may require several weeks at a therapeutic dosage before improvement is noted. Calcium-channel blockers are not as effective as beta-blockers for prevention but may be more appropriate for some patients, such as those with bradycardia, diabetes mellitus, or asthma (Goadsby et al., 2002).

Alcohol, nitrites, vasodilators, and histamines may precipitate cluster headaches. Elimination of these factors helps prevent the headaches. Prophylactic medication therapy may include beta-blockers, ergotamine tartrate (occasionally), lithium, naproxen (Naprosyn), and methysergide (Sansert); such therapy is effective in 20% to 70% of cases (Hickey, 2003).

Medical Management

Therapy for migraine headache is divided into abortive (symptomatic) and preventive approaches. The abortive approach, best employed in those patients who have less frequent attacks, is aimed at relieving or limiting a headache at the onset or while it is in progress. The preventive approach is used in patients who experience more frequent attacks at regular or predictable intervals and may have a medical condition that precludes the use of abortive therapies (Bader & Littlejohns, 2004; Hickey, 2003).

The triptans, serotonin receptor agonists, are the most specific antimigraine agents available. These agents cause vasoconstriction, reduce inflammation, and may reduce pain transmission. The five triptans in routine clinical use include sumatriptan (Imitrex), naratriptan (Amerge), rizatriptan (Maxalt), zolmitriptan (Zomig), and almotriptan (Goadsby et al., 2002). Numerous serotonin receptor agonists are under study.

Perhaps the most widely used triptan is sumatriptan succinate (Imitrex); it is available in oral, intranasal, and subcutaneous preparations and is effective for the treatment of acute migraine and cluster headaches in adults (Bader & Littlejohns, 2004; Hickey, 2003). The subcutaneous form usually relieves symptoms within 1 hour and is available in an autoinjector for immediate patient use, although this form is expensive. Sumatriptan has been found to be effective in relieving moderate to severe migraine headaches in a large number of adult patients. Sumatriptan can cause chest pain and is contraindicated in patients with ischemic heart disease (Goadsby et al., 2002). Careful administration and dosing instructions to patients are important to prevent adverse reactions such as increased blood pressure, drowsiness, muscle pain, sweating, and anxiety. Interactions are possible if the medication is taken in conjunction with St. John's wort (Karch, 2005).

Many of the triptan medications are available in a variety of formulations, such as nasal sprays, inhalers, suppositories, or injections; however, 80% of patients prefer the oral formulations (Goadsby et al., 2002). None of these medications should be taken concurrently with medications containing ergotamine, because of the potential for a prolonged vasoactive reaction (Karch, 2005).

Ergotamine preparations (taken orally, sublingually, subcutaneously, intramuscularly, by rectum, or by inhalation) may be effective in aborting the headache if taken early in the migraine process. They are low in cost. Ergotamine tartrate acts on smooth muscle, causing prolonged constriction of the cranial blood vessels. Each patient's dosage is based on individual needs. Side effects include aching muscles, paresthesias (numbness and tingling), nausea, and vomiting. Cafergot, a combination of ergotamine and caffeine, can arrest or reduce the severity of the headache if it is taken at the first sign of an attack (Karch, 2005).

Researchers are evaluating several antiepileptic medications for migraine prevention. Topiramate was effective in migraine prevention during the first month of treatment in 483 patients but needs to be tested for longer than 1 month (Brandes, Saper, Diamond, et al., 2004). Use of topiramate and gabapentin for migraine prevention may have a side effect of impairing cognitive ability (Salinsky, Strorzbach, Spencer, et al., 2005).

The medical management of an acute attack of cluster headaches may include 100% oxygen by face mask for 15 minutes, ergotamine tartrate, sumatriptan, corticosteroids, or a percutaneous sphenopalatine ganglion blockade (Bader & Littlejohns, 2004; Hickey, 2003).

The medical management of cranial arteritis consists of early administration of a corticosteroid to prevent the possibility of loss of vision due to vascular occlusion or rupture of the involved artery. The patient is instructed not to stop the medication abruptly, because this can lead to relapse. Analgesic agents are prescribed for comfort.

Nursing Management

When migraine or the other types of headaches have been diagnosed, the goals of nursing management is to enhance pain relief. It is reasonable to try nonpharmacologic interventions first, but the use of pharmacologic agents should not be delayed. The goal is to treat the acute event of the headache and to prevent recurrent episodes. Prevention involves patient education regarding precipitating factors, possible lifestyle or habit changes that may be helpful, and pharmacologic measures.

Relieving Pain

Individualized treatment depends on the type of headache and differs for migraine, cluster headaches, cranial arteritis, and tension headache (Bader & Littlejohns, 2004; Hickey, 2003). Nursing care is directed toward treatment of the acute episode. A migraine or a cluster headache in the early phase requires abortive medication therapy instituted as soon as possible. Some headaches can be prevented if the appropriate medications are taken before the onset of pain. Nursing care during a fully developed attack includes comfort measures such as a quiet, dark environment and elevation of the head of the bed to 30 degrees. In addition, symptomatic treatment such as antiemetics may be indicated (Goadsby et al., 2002).

Symptomatic pain relief for tension headache may be obtained by application of local heat or massage. Additional strategies may include the use of analgesic agents, antidepressant medications, and muscle relaxants.

Promoting Home and Community-Based Care

TEACHING PATIENTS SELF-CARE

Headaches, especially migraines, are more likely to occur when the patient is ill, overly tired, or stressed. Nonpharmacologic therapies are important and include patient education about the type of headache, its mechanism (if known), and appropriate changes in lifestyle to avoid triggers. Regular sleep, meals, exercise, relaxation, and avoidance of dietary triggers may be helpful in avoiding headaches (Goadsby et al., 2002).

The patient with tension headaches needs teaching and reassurance that the headache is not the result of a brain tumor; this is a common unspoken fear. Stress reduction techniques, such as biofeedback, exercise programs, and meditation, are examples of nonpharmacologic therapies that may prove helpful. The patient and family need to be reminded of the importance of following the prescribed treatment regimen for headache and keeping follow-up appointments. In addition, the patient is reminded of the importance of participating in health promotion activities and recommended health screenings to promote a healthy lifestyle. Chart 61-7 presents a home care checklist for the patient with migraine headaches.

CONTINUING CARE

The National Headache Foundation (see Resources) provides a list of clinics in the United States and the names of physicians who specialize in headache and who are members of the American Association for the Study of Headache.

CHART 61-7

HOME CARE CHECKLIST • The Patient With Migraine Headaches

At the completion of the home instruction, the patient or caregiver will be able to:	Patient	Caregiver
• Define migraine headaches and describe characteristics and manifestations.	✔	✔
• Identify triggers of migraine headaches and how to avoid such triggers as:	✔	✔
• Foods that contain tyramine, such as chocolate, cheese, coffee, dairy products		
• Dietary habits that result in long periods between meals		
• Menstruation and ovulation (causes hormone fluctuation)		
• Alcohol (causes vasodilation of blood vessels)		
• Fatigue and fluctuations in sleep patterns		
• State importance of developing and using a headache diary.	✔	✔
• State stress management and lifestyle changes to minimize the frequency of headaches.	✔	✔
• State pharmacologic management: acute therapy and prophylaxis, to include medication regimen and side effects.	✔	✔
• Identify comfort measures during headache attacks, such as resting in a quiet and dark environment, applying cold compresses to the painful area, and elevating the head.	✔	✔
• Identify resources for education and support, such as the National Headache Foundation.	✔	✔

Critical Thinking Exercises

1 ebp Your 25-year-old patient with a brain tumor has early signs of increased ICP. Describe the medical management you would anticipate to control the ICP and the nursing measures that are indicated. How would you determine whether your interventions were effective in alleviating the increased ICP? What is the evidence base for practices to decrease ICP? Identify the criteria used to evaluate the strength of the evidence for these practices.

2 A patient is admitted to your unit after undergoing intracranial surgery for a brain tumor. Describe the major complications to assess for, along with the signs and symptoms of each. Describe the pharmacologic treatment and nursing measures that are indicated postoperatively. What patient and family teaching is important for the patient and family? How would you modify your teaching and discharge planning if the patient understands little English?

3 ebp You are caring for a 35-year-old patient who is admitted to the hospital for evaluation of her headaches. What resources would you use to identify the current guidelines for classification and treatment of headaches? What is the evidence base for headache treatment practices? Identify the criteria used to evaluate the strength of the evidence for these practices.

REFERENCES AND SELECTED READINGS

BOOKS

American Association of Neuroscience Nurses (AANN). (2005). *Guide to the care of the patient with intracranial pressure monitoring: AANN reference series for clinical practice.* Glenview, IL: Author.

Bader, M. K. & Littlejohns, L. R. (2004) *AANN core curriculum for neuroscience nursing* (4th ed.). St. Louis: Elsevier.

Brain Trauma Foundation (2003). *Guidelines for the management of severe traumatic brain injury.* New York: Brain Trauma Foundation.

Dudek, S. G. (2006). *Nutrition essentials for nursing practice* (5th ed.). Philadelphia: Lippincott Williams & Wilkins.

Elisevich, K. & Smith, B. J. (2002). *Epilepsy surgery: Case studies and commentaries.* Philadelphia: Lippincott Williams & Wilkins.

Fischbach, F. (2005). *Nurses' quick reference to common laboratory and diagnostic tests* (4th ed.). Philadelphia: Lippincott Williams & Wilkins.

Hickey, J. V. (2003). *The clinical practice of neurologic and neurosurgical nursing* (5th ed.). Philadelphia: Lippincott Williams & Wilkins.

Karch, A. (2005). *Lippincott's nursing drug guide.* Philadelphia: Lippincott Williams & Wilkins.

Luders, H. O. (2004). *Deep brain stimulation and epilepsy.* New York: Martin Dunitz, Taylor & Francis Group.

Porth, C. M. (2005). *Pathophysiology: Concepts of altered health states* (7th ed.) Philadelphia: Lippincott Williams & Wilkins.

Rice, J., Robichaux, C. & Leonard, A. (2005) Nervous system alteration. In Sole, M., Klein, D. & Mosely, M. (eds.) *Introduction to critical care nursing* (4th ed.). St. Louis, MO: Elsevier Saunders.

Rho, J. M., Sankar, R. & Cavazos, J. E. (2004). *Epilepsy: Scientific foundations of clinical practice.* New York: Marcel Dekker.

Ropper, A. H., Gress, D., Diringer, M. N., et al. (2004). *Neurological and neurosurgical intensive care* (4th ed.). Philadelphia: Lippincott, Williams & Wilkins.

Seidel, H., Ball, J., Dains, J. et al. (2003). *Mosby's guide to physical examination* (5th ed.). St. Louis: Mosby.

Somjen, G. (2004). *Ions in the brain: Normal function, seizures and stroke.* Oxford: Oxford University Press.

Stafstrom, C. E. & Rho, J. M. (2004). *Epilepsy and the ketogenic diet.* Totowa, NJ: Humana Press.

Suarez, J. (2004). *Critical care neurology and neurosurgery.* Totowa, NJ: Humana Press.

Worthington, P. H. (2004). *Practical aspects of nutritional support.* Philadelphia: Saunders.

JOURNALS

**Asterisks indicate nursing research articles.*

General

*Bond, A., Draeger, C., Mandleco, B., et al. (2003). Needs of family members of patients with severe traumatic brain injury. *Critical Care Nurse, 23*(4), 63–72.

Diringer, M. N. (2004). Treatment of fever in the neurologic intensive care unit with a catheter-based heat exchange system. *Critical Care Medicine, 32*(2), 559–564.

Henneman, E. A. & Karras, G. E. (2004). Determining brain death in adults: A guideline for use in critical care. *Critical Care Nurse, 24*(5), 50–56.

Holcomb, S. (2002). Diabetes insipidus. *Dimensions of Critical Care Nursing, 21*(3), 94–97.

Kurtoglu, M., Yanar, H., Bilsel, Y., et al. (2004). Venous thromboembolism prophylaxis after head and spinal trauma: Intermittent pneumatic compression devices versus low molecular weight heparin. *World Journal of Surgery, 28*(8), 807–811.

*Meeker, M., Du, R., Bacchetti, P., et al. (2005). Pupil examination: Validity and clinical utility of an automated pupillometer. *Journal of Neuroscience Nursing, 37*(1), 34–40.

*O'Farrell, B., Vandervoort, M., Bisnaire, D., et al. (2001). Evaluation of portable bladder ultrasound: Accuracy and effect on nursing practice in an acute care neuroscience unit. *Journal of Neuroscience Nursing, 33*(6), 301–309.

Park, P., Garton, H., Kocan, M., et al. (2004). Risk of infection with prolonged ventricular catheterization. *Neurosurgery, 55*(3), 594–601.

Headache

Brandes, J. L., Saper, J. R., Diamond, M., et al. (2004). Topiramate for migraine prevention: A randomized controlled trial. *Journal of the American Medical Association, 291*(8), 965–973.

Goadsby, P. J., Lipton, R. & Ferrari, M. (2002). Migraine: Current understanding and treatment. *New England Journal of Medicine, 346*(4), 257–270.

Headache Classification Subcommittee of the International Headache Society. (2004). International classification of headache disorders (2nd ed.). *Cephalalgia, 24*(Suppl. 1), 1–150.

Lipton, R., Bigal, M., Steiner, T., et al. (2004). Classification of primary headaches. *Neurology, 63*(3), 427–435.

Salinsky, M. C., Strorzbach, D., Spencer, D. C., et al. (2005). Effects of topiramate and gabapentin on cognitive abilities in healthy volunteers. *Neurology, 64*(3), 792–798.

Increased Intracranial Pressure

Alderson, P., Gadkary, C. & Signorini, D. F. (2004). Therapeutic hypothermia for head injury. *The Cochrane Database of Systematic Reviews,* (4), CD001048.

Bader, M., Littlejohns, L. & March, K. (2003). Brain tissue oxygen monitoring in severe brain injury: II. Implications for critical care teams and case study. *Critical Care Nurse, 23*(4), 29–43.

Censullo, J. & Sebastian, S. (2003). Pentobarbital sodium coma for refractory intracranial hypertension. *Journal of Neuroscience Nursing, 35*(5), 252–256.

Fan, J. (2004). Effects of backrest position on intracranial pressure and cerebral perfusion pressure in people with brain injury: A systematic review. *Journal of Neuroscience Nursing, 36*(5). 278–288.

Johnston, A., Steiner, L., Coles, J., et al. (2005). Effect of cerebral perfusion pressure augmentation on regional oxygenation and metabolism after head injury. *Critical Care Medicine, 33*(1), 198–195.

Littlejohns, L. R., Bader, M. K. & March, K. (2003). Brain tissue oxygen monitoring in severe brain injury, I. Research and usefulness in critical care. *Critical Care Nurse, 23*(4), 17–25.

Nelson, D., Bellander, B., MacCallum, R., et al. (2004). Cerebral microdialysis of patients with severe traumatic brain injury exhibits highly individualistic patterns as visualized by cluster analysis with self-organizing maps. *Critical Care Medicine, 32*(12), 2428–2436.

Polderman, K. (2004). Application of therapeutic hypothermia in the ICU: Opportunities and pitfalls of a promising treatment modality—Indications and evidence. *Intensive Care Medicine, 30*(4), 556–575.

Stevens, W. (2004). Multimodal monitoring: Head injury management using SJvO2 and LICOX. *Journal of Neuroscience Nursing, 36*(6), 332–339.

Stocchetti, N., Canavesi, K., Magnoni, S., et al. (2004). Arterio-jugular difference of oxygen content and outcome after head injury. *Anesthesia and Analgesia, 99*(1), 230–234.

Neurosurgical Care

Fukunaga, A., Naritaka, H., Fukaya, R., et al. (2004). Povidone-iodine ointment and gauze dressings associate with reduced catheter-related infection in seriously ill neurosurgical patients. *Infection Control and Hospital Epidemiology, 25*(8), 696–698.

Petrovich, Z., Jozsef, G., Yu, C., et al. (2003). Radiotherapy and stereotactic radiosurgery for pituitary tumors. *Neurosurgery Clinics of North America, 14*(1), 147–166.

Pickett, C. A. (2003). Diagnosis and management of pituitary tumors: Recent advances. *Primary Care Clinical Office Practice, 30*(4), 765–789.

Roberts, G. (2004). A review of the efficacy and safety of opioid analgesics post-craniotomy. *Nursing in Critical Care, 9*(6), 277–283.

Stapelfeldt, C., Lobo, E., Brown, R., et al. (2005). Intraoperative clonidine administration to neurosurgical patients. *Anesthesia and Analgesia, 100*(1), 226–232.

Seizures and Epilepsy

Cascino, G. B., Buchhalter, J. & Mullan, B. (2004). The current place of single photon emission computed tomography in epilepsy evaluations. *Neuroimaging Clinics of North America, 14*(3), 553–561.

Chang, B. S. & Lowenstein, D. H. (2003). Mechanism of disease: Epilepsy. *New England Journal of Medicine, 349*(13), 1257–1266.

French, J., Kanner, A., Bautista, J., et al. (2004). Efficacy and tolerability of new antileptic drugs: Treatment of refractory epilepsy. *Neurology, 62*(8), 1261–1273.

Gross, R., Gidal, B. & Pack, A. (2004). Antiseizure drugs and reduced bone density. *Neurology, 62*(11), E24–E25.

Murphy, P. W., Chesson, A., Berman, S. A., et al. (2001). Neurology patient education materials: Do our educational aids fit our patients' needs? *Journal of Neuroscience Nursing, 33*(2), 99–112.

Parmet, S., Lynm, C. & Glass, R. M. (2004). Epilepsy: JAMA patient page. *Journal of the American Medical Association, 291*(5), 654.

Pena, C. (2003). Seizure: A calm response and careful observation are crucial. *American Journal of Nursing, 103*(11), 73–81.

Spencer, S., Berg, A., Vickrey, B., et al. (2003). Initial outcomes in the multicenter study of epilepsy surgery. *Neurology, 61*(12), 1680–1685.

Unconsciousness and Coma

Booth, C. M., Boone, R. H., Tomlinson, G., et al. (2004). Is this patient dead, vegetative, or severely neurologically impaired? *Journal of the American Medical Association, 291*(7), 870–879.

*Davis, A. & Giminez, A. (2003). Cognitive-behavioral recovery in comatose patients following auditory sensory stimulation. *Journal of Neuroscience Nursing*, 35(4), 202–209.

RESOURCES

American Headache Society, 19 Mantua Rd., Mount Royal, NJ 08061; 856-423-0043; http://www.ahsnet.org. Accessed June 23, 2006.

Brain Injury Association, 105 North Alfred St., Alexandria, VA 22314; 703-235-6000; http://www.biausa.org. Accessed June 23, 2006.

Brain Trauma Foundation, 523 E. 72nd Street, New York, NY 10021; 212-772-0608; http://www.braintrauma.org. Accessed June 23, 2006.

Epilepsy Foundation, 4351 Garden City Dr., Landover, MD 20785-2223; 301-459-3700; http://www.epilepsyfoundation.org. Accessed June 23, 2006.

Hydrocephalus Association, 870 Market St., Suite 705, San Francisco, CA 94102; 415-732-7040; fax 415-732-7044; e-mail: hydroassoc@aol.com.

National Headache Foundation, 428 W St. James Pl., 2nd floor, Chicago, IL 60614-2750; 1-888-NHF-5552; http://www.headaches.org. Accessed June 23, 2006.

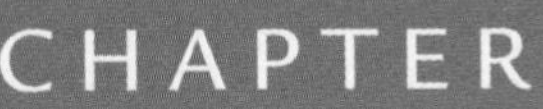

CHAPTER 62

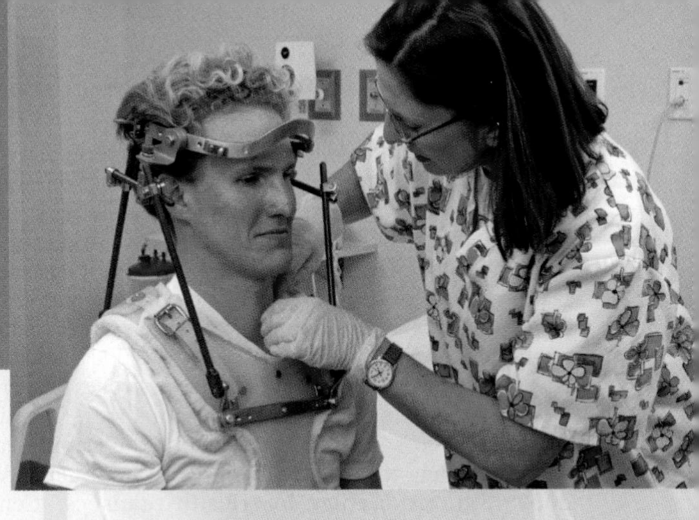

Management of Patients With Cerebrovascular Disorders

Learning Objectives

On completion of this chapter, the learner will be able to:

1. Describe the incidence and social impact of cerebrovascular disorders.
2. Identify the risk factors for cerebrovascular disorders and related measures for prevention.
3. Compare the various types of cerebrovascular disorders: their causes, clinical manifestations, and medical management.
4. Relate the principles of nursing management to the care of a patient in the acute stage of an ischemic stroke.
5. Use the nursing process as a framework for care of a patient recovering from an ischemic stroke.
6. Use the nursing process as a framework for care of a patient with a cerebral aneurysm.
7. Identify essential elements for family teaching and preparation for home care of the patient who has had a stroke.

"Cerebrovascular disorders" is an umbrella term that refers to a functional abnormality of the central nervous system (CNS) that occurs when the normal blood supply to the brain is disrupted. Stroke is the primary cerebrovascular disorder in the United States and in the world; it is the third leading cause of death behind heart disease and cancer. Approximately 700,000 people experience a stroke each year in the United States. Approximately 500,000 of these are new strokes, and 200,000 are recurrent strokes (American Heart Association [AHA], 2006). With about 4.8 million stroke survivors alive today, stroke is the leading cause of serious, long-term disability in the United States (AHA, 2006; National Center for Health Statistics, Centers for Disease Control, 2002). The financial impact of stroke is profound, with estimated direct and indirect costs of $53.6 billion in 2004 (AHA, 2006).

Strokes can be divided into two major categories: ischemic (85%) in which vascular occlusion and significant hypoperfusion occur, and hemorrhagic (15%), in which there is extravasation of blood into the brain or subarachnoid space (Albers, Amarenco, Easton, et al., 2004). Although there are some similarities between the two broad types of stroke, differences exist in etiology, pathophysiology, medical management, surgical management, and nursing care. Table 62-1 compares ischemic and hemorrhagic strokes.

CONCEPTS in action ANIMATION

Ischemic Stroke

An ischemic stroke, cerebrovascular accident (CVA), or "brain attack" is a sudden loss of function resulting from disruption of the blood supply to a part of the brain. The term "brain attack" is being used to suggest to health care practitioners and the public that a stroke is an urgent health care issue similar to a heart attack. With the approval of thrombolytic therapy for the treatment of acute ischemic stroke in 1996 came a revolution in the care of patients after a stroke. Early treatment with thrombolytic therapy for ischemic stroke results in fewer stroke symptoms and less loss of function (National Institute of Neurologic Disorders and Stroke [NINDS], 1995). Currently approved thrombolytic therapy has a treatment window of only 3 hours after the onset of a stroke. Urgency is needed on the part of the public and health care practitioners for rapid transport of the patient to a hospital for assessment and administration of the medication.

Ongoing research is focusing on acute ischemic stroke. The most recent advance is the approval by the U.S. Food and Drug Administration (FDA) of a clot retrieval device that opens the blocked artery and restores blood flow to the brain (Felton, Ogden, Pena, et al., 2005). The device has been used in a small number of cases, and research on clinical outcomes continues.

Ischemic strokes are subdivided into five different types based on the cause (Albers et al., 2004): (1) large artery thrombotic strokes (20%), (2) small penetrating artery thrombotic strokes (25%), (3) cardiogenic embolic strokes (20%), (4) cryptogenic strokes (30%), and (5) other (5%) (see Table 62-1).

Large artery thrombotic strokes are caused by atherosclerotic plaques in the large blood vessels of the brain. Thrombus formation and occlusion at the site of the atherosclerosis result in ischemia and **infarction** (deprivation of blood supply).

Small penetrating artery thrombotic strokes affect one or more vessels and are the most common type of ischemic stroke. Small artery thrombotic strokes are also called lacunar strokes because of the cavity that is created after the death of infarcted brain tissue.

Cardiogenic embolic strokes are associated with cardiac dysrhythmias, usually atrial fibrillation. Embolic strokes can also be associated with valvular heart disease and thrombi in the left ventricle. Emboli originate from the heart and circulate to the cerebral vasculature, most commonly the left middle cerebral artery, resulting in a stroke. Embolic strokes may be prevented by the use of anticoagulation therapy in patients with atrial fibrillation.

The last two classifications of ischemic strokes are cryptogenic strokes, which have no known cause, and strokes from other causes, such as illicit drug use, coagulopathies, migraine, and spontaneous dissection of the carotid or vertebral arteries (Albers et al., 2004).

Glossary

agnosia: failure to recognize familiar objects perceived by the senses
aneurysm: a weakening or bulge in an arterial wall
aphasia: inability to express oneself or to understand language
apraxia: inability to perform previously learned purposeful motor acts on a voluntary basis
ataxia: impaired ability to coordinate movement, often seen as a staggering gait or postural imbalance
dysarthria: defects of articulation due to neurologic causes
expressive aphasia: inability to express oneself; often associated with damage to the left frontal lobe area
hemianopsia: blindness of half of the field of vision in one or both eyes
hemiplegia/hemiparesis: weakness/paralysis of one side of the body, or part or it, due to an injury to the motor areas of the brain
infarction: a zone of tissue deprived of blood supply
Korsakoff's syndrome: personality disorder characterized by psychosis, disorientation, delirium, insomnia, and hallucinations
penumbra region: area of low cerebral blood flow
receptive aphasia: inability to understand what someone else is saying; often associated with damage to the temporal lobe area

TABLE 62-1 Comparison of Major Types of Stroke

Item	Ischemic	Hemorrhagic
Causes	Large artery thrombosis Small penetrating artery thrombosis Cardiogenic embolic Cryptogenic (no known cause) Other	Intracerebral hemorrhage Subarachnoid hemorrhage Cerebral aneurysm Arteriovenous malformation
Main Presenting Symptoms	Numbness or weakness of the face, arm, or leg, especially on one side of the body	"Exploding headache" Decreased level of consciousness
Functional Recovery	Usually plateaus at 6 months	Slower, usually plateaus at about 18 months

Pathophysiology

In an ischemic brain attack, there is disruption of the cerebral blood flow due to obstruction of a blood vessel. This disruption in blood flow initiates a complex series of cellular metabolic events referred to as the ischemic cascade (Fig. 62-1).

The ischemic cascade begins when cerebral blood flow decreases to less than 25 mL per 100 g per minute. At this point, neurons are no longer able to maintain aerobic respiration. The mitochondria must then switch to anaerobic respiration, which generates large amounts of lactic acid, causing a change in the pH level. This switch to the less efficient anaerobic respiration also renders the neuron incapable of producing sufficient quantities of adenosine triphosphate (ATP) to fuel the depolarization processes. The membrane pumps that maintain electrolyte balances begin to fail, and the cells cease to function.

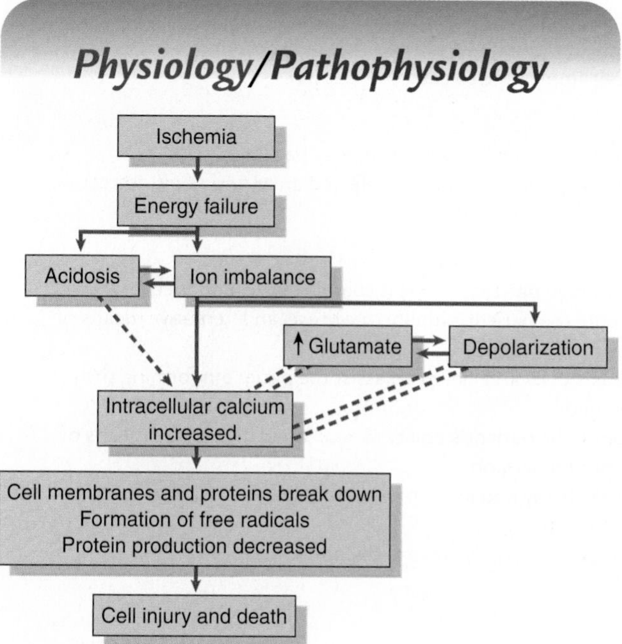

FIGURE 62-1. Processes contributing to ischemic brain cell injury. Courtesy of National Stroke Association, Englewood, Colorado.

Early in the cascade, an area of low cerebral blood flow, referred to as the **penumbra region**, exists around the area of infarction. The penumbra region is ischemic brain tissue that may be salvaged with timely intervention. The ischemic cascade threatens cells in the penumbra because membrane depolarization of the cell wall leads to an increase in intracellular calcium and the release of glutamate. The influx of calcium and the release of glutamate, if continued, activate a number of damaging pathways that result in the destruction of the cell membrane, the release of more calcium and glutamate, vasoconstriction, and the generation of free radicals. These processes enlarge the area of infarction into the penumbra, extending the stroke.

Each step in the ischemic cascade represents an opportunity for intervention to limit the extent of secondary brain damage caused by a stroke. The penumbra area may be revitalized by administration of tissue plasminogen activator (t-PA). Medications that protect the brain from secondary injury are called neuroprotectants. A number of ongoing clinical trials focus on neuroprotective medications and strategies to improve stroke recovery and survival (Hinkle & Bowman, 2003).

Clinical Manifestations

An ischemic stroke can cause a wide variety of neurologic deficits, depending on the location of the lesion (which vessels are obstructed), the size of the area of inadequate perfusion, and the amount of collateral (secondary or accessory) blood flow (see Chapter 60 for discussion of anatomy and brain blood supply). The patient may present with any of the following signs or symptoms:

- Numbness or weakness of the face, arm, or leg, especially on one side of the body
- Confusion or change in mental status
- Trouble speaking or understanding speech
- Visual disturbances
- Difficulty walking, dizziness, or loss of balance or coordination
- Sudden severe headache

Motor, sensory, cranial nerve, cognitive, and other functions may be disrupted. Table 62-2 reviews the neurologic deficits frequently seen in patients with strokes. Table 62-3 compares the symptoms and behaviors seen in right hemispheric stroke with those seen in left hemispheric stroke.

TABLE 62-2 Neurologic Deficits of Stroke: Manifestations and Nursing Implications

Neurologic Deficit	Manifestation	Nursing Implications/Patient Teaching Applications
Visual Field Deficits		
Homonymous hemianopsia (loss of half of the visual field)	• Unaware of persons or objects on side of visual loss • Neglect of one side of the body • Difficulty judging distances	Place objects within intact field of vision. Approach the patient from side of intact field of vision. Instruct/remind the patient to turn head in the direction of visual loss to compensate for loss of visual field. Encourage the use of eyeglasses if available. When teaching the patient, do so within patient's intact visual field.
Loss of peripheral vision	• Difficulty seeing at night • Unaware of objects or the borders of objects	Place objects in center of patient's intact visual field. Encourage the use of a cane or other object to identify objects in the periphery of the visual field. Driving ability will need to be evaluated.
Diplopia	• Double vision	Explain to the patient the location of an object when placing it near the patient. Consistently place patient care items in the same location.
Motor Deficits		
Hemiparesis	• Weakness of the face, arm, and leg on the same side (due to a lesion in the opposite hemisphere)	Place objects within the patient's reach on the nonaffected side. Instruct the patient to exercise and increase the strength on the unaffected side.
Hemiplegia	• Paralysis of the face, arm, and leg on the same side (due to a lesion in the opposite hemisphere)	Encourage the patient to provide range-of-motion exercises to the affected side. Provide immobilization as needed to the affected side. Maintain body alignment in functional position. Exercise unaffected limb to increase mobility, strength, and use.
Ataxia	• Staggering, unsteady gait • Unable to keep feet together; needs a broad base to stand	Support patient during the initial ambulation phase. Provide supportive device for ambulation (walker, cane). Instruct the patient not to walk without assistance or supportive device.
Dysarthria	• Difficulty in forming words	Provide the patient with alternative methods of communicating. Allow the patient sufficient time to respond to verbal communication. Support patient and family to alleviate frustration related to difficulty in communicating.
Dysphagia	• Difficulty in swallowing	Test the patient's pharyngeal reflexes before offering food or fluids. Assist the patient with meals. Place food on the unaffected side of the mouth. Allow ample time to eat.
Sensory Deficits		
Paresthesia (occurs on the side opposite the lesion)	• Numbness and tingling of extremity • Difficulty with proprioception	Instruct patient that sensation may be altered. Provide range of motion to affected areas and apply corrective devices as needed.
Verbal Deficits		
Expressive aphasia	• Unable to form words that are understandable; may be able to speak in single-word responses	Encourage patient to repeat sounds of the alphabet. Explore the patient's ability to write as an alternative means of communication.
Receptive aphasia	• Unable to comprehend the spoken word; can speak but may not make sense	Speak slowly and clearly to assist the patient in forming the sounds. Explore the patient's ability to read as an alternative means of communication.
Global (mixed) aphasia	• Combination of both receptive and expressive aphasia	Speak clearly and in simple sentences; use gestures or pictures when able. Establish alternative means of communication.

TABLE 62-2 Neurologic Deficits of Stroke: Manifestations and Nursing Implications (Continued)

Neurologic Deficit	Manifestation	Nursing Implications/Patient Teaching Applications
Cognitive Deficits		
	• Short- and long-term memory loss	Reorient patient to time, place, and situation frequently.
	• Decreased attention span	Use verbal and auditory cues to orient patient.
	• Impaired ability to concentrate	Provide familiar objects (family photographs, favorite objects).
	• Poor abstract reasoning	Use noncomplicated language.
	• Altered judgment	Match visual tasks with a verbal cue; holding a toothbrush, simulate brushing of teeth while saying, "I would like you to brush your teeth now." Minimize distracting noises and views when teaching the patient. Repeat and reinforce instructions frequently.
Emotional Deficits		
	• Loss of self-control	Support patient during uncontrollable outbursts.
	• Emotional lability	Discuss with the patient and family that the outbursts are due to the disease process.
	• Decreased tolerance to stressful situations	Encourage patient to participate in group activity.
	• Depression	Provide stimulation for the patient.
	• Withdrawal	Control stressful situations, if possible.
	• Fear, hostility, and anger	Provide a safe environment.
	• Feelings of isolation	Encourage patient to express feelings and frustrations related to disease process.

Motor Loss

A stroke is an upper motor neuron lesion and results in loss of voluntary control over motor movements. Because the upper motor neurons decussate (cross), a disturbance of voluntary motor control on one side of the body may reflect damage to the upper motor neurons on the opposite side of the brain. The most common motor dysfunction is **hemiplegia** (paralysis of one side of the body) caused by a lesion of the opposite side of the brain. **Hemiparesis**, or weakness of one side of the body, is another sign. The concept of upper and lower motor neuron lesions is described in more detail in Table 60-4 in Chapter 60.

In the early stage of stroke, the initial clinical features may be flaccid paralysis and loss of or decrease in the deep tendon reflexes. When these deep reflexes reappear (usually by 48 hours), increased tone is observed along with spasticity (abnormal increase in muscle tone) of the extremities on the affected side.

TABLE 62-3 Comparison of Left and Right Hemispheric Strokes

Left Hemispheric Stroke	Right Hemispheric Stroke
Paralysis or weakness on right side of body	Paralysis or weakness on left side of body
Right visual field deficit	Left visual field deficit
Aphasia (expressive, receptive, or global)	Spatial-perceptual deficits
Altered intellectual ability	Increased distractibility
Slow, cautious behavior	Impulsive behavior and poor judgment
	Lack of awareness of deficits

Communication Loss

Other brain functions affected by stroke are language and communication. In fact, stroke is the most common cause of aphasia. The following are dysfunctions of language and communication:

- **Dysarthria** (difficulty in speaking), caused by paralysis of the muscles responsible for producing speech
- Dysphasia (impaired speech) or **aphasia** (loss of speech), which can be **expressive aphasia**, **receptive aphasia**, or global (mixed) aphasia
- **Apraxia** (inability to perform a previously learned action), as may be seen when a patient makes verbal substitutions for desired syllables or words

Perceptual Disturbances

Perception is the ability to interpret sensation. Stroke can result in visual-perceptual dysfunctions, disturbances in visual-spatial relations, and sensory loss.

Visual-perceptual dysfunctions are caused by disturbances of the primary sensory pathways between the eye and visual cortex. Homonymous **hemianopsia** (loss of half of the visual field) may occur from stroke and may be temporary or permanent. The affected side of vision corresponds to the paralyzed side of the body.

Disturbances in visual-spatial relations (perceiving the relationship of two or more objects in spatial areas) are frequently seen in patients with right hemispheric damage.

Sensory Loss

The sensory losses from stroke may take the form of slight impairment of touch, or it may be more severe, with loss of proprioception (ability to perceive the position and motion of body parts) as well as difficulty in interpreting visual, tactile, and auditory stimuli. **Agnosias** are deficits in the ability to recognize previously familiar objects perceived by one or more of the senses.

Cognitive Impairment and Psychological Effects

If damage has occurred to the frontal lobe, learning capacity, memory, or other higher cortical intellectual functions may be impaired. Such dysfunction may be reflected in a limited attention span, difficulties in comprehension, forgetfulness, and a lack of motivation. These changes can cause the patient to become easily frustrated during rehabilitation. Depression is common and may be exaggerated by the patient's natural response to this catastrophic event. Emotional lability, hostility, frustration, resentment, lack of cooperation, and other psychological problems may occur.

Assessment and Diagnostic Findings

Any patient with neurologic deficits needs a careful history and a complete physical and neurologic examination. Initial assessment focuses on airway patency, which may be compromised by loss of gag or cough reflexes and altered respiratory pattern; cardiovascular status (including blood pressure, cardiac rhythm and rate, carotid bruit); and gross neurologic deficits.

Patients may present to the acute care facility with temporary neurologic symptoms. A transient ischemic attack (TIA) is a neurologic deficit lasting less than 24 hours, with most episodes resolving in less than 1 hour. A TIA is manifested by a sudden loss of motor, sensory, or visual function. The symptoms result from temporary ischemia (impairment of blood flow) to a specific region of the brain. A TIA may serve as a warning of impending stroke. Lack of evaluation and treatment of a patient who has experienced previous TIAs may result in a stroke and irreversible deficits (Hinkle, 2005).

The initial diagnostic test for a stroke is a noncontrast computed tomography (CT) scan performed emergently to determine if the event is ischemic or hemorrhagic (the category of stroke determines treatment). Further diagnostic workup for ischemic stroke involves attempting to identify the source of the thrombi or emboli. A 12-lead electrocardiogram (ECG) and a carotid ultrasound are standard tests. Other studies may include cerebral angiography; transcranial Doppler flow studies; transthoracic or transesophageal echocardiography; magnetic resonance imaging (MRI) of the brain, neck, or both; xenon-enhanced CT scan; and single photon emission CT (SPECT) scan (Adams, Adams, Brott, et al., 2003).

Prevention

Primary prevention of ischemic stroke remains the best approach. Stroke risk screenings are an ideal opportunity to lower stroke risk by identifying people or groups of people who are at high risk for stroke and by educating patients and the community about recognition and prevention of stroke (DeLemos, Atkinson, Croopnick, et al., 2003). Recent research findings suggest that low-dose aspirin may lower the risk of stroke in women (Ridker, Cook, Lee, et al., 2005).

Advanced age, gender, and race are well-known nonmodifiable risk factors for stroke. High-risk groups include people older than 55 years of age; the incidence of stroke more than doubles in each successive decade. Men have a higher rate of stroke than women do. Another high-risk group is African Americans; the incidence of first stroke in African Americans is almost twice that in Caucasian Americans (AHA, 2003).

Modifiable risk factors for ischemic stroke include hypertension, atrial fibrillation, hyperlipidemia, obesity, smoking, and diabetes (Chart 62-1). For people who are at high risk, interventions that alter modifiable factors, such as treating hypertension and hyperglycemia and stopping smoking, will reduce stroke risk. Other treatable conditions that increase risk for stroke are asymptomatic carotid stenosis and valvular heart disease (eg, endocarditis, prostatic heart valves). Periodontal disease has also been linked to stroke risk. The association between periodontal disease and stroke may result from the host inflammatory response and the chronic bacterial infection. However, the exact mechanism is not fully understood (Grau, Becher, Zigler, et al., 2004). Periodontal disease is a treatable and preventable condition. Many health promotion efforts encourage a healthy lifestyle with appropriate health maintenance; eating a low-fat, low-cholesterol diet; and increasing exercise.

Several methods of preventing recurrent stroke have been identified for patients with TIAs or ischemic stroke. Patients with moderate to severe carotid stenosis are treated with carotid endarterectomy (Rothwell, Eliasziw, Gutnikov, et al., 2004). In patients with atrial fibrillation, which increases the risk for emboli, administration of warfarin (Coumadin), an anticoagulant that inhibits clot formation, may prevent both thrombotic and embolic strokes.

Medical Management

Patients who have experienced a TIA or stroke should have medical management for secondary prevention. Those with atrial fibrillation (or cardioembolic strokes) are treated with dose-adjusted warfarin sodium (Coumadin) unless contraindicated. The international normalized ratio (INR) target is 2.5. If warfarin is contraindicated, aspirin is the best

CHART 62-1

Modifiable Risk Factors for Ischemic Stroke

- Hypertension (controlling hypertension, the major risk factor, is the key to preventing stroke)
- Atrial fibrillation
- Hyperlipidemia
- Diabetes mellitus (associated with accelerated atherogenesis)
- Smoking
- Asymptomatic carotid stenosis
- Obesity
- Excessive alcohol consumption

NURSING RESEARCH PROFILE

Education About Stroke Risk

Miller, E. T. & Spilker, J. (2003). Readiness to change and brief educational interventions: Successful strategies to reduce stroke risk. *Journal of Neuroscience Nursing, 35*(4), 215–222.

Purpose

Despite advances in stroke treatment and prevention, the public's knowledge of the signs and symptoms of a stroke, the importance of seeking stroke treatment early, and stroke risk reduction behaviors remains limited. The purpose of the study was to determine whether a brief educational intervention, tailored to the patient's stage of readiness to change, could affect the initiation and achievement of stroke risk-reducing behaviors for an at-risk population.

Design

This pilot study consisted of a repeated-measures design that involved three groups: control, simple advice, and brief educational intervention (BI). Sixty patients participated in the study, and the mean age was 68 years. All groups received a face-to-face interview for 30 minutes that included assessment of the following: knowledge of stroke risk factors, stroke symptoms, and risk reduction behaviors; readiness to change; functional status; depression; and quality of life. The control group received only the initial interview. The simple advice group received additional review of stroke risk reduction and symptoms, received "firm advice" about strategies to change based on the readiness stage, and were asked to set one goal for change. The BI group received the same interventions as the simple advice group, plus motivational counseling targeted to the person's specific goals for risk reduction and the stage of readiness to change for each behavior. The BI group also received another 15-minute interview at 4 to 6 weeks after the initial interview to evaluate progress in achieving goals. All three groups were evaluated at 3 months after the initial interview, using the same assessments as at the initial interview.

Findings

Results of this study support the use of the BI to reduce modifiable risk factors for stroke and to increase stroke knowledge. The BI group had a higher number of newly initiated behaviors ($p = .005$), achieved stroke risk reduction behaviors ($p = .006$), and achieved changes in knowledge of stroke symptoms and risks ($p = .001$). There were significant positive correlations between the "action" stage of readiness to change and the initiation and achievement of the new stroke risk reduction behaviors ($p = .002$).

Nursing Implications

This study reaffirms the value of nurses educating patients about stroke risk-reducing behaviors and improving stroke knowledge. Contact with patients can occur in many different settings (hospital, rehabilitation, home, community, occupational, outpatient), and the opportunity for education exists in each setting. Nurses are able to identify modifiable stroke risk factors, assess patients' knowledge deficits, and set realistic goals based on the patients' readiness to change.

option, although other medications may be used if both are contraindicated (Albers et al., 2004).

Platelet-inhibiting medications, including aspirin, extended-release dipyridamole (Persantine) plus aspirin, clopidogrel (Plavix), and ticlopidine (Ticlid), decrease the incidence of cerebral infarction in patients who have experienced TIAs and stroke from suspected embolic or thrombotic causes. The specific medication that is used is based on the patient's health history.

Medications classified as 3-hydroxy-2-methyl-glutaryl-coenzyme A reductase inhibitors (also known as statins) have been found in many studies to reduce coronary events and strokes. Benefits were found to be independent of cholesterol levels, and they are now widely used for stroke prevention. The indications for a statin medication, such as simvastatin (Zocor), have recently been updated by the FDA to include secondary stroke prevention (American Heart Association & American Stroke Association, 2004; Fisher & Davalos, 2004). After the acute stroke period, antihypertensive medications are also used, if indicated, for secondary stroke prevention. Benefits have been observed with the use of angiotensin-converting enzyme (ACE) inhibitors and thiazide diuretics (Chobanian, Bakris, Black, et al., 2003; Fisher & Davalos, 2004).

Thrombolytic Therapy

Thrombolytic agents are used to treat ischemic stroke by dissolving the blood clot that is blocking blood flow to the brain. Recombinant t-PA is a genetically engineered form of t-PA, a thrombolytic substance made naturally by the body. It works by binding to fibrin and converting plasminogen to plasmin, which stimulates fibrinolysis of the atherosclerotic lesion. Rapid diagnosis of stroke and initiation of thrombolytic therapy (within 3 hours) in patients with ischemic stroke leads to a decrease in the size of the stroke and an overall improvement in functional outcome after 3 months (Adams et al., 2003; NINDS, 1995). Ongoing clinical trials continue to investigate other thrombolytic agents (Haley, Lyden, Johnson, et al., 2005).

To realize the full potential of thrombolytic therapy, community education directed at recognizing the symptoms of stroke and obtaining appropriate emergency care is necessary to ensure rapid transport to a hospital and initiation of therapy within the 3-hour period. Delays make the patient ineligible for thrombolytic therapy, because revascularization of necrotic tissue (which develops after 3 hours) increases the risk for cerebral edema and hemorrhage.

ENHANCING PROMPT DIAGNOSIS

After being notified by emergency medical service personnel, the emergency department contacts the appropriate staff (neurologist, neuroradiologist, radiology department, nursing staff, ECG, and laboratory technicians) and informs them of the patient's imminent arrival at the hospital. Many institutions have brain attack teams that respond rapidly, ensuring that treatment occurs within the allotted period.

Initial management requires the definitive diagnosis of an ischemic stroke by CT scanning and determination of whether the patient meets the criteria for t-PA therapy (Chart 62-2). Some of the absolute contraindications for thrombolytic therapy include symptom onset greater than 3 hours before admission, a patient who is anticoagulated, or a patient who has recently had any type of intracranial pathology (eg, previous stroke, head injury, trauma). Once it is determined that the patient is a candidate for t-PA therapy, no anticoagulants are administered for the next 24 hours.

Before receiving t-PA, the patient is assessed using the National Institutes of Health Stroke Scale (NIHSS), a standardized assessment tool that helps evaluate stroke severity (Table 62-4). Total NIHSS scores range from 0 (normal) to 42 (severe stroke). Certification in the administration of the scale is recommended and is available for nurses and other health care professionals.

CHART 62-2

Eligibility Criteria for t-PA Administration

- Age 18 years or older
- Clinical diagnosis of ischemic stroke
- Time of onset of stroke known and is 3 hours or less
- Systolic blood pressure ≤185 mm Hg; diastolic ≤110 mm Hg
- Not a minor stroke or rapidly resolving stroke
- No seizure at onset of stroke
- Not taking warfarin (Coumadin)
- Prothrombin time ≤15 seconds or INR ≤1.7
- Not receiving heparin during the past 48 hours with elevated partial thromboplastin time
- Platelet count ≥100,000/mm^3
- No prior intracranial hemorrhage, neoplasm, arteriovenous malformation, or aneurysm
- No major surgical procedures within 14 days
- No stroke, serious head injury, or intracranial surgery within 3 months
- No gastrointestinal or urinary bleeding within 21 days

DOSAGE AND ADMINISTRATION

The patient is weighed to determine the dose of t-PA. The dosage for t-PA is 0.9 mg/kg, with a maximum dose of 90 mg. Ten percent of the calculated dose is administered as an intravenous (IV) bolus over 1 minute. The remaining dose (90%) is administered by IV over 1 hour via an infusion pump.

The patient is admitted to the intensive care unit or an acute stroke unit, where continuous cardiac monitoring and frequent neurologic assessments are conducted. Vital signs are obtained frequently, with particular attention to blood pressure (with the goal of lowering the risk of intracranial hemorrhage). An example of a standard protocol would be to obtain vital signs every 15 minutes for the first 2 hours, every 30 minutes for the next 6 hours, then every hour until 24 hours after treatment. Blood pressure should be maintained with the systolic pressure less than 180 mm Hg and the diastolic pressure less than 105 mm Hg (Adams et al., 2003). Airway management is instituted based on the patient's clinical condition and arterial blood gas values.

SIDE EFFECTS

Bleeding is the most common side effect of t-PA administration, and the patient is closely monitored for any bleeding (IV insertion sites, urinary catheter site, endotracheal tube, nasogastric tube, urine, stool, emesis, other secretions). A 24-hour delay in placement of nasogastric tubes, urinary catheters, and intra-arterial pressure catheters is recommended. Intracranial bleeding is a major complication that occurred in approximately 6.4% of patients in the initial t-PA study (NINDS, 1995). A number of factors were associated with the occurrence of symptomatic intracranial bleeding: age greater than 70 years, baseline NIHSS score greater than 20, serum glucose concentration 300 mg/dL or higher, and edema or mass effect observed on the patient's initial CT scan (Ingall, O'Fallen, Asplund, et al., 2004).

Therapy for Patients With Ischemic Stroke Not Receiving t-PA

Not all patients are candidates for t-PA therapy. Other treatments may include anticoagulant administration (IV heparin or low-molecular-weight heparin). Because of the risks associated with anticoagulation, their general use is no longer recommended for patients with acute ischemic stroke, whether treated with t-PA or not (Albers et al., 2004).

Careful maintenance of cerebral hemodynamics to maintain cerebral perfusion is extremely important after a stroke. Increased intracranial pressure (ICP) from brain edema, and associated complications, may occur after a large ischemic stroke. Interventions during this period include measures to reduce ICP, such as administering an osmotic diuretic (eg, mannitol), maintaining the partial pressure of carbon dioxide ($PaCO_2$) within the range of 30 to 35 mm Hg, and positioning to avoid hypoxia. Other treatment measures include the following:

- Elevation of the head of the bed to promote venous drainage and to lower increased ICP
- Intubation with an endotracheal tube to establish a patent airway, if necessary

TABLE 62-4 Summary of National Institutes of Health Stroke Scale (NIHSS)

Category	Description	Score
1a. Level of consciousness (LOC)	Alert	0
	Arousable by minor stimulation	1
	Obtunded, strong stimulation to attend	2
	Unresponsive, or reflexic responses only	3
1b. LOC questions (month, age)	Answers both correctly	0
	Answers one correctly	1
	Both incorrect	2
1c. LOC, commands (open, close eyes; make fist, let go)	Obeys both correctly	0
	Obeys one correctly	1
	Both incorrect	2
2. Best gaze (eyes open—patient follows examiner's finger or face)	Normal	0
	Partial gaze palsy	1
	Forced deviation	2
3. Visual (Introduce visual stimulus/threat to patient's visual field quadrants)	No visual loss	0
	Partial hemianopia	1
	Complete hemianopia	2
	Bilateral hemianopia	3
4. Facial palsy (show teeth, raise eyebrows and squeeze eyes shut)	Normal	0
	Minor	1
	Partial	2
	Complete	3
5a. Motor; arm—left (elevate extremity to 90° and score drift/movement)	No drift	0
	Drift but maintains in air	1
	Unable to maintain in air	2
	No effort against gravity	3
	No movement	4
	Amputation, joint fusion (explain)	N/A
5b. Motor; arm—right (elevate extremity to 90° and score drift/movement)	No drift	0
	Drift but maintains in air	1
	Unable to maintain in air	2
	No effort against gravity	3
	No movement	4
	Amputation, joint fusion (explain)	N/A
6a. Motor; leg—left (elevate extremity to 30° and score drift/movement)	No drift	0
	Drift but maintains in air	1
	Unable to maintain in air	2
	No effort against gravity	3
	No movement	4
	Amputation, joint fusion (explain)	N/A
6b. Motor; leg—right (elevate extremity to 30° and score drift/movement)	No drift	0
	Drift but maintains in air	1
	Unable to maintain in air	2
	No effort against gravity	3
	No movement	4
	Amputation, joint fusion (explain)	N/A
7. Limb ataxia (finger-to-nose and heel-to-shin testing)	Absent	0
	Present in one limb	1
	Present in two limbs	2
8. Sensory (pin prick to face, arm, trunk and leg—compare side to side)	Normal	0
	Mild to moderate loss	1
	Severe to total loss	2
9. Best language (name items, describe a picture and read sentences)	No aphasia	0
	Mild to moderate aphasia	1
	Severe aphasia	2
	Mute	3

continued >

TABLE 62-4 Summary of National Institutes of Health Stroke Scale (NIHSS) (Continued)

Category	Description	Score
10. Dysarthria (evaluate speech clarity by having patient repeat words)	Normal	0
	Mild to moderate dysarthria	1
	Severe dysarthia, mostly unintelligible or worse	2
	Intubated or other physical barrier	N/A
11. Extinction and inattention (use information from prior testing to score)	No abnormality	0
	Visual, tactile, auditory, or other extinction to bilateral simulataneous stimulation	1
	Profound hemiattention or extinction to more than one modality.	2
Total score		

Adapted from the version available at the National Institute of Neurological Disorders and Stroke, National Institutes of Health, Bethesda, MD 20892, http://www.ninds.nih.gov/doctors/NIH_Stroke_Scale.pdf. It is recommended that the full scale with all instructions be used.

- Continuous hemodynamic monitoring (the goals for blood pressure remain controversial for a patient who has not received thrombolytic therapy; antihypertensive treatment may be withheld unless the systolic blood pressure exceeds 220 mm Hg or the diastolic blood pressure exceeds 120 mm Hg)
- Neurologic assessment to determine whether the stroke is evolving and whether other acute complications are developing; such complications may include seizures, bleeding from anticoagulation, or medication-induced bradycardia, which can result in hypotension and subsequent decreases in cardiac output and cerebral perfusion pressure
- Acute ischemic stroke clinical guidelines are given in Appendix B.

Managing Potential Complications

Adequate cerebral blood flow is essential for cerebral oxygenation. If cerebral blood flow is inadequate, the amount of oxygen supplied to the brain will decrease, and tissue ischemia will result. Adequate oxygenation begins with pulmonary care, maintenance of a patent airway, and administration of supplemental oxygen as needed. The importance of adequate gas exchange in these patients cannot be overemphasized. Many are at risk for aspiration pneumonia, which can interfere with gas exchange.

Other potential complications after a stroke include urinary tract infections, cardiac dysrhythmias, and complications of immobility.

Surgical Prevention of Ischemic Stroke

The main surgical procedure for selected patients with TIAs and mild stroke is carotid endarterectomy, which is currently the most frequently performed noncardiac vascular procedure. A carotid endarterectomy is the removal of an atherosclerotic plaque or thrombus from the carotid artery to prevent stroke in patients with occlusive disease of the extracranial cerebral arteries (Fig. 62-2). This surgery is indicated for patients with symptoms of TIA or mild stroke found to be caused by severe (70% to 99%) carotid artery stenosis or moderate (50% to 69%) stenosis with other significant risk factors (Rothwell et al., 2004).

Carotid stenting is a less invasive procedure that is used, at times, for severe stenosis. A study including 334 patients with severe carotid artery stenosis who underwent stenting with the use of an emboli-protection device demonstrated that this procedure was not inferior to carotid endarterectomy (Yadav, Wholey, Kuntz, et al., 2004). Carotid stenting is used for selected patients who are at high risk for surgery, and its efficacy continues to be investigated.

NURSING MANAGEMENT

The primary complications of carotid endarterectomy are stroke, cranial nerve injuries, infection or hematoma at the incision, and carotid artery disruption. It is important to maintain adequate blood pressure levels in the immediate postoperative period. Hypotension is avoided to prevent cerebral ischemia and thrombosis. Uncontrolled hyper-

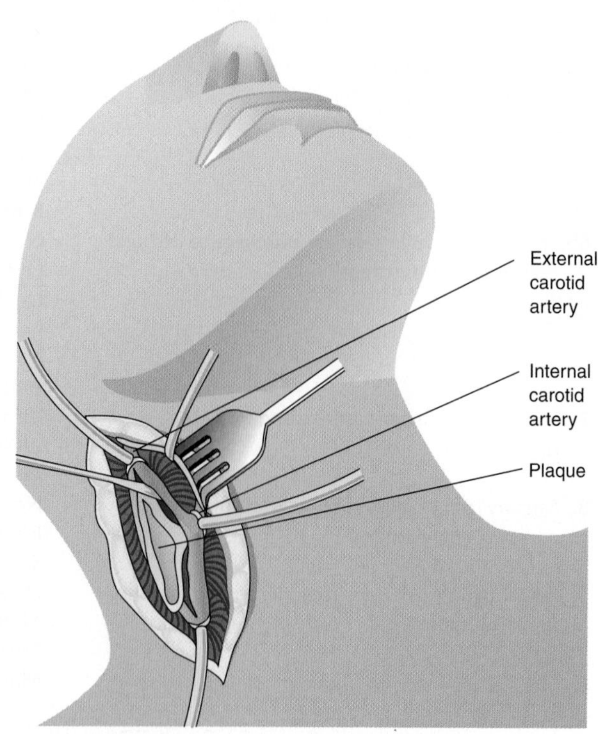

FIGURE 62-2. Plaque, a potential source of emboli in TIA and stroke, is surgically removed from the carotid artery.

tension may precipitate cerebral hemorrhage, edema, hemorrhage at the surgical incision, or disruption of the arterial reconstruction. Sodium nitroprusside is commonly used to reduce the blood pressure to previous levels. Close cardiac monitoring is necessary, because these patients have a high incidence of coronary artery disease.

After carotid endarterectomy, a neurologic flow sheet is used to monitor and document assessment parameters for all body systems, with particular attention to neurologic status. The neurosurgeon is notified immediately if a neurologic deficit develops. Formation of a thrombus at the site of the endarterectomy is suspected if there is a sudden increase in neurologic deficits, such as weakness on one side of the body. The patient should be prepared for repeat endarterectomy.

Difficulty in swallowing, hoarseness, or other signs of cranial nerve dysfunction must be assessed. The nurse focuses on assessment of the following cranial nerves: facial (VII), vagus (X), spinal accessory (XI), and hypoglossal (XII). Some edema in the neck after surgery is expected; however, extensive edema and hematoma formation can obstruct the airway. Emergency airway supplies, including those needed for a tracheostomy, must be available. Table 62-5 provides more information about potential complications of carotid surgery.

Nursing Process

The Patient Recovering From an Ischemic Stroke

The acute phase of an ischemic stroke may last 1 to 3 days, but ongoing monitoring of all body systems is essential as long as the patient requires care. The patient who has had a stroke is at risk for multiple complications, including deconditioning and other musculoskeletal problems, swallowing difficulties, bowel and bladder dysfunction, inability to perform self-care, and skin breakdown. After the stroke is complete, management focuses on the prompt initiation of rehabilitation for any deficits.

Assessment

During the acute phase, a neurologic flow sheet is maintained to provide data about the follow-

TABLE 62-5 Selected Complications of Carotid Endarterectomy and Nursing Interventions

Complication	Characteristics	Nursing Interventions
Incision hematoma	Occurs in 5.5% of patients. Large or rapidly expanding hematomas require emergency treatment. If the airway is obstructed by the hematoma, the incision may be opened at the bedside.	Monitor neck discomfort and wound expansion. Report swelling, subjective feelings of pressure in the neck, difficulty breathing.
Hypertension	Poorly controlled hypertension increases the risk of postoperative complications, including hematoma and hyperperfusion syndrome. There is an increased incidence of neurologic impairment and death due to intracerebral hemorrhage. May be related to surgically induced abnormalities of carotid baroreceptor sensitivity.	Risk is highest in the first 48 hours after surgery. Check blood pressure frequently and report deviations from baseline. Observe for and report new onset of neurologic deficits.
Postoperative hypotension	Occurs in approximately 5% of patients. Treated with fluids and low-dose phenylephrine infusion. Usually resolves in 24 to 48 hours. Patients with hypotension should have serial ECGs to rule out myocardial infarction.	Monitor blood pressure and observe for signs and symptoms of hypotension.
Hyperperfusion syndrome	Occurs when cerebral vessel autoregulation fails. Arteries accustomed to diminished blood flow may be permanently dilated; increased blood flow after endarterectomy coupled with insufficient vasoconstriction leads to capillary bed damage, edema, and hemorrhage.	Observe for severe unilateral headache improved by sitting upright or standing.
Intracerebral hemorrhage	Occurs infrequently, but is often fatal (60%) or results in serious neurologic impairment. Can occur secondary to hyperperfusion syndrome. Increased risk with advanced age, hypertension, presence of high-grade stenosis, poor collateral flow, and slow flow in the region of the middle cerebral artery.	Monitor neurologic status and report any changes in mental status or neurologic functioning immediately.

ing important measures of the patient's clinical status:

- Change in level of consciousness or responsiveness as evidenced by movement, resistance to changes of position, and response to stimulation; orientation to time, place, and person
- Presence or absence of voluntary or involuntary movements of the extremities; muscle tone; body posture; and position of the head
- Stiffness or flaccidity of the neck
- Eye opening, comparative size of pupils and pupillary reactions to light, and ocular position
- Color of the face and extremities; temperature and moisture of the skin
- Quality and rates of pulse and respiration; arterial blood gas values as indicated, body temperature, and arterial pressure
- Ability to speak
- Volume of fluids ingested or administered; volume of urine excreted each 24 hours
- Presence of bleeding
- Maintenance of blood pressure within the desired parameters

After the acute phase, the nurse assesses mental status (memory, attention span, perception, orientation, affect, speech/language), sensation/perception (usually the patient has decreased awareness of pain and temperature), motor control (upper and lower extremity movement), swallowing ability, nutritional and hydration status, skin integrity, activity tolerance, and bowel and bladder function. Ongoing nursing assessment continues to focus on any impairment of function in the patient's daily activities, because the quality of life after stroke is closely related to the patient's functional status.

Diagnosis

Nursing Diagnoses

Based on the assessment data, the major nursing diagnoses for a patient with a stroke may include the following:

- Impaired physical mobility related to hemiparesis, loss of balance and coordination, spasticity, and brain injury
- Acute pain (painful shoulder) related to hemiplegia and disuse
- Self-care deficits (bathing, hygiene, toileting, dressing, grooming, and feeding) related to stroke sequelae
- Disturbed sensory perception related to altered sensory reception, transmission, and/or integration
- Impaired swallowing
- Total urinary incontinence related to flaccid bladder, detrusor instability, confusion, or difficulty in communicating
- Disturbed thought processes related to brain damage, confusion, or inability to follow instructions
- Impaired verbal communication related to brain damage
- Risk for impaired skin integrity related to hemiparesis, hemiplegia, or decreased mobility
- Interrupted family processes related to catastrophic illness and caregiving burdens
- Sexual dysfunction related to neurologic deficits or fear of failure

Collaborative Problems/Potential Complications

Potential complications include:

- Decreased cerebral blood flow due to increased ICP
- Inadequate oxygen delivery to the brain
- Pneumonia

Planning and Goals

Although rehabilitation begins on the day the patient has the stroke, the process is intensified during convalescence and requires a coordinated team effort. It is helpful for the team to know what the patient was like before the stroke: his or her illnesses, abilities, mental and emotional state, behavioral characteristics, and activities of daily living (ADLs). It is also helpful for clinicians to be knowledgeable about the relative importance of predictors of stroke outcome (age, NIHSS score, and level of consciousness at time of admission) in order to provide stroke survivors and their families with realistic goals (Adams et al., 2003; Cucchiara, Kasner, Wolk, et al., 2004).

The major goals for the patient (and family) may include improved mobility, avoidance of shoulder pain, achievement of self-care, relief of sensory and perceptual deprivation, prevention of aspiration, continence of bowel and bladder, improved thought processes, achieving a form of communication, maintaining skin integrity, restored family functioning, improved sexual function, and absence of complications.

Nursing Interventions

Nursing care has a significant impact on the patient's recovery. Often, many body systems are impaired as a result of the stroke, and conscientious care and timely interventions can prevent debilitating complications. During and after the acute phase, nursing interventions focus on the whole person. In addition to providing physical care, the nurse encourages and fosters recovery by listening to the patient and asking questions to elicit the meaning of the stroke experience.

Improving Mobility and Preventing Joint Deformities

A patient with hemiplegia has unilateral paralysis (paralysis on one side). When control of the voluntary muscles is lost, the strong flexor muscles exert control over the extensors. The arm tends to adduct (adductor muscles are stronger than abductors) and to rotate internally. The elbow and the wrist tend to flex, the affected leg tends to rotate externally at the hip joint and flex at the knee, and the foot at the ankle joint supinates and tends toward plantar flexion.

Correct positioning is important to prevent contractures; measures are used to relieve pressure, assist in maintaining good body alignment, and prevent compressive neuropathies, especially of the ulnar and peroneal nerves. Because flexor muscles are stronger than extensor muscles, a posterior splint applied at night to the affected extremity may prevent flexion and maintain correct positioning during sleep. (See Chapter 11 for additional information.)

PREVENTING SHOULDER ADDUCTION

To prevent adduction of the affected shoulder while the patient is in bed, a pillow is placed in the axilla when there is limited external rotation; this keeps the arm away from the chest. A pillow is placed under the arm, and the arm is placed in a neutral (slightly flexed) position, with distal joints positioned higher than the more proximal joints (ie, the elbow is positioned higher than the shoulder and the wrist higher than the elbow). This helps to prevent edema and the resultant joint fibrosis that will limit range of motion if the patient regains control of the arm (Fig. 62-3).

POSITIONING THE HAND AND FINGERS

The fingers are positioned so that they are barely flexed. The hand is placed in slight supination (palm faces upward), which is its most functional position. If the upper extremity is flaccid, a volar resting splint can be used to support the wrist and hand in a functional position. If the upper extremity is spastic, a hand roll is not used, because it stimulates the grasp reflex. In this instance a dorsal wrist splint is useful in allowing the palm to be free of pressure. Every effort is made to prevent hand edema.

Spasticity, particularly in the hand, can be a disabling complication after stroke. Researchers reported that repeated intramuscular injections of botulinum toxin A into wrist and finger muscles reduced upper limb spasticity after stroke, resulting in significant and sustained improvements in muscle tone (Gordon, Brashear, Elovic, et al., 2004).

CHANGING POSITIONS

The patient's position should be changed every 2 hours. To place a patient in a lateral (side-lying) position, a pillow is placed between the legs before the patient is turned. To promote venous return and prevent edema, the upper thigh should not be acutely flexed. The patient may be turned from side to side, but if sensation is impaired, the amount of time spent on the affected side should be limited.

If possible, the patient is placed in a prone position for 15 to 30 minutes several times a day. A small pillow or a support is placed under the pelvis, extending from the level of the umbilicus to the upper third of the thigh (Fig. 62-4). This position helps to promote hyperextension of the hip joints, which is essential for normal gait and helps prevent knee and hip flexion contractures. The prone position also helps to drain bronchial secretions and prevents contractural deformities of the shoulders and knees. During positioning, it is important to reduce pressure and change position frequently to prevent pressure ulcers.

ESTABLISHING AN EXERCISE PROGRAM

The affected extremities are exercised passively and put through a full range of motion four or five times a day to maintain joint mobility, regain motor control, prevent contractures in the paralyzed extremity, prevent further deterioration of the neuromuscular system, and enhance circulation. Exercise is helpful in preventing venous stasis, which may predispose the patient to thrombosis and pulmonary embolus.

Repetition of an activity forms new pathways in the CNS and therefore encourages new patterns of motion. At first, the extremities are usually flaccid. If tightness occurs in any area, the range-of-motion exercises should be performed more frequently (see Chapter 11).

The patient is observed for signs and symptoms that may indicate pulmonary embolus or excessive cardiac workload during exercise; these include shortness of breath, chest pain, cyanosis, and increasing pulse rate with exercise. Frequent short periods of exercise always are preferable to longer periods at infrequent intervals. Regularity in exercise is most important. Improvement in muscle strength and maintenance of range of motion can be achieved only through daily exercise.

The patient is encouraged and reminded to exercise the unaffected side at intervals throughout the day. It is helpful to develop a written schedule to remind the patient of the exercise activities. The nurse supervises and supports the patient during these activities. The patient can be taught to put the unaffected leg under the affected one to assist in moving it when turning

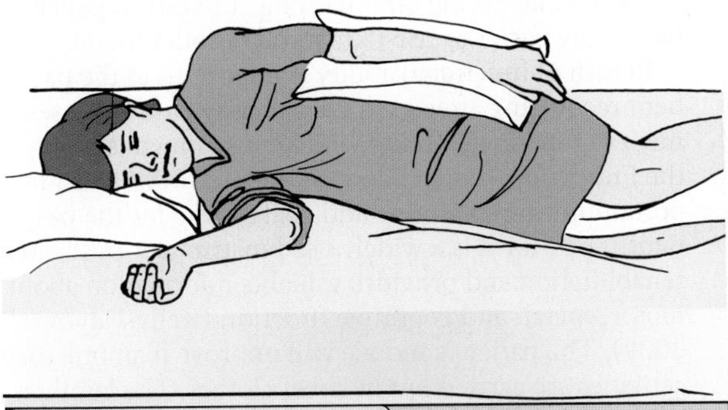

FIGURE 62-3. Correct positioning to prevent shoulder adduction.

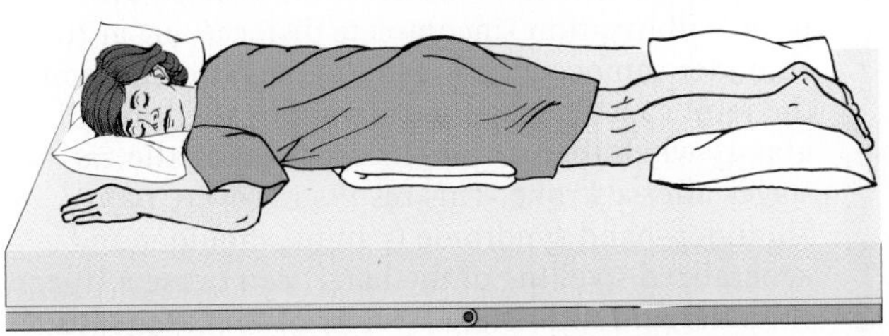

FIGURE 62-4. Prone position with pillow support helps prevent hip flexion.

and exercising. Flexibility, strengthening, coordination, endurance, and balancing exercises prepare the patient for ambulation. Quadriceps muscle setting and gluteal setting exercises are started early to improve the muscle strength needed for walking; these are performed at least five times daily for 10 minutes at a time.

PREPARING FOR AMBULATION

As soon as possible, the patient is assisted out of bed. Usually an active rehabilitation program is started as soon as the patient regains consciousness. The patient is first taught to maintain balance while sitting and then to learn to balance while standing. If the patient has difficulty in achieving standing balance, a tilt table, which slowly brings the patient to an upright position, can be used. Tilt tables are especially helpful for patients who have been on bed rest for prolonged periods and have orthostatic blood pressure changes.

If the patient needs a wheelchair, the folding type with hand brakes is the most practical because it allows the patient to manipulate the chair. The chair should be low enough to allow the patient to propel it with the uninvolved foot and narrow enough to permit it to be used in the home. When the patient is transferred from the wheelchair, the brakes must be applied and locked on both sides of the chair.

The patient is usually ready to walk as soon as standing balance is achieved. Parallel bars are useful in these first efforts. A chair or wheelchair should be readily available in case the patient suddenly becomes fatigued or feels dizzy.

The training periods for ambulation should be short and frequent. As the patient gains strength and confidence, an adjustable cane can be used for support. Generally, a three- or four-pronged cane provides a stable support in the early phases of rehabilitation.

Preventing Shoulder Pain

As many as 70% of stroke patients suffer severe pain in the shoulder that prevents them from learning new skills. Shoulder function is essential in achieving balance and performing transfers and self-care activities. Three problems can occur: painful shoulder, subluxation of the shoulder, and shoulder–hand syndrome.

A flaccid shoulder joint may be overstretched by the use of excessive force in turning the patient or from overstrenuous arm and shoulder movement. To prevent shoulder pain, the nurse should never lift the patient by the flaccid shoulder or pull on the affected arm or shoulder. If the arm is paralyzed, subluxation (incomplete dislocation) at the shoulder can occur as a result of overstretching of the joint capsule and musculature by the force of gravity when the patient sits or stands in the early stages after a stroke. This results in severe pain. Shoulder–hand syndrome (painful shoulder and generalized swelling of the hand) can cause a frozen shoulder and ultimately atrophy of subcutaneous tissues. When a shoulder becomes stiff, it is usually painful.

Many shoulder problems can be prevented by proper patient movement and positioning. The flaccid arm is positioned on a table or with pillows while the patient is seated. Some clinicians advocate the use of a properly worn sling when the patient first becomes ambulatory, to prevent the paralyzed upper extremity from dangling without support. Range-of-motion exercises are important in preventing painful shoulder. Overstrenuous arm movements are avoided. The patient is instructed to interlace the fingers, place the palms together, and push the clasped hands slowly forward to bring the scapulae forward; he or she then raises both hands above the head. This is repeated throughout the day. The patient is instructed to flex the affected wrist at intervals and move all the joints of the affected fingers. He or she is encouraged to touch, stroke, rub, and look at both hands. Pushing the heel of the hand firmly down on a surface is useful. Elevation of the arm and hand is also important in preventing dependent edema of the hand. Patients with continuing pain after attempted movement and positioning may require the addition of analgesia to their treatment program.

Medications are helpful in the management of poststroke pain. Amitriptyline hydrochloride (Elavil) has been used, but it can cause cognitive problems, has a sedating effect, and is not effective in all patients. The antiseizure medication lamotrigine (Lamictal) has been found to be effective for poststroke pain, and it may serve as an alternative for patients who cannot tolerate amitriptyline (Nicholson, 2004).

Enhancing Self-Care

As soon as the patient can sit up, personal hygiene activities are encouraged. The patient is helped to set realistic goals; if feasible, a new task is added daily. The first step is to carry out all self-care activities on the unaffected side. Such activities as combing the hair, brushing the teeth, shaving with an electric razor, bathing, and eating can be carried out with one hand and are suitable for self-care. Although the patient may feel awkward at first, the various motor skills can be learned by repetition, and the unaffected side will become stronger with use. The nurse must be sure that the patient does not neglect the affected side. Assistive devices will help make up for some of the patient's deficits (Chart 62-3). A small towel is easier to control while drying after bathing, and boxed paper tissues are easier to use than a roll of toilet tissue.

Return of functional ability is important to the patient recovering after a stroke. An early baseline assessment of functional ability with an instrument such as the Functional Independence Measure (FIM™) is important in team planning and goal setting for the patient. The FIM™ is a widely used instrument in stroke rehabilitation and provides valuable information about motor, social, and cognitive function (Kelly-Hayes, 2004). The patient's morale will improve if ambulatory activities are carried out in street clothes. The family is instructed to bring in clothing that is preferably a size larger than that normally worn. Clothing fitted with

NURSING RESEARCH PROFILE

Long-Term Pain After a Stroke

Widar, M., Ahlström, G. & Ek, A. (2004). Health-related quality of life in persons with long-term pain after a stroke. *Journal of Clinical Nursing, 13*(4), 497–505.

Purpose

There is a lack of knowledge and awareness about pain conditions after stroke. Pain after a stroke can occur in a variety of forms, can go unnoticed by relatives and health care personnel, and can affect the quality of life. The purpose of this study was to describe health-related quality of life in people with long-term pain after a stroke, and to compare different types of pain conditions (central post-stroke pain, pain in the shoulder and/or arm, tension-type headache) by demographic data.

Design

This study combined qualitative and quantitative methods. Forty-three participants with long-term pain (pain lasting longer than 6 months) after a stroke were included. A qualitative interview was conducted, and two self-reported questionnaires (SF-36 and the Hospital Anxiety and Depression [HAD] Scale) were administered.

Findings

Mean duration of pain was 20 months, and the majority of participants were men ($n = 30$). Physical and cognitive functioning, financial security, good relationships and support, and having the ability to be together with family and friends were important factors associated with experiencing a good quality of life. The participants in this study rated their quality of life lower as compared with other stroke survivors. No significant differences were found on the SF-36 or the HAD with regard to the types of pain reported by participants.

Nursing Implications

Nurses in all settings who are involved with patients who have had a stroke and their families can use this information to better understand pain in patients who have experienced stroke and how it affects their quality of life. Assessment of quality of life is important for all patients who have had a stroke, especially for those with long-term pain. This study reinforces the importance of support and resources in stroke recovery. Nurses can provide better supportive care when they appreciate and understand the person's perceptions and transitions that accompany life after stroke.

CHART 62-3

Assistive Devices to Enhance Self-Care After Stroke

EATING DEVICES

- Nonskid mats to stabilize plates
- Plate guards to prevent food from being pushed off plate
- Wide-grip utensils to accommodate a weak grasp

BATHING AND GROOMING DEVICES

- Long-handled bath sponge
- Grab bars, nonskid mats, hand-held shower heads
- Electric razors with head at 90 degrees to handle
- Shower and tub seats, stationary or on wheels

TOILETING AIDS

- Raised toilet seat
- Grab bars next to toilet

DRESSING AIDS

- Velcro closures
- Elastic shoelaces
- Long-handled shoe horn

MOBILITY AIDS

- Canes, walkers, wheelchairs
- Transfer devices such as transfer boards and belts

front or side fasteners or Velcro closures is the most suitable. The patient has better balance if most of the dressing activities are carried out while seated.

Perceptual problems may make it difficult for the patient to dress without assistance because of an inability to match the clothing to the body parts. To assist the patient, the nurse can take steps to keep the environment organized and uncluttered, because the patient with a perceptual problem is easily distracted. The clothing is placed on the affected side in the order in which the garments are to be put on. Using a large mirror while dressing promotes the patient's awareness of what he or she is putting on the affected side. Each garment is put on the affected side first. The patient has to make many compensatory movements when dressing; these can produce fatigue and painful twisting of the intercostal muscles. Support and encouragement are provided to prevent the patient from becoming overly fatigued and discouraged. Even with intensive training, not all patients can achieve independence in dressing.

Managing Sensory-Perceptual Difficulties

Patients with a decreased field of vision should be approached on the side where visual perception is intact. All visual stimuli (eg, clock, calendar, television) should be placed on this side. The patient can be taught to turn the head in the direction of the defective visual field to compensate for this loss. The nurse should make eye contact with the patient and draw his or her attention to the affected side by encouraging the patient to move the head. The nurse may also want to stand at a position that encourages the patient to move or turn to visualize who is in the room. Increasing the natural or artificial lighting in the room and providing eyeglasses are important aids to increasing vision.

The patient with homonymous hemianopsia (loss of half of the visual field) turns away from the affected side of the body and tends to neglect that side and the space on that side; this is called amorphosynthesis. In such instances, the patient cannot see food on half of the tray, and only half of the room is visible. It is important for the nurse to constantly remind the patient of the other side of the body, to maintain alignment of the extremities, and, if possible, to place the extremities where the patient can see them.

Assisting With Nutrition

Stroke can result in swallowing problems (dysphagia) due to impaired function of the mouth, tongue, palate, larynx, pharynx, or upper esophagus. Patients must be observed for paroxysms of coughing, food dribbling out of or pooling in one side of the mouth, food retained for long periods in the mouth, or nasal regurgitation when swallowing liquids. The use of an algorithm may be helpful in the dietary management of dysphagia (Runions, Rodrigue & White, 2004). Swallowing difficulties place the patient at risk for aspiration, pneumonia, dehydration, and malnutrition.

A speech therapist will evaluate the patient's gag reflexes and ability to swallow. Even if swallowing function is partially impaired, it may return in some patients over time, or the patient may be taught alternative swallowing techniques, advised to take smaller boluses of food, and taught about types of foods that are easier to swallow. The patient may be started on a thick liquid or purèed diet, because these foods are easier to swallow than thin liquids. Having the patient sit upright, preferably out of bed in a chair, and instructing him or her to tuck the chin toward the chest as he or she swallows will help prevent aspiration. The diet may be advanced as the patient becomes more proficient at swallowing. If the patient cannot resume oral intake, a gastrointestinal feeding tube will be placed for ongoing tube feedings.

Enteral tubes can be either nasogastric (placed in the stomach) or nasoenteral (placed in the duodenum) to reduce the risk of aspiration. Nursing responsibilities in feeding include elevating the head of the bed at least 30 degrees to prevent aspiration, checking the position of the tube before feeding, ensuring that the cuff of the tracheostomy tube (if in place) is inflated, and giving the tube feeding slowly. The feeding tube is aspirated periodically to ensure that the feedings are passing through the gastrointestinal tract. Retained or residual feedings increase the risk for aspiration. Patients with retained feedings may benefit from the placement of a gastrostomy tube or a percutaneous endoscopic gastrostomy tube. In a patient with a nasogastric tube, the feeding tube should be placed in the duodenum to reduce the risk of aspiration. For long-term feedings, a gastrostomy tube is preferred. Management of patients with tube feedings is discussed in Chapter 36.

Attaining Bowel and Bladder Control

After a stroke, the patient may have transient urinary incontinence due to confusion, inability to communicate needs, and inability to use the urinal or bedpan because of impaired motor and postural control. Occasionally after a stroke, the bladder becomes atonic, with impaired sensation in response to bladder filling. Sometimes control of the external urinary sphincter is lost or diminished. During this period, intermittent catheterization with sterile technique is carried out. After muscle tone increases and deep tendon reflexes return, bladder tone increases and spasticity of the bladder may develop. Because the patient's sense of awareness is clouded, persistent urinary incontinence or urinary retention may be symptomatic of bilateral brain damage. The voiding pattern is analyzed, and the urinal or bedpan is offered on this pattern or schedule. The upright posture and standing position are helpful for male patients during this aspect of rehabilitation.

Patients may have problems with bowel control, particularly constipation. Unless contraindicated, a high-fiber diet and adequate fluid intake (2 to 3 L per day) should be provided and a regular time (usually after breakfast) should be established for toileting. See Chapter 11 for additional information about bowel and bladder retraining programs.

Improving Thought Processes

After a stroke, the patient may have problems with cognitive, behavioral, and emotional deficits related to brain damage. However, in many instances, a considerable degree of function can be recovered, because not all areas of the brain are equally damaged; some remain more intact and functional than others.

After assessment that delineates the patient's deficits, the neuropsychologist, in collaboration with the primary care physician, psychiatrist, nurse, and other professionals, structures a training program using cognitive-perceptual retraining, visual imagery, reality orientation, and cueing procedures to compensate for losses.

The role of the nurse is supportive. The nurse reviews the results of neuropsychological testing, observes the patient's performance and progress, gives positive feedback, and, most importantly, conveys an attitude of confidence and hope. Interventions capitalize on the patient's strengths and remaining abilities while attempting to improve performance of affected functions. Other interventions are similar to those for improving cognitive functioning after a head injury (see Chapter 63).

Improving Communication

Aphasia, which impairs the patient's ability to express himself or herself and to understand what is being said, may become apparent in various ways. The cortical area that is responsible for integrating the myriad pathways required for the comprehension and formulation of language is called Broca's area. It is located in a convolution adjoining the middle cerebral artery. This area is responsible for control of the combinations of muscular movements needed to speak each word. Broca's area is so close to the left motor area that a disturbance in the motor area often affects the speech area. This is why so many patients who are paralyzed on the right side (due to damage or injury to the left side of the brain) cannot speak, whereas those paralyzed on the left side are less likely to have speech disturbances.

The speech therapist assesses the communication needs of the stroke patient, describes the precise deficit, and suggests the best overall method of communication. Most language intervention strategies can be tailored for the individual patient. The patient is expected to take an active part in establishing goals.

A person with aphasia may become depressed. The inability to talk on the telephone, answer a question, or participate in conversation often causes anger, frustration, fear of the future, and hopelessness. Nursing interventions include strategies to make the atmosphere conducive to communication. This includes being sensitive to the patient's reactions and needs and responding to them in an appropriate manner, while always treating the patient as an adult. The nurse provides strong emotional support and understanding to allay anxiety and frustration.

A common pitfall is for the nurse or other health care team member to complete the thoughts or sentences of the patient. This should be avoided, because it causes the patient to become more frustrated at not being allowed to speak and may deter efforts to practice putting thoughts together and completing sentences. A consistent schedule, routines, and repetition help the patient to function despite significant deficits. A written copy of the daily schedule, a folder of personal information (birth date, address, names of relatives), checklists, and an audiotaped list help improve the patient's memory and concentration. The patient may also benefit from a communication board, which has pictures of common needs and phrases. The board may be translated into several languages.

When talking with the patient, it is important for the nurse to gain the patient's attention, speak slowly, and keep the language of instruction consistent. One instruction is given at a time, and time is allowed for the patient to process what has been said. The use of gestures may enhance comprehension. Speaking is thinking out loud, and the emphasis is on thinking. Listening and sorting out incoming messages requires mental effort; the patient must struggle against mental inertia and needs time to organize a response.

In working with the patient with aphasia, the nurse must remember to talk to the patient during care activities. This provides social contact for the patient. Chart 62-4 describes points to keep in mind when communicating with the patient with aphasia.

CHART 62-4

Communicating With the Patient With Aphasia

- Face the patient and establish eye contact.
- Speak in a normal manner and tone.
- Use short phrases, and pause between phrases to allow the patient time to understand what is being said.
- Limit conversation to practical and concrete matters.
- Use gestures, pictures, objects, and writing.
- As the patient uses and handles an object, say what the object is. It helps to match the words with the object or action.
- Be consistent in using the same words and gestures each time you give instructions or ask a question.
- Keep extraneous noises and sounds to a minimum. Too much background noise can distract the patient or make it difficult to sort out the message being spoken.

Maintaining Skin Integrity

The patient who has had a stroke may be at risk for skin and tissue breakdown because of altered sensation and inability to respond to pressure and discomfort by turning and moving. Preventing skin and tissue breakdown requires frequent assessment of the skin, with emphasis on bony areas and dependent parts of the body. During the acute phase, a specialty bed (eg, low-air-loss bed) may be used until the patient can move independently or assist in moving.

A regular turning schedule (at least every 2 hours) must be adhered to even if pressure-relieving devices are used to prevent tissue and skin breakdown. When the patient is positioned or turned, care must be used to minimize shear and friction forces, which cause damage to tissues and predispose the skin to breakdown.

The patient's skin must be kept clean and dry; gentle massage of healthy (nonreddened) skin and adequate nutrition are other factors that help to maintain normal skin and tissue integrity (see Chapter 11).

Improving Family Coping

Family members play an important role in the patient's recovery. Family members are encouraged to participate in counseling and to use support systems that will help with the emotional and physical stress of caring for the patient. Involving others in the patient's care and teaching stress management techniques and methods for maintaining personal health also facilitate family coping.

The family may have difficulty accepting the patient's disability and may be unrealistic in their expectations. They are given information about the expected outcomes and are counseled to avoid doing activities for the patient that he or she can do. They are assured that their love and interest are part of the patient's therapy.

The family needs to be informed that the rehabilitation of the hemiplegic patient requires many months and that progress may be slow. The gains made by the patient in the hospital or rehabilitation unit must be maintained. All caregivers should approach the patient with a supportive and optimistic attitude, focusing on the patient's remaining abilities. The rehabilitation team, the medical and nursing team, the patient, and the family must all be involved in developing attainable goals for the patient at home.

Most relatives of patients with stroke handle the physical changes better than the emotional aspects of care. The family should be prepared to expect occasional episodes of emotional lability. The patient may laugh or cry easily and may be irritable and demanding or depressed and confused. The nurse can explain to the family that the patient's laughter does not necessarily connote happiness, nor does crying reflect sadness, and that emotional lability usually improves with time.

Helping the Patient Cope With Sexual Dysfunction

Sexual functioning can be profoundly altered by stroke. Although research in this area of stroke management is limited, it appears that patients who have had a stroke consider sexual function to be important, and many have sexual dysfunction. Sexual dysfunction after stroke is multifactorial. There may be medical reasons for the dysfunction (neurologic and cognitive deficits, previous diseases, medications), as well as various psychosocial factors. A stroke is such a catastrophic illness that the patient experiences loss of self-esteem and value as a sexual being. These psychosocial factors play an important role in determining sexual drive, activity, and satisfaction after a stroke (Murray & Harrison, 2004).

Nurses in the rehabilitation setting play a crucial role in beginning a dialogue between the patient and his or her partner about sexuality after a stroke. In-depth assessments to determine sexual history before and after the stroke should be followed by appropriate interventions. Interventions for the patient and partner focus on providing relevant information, education, reassurance, adjustment of medications, counseling regarding coping skills, suggestions for alternative sexual positions, and a means of sexual expression and satisfaction.

Promoting Home and Community-Based Care

TEACHING PATIENTS SELF-CARE

Patient and family education is a fundamental component of rehabilitation. The nurse provides teaching about stroke, its causes and prevention, and the rehabilitation process. In both acute care and rehabilitation facilities, the focus is on teaching the patient to resume as much self-care as possible. This may entail using assistive devices or modifying the home environment to help the patient live with a disability.

An occupational therapist may be helpful in assessing the home environment and recommending modifications to help the patient become more independent. For example, a shower is more convenient than a tub for the patient with hemiplegia because most patients do not gain sufficient strength to get up and down from a tub. Sitting on a stool of medium height with rubber suction tips allows the patient to wash with greater ease. A long-handled bath brush with a soap container is helpful to the patient who has only one functional hand. If a shower is not available, a stool may be placed in the tub and a portable shower hose attached to the faucet. Handrails may be attached alongside the bathtub and the toilet. Other assistive devices include special utensils for eating, grooming, dressing, and writing (see Chart 62-3).

A program of physical therapy can be beneficial in the home environment. Recent research has focused on a number of techniques using robotics. One technique that was shown to result in a reduction in motor impairment concentrates on enhanced exercise of the affected limb. Another technique that showed positive outcomes uses sensorimotor training of the upper limb and the wrist (Volpe, Ferraro, Lynch, et al., 2004).

CONTINUING CARE

The recovery and rehabilitation process after stroke may be prolonged and requires patience and perseverance on the part of both the patient and the family. Depending on the specific neurologic deficits resulting from the stroke, the patient at home may require the services of a number of health care professionals. The nurse often coordinates the care of the patient at home and considers the many educational needs of caregivers and patients (O'Connell, Baker & Prosser, 2003). The family (often the spouse) will require education as well as assistance in planning and providing care. The caregiver often requires reminders to attend to his or her own health concerns and well-being.

The family is advised that the patient may tire easily, may become irritable and upset by small events, and is likely to show less interest in things. Because a stroke frequently occurs in the later stages of life, there is the possibility of intellectual decline related to dementia.

Emotional problems associated with stroke are often related to speech dysfunction and the frustrations of being unable to communicate. A speech therapist who visits the home allows the family to be involved and gives the family practical instructions to help the patient between therapy sessions.

Depression is a common and serious problem in the patient who has had a stroke. Antidepressant therapy may help if depression dominates the patient's life. As progress is made in the rehabilitation program, some problems will diminish. The family can help by continuing to support the patient and by giving positive reinforcement for the progress that is being made.

Community-based stroke support groups may allow the patient and family to learn from others with similar problems and to share their experiences. Support groups take the form of in-person meetings as well as Web-based support programs (Pierce, Steiner, Govoni, et al., 2004). The patient is encouraged to continue hobbies and recreational and leisure interests and to maintain contact with friends to prevent social isolation. All nurses coming in contact with the patient should encourage the patient to keep active, adhere to the exercise program, and remain as self-sufficient as possible.

The nurse should recognize the potential effects of caregiving on the family. Not all families have the adaptive coping skills and adequate psychological functioning necessary for the long-term care of another person. The patient's spouse may be elderly, with his or her own health concerns; in some instances the patient may have been the provider of care to the spouse. Even healthy caregivers may find it difficult to maintain a schedule that includes being available around the clock. A study found that poststroke changes in behavior and memory, in combination with poor motor function, were particularly taxing for caregivers and affected their perceived mental health (Clark, Dunbar, Shields, et al., 2004).

Another study found that the tasks perceived by caregivers as most time-consuming and difficult (managing finances, managing behaviors of the stroke survivor, and providing emotional support) were also predictive of depressed mood in caregivers (Bakas, Austin, Jessup, et al., 2004). Depressed caregivers are more likely to resort to physical or emotional abuse of the patient and are more likely to place the patient in a nursing home. Respite care (planned short-term care to relieve the family from having to provide continuous 24-hour care) may be available from an adult day care center. Some hospitals also offer weekend respite care that can provide caregivers with needed time for themselves. The nurse encourages the family to arrange for such services and provides information to assist them.

The nurse involved in home and continuing care also needs to remind the patient and family of the need for continuing health promotion and screening practices. Patients who have not been involved in these practices in the past are educated about their importance and are referred to appropriate health care providers, if indicated.

Evaluation

Expected Patient Outcomes

Expected patient outcomes may include the following:

1. Achieves improved mobility
   a. Avoids deformities (contractures and footdrop)
   b. Participates in prescribed exercise program
   c. Achieves sitting balance
   d. Uses unaffected side to compensate for loss of function of hemiplegic side
2. Reports absence of shoulder pain
   a. Demonstrates shoulder mobility; exercises shoulder
   b. Elevates arm and hand at intervals
3. Achieves self-care; performs hygiene care; uses adaptive equipment
4. Turns head to see people or objects
5. Demonstrates improved swallowing ability
6. Achieves normal bowel and bladder elimination
7. Participates in cognitive improvement program
8. Demonstrates improved communication
9. Maintains intact skin without breakdown
   a. Demonstrates normal skin turgor
   b. Participates in turning and positioning activities
10. Family members demonstrate a positive attitude and coping mechanisms
    a. Encourage patient in exercise program
    b. Take an active part in rehabilitation process
    c. Contact respite care programs or arrange for other family members to assume some responsibilities for care
11. Develops alternative approaches to sexual expression

Hemorrhagic Stroke

Hemorrhagic strokes account for 15% to 20% of cerebrovascular disorders and are primarily caused by intracranial or subarachnoid hemorrhage. Hemorrhagic strokes are caused by bleeding into the brain tissue, the ventricles, or the subarachnoid space. Primary intracerebral hemorrhage from a spontaneous rupture of small vessels accounts for approximately 80% of hemorrhagic strokes and is caused chiefly by uncontrolled hypertension. Subarachnoid hemorrhage results from a ruptured intracranial **aneurysm** (a weakening in the arterial wall) in about half the cases (Bader & Littlejohns, 2004).

Another common cause of intracerebral hemorrhage in the elderly is cerebral amyloid angiopathy, which involves damage caused by the deposit of beta-amyloid protein in the small and medium-sized blood vessels of the brain. Secondary intracerebral hemorrhage is associated with arteriovenous malformations (AVMs), intracranial aneurysms, intracranial neoplasms, or certain medications (eg, anticoagulants, amphetamines) (Bader & Littlejohns, 2004; Hickey, 2003). The mortality rate has been reported to be as high as 43% at 30 days after an intracranial hemorrhage (Bader & Littlejohns, 2004). Patients who survive the acute phase of care usually have more severe deficits and a longer recovery time compared to those with ischemic stroke.

Pathophysiology

The pathophysiology of hemorrhagic stroke depends on the cause and type of cerebrovascular disorder. Symptoms are produced when a primary hemorrhage, aneurysm, or AVM presses on nearby cranial nerves or brain tissue or, more dramatically, when an aneurysm or AVM ruptures, causing subarachnoid hemorrhage (hemorrhage into the cranial subarachnoid space). Normal brain metabolism is disrupted by the brain's being exposed to blood; by an increase in ICP resulting from the sudden entry of blood into the subarachnoid space, which compresses and injures brain tissue; or by secondary ischemia of the brain resulting from the reduced perfusion pressure and vasospasm that frequently accompany subarachnoid hemorrhage.

Intracerebral Hemorrhage

An intracerebral hemorrhage, or bleeding into the brain substance, is most common in patients with hypertension and cerebral atherosclerosis, because degenerative changes from these diseases cause rupture of the blood vessel. An intracerebral hemorrhage may also result from certain types of arterial pathology, brain tumors, and the use of medications (oral anticoagulants, amphetamines, and illicit drug use).

Bleeding occurs most commonly in the cerebral lobes, basal ganglia, thalamus, brain stem (mostly the pons), and cerebellum (Hickey, 2003). Occasionally, the bleeding ruptures the wall of the lateral ventricle and causes intraventricular hemorrhage, which is frequently fatal.

Intracranial (Cerebral) Aneurysm

An intracranial (cerebral) **aneurysm** is a dilation of the walls of a cerebral artery that develops as a result of weakness in the arterial wall. The cause of aneurysms is unknown, although research is ongoing. An aneurysm may be due to atherosclerosis, which results in a defect in the vessel wall with subsequent weakness of the wall; a congenital defect of the vessel wall; hypertensive vascular disease; head trauma; or advancing age.

Any artery within the brain can be the site of a cerebral aneurysm, but these lesions usually occur at the bifurcations of the large arteries at the circle of Willis (Fig. 62-5). The cerebral arteries most commonly affected by an aneurysm are the internal carotid artery (ICA), anterior cerebral artery (ACA), anterior communicating artery (ACoA), posterior communicating artery (PCoA), posterior cerebral artery (PCA), and middle cerebral artery (MCA). Multiple cerebral aneurysms are not uncommon.

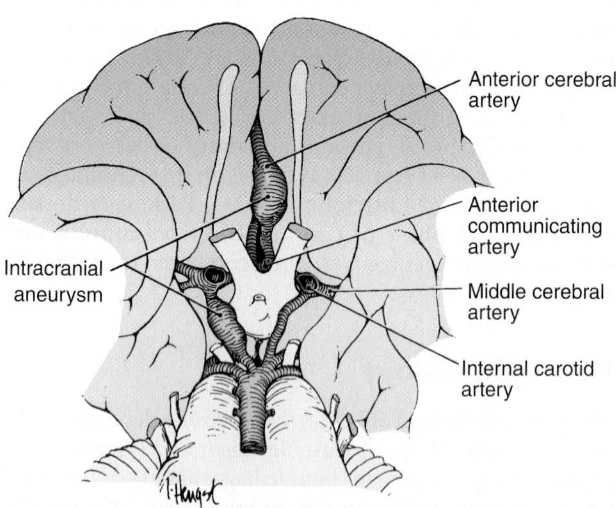

FIGURE 62-5. Intracranial aneurysms.

Arteriovenous Malformations

An AVM is caused by an abnormality in embryonal development that leads to a tangle of arteries and veins in the brain that lacks a capillary bed. The absence of a capillary bed leads to dilation of the arteries and veins and eventual rupture. AVM is a common cause of hemorrhagic stroke in young people.

Subarachnoid Hemorrhage

A subarachnoid hemorrhage (hemorrhage into the subarachnoid space) may occur as a result of an AVM, intracranial aneurysm, trauma, or hypertension. The most common causes are a leaking aneurysm in the area of the circle of Willis and a congenital AVM of the brain.

Clinical Manifestations

The patient with a hemorrhagic stroke can present with a wide variety of neurologic deficits, similar to the patient with ischemic stroke. The conscious patient most commonly reports a severe headache. A comprehensive assessment reveals the extent of the neurologic deficits. Many of the same motor, sensory, cranial nerve, cognitive, and other functions that are disrupted after ischemic stroke are also altered after a hemorrhagic stroke. Table 62-2 reviews the neurologic deficits frequently seen in stroke patients. Table 62-3 compares the symptoms seen in right hemispheric stroke with those seen in left hemispheric stroke. Other symptoms that may be observed more frequently in patients with acute intracerebral hemorrhage (compared with ischemic stroke) are vomiting, an early sudden change in level of consciousness, and possibly focal seizures due to frequent brain stem involvement (Hickey, 2003).

In addition to the neurologic deficits that are similar to those of ischemic stroke, the patient with an intracranial aneurysm or AVM can have some unique clinical manifestations. Rupture of an aneurysm or AVM usually produces a sudden, unusually severe headache and often loss of consciousness for a variable period of time. There may be pain and rigidity of the back of the neck (nuchal rigidity) and spine due to meningeal irritation. Visual disturbances (visual loss, diplopia, ptosis) occur if the aneurysm is adjacent to the oculomotor nerve. Tinnitus, dizziness, and hemiparesis may also occur.

At times, an aneurysm or AVM leaks blood, leading to the formation of a clot that seals the site of rupture. In this instance, the patient may show little neurologic deficit. In other cases, severe bleeding occurs, resulting in cerebral damage, followed rapidly by coma and death.

Prognosis depends on the neurologic condition of the patient, the patient's age, associated diseases, and the extent and location of the hemorrhage or intracranial aneurysm. Subarachnoid hemorrhage from an aneurysm is a catastrophic event with significant morbidity and mortality. Chart 62-5 presents ethical issues related to the patient with a severe hemorrhagic stroke.

CHART 62-5

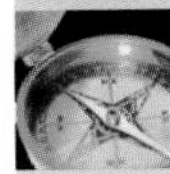

Ethics and Related Issues

What Are the Ethical Issues Related to DNR Orders After Severe Stroke?

SITUATION

An 85-year-old patient is admitted with a large intracerebral hemorrhage, severe neurologic deficits, and a past medical history of coronary artery bypass graft surgery, hypertension, atrial fibrillation, and gout. The patient does not have an advanced directive. The attending physician suggests a do-not-resuscitate (DNR) order to the family.

DILEMMA

The principle of autonomy for the patient (including death with dignity) conflicts with the principle of beneficence for the health care providers.

DISCUSSION

1. What arguments would you pose in favor of the DNR order?
2. What arguments would you pose against the DNR order?
3. Does the family have the right to refuse?
4. Is a DNR order an example of "patient abandonment" by health care workers, or an attempt to limit treatment and avoid CPR in a patient with an anticipated poor outcome?

Assessment and Diagnostic Findings

Any patient with suspected stroke should undergo a CT scan to determine the type of stroke, the size and location of the hematoma, and the presence or absence of ventricular blood and hydrocephalus. CT scan and cerebral angiography confirm the diagnosis of an intracranial aneurysm or AVM. These tests show the location and size of the lesion and provide information about the affected arteries, veins, adjoining vessels, and vascular branches. Lumbar puncture is performed if there is no evidence of increased ICP, the CT scan results are negative, and subarachnoid hemorrhage must be confirmed. Lumbar puncture in the presence of increased ICP could result in brain stem herniation or rebleeding. When diagnosing a hemorrhagic stroke in a patient younger than 40 years of age, some clinicians obtain a toxicology screen for illicit drug use.

The Hunt-Hess classification system guides the physician in diagnosing the severity of subarachnoid hemorrhage after an aneurysmal bleed (Table 62-6). Classification of the patient by severity of neurologic deficit provides a baseline for future comparisons.

TABLE 62-6 Hunt-Hess Classification of Subarachnoid Hemorrhages

Grade	Description
0	Unruptured aneurysm
1	Asymptomatic, or mild headache and slight nuchal rigidity
1a	No acute meningeal or brain reaction, but with fixed neurologic deficit
2	Cranial nerve (CN) palsy (eg, oculomotor [CN III], abducens [CN VI]), moderate-to-severe headache, nuchal rigidity
3	Mild focal deficit, lethargy, or confusion
4	Stupor, moderate to severe hemiparesis, early decerebrate rigidity
5	Deep coma, decerebrate rigidity, moribund appearance
	Add one grade for serious systemic disease (eg, hypertension, chronic obstructive pulmonary disease) or severe vasospasm on angiography

Adapted from Hickey, J. V. (2003). *The clinical practice of neurological and neurosurgical nursing* (5th ed., p. 527). Philadelphia: Lippincott Williams & Wilkins.

Prevention

Primary prevention of hemorrhagic stroke is the best approach and includes managing hypertension and ameliorating other significant risk factors. Control of hypertension, especially in people older than 55 years of age, clearly reduces the risk for hemorrhagic stroke (Bader & Littlejohns, 2004). Additional risk factors are increased age, male gender, and excessive alcohol intake (Ariesen, Claus, Rinkel, et al., 2003). Stroke risk screenings provide an ideal opportunity to lower hemorrhagic stroke risk by identifying high-risk individuals or groups and educating patients and the community about recognition and prevention.

A prevention effort unique to hemorrhagic stroke is to increase the public's awareness about the association between phenylpropanolamine (PPA, an ingredient found in appetite suppressants as well as cold and cough agents) and hemorrhagic stroke. The FDA requested that pharmaceutical companies voluntarily discontinue marketing products containing PPA, because research found that PPA was an independent risk factor for hemorrhagic stroke (Cantu, Arauz, Murillo-Bonilla, et al., 2003). Many products have been removed voluntarily from the market, but consumers should continue to look for this ingredient on labels.

Complications

Potential complications of hemorrhagic stroke include rebleeding; cerebral vasospasm resulting in cerebral ischemia; acute hydrocephalus, which results when free blood obstructs the reabsorption of cerebrospinal fluid (CSF) by the arachnoid villi; and seizures.

Cerebral Hypoxia and Decreased Blood Flow

Immediate complications of a hemorrhagic stroke include cerebral hypoxia, decreased cerebral blood flow, and extension of the area of injury. Providing adequate oxygenation of blood to the brain minimizes cerebral hypoxia. Brain function depends on delivery of oxygen to the tissues.

Administering supplemental oxygen and maintaining the hemoglobin and hematocrit at acceptable levels will assist in maintaining tissue oxygenation.

Cerebral blood flow is dependent on the blood pressure, cardiac output, and integrity of cerebral blood vessels. Adequate hydration (IV fluids) must be ensured to reduce blood viscosity and improve cerebral blood flow. Extremes of hypertension or hypotension need to be avoided to prevent changes in cerebral blood flow and the potential for extending the area of injury.

A seizure can also compromise cerebral blood flow, resulting in further injury to the brain. Observing for seizure activity and initiating appropriate treatment are important components of care after a hemorrhagic stroke.

Vasospasm

The development of cerebral vasospasm (narrowing of the lumen of the involved cranial blood vessel) is a serious complication of subarachnoid hemorrhage and accounts for 40% to 50% of the morbidity and mortality of those who survive the initial intracranial bleed. The mechanism responsible for the spasm is not clear, but vasospasm is associated with increasing amounts of blood in the subarachnoid cisterns and cerebral fissures, as visualized by CT scan. Monitoring for vasospasm may be performed through the use of bedside transcranial Doppler ultrasonography (TCD) or follow-up cerebral angiography (Oyama & Criddle, 2004).

Vasospasm leads to increased vascular resistance, which impedes cerebral blood flow and causes brain ischemia and infarction. The signs and symptoms reflect the areas of the brain involved. Vasospasm is often heralded by a worsening headache, a decrease in level of consciousness (confusion, lethargy, and disorientation), or a new focal neurologic deficit (aphasia, hemiparesis).

Vasospasm frequently occurs 4 to 14 days after initial hemorrhage, when the clot undergoes lysis (dissolution), and increases the chances of rebleeding. It is believed that early surgery to clip the aneurysm prevents rebleeding and that removal of blood from the basal cisterns around the major cerebral arteries may prevent vasospasm. The administration of calcium-channel blockers such as nimodipine (Nimotop) during the critical period in which vasospasm may occur can prevent delayed ischemic deterioration. Advances in technology have led to the introduction of interventional neuroradiology for the treatment of aneurysms. Endovascular techniques may be used in selected patients to occlude the artery supplying the aneurysm with a balloon or to occlude the aneurysm itself. As more studies on these techniques are completed, their use will increase.

Management of vasospasm remains difficult and controversial. Based on one theory, that vasospasm is caused by an increased influx of calcium into the cell, medication therapy may be used to block or antagonize this action and prevent or reverse the action of vasospasm if already present. Calcium-channel blockers may include nimodipine (Nimotop), verapamil (Isoptin), and nifedipine (Procardia). Another therapy for vasospasm, referred to as "triple-H therapy," is aimed at minimizing the deleterious effects of the associated cerebral ischemia and includes (1) fluid volume expanders (hypervolemia), (2) induced arterial hypertension, and (3) hemodilution (Sen, Belli, Albon, et al., 2003).

Increased ICP

An increase in ICP can occur after either an ischemic or a hemorrhagic stroke but almost always follows a subarachnoid hemorrhage, usually because of disturbed circulation of CSF caused by blood in the basal cisterns. If the patient shows evidence of deterioration from increased ICP (due to cerebral edema, herniation, hydrocephalus, or vasospasm), CSF drainage may be instituted by cautious lumbar puncture or ventricular catheter drainage, and mannitol is administered to reduce ICP. When mannitol is used as a long-term measure to control ICP, dehydration and disturbances in electrolyte balance (hyponatremia or hypernatremia; hypokalemia or hyperkalemia) may occur. Mannitol pulls water out of the brain tissue by osmosis and reduces total-body water through diuresis. The patient is monitored for signs of dehydration and for rebound elevation of ICP.

Systemic Hypertension

Preventing sudden systemic hypertension is critical in the management of intracerebral hemorrhage. Although specific goals for blood pressure management are individualized for each patient, systolic blood pressure may be lowered to less than 150 mm Hg to prevent hematoma enlargement (Ohwaki, Yano, Nagashima, et al., 2004). If blood pressure is elevated, antihypertensive therapy (labetalol [Normodyne], nicardipine [Cardene], nitroprusside [Nitropress]) may be prescribed. During the administration of antihypertensives, arterial hemodynamic monitoring is important to detect and avoid a precipitous drop in blood pressure, which can produce brain ischemia. Because seizures cause elevation of blood pressure, antiseizure agents are often administered prophylactically. Stool softeners are used to prevent straining, which can also elevate the blood pressure.

Medical Management

The goals of medical treatment for hemorrhagic stroke are to allow the brain to recover from the initial insult (bleeding), to prevent or minimize the risk for rebleeding, and to prevent or treat complications. Ongoing clinical trials are investigating whether the use of recombinant activated factor VII can reduce the bleeding after intracerebral hemorrhage (Mayer, Brun, Begtrup, et al., 2005).

Management is primarily supportive and consists of bed rest with sedation to prevent agitation and stress, management of vasospasm, and surgical or medical treatment to prevent rebleeding. Analgesics (codeine, acetaminophen) may be prescribed for head and neck pain. The patient is fitted with sequential compression devices to prevent deep vein thrombosis (DVT) (Farray, Carman & Fernandez, 2004).

Surgical Management

In many cases, a primary intracerebral hemorrhage is not treated surgically. However, if the diameter of the hematoma exceeds 3 cm and the Glasgow Coma Scale score decreases, surgical evacuation is strongly recommended for the patient with a cerebellar hemorrhage (Hickey, 2003). Surgical evacuation is most frequently accomplished via a craniotomy (see Chapter 61).

The patient with an intracranial aneurysm is prepared for surgical intervention as soon as his or her condition is considered stable. The Hunt-Hess classification system guides the physician in diagnosing the severity of subarachnoid hemorrhage after an aneurysm bleeds and in appropriate timing of the surgery (see Table 62-6). Morbidity and mortality from surgery are high if the patient is stuporous or comatose (Hunt-Hess grade 4 or 5). Surgical treatment of the patient with an unruptured aneurysm is an option.

The goal of surgery is to prevent bleeding in an unruptured aneurysm or further bleeding in an already ruptured aneurysm. This objective is accomplished by isolating the aneurysm from its circulation or by strengthening the arterial wall. An aneurysm may be excluded from the cerebral circulation by means of a ligature or a clip across its neck. If this is not anatomically possible, the aneurysm can be reinforced by wrapping it with some substance to provide support and induce scarring. Ongoing research is investigating intraoperative techniques, such as hypothermia, that may help to improve the outcome of patients with aneurysmal subarachnoid hemorrhage (Todd, Hindman, Clarke, et al. 2005).

Several less invasive endovascular treatments are now being used for aneurysms. These procedures are performed by neurosurgeons in neurointerventional radiology facilities. Two procedures are endovascular treatment (occlusion of the parent artery) and aneurysm coiling (obstruction of the aneurysm site with a coil). Although these techniques are associated with lower risks than intracranial surgery in general, secondary stroke and rupture of the aneurysm are still potential complications (Bader & Littlejohns, 2004).

Postoperative complications include psychological symptoms (disorientation, amnesia, **Korsakoff's syndrome**, personality changes), intraoperative embolization, postoperative internal artery occlusion, fluid and electrolyte disturbances (from dysfunction of the neurohypophyseal system), and gastrointestinal bleeding.

Nursing Process

The Patient With a Hemorrhagic Stroke

Assessment

A complete neurologic assessment is performed initially and includes evaluation for the following:

- Altered level of consciousness
- Sluggish pupillary reaction
- Motor and sensory dysfunction
- Cranial nerve deficits (extraocular eye movements, facial droop, presence of ptosis)
- Speech difficulties and visual disturbance
- Headache and nuchal rigidity or other neurologic deficits

All patients should be monitored in the intensive care unit after an intracerebral or subarachnoid hemorrhage. Neurologic assessment findings are documented and reported as indicated. The frequency of these assessments varies depending on the patient's condition. Any changes in the patient's condition require reassessment and thorough documentation; changes should be reported immediately.

Alteration in level of consciousness often is the earliest sign of deterioration in a patient with a hemorrhagic stroke. Because nurses have the most frequent contact with patients, they are in the best position to detect subtle changes. Mild drowsiness and slight slurring of speech may be early signs that the level of consciousness is deteriorating.

Diagnosis

Nursing Diagnoses

Based on the assessment data, the patient's major nursing diagnoses may include the following:

- Ineffective tissue perfusion (cerebral) related to bleeding or vasospasm
- Disturbed sensory perception related to medically imposed restrictions (aneurysm precautions)
- Anxiety related to illness and/or medically imposed restrictions (aneurysm precautions)

Collaborative Problems/ Potential Complications

Based on the assessment data, potential complications that may develop include the following:

- Vasospasm
- Seizures
- Hydrocephalus
- Rebleeding
- Hyponatremia

Planning and Goals

The goals for the patient may include improved cerebral tissue perfusion, relief of sensory and perceptual deprivation, relief of anxiety, and the absence of complications.

Nursing Interventions

Optimizing Cerebral Tissue Perfusion

The patient is closely monitored for neurologic deterioration resulting from recurrent bleeding, increasing ICP, or vasospasm. A neurologic flow record is maintained. The blood pressure, pulse, level of consciousness (an indicator of cerebral perfusion), pupillary responses, and motor function are checked hourly. Respiratory status is monitored, because a reduction in oxygen in areas of the brain with impaired autoregulation increases the chances of a cerebral infarction. Any changes are reported immediately.

IMPLEMENTING ANEURYSM PRECAUTIONS

Cerebral aneurysm precautions are implemented for the patient with a diagnosis of aneurysm to provide a nonstimulating environment, prevent increases in ICP, and prevent further bleeding. The patient is placed on immediate and absolute bed rest in a quiet, nonstressful environment, because activity, pain, and anxiety elevate the blood pressure, which increases the risk for bleeding. Visitors, except for family, are restricted.

The head of the bed is elevated 15 to 30 degrees to promote venous drainage and decrease ICP. Some neurologists, however, prefer that the patient remain flat to increase cerebral perfusion.

Any activity that suddenly increases the blood pressure or obstructs venous return is avoided. This includes the Valsalva maneuver, straining, forceful sneezing, pushing oneself up in bed, acute flexion or rotation of the head and neck (which compromises the jugular veins), and cigarette smoking. Any activity requiring exertion is contraindicated. The patient is instructed to exhale through the mouth during voiding or defecation to decrease strain. No enemas are permitted, but stool softeners and mild laxatives are prescribed. Both prevent constipation, which would cause an increase in ICP, as would enemas. Dim lighting is helpful, because photophobia (visual intolerance of light) is common. Coffee and tea, unless decaffeinated, are usually eliminated.

Thigh-high elastic compression stockings or sequential compression boots may be prescribed to decrease the incidence of DVT resulting from immobility. The legs are observed for signs and symptoms of DVT (tenderness, redness, swelling, warmth, and edema), and abnormal findings are reported.

The nurse administers all personal care. The patient is fed and bathed to prevent any exertion that might increase the blood pressure. External stimuli are kept to a minimum, including no television, no radio, and no reading. Visitors are restricted in an effort to keep the patient as quiet as possible. This precaution must be individualized based on the patient's condition and response to visitors. A sign indicating this restriction should be placed on the door of the room, and the restrictions should be discussed with both patient and family. The purpose of aneurysm precautions should be thoroughly explained to both the patient (if possible) and family.

Relieving Sensory Deprivation and Anxiety

Sensory stimulation is kept to a minimum for patients on aneurysm precautions. For patients who are awake, alert, and oriented, an explanation of the restrictions helps reduce the patient's sense of isolation. Reality orientation is provided to help maintain orientation.

Keeping the patient well informed of the plan of care provides reassurance and helps minimize anxiety. Appropriate reassurance also helps relieve the patient's fears and anxiety. The family also requires information and support.

Monitoring and Managing Potential Complications

VASOSPASM

The patient is assessed for signs of possible vasospasm: intensified headaches, a decrease in level of responsiveness (confusion, disorientation, lethargy), or evidence of aphasia or partial paralysis. These signs may develop several days after surgery or on the initiation of treatment and must be reported immediately. If vasospasm is diagnosed, calcium-channel blockers or fluid volume expanders may be prescribed.

SEIZURES

Seizure precautions are maintained for every patient who may be at risk for seizure activity. Should a seizure occur, maintaining the airway and preventing injury are the primary goals. Medication therapy is initiated at this time, if not already prescribed. The medication of choice for many years has been phenytoin (Dilantin). Its use is being questioned due to the results of research including 527 patients, which suggested that phenytoin may increase functional and cognitive disability after subarachnoid hemorrhage (Naidech, Kreiter, Janjua, et al., 2005).

HYDROCEPHALUS

Blood in the subarachnoid space or ventricles impedes the circulation of CSF, resulting in hydrocephalus. A CT scan that indicates dilated ventricles confirms the diagnosis. Hydrocephalus can occur within the first 24 hours (acute) after subarachnoid hemorrhage or several days (subacute) to several weeks (delayed) later. Symptoms vary according to the time of onset and may be nonspecific. Acute hydrocephalus is characterized by sudden onset of stupor or coma and is managed with a ventriculostomy drain to decrease ICP. Symptoms of subacute and delayed hydrocephalus include gradual onset of drowsiness, behavioral changes, and ataxic gait. A ventriculoperitoneal shunt is surgically placed to treat chronic hydrocephalus. Changes in patient responsiveness are reported immediately.

REBLEEDING

The rate of recurrent hemorrhage is approximately 2% after a primary intracerebral hemorrhage. Hypertension is the most serious risk factor, suggesting the importance of appropriate antihypertensive treatment (Bader & Littlejohns, 2004).

Aneurysm rebleeding occurs most frequently during the first 2 weeks after the initial hemorrhage and is considered a major complication. Symptoms of rebleeding include sudden severe headache, nausea, vomiting, decreased level of consciousness, and neurologic deficit. Rebleeding is confirmed by CT scan. Blood pressure is carefully maintained with medications. The most effective preventive treatment is to secure the aneurysm if the patient is a candidate for surgery or endovascular treatment.

HYPONATREMIA

After subarachnoid hemorrhage, hyponatremia is found in 10% to 40% of patients (Dooling & Winkelman, 2004). Laboratory data must be checked frequently, and hyponatremia (defined as a serum sodium concentration of less than 135 mEq/L) must be identified as early as possible. The physician needs to be notified of a low serum sodium level that has persisted for 24 hours or longer (Dooling & Winkelman, 2004). The patient will then be evaluated for syndrome of inappropriate antidiuretic hormone (SIADH) or cerebral salt-wasting phenomenon. (SIADH is described in Chapter 14.) Cerebral salt-wasting phenomenon occurs when the kidneys are unable to conserve sodium; the treatment most often is the use of hypertonic 3% saline (Dooling & Winkelman, 2004).

Promoting Home and Community-Based Care

TEACHING PATIENTS SELF-CARE

The patient and family are provided with information that will enable them to cooperate with the care and restrictions required during the acute phase of hemorrhagic stroke and to prepare them to return home. Patient and family teaching includes information about the causes of hemorrhagic stroke and its possible consequences. In addition, the patient and family are informed about the medical treatments that are implemented, including surgical intervention if warranted, and the importance of interventions taken to prevent and detect complications (ie, aneurysm precautions, close monitoring of the patient). Depending on the presence and severity of neurologic impairment and other complications resulting from the stroke, the patient may be transferred to a rehabilitation unit or center for additional patient and family teaching about strategies to regain self-care ability. Teaching addresses the use of assistive devices or modification of the home environment to help the patient live with the disability. Modifications of the home may be required to provide a safe environment.

CONTINUING CARE

The acute and rehabilitation phase of care focuses on obvious needs, issues, and deficits for the patient with a hemorrhagic stroke. The patient and family are reminded of the importance of following recommendations to prevent further hemorrhagic stroke and keeping follow-up appointments with health care providers for monitoring of risk factors. Referral for home care may be warranted to assess the home environment and the ability of the patient and to ensure that the patient and family are able to manage at home. Home visits provide opportunities to monitor the physical and psychological status of the patient and the ability of the family to cope with any alterations in the patient's status. In addition, the home care nurse reminds the patient and family of the importance of continuing health promotion and screening practices. Chart 62-6 lists teaching points for the patient recovering from a stroke.

CHART 62-6

HOME CARE CHECKLIST • The Patient Recovering From a Stroke

At the completion of the home care instruction, the patient or caregiver will be able to:	Patient	Caregiver
• Discuss measures to prevent subsequent strokes.	✔	✔
• Identify signs and symptoms of specific complications.	✔	✔
• Identify potential complications and discuss measures to prevent them (blood clots, aspiration, pneumonia, urinary tract infection, fecal impaction, skin breakdown, contracture).	✔	✔
• Identify psychosocial consequences of stroke and appropriate interventions.	✔	✔
• Identify safety measures to prevent falls.	✔	✔
• State names, doses, indications, and side effects of medications.	✔	✔
• Demonstrate adaptive techniques for accomplishing ADLs.	✔	✔
• Demonstrate swallowing techniques (for patients with dysphagia).	✔	✔
• Demonstrate care of enteric feeding tube, if applicable.	✔	✔
• Demonstrate home exercises, use of splints or orthotics, proper positioning, and frequent repositioning.	✔	✔
• Describe procedures for maintaining skin integrity.	✔	✔
• Demonstrate indwelling catheter care, if applicable. Describe a bowel and bladder elimination program as appropriate.	✔	✔
• Identify appropriate recreational or diversional activities, support groups, and community resources.	✔	✔

Evaluation

Expected Patient Outcomes

Expected patient outcomes may include the following:

1. Demonstrates intact neurologic status and normal vital signs and respiratory patterns
   a. Is alert and oriented to time, place, and person
   b. Demonstrates normal speech patterns and intact cognitive processes
   c. Demonstrates normal and equal strength, movement, and sensation of all four extremities
   d. Exhibits normal deep tendon reflexes and pupillary responses
2. Demonstrates normal sensory perceptions
   a. States rationale for aneurysm precautions
   b. Exhibits clear thought processes
3. Exhibits reduced anxiety level
   a. Is less restless
   b. Exhibits absence of physiologic indicators of anxiety (eg, has normal vital signs; normal respiratory rate; absence of excessive, fast speech)
4. Is free of complications
   a. Exhibits absence of vasospasm
   b. Exhibits normal vital signs and neuromuscular activity without seizures
   c. Verbalizes understanding of seizure precautions
   d. Exhibits normal mental status and normal motor and sensory status
   e. Reports no visual changes

Critical Thinking Exercises

1 Your patient had symptoms of an ischemic stroke approximately 1 hour ago and is undergoing a confirmatory CT scan in 30 minutes. What are the time frame and criteria for t-PA administration? What nursing actions would you take? What is your rationale for these actions?

2 Your patient has expressive aphasia following an ischemic stroke. How would you explain this phenomenon to the patient and family? Describe appropriate techniques for communicating with a patient with this type of aphasia.

3 ebp Your patient is admitted with hemorrhagic stroke and is at high risk for DVT. What measures should be implemented for DVT prophylaxis? Identify the evidence for and the criteria used to evaluate the strength of the evidence for the specific measures identified for DVT prophylaxis.

4 A 70-year-old patient with a history of diabetes is expected to be discharged to home today after a 5-day stay for an ischemic stroke. She has some residual right-sided weakness. What teaching would be indicated to prevent another stroke? What resources may be needed to enable her to go home as scheduled?

REFERENCES AND SELECTED READINGS

BOOKS AND PAMPHLETS

American Association of Neuroscience Nurses. (2004). *Guide to the care of the patient with ischemic stroke: AANN reference series for clinical practice.* Glenview, IL: Author.

American Heart Association. (2006). *American Heart Association heart and stroke statistics—2006 update.* Dallas, TX: Author.

Babikiam, V. L., Wesler, L. R. & Higashida, R. T. (2003). *Imaging cerebrovascular disease.* Philadelphia: Elsevier.

Bader, M. K. & Littlejohns, J. R. (2004). *AANN core curriculum for neuroscience nursing* (4th ed.). St. Louis: Elsevier.

Diepenbrock, N. H. (2004). *Quick reference to critical care* (2nd ed.). Philadelphia: Lippincott Williams & Wilkins.

Furic, K. L. & Kelly, P. J. (2004). *Handbook of stroke prevention in clinical practice.* Totowa, NJ: Humana Press.

Hickey, J. V. (2003). *The clinical practice of neurological and neurosurgical nursing* (5th ed.). Philadelphia: Lippincott Williams & Wilkins.

LeRoux, P. D., Winn, H. R. & Newell, D. W. (2004). *Management of cerebral aneurysms.* Philadelphia: Elsevier.

Porth, C. M. (2005). *Pathophysiology: Concepts of altered health states* (7th ed.). Philadelphia: Lippincott Williams & Wilkins.

Read, S. J. & Virley, D. (2005). *Stroke genomics: Methods and reviews.* Totowa, NJ: Humana Press.

Ropper, A. H., Gress, D., Diringer, M. N., et al. (2004). *Neurological and neurosurgical intensive care* (4th ed.). Philadelphia: Lippincott Williams & Wilkins.

Somjen, G. (2004). *Ions in the brain: Normal function, seizures and stroke.* Oxford: Oxford University Press.

Winn, H. R. (2003). *Youman's neurological surgery* (5th ed.). Philadelphia: W. B. Saunders.

United States Department of Health and Human Services. (2003). *A public health action plan to prevent heart disease and stroke.* Atlanta: U.S. Department of Health and Human Services, Centers for Disease Control and Prevention.

JOURNALS

**Asterisks indicate nursing research articles.*

Adams, H. P., Adams, R. J., Brott, T., et al. (2003). Guidelines for the early management of patients with ischemic stroke. A scientific statement from the Stroke Council of the American Stroke Association. *Stroke, 34*(4), 1056–1083.

Albers, G. W., Amarenco, P., Easton, D. J., et al. (2004). Antithrombotic and thrombolytic therapy for ischemic stroke: The seventh ACCP conference on antithrombotic and thrombolytic therapy. *Chest, 126*(3 Suppl.), 483S–512S.

American Heart Association & American Stroke Association. (2004). Statins after ischemic stroke and transient ischemic attack. An advisory statement from the Stroke Council, American Heart Association and American Stroke Association. *Stroke, 35*(4), 1023.

Ariesen, M. J., Claus, S. P., Rinkel, G. J. E., et al. (2003). Risk factors for intracerebral hemorrhage in the general population: A systematic review. *Stroke, 34*(8), 2060–2066.

*Bakas, T., Austin, J. K., Jessup, S. L., et al. (2004). Time and difficulty of tasks provided by family caregivers of stroke survivors. *Journal of Neuroscience Nursing, 36*(2), 95–106.

Cantu, C., Arauz, A., Murillo-Bonilla, L. M., et al. (2003). Stroke associated with sympathomimetics contained in over-the-counter cough and cold drugs. *Stroke, 34*(7), 1667–1673.

Chobanian, A. V., Bakris, G. L., Black, H. R., et al. (2003). The seventh report of the Joint National Committee on Prevention, Detection, Evaluation, and Treatment of High Blood Pressure: The JNC 7 report. *Journal of the American Medical Association, 289*(19), 2560–2572.

*Clark, P. C., Dunbar, S. B., Shields, C. G., et al. (2004). Influence of stroke survivor characteristics and family conflict surrounding recovery on caregivers' mental and physical health. *Nursing Research, 53*(6), 406–413.

Cucchiara, B. L., Kasner, S. E., Wolk, D. A., et al. (2004). CLASS-I Investigators. Early impairment in consciousness predicts mortality after hemispheric ischemic stroke. *Critical Care Medicine, 32*(1), 241–245.

DeLemos, C. D., Atkinson, R. P., Croopnick, S. L., et al. (2003). How effective are "community" stroke screening programs at improving stroke knowledge and prevention practices? Results of a 3-month follow-up study. *Stroke, 34*(12), e247–e249.

Dooling, E. & Winkelman, S. (2004). Hyponatremia in the patient with subarachnoid hemorrhage. *Journal of Neuroscience Nursing, 36*(3), 130–135.

Farray, D., Carman, T. L. & Fernandez, B. B. (2004). The treatment and prevention of deep vein thrombosis in the preoperative management of patients who have neurologic diseases. *Neurologic Clinics of North America, 22*(2), 423–439.

Felton, R. P., Ogden, N. R. P., Pena, C., et al., (2005). The Food and Drug Administration medical device review process: Clearance of a clot retriever for use in ischemic stroke. *Stroke, 36*(2), 404–406.

Fisher M. & Davalos, A. (2004). Emerging therapies for cerebrovascular disorders. *Stroke, 35*(2), 367–369.

Gordon, M. F., Brashear, A, Elovic, E., et al. For the BOTOX Poststroke Spasticity Study Group. (2004). Repeated dosing of botulinum toxin type A for upper limb spasticity following stroke. *Neurology, 63*(10), 1971–1973.

Grau, A. J., Becher, H., Zigler, C. M., et al. (2004). Periodontal disease as a risk factor for ischemic stroke. *Stroke, 35*(2), 496–501.

Haley, E. C., Lyden, P. D., Johnson, K. C., et al. (2005). A pilot dose-escalation safety study of tenecteplase in acute ischemic stroke. *Stroke, 36*(3), 607–612.

Haymore, J. (2004). A neuron in a haystack: Advanced neurological assessment. *AACN Clinical Issues, 15*(4), 568–581.

Hinkle, J. L. (2005). An update on transient ischemic attacks. *Journal of Neuroscience Nursing, 37*(5), 243–248.

Hinkle, J. L. & Bowman, L. (2003). Neuroprotection for ischemic stroke. *Journal of Neuroscience Nursing, 35*(2), 114–118.

Ingall, T. J., O'Fallen, W. M., Asplund, K., et al. (2004). Findings from the reanalysis of the NINDS tissue plasminogen activator for acute ischemic stroke treatment trial. *Stroke, 35*(10), 2418–2424.

Kelly-Hayes, M. (2004). Stroke outcomes measures. *Journal of Cardiovascular Nursing, 19*(5), 301–307.

Mayer, S. A., Brun, N. C., Begtrup, K., et al. (2005). Recombinant activated factor VII for acute intracerebral hemorrhage. *New England Journal of Medicine, 352*(8), 777–785.

*Miller, E. T. & Spilker, J. (2003). Readiness to change and brief educational interventions: Successful strategies to reduce stroke risk. *Journal of Neuroscience Nursing, 35*(4), 215–222.

Miller, K. L., Liebowitz, R. S. & Newby, K. L. (2004). Complementary and alternative medicine in cardiovascular disease: A review of biologically based approaches. *American Heart Journal, 147*(3), 401–411.

Murray, C. D. & Harrison, B. (2004). The meaning and experience of being a stroke survivor: An interpretative and phenomenological analysis. *Disability and Rehabilitation, 26*(13), 808–816.

Naidech, A. M., Kreiter, K. T., Janjua, N., et al., (2005). Phenytoin exposure is associated with functional and cognitive disability after subarachnoid hemorrhage. *Stroke, 36*(3), 583–587.

National Center for Health Statistics, Centers for Disease Control and Prevention. (2002). Fast stats A to Z: Stroke. Available at: http://www.cdc.gov/nchs/fastats/stroke.htm (accessed June 23, 2006).

National Institute of Neurologic Disorders and Stroke (NINDS), rt-PA Stroke Study Group. (1995). Tissue plasminogen activator for acute ischemic stroke. *New England Journal of Medicine, 333*(24), 1581–1587.

Nicholson, B. D. (2004). Evaluation and treatment of central pain syndromes. *Neurology, 62*(Suppl 2), S30–S35.

*O'Connell, B., Baker, L. & Prosser, A. (2003). The educational needs of caregivers of stroke survivors in acute and community settings. *Journal of Neuroscience Nursing, 35*(1), 21–28.

Ohwaki, K., Yano, E., Nagashima, H., et al. (2004). Blood pressure management in acute intracerebral hemorrhage. *Stroke, 35*(6), 1364–1367.

Oyama, K. & Criddle, L. (2004). Vasospasm after aneurysmal subarachnoid hemorrhage. *Critical Care Nurse, 24*(5), 58–67.

*Pierce, L. L., Steiner, V., Govoni, A. L., et al. (2004). Caregivers dealing with stroke pull together and feel connected. *Journal of Neuroscience Nursing, 36*(1), 32–39.

Ridker, P. M., Cook, N. R., Lee, I., et al. (2005). A randomized trial of low-dose aspirin in the primary prevention of cardiovascular disease in women. *New England Journal of Medicine, 353*(13), 1293–1304.

Rothwell, P. M., Eliasziw, M., Gutnikov, S. A., et al. (2004). Endarterectomy for symptomatic carotid stenosis in relation to clinical subgroups and timing of surgery. *Lancet, 363*(9413), 915–924.

Runions, S., Rodrigue, N. & White, C. (2004). Practice on an acute stroke unit after implementation of a decision-making algorithm for dietary management of dysphagia. *Journal of Neuroscience Nursing, 36*(4), 200–207.

Sen, J., Belli, A., Albon, H., et al. (2003). Triple-H therapy in the management of aneurysmal subarachnoid haemorrhage. *Lancet Neurology, 2*(10), 614–620.

Todd, M. M., Hindman, B. J., Clarke, W. R., et al. (2005). Mild intraoperative hypothermia during surgery for intracranial aneurysm. *New England Journal of Medicine, 352*(2), 135–145.

Volpe, B. T., Ferraro, M., Lynch, D., et al., (2004). Robotics and other devices in the treatment of patients recovering from stroke. *Current Atherosclerosis Reports, 6*(4), 314–319.

*Widar, M., Ahlström, G. & Ek, A. (2004). Health-related quality of life in persons with long-term pain after a stroke. *Journal of Clinical Nursing, 13*(4), 497–505.

Yadav, J. S., Wholey, M. H., Kuntz, R. E., et al. (2004). Protected carotid-artery stenting versus endarterectomy in high-risk patients. *New England Journal of Medicine, 351*(15), 1493–1501.

RESOURCES

American Stroke Association, a Division of the American Heart Association, 7272 Greenville Avenue, Dallas, TX 75231-5129; 888-4-STROKE or 888-478-7653; http://www.strokeassociation.org. Accessed June 23, 2006.

National Institute of Neurological Disorders and Stroke, National Institutes of Health, Bethesda, MD 20892; http://www.ninds.nih.gov. Accessed June 23, 2006.

National Stroke Association, 9707 Easter Lane, Englewood, CO 80112-3754; 800-787-6537 or 303-649-9299, fax 303-649-1328; http://www.stroke.org. Accessed June 23, 2006.

CHAPTER 63

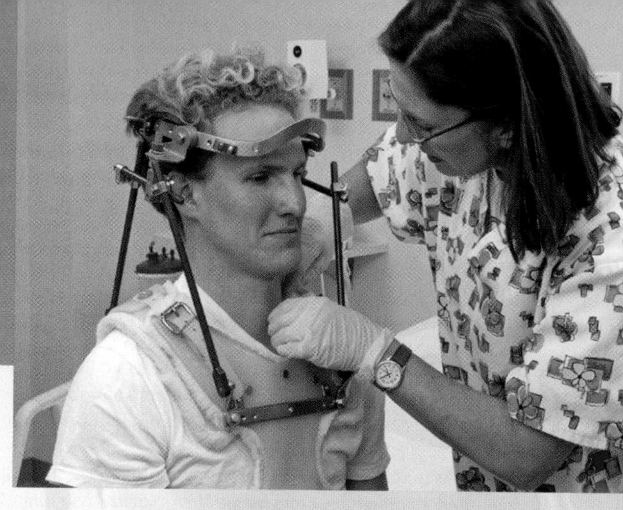

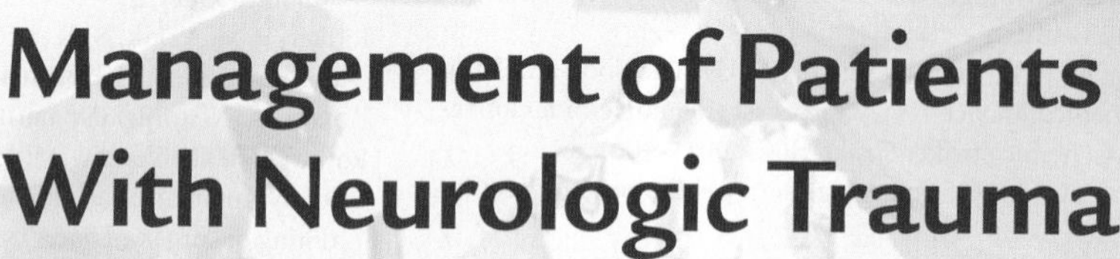

Management of Patients With Neurologic Trauma

Learning Objectives

On completion of this chapter, the learner will be able to:

1. Differentiate among patients with head injuries according to mechanism of injury, clinical signs and symptoms, diagnostic testing, and treatment options.
2. Describe the nursing management of patients with head injury.
3. Use the nursing process as a framework for care of patients with brain injury.
4. Identify the population at risk for spinal cord injury.
5. Describe the clinical features and management of the patient with neurogenic shock.
6. Discuss the pathophysiology of autonomic dysreflexia and describe the appropriate nursing interventions.
7. Use the nursing process as a framework for care of patients with spinal cord injury.

Trauma involving the central nervous system can be life-threatening. Even if it is not life-threatening, brain and spinal cord injury may result in major physical and psychological dysfunction and can alter the patient's life completely. Neurologic trauma affects the patient, the family, the health care system, and society as a whole because of its major sequelae and the costs of acute and long-term care of patients with trauma to the brain and spinal cord.

Head Injuries

Head injury is a broad classification that includes injury to the scalp, skull, or brain. It is the most common cause of death from trauma in the United States. Approximately 1.4 million people receive treatment for head injuries every year. Of these, 235,000 are hospitalized, 80,000 have permanent disabilities, and 50,000 people die. Traumatic brain injury is the most serious form of head injury. The most common causes of traumatic brain injury are motor vehicle crashes, violence, and falls. Groups at highest risk for traumatic brain injury are people between the ages of 15 and 24 years and males, who suffer traumatic brain injury at a rate almost twice that of females. The very young (younger than 5 years) and the very old (older than 75 years) are also at increased risk. An estimated 5.3 million Americans today are living with a disability as a result of a traumatic brain injury (Langlois, Rutland-Brown, & Thomas, 2004). The best approach to head injury is prevention (Chart 63-1).

CHART 63-1

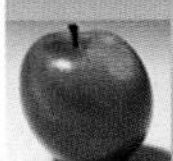

Health Promotion

Preventing Head and Spinal Cord Injuries

- Advise drivers to obey traffic laws, and to avoid speeding or driving when under the influence of drugs or alcohol.
- Advise all drivers and passengers to wear seat belts and shoulder harnesses. Children younger than 12 years of age should be restrained in an age/size-appropriate system in the back seat.
- Caution passengers against riding in the back of pickup trucks.
- Advise motorcyclists, scooter riders, bicyclists, skateboarders, and roller skaters to wear helmets.
- Promote educational programs that are directed toward violence and suicide prevention in the community.
- Provide water safety instruction.
- Teach patients steps that can be taken to prevent falls, particularly in the elderly.
- Advise athletes to use protective devices. Recommend that coaches be educated in proper coaching techniques.
- Advise owners of firearms to keep them locked in a secure area where children cannot access them.

Glossary

autonomic dysreflexia: a life-threatening emergency in spinal cord injury patients that causes a hypertensive emergency; also called autonomic hyperreflexia

brain injury: an injury to the skull or brain that is severe enough to interfere with normal functioning

brain injury, closed (blunt): occurs when the head accelerates and then rapidly decelerates or collides with another object and brain tissue is damaged, but there is no opening through the skull and dura

brain injury, open: occurs when an object penetrates the skull, enters the brain, and damages the soft brain tissue in its path (penetrating injury), or when blunt trauma to the head is so severe that it opens the scalp, skull, and dura to expose the brain

concussion: a temporary loss of neurologic function with no apparent structural damage to the brain

contusion: bruising of the brain surface

complete spinal cord lesion: a condition that involves total loss of sensation and voluntary muscle control below the lesion

halo vest: a lightweight vest with an attached halo that stabilizes the cervical spine

head injury: an injury to the scalp, skull, and/or brain

incomplete spinal cord lesion: a condition where there is preservation of the sensory or motor fibers, or both, below the lesion

neurogenic bladder: bladder dysfunction that results from a disorder or dysfunction of the nervous system; may result in either urinary retention or bladder overactivity

paraplegia: paralysis of the lower extremities with dysfunction of the bowel and bladder from a lesion in the thoracic, lumbar, or sacral regions of the spinal cord

secondary injury: an insult to the brain subsequent to the original traumatic event

spinal cord injury (SCI): an injury to the spinal cord, vertebral column, supporting soft tissue, or intervertebral disks caused by trauma

tetraplegia (quadriplegia): paralysis of both arms and legs, with dysfunction of bowel and bladder from a lesion of the cervical segments of the spinal cord

transection: severing of the spinal cord itself; transection can be complete (all the way through the cord) or incomplete (partially through)

Pathophysiology

Research suggests that not all brain damage occurs at the moment of impact. Damage to the brain from traumatic injury takes two forms: primary injury and secondary injury. Primary injury is the initial damage to the brain that results from the traumatic event. This may include contusions, lacerations, and torn blood vessels due to impact, acceleration/deceleration, or foreign object penetration (Porth, 2005). **Secondary injury** evolves over the ensuing hours and days after the initial injury and is due primarily to unchecked cerebral edema, ischemia, and the chemical changes associated with direct trauma to the brain (Littlejohns, Bader, & March, 2003).

An injured brain is different from other injured body areas because of its unique characteristics. It resides within the skull, which is a rigid, closed compartment (Hickey, 2003). Unlike an injured ankle, in which the covering skin expands with swelling, the confines of the skull do not allow for the expansion of cranial contents. Any bleeding or swelling within the skull increases the volume of contents within a container of fixed size and therefore can cause increased intracranial pressure (ICP) (see Chapter 61). If the increased pressure is high enough, it can cause displacement of the brain through or against the rigid structures of the skull. This causes restriction of blood flow to the brain, decreasing oxygen delivery and waste removal. Cells within the brain become anoxic and cannot metabolize properly, producing ischemia, infarction, irreversible brain damage, and, eventually, brain death (Fig. 63-1).

Scalp Injury

Isolated scalp trauma is generally classified as a minor injury. Because its many blood vessels constrict poorly, the scalp bleeds profusely when injured. Trauma may result in an abrasion (brush wound), contusion, laceration, or hematoma beneath the layers of tissue of the scalp (subgaleal hematoma). A large avulsion (tearing away) of the scalp may be potentially life-threatening and is a true emergency. Diagnosis of a scalp injury is based on physical examination, inspection, and palpation. Scalp wounds are potential portals of entry for organisms that cause intracranial infections. Therefore, the area is irrigated before the laceration is sutured, to remove foreign material and to reduce the risk for infection. Subgaleal hematomas (hematomas below the outer covering of the skull) usually absorb on their own and do not require any specific treatment.

Skull Fractures

A skull fracture is a break in the continuity of the skull caused by forceful trauma. It may occur with or without damage to the brain. Skull fractures can be classified as simple, comminuted, depressed, or basilar. A simple (linear) fracture is a break in the continuity of the bone. A comminuted skull fracture refers to a splintered or multiple fracture line. When bone fragments are embedded into brain tissue, the fracture is depressed. A fracture of the base of the skull is called a basilar skull fracture (Fig. 63-2) (Porth, 2005). A fracture may be open, indicating a scalp laceration or tear in the dura (for example, from a bullet or an ice pick), or closed, in which case the dura is intact.

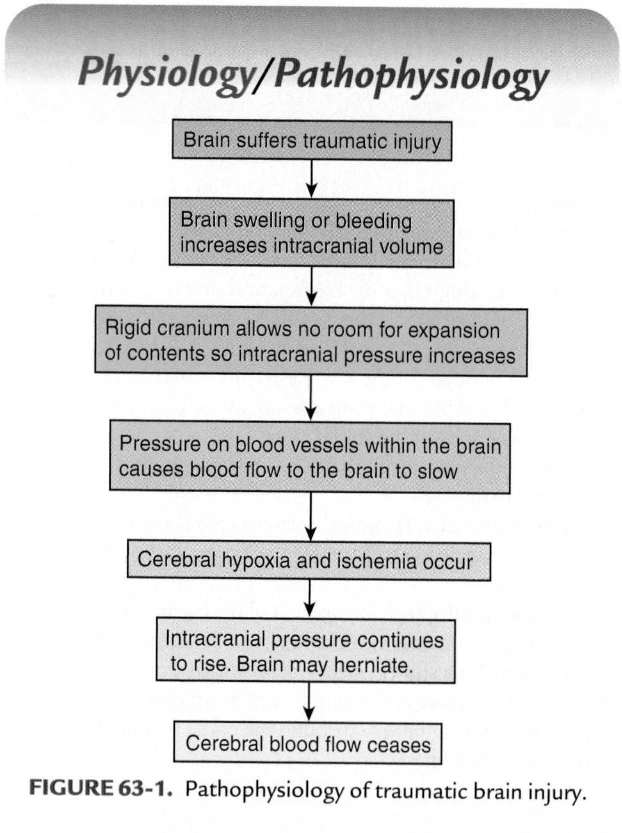

Physiology/Pathophysiology

Brain suffers traumatic injury
↓
Brain swelling or bleeding increases intracranial volume
↓
Rigid cranium allows no room for expansion of contents so intracranial pressure increases
↓
Pressure on blood vessels within the brain causes blood flow to the brain to slow
↓
Cerebral hypoxia and ischemia occur
↓
Intracranial pressure continues to rise. Brain may herniate.
↓
Cerebral blood flow ceases

FIGURE 63-1. Pathophysiology of traumatic brain injury.

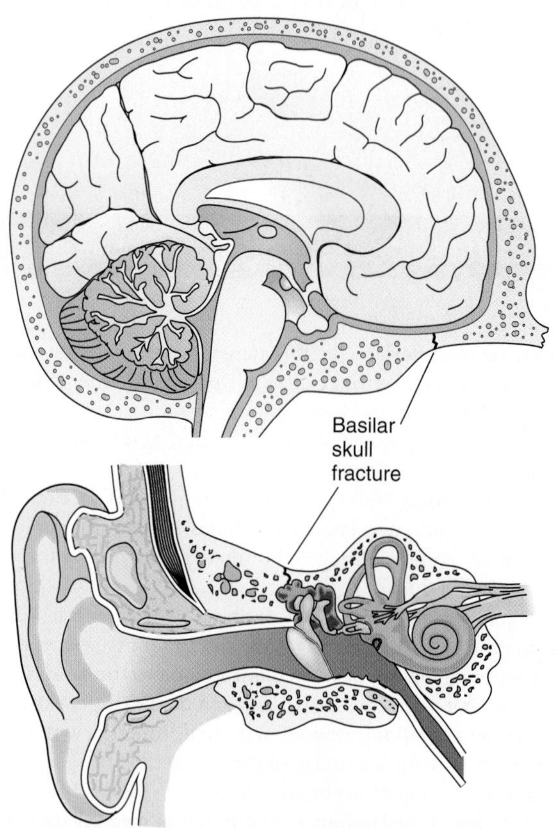

FIGURE 63-2. Basilar fractures allow cerebrospinal fluid to leak from the nose and ears. Adapted from Hickey, J. V. (2003). *The clinical practice of neurological and neurosurgical nursing* (5th ed.). Philadelphia: Lippincott Williams & Wilkins.

Clinical Manifestations

The symptoms, apart from those of the local injury, depend on the severity and the distribution of the underlying brain injury. Persistent, localized pain usually suggests that a fracture is present. Fractures of the cranial vault may or may not produce swelling in the region of the fracture; therefore, an x-ray is needed for diagnosis.

Fractures of the base of the skull tend to traverse the paranasal sinus of the frontal bone or the middle ear located in the temporal bone (see Fig. 63-2). Therefore, they frequently produce hemorrhage from the nose, pharynx, or ears, and blood may appear under the conjunctiva. An area of ecchymosis (bruising) may be seen over the mastoid (Battle's sign). Basilar skull fractures are suspected when cerebrospinal fluid escapes from the ears (CSF otorrhea) and the nose (CSF rhinorrhea). A halo sign (a blood stain surrounded by a yellowish stain) may be seen on bed linens or on the head dressing and is highly suggestive of a CSF leak. Drainage of CSF is a serious problem, because meningeal infection can occur if organisms gain access to the cranial contents via the nose, ear, or sinus through a tear in the dura. Bloody CSF suggests an associated brain laceration or contusion (Bader & Littlejohns, 2004).

Assessment and Diagnostic Findings

Radiologic examination confirms the presence and extent of a skull fracture (Porth, 2005). A rapid physical examination and evaluation of neurologic status detects obvious brain injuries, and a computed tomography (CT) scan uses high-speed x-ray scanning to detect less apparent abnormalities. It is a fast, accurate, and safe diagnostic procedure that shows the presence, nature, location, and extent of acute lesions. It is also helpful in the ongoing management of head injury, because it can disclose cerebral edema, contusion, intracerebral or extracerebral hematoma, subarachnoid and intraventricular hemorrhage, and late changes (infarction, hydrocephalus) (Torpy, Lynm & Glass, 2005).

Magnetic resonance imaging (MRI) is used to evaluate patients with head injury when a more accurate picture of the anatomic nature of the injury is warranted and when the patient is stable enough to undergo this longer diagnostic procedure (Torpy et al., 2005).

Cerebral angiography may also be used; it identifies supratentorial, extracerebral, and intracerebral hematomas and cerebral contusions. Lateral and anteroposterior views of the skull are obtained.

Gerontologic Considerations

Elderly patients must be assessed very carefully (Scheetz, 2005). Even with similar types of injury, an elderly person often suffers more severe injury than a young person and often recovers more slowly and with more complications (Bader & Littlejohns, 2004). The elderly patient with confusion or behavioral disturbances should be assessed for head injury, because unrecognized "minor" head trauma may account for behavioral and confusional episodes in some elderly people (Brewer, 2003). A misdiagnosed or untreated episode of confusion in an elderly patient may result in long-term disability that might have been avoided if the injury had been detected and treated promptly. Older patients with head injuries differ from those who are younger by etiology of injury, higher mortality rates, and poorer functional outcomes (Flanagan, Hibbard & Gordon, 2005).

Medical Management

Nondepressed skull fractures generally do not require surgical treatment; however, close observation of the patient is essential. Nursing personnel may observe the patient in the hospital, but if no underlying brain injury is present, the patient may be allowed to return home. If the patient is discharged home, specific instructions must be given to the family (see later discussion of concussion).

Depressed skull fractures usually require surgery, particularly if contaminated or deformed fractures are present (Ropper, Gress, Diringer, et al., 2004). Before the surgery, the scalp is shaved and cleansed with copious amounts of saline to remove debris. The fracture is exposed, skull fragments are elevated, any underlying dural laceration is repaired, and any accompanying hematoma is evacuated (Ropper et al., 2004). Large defects can be repaired immediately with bone or artificial grafts; if significant cerebral edema is present, repair of the defect may be delayed for 3 to 6 months. Penetrating wounds require surgical débridement to remove foreign bodies and devitalized brain tissue and to control hemorrhage (Winn, 2003). IV antibiotic treatment is instituted immediately, particularly with a dural laceration, and blood component therapy is administered if indicated.

As stated previously, fractures of the base of the skull are serious because they are usually open (involving the paranasal sinuses or the middle or external ear) and result in CSF leakage. The nasopharynx and the external ear should be kept clean. Usually a piece of sterile cotton is placed loosely in the ear, or a sterile cotton pad may be taped loosely under the nose or against the ear to collect the draining fluid. The patient who is conscious is cautioned not to blow his or her nose. The head is elevated 30 degrees to reduce ICP and promote spontaneous closure of the leak (Bader & Littlejohns, 2004; Hickey, 2003). Some neurosurgeons, however, prefer that the bed be kept flat (Fan, 2004). Persistent CSF rhinorrhea or otorrhea usually requires surgical intervention.

Brain Injury

The most important consideration in any head injury is whether the brain is injured. Even seemingly minor injury can cause significant brain damage secondary to obstructed blood flow and decreased tissue perfusion. The brain cannot store oxygen or glucose to any significant degree. Because the cerebral cells need an uninterrupted blood supply to obtain these nutrients, irreversible brain damage and cell death occur if the blood supply is interrupted for even a few minutes. Clinical manifestations of **brain injury** (injury to the brain that is severe enough to interfere with normal functioning) are listed in Chart 63-2. **Closed (blunt) brain injury** occurs when the head accelerates and then rapidly

CHART 63-2

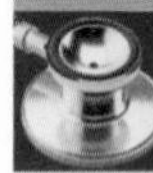

Assessing Traumatic Brain Injury

Be on the alert for the following signs and symptoms:
- Altered level of consciousness
- Confusion
- Pupillary abnormalities (changes in shape, size, and response to light)
- Altered or absent gag reflex
- Absent corneal reflex
- Sudden onset of neurologic deficits
- Changes in vital signs (altered respiratory pattern, widened pulse pressure, bradycardia, tachycardia, hypothermia or hyperthermia)
- Vision and hearing impairment
- Sensory dysfunction
- Headache
- Seizures

decelerates or collides with another object (eg, a wall, the dashboard of a car) and brain tissue is damaged but there is no opening through the skull and dura. **Open brain injury** occurs when an object penetrates the skull, enters the brain, and damages the soft brain tissue in its path (penetrating injury), or when blunt trauma to the head is so severe that it opens the scalp, skull, and dura to expose the brain.

Types of Brain Injury

Concussion

A cerebral **concussion** after head injury is a temporary loss of neurologic function with no apparent structural damage. A concussion (also referred to as a mild traumatic brain injury) generally involves a period of unconsciousness lasting from a few seconds to a few minutes. The jarring of the brain may be so slight as to cause only dizziness and spots before the eyes ("seeing stars"), or it may be severe enough to cause complete loss of consciousness for a time (McCrea, Guskiewicz, Marshall, et al., 2003). If the brain tissue in the frontal lobe is affected, the patient may exhibit bizarre irrational behavior, whereas involvement of the temporal lobe can produce temporary amnesia or disorientation.

The patient may be hospitalized overnight for observation or discharged from the hospital in a relatively short time after a concussion. Treatment involves observing the patient for headache, dizziness, lethargy, irritability, and anxiety. The occurrence of these symptoms after injury is referred to as postconcussion syndrome. Giving the patient information, explanations, and encouragement may reduce some of the problems of postconcussion syndrome. The patient is advised to resume normal activities slowly; the exact recovery time is not known (McCrea et al., 2003). The family is instructed to observe for the following signs and symptoms and to notify the physician or clinic (or bring the patient to the emergency department) if they occur:

- Difficulty in awakening
- Difficulty in speaking
- Confusion
- Severe headache
- Vomiting
- Weakness of one side of the body

A concussion was once thought of as a minor head injury without significant sequelae. However, studies have demonstrated that there are often disturbing and sometimes residual effects, including headache, lethargy, personality and behavior changes, attention deficits, difficulty with memory, and disruption in work habits (Brewer, 2003).

Contusion

In cerebral **contusion**, a more severe injury than concussion, the brain is bruised, with possible surface hemorrhage. The patient is unconscious for more than a few seconds or minutes. Clinical signs and symptoms depend on the size of the contusion and the amount of associated cerebral edema. The patient may lie motionless, with a faint pulse, shallow respirations, and cool, pale skin. Often involuntary evacuation of the bowels and the bladder occurs. The patient may be aroused with effort but soon slips back into unconsciousness. The blood pressure and the temperature are subnormal, and the clinical picture is somewhat similar to that of shock. In general, patients with severe brain injury who have abnormal motor function, abnormal eye movements, and elevated ICP have poor outcomes—brain damage, disability, or death. Conversely, patients may recover consciousness but pass into a stage of cerebral irritability. In this stage, the patient is conscious and easily disturbed by any form of stimulation, such as noises, light, and voices; he or she may become hyperactive at times. Gradually, the pulse, respirations, temperature, and other body functions return to normal, but full recovery can be delayed for months. Residual headache and vertigo are common, and impaired mental function or seizures may occur as a result of irreparable cerebral damage.

Diffuse Axonal Injury

Diffuse axonal injury involves widespread damage to axons in the cerebral hemispheres, corpus callosum, and brain stem. It can be seen with mild, moderate, or severe head trauma. The patient experiences no lucid intervals, immediate coma, decorticate and decerebrate posturing (see Fig. 61-1 in Chapter 61 and the discussion in Chapter 60), and global cerebral edema. Diagnosis is made by clinical signs in conjunction with a CT or MRI scan. Recovery depends on the severity of the axonal injury.

Intracranial Hemorrhage

Hematomas (collections of blood) that develop within the cranial vault are the most serious brain injuries (Bader & Littlejohns, 2004; Hickey, 2003). A hematoma may be epidural (above the dura), subdural (below the dura), or intracerebral (within the brain) (Fig. 63-3). Major symptoms are frequently delayed until the hematoma is large enough to cause distortion of the brain and increased ICP. The signs and symptoms of cerebral ischemia resulting from

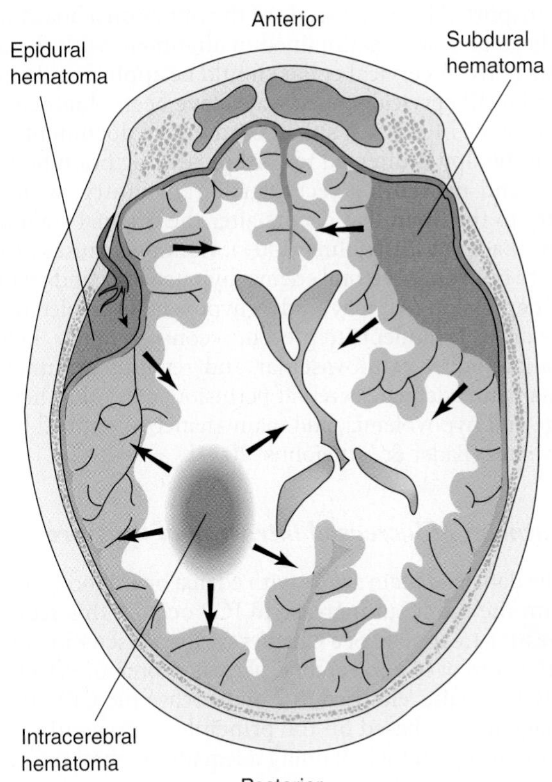

FIGURE 63-3. Location of epidural, subdural, and intracerebral hematomas.

compression by a hematoma are variable and depend on the speed with which vital areas are affected and the area that is injured (American Association of Neuroscience Nurses [AANN], 2005). In general, a rapidly developing hematoma, even if small, may be fatal, whereas a larger but slowly developing one may allow compensation for increases in ICP.

EPIDURAL HEMATOMA (EXTRADURAL HEMATOMA OR HEMORRHAGE)

After a head injury, blood may collect in the epidural (extradural) space between the skull and the dura. This can result from a skull fracture that causes a rupture or laceration of the middle meningeal artery, the artery that runs between the dura and the skull inferior to a thin portion of temporal bone. Hemorrhage from this artery causes rapid pressure on the brain.

Symptoms are caused by the expanding hematoma. Usually, a momentary loss of consciousness occurs at the time of injury, followed by an interval of apparent recovery (lucid interval). Although the lucid interval is considered a classic characteristic of an epidural hematoma, no lucid interval has been reported in many patients with this lesion (Bader & Littlejohns, 2004; Hickey, 2003), and therefore it should not be considered a critical defining criterion. During the lucid interval, compensation for the expanding hematoma takes place by rapid absorption of CSF and decreased intravascular volume, both of which help maintain a normal ICP. When these mechanisms can no longer compensate, even a small increase in the volume of the blood clot produces a marked elevation in ICP. Then, often suddenly, signs of compression appear (usually deterioration of consciousness and signs of focal neurologic deficits, such as dilation and fixation of a pupil or paralysis of an extremity), and the patient's condition deteriorates rapidly.

An epidural hematoma is considered an extreme emergency; marked neurologic deficit or even respiratory arrest can occur within minutes. Treatment consists of making openings through the skull (burr holes) to decrease ICP emergently, remove the clot, and control the bleeding. A craniotomy may be required to remove the clot and control the bleeding. A drain is usually inserted after creation of burr holes or a craniotomy to prevent reaccumulation of blood.

SUBDURAL HEMATOMA

A subdural hematoma is a collection of blood between the dura and the brain, a space normally occupied by a thin cushion of fluid. The most common cause of subdural hematoma is trauma, but it can also occur as a result of coagulopathies or rupture of an aneurysm. A subdural hemorrhage is more frequently venous in origin and is caused by the rupture of small vessels that bridge the subdural space (Porth, 2005). The subdural hematoma that results may be acute, subacute, or chronic, depending on the size of the involved vessel and the amount of bleeding.

Acute and Subacute Subdural Hematoma

Acute subdural hematomas are associated with major head injury involving contusion or laceration. Clinical symptoms develop over 24 to 48 hours. Signs and symptoms include changes in the level of consciousness (LOC), pupillary signs, and hemiparesis. There may be minor or even no symptoms with small collections of blood. Coma, increasing blood pressure, decreasing heart rate, and slowing respiratory rate are all signs of a rapidly expanding mass requiring immediate intervention. Subacute subdural hematomas are the result of less severe contusions and head trauma. Clinical manifestations usually appear between 48 hours and 2 weeks after the injury. Signs and symptoms are similar to those of an acute subdural hematoma.

If the patient can be transported rapidly to the hospital, an immediate craniotomy is performed to open the dura, allowing the subdural clot to be evacuated. Successful outcome also depends on the control of ICP and careful monitoring of respiratory function (see the discussion of intracranial surgery in Chapter 61). The mortality rate for patients with acute or subacute subdural hematoma is high because of associated brain damage.

Chronic Subdural Hematoma

Chronic subdural hematomas can develop from seemingly minor head injuries and are seen most frequently in the elderly. The elderly are prone to this type of head injury secondary to brain atrophy, which is a frequent consequence of the aging process. Seemingly minor head trauma may produce enough impact to shift the brain contents abnormally. The time between injury and onset of symptoms can be lengthy (eg, 3 weeks to months), so the actual injury may be forgotten.

A chronic subdural hematoma can resemble other conditions; for example, it may be mistaken for a stroke. The bleeding is less profuse, but compression of the intracranial contents still occurs. The blood within the brain changes in character in 2 to 4 days, becoming thicker and darker. In a few weeks, the clot breaks down and has the color and consistency of motor oil. Eventually, calcification or ossification of the clot takes place. The brain adapts to this foreign body invasion, and the clinical signs and symptoms fluctuate. Symptoms include severe headache, which tends to come and go; alternating focal neurologic signs; personality changes; mental deterioration; and focal seizures. The patient may be labeled neurotic or psychotic if the cause is overlooked.

The treatment of a chronic subdural hematoma consists of surgical evacuation of the clot. The procedure may be carried out through multiple burr holes, or a craniotomy may be performed for a sizable subdural mass that cannot be suctioned or drained through burr holes.

INTRACEREBRAL HEMORRHAGE AND HEMATOMA

Intracerebral hemorrhage is bleeding into the substance of the brain. It is commonly seen in head injuries when force is exerted to the head over a small area (eg, missile injuries, bullet wounds, stab injuries). These hemorrhages within the brain may also result from

- Systemic hypertension, which causes degeneration and rupture of a vessel
- Rupture of a saccular aneurysm
- Vascular anomalies
- Intracranial tumors
- Bleeding disorders such as leukemia, hemophilia, aplastic anemia, and thrombocytopenia
- Complications of anticoagulant therapy

Nontraumatic causes of intracerebral hemorrhage are discussed in Chapter 62.

The onset may be insidious, beginning with the development of neurologic deficits followed by headache. Management includes supportive care, control of ICP, and careful administration of fluids, electrolytes, and antihypertensive medications. Surgical intervention by craniotomy or craniectomy permits removal of the blood clot and control of hemorrhage but may not be possible because of the inaccessible location of the bleeding or the lack of a clearly circumscribed area of blood that can be removed.

Management of Brain Injuries

Assessment and diagnosis of the extent of injury are accomplished by the initial physical and neurologic examinations. CT and MRI scans are the primary neuroimaging diagnostic tools and are useful in evaluating the brain structure. Positron emission tomography (PET) is available in some trauma centers; this method of scanning examines brain function rather than structure. A flowchart developed by the Brain Trauma Foundation (2003) for the initial management of brain injury is presented in Figure 63-4.

Any patient with a head injury is presumed to have a cervical spine injury until proven otherwise. The patient is transported from the scene of the injury on a board with the head and neck maintained in alignment with the axis of the body. A cervical collar should be applied and maintained until cervical spine x-rays have been obtained and the absence of cervical spinal cord injury documented.

All therapy is directed toward preserving brain homeostasis and preventing secondary brain injury, which is injury to the brain that occurs after the original traumatic event (Bader & Littlejohns, 2004). Common causes of secondary injury are cerebral edema, hypotension, and respiratory depression that may lead to hypoxemia and electrolyte imbalance. Treatments to prevent secondary injury include stabilization of cardiovascular and respiratory function to maintain adequate cerebral perfusion, control of hemorrhage and hypovolemia, and maintenance of optimal blood gas values (Bader & Littlejohns, 2004).

Treatment of Increased Intracranial Pressure

As the damaged brain swells with edema or as blood collects within the brain, an increase in ICP occurs; this requires aggressive treatment. See Chapter 61 for a discussion of the relationship of ICP to cerebral perfusion pressure (CPP). If the ICP remains elevated, it can decrease the CPP. Initial management is based on the principle of preventing secondary injury and maintaining adequate cerebral oxygenation (see Fig. 63-4).

Surgery is required for evacuation of blood clots, débridement and elevation of depressed fractures of the skull, and suture of severe scalp lacerations. ICP is monitored closely; if increased, it is managed by maintaining adequate oxygenation, elevating the head of the bed, and maintaining normal blood volume. Devices to monitor ICP or drain CSF can be inserted during surgery or at the bedside using aseptic technique. The patient is cared for in the intensive care unit, where expert nursing care and medical treatment are readily available (AANN, 2005).

Supportive Measures

Treatment also includes ventilatory support, seizure prevention, fluid and electrolyte maintenance, nutritional support, and management of pain and anxiety. Comatose patients are intubated and mechanically ventilated to ensure adequate oxygenation and protect the airway.

Because seizures can occur after head injury and can cause secondary brain damage from hypoxia, antiseizure agents may be administered. If the patient is very agitated, benzodiazepines may be prescribed to calm the patient without decreasing LOC. These medications do not affect ICP or CPP, making them good choices for the patient with head injury. A nasogastric tube may be inserted, because reduced gastric motility and reverse peristalsis are associated with head injury, making regurgitation and aspiration common in the first few hours.

Brain Death

When a patient has sustained a severe head injury incompatible with life, the patient is a potential organ donor.

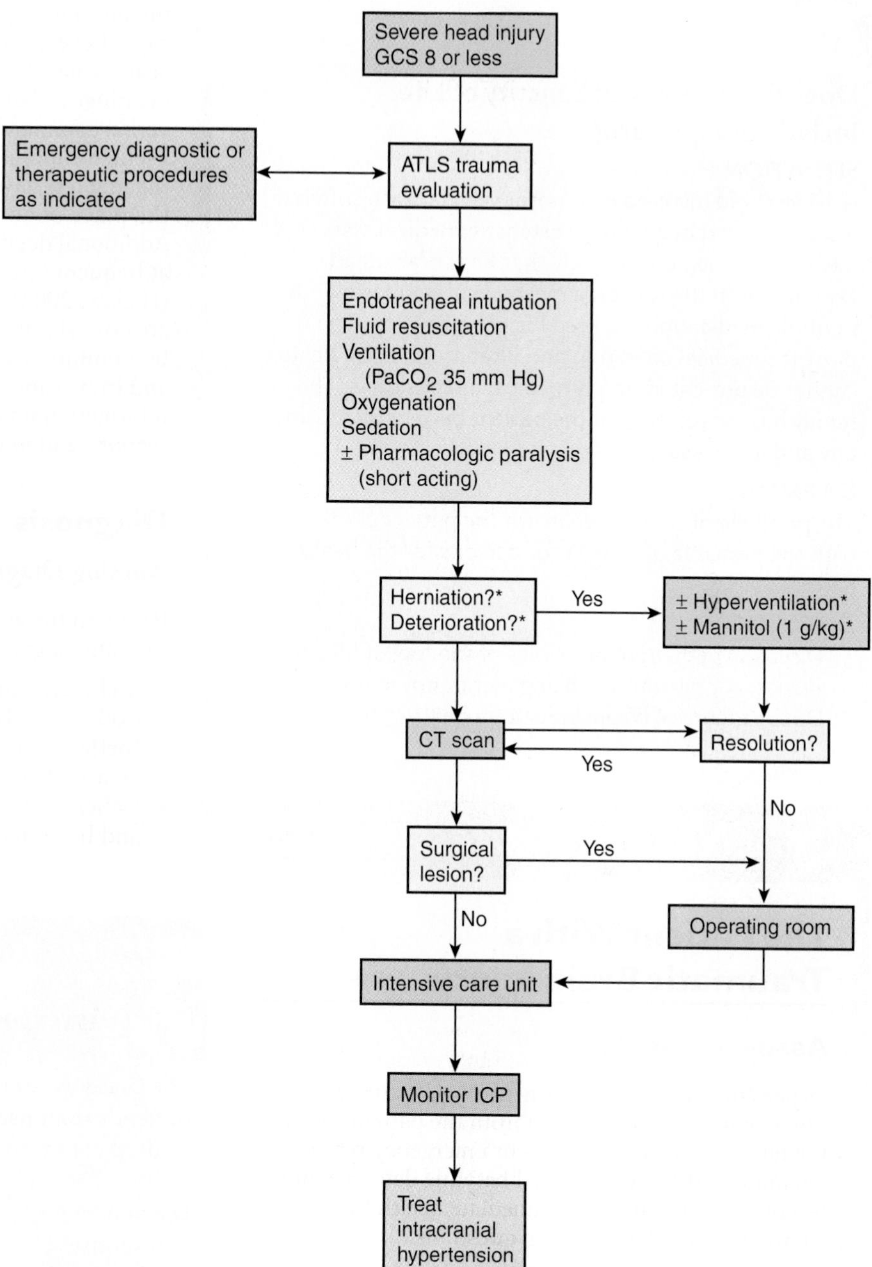

FIGURE 63-4. Initial management of the patient with severe head injury (treatment option). Copyright © 2003 Brain Trauma Foundation, Inc.

The nurse may assist in the clinical examination for determination of brain death and in the process of organ procurement. Since 1981, all 50 states have recognized the Uniform Determination of Brain Death Act. This act states that death will be determined with accepted medical standards and that death will indicate irreversible loss of all brain function (Henneman & Karras, 2004). The three cardinal signs of brain death on clinical examination are coma, the absence of brain-stem reflexes, and apnea (Haymore, 2004). Adjunctive tests such as EEG and cerebral blood flow (CBF) studies are often used to confirm brain death (Hickey, 2003). The health care team provides information to the family and assists them with the decision-making process about organ donation. Chart 63-3 poses an ethical dilemma related to stopping life support.

CHART 63-3

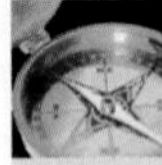

Ethics and Related Issues

Does the Principle of Sanctity of Life Include Brain Death?

SITUATION

A 16-year-old involved in a motor vehicle crash suffered a severe closed head injury. Extensive medical tests have determined conclusively that he is brain dead. He remains in the ICU on a mechanical ventilator with multiple medications to keep his heart beating. The patient's medical condition and ultimate physical death cannot be prevented by any medical interventions. The family has requested that the patient be kept alive using any and all measures.

DILEMMA

The principle of sanctity of life for the patient conflicts with the principle of respect for persons for the health care providers.

DISCUSSION

1. Discuss whether the principles of sanctity of life and respect for persons are being met or not met.
2. Does sanctity of life include brain death?

Nursing Process

The Patient With a Traumatic Brain Injury

Assessment

Depending on the patient's neurologic status, the nurse may elicit information from the patient, from the family, or from witnesses or emergency rescue personnel. Although all usual baseline data may not be collected initially, the immediate health history should include the following questions:

- When did the injury occur?
- What caused the injury? A high-velocity missile? An object striking the head? A fall?
- What was the direction and force of the blow?

A history of unconsciousness or amnesia after a head injury indicates a significant degree of brain damage, and changes that occur minutes to hours after the initial injury can reflect recovery or indicate the development of secondary brain damage. Therefore, the nurse also should try to determine if there was a loss of consciousness, what the duration of the unconscious period was, and whether the patient could be aroused.

In addition to asking questions that establish the nature of the injury and the patient's condition immediately after the injury, the nurse examines the patient thoroughly. This assessment includes determining the patient's LOC using the Glasgow Coma Scale and assessing the patient's response to tactile stimuli (if unconscious), pupillary response to light, corneal and gag reflexes, and motor function. The Glasgow Coma Scale (Chart 63-4) is based on the three criteria of eye opening, verbal responses, and motor responses to verbal commands or painful stimuli. It is particularly useful for monitoring changes during the acute phase, the first few days after a head injury. It does not take the place of an in-depth neurologic assessment. Additional detailed assessments are made initially and at frequent intervals throughout the acute phase of care (Hickey, 2003). The baseline and ongoing assessments are critical nursing interventions for the patient with brain injury, whose condition can worsen dramatically and irrevocably if subtle signs are overlooked. More information on assessment is provided in the following sections and in Figure 63-5 and Table 63-1.

Diagnosis

Nursing Diagnoses

Based on the assessment data, the patient's major nursing diagnoses may include the following:

- Ineffective airway clearance and impaired gas exchange related to brain injury
- Ineffective cerebral tissue perfusion related to increased ICP, decreased CPP, and possible seizures
- Deficient fluid volume related to decreased LOC and hormonal dysfunction

CHART 63-4

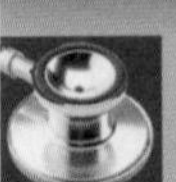

Assessment for Glasgow Coma Scale

The Glasgow Coma Scale is a tool for assessing a patient's response to stimuli. Scores range from 3 (deep coma) to 15 (normal).

Eye opening response	Spontaneous	4
	To voice	3
	To pain	2
	None	1
Best verbal response	Oriented	5
	Confused	4
	Inappropriate words	3
	Incomprehensible sounds	2
	None	1
Best motor response	Obeys command	6
	Localizes pain	5
	Withdraws	4
	Flexion	3
	Extension	2
	None	1
Total		3 to 15

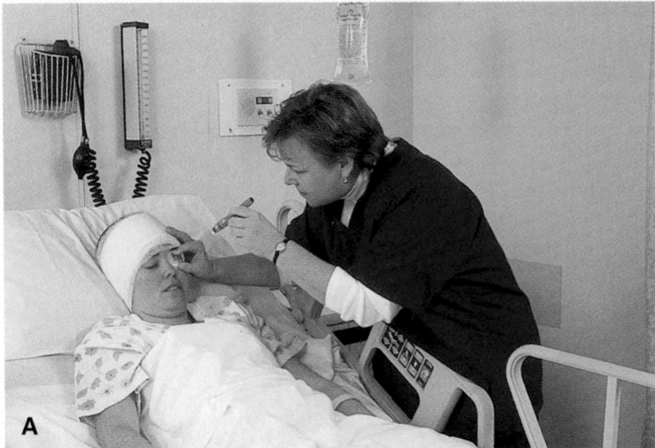

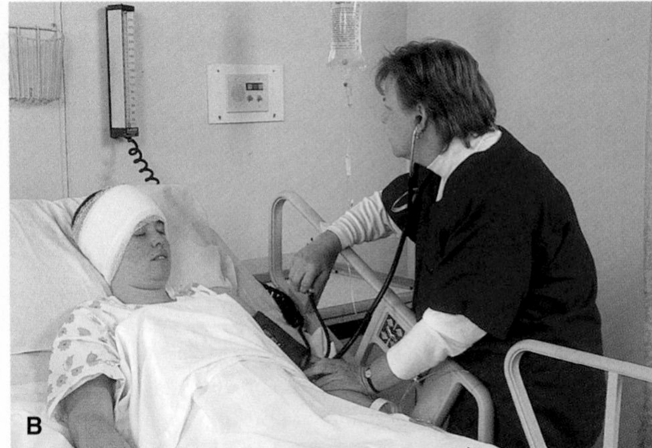

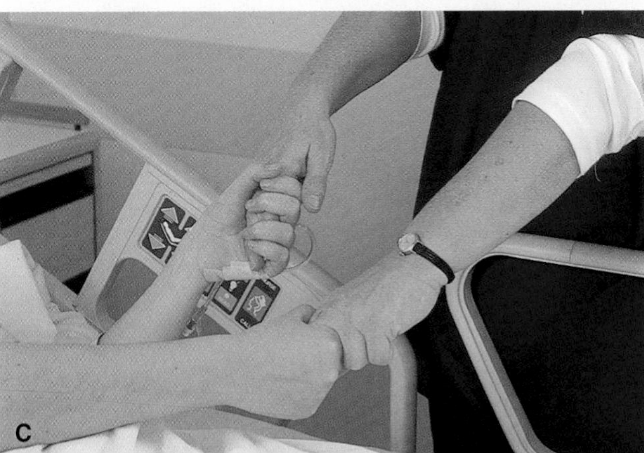

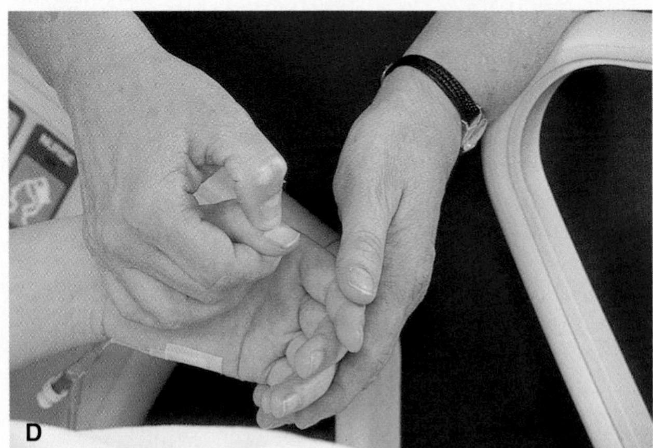

FIGURE 63-5. Assessment parameters for the patient with a head injury include (**A**) eye opening and responsiveness, (**B**) vital signs, and (**C, D**) motor response reflected in hand strength or response to painful stimulus. Photo © B. Proud.

- Imbalanced nutrition, less than body requirements, related to increased metabolic demands, fluid restriction, and inadequate intake
- Risk for injury (self-directed and directed at others) related to seizures, disorientation, restlessness, or brain damage
- Risk for imbalanced body temperature related to damaged temperature-regulating mechanisms in the brain
- Risk for impaired skin integrity related to bed rest, hemiparesis, hemiplegia, immobility, or restlessness
- Disturbed thought processes (deficits in intellectual function, communication, memory, information processing) related to brain injury
- Disturbed sleep pattern related to brain injury and frequent neurologic checks
- Interrupted family processes related to unresponsiveness of patient, unpredictability of outcome, prolonged recovery period, and the patient's residual physical disability and emotional deficit
- Deficient knowledge about brain injury, recovery, and the rehabilitation process

The nursing diagnoses for the unconscious patient and the patient with increased ICP also apply (see Chapter 61).

Collaborative Problems/ Potential Complications

Based on all the assessment data, the major complications include the following:

- Decreased cerebral perfusion
- Cerebral edema and herniation
- Impaired oxygenation and ventilation
- Impaired fluid, electrolyte, and nutritional balance
- Risk of posttraumatic seizures

Planning and Goals

The goals for the patient may include maintenance of a patent airway, adequate CPP, fluid and electrolyte balance, adequate nutritional status, prevention of secondary injury, maintenance of normal body temperature, maintenance of skin integrity, improvement of cognitive function, prevention of sleep deprivation,

TABLE 63-1 Summary of Multisystem Assessment Measures for the Patient With Traumatic Brain Injury

System-Specific Considerations	Assessment Data
Neurologic System	
• Severe head injury results in unconsciousness and alters many neurologic functions. • All body functions must be supported. • Increased ICP and herniation syndromes are life-threatening • Measures are instituted to control elevated ICP.	• Assessment of neurologic signs • Assessment for signs and symptoms of ICP elevation • Calculation of cerebral perfusion pressure if ICP monitor is in place • Monitoring of antiseizure medication blood levels
Integumentary System (Skin and Mucous Membranes)	
• Immobility secondary to injury and unconsciousness contributes to the development of pressure areas and skin breakdown. • Intubation causes irritation of the mucous membrane.	• Assessment of skin integrity and character of the skin • Assessment of oral mucous membrane
Musculoskeletal System	
• Immobility contributes to musculoskeletal changes. • Decerebrate or decorticate posturing makes proper positioning difficult.	• Assessment of range of motion of joints and development of deformities or spasticity
Gastrointestinal System	
• Administration of corticosteroids places the patient at high risk for GI hemorrhage. • Injury to the GI tract can result in paralytic ileus. • Constipation can result from bed rest, NPO status, fluid restriction, and opioids given for pain control. • Bowel incontinence is related to the patient's unconscious state or altered mental state.	• Assessment of abdomen for bowel sounds and distention • Monitoring for decreased hemoglobin
Genitourinary System	
• Fluid restriction or use of diuretics can alter the amount of urinary output. • Urinary incontinence is related to the patient's unconscious state.	• Intake and output record
Metabolic (Nutritional) System	
• The patient receives all fluids IV for the first few days until the GI tract is functioning. • A nutritional consultation is initiated within the first 24–48 h; parenteral or enteral nutrition may be started.	• Assessment of fluid and electrolyte balance • Recording of weight, if possible • Hematocrit • Electrolyte studies
Respiratory System	
• Complete or partial airway obstruction will compromise the oxygen supply to the brain. • An altered respiratory pattern can result in cerebral hypoxia. • A short period of apnea at the moment of impact can result in spotty atelectasis. • Systemic disturbances from head injury can cause hypoxemia. • Brain injury can alter brain stem respiratory function. • Shunting of blood to the lungs as a result of a sympathetic discharge at the time of injury can cause neurogenic pulmonary edema.	• Assessment of respiratory function – Auscultate chest for breath sounds. – Note the respiratory pattern if possible (not possible if a ventilator is being used). – Note the respiratory rate – Note whether the cough reflex is intact. • Arterial blood gas levels • Complete blood count • Chest x-ray studies • Sputum cultures • O_2 saturation using pulse oximetry
Cardiovascular System	
• The patient may develop cardiac dysrhythmias, tachycardia, or bradycardia. • The patient may develop hypotension or hypertension. • Because of immobility and unconsciousness, the patient is at high risk for deep vein thromboses and pulmonary emboli.	• Assessment of vital signs • Monitoring for cardiac dysrhythmias • Assessment for deep vein thromboses of legs • Electrocardiogram • Electrolyte studies

TABLE 63-1 Summary of Multisystem Assessment Measures for the Patient With Traumatic Brain Injury (Continued)

System-Specific Considerations	Assessment Data
• Fluid and electrolyte imbalance can be related to several problems, including alterations in antidiuretic hormone (ADH) secretion, the stress response, or fluid restriction. • Specific conditions may occur: – Diabetes insipidus (DI) – Syndrome of inappropriate secretion of ADH (SIADH) – Electrolyte imbalance – Hyperosmolar nonketotic hyperglycemia	• Blood coagulation studies • I^{125} fibrinogen scan of legs • Blood glucose level • Blood acetone level • Blood osmolality • Urine specific gravity
Psychological/Emotional Response	
• The traumatic head-injured patient is unconscious. • The family needs emotional support to deal with the crisis.	• Collection of information about the family and the role of the head-injured person within the family • Assessment of the family to determine how functional it was before the injury occurred

effective family coping, increased knowledge about the rehabilitation process, and absence of complications.

Nursing Interventions

The nursing interventions for the patient with a head injury are extensive and diverse; they include making nursing assessments, setting priorities for nursing interventions, anticipating needs and complications, and initiating rehabilitation.

Monitoring for Declining Neurologic Function

The importance of ongoing assessment and monitoring of the patient with brain injury cannot be overstated. The following parameters are assessed initially and as frequently as the patient's condition requires. As soon as the initial assessment is made, the use of a neurologic flow chart is started and maintained.

LEVEL OF CONSCIOUSNESS

The Glasgow Coma Scale is used to assess LOC at regular intervals, because changes in the LOC precede all other changes in vital and neurologic signs. The patient's best responses to predetermined stimuli are recorded (see Chart 63-4). Each response is scored (the greater the number, the better the functioning), and the sum of these scores gives an indication of the severity of coma and a prediction of possible outcome. The lowest score is 3 (least responsive); the highest is 15 (most responsive). A score of 8 or less is generally accepted as indicating a severe head injury (Haymore, 2004).

VITAL SIGNS

Although a change in LOC is the most sensitive neurologic indication of deterioration of the patient's condition, vital signs also are monitored at frequent intervals to assess the intracranial status. Table 63-1 depicts the general assessment parameters for the patient with a head injury.

Signs of increasing ICP include slowing of the heart rate (bradycardia), increasing systolic blood pressure, and widening pulse pressure. As brain compression increases, respirations become rapid, the blood pressure may decrease, and the pulse slows further. This is an ominous development, as is a rapid fluctuation of vital signs (Hickey, 2003). A rapid increase in body temperature is regarded as unfavorable because hyperthermia increases the metabolic demands of the brain and may indicate brain stem damage, a poor prognostic sign. The temperature is maintained at less than 38°C (100.4°F). Tachycardia and arterial hypotension may indicate that bleeding is occurring elsewhere in the body.

MOTOR FUNCTION

Motor function is assessed frequently by observing spontaneous movements, asking the patient to raise and lower the extremities, and comparing the strength and equality of the upper and lower extremities at periodic intervals. To assess upper extremity strength, the nurse instructs the patient to squeeze the examiner's fingers tightly. The nurse assesses lower extremity motor strength by placing the hands on the soles of the patient's feet and asking the patient to push down against the examiner's hands. Examination of the motor system is discussed in Chapter 60 in more detail. The presence or absence of spontaneous movement of each extremity is also noted, and speech and eye signs are assessed.

If the patient does not demonstrate spontaneous movement, responses to painful stimuli are assessed (Haymore, 2004). Motor response to pain is assessed by applying a central stimulus, such as pinching the pectoralis major muscle, to determine the patient's best response. Peripheral stimulation may provide inaccurate assessment data because it may result in a reflex movement rather than a voluntary motor response. Abnormal responses (lack of motor response; extension responses) are associated with a poorer prognosis.

OTHER NEUROLOGIC SIGNS

In addition to the patient's spontaneous eye opening, evaluated with the Glasgow Coma Scale, the size and equality of the pupils and their reaction to light are assessed. A unilaterally dilated and poorly responding pupil may indicate a developing hematoma, with subsequent pressure on the third cranial nerve due to shifting of the brain. If both pupils become fixed and dilated, this indicates overwhelming injury and intrinsic damage to the upper brain stem and is a poor prognostic sign (Arbour, 2004; Hickey, 2003).

The patient with a head injury may develop deficits such as anosmia (lack of sense of smell), eye movement abnormalities, aphasia, memory deficits, and posttraumatic seizures or epilepsy. Patients may be left with residual psychological deficits (impulsiveness, emotional lability, or uninhibited, aggressive behaviors) and, as a consequence of the impairment, may lack insight into their emotional responses.

Maintaining the Airway

One of the most important nursing goals in the management of head injury is to establish and maintain an adequate airway. The brain is extremely sensitive to hypoxia, and a neurologic deficit can worsen if the patient is hypoxic. Therapy is directed toward maintaining optimal oxygenation to preserve cerebral function. An obstructed airway causes carbon dioxide retention and hypoventilation, which can produce cerebral vessel dilation and increased ICP.

Interventions to ensure an adequate exchange of air are discussed in Chapter 61 and include the following:

- Maintain the unconscious patient in a position that facilitates drainage of oral secretions, with the head of the bed elevated about 30 degrees to decrease intracranial venous pressure (Fan, 2004).
- Establish effective suctioning procedures (pulmonary secretions produce coughing and straining, which increase ICP).
- Guard against aspiration and respiratory insufficiency.
- Closely monitor arterial blood gas values to assess the adequacy of ventilation. The goal is to keep blood gas values within the normal range to ensure adequate cerebral blood flow.
- Monitor the patient who is receiving mechanical ventilation.
- Monitor for pulmonary complications such as acute respiratory distress syndrome (ARDS) and pneumonia (Bader & Littlejohns, 2004).

Monitoring Fluid and Electrolyte Balance

Brain damage can produce metabolic and hormonal dysfunctions. The monitoring of serum electrolyte levels is important, especially in patients receiving osmotic diuretics, those with syndrome of inappropriate antidiuretic hormone (SIADH), and those with posttraumatic diabetes insipidus.

Serial studies of blood and urine electrolytes and osmolality are carried out, because head injuries may be accompanied by disorders of sodium regulation. Hyponatremia is common after head injury due to shifts in extracellular fluid, electrolytes, and volume. Hyperglycemia, for example, can cause an increase in extracellular fluid that lowers sodium (Hickey, 2003). Hypernatremia may also occur as a result of sodium retention that may last several days, followed by sodium diuresis. Increasing lethargy, confusion, and seizures may be due to electrolyte imbalance.

Endocrine function is evaluated by monitoring serum electrolytes, blood glucose values, and intake and output. Urine is tested regularly for acetone. A record of daily weights is maintained, especially if the patient has hypothalamic involvement and is at risk for the development of diabetes insipidus.

Promoting Adequate Nutrition

Head injury results in metabolic changes that increase calorie consumption and nitrogen excretion. Protein demand increases. Early initiation of nutritional therapy has been shown to improve outcomes in patients with head injury. Parenteral nutrition via a central line or enteral feedings administered via a nasogastric or nasojejunal feeding tube should be started within 48 hours after admission (Bader, Littlejohns & March, 2003). If CSF rhinorrhea occurs, an oral feeding tube should be inserted instead of a nasal tube.

Laboratory values should be monitored closely in patients receiving parenteral nutrition. Elevating the head of the bed and aspirating the enteral tube for evidence of residual feeding before administering additional feedings can help prevent distention, regurgitation, and aspiration. A continuous-drip infusion or pump may be used to regulate the feeding. The principles and technique of enteral feedings are discussed in Chapter 36. Enteral or parenteral feedings are usually continued until the swallowing reflex returns and the patient can meet caloric requirements orally.

Preventing Injury

Often, as the patient emerges from coma, a period of lethargy and stupor is followed by a period of agitation. Each phase is variable and depends on the individual, the location of the injury, the depth and duration of coma, and the patient's age. The patient emerging from a coma may become increasingly agitated toward the end of the day. Restlessness may be caused by hypoxia, fever, pain, or a full bladder. It may indicate injury to the brain but may also be a sign that the patient is regaining consciousness. (Some restlessness may be beneficial because the lungs and extremities are exercised.) Agitation may also be due to discomfort from catheters, IV lines, restraints, and repeated neurologic checks. Alternatives to restraints must be used whenever possible.

Strategies to prevent injury include the following:

- The patient is assessed to ensure that oxygenation is adequate and the bladder is not distended. Dressings and casts are checked for constriction.
- Padded side rails are used or the patient's hands are wrapped in mitts to protect the patient from self-

injury and dislodging of tubes (Fig. 63-6). Restraints are avoided, because straining against them can increase ICP or cause other injury. Enclosed or floor-level specialty beds may be indicated.
- Opioids are avoided as a means of controlling restlessness, because these medications depress respiration, constrict the pupils, and alter responsiveness.
- Environmental stimuli are reduced by keeping the room quiet, limiting visitors, speaking calmly, and providing frequent orientation information (eg, explaining where the patient is and what is being done).
- Adequate lighting is provided to prevent visual hallucinations.
- Efforts are made to minimize disruption of the patient's sleep/wake cycles.
- The patient's skin is lubricated with oil or emollient lotion to prevent irritation due to rubbing against the sheet.
- If incontinence occurs, an external sheath catheter may be used on a male patient. Because prolonged use of an indwelling catheter inevitably produces infection, the patient may be placed on an intermittent catheterization schedule.

Maintaining Body Temperature

An increase in body temperature in the patient with a head injury can be the result of damage to the hypothalamus, cerebral irritation from hemorrhage, or infection. The nurse monitors the patient's temperature every 2 to 4 hours. If the temperature increases, efforts are made to identify the cause and to control it using acetaminophen and cooling blankets to maintain normothermia (Bader & Littlejohns, 2004; Diringer, 2004). Cooling blankets should be used with caution so as not to induce shivering, which increases ICP. If infection is suspected, potential sites of infection are cultured and antibiotics are prescribed and administered.

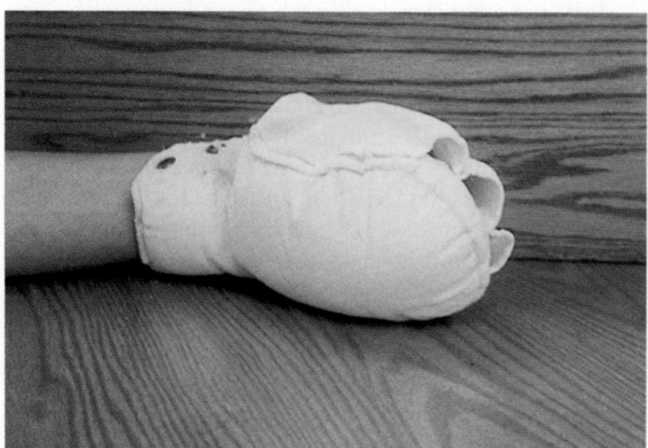

FIGURE 63-6. Hands of the patient with a head injury may be placed in a Posey mitt to prevent self-injury. This mitt has finger holes so that circulation can be assessed without removing the mitt. Photo courtesy of Sarah Trainer, RN, Roxborough Memorial Hospital, Philadelphia.

Use of mild hypothermia to 34° to 35° C (94° to 96° F) has been tested in small randomized controlled trials for at least 12 hours versus normothermia (control) in patients with closed head injury (Alderson, Gadkary & Signorini, 2005). The clinical trials with small samples showed improvement in patient outcomes but need to be repeated in larger trials. Because hypothermia increases the risk of pneumonia and has other side effects, this treatment is not currently recommended outside of controlled clinical trials.

Maintaining Skin Integrity

Patients with traumatic head injury often require assistance in turning and positioning because of immobility or unconsciousness. Prolonged pressure on the tissues decreases circulation and leads to tissue necrosis. Potential areas of breakdown need to be identified early to avoid the development of pressure ulcers. Specific nursing measures include the following:

- Assessing all body surfaces and documenting skin integrity every 8 hours
- Turning and repositioning the patient every 2 hours
- Providing skin care every 4 hours
- Assisting the patient to get out of bed to a chair three times a day

Improving Cognitive Functioning

Although many patients with head injury survive because of resuscitative and supportive technology, they frequently have significant cognitive sequelae that may not be detected during the acute phase of injury. Cognitive impairment includes memory deficits, decreased ability to focus and sustain attention to a task (distractibility), reduced ability to process information, and slowness in thinking, perceiving, communicating, reading, and writing. Psychiatric, emotional, and relationship problems develop in many patients after head injury (Hsueh-Fen & Stuifbergen, 2004). Resulting psychosocial, behavioral, emotional, and cognitive impairments are devastating to the family as well as to the patient (Davis & Gimenez, 2004; Hsueh-Fen & Stuifbergen, 2004).

These problems require collaboration among many disciplines. A neuropsychologist (specialist in evaluating and treating cognitive problems) plans a program and initiates therapy or counseling to help the patient reach maximal potential (Eslinger, 2002). Cognitive rehabilitation activities help the patient to devise new problem-solving strategies. The retraining is carried out over an extended period and may include the use of sensory stimulation and reinforcement, behavior modification, reality orientation, computer-training programs, and video games. Assistance from many disciplines is necessary during this phase of recovery. Even if intellectual ability does not improve, social and behavioral abilities may.

The patient recovering from a traumatic brain injury may experience fluctuations in the level of cognitive function, with orientation, attention, and memory frequently affected. Many types of sensory stimulation

NURSING RESEARCH PROFILE

Mother–Child Relationship After Traumatic Brain Injury

Hsueh-Fen, S. & Stuifbergen, A. K. (2004). Love and load: The lived experience of the mother–child relationship among young adult traumatic brain-injured survivors. *Journal of Neuroscience Nursing, 36*(2), 73–81.

Purpose

Traumatic brain injury (TBI) is a leading cause of death and disability across all age groups in the United States. The aim of this qualitative study was to describe the meaning of the relationship between young adult TBI survivors and their mothers.

Design

A phenomenologic approach was used to explore the meaning of the lived experience of young adult survivors of TBI and their maternal caregivers. Data saturation was reached with 12 mother–child dyads including 9 male and 3 female TBI survivors ranging in age from 18 to 25 years. The maternal caregivers were between 44 and 54 years of age. A one-time interview lasting 2 to 4 hours using an interview guide with predetermined questions was used to collect the data from mothers and children. The interviews were conducted an average of 3.6 years after injury.

Findings

The major themes identified included a sense of abnormality for both mothers and children about meeting societal and family expectations of normal young adulthood and a period of uncertainty waiting for the survivors' conditions to improve. Mother–child relationship themes included dependence and autonomy, marital threat, and maintaining harmony. The final theme was a series of changes in the interaction between TBI and family relationships.

Nursing Implications

Long-term community interventions are needed to help TBI survivors and their families decrease the burden of injury and the resulting stress. Nurses need to be instrumental in helping design and test innovative intervention programs. Specific interventions are needed to increase the survivors' self-esteem and improve quality of life for both survivors and their families.

programs have been tried, and research on these programs is ongoing (Davis & Gimeniz, 2004). When pushed to a level greater than the impaired cortical functioning allows, the patient may show symptoms of fatigue, anger, and stress (headache, dizziness). The Rancho Los Amigos Level of Cognitive Function is a scale frequently used to assess cognitive function and evaluate ongoing recovery from head injury. Nursing management and a description of each level are included in Table 63-2. Progress through the levels of cognitive function can vary widely for individual patients.

Preventing Sleep Pattern Disturbance

Patients who require frequent monitoring of neurologic status may experience sleep deprivation as they are awakened hourly for assessment of LOC. To allow the patient longer times of uninterrupted sleep and rest, the nurse can group nursing care activities so that the patient is disturbed less frequently. Environmental noise is decreased, and the room lights are dimmed. Back rubs and other measures to increase comfort can assist in promoting sleep and rest.

Supporting Family Coping

Having a loved one sustain a serious head injury can produce a great deal of prolonged stress in the family. This stress can result from the patient's physical and emotional deficits, the unpredictable outcome, and altered family relationships. Families report difficulties in coping with changes in the patient's temperament, behavior, and personality. Such changes are associated with disruption in family cohesion, loss of leisure pursuits, and loss of work capacity, as well as social isolation of the caretaker. The family may experience marital disruptions, anger, grief, guilt, and denial in recurring cycles (Hsueh-Fen & Stuifbergen, 2004).

To promote effective coping, the nurse can ask the family how the patient is different now, what has been lost, and what is most difficult about coping with this situation. Helpful interventions include providing family members with accurate and honest information and encouraging them to continue to set well-defined short-term goals. Family counseling helps address the family members' overwhelming feelings of loss and helplessness and gives them guidance for the management of inappropriate behaviors. Support groups help the family members share problems, develop insight, gain information, network, and gain assistance in maintaining realistic expectations and hope.

The Brain Injury Association (see Resources) serves as a clearinghouse for information and resources for patients with head injuries and their families, including specific information on coma, rehabilitation, behavioral consequences of head injury, and family issues. This organization can provide names of facilities and professionals who work with patients with head injuries and can assist families in organizing local support groups.

TABLE 63-2 Rancho Los Amigos Scale: Levels of Cognitive Function

Cognitive Level	Description	Nursing Management
	For levels I–III, the key approach is to *provide stimulation*.	
I: No response	Completely unresponsive to all stimuli, including painful stimuli	Multiple modalities of sensory input should be used. Examples are listed here, but management should be individualized and expanded based on available materials and patient preferences (determined by obtaining information from the family).
II: Generalized response	Nonpurposeful response; responds to pain, but in a nonpurposeful manner	*Olfactory:* perfumes, flowers, shaving lotion *Visual:* family pictures, card, personal items
III: Localized response	Responses more focused: withdraws to pain; turns toward sound; follows moving objects that pass within visual field; pulls on sources of discomfort (eg, tubes, restraints); may follow simple commands but inconsistently and in a delayed manner	*Auditory:* radio, television, tapes of family voices or favorite recordings, talking to patient (nurse, family members). The nurse should tell patient what is going to be done, discuss the environment, provide encouragement. *Tactile:* touching of skin, rubbing various textures on skin *Movement:* range of motion exercises, turning, repositioning, use of water mattress
	For levels IV–VI, the key approach is to *provide structure*.	
IV: Confused, agitated response	Alert, hyperactive state in which patient responds to internal confusion/agitation; behavior non-purposeful in relation to the environment; aggressive, bizarre behavior common	For level IV, which lasts 2–4 weeks, interventions are directed at decreasing agitation, increasing environmental awareness, and promoting safety. • Approach patient in a calm manner, and use a soft voice. • Screen patient from environmental stimuli (eg, sounds, sights); provide a quiet, controlled environment. • Remove devices that contribute to agitation (eg, tubes), if possible. • Functional goals cannot be set, because the patient is unable to cooperate.
V: Confused, inappropriate response	When agitation occurs, it is the result of external rather than internal stimuli; focused attention is difficult; memory is severely impaired; responses are fragmented and inappropriate to the situation; there is no carryover of learning from one situation to the other.	For levels V and VI, interventions are directed at decreasing confusion, improving cognitive function, and improving independence in performing ADLs. • Provide supervision. • Use repetition and cues to teach ADLs. Focus the patient's attention and help to increase his or her concentration.
VI: Confused, appropriate response	Follows simple directions consistently but is inconsistently oriented to time and place; short-term memory worse than long-term memory; can perform some ADLs	• Help the patient organize activity. • Clarify misinformation and reorient when confused. • Provide a consistent, predictable schedule (eg, post daily schedule on large poster board).
	For levels VII–X, the key approach is *integration into the community*.	
VII: Automatic, appropriate response	Appropriately responsive and oriented within the hospital setting; needs little supervision in ADLs; some carryover of learning; patient has superficial insight into disabilities; has decreased judgment and problem-solving abilities; lacks realistic planning for future	For levels VII–X, interventions are directed at increasing the patient's ability to function with minimal or no supervision in the community. • Reduce environmental structure. • Help the patient plan for adapting ADLs for self into the home environment. • Discuss and adapt home living skills (eg, cleaning, cooking) to patient's ability.

continued >

TABLE 63-2 Rancho Los Amigos Scale: Levels of Cognitive Function (Continued)

Cognitive Level	Description	Nursing Management
VIII: Purposeful, appropriate	Alert, oriented, intact memory; has realistic goals for the future. Able to complete familiar tasks for 1 hour in a distracting environment; overestimates or underestimates abilities, argumentative, easily frustrated, self-centered. Uncharacteristically dependent/independent.	• Provide stand-by assistance as needed for ADLs and home living skills.
IX: Purposeful, appropriate	Independently shifts back and forth between tasks and completes them accurately for at least two consecutive hours. Uses assistive memory devices to recall schedule and activities. Aware of and acknowledges impairments and disabilities when they interfere with task completion. Depression may continue. May be easily irritable and have a low frustration tolerance.	• Provide assistance on request for adapting ADLs and home living skills.
X: Purposeful, appropriate	Able to handle multiple tasks simultaneously in all environments but may require periodic breaks. Independently initiates and carries out familiar and unfamiliar tasks but may require more than usual amount of time and/or compensatory strategies to complete them. Accurately estimates abilities and independently adjusts to task demands. Periodic periods of depression may occur. Irritability and low frustration tolerance when sick, fatigued and/or under stress.	• Monitor for signs and symptoms of depression. • Help the patient plan, anticipate concerns, and solve problems.

Used with permission from Los Amigos Research and Education Institute, Inc., Downey, CA 2002.

Many patients with severe head injury die of their injuries, and many of those who survive experience long-term disabilities that prevent them from resuming their previous roles and functions. During the most acute phase of injury, family members need support and facts from the health care team.

Many patients with severe head injuries that result in brain death are young and otherwise healthy and are therefore considered for organ donation. Family members of patients with such injuries need support during this extremely stressful time and assistance in making decisions to end life support and permit donation of organs. They need to know that the patient who is brain dead and whose respiratory and cardiovascular systems are maintained through life support is not going to survive and that the severe head injury, not the removal of the patient's organs or the removal of life support, is the cause of the patient's death. Bereavement counselors and members of the organ procurement team are often very helpful to family members in making decisions about organ donation and in helping them cope with stress.

Monitoring and Managing Potential Complications

DECREASED CEREBRAL PERFUSION PRESSURE

Maintenance of adequate CPP is important to prevent serious complications of head injury due to decreased cerebral perfusion (Bader et al., 2003; Littlejohns et al., 2003). Adequate CPP is greater than 70 mm Hg. Any decrease in this pressure can impair cerebral perfusion and cause brain hypoxia and ischemia, leading to permanent damage. Therapy (eg, elevation of the head of the bed and increased IV fluids) is directed toward decreasing cerebral edema and increasing venous outflow from the brain. Systemic hypotension, which causes vasoconstriction and a significant decrease in CPP, is treated with increased IV fluids.

CEREBRAL EDEMA AND HERNIATION

The patient with a head injury is at risk for additional complications such as increased ICP and brain stem herniation. Cerebral edema is the most common cause of increased ICP in the patient with a head injury, with the swelling peaking approximately 48 to 72 hours after injury. Bleeding also may increase the volume of contents within the rigid, closed compartment of the skull, causing increased ICP and herniation of the brain stem and resulting in irreversible brain anoxia and brain death (Arbour, 2004; Censullo & Sebastian, 2004). Measures to control ICP are discussed in Chapter 61 and listed in Chart 63-5.

IMPAIRED OXYGENATION AND VENTILATION

Impaired oxygen and ventilation may require mechanical ventilatory support. The patient must be monitored for a patent airway, altered breathing patterns, and

CHART 63-5

Controlling Intracranial Pressure in Patients With Severe Brain Injury

- Elevate the head of the bed as prescribed.
- Maintain the patient's head and neck in neutral alignment (no twisting or flexing the neck).
- Initiate measures to prevent the Valsalva maneuver (eg, stool softeners).
- Maintain normal body temperature.
- Administer O_2 to maintain PaO_2 >90 mm Hg.
- Maintain fluid balance with normal saline solution.
- Avoid noxious stimuli (eg, excessive suctioning, painful procedures).
- Administer sedation to reduce agitation.
- Maintain cerebral perfusion pressure >70 mm Hg.

hypoxemia and pneumonia. Interventions may include endotracheal intubation, mechanical ventilation, and positive end-expiratory pressure. These topics are discussed in further detail in Chapters 25 and 61.

IMPAIRED FLUID, ELECTROLYTE, AND NUTRITIONAL BALANCE

Fluid, electrolyte, and nutritional imbalances are common in the patient with a head injury. Common imbalances include hyponatremia, which is often associated with SIADH (see Chapters 14 and 42), hypokalemia, and hyperglycemia (Hickey, 2003). Modifications in fluid intake with tube feedings or IV fluids, including hypertonic saline, may be necessary to treat these imbalances (Johnson & Criddle, 2004). Insulin administration may be prescribed to treat hyperglycemia.

Undernutrition is also a common problem in response to the increased metabolic needs associated with severe head injury. If the patient cannot eat, enteral feedings or parenteral nutrition may be initiated within 48 hours after the injury to provide adequate calories and nutrients (Bader et al., 2003). Nutritional support in the form of early feeding after head injury is associated with better survival outcomes and decreased disability (Yanagawa, Bunn, Roberts, et al., 2002).

POST-TRAUMATIC SEIZURES

Patients with head injury are at an increased risk for post-traumatic seizures. Post-traumatic seizures are classified as immediate (within 24 hours after injury), early (within 1 to 7 days after injury), or late (more than 7 days after injury) (Somjen, 2004). Seizure prophylaxis is the practice of administering antiseizure medications to patients with head injury to prevent seizures. It is important to prevent post-traumatic seizures, especially in the immediate and early phase of recovery, because seizures may increase ICP and decrease oxygenation. However, many antiseizure medications impair cognitive performance and can prolong the duration of rehabilitation. Therefore, it is important to weigh the overall benefit of these medications against their side effects. Research evidence supports the use of prophylactic antiseizure agents to prevent immediate and early seizures after head injury, but not for prevention of late seizures (Somjen, 2004).

The nurse must assess the patient carefully for the development of post-traumatic seizures. Risk factors that increase the likelihood of seizures are brain contusion with subdural hematoma, skull fracture, loss of consciousness or amnesia of 1 day or more, and age older than 65 years (Somjen, 2004). The nursing management of seizures is addressed in Chapter 61.

Other complications after traumatic head injury include systemic infections (pneumonia, urinary tract infection [UTI], septicemia), neurosurgical infections (wound infection, osteomyelitis, meningitis, ventriculitis, brain abscess), and heterotrophic ossification (painful bone overgrowth in weight-bearing joints).

Promoting Home and Community-Based Care

TEACHING PATIENTS SELF-CARE

Teaching early in the course of head injury often focuses on reinforcing information given to the family about the patient's condition and prognosis. As the patient's status and expected outcome change over time, family teaching may focus on interpretation and explanation of changes in the patient's physical and psychological responses.

If the patient's physical status allows discharge to home, the patient and family are instructed about limitations that can be expected and complications that may occur. The nurse explains to the patient and family, verbally and in writing, how to monitor for complications that merit contacting the neurosurgeon. Depending on the patient's prognosis and physical and cognitive status, the patient may be included in teaching about self-care management strategies.

If the patient is at risk for late posttraumatic seizures, antiseizure medications may be prescribed at discharge. The patient and family require instruction about the side effects of these medications and the importance of continuing to take them as prescribed.

CONTINUING CARE

Rehabilitation of the patient with a head injury begins at the time of injury and continues into the home and community. Depending on the degree of brain damage, the patient may be referred to a rehabilitation setting that specializes in cognitive restructuring after brain injury (Ashley, 2004). The patient is encouraged to continue the rehabilitation program after discharge, because improvement in status may continue 3 or more years after injury. Changes in the patient with a head injury and the effects of long-term rehabilitation on the family and their coping abilities need frequent assessment. Continued teaching and support of the patient and family are essential as their needs and the patient's status change. Teaching points to address with the family of the patient who is about to return home are described in Chart 63-6.

CHART 63-6

HOME CARE CHECKLIST • The Patient With a Traumatic Brain Injury

At the completion of the home care instruction, the patient or caregiver will be able to:	Patient	Caregiver
• Explain the need for monitoring for changes in neurologic status and for complications	✔	✔
• Identify changes in neurologic status and signs and symptoms of complications that should be reported to the neurosurgeon or nurse		✔
• Demonstrate safe techniques to assist patient with self-care, hygiene, and ambulation		✔
• Demonstrate safe technique for eating, feeding patient, or assisting patient with eating	✔	✔
• Explain rationale for taking medications as prescribed	✔	✔
• Identify need for close monitoring of behavior due to changes in cognitive functioning		✔
• Describe household modifications needed to ensure safe environment for the patient		✔
• Describe strategies for reinforcing positive behaviors		✔
• State importance of continuing follow-up by health care team	✔	✔

Depending on his or her status, the patient is encouraged to return to normal activities gradually. Referral to support groups and to the Brain Injury Association may be warranted.

During the acute and rehabilitation phases of care, the focus of teaching is on obvious needs, issues, and deficits. The nurse needs to remind the patient and family of the need for continuing health promotion and screening practices after these initial phases. Patients who have not been involved in these practices in the past are educated about their importance and are referred to appropriate health care providers.

Evaluation

Expected Patient Outcomes

Expected patient outcomes may include the following:

1. Attains or maintains effective airway clearance, ventilation, and brain oxygenation
   a. Achieves normal blood gas values and has normal breath sounds on auscultation
   b. Mobilizes and clears secretions
2. Achieves satisfactory fluid and electrolyte balance
   a. Demonstrates serum electrolytes within normal range
   b. Has no clinical signs of dehydration or overhydration
3. Attains adequate nutritional status
   a. Has less than 50 mL of aspirate in stomach before each tube feeding
   b. Is free of gastric distention and vomiting
   c. Shows minimal weight loss
4. Avoids injury
   a. Shows lessening agitation and restlessness
   b. Is oriented to time, place, and person
5. Maintains normal body temperature
   a. Absence of fever
   b. Absence of hypothermia
6. Demonstrates intact skin integrity
   a. Exhibits no redness or breaks in skin integrity
   b. Exhibits no pressure ulcers
7. Shows improvement in cognitive function and improved memory
8. Demonstrates normal sleep/wake cycle
9. Demonstrates absence of complications
   a. Exhibits normal vital signs and body temperature, and increasing orientation to time, place, and person
   b. Demonstrates normal or reduced ICP
10. Experiences no posttraumatic seizures
    a. Takes antiseizure medications as prescribed
    b. Identifies side effects/adverse effects of antiseizure medications
11. Family demonstrates adaptive family processes
    a. Joins support group
    b. Shares feelings with appropriate health care personnel
    c. Makes end-of-life decisions, if needed
12. Participates in rehabilitation process as indicated for patient and family members
    a. Takes active role in identifying rehabilitation goals and participating in recommended patient care activities
    b. Prepares for discharge

Spinal Cord Injury

Spinal cord injury (SCI) is a major health problem. Almost 200,000 people in the United States live each day with a disability from SCI, and an estimated 12,000 to 14,000 new injuries occur each year (Mendel, Hentschel & Guiot, 2005). SCI occurs more often in males (82%) than in females (18%) (Bader & Littlejohns, 2004; Scivoletto & Morganti, 2004). Young people between the ages of 16 and 30 years account for more than half of the new SCIs each year. African

Americans are at a higher risk than Caucasian Americans, with the incidence rising in recent years. The most common cause of SCI is motor vehicle crashes, which account for 35% of the injuries. Violence-related injuries account for almost as many SCIs (24%), with falls causing 22% and sports-related injuries causing 8% (Bader & Littlejohns, 2004). The frequency of associated injuries and medical complications is high.

The predominant risk factors for SCI include age, gender, and alcohol and drug use. The frequency with which these risk factors are associated with SCI serves to emphasize the importance of primary prevention. The same interventions suggested earlier in this chapter for head injury prevention serve to decrease the incidence of SCI as well (see Chart 63-1) (Liu, Ivers, Norton, et al., 2004).

The vertebrae most frequently involved in SCI are the 5th, 6th, and 7th cervical (neck) vertebrae (C5–C7), the 12th thoracic vertebra (T12), and the 1st lumbar vertebra (L1). These vertebrae are most susceptible because there is a greater range of mobility in the vertebral column in these areas (Porth, 2005).

Pathophysiology

Damage to the spinal cord ranges from transient concussion (from which the patient fully recovers) to contusion, laceration, and compression of the cord substance (either alone or in combination), to complete **transection** (severing) of the cord (which renders the patient paralyzed below the level of the injury).

SCIs can be separated into two categories: primary injuries and secondary injuries (Porth, 2005). Primary injuries are the result of the initial insult or trauma and are usually permanent. Secondary injuries are usually the result of a contusion or tear injury, in which the nerve fibers begin to swell and disintegrate. A secondary chain of events produces ischemia, hypoxia, edema, and hemorrhagic lesions, which in turn result in destruction of myelin and axons (Hickey, 2003). These secondary reactions, believed to be the principal causes of spinal cord degeneration at the level of injury, are now thought to be reversible during the first 4 to 6 hours after injury. Therefore, if the cord has not suffered irreparable damage, some method of early treatment is needed to prevent partial damage from developing into total and permanent damage (Bader & Littlejohns, 2004) (see later discussion).

Clinical Manifestations

Manifestations of SCI depend on the type and level of injury (Chart 63-7). The type of injury refers to the extent of injury to the spinal cord itself. **Incomplete spinal cord lesions** (the sensory or motor fibers, or both, are preserved below the lesion) are classified according to the area of spinal cord damage: central, lateral, anterior, or peripheral. The American Spinal Injury Association (ASIA) provides another standard classification of SCI according to the degree of sensory and motor function present after injury (Chart 63-8). "Neurologic level" refers to the lowest level at which sensory and motor functions are normal. Below the neurologic level, there is total sensory and motor paralysis, loss of bladder and bowel control (usually with urinary retention and bladder distention), loss of sweating and vasomotor tone, and marked reduction of blood pressure from loss of peripheral vascular resistance. A **complete spinal cord lesion** (total loss of sensation and voluntary muscle control below the lesion) can result in **paraplegia** (paralysis of the lower body) or tetraplegia (formerly **quadriplegia**—paralysis of all four extremities).

If conscious, the patient usually complains of acute pain in the back or neck, which may radiate along the involved nerve. However, absence of pain does not rule out spinal injury, and a careful assessment of the spine should be conducted if there has been a significant force and mechanism of injury (ie, concomitant head injury). Often the patient speaks of fear that the neck or back is broken.

Respiratory dysfunction is related to the level of injury. The muscles contributing to respiration are the abdominals and intercostals (T1 to T11) and the diaphragm (C4). In high cervical cord injury, acute respiratory failure is the leading cause of death. Functional abilities by level of injury are described in Table 63-3.

Assessment and Diagnostic Findings

A detailed neurologic examination is performed. Diagnostic x-rays (lateral cervical spine x-rays) and CT scanning are usually performed initially. An MRI scan may be ordered as a further work-up if a ligamentous injury is suspected, because significant spinal cord damage may exist even in the absence of bony injury. If an MRI scan is contraindicated, a myelogram may be used to visualize the spinal axis (Bader & Littlejohns, 2004). An assessment is made for other injuries, because spinal trauma often is accompanied by concomitant injuries, commonly to the head and chest. Continuous ECG monitoring may be indicated if a spinal cord injury is suspected, because bradycardia (slow heart rate) and asystole (cardiac standstill) are common in patients with acute spinal cord injuries.

Emergency Management

The immediate management at the scene of the injury is critical, because improper handling of the patient can cause further damage and loss of neurologic function. Any patient who is involved in a motor vehicle crash, a diving or contact sports injury, a fall, or any direct trauma to the head and neck must be considered to have SCI until such an injury is ruled out. Initial care must include a rapid assessment, immobilization, extrication, stabilization or control of life-threatening injuries, and transportation to the most appropriate medical facility (Baker & Saulino, 2002).

At the scene of the injury, the patient must be immobilized on a spinal (back) board, with head and neck in a neutral position, to prevent an incomplete injury from becoming complete. One member of the team must assume control of the patient's head to prevent flexion, rotation, or extension; this is done by placing the hands on both sides of the patient's head at about ear level to limit movement and maintain alignment while a spinal board or cervical immobilizing device is applied. If possible, at least four people should slide the patient carefully onto a board for transfer to the hospital.

CHART 63-7

Effects of Spinal Cord Injuries

CENTRAL CORD SYNDROME

- Characteristics: Motor deficits (in the upper extremities compared to the lower extremities; sensory loss varies but is more pronounced in the upper extremities); bowel/bladder dysfunction is variable, or function may be completely preserved.
- Cause: Injury or edema of the central cord, usually of the cervical area. May be caused by hyperextension injuries.

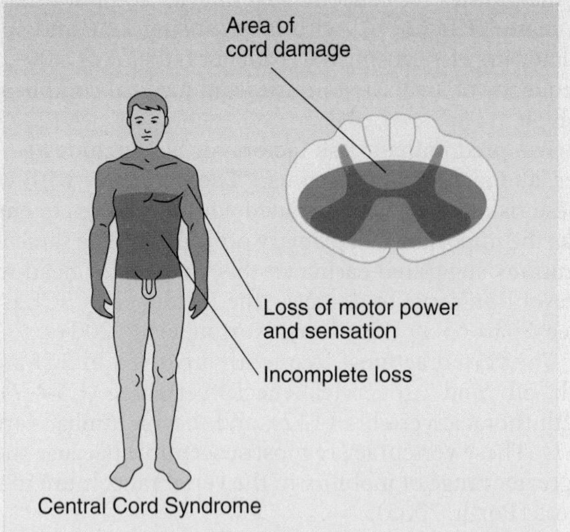

Central Cord Syndrome

ANTERIOR CORD SYNDROME

- Characteristics: Loss of pain, temperature, and motor function is noted below the level of the lesion; light touch, position, and vibration sensation remain intact.
- Cause: The syndrome may be caused by acute disk herniation or hyperflexion injuries associated with fracture-dislocation of vertebra. It also may occur as a result of injury to the anterior spinal artery, which supplies the anterior two thirds of the spinal cord.

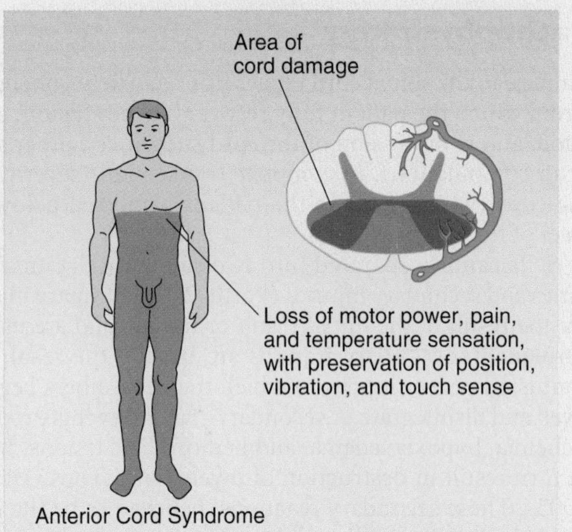

Anterior Cord Syndrome

BROWN-SÉQUARD SYNDROME (LATERAL CORD SYNDROME)

- Characteristics: Ipsilateral paralysis or paresis is noted, together with ipsilateral loss of touch, pressure, and vibration and contralateral loss of pain and temperature.
- Cause: The lesion is caused by a transverse hemisection of the cord (half of the cord is transected from north to south), usually as a result of a knife or missile injury, fracture-dislocation of a unilateral articular process, or possibly an acute ruptured disk.

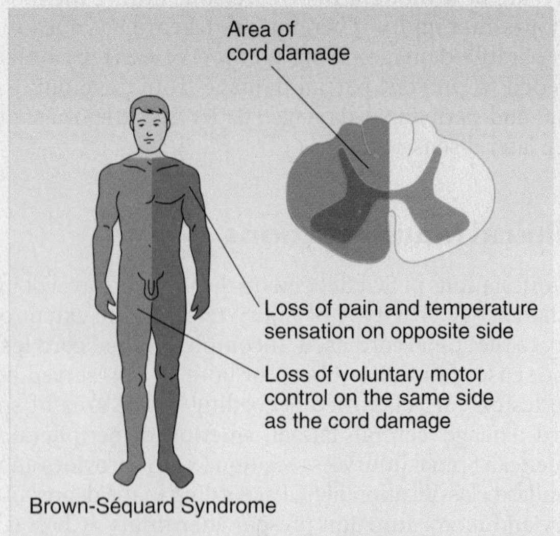

Brown-Séquard Syndrome

Adapted from Hickey, L. (2003). *The clinical practice of neurological and neurosurgical nursing* (5th ed., pp. 419–421). Philadelphia: Lippincott Williams & Wilkins.

CHART 63-8

ASIA Impairment Scale

A = Complete: No motor or sensory function is preserved in the sacral segments S4-S5.
B = Incomplete: Sensory but not motor function is preserved below the neurologic level, and includes the sacral segments S4–S5.
C = Incomplete: Motor function is preserved below the neurologic level, and more than half of key muscles below the neurologic level have a muscle grade less than 3.
D = Incomplete: Motor function is preserved below the neurologic level, and at least half of key muscles below the neurologic level have a muscle grade of 3 or greater.
E = Normal: Motor and sensory function are normal.

Used with permission of American Spinal Injury Association.

Any twisting movement may irreversibly damage the spinal cord by causing a bony fragment of the vertebra to cut into, crush, or sever the cord completely.

The standard of care is that the patient is referred to a regional spinal injury or trauma center because of the multidisciplinary personnel and support services required to counteract the destructive changes that occur in the first 24 hours after injury. However, no randomized controlled trials have been conducted to confirm that referral results in better outcomes for the patient with SCI (Jones & Bagnall, 2004). During treatment in the emergency and x-ray departments, the patient is kept on the transfer board. The patient must always be maintained in an extended position. No part of the body should be twisted or turned, nor should the patient be allowed to sit up. Once the extent of the injury has been determined, the patient may be placed on a rotating bed (Fig. 63-7) or in a cervical collar (Fig. 63-8). Later, if SCI and bone instability have been ruled out, the patient may be moved to a conventional bed or the collar may be removed without harm. If a rotating bed is needed but not available, the patient should be placed in a cervical collar and on a firm mattress.

TABLE 63-3 Functional Abilities by Level of Cord Injury

Injury Level	Segmental Sensorimotor Function	Dressing, Eating	Elimination	Mobility*
C1	Little or no sensation or control of head and neck; no diaphragm control; requires continuous ventilation	Dependent	Dependent	Limited. Voice or sip-n-puff controlled electric wheelchair
C2 to C3	Head and neck sensation; some neck control; independent of mechanical ventilation for short periods	Dependent	Dependent	Same as for C1
C4	Good head and neck sensation and motor control; some shoulder elevation; diaphragm movement	Dependent, may be able to eat with adaptive sling	Dependent	Limited to voice, mouth, head, chin, or shoulder-controlled electric wheelchair
C5	Full head and neck control; shoulder strength; elbow flexion	Independent with assistance	Maximal assistance	Electric or modified manual wheelchair, needs transfer assistance
C6	Fully innervated shoulder; wrist extension or dorsiflexion	Independent or with minimal assistance	Independent or with minimal assistance	Independent in transfers and wheelchair
C7 to C8	Full elbow extension; wrist plantar flexion; some finger control	Independent	Independent	Independent; manual wheelchair
T1 to T5	Full hand and finger control; use of intercostal and thoracic muscles	Independent	Independent	Independent; manual wheelchair
T6 to T10	Abdominal muscle control, partial to good balance with trunk muscles	Independent	Independent	Independent; manual wheelchair
T11 to L5	Hip flexors, hip abductors (L1–L3); knee extension (L2–4); knee flexion and ankle dorsiflexion (L4–5)	Independent	Independent	Short distance to full ambulation with assistance
S1 to S5	Full leg, foot, and ankle control; innervation of perineal muscles for bowel, bladder, and sexual function (S2–4)	Independent	Normal to impaired bowel and bladder function	Ambulate independently with or without assistance

* Assistance refers to adaptive equipment, setup, or physical assistance.
From Porth, C. M. (2005). *Pathophysiology: Concepts of altered health states* (7th ed.,Table 51-2). Philadelphia: Lippincott Williams & Wilkins.

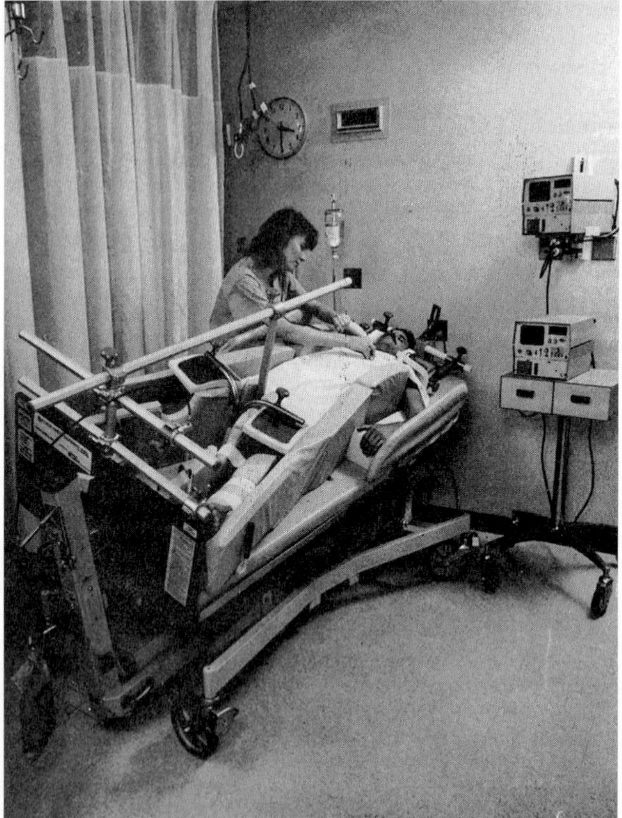

FIGURE 63-7. Roto Rest bed. Courtesy of Kinetic Concepts, San Antonio, TX.

Medical Management (Acute Phase)

The goals of management are to prevent further SCI and to observe for symptoms of progressive neurologic deficits. The patient is resuscitated as necessary, and oxygenation and cardiovascular stability are maintained. Many changes in the treatment of SCI have occurred during the past 20 years. Treatments such as hypothermia, corticosteroids, and naloxone were investigated and used during the 1980s; of these, high-dose corticosteroids have shown the most promise, but their use remains controversial (McCutcheon, Selassie, Gu, et al., 2004). Currently, new pharmacologic agents are being investigated for the acute and chronic phases of SCI (Grijaiva, Guizar-Sahagun, Castaneda-Hernandez, et al., 2003; McCutcheon et al., 2004). This injury continues to be a devastating event, and new treatment methods are continually being investigated.

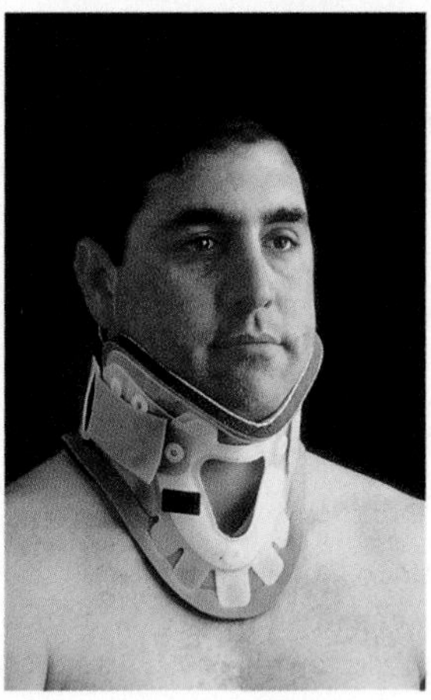

FIGURE 63-8. Cervical collar. Courtesy of Aspen Medical Products.

Pharmacologic Therapy

In some studies, the administration of high-dose corticosteroids, specifically methylprednisolone, has been found to improve motor and sensory outcomes at 6 weeks, 6 months, and 1 year if given within 8 hours after injury (Hickey, 2003). Another study of 1224 patients found that acute care hospital charges and length of stay were significantly higher for those receiving methylprednisolone compared to those who did not receive the medication (McCutcheon et al., 2004). Despite the ongoing discussion of the cost–benefit ratio of the practice, the use of high-dose methylprednisolone is accepted as standard therapy in many countries and remains an established clinical practice in most trauma centers in the United States (Hickey, 2003; McCutcheon et al., 2004).

Respiratory Therapy

Oxygen is administered to maintain a high partial pressure of oxygen (PaO_2), because hypoxemia can create or worsen a neurologic deficit of the spinal cord. If endotracheal intubation is necessary, extreme care is taken to avoid flexing or extending the patient's neck, which can result in extension of a cervical injury.

In high cervical spine injuries, spinal cord innervation to the phrenic nerve, which stimulates the diaphragm, is lost. Diaphragmatic pacing (electrical stimulation of the phrenic nerve) attempts to stimulate the diaphragm to help the patient breathe (Rice, Robichaux & Leonard, 2005). Intramuscular diaphragmatic pacing is currently in the clinical trial phase for the patient with a high cervical injury. This is implanted via laparoscopic surgery, usually after the acute phase (Bader & Littlejohns, 2004).

Skeletal Fracture Reduction and Traction

Management of SCI requires immobilization and reduction of dislocations (restoration of normal position) and stabilization of the vertebral column.

Cervical fractures are reduced, and the cervical spine is aligned with some form of skeletal traction, such as skeletal tongs or calipers, or with use of the halo device (Rice et al., 2005). A variety of skeletal tongs are available, all of which involve fixation in the skull in some manner. The Gardner-Wells tongs require no predrilled holes in the skull. Crutchfield and Vinke tongs are inserted through holes made in the skull with a special drill under local anesthesia.

Traction is applied to the skeletal traction device by weights, the amount depending on the size of the patient and the degree of fracture displacement. The traction force is exerted along the longitudinal axis of the vertebral bodies, with the patient's neck in a neutral position. The traction is then gradually increased by adding more weights. As the amount of traction is increased, the spaces between the intervertebral disks widen and the vertebrae are given a chance to slip back into position. Reduction usually takes place after correct alignment has been restored. Once reduction is achieved, as verified by cervical spine x-rays and neurologic examination, the weights are gradually removed until the amount of weight needed to maintain the alignment is identified. The weights should hang freely so as not to interfere with the traction. Traction is sometimes supplemented with manual manipulation of the neck by a surgeon to help achieve realignment of the vertebral bodies.

A halo device may be used initially with traction, or may be applied after removal of the tongs. It consists of a stainless-steel halo ring that is fixed to the skull by four pins. The ring is attached to a removable **halo vest**, a device that suspends the weight of the unit circumferentially around the chest. A metal frame connects the ring to the chest. Halo devices provide immobilization of the cervical spine while allowing early ambulation (Fig. 63-9).

Thoracic and lumbar injuries are usually treated with surgical intervention followed by immobilization with a fitted brace. Traction is not indicated either before or after surgery, due to the relative stability of the spine in these regions.

NURSING ALERT

The patient's vital organ functions and body defenses must be supported and maintained until spinal and neurogenic shock abates and the neurologic system has recovered from the traumatic insult; this can take up to 4 months (Hickey, 2003).

Surgical Management

Surgery is indicated in any of the following instances:

- Compression of the cord is evident.
- The injury results in a fragmented or unstable vertebral body.
- The injury involves a wound that penetrates the cord.
- Bony fragments are in the spinal canal.
- The patient's neurologic status is deteriorating.

Surgery is performed to reduce the spinal fracture or dislocation or to decompress the cord. A laminectomy (excision of the posterior arches and spinous processes of a vertebra) may be indicated in the presence of progressive neurologic deficit, suspected epidural hematoma, bony fragments, or penetrating injuries that require surgical débridement, or to permit direct visualization and exploration of the cord. Various techniques (ie, fusion or fixation) are used to create a stable spinal column (Bader & Littlejohns, 2004).

Management of Acute Complications of Spinal Cord Injury

Spinal and Neurogenic Shock

The spinal shock associated with SCI reflects a sudden depression of reflex activity in the spinal cord (areflexia) below the level of injury. The muscles innervated by the

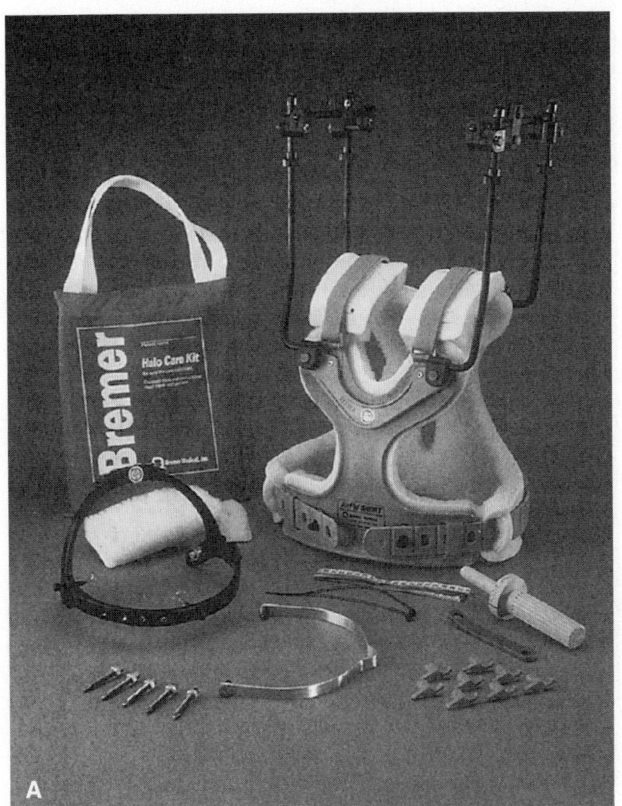

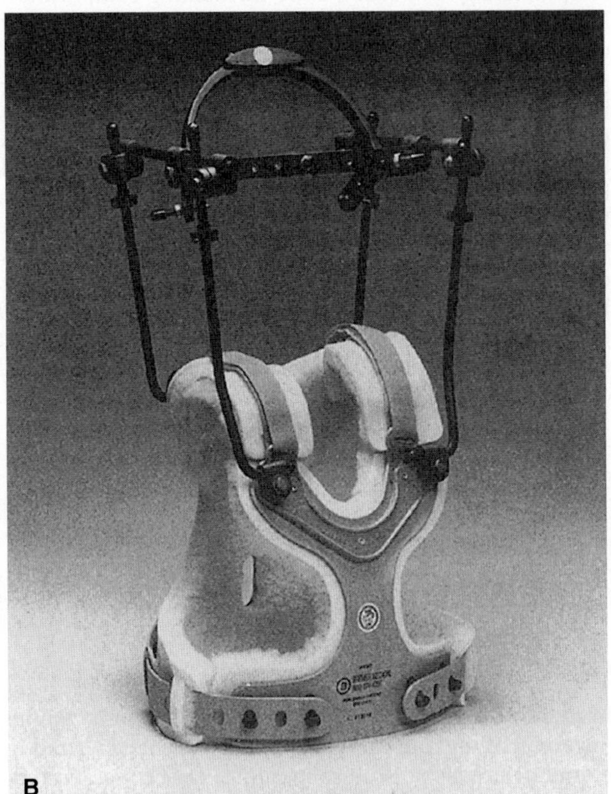

FIGURE 63-9. Halo systems for cervical and thoracic vertebral injuries. (**A**) Halo cervical skeletal traction and vest. Courtesy of Bremer Medical, Inc., Darwin Road, Jacksonville, FL. (**B**) Halo and vest. Courtesy of Acromed Corp., Cleveland, OH.

part of the spinal cord segment below the level of the lesion are without sensation, paralyzed, and flaccid, and the reflexes are absent. In particular, the reflexes that initiate bladder and bowel function are affected. Bowel distention and paralytic ileus can be caused by depression of the reflexes and are treated with intestinal decompression by insertion of a nasogastric tube (Hickey, 2003).

Neurogenic shock develops due to the loss of autonomic nervous system function below the level of the lesion (Hickey, 2003). The vital organs are affected, causing the blood pressure and heart rate to decrease. This loss of sympathetic innervation causes a variety of other clinical manifestations, including a decrease in cardiac output, venous pooling in the extremities, and peripheral vasodilation. In addition, the patient does not perspire on the paralyzed portions of the body, because sympathetic activity is blocked; therefore, close observation is required for early detection of an abrupt onset of fever. Further discussion of neurogenic shock can be found in Chapter 15.

With injuries to the cervical and upper thoracic spinal cord, innervation to the major accessory muscles of respiration is lost and respiratory problems develop. These include decreased vital capacity, retention of secretions, increased $PaCO_2$ levels and decreased oxygen levels, respiratory failure, and pulmonary edema.

Deep Vein Thrombosis

Deep vein thrombosis (DVT) is a potential complication of immobility and is common in patients with SCI (Bader & Littlejohns, 2004). Patients who develop DVT are at risk for pulmonary embolism, a life-threatening complication. Manifestations of pulmonary embolism include pleuritic chest pain, anxiety, shortness of breath, and abnormal blood gas values (increased $PaCO_2$ and decreased PaO_2). The patient should be assessed for a low-grade fever, which may be the first sign of a DVT, and thigh and calf measurements are made daily. The patient is evaluated for the presence of DVT if the circumference of one extremity increases significantly. Low-dose anticoagulation therapy usually is initiated to prevent DVT and PE, along with the use of thigh-high elastic compression stockings or pneumatic compression devices. In some cases, permanent indwelling filters (see Chapter 23) may be placed prophylactically in the vena cava to prevent emboli (dislodged clots) from migrating to the lungs and causing pulmonary emboli (Bader & Littlejohns, 2004).

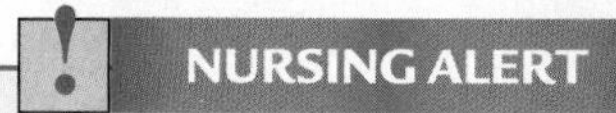

Never massage the calves or thighs, because of the danger of dislodging an undetected DVT.

Other Complications

In addition to respiratory complications (respiratory failure, pneumonia) and **autonomic dysreflexia** (characterized by pounding headache, profuse sweating, nasal congestion, piloerection ["goose bumps"], bradycardia, and hypertension), other complications that may occur include pressure ulcers and infection (urinary, respiratory, and local infection at the skeletal traction pin sites) (Rice et al., 2005).

Nursing Process

The Patient With Acute Spinal Cord Injury

Assessment

The breathing pattern is observed, the strength of the cough is assessed, and the lungs are auscultated, because paralysis of abdominal and respiratory muscles diminishes coughing and makes clearing of bronchial and pharyngeal secretions difficult. Reduced excursion of the chest also results.

The patient is monitored closely for any changes in motor or sensory function and for symptoms of progressive neurologic damage. In the early stages of SCI, determining whether the cord has been severed may be impossible, because signs and symptoms of cord edema are indistinguishable from those of cord transection. Edema of the spinal cord may occur with any severe cord injury and may further compromise spinal cord function.

Motor and sensory functions are assessed through careful neurologic examination. These findings usually are recorded on a flow sheet so that changes in the baseline neurologic status can be monitored closely and accurately. The ASIA classification is commonly used to describe level of function for SCI patients. Chart 63-7 gives examples of the effects of altered spinal cord function. At the minimum:

- Motor ability is tested by asking the patient to spread the fingers, squeeze the examiner's hand, and move the toes or turn the feet.
- Sensation is evaluated by gently pinching the skin or touching it lightly with an object such as a tongue blade, starting at shoulder level and working down both sides of the extremities. The patient should have both eyes closed so that the examination reveals true findings, not what the patient hopes to feel. The patient is asked where the sensation is felt.
- Any decrease in neurologic function is reported immediately.

The patient is also assessed for spinal shock, a complete loss of all reflex, motor, sensory, and autonomic activity below the level of the lesion that causes bladder paralysis and distention. The lower abdomen is palpated for signs of urinary retention and overdistention of the bladder. Further assessment is made for gastric dilation and ileus caused by an atonic bowel, a result of autonomic disruption.

Temperature is monitored, because the patient may have periods of hyperthermia as a result of alteration in temperature control due to autonomic disruption.

Diagnosis

Nursing Diagnoses

Based on the assessment data, the patient's major nursing diagnoses may include the following:

- Ineffective breathing patterns related to weakness or paralysis of abdominal and intercostal muscles and inability to clear secretions
- Ineffective airway clearance related to weakness of intercostal muscles
- Impaired bed and physical mobility related to motor and sensory impairments
- Disturbed sensory perception related to motor and sensory impairment
- Risk for impaired skin integrity related to immobility and sensory loss
- Impaired urinary elimination related to inability to void spontaneously
- Constipation related to presence of atonic bowel as a result of autonomic disruption
- Acute pain and discomfort related to treatment and prolonged immobility

Collaborative Problems/ Potential Complications

Based on the assessment data, potential complications that may develop include:

- DVT
- Orthostatic hypotension
- Autonomic dysreflexia

Planning and Goals

The goals for the patient may include improved breathing pattern and airway clearance, improved mobility, improved sensory and perceptual awareness, maintenance of skin integrity, relief of urinary retention, improved bowel function, promotion of comfort, and absence of complications.

Nursing Interventions

Promoting Adequate Breathing and Airway Clearance

Possible impending respiratory failure is detected by observing the patient, measuring vital capacity, monitoring oxygen saturation through pulse oximetry, and monitoring arterial blood gas values. Early and vigorous attention to clearing bronchial and pharyngeal secretions can prevent retention of secretions and atelectasis. Suctioning may be indicated, but caution must be used, because this procedure can stimulate the vagus nerve, producing bradycardia, which can result in cardiac arrest.

If the patient cannot cough effectively because of decreased inspiratory volume and inability to generate sufficient expiratory pressure, chest physical therapy and assisted coughing may be indicated. Specific breathing exercises are supervised by the nurse to increase the strength and endurance of the inspiratory muscles, particularly the diaphragm. Assisted coughing promotes clearing of secretions from the upper respiratory tract and is similar to the use of abdominal thrusts to clear an airway (see Chapter 25). Ensuring proper humidification and hydration is important to prevent secretions from becoming thick and difficult to remove even with coughing. The patient is assessed for signs of respiratory infection (cough, fever, dyspnea). Smoking is discouraged, because it increases bronchial and pulmonary secretions and impairs ciliary action.

Ascending edema of the spinal cord in the acute phase may cause respiratory difficulty that requires immediate intervention. Therefore, the patient's respiratory status must be monitored frequently.

Improving Mobility

Proper body alignment is maintained at all times. The patient is repositioned frequently and is assisted out of bed as soon as the spinal column is stabilized. The feet are prone to footdrop; therefore, various types of splints are used to prevent footdrop. When used, the splints are removed and reapplied every 2 hours. Trochanter rolls, applied from the crest of the ilium to the midthigh of both legs, help prevent external rotation of the hip joints.

Patients with lesions above the midthoracic level have loss of sympathetic control of peripheral vasoconstrictor activity, leading to hypotension. These patients may tolerate changes in position poorly and require monitoring of blood pressure when positions are changed. Usually, the patient is turned every 2 hours. If not on a rotating bed, the patient should not be turned unless the spine is stable and the physician has indicated that it is safe to do so.

Contractures develop rapidly with immobility and muscle paralysis. A joint that is immobilized too long becomes fixed as a result of contractures of the tendon and joint capsule. Atrophy of the extremities results from disuse. Contractures and other complications may be prevented by range-of-motion exercises that help preserve joint motion and stimulate circulation. Passive range-of-motion exercises should be implemented as soon as possible after injury. Toes, metatarsals, ankles, knees, and hips should be put through a full range of motion at least four, and ideally five, times daily.

For most patients who have a cervical fracture without neurologic deficit, reduction in traction followed by rigid immobilization for 6 to 8 weeks restores skeletal integrity. These patients are allowed to move gradually to an erect position. A four-poster neck brace or molded collar is applied when the patient is mobilized after traction is removed (see Fig. 63-8).

Promoting Adaptation to Sensory and Perceptual Alterations

The nurse assists the patient to compensate for sensory and perceptual alterations that occur with SCI. The intact senses above the level of the injury are stimulated through touch, aromas, flavorful food and beverages, conversation, and music. Additional strategies include the following:

- Providing prism glasses to enable the patient to see from the supine position

- Encouraging use of hearing aids, if indicated, to enable the patient to hear conversations and environmental sounds
- Providing emotional support to the patient
- Teaching the patient strategies to compensate for or cope with these deficits

Maintaining Skin Integrity

Because patients with SCI are immobilized and have loss of sensation below the level of the lesion, they have the highest prevalence of pressure ulcers in the United States (Phillips, 2003). Pressure ulcers have developed within 6 hours in areas of local tissue ischemia, where there is continuous pressure and where the peripheral circulation is inadequate as a result of spinal shock and a recumbent position. Prolonged immobilization of the patient on a transfer board also increases the risk for pressure ulcers. The most common sites are over the ischial tuberosity, the greater trochanter, the sacrum, and the occiput (back of head). Patients who wear cervical collars for prolonged periods may develop breakdown from the pressure of the collar under the chin, on the shoulders, and at the occiput.

The patient's position is changed at least every 2 hours. Turning not only assists in the prevention of pressure ulcers but also prevents pooling of blood and edema in the dependent areas.

Careful inspection of the skin is made each time the patient is turned. The skin over the pressure points is assessed for redness or breaks; the perineum is checked for soilage, and the catheter is observed for adequate drainage. The patient's general body alignment and comfort are assessed. Special attention should be given to pressure areas in contact with the transfer board.

The patient's skin should be kept clean by washing with a mild soap, rinsing well, and blotting dry. Pressure-sensitive areas should be kept well lubricated and soft with hand cream or lotion. To increase understanding of the reasons for preventive measures, the patient is educated about the danger of pressure ulcers and is encouraged to take control and make decisions about appropriate skin care (Kinder, 2005). See Chapter 11 for other aspects of the prevention of pressure ulcers.

Maintaining Urinary Elimination

Immediately after SCI, the urinary bladder becomes atonic and cannot contract by reflex activity. Urinary retention is the immediate result. Because the patient has no sensation of bladder distention, overstretching of the bladder and detrusor muscle may occur, delaying the return of bladder function.

Intermittent catheterization is carried out to avoid overdistention of the bladder and UTI. If this is not feasible, an indwelling catheter is inserted temporarily. At an early stage, family members are shown how to carry out intermittent catheterization and are encouraged to participate in this facet of care, because they will be involved in long-term follow-up and must be able to recognize complications so that treatment can be instituted.

The patient is taught to record fluid intake, voiding pattern, amounts of residual urine after catheterization, characteristics of urine, and any unusual sensations that may occur. The management of a **neurogenic bladder** (bladder dysfunction that results from a disorder or dysfunction of the nervous system) is discussed in detail in Chapter 11.

Improving Bowel Function

Immediately after SCI, a paralytic ileus usually develops due to neurogenic paralysis of the bowel; therefore, a nasogastric tube is often required to relieve distention and to prevent vomiting and aspiration.

Bowel activity usually returns within the first week. As soon as bowel sounds are heard on auscultation, the patient is given a high-calorie, high-protein, high-fiber diet, with the amount of food gradually increased. The nurse administers prescribed stool softeners to counteract the effects of immobility and analgesic agents. A bowel program is instituted as early as possible.

Providing Comfort Measures

A patient who has had pins, tongs, or calipers placed for cervical stabilization may have a slight headache or discomfort for several days after the pins are inserted. Patients initially may be bothered by the rather startling appearance of these devices, but usually they readily adapt to it because the device provides comfort for the unstable neck. The patient may complain of being caged in and of noise created by any object coming in contact with the steel frame of a halo device, but he or she can be reassured that adaptation to such annoyances will occur.

THE PATIENT IN HALO TRACTION

The areas around the four pin sites of a halo device are cleaned daily and observed for redness, drainage, and pain. The pins are observed for loosening, which may contribute to infection. If one of the pins becomes detached, the head is stabilized in a neutral position by one person while another notifies the neurosurgeon. A torque screwdriver should be readily available in case the screws on the frame need tightening.

The skin under the halo vest is inspected for excessive perspiration, redness, and skin blistering, especially on the bony prominences. The vest is opened at the sides to allow the torso to be washed. The liner of the vest should not become wet, because dampness causes skin excoriation. Powder is not used inside the vest, because it may contribute to the development of pressure ulcers. The liner should be changed periodically to promote hygiene and good skin care. If the patient is to be discharged with the vest, detailed instructions must be given to the family, with time allowed for them to return demonstrate the necessary skills of halo vest care (Chart 63-9).

CHART 63-9

HOME CARE CHECKLIST • The Patient With a Halo Vest

At the completion of the home care instruction, the patient or caregiver will be able to:	Patient	Caregiver
• Describe the rationale for use of the halo vest	✔	✔
• Demonstrate assessment of frame, traction, tongs, and pins		✔
• Describe emergency measures if respiratory or other complications develop while patient is in halo vest or if frame becomes dislodged		✔
• Demonstrate pin care using correct technique		✔
• Identify signs and symptoms of infection	✔	✔
• Assess the skin for reddened or irritated areas and breakdown		✔
• Demonstrate care of skin		✔
• Explain the reasons for and the method for changing the vest liner	✔	✔
• Demonstrate safe techniques to assist patient with self-care, hygiene, and ambulation		✔
• Identify signs and symptoms of complications (DVT, respiratory impairment, urinary tract infection)		✔

Monitoring and Managing Potential Complications

THROMBOPHLEBITIS

Thrombophlebitis is a relatively common complication in patients after SCI. DVT occurs in a high percentage of SCI patients, placing them at risk for PE. The patient must be assessed for symptoms of thrombophlebitis and PE: chest pain, shortness of breath, and changes in arterial blood gas values must be reported promptly to the physician. The circumferences of the thighs and calves are measured and recorded daily; further diagnostic studies are performed if a significant increase is noted. Patients remain at high risk for thrombophlebitis for several months after the initial injury. Patients with paraplegia or tetraplegia are at increased risk for the rest of their lives. Immobilization and the associated venous stasis, as well as varying degrees of autonomic disruption, contribute to the high risk and susceptibility for DVT (Farray, Carman & Fernandez, 2004).

Anticoagulation is initiated once head injury and other systemic injuries have been ruled out. Low-dose fractionated or unfractionated heparin may be followed by long-term oral anticoagulation (ie, warfarin) or subcutaneous fractionated heparin injections. Additional measures such as range-of-motion exercises, thigh-high elastic compression stockings, and adequate hydration are important preventive measures. Pneumatic compression devices may also be used to reduce venous pooling and promote venous return. It is also important to avoid external pressure on the lower extremities that may result from flexion of the knees while the patient is in bed.

ORTHOSTATIC HYPOTENSION

For the first 2 weeks after SCI, the blood pressure tends to be unstable and quite low. It gradually returns to preinjury levels, but periodic episodes of severe orthostatic hypotension frequently interfere with efforts to mobilize the patient. Interruption in the reflex arcs that normally produce vasoconstriction in the upright position, coupled with vasodilation and pooling in abdominal and lower extremity vessels, can result in blood pressure readings of 40 mm Hg systolic and 0 mm Hg diastolic. Orthostatic hypotension is a particularly common problem for patients with lesions above T7. In some patients with tetraplegia, even slight elevations of the head can result in dramatic changes in blood pressure.

A number of techniques can be used to reduce the frequency of hypotensive episodes. Close monitoring of vital signs before and during position changes is essential. Vasopressor medication can be used to treat the profound vasodilation. Thigh-high elastic compression stockings should be applied to improve venous return from the lower extremities. Abdominal binders may also be used to encourage venous return and provide diaphragmatic support when the patient is upright. Activity should be planned in advance, and adequate time should be allowed for a slow progression of position changes from recumbent to sitting and upright. Tilt tables frequently are helpful in assisting patients to make this transition.

AUTONOMIC DYSREFLEXIA

Autonomic dysreflexia (autonomic hyperreflexia) is an acute emergency that occurs as a result of exaggerated autonomic responses to stimuli that are harmless in normal people. It occurs only after spinal shock has resolved. This syndrome is characterized by a severe, pounding headache with paroxysmal hypertension, profuse diaphoresis (most often of the forehead), nausea, nasal congestion, and bradycardia. It occurs among patients with cord lesions above T6 (the sympathetic visceral outflow level) after spinal shock has subsided. The sudden increase in blood pressure may cause a rupture of one or more cerebral blood vessels or lead to increased ICP. A number of stimuli may trigger this reflex: distended bladder (the most common cause); distention or contraction of the visceral organs, especially the bowel (from constipation, impaction); or stimulation of the skin (tactile, pain, thermal stimuli, pressure ulcer). Because this is an emergency situation, the objectives are to remove the triggering stimulus and to avoid the possibly serious complications.

The following measures are carried out:

- The patient is placed immediately in a sitting position to lower blood pressure.
- Rapid assessment is performed to identify and alleviate the cause.
- The bladder is emptied immediately via a urinary catheter. If an indwelling catheter is not patent, it is irrigated or replaced with another catheter.
- The rectum is examined for a fecal mass. If one is present, a topical anesthetic is inserted 10 to 15 minutes before the mass is removed, because visceral distention or contraction can cause autonomic dysreflexia.
- The skin is examined for any areas of pressure, irritation, or broken skin.
- Any other stimulus that could be the triggering event, such as an object next to the skin or a draft of cold air, must be removed.
- If these measures do not relieve the hypertension and excruciating headache, a ganglionic blocking agent (hydralazine hydrochloride [Apresoline]) is prescribed and administered slowly by the IV route.
- The medical record or chart is labeled with a clearly visible note about the risk for autonomic dysreflexia.
- The patient is instructed about prevention and management measures.
- Any patient with a lesion above the T6 segment is informed that such an episode is possible and may occur even many years after the initial injury.

Promoting Home and Community-Based Care

TEACHING PATIENTS SELF-CARE

In most cases, patients with SCI (ie, patients with tetraplegia or paraplegia) need long-term rehabilitation. The process begins during hospitalization, as acute symptoms begin to subside or come under better control and the overall deficits and long-term effects of the injury become clear. The goals begin to shift from merely surviving the injury to learning strategies necessary to cope with the alterations that the injury imposes on activities of daily living (ADLs). The emphasis shifts from ensuring that the patient is stable and free of complications to specific assessment and planning designed to meet the patient's rehabilitation needs. Patient teaching may initially focus on the injury and its effects on mobility, dressing, and bowel, bladder, and sexual function. As the patient and family acknowledge the consequences of the injury and the resulting disability, the focus of teaching broadens to address issues necessary for carrying out the tasks of daily living and taking charge of their lives (Kinder, 2005). Teaching begins in the acute phase and continues throughout rehabilitation and throughout the patient's life as changes occur, the patient ages, and problems arise (Capoor & Stein, 2005).

Caring for the patient with SCI at home may at first seem a daunting task to the family. They will require dedicated nursing support to gradually assume full care of the patient.

Although maintaining function and preventing complications will remain important, goals regarding self-care and preparation for discharge will assist in a smooth transition to rehabilitation and eventually to the community.

CONTINUING CARE

The ultimate goal of the rehabilitation process is independence. The nurse becomes a support to both the patient and the family, assisting them to assume responsibility for increasing aspects of patient care and management. Care for the patient with SCI involves members of all the health care disciplines, which may include nursing, medicine, rehabilitation, respiratory therapy, physical and occupational therapy, case management, and social services. The nurse often serves as coordinator of the management team and as a liaison with rehabilitation centers and home care agencies. The patient and family often require assistance in dealing with the psychological impact of the injury and its consequences; referral to a psychiatric clinical nurse specialist or other mental health care professional often is helpful.

The nurse should reassure female patients with SCI that pregnancy is not contraindicated, but that pregnant women with acute or chronic SCI pose unique management challenges (Jackson, Lindsey, Klebine, et al., 2004). The normal physiologic changes of pregnancy may predispose women with SCI to many potentially life-threatening complications, including autonomic dysreflexia, pyelonephritis, respiratory insufficiency, thrombophlebitis, PE, and unattended delivery. Preconception assessment and counseling are strongly recommended to ensure that the woman is in optimal health and to increase the likelihood of an uneventful pregnancy and healthy outcomes.

As more patients survive acute SCI, they face the changes associated with aging with a disability. Therefore, teaching in the home and community focuses on health promotion and addresses the need to minimize risk factors (eg, smoking, alcohol and drug abuse, obesity) (Mastrogiovanni, Phillips & Fine, 2003). Home care nurses and others who have contact with patients with SCI are in a position to teach patients about healthy lifestyles, remind them of the need for health screenings, and make referrals as appropriate. Assisting patients to identify accessible health care providers, clinical facilities, and imaging centers may increase the likelihood that they will participate in health screening.

Evaluation

Expected Patient Outcomes

Expected patient outcomes may include the following:

1. Demonstrates improvement in gas exchange and clearance of secretions, as evidenced by normal breath sounds on auscultation
   a. Breathes easily without shortness of breath
   b. Performs hourly deep-breathing exercises, coughs effectively, and clears pulmonary secretions
   c. Is free of respiratory infection (ie, has normal temperature, respiratory rate, and pulse, normal breath sounds, absence of purulent sputum)
2. Moves within limits of the dysfunction and demonstrates completion of exercises within functional limitations
3. Demonstrates adaptation to sensory and perceptual alterations
   a. Uses assistive devices (eg, prism glasses, hearing aids, computers) as indicated
   b. Describes sensory and perceptual alterations as a consequence of injury
4. Demonstrates optimal skin integrity
   a. Exhibits normal skin turgor; skin is free of reddened areas or breaks
   b. Participates in skin care and monitoring procedures within functional limitations
5. Regains urinary bladder function
   a. Exhibits no signs of UTI (ie, has normal temperature; voids clear, dilute urine)
   b. Has adequate fluid intake
   c. Participates in bladder training program within functional limitations
6. Regains bowel function
   a. Reports regular pattern of bowel movement
   b. Consumes adequate dietary fiber and oral fluids
   c. Participates in bowel training program within functional limitations
7. Reports absence of pain and discomfort
8. Is free of complications
   a. Demonstrates no signs of thrombophlebitis or DVT
   b. Exhibits no manifestations of pulmonary embolism (eg, no chest pain or shortness of breath; arterial blood gas values are normal)
   c. Maintains blood pressure within normal limits
   d. Reports no lightheadedness with position changes
   e. Exhibits no manifestations of autonomic dysreflexia (ie, absence of headache, diaphoresis, nasal congestion, bradycardia, or diaphoresis)

Medical Management of Long-Term Complications of Spinal Cord Injury

Tetraplegia refers to the loss of movement and sensation in all four extremities and the trunk, associated with injury to the cervical spinal cord (Bader & Littlejohns, 2004). Paraplegia refers to loss of motion and sensation in the lower extremities and all or part of the trunk as a result of damage to the thoracic or lumbar spinal cord or to the sacral root. Both conditions most frequently follow trauma such as falls, injuries, and gunshot wounds, but they may also be the result of spinal cord lesions (intervertebral disk, tumor, vascular lesions), multiple sclerosis, infections and abscesses of the spinal cord, and congenital disorders such as spina bifida.

The patient faces a lifetime of disability, requiring ongoing follow-up and care and the expertise of a number of health professionals, including physicians (specifically a physiatrist), rehabilitation nurses, occupational therapists, physical therapists, psychologists, social workers, rehabilitation engineers, and vocational counselors at different times as the need arises.

As the years go by, these patients also have the same medical problems as others in the aging population. In addition, they face the threat of complications associated with their disability (Charlifue, Lammertse & Adkins, 2004). Usually, the patient is encouraged to attend a spinal clinic when complications and other issues arise. Lifetime care includes assessment of the urinary tract at prescribed intervals, because there is the likelihood of continuing alteration in detrusor and sphincter function, and the patient is prone to UTI.

Long-term problems and complications of SCI include premature aging, disuse syndrome, autonomic dysreflexia (discussed earlier), bladder and kidney infections, spasticity, and depression (Capoor & Stein, 2005). Pressure ulcers with potential complications of sepsis, osteomyelitis, and fistulas occur in about 10% of patients. Spasticity may be particularly disabling. Heterotopic ossification (overgrowth of bone) in the hips, knees, shoulders, and elbows occurs in many patients after SCI. Both of these complications are painful and can produce a loss of range of motion (Bader & Littlejohns, 2004). Management includes observing for and addressing any alteration in physiologic status and psychological outlook, as well as the prevention and treatment of long-term complications. The nursing role involves emphasizing the need for vigilance in self-assessment and care.

Nursing Process

The Patient With Tetraplegia or Paraplegia

Assessment

Assessment focuses on the patient's general condition, complications, and how the patient is managing at that particular point in time. A head-to-toe assessment and review of systems should be part of the database, with emphasis on the areas that are prone to problems in this population. A thorough inspection of all areas of the skin for redness or breakdown is critical. The nurse reviews the established bowel and bladder program with the patient, because the program must continue uninterrupted. Patients with tetraplegia or paraplegia have varying degrees of loss of motor power, deep and superficial sensation, vasomotor control, bladder and bowel control, and sexual function. They are faced with potential complications related to immobility, skin breakdown and pressure ulcers, recurring UTIs, contractures, and disruptions. Knowledge about these particular issues can further guide the assessment in any setting. Nurses in all settings, including home care, must be aware of these potential complications in the lifetime management of these patients.

An understanding of the emotional and psychological responses to tetraplegia or paraplegia is achieved by observing the responses and behaviors of the patient and family and by listening to their concerns. Documenting these assessments and reviewing the plan with the entire team on a regular basis provide insight into how both the patient and the family are coping with the changes in lifestyle and body functioning. Additional information frequently can be gathered from the social worker or psychiatric/mental health worker.

It takes time for the patient and family to comprehend the magnitude of the disability. They may go through stages of grief, including shock, disbelief, denial, anger, depression, and acceptance. During the acute phase of the injury, denial can be a protective mechanism to shield the patient from the overwhelming reality of what has happened. As the patient realizes the permanent nature of paraplegia or tetraplegia, the grieving process may be prolonged and all-encompassing because of the recognition that long-held plans and expectations are interrupted or permanently altered. A period of depression often follows as the patient experiences a loss of self-esteem in areas of self-identity, sexual functioning, and social and emotional roles. Exploration and assessment of these issues can assist in developing a meaningful plan of care.

Diagnosis

Nursing Diagnoses

Based on the assessment data, the major nursing diagnoses of the patient with tetraplegia or paraplegia may include the following:

- Impaired bed and physical mobility related to loss of motor function
- Risk for disuse syndrome
- Risk for impaired skin integrity related to permanent sensory loss and immobility
- Impaired urinary elimination related to level of injury
- Constipation related to effects of spinal cord disruption
- Sexual dysfunction related to neurologic dysfunction
- Ineffective coping related to impact of disability on daily living
- Deficient knowledge about requirements for long-term management

Collaborative Problems/ Potential Complications

Based on all the assessment data, potential complications of tetraplegia or paraplegia that may develop include:

- Spasticity
- Infection and sepsis

Planning and Goals

The goals for the patient may include attainment of some form of mobility; maintenance of healthy, intact skin; achievement of bladder management without infection; achievement of bowel control; achievement of sexual expression; strengthening of coping mechanisms; and absence of complications.

Nursing Interventions

The patient requires extensive rehabilitation, which is less difficult if appropriate nursing management has been carried out during the acute phase of the injury or illness. Nursing care is one of the key factors determining the success of the rehabilitation program. The main objective is for the patient to live as independently as possible in the home and community.

Increasing Mobility

EXERCISE PROGRAMS

The unaffected parts of the body are built up to optimal strength to promote maximal self-care. The muscles of the hands, arms, shoulders, chest, spine, abdomen, and neck must be strengthened in the patient with paraplegia, because he or she must bear full weight on these muscles to ambulate. The triceps and the latissimus dorsi are important muscles used in crutch walking. The muscles of the abdomen and the back also are necessary for balance and for maintaining the upright position.

To strengthen these muscles, the patient can do push-ups when in a prone position and sit-ups when in a sitting position. Extending the arms while holding weights (traction weights can be used) also develops muscle strength. Squeezing rubber balls or crumbling newspaper promotes hand strength.

With encouragement from all members of the rehabilitation team, the patient with paraplegia can develop the increased exercise tolerance needed for gait training and ambulation activities. The importance of maintaining cardiovascular fitness is stressed to the patient. Alternative exercises to increase the heart rate to target levels must be designed within the patient's abilities.

MOBILIZATION

After the spine is stable enough to allow the patient to assume an upright posture, mobilization activities are initiated. A brace or vest may be used, depending on the level of the lesion. A patient whose paralysis is a result of complete transection of the cord can begin weight-bearing early, because no further damage can be incurred. The sooner muscles are used, the less chance there is of disuse atrophy. The earlier the patient is brought to a standing position, the less opportunity for osteoporotic changes to take place in the long bones. Weight-bearing also reduces the possibility of renal calculi and enhances many other metabolic processes.

Braces and crutches enable some patients with paraplegia to ambulate for short distances. Ambulation using crutches requires a high expenditure of energy. Motorized wheelchairs and specially equipped vans can provide greater independence and mobility for patients with high-level SCI or other lesions. Every effort should be made to encourage the patient to be as mobile and active as possible.

Preventing Disuse Syndrome

Patients are at high risk for development of contractures as a result of disuse syndrome due to the musculoskeletal system changes (atrophy) brought about by the loss of motor and sensory functions below the level of injury. Range-of-motion exercises must be provided at least four times a day, and care is taken to stretch the Achilles tendon with exercises (Hickey, 2003). The patient is repositioned frequently and is maintained in proper body alignment whether in bed or in a wheelchair (Hickey, 2003).

Contractures can complicate day-to-day care, increasing the difficulty of positioning and decreasing mobility. A number of surgical procedures have been tried with varying degrees of success. These techniques are used if more conservative approaches fail, but the best treatment is prevention.

Promoting Skin Integrity

Because these patients spend a great portion of their lives in wheelchairs, pressure ulcers are an ever-present threat. Contributing factors are permanent sensory loss over pressure areas; immobility, which makes relief of pressure difficult; trauma from bumps (against the wheelchair, toilet, furniture, and so forth) that cause unnoticed abrasions and wounds; loss of protective function of the skin from excoriation and maceration due to excessive perspiration and possible incontinence; and poor general health (anemia, edema, malnutrition), leading to poor tissue perfusion. The prevention and management of pressure ulcers are discussed in detail in Chapter 11.

The person with tetraplegia or paraplegia must take responsibility for monitoring (or directing monitoring) of his or her skin status. This involves relieving pressure and not remaining in any position for longer than 2 hours, in addition to ensuring that the skin receives meticulous attention and cleansing. The patient is taught that ulcers develop over bony prominences that are exposed to unrelieved pressure in the lying and sitting positions. The most vulnerable areas are identified. The patient with paraplegia is instructed to use mirrors, if possible, to inspect these areas morning and night, observing for redness, slight edema, or any abrasions. While in bed, the patient should turn at 2-hour intervals and then inspect the skin again for redness that does not fade on pressure. The bottom sheet should be checked for wetness and for creases. The patient with tetraplegia or paraplegia who cannot perform these activities is encouraged to direct others to check these areas and prevent ulcers from developing.

The patient is taught to relieve pressure while in the wheelchair by doing push-ups, leaning from side to side to relieve ischial pressure, and tilting forward while leaning on a table. The caregiver for the patient with tetraplegia will need to perform these activities if the patient cannot do so independently. A wheelchair cushion is prescribed to meet individual needs, which may change in time with changes in posture, weight, and skin tolerance. A referral can be made to a rehabilitation engineer, who can measure pressure levels while the patient is sitting and then tailor the cushion and other necessary aids and assistive devices to the patient's needs.

The diet for the patient with tetraplegia or paraplegia should be high in protein, vitamins, and calories to ensure minimal wasting of muscle and the maintenance of healthy skin, and high in fluids to maintain well-functioning kidneys. Excessive weight gain and obesity should be avoided, because they limit mobility (Mastrogiovanni et al., 2003).

Improving Bladder Management

The effect of the spinal cord lesion on the bladder depends on the level of injury, the degree of cord damage, and the length of time after injury. A patient with tetraplegia or paraplegia usually has either a reflex or a nonreflex bladder (see Chapters 11 and 44). Both bladder types increase the risk of UTI.

The nurse emphasizes the importance of maintaining an adequate flow of urine by encouraging a fluid intake of about 2.5 L daily. The patient should empty the bladder frequently so that there is minimal residual urine and should pay attention to personal hygiene, because infection of the bladder and kidneys almost always occurs by the ascending route. The perineum must be kept clean and dry, and attention must be given to the perianal skin after defecation. Underwear should be cotton (which is more absorbent) and should be changed at least once a day.

If an external catheter (condom catheter) is used, the sheath is removed nightly; the penis is cleansed to remove urine and is dried carefully, because warm urine on the periurethral skin promotes the growth of bacteria. Attention also is given to the collection bag. The nurse emphasizes the importance of monitoring for signs of UTI: cloudy, foul-smelling urine or hematuria (blood in the urine), fever, or chills.

The female patient who cannot achieve reflex bladder control or self-catheterization may need to wear pads or waterproof undergarments. Surgical intervention may be indicated in some patients to create a urinary diversion.

Establishing Bowel Control

The objective of a bowel training program is to establish bowel evacuation through reflex conditioning, a technique described in Chapter 38. If a cord injury occurs above the sacral segments or nerve roots and there is reflex activity, the anal sphincter may be massaged (digital stimulation) to stimulate defecation. If the cord lesion involves the sacral segment or nerve roots, anal massage is not performed, because the anus may be relaxed and lack tone. Massage is also contraindicated if there is spasticity of the anal sphincter. The anal sphincter is massaged by inserting a gloved finger (which has been adequately lubricated) 2.5 to 3.7 cm (1 to 1.5 in) into the rectum and moving it in a circular motion or from side to side. It soon becomes apparent which area triggers the defecation response. This procedure should be performed at regular time intervals (usually every 48 hours), after a meal, and at a time that will be convenient for the patient at home. The patient also is taught the symptoms of impaction (frequent loose stools; constipation) and is cautioned to watch for hemorrhoids. A diet with sufficient fluids and fiber is essential to developing a successful bowel training program, avoiding constipation, and decreasing the risk of autonomic dysreflexia.

Counseling on Sexual Expression

Many patients with tetraplegia and paraplegia can have some form of meaningful sexual relationship, although modifications are necessary. The patient and partner benefit from counseling about the range of sexual expression possible, special techniques and positions, exploration of body sensations offering sensual feelings, and urinary and bowel hygiene as related to sexual activity. For men with erectile failure, penile prostheses enable them to have and sustain an erection, and impotence drugs may be helpful. Sildenafil (Viagra), vardenafil (Levitra), and tadalafil (Cialis), for example, are oral smooth muscle relaxants that cause blood to flow into the penis, resulting in an erection (see Chapter 49).

Sexual education and counseling services are included in the rehabilitation services at spinal centers. Small-group meetings in which patients can share their feelings, receive information, and discuss sexual concerns and practical aspects are helpful in producing effective attitudes and adjustments (Bader & Littlejohns, 2004).

Enhancing Coping Mechanisms

The impact of the disability and loss becomes marked when the patient returns home. Each time something new enters the patient's life (eg, a new relationship, going to work), the patient is reminded anew of his or her limitations. Grief reactions and depression are common.

To work through this depression, the patient must have some hope for relief in the future. The nurse can encourage the patient to feel confident in his or her ability to achieve self-care and relative independence. The role of the nurse ranges from caretaker during the acute phase to teacher, counselor, and facilitator as the patient gains mobility and independence.

The patient's disability affects not only the patient, but also the entire family. In many cases, family therapy is helpful in working through issues as they arise.

Adjustment to the disability leads to the development of realistic goals for the future, making the best of the abilities that are left intact and reinvesting in other activities and relationships. Rejection of the disability causes self-destructive neglect and noncompliance with the therapeutic program, which leads to more frustration and depression. Crises for which interventions may be sought include social, psychological, marital, sexual, and psychiatric problems. The family usually requires counseling, social services, and other support systems to help them cope with the changes in their lifestyle and socioeconomic status.

A major goal of nursing management is to help the patient overcome his or her sense of futility and to encourage the patient in the emotional adjustment that must be made before he or she is willing to venture into the outside world. However, an excessively sympathetic attitude on the part of the nurse may cause the patient to develop an overdependence that defeats the purpose of the entire rehabilitation program. The patient is taught and assisted when necessary, but the nurse should avoid performing activities that the patient can do independently with a little effort. This approach to care more than repays itself in the satisfaction of seeing a completely demoralized and helpless patient become independent and find meaning in a newly emerging lifestyle.

Monitoring and Managing Potential Complications

SPASTICITY

Muscle spasticity is one of the most problematic complications of tetraplegia and paraplegia. These incapacitating flexor or extensor spasms, which occur below the level of the spinal cord lesion, interfere with both the rehabilitation process and ADLs. Spasticity results from an imbalance between the facilitatory and inhibitory effects on neurons that exist normally. The area of the cord distal to the site of injury or lesion becomes disconnected from the higher inhibitory centers located in the brain, so facilitatory impulses, which originate from muscles, skin, and ligaments, predominate.

Spasticity is defined as a condition of increased muscle tone in a muscle that is weak. Initial resistance to stretching is quickly followed by sudden relaxation. The stimulus that precipitates spasm can be obvious, such as movement or a position change, or subtle, such as a slight jarring of the wheelchair. Most patients with tetraplegia or paraplegia have some degree of spasticity. With SCI, the onset of spasticity usually occurs from a few weeks to 6 months after the injury. The same muscles that are flaccid during the period of spinal shock develop spasticity during recovery. The intensity of spasticity tends to peak approximately 2 years after the injury, after which the spasms tend to regress.

Management of spasticity is based on the severity of symptoms and the degree of incapacitation. The antispasmodic medication baclofen (Lioresal) is one of the most commonly used agents because it is available in an oral and an intrathecal form (Rawlins, 2004; Staal, Arends & Ho, 2003). Other medications such as diazepam (Valium) and dantrolene (Dantrium) are also effective in controlling spasm. All of the antispasmodic medications cause drowsiness, weakness, and vertigo in some patients. Passive range-of-motion exercises and frequent turning and repositioning are helpful, because stiffness tends to increase spasticity. These activities also are essential in the prevention of contractures, pressure ulcers, and bowel and bladder dysfunction.

INFECTION AND SEPSIS

Patients with tetraplegia and paraplegia are at increased risk for infection and sepsis from a variety of sources: urinary tract, respiratory tract, and pressure ulcers. Sepsis remains a major cause of complications and death in these patients. Prevention of infection and sepsis is essential through maintenance of skin integrity, complete emptying of the bladder at regular intervals, and prevention of urinary and fecal incontinence. The risk for respiratory infection can be decreased by avoiding contact with people who have symptoms of respiratory infection, performing coughing and deep-breathing exercises to prevent pooling of respiratory secretions, receiving yearly influenza vaccines, and giving up smoking. A high-protein diet is important in maintaining an adequate immune system, as is avoiding factors that may reduce immune system function, such as excessive stress, drug abuse, and excessive alcohol intake.

If infection occurs, the patient requires thorough assessment and prompt treatment. Antibiotic therapy and adequate hydration, in addition to local measures (depending on the site of infection), are initiated immediately.

UTIs are minimized or prevented by

- Aseptic technique in catheter management
- Adequate hydration
- Bladder training program
- Prevention of overdistention of the bladder and urinary stasis

Skin breakdown and infection are prevented by

- Maintenance of a turning schedule
- Frequent back care
- Regular assessment of all skin areas
- Regular cleaning and lubrication of the skin
- Passive range-of-motion exercise to prevent contractures
- Pressure relief, particularly over broken skin areas, bony prominences, and heels
- Wrinkle-free bed linen

Pulmonary infections are managed and prevented by

- Frequent coughing, turning, and deep-breathing exercises and chest physiotherapy
- Aggressive respiratory care and suctioning of the airway if a tracheostomy is present
- Assisted coughing
- Adequate hydration

Infections of any kind can be life-threatening. Aggressive nursing interventions are key to their prevention and management.

Promoting Home and Community-Based Care

TEACHING PATIENTS SELF-CARE

Patients with tetraplegia or paraplegia are at risk for complications for the rest of their lives. Therefore, a major aspect of nursing care is teaching the patient and family about these complications and about strategies to minimize risks. UTIs, contractures, infected pressure ulcers, and sepsis may necessitate hospitalization. Other late complications that may occur include lower extremity edema, joint contractures, respiratory dysfunction, and pain. To avoid these and other complications, the patient and a family member are taught skin care, catheter care, range-of-motion exercises, breathing exercises, and other care techniques. Teaching is initiated as soon as possible and extends into the rehabilitation or long-term care facility and home. In all aspects of care, it is important for the nurse and patient to set mutual goals and discuss the tasks the patient is capable of doing independently and which tasks the patient needs assistance to complete (See Chapter 11 for a more detailed discussion of rehabilitation.)

CONTINUING CARE

Referral for home care is often appropriate for assessment of the home setting, patient teaching, and evaluation of the patient's physical and emotional status. During visits by the home care nurse, teaching about strategies to prevent or minimize potential complications is reinforced. The home environment is assessed for adequacy for care and for safety. Environmental modifications are made, and specialized equipment is obtained, ideally before the patient goes home.

The home care nurse also assesses the patient's and the family's adherence to recommendations and their use of coping strategies. The use of inappropriate coping strategies (eg, drug and alcohol use) is assessed, and referrals to counseling are made for the patient and family. Appropriate and effective coping strategies are reinforced. The nurse reviews previous teaching and determines the need for further physical or psychological assistance. The patient's self-esteem and body image may be very poor at this time. Because people with high levels of social support often report feelings of well-being despite major physical disability, it is beneficial for the nurse to assess and promote further development of the support system and effective coping strategies for each patient.

The patient requires continuing, lifelong follow-up by the physician, physical therapist, and other rehabilitation team members, because the neurologic deficit is usually permanent and new deficits, complications, and secondary conditions can develop. These require prompt attention before they take their toll in additional physical impairment, time, morale, and financial costs. The local counselor for the Office of Vocational Rehabilitation works with the patient with respect to job placement or additional educational or vocational training.

The nurse is in a good position to remind patients and family members of the need for continuing health promotion and screening practices. Referral to accessible health care providers and imaging centers is important in health promotion and health screening. Chapter 10 has more information on chronic illness and disability.

Evaluation

Expected Patient Outcomes

Expected patient outcomes may include the following:

1. Attains some form of mobility
2. Contractures do not develop
3. Maintains healthy, intact skin
4. Achieves bladder control, absence of UTI
5. Achieves bowel control
6. Reports sexual satisfaction
7. Shows improved adaptation to environment and others
8. Exhibits reduction in spasticity
   a. Reports understanding of the precipitating factors
   b. Uses measures to reduce spasticity
9. Describes long-term management required
10. Exhibits absence of complications

Critical Thinking Exercises

1 A 70-year-old patient was brought to the emergency department after he fell and hit his head and was unconscious for about 2 minutes. He now seems alert and oriented. What type of injury has he most likely sustained? What discharge instructions are warranted for this patient's family or caregiver? How would you modify your discharge instructions if the patient lives alone?

2 A 19-year-old patient is admitted with a severe closed head injury. What are the pertinent nursing diagnoses, goals, and expected outcomes for the patient? What health promotion strategies are relevant to teach the patient and family before discharge?

3 ebp A 47-year-old man with paraplegia secondary to spinal cord injury, diabetes, and obesity is admitted. What resources would you use to identify recommendations to reduce skin breakdown? What is the evidence base for these recommendations? Discuss the strength of the evidence, and identify the criteria used to evaluate the strength of the evidence for these recommendations.

REFERENCES AND SELECTED READINGS

BOOKS

American Association of Neuroscience Nurses (AANN). (2005). *Guide to the care of the patient with intracranial pressure monitoring: AANN reference series for clinical practice.* Glenview, IL: Author.

Ashley, M. J. (2004). *Traumatic brain injury: Rehabilitative treatment and case management* (2nd ed.). Boca Raton: CRC Press.

Bader, M. K. & Littlejohns, L. R. (2004). *AANN core curriculum for neuroscience nursing* (4th ed.). St. Louis: Elsevier.

Diepenbrock, N. H. (2004). *Quick reference to critical care* (2nd ed.). Philadelphia: Lippincott.

Eslinger, P. J. (Ed.). (2002). *Neuropsychological interventions: Clinical research and practice.* New York: Guilford Press.

Hickey, J. V. (2003). *The clinical practice of neurological and neurosurgical nursing* (5th ed.). Philadelphia: Lippincott Williams & Wilkins.

Langlois, J. A., Rutland-Brown, W. & Thomas, K. E. (2004). *Traumatic brain injury in the United States: Emergency department visits, hospitalizations and deaths.* Atlanta: Centers for Disease Control and Prevention, National Center for Injury Prevention and Control.

Mendel, E., Hentschel, S. J. & Guiot, B. H. (2005). Injuries to the cervical spine. In Rengachary, S. S. & Ellenbogen, R. G. (Eds.). *Principles of neurosurgery* (2nd ed.). Philadelphia: Elsevier Mosby.

Porth, C. M. (2005). *Pathophysiology: Concepts of altered health states* (7th ed.). Philadelphia: Lippincott Williams & Wilkins.

Rice, J. N., Robichaux, C. & Leonard, A. (2005). Nervous system alterations. In Sole, M. L., Klein, D. G. & Moseley, M. J. (Eds.). *Introduction to critical care nursing.* St. Louis: Elsevier Saunders.

Ropper, A. H., Gress, D., Diringer, M. N., et al. (2004). *Neurological and neurosurgical intensive care* (4th ed.). Philadelphia: Lippincott, Williams & Wilkins.

Somjen, G. (2004). *Ions in the brain: Normal function, seizures and stroke.* Oxford: Oxford University Press.

The Brain Trauma Foundation. (2003). *Guidelines for the management of severe head injury.* New York: The Brain Trauma Foundation.

Vaccaro, A. R. (2003). *Fractures of the cervical, thoracic, and lumbar spine.* New York: Marcel Dekker.

Winn, H. R. (2003). *Youman's neurological surgery* (5th ed., Vols. 1–4). Philadelphia: W. B. Saunders.

JOURNALS

**Asterisks indicate nursing research articles.*

Head Injury

Alderson, P., Gadkary, C. & Signorini, D. F. (2004). Therapeutic hypothermia for head injury. *The Cochrane Database of Systematic Reviews*, (4), CD001048.

Arbour, R. (2004). Intracranial hypertension: Monitoring and assessment. *Critical Care Nurse, 24*(5), 19–34.

Bader, M. K., Littlejohns, L. R. & March, K. (2003). Brain tissue oxygen monitoring in severe brain injury: Part II. Implications for critical care teams and case study. *Critical Care Nurse, 23*(4), 29–43.

Brewer, T. (2003). Are you paying attention? *American Journal of Nursing, 103*(7), 58–63.

Censullo, J. L. & Sebastian, S. (2004). Pentobarbital sodium coma for refractory intracranial hypertension. *Journal of Neuroscience Nursing, 35*(5), 252–262.

*Davis, A. E. & Gimeniz, A. (2004). Cognitive-behavioral recovery in comatose patients following auditory sensory stimulation. *Journal of Neuroscience Nursing, 35*(4), 202–209.

Diringer, M. N. (2004). Treatment of fever in the neurologic intensive care unit with a catheter-based heat exchange system. *Critical Care Medicine, 32*(2), 559–564.

Fan, J. Y. (2004). Effect of backrest position on intracranial pressure and cerebral perfusion pressure in individuals with brain injury: A systematic review. *Journal of Neuroscience Nursing, 36*(5), 278–288.

Flanagan, S. R., Hibbard, M. R. & Gordon, W. A. (2005). The impact of age on traumatic brain injury. *Physical Medicine and Rehabilitation Clinics of North America, 16*(1), 163–178.

Hagen, C., Malkmus, D., & Durham, P. (1972). *Rancho Los Amigos Level of Cognitive Function scale.* Communication Disorders Service, Rancho Los Amigos Hospital, Downey, CA, 1972. Revised 11/15/74 by Danese Malkmus, M. A., and Kathryn Stenderup.

Haymore, J. (2004). A neuron in a haystack: Advanced neurological assessment. *AACN Clinical Issues, 15*(4), 568–581.

Henneman, E. A. & Karras, G. E. (2004). Determining brain death in adults: A guideline for use in critical care. *Critical Care Nurse, 24*(5), 50–56.

*Hsueh-Fen, S. & Stuifbergen, A. K. (2004). Love and load: The lived experience of the mother-child relationship among young adult traumatic brain-injured survivors. *Journal of Neuroscience Nursing, 36*(2), 73–81.

Johnson, A. L. & Criddle, L. M. (2004). Pass the salt: Indications for and implications of using hypertonic saline. *Critical Care Nurse, 24*(5), 36–48.

Lempe, D. M. (2004). Riding out the storm: Sympathetic storming after traumatic brain injury. *Journal of Neuroscience Nursing, 36*(1), 4–9.

Littlejohns, L. R., Bader, M. K., & March, K. (2003). Brain tissue oxygen monitoring in severe brain injury, Part I: Research and usefulness in critical care. *Critical Care Nurse, 23*(4), 17–25.

McCrea, M., Guskiewicz, K. M., Marshall, S. W., et al. (2003). Acute effects and recovery time following concussion in collegiate football players: The NCAA concussion study. *Journal of the American Medical Association, 290*(19), 2556–2563.

*Scheetz, L. J. (2005). Relationship of age, injury severity, injury types, comorbid conditions, level of care, and survival among older motor vehicle trauma patients. *Research in Nursing and Health, 28*(3), 198–209.

Torpy, J. M., Lynm, C. & Glass, R. M. (2005). Head injury. *Journal of the American Medical Association, 294*(12), 1580.

Yanagawa, T., Bunn, F., Roberts, I., et al. (2005). Nutritional support for head-injured patients. *The Cochrane Database of Systematic Reviews,* (3), CD001530.

Spinal Cord Injury

Baker, E. & Saulino, P. (2002). First-ever guidelines for spinal cord injuries. *RN, 65*(10), 32–37.

Capoor, J. & Stein, A. B. (2005). Aging with spinal cord injury. *Physical Medicine and Rehabilitation Clinics of North America, 16*(1), 129–162.

Charlifue, S., Lammertse, D. P. & Adkins, R. H. (2004). Aging with spinal cord injury: Changes in selected health indices and life satisfaction. *Archives of Physical Medicine and Rehabilitation, 85*(11), 1848–1853.

Farray, D., Carman, T. L. & Fernandez, B. B. (2004). The treatment and prevention of deep vein thrombosis in the preoperative management of patients who have neurologic diseases. *Neurologic Clinics of North America, 22*(2), 423–439.

Grijaiva, I., Guizar-Sahagun, G., Castaneda-Hernandez, G., et al. (2003). Efficacy and safety of 4-aminopyridine in patients with long-term spinal cord injury: A randomized, double-blind, placebo-controlled trial. *Pharmacotherapy, 23*(7), 823–834.

Jackson, A. B., Lindsey, L. L., Klebine, P. L., et al. (2004). Reproductive health for women with spinal cord injury: Pregnancy and delivery. *SCI Nursing, 21*(2), 88–91.

Jones, L. & Bagnall, A. (2005). Spinal injuries centers (SCIs) for acute traumatic spinal cord injury. *The Cochrane Database of Systematic Reviews,* (4), CD004442.

*Kinder, R. A. (2005). Psychological hardiness in women with paraplegia. *Rehabilitation Nursing, 30*(2), 68–72.

Mastrogiovanni, D., Phillips, E. M. & Fine, C. F. (2003). The bariatric spinal cord injured person: Challenges in preventing and healing skin problems. *Topics in Spinal Cord Injury Rehabilitation, 9*(2), 38–44.

McCutcheon, E. P., Selassie, A. W., Gu, J. K., et al. (2004). Acute traumatic spinal cord injury, 1993–2000: A population-based assessment of methylprednisolone administration and hospitalization. *Journal of Trauma, 56*(5), 1076–1083.

Phillips, E. M. (2003). Evidence-based practice: Pressure ulcer management guidelines for spinal cord injury. *Topics in Spinal Cord Injury Rehabilitation, 9*(2), 16–19.

Rawlins, P. K. (2004). Intrathecal baclofen therapy over 10 years. *Journal of Neuroscience Nursing, 61*(6), 322–327.

Scivoletto, G. & Morganti, B. (2004). Sex-related differences of rehabilitation outcomes of spinal cord lesions patients. *Clinical Rehabilitation, 18*(6), 709–713.

Smits, M., Dippel, D. W., Haan, H., et al. (2005). External validation of the Canadian CT head rule and the New Orleans criteria for CT scanning in patients with minor head injuries. *Journal of American Medical Association, 294*(12), 1519–1525.

*Staal, C., Arends, A., & Ho, S. (2003). A self-report of quality of life of patients receiving intrathecal baclofen therapy. *Rehabilitation Nursing, 28*(5), 159–162.

Prevention

Liu, B., Ivers R., Norton, R., et al. (2004). Helmets for preventing injury in motorcycle riders. *The Cochrane Library,* (2), CD004333.

RESOURCES

American Association of Neuroscience Nurses (AANN), 4700 W. Lake Ave, Chicago, IL 60025-1485; 847-375-4733 or 888-557-2266; http://www.aann.org. Accessed June 23, 2006.

American Association of Spinal Cord Injury Nurses (AASCIN), 75-20 Astoria Blvd., Jackson Heights, NY 11370-1177; 718-803-3782; http://www.aascin.org. Accessed June 23, 2006.

American Paralysis/Spinal Cord Hotline, 800-526-3456.

Association of Rehabilitation Nurses, 5700 Old Orchard Rd., Skokie, IL 60077; 708-966-8673; http://www.rehabnurse.org. Accessed June 23, 2006.

The Brain Injury Association, Inc., 8201 Greensboro Drive, Suite 611, McLean, VA 22102; 703-761-0659; family help line: 800-444-6443; http://www.biausa.org. Accessed June 23, 2006.

The Brain Trauma Foundation, 523 East 72d Street, New York, NY 10021; 212-772-0608; http://wtrauma.org. Accessed June 23, 2006.

Centers for Disease Control and Prevention, National Center for Injury Prevention and Control, Mailstop K65, 4770 Buford Highway NE, Atlanta, GA 30341-3724; 770-488-1506; http://wov/ncipc/ncipchm.htm. Accessed June 23, 2006.

Information Center for Individuals with Disabilities, Fort Point Place, 27-43 Wormwood St., Boston, MA 02210-1606; 617-727-5540; http://www.disability.net. Accessed June 23, 2006.

The Library of Congress, Division of the Blind and Physically Handicapped, 1291 Taylor St., NW, Washington, DC 20542; 202-707-5100; http://www.loc.gov/access/. Accessed June 23, 2006.

National Rehabilitation Information Center, 1010 Wayne Avenue, Suite 800, Silver Spring, MD 20910; 800-346-2742, TTY 301-495-5626; http://www.naric.com. Accessed June 23, 2006.

National Spinal Cord Injury Association, 8300 Colesville Rd., Silver Spring, MD 20910; 301-588-6959; http://www.spinalcord.org. Accessed June 23, 2006.

Paralyzed Veterans of America, 801 18th St., NW, Washington, DC 20006; 202-872-1300; http://www.pva.org. Accessed June 23, 2006.

Rehabilitation Services Administration, Department of Human Services, 605 G Street, NW, Room 101M, Washington, DC 20001; 202-727-3211; http://www.ed.gov/offices/OSERS/RSA/rsa.html. Accessed June 23, 2006.

Waiting.com, run by and for the families of traumatic brain injury; for legal questions: Attorney Gordon S. Johnson, Jr., 800-992-9447; http://www.waiting.com. Accessed June 23, 2006.

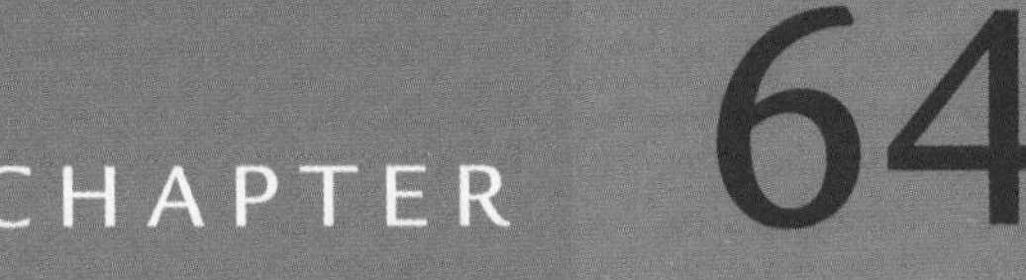
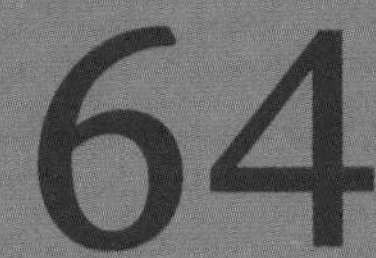

CHAPTER 64

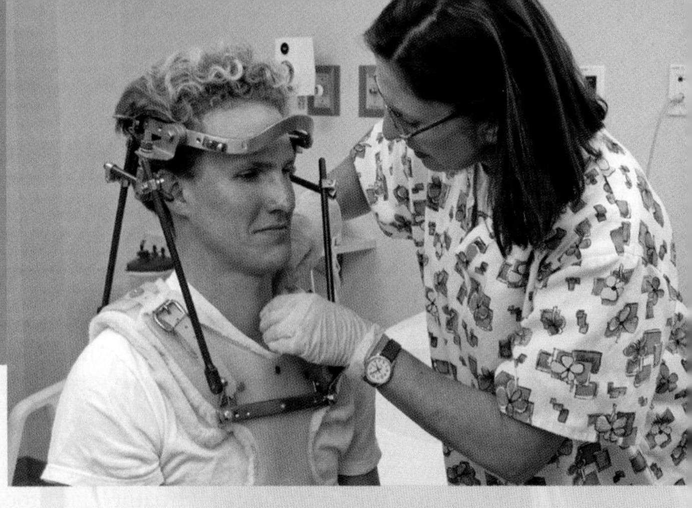

Management of Patients With Neurologic Infections, Autoimmune Disorders, and Neuropathies

Learning Objectives

On completion of this chapter, the learner will be able to:

1. Differentiate among the infectious disorders of the nervous system according to causes, manifestations, medical care, and nursing management.
2. Describe the pathophysiology, clinical manifestations, and medical and nursing management of multiple sclerosis, myasthenia gravis, and Guillain-Barré syndrome.
3. Use the nursing process as a framework for care of patients with multiple sclerosis, myasthenia gravis, and Guillain-Barré syndrome.
4. Describe disorders of the cranial nerves, their manifestations, and indicated nursing interventions.
5. Develop a plan of nursing care for the patient with a cranial nerve disorder.

The diverse group of neurologic disorders that make up infectious and autoimmune disorders and cranial and peripheral neuropathies presents unique challenges for nursing care. Infectious processes of the nervous system sometimes cause death or permanent dysfunction. Autoimmune disorders usually have a slow, progressive course, requiring the nurse to manage symptoms and facilitate the patient's and family's understanding of the disease process and treatment approaches. Cranial and peripheral nerve disorders may affect the patient's comfort, functional independence, and self-esteem.

The nurse who cares for patients with these disorders must have a clear understanding of the pathologic processes and the clinical outcomes. Some of the issues nurses must help patients and families confront include adaptation to the effects of the disease, potential changes in family dynamics, and, possibly, end-of-life issues.

Infectious Neurologic Disorders

The infectious disorders of the nervous system include meningitis, brain abscesses, various types of encephalitis, and Creutzfeldt-Jakob and variant Creutzfeldt-Jakob disease. The clinical manifestations, assessment, and diagnostic findings as well as the medical and nursing management are related to the specific infectious process.

Meningitis

Meningitis is an inflammation of the pia mater, the arachnoid, and the cerebrospinal fluid (CSF)–filled subarachnoid space (Porth, 2005). Meningitis is classified as septic or aseptic. Septic meningitis is caused by bacteria. In aseptic meningitis, the cause is viral or secondary to lymphoma, leukemia, or human immunodeficiency virus (HIV). The most common pathogens causing septic meningitis in the United States are *Streptococcus pneumoniae* and *Neisseria meningitidis* (Goetz, 2003). *Haemophilus influenzae* was once a common cause of meningitis in children, but, because of vaccination, infection with this organism is now rare in the United States. Outbreaks of *N. meningitidis* infection are most likely to occur in dense community groups, such as college campuses and military installations. Although infections occur year round, the peak incidence is in the winter and early spring. Factors that increase the risk for bacterial meningitis include tobacco use and viral upper respiratory infection, because they increase the amount of droplet production. Otitis media and mastoiditis increase the risk for bacterial meningitis, because the bacteria can cross the epithelial membrane and enter the subarachnoid space. People with immune system deficiencies are also at greater risk for development of bacterial meningitis.

Pathophysiology

Meningeal infections generally originate in one of two ways: through the bloodstream as a consequence of other infections, or by direct spread, such as might occur after a traumatic injury to the facial bones or secondary to invasive procedures.

N. meningitidis concentrates in the nasopharynx and is transmitted by secretion or aerosol contamination. Bacterial or meningococcal meningitis also occurs as an opportunistic infection in patients with acquired immunodeficiency syndrome (AIDS) and as a complication of Lyme disease (Chart 64-1).

Once the causative organism enters the bloodstream, it crosses the blood–brain barrier and proliferates in the CSF. The host immune response stimulates the release of cell wall fragments and lipopolysaccharides, facilitating inflammation of the subarachnoid and pia mater. Because the cranial vault contains little room for expansion, the inflammation may cause increased intracranial pressure (ICP). CSF circulates through the subarachnoid space, where inflammatory cellular materials from the affected meningeal tissue enter and accumulate. CSF studies demonstrate decreased glucose, increased protein levels, and increased white blood cell count (Spach, 2003).

The prognosis for bacterial meningitis depends on the causative organism, the severity of the infection and illness, and the timeliness of treatment. Acute fulminant presentation may include adrenal damage, circulatory collapse, and widespread hemorrhages (Waterhouse-Friderichsen syndrome). This syndrome is the result of endothelial damage and vascular necrosis caused by the bacteria. Complications

Glossary

ataxia: impaired coordination of movements

bulbar paralysis: immobility of muscles innervated by cranial nerves with their cell bodies in the lower portion of the brain stem

diplopia: double vision, or the awareness of two images of the same object occurring in one or both eyes

dyskinesia: impaired ability to execute voluntary movements

dysphagia: difficulty swallowing, causing the patient to be at risk for aspiration

dysphonia: voice impairment or altered voice production

neuropathy: general term indicating a disorder of the nervous system

paresthesia: a sensation of numbness or tingling or a "pins and needles" sensation

prion: a particle smaller than a virus that is resistant to standard sterilization procedures

spasticity: muscular hypertonicity with increased resistance to stretch often associated with weakness, increased deep tendon reflexes, and diminished superficial reflexes

spongiform: having the appearance or quality of a sponge

CHART 64-1

Meningitis in Specific Populations

Meningitis can occur as a complication of other diseases and is an opportunistic infection seen with greater frequency in patients who are immunocompromised.

MENINGITIS IN PATIENTS WITH AIDS

- Aseptic, cryptococcal, and tuberculous forms of meningitis have been reported in patients with AIDS.
- Acute and chronic forms of aseptic meningitis may occur with AIDS; both are accompanied by headache, but signs of meningeal irritation usually occur with the acute form.
- Aseptic meningitis may be accompanied by cranial nerve palsies. The meningitis is thought to be related to direct infection of the central nervous system by human immunodeficiency virus (HIV) because it can be isolated from the cerebrospinal fluid (CSF).
- Cryptococcal meningitis is the most common fungal infection of the central nervous system in patients with AIDS. Patients may experience headache, nausea, vomiting, seizures, confusion, and lethargy. Treatment consists of IV administration of amphotericin B followed by fluconazole. Maintenance therapy with fluconazole may be necessary to prevent relapse.
- Some immunosuppressed patients develop few if any symptoms because of blunted inflammatory responses; others develop atypical features.

MENINGITIS IN PATIENTS WITH LYME DISEASE

- Lyme disease is a multisystem inflammatory process caused by the tick-transmitted spirochete *Borrelia burgdorferi.*
- Neurologic abnormalities are seen in later stages (stages 2 or 3). Stage 2 occurs with the start of a characteristic rash or 1 to 6 months after the rash has disappeared.
- Neurologic abnormalities include aseptic meningitis, chronic lymphocytic meningitis, and encephalitis.
- Cranial nerve inflammation, including Bell's palsy and other peripheral neuropathies, is common.
- Stage 3 (the chronic form of the disease) begins years after the initial tick infection and is characterized by arthritis, skin lesions, and neurologic abnormalities.
- Most patients with stage 2 and 3 Lyme disease are treated with IV antibiotics, usually ceftriaxone or penicillin G.
- Meningeal and systemic symptoms begin to improve within days, although other symptoms, such as headache, may persist for weeks.

include visual impairment, deafness, seizures, paralysis, hydrocephalus, and septic shock.

Clinical Manifestations

Headache and fever are frequently the initial symptoms. Fever tends to remain high throughout the course of the illness. The headache is usually either steady or throbbing and very severe as a result of meningeal irritation (Bickley & Szilagyi, 2003). Meningeal irritation results in a number of other well-recognized signs common to all types of meningitis:

- Nuchal rigidity (stiff neck): This is an early sign (Diepenbrock, 2004). Any attempts at flexion of the head are difficult because of spasms in the muscles of the neck. Forceful flexion causes severe pain.
- Positive Kernig's sign: When the patient is lying with the thigh flexed on the abdomen, the leg cannot be completely extended (Fig. 64-1).
- Positive Brudzinski's sign: When the patient's neck is flexed (after ruling out cervical trauma or injury), flexion of the knees and hips is produced; when the lower extremity of one side is passively flexed, a similar movement is seen in the opposite extremity (see Fig. 64-1). Brudzinski's sign is a more sensitive indicator of meningeal irritation than Kernig's sign (Pullen, 2004).
- Photophobia (extreme sensitivity to light): This finding is common, although the cause is unclear.

A rash can be a striking feature of *N. meningitidis* infection, occurring in about half of patients with this type of meningitis. Skin lesions develop, ranging from a petechial rash with purpuric lesions to large areas of ecchymosis.

Disorientation and memory impairment are common early in the course of the illness. The changes depend on the severity of the infection as well as the individual response to the physiologic processes. Behavioral manifestations are also common. As the illness progresses, lethargy, unresponsiveness, and coma may develop.

Seizures occur in 30% of adults with *S. pneumoniae* meningitis and are the result of areas of irritability in the brain (Goetz, 2003). ICP increases secondary to the accumulation of purulent exudate. The initial signs of increased ICP include decreased level of consciousness and focal motor deficits. If ICP is not controlled, the uncus of the temporal lobe may herniate through the tentorium, causing pressure on the brain stem. Brain stem herniation is a life-threatening event that causes cranial nerve dysfunction and depresses the centers of vital functions, such as the medulla. See Chapter 61 for discussion of the patient with a change in level of consciousness (LOC) or increased ICP.

An acute fulminant infection occurs in about 10% of patients with meningococcal meningitis, producing signs of

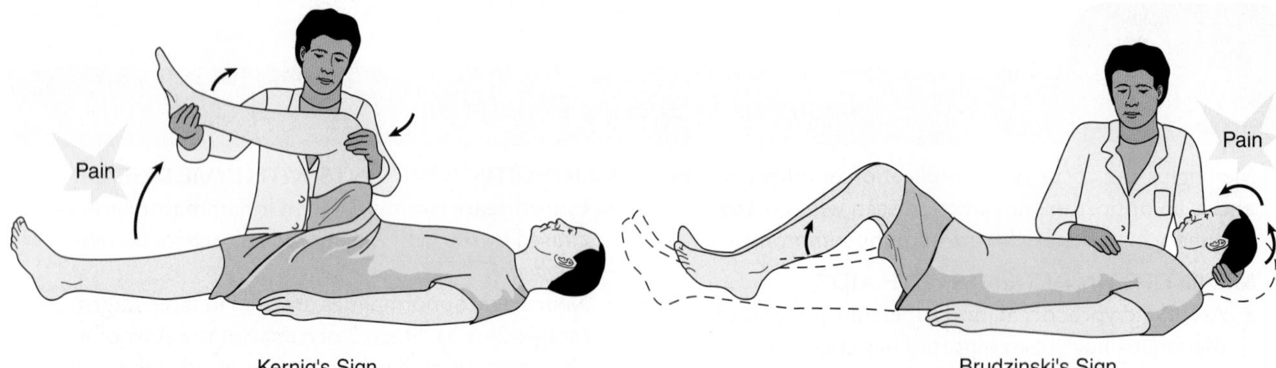

FIGURE 64-1. Testing for meningeal irritation. (**A**) Kernig's sign. (**B**) Brudzinski's sign.

overwhelming septicemia: an abrupt onset of high fever, extensive purpuric lesions (over the face and extremities), shock, and signs of disseminated intravascular coagulopathy (DIC). Death may occur within a few hours after onset of the infection.

Assessment and Diagnostic Findings

If the clinical presentation suggests meningitis, diagnostic testing is conducted to identify the causative organism. Bacterial culture and Gram staining of CSF and blood are key diagnostic tests (Fischbach, 2002). The presence of polysaccharide antigen in CSF further supports the diagnosis of bacterial meningitis (Porth, 2005).

Prevention

Since 1971, the military has vaccinated all new recruits against meningococcal meningitis, resulting in a dramatic decrease in its incidence. Researchers have suggested vaccination of college freshman, because surveillance studies indicate that freshmen living in dormitories are at highest risk for development of meningococcal meningitis. Vaccination is not a universal requirement for college freshmen, however; the policy is determined by the college or university. The American Academy of Pediatrics provides information to college freshmen and their parents about the risk of disease and the availability of vaccination (Spiro & Spiro, 2004).

People in close contact with patients with meningococcal meningitis should be treated with antimicrobial chemoprophylaxis using rifampin (Rifadin), ciprofloxacin hydrochloride (Cipro), or ceftriaxone sodium (Rocephin) (Bader & Littlejohns, 2004). Therapy should be started within 24 hours after exposure because a delay in the initiation of therapy will limit the effectiveness of the prophylaxis (Spach, 2003). Vaccination should also be considered as an adjunct to antibiotic chemoprophylaxis for anyone living with a person who develops meningococcal infection. Vaccination against *H. influenzae* and *S. pneumoniae* should be encouraged for children and at-risk adults.

Medical Management

Successful outcomes depend on the early administration of an antibiotic that crosses the blood–brain barrier into the subarachnoid space in sufficient concentration to halt the multiplication of bacteria. Penicillin antibiotics (eg, ampicillin, piperacillin) or one of the cephalosporins (eg, ceftriaxone sodium, cefotaxime sodium) may be used. Vancomycin hydrochloride alone or in combination with rifampin may be used if resistant strains of bacteria are identified. High doses of the appropriate antibiotic are administered IV.

Dexamethasone has been shown to be beneficial as adjunct therapy in the treatment of acute bacterial meningitis and in pneumococcal meningitis if it is administered 15 to 20 minutes before the first dose of antibiotic and every 6 hours for the next 4 days. Studies indicate that dexamethasone improves the outcome in adults and does not increase the risk for gastrointestinal bleeding (de Gans & van de Beek, 2002).

Dehydration and shock are treated with fluid volume expanders. Seizures, which may occur early in the course of the disease, are controlled with phenytoin (Dilantin). Increased ICP is treated as necessary (see Chapter 61).

Nursing Management

The patient with meningitis is critically ill; therefore, many of the nursing interventions are collaborative with the physician, respiratory therapist, and other members of the health care team. The patient's safety and well-being depend on sound nursing judgment.

Neurologic status and vital signs are continually assessed. Pulse oximetry and arterial blood gas values are used to quickly identify the need for respiratory support if increasing ICP compromises the brain stem. Insertion of a cuffed endotracheal tube (or tracheotomy) and mechanical ventilation may be necessary to maintain adequate tissue oxygenation.

Arterial blood pressures are monitored to assess for incipient shock, which precedes cardiac or respiratory failure. Rapid IV fluid replacement may be prescribed, but care is taken to prevent fluid overload. Fever also increases the workload of the heart and cerebral metabolism. ICP will increase in response to increased cerebral metabolic demands. Therefore, measures are taken to reduce body temperature as quickly as possible.

Other important components of nursing care include the following measures:

- Protecting the patient from injury secondary to seizure activity or altered LOC

- Monitoring daily body weight; serum electrolytes; and urine volume, specific gravity, and osmolality, especially if syndrome of inappropriate antidiuretic hormone (SIADH) is suspected
- Preventing complications associated with immobility, such as pressure ulcers and pneumonia
- Instituting infection control precautions until 24 hours after initiation of antibiotic therapy (oral and nasal discharge is considered infectious)

Any sudden, critical illness can be devastating to the family. Because the patient's condition is often critical and the prognosis guarded, the family needs to be informed about the patient's condition. Periodic family visits are essential to facilitate coping of the patient and family. An important aspect of the nurse's role is to support the family and assist them in identifying others who can be supportive to them during the crisis.

CHART 64-2

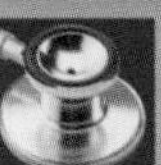

Assessing for Brain Abscesses

Be on the alert for the folowing signs and symptoms:

FRONTAL LOBE
Hemiparesis
Aphasia (expressive)
Seizures
Frontal headache

TEMPORAL LOBE
Localized headache
Changes in vision
Facial weakness
Aphasia

CEREBELLAR ABSCESS
Occipital headache
Ataxia (inability to coordinate movements)
Nystagmus (rhythmic, involuntary movements of the eye)

Adapted from Hickey, J. V. (2003). *The clinical practice of neurological and neurosurgical nursing* (5th ed.). Philadelphia: Lippincott Williams & Wilkins.

Brain Abscess

Brain abscesses account for approximately 1% of space-occupying brain lesions in the United States and are more common in males during the first two decades of life (Bader & Littlejohns, 2004). Brain abscess is rare in immunocompetent people; it is more frequently diagnosed in people who are immunosuppressed as a result of an underlying disease or use of immunosuppressive mediations.

Pathophysiology

A brain abscess is a collection of infectious material within the tissue of the brain. Bacteria are the most common causative organisms (Hickey, 2003). The most common predisposing conditions for abscesses among immunocompetent adults are otitis media and sinusitis (Goetz, 2003). An abscess can result from intracranial surgery, penetrating head injury, or tongue piercing (Armstrong, 2004). Organisms causing brain abscess may reach the brain by hematologic spread from the lungs, gums, tongue, or heart, or from a wound or intra-abdominal infection (Hickey, 2003). Brain abscesses in immunocompromised people may result from various pathogens. To prevent brain abscess, otitis media, mastoiditis, sinusitis, dental infections, and systemic infections should be treated promptly.

Clinical Manifestations

The clinical manifestations of a brain abscess result from alterations in intracranial dynamics (edema, brain shift), infection, or the location of the abscess (Chart 64-2).

Headache, usually worse in the morning, is the most prevailing symptom. Fever, vomiting and focal neurologic deficits occur as well. Focal deficits such as weakness and decreasing vision reflect the area of brain that is involved. As the abscess expands, symptoms of increased ICP such as decreasing LOC and seizures are observed.

Assessment and Diagnostic Findings

Neuroimaging studies such as magnetic resonance imaging (MRI) and computed tomography (CT) identify the size and location of the abscess. The MRI and CT scans demonstrate a ring around a hypodense area. Aspiration of the abscess, guided by CT or MRI, is the best method to culture and identify the infectious organism. Blood cultures are obtained if the abscess is believed to arise from a distant source. Chest x-ray is performed to rule out predisposing lung infections. A CT scan of the head is performed to evaluate the bony structure of the middle ear and sinuses (Goetz, 2003).

Medical Management

Treatment is aimed at controlling increased ICP, draining the abscess, and providing antimicrobial therapy directed at the abscess and the primary source of infection. Large IV doses of antibiotics are administered to penetrate the blood–brain barrier and reach the abscess. The choice of the specific antibiotic medication is based on culture and sensitivity testing and directed at the causative organism (Bader & Littlejohns, 2004). Corticosteroids may be prescribed to help reduce the inflammatory cerebral edema if the patient shows evidence of an increasing neurologic deficit. Antiseizure medications (phenytoin, phenobarbital) may be prescribed to prevent or treat seizures.

Nursing Management

Nursing care focuses on continuing to assess the neurologic status, administering medications, assessing the response to treatment, and providing supportive care.

Ongoing neurologic assessment alerts the nurse to changes in ICP, which may indicate a need for more aggressive intervention. The nurse also assesses and documents the responses to medications. Blood laboratory test results, specifically blood glucose and serum potassium levels, need to be closely monitored when corticosteroids are prescribed. Administration of insulin or electrolyte replacement may be required to return these values to normal or acceptable levels.

Patient safety is another key nursing responsibility. Injury may result from decreased LOC or falls related to motor weakness or seizures.

The patient with a brain abscess is extremely ill, and neurologic deficits, such as hemiparesis, seizures, visual deficits, and cranial nerve palsies, may remain after treatment. Focal seizures are the most common sequelae, occurring in about 30% of patients (Hickey, 2003). The nurse must assess the family's ability to express distress at the patient's condition, cope with the patient's illness and deficits, and obtain support.

Herpes Simplex Virus Encephalitis

Encephalitis is an acute inflammatory process of the brain tissue. Herpes simplex virus (HSV) is the most common cause of acute encephalitis in the United States (Crumpacker, Gonzalez & Makar, 2003). There are two herpes simplex viruses, HSV-1 and HSV-2. HSV-1 typically affects children and adults. HSV-2 most commonly affects neonates and is discussed in pediatric textbooks.

Pathophysiology

HSV-1 causes encephalitis by following a retrograde intraneuronal path to the brain. The olfactory and trigeminal nerves are the most commonly involved paths. Researchers also believe that latent virus in brain tissue may reactivate and result in encephalitis (Whitley & Gnann, 2002).

Clinical Manifestations

HSV-1 encephalitis causes inflammation and hemorrhagic necrosis of the temporal lobe, differentiating HSV-1 from other agents that cause encephalitis (Crumpacker et al., 2003). The initial symptoms include fever, headache, and confusion. Focal neurologic symptoms reflect the areas of cerebral inflammation and necrosis and include behavioral changes, focal seizures, dysphasia, hemiparesis, and altered LOC (Whitley & Gnann, 2002).

Assessment and Diagnostic Findings

Neuroimaging studies, electroencephalography (EEG), and CSF examination are used to diagnose HSV encephalitis. MRI is the neuroimaging study of choice for detection of early changes caused by HSV-1; the study will show edema in the temporal lobe (Crumpacker et al., 2003). The EEG demonstrates periodic high-voltage spikes originating in the temporal lobe. Lumbar puncture often reveals a high opening pressure and low glucose and high protein levels in CSF samples. Viral cultures are almost always negative. The polymerase chain reaction (PCR) is the standard test for early diagnosis of HSV-1 encephalitis. PCR identifies the DNA bands of HSV-1 in the CSF (Raschilas, Wolff, Delatour, et al., 2002). The validity of PCR is very high between the third and tenth days after symptom onset.

Medical Management

Acyclovir (Zovirax), an antiviral agent, is the medication of choice in the treatment of HSV (Karch, 2005). Studies have indicated that early administration of acyclovir improves the prognosis associated with HSV-1 encephalitis (Raschilas et al., 2002). The mode of action is inhibition of viral DNA replication. Acyclovir usually is well tolerated by the patient. To prevent relapse, treatment should continue for up to 3 weeks. Slow IV administration over 1 hour prevents crystallization of the medication in the urine. The usual dose of acyclovir is decreased if the patient has a history of renal insufficiency (Karch, 2005). Studies are in progress to determine the effectiveness of an oral agent, valacyclovir hydrochloride (Valtrex), in the treatment of HSV-1 encephalitis (Crumpacker et al., 2003).

Nursing Management

Assessment of neurologic function is key to monitoring the progression of disease. Comfort measures to reduce headache include dimming the lights, limiting noise, and administering analgesic agents. Opioid analgesic medications may mask neurologic symptoms; therefore, they are used cautiously. Focal seizures and altered LOC require care directed at injury prevention and safety. Nursing care addressing patient and family anxieties is ongoing throughout the illness. Monitoring of blood chemistry test results and urinary output will alert the nurse to the presence of renal complications related to acyclovir therapy.

Arthropod-Borne Virus Encephalitis

Arthropod vectors transmit several types of viruses that cause encephalitis. The primary vector in North America is the mosquito. In cases of West Nile virus, humans are the secondary host; birds are the primary host (Morgan, 2004). Arbovirus infection (transmitted by arthropod vectors) occurs in specific geographic areas during the summer and fall. In the United States, West Nile and St. Louis are the most common types of arboviral encephalitis; both are members of the Japanese encephalitis serogroup (Solomon, 2004). West Nile virus was first observed in the United States in 1999; encephalitis develops in 1 out of 150 cases (Morgan, 2004).

Pathophysiology

Viral replication occurs at the site of the mosquito bite. The host immune response attempts to control viral replication. If the immune response is inadequate, viremia will ensue. The virus gains access to the central nervous system (CNS) via the cerebral capillaries, resulting in encephalitis. It spreads from neuron to neuron, predominantly affecting the cortical gray matter, the brain stem, and the thalamus. Meningeal exudates compound the clinical presentation by irritating the meninges and increasing ICP (Solomon, 2004).

Clinical Manifestations

St. Louis and West Nile encephalitis most commonly affect adults. Climate, an environment conducive to arthropod proliferation, and human behavior contribute to the occurrence of St. Louis and West Nile encephalitis. An arboviral encephalitis begins with early flu-like symptoms, but specific neurologic manifestations depend on the viral type. A unique clinical feature of St. Louis encephalitis is SIADH with hyponatremia. Signs and symptoms specific to West Nile encephalitis include a maculopapular or morbilliform rash on the neck, trunk, arms, and legs and flaccid paralysis (Morgan, 2004). Both West Nile and St. Louis encephalitis can result in Parkinsonian-like movements, reflecting inflammation of the basal ganglia. Seizures, a poor prognostic indicator, are present in both types of encephalitis but are more common in the St. Louis type (Solomon, 2004).

Assessment and Diagnostic Findings

After a brief febrile prodrome, neurologic symptoms will reflect the area of the brain that is involved. Neuroimaging and CSF evaluation are useful in the diagnosis of arboviral encephalitis. The MRI scan demonstrates inflammation of the basal ganglia in cases of St. Louis encephalitis and inflammation in the periventricular area in cases of West Nile encephalitis. Immunoglobulin M antibodies to West Nile Virus are observed in serum and CSF (Morgan, 2004). Serum cultures are not useful, because the viremia is brief. PCR evaluation of CSF may demonstrate viral RNA (Solomon, 2004).

Medical Management

No specific medication for arboviral encephalitis exists. Medical management is aimed at controlling the seizures and the increased ICP. Studies indicate that interferon may be useful in treating St. Louis encephalitis. Ribavirin and interferon alpha-2b show some effect against West Nile virus but have not been evaluated in controlled studies (Morgan, 2004). Neuropsychiatric complications, such as emotional outbursts and other behavior changes, occur frequently. Although no vaccine is available for St. Louis encephalitis, evidence suggests that a vaccine may decrease the risk of acquiring West Nile encephalitis (Solomon, 2004).

Nursing Management

If the patient is very ill, hospitalization may be required. The nurse carefully assesses neurologic status and identifies improvement or deterioration in the patient's condition. Injury prevention is key in light of the potential for falls or seizures. Arboviral encephalitis may result in death or life-long residual health issues such as neurologic deficits and seizures. The family will need support and teaching to cope with these outcomes.

Public education addressing the prevention of arboviral encephalitis is a key nursing role. Clothing that provides coverage and insect repellents containing 25% to 30% diethyltoluamide (DEET) should be used on exposed clothing and skin in high-risk areas to decrease mosquito and tick bites (Bader & Littlejohns, 2004). Screens should be in good repair in the home, and standing water should be removed. Blood donation centers screen all blood for West Nile virus. Cases of West Nile virus must be reported to the Centers for Disease Control and Prevention (CDC) (Morgan, 2004).

Fungal Encephalitis

Fungal infections of the CNS occur rarely in healthy people. The presentation of fungal encephalitis is related to geographic area or to an immune system that is compromised due to disease or immunosuppressive medication. When fungal infections occur in immunocompetent people, the causative organism is usually *Cryptococcus neoformans* or *Blastomyces dermatitidis*. Other fungi that cause neurologic infection include *Histoplasma capsulatum, Aspergillus fumigatus, Candida,* and *Coccidioides immitis* (Goetz, 2003). *C. immitis* is found mainly in California, Arizona, New Mexico, and Texas. *B. dermatitidis* exists in the southeastern United States and in the Ohio, St. Lawrence, and Mississippi River basins. It is a risk for coal miners, construction workers, and farmers. *C. neoformans* is associated with exposure to bird droppings and may be seen in bird handlers.

Pathophysiology

The fungal spores enter the body via inhalation. They initially infect the lungs, causing vague respiratory symptoms or pneumonitis. The fungi may enter the bloodstream, causing a fungemia. If the fungemia overwhelms the person's immune system, the fungus may spread to the CNS. The fungal invasion may cause meningitis, encephalitis, or brain abscess (Goetz, 2003).

Clinical Manifestations

The common symptoms of fungal encephalitis include fever, malaise, headache, meningeal signs, and change in LOC or cranial nerve dysfunction. Symptoms of increased ICP related to hydrocephalus often occur. *C. neoformans* and *C. immitis* are associated with specific skin lesions. *H. capsulatum* is associated with seizures, and *A. fumigatus* may cause ischemic or hemorrhagic strokes (Goetz, 2003).

Assessment and Diagnostic Findings

A history of immunosuppression associated with AIDS or use of immunosuppressive medications may indicate fungal disease of the brain. Occupational and travel history may point to a fungal cause of CNS infection. Infections caused by *H. capsulatum* and *C. immitis* will demonstrate fungal antibodies in serologic tests. The CSF usually demonstrates elevated white cell and protein levels; glucose levels are decreased. *C. neoformans* is easily identified in CSF fungal cultures. *Candida* may be cultured from the blood or CSF. Cisternal or ventricular cultures of CSF may need to be obtained to identify *B. dermatitidis. A. fumigatus* is difficult to isolate in CSF and is diagnosed by lung biopsy (Goetz, 2003). Neuroimaging is used to identify CNS changes related to fungal infection. MRI is the study of choice; it demonstrates areas of hemorrhage, abscess, or enhanced meninges indicating inflammation.

Medical Management

Medical management is directed at the causative fungus and the neurologic consequences of the infection. Seizures are controlled by standard antiseizure medications. Increased

ICP is controlled by repeated lumbar punctures or shunting of CSF.

Antifungal agents are administered for a specific period to cure the infection in patients with competent immune systems. Patients with compromised immune systems receive antifungal therapy until the infection is controlled, after which they receive a maintenance dose of the medication for an indefinite period.

Although the dose and duration of treatment depend on the causative fungi, amphotericin B is the standard antifungal agent used in treatment (Karch, 2005). Dosing depends on the causative organism, and it is usually administered IV. The most common adverse reactions are fever, chills, body aches, and hypotension. Renal insufficiency is a serious reaction to amphotericin B that can occur. Fluconazole (Diflucan) or flucytosine (Ancobon) may be administered orally in conjunction with amphotericin B as maintenance therapy. Potential side effects of fluconazole include nausea, vomiting, and a transient increase in liver enzymes. The most common adverse reaction to flucytosine is bone marrow suppression. Therefore, patients receiving flucytosine should have leukocyte and platelet counts monitored regularly.

Nursing Management

The ICP will increase if hydrocephalus develops and the inflammatory response progresses. Nursing assessment aimed at early identification of increased ICP is necessary to ensure early control and management. (See Chapter 61 for management of the patient with increased ICP.) Administering nonopioid analgesics, limiting environmental stimuli, and positioning may optimize patient comfort. Administering diphenhydramine (Benadryl) and acetaminophen (Tylenol) approximately 30 minutes before giving amphotericin B may prevent flu-like side effects. If renal insufficiency develops, the dose may need to be reduced. Increasing levels of serum creatinine and blood urea nitrogen (BUN) may alert the nurse to the development of renal insufficiency and the need to address the patient's renal status.

Providing support assists the patient and family to cope with the illness. Work-up of the patient for immunodeficiency diseases such as AIDS may put additional stress on the family. The nurse may need to mobilize community support systems for the patient and family, because the recovery may be long.

Creutzfeldt-Jakob and Variant Creutzfeldt-Jakob Disease

Creutzfeldt-Jakob disease (CJD) and variant Creutzfeldt-Jakob (vCJD) disease belong to a group of degenerative, infectious neurologic disorders called transmissible spongiform encephalopathies (TSE). CJD is very rare and has no identifiable cause. vCJD is the human variation of bovine spongiform encephalopathy (BSE); it results from the ingestion by humans of prions in infected beef. TSEs are caused by **prions**, proteinaceous particles that are smaller than a virus and are resistant to standard methods of sterilization. Although CJD and vCJD have distinct clinical features, one characteristic they share is a lack of CNS inflammation. CJD may lie dormant for decades before causing neurologic degeneration. The incubation period of vCJD seems to be shorter (less than 10 years). It is not known whether an increased number of cases will appear in the future. In both diseases, the symptoms are progressive, there is no definitive treatment, and the outcome is fatal.

The risk of vCJD in the United States is thought to be low, because cattle are fed primarily with soy-derived feed, as opposed to feed containing animal parts. By December 2002, 121 people had died in Europe from vCJD; the number of cases has decreased since that time (Andrews, Farrington, Ward, et al., 2003).

Pathophysiology

The prion is a unique pathogen because it lacks nucleic acid, which enables the organism to withstand conventional means of sterilization. The ability of the prion to replicate in the absence of nucleic acid remains a mystery (Glatzel, Stoeck, Seeger, et al., 2005). In both CJD and vCJD, the prion crosses the blood–brain barrier and is deposited in brain tissue. The prion causes degeneration of brain tissue. Cell death occurs, and spongy vacuoles are produced in the brain (**spongiform** changes). The spongiform vacuoles are surrounded by amyloid plaque, a condition unique to vCJD.

Ninety percent of the cases of CJD appear sporadically; the incidence is 1 case per 1 million people (Goetz, 2003). Although it is not transmittable by typical human contact, 5% of cases of sporadic CJD result from contaminated neurosurgical instruments, cadaver-derived growth factor, or corneal transplants (Goetz, 2003).Ten percent of cases appear to be familial.

In the mid-1980s, BSE was identified in dairy cattle herds in the United Kingdom. One third of the cattle were infected, and 200,000 animals died of the disease. Researchers believed that BSE would not be transmitted to humans; however, in 1996 the first case of vCJD was described (Belkin, 2003). The mode of transmission was linked to the ingestion of beef contaminated with neurologic tissue. All of the people who have developed vCJD have a specific, shared genotype (Goetz, 2003).

In 1998, additional concerns were raised about the safety of the blood supply in the United Kingdom. The prion exists in lymphoid tissue and blood in both vCJD and CJD. Both prion diseases are believed to be bloodborne. No method is available to screen blood for infectivity. The American Red Cross will not accept blood from anyone who has traveled to Europe in the past 6 months (Fontenot, 2003).

Clinical Manifestations

CJD and vCJD have several clinically distinct features. Psychiatric symptoms occur early in vCJD, whereas they are a late symptom in CJD. The mean age at onset of vCJD is 27 years, whereas the mean age for CJD onset is 50 years (Belkin, 2003). The presenting symptoms of vCJD include affective symptoms, sensory disturbance, and limb pain. Muscle spasms and rigidity, dysarthria, incoordination, cognitive impairment, and sleep disturbances follow (Fontenot, 2003; Goetz, 2003). Patients with sporadic CJD present with mental deterioration, ataxia, and visual disturbance. Memory loss, involuntary movement, paralysis, and mutism occur as the disease progresses. After clinical presentation, people with vCJD survive an average of 14 months. The patient with CJD survives about 6 months after clinical presentation (Belkin, 2003; Goetz, 2003).

Assessment and Diagnostic Findings

Historically, brain biopsy was used to diagnose CJD. The three diagnostic tests currently used in suspicious clinical presentations to support the diagnosis of CJD are immunologic assessment, electroencephalography, and MRI scanning. Immunologic assessment of CSF detects a protein kinase inhibitor called 14-3-3. The presence of this inhibitor indicates neuronal cell death, which is not specific to CJD but does support the diagnosis. The electroencephalogram (EEG) reveals a characteristic pattern over the duration of the disease. After initial slowing, the EEG shows periodic activity. Later in the course of the disease, the EEG shows burst-suppressions characterized by periodic spikes alternating with slow periods. The MRI scan demonstrates symmetric or unilateral hyperintense signals arising from the basal ganglia.

Patients with vCJD do not demonstrate EEG or CSF changes, and the MRI scan shows bilateral hyperintensity of the posterior thalamus (Goetz, 2003). The prion associated with vCJD has been shown to accumulate in the tonsils and other lymphoreticular tissues; therefore, tonsillar biopsy may be used in the diagnosis of vCJD (Belkin, 2003).

Medical Management

After the onset of specific neurologic symptoms, progression of disease occurs quickly. There is no effective treatment for CJD or vCJD. The care of the patient is supportive and palliative. Goals of care include prevention of injury related to immobility and dementia, promotion of patient comfort, and provision of support and education for the family.

Nursing Management

The nursing care of patients is primarily supportive and palliative. Psychological and emotional support of the patient and family throughout the course of the illness is needed. Care extends to providing for a dignified death and supporting the family through the processes of grief and loss. Hospice services are appropriate either at home or at an inpatient facility. See Chapter 17 for an in-depth discussion of end-of-life issues.

Prevention of disease transmission is an important part of nursing care. Although patient isolation is not necessary, use of standard precautions is important. Institutional protocols are followed for blood and body fluid exposure and decontamination of equipment. In the operating room, it is recommended that disposable instruments be used and then incinerated, because conventional methods of sterilization do not destroy the prion (Bader & Littlejohns, 2004). The World Health Organization has guidelines that outline the stringent sterilization methods that must be used to destroy prions on surfaces (Brown & Merritt, 2003).

Autoimmune Processes

Autoimmune nervous system disorders include multiple sclerosis, myasthenia gravis, and Guillain-Barré syndrome.

Multiple Sclerosis

Multiple sclerosis (MS) is an immune-mediated, progressive demyelinating disease of the CNS. Demyelination refers to the destruction of myelin, the fatty and protein material that surrounds certain nerve fibers in the brain and spinal cord; it results in impaired transmission of nerve impulses (Fig. 64-2). MS may occur at any age but typically manifests in young adults between the ages of 20 and 40 years; it affects women more frequently than men (Holland & Madonna, 2005).

The cause of MS is an area of ongoing research. Autoimmune activity results in demyelination, but the sensitized antigen has not been identified. Multiple factors play a role in the initiation of the immune process. Geographic prevalence is highest in all of Europe, New Zealand, southern Australia, the northern United States, and southern Canada (Olek, 2005). Researchers believe that some environmental exposure at a young age may play a role in the development of MS later in life.

Genetic predisposition is indicated by the presence of a specific cluster (haplotype) of human leukocyte antigens

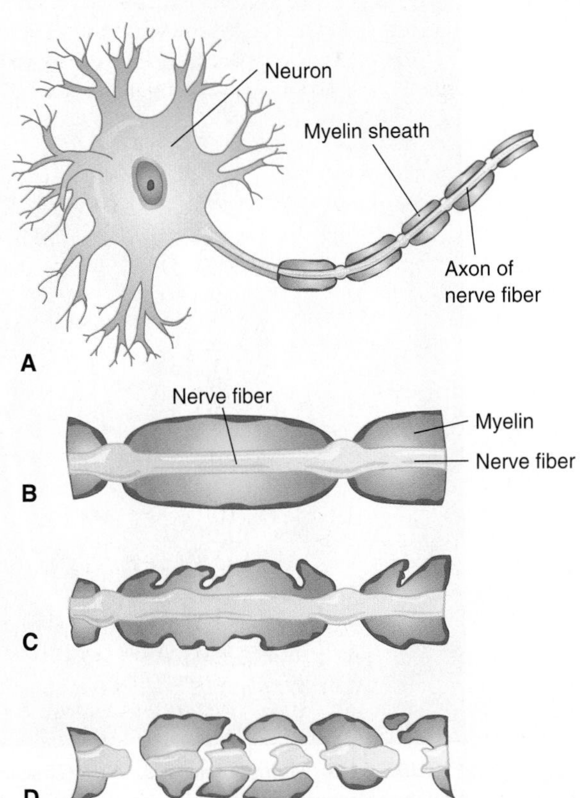

FIGURE 64-2. The process of demyelination. **A** and **B** depict a normal nerve cell and axon with myelin. **C** and **D** show the slow disintegration of myelin, resulting in a disruption in axon function.

(HLA) on the cell wall. The presence of this haplotype may promote susceptibility to factors, such as viruses, that trigger the autoimmune response activated in MS. A specific virus capable of initiating the autoimmune response has not been identified. It is believed that DNA on the virus mimics the amino acid sequence of myelin, resulting in an immune system cross-reaction in the presence of a defective immune system (Holland & Madonna, 2005).

Pathophysiology

Sensitized T cells typically cross the blood–brain barrier; their function is to check the CNS for antigens and then leave. In MS, the sensitized T cells remain in the CNS and promote the infiltration of other agents that damage the immune system (Rosen & Geha, 2004). The immune system attack leads to inflammation that destroys myelin (which normally insulates the axon and speeds the conduction of impulses along the axon) and the oligodendroglial cells that produce myelin in the CNS.

Demyelination interrupts the flow of nerve impulses and results in a variety of manifestations, depending on the nerves affected. Plaques appear on demyelinated axons, further interrupting the transmission of impulses. Demyelinated axons are scattered irregularly throughout the CNS (Fig. 64-3). The areas most frequently affected are the optic nerves, chiasm, and tracts; the cerebrum; the brain stem and cerebellum; and the spinal cord. Eventually, the axons themselves begin to degenerate, resulting in permanent and irreversible damage (Holland & Madonna, 2005).

Clinical Manifestations

The course of MS may assume many different patterns (Fig. 64-4) (Lublin & Reingold, 1996). In some patients, the disease follows a benign course and symptoms are so mild that the patient does not seek health care or treatment. Between 80% and 85% of patients with MS have a relapsing remitting (RR) course. With each relapse, recovery is usually complete; however residual deficits may occur and accumulate over time, contributing to functional decline. Fifty percent of those with the RR course of MS progress to a secondary progressive course, in which disease progression occurs with or without relapses. Ten percent of patients have a primary progressive course, in which disabling symptoms steadily increase, with rare plateaus and temporary improvement (Cohen & Rudick, 2003). Primary progressive MS may result in quadriparesis, cognitive dysfunction, visual loss, and brain stem syndromes. The least common presentation (about 5% of cases) is the progressive relapsing course. It is characterized by relapses with continuous disabling progression between exacerbations (Kieseier & Hartung, 2003).

The signs and symptoms of MS are varied and multiple, reflecting the location of the lesion (plaque) or combination of lesions. The primary symptoms most commonly reported

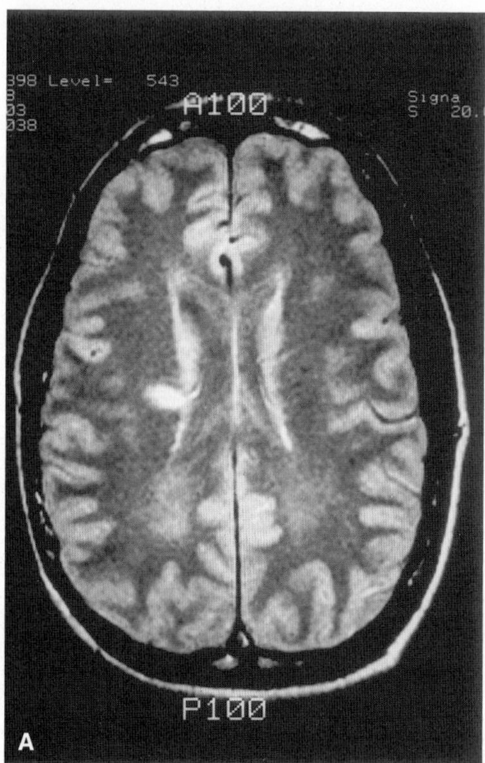

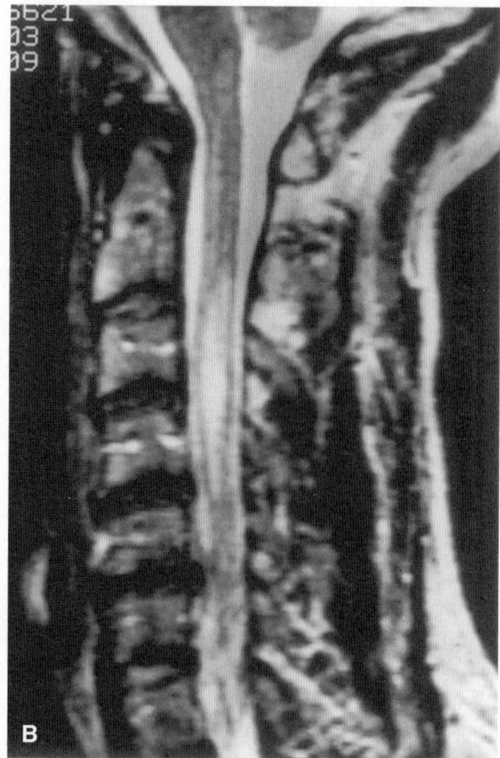

FIGURE 64-3. Multiple sclerosis. (**A**) A CT scan of brain demonstrates an area of demyelination in the periventricular white matter of the right frontal lobe. The plaque is perpendicular to the lateral ventricle, a typical finding in MS. (**B**) An MRI of the spinal cord in the same patient highlights another typical finding: a flame-shaped area of demyelination within the midcervical region of the spinal cord. Courtesy of the Danbury Hospital Department of Radiology.

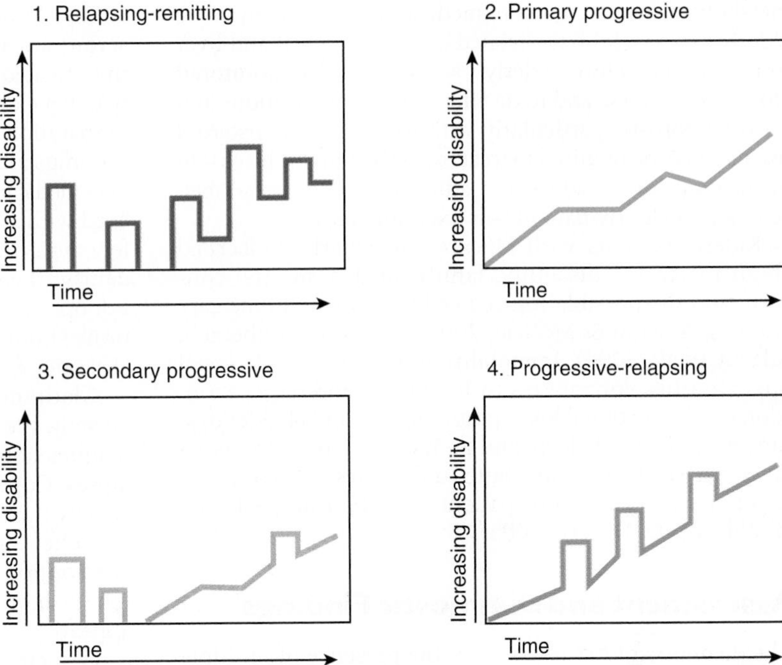

FIGURE 64-4. Types and courses of MS. 1. Relapsing remitting (RR) MS is characterized by clearly acute attacks with full recovery or with sequelae and residual deficit upon recovery. Periods between disease relapses are characterized by lack of disease progression. 2. Primary progressive (PP) MS is characterized by disease showing progression of disability from onset, without plateaus or remissions or with occasional plateaus and temporary minor improvements. 3. Secondary progressive (SP) MS begins with an initial RR course, followed by progression of variable rate, which may also include occasional relapses and minor remissions. 4. Progressive-relapsing (PR) MS shows progression from onset but with clear acute relapses with or without recovery. From Lublin, F. D. & Reingold, F. C. (1996). Defining the clinical course of multiple sclerosis: Results of an international survey. *Neurology, 46*(64), 907–911. Used with permission from Lippincott Williams & Wilkins.

are fatigue, depression, weakness, numbness, difficulty in coordination, loss of balance, and pain. Visual disturbances due to lesions in the optic nerves or their connections may include blurring of vision, **diplopia** (double vision), patchy blindness (scotoma), and total blindness.

Fatigue affects 87% of people with MS; 40% of that group indicate that fatigue is the most disabling symptom (Racke, Hawker & Frohman, 2004). Fatigue is defined as a subjective lack of physical or mental energy that interferes with desired activity. Depression, heat, anemia, deconditioning, and medication may contribute to fatigue. Recent studies indicate that the degree of axonal damage correlates with fatigue; therefore, medications that reduce the frequency of relapse may control the feeling of fatigue (Tartaglia, Narayanan, Francis, et al., 2004). Avoiding hot temperatures, effective treatment of depression and anemia, and physical therapy may control fatigue.

Like fatigue, pain is a symptom that can contribute to social isolation. The report of pain among patients with MS is variable, between 30% and 90% (Svendsen, Jensen, Overvad, et al., 2003). Lesions on the sensory pathways cause pain. Additional sensory manifestations include paresthesias, dysesthesias, and proprioception loss (Stern, 2005). Many people with MS need daily analgesics. In some cases, pain is managed with opioids, antiseizure medication, or antidepressants. Rarely, surgery may be needed to interrupt pain pathways.

Among perimenopausal women, those with MS are more likely to have pain related to osteoporosis. In addition to estrogen loss, immobility and corticosteroid therapy play a role in the development of osteoporosis among women with MS. Bone mineral density testing is recommended for this high-risk group (Smeltzer, Zimmerman & Capriotti, 2005). Diagnosis and treatment of osteoporosis are discussed in Chapter 68.

Spasticity (muscle hypertonicity) of the extremities and loss of the abdominal reflexes result from involvement of the main motor pathways (pyramidal tracts) of the spinal cord. Disruption of the sensory axons may produce sensory dysfunction (paresthesias, pain). Cognitive and psychosocial problems may reflect frontal or parietal lobe involvement. Some degree of cognitive change (eg, memory loss, decreased concentration) occurs in about half of patients, but severe cognitive changes with dementia (progressive organic mental disorder) are rare.

Involvement of the cerebellum or basal ganglia can produce **ataxia** (impaired coordination of movements) and tremor. Loss of the control connections between the cortex and the basal ganglia may occur and cause emotional lability and euphoria. Bladder, bowel, and sexual dysfunctions are common.

Secondary complications of MS include urinary tract infections, constipation, pressure ulcers, contracture deformities, dependent pedal edema, pneumonia, reactive depression, and decreased bone density. Emotional, social, marital, economic, and vocational problems may also be a consequence of the disease.

Exacerbations and remissions are characteristic of MS. During exacerbations, new symptoms appear and existing ones worsen; during remissions, symptoms decrease or disappear. Relapses may be associated with periods of emotional and physical stress (Holland & Madonna, 2005).

Gerontologic Considerations

The life expectancy for patients with MS is not dramatically different from that of patients without MS; 45% of people with MS are older than 55 years of age (Finlayson, Denend & Hudson, 2004). Patients with MS who are elderly have specific physical and psychosocial challenges. They may have chronic health problems, for which they may be taking additional medications that could interact with medications prescribed for MS. The absorption, distribution, metabolism, and excretion of medications are altered in the elderly as a result of age-related changes in renal and liver functions. Therefore, elderly patients must be monitored closely for adverse and toxic effects of MS medications and for osteoporosis (particularly with frequent corticosteroid use that may be required to treat exacerbations). The cost of medications may lead to poor adherence to the prescribed regimen in elderly patients on fixed incomes.

Elderly patients with MS are particularly concerned about increasing disability, family burden, marital concern, and the possible future need for nursing home care (Courts, Newton & McNeal, 2005; Harrison, Stuifbergen, Adachi, et al., 2004). Immobility resulting in fewer social opportunities contributes to loneliness and depression. Along with functional loss, spasticity, pain and bladder dysfunction, impaired sleep, and an increased need for assistance with self-care contribute to the physical challenges experienced by the elderly patient with MS (Klingbeil, Baer & Wilson, 2004; Stern, 2005).

Assessment and Diagnostic Findings

The diagnosis of MS is based on the presence of multiple plaques in the central nervous system observed with MRI (Kieseier & Hartung, 2003). Electrophoresis of CSF identifies the presence of oligoclonal banding (several bands of immunoglobulin G bonded together, indicating an immune system abnormality). Evoked potential studies can help define the extent of the disease process and monitor changes. Underlying bladder dysfunction is diagnosed by urodynamic studies. Neuropsychological testing may be indicated to assess cognitive impairment. A sexual history helps to identify changes in sexual function.

Medical Management

No cure exists for MS. An individual treatment program is indicated to relieve the patient's symptoms and provide continuing support, particularly for patients with cognitive changes, who may need more structure and support. The goals of treatment are to delay the progression of the disease, manage chronic symptoms, and treat acute exacerbations. Many patients with MS have a stable disease course and require only intermittent treatment, whereas others experience steady progression of their disease. Symptoms requiring intervention include spasticity, fatigue, bladder dysfunction, and ataxia. Management strategies target the various motor and sensory symptoms and effects of immobility that can occur.

Pharmacologic Therapy

Medications prescribed for MS include those for disease modification and those for symptom management. The disease-modifying therapies available to treat MS include immunomodulating therapies and immunosuppressive agents (Burks, 2005).

DISEASE-MODIFYING THERAPIES

The disease-modifying medications reduce the frequency of relapse, the duration of relapse, and the number and size of plaques observed on MRI. All of the medications require injection.

Interferon beta-1a (Rebif) and interferon beta-1b (Betaseron) are administered subcutaneously. Researchers have investigated the clinical effectiveness of beta-1b compared with beta-1a (Barbero, Verdun, Bergui, et al., 2004). Another preparation of interferon beta-1a, Avonex, is administered intramuscularly once a week. Side effects of all the interferon beta medications include flu-like symptoms that can be managed with acetaminophen and ibuprofen and resolve after a few months. Additional side effects include potential liver damage, fetal abnormalities, and depression (Burks, 2005). For optimal control of disability, disease-modifying medications should be started early in the course of the disease (Kieseier & Hartung, 2003; Olek, 2005).

Glatiramer acetate (Copaxone) reduces the rate of relapse in the RR course of MS. It decreases the number of plaques noted on MRI and increases the time between relapses. Copaxone is administered subcutaneously daily. It acts by increasing the antigen-specific suppressor T cells. Side effects and injection site reactions are rare. Copaxone is an option for those with an RR course; however, it may take 6 months for evidence of an immune response to appear.

IV methylprednisolone, the key agent in treating acute relapse in the RR course, shortens the duration of relapse. It exerts anti-inflammatory effects by acting on T cells and cytokines. One gram is administered IV daily for 3 days, followed by an oral taper of prednisone (Kieseier & Hartung, 2003). Side effects include mood swings, weight gain, and electrolyte imbalances.

The medication mitoxantrone (Novantrone) is administered via IV infusion every 3 months. Novantrone can reduce the frequency of clinical relapses in patients with secondary-progressive or worsening relapsing-remitting MS. Patients must be very closely monitored for side effects, especially cardiac toxicity (Karch, 2005).

SYMPTOM MANAGEMENT

Medications are also prescribed for management of specific symptoms. Baclofen (Lioresal), a gamma-aminobutyric acid (GABA) agonist, is the medication of choice for treating spasticity. It can be administered orally or by intrathecal injection. Benzodiazepines (Valium), tizanidine (Zanaflex), and dantrolene (Dantrium) may also be used to treat spasticity. Patients with disabling spasms and contractures may require nerve blocks or surgical intervention. Fatigue that interferes with activities of daily living (ADLs) may be treated with amantadine (Symmetrel), pemoline (Cylert), or fluoxetine (Prozac). Ataxia is a chronic problem most resistant to treatment. Medications used to treat ataxia include beta-adrenergic blockers (Inderal), antiseizure agents (Neurontin), and benzodiazepines (Klonopin).

Bladder and bowel problems are often among the most difficult ones for patients, and a variety of medications (anticholinergics, alpha-adrenergic blockers, antispasmodic agents) may be prescribed. Nonpharmacologic strategies also assist in establishing effective bowel and bladder elimination (see later discussion).

Urinary tract infection is often superimposed on the underlying neurologic dysfunction. Ascorbic acid (vitamin C) may be prescribed to acidify the urine, making bacterial growth less likely. Antibiotics are prescribed when appropriate.

Nursing Process

The Patient With Multiple Sclerosis

Assessment

Nursing assessment addresses actual and potential problems associated with the disease, including neurologic deficits, secondary complications, and the impact of the disease on the patient and family. The patient's mobility and balance are observed to determine whether there is danger of falling. Assessment of function is carried out both when the patient is well rested and when he or she is fatigued. The patient is assessed for weakness, spasticity, visual impairment, incontinence, and disorders of swallowing and speech. Additional areas of assessment include the following:

- How has MS affected the patient's lifestyle?
- How well is the patient coping?
- What would the patient like to do better?

Diagnosis

Nursing Diagnoses

Based on the assessment data, the patient's major nursing diagnoses may include the following:

- Impaired bed and physical mobility related to weakness, muscle paresis, spasticity
- Risk for injury related to sensory and visual impairment
- Impaired urinary and bowel elimination (urgency, frequency, incontinence, constipation) related to nervous system dysfunction
- Impaired verbal communication and risk for aspiration related to cranial nerve involvement
- Disturbed thought processes (loss of memory, dementia, euphoria) related to cerebral dysfunction
- Ineffective individual coping related to uncertainty of course of MS
- Impaired home maintenance management related to physical, psychological, and social limits imposed by MS
- Potential for sexual dysfunction related to lesions or psychological reaction

Planning and Goals

The major goals for the patient may include promotion of physical mobility, avoidance of injury, achievement of bladder and bowel continence, promotion of speech and swallowing mechanisms, improvement of cognitive function, development of coping strengths, improved home maintenance management, and adaptation to sexual dysfunction.

Nursing Interventions

An individualized program of physical therapy, rehabilitation, and education is combined with emotional support. An educational plan of care is developed to enable the person with MS to deal with the physiologic, social, and psychological problems that accompany chronic disease.

Promoting Physical Mobility

Relaxation and coordination exercises promote muscle efficiency. Progressive resistive exercises are used to strengthen weak muscles, because diminishing muscle strength is often significant in MS.

EXERCISES

Walking improves the gait, particularly the problem of loss of position sense of the legs and feet. If certain muscle groups are irreversibly affected, other muscles can be trained to compensate. Instruction in the use of assistive devices may be needed to ensure their safe and correct use.

MINIMIZING SPASTICITY AND CONTRACTURES

Muscle spasticity is common and, in its later stages, is characterized by severe adductor spasm of the hips with flexor spasm of the hips and knees. Without relief, fibrous contractures of these joints will occur. Warm packs may be beneficial, but hot baths should be avoided because of risk for burn injury secondary to sensory loss and increasing symptoms that may occur with elevation of the body temperature.

Daily exercises for muscle stretching are prescribed to minimize joint contractures. Special attention is given to the hamstrings, gastrocnemius muscles, hip adductors, biceps, and wrist and finger flexors. Muscle spasticity is common and interferes with normal function. A stretch–hold–relax routine is helpful for relaxing and treating muscle spasticity. Swimming and stationary bicycling are useful, and progressive weight bearing can relieve spasticity in the legs. The patient should not be hurried in any of these activities, because this often increases spasticity.

ACTIVITY AND REST

The patient is encouraged to work and exercise to a point just short of fatigue. Very strenuous physical exercise is not advisable, because it raises the body temperature and may aggravate symptoms. The patient is advised to take frequent short rest periods, preferably lying down. Extreme fatigue may contribute to the exacerbation of symptoms.

MINIMIZING EFFECTS OF IMMOBILITY

Because of the decrease in physical activity that often occurs with MS, complications associated with immobility, including pressure ulcers, expiratory muscle weakness, and accumulation of bronchial secretions, need to be considered and steps taken to prevent them. Measures to prevent such complications include assessing and maintaining skin integrity and having the patient perform coughing and deep-breathing exercises.

Preventing Injury

If motor dysfunction causes problems of incoordination and clumsiness, or if ataxia is apparent, the patient is at risk for falling. To overcome this disability, the patient is taught to walk with feet apart to widen the base of support and to increase walking stability. If loss of position sense occurs, the patient is taught to watch the feet while walking. Gait training may require assistive devices (walker, cane, braces, crutches, parallel bars) and instruction about their use by a physical therapist. If the gait remains inefficient, a wheelchair or motorized scooter may be the solution. The occupational therapist is a valuable resource person in suggesting and securing aids to promote independence. If incoordination is a problem and tremor of the upper extremities occurs when voluntary movement is attempted (intention tremor), weighted bracelets or wrist cuffs are helpful. The patient is trained in transfer and activities of daily living (ADLs).

Because sensory loss may occur in addition to motor loss, pressure ulcers are a continuing threat to skin integrity. The need to use a wheelchair continuously increases the risk. See Chapter 11 for a discussion of the prevention and treatment of pressure ulcers.

Enhancing Bladder and Bowel Control

Generally, bladder symptoms fall into the following categories: (1) inability to store urine (hyperreflexic, uninhibited); (2) inability to empty the bladder (hyporeflexic, hypotonic); and (3) a mixture of both types. The patient with urinary frequency, urgency, or incontinence requires special support. The sensation of the need to void must be heeded immediately, so the bedpan or urinal should be readily available. A voiding time schedule is set up (every 1.5 to 2 hours initially, with gradual lengthening of the interval). The patient is instructed to drink a measured amount of fluid every 2 hours and then attempt to void 30 minutes after drinking. Use of a timer or wristwatch with an alarm may be helpful for the patient who does not have enough sensation to signal the need to empty the bladder. The nurse encourages the patient to take the prescribed medications to treat bladder spasticity, because this allows greater independence. Intermittent self-catheterization (see Chapter 11) has been successful in maintaining bladder control in patients with MS. If a female patient has permanent urinary incontinence, urinary diversion procedures may be considered. The male patient may wear a condom appliance for urine collection.

Bowel problems include constipation, fecal impaction, and incontinence. Adequate fluids, dietary fiber, and a bowel-training program are frequently effective in solving these problems. See Chapter 11 for a discussion of promoting bowel continence.

Enhancing Communication and Managing Swallowing Difficulties

If the cranial nerves that control the mechanisms of speech and swallowing are affected, dysarthrias (defects of articulation) marked by slurring, low volume of speech, and difficulties in phonation may occur. **Dysphagia** (difficulty swallowing) may also occur. A speech therapist evaluates speech and swallowing and instructs the patient, family, and health team members about strategies to compensate for speech and swallowing problems. The nurse reinforces this instruction and encourages the patient and family to adhere to the plan. Impaired swallowing increases the patient's risk for aspiration; therefore, strategies are needed to reduce that risk. Such strategies include having suction apparatus available, careful feeding, and proper positioning for eating.

Improving Sensory and Cognitive Function

Measures may be taken if visual defects or changes in cognitive status occur.

VISION

The cranial nerves affecting vision may be affected by MS. An eye patch or a covered eyeglass lens may be used to block the visual impulses of one eye if the patient has diplopia (double vision). Prism glasses may be helpful for patients who are confined to bed and have difficulty reading in the supine position. People who are unable to read regular-print materials are eligible for the free "talking book" services of the Library of Congress or may obtain large-print or audio books from local libraries.

COGNITION AND EMOTIONAL RESPONSES

Cognitive impairment and emotional lability occur early in MS in some patients and may impose numerous stresses on the patient and family. Some patients with MS are forgetful and easily distracted and may exhibit emotional lability.

Patients adapt to illness in a variety of ways, including denial, depression, withdrawal, and hostility. Emotional support assists patients and their families to adapt to the changes and uncertainties associated with MS and to cope with the disruption in their lives. The patient is assisted to set meaningful and realistic goals, to remain as active as possible, and to keep up social interests and activities. Hobbies may help the patient's morale and provide satisfying interests if the disease progresses to the stage in which formerly enjoyed activities can no longer be pursued.

The family should be made aware of the nature and degree of cognitive impairment. The environment is kept structured, and lists and other memory aids are used to help the patient with cognitive changes to maintain a daily routine. The occupational therapist can be helpful in formulating a structured daily routine.

STRENGTHENING COPING MECHANISMS

The diagnosis of MS is always distressing to the patient and family. They need to know that no two patients with MS have identical symptoms or courses of illness. Although some patients do experience significant disability early, others have a near-normal lifespan with minimal disability. Some families, however, face overwhelming frustrations and problems. MS affects people who are often in a productive stage of life and concerned about career and family responsibilities. Family conflict, disintegration, separation, and divorce are not uncommon. Often, very young family members assume the responsibility of caring for a parent with MS. Nursing interventions in this area include alleviating stress and making appropriate referrals for counseling and support to minimize the adverse effects of dealing with chronic illness.

The nurse, mindful of these complex problems, initiates home care and coordinates a network of services, including social services, speech therapy, physical therapy, and homemaker services. To strengthen the patient's coping skills, as much information as possible is provided. Patients need an updated list of available assistive devices, services, and resources.

Coping through problem solving involves helping the patient define the problem and develop alternatives for its management. Careful planning and maintaining flexibility and a hopeful attitude are useful for psychological and physical adaptation.

Improving Home Management

MS can affect every facet of daily living. Certain abilities are often impossible to regain after they are lost. Physical function may vary from day to day. Modifications that allow independence in home management should be implemented (eg, assistive eating devices, raised toilet seat, bathing aids, telephone modifications, long-handled comb, tongs, modified clothing). Exposure to heat increases fatigue and muscle weakness, so air conditioning is recommended in at least one room. Exposure to extreme cold may increase spasticity.

Promoting Sexual Functioning

Patients with MS and their partners face problems that interfere with sexual activity, both as a direct consequence of nerve damage and also from psychological reactions to the disease. Easy fatigability, conflicts arising from dependency and depression, emotional lability and loss of self-esteem compound the problem. Erectile and ejaculatory disorders in men and orgasmic dysfunction and adductor spasms of the thigh muscles in women can make sexual intercourse difficult or impossible. Bladder and bowel incontinence and urinary tract infections add to the difficulties.

An experienced sexual counselor helps bring into focus the patient's or partner's sexual resources and suggests relevant information and supportive therapy. Sharing and communicating feelings, planning for sexual activity (to minimize the effects of fatigue), and exploring alternative methods of sexual expression may open up a wide range of sexual enjoyment and experiences.

Promoting Home and Community-Based Care

TEACHING PATIENTS SELF-CARE

As the disease progresses, the patient and family need to learn new strategies to maintain optimal independence. Teaching of new self-care techniques may be initiated in the hospital or clinic setting and reinforced in the home. Self-care education may address the use of assistive devices, self-catheterization, and administration of medications that affect the course of the disease or treat complications. A teaching plan that addresses intramuscular or subcutaneous administration of medications is developed for the patient and his or her family. Exercises that enable the patient to continue some form of activity or that maintain or improve swallowing, speech, or respiratory function may be taught to the patient and family (Chart 64-3).

CONTINUING CARE

After discharge, the home care nurse often provides teaching and reinforcement of new interventions in the patient's home. Nurses in the home setting assess for changes in the patient's physical and emotional status, provide physical care to the patient if required, coordinate outpatient services and resources, and encourage health promotion, appropriate health screenings, and adaptation. Research has identified decreased financial and interpersonal resources as barriers to health promotion (Becker & Stuifbergen, 2004). If changes in the disease or its course are noted, the home care nurse encourages the patient to contact the primary care provider, because treatment of an acute exacerbation or new problem may be indicated. Continuing health care and follow-up are recommended.

The patient with MS is encouraged to contact the local chapter of the National Multiple Sclerosis Society for services, publications, and contact with others who have MS (see Resources). Local chapters also provide direct services to patients. Through group participation, the patient has an opportunity to meet others with similar problems, share experiences, and learn self-help methods in a social environment.

Evaluation

Expected Patient Outcomes

Expected patient outcomes may include the following:

1. Improves physical mobility
   a. Participates in gait-training and rehabilitation program
   b. Establishes a balanced program of rest and exercise
   c. Uses assistive devices correctly and safely
2. Is free of injury
   a. Uses visual cues to compensate for decreased sense of touch or position
   b. Asks for assistance when necessary

NURSING RESEARCH PROFILE

The Influence of Marriage in People With Multiple Sclerosis

Harrison, T., Stuifbergen, A., Adachi, E., et al. (2004). Marriage, impairment, and acceptance in persons with multiple sclerosis. *Western Journal of Nursing Research, 26*(3), 266–285.

Purpose

Multiple sclerosis (MS) is a stressful disease for individuals and their marital partners. This study was designed to investigate the relationships between marital status, marital concern, perceived impairment, health-promoting behaviors, and acceptance of disability in people with MS.

Design

This was a longitudinal design using mailed questionnaires. The sample population for this study consisted of 454 people with MS who responded at five time points over a 6-year period. The mean age of men was 50 years, and that of women 47 years. Over the 6-year period 66% ($n = 248$) of women and 72% ($n = 55$) of the men were consistently married. Instruments used included the Acceptance of Illness Scale, Incapacity Status Scale (ISS), Health Promoting Lifestyle Profile–II (HPLP-II), and the Marital Concern Scale. The data were analyzed with Pearson correlations, independent sample *t* tests, and repeated-measures ANOVA.

Findings

The findings indicated that both acceptance of disability and perceived impairment increase significantly over time for men and women ($p \leq .001$). For men, being married was associated with a greater acceptance of disability and less perceived impairment ($p = .02$). Men were more concerned than women about how MS affected their sexual relationships.

Nursing Implications

Nurses working with patients who have MS should be aware that the findings of this study suggest that there is a benefit from being in a marital relationship. Many psychological aspects of chronic illness appear to be handled within the context of the marital relationship. This study also reported that men and women have different marital concerns; for example, men were more concerned than women about how MS affected their sexual relationships. Those who remain married may have a higher acceptance of disability compared to those not consistently married.

CHART 64-3

HOME CARE CHECKLIST • The Patient With Multiple Sclerosis

At the completion of the home care instruction, the patient or caregiver will be able to:	Patient	Caregiver
• State how to access the local chapter of the National MS Society and available resources.	✔	✔
• Discuss the clinical course of MS.	✔	✔
• Identify strategies to manage symptoms (pain, cognitive responses, dysphagia, tremors, visual disturbances).	✔	✔
• State how to prevent complications (pressure ulcers, pneumonia, depression).	✔	✔
• Identify coping strategies.	✔	✔
• Identify ways to minimize fatigue.	✔	✔
• Explain how to prevent injury.	✔	✔
• State ways to adapt to sexual dysfunction.	✔	✔
• Discuss ways to control bowel and bladder function.	✔	✔
• Name benefits of exercise and physical activity.	✔	✔
• Identify ways to minimize immobility and spasticity.	✔	✔
• Describe medication regimen and potential adverse effects.	✔	✔
• Demonstrate correct techniques of administering injectable medications, if prescribed.	✔	✔

3. Attains or maintains control of bladder and bowel patterns
   a. Monitors self for urine retention and employs intermittent self-catheterization technique, if indicated
   b. Identifies the signs and symptoms of urinary tract infection
   c. Maintains adequate fluid and fiber intake
4. Participates in strategies to improve speech and swallowing
   a. Practices exercises recommended by speech therapist
   b. Maintains adequate nutritional intake without aspiration
5. Compensates for altered thought processes
   a. Uses lists and other aids to compensate for memory losses
   b. Discusses problems with trusted advisor or friend
   c. Substitutes new activities for those that are no longer possible
6. Demonstrates effective coping strategies
   a. Maintains sense of control
   b. Modifies lifestyle to fit goals and limitations
   c. Verbalizes desire to pursue goals and developmental tasks of adulthood
7. Adheres to plan for home maintenance management
   a. Uses appropriate techniques to maintain independence
   b. Engages in health promotion activities and health screenings as appropriate
8. Adapts to changes in sexual function
   a. Is able to discuss problem with partner and appropriate health professional
   b. Identifies alternative means of sexual expression

Myasthenia Gravis

Myasthenia gravis, an autoimmune disorder affecting the myoneural junction, is characterized by varying degrees of weakness of the voluntary muscles. Approximately 60,000 people have myasthenia gravis in the United States (Phillips, 2004). Women are affected more frequently than men, and they tend to develop the disease at an earlier age (20 to 40 years of age, versus 60 to 70 years for men) (Scherer, Bedlack & Simel, 2005).

Pathophysiology

Normally, a chemical impulse precipitates the release of acetylcholine from vesicles on the nerve terminal at the myoneural junction. The acetylcholine attaches to receptor sites on the motor endplate and stimulates muscle contraction. Continuous binding of acetylcholine to the receptor site is required for muscular contraction to be sustained.

In myasthenia gravis, antibodies directed at the acetylcholine receptor sites impair transmission of impulses across the myoneural junction (Rosen & Geha, 2004). Therefore, fewer receptors are available for stimulation, resulting in voluntary muscle weakness that escalates with continued activity (Fig. 64-5). These antibodies are found in 80% to 90% of the people with myasthenia gravis (Scherer et al., 2005). Eighty percent of people with myasthenia gravis have either thymic hyperplasia or a thymic tumor, and the thymus gland is believed to be the site of antibody production (Keesey, 2002). In patients who are antibody negative, researchers believe that the offending antibody is directed at a portion of the receptor site rather than the whole complex.

Clinical Manifestations

The initial manifestation of myasthenia gravis usually involves the ocular muscles. Diplopia (double vision) and ptosis (drooping of the eyelids) are common. However, the majority of patients also experience weakness of the muscles of the face and throat (bulbar symptoms) and generalized weakness. Weakness of the facial muscles results in a bland facial expression. Laryngeal involvement produces **dysphonia** (voice impairment) and increases the patient's risk for choking and aspiration. Generalized weakness affects all the extremities and the intercostal muscles, resulting in decreasing vital capacity and respiratory failure. Myasthenia gravis is purely a motor disorder with no effect on sensation or coordination.

Assessment and Diagnostic Findings

An acetylcholinesterase inhibitor test is used to diagnose myasthenia gravis. The acetylcholinesterase inhibitor stops the breakdown of acetylcholine, thereby increasing availability at the neuromuscular junction. Edrophonium chloride (Tensilon), a fast-acting acetylcholinesterase inhibitor, is administered IV to diagnose myasthenia gravis (Scherer et al., 2005). Thirty seconds after injection, facial

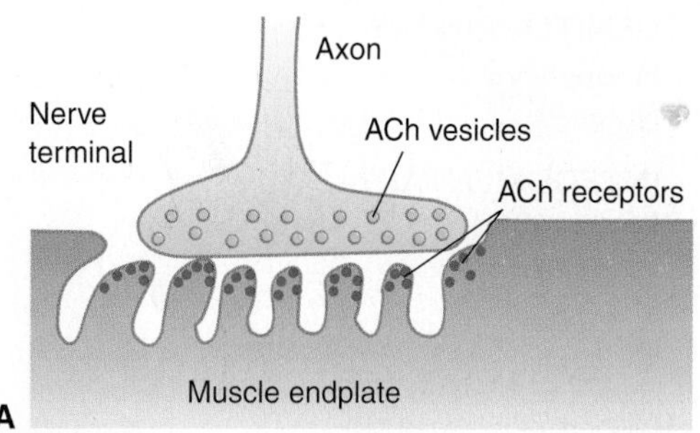

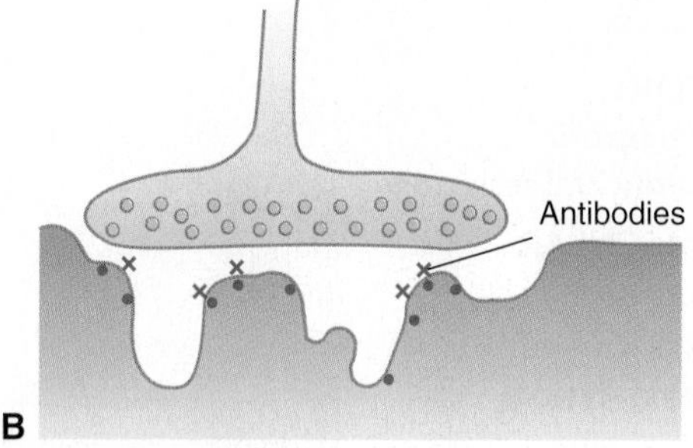

FIGURE 64-5. Myasthenia gravis. (**A**) Normal ACh receptor site. (**B**) ACh receptor site in myasthenia gravis. ACh = acetylcholine.

muscle weakness and ptosis should resolve for about 5 minutes. Immediate improvement in muscle strength after administration of this agent represents a positive test and usually confirms the diagnosis. Atropine should be available to control the side effects of edrophonium, which include bradycardia, sweating, and cramping (Scherer et al., 2005).

The presence of acetylcholine receptor antibodies is identified in serum. Repetitive nerve stimulation demonstrates a decrease in successive action potentials. The thymus gland, a site of acetylcholine receptor antibody production, may be enlarged in myasthenia gravis. An MRI scan is used to identify an enlarged thymus gland (Juel, 2004).

Medical Management

Management of myasthenia gravis is directed at improving function and reducing and removing circulating antibodies. Therapeutic modalities include administration of anticholinesterase medications and immunosuppressive therapy, plasmapheresis, and thymectomy.

Pharmacologic Therapy

Pyridostigmine bromide (Mestinon), an anticholinesterase medication, is the first line of therapy. It provides symptomatic relief by inhibiting the breakdown of acetylcholine and increasing the relative concentration of available acetylcholine at the neuromuscular junction. The dosage is gradually increased to a daily maximum and is administered in divided doses (usually four times a day). Adverse effects of anticholinesterase medications include fasciculations, abdominal pain, diarrhea, and increased oropharyngeal secretions (Saperstein & Barohn, 2004). Pyridostigmine tends to have fewer side effects than other anticholinesterase medications (Chart 64-4).

If pyridostigmine bromide does not improve muscle strength and control fatigue, the next agents used are the immunomodulating drugs. The goal of immunosuppressive therapy is to reduce production of the antibody. Corticosteroids suppress the patient's immune response, decreasing the amount of antibody production, and this correlates with clinical improvement. An initial dose of prednisone is given daily; as symptoms improve, the medication is tapered and a maintenance dose may be given indefinitely (Saperstein & Barohn, 2004). As the corticosteroid dosage is gradually increased, the anticholinesterase dosage is lowered. Cytotoxic medications are used to treat myasthenia gravis if there is inadequate response to steroids. Azathioprine (Imuran) inhibits T lymphocytes and reduces acetylcholine receptor antibody levels. Therapeutic effects may not be evident for 3 to 12 months. Leukopenia and hepatotoxicity are serious adverse effects, so monthly evaluation of liver enzymes and white blood cell count is necessary. Cyclosporine (Neoral) and cyclophosphamide (Cytoxan) may be used, but their side effects are a significant limiting factor (Saperstein & Barohn, 2004).

A number of medications are contraindicated for patients with myasthenia gravis because they exacerbate the symptoms. The physician and the patient should weigh risks and benefits before any new medications are prescribed, including antibiotics, cardiovascular medications, antiseizure and psychotropic medications, morphine, quinine and related agents, beta-blockers, and nonprescription medications. Procaine (Novocain) should be avoided, and the patient's dentist is advised of the diagnosis of myasthenia gravis.

CHART 64-4

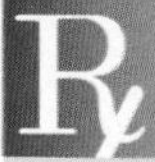

PHARMACOLOGY • *Potential Adverse Effects of Anticholinesterase Medications*

CENTRAL NERVOUS SYSTEM
Irritability
Anxiety
Insomnia
Headache
Dysarthria
Syncope
Seizures
Coma
Diaphoresis

RESPIRATORY
Bronchial relaxation
Increased bronchial secretions

CARDIOVASCULAR
Tachycardia
Hypotension

GASTROINTESTINAL
Abdominal cramps
Nausea
Vomiting
Diarrhea
Anorexia
Increased salivation

SKELETAL MUSCLES
Fasciculations
Spasms
Weakness

GENITOURINARY
Frequency
Urgency

INTEGUMENTARY
Rash
Flushing

Plasmapheresis

Plasmapheresis (plasma exchange) is a technique used to treat exacerbations. The patient's plasma and plasma components are removed through a centrally placed large-bore double-lumen catheter. The blood cells and antibody-containing plasma are separated, after which the cells and a plasma substitute are reinfused. Plasma exchange produces a temporary reduction in the level of circulating antibodies. The typical course of plasmapheresis consists of daily or alternate-day treatment, and the number of treatments is determined by the patient's response. Plasma exchange improves symptoms in 75% of patients; however, improvement lasts only a few weeks after treatment is completed. Cholinesterase inhibitors, corticosteroids, immunosuppressive drugs, or a combination of these are used to sustain improvement (Bader & Littlejohns, 2004). Intravenous immune globulin (IVIG) is also used to treat exacerbations (Dalakas, 2004). Although IVIG is easier than plasmapheresis to administer, the response to plasmapheresis is more rapid. No treatments cure myasthenia gravis, because they do not stop the production of the acetylcholine receptor antibodies.

Surgical Management

Thymectomy (surgical removal of the thymus gland) can produce antigen-specific immunosuppression and result in clinical improvement. The procedure results in either partial or complete remission. A course of preoperative plasmapheresis decreases the time needed for postoperative mechanical ventilation (Juel, 2004). The entire gland must be removed for optimal clinical outcomes; therefore, surgeons prefer the transsternal surgical approach. After surgery, the patient is monitored in an intensive care unit, with special attention to respiratory function. The patient is weaned from mechanical ventilation after thorough respiratory assessment. After the thymus gland is removed, it may take up to 3 years for the patient to benefit from the procedure, because of the long life of circulating T cells (Saperstein & Barohn, 2004).

Complications

Respiratory Failure

A myasthenic crisis is an exacerbation of the disease process characterized by severe generalized muscle weakness and respiratory and bulbar weakness that may result in respiratory failure. Crisis may result from disease exacerbation or a specific precipitating event. The most common precipitator is respiratory infection; others include medication change, surgery, pregnancy, and medications that exacerbate myasthenia. The edrophonium chloride (Tensilon) test is no longer used to diagnose crisis, because it is associated with an increased risk of respiratory arrest in a crisis (Juel, 2004). A cholinergic crisis caused by overmedication with cholinesterase inhibitors is rare; atropine sulfate should be on hand to treat bradycardia or respiratory distress (Juel, 2004).

Neuromuscular respiratory failure is the critical complication in myasthenic and cholinergic crises. Respiratory muscle and bulbar weakness combine to cause respiratory compromise. Weak respiratory muscles do not support inhalation. An inadequate cough and an impaired gag reflex, caused by bulbar weakness, result in poor airway clearance. A downward trend of two respiratory function tests, the negative inspiratory force and vital capacity, is the first clinical sign of respiratory compromise.

Endotracheal intubation and mechanical ventilation may be needed (see Chapter 25). Noninvasive positive-pressure ventilation uses an external device that provides respiratory support without endotracheal intubation (Rabinstein & Wijdicks, 2003). Cholinesterase inhibitors are stopped when respiratory failure occurs and gradually restarted after the patient demonstrates improvement with a course of plasmapheresis or IVIG (Bader & Littlejohns, 2004; Juel, 2004). Nutritional support may be needed if the patient is intubated for a long period.

Nursing Management

Because myasthenia gravis is a chronic disease and most patients are seen on an outpatient basis, much of the nursing care focuses on patient and family teaching. Educational topics for outpatient self-care include medication management, energy conservation, strategies to help with ocular manifestations, and prevention and management of complications.

Medication management is a crucial component of ongoing care. Understanding the actions of the medications and taking them on schedule is emphasized, as are the consequences of delaying medication and the signs and symptoms of myasthenic and cholinergic crises. The patient can determine the best times for daily dosing by keeping a diary to determine fluctuation of symptoms and to learn when the medication is wearing off. The medication schedule can then be manipulated to maximize strength throughout the day.

NURSING ALERT

Maintenance of stable blood levels of anticholinesterase medications is imperative to stabilize muscle strength. Therefore, the anticholinesterase medications must be administered on time. Any delay in administration of medications may exacerbate muscle weakness and make it impossible for the patient to take medications orally.

The patient is also taught strategies to conserve energy. To do this, the nurse helps the patient identify the optimal times for rest throughout the day. If the patient lives in a two-story home, the nurse can suggest that frequently used items (eg, hygiene products, cleaning products, snacks) be kept on each floor to minimize travel between floors. The patient is encouraged to apply for a handicapped license plate, to minimize walking from parking spaces, and to schedule activities to coincide with peak energy and strength levels.

To minimize the risk of aspiration, mealtimes should coincide with the peak effects of anticholinesterase medication. In addition, rest before meals is encouraged, to reduce muscle fatigue. The patient is advised to sit upright during meals, with the neck slightly flexed to facilitate swallowing. Soft foods in gravy or sauces can be swallowed more easily;

if choking occurs frequently, the nurse can suggest puréed food with a pudding-like consistency. Suction should be available at home, with the patient and family instructed in its use. Supplemental feedings may be necessary in some patients to ensure adequate nutrition.

Impaired vision results from ptosis of one or both eyelids, decreased eye movement, or double vision. To prevent corneal damage when the eyelids do not close completely, the patient is instructed to tape the eyes closed for short intervals and to regularly instill artificial tears. Patients who wear eyeglasses can have "crutches" attached to help lift the eyelids. Patching of one eye can help with double vision.

The patient is reminded of the importance of maintaining health promotion practices and of following health care screening recommendations. Factors that exacerbate symptoms and potentially cause crisis should be noted and avoided: emotional stress, infections (particularly respiratory infections), vigorous physical activity, some medications, and high environmental temperature. The Myasthenia Gravis Foundation of America provides support groups, services, and educational materials for patients, families, and health care providers (see Resources).

Myasthenic Crisis

Respiratory distress and varying degrees of dysphagia (difficulty swallowing), dysarthria (difficulty speaking), eyelid ptosis, diplopia, and prominent muscle weakness are symptoms of myasthenic crisis. The patient is placed in an intensive care unit for constant monitoring because of associated intense and sudden fluctuations in clinical condition.

Providing ventilatory assistance takes precedence in the immediate management of the patient with myasthenic crisis. Ongoing assessment for respiratory failure is essential. The nurse assesses the respiratory rate, depth, and breath sounds and monitors pulmonary function parameters (vital capacity and negative inspiratory force) to detect pulmonary problems before respiratory dysfunction progresses. Blood is drawn for arterial blood gas analysis. Endotracheal intubation and mechanical ventilation may be needed (see Chapter 25).

If the abdominal, intercostal, and pharyngeal muscles are severely weak, the patient cannot cough, take deep breaths, or clear secretions. Chest physical therapy, including postural drainage to mobilize secretions and suctioning to remove secretions, may have to be performed frequently. (Postural drainage should not be performed for 30 minutes after feeding.)

Assessment strategies and supportive measures include the following:

- Arterial blood gases, serum electrolytes, input and output, and daily weight are monitored.
- If the patient cannot swallow, nasogastric tube feedings may be prescribed.
- Sedatives and tranquilizers are avoided, because they aggravate hypoxia and hypercapnia and can cause respiratory and cardiac depression.

Guillain-Barré Syndrome

Guillain-Barré syndrome is an autoimmune attack on the peripheral nerve myelin. The result is acute, rapid segmental demyelination of peripheral nerves and some cranial nerves, producing ascending weakness with **dyskinesia** (inability to execute voluntary movements), hyporeflexia, and **paresthesias** (numbness). An antecedent event (most often a viral infection) precipitates clinical presentation. *Campylobacter jejuni,* cytomegalovirus, Epstein-Barr virus, *Mycoplasma pneumoniae, Haemophilus influenzae,* and human immunodeficiency virus (HIV) are the most common infectious agents that are associated with the development of Guillain-Barré syndrome (Kieseier & Hartung, 2003). An increased incidence of Guillain-Barré syndrome occurred after influenza vaccination in 1976–1977; therefore, the syndrome continues to be tracked in the vaccine adverse events reporting system (Haber, DeStefano, Angulo, et al., 2004).

The annual worldwide incidence of Guillain-Barré syndrome is 0.6 to 1.4 cases per 100,000, and it is more frequent in males between 16 and 25 years of age and between 45 and 60 years of age (Whyte, 2003). Results of studies on recovery rates differ, but most indicate that 60% to 75% of patients recover completely. Residual deficits of varying degree occur in 20% to 25% of patients (Cook & Orb, 2003). Residual deficits are most likely in patients with rapid disease progression, those who require mechanical ventilation, and those 60 years of age or older. Death occurs in 5% of cases, resulting from respiratory failure, autonomic dysfunction, sepsis, or pulmonary emboli (Whyte, 2003).

Pathophysiology

Myelin is a complex substance that covers nerves, providing insulation and speeding the conduction of impulses from the cell body to the dendrites. The cell that produces myelin in the peripheral nervous system is the Schwann cell. In Guillain-Barré syndrome, the Schwann cell is spared, allowing for remyelination in the recovery phase of the disease.

Guillain-Barré syndrome is the result of a cell-mediated and humoral immune attack on peripheral nerve myelin proteins that causes inflammatory demyelination. The best-accepted theory of cause is molecular mimicry (Kieseier & Hartung, 2003), in which an infectious organism contains an amino acid that mimics the peripheral nerve myelin protein. The immune system cannot distinguish between the two proteins and attacks and destroys peripheral nerve myelin. The exact location of the immune attack within the peripheral nervous system is the ganglioside GM1b. With the autoimmune attack, there is an influx of macrophages and other immune-mediated agents that attack myelin, cause inflammation and destruction, and leave the axon unable to support nerve conduction (Bader & Littlejohns, 2004).

Clinical Manifestations

Guillain-Barré syndrome typically begins with muscle weakness and diminished reflexes of the lower extremities. Hyporeflexia and weakness may progress to tetraplegia. Demyelination of the nerves that innervate the diaphragm and intercostal muscles results in neuromuscular respiratory failure. Sensory symptoms include paresthesias of the hands and feet and pain related to the demyelination of sensory fibers.

The antecedent event usually occurs 2 weeks before symptoms begin. Weakness usually begins in the legs and progresses upward. Maximum weakness, the plateau, varies in length but usually includes neuromuscular respiratory failure and bulbar weakness. The duration of the symptoms is variable; complete functional recovery may take up to 2 years (Hickey, 2003). Any residual symptoms are permanent and reflect axonal damage from demyelination.

Cranial nerve demyelination can result in a variety of clinical manifestations. Optic nerve demyelination may result in blindness. Bulbar muscle weakness related to demyelination of the glossopharyngeal and vagus nerves results in the inability to swallow or clear secretions. Vagus nerve demyelination results in autonomic dysfunction, manifested by instability of the cardiovascular system. The presentation is variable and may include tachycardia, bradycardia, hypertension, or orthostatic hypotension. The symptoms of autonomic dysfunction occur and resolve rapidly. Guillain-Barré syndrome does not affect cognitive function or level of consciousness.

Although the classic clinical features include areflexia and ascending weakness, variation in presentation occurs. There may be a sensory presentation, with progressive sensory symptoms, an atypical axonal destruction, or the Miller-Fisher variant, which includes paralysis of the ocular muscles, ataxia, and areflexia (Kieseier & Hartung, 2003).

Assessment and Diagnostic Findings

The patient presents with symmetric weakness, diminished reflexes, and upward progression of motor weakness. A history of a viral illness in the previous few weeks suggests the diagnosis. Changes in vital capacity and negative inspiratory force are assessed to identify impending neuromuscular respiratory failure. Serum laboratory tests are not useful in the diagnosis. However, elevated protein levels are detected in CSF evaluation, without an increase in other cells. Evoked potential studies demonstrate a progressive loss of nerve conduction velocity.

Medical Management

Because of the possibility of rapid progression and neuromuscular respiratory failure, Guillain-Barré syndrome is a medical emergency, requiring management in an intensive care unit. After baseline values are identified, assessment of changes in muscle strength and respiratory function alert the clinician to the physical and respiratory needs of the patient. Respiratory therapy or mechanical ventilation may be necessary to support pulmonary function and adequate oxygenation. Some clinicians recommend elective intubation before the onset of extreme respiratory muscle fatigue. Emergent intubation may result in autonomic dysfunction (Rabinstein & Wijdicks, 2003). Mechanical ventilation may be required for an extended period. The patient is weaned from mechanical ventilation after the respiratory muscles can again support spontaneous respiration and maintain adequate tissue oxygenation.

Other interventions are aimed at preventing the complications of immobility. These may include the use of anticoagulant agents and thigh-high elastic compression stockings or sequential compression boots to prevent thrombosis and pulmonary emboli.

Plasmapheresis and IVIG are used to affect directly the peripheral nerve myelin antibody level. Both therapies decrease circulating antibody levels and reduce the amount of time the patient is immobilized and dependent on mechanical ventilation. Studies indicate that IVIG and plasmapheresis are equally effective in treating Guillain-Barré syndrome; however, IVIG is currently the therapy of choice because it is associated with fewer side effects (Dalakas, 2004; Whyte, 2003). The cardiovascular risks posed by autonomic dysfunction require continuous electrocardiographic (ECG) monitoring. Tachycardia and hypertension are treated with short-acting medications such as alpha-adrenergic blocking agents. The use of short-acting agents is important, because autonomic dysfunction is very labile. Hypotension is managed by increasing the amount of IV fluid administered.

Nursing Process

The Patient With Guillain-Barré Syndrome

Assessment

Ongoing assessment for disease progression is critical. The patient is monitored for life-threatening complications (respiratory failure, cardiac dysrhythmias, deep vein thrombosis [DVT]), so that appropriate interventions can be initiated. Because of the threat to the patient in this sudden, potentially life-threatening disease, the nurse must assess the patient's and family's ability to cope and their use of coping strategies.

Diagnosis

Nursing Diagnoses

Based on the assessment data, the patient's major nursing diagnoses may include the following:

- Ineffective breathing pattern and impaired gas exchange related to rapidly progressive weakness and impending respiratory failure
- Impaired bed and physical mobility related to paralysis
- Imbalanced nutrition, less than body requirements, related to inability to swallow
- Impaired verbal communication related to cranial nerve dysfunction
- Fear and anxiety related to loss of control and paralysis

Collaborative Problems/ Potential Complications

Based on the assessment data, potential complications that may develop include the following:

- Respiratory failure
- Autonomic dysfunction

Planning and Goals

The major goals for the patient may include improved respiratory function, increased mobility, improved nutritional status, effective communication, decreased fear and anxiety, and absence of complications.

Nursing Interventions

Maintaining Respiratory Function

Respiratory function can be maximized with incentive spirometry and chest physiotherapy. Monitoring for changes in vital capacity and negative inspiratory force are key to early intervention for neuromuscular respiratory failure. Mechanical ventilation is required if the vital capacity falls, making spontaneous breathing impossible and tissue oxygenation inadequate.

Parameters for determining the appropriate time to begin mechanical ventilation include a vital capacity of less than 15 mL/kg, partial pressure of oxygen (PaO_2) lower than 70 mm Hg, and progressive bulbar weakness (Rabinstein & Wijdicks, 2003). The potential need for mechanical ventilation should be discussed with the patient and family on admission, to provide time for psychological preparation and decision-making. Intubation and mechanical ventilation will result in less anxiety if it is initiated on a nonemergency basis to a well-informed patient. The patient may require mechanical ventilation for a long period. Nursing management of the patient requiring mechanical ventilation is discussed in Chapter 25.

Bulbar weakness that impairs the ability to swallow and clear secretions is another factor in the development of respiratory failure in the patient with Guillain-Barré syndrome. Suctioning may be needed to maintain a clear airway.

The nurse assesses the blood pressure and heart rate frequently to identify autonomic dysfunction, so that interventions can be initiated quickly if needed. Medications are administered or a temporary pacemaker is placed for clinically significant bradycardia (Winer, 2002).

Enhancing Physical Mobility

Nursing interventions to enhance physical mobility and prevent the complications of immobility are key to the function and survival of these patients. The paralyzed extremities are supported in functional positions, and passive range-of-motion exercises are performed at least twice daily. DVT and pulmonary embolism are threats to the paralyzed patient. Nursing interventions are aimed at preventing DVT. Range-of-motion exercises, position changes, anticoagulation, the use of thigh-high elastic compression stockings or sequential compression boots, and adequate hydration decrease the risk for DVT.

Padding may be placed over bony prominences, such as the elbows and heels, to reduce the risk for pressure ulcers. The need for consistent position changes every 2 hours cannot be overemphasized. The nurse evaluates laboratory test results that may indicate malnutrition or dehydration, both of which increase the risk for pressure ulcers. The nurse collaborates with the physician and dietitian to develop a plan to meet the patient's nutritional and hydration needs.

Providing Adequate Nutrition

Paralytic ileus may result from insufficient parasympathetic activity. In this event, the nurse administers IV fluids and parenteral nutrition as prescribed and monitors for the return of bowel sounds. If the patient cannot swallow due to **bulbar paralysis** (immobility of muscles), a gastrostomy tube may be placed to administer nutrients. The nurse carefully assesses the return of the gag reflex and bowel sounds before resuming oral nutrition.

Improving Communication

Because of paralysis, the patient cannot talk, laugh, or cry and therefore has no method for communicating needs or expressing emotion. Establishing some form of communication with picture cards or an eye blink system provides a means of communication. Collaboration with the speech therapist may be helpful in developing a communication mechanism that is most effective for a specific patient.

Decreasing Fear and Anxiety

The patient and family are faced with a sudden, potentially life-threatening disease, and anxiety and fear are constant themes for them. The impact of disease on the family depends on the patient's role within the family. Referral to a support group may provide information and support to the patient and family.

The family may feel helpless in caring for the patient. Mechanical ventilation and monitoring devices may frighten and intimidate them. Family members often want to participate in physical care; with instruction and support by the nurse, they should be allowed to do so.

In addition to fear, the patient may experience isolation, loneliness, and lack of control. Nursing interventions that increase the patient's sense of control include providing information about the condition, emphasizing a positive appraisal of coping resources, and teaching relaxation exercises and distraction techniques. The positive attitude and atmosphere of the multidisciplinary team are important to promote a sense of well-being.

Diversional activities are encouraged to decrease loneliness and isolation. Encouraging visitors, engaging visitors or volunteers to read to the patient, listening to music or books on tape, and watching television are ways to alleviate the patient's sense of isolation.

Monitoring and Managing Potential Complications

Thorough assessment of respiratory function at regular and frequent intervals is essential, because respiratory insufficiency and subsequent failure due to weakness or paralysis of the intercostal muscles and diaphragm may develop quickly. Respiratory failure is the major cause of mortality, which is reported to be as high as 20% (Rabinstein & Wijdicks, 2003). In addition to the respiratory rate and the quality of respirations, vital capacity is monitored frequently and at regular intervals, so that respiratory insufficiency can be anticipated. Decreasing vital capacity associated with weakness of the muscles used in swallowing, which causes difficulty in both coughing and swallowing, indicates impending respiratory failure. Signs and symptoms include breathlessness while speaking, shallow and irregular breathing, use of accessory muscles, tachycardia, and changes in respiratory pattern.

Parameters for determining the onset of respiratory failure are established on admission, allowing intubation and the initiation of mechanical ventilation on a nonemergent basis. This also allows the patient to be prepared for the procedure in a controlled manner, which reduces anxiety and complications.

Other complications include cardiac dysrhythmias, which necessitate ECG monitoring; transient hypertension; orthostatic hypotension; DVT; pulmonary embolism; urinary retention; and other threats to any immobilized and paralyzed patient. These require monitoring and attention to prevent them and prompt treatment if indicated.

Promoting Home and Community-Based Care

TEACHING PATIENTS SELF-CARE

Patients with Guillain-Barré syndrome and their families are usually frightened by the sudden onset of life-threatening symptoms and their severity. Therefore, teaching the patient and family about the disorder and its generally favorable prognosis is important (Chart 64-5).

During the acute phase of the illness, the patient and family are instructed about strategies they can implement to minimize the effects of immobility and other complications. As function begins to return, family members and other home care providers are instructed about care of the patient and their role in the rehabilitation process. Preparation for discharge is an interdisciplinary effort requiring family or caregiver education by all team members, including the nurse, physician, occupational and physical therapists, speech therapist, and respiratory therapist.

CONTINUING CARE

Most patients with Guillain-Barré syndrome experience complete recovery. Patients who have experienced total or prolonged paralysis require intensive rehabilitation; the extent depends on the patient's needs. Approaches include a comprehensive inpatient program if deficits are significant, an outpatient program if the patient can travel by car, or a home program of

CHART 64-5

HOME CARE CHECKLIST • The Patient With Guillain-Barré Syndrome

At the completion of the home care instruction, the patient or caregiver will be able to:	Patient	Caregiver
• Describe the disease process of Guillain-Barré syndrome.	✔	✔
• Manage respiratory needs: tracheostomy care, suctioning.		✔
• Demonstrate proper body mechanics regarding lifting and transfers.		✔
• Practice gait training and strength endurance.	✔	✔
• Perform range-of-motion exercises.	✔	✔
• Perform activities of daily living and manage self-care:		
• Nutrition	✔	✔
• Bowel and bladder management	✔	✔
• Skin care	✔	✔
• Adaptive equipment for bathing, hygiene, grooming, dressing	✔	✔
• Operate and explain function of medical equipment and mobility aids: walkers, wheelchairs, bedside commodes, tub transfer benches, adaptive devices	✔	✔
• Use coping mechanisms and diversional activities appropriately.	✔	✔
• Implement safety measures in the home.	✔	✔
• Know how to contact and use community resources and the Guillain-Barré Syndrome Foundation International.	✔	✔

physical and occupational therapy. The recovery phase may be long and requires patience as well as involvement on the part of the patient and family.

During acute care, the focus is on immediate issues and deficits. The nurse needs to remind or instruct patients and family members of the need for continuing health promotion and screening practices after this initial phase of care.

Evaluation

Expected Patient Outcomes

Expected patient outcomes may include the following:

1. Maintains effective respirations and airway clearance
   a. Has normal breath sounds on auscultation
   b. Demonstrates gradual improvement in respiratory function
2. Shows increasing mobility
   a. Regains use of extremities
   b. Participates in rehabilitation program
   c. Demonstrates no contractures and minimal muscle atrophy
3. Receives adequate nutrition and hydration
   a. Consumes diet adequate to meet nutritional needs
   b. Swallows without aspiration
4. Demonstrates recovery of speech
   a. Can communicate needs through alternative strategies
   b. Practices exercises recommended by the speech therapist
5. Shows lessening fear and anxiety
6. Absence of complications
   a. Breathes spontaneously
   b. Has vital capacity within normal range
   c. Exhibits normal arterial blood gases and pulse oximetry

Cranial Nerve Disorders

Because the brain stem and cranial nerves involve vital motor, sensory, and autonomic functions of the body, these nerves may be affected by conditions arising primarily within these structures or in secondary extension from adjacent disease processes. The cranial nerves (Fig. 64-6) are examined separately and in sequence (see Chapter 60). Some cranial nerve deficits can be detected by observing the patient's face, eye movements, speech, and swallowing. Electromyography (EMG) is used to investigate motor and sensory dysfunction. An MRI scan is used to obtain images of the cranial nerves and brain stem. An overview of disorders that may affect each of the cranial nerves, including clinical manifestations and nursing interventions, is presented in Table 64-1. The following discussion centers on the most common disorders of the cranial nerves: trigeminal neuralgia, a condition affecting the fifth cranial nerve, and Bell's palsy, caused by involvement of the seventh cranial nerve.

Trigeminal Neuralgia (Tic Douloureux)

Trigeminal neuralgia is a condition of the fifth cranial nerve that is characterized by paroxysms of pain in the area innervated by any of the three branches, but most commonly the second and third branches of the trigeminal nerve (Filipchuk, 2003) (Fig. 64-7). The pain ends as abruptly as it starts and is described as a unilateral shooting and stabbing sensation. The unilateral nature of the pain is an important diagnostic characteristic (Bader & Littlejohns, 2004). Associated involuntary contraction of the facial muscles can cause sudden closing of the eye or twitching of the mouth, hence the name *tic douloureux* (painful twitch). Although the cause is

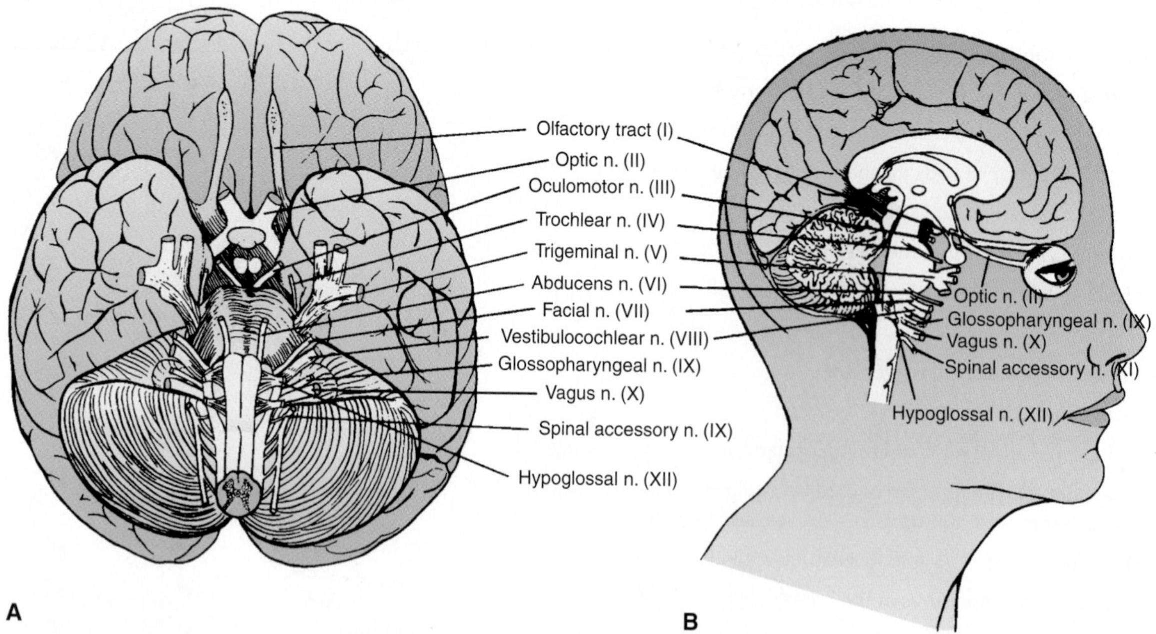

FIGURE 64-6. The cranial nerves. (**A**) Inferior view of the brain showing the cranial nerves. (**B**) Lateral view showing a schematic version of the cranial nerves.

TABLE 64-1 Disorders of Cranial Nerves

Disorder	Clinical Manifestations	Nursing Interventions
Olfactory Nerve—I		
Head trauma Intracranial tumor Intracranial surgery	Unilateral or bilateral anosmia (temporary or persistent) Diminished taste for food	Assess sense of smell. Assess for cerebrospinal fluid rhinorrhea if patient has sustained head trauma.
Optic Nerve—II		
Optic neuritis Increased intracranial pressure Pituitary tumor	Lesions of optic tract producing homonymous hemianopsia	Assess visual acuity. Restructure environment to prevent injuries. Teach patient to accommodate for visual loss.
Oculomotor Nerve—III **Trochlear Nerve—IV** **Abducens Nerve—VI**		
Vascular Brain stem ischemia Hemorrhage and infarction Neoplasm Trauma Infection	Dilation of pupil with loss of light reflex on one side Impairment of ocular movement Diplopia Gaze palsies Ptosis of eyelid	Assess extraocular movement and for nonreactive pupil.
Trigeminal Nerve—V		
Trigeminal neuralgia Head trauma Cerebellopontine lesion Sinus tract tumor and metastatic disease Compression of trigeminal root by tumor	Pain in face Diminished or loss of corneal reflex Chewing dysfunction	Assess for pain and triggering mechanisms for pain. Assess for difficulty in chewing. Discuss trigger zones and pain precipitants with patient. Protect cornea from abrasion. Ensure good oral hygiene. Educate patient about medication regimen.
Facial Nerve—VII		
Bell's palsy Facial nerve tumor Intracranial lesion Herpes zoster	Facial dysfunction; weakness and paralysis Hemifacial spasm Diminished or absent taste Pain	Recognize facial paralysis as emergency; refer for treatment as soon as possible. Teach protective care for eyes. Select easily chewed foods; patient should eat and drink from unaffected side of mouth. Emphasize importance of oral hygiene. Provide emotional support for changed appearance of face.
Vestibulocochlear Nerve—VIII		
Tumors and acoustic neuroma Vascular compression of nerve Ménière's syndrome	Tinnitus Vertigo Hearing difficulties	Assess pattern of vertigo. Provide for safety measures to prevent falls. Ensure that patient can obtain balance before ambulating. Caution patient to change positions slowly. Assist with ambulation. Encourage use of activity of daily living aids.
Glossopharyngeal Nerve—IX		
Glossopharyngeal neuralgia from neurovascular compression of cranial nerves IX and X Trauma Inflammatory conditions Tumor Vertebral artery aneurysms	Pain at base of tongue Difficulty in swallowing Loss of gag reflex Palatal, pharyngeal, and laryngeal paralysis	Assess for paroxysmal pain in throat, decreased or absent swallowing, gag and cough reflexes. Monitor for dysphagia, aspiration, nasal dysarthric speech. Position patient upright for eating or tube feeding.

continued >

TABLE 64-1 Disorders of Cranial Nerves (Continued)

Disorder	Clinical Manifestations	Nursing Interventions
Vagus Nerve—X		
Spastic palsy of larynx; bulbar paralysis; high vagal paralysis Guillain-Barré syndrome Vagal body tumors Nerve paralysis from malignancy, surgical trauma such as carotid endarterectomy	Voice changes (temporary or permanent hoarseness) Vocal paralysis Dysphagia	Assess for airway obstruction/provide airway management. Prevent aspiration. Support patient having voice reconstruction procedures.
Spinal Accessory Nerve—XI		
Spinal cord disorder Amyotrophic lateral sclerosis Trauma Guillain-Barré syndrome	Drooping of affected shoulder with limited shoulder movement Weakness or paralysis of head rotation, flexion, extension; shoulder elevation	Support patient undergoing diagnostic tests.
Hypoglossal Nerve—XII		
Medullary lesions Amyotrophic lateral sclerosis Polio and motor system disease, which may destroy hypoglossal nuclei Multiple sclerosis Trauma	Abnormal movements of tongue Weakness or paralysis of tongue muscles Difficulty in talking, chewing, and swallowing	Observe swallowing ability. Observe speech pattern. Be aware of swallowing or vocal difficulties. Prepare for alternate feeding methods (tube feeding) to maintain nutrition.

not certain, vascular compression and pressure are suggested causes. As the brain changes with age, a loop of a cerebral artery or vein may compress the nerve root entry point. Some evidence also suggests that demyelination of the trigeminal root may occur (Filipchuk, 2003).

Trigeminal neuralgia is most likely to occur in the fifth or sixth decade of life, and it is more common among women and in people with MS compared to the general population (Bader & Littlejohns, 2004; Filipchuk, 2003). Pain-free intervals may be measured in terms of minutes, hours, days, or

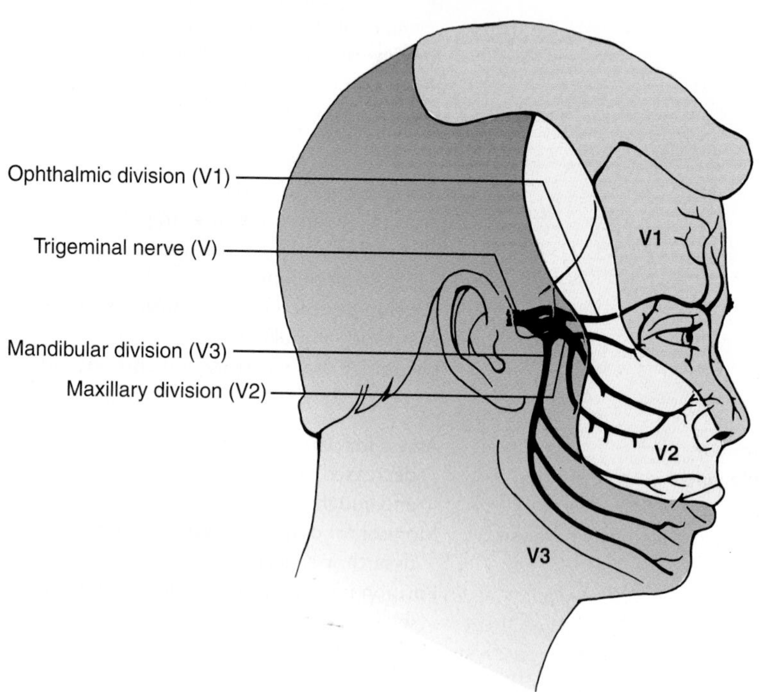

FIGURE 64-7. Distribution of trigeminal nerve branches.

longer. With advancing years, the painful episodes tend to become more frequent and agonizing. The patient lives in constant fear of attacks.

Paroxysms can occur with any stimulation of the terminals of the affected nerve branches, such as washing the face, shaving, brushing the teeth, eating, and drinking. A draft of cold air or direct pressure against the nerve trunk may also cause pain. Certain areas are called trigger points because the slightest touch immediately starts a paroxysm or episode. To avoid stimulating these areas, patients with trigeminal neuralgia try not to touch or wash their faces, shave, chew, or do anything else that might cause an attack. These behaviors are a clue to the diagnosis.

Medical Management

Pharmacologic Therapy

Antiseizure agents, such as carbamazepine (Tegretol), relieve pain in most patients with trigeminal neuralgia by reducing the transmission of impulses at certain nerve terminals. Carbamazepine is taken with meals. Serum levels must be monitored to avoid toxicity in patients who require high doses to control the pain. Side effects include nausea, dizziness, drowsiness, and aplastic anemia. The patient is monitored for bone marrow depression during long-term therapy. Gabapentin (Neurontin) and baclofen (Lioresal) are also used for pain control. If pain control is still not achieved, phenytoin (Dilantin) may be used as adjunctive therapy.

Surgical Management

If pharmacologic management fails to relieve pain, a number of surgical options are available. The choice of procedure depends on the patient's preference and health status.

MICROVASCULAR DECOMPRESSION OF THE TRIGEMINAL NERVE

An intracranial approach is used to relieve the contact between the cerebral vessel and the trigeminal nerve root entry (Filipchuk, 2003). With the aid of an operating microscope, the artery loop is lifted from the nerve to relieve the pressure, and a small prosthetic device is inserted to prevent recurrence of impingement on the nerve. Although this procedure relieves facial pain while preserving normal sensation, the pain-free interval averages only 1.9 years, with pain reoccurring in 47% of patients within 1 year after surgery (Filipchuk, 2003). The postoperative management is the same as for other intracranial surgeries (see Chapter 61).

RADIOFREQUENCY THERMAL COAGULATION

Percutaneous radiofrequency produces a thermal lesion on the trigeminal nerve. Although immediate pain relief is experienced, dysesthesia of the face and loss of the corneal reflex may occur. The pain recurrence rate is 25% to 37% within 5 years (Filipchuk, 2003). Use of stereotactic MRI for identification of the trigeminal nerve followed by gamma knife radiosurgery is being used at some medical centers.

PERCUTANEOUS BALLOON MICROCOMPRESSION

Percutaneous balloon microcompression disrupts large myelinated fibers in all three branches of the trigeminal nerve. After its placement, the balloon is filled with a contrast material for fluoroscopic identification. The balloon compresses the nerve root for 1 minute and provides microvascular decompression. This procedure provides immediate pain relief with a recurrence rate of 25% within 3 years, but masseter muscle weakness and facial dysesthesia may result postoperatively (Filipchuk, 2003).

Nursing Management

Preventing Pain

Preoperative management of a patient with trigeminal neuralgia occurs mostly on an outpatient basis and includes recognizing factors that may aggravate excruciating facial pain, such as food that is too hot or too cold or jarring of the patient's bed or chair. Even washing the face, combing the hair, or brushing the teeth may produce acute pain. The nurse can assist the patient in preventing or reducing this pain by providing instructions about preventive strategies. Providing cotton pads and room-temperature water for washing the face, instructing the patient to rinse with mouthwash after eating if toothbrushing causes pain, and performing personal hygiene during pain-free intervals are all effective strategies. The patient is instructed to take food and fluids at room temperature, to chew on the unaffected side, and to ingest soft foods. The nurse recognizes that anxiety, depression, and insomnia often accompany chronic painful conditions and uses appropriate interventions and referrals. See Chapter 13 for management of patients with chronic pain.

Providing Postoperative Care

Postoperative neurologic assessments are conducted to evaluate the patient for facial motor and sensory deficits in each of the three branches of the trigeminal nerve. If the surgery results in sensory deficits to the affected side of the face, the patient is instructed not to rub the eye, because the pain of a resulting injury will not be detected. The eye is assessed for irritation or redness. Artificial tears may be prescribed to prevent dryness in the affected eye. The patient is cautioned not to chew on the affected side until numbness has diminished. The patient is observed carefully for any difficulty in eating or swallowing foods of different consistencies.

Bell's Palsy

Bell's palsy (facial paralysis) is caused by unilateral inflammation of the seventh cranial nerve, which results in weakness or paralysis of the facial muscles on the affected side (Fig. 64-8). Although the cause is unknown, theories about

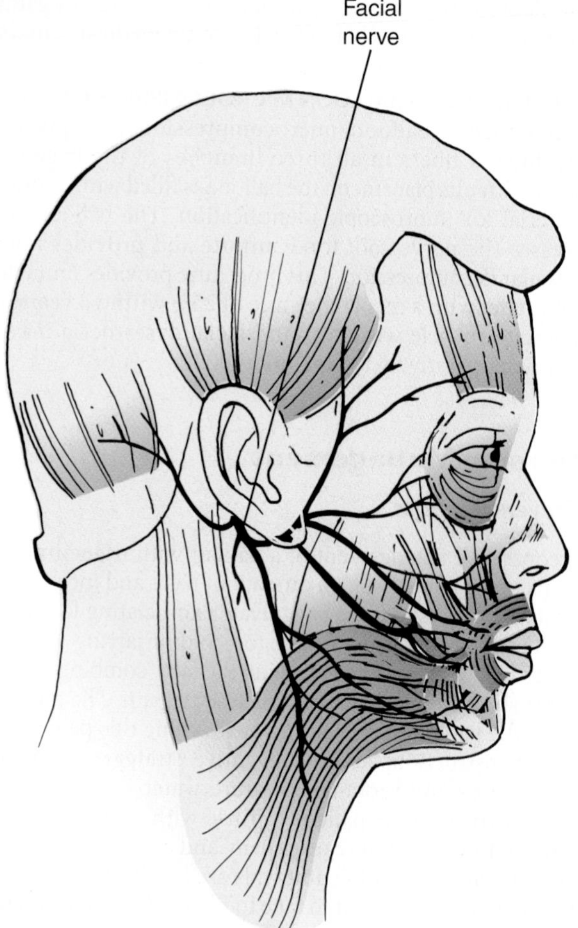

FIGURE 64-8. Distribution of facial nerve.

causes include vascular ischemia, viral disease (herpes simplex, herpes zoster), autoimmune disease, or a combination of all of these factors. The incidence is 13 to 34 cases per 100,000; it increases with age and among pregnant women in the third trimester (Campbell & Brundage, 2002; Shmorgun, Chan & Ray, 2002).

Bell's palsy may be a type of pressure paralysis. The inflamed, edematous nerve becomes compressed to the point of damage, or its blood supply is occluded, producing ischemic necrosis of the nerve. The face is distorted from paralysis of the facial muscles; increased lacrimation (tearing); and painful sensations in the face, behind the ear, and in the eye. The patient may experience speech difficulties and may be unable to eat on the affected side because of weakness or paralysis of the facial muscles. Most patients recover completely, and Bell's palsy rarely recurs (Gilden, 2004).

Medical Management

The objectives of treatment are to maintain the muscle tone of the face and to prevent or minimize denervation. The patient should be reassured that no stroke has occurred and that spontaneous recovery occurs within 3 to 5 weeks in most patients.

Corticosteroid therapy (prednisone) may be prescribed to reduce inflammation and edema; this reduces vascular compression and permits restoration of blood circulation to the nerve. Early administration of corticosteroid therapy appears to diminish the severity of the disease, relieve the pain, and prevent or minimize denervation.

Facial pain is controlled with analgesic agents. Heat may be applied to the involved side of the face to promote comfort and blood flow through the muscles. Electrical stimulation may be applied to the face to prevent muscle atrophy. Although most patients recover with conservative treatment, surgical exploration of the facial nerve may be indicated if a tumor is suspected, for surgical decompression of the facial nerve, or for surgical treatment of a paralyzed face.

Nursing Management

While the paralysis lasts, nursing care involves protection of the eye from injury. Frequently, the eye does not close completely and the blink reflex is diminished, so the eye is vulnerable to injury from dust and foreign particles. Corneal irritation and ulceration may occur. Distortion of the lower lid alters the proper drainage of tears. To prevent injury, the eye should be covered with a protective shield at night. The eye patch may abrade the cornea, however, because there is some difficulty in keeping the partially paralyzed eyelids closed. Eye ointment may be applied at bedtime to promote adherence of the eyelids to prevent injury during sleep. The patient can be taught to close the paralyzed eyelid manually before going to sleep. Wrap-around sunglasses or goggles may be worn during the day to decrease normal evaporation from the eye.

After the sensitivity of the nerve to touch decreases and the patient can tolerate touching the face, the nurse can suggest massaging the face several times daily, using a gentle upward motion, to maintain muscle tone. Facial exercises, such as wrinkling the forehead, blowing out the cheeks, and whistling, may be performed with the aid of a mirror to prevent muscle atrophy. Exposure of the face to cold and drafts is avoided.

Disorders of the Peripheral Nervous System

Peripheral Neuropathies

A peripheral **neuropathy** (disorder of the nervous system) is a disorder affecting the peripheral motor and sensory nerves. Peripheral nerves connect the spinal cord and brain to all other organs. They transmit motor impulses from the brain and relay sensory impulses to the brain. Peripheral neuropathies are characterized by bilateral and symmetric disturbance of function, usually beginning in the feet and hands. The most common cause of peripheral neuropathy is diabetes with poor glycemic control (Tesfaye, Chaturvedi, Simon, et al., 2005). The major symptoms of peripheral nerve disorders are loss of sensation, muscle atrophy, weakness, diminished reflexes, pain, and paresthesia (numbness, tingling) of the extremities.

Peripheral nerve disorders are diagnosed by history, physical examination, and electrodiagnostic studies such as electroencephalography. The diagnosis of peripheral neuropathy in the geriatric population is challenging because many symptoms, such as decreased reflexes, can be associated with the normal aging process (Richardson, 2002).

No specific treatment exists for peripheral neuropathy. Elimination or control of the cause may slow progression. Patients with peripheral neuropathy are at risk for falls, thermal injuries, and skin breakdown. The plan of care includes inspection of the lower extremities for skin breakdown. Assistive devices such as a walker or cane may decrease the risk of falls. Bath water temperature is checked to avoid thermal injury. Footwear should be accurately sized. Driving may be limited or eliminated, thereby disrupting the patient's sense of independence.

Mononeuropathy

Mononeuropathy is limited to a single peripheral nerve and its branches. It arises when the trunk of the nerve is compressed or entrapped (as in carpal tunnel syndrome), traumatized (as when bruised by a blow), overstretched (as in joint dislocation), punctured by a needle used to inject a drug or damaged by the drugs thus injected, or inflamed because an adjacent infectious process extends to the nerve trunk. Mononeuropathy is frequently seen in patients with diabetes.

Pain is seldom a major symptom of mononeuropathy when the condition is due to trauma, but in patients with complicating inflammatory conditions such as arthritis, pain is prominent. Pain is increased by all body movements that tend to stretch, strain, or cause pressure on the injured nerve and by sudden jarring of the body (eg, from coughing or sneezing). The skin in the areas supplied by nerves that are injured or diseased may become reddened and glossy, the subcutaneous tissue may become edematous, and the nails and hair in this area are altered. Chemical injuries to a nerve trunk, such as those caused by drugs injected into or near it, are often permanent.

The objective of treatment of mononeuropathy is to remove the cause, if possible (eg, freeing the compressed nerve). Local corticosteroid injections may reduce inflammation and the pressure on the nerve. Aspirin or codeine may be used to relieve pain.

Nursing care involves protection of the affected limb or area from injury, as well as appropriate patient teaching about mononeuropathy and its treatment.

Critical Thinking Exercises

1 A 19-year-old college student is admitted with suspected meningococcal meningitis. Identify two neurologic changes that may reflect increased ICP. What interventions would be included in your plan of care to protect the patient from injury? The patient's family has many questions about the disease and their risk of contracting meningitis. Develop a teaching plan that would describe meningococcal meningitis and prophylactic therapy for the patient's family and close contacts.

2 ebp Your patient has been receiving a new medication for the treatment of MS for about 6 months. She reports that she is becoming very discouraged because the medication does not seem to improve her symptoms. What resources would you use to identify the current guidelines for pharmacologic treatment of MS? What is the current evidence base for disease-modifying therapies? Identify the criteria used to evaluate the strength of the evidence for disease-modifying therapies. How would you use this information in developing a plan of care for this patient?

3 Your 40-year-old patient has myasthenia gravis. Her condition has been stable and she has been able to manage without assistance, but she reports increasing weakness and fatigue. What nursing assessments and interventions are warranted for her? What discharge plans are indicated if she is to return home to the care of her family? How would your discharge planning change if she lived alone in an apartment on the third floor of a building without an elevator?

4 Your patient has been admitted to the intensive care unit with a diagnosis of possible Guillain-Barré syndrome. Identify the priorities of assessment for this patient and the nursing and medical interventions that you would anticipate. What medications should you have readily available for this patient?

REFERENCES AND SELECTED READINGS

BOOKS

Bader, M. K. & Littlejohns, J. R. (2004). *AANN core curriculum for neuroscience nursing* (4th ed.). St. Louis: Elsevier.

Bickley, L. S. & Szilagyi, P. G. (2003). *Bates' guide to physical examination and history taking* (8th ed.). Philadelphia: Lippincott Williams & Wilkins.

Cohen, J. A. & Rudick, R. A. (2003). *Multiple sclerosis therapeutics* (2nd ed.). New York: Martin Dunitz.

Diepenbrock, N. H. (2004). *Quick reference to critical care* (2nd ed.). Philadelphia: Lippincott Williams & Wilkins.

Fischbach, F. (2002). *Common laboratory and diagnostic tests* (3rd ed.). Philadelphia: Lippincott Williams & Wilkins.

Goetz, C. (2003). *Textbook of clinical neurology* (2nd ed.). Philadelphia: Saunders.

Hickey, J. (2003). *Clinical practice of neurologic and neurosurgical nursing* (4th ed.). Philadelphia: Lippincott Williams & Wilkins.

Karch, A. (2005). *Lippincott's nursing drug guide*. Philadelphia: Lippincott Williams & Wilkins.

Keesey, J. C. (2002). *Myasthenia gravis: An illustrated history*. Roseville, CA: Publishers Design Group.

Olek, M. J. (2005). *Multiple sclerosis: Etiology, diagnosis and new treatment strategies*. Totowa, NJ: Humana Press.

Porth, C. M. (2005). *Pathophysiology: Concepts of altered health states.* (7th ed.) Philadelphia: Lippincott Williams & Wilkins.

Ropper, A. H., Gress, D., Diringer, M. N., et al. (2004). *Neurological and neurosurgical intensive care* (4th ed.). Philadelphia: Lippincott Williams & Wilkins.

Rosen, F. & Geha, R. (2004). *Case studies in immunology: A clinical companion* (4th ed.). New York: Garland Publishing.

JOURNALS

**Asterisks indicate nursing research articles.*

CNS Infections

Armstrong, M. L. (2004). Caring for the patient with piercings. *RN, 67*(6), 46–53.

Crumpacker, C., Gonzalez, R. & Makar, R. (2003). Case 26-2003: A 50-year-old Colombian man with fever and seizures. *New England Journal of Medicine, 349*(8), 789–796.

de Gans, J. & van de Beek, D. (2002). Dexamethasone in adults with bacterial meningitis. *New England Journal of Medicine, 347*(20), 1549–1556.

Morgan, R. (2004). West Nile viral encephalitis: A case study. *Journal of Neuroscience Nursing, 36*(4), 185–189.

Pullen, R. (2004). Assessing for signs of meningitis. *Nursing, 34*(5), 18.

Raschilas, F., Wolff, M., Delatour, F., et al. (2002). Outcome of and prognostic factors for herpes simplex encephalitis in adult patients: Results of a multi-center study. *Clinical Infectious Disease,* 35(3), 254–260.

Solomon, T. (2004). Flavivirus encephalitis. *New England Journal of Medicine,* 351(4), 370–377.

Spach, D. (2003). New issues in bacterial meningitis in adults. *Postgraduate Medicine, 114*(5), 1–9.

Spiro, C. & Spiro, D. (2004). Acute meningitis. *Clinician Reviews, 14*(3), 53–60.

Whitley, R. & Gnann, J. (2002). Viral encephalitis: Familiar infections and emerging pathogens. *Lancet, 359*(9305), 507–515.

Creutzfeldt-Jakob Disease

Andrews, N., Farrington, C., Ward, H., et al. (2003). Death from variant Creutzfeldt-Jakob disease in the UK. *The Lancet, 361*(9359), 751–752.

Belkin, N. (2003). Creutzfeldt-Jakob disease: Identifying prions and carriers. *AORN, 78*(2), 204–208.

Brown, S. A. & Merritt, K. (2003). Use of containment pans and lids for autoclaving caustic solutions. *American Journal of Infection Control, 31*(4), 257–260.

Fontenot, A. (2003). The fundamentals of variant Creutzfeldt-Jakob disease. *Journal of Neuroscience Nursing,* 35(6), 327–331.

Glatzel, M., Stoeck, K., Seeger, H., et al. (2005). Human prion diseases: Molecular and clinical aspects. *Archives of Neurology, 62*(4), 545–552.

Multiple Sclerosis

Barbero, P., Verdun, E., Bergui, M., et al. (2004). High dose, frequently administered interferon beta therapy for relapsing remitting multiple sclerosis must be maintained over the long term: The interferon beta dose reduction study. *Journal of the Neurological Sciences, 222*(1–2), 13–19.

*Becker, H. & Stuifbergen, A. (2004). What makes it so hard? Barriers to health promotion experienced by people with multiple sclerosis and polio. *Family Community Health, 27*(1), 75–85.

Burks, J. S. (2005). A practical approach to immunomodulatory therapy for multiple sclerosis. *Physical Medicine and Rehabilitation Clinics of North America, 16*(2), 449–466.

Courts, N. F., Newton, A. N. & McNeal, L. J. (2005). Husbands and wives living with multiple sclerosis. *Journal of Neuroscience Nursing, 37*(1), 20–27.

*Finlayson, M., Denend, T. & Hudson, E. (2004). Aging with multiple sclerosis. *Journal of Neuroscience Nursing, 36*(5), 245–251.

*Harrison, T., Stuifbergen, A., Adachi, E., et al. (2004). Marriage, impairment, and acceptance in persons with multiple sclerosis. *Western Journal of Nursing Research, 26*(3), 266–285.

Holland, N. & Madonna, M. (2005). Nursing grand rounds: Multiple sclerosis. *Journal of Neuroscience Nursing, 37*(1), 15–19.

Kieseier, B. C. & Hartung, H. (2003). Current disease modifying therapies in multiple sclerosis. *Seminars in Neurology, 23*(2), 133–142.

Klingbeil, H., Baer, H. R., & Wilson, P. E. (2004). Aging with a disability. *Archives of Physical Medicine and Rehabilitation, 85*(7), S68–S73.

Lublin, F. D. & Reingold, S. C. (1996). Defining the clinical course of multiple sclerosis: Results of an international study. *Neurology, 46*(4), 907–911.

Racke, M., Hawker, K. & Frohman, E. M. (2004). Fatigue in multiple sclerosis. *Archives of Neurology, 61*(2), 176–177.

*Smeltzer, S. C. (2002). Reproductive decision making in women with multiple sclerosis. *Journal of Neuroscience Nursing, 34*(3), 145–157.

*Smeltzer, S. C., Zimmerman, V. & Capriotti, T. (2005). Osteoporosis risk and bone mineral density in women with physical disabilities. *Archives of Physical Medicine and Rehabilitation, 86*(3), 582–586.

Stern, M. (2005). Aging with multiple sclerosis. *Physical Medicine and Rehabilitation Clinics of North America, 16*(1), 219–234.

Svendsen, K. B., Jensen, T. S., Overvad, K., et al. (2003). Pain in patients with multiple sclerosis. *Archives of Neurology, 60*(8), 1089–1094.

Tartaglia, M., Narayanan, S., Francis, S., et al. (2004). The relationship between diffuse axonal damage and fatigue in multiple sclerosis. *Archives of Neurology, 61*(2), 201–207.

Myasthenia Gravis

Dalakas, M. C. (2004). Intravenous immunoglobulin in autoimmune neuromuscular diseases. *Journal of the American Medical Association, 291*(19), 2367–2375.

Juel, V. (2004). Myasthenia gravis: Management of myasthenic crisis and the perioperative care. *Seminars in Neurology, 24*(1), 75–80.

Phillips, L. H. (2004). The epidemiology of myasthenia gravis. *Seminars in Neurology, 24*(1), 17–20.

Rabinstein, A. & Wijdicks, E. (2003). Warning signs of imminent respiratory failure in neurological patients. *Seminars in Neurology, 23*(1), 97–103.

Saperstein, D. & Barohn, R. (2004). Management of myasthenia gravis. *Seminars in Neurology, 24*(1), 41–46.

Scherer, K., Bedlack, R. S., & Simel, D. L. (2005). Does this patient have myasthenia gravis? *Journal of the American Medical Association, 293*(15), 1906–1914.

Guillain-Barré Syndrome

Cooke, J. & Orb, A. (2003). The recovery phase in Guillain-Barré syndrome: Moving from dependency to independence. *Rehabilitation Nursing, 28*(4), 105–109.

Haber, P., DeStefano, F., Angulo, F., et al. (2004). Guillain-Barré syndrome following influenza vaccination. *Journal of the American Medical Association, 292*(20), 2478–2481.

Kieseier, B. & Hartung, H. (2003). Therapeutic strategies in the Guillain-Barré syndrome. *Seminars in Neurology, 23*(2), 159–165.

Whyte, J. (2003). Guillain-Barré: A case of muscular weakness and ambulatory difficulty. *Nurse Practitioner, 28*(3), 58–61.

Winer, J. B. (2002). Treatment of Guillain-Barré syndrome. *QJM: An International Journal of Medicine, 95*(11), 717–721.

Trigeminal Neuralgia and Neuropathies

Campbell, K. E., & Brundage, J. F. (2002). Effects of climate, latitude, and season on the incidence of Bell's palsy in the U.S. Armed Forces, October 1997 to September 1999. *American Journal of Epidemiology, 156*(1), 32–39.

Filipchuk, D. (2003). Classic trigeminal neuralgia: A surgical perspective. *Journal of Neuroscience Nursing, 35*(2), 82–86.

Gilden, D. H. (2004). Clinical practice: Bell's palsy. *New England Journal of Medicine, 351*(13), 1323–1331.

Richardson, J. K. (2002). The clinical identification of peripheral neuropathy among older persons. *Archives of Physical Medicine and Rehabilitation, 83*(3), 1553–1558.

Shmorgun, D., Chan, W. S. & Ray, J. G. (2002). Association between Bell's palsy in pregnancy and pre-eclampsia. *QJM: An International Journal of Medicine, 95*(6), 359–362.

Tesfaye, S., Chaturvedi, N., Simon, E. M., et al. (2005). Vascular risk factors and diabetic neuropathy. *New England Journal of Medicine, 352*(4), 341–350.

RESOURCES

Guillain-Barré Syndrome Foundation International, P.O. Box 262, Wynnewood, PA 19096; 610-667-0131, fax 610-667-7036; http://www.guillain-barre.com/. Accessed June 23, 2006.

Journal of the American Medical Association Patient Pages; http://www.jama.ama-assn.org/cgi/collectionpatient_page. Accessed June 23, 2006.

Myasthenia Gravis Foundation of America, 222 S. Riverside Plaza, Suite 1540, Chicago, IL 60606; 800-541-5454, 312-258-0522, fax 312-258-0461; http://www.myasthenia.org. Accessed June 23, 2006.

National Multiple Sclerosis Society, 733 Third Avenue, New York, NY 10017; 800-344-4867; http://www.nmss.org. Accessed June 23, 2006.

The Neuropathy Association, Inc.; P.O. Box 26226, New York, NY 10117; 212-692-0662; http://www.neuropathy.org. Accessed June 23, 2006.

CHAPTER 65

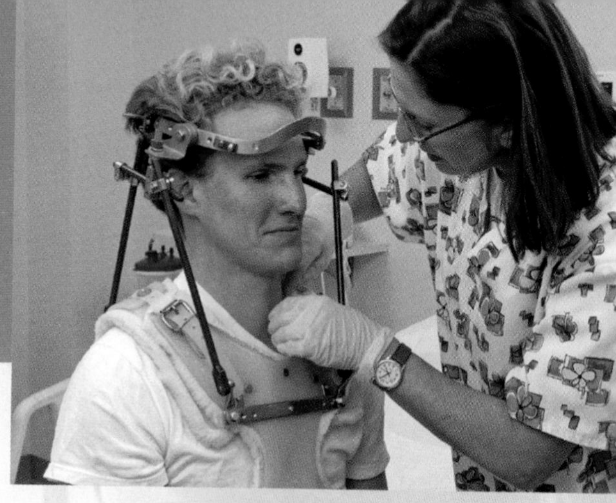

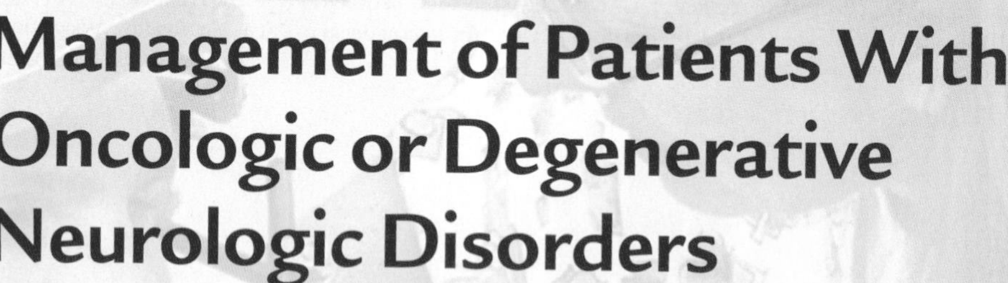

Management of Patients With Oncologic or Degenerative Neurologic Disorders

Learning Objectives

On completion of this chapter, the learner will be able to:

1. Identify the pathophysiologic processes responsible for oncologic disorders.
2. Describe brain and spinal cord tumors: their classification, clinical manifestations, diagnosis, and medical and nursing management.
3. Use the nursing process as a framework for care of patients with cerebral metastases or inoperable brain tumors.
4. Identify the pathophysiologic processes responsible for various degenerative neurologic disorders.
5. Use the nursing process as a framework for care of patients with degenerative neurologic disorders.
6. Identify resources for patients and families with oncologic and degenerative neurologic disorders.

The occurrence of oncologic or degenerative disease processes in the neurologic system produces a unique set of nursing management challenges. Oncologic disorders include brain and spinal cord tumors. Degenerative neurologic disorders include Parkinson's disease, Huntington's disease, Alzheimer's disease, amyotrophic lateral sclerosis, muscular dystrophies, and degenerative disc disease. Postpolio syndrome is thought to be degenerative in nature and is included in this chapter.

Oncologic Disorders of the Brain and Spinal Cord

Oncologic disorders in the brain and spinal cord include several types of neoplasms, each with its own biology, prognosis, and treatment options. Because of the unique anatomy and physiology of the central nervous system (CNS), this collection of neoplasms is challenging to diagnose and treat.

Primary Brain Tumors

A brain tumor is a localized intracranial lesion that occupies space within the skull. A tumor usually grows as a spherical mass, but it also can grow diffusely and infiltrate tissue. The effects of neoplasms are caused by the compression and infiltration of tissue. A variety of physiologic changes result, causing any or all of the following pathophysiologic events:

- Increased intracranial pressure (ICP) and cerebral edema
- Seizure activity and focal neurologic signs
- Hydrocephalus
- Altered pituitary function

Primary brain tumors originate from cells and structures within the brain. Secondary, or metastatic, brain tumors develop from structures outside the brain and occur in 10% to 20% of patients with cancer (Bader & Littlejohns, 2004). Brain tumors rarely metastasize outside the CNS, but metastatic lesions to the brain occur commonly from the lung, breast, lower gastrointestinal tract, pancreas, kidney, and skin (melanomas).

The cause of primary brain tumors is unknown. The only known risk factor is exposure to ionizing radiation. Both glial and meningeal neoplasms have been linked to irradiation of the cranium, with a latency period of 10 to 20 years after exposure (American Brain Tumor Association [ABTA], 2006). Additional possible causes have been investigated, but results of studies are conflicting and unconvincing; suggested causes have included use of cellular telephones, exposure to high-tension wires, use of hair dyes, head trauma, and dietary exposure to such factors as nitrates (found in some processed and barbecued foods).

The incidence of brain tumors appears to have increased in the past few decades. Epidemiologic data, however, suggest that this is due to more aggressive and more accurate diagnosis rather than an actual rise in incidence. An estimated 18,000 new cases of malignant brain tumors occur per year: 14.2 per 100,000 men and 13.9 per 100,000 women (ABTA, 2006). Secondary tumors or metastases to the brain from a systemic primary cancer are more common. The highest incidence of brain tumors in adults occurs in the fifth, sixth, and seventh decades, with a slightly higher incidence in men (Bader & Littlejohns, 2004). In adults, most brain tumors originate from glial cells (cells that make up the structure and support system of the brain and spinal cord) and are supratentorial (located above the covering of the cerebellum). Neoplastic lesions in the brain ultimately cause death by impairing vital functions, such as respiration, or by increasing ICP.

Types of Primary Brain Tumors

Brain tumors may be classified into several groups: those arising from the coverings of the brain (eg, dural meningioma), those developing in or on the cranial nerves (eg, acoustic neuroma), those originating within brain tissue (eg, glioma), and metastatic lesions originating elsewhere in the body. Tumors of the pituitary and pineal glands and of cerebral blood vessels are also types of brain tumors. Relevant clinical considerations include the location and the histologic character of the tumor. Tumors may be benign or malignant. A benign tumor can occur in a vital area and can grow large enough to have effects as serious as those of a malignant tumor.

Glossary

akathisia: restlessness, urgent need to move around, and agitation
bradykinesia: very slow voluntary movements and speech
chorea: rapid, jerky, involuntary, purposeless movements of the extremities or facial muscles, including facial grimacing
dementia: a progressive organic mental disorder characterized by personality changes, confusion, disorientation, and deterioration of intellect associated with impaired memory and judgment
dyskinesia: impaired ability to execute voluntary movements
dysphonia: abnormal voice quality caused by weakness and incoordination of muscles responsible for speech
micrographia: small and often illegible handwriting
neurodegenerative: a disease, process, or condition that leads to deterioration of normal cells or function of the nervous system
papilledema: edema of the optic nerve
paresthesia: a sensation of numbness, tingling, or a "pins and needles" sensation
radiculopathy: disease of a spinal nerve root, often resulting in pain and extreme sensitivity to touch
sciatica: inflammation of the sciatic nerve, resulting in pain and tenderness along the nerve through the thigh and leg
spondylosis: ankylosis or stiffening of the cervical or lumbar vertebrae

Gliomas

Glial tumors, the most common type of intracerebral brain neoplasm, are divided into many categories. See Chart 65-1 for the classification of these and other brain tumors. Astrocytomas are the most common type of glioma and are graded from I to IV, indicating the degree of malignancy (Diepenbrock, 2004). The grade is based on cellular density, cell mitosis, and appearance. Usually, these tumors spread by infiltrating into the surrounding neural connective tissue and therefore cannot be totally removed without causing considerable damage to vital structures.

Oligodendroglial tumors represent 20% of gliomas and are categorized as low-grade or high-grade (anaplastic). The histologic distinction between astrocytomas and oligodendrogliomas is difficult to make but important, because recent research shows that oligodendrogliomas are more sensitive than astrocytomas to chemotherapy (Eskandar, Loeffler, O'Neill, et al., 2004).

Meningiomas

Meningiomas, which represent 15% to 20% of all primary brain tumors, are common benign encapsulated tumors of arachnoid cells on the meninges (Diepenbrock, 2004). They are slow-growing and occur most often in middle-aged adults (more often in women). Meningiomas most often occur in areas proximal to the venous sinuses. Manifestations depend on the area involved and are the result of compression rather than invasion of brain tissue. Standard treatment is surgery with complete removal or partial dissection.

Acoustic Neuromas

An acoustic neuroma is a tumor of the eighth cranial nerve, the cranial nerve most responsible for hearing and balance. It usually arises just within the internal auditory meatus, where it frequently expands before filling the cerebellopontine recess. An acoustic neuroma may grow slowly and attain considerable size before it is correctly diagnosed. The patient usually experiences loss of hearing, tinnitus, and episodes of vertigo and staggering gait. As the tumor becomes larger, painful sensations of the face may occur on the same side, as a result of the tumor's compression of the fifth cranial nerve. Most acoustic neuromas are benign, can be surgically removed, and have a good prognosis (Diepenbrock, 2004). Some acoustic neuromas may be suitable for stereotactic radiotherapy rather than open craniotomy (Bohan & Glass-Macenka, 2004). Stereotactic radiotherapy is discussed later in this chapter.

CHART 65-1

Classification of Brain Tumors in Adults

- **I. Intracerebral Tumors**
  - A. Gliomas—infiltrate any portion of the brain; most common type of brain tumor
    1. Astrocytomas (grades I and II)
    2. Glioblastoma multiforme (astrocytoma grades III and IV)
    3. Oligodendrocytoma (low and high grades)
    4. Ependymoma (grades I to IV)
    5. Medulloblastoma
- **II. Tumors Arising From Supporting Structures**
  - A. Meningiomas
  - B. Neuromas (acoustic neuroma, schwannoma)
  - C. Pituitary adenomas
- **III. Developmental Tumors**
  - A. Angiomas
  - B. Dermoid, epidermoid, teroma, craniopharyngioma
- **IV. Metastatic Lesions**

Pituitary Adenomas

Pituitary tumors represent about 7% to 12% of all brain tumors and cause symptoms as a result of pressure on adjacent structures or hormonal changes (hyperfunction or hypofunction of the pituitary). The pituitary gland, also called the hypophysis, is a relatively small gland located in the sella turcica. It is attached to the hypothalamus by a short stalk (hypophyseal stalk) and is divided into two lobes: the anterior lobe (adenohypophysis) and the posterior lobe (neurohypophysis).

PRESSURE EFFECTS OF PITUITARY ADENOMAS

Pressure from a pituitary adenoma may be exerted on the optic nerves, optic chiasm, or optic tracts or on the hypothalamus or the third ventricle if the tumor invades the cavernous sinuses or expands into the sphenoid bone. These pressure effects produce headache, visual dysfunction, hypothalamic disorders (disorders of sleep, appetite, temperature, and emotions), increased ICP, and enlargement and erosion of the sella turcica.

HORMONAL EFFECTS OF PITUITARY ADENOMAS

Functioning pituitary tumors can produce one or more hormones normally produced by the anterior pituitary. There are prolactin-secreting pituitary adenomas (prolactinomas), growth hormone-secreting pituitary adenomas that produce acromegaly in adults, and adrenocorticotropic hormone (ACTH)-producing pituitary adenomas that result in Cushing's disease. Adenomas that secrete thyroid-stimulating hormone or follicle-stimulating hormone and luteinizing hormone occur infrequently, whereas adenomas that produce both growth hormone and prolactin are relatively common.

The female patient whose pituitary gland is secreting excessive quantities of prolactin presents with amenorrhea or galactorrhea (excessive or spontaneous flow of milk). Male patients with prolactinomas may present with impotence and hypogonadism. Acromegaly, caused by excess growth hormone, produces enlargement of the hands and feet, distortion of the facial features, and pressure on peripheral nerves (entrapment syndromes). The clinical features of Cushing's disease, a condition associated with prolonged overproduction of cortisol, occur with excessive production of ACTH. Manifestations include a form of obesity with redistribution of fat to the facial, supraclavicular, and abdominal areas; hypertension; purple striae and ecchymoses; osteoporosis; elevated blood glucose levels; and emotional disorders. Endocrine disorders resulting from these tumors are discussed in Chapter 42.

Angiomas

Brain angiomas (masses composed largely of abnormal blood vessels) are found either in or on the surface of the brain. They occur in the cerebellum in 83% of cases. Some persist throughout life without causing symptoms; others cause symptoms of a brain tumor. Occasionally, the diagnosis is suggested by the presence of another angioma somewhere in the head or by a bruit (an abnormal sound) that is audible over the skull. Because the walls of the blood vessels in angiomas are thin, these patients are at risk for hemorrhagic stroke. In fact, cerebral hemorrhage in people younger than 40 years of age should suggest the possibility of an angioma.

Gerontologic Considerations

The most frequent tumor types in the elderly are anaplastic astrocytoma, glioblastoma multiforme, and cerebral metastases from other sites. The incidence of primary brain tumors and the likelihood of malignancy increase with age (Bader & Littlejohns, 2004). Intracranial tumors can produce personality changes, confusion, speech dysfunction, or disturbances of gait. In elderly patients, early signs and symptoms of intracranial tumors can be easily overlooked or incorrectly attributed to cognitive and neurologic changes associated with normal aging. Neurologic signs and symptoms in the elderly must be carefully evaluated, because 10% of brain metastases occur in patients with a history of prior cancer.

Clinical Manifestations

Brain tumors can produce either focal or generalized neurologic signs and symptoms. Generalized symptoms reflect increased ICP, and the most common focal or specific signs and symptoms result from tumors that interfere with functions in specific brain regions. Figure 65-1 indicates common tumor sites in the brain.

Increased Intracranial Pressure

As discussed in Chapter 61, the skull is a rigid compartment containing essential noncompressible contents: brain matter, intravascular blood, and cerebrospinal fluid (CSF).

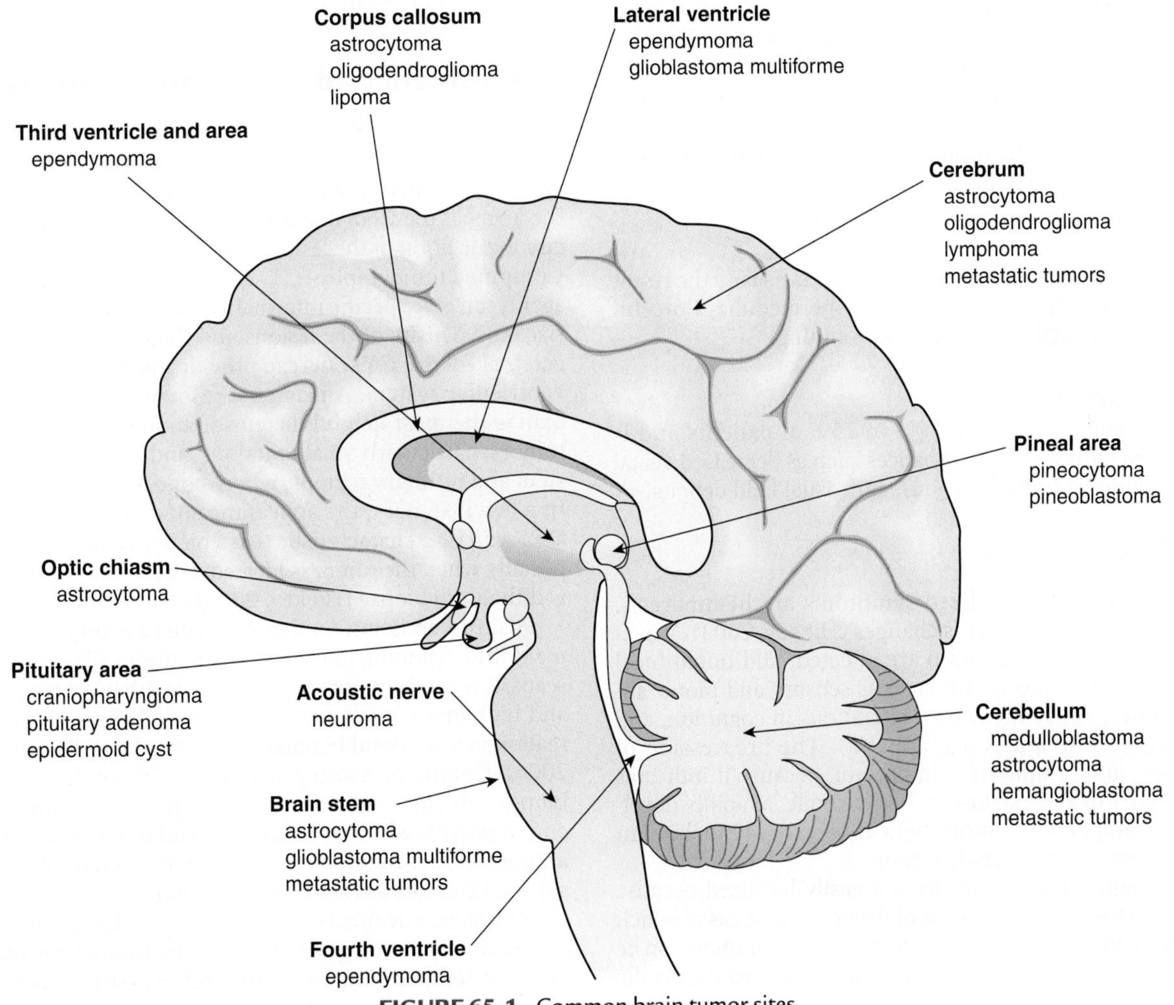

FIGURE 65-1. Common brain tumor sites.

According to the modified Monro-Kellie hypothesis, if any one of these skull components increases in volume, ICP increases unless one of the other components decreases in volume. Consequently, any change in volume occupied by the brain (as occurs with disorders such as brain tumor or cerebral edema) produces signs and symptoms of increased ICP.

Symptoms of increased ICP result from a gradual compression of the brain by the enlarging tumor. The effect is a disruption of the equilibrium that exists between the brain, the CSF, and the cerebral blood. As the tumor grows, compensatory adjustments may occur through compression of intracranial veins, reduction of CSF volume (by increased absorption or decreased production), a modest decrease in cerebral blood flow, or reduction of intracellular and extracellular brain tissue mass. When these compensatory mechanisms fail, the patient develops signs and symptoms of increased ICP, most often including headache, nausea with or without vomiting, and **papilledema** (edema of the optic disk) (Bohan & Glass-Macenka, 2004; Hickey, 2003). Personality changes and a variety of focal deficits, including motor, sensory, and cranial nerve dysfunction, are common.

HEADACHE

Headache, although not always present, is most common in the early morning and is made worse by coughing, straining, or sudden movement. It is thought to be caused by the tumor's invading, compressing, or distorting the pain-sensitive structures or by edema that accompanies the tumor. Headaches are usually described as deep or expanding or as dull but unrelenting. Frontal tumors usually produce a bilateral frontal headache; pituitary gland tumors produce pain radiating between the two temples (bitemporal); in cerebellar tumors, the headache may be located in the suboccipital region at the back of the head.

VOMITING

Vomiting, seldom related to food intake, is usually the result of irritation of the vagal centers in the medulla. Forceful vomiting is described as projectile vomiting.

VISUAL DISTURBANCES

Papilledema is present in 70% to 75% of patients and is associated with visual disturbances such as decreased visual acuity, diplopia (double vision), and visual field deficits.

Localized Symptoms

Common focal or localized symptoms are hemiparesis, seizures, and mental status changes (Hickey, 2003). When specific regions of the brain are affected, additional local signs and symptoms occur, such as sensory and motor abnormalities, visual alterations, alterations in cognition, and language disturbances (eg, aphasia). The progression of the signs and symptoms is important, because it indicates tumor growth and expansion. For example, a rapidly developing hemiparesis is more typical of a highly malignant glioma than of a low-grade tumor.

Although some tumors are not easily localized because they lie in so-called silent areas of the brain (ie, areas in which functions are not definitely determined), many tumors can be localized by correlating the signs and symptoms to specific areas in the brain, as follows:

- A motor cortex tumor produces seizure-like movements localized on one side of the body, called Jacksonian seizures.
- An occipital lobe tumor produces visual manifestations: contralateral homonymous hemianopsia (visual loss in half of the visual field on the opposite side of the tumor) and visual hallucinations.
- A cerebellar tumor causes dizziness, an ataxic or staggering gait with a tendency to fall toward the side of the lesion, marked muscle incoordination, and nystagmus (involuntary rhythmic eye movements), usually in the horizontal direction.
- A frontal lobe tumor frequently produces personality disorders, changes in emotional state and behavior, and an apathetic mental attitude. The patient often becomes extremely untidy and careless and may use obscene language.
- A cerebellopontine angle tumor usually originates in the sheath of the acoustic nerve and gives rise to a characteristic sequence of symptoms. Tinnitus and vertigo appear first, soon followed by progressive nerve deafness (eighth cranial nerve dysfunction). Numbness and tingling of the face and tongue occur (due to involvement of the fifth cranial nerve). Later, weakness or paralysis of the face develops (seventh cranial nerve involvement). Finally, because the enlarging tumor presses on the cerebellum, abnormalities in motor function may be present.

Assessment and Diagnostic Findings

The history of the illness and the manner and time frame in which the symptoms evolved are key components in the diagnosis of brain tumors. A neurologic examination indicates the areas of the CNS that are involved. To assist in the precise localization of the lesion, a battery of tests is performed. Computed tomography (CT) scans, enhanced by a contrast agent, can give specific information concerning the number, size, and density of the lesions and the extent of secondary cerebral edema. CT scans can provide information about the ventricular system. A magnetic resonance imaging (MRI) scan is the most helpful diagnostic tool for detecting brain tumors, particularly smaller lesions, and tumors in the brain stem and pituitary regions, where bone is thick (Fig. 65-2). In a few instances, the appearance of a brain tumor on an MRI scan is so characteristic that a biopsy is unnecessary, especially when the tumor is located in a part of the brain that is difficult to biopsy (Hickey, 2003).

Positron emission tomography (PET) is used to supplement MRI scanning in centers where it is available. On PET scans, low-grade tumors are associated with hypometabolism and high-grade tumors show hypermetabolism. This information can be useful in making treatment decisions (ABTA, 2006). Computer-assisted stereotactic (three-dimensional) biopsy is being used to diagnose deep-seated brain tumors and to provide a basis for treatment and prognosis. Cerebral angiography provides visualization of cerebral blood vessels and can localize most cerebral tumors.

An electroencephalogram (EEG) can detect an abnormal brain wave in regions occupied by tumor; it is used to evaluate temporal lobe seizures and to assist in ruling out other disorders.

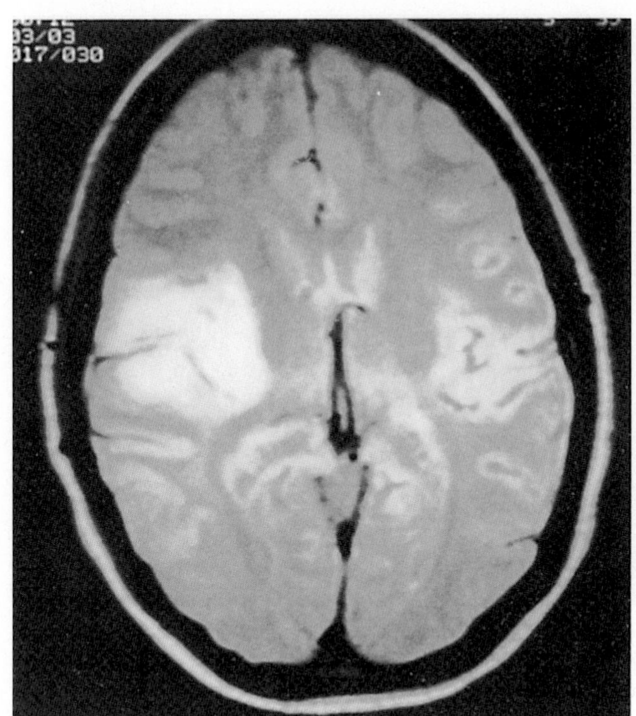

FIGURE 65-2. Low-grade glioma. MRI of the brain shows an abnormal density in the right temporal lobe. Courtesy of the Hospital of the University of Pennsylvania, Nuclear Medicine Section, Philadelphia, PA.

Cytologic studies of the CSF may be performed to detect malignant cells, because CNS tumors can shed cells into the CSF.

Medical Management

A variety of medical treatment modalities, including chemotherapy and external-beam radiation therapy, are used alone or in combination with surgical resection. Radiation therapy, the cornerstone of treatment for many brain tumors, decreases the incidence of recurrence of incompletely resected tumors. Brachytherapy (the surgical implantation of radiation sources to deliver high doses at a short distance) has had promising results for primary malignancies. It is usually used as an adjunct to conventional radiation therapy or as a rescue measure for recurrent disease.

Intravenous (IV) autologous bone marrow transplantation is used in some patients who will receive chemotherapy or radiation therapy, because it can "rescue" the patient from the bone marrow toxicity associated with high doses of chemotherapy and radiation. A fraction of the patient's bone marrow is aspirated, usually from the iliac crest, and stored. The patient receives large doses of chemotherapy or radiation therapy to destroy large numbers of malignant cells. The marrow is then reinfused intravenously after treatment is completed.

Corticosteroids may be used before and after treatment to reduce cerebral edema and promote a smoother, more rapid recovery.

Gene transfer therapy uses retroviral vectors to carry genes to the tumor, reprogramming the tumor tissue for susceptibility to treatment. This approach is being tested (ABTA, 2006).

A new technique being investigated is photodynamic therapy. This is a treatment of primary malignant brain tumors that delivers targeted photodynamic therapy while conserving healthy brain tissue (Schmidt, Meyer, Reichert, et al., 2004).

Surgical Management

The objective of surgical management is to remove or destroy the entire tumor without increasing the neurologic deficit (paralysis, blindness) or to relieve symptoms by partial removal (decompression). A variety of treatment modalities may be used; the specific approach depends on the type of tumor, its location, and its accessibility. In many patients, combinations of these modalities are used. Most pituitary adenomas are treated by transsphenoidal microsurgical removal (see Chapter 61), and the remainder of tumors that cannot be removed completely are treated by radiation (Pickett, 2003). An untreated brain tumor ultimately leads to death, either from increasing ICP or from the damage the tumor causes to brain tissue.

Conventional surgical approaches require a craniotomy (incision into the skull). See Chapter 61 for a discussion of care of the patient who has undergone a craniotomy. This approach is used in patients with meningiomas, acoustic neuromas, cystic astrocytomas of the cerebellum, colloid cysts of the third ventricle, congenital tumors such as dermoid cyst, and some of the granulomas. With improved imaging techniques and the availability of the operating microscope and microsurgical instrumentation, even large tumors can be removed through a relatively small craniotomy. For patients with malignant glioma, complete removal of the tumor and cure are not possible, but the rationale for resection includes relief of ICP, removal of any necrotic tissue, and reduction in the bulk of the tumor, which theoretically leaves behind fewer cells to become resistant to radiation or chemotherapy.

Stereotactic approaches involve the use of a three-dimensional frame that allows very precise localization of the tumor; a stereotactic frame and multiple imaging studies (x-rays, CT scans) are used to localize the tumor and verify its position (Fig. 65-3). New brain-mapping technology helps determine how close diseased areas of the brain are to structures essential for normal brain function. Lasers or radiation can be delivered with stereotactic approaches. Radioisotopes such as iodine 131 (^{131}I) can also be implanted directly into the tumor to deliver high doses of radiation to the tumor (brachytherapy) while minimizing effects on surrounding brain tissue.

Stereotactic procedures may be performed using a linear accelerator or gamma knife to perform radiosurgery. These procedures allow treatment of deep, inaccessible tumors, often in a single session. Precise localization of the tumor is accomplished by the stereotactic approach and by minute measurements and precise positioning of the patient. Multiple narrow beams then deliver a very high dose of radiation. An advantage of this method is that no surgical incision is needed; a disadvantage is the lag time between treatment and the desired result (Gnanadurai, Purushothamam, Rajshekhar, et al., 2004).

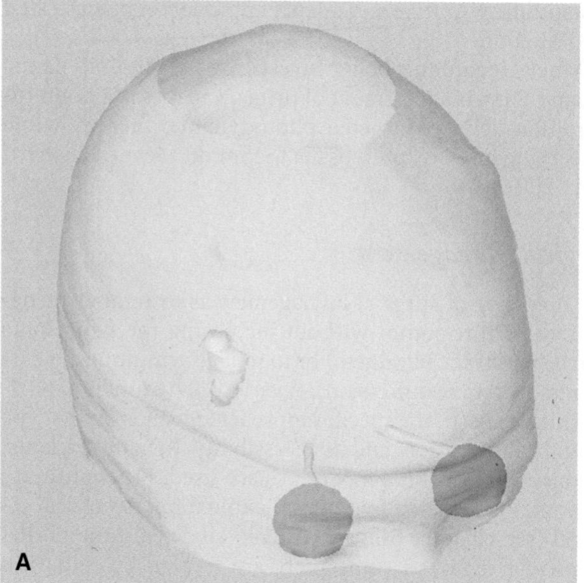

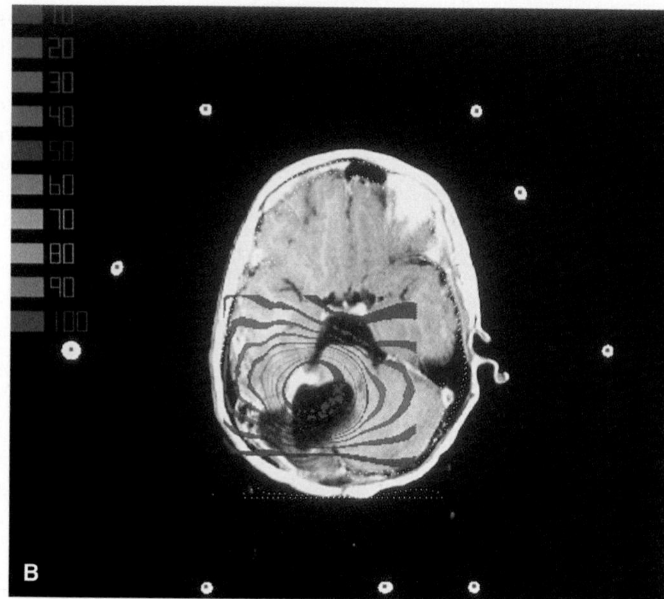

FIGURE 65-3. (**A**) Using stereotactic or "brain-mapping" guided approach, a 3-D computer image fuses the CT and MRI to pinpoint the exact location of the brain tumor. This low-grade astrocytoma is localized adjacent to the brain stem, is nonoperable, and is treated with radiation. Note the optic chasm and optic nerves. (**B**) Computerized image of the prescribed radiation dose.

Nursing Management

The patient with a brain tumor may be at increased risk for aspiration due to cranial nerve dysfunction. Preoperatively, the gag reflex and ability to swallow are evaluated. In patients with diminished gag response, care includes teaching the patient to direct food and fluids toward the unaffected side, having the patient sit upright to eat, offering a semisoft diet, and having suction readily available. Function should be reassessed postoperatively, because changes can occur.

The effects of increased ICP caused by the tumor mass are reviewed in Chapter 61. The nurse performs neurologic checks, monitors vital signs, maintains a neurologic flow chart, spaces nursing interventions to prevent rapid increase in ICP, and reorients the patient when necessary to person, time, and place. Patients with changes in cognition caused by their lesion require frequent reorientation and the use of orienting devices (eg, personal possessions, photographs, lists, a clock), supervision of and assistance with self-care, and ongoing monitoring and intervention for prevention of injury. Patients with seizures are carefully monitored and protected from injury.

Motor function is checked at intervals, because specific motor deficits may occur, depending on the tumor's location. Sensory disturbances are assessed. Speech is evaluated. Eye movement and pupillary size and reaction may be affected by cranial nerve involvement. One study that examined the experience of patients with brain tumors 3 to 5 days postoperatively found that the basic needs of patients were met but suggested changes such as minimizing the atmosphere of urgency and hurry, appointing a primary nurse for each patient, and giving more postoperative information (Lepola, Toljamo, Ahi, et al., 2001). The nursing process for patients undergoing neurosurgery is discussed in Chapter 61.

Cerebral Metastases

A significant number of patients with cancer experience neurologic deficits caused by metastasis to the brain. Metastatic lesions to the brain constitute the most common neurologic complication, occurring in 25% of patients with cancer (Ropper, Gress, Diringer, et al., 2004). This occurrence becomes important clinically as more patients with all forms of cancer live longer because of improved therapies. Neurologic signs and symptoms include headache, gait disturbances, visual impairment, personality changes, altered mentation (memory loss and confusion), focal weakness, paralysis, aphasia, and seizures. These signs and symptoms can be devastating to both patient and family.

Medical Management

The treatment of metastatic brain cancer is palliative and involves eliminating or reducing serious symptoms. Even when palliation is the goal, distressing signs and symptoms can be relieved, thereby improving the quality of life for both patient and family. Patients with intracerebral metastases who are not treated have a steady downhill course with a limited survival time, whereas those who are treated may survive for slightly longer periods. The median survival time for patients with no treatment for brain metastases is 1 month; with corticosteroid treatment alone it is 2 months; radiation therapy extends the median survival time to 3 to 6 months.

The therapeutic approach includes radiation therapy (the foundation of treatment), surgery (usually for a single intracranial metastasis), and chemotherapy; more often, some combination of these treatments is the optimal method. Gamma knife radiosurgery is considered if three or fewer lesions are present.

Pharmacologic Therapy

Corticosteroids are useful in relieving headache and alterations in level of consciousness. Researchers believe that corticosteroids such as dexamethasone (Decadron) and prednisone (Deltasone) reduce inflammation around the metastatic deposits and decrease the edema surrounding them (Nahaczewski, Fowler & Hariharan, 2004). Other medications used include osmotic diuretics (eg, mannitol [Osmitrol]) to decrease the fluid content of the brain, which leads to a decrease in ICP. Antiseizure agents (eg, phenytoin [Dilantin]) are used to prevent and treat seizures (Ropper et al., 2004). Venous thromboembolic events, such as deep vein thrombosis (DVT) and pulmonary embolism (PE), occur in about 15% of patients and are associated with significant morbidity. Anticoagulants usually are not prescribed because of the risk for CNS hemorrhage; however, prophylactic therapy with low-molecular-weight heparin is under investigation.

Chemotherapy plays a small role in managing brain metastasis because of poor penetration across the blood–brain barrier. Drug penetration and sensitivity of brain cells are two factors that determine the responsiveness of metastatic brain tumors to chemotherapy. Research is being directed at multidrug regimens and drug resistance (ABTA, 2006). Encouraging results have been seen with chemotherapeutic agents such as carmustine (BCNU), lomustine (CCNU), and PCV (a triple-drug combination of procarbazine hydrochloride, lomustine, and vincristine). Promising results have been seen with the use of topotecan (Hycamtin), another chemotherapy agent.

Pain is managed by means of a stepped progression in the doses and type of analgesic agents needed for relief. If the patient has severe pain, morphine can be infused into the epidural or subarachnoid space through a spinal needle and a catheter placed as near as possible to the spinal segment where the pain is projected. Small doses of morphine are administered at prescribed intervals (see Chapter 13).

Nursing Process

The Patient With Cerebral Metastases or Incurable Brain Tumor

Assessment

The nursing assessment includes a baseline neurologic examination and focuses on how the patient is functioning, moving, and walking; adapting to weakness or paralysis and to loss of vision and speech; and dealing with seizures. Assessment addresses symptoms that cause distress to the patient, including pain, respiratory problems, bowel and bladder disorders, sleep disturbances, and impairment of skin integrity, fluid balance, and temperature regulation. Tumor invasion, compression, or obstruction may cause these disorders.

Nutritional status is assessed, because cachexia (weak and emaciated condition) is common in patients with metastases. The nurse explores changes associated with poor nutritional status (anorexia, pain, weight loss, altered metabolism, muscle weakness, malabsorption, and diarrhea) and asks the patient about altered taste sensations that may be secondary to dysphagia, weakness, and depression and about distortions and impaired sense of smell (anosmia).

The nurse takes a dietary history to assess food intake, intolerance, and preferences. Calculation of body mass index can confirm the loss of subcutaneous fat and lean body mass (see Chapter 5). Biochemical measurements (albumin, transferrin, total lymphocyte count, creatinine index, and urinary tests) are reviewed to assess the degree of malnutrition, impaired cellular immunity, and electrolyte balance. A dietitian assists in determining the caloric needs of the patient.

The nurse works with other members of the health care team to assess the impact of the illness on the family in terms of home care, altered relationships, financial problems, time pressures, and family problems. This information is important in helping family members cope with the diagnosis and the changes associated with it.

Diagnosis

Nursing Diagnoses

Based on the assessment data, the patient's major nursing diagnoses may include the following:

- Self-care deficit (feeding, bathing, and toileting) related to loss or impairment of motor and sensory function and decreased cognitive abilities
- Imbalanced nutrition, less than body requirements, related to cachexia due to treatment and tumor effects, decreased nutritional intake, and malabsorption
- Anxiety related to fear of dying, uncertainty, change in appearance, or altered lifestyle
- Interrupted family processes related to anticipatory grief and the burdens imposed by the care of the person with a terminal illness

Other nursing diagnoses of the patient with cerebral metastases may include acute pain related to tumor compression; impaired gas exchange related to dyspnea; constipation related to decreased fluid and dietary intake and medications; impaired urinary elimination related to reduced fluid intake, vomiting, and reactions to medications; sleep pattern disturbances related to discomfort and fear of dying; impairment of skin integrity related to cachexia, poor tissue perfusion, and decreased mobility; deficient fluid volume related to fever, vomiting, and low fluid intake; and ineffective thermoregulation related to hypothalamic involvement, fever, and chills. See Chapter 16 for assessment and nursing interventions for the patient with cancer.

Planning and Goals

The goals for the patient may include compensating for self-care deficits, improving nutrition, reducing anxiety, enhancing family coping skills, and absence of complications.

Nursing Interventions

Compensating for Self-Care Deficits

The patient may have difficulty participating in goal setting as the tumor metastasizes and affects cognitive function. The nurse should encourage the family to keep the patient as independent as possible for as long as possible. Increasing assistance with self-care activities is required. Because the patient with cerebral metastasis and the family live with uncertainty, they are encouraged to plan for each day and to make the most of each day. The tasks and challenges are to assist the patient to find useful coping mechanisms, adaptations, and compensations for solving problems that arise. This helps patients maintain some sense of control. An individualized exercise program helps maintain strength, endurance, and range of motion. Eventually, referral for home or hospice care may be necessary (see Chapter 17).

Improving Nutrition

Patients with nausea, vomiting, diarrhea, breathlessness, and pain are rarely interested in eating. These symptoms are managed or controlled through assessment, planning, and care. The nurse teaches the family how to position the patient for comfort during meals. Meals are planned for times when the patient is rested and in less distress from pain or the effects of treatment.

The patient needs to be clean, comfortable, and free of pain for meals, in an environment that is as attractive as possible. Oral hygiene before meals helps to improve intake. Offensive sights, sounds, and odors are eliminated. Creative strategies may be required to make food more palatable, provide enough fluids, and increase opportunities for socialization during meals. The family may be asked to keep a daily weight chart and to record the quantity of food eaten to determine the daily calorie count. Dietary supplements, if acceptable to the patient, can be provided to meet increased caloric needs. If the patient is not interested in most usual foods, those foods preferred by the patient should be offered. When the patient shows marked deterioration as a result of tumor growth and effects, some other form of nutritional support (eg, tube feeding, parenteral nutrition) may be indicated if consistent with the patient's end-of-life preferences (Dudek, 2006; Worthington, 2004). Nursing interventions include assessing the patency of the central and IV lines or feeding tube, monitoring the insertion site for infection, checking the infusion rate, monitoring intake and output, and changing the IV tubing and dressing. Family members are instructed in these techniques if they will be providing care at home. Parenteral nutrition can be provided at home if indicated.

The patient's quality of life may guide the selection, initiation, maintenance, and discontinuation of nutritional support. The nurse and family should not place too much emphasis on eating or on discussions about food, because the patient may not desire aggressive nutritional intervention. The subsequent course of action must be congruent with the wishes and choices of the patient and family.

Relieving Anxiety

Patients with cerebral metastases may be restless, with changing moods that may include intense depression, euphoria, paranoia, and severe anxiety. The response of patients to terminal illness reflects their pattern of reaction to other crisis situations. Serious illness imposes additional strains that often bring other unresolved problems to light. The patient's own coping strategies can help deal with anxious and depressed feelings. Health care providers need to be sensitive to the patient's concerns and fears.

Patients need the opportunity to exercise some control over their situation. A sense of mastery can be gained as they learn to understand the disease and its treatment and how to deal with their feelings. The presence of family, friends, a spiritual advisor, and health professionals may be supportive. Support groups such as the Brain Tumor Support Group may provide a feeling of support and strength.

Spending time with patients allows them time to talk and to communicate their fears and concerns. Open communication and acknowledgment of fears are often therapeutic. Touch is also a form of communication. These patients need reassurance that continuing care will be provided and that they will not be abandoned. The situation becomes more endurable when others share in the experience of dying. If a patient's emotional reactions are very intense or prolonged, additional help from a spiritual advisor, social worker, or mental health professional may be indicated.

Enhancing Family Processes

The family needs to be reassured that their loved one is receiving optimal care and that attention will be paid to the patient's changing symptoms and concerns. When the patient can no longer carry out self-care, the family and additional support systems (social worker, home health aid, home care nurse, hospice nurse) may be needed. A nursing goal is to keep the patient's and family's anxiety at a manageable level.

Promoting Home and Community-Based Care

TEACHING PATIENTS SELF-CARE

The patient and family often have major responsibility for care at home. Therefore, teaching includes pain management strategies, prevention of complications related to treatment strategies, and methods to ensure adequate fluid and food intake (Chart 65-2). Teaching needs of the patient and family regarding care priorities are likely to change as the disease progresses. The nurse should assess the changing needs of the patient and the family and inform them about resources and services early, to assist them in dealing with changes in the patient's condition.

CHART 65-2

HOME CARE CHECKLIST • The Patient With Cerebral Metastases

At the completion of the home care instruction, the patient or caregiver will be able to:	Patient	Caregiver
• State effects of the tumor according to its type and location in the brain.	✔	✔
• Describe side effects of treatment.	✔	✔
• Identify community resources, including:		
— Home health services	✔	✔
— Hospices	✔	✔
— Support groups	✔	✔
— American Brain Tumor Association	✔	✔
• Identify coping strategies, such as:		
— Taking control, setting daily goals, and staying positive	✔	✔
— Rehabilitation to improve self-care	✔	
— Relaxation techniques	✔	✔
— Family support		✔
• Verbalize an understanding of the treatment plan for:		
— Medications and pain control	✔	✔
— Nutritional needs	✔	✔
— Contacting the health care provider	✔	✔

CONTINUING CARE

Home care nursing and hospice services are valuable resources that should be made available to the patient and the family early in the course of a terminal illness. Anticipating needs before they occur can assist in smooth initiation of services. Home care needs and interventions focus on four major areas: palliation of symptoms and pain control, assistance in self-care, control of treatment complications, and administration of specific forms of treatment, such as parenteral nutrition. The home care nurse assesses pain management, respiratory status, complications of the disorder and its treatment, and the patient's cognitive and emotional status. Additionally, the nurse assesses the family's ability to perform necessary care and notifies the physician about changing needs or complications if indicated.

The patient and family who elect to care for the patient at home as the disease progresses benefit from the care and support provided through hospice services. Steps to initiate hospice care, including discussion of hospice care as an option, should not be postponed until death is imminent. Exploration of hospice care as an option should be initiated at a time when hospice services can provide support and care to the patient and family consistent with their end-of-life decisions and can assist in allowing death with dignity. End-of-life care is further described in Chapter 17.

Evaluation

Expected Patient Outcomes

Expected patient outcomes may include the following:

1. Engages in self-care activities as long as possible
   a. Uses assistive devices or accepts assistance as needed
   b. Schedules periodic rest periods to permit maximal participation in self-care
2. Maintains as optimal a nutritional status as possible
   a. Eats and accepts food within limits of condition and preferences
   b. Accepts alternative methods of providing nutrition if indicated
3. Reports being less anxious
   a. Is less restless and is sleeping better
   b. Verbalizes concerns and fears about death
   c. Participates in activities of personal importance as long as feasible
4. Family members seek help as needed
   a. Demonstrate ability to bathe, feed, and care for the patient and participate in pain management and prevention of complications
   b. Express feelings and concerns to appropriate health professionals
   c. Discuss and seek hospice care as an option

Spinal Cord Tumors

Tumors within the spine are classified according to their anatomic relation to the spinal cord. They include intramedullary lesions (within the spinal cord), extramedullary-intradural lesions (within or under the spinal dura), and extramedullary-extradural lesions (outside the dural membrane). Tumors that occur within the spinal cord or exert pressure on it cause symptoms ranging from localized or shooting pains and weakness and loss of reflexes above the tumor level to progressive loss of motor function and paralysis. Usually, sharp pain occurs in the area innervated by the spinal roots that arise from the cord in the region of the tumor. In addition, increasing sensory deficits develop below the level of the lesion.

Assessment and Diagnostic Findings

Neurologic examination and diagnostic studies are used to make the diagnosis. Neurologic examination includes assessment of pain, loss of reflexes, loss of sensation or motor function, and the presence of weakness and paralysis. Additional assessment findings usually include pain duration for longer than 1 month and an elevated erythrocyte sedimentation rate (Derebery & Anderson, 2002). Helpful diagnostic studies include x-rays, radionuclide bone scans, CT scans, MRI scans, and biopsy. The MRI scan is the most commonly used and the most sensitive diagnostic tool, and it is particularly helpful in detecting epidural spinal cord compression and metastases (Bader & Littlejohns, 2004).

CHART 65-3

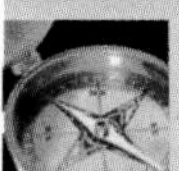

Ethics and Related Issues

What Constitutes Assisted Suicide?

SITUATION

A 76-year-old man is admitted to the hospital with a metastatic spinal cord tumor. He is in respiratory distress and near death. The patient and family state they want no heroic measures and the physician writes a "do not resuscitate" order on the chart.

DILEMMA

The principle of beneficence and the nurse's duty to care conflict with the principle of respect for the person and the patient's right to death with dignity.

DISCUSSION

1. Is the "do not resuscitate" order an act of assisted suicide?
2. Is it active or passive euthanasia? What is the nurse's role in caring for the patient if this action conflicts with his/her personal beliefs?
3. If no other nurse is available to provide care, does the nurse have the right to refuse? Is this patient abandonment?

Medical Management

Treatment of specific intraspinal tumors depends on the type and location of the tumor and the presenting symptoms and physical status of the patient. Surgical intervention is the primary treatment for most spinal cord tumors. Other treatment modalities include partial removal of the tumor, decompression of the spinal cord, chemotherapy, and radiation therapy, particularly for intramedullary tumors and metastatic lesions (Bader & Littlejohns, 2004).

Epidural spinal cord compression occurs in 5% to 7% of patients who die of cancer and is considered a neurologic emergency (Held-Warmkessel, 2005). For the patient with epidural spinal cord compression resulting from metastatic cancer (most commonly from breast, prostate, or lung), high-dose dexamethasone (Decadron) combined with radiation therapy is effective in relieving pain (Held-Warmkessel, 2005). See Chapter 16 for a discussion of care of the patient with spinal cord compression. Palliative care may be an option for the medical management of some patients. Chart 65-3 explores an ethical issue related to end-of-life care for a patient with a metastatic spinal cord tumor.

Surgical Management

Tumor removal is desirable but not always possible. The goal is to remove as much tumor as possible while sparing uninvolved portions of the spinal cord. Microsurgical techniques have improved the prognosis for patients with intramedullary tumors. Prognosis is related to the degree of neurologic impairment at the time of surgery, the speed with which symptoms occurred, and the origin of the tumor. Patients with extensive neurologic deficits before surgery usually do not make significant functional recovery even after successful tumor removal.

Nursing Management

Providing Preoperative Care

The objectives of preoperative care include recognition of neurologic changes through ongoing assessments, pain control, and management of altered activities of daily living (ADLs) resulting from sensory and motor deficits and bowel and bladder dysfunction. The nurse assesses for weakness, muscle wasting, spasticity, sensory changes, bowel and bladder dysfunction, and potential respiratory problems, especially if a cervical tumor is present. The patient is also evaluated for coagulation deficiencies. A history of aspirin intake is obtained and reported, because the use of aspirin may impede hemostasis postoperatively. Breathing exercises are taught and demonstrated preoperatively. Postoperative pain management strategies are discussed with the patient before surgery.

Assessing the Patient After Surgery

The patient is monitored for deterioration in neurologic status. A sudden onset of neurologic deficit is an ominous sign and may be due to vertebral collapse associated with spinal cord infarction. Frequent neurologic checks are carried out, with emphasis on movement, strength, and sensation of the upper and lower extremities. Assessment of sensory function involves pinching the skin of the arms, legs, and trunk to determine if there is loss of feeling and, if so, at what level. Vital signs are monitored at regular intervals.

Managing Pain

The prescribed pain medication should be administered in adequate amounts and at appropriate intervals to relieve pain and prevent its recurrence. Pain is the hallmark of spinal metastasis. Patients with sensory root involvement or vertebral collapse may suffer excruciating pain, which requires effective pain management (Herndon, 2003).

The bed is usually kept flat initially. The nurse turns the patient as a unit, keeping shoulders and hips aligned and the back straight. The side-lying position is usually the most comfortable, because this position imposes the least pressure on the surgical site. Placement of a pillow between the knees of the patient in a side-lying position helps to prevent extreme knee flexion.

Monitoring and Managing Potential Complications

If the tumor was in the cervical area, the possibility of postoperative respiratory compromise arises. The nurse monitors the patient for asymmetric chest movement, abdominal breathing, and abnormal breath sounds. For a high cervical lesion, the endotracheal tube remains in place until adequate respiratory function is ensured. The patient is encouraged to perform deep-breathing and coughing exercises.

The area over the bladder is palpated or a bladder scan is performed to assess for urinary retention. The nurse also monitors for incontinence, because urinary dysfunction usually implies significant decompensation of spinal cord function. An intake and output record is maintained. Additionally, the abdomen is auscultated for bowel sounds.

Staining of the dressing may indicate leakage of CSF from the surgical site, which may lead to serious infection or to an inflammatory reaction in the surrounding tissues that can cause severe pain in the postoperative period.

Promoting Home and Community-Based Care

TEACHING PATIENTS SELF-CARE

In preparation for discharge, the patient is assessed for the ability to function independently in the home and for the availability of resources such as family members to assist in caregiving. Patients with residual sensory involvement are cautioned about the dangers of extremes in temperature. They should be alerted to the dangers of heating devices (eg, hot water bottles, heating pads, space heaters). The patient is taught to check skin integrity daily. Patients with impaired motor function related to motor weakness or paralysis may require training in ADLs and safe use of assistive devices, such as a cane, walker, or wheelchair.

The patient and family members are instructed about pain management strategies, bowel and bladder management, and assessment for signs and symptoms that should be reported promptly.

CONTINUING CARE

Referral for inpatient or outpatient rehabilitation may be warranted to improve self-care abilities. A home care referral may be indicated and provides the home care nurse with the opportunity to assess the patient's physical and psychological status and the patient's and family's ability to adhere to recommended management strategies. During the home visit, the nurse determines whether changes in neurologic function have occurred. The patient's respiratory status and nutritional status are assessed. The adequacy of pain management is assessed, and modifications are made to ensure adequate pain relief. The need for hospice services or placement in an extended-care facility is discussed with the patient and family if warranted, and the patient is asked about preferences for end-of-life care. Additionally, social workers may be consulted to assist the patient and family members in identifying support groups and agencies that can provide help in coping with the disease process.

Degenerative Disorders

Disorders of the central and peripheral nervous system that are **neurodegenerative** (leading to deterioration of normal cells or function of the nervous system) are characterized by the slow onset of signs and symptoms. Patients are managed at home for as long as possible and are admitted to the acute care setting for exacerbations, treatments, and surgical interventions as needed.

Parkinson's Disease

Parkinson's disease is a slowly progressing neurologic movement disorder that eventually leads to disability. The degenerative or idiopathic form is the most common; there is also a secondary form with a known or suspected cause. Although the cause of most cases is unknown, research suggests several causative factors, including genetics, atherosclerosis, excessive accumulation of oxygen free radicals, viral infections, head trauma, chronic use of antipsychotic medications, and some environmental exposures. Parkinsonian symptoms usually first appear in the fifth decade of life; however, cases have been diagnosed as early as 30 years of age. It is the fourth most common neurodegenerative disease. Parkinson's disease affects men more frequently than women. It affects 1% of the population older than 65 years of age, and 2% of those older than 85 years (Rao, Fisch, Srinivasan, et al., 2003).

Pathophysiology

Parkinson's disease is associated with decreased levels of dopamine resulting from destruction of pigmented neuronal cells in the substantia nigra in the basal ganglia region of the brain (Fig. 65-4). Fibers or neuronal pathways project from the substantia nigra to the corpus striatum, where neurotransmitters are key to the control of complex body movements. Through the neurotransmitters acetylcholine (excitatory) and dopamine (inhibitory), striatal neurons relay messages to the higher motor centers that control and refine motor movements. The loss of dopamine stores in this area of the brain results in more excitatory neurotransmitters than inhibitory neurotransmitters, leading to an imbalance that affects voluntary movement.

Clinical symptoms do not appear until 60% of the pigmented neurons are lost and the striatal dopamine level is decreased by 80%. Cellular degeneration impairs the extrapyramidal tracts that control semiautomatic functions and coordinated movements; motor cells of the motor cortex and the pyramidal tracts are not affected. Researchers are working on uncovering the exact mechanism of neurodegeneration; current theories are that it is caused by oxidative stress in a portion of the neuron known as

Physiology/Pathophysiology

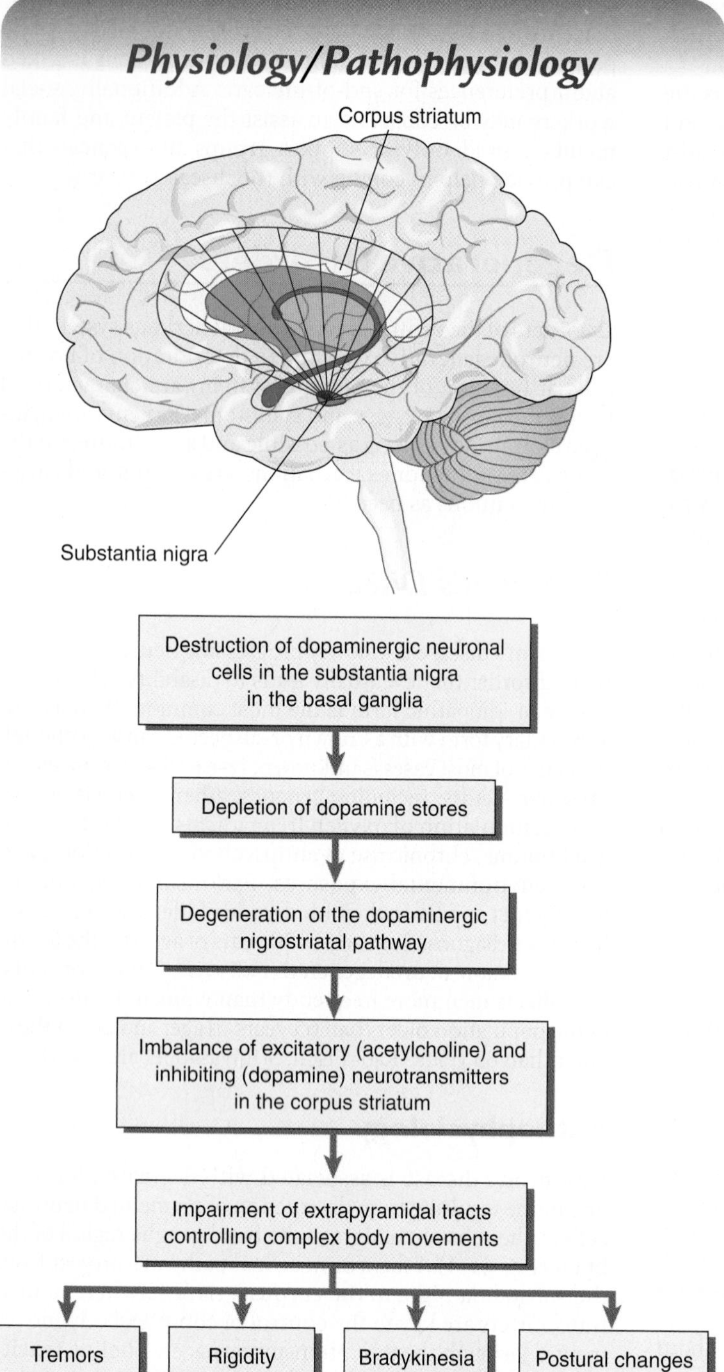

FIGURE 65-4. Pathophysiology of Parkinson's disease. The nuclei in the substantia nigra project fibers to the corpus striatum. The nerve fibers carry dopamine to the corpus striatum. The loss of dopamine nerve cells from the brain's substantia nigra is thought to be responsible for the symptoms of parkinsonism.

Lewy bodies (Andersen, 2004), by protein aggregation, or by a combination of the two mechanisms (Ross & Poirier, 2004).

Clinical Manifestations

Parkinson's disease has a gradual onset, and symptoms progress slowly over a chronic, prolonged course. The cardinal signs are tremor, rigidity, **bradykinesia** (abnormally slow movements), and postural instability (Torpy, Lynm & Glass, 2004).

Tremor

Although symptoms are variable, a slow, unilateral resting tremor is present in 75% of patients at the time of diagnosis (Rao et al., 2003). Resting tremor characteristically disappears with purposeful movement but is evident when the extremities are motionless. The tremor may manifest as a rhythmic, slow turning motion (pronation–supination) of the forearm and the hand and a motion of the thumb against the fingers as if rolling a pill between the fingers. Tremor is present while the patient is at rest; it increases when the patient is walking, concentrating, or feeling anxious.

Rigidity

Resistance to passive limb movement characterizes muscle rigidity. Passive movement of an extremity may cause the limb to move in jerky increments, referred to as cogwheeling (Rao et al., 2003). Involuntary stiffness of the passive extremity increases when another extremity is engaged in voluntary active movement. Stiffness of the arms, legs, face, and posture are common (Torpy et al., 2004). Early in the disease, the patient may complain of shoulder pain due to rigidity.

Bradykinesia

One of the most common features of Parkinson's disease is bradykinesia, which refers to the overall slowing of active movement (Rao et al., 2003). Patients may also take longer to complete activities and have difficulty initiating movement, such as rising from a sitting position or turning in bed.

Postural Instability

The patient commonly develops postural and gait problems (Rao et al., 2003). A loss of postural reflexes occurs, and the patient stands with the head bent forward and walks with a propulsive gait. The posture is caused by the forward flexion of the neck, hips, knees, and elbows. The patient may walk faster and faster, trying to move the feet forward under the body's center of gravity (shuffling gait). Difficulty in pivoting that causes loss of balance (either forward or backward) places the patient at risk for falls.

Other Manifestations

The effect of Parkinson's disease on the basal ganglia often produces autonomic symptoms that include excessive and uncontrolled sweating, paroxysmal flushing, orthostatic hypotension, gastric and urinary retention, constipation, and sexual dysfunction. Psychiatric changes are often interrelated and may be predictive of one another. They include depression, **dementia** (progressive mental deterioration), sleep disturbances, and hallucinations (Press, 2004). Depression is common; whether it is a reaction to the disorder or is related to a biochemical abnormality is uncertain. Mental changes may appear in the form of cognitive, perceptual, and memory deficits, although intellect is not usually affected. A number of psychiatric manifestations (personality changes, psychosis, dementia, and acute confusion) are common in elderly patients with Parkinson's disease. The prevalence of dementia is between 40% and 70%, and the pattern is similar to that of patients with Alzheimer's disease (Press, 2004).

Approximately 75% of patients with Parkinson's disease experience sleep disturbances (Bader & Littlejohns, 2004). This may be related to depression, dementia, or medications. Auditory and visual hallucinations have been reported in approximately 37% of people with Parkinson's disease and may be associated with depression, dementia, lack of sleep, or adverse effects of medications.

Hypokinesia (abnormally diminished movement) is also common and may appear after the tremor. The freezing phenomenon refers to a transient inability to perform active movement and is thought to be an extreme form of bradykinesia. Additionally, the patient tends to shuffle and exhibits a decreased arm swing. As dexterity declines, **micrographia** (small handwriting) develops. The face becomes increasingly mask-like and expressionless, and the frequency of blinking decreases. **Dysphonia** (soft, slurred, low-pitched, and less audible speech) may occur due to weakness and incoordination of the muscles responsible for speech. In many cases, the patient develops dysphagia, begins to drool, and is at risk for choking and aspiration.

Complications associated with Parkinson's disease are common and are typically related to disorders of movement. As the disease progresses, patients are at risk for respiratory and urinary tract infection, skin breakdown, and injury from falls. The adverse effects of medications used to treat the symptoms are associated with numerous complications such as dyskinesia or orthostatic hypotension (Karch, 2005).

Assessment and Diagnostic Findings

Although laboratory tests and imaging studies are not helpful to the clinician in diagnosing Parkinson's disease, ongoing research with PET and single photon emission computed tomography (SPECT) scanning has been helpful in understanding the disease and advancing treatment (Bader & Littlejohns, 2004). Currently, the disease is diagnosed clinically from the patient's history and the presence of two of the four cardinal manifestations: tremor, rigidity, bradykinesia, and postural changes.

Early diagnosis can be difficult, because patients rarely are able to pinpoint when the symptoms started. Often, a family member notices a change such as stooped posture, a stiff arm, a slight limp, tremor, or slow, small handwriting. The medical history, presenting symptoms, neurologic examination, and response to pharmacologic management are carefully evaluated when making the diagnosis.

Medical Management

Treatment is directed at controlling symptoms and maintaining functional independence, because no medical or surgical approaches in current use prevent disease progression. Care is individualized for each patient based on presenting symptoms and social, occupational, and emotional needs. Pharmacologic management is the mainstay of treatment, although advances in research have led to increased surgical options. Patients are usually cared for at home and are admitted to the hospital only for complications or to initiate new treatments.

Pharmacologic Therapy

Antiparkinsonian medications act by (1) increasing striatal dopaminergic activity; (2) reducing the excessive influence of excitatory cholinergic neurons on the extrapyramidal tract, thereby restoring a balance between dopaminergic and cholinergic activities; or (3) acting on neurotransmitter pathways other than the dopaminergic pathway.

ANTIPARKINSONIAN MEDICATIONS

Levodopa (Larodopa) is the most effective agent and the mainstay of treatment. Levodopa is thought to precipitate oxidation, and there is ongoing debate as to whether this further damages the substantia nigra and speeds disease progression (Parkinson Study Group, 2004). Levodopa is converted to dopamine in the basal ganglia, producing symptom relief. The beneficial effects of levodopa are most pronounced in the first few years of treatment. Benefits begin to wane and adverse effects become more severe over time. Confusion, hallucinations, depression, and sleep alterations are associated with prolonged use. Levodopa is usually administered in combination with carbidopa (Sinemet), an amino acid decarboxylase inhibitor that helps to maximize the beneficial effects of levodopa by preventing its breakdown outside the brain and reducing its adverse effects (Parkinson Study Group, 2004).

Within 5 to 10 years, most patients develop a response to the medication characterized by **dyskinesia** (abnormal involuntary movements), including facial grimacing, rhythmic jerking movements of the hands, head bobbing, chewing and smacking movements, and involuntary movements of the trunk and extremities. The patient may experience an on–off syndrome in which sudden periods of near-immobility ("off effect") are followed by a sudden return of effectiveness of the medication ("on effect"). Various adjunctive therapies are used to minimize dyskinesias (Bader & Littlejohns, 2004). Another potential complication of long-term dopaminergic medication use is neuroleptic malignant syndrome, which is characterized by severe rigidity, stupor, and hyperthermia (Ward, 2005).

ANTICHOLINERGIC THERAPY

Anticholinergic agents (eg, trihexyphenidyl hydrochloride [Apo-Trihex], benztropine mesylate [Cogentin]) are effective in controlling tremor and rigidity (Bader & Littlejohns, 2004). They may be used in combination with levodopa. They counteract the action of the neurotransmitter acetylcholine. Because the side effects include blurred vision, flushing, rash, constipation, urinary retention, and acute confusional states, these medications are often poorly tolerated in elderly patients. Intraocular pressure must be closely monitored; these medications are contraindicated in patients with narrow-angle glaucoma. Patients with prostate hyperplasia are monitored for signs of urinary retention.

ANTIVIRAL THERAPY

Amantadine hydrochloride (Symmetrel) is an antiviral agent used in the treatment of early Parkinson's disease to reduce rigidity, tremor, bradykinesia, and postural changes (Bader & Littlejohns, 2004). It is thought to act by releasing dopamine from neuronal storage sites, but the exact mechanism is not known; it may have antiglutamatergic properties that affect the glutamatergic pathway, thus improving levodopa-induced dyskinesias (Bader & Littlejohns, 2004). Amantadine hydrochloride has a low incidence of side effects, which include psychiatric disturbances (mood changes, confusion, depression, hallucinations), lower extremity edema, nausea, epigastric distress, urinary retention, headache, and visual impairment.

DOPAMINE AGONISTS

Bromocriptine mesylate (Parlodel) and pergolide (Permax) are dopamine receptor agonists that can be useful in postponing the initiation of carbidopa or levodopa therapy. Alternatively, dopamine agonists are added to the medication regimen after carbidopa or levodopa loses effectiveness. Pergolide is 10 times more potent than bromocriptine mesylate, although this provides no therapeutic advantage. Adverse reactions to these medications include nausea, vomiting, diarrhea, lightheadedness, hypotension, impotence, and psychiatric effects.

Two new dopamine agonists, ropinirole hydrochloride (Requip) and pramipexole (Mirapex), both nonergot derivatives, are first-line treatment for patients in the early stages of Parkinson's disease and are not expected to have the potentially serious adverse effects of pergolide and bromocriptine mesylate (Bader & Littlejohns, 2004). Pramipexole can be used without levodopa for treatment of early disease and with levodopa in advanced stages. Cabergoline (Dostinex), an ergot alkaloid with a long duration of action, also has been approved for use.

MONOAMINE OXIDASE INHIBITORS

Of the monoamine oxidase (MAO) inhibitors, selegiline (Eldepryl) is a promising development in the pharmacotherapy of Parkinson's disease. This medication inhibits dopamine breakdown and is thought to slow the progression of the disease (Bader & Littlejohns, 2004). Selegiline is currently used in combination with a dopamine agonist to delay the use of carbidopa or levodopa therapy. Adverse effects are similar to those of levodopa.

CATECHOL-*O*-METHYLTRANSFERASE INHIBITORS

Clinical trials suggest that the catechol-*O*-methyltransferase (COMT) inhibitors entacapone (Comtan) and tolcapone (Tasmar) have little effect on parkinsonian symptoms when given alone but can increase the duration of action of carbidopa or levodopa when given in combination with them (Bader & Littlejohns, 2004). COMT inhibitors block an enzyme that metabolizes levodopa, making more levodopa available for conversion to dopamine in the brain. Entacapone and tolcapone reduce motor fluctuations in patients with advanced Parkinson's disease.

ANTIDEPRESSANTS

Tricyclic antidepressants may be prescribed to alleviate the depression that is so common in patients with Parkinson's disease. The usual dosage is one third to one half of the dosage used in depressed patients without Parkinson's disease. Amitriptyline hydrochloride (Elavil) is typically prescribed because of its anticholinergic and antidepressant effects. Serotonin reuptake inhibitors, such as fluoxetine hydrochloride (Prozac) and bupropion hydrochloride (Wellbutrin), are effective for treating depression but may aggravate symptoms of Parkinson's disease.

ANTIHISTAMINES

Diphenhydramine hydrochloride (Benadryl), orphenadrine citrate (Banflex), and phenindamine hydrochloride (Neo-Synephrine) have mild central anticholinergic and sedative effects and may reduce tremors.

Surgical Management

The limitations of levodopa therapy, improvements in stereotactic surgery, and new approaches in transplantation have renewed interest in the surgical treatment of Parkinson's disease. In patients with disabling tremor, rigidity, or severe levodopa-induced dyskinesia, surgery may be considered. Although surgery provides some relief in selected patients, it has not been shown to alter the course of the disease or to produce permanent improvement (Bader & Littlejohns, 2004).

STEREOTACTIC PROCEDURES

Thalamotomy and pallidotomy are effective in relieving many of the symptoms of Parkinson's disease. Patients eligible for these procedures are those who have had an inadequate response to medical therapy; they must meet strict criteria to be eligible. Candidates eligible for these procedures are patients with idiopathic Parkinson's disease who are taking maximum doses of antiparkinsonian medications. Patients with dementia and atypical Parkinson's disease are usually not considered for stereotactic procedures. Parkinson's disease rating scales and specific neurologic tests are used to identify eligible patients.

The intent of thalamotomy and pallidotomy is to interrupt the nerve pathways and thereby alleviate tremor or rigidity. During thalamotomy, a stereotactic electrical stimulator destroys part of the ventrolateral portion of the thalamus in an attempt to reduce tremor; the most common complications are ataxia and hemiparesis. Pallidotomy involves destruction of part of the ventral aspect of the medial globus pallidus through electrical stimulation in patients with advanced disease. The procedure is effective in reducing rigidity, bradykinesia, and dyskinesia, thus improving motor function and ADLs in the immediate postoperative course (Bader & Littlejohns, 2004). Potential complications include hemiparesis and stroke, as well as cognitive, speech, swallowing, and visual changes.

A CT scan, x-ray, MRI scan, or angiogram is used to localize the appropriate surgical site in the brain. Then the patient's head is positioned in a stereotactic frame (Fig. 65-5). After the surgeon makes an incision in the skin and a burr hole, an electrode is passed through to the target area in the thalamus or globus pallidum. The desired response of the patient to the electrical stimulation (ie, a decrease in rigidity) is the basis for the selection of the area of the brain to be destroyed. Stereotactic procedures are completed on one side of the brain at a time. If rigidity or tremor is bilateral, a 6-month interval is suggested between procedures.

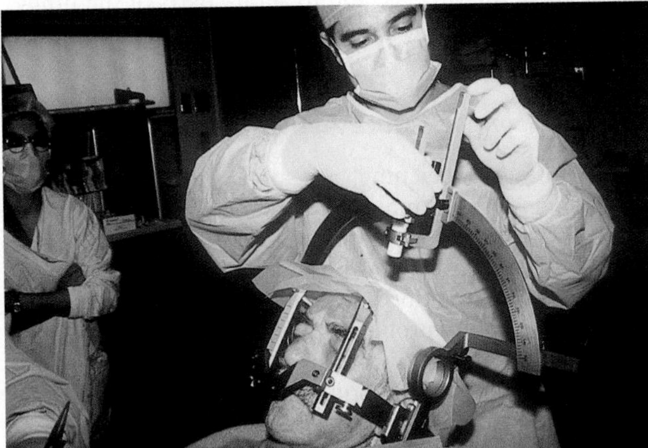

FIGURE 65-5. A stereotactic frame is applied to a patient's head in preparation for pallidotomy. The frame immobilizes the head.

NEURAL TRANSPLANTATION

Ongoing research is exploring transplantation of porcine neuronal cells, human fetal cells, and stem cells (Bader & Littlejohns 2004). Legal, ethical, and political concerns surrounding the use of fetal brain cells and stem cells have limited the implementation of these procedures.

DEEP BRAIN STIMULATION

Pacemaker-like brain implants are used to relieve tremors. The stimulation can be bilateral or unilateral; bilateral stimulation of the subthalamic nucleus is thought to be of greater benefit to patients than results achieved with thalamotomy, pallidotomy, or fetal nigral transplantation (Bader & Littlejohns, 2004). In deep brain stimulation, an electrode is placed in the thalamus and connected to a pulse generator that is implanted in a subcutaneous subclavicular or abdominal pouch. The battery-powered pulse generator sends high-frequency electrical impulses through a wire placed under the skin to a lead anchored to the skull (Fig. 65-6). The electrode blocks nerve pathways in the brain that cause tremors. These devices are not without complications, both from the surgical procedure needed for implantation and from complications (eg, lead leakage) of the device itself (Stewart, Desaloms, & Sanghera, 2005).

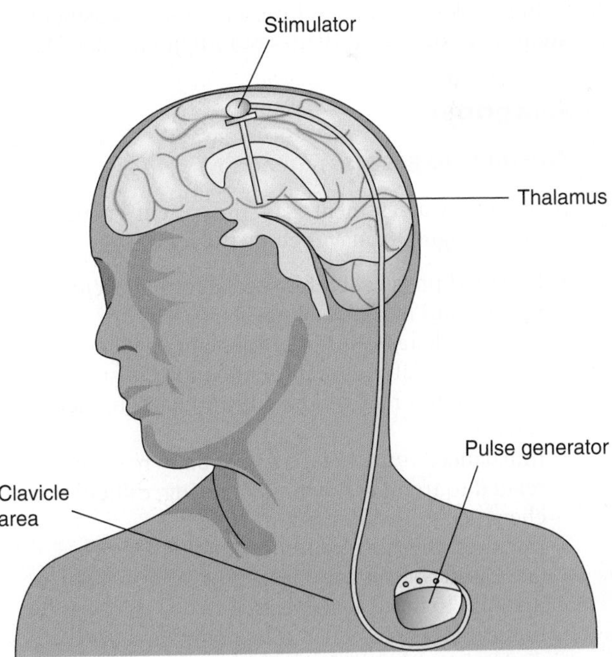

FIGURE 65-6. Deep brain stimulation is provided by a pulse generator surgically implanted in a pouch beneath the clavicle. The generator sends high-frequency electrical impulses to the thalamus, thereby blocking the nerve pathways associated with tremors in Parkinson's disease.

Nursing Process

The Patient With Parkinson's Disease

Assessment

Assessment focuses on how the disease has affected the patient's ADLs and functional abilities. The patient is observed for degree of disability and functional changes that occur throughout the day, such as responses to medication. Almost every patient with a movement disorder has some functional alteration and may have some type of behavioral dysfunction. The following questions may be useful to assess alterations:

- Do you have leg or arm stiffness?
- Have you experienced any irregular jerking of your arms or legs?
- Have you ever been "frozen" or rooted to the spot and unable to move?
- Does your mouth water excessively? Have you (or others) noticed yourself grimacing or making faces or chewing movements?
- What specific activities do you have difficulty doing?

During this assessment, the nurse observes the patient for quality of speech, loss of facial expression, swallowing deficits (drooling, poor head control, coughing), tremors, slowness of movement, weakness, forward posture, rigidity, evidence of mental slowness, and confusion. Parkinson's symptoms, as well as side effects of medications, put these patients at high risk of falls; therefore, a fall risk assessment should be conducted (Bader & Littlejohns, 2004).

Diagnosis

Nursing Diagnoses

Based on the assessment data, the patient's major nursing diagnoses may include the following:

- Impaired physical mobility related to muscle rigidity and motor weakness
- Self-care deficits (feeding, dressing, hygiene, and toileting) related to tremor and motor disturbance
- Constipation related to medication and reduced activity
- Imbalanced nutrition, less than body requirements, related to tremor, slowness in eating, difficulty in chewing and swallowing
- Impaired verbal communication related to decreased speech volume, slowness of speech, inability to move facial muscles
- Ineffective coping related to depression and dysfunction due to disease progression

Other nursing diagnoses may include sleep pattern disturbances, deficient knowledge, risk for injury, risk for activity intolerance, disturbed thought processes, and compromised family coping.

Planning and Goals

The goals for the patient may include improving functional mobility, maintaining independence in ADLs, achieving adequate bowel elimination, attaining and maintaining acceptable nutritional status, achieving effective communication, and developing positive coping mechanisms.

Nursing Interventions

Improving Mobility

A progressive program of daily exercise will increase muscle strength, improve coordination and dexterity, reduce muscular rigidity, and prevent contractures that occur when muscles are not used. Walking, riding a stationary bicycle, swimming, and gardening are all exercises that help maintain joint mobility. Stretching (stretch–hold–relax) and range-of-motion exercises promote joint flexibility. Postural exercises are important to counter the tendency of the head and neck to be drawn forward and down. A physical therapist may be helpful in developing an individualized exercise program and can provide instruction to the patient and caregiver on exercising safely. Faithful adherence to an exercise and walking program helps to delay the progress of the disease. Warm baths and massage, in addition to passive and active exercises, help relax muscles and relieve painful muscle spasms that accompany rigidity.

Balance may be adversely affected because of the rigidity of the arms (arm swinging is necessary in normal walking). Special walking techniques must be learned to offset the shuffling gait and the tendency to lean forward. The patient is taught to concentrate on walking erect, to watch the horizon, and to use a wide-based gait (ie, walking with the feet separated). A conscious effort must be made to swing the arms, raise the feet while walking, and use a heel-toe placement of the feet with long strides. The patient is advised to practice walking to marching music or to the sound of a ticking metronome, because this provides sensory reinforcement. Doing breathing exercises while walking helps to move the rib cage and to aerate parts of the lungs. Frequent rest periods aid in preventing frustration and fatigue.

Enhancing Self-Care Activities

Encouraging, teaching, and supporting the patient during ADLs promote self-care (Stewart et al., 2005). See Chapter 11 for rehabilitation techniques.

Environmental modifications are necessary to compensate for functional disabilities. Patients may have severe mobility problems that make normal activities impossible. Adaptive or assistive devices may be useful. A hospital bed at home with bedside rails, an overbed frame with a trapeze, or a rope tied to the foot of the bed can provide assistance in pulling up without help. An occupational therapist can evaluate the patient's needs in the home, make recommendations regarding adaptive devices, and teach the patient and caregiver how to improvise.

Improving Bowel Elimination

The patient may have severe problems with constipation. Among the factors causing constipation are weakness of the muscles used in defecation, lack of exercise, inadequate fluid intake, and decreased autonomic nervous system activity. The medications used for the treatment of the disease also inhibit normal intestinal secretions. A regular bowel routine may be established by encouraging the patient to follow a regular time pattern, consciously increase fluid intake, and eat foods with a moderate fiber content. Laxatives should be avoided. Psyllium (Metamucil), for example, decreases constipation but carries the risk of bowel obstruction (Karch, 2005). A raised toilet seat is useful, because the patient has difficulty in moving from a standing to a sitting position.

Improving Nutrition

Patients may have difficulty maintaining their weight. Eating becomes a very slow process, requiring concentration due to a dry mouth from medications and difficulty chewing and swallowing. These patients are at risk for aspiration because of impaired swallowing and the accumulation of saliva. They may be unaware that they are aspirating; subsequently, bronchopneumonia may develop.

Monitoring weight on a weekly basis indicates whether caloric intake is adequate. Supplemental feedings increase caloric intake. As the disease progresses, a nasogastric tube or percutaneous endoscopic gastroscopy may be necessary to maintain adequate nutrition. A dietitian can be consulted regarding nutritional needs.

Enhancing Swallowing

Swallowing difficulties are common in Parkinson's disease (Galvez-Jimenez & Lang, 2004). These can lead to problems with poor head control, tongue tremor, hesitancy in initiating swallowing, difficulty in shaping food into a bolus, and disturbances in pharyngeal motility. To offset these problems, the patient should sit in an upright position during mealtime. A semisolid diet with thick liquids is easier to swallow than solids; thin liquids should be avoided. Thinking through the swallowing sequence is helpful. The patient is taught to place the food on the tongue, close the lips and teeth, lift the tongue up and then back, and swallow. The patient is encouraged to chew first on one side of the mouth and then on the other. To control the buildup of saliva, the patient is reminded to hold the head upright and make a conscious effort to swallow. Massaging the facial and neck muscles before meals may be beneficial.

Encouraging the Use of Assistive Devices

An electric warming tray keeps food hot and allows the patient to rest during the prolonged time that it may take to eat. Special utensils also assist at mealtime. A plate that is stabilized, a nonspill cup, and eating utensils with built-up handles are useful self-help devices. The occupational therapist can assist in identifying appropriate adaptive devices.

Improving Communication

Speech disorders are present in most patients with Parkinson's disease. Their low-pitched, monotonous, soft speech requires that they make a conscious effort to speak slowly, with deliberate attention to what they are saying. The patient is reminded to face the listener, exaggerate the pronunciation of words, speak in short sentences, and take a few deep breaths before speaking. A speech therapist may be helpful in designing speech improvement exercises and assisting the family and health care personnel to develop and use a method of communication that meets the patient's needs. A small electronic amplifier is helpful if the patient has difficulty being heard.

Supporting Coping Abilities

Support can be given by encouraging the patient and pointing out that activities will be maintained through active participation. A combination of physiotherapy, psychotherapy, medication therapy, and support group participation may help reduce the depression that often occurs.

Patients often feel embarrassed, apathetic, inadequate, bored, and lonely. These feelings may be due, in part, to physical slowness and the great effort that even small tasks require. The patient is assisted and encouraged to set achievable goals (eg, improvement of mobility).

Because Parkinson's disease can lead to withdrawal and depression, patients must be active participants in their therapeutic program, including social and recreational events. A planned program of activity throughout the day prevents too much daytime sleeping as well as disinterest and apathy.

Every effort should be made to encourage patients to carry out the tasks involved in meeting their own daily needs and to remain independent. Doing things for the patient merely to save time undermines the basic goal of improving coping abilities and promoting a positive self-concept.

Promoting Home and Community-Based Care

TEACHING PATIENTS SELF-CARE

Patient and family education is important in the management of Parkinson's disease. Teaching needs depend on the severity of symptoms and the stage of the disease. Care must be taken not to overwhelm the patient and family with too much information early in the disease process. The patient's and family's need for information is ongoing as adaptations become necessary. The education plan should include a clear explanation of the disease and the goal of assisting the patient to remain functionally independent as long as possible. Every effort is made to explain the nature of the disease and its management, to offset disabling anxieties and fears. The patient and family must be taught about the effects and side effects of medications and about the importance of reporting side effects to the physician (Chart 65-4).

CONTINUING CARE

In the early stages, the patient can be managed well at home. Family members often serve as caregivers, with home care or community services available to assist in meeting health care needs as the disease progresses. The family caregiver may be under considerable stress from living with and caring for a person with a significant disability. Providing information about treatment and care prevents many unnecessary problems. The caregiver is included in the plan and may be advised to learn stress reduction techniques, to include others in the caregiving process, to obtain periodic relief from responsibilities, and to have a yearly health assessment. Allowing family members to express feelings of frustration, anger, and guilt is often helpful to them.

The patient should be evaluated in the home for adaptation and safety needs and compliance with the plan of care. In the advanced stages, patients usually enter long-term care facilities if family support is absent. Periodically, admission to an acute care facility may be necessary for changes in medical management or treatment of complications. Nurses provide support, education, and monitoring of patients over the course of the illness.

The nurse involved in home and continuing care needs to remind the patient and family members of the importance of addressing health promotion needs such as screening for hypertension and stroke risk assessments in this predominantly elderly population. Patients are taught about the importance of these activities and are referred to appropriate health care providers. Informational booklets and a newsletter for patient education are published by the National Parkinson's Foundation, Inc., and the American Parkinson's Disease Association (see Resources).

Evaluation

Expected Patient Outcomes

Expected patient outcomes may include the following:

1. Strives toward improved mobility
   a. Participates in exercise program daily
   b. Walks with wide base of support; exaggerates arm swinging when walking
   c. Takes medications as prescribed

CHART 65-4

HOME CARE CHECKLIST • The Patient With Parkinson's Disease

At the completion of the home care instruction, the patient or caregiver will be able to:	Patient	Caregiver
• Define Parkinson's disease and discuss its long-term effects.	✔	✔
• Identify the medication regimen and name adverse effects, and precautions.	✔	✔
• Discuss the risk for injury; prevent falls; implement adaptive measures in the home.	✔	✔
• Describe nutritional needs, dietary restrictions, dysphagia management, and ways to prevent aspiration.	✔	✔
• Manage constipation: fluid intake, bowel routine.	✔	✔
• Manage urinary problems: functional incontinence, retention (indwelling urinary catheter care, suprapubic catheter care).	✔	✔
• Explain effects of immobility and define preventive care: skin breakdown (frequent turning, pressure release, skin care), pneumonia (deep breathing, movement), contractures (range-of-motion exercises).	✔	✔
• Define benefits of daily exercise program.	✔	✔
• Walk and balance safely.	✔	
• Demonstrate speech and communication skills: speech exercises, communication techniques, breathing exercises.	✔	
• Name signs and symptoms of infection (urinary and respiratory) and state when health care provider should be notified.	✔	✔
• Describe strategies to promote self-care activities and independence.	✔	✔
• Identify resources: American Parkinson's Disease Association, National Parkinson's Disease Foundation, and local support groups.	✔	✔

2. Progresses toward self-care
   a. Allows time for self-care activities
   b. Uses self-help devices
3. Maintains bowel function
   a. Consumes adequate fluid
   b. Increases dietary intake of fiber
   c. Reports regular pattern of bowel function
4. Attains improved nutritional status
   a. Swallows without aspiration
   b. Takes time while eating
5. Achieves a method of communication
   a. Communicates needs
   b. Practices speech exercises
6. Copes with effects of Parkinson's disease
   a. Sets realistic goals
   b. Demonstrates persistence in meaningful activities
   c. Verbalizes feelings to appropriate person

Huntington's Disease

Huntington's disease is a chronic, progressive, hereditary disease of the nervous system that results in progressive involuntary choreiform movement and dementia in approximately 1 in 10,000 individuals (Bossy-Wetzel, Schwarzenbacher & Lipton, 2004). It can affect men and women of any race at midlife (Bader & Littlejohns, 2004). Because it is transmitted as an autosomal dominant genetic disorder, each child of a parent with Huntington's disease has a 50% risk of inheriting the disorder.

Pathophysiology

The basic pathology involves premature death of cells in the striatum (caudate and putamen) of the basal ganglia, the region deep within the brain that is involved in the control of movement (Bossy-Wetzel et al., 2004). Cells also are lost in the cortex, the region of the brain associated with thinking, memory, perception, and judgment, and in the cerebellum, the area that coordinates voluntary muscle activity. Researchers now believe that a building block for protein called glutamine abnormally collects in the cell nucleus, causing cell death. Why the protein destroys only certain brain cells is unknown, but several theories have been proposed to explain the phenomenon (Bader & Littlejohns, 2004; Bossy-Wetzel et al., 2004).

Onset usually occurs between the ages of 35 and 45 years, although about 10% of patients are children. The disease progresses slowly. Despite a ravenous appetite, patients usually become emaciated and exhausted (Mahant, McCusker, Byth, et al., 2003). Patients succumb in 10 to 20 years to heart failure, pneumonia, or infection, or as a result of a fall or choking.

Clinical Manifestations

The most prominent clinical features of the disease are **chorea** (abnormal involuntary movements), intellectual decline, and, often, emotional disturbance. As the disease progresses, a constant writhing, twisting, uncontrollable movement may involve the entire body. These motions are devoid of purpose or rhythm, although patients may try to turn them into purposeful movement. All of the body musculature is involved. Facial movements produce tics and grimaces. Speech becomes slurred, hesitant, often explosive, and eventually unintelligible. Chewing and swallowing are difficult, and there is a constant danger of choking and aspiration. Choreiform movements persist during sleep but are diminished (Mahant et al., 2003).

As with speech, the gait becomes disorganized to the point that ambulation eventually is impossible. Although independent ambulation should be encouraged for as long as possible, a wheelchair usually becomes necessary. Eventually, the patient is confined to bed when the chorea interferes with walking, sitting, and all other activities (Rosenblatt, Abbott, Gourley, et al., 2003). Bladder and bowel control is lost. Cognitive function is usually affected, with dementia usually occurring (Rosenblatt et al., 2003). Initially, the patient is aware that the disease is responsible for the myriad dysfunctions that are occurring. The mental and emotional changes that occur may be more devastating to the patient and family than the abnormal movements. Personality changes may result in nervous, irritable, or impatient behaviors. In the early stages, patients are particularly subject to uncontrollable fits of anger; profound, often suicidal depression; apathy; anxiety; psychosis; or euphoria (Bader & Littlejohns, 2004). Judgment and memory are impaired, and dementia eventually ensues. Hallucinations, delusions, and paranoid thinking may precede the appearance of disjointed movements. Emotional and cognitive symptoms often become less acute as the disease progresses.

Assessment and Diagnostic Findings

The diagnosis is made based on the clinical presentation of characteristic symptoms, a positive family history, and exclusion of other causes. A genetic marker for Huntington's disease has been identified through the use of recombinant DNA technology (Bader & Littlejohns, 2004). As a result, researchers can now identify presymptomatic individuals who will develop this disease. Although this presymptomatic test can remove the uncertainty, it offers no hope of cure or even specific prediction of the timing of its onset. Researchers continue to study the genetic causes that lead to the death of brain cells (Bossy-Wetzel et al., 2004).

Management

Although no treatment halts or reverses the underlying process, several medications reduce chorea. Thiothixene hydrochloride (Navane) and haloperidol decanoate (Haldol), which predominantly block dopamine receptors, improve the chorea in many patients. A double-blind multicenter study of riluzole (Rilutek) showed chorea was reduced in the group that received 200 mg/day compared with those who received a placebo or 100 mg/day of the medication (Huntington Study Group, 2003). Motor signs must be assessed and evaluated on an ongoing basis so that optimal therapeutic drug levels can be reached. **Akathisia** (motor restlessness) in the overmedicated patient is dangerous because it may be mistaken for the restless fidgeting of the illness and consequently may be overlooked.

In certain types of the disease, hypokinetic motor impairment resembles parkinsonism. In patients who present with rigidity, some temporary benefit may be obtained from antiparkinson medications, such as levodopa (Larodopa).

Patients who have emotional disturbances, particularly depression, may be helped by antidepressant medications. The threat of suicide is always present. Psychotic symptoms usually respond to antipsychotic medications (Bader & Littlejohns, 2004). Psychotherapy aimed at allaying anxiety and reducing stress may be beneficial. Nurses must look beyond the disease to focus on the patient's needs and capabilities (Chart 65-5). One study showed improved physical, mental, and social functioning in a small group of patients with Huntington's disease using remotivation therapy and a more stimulating environment (Sullivan, Bird, Alpay, et al., 2001).

Promoting Home and Community-Based Care

TEACHING PATIENTS SELF-CARE

The needs of the patient and family for education depend on the nature and severity of the physical, cognitive, and psychological changes experienced by the patient. The patient and family members are taught about the medications prescribed and about signs indicating a need for change in medication or dosage. The teaching plan addresses strategies to manage symptoms such as chorea, swallowing problems, limitations in ambulation, and loss of bowel and bladder function. Consultation with a speech therapist may be indicated to assist in identifying alternative communication strategies if speech is affected.

Patients of childbearing age often seek information about their risk for transmitting the disease. Even though the gene was mapped in 1983 and presymptomatic testing has been offered since 1986, many patients choose not to be tested (Bader & Littlejohns, 2004). For most people, the benefits of testing are unclear because of ethical issues and concerns about confidentiality. Genetic counseling is crucial after testing, and patients and their families may require long-term psychological counseling and emotional, financial, and legal support.

CONTINUING CARE

A program combining medical, nursing, psychological, social, occupational, speech, and physical rehabilitation services and palliative care is needed to help the patient and family cope with this severely disabling illness (Olson & Cristian, 2005). Huntington's disease exacts enormous emotional, physical, social, and financial tolls on every member of the patient's family. The family needs supportive care as they adjust to the impact of the illness (Dawson, Kristjanson, Toye, et al., 2004). Regular follow-up visits help to allay the fear of abandonment.

Home care assistance, day care centers, respite care, and eventually skilled long-term care can assist the patient and family in coping with the constant strain of the illness. Although the relentless progression of the disease cannot be halted, families can benefit from supportive care.

Voluntary organizations can be major aids to families and have been largely responsible for bringing the illness to national attention. The Huntington's Disease Foundation of America helps patients and families by providing information, referrals, family and public education, and support for research.

Alzheimer's Disease

Alzheimer's disease, or senile dementia of the Alzheimer's type, is a chronic, progressive, and degenerative brain disorder that is accompanied by profound effects on memory, cognition, and ability for self-care. Approximately 4.5 million people in the United States are affected (Tariot, Farlow, Grossberg, et al., 2004). Research suggests that oxidative stress, primarily in the hippocampus and neocortex of people with this type of dementia, plays a role in the pathophysiology of the disease (Andersen, 2004). Alzheimer's disease is one of the most feared disorders of modern times because of its catastrophic consequences for the patient and family, who are faced with many crucial end-of-life decisions (Schulz, Mendelsohn, Haley, et al., 2003). Chapter 12 discusses the manifestations, management, and nursing care of the patient with Alzheimer's disease.

Amyotrophic Lateral Sclerosis

Amyotrophic lateral sclerosis (ALS) is a disease of unknown cause in which there is a loss of motor neurons (nerve cells controlling muscles) in the anterior horns of the spinal cord and the motor nuclei of the lower brain stem. It is often referred to as Lou Gehrig's disease after the famous baseball player who suffered from it (Bossy-Wetzel et al., 2004). As motor neuron cells die, the muscle fibers that they supply undergo atrophic changes. Neuronal degeneration may occur in both the upper and lower motor neuron systems. Theories about the cause of ALS include autoimmune disease, free radical damage, and oxidative stress (Andersen, 2004). The leading theory held by researchers is that overexcitation of nerve cells by the neurotransmitter glutamate leads to cell injury and neuronal degeneration.

The incidence of ALS is 1.5 cases per 100,000 in the general population; it affects more men than women, with onset occurring usually in the fifth or sixth decade (Klingbeil, Baer & Wilson, 2004). Cigarette smoking has been proposed as a risk factor for ALS; one prospective study found that cigarette smoking was associated with increased death rates in women with the disease, compared to men (Weisskopt, McCullough, Calle, et al., 2004).

Clinical Manifestations

Clinical manifestations depend on the location of the affected motor neurons, because specific neurons activate specific muscle fibers. The chief symptoms are fatigue, progressive muscle weakness, cramps, fasciculations (twitching), and incoordination (Bader & Littlejohns, 2004). Loss

CHART 65-5

Care of the Patient With Huntington's Disease

NURSING DIAGNOSIS

Risk for injury from falls and possible skin breakdown (pressure ulcers, abrasions), resulting from constant movement

NURSING INTERVENTIONS

Pad the sides and head of the bed; ensure that the patient can see over the sides of bed.

Use padded heel and elbow protectors.

Keep the skin meticulously clean.

Apply emollient cleansing agent and skin lotion frequently.

Use soft sheets and bedding.

Have patient wear football padding or other forms of padding.

Encourage ambulation with assistance to maintain muscle tone.

Secure the patient (only if necessary) in bed or chair with padded protective devices, making sure that they are loosened frequently.

NURSING DIAGNOSIS

Imbalanced nutrition, less than body requirements, due to inadequate intake and dehydration resulting from swallowing or chewing disorders and danger of choking or aspirating food

NURSING INTERVENTIONS

Administer phenothiazines as prescribed before meals (appears to calm some patients).

Use a warming tray.

Talk to the patient before mealtime to promote relaxation; use mealtime for social interaction. Provide undivided attention. Help the patient enjoy the mealtime experience.

Learn the position that is best for *this* patient. Keep patient as close to upright as possible while feeding. Stabilize patient's head gently with one hand while feeding.

Show the food and tell the patient what the foods are (eg, whether hot or cold).

Encircle the patient with one arm and get as close as possible to provide stability and support while feeding. Use pillows and wedges for additional support.

Do not interpret stiffness, turning away, or sudden turning of the head as rejection; these are uncontrollable choreiform movements.

For feeding, use a long-handled spoon (iced-tea spoon). Place spoon on middle of tongue and exert slight pressure.

Place bite-sized food between patient's teeth. Serve stews, casseroles, thick liquids; avoid too many milk drinks (produces mucus).

Disregard messiness. Treat the person with dignity.

Wait for the patient to chew and swallow before introducing another spoonful. Make sure that bite-sized food is small.

Give between-meal feedings. Constant movement expends more calories. Patients often have voracious appetites, particularly for sweets.

Use blenderized meals if patient cannot chew; do not repeatedly give the same strained baby foods; gradually introduce increased textures and consistencies to the diet.

For swallowing difficulties:

- Apply gentle deep pressure around the patient's mouth.
- Rub fingers in circles on the patient's cheeks.
- Rub fingers simultaneously down each side of the patient's throat.

Develop skill in Heimlich maneuver (to be used in the event of choking).

NURSING DIAGNOSIS

Anxiety and impaired communication from excessive grimacing and unintelligible speech

NURSING INTERVENTIONS

Read to the patient.

Employ biofeedback and relaxation therapy to reduce stress.

Consult with speech therapist to help maintain and prolong communication abilities.

Try to devise a communication system, perhaps using cards with words or pictures of familiar objects, before verbal communication becomes too difficult. Patients can indicate correct card by hitting it with hand, grunting, or blinking the eyes.

Learn how this particular patient expresses needs and wants—particularly nonverbal messages (widening of eyes, responses).

Patients can understand even if unable to speak. Do not isolate patients by ceasing to communicate with them.

NURSING DIAGNOSIS

Disturbed thought processes and impaired social interaction

NURSING INTERVENTIONS

Have clock, calendar, and wall posters in view.

Interact with the patient in a creative manner.

Use every opportunity for one-to-one contact.

Use music for relaxation.

Reorient the patient after awakening.

Have the patient wear an identification bracelet with name, telephone number, and "memory impaired" on it.

Keep the patient in the social mainstream.

Recruit and train volunteers for social interaction. Role model appropriate interactions.

Do not abandon a patient because the disease is eventually terminal. Patients are *living* until the end.

NURSING RESEARCH PROFILE

Testing an Intervention for Caregivers of People With Dementia

Maas, M. L., Reed, D., Park, M., et al., (2004). Outcomes of family involvement in care intervention for caregivers of individuals with dementia. *Nursing Research, 53*(2), 76–86.

Purpose

Many patients with neurodegenerative diseases develop dementia and are relocated from home to a nursing home for care. This relocation results in many changes for the family, especially the caregiver. The purpose of this study was to test the effects of an intervention on the perceptions of family members about their caregiving role, the relationships with staff, and satisfaction with the care of relatives with dementia.

Design

A quasi-experimental design with nonequivalent groups was used to test the effects of the Family Involvement in Care (FIC) partnership intervention. The FIC intervention was 9 months in length and involved negotiated written partnerships between family and staff caregivers. The samples from 14 nursing homes included 185 family members with an average age of 61 years and 895 staff members with an average age of 37 years. The special dementia care units were matched by age and staff turnover and were randomized from matched pairs to experimental and control conditions; repeated pretest and posttest measures were used to test the effects of the intervention.

Findings

Beneficial intervention effects were found for family members in three areas of the family caregiver outcomes: emotional reactions to the caregiving role, perceptions of relationships with staff, and perceptions of care for relatives. Beneficial intervention effects were found in one area of family caregiver outcomes for staff, that of staff perceptions of the family caregiving role. Some of the effects of the intervention were found only for caregivers who were of the same generation as the nursing home resident.

Nursing Implications

This study is of particular interest for nurses working in nursing homes or assisting families to make the transition of placement of a family member in a nursing home. The intervention used in the study improved the caregiving experience of family members in nursing homes as well as the attitudes of nursing home staff toward family members. More research is needed, because the intervention did not influence perceived conflict with staff on the part of family caregivers or the perception of a partnership with family caregivers on the part of staff.

of motor neurons in the anterior horns of the spinal cord results in progressive weakness and atrophy of the muscles of the arms, trunk, or legs. Spasticity usually is present, and the deep tendon stretch reflexes become brisk and overactive. Usually, the function of the anal and bladder sphincters remains intact, because the spinal nerves that control muscles of the rectum and urinary bladder are not affected.

In about 25% of patients, weakness starts in the muscles supplied by the cranial nerves, and difficulty in talking, swallowing, and ultimately breathing occurs. When the patient ingests liquids, soft palate and upper esophageal weakness causes the liquid to be regurgitated through the nose. Weakness of the posterior tongue and palate impairs the ability to laugh, cough, or even blow the nose. If bulbar muscles are impaired, speaking and swallowing are progressively difficult, and aspiration becomes a risk. The voice assumes a nasal sound, and articulation becomes so disrupted that speech is unintelligible. Some emotional liability may be present, but intellectual function is not impaired. Eventually, respiratory function is compromised.

The prognosis generally is based on the area of CNS involvement and the speed with which the disease progresses. Death usually occurs as a result of infection, respiratory failure, or aspiration.

Assessment and Diagnostic Findings

ALS is diagnosed on the basis of the signs and symptoms, because no clinical or laboratory tests are specific for this disease. Electromyography and muscle biopsy studies of the affected muscles indicate reduction in the number of functioning motor units (Bader & Littlejohns, 2004). An MRI scan may show high signal intensity in the corticospinal tracts; this differentiates ALS from a multifocal motor neuropathy.

Management

No specific therapy exists for ALS. The main focus of medical and nursing management is on interventions to maintain or improve function, well-being, and quality of life. The median survival time from onset is 25 months. Among newly diagnosed cases, there was a decline in survival rates when 1226 patients were studied over a 10-year period (Forbes, Colville, Cran, et al., 2004).

The medication riluzole (Rilutek), a glutamate antagonist, was approved by the U.S. Food and Drug Administration in 1995 after clinical trials found that it slows the deterioration of motor neurons. The action of riluzole is not clear, but its pharmacologic properties suggest that it may have a neuroprotective effect in the early stages of ALS. Two randomized controlled drug trials showed that a dose of 100 mg riluzole per day was modestly effective in prolonging survival time (Miller, Mitchell, Lyon, et al., 2002).

Symptomatic treatment and rehabilitative measures are employed to support the patient and improve the quality of life. Baclofen (Lioresal), dantrolene sodium (Dantrium), or diazepam (Valium) may be useful for patients troubled by spasticity, which causes pain and interferes with self-care. Research evaluating the effect of ceftriaxone sodium (Rocephin) found that it slows the course of the disease in mice, but it has not been tested yet in humans (Brown, 2005).

Most patients with ALS are managed at home and in the community, with hospitalization for acute problems. The most common reasons for hospitalization are dehydration and malnutrition, pneumonia, and respiratory failure; recognizing these problems at an early stage in the illness allows for the development of preventive strategies. End-of-life issues include pain, dyspnea, and delirium (Olson & Cristian, 2005).

A patient experiencing problems with aspiration and swallowing may require enteral feeding. The American Academy of Neurology practice guidelines suggest the placement of a percutaneous endoscopic gastrostomy tube before the forced vital capacity drops below 50% of the predicted value. The tube can be safely placed in patients who are using noninvasive positive-pressure ventilation for ventilatory support (Boitano, Jordan & Benditt, 2001).

Mechanical ventilation (using negative-pressure ventilators) is an option if alveolar hypoventilation develops. Noninvasive positive-pressure ventilation is also an option (Bader & Littlejohns, 2004). The use of noninvasive positive-pressure ventilation is particularly helpful at night and postpones the decision of whether to undergo a tracheotomy for long-term mechanical ventilation.

Decisions about life support measures are made by the patient and family and should be based on a thorough understanding of the disease, the prognosis, and the implications of initiating such therapy. Patients are encouraged to complete an advance directive or "living will" to preserve their autonomy in decision making. In locations where physician-assisted suicide is an option, about 20% of patients with ALS chose this option (Appel, 2004). See Chapter 17 for additional discussion of end-of-life care.

The Amyotrophic Lateral Sclerosis Association has broad programs of research funding, patient and clinical services, patient information and support, and medical and public information. The *ALS Association Quarterly Newsletter* is a source of practical information (see Resources).

Muscular Dystrophies

The muscular dystrophies are a group of incurable muscle disorders characterized by progressive weakening and wasting of the skeletal or voluntary muscles. Most of these diseases are inherited. Duchenne muscular dystrophy, the most common type, occurs in 1 of every 3300 male births (Bader & Littlejohns, 2004). The pathologic features include degeneration and loss of muscle fibers, variation in muscle fiber size, phagocytosis and regeneration, and replacement of muscle tissue by connective tissue. The common characteristics of these diseases include varying degrees of muscle wasting and weakness and abnormal elevation in serum levels of muscle enzymes (Mathews, 2003). Differences among these diseases center on the genetic pattern of inheritance, the muscles involved, the age at onset, and the rate of disease progression. The unique needs of these patients, who in the past did not live to adulthood, must be addressed as they live longer due to better supportive care (Klingbeil et al., 2004; Mathews, 2003).

Medical Management

Treatment of the muscular dystrophies at this time focuses on supportive care and prevention of complications in the absence of a cure or specific pharmacologic interventions (Mathews, 2003). The goal of supportive management is to keep the patient active and functioning as normally as possible and to minimize functional deterioration. An individualized therapeutic exercise program is prescribed to prevent muscle tightness, contractures, and disuse atrophy. Night splints and stretching exercises are used to delay contractures of the joints, especially the ankles, knees, and hips. Braces may compensate for muscle weakness.

Spinal deformity is a severe problem. Weakness of trunk muscles and spinal collapse occur almost routinely in patients with severe neuromuscular disease. To help prevent spinal deformity, the patient is fitted with an orthotic jacket to improve sitting stability and reduce trunk deformity. This measure also supports cardiovascular status. In time, spinal fusion is performed to maintain spinal stability. Other procedures may be carried out to correct deformities.

Compromised pulmonary function may result either from progression of the disease or from deformity of the thorax secondary to severe scoliosis. Intercurrent illnesses, upper respiratory infections, and fractures from falls must be vigorously treated in a way that minimizes immobilization, because joint contractures become worse when the patient's activities are more restricted than usual.

Other difficulties may be manifested in relation to the underlying disease. Dental and speech problems may result from weakness of the facial muscles, which makes it difficult to attend to dental hygiene and to speak coherently. Gastrointestinal tract problems may include gastric dilation, rectal prolapse, and fecal impaction. Finally, cardiomyopathy appears to be a common complication in all forms of muscular dystrophy.

Genetic counseling is advised for parents and siblings of the patient because of the genetic nature of this disease. The Muscular Dystrophy Association works to combat neuromuscular disease through research, programs of patient services and clinical care, and professional and public education (see Resources).

Nursing Management

The goals of the patient and the nurse are to maintain function at optimal levels and to enhance the quality of life. Therefore, the patient's physical requirements, which are considerable, are addressed without losing sight of emotional and developmental needs. The patient and family are actively involved in decision-making, including end-of-life decisions (Bostrom & Ahlstrom, 2004).

During hospitalization for treatment of complications, the knowledge and expertise of the patient and family members responsible for caregiving in the home are assessed. Because the patient and family caregivers often have developed caregiving strategies that work effectively for them, these strategies need to be acknowledged and accepted, and provisions must be made to ensure that they are maintained during hospitalization.

Families of adolescents and young adults with muscular dystrophy need assistance to shift the focus of care from pediatric to adult care and to understand the usual disease course (Bostrom & Ahlstrom, 2004). Nursing goals include assisting the adolescent to make the transition to adult values and expectations while providing age-appropriate ongoing care. The nurse may need to help build the confidence of an older adolescent or adult patient by encouraging him or her to pursue job training to become economically independent. Other nursing interventions might include guidance in accessing adult health care and finding appropriate programs in sex education.

Promoting Home and Community-Based Care

TEACHING PATIENTS SELF-CARE

The management goals are addressed in special rehabilitation programs or in the patient's home and community (Bader & Littlejohns, 2004). Therefore, the patient and family require information and instruction about the disorder, its anticipated course, and care and management strategies that will optimize the patient's growth and development and physical and psychological status. Members of a variety of health-related disciplines are involved in patient and family teaching; recommendations are communicated to all members of the health care team so that they may work toward common goals.

CONTINUING CARE

Both the neuromuscular disease and the associated deformities may progress in adolescence and adulthood. Self-help and assistive devices can aid in maintaining maximum independence. These devices, recommended by physical and occupational therapists, often become necessary as more muscle groups are affected.

The family is taught to monitor the patient for respiratory problems, because respiratory infection and cardiac failure are the most common causes of death (Bader & Littlejohns, 2004). As respiratory difficulties develop, patients and their families need information regarding respiratory support (Mathews, 2003). Options currently exist that can provide ventilatory support (eg, negative-pressure devices, positive-pressure ventilators) while allowing mobility. Patients can remain relatively independent in a wheelchair, for example, while being maintained on a ventilator at home for many years.

The patient is encouraged to continue with range-of-motion exercises to prevent contractures, which are particularly disabling. Practical adaptations must be made, however, to cope with the effects of chronic neuromuscular disability. The patient at various stages of the disease may require a manual or an electric wheelchair, gait aids, upper and lower extremity and spinal orthoses, seating systems, bathroom equipment, lifts, ramps, and additional assistive devices, all of which require a team approach. The home care nurse assesses how the patient and family are managing, makes referrals, and coordinates the activities of the physical therapist, occupational therapist, and social services.

The patient is greatly concerned about issues surrounding the threat of increasing disability and dependence on others, accompanied by a significant deterioration in health-related quality of life. The patient is faced with a progressive loss of function, leading eventually to death (Bostrom & Ahlstrom, 2004). Feelings of helplessness and powerlessness are common. Each functional loss is accompanied by grief and mourning. The patient and family are assessed for depression, anger, or denial. The patient and family are assisted and encouraged to address decisions about end-of-life options before their need arises.

A psychiatric nurse clinician or other mental health professional may assist the patient to cope and adapt to the disease. By understanding and addressing the physical and psychological needs of the patient and family, the nurse provides a hopeful, supportive, and nurturing environment.

Degenerative Disk Disease

Low back pain is a significant public health disorder in the United States, although its prevalence is difficult to quantify. Current estimates are that between 22% and 65% of people have an episode of back pain in any given year, and between 11% and 84% of adults have an episode within their lifetime. This results in significant economic and social costs, with health care expenditures in the United States approaching $26 billion annually (Luo, Pietrobon, Sun, et al., 2004). Acute low back pain lasts less than 3 months, whereas chronic or degenerative disease has a duration of 3 months or longer. Most back problems are related to disk disease.

Pathophysiology

The intervertebral disk is a cartilaginous plate that forms a cushion between the vertebral bodies (Fig. 65-7A). This tough, fibrous material is incorporated in a capsule. A ball-like cushion in the center of the disk is called the nucleus pulposus. In herniation of the intervertebral disk (ruptured disk), the nucleus of the disk protrudes into the annulus (the fibrous ring around the disk), with subsequent nerve compression. Protrusion or rupture of the nucleus pulposus usually is preceded by degenerative changes that occur with aging. Loss of protein polysaccharides in the disk decreases the water content of the nucleus pulposus. The development of radiating cracks in the annulus weakens resistance to nucleus herniation. After trauma (falls and repeated minor stresses such as lifting incorrectly), the cartilage may be injured.

For most patients, the immediate symptoms of trauma are short-lived, and those resulting from injury to the disk do not appear for months or years. Then, with degeneration in the disk, the capsule pushes back into the spinal canal, or it may rupture and allow the nucleus pulposus to be pushed back against the dural sac or against a spinal nerve as it emerges from the spinal column (see Fig. 65-7B). This sequence produces pain due to **radiculopathy** (pressure in the area of dis-

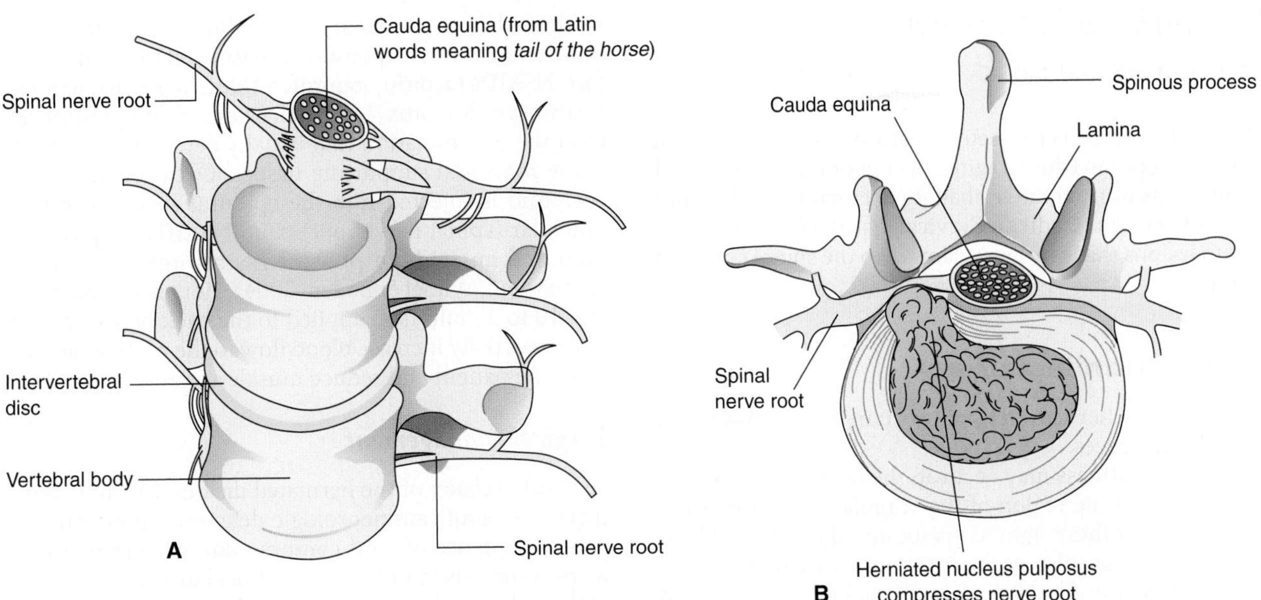

FIGURE 65-7. (**A**) Normal lumbar spine vertebrae, invertebral disks, and spinal nerve root; (**B**) ruptured vertebral disk.

tribution of the involved nerve endings). Continued pressure may produce degenerative changes in the involved nerve, such as changes in sensation and deep tendon reflexes.

Clinical Manifestations

A herniated disk with accompanying pain may occur in any portion of the spine: cervical, thoracic (rare), or lumbar. The clinical manifestations depend on the location, the rate of development (acute or chronic), and the effect on the surrounding structures.

Assessment and Diagnostic Findings

A thorough health history and physical examination are important to rule out potentially serious conditions that may manifest as low back pain, including fracture, tumor, infection, or cauda equina syndrome (Derebery & Anderson, 2002).

The MRI scan has become the diagnostic tool of choice for localizing even small disk protrusions, particularly for lumbar spine disease. If the clinical symptoms are not consistent with the pathology seen on MRI, CT scanning and myelography are performed. A neurologic examination is carried out to determine whether reflex, sensory, or motor impairment from root compression is present and to provide a baseline for future assessment. Electromyography may be used to localize the specific spinal nerve roots involved.

Medical Management

Herniations of the cervical and the lumbar disks occur most commonly and are usually managed conservatively with bed rest and medication (Derebery & Anderson, 2002). Surgery is sometimes necessary.

Surgical Management

In general, surgical excision of a herniated disk is performed if there is evidence of a progressing neurologic deficit (muscle weakness and atrophy, loss of sensory and motor function, loss of sphincter control) and continuing pain or **sciatica** (leg pain resulting from sciatic nerve involvement) that are unresponsive to conservative management. The goal of surgical treatment is to reduce the pressure on the nerve root to relieve pain and reverse neurologic deficits (Bader & Littlejohns, 2004). Microsurgical techniques make it possible to remove only the amount of tissue that is necessary, which preserves the integrity of normal tissue better and imposes less trauma on the body. During these procedures, spinal cord function can be monitored electrophysiologically.

To achieve the goal of pain relief, several surgical techniques are used, depending on the type of disk herniation, surgical morbidity, and overall results of previous surgery:

- Discectomy: removal of herniated or extruded fragments of intervertebral disk
- Laminectomy: removal of the bone between the spinal process and facet pedicle junction to expose the neural elements in the spinal canal (Bader & Littlejohns, 2004); this allows the surgeon to inspect the spinal canal, identify and remove pathologic tissue, and relieve compression of the cord and roots
- Hemilaminectomy: removal of part of the lamina and part of the posterior arch of the vertebra
- Partial laminectomy or laminotomy: creation of a hole in the lamina of a vertebra
- Discectomy with fusion: a bone graft (from iliac crest or bone bank) is used to fuse the vertebral spinous process; the object of spinal fusion is to bridge over the defective disk to stabilize the spine and reduce the rate of recurrence
- Foraminotomy: removal of the intervertebral foramen to increase the space for exit of a spinal nerve, resulting in reduced pain, compression, and edema

Herniation of a Cervical Intervertebral Disk

The cervical spine is subjected to stresses that result from disk degeneration (due to aging, occupational stresses) and **spondylosis** (degenerative changes occurring in a disk and adjacent vertebral bodies). Cervical disk degeneration may lead to lesions that can cause damage to the spinal cord and its roots.

Clinical Manifestations

A cervical disk herniation usually occurs at the C5–C6 and C6–C7 interspaces.

Pain and stiffness may occur in the neck, the top of the shoulders, and the region of the scapulae. Sometimes patients interpret these signs as symptoms of heart trouble or bursitis. Pain may also occur in the upper extremities and head, accompanied by **paresthesia** (tingling or a "pins and needles" sensation) and numbness of the upper extremities. Cervical MRI usually confirms the diagnosis.

Medical Management

The goals of treatment are to rest and immobilize the cervical spine to give the soft tissues time to heal and to reduce inflammation in the supporting tissues and the affected nerve roots in the cervical spine. Bed rest (usually 1 to 2 days) is important because it eliminates the stress of gravity and relieves the cervical spine of the need to support the head. It also reduces inflammation and edema in soft tissues around the disk, relieving pressure on the nerve roots. Proper positioning on a firm mattress may bring dramatic relief from pain.

The cervical spine may be rested and immobilized by a cervical collar, cervical traction, or a brace. A collar allows maximal opening of the intervertebral foramina and holds the head in a neutral or slightly flexed position. The patient may have to wear the collar 24 hours a day during the acute phase. The skin under the collar is inspected for irritation. After the patient is free of pain, cervical isometric exercises are started to strengthen the neck muscles.

The effectiveness of cervical traction is still being evaluated, but when used it is accomplished by means of a head halter attached to a pulley and weight (Derebery & Anderson, 2002). It increases vertebral separation and thus relieves pressure on the nerve roots. The head of the bed is elevated to provide countertraction (see Chapter 67). If the skin becomes irritated, the halter can be padded. A male patient may suffer more skin irritation if he shaves, because a beard offers a natural form of padding.

Pharmacologic Therapy

Analgesic agents (nonsteroidal anti-inflammatory agents [NSAIDs], propoxyphene [Darvon], oxycodone [Tylox], or hydrocodone [Vicodin]) are prescribed during the acute phase to relieve pain, and sedatives may be administered to control the anxiety that is often associated with cervical disk disease. Muscle relaxants (cyclobenzaprine [Flexeril], methocarbamol [Robaxin], metaxalone [Skelaxin]) are administered to interrupt muscle spasm and to promote comfort. NSAIDs (aspirin, ibuprofen [Motrin, Advil], naproxen [Naprosyn, Anaprox]) or corticosteroids are prescribed to treat the inflammation that usually occurs in the affected nerve roots and supporting tissues. Occasionally, a corticosteroid is injected into the epidural space for relief of radicular (spinal nerve root) pain. NSAIDs are given with food and antacids to prevent gastrointestinal irritation (Borenstein, Wiesel & Boden, 2004). Hot, moist compresses (for 10 to 20 minutes) applied to the back of the neck several times daily increase blood flow to the muscles and help relax the patient and reduce muscle spasm.

Surgical Management

Surgical excision of the herniated disk may be necessary if there is a significant neurologic deficit, progression of the deficit, evidence of cord compression, or pain that either worsens or fails to improve. A cervical discectomy, with or without fusion, may be performed to alleviate symptoms (Fowler, Anthony-Phillips, Mehta, et al., 2005). An anterior surgical approach may be used through a transverse incision to remove disk material that has herniated into the spinal canal and foramina, or a posterior approach may be used at the appropriate level of the cervical spine. Potential complications with the anterior approach include carotid or vertebral artery injury, recurrent laryngeal nerve dysfunction, esophageal perforation, and airway obstruction. Complications of the posterior approach include damage to the nerve root or the spinal cord due to retraction or contusion of either of these structures, resulting in weakness of muscles supplied by the nerve root or cord.

Microsurgery, such as endoscopic microdiscectomy, may be performed in selected patients through a small incision and using magnification techniques. The patient who undergoes microsurgery usually has less tissue trauma and pain and consequently a shorter hospital stay than after conventional surgical approaches.

Nursing Process

The Patient Undergoing a Cervical Discectomy

Assessment

The patient is asked about past injuries to the neck (whiplash), because unresolved trauma can cause persistent discomfort, pain and tenderness, and symptoms of arthritis in the injured joint of the cervical spine. Assessment includes determining the onset, location, and radiation of pain and assessing for paresthesias, limited movement, and diminished function of the neck, shoulders, and upper extremities. It is important to determine whether the symptoms are bilateral; with large herniations, bilateral symptoms may be caused by cord compression. The area around the cervical spine is palpated to assess muscle tone and tenderness. Range of motion in the neck and shoulders is evaluated.

The patient is asked about any health issues that may influence the postoperative course and quality of life (Fowler et al., 2005). The nurse determines the patient's need for information about the surgical procedure and reinforces what the physician has explained. Strategies for pain management are discussed with the patient.

Diagnosis

Nursing Diagnoses

Based on the assessment data, the patient's major nursing diagnoses may include the following:

- Acute pain related to the surgical procedure
- Impaired physical mobility related to the postoperative surgical regimen
- Deficient knowledge about the postoperative course and home care management

Other nursing diagnoses may include preoperative anxiety, postoperative constipation, urinary retention related to the surgical procedure, self-care deficits related to use of a neck orthosis, and sleep pattern disturbance related to disruption in lifestyle.

Collaborative Problems/ Potential Complications

Based on all the assessment data, the potential complications may include the following:

- Hematoma at the surgical site, resulting in cord compression and neurologic deficit
- Recurrent or persistent pain after surgery

Planning and Goals

The goals for the patient may include relief of pain, improved mobility, increased knowledge and self-care ability, and prevention of complications.

Nursing Interventions

Relieving Pain

The patient may be kept flat in bed for 12 to 24 hours. If the patient has had a bone fusion with bone removed from the iliac crest, considerable pain may be experienced at the donor site. Interventions consist of monitoring the donor site for hematoma formation, administering the prescribed postoperative analgesic agent, positioning for comfort, and reassuring the patient that the pain can be relieved. If the patient experiences a sudden increase in pain, extrusion of the graft may have occurred, requiring reoperation. A sudden increase in pain should be promptly reported to the surgeon.

The patient may experience a sore throat, hoarseness, and dysphagia due to temporary edema. These symptoms are relieved by throat lozenges, voice rest, and humidification. A puréed diet may be given if the patient has dysphagia.

Improving Mobility

Postoperatively, a cervical collar (neck orthosis) is usually worn, which contributes to limited neck motion and altered mobility. The patient is instructed to turn the body instead of the neck when looking from side to side. The neck should be kept in a neutral (midline) position. The patient is assisted during position changes, to make sure that head, shoulders, and thorax are kept aligned. When assisting the patient to a sitting position, the nurse supports the patient's neck and shoulders. To increase stability, the patient should wear shoes when ambulating.

Monitoring and Managing Potential Complications

The patient is evaluated for bleeding and hematoma formation by assessing for excessive pressure in the neck or severe pain in the incision area. The dressing is inspected for serosanguineous drainage, which suggests a dural leak. If this occurs, meningitis is a threat. A complaint of headache requires careful evaluation. Neurologic checks are made for swallowing deficits and upper and lower extremity weakness, because cord compression may produce rapid or delayed onset of paralysis. The patient who has had an anterior cervical discectomy is also assessed for a sudden return of radicular (spinal nerve root) pain, which may indicate instability of the spine.

Throughout the postoperative course, the patient is monitored frequently to detect any signs of respiratory difficulty, because retractors used during surgery may injure the recurrent laryngeal nerve, resulting in hoarseness and the inability to cough effectively and clear pulmonary secretions. In addition, the blood pressure and pulse are monitored to evaluate cardiovascular status.

Bleeding at the surgical site and subsequent hematoma formation may occur. Severe localized pain not relieved by analgesic agents should be reported to the surgeon. A change in neurologic status (motor or sensory function) should be reported promptly, because it suggests hematoma formation that may necessitate surgery to prevent irreversible motor and sensory deficits.

Promoting Home and Community-Based Care

TEACHING PATIENTS SELF-CARE

The patient's hospital stay is likely to be short; therefore, the patient and family should understand the care that is important for a smooth recovery. A cervical collar is usually worn for about 6 weeks. The patient is instructed in use and care of the cervical collar. The patient is instructed to alternate tasks that involve minimal body movement (e.g., reading) with tasks that require greater body movement.

The patient is instructed about strategies for pain management and about signs and symptoms that may indicate complications that should be reported to the physician. The nurse assesses the patient's understanding of these management strategies, limitations, and recommendations. Additionally, the nurse assists the patient in identifying strategies to cope with ADLs (eg, self-care, childcare) and minimize risks to the surgical site (Chart 65-6). A discharge teaching plan is developed collaboratively by members of the health care team to decrease the risk for recurrent disk herniation. Topics include those previously discussed as well as proper body mechanics, maintenance of optimal weight, proper exercise techniques, and modifications in activity.

CONTINUING CARE

The patient is instructed to see the physician at prescribed intervals so that the physician can document the disappearance of old symptoms and assess the range of motion of the neck. Recurrent or persistent pain may occur despite removal of the offending disk or disk fragments. Patients who undergo discectomy usually have consented to surgery after prolonged pain; they have often undergone repeated courses of ineffective conservative management and previous surgeries to relieve the pain. Therefore, the recurrence or persistence of symptoms postoperatively, including pain and sensory deficits, is often discouraging for the patient and family. The patient who experiences recurrence of symptoms requires emotional support and

CHART 65-6

HOME CARE CHECKLIST • The Patient With Cervical Discectomy and Cervical Collar

At the completion of the home care instruction, the patient or caregiver will be able to:	Patient	Caregiver
• Care for the surgical incision site.		
— Keep staples or sutures clean and dry and cover with dry dressing.		✔
— Notify physician if any signs or symptoms of infection occur, such as fever, redness or irritation, drainage, increased pain.	✔	✔
• Demonstrate proper body mechanics and prescribed exercise techniques.	✔	
• Modify activity:		
— Avoid sitting or standing for more than 30 minutes.	✔	
— Avoid twisting, flexing, extending, or rotating the neck.	✔	
— Avoid long automobile rides.	✔	
— Avoid sleeping in a prone position or use of pillows, to minimize neck flexion in bed; keep head in a neutral position.	✔	
— Use adequate mattress and chair support.	✔	
— Wear low-heeled shoes.	✔	
• Follow physician's instructions regarding lifting, climbing stairs, driving a car, sexual activity, sports, exercise, and return to work.	✔	
• Practice stress reduction and relaxation techniques.	✔	
• Care of the cervical collar:		
— Wear the collar at all times until directed otherwise by the physician.	✔	
— Wash the neck twice a day with mild soap.	✔	✔
— Keep the neck still while the collar is open.	✔	
• With the assistance of a helper, wash the neck in steps:		
— Lie flat and supine.	✔	
— Open the Velcro tabs on each side of the collar and remove its front portion.		✔
— Gently wash and dry the neck.		✔
— Replace the front part of the collar and refasten the tabs.		✔
— Turn to one side with a thin pillow under the head.	✔	
— Open one tab.	✔	
— Gently wash and dry the back of the neck. Refasten the tab.		✔
— Turn to the other side and wash and dry this side. Refasten the tab.		✔
• Place a wrinkle-free silk scarf under the collar to increase comfort.	✔	✔
• ***For men:*** Shave without twisting or moving the neck. This may be done with help while lying flat or sitting. Remove only the front part of the collar for shaving.	✔	✔

understanding. Additionally, the patient is assisted in modifying activities and in considering options for subsequent treatment.

The patient with degenerative disk disease tends to focus on obvious needs, issues, and deficits. Therefore, the nurse needs to remind the patient and family members of the need to participate in health promotion and health screening practices.

Evaluation

Expected Patient Outcomes

Expected patient outcomes may include the following:

1. Reports decreasing frequency and severity of pain
2. Demonstrates improved mobility
   a. Demonstrates progressive participation in self-care activities
   b. Identifies prescribed activity limitations and restrictions
   c. Demonstrates proper body mechanics
3. Is knowledgeable about postoperative course, medications, and home care management.
   a. Lists the signs and symptoms to be reported postoperatively
   b. Identifies dose, action, and potential side effects of medications
   c. Identifies appropriate home care management activities and any restrictions
4. Has absence of complications
   a. Reports no increase in incision pain or sensory symptoms
   b. Demonstrates normal findings on neurologic assessment

Herniation of a Lumbar Disk

Most lumbar disk herniations occur at the L4–L5 or the L5–S1 interspace (Borenstein et al., 2004). A herniated lumbar disk produces low back pain accompanied by varying degrees of sensory and motor impairment.

Clinical Manifestations

The patient complains of low back pain with muscle spasms, followed by radiation of the pain into one hip and down into the leg (sciatica). Pain is aggravated by actions that increase intraspinal fluid pressure, such as bending, lifting, or straining (as in sneezing or coughing), and usually is relieved by bed rest. Usually there is some type of postural deformity, because pain causes an alteration of the normal spinal mechanics. If the patient lies on the back and attempts to raise a leg in a straight position, pain radiates into the leg; this maneuver, called the straight leg-raising test, stretches the sciatic nerve. Additional signs include muscle weakness, alterations in tendon reflexes, and sensory loss.

Assessment and Diagnostic Findings

The diagnosis of lumbar disk disease is based on the history and physical findings and the use of imaging techniques such as MRI, CT, and myelography.

Medical Management

The objectives of treatment are to relieve pain, slow disease progression, and increase the patient's functional ability. Bed rest, previously a standard in back pain treatment, is no longer recommended (Derebery & Anderson, 2002).

Because muscle spasm is prominent during the acute phase, muscle relaxants are used. NSAIDs and systemic corticosteroids may be administered to counter the inflammation that usually occurs in the supporting tissues and the affected nerve roots. Moist heat and massage help to relax muscles. Antidepressant agents appear to help in low back pain that is neuropathic in origin (Derebery & Anderson, 2002).

Strategies for increasing the patient's functional ability include weight reduction, physical therapy, and biofeedback. While not fully tested in clinical trials, yoga has been found to be beneficial for some patients by decreasing depression, increasing motivation, and fostering increased body awareness (Jacobs, Mehling, Goldberg et al., 2004). Chapter 13 describes nursing interventions for the patient with pain.

Surgical Management

In the lumbar region, surgical treatment includes lumbar disk excision through a posterolateral laminotomy and the newer techniques of microdiscectomy and percutaneous discectomy. In microdiscectomy, an operating microscope is used to visualize the offending disk and compressed nerve roots; it permits a small incision (2.5 cm [1 inch]) and minimal blood loss and takes about 30 minutes of operating time. Generally, the hospital stay is short, and the patient makes a rapid recovery. Percutaneous discectomy is an alternative treatment for herniated intervertebral disks of the lumbar spine at the L4–L5 level (Bader & Littlejohns, 2004). One approach in current use is through a 2.5-cm (1-inch) incision just above the iliac crest. A tube, trocar, or cannula is inserted under x-ray guidance through the retroperitoneal space to the involved disk space. Special instruments are used to remove the disk. The operating time is about 15 minutes. Blood loss and postoperative pain are minimal, and usually the patient is discharged within 2 days after surgery. The disadvantage of this procedure is the possibility of damage to structures in the surgical pathway.

COMPLICATIONS OF DISK SURGERY

A patient undergoing a disk procedure at one level of the vertebral column may have a degenerative process at other levels. A herniation relapse may occur at the same level or elsewhere, so the patient may become a candidate for another disk procedure. Arachnoiditis (inflammation of the arachnoid membrane) may occur after surgery (and after myelography); it involves an insidious onset of diffuse, frequently burning pain in the lower back, radiating into the buttocks. Disk excision can leave adhesions and scarring around the spinal nerves and dura, which then produce inflammatory changes that create chronic neuritis and neurofibrosis. Disk surgery may relieve pressure on the spinal nerves, but it does not reverse the effects of neural injury and scarring and the pain that results. Failed disk syndrome (recurrence of sciatica after lumbar discectomy) remains a common cause of disability (Borenstein et al., 2004).

Nursing Management

Providing Preoperative Care

Most patients fear surgery on any part of the spine and therefore need explanations about the surgery and reassurance that it will not weaken the back. When data are being collected for the health history, any reports of pain, paresthesia, or muscle spasm are recorded to provide a baseline for comparison after surgery. Preoperative assessment also includes an evaluation of movement of the extremities as well as bladder and bowel function. To facilitate the postoperative turning procedure, the patient is taught to turn as a unit (called logrolling) as part of the preoperative preparation (Fig. 65-8). Before surgery, the patient is also encouraged to take deep breaths, cough, and perform muscle-setting exercises to maintain muscle tone.

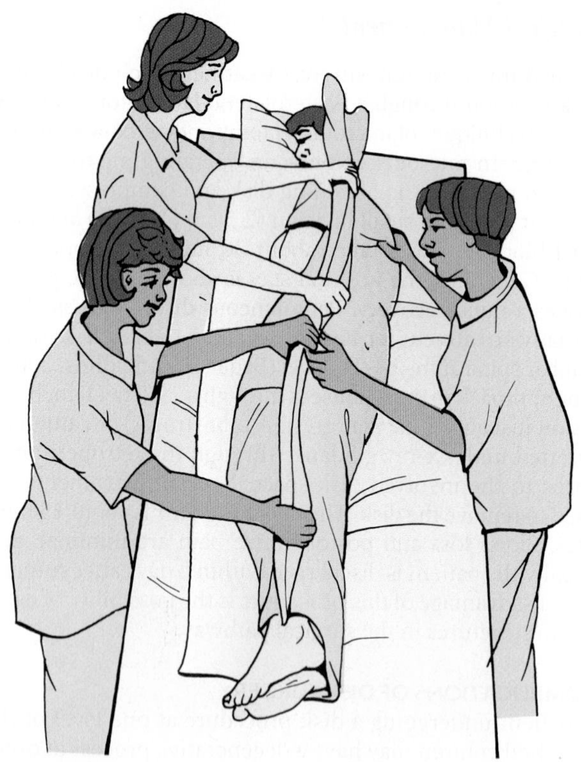

FIGURE 65-8. Before the patient undergoes laminectomy surgery, the logrolling technique that will be used for turning the patient should be demonstrated. The patient's arms will be crossed and the spine aligned. To avoid twisting the spine, the head, shoulders, knees, and hips are turned at the same time so that the patient rolls over like a log. When in a side-lying position, the patient's back, buttocks, and legs are supported with pillows.

Assessing the Patient After Surgery

After lumbar disk excision, vital signs are checked frequently and the wound is inspected for hemorrhage, because vascular injury is a complication of disk surgery. Because postoperative neurologic deficits may occur from nerve root injury, the sensation and motor strength of the lower extremities are evaluated at specified intervals, along with the color and temperature of the legs and sensation of the toes. It is important to assess for urinary retention, another sign of neurologic deterioration.

In discectomy with fusion, the patient has an additional surgical incision if bone fragments were taken from the iliac crest or fibula to serve as wedges in the spine. The recovery period is longer than for those patients who underwent discectomy without spinal fusion, because bony union must take place.

Positioning the Patient

To position the patient, a pillow is placed under the head, and the knee rest is elevated slightly to relax the back muscles. When the patient is lying on one side, however, extreme knee flexion must be avoided. The patient is encouraged to move from side to side to relieve pressure and is reassured that no injury will result from moving. When the patient is ready to turn, the bed is placed in a flat position and a pillow is placed between the patient's legs. The patient turns as a unit (logrolls) without twisting the back.

To get out of bed, the patient lies on one side while pushing up to a sitting position. At the same time, the nurse or family member eases the patient's legs over the side of the bed. Coming to a sitting or standing posture is accomplished in one long, smooth motion. Most patients walk to the bathroom on the same day as the surgery. Sitting is discouraged except for defecation.

Promoting Home and Community-Based Care

TEACHING PATIENTS SELF-CARE

The patient is advised to increase activity gradually, as tolerated, because it takes up to 6 weeks for the ligaments to heal. Excessive activity may result in spasm of the paraspinal muscles.

Activities that produce flexion strain on the spine (eg, driving a car) should be avoided until healing has taken place. Heat may be applied to the back to relax muscle spasms. Scheduled rest periods are important, and the patient is advised to avoid heavy work for 2 to 3 months after surgery. Exercises are prescribed to strengthen the abdominal and erector spinal muscles. A back brace or corset may be necessary if back pain persists.

CONTINUING CARE

Referral for inpatient or outpatient rehabilitation may be warranted to improve self-care abilities after medical or surgical treatment for herniation of a lumbar disk. A home care referral may be indicated and provides the home care nurse with the opportunity to assess the patient's physical and psychological status, as well as his or her ability to adhere to recommended management strategies. During the home visit, the nurse determines whether changes in neurologic function have occurred. The adequacy of pain management is assessed, and modifications are made to ensure adequate pain relief.

Postpolio Syndrome

Patients who survived the polio epidemic of the 1950s, many of whom are now elderly, are developing new symptoms of weakness, fatigue, and musculoskeletal pain. Researchers estimate that between 60% and 80% of the 640,000 polio survivors are experiencing the phenomenon known as postpolio syndrome; men and women appear to be equally at risk (Bartels & Omura, 2005).

Pathophysiology

The exact cause of postpolio syndrome is not known, but researchers suspect that, with aging or muscle overuse, the neurons not destroyed originally by the poliovirus cannot continue generating axon sprouts (Bartels & Omura, 2005). These new terminal axon sprouts reinnervated the affected muscles after the initial insult but may be more vulnerable as the body ages.

Assessment and Diagnostic Findings

No specific diagnostic test exists for this syndrome. The clinical diagnosis is made on the basis of the history and physical examination and exclusion of other medical conditions that could be causing the new symptoms. Patients report a history of paralytic poliomyelitis followed by partial or complete recovery of function, with a plateau of function and then the recurrence of symptoms. Signs and symptoms may occur 30 to 40 years after the original onset of poliomyelitis (Klingbeil et al., 2004).

Management

No specific medical or surgical treatment is available for this syndrome, and therefore nurses play a pivotal role in the team approach to assisting patients and families in dealing with the symptoms of progressive loss of muscle strength and significant fatigue. Other health care professionals who may assist in patient care include physical, occupational, speech, and respiratory therapists. Nursing interventions are aimed at slowing the loss of strength and maintaining the patient's physical, psychological, and social well-being.

The patient needs to plan and coordinate activities to conserve energy and reduce fatigue. Rest periods should be planned and assistive devices used to reduce weakness and fatigue. Important activities should be planned for the morning, because fatigue often increases in the afternoon and evening (Bartels & Omura, 2005).

One study proposed an explanatory model of health promotion and quality of life in patients with postpolio syndrome (Stuifbergen, Seraphine, Harrison, et al., 2005). The results suggested that quality of life is the result of a complex interplay among contextual factors such as severity of impairment, antecedent variables, and health-promoting behaviors. Other researchers reported an increase in function and self-care activities in postpolio patients after a 12-week program of yoga and meditation (DeMayo, Singh, Duryea, et al., 2004).

Pain in muscles and joints may be a problem. Nonpharmacologic techniques such as the application of heat and cold are most appropriate, because these elderly patients may not tolerate or have strong reactions to medications.

Maintaining a balance between having adequate nutritional intake and avoiding excess calories that can lead to obesity in this sedentary group of patients is a challenge. Pulmonary hygiene and adequate fluid intake can help with airway management. Several interventions can improve sleep, including limiting caffeine intake before bedtime and assessing for nocturia. If nocturia is an issue, the patient needs to be evaluated for obstructive sleep apnea. Supportive ventilation may be appropriate, with continuous positive airway pressure if sleep apnea is a problem.

Bone density testing in patients with postpolio syndrome has revealed low bone mass and osteoporosis (Smeltzer, Zimmeman & Capriotti, 2005). Therefore, the importance of identifying risks, preventing falls, and treating osteoporosis must be discussed with patients and families. The nurse also needs to remind patients and family members of the need for health promotion activities and health screening.

Critical Thinking Exercises

1 A 68-year-old patient with known cerebral metastases is admitted to the hospital. He reports new-onset right-sided weakness and headache. What immediate action should you take? What medical treatments can you anticipate? What surgical treatment (if any) would be anticipated? What teaching for the patient and the family is warranted, and why?

2 A 50-year-old man newly diagnosed with Parkinson's disease asks what type of medication he will be given. What are the possible medications that will be used to treat his disease, and the long-term effects of each? How would your discharge teaching targeted toward medications be modified if the patient lives alone?

3 ebp A 35-year-old woman has a history of low back pain. She has been on bed rest for the last 3 days at home. What resources would you use to identify the current guidelines for treatment of low back pain? What is the current evidence base for bed rest? Identify the criteria used to evaluate the strength of the evidence for bed rest.

4 A 60-year-old patient with postpolio syndrome is having difficulty with fatigue and pain. What interventions and actions would you suggest to assist in the management of these symptoms? What strategies would you advise the patient to avoid? What is the rationale for your suggestions? State the types of health promotion activities you would recommend to this patient and the rationale for your recommendations.

REFERENCES AND SELECTED READINGS

BOOKS

Bader, M. K. & Littlejohns, L. R. (2004). *AANN core curriculum for neuroscience nursing* (4th ed.). St. Louis: Elsevier.

Borenstein, D. G., Wiesel, S. W. & Boden, S. D. (2004). *Low back and neck pain: Comprehensive diagnosis and management* (3rd ed.). Philadelphia: Saunders.

Derebery, J. & Anderson, J. R. (2002). *Low back pain: An evidence based, biopsychosocial model for clinical management.* Beverly Farms, MA: OEM Press.

Diepenbrock, N. H. (2004). *Quick reference to critical care* (2nd ed.). Philadelphia: Lippincott Williams & Wilkins.

Dudek, S. G. (2006). *Nutrition essentials for nursing practice* (5th ed.). Philadelphia: Lippincott Williams & Wilkins.

Hickey, J. (2003). *Clinical practice of neurologic and neurosurgical nursing* (5th ed.). Philadelphia: Lippincott Williams & Wilkins.

Karch, A. (2005). *Lippincott's nursing drug guide.* Philadelphia: Lippincott Williams & Wilkins.

Porth, C. M. (2005). *Pathophysiology: Concepts of altered health states* (7th ed.). Philadelphia: Lippincott Williams & Wilkins.

Rice, J. N., Robichaux, C. & Leonard, A. (2005). Nervous system alterations. In Ropper, A. H., Gress, D., Diringer, M. N., et al. *Neurological and neurosurgical intensive care* (4th ed.). Philadelphia: Lippincott Williams & Wilkins.

Ropper, A. H., Gress, D., Diringer, M. N., et al. (2004). *Neurological and neurosurgical intensive care* (4th ed.). Philadelphia: Lippincott Williams & Wilkins.

Sole, M., Klein, D. G., & Moseley, M. J. (Eds.). (2005). *Introduction to critical care nursing* (4th ed.). St. Louis: Elsevier Saunders.

Worthington, P. H. (2004). *Practical aspects of nutritional support.* Philadelphia: Saunders.

JOURNALS

**Asterisks indicate nursing research articles.*

General

Andersen, J. (2004). Oxidative stress in neurodegeneration: Cause or consequence? *Nature Reviews: Neuroscience, 5*(Suppl), S18–S25.

Bossy-Wetzel, E., Schwarzenbacher, R. & Lipton, S. A. (2004). Molecular pathways to neurodegeneration. *Nature Reviews: Neuroscience, 5*(Suppl), S2–S8.

Klingbeil, H., Baer, H. R. & Wilson, P. E. (2004). Aging with a disability. *Archives of Physical Medicine and Rehabilitation, 85*(7), S68–S73.

Olson, E. & Cristian, A. (2005). The role of rehabilitation medicine and palliative care in the treatment of patients with end-stage disease. *Physical Medicine and Rehabilitation Clinics of North America, 16*(1), 285–305.

Ross, C. A. & Poirier, M. A. (2004). Protein aggregation and neurodegenerative disease. *Nature Reviews: Neuroscience, 5*(Suppl), S10–S17.

*Smeltzer, S. C., Zimmerman, V. & Capriotti, T. (2005). Osteoporosis risk and bone mineral density in women with physical disabilities. *Archives of Physical Medicine and Rehabilitation,* 86(3), 582–586.

Alzheimer's Disease

*Maas, M. L., Reed, D., Park, M., et al. (2004). Outcomes of family involvement in care intervention for caregivers of individuals with dementia. *Nursing Research, 53*(2), 76–86.

Schulz, R., Mendelsohn, A. B., Haley, W. A., et al. (2003). End-of-life care and the effects of bereavement on family caregivers of persons with dementia. *New England Journal of Medicine, 349*(20), 1936–1942.

Tariot, P. N., Farlow, M. R., Grossberg, G. T., et al. (2004). Memantine treatment in patients with moderate to severe Alzheimer disease already receiving donepezil. *Journal of the American Medical Association, 291*(3), 317–324.

*Ward-Smith, P. & Forred, D. (2005). Participation in a dementia evaluation program: Perceptions of family members. *Journal of Neuroscience Nursing, 37*(2), 92–96.

Amyotrophic Lateral Sclerosis

Appel, S. H. (2004). Euthanasia and physician-assisted suicide in ALS: A commentary. *American Journal of Hospice and Palliative Medicine, 21*(6), 405–406.

Boitano, L. J., Jordan, T. & Benditt, J. O. (2001). Noninvasive ventilation allows gastrostomy tube placement in patients with advanced ALS. *Neurology, 56*(3), 413–414.

Brown, R. H. (2005). Amyotrophic lateral sclerosis: A new role for old drugs. *New England Journal of Medicine, 352*(13), 1376–1378.

*Dobratz, M. (2004). A comparative study of variables that have an impact on noncancer end-of-life diagnoses. *Clinical Nursing Research, 13*(4), 309–325.

Forbes, R. B., Colville, S., Cran, G. W., et al. (2004). Unexpected decline in survival from amyotrophic lateral sclerosis/motor neuron disease. *Journal of Neurology, Neurosurgery and Psychiatry, 75*(12), 1753–1755.

Miller, R. G., Mitchell, J. D., Lyon, M., et al. (2002). Riluzole for amyotrophic lateral sclerosis. *The Cochrane Library,* (2), CD001447.

Weisskopt, M. G., McCullough, M. L., Calle, E. E., et al. (2004). Prospective study of cigarette smoking and amyotrophic lateral sclerosis. *American Journal of Epidemiology, 160*(1), 26–33.

Degenerative Disk Disease

*Fowler, S., Anthony-Phillips, P., Mehta, D., et al. (2005). Health-related quality of life in patients undergoing anterior cervical discectomy. *Journal of Neuroscience Nursing, 37*(2), 97–100.

Jacobs, B. P., Mehling, W., Goldberg, H., et al. (2004). Feasibility of conducting a clinical trial on hatha yoga for chronic low back pain: Methodological lesions. *Alternative Therapies, 10*(2), 80–83.

Luo, X., Pietrobon, R., Sun, S. X., et al. (2004). Estimates and patterns of direct healthcare expenditures among individuals with back pain in the United States. *Spine, 29*(1), 79–86.

Huntington's Disease

*Dawson, S., Kristjanson, L., Toye, C., et al. (2004). Living with Huntington's disease: Need for supportive care. *Nursing and Health Sciences, 6*(2), 123–130.

Ho, A. K., Sahakian, B. J., Brown, R. G., et al. (2003). Profile of cognitive progression in early Huntington's disease. *Neurology, 61*(12), 1702–1706.

Huntington Study Group. (2003). Dosage effects of riluzole in Huntington's disease: A multicenter placebo-controlled study. *Neurology, 61*(11), 1551–1556.

Mahant, N., McCusker, E. A., Byth, K., et al. (2003). Huntington's disease: Clinical correlates of disability and progression. *Neurology, 61*(8), 1085–1092.

Rosenblatt, A., Abbott, M. H., Gourley, L. M., et al. (2003). Predictors of neuropathological severity in 100 patients with Huntington's disease. *Annals of Neurology, 54*(4), 488–493.

Sullivan, F., Bird, E., Alpay, M., et al. (2001). Remotivation therapy and Huntington's disease. *Journal of Neuroscience Nursing, 33*(3), 136–142.

Muscular Dystrophy

Bostrom, K. & Ahlstrom, G. (2004). Living with a chronic deteriorating disease: The trajectory with muscular dystrophy over ten years. *Disability and Rehabilitation, 26*(23), 1388–1398.

Mathews, K. D. (2003). Muscular dystrophy overview: Genetics and diagnosis. *Neurologic Clinics of North America, 21*(4), 795–816.

Oncologic Disorders

American Brain Tumor Association (ABTA). (2006). *A primer of brain tumors: A patient's reference manual* (8th ed.). Available at: http://www.abta.org (accessed June 23, 2006).

Bohan, E. & Glass-Macenka, D. (2004). Surgical management of patients with primary brain tumors. *Seminars in Oncology Nursing, 20*(4), 240–252.

Coles, M. C. (2004). S1 radiculopathy due to adenocarcinoma: A case study. *Journal of Neuroscience Nursing, 36*(1), 40–41.

Eskandar, E. N., Loeffler, J. S., O'Neill, A. M., et al. (2004). Case 33-2004: A 34-year-old man with a seizure and frontal-lobe brain lesion. *New England Journal of Medicine, 351*(18), 1875–1882.

Gnanadurai, A., Purushothamam, L., Rajshekhar, V., et al. (2004). Stereotactic radiosurgery for brain lesions: An observation and follow-up. *Journal of Neuroscience Nursing, 36*(4), 225–227.

Held-Warmkessel, J. (2005). Managing critical cancer complications. *Nursing, 35*(1), 58–63.

Herndon, C. (2003). Pharmacological management of cancer pain. *Journal of Neuroscience Nursing, 35*(6), 321–326.

*Lepola, I., Toljamo, M., Ahi, R., et al. (2001). Being a brain tumor patient: A descriptive study of patient's experiences. *Journal of Neuroscience Nursing, 33*(3), 143–147.

Nahaczewski, A. E., Fowler, S. & Hariharan, S. (2004). Dexamethasone therapy in patients with brain tumors: A focus on tapering. *Journal of Neuroscience Nursing, 36*(6), 340–343.

Pickett, C. A. (2003). Diagnosis and management of pituitary tumors: Recent advances. *Primary Care Clinical Office Practice, 30*(4), 765–789.

Schmidt, M. H., Meyer, G. A., Reichert, K. W., et al. (2004). Evaluation of photodynamic therapy near functional brain tissue in patients with recurrent brain tumors. *Journal of Neuro-Oncology, 67*(1–2), 201–207.

Parkinson's Disease

Emre, M., Aarsland, D., Albanese, A., et al. (2004). Rivastigmine for dementia associated with Parkinson's disease. *New England Journal of Medicine, 351*(24), 2509–2518.

Galvez-Jimenez, N. & Lang, A. (2004). The perioperative management of Parkinson's disease revisited. *Neurologic Clinics of North America, 22*(2), 367–377.

Press, D. Z. (2004). Parkinson's disease dementia: A first step? *New England Journal of Medicine, 351*(24), 2547–2549.

Rao, G., Fisch, L., Srinivasan, S., et al. (2003). Does this patient have Parkinson disease? *Journal of the American Medical Association, 289*(3), 347–353.

Stewart, R. M., Desaloms, J. M., & Sanghera, M. K. (2005). Stimulation of the subthalamic nucleus for the treatment of Parkinson's disease: Postoperative management programming and rehabilitation. *Journal of Neuroscience Nursing, 37*(2), 108–114.

The Parkinson Study Group. (2004). Levodopa and the progression of Parkinson's disease. *New England Journal of Medicine, 351*(24), 2498–2508.

Torpy, J. M., Lynm, C. & Glass, R. M. (2004). Parkinson disease. *Journal of the American Medical Association, 291*(3), 390.

Ward, C. (2005). Neuroleptic malignant syndrome in a patient with Parkinson's disease: A case study. *Journal of Neuroscience Nursing, 37*(3), 160–162.

Postpolio Syndrome

Bartels, M. N. & Omura, A. (2005). Aging in polio. *Physical Medicine and Rehabilitation Clinics of North America, 16*(1), 197–218.

*Becker, H. & Stuifbergen, A. (2004). What makes it so hard? Barriers to health promotion experienced by people with multiple sclerosis and polio. *Family Community Health, 27*(1), 75–85.

DeMayo, W., Singh, B., Duryea, B., et al. (2004). Hatha yoga and meditation in patients with post-polio syndrome. *Alternative Therapies, 10*(2), 24–25.

*Stuifbergen, A., Seraphine, A., Harrison, T., et al. (2005). An explanatory model of health promotion and quality of life for persons with post-polio syndrome. *Social Science and Medicine, 60*(2), 383–393.

RESOURCES

American Brain Tumor Association, 2720 River Rd., Des Plaines, IL 60018; 847-827-9910; http://www.abta.org. Accessed June 23, 2006.

American Cancer Society, 1599 Clifton Road NE, Atlanta, GA 30329; 800-227-2345; http://www.cancer.org. Accessed June 23, 2006.

American Parkinson's Disease Association, 1250 Hyland Blvd. Suite 4B, Staten Island, NY 10305-1945; 800-223-2732; http://www.apdaparkinson.org. Accessed June 23, 2006.

Amyotrophic Lateral Sclerosis Association, 27001 Agoura Road, Suite 150, Calabasas Hills, CA 91301; 800-782-4747; 818-880-9007 (patients only); http://www.alsa.org. Accessed June 23, 2006.

Huntington's Disease Society of America, 158 W. 29th Street, 7th Floor, New York, NY 10001-5300; 800-345-4372 or 212-242-1968; http://www.hdsa.org. Accessed June 23, 2006.

Muscular Dystrophy Association—USA, National Headquarters, 3300 East Sunrise Drive, Tucson, AZ 85718; 800-572-1717: http://www.mdausa.org. Accessed June 23, 2006.

National Brain Tumor Foundation, 414 Thirteenth Street, Suite 700, Oakland, CA 94612-2603; 800-934-CURE; http://www.braintumor.org. Accessed June 23, 2006.

National Parkinson Foundation, Inc., Bob Hope Parkinson Research Center, 1501 NW 9th Ave., Bob Hope Road, Miami, FL 33136-1494; 800-327-4545; http://www.parkinson.org. Accessed June 23, 2006.

UNIT 15

Musculoskeletal Function

Case Study

Applying Concepts from NANDA, NIC, and NOC

A Patient With Musculoskeletal Limitations Complicated by a Medical Illness

Mrs. Waterman is a 70-year-old woman with severe osteoarthritis of the spine and a recent history of left total hip replacement. She has been attending outpatient physical therapy sessions three times a week and uses a rolling walker at home. She has been admitted to the hospital with a partial small bowel obstruction. The health care team anticipates that the obstruction will resolve with medical treatment, and her expected length of stay is 5 to 7 days. Currently she is allowed nothing by mouth, has a Salem sump tube in place, and is receiving peripheral parenteral nutrition. The nurse is concerned that Mrs. Waterman's already impaired physical mobility will decline further secondary to her illness and the medical treatments that make independent ambulation difficult.

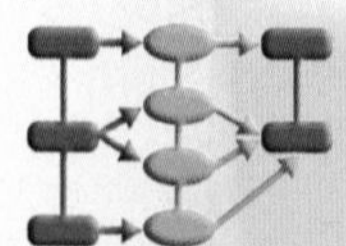

Turn to Appendix C to see a concept map that illustrates the relationships that exist between the nursing diagnoses, interventions, and outcomes for the patient's clinical problems.

Nursing Classifications and Languages

NANDA Nursing Diagnoses	NIC Nursing Interventions	NOC Nursing Outcomes Return to functional baseline status, stabilization of, or improvement in:
Impaired Physical Mobility—Limitation in independent, purposeful physical movement of the body or of one or more extremities	**Exercise Promotion**—Facilitation of regular physical exercise to maintain or advance a higher degree of fitness	**Mobility Level**—Ability to move purposefully in own environment independently with or without assistive device
Risk for Disuse Syndrome—At risk for deterioration of body systems as the result of prescribed or unavoidable musculoskeletal inactivity	**Exercise Promotion: Strength Training**—Facilitating regular resistive muscle training to retain or increase muscle strength	**Immobility Consequences: Physiological**—Severity of compromise in physiological functioning due to impaired physical mobility
	Embolus Precautions—Reduction of the risk of embolus in a patient with thrombi or at risk for developing thrombus formation	
	Pressure Ulcer Prevention—Prevention of pressure ulcers for an individual at high risk for developing them	
	Surveillance—Purposeful and ongoing acquisition, interpretation, and synthesis of patient data for clinical decision-making	

NANDA International (2005). *Nursing diagnoses: Definitions & classification 2005–2006.* Philadelphia: North American Nursing Diagnosis Association.

Dochterman, J. M., & Bulechek, G. M. (2004). *Nursing interventions classification (NIC)* (4th ed.). St. Louis: Mosby.

Iowa Outcomes Project (2004). In Moorhead, S., Johnson, M., & Maas, M. (2004). *Nursing outcomes classification (NOC)* (3rd ed.). St. Louis: Mosby.

Dochterman, J. M., & Jones, D. A. (2003). *Unifying nursing languages: The harmonization of NANDA, NIC, and NOC.* Washington, DC: American Nurses Association.

CHAPTER 66

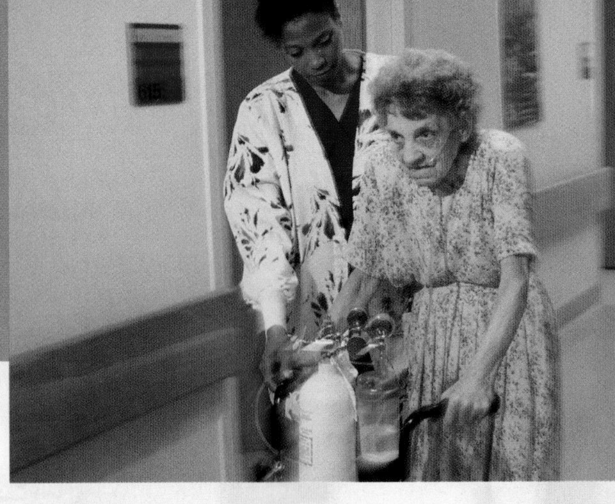

Assessment of Musculoskeletal Function

Learning Objectives

On completion of this chapter, the learner will be able to:

1. Describe the basic structure and function of the musculoskeletal system.
2. Discuss the significance of the health history to the assessment of musculoskeletal health.
3. Describe the significance of physical assessment to the diagnosis of musculoskeletal dysfunction.
4. Specify the diagnostic tests used for assessment of musculoskeletal function.

The musculoskeletal system includes the bones, joints, muscles, tendons, ligaments, and bursae of the body. The functions of these components are highly integrated; therefore, disease in or injury to one component adversely affects the others. For instance, an infection in a joint (septic arthritis) causes degeneration of the articular surfaces of the bones within the joint and local muscle atrophy.

Diseases and injuries that involve the musculoskeletal system are commonly implicated in disability and death. The leading cause of disability in the United States is arthritis (Centers for Disease Control and Prevention, 2002). Falls account for more than 420,000 hospitalizations yearly among the elderly. Hip fracture is the most common musculoskeletal condition that necessitates hospitalization in patients who are at least 65 years of age (U.S. Department of Health and Human Services [DHHS], 2004). Musculoskeletal diseases and injuries can significantly affect overall productivity, independence, and quality of life in people of all ages. Nurses in all practice areas encounter patients with disruption in musculoskeletal function.

Anatomic and Physiologic Overview

The health and proper functioning of the musculoskeletal system is interdependent with that of the other body systems. The musculoskeletal system has important functions. It provides protection for vital organs, including the brain, heart, and lungs, and provides a sturdy framework to support body structures. It also makes mobility possible. Joints hold the bones together and allow the body to move. The muscles attached to the skeleton contract, moving the bones and producing heat that helps maintain body temperature. Movement facilitates the return of deoxygenated blood to the right side of the heart by massaging the venous vasculature. In addition, the musculoskeletal system serves as a reservoir for immature blood cells and essential minerals, including calcium, phosphorus, magnesium, and fluoride. More than 98% of total body calcium is present in bone. In addition, the red bone marrow located within bone cavi-

Glossary

atonic: without tone; denervated muscle that atrophies
atrophy: shrinkage-like decrease in the size of a muscle
bursa: fluid-filled sac found in connective tissue, usually in the area of joints
callus: cartilaginous/fibrous tissue at fracture site
cancellous bone: lattice-like bone structure; trabecular bone
cartilage: tough, elastic, avascular tissue at ends of bone
clonus: rhythmic contraction of muscle
contracture: abnormal shortening of muscle or joint, or both; fibrosis
cortical bone: compact bone
crepitus: grating or crackling sound or sensation; may occur with movement of ends of a broken bone or irregular joint surface
diaphysis: shaft of long bone
effusion: excess fluid in joint
endosteum: a thin, vascular membrane covering the marrow cavity of long bones and the spaces in cancellous bone
epiphysis: end of long bone
fascia (epimysium): fibrous tissue that covers, supports, and separates muscles
fasciculation: involuntary twitch of muscle fibers
flaccid: limp; without muscle tone
hypertrophy: enlargement; increase in size of muscle
isometric contraction: muscle tension increased, length unchanged, no joint motion
isotonic contraction: muscle tension unchanged, muscle shortened, joint moved
joint: area where bone ends meet; provides for motion and flexibility
joint capsule: fibrous tissue that encloses bone ends and other joint surfaces
kyphosis: increase in the convex curvature of the spine
lamellae: mature compact bone structures that form concentric rings of bone matrix; lamellar bone
ligament: fibrous band connecting bones
lordosis: increase in lumbar curvature of the spine
ossification: process in which minerals (calcium) are deposited in bone matrix
osteoarthritis: degenerative joint disease characterized by destruction of the articular cartilage and overgrowth of bone
osteoblast: bone-forming cell
osteoclast: bone resorption cell
osteocyte: mature bone cell
osteogenesis: bone formation
osteoid: pertaining to bone matrix tissue; "pre-bone"
osteon: microscopic functional bone unit
osteoporosis: significant loss of bone mass and strength with increased risk for fracture
paralysis: absence of muscle movement suggesting nerve damage
paresthesia: abnormal sensation (eg, burning, tingling, numbness)
periosteum: fibrous connective tissue covering bone
remodeling: process that ensures bone maintenance through simultaneous bone resorption and formation
resorption: removal/destruction of tissue, such as bone
scoliosis: lateral curving of the spine
spastic: having greater than normal muscle tone
synovium: membrane in joint that secretes lubricating fluid
tendon: cord of fibrous tissue connecting muscle to bone
tone (tonus): normal tension (resistance to stretch) in resting muscle
trabeculae: lattice-like bone structure; cancellous bone

ties produces red blood cells, white blood cells, and platelets through a process referred to as hematopoiesis.

Structure and Function of the Skeletal System

There are 206 bones in the human body, divided into four categories:

- Long bones (eg, femur)
- Short bones (eg, metacarpals)
- Flat bones (eg, sternum)
- Irregular bones (eg, vertebrae)

The shape and construction of a specific bone are determined by its function and the forces exerted on it. Bones are constructed of **cancellous** (trabecular) or **cortical** (compact) bone tissue. Long bones are shaped like rods or shafts with rounded ends (Fig. 66-1). The shaft, known as the **diaphysis**, is primarily cortical bone. The ends of the long bones, called **epiphyses**, are primarily cancellous bone. The epiphyseal plate separates the epiphyses from the diaphysis and is the center for longitudinal growth in children. It is calcified in adults. The ends of long bones are covered at the joints by articular **cartilage**, which is tough, elastic, avascular tissue. Long bones are designed for weight bearing and movement. Short bones consist of cancellous bone covered by a layer of compact bone. Flat bones are important sites of hematopoiesis and frequently provide vital organ protection. They are made of cancellous bone layered between compact bone. Irregular bones have unique shapes related to their function. Generally, irregular bone structure is similar to that of flat bones.

Bone is composed of cells, protein matrix, and mineral deposits. The cells are of three basic types—**osteoblasts, osteocytes**, and **osteoclasts.** Osteoblasts function in bone formation by secreting bone matrix. The matrix consists of collagen and ground substances (glycoproteins and proteoglycans) that provide a framework in which inorganic mineral salts are deposited. These minerals are primarily composed of calcium and phosphorus. Osteocytes are mature bone cells involved in bone maintenance; they are lo-

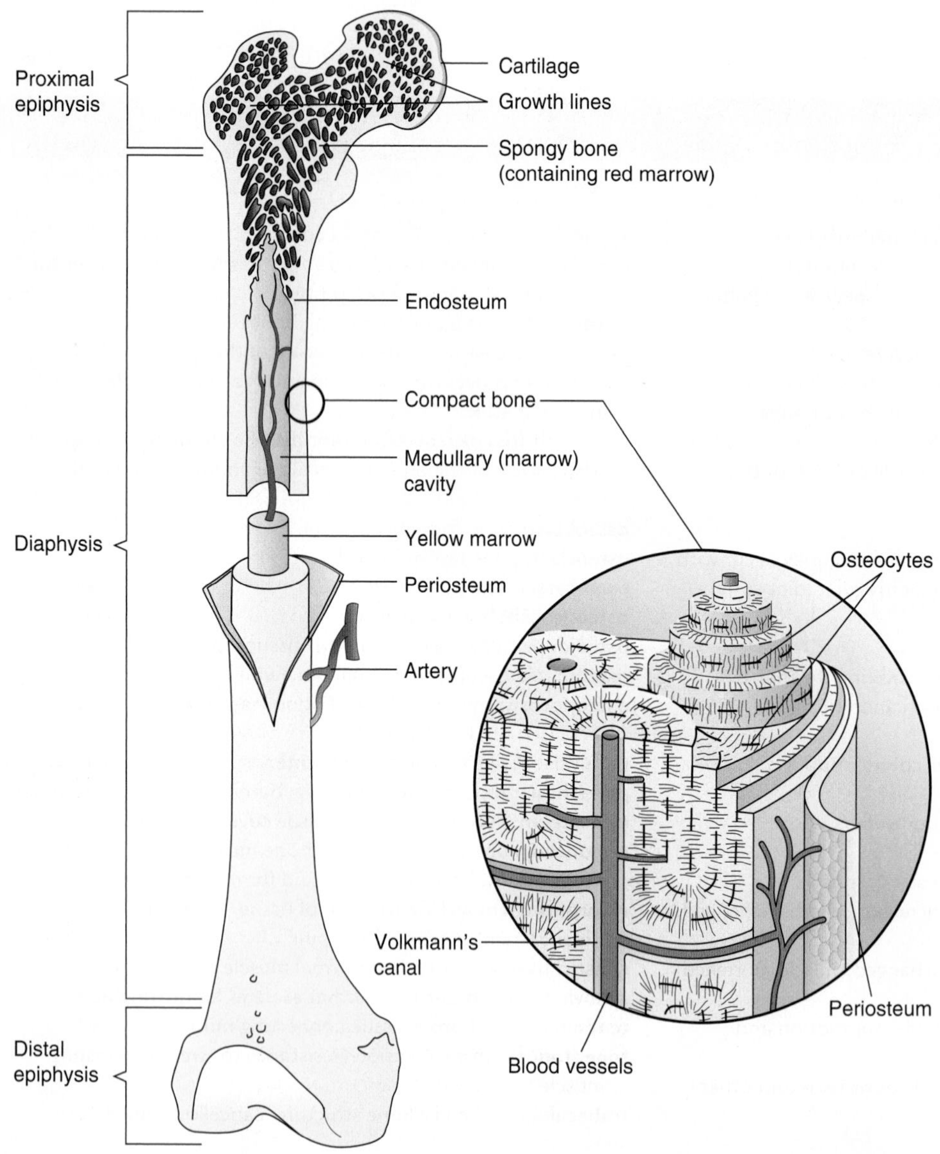

FIGURE 66-1. Structure of a long bone; composition of compact bone.

cated in lacunae (bone matrix units). Osteoclasts, located in shallow Howship's lacunae (small pits in bones), are multinuclear cells involved in dissolving and resorbing bone. The microscopic functioning unit of mature cortical bone is the **osteon** (Haversian system). The center of the osteon, the Haversian canal, contains a capillary. Around the capillary are circles of mineralized bone matrix called **lamellae.** Within the lamellae are lacunae that contain osteocytes. These are nourished through tiny structures, canaliculi (canals), that communicate with adjacent blood vessels within the Haversian system.

Lacunae in cancellous bone are layered in an irregular lattice network (**trabeculae**). Red bone marrow fills the lattice network. Capillaries nourish the osteocytes located in the lacunae.

Covering the bone is a dense, fibrous membrane known as the **periosteum.** This membranous structure nourishes bone and facilitates its growth. The periosteum contains nerves, blood vessels, and lymphatics. It also provides for the attachment of tendons, which connect muscles to bones, and ligaments, which connect bones to bones.

The **endosteum** is a thin, vascular membrane that covers the marrow cavity of long bones and the spaces in cancellous bone. Osteoclasts, which dissolve bone to maintain the marrow cavity, are located near the endosteum in Howship's lacunae.

Bone marrow is a vascular tissue located in the medullary (shaft) cavity of long bones and in flat bones. Red bone marrow, located mainly in the sternum, ilium, vertebrae, and ribs in adults, is responsible for producing red blood cells, white blood cells, and platelets. In adults, the long bone is filled with fatty, yellow marrow.

Bone tissue is well vascularized. Cancellous bone receives a rich blood supply through metaphyseal and epiphyseal vessels. Periosteal vessels carry blood to compact bone through minute Volkmann's canals. In addition, nutrient arteries penetrate the periosteum and enter the medullary cavity through foramina (small openings). Nutrient arteries supply blood to the marrow and bone. The venous system may accompany arteries or may exit independently.

Bone Formation

Osteogenesis (bone formation) begins long before birth. **Ossification** is the process by which the bone matrix (collagen fibers and ground substance) is formed and hard mineral crystals composed of calcium and phosphorus (eg, hydroxyapatite) are bound to the collagen fibers. The mineral components of the bone give it its characteristic strength, whereas the proteinaceous collagen gives bone its resilience.

There are two basic processes of ossification: endochondral and intramembranous. Most bones in the body are formed by endochondral ossification, in which a cartilage-like tissue (**osteoid**) is formed, resorbed, and replaced by bone. Intramembranous ossification occurs when bone develops within membrane, as in the bones of the face and skull.

Bone Maintenance

Bone is a dynamic tissue in a constant state of turnover. During childhood, bones grow and form by a process called modeling. By early adulthood (ie, early 20s), **remodeling** is the primary process that occurs. Remodeling maintains bone structure and function through simultaneous **resorption** and osteogenesis, and as a result, complete skeletal turnover occurs every 10 years (DHHS, 2004).

The balance between bone resorption and formation is influenced by the following factors: physical activity; dietary intake of certain nutrients, especially calcium; and several hormones, including calcitriol (ie, active vitamin D), parathormone (parathyroid hormone), calcitonin, thyroid hormone, cortisol, growth hormone, and the sex hormones estrogen and testosterone (DHHS, 2004).

Physical activity, particularly weight-bearing activity, acts to stimulate bone formation and remodeling. Bones subjected to continued weight-bearing tend to be thick and strong. Conversely, people who are unable to engage in regular weight-bearing activities, such as those on prolonged bed rest or those with disabilities, have increased bone resorption from calcium loss, and their bones become osteopenic and weak. These weakened bones may fracture easily.

Good dietary habits are integral to bone health. In particular, absorption of approximately 1500 mg of calcium daily is essential to maintaining adult bone mass. This may be achieved through ingesting calcium-rich foods on a daily basis (eg, through drinking 16 to 24 ounces of milk daily).

Several hormones are vital in ensuring that calcium is properly absorbed and available for bone mineralization and matrix formation. Biologically active vitamin D (calcitriol) functions to increase the amount of calcium in the blood by promoting absorption of calcium from the gastrointestinal tract. It also facilitates mineralization of osteoid tissue. A deficiency of vitamin D results in bone mineralization deficit, deformity, and fracture.

Parathormone and calcitonin are the major hormonal regulators of calcium homeostasis. Parathormone regulates the concentration of calcium in the blood, in part by promoting movement of calcium from the bone. In response to low calcium levels in the blood, increased levels of parathormone prompt the mobilization of calcium, the demineralization of bone, and the formation of bone cysts. Calcitonin, secreted by the thyroid gland in response to elevated blood calcium levels, inhibits bone resorption and increases the deposit of calcium in bone.

Both thyroid hormone and cortisol have multiple systemic effects with specific effects on bones. Excessive thyroid hormone production in adults (eg, Graves' disease) can result in increased bone resorption and decreased bone formation. Increased levels of cortisol have these same effects. Patients receiving long-term synthetic cortisol or corticosteroids (ie, prednisone [Deltasone, Prednicot]) are at increased risk for steroid-induced osteopenia and fractures.

Growth hormone has direct and indirect effects on skeletal growth and remodeling. It stimulates the liver and to a lesser degree the bones to produce insulin-like growth factor-1 (IGF-I), which accelerates bone modeling in children and adolescents. Growth hormone also directly stimulates skeletal growth in children and adolescents. It is believed that the low levels of both growth hormone and IGF-I that occur with aging may be partly responsible for decreased bone formation and resultant osteopenia.

The sex hormones testosterone and estrogen have important effects on bone remodeling. Estrogen stimulates osteoblasts and inhibits osteoclasts; therefore, bone formation is enhanced and resorption is inhibited. Testosterone has both direct and indirect effects on bone growth and formation. It directly causes skeletal growth in adolescence and has continued effects on skeletal muscle growth throughout the lifespan. Increased muscle mass results in greater weight-bearing stress on bones, resulting in increased bone formation. In addition, testosterone converts to estrogen in adipose tissue, providing an additional source of bone-preserving estrogen for aging men.

Recent research findings suggest that low levels of estrogen or increased levels of corticosteroids cause disruption in normal osteoclast and osteoblast homeostasis. In particular, these factors and perhaps others (ie, either primary or metastatic bone tumors and heightened T-cell activation in rheumatoid arthritis) promote the activity of nuclear factor B ligand (RANKL). RANKL is a cytokine that promotes the formation and activation of osteoclasts. Increased activity of RANKL results in accelerated bone resorption, which leads to bone loss and fractures. Promising research is currently focused on developing medications that block the effects of RANKL and on developing useful laboratory tests of RANKL levels that may guide therapy aimed at reducing the risk of fractures (Hofbauer & Schoppet, 2004; Schett, Kiechl, Redlich, et al., 2004).

Blood supply to the bone also affects bone formation. With diminished blood supply or hyperemia (congestion), osteogenesis and bone density decrease. Bone necrosis occurs when the bone is deprived of blood.

Bone Healing

Most fractures heal through a combination of intramembranous and endochondral ossification processes. When a bone is fractured, the bone fragments are not merely patched together with scar tissue. Instead, the bone regenerates itself.

Fracture healing occurs in four areas:

- Bone marrow, where endothelial cells rapidly undergo transformation and become osteoblastic bone-forming cells
- Bone cortex, where new osteons are formed
- Periosteum, where a hard callus/bone is formed through intramembranous ossification peripheral to the fracture, and where a cartilage model is formed through endochondral ossification adjacent to the fracture site
- External soft tissue, where a bridging **callus** (fibrous tissue) stabilizes the fracture

The process of fracture healing occurs via six stages, each stimulated by the release and activation of biologic regulators and signaling molecules (Buckwalter, Einhorn, & Sheldon, 2000):

1. *Hematoma and inflammation:* The body's response is similar to that after injury elsewhere in the body. There is bleeding into the injured tissue and formation of a fracture hematoma. The hematoma is a source of signaling molecules, such as cytokines, transforming growth factor-beta (TGF-β), and platelet-derived growth factor (PDGF), which initiate the fracture healing processes. The fracture fragment ends become devitalized because of the interrupted blood supply. The injured area is invaded by macrophages (large phagocytic white blood cells), which débride the area. Inflammation, swelling, and pain are present. The inflammatory stage lasts several days and resolves with a decrease in pain and swelling.
2. *Angiogenesis and cartilage formation:* Under the influence of signaling molecules, cell proliferation and differentiation occur. Blood vessels and cartilage overlie the fracture.
3. *Cartilage calcification:* Chondrocytes in the cartilage callus form matrix vesicles, which regulate calcification of the cartilage. Enzymes within these matrix vesicles prepare the cartilage for calcium release and deposit.
4. *Cartilage removal:* The calcified cartilage is invaded by blood vessels and becomes resorbed by chondroblasts and osteoclasts. It is replaced by woven bone similar to that of the growth plate.
5. *Bone formation:* Minerals continue to be deposited until the bone is firmly reunited. With major adult long bone fractures, ossification takes 3 to 4 months.
6. *Remodeling:* The final stage of fracture repair consists of remodeling the new bone into its former structural arrangement. Remodeling may take months to years, depending on the extent of bone modification needed, the function of the bone, and the functional stresses on the bone. Cancellous bone heals and remodels more rapidly than does compact cortical bone.

Serial x-rays are used to monitor the progress of bone healing. The type of bone fractured, the adequacy of blood supply, the surface contact of the fragments, and the age and general health of the person influence the rate of fracture healing. Adequate immobilization is essential until there is x-ray evidence of bone formation with ossification.

BONE HEALING WITH FRAGMENTS FIRMLY APPROXIMATED

When fractures are treated with open rigid compression plate fixation techniques, the bony fragments can be placed in direct contact. Primary bone healing occurs through cortical bone (Haversian) remodeling. Little or no cartilaginous callus develops. Immature bone develops from the endosteum. There is an intensive regeneration of new osteons, which develop in the fracture line by a process similar to normal bone maintenance. Fracture strength is obtained when the new osteons have become established.

Structure and Function of the Articular System

The junction of two or more bones is called a **joint** (articulation). There are three basic kinds of joints: synarthrosis, amphiarthrosis, and diarthrosis joints. Synarthrosis joints are immovable (eg, the skull sutures). Amphiarthrosis joints (eg, the vertebral joints and the symphysis pubis) allow limited motion; the bones of amphiarthrosis joints are joined by fibrous cartilage. Diarthrosis joints are freely movable joints (Fig. 66-2).

There are several types of diarthrosis joints:

- *Ball-and-socket* joints (eg, the hip and the shoulder) permit full freedom of movement.
- *Hinge* joints permit bending in one direction only (eg, the elbow and the knee).

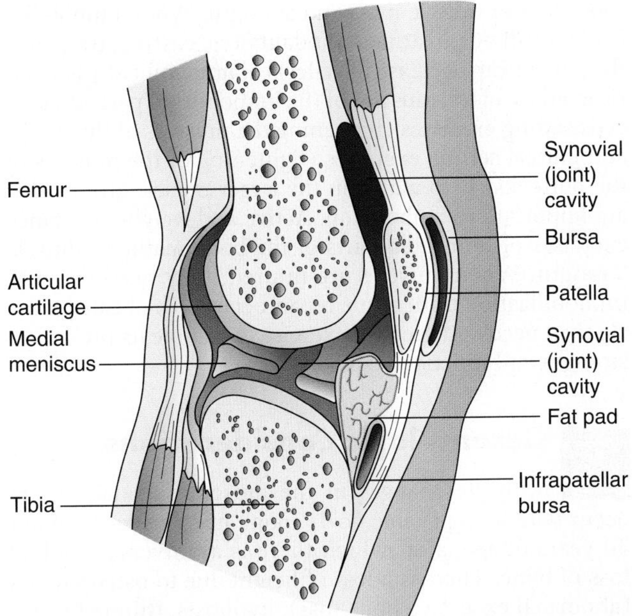

FIGURE 66-2. Hinge joint of the knee.

- *Saddle* joints allow movement in two planes at right angles to each other. The joint at the base of the thumb is a saddle, biaxial joint.
- *Pivot* joints are characterized by the articulation between the radius and the ulna. They permit rotation for such activities as turning a doorknob.
- *Gliding* joints allow for limited movement in all directions and are represented by the joints of the carpal bones in the wrist.

The ends of the articulating bones of a typical movable joint are covered with smooth hyaline cartilage. A tough, fibrous sheath called the **joint capsule** surrounds the articulating bones. The capsule is lined with a membrane, the **synovium**, which secretes the lubricating and shock-absorbing synovial fluid into the joint capsule. Therefore, the bone surfaces are not in direct contact. In some synovial joints (eg, the knee), fibrocartilage disks (eg, medial meniscus) are located between the articular cartilage surfaces. These disks provide shock absorption.

Ligaments (fibrous connective tissue bands) bind the articulating bones together. Ligaments and muscle tendons, which pass over the joint, provide joint stability. In some joints, interosseous ligaments (eg, the cruciate ligaments of the knee) are found within the capsule and add stability to the joint.

A **bursa** is a sac filled with synovial fluid that cushions the movement of tendons, ligaments, and bones at a point of friction. Bursae are found at the elbow, shoulder, knee, and some other joints.

Structure and Function of the Skeletal Muscle System

Muscles are attached by **tendons** (cords of fibrous connective tissue) or aponeuroses (broad, flat sheets of connective tissue) to bones, connective tissue, other muscles, soft tissue, or skin. The muscles of the body are composed of parallel groups of muscle cells (fasciculi) encased in fibrous tissue called **fascia** or **epimysium.** The more fasciculi contained in a muscle, the more precise the movements. Muscles vary in shape and size according to the activities for which they are responsible. Skeletal (striated) muscles are involved in body movement, posture, and heat-production functions. Muscles contract to bring the two points of attachment closer together, resulting in movement.

Skeletal Muscle Contraction

CONCEPTS in action ANIMATION

Each muscle cell (also referred to as a muscle fiber) contains myofibrils, which in turn are composed of a series of sarcomeres, the actual contractile units of skeletal muscle. Sarcomeres contain thick myosin and thin actin filaments.

Muscle cells contract in response to electrical stimulation delivered by an effector nerve cell at the motor end plate. When stimulated, the muscle cell depolarizes and generates an action potential in a manner similar to that described for nerve cells. These action potentials propagate along the muscle cell membrane and lead to the release of calcium ions that are stored in specialized organelles called sarcoplasmic reticula. When there is a local increase in calcium ion concentration, the myosin and actin filaments slide across one another. Shortly after the muscle cell membrane is depolarized, it recovers its resting membrane voltage. Calcium is rapidly removed from the sarcomeres by active reaccumulation in the sarcoplasmic reticulum. When the calcium concentration in the sarcomere decreases, the myosin and actin filaments cease to interact, and the sarcomere returns to its original resting length (relaxation). Actin and myosin do not interact in the absence of calcium.

Energy is consumed during muscle contraction and relaxation. The primary source of energy for the muscle cells is adenosine triphosphate (ATP), which is generated through cellular oxidative metabolism. At low levels of activity (ie, sedentary activity), the skeletal muscle synthesizes ATP from the oxidation of glucose to water and carbon dioxide. During periods of strenuous activity, when sufficient oxygen may not be available, glucose is metabolized primarily to lactic acid, an inefficient process compared with that of oxidative pathways. Stored muscle glycogen is used to supply glucose during periods of activity. Muscle fatigue is thought to be caused by depletion of glycogen and accumulation of lactic acid. As a result, the cycle of muscle contraction and relaxation cannot continue.

During muscle contraction, the energy released from ATP is not completely used. The excess energy is dissipated in the form of heat. During isometric contraction, almost all of the energy is released in the form of heat; during isotonic contraction, some of the energy is expended in mechanical work. In some situations, such as shivering because of cold, the need to generate heat is the primary stimulus for muscle contraction.

The contraction of muscle fibers can result in either isotonic or isometric contraction of the muscle. In **isometric contraction**, the length of the muscles remains constant but the force generated by the muscles is increased; an example of this is pushing against an immovable wall. **Isotonic contraction**, on the other hand, is characterized by shortening of the muscle with no increase in tension within the muscle; an example of this is flexing the forearm. In normal activities, many muscle movements are a combination of isometric and isotonic contraction. For example, during walking, isotonic contraction results in shortening of the leg, and isometric contraction causes the stiff leg to push against the floor.

The speed of the muscle contraction is variable. Myoglobulin is a hemoglobin-like protein pigment present in striated muscle cells that transports oxygen. Muscles containing large quantities of myoglobulin (red muscles) have been observed to contract slowly and powerfully (eg, respiratory and postural muscles). Muscles containing little myoglobulin (white muscles) contract quickly (eg, extraocular eye muscles). Most muscles contain both red and white muscle fibers (Porth, 2005).

Muscle Tone

Relaxed muscles demonstrate a state of readiness to respond to contraction stimuli. This state of readiness, known as muscle **tone (tonus)**, is produced by the maintenance of some of the muscle fibers in a contracted state. Muscle spindles, which are sense organs in the muscles, monitor muscle tone. Muscle tone is minimal during sleep and is increased when the person is anxious. A muscle that is limp and without tone is described as **flaccid**; a muscle with greater-than-normal tone is described as **spastic.** In conditions characterized by lower motor neuron destruction (eg, polio), denervated muscle becomes **atonic** (soft and flabby) and atrophies.

Muscle Actions

Muscles accomplish movement by contraction. Through the coordination of muscle groups, the body is able to perform a wide variety of movements (Chart 66-1). The prime mover is the muscle that causes a particular motion. The muscles assisting the prime mover are known as synergists. The muscles causing movement opposite to that of the prime mover are known as antagonists. An antagonist must relax to allow the prime mover to contract, producing motion. For example, when contraction of the biceps causes flexion of the elbow joint, the biceps are the prime movers, and the triceps are the antagonists. A person with muscle **paralysis** (a loss of movement, possibly from nerve damage) may be able to retrain functioning muscles within the synergistic group to produce the needed movement. Muscles of the synergistic group then become the prime movers.

Exercise, Disuse, and Repair

Muscles need to be exercised to maintain function and strength. When a muscle repeatedly develops maximum or close to maximum tension over a long time, as in regular exercise with weights, the cross-sectional area of the muscle increases. This enlargement, known as **hypertrophy**, results from an increase in the size of individual muscle fibers without an increase in their number. Hypertrophy persists only if the exercise is continued. The opposite phenomenon occurs with disuse of muscle over a long period of time. Age and disuse cause loss of muscular function as fibrotic tissue replaces the contractile muscle tissue. The decrease in the size of a muscle is called **atrophy.** Bed rest and immobility cause loss of muscle mass and strength. When immobility is the result of a treatment modality (eg, casting, traction), the patient can decrease the effects of immobility by isometric exercise of the muscles of the immobilized part. Quadriceps setting exercises (tightening the muscles of the thigh) and gluteal setting exercises (tightening of the muscles of the buttocks) help maintain the larger muscle groups that are important in ambulation. Active and weight-resistance exercises of uninjured parts of the body maintain muscle strength. When muscles are injured, they need rest and immobilization until tissue repair occurs. The healed muscle then needs progressive exercise to resume its pre-injury strength and functional ability.

Gerontologic Considerations

Multiple changes in the musculoskeletal system occur with aging (Table 66-1). Bone mass peaks by about 30 years of age, after which there is a universal gradual loss of bone. There is a loss of height due to **osteoporosis** (abnormal excessive bone loss), kyphosis, thinned intervertebral disks, and flexion of the knees and hips. Numerous metabolic changes, including menopausal withdrawal of estrogen and decreased activity, contribute to **osteoporosis.** Women lose more bone mass than men. In addition, bones change in shape and have reduced strength. Fractures are common. In the elderly, collagen structures are less able to absorb energy. Ligaments become weak. The articular cartilage degenerates in weight-bearing areas and heals less readily. This contributes to the development of **osteoarthritis** (degenerative joint disease). Joints enlarge and range of motion decreases. Muscle mass and strength are also diminished. There is also an actual loss in the size and number of muscle fibers due to myofibril atrophy with fibrous tissue replacement. Increased inactivity, diminished neuron stimulation, and nutritional deficiencies contribute to loss of muscle strength. In addition, remote musculoskeletal problems for which the patient has compensated may become new problems with age-related changes. For example, people who have had polio and who have been able to function normally by using synergistic muscle groups may discover increasing incapacity because of a reduced compensatory ability. However, many of the effects of aging can be slowed if the body is kept healthy and active through positive lifestyle behaviors.

Assessment

Health History

The nursing assessment of the patient with musculoskeletal dysfunction includes an evaluation of the effects of the musculoskeletal problem on the patient. The nurse is concerned with assisting patients who have musculoskeletal problems to maintain their general health, accomplish their activities of daily living, and manage their treatment programs. The nurse encourages optimal nutrition and prevents problems related to immobility. Through an individualized plan of nursing care, the nurse helps the patient achieve maximum health.

CHART 66-1

Body Movements Produced by Muscle Contraction

Flexion—bending at a joint (eg, elbow)
Extension—straightening at a joint
Abduction—moving away from midline
Adduction—moving toward midline
Rotation—turning around a specific axis (eg, shoulder joint)
Circumduction—cone-like movement
Supination—turning upward
Pronation—turning downward
Inversion—turning inward
Eversion—turning outward
Protraction—pushing forward
Retraction—pulling backward

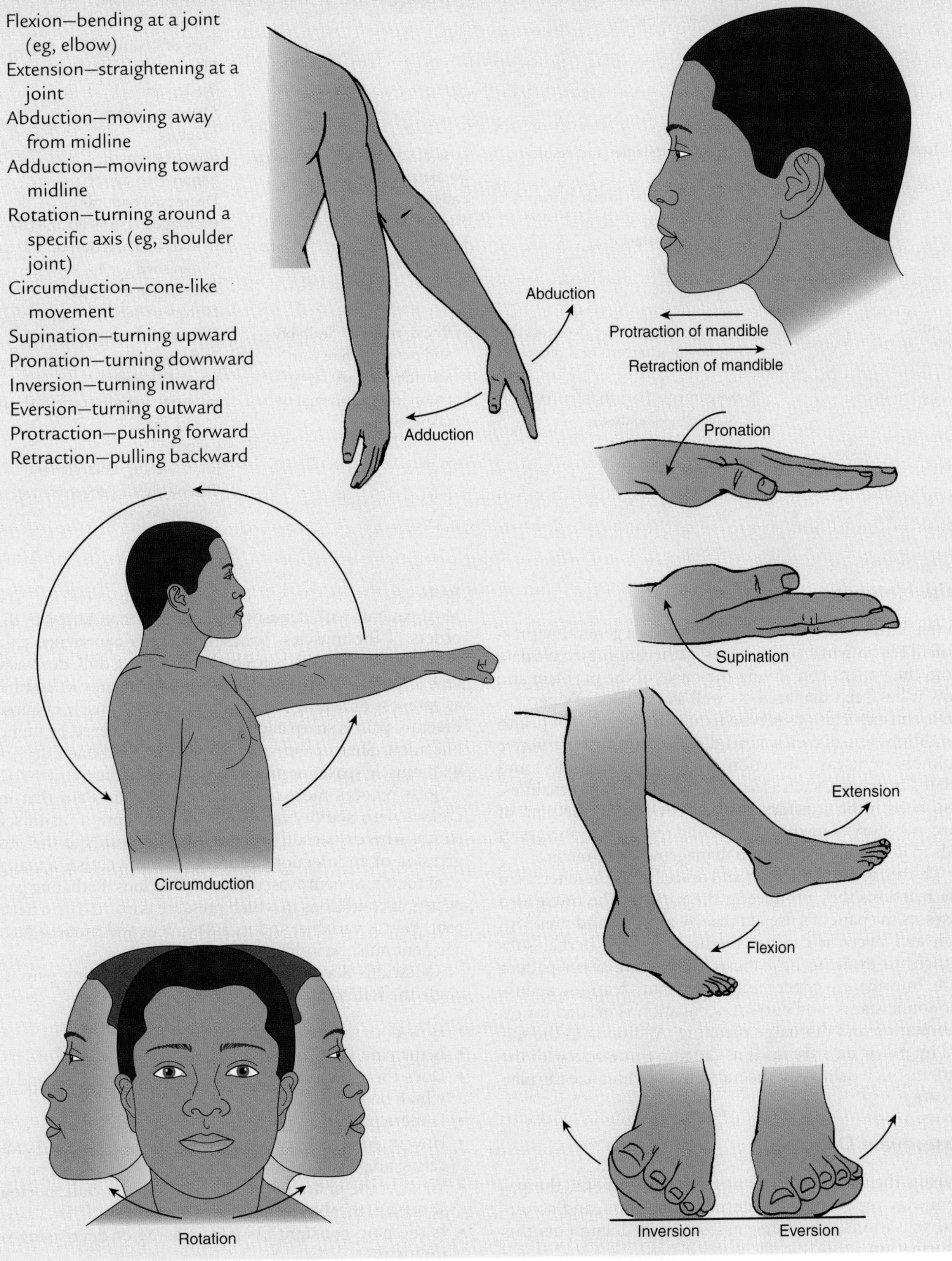

TABLE 66-1 Age-Related Changes of the Musculoskeletal System

Musculoskeletal System	Structural Changes	Functional Changes	History and Physical Findings
Bones	Gradual, progressive loss of bone mass after age 30 yr Vertebrae collapse	Bones fragile and prone to fracture: vertebrae, hip, wrist	Loss of height Posture changes Kyphosis Loss of flexibility Flexion of hips and knees Back pain Osteoporosis Fracture
Muscles	Increase in collagen and resultant fibrosis Muscles diminish in size (atrophy); wasting Tendons less elastic	Loss of strength and flexibility Weakness Fatigue Stumbling Falls	Loss of strength Diminished agility Decreased endurance Prolonged response time (diminished reaction time) Diminished tone Broad base of support History of falls
Joints	Cartilage—progressive deterioration Thinning of intervertebral discs	Stiffness, reduced flexibility, and pain interfere with activities of daily living	Diminished range of motion Stiffness Loss of height
Ligaments	Lax ligaments (less than normal strength; weakness)	Postural joint abnormality Weakness	Joint pain on motion; resolves with rest Crepitus Joint swelling/enlargement Osteoarthritis (degenerative joint disease)

Initial Interview

In the initial interview, the nurse obtains a general impression of the patient's health status, gathering subjective data from the patient concerning the onset of the problem and how it has been managed, as well as the patient's perceptions and expectations related to health. Concurrent health conditions (eg, diabetes, heart disease, chronic obstructive pulmonary disease, infection, preexisting disability) and related problems, such as familial or genetic abnormalities, also need to be considered when developing the plan of care. A history of medication use and response to analgesics aids in designing medication management regimens.

The nurse notes allergies and describes them in terms of the reactions they produce in the patient. The nurse also assesses the patient's use of tobacco, alcohol, and prescription and over-the-counter medications and herbal substances to evaluate how these agents may affect patient care. Information concerning the patient's learning ability, economic status, and current occupation is needed for rehabilitation and discharge planning. Additions to the initial interview data are made as the nurse interacts with the patient. Such data assist the nurse to individualize the plan of care.

Assessment Data

During the interview and physical assessment, the patient may report pain, tenderness, tightness, and abnormal sensations. The nurse assesses and documents this information.

PAIN

Most patients with diseases and traumatic conditions or disorders of the muscles, bones, and joints experience pain. Bone pain is characteristically described as a dull, deep ache that is "boring" in nature, whereas muscular pain is described as soreness or aching and is referred to as "muscle cramps." Fracture pain is sharp and piercing and is relieved by immobilization. Sharp pain may also result from bone infection with muscle spasm or pressure on a sensory nerve.

Rest relieves most musculoskeletal pain. Pain that increases with activity may indicate joint sprain or muscle strain, whereas steadily increasing pain points to the progression of an infectious process (osteomyelitis), a malignant tumor, or neurovascular complications. Radiating pain occurs in conditions in which pressure is exerted on a nerve root. Pain is variable, and its assessment and nursing management must be individualized.

Questions that the nurse should ask regarding pain include the following:

- How does the patient describe the pain?
- Is the pain localized?
- Does the pain radiate? If so, in which direction and to which body parts?
- Is there pain in any other part of the body?
- How intense is the pain on a scale of 0 to 10 (with 0 indicating no pain and 10 indicating the worst possible pain)?
- What is the character of the pain (sharp, dull, boring, shooting, throbbing, cramping)?
- Is the pain constant? Is it increasing or decreasing in intensity?

GENETICS IN NURSING PRACTICE

Musculoskeletal Disorders

When assessing a patient with musculoskeletal complaints, nurses must not overlook the possibility of a genetic component to the patient's problems

MUSCULOSKELETAL IMPAIRMENTS INFLUENCED BY GENETIC FACTORS

- Achondroplasia
- Congenital talipes equinovarus (clubfoot)
- Developmental dysplasia of the hip (DDH) (congenital hip dysplasia)
- Ehlers-Danlos syndrome
- Marfan syndrome
- Stickler syndrome
- Osteogenesis imperfecta
- Osteoporosis
- Scoliosis

NURSING ASSESSMENTS

Family History

- Assess for other similarly affected family members.
- Assess for the presence of other related genetic conditions (eg, hematologic, cardiac, integumentary conditions).
- Determine the age at onset (eg, fractures present at birth as in osteogenesis imperfecta, hip dislocation present at birth in DDH, or early-onset osteoporosis).

Patient Assessment

- Assess stature for general screening purposes (unusually short stature may be related to achondroplasia; unusually tall stature may be related to Marfan syndrome).
- Assess for disease-specific skeletal findings (eg, pectus excavatum, scoliosis, long fingers [Marfan syndrome], osteoarthritis of the hip and waddling gait [DDH]).
- Assess for disease-specific skin findings (eg, velvety texture with unusual scarring and/or thin fragile skin [Ehlers-Danlos syndrome]).
- Assess for other common disease-specific findings (eg, vision impairment [Stickler syndrome, Marfan syndrome], blue/gray sclerae, opalescent dentin, hearing impairment [osteogenesis imperfecta]).

MANAGEMENT ISSUES SPECIFIC TO GENETICS

- Inquire whether DNA gene mutation or other genetic testing has been performed on affected family members.
- If indicated, refer patient for further genetic counseling and evaluation so that family members can discuss inheritance, risk to other family members, and the availability of genetic testing and gene-based interventions.
- Offer appropriate genetics information and resources.
- Assess patient's understanding of genetics information.
- Provide support to families with newly diagnosed genetic-related musculoskeletal disorders.
- Participate in management and coordination of care of patients with genetic conditions and people predisposed to develop or pass on a genetic condition.

GENETICS RESOURCES

Genetic Alliance—a directory of support groups for patients and families with genetic conditions; http://www.geneticalliance.org. Accessed August 10, 2006.

Gene Clinics—a listing of common genetic disorders with up-to-date clinical summaries, genetic counseling and testing information; http://www.geneclinics.org. Accessed August 10, 2006.

National Organization of Rare Disorders—a directory of support groups and information for patients and families with rare genetic disorders; http://www.rarediseases.org. Accessed August 10, 2006.

OMIM: Online Mendelian Inheritance in Man—a complete listing of inherited genetic conditions; http://www.ncbi.nlm.nih.gov/entrez/query.fcgi?db=OMIM. Accessed August 10, 2006.

- What relieves the pain?
- What makes the pain worse?
- What was the patient doing before the pain occurred?
- What was the manner of onset (ie, how did the pain develop)?
- Does the patient experience increased discomfort when overly tired from lack of sleep, exciting stimuli, or too much activity?

Assessments that the nurse should make regarding the pain include the following:

- Is the body in proper alignment?
- Is there pressure from traction, bed linens, a cast, or other appliances?
- Is there tension on the skin at a pin site?

It is important that the patient's pain and discomfort be managed successfully. Not only is pain exhausting, but, if prolonged, it can force the patient to become increasingly preoccupied and dependent (see Chapter 13).

ALTERED SENSATIONS

Sensory disturbances are frequently associated with musculoskeletal problems. The patient may describe **paresthesias**, which are burning, tingling sensations or numbness.

These sensations may be caused by pressure on nerves or by circulatory impairment. Soft tissue swelling or direct trauma to these structures can impair their function. The nurse assesses the neurovascular status of the involved musculoskeletal area.

Questions that the nurse should ask regarding altered sensations include the following:

- Is the patient experiencing any abnormal sensations or numbness?
- If the abnormal sensation or feeling of numbness involves an extremity, how does this feeling compare to sensation in the unaffected extremity?
- When did the condition begin? Is it getting worse?
- Does the patient also have pain? (If the patient has pain, then the questions and assessments for pain discussed previously should be followed.)

Assessments that the nurse should make regarding the altered sensations include the following:

- If the affected part is an extremity, how does its overall appearance compare to the unaffected extremity?
- Can the patient move the affected part?
- What is the color of the part distal to the affected area? Is it pale? Dusky? Mottled? Cyanotic?
- Does rapid capillary refill occur? (The nurse can gently squeeze a nail until it blanches, then release the pressure. The amount of time for the color under the nail to return to normal is noted. Color normally returns within 3 seconds. The return of color is evidence of capillary refill.)
- Is a pulse palpable distal to the affected area? If the affected area is an extremity, how does the pulse compare to that felt in the unaffected extremity?
- Is edema present?
- Is any constrictive device or clothing causing nerve or vascular compression?
- Does elevating the affected part or modifying its position affect the symptoms?

Physical Assessment

An examination of the musculoskeletal system ranges from a basic assessment of functional capabilities to sophisticated physical examination maneuvers that facilitate diagnosis of specific bone, muscle, and joint disorders (Chart 66-2). The extent of assessment depends on the patient's physical complaints, health history, and physical clues that warrant further exploration. The nursing assessment is primarily a functional evaluation, focusing on the patient's ability to perform activities of daily living.

Techniques of inspection and palpation are used to evaluate the patient's posture, gait, bone integrity, joint function, and muscle strength and size. In addition, assessing the skin and neurovascular status is an important part of a complete musculoskeletal assessment. The nurse also should understand and be able to perform correct assessment techniques on patients with musculoskeletal trauma. When specific symptoms or physical findings of musculoskeletal dysfunction are apparent, the nurse carefully documents the examination findings and shares the information with the physician, who may decide that a more extensive examination and a diagnostic workup are necessary.

CHART 66-2

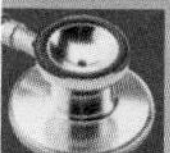

Assessing for Peripheral Nerve Function

Assessment of peripheral nerve function has two key elements: evaluation of sensation and evaluation of motion. The nurse may perform one or all of the following during a musculoskeletal assessment.

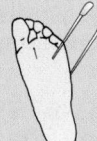

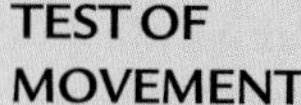

NERVE	TEST OF SENSATION	TEST OF MOVEMENT
Peroneal nerve	Prick the skin midway between the great and second toe. 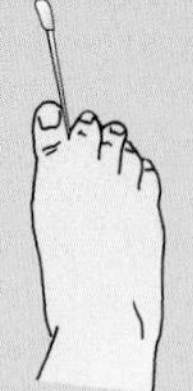	Ask the patient to dorsiflex the ankle and extend the toes. 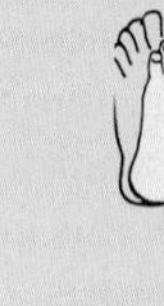
Tibial nerve	Prick the medial and lateral surface of the sole.	Ask the patient to plantar flex toes and ankle. 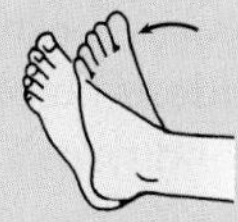
Radial nerve	Prick the skin midway between the thumb and second finger. 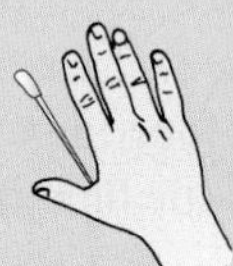	Ask the patient to stretch out the thumb, then the wrist, and then the fingers at the metacarpal joints.
Ulnar nerve	Prick the distal fat pad of the small finger. 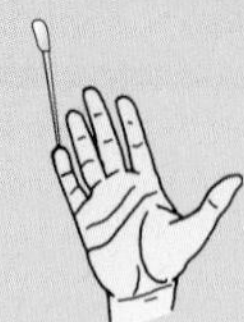	Ask the patient to abduct all fingers. 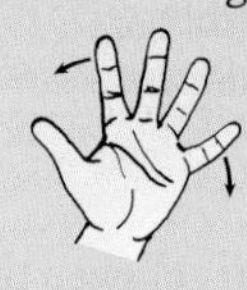
Median nerve	Prick the top or distal surface of the index finger. 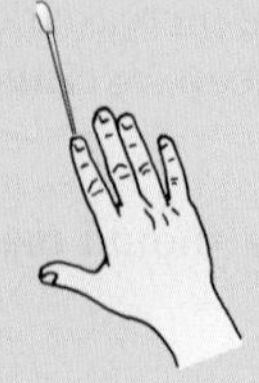	Ask the patient to touch the thumb to the little finger. Also observe whether the patient can flex the wrist. 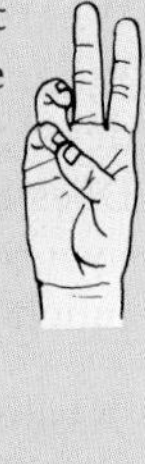

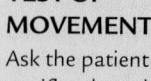

Posture

The normal curvature of the spine is convex through the thoracic portion and concave through the cervical and lumbar portions. Common deformities of the spine include **kyphosis**, an increased forward curvature of the thoracic spine; **lordosis**, or swayback, an exaggerated curvature of the lumbar spine; and **scoliosis**, a lateral curving deviation of the spine (Fig. 66-3). Kyphosis is frequently seen in elderly patients with osteoporosis and in some patients with neuromuscular diseases. Scoliosis may be congenital, idiopathic (without an identifiable cause), or the result of damage to the paraspinal muscles, as in polio. Lordosis is frequently seen during pregnancy as the woman adjusts her posture in response to changes in her center of gravity.

During inspection of the spine, the entire back, buttocks, and legs are exposed. The examiner inspects the spinal curves and trunk symmetry from posterior and lateral views. Standing behind the patient, the examiner notes any differences in the height of the shoulders or iliac crests. The gluteal folds are normally symmetric. Shoulder and hip symmetry, as well as the line of the vertebral column, are inspected with the patient erect and with the patient bending forward (flexion). Scoliosis is evidenced by an abnormal lateral curve in the spine, shoulders that are not level, an asymmetric waistline, and a prominent scapula, accentuated by bending forward. Older adults experience a loss in height due to loss of vertebral cartilage and osteoporosis-related vertebral fractures. Therefore, an adult's height should be measured periodically.

Gait

Gait is assessed by having the patient walk away from the examiner for a short distance. The examiner observes the patient's gait for smoothness and rhythm. Any unsteadiness or irregular movements (frequently noted in elderly patients) are considered abnormal. When a limping motion is noted, it is most frequently caused by painful weight bearing. In such instances, the patient can usually pinpoint the area of discomfort, thus guiding further examination. If one extremity is shorter than another, a limp may also be observed as the patient's pelvis drops downward on the affected side with each step. Limited joint motion may affect gait. In addition, a variety of neurologic conditions are associated with abnormal gaits, such as a spastic hemiparesis gait (stroke), steppage gait (lower motor neuron disease), and shuffling gait (Parkinson's disease).

Bone Integrity

The bony skeleton is assessed for deformities and alignment. Symmetric parts of the body, such as extremities, are compared. Abnormal bony growths due to bone tumors may be observed. Shortened extremities, amputations, and body parts that are not in anatomic alignment are noted. Fracture findings may include abnormal angulation of long bones, motion at points other than joints, and crepitus (a grating sound) at the point of abnormal motion. Movement of fracture fragments must be minimized to avoid additional injury.

Joint Function

The articular system is evaluated by noting range of motion, deformity, stability, and nodular formation. Range of motion is evaluated both actively (the joint is moved by the muscles surrounding the joint) and passively (the joint is moved by the examiner). The examiner is familiar with the normal range of motion of major joints (see Chapter 11).

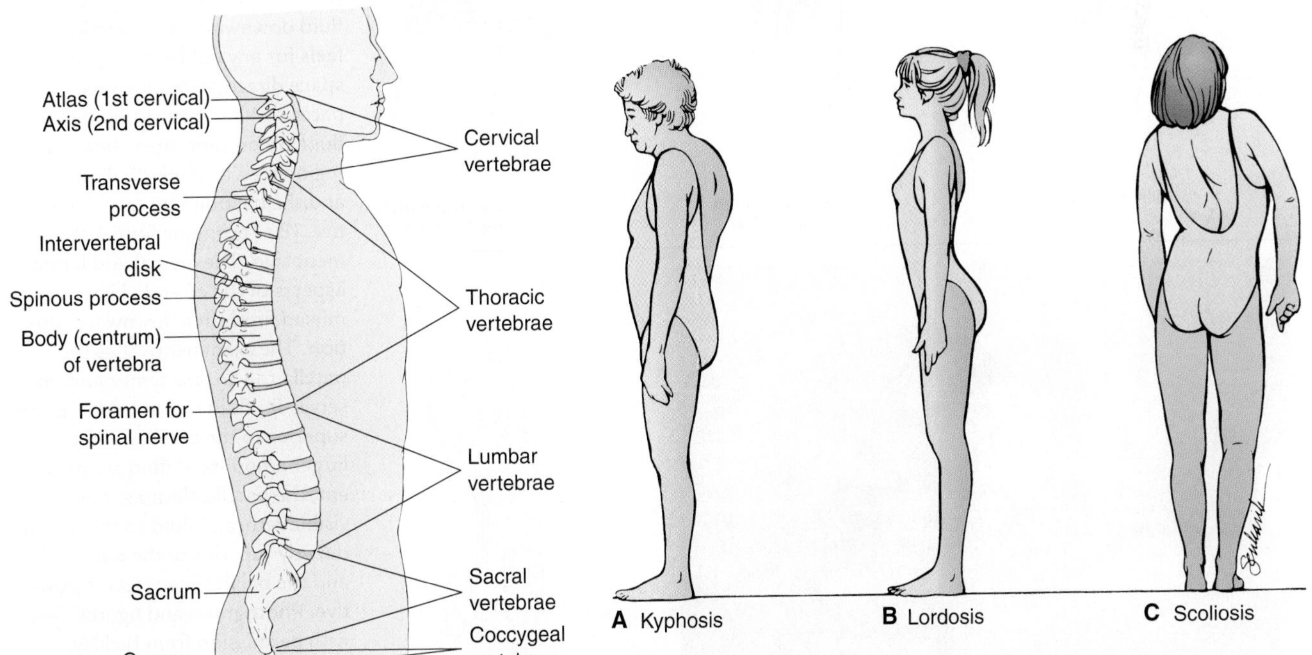

FIGURE 66-3. A normal spine and three abnormalities. (**A**) Kyphosis: an increased convexity or roundness of the spine's thoracic curve. (**B**) Lordosis: swayback; exaggeration of the lumbar spine curve. (**C**) Scoliosis: a lateral curvature of the spine.

Precise measurement of range of motion can be made by a goniometer (a protractor designed for evaluating joint motion). Limited range of motion may be the result of skeletal deformity, joint pathology, or **contracture** (shortening of surrounding joint structures) of the surrounding muscles, tendons, and joint capsule. In elderly patients, limitations of range of motion associated with osteoarthritis may reduce their ability to perform activities of daily living.

If joint motion is compromised or the joint is painful, the joint is examined for **effusion** (excessive fluid within the capsule), swelling, and increased temperature that may reflect active inflammation. An effusion is suspected if the joint is swollen and the normal bony landmarks are obscured. The most common site for joint effusion is the knee. If large amounts of fluid are present in the joint spaces beneath the patella, it may be identified by assessing for the balloon sign and for ballottement of the knee (Fig. 66-4). If inflammation or fluid is suspected in a joint, consultation with a physician is indicated.

Joint deformity may be caused by contracture, dislocation (complete separation of joint surfaces), subluxation (partial separation of articular surfaces), or disruption of structures surrounding the joint. Weakness or disruption of joint-supporting structures may result in a weak joint that requires an external supporting appliance (eg, brace).

Palpation of the joint while it is passively moved provides information about the integrity of the joint. Normally, the joint moves smoothly. A snap or crack may indicate that a ligament is slipping over a bony prominence. Slightly roughened surfaces, as in arthritic conditions, result in **crepitus** (grating, crackling sound or sensation) as the irregular joint surfaces move across one another.

The tissues surrounding joints are examined for nodule formation. Rheumatoid arthritis, gout, and osteoarthritis may produce characteristic nodules. The subcutaneous nodules of rheumatoid arthritis are soft and occur within and along tendons that provide extensor function to the joints. The nodules of gout are hard and lie within and immediately adjacent to the joint capsule itself. They may rupture, exuding white uric acid crystals onto the skin surface. Osteoarthritic nodules are hard and painless and represent bony overgrowth that has resulted from destruction of the cartilaginous surface of bone within the joint capsule. They are frequently seen in older adults.

Often, the size of the joint is exaggerated by atrophy of the muscles proximal and distal to that joint. This is seen in

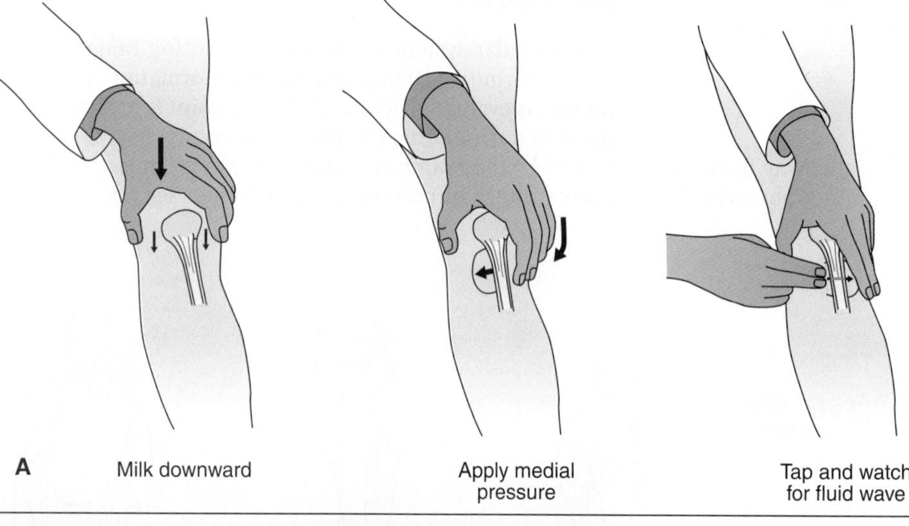

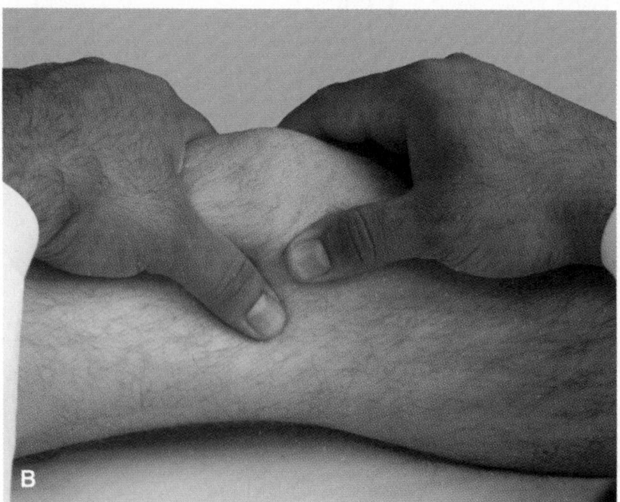

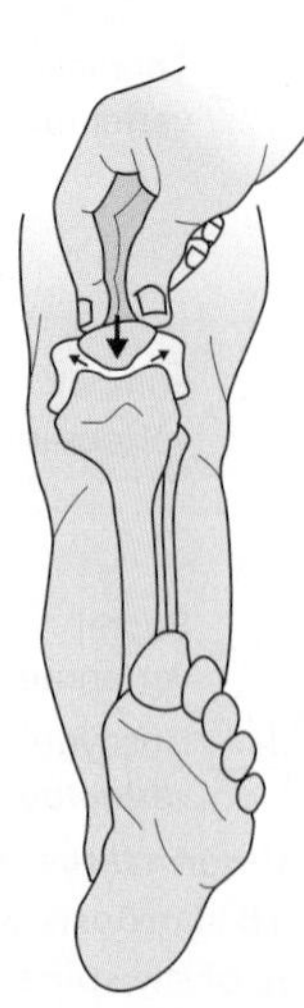

FIGURE 66-4. Tests for detecting fluid in the knee. (**A**) Technique for balloon sign. The medial and lateral aspects of the extended knee are milked firmly in a downward motion, which displaces any fluid downward. The examiner feels for any fluid entering the space directly inferior to the patella. When larger amounts of fluid are present, the subpatellar region feels as if it is "ballooning," and the balloon sign test is positive. (**B**) Technique for ballottement sign. The medial and lateral aspects of the extended knee are milked firmly in a downward motion. The examiner pushes the patella toward the femur and observes for fluid return to the region superior to the patella. When larger amounts of fluid are present, the patella elevates, there is visible return of fluid to the region directly superior to the patella, and the ballottement test is positive. Photograph and figures used with permission from Bickley, L. S., & Szilagyi, P. G. (2003). *Bates' guide to physical examination and history taking* (9th ed.). Philadelphia: Lippincott Williams & Wilkins.

rheumatoid arthritis of the knees, in which the quadriceps muscle may atrophy dramatically. In rheumatoid arthritis, joint involvement assumes a symmetric pattern (Figure 66-5). (See Chapter 54 for further information about rheumatoid arthritis.)

Muscle Strength and Size

The muscular system is assessed by noting muscular strength and coordination, the size of individual muscles, and the patient's ability to change position. Weakness of a group of muscles might indicate a variety of conditions, such as polyneuropathy, electrolyte disturbances (particularly potassium and calcium), myasthenia gravis, poliomyelitis, and muscular dystrophy. By palpating the muscle while passively moving the relaxed extremity, the nurse can determine the muscle tone. The nurse assesses muscle strength by having the patient perform certain maneuvers with and without added resistance. For example, when the biceps are tested, the patient is asked to extend the arm fully and then to flex it against resistance applied by the nurse. A simple handshake may provide an indication of grasp strength.

The nurse may elicit muscle **clonus** (rhythmic contractions of a muscle) in the ankle or wrist by sudden, forceful, sustained dorsiflexion of the foot or extension of the wrist. **Fasciculation** (involuntary twitching of muscle fiber groups) may be observed.

The nurse measures the girth of an extremity to monitor increased size due to exercise, edema, or bleeding into the muscle. Girth may decrease due to muscle atrophy. The unaffected extremity is measured and used as the reference standard for the affected extremity. Measurements are taken at the maximum circumference of the extremity. It is important that the measurements be taken at the same location on the extremity, and with the extremity in the same position, with the muscle at rest. Distance from a specific anatomic landmark (eg, 10 cm below the medial aspect of the knee for measurement of the calf muscle) should be indicated in the patient's record so that subsequent measurements can be made at the same point. For ease of serial assessment, the nurse may indicate the point of measurement by marking the skin. Variations in size greater than 1 cm are considered significant.

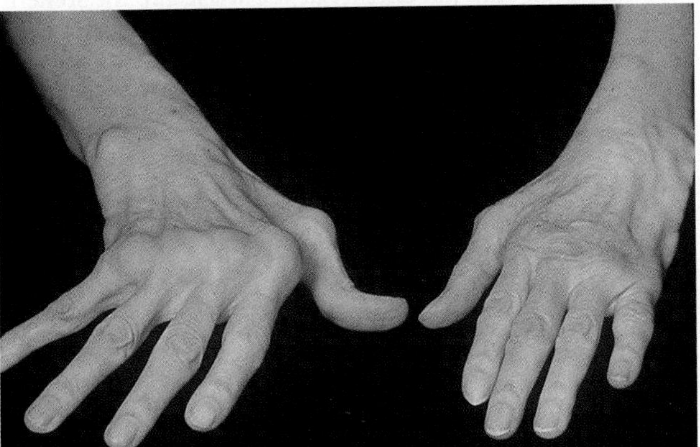

FIGURE 66-5. Rheumatoid arthritis joint deformity with ulnar deviation of fingers and "swan-neck" deformity of fingers (ie, hyperextension of proximal interphalangeal joints with flexion of distal interphalangeal joints).

Skin

In addition to assessing the musculoskeletal system, the nurse inspects the skin for edema, temperature, and color. Palpation of the skin can reveal whether any areas are warmer, suggesting increased perfusion or inflammation, or cooler, suggesting decreased perfusion, and whether edema is present. Cuts, bruises, skin color, and evidence of decreased circulation or inflammation can influence nursing management of musculoskeletal conditions.

Neurovascular Status

It is important for the nurse to perform frequent neurovascular assessments of patients with musculoskeletal disorders (especially of those with fractures) because of the risk for tissue and nerve damage. One complication that the nurse needs to be alert for when assessing the patient is compartment syndrome, which is described in detail later in this unit. This major neurovascular problem is caused by pressure within a muscle compartment that increases to such an extent that microcirculation diminishes, leading to nerve and muscle anoxia and necrosis. Function can be permanently lost if the anoxic situation continues for longer than 6 hours. Assessment of neurovascular status (Chart 66-3) is frequently referred to as assessment of CMS (circulation, motion, and sensation).

The Patient With Musculoskeletal Injury

Special precautions must be taken when assessing a patient who has sustained trauma. If there is injury to an extremity, it is important to assess for soft tissue trauma, deformity, and neurovascular status. If the patient might have a cervical spine injury and is wearing a cervical collar, the collar must not be removed until the absence of spinal cord injury is confirmed by x-ray. When the collar is removed, the cervical spine area is gently assessed for swelling, tenderness, and deformity. With pelvic trauma, abdominal organ injuries may occur. The patient is assessed for abdominal pain, tenderness, hematomas, and the presence or

CHART 66-3

Indicators of Peripheral Neurovascular Dysfunction

Circulation

Color: Pale, cyanotic, or mottled
Temperature: Cool
Capillary refill: More than 3 seconds

Motion

Weakness
Paralysis

Sensation

Paresthesia
Unrelenting pain
Pain on passive stretch
Absence of feeling

absence of femoral pulses. If blood is present at the urinary meatus, the nurse should suspect bladder and urethral injury, and the patient should not be catheterized. Instead, such findings should be reported immediately to the emergency department physician or the surgeon.

Diagnostic Evaluation

Imaging Procedures

Types of Imaging Procedures

X-RAY STUDIES

X-ray studies are important in evaluating patients with musculoskeletal disorders. Bone x-rays determine bone density, texture, erosion, and changes in bone relationships. X-ray study of the cortex of the bone reveals any widening, narrowing, or signs of irregularity. Joint x-rays reveal fluid, irregularity, spur formation, narrowing, and changes in the joint structure. Multiple x-rays are needed for full assessment of the structure being examined. Serial x-rays may be indicated to determine if healing of a fractured bone is progressing normally or to determine if a bone affected by a degenerative disease (eg, osteoarthritis) is responding to prescribed therapy. After being positioned for the study, the patient must remain still while the x-rays are taken.

COMPUTED TOMOGRAPHY

A computed tomography (CT) scan shows in detail a specific plane of involved bone and can reveal tumors of the soft tissue or injuries to the ligaments or tendons. It is used to identify the location and extent of fractures in areas that are difficult to evaluate (eg, acetabulum). CT studies, which may be performed with or without the use of contrast agents, last about 1 hour. The patient must remain still during the procedure.

MAGNETIC RESONANCE IMAGING

Magnetic resonance imaging (MRI) is a noninvasive imaging technique that uses magnetic fields, radiowaves, and computers to demonstrate abnormalities (ie, tumors or narrowing of tissue pathways through bone) of soft tissues such as muscle, tendon, cartilage, nerve, and fat. Because an electromagnet is used, patients with any metal implants, clips, or pacemakers are not candidates for MRI.

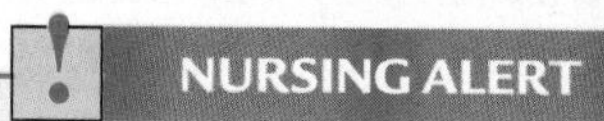

Jewelry, hair clips, hearing aids, credit cards with magnetic strips, and other metal-containing objects must be removed before the MRI is performed; otherwise they can become dangerous projectile objects or cause burns. Credit cards with magnetic strips may be erased, and non-removable cochlear devices can become inoperable. Also, transdermal patches (eg, NicoDerm, Transderm-Nitro, Transderm Scopolamine, Catapres-TTS [clonidine]) that have a thin layer of aluminized backing must be removed before MRI because they can cause burns. The physician should be notified before the patches are removed.

To enhance visualization of anatomic structures, intravenous (IV) contrast agent may be used. During the MRI, the patient needs to lie still for 1 to 2 hours and hears a rhythmic knocking sound. Patients who experience claustrophobia may be unable to tolerate the confinement of closed MRI equipment without sedation. Open MRI systems are available, but they use lower-intensity magnetic fields, which reduces the quality of the imaging; thus, repeated imaging may be required. Advantages of open MRI include increased patient comfort, reduced problems with claustrophobic reactions, and reduced noise.

ARTHROGRAPHY

Arthrography is useful in identifying acute or chronic tears of the joint capsule or supporting ligaments of the knee, shoulder, ankle, hip, or wrist. A radiopaque contrast agent or air is injected into the joint cavity to outline soft tissue structures and the contour of the joint. The joint is put through its range of motion to distribute the contrast agent while a series of x-rays is obtained. If a tear is present, the contrast agent leaks out of the joint and is evident on the x-ray image.

After an arthrogram, a compression elastic bandage is applied as prescribed and the joint is usually rested for 12 hours. The nurse provides additional comfort measures (mild analgesia, ice) as appropriate. The nurse explains to the patient that it is normal to experience clicking or crackling in the joint for a day or two after the procedure, until the contrast agent or air is absorbed.

Nursing Interventions

Before the patient undergoes an imaging study, the nurse assesses for conditions that may require special consideration during the study or that may be contraindications to the study (eg, pregnancy; claustrophobia; inability to tolerate required positioning due to age, debility, or disability; metal implants). If contrast agents will be used for CT scan, MRI, or arthrography, the nurse carefully assesses the patient for possible allergy.

Bone Densitometry

Bone densitometry is used to estimate bone mineral density (BMD). This can be performed through the use of x-rays or ultrasound. Dual-energy x-ray absorptiometry (DEXA) determines bone mineral density at the wrist, hip, or spine to estimate the extent of osteoporosis and to monitor a patient's response to treatment for osteoporosis. Although heel bone sonometry (ultrasound) and peripheral DEXAs are cost-effective, readily available screening tools for osteoporosis, hip BMD testing is considered the most accurate test for osteoporosis and for predicting risk of hip fracture. Therefore, evidence-based guidelines espouse using hip BMD as the first-line test for osteoporosis (Bates, Black, & Cummings, 2002). In particular, hip BMD is recommended as an osteoporosis screening for all Caucasian women older than 65 years and for other people at increased risk for osteoporosis-related fractures (Cummings, Bates, & Black, 2002). (See Chapter 68 for a further discussion of osteoporosis risks.)

Nuclear Studies

Bone Scan

A bone scan is performed to detect metastatic and primary bone tumors, osteomyelitis, certain fractures, and aseptic necrosis. A bone-seeking radioisotope is injected IV. The scan is performed 2 to 3 hours after the injection. At this point, distribution and concentration of the isotope in the bone are measured. The degree of nuclide uptake is related to the metabolism of the bone. An increased uptake of isotope is seen in primary skeletal disease (osteosarcoma), metastatic bone disease, inflammatory skeletal disease (osteomyelitis), and certain types of fractures.

NURSING INTERVENTIONS

Before the patient undergoes a bone scan, the nurse inquires about possible allergy to the radioisotope and assesses for any condition that would contraindicate performing the procedure (eg, pregnancy). In addition, the nurse encourages the patient to drink plenty of fluids to help distribute and eliminate the isotope. Before the scan, the nurse asks the patient to empty the bladder, because a full bladder interferes with accurate scanning of the pelvic bones.

Endoscopic Studies

Arthroscopy

Arthroscopy is a procedure that allows direct visualization of a joint to diagnose joint disorders. Treatment of tears, defects, and disease processes may be performed through the arthroscope. The procedure is performed in the operating room under sterile conditions; injection of a local anesthetic into the joint or general anesthesia is used. A large-bore needle is inserted, and the joint is distended with saline. The arthroscope is introduced, and joint structures, synovium, and articular surfaces are visualized. After the procedure, the puncture wound is closed with adhesive strips or sutures and covered with a sterile dressing. Complications are rare but may include infection, hemarthrosis, neurovascular compromise, thrombophlebitis, stiffness, effusion, adhesions, and delayed wound healing.

NURSING INTERVENTIONS

The joint is wrapped with a compression dressing to control swelling. In addition, ice may be applied to control edema and discomfort. Frequently, the joint is kept extended and elevated to reduce swelling. It is important to monitor neurovascular status. The nurse administers prescribed analgesics to control discomfort. The nurse explains when the patient can resume activity and what weight-bearing limits to follow, as prescribed by the orthopedic surgeon. The nurse also explains to the patient and family the symptoms (eg, swelling, numbness, cool skin) to watch for in order to determine whether complications are occurring and the importance of notifying the physician of these observations. Finally, the nurse explains the physician's prescription for analgesic medication.

Other Studies

Arthrocentesis

Arthrocentesis (joint aspiration) is carried out to obtain synovial fluid for purposes of examination or to relieve pain due to effusion. Examination of synovial fluid is helpful in the diagnosis of septic arthritis and other inflammatory arthropathies and reveals the presence of hemarthrosis (bleeding into the joint cavity), which suggests trauma or a bleeding disorder. Normally, synovial fluid is clear, pale, straw-colored, and scanty in volume. Using aseptic technique, the physician inserts a needle into the joint and aspirates fluid. Anti-inflammatory medications may be injected into the joint. A sterile dressing is applied after aspiration. There is a risk of infection after this procedure.

Electromyography

Electromyography (EMG) provides information about the electrical potential of the muscles and the nerves leading to them. The test is performed to evaluate muscle weakness, pain, and disability. The purpose of the procedure is to determine any abnormality of function and to differentiate muscle and nerve problems. Needle electrodes are inserted into selected muscles, and responses to electrical stimuli are recorded on an oscilloscope. Warm compresses may relieve residual discomfort after the study.

Biopsy

Biopsy may be performed to determine the structure and composition of bone marrow, bone, muscle, or synovium to help diagnose specific diseases. The nurse prepares the patient by providing teaching about the procedure and assuring the patient that analgesic agents will be provided. The nurse monitors the biopsy site for edema, bleeding, pain, and infection. Ice is applied as prescribed to control bleeding and edema. In addition, analgesics are administered as prescribed for comfort.

Laboratory Studies

Examination of the patient's blood and urine can provide information about a primary musculoskeletal problem (eg, Paget's disease), a developing complication (eg, infection), the baseline for instituting therapy (eg, anticoagulant therapy), or the response to therapy. The complete blood count includes the hemoglobin level (which is frequently lower after bleeding associated with trauma and surgery) and the white blood cell count (which is elevated with any inflammatory condition, including acute infections, trauma, acute hemorrhage, and tissue necrosis). Before surgery, coagulation studies are performed to detect bleeding tendencies (because bone is very vascular tissue).

Blood chemistry studies provide data about a wide variety of musculoskeletal conditions. Serum calcium levels are altered in patients with osteomalacia, parathyroid dysfunction, Paget's disease, metastatic bone tumors, or prolonged immobilization. Serum phosphorus levels are inversely related to calcium levels and are diminished in osteomalacia associated with malabsorption syndrome. Acid phosphatase is elevated in Paget's disease and metastatic cancer. Alkaline phosphatase is elevated during early fracture healing and in diseases with increased osteoblastic activity (eg, metastatic bone tumors). Bone metabolism may be evaluated through thyroid studies and determination of calcitonin, parathormone, and vitamin D levels. Serum enzyme levels of creatine kinase and aspartate aminotransferase become elevated with muscle damage. Serum osteocalcin (bone GLA protein) indicates the rate of bone turnover. Urine calcium levels increase with bone destruction (eg, parathyroid dysfunction, metastatic bone tumors, multiple myeloma).

Specific serum biochemical markers can be used to provide information about bone formation; these include bone-specific alkaline phosphatase and osteocalcin from osteoblasts, and procollagen 1 carboxyterminal propeptide and procollagen 1 aminoterminal propeptide from the bone matrix. Specific serum biochemical markers that provide information about bone resorption include tartrate-resistant acid phosphatase and bone sialoprotein from osteoclasts, and aminoterminal telopeptide of type 1 collagen and carboxyterminal telopeptide of type 1 collagen from bone matrix. Biochemical markers of bone resorption in the urine include pyridinoline and deoxypyridinoline cross-links, aminoterminal telopeptide of type 1 collagen, and hydroxyproline from collagen degradation from bone matrix (Koopman & Moreland, 2004).

Nursing Implications

Determining the patient's functional status and health care needs is an integral part of the nursing assessment. Nursing diagnoses and the nursing plan of care are developed and modified according to the patient's needs.

During the period of assessment, the patient requires support and nursing care, including physical and psychological preparation for examinations and tests. Patient education before the tests (what is to be done; why it is being done; what the patient can expect to experience, including tactile, visual, and auditory sensations; and what patient participation is expected) reduces anxiety and enables the patient to be an active participant in care.

The resulting medical diagnosis and prescribed treatment regimen affect the nursing management of the patient. The nursing plan of care includes nursing measures to facilitate the resolution of the patient's health problems and promotion of health. The nursing assessment enables the nurse to identify the health problems that can be improved by nursing interventions. In collaboration with the patient, health goals and nursing strategies are formulated to resolve the identified nursing diagnoses.

Critical Thinking Exercises

1 ebp A 62-year-old Caucasion woman presents to the family practice clinic where you are the nurse manager for her annual wellness examination. She asks you if she should have "a type of bone scan" because her younger sister had recently had a hip fracture. She also tells you that her mother died of pneumonia at age 68 after she fell and broke her hip. What is the evidence base that indicates that this woman may be at increased risk of osteoporosis-related fractures? What other risk factors for osteoporosis might you assess? What recommendations might be made for appropriate testing in this patient?

2 A young man is an inpatient on the orthopedic unit where you work as a staff nurse. He is in traction after surgery to treat a fracture of the femur. What nursing interventions will you plan to implement that might prevent muscle atrophy?

3 ebp You are teaching a class at a senior center on age-associated changes in the musculoskeletal system. The participants have experienced many of the changes you identify and ask you what they can do about them. What is the evidence base that supports the strategies that these elderly citizens might implement to minimize these changes and maximize musculoskeletal health? What is the strength of the evidence of the effectiveness of these strategies? Focus your teaching strategies on prevention of falls and on prevention of osteoporosis.

REFERENCES AND SELECTED READINGS

BOOKS

Bickley, L. S., & Szilagyi, P. G. (2005). *Bates' guide to physical examination and history taking* (9th ed.). Philadelphia: Lippincott Williams & Wilkins.

Buckwalter, J. A., Einhorn, T. A., & Sheldon, R. S. (2000). *Orthopaedic basic science: Biology and biomechanics of the musculoskeletal system* (2nd ed.). Rosemont, IL: American Academy of Orthopaedic Surgeons.

Fischbach, F. T., & Dunning, M. B. (2004). *A manual of laboratory and diagnostic tests* (7th ed.). Philadelphia: Lippincott Williams & Wilkins.

Koopman, W. J., & Moreland, L. W. (2004). *Arthritis and allied conditions* (15th ed.). Philadelphia: Lippincott Williams & Wilkins.

Maher, A., Salmond, S. W., & Pellino, T. A. (2002). *Orthopaedic nursing* (3rd ed.). St. Louis: Elsevier.

Porth, C. M. (2005). *Pathophysiology: Concepts of altered health states* (7th ed.). Philadelphia: Lippincott Williams & Wilkins.

Reider, B. (2005). *The orthopaedic physical examination* (2nd ed.). St. Louis: Elsevier.

Weber, J. W., & Kelley, J. (2003). *Health assessment in nursing* (2nd ed.). Philadelphia: Lippincott Williams & Wilkins.

U.S. Department of Health and Human Services (2004). *Bone health and osteoporosis: A report of the Surgeon General.* U.S. Department of Health and Human Services/Public Health Service, Office of the Surgeon General, Rockville, MD.

JOURNALS

Altizer, L. (2002). Neurovascular assessment. *Orthopaedic Nursing, 21*(4), 48–50.

Bates, D. W., Black, D. M., & Cummings, S. W. (2002). Clinical use of bone densitometry: Clinical applications. *Journal of American Medical Association, 288*(15), 1898–1901.

Centers for Disease Control and Prevention. (2002). Prevalence of self-reported arthritis or chronic joint symptoms among adults. *Morbidity and Mortality Weekly Report, 51*(42), 948–950.

Cummings, S. R., Bates, D., & Black, D. M. (2002). Clinical use of bone densitometry: Scientific review. *Journal of American Medical Association, 288*(15), 1889–1897.

Hofbauer, L. C., & Schoppet, M. (2004). Clinical implications of the osteoprotegerin/RANKL/RANK system for bone and vascular diseases. *Journal of the American Medical Association, 292*(4), 490–495.

National Association of Orthopedic Nurses (NAON). (2005). Palliative care: Improving the quality of care for patients with chronic, incurable musculoskeletal conditions: Consensus document. *Orthopaedic Nursing, 24*(1), 8–11.

Ory, P. A. (2003). Radiography in the assessment of musculoskeletal conditions. *Best Practices and Research in Clinical Rheumatology, 17*(3), 495–512.

Reid, M. C., Williams, C. S., & Gill, T. M. (2003). The relationship between psychological factors and disabling musculoskeletal pain in community-dwelling older persons. *Journal of the American Geriatrics Society, 51*(8), 1092–1098.

Schett, G., Kiechl, S., Redlich, K., et al. (2004). Soluble RANKL and risk of nontraumatic fractures. *Journal of American Medical Association, 291*(9), 1108–1113.

Watters, C. L., Harvey, C. V., Meehan, A. J., et al. (2005). Palliative care: A challenge for orthopaedic nursing care. *Orthopaedic Nursing, 24*(1), 4–7.

RESOURCES

American College of Sports Medicine, 401 W. Michigan Street, Indianapolis, IN 46202-3233; (317) 637-9200; http://www.acsm.org. Accessed August 10, 2006.

National Association of Orthopaedic Nurses (NAON), East Holly Avenue, Box 56, Pitman, NJ 08071-0056; (856) 256-2310; http://www.orthonurse.com. Accessed August 10, 2006.

National Institute of Arthritis and Musculoskeletal and Skin Diseases, Information Clearing House, National Institutes of Health, 1 AMS Circle, Bethesda, MD 20892-3675; 1-877-22-NIAMS (toll free); http://www.niams.nih.gov. Accessed August 10, 2006.

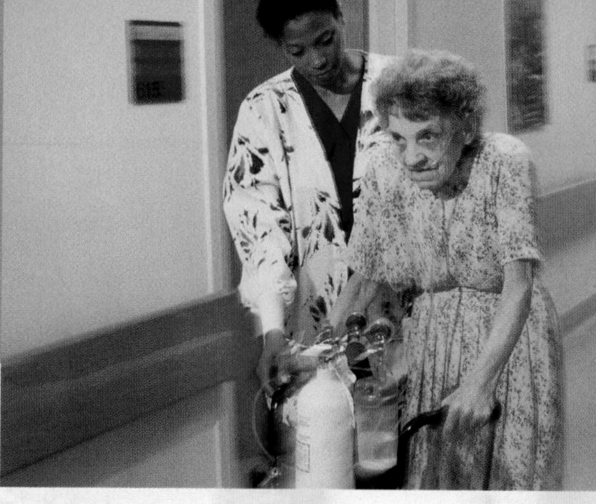

CHAPTER 67

Musculoskeletal Care Modalities

Learning Objectives

On completion of this chapter, the learner will be able to:

1. Describe the preventive and health teaching needs of the patient with a cast.
2. Use the nursing process as a framework for care of the patient with a cast.
3. Describe the various types of traction and the principles of effective traction.
4. Identify the preventive nursing care needs of the patient in traction.
5. Use the nursing process as a framework for care of the patient in traction.
6. Compare the nursing needs of the patient undergoing total hip replacement with those of the patient undergoing total knee replacement.
7. Use the nursing process as a framework for care of the patient undergoing orthopedic surgery.

The management of musculoskeletal injuries and disorders frequently includes the use of casts, traction, artificial joint replacement, surgery, or a combination of these. Patient education is essential for optimal outcomes. The nurse prepares the patient for immobilization with casts or traction, for surgery, and for joint replacement when indicated. Nursing care is planned to maximize the effectiveness of these treatment modalities and to prevent potential complications associated with each of the interventions. The patient is taught to manage his or her care at home and how to safely resume activities.

The Patient in a Cast

A **cast** is a rigid external immobilizing device that is molded to the contours of the body. A cast is used specifically to immobilize a reduced **fracture**, to correct a deformity, to apply uniform pressure to underlying soft tissue, or to support and stabilize weakened joints (Altizer, 2004a). Generally, casts permit mobilization of the patient while restricting movement of a body part.

The condition being treated influences the type and thickness of the cast applied. Generally, the joints proximal and distal to the area to be immobilized are included in the cast. However, with some fractures, cast construction and molding may allow movement of a joint while immobilizing a fracture (eg, three-point fixation in a patellar tendon weight-bearing cast). Various types of casts include the following:

Short-arm cast: Extends from below the elbow to the palmar crease, secured around the base of the thumb. If the thumb is included, it is known as a *thumb spica* or *gauntlet* cast.

Long-arm cast: Extends from the axillary fold to the proximal palmar crease. The elbow usually is immobilized at a right angle.

Short-leg cast: Extends from below the knee to the base of the toes. The foot is flexed at a right angle in a neutral position.

Long-leg cast: Extends from the junction of the upper and middle third of the thigh to the base of the toes. The knee may be slightly flexed.

Walking cast: A short- or long-leg cast reinforced for strength.

Body cast: Encircles the trunk.

Shoulder spica cast: A body jacket that encloses the trunk and the shoulder and elbow.

Hip spica cast: Encloses the trunk and a lower extremity. A double hip spica cast includes both legs.

Figure 67-1 illustrates the long-arm and long-leg casts and areas in which pressure problems commonly occur with these casts.

Many injuries that were previously treated with casts may now be treated with other immobilization devices (eg, immobilizers).

Casting Materials

Nonplaster

Generally referred to as fiberglass casts, these water-activated polyurethane materials have the versatility of plaster (see later discussion) but are lighter in weight, stronger, water resistant, and durable. They consist of an open-weave, nonabsorbent fabric impregnated with cool water-activated hardeners that bond and reach full rigid strength in minutes.

Nonplaster casts are porous and therefore diminish skin problems. They do not soften when wet, which allows for hydrotherapy (use of water for treatment) when appropriate. When wet, they are dried with a hair dryer on a cool setting; thorough drying is important to prevent skin break-

Glossary

abduction: movement away from the center or median line of the body

adduction: movement toward the center or median line of the body

arthrodesis: surgical fusion of a joint

arthroplasty: surgical repair of a joint; joint replacement

avascular necrosis: death of tissue due to insufficient blood supply

brace: externally applied device to support the body or a body part, control movement, and prevent injury

cast: rigid external immobilizing device molded to contours of body part

cast syndrome: psychological (claustrophobic reaction) or physiologic (superior mesenteric artery syndrome) responses to confinement in body cast

continuous passive motion (CPM) device: a device that promotes range of motion, circulation, and healing

edema: soft tissue swelling due to fluid accumulation

external fixator: external metal frame attached to bone fragments to stabilize them

fasciotomy: surgical procedure to release constricting muscle fascia so as to relieve muscle tissue pressure

fracture: a break in the continuity of the bone

heterotopic ossification: misplaced formation of bone

neurovascular status: neurologic (motor and sensory components) and circulatory functioning of a body part

open reduction with internal fixation (ORIF): open surgical procedure to repair and stabilize a fracture

osteomyelitis: infection of the bone

osteotomy: surgical cutting of bone

sling: bandage used to support an arm

splint: device designed specifically to support and immobilize a body part in a desired position

traction: application of a pulling force to a part of the body

trapeze: overhead assistive device to promote patient mobility in bed

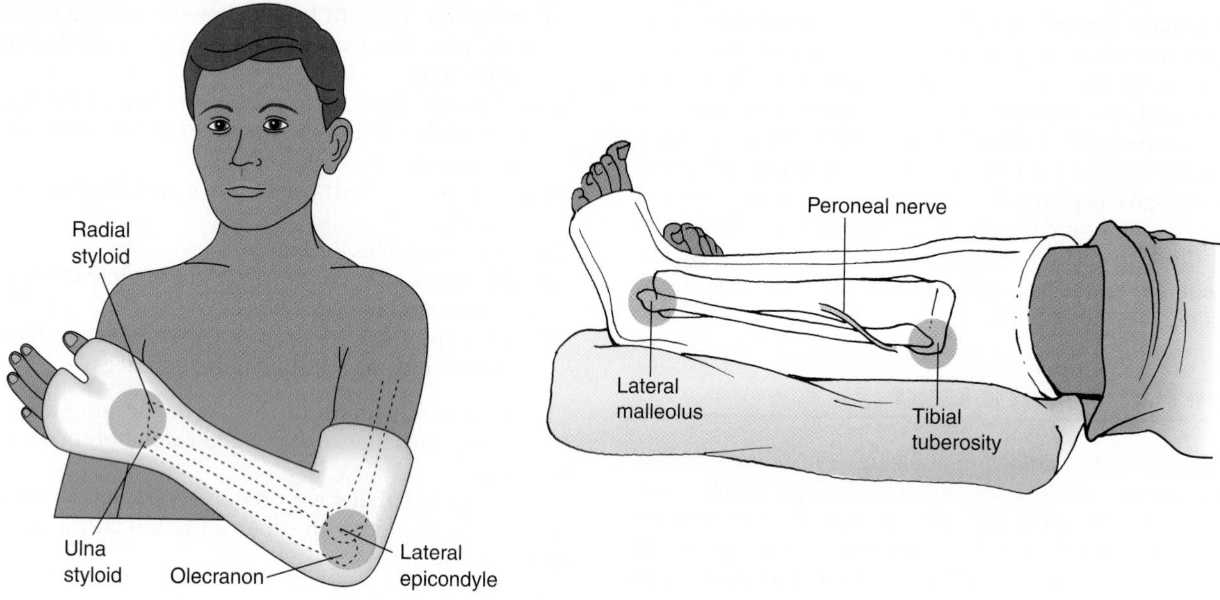

FIGURE 67-1. Pressure areas in common types of casts. *Left,* long-arm cast; *right,* short-leg cast.

down. They are used for nondisplaced fractures with minimal swelling and for long-term wear (Maher, Salmond, & Pellino, 2002).

Plaster

The traditional cast is made of plaster. Rolls of plaster bandage are wet in cool water and applied smoothly to the body. A crystallizing reaction occurs, and heat is given off (an exothermic reaction). The heat given off during this reaction can be uncomfortable, and the nurse should inform the patient about the sensation of increasing warmth so that the patient does not become alarmed. Additionally, the nurse should explain that the cast needs to be exposed to air (ie, uncovered) to allow maximum dissipation of the heat and that most casts cool after about 15 minutes.

The crystallization process produces a rigid dressing. The speed of the reaction varies from a few minutes to 15 to 20 minutes. The orthopedist (orthopedic surgeon) prescribes the plaster setting speed appropriate for the cast being applied by determining the mix and temperature of the cast medium. After the plaster sets, the cast remains wet and somewhat soft. It does not have its full strength until it is dry. While the cast is damp, it can be dented. Therefore, it must be handled with the palms of the hand and not allowed to rest on hard surfaces or sharp edges. Cast dents may press on the skin, causing irritation and skin breakdown. The plaster cast requires 24 to 72 hours to dry completely, depending on its thickness and the environmental drying conditions. A freshly applied cast should be exposed to circulating air to dry and should not be covered with clothing or bed linens or placed on plastic-coated mats or bedding. A wet plaster cast appears dull and gray, sounds dull on percussion, feels damp, and smells musty. A dry plaster cast is white and shiny, resonant to percussion, odorless, and firm (Maher et al., 2002).

Nursing Process

The Patient in a Cast

Assessment

Before the cast is applied, the nurse completes an assessment of the patient's general health, presenting signs and symptoms, emotional status, understanding of the need for the cast, and condition of the body part to be immobilized in the cast. Physical assessment of the part to be immobilized must include assessment of the **neurovascular status** (neurologic and circulatory functioning) of the body part, degree and location of swelling, bruising, and skin abrasions.

Diagnosis

Nursing Diagnoses

Based on the assessment data, major nursing diagnoses for the patient with a cast may include the following:

- Deficient knowledge related to the treatment regimen
- Acute pain related to the musculoskeletal disorder
- Impaired physical mobility related to the cast
- Self-care deficit: bathing/hygiene, feeding, dressing/grooming, or toileting due to restricted mobility
- Impaired skin integrity related to lacerations and abrasions
- Risk for peripheral neurovascular dysfunction related to physiologic responses to injury and compression effect of cast

Collaborative Problems/ Potential Complications

Based on the assessment data, potential complications that may develop include the following:

- Compartment syndrome
- Pressure ulcer
- Disuse syndrome
- Delayed union or nonunion of the fracture(s) (see Chapter 69)

Planning and Goals

The major goals for the patient with a cast include knowledge of the treatment regimen, relief of pain, improved physical mobility, achievement of maximum level of self-care, healing of any trauma-associated lacerations and abrasions, maintenance of adequate neurovascular function, and absence of complications.

Nursing Interventions

Explaining the Treatment Regimen

Prior to cast application, the patient needs information about the underlying pathologic condition and the purpose and expectations of the prescribed treatment regimen. This knowledge promotes the patient's active participation in and adherence to the treatment program. It is important to prepare the patient for the application of the cast by describing the anticipated sights, sounds, and sensations (eg, heat from the hardening reaction of the plaster). The patient needs to know what to expect during application and that the body part will be immobilized after casting (Chart 67-1).

Relieving Pain

The nurse must carefully evaluate pain associated with musculoskeletal conditions, asking the patient to indicate the exact site and to describe the character and intensity of the pain to help determine its cause. Most pain can be relieved by elevating the involved part, applying cold packs as prescribed, and administering analgesics.

NURSING ALERT

A patient's unrelieved pain must be immediately reported to the physician to avoid possible paralysis and necrosis.

Pain associated with the underlying condition (eg, fracture) is frequently controlled by immobilization. Pain due to **edema** that is associated with trauma, surgery, or bleeding into the tissues can frequently be controlled by elevation and, if prescribed, intermittent application of cold packs. Ice bags (one-third to one-half full) or cold application devices are placed on each side of the cast, if prescribed, making sure not to indent the cast.

Pain may be indicative of complications. Pain associated with compartment syndrome (see Chapter 66 and the discussion later in this chapter) is relentless and is not controlled by modalities such as elevation, application of cold if prescribed, and usual dosages of analgesics. Severe pain over a bony prominence warns of an impending pressure ulcer. Pain decreases when ulceration occurs. Discomfort due to pressure on the skin may be relieved by elevation that controls edema or by positioning that alters pressure. It may be necessary to modify the cast or to apply a new cast.

NURSING ALERT

The nurse must never ignore complaints of pain from the patient in a cast because of the possibility of problems, such as impaired tissue perfusion or pressure ulcer formation.

Improving Mobility

Every joint that is not immobilized should be exercised and moved through its range of motion to maintain function. If the patient has a leg cast, the nurse encourages toe exercises. If the patient has an arm cast, the nurse encourages finger exercises.

Promoting Healing of Skin Abrasions

To promote healing, it is important to treat any skin lacerations and abrasions that may have occurred as a result of the trauma that caused the fracture before the cast is applied. The nurse thoroughly cleans the skin and treats it as prescribed. The patient may require a tetanus booster if the wound is dirty and if the last known booster was administered more than 5 years ago. Sterile dressings are used to cover the injured skin. If the skin wounds are extensive, an alternative method (eg, external fixator) may be chosen to immobilize the body part. While the cast is on, the nurse observes the patient for systemic signs of infection, odors from the cast, and purulent drainage staining the cast. It is important to notify the physician if any of these occur.

Maintaining Adequate Neurovascular Function

Edema is a natural response of the tissue to trauma. The patient may complain that the cast is too tight. Vascular insufficiency and nerve compression due to unrelieved swelling can result in compartment syndrome (Fig. 67-2). The nurse monitors circulation, motion, and sensation of the affected extremity, assessing the fingers or toes of the casted extremity and comparing them with those of the opposite extremity. Normal findings include minimal edema, minimal discomfort, pink color, warm to touch, rapid

CHART 67-1 Guidelines for Applying a Cast

Application of a cast involves the following procedures:

NURSING ACTIONS	RATIONALE
1. Support extremity or body part to be casted.	1. Minimizes movement; maintains reduction and alignment; increases comfort.
2. Position and maintain part to be casted in position indicated by physician during casting procedure.	2. Facilitates casting; reduces incidence of complications (eg, malunion, nonunion, contracture).
3. Drape patient.	3. Avoids undue exposure; protects other body parts from contact with casting materials.
4. Wash and dry part to be casted.	4. Reduces incidence of skin breakdown.
5. Place knitted material* (eg, stockinette) over part to be casted.	5. Protects skin from casting materials.
• Apply in smooth and nonconstrictive manner.	Protects skin from pressure.
• Allow additional material.	Folds over edges of cast when finishing application; creates smooth, padded edge; protects skin from abrasion.
6. Wrap soft, nonwoven roll padding* smoothly and evenly around part.	6. Protects skin from pressure of cast.
• Use additional padding around bony prominences to protect superficial nerves (eg, head of fibula, olecranon process).	Protects skin at bony prominences. Protects superficial nerves.
7. Apply plaster or nonplaster casting material evenly on body part.	7. Creates smooth, solid, well-contoured cast.
• Choose appropriate width bandage.	Facilitates smooth application.
• Overlap preceding turn by half the width of the bandage.	Creates smooth, solid, immobilizing cast.
• Use continuous motion, maintaining constant contact with body part.	Shapes cast properly for adequate support.
• Use additional casting material (splints) at joints and at points of anticipated cast stress.	Strengthens cast.
8. "Finish" cast:	8.
• Smooth edges.	Protects skin from abrasion.
• Trim and reshape with cast knife or cutter.	Allows full range of motion of adjacent joints.
9. Remove particles of casting materials from skin.	9. Prevents particles from loosening and sliding underneath cast.
10. Support cast during hardening.	10. Casting materials begin to harden in minutes.
• Handle hardening casts with palms of hands.	Maximum hardness of nonplaster cast occurs in minutes. Maximum hardness of plaster cast occurs with drying (24 to 72 hours, depending on environment and thickness of cast).
• Support cast on firm smooth surface.	
• Do not rest cast on hard surfaces or on sharp edges.	
• Avoid pressure on cast.	Avoids denting of cast and development of pressure areas.
11. Promote drying of cast.	11. Facilitates drying.
• Leave cast uncovered and exposed to air.	
• Turn patient every 2 hours supporting major joints.	
• Fans may be used to increase air flow and speed drying.	

* Nonabsorbent materials are used with nonplaster casts.

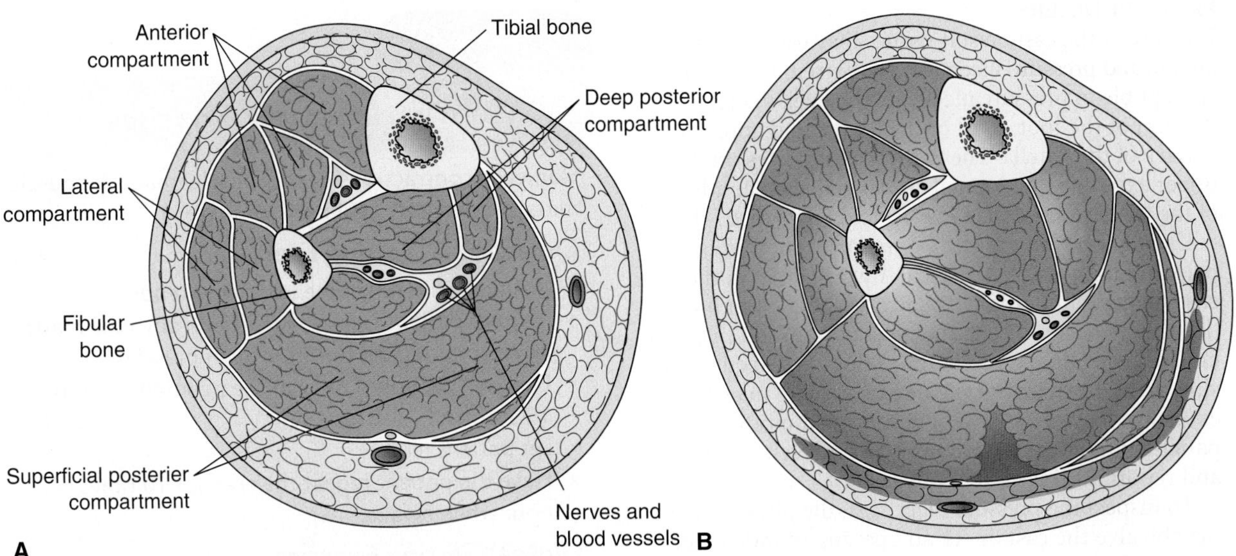

FIGURE 67-2. (**A**) Cross-section of normal lower leg with muscle compartments. (**B**) Cross-section of lower leg with compartment syndrome. Swelling of muscles causes compression of nerves and blood vessels.

capillary refill response, normal sensations, and ability to exercise fingers or toes. The nurse encourages the patient to move fingers or toes hourly when awake to stimulate circulation (Maher et al., 2002).

It is important to perform frequent, regular assessments of neurovascular status. The "five P's" that require assessment are symptoms of neurovascular compromise and compartment syndrome: *p*ain, *p*allor, *p*ulselessness, *p*aresthesia, and *p*aralysis. Early recognition of diminished circulation and nerve function is essential to prevent loss of function. The nurse adjusts the extremity so that it is no higher than heart level to enhance arterial perfusion and control edema and notifies the physician at once if signs of compromised neurovascular status are present.

Monitoring and Managing Potential Complications

Fractures may require weeks and sometimes months to heal. When fracture healing is disrupted, bone union may be delayed or stopped completely. Complications of fracture healing fall into two categories—early and delayed. Early complications include shock, fat embolism syndrome, compartment syndrome, and thromboembolic complications such as deep vein thrombosis (DVT) and pulmonary embolus (PE). Delayed complications include delayed union and nonunion, avascular necrosis, complex regional pain syndrome, and heterotopic ossification (see Chapter 69).

COMPARTMENT SYNDROME

Compartment syndrome occurs when there is increased tissue pressure within a limited space (eg, cast, muscle compartment) that compromises the circulation and the function of the tissue within the confined area. To relieve the pressure, the cast must be bivalved (cut in half longitudinally) while maintaining alignment, and the extremity must be elevated no higher than heart level to ensure arterial perfusion (Chart 67-2). If pressure is not relieved and circulation is not restored, a **fasciotomy** may be necessary to relieve the pressure within the muscle compartment. The nurse closely monitors the patient's response to conservative and surgical management of compartment syndrome. The nurse records neurovascular responses and promptly reports changes to the physician.

CHART 67-2

Procedure for Bivalving a Cast

The following procedure is followed when a cast is bivalved.

1. With a cast cutter, a longitudinal cut is made to divide the cast in half.
2. The underpadding is cut with scissors.
3. The cast is spread apart with cast spreaders to relieve pressure and to inspect and treat the skin without interrupting the reduction and alignment of the bone.
4. After the pressure is relieved, the anterior and posterior parts of the cast are secured together with an elastic compression bandage to maintain immobilization.
5. To control swelling and promote circulation, the extremity is elevated (but no higher than heart level, to minimize the effect of gravity on perfusion of the tissues).

PRESSURE ULCERS

Pressure of the cast on soft tissues may cause tissue anoxia and pressure ulcers. Lower extremity sites most susceptible to pressure ulcers are the heel, malleoli, dorsum of the foot, head of the fibula, and anterior surface of the patella. The main pressure sites on the upper extremity are located at the medial epicondyle of the humerus and the ulnar styloid (see Fig. 67-1).

Usually, the patient with a pressure ulcer reports pain and tightness in the area. A warm area on the cast suggests underlying tissue erythema. Skin breakdown may occur. The drainage may stain the cast and emit an odor. Even if discomfort does not occur with skin breakdown and tissue necrosis, there may still be extensive loss of tissue. The nurse must monitor the patient with a cast for pressure ulcer development and report findings to the physician.

To inspect the pressure ulcer area, the physician may bivalve the cast or cut an opening (window) in the cast. If the physician elects to create a window to inspect the pressure site, a portion of the cast is cut out. The affected area is inspected and possibly treated. The portion of the cast is replaced and held in place by an elastic compression dressing or tape. This prevents the underlying tissue from swelling through the window and creating pressure areas around its margins (Maher et al., 2002).

DISUSE SYNDROME

While in a cast, the patient needs to learn to tense or contract muscles (eg, isometric muscle contraction) without moving the part. This helps reduce muscle atrophy and maintain muscle strength. The nurse teaches the patient with a leg cast to "push down" the knee and teaches the patient in an arm cast to "make a fist." Muscle-setting exercises (eg, quadriceps-setting and gluteal-setting exercises) are important in maintaining muscles essential for walking (Chart 67-3). Isometric exercises should be performed hourly while the patient is awake.

CHART 67-3

Muscle-Setting Exercises

Isometric contractions of the muscle maintain muscle mass and strength and prevent atrophy.

Quadriceps-Setting Exercise

- Position patient supine with leg extended.
- Instruct patient to push knee back onto the mattress by contracting the anterior thigh muscles.
- Encourage patient to hold the position for 5 to 10 seconds.
- Let patient relax.
- Have the patient repeat the exercise 10 times each hour when awake.

Gluteal-Setting Exercise

- Position the patient supine with legs extended, if possible.
- Instruct the patient to contract the muscles of the buttocks.
- Encourage the patient to hold the contraction for 5 to 10 seconds.
- Let the patient relax.
- Have the patient repeat the exercise 10 times each hour when awake.

Promoting Home and Community-Based Care

TEACHING THE PATIENT SELF-CARE

Self-care deficits occur when a portion of the body is immobilized. The nurse encourages the patient to participate actively in personal care and to use assistive devices safely. The nurse must assist the patient in identifying areas of self-care deficit and in developing strategies to achieve independence in activities of daily living (ADLs) (Chart 67-4). The patient's participation in planning and accomplishing ADLs is an important aspect of self-care, independence, maintaining control, and avoiding untoward psychological reactions, such as depression.

When the cast is dry, the nurse instructs the patient as follows:

- Move about as normally as possible, but avoid excessive use of the injured extremity, and avoid walking on wet, slippery floors or sidewalks.
- Perform prescribed exercises regularly, as prescribed.
- Elevate the casted extremity to heart level frequently to prevent swelling.
- Do not attempt to scratch the skin under the cast. This may cause a break in the skin and result in the formation of a skin ulcer. Cool air from a hair dryer may alleviate an itch. Do not insert objects such as coat hangers inside the cast to scratch itching skin. If itching persists, contact your physician.
- Cushion rough edges of the cast with tape.
- Keep the cast dry but do not cover it with plastic or rubber, because this causes condensation, which dampens the cast and skin. Moisture softens a plaster cast. (A wet fiberglass cast must be dried thoroughly with a hair dryer on a cool setting to avoid skin burns.)
- Report any of the following to the physician: persistent pain, swelling that does not respond to elevation, changes in sensation, decreased ability to move exposed fingers or toes, and changes in skin color and temperature.
- Note odors around the cast, stained areas, warm spots, and pressure areas. Report them to the physician.
- Report a broken cast to the physician; do not attempt to fix it yourself.

CONTINUING CARE

The nurse prepares the patient for cast removal or cast changes by explaining what to expect (Chart 67-5). The

CHART 67-4

HOME CARE CHECKLIST • The Patient With a Cast

At the completion of the home care instruction, the patient or caregiver will be able to:	Patient	Caregiver
• Describe techniques to promote cast drying (eg, do not cover, leave exposed to circulating air; handle damp plaster cast with palms of hands and do not rest the cast on hard surfaces or sharp edges that can dent soft cast)	✔	✔
• Describe approaches to controlling swelling and pain (eg, elevate casted extremity to heart level, apply intermittent ice bag if prescribed, take analgesics as prescribed)	✔	✔
• Report pain uncontrolled by elevating the casted limb and by analgesics (may be an indicator of impaired tissue perfusion—compartment syndrome or pressure ulcer)	✔	
• Demonstrate ability to transfer (eg, from a bed to a chair)	✔	
• Use mobility aids safely	✔	
• Avoid excessive use of injured extremity; observe prescribed weight-bearing limits	✔	
• Manage minor irritations from cast (eg, for skin irritation from cast edge, pad rough edges with tape; to relieve itching, blow cool air from hair drier)	✔	✔
• Demonstrate exercises to promote circulation and minimize disuse syndrome	✔	
• State indicators of complications to report promptly to physician (eg, uncontrolled swelling and pain; cool, pale fingers or toes; paresthesia; paralysis; purulent drainage staining casts; signs of systemic infection; cast breaks)	✔	✔
• Describe care of extremity following cast removal (eg, skin care; gradual resumption of normal activities to protect limb from undue stresses; management of swelling)	✔	✔

CHART 67-5

Guidelines for Removing a Cast

The following procedure is followed when a cast is removed:

NURSING ACTIONS	RATIONALE
1. Inform the patient about the procedure.	1. Facilitates cooperation and reduces fear about the procedure.
2. Reassure patient that the electric saw or cast cutter will not cut skin. (Explain that blade oscillates to cut cast and vibrations will be felt.)	2. Reduces anxiety.
3. Wear eye protection (patient and operator of the cast cutter).	3. Protects eyes from flying cast particles.
4. Bivalve cast using a series of alternating pressures and linear movements of blade along the line to be cut.	4. Cuts cast in halves. Avoids burning sensation from prolonged contact of oscillating blade with padding.
5. Cut padding with scissors.	5. Releases all of the casting materials.
6. Support body part as it is removed from the cast.	6. Reduces stresses on body part that has been immobilized.
7. Gently wash and dry area that has been immobilized.* Apply emollient lotion.	7. Removes dead skin that has accumulated during immobilization. Keeps skin supple.
8. Teach patient to avoid rubbing and scratching skin.	8. Prevents skin breakdown.
9. Collaborate with physical therapist to teach patient to resume active use of body part gradually within the guidelines of prescribed therapeutic regimen.	9. Protects weakened part from excessive stress. Progressive exercises reduce stiffness, restore muscle strength and function.
10. Teach patient to control swelling by elevating the extremity or using elastic bandage if prescribed.	10. Facilitates circulation (ie, venous return) and controls fluid pooling.

* If a new cast is to be applied, follow guidelines for application of a cast and associated nursing care.

cast is cut with a cast cutter, which vibrates. The patient can feel the vibration and pressure during its use. The cutter does not penetrate deeply enough to hurt the patient's skin. The cast padding is cut with scissors.

The formerly casted body part is weak from disuse, is stiff, and may appear atrophied. There may be extreme stiffness even after only a few weeks of immobilization. Therefore, support is needed when the cast is removed. The skin, which is usually dry and scaly from accumulated dead skin, is vulnerable to injury from scratching. The skin needs to be washed gently and lubricated with an emollient lotion.

The nurse and physical therapist teach the patient to resume activities gradually within the prescribed therapeutic regimen. Exercises prescribed to help the patient regain joint motion are explained and demonstrated. Because the muscles are weak from disuse, the body part that has been casted cannot withstand normal stresses immediately. In addition, the nurse teaches the patient with noticeable swelling of the affected extremity after cast removal to continue to elevate the extremity to control swelling until normal muscle tone and use are reestablished.

Evaluation

Expected Patient Outcomes

Expected patient outcomes may include:

1. Understands the therapeutic regimen
   a. Elevates affected extremity
   b. Exercises according to instructions
   c. Keeps cast dry
   d. Reports any complications that develop
   e. Keeps follow-up clinic or physician appointments
2. Reports less pain
   a. Elevates extremity that is in the cast
   b. Repositions self
   c. Uses prescribed oral analgesic as needed
3. Demonstrates increased mobility
   a. Uses assistive devices safely
   b. Exercises to increase strength
   c. Changes position frequently
   d. Performs range-of-motion exercises of joints not in the cast
4. Exhibits healing of abrasions and lacerations
   a. Demonstrates no local signs of infection (ie, local discomfort, purulent drainage, cast staining, or odor from cast)
   b. Demonstrates no systemic signs or symptoms of infection
   c. Exhibits intact skin when cast is removed
5. Maintains adequate neurovascular function of affected extremity
   a. Exhibits normal skin color and temperature
   b. Experiences minimal swelling
   c. Exhibits satisfactory capillary refill on testing
   d. Demonstrates active movement of fingers or toes if they are not casted
   e. Reports normal sensations in casted body part
   f. Reports that pain is controllable
6. Exhibits absence of complications
   a. Demonstrates normal neurovascular status of casted extremity
   b. Develops no pressure ulcers
   c. Exhibits minimal muscle wasting
7. Participates in self-care activities
   a. Performs hygiene and grooming activities independently or with minimal assistance
   b. Performs ADLs independently or with minimal assistance
   c. Complies with prescribed exercise regimen

Care of the Patient With an Arm Cast

The patient whose arm is immobilized in a cast must readjust to many routine tasks. The unaffected arm must assume all the upper extremity activities. The nurse, in consultation with an occupational therapist, suggests devices designed to aid one-handed activities. The patient may experience fatigue due to modified activities and the weight of the cast. Frequent rest periods are necessary.

To control swelling, the immobilized arm is elevated. When the patient is lying down, the arm is elevated so that each joint is positioned higher than the preceding proximal joint (eg, elbow higher than the shoulder, hand higher than the elbow).

A **sling** may be used when the patient ambulates. To prevent pressure on the cervical spinal nerves, the sling should distribute the supported weight over a large area and not on the back of the neck. The nurse encourages the patient to remove the arm from the sling and elevate it frequently.

Circulatory disturbances in the hand may become apparent with signs of cyanosis, swelling, and an inability to move the fingers. One serious effect of impaired circulation in the arm is Volkmann's contracture, a specific type of compartment syndrome. Contracture of the fingers and wrist occurs as the result of obstructed arterial blood flow to the forearm and hand. The patient is unable to extend the fingers, describes abnormal sensation (eg, unrelenting pain, pain on passive stretch), and exhibits signs of diminished circulation to the hand. Permanent damage develops within a few hours if action is not taken (see Chart 69-4).

This serious complication can be prevented with nursing surveillance and proper care. Neurovascular checks must be done frequently (see Chapter 66). Compartment syndrome is managed in part by bivalving (cutting) the cast to release the constricting cast and dressings. A fasciotomy may be necessary to improve vascular status.

Care of the Patient With a Leg Cast

The application of a leg cast imposes a degree of immobility on the patient. The cast may be a short-leg cast, extending to the knee, or a long-leg cast, extending to the groin. The fresh cast must be handled in a manner that will not cause denting or disruption of the cast.

The patient's leg must be supported on pillows to heart level to control swelling, and ice packs should be applied as prescribed over the fracture site for 1 or 2 days. The patient is taught to elevate the casted leg when seated. The patient should also assume a recumbent position several times a day with the casted leg elevated to promote venous return and control swelling.

The nurse assesses circulation by observing the color, temperature, and capillary refill of the exposed toes. Nerve function is assessed by observing the patient's ability to move the toes and by asking about the sensations in the foot. Numbness, tingling, and burning may be caused by peroneal nerve injury from pressure at the head of the fibula.

NURSING ALERT

Injury to the peroneal nerve as a result of pressure is a cause of footdrop (the inability to maintain the foot in a normally flexed position). Consequently, the patient drags the foot when ambulating.

When the cast is hard and dry, the nurse and physical therapist teach the patient how to transfer and ambulate safely with assistive devices (eg, crutches, walker). The gait to be used depends on whether the patient is permitted to bear weight. If weight-bearing is allowed, the cast is reinforced to withstand the body weight. A cast boot, worn over the casted foot, provides a broad, nonskid walking surface.

Care of the Patient With a Body or Spica Cast

Casts that encase the trunk (body cast) and portions of one or two extremities (spica cast) require special nursing strategies. Body casts are used to immobilize the spine. Hip spica casts are used for some femoral fractures and after some hip joint surgeries, and shoulder spica casts are used for some humeral neck fractures.

Nursing responsibilities include preparing and positioning the patient, assisting with skin care and hygiene, and monitoring for **cast syndrome**, which occurs as a result of psychological and physiologic responses to confinement to a cast (Maher et al., 2002). Explaining the procedure helps reduce the patient's apprehension about being encased in a large cast. The nurse reassures the patient that several people will provide care during the application, that support for the injured area will be adequate, and that care providers will be as gentle as possible. Medications for pain relief and relaxation administered before the procedure enable the patient to cooperate during application of the cast.

Cracking or denting of the cast is prevented by supporting the patient on a firm mattress and with flexible, waterproof pillows until the cast dries. The nurse positions the pillows next to each other, because spaces between pillows allow the damp cast to sag, become weak, and possibly break. A pillow is not placed under the head and shoulders of a patient in a body cast while the cast is drying, because doing so causes pressure on the chest.

The nurse turns the patient as a unit toward the uninjured side every 2 hours to relieve pressure and to allow the cast to dry. It is important to avoid twisting the patient's body within the cast. Sufficient personnel (at least three people) are needed when the patient is turned so that the fresh cast can be adequately supported with the palms of the hands at vulnerable points (ie, body joints) to prevent cracking. The nurse encourages the patient to assist in the repositioning, if not contraindicated, by use of the **trapeze** or bed rail. A stabilizing abduction bar incorporated into a spica cast should never be used as a turning device. The nurse adjusts the pillows to provide support without creating areas of pressure.

The nurse turns the patient to a prone position, twice daily if tolerated, to provide postural drainage of the bronchial tree and to relieve pressure on the back. A small pillow under the abdomen enhances comfort. The nurse can either place a pillow lengthwise under the dorsa of the feet or allow the toes to hang over the edge of the bed to prevent the toes from being forced into the mattress.

The nurse inspects the skin around the edges of the cast frequently for signs of irritation. The nurse can inspect some of the skin under the cast by pulling the skin taut and using a flashlight. The skin can be bathed and massaged by reaching under the cast edges with the fingers.

The perineal opening must be large enough for hygienic care. To protect the cast from soiling, the nurse can insert clean dry plastic sheeting under the dry cast and over the cast edge before elimination by the patient. Usually, fracture bedpans are easier to use than regular bedpans for patients with a hip spica cast.

Patients immobilized in large casts may develop cast syndrome that may include psychological or physiologic manifestations. The psychological component is similar to a claustrophobic reaction. The patient exhibits an acute anxiety reaction characterized by behavioral changes and autonomic responses (eg, increased respiratory rate, diaphoresis, dilated pupils, increased heart rate, elevated blood pressure). The nurse needs to recognize the anxiety reaction and provide an environment in which the patient feels secure.

The physiologic cast syndrome responses (superior mesenteric artery syndrome) are associated with immobility in a body cast. With decreased physical activity, gastrointestinal motility decreases, intestinal gases accumulate, intestinal pressure increases, and ileus may occur. The patient exhibits abdominal distention, abdominal discomfort, nausea, and vomiting. As with other instances of adynamic ileus, the patient is treated conservatively with decompression (nasogastric intubation connected to suction) and intravenous (IV) fluid therapy until gastrointestinal motility is restored. If the cast restricts the abdomen, the abdominal window must be enlarged. After the ileus resolves and bowel sounds resume, the patient gradually resumes an oral diet. Rarely, the distention places traction on the superior mesenteric artery, reducing the blood supply to the bowel. The bowel may become gangrenous, which requires surgical intervention. The nurse monitors the patient in a large body cast for potential cast syndrome, noting bowel sounds every 4 to 8 hours, and reports distention, nausea, and vomiting to the physician.

The patient with a body or spica cast is often cared for in the home. The nurse teaches family members how to care for the patient, which includes providing hygienic and skin care, ensuring proper positioning, preventing complications, and recognizing symptoms that should be reported to the health care provider.

The Patient with Splints or Braces

Contoured **splints** of plaster or pliable thermoplastic materials may be used for conditions that do not require rigid immobilization, for those in which swelling may be anticipated, and for those that require special skin care. The splint needs to immobilize and support the body part in a functional position. The splint must be well padded to prevent pressure, skin abrasion, and skin breakdown. The splint is overwrapped with an elastic bandage applied in a spiral fashion and with pressure uniformly distributed so that circulation is not restricted. The nurse frequently assesses the neurovascular status and skin integrity of the splinted extremity.

Soft immobilizers may be used to support an injured body part. Usually, the extremity is wrapped with an elastic bandage and then secured in a padded, contoured, canvas immobilizer. Rigid immobilization is not achieved. The nurse provides skin care and makes adjustments for swelling.

For long-term use, **braces** (orthoses) are used to provide support, control movement, and prevent additional injury. They are custom fitted to various parts of the body. Braces may be constructed of plastic materials, canvas, leather, or metal. The orthotist adjusts the brace for fit, positioning, and motion so that movement is enhanced, any deformities are corrected, and discomfort is minimized.

The nurse helps the patient learn to apply the brace and to protect the skin from irritation and breakdown. The nurse also assesses neurovascular integrity and comfort when the patient is wearing the brace, encourages the patient to wear the brace as prescribed, and reassures the patient that minor adjustments of the brace by the orthotist will increase comfort and minimize problems associated with its long-term use.

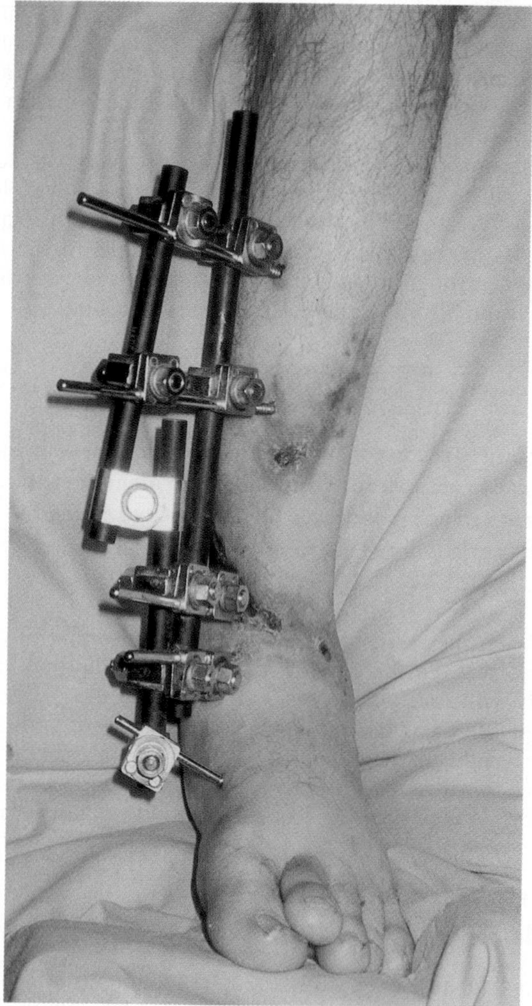

FIGURE 67-3. External fixation device. Pins are inserted into bone. The fracture is reduced and aligned and then stabilized by attaching the pins to a rigid portable frame. The device facilitates treatment of soft tissue damaged in complex fractures.

The Patient with an External Fixator

External fixators are used to manage open fractures with soft tissue damage. They provide stable support for severe comminuted (crushed or splintered) fractures while permitting active treatment of damaged soft tissues (Fig. 67-3). Complicated fractures of the humerus, forearm, femur, tibia, and pelvis are managed with external skeletal fixators. The fracture is reduced, aligned, and immobilized by a series of pins inserted in the bone. Pin position is maintained through attachment to a portable frame. The fixator facilitates patient comfort, early mobility, and active exercise of adjacent uninvolved joints; thus, complications due to disuse and immobility are minimized.

Nursing Interventions

It is important to prepare the patient psychologically for application of the external fixator. The apparatus looks clumsy and foreign. Reassurance that the discomfort associated with the device is minimal and that early mobility is anticipated promotes acceptance of the device.

After the external fixator is applied, the extremity is elevated to reduce swelling. If there are sharp points on the fixator or pins, they are covered with cork or tape to prevent device-induced injuries. The nurse monitors the neurovascular status of the extremity every 2 to 4 hours and assesses each pin site for redness, drainage, tenderness, pain, and loosening of the pin. Some serous drainage from the pin sites is to be expected. The nurse must be alert for potential problems caused by pressure from the device on the skin, nerves, or blood vessels and for the development of compartment syndrome (see Chapter 69). The nurse carries out pin care as prescribed to prevent pin tract infection. This typically includes cleaning each pin site separately one or two times a day with cotton-tipped applicators soaked in chlorhexidine solution. If signs of infection are present or if the pins or clamps seem loose, the nurse notifies the physician.

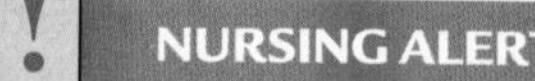

NURSING ALERT

The nurse never adjusts the clamps on the external fixator frame. It is the physician's responsibility to do so.

The nurse encourages isometric and active exercises as tolerated. When the swelling subsides, the nurse helps the patient become mobile within the prescribed weight-bearing limits (non–weight-bearing to full weight-bearing). Adherence to weight-bearing instructions minimizes the chance of loosening of the pins when stress is applied to the bone–pin interface. The fixator is removed after the soft tissue heals. The fracture may require additional stabilization by a cast or molded orthosis while healing.

The Ilizarov external fixator is a special device used to correct angulation and rotational defects, to treat nonunion (failure of bone fragments to heal), and to lengthen limbs. Tension wires are attached to fixator rings, which are joined by telescoping rods. Bone formation is stimulated by prescribed daily adjustment of the telescoping rods. It is important to teach the patient how to adjust the telescoping rods and how to perform skin care. Generally, the nurse can encourage weight-bearing. After the desired correction has been achieved, no additional adjustments are made, and the fixator is left in place until the bone heals.

Promoting Home and Community-Based Care

TEACHING THE PATIENT SELF-CARE

The nurse teaches the patient to perform pin site care according to the prescribed protocol (clean technique can be used at home [Holmes & Brown, 2005]) and to report promptly any signs of pin site infection: redness, tenderness, increased or purulent pin site drainage, or fever. The nurse also instructs the patient and family to monitor neurovascular status and report any changes promptly. The nurse teaches the patient or family member to check the integrity of the fixator frame daily and to report loose pins or clamps. A physical therapy referral is helpful in teaching the patient how to transfer, use ambulatory aids safely, and adjust to weight-bearing limits and altered gait patterns (Chart 67-6).

The Patient in Traction

Traction is the application of a pulling force to a part of the body. Traction is used to minimize muscle spasms; to reduce, align, and immobilize fractures; to reduce deformity; and to increase space between opposing surfaces. Traction must be applied in the correct direction and magnitude to obtain its therapeutic effects. As muscle and soft tissues relax, the amount of weight used may be changed to obtain the desired effect (Maher et al., 2002).

At times, traction needs to be applied in more than one direction to achieve the desired line of pull. When this is done, one of the lines of pull counteracts the other. These lines of pull are known as the vectors of force. The actual resultant pulling force is somewhere between the two lines of pull (Fig. 67-4). The effects of traction are evaluated with x-ray studies, and adjustments are made if necessary.

Traction is used primarily as a short-term intervention until other modalities, such as external or internal fixation, are possible. This reduces the risk of disuse syndrome and minimizes the length of hospitalization, often allowing the patient to be cared for in the home setting (Maher et al., 2002).

Principles of Effective Traction

Whenever traction is applied, countertraction must be used to achieve effective traction. Countertraction is the force acting in the opposite direction. Usually, the patient's body

CHART 67-6

HOME CARE CHECKLIST • The Patient With an External Fixator

At the completion of the home care instruction, the patient or caregiver will be able to:	Patient	Caregiver
• Demonstrate prescribed pin site care	✔	✔
• State signs of pin site infection (eg, redness, tenderness, increased or purulent pin site drainage) to be reported promptly	✔	✔
• Describe approaches to controlling swelling and pain (eg, elevate extremity to heart level, take analgesics as prescribed)	✔	✔
• Report pain uncontrolled by elevation and analgesics (may be an indicator of impaired tissue perfusion, compartment syndrome, or pin tract infection)	✔	
• Demonstrate ability to transfer	✔	
• Use mobility aids safely	✔	
• Avoid excessive use of injured extremity; observe prescribed weight-bearing limits	✔	
• State indicators of complications to report promptly to physician (eg, uncontrolled swelling and pain; cool, pale fingers or toes; paresthesia; paralysis; purulent drainage; signs of systemic infection; loose fixator pins or clamps)	✔	✔
• Describe care of extremity after fixator removal (eg, gradual resumption of normal activities to protect limb from undue stresses)	✔	✔

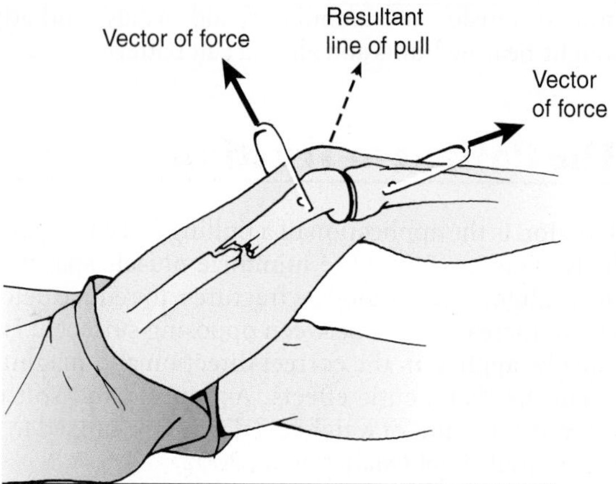

FIGURE 67-4. Traction may be applied in different directions to achieve the desired therapeutic line of pull. Adjustments in applied forces may be prescribed over the course of treatment.

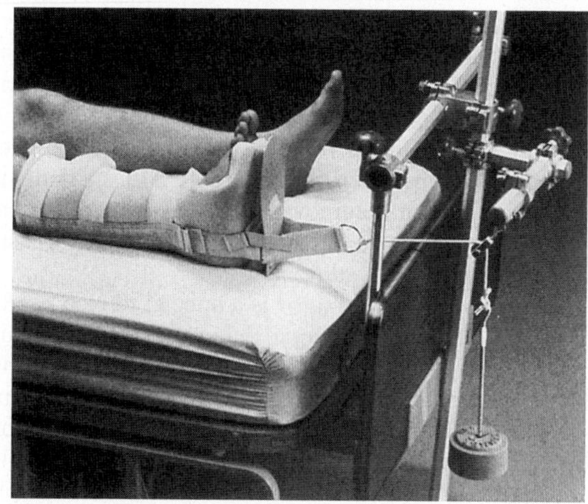

FIGURE 67-5. Buck's extension traction. Lower extremity in unilateral Buck's extension traction is aligned in a foam boot and traction applied by the free-hanging weight.

weight and bed position adjustments supply the needed countertraction.

> **NURSING ALERT**
>
> **Countertraction must be maintained for effective traction.**

The following are additional principles to follow when caring for the patient in traction:

- Traction must be continuous to be effective in reducing and immobilizing fractures.
- Skeletal traction is *never* interrupted.
- Weights are not removed unless intermittent traction is prescribed.
- Any factor that might reduce the effective pull or alter its resultant line of pull must be eliminated:
  - The patient must be in good body alignment in the center of the bed when traction is applied.
  - Ropes must be unobstructed.
  - Weights must hang freely and not rest on the bed or floor.
  - Knots in the rope or the footplate must not touch the pulley or the foot of the bed.

There are several types of traction. *Straight* or *running traction* applies the pulling force in a straight line with the body part resting on the bed. Buck's extension traction (Fig. 67-5) is an example of straight traction. *Balanced suspension traction* (Fig. 67-6) supports the affected extremity off the bed and allows for some patient movement without disruption of the line of pull.

Traction may be applied to the skin (*skin traction*) or directly to the bony skeleton (*skeletal traction*). The mode of application is determined by the purpose of the traction. Traction can be applied with the hands (*manual traction*). This is temporary traction that may be used when applying a cast, giving skin care under a Buck's extension foam boot, or adjusting the traction apparatus.

Skin Traction

Skin traction is used to control muscle spasms and to immobilize an area before surgery. Skin traction is accomplished by using a weight to pull on traction tape or on a foam boot attached to the skin. The amount of weight applied must not exceed the tolerance of the skin. No more than 2 to 3.5 kg (4.5 to 8 lb) of traction can be used on an extremity. Pelvic traction is usually 4.5 to 9 kg (10 to 20 lb), depending on the weight of the patient.

Types of skin traction used for adults include Buck's extension traction (applied to the lower leg), the cervical head halter (occasionally used to treat neck pain), and the pelvic belt (sometimes used to treat back pain).

Buck's Extension Traction

Buck's extension traction (unilateral or bilateral) is skin traction to the lower leg. The pull is exerted in one plane when partial or temporary immobilization is desired (see Fig. 67-5). It is used to immobilize fractures of the proximal femur before surgical fixation.

Before the traction is applied, the nurse inspects the skin for abrasions and circulatory disturbances. The skin and circulation must be in healthy condition to tolerate the traction. The extremity should be clean and dry before the foam boot or traction tape is applied.

To apply Buck's traction, one nurse elevates and supports the extremity under the patient's heel and knee while another nurse places the foam boot under the leg, with the patient's heel in the heel of the boot. Next, the nurse secures Velcro straps around the leg. Traction tape overwrapped with elastic bandage in a spiral fashion may be used instead of the boot. Excessive pressure is avoided over the malleolus and proximal fibula during application to prevent pressure ulcers and nerve damage. The nurse then passes the rope affixed to the spreader or footplate over a pulley fastened to the end

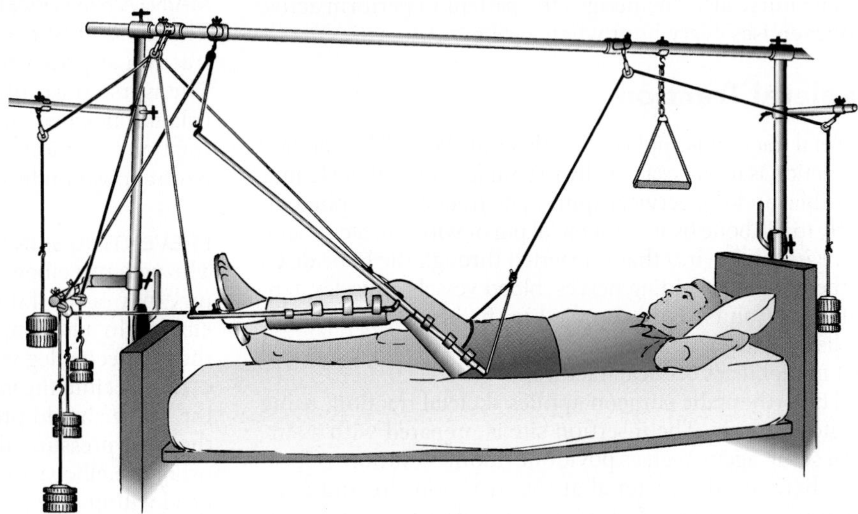

FIGURE 67-6. Balanced suspension skeletal traction with Thomas leg splint. The patient can move vertically as long as the resultant line of pull is maintained.

of the bed and attaches the weight—usually 5 to 8 pounds—to the rope.

Potential Complications

Skin breakdown, nerve pressure, and circulatory impairment are complications that may develop as a result of skin traction. Skin breakdown results from irritation caused by contact of the skin with the tape or foam and shearing forces. Older adults are at greater risk for this complication because of their sensitive, fragile skin.

Nerve damage can result from pressure on the peripheral nerves. Footdrop may occur if pressure is applied to the peroneal nerve at the point at which it passes around the neck of the fibula just below the knee.

Circulatory impairment is manifested by cold skin temperature, decreased peripheral pulses, slow capillary refill time, and bluish skin. DVT, a serious circulatory impairment, may be manifested by unilateral calf tenderness, warmth, redness, and swelling (see Chapter 31).

Nursing Interventions

ENSURING EFFECTIVE TRACTION

To ensure effective skin traction, it is important to avoid wrinkling and slipping of the traction bandage and to maintain countertraction. Proper positioning must be maintained to keep the leg in a neutral position. To prevent bony fragments from moving against one another, the patient should not turn from side to side; however, the patient may shift position slightly with assistance.

MONITORING AND MANAGING POTENTIAL COMPLICATIONS

Skin Breakdown

During the initial assessment, the nurse identifies sensitive, fragile skin (common in older adults). The nurse also closely monitors the status of the skin in contact with tape or foam to ensure that shearing forces are avoided. The nurse performs the following procedures to monitor and prevent skin breakdown:

- removes the foam boots to inspect the skin, the ankle, and the Achilles tendon three times a day. A second nurse is needed to support the extremity during the inspection and skin care.
- palpates the area of the traction tapes daily to detect underlying tenderness.
- provides back care at least every 2 hours to prevent pressure ulcers. The patient who must remain in a supine position is at increased risk for development of a pressure ulcer.
- uses special mattress overlays (eg, air-filled, high-density foam) to prevent pressure ulcers.

Nerve Damage

Skin traction can place pressure on peripheral nerves. When traction is applied to the lower extremity, care must be taken to avoid pressure on the peroneal nerve at the point at which it passes around the neck of the fibula just below the knee. Pressure at this point can cause footdrop. The nurse questions the patient about sensation and asks the patient to move the toes and foot. Dorsiflexion of the foot demonstrates function of the peroneal nerve. Weakness of dorsiflexion or foot movement and inversion of the foot might indicate pressure on the common peroneal nerve. Plantar flexion demonstrates function of the tibial nerve.

The following are important points to keep in mind when caring for the patient in traction:

- Regularly assess sensation and motion.
- Immediately investigate any complaint of a burning sensation under the traction bandage or boot.
- Promptly report altered sensation or impaired motor function.

Circulatory Impairment

After skin traction is applied, the nurse assesses circulation of the foot or hand within 15 to 30 minutes and then every 1 to 2 hours. Circulatory assessment consists of the following:

- Peripheral pulses, color, capillary refill, and temperature of the fingers or toes
- Indicators of DVT, including unilateral calf tenderness, warmth, redness, and swelling

The nurse also encourages the patient to perform active foot exercises every hour when awake.

Skeletal Traction

Skeletal traction is applied directly to the bone. This method of traction is used occasionally to treat fractures of the femur, the tibia, and the cervical spine. The traction is applied directly to the bone by use of a metal pin or wire (eg, Steinmann pin, Kirschner wire) that is inserted through the bone distal to the fracture, avoiding nerves, blood vessels, muscles, tendons, and joints. Tongs applied to the head (eg, Gardner-Wells or Vinke tongs) are fixed to the skull to apply traction that immobilizes cervical fractures.

The orthopedic surgeon applies skeletal traction, using surgical asepsis. The insertion site is prepared with a surgical scrub agent such as povidone–iodine solution. A local anesthetic is administered at the insertion site and periosteum. The surgeon makes a small skin incision and drills the sterile pin or wire through the bone. The patient feels pressure during this procedure and possibly some pain when the periosteum is penetrated.

After insertion, the pin or wire is attached to the traction bow or caliper. The ends of the pin or wire are covered with corks or tape to prevent injury to the patient or caregivers. The weights are attached to the pin or wire bow by a rope-and-pulley system that exerts the appropriate amount and direction of pull for effective traction. Skeletal traction frequently uses 7 to 12 kg (15 to 25 lb) to achieve the therapeutic effect. The weights applied initially must overcome the shortening spasms of the affected muscles. As the muscles relax, the traction weight is reduced to prevent fracture dislocation and to promote healing.

Often, skeletal traction is balanced traction, which supports the affected extremity, allows for some patient movement, and facilitates patient independence and nursing care while maintaining effective traction. The Thomas splint with a Pearson attachment is frequently used with skeletal traction for fractures of the femur (see Fig. 67-6). Because upward traction is required, an overbed frame is used.

When skeletal traction is discontinued, the extremity is gently supported while the weights are removed. The pin is cut close to the skin and removed by the physician. Internal fixation, casts, or splints are then used to immobilize and support the healing bone.

Nursing Interventions

MAINTAINING EFFECTIVE TRACTION

When skeletal traction is used, the nurse checks the traction apparatus to see that the ropes are in the wheel grooves of the pulleys, that the ropes are not frayed, that the weights hang freely, and that the knots in the rope are tied securely. The nurse also evaluates the patient's position, because slipping down in bed results in ineffective traction.

> **! NURSING ALERT**
>
> **The nurse must never remove weights from skeletal traction unless a life-threatening situation occurs. Removal of the weights completely defeats their purpose and may result in injury to the patient.**

MAINTAINING POSITIONING

The nurse must maintain alignment of the patient's body in traction as prescribed to promote an effective line of pull. The nurse positions the patient's foot to avoid footdrop (plantar flexion), inward rotation (inversion), and outward rotation (eversion). The patient's foot may be supported in a neutral position by orthopedic devices (eg, foot supports).

PREVENTING SKIN BREAKDOWN

The patient's elbows frequently become sore, and nerve injury may occur if the patient repositions by pushing on the elbows. In addition, patients frequently push on the heel of the unaffected leg when they raise themselves. This digging of the heel into the mattress may injure the tissues. Therefore, the nurse should protect the elbows and heels and inspect them for pressure ulcers. To encourage movement without using the elbows or heel, a trapeze can be suspended overhead within easy reach of the patient. The trapeze helps the patient move about in bed and move on and off the bedpan.

Specific pressure points are assessed for redness and skin breakdown. Areas that are particularly vulnerable to pressure caused by a traction apparatus applied to the lower extremity include the ischial tuberosity, popliteal space, Achilles tendon, and heel. If the patient is not permitted to turn on one side or the other, the nurse must make a special effort to provide back care and to keep the bed dry and free of crumbs and wrinkles. The patient can assist by holding the overhead trapeze and raising the hips off the bed. If the patient cannot do this, the nurse can push down on the mattress with one hand to relieve pressure on the back and bony prominences and to provide for some shifting of weight. A pressure-relieving air-filled or high-density foam mattress overlay may reduce the risk of pressure ulcer.

For change of bed linens, the patient raises the torso while nurses on both sides of the bed roll down and replace the upper mattress sheet. Then, as the patient raises the buttocks off the mattress, the nurses slide the sheets under the buttocks. Finally, the nurses replace the lower section of the bed linens while the patient rests on the back. Sheets and blankets are placed over the patient in such a way that the traction is not disrupted.

MONITORING NEUROVASCULAR STATUS

The nurse assesses the neurovascular status of the immobilized extremity at least every hour initially and then every 4 hours. The nurse instructs the patient to report any changes in sensation or movement immediately so that they can be promptly evaluated. DVT is a significant risk for the immobilized patient. The nurse encourages the patient to do active flexion–extension ankle exercises and isometric contraction of the calf muscles (calf-pumping exercises) 10 times an hour while awake to decrease venous stasis. In addition, elastic stockings, compression devices, and anticoagulant therapy may be prescribed to help prevent thrombus formation.

Prompt recognition of a developing neurovascular problem is essential so that corrective measures can be instituted promptly.

PROVIDING PIN SITE CARE

The wound at the pin insertion site requires attention. The goal is to avoid infection and development of **osteomyelitis.**

For the first 48 hours after insertion, the site is covered with a sterile absorbent nonstick dressing and a rolled gauze or Ace-type bandage. After this time, a loose cover dressing or no dressing is recommended. (A bandage is necessary if the patient is exposed to airborne dust.) Pin site care is individually prescribed and performed initially one or two times a day. The frequency of pin care needs to be increased if mechanical looseness of pins or early signs of infection are present (eg, edema, purulent drainage, erythema, tenderness). Chlorhexidine solution is recommended as the most effective cleansing solution; however, water and saline are alternate choices. Hydrogen peroxide and Betadine solutions have been used, but they are believed to be cytotoxic to osteoblasts and may actually damage healthy tissue (Rabenberg, Ingersoll, Sandrey, et al., 2002).

The nurse must inspect the pin sites daily for reaction (ie, normal changes that occur at the pin site after insertion) and infection. Signs of reaction may include redness, warmth, and serous or slightly sanguinous drainage at the site. These signs subside after 72 hours. Signs of infection may mirror those of reaction but also include the presence of purulent drainage, pin loosening, and odor. Minor infections may be readily treated with antibiotics, whereas infections that result in systemic manifestations may additionally warrant pin removal until the infection resolves (Holmes & Brown, 2005). When pins are mechanically stable (after 48 to 72 hours), weekly pin site care is recommended.

Crusting may occur at the pin site and should remain undisturbed unless there are concomitant signs of infection. Crusts provide a normal protective barrier, and their removal may disturb healing tissue and make it more vulnerable to infection (Holmes & Brown, 2005).

The patient should be taught to perform pin site care prior to discharge from the hospital and should be provided with written follow-up instructions that include the signs and symptoms of infection. The patient is permitted to take showers within 5 to 10 days of pin insertion and is encouraged to leave the pins open to water flow. The sites are dried with a clean towel and left open to air.

NURSING ALERT

The nurse must inspect the pin site at least every 8 hours for signs of inflammation and evidence of infection.

PROMOTING EXERCISE

Patient exercises, within the therapeutic limits of the traction, assist in maintaining muscle strength and tone and in promoting circulation. Active exercises include pulling up on the trapeze, flexing and extending the feet, and range-of-motion and weight-resistance exercises for noninvolved joints. Isometric exercises of the immobilized extremity (quadriceps-setting and gluteal-setting exercises) are important for maintaining strength in major ambulatory muscles (see Chart 67-3). Without exercise, the patient will lose muscle mass and strength, and rehabilitation will be greatly prolonged.

Nursing Process

The Patient in Traction

Assessment

The nurse must consider the psychological and physiologic impact of the musculoskeletal problem, traction device, and immobility. Traction restricts mobility and independence. The equipment often looks threatening, and its application can be frightening. Confusion, disorientation, and behavioral problems may develop in patients who are confined in a limited space for an extended time. Therefore, the nurse must assess and monitor the patient's anxiety level and psychological responses to traction.

It is important to evaluate the body part to be placed in traction and its neurovascular status (ie, color, temperature, capillary refill, edema, pulses, ability to move, and sensations) and compare it to the unaffected extremity. The nurse also assesses skin integrity along with body system functioning for baseline data. Ongoing assessment is indicated for the patient in traction. Immobility-related complications may include pressure ulcers, atelectasis, pneumonia, constipation, loss of appetite, urinary stasis, urinary tract infections, and venous thromboemboli formation. Early identification of preexisting or developing conditions facilitates prompt interventions to resolve them.

Diagnosis

Nursing Diagnoses

Based on the nursing assessment, the patient's major nursing diagnoses related to traction may include the following:

- Deficient knowledge related to the treatment regimen
- Anxiety related to health status and the traction device
- Acute pain related to musculoskeletal disorder
- Self-care deficit: feeding, bathing/hygiene, dressing/grooming, and/or toileting related to traction
- Impaired physical mobility related to musculoskeletal disorder and traction

Collaborative Problems/ Potential Complications

Based on the assessment data, potential complications that may develop include the following:

- Pressure ulcer
- Atelectasis
- Pneumonia
- Constipation
- Anorexia
- Urinary stasis and infection
- Venous thromboemboli with DVT or PE

Planning and Goals

The major goals for the patient in traction may include understanding of the treatment regimen, reduced anxiety, maximum comfort, maximum level of self-care, maximum mobility within the therapeutic limits of traction, and absence of complications.

Nursing Interventions

Promoting Understanding of the Treatment Regimen

The patient must understand the condition being treated and the rationale for the traction therapy. The nurse may need to repeat and reinforce the information. With increased understanding of the therapy, the patient becomes an active participant in health care and more likely to cooperate with treatment.

Reducing Anxiety

Before any traction is applied, the patient needs to be informed about the procedure, its purpose, and its implications. The nurse encourages the patient to participate in decisions that affect care. Increasing the patient's sense of control reduces feelings of helplessness, allays apprehension, and fosters coping.

After being in traction for a while, the patient may react to being confined to a limited space. Frequent visits by the nurse can reduce feelings of isolation and confinement. The nurse should encourage family and friends to visit frequently for the same reason. The nurse encourages diversional activities that can be performed within the limits of the traction.

Achieving a Maximum Level of Comfort

Because the patient is immobilized in bed, the mattress needs to be firm. Special mattresses or mattress overlays designed to prevent pressure ulcers may be placed on the bed before the traction is applied. The nurse can relieve pressure on dependent body parts by turning and positioning the patient for comfort within the limits of the traction and by making sure the bed linens remain wrinkle-free and dry.

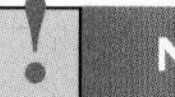

NURSING ALERT

The nurse must promptly investigate every report of discomfort expressed by the patient in traction.

Achieving Maximum Self-Care

Initially, the patient may require assistance with self-care activities. The nurse helps the patient eat, bathe, dress, and toilet. Convenient arrangement of items such as the telephone, tissues, water, and assistive devices (eg, reachers, overbed trapeze) may facilitate self-care. With resumption of self-care activities, the patient feels less dependent and less frustrated and experiences improved self-esteem.

Because some assistance is required throughout the period of immobility, the nurse and the patient can creatively develop routines that maximize the patient's independence.

Attaining Maximum Mobility With Traction

During traction therapy, the nurse encourages the patient to exercise muscles and joints that are not in traction to prevent deterioration and deconditioning. The physical therapist can design bed exercises that minimize loss of muscle strength. During the patient's exercise, the nurse ensures that traction forces are maintained and that the patient is properly positioned to prevent complications resulting from poor alignment.

Monitoring and Managing Potential Complications

PRESSURE ULCERS

The nurse examines the patient's skin frequently for evidence of pressure or friction, paying special attention to bony prominences. It is helpful to reposition the patient frequently and to use protective devices (eg, elbow protectors) to relieve pressure. If the risk of skin breakdown is high, as in a patient with multiple trauma or a debilitated elderly patient, use of a specialized bed is considered to prevent skin breakdown. If a pressure ulcer develops, the nurse consults with the physician and the wound-ostomy-continence nurse.

ATELECTASIS AND PNEUMONIA

The nurse auscultates the patient's lungs every 4 to 8 hours to assess respiratory status and teaches the patient deep-breathing and coughing exercises to aid in fully expanding the lungs and moving pulmonary secretions. If the patient history and baseline assessment indicate that the patient is at risk for development of respiratory complications, specific therapies (eg, use of incentive spirometer) may be indicated. If a respiratory complication develops, prompt institution of prescribed therapy is needed.

CONSTIPATION AND ANOREXIA

Reduced gastrointestinal motility results in constipation and anorexia. A diet high in fiber and fluids may help stimulate gastric motility. If constipation develops, therapeutic measures may include stool softeners, laxatives, suppositories, and enemas. To improve the patient's appetite, the nurse identifies and includes the patient's food preferences, as appropriate, within the prescribed therapeutic diet.

URINARY STASIS AND INFECTION

Incomplete emptying of the bladder related to positioning in bed can result in urinary stasis and infection.

In addition, the patient may find use of the bedpan uncomfortable and may limit fluids to minimize the frequency of urination. The nurse monitors the fluid intake and the character of the urine. The nurse teaches the patient to consume adequate amounts of fluid and to void every 3 to 4 hours. If the patient exhibits signs or symptoms of urinary tract infection, the nurse notifies the physician.

VENOUS THROMBOEMBOLISM

Venous stasis that predisposes the patient to venous thromboembolism occurs with immobility. The nurse teaches the patient to perform ankle and foot exercises within the limits of the traction therapy every 1 to 2 hours when awake to prevent DVT. The patient is encouraged to drink fluids to prevent dehydration and associated hemoconcentration, which contribute to stasis. The nurse monitors the patient for signs of DVT, including unilateral calf tenderness, warmth, redness, and swelling (increased calf circumference). The nurse promptly reports findings to the physician for definitive evaluation and therapy.

Evaluation

Expected Patient Outcomes

Expected patient outcomes may include:

1. Demonstrates knowledge of traction therapy
   a. Describes purpose of traction
   b. Participates in plan of care
2. Exhibits reduced anxiety
   a. Appears relaxed
   b. Uses effective coping mechanisms
   c. Verbalizes concerns and feelings
   d. Engages in diversional activities
3. States increased level of comfort
   a. Requests oral analgesia as needed
   b. Repositions self frequently
4. Performs self-care activities
   a. Requires minimal assistance with feeding, bathing/hygiene, dressing/grooming, and/or toileting
   b. Uses assistive devices safely
5. Demonstrates increased mobility
   a. Performs prescribed exercises
   b. Repositions self within limits of traction
6. Experiences no complications
   a. Has intact skin
   b. Has clear lungs
   c. Does not report shortness of breath
   d. Does not have a productive cough
   e. Exhibits a regular bowel evacuation pattern
   f. Has a normal appetite
   g. Voids clear, yellow, nonconcentrated urine of adequate amount
   h. Does not exhibit signs or symptoms of venous thromboembolism

The Patient Undergoing Orthopedic Surgery

Many patients with musculoskeletal dysfunction undergo surgery to correct the condition. Conditions that may be corrected by surgery include unstabilized fracture, deformity, joint disease, necrotic or infected tissue, and tumors. Frequent surgical procedures include **open reduction with internal fixation (ORIF)** and closed reduction with internal fixation (fracture fragments are not surgically exposed) for fractures; arthroplasty, meniscectomy, and joint replacement for joint conditions; amputation for severe extremity conditions (eg, gangrene, massive trauma); bone graft for joint stabilization, defect filling, or stimulation of bone healing; and tendon transfer for improving motion. The goals include improving function by restoring motion and stability and relieving pain and disability. Chart 67-7 describes orthopedic surgeries.

Joint surgery is one the most frequently performed orthopedic surgeries. Joint disease or deformity may necessitate surgical intervention to relieve pain, improve stability, and improve function. Surgical procedures include excision

CHART 67-7

Orthopedic Surgeries

Open reduction: the correction and alignment of the fracture after surgical dissection and exposure of the fracture

Internal fixation: the stabilization of the reduced fracture by the use of metal screws, plates, wires, nails, and pins

Arthroplasty: the repair of joint problems through the operating arthroscope (an instrument that allows the surgeon to operate within a joint without a large incision) or through open joint surgery

Hemiarthroplasty: the replacement of one of the articular surfaces (eg, in a hip hemiarthroplasty, the femoral head and neck are replaced with a femoral prosthesis—the acetabulum is not replaced)

Joint arthroplasty or replacement: the replacement of joint surfaces with metal or synthetic materials

Total joint arthroplasty or replacement: the replacement of both articular surfaces within a joint with metal or synthetic materials

Meniscectomy: the excision of damaged joint fibrocartilage

Amputation: the removal of a body part

Bone graft: the placement of bone tissue (autologous or homologous grafts) to promote healing, to stabilize, or to replace diseased bone

Tendon transfer: the movement of tendon insertion to improve function

Fasciotomy: the incision and diversion of the muscle fascia to relieve muscle constriction, as in compartment syndrome, or to reduce fascia contracture

of damaged and diseased tissue, repair of damaged structures (eg, ruptured tendon), removal of loose bodies (débridement), **arthroplasty** (replacement of all or part of the joint surfaces), and **arthrodesis** (immobilizing fusion of a joint).

The procedure is based on the patient's age, underlying orthopedic condition, and general physical health and the impact of joint disability on daily activities. Timing of these procedures is important to ensure maximum function. Surgery should be performed before surrounding muscles become contracted and atrophied and serious structural abnormalities occur. The physician carefully evaluates the patient so that the most appropriate procedure is performed.

Because these are elective procedures, many patients donate their own blood during the weeks preceding their surgery. This blood is used to replace blood lost during surgery. Autologous blood transfusions eliminate many of the risks of transfusion therapy.

Blood is conserved during surgery to minimize loss. A pneumatic tourniquet may be applied after exsanguination of the limb with bandages to produce a "bloodless field." This technique has the advantages of keeping the surgical field dry, minimizing blood loss, and providing some additional limb anesthesia (McEwen, Kelly, Jardanowski, et al., 2002). Intraoperative blood salvage with reinfusion is used when a large volume of blood loss is anticipated. Postoperative blood salvage with intermittent autotransfusion also reduces the need for blood transfusion.

Joint Replacement

Patients with severe joint pain and disability may undergo joint replacement. Conditions contributing to joint degeneration include osteoarthritis (degenerative joint disease), rheumatoid arthritis, trauma, and congenital deformity. Some fractures (eg, femoral neck fracture) may cause disruption of the blood supply and subsequent **avascular necrosis;** management with joint replacement may be elected over ORIF. Joints frequently replaced include the hip, knee (Fig. 67-7), and finger joints. Less frequently, more complex joints (shoulder, elbow, wrist, ankle) are replaced.

Most joint replacements consist of metal and high-density polyethylene components. Finger prostheses are usually Silastic. The joint implants may be cemented in the prepared bone with polymethyl methacrylate (PMMA), a bone-bonding agent that has properties similar to bone. Loosening of the prosthesis due to cement–bone interface failure is a common reason for prosthesis failure. Press-fit, ingrowth prostheses (porous-coated, cementless artificial joint components) that allow the patient's bone to grow into and securely fix the prosthesis in the bone are alternatives to cemented prostheses. Accurate fitting and the presence of healthy bone with adequate blood supply are important in the use of cementless components. Much progress has been made in reducing prosthesis failure rate through improved techniques, improved materials, and use of bone grafts.

With joint replacement, excellent pain relief is obtained in most patients. Return of motion and function depends on preoperative soft tissue condition, soft tissue reactions, and general muscle strength. Early failure of joint replacement is associated with excessive activity and preoperative joint and bone pathology.

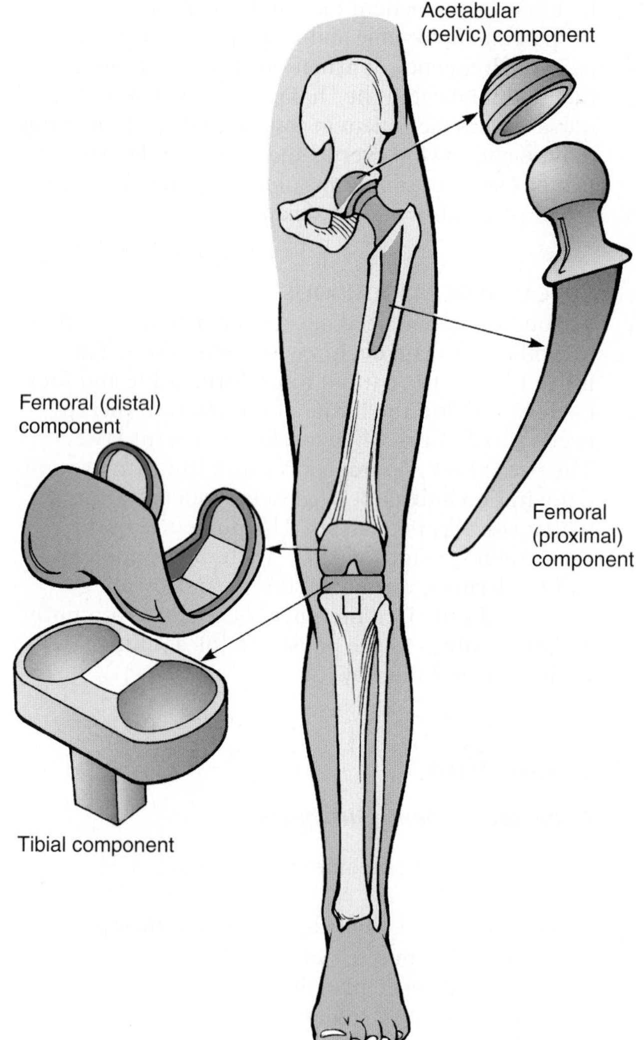

FIGURE 67-7. Examples of hip and knee replacement.

Nursing Interventions

Assessment of the patient and preoperative management are aimed at having the patient in optimal health at the time of surgery. Preoperatively, it is important to evaluate cardiovascular, respiratory, renal, and hepatic functions. Age, obesity, preoperative leg edema, a history of any venous thromboemboli, and varicose veins increase the risk for postoperative DVT and PE. In patients older than 60 years undergoing total hip replacement, these complications are the most common causes of postoperative mortality, and every effort is made to prevent them.

Preoperatively, it is important to assess the neurovascular status of the extremity undergoing joint replacement. Postoperative assessment data are compared with preoperative assessment data to identify changes and deficits. For example, an absent pulse postoperatively is of concern unless the pulse was also absent preoperatively. Nerve palsy could occur as a result of surgery.

PREVENTING INFECTION

Preoperative assessment of the patient for infections, including urinary tract infection, is necessary because of the risk for postoperative infection. Any infection 2 to 4 weeks before planned surgery may result in postponement of surgery. Preoperative skin preparation frequently begins 1 or 2 days before the surgery. Airborne bacteria that contaminate the wound at the time of surgery cause most deep infections. Therefore, as with any surgery, there is strict adherence to aseptic principles, and the operating area is controlled and made as bacteria free as possible.

Prophylactic antibiotics are administered as a single preoperative or short perioperative course (Geier, 2000). Culture of the joint during surgery, before intraoperative antibiotic therapy is begun, may be important in identifying and treating subsequent infections.

If osteomyelitis develops, it is difficult to treat. Persistent infection at the site of the prosthesis usually requires removal of the implant and joint revision, which is a complex procedure. Also, it is not always possible to achieve a functional joint when the reconstruction procedure has to be repeated.

PROMOTING AMBULATION

Patients with total hip or total knee replacement begin ambulation with a walker or crutches within a day after surgery. The nurse and the physical therapist assist the patient in achieving the goal of independent ambulation. At first, the patient may be able to stand for only a brief period because of orthostatic hypotension. Specific weight-bearing limits on the prosthesis are determined by the physician and are based on the patient's condition, the procedure, and the fixation method. Usually, patients with cemented prostheses can proceed to weight-bearing as tolerated. If the patient has a press-fit, cementless, ingrowth prosthesis, weight-bearing immediately after surgery may be limited to minimize micromotion of the prosthesis in the bone. As the patient is able to tolerate more activity, the nurse encourages transferring to a chair several times a day for short periods and walking for progressively greater distances.

Total Hip Replacement

Total hip replacement is the replacement of a severely damaged hip with an artificial joint. Indications for this surgery include arthritis (osteoarthritis, rheumatoid arthritis), femoral neck fractures, failure of previous reconstructive surgeries (failed prosthesis, **osteotomy**), and conditions resulting from congenital hip disease (developmental dysplasia of the hip [DDH]). A variety of total hip prostheses are available. Most consist of a metal femoral component topped by a spherical ball fitted into a plastic acetabular socket (see Fig. 67-7).

The surgeon selects the prosthesis that is best suited to the individual patient, considering various factors, including skeletal structure and activity level. The patient has irreversibly damaged hip joints, and the potential benefits, including improved quality of life, outweigh the surgical risks. With the advent of improved prosthetic materials and operative techniques, the life of the prosthesis has been extended, and today younger patients with severely damaged and painful hip joints are undergoing total hip replacement.

Nursing Interventions

The nurse must be aware of and monitor for specific potential complications associated with total hip replacement. Complications that may occur include dislocation of the hip prosthesis, excessive wound drainage, thromboembolism, infection, and heel pressure ulcer. Other complications for which the nurse must monitor include those associated with immobility, **heterotopic ossification** (formation of bone in the periprosthetic space), avascular necrosis (bone death caused by loss of blood supply), and loosening of the prosthesis.

PREVENTING DISLOCATION OF THE HIP PROSTHESIS

Maintenance of the femoral head component in the acetabular cup is essential. The nurse teaches the patient about positioning the leg in **abduction**, which helps prevent dislocation of the prosthesis. The use of an abduction splint, a wedge pillow (Fig. 67-8), or two or three pillows between the legs keeps the hip in abduction. When the nurse turns the patient in bed, it is important to keep the operative hip in abduction. Depending on the surgeon's preference, some patients are not permitted to be turned onto the affected side, whereas others may be turned to either side.

The patient's hip is never flexed more than 90 degrees. To prevent hip flexion, the nurse does not elevate the head of the bed more than 60 degrees. For use of the fracture bedpan, the nurse instructs the patient to flex the unaffected hip and to use the trapeze to lift the pelvis onto the pan. The patient is also reminded not to flex the affected hip.

Limited flexion is maintained during transfers and when sitting. When the patient is initially assisted out of bed, an abduction splint or pillows are kept between the legs. The nurse encourages the patient to keep the affected hip in extension, instructing the patient to pivot on the unaffected leg with assistance by the nurse, who protects the affected hip from **adduction**, flexion, internal or external rotation, and excessive weight-bearing.

High-seat (orthopedic) chairs, semireclining wheelchairs, and raised toilet seats may be used to minimize hip joint flexion. When sitting, the patient's hips should be higher than the knees. The patient's affected leg should not be elevated when sitting. The patient may flex the knee.

The nurse teaches the patient protective positioning, which includes maintaining abduction and avoiding internal and external rotation, hyperextension, and acute flexion. A cradle boot may be used to prevent leg rotation and to support the heel off the bed, preventing development of a pressure ulcer. The patient should use pillows between the legs when in a supine or side-lying position and when turning. Generally, the nurse instructs the patient not to sleep on the

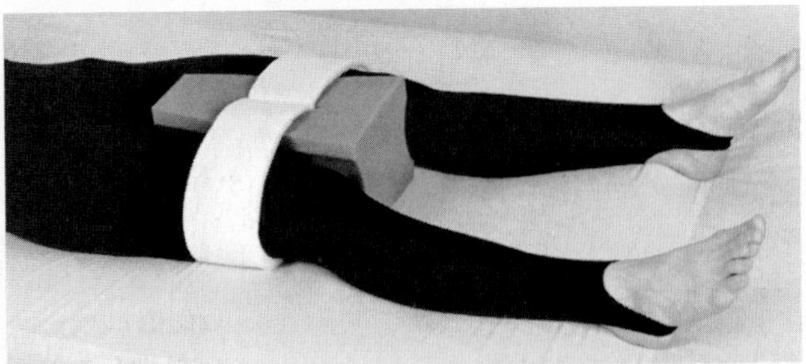

FIGURE 67-8. An abduction pillow may be used after a total hip replacement to prevent dislocation of the prosthesis.

side on which the surgery was performed without consulting the surgeon. At no time should the patient cross his or her legs. The patient must avoid acute flexion of the hip. The patient should not bend at the waist to put on shoes and socks. Occupational therapists can provide the patient with devices to assist with dressing below the waist. Hip precautions should be enforced for 4 or more months after surgery (Chart 67-8).

Dislocation may occur with positioning that exceeds the limits of the prosthesis. The nurse must recognize dislocation of the prosthesis. Indicators are as follows:

- Increased pain at the surgical site, swelling, and immobilization
- Acute groin pain in the affected hip or increased discomfort
- Shortening of the leg
- Abnormal external or internal rotation
- Restricted ability or inability to move the leg
- Reported "popping" sensation in the hip

If a prosthesis becomes dislocated, the nurse (or the patient, if at home) immediately notifies the surgeon, because the hip must be reduced and stabilized promptly so that the leg does not sustain circulatory and nerve damage. After closed reduction, the hip may be stabilized with Buck's traction or a brace to prevent recurrent dislocation. As the muscles and joint capsule heal, the chance of dislocation diminishes. Stresses to the new hip joint should be avoided for the first 3 to 6 months.

MONITORING WOUND DRAINAGE

Fluid and blood accumulating at the surgical site are usually drained with a portable suction device. This prevents accumulation of fluid, which could contribute to discomfort and provide a site for infection. Drainage of 200 to 500 mL in the first 24 hours is expected; by 48 hours postoperatively, the total drainage in 8 hours usually decreases to 30 mL or less, and the suction device is then removed. The nurse promptly notifies the physician of any drainage volumes greater than anticipated.

If extensive blood loss is anticipated after total joint replacement surgery, an autotransfusion drainage system (in which the drained blood is filtered and reinfused into the patient during the immediate postoperative period) may be used to decrease the need for homologous blood transfusions (Warner, 2001).

CHART 67-8

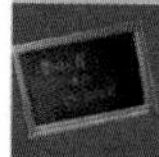

Patient Education

Avoiding Hip Dislocation After Replacement Surgery

Until the hip prosthesis stabilizes after hip replacement surgery, it is necessary to follow instructions for proper positioning so that the prosthesis remains in place. Dislocation of the hip is a serious complication of surgery that causes pain and loss of function and necessitates reduction under anesthesia to correct the dislocation. Desirable positions include abduction, neutral rotation, and flexion of less than 90 degrees. When you are seated, the knees should be lower than the hip.

Methods for avoiding displacement include the following:

- Keep the knees apart at all times.
- Put a pillow between the legs when sleeping.
- Never cross the legs when seated.
- Avoid bending forward when seated in a chair.
- Avoid bending forward to pick up an object on the floor.
- Use a high-seated chair and a raised toilet seat.
- Do not flex the hip to put on clothing such as pants, stockings, socks, or shoes. Positions to avoid after total hip replacement are illustrated below.

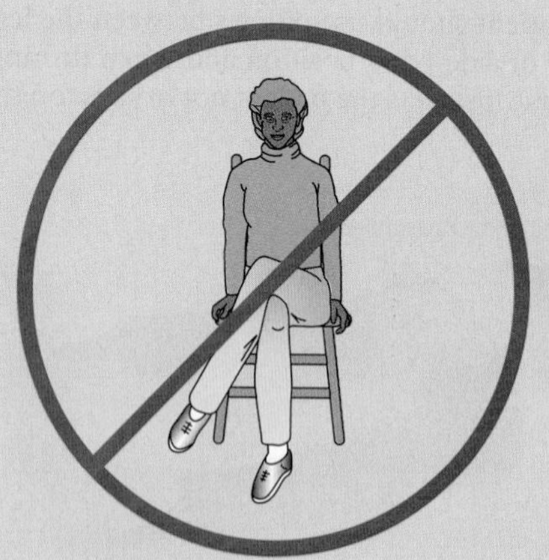

Affected leg should not cross the center of the body

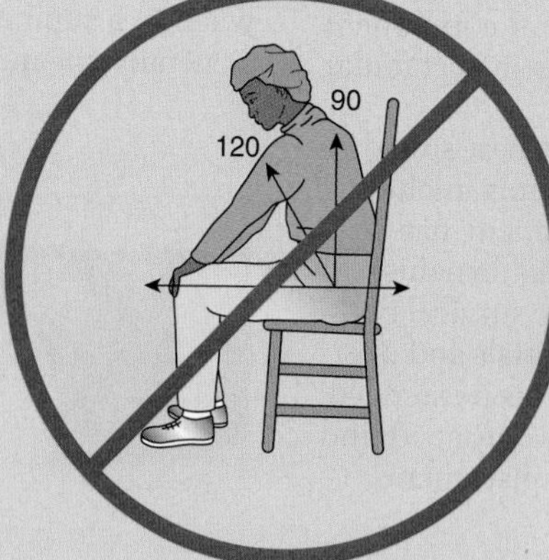

Hip should not bend more than 90 degrees

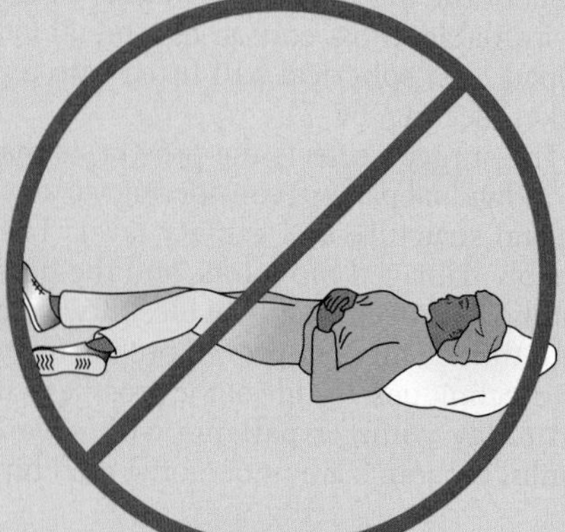

Affected leg should not turn inward

PREVENTING DEEP VEIN THROMBOSIS

The risk of venous thromboembolism is particularly great after reconstructive hip surgery. The incidence of DVT is 45% to 70%. The peak occurrence is 5 to 7 days after surgery. About 20% of patients with DVT develop PE, of which about 1% to 3% of cases are fatal (Morris, 2004). Therefore, the nurse must institute preventive measures and monitor the patient closely for the development of DVT and PE. Signs of DVT include calf pain, swelling, and tenderness. Measures to promote circulation and decrease venous stasis are priorities for the patient undergoing hip reconstruction. The nurse encourages the patient to consume adequate amounts of fluids, to perform ankle and foot exercises hourly while awake, to use elastic stockings and sequential compression devices as prescribed, and to transfer out of bed and ambulate with assistance beginning on the first postoperative day. Low-molecular-weight heparin (eg, enoxaparin [Lovenox], dalteparin [Fragmin]) or sometimes unfractionated heparin is frequently prescribed as prophylaxis for DVT after hip replacement surgery.

PREVENTING INFECTION

Infection, a serious complication of total hip replacement, may necessitate removal of the implant. Patients who are elderly, obese, or poorly nourished and patients who have diabetes, rheumatoid arthritis, concurrent infections (eg, urinary tract infection, dental abscess), or large hematomas are at high risk for infection.

Because total joint infections are so disastrous, all efforts are made to prevent them. Potential sources of infection are avoided. Prophylactic antibiotics are prescribed. If indwelling urinary catheters or portable wound suction devices are used, they are removed as soon as possible to avoid infection. Prophylactic antibiotics are prescribed if the patient needs any future surgical or invasive procedures, such as tooth extraction or cystoscopic examination.

Acute infections may occur within 3 months after surgery and are associated with progressive superficial infections or hematomas. Delayed surgical infections may appear 4 to 24 months after surgery and may cause return of discomfort in the hip. Infections occurring more than 2 years after surgery are attributed to the spread of infection through the bloodstream from another site in the body. If an infection occurs, antibiotics are prescribed. Severe infections may require surgical débridement or removal of the prosthesis.

PROMOTING HOME AND COMMUNITY-BASED CARE

Teaching the Patient Self-Care

Before the patient prepares to leave the acute care setting, the nurse provides thorough teaching to promote continuity of the therapeutic regimen and active participation in the rehabilitation process (Chart 67-9). The nurse advises the patient of the importance of the daily exercise program in maintaining the functional motion of the hip joint and strengthening the abductor muscles of the hip, and reminds the patient that it will take time to strengthen and retrain the muscles.

Assistive devices (crutches, walker, or cane) are used for a time. After sufficient muscle tone has developed to permit a normal gait without discomfort, these devices are not necessary. In general, by 3 months, the patient can resume routine ADLs. Stair climbing is permitted as prescribed but is kept to a minimum for 3 to 6 months. Frequent walks, swimming, and use of a high rocking chair are excellent for hip exercises. Sexual intercourse should be carried out with the patient in the dependent position (flat on the back) for 3 to 6 months to avoid excessive adduction and flexion of the new hip.

At no time during the first 4 months should the patient cross the legs or flex the hip more than 90 degrees. Assistance in putting on shoes and socks may be needed. The patient should avoid low chairs and sitting for longer than 45 minutes at a time. These precautions minimize hip flexion and the risks of prosthetic dislocation, hip stiffness, and flexion contracture. Traveling long distances should be avoided unless frequent position changes are possible. Other activities to avoid include tub baths, jogging, lifting heavy loads, and excessive bending and twisting (eg, lifting, shoveling snow, forceful turning).

Continuing Care

The nurse may make a home visit to assess for potential problems and to monitor wound healing (see Chart 67-9). The nurse, physical therapist, or occupational therapist assesses the home environment for physical barriers that may impede the patient's rehabilitation. In addition, the nurse or therapist may need to assist the patient in acquiring devices such as reachers or long-handled tongs to help with dressing, or toilet seat extenders.

After successful surgery and rehabilitation, the patient can expect a hip joint that is free or almost free of pain, has good motion, is stable, and permits normal or near-normal ambulation. Chart 67-10 is a plan of nursing care for the patient with a total hip replacement.

Total Knee Replacement

Total knee replacement surgery is considered for patients who have severe pain and functional disabilities related to destruction of joint surfaces by arthritis (osteoarthritis, rheumatoid arthritis, posttraumatic arthritis) or bleeding into the joint (eg, hemarthrosis), such as may result from hemophilia. Metal and acrylic prostheses designed to provide the patient with a functional, painless, stable joint may be used. If the patient's ligaments have weakened, a fully constrained (hinged) or semiconstrained prosthesis may be used to provide joint stability. A nonconstrained prosthesis depends on the patient's ligaments for joint stability.

Nursing Interventions

Postoperatively, the knee is dressed with a compression bandage. Ice may be applied to control edema and bleeding. The nurse assesses the neurovascular status of the leg. It is important to encourage active flexion of the foot every hour when the patient is awake. Efforts are directed at preventing complications (thromboembolism, peroneal nerve palsy, infection, limited range of motion).

A wound suction drain removes fluid accumulating in the joint. Drainage ranges from 200 to 400 mL during the first 24 hours after surgery and diminishes to less than 25 mL by 48 hours. Then the surgeon removes the drains. If extensive bleeding is anticipated, an autotransfusion drainage system may be used during the immediate postoperative period. The

CHART 67-9

Providing Home Care After Hip Replacement

Considerations

- Pain management
- Wound care
- Mobility
- Self-care (activities of daily living)
- Potential problems

Nursing Interventions

Discuss with patient methods to reduce pain:

- Periodic rest
- Distraction and relaxation techniques
- Medication therapy (eg, nonsteroidal anti-inflammatory drugs, opioid analgesics): actions of medications, administration, schedule, side effects

Instruct patient in the following:

- Keeping incision clean and dry
- Taking care of the wound and changing the dressing
- Recognizing signs of wound infection (eg, pain, swelling, drainage, fever)

Explain that sutures or staples will be removed 10 to 14 days after surgery.

Teach patient about the following:

- Safe use of assistive devices
- Weight-bearing limits
- How to change positions frequently
- Limitations on hip flexion and adduction (eg, avoid acute flexion and crossing legs)
- How to stand without flexing hip acutely
- Avoidance of low-seated chairs
- Sleeping with pillow between legs to prevent adduction
- Gradual increase in activities and participation in prescribed exercise regimen
- Use of important medications such as warfarin (Coumadin) and aspirin

Assess home environment for physical barriers.

Instruct patient to use elevated toilet seat and to use reachers to aid in dressing.

Encourage patient to accept assistance with activities of daily living during early convalescence until mobility and strength improve.

Arrange services and accommodations to address the patient's disability or illness, as appropriate.

Assess patient for development of potential problems, and instruct patient to report signs of potential problems:

- Dislocation of prosthesis (eg, increased pain, shortening of leg, inability to move leg, popping sensation in hip, abnormal rotation)
- Deep vein thrombosis (eg, calf pain, swelling)
- Wound infection (eg, swelling, purulent drainage, pain, fever)
- Pulmonary emboli (eg, sudden dyspnea, tachypnea, pleuritic chest pain)

Discuss with patient the need to continue regular health care (routine physical examinations) and screenings.

color, type, and amount of drainage are documented, and any excessive drainage or change in characteristics of the drainage is promptly reported to the physician.

Frequently, a **continuous passive motion (CPM) device** is used. The patient's leg is placed in this device, which increases circulation and range of motion of the knee joint. The rate and amount of extension and flexion are prescribed. Usually, 10 degrees of extension and 50 degrees of flexion are prescribed initially, increasing to 90 degrees of flexion with full extension (0 degrees) by discharge (Fig. 67-9).

The nurse encourages the patient to use the CPM device most of the time. The physical therapist supervises exercises for strength and range of motion. If satisfactory flexion is not achieved, gentle manipulation of the knee joint under general anesthesia may be necessary about 2 weeks after surgery.

The nurse assists the patient to get out of bed on the evening or the day after surgery. The knee is usually protected with a knee immobilizer (splint, cast, or brace) and is elevated when the patient sits in a chair. The physician prescribes weight-bearing limits. Progressive ambulation, using assistive devices and within the prescribed weight-bearing limits, begins on the day after surgery.

After discharge from the hospital, the patient may continue to use the CPM device at home and may undergo physical therapy on an outpatient basis. Late complications that may occur include infection and loosening and wear of prosthetic components. Patients usually can achieve a pain-free, functional joint and participate more fully in life activities than before the surgery.

Nursing Process

Preoperative Care of the Patient Undergoing Orthopedic Surgery

Assessment

Assessment of the patient is focused on hydration status, current medication history, and possible infection. Adequate hydration is an important goal for orthopedic

(text continues on page 2382)

CHART 67-10

Plan of Nursing Care The Patient With a Total Hip Replacement

Nursing Diagnosis: Pain related to total hip replacement
Goal: Relief of pain

NURSING INTERVENTIONS	RATIONALE	EXPECTED OUTCOMES
1. Assess patient for pain using a standard pain intensity scale.	1. Pain is expected after a surgical procedure because of the surgical trauma and tissue response. Muscle spasms occur after total hip replacements. Immobility causes discomfort at pressure points.	• Patient describes discomfort • Expresses confidence in efforts to control pain • States pain is reduced; pain intensity scores are decreasing • Appears comfortable and relaxed • Uses physical, psychological, and pharmacologic measures to reduce pain and discomfort
2. Ask patient to describe discomfort.	2. Pain characteristics may help to determine the cause of discomfort. Pain may be due to complications (hematoma, infection, dislocation). Pain is an individual experience—it means different things to different people.	
3. Acknowledge existence of pain; inform patient of available analgesics or muscle relaxants.	3. The nurse can reduce the stress experienced by patient by communicating concern and availability of assistance to help the patient deal with the pain	
4. Use pain-modifying techniques.	4.	
a. Administer analgesics as prescribed.	a. Patient will require parenteral opioids during the first 24–48 hours, and then will progress to oral analgesics.	
b. Change position within prescribed limits.	b. Use of pillows to provide adequate support and relief of pressure on bony prominences assists in minimizing pain.	
c. Modify environment.	c. Interactions with others, distractions, and sensory overload or deprivation may affect pain experience.	
d. Notify surgeon about persistent pain.	d. Surgical intervention may be necessary if pain is due to hematoma or excessive edema.	
5. Evaluate and record discomfort and effectiveness of pain-modifying techniques.	5. Effectiveness of action is based on experience; data provide a baseline about pain experiences, management, and pain relief.	

continued >

CHART 67-10

Plan of Nursing Care — The Patient With a Total Hip Replacement (Continued)

Nursing Diagnosis: Impaired physical mobility related to positioning, weight-bearing, and activity restrictions after hip replacement
Goal: Achieves pain-free, functional, stable hip joint

NURSING INTERVENTIONS	RATIONALE	EXPECTED OUTCOMES
1. Maintain proper positioning of hip joint (abduction, neutral rotation, limited flexion).	1. Prevents dislocation of hip prosthesis.	• Prescribed position maintained • No heel pressure • Patient assists in position changes • Shows increased independence in transfers • Exercises hourly • Participates in progressive ambulation program • Actively participates in exercise regimen • Uses ambulatory aids correctly and safely
2. Keep pressure off heel.	2. Prevents pressure ulcer on heel.	
3. Instruct and assist in position changes and transfers.	3. Encourages patient's active participation while preventing dislocation.	
4. Instruct and supervise isometric quadriceps- and gluteal-setting exercises.	4. Strengthens muscles needed for walking.	
5. In consultation with physical therapist, instruct and supervise progressive safe ambulation within limitations of weight-bearing prescription.	5. Amount of weight-bearing depends on patient's condition and prosthesis; ambulatory aids are used to assist the patient with non–weight-bearing and partial weight-bearing ambulation.	
6. Offer encouragement and support exercise regimen.	6. Reconditioning exercises can be uncomfortable and fatiguing; encouragement helps patient comply with exercise program.	
7. Instruct and supervise safe use of ambulatory aids.	7. Prevents injury from unsafe use and prevents falls.	

Collaborative Problems: Hemorrhage; neurovascular compromise; dislocation of prosthesis; deep vein thrombosis; infection related to surgery
Goal: Absence of complications

NURSING INTERVENTIONS	RATIONALE	EXPECTED OUTCOMES
Hemorrhage		
1. Monitor vital signs, observing for shock.	1. Changes in pulse, blood pressure, and respirations may indicate development of shock. Blood loss and stress of surgery may contribute to development of shock.	• Vital signs stabilize within normal limits • Amount of drainage decreases • No bright red bloody drainage • Hematology values are within normal limits
2. Note character and amount of drainage.	2. Within 48 hours, bloody drainage collected in portable suction device should decrease to 25–30 mL per 8 hours. Excessive drainage (more than 250 mL in first 8 hours after surgery) and bright red drainage may indicate active bleeding.	

CHART 67-10

Plan of Nursing Care The Patient With a Total Hip Replacement (Continued)

NURSING INTERVENTIONS	RATIONALE	EXPECTED OUTCOMES
3. Notify surgeon if patient develops shock or excessive bleeding and prepare for administration of fluids, blood component therapy, and medications.	3. Corrective measures need to be instituted.	
4. Monitor hemoglobin and hematocrit values.	4. Anemia due to blood loss may develop. Blood replacement or iron supplementation may be needed.	
Neurovascular Dysfunction		
1. Assess affected extremity for color and temperature.	1. The skin becomes pale and feels cool with decreased tissue perfusion. Venous congestion may produce cyanosis.	• Color normal • Extremity warm • Normal capillary refill • Moderate edema and swelling; tissue not palpably tense • Pain controllable • No pain with passive dorsiflexion • Normal sensations • No paresthesia • Normal motor abilities • No paresis or paralysis • Pulses strong and equal
2. Assess toes for capillary refill response.	2. After compression of the nail, rapid return of pink color indicates good capillary perfusion.	
3. Assess extremity for edema and swelling. Report patient complaints of leg tightness.	3. The trauma of surgery will cause edema. Excessive swelling and hematoma formation can compromise circulation and function.	
4. Elevate extremity (keep leg lower than hip when in chair).	4. Minimizes dependent edema.	
5. Assess for deep, throbbing, unrelenting pain.	5. Surgical pain can be controlled; pain due to neurovascular compromise is not relieved by treatment.	
6. Assess for pain on passive flexion of foot.	6. With nerve ischemia, there will be pain on passive stretch. Additionally, pain or tenderness may indicate deep vein thrombosis.	
7. Assess for change in sensations and numbness.	7. Diminished pain and sensory function may indicate nerve damage. Sensation in web between great and second toe—peroneal nerve; sensation on sole of foot—tibial nerve.	
8. Assess ability to move foot and toes.	8. Dorsiflexion of ankle and extension of toes indicate function of peroneal nerve. Plantar flexion of ankle and flexion of toes indicate function of tibial nerve.	
9. Assess pedal pulses in both feet.	9. Indicator of extremity circulation.	
10. Notify surgeon if altered neurovascular status is noted.	10. Function of extremity needs to be preserved.	

continued >

CHART 67-10

Plan of Nursing Care The Patient With a Total Hip Replacement (Continued)

NURSING INTERVENTIONS	RATIONALE	EXPECTED OUTCOMES
Dislocation of Prosthesis		
1. Position patient as prescribed.	1. Hip component positioning (femoral component in acetabular component) needs to be maintained.	• Prosthesis not dislocated • Adheres to recommendations to prevent dislocation
2. Use abductor splint or pillows to maintain position and to support extremity.	2. Keep hip in abduction and in a neutral rotation to prevent dislocation.	
3. Support leg and place pillows between legs when patient is turning and side-lying; turn to the unaffected side.	3–5. Prevent dislocation.	
4. Avoid acute flexion of hip (head of bed at 60 degrees or less).		
5. Avoid crossing legs.		
6. Assess for dislocation of prosthesis (extremity shortens, internally or externally rotated, severe hip pain, patient unable to move extremity)	6. Findings may indicate dislocation of prosthesis.	
7. Notify surgeon of possible dislocation.	7. Joint dislocations compromise neurovascular status and future function of extremity.	
Deep Vein Thrombosis		
1. Use elastic compression stocking or sequential compression device as prescribed.	1. Aid in venous blood return and prevent stasis.	• Wears elastic stockings; uses compression device • No skin breakdown • Pulses equal and strong • Skin temperature normal • No calf pain or tenderness • Changes position with assistance and supervision • Participates in exercise regimen • Well hydrated • No chest pain; lungs clear to auscultation; no evidence of pulmonary emboli
2. Remove stocking for 20 minutes twice a day and provide skin care.	2. Skin care is necessary to avoid breakdown. Extended removal of stockings defeats purpose of stockings.	
3. Assess popliteal, dorsalis pedis, and posterior tibial pulses.	3. Pulses indicate arterial perfusion of extremity.	
4. Assess skin temperature of legs.	4. Local inflammation will increase local skin temperature.	
5. Assess for unilateral calf pain or tenderness every 8 hours.	5. Pain on dorsiflexion of ankle may indicate deep vein thrombosis.	
6. Avoid pressure on popliteal blood vessels from equipment (eg, abductor splint straps, sequential compression stockings) or pillows.	6. Compression of blood vessels diminishes blood flow.	
7. Change position and increase activity as prescribed.	7. Activity promotes circulation and diminishes venous stasis.	
8. Supervise ankle exercises hourly.	8. Muscle exercise promotes circulation.	
9. Monitor body temperature.	9. Body temperature increases with inflammation.	
10. Encourage fluids.	10. Dehydration increases blood viscosity	

CHART 67-10

Plan of Nursing Care — The Patient With a Total Hip Replacement (Continued)

NURSING INTERVENTIONS	RATIONALE	EXPECTED OUTCOMES
Infection		• Vital signs normal • Well-approximated incision without drainage or excessive inflammatory response • Minimal discomfort; no hematoma • Patient tolerates antibiotics
1. Monitor vital signs.	1. Temperature, pulse, and respirations increase in response to infection. (Magnitude of response may be minimal in an elderly patient.)	
2. Use aseptic technique for dressing changes and emptying of portable drainage.	2. Avoids introducing organisms.	
3. Assess wound appearance and character of drainage.	3. Red, swollen, draining incision is indicative of infection.	
4. Assess complaints of pain.	4. Pain may be due to wound hematoma—a possible locus of infection—that needs to be surgically evacuated.	
5. Administer prophylactic antibiotics if prescribed, and observe for side effects.	5. Infected prosthesis is avoided.	

Nursing Diagnosis: Risk for ineffective health maintenance related to total hip replacement
Goal: Cares for self at home

NURSING INTERVENTIONS	RATIONALE	EXPECTED OUTCOMES
1. Assess home environment for discharge planning.	1. Physical barriers (especially stairs, bathrooms) may limit patient's ability to ambulate and care for self at home.	• Home is accessible for patient at time of discharge. • Patient appears relaxed and develops strategies to deal with identified problems. • Personal assistance is available. • Patient demonstrates ability to provide necessary assistance within therapeutic prescription. • Patient complies with home care program. • Patient keeps follow-up health care appointments.
2. Encourage patient to express concerns about care at home; explore together possible solutions to the problem.	2. Patient may have special problems that need to be identified and resolved.	
3. Assess availability of physical assistance for health care activities.	3. Because of limitation of mobility and limited hip range of motion, patient may require some assistance in routine health care.	
4. Teach home health care regimen to caregiver.	4. Understanding of rehabilitative regimen is necessary for compliance.	
5. Instruct patient on posthospital care: a. Activity limitations (hip precautions, weight-bearing limits) b. Exercise instructions c. Safe use of ambulatory aids d. Wound care e. Measures to promote healing f. Medications, if any g. Potential problems h. Continuing health care supervision and management	5. Lack of knowledge and poor preparation for care at home contribute to patient anxiety, insecurity, and nonadherence to therapeutic regimen.	

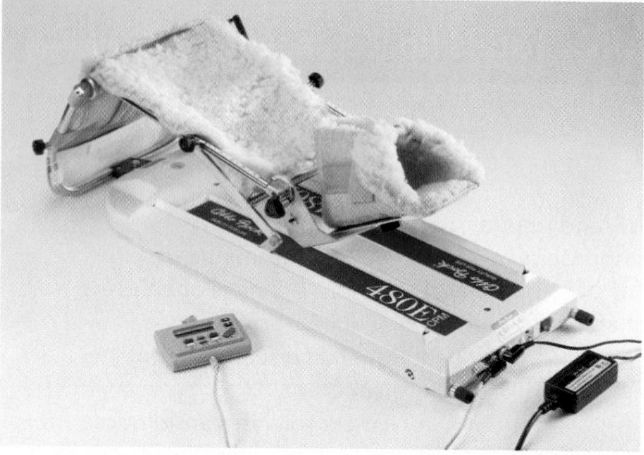

FIGURE 67-9. Lower-limb continuous passive motion (CPM) device. The Otto Bock 480E Knee CPM is 11 kg (24 lb) and combines durable construction with portability and ease of operation. CPM is best applied immediately after surgery and continued, uninterrupted, for up to 6 weeks as prescribed by the physician. Photo courtesy of Otto Bock Healthcare, Minneapolis, MN.

patients. Immobilization and bed rest contribute to the following complications: DVT, PE, urinary stasis and associated bladder infections, and kidney stone formation. Adequate hydration decreases blood viscosity and venous stasis and ensures adequate urine flow. To determine preoperative hydration status, the nurse assesses the skin and mucous membranes, vital signs, urinary output, and laboratory values.

The medication history provides information for perioperative management. The patient with chronic illness (eg, adrenal insufficiency, rheumatoid arthritis, chronic pulmonary disease, multiple sclerosis) or with a transplanted organ frequently has received long-term administration of corticosteroid medications to control disease symptoms or prevent rejection. The corticosteroid should be administered preoperatively, intraoperatively, and postoperatively as prescribed to prevent the occurrence of acute adrenal insufficiency from suppressed adrenal function. The patient's use of other medications, such as anticoagulants, cardiovascular agents, or insulin, needs to be documented and discussed with the surgeon and anesthesiologist to ensure adequate management.

The nurse asks the patient specifically about the occurrence of colds, dental problems, urinary tract infections, and other infections within the 2 weeks before surgery. Osteomyelitis could develop through hematologous spread. Permanent disability can result if infection occurs within a bone or joint. Preexisting infections must be resolved before elective orthopedic surgery is performed.

Other areas of preoperative assessment are similar to those for any patient undergoing surgery. Intramuscular medications are injected into a site other than the surgical site, because tissue absorption is better in nontraumatized tissues.

Nursing Diagnoses

Based on the nursing assessment data, the patient's major preoperative nursing diagnoses related to orthopedic status may include the following:

- Acute pain related to fracture, joint degeneration, swelling, or inflammation
- Risk for peripheral neurovascular dysfunction related to swelling, constricting devices, or impaired venous return
- Risk for ineffective therapeutic regimen management related to insufficient knowledge or lack of available support and resources
- Impaired physical mobility related to pain, swelling, and possible presence of an immobilization device
- Risk for situational low self-esteem and/or disturbed body image related to impact of musculoskeletal disorder

Planning and Goals

The major goals for the patient before orthopedic surgery may include relief of pain, adequate neurovascular function, health promotion, improved mobility, and positive self-esteem.

Nursing Interventions

Relieving Pain

Physical, pharmacologic, and psychological strategies to control pain are useful in the preoperative period. Specific strategies are tailored to the individual patient and based on assessment of the intensity, type, and duration of pain. Discomfort is decreased with immobilization of a fractured bone or an injured, inflamed joint. Elevation of an edematous extremity promotes venous return and reduces associated discomfort. Ice, if prescribed, relieves swelling and reduces discomfort by diminishing nerve stimulation.

Pain assessment is as important as assessing the patient's temperature, pulse, respirations, and blood pressure. In fact, assessment of pain is referred to as the "fifth vital sign." Location, quality, and intensity of pain are three important parameters to assess. The nurse asks the patient to identify the exact location of pain; this may provide essential diagnostic clues. For instance, a patient with compartment syndrome might identify the location of pain as distal to the fracture or surgical repair site. (Compartment syndrome was discussed earlier in this chapter, and in Chapter 66.) Quality of pain is determined by asking for a description of the pain (eg, "burning," "throbbing," or "stabbing"). Intensity of pain might be described as mild to excruciating and is rated using a variety of intensity pain scales, such as the numeric pain scale or FACES pain scale. (See Chapter 13 for a discussion of pain intensity scales.)

Analgesics are frequently prescribed to control the acute pain of musculoskeletal injury or surgery and associated muscle spasm. During the immediate post-operative period, the nurse needs to discuss and coor-

NURSING RESEARCH PROFILE

Ensuring Preoperative Education in Rural Populations

Thomas, K., Burton, D., Withrow, L., et al. (2004). Impact of a preoperative education program via interactive telehealth network for rural patients having total joint replacement. *Orthopaedic Nursing, 23*(1), 39–44.

Purpose

Traditional preoperative education programs have beneficial effects for orthopedic patients. However, patients who live in rural areas that are geographically distant from major health care facilities may not be able to travel great distances to attend the classes. The purpose of this pilot project was to determine the effectiveness of providing preoperative education programs via an interactive telehealth network to rural patients having total joint replacements at a regional medical center.

Design

A clinical coordinator conducted a traditional preoperative class on total joint replacement surgery with participants at a regional medical center concurrently with participants at a remote telehealth site. This class was conducted so that it mirrored previously offered non-telehealth preoperative classes. Patient education materials were mailed to the 46 telehealth participants' homes before the class, and they were asked to bring these materials to the telehealth sites on the day of the class. At the remote sites, trained on-site coordinators escorted participants and their families to the telehealth rooms. They were given instructions about how to ask questions or make comments to the presenter at the medical center. Efforts were made to actively involve the participants at the telehealth sites by addressing them individually during the class. All participants were asked to complete an evaluation of the class at its conclusion.

Findings

At the conclusion of the program, the evaluative survey data were analyzed. Findings included the following:

- Twenty of a total of 46 of the evaluation forms were returned, a response rate of 43%, which is an above-average survey response rate.
- All 20 of the respondents confirmed that the use of the telehealth network was an acceptable way to obtain the educational information.
- The average length of stay before and after implementation of interactive telehealth education classes decreased for total hip arthroplasty surgery from 6.3 to 5.6 days and for total knee arthroplasty from 5.4 to 4.8 days. These findings suggest that attendance at these classes may have been associated with shorter hospital length of stay and hence decreased costs.

Nursing Implications

This medical center continues to use telehealth education for total joint preoperative education for rural patients and their families. Nurses are key players in the development of these types of alternative educational programs for patients without ready access to medical centers.

dinate the administration of effective analgesic medications (eg, opioids, nonsteroidal anti-inflammatory drugs) with the anesthesiologist, anesthetist, and surgeon. Alternative methods of achieving analgesia (eg, distraction, focusing, guided imagery, quiet environment, back rubs) may be used to decrease pain. The nurse assesses and documents the pain location, quality, and intensity both before and after administering analgesic medications in order to gauge their effectiveness at achieving pain relief.

Maintaining Adequate Neurovascular Function

Trauma, edema, or immobilization devices may interrupt tissue perfusion. The nurse must frequently assess neurovascular status (ie, color, temperature, capillary refill, pulses, edema, pain, sensation, motion) of the extremity and document the findings. If circulation is compromised, the nurse institutes measures to restore adequate circulation. These include promptly notifying the physician, elevating the extremity, and releasing constricting wraps or assisting with bivalving constrictive casts as prescribed.

Promoting Health

The nurse assists the patient in performing activities that promote health during the perioperative period. The nurse assesses nutritional status and hydration. The preoperative fasting regimen is usually tolerated well. If the patient has diabetes, is elderly and frail, or has experienced multiple trauma, special fluid and nutritional provisions may be necessary.

The nurse monitors fluid intake, urinary output, and urinalysis findings. At times, patients may limit their fluid intake to minimize the use of a bedpan. A small fracture bedpan may be more comfortable for the patient to use. An indwelling catheter should be used only when necessary to minimize the risk of urinary tract infection. A preexisting urinary tract infection must be effectively treated prior to surgery.

Coughing, deep breathing, and use of the incentive spirometer are practiced preoperatively for improved respiratory function during the postoperative period. Preoperative teaching facilitates postoperative adherence to respiratory exercises. Smoking should be stopped during the preoperative period to facilitate optimal respiratory function.

The nurse provides skin care, paying special attention to pressure points. It is important to institute the use of pressure-reducing surfaces (ie, special mattresses) before surgery for patients who are at high risk for skin breakdown.

To minimize the risk of infection, the nurse meticulously and gently cleans the skin with soap and water on the day before surgery. If the surgery is elective, the orthopedic surgeon may instruct the patient to use a germicidal soap for several days before hospitalization. The patient may be asked to mark the operative site prior to surgery to minimize the risk that the wrong site is selected in the operating room.

The nurse discusses with the patient and the family the need for assistance with ADLs and the therapeutic regimen during convalescence so that adequate support is available when the patient is discharged. Modification of the home environment may be necessary to accommodate the altered mobility of the patient after surgery. Referral to the social worker and the case manager may be needed to ensure a smooth transition to home care.

Improving Mobility

Preoperatively, the patient's mobility may be impaired by pain, swelling, and immobilizing devices (eg, splints, casts, traction). The nurse should elevate and adequately support edematous extremities with pillows. It is important to control pain before an injured part is moved by administering analgesic medication in time for it to take effect. The injured part is supported when it is moved. The nurse encourages movement within the limits of therapeutic immobility. The patient should perform active range-of-motion exercises of uninvolved joints, and, unless contraindicated, the nurse teaches gluteal-setting and quadriceps-setting isometric exercises to maintain the muscles needed for ambulation (see Chart 67-3). The patient who will be using assistive devices postoperatively may exercise to strengthen the upper extremities and shoulders. If the use of assistive devices (eg, crutches, walker, wheelchair) is anticipated, the nurse encourages the patient to practice with them preoperatively to facilitate their safe use and to promote earlier independent mobility.

Helping the Patient Maintain Self-Esteem

Preoperatively, orthopedic patients may need assistance in accepting changes in body image, diminished self-esteem, or inability to perform their roles and responsibilities. The degree of assistance required in this area varies greatly, depending on the events preceding hospitalization, the surgery and rehabilitation planned, and the temporary or permanent nature of the problems. The nurse promotes a trusting relationship so that the patient feels comfortable expressing concerns and anxieties, and helps the patient examine his or her feelings about changes in self-concept. The nurse clarifies any misconceptions the patient may have and helps the patient work through modifications needed to adapt to alterations in physical capacity and to reestablish positive self-esteem.

Evaluation

Expected Patient Outcomes

Expected patient outcomes may include:

1. Reports relief of pain
    a. Uses multiple approaches to reduce pain
    b. States that medication is effective in relieving pain
    c. Moves with increasing comfort
2. Exhibits adequate neurovascular function
    a. Exhibits normal skin color
    b. Has warm skin
    c. Has normal capillary refill response
    d. Reports normal sensation and demonstrates joint motion
    e. Demonstrates reduced swelling
3. Promotes health
    a. Eats balanced diet appropriate to meet nutritional needs
    b. Maintains adequate hydration
    c. Abstains from smoking
    d. Practices respiratory exercises
    e. Repositions self to relieve skin pressure
    f. Engages in strengthening and preventive exercises
    g. Plans for assistance during convalescence at home
4. Maximizes mobility within therapeutic limits
    a. Requests assistance when moving
    b. Elevates edematous extremity after transfer
    c. Uses immobilizing devices and assistive devices safely as prescribed
5. Expresses positive self-esteem
    a. Acknowledges temporary or permanent changes in body image
    b. Discusses role performance changes
    c. Participates in decisions about care

Nursing Process

Postoperative Care of the Patient Undergoing Orthopedic Surgery

Assessment

After orthopedic surgery, the nurse continues the preoperative care plan, modifying it to match the patient's current postoperative status. The nurse reassesses the patient's needs related to pain, neurovascular status, health promotion, mobility, and self-esteem. Skeletal trauma and surgery performed on bones, muscles, or joints can produce significant pain, especially during the first 1 or 2 postoperative days. Tissue perfusion must be monitored closely, because edema and bleeding into the tissues can compromise circulation and result in compartment syndrome. Inactivity contributes to venous stasis and the development of venous thromboemboli that may include DVTs or PEs. General anesthesia, analgesia, and immobility can result in altered functioning of the respiratory, gastrointestinal, and urinary systems.

The nurse notes the prescribed limits on mobility and assesses the patient's understanding of the mobility restrictions. The nurse discusses the plan of care with the patient and encourages his or her active participation in the plan.

In addition, the nurse assesses and monitors the patient for potential problems related to the surgery. Frequent assessment of vital signs including pain, level of consciousness, neurovascular status, wound drainage, breath sounds, bowel sounds, and fluid balance provides the nurse with data that may suggest the possible development of complications. The nurse reports abnormal findings to the physician promptly.

With major orthopedic surgery, there is a risk for hypovolemic shock because of blood loss. Muscle dissection frequently produces wounds in which hemostasis is poor. Wounds that are closed under tourniquet control may bleed during the postoperative period. The nurse must be alert for signs of hypovolemic shock.

Changes in the patient's pulse rate, respiratory rate, or color of the skin or mucous membranes may indicate pulmonary or cardiovascular complications. Atelectasis and pneumonia are common and may be related to preexisting pulmonary disease, deep anesthesia, decreased activity, and reduced respiratory reserve due to advanced age or an underlying musculoskeletal disorder (eg, restrictive lung expansion secondary to kyphosis, rheumatoid arthritis, or osteoporosis).

Voiding in unnatural positions may contribute to urinary retention. In addition, elderly men usually have some degree of prostate enlargement and may already have difficulty voiding. Therefore, it is important to monitor urinary output.

Temperature elevations within the first 48 hours are frequently related to atelectasis or other respiratory problems. Temperature elevations during the next few days are frequently associated with urinary tract infections. Superficial wound infections take 4 to 6 days to develop. Fever from phlebitis usually occurs during the end of the first week through the second week.

Venous thromboembolus (see discussions of DVT in Chapter 31 and PE in Chapter 23) is one of the most common and most dangerous of all complications occurring in the postoperative orthopedic patient. Advanced age, venous stasis, lower extremity orthopedic surgery, and immobilization are significant risk factors. The nurse assesses the patient daily for unilateral calf swelling, tenderness, warmth, and redness. The nurse promptly reports abnormal findings to the physician.

In addition, fat emboli syndrome (FES) (see Chapter 69) may occur with orthopedic surgery. The nurse must be alert to any signs and symptoms that may suggest the development of FES. These may include respiratory distress; onset of delirium or any acute change in level of consciousness; and development of unusual skin rashes, especially a papular rash on the upper torso.

Diagnosis

Nursing Diagnoses

Based on all assessment data, the patient's major nursing diagnoses after orthopedic surgery may include the following:

- Acute pain related to the surgical procedure, swelling, and immobilization
- Risk for peripheral neurovascular dysfunction related to swelling, constricting devices, or impaired circulation
- Risk for ineffective therapeutic regimen management related to insufficient knowledge or available support and resources
- Impaired physical mobility related to pain, edema, or the presence of an immobilizing device (eg, splint, cast, or brace)
- Risk for situational low self-esteem, disturbed body image or ineffective role performance related to impact of the musculoskeletal disorder

Collaborative Problems/ Potential Complications

Based on the assessment data, potential complications may include the following:

- Hypovolemic shock
- Atelectasis; pneumonia
- Urinary retention
- Infection
- Venous thromboembolism, including DVT or PE
- Constipation and fecal impaction

Planning and Goals

The major goals for the patient after orthopedic surgery may include relief of pain, adequate neurovascular function, health promotion, improved mobility, positive self-esteem, and absence of complications.

Nursing Interventions

Relieving Pain

After orthopedic surgery, pain can be intense. Edema, hematomas, and muscle spasms contribute to the pain. Some patients report that the pain is less than that experienced preoperatively, and only moderate amounts of analgesics are needed. The nurse assesses the patient's level of pain, evaluates the patient's response to therapeutic measures, and makes every effort to relieve the pain and discomfort. Pain assessment must occur on an ongoing basis and take place at least as often as vital signs are assessed.

Multiple pharmacologic approaches to pain management exist. Patient-controlled analgesia (PCA) and epidural analgesia may be prescribed to relieve the pain. If the patient is receiving preemptive analgesia on an ongoing basis via a PCA IV pump, the nurse ensures that the patient receives boluses of the analgesic agent prior to performing planned physical activities. If intramuscular and oral analgesics are prescribed on an as-needed basis (PRN), the nurse should administer medications on a preventive basis within the prescribed intervals if the onset of pain can be predicted (eg, 30 minutes before planned activity such as transfer or exercise). The nurse should offer the medication at set intervals. The nurse rotates intramuscular injection sites, avoiding the operative hip and thigh.

In addition to pharmacologic approaches to controlling pain, elevation of the operative extremity and application of cold packs, if prescribed, help control edema and pain. Surgical drains inserted in the wound decrease fluid accumulation and hematoma formation. The nurse may find that repositioning, relaxation, distraction, and guided imagery help in reducing the patient's pain.

The nurse should report increasing and uncontrollable pain to the orthopedic surgeon for evaluation. Pain should diminish rapidly after the initial postoperative period. After 2 to 3 days, most patients require only occasional oral analgesia for residual muscle soreness and spasm.

Maintaining Adequate Neurovascular Function

The nurse continues the preoperative plan of care. The nurse monitors the neurovascular status of the involved body part and notifies the physician promptly of any indications of diminished tissue perfusion. The patient is reminded to perform muscle-setting, ankle, and calf-pumping exercises hourly while awake to enhance circulation.

Maintaining Health

The nurse continues the preoperative plan of care. It is important to encourage the patient to participate in the postoperative treatment regimen.

A well-balanced diet with adequate protein and vitamins is essential for wound healing. The patient progresses to a regular diet as soon as possible. However, large amounts of milk should not be given to orthopedic patients who are on bed rest, because this may increase serum calcium levels and require the kidneys to excrete more calcium, which increases the risk of urinary calculi.

The nurse assesses the patient for early manifestations of pressure ulcers (eg, redness over bony prominences), which are a threat to any patient who must spend an extended time in bed or who is elderly, malnourished, or unable to move without assistance. Turning the patient frequently at preset intervals (eg, every 2 hours), washing and drying the skin, and minimizing pressure over bony prominences are necessary to avoid skin breakdown.

Improving Physical Mobility

Patients are frequently reluctant to move after orthopedic surgery. Preoperative education about the planned postoperative treatment regimen promotes patient adherence to an optimal rehabilitation regimen. Patients often increase their mobility once they have been reassured that movement within therapeutic limits is beneficial, that the nurse will provide assistance, and that discomfort can be controlled.

Metal pins, screws, rods, and plates used for internal fixation are designed to maintain the position of the bone until ossification occurs. They are not designed to support the body's weight, and they can bend, loosen, or break if stressed. The estimated strength of the bone, the stability of the fracture, reduction and fixation, and the amount of bone healing are important considerations in determining weight-bearing limits. Although the incision may appear healed, the underlying bone requires more time to repair and regain normal strength. Some orthopedic procedures require weight-bearing restrictions. The orthopedic surgeon will prescribe the weight-bearing limits and the use of protective devices (orthoses), if necessary, after surgery.

The physical therapist tailors the rehabilitation program to each patient's needs. The goal is the patient's return to the highest level of function in the shortest time possible. Rehabilitation involves progressive increases in the patient's activities and exercises. Assistive devices (crutches, walker) may be used for postoperative mobility. Preoperative practice with assistive devices helps the patient use them appropriately postoperatively. The nurse makes sure that the patient uses these devices safely (see discussions of crutch walking and use of a walker in Chapter 11).

Maintaining Self-Esteem

The nurse continues the preoperative plan of care. The nurse and the patient set realistic goals. Increased ability to perform self-care activities within the limits of the therapeutic regimen and resumption of roles facilitate the patient's recognition of abilities and promote self-esteem, personal identity, and role performance. Acceptance of altered body image is facilitated by support provided by the nurse, family, and others.

Monitoring and Managing Potential Complications

HYPOVOLEMIC SHOCK

Excessive loss of blood during or after surgery can result in shock. The nurse monitors the patient for signs and symptoms of hypovolemic shock: increased pulse rate (eg, >100 bpm), decreased blood pressure (eg, <90/60 mm Hg), narrowed pulse pressure (eg, <20 mm Hg), urine output less than 30 mL per hour, restlessness, change in mentation, thirst, and decreased hemoglobin and hematocrit. The nurse reports these findings to the orthopedic surgeon and assists in appropriate management. (See Chapter 15 for a discussion of managing shock.)

ATELECTASIS AND PNEUMONIA

The nurse monitors the patient's breath sounds and encourages deep-breathing and coughing exercises. Full expansion of the lungs prevents the accumulation of pulmonary secretions and the development of atelectasis and pneumonia. Incentive spirometry use is encouraged. If signs of respiratory problems develop (eg, increased respiratory rate, productive cough, diminished or adventitious breath sounds, fever), the nurse reports the findings to the surgeon.

URINARY RETENTION

The nurse closely monitors the patient's urinary output after surgery. The nurse encourages the patient to void every 3 to 4 hours to prevent urinary retention and bladder distention. It is important to provide privacy during toileting. Because the patient may need to void in an unusual position, the nurse assists the patient with positioning. Fracture bedpans may be more comfortable to use than other bedpans. Voiding in the side-lying position may be helpful to the male patient. Some male patients can void only if standing, and clarification with the surgeon of the activity prescription may be needed before the patient is assisted to a standing position.

If the patient cannot void, intermittent catheterizations may be prescribed until the patient can void independently. Indwelling urinary catheters should be used only when necessary and should be removed as soon as possible. The patient may follow a catheterization protocol that incorporates the use of a bladder scanner to estimate the amount of urine in the bladder, thereby determining if catheterization is necessary. Catheterization protocol use has decreased the number of nosocomial urinary tract infections created by unnecessary catheterizations (Frederickson, Neitzel, Miller, et al., 2000).

INFECTION

Infection is a risk after any surgery, but it is of particular concern for the postoperative orthopedic patient because of the high risk of osteomyelitis. Osteomyelitis often requires prolonged courses of IV antibiotics. At times, the infected bone and prosthesis or internal fixation device must be surgically removed. Therefore, prophylactic systemic antibiotics are usually prescribed during the perioperative and immediate postoperative period. The nurse assesses the patient's response to these antibiotics. When changing dressings and emptying wound drainage devices, aseptic technique is essential. The nurse monitors the patient's vital signs, incision, and drainage. The nurse monitors the patient for signs of urinary tract infection. Prompt assessment for and treatment of infection are essential.

VENOUS THROMBOEMBOLISM AND DEEP VEIN THROMBOSIS

Prevention of DVT requires use of ankle and calf-pumping exercises, elastic compression stockings, and sequential compression devices. Adequate hydration and early mobilization are equally important. Prophylactic warfarin (Coumadin), low-molecular-weight heparin (eg, enoxaparin [Lovenox], dalteparin [Fragmin]), or low-dose unfractionated heparin may be prescribed in the immediate postoperative period. Typically, either warfarin or aspirin is prescribed during the later rehabilitation period for DVT prophylaxis (Rice & Walsh, 2001). The nurse monitors the patient for signs of DVT and promptly reports findings to the physician for management.

CONSTIPATION

Constipation is a frequently overlooked complication, because patients are discharged to a rehabilitation or home setting in 3 or 4 days. Constipation occurs because of decreased mobility and hydration, coupled with the use of opioids. Prevention of constipation requires continual monitoring of bowel function. Adequate hydration, early mobilization, and stool softeners may be prescribed to prevent fecal impaction (see Chapter 38).

PROMOTING HOME AND COMMUNITY-BASED CARE

Teaching the Patient Self-Care

Because the length of stay in the hospital after orthopedic surgery is usually 3 or 4 days, most convalescence and rehabilitation take place at home or in a nonacute care setting. The nurse teaches the patient and the family to recognize complications that must be reported promptly to the orthopedic surgeon. The patient must understand the prescribed medication regimen. The nurse should demonstrate proper wound care. The patient gradually resumes physical activities and adheres to weight-bearing limits. The patient must be able to perform transfers and to use mobility aids safely. If the patient has a cast or other immobilizing device, family members should be instructed about how to assist the patient in a way that is safe for the patient and for the family member (eg, using proper body mechanics when assisting the patient). Specific exercises need to be taught and practiced before discharge. The nurse discusses recovery and health promotion, emphasizing a healthy lifestyle and diet.

Continuing Care

If special equipment or home modifications are needed for safe care at home, they must be in place before the patient is discharged home. Discharge planning begins immediately after surgery. The nurse, physical therapist, and social worker can assist the patient and family in identifying their needs and in getting ready to care for the patient at home.

CHART 67-11

HOME CARE CHECKLIST • The Patient Who Has Had Orthopedic Surgery

At the completion of the home care instruction, the patient or caregiver will be able to:	Patient	Caregiver
• Describe wound care	✔	✔
• State indicators of wound infections (eg, redness, swelling, tenderness, purulent drainage, fever)	✔	✔
• Consume a healthy diet to promote wound and bone healing	✔	
• Participate in prescribed exercise regimen to promote circulation and mobility	✔	
• Use mobility aids safely	✔	
• Observe prescribed weight-bearing and activity limits	✔	
• Take prescribed therapeutic and prophylactic medications (eg, antibiotics, anticoagulants, analgesics)	✔	
• State indicators of complications to report promptly to physician (eg, uncontrolled swelling and pain; cool, pale fingers or toes; paresthesia; paralysis; purulent drainage; signs of systemic infection; signs of deep vein thrombosis or pulmonary emboli)	✔	✔
• Identify modifications of home environment to promote safe environment and independence during recovery and rehabilitation	✔	✔

Frequently, home health nursing and home physical therapy are part of the discharge plan of care. These referrals provide resources and help the patient and the family cope with the demands of care during convalescence and rehabilitation. The nurse can explore problems that the patient and family identify during the home care visit. The nurse assesses the patient's progress and monitors for possible complications. Regular medical follow-up care after discharge needs to be arranged (Chart 67-11).

Because patients and their family members and health care providers tend to focus on the most obvious needs and issues, the nurse reminds the patient and family about the importance of continuing health promotion and screening practices. Patients who have not been involved in these practices in the past are educated about their importance and are referred to appropriate health care providers.

Evaluation

Expected Patient Outcomes

Expected patient outcomes may include:

1. Reports decreased level of pain
   a. Uses multiple approaches to reduce pain
   b. Uses occasional oral analgesic medication to control discomfort
   c. Elevates extremity to control edema and discomfort
   d. Moves with greater comfort
2. Exhibits adequate neurovascular function
   a. Exhibits normal color and temperature of skin
   b. Has warm skin
   c. Has normal capillary refill response
   d. Demonstrates intact sensory and motor function
   e. Demonstrates reduced swelling
3. Promotes health
   a. Eats diet appropriate for nutritional needs
   b. Maintains adequate hydration
   c. Abstains from smoking
   d. Practices respiratory exercises
   e. Repositions self to relieve pressure on skin
   f. Engages in strengthening and preventive exercises
4. Maximizes mobility within the therapeutic limits
   a. Requests assistance when moving
   b. Elevates edematous extremity after transfer
   c. Uses immobilizing devices as prescribed
   d. Complies with prescribed weight-bearing limitation
5. Expresses positive self-esteem
   a. Discusses temporary or permanent changes in body image
   b. Discusses role performance
   c. Views self as capable of assuming responsibilities
   d. Actively participates in planning care and in the therapeutic regimen
6. Exhibits absence of complications
   a. Does not experience shock
   b. Maintains normal vital signs and blood pressure
   c. Has clear lung sounds
   d. Demonstrates wound healing without signs of infection
   e. Does not experience urinary retention
   f. Voids clear urine
   g. Exhibits no signs of DVT or PE
   h. Does not experience constipation

Critical Thinking Exercises

1 An 84-year-old woman has had an internal fixation for her fractured hip. On her second postoperative day, she complains that her elastic stockings feel tight and hot and asks you to remove them. How would you respond to this request? What is the rationale for your action? Role-play your explanation to her regarding the purpose of the stockings.

2 A 68-year-old man has had a repair of a fracture of his right tibia. During the evening of his second postoperative day, he complains of increasing pain and slight paresthesias of his right toes. Opioid analgesics have only moderately relieved his pain. The night-shift nurse documents her findings and asks you, as the oncoming day-shift nurse, to report these findings to the orthopedic surgeon when he makes his rounds. You assess the patient after report and find that he now describes his right lower leg as "feeling tight" and that he has sensations of "pins and needles." His right lower leg is shiny, capillary refill is longer than 3 seconds, and his right toes feel much cooler than the left toes. What additional assessments might you make at this time? What is your priority nursing diagnosis and intervention?

3 ebp You are an experienced orthopedic nurse and you note that different orthopedic surgical groups at the orthopedic unit where you work have different protocols for knee and hip surgery redressings. One group prescribes an antibiotic ointment (eg, Neosporin) with a clean dressing applied to the surgical site, a second group uses no dressing or ointment to the surgical site, and a third group prescribes Betadine and a sterile dressing applied to the surgical site. What is the strength of the evidence that identifies whether one type of surgical site dressing is superior to the others?

4 An 80-year-old woman with multiple trauma has had open reduction with internal fixation (ORIF) of her right hip. On the second postoperative day, a physical therapy assistant helps the patient get out of bed. She has been sitting out of bed for approximately an hour and a half when she requests to be placed back in bed. What is the best way to accomplish this transfer from chair to bed? What specific precautions might you follow?

REFERENCES AND SELECTED READINGS

BOOKS

Kneale, J. (2005). *Orthopaedic nursing* (2nd ed.). Philadelphia: Elsevier.

Kneale, J., & Davis, P. (2004). *Orthopaedic and trauma nursing*. Philadelphia: Elsevier.

Magee, D. (2002). *Orthopedic physical assessment* (4th ed.). Philadelphia: Elsevier.

Maher, A., Salmond, S., & Pellino, T. (2002). *Orthopaedic nursing* (3rd ed.). Philadelphia: Elsevier.

Marcus, J., & Lawrence, K. (2001). *Orthopaedic patient education resource manual*. Gaithersburg, MD: Aspen Publishers.

Mercier, L. (2000). *Practical orthopedics* (5th ed.). St. Louis: Mosby.

Miller, M. (2004). *Review of orthopaedics*. Philadelphia: Elsevier.

Moehring, H., & Greenspan, A. (2000). *Fractures: Diagnosis and treatment*. New York: McGraw-Hill.

Munziger, U. (2004). *Primary knee arthroplasty*. New York: Springer-Verlag.

Schoen, D. (2000). *Adult orthopaedic nursing*. Philadelphia: Lippincott Williams & Wilkins.

Schoen, D. (2000). *Clinical orthopaedic nursing: An illustrated guide*. Philadelphia: Lippincott Williams & Wilkins.

Schoen, D. (Ed.). (2001). *NAON core curriculum for orthopaedic nursing* (4th ed.). Pitman, NJ: National Association of Orthopaedic Nurses.

U.S. Department of Health and Human Services. (2004). *Bone health and osteoporosis: A report of the Surgeon General*. Rockville, MD: U.S. Department of Health and Human Services, Office of the Surgeon General.

JOURNALS

**An asterisk indicates nursing research articles.*

Altizer, L. (2004a). Casting for immobilization. *Orthopaedic Nursing, 23*(2), 136–141.

Altizer, L. (2004b). Patient education for total hip or knee replacement. *Orthopaedic Nursing, 23*(4), 283–288.

Bisaillon, S., Faraone, J., Elliott, K., et al. (2004). Improving care for orthopaedic patients undergoing surgery for hip fracture and total knee replacement through best practice. *Orthopaedic Nursing, 8*(4), 215–220.

Bernardo, L. M. (2001). EBP for pin site care in injured children. *Orthopaedic Nursing, 20*(5), 29–34.

Best, J. (2005). Revision total hip and total knee arthroplasty. *Orthopaedic Nursing, 24*(3), 174–181.

Davis, P. (2004). A critical exploration of practice improvement in orthopaedic nursing with reference to venous thromboembolism prevention. *Journal of Orthopaedic Nursing, 8*(4), 208–214.

Doheny, M. O., & Deuchec, M. J. (2001). Healthy People 2010: Implications for orthopaedic nurses. *Orthopaedic Nursing, 20*(4), 59–65.

*Feldt, K. S., & Gunderson, J. (2002). Treatment of pain for older hip fracture patients across settings. *Orthopaedic Nursing, 21*(5), 63–71.

*Frederickson, M., Neitzel, J., Miller, E. H., et al. (2000). The implementation of bedside bladder ultrasound technology: Effects of patient and cost postoperative outcomes in tertiary care. *Orthopaedic Nursing, 19*(3), 79–87.

Geier, K. (2000). Improving outcomes in elective orthopaedic surgery: A guide for nurses and total joint arthroplasty patients. *Orthopaedic Nursing, 19*(suppl.), 4–31.

Harvey, C. (2001). Compartment syndrome: When it is least expected. *Orthopaedic Nursing, 20*(3), 15–26.

Hohlt, T. (2000). Deep-vein thrombosis prevention in orthopaedic patients: Affecting outcomes through interdisciplinary education. *Orthopaedic Nursing, 19*(5), 73–78.

Holmes, S. B., & Brown, S. J. (2005). Skeletal pin site care: National Association of Orthopaedic Nurses guidelines for orthopaedic nursing. *Orthopaedic Nursing, 24*(2), 99–107.

McEwen, J. A., Kelly, D. L., Jardanowski, T., et al. (2002). Tourniquet safety in lower leg application. *Orthopaedic Nursing, 21*(5), 55–62.

*Moon, L., & Backer, J. (2000). Relationships among self-efficacy, outcome expectancy, and postoperative behaviors in total joint replacement patients. *Orthopaedic Nursing, 19*(2), 77–85.

*Morris, B. (2004). Nursing initiatives for deep vein thrombosis prophylaxis: Pragmatic timing of administration. *Orthopaedic Nursing, 23*(2), 142–149.

Rabenberg, V. S., Ingersoll, C. D., Sandrey, M. A., et al. (2002). The bactericidal and cytotoxic effects of antimicrobial wound cleansers. *Journal of Athletic Training, 37*(1), 51–54.

Rice, K. L., & Walsh, E. M. (2001). Minimizing venous thromboembolic complications in the orthopaedic patient. *Orthopaedic Nursing, 20*(6), 21–27.

*Ridge, R., & Goodson, A. (2000). The relationship between multidisciplinary discharge outcomes and functional status after total hip replacement. *Orthopaedic Nursing, 19*(1), 71–82.

Schoen, D. C. (2003). Hip fracture. *Orthopaedic Nursing, 22*(4), 307–309.

*Slowikowski, R., & Flaherty, J. (2000). Epidural analgesia for postoperative orthopaedic pain. *Orthopaedic Nursing, 19*(1), 23–32.

*Thomas, K., Burton, D., Withrow, L., et al. (2004). Impact of a preoperative education program via interactive telehealth network for rural patients having total joint replacement. *Orthopaedic Nursing, 23*(1), 39–44.

Turkoski, B. (2000). Preventing DVT in orthopaedic patients. *Orthopaedic Nursing, 19*(5), 93–99.

Warner, C. (2001). The use of the orthopaedic perioperative autotransfusion (OrthoPAT) system in total joint replacement surgery. *Orthopaedic Nursing, 20*(6), 29–32.

RESOURCES

National Association of Orthopaedic Nurses (NAON), East Holly Avenue, Box 56, Pitman, NJ 08071; http://www.orthonurse.org. Accessed August 4, 2006.

National Institute of Arthritis and Musculoskeletal and Skin Diseases, National Institutes of Health, 1 AMS Circle, Bethesda, MD 20892; http://www.niams.nih.gov. Accessed August 4, 2006.

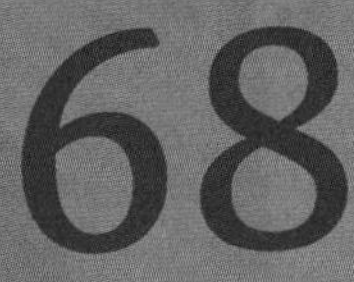

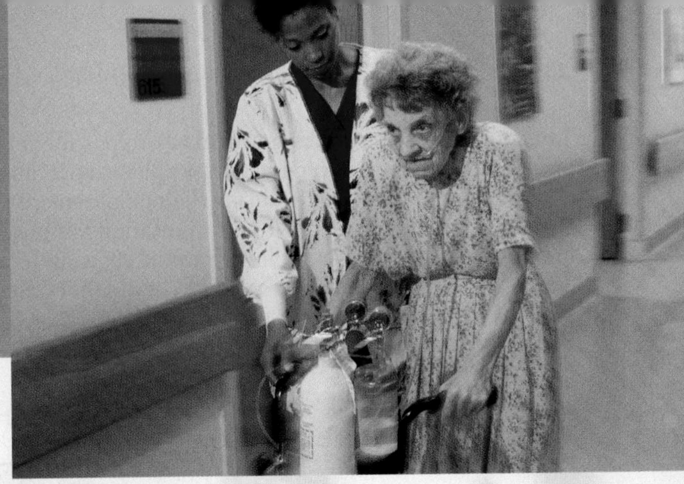

CHAPTER 68

Management of Patients With Musculoskeletal Disorders

Learning Objectives

On completion of this chapter, the learner will be able to:

1. Use the nursing process as a framework for care of the patient with low back pain.
2. Describe the rehabilitation and health education needs of the patient with low back pain.
3. Describe common conditions of the upper extremities and nursing care of the patient undergoing surgery of the hand or wrist.
4. Use the nursing process as a framework for care of the patient undergoing foot surgery.
5. Explain the pathophysiology, pathogenesis, prevention, and management of osteoporosis.
6. Identify the causes and related medical management of osteomalacia.
7. Describe medication modalities for the patient with Paget's disease.
8. Use the nursing process as a framework for care of the patient with osteomyelitis.
9. Use the nursing process as a framework for care of the patient with a bone tumor.

Musculoskeletal disorders, particularly impairment of the back and spine, are leading health problems and causes of disability, mainly in people during their employment years. The functional and psychological limitations imposed on the patient may be severe. The economic costs, in terms of loss of productivity, medical expenses, and other costs that are not compensated, are estimated to exceed $20 billion annually in the United States (Pai & Sundaram, 2004).

Acute Low Back Pain

The number of visits to primary care providers resulting from low back pain is second only to the number of visits for upper respiratory illnesses (Pai & Sundaram, 2004). Most low back pain is caused by one of many musculoskeletal problems, including acute lumbosacral strain, unstable lumbosacral ligaments and weak muscles, osteoarthritis of the spine, spinal stenosis, intervertebral disk problems, and unequal leg length.

Older patients may experience back pain associated with osteoporotic vertebral fractures or bone metastasis. Other causes include kidney disorders, pelvic problems, retroperitoneal tumors, and abdominal aortic aneurysms.

In addition, obesity, stress, and occasionally depression may contribute to low back pain. Back pain due to musculoskeletal disorders usually is aggravated by activity, whereas pain due to other conditions is not. Patients with chronic low back pain may develop a dependence on alcohol or analgesics used to cope with and self-treat the pain.

Pathophysiology

The spinal column can be considered as an elastic rod constructed of rigid units (vertebrae) and flexible units (intervertebral disks) held together by complex facet joints, multiple ligaments, and paravertebral muscles. Its unique construction allows for flexibility while providing maximum protection for the spinal cord. The spinal curves absorb vertical shocks from running and jumping. The trunk muscles help stabilize the spine. The abdominal and thoracic muscles are important in lifting activities, working together to minimize stress on the spinal units. Disuse weakens these supporting muscular structures. Obesity, postural problems, structural problems, and overstretching of the spinal supports may result in back pain.

The intervertebral disks change in character as a person ages. A young person's disks are mainly fibrocartilage with a gelatinous matrix. As a person ages, the fibrocartilage becomes dense and irregularly shaped. Disk degeneration is a common cause of back pain. The lower lumbar disks, L4–L5 and L5–S1, are subject to the greatest mechanical stress and the greatest degenerative changes. Disk protrusion (herniated nucleus pulposus) or facet joint changes can cause pressure on nerve roots as they leave the spinal canal, which results in pain that radiates along the nerve. Management of intervertebral disk disease is discussed in Chapter 65.

Clinical Manifestations

The typical patient reports either acute back pain (lasting less than 3 months) or chronic back pain (lasting more than 3 months without improvement) and fatigue. The patient may report pain radiating down the leg, which is known as **radiculopathy** or **sciatica**; presence of this symptom suggests nerve root involvement. The patient's gait, spinal mobility, reflexes, leg length, leg motor strength, and sensory perception may be affected. Physical examination may disclose paravertebral muscle spasm (greatly increased muscle tone of the back postural muscles) with a loss of the normal lumbar curve and possible spinal deformity.

Assessment and Diagnostic Findings

The Agency for Heathcare Research and Quality (1994) developed guidelines for assessment and management of acute low back pain. These safe, conservative, cost-effective, and evidence-based guidelines were developed to help reduce the use of noneffective therapeutic interventions, including prolonged bed rest.

The initial evaluation of acute low back pain includes a focused history and physical examination, including general observation of the patient, back examination, and neurologic testing (reflexes, sensory impairment, straight-leg raising, muscle strength, and muscle atrophy). The findings suggest either nonspecific back symptoms or potentially serious problems, such as sciatica, spine fracture, cancer, infection, or rapidly progressing neurologic deficit. If the initial examination does not suggest a serious condition, no additional testing is performed during the first 4 weeks of symptoms.

The diagnostic procedures described in Chart 68-1 may be indicated for the patient with potentially serious or prolonged low back pain. The nurse prepares the patient for these studies, provides the necessary support during the testing period, and monitors the patient for any adverse responses to the procedures.

Glossary

bursitis: inflammation of a fluid-filled sac in a joint
contracture: abnormal shortening of muscle or fibrosis of joint structures
involucrum: new bone growth around a sequestrum
radiculopathy: disease of a nerve root
sciatica: sciatic nerve pain; pain travels down back of thigh into foot
sequestrum: dead bone in abscess cavity
tendinitis: inflammation of muscle tendons

CHART 68-1

Diagnostic Procedures for Low Back Pain

X-ray of the spine—may demonstrate a fracture, dislocation, infection, osteoarthritis, or scoliosis
Bone scan and blood studies—may disclose infections, tumors, and bone marrow abnormalities
Computed tomography (CT)—useful in identifying underlying problems, such as obscure soft tissue lesions adjacent to the vertebral column and problems of vertebral disks
Magnetic resonance imaging (MRI)—permits visualization of the nature and location of spinal pathology
Electromyogram (EMG) and nerve conduction studies—used to evaluate spinal nerve root disorders (radiculopathies)

Medical Management

Most back pain is self-limited and resolves within 4 weeks with analgesics, rest, stress reduction, and relaxation. Based on initial assessment findings, the patient is reassured that the assessment indicates that the back pain is not due to a serious condition. Management focuses on relief of pain and discomfort, activity modification, and patient education.

Nonprescription analgesics (eg, acetaminophen [Tylenol], ibuprofen [Motrin]) are usually effective in achieving pain relief. At times, a patient may require the addition of muscle relaxants or opioids. Heat or cold therapy frequently provides temporary relief of symptoms. In the absence of symptoms of disease (radiculopathy of the roots of spinal nerves), spinal manipulation performed by a chiropractor or an osteopath may be helpful. Laser therapy using a handheld device that emits electromagnetic radiation directly to the lower back is effective in alleviating symptoms over the short term, but its long-term efficacy is unknown. Recent evidence suggests that massage may be therapeutic. Other physical modalities, including traction, hydrotherapy, ultrasound, biofeedback, transcutaneous electrical nerve stimulation, and use of magnets, have no proven efficacy in treating acute low back pain (Maher, 2004).

Most patients need to alter their activity patterns to avoid aggravating the pain. Twisting, bending, lifting, and reaching, all of which stress the back, are avoided. The patient is taught to change position frequently. Sitting should be limited to 20 to 50 minutes based on level of comfort. Bed rest is recommended for 1 to 2 days, with a maximum of 4 days and *only* if pain is severe. A gradual return to activities and low-stress aerobic exercise is recommended. Conditioning exercises for the trunk muscles are begun after about 2 weeks.

If there is no improvement within 1 month, additional assessments for physiologic abnormalities are performed. Management is based on findings.

Nursing Process

The Patient With Acute Low Back Pain

Assessment

The nurse asks the patient with low back pain to describe the discomfort (eg, location, severity, duration, characteristics, radiation, associated weakness in the legs). Descriptions of how the pain occurred—with a specific action (eg, opening a garage door) or with an activity in which weak muscles were overused (eg, weekend gardening)—and how the patient has dealt with the pain often suggest areas for intervention and patient teaching.

If back pain is a recurrent problem, information about previous successful pain control methods helps in planning current management. The nurse also asks how the back pain affects the patient's lifestyle. Information about work and recreational activities helps identify areas for back health education. Because stress and anxiety can evoke muscle spasms and pain, the nurse assesses environmental variables, work situations, and family relationships. In addition, the nurse assesses the effect of chronic pain on the emotional well-being of the patient. Referral to a psychiatric advanced practice nurse for assessment and management of stressors contributing to the low back pain and related depression may be appropriate.

During the interview, the nurse observes the patient's posture, position changes, and gait. Often, the patient's movements are guarded, with the back kept as still as possible. The patient often selects a chair of standard seat height with arms for support. The patient may sit and stand in an unusual position, leaning away from the most painful side, and may ask for assistance when undressing for the physical examination.

On physical examination, the nurse assesses the spinal curve, any leg length discrepancy, and pelvic crest and shoulder symmetry. The nurse palpates the paraspinal muscles and notes spasm and tenderness. When the patient is in a prone position, the paraspinal muscles relax, and any deformity caused by spasm subsides. The patient is asked to bend forward and then laterally, and any discomfort or limitations in movement are noted. It is important to determine the effect of these limitations in movement on activities of daily living (ADLs). The nurse evaluates nerve involvement by assessing deep tendon reflexes, sensations (eg, paresthesia), and muscle strength. Back and leg pain on straight-leg raising (with the patient supine, the patient's leg is lifted upward with the knee extended) suggests nerve root involvement. Obesity can contribute to low back pain. If the patient is obese, the nurse completes a nutritional assessment.

Nursing Diagnoses

Based on the assessment data, the patient's major nursing diagnoses may include the following:

- Acute pain related to musculoskeletal problems
- Impaired physical mobility related to pain, muscle spasms, and decreased flexibility
- Deficient knowledge related to back-conserving techniques of body mechanics
- Risk for situational low self-esteem related to impaired mobility, chronic pain, and altered role performance
- Imbalanced nutrition: more than body requirements related to obesity

Planning and Goals

The major goals for the patient may include relief of pain, improved physical mobility, use of back-conserving techniques of body mechanics, improved self-esteem, and weight reduction (Chart 68-2).

Nursing Interventions

Relieving Pain

To relieve pain, the nurse encourages the patient to reduce stress on the back muscles and to change position frequently. The patient is taught to control and modify the perceived pain through behavioral therapies that reduce muscular and psychological tension. Diaphragmatic breathing and relaxation help reduce muscle tension contributing to low back pain. Diverting the patient's attention from the pain to another activity (eg, reading, conversation, watching television) may be helpful in some instances. Guided imagery, in which the relaxed patient learns to focus on a pleasant event, may be used along with other pain-relief strategies (see Chart 68-2).

If medication is prescribed, the nurse assesses the patient's response to each medication. As the acute pain subsides, medication dosages are reduced as prescribed. Self-applied intermittent heat or cold may reduce the pain. The nurse evaluates and notes the patient's response to various pain management modalities.

Improving Physical Mobility

Physical mobility is monitored through continuing assessments. The nurse assesses how the patient moves and stands. As the back pain subsides, self-care activities are resumed with minimal strain on the injured structures. Position changes should be made slowly and carried out with assistance as required. Twisting and jarring motions are avoided. The nurse encourages the patient to alternate lying, sitting, and walking activities frequently and advises the patient to avoid sitting, standing, or walking for long periods. The patient may find that sitting in a chair with arm rests to support some of the body weight and a soft support at the small of the back provides comfort.

CHART 68-2

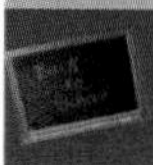

Patient Education

Strategies for Managing Low Back Pain

PAIN MANAGEMENT

- Limit bed rest; keep your knees flexed to decrease strain on your back.
- Try *nonpharmacologic approaches* such as distraction, relaxation, imagery, thermal interventions (eg, ice or heat), and stress reduction.
- *Pharmacologic approaches:* take nonsteroidal anti-inflammatory drugs, analgesics, muscle relaxants as prescribed.

EXERCISE

- Stretch to enhance flexibility. Do strengthening exercises.
- Perform prescribed back exercises to increase function, gradually increasing time and repetitions.

BODY MECHANICS

- Practice good posture.
- Avoid twisting your body.
- Push objects rather than pull them.
- Keep load close to your body when lifting.
- Bend your knees and tighten abdominal muscles when lifting.
- Avoid overreaching.
- Use a wide base of support.
- Use a back brace to protect your back.

WORK MODIFICATIONS

- Adjust work area to avoid stress on back.
- Adjust height of chair or work table.
- Use lumbar support in chair.
- Avoid prolonged standing and repetitive tasks.
- Avoid bending, twisting, and lifting heavy objects.
- Avoid work involving continuous vibrations.

STRESS REDUCTION

- Understand that stress and anxiety can lead to muscle tension and pain.
- Explore effective coping mechanisms.
- Learn and practice stress reduction techniques.
- Follow through on referral to back clinic.

With severe pain, the patient is instructed to limit activities for 1 to 2 days. Extended periods of inactivity are not effective and result in deconditioning. A firm, nonsagging mattress (a bed board may be used) is recommended. Lumbar flexion is increased by elevating the head and thorax 30 degrees using pillows or a foam wedge and slightly flexing the knees supported on a pillow. Alternatively, the patient can assume a lateral position with knees and hips flexed (curled position) with a pillow between the knees and legs and a pillow supporting the head (Fig. 68-1). A prone position should be avoided because it accentuates lordosis. The nurse instructs the patient to get out of bed by rolling to one side and placing the legs down while pushing the torso up, keeping the back straight.

As the patient achieves comfort, activities are gradually resumed, and an exercise program is initiated. Initially, low-stress aerobic exercises, such as short walks or swimming, are suggested. After 2 weeks, conditioning exercises for the abdominal and trunk muscles are started. The physical therapist designs an exercise program for the individual patient to reduce lordosis, increase flexibility, and reduce strain on the back. It may include hyperextension exercises to strengthen the paravertebral muscles, flexion exercises to increase back movement and strength, and isometric flexion exercises to strengthen trunk muscles. Each exercise period begins with relaxation. Exercise begins gradually and increases as the patient recovers.

The nurse encourages the patient to adhere to the prescribed exercise program. Erratic exercising is ineffective. For most exercise programs, it is suggested that the person exercise twice a day for 30 minutes at a time, increasing the number of exercises gradually. Some patients may find it difficult to adhere to a program of prescribed exercises for a long period. These patients are encouraged to improve their posture, use good body mechanics on a regular basis, and engage in regular exercise activities (eg, walking, swimming) to maintain a healthy back. Activities should not cause excessive lumbar strain, twisting, or discomfort; for example, activities such as horseback riding and weight-lifting should be avoided.

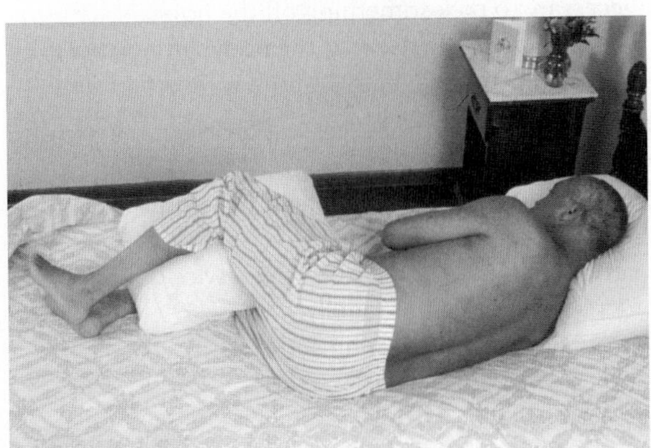

FIGURE 68-1. Positioning to promote lumbar flexion. © B. Proud.

Using Proper Body Mechanics

Good body mechanics and posture are essential to avoid recurrence of back pain. The patient must be taught how to stand, sit, lie, and lift properly (Figs. 68-2 and 68-3). Providing the patient with a list of suggestions helps in making these long-term changes (Chart 68-3). The patient who wears high heels is encouraged to change to low heels with good arch support. The patient who is required to stand for long periods should shift weight frequently and should rest one foot on a low stool, which decreases lumbar lordosis. Patients who stand in place for a long period of time (eg, cashiers) should stand on a foot cushion made of foam or rubber. The proper posture can be verified by looking in a mirror to see whether the chest is up, the abdomen is tucked in, and the shoulders are down and relaxed. Locking the knees when standing is avoided, as is bending forward for long periods.

When the patient is sitting, the knees and hips should be flexed, and the knees should be level with the hips or higher to minimize lordosis. The feet should be flat on the floor. The back needs to be supported, so patients should avoid sitting on stools or chairs that do not provide firm back support. The patient should sleep on the side with knees and hips flexed, or supine with knees supported in a flexed position. Sleeping prone should be avoided.

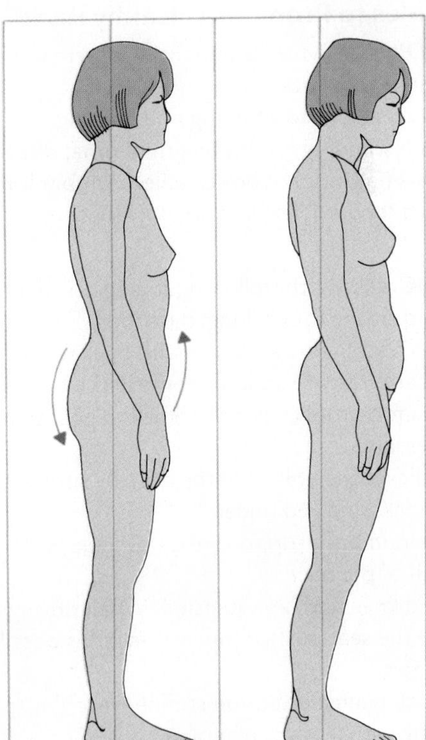

FIGURE 68-2. Proper and improper standing postures. (*Left*) Abdominal muscles contracted, giving a feeling of upward pull, and gluteal muscles contracted, giving a downward pull. (*Right*) Slouch position, showing abdominal muscles relaxed and body out of proper alignment.

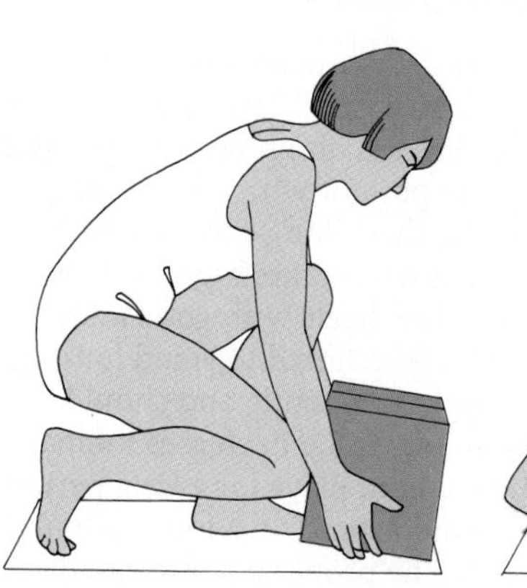
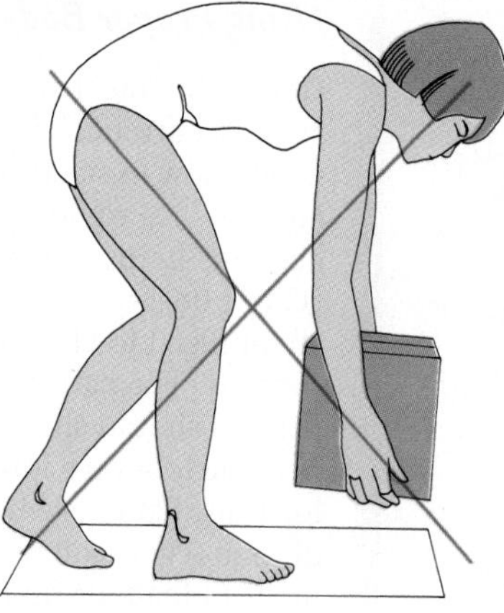

FIGURE 68-3. Proper and improper lifting techniques. (*Left*) Correct position for lifting. This person is using the long and strong muscles of the arms and legs and holding the object so that the line of gravity falls within the base of support. (*Right*) Incorrect position for lifting because pull is exerted on the back muscles and leaning causes the line of gravity to fall outside the base.

The nurse instructs the patient in the safe and correct way to lift objects—using the strong quadriceps muscles of the thighs, with minimal use of weak back muscles. With feet placed hip-width apart to provide a wide base of support, the patient should bend the knees, tighten the abdominal muscles, and lift the object close to the body with a smooth motion, avoiding twisting and jarring motions. To prevent recurrence of acute low back pain, the nurse may instruct the patient to avoid lifting more than one third of his or her weight without help.

It takes about 6 months for a person to readjust postural habits. Practicing these protective and defensive postures, positions, and body mechanics results

CHART 68-3

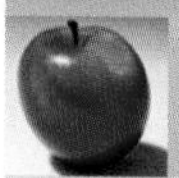

Health Promotion

Activities to Promote a Healthy Back

STANDING. Advise the patient to adhere to the following guidelines:

- Avoid prolonged standing and walking.
- When standing for any length of time, rest one foot on a small stool or box to relieve lumbar lordosis.
- Avoid forward flexion work positions.
- Avoid high heels.

SITTING. Discuss the following strategies with the patient:

- Avoid sitting for prolonged periods.
- Sit in a straight-back chair with back well supported and arm rests to support some of the body weight; use a footstool to position knees higher than hips if necessary.
- Eradicate the hollow of the back by sitting with the buttocks "tucked under."
- Maintain back support; use a soft support at the small of the back.
- Avoid knee and hip extension. When driving a car, have the seat pushed forward as far as possible for comfort.
- Guard against extension strains–reaching, pushing, sitting with legs straight out.
- Alternate periods of sitting with walking.

LYING. Encourage the patient to do the following:

- Rest at intervals; fatigue contributes to spasm of the back muscles.
- Place a firm bed board under the mattress.
- Avoid sleeping in a prone position.
- When lying on the side, place a pillow under the head and one between the legs, with the legs flexed at the hips and knees.
- When supine, use a pillow under the knees to decrease lordosis.

LIFTING. Emphasize the importance of the following strategies:

- When lifting, keep the back straight and hold the load as close to the body as possible.
- Lift with the large leg muscles, not the back muscles.
- Use trunk muscles to stabilize the spine.
- Squat while keeping the back straight when it is necessary to pick something off the floor.
- Avoid twisting the trunk of the body, lifting above waist level, and reaching up for any length of time.

EXERCISING. Daily exercise is important in the prevention of back problems.

- Walk daily and gradually increase the distance and pace of walking.
- Perform prescribed back exercises twice daily, increasing exercise gradually.
- Avoid jumping and jarring activities.

in natural strengthening of the back and diminishes the chance that back pain will recur.

Improving Self-Esteem

Because of the immobility associated with low back pain, the patient may depend on other people to do various tasks. Dependency may continue beyond physiologic needs and become a way to fulfill psychosocial needs. Assisting both the patient and support people to recognize continued dependency helps the patient identify and cope with the underlying reason for the dependency.

Role-related responsibilities may have been modified with the onset of low back pain. As recovery from acute low back pain and immobility progresses, the patient may resume former role-related responsibilities.

However, if these activities contributed to the development of low back pain, it may be difficult to resume them without the development of chronic low back pain syndrome, with associated disability and depression. If the patient experiences secondary gains associated with low back disability (eg, worker's compensation, easier lifestyle or workload, increased emotional support), a "low back neurosis" may develop. The patient may need help in coping with specific stressors and in learning how to control stressful situations. When people successfully deal with stress, they develop confidence in their abilities to manage other stressful situations. Psychotherapy or counseling may be needed to assist the person in resuming a full, productive life. Back clinics use multidisciplinary approaches to help the patient with pain and with resumption of role-related responsibilities.

Modifying Nutrition for Weight Reduction

Obesity contributes to back strain by stressing the relatively weak back muscles. Exercises are less effective and more difficult to perform when the patient is overweight. Weight reduction through diet modification may prevent recurrence of back pain. Weight reduction is based on a sound nutritional plan that includes a change in eating habits to maintain desirable weight. Monitoring weight reduction, noting achievement, and providing encouragement and positive reinforcement facilitate adherence. Frequently, back problems resolve as optimal weight is achieved.

Evaluation

Expected Patient Outcomes

Expected patient outcomes may include the following:

1. Experiences pain relief
   a. Rests comfortably
   b. Changes positions comfortably
   c. Obtains relief through use of physical modalities, psychological techniques, and medications
   d. Avoids drug dependency
2. Demonstrates resumption of physical mobility
   a. Resumes activities gradually
   b. Avoids positions that cause discomfort and muscle spasm
   c. Plans recumbent rest periods throughout the day
3. Demonstrates back-conserving body mechanics
   a. Improves posture
   b. Positions self to minimize stress on the back
   c. Demonstrates use of good body mechanics
   d. Participates in exercise program
4. Resumes role-related responsibilities
   a. Uses coping techniques to deal with stressful situations
   b. Demonstrates decreased dependence on others for self-care
   c. Resumes role responsibilities as low back pain resolves
   d. Resumes full, productive lifestyle
5. Achieves desired weight
   a. Identifies need to lose weight if appropriate
   b. Sets realistic goals
   c. Participates in development of weight-reduction plan
   d. Complies with weight-reduction regimen

Common Upper Extremity Problems

The structures in the upper extremities are frequently the sites of painful syndromes. The structures most frequently affected are the shoulder, wrist, and hand.

Bursitis and Tendinitis

Bursitis and **tendinitis** are inflammatory conditions that commonly occur in the shoulder. Bursae are fluid-filled sacs that prevent friction between joint structures during joint activity. When inflamed, they are painful. Similarly, muscle tendon sheaths become inflamed with repetitive stretching. The inflammation causes proliferation of synovial membrane and pannus formation, which restricts joint movement. Conservative treatment includes rest of the extremity, intermittent ice and heat to the joint, and nonsteroidal anti-inflammatory drugs (NSAIDs) to control the inflammation and pain. Arthroscopic synovectomy may be considered if shoulder pain and weakness persist.

Loose Bodies

Loose bodies may occur in a joint as a result of articular cartilage wear and bone erosion. These fragments interfere with joint movement, locking the joint, resulting in painful movement. Loose bodies are removed by arthroscopic surgery.

Impingement Syndrome

Overuse (microtrauma) may produce an impingement syndrome in the shoulder. The supraspinatus and biceps tendons become irritated and edematous and press against the acromion process, limiting shoulder motion. The patient experiences pain, shoulder tenderness, limited movement, muscle spasm, and atrophy. The process may progress to a rotator cuff tear. Conservative treatment includes rest, NSAIDs, joint injections, and physical therapy (Chart 68-4). Arthroscopic débridement (a minimally invasive surgical procedure that permits evacuation of joint debris) is used for persistent pain. Gentle joint motion is begun after surgery. (See Chapter 69 for a discussion of rotator cuff injury.)

Carpal Tunnel Syndrome

Carpal tunnel syndrome is an entrapment neuropathy that occurs when the median nerve at the wrist is compressed by a thickened flexor tendon sheath, skeletal encroachment, edema, or a soft tissue mass. The syndrome is commonly caused by repetitive hand and wrist movements, but it may also be associated with arthritis, hypothyroidism, or pregnancy. Patients who perform repetitive movements or those whose hands are repeatedly exposed to cold temperatures, vibrations, or extreme direct pressure are at a greater risk for carpal tunnel syndrome. The patient experiences pain, numbness, paresthesia, and possibly weakness along the median nerve (thumb, index, and middle fingers). Tinel's sign may be used to help identify carpal tunnel syndrome (Fig. 68-4). Night pain is common.

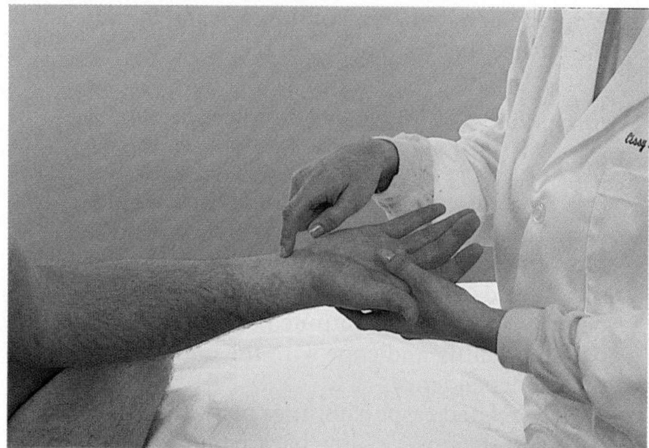

FIGURE 68-4. Tinel's sign may be elicited in patients with carpal tunnel syndrome by percussing lightly over the median nerve, located on the inner aspect of the wrist. If the patient reports tingling, numbness, and pain, the test for Tinel's sign is considered positive. From Weber, J. W., & Kelley, J. (2006). *Health assessment in nursing* (3rd ed.). Philadelphia: Lippincott Williams & Wilkins. © B. Proud.

CHART 68-4

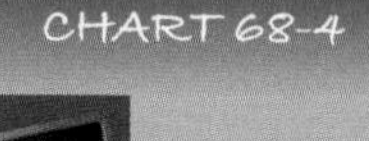

Patient Education

Measures to Promote Shoulder Healing of Impingement Syndrome

- Rest the joint in a position that minimizes stress on the joint structures, to prevent further damage and the development of adhesions.
- Support the affected arm on pillows while sleeping, to keep from turning onto the shoulder.
- For the first 24 to 48 hours of the acute phase, apply cold to reduce swelling and discomfort; then, according to the treatment plan, apply heat intermittently to promote circulation and healing.
- Gradually resume motion and use of the joint. Assistance with dressing and other activities of daily living may be needed.
- Avoid working and lifting above shoulder level or pushing an object against a "locked" shoulder.
- Perform the prescribed daily range-of-motion and strengthening exercises.

Treatment of carpal tunnel syndrome is based on the cause of the condition. Wrist splints to prevent hyperextension and prolonged flexion of the wrist, avoidance of repetitive flexion of the wrist (eg, making ergonomic changes at work to reduce wrist strain), NSAIDs, and carpal canal cortisone injections may relieve the symptoms. Specific yoga postures, relaxation, and acupuncture may be nontraditional alternatives to relieve carpal tunnel symptoms.

Traditional open nerve release or endoscopic laser surgery are the two most common surgical management options for treatment of carpal tunnel syndrome. Both of these procedures are performed under local anesthesia and involve making small incisions into the affected wrist, cutting the carpal ligament so that the carpal tunnel is widened. Smaller incisions are made with the endoscopic laser procedure, and there is less scar formation and a shorter recovery time than with the open method. Following either of these procedures, the patient wears a hand splint and limits hand use during healing. The patient may need assistance with personal care and ADLs. Full recovery of motor and sensory function after either type of nerve release surgery may take several weeks or months.

Ganglion

A ganglion, a collection of gelatinous material near the tendon sheaths and joints, appears as a round, firm, cystic swelling, usually on the dorsum of the wrist. It most frequently occurs in women younger than 50 years. The ganglion is locally tender and may cause an aching pain. When a tendon sheath is involved, weakness of the finger occurs. Treatment may include aspiration, corticosteroid injection, or surgical excision. After treatment, a compression dressing and immobilization splint are used.

Dupuytren's Disease

Dupuytren's disease results in is a slowly progressive **contracture** of the palmar fascia, called Dupuytren's contracture, which causes flexion of the fourth and fifth fingers, and frequently the middle finger. This renders the fingers more or less useless (Fig. 68-5). It is caused by an inherited autosomal dominant trait and occurs most frequently in men who are older than 50 years and who are of Scandinavian or Celtic origin. It is also associated with arthritis, diabetes, gout, and alcoholism (Childs, 2005). It starts as a nodule of the palmar fascia. The nodule may not change, or it may progress so that the fibrous thickening extends to involve the skin in the distal palm and produces a contracture of the fingers. The patient may experience dull aching discomfort, morning numbness, cramping, and stiffness in the affected fingers. This condition starts in one hand, but eventually both hands are affected symmetrically. Initially, finger-stretching exercises may prevent contractures. With contracture development, palmar and digital fasciectomies are performed to improve function. Finger exercises are begun on postoperative day 1 or 2.

Nursing Process

The Patient Undergoing Surgery of the Hand or Wrist

Assessment

Surgery of the hand or wrist, unless related to major trauma, is generally an ambulatory procedure. Before surgery, the nurse assesses the patient's level and type of discomfort and limitations in function caused by the ganglion, carpal tunnel syndrome, Dupuytren's contracture, or other condition of the hand.

Nursing Diagnoses

Based on the assessment data, the nursing diagnoses for the patient undergoing surgery of the hand or wrist may include the following:

- Risk for peripheral neurovascular dysfunction related to surgical procedure
- Acute pain related to inflammation and edema
- Self-care deficit: bathing/hygiene, dressing/grooming, feeding, and/or toileting related to bandaged hands
- Risk for infection related to surgical procedure

Planning and Goals

The goals of the patient may include relief of pain, improved self-care, and absence of infection.

Nursing Interventions

Promoting Neurovascular Function

Neurovascular assessment of the exposed fingers every hour for the first 24 hours is essential for monitoring function of the nerves and perfusion of the hand. The nurse compares the affected hand with the unaffected hand and the postoperative status with the documented preoperative status. The nurse asks the patient to describe the sensations in the hands and to demonstrate finger mobility. With tendon repairs and nerve, vascular, or skin grafts, motor function is tested as necessary. The nurse assesses the temperature of the affected hand. Dressings provide support but are nonconstrictive. Pain uncontrolled by analgesics suggests compromised neurovascular functioning.

Relieving Pain

Pain may be related to surgery, edema, hematoma formation, or restrictive bandages. To control swelling that may increase the patient's pain and discomfort, the nurse elevates the hand to heart level with pillows. When higher elevation is prescribed, an elevating sling may be attached to an intravenous (IV) pole or to an overhead frame. If the patient is ambulatory, the arm is elevated in a conventional sling with the hand at heart level.

Intermittent use of ice packs to the surgical area during the first 24 to 48 hours may be prescribed to control edema. Unless contraindicated, active extension and flexion of the fingers to promote circulation are encouraged, even though movement is limited by the bulky dressing.

Generally, the pain and discomfort can be controlled by oral analgesics. The nurse evaluates the patient's response to analgesics and to other pain control measures. Patient education concerning analgesics is important.

Improving Self-Care

During the first few days after surgery, the patient needs assistance with ADLs because one hand is bandaged and independent self-care is impaired. The patient may need to arrange for assistance with feeding, bathing and hygiene, dressing, grooming, and toileting. Within a few days, the patient develops skills in one-handed ADLs and is usually able to function with minimal assistance and use of assistive devices. The nurse encourages use of the involved hand, unless

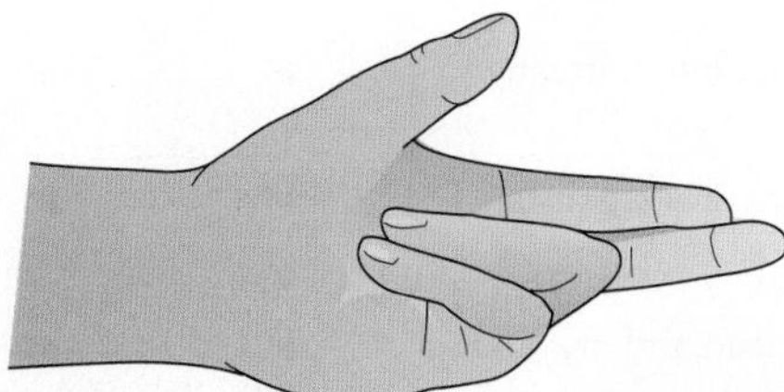

FIGURE 68-5. Dupuytren's contracture, a flexion deformity caused by an inherited trait, is a slowly progressive contracture of the palmar fascia, which severely impairs the function of the fourth, fifth, and sometimes, the middle finger.

contraindicated, within the limits of discomfort. As rehabilitation progresses, the patient resumes use of the injured hand. Physical or occupational therapy–directed exercises may be prescribed. The nurse emphasizes adherence to the therapeutic regimen.

Preventing Infection

As with all surgery, there is a risk of infection. The nurse teaches the patient to monitor temperature and signs and symptoms that suggest an infection. It also is important to instruct the patient to keep the dressing clean and dry and to report any drainage, foul odor, or increased pain and swelling. Patient education includes aseptic wound care as well as education related to prescribed prophylactic antibiotics.

Promoting Home and Community-Based Care

TEACHING PATIENTS SELF-CARE

After the patient has undergone hand surgery, the nurse teaches the patient how to monitor neurovascular status and the signs of complications that need to be reported to the surgeon (eg, paresthesia, paralysis, uncontrolled pain, coolness of fingers, extreme swelling, excessive bleeding, purulent drainage, fever). The nurse discusses prescribed medications with the patient. In addition, the nurse teaches the patient to elevate the hand above the elbow and to apply ice (if prescribed) to control swelling. Unless contraindicated, the nurse encourages extension and flexion exercises of the fingers to promote circulation. The use of assistive devices is encouraged if they would be helpful in promoting accomplishment of ADLs. For bathing, the nurse instructs the patient to keep the dressing dry by covering it with a secured plastic bag. Generally, the wound is not redressed until the patient's follow-up visit with the surgeon (Chart 68-5).

Evaluation

Expected Patient Outcomes

Expected patient outcomes may include:

1. Maintains peripheral tissue perfusion
   a. Demonstrates normal skin temperature and capillary refill
   b. Exhibits normal sensations
   c. Exhibits acceptable motor function
2. Achieves pain relief
   a. Reports increased comfort
   b. Controls edema through elevation of the hand
   c. Experiences no discomfort with movement
3. Demonstrates independent self-care
   a. Secures assistance with ADLs during first few days postoperatively
   b. Adapts to one-handed ADLs
   c. Uses injured hand within its functional capability
4. Demonstrates absence of wound infection
   a. Adheres to treatment protocol and prevention strategies
   b. Reports temperature and pulse within normal limits
   c. Experiences no purulent wound drainage
   d. Experiences no wound inflammation

Common Foot Problems

Disabilities of the foot are commonly caused by poorly fitting shoes. Fashion, vanity, and eye appeal, rather than function and physiology of the foot, are the determining factors

CHART 68-5

HOME CARE CHECKLIST • Hand Surgery

At the completion of the home care instruction, the patient or caregiver will be able to:	Patient	Caregiver
• Demonstrate how to assess neurovascular status	✔	✔
• State abnormal findings (eg, unrelenting pain; paralysis; paresthesia; cool, nonblanching fingers) to report to physician promptly	✔	✔
• Demonstrate control of edema by elevating hand above elbow and applying ice intermittently if prescribed	✔	✔
• Identify signs and symptoms of infection (eg, elevated temperature, purulent drainage)	✔	✔
• Demonstrate finger exercises to promote circulation, unless contraindicated	✔	
• Describe methods to prevent wound infection (eg, keeping hand dressing clean and dry during activities of daily living)	✔	✔
• Describe use of prescribed medications	✔	✔
• Demonstrate use of assistive devices, if appropriate	✔	

in the design of footwear. Ill-fitting shoes distort normal anatomy while inducing deformity and pain.

Several systemic diseases affect the feet. Patients with diabetes are prone to develop corns and peripheral neuropathies with diminished sensation, leading to ulcers at pressure points of the foot. Patients with peripheral vascular disease and arteriosclerosis complain of burning and itching feet, resulting in scratching and skin breakdown. Foot deformities may occur with rheumatoid arthritis. Dermatologic problems commonly affect the feet in the form of fungal infections and plantar warts.

The discomforts of foot strain are treated with rest, elevation, physiotherapy, supportive strappings, and orthotic devices. The patient must inspect the foot and skin under pads and orthotic devices for pressure and skin breakdown daily. If a "window" is cut into shoes to relieve pressure over a bony deformity, the skin must be monitored daily for breakdown from pressure exerted at the "window" area. Active foot exercises promote circulation and help strengthen the feet. Walking in properly fitting shoes is considered the ideal exercise.

Plantar Fasciitis

Plantar fasciitis, an inflammation of the foot-supporting fascia, presents as an acute onset of heel pain experienced with the first steps in the morning. The pain is localized to the anterior medial aspect of the heel and diminishes with gentle stretching of the foot and Achilles tendon. Management includes stretching exercises, wearing shoes with support and cushioning to relieve pain, orthotic devices (eg, heel cups, arch supports), and NSAIDs. Unresolved plantar fasciitis may progress to fascial tears at the heel and eventual development of heel spurs.

Corn

A corn is an area of hyperkeratosis (overgrowth of a horny layer of epidermis) produced by internal pressure (the underlying bone is prominent because of a congenital or acquired abnormality, commonly arthritis) or external pressure (ill-fitting shoes). The fifth toe is most frequently involved, but any toe may be involved.

Corns are treated by soaking and scraping off the horny layer by a podiatrist, by application of a protective shield or pad, or by surgical modification of the underlying offending osseous structure. Soft corns are located between the toes and are kept soft by moisture. Treatment consists of drying the affected spaces and separating the affected toes with lamb's wool or gauze. A wider shoe may be helpful. Usually, a podiatrist is consulted to treat the underlying cause.

Callus

A callus is a discretely thickened area of the skin that has been exposed to persistent pressure or friction. Faulty foot mechanics usually precede the formation of a callus. Treatment consists of eliminating the underlying causes and having the callus treated by a podiatrist if it is painful. A keratolytic ointment may be applied and a thin plastic cup worn over the heel if the callus is on this area. Felt padding with an adhesive backing is also used to prevent and relieve pressure. Orthotic devices can be made to remove the pressure from bony protuberances, or the protuberance may be excised.

Ingrown Toenail

An ingrown toenail (onychocryptosis) is a condition in which the free edge of a nail plate penetrates the surrounding skin, either laterally or anteriorly. A secondary infection or granulation tissue may develop. This painful condition is caused by improper self-treatment, external pressure (tight shoes or stockings), internal pressure (deformed toes, growth under the nail), trauma, or infection. Trimming the nails properly (clipping them straight across and filing the corners consistent with the contour of the toe) can prevent this problem. Active treatment consists of washing the foot twice a day, followed by the application of a local antibiotic ointment, and relieving the pain by decreasing the pressure of the nail plate on the surrounding soft tissue. Warm, wet soaks help drain an infection. A toenail may need to be excised by the podiatrist if there is severe infection.

Hammer Toe

Hammer toe is a flexion deformity of the interphalangeal joint, which may involve several toes (Fig. 68-6A). The condition is usually an acquired deformity. Tight socks or shoes may push an overlying toe back into the line of the other toes. The toes usually are pulled upward, forcing the metatarsal joints (ball of the foot) downward. Corns develop on top of the toes, and tender calluses develop under the metatarsal area. The treatment consists of conservative measures: wearing open-toed sandals or shoes that conform to the shape of the foot, carrying out manipulative exercises, and protecting the protruding joints with pads. Surgery (osteotomy) may be used to correct a resulting deformity.

Hallux Valgus

Hallux valgus (commonly called a bunion) is a deformity in which the great toe deviates laterally (see Fig. 68-6C). Associated with this is a marked prominence of the medial aspect of the first metatarsophalangeal joint. There is also osseous enlargement (exostosis) of the medial side of the first metatarsal head, over which a bursa may form (secondary to pressure and inflammation). Acute bursitis symptoms include a reddened area, edema, and tenderness.

Factors contributing to bunion formation include heredity, ill-fitting shoes, and gradual lengthening and widening of the foot associated with aging. Osteoarthritis is frequently associated with hallux valgus. Treatment depends on the patient's age, the degree of deformity, and the severity of symptoms. If a bunion deformity is uncomplicated, wearing a shoe that conforms to the shape of the foot or that is molded to the foot to prevent pressure on the protruding portions may be the only treatment needed. Corticosteroid injections

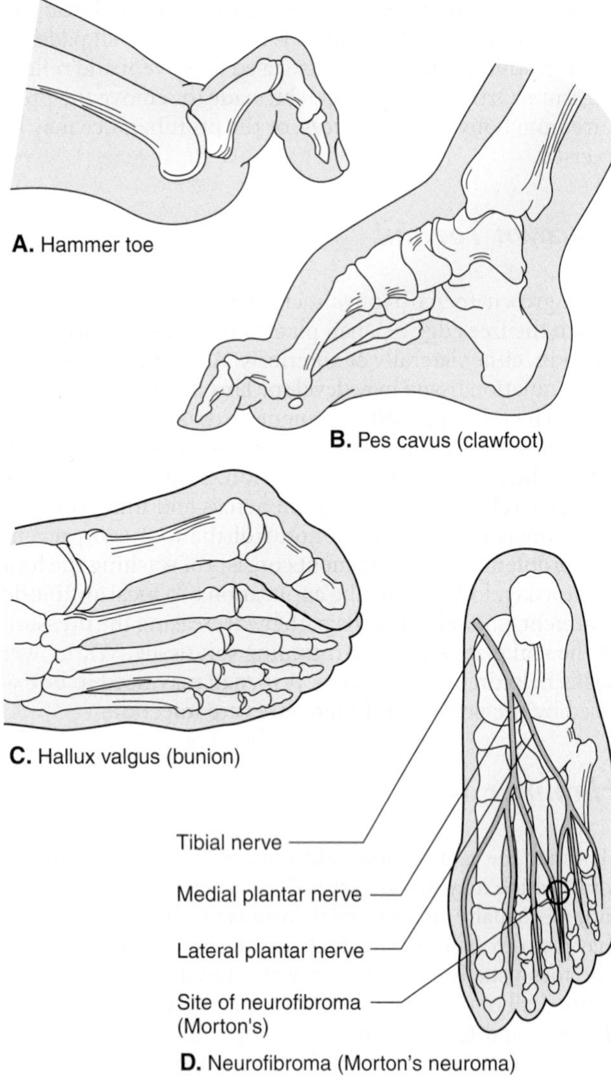

FIGURE 68-6. Common foot deformities.

control acute inflammation. Surgical removal of the bunion (exostosis) and osteotomies to realign the toe may be required to improve function and appearance. Complications related to bunionectomy include limited range of motion, paresthesias, tendon injury, and recurrence of deformity.

Postoperatively, the patient may have intense throbbing pain at the operative site, requiring liberal doses of analgesic medication. The foot is elevated to the level of the heart to decrease edema and pain. The neurovascular status of the toes is assessed. The duration of immobility and initiation of ambulation depend on the procedure used. Toe flexion and extension exercises are initiated to facilitate walking. Shoes that fit the shape and size of the foot are recommended.

Pes Cavus

Pes cavus (clawfoot) refers to a foot with an abnormally high arch and a fixed equinus deformity of the forefoot (see Fig. 68-6B). The shortening of the foot and increased pressure produce calluses on the metatarsal area and on the dorsum of the foot. Charcot-Marie-Tooth disease (a peripheral neuromuscular disease associated with a familial degenerative disorder), diabetes mellitus, and tertiary syphilis are common causes of pes cavus. Exercises are prescribed to manipulate the forefoot into dorsiflexion and relax the toes. Bracing to protect the foot may be used. In severe cases, arthrodesis (fusion) is performed to reshape and stabilize the foot.

Morton's Neuroma

Morton's neuroma (plantar digital neuroma, neurofibroma) is a swelling of the third (lateral) branch of the median plantar nerve (see Fig. 68-6D). The third digital nerve, which is located in the third intermetatarsal (web) space, is most commonly involved. Microscopically, digital artery changes cause an ischemia of the nerve.

The result is a throbbing, burning pain in the foot that is usually relieved when the patient rests. Conservative treatment consists of inserting innersoles and metatarsal pads designed to spread the metatarsal heads and balance the foot posture. Local injections of hydrocortisone and a local anesthetic may provide relief. If these fail, surgical excision of the neuroma is necessary. Pain relief and loss of sensation are immediate and permanent.

Flatfoot

Flatfoot (pes planus) is a common disorder in which the longitudinal arch of the foot is diminished. It may be caused by congenital abnormalities or associated with bone or ligament injury, muscle and posture imbalances, excessive weight, muscle fatigue, poorly fitting shoes, or arthritis. Symptoms include a burning sensation, fatigue, clumsy gait, edema, and pain.

Exercises to strengthen the muscles and to improve posture and walking habits are helpful. A number of foot orthoses are available to give the foot additional support.

Nursing Process

The Patient Undergoing Foot Surgery

Assessment

Surgery of the foot may be necessary because of various conditions, including neuromas and foot deformities (bunion, hammer toe, clawfoot). Generally, foot surgery is performed on an outpatient basis. Before surgery, the nurse assesses the patient's ambulatory ability and balance and the neurovascular status of the foot. Additionally, the nurse considers the availability of assistance at home and the structural characteristics of the home in planning for care during the first few days after surgery. The nurse uses these data, in addition to knowledge of the usual medical management of the condition, to formulate appropriate nursing diagnoses.

Nursing Diagnoses

Based on the assessment data, the nursing diagnoses for the patient undergoing foot surgery may include the following:

- Risk for ineffective peripheral tissue perfusion related to edema
- Acute pain related to surgery, inflammation, and edema
- Impaired physical mobility related to the foot-immobilizing device
- Risk for infection related to the surgical procedure/surgical incision

Planning and Goals

The goals for the patient may include adequate tissue perfusion, relief of pain, improved mobility, and absence of infection.

Nursing Interventions

Promoting Tissue Perfusion

Neurovascular assessment of the exposed toes every 1 to 2 hours for the first 24 hours is essential to monitor the function of the nerves and the perfusion of the tissues. If the patient is discharged within several hours after the surgery, the nurse teaches the patient and family how to assess for edema and neurovascular status (circulation, motion, sensation). Compromised neurovascular function can increase the patient's pain (see Chart 66-3 in Chapter 66).

Relieving Pain

Pain experienced by patients who undergo foot surgery is related to inflammation and edema. Formation of a hematoma may contribute to the discomfort. To control the edema, the foot should be elevated on several pillows when the patient is sitting or lying. Ice packs applied intermittently to the surgical area during the first 24 to 48 hours may be prescribed to control edema and provide some pain relief. As activity increases, the patient may find that dependent positioning of the foot is uncomfortable. Simply elevating the foot often relieves the discomfort. Oral analgesics may be used to control the pain. The nurse instructs the patient and family about appropriate use of these medications.

Improving Mobility

After surgery, the patient will have a bulky dressing on the foot, protected by a light cast or a special protective boot. Limits for weight-bearing on the foot will be prescribed by the surgeon. Some patients are allowed to walk on the heel and progress to weight-bearing as tolerated; other patients are restricted to non–weight-bearing activities. Assistive devices (eg, crutches, walker) may be needed. The choice of the devices depends on the patient's general condition and balance and on the weight-bearing prescription. Safe use of the assistive devices must be ensured through adequate patient education and practice before discharge. Strategies to move around the house safely while using assistive devices are discussed with the patient. As healing progresses, the patient gradually resumes ambulation within prescribed limits. The nurse emphasizes adherence to the therapeutic regimen.

Preventing Infection

Any surgery carries a risk of infection. In addition, percutaneous pins may be used to hold bones in position, and these pins serve as potential sites for infection. Care must be taken to protect the surgical wound from dirt and moisture. When bathing, the patient can secure a plastic bag over the dressing to prevent it from getting wet. Patient instructions concerning aseptic wound care and pin care may be necessary.

The nurse teaches the patient to monitor for temperature changes and infection. Drainage on the dressing, a foul odor, or increased pain and swelling could indicate infection. The nurse instructs the patient to promptly report any of these findings to the physician. If prophylactic antibiotics are prescribed, the nurse provides instruction about their correct use.

Promoting Home and Community-Based Care

TEACHING PATIENTS SELF-CARE

The nurse plans patient teaching for home care, focusing on neurovascular status, pain management, mobility, and wound care (Chart 68-6).

Evaluation

Expected Patient Outcomes

Expected patient outcomes may include:

1. Maintains peripheral tissue perfusion
   a. Demonstrates normal skin temperature and capillary refill
   b. Exhibits normal sensations
   c. Exhibits acceptable motor function
2. Obtains pain relief
   a. Elevates foot to control edema
   b. Applies ice to foot as prescribed
   c. Uses oral analgesics as needed and prescribed
   d. Reports decreased pain and increased comfort
3. Demonstrates increased mobility
   a. Uses assistive devices safely
   b. Resumes weight-bearing gradually as prescribed

CHART 68-6

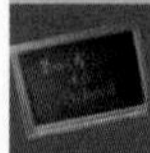

Patient Education

Self-Care After Foot Surgery

NEUROVASCULAR STATUS

The following signs and symptoms indicate impaired circulation and should be reported to your health care provider right away:

- Change in sensation
- Inability to move toes
- Toes or foot cool to touch
- Color changes

PAIN MANAGEMENT

Methods to reduce pain include the following:

- Elevate foot to heart level.
- Apply ice as prescribed.
- Use analgesics as prescribed.
- Report pain that is not relieved.

MOBILITY

- Use assistive devices safely.
- Comply with prescribed weight-bearing limits.
- Wear special protective shoe over the dressing.

WOUND CARE

- Keep the dressing or cast clean and dry.
- Report signs of wound infection (eg, pain, drainage, fever) immediately.
- Follow the prescribed antibiotic regimen.
- Keep your appointment with the surgeon for the initial dressing change.

    c. Exhibits diminished disability associated with preoperative condition
4. Develops no infection
    a. Reports temperature and pulse within normal limits
    b. Reports no purulent drainage or signs of wound inflammation
    c. Maintains clean and dry dressing
    d. Takes prophylactic antibiotics as prescribed

Metabolic Bone Disorders

Osteoporosis

The bone disease osteoporosis is a costly disorder not only in terms of health care dollars but also in terms of human suffering, pain, disability, and death. It is estimated that osteoporosis and its precursor, osteopenia, will affect approximately 40 million Americans older than 50 years by 2010 (U.S. Department of Health and Human Services [DHHS], 2004).

Characteristics of osteoporosis include a reduction of bone density and a change in bone structure, both of which increase susceptibility to fracture. The normal homeostatic bone turnover is altered; the rate of bone resorption is greater than the rate of bone formation, resulting in a reduced total bone mass. Suboptimal bone mass development in children and teens contributes to the development of osteoporosis. With osteoporosis, the bones become progressively porous, brittle, and fragile; they fracture easily under stresses that would not break normal bone. Osteoporosis frequently results in compression fractures (Fig. 68-7) of the thoracic and lumbar spine, fractures of the neck and intertrochanteric region of the femur, and Colles' fractures of the wrist. These fractures may be the first clinical manifestation of osteoporosis. Fracture risk increases with increasing age and is greatest in Caucasian women. It is projected that 40% of Caucasian American women older than 50 years will experience an osteoporosis-related fracture in their lifetimes (DHHS, 2004). Multiple compression fractures of the vertebrae result in skeletal deformity.

The gradual collapse of a vertebra may be asymptomatic; it is observed as progressive kyphosis. With the development of kyphosis ("dowager's hump"), there is an associated loss of height (Fig. 68-8). Frequently, postmenopausal women lose height from vertebral collapse. The postural changes result in relaxation of the abdominal muscles and a protruding abdomen. The deformity may also produce pulmonary insufficiency. Many patients complain of fatigue.

Prevention

It is thought that 60% to 80% of a person's peak bone mass is genetically determined. Up to 90% of peak adult bone

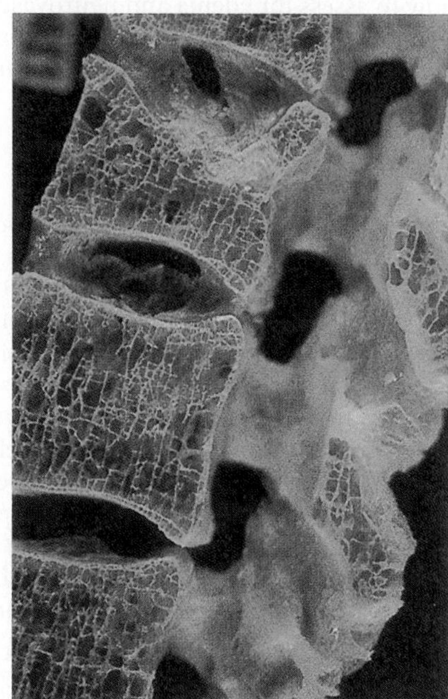

FIGURE 68-7. Progressive osteoporotic bone loss and compression fractures. From Rubin, E., Gorstein, F., Schwarting, R., et al. (2004). *Pathology* (4th ed.). Philadelphia: Lippincott Williams & Wilkins.

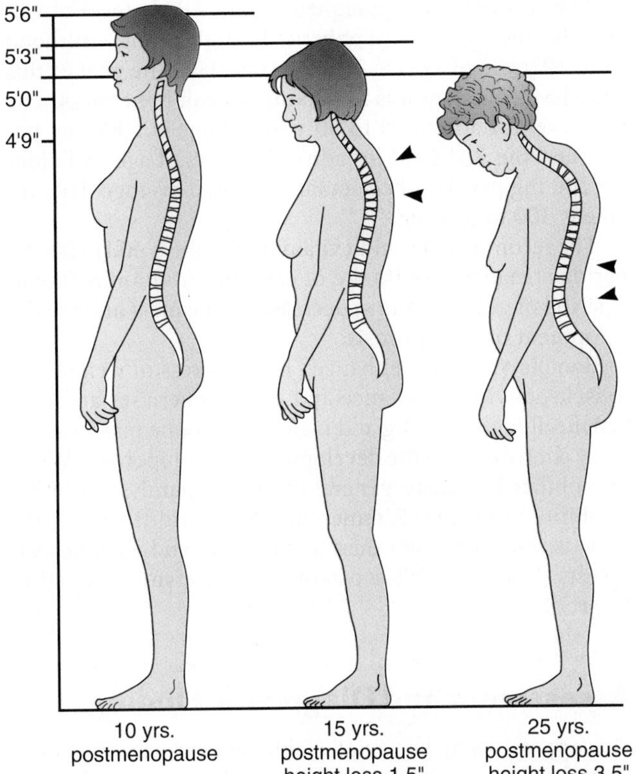

FIGURE 68-8. Typical loss of height associated with osteoporosis and aging.

mass is achieved between the ages of 18 and 20 years in females and males, respectively; this can be affected by factors such as diet, physical activity, and medications (Hampton, 2004). Primary osteoporosis occurs in women after menopause (usually between the ages of 45 and 55 years) and in men later in life, but it is not merely a consequence of aging. Failure to develop optimal peak bone mass during childhood, adolescence, and young adulthood contributes to the development of osteoporosis without resultant bone loss. Early identification of at-risk teenagers and young adults, increased calcium intake, participation in regular weight-bearing exercise, and modification of lifestyle (eg, reduced use of caffeine, cigarettes, carbonated soft drinks, and alcohol) are interventions that decrease the risk of osteoporosis, fractures, and associated disability later in life. Secondary osteoporosis is the result of medications or other conditions and diseases that affect bone metabolism. Specific disease states (eg, celiac disease, hypogonadism) and medications (eg, corticosteroids, antiseizure medications) that place patients at risk need to be identified and therapies instituted to reverse the development of osteoporosis.

Gerontologic Considerations

The prevalence of osteoporosis in women older than 80 years is 50% (DHHS, 2004). The average 75-year-old woman has lost 25% of her cortical bone and 40% of her trabecular bone. With the aging of the population, the incidence of fractures (more than 1.5 million osteoporotic fractures per year), pain, and disability associated with osteoporosis is increasing. Most residents of long-term care facilities have a low bone mineral density (BMD) and are at risk for bone fracture. Osteoporotic-related fractures account for more than 800,000 emergency department visits, more than 2,600,000 outpatient visits, and the placement of more than 180,000 people in long-term care facilities annually in the United States (DHHS, 2004). Hip protectors had been thought to reduce the incidence of hip fracture in the elderly; however, recent evidence suggests that they are not effective in preventing fractures (Parker, Gillespie, & Gillespie, 2004; Van Schoor, Smit, Twisk, et al., 2003).

Elderly people absorb dietary calcium less efficiently and excrete it more readily through their kidneys; therefore, postmenopausal women and the elderly need to consume liberal amounts of calcium. As much as 1500 mg daily for postmenopausal women may be prescribed.

Pathophysiology

Normal bone remodeling in the adult results in gradually increased bone mass until the early 30s. Gender, race, genetics, aging, low body weight and body mass index, nutrition, lifestyle choices (eg, smoking, caffeine, consumption of carbonated soft drinks and alcohol), and physical activity influence peak bone mass and the development of osteoporosis (Fig. 68-9). Although the consequences of osteoporosis (eg, fractures) occur with aging, osteoporosis is not a disease of the elderly. Rather, its onset occurs earlier in life, when bone mass peaks and then begins to decline.

Loss of bone mass is a universal phenomenon associated with aging. Age-related loss begins soon after the peak bone mass is achieved (ie, in the fourth decade). Calcitonin, which inhibits bone resorption and promotes bone formation, is decreased. Estrogen, which inhibits bone breakdown, decreases with aging. On the other hand, parathyroid hormone (PTH) increases with aging, increasing bone turnover and resorption. The consequence of these changes is net loss of bone mass over time.

The withdrawal of estrogens at menopause or with oophorectomy causes an accelerated bone resorption that continues during the postmenopausal years. Women develop osteoporosis more frequently and more extensively than men because of lower peak bone mass and the effect of estrogen loss during menopause. More than half of all women older than 50 years show evidence of osteopenia. World Health Organization (WHO) diagnostic categories for osteoporosis are based on BMD scan findings (WHO, 2003).

Secondary osteoporosis is associated with many disease states, nutritional deficiencies, and medications. Coexisting medical conditions (eg, malabsorption syndromes, lactose intolerance, alcohol abuse, renal failure, liver failure, Cushing's syndrome, hyperthyroidism, and hyperparathyroidism) contribute to bone loss and the development of osteoporosis. Medications (eg, corticosteroids, antiseizure medications, heparin, tetracycline, aluminum-containing antacids, and thyroid supplements) affect the body's use and metabolism of calcium. The degree of osteoporosis is related to the duration of medication therapy. When the therapy is discontinued or the metabolic problem is corrected, the progression of osteoporosis is halted, but restoration of lost bone mass usually does not occur.

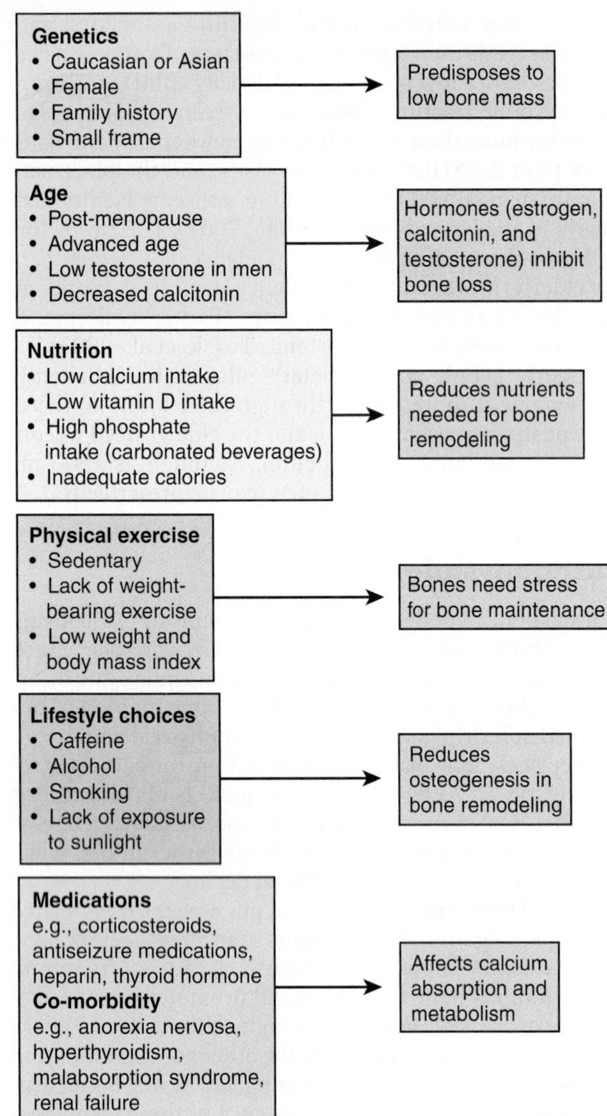

FIGURE 68-9. Risk factors for osteoporosis, and the effects of these factors on bone.

Risk Factors

Small-framed, nonobese Caucasian women are at greatest risk for osteoporosis. Also, Asian women of slight build are at risk for low peak BMD. African-American women, who have a greater bone mass than Caucasian women, are less susceptible to osteoporosis. Men have a greater peak bone mass and do not experience sudden estrogen reduction. As a result, osteoporosis occurs in men at a lower rate and at an older age (about one decade later). It is believed that testosterone and estrogen are important in achieving and maintaining bone mass in men.

Nutritional factors contribute to the development of osteoporosis. A diet that includes adequate calories and nutrients needed to maintain bone, calcium, and vitamin D must be consumed. Vitamin D is necessary for calcium absorption and for normal bone mineralization. Dietary calcium and vitamin D must be adequate to maintain bone remodeling and body functions. The best source of calcium and vitamin D is fortified milk. A cup of milk or calcium-fortified orange juice contains about 300 mg of calcium.

The recommended adequate intake (RAI) level of calcium for the age range of puberty through young adulthood (9 to 19 years of age) is 1300 mg per day. The goal of this daily level of calcium is to maximize peak bone mass. The RAI level for adults 19 to 50 years of age is 1000 mg per day, and the RAI level for adults 51 years of age and older is 1200 mg per day. The actual estimated average daily intake is 300 to 500 mg.

The recommended adult vitamin D intake is 400 to 600 IU per day. Inadequate intake of calcium or vitamin D over a period of years results in decreased bone mass and the development of osteoporosis.

Bone formation is enhanced by the stress of weight and muscle activity. Resistance and impact exercises are most beneficial in developing and maintaining bone mass. Immobility contributes to the development of osteoporosis. When immobilized by casts, general inactivity, paralysis or other disability (Smeltzer, Zimmerman, & Capriotti, 2005), the bone is resorbed faster than it is formed, and osteoporosis results. Risk factors for osteoporosis are summarized in Chart 68-7.

Assessment and Diagnostic Findings

Osteoporosis may be undetectable on routine x-rays until there has been 25% to 40% demineralization, resulting in radiolucency of the bones. When the vertebrae collapse, the

CHART 68-7

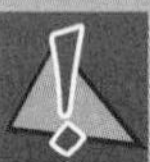

Risk Factors and Risk-Lowering Strategies for Osteoporosis

Individual Risk Factors

- Female
- Caucasian, non-Hispanic, or Asian
- Increased age
- Low weight and body mass index
- Estrogen deficiency or menopause
- Family history
- Low initial bone mass
- Contributing, coexisting medical conditions (eg, celiac disease) and medications (eg, corticosteroids, antiseizure medications), thyroid hormone

Lifestyle Risk Factors

- Diet low in calcium and vitamin D
- Cigarette smoking
- Use of alcohol and/or caffeine
- Lack of weight-bearing exercise
- Lack of exposure to sunshine

Risk-Lowering Strategies

- Increased dietary calcium and vitamin D intake
- Smoking cessation
- Alcohol and caffeine consumption in moderation
- Regular weight-bearing exercise regimen
- Outdoor activity

thoracic vertebrae become wedge-shaped and the lumbar vertebrae become biconcave. Osteoporosis is diagnosed by dual-energy x-ray absorptiometry (DEXA), which provides information about BMD at the spine and hip. The DEXA scan data are analyzed and reported as T-scores (the number of standard deviations [SDs] above or below the average BMD value for a young, healthy Caucasian woman). A normal BMD is less than 1 SD below the young adult mean value. WHO (2003) defines osteoporosis as being present when the T-score is at least 2.5 SD below the young adult mean value. Osteopenia is diagnosed when the BMD T-score is between 1 and 2.5 SD below the young adult mean value. Fracture risk increases progressively as the SD of the T-score falls below the mean value.

Quantitative ultrasound studies of the heel and DEXA of the wrist, hip, or spine are used to screen for osteoporosis and to predict the risk of hip and nonvertebral fracture. Current evidence-based guidelines recommend the use of hip BMD as the first-line screening test for osteoporosis (Bates, Black, & Cummings, 2002). In particular, hip BMD is recommended as a screening tool for all Caucasian women older than 65 years and for others thought to be at increased risk for osteoporotic fractures.

BMD studies are useful in identifying osteopenic and osteoporotic bone and in assessing response to therapy. Through early screening (using both assessment of risk factors and BMD scans), promotion of adequate dietary intake of calcium and vitamin D, encouragement of lifestyle changes, and early institution of preventive medications, bone loss and osteoporosis can be reduced, resulting in a reduced incidence of fracture.

Laboratory studies (eg, serum calcium, serum phosphate, serum alkaline phosphatase, urine calcium excretion, urinary hydroxyproline excretion, hematocrit, erythrocyte sedimentation rate [ESR]) and x-ray studies are used to exclude other possible medical diagnoses (eg, multiple myeloma, osteomalacia, hyperparathyroidism, malignancy) that contribute to bone loss.

NURSING RESEARCH PROFILE

Predicting the Risk of Osteoporosis in Women with Disabilities

Smeltzer, S. C., & Zimmerman, V. L. (2005). Usefulness of the SCORE index as a predictor of osteoporosis in women with disabilities. *Orthopaedic Nursing, 24*(1), 33–39.

Purpose

Osteoporosis is a major cause of morbidity in perimenopausal women. Studies to date have not evaluated osteoporosis risk predictors in women with disabilities. Prior studies have focused on nondisabled women and their measures of bone mineral density (BMD). The purpose of this study was to evaluate the usefulness of the Simple Calculated Osteoporosis Risk Estimation (SCORE) index in the identification of women with disabilities who might be at risk for osteoporosis.

Design

A convenience sample (N = 307) of women with a variety of disabilities was recruited from a variety of settings (eg, health fairs, educational programs). Disability was determined by self-report. Participants completed the 6-item SCORE index and underwent peripheral BMD measurement.

Individuals' responses to questions about age, history of atraumatic fracture, history of rheumatoid arthritis, race, estrogen use, and weight are used to calculate the SCORE index; a value of 6 or higher indicates the need for BMD testing. Results of the SCORE index were then analyzed to determine the sensitivity, specificity, and accuracy in predicting low BMD in the sample of women with disabilities. BMD measurements were reported as T-scores. The World Health Organization (WHO) criteria for osteoporosis is a T-score ≤ 2.5.

Findings

According to the BMD T-scores, 44.6% of the women in the sample had a normal BMD, with the remainder classified as having either osteopenia or osteoporosis. The group mean of the SCORE index was 3.9 (± 5.9), suggesting an absence of osteoporosis risk. The sensitivity, specificity, and accuracy of the SCORE index in predicting a BMD of 2.5 or less (osteoporosis) were 65.7%, 61.1%, and 62.2%, respectively. The sensitivity, specificity, and accuracy of the SCORE index in predicting a BMD of 2.0 or less (osteopenia) were 62.6%, 63%, and 62.9%, respectively. The low sensitivity, specificity, and accuracy of the SCORE index in predicting osteoporosis do not support the clinical use of this index with women with disabilities. Further studies to develop a screening index that is sensitive, specific, and accurate in identifying osteoporosis risk in women with disabilities are necessary.

Nursing Implications

The SCORE index is not a useful osteoporosis screening tool for women with disabilities. This may be because the SCORE index was not developed to take into account disabilities and the osteoporosis-related risks that tend to be associated with disabilities. Currently, no osteoporosis screening tools take into account disabilities that women may have in their guidelines for assessment. Therefore, women with disabilities should be individually assessed for risk factors for osteoporosis risk and not screened by either the SCORE index or other current osteoporosis screening tools.

Medical Management

A diet rich in calcium and vitamin D throughout life, with an increased calcium intake during adolescence, young adulthood, and the middle years, protects against skeletal demineralization. Such a diet includes three glasses of skim or whole vitamin D–enriched milk or other foods high in calcium (eg, cheese and other dairy products, steamed broccoli, canned salmon with bones) daily. To ensure adequate calcium intake, a calcium supplement (eg, Caltrate, Citracal) with Vitamin D may be prescribed and taken with meals or with a beverage high in vitamin C to promote absorption. The recommended daily dose should be split and not taken as a single dose. Common side effects of calcium supplements are abdominal distention and constipation.

Regular weight-bearing exercise promotes bone formation. From 20 to 30 minutes of aerobic exercise (eg, walking), 3 days or more a week, is recommended. Weight training stimulates an increase in BMD. In addition, exercise improves balance, reducing the incidence of falls and fractures (Chart 68-8).

Pharmacologic Therapy

At natural or surgical menopause, hormone therapy with estrogen and progesterone had been the mainstay of therapy

CHART 68-8

HOME CARE CHECKLIST • Osteoporosis

At the completion of the home care instruction, the patient or caregiver will be able to:	Patient	Caregiver
Adolescents and Young Adults		
• List risk factors for osteoporosis	✔	✔
• Identify calcium- and vitamin D-rich foods	✔	
• Consume diet with adequate calcium (1000–1300 mg/day) and vitamin D	✔	
• Engage in weight-bearing exercise daily	✔	
• Modify lifestyle choices—avoid smoking, alcohol, caffeine, and carbonated beverages	✔	
Menopausal and Postmenopausal Women		
• List risk factors for osteoporosis	✔	✔
• Identify calcium- and vitamin D-rich foods	✔	
• Consume diet with adequate calcium (1200–1500 mg/day) and vitamin D	✔	
• Discuss calcium supplements	✔	
• Engage in weight-bearing exercise at least 3 times weekly	✔	
• Engage in exercise that improves balance to reduce the incidence of falls	✔	
• Demonstrate good body mechanics	✔	
• Modify lifestyle choices—avoid smoking, alcohol, caffeine, and carbonated beverages	✔	
• Discuss pharmacologic agents to maintain and enhance bone mass	✔	
• Review concurrent medical conditions and medications with health care provider to identify factors that contribute to bone mass loss	✔	✔
• Assess home environment for hazards contributing to falls	✔	✔
Men		
• List risk factors associated with osteoporosis in men, including medications (eg, corticosteroids, antiseizure medications, aluminum-containing antacids); chronic diseases (eg, kidney, lung, gastrointestinal); and undiagnosed low testosterone levels	✔	✔
• Modify lifestyle choices—avoid smoking, alcohol, caffeine, and carbonated beverages	✔	
• Engage in weight-bearing exercise daily, such as walking, weightlifting, and resistance exercise	✔	
• Consume diet with adequate calcium (1000–1200 mg/day) and vitamin D (400 IU/day)	✔	
• Participate in screening for osteoporosis	✔	
• Talk with health care provider about use of medications (eg, alendronate) to enhance bone mass or to correct testosterone deficiency	✔	
• Assess home environment for hazards contributing to falls	✔	✔

to retard bone loss and prevent occurrence of fractures. Estrogen replacement decreases bone resorption and increases bone mass, reducing the incidence of osteoporotic fractures. However, recent studies have demonstrated greater risks, including strokes, venous thromboemboli, and breast cancer, than the benefits of osteoporosis preventive treatment could justify. Experts now urge that postmenopausal women take hormone therapy only if they have a high risk for osteoporosis and if they cannot take other medications to treat osteoporosis (Cauley, Robbins, Chen, et al., 2003).

Selective estrogen receptor modulators (SERMs), such as raloxifene (Evista), reduce the risk of osteoporosis by preserving BMD without estrogenic effects on the uterus. They are indicated for both prevention and treatment of osteoporosis.

Medications commonly prescribed to treat osteoporosis include bisphosphonates (eg, alendronate [Fosamax], risedronate [Actonel], ibandronate [Boniva]) and calcitonin. Bisphosphonates reduce spine and hip fractures associated with osteoporosis through increasing bone mass and decreasing bone loss by inhibiting osteoclast function. Alendronate and risedronate are approved for the prevention and treatment of corticosteroid-induced osteoporosis in men and women. Alendronate, given weekly, has been shown to be as effective as previously used daily dosing. Ibandronate is a newer agent that requires only once-monthly administration. Adequate calcium and vitamin D intake is needed for maximum effect, but these supplements should not be taken at the same time of day as bisphosphonates. Side effects of bisphosphonates include gastrointestinal symptoms (eg, dyspepsia, nausea, flatulence, diarrhea, constipation), and some patients may develop esophageal ulcers, gastric ulcers, or osteonecrosis of the jaw related to bisphosphonate use (Ruggiero, Mehrotra, Rosenberg, et al., 2004). Patients must take these medications on an empty stomach on arising in the morning with a full glass of water and must sit upright for 30 to 60 minutes after their administration.

Calcitonin (Miacalcin) directly inhibits osteoclasts, thereby reducing bone loss and increasing BMD. Calcitonin is administered by nasal spray or by subcutaneous or intramuscular injection. Side effects include nasal irritation, flushing, gastrointestinal disturbances, and urinary frequency.

Teriparatide (Forteo), a subcutaneously administered medication that is given once daily, has recently been approved by the Food and Drug Administration for the treatment of osteoporosis. As a recombinant PTH, it stimulates osteoblasts to build bone matrix and facilitates overall calcium absorption (Achenbrenner, Robbins, Chen, et al., 2003).

In addition, antilipid medications, such as statins (HMG-CoA reductase inhibitors), reduce the incidence of fractures in patients who take these medications to control their hyperlipidemia. The statins promote bone growth, thereby preventing the development of osteoporosis.

Fracture Management

Fractures of the hip are managed surgically by joint replacement or by closed or open reduction with internal fixation (eg, hip pinning). Surgery, early ambulation, intensive physical therapy, and adequate nutrition result in decreased morbidity and improved outcomes. In addition, patients need to be evaluated for osteoporosis and treated, if indicated.

Osteoporotic compression fractures of the vertebra are managed conservatively. Additional vertebral fractures and progressive kyphosis are common. Pharmacologic and dietary treatments are aimed at increasing vertebral bone density. Percutaneous vertebroplasty/kyphoplasty (injection of polymethylmethacrylate bone cement into the fractured vertebra, followed by inflation of a pressurized balloon to restore the shape of the affected vertebra) can provide rapid relief of acute pain and improve quality of life. The long-term effect of this procedure is unknown. Patients who have not responded to first-line approaches to the treatment of vertebral compression fracture can be considered for the procedure. It is contraindicated in the presence of infection, old fractures, and certain coagulopathies (Hayne, 2003).

Nursing Process

The Patient With a Spontaneous Vertebral Fracture Related to Osteoporosis

Assessment

Health promotion, identification of people at risk for osteoporosis, and recognition of problems associated with osteoporosis form the basis for nursing assessment. The health history includes questions concerning the occurrence of osteopenia and osteoporosis and focuses on family history, previous fractures, dietary consumption of calcium, exercise patterns, onset of menopause, and use of corticosteroids as well as alcohol, smoking, and caffeine intake. Any symptoms the patient is experiencing, such as back pain, constipation, or altered body image, are explored.

Physical examination may disclose a fracture, kyphosis of the thoracic spine, or shortened stature. Problems in mobility and breathing may exist as a result of changes in posture and weakened muscles.

Nursing Diagnoses

Based on the assessment data, the major nursing diagnoses for the patient who experiences a spontaneous vertebral fracture related to osteoporosis may include the following:

- Deficient knowledge about the osteoporotic process and treatment regimen
- Acute pain related to fracture and muscle spasm
- Risk for constipation related to immobility or development of ileus (intestinal obstruction)
- Risk for injury: additional fractures related to osteoporosis

Planning and Goals

The major goals for the patient may include knowledge about osteoporosis and the treatment regimen, relief of pain, improved bowel elimination, and absence of additional fractures.

Nursing Interventions

Promoting Understanding of Osteoporosis and the Treatment Regimen

Patient teaching focuses on factors influencing the development of osteoporosis, interventions to arrest or slow the process, and measures to relieve symptoms. Adequate dietary or supplemental intake of calcium and vitamin D, regular weight-bearing exercise, and modification of lifestyle, if necessary (eg, cessation of smoking and reduced use of caffeine, carbonated soft drinks, and alcohol), help maintain bone mass. Diet, exercise, and physical activity are the primary keys to developing high-density bones that are resistant to osteoporosis. It is emphasized that all people continue to need sufficient calcium, vitamin D, sunshine, and weight-bearing exercise to slow the progression of osteoporosis.

Patient teaching related to medication therapy is important. Because gastrointestinal symptoms and abdominal distention are frequent side effects of calcium supplements, the nurse instructs the patient to take the calcium supplements with meals. Also, it is important to teach the patient to drink adequate fluids to reduce the risk of renal calculi. Bisphosphonate therapy requires adherence to prevent side effects, including esophageal and gastrointestinal disturbances. Bisphosphonates must be taken on an empty stomach with a full glass of water, and then the patient must not consume foods or liquids or assume a reclining position for 30 to 60 minutes. Nasal calcitonin is administered daily, alternating the nares to prevent nasal mucosal dryness. An adequate daily intake of dietary calcium and vitamin D is needed along with these prescribed medications.

Relieving Pain

Relief of back pain resulting from compression fracture may be accomplished by resting in bed in a supine or side-lying position several times a day. The mattress should be firm and nonsagging. Knee flexion increases comfort by relaxing back muscles. Intermittent local heat and back rubs promote muscle relaxation. The nurse instructs the patient to move the trunk as a unit and to avoid twisting. The nurse encourages good posture and teaches body mechanics. When the patient is assisted out of bed, a lumbosacral corset may be worn for temporary support and immobilization, although such a device is frequently uncomfortable and is poorly tolerated by many elderly patients. The patient gradually resumes activities as pain diminishes.

Improving Bowel Elimination

Constipation is a problem related to immobility and medications. Early institution of a high-fiber diet, increased fluids, and the use of prescribed stool softeners help prevent or minimize constipation. If the vertebral collapse involves the T10–L2 vertebrae, the patient may develop a paralytic ileus. The nurse therefore monitors the patient's intake, bowel sounds, and bowel activity.

Preventing Injury

Physical activity is essential to strengthen muscles, improve balance, prevent disuse atrophy, and retard progressive bone demineralization. Isometric exercises can strengthen trunk muscles. The nurse encourages walking, good body mechanics, and good posture. Daily weight-bearing activity, preferably outdoors in the sunshine to enhance the body's ability to produce vitamin D, is encouraged. Sudden bending, jarring, and strenuous lifting are avoided.

GERONTOLOGIC CONSIDERATIONS

Elderly people fall frequently as a result of environmental hazards, neuromuscular disorders, diminished senses and cardiovascular responses, and responses to medications. The patient and family need to be included in planning for care and preventive management regimens. For example, the home environment should be assessed for safety and elimination of potential hazards (eg, scatter rugs, cluttered rooms and stairwells, toys on the floor, pets underfoot). A safe environment can then be created (eg, well-lighted staircases with secure hand rails, grab bars in the bathroom, properly fitting footwear).

Evaluation

Expected Patient Outcomes

Expected patient outcomes may include:

1. Acquires knowledge about osteoporosis and the treatment regimen
   a. States relationship of calcium and vitamin D intake and exercise to bone mass
   b. Consumes adequate dietary calcium and vitamin D
   c. Increases level of exercise
   d. Takes prescribed medications, following instructions for administration
   e. Adheres to prescribed screening and monitoring procedures
2. Achieves pain relief
   a. Experiences pain relief at rest
   b. Experiences minimal discomfort during ADLs
   c. Demonstrates diminished tenderness at fracture site
3. Demonstrates normal bowel elimination
   a. Has active bowel sounds
   b. Reports regular pattern of bowel movements

4. Experiences no new fractures
   a. Maintains good posture
   b. Uses good body mechanics
   c. Consumes a diet high in calcium and vitamin D
   d. Engages in weight-bearing exercises (walks daily)
   e. Rests by lying down several times a day
   f. Participates in outdoor activities
   g. Creates a safe home environment
   h. Accepts assistance and supervision as needed

Osteomalacia

Osteomalacia is a metabolic bone disease characterized by inadequate mineralization of bone. As a result of faulty mineralization, there is softening and weakening of the skeleton, causing pain, tenderness to touch, bowing of the bones, and pathologic fractures. On physical examination, skeletal deformities (spinal kyphosis and bowed legs) give patients an unusual appearance and a waddling or limping gait. These patients may be uncomfortable with their appearance. As a result of calcium deficiency, muscle weakness, and unsteadiness, there is an increased risk for falls and fractures.

Pathophysiology

The primary defect in osteomalacia is a deficiency of activated vitamin D (calcitriol), which promotes calcium absorption from the gastrointestinal tract and facilitates mineralization of bone. The supply of calcium and phosphate in the extracellular fluid is low. Without adequate vitamin D, calcium and phosphate are not moved to calcification sites in bones.

Osteomalacia may result from failed calcium absorption (eg, malabsorption syndrome) or from excessive loss of calcium from the body. Gastrointestinal disorders (eg, celiac disease, chronic biliary tract obstruction, chronic pancreatitis, small bowel resection) in which fats are inadequately absorbed are likely to produce osteomalacia through loss of vitamin D (along with other fat-soluble vitamins) and calcium, the latter being excreted in the feces with fatty acids. In addition, liver and kidney diseases can produce a lack of vitamin D because these are the organs that convert vitamin D to its active form.

Severe renal insufficiency results in acidosis. The body uses available calcium to combat the acidosis, and PTH stimulates the release of skeletal calcium in an attempt to reestablish a physiologic pH. During this continual drain of skeletal calcium, bony fibrosis occurs, and bony cysts form. Chronic glomerulonephritis, obstructive uropathies, and heavy metal poisoning result in a reduced serum phosphate level and demineralization of bone.

Hyperparathyroidism leads to skeletal decalcification and thus to osteomalacia by increasing phosphate excretion in the urine. Prolonged use of antiseizure medication (eg, phenytoin, phenobarbital) poses a risk of osteomalacia, as does insufficient vitamin D (dietary, sunlight).

Osteomalacia that results from malnutrition (deficiency in vitamin D often associated with poor intake of calcium) is a result of poverty, poor dietary habits, and lack of knowledge about nutrition. It occurs most frequently in parts of the world where vitamin D is not added to food, where dietary deficiencies exist, and where sunlight is rare.

Gerontologic Considerations

A nutritious diet is particularly important in elderly people. Adequate intake of calcium and vitamin D is promoted. Because sunlight is necessary for synthesizing vitamin D, people should be encouraged to spend some time in the sun. Prevention, identification, and management of osteomalacia in the elderly are essential to reduce the incidence of fractures. When osteomalacia is combined with osteoporosis, the incidence of fracture increases.

Assessment and Diagnostic Findings

On x-ray studies, generalized demineralization of bone is evident. Studies of the vertebrae may show a compression fracture with indistinct vertebral endplates. Laboratory studies show low serum calcium and phosphorus levels and a moderately elevated alkaline phosphatase concentration. Urine excretion of calcium and creatinine is low. Bone biopsy demonstrates an increased amount of osteoid, a demineralized, cartilaginous bone matrix that is sometimes referred to as “pre-bone.”

Medical Management

Physical, psychological, and pharmaceutical measures are used to reduce the patient’s discomfort and pain. When assisting the patient to change positions, the nurse handles the patient gently, and pillows are used to support the body. As the patient responds to therapy, the skeletal discomfort diminishes.

If possible, the underlying cause of osteomalacia is corrected. Frequently, skeletal problems associated with osteomalacia resolve themselves when the underlying nutritional deficiency or pathologic process is adequately treated.

If osteomalacia is caused by malabsorption, increased doses of vitamin D, along with supplemental calcium, are usually prescribed. Exposure to sunlight may be recommended; ultraviolet radiation transforms a cholesterol substance (7-dehydrocholesterol) present in the skin into vitamin D.

If osteomalacia is dietary in origin, a diet with adequate protein and increased calcium and vitamin D is provided. The patient is instructed about dietary sources of calcium and vitamin D (eg, fortified milk and cereals, eggs, chicken livers). The safe use of supplements is reviewed. Because high doses of vitamin D are toxic and increase the risk for hypercalcemia, the importance of monitoring serum calcium levels is stressed. Vitamin D raises the concentrations of calcium and phosphorus in the extracellular fluid and thus makes these ions available for mineralization of bone.

Long-term monitoring of the patient is appropriate to ensure stabilization or reversal of osteomalacia. Some persistent orthopedic deformities may need to be treated with braces or surgery (eg, osteotomy may be performed to correct long bone deformity).

Paget’s Disease

Paget’s disease (osteitis deformans) is a disorder of localized rapid bone turnover, most commonly affecting the skull, femur, tibia, pelvic bones, and vertebrae. The disease occurs in about 2% to 3% of the population older than 50 years. The incidence is slightly greater in men than in women and increases with aging. A family history has been noted, with siblings often developing the disease. The cause of Paget's disease is not known.

Pathophysiology

In Paget's disease, there is a primary proliferation of osteoclasts, which produces bone resorption. This is followed by a compensatory increase in osteoblastic activity that replaces the bone. As bone turnover continues, a classic mosaic (disorganized) pattern of bone develops. Because the diseased bone is highly vascularized and structurally weak, pathologic fractures occur. Structural bowing of the legs causes malalignment of the hip, knee, and ankle joints, which contributes to the development of arthritis and back and joint pain.

Clinical Manifestations

Paget's disease is insidious; most patients never experience symptoms. Some patients do not experience symptoms but have skeletal deformity. A few patients have symptomatic deformity and pain. The condition is most frequently identified on x-ray studies performed during a routine physical examination or during a workup for another problem. Sclerotic changes, skeletal deformities (eg, bowing of the femur and tibia, enlargement of the skull, deformity of pelvic bones), and cortical thickening of the long bones occur.

In most patients, skeletal deformity involves the skull or long bones. The skull may thicken, and the patient may report that a hat no longer fits. In some cases, the cranium, but not the face, is enlarged. This gives the face a small, triangular appearance. Most patients with skull involvement have impaired hearing from cranial nerve compression and dysfunction. Other cranial nerves may also be compressed.

The femurs and tibiae tend to bow, producing a waddling gait. The spine is bent forward and is rigid; the chin rests on the chest. The thorax is compressed and immobile on respiration. The trunk is flexed on the legs to maintain balance and the arms are bent outward and forward and appear long in relation to the shortened trunk.

Pain, tenderness, and warmth over the bones may be noted. The pain is mild to moderate, deep, and aching; it increases with weight-bearing if the lower extremities are involved. Pain and discomfort may precede skeletal deformities of Paget's disease by years and are often wrongly attributed by the patient to old age or arthritis.

The temperature of the skin overlying the affected bone increases because of increased bone vascularity. Patients with large, highly vascular lesions may develop high-output cardiac failure because of the increased vascular bed and metabolic demands.

Assessment and Diagnostic Findings

Elevated serum alkaline phosphatase concentration and urinary hydroxyproline excretion reflect increased osteoblastic activity. Higher values suggest more active disease. Patients with Paget's disease have normal blood calcium levels. X-rays confirm the diagnosis of Paget's disease. Local areas of demineralization and bone overgrowth produce characteristic mosaic patterns and irregularities. Bone scans demonstrate the extent of the disease. Bone biopsy may aid in the differential diagnosis.

Medical Management

Pain usually responds to NSAIDs. Gait problems from bowing of the legs are managed with walking aids, shoe lifts, and physical therapy. Weight is controlled to reduce stress on weakened bones and malaligned joints. Asymptomatic patients may be managed with diets adequate in calcium and vitamin D and periodic monitoring.

Fractures, arthritis, and hearing loss are complications of Paget's disease. Fractures are managed according to location. Healing occurs if fracture reduction, immobilization, and stability are adequate. Severe degenerative arthritis may require total joint replacement. Loss of hearing is managed with hearing aids and communication techniques used with hearing-impaired people (eg, speech reading, body language).

Pharmacologic Therapy

Patients with moderate to severe disease may benefit from specific antiosteoclastic therapy. Several medications reduce bone turnover, reverse the course of the disease, relieve pain, and improve mobility.

Calcitonin, a polypeptide hormone, retards bone resorption by decreasing the number and availability of osteoclasts. Calcitonin therapy facilitates remodeling of abnormal bone into normal lamellar bone, relieves bone pain, and helps alleviate neurologic and biochemical signs and symptoms. Calcitonin is administered subcutaneously or by nasal inhalation. Side effects include flushing of the face and nausea. The effect of calcitonin therapy is evident in 3 to 6 months through reduction of bone loss and pain.

Bisphosphonates, such as etidronate disodium (Didronel) and alendronate sodium (Fosamax), produce rapid reduction in bone turnover and relief of pain. They also reduce serum alkaline phosphatase and urinary hydroxyproline levels. Food inhibits absorption of these medications. Adequate daily intake of calcium (1500 mg) and vitamin D (400 to 600 IU) is required during therapy.

Plicamycin (Mithracin), a cytotoxic antibiotic, may be used to control the disease. This medication is reserved for severely affected patients with neurologic compromise and for those whose disease is resistant to other therapy. This medication has dramatic effects on pain reduction and on serum calcium, alkaline phosphatase, and urinary hydroxyproline levels. It is administered by IV infusion; hepatic, renal, and bone marrow function must be monitored during therapy. Clinical remissions may continue for months after the medication is discontinued.

Gerontologic Considerations

Because Paget's disease tends to affect elderly people, careful assessment of a patient's pain and discomfort is necessary. Patient teaching helps the patient understand the treatment regimen, the need for a diet with adequate calcium and vitamin D, and how to compensate for altered musculoskeletal functioning. The home environment is assessed for safety to prevent falls and to reduce the risk of fracture. Strategies for coping with a chronic health problem and its effect on quality of life need to be developed.

Musculoskeletal Infections

Osteomyelitis

Osteomyelitis is an infection of the bone. The bone becomes infected in one of three ways:

- Extension of soft tissue infection (eg, infected pressure or vascular ulcer, incisional infection)
- Direct bone contamination from bone surgery, open fracture, or traumatic injury (eg, gunshot wound)
- Hematogenous (bloodborne) spread from other sites of infection (eg, infected tonsils, boils, infected teeth, upper respiratory infections). Osteomyelitis resulting from hematogenous spread typically occurs in a bone in an area of trauma or lowered resistance, possibly from subclinical (nonapparent) trauma.

Patients who are at high risk for osteomyelitis include those who are poorly nourished, elderly, or obese. Other patients at risk include those with impaired immune systems, those with chronic illnesses (eg, diabetes, rheumatoid arthritis), and those receiving long-term corticosteroid therapy or immunosuppressive agents.

Postoperative surgical wound infections occur within 30 days after surgery. They are classified as incisional (superficial, located above the deep fascia layer) or deep (involving tissue beneath the deep fascia). If an implant has been used, deep postoperative infections may occur within a year. Deep sepsis after arthroplasty may be classified as follows:

- Stage 1, acute fulminating: occurring during the first 3 months after orthopedic surgery; frequently associated with hematoma, drainage, or superficial infection
- Stage 2, delayed onset: occurring between 4 and 24 months after surgery
- Stage 3, late onset: occurring 2 or more years after surgery, usually as a result of hematogenous spread

Bone infections are more difficult to eradicate than soft tissue infections because the infected bone is mostly avascular and not accessible to the body's natural immune response. Also, there is decreased penetration by antibiotics. Osteomyelitis may become chronic and may affect the patient's quality of life.

Pathophysiology

Between 70% and 80% of bone infections are caused by *Staphylococcus aureus*. Other pathogenic organisms that are frequently found in osteomyelitis include *Proteus* and *Pseudomonas* species and *Escherichia coli*. The incidence of penicillin-resistant, nosocomial, gram-negative, and anaerobic infections is increasing.

The initial response to infection is inflammation, increased vascularity, and edema. After 2 or 3 days, thrombosis of the blood vessels occurs in the area, resulting in ischemia with bone necrosis. The infection extends into the medullary cavity and under the periosteum and may spread into adjacent soft tissues and joints. Unless the infective process is treated promptly, a bone abscess forms. The resulting abscess cavity contains dead bone tissue (the **sequestrum**), which does not easily liquefy and drain. Therefore, the cavity cannot collapse and heal, as it does in soft tissue abscesses. New bone growth (the **involucrum**) forms and surrounds the sequestrum. Although healing appears to take place, a chronically infected sequestrum remains and produces recurring abscesses throughout the patient's life. This is referred to as chronic osteomyelitis.

Clinical Manifestations

When the infection is bloodborne, the onset is usually sudden, occurring often with the clinical and laboratory manifestations of sepsis (eg, chills, high fever, rapid pulse, general malaise). The systemic symptoms at first may overshadow the local signs. As the infection extends through the cortex of the bone, it involves the periosteum and the soft tissues. The infected area becomes painful, swollen, and extremely tender. The patient may describe a constant, pulsating pain that intensifies with movement as a result of the pressure of the collecting pus. When osteomyelitis occurs from spread of adjacent infection or from direct contamination, there are no symptoms of sepsis. The area is swollen, warm, painful, and tender to touch.

The patient with chronic osteomyelitis presents with a continuously draining sinus or experiences recurrent periods of pain, inflammation, swelling, and drainage. The low-grade infection thrives in scar tissue, because it has a reduced blood supply.

Assessment and Diagnostic Findings

In acute osteomyelitis, early x-ray findings demonstrate soft tissue swelling. In about 2 weeks, areas of irregular decalcification, bone necrosis, periosteal elevation, and new bone formation are evident. Radioisotope bone scans, particularly the isotope-labeled white blood cell (WBC) scan, and magnetic resonance imaging (MRI) help with early definitive diagnosis. Blood studies reveal leukocytosis and an elevated ESR. Wound and blood culture studies are performed to identify appropriate antibiotic therapy.

With chronic osteomyelitis, large, irregular cavities, raised periosteum, sequestra, or dense bone formations are seen on x-ray. Bone scans may be performed to identify areas of infection. The ESR and the WBC count are usually normal. Anemia, associated with chronic infection, may be evident. The abscess is cultured to determine the infective organism and appropriate antibiotic therapy.

Prevention

Prevention of osteomyelitis is the goal. Elective orthopedic surgery should be postponed if the patient has a current infection (eg, urinary tract infection, sore throat) or a recent history of infection. During orthopedic surgery, careful attention is paid to the surgical environment and to techniques to decrease direct bone contamination. Prophylactic antibiotics, administered to achieve adequate tissue levels at the time of surgery and for 24 hours after surgery, are helpful. Urinary catheters and drains are removed as soon as possible to decrease the incidence of hematogenous spread of infection.

Treatment of focal infections diminishes hematogenous spread. Aseptic postoperative wound care reduces the incidence of superficial infections and osteomyelitis. Prompt management of soft tissue infections reduces extension of infection to the bone. When patients who have had joint replacement surgery undergo dental procedures or other invasive procedures (eg, cystoscopy), prophylactic antibiotics are frequently recommended.

Medical Management

The initial goal of therapy is to control and halt the infective process. Antibiotic therapy depends on the results of blood and wound cultures. Frequently, the infection is caused by more than one pathogen. General supportive measures (eg, hydration, diet high in vitamins and protein, correction of anemia) should be instituted. The area affected with osteomyelitis is immobilized to decrease discomfort and to prevent pathologic fracture of the weakened bone. Warm wet soaks for 20 minutes several times a day may be prescribed to increase circulation to the affected area.

Pharmacologic Therapy

As soon as the culture specimens are obtained, IV antibiotic therapy begins, based on the assumption that infection results from a staphylococcal organism that is sensitive to a semisynthetic penicillin or cephalosporin. The aim is to control the infection before the blood supply to the area diminishes as a result of thrombosis. Around-the-clock dosing is necessary to achieve a sustained high therapeutic blood level of the antibiotic. After results of the culture and sensitivity studies are known, an antibiotic to which the causative organism is sensitive is prescribed. IV antibiotic therapy continues for 3 to 6 weeks. After the infection appears to be controlled, the antibiotic may be administered orally for up to 3 months. To enhance absorption of the orally administered medication, antibiotics should not be administered with food.

Surgical Management

If the infection is chronic, surgical débridement is indicated but is reserved for patients with acute osteomyelitis that does not respond to antibiotic therapy. The infected bone is surgically exposed, the purulent and necrotic material is removed, and the area is irrigated with sterile saline solution. Antibiotic-impregnated beads may be placed in the wound for direct application of antibiotics for 2 to 4 weeks. IV antibiotic therapy is continued.

In chronic osteomyelitis, antibiotics are adjunctive therapy to surgical débridement. A sequestrectomy (removal of enough involucrum to enable the surgeon to remove the sequestrum) is performed. In many cases, sufficient bone is removed to convert a deep cavity into a shallow saucer (saucerization). All dead, infected bone and cartilage must be removed before permanent healing can occur. A closed suction irrigation system may be used to remove debris. Wound irrigation using sterile physiologic saline solution may be performed for 7 to 8 days.

The wound is either closed tightly to obliterate the dead space or packed and closed later by granulation or possibly by grafting. The débrided cavity may be packed with cancellous bone graft to stimulate healing. With a large defect, the cavity may be filled with a vascularized bone transfer or muscle flap (in which a muscle is moved from an adjacent area with blood supply intact). These microsurgery techniques enhance the blood supply. The improved blood supply facilitates bone healing and eradication of the infection. These surgical procedures may be staged over time to ensure healing. Because surgical débridement weakens the bone, internal fixation or external supportive devices may be needed to stabilize or support the bone to prevent pathologic fracture.

Nursing Process

The Patient With Osteomyelitis

Assessment

The patient reports an acute onset of signs and symptoms (eg, localized pain, edema, erythema, fever) or recurrent drainage of an infected sinus with associated pain, edema, and low-grade fever. The nurse assesses the patient for risk factors (eg, older age, diabetes, long-term corticosteroid therapy) and for a history of previous injury, infection, or orthopedic surgery. The patient avoids pressure on the area and guards movement. In acute hematogenous osteomyelitis, the patient exhibits generalized weakness due to the systemic reaction to the infection.

Physical examination reveals an inflamed, markedly edematous, warm area that is tender. Purulent drainage may be noted. The patient has an elevated temperature. With chronic osteomyelitis, the temperature elevation may be minimal, occurring in the afternoon or evening.

Nursing Diagnoses

Based on the nursing assessment data, nursing diagnoses for the patient with osteomyelitis may include the following:

- Acute pain related to inflammation and edema
- Impaired physical mobility related to pain, use of immobilization devices, and weight-bearing limitations
- Risk for extension of infection: bone abscess formation
- Deficient knowledge related to the treatment regimen

Planning and Goals

The patient's goals may include relief of pain, improved physical mobility within therapeutic limitations, control and eradication of infection, and knowledge of the treatment regimen.

Nursing Interventions

Relieving Pain

The affected part may be immobilized with a splint to decrease pain and muscle spasm. The nurse monitors the neurovascular status of the affected extremity. The wounds are frequently very painful, and the extremity must be handled with great care and gentleness. Elevation reduces swelling and associated discomfort. Pain is controlled with prescribed analgesics and other pain-reducing techniques.

Improving Physical Mobility

Treatment regimens restrict activity. The bone is weakened by the infective process and must be protected by immobilization devices and by avoidance of stress on the bone. The patient must understand the rationale for the activity restrictions. The joints above and below the affected part should be gently moved through their range of motion. The nurse encourages full participation in ADLs within the physical limitations to promote general well-being.

Controlling the Infectious Process

The nurse monitors the patient's response to antibiotic therapy and observes the IV access site for evidence of phlebitis, infection, or infiltration. With long-term, intensive antibiotic therapy, the nurse monitors the patient for signs of superinfection (eg, oral or vaginal candidiasis, loose or foul-smelling stools).

If surgery is necessary, the nurse takes measures to ensure adequate circulation to the affected area (wound suction to prevent fluid accumulation, elevation of the area to promote venous drainage, avoidance of pressure on the grafted area), to maintain needed immobility, and to ensure the patient's adherence to weight-bearing restrictions. The nurse changes dressings using aseptic technique to promote healing and to prevent cross-contamination.

The nurse continues to monitor the general health and nutrition of the patient. A diet high in protein and vitamin C promotes a positive nitrogen balance and healing. The nurse encourages adequate hydration as well.

Promoting Home and Community-Based Care

TEACHING PATIENTS SELF-CARE

The patient and family are taught about the importance of strictly adhering to the therapeutic regimen of antibiotics and preventing falls or other injuries that could result in bone fracture. They need to learn to maintain and manage the IV access and IV administration equipment in the home. Teaching includes medication name, dosage, frequency, administration rate, safe storage and handling, adverse reactions, and necessary laboratory monitoring. In addition, aseptic dressing and warm compress techniques are taught.

The nurse carefully monitors the patient for the development of additional sites that are painful or sudden increases in body temperature. The nurse instructs the patient and family to observe for and report elevated temperature, drainage, odor, signs of increased inflammation, adverse reactions, and signs of superinfection.

CONTINUING CARE

Management of osteomyelitis, including wound care and IV antibiotic therapy, is usually performed at home. The patient must be medically stable and physically able and motivated to adhere strictly to the therapeutic regimen of antibiotic therapy. The home care environment needs to be conducive to the promotion of health and to the requirements of the therapeutic regimen.

If warranted, the nurse completes a home assessment to determine the patient's and family's abilities regarding continuation of the therapeutic regimen. If the patient's support system is questionable or if the patient lives alone, a home care nurse may be needed to assist with IV administration of the antibiotics. The nurse monitors the patient for response to the treatment, signs and symptoms of superinfections, and adverse drug reactions. The nurse stresses the importance of follow-up health care appointments and recommends age-appropriate health screening (Chart 68-9).

Evaluation

Expected Patient Outcomes

Expected patient outcomes may include:

1. Experiences pain relief
   a. Reports decreased pain
   b. Experiences no tenderness at site of previous infection
   c. Experiences no discomfort with movement
2. Increases physical mobility
   a. Participates in self-care activities
   b. Maintains full function of unimpaired extremities
   c. Demonstrates safe use of immobilizing and assistive devices
   d. Modifies environment to promote safety and to avoid falls
3. Shows absence of infection
   a. Takes antibiotic as prescribed
   b. Reports normal temperature
   c. Exhibits no edema
   d. Reports absence of drainage
   e. Laboratory results indicate normal white blood cell count and erythrocyte sedimentation rate.
   f. Wound cultures are negative.

CHART 68-9

HOME CARE CHECKLIST • Osteomyelitis

At the completion of the home care instruction, the patient or caregiver will be able to:	Patient	Caregiver
• Describe osteomyelitis	✔	✔
• Relieve pain with pharmacologic and nonpharmacologic interventions	✔	
• State weight-bearing and activity restrictions	✔	✔
• Demonstrate safe use of ambulatory aids and assistive devices	✔	
• Describe use of prescribed medications	✔	✔
• Comply with antibiotic regimen	✔	
• Promote healing through aseptic dressing changes	✔	✔
• Demonstrate proper wound care	✔	✔
• Report signs and symptoms of continuing infection or superinfection	✔	✔

4. Adheres to therapeutic plan
   a. Takes medications as prescribed
   b. Protects weakened bones
   c. Demonstrates proper wound care
   d. Reports signs and symptoms of complications promptly
   e. Consumes a diet high in protein and vitamin C
   f. Keeps follow-up health care appointments
   g. Reports increased strength
   h. Reports no elevation of temperature or recurrence of pain, edema, or other symptoms at the site

Septic (Infectious) Arthritis

Joints can become infected through spread of infection from other parts of the body (hematogenous spread) or directly through trauma or surgical instrumentation. Previous trauma to joints, joint replacement, coexisting arthritis, and diminished host resistance contribute to the development of an infected joint. *S. aureus* causes most adult joint infections, followed by streptococci and gonococci (Issa & Thompson, 2003). Prompt recognition and treatment of an infected joint are important because accumulating purulent material results in chondrolysis (destruction of hyaline cartilage).

Clinical Manifestations

The patient with acute septic arthritis usually presents with a warm, painful, swollen joint with decreased range of motion. Systemic chills, fever, and leukocytosis are present. Risk factors include advanced age, diabetes mellitus, rheumatoid arthritis, and preexisting joint disease or joint replacement. Elderly patients and patients taking corticosteroids or immunosuppressive medications may not exhibit typical clinical manifestations of infection. Therefore, they require ongoing assessment to detect infection as early as possible in the infectious process.

Assessment and Diagnostic Findings

An assessment for the source and cause of infection is performed. Diagnostic studies include aspiration, examination, and culture of the synovial fluid. Computed tomography (CT) and MRI may reveal damage to the joint lining. Radioisotope scanning may be useful in localizing the infectious process.

Management

Prompt treatment is essential and may save a joint prosthesis for patients who have one. Broad-spectrum IV antibiotics are started promptly and then changed to organism-specific antibiotics after culture results are available. The IV antibiotics are continued until symptoms disappear. The synovial fluid is monitored for sterility and decrease in WBCs.

In addition to prescribing antibiotics, the physician may aspirate the joint with a needle to remove excessive joint fluid, exudate, and debris. This promotes comfort and decreases joint destruction caused by the action of proteolytic enzymes in the purulent fluid. Occasionally, arthrotomy or arthroscopy is used to drain the joint and remove dead tissue.

The inflamed joint is supported and immobilized in a functional position by a splint that increases the patient's comfort. Analgesics, such as codeine, may be prescribed to relieve pain. After the infection has responded to antibiotic therapy, NSAIDs may be prescribed to limit joint damage. The patient's nutrition and fluid status is monitored. Progressive range-of-motion exercises are prescribed after the infection subsides.

If septic joints are treated promptly, recovery of normal function is expected. The patient is assessed periodically for recurrence. If the articular cartilage was damaged during the inflammatory reaction, joint fibrosis and diminished function may result.

The nurse describes the septic arthritis process to the patient and teaches the patient how to relieve pain using pharmacologic and nonpharmacologic interventions. The nurse also explains the importance of supporting the affected joint, adhering to the prescribed antibiotic regimen, and observing weight-bearing and activity restrictions. Additionally, the nurse demonstrates and encourages the patient to practice safe use of ambulatory aids and assistive devices.

The nurse teaches the patient strategies to promote healing through aseptic dressing changes and proper wound care. The patient is then encouraged to perform range-of-motion exercises after the infection subsides.

Bone Tumors

Neoplasms of the musculoskeletal system are of various types, including osteogenic, chondrogenic, fibrogenic, muscle (rhabdomyogenic), and marrow (reticulum) cell tumors as well as nerve, vascular, and fatty cell tumors. They may be primary tumors or metastatic tumors from primary cancers elsewhere in the body (eg, breast, lung, prostate, kidney). Metastatic bone tumors are more common than primary bone tumors.

Benign Bone Tumors

Benign tumors of the bone and soft tissue are more common than malignant primary bone tumors. Benign bone tumors generally are slow-growing, well circumscribed, and encapsulated; present few symptoms; and are not a cause of death.

Benign primary neoplasms of the musculoskeletal system include osteochondroma, enchondroma, bone cyst (eg, aneurysmal bone cyst), osteoid osteoma, rhabdomyoma, and fibroma. Some benign tumors, such as giant cell tumors, have the potential to become malignant.

Osteochondroma is the most common benign bone tumor. It usually occurs as a large projection of bone at the end of long bones (at the knee or shoulder). It develops during growth and then becomes a static bony mass. In fewer than 1% of patients, the cartilage cap of the osteochondroma may undergo malignant transformation after trauma, and a chondrosarcoma or osteosarcoma may develop.

Enchondroma is a common tumor of the hyaline cartilage that develops in the hand, femur, tibia, or humerus. Usually, the only symptom is a mild ache. Pathologic fractures may occur.

Bone cysts are expanding lesions within the bone. Aneurysmal (widening) bone cysts are seen in young adults, who present with a painful, palpable mass of the long bones, vertebrae, or flat bone. Unicameral (single cavity) bone cysts occur in children and cause mild discomfort and possible pathologic fractures of the upper humerus and femur, which may heal spontaneously.

A painful tumor that occurs in children and young adults is the osteoid osteoma. The neoplastic tissue is surrounded by reactive bone formation that can be identified by x-ray.

Giant cell tumors (osteoclastomas) are benign for long periods but may invade local tissue and cause destruction. They occur in young adults and are soft and hemorrhagic. Eventually, giant cell tumors may undergo malignant transformation and metastasize.

Malignant Bone Tumors

Primary malignant musculoskeletal tumors are relatively rare and arise from connective and supportive tissue cells (sarcomas) or bone marrow elements (multiple myeloma; see Chapter 33). Malignant primary musculoskeletal tumors include osteosarcoma, chondrosarcoma, Ewing's sarcoma, and fibrosarcoma. Soft tissue sarcomas include liposarcoma, fibrosarcoma of soft tissue, and rhabdomyosarcoma. Bone tumor metastasis to the lungs is common.

Osteogenic sarcoma (osteosarcoma) is the most common and most often fatal primary malignant bone tumor. Prognosis depends on whether the tumor has metastasized to the lungs at the time the patient seeks health care. Osteogenic sarcoma appears most frequently in males between the ages of 10 and 25 years (in bones that grow rapidly), in older people with Paget's disease, and as a result of radiation exposure. Clinical manifestations include pain, edema, limited motion, and weight loss (which is considered an ominous finding). The bony mass may be palpable, tender, and fixed, with an increase in skin temperature over the mass and venous distention. The primary lesion may involve any bone, but the most common sites are the distal femur, the proximal tibia, and the proximal humerus.

Malignant tumors of the hyaline cartilage are called chondrosarcomas. These tumors are the second most common primary malignant bone tumor. They are large, bulky, slow-growing tumors that affect adults. The usual tumor sites include the pelvis, femur, humerus, spine, scapula, and tibia. Metastasis to the lungs occurs in fewer than half of patients. When these tumors are well differentiated, large bloc excision or amputation of the affected extremity results in increased survival rates. These tumors may recur.

Metastatic Bone Disease

Metastatic bone disease (secondary bone tumor) is more common than any primary bone tumor. Tumors arising from tissues elsewhere in the body may invade the bone and produce localized bone destruction (lytic lesions) or bone overgrowth (blastic lesions). The most common primary sites of tumors that metastasize to bone are the kidney, prostate, lung, breast, ovary, and thyroid. Metastatic tumors most frequently attack the skull, spine, pelvis, femur, and humerus and often involve more than one bone (polyostotic).

Pathophysiology

A tumor in the bone causes the normal bone tissue to react by osteolytic response (bone destruction) or osteoblastic response (bone formation). Primary tumors cause bone destruction, which weakens the bone, resulting in bone fractures. Adjacent normal bone responds to the tumor by altering its normal pattern of remodeling. The bone's surface changes and the contours enlarge in the tumor area.

Malignant bone tumors invade and destroy adjacent bone tissue. Benign bone tumors, in contrast, have a symmetric, controlled growth pattern and place pressure on adjacent bone tissue. Malignant invading bone tumors weaken the structure of the bone until it can no longer withstand the stress of ordinary use; pathologic fracture commonly results.

Clinical Manifestations

Patients with metastatic bone tumor may have a wide range of associated clinical manifestations. They may be symptom-free or have pain (mild and occasional to constant and severe), varying degrees of disability, and, at times, obvious bone growth. Weight loss, malaise, and fever may be present. The tumor may be diagnosed only after pathologic fracture has occurred.

With spinal metastasis, spinal cord compression may occur. It can progress rapidly or slowly. Neurologic deficits (eg, progressive pain, weakness, gait abnormality, paresthesia, paraplegia, urinary retention, loss of bowel or bladder control) must be identified early and treated with decompressive laminectomy to prevent permanent spinal cord injury.

Assessment and Diagnostic Findings

The differential diagnosis is based on the history, physical examination, and diagnostic studies, including CT, bone scans, myelography, arteriography, MRI, biopsy, and biochemical assays of the blood and urine. Serum alkaline phosphatase levels are frequently elevated with osteogenic sarcoma. With metastatic carcinoma of the prostate, serum acid phosphatase levels are elevated. Hypercalcemia is present with bone metastases from breast, lung, or kidney cancer. Symptoms of hypercalcemia include muscle weakness, fatigue, anorexia, nausea, vomiting, polyuria, cardiac dysrhythmias, seizures, and coma. Hypercalcemia must be identified and treated promptly. A surgical biopsy is performed for histologic identification. Extreme care is taken during the biopsy to prevent seeding and resultant recurrence after excision of the tumor.

Chest x-rays are performed to determine the presence of lung metastasis. Surgical staging of musculoskeletal tumors is based on tumor grade and site (intracompartmental or extracompartmental), as well as on metastasis. Staging is used for planning treatment.

During the diagnostic period, the nurse explains the diagnostic tests and provides psychological and emotional support to the patient and family. The nurse assesses coping behaviors and encourages use of support systems.

Medical Management

Primary Bone Tumors

The goal of primary bone tumor treatment is to destroy or remove the tumor. This may be accomplished by surgical excision (ranging from local excision to amputation and disarticulation), radiation therapy if the tumor is radiosensitive, and chemotherapy (preoperative, intraoperative [neoadjuvant], postoperative, and adjunctive for possible micrometastases). Major gains are being made in the use of wide bloc excision with restorative grafting technique (Muscolo, Ayerza, Aponte-Tinao, et al., 2005). Survival and quality of life are important considerations in procedures that attempt to save the involved extremity (Zahlten-Hingurange, Bernd, Ewerbeck, et al., 2004).

Limb-sparing (salvage) procedures are used to remove the tumor and adjacent tissue. A customized prosthesis, total joint arthroplasty, or bone tissue from the patient (autograft) or from a cadaver donor (allograft) replaces the resected tissue. Soft tissue and blood vessels may need grafting because of the extent of the excision. Complications may include infection, loosening or dislocation of the prosthesis, allograft nonunion, fracture, devitalization of the skin and soft tissues, joint fibrosis, and recurrence of the tumor. Function and rehabilitation after limb salvage depend on positive encouragement and reducing the risk of complications.

Surgical removal of the tumor may require amputation of the affected extremity, with the amputation extending well above the tumor to achieve local control of the primary lesion (see Nursing Process: The Patient Undergoing an Amputation in Chapter 69).

Because of the danger of metastasis with malignant bone tumors, combined chemotherapy is started before and continued after surgery in an effort to eradicate micrometastatic lesions. The goal of combined chemotherapy is greater therapeutic effect at a lower toxicity rate with reduced resistance to the medications. There is an improved long-term survival rate when a localized osteosarcoma is removed and chemotherapy is initiated. Soft tissue sarcomas are treated with radiation, limb-sparing excision, and adjuvant chemotherapy (see Chapter 16).

Secondary Bone Tumors

The treatment of metastatic bone cancer is palliative. The therapeutic goal is to relieve the patient's pain and discomfort while promoting quality of life.

If metastatic disease weakens the bone, structural support and stabilization are needed to prevent pathologic fracture. At times, large bones with metastatic lesions are strengthened by prophylactic internal fixation. Internal fixation of pathologic fractures, arthroplasty, or methylmethacrylate (bone cement) reconstruction minimizes associated disability and pain. Patients with metastatic disease are at higher risk than other patients for postoperative pulmonary congestion, hypoxemia, deep vein thrombosis, and hemorrhage.

Hypercalcemia results from breakdown of bone. It needs to be recognized promptly. Treatment includes hydration with IV administration of normal saline solution; diuresis; mobilization; and medications such as bisphosphonates, pamidronate, and calcitonin. Because inactivity leads to loss of bone mass and increased calcium in the blood, the nurse assists the patient to increase activity and ambulation.

Hematopoiesis is frequently disrupted by tumor invasion of the bone marrow or by treatment (chemotherapy or radiation). Blood component therapy restores hematologic factors. Pain can result from multiple factors, including the osseous metastasis, surgery, chemotherapy or radiation side effects, and arthritis. Pain must be assessed accurately and managed with adequate and appropriate opioid, nonopioid, and nonpharmaceutical interventions. External beam radiation to involved metastatic sites may be used. Patients with multiple bony metastases may achieve pain control with systemically administered "bone-seeking" isotopes (eg, strontium 89). See Chapter 13 for more information about pain management.

Additional therapies are used to treat the original cancer. Radiation and hormonal therapy may be effective in promoting healing of osteolytic lesions. Chemotherapy is used to control the primary disease (see Chapter 16).

Nursing Process

The Patient With a Bone Tumor

Assessment

The nurse asks the patient about the onset and course of symptoms. During the interview, the nurse assesses the patient's understanding of the disease process, how the patient and the family have been coping, and how the patient has managed the pain. On physical examination, the nurse gently palpates the mass and notes its size and associated soft tissue swelling, pain, and tenderness. Assessment of the neurovascular status and range of motion of the extremity provides baseline data for future comparisons. The nurse evaluates the patient's mobility and ability to perform ADLs.

Diagnosis

Nursing Diagnoses

Based on the nursing assessment data, the major nursing diagnoses for the patient with a bone tumor may include the following:

- Deficient knowledge related to the disease process and the therapeutic regimen
- Acute and chronic pain related to pathologic process and surgery
- Risk for injury: pathologic fracture related to tumor and metastasis
- Ineffective coping related to fear of the unknown, perception of disease process, and inadequate support system
- Risk for situational low self-esteem related to loss of body part or alteration in role performance

Collaborative Problems/ Potential Complications

Potential complications may include the following:

- Delayed wound healing
- Nutritional deficiency
- Infection
- Hypercalcemia

Planning and Goals

The major goals for the patient include knowledge of the disease process and treatment regimen, control of pain, absence of pathologic fractures, effective patterns of coping, improved self-esteem, and absence of complications.

Nursing Interventions

The nursing care of a patient who has undergone excision of a bone tumor is similar in many respects to that of other patients who have had skeletal surgery. Vital signs are monitored; blood loss is assessed; and observations are made to assess for the development of complications such as deep vein thrombosis, pulmonary emboli, infection, contracture, and disuse atrophy. The affected part is elevated to reduce edema, and the neurovascular status of the extremity is assessed.

Promoting Understanding of the Disease Process and Treatment Regimen

Patient and family teaching about the disease process and diagnostic and management regimens is essential. Explanation of diagnostic tests, treatments (eg, wound care), and expected results (eg, decreased range of motion, numbness, change of body contours) helps the patient deal with the procedures and changes. Cooperation and adherence to the therapeutic regimen are enhanced through understanding. The nurse can most effectively reinforce and clarify information provided by the physician by being present during these discussions.

Relieving Pain

Accurate pain assessment is the foundation for pain management. Pharmacologic and nonpharmacologic pain management techniques are used to relieve pain and increase the patient's comfort level. The nurse works with the patient in designing the most effective pain management regimen, thereby increasing the patient's control over the pain. The nurse prepares the patient and gives support during painful procedures. Prescribed IV or epidural analgesics are used during the early postoperative period. Later, oral or transdermal opioid or nonopioid analgesics are indicated to alleviate pain. In addition, external radiation or systemic radioisotopes (eg, strontium 89) may be used to control pain. See Chapter 13 for further discussion of pain management.

Preventing Pathologic Fracture

Bone tumors weaken the bone to a point at which normal activities or even position changes can result in fracture. During nursing care, the affected extremities must be supported and handled gently. External supports (eg, splints) may be used for additional protection. At times, the patient may elect to have surgery (eg, open reduction with internal fixation, joint replacement) in an attempt to prevent pathologic fracture. Prescribed weight-bearing restrictions must be followed. The nurse and physical therapist teach the patient how to use assistive devices safely and how to strengthen unaffected extremities.

Promoting Coping Skills

The nurse encourages the patient and family to verbalize their fears, concerns, and feelings. They need to be supported as they deal with the impact of the malignant bone tumor. Feelings of shock, despair, and grief are expected. Referral to a psychiatric advanced practice nurse, psychologist, counselor, or spiritual advisor may be indicated for specific psychological help and emotional support.

Promoting Self-Esteem

Independence versus dependence is an issue for the patient who has a malignancy. Lifestyle is dramatically changed, at least temporarily. It is important to support the family in working through the adjustments that must be made. The nurse assists the patient in dealing with changes in body image due to surgery and possible amputation. It is helpful to provide realistic reassurance about the future and resumption of role-related activities and to encourage self-care and socialization. The patient participates in planning daily activities. The nurse encourages the patient to be as independent as possible. Involvement of the patient and family throughout treatment encourages confidence, restoration of self-concept, and a sense of being in control of one's life.

Monitoring and Managing Potential Complications

DELAYED WOUND HEALING

Wound healing may be delayed because of tissue trauma from surgery, previous radiation therapy, inadequate nutrition, or infection. The nurse minimizes pressure on the wound site to promote circulation to the tissues. An aseptic, nontraumatic wound dressing promotes healing. Monitoring and reporting of laboratory findings facilitate initiation of interventions to promote homeostasis and wound healing.

Repositioning the patient at frequent intervals reduces the incidence of skin breakdown and pressure ulcers. Special therapeutic beds may be needed to prevent skin breakdown and to promote wound healing after extensive surgical reconstruction and skin grafting.

INADEQUATE NUTRITION

Because loss of appetite, nausea, and vomiting are frequent side effects of chemotherapy and radiation therapy, it is necessary to provide adequate nutrition for healing and health promotion. Antiemetics and relaxation techniques reduce the adverse gastrointestinal effects of chemotherapy. Stomatitis is controlled with anesthetic or antifungal mouthwash (see Chapter 16). Adequate hydration is essential. Nutritional supplements or parenteral nutrition may be prescribed to achieve adequate nutrition.

OSTEOMYELITIS AND WOUND INFECTIONS

Prophylactic antibiotics and strict aseptic dressing techniques are used to diminish the occurrence of osteomyelitis and wound infections. During healing, other infections (eg, upper respiratory infections) need to be prevented so that hematogenous spread does not result in osteomyelitis. If the patient is receiving chemotherapy, it is important to monitor the WBC count and to instruct the patient to avoid contact with people who have colds or other infections.

HYPERCALCEMIA

Hypercalcemia is a dangerous complication of bone cancer. The symptoms must be recognized and treatment initiated promptly. Symptoms include muscular weakness, incoordination, anorexia, nausea and vomiting, constipation, electrocardiographic changes (eg, shortened QT interval and ST segment, bradycardia, heart blocks), and altered mental states (eg, confusion, lethargy, psychotic behavior). See Chapter 14 for a discussion of hypercalcemia and its management.

Promoting Home and Community-Based Care

TEACHING PATIENTS SELF-CARE

Preparation for and coordination of continuing health care are begun early as a multidisciplinary effort. Patient teaching addresses medication, dressing, treatment regimens, and the importance of physical and occupational therapy programs. The nurse teaches weight-bearing limitations and special handling to prevent pathologic fractures. It is important that the patient and family know the signs and symptoms of possible complications as well as resources available for continuing care (Chart 68-10).

CONTINUING CARE

Frequently, arrangements are made with a home health care agency for home care supervision and follow-up. The home care nurse assesses the patient's and family's abilities to meet the patient's needs and determines whether the services of other agencies are needed. The nurse advises the patient to have readily available the telephone numbers of people to contact in case concerns arise.

The nurse emphasizes the need for long-term health supervision to ensure cure or to detect tumor recurrence or metastasis and the need for recommended health screening. If the patient has metastatic disease, end-of-life issues may need to be explored. Referral for hospice care is made if appropriate.

CHART 68-10

HOME CARE CHECKLIST • Bone Tumor

At the completion of the home care instruction, the patient or caregiver will be able to:	Patient	Caregiver
• Describe tumor growth process	✔	✔
• Control pain with pharmacologic and nonpharmacologic interventions	✔	✔
• Support affected musculoskeletal area	✔	
• Describe use of prescribed medications	✔	✔
• Comply with medication regimen	✔	
• Consume diet to promote healing and health	✔	
• State weight-bearing and activity restrictions	✔	✔
• Demonstrate safe use of ambulatory aids and assistive devices	✔	
• Protect affected bone from pathologic fracture	✔	✔
• Identify complications of tumor and therapy	✔	✔
• Report signs and symptoms of complications promptly	✔	✔
• Use effective coping strategies	✔	
• Maintain role performance	✔	

Evaluation

Expected Patient Outcomes

Expected patient outcomes may include:

1. Describes disease process and treatment regimen
   a. Describes pathologic condition
   b. States goals of the therapeutic regimen
   c. Seeks clarification of information
2. Achieves control of pain
   a. Uses multiple pain control techniques, including prescribed medications
   b. Experiences no pain or decreased pain at rest, during ADLs, or at surgical sites
3. Experiences no pathologic fracture
   a. Avoids stress to weakened bones
   b. Uses assistive devices safely and appropriately
   c. Strengthens uninvolved extremities with exercise
4. Demonstrates effective coping patterns
   a. Verbalizes feelings
   b. Identifies strengths and abilities
   c. Makes decisions
   d. Requests assistance as needed
5. Demonstrates positive self-concept
   a. Identifies home and family responsibilities that can be accomplished
   b. Exhibits confidence in own abilities
   c. Demonstrates acceptance of altered body image
   d. Demonstrates independence in ADLs
6. Exhibits absence of complications
   a. Demonstrates wound healing
   b. Experiences no skin breakdown
   c. Maintains or increases body weight
   d. Experiences no infections
   e. Does not experience hypercalcemia
   f. Manages side effects of therapies
   g. Reports symptoms of medication toxicity or complications
7. Participates in continuing health care at home
   a. Adheres to prescribed regimen (ie, takes prescribed medications, continues physical and occupational therapy programs)
   b. Acknowledges need for long-term health supervision
   c. Keeps follow-up health care appointments
   d. Reports occurrence of symptoms or complications

Critical Thinking Exercises

1 Your elderly aunt, an avid gardener and knitter, calls to tell you that she is awakened nearly every night with pain and numbness in both of her hands. What other questions would you ask her to try to determine the cause of her pain? What is the rationale for obtaining this information? What advice would you provide her for further investigation of this problem?

2 ebp At the general medical clinic where you are a nurse, a 64-year-old woman presents with acute onset of low back pain. You discover that she has a history of long-term alcohol use and has smoked one pack of cigarettes daily for the past 45 years. What musculoskeletal condi-

tions is she at risk of developing? What specific questions would you ask her to determine the status of her bone health? Discuss the strength of the evidence that supports any risk factor reduction strategies you consider implementing.

3 ebp You are a home care nurse who is about to visit a 26-year-old patient with osteomyelitis that occurred after a fracture to the left tibia and fibula sustained in a motorcycle crash. What is the strength of the evidence that identifies factors that affect bone healing? Discuss the significance of these factors in determining your health teaching strategies for this patient.

4 You are caring for an elderly patient who has advanced cancer. During the afternoon, she complains of muscle weakness, extreme fatigue, anorexia, and nausea. Her urinary output is also elevated. What laboratory value would you assess? What nursing interventions would you implement in light of her new symptoms? What might be the pathophysiology behind these new symptoms?

REFERENCES AND SELECTED READINGS

BOOKS

Agency for Healthcare Research and Quality (1994). *Acute low back problems in adults: Clinical practice guidelines.* (AHRQ Pub. No. 95-0643). Rockville, MD: U.S. Department of Health and Human Services, Public Health Service. Author.

American Academy of Family Physicians (2002). *Osteoporosis: Nutrition management for older adults.* Washington, DC: Nutrition Screening Initiative.

Baxter, R. E. (2003). *Pocket guide to musculoskeletal assessment.* Philadelphia: WB Saunders.

Bickley, L. S., & Szilagyi, P. G. (2006). *Bates' guide to physical assessment* (9th ed.). Philadelphia: Lippincott Williams & Wilkins.

DeGowin, R. L., & Brown, D. D. (2004). *DeGowin's diagnostic examination* (8th ed.). New York: McGraw-Hill.

Dunphy, L. M., & Winland-Brown, J. E. (2001). *Primary care: The art and science of advanced practice nursing.* Philadelphia: F. A. Davis Company.

Konin, J. G. (2002). *Special tests for orthopedic examination* (2nd ed.). Clifton Park, NY: Delmar Learning.

Maher, A. B., Salmond, S. W., & Pellino, T. (Eds.). (2002). *Orthopedic nursing* (2nd ed.). Philadelphia: W. B. Saunders.

McGee, D. J. (2002). *Orthopedic physical assessment* (4th ed.). Philadelphia: W. B. Saunders.

Miller, C. A. (2004). *Nursing for wellness in older adults: Theory and practice* (4th ed.). Philadelphia: Lippincott Williams & Wilkins.

National Osteoporosis Foundation (2002). *America's bone health: The state of osteoporosis and low bone mass in our nation.* Washington, DC: National Osteoporosis Foundation.

Porth, C. M. (2005). *Pathophysiology: Concepts of altered health states* (7th ed.). Philadelphia: Lippincott Williams & Wilkins.

Rubin, E., Gorstein, F., Schwarting, R., et al. (2004). *Pathology* (4th ed.). Philadelphia: Lippincott Williams & Wilkins.

Shoen, D. C. (2000). *Adult orthopedic nursing.* Philadelphia: Lippincott Williams & Wilkins.

Skinner, H. (2003). *Current diagnosis and treatment in orthopedics.* New York: McGraw-Hill.

U.S. Department of Health and Human Services (2004). *Bone health and osteoporosis: A report of the Surgeon General.* U.S. Department of Health and Human Services/Public Health Services, Office of the Surgeon General, Rockville, MD.

Weber, J. W., & Kelley, J. (2006). *Health assessment in nursing* (3rd ed.). Philadelphia: Lippincott Williams & Wilkins.

World Health Organization (2003). *Prevention and management of osteoporosis.* Geneva, Switzerland: World Health Organization.

JOURNALS

**Asterisks indicates nursing research articles.*

Achenbrenner, J. A., Robbins, J., Chen, Z., et al. (2003). Effects of estrogen plus progestin on risk of fracture and bone mineral density: The Women's Health Initiative randomized trial. *Journal of American Medical Association, 290*(13), 1729–1738.

Alam, N. M., Archer, J. A., & Lee, E. (2004). Osteoporotic fragility fractures in African Americans: Under-recognized and undertreated. *Journal of the National Medical Association, 96*(12), 1640–1645.

Bates, D. W., Black, D. M., & Cummings, S. W. (2002). Clinical use of bone densitometry: Clinical applications. *Journal of American Medical Association, 288*(15), 1898–1901.

Binkley, N., & Krueger, D. (2005). Current osteoporosis prevention and management. *Topics in Geriatric Rehabilitation, 21*(1), 17–29.

Bonnick, S. L. (2005). Bone mass measurement techniques in clinical practice: Methods, applications, and interpretation. *Topics in Geriatric Rehabilitation, 21*(1), 30–41.

Cauley, J. A., Robbins, J., Chen, Z., et al. (2003). Effects of estrogen plus progestin on risk of fracture and bone mineral density: The Women's Health Initiative randomized trial. *Journal of American Medical Association, 290*(13), 1729–1738.

Childs, S. G. (2005). Dupuytren's disease. *Orthopaedic Nursing, 24*(2), 160–163.

Colon-Emeric, C. S., Caebeer, L., Saag, K., et al. (2004). Barriers to providing osteoporosis care in skilled nursing facilities: Perceptions of medical directors and directors of nursing. *Journal of the American Medical Directors Association, 6*(3 suppl.), S61–S66.

Dincbas, F. O., Koca, S., Mandel, N. M., et al. (2005). The role of preoperative radiotherapy in nonmetastatic high-grade osteosarcoma of the extremities for limb-sparing surgery. *International Journal of Radiation Oncology, Biology, Physics, 62*(3), 820–828.

Francis, R. (2005). Osteoporosis management in older people. *Geriatric Medicine, 35*(3), 71–74.

Hampton, T. (2004). Experts urge early investment in bone health. *Journal of American Medical Association, 291*(7), 811–812.

Hayne, J. B. (2003). Vertebroplasty and kyphoplasty: New treatments for painful osteoporotic vertebral fractures. *American Journal of Nursing, 103*(9), 64CC–64FF.

Hoffmeister, E. (2005). Preventing fractures: Different approaches for patients with osteoporosis. *Bone and Joint, 11*(4), 37–39.

Issa, N. C., & Thompson, R. L. (2003). Diagnosing and managing septic arthritis: A practical approach. *Journal of Musculoskeletal Medicine, 20*(2), 70–75.

Lemke, D. M. (2005). Vertebroplasty and kyphoplasty for treatment of painful osteoporotic compression fractures. *Journal of the American Academy of Nurse Practitioners, 17*(7), 268–276.

Lew, D. P., & Waldvogel, F. A. (2004). Osteomyelitis. *Lancet, 364*(9431), 369–379.

Maher, C. G. (2004). Effective physical treatment for chronic low back pain. *Orthopaedic Clinics of North America, 35*(1), 57–64.

Malanga, G. A., & Dennis, R. L. (2005). Treatment of acute low back pain: Use of medications. *Journal of Musculoskeletal Medicine, 22*(2), 79–84.

*Marrs, J. (2005). Case analysis: Osteoporosis in the oncology setting. *Clinical Journal of Oncology Nursing, 9*(2), 261–263.

McGraw, K. J., Lippert, J. A., Minkus, K. D., et al. (2002). Prospective evaluation of pain relief in 100 patients undergoing percutaneous vertebroplasty: Results and follow-up. *Journal of Vascular and Interventional Radiology, 13*(9), 883–886.

McGuire, K. J., Bernstein, J., Polsky, D., et al. (2004). Delays until surgery after hip fracture increases mortality. *Clinical Orthopaedics and Related Research, 428*(11), 294–301.

Muscolo, D. L., Ayerza, M. A., Aponte-Tinao, L. A., et al. (2005). Use of distal femoral osteoarticular allografts in limb salvage surgery. *Journal of Bone and Joint Surgery, 87A*(11), 2449–2455.

Osteoporosis prevention, diagnosis, and therapy (Consensus Conference). (2001). *Journal of American Medical Association, 285*(6), 785–794.

Pai, S., & Sundaram, L. J. (2004). Low back pain: An economic assessment in the United States. *Orthopaedic Clinics of North America, 35*(1), 1–5.

Parker, M. J., Gillespie, L. D., & Gillespie, W. J. (2004). Hip protectors for preventing hip fractures in the elderly. *Cochrane Database System Review*, 3: CD001255.

Pollock, R., Stalley, P., Lee, K., et al. (2005). Free vascularized fibula grafts in limb salvage surgery. *Journal of Reconstructive Microsurgery, 21*(2), 79–84.

Predey, T. A., Sewall, L. E., & Smith, S. J. (2002). Percutaneous vertebroplasty: New treatment for vertebral compression fractures. *American Family Physician, 66*(4), 611–615.

Ruggiero, S. L., Mehrotra, B., Rosenberg, T. J., et al. (2004). Osteonecrosis of the jaws associated with the use of bisphosphonates: A review of 63 cases. *Journal of Oral Maxillofacial Surgery, 62*(5), 527–534.

*Sedlak, C. A., Doheny, M. O., Estok, P. J., et al. (2005). Tailored interventions to enhance osteoporosis prevention in women. *Orthopaedic Nursing, 24*(4), 270–276.

*Smeltzer, S. C., & Zimmerman, V. L. (2005). Usefulness of the SCORE Index as a predictor of osteoporosis in women with disabilities. *Orthopaedic Nursing, 24*(1), 33–39.

*Smeltzer, S. C., Zimmerman, V. L., & Capriotti, T. (2005). Osteoporosis risk and low bone mineral density in women with physical disabilities. *Archives of Physical Medicine and Rehabilitation, 86*(3), 582–586.

Sunyecz, J. A., & Weisman, S. M. (2005). The role of calcium in osteoporosis drug therapy. *Journal of Women's Health, 14*(2), 180–192.

*Thornton, M. J., Sedlak, C. A., & Doheny, M. O. (2004). Height change and bone mineral density: Revisited. *Orthopaedic Nursing, 23*(5), 315–320.

Van Schoor, N. M., Smit, J. H., Twisk, J. W., et al. (2003). Prevention of hip fractures by external hip protectors: A randomized controlled trial. *Journal of American Medical Association, 289*(15), 1957–1962.

Zahlten-Hingurange, A., Bernd, L., Ewerbeck, V., et al. (2004). Equal quality of life after limb-sparing or ablative surgery for lower extremity sarcomas. *British Journal of Cancer, 91*(6), 1012–1014.

*Ziccardi, S. L., Sedlak, C. A., & Doheny, M. O. (2004). Knowledge and health beliefs of osteoporosis in college nursing students. *Orthopaedic Nursing, 23*(2), 128–133.

Zoarski, G. H., Snow, P., & Olan, W. J. (2002). Percutaneous vertebroplasty for osteoporotic compression fractures: Quantitative prospective evaluation of long-term outcomes. *Journal of Vascular and Interventional Radiology, 13*(2), 139–148.

RESOURCES

Arthritis Foundation; P.O. Box 7669, Atlanta, GA 30357; (800) 568-4045; http://www.arthritis.org. Accessed August 10, 2006.

National Institute of Arthritis and Musculoskeletal and Skin Diseases, Office of Communications and Public Liaison, Bldg. 31/Rm.CO5, 31 Center Drive, MSC 2350, Bethesda, MD 10892; (301) 496-8190; http://www.niams.nih.gov. Accessed August 10, 2006.

National Osteoporosis Foundation; 1232 22nd Street NW, Washington, DC, 20037; (202) 223-2226; http://www.nof.org. Accessed August 10, 2006.

Paget Foundation; 120 Wall Street, Suite 1602, New York, NY 10005; (212) 509-5335; http://www.paget.org. Accessed August 10, 2006.

Society for Interventional Radiology; 3975 Fair Ridge Drive, Suite 400 North, Fairfax, VA 22033; (800) 488-7284; http://www.sirweb.org. Accessed August 10, 2006.

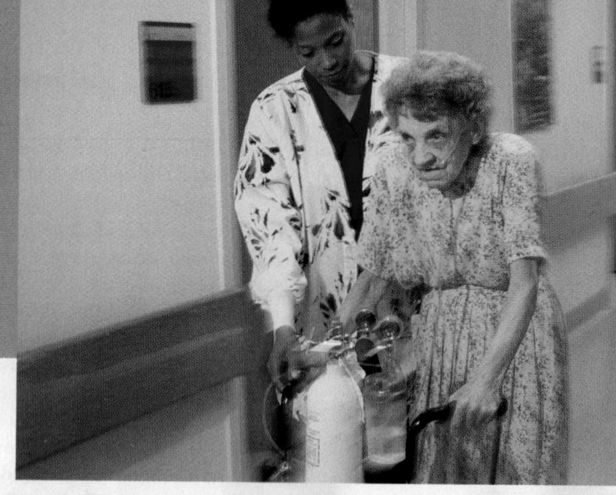

CHAPTER 69

Management of Patients With Musculoskeletal Trauma

Learning Objectives

On completion of this chapter, the learner will be able to:

1. Differentiate between contusions, strains, sprains, and dislocations.
2. Describe selected sport and occupational injuries and injury-prevention strategies.
3. Specify the clinical manifestations of a fracture and the emergency management of the patient with a fracture.
4. Describe the principles and methods of fracture reduction, fracture immobilization, and management of open fractures.
5. Use the nursing process as a framework for care of the patient with a simple fracture.
6. Describe the prevention and management of immediate and delayed complications of fractures.
7. Describe the rehabilitation needs of patients with fractures of the clavicle, upper and lower extremities, pelvis, hips, ribs, and thoracolumbar spine.
8. Use the nursing process as a framework for care of the elderly patient with a fracture of the hip.
9. Describe the rehabilitation and health education needs of the patient who has had an amputation.
10. Use the nursing process as a framework for care of the patient with an amputation.

Injury to one part of the musculoskeletal system results in injury or dysfunction of adjacent structures and of the structures enclosed or supported by them. If a bone is broken, the adjacent muscles cannot function, and blood vessels and nerves in the vicinity of the fracture may be injured. If motor nerves do not send impulses to the muscles, the muscles do not contract and the bones cannot move. If joint surfaces do not articulate normally, neither the bones nor the muscles can function properly.

Treatment of injury to the musculoskeletal system involves providing support to the injured part until healing is complete. Support may be provided by externally applied bandages, adhesive strapping, splints, or casts. Alternatively, support may be applied directly to the bone in the form of pins or plates. At times, traction must be applied to prevent or correct deformity or shortening. Pain relief is important during treatment to facilitate healing. Anti-inflammatory medications, muscle relaxants, and analgesics may help diminish edema and relax muscles at risk for spasm that can cause further injury to inflamed muscles or to fractured bones.

After the immediate and painful effects of the injury have passed, treatment efforts are focused on preventing fibrosis and atrophy or degeneration of the injured muscles and joint structures, respectively. Proper exercise guards against these complications. In some cases, the medications administered and the support applied permit earlier activity and promote healing. Various forms of physical and occupational therapy may hasten the healing process and recovery of function.

Contusions, Strains, and Sprains

A **contusion** is a soft tissue injury produced by blunt force, such as a blow, kick, or fall. Many small blood vessels rupture and bleed into soft tissues (ecchymosis, or bruising). A hematoma develops when the bleeding is sufficient to cause an appreciable collection of blood. Local symptoms (pain, swelling, and discoloration) are controlled with intermittent application of cold packs. Most contusions resolve in 1 to 2 weeks.

A **strain**, or a "pulled muscle," is an injury to a musculotendinous unit caused by overuse, overstretching, or excessive stress. Strains are graded along a continuum based on post-injury symptoms and loss of function, and reflect the degree of injury. Three types of strain are recognized:

- A first-degree strain reflects tearing of few muscle fibers and is accompanied by minor edema, tenderness, and mild muscle spasm, without noticeable loss of function.
- A second-degree strain involves tearing of more muscle fibers and is manifested by notable loss of load-bearing strength with accompanying edema, tenderness, muscle spasm, and ecchymosis.
- A third-degree strain is the most severe type and involves complete disruption of at least one musculotendinous unit that involves separation of muscle from muscle, muscle from tendon, or tendon from bone. A patient with this type of strain presents with significant pain, muscle spasm, ecchymosis, edema, and loss of function. An x-ray should be obtained to rule out bone injury, because an avulsion fracture (in which a bone fragment is pulled away from the bone by a tendon) may be associated with a third-degree strain.

A **sprain** is an injury to the ligaments and supporting muscle fibers that surround a joint. It is caused by a wrenching or twisting motion. The function of a ligament is to stabilize the articulating bones of a joint while permitting mobility. A torn ligament loses its stabilizing ability. Blood vessels rupture and edema occurs; the joint is tender, and movement of the joint becomes painful. The degree of disability and pain increases during the first 2 to 3 hours after the injury because of the associated swelling

Glossary

allograft: tissue harvested from a donor for use in another person

amputation: removal of a body part, usually a limb or part of a limb

arthroscope: surgical instrument used to examine internal joint structures

autograft: tissue harvested from one area of the body and used for transplantation to another area of the body

avascular necrosis: death of tissue secondary to poor perfusion and hypoxemia

contusion: blunt force injury to soft tissue

crepitus: a grating sound heard by rubbing bony fragments together or a grating sensation felt, also by rubbing bony fragments together

débridement: surgical removal of contaminated and devitalized tissues and foreign material

delayed union: prolongation of expected healing time for a fracture

disarticulation: amputation through a joint

dislocation: separation of joint surfaces

fracture: a break in the continuity of a bone

fracture reduction: restoration of fracture fragments into anatomic alignment and rotation

malunion: healing of a fractured bone in a malaligned position

meniscus: crescent-shaped fibrocartilage found in certain joints, such as the knee joint

nonunion: failure of fragments of a fractured bone to heal together

phantom limb pain: pain perceived as being in the amputated limb

RICE: acronym for *R*est, *I*ce, *C*ompression, *E*levation

rotator cuff: shoulder muscles (supraspinatus, subscapularis, infraspinatus, and teres minor) and their tendons

sprain: an injury to ligaments and other soft tissues at a joint

strain: a musculotendinous injury

subluxation: partial separation or dislocation of joint surfaces

tendinitis: inflammation of a tendon

and bleeding. Sprains are graded in a manner similar to the grading system used for strains:

- A first-degree sprain is caused by tearing of a few ligamentous fibers. It is manifested by mild edema, local tenderness, and pain that is elicited when the joint is moved; however, there is no appreciable joint instability.
- A second-degree sprain involves tearing of more fibers. It results in increased edema, tenderness, pain with motion, joint instability, and partial loss of normal joint function.
- A third-degree sprain occurs when a ligament is completely torn. It is manifested by severe pain, tenderness, increased edema, and abnormal joint motion.

Management

Treatment of contusions, strains, and sprains consists of resting and elevating the affected part, applying cold, and using a compression bandage. (The acronym **RICE**—*R*est, *I*ce, *C*ompression, *E*levation—is helpful for remembering treatment interventions.) Rest prevents additional injury and promotes healing. Intermittent application of moist or dry cold packs for 20 to 30 minutes during the first 24 to 48 hours after injury produces vasoconstriction, which decreases bleeding, edema, and discomfort. Care must be taken to avoid skin and tissue damage from excessive cold. An elastic compression bandage controls bleeding, reduces edema, and provides support for the injured tissues. Elevation controls the swelling. If the sprain or strain is third-degree, surgical repair or immobilization by cast may be necessary so that the joint will not lose its stability. The neurovascular status (circulation, motion, sensation) of the injured extremity is monitored frequently.

After the acute inflammatory stage (eg, 24 to 48 hours after injury), heat may be applied intermittently (for 15 to 30 minutes, four times a day) to relieve muscle spasm and to promote vasodilation, absorption, and repair. Depending on the severity of injury, progressive passive and active exercises may begin in 2 to 5 days. Severe sprains and strains may require 1 to 3 weeks of immobilization before exercises are initiated. Excessive exercise early in the course of treatment delays recovery. Strains and sprains take weeks or months to heal, because ligaments and tendons are relatively avascular. Splinting may be used to prevent reinjury.

Joint Dislocations

A **dislocation** of a joint is a condition in which the articular surfaces of the bones forming the joint are no longer in anatomic contact. The bones are literally "out of joint." A **subluxation** is a partial dislocation of the articulating surfaces. Traumatic dislocations are orthopedic emergencies because the associated joint structures, blood supply, and nerves are distorted and severely stressed. If the dislocation is not treated promptly, **avascular necrosis** (AVN; tissue death due to anoxia and diminished blood supply) and nerve palsy may occur.

Dislocations may be congenital, or present at birth (eg, developmental dysplasia of the hip [DDH]); spontaneous or pathologic, caused by disease of the articular or periarticular structures; or traumatic, resulting from injury in which the joint is disrupted by force.

Signs and symptoms of a traumatic dislocation include acute pain, change in contour of the joint, change in the length of the extremity, loss of normal mobility, and change in the axis of the dislocated bones. X-rays confirm the diagnosis and reveal any associated fracture.

Medical Management

The affected joint needs to be immobilized while the patient is transported to the hospital. The dislocation is promptly reduced (ie, displaced parts are brought into normal position) to preserve joint function. Analgesia, muscle relaxants, and possibly anesthesia are used to facilitate closed reduction (eg, noninvasive or nonsurgical reduction). The joint is immobilized by bandages, splints, casts, or traction and is maintained in a stable position. Neurovascular status is monitored. After reduction, if the joint is stable, gentle, progressive, active and passive movement is begun to preserve range of motion (ROM) and restore strength. The joint is supported between exercise sessions.

Nursing Management

Nursing care is directed at providing comfort, evaluating the patient's neurovascular status, and protecting the joint during healing. The nurse teaches the patient how to manage the immobilizing devices, how to protect the joint from reinjury, and how to use assistive or adaptive devices for carrying out activities of daily living.

Sports-Related Injuries

Many people participate in recreational sports. These recreational athletes may push themselves beyond the level of their physical conditioning and incur injuries. Professional athletes are also susceptible to injury, even though their training is supervised closely to minimize the occurrence of injury.

Injuries to the musculoskeletal system may be acute (eg, sprains, strains, dislocations, fractures), or they may be gradual, resulting from overuse (eg, chondromalacia patella, tendinitis, stress fractures). These injuries include the following:

- Contusions result from direct falls or blows. The initial dull pain becomes greater, with edema and stiffness occurring by the next day.
- Sprains occur most commonly in the ankles but may also occur in fingers and knees. Ankle sprains account for 25% of all sports-related injuries (Schoen, 2005). If the

sprain is third-degree, the joint becomes unstable, and surgical repair may be required.

- Strains manifest with a sharp, stabbing pain caused by bleeding and immediate muscle spasm. Tennis players often suffer calf muscle strains; soccer players often experience quadriceps strains; and swimmers, weightlifters, and tennis players often suffer shoulder strains.
- **Tendinitis** (inflammation of a tendon) is caused by overuse and is seen in tennis players (epicondylar tendinitis, or "tennis elbow"), runners and gymnasts (Achilles tendinitis), and basketball players (infrapatellar tendinitis).
- Meniscal injuries of the knee occur with excessive rotational stress.
- Dislocations are seen with sports that involve throwing or lifting.
- Traumatic fractures occur with falls. Skaters and bikers frequently suffer Colles' fractures of the wrist when they fall on outstretched arms, and ballet dancers and track and field athletes may experience metatarsal fractures.
- Stress fractures occur with repeated bone trauma from activities such as running, jumping, and throwing as well as from sports that include track and field, gymnastics, basketball, rowing, baseball, and tennis. Track and field–related injuries account for more than 50% of stress fractures in men and more than 64% of stress fractures in women (Sanderlin & Raspa, 2003). The tibia and metatarsals are most vulnerable. In general, stress fractures of other bones occur less often, but certain types of stress fractures are more likely to occur in some athletes than in others. For example, rowers are vulnerable to stress fractures of the ribs, and baseball or tennis players are more vulnerable to stress fractures of the upper extremities.

Management

Management of sprains, strains, fractures, and tendinitis is described in this chapter. Management of low back pain is described in Chapter 68. Patients who have experienced sports-related injuries are often highly motivated to return to their previous level of activity. Compliance with restriction of activities and gradual resumption of activities may be a significant problem for them. They need to be taught how to avoid further injury or a new injury. Injured athletes are at risk for reinjury; 60% of athletes diagnosed with a new stress fracture have had a previous stress fracture (Sandelin & Raspa, 2003). With recurrence of symptoms, athletes need to diminish their level and intensity of activity to a comfortable level and to treat symptoms with RICE. The time required to recover from a sports-related injury can be as short as a few days or considerably longer than 6 weeks, depending on the severity of the injury.

Prevention

Sports-related injuries can often be prevented by using proper equipment (eg, running shoes for joggers, wrist guards for skaters) and by effectively training and conditioning the body. Specific training needs to be tailored to the person and the sport. Stretching prior to engaging in sports or exercise had long been recommended; however, recent studies suggest that stretching may not prevent injury (Hart, 2005; Thacker, Gilchrist, Stroup, et al., 2004).

After exercise, the body needs to cool off to prevent cardiovascular problems such as hypotension, syncope, and dysrhythmias. Changes in activities and stresses should occur gradually. In addition, the athlete needs to be taught to "tune in" to body symptoms that indicate stress and to modify activities to minimize injury and to promote healing.

Occupation-Related Injuries

According to the U.S. Department of Labor, occupation-related musculoskeletal disorders are injuries or illnesses of the muscles, nerves, tendons, joints, cartilage, and bones that occur because of exposure to work-related risks (U.S. Department of Labor Bureau of Labor Statistics [BLS], 2003). In 2003, more than 4,351,000 cases of nonfatal musculoskeletal injuries and illnesses occurred in the workplace in the private sector (eg, not including the military or government agencies); of these, 1,315,000 injuries resulted in lost work days.

The most frequent types of single injuries that occurred were sprains, strains, and tears (5,639,000); bruises and contusions (1,188,000); fractures (949,600); soreness and pain (664,000); back injuries (374,000); amputations (81,500); and tendinitis (77,300) (BLS, 2003). Management of sprains, strains, fractures, amputations, and tendinitis is described in this chapter; management of low back pain is described in Chapter 68.

Injuries to the hand and wrist generally accounted for the greatest number of lost work days (Barr, Barbe, & Clark, 2004). People who have the greatest risk of occupation-related injuries and lost work days are farmers, general contractors, steelworkers, autoworkers, truck drivers, and nursing personnel (BLS, 2003).

Prevention of Injuries in Nursing Personnel

Nursing is consistently ranked among the top ten occupations that are most involved in occupation-related injuries and lost work days. Whereas the rates of other occupation-related injuries have tended to decrease over the past decade, the rates of injuries among all nursing personnel, including registered nurses, licensed practical nurses/licensed vocational nurses, and unlicensed assistive personnel, have continued to increase. Most of these injuries have occurred during patient handling and movement activities (Nelson & Baptiste, 2004; Nelson, Owen, Lloyd, et al., 2003). Traditional, nonevidence-based methods to prevent musculoskeletal injuries among nursing personnel during patient handling and moving have revolved around training sessions on proper body mechanics and "safe" lifting of patients and use of back belts. Nelson and colleagues (Nelson & Baptiste, 2004; Nelson et al., 2003) advocate the following evidence-based methods to deter occupational-related injuries among nursing personnel:

- Hospitals, long-term care facilities, and other health care organizations should purchase patient handling equipment (eg, Hoyer lifts) and train nursing personnel in their appropriate use.
- Health care organizations should institute "no lift" policies for individual nursing personnel. Rather, patient lift teams should be organized.
- Health care organizations should devise methods to assess their patient care ergonomic risks and develop algorithms

NURSING RESEARCH PROFILE

Musculoskeletal Problems in Nurses

Lipscomb, J., Trinkoff, A., Brady, B., et al. (2004). Health care system changes and reported musculoskeletal disorders among registered nurses. *American Journal of Public Health, 94*(8), 1431–1441.

Purpose

During the past two decades, changes within the American health care system to a managed care model have resulted in shorter hospital stays and higher acuity levels in hospitalized patients. During this same time, the number of nursing personnel in hospitals declined by 7.3%. Hospitals rank sixth overall in the reported incidence of nonfatal occupational injuries, and nurses who work in hospitals experience a host of occupation-related musculoskeletal injuries, particularly to the back, shoulder, and neck. This research study examined whether changes in the health care system are associated with an increase in occupation-related injuries in hospital nurses.

Design

This descriptive study used a cross-sectional survey design. A sample of 2000 registered nurses (RNs) was selected for potential participation from two state board of nursing database registries with known ethnic diversity. Of these, 1163 RNs consented and were eligible to participate. All study participants were currently employed as nurses, had been in their current positions for at least 1 year, and had not experienced an injury for at least 3 months prior to completing the survey.

Data were anonymously collected using an eight-page survey that included questions about back, shoulder, and neck problems using selected items from the Nordic Questionnaire of Musculoskeletal Symptoms; questions about staffing levels, patient acuity, and delivery of care using a modified Shindul-Rothchild tool that surveyed reported health care system changes over the past year; and questions about work-related psychological effects using the Job Content Questionnaire. Other variables, including age, body mass index, ethnicity, having children younger than 4 years of age, and caring for other dependents, were analyzed and then controlled as covariates within the logistic regression model.

Findings

Among the study participants, the reported prevalences of back, shoulder, and neck musculoskeletal disorders were 29%, 17%, and 20%, respectively.

Reported health care system changes were highly associated with moderate levels of change (defined as at least four system changes within the past year) and musculoskeletal disorders, including back musculoskeletal disorders, with an odds ratio (OR) of 2.60 (95% confidence interval [CI] = 1.53, 4.42); shoulder musculoskeletal disorders, with an OR of 1.16 (95% CI = 0.68, 1.98); and neck musculoskeletal disorders, with an OR of 2.41 (95% CI = 1.37, 4.22).

When adjusted for demographic and lifestyle variables, work characteristics, and psychological work-related demands, logistic regression revealed a distinct association between high levels of change (defined as more than six system changes in the past year) and musculoskeletal disorders, including back musculoskeletal disorders, with an OR of 3.42 (95% CI = 1.61, 7.27); shoulder musculoskeletal disorders, with an OR of 2.63 (95% CI = 1.17, 5.91); and neck musculoskeletal disorders, with an OR of 4.45 (95% CI = 1.97, 10.08).

Nursing Implications

The findings of this study suggest that RNs who reported working in a health care system with more than six system changes within the past year that may have included increased work responsibilities, increased patient acuity, more unfilled nursing positions, heavier workloads, and increased "floating" responsibilities had 3.42 times greater odds of having a back disorder, 2.63 times greater odds of having a shoulder disorder, and 4.45 times greater odds of having a neck disorder than a colleague who worked in a health care system without any of these changes within the past year.

These results demonstrate that nurses who work in settings in which there are changes that include higher patient acuity, greater workloads, and increased work-related responsibilities have a greater likelihood of experiencing musculoskeletal disorders than nurses who work in settings without these types of changes. Nurses must advocate for improved staffing methods and workloads to avoid injuries and preserve their own livelihood and health.

for patient handling and movement that include patient transfer and movement activities.

Specific Musculoskeletal Injuries

Rotator Cuff Tears

Rotator cuff tears may result from an acute injury or from chronic joint stresses. Patients complain of pain, limited ROM, and some joint dysfunction, including muscle weakness. In many cases, the patient with a rotator cuff tear experiences night pain and cannot sleep on the involved side. The patient cannot perform over-the-head activities. The acromioclavicular joint is tender. X-rays are helpful in evaluating the joint. Arthrography and magnetic resonance imaging (MRI) are used to determine soft tissue pathology and the extent of the rotator cuff tear.

Initial conservative management includes use of nonsteroidal anti-inflammatory drugs (NSAIDs), rest with modification of activities, injection of a corticosteroid into the shoulder joint, and progressive stretching, ROM, and strengthening exercises. Some rotator cuff tears require arthroscopic **débridement** (removal of devitalized tissue) or arthroscopic or open acromioplasty with tendon repair. Postoperatively, the shoulder is immobilized for several days to 4 weeks. Physical therapy with shoulder exercises is begun as prescribed, and the patient is instructed in how to perform the exercises at home. Full recovery is expected in 6 to 12 months.

Epicondylitis (Tennis Elbow)

Epicondylitis is a chronic, painful condition that is caused by excessive, repetitive extension, flexion, pronation, and supination activities of the forearm. These excessive, repetitious activities result in inflammation (tendinitis) and minor tears in the tendons at the origin of the muscles on the medial or lateral epicondyles. Activities contributing to the development of epicondylitis include tennis, other racket sports, pitching, gymnastics, and repetitive use of a screwdriver. The pain characteristically radiates down the extensor (dorsal) surface of the forearm. The patient may have a weakened grasp. Most often, relief is obtained by rest and avoidance of the aggravating activity.

Application of ice after the activity and administration of NSAIDs usually relieve the pain. In some instances, the arm is immobilized in a molded splint or cast. Because of its degenerative effects on tendons, local injection of a corticosteroid is reserved for patients with severe pain who do not respond to NSAIDs and immobilization. After pain subsides, rehabilitation exercises include gentle and gradual increased stretching of the tendons. A tennis elbow counterforce strap that limits extension of the elbow may be prescribed when activity is resumed. Occasionally, surgery may be needed to release strictures or to débride the joint.

Lateral and Medial Collateral Ligament Injury

Lateral and medial collateral ligaments of the knee (Fig. 69-1) provide stability lateral and medial to the knee. Injury to these ligaments occurs when the foot is firmly planted and the knee is struck—either medially, causing stretching and tearing injury to the lateral collateral ligament, or laterally, causing stretching and tearing injury to the medial collateral ligament (more common occurrence). The patient experiences an acute onset of pain, point tenderness (eg, tenderness at the site of injury), joint instability, and inability to walk without assistance.

Medical Management

Early management includes RICE. The joint is evaluated for fracture. Hemarthrosis (bleeding into the joint) may develop, contributing to the pain. The joint fluid may be aspirated to relieve pressure.

The treatment depends on the severity of the sprain. Conservative management includes limited weight bearing and use of protective elastic bandaging or a brace. As pain subsides, ROM exercise is encouraged. The patient's return to full activities, including sports, depends on return of motion, functional stability of the joint, and muscle strength.

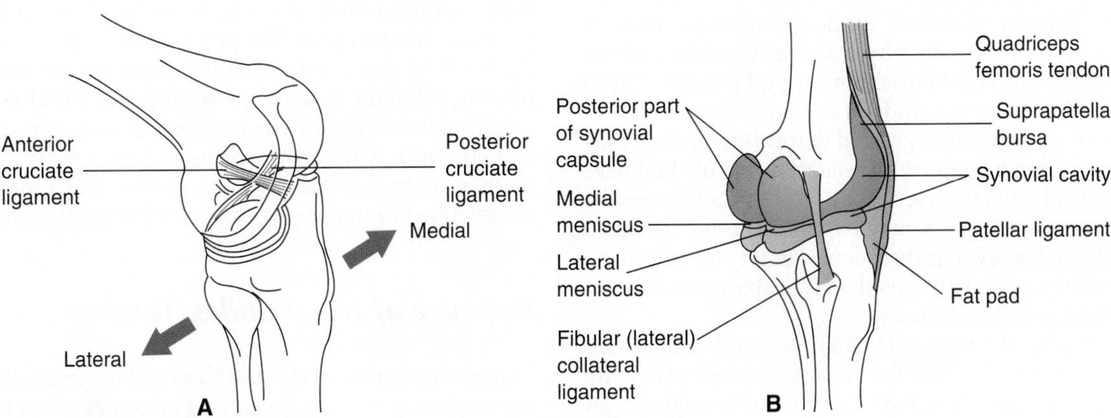

FIGURE 69-1. Knee ligaments, tendons, and menisci. (**A**) Anterolateral view. (**B**) Posterolateral view.

If needed, surgical reconstruction may be performed immediately, or it may be delayed. Generally, the leg is immobilized, and weight bearing is restricted for 6 to 8 weeks. A progressive rehabilitation program helps restore the function and strength of the knee. Rehabilitation occurs over many months, and the patient may need to wear a derotational brace while engaging in sports.

Nursing Management

The nurse provides patient teaching about proper use of ambulatory devices, the healing process, and activity limitation to promote healing. The nurse teaches the surgical patient about pain management, medications (analgesics, antibiotics), brace use, wound care, possible complications (eg, altered neurovascular status, infection, skin breakdown), and self-care.

Anterior and Posterior Cruciate Ligament Injury

The anterior cruciate ligament (ACL) and the posterior cruciate ligament (PCL) of the knee stabilize forward and backward motion of the femur and tibia (see Fig. 69-1). These ligaments cross in the center of the knee. Injury occurs when the foot is firmly planted, the knee is hyperextended, and the person twists the torso and femur. The patient reports hearing a "pop" or feeling a tearing sensation with this twisting injury. If the patient exhibits significant swelling of the joint within 2 hours after the injury, the ACL may be torn. The patient experiences pain, joint instability, and pain with ambulation.

Immediate postinjury management includes RICE. The joint is evaluated for fracture. Joint effusion and hemarthrosis require joint aspiration and wrapping with a compression elastic dressing.

Treatment depends on the severity of the injury and the effect of the injury on daily activities. Early treatment involves application of a brace, physical therapy, and avoidance of jumping activities. Surgical ACL reconstruction may be scheduled after near-normal joint ROM is achieved and includes tendon repair with grafting. This is typically performed as ambulatory arthroscopic surgery, a procedure in which the surgeon uses an **arthroscope** to visualize and repair the damage. The best surgical candidates include patients who are young and physically active; older and less active patients may benefit from nonsurgical therapy (Alford & Bach, 2004). A recent study of the outcomes of arthroscopic knee surgery has suggested that this treatment may be ineffective for patients with osteoarthritis of the knees (Moseley, O'Malley, Petersen, et al., 2002). Candidates for arthroscopic knee surgery may be reluctant to consent to the treatment; however, arthroscopic surgery for traumatic injuries to the knee is still considered a viable treatment option, with an excellent outcome.

After surgery, the patient is taught to control pain with oral opioid analgesics, NSAIDs, and cryotherapy (a cooling pad incorporated in a dressing). The patient is taught about monitoring the neurovascular status of the leg, wound care, and signs of complications that need to be reported promptly to the surgeon. Exercises (ankle pumps, quadriceps sets, and hamstring sets) are encouraged during the early postoperative period. The nurse reinforces instruction about weight-bearing limits, exercise restrictions, and the use of a knee brace or immobilizer. The patient must protect the graft by complying with exercise restrictions. The physical therapist supervises progressive ROM and weight bearing (as permitted). Continuous passive motion may be helpful in restoring full ROM. Rehabilitation after surgery typically takes 6 to 12 months.

Meniscal Injuries

Two crescent-shaped (semilunar) cartilages in the knee, called menisci, are attached to the edge of the shallow articulating surface of the head of the tibia (see Fig. 69-1). Each **meniscus** moves slightly backward and forward to accommodate the condyles of the femur when the leg is flexed or extended. Normally, little twisting movement is permitted in the knee joint. Twisting of the knee or repetitive squatting and impact may result in either tearing or detachment of the cartilage from its attachment to the head of the tibia.

These injuries leave loose cartilage in the knee joint that may slip between the femur and the tibia, preventing full extension of the leg. If this happens during walking or running, the patient often describes the leg as "giving way." The patient may hear or feel a click in the knee when walking, especially when extending the leg that is bearing weight, as in going upstairs. When the cartilage is attached to the front and back of the knee but torn loose laterally (bucket-handle tear), it may slide between the bones to lie between the condyles and prevent full flexion or extension. As a result, the knee "locks." Meniscal injuries produce pain and disability because the patient never knows when the knee will malfunction. Also, the torn cartilage is an irritant in the joint, causing inflammation, chronic synovitis, and effusion.

Initial conservative treatment includes immobilization of the knee, use of crutches, anti-inflammatory agents, analgesics, and modification of activities to avoid those that cause the symptoms. If symptoms persist, the extent of meniscal injury is evaluated by MRI. Damaged cartilage is surgically removed (meniscectomy) arthroscopically. After surgery, a pressure dressing is applied, and a knee-immobilizing splint may be recommended. The most common complication is an effusion into the knee joint, which produces marked pain. The physician may need to aspirate the joint to remove fluid and relieve the pressure. The patient is taught quadriceps-setting and ROM exercises. Additional exercises help restore full function, stability, and strength. After arthroscopic meniscectomy, most patients resume activities in a day or two, and sports can be resumed in several weeks, as prescribed by the physician.

Rupture of the Achilles Tendon

Traumatic rupture of the Achilles tendon, generally within the tendon sheath, occurs during activities when there is a sudden contraction of the calf muscle with the foot fixed firmly to the floor or ground. The patient experiences sharp pain and cannot plantar flex the foot. Immediate surgical repair of complete Achilles tendon ruptures is usually recommended to obtain satisfactory results. After surgery, a cast or brace is used to immobilize the joint. In some situations, conservative management with a plantar-flexed cast for 6 to 8 weeks may be used. After immobilization, a heel lift is worn and progressive physical therapy to promote ankle ROM and strength is begun.

Fractures

A **fracture** is a break in the continuity of bone and is defined according to its type and extent. Fractures occur when the bone is subjected to stress greater than it can absorb. Fractures are caused by direct blows, crushing forces, sudden twisting motions, and extreme muscle contractions. When the bone is broken, adjacent structures are also affected, resulting in soft tissue edema, hemorrhage into the muscles and joints, joint dislocations, ruptured tendons, severed nerves, and damaged blood vessels. Body organs may be injured by the force that caused the fracture or by fracture fragments.

Types of Fractures

A *complete fracture* involves a break across the entire cross-section of the bone and is frequently displaced (removed from its normal position). An *incomplete fracture* (eg, greenstick fracture) involves a break through only part of the cross-section of the bone. A *comminuted* fracture is one that produces several bone fragments. A *closed fracture* (simple fracture) is one that does not cause a break in the skin. An *open fracture* (compound, or complex, fracture) is one in which the skin or mucous membrane wound extends to the fractured bone. Open fractures are graded according to the following criteria:

- Grade I is a clean wound less than 1 cm long.
- Grade II is a larger wound without extensive soft tissue damage.
- Grade III is highly contaminated, has extensive soft tissue damage, and is the most severe.

Fractures may also be described according to the anatomic placement of fragments. Specific types of fractures are reviewed in Chart 69-1.

Clinical Manifestations

The clinical manifestations of a fracture include acute pain, loss of function, deformity, shortening of the extremity, crepitus, and local swelling and discoloration. Not all of these clinical manifestations are present in every fracture. For example, many are not present with linear or fissure fractures or with impacted fractures. The diagnosis of a fracture is based on the patient's symptoms, the physical signs, and the x-ray findings. Usually, the patient reports having sustained an injury to the area.

Pain

The pain is continuous and increases in severity until the bone fragments are immobilized. The muscle spasms that accompany a fracture begin within 20 minutes after the injury and result in more intense pain than the patient reports at the time of injury. The muscle spasms can minimize further movement of the fracture fragments or can result in further bony fragmentation or malalignment.

Loss of Function

After a fracture, the extremity cannot function properly because normal function of the muscles depends on the integrity of the bones to which they are attached. Pain contributes to the loss of function. In addition, abnormal movement (false motion) may be present.

Deformity

Displacement, angulation, or rotation of the fragments in a fracture of the arm or leg causes a deformity (either visible or palpable) that is detectable when the limb is compared with the uninjured extremity. Deformity also results from soft tissue swelling.

Shortening

In fractures of long bones, there is actual shortening of the extremity because of the contraction of the muscles that are attached distal and proximal to the site of the fracture. The fragments often overlap by as much as 2.5 to 5 cm (1 to 2 inches).

Crepitus

When the extremity is examined with the hands, a grating sensation, called **crepitus,** can be felt. It is caused by the rubbing of the bone fragments against each other.

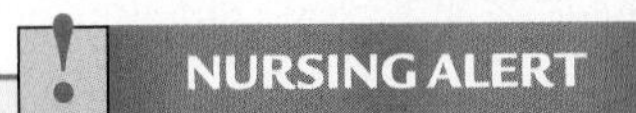

Testing for crepitus can produce further tissue damage and should be avoided.

Swelling and Discoloration

Localized edema and discoloration of the skin (ecchymosis) occur after a fracture as a result of trauma and bleeding into the tissues. These signs may not develop for several hours after the injury.

Emergency Management

Immediately after injury, whenever a fracture is suspected, it is important to immobilize the body part before the patient is moved. If an injured patient must be removed from a vehicle before splints can be applied, the extremity is supported distal and proximal to the fracture site to prevent rotation as well as angular motion.

Adequate splinting is essential. Joints proximal and distal to the fracture must be immobilized to prevent movement of fracture fragments that can cause additional pain, soft tissue damage, and bleeding. Temporary, well-padded

CHART 69-1

Specific Types of Fractures

Avulsion: a fracture in which a fragment of bone has been pulled away by a tendon and its attachment
Comminuted: a fracture in which bone has splintered into several fragments
Compound: a fracture in which damage also involves the skin or mucous membranes; also called an open fracture
Compression: a fracture in which bone has been compressed (seen in vertebral fractures)
Depressed: a fracture in which fragments are driven inward (seen frequently in fractures of skull and facial bones)
Epiphyseal: a fracture through the epiphysis
Greenstick: a fracture in which one side of a bone is broken and the other side is bent
Impacted: a fracture in which a bone fragment is driven into another bone fragment
Oblique: a fracture occurring at an angle across the bone (less stable than a transverse fracture)
Pathologic: a fracture that occurs through an area of diseased bone (eg, osteoporosis, bone cyst, Paget's disease, bony metastasis, tumor); can occur without trauma or a fall
Simple: a fracture that remains contained, with no disruption of the skin integrity
Spiral: a fracture that twists around the shaft of the bone
Stress: a fracture that results from repeated loading without bone and muscle recovery
Transverse: a fracture that is straight across the bone shaft

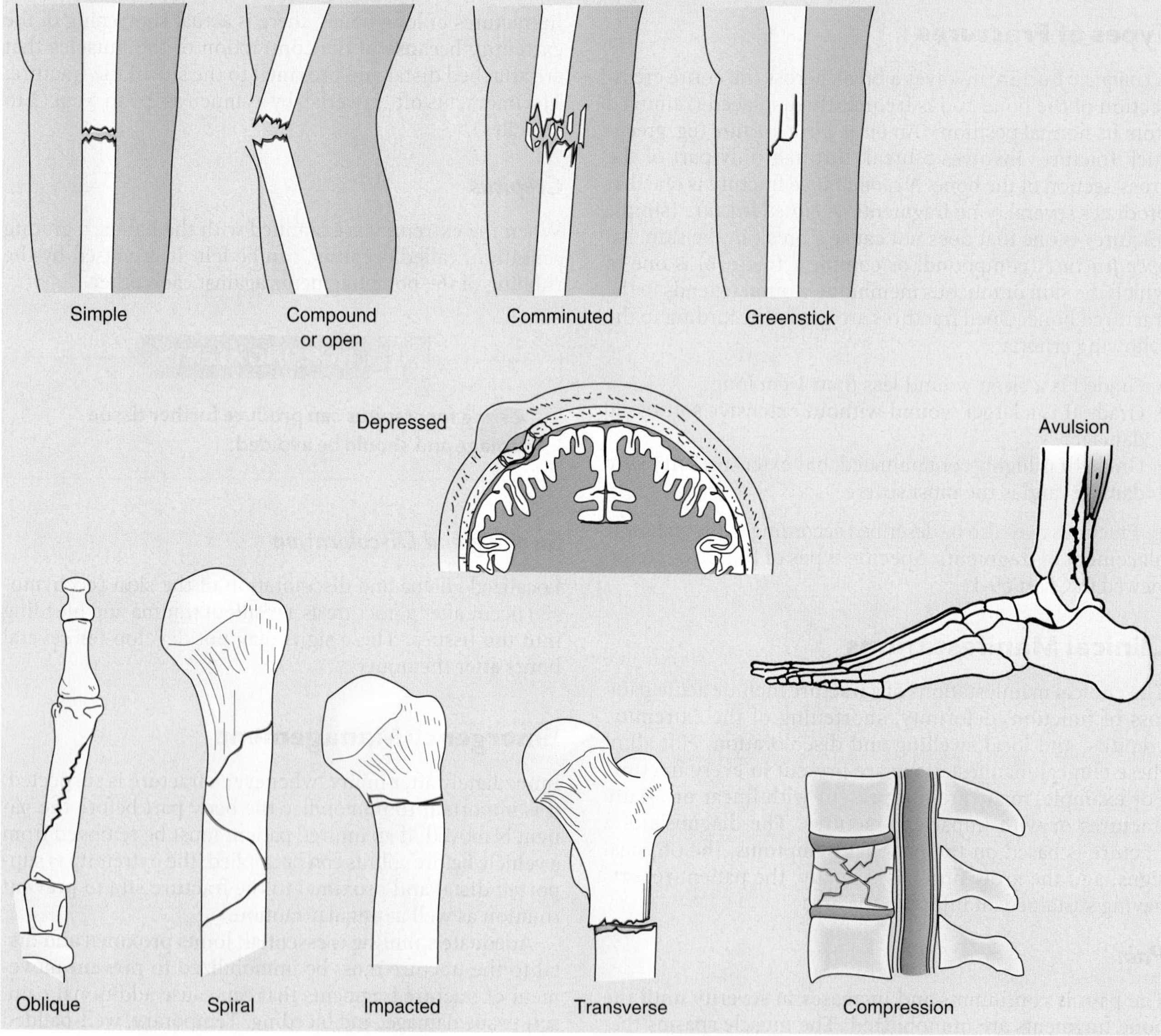

splints, firmly bandaged over clothing, serve to immobilize the fracture. Immobilization of the long bones of the lower extremities may be accomplished by bandaging the legs together, with the unaffected extremity serving as a splint for the injured one. In an upper extremity injury, the arm may be bandaged to the chest, or an injured forearm may be placed in a sling. The neurovascular status distal to the injury should be assessed both before and after splinting to determine the adequacy of peripheral tissue perfusion and nerve function.

With an *open fracture,* the wound is covered with a sterile dressing to prevent contamination of deeper tissues. No attempt is made to reduce the fracture, even if one of the bone fragments is protruding through the wound. Splints are applied for immobilization.

In the emergency department, the patient is evaluated completely. The clothes are gently removed, first from the uninjured side of the body and then from the injured side. The patient's clothing may be cut away. The fractured extremity is moved as little as possible to avoid more damage.

Medical Management

The principles of fracture treatment include reduction, immobilization, and regaining of normal function and strength through rehabilitation.

Reduction

Reduction of a fracture ("setting" the bone) refers to restoration of the fracture fragments to anatomic alignment and rotation. Either closed reduction or open reduction may be used to reduce a fracture. The specific method selected depends on the nature of the fracture; however, the underlying principles are the same. Usually, the physician reduces a fracture as soon as possible to prevent loss of elasticity from the tissues through infiltration by edema or hemorrhage. In most cases, **fracture reduction** becomes more difficult as the injury begins healing.

Before fracture reduction and immobilization, the patient is prepared for the procedure; permission for the procedure is obtained, and an analgesic is administered as prescribed. Anesthesia may be administered. The injured extremity must be handled gently to avoid additional damage.

CLOSED REDUCTION

In most instances, closed reduction is accomplished by bringing the bone fragments into apposition (ie, placing the ends in contact) through manipulation and manual traction. The extremity is held in the desired position while the physician applies a cast, splint, or other device. Reduction under anesthesia with percutaneous pinning may be used. The immobilizing device maintains the reduction and stabilizes the extremity for bone healing. X-rays are obtained to verify that the bone fragments are correctly aligned.

Traction (skin or skeletal) may be used to effect fracture reduction and immobilization. Traction may be used until the patient is physiologically stable and able to withstand surgical fixation. Use of traction and the nursing management of a patient in traction are discussed more fully in Chapter 67.

OPEN REDUCTION

Some fractures require open reduction. Through a surgical approach, the fracture fragments are reduced. Internal fixation devices (metallic pins, wires, screws, plates, nails, or rods) may be used to hold the bone fragments in position until solid bone healing occurs. These devices may be attached to the sides of bone, or they may be inserted through the bony fragments or directly into the medullary cavity of the bone (Fig. 69-2). Internal fixation devices ensure firm approximation and fixation of the bony fragments.

Immobilization

After the fracture has been reduced, the bone fragments must be immobilized, or held in correct position and alignment, until union occurs. Immobilization may be accomplished by external or internal fixation. Methods of external fixation include bandages, casts, splints, continuous traction, and external fixators. Metal implants used for internal fixation serve as internal splints to immobilize the fracture.

Maintaining and Restoring Function

Reduction and immobilization are maintained as prescribed to promote bone and soft tissue healing. Edema is

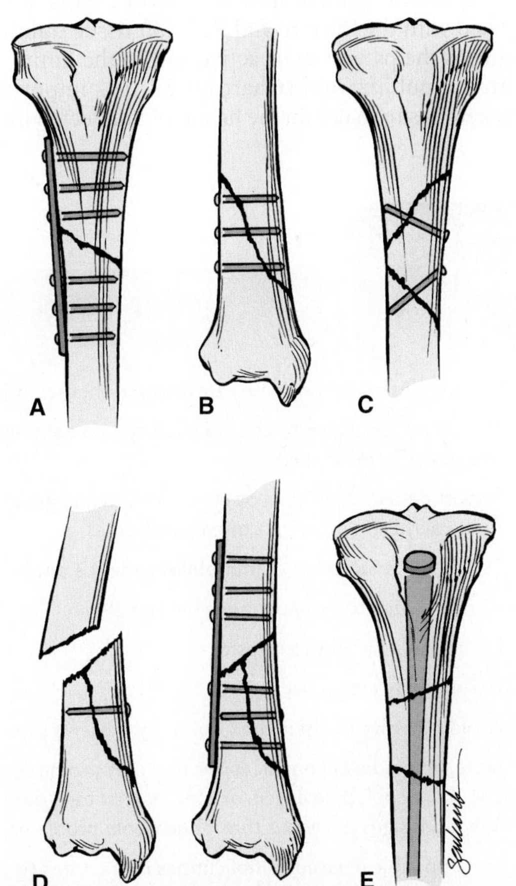

FIGURE 69-2. Techniques of internal fixation. (**A**) Plate and six screws for a transverse or short oblique fracture. (**B**) Screws for a long oblique or spiral fracture. (**C**) Screws for a long butterfly fragment. (**D**) Plate and six screws for a short butterfly fragment. (**E**) Medullary nail for a segmental fracture.

controlled by elevating the injured extremity and applying ice as prescribed. Neurovascular status (circulation, movement, sensation) is monitored, and the orthopedic surgeon is notified immediately if signs of neurovascular compromise are identified. Restlessness, anxiety, and discomfort are controlled with a variety of approaches, such as reassurance, position changes, and pain relief strategies, including use of analgesics. Isometric and muscle-setting exercises are encouraged to minimize disuse atrophy and to promote circulation. Participation in activities of daily living (ADLs) is encouraged to promote independent functioning and self-esteem. Gradual resumption of activities is promoted within the therapeutic prescription. With internal fixation, the surgeon determines the amount of movement and weight-bearing stress the extremity can withstand and prescribes the level of activity. (See Nursing Process sections in Chapter 67 for more information about caring for patients who have a cast, are in traction, or are undergoing orthopedic surgery.)

Nursing Management

Patients With Closed Fractures

The nurse encourages patients with closed (simple) fractures to return to their usual activities as rapidly as possible. The nurse teaches the patient how to control edema and pain associated with the fracture and with soft tissue trauma and encourages the patient to be active within the limits of the fracture immobilization (Chart 69-2). It is important to teach exercises to maintain the health of unaffected muscles and to increase the strength of muscles needed for transferring and for using assistive devices (eg, crutches, walker, special utensils). The nurse and physical therapist teach patients how to use assistive devices safely. Plans are made to help patients modify their home environment as needed and to secure personal assistance if necessary. Patient teaching includes self-care, medication information, monitoring for potential complications, and the need for continuing health care supervision. Fracture healing and restoration of full strength and mobility may take many months.

Patients With Open Fractures

In an open fracture, there is a risk for osteomyelitis, tetanus, and gas gangrene. The objectives of management are to prevent infection of the wound, soft tissue, and bone and to promote healing of soft tissue and bone. The nurse administers tetanus prophylaxis if indicated. Serial irrigation and débridement are used to remove anaerobic organisms. Intravenous (IV) antibiotics are prescribed to prevent or treat infection.

Prompt, thorough wound irrigation and débridement in the operating room are necessary. The wound is cultured and devitalized bone fragments are removed. The fracture is carefully reduced and stabilized by external fixation (see Chapter 67) or intramedullary nails. Any damage to blood vessels, soft tissue, muscles, nerves, and tendons is treated.

With open fractures, primary wound closure is usually delayed. Heavily contaminated wounds are left unsutured and dressed with sterile gauze to permit edema and wound drainage. Wound irrigation and débridement may be repeated, removing infected and devitalized tissue and increas-

CHART 69-2

HOME CARE CHECKLIST • Closed Fracture

At the completion of the home care instruction, the patient or caregiver will be able to:	Patient	Caregiver
• Describe approaches to control swelling and pain (eg, elevate extremity to heart level; take analgesics as prescribed)	✔	✔
• Report pain uncontrolled by elevation and analgesics (may be an indicator of impaired tissue perfusion or compartment syndrome)	✔	✔
• Describe management of immobilizing device or care of incision	✔	✔
• Consume diet to promote bone healing	✔	
• Demonstrate ability to transfer	✔	
• Use mobility aids safely	✔	
• Avoid excessive use of injured extremity; observe prescribed weight-bearing limits	✔	
• State indicators of complications to report promptly to physician (eg, uncontrolled swelling and pain; cool, pale fingers or toes; paresthesia; paralysis; signs of local and systemic infection; signs of venous thromboemboli; problems with immobilization device)	✔	✔
• State possible delayed complications of fractures (ie, delayed union; nonunion; avascular necrosis; reaction to internal fixation device; complex regional pain syndrome (CRPS), formally called reflex sympathetic dystrophy syndrome; heterotopic ossification)	✔	
• Describe gradual resumption of normal activities when medically cleared, and discuss how to protect fracture site from undue stresses	✔	✔

ing vascularity in the region. After it has been determined that infection is not present, the wound is closed in 5 to 7 days, and all dead space is obliterated by grafting of autogenous skin or a flap.

The nurse elevates the extremity to minimize edema. It is important to assess neurovascular status frequently. The nurse measures the patient's temperature at regular intervals and monitors the patient for signs of infection (or instructs the patient or family to do so). In 4 to 8 weeks, bone grafting may be necessary to bridge bone defects and to stimulate bone healing.

Fracture Healing and Complications

Weeks to months are required for most fractures to heal. Many factors influence the speed with which fractures heal (Chart 69-3). The reduction of fracture fragments must be accurate and maintained to ensure healing. The affected bone must have an adequate blood supply. The type of fracture also affects healing time. In general, fractures of flat bones (pelvis, scapula) heal rapidly. Fractures at the ends of long bones, where the bone is more vascular and cancellous, heal more quickly than do fractures in areas where the bone is dense and less vascular (midshaft). Weight bearing stimulates healing of stabilized fractures of the long bones in the lower extremities.

If fracture healing is disrupted, bone union may be delayed or stopped completely. Factors that can impair fracture healing include inadequate fracture immobilization, inadequate blood supply to the fracture site or adjacent tissue, extensive space between bone fragments, interposition of soft tissue between bone ends, infection, and metabolic problems.

Complications of fractures fall into two categories—early and delayed. Early complications include shock, fat embolism, compartment syndrome, venous thromboemboli (deep vein thrombosis [DVT], pulmonary embolism [PE]), disseminated intravascular coagulation, and infection. Delayed complications include delayed union, malunion, nonunion, AVN of bone, reaction to internal fixation devices, complex regional pain syndrome (CRPS, formerly called reflex sympathetic dystrophy [RSD]), and heterotopic ossification.

CHART 69-3

Factors That Affect Fracture Healing

Factors That Enhance Fracture Healing

- Immobilization of fracture fragments
- Maximum bone fragment contact
- Sufficient blood supply
- Proper nutrition
- Exercise: weight bearing for long bones
- Hormones: growth hormone, thyroid, calcitonin, vitamin D, anabolic steroids
- Electric potential across fracture

Factors That Inhibit Fracture Healing

- Extensive local trauma
- Bone loss
- Inadequate immobilization
- Space or tissue between bone fragments
- Infection
- Local malignancy
- Metabolic bone disease (eg, Paget's disease)
- Irradiated bone (radiation necrosis)
- Avascular necrosis
- Intra-articular fracture (synovial fluid contains fibrolysins, which lyse the initial clot and retard clot formation)
- Age (elderly persons heal more slowly)
- Corticosteroids (inhibit the repair rate)

Early Complications

Shock

Hypovolemic shock resulting from hemorrhage (both visible and nonvisible blood loss) and from loss of intravascular volume into the interstitial space, particularly within damaged tissues, may occur in fractures of the extremities, thorax, pelvis, or spine. Because the bone is very vascular, large quantities of blood may be lost as a result of trauma, especially in fractures of the femur and pelvis. Treatment of shock consists of stabilizing the fracture to prevent further hemorrhage, restoring blood volume and circulation, relieving the patient's pain, providing adequate splinting, and protecting the patient from further injury and other complications. (See Chapter 15 for a discussion of shock.)

Fat Embolism Syndrome

After fracture of long bones or pelvic bones, multiple fractures, or crush injuries, fat emboli may develop. Fat embolism syndrome occurs most frequently in young adults (typically in those 20 to 30 years of age) and elderly adults who experience fractures of the proximal femur (ie, hip fracture). At the time of fracture, fat globules may diffuse into the vascular compartment because the marrow pressure is greater than the capillary pressure or because catecholamines elevated by the patient's stress reaction mobilize fatty acids and promote the development of fat globules in the bloodstream (Porth, 2005). The fat globules (emboli) may occlude the small blood vessels that supply the lungs, brain, kidneys, and other organs. The onset of symptoms is rapid, usually within 24 to 72 hours of injury, but may occur up to a week after injury (Porth, 2005).

Clinical Manifestations

Presenting features include hypoxia, tachypnea, tachycardia, and pyrexia. The respiratory distress response includes tachypnea, dyspnea, crackles, wheezes, precordial chest pain, cough, large amounts of thick white sputum, and tachycardia. Occlusion of a large number of small vessels causes the pulmonary pressure to rise. Edema and hemorrhages in the alveoli impair oxygen transport, leading to hypoxia. Arterial blood gas values show the partial pressure of oxygen (PaO_2) to be less than 60 mm Hg, with an early respiratory alkalosis and later respiratory acidosis. The chest x-ray shows a typical "snowstorm" infiltrate. Without prompt, definitive treatment, acute pulmonary edema, acute respiratory distress syndrome (ARDS), and heart failure may develop.

Cerebral disturbances (due to hypoxia and the lodging of fat emboli in the brain) are manifested by mental status changes varying from headache and mild agitation to delirium and coma.

NURSING ALERT

Subtle personality changes, restlessness, irritability, or confusion in a patient who has sustained a fracture are indications for immediate arterial blood gas studies.

With systemic embolization, the patient appears pale. Petechiae, possibly due to a transient thrombocytopenia, are noted in the buccal membranes and conjunctival sacs, on the hard palate, and over the chest and anterior axillary folds. The patient develops a fever greater than 39.5°C (about 103°F). Free fat may be found in the urine if emboli are filtered by the renal tubules. Acute tubular necrosis and renal failure may develop.

Prevention and Management

Immediate immobilization of fractures (including early surgical fixation), minimal fracture manipulation, adequate support for fractured bones during turning and positioning, and maintenance of fluid and electrolyte balance are measures that may reduce the incidence of fat emboli. The nurse monitors high-risk patients (adults between 20 and 30 years of age with long bone, pelvic, or multiple fractures or crush injuries, and elderly patients with hip fractures) to identify this complication. Prompt initiation of respiratory support is essential.

The objectives of management are to support the respiratory system, to prevent respiratory failure, and to correct homeostatic disturbances (Porth, 2005). Acute pulmonary edema and ARDS are the most common causes of death. Respiratory support is provided with high-flow oxygen. Controlled-volume ventilation with positive end-expiratory pressure (PEEP) may be used to prevent or treat pulmonary edema. Corticosteroids may be administered IV to treat the inflammatory lung reaction and to control cerebral edema (Porth, 2005). Vasopressor medications to support cardiovascular function are administered IV to prevent hypotension, shock, and interstitial pulmonary edema. Accurate fluid intake and output records facilitate adequate fluid replacement therapy. Morphine may be prescribed for pain for the patient who is on a ventilator, and an IV benzodiazepine (eg, midazolam [Versed]) may be prescribed to relieve anxiety. In addition, the nurse provides calm reassurance to allay apprehension. The patient's response to therapy is closely monitored (see Chapter 23 for the nursing management of respiratory failure and Chapter 25 for care of the patient on a ventilator).

Fat emboli are a major cause of death for patients with fractures. Therefore, the nurse must recognize early indications of fat embolism syndrome and report them promptly to the physician. Respiratory support must be instituted early.

Compartment Syndrome

An anatomic compartment is an area of the body encased by bone or fascia (eg, the fibrous membrane that covers and separates muscles) that contains muscles, nerves, and blood vessels. The human body has 46 anatomic compartments, and 36 of these are located in the extremities. Compartment syndrome is a complication that develops when pressure within a compartment is greater than normal. There are three types of compartment syndromes: acute compartment syndrome, chronic compartment syndrome, and crush compartment syndrome. Acute compartment syndrome involves a sudden and severe decrease in blood flow to the tissues distal to an area of injury that results in ischemic necrosis if prompt, decisive intervention does not occur. Chronic compartment syndrome is characterized by pain, aching, and tightness in a muscle or muscle group that has been subjected to inordinate stress or exercise. In this instance, muscle volume increases by as much as 20% within a short time, resulting in stretching of the fascia and inflammation. Crush compartment syndrome is caused by massive external compression or crushing of a compartment; for instance, this may occur when a car jack fails and a car falls on a mechanic. This type of massive injury results in systemic effects that include rhabdomyolysis that causes acute renal failure and that may eventually lead to multiple organ dysfunction syndrome (MODS) (Altizer, 2004).

The following discussion focuses on acute compartment syndrome. The patient complains of deep, throbbing, unrelenting pain, which continues to increase despite the administration of opioids and seems out of proportion to the injury. A hallmark sign is pain that occurs or intensifies with passive ROM. This pain can be caused by (1) a reduction in the size of the muscle compartment because the enclosing muscle fascia is too tight or a cast or dressing is constrictive or (2) an increase in compartment contents because of edema or hemorrhage (eg, fractures, venomous snake bites, burns). The lower leg is most frequently involved, but the forearm is also at risk (Fig. 69-3). The pressure within a muscle compartment may increase to such an extent as to decrease microcirculation, causing nerve and muscle anoxia and necrosis. Permanent function can be lost if the anoxic situation continues for longer than 6 hours (Altizer, 2004).

Assessment and Diagnostic Findings

Frequent assessment of neurovascular function after a fracture is essential and focuses on the "5 P's:" *p*ain, *p*aralysis, *p*aresthesias, *p*allor, and *p*ulselessness. Sensory deficits include deep, throbbing, escalating pain that increases with

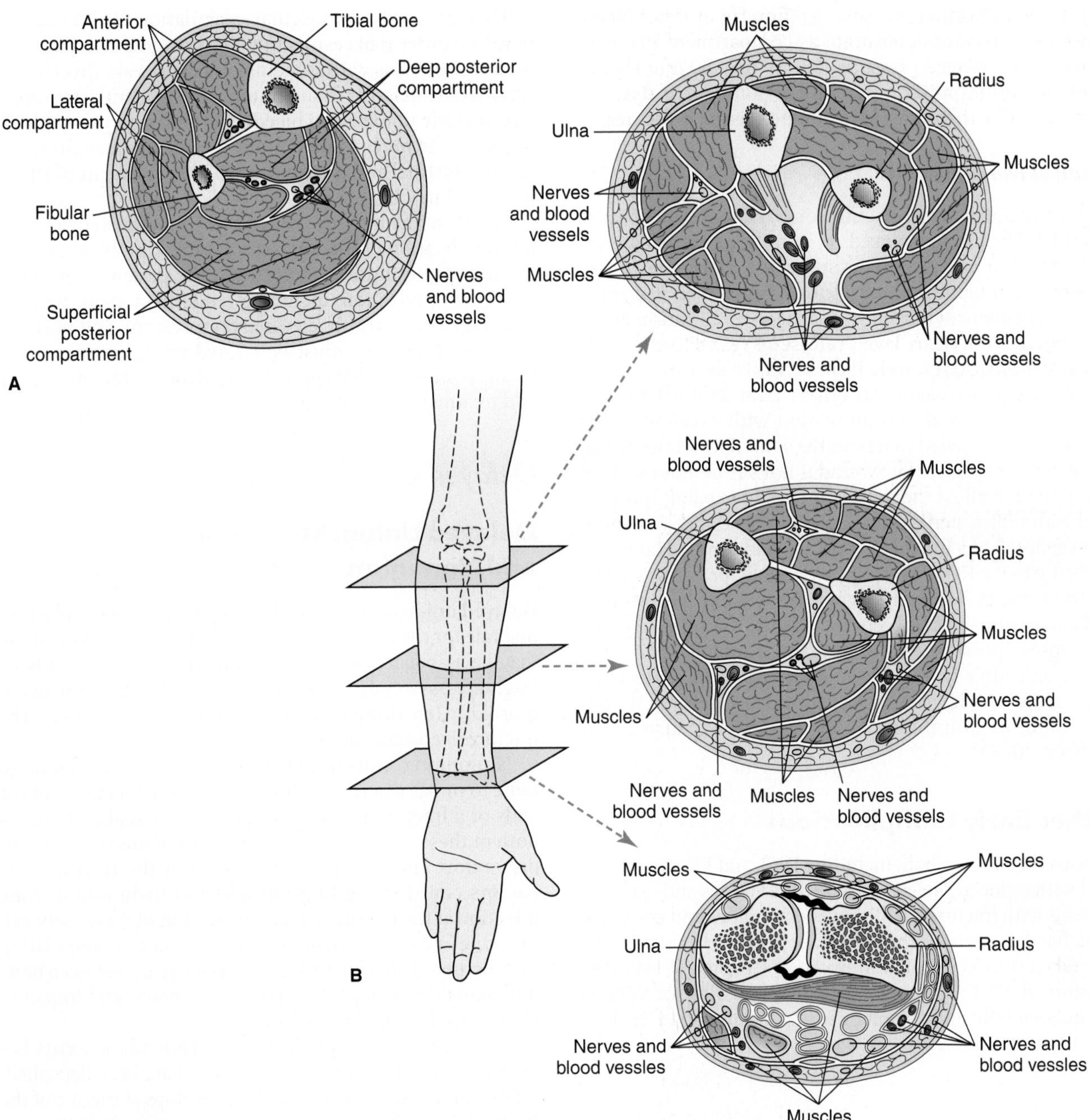

FIGURE 69-3. Cross-sections of anatomic compartments. (**A**) Compartments of the left lower leg. (**B**) Compartments of the left forearm. From Chapman, M. W., Szabo, R. M., & Marder, R. A. (2000). *Chapman's orthopaedic surgery* (3rd ed., pp. 395–396). Philadelphia: Lippincott Williams & Wilkins.

passive stretching. Paresthesia (burning or tingling sensation) and numbness are early signs of nerve involvement. Motion is evaluated by asking the patient to move the fingers or toes distal to the potential problem. With continued nerve ischemia and edema, the patient experiences sensations of hypoesthesia (diminished sensitivity to stimulation) and then absence of feeling. Motor weakness may occur as a late sign of nerve ischemia. No movement (paralysis) suggests nerve damage.

Peripheral circulation is evaluated by assessing color, temperature, capillary refill time, swelling, and pulses. Edema reduces tissue perfusion. Cyanotic (blue-tinged) nail beds suggest venous congestion. Pallor or dusky and cold fingers or toes and prolonged capillary refill time suggest diminished arterial perfusion. Edema may obscure the presence of arterial pulsation, and Doppler ultrasonography may be used to verify a pulse. Pulselessness is a very late sign that may signify lack of distal tissue perfusion (Altizer, 2004).

Palpation of the muscle, if possible, reveals it to be swollen and hard. The orthopedic surgeon may measure the actual tissue pressure by inserting a tissue pressure-monitoring device, such as a Wick catheter, into the muscle compartment

(Fig. 69-4). (Normal pressure is 8 mm Hg or less.) Nerve and muscle tissues deteriorate as compartment pressure increases. Prolonged pressure of more than 30 mm Hg can result in compromised microcirculation. Nerve tissue is more sensitive than muscle to elevated tissue pressures.

Medical Management

Prompt management of acute compartment syndrome is essential. The physician needs to be notified immediately if neurovascular compromise is suspected. Delay may result in permanent nerve and muscle damage or even necrosis.

Compartment syndrome is managed by elevation of the extremity to the heart level, release of restrictive devices (dressings or cast), or both. If conservative measures do not restore tissue perfusion and relieve pain within 1 hour, a fasciotomy (surgical decompression with excision of the fascia) may be needed to relieve the constrictive muscle fascia. After fasciotomy, the wound is not sutured but instead is left open to allow the muscle tissues to expand; it is covered with moist, sterile saline dressings. The affected arm or leg is splinted in a functional position and elevated, and prescribed passive ROM exercises are usually performed every 4 to 6 hours. In 3 to 5 days, when the swelling has resolved and tissue perfusion has been restored, the wound is débrided and closed (possibly with skin grafts). Complications that may occur after fasciotomy include AVN and infection. In patients who have sustained a fracture, delayed union, malunion, or nonunion of the fracture may also occur (Altizer, 2004).

Other Early Complications

Venous thromboemboli, including DVT and PE, are associated with reduced skeletal muscle contractions and bed rest. Patients with fractures of the lower extremities and pelvis are at high risk for venous thromboemboli. PEs may cause death several days to weeks after injury. (See Chapter 31 for a discussion of DVT; Chapter 30 for a discussion of venous thromboemboli; and Chapter 23 for a discussion of PE.)

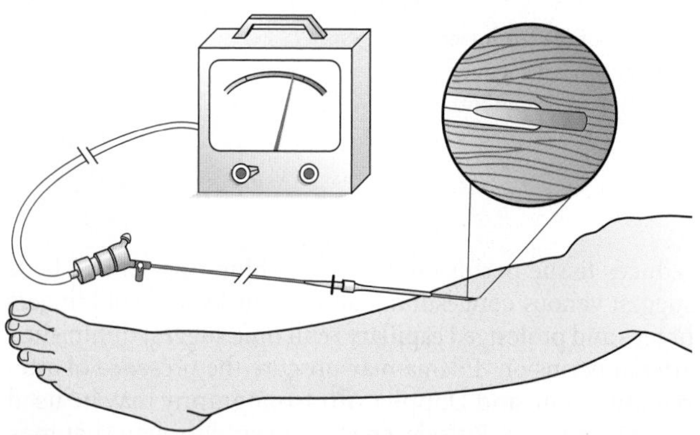

FIGURE 69-4. The Wick catheter is inserted into a muscle compartment and continuously monitors compartment pressure. From Chapman, M. W., Szabo, R. M., & Marder, R. A. (2000). *Chapman's orthopaedic surgery* (3rd ed., p. 401). Philadelphia: Lippincott Williams & Wilkins.

Disseminated intravascular coagulation (DIC) is a systemic disorder that results in widespread hemorrhage and microthrombosis with ischemia. Its causes are diverse and can include massive tissue trauma. Early manifestations of DIC include unexpected bleeding after surgery, and bleeding from the mucous membranes, venipuncture sites, and gastrointestinal and urinary tracts. The treatment of DIC is discussed in Chapter 33.

All open fractures are considered contaminated. Surgical internal fixation of fractures carries a risk of infection. The nurse must monitor for and teach the patient to monitor for signs of infection, including tenderness, pain, redness, swelling, local warmth, elevated temperature, and purulent drainage. Infections must be treated promptly. Antibiotic therapy must be appropriate and adequate for prevention and treatment of infection.

Delayed Complications

Delayed Union, Malunion, and Nonunion

Delayed union occurs when healing does not occur at a normal rate for the location and type of fracture. Delayed union may be associated with distraction (pulling apart) of bone fragments, systemic or local infection, poor nutrition, or comorbidity (eg, diabetes mellitus, autoimmune disease). The fracture eventually heals.

Nonunion results from failure of the ends of a fractured bone to unite, whereas **malunion** results from failure of the ends of a fractured bone to unite in normal alignment. In both of these instances, the patient complains of persistent discomfort and abnormal movement at the fracture site. Factors contributing to nonunion and malunion include infection at the fracture site, interposition of tissue between the bone ends, inadequate immobilization or manipulation that disrupts callus formation, excessive space between bone fragments (bone gap), limited bone contact, and impaired blood supply resulting in AVN.

In nonunion, fibrocartilage or fibrous tissue exists between the bone fragments; no bone salts have been deposited. A false joint (pseudarthrosis) often develops at the site of the fracture. Nonunion most commonly occurs with fractures of the middle third of the humerus, the lower third of the tibia, and, in elderly people, the neck of the femur.

Medical Management

The physician treats nonunion with internal fixation, bone grafting, electrical bone stimulation, or a combination of these therapies. Internal fixation stabilizes the bone fragments and ensures bone contact.

Bone grafts provide for osteogenesis, osteoconduction, or osteoinduction. *Osteogenesis* (bone formation) occurs after transplantation of bone containing osteoblasts. *Osteoconduction* is provision by the graft of the structural matrix for ingrowth of blood vessels and osteoblasts. *Osteoinduction* is the stimulation of host stem cells to differentiate into osteoblasts by several growth factors, including bone morphogenetic proteins (BMPs), particularly BMP-2, BMP-6, and BMP-9 (Boden, 2005).

Grafted bone undergoes a reconstructive process that results in a gradual replacement of graft with new bone. During surgery the bone fragments are trimmed, infection (if present) is removed, and a bone graft is placed in the bony defect. The bone graft may be an **autograft** (tissue, frequently from the iliac crest, harvested from the patient for his or her own use) or an **allograft** (tissue harvested from a donor for a recipient). The bone graft fills the bone gap, provides a lattice structure for invasion by bone cells, and actively promotes bone growth. The type of bone selected for grafting depends on function: cortical bone is used for structural strength, cancellous bone for osteogenesis, and corticocancellous bone for strength and rapid incorporation. Bone grafts may be chips, wedges, blocks, bone segments, or demineralized bone matrix. At times, autograft bone, allograft bone, and demineralized cortical matrix are combined to optimize graft incorporation and bone healing. Free vascularized bone autografts are grafted with their own blood supply, allowing for primary fracture healing.

After grafting, immobilization and non–weight-bearing exercises are required while the bone graft becomes incorporated and the fracture or defect heals. Depending on the type of bone grafted, healing may take from 6 to 12 months or longer. Bone grafting problems include wound or graft infection, fracture of the graft, and nonunion (Boden, 2005). Specific problems associated with autografts include a limited quantity of bone available for harvest and harvest site pain that may persist for up to 2 years after harvest (Boden, 2005). Infrequent specific allograft problems include partial acceptance (lack of host and donor histocompatibility, which retards graft incorporation), graft rejection (rapid and complete resorption of the graft), and transmission of disease (rare).

Osteogenesis in nonunion may be stimulated by electrical impulses; the effectiveness is similar to that of bone grafting. Use of electrical impulses is not effective with large bone gaps or synovial pseudarthrosis. The electrical stimulation modifies the tissue environment, making it electronegative, which enhances mineral deposition and bone formation that promotes bone growth.

In some situations, pins that act as cathodes are inserted percutaneously, directly into the fracture site, and electrical impulses are directed to the fracture continuously. Direct current methods cannot be used when infection is present.

Another method for stimulating osteogenesis is noninvasive inductive coupling. Pulsing electromagnetic fields are delivered to the fracture for approximately 10 hours each day by an electromagnetic coil over the nonunion site (Fig. 69-5). During the electrical stimulation treatment period, which takes 3 to 6 months or longer, rigid fracture fixation with adequate support is needed.

Nursing Management

The patient with a nonunion has experienced an extended time in fracture treatment and frequently becomes frustrated with prolonged therapy. The nurse provides emotional support and encouragement to the patient and encourages compliance with the treatment regimen. The orthopedic

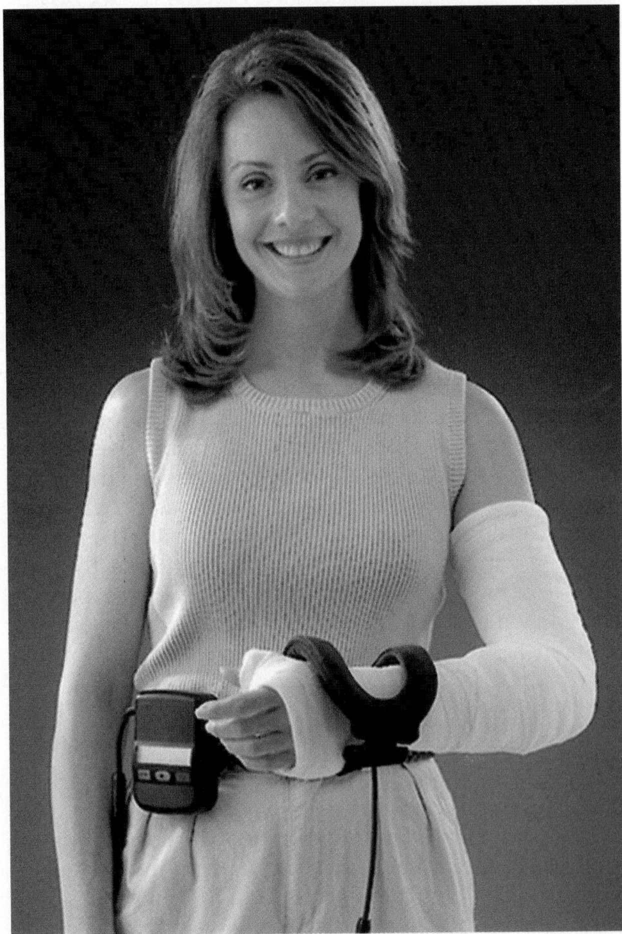

FIGURE 69-5. Bone healing stimulator applied to the arm. (Courtesy of EBI Medical Systems, Parsippany, NJ)

surgeon evaluates the progression of bone healing with periodic x-rays.

Nursing care for the patient with a bone graft includes pain management, monitoring the patient for signs of infection at the harvest and recipient sites, and patient education. The nurse needs to reinforce information concerning the objectives of the bone graft, immobilization, non–weight-bearing exercises, wound care, signs of infection, and the importance of follow-up care with the orthopedic surgeon.

Nursing care for the patient with electrical bone stimulation focuses on patient education that addresses immobilization, weight-bearing restrictions, and correct daily use of the stimulator as prescribed.

Avascular Necrosis of Bone

Avascular necrosis (AVN) occurs when the bone loses its blood supply and dies. It may occur after a fracture with disruption of the blood supply (especially of the femoral neck). It is also seen with dislocations, bone transplantation, prolonged high-dose corticosteroid therapy, chronic renal disease, sickle cell anemia, and other diseases. The devitalized bone may collapse or reabsorb. The patient develops pain and experiences limited movement. X-rays reveal loss of mineralized matrix and structural collapse. Treatment generally consists of attempts to revitalize the bone with bone grafts, prosthetic replacement, or arthrodesis (joint fusion).

Reaction to Internal Fixation Devices

Internal fixation devices may be removed after bony union has taken place. However, in most patients, the device is not removed unless it produces symptoms. Pain and decreased function are the prime indications that a problem has developed. Problems may include mechanical failure (inadequate insertion and stabilization); material failure (faulty or damaged device); corrosion of the device, causing local inflammation; allergic response to the metallic alloy used; and osteoporotic remodeling adjacent to the fixation device (in which stress needed for bone strength is transferred to the device, causing a disuse osteoporosis) (Bucholz, Heckman, Court-Brown, et al., 2005). If the device is removed, the bone needs to be protected from refracture related to osteoporosis, altered bone structure, and trauma. Bone remodeling reestablishes the bone's structural strength.

Complex Regional Pain Syndrome

Complex regional pain syndrome (CRPS), formerly called RSD, is a painful sympathetic nervous system problem. It occurs infrequently. When it does occur, it is most often in an upper extremity after trauma and is seen more often in women. Clinical manifestations of CRPS include severe burning pain, local edema, hyperesthesia, stiffness, discoloration, vasomotor skin changes (ie, fluctuating warm, red, dry and cold, sweaty, cyanotic), and trophic changes (ie, glossy, shiny skin; increased hair and nail growth). This syndrome is frequently chronic, with extension of symptoms to adjacent areas of the body. Disuse muscle atrophy and bone deossification (osteoporosis) occur with persistence of CRPS. Patients may exhibit ineffective individual coping related to the chronic pain.

Management

Prevention may include elevation of the extremity after injury or surgery and selection of an immobilization device (eg, external fixator) that allows for the greatest ROM and functional use of the rest of the extremity. Early effective pain relief is the focus of management. Pain may need to be controlled with analgesics, anesthetic nerve blocks, or IV bisphosphonate pamidronate (Aredia). NSAIDs, corticosteroids, muscle relaxants, and antidepressants also may be used. With pain relief, the patient can participate in ROM exercises and functional use of the affected area. The nurse needs to help the patient cope with CRPS manifestations and explore multiple ways to control pain (see Chapter 13). The nurse avoids using the involved extremity for blood pressure measurements and venipunctures.

Heterotopic Ossification

Heterotopic ossification (myositis ossificans) is the abnormal formation of bone, near bones or in muscle, in response to soft tissue trauma after blunt trauma, fracture, or total joint replacement. The muscle is painful, and normal muscular contraction and movement are limited. Early mobilization may prevent its occurrence. NSAIDs (eg, ibuprofen [Advil, Motrin]) may be used prophylactically if deep muscle contusion has occurred. Usually, the bone lesion resorbs over time, but the abnormal bone eventually may need to be excised if symptoms persist.

Fractures of Specific Sites

Injuries to the skeletal structure may vary from a simple linear fracture to a severe crushing injury. The type and location of the fracture and the extent of damage to surrounding structures determine the therapeutic management. Maximum functional recovery is the goal of management.

Clavicle

Fracture of the clavicle (collar bone) is a common injury that results from a fall or a direct blow to the shoulder. Head or cervical spine injuries may accompany these fractures. The clavicle helps hold the shoulder upward, outward, and backward from the thorax. Therefore, when the clavicle is fractured, the patient assumes a protective position, slumping the shoulders and immobilizing the arm to prevent shoulder movements. The treatment goal is to align the shoulder in its normal position by means of closed reduction and immobilization.

More than 80% of these fractures occur in the middle third of the clavicle. A clavicular strap, also called a *figure-eight bandage* (Fig. 69-6), may be used to pull the shoulders back, reducing and immobilizing the fracture. When a clavicular strap is used, the axillae are well padded to prevent a compression injury to the brachial plexus and the axillary artery. The nurse monitors the circulation and nerve function of both arms. A sling may be used to support the arm and to relieve pain. The patient may be permitted to use the arm for light activities within the range of comfort.

Fracture of the distal third of the clavicle, without displacement and ligament disruption, is treated with a sling and restricted motion of the arm. When a fracture in the distal third is accompanied by a disruption of the coracoclavicular ligament that connects the coracoid process of the scapula and the inferior surface of the clavicle, the bony fragments are frequently displaced. This type of injury may be treated by open reduction with internal fixation (ORIF).

The nurse cautions the patient not to elevate the arm above shoulder level until the ends of the bone have united (about 6 weeks) but encourages the patient to exercise the elbow, wrist, and fingers as soon as possible. When prescribed, shoulder exercises (Fig. 69-7) are performed to obtain full shoulder motion. Vigorous activity is limited for 3 months.

Complications of clavicular fractures include trauma to the nerves of the brachial plexus, injury to the subclavian vein or artery from a bony fragment, and malunion. Malunion may be a cosmetic problem (eg, when low-neckline clothing is worn).

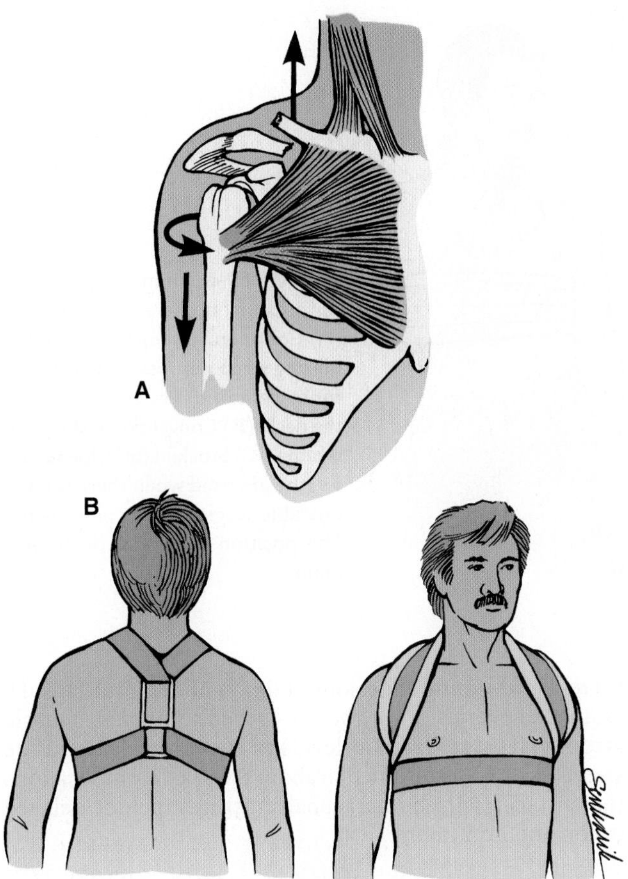

FIGURE 69-6. Fracture of the clavicle. (**A**) Anteroposterior view shows typical displacement in midclavicular fracture. (**B**) Immobilization is accomplished with a clavicular strap.

Humeral Neck

Fractures of the proximal humerus may occur through either the anatomic or the surgical neck of the humerus. The anatomic neck is located just below the humeral head. The surgical neck is the region below the tubercles. Impacted fractures of the surgical neck of the humerus are seen most frequently in older women after a fall on an outstretched arm. These are essentially nondisplaced fractures. Active middle-aged patients who are injured in a fall may suffer severely displaced humeral neck fractures with associated rotator cuff damage.

The patient presents with the affected arm hanging limp at the side or supported by the uninjured hand. Neurovascular assessment of the extremity is essential to evaluate fully the extent of injury and the possible involvement of the neurovascular bundle (nerves and blood vessels) of the arm.

Many impacted fractures of the surgical neck of the humerus are not displaced and do not require reduction. The arm is supported and immobilized by a sling and swathe that secure the supported arm to the trunk (Fig. 69-8). A soft pad is placed in the axilla to absorb moisture and prevent skin breakdown. Limitation of motion and stiffness of the shoulder occur with disuse. Therefore, pendulum exercises are begun as soon as tolerated by the patient. (In pendulum or circumduction exercises, the nurse or physical therapist instructs the patient to lean forward and allow the affected arm to abduct and rotate [see Fig. 69-7].) Early motion of the joint does not displace the fragments if motion is carried out within the limits imposed by pain.

These fractures require 6 to 10 weeks to heal, and the patient should avoid vigorous activity (eg, tennis) for an

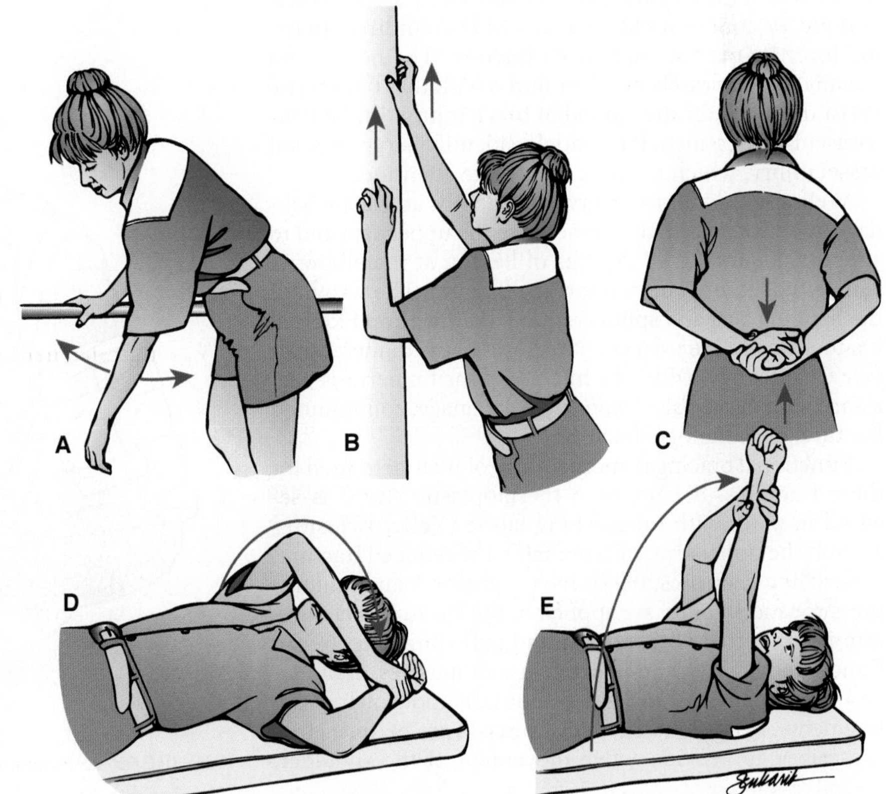

FIGURE 69-7. Exercises that promote shoulder range of motion include (**A**) pendulum exercise and (**B**) wall climbing. The unaffected arm is used to assist with (**C**) internal rotation, (**D**) external rotation, and (**E**) elevation. In C, D, and E, the unaffected arm is used for power.

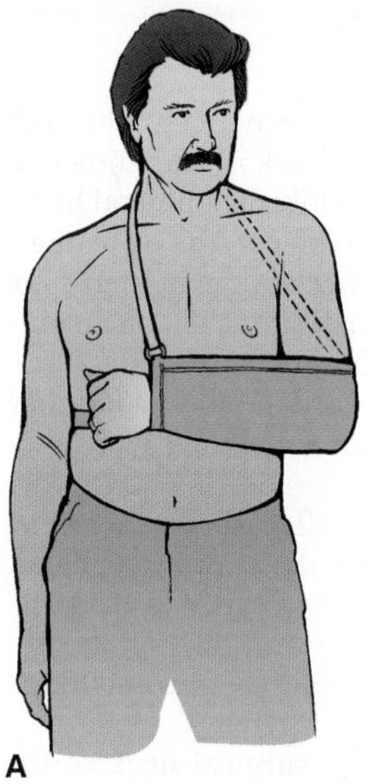

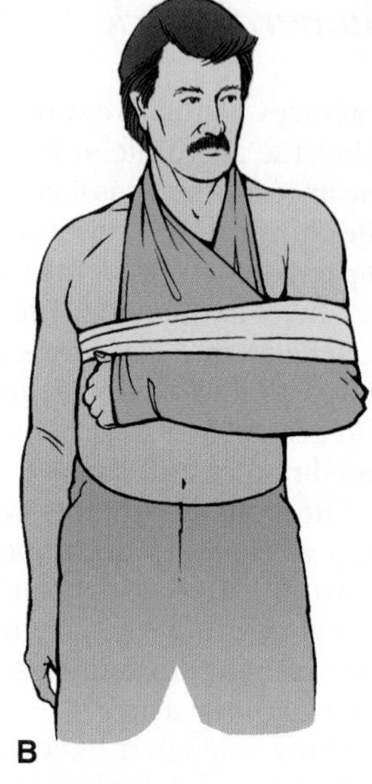

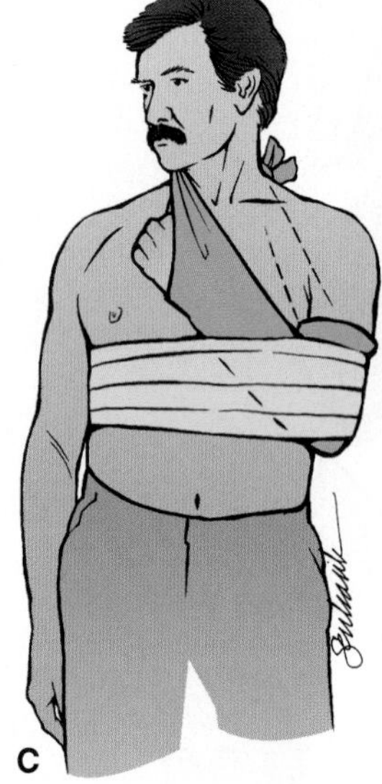

FIGURE 69-8. Immobilizers for proximal humeral fractures. (**A**) Commercial sling with immobilizing strap permits easy removal for hygiene and is comfortable on the neck. (**B**) Conventional sling and swathe. (**C**) Stockinette Velpeau and swathe are used when there is an unstable surgical neck component. This position relaxes the pectoralis major.

additional 4 weeks. Residual stiffness, aching, and some limitation of ROM may persist for 6 months or longer.

When a humeral neck fracture is displaced, treatment consists of closed reduction, ORIF, or replacement of the humeral head with a prosthesis. In this type of fracture, exercises are started only after a prescribed period of immobilization.

Humeral Shaft

Fractures of the shaft of the humerus are most frequently caused by (1) direct trauma that results in a transverse, oblique, or comminuted fracture or (2) an indirect twisting force that results in a spiral fracture. The nerves and brachial blood vessels may be injured with these fractures. Wrist drop is indicative of radial nerve injury. Initial neurovascular assessment is essential to identify nerve or blood vessel injury, which requires immediate attention.

Well-padded splints, overwrapped with an elastic bandage, are used to initially immobilize the upper arm and to support the arm in 90 degrees of flexion at the elbow. A sling or collar and cuff support the forearm. The weight of the hanging arm and splints reduces the fracture. External fixators are used to treat open fractures of the humeral shaft (see Chapter 67). ORIF of a fracture of the humerus is necessary with nerve palsy, blood vessel damage, comminuted fracture, or pathologic fracture.

Functional bracing is another form of treatment used for these fractures. A contoured thermoplastic sleeve is secured in place with interlocking fabric (Velcro) closures around the upper arm, immobilizing the reduced fracture. As swelling decreases, the sleeve is tightened, and uniform pressure and stability are applied to the fracture. The forearm is supported with a collar and cuff sling (Fig. 69-9). Functional bracing allows active use of muscles, shoulder and elbow motion, and good approximation of fracture fragments. Pendulum shoulder exercises are performed as prescribed to provide active movement of the shoulder, thereby preventing adhesions of the shoulder joint capsule. Isometric exercises may be prescribed to prevent muscle atrophy. The callus that develops is substantial, and the sleeve can be discontinued in about 8 weeks. Complications that are seen with humeral shaft fractures include delayed union and nonunion.

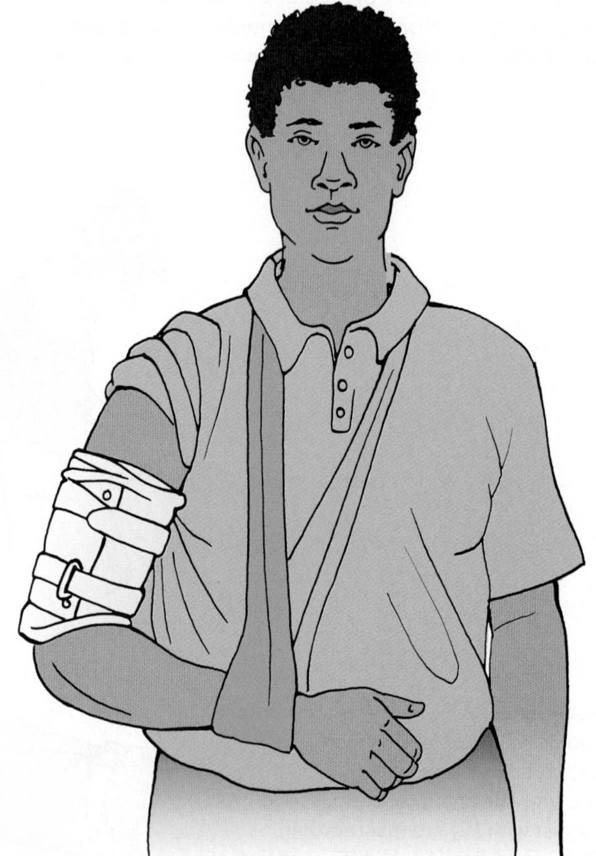

FIGURE 69-9. Functional humeral brace with collar and cuff sling.

Elbow

Fractures of the distal humerus result from motor vehicle crashes, falls on the elbow (in the extended or flexed position), or a direct blow. These fractures may result in injury to the median, radial, or ulnar nerves.

The patient is evaluated for paresthesia and signs of compromised circulation in the forearm and hand. The most serious complication of a supracondylar fracture of the humerus is Volkmann's contracture (an acute compartment syndrome), which results from antecubital swelling or damage to the brachial artery (Chart 69-4). The nurse needs to monitor the patient regularly for compromised neurovascular status and signs and symptoms of acute compartment syndrome.

Other potential complications are damage to the joint articular surfaces and hemarthrosis (blood in the joint). If hemarthrosis is present, the physician may aspirate the joint to remove the blood, thereby relieving the pressure and pain.

The goal of therapy is prompt reduction and stabilization of the distal humerus fracture, followed by controlled active motion after swelling has subsided and healing has begun. If the fracture is not displaced, the arm is immobilized in a cast or posterior splint with the elbow at 45 to 90 degrees of flexion and placed in a sling. A thermoplastic splint is used to support the fracture, and rehabilitation exercises continue for 4 to 6 weeks.

Usually, a displaced fracture is treated with ORIF. Excision of bone fragments may be necessary. Additional external support with a splint is then applied. Active finger exercises are encouraged. Gentle ROM exercise of the injured joint is begun about 1 week after internal fixation. Motion promotes healing of injured joints by producing movement of synovial fluid into the articular cartilage. Active exercise of the elbow to prevent residual limitation of motion is performed as prescribed.

CHART 69-4

Volkmann's Contracture

- Observe the distal part of the extremity for swelling, skin color, nail bed capillary refill, and temperature. Compare affected and unaffected hands.
- Assess radial pulse.
- Assess for paresthesia (tingling and burning sensations) in the hand, which may indicate nerve injury or impending ischemia.
- Evaluate the patient's ability to move the fingers.
- Explore the intensity and character of the pain.
- Directly measure tissue pressure as prescribed.
- Report indications of diminished nerve function or diminished circulatory perfusion promptly before irreparable damage occurs; fasciotomy may become necessary.

Radial Head

Radial head fractures are common and are usually produced by a fall on an outstretched hand with the elbow extended. If blood has collected in the elbow joint (hemarthrosis), it is aspirated to relieve pain and to allow early active elbow and forearm ROM exercises. Immobilization for undisplaced fractures is accomplished with a splint. The patient is instructed not to lift with the arm for approximately 4 weeks. If the fracture is displaced, surgery is typically indicated, with excision of the radial head when necessary. Postoperatively, the arm is immobilized in a posterior plaster splint and sling. The patient is encouraged to carry out a program of active motion of the elbow and forearm when prescribed.

Radial and Ulnar Shafts

Fractures of the shaft of the bones of the forearm occur most frequently in children. The radius or the ulna may be fractured at any level. Frequently, displacement occurs when both bones are broken. The forearm's unique functions of pronation and supination must be preserved with good anatomic position and alignment.

If the fragments are not displaced, the fracture is treated by closed reduction with a long-arm cast applied from the upper arm to the proximal palmar crease. A loop may be incorporated in the cast near the elbow and a sling pulled through it to prevent the cast from sagging against the forearm.

The circulation, motion, and sensation of the hand are assessed after the cast is applied. The arm is elevated to control edema. Frequent finger flexion and extension are encouraged to reduce edema. Active motion of the involved shoulder is essential. The reduction and alignment are monitored closely by x-rays to ensure adequate immobilization. The fracture is immobilized for about 12 weeks; during the last 6 weeks, the arm may be in a functional forearm brace that allows exercise of the wrist and elbow. Lifting and twisting are avoided.

Displaced fractures are managed by ORIF, using a compression plate with screws, intramedullary nails, or rods. The arm is usually immobilized in a plaster splint or cast. Open fractures may be managed with external fixation devices. The arm is elevated to control swelling. Neurovascular status is monitored. Elbow, wrist, and hand exercises are begun as permitted by the immobilization device.

Wrist

Fractures of the distal radius (Colles' fracture) are common and are usually the result of a fall on an open, dorsiflexed hand. This fracture is frequently seen in elderly women with osteoporotic bones and weak soft tissues that do not dissipate the energy of the fall. The patient presents with a deformed wrist, radial deviation, pain, swelling, weakness, limited finger ROM, and numbness.

Treatment usually consists of closed reduction and immobilization with a short-arm cast. For fractures with extensive comminution or impaction, ORIF, arthroscopic percutaneous pinning, or external fixation is used to achieve and maintain reduction and to allow for early functional rehabilitation. The wrist and forearm are elevated for 48 hours after reduction to control swelling.

Active motion of the fingers and shoulder should begin promptly. The patient is taught to perform the following exercises to reduce swelling and prevent stiffness:

- Hold the hand at the level of the heart.
- Move the fingers from full extension to flexion. Hold and release. (Repeat at least 10 times every hour when awake.)
- Use the hand in functional activities.
- Actively exercise the shoulder and elbow, including complete ROM exercises of both joints.

The fingers may swell due to diminished venous and lymphatic return. The nurse assesses the sensory function of the median nerve by pricking the distal aspect of the index finger. The motor function is assessed by the patient's ability to touch the thumb to the little finger. Diminished circulation and nerve function must be treated promptly by release of constricting bandages.

Hand

Trauma to the hand often requires extensive reconstructive surgery. The objective of treatment is always to regain maximum function of the hand.

For an undisplaced fracture of the phalanx (finger bone), the finger is splinted for 3 to 4 weeks to relieve pain and to protect the finger from further trauma. Displaced fractures and open fractures may require ORIF, using wires or pins.

The neurovascular status of the injured hand is evaluated. Swelling is controlled by elevation of the hand. Functional use of the uninvolved portion of the hand is encouraged. Assistive devices might be recommended to aid the patient in performing ADLs until the hand has healed and functional status returns.

Pelvis

The sacrum, ilium, pubis, and ischium bones form the pelvic bone, a fused, stable, bony ring in adults (Fig. 69-10). Falls, motor vehicle crashes, and crush injuries can cause pelvic fractures. Pelvic fractures are serious because at least two thirds of affected patients have significant and multiple injuries. Management of severe, life-threatening pelvic fractures is coordinated with the trauma team. Hemorrhage and thoracic, intra-abdominal, and cranial injuries have priority over treatment of fractures. There is a high mortality rate associated with pelvic fractures, related to hemorrhage, pulmonary complications, fat emboli, thromboembolic complications, and infection.

Signs and symptoms of pelvic fracture include ecchymosis; tenderness over the symphysis pubis, anterior iliac spines, iliac crest, sacrum, or coccyx; local edema; numbness or tingling of the pubis, genitals, and proximal thighs; and inability to bear weight without discomfort. Computed tomography (CT) of the pelvis helps determine the extent of injury by demonstrating sacroiliac joint disruption, soft tissue trauma, pelvic hematoma, and fractures. Neurovascular assessment of the lower extremities is completed to detect injury to pelvic blood vessels and nerves.

Hemorrhage and shock are two of the most serious consequences that may occur. Bleeding arises from the cancellous surfaces of the fracture fragments, from laceration of veins and arteries by bone fragments, and possibly from a torn iliac artery. The peripheral pulses of both lower extremities are palpated; absence of a pulse may indicate a tear in the iliac artery or one of its branches. Peritoneal lavage or abdominal CT may be performed to detect intra-abdominal hemorrhage. The patient is handled gently to minimize further bleeding and shock (Bucholz et al., 2005).

The nurse assesses for injuries to the bladder, rectum, intestines, other abdominal organs, and pelvic vessels and nerves. To assess for urinary tract injury, the patient's urine is examined for blood. A voiding cystourethrogram and an IV urogram may be performed. Laceration of the urethra is

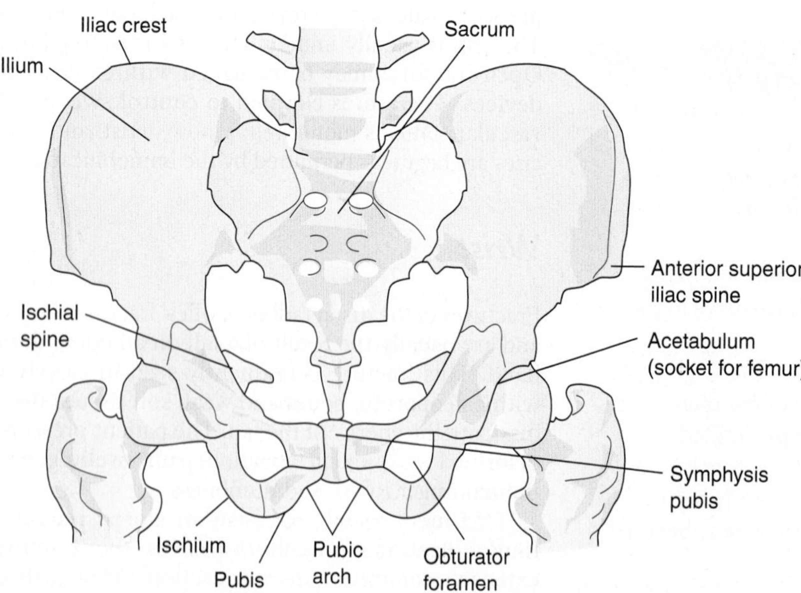

FIGURE 69-10. Pelvic bones.

suspected in males with anterior fracture of the pelvis and blood at the urethral meatus (Bucholz et al., 2005). Females rarely experience a lacerated urethra. A urinary drainage catheter should not be inserted until the status of the urethra is known. Diffuse and intense abdominal pain, hyperactive or absent bowel sounds, and abdominal rigidity and resonance (free air) or dullness to percussion (blood) suggest injury to the intestines or abdominal bleeding.

Numerous classification systems have been used to describe pelvic fractures in relation to anatomy, stability, and mechanism of injury. Some fractures of the pelvis do not disrupt the pelvic ring; others disrupt the ring, which may be rotationally or vertically unstable. The severity of pelvic fractures varies. Long-term complications of pelvic fractures include malunion, nonunion, residual gait disturbances, and back pain from ligament injury.

Stable Pelvic Fractures

Stable fractures of the pelvis (Fig. 69-11) include fracture of a single pubic or ischial ramus, fracture of ipsilateral pubic and ischial rami, fracture of the pelvic wing of the ilium (Duverney's fracture), and fracture of the sacrum or coccyx. If injury results in only a slight widening of the pubic symphysis or the anterior sacroiliac joint and the pelvic ligaments are intact, the disrupted pubic symphysis is likely to heal spontaneously with conservative management. Most fractures of the pelvis heal rapidly because the pelvic bones are mostly cancellous bone, which has a rich blood supply.

Stable pelvic fractures are treated with a few days of bed rest and symptom management until the pain and discomfort are controlled. The patient on bed rest is at risk for complications from immobility, including constipation, venous thromboemboli, pressure ulcers, and atelectasis and pneumonia. Fluids, dietary fiber, ankle and leg exercises, elastic compression stockings to aid venous return, logrolling, coughing and deep breathing, and skin care reduce the risk of complications and increase the patient's comfort. The patient with a fractured sacrum is at risk for paralytic ileus, and bowel sounds should be monitored.

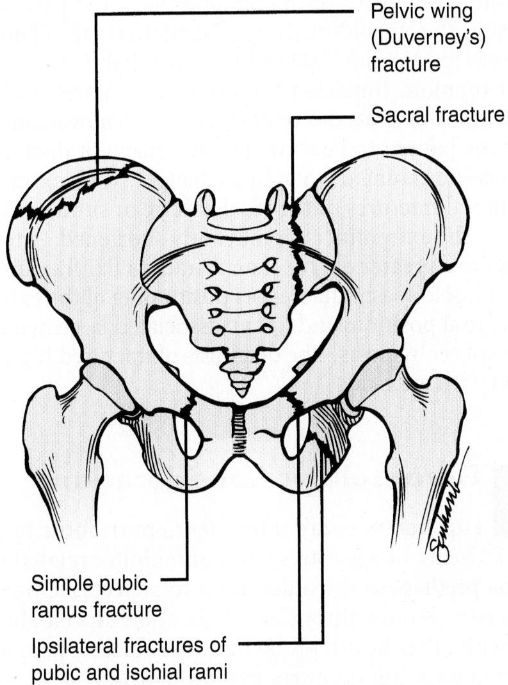

FIGURE 69-11. Stable pelvic fractures.

The patient with a fracture of the coccyx experiences pain on sitting and with defecation. Sitz baths may be prescribed to relieve pain, and stool softeners may be given to prevent the need to strain on defecation. As pain resolves, activity is gradually resumed with the use of ambulatory aids (eg, crutches, walker) for protected weight bearing. Early mobilization reduces problems related to immobility.

Unstable Pelvic Fractures

Unstable fractures of the pelvis (Fig. 69-12) may result in rotational instability (eg, the "open book" type, in which a separation occurs at the symphysis pubis with sacral ligament disruption), vertical instability (eg, the vertical shear type, with superior–inferior displacement), or a combination of both. Lateral or anterior–posterior compression of the pelvis produces rotationally unstable pelvic fractures. Vertically unstable pelvic fractures occur when force is exerted on the pelvis vertically, as when the person falls from a height onto extended legs or is struck from above by a falling object. Vertical shear pelvic fractures involve the anterior and posterior pelvic ring with vertical displacement, usually through the sacroiliac joint. There is generally complete disruption of the posterior sacroiliac, sacrospinous, and sacrotuberous ligaments. Vertical displacement of the hemipelvis is usually evident.

Immediate treatment in the emergency department of a patient with an unstable pelvic fracture includes stabilizing the pelvic bones and tamponading or compressing bleeding vessels with a pelvic binder. If major vessels are lacerated, the bleeding may be stopped through emergent embolization using interventional radiology techniques prior to surgery. Approximately 20% of patients with unstable pelvic fractures bleed excessively, requiring more than 15 units of blood products within the first 24 hours after injury (Bongiovannie, Bradley, & Kelley, 2005). These patients are at risk for hemorrhagic shock (see Chapter 15 for nursing management of the patient in shock). After the patient is hemodynamically stable, treatment generally involves external fixation or ORIF. These measures promote hemostasis, hemodynamic stability, comfort, and early mobilization.

Acetabulum

Drivers and passengers sitting in the right front seat in motor vehicle crashes may forcibly propel their knees into the dashboard, injuring the knee-thigh-hip complex (Rupp & Schneider, 2004). The acetabulum is particularly vulnerable to fracture with these types of injuries. Treatment depends on the pattern of fracture. Stable, nondisplaced fractures may be managed with traction and protective (toe-touch) weight bearing so that the affected foot is only placed on the floor for balance. Displaced and unstable acetabular fractures are treated with open reduction, joint débridement, and internal fixation or arthroplasty. Internal fixation permits early non–weight-bearing ambulation and ROM exercise. Complications seen with acetabular fractures

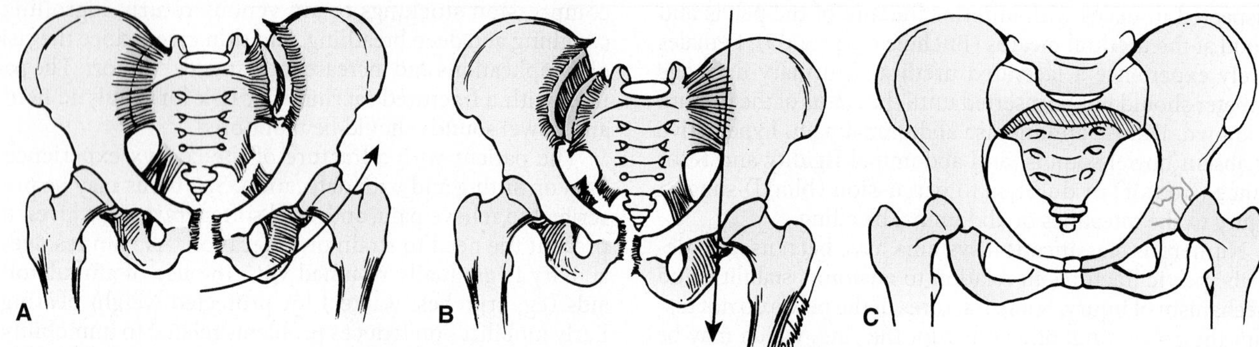

FIGURE 69-12. Unstable pelvic fracture. (**A**) Rotationally unstable fracture. The symphysis pubis is separated and the anterior sacroiliac, sacrotuberous, and sacrospinous ligaments are disrupted. (**B**) Vertically unstable fracture. The hemipelvis is displaced anteriorly and posteriorly through the symphysis pubis, and the sacroiliac joint ligaments is disrupted. (**C**) Undisplaced fracture of the acetabulum.

include nerve palsy, heterotopic ossification, and posttraumatic arthritis.

Femur

Elderly people (particularly women) who have brittle bones from osteoporosis and who tend to fall frequently have a high incidence of hip fracture. Weak quadriceps muscles, general frailty due to age, and conditions that produce decreased cerebral arterial perfusion (transient ischemic attacks, anemia, emboli, cardiovascular disease, effects of medications) contribute to the incidence of falls. The patient who has sustained a hip fracture frequently has a comorbid condition (eg, cardiovascular, pulmonary, renal, endocrine). Often, a fractured hip is a catastrophic event that has a negative impact on the patient's lifestyle and quality of life.

There are two major types of hip fracture. *Intracapsular fractures* are fractures of the neck of the femur. *Extracapsular fractures* are fractures of the trochanteric region (between the base of the neck and the lesser trochanter of the femur) and of the subtrochanteric region (Fig. 69-13). Fractures of the neck of the femur may damage the vascular system that supplies blood to the head and the neck of the femur, and the bone may become ischemic. For this reason, AVN is common in patients with femoral neck fractures.

Extracapsular intertrochanteric fractures have an excellent blood supply and heal readily. However, extensive soft tissue damage may have occurred at the time of injury. It is not uncommon for the fracture to be comminuted and unstable. The elderly are particularly vulnerable to intertrochanteric fractures and generally have a much worse prognosis than younger patients.

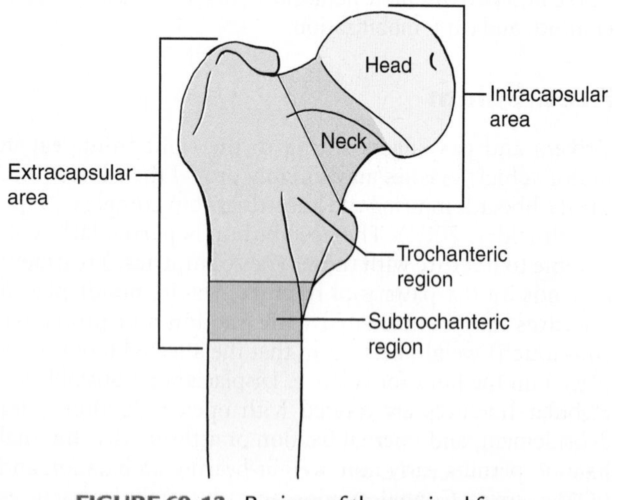

FIGURE 69-13. Regions of the proximal femur.

Clinical Manifestations

With fractures of the femoral neck, the leg is shortened, adducted, and externally rotated. The patient complains of pain in the hip and groin or in the medial side of the knee. With most fractures of the femoral neck, the patient cannot move the leg without a significant increase in pain. The patient is most comfortable with the leg slightly flexed in external rotation. Impacted intracapsular femoral neck fractures cause moderate discomfort (even with movement), may allow the patient to bear weight, and may not demonstrate obvious shortening or rotational changes. With extracapsular femoral fractures of the trochanteric or subtrochanteric regions, the extremity is significantly shortened, externally rotated to a greater degree than intracapsular fractures, exhibits muscle spasm that resists positioning of the extremity in a neutral position, and has an associated large hematoma or area of ecchymosis. The diagnosis of fractured hip is confirmed with an x-ray.

Gerontologic Considerations

Hip fractures are a frequent contributor to death after 75 years of age. Stress and immobility related to the trauma predispose the older adult to atelectasis, pneumonia, sepsis, venous thromboemboli, and reduced ability to cope with other health problems. Many elderly people hospitalized with hip fractures exhibit delirium as a result of the stress of the trauma, unfamiliar surroundings, sleep deprivation, and medications. Preoperative predictors of postoperative delirium include age older than 70 years; a history of alcohol abuse; impaired cognitive status; poor functional status; and markedly abnormal serum sodium, potassium, or glucose concentrations. In addition, delirium that develops in some elderly patients may be caused by mild cerebral ischemia or mild hypoxemia. Other factors associated with delirium include responses to medications and anesthesia, malnutrition, dehydration, infectious processes, mood disturbances, and blood loss.

To prevent complications, the nurse must assess the elderly patient for chronic conditions that require close monitoring. Examination of the legs may reveal edema due to heart failure or peripheral pulselessness from peripheral vascular disease. Similarly, chronic respiratory problems may be present and may contribute to the possible development of atelectasis or pneumonia. Coughing and deep-breathing exercises are encouraged. Frequently, elderly people are taking cardiac, antihypertensive, or respiratory medications that need to be continued. The patient's responses to these medications should be monitored.

Dehydration and poor nutrition may be present. At times, elderly people who live alone cannot summon help at the time of injury. A day or two may pass before assistance is provided, and as a result dehydration occurs. Dehydration contributes to hemoconcentration and predisposes the patient to the development of venous thromboemboli. Therefore, the patient needs to be encouraged to consume adequate fluids and a healthy diet.

Muscle weakness and wasting may have initially contributed to the fall and fracture. Bed rest and immobility cause an additional loss of muscle strength unless the nurse encourages the patient to move all joints except the involved hip and knee. Patients are encouraged to use their arms and the overhead trapeze to reposition themselves. This strengthens the arms and shoulders, which facilitates walking with assistive devices.

Medical Management

Buck's extension traction, a type of temporary skin traction, may be applied to reduce muscle spasm, to immobilize the extremity, and to relieve pain. The goal of surgical treatment of hip fractures is to obtain a satisfactory fixation so that the patient can be mobilized quickly and avoid secondary medical complications. Surgical treatment consists of (1) open or closed reduction of the fracture and internal fixation, (2) replacement of the femoral head with a prosthesis (hemiarthroplasty), or (3) closed reduction with percutaneous stabilization for an intracapsular fracture. Surgical intervention is carried out as soon as possible after injury. The preoperative objective is to ensure that the patient is in as favorable a condition as possible for the surgery. Displaced femoral neck fractures may be treated as emergencies, with reduction and internal fixation performed within 12 to 24 hours after fracture. This minimizes the effects of diminished blood supply and reduces the risk of AVN.

After general or spinal anesthesia, the hip fracture is reduced under x-ray visualization using an image intensifier. A stable fracture is usually fixed with nails, a nail-and-plate combination, multiple pins, or compression screw devices (Fig. 69-14). The orthopedic surgeon determines the specific fixation device based on the fracture site or sites. Adequate reduction is important for fracture healing: the better the reduction, the better the healing.

Hemiarthroplasty (replacement of the head of the femur with a prosthesis) is usually reserved for fractures that cannot be satisfactorily reduced or securely nailed or to avoid complications of nonunion and AVN of the head of the femur. Total hip replacement (see Chapter 67) may be used in selected patients with acetabular defects.

Nursing Management

The immediate postoperative care for a patient with a hip fracture is similar to that for other patients undergoing major

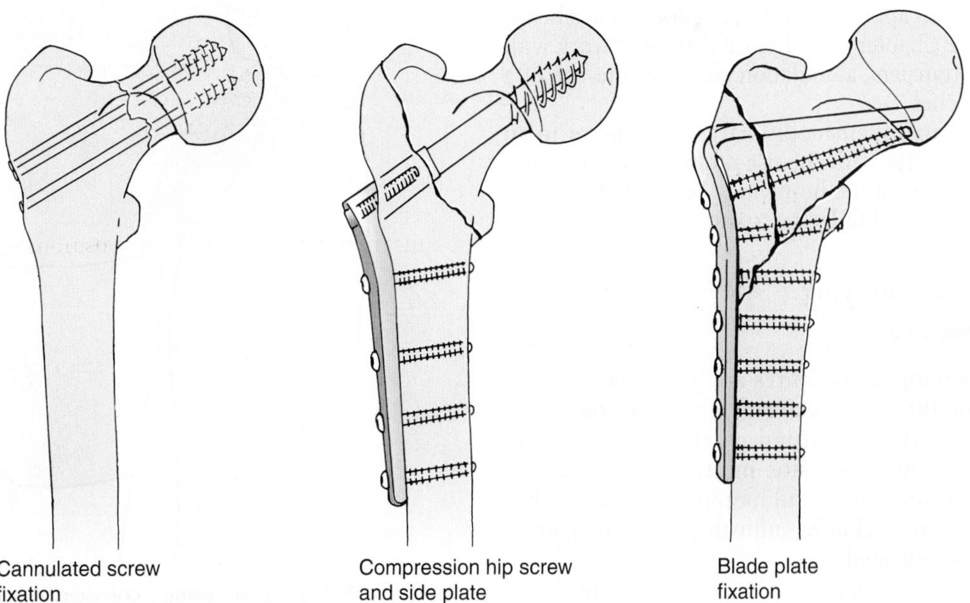

FIGURE 69-14. Examples of internal fixation for hip fractures. Internal fixation is achieved through the use of screws and plates specifically designed for stability and fixation.

surgery (see Care of the Patient Undergoing Orthopedic Surgery in Chapter 20 and Chapter 67). Attention is given to pain management, prevention of secondary medical problems, and early mobilization of the patient so that independent functioning can be restored.

During the first 24 to 48 hours, relief of pain and prevention of complications are priorities. The nurse encourages deep-breathing, coughing, and foot flexion exercises every 1 to 2 hours. Thigh-high elastic compression stockings and pneumatic compression devices are used and anticoagulants are administered to prevent the formation of venous thromboemboli. The nurse administers prescribed prophylactic IV antibiotics and monitors the patient's hydration, nutritional status, and urine output. A pillow is placed between the legs to maintain abduction and alignment and to provide needed support when turning the patient.

Repositioning the Patient

The nurse may turn the patient onto the affected or unaffected extremity as prescribed by the physician. The standard method involves placing a pillow between the patient's legs to keep the affected leg in an abducted position. The patient is then turned onto the side while proper alignment and supported abduction are maintained.

Promoting Exercise

The patient is encouraged to exercise as much as possible by means of the overbed trapeze. This device helps strengthen the arms and shoulders in preparation for protected ambulation (eg, toe touch, partial weight bearing). On the first postoperative day, the patient transfers to a chair with assistance and begins assisted ambulation. The amount of weight bearing that can be permitted depends on the stability of the fracture reduction. The physician prescribes the degree of weight bearing and the rate at which the patient can progress to full weight bearing. In general, hip flexion and internal rotation restrictions apply only if the patient has had a hemiarthroplasty (see Chapter 67). Physical therapists work with the patient on transfers, ambulation, and the safe use of a walker and crutches.

The patient can anticipate discharge to home or to an extended care facility with the use of an ambulatory aid. Some modifications in the home may be needed, such as installation of elevated toilet seats and grab bars.

Monitoring and Managing Potential Complications

Elderly people with hip fractures are particularly prone to complications that may require more vigorous treatment than the fracture. In some instances, shock proves fatal. Achievement of homeostasis after injury and after surgery is accomplished through careful monitoring and collaborative management, including adjustment of therapeutic interventions as indicated.

Neurovascular complications may occur from direct injury to nerves and blood vessels or from increased tissue pressure. With hip fracture, bleeding into the tissues is expected. Excessive swelling may be observed. Therefore, the nurse must monitor the neurovascular status of the affected leg.

DVT is the most common complication. To prevent DVT, the nurse encourages intake of fluids and ankle and foot exercises. Elastic compression stockings, sequential compression devices, and prophylactic anticoagulant therapy may be prescribed. The nurse assesses the patient's legs at least every 4 hours for signs of DVT, which may include unilateral calf tenderness, warmth, redness, and swelling.

Pulmonary complications, which commonly include atelectasis and pneumonia, are a threat to elderly patients undergoing hip surgery. Deep-breathing exercises, a change of position at least every 2 hours, and the use of an incentive spirometer help prevent respiratory complications. Pain must be treated with analgesic agents, typically opioids; otherwise, the patient may not be able to readily cough, deep breathe, or engage in prescribed activities. The nurse assesses breath sounds at least every 4 hours to detect adventitious or diminished sounds.

Skin breakdown is often seen in elderly patients with hip fracture. Blisters caused by tape are related to the tension of soft tissue edema under the nonelastic tape. An elastic hip spica wrap dressing (Fig. 69-15) or elastic tape applied in a

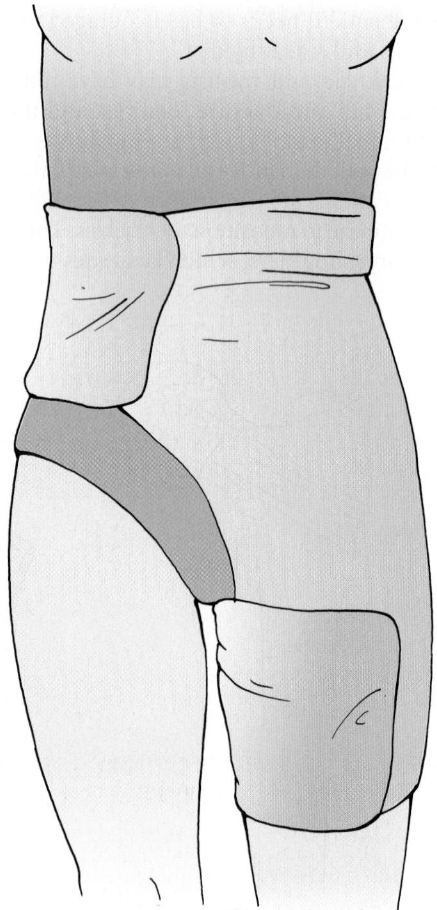

FIGURE 69-15. Patient using a commercial single-piece stretch spica wrap.

vertical fashion may reduce the incidence of tape blisters. In addition, patients with hip fractures tend to remain in one position and may develop pressure ulcers. Proper skin care, especially on the heels, back, sacrum, and shoulders, helps to relieve pressure. High-density foam, static air, or another type of special mattress may provide protection by distributing pressure evenly.

Loss of bladder control (incontinence or retention) may occur. In general, the routine use of an indwelling catheter is avoided because of the high risk for urinary tract infection. If a catheter is inserted at the time of surgery, it usually is removed on the morning of the first postoperative day. Because urinary retention is common after surgery, the nurse must assess the patient's voiding patterns. To ensure proper urinary tract function, the nurse encourages liberal fluid intake if the patient has no preexisting cardiac disease (eg, heart failure, coronary artery disease).

Delayed complications of hip fractures include infection, nonunion, AVN of the femoral head (particularly with femoral neck fractures), and fixation device problems (eg, protrusion of the fixation device through the acetabulum, loosening of hardware). Infection is suspected if the patient complains of persistent, moderate discomfort in the hip and has an elevated erythrocyte sedimentation rate.

The nursing management of the elderly patient with a hip fracture is summarized in the Plan of Nursing Care (Chart 69-5).

Health Promotion

Osteoporosis screening of patients who have experienced hip fracture is important for prevention of future fractures. With dual-energy x-ray absorptiometry (DEXA) scan testing, the risk for additional fracture can be predicted. Specific patient education regarding dietary requirements, lifestyle changes, and weight-bearing exercise to promote bone health is needed. Specific therapeutic interventions need to be initiated to retard additional bone loss and to build bone mineral density. (Refer to Chapter 68 for management of osteoporosis.) Prevention of falls is also important and may be achieved through exercises to improve muscle tone and balance and through the elimination of environmental hazards.

Femoral Shaft

Considerable force is required to break the shaft of the femur in adults. Most femoral fractures are seen in young adults who have been involved in a motor vehicle crash or who have fallen from a high place. Frequently, these patients have associated multiple injuries.

The patient presents with an enlarged, deformed, painful thigh and cannot move the hip or the knee. The fracture may be transverse, oblique, spiral, or comminuted. Frequently, the patient develops shock, because the loss of 2 to 3 units of blood into the tissues is common with these fractures. An expanding diameter of the thigh may indicate continued bleeding. Types of femoral fractures are illustrated in Figure 69-16A.

Assessment and Diagnostic Findings

Assessment includes checking the neurovascular status of the extremity, especially circulatory perfusion of the lower leg and foot (popliteal, posterior tibial, and pedal pulses and toe capillary refill time). A Doppler ultrasound monitoring device may be needed to assess blood flow. Dislocation of the hip and knee may accompany these fractures. Knee effusion suggests ligament damage and possible instability of the knee joint.

Medical Management

Continued neurovascular monitoring is needed. The fracture is immobilized so that additional soft tissue damage does not occur. Generally, skeletal traction (see Fig. 69-16B and C) or splinting is used to immobilize fracture fragments until the patient is physiologically stable and ready for ORIF procedures.

Internal fixation usually is carried out within a few days after injury. Intramedullary locking nail devices are used for midshaft (diaphyseal) fractures. Depending on the supracondylar fracture pattern, intramedullary nailing or screw plate fixation may be used. Internal fixation permits early mobilization. A thigh cuff orthosis may be used for external support. To preserve muscle strength, the patient is instructed to exercise the hip and the lower leg, foot, and toes on a regular basis. Active muscle movement enhances healing by increasing blood supply and electrical potentials at the fracture site. Prescribed weight-bearing limits are based on the type of fracture. Physical therapy includes ROM and strengthening exercises, safe use of ambulatory aids, and gait training. Functional ambulation stimulates fracture healing. Healing time is 4 to 6 months.

Compression plates and intramedullary nails may need to be removed after 12 to 18 months due to loosening. After the plates are removed, a thigh cuff orthosis is used for several months to provide support while bone remodeling occurs.

Infrequently, because of patient risks associated with anesthesia and surgery, middle shaft and distal (supracondylar) fractures may be managed with skeletal traction. Between 2 and 4 weeks after injury, when pain and swelling have subsided, skeletal traction is removed and the patient is placed in a cast brace. The cast brace is a total contact device (ie, encircles the limb) and holds the reduced fracture. The muscle, through hydrodynamic compression, stabilizes the bone and stimulates healing. Minimal partial weight bearing is begun and is progressed to full weight bearing as tolerated. The cast brace is worn for 12 to 14 weeks.

(text continues on page 2458)

CHART 69-5

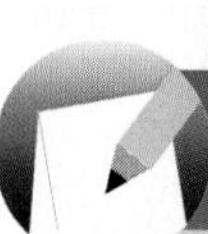

Plan of Nursing Care Care of the Elderly Patient With a Fractured Hip

Nursing Diagnosis: Acute pain related to fracture, soft tissue damage, muscle spasm, and surgery
Goal: Relief of pain

NURSING INTERVENTIONS	RATIONALE	EXPECTED OUTCOMES
1. Assess type and location of patient's pain whenever vital signs are obtained and as needed.	1. Pain is expected after fracture; soft tissue damage and muscle spasm contribute to discomfort; pain is subjective and is evaluated through description of characteristics and location, which are important for determining cause of discomfort and for proposing interventions. Continuing pain may indicate development of neurovascular problems. Pain must be assessed periodically to gauge effectiveness of continuing analgesic therapy.	• Patient describes discomfort • Expresses confidence in efforts to control pain • Expresses little discomfort with position changes • Expresses comfort when leg is positioned and immobilized • Minimizes movement of extremity before reduction and fixation • Uses physical, psychological, and pharmacologic measures to reduce discomfort • Describes a decrease in pain in 24–48 hours after surgery • Requests pain medications and uses pain relief measures early in pain cycle • States that positioning provides comfort • Appears comfortable and relaxed • Moves with increasing comfort as healing progresses
2. Acknowledge existence of pain; inform patient of available analgesics; record patient's baseline discomfort.	2. Reduces stress experienced by the patient by communicating concern and availability of help in dealing with pain. Documentation provides baseline data.	
3. Handle the affected extremity gently, supporting it with hands or pillow.	3. Movement of bone fragments is painful; muscle spasms occur with movement; adequate support diminishes soft tissue tension.	
4. Apply Buck's traction as prescribed. Use trochanter roll.	4. Immobilizes fracture to decrease pain, muscle spasm, and external rotation of hip.	
5. Use pain-modifying strategies.	5. Pain perception can be diminished by distraction and refocusing of attention.	
a. Modify the environment.	a. Interaction with others, distraction, and environmental stimuli may modify pain experiences.	
b. Administer prescribed analgesics as needed.	b. Analgesics reduce the pain; muscle relaxants may be prescribed to decrease discomfort associated with muscle spasm.	
c. Encourage patient to use pain relief measures to keep pain tolerable.	c. Mild pain is easier to control than severe pain.	

CHART 69-5

Plan of Nursing Care Care of the Elderly Patient With a Fractured Hip (Continued)

NURSING INTERVENTIONS	RATIONALE	EXPECTED OUTCOMES
d. Evaluate patient's response to medications and other pain-reduction techniques.	d. Assessment of effectiveness of measures provides basis for future management interventions; early identification of adverse reactions is necessary for corrective measures and care plan modifications.	
e. Consult with physician if relief of pain is not obtained.	e. Change in treatment plan may be necessary.	
6. Position for comfort and function.	6. Alignment of body facilitates comfort; positioning for function diminishes stress on musculoskeletal system.	
7. Assist with frequent changes in position.	7. Change of position relieves pressure and associated discomfort.	

Nursing Diagnosis: Impaired physical mobility related to fractured hip
Goal: Achieves pain-free, functional, stable hip

NURSING INTERVENTIONS	RATIONALE
1. Maintain neutral positioning of hip.	1. Prevents stress at the site of fixation.
2. Use trochanter roll.	2. Minimizes external rotation.
3. Place pillow between legs when turning.	3. Supports leg; prevents adduction.
4. Instruct and assist in position changes and transfers.	4. Encourages patient's active participation while preventing stress on hip fixation.
5. Instruct in and supervise isometric, quadriceps-setting, and gluteal-setting exercises.	5. Strengthens muscles needed for walking.
6. Encourage use of trapeze.	6. Strengthens shoulder and arm muscles necessary for use of ambulatory aids.
7. In consultation with physical therapist, instruct in and supervise progressive safe ambulation within limitations of weight-bearing prescription.	7. Amount of weight-bearing depends on the patient's condition, fracture stability, and fixation device; ambulatory aids are used to assist the patient with non-weight-bearing and partial-weight-bearing ambulation.
8. Offer encouragement and support exercise regimen.	8. Reconditioning exercises can be uncomfortable and fatiguing; encouragement helps patient comply with the program.
9. Instruct in and supervise safe use of ambulatory aids.	9. Prevents injury from unsafe use.

EXPECTED OUTCOMES

- Patient engages in therapeutic positioning
- Uses pillow between legs when turning
- Assists in position changes; shows increased independence in transfers
- Exercises every 2 hours while awake
- Uses trapeze
- Participates in progressive ambulation program
- Actively participates in exercise regimen
- Uses ambulatory aids correctly and safely

continued >

CHART 69-5

Plan of Nursing Care — Care of the Elderly Patient With a Fractured Hip (Continued)

Nursing Diagnosis: Impaired skin integrity related to surgical incision
Goal: Achieves wound healing

NURSING INTERVENTIONS	RATIONALE	EXPECTED OUTCOMES
1. Monitor vital signs.	1. Temperature, pulse, and respiration increase in response to infection. (Magnitude of response may be minimal in elderly patients.)	• Patient maintains vital signs within normal range • Exhibits well-approximated incision without drainage or excessive inflammatory response • Relates minimal discomfort; demonstrates no hematoma • Tolerates antibiotics; exhibits no evidence of osteomyelitis
2. Perform aseptic dressing changes.	2. Avoids introducing infectious organisms.	
3. Assess wound appearance and character of drainage.	3. Red, swollen, draining incision is indicative of infection.	
4. Assess report of pain.	4. Pain may be due to wound hematoma, a possible locus of infection, which needs to be surgically evacuated.	
5. Administer prophylactic antibiotic if prescribed, and observe for side effects.	5. Antibiotics reduce the risk for infection.	

Nursing Diagnosis: Risk for impaired urinary elimination related to immobility
Goal: Maintains normal urinary elimination patterns

NURSING INTERVENTIONS	RATIONALE	EXPECTED OUTCOMES
1. Monitor intake and output.	1. Adequate fluid intake ensures hydration; adequate urinary output minimizes urinary stasis.	• Intake and output are adequate; patient exhibits normal voiding patterns • Demonstrates no evidence of urinary tract infection
2. Avoid/minimize use of indwelling catheter.	2. Source of bladder infection.	
3. Perform intermittent catheterization for urinary retention	3. Empties bladder; reduces urinary tract infections	

Nursing Diagnosis: Risk for ineffective coping related to injury, anticipated surgery, and dependence
Goal: Uses effective coping mechanisms to modify stress

NURSING INTERVENTIONS	RATIONALE	EXPECTED OUTCOMES
1. Encourage patient to express concerns and to discuss the possible impact of fractured hip.	1. Verbalization helps patient deal with problems and feelings. Clarification of thoughts and feelings promotes problem-solving.	• Patient describes feelings concerning fractured hip and implications for lifestyle • Uses available resources and coping mechanisms; develops health promotion strategies • Uses community resources as needed
2. Support use of coping mechanisms. Involve significant others and support services as needed.	2. Coping mechanisms modify disabling effects of stress; sharing concerns lessens the burden and facilitates necessary modification.	

CHART 69-5

Plan of Nursing Care — Care of the Elderly Patient With a Fractured Hip (Continued)

NURSING INTERVENTIONS	RATIONALE	EXPECTED OUTCOMES
3. Contact social services, if needed.	3. Anxiety may be related to financial or social problems; facilitates management of problems associated with continuing care.	• Participates in development of health care plan
4. Explain anticipated treatment regimen and routines to facilitate positive attitude in relation to rehabilitation.	4. Understanding of plan of care helps to diminish fears of the unknown.	
5. Encourage patient to participate in planning.	5. Participating in care provides for some control of self and environment.	

Nursing Diagnosis: Risk for disturbed thought process related to age, stress of trauma, unfamiliar surroundings, and medication therapy
Goal: Remains oriented and participates in decision making

NURSING INTERVENTIONS	RATIONALE	EXPECTED OUTCOMES
1. Assess orientation status.	1. Evaluate presenting orientation of patient; confusion may result from stress of fracture, unfamiliar surroundings, coexisting systemic disease, cerebral ischemia, hypoxemia, or other factors. Baseline data are important for determining change.	• Patient establishes effective communication • Demonstrates orientation to time, place, and person • Participates in self-care activities • Remains mentally alert • Avoids episodes of confusion
2. Interview family regarding patient's orientation and cognitive abilities before injury.	2. Provides data for evaluation of current findings.	
3. Assess patient for auditory and visual deficits.	3. Diminished vision and auditory acuity frequently occur with aging; glasses and hearing aid may increase patient's ability to interact with environment.	
a. Assist patient with use of sensory aids (eg, glasses, hearing aid)	a. Aids must be in good working order and available for use.	
b. Control environmental distractors	b. Facilitates communication.	
4. Orient to and stabilize environment	4.	
a. Use orientation activities and aids (eg, clock, calendar, pictures, introduction of self).	a. Short-term memory may be faulty in the elderly; frequent reorientation helps.	
b. Minimize number of staff working with patient.	b. Consistency of caregivers promotes trust.	

continued >

CHART 69-5

Plan of Nursing Care Care of the Elderly Patient With a Fractured Hip (Continued)

NURSING INTERVENTIONS	RATIONALE	EXPECTED OUTCOMES
5. Give simple explanations of procedures and plan of care.	5. Promotes understanding and active participation.	
6. Encourage participation in hygiene and nutritional activities.	6. Participation in routine activities promotes orientation, increases awareness of self.	
7. Provide for safety. a. Keep side rails up when patient is in bed. b. Keep light on at night. c. Have call bell available. d. Provide prompt response to requests for assistance.	7. Side rails decrease chance for additional injury from falls; mechanism for securing assistance is available to patient; independent activities based on faulty judgment may result in injury.	
8. Assess mental responses to medications, especially sedatives and analgesics.	8. Elderly people tend to be more sensitive to medications; abnormal responses (eg, hallucinations, depression) may occur.	

Collaborative Problems: Hemorrhage; peripheral neurovascular dysfunction; deep vein thrombosis; pulmonary complications; pressure ulcers related to surgery and immobility
Goal: Absence of complications

NURSING INTERVENTIONS	RATIONALE	EXPECTED OUTCOMES
Hemorrhage		
1. Monitor vital signs, observing for shock.	1. Changes in pulse, blood pressure, and respirations may indicate development of shock; blood loss and stress may contribute to development of shock.	• Vital signs are stabilized within normal limits • Experiences no excessive or bright red drainage • Exhibits stable postoperative hemoglobin and hematocrit values
2. Consider preinjury blood pressure values and management of coexisting hypertension, if present.	2. Necessary for interpretation of current blood pressure determinations.	
3. Note character and amount of drainage.	3. Excessive drainage and bright red drainage may indicate active bleeding.	
4. Notify surgeon if patient develops shock or excessive bleeding.	4. Corrective measures need to be instituted.	
5. Note hemoglobin and hematocrit values, and report decreases in values.	5. Anemia due to blood loss may develop; bleeding into tissues after hip fracture may be extensive; blood replacement may be needed.	

CHART 69-5

Plan of Nursing Care Care of the Elderly Patient With a Fractured Hip (Continued)

NURSING INTERVENTIONS	RATIONALE	EXPECTED OUTCOMES
Pulmonary Complications		
1. Assess respiratory status: respiratory rate, depth, and duration, breath sounds, sputum. Monitor temperature.	1. Anesthesia and bed rest diminish respiratory effort and cause pooling of respiratory secretions. Adventitious breath sounds, pain on respiration, shortness of breath, blood tinged sputum, cough, etc., indicate pulmonary dysfunction.	• Patient has clear breath sounds • Breath sounds present in all fields • Exhibits no shortness of breath, chest pain, or elevated temperature • PaO_2 on room air within normal limits • Performs respiratory exercises; uses incentive spirometer as instructed • Changes position frequently • Consumes adequate fluids
2. Report adventitious and diminished breath sounds and elevated temperature.	2. Elevated temperature in the early postoperative period may be due to atelectasis or pneumonia.	
3. Supervise deep breathing and coughing exercises. Encourage use of incentive spirometer if prescribed.	3. Promote optimal ventilation. Coexisting respiratory conditions diminish lung expansion.	
4. Administer oxygen as prescribed.	4. Reduced ventilatory efforts may diminish PaO_2 when patient is breathing room air.	
5. Turn and reposition patient at least every 2 hours. Mobilize patient (assist patient out of bed) as soon as possible.	5. Promotes optimal ventilation. Diminishes pooling of respiratory secretions.	
6. Ensure adequate hydration.	6. Liquefies respiratory secretions. Facilitates expectoration.	
Peripheral Neurovascular Dysfunction		
1. Assess affected extremity for color and temperature.	1. The skin becomes pale and feels cool with decreased tissue perfusion. Venous congestion may cause cyanosis.	• Patient has normal color and the extremity is warm • Demonstrates normal capillary refill response • Exhibits moderate swelling; tissue not palpably tense • States pain is tolerable • Reports no pain with passive dorsiflexion • Reports normal sensations and no paresthesia • Demonstrates normal motor abilities and no paresis or paralysis • Has strong and equal pulses
2. Assess toes for capillary refill response.	2. After compression of the nail, rapid return of pink color indicates good capillary perfusion.	
3. Assess affected extremity for edema and swelling.	3. The trauma of surgery will cause swelling; excessive swelling and hematoma formation can compromise circulation and function; edema may be due to coexisting cardiovascular disease.	
4. Elevate affected extremity.	4. Minimizes dependent edema.	
5. Assess for deep, throbbing, unrelenting pain.	5. Surgical pain can be controlled; pain due to neurovascular compromise is refractory to treatment with analgesics.	

continued >

CHART 69-5

Plan of Nursing Care: Care of the Elderly Patient With a Fractured Hip (Continued)

NURSING INTERVENTIONS	RATIONALE	EXPECTED OUTCOMES
6. Assess for pain on passive flexion of foot.	6. With nerve ischemia, there will be pain on passive stretch.	
7. Assess for sensations and numbness.	7. Diminished pain and paresthesia may indicate nerve damage. Sensation in web between great and second toe—peroneal nerve; sensation on sole of foot—tibial nerve.	
8. Assess ability to move foot and toes.	8. Dorsiflexion of ankle and extension of toes indicate function of peroneal nerve. Plantar flexion of ankle and flexion of toes indicate functioning of tibial nerve.	
9. Assess pedal pulses in both feet.	9. Indicates circulatory status of extremities.	
10. Notify surgeon if diminished neurovascular status occurs.	10. Function of extremity needs to be preserved.	
Deep Vein Thrombosis		
1. Apply thigh-high elastic compression stockings and/or sequential compression device as prescribed.	1. Compression aids venous blood return and prevents stasis.	• Wears thigh-high elastic compression stockings • Uses sequential compression device • Experiences no more warmth than usual in skin areas • Exhibits no increase in calf circumference • Demonstrates no evidence of calf tenderness, warmth, redness, or swelling • Changes position with assistance and supervision • Participates in exercise regimen • Experiences no chest pain; has lungs clear to auscultation; presents no evidence of pulmonary emboli • Exhibits no signs of dehydration; has normal hematocrit • Maintains normal body temperature
2. Remove stockings for 20 minutes twice a day, and provide skin care.	2. Skin care is necessary to avoid skin breakdown. Extended removal of stocking or device defeats purpose.	
3. Assess popliteal, dorsalis pedis, and posterior tibial pulses.	3. Pulses indicate arterial perfusion of extremity. With coexisting arteriosclerotic vascular disease, pulses may be diminished or absent.	
4. Assess skin temperature of legs.	4. Local inflammation increases local skin temperature.	
5. Assess calf every 4 hours for tenderness, warmth, redness, and swelling.	5. Unilateral calf tenderness, warmth, redness, and swelling may indicate deep vein thrombosis.	
6. Measure calf circumference twice daily.	6. Increased calf circumference indicates edema or altered perfusion.	
7. Avoid pressure on popliteal blood vessels from appliances or pillows.	7. Compression of blood vessels diminishes blood flow.	
8. Change patient's position and increase activity as prescribed.	8. Activity promotes circulation and diminishes venous stasis.	

CHART 69-5

Plan of Nursing Care Care of the Elderly Patient With a Fractured Hip (Continued)

NURSING INTERVENTIONS	RATIONALE	EXPECTED OUTCOMES
9. Supervise ankle exercises hourly while patient is awake.	9. Muscle exercise promotes circulation.	
10. Ensure adequate hydration.	10. Elderly people may become dehydrated because of low fluid intake, resulting in hemoconcentration.	
11. Monitor body temperature.	11. Body temperature increases with inflammation (magnitude of response minimal in elderly people).	
Pressure Ulcers		
1. Monitor condition of skin at pressure points (eg, heels, sacrum, shoulders); inspect heels at least twice a day.	1. Elderly patients are subject to skin breakdown at points of pressure because of diminished subcutaneous tissue.	• Patient exhibits no signs of skin breakdown • Skin remains intact • Repositions self frequently • Uses protective devices
2. Reposition patient at least every 2 hours. Avoid skin shearing.	2. Avoids prolonged pressure and trauma to the skin.	
3. Administer skin care, especially to pressure points.	3. Immobility causes pressure at bony prominences; position changes relieve pressure.	
4. Use special care mattress and other protective devices (eg, heel protectors); support heel off the mattress.	4. Devices minimize pressure on skin at bony prominences.	
5. Institute care according to protocol at first indication of potential skin breakdown.	5. Early interventions prevent tissue destruction and prolonged rehabilitation.	

Nursing Diagnosis: Risk for ineffective health maintenance related to fractured hip and impaired mobility
Goal: Exhibits health maintenance/promotion behaviors

NURSING INTERVENTIONS	RATIONALE	EXPECTED OUTCOMES
1. Assess home environment for discharge planning.	1. Physical barriers (especially stairs, bathrooms) may limit patient's ability to ambulate and care for self at home.	• Home is accessible for patient at time of discharge • Patient appears relaxed and develops strategies to deal with identified problems • Has personal assistance available • Demonstrates ability to use necessary assistive devices within therapeutic prescription • Complies with home care program; keeps follow-up health care appointments
2. Encourage patient to express concerns about care at home; explore with patient possible solutions to problems.	2. Patient may have special problems that need to be identified so that solutions might be identified.	
3. Assess availability of physical assistance for ADLs and health care activities.	3. Because of limitation of mobility, patient requires some assistance in ADLs and routine health care.	

continued >

CHART 69-5

Plan of Nursing Care — Care of the Elderly Patient With a Fractured Hip (Continued)

NURSING INTERVENTIONS	RATIONALE	EXPECTED OUTCOMES
4. Teach caregiver the home health care regimen.	4. Understanding of rehabilitative regimen is necessary for compliance.	
5. Instruct patient in posthospital care: a. Activity limitations b. Reinforce exercise instructions c. Safe use of ambulatory aids d. Wound care e. Measures to promote healing (nutrition, wound care) f. Medications g. Potential problems h. Continuing health care supervision	5. Lack of knowledge and poor preparation for care at home contribute to patient anxiety, insecurity, and nonadherence to therapeutic regimen.	

An external fixator may be used if the patient has experienced an open fracture, has extensive soft tissue trauma, has lost bone, has an infection, or has hip and tibial fractures.

A common complication after fracture of the femoral shaft is restriction of knee motion. Active and passive knee exercises begin as soon as possible, depending on the management approach and the stability of the fracture and knee ligaments. Other complications include malunion, delayed union or nonunion, pudendal nerve palsy, and infection.

Knee

Fracture to the most distal portion of the femur, the patella (kneecap), and fracture to the most proximal portion of the tibia (tibial plateau, shinbone) may be defined as fractures of the knee. These fractures may be caused by motor vehicle crashes (eg, knee forcibly banging into the dashboard), direct blows to the knee from contact sports or intentionally inflicted trauma, or falls. The patient typically presents with acute pain to the affected knee and can-

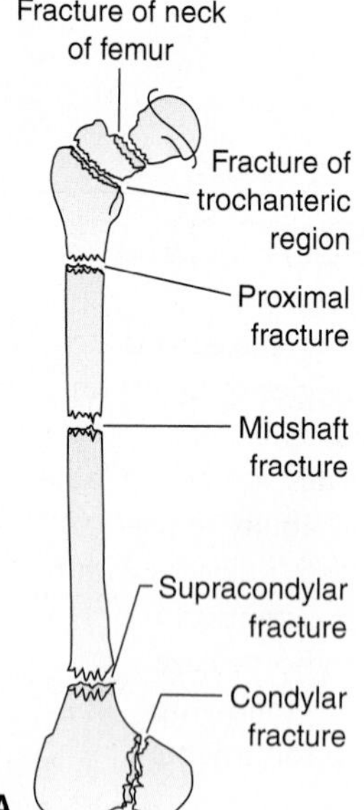

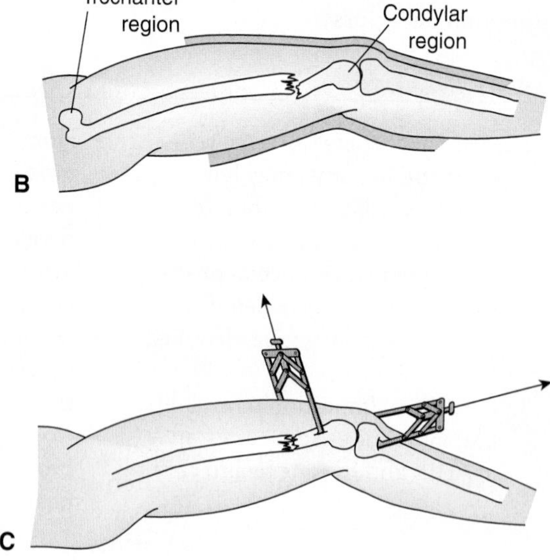

FIGURE 69-16. (A) Types of femoral fractures. (B) Example of deformity on admission to hospital. (C) Adequate reduction is achieved when additional wire is inserted in the lower femoral fragment and vertical lift is secured.

not ambulate or bear weight on the affected extremity. Theaffected knee is notably edematous. As few as 6% of all cases of acute knee pain may reflect a knee fracture (Jackson, O'Malley, & Kroenke, 2003).

Assessment and Diagnostic Findings

Most physicians and nurse practitioners follow the Ottawa decision rules when they assess and diagnose patients with suspected knee fractures (Jackson et al., 2003). The Ottawa decision rules specify that if a patient presents with acute knee pain that occurs as a result of an injury (such as a fall or direct blow to the knee) and if the patient is also older than 55 years, or complains of knee tenderness, or cannot take four steps while bearing weight on the injured knee, or cannot flex the knee 90 degrees, an x-ray of the knee should be obtained (Jackson et al., 2003). If there is suspected fracture of the tibial plateau, a CT scan may be indicated to determine the extent of injury.

Medical Management

Patients with significant joint effusions may benefit from arthrocentesis to provide relief of intra-articular pressure. Most patients also benefit from the anti-inflammatory and analgesic effects of NSAIDs such as ibuprofen (Motrin, Advil). Other treatment that may be prescribed depends on the knee bone that is fractured and the extent of the injury, including whether the fracture is displaced or nondisplaced. Nondisplaced fractures may be effectively treated with 6 weeks of immobilization and gradual increases in weight bearing, while displaced fractures typically require ORIF surgical procedures.

Tibia and Fibula

The most common fractures below the knee are tibia and fibula fractures. Fractures of the tibia and fibula often occur in association with each other and tend to result from a direct blow, falls with the foot in a flexed position, or a violent twisting motion. The patient presents with pain, deformity, obvious hematoma, and considerable edema. Frequently, these fractures are open and involve severe soft tissue damage because there is little subcutaneous tissue in the area.

Assessment and Diagnostic Findings

The peroneal nerve is assessed for damage. If nerve function is impaired, the patient cannot dorsiflex the great toe and has diminished sensation in the first web space. The tibial artery is assessed for damage by evaluating pulses, skin temperature, and color and by testing the capillary refill response. Hemiarthrosis or ligament damage may occur with fracture near the joint.

The patient is monitored for an anterior acute compartment syndrome. Signs and symptoms include pain that escalates despite opioid analgesics and that increases with plantar flexion, a palpably tense and tender muscle lateral to the tibial crest, and complaints of paresthesias.

Medical Management

Most closed tibial fractures are treated with closed reduction and initial immobilization in a long-leg walking cast or a patellar tendon–bearing cast. Reduction must be relatively accurate in relation to angulation and rotation. As with other lower extremity fractures, the leg is elevated to control edema. Partial weight bearing is usually prescribed after 7 to 10 days. Activity decreases edema and increases circulation. The cast is changed to a short-leg cast or brace in 3 to 4 weeks, which allows for knee motion. Fracture healing takes 6 to 10 weeks. At times it is difficult to maintain reduction, and percutaneous pins may be placed in the bone and held in position by an external fixator.

Comminuted fractures may be treated with skeletal traction, internal fixation with intramedullary nails or plates and screws, or external fixation. External support may be used with internal fixation. Hip, foot, and knee exercises are encouraged within the limits of the immobilizing device. Partial weight bearing is begun when prescribed and is progressed as the fracture heals in 4 to 8 weeks.

Open fractures are treated with external fixation. Distal fractures with extensive soft tissue damage heal slowly and may require bone grafting.

Continued neurovascular evaluation is needed. The development of acute compartment syndrome requires prompt recognition and resolution to prevent permanent functional deficit. Other complications include delayed union, infection, impaired wound edge healing due to limited soft tissue, and loosening of the internal fixation hardware.

Rib

Uncomplicated fractures of the ribs occur frequently in adults and usually result in no impairment of function. Because these fractures cause pain with respiratory effort, the patient tends to decrease respiratory excursions and refrains from coughing. As a result, tracheobronchial secretions are not mobilized, aeration of the lung is diminished, and a predisposition to atelectasis and pneumonia results. To help the patient cough and take deep breaths, the nurse may splint the chest with his or her hands. Occasionally, an anesthesia care provider administers intercostal nerve blocks to relieve pain and to permit productive coughing.

Chest strapping to immobilize the rib fracture is not used, because decreased chest expansion may result in atelectasis and pneumonia. The pain associated with rib fracture diminishes significantly in 3 or 4 days, and the fracture heals within 6 weeks. In addition to atelectasis and pneumonia, complications may include a flail chest, pneumothorax, and hemothorax. The assessment and management of patients with these conditions is discussed in Chapter 23.

Thoracolumbar Spine

Fractures of the thoracolumbar spine may involve (1) the vertebral body, (2) the laminae and articulating processes, and (3) the spinous processes or transverse processes. The T12 to L2 area of the spine is most vulnerable to fracture. Fractures generally result from indirect trauma caused by excessive loading, sudden muscle contraction, or excessive motion beyond physiologic limits. Osteoporosis contributes to vertebral body collapse (compression fracture) (Bucholz et al., 2005).

Stable spinal fractures are caused by flexion, extension, lateral bending, or vertical loading. The anterior structural column (vertebral bodies and disks) or the posterior structural column (neural arch, articular processes, ligaments) are disrupted. Unstable fractures occur with fracture-dislocations and exhibit disruption of both anterior and posterior structural columns. The potential for neural damage (eg, spinal cord injury) exists.

The patient with a spinal fracture presents with acute tenderness, swelling, paravertebral muscle spasm, and change in the normal curves or in the gap between spinous processes. Pain is greater with moving, coughing, or weight bearing. Immobilization is essential until initial assessments have determined whether there is any spinal cord injury and whether the fracture is stable or unstable. (Refer to Chapter 63 for discussion of immobilization.) If spinal cord injury with neurologic deficit does occur, it usually requires immediate surgery (laminectomy with spinal fusion) to decompress the spinal cord.

Stable spinal fractures are treated conservatively with limited bed rest. The head of the bed is elevated less than 30 degrees until the acute pain subsides (several days). Analgesics are prescribed for pain relief. The patient is monitored for a transient paralytic ileus caused by associated retroperitoneal hemorrhage. Sitting is avoided until the pain subsides. A spinal brace or plastic thoracolumbar orthosis may be applied for support during progressive ambulation and resumption of activities.

The patient with an unstable fracture is treated with bed rest, possibly with the use of a special turning device or bed (eg, Circ-O-Lectric bed) to maintain spinal alignment. Neurologic status is monitored closely during the preoperative and postoperative periods. Within 24 hours after fracture, open reduction, decompression, and fixation with spinal fusion and instrument stabilization are usually accomplished. Postoperatively, the patient may be cared for on the turning device or in a bed with a firm mattress. Progressive ambulation is begun a few days after surgery, with the patient using a body brace orthosis. Patient teaching emphasizes good posture, good body mechanics, and, after healing is sufficient, back-strengthening exercises. (Spinal cord injury is discussed in Chapter 63.)

Amputation

Amputation is the removal of a body part, usually an extremity. Amputation of a lower extremity is often necessary because of progressive peripheral vascular disease (often a sequela of diabetes mellitus), fulminating gas gangrene, trauma (crushing injuries, burns, frostbite, electrical burns), congenital deformities, chronic osteomyelitis, or malignant tumor. Of all these causes, peripheral vascular disease accounts for most amputations of lower extremities. (See Chapter 31 for more information about peripheral vascular disease.) Amputation of an upper extremity occurs less frequently than amputation of a lower extremity and is most often necessary because of either traumatic injury or a malignant tumor. It is estimated that one of every 200 Americans has had an amputation (National Lower Limb Information Center, 2006).

Amputation is used to relieve symptoms, to improve function, and, most importantly, to save or improve the patient's quality of life. If the health care team communicates a positive attitude, the patient adjusts to the amputation more readily and actively participates in the rehabilitative plan, learning how to modify activities and how to use assistive devices for ADLs and mobility.

Levels of Amputation

Amputation is performed at the most distal point that will heal successfully. The site of amputation is determined by two factors: circulation in the part and functional usefulness (ie, meets the requirements for the use of a prosthesis).

The circulatory status of the extremity is evaluated through physical examination and diagnostic studies. Muscle and skin perfusion is important for healing. Doppler flow studies with duplex ultrasound, segmental blood pressure determinations, and transcutaneous partial pressure of oxygen (PaO_2) are valuable diagnostic aids. Angiography is performed if revascularization is considered an option.

The objective of surgery is to conserve as much extremity length as needed to preserve function and possibly to achieve a good prosthetic fit. Preservation of knee and elbow joints is desired. Figure 69-17 shows the levels at which an extremity may be amputated. Most amputations involving extremities can be eventually fitted with a prosthesis.

The amputation of toes and portions of the foot causes minor changes in gait and balance. A Syme amputation (modified ankle **disarticulation** amputation) is performed most frequently for extensive foot trauma and produces a painless, durable extremity end that can withstand full weight-bearing. Below-knee amputation (BKA) is preferred to above-knee amputation (AKA) because of the importance of the knee joint and the energy requirements for walking. Knee disarticulations are most successful with young, active patients who can develop precise control of the prosthesis. When AKAs are performed, all possible length is preserved, muscles are stabilized and shaped, and hip contractures are prevented for maximum ambulatory potential. Most people who have a hip disarticulation amputation must rely on a wheelchair for mobility.

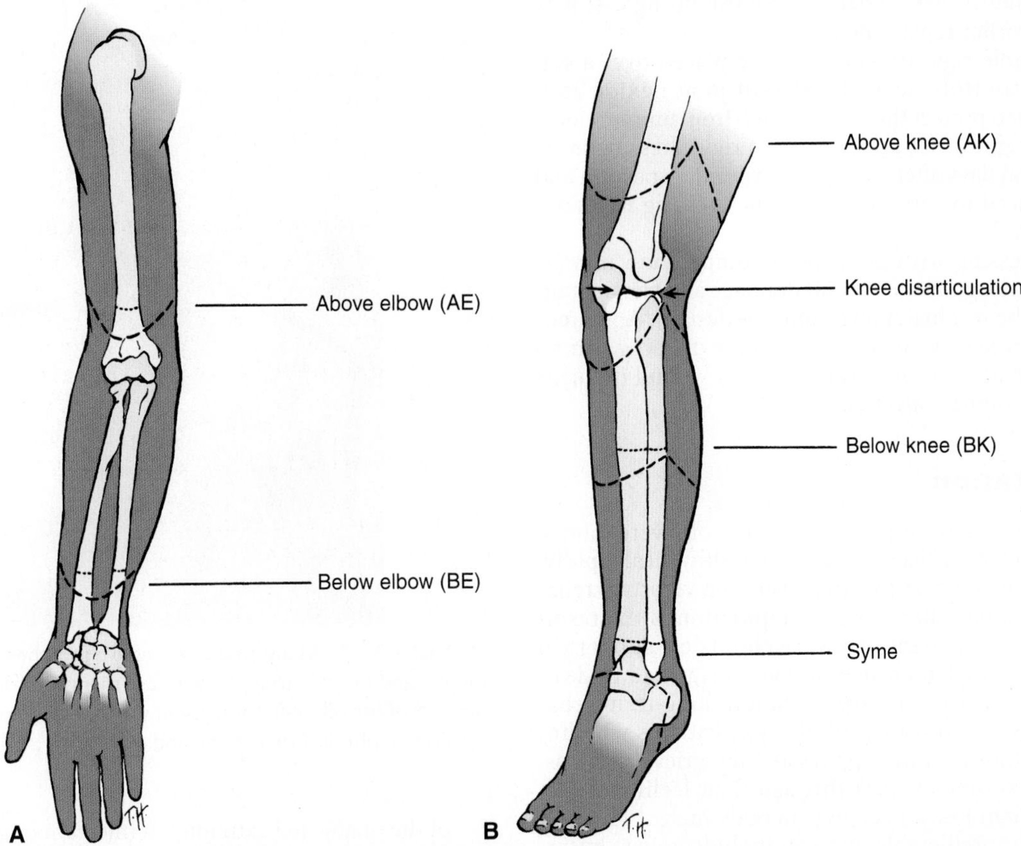

FIGURE 69-17. Levels of amputation are determined by circulatory adequacy, type of prosthesis, function of the part, and muscle balance. (**A**) Levels of amputation of upper extremity. (**B**) Levels of amputation of lower extremity.

Upper extremity amputations are performed with the goal of preserving the maximum functional length. The prosthesis is fitted early for maximum function.

A *staged amputation* may be used when gangrene and infection exist. Initially, a guillotine amputation (eg, nonclosed stump) is performed to remove the necrotic and infected tissue. The wound is débrided and allowed to drain. Sepsis is treated with systemic antibiotics. In a few days, after the infection has been controlled and the patient's condition has stabilized, a definitive amputation with skin closure is performed.

Complications

Complications that may occur with amputation include hemorrhage, infection, skin breakdown, phantom limb pain, and joint contracture. Because major blood vessels have been severed, massive bleeding may occur. Infection is a risk with all surgical procedures. The risk of infection increases with contaminated wounds after traumatic amputation. Skin irritation caused by the prosthesis may result in skin breakdown. **Phantom limb pain** is caused by the severing of peripheral nerves. Joint contracture is caused by positioning and a protective flexion withdrawal pattern associated with pain and muscle imbalance.

Medical Management

The objective of treatment is to achieve healing of the amputation wound, the result being a nontender residual limb (stump) with healthy skin for prosthesis use. Healing is enhanced by gentle handling of the residual limb, control of residual limb edema through rigid or soft compression dressings, and use of aseptic technique in wound care to avoid infection.

A closed rigid cast dressing is frequently used to provide uniform compression, to support soft tissues, to control pain, and to prevent joint contractures. Immediately after surgery, a sterilized residual limb sock is applied to the residual limb. Felt pads are placed over pressure-sensitive areas. The residual limb is wrapped with elastic plaster-of-paris bandages while firm, even pressure is maintained. Care is taken not to constrict circulation.

For the patient with a lower extremity amputation, the plaster cast may be equipped to attach a temporary prosthetic extension (pylon) and an artificial foot. This rigid dressing technique is used as a means of creating a socket for immediate postoperative prosthetic fitting. The length of the prosthesis is tailored to the individual patient. Early minimal weight bearing on the residual limb with a rigid cast dressing and a pylon attached produces little discomfort. The cast is changed in about 10 to 14 days. Elevated body temperature, severe pain, or a loose-fitting cast may necessitate earlier replacement.

A removable rigid dressing may be placed over a soft dressing to control edema, to prevent joint flexion contracture, and to protect the residual limb from unintentional trauma during transfer activities. This rigid dressing is removed several days after surgery for wound inspection and is then replaced to control edema. The dressing facilitates residual limb shaping.

A soft dressing with or without compression may be used if there is significant wound drainage and frequent inspection of the residual limb (stump) is desired. An immobilizing splint may be incorporated in the dressing. Stump (wound) hematomas are controlled with wound drainage devices to minimize infection.

Rehabilitation

Patients who require amputation because of severe trauma are usually, but not always, young and healthy, heal rapidly, and are physically able to participate in a vigorous rehabilitation program. Because the amputation is the result of an injury, the patient needs psychological support in accepting the sudden change in body image and in dealing with the stresses of hospitalization, long-term rehabilitation, and modification of lifestyle. Patients who undergo amputation need support as they grieve the loss, and they need time to work through their feelings about their permanent loss and change in body image. Their reactions are unpredictable and can include anger, bitterness, and hostility.

The multidisciplinary rehabilitation team (patient, nurse, physician, social worker, physical therapist, occupational therapist, psychologist, prosthetist, vocational rehabilitation worker) helps the patient achieve the highest possible level of function and participation in life activities (Fig. 69-18). Prosthetic clinics and amputee support groups facilitate this rehabilitation process. Vocational counseling and job retraining may be necessary to help patients return to work.

Psychological issues (eg, denial, withdrawal) may be influenced by the type of support the patient receives from the rehabilitation team and by how quickly ADLs and use of the prosthesis are learned. Knowing the full options and capabilities available with the various prosthetic devices can give the patient a sense of control over the resulting disability.

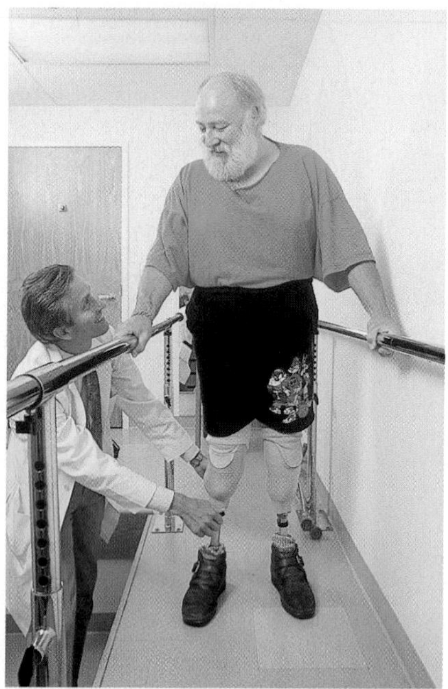

FIGURE 69-18. Many amputees receive prostheses soon after surgery and begin learning how to use them with the help and support of the rehabilitation team, which includes nurses, physicians, physical therapists, and others.

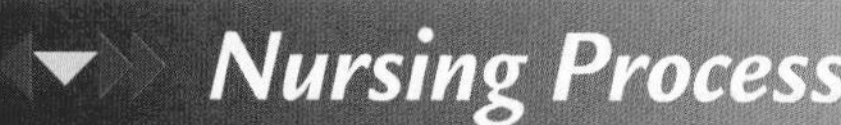

The Patient Undergoing an Amputation

Assessment

Before surgery, the nurse must evaluate the neurovascular and functional status of the extremity through history and physical assessment. If the patient has experienced a traumatic amputation, the nurse assesses the function and condition of the residual limb. The nurse also assesses the circulatory status and function of the unaffected extremity. If infection or gangrene develops, the patient may have associated enlarged lymph nodes, fever, and purulent drainage. A culture is taken to determine the appropriate antibiotic therapy.

The nurse evaluates the patient's nutritional status and creates a plan for nutritional care in consultation with a dietitian or metabolic support team, if indicated. For wound healing, a diet with adequate protein and vitamins is essential.

Any concurrent health problems (eg, dehydration, anemia, cardiac insufficiency, chronic respiratory problems, diabetes mellitus) need to be identified and treated so that the patient is in the best possible condition to withstand the trauma of surgery. The use of corticosteroids, anticoagulants, vasoconstrictors, or vasodilators may influence management and prolong or deter wound healing.

The nurse assesses the patient's psychological status. Determination of the patient's emotional reaction to amputation and resulting disability is essential for nursing care. Grief responses to permanent alterations in body image, function, and mobility are normal. An adequate support system and professional counseling can help the patient cope in the aftermath of amputation surgery.

Diagnosis

Nursing Diagnoses

Based on the assessment data, the patient's major nursing diagnoses may include the following:

- Acute pain related to amputation
- Risk for disturbed sensory perception: phantom limb pain related to amputation

NURSING RESEARCH PROFILE

The Effect of Upper Extremity Amputation on Farmers

Reed, D. (2004). Understanding and meeting the needs of farmers with amputations. *Orthopaedic Nursing, 23*(6), 397–405.

Purpose

Farming is a hazardous occupation: nearly 200,000 significant farming injuries occur yearly, and more than 5% of these result in permanent injury or disability. Eleven percent of these significant injuries involve traumatic amputations, most frequently to the upper extremities. Most farmers who are subjected to traumatic upper extremity amputations return to farming, yet little is known about their specific psychological, social, and vocational needs. The purpose of this study was to identify these specific needs so that nurses who provide care for them can more ably assist them to resume their lives of farming.

Design

A purposive sample of 16 farmers who were at least 1 year post-traumatic above-the-wrist amputation participated in this qualitative study. All participants were male, with a mean age of 49.7 years (range, 20 to 82 years). The mean age at injury was 35 years. Fifteen of these participants owned at least one prosthesis.

Participants were interviewed regarding their injury event, rehabilitation process, and current work status using the constant comparative analysis technique of grounded theory. Transcripts were continuously analyzed and coded until data saturation occurred (ie, until no new data were found). Three participants and a panel of peer reviewers audited the completed analysis and confirmed its accuracy and veracity.

Findings

All participants blamed themselves for their traumatic injuries, with most of them attributing their injuries to their own "carelessness;" however, they also acknowledged that the actions that led to their traumatic amputations were common practices among farmers. Participants reported significant disruption in the lives and the livelihood of their families as a result of the amputation. In particular, many wives were burdened with taking on farming tasks that they were unprepared to assume. Several reported loss of wages and livelihood during the rehabilitation process. All participants reported frustration with being unable to quickly resume farming, and two reported experiencing clinical depression.

Participants related that health care professionals were ill prepared to help them in their vocational rehabilitation because they did not understand farming. As a consequence, none of the participants completed their prescribed physical or occupational therapy regimen. All participants reported another injury soon after their return to farming, as well as frequent falls, disturbing phantom limb pain, and feeling unprepared for "what to expect" post-amputation.

Only 8 of the 15 participants who had a prosthesis ever used it. In particular, cosmetic prostheses that were designed to look like a human hand were reported as not functional for farming. In many instances, the prosthesis was called a "nuisance" and thought to provide a greater risk of further injury during day-to-day farming.

Nursing Implications

Farmers with traumatic upper extremity amputations have unique psychological, social, and vocational rehabilitative needs. Most modern farms are family-owned; therefore, when a farmer experiences any traumatic injury, it has a profound impact on the entire family. The nurse must provide support to the injured farmer and to the farmer's family, providing referrals to amputee support groups and agricultural health and safety center support groups. Providing anticipatory guidance regarding rehabilitation, prosthetic function and fit, occupation-related frustrations, and phantom limb pain may help the farmer and the farmer's family cope with these issues. Rehabilitation must be interdisciplinary and tailored to the specific needs of the injured farmer so that he or she can resume his or her chosen vocation without risking additional injury.

- Impaired skin integrity related to surgical amputation
- Disturbed body image related to amputation of body part
- Ineffective coping, related to failure to accept loss of body part and resulting disability
- Risk for anticipatory and/or dysfunctional grieving related to loss of body part and resulting disability
- Self-care deficit: feeding, bathing/hygiene, dressing/grooming, or toileting, related to loss of extremity
- Impaired physical mobility related to loss of extremity

Collaborative Problems/ Potential Complications

Based on the assessment data, potential complications that may develop include the following:

- Postoperative hemorrhage
- Infection
- Skin breakdown

Planning and Goals

The major goals of the patient may include relief of pain, absence of altered sensory perceptions, wound healing, acceptance of altered body image, resolution of the grieving process, independence in self-care, restoration of physical mobility, and absence of complications.

Nursing Interventions

Relieving Pain

Surgical pain can be effectively controlled with opioid analgesics that may be accompanied with adjuvant nonpharmaceutical interventions, or evacuation of a hematoma or accumulated fluid. Pain may be incisional or may be caused by inflammation, infection, pressure on a bony prominence, or hematoma. Muscle spasms may add to the patient's discomfort. Changing the patient's position or placing a light sandbag on the residual limb to counteract the muscle spasm may improve the patient's level of comfort. Evaluation of the patient's pain and responses to interventions is an important part of the nurse's role in pain management. The pain may be an expression of grief and alteration of body image.

Minimizing Altered Sensory Perceptions

A person who has had an amputation may experience phantom limb pain soon after surgery or 2 to 3 months after amputation. It occurs more frequently in patients who have had AKAs. The patient describes pain or unusual sensations, such as numbness, tingling, or muscle cramps, as well as a feeling that the extremity is present, crushed, cramped, or twisted in an abnormal position. When a patient describes phantom pains or sensations, the nurse acknowledges these feelings and helps the patient modify these perceptions.

Phantom sensations diminish over time. The pathogenesis of the phantom limb phenomenon is unknown. Keeping the patient active helps decrease the occurrence of phantom limb pain. Early intensive rehabilitation and stump desensitization with kneading massage bring relief. Distraction techniques and activity are helpful. In addition to the nursing interventions, transcutaneous electrical nerve stimulation (TENS), ultrasound, or local anesthetics may provide relief for some patients. In addition, beta-blockers may relieve dull, burning discomfort; antiseizure medications control stabbing and cramping pain; and tricyclic antidepressants are used to improve mood and coping ability.

Promoting Wound Healing

The residual limb must be handled gently. Whenever the dressing is changed, aseptic technique is required to prevent wound infection and possible osteomyelitis.

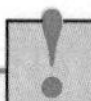

NURSING ALERT

If the cast or elastic dressing inadvertently comes off, the nurse must immediately wrap the residual limb with an elastic compression bandage. If this is not done, excessive edema will develop in a short time, resulting in a delay in rehabilitation. The nurse notifies the surgeon if a cast dressing comes off, so that another cast can be applied promptly.

Residual limb shaping is important for prosthesis fitting. The nurse instructs the patient and family in wrapping the residual limb with elastic dressings (Figs. 69-19 and 69-20). After the incision is healed, the nurse teaches the patient to care for the residual limb.

Enhancing Body Image

Amputation is a reconstructive procedure that alters the patient's body image. The nurse who has established a trusting relationship with the patient is better able to communicate acceptance of the patient who has experienced an amputation. The nurse encourages the patient to look at, feel, and care for the residual limb. It is important to identify the patient's strengths and resources to facilitate rehabilitation. The nurse helps the patient regain the previous level of independent functioning. The patient who is accepted as a whole person is more readily able to resume responsibility for self-care; self-concept improves, and body-image changes are accepted. Even with highly motivated patients, this process may take months.

Helping the Patient to Resolve Grieving

The loss of an extremity (or part of one) may come as a shock even if the patient was prepared preoperatively. The patient's behavior (eg, crying, withdrawal, apathy, anger) and expressed feelings (eg, depression, fear, helplessness) reveal how the patient is coping with the loss and working through the grieving process. The nurse acknowledges the loss by listening and providing support.

The nurse creates an accepting and supportive atmosphere in which the patient and family are encouraged to express and share their feelings and work through the grief process. The support from family and friends promotes the patient's acceptance of the loss. The nurse helps the patient deal with immediate needs and become oriented to realistic rehabilitation goals and future independent functioning. Mental health and support group referrals may be appropriate.

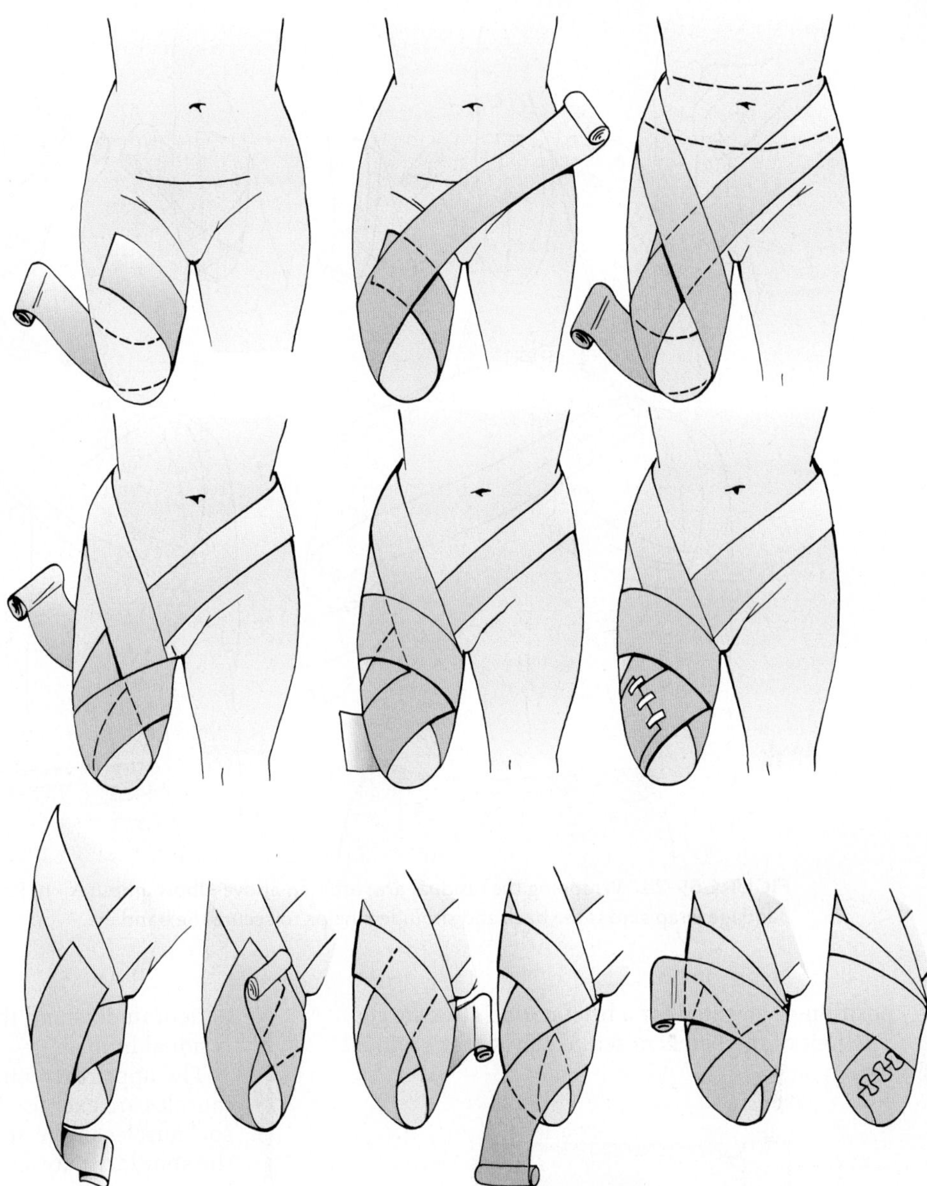

FIGURE 69-19. Wrapping the residual leg after an above-knee amputation (AKA). Elastic bandaging minimizes edema and shapes the stump in a firm conical form to fit a prosthesis.

Promoting Independent Self-Care

Amputation of an extremity affects the patient's ability to provide adequate self-care. The patient is encouraged to be an active participant in self-care. The patient needs time to accomplish these tasks and must not be rushed. Practicing an activity with consistent, supportive supervision in a relaxed environment enables the patient to learn self-care skills. The patient and the nurse need to maintain positive attitudes and to minimize fatigue and frustration during the learning process.

Independence in dressing, toileting, and bathing (shower or tub) depends on balance, transfer abilities, and physiologic tolerance of the activities. The nurse works with the physical therapist and occupational therapist to teach and supervise the patient in these self-care activities.

The patient with an upper extremity amputation has self-care deficits in feeding, bathing, and dressing. Assistance is provided only as needed; the nurse encourages the patient to learn to do these tasks, using assistive feeding and dressing aids when needed. The nurse, therapists, and prosthetist work with the patient to achieve maximum independence.

Helping the Patient to Achieve Physical Mobility

Proper positioning prevents the development of hip or knee joint contracture in the patient with a lower extremity amputation. Abduction, external rotation, and flexion of the lower extremity are avoided. Depending on the surgeon's preference, the residual limb may be placed in an extended

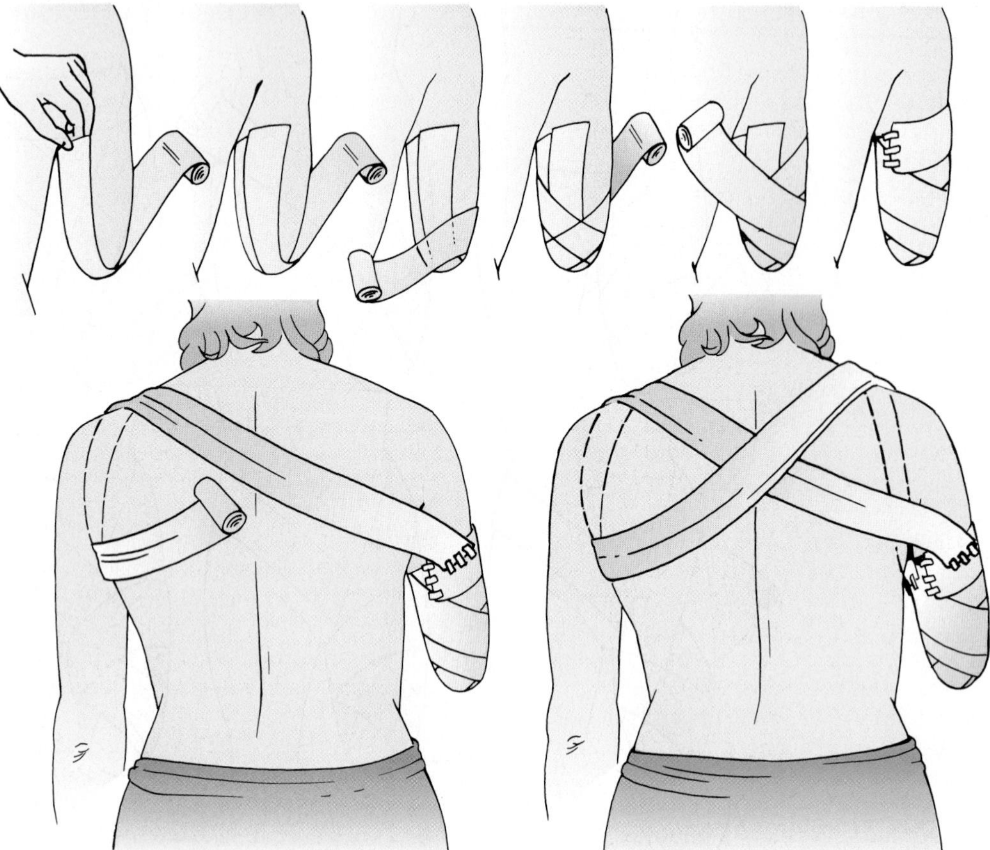

FIGURE 69-20. Wrapping the residual arm after an above-elbow amputation. Passing the bandage wrap across the back and shoulders helps to secure the bandage.

position or elevated for a brief period after surgery. The foot of the bed is raised to elevate the residual limb.

NURSING ALERT

The residual limb should not be placed on a pillow, because a flexion contracture of the hip may result.

The nurse encourages the patient to turn from side to side and to assume a prone position, if possible, to stretch the flexor muscles and to prevent flexion contracture of the hip. The nurse discourages sitting for prolonged periods, to prevent flexion contracture. The legs should remain close together to prevent an abduction deformity. The nurse encourages the patient to use assistive devices (eg, reachers) to more readily perform self-care activities and to identify what home modifications, if any, should be made to perform these activities in the home environment.

Postoperative ROM exercises are started early because contracture deformities develop rapidly. ROM exercises include hip and knee exercises for BKAs and hip exercises for AKAs. It is important that the patient understand the importance of exercising the residual limb.

The upper extremities, trunk, and abdominal muscles are exercised and strengthened. The extensor muscles in the arm and the depressor muscles in the shoulder play an important part in crutch walking. The patient uses an overhead trapeze to change position and strengthen the biceps. The patient may flex and extend the arms while holding weights. Doing push-ups while seated strengthens the triceps muscles. Exercises (such as hyperextension of the residual limb), conducted under the supervision of the physical therapist, also aid in strengthening muscles as well as increasing circulation, reducing edema, and preventing atrophy.

Because a patient who has had an upper extremity amputated uses both shoulders to operate the prosthesis, the muscles of both shoulders are exercised. A patient with an above-the-elbow amputation or shoulder disarticulation is likely to develop a postural abnormality caused by loss of the weight of the amputated extremity. Postural exercises are helpful.

Strength and endurance are assessed, and activities are increased gradually to prevent fatigue. As the patient progresses to independent use of the wheelchair, use of ambulatory aids, or ambulation with a prosthesis, the nurse emphasizes safety considerations. Environmental barriers (eg, steps, inclines, doors, throw rugs, wet surfaces) are identified, and methods of managing them are practiced. It is important to anticipate, identify, and manage problems associated with the use of the mobility aids (eg, pressure on the axillae from crutches, skin irritation of the hands from wheelchair use, residual limb irritation from a prosthesis).

Amputation of the leg changes the center of gravity; therefore, the patient may need to practice position changes (eg, standing from sitting, standing on one foot). The patient is taught transfer techniques early and is reminded to maintain good posture when getting out of bed. A well-fitting shoe with a nonskid sole should be worn. During position changes, the patient should be guarded and stabilized with a transfer belt at the waist to prevent falling.

As soon as possible, the patient with a lower extremity amputation is assisted to stand between parallel bars to allow extension of the temporary prosthesis to the floor with minimal weight bearing. How soon after surgery the patient is allowed to bear full body weight on the artificial foot depends on the patient's physical status and wound healing. As endurance increases and balance is achieved, ambulation is started with the use of parallel bars or crutches. The patient learns to use a normal gait, with the residual limb moving back and forth while walking with the crutches. To prevent a permanent flexion deformity from occurring, the residual limb should *not* be held up in a flexed position.

The patient with an upper extremity amputation is taught how to carry out ADLs with one arm. The patient is started on one-handed self-care activities as soon as possible. The use of a temporary prosthesis is encouraged. The patient who learns to use the prosthesis soon after the amputation is less dependent on one-handed self-care activities.

The patient with an upper extremity amputation may wear a cotton T-shirt to prevent contact between the skin and shoulder harness and to promote absorption of perspiration. The prosthetist advises about cleaning the washable portions of the harness. Periodically, the prosthesis is inspected for potential problems.

The residual limb must be conditioned and shaped into a conical form to permit accurate fit, maximum comfort, and function of the prosthetic device. Elastic bandages, an elastic residual limb shrinker, or an air splint is used to condition and shape the residual limb. The nurse teaches the patient or a member of the family the correct method of bandaging.

Bandaging supports the soft tissue and minimizes the formation of edema while the residual limb is in a dependent position. The bandage is applied in such a manner that the remaining muscles required to operate the prosthesis are as firm as possible, whereas those muscles that are no longer useful atrophy. An improperly applied elastic bandage contributes to circulatory problems and a poorly shaped residual limb.

Effective preprosthetic care is important to ensure proper fitting of the prosthesis. The major problems that can delay prosthetic fitting during this period are (1) flexion deformities, (2) nonshrinkage of the residual limb, and (3) abduction deformities of the hip.

The physician usually prescribes activities to condition or "toughen" the residual limb in preparation for a prosthesis. The patient begins by pushing the residual limb into a soft pillow, then into a firmer pillow, and finally against a hard surface. The patient is taught to massage the residual limb to mobilize the surgical incision site, decrease tenderness, and improve vascularity. Massage is usually started once healing has occurred and is first performed by the physical therapist. Skin inspection and preventive care are taught.

The prosthesis socket is custom molded to the residual limb by the prosthetist. Prostheses are designed for specific activity levels and patient abilities. Types of prostheses include hydraulic, pneumatic, biofeedback-controlled, myoelectrically controlled, and synchronized prostheses.

Adjustments of the prosthetic socket are made by the prosthetist to accommodate the residual limb changes that occur during the first 6 months to 1 year after surgery. A light plaster cast, an elastic bandage, or a shrinking sock is used to limit edema during periods when the patient is not wearing the permanent prosthesis.

Some patients are not candidates for a prosthesis and are thus nonambulatory amputees. If use of a prosthesis is not possible, the patient is instructed in the use of a wheelchair to achieve independence. A special wheelchair designed for patients who have had amputations is recommended. Because of the decreased weight in the front, a regular wheelchair may tip backward when the patient sits in it. In wheelchairs designed for patients who have had amputations, the rear axle is set back about 5 cm (2 inches) to compensate for the change in weight distribution.

Monitoring and Managing Potential Complications

After any surgery, efforts are made to reestablish homeostasis and to prevent complications related to surgery, anesthesia, and immobility. The nurse assesses body systems (eg, respiratory, hematological, gastrointestinal, genitourinary, skin) for problems associated with immobility (eg, atelectasis, pneumonia, DVT, PE, anorexia, constipation, urinary stasis, pressure ulcer) and institutes corrective management. Avoiding problems associated with immobility and restoring physical activity are necessary for maintenance of health.

Massive hemorrhage due to a loosened suture is the most threatening problem. The nurse monitors the patient for any signs or symptoms of bleeding. It is also important to monitor the patient's vital signs and to observe the suction drainage.

NURSING ALERT

Immediate postoperative bleeding may develop slowly or may take the form of a massive hemorrhage resulting from a loosened suture. A large tourniquet should be in plain sight at the patient's bedside so that, if severe bleeding occurs, it can be applied to the residual limb to control the hemorrhage. The nurse immediately notifies the surgeon in the event of excessive bleeding.

Infection is a common complication of amputation. Patients who have undergone traumatic amputation have a contaminated wound. The nurse administers antibiotics as prescribed. It is important to monitor the incision, dressing, and drainage for indications of infection (eg, change in color, odor, or consistency of drainage; increasing discomfort). The nurse also assesses for systemic indicators of infection (eg, elevated temperature, leukocytosis with an increase of >10% bands on the differential) and promptly reports indications of infection to the surgeon.

Skin breakdown may result from immobilization or from pressure from various sources. The prosthesis may cause pressure areas to develop. The nurse and the patient assess for breaks in the skin. Careful skin hygiene is essential to prevent skin irritation, infection, and breakdown. The healed residual limb is washed and dried (gently) at least twice daily. The skin is inspected for pressure areas, dermatitis, and blisters. If they are present, they must be treated before further skin breakdown occurs. Usually, a residual limb sock is worn to absorb perspiration and to prevent direct contact between the skin and the prosthetic socket. The sock is changed daily and must fit smoothly to prevent irritation caused by wrinkles. The socket of the prosthesis is washed with a mild detergent, rinsed, and dried thoroughly with a clean cloth. It must be thoroughly dry before the prosthesis is applied.

Promoting Home and Community-Based Care

TEACHING THE PATIENT TO MANAGE SELF-CARE

Before the patient is discharged to the home or to a rehabilitation facility, the patient and family are encouraged to become active participants in care. They participate in care of the skin, residual limb, and prosthesis as appropriate. The patient receives ongoing instructions and practice sessions in learning how to transfer and how to use mobility aids and other assistive devices safely. The nurse explains the signs and symptoms of complications that must be reported to the physician (Chart 69-6).

CHART 69-6

HOME CARE CHECKLIST • Amputation

At the completion of the home care instruction, the patient or caregiver will be able to:	Patient	Caregiver
• Describe approaches to controlling pain (eg, take analgesics as prescribed; use nonpharmacologic interventions)	✔	✔
• Report pain that is uncontrolled by analgesics and other pain management techniques	✔	
• Describe care of residual limb and conditioning for prosthesis	✔	✔
• Consume healthy diet to promote wound healing	✔	
• Demonstrate ability to transfer	✔	
• Use mobility and activity aids safely	✔	
• Participate in rehabilitation program to regain functional independence	✔	
• State indicators of complications to report promptly to physician (eg, uncontrolled pain; signs of local or systemic infection; residual limb skin breakdown)	✔	✔
• Identify professionals and community agencies to help with transition to home	✔	✔
• Identify support group to facilitate rehabilitation	✔	✔
• Describe effects of amputation on self-image	✔	
• Acknowledge grieving as part of coping process	✔	✔
• Identify modifications of home environment to promote safe environment and independence during rehabilitation	✔	✔
• Identify the importance of keeping follow-up appointments and participating in health screening and health promotion activities, including exercises	✔	✔

CONTINUING CARE IN THE HOME AND COMMUNITY

After the patient has achieved physiologic homeostasis and has demonstrated achievement of major health care goals, rehabilitation continues either in a rehabilitation facility or at home. Continued support and supervision by the home care nurse are essential.

The patient's home environment should be assessed prior to discharge. Modifications are made to ensure the patient's continuing care, safety, and mobility. An overnight or weekend experience at home may be tried to identify problems that were not identified on the assessment visit. Physical therapy and occupational therapy may continue in the home or on an outpatient basis. Transportation to continuing health care appointments must be arranged. The social service department of the hospital or the community agency managing continued health care may be of great assistance in securing personal assistance and transportation services.

During follow-up health visits, the nurse evaluates the patient's physical and psychosocial adjustment. Periodic preventive health assessments are necessary. Frequently, an elderly spouse cannot provide the assistance required, and additional help at home is needed. Modifications in the plan of care are made on the basis of such findings. Often, the patient and family find involvement in an amputee support group to be of value; here, they can share problems, solutions, and resources. Talking with those who have successfully dealt with a similar problem may help the patient develop a satisfactory solution.

Because patients and their family members and health care providers tend to focus on the most obvious needs and issues, the nurse reminds the patient and family about the importance of continuing health promotion and screening practices, such as regular physical examinations and diagnostic screening tests. Accessible facilities for screening, health care, and exercise are identified. Patients who have not been involved in these practices in the past are instructed in their importance and are referred to appropriate health care providers.

Evaluation

Expected Patient Outcomes

Expected patient outcomes may include:

1. Experiences absence of pain
   a. Appears relaxed
   b. Verbalizes comfort
   c. Uses measures to increase comfort
   d. Participates in self-care and rehabilitative activities
2. Experiences absence of phantom limb pain
   a. Reports diminished phantom sensations
   b. Uses distraction techniques
   c. Performs stump desensitization massage
3. Achieves wound healing
   a. Controls residual limb edema
   b. Exhibits healed, nontender, nonadherent scar
   c. Demonstrates residual limb care
4. Demonstrates improved body image and effective coping
   a. Acknowledges change in body image
   b. Participates in self-care activities
   c. Demonstrates increasing independence
   d. Projects self as a whole person
   e. Resumes role-related responsibilities
   f. Reestablishes social contacts
   g. Demonstrates confidence in abilities
5. Exhibits resolution of grieving
   a. Expresses grief
   b. Works through feelings with family and friends
   c. Focuses on future functioning
   d. Participates in support group
6. Achieves independent self-care
   a. Asks for assistance when needed
   b. Uses aids and assistive devices to facilitate self-care
   c. Verbalizes satisfaction with abilities to perform ADLs
7. Achieves maximum independent mobility
   a. Avoids positions contributing to contracture development
   b. Demonstrates full active ROM
   c. Maintains balance when sitting and transferring
   d. Increases strength and endurance
   e. Demonstrates safe transferring technique
   f. Achieves functional use of prosthesis
   g. Overcomes environmental barriers to mobility
   h. Uses community services and resources as needed
8. Exhibits absence of complications of hemorrhage, infection, skin breakdown
   a. Does not experience excessive bleeding
   b. Maintains normal blood values
   c. Is free of local or systemic signs of infection
   d. Repositions self frequently
   e. Is free of pressure-related problems
   f. Reports any skin discomfort and irritations promptly

Critical Thinking Exercises

1 ebp You volunteer to help provide field first aid for your neighborhood's softball league. Common injuries you expect include sprains, strains, and possibly dislocations and fractures. What specific assessment would you make to differentiate these problems? Describe the evidence base that supports the best emergency management practices for each of these problems. What is the strength of the evidence that supports your proposed interventions?

2 You are the nurse manager of an orthopedic surgery unit. This past month you have noted an increased incidence of occupation-related musculoskeletal injuries among the nursing personnel assigned to your unit. What type of assessments would you perform to determine the cause and severity of these injuries? What are some potential strategies you might implement to prevent further injuries among your nursing personnel?

3 You are a staff nurse in an outpatient orthopedic clinic that has its own same-day surgery center and rehabilitation services. A 34-year-old man presents with a tear of his ACL that occurred during a game of "pick-up" basketball. The orthopedic surgeon recommends arthroscopic surgery. The patient asks you why surgery is needed—his father tore his ACL last year and did not have surgery. He also notes that he heard on the news that arthroscopic surgery of the knees does not improve patient outcomes. What can this patient expect in terms of functional outcomes if he consents to arthroscopic surgery versus if he elects not to have the surgery? Describe this patient's anticipated postarthroscopic care, monitoring to prevent complications, and activity restrictions.

4 ebp You make a home health care visit to a middle-aged farmer who had a traumatic amputation of his left forearm 3 weeks ago. What is the evidence base that guides you in your assessment of this patient? How do you determine his progress? What findings might suggest that the patient is developing a problem? Describe your plan of action. In addition, what environmental and social support factors should you include in your assessment of the home care situation?

REFERENCES AND SELECTED READINGS

BOOKS

Bickley, L. S., & Szilagyi, P. G. (2006). *Bates' guide to physical assessment* (9th ed.). Philadelphia: Lippincott Williams & Wilkins.

Bucholz, R. W., Heckman, J. D., Court-Brown, C., et al. (2005). *Rockwood and Green's fractures in adults* (6th ed.). Philadelphia: Lippincott Williams & Wilkins.

Chapman, M. W., Szabo, R. M., & Marder, R. A. (2000). *Chapman's orthopaedic surgery* (3rd ed.). Philadelphia: Lippincott Williams & Wilkins.

Fischbach, F. T., & Dunning, M. B. (2004). *A manual of laboratory and diagnostic tests* (7th ed.). Philadelphia: Lippincott Williams & Wilkins.

Maher, A., Salmond, S. W., & Pellino, T. A. (2002). *Orthopaedic nursing* (3rd ed.). St. Louis: Elsevier.

National Lower Limb Information Center (2006). *Fact sheet: Amputation statistics by cause: Limb loss in the United States.* Available at: http://www.amputee-coalition.org/fact_sheets/amp_stats_cause.html. Accessed August 10, 2006.

Porth, C. M. (2005). *Pathophysiology: Concepts of altered health states* (7th ed.). Philadelphia: Lippincott Williams & Wilkins.

U.S. Department of Health and Human Services (2004). *Bone health and osteoporosis: A report of the Surgeon General.* U.S. Department of Health and Human Services/Public Health Service, Office of the Surgeon General, Rockville, MD.

U.S. Department of Labor, Bureau of Labor Statistics (2003). *Workplace injuries and illnesses.* Available at: http://www.bls.gov/iif/home.htm. Accessed August 10, 2006.

JOURNALS

**Asterisks indicate nursing research articles.*

Alford, J. W., & Bach, B. B. (2004). Managing ACL tears: When to treat, when to refer. *Journal of Musculoskeletal Medicine, 21*(1), 520–526.

Altizer, L. (2004). Compartment syndrome. *Orthopaedic Nursing, 23*(6), 391–396.

Barr, A. B., Barbe, M. F., & Clark, B. D. (2004). Work-related musculoskeletal disorders of the hand and wrist: Epidemiology, pathophysiology, and sensorimotor changes. *Journal of Orthopaedic and Sports Physical Therapy, 34*(6), 610–627.

Bedi, A., & Le, T. T. (2004). Subtrochanteric femur fractures. *Orthopedic Clinics of North America, 35*(4), 473–483.

Birmingham, T. B., Kramer, J. F., & Kirkley, A. (2002). Effect of a functional knee brace on knee flexion and extension strength after anterior cruciate ligament reconstruction. *Archives of Physical Medicine and Rehabilitation, 83*(10), 1472–1475.

Boden, S. D. (2005). The ABCs of BMPs. *Orthopaedic Nursing, 24*(1), 49–52.

Bongiovanni, M. S., Bradley, S. L., & Kelley, D. M. (2005). Orthopedic trauma: Critical care nursing issues. *Critical Care Nursing Quarterly, 28*(1), 60–71.

Calmbach, W. L., & Hutchens, M. (2003). Evaluation of patients presenting with knee pain: Part II: Differential diagnosis. *American Family Physician, 68*(5), 917–922.

Ditmyer, M. M., Topp, R., & Pifer, M. (2002). Prehabilitation in preparation for orthopaedic surgery, *Orthopaedic Nursing, 21*(5), 43–51.

Hardy, M. A. (2004). Principles of metacarpal and phalangeal fracture management: A review of rehabilitation concepts. *Journal of Orthopaedic and Sports Physical Therapy, 34*(12), 781–799.

Hart, L. (2005). Effect of stretching on sport injury risk: A review. *Clinical Journal of Sports Medicine, 15*(2), 113.

Hoffman, D., Saltzman, C. L., & Buckwalter, J. A. (2002). Outcome of lower extremity malignancy survivors treated with transfemoral amputation. *Archives of Physical Medicine and Rehabilitation, 83*(1), 177–182.

Jackson, J. L., O'Malley, P. G., & Kroenke, K. (2003). Evaluation of acute knee pain in primary care. *Annals of Internal Medicine, 139*(7), 575–588.

Levin, A. Z. (2004). Functional outcome following amputation. *Topics in Geriatric Rehabilitation, 20*(4), 253–261.

*Lipscomb, J., Trinkoff, A., Brady, B., et al. (2004). Health care system changes and reported musculoskeletal disorders among registered nurses. *American Journal of Public Health, 94*(8), 1431–1435.

Marzen-Groller, K., & Bartman, K. (2005). Building a successful support group for post-amputation patients. *Journal of Vascular Nursing, 23*(2), 42–45.

Merrick, M. A. (2002). Secondary injury after musculoskeletal trauma: A review and update. *Journal of Athletic Training, 37*(2), 209–217.

Moseley, J. B., O'Malley, K., Petersen, N. J., et al. (2002). A controlled trial of arthroscopic surgery for osteoarthritis of the knee. *New England Journal of Medicine, 347*(2), 81–88.

National Association of Orthopedic Nurses (2005). Palliative care: Improving the quality of care for patients with chronic, incurable musculoskeletal conditions: Consensus document. *Orthopaedic Nursing, 24*(1), 8–11.

*Nelson, A., & Baptiste, A. (2004). Evidence-based practices for safe patient handling and movement. *Online Journal of Issues in Nursing, 9*(3), manuscript 3, 1–26. Available at: www.nursingworld.org/ojin/topic25/tpc_3.htm. Accessed August 10, 2006.

Nelson, A., Owen, B., Lloyd, J. D., et al. (2003). Safe patient handling and movement. *American Journal of Nursing, 103*(3), 32–43.

Peer, K. S. (2004). Bone health in athletes: Factors and future considerations. *Orthopaedic Nursing, 23*(3), 174–181.

*Reed, D. (2004). Understanding and meeting the needs of farmers with amputations. *Orthopaedic Nursing, 23*(6), 397–405.

Rupp, J. D., & Schneider, L. W. (2004). Injuries to the hip joint in frontal motor-vehicle crashes: Biomechanical and real-world perspectives. *Orthopedic Clinics of North America, 35*(4), 493–504.

Sanderlin, B. W., & Raspa, R. F. (2003). Common stress fractures. *American Family Physician, 68*(8), 1527–1532.

Schoen, D. C. (2005). The mystery of ankle problems. *Orthopaedic Nursing, 24*(2), 166–169.

Stolz, D., Miller, M., Bannerman, E., et al. (2002). Nutrition screening and assessment of patients attending a multidisciplinary falls clinic. *Nutrition and Dietetics, 59*(4), 234–239.

Thacker, S. B., Gilchrist, J., Stroup, D. F., et al. (2004). The impact of stretching on sports injury risk: A systematic review of the literature. *Medicine and Science in Sports and Exercise, 36*(3), 371–378.

RESOURCES

AgrAbility Project of America, Purdue University, 1146 ABE Building, West Lafayette, IN 47907; (800) 825-4264 (toll free); http://www.agrability.org. Accessed August 10, 2006.

American College of Sports Medicine, 401 W. Michigan Street, Indianapolis, IN 46202; (317) 637-9200; http://www.acsm.org. Accessed August 10, 2006.

Amputee Resource Foundation of America, Inc., 2324 Wildwood Trail, Suite F104, Minnetonka, MN 55305; http://www.amputeeresource.org. Accessed August 10, 2006.

National Amputation Foundation, 73 Church Street, Malverne, NY 11565; (516) 887-3600; http://www.nationalamputation.org. Accessed August 10, 2006.

National Association of Orthopaedic Nurses (NAON), East Holly Avenue, Box 56, Pitman, NJ 08071; (856) 256-2310; http://www.orthonurse.com. Accessed August 10, 2006.

National Institute for Occupational Safety and Health, 1600 Clifton Road, Atlanta, GA 30333; (800)356-4674 (toll free); http://www.cdc.gov.niosh.html. Accessed August 10, 2006.

National Institute of Arthritis and Musculoskeletal and Skin Diseases, Information Clearing House, National Institutes of Health, 1 AMS Circle, Bethesda, MD 20892; (877) 22-NIAMS (toll free); http://www.niams.nih.gov. Accessed August 10, 2006.

U.S. Department of Labor, Occupational Safety and Health Administration, Room N3641, 200 Constitution Avenue, Washington, DC 20210; (800)321-6742 (toll free); http://www.osha.gov. Accessed August 10, 2006.

UNIT 16

Other Acute Problems

Case Study

Applying Concepts from NANDA, NIC, and NOC

A Patient With Multiple Trauma Resulting in Hemorrhage and Risk for Shock

Rescue personnel bring 19-year-old **Anna Woo** to the Emergency Department (ED) after a motorcycle crash. She has facial contusions and lacerations, a fractured sternum, three fractured ribs, a hemothorax, a dislocated hip and fractured pelvis, and multiple minor lacerations. She is moaning but responds to her name. Initial findings include an unobstructed airway with absent breath sounds in the right basilar lung field, tachypnea with 32 shallow respirations per minute, and ABG values as follows: pH 7.29; pCO_2 48; SaO_2 90%; HCO_3^- 24. Blood pressure is 94/70; skin is cool and clammy; heart rate is 100; and peripheral pulses are intact. After a preliminary survey and placement of intravenous access lines, a chest tube is inserted. Immediately, 300 mL of bloody fluid drains into the collection chamber. Grossly bloody fluid continues to drain from the chest tube at a rate of 20 mL every 15 minutes.

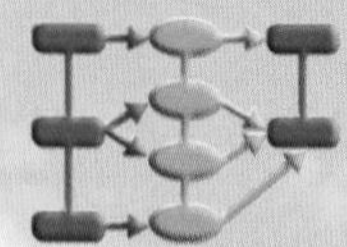

Turn to Appendix C to see a concept map that illustrates the relationships that exist between the nursing diagnoses, interventions, and outcomes for the patient's clinical problems.

Nursing Classifications and Languages

NANDA Nursing Diagnoses	NIC Nursing Interventions	NOC Nursing Outcomes Return to functional baseline status, stabilization of, or improvement in:
Ineffective Breathing Pattern—Inspiration and/or expiration that does not provide adequate ventilation	**Airway Management**—Facilitation of patency of air passages	**Respiratory Status: Airway Patency**—Open, clear tracheobronchial passages for air exchange
Impaired Gas Exchange—Excess or deficit in oxygenation and/or carbon dioxide elimination at the alveolar-capillary membrane	**Respiratory Monitoring**—Collection and analysis of patient data to ensure airway patency and adequate gas exchange	**Respiratory Status: Ventilation**—Movement of air in and out of the lungs
Deficient Fluid Volume—Decreased intravascular, interstitial, and/or intracellular fluid	**Oxygen Therapy**—Administration of oxygen and monitoring of its effectiveness	**Respiratory Status: Gas Exchange**—Alveolar exchange of carbon dioxide and oxygen to maintain arterial blood gas concentrations
Decreased Cardiac Output—Inadequate blood pumped by the heart to meet metabolic demands of the body	**Acid-Base Management**—Promotion of acid-base balance and prevention of complications resulting from acid-base imbalance	**Electrolyte and Acid/Base Balance**—Balance of electrolytes and nonelectrolytes in the intracellular and extracellular compartments of the body
	Hemorrhage Control—Reduction or elimination of rapid and excessive blood loss	**Circulation Status**—Unobstructed, unidirectional blood flow at an appropriate pressure through large vessels of the systemic and pulmonary circuits
	IV Insertion—Insertion of a needle into a peripheral or central vein for the purpose of administering fluids, blood, or medications	**Vital Signs**—Extent to which temperature, pulse, respiration, and blood pressure are within normal range for the individual
	Hypovolemia Management—Expansion of intravascular fluid volume in a patient who is volume-depleted	**Cardiac Pump Effectiveness**—Adequacy of blood volume ejected from the left ventricle to support systolic perfusion pressure
	Blood Products Administration—Administration of blood or blood products and monitoring of patient's response	
	Vital Signs Monitoring—Collection and analysis of cardiovascular, respiratory, and body temperature data to determine and prevent complications	
	Shock Prevention—Detecting and treating a patient at risk for impending shock	
	Shock Management—Facilitation of the delivery of oxygen and nutrients to systemic tissue with removal of cellular waste products in a patient with severely altered tissue perfusion	

NANDA International (2005). *Nursing diagnoses: Definitions & Classification 2005–2006.* Philadelphia: North American Nursing Diagnosis Association.

Dochterman, J. M., & Bulechek, G. M. (2004). *Nursing interventions classification (NIC)* (4th ed.). St. Louis: Mosby.

Iowa Outcomes Project (2004). In Moorhead, S., Johnson, M., & Maas, M. (2004). *Nursing outcomes classification (NOC)* (3rd ed.). St. Louis: Mosby.

Dochterman, J. M., & Jones, D. A. (2003). *Unifying nursing languages: The harmonization of NANDA, NIC, and NOC.* Washington, DC: American Nurses Association.

CHAPTER 70

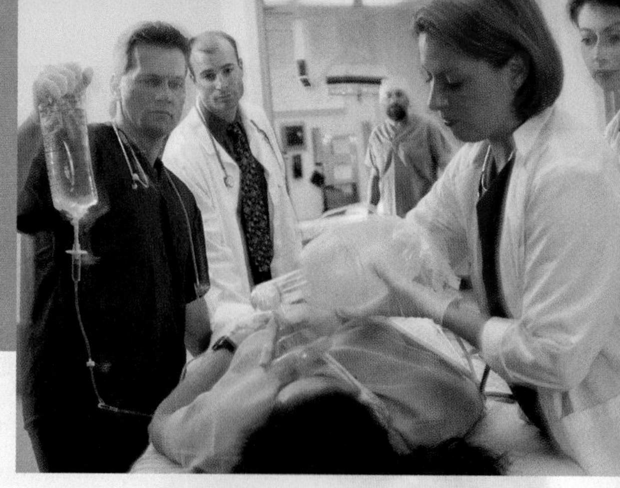

Management of Patients With Infectious Diseases

Learning Objectives

On completion of this chapter, the learner will be able to:

1. Differentiate between colonization, infection, and disease.
2. Use information obtained from the microbiology report to interpret infectious disease evidence.
3. Identify federal and local resources available to the nurse seeking information about infectious diseases.
4. Identify the merit of vaccines recommended for health care workers.
5. Identify the reasons for Standard and Transmission-Based Precautions and discuss the elements of these standards.
6. Describe the concept of emerging infectious diseases and factors that lead to the development of these diseases.
7. Use the nursing process as a framework for care of patients with sexually transmitted disease.
8. Describe home health care measures that reduce the risk of infection.
9. Use the nursing process as a framework for care of patients with infectious diseases.

An infectious disease is any disease caused by the growth of pathogenic microbes in the body. It may or may not be communicable (ie, contagious). Modern science has controlled, eradicated, or decreased the incidence of many infectious diseases. However, increases in other infections, such as those caused by antibiotic-resistant organisms and emerging infectious diseases, are of great and growing concern. Examples of these infectious diseases are presented in this chapter. Other infectious diseases are discussed in the appropriate chapters (for example, see Chapter 23 for information on tuberculosis [TB]). It is important to understand infectious causes and the treatment of contagious, serious, and common infections. Table 70-1 presents an overview of many infectious diseases, their causative organisms, mode of transmission, and usual **incubation periods** (time between contact and development of the first signs and symptoms).

The nurse plays an important role in infection control and prevention. Educating patients may decrease their risk of becoming infected or may decrease the sequelae of infection. Using appropriate barrier precautions, observing prudent hand hygiene, and ensuring aseptic care of intravenous (IV) catheters and other invasive equipment also assists in reducing infections.

The Infectious Process

The Chain of Infection

A complete chain of events is necessary for infection to occur. Figure 70-1 illustrates the elements of the chain and identifies points where health care workers can intervene to interrupt the chain. The necessary elements for infection to occur are the following:

- A causative organism
- A reservoir of available organisms
- A portal or mode of exit from the reservoir
- A mode of transmission from reservoir to host
- A susceptible host
- A mode of entry to host

(text continues on page 2478)

Glossary

bacteremia: laboratory-proven presence of bacteria in the bloodstream

carrier: person who carries an organism without apparent signs and symptoms; one who is able to transmit an infection to others

Centers for Disease Control and Prevention (CDC): federal agency responsible for monitoring endemic and epidemic disease, for recommending strategies to decrease disease incidence, and for developing guidelines to reduce risk to patients and health care workers

colonization: microorganisms present in or on a host, without host interference or interaction and without eliciting symptoms in the host

emerging infectious diseases: human infectious diseases with incidence increased within the past two decades or potential increase in the near future

fungemia: a bloodstream infection caused by a fungal organism

health care–associated infection (HAI): an infection not present or incubating at the time of admission to the health care setting; this term is replacing the term "nosocomial infection."

host: person who provides living conditions to support a microorganism

immune: person with protection from a previous infection or immunization who resists reinfection when re-exposed to the same agent

incubation period: time between contact and onset of signs and symptoms

infection: condition in which the host interacts physiologically and immunologically with a microorganism

infectious disease: the consequences that result from invasion of the body by microorganisms that can produce harm to the body and potentially death.

latency: time interval after primary infection when a microorganism lives within the host without producing clinical evidence

methicillin-resistant *Staphylococcus aureus* (MRSA): *Staphylococcus aureus* bacterium that is not susceptible to extended-penicillin antibiotic formulas, such as methicillin, oxacillin, or nafcillin

normal flora: persistent nonpathogenic organisms colonizing a host

nosocomial infection: infection acquired in the hospital that was not present or incubating at the time of hospital admission

reservoir: any person, plant, animal, substance, or location that provides living conditions for microorganisms and that enables further dispersal of the organism

Standard Precautions: strategy of assuming all patients may carry infectious agents and using appropriate barrier precautions for all health care worker–patient interactions

susceptible: not possessing immunity to a particular pathogen

transient flora: organisms that have been recently acquired and are likely to be shed in a relatively short period

Transmission-Based Precautions: precautions used in addition to Standard Precautions when contagious or epidemiologically significant organisms are recognized. The three types of Transmission-Based Precautions are Airborne, Droplet, and Contact Precautions.

vancomycin-resistant *Staphylococcus aureus* (VRSA): *Staphylococcus aureus* bacterium that is not susceptible to vancomycin

vancomycin-resistant *Enterococcus* (VRE): *Enterococcus* bacterium that is resistant to the antibiotic vancomycin

virulence: degree of pathogenicity of an organism

TABLE 70-1 Infectious Diseases, Causative Organisms, Modes of Transmission, and Usual Incubation Periods

Disease or Condition	Organism	Usual Mode of Transmission	Usual Incubation Period (Infection to First Symptom)
Acquired immunodeficiency syndrome (AIDS)	Human immunodeficiency virus (HIV)	Sexual; percutaneous; perinatal	Median of 10 yr
Amebiasis	*Entamoeba histolytica*	Contaminated water	2–4 wk
Anthrax	*Bacillus anthracis*	Airborne or contact	2–60 days
Chancroid	*Haemophilus ducreyi*	Sexual	3–5 days
Chickenpox	Varicella zoster	Airborne or contact	About 14 days
Cholera	*Vibrio cholerae*	Ingestion of water contaminated with human waste	A few hours to 5 days
Cryptococcosis	*Cryptococcus neoformans*	Probably by inhalation	Unknown
Cryptosporidiosis	*Cryptosporidium* species	Ingestion of contaminated water; direct contact with carrier	Probably 1–12 days
Cytomegalovirus (CMV) infection	Cytomegalovirus	Transfusion and transplantation; sexual; perinatal	Highly variable: 3–8 wk after transfusion, 3–12 wk after delivery of newborn
Diarrheal disease (common causes)	*Campylobacter* species	Ingestion of contaminated food	3–5 days
	Clostridium difficile	Fecal-oral	Variable; in part related to the influence of antibiotics
	Salmonella species	Ingestion of contaminated food or drink	12–36 hr
	Shigella species	Ingestion of contaminated food or drink; direct contact with carrier	1–3 days
	Yersinia species	Ingestion of contaminated food or drink; direct contact with carrier	1–3 days
Ebola	Ebola virus	Contact with blood or body fluids	2–21 days
Gonorrhea	*Neisseria gonorrhoeae*	Sexual; perinatal	2–7 days
Hand, foot, and mouth disease	Coxsackievirus	Direct contact with nose and throat secretions and with feces of infected people	3–5 days
Hantavirus pulmonary syndrome (HPS)	Sin nombre virus	Contact (direct or indirect) with rodents	Unclear
Foodborne hepatitis	Hepatitis A virus	Ingestion of contaminated food or drink; direct contact with carrier	15–50 days
	Hepatitis E virus	Ingestion of contaminated food or drink; direct contact with carrier	Unclear
Bloodborne hepatitis	Hepatitis B virus	Sexual; perinatal; percutaneous	45–160 days
	Hepatitis C virus	Sexual; perinatal; percutaneous	6–9 mo
	Hepatitis D	Sexual; perinatal; percutaneous	Unclear
	Hepatitis G	Percutaneous	Unclear
Herpangina	Coxsackievirus	Direct contact with nose and throat secretions and feces of infected people	3–5 days
Herpes simplex	Human herpesvirus 1 and 2	Contact with mucous membrane secretions	2–12 days
Histoplasmosis	*Histoplasma capsulatum*	Inhalation of airborne spores	5–18 days
Hookworm disease	*Necator americanus; Ancyclostoma duodenale*	Contact with soil contaminated with human feces	A few weeks to many months
Impetigo	*Staphylococcus aureus*	Contact with *S. aureus* carrier	4–10 days
Influenza	Influenza virus A, B, or C	Droplet spread	24–72 hr
Lassa fever	Lassa virus	Contact with animal droppings; direct contact with blood or body fluids	7–21 days
Legionnaires' disease	*Legionella pneumophila*	Airborne from water source	2–10 days
Listeriosis	*Listeria monocytogenes*	Foodborne; perinatal	Unclear; probably 3–70 days
Lyme disease	*Borrelia burgdorferi*	Tick bite	14–23 days
Lymphogranuloma venereum	*Chlamydia inguinale*	Sexual	Weeks to years
Malaria	*Plasmodium vivax; Plasmodium malariae; Plasmodium falciparum; Plasmodium ovale*	Bite from *Anopheles* species mosquito	12–30 days

TABLE 70-1 Infectious Diseases, Causative Organisms, Modes of Transmission, and Usual Incubation Periods (Continued)

Disease or Condition	Organism	Usual Mode of Transmission	Usual Incubation Period (Infection to First Symptom)
Marburg hemorrhagic fever	Marburg virus	Unknown route of transmission from animals to humans; person-to-person by droplets and direct contact	5–10 days
Meningococcal meningitis or bacteremia	*Neisseria meningitidis*	Contact with pharyngeal secretions; perhaps airborne	2–10 days
Mononucleosis	Epstein-Barr virus	Contact with pharyngeal secretions	4–6 weeks
Mycobacterial diseases (nontuberculosis *Mycobacterium* species)	*Mycobacterium avium; Mycobacterium kansasii; Mycobacterium fortuitum; Mycobacterium gordonae;* other *Mycobacterium* species	Variable; probably contact with soil, water, or other environmental source; none is transmissible person-to-person	Variable
Mycoplasmal pneumonia	*Mycoplasma pneumoniae*	Droplet inhalation	14–21 days
Norovirus	*Norovirus*	Fecal–oral by food or water or by person-to-person spread	24–48 hours
Pediculosis	*Pediculus humanus capitis* (head louse); *Phthirus pubis* (crab louse)	Direct contact	1–2 wk
Pinworm disease	*Enterobius vermicularis*	Direct contact with egg-contaminated articles	4- to 6-wk life cycle; often takes months of infection before recognition
Pneumocystis jiroveci pneumonia	*Pneumocystis jiroveci*	Unknown; not transmitted person-to-person	Infants: 1–2 mo; adults: unclear
Pneumococcal pneumonia	*Streptococcus pneumoniae*	Droplet spread	Probably 1–3 days
Rabies	Rabies virus	Bite from rabid animal	2–8 wk
Respiratory syncytial disease	Respiratory syncytial virus	Self-inoculation by mouth or nose after contact with infectious respiratory secretions	3–7 days
Ringworm	*Microsporum* species; Trychophyton species	Direct and indirect contact with lesions	4–10 days
Rocky mountain spotted fever	*Rickettsia ricketsii*	Bite from infected tick	3–14 days
Roseola infantum	Human herpes virus 6	Saliva	10–15 days
Rotavirus gastroenteritis	Rotavirus	Fecal–oral route	About 48 hr
Rubella	Rubella virus	Droplet spread; direct contact	14–21 days
Scabies	*Sarcoptes scabei*	Direct skin contact	2–6 wk
Severe acute respiratory syndrome (SARS)	SARS-associated coronavirus (SARS-CoV)	Droplet; direct contact; occasionally airborne	2–10 days
Smallpox	*Variola major*	Airborne and contact	7–14 days
Syphilis	*Treponema pallidum*	Sexual; perinatal	10 days to 10 wk
Tetanus	*Clostridium tetani*	Puncture wound	4–21 days
Trichinosis	*Trichinella spiralis*	Ingestion of insufficiently cooked foods, especially pork and beef	10–14 days
Tuberculosis	*Mycobacterium tuberculosis*	Airborne	4–12 wk to the formation of primary lesion
West Nile virus	West Nile virus	Bite of infected mosquitoes; from transfusions and transplants; perinatal	3–14 days

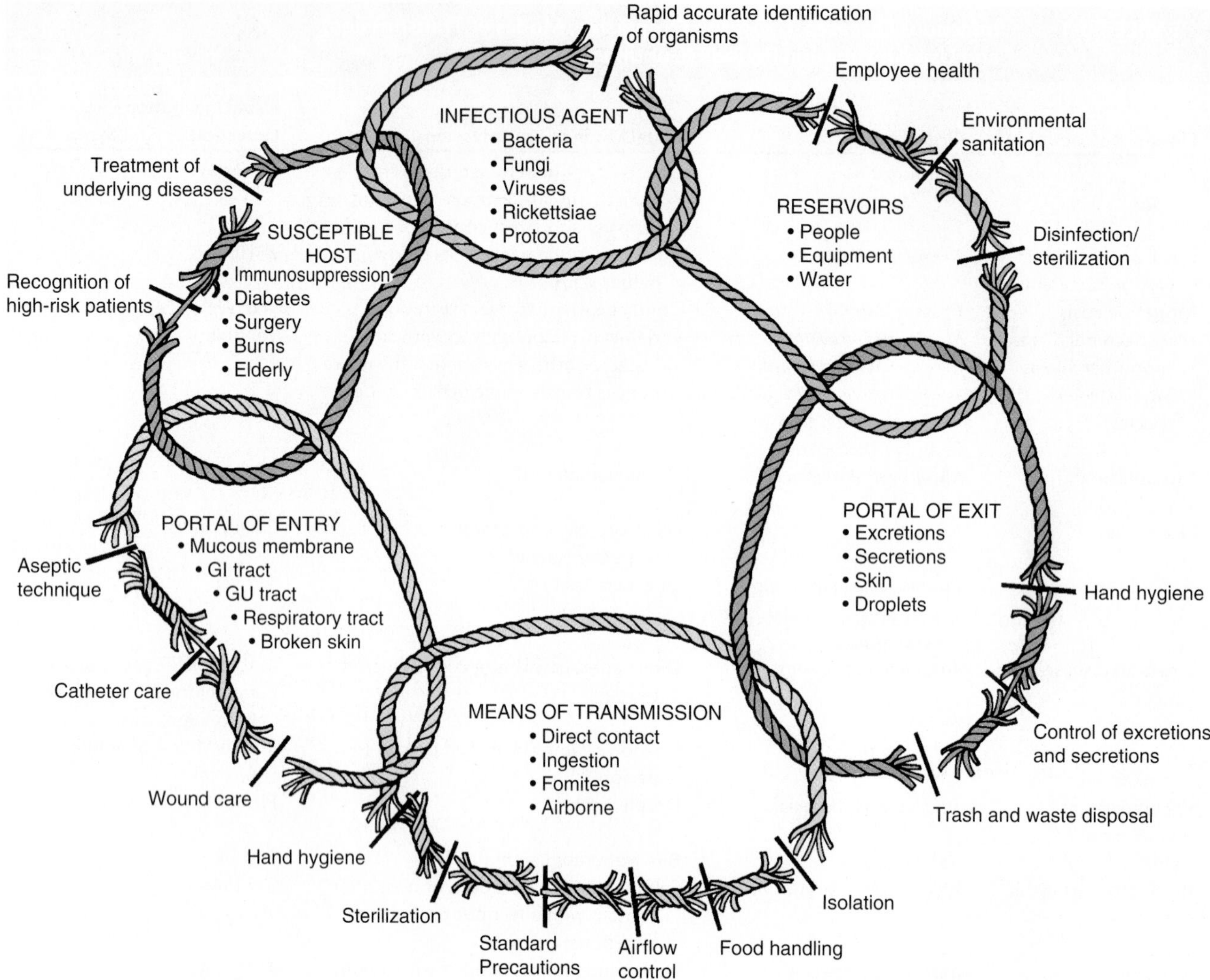

FIGURE 70-1. Health care workers' interventions used to break the chain of infection transmission.

Causative Organism

The types of microorganisms that cause infections are bacteria, rickettsiae, viruses, protozoa, fungi, and helminths.

Reservoir

Reservoir is the term used for any person, plant, animal, substance, or location that provides nourishment for microorganisms and enables further dispersal of the organism. Infections may be prevented by eliminating the causative organisms from the reservoir.

Mode of Exit

The organism must have a mode of exit from a reservoir. An infected host must shed organisms to another or to the environment before transmission can occur. Organisms exit through the respiratory tract, the gastrointestinal tract, the genitourinary tract, or the blood.

Route of Transmission

A route of transmission is necessary to connect the infectious source with its new host. Organisms may be transmitted through sexual contact, skin-to-skin contact, percutaneous injection, or infectious particles carried in the air. A person who carries or transmits an organism but does not have apparent signs and symptoms of infection is called a **carrier.**

It is important to recognize that specific organisms require specific routes of transmission for infection to occur. For example, *Mycobacterium tuberculosis* is almost always transmitted by the airborne route. Health care providers do not "carry" *M. tuberculosis* bacteria on their hands or clothing. In contrast, bacteria such as *Staphylococcus aureus* are easily transmitted from patient to patient on the hands of health care providers.

When appropriate, the nurse should explain routes of disease transmission to patients. For example, a nurse may explain that sharing a room with a patient who is infected with human immunodeficiency virus (HIV) does not pose a risk because intimate contact (ie, sexual or parenteral) is necessary for transmission to occur.

Susceptible Host

For infection to occur, the **host** must be **susceptible** (not possessing immunity to a particular pathogen). Previous infection or vaccine administration may render the host

immune (not susceptible) to further infection with an agent. Although exposure to potentially infectious microorganisms occurs essentially on a constant basis, our elaborate immune systems generally prevent infection from occurring. A person who is immunosuppressed has much greater susceptibility to infection than a healthy person.

Portal of Entry

A portal of entry is needed for the organism to gain access to the host. Again, specific organisms may require specific portals of entry for infection to occur. For example, airborne *M. tuberculosis* does not cause disease when it settles on the skin of an exposed host; the only entry route for *M. tuberculosis* is through the respiratory tract.

Colonization, Infection, and Infectious Disease

Relatively few anatomic sites (eg, brain, blood, bone, heart, vascular system) are sterile. Bacteria found throughout the body usually provide beneficial **normal flora** to compete with potential pathogens, to facilitate digestion, or to work in other ways symbiotically with the host.

Colonization

The term **colonization** is used to describe microorganisms present without host interference or interaction. Organisms reported in microbiology test results often reflect colonization rather than infection. The nurse and other members of the patient's health care team must interpret microbiology test results accurately to ensure appropriate treatment.

Infection

Infection indicates a host interaction with an organism. A patient colonized with *S. aureus* may have staphylococci on the skin without any skin interruption or irritation. However, if the patient had an incision, *S. aureus* could enter the wound, resulting in an immune system reaction of local inflammation and migration of white cells to the site. Clinical evidence of redness, heat, and pain and laboratory evidence of white blood cells on the wound specimen smear suggest infection. In this example, the host identifies the staphylococci as *foreign*. Infection is recognized by the host reaction (manifested by signs and symptoms) and by laboratory-based organism identification.

Infectious Disease

It is important to recognize the difference between infection and infectious disease. **Infectious disease** is the state in which the infected host displays a decline in wellness due to the infection. When the host interacts immunologically with an organism but remains symptom free, the definition of infectious disease has not been met. For example, when a person is first infected with *M. tuberculosis*, infection can be detected by a positive tuberculin skin test, which demonstrates immunologic recognition. Most people who are infected with *M. tuberculosis* have latent infection, but few people (approximately 10%) actually become ill and demonstrate symptoms of TB (fever, weight loss, and advancing pneumonia). Figure 70-2 depicts response to bacterial infection at the cellular level and at the host level.

The primary source of information about most bacterial infections is the microbiology laboratory report. The microbiology laboratory report should be viewed as a tool to be

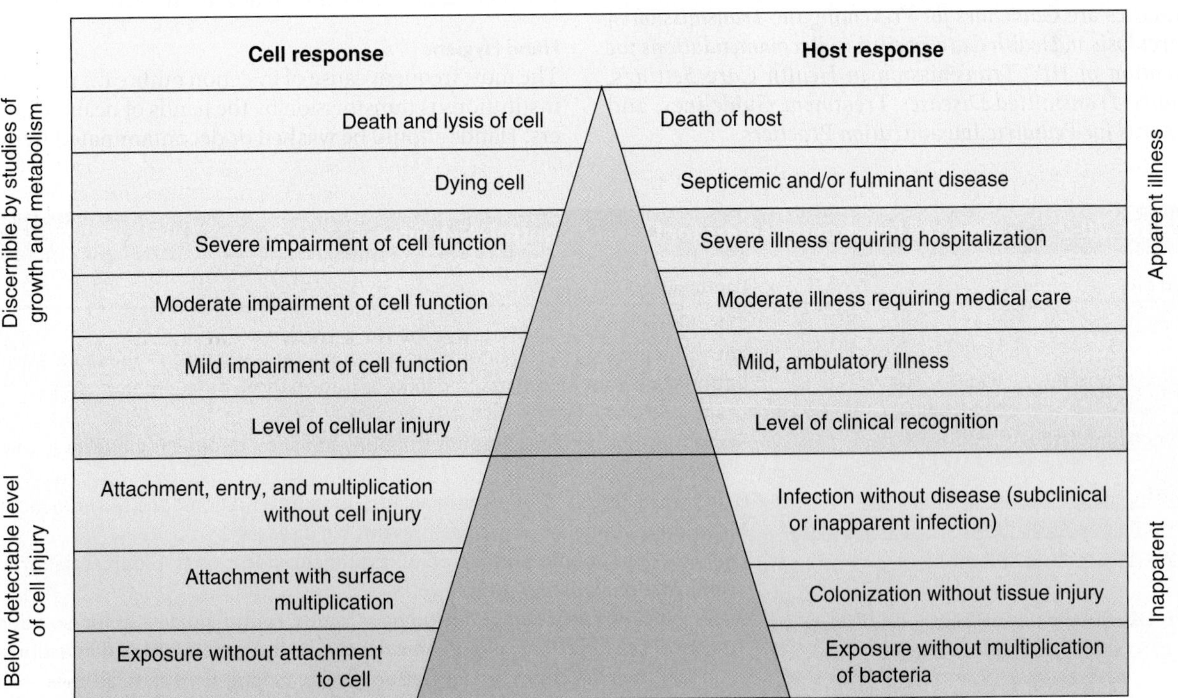

FIGURE 70-2. Biologic spectrum of response to bacterial infection at the cellular level (*left*) and of the intact host (*right*). Redrawn from Evans, A. S., & Brachman, P. S. (1998). *Bacterial infections in humans.* New York: Plenum.

used along with clinical indicators to determine whether a patient is colonized, infected, or diseased. Microbiology reports from clinical specimens usually show three components: the smear and stain, the culture and organism identification, and the antimicrobial susceptibility (ie, sensitivity). As a marker for the likelihood of infection, the smear and stain generally provide the most helpful information because they describe the mix of cells present at the anatomic site at the time of specimen collection. Culture and sensitivity results specify which organisms are recognized and which antibiotics actively affect the bacteria.

Infection Control and Prevention

The World Health Organization (WHO) and the **Centers for Disease Control and Prevention** (CDC) are the principal agencies involved in setting guidelines about infection prevention. In recent years, attention to **health care–associated infections (HAIs)**, formerly referred to as **nosocomial infections**, has grown with increased guidance from the Joint Commission for Accreditation for Healthcare Organizations (JCAHO), the Institute for Healthcare Improvement (IHI), and Medicare.

The impact of infectious diseases changes through time as microorganisms mutate, as human behavior patterns shift, or as therapeutic options change. The CDC serves an important function in providing timely scientific recommendations about many of the situations that a nurse may face when caring for or teaching a patient with an infectious disease. The CDC routinely publishes recommendations, guidelines, and summaries. Through its Internet site (http://www.cdc.gov) and its weekly journal, the *Morbidity and Mortality Weekly Report* (MMWR), the CDC reports significant cases, outbreaks, environmental hazards, or other public health problems. Examples of important CDC guidelines and summaries are *Guidelines for Preventing the Transmission of Tuberculosis in Health Care Facilities*, *Recommendations for Prevention of HIV Transmission in Health Care Settings*, *Sexually Transmitted Diseases Treatment Guidelines*, and *Standards for Pediatric Immunization Practices*.

This chapter summarizes several aspects of infectious diseases. However, the field of infection control and prevention is changing very rapidly. Health care workers should seek the most current information when they address patient care concerns or make infection control policies. Table 70-2 presents an overview of selected CDC web sites.

Preventing Infection in the Hospital

Isolation Precautions

Isolation precautions are guidelines created to prevent transmission of microorganisms in hospitals. The Hospital Infection Control Practices Advisory Committee (HICPAC) of the CDC recommends two tiers of isolation precautions. The first tier, called Standard Precautions, is designed for the care of *all* patients in the hospital and is the primary strategy for preventing HAIs. The second tier, called Transmission-Based Precautions, is designed for care of patients with known or suspected infectious diseases spread by airborne, droplet, or contact routes.

STANDARD PRECAUTIONS

The tenets of **Standard Precautions** are that all patients are colonized or infected with microorganisms, whether or not there are signs or symptoms, and that a uniform level of caution should be used in the care of all patients. The elements of Standard Precautions include hand hygiene, use of gloves and other barriers (eg, mask, eye protection, face shield, gown), proper handling of patient care equipment and linen, environmental control, prevention of injury from sharps devices, and patient placement (ie, room assignments) within health care facilities. Hand hygiene, glove use, needlestick prevention, and avoidance of splash or spray of body fluids are discussed in the following sections. Chart 52-3 in Chapter 52 describes the Standard Precautions in detail.

Hand Hygiene

The most frequent cause of infection outbreaks in health care institutions is transmission by the hands of health care workers. Hands should be washed or decontaminated frequently

TABLE 70-2 Selected Important Centers for Disease Control Web Sites

Web Site	Features
www.cdc.gov	CDC home page Entry point to other sites; information about current situations in infectious diseases
www.cdc.gov/flu	Information about influenza and links to information, data, recommendations, and updates
www.cdc.gov/std	Sexually transmitted diseases information, statistics, treatment guidelines, and laboratory guidelines
www.bt.cdc.gov/agent/agentlist.asp	Bioterrorism history, bioterrorism agents, updates, situations, and recommendations
www.cdc.gov/node.do/id/0900f3ec8005df/f	Menu-driven overview of vaccine-preventable diseases
www.cdc.gov/drugresistance/	Overview of antibiotic/antimicrobial resistance, educational resources, laboratory information, and fact sheets
www.cdc.gov/nicidod/dhqp/index.html	Issues in health care settings, including infection control guidelines for isolation, surgical site infections, pneumonia, intravascular catheter–related infections, urinary tract infections, and infection control in long-term care facilities
www.cdc.gov/hiv/	Information about the epidemiology of HIV/AIDS, including fact sheets, slide sets, and statistics

CHART 70-1

Hand Hygiene Methods

Hand Decontamination with Alcohol-Based Product

- After contact with body fluids, excretions, mucous membranes, nonintact skin, or wound dressings as long as hands are not visibly soiled
- After contact with a patient's intact skin (as after taking pulse or blood pressure or lifting a patient)
- In patient care, when moving from a contaminated body site to a clean body site
- After contact with inanimate objects in the patient's immediate vicinity
- Before caring for patients with severe neutropenia or other forms of severe immune suppression
- Before donning sterile gloves when inserting central catheters
- Before inserting urinary catheters or other devices that do not require a surgical procedure
- After removing gloves

Hand Washing

- When hands are visibly dirty or contaminated with biologic material from patient care
- When health care workers do not tolerate waterless alcohol product

during patient care. Chart 70-1 describes the recommended hand hygiene methods.

When hands are visibly dirty or contaminated with biologic material from patient care, hands should be washed with soap and water. In intensive care units and other locations in which virulent or resistant organisms are likely to be present, antimicrobial agents (eg, chlorhexidine gluconate, iodophors, chloroxylenol, and triclosan) may be used. Effective hand washing requires at least *15 seconds of vigorous scrubbing*, with special attention to the area around nail beds and between fingers, where there is a high bacterial load. Hands should be thoroughly rinsed after washing.

If hands are not visibly soiled, health care providers are strongly encouraged to use alcohol-based, waterless antiseptic agents for routine hand decontamination. These solutions are superior to soap or antimicrobial handwashing agents in their speed of action and effectiveness against microorganisms. Because they are formulated with emollients, they are usually better tolerated than other agents, and because they can be used without sinks and towels, health care workers have been found to be more compliant with their use. Nurses working in home health care or other settings where they are relatively mobile should carry pocket-sized containers of alcohol-based solutions (Rhinehart & McGoldrick, 2005).

Normal skin flora usually consist of coagulase-negative staphylococci or diphtheroids. In the health care setting, workers may temporarily carry other bacteria (ie, **transient flora**) such as *S. aureus*, *Pseudomonas aeruginosa*, or other organisms with increased pathogenic potential. Generally, transient flora are superficially attached and are shed with hand hygiene and skin regeneration.

Hand washing or disinfection reduces the bacterial load and decreases the risk of transfer to other patients. All health care settings should have mechanisms to evaluate compliance with hand disinfection by all who care for patients.

Nurses should not wear artificial fingernails or nail extenders when providing patient care. These items have been epidemiologically linked to several significant outbreaks of infections. Natural nails should be kept less than 0.25 inches (0.6 cm) long, and nail polish should be removed when chipped, because it can support increased bacterial growth (CDC, 2002a).

Glove Use

Gloves provide an effective barrier for hands from the microflora associated with patient care. Gloves should be worn when a health care worker has contact with any patient's secretions or excretions and must be discarded after each patient care contact. Because microbial organisms colonizing health care workers' hands can proliferate in the warm, moist environment provided by gloves, hands must be thoroughly washed with soap or an antimicrobial agent after gloves are removed. As patient advocates, nurses have an important role in promoting hand washing and glove use by other hospital workers, such as laboratory personnel, technicians, and others who have contact with patients.

Latex gloves are often preferred over vinyl gloves because of greater comfort and fit and because some studies indicate that they afford greater protection from exposure. However, their increased use in recent years has been accompanied by increased reports of allergic reactions to latex among health care workers. Reactions range from local skin irritation to more severe reactions, including generalized dermatitis, conjunctivitis, asthma, angioedema, and anaphylaxis (see Chapter 53).

The nurse who experiences irritation or an allergic reaction associated with exposure to latex should report symptoms to an occupational health specialist or physician. Suggested methods for reducing the incidence of such reactions include the use of vinyl gloves, powder-free gloves, or "low-protein" latex gloves.

Needlestick Prevention

The most important aspect of reducing the risk of bloodborne infection is avoidance of percutaneous injury. Extreme care is essential in all situations in which needles, scalpels, and other sharp objects are handled. Used needles should not be recapped. Instead, they are placed directly into puncture-resistant containers near the place where they are used. If a situation dictates that a needle must be recapped, the nurse must use a mechanical device to hold the cap or use a one-handed approach to decrease the likelihood of skin puncture. Since 2001, the Occupational Safety and Health Administration (OSHA) has required nurses to use needleless devices and other instruments designed to prevent injury from sharps when appropriate (OSHA, 2001).

Avoidance of Splash and Spray

When the health care provider is involved in an activity in which body fluids may be sprayed or splashed, appropriate barriers must be used. If a splash to the face may occur, goggles and a face mask are warranted. If the health care worker is handling material that may soil clothing or is involved in a procedure in which clothing may be splashed with biologic material, a cover gown should be worn.

TRANSMISSION-BASED PRECAUTIONS

Some microbes are so contagious or epidemiologically significant that precautions in addition to the Standard Precautions should be used when such organisms are recognized. The CDC recommends a second tier of precautions, called **Transmission-Based Precautions.** The additional isolation categories are Airborne, Droplet, and Contact Precautions (CDC, 2004g).

Airborne Precautions are required for patients with presumed or proven pulmonary TB, chickenpox, or other airborne pathogen. Airborne precautions are also advised if a patient is infected with smallpox (eg, as a result of a bioterrorist attack). When hospitalized, patients should be in rooms with negative air pressure; the door should remain closed, and health care providers should wear an N-95 respirator (ie, protective mask) at all times while in the patient's room.

Droplet Precautions are used for organisms that can be transmitted by close, face-to-face contact, such as influenza or meningococcal meningitis. While taking care of a patient requiring Droplet Precautions, the nurse should wear a face mask, but because the risk of transmission is limited to close contact, the door may remain open.

Contact Precautions are used for organisms that are spread by skin-to-skin contact, such as antibiotic-resistant organisms or *Clostridium difficile.* Contact Precautions are designed to emphasize cautious technique and the use of barriers for organisms that have serious epidemiologic consequences or those easily transmitted by contact between health care worker and patient. When possible, the patient requiring contact isolation is placed in a private room to facilitate hand hygiene and decreased environmental contamination. Masks are not needed, and doors do not need to be closed (Chart 70-2).

Specific Organisms with Health Care–Associated Infection Potential

CLOSTRIDIUM DIFFICILE

This spore-forming bacterium has significant HAI potential. Infection is usually preceded by antibiotics that disrupt normal intestinal flora and allow the antibiotic-resistant *C. difficile* spores to proliferate within the intestine. The organism causes pathology by releasing toxins into the lumen of the bowel. In pseudomembranous colitis, the most extreme form of *C. difficile* infection, debris from the injured lumen of the bowel and from white blood cells accumulates in the form of pseudomembranes or studded areas of the colon. The destruction of such a large anatomic area can produce profound sepsis.

Because antibiotics are used so extensively in the health care setting, many patients are at risk for infection with *C. difficile.* The nosocomial potential is increased because the spore is relatively resistant to disinfectants and can be spread on the hands of health care providers after contact with equipment that has previously been contaminated with *C. difficile.* Control is best achieved by using Contact Precautions for infected patients. Glove use and hand hygiene are stressed for all care workers. In addition, the CDC recommends an intensified environmental cleaning using a 1:10 bleach:water solution. Equipment should be cleaned whenever visibly soiled. Items close to the patient (such as the overbed table and side rails) should be cleaned daily. IV poles and other peripheral items should be cleaned when the patient is discharged.

METHICILLIN-RESISTANT *STAPHYLOCOCCUS AUREUS*

Methicillin-resistant *Staphylococcus aureus* (MRSA), a common human pathogen, refers to *S. aureus* that is resistant to methicillin or its comparable pharmaceutical agents, oxacillin and nafcillin. Soon after penicillin was discovered in the 1940s, *S. aureus* became all but universally penicillin resistant. Alternative therapies in the form of cephalosporins and synthetic penicillin solutions such as methicillin were introduced. However, since the late 1970s, MRSA has become increasingly more prevalent, and transmission within hospitals and nursing homes has been well documented.

Vancomycin (Vancocin) and linezolid (Zyvox) are the preferred alternative treatments for serious MRSA infection. However, there is concern that MRSA will eventually also become resistant to these medications because they are used so commonly. Since 2002, a very small but disturbing number of patients have been diagnosed with *S. aureus* infections that are completely resistant to vancomycin (ie, **vancomycin-resistant *Staphylococcus aureus* [VRSA]**). The threat of VRSA is considered a very serious public health concern because of the pathogenicity of *S. aureus.* Without effective antibiotics, many patients with *S. aureus* infections would have a poor outcome (CDC, 2002b). Control of MRSA alone is an important goal, and it may also make the emergence of VRSA strains less likely.

Health care providers can and do transmit MRSA to patients easily because *S. aureus* commonly colonizes skin. Although there is little evidence that MRSA is more virulent than other strains of staphylococci, the colonized patient has an increased probability of true infection with MRSA, especially when invasive procedures, such as IV therapy, respiratory therapy, or surgery, are performed. The patient colonized with MRSA also serves as a reservoir of resistant organisms that can be transmitted to others. MRSA acquired in the hospital may persist as normal flora in the patient for extended periods. Colonization is seldom recognized; thus, the health care provider must assume that *every* patient contact offers the possibility of MRSA exposure.

VANCOMYCIN-RESISTANT *ENTEROCOCCUS*

Vancomycin-resistant *Enterococcus* (VRE) is the second most frequently isolated source of HAIs in the United States. This gram-positive bacterium, which is part of the normal flora of the gastrointestinal tract, can produce significant disease when it infects blood, wounds, or urine.

Enterococcus has several traits that make it an easily transmittable HAI organism. It is a normal part of the gastrointestinal flora of the host; it is bile-resistant and able to withstand harsh anatomic sites, such as the intestine; and it endures well on the hands of health care providers and on environmental objects.

As a relatively resistant organism at baseline, therapy for *Enterococcus* is limited to penicillin formulations (eg, ampicillin), vancomycin in combination with an aminoglyco-

CHART 70-2

Summary of Types of Precautions and Patients Requiring the Precautions

Standard Precautions

Use Standard Precautions for the care of all patients.

Airborne Precautions

In addition to Standard Precautions, use Airborne Precautions for patients known or suspected to have serious illnesses transmitted by airborne droplet nuclei. Examples of such illnesses include the following:

- Measles
- Varicella (including disseminated zoster)*
- Tuberculosis

Droplet Precautions

In addition to Standard Precautions, use Droplet Precautions for patients known or suspected to have serious illnesses transmitted by large particle droplets. Examples of such illnesses include:

- Invasive *Haemophilus influenzae* type b disease, including meningitis, pneumonia, epiglottitis, and sepsis
- Invasive *Neisseria meningitidis* disease, including meningitis, pneumonia, and sepsis
- Other serious bacterial respiratory infections spread by droplet transmission, including:
  - Diphtheria (pharyngeal)
  - Primary atypical pneumonia (*Mycoplasma pneumoniae*)
  - Pertussis
  - Pneumonic plague
  - Streptococcal (group A) pharyngitis, pneumonia, or scarlet fever in infants and young children
- Serious viral infections spread by droplet transmission, including:
  - Adenovirus*
  - Influenza
  - Mumps
  - Parvovirus B19
  - Rubella

Contact Precautions

In addition to Standard Precautions, use Contact Precautions for patients known or suspected to have serious illnesses easily transmitted by direct patient contact or by contact with items in the patient's environment. Examples of such illnesses include:

- Gastrointestinal, respiratory, skin, or wound infections or colonization with multidrug-resistant bacteria judged by the infection control program, based on current state, regional, or national recommendations, to be of special clinical and epidemiologic significance
- Enteric infections with a low infectious dose or prolonged environmental survival, including:
  - *Clostridium difficile*
  - For diapered or incontinent patients: enterohemorrhagic *Escherichia coli* O157:H7, *Shigella* species, hepatitis A, or rotavirus
- Respiratory syncytial virus, parainfluenza virus, or enteroviral infections in infants and young children
- Skin infections that are highly contagious or that may occur on dry skin, including:
  - Diphtheria (cutaneous)
  - Herpes simplex virus (neonatal or mucocutaneous)
  - Impetigo
  - Major (noncontained) abscesses, cellulitis, or pressure ulcers
  - Pediculosis
  - Scabies
  - Staphylococcal furunculosis in infants and young children
  - Zoster (disseminated or in the immunocompromised host)*
- Viral and hemorrhagic conjunctivitis
- Viral hemorrhagic infections (Ebola, Lassa, or Marburg)

*Certain infections require more than one type of precaution.
From Centers for Disease Control and Prevention, Atlanta, GA, 1997.

side (eg, gentamicin), or more recently linezolid (Zyvox). Between 1994 and 2003, the CDC recorded an increase of more than 62% in the number of cases of VRE infections in patients in intensive care units (CDC, 2004a). This rapid increase has serious implications. Because many strains of VRE are resistant to all other antimicrobial therapies, clinicians are left with few choices for effective therapy. Equally important, VRE colonization and infection may serve as a reservoir of vancomycin-resistant coded genes that may be transferred to the more virulent *S. aureus* (CDC, 2002b).

Preventing Health Care-Associated Bloodstream Infections (Bacteremia and Fungemia)

Reducing the risk of health care–associated bloodstream infections requires preventive activities in addition to Standard Precautions. If a nosocomial bloodstream infection occurs, early diagnosis is important to prevent complications, such as endocarditis and brain abscess. Mortality rates associated with infection by some organisms may be as high as 25%. The estimated cost attributed to catheter-related bloodstream infections is $3700 to $29,000 per case (Mermel, 2000).

Bacteremia is defined as the laboratory-confirmed presence of bacteria in the bloodstream. **Fungemia** is a bloodstream infection caused by a fungal organism. Any vascular access device (VAD) can serve as the source for a bloodstream infection. Most hospitalized patients receive VADs, and increasingly, long-term central catheters are used to provide IV therapy to outpatients in clinic or home settings. In all instances, the nurse must use appropriate care to reduce the risk of bacteremia and to be alert for signs of bacteremia. Chart 70-3 identifies conditions that suggest the presence of nosocomial VAD-related bacteremia or fungemia.

Hand hygiene and strict attention to aseptic technique are essential during the insertion of all VADs. Health care personnel who insert central catheters should use surgical technique, including sterile gloves, sterile gowns with long sleeves, masks, and a large drape over the patient.

DISINFECTING SKIN

The patient's own flora, traversing the exterior of a peripherally inserted catheter or contaminating the central catheter hub, is the most common bacterial source of catheter-related bacteremia (CDC, 2002e). Rarely, IV fluid itself can become contaminated and serve as a source of infection. The preferred solution for disinfection of the insertion site is chlorhexidine gluconate (CHG). Alternative solutions are povidone–iodine or alcohol. Triple-antibiotic ointment should not be used on the insertion site because it has been shown to lead to increased colonization with *Candida* species (Mermel, 2000).

There is no apparent difference in risk or benefit when comparing transparent polyurethane dressings and gauze dressings. However, if blood is oozing from the catheter insertion site, a gauze dressing should be used. Most importantly, the dressing should be applied using aseptic technique and should be sealed along its entire perimeter (CDC, 2002e). A highly absorbent CHG-impregnated dressing (Biopatch Antimicrobial Dressing), which releases disinfectant for up to 7 days, has been shown to reduce the incidence of HAI bacteremia by 60% (Maki, Mermel, & Lugar, 2000).

CHANGING INFUSION SETS, CAPS, AND SOLUTIONS

Infusion sets and stopcock caps should be changed no more frequently than every 3 days, unless an infusion set is used for the delivery of blood or lipid solutions. Infusion sets and tubing for blood, blood products, or lipid emulsions should be changed within 24 hours of initiating the infusion. Blood infusions should finish within 4 hours of hanging the blood; lipid solutions should be completed within 24 hours of hanging. There are no guidelines for the appropriate intervals for the hang time of other solutions. Injection ports should be cleaned with 70% alcohol or an iodophor before accessing the system (CDC, 2002e).

CHART 70-3

Conditions That Suggest the Presence of Nosocomial Vascular Access Device-Related Bacteremia or Fungemia

- The patient has catheter in place, appears septic, but has no obvious reason to suggest predisposition to sepsis.
- There is no infection at another body site to indicate probable source of sepsis.
- The site of vascular line insertion is red, swollen, or draining (especially purulent drainage).
- The patient has a central vascular line in place at the onset of sepsis.
- The bloodstream infection is caused by *Candida* species or by common skin organisms such as coagulase-negative staphylococci, *Bacillus* species, or *Corynebacterium* species.
- The patient remains septic after appropriate therapy without removal of the vascular access device.

Preventing Infection in the Community

The CDC and state and local public health departments share responsibility for prevention and control of infection in the community. Methods of infection prevention include sanitation techniques (eg, water purification, disposal of sewage and other potentially infectious materials), regulated health practices (eg, the handling, storage, packaging, and preparation of food by institutions), and immunization programs. In the United States, immunization programs have markedly decreased the incidence of infectious diseases.

Vaccination Programs

The goal of vaccination programs is to use wide-scale efforts to prevent specific infectious diseases from occurring in a population. Public health decisions about vaccine campaign implementation efforts are complex. Risks and benefits for the person and the community must be evaluated in terms of morbidity, mortality, and financial cost and benefit.

The most successful vaccine programs have been those for the prevention of smallpox, measles, mumps, rubella, polio, diphtheria, pertussis, and tetanus. In 2002, concerns that smallpox could be reintroduced as an act of biowarfare led to a decision that medical first responders and selected others should again receive smallpox vaccine (Donnellson, 2003). Bioterrorism is addressed in Chapter 72.

More than 25 vaccines are currently licensed in the United States. Vaccines are suspensions of antigen preparations, intended to produce a human immune response to protect the host from future encounters with the organism. Because no vaccine is completely safe for all recipients, contraindications on package inserts of a vaccine must be heeded. These guidelines provide details about studied experiences with allergy and other complications and provide crucial information about refrigeration, storage, dosage, and administration. The most common adverse effects are allergy to the antigen or carrier solution and the occurrence of the actual disease (often in modified form) when live vaccine is used.

The standard recommended immunization schedules for adults as developed by the CDC are shown in Table 70-3.

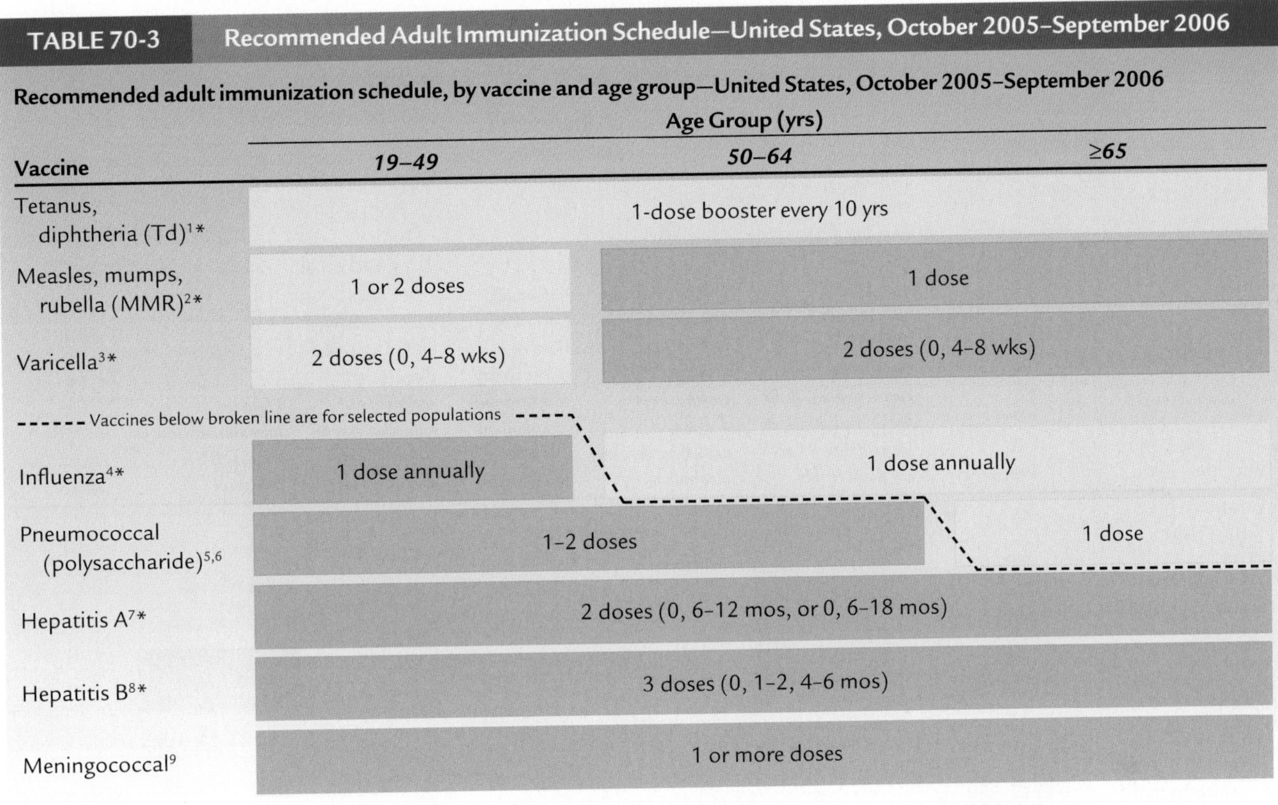

TABLE 70-3 Recommended Adult Immunization Schedule—United States, October 2005–September 2006

Recommended adult immunization schedule, by vaccine and age group—United States, October 2005–September 2006

<table>
<tr><th rowspan="2">Vaccine</th><th colspan="3">Age Group (yrs)</th></tr>
<tr><th>19–49</th><th>50–64</th><th>≥65</th></tr>
<tr><td>Tetanus, diphtheria (Td)[1]*</td><td colspan="3">1-dose booster every 10 yrs</td></tr>
<tr><td>Measles, mumps, rubella (MMR)[2]*</td><td>1 or 2 doses</td><td colspan="2">1 dose</td></tr>
<tr><td>Varicella[3]*</td><td>2 doses (0, 4–8 wks)</td><td colspan="2">2 doses (0, 4–8 wks)</td></tr>
<tr><td colspan="4">------ Vaccines below broken line are for selected populations ------</td></tr>
<tr><td>Influenza[4]*</td><td>1 dose annually</td><td colspan="2">1 dose annually</td></tr>
<tr><td>Pneumococcal (polysaccharide)[5,6]</td><td colspan="2">1–2 doses</td><td>1 dose</td></tr>
<tr><td>Hepatitis A[7]*</td><td colspan="3">2 doses (0, 6–12 mos, or 0, 6–18 mos)</td></tr>
<tr><td>Hepatitis B[8]*</td><td colspan="3">3 doses (0, 1–2, 4–6 mos)</td></tr>
<tr><td>Meningococcal[9]</td><td colspan="3">1 or more doses</td></tr>
</table>

[Light shading] For all persons in this category who meet the age requirements and who lack evidence of immunity (eg, lack documentation of vaccination or have no evidence of prior infection)

[Dark shading] Recommended if some other risk factor is present (eg, on the basis of medical, occupational, lifestyle, or other indications)

* Covered by the Vaccine Injury Compensation Program.

NOTE: These recommendations must be read along with the footnotes, which can be found below.

Approved by the Advisory Committee on Immunization Practices, the American College of Obstetricians and Gynecologists, and the American Academy of Family Physicians

1. Tetanus and diphtheria (Td) vaccination. Adults with uncertain histories of a complete primary vaccination series with diphtheria and tetanus toxoid-containing vaccines should receive a primary series using combined Td toxoid. A primary series for adults is 3 doses; administer the first 2 doses at least 4 weeks apart and the third dose 6–12 months after the second. Administer 1 dose if the person received the primary series and if the last vaccination was received ≥10 years previously. Consult the ACIP statement for recommendations for administering Td as prophylaxis in wound management (http://www.cdc.gov/mmwr/preview/mmwrhtml/00041645.htm). The American College of Physicians Task Force on Adult Immunization supports a second option for Td use in adults: a single Td booster at age 50 years for persons who have completed the full pediatric series, including the teenage/young adult booster. A newly licensed tetanus-diphtheria—acellular-pertussis vaccine is available for adults. ACIP recommendations for its use will be published.

2. Measles, mumps, rubella (MMR) vaccination. *Measles component:* adults born before 1957 can be considered immune to measles. Adults born during or after 1957 should receive ≥1 dose of MMR unless they have a medical contraindication, documentation of ≥1 dose, history of measles based on health care provider diagnosis, or laboratory evidence of immunity. A second dose of MMR is recommended for adults who 1) were recently exposed to measles or in an outbreak setting; 2) were previously vaccinated with killed measles vaccine; 3) were vaccinated with an unknown type of measles vaccine during 1963–1967; 4) are students in postsecondary educational institutions; 5) work in a health care facility; or 6) plan to travel internationally. Withhold MMR or other measles-containing vaccines from HIV-infected persons with severe immunosuppression. *Mumps component:* 1 dose of MMR vaccine should be adequate for protection for those born during or after 1957 who lack a history of mumps based on health care provider diagnosis or who lack laboratory evidence of immunity. *Rubella component:* administer 1 dose of MMR vaccine to women whose rubella vaccination history is unreliable or who lack laboratory evidence of immunity. For women of childbearing age, regardless of birth year, routinely determine rubella immunity and counsel women regarding congenital rubella syndrome. Do not vaccinate women who are pregnant or who might become pregnant within 4 weeks of receiving vaccine. Women who do not have evidence of immunity should receive MMR vaccine upon completion or termination of pregnancy and before discharge from the health care facility.

3. Varicella vaccination. Varicella vaccination is recommended for all adults without evidence of immunity to varicella. Special consideration should be given to those who 1) have close contact with persons at high risk for severe disease (health-care workers and family contacts of immunocompromised persons) or 2) are at high risk for exposure or transmission (eg, teachers of young children; child care employees; residents and staff members of institutional settings, including correctional institutions; college students; military personnel; adolescents and adults living in households with children; nonpregnant women of childbearing age; and international travelers). Evidence of immunity to varicella in adults includes any of the following: 1) documented age-appropriate varicella

continued >

TABLE 70-4 Recommended Adult Immunization Schedule by Vaccine and Medical and Other Indications—United States, October 2005–September 2006

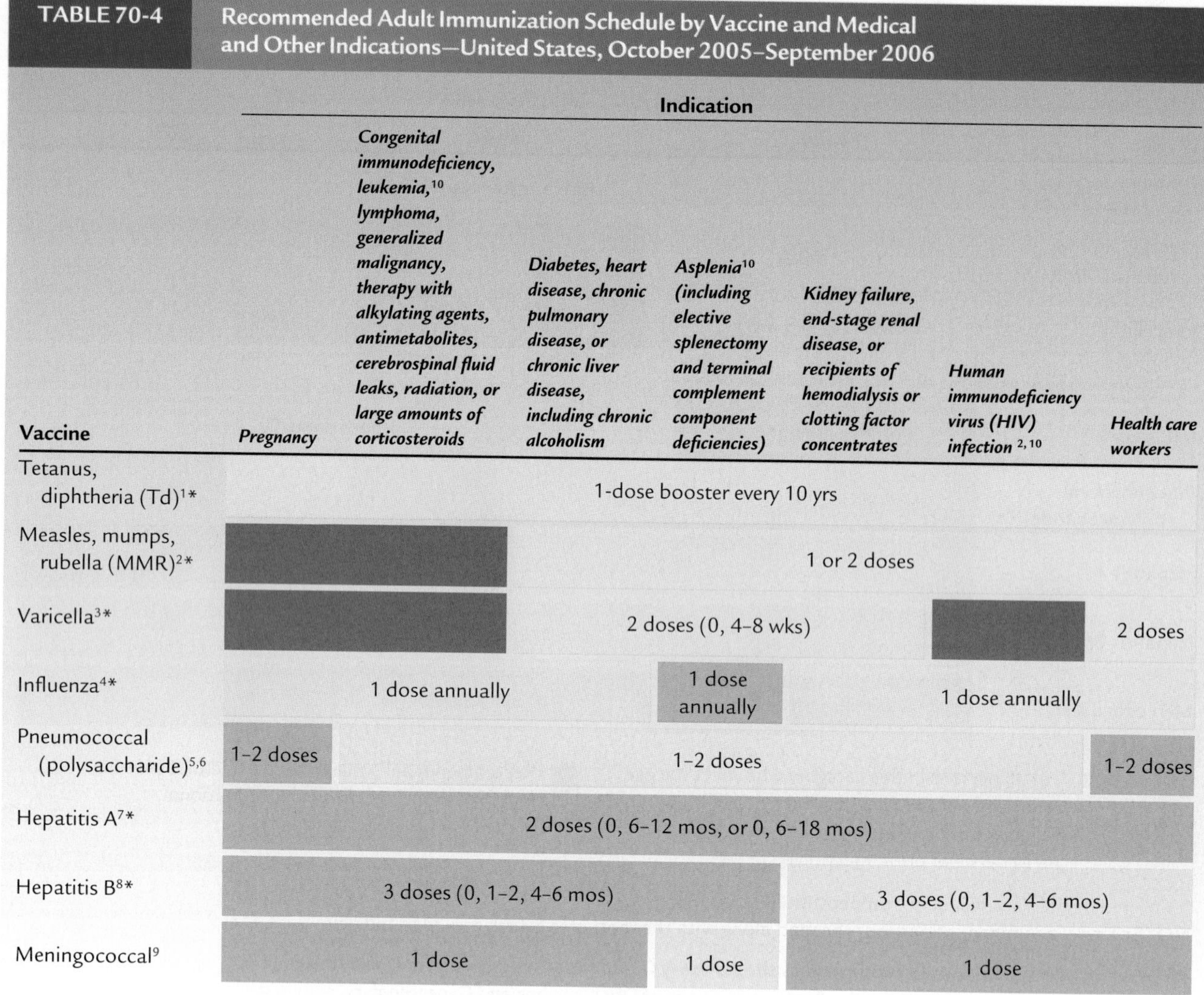

<table>
<tr><th></th><th colspan="7">Indication</th></tr>
<tr><th>Vaccine</th><th>Pregnancy</th><th>Congenital immunodeficiency, leukemia,[10] lymphoma, generalized malignancy, therapy with alkylating agents, antimetabolites, cerebrospinal fluid leaks, radiation, or large amounts of corticosteroids</th><th>Diabetes, heart disease, chronic pulmonary disease, or chronic liver disease, including chronic alcoholism</th><th>Asplenia[10] (including elective splenectomy and terminal complement component deficiencies)</th><th>Kidney failure, end-stage renal disease, or recipients of hemodialysis or clotting factor concentrates</th><th>Human immunodeficiency virus (HIV) infection [2, 10]</th><th>Health care workers</th></tr>
<tr><td>Tetanus, diphtheria (Td)[1]*</td><td colspan="7">1-dose booster every 10 yrs</td></tr>
<tr><td>Measles, mumps, rubella (MMR)[2]*</td><td colspan="2"></td><td colspan="5">1 or 2 doses</td></tr>
<tr><td>Varicella[3]*</td><td colspan="2"></td><td colspan="3">2 doses (0, 4–8 wks)</td><td></td><td>2 doses</td></tr>
<tr><td>Influenza[4]*</td><td colspan="3">1 dose annually</td><td>1 dose annually</td><td colspan="3">1 dose annually</td></tr>
<tr><td>Pneumococcal (polysaccharide)[5,6]</td><td>1–2 doses</td><td colspan="5">1–2 doses</td><td>1–2 doses</td></tr>
<tr><td>Hepatitis A[7]*</td><td colspan="7">2 doses (0, 6–12 mos, or 0, 6–18 mos)</td></tr>
<tr><td>Hepatitis B[8]*</td><td colspan="4">3 doses (0, 1–2, 4–6 mos)</td><td colspan="3">3 doses (0, 1–2, 4–6 mos)</td></tr>
<tr><td>Meningococcal[9]</td><td colspan="3">1 dose</td><td>1 dose</td><td colspan="3">1 dose</td></tr>
</table>

For all persons in this category who meet the age requirements and who lack evidence of immunity (eg, lack documentation of vaccination or have no evidence of prior infection

Recommended if some other risk factor is present (eg, on the basis of medical, occupational, lifestyle, or other indications)

Contraindicated

* Covered by the Vaccine Injury Compensation Program.

NOTE: These recommendations must be read along with the footnotes, which can be found below.

vaccination (i.e., receipt of 1 dose before age 13 years or receipt of 2 doses [administered at least 4 weeks apart] after age 13 years); 2) U.S.-born before 1966 or history of varicella disease before 1966 for non-U.S.-born persons; 3) history of varicella based on health care provider diagnosis or parental or self-report of typical varicella disease for persons born during 1966–1967 (for a patient reporting a history of an atypical, mild case, health care providers should seek either an epidemiologic link with a typical varicella case or evidence of laboratory confirmation, if it was performed at the time of acute disease); 4) history of herpes zoster based on health care provider diagnosis; or 5) laboratory evidence of immunity. Do not vaccinate women who are pregnant or who might become pregnant within 4 weeks of receiving the vaccine. Assess pregnant women for evidence of varicella immunity. Women who do not have evidence of immunity should receive dose 1 of varicella vaccine upon completion or termination of pregnancy and before discharge from the health care facility. Dose 2 should be administered 4–8 weeks after dose 1.

4. Influenza vaccination. *Medical indications:* chronic disorders of the cardiovascular or pulmonary systems, including asthma; chronic metabolic diseases, including diabetes mellitus, renal dysfunction, hemoglobinopathies, or immunosuppression (including immunosuppression caused by medications or HIV); any condition (eg, cognitive dysfunction, spinal cord injury, seizure disorder, or other neuromuscular disorder) that compromises respiratory function or the handling of respiratory secretions or that can increase the risk for aspiration; and pregnancy during the influenza season. No data exist on the risk for severe or complicated influenza disease among persons with asplenia; however, influenza is a risk factor for secondary bacterial infections that can cause severe disease among persons with asplenia. *Occupational indications:* health care workers and employees of long-term—care and assisted living facilities. *Other indications:* residents of nursing homes and other long-term—care and assisted living facilities; persons likely to transmit influenza to persons at high risk (ie, in-home household contacts and caregivers of children aged 0–23 months, or persons of all ages with high-risk conditions), and anyone who wishes to be vaccinated. For healthy, nonpregnant persons aged 5–49 years without high-risk conditions who are not contacts of severely immunocompromised persons in special care units, intranasally administered influenza vaccine (FluMist®) may be administered in lieu of inactivated vaccine.

The schedule is revised as epidemiologic evidence warrants, and nurses are advised to consult the CDC to determine the most recent schedule. Variations to the recommended immunization schedule should be made on a case-by-case basis, depending on the patient's risk factors. The recommended vaccines for adults are designed to protect those with underlying diseases that increase infection risk, those with potential for occupational exposure, and those who may be exposed to infectious agents during travel. Immunosuppressed adults (including those who have had a splenectomy) should be vaccinated for pneumococcus (*Streptococcus pneumoniae*), meningococcus (*Neisseria meningitidis*), and *Haemophilus influenzae*. All health care workers should be immune to measles, mumps, rubella, hepatitis B, and varicella. An annual influenza vaccine is recommended for people with chronic conditions such as immune suppression, asthma, and cardiac or respiratory diseases, as well as for all health care workers.

Information about individual vaccines and vaccine-preventable diseases can be found on the Internet at http://www.cdc.gov/nip/diseases/disease-chart-hcp.htm. The CDC also provides a 24-hour telephone hotline (800-232-2522) for routine pediatric or adult vaccine advice. Advice about optimal vaccinations for travelers is available on the Internet at http://www.cdc.gov/nip/travel/vaccinat.htm and by phone (877-FYI-TRIP).

The incidence of vaccine-preventable diseases, such as measles, mumps, rubella, and diphtheria, is affected by immigration from developing countries. Vaccine campaigns in developing countries are often financially and logistically constrained, and immigrants from such areas may be more likely than U.S. residents to be unprotected. Individual risk and epidemic risk are reduced when vaccination campaigns reach all communities, including those with a high proportion of immigrants.

COMMON VACCINES

Measles, Mumps, and Rubella Vaccine

Since the measles, mumps, and rubella (MMR) vaccines were licensed, endemic rubella has been eliminated in the United States (CDC, 2005b), and mumps and rubella have decreased by more than 99%. To maintain this effective public health strategy, routine MMR vaccination should be administered to children at 12 to 15 months of age, with repeat dosing at 4 to 6 years of age (Atkinson, Gantt, Mayfield, et al., 2004). All health care workers should demonstrate immunity to these three viruses by one of the following: birth date before 1957, documented administration of two doses of vaccine, laboratory evidence of immunity, or documentation of physician-diagnosed measles or mumps.

---

5. Pneumococcal polysaccharide vaccination. *Medical indications:* chronic disorders of the pulmonary system (excluding asthma); cardiovascular diseases; diabetes mellitus; chronic liver diseases, including liver disease as a result of alcohol abuse (eg, cirrhosis); chronic renal failure or nephrotic syndrome; functional or anatomic asplenia (eg, sickle cell disease or splenectory [if elective splenectomy is planned, vaccinate at least 2 weeks before surgery]); immunosuppressive conditions (eg, congenital immunodeficiency, HIV infection [vaccinate as close to diagnosis as possible when CD4 cell counts are highest], leukemia, lymphoma, multiple myeloma, Hodgkin disease, generalized malignancy, or organ or bone marrow transplantation); chemotherapy with alkylating agents, antimetabolites, or long-term systemic corticosteroids; and cochlear implants. *Other indications:* Alaska Natives and certain American Indian populations; residents of nursing homes and other long-term—care facilities.

6. Revaccination with pneumococcal polysaccharide vaccine. One-time revaccination after 5 years for person with chronic renal failure or nephritic syndrome; functional or anatomic asplenia (eg, sickle cell disease or splenectomy); immunosuppressive conditions (eg, congenital immunodeficiency, HIV infection, leukemia, lymphoma, multiple myeloma, Hodgkin disease, generalized malignancy, or organ or bone marrow transplantation); or chemotherapy with alkylating agents, antimetabolites, or long-term systemic corticosteroids. For persons aged ≥65 years, one-time revaccination if they were vaccinated ≥5 years previously and were aged <65 years at the time of primary vaccination.

7. Hepatitis A vaccination. *Medical indications:* persons with clotting-factor disorders or chronic liver disease. *Behavioral indications:* men who have sex with men or users of illegal drugs. *Occupational indications:* Persons working with hepatitis A virus (HAV)–infected primate or with HAV in a research laboratory setting. *Other indications:* persons traveling to or working in countries that have high or intermediate endemicity of hepatitis A (for list of countries, see http://www.cdc.gov/travel/diseases.htm#hepa) as well as any person wishing to obtain immunity. Current vaccines should be administered in a 2-dose series at either 0 and 6–12 months, or 0 and 6–18 months. If the combined hepatitis A and hepatitis B vaccine is used, administer 3 doses at 0, 1, and 6 months.

8. Hepatitis B vaccination. *Medical indications:* hemodialysis patients (use special formulation [40 μg/mL] or two 20–μg/mL doses) or patients who receive clotting-factor concentrates. *Occupational indications:* health care workers and public-safety workers who have exposure to blood in the workplace and persons in training in schools of medicine, dentistry, nursing, laboratory technology, and other allied health professions. *Behavioral indications:* injection-drug users; persons with more than one sex partner during the previous 6 months; persons with a recently acquired sexually transmitted disease (STD); and men who have sex with men. *Other indications:* household contacts and sex partners or persons with chronic hepatitis B virus (HBV) infection; clients and staff members of institutions for developmentally disabled persons; all clients of STD clinics; inmates of correctional facilities; and international travelers who will be in countries with high or intermediate prevalence of chronic HBV infection for more than 6 months (for list of countries, see http://www.cdc.gov/travel/diseases.htm#hepa).

9. Meningococcal vaccination. *Medical indications:* adults with anatomic or functional asplenia or terminal complement component deficiencies. *Other indications:* first-year college students living in dormitories; microbiologists who are routinely exposed to isolates of *Neisseria meningitidis;* military recruits; and persons who travel to or reside in countries in which meningococcal disease is hyperendemic or epidemic (eg, the "meningitis belt" of sub-Saharan Africa during the dry season [December–June]), particularly if contact with local populations will be prolonged. Vaccination is required by the government of Saudi Arabia for all travelers to Mecca during the annual Hajj. Meningococcal conjugate vaccine is preferred for adults meeting any of the above indications who are aged ≤55 years, although meningococcal polysaccharide vaccine (MPSV4) is an acceptable alternative. Revaccination after 5 years might be indicated for adults previously vaccinated with MPSV4 who remain at high risk for infection (eg, persons residing in areas in which disease is epidemic).

10. Selected conditions for which *Haemophilus influenza* type b (Hib) vaccine may be used. Hib conjugate vaccines are licensed for children aged 6–71 months. No efficacy data are available on which to base a recommendation concerning use of Hib vaccine for older children and adults with the chronic conditions associated with an increased risk for Hib disease. However, studies suggest good immunogenicity in patients who have sickle cell disease, leukemia, or HIV infection or who have had splenectomies; administering vaccine to these patients is not contraindicated.

Patients should be advised that fever, transient lymphadenopathy, or hypersensitivity reaction might occur following an MMR vaccination. The risk of side effects is greater in vaccine recipients who have not previously received the vaccine than in those who have received repeat doses. Antipyretics may be used to decrease the risk of fever, but aspirin should be avoided in infants and children because of the risk for Reye's syndrome.

Varicella (Chickenpox) Vaccine

Varicella zoster is the virus that causes chickenpox and herpes zoster. In its natural state, the varicella virus attacks most people as children, causing disseminated disease in the form of chickenpox. This disease is often more severe in adults. Transmission occurs by the airborne and contact routes. With rare exception, varicella infects a person only once. The incubation period is about 2 weeks (range, 10 to 21 days). During a prodrome of general malaise (often noticed about 2 days before the rash develops), the newly infected host is capable of transmitting the virus to other susceptible contacts. Typically, the vesicular, pustular rash spreads rapidly from few to many lesions in a matter of hours. New lesion formation continues for 2 to 3 days, with lesions appearing at different stages throughout this time. By the fourth symptomatic day, the lesions begin to dry, and new lesions usually do not develop. Fever is common during the 4 to 6 days of rash progression. When the lesions have crusted, the patient is no longer contagious.

Herpes zoster, also known as shingles, is a localized rash caused by recurrent varicella. Vesicles are restricted to areas supplied by single associated nerve groups. Varicella may be transmitted from the rash of those with shingles to people who are susceptible to varicella. In May 2006, the FDA approved Zostavax, a vaccine to reduce the risk of shingles. In people over 60 years of age, the vaccine has been found to reduce the risk of shingles by approximately 50%.

The varicella vaccine was first recommended as part of the routine vaccine schedule in the United States in 1996. The vaccine is effective in preventing chickenpox in approximately 85% of people vaccinated and significantly reduces the severity in almost all those who get the disease despite vaccination (Atkinson et al., 2004). The vaccine should not be given to those who have depressed immune function, are pregnant, have received blood products in the past 6 months, or have demonstrated allergy to varicella vaccine.

Influenza Vaccine

Influenza is an acute viral respiratory disease that predictably and periodically causes worldwide epidemics known as pandemics. Epidemics occur every 2 to 3 years, with a highly variable degree of severity. Between 1990 and 1999, an estimated 36,000 deaths per year have been attributed to influenza or its sequelae (ie, pneumonia, cardiopulmonary collapse) (CDC, 2004b).

Each year, a new vaccine is composed of the three virus strains (two type A influenza strains and one type B influenza strain) considered most likely to occur in the coming season. When the presumed influenza agents have been correctly anticipated and included in that year's vaccine, the vaccine offers approximately 70% to 90% protection for healthy children and young adults. Although less effective in preventing disease in the elderly, it decreases the severity of illness in those who do become infected. In extended care facilities, the vaccine is approximately 80% effective in preventing death and 50% to 60% effective in preventing pneumonia or hospitalization (CDC, 2004b). The vaccine is administered as an injection with inactivated virus or as a nasal spray with live attenuated virus.

The Advisory Committee for Immunization Practices of the Public Health Service recommends annual influenza vaccinations for the following groups: people older than 50 years of age, children 6 to 23 months of age, pregnant women, residents of extended care facilities, and those with chronic medical diseases or disabilities. In addition, health care providers and household members of those in high-risk groups should receive the vaccine to reduce the risk of transmission to people vulnerable to influenza sequelae. Vaccine campaigns among health care workers and patients should be intensified when there is evidence of community influenza.

REPORTING PROBLEMS WITH VACCINES

Nurses should ask parents or adult vaccine recipients to provide information about any problems encountered after vaccination. As mandated by law, a Vaccine Adverse Event Reporting System (VAERS) form must be completed with the following information: type of vaccine received, timing of vaccination, onset of the adverse event, current illnesses or medication, history of adverse events after vaccination, and demographic information about the recipient. Forms are obtained by telephone (1-800-822-7967) or via the Internet (http://www.vaers.hhs.gov). The form can also be submitted online at http://secure.vaers.org/VaersDataEntryintro.htm.

CONTRAINDICATIONS TO VACCINES

Patients who have developed encephalopathy within 7 days of a previous diphtheria, tetanus, and pertussis (DTP) dose, and those who have developed anaphylaxis or other moderate or severe sequelae after a previous dose, should not receive further doses. DTP is often deferred for the child who previously developed a fever higher than 40°C (104°F) within 48 hours of vaccination or who had a seizure or developed a shock-like state within 3 days of previous vaccination. Live vaccines usually are contraindicated for patients or close contacts of patients with severe immunosuppression (eg, HIV infection, leukemia, lymphoma, generalized malignancy, significant corticosteroid use, or use of immunosuppressive medications to prevent transplant rejection). The MMR vaccine should not be administered to pregnant women.

Planning for an Influenza Pandemic

A pandemic is a global outbreak of a disease. For example, influenza caused three pandemics in the 20th century. In the United States, the disease caused more than 500,000 deaths in the 1918 "Spanish flu" pandemic, about 70,000 deaths in 1957 in the "Asian flu" pandemic, and about 34,000 deaths in 1968 in the "Hong Kong flu" pandemic.

There are many subtypes of influenza viruses that have pandemic potential because they constantly change within animals and secondarily within humans. As a result of these changes, essentially new viruses can "emerge" and can expose entire populations who are immunologically unprotected.

Influenza pandemics are likely to be more catastrophic than other anticipated public health problems because they last longer than other emergency events, they often occur in "waves," they deplete the available health care workforce, and they reduce the supply of medical equipment because of their widespread nature. Although public health experts cannot predict exactly when the next influenza pandemic will occur, they believe that it is just a matter of time until another one occurs. The severity cannot be accurately predicted, but models suggest that a medium-intensity pandemic could cause more than 200,000 deaths in the United States and quickly overwhelm the existing health care infrastructure. The CDC encourages all health care institutions to have a pandemic plan and to test the components of the plan regularly. A tool to help estimate the number of hospitalizations that will occur, the need for intensive care unit beds, and the need for ventilators can be found at http://www.cdc.gov/flu/flusurge.htm.

AVIAN INFLUENZA PANDEMIC

Avian influenza (bird flu) is an infection caused by influenza viruses that chiefly infect birds and poultry. The H5N1 strain (named for the characteristics of the viral surface proteins hemagglutinin and neuraminidase) is of particular concern. It has caused a number of outbreaks in poultry since 2003, and the increase seems to be ongoing as flocks of migratory birds have rapidly disseminated the virus throughout much of the world. While many avian influenza viruses are natural and nonpathogenic in birds, H5N1 is unusual because of its high mortality rate in birds and because it has shown a limited ability to be transmitted from a bird source to mammals, including humans. The human mortality rate for H5N1 avian influenza has been approximately 50%. The majority of human cases of H5N1 are attributed to direct contact with poultry, but there are rare instances that suggest occasional human-to-human transmission.

Scientists are especially concerned that avian influenza H5N1 may change, either through mutation or reassortment, to become easily transmitted from human to human. The mutation threat is that the virus could be naturally altered in a mammalian host. The reassortment threat is that a person could be coinfected with both the human strain and the avian strain, creating an essentially new strain with the pathogenicity of H5N1 and the transmissibility of the human influenza virus. In either scenario, if H5N1 were easily transmissible to humans, it would be likely to cause a severe pandemic because the human population has no immunity to the virus and because development of an appropriate vaccine would take too long to effectively stop the pandemic waves (CDC, 2006).

The symptoms associated with H5N1 avian influenza in humans have ranged from the symptoms typically seen with seasonal influenza (cough, fever, and muscle aches) to severe pneumonia and multiorgan failure. It is not yet clear whether the typical influenza antivirals (ie, oseltamivir and zanamivir) would be effective to treat humans infected with H5N1. However, these medications are being mass produced and stockpiled as part of a national strategy to prepare for the possibility of an H5N1 avian influenza pandemic. Simple infection control strategies using careful hand hygiene and masks will be especially important in an avian influenza pandemic. Health departments throughout the country are also planning how to implement isolation programs to keep symptomatic people away from schools and workplaces (CDC, 2006).

Home-Based Care of the Patient with an Infectious Disease

The nurse who cares for the patient with an infectious disease in the home should provide information about infection risk prevention to the patient, the family, and the caregiver (Chart 70-4). Recognizing that a health history may not identify all active or latent infections, the caregiver should carefully follow Standard Precautions in the home. The nurse should establish a work environment that facilitates hand disinfection and aseptic technique.

Family caregivers should receive an annual influenza vaccine. This is especially true if the caregiver or the patient is older than 50 years, has underlying cardiac or pulmonary disease, or has underlying immunosuppression.

CHART 70-4

HOME CARE CHECKLIST • Prevention of Infection in the Home Care Setting

At the completion of the home care instruction, the patient or caregiver will be able to:	Patient	Caregiver
• Demonstrate aseptic technique in the care of technical equipment such as intravenous catheter and indwelling urinary catheter.	✔	✔
• Demonstrate thorough hand hygiene after patient care. (Use alcohol-based disinfectant *or* handwashing.)	✔	✔
• Complies with antibiotic regimen (patient) or with completion of vaccination series (patient and caregiver).	✔	✔
• State the rationale for thoroughly cooking all foods and storing meat products separate from other food groups.	✔	✔
• Use separate eating utensils and towels.	✔	✔
• Avoid contact with someone who has a known infectious disease.	✔	✔

Patients requiring home care are often people with immunosuppression from underlying conditions, such as HIV infection or cancer, or those who have therapy-induced immunosuppression, as occurs with many antineoplastic agents. Careful assessment for signs of infection is important.

Reducing Risk to the Patient

Equipment Care

All caregivers must pay careful attention to disinfection and aseptic technique while using medical equipment. Catheter-related sepsis should be suspected in a patient who has unexplained fever, redness, swelling, and drainage around a vascular catheter insertion site.

Indwelling urinary catheters should be discontinued whenever possible, because each day of use increases the risk of infection. The nurse should promptly report signs of urinary tract infection or of generalized sepsis to the patient's physician.

Patient Teaching

When assessing the infectious risk of the immunosuppressed patient in the home environment, it is important to realize that intrinsic colonizing bacteria and latent viral infections present a greater risk than do extrinsic environmental contaminants. The patient and family need reassurance that their home should be clean but not sterile. Common-sense approaches to cleanliness and risk reduction are helpful.

For patients with neutropenia or with T-cell dysfunction (eg, patients with acquired immunodeficiency syndrome [AIDS]), it is wise to restrict visits of people with potentially contagious illnesses. The patient who is severely neutropenic should not eat uncooked fruits and vegetables. The immunosuppressed patient is vulnerable to acquiring bacterial infection with enteric pathogens from food; therefore, family members should be reminded about the need to follow recommendations for hygiene and safe cooking times and temperatures.

Reducing Risk to Household Members

Establishing reasonable barriers to infection transmission in the household is an important part of home care. The route of transmission of the organism in question must first be determined. The nurse can then teach household members strategies to reduce their risk of becoming infected. If the patient has active pulmonary TB, the public health department should be contacted to provide screening and treatment for family members. If the patient has shingles (herpes zoster), family members who have had varicella vaccine or who have previously had chickenpox are considered immune and need no precautions. However, if a family member is immunosuppressed or otherwise susceptible to varicella, maintaining physical separation may be an important strategy during the time when the patient has draining lesions. When the patient is infected with *Shigella, Salmonella, C. difficile,* hepatitis A, or other enteric organisms, the family should be reassured that common household disinfectants are effective in controlling environmental contamination.

Family members who assist in the care of a patient with a bloodborne infection such as HIV or hepatitis C can prevent transmission by carefully handling any sharp objects that are contaminated with blood. Family teaching may include discussion about the need for caution when shaving the patient; performing dressing changes; or administering any IV, intramuscular, or subcutaneous medication. To collect and dispose of used needles, syringes, and vascular access equipment, the family should use containers designed for sharps disposal. With the exception of TB, the opportunistic infections associated with AIDS do not usually pose a risk to the healthy family member. Family members should be reassured that dishes are safe to use after being washed with hot water and that linens and clothing are safe to use after being washed in a hot-water cycle.

Nursing Process

The Patient With an Infectious Disease

Assessment

The health history and physical examination and the use of diagnostic tests are important for determining the presence of infection and infectious diseases. Symptoms of infectious diseases vary significantly between and within diseases. For some infections, visible symptoms such as rash, redness, or swelling provide early warnings of infection. In other infections, such as TB and HIV, asymptomatic latency is prolonged, and infection must be determined through diagnostic procedures.

The goals of history taking are to establish the likelihood and probable source of infection as well as the degree of associated pathology and symptoms. The patient's previous medical record is reviewed when possible. In obtaining a health history, some of the following questions may be asked:

- Does the patient have a history of previous or recurrent infections?
- Has there been fever? How high has the patient's temperature been? What is the fever pattern? Is the temperature constant, or does it rise and fall? Has fever been associated with chills? Has the patient taken medication to relieve fever?
- Is there cough? Is the cough chronic or acute? Is it associated with shortness of breath? Does the cough produce sputum? Is the sputum bloody? Has the patient had a tuberculin skin test (TST) recently? If so, what were the results? Has the patient been given isoniazid (INH) prophylaxis for TB infection? Has the patient been treated for TB in the past?
- Is there pain? Where is the pain? What is the nature of the pain? Does the patient have sore throat, headache, myalgias, or arthralgias? Is there pain on urination or other activity?

- Is there edema? Is there drainage associated with the edema? Is the edematous area warm to touch?
- Is there a draining lesion? Is the drainage associated with trauma or a previous procedure? Is the drainage purulent or clear?
- Does the patient have diarrhea, vomiting, or abdominal pain?
- Is there rash? What is the nature of the rash—is it flat, raised, red, crusted, purulent, or lace-like?
- What is the patient's vaccination history?
- Has the patient taken medications that could induce rash?
- Has there been exposure to another person who has an identified infectious disease or rash?
- Has there been an insect or animal bite? Has there been an animal scratch or other exposure to pets, farm animals, or experimental animals?
- What medications are used? Have antibiotics been taken recently or long term? Is the patient being treated with corticosteroids, immunosuppressive agents, or chemotherapy?
- Is there a history of substance abuse?
- Has the patient been treated in the past for other infectious diseases? Has the patient been hospitalized for infectious diseases?
- If sexual history is pertinent, has there been sexual exposure to another person with a known sexually transmitted disease (STD)? Has the patient been treated for STDs in the past? Is the patient pregnant, or has she recently been pregnant? Has the patient been tested for HIV?
- Has the patient traveled to or from a developing country or abroad? What was the immunization or antimicrobial prophylaxis used for protection while traveling?
- What is the patient's occupation? What are the patient's recreational activities? Hobbies?

Because infection may occur in any body system, physical examination may reveal signs of infection at any body site. Generalized signs of chronic infection may include significant weight loss or pallor associated with anemia of chronic diseases. Acute infection may manifest with fever, chills, lymphadenopathy, or rash. Localized signs vary by source of infection. Purulent drainage, pain, edema, and redness are strongly associated with localized infection. Cough and shortness of breath may be caused by influenza, pneumonia, or TB, as well as many noninfectious causes.

Diagnosis

Nursing Diagnoses

Based on assessment data, the patient's major nursing diagnoses related specifically to infection may include the following:

- Risk for infection transmission
- Deficient knowledge about the disease, cause of infection, treatment, and prevention measures
- Risk for ineffective thermoregulation (fever) related to the presence of infection

Infection may interrupt the normal function of any affected body system. These system alterations can be found in the appropriate chapters.

Collaborative Problems/ Potential Complications

Based on the assessment data, potential complications that may develop include the following:

- Septicemia, bacteremia, or sepsis
- Septic shock
- Dehydration
- Abscess formation
- Endocarditis
- Infectious disease–related cancers
- Infertility
- Congenital abnormalities

Planning and Goals

Major goals for the patient may include prevention of spread of infection, increased knowledge about the infection and its treatment, control of fever and related discomforts, and absence of complications.

Nursing Interventions

Preventing Infection Transmission

Preventing the spread of infection requires an understanding of the usual routes of transmission of the organism. The hospitalized patient may pose a contagious risk to others if the disease is easily spread (such as *C. difficile*) or is spread through an airborne route (such as TB). In these situations, strict adherence to isolation measures is important in reducing the opportunity for spread. Preventing transmission of organisms from patient to patient usually requires participation of the health care team. Transmission of organisms on the hands and gloves of health care workers remains a common source of cross-infection in the hospital or clinic setting.

Nurses serve an important role in preventing the transfer of organisms in two ways. First, as the health professionals who often spend the most time with patients, nurses have a greater opportunity for spreading organisms. It is imperative that nurses disinfect their hands before and after contact with patients and after performing a potentially hand-contaminating activity. Hands must be disinfected each time gloves are removed. For example, the nurse who has performed endotracheal suctioning should remove the gloves, wash the hands, and put on a new pair of gloves before performing wound care on the same patient.

The second way that nurses reduce hand-to-hand spread is to serve as patient advocates. With the number of health care workers involved in patient care each day, there is a significant opportunity for breaks in hand-hygiene technique. To the degree feasible, the nurse should observe the hand-hygiene activities of other professionals and discuss with them any lapses in technique that are observed.

Teaching About the Infectious Process

Interruption of transmission requires diagnosis and patient compliance with the treatment regimen. The nurse's role is to educate the patient and, in some situations, to report the case to public health officials for contact tracing and verification of follow-up.

The nurse must stress the importance of immunization to parents of young children and to others for whom vaccines are recommended, such as patients who are elderly, are immunosuppressed, or have chronic illnesses or disabilities. Nurses should recognize their personal responsibility to receive the hepatitis B vaccine and an annual influenza vaccine to reduce potential transmission to themselves and vulnerable patient groups.

Infectious diseases often seem mysterious and frequently are socially stigmatizing. Patient teaching efforts require empathy and sensitivity. For example, in the past, TB was a stigmatizing disease. The nurse may need to provide core information to the patient who needs INH prophylaxis to promote understanding and allay guilt that the patient may feel.

Controlling Fever and Accompanying Discomforts

Fever must always be investigated to determine whether infection is the source. Evidence indicates that fever, mediated by the hypothalamus, may potentiate beneficial functions in the syndrome of reactions known as *acute-phase reaction.* These reactions include changes in liver protein synthesis; alterations in serum metals, such as iron; and increased production of certain classes of white blood cells and other cells of the immune system. Most fevers are physiologically controlled so that the temperature remains below 105.8°F (41°C). However, severe fever, as occurs with meningococcal meningitis, may cause heat stroke and other complications. Even milder fevers accompanied by fatigue, chills, and diaphoresis are often uncomfortable for the patient. Whether fever is treated or untreated, adequate fluid intake is important during febrile episodes.

NURSING ALERT

Because fever offers clues about infection severity and the success of antibiotic therapy, outpatients with fever should be taught to obtain accurate temperature readings. Frequently, parents know that a child has warm skin but do not disturb the child by taking a temperature reading. Body temperature information can be very helpful in adjusting therapy or in reevaluating a preliminary diagnosis.

Monitoring and Managing Potential Complications

The patient with a rapidly progressive infectious disease should have vital signs and level of consciousness closely monitored. X-ray findings and microbiologic, immunologic, hematologic, cytologic, and parasitologic laboratory values must be interpreted in the context of other clinical findings to assess the course of the infectious disease.

Antibiotic therapy is frequently complex, and modifications are necessary because of sensitivity test results and disease progression. It is important to initiate antibiotic therapy as soon as it is prescribed rather than waiting until routine medication scheduling times. This ensures that therapeutic blood levels can be attained as quickly as possible. The Plan of Nursing Care in Chart 70-5 describes nursing interventions for specific complications of infection.

Evaluation

Expected Patient Outcomes

Expected patient outcomes may include the following:

1. Uses appropriate methods to prevent the spread of infection
2. Acquires knowledge about the infectious process
3. Exhibits absence of elevated body temperature

Diarrheal Diseases

Diarrheal diseases, which are especially prevalent in the developing world, cause significant morbidity and mortality. Each year, diarrheal diseases kill about 2 million children younger than 5 years of age. The most important cause of death associated with these diseases is dehydration, and the most important treatment that decreases death rates is rehydration therapy (Guerrant, Kosek, Moore, et al., 2002).

In the United States, the epidemiology of diarrheal diseases is changing constantly. Water disinfection, pasteurization, and appropriate food packaging have decreased the incidence of diseases such as typhoid and cholera. However, importation of foreign foods, environmental and ecological changes, and changes in diagnostic test modalities have led to recognition of important new trends and outbreaks.

Transmission

The portal of entry of all diarrheal pathogens is oral ingestion. Although the food we eat is far from sterile, the high acidity of the stomach and the antibody-producing cells of the small bowel generally serve to decrease the potential of pathogens. Infection can occur when the infectious dose is high enough, or if the food neutralizes the acidic environment. Decreased gastric acidity with disruption of normal bowel flora (as occurs after surgery), use of antimicrobial agents, and the immune dysfunction of AIDS all decrease intestinal defenses.

(text continues on page 2501)

CHART 70-5

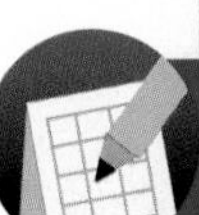

Plan of Nursing Care Care of the Patient With An Infectious Disease

Nursing Diagnosis: Risk for infection transmission
Goal: Prevention of transmission of infectious agents

NURSING INTERVENTIONS	RATIONALE	EXPECTED OUTCOMES
1. Prevent patient-to-patient infection spread.	1. Organisms that are spread through an airborne route or are very contagious through direct contact can be transmitted in a health care setting.	• No evidence of patient-to-patient transmission of infection • No evidence of transmission via health care workers • No occupationally acquired infections in nurses and other health care workers • No evidence of transmission due to contaminated equipment • Absence of bacteremia, septicemia, and sepsis • Absence of urinary tract infections • Absence of pneumonia
a. Provide isolation according to CDC guidelines and Standard Precautions.	a. CDC isolation strategies are developed to reduce the likelihood of transmission from patient to patient.	
b. Ensure that patients with airborne infections remain in private rooms during hospital stay. If they must leave their rooms, arrangements should be made to decrease the likelihood of contact with other patients. Rooms should be ventilated according to CDC criteria. Personal protective equipment in the form of N95 respirators should be worn as indicated. The N95 respirator is the minimal level of personal protection for tuberculosis control. The "N" indicates the filter resistance to oil aerosols; and the "95" indicates that the respirator has 95% effectiveness in filtering test particles (CDC, 1998c). In any care setting where patients may have increased risk for the sequelae of influenza, annual influenza vaccination should be encouraged for personnel and patients.	b. Engineering controls are important in the prevention of airborne diseases. Influenza vaccine safely reduces risk of illness associated with this highly communicable, and frequently virulent, condition.	
c. Ensure that patients with highly transmissible, nonairborne organisms such as *Clostridium difficile* and *Shigella* species are physically separated from other patients if hygiene or institutional policy dictates.	c. Increased prevention strategies are needed when the organism has high epidemic potential.	

continued >

CHART 70-5

Plan of Nursing Care — Care of the Patient With An Infectious Disease (Continued)

NURSING INTERVENTIONS	RATIONALE	EXPECTED OUTCOMES
2. Prevent health care workers' transfer of organisms from patient to patient.	2. Transfer of organisms on the hands of health care workers is a common route of transmission. Hospital organisms colonizing the hands of health care workers may be virulent.	
a. Perform hand hygiene (by hand washing or by use of alcohol-based solution) consistently and thoroughly, disinfecting hands before and after each patient contact, and after procedures that offer contamination risk while caring for an individual patient.	a. Hand hygiene is important in reducing transient flora on outer epidermal layers of skin. Alcohol-based hand disinfectants are effective methods to reduce transient flora.	
b. Use gloves when handling any body fluid from any patient. Change gloves between patient care activities, and disinfect hands after gloves are removed.	b. Gloves provide effective barrier protection. Gloves quickly become contaminated and then become a potential vehicle for the transfer of organisms between patients. Microflora on hands are likely to proliferate while gloves are worn.	
c. Avoid wearing artificial fingernails or extenders when providing patient care. Keep natural nails less than ¼ inch long.	c. Artificial fingernails and extenders harbor microorganisms.	
d. Monitor the hand hygiene and glove use behaviors of health care professionals caring for the patient.	d. Poor compliance with hand hygiene among health care workers has been well documented and should be anticipated. It is important for the nurse as the patient's advocate to communicate protective behavior.	
3. Prevent patient-to-health care worker transmission of infection.	3. Health care workers may acquire infections occupationally due to close contact with patients.	
a. Avoid risk of infection with tuberculosis.	a. The most important element in the reduction of tuberculosis is early identification. Many of the symptoms of tuberculosis are subtle, and may be first observed by the nurse who has prolonged contact with the patient.	

CHART 70-5

Plan of Nursing Care Care of the Patient With An Infectious Disease (Continued)

NURSING INTERVENTIONS	RATIONALE	EXPECTED OUTCOMES
(1) Participate in the early identification of patients with active disease. Patients will be asked about risk factors, symptoms, previous exposure, and TST status.	(1) Identification of patients at risk can help to prevent exposure.	
(2) Expedite diagnostic work-up with chest x-ray, sputum analysis for organisms, and TST administration as appropriate.	(2) Confirmation of diagnosis facilitates development of an appropriate treatment plan, including prevention of spread of infection.	
(3) Maintain engineering controls. Keep the patient in a private room with a closed door.	(3) Confining airflow to the immediate vicinity of the patient and exhausting air to the outside reduce the likelihood of transmission to health care workers in areas outside of the patient room.	
(4) Use protection in isolation room or when participating in procedures that are likely to generate cough, such as suctioning, intubation, or administering nebulized medications.	(4) N95 respirators are designed to reduce health care workers' risk.	
b. Avoid risk of transmission of blood-borne diseases such as hepatitis B, hepatitis C, and the human immunodeficiency virus.	b. Health care workers can contract blood-borne diseases via percutaneous injury such as needlestick or by contact with blood or body fluids to mucous membranes, such as eyes and mouth.	
(1) Get hepatitis B vaccination.	(1) Hepatitis B vaccine should be administered to reduce risk from this contagious bloodborne virus.	
(2) Use Standard Precautions as defined by the CDC.	(2) Standard Precautions are based on the recognition that most patients are not identified as infected by physical assessment or history taking. Health care workers must	

continued >

CHART 70-5

Plan of Nursing Care Care of the Patient With An Infectious Disease (Continued)

NURSING INTERVENTIONS	RATIONALE	EXPECTED OUTCOMES
	assume that all patients may be infected with bloodborne or other infection and must use barrier precautions appropriately for *all* patients.	
(3) Use "needleless" syringes and other injury-preventing devices.	(3) Use of injury-preventing devices decreases risk of transmission of bloodborne diseases.	
c. Avoid risk of airborne diseases. (1) Get influenza vaccination annually. (2) Get vaccinated or produce proof of immunity to measles, mumps, rubella, and varicella.	c. Influenza vaccine is recommended for health care workers to reduce the likelihood of transmission in health care settings where immunocompromised patients can be exposed.	
4. Prevent patient exposure to contaminated medical equipment.	4. Technologic advances offer increased opportunity for invasive procedures. Equipment may be complex and difficult to clean.	
a. Ensure that equipment that is inserted through intact skin is sterilized between patient uses.	a. Sterilization renders equipment free of all microorganisms.	
b. Ensure that equipment that has contact with mucous membranes is sterilized or receives "high-level disinfection" between patient uses.	b. High-level disinfection renders an object free of all microorganisms with the possible exception of spore-producing organisms.	
c. Ensure that equipment used against intact skin is thoroughly cleaned and receives "low-level disinfection" between patient uses.	c. The disinfection goal for low-level disinfection is to reduce the load of microorganisms to a level that is not threatening to the host with intact skin.	
5. Follow established guidelines for the routine removal and replacement of intravenous devices.	5. Indwelling intravenous devices can serve as a conduit for organisms to migrate into the bloodstream.	
6. Remove urinary catheters at the earliest time possible.	6. The risk of urinary tract infections is directly proportional to the length of time that a urinary catheter remains in place.	
7. Remove endotracheal and nasogastric tubes as soon as possible.	7. The risk for pneumonia is increased as the use of indwelling equipment increases.	

CHART 70-5

Plan of Nursing Care — Care of the Patient With An Infectious Disease (Continued)

Nursing Diagnosis: Deficient knowledge about disease, cause of infection, and preventive measures
Goal: Acquisition of knowledge about the infectious process

NURSING INTERVENTIONS	RATIONALE	EXPECTED OUTCOMES
1. Listen carefully to what the patient says about illness and previous treatment.	1. Listening facilitates detection of misunderstanding and misinformation and provides opportunity for education.	• Patient actively participates in treatment • Patient complies with infection control measures
2. Provide pertinent explanations about: a. Organism and route of transmission b. Treatment goals c. Follow-up schedule d. Prevention of transmission to others	2. Knowledge about specific diagnoses and treatments may increase compliance.	
3. Allow opportunities for questions and discussions.	3. The patient's questions indicate issues that need clarification.	
4. Teach the patient and family about: a. Prophylaxis or immunization, if recommended b. Community resources, if necessary c. Means of preventing transmission within the home	4. Understanding of the risks and precautions associated with an infectious disease may reduce the opportunity for further spread.	

Nursing Diagnosis: Risk for imbalanced body temperature (fever) related to the presence of infection
Goal: Patient comfort and return of normal temperature

NURSING INTERVENTIONS	RATIONALE	EXPECTED OUTCOMES
1. Monitor temperature, pulse, and respirations at regular intervals.	1. Graph fever curve to help evaluate when fever occurs, how long it lasts, and whether it responds to therapy.	• Body temperature within normal limits • Maintenance of fluid and electrolyte balance • Patient comfortable

continued >

CHART 70-5

Plan of Nursing Care — Care of the Patient With An Infectious Disease (Continued)

Collaborative Problems: Among potential complications are septicemia, bacteremia, or sepsis, septic shock, dehydration, abscess formation, endocarditis, infectious disease–related cancers, and infertility.
Goal: Absence of complications

NURSING INTERVENTIONS	RATIONALE	EXPECTED OUTCOMES
Septicemia, Bacteremia, Sepsis		
1. Monitor patient for evidence of infection at any location.	1. Vigilance for bacterial or fungal infection at any site promotes early recognition and treatment and reduces the likelihood of secondary infections.	• No episode of infection • Effective treatment of identified bacterial and fungal infections without progression to bloodstream infection • Early improvement in septic course
2. Assess treatment effectiveness of all identified infections.	2. The natural course of some infections may be rapid unless antibiotics are administered promptly.	
3. Administer antibiotics as prescribed with first dose given at the earliest time possible.	3. Prompt treatment will improve outcomes.	
Septic Shock		
1. Routinely, and as warranted, monitor vital signs for patients with recognized infections and severely immunosuppressed patients at risk for shock. In particular, be alert for signs of: a. Fever b. Tachycardia (more than 90 bpm) c. Tachypnea (more than 20 breaths/min) d. Evidence of decreased perfusion or dysfunction of vital organs in the form of (1) Change of mental status (2) Hypoxemia as measured by arterial blood gases (3) Elevated lactate levels (4) Urine output (less than 30 mL/h)	1. Early recognition of the signs and prompt treatment of impending shock may reduce the associated severity or mortality.	• Absence of symptoms of septic shock • Hemodynamic and respiratory status within normal range
2. Administer antibiotics, fluid replacement, vasopressors, and oxygen as prescribed.	2. Therapeutic maintenance of hemodynamic and respiratory status is necessary until infection is effectively treated with antimicrobial regimen.	

CHART 70-5

Plan of Nursing Care — Care of the Patient With An Infectious Disease (Continued)

NURSING INTERVENTIONS	RATIONALE	EXPECTED OUTCOMES
Dehydration		
1. Assess for dehydration (thirst, dryness of mucous membranes, loss of skin turgor, reduced peripheral pulses, urine output less than 30 mL/h).	1. Signs of dehydration provide a basis for fluid replacement and suggest possible further complications of circulatory collapse.	• Attains fluid balance (output approximates intake: body weight unchanged) • Mucous membranes appear moist; normal skin turgor • Serum electrolytes are within normal limits
2. Monitor weight.	2. Rapid changes in weight indicate fluid volume changes.	
3. Monitor intake and output and serum electrolyte levels.	3. Dehydration produces a deficit in some electrolytes. Decreased urine production may indicate hypovolemia and decreased renal perfusion.	
4. Replace fluids as needed. If the patient can tolerate oral fluids, offer fluids every 2–4 hours. Administer intravenous fluids as prescribed.	4. When possible, oral hydration is preferable because the patient can select the beverage, control the rate and interval of replacement, and care for self at home. Additionally, the risks associated with vascular devices are avoided. If intravenous fluid is required, intravenous solutions are selected to facilitate intestinal reabsorption of fluid and electrolytes.	
Abscess Formation		
1. Assess vascular access sites, wound sites, pressure ulcers, and other appropriate sites for apparent collections of purulent material.	1. Collections of purulent material often require drainage before antimicrobial therapy is effective.	• Absence of abscess • Takes antibiotics as prescribed.
2. Assess the patient who has had abdominal surgery or trauma to abdominal area for localized signs of intra-abdominal abscess. These signs include: a. Low-grade fever b. Elevated peripheral white blood cell count c. Localized pain d. Abdominal tenderness e. Visible or palpable mass f. Postoperative diarrhea g. GI bleeding	2. Intra-abdominal abscess formation is most common following traumatic or surgical disruption of the GI tract. Signs are often initially subtle.	

continued >

CHART 70-5

Plan of Nursing Care — Care of the Patient With An Infectious Disease (Continued)

NURSING INTERVENTIONS	RATIONALE	EXPECTED OUTCOMES
3. Assess patient who has had percutaneous abscess drainage to determine whether drainage has been successful. Be alert for all of the above signs and symptoms.	3. After percutaneous drainage, recurrent or persistent signs of abscess may indicate the need for surgical treatment.	
4. Administer antibiotics as prescribed	4. Antibiotics, along with drainage, are the most important elements of intra-abdominal abscess management.	
Endocarditis		
Prevention		
1. Teach patients with the following conditions about the importance of antibiotic prophylaxis for events and procedures that may introduce the risk of endocarditis: a. Valvular disease b. Congenital heart disease c. Intracardiac prosthesis d. Previous endocarditis	1. Patients with underlying valvular disease and other cardiac abnormalities are at increased risk for "seeding" of the cardiac valves during procedures that can cause bacteremia.	• Informs health care professionals of cardiac conditions that require antibiotic prophylaxis before invasive procedures • Takes prophylactic antibiotics as prescribed
Management		
1. Obtain blood cultures as prescribed; carefully record results. Note persistent bloodstream infections with a particular organism.	1. A definitive diagnosis of endocarditis requires blood culture confirmation.	• Endocarditis is diagnosed, treated, and cured.
2. Obtain a detailed history about the duration of fever in the absence of well-recognized cause.	2. Endocarditis should be suspected in patients who report an unexplained fever of more than 1 week's duration	
3. Administer intravenous antibiotic therapy at prescribed time schedule.	3. Intravenous therapy is usually required for cure. The goal of therapy is complete eradication of all organisms. Careful adherence to following the scheduled administration is therefore essential.	

Infectious Disease-Related Cancers and Infertility

These potential complications of infectious diseases are prevented by primary avoidance of infection. Management of them is directed toward treating each of them as a non-infectious entity. For example, the management of cancer secondary to hepatitis B is handled as an oncology issue, not as an infectious disease issue.

Causes

There are many bacterial, viral, and parasitic causes of diarrheal diseases. Common causes of bacterial infection include *Escherichia coli* and *Salmonella, Shigella, Campylobacter,* and *Yersinia* species. The most significant viral causes of diarrhea are *Rotavirus,* which commonly results in diarrhea in young children, and *Calcivirus* (often called *Norovirus*), a virus associated with outbreaks in long-term care facilities and cruise ships. Parasitic infections of importance include *Giardia* and *Cryptosporidium* species and *Entamoeba histolytica.*

Campylobacter Infections

Campylobacter species are the most frequent cause of diarrheal disease worldwide. The bacterium, which is abundant in animal foods, is especially common in poultry but can also be found in beef and pork. Direct person-to-person transmission appears to be less common than in other enteric pathogens, such as *Shigella.* Guillain-Barré syndrome, a neurologic disorder characterized by temporary paralysis, is a complication of approximately 1 of 1000 cases of *Campylobacter* infection.

Cooking and storing food at appropriate temperatures protects against *Campylobacter.* It is important that kitchen utensils used in meat preparation be kept away from other food to prevent *Campylobacter* transmission.

After a person is infected, the bacterium directly attacks the lumen of the intestine and may cause disease through enterotoxin release. Symptoms can range from mild abdominal cramping and minimal diarrhea to severe disease with profuse watery bloody diarrhea and debilitating abdominal cramping. Antimicrobial therapy is recommended only for patients who are seriously ill (CDC, 2005c).

Salmonella Infection

Salmonella is a gram-negative bacillus with many species, including the very pathogenic *Salmonella typhi* (ie, typhoid fever). Of the nontyphi species, most organisms are prevalent in animal food sources. *Salmonella* species contaminate more than 50% of commercially available chicken products and are frequently found in eggs (intact and with broken shells), in raw milk, and occasionally in beef (Crump, Griffin, & Angulo, 2002). Approximately 40% of the deaths caused by *Salmonella* occur in nursing home residents. The high mortality rate reflects the seriousness of the infection in the elderly, who often have weakened immune systems (CDC, 2000a).

Variable symptoms are associated with *Salmonella* species infection, including an asymptomatic carrier state, gastroenteritis, and systemic infection. Diarrhea with gastroenteritis is common. Disseminated disease and bacteremia, sometimes accompanied by diarrhea, are less common.

The person with *Salmonella*-caused diarrhea can be a source for transmission to others. The importance of good hygiene should be emphasized, and health care workers should use special care when handling bedpans, stool specimens, or other objects that may be contaminated with feces. Hand hygiene is imperative after any contact with a person with *Salmonella* diarrhea. Although patients with systemic salmonellosis require antimicrobial therapy, those with gastroenteritis only are not usually treated, because antibiotic use may increase the period of time that the patient carries the bacteria while not improving the clinical outcome.

Shigella Infection

The *Shigella* species is a gram-negative organism that invades the lumen of the intestine and causes disease and severe watery (possibly bloody) diarrhea. *Shigella* species are spread through the fecal–oral route, with easy transmission from one person to another. *Shigella* exhibits high levels of **virulence** (degree of pathogenicity of an organism); infection with a very small number of organisms can cause disease. Because transmission occurs easily with improper hygiene, it is not surprising that *Shigella* organisms disproportionately affect pediatric populations. Disease in the very young may infrequently be complicated by pulmonary or neurologic symptoms.

Antimicrobial therapy should be instituted early. Frequently, initial therapy choices must be altered when final microbiologic testing reveals the organism's sensitivity.

Escherichia coli

E. coli is the most common aerobic organism colonizing the large bowel. When *E. coli* bacteria are cultured from fecal specimens, the results usually reflect normal flora. However, certain strains of *E. coli* with increased virulence have been responsible for significant outbreaks of diarrheal disease in recent years. These stronger pathologic strains are subgrouped as enterotoxigenic *E. coli* (ETEC) because of their production of enterotoxins. ETEC strains often cause cholera-like disease, with rapid, severe dehydration and an increased risk of death.

Several recent outbreaks of an *E. coli* species, 0157:H7, have been linked to the ingestion of undercooked beef. This bacterium lives in the intestines of cattle and can be introduced into meat at the time of slaughter. Prevention of disease from *E. coli* 0157:H7 is aimed at teaching the public to cook ground beef thoroughly (ie, until the meat is no longer pink and the juices run clear).

Calcivirus (Norwalk-like Virus; Norovirus)

Calcivirus, which is often referred to as the Norwalk-like virus or the *Norovirus,* is a very common cause of foodborne illness. This agent has been associated with important diarrheal outbreaks in long-term care facilities, hospitals, and cruise ships. Onset of illness is usually acute, with vomiting and watery diarrhea that generally last for approximately 2 days. Dehydration is the most common complication.

Calcivirus is transmitted easily from person to person by direct contact and by ingesting contaminated food. Water-borne outbreaks have been associated with sewage-contaminated wells and with contaminated swimming pools. Although people with *Calcivirus* infection typically recover within 2 to 3 days, they may continue to transmit the virus to others for approximately 2 more weeks.

In the past, because of the poor availability of laboratory tests, most cases of *Calcivirus* were not diagnosed. However, in recent years, public health laboratories have improved their ability to diagnose *Calcivirus* by using reverse transcriptase polymerase chain reaction (RT-PCR) tests. These tests can confirm the presence of the virus from stool, emesis, or environmental samples.

Calciviruses can withstand environmental extremes of heat or cold and are resistant to chemical disinfection, which are significant reasons for their epidemic potential. Control of *Calcivirus* in health care facilities requires a coordinated program with decisions about isolation, environmental disinfection, diagnosis, and coordination with public health officials. Contact precautions should be used when caring for patients with incontinence and during outbreaks of the virus. Workers should wear masks if they are cleaning heavily soiled areas, or caring for a patient who is actively vomiting. No Environmental Protection Agency (EPA)–approved disinfectants have specific claims about effectiveness for *Calcivirus*. Therefore, the CDC recommends that surface disinfection be accomplished with a freshly prepared solution of 1 part bleach to 50 parts water or with the peroxygen compound Virkon-S, which has been approved for feline *Calcivirus* and may be similarly effective for human viruses. The CDC guide, *Norovirus in Healthcare Facilities—April 2005,* is available at www.cdc.gov/ncidod/dhqp/id_norovirusFS.htm (CDC, 2005d).

Giardia lamblia

Transmission of the protozoan *Giardia lamblia* occurs when food or drink is contaminated with viable cysts of the organism. People often become infected while traveling to endemic areas or by drinking contaminated water from mountain streams within the United States. The organism can be transmitted by close contact, as occurs in day care settings. Transmission by sexual contact has also been documented.

Frequently, the infection goes unnoticed. Infection is often recognized more easily in children than in adults. In extreme cases, the patient may experience abdominal pain and chronic diarrhea, usually described as containing mucus and fat but not blood. Microscopic examination of stool specimens reveals the trophozoite or cyst stages of the parasitic life cycle.

Metronidazole (Flagyl) is commonly used to treat *Giardia,* but success rates for this and alternative therapies are inconsistent. Patients with *Giardia* infections should be instructed that the organism can be easily transmitted in family or group settings. Personal hygiene measures should be reinforced, and those who travel or camp where water is not treated and filtered should be advised to avoid local water supplies unless water is purified before drinking or using it in cooking.

Vibrio cholerae

Although reported cases of cholera have been rare in the United States in recent decades, no discussion of infectious diarrhea is complete without mention of this very serious infectious disease. Historically, epidemics of cholera have influenced all aspects of life—from medical to political—and infection rates have been significant enough to destroy governments and armies. Cholera is always a concern when wars or natural disasters result in inadequately processed waste water. *Vibrio cholerae* also may be found naturally in brackish rivers and coastal waters.

V. cholerae is a gram-negative organism with several different serotypes. The type usually associated with epidemics is toxigenic *V. cholerae* 01. The organism is transmitted by contaminated food or water. Most recent cases in the United States have been from contaminated shellfish found in the Gulf of Mexico or from contaminated shellfish brought into the United States by visitors.

Cholera causes disease with a very rapid onset of copious diarrhea in which up to 1 L of fluid per hour can be lost. Dehydration, with subsequent cardiopulmonary collapse, may cause rapid progression from onset of signs and symptoms to death. The principal therapy is rehydration. Rehydration efforts should be vigorous and sustained. If oral rehydration cannot be accomplished, the patient needs IV therapy.

In the United States, cholera should be suspected in patients who have watery diarrhea after eating shellfish harvested from the Gulf of Mexico. Confirmation of the causative organism can be made by stool culture. It is imperative that all cases are reported to local and state public health authorities. People traveling to areas where cholera occurs regularly should remember the simple rule of thumb: "boil it, cook it, peel it, or forget it."

Nursing Process

The Patient With Infectious Diarrhea

Assessment

The most important element of assessment in the patient with diarrhea is to determine hydration status. The goal of rehydration is to correct the dehydration. Assessment includes evaluation for thirst, dryness of oral mucous membranes, sunken eyes, a weakened pulse, and loss of skin turgor. Careful observation for these signs is especially important in cases of rapidly dehydrating diseases (most notably cholera) and in younger children.

Intake and output measurements are crucial in determining fluid balance. Liquid stool should be measured and recorded, along with the frequency of stools. It is important to note the consistency and appearance of stool as key indicators of the type and severity of the diarrheal disease. The presence of mucus or blood should also be documented.

When conducting a health history, the nurse asks if the patient has recently traveled, if the patient is being treated with antibiotics, if the patient has been in contact with anyone who has recently had diarrheal disease, and what the patient has recently eaten. Frequently, patients attribute the most recent meal eaten as the cause of symptoms. However, the incubation period for most diarrheal conditions is longer than the time interval between meals, and the nurse needs to get detailed information about the meal preceding the illness and about all food intake in the previous 3 to 4 days. When eliciting this kind of history, it is helpful to ask the patient to list every food tasted. The nurse also asks the patient if he or she is employed in a food preparation service, because the local public health departments should be notified about any person with infectious diarrhea who works in the food industry.

Diagnosis

Nursing Diagnoses

Based on the assessment data, the patient's major nursing diagnoses may include the following:

- Deficient fluid volume related to fluid lost through diarrhea
- Deficient knowledge about the infection and the risk of transmission to others

Collaborative Problems/ Potential Complications

Based on the assessment data, potential complications that may develop include the following:

- Bacteremia
- Hypovolemic shock

Planning and Goals

The most important goals are maintenance of fluid and electrolyte balance, increased knowledge about the disease and risk of transmission, and absence of complications.

Nursing Interventions

Correcting Dehydration Associated with Diarrhea

The patient is assessed to determine the degree of dehydration. This assessment helps determine the amount and route of rehydration needed. Oral rehydration therapy is a strategy used to reduce the severe complications of diarrheal disease regardless of causative agent. It is inexpensive and effective for most patients, but it is often underused because of sustained cultural beliefs discouraging oral intake during episodes of diarrhea. After much refinement of the formula, the World Health Organization (WHO) and the United Nations International Children's Emergency Fund (UNICEF) agreed on the makeup of a single solution for the treatment of dehydration and electrolyte imbalance associated with cholera and other forms of diarrheal disease. The solution contains (in millimoles per liter) sodium, 90; potassium, 20; chloride, 80; citrate, 10; and glucose, 111.

MILD DEHYDRATION

The patient exhibits dry oral mucous membranes of the mouth and increased thirst. The rehydration goal at this level of dehydration is to deliver about 50 mL of oral rehydration solution (ORS) per 1 kg of weight over a 4-hour interval.

MODERATE DEHYDRATION

Common findings are sunken eyes, loss of skin turgor, increased thirst, and dry oral mucous membranes. The rehydration goal at this level of dehydration is to deliver about 100 mL/kg of ORS over 4 hours.

SEVERE DEHYDRATION

The patient with severe dehydration shows signs of shock (ie, rapid thready pulse, cyanosis, cold extremities, rapid breathing, lethargy, or coma) and should receive IV replacement until hemodynamic and mental status return to normal. When improvement is evident, the patient can be treated with ORS.

Administering Rehydration Therapy

In the United States, commercially available preparations, such as CeraLyte, Pedialyte, and Oralyte, have been effective fluid and electrolyte replacements for children with viral diarrheal disorders common in this country. However, when diarrheal losses are very high (>10 mL/kg per hour), the lower sodium concentrations of these formulas make them less appropriate than the WHO formula.

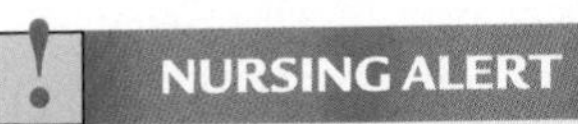

Sports drinks do not replace fluid losses correctly and should not be used.

For the hospitalized child, diarrheal fluid loss should be weighed, and ORS should be administered at a rate of 1 mL for each gram of diarrheal stool. Stool losses can be estimated so that the patient receives about 10 mL/kg of ORS for each diarrheal stool.

It is important for children and adults with acute diarrheal symptoms to maintain caloric intake. Recommended foods include starches, cereals, yogurt, fruits, and vegetables. Foods that are high in simple sugars, such as undiluted apple juice or gelatin, should be avoided.

Because diarrheal episodes are often accompanied by vomiting, rehydration and refeeding can be difficult. Oral rehydration therapy should be delivered frequently in small amounts. When they are persistently vomiting, small children often require frequent administration of fluids by spoonfuls rather than by drinking from a bottle or a cup. IV therapy is necessary for the patient who is severely dehydrated or in shock.

Increasing Knowledge and Preventing Spread of Infection

Public health nurses, school nurses, and others who are involved in patient teaching should emphasize principles of safe food preparation, with special attention to meat preparation and cooking. Ground beef should be cooked until no longer pink, and all meat should be maintained at temperatures below 40°F or above 140°F. In planning events for groups of people, adequate provision for storage and reheating to temperature thresholds is important. When preparing food, it is important to use different surfaces, knives, and other equipment for meat and nonmeat items.

Diarrheal diseases discussed in this section must be reported to local or state health departments. The goal of reporting is to provide information for determining incidence trends and promptly identifying any restaurants or other food preparation establishments that have served contaminated food.

The need for rehydration and refeeding should be taught to parents of children with diarrheal disease. Beliefs about illness and food patterns may have a traditional or cultural basis, and any teaching of health facts requires cultural sensitivity.

In both homes and health care delivery settings, good hygiene and principles of Standard Precautions should be emphasized.

Monitoring and Managing Potential Complications

BACTEREMIA

E. coli, Salmonella, and *Shigella* are organisms that can enter the bloodstream and disseminate to other organs. Blood cultures are necessary in the acutely febrile patient with diarrhea. If initial smear results reveal gram-negative organisms, antibiotic therapy is instituted.

HYPOVOLEMIC SHOCK

Shock associated with diarrheal diseases demands accurate intake and output assessment and vigorous fluid replacement. In rare instances, patients with severe fluid imbalance require intensive care nursing support with aggressive hemodynamic monitoring. For further information, see Chapter 15.

Evaluation

Expected Patient Outcomes

Expected patient outcomes may include the following:

1. Attains fluid balance
   a. Output approximates intake
   b. Mucous membranes appear moist
   c. Skin turgor is normal
   d. Adequate amounts of fluids and calories ingested
   e. Absence of vomiting
   f. Stools are of normal color and consistency
2. Acquires knowledge and understanding about infectious diarrhea and transmission potential
   a. Takes proper precautions to prevent spread of infection to others
   b. Describes principles and techniques of safe food storage, preparation, and cooking
3. Absence of complications
   a. Temperature is within normal range
   b. Blood culture reports are negative
   c. Fluid balance is achieved

Sexually Transmitted Diseases (STD)

An STD (also known as a sexually transmitted infection [STI]) is a disease acquired through sexual contact with an infected person. Table 70-4 identifies diseases that can be classified as STDs. Infections caused by organisms not generally considered STDs can also be transmitted during sexual contact, eg, *G. lamblia,* usually associated with contaminated water, can be transmitted through sexual exposure.

STDs are the most common infectious diseases in the United States and are epidemic in most parts of the world. Portals of entry of STD-causing microorganisms and sites of infection include the skin and mucosal linings of the urethra, cervix, vagina, rectum, and oropharynx.

Approximately 19 million Americans become infected with STDs annually. STDs have severe health consequences. In addition, they represent a financial burden estimated to be as high as $15.5 billion per year (CDC, 2004h). To determine the most effective methods for communicating information about STDs to people between 25 and 45 years of age (those who are most at risk for STDS), the CDC sought the help of focus groups. These groups proposed that using straightforward language and personal testimonials, developing materials for targeted audiences (eg, people who want information about protecting themselves), and conducting presentations in trusted establishments (eg, churches, health care facilities) might be effective. These suggestions could serve as a resource to all health care personnel who specialize in the prevention of STDs (CDC, 2004i).

TABLE 70-5 Conditions Classified as Sexually Transmitted Diseases (STDs) and Their Routes of Transmission

Disease	Route(s) of Transmission
Chancroid, *Lymphogranuloma venereum,* and *Granuloma inguinale*	Sexual
Chlamydia	Sexual
Cytomegalovirus (CMV)	Sexual, less intimate contact
Gonorrhea	Sexual, perinatal
Hepatitis B (HBV)	Sexual, percutaneous, perinatal
Hepatitis C (HCV)	Percutaneous, probably sexual, probably perinatal
Herpes simplex	Sexual
HIV infection/AIDS	Sexual, percutaneous, perinatal
Human papillomavirus (HPV)	Sexual
Syphilis	Sexual, perinatal

Education about prevention of STDs includes information about risk factors and behaviors that can lead to infection. Included in this education is information about the relative value of condoms in reducing risk of infection. The use of a condom to provide a protective barrier from transmission of STD-related organisms has been broadly promoted, especially since the recognition of HIV/AIDS. At first referred to as a method to ensure *safe sex*, the use of condoms has been shown to reduce but not eliminate the risk of transmission of HIV and other STDs. Thus, the term *safer sex* more appropriately connotes the public health message to be used when promoting the use of condoms.

STDs provide a unique set of challenges for nurses, physicians, and public health officials. Because of perceived stigma and possible threat to emotional relationships, people with symptoms of STDs are often reluctant to seek health care in a timely fashion. Similar to many other infectious diseases, STDs may progress without symptoms. A delay in diagnosis and treatment is potentially harmful because the risk of complications for the infected person and the risk of transmission to others increase over time.

Infection with one STD suggests the possibility of infection with other diseases as well. After one STD is identified, diagnostic evaluation for others should be performed. The possibility of HIV infection should be pursued when any STD is diagnosed.

Human Immunodeficiency Virus

HIV is the causative agent of AIDS. The definition of AIDS, as determined by the CDC, sets a point in the continuum of HIV pathogenesis in which the host has clinically demonstrated profound immune dysfunction. Since 1993, the AIDS definition has also included a CD4-positive (CD4+) cell count of less than 200 cells/mm^3 as a threshold criterion. CD4+ cells are a subset of lymphocytes and one of the targets of HIV infection. Many opportunistic infections and neoplasms serve as more qualitative markers of immunosuppression severity.

HIV is transmitted through sexual contact or percutaneous injection of contaminated blood, or perinatally from infected mother to fetus. Most people infected by the percutaneous route are IV or injecting drug users who share contaminated needles, but transmission is also remotely possible through contaminated blood transfusion. Since 1985, all blood transfusions have been screened, and transfusion-related transmission of HIV is now extremely unlikely. Additional information about HIV is provided in Chapter 52.

Risk to Health Care Workers

Health care workers can be infected through the percutaneous route if needlestick or other injury from a sharp object introduces contaminated blood. Prospective studies of this risk demonstrate that less than 1% of such occupational exposures (in which the source patient is infected with HIV) lead to transmission (CDC, 2001a). Despite the rarity of transmission, health care workers are advised to take extreme care to avoid needlestick or mucous membrane exposure to blood from all patients. Needlesticks and percutaneous injuries are the most frequently reported exposure for those rare employees who have had occupationally acquired infection (Do, Ciesielski, Metler, et al., 2003). Employers in health care facilities are required to provide devices designed to reduce the risk of needlestick and other injuries. Since 1996, the CDC has recommended postexposure prophylaxis for significant occupational exposures to HIV. Counseling about the advisability of prophylaxis, appropriate combination of drugs, and dosing should be made on a case-by-case basis. Table 70-5 provides the recommended algorithm to determine which combination of antiretroviral agents should be offered to the exposed health care worker. All health care workers should understand the need to report a needlestick or other percutaneous exposure immediately.

Syphilis

Syphilis is an acute and chronic infectious disease caused by the spirochete *Treponema pallidum*. It is acquired through sexual contact or may be congenital in origin.

Stages of Syphilis

In the untreated person, the course of syphilis can be divided into three stages: primary, secondary, and tertiary. These stages reflect the time from infection and the clinical manifestations observed in that period and are the basis for treatment decisions.

Primary syphilis occurs 2 to 3 weeks after initial inoculation with the organism. A painless lesion at the site of infection is called a *chancre*. Untreated, these lesions usually resolve spontaneously within about 2 months.

Secondary syphilis occurs when the hematogenous spread of organisms from the original chancre leads to generalized infection. The rash of secondary syphilis occurs about 2 to 8 weeks after the chancre and involves the trunk and the extremities, including the palms of the hands and the soles of the feet. Transmission of the organism can occur through contact with these lesions. Generalized signs of infection may include lymphadenopathy, arthritis, meningitis, hair loss, fever, malaise, and weight loss.

After the secondary stage, there is a period of **latency**, when the infected person has no signs or symptoms of syphilis. Latency can be interrupted by a recurrence of secondary syphilis.

Tertiary syphilis is the final stage in the natural history of the disease. It is estimated that between 20% and 40% of those infected do not exhibit signs and symptoms in this final stage. Tertiary syphilis presents as a slowly progressive inflammatory disease with the potential to affect multiple organs. The most common manifestations at this level are aortitis and neurosyphilis, as evidenced by dementia, psychosis, paresis, stroke, or meningitis.

Assessment and Diagnostic Findings

Because syphilis shares symptoms with many diseases, clinical history and laboratory evaluation are important.

TABLE 70-6 Recommended Algorithm to Determine HIV Post-Exposure Prophylaxis (PEP)

Exposure Type	Source HIV Positive Asymptomatic or Viral Load <1,500 RNA Copies/Ml	Source HIV Positive Symptomatic or Known High Viral Load	Source with Unknown HIV Status	Unknown Source	Source HIV Negative
Less severe percutaneous exposure (solid needle and superficial injury)	Basic two-drug regimen*	Basic two-drug regimen* and one drug from expanded drug list†	Generally, no PEP warranted, but consider basic two-drug regimen* if source has HIV risk factors	Generally, no PEP warranted, but consider basic two-drug regimen* in settings where exposure to HIV-infected persons is likely	No prophylaxis is warranted
More severe percutaneous exposure (large-bore hollow needle, deep puncture, visible blood on device, needle used in patient's artery or vein)	Basic two-drug regimen* and one drug from expanded drug list†	Basic two-drug regimen* and one drug from expanded drug list†	Same as above	Same as above	Same as above
Small-volume mucous membrane exposure or nonintact skin exposure (a few drops)	Basic two-drug regimen*	Basic two-drug regimen*	Same as above	Same as above	Same as above
Large-volume mucous membrane exposure or nonintact skin exposure (large-volume splash or spray)	Basic two-drug regimen*	Basic two-drug regimen* and one drug from expanded drug list†	Same as above	Same as above	Same as above

d4T, stavudine (Zerit); ddI, didanosine (Videx); 3TC, lamivudine (Epivir); ZDV, zidovudine (Retrovir [AZT])
*Basic two-drug regimen = (ZDV and 3TC) *or* (3TC and d4T) *or* (d4T and ddI).
†Expanded drug list: indinavir (Crixivan), nelfinavir (Viracept), abacavir (Ziagen), efavirenz (Sustiva)
Recommendations based on: Centers for Disease Control and Prevention. (2001). Updated U.S. Public Health Service guidelines for the management of occupational exposures to HBV, HCV, and HIV and recommendations for postexposure prophylaxis. *Morbidity and Mortality Weekly Report, 50* (RR-11), 1–42.

The conclusive diagnosis of syphilis can be made by direct identification of the spirochete obtained from the chancre lesions of primary syphilis. Serologic tests used in the diagnosis of secondary and tertiary syphilis require clinical correlation in interpretation. The serologic tests are summarized as follows:

- *Nontreponemal* or *reagin tests*, such as the Venereal Disease Research Laboratory (VDRL) or the rapid plasma reagin circle card test (RPR-CT), are generally used for screening and diagnosis. After adequate therapy, the test result is expected to decrease quantitatively until it is read as negative, usually about 2 years after therapy is completed.
- *Treponemal tests*, such as the fluorescent treponemal antibody absorption test (FTA-ABS) and the microhemagglutination test (MHA-TP), are used to verify that the screening test did not represent a false-positive result. Positive results usually are positive for life and therefore are not appropriate to determine therapeutic effectiveness.

Medical Management

Treatment of all stages of syphilis is administration of antibiotics. Penicillin G benzathine is the medication of choice for early syphilis or early latent syphilis of less than 1 year's duration. It is administered by intramuscular injection at a single session. Patients with late latent or latent syphilis of unknown duration should receive three injections at 1-week intervals. Patients who are allergic to penicillin are usually treated with doxycycline. The patient treated with penicillin is monitored for 30 minutes after the injection to observe for a possible allergic reaction.

Treatment guidelines established by the CDC are updated on a regular basis. Recommendations provide special guidelines for treatment in the setting of pregnancy, allergy,

HIV infection, pediatric infection, congenital infection, and neurosyphilis (CDC, 2002d).

Nursing Management

Syphilis is a reportable communicable disease. In any health care facility, a mechanism must be in place to ensure that all diagnosed patients are reported to the state or local public health department to ensure community follow-up. The public health department is responsible for identification of sexual contacts, contact notification, and contact screening.

Lesions of primary and secondary syphilis may be highly infective. Gloves are worn when direct contact with lesions is likely, and hand hygiene is performed after gloves are removed. Isolation in a private room is not required (Chart 70-6).

Chlamydia trachomatis *and* Neisseria gonorrhoeae

Chlamydia trachomatis and *Neisseria gonorrhoeae* are the most commonly reported STDs. Coinfection with *C. trachomatis* often occurs in patients infected with *N. gonorrhoeae*. The group with the greatest risk for *C. trachomatis* infection is young women between the ages of 16 and 24 years.

Transmission of *C. trachomatis* from a pregnant woman to her infant during a vaginal birth is common. Transmission of *N. gonorrhoeae* can also occur as a result of contact with the vaginal mucosa during birth. About 20% to 50% of infants born to mothers with *C. trachomatis* infection develop chlamydial conjunctivitis, and about 20% develop chlamydial pneumonia (Schacter & Grossman, 2001). Infants of mothers with *N. gonorrhoeae* infection are at risk for conjunctivitis, arthritis, meningitis, scalp abscesses (because of fetal monitoring electrodes), and generalized sepsis.

CHART 70-6

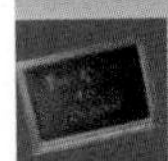

Patient Education

Preventing the Spread of Syphilis

- If multiple penicillin injections are required, complete the full course of therapy.
- Refrain from sexual contact with previous or current partners until the partners have been treated.
- If you have primary or secondary syphilis, be aware that with proper treatment, skin lesions and other sequelae of infection will improve, and serology eventually will reflect cure.
- Condoms significantly reduce the risk of transmission of syphilis and other sexually transmitted diseases.
- Having multiple sexual partners increases the risk of acquiring syphilis and other sexually transmitted diseases.

Clinical Manifestations

Women

Both *C. trachomatis* and *N. gonorrhoeae* infections frequently do not cause symptoms in women. When symptoms are present, mucopurulent cervicitis with exudates in the endocervical canal is the most frequent finding. Women with gonorrhea can also present with symptoms of urinary tract infection or vaginitis.

Men

Although men are more likely than women to have symptoms when infected, infection with *N. gonorrhoeae* and/or *C. trachomatis* can be asymptomatic. When symptoms are present, they may include burning during urination and penile discharge. Patients with *N. gonorrhoeae* infection may also report painful swollen testicles.

Complications

In women, pelvic inflammatory disease (PID), ectopic pregnancy, endometritis, and infertility are possible complications of either *N. gonorrhoeae* or *C. trachomatis* infection. In men, epididymitis, a painful disease that may lead to infertility, may result from infection with either bacterium. In people of either gender, *N. gonorrhoeae* may cause arthritis or bloodstream infection.

Assessment and Diagnostic Findings

The patient is assessed for fever, discharge (urethral, vaginal, or rectal), and signs of arthritis. Diagnostic methods used in *N. gonorrhoeae* infection include Gram stain (appropriate only for male urethral samples), culture, and nucleic acid amplification tests (NAATs). Gram stain and the direct fluorescent antibody test can be used in chlamydia. NAATs are also available for *C. trachomatis* but demand strict attention to laboratory procedures to ensure test reliability. In the male patient, specimens are obtained from the urethra, anal canal, and pharynx. In the female patient, samples are obtained from the endocervix, anal canal, and pharynx. Because *N. gonorrhoeae* organisms are susceptible to environmental changes, specimens for culture must be delivered to the laboratory immediately after they are obtained.

Because as many as 70% of chlamydial infections are asymptomatic, the CDC recommends that all pregnant women and all sexually active women younger than 26 years of age be routinely tested for chlamydial infection. Systematic audits have demonstrated poor compliance with recommended screening, probably because of inconsistent availability of laboratory facilities, misperceptions about the risk to young women, and discomfort associated with sexual history taking (CDC, 2004d).

Medical Management

Because patients are often coinfected with both gonorrhea and chlamydia, the CDC recommends dual therapy even if only gonorrhea has been laboratory-proven. The CDC-recommended treatment for chlamydia is either doxycycline (Adoxa) or azithromycin (Zithromax) and one of the following for gonorrhea: ceftriaxone (Rocephin), cefixime (Suprax), ciprofloxacin (Cipro), or ofloxacin (Floxin). These antibiotics are not recommended during pregnancy. CDC guidelines should be used to determine alternative therapy for the patient who is pregnant or allergic or who has a complicated chlamydial infection.

Patients with uncomplicated gonorrhea who are treated with CDC-recommended therapy do not routinely need to return for a proof-of-cure visit. If the patient reports a new episode of symptoms or tests are positive for gonorrhea again, the most likely explanation is reinfection rather than treatment failure. Serologic testing for syphilis and HIV should be offered to patients with gonorrhea or chlamydia, because any STD increases the risk of other STD infections.

Nursing Management

Gonorrhea and chlamydia are reportable communicable diseases. In any health care facility, a mechanism should be in place to ensure that all diagnosed patients are reported to the local public health department to ensure follow-up of the patient. The public health department also is responsible for interviewing the patient to identify sexual contacts, so that contact notification and screening can be initiated.

The target group for preventive patient teaching about gonorrhea and chlamydia is the adolescent and young adult population. Along with reinforcing the importance of abstinence, when appropriate, education should address postponing the age of initial sexual exposure, limiting the number of sexual partners, and use of condoms for barrier protection. Young women and pregnant women should also be instructed about the importance of routine screening for chlamydia.

Nursing Process

The Patient With a Sexually Transmitted Disease

Assessment

Protecting confidentiality is important when discussing sexual issues. When a detailed sexual history is necessary, it is important to respect the patient's right to privacy. The patient should be asked to describe the onset and progression of symptoms and to characterize any lesions by location and by describing drainage, if present. Brief explanations of why the information is needed are often helpful. Clarification of terms may be necessary if either the patient or nurse uses words that are unfamiliar to the other.

Asking specific information about sexual contacts usually should be done only when the nurse is part of a team that will conduct partner notification. The nurse should describe to the patient the public health notification process and resources that are available to assist sexual partners and/or infants and children.

During the physical examination, the examiner looks for rashes, lesions, drainage, discharge, or swelling. Inguinal nodes are palpated to elicit tenderness and to assess swelling. Women are examined for abdominal or uterine tenderness. The mouth and throat are examined for signs of inflammation or exudate. The nurse wears gloves while examining the mucous membranes, and gloves are changed and replaced after vaginal or rectal examination.

Diagnosis

Nursing Diagnoses

Based on assessment data, the patient's major nursing diagnoses may include the following:

- Deficient knowledge about the disease and risk for spread of infection and reinfection
- Anxiety related to anticipated stigmatization and to prognosis and complications
- Noncompliance with treatment

Collaborative Problems/ Potential Complications

Based on assessment data, potential complications that may develop include the following:

- Increased risk for ectopic pregnancy
- Infertility
- Transmission of infection to fetus, resulting in congenital abnormalities and other outcomes
- Neurosyphilis
- Gonococcal meningitis
- Gonococcal arthritis
- Syphilitic aortitis
- HIV-related complications

Planning and Goals

Major goals are increased patient understanding of the natural history and treatment of the infection, reduction in anxiety, increased compliance with therapeutic and preventive goals, and absence of complications.

Nursing Interventions

Increasing Knowledge and Preventing Spread of Disease

Education about STDs and prevention of the spread to others is often accomplished simultaneously. The infected patient should be told what the causative organism is and should receive an explanation of the usual course of the infection (including the interval of potential communicability to others) and possible complications. The nurse should stress the importance of following therapy as prescribed and the need to report any side effects or symptom progression.

Discussion should emphasize that the same behaviors that led to infection with one STD increase the risk for any other STD, including HIV. Methods used to contact sexual partners should be discussed. The patient should understand that until the partner has been treated, continued sexual exposure to the same person may lead to reinfection. The relative value of condoms in reducing the risk for infection with STDs should be addressed. When appropriate, the patient should be encouraged to discuss any reasons for resistance to condom use to promote thoughtful decision making about this preventive method.

Reducing Anxiety

When appropriate, the patient is encouraged to discuss anxieties and fear associated with the diagnosis, treatment, or prognosis. By individualizing teaching efforts, factual information applied to specific needs may offer reassurance. Patients may need help in planning discussion with partners. If the patient is especially apprehensive about this aspect, referral to a social worker or other specialist may be appropriate. For example, such support is especially important when the patient has newly diagnosed HIV infection. Patients with HIV may benefit from programs that combine support, education, counseling, and therapeutic goals. Such programs are designed to offer coordinated care throughout the course of disease progression.

Increasing Compliance

In group settings (eg, an outpatient obstetric setting) or in a one-to-one setting, open discussion about STD information facilitates patient teaching. Discomfort can be reduced by factual explanation of causes, consequences, treatments, prevention, and responsibilities. Because most communities have expanded STD prevention resources, referrals to appropriate agencies can complement individual educational efforts and ensure that later questions or uncertainties can be addressed by experts. Patients can obtain more information by accessing the CDC web site (http://www.cdc.gov/nchstp/dstd/disease_info.htm) or by calling 1-888-CDC-FACT.

Monitoring and Managing Potential Complications

INFERTILITY AND INCREASED RISK OF ECTOPIC PREGNANCY

STDs may lead to PID and, with it, increased risk for ectopic pregnancy and infertility. For additional information, see Chapter 47.

CONGENITAL INFECTIONS

All STDs can be transmitted to infants in utero or at the time of birth. Complications of congenital infection can range from localized infection (eg, throat infection with *N. gonorrhoeae*), to congenital abnormalities (eg, stunting of growth or deafness from congenital syphilis), to life-threatening disease (eg, congenital herpes simplex virus).

NEUROSYPHILIS, GONOCOCCAL MENINGITIS, GONOCOCCAL ARTHRITIS, AND SYPHILITIC AORTITIS

STDs can cause disseminated infection. The central nervous system may be infected, as seen in cases of neurosyphilis or gonococcal meningitis. Gonorrhea that infects the skeletal system may result in gonococcal arthritis. Syphilis can infect the cardiovascular system by forming vegetative lesions on the mitral or aortic valves.

HIV-RELATED COMPLICATIONS

HIV infection leads to the profound immunosuppression characteristic of AIDS. Complications of HIV infection include many opportunistic infections, including *Pneumocystis jiroveci, Cryptococcus neoformans*, cytomegalovirus, and *Mycobacterium avium* (see Chapter 52).

Evaluation

Expected Patient Outcomes

Expected patient outcomes may include the following:

1. Exhibits knowledge about STDs and their transmission
2. Demonstrates a less anxious demeanor
   a. Discusses anxieties and goals for treatment
   b. Inspects self for lesions, rashes, and discharge
   c. Accepts support, education, and counseling when indicated
   d. Assists with sharing information about infection with sexual partners
   e. Discusses risk-reduction behaviors and safer sex practices
3. Complies with treatment
4. Achieves effective treatment
5. Reports for follow-up examinations if necessary
6. Absence of complications

Emerging Infectious Diseases

As defined by the CDC, **emerging infectious diseases** are human diseases of infectious origin that have increased within the past two decades or that are likely to increase in the near future. Examples of emerging infectious diseases presented here include severe acute respiratory syndrome (SARS), West Nile virus, Legionnaires' disease, hantavirus pulmonary syndrome, and viral hemorrhagic fevers. Table 70-1 provides an overview of infectious diseases, including emerging infectious diseases.

Many factors contribute to newly emerging or re-emerging infectious diseases. These include travel, globalization of food supply and central processing of food, population growth, increased urban crowding, population movements (eg, those that result from war, famine, or disaster), ecologic changes, human behavior (eg, risky sexual behavior, IV/injection drug use), antimicrobial resistance, and breakdown in public health measures.

These diseases are important from an epidemiologic standpoint because their incidence has not yet stabilized. When the pattern of disease in a community is not well understood in the medical-scientific community, patients, families, and others in the community often become alarmed about these diseases. During times of increased concern about bioterrorism, whether triggered by actual events or by hoaxes, nurses have responsibility to rationally separate facts from fears. In discussions with patients and other caregivers, it is important to keep the focus on what is known and to clarify the plan for diagnosis, treatment, and containment.

Severe Acute Respiratory Syndrome

In March 2003, WHO issued a global warning about the sudden appearance of an epidemic of influenza-like disease in Asia, which was called severe acute respiratory syndrome (SARS). The disease is caused by a member of the coronavirus family that was also first recognized in 2003. SARS occurred in more than 15 other countries within a number of weeks.

The worldwide dissemination was largely attributed to travel, because of strong epidemiologic evidence that patients from many countries had originally shared common exposures in Hong Kong. SARS is as an example of how suddenly benign microorganisms, especially viruses, can mutate to become important human pathogens. The epidemic and its relatively quick resolution illustrate the important role of public health and need for consistent attention to infection control principles. Before SARS came to the attention of WHO, transmission to nurses and other health care professionals occurred frequently. Once patients were appropriately isolated, with health care workers using barrier precautions and cleaning contaminated surfaces carefully, transmission was effectively reduced or prevented.

Initially, patients with SARS present with fever and cough. A minority of those infected progress to experience respiratory distress. Because fever and cough are such common and nonspecific symptoms, health care providers need to establish careful methods to screen patients for both this clinical presentation and potential exposure.

The 2003 SARS outbreak demonstrated that careful patient screening, use of infection control behaviors, and amplified protection (use of N-95 respirator, goggles, and full garment covering) during aerosol-producing procedures (eg, intubation, extubation, suctioning, manual bagging) were protective for health care workers (Bell, 2004; Loutfy, Wallington, Rutledge, et al., 2004).

West Nile Virus

The West Nile virus was first recognized in the 1930s in Africa and was first seen in humans in the United States in 1999. Although most human infections are mild or asymptomatic, a range of presentations is possible. Approximately 20% of people infected have a mild disease; headache and fever are frequently reported. Fewer than 1 in 150 infections develop into more severe illness, including encephalitis (Petersen & Marfin, 2002).

The incubation period (ie, from mosquito bite to onset of symptoms) is between 3 and 14 days. Currently, there is no treatment for West Nile virus infection. Medical and nursing management consists of fluid replacement, airway management, and supportive nursing care when meningitis symptoms are present.

Birds are the natural reservoir for the virus, and since 1999, the population of infected birds in the eastern United States has increased steadily. Mosquitoes become infected when feeding on birds and can transmit the virus to animals and humans. There is no human-to-human transmission of the virus and no evidence of transfer from infected birds to humans. However, as a precaution, it is wise to teach people in affected areas to wear gloves when handling dead birds (CDC, 2002c).

Legionnaires' Disease

Legionnaires' disease is a multisystem illness that usually includes pneumonia and is caused by the gram-negative bacterium *Legionella pneumophila.* Named after an outbreak among people attending a convention of the American Legion in 1976, its potential to cause outbreaks has been demonstrated repeatedly in hospitals and other settings. It continues to be considered an emerging infectious disease because there are new presentations in recent years, and increasing incidence. For example, in recent years, outbreaks have been associated with the use of whirlpools, decorative fountains, and water used for flower shows.

Legionella organisms are found in many man-made and naturally occurring water sources. Although the organisms may initially be introduced to the plumbing system in low numbers, growth is enhanced by water storage, sediment, temperatures ranging from 25° to 42°C (77° to 107°F), and certain amoebae frequently present in water that can support intracellular growth of legionellae.

Pathophysiology

L. pneumophila is transmitted by the aerosolized route from an environmental source to a person's respiratory tract. It is not transmitted from person to person. In hospitals, patients may be exposed to aerosols created by cooling towers, water exposure from in-room plumbing, and respiratory therapy equipment. Because underlying medical conditions can increase host susceptibility and subsequent severity of disease and because hospital plumbing systems are often very complex, outbreaks occur in hospitals more frequently than at other centers within the community. The mortality rate for all people diagnosed with Legionnaires' disease is approximately 12% (CDC, 2004c).

Risk Factors

Risk factors for *Legionella* infection include diseases that lead to severe immunosuppression, such as AIDS, hematologic malignancy, end-stage renal disease, or use of immunosuppressive agents. Other factors associated with increased risk include advanced age, diabetes, alcohol abuse, smoking, and other pulmonary disease.

Clinical Manifestations

The lungs are the principal organs of infection; however, other organs may also be involved. The incubation period ranges from 2 to 10 days. Early symptoms may include malaise, myalgias, headache, and dry cough. The patient develops increasing pulmonary symptoms, including productive cough, dyspnea, and chest pain. Patients are usually febrile, and body temperatures may reach or exceed 39.4°C (103°F). Diarrhea and other gastrointestinal symptoms are common. In severe cases, multiorgan involvement and failure may follow.

Assessment and Diagnostic Findings

The diagnostic approach generally involves accumulation of information obtained from the history, physical examination, x-rays, laboratory findings, and assessment of therapeutic effectiveness. Chest x-ray abnormalities may vary in severity and in location within the lungs. Laboratory tests available for the diagnosis of *Legionella* include culture or tests that detect either antigen or antibody. The most frequently used test is the urinary antigen. The greatest limitation of the test is that it detects only one subgroup of one of the several species of *Legionella*. The CDC recommends using multiple tests when Legionnaires' disease is suspected, because none of the tests is completely accurate.

Medical Management

Azithromycin (Zithromax) is considered the antibiotic of choice. Other options include clarithromycin (Biaxin), erythromycin (Ilotycin), and levofloxacin (Levaquin).

Nursing Management

The nursing management described for the patient with any pneumonia (see Chapter 23) should form the basis of care for the patient with *Legionella* pneumonia. Isolation is not required because *Legionella* is not transmitted between humans. When the patient has acquired the infection in a health care facility, water cultures should be performed to determine if the water supply is contaminated.

Hantavirus Pulmonary Syndrome

Hantavirus pulmonary syndrome (HPS) is caused by a member of the Hantavirus family of viruses. In the United States, the Sin Nombre hantavirus causes severe cardiopulmonary illness, with a case mortality rate of approximately 50%. It occurs most frequently in the western United States, but the rodents known to carry the virus are found throughout the country (Vaheri & Calisher, 2002).

The diagnosis of HPS should be suspected in patients who live in rural areas; who may have had exposure to rodents; and who report fever, aching muscles, and nausea. Thrombocytopenia and hemoconcentration are also common.

No specific treatment for HPS has been approved. Early identification, assessment, and maintenance of respiratory status are the most important aspects of care for patients with the disease. Intake and output should be monitored closely because overhydration is possible, with resultant cardiopulmonary compromise.

Prevention requires strategies to reduce human contact with rodents and their droppings. Public health programs and clinics in rural areas should regularly teach people to eliminate rodent food sources that are in areas close to humans. Openings in walls or cabinets should be sealed. Traps should be used in areas such as sheds and barns in which humans work and rodents may enter. Gloves should be worn when removing an animal from a trap, and the trap should be disinfected with a 1:10 bleach solution. People entering such areas should be taught to avoid stirring up dust or breathing potentially contaminated dust. Brooms and vacuum cleaners should be used with caution; areas that may emit dust while being cleaned should be first dampened with a bleach solution to reduce viral contaminants and the potential for dust dispersion.

Viral Hemorrhagic Fevers

Viral hemorrhagic fevers are a group of illnesses caused by several families of viruses (the arenaviruses, filoviruses, bunyaviruses, and flaviviruses). These viruses cause a syndrome characterized by multisystem involvement resulting in a damaged vascular system. Although most cases of hemorrhagic fever are severe, some cases are less acute. The viruses as a whole can be found throughout the world; however, each virus usually causes disease only in its own limited geographic area.

The Ebola and Marburg viruses, which both belong to the filovirus family, are the best-known viral hemorrhagic fever viruses. Since the 1960s, they have been the source of an irregular pattern of sporadic outbreaks. The clinical course differs among patients but often includes fever, hemorrhage, vomiting, diarrhea, cough, and jaundice. Symptoms usually occur rapidly, and the course of the illness often progresses rapidly to profound hemorrhage, organ destruction, and shock. The mortality rate ranges from 25% to 80%. When patients survive, the recovery period is often prolonged, and weakness, malaise, and cachexia are common.

Nonhuman animals or insects appear to be the natural reservoirs of the viruses. Humans usually become infected when exposed to the natural reservoir—for example, after exposure to an unrecognized host or an insect bite. However, human-to-human transmission occurs occasionally; it involves close contact and usually occurs via the bloodborne route after exposure to blood or other body fluid. Percutaneous exposure requires only a very low inoculum of contaminated blood for transmission to occur. Mucous membrane exposure is another method of transmission. Although airborne transmission does not appear to be likely, the possibility has not been entirely eliminated.

A diagnosis of Ebola or Marburg should be considered in a patient who has a febrile, hemorrhagic illness after traveling to Asia or Africa or who has handled animals or animal carcasses from those parts of the world. The CDC should be contacted immediately when Ebola and Marburg viruses are suspected because hospital and local public health laboratories would not be able to confirm a diagnosis. Because no cases of Ebola or Marburg have been diagnosed in the United States to date, more likely diagnoses should also be considered whenever one of these diseases is a diagnostic possibility.

All health care workers who are involved in caring for patients with filoviruses must adhere to strict infection control measures. Systems must be set up to have objective observers ensure that each worker wears complete protective equipment in the form of cap, goggles, mask, gown, gloves, and shoe covers.

Treatment is largely supportive maintenance of the circulatory system and respiratory systems. It is likely that the infected patient will need ventilator and dialysis support during the acute phases of illness (CDC, 2005b). Supportive care for a patient with such a devastating disease requires psychological support for the patient and family. The patient, family, health care workers, and others in the community will need substantial, coordinated education about the known elements and approach. Intervention may be required from those trained to provide psychological support for traumatic or terrorist events.

Travel and Immigration

Travel, trade, migration, and wars have led to many epidemics throughout history. The potential for epidemics is greatest when travelers and immigrants introduce microorganisms to which the host population has little or no immunity. Examples of important epidemics in the Western Hemisphere have included yellow fever, malaria, hookworm, leprosy, smallpox, measles, mumps, and syphilis. The HIV epidemic demonstrates the way that travel and immigration allow a disease to spread undetected worldwide. The SARS outbreak demonstrates the way that global travel contributed to a rapidly occurring epidemic involving an unrecognized pathogen.

In the United States, an infrastructure with enforced vaccination, clean water, and insect and rodent control decreases the risk that epidemics will progress even when travel may introduce exotic microorganisms. However, the recent experience with West Nile virus reinforced knowledge that insect transmission can lead to significant human outbreaks. Thus, the concern grows that vector-borne diseases such as dengue and malaria may increase in the United States as mosquitoes can transmit disease locally when a reservoir of infected humans is established (CDC, 2004e). The CDC maintains an active surveillance system to monitor and halt the incidence of many diseases prospectively.

Immigration and Acquired Immunodeficiency Disease Syndrome

The fact that AIDS reached pandemic proportions in less than a decade after its recognition attests to the efficiency of world travel in spreading disease. Such rapid transmission rates are especially dramatic because HIV essentially requires intimate contact between two people through sexual activity or sharing blood through needles.

HIV/AIDS is now an international health disaster. Since the start of the epidemic, more than 60 million people have become infected with HIV and more than 20 million have died of AIDS. Control of the epidemic anywhere in the world requires control everywhere. More than 95% of the current burden is felt in economically depressed countries, which means that the control of the disease, using antiretroviral therapy and public health education, requires investment from nations, corporations, and people throughout the world, especially the wealthy nations (UNAIDS, 2004).

Immigration and Tuberculosis

Although there are substantive efforts to eliminate TB in the United States, TB remains a growing epidemic in developing nations. Approximately one third of the world's population is currently infected with TB. Between 5% and 10% of those infected eventually develop disease; therefore, approximately 8 million people per year become ill with TB (WHO, 2005). Immigration has always been an important influence in the dynamic epidemiology of TB in the United States. In 2003, the incidence of TB in the United States was eight times greater in foreign-born people than in native-born people (CDC, 2004f).

The association between immigration and transmission risk is greatest in urban areas, because these locations are frequently heavily populated and visited by foreign-born people. These locales are also often the epicenter of the HIV epidemic. Because HIV infection depletes T cells, which are necessary for TB protection, the geographic closeness of these two microorganisms potentiates increased rates of both diseases.

A positive tuberculin skin test (TST) establishes that TB infection has occurred at some time in a person's life but does not provide information about current infectivity. The reliability of TST interpretation is decreased among foreign-born people because the bacille Calmette-Guérin (BCG) vaccine is used in many countries. After receiving BCG, people often have some degree of TST reactivity for a prolonged time.

Immigration and Vector-Borne Diseases

Malaria and dengue are diseases that cause significant morbidity and mortality throughout the developing world. These diseases may be "imported" to the United States via travel, immigration, or commerce. They are caused by microorganisms that can be spread to humans by mosquitoes in the United States that thrive in tropical zones and breed in stagnant water sources. Although malaria was eradicated in the United States in the 1950s, limited local outbreaks have occurred regularly when mosquitoes acquire the bacteria from a person recently traveling from an area in which malaria is endemic and transmit it to a small number of people (Fig. 70-3). Similarly, an increase of dengue virus in the Caribbean has caused concern that outbreaks may occur in the United States.

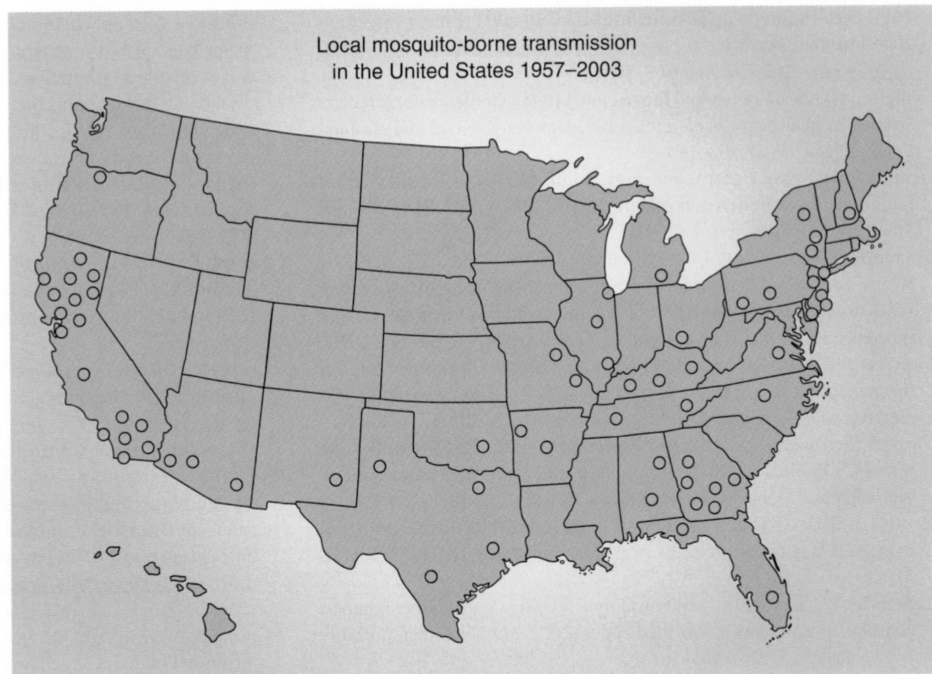

FIGURE 70-3. Episodes of local transmission of malaria in the United States, 1957–2003. (Redrawn from map available at: http://www.cdc.gov/malaria/features/prevent_reintroduction.htm)

Critical Thinking Exercises

1 The hospital where you work has very few private rooms; often there are not enough available for patients who have MRSA. What methods can you recommend that will allow contact precautions to be followed in the absence of private rooms? What behaviors of health care personnel can be audited to measure compliance with contact precautions? How do you reassure personnel, patients, and visitors that a safe environment is being provided? What products or equipment can be helpful?

2 ebp The health care facility where you work is located in an area that has recently been flooded. There are local concerns about contaminated municipal water. How do you ensure that hand hygiene can continue in your setting? As patients are being admitted for diarrheal diseases, how do you assess their status? What methods can you use to decrease hospital transmission of infections? What is the evidence base for these methods? What criteria would you use to evaluate the strength of that evidence?

3 The incidence of influenza has reportedly increased throughout the world. Your health care facility is preparing for cases in your region. As influenza vaccine is promoted, what measures can be used to increase the acceptance of the vaccine by reluctant personnel? What additional protective measures can be used to decrease the chance of an outbreak? What resources are available to keep the health care staff aware of changing conditions?

REFERENCES AND SELECTED READINGS

BOOKS

Atkinson, W., Gantt, J., Mayfield, M., Furphy, L., & Centers for Disease Control and Prevention (Eds.). (2004). *Epidemiology and prevention of vaccine preventable diseases* (8th ed., pp. 97–113). Atlanta: Centers for Disease Control and Prevention.

Centers for Disease Control and Prevention (2000b). *Tracking the hidden epidemics: Trends in STDs in the United States* [on-line]. Available at http://www.cdc.gov/nchstp/dstd/stats_trends2000.pdf. (Accessed August 9, 2006)

Chin, J. (2000). *Control of communicable diseases in man.* Washington, DC: American Public Health Association

Gorbach, S. L., Bartlett, J., & Blacklow, N. R. (2003). *Infectious diseases.* Philadelphia: W. B. Saunders.

Guerrant, R. L., & Steiner, T. S. (2005). Principles and syndromes of enteric infection. In Mandell, G. L., Douglas, R. G., & Bennett, J. E. (Eds.), *Principles and practice of infectious diseases.* New York: Churchill Livingstone.

Mayhall, C. G. (2004). *Hospital epidemiology and infection control.* Philadelphia: Lippincott Williams & Wilkins.

Rhinehart, E., & McGoldrick, M. (2005). *Infection control in home care and hospice* (2nd ed.). Boston: Jones and Bartlett Publishers, Inc.

Satcher, D. (2001). *The Surgeon General's call to action to promote sexual health and responsible sexual behavior* [on-line]. Available at http://www.surgeongeneral.gov/library/sexualhealth. (Accessed August 9, 2006)

Schacter, J., & Grossman, M. (2001). *Chlamydia.* In Remington, J. S., & Klein, J. O. (Eds.), *Infectious diseases of the fetus and newborn infant.* Philadelphia: W. B. Saunders.

Wenzel, R. P. (2003). *Prevention and control of nosocomial infections.* Philadelphia: Lippincott Williams & Wilkins.

JOURNALS

**Asterisks indicate nursing research articles.*

Bell, D. M. (2004). World Health Organization Working Group on Prevention of International and Community Transmission of SARS.

Public health interventions and SARS spread, 2003. Emerg Infect Dis 2004 [on-line]. Available at http://www.cdc.gov/ncidod/EID/vol10no11/04-0729.htm. Accessed August 9, 2006.

Centers for Disease Control and Prevention. (1998). Guideline for infection control in healthcare personnel, 1998. *Infection Control and Hospital Epidemiology, 19*(6), 407–463.

Centers for Disease Control and Prevention. (2000a). Surveillance for foodborne disease outbreaks—United States, 1993–1997. *Morbidity and Mortality Weekly Report, 49*(SS-01), 1–51.

Centers for Disease Control and Prevention. (2001a). Updated U.S. Public Health Service guidelines for the management of occupational exposures to HBV, HCV, and HIV and recommendations for postexposure prophylaxis. *Morbidity and Mortality Weekly Report, 50*(RR-11), 1–42.

Centers for Disease Control and Prevention. (2001b). Recommendations for preventing transmission of infections among chronic hemodialysis patients. *Morbidity and Mortality Weekly Report, 50*(RR05), 1–43.

Centers for Disease Control and Prevention. (2001c). "Norwalk-Like viruses." Public health consequences and outbreak management. *Morbidity and Mortality Weekly Report, 50*(RR09), 1–18.

Centers for Disease Control and Prevention. (2002a). Guideline for hand hygiene in health care settings. *Morbidity and Mortality Weekly Report, 51*(RR-16), 1–56.

Centers for Disease Control and Prevention. (2002b). *Staphylococcus aureus* resistant to vancomycin—United States, 2002. *Morbidity and Mortality Weekly Report, 51*(26), 565–567.

Centers for Disease Control and Prevention. (2002c). West Nile virus—2001. *Morbidity and Mortality Weekly Report, 51*(23), 497–501.

Centers for Disease Control and Prevention. (2002d). Sexually transmitted diseases: Treatment guidelines, 2002. *Morbidity and Mortality Weekly Report, 51*(RR06), 1–80.

Centers for Disease Control and Prevention. (2002e). Guidelines for the prevention of intravascular catheter-related infections. *Morbidity and Mortality Weekly Report, 51*(RR-10), 1–28.

Centers for Disease Control and Prevention. (2003). Epidemic/epizootic West Nile virus control in the United States: Revised guidelines for prevention, surveillance and control. 1–77. Available at http://www.cdc.gov/ncidod/dvbid/westnile/resources/wnv-guidelines-aug-2003.pdf. Accessed August 9, 2006.

Centers for Disease Control and Prevention. (2004a). National Nosocomial Infections Surveillance System report: Data summary, from January 1992–June 2004, issued October 2004. *American Journal of Infection Control, 32*(8), 470–485.

Centers for Disease Control and Prevention. (2004b). Prevention and control of influenza: Recommendations of the Advisory Committee on Immunization Practices. *Morbidity and Mortality Weekly Report: CDC Surveillance Summaries, 53*(RR06), 1–40.

Centers for Disease Control and Prevention. (2004c). Healthcare Infection Control Practices Advisory Committee: Guidelines for preventing healthcare-associated pneumonia, 2003. *Morbidity and Mortality Weekly Report, 53*(RR-03), 1–36.

Centers for Disease Control and Prevention. (2004d). Chlamydia screening among sexually active young female enrollees of health plans—United States 1991–2001, 2004. *Morbidity and Mortality Weekly Report, 53*(42), 983–1004.

Centers for Disease Control and Prevention. (2004e). Multifocal autochthonous transmission of malaria—Florida, 2003–2004. *Morbidity and Mortality Weekly Report, 53*(19), 412–413.

Centers for Disease Control and Prevention. (2004f). Reported tuberculosis in the United States, 2003. Atlanta, GA: U.S. Department of Health and Human Services, CDC, September 2004. Available at www.cdc.gov/nchstp/tb/surv/surv2003/default.htm.

Centers for Disease Control and Prevention. (2004g). Healthcare Infection Control Practices Advisory Committee. Draft guideline for isolation precautions: Preventing transmission of infectious agents in healthcare settings 2004. *Federal Register, 69*(113).

Centers for Disease Control and Prevention. (2004h). Trends in reportable sexually transmitted diseases in the United States, 2003: National data on chlamydia, gonorrhea, and syphilis. Available at www.cdc.gov/std/stats/trends2003.htm.

Centers for Disease Control and Prevention. (2004i). STD Communications Database. General public focus group findings. February 2004. Available at www.cdc.gov/std/HealthComm/ExecSumHPVGenPub2004.pdf.

Centers for Disease Control and Prevention. (2005a). Achievements in public health: Elimination of rubella and congenital rubella syndrome—United States, 1969–2004. *Morbidity and Mortality Weekly Report, 54*(11), 279–282.

Centers for Disease Control and Prevention. (2005b). Brief report: Outbreak of Marburg virus hemorrhagic fever—Angola, October 1, 2004–March 29, 2005. *Morbidity and Mortality Weekly Report, 54* (Dispatch), 1–2.

Centers for Disease Control and Prevention. (2005c). Foodborne illness; frequently asked questions. 2005. Available at http://www.cdc.gov/ncidod/dbmd/diseaseinfo/foodborneinfections_g.htm. Accessed August 9, 2006.

Centers for Disease Control and Prevention. (2005d). Norovirus in healthcare facilities. Available at http://www.cdc.gov/ncidod/dhqp/id_norovirusfs.html. Accessed August 9, 2006.

Centers for Disease Control and Prevention. (2006). Key facts about avian influenza (bird flu) and avian influenza A (H5N1) virus. Available at http://www.cdc.gov/flu/avian/gen-info/facts.htm. Accessed August 9, 2006.

Crump, J. A., Griffin, P. M., & Angulo, F. (2002). Bacterial contamination of animal feed and its relationship to human foodborne illness. *Clinical Infectious Diseases, 35,* 859–865.

Do, A., Ciesielski, C. A., Metler, R. P., et al. (2003). Occupationally acquired human immunodeficiency virus (HIV) infection: National case surveillance data during 20 Years of the HIV epidemic in the United States. *Infection Control Hospital Epidemiology, 24*(2), 86–96.

Donnellson, C. (2003). Smallpox legislation introduced. *American Journal of Nursing, 103*(4), 29.

Drinka, P., Faulks, J. T., Gauerke, C., et al. (2001). Adverse events associated with methicillin-resistant *Staphylococcus aureus* in a nursing home. *Archives of Internal Medicine, 161*(19), 2371–2377.

Guerrant, R. L., Kosek, M., Moore, S. et al. (2002) Magnitude and impact of diarrheal diseases. *Archives of Medical Research, 33*(4), 351–355.

*Harris, J. R., & Miller, T. H. (2000). Preventing nosocomial pneumonia: Evidence-based practice. *Critical Care Nurse, 20*(1), 51–66.

Jarvis, W. R. (2001). Infection control and changing health-care delivery systems. *Emerging Infectious Diseases, 7*(3), 170–173.

Jarvis, W. R. (2004). The state of the science of health care epidemiology, infection control, and patient, 2004. *American Journal of Infection Control, 32*(8), 496–504.

*Larson, E., Silberger, M., Jakob, K., et al. (2000). Assessment of alternative hand hygiene regimens to improve skin health among neonatal intensive care unit nurses. *Heart & Lung, 29*(1), 136–142.

Loutfy, M. R., Wallington, T., Rutledge, T., et al. (2004). Hospital preparedness and SARS. *Emerging Infectious Diseases* 2004. Available at http://www.cdc.gov/ncidod/EID/vol10no5/03-0717.htm. Accessed August 9, 2006.

Maki, D. G., Mermel, L. A., & Lugar, D. (2000). The efficacy of a chlorhexidine impregnated sponge (Biopatch) for the prevention of intravascular catheter related infection: A prospective randomized controlled multicenter study [abstract]. Presented at the Interscience Conference on Antimicrobial Agents and Chemotherapy. Toronto, Ontario, Canada: American Society for Microbiology.

Mangram, A. J., Horan, T. C., Pearson, M. L., et al. (1999). Guideline for the prevention of surgical site infection, 1999. *Infection Control and Hospital Epidemiology, 20*(4), 250–278.

Mermel, L. A. (2000). Prevention of intravascular catheter-related infections. *Annals of Internal Medicine, 132*(5), 391–402.

Mermel, L. A., Farr, B. M., Sherertz, R. J., et al (2001). Guidelines for the management of intravascular catheter-related infections. *Journal of Intravenous Nursing 24*(3), 180–207.

Michael, P. A. (2002). Preventing and treating meningococcal meningitis. *MedSurg Nursing, 11*(1), 9–12.

Occupational Safety and Health Administration (OSHA). (2001). Occupational exposure to bloodborne pathogens: Needlestick and other sharps injuries. Final rule. *Federal Register, 66,* 5317–5325.

Petersen, L. R., & Marfin, A. A. (2002) West Nile Virus: A primer for the clinician. *Annals of Internal Medicine, 137*(3), 173–179.

Scheckler, W. E., Brimhall, D., Buck, A. S., et al. (1998). Requirements for infrastructure and essential activities in infection control and epidemiology in hospitals: A consensus panel report. *Infection Control and Hospital Epidemiology, 26*(1), 46–60.

Shlaes, D. M., Gerding, D. N., John, J. F., et al. (1997). Society for Healthcare Epidemiology of America and the Infectious Diseases Society of America Joint Committee on the Prevention of Antimicrobial Resistance. Guidelines for the prevention of antimicrobial resistance in hospitals. *Infection Control and Hospital Epidemiology, 18*(11), 275–291.

Tsiodras, S., Gold, H. S., Sakoulas, G., et al. (2001). Linezolid resistance in a clinical isolate of *Staphylococcus aureus. Lancet, 358*(9277), 207–208.

UNAIDS. Global AIDS Report 2004. 2004. Available at http:www.unaids.org/bankok2004/GAR_html. Accessed August 9, 2006.

Vaheri, A., & Calisher, C. (2002). Conference summary: The fifth international conference on hemorrhagic fever with renal syndrome, hantavirus pulmonary syndrome, and hantaviruses. *Emerging Infectious Diseases, 8*(1), 109.

WHO. (2005). Global tuberculosis control: Surveillance, planning and financing. Available at http:/www.who.int/tb/publications/global_report/2005/pdf. Accessed August 9, 2006.

Writing Committee of the World Health Organization (WHO) Consultation on Human Influenza A/H5. (2005). Avian influenza A (H5N1) infection in humans. *New England Journal of Medicine, 353*(13), 1374–1385.

Zaragoza, M., Salles, M., Gomez, J., et al. (1999). Handwashing with soap or alcoholic solutions? A randomized clinical trial of its effectiveness. *American Journal of Infection Control, 27*(3), 258–261.

RESOURCES

American Lung Association, 61 Broadway, 6th Floor, New York, NY 10006; (800) 548-8252; http://www.lungusa.org. Accessed August 9, 2006.

American Public Health Association (APHA), 800 I St. NW, Washington, DC 20001; (202) 777-2742; http://www.apha.org. Accessed August 9, 2006.

Association for Professionals in Infection Control and Epidemiology (APIC), Inc., 1275 K St. NW, Suite 1000, Washington, DC 20005; (202) 789-1890; http://www.apic.org. Accessed August 9, 2006.

Centers for Disease Control and Prevention (CDC), 1600 Clifton Road NE, Atlanta, GA 30333; (404) 639-3311; http://www.cdc.gov. Accessed August 9, 2006.

Department of Infectious and Parasitic Disease Pathology, Armed Forces Institute of Pathology (AFIP), 6825 16th Street NW, Washington, DC 20306; (202) 782-2100; http://www.afip.org. Accessed August 9, 2006.

Infectious Diseases Society of America (IDSA), 66 Canal Center Plaza, Suite 600, Alexandria, VA 22314; (703) 684-1006; www.idsociety.org. Accessed August 9, 2006.

National Foundation for Infectious Diseases (NFID), 4733 Bethesda Avenue, Suite 750, Bethesda, MD 20814; (301) 656-0003; http://www.nfid.org. Accessed August 9, 2006.

National Institute of Allergy and Infectious Diseases (NIAID), National Institutes of Health, 6610 Rockledge Drive, MSC 6612, Bethesda, MD 20892; (301) 402-1663; http://www.niaid.nih.gov/default.htm. Accessed August 9, 2006.

Occupational Safety and Health Administration (OSHA), 200 Constitution Ave. NW, Washington, DC 20210; (877) 889-5627; http://www.osha.gov. Accessed August 9, 2006.

Society for Healthcare Epidemiology of America (SHEA), 66 Canal Center Plaza, Suite 600, Alexandria, VA 22314; (703) 684-1006; http://www.shea-online.org. Accessed August 9, 2006.

World Health Organization (WHO), Avenue Appia 20, 1211 Geneva 27, Switzerland; (4 122) 791-222; http://www.who.int/home-page. Accessed August 9, 2006.

CHAPTER 71

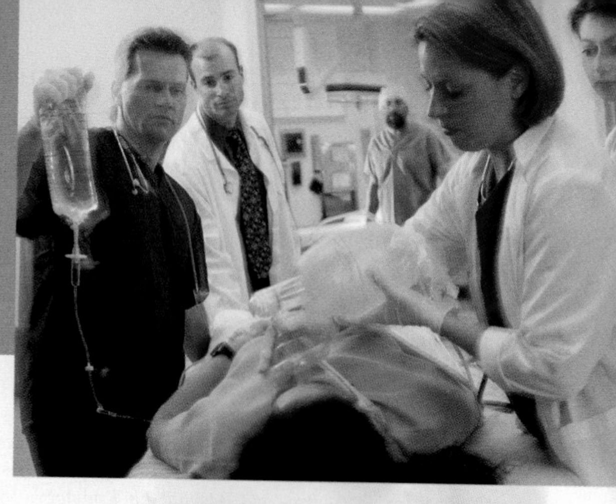

Emergency Nursing

Learning Objectives

On completion of this chapter, the learner will be able to:

1. Describe emergency care as a collaborative, holistic approach that includes the patient, the family, and significant others.
2. Discuss priority emergency measures instituted for any patient with an emergency condition.
3. Describe the emergency management of patients with intra-abdominal injuries.
4. Identify the priorities of care for the patient with multiple injuries.
5. Compare and contrast the emergency management of patients with heat stroke, frostbite, and hypothermia.
6. Specify the similarities and differences of the emergency management of patients with swallowed or inhaled poisons, skin contamination, and food poisoning.
7. Discuss the emergency management of patients with drug overdose and with acute alcohol intoxication.
8. Describe the significance of crisis intervention in the care of rape victims.
9. Differentiate between the emergency care of patients who are overactive, those who are violent, those who are depressed, and those who are suicidal.

The term *emergency management* traditionally refers to care given to patients with urgent and critical needs. However, because many people lack access to health care, the emergency department (ED) is increasingly used for nonurgent problems. Therefore, the philosophy of emergency management has broadened to include the concept that an emergency is whatever the patient or the family considers it to be.

Large numbers of people seek emergency care for serious life-threatening cardiac conditions, such as acute coronary syndrome (ACS), acute heart failure, pulmonary edema, and cardiac dysrhythmias. Priorities for managing these cardiac conditions are discussed in Chapters 27, 28, and 30. Emergency management of trauma and other conditions not found elsewhere in this book are discussed in this chapter. It is assumed that care and treatment are provided under the direction of a physician or emergency nurse practitioner. Facts about ED visits in the United States are presented in Chart 71-1.

CHART 71-1

Facts About Emergency Department Visits

In 2003, there were 114 million visits to emergency departments (EDs), a 26% increase from 1993. This increase is a result of overall population growth (by 12.3%) and an increase in the number of seniors (by 9.6%).

- People 65 years and older had the highest rate of ED visits; these rates were five times higher for nursing home residents. More than one third of all ED visits are by people older than 65 years.
- More than 14% of patients arrived at the ED by ambulance.
- Patients with Medicaid used EDs four times more often than patients with private health insurance.
- Injuries, poisonings, and adverse effects of medical treatments accounted for 35% of all ED visits.
- The leading causes of injuries, including falls, being unintentionally struck, and motor vehicle crashes, accounted for 41% of injury-related ED visits.
- The average ED waiting time before being seen by a health care provider for definitive treatment was 46.5 minutes.

Source: National Hospital Ambulatory Medical Care Survey. (2003). *2003 Emergency department summary.* Advance Data No. 358. Available online: http://www.cdc.gov/nchs/pressroom/05news/emergencydept.html. Accessed August 10, 2006.

Scope and Practice of Emergency Nursing

The emergency nurse has had specialized education, training, experience, and expertise in assessing and identifying patients' health care problems in crisis situations. In addition, the emergency nurse establishes priorities, monitors and continuously assesses acutely ill and injured patients, supports and attends to families, supervises allied health personnel, and teaches patients and families within a time-limited, high-pressured care environment. Nursing interventions are accomplished interdependently, in

Glossary

antivenin: antitoxin manufactured from venom of poisonous snakes to assist the patient's immune system response to an envenomation

carboxyhemoglobin: hemoglobin that is bound to carbon monoxide and therefore is unable to bind with oxygen, resulting in hypoxemia

corrosive poison: alkaline or acidic agent; causes tissue destruction after contact

cricothyroidotomy: surgical opening of the cricothyroid membrane to obtain an airway that is maintained with a tracheostomy or endotracheal tube

diagnostic peritoneal lavage: instillation of lactated Ringer's or normal saline solution into the abdominal cavity to detect red blood cells, white blood cells, bile, bacteria, amylase, or gastrointestinal contents indicative of abdominal injury

emergent: triage category signifying potentially life-threatening injuries or illnesses requiring immediate treatment

envenomation: injection of a poisonous material by sting, spine, bite, or other means

fasciotomy: surgical incision of the extremity to the level of the fascia to relieve pressure and restore neurovascular function to the extremity

Hare traction: portable in-line traction applied to the lower extremity to manage femur or hip fractures or dislocations

minor: triage category signifying non–life-threatening injuries or illnesses that can be routinely managed in a clinic or physician's office or that require no medical care

nonurgent: triage category signifying episodic or minor injury or illness in which treatment may be delayed several hours or longer without increased morbidity

resuscitation: triage category signifying life-threatening injuries or illnesses requiring immediate intervention

triage: process of assessing patients to determine management priorities

urgent: triage category signifying serious illness or injury that is not immediately life-threatening

consultation with or under the direction of a physician or nurse practitioner. The strengths of nursing and medicine are complementary in an emergency situation. Appropriate nursing and medical interventions are anticipated based on assessment data. The emergency health care staff members work as a team in performing the highly technical, hands-on skills required to care for patients in emergency situations.

The nursing process provides a logical framework for problem solving in this environment. Patients in the ED have a wide variety of actual or potential problems, and their condition may change constantly. Therefore, nursing assessment must be continuous, and nursing diagnoses change with the patient's condition. Although a patient may have several diagnoses at a given time, the focus is on the most life-threatening ones; often, both independent and interdependent nursing interventions are required.

Issues in Emergency Nursing Care

Emergency nursing is demanding because of the diversity of conditions and situations that present unique challenges. These challenges include legal issues, occupational health and safety risks for ED staff, and the challenge of providing holistic care in the context of a fast-paced, technology-driven environment in which serious illness and death are confronted on a daily basis. Another dimension of emergency nursing is nursing in disasters. With the increasing use of weapons of terror and mass destruction, the emergency nurse must expand his or her knowledge base to encompass recognizing and treating patients exposed to biologic and other terror weapons and anticipate nursing care in the event of a mass casualty incident. See Chapter 72 for a full discussion of nursing care in disasters, including caring for patients injured by acts of terrorism.

Documentation of Consent and Privacy

Consent to examine and treat the patient is part of the ED record. The patient must consent to invasive procedures (eg, angiography, lumbar puncture) unless he or she is unconscious or in critical condition and unable to make decisions. If the patient is unconscious and brought to the ED without family or friends, this fact should be documented. Monitoring of the patient's condition, as well as all instituted treatments and the times at which they were performed, must be documented. After treatment, a notation is made on the record about the patient's condition on discharge or transfer and about instructions given to the patient and family for follow-up care.

At the time of consent, the patient is usually also provided a statement of the privacy policy of the health care agency, according to federal law. Patients involved in violent events are often provided with an alias and access to the medical record, both paper and electronic, is limited to protect the privacy of the patient. A patient may also request extra privacy by limiting access to his or her room and by choosing not to receive phone calls, mail, flowers, other gifts, or certain visitors. These practices relate to the federally mandated privacy policy stipulated in the Health Insurance Portability and Accountability Act (HIPAA).

Limiting Exposure to Health Risks

Because of the increasing numbers of people infected with hepatitis B and C and with human immunodeficiency virus (HIV), health care providers are at an increased risk for exposure to communicable diseases through blood or other body fluids. This risk is further compounded in the ED because of the common use of invasive treatments in patients who may have a wide range of conditions and who frequently cannot provide a comprehensive medical history. All emergency health care providers must adhere strictly to Standard Precautions for minimizing exposure.

The reemergence of tuberculosis as a major health problem is complicated by multi–drug-resistant tuberculosis and by tuberculosis concomitant with HIV infection. Early identification and adherence to transmission-based precautions for patients who are potentially infectious are crucial. Nurses in the ED are usually fitted with personal high-efficiency particulate air (HEPA) filter masks to use when treating patients with airborne diseases.

The potential for exposure to highly contagious organisms, hazardous chemicals or gases, and radiation related to acts of terrorism or natural or manmade disasters presents additional risks to ED staff. Refer to Chapter 72 for information about decontamination procedures.

Violence in the Emergency Department

Not only do ED staff members encounter patients who are violent from substance abuse, injury, or other emergencies, but they may also encounter violent situations in the rest of the environment. Patients and families waiting for assistance are frequently emotionally volatile. Often, waiting rooms are the sites where feelings of dissatisfaction, fear, and anger are channeled violently. Some EDs assign security officers to the area and have installed metal detectors to identify weapons and protect patients, families, and staff. It is not unusual for a patient or family member to come to the ED armed. Nurses and other personnel must be prepared to deal with such circumstances.

Safety is the first priority. Protecting the ED on a daily basis prevents any untoward events from occurring. Protection of the department provides protection for the patients, families, and staff. It is essential that all nurses be aware of the environment in which they are working.

Metal detectors, silent alarm systems, and secured entry into the department assist in maintaining safety. Members of gangs and feuding families need to be separated in the ED, in the waiting room, and later in the inpatient nursing unit to avoid angry confrontations. Security officers should be ready to assist at all times. The ED should be able to be locked against entry if security is at all in question.

Patients from prison and those who are under guard need to be handcuffed to the bed and appropriately assessed to ensure the safety of hospital staff and other patients. The same assessment and care that are provided to patients with hand or ankle restraints are provided to patients with handcuffs. In addition, the following precautions are taken:

- Never release the hand or ankle restraint (handcuff).
- Always have a guard present in the room.
- Place the patient face down on the stretcher to avoid injury from head-butting, spitting, or biting.

- Use restraints on any violent patient as needed.
- Administer medication if necessary to control violent behavior until definitive treatment can be obtained.

In the case of gunfire in the ED, self-protection is a priority. There is no advantage to protecting others if the caregivers are also injured. Security officers and police must gain control of the situation first, and then care is provided to the injured.

Providing Holistic Care

Sudden illness or trauma is a stress to physiologic and psychological homeostasis that requires physiologic and psychological healing. Patients and families experiencing sudden injury or illness often are overwhelmed by anxiety because they have not had time to adapt to the crisis. They experience real and terrifying fear of death, mutilation, immobilization, and other assaults on their personal identity and body integrity. When confronted with trauma, severe disfigurement, severe illness, or sudden death, the family experiences several stages of crisis. The stages begin with anxiety and progress through denial, remorse and guilt, anger, grief, and reconciliation. The initial goal for the patient and family is anxiety reduction, a prerequisite to effective and appropriate coping. During this stressful time, safety is of prime importance. Close observation and preplanning are essential and security personnel are stationed nearby in the event that a patient or family member responds to stress with physical violence.

Assessment of the patient and family's psychological function includes evaluating emotional expression, degree of anxiety, and cognitive functioning. Possible nursing diagnoses include anxiety related to uncertain potential outcomes of the illness or trauma and ineffective individual coping related to acute situational crisis. In addition to anxiety, possible nursing diagnoses for the family include anticipatory grieving, alterations in family processes, and ineffective family coping related to acute situational crises.

PATIENT-FOCUSED INTERVENTIONS

Clinicians caring for the patient should act confidently and competently to relieve anxiety. Responding to the patient in a warm manner promotes a sense of security. Explanations should be given on a level that the patient can understand, because an informed patient is better able to cope positively with stress. Human contact and reassuring words reduce the panic of the severely injured or ill person and aid in dispelling fear of the unknown.

The unconscious patient should be treated as if conscious; that is, the patient should be touched, called by name, and given an explanation of every procedure that is performed. As the patient regains consciousness, the nurse should orient the patient by stating his or her name, the date, and the location. This basic information should be provided repeatedly, as needed, in a reassuring way.

FAMILY-FOCUSED INTERVENTIONS

The family is kept informed about where the patient is, how he or she is doing, and the care that is being given. Allowing the family to stay with the patient, when possible, also helps allay their anxieties. Additional interventions are based on the assessment of the stage of crisis that the family is experiencing. Measures to help family members cope with sudden death are presented in Chart 71-2.

Anxiety and Denial. During these crises, family members are encouraged to recognize and talk about their feelings of anxiety. Asking questions is encouraged. Honest answers given at the level of the family's understanding must be provided. Although denial is an ego-defense mechanism that protects one from recognizing painful and disturbing aspects of reality, prolonged denial is not encouraged or supported. The family must be prepared for the reality of what has happened and what may come.

Remorse and Guilt. Expressions of remorse and guilt are common, with family members accusing themselves (or each other) of negligence or minor omissions. Family members are urged to verbalize their feelings until they realize that there was probably little that they could have done to prevent the injury or illness.

CHART 71-2

Helping Family Members Cope With Sudden Death

- Take the family to a private place.
- Talk to the family together, so that they can mourn together.
- Reassure the family that everything possible was done; inform them of the treatment rendered.
- Avoid using euphemisms such as "passed on." Show the family that you care by touching, offering coffee, water, and the services of a chaplain.
- Encourage family members to support each other and to express emotions freely (grief, loss, anger, helplessness, tears, disbelief).
- Avoid giving sedation to family members; this may mask or delay the grieving process, which is necessary to achieve emotional equilibrium and to prevent prolonged depression.
- Encourage the family to view the body if they wish; this action helps to integrate the loss. Cover disfigured and injured areas before the family sees the body. Go with the family to see the body. Show acceptance by touching the body to give the family "permission" to touch.
- Spend time with the family, listening to them and identifying any needs that they may have for which the nursing staff can be helpful.
- Allow family members to talk about the deceased and what he or she meant to them; this permits ventilation of feelings of loss. Encourage the family to talk about events preceding admission to the emergency department. Do not challenge initial feelings of anger or denial.
- Avoid volunteering unnecessary information (eg, the patient was drinking).

Anger. Expressions of anger, common in crisis situations, are a way of handling anxiety and fear. Anger is frequently directed by the family at the patient, but it is also often expressed toward the physician, the nurse, or admitting personnel. The therapeutic approach is to allow the anger to be ventilated, then assist the family members to identify their feelings of frustration.

Grief. Grief is a complex emotional response to anticipated or actual loss. The key nursing intervention is to help family members work through their grief and to support their coping mechanisms, letting them know that it is normal and acceptable for them to cry, feel pain, and express loss. The hospital chaplain and social services staff both serve as invaluable members of the team when assisting families to work through their grief.

Emergency Nursing and the Continuum of Care

As stated previously, one principle underlying emergency care is that the patient is rapidly assessed, treated, and referred to the appropriate setting for ongoing care. This makes the ED a very temporary point on the continuum of care. Most patients who receive emergency care are discharged directly from the ED to their homes, and emergency nurses must plan and facilitate the patient's safe discharge and follow-up care in the home and the community.

Discharge Planning

Before discharge, instructions for continuing care are given to the patient and the family or significant others. All instructions should be given not only verbally but also in writing, so that the patient can refer to them later. Many EDs have preprinted standard instruction sheets for the more common conditions. These instructions are then individualized for each patient. These instructions may be available in a variety of languages. If they are not available in a language that the patient speaks, an interpreter should be used. Instructions should include information about prescribed medications, treatments, diet, activity, and when to contact a health care provider or schedule follow-up appointments. It is imperative that instructions are written legibly, use simple language, and are clear in their teaching. When providing discharge instructions, the nurse also considers any special needs the patient may have related to hearing or visual impairments. Alternate formats of instruction (eg, large print, Braille, audiotape) should be available to meet the needs of patients with hearing or visual impairments.

Community Services

Before discharge, some patients require the services of a social worker to help them meet continuing health care needs. For patients and families who cannot provide care at home, community agencies (eg, home care nursing services, Visiting Nurse Association) may be contacted before discharge to arrange services. This is particularly important for elderly patients who need assistance. Identifying continuing health care needs and making arrangements for meeting these needs can prevent return visits to the ED and readmission to the hospital.

For patients who are returning to extended care facilities and for those who already rely on community agencies for continuing health care, communication about the patient's condition and any changes in health care needs that have occurred must be provided to the appropriate facilities or agencies. This communication is essential to promote continuity of care and to ensure ongoing care to meet the patient's changing health care needs.

Gerontologic Considerations

The ED is a common point of entry into the health care system for patients 65 years and older. In fact, patients in this age group account for more than 99 million visits to emergency facilities each year (National Hospital Ambulatory Medical Care Survey, 2003) (see Chart 71-1). Elderly patients typically arrive with one or more presenting conditions. Nonspecific symptoms, such as weakness and fatigue, episodes of falling, incontinence, and change in mental status, may be manifestations of acute, potentially life-threatening illness in the elderly person. Emergencies in this age group may be more difficult to manage because elderly patients may have an atypical presentation, an altered response to treatment, a greater risk of developing complications, or a combination of these factors.

The elderly patient may perceive the emergency as a crisis signaling the end of an independent lifestyle or even resulting in death. The nurse should give attention to the patient's feelings of anxiety and fear.

The older patient may have fewer sources of social and financial support in addition to frail health. The nurse should assess the psychosocial resources of the patient (and of the caregiver, if necessary) and anticipate discharge needs. Referrals for support services (eg, to the social service department or a gerontologic nurse specialist) may be necessary.

Principles of Emergency Care

By definition, emergency care is care that must be rendered without delay. In an ED, several patients with diverse health problems—some life-threatening, some not—may present to the ED simultaneously. One of the first principles of emergency care is triage.

Triage

The word **triage** comes from the French word *trier,* meaning "to sort." In the daily routine of the ED, triage is used to sort patients into groups based on the severity of their health problems and the immediacy with which these problems must be treated.

EDs use various triage systems with differing terminology, but all share this characteristic of a hierarchy based on the potential for loss of life. A basic and widely used triage system that has been in use for many years has three categories: emergent, urgent, and nonurgent (Berner, 2005). **Emergent** patients have the highest priority—their conditions are life-threatening and they must be seen immediately. **Urgent** patients have serious health problems but not immediately life-threatening ones; they must be seen within 1 hour. **Nonurgent** patients have episodic illnesses that can be addressed within 24 hours without increased morbidity (Berner, 2005). A fourth class that is increasingly used is "fast-track." These patients require simple first aid or basic primary care and may be treated in the ED or safely referred to a clinic or physician's office.

A more refined comprehensive triage system has been implemented to incorporate the changes in the use of the ED for both emergency and routine health care. This system has five levels: resuscitation, emergent, urgent, nonurgent, and minor (Tanabe, Gimbel, Yarnold, et al., 2004). The increased number of triage levels assists the triage nurse to more precisely determine the needs of the patient and the urgency for treatment. This five-level triage system is currently used throughout the United States, Australia, the United Kingdom, and Canada.

In the five-level system, patients in the emergent category identified in the previously used three-level system have been divided into two distinct groupings, resuscitation and emergent. Patients in the **resuscitation** category need treatment immediately to prevent death. Patients in the emergent category may deteriorate rapidly and develop a major life-threatening situation or require time-sensitive treatment. Patients in the urgent category have non–life-threatening conditions but require two or more resources (defined below) to provide their care. If these patients' vital signs deviate significantly from their baseline, they may require "up-triaging" to the emergent category. Patients in the nonurgent category have non–life-threatening conditions and likely need only one resource to provide for their needs. Patients in the **minor** category have no life-threatening condition and likely require no resources to provide their evaluation and management.

Resources are defined as imaging studies, medications administered by intravenous (IV) or intramuscular (IM) routes, and invasive procedures. Insertion of an indwelling catheter is an example of a one-resource procedure. Moderate sedation would be classified as a two-resource procedure because it requires frequent monitoring and IV medications.

Triage is an advanced skill. Emergency nurses spend many hours learning to classify different illnesses and injuries to ensure that patients most in need of care do not needlessly wait to receive it. Protocols may be followed to initiate laboratory or x-ray studies while the patient is in the triage area awaiting a bed in the ED. Collaborative protocols are developed and used by the triage nurse based on his or her level of experience. Nurses in the triage area collect additional crucial baseline data: full vital signs including pain assessment, history of the current event and past medical history, neurologic assessment findings, weight, allergies (especially latex), domestic violence screening, and necessary diagnostic data. Some facilities collect these data in a computerized system, which helps guide the nurse through the assessment and documentation. The following questions reflect the minimum information that should be obtained from the patient or from the person who accompanied the patient to the ED. (Of course, all answers are documented for reference by other health care providers.)

- What were the circumstances, precipitating events, location, and time of the injury or illness?
- When did the symptoms appear?
- Was the patient unconscious after the injury or onset of illness?
- How did the patient get to the ED?
- What was the health status of the patient before the injury or illness?
- Is there a history of medical illness or previous surgeries? A history of admissions to the hospital?
- Is the patient currently taking any medications, especially hormones, insulin, digitalis, or anticoagulants?
- Does the patient have any allergies, especially to eggs, latex, medications, or nuts?
- Does the patient have any fears? Does the patient feel that he or she is in a situation in which he or she is unsafe?
- When was the last meal eaten? (This is important if general anesthesia is to be given or if the patient is unconscious.)
- When was the last menstrual period?
- Is the patient under a physician's care? What are the name and location of the physician?
- What was the date of the patient's most recent tetanus immunization?

Routine ED triage protocols differ significantly from the triage protocols used in disasters and mass casualty incidents (field triage). Routine triage directs all available resources to the patients who are most critically ill, regardless of potential outcome. In field triage (or hospital triage during a disaster), scarce resources must be used to benefit the most people possible. This distinction affects triage decisions. See Chapter 72 for a discussion of triage in mass casualty situations.

Assess and Intervene

For the patient assigned to a resuscitation, emergent, or urgent triage category, stabilization, provision of critical treatments, and prompt transfer to the appropriate setting (intensive care unit, operating room, general care unit) are the priorities of emergency care. Although treatment is initiated in the ED, ongoing definitive treatment of the underlying problem is provided in other settings, and the sooner the patient is stabilized and moved to that area, the better the outcome.

A systematic approach to effectively establishing and treating health priorities is the primary survey/secondary survey approach. The primary survey focuses on stabilizing life-threatening conditions. The ED staff work collaboratively and follow the ABCD (**a**irway, **b**reathing, **c**irculation, **d**isability) method:

- Establish a patent airway.
- Provide adequate ventilation, employing resuscitation measures when necessary. (Trauma patients must have the cervical spine protected and chest injuries assessed first.)
- Evaluate and restore cardiac output by controlling hemorrhage, preventing and treating shock, and maintaining or restoring effective circulation. This includes the prevention and management of hypothermia.
- Determine neurologic disability by assessing neurologic function using the Glasgow Coma Scale (see Chapter 65).

After these priorities have been addressed, the ED team proceeds with the secondary survey. This includes the following:

- A complete health history and head-to-toe assessment
- Diagnostic and laboratory testing
- Insertion or application of monitoring devices such as electrocardiogram (ECG) electrodes, arterial lines, or urinary catheters
- Splinting of suspected fractures
- Cleansing, closure, and dressing of wounds
- Performance of other necessary interventions based on the patient's condition

Once the patient has been assessed, stabilized, and tested, appropriate medical and nursing diagnoses are formulated, initial important treatment is started, and plans for the proper disposition of the patient are made. Many emergent and urgent conditions and priority emergency interventions are discussed in detail in the remaining sections of this chapter.

In addition to the management of the illness or injury, the ED nurse must also focus on providing comfort and emotional support to the patient and family. Included in this is pain management. Effective pain management must be instituted early and should include rapid-acting agents that result in minimal sedation so that the patient can continue to interact with the staff for continued assessment. Moderate sedation can help facilitate short procedures in the ED; the patient will not remember the procedure later. The patient is closely monitored during the procedure and then rapidly awakens when it is complete (see Chapter 19).

Family crisis intervention is essential for all ED patients. Even if a patient's condition is not emergent, the situation may be perceived as such by the family. Every family needs attention and support. The chaplain and social worker may be available to assist with interventions.

Airway Obstruction

Acute upper airway obstruction is a life-threatening medical emergency.

Pathophysiology

The airway may be partially or completely occluded. Partial obstruction of the airway can lead to progressive hypoxia, hypercarbia, and respiratory and cardiac arrest. If the airway is completely obstructed, permanent brain injury or death will occur within 3 to 5 minutes secondary to hypoxia. Air movement is absent in the presence of complete airway obstruction. Oxygen saturation of the blood decreases rapidly because the obstructed airway prevents entry of air into the lungs. Oxygen deficit occurs in the brain, resulting in unconsciousness, with death following rapidly.

Upper airway obstruction has a number of causes, including aspiration of foreign bodies, anaphylaxis, viral or bacterial infection, trauma, and inhalation or chemical burns. For elderly patients, especially those in extended-care facilities, sedatives and hypnotic medications, diseases affecting motor coordination (eg, Parkinson's disease), and mental dysfunction (eg, dementia, mental retardation) are risk factors for asphyxiation by food. In adults, aspiration of a bolus of meat is the most common cause of airway obstruction. In children, small toys, buttons, coins, and other objects are commonly aspirated in addition to food. Peritonsillar abscesses, epiglottitis, and other acute infectious processes of the posterior pharynx can also result in airway obstruction.

Clinical Manifestations

Typically, a person with a foreign body airway obstruction cannot speak, breathe, or cough. The patient may clutch the neck between the thumb and fingers (*universal distress signal*). Other common signs and symptoms include choking, apprehensive appearance, inspiratory and expiratory stridor, labored breathing, use of accessory muscles (suprasternal and intercostal retraction), flaring nostrils, increasing anxiety, restlessness, and confusion. Cyanosis and loss of consciousness develop as hypoxia worsens.

Assessment and Diagnostic Findings

Assessment of the patient who has a foreign object occluding the airway may involve simply asking the person whether he or she is choking and requires help. If the person is unconscious, inspection of the oropharynx may reveal the offending object. X-rays, laryngoscopy, or bronchoscopy also may be performed.

Management

If the patient can breathe and cough spontaneously, a partial obstruction should be suspected. The victim is encouraged to cough forcefully and to persist with spontaneous coughing and breathing efforts as long as good air exchange exists. There may be some wheezing between coughs. If the patient demonstrates a weak, ineffective cough, high-pitched noise while inhaling, increased respiratory difficulty, or cyanosis, the patient should be managed as if there were complete airway obstruction.

After the obstruction is removed, rescue breathing is initiated. If the patient has no pulse, cardiac compressions are instituted. These measures provide oxygen to the brain, heart, and other vital organs until definitive medical treatment can restore and support normal heart and ventilatory activity.

ESTABLISHING AN AIRWAY

Establishing an airway may be as simple as repositioning the patient's head to prevent the tongue from obstructing the pharynx. Alternatively, other maneuvers, such as abdominal thrusts, the head-tilt–chin-lift maneuver, the jaw-thrust maneuver, or insertion of specialized equipment, may be needed to open the airway, remove a foreign body, or maintain the airway. In all maneuvers, the cervical spine must be protected from injury. After these maneuvers are performed, the patient is assessed for breathing by watching for chest movement and listening and feeling for air movement. In such a case, nursing diagnoses would include ineffective airway clearance related to obstruction of the tongue, object, or fluids (blood, saliva). The nursing diagnosis may also be ineffective breathing pattern related to obstruction or injury.

Abdominal Thrusts

The terms *subdiaphragmatic abdominal thrusts* and *abdominal thrusts* are used interchangeably, depending on the circumstances. A subdiaphragmatic abdominal thrust, by elevating the diaphragm, can force air from the lungs to create an artificial cough intended to move and expel an obstructing foreign body from the airway. The term *Heimlich maneuver* is used for the sake of uniformity. Chart 71-3 describes how to manage a foreign body obstruction using abdominal or chest thrusts.

Head-Tilt–Chin-Lift Maneuver

The patient is placed supine on a firm, flat surface. If the patient is lying face down, the body is turned as a unit so that the head, shoulders, and torso move simultaneously with no twisting. Next, the airway is opened using either the head-tilt–chin-lift maneuver or the jaw-thrust maneuver. In the head-tilt–chin-lift maneuver, one hand is placed on the victim's forehead, and firm backward pressure is applied with the palm to tilt the head back. The fingers of the other hand are placed under the bony part of the lower jaw near the chin and lifted up. The chin and the teeth are brought forward almost to occlusion to support the jaw.

CHART 71-3

Managing a Foreign Body Airway Obstruction

Assess for Indications of Airway Obstruction

- Person may clutch the neck between thumb and fingers
- Weak, ineffective cough; high-pitched noises on inspiration
- Increased respiratory distress
- Inability to speak, breathe, or cough
- Collapse

Heimlich Maneuver (subdiaphragmatic abdominal thrusts)

FOR STANDING OR SITTING CONSCIOUS PATIENT:

Stand behind the patient, wrap your arms around the patient's waist, and proceed as follows:

1. Make a fist with one hand, placing the thumb side of the fist against the patient's abdomen, in the midline slightly above the umbilicus and well below the xiphoid process. Grasp the fist with the other hand.
2. Press your fist into the patient's abdomen with a quick inward and upward thrust. Each new thrust should be a separate and distinct maneuver.

FOR PATIENT LYING DOWN (UNCONSCIOUS):

1. Position patient on the back.
2. Kneel astride the patient's thighs, facing the head.
3. Place the heel of one hand against the patient's abdomen, in the midline slightly above the umbilicus and well below the tip of the xiphoid; place the second hand directly on top of the first.
4. Press into the abdomen with a quick upward thrust.

FINGER SWEEP:

1. Open the adult patient's mouth by grasping both the tongue and lower jaw between the thumb and fingers and lifting the mandible (tongue–jaw lift). This maneuver is to be used *only in the unconscious adult patient.* This action draws the tongue away from the back of the throat and away from the foreign body that may be lodged there.
2. Insert the index finger of the other hand down along the inside of the cheek and scrape across the back of the throat.
3. Use a hooking action to dislodge the foreign body and maneuver it into the mouth for removal. Care is used to avoid forcing the object deeper into the throat.

CHEST THRUSTS WITH CONSCIOUS PATIENT STANDING OR SITTING (this technique is to be used *only in the patient in advanced stages of pregnancy or in the markedly obese person):*

1. Stand behind the patient with your arms under the patient's axillae to encircle the patient's chest.
2. Place the thumb side of your fist on the middle of the patient's sternum, taking care to avoid the xiphoid process and the margins of the rib cage.
3. Grasp your fist with the other hand and perform backward thrusts until the foreign body is expelled or the patient becomes unconscious. Each thrust should be administered with the intent of relieving the obstruction.

CHEST THRUST WITH PATIENT LYING (unconscious). This maneuver is *used only in the patient in advanced stages of pregnancy or when the rescuer cannot apply the Heimlich maneuver effectively to the unconscious, markedly obese person:*

1. Place the patient on the back and kneel close to the side of the patient's body.
2. Place the heel of your hand on the lower half of the sternum.
3. Deliver each chest thrust slowly and distinctly with the intent of relieving the obstruction.

Adapted from American Heart Association. (2005). *BLS for healthcare providers.* (2005). American Heart Association. Available online: http://www.americanheart.org. Accessed August 9, 2006.

NURSING ALERT

The head-tilt–chin-lift maneuver, which helps tilt the head back, should be used only if it is determined that the patient's cervical spine is not injured.

Jaw-Thrust Maneuver

After one hand is placed on each side of the patient's jaw, the angles of the patient's lower jaw are grasped and lifted, displacing the mandible forward. This is a safe approach to opening the airway of a patient with suspected neck injury because it can be accomplished without extending the neck.

Oropharyngeal Airway Insertion

An oropharyngeal airway is a semicircular tube or tube-like plastic device that is inserted over the back of the tongue into the lower posterior pharynx in a patient who is breathing spontaneously but who is unconscious (Chart 71-4). This type of airway prevents the tongue from falling back against the posterior pharynx and obstructing the airway. It also allows health care providers to suction secretions.

Endotracheal Intubation

The purpose of endotracheal intubation is to establish and maintain the airway in patients with respiratory insufficiency or hypoxia. Endotracheal intubation is indicated for the following reasons: (1) to establish an airway for a patient who cannot be adequately ventilated with an oropharyngeal airway, (2) to bypass an upper airway obstruction, (3) to prevent aspiration, (4) to permit connection of the patient to a resuscitation bag or mechanical ventilator, and (5) to facilitate the removal of tracheobronchial secretions (Fig. 71-1). Because the procedure requires skill, endotracheal intubation is performed only by those who have had extensive training. These include physicians, nurse anesthetists, respiratory therapists, flight nurses, and nurse practitioners. However, the emergency nurse is commonly called on to assist with intubation.

Intubation With a Combitube

If the patient is not hospitalized and cannot be intubated in the field, emergency medical personnel may insert a Combitube. The tube rapidly provides pharyngeal ventilation. When the tube is inserted into the trachea, it functions like an endotracheal tube (Fig. 71-2).

The two balloons that surround the tube are inflated after the tube is inserted. One balloon is large (100 mL) and occludes the oropharynx. This permits ventilation by forcing air through the larynx. The smaller balloon is inflated with 15 mL of air and can occlude the trachea if it is inadvertently placed there. Breath sounds are auscultated after balloon inflation to make sure that the oropharyngeal

CHART 71-4

Inserting an Oropharyngeal Airway

1. Measure the oral airway alongside the head. The airway should reach from lip to ear.
2. Extend the patient's head by placing one hand under the bony chin (*only if the cervical spine is uninjured*). With the other hand, tilt the head backward by applying pressure to the forehead while simultaneously lifting the chin forward.
3. Open the patient's mouth.
4. (**A**) Insert the oropharyngeal airway with the tip facing up toward the roof of the mouth until it passes the uvula. (**B**) Rotate the tip 180 degrees so that the tip is pointed down toward the pharynx. This displaces the tongue anteriorly, and the patient then breathes through and around the airway.
5. The distal end of the oropharyngeal airway is in the hypopharynx, and the flange is approximately at the patient's lips. Make sure that the tongue has not been pushed into the airway.

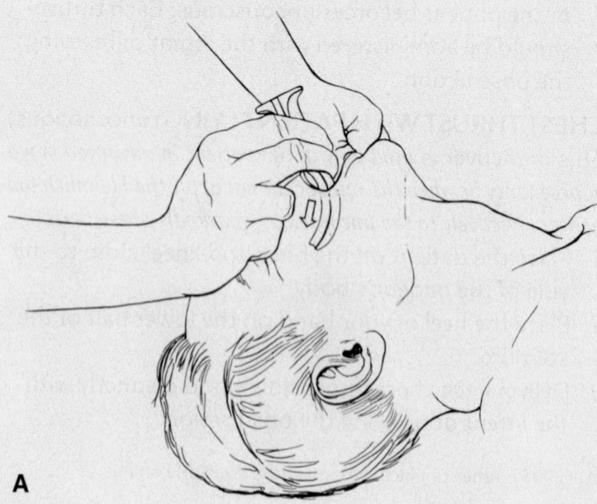

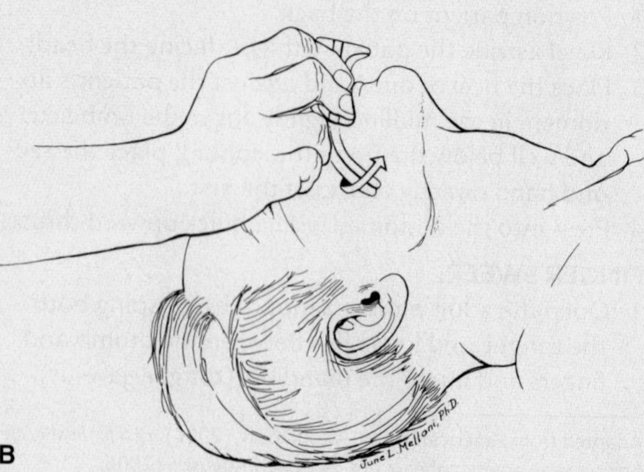

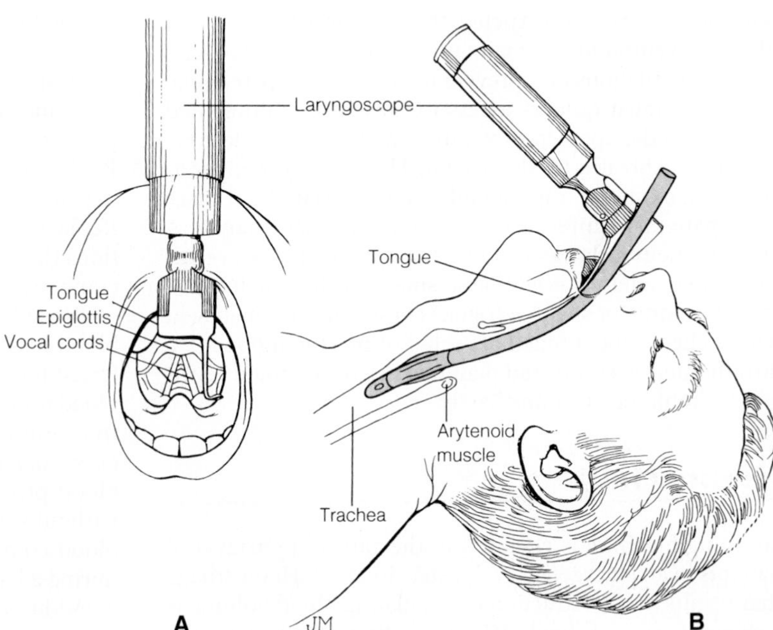

FIGURE 71-1. Endotracheal intubation in a patient without a cervical spine injury. (**A**) The primary glottic landmarks for tracheal intubation as visualized with proper placement of the laryngoscope. (**B**) Positioning the endotracheal tube.

balloon (or cuff) does not obstruct the glottis. The patient can be ventilated through either one of the two ports (eg, tracheal or esophageal) of the tube, depending on whether the tube is placed in the trachea or esophagus.

Cricothyroidotomy (Cricothyroid Membrane Puncture)

Cricothyroidotomy is the opening of the cricothyroid membrane to establish an airway. This procedure is used in emergency situations in which endotracheal intubation is either not possible or contraindicated, as in airway obstruction from extensive maxillofacial trauma, cervical spine injuries, laryngospasm, laryngeal edema (after an allergic reaction or extubation), hemorrhage into neck tissue, or obstruction of the larynx.

MAINTAINING VENTILATION

Only a few conditions, such as an obstructed airway or a sucking wound of the chest, take precedence over the immediate control of hemorrhage. After the airway is

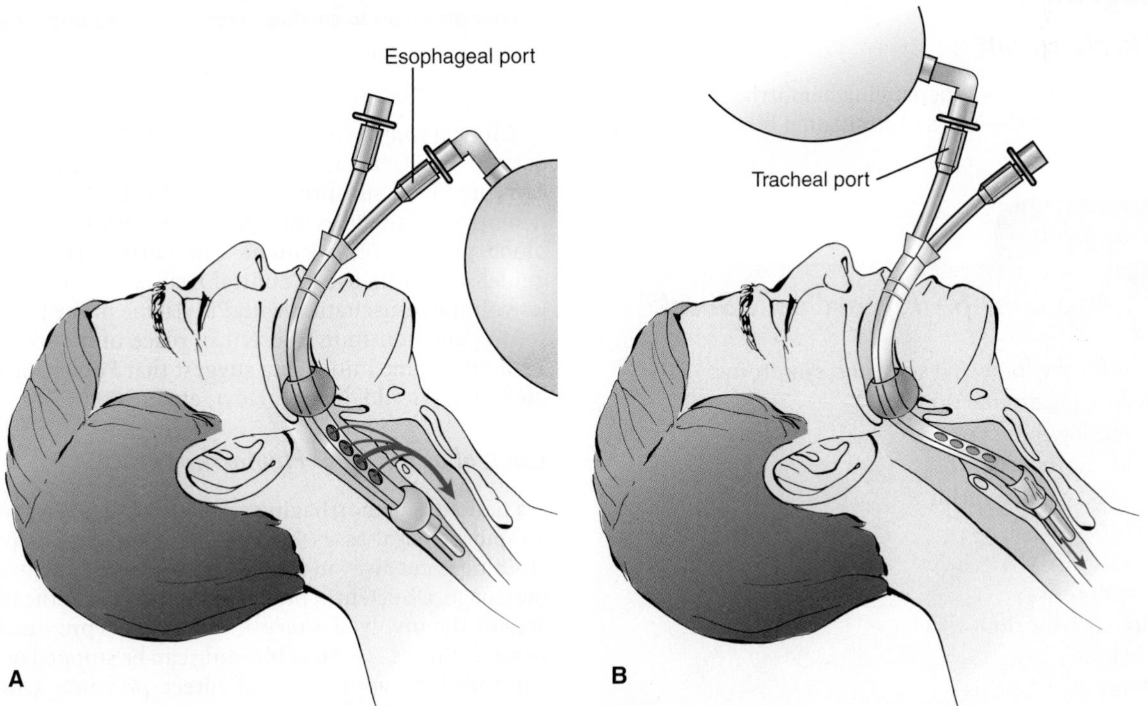

FIGURE 71-2. Combitube (**A**) in esophageal position and (**B**) in tracheal position.

determined to be unobstructed, the nurse must ensure that adequate ventilation is maintained. Satisfactory management of ventilations may prevent hypoxia and hypercapnia. The nurse must quickly assess for absent or diminished breath sounds, open chest wounds, and difficulty delivering artificial breaths for the patient. The nurse should monitor pulse oximetry, capnography, and arterial blood gases if the patient requires airway or ventilatory assistance. A tension pneumothorax can mimic hypovolemia, so ventilatory assessment precedes assessment for hemorrhage. A pneumothorax or sucking (open) chest wound is managed with a chest tube; immediate relief of increasing positive intrathoracic pressure and maintenance of adequate ventilation should occur immediately.

Hemorrhage

Stopping bleeding is essential to the care and survival of patients in an emergency or disaster situation. Hemorrhage that results in the reduction of circulating blood volume is a primary cause of shock. Minor bleeding, which is usually venous, generally stops spontaneously unless the patient has a bleeding disorder or has been taking anticoagulants.

The patient is assessed for signs and symptoms of shock: cool, moist skin (resulting from poor peripheral perfusion), decreasing blood pressure, increasing heart rate, delayed capillary refill, and decreasing urine volume (Chart 71-5). The goals of emergency management are to control the bleeding, maintain adequate circulating blood volume for tissue oxygenation, and prevent shock. Patients who hemorrhage are at risk for cardiac arrest caused by hypovolemia with secondary anoxia. Nursing interventions are carried out collaboratively with other members of the emergency health care team.

Management

Fluid Replacement

Whenever a patient is experiencing hemorrhage—whether external or internal—a loss of circulating blood results in a fluid volume deficit and decreased cardiac output. Therefore, fluid replacement is imperative to maintain circulation. Typically, two large-gauge IV catheters are inserted to provide a means for fluid and blood replacement, and blood samples are obtained for analysis, typing, and cross-matching. Replacement fluids are administered as prescribed, depending on clinical estimates of the type and volume of fluid lost. Replacement fluids may include isotonic electrolyte solutions (lactated Ringer's, normal saline), colloids, and blood component therapy.

Packed red blood cells are infused when there is massive blood loss. In emergencies, type O-negative blood is preferred for women of childbearing age and type O-positive blood is preferred for men and for postmenopausal women. In a resuscitation situation, there is not time to type and cross-match or type and screen blood. Type O-negative blood provides safe administration of blood immediately without sensitizing an Rh-negative woman to Rh-positive blood (sensitization can result in neonatal complications during a later pregnancy).

Additional platelets and clotting factors are given when large amounts of blood are needed, because transfused packed red blood cells are deficient in clotting factors. These additional products are given based on the results of coagulation studies that suggest a platelet or clotting deficiency.

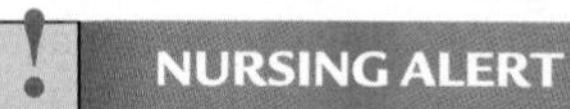

The infusion rate is determined by the severity of the blood loss and the clinical evidence of hypovolemia. If massive blood replacement is necessary, the blood must be warmed in a commercial blood warmer, because administration of large amounts of blood that has been refrigerated has a core cooling effect that may lead to cardiac arrest and coagulopathy.

Clinical trials using artificial blood (PolyHeme) are underway. PolyHeme is a human hemoglobin-based oxygen-carrying blood substitute that may be used for patients in hemorrhagic shock as interim therapy prior to surgery and blood product replacement. The current recommended guidelines for its use in clinical trials are to initiate vascular volume resuscitation with PolyHeme in the prehospital setting and continue to use it in place of blood for up to 12 hours. Some initial data suggest that PolyHeme may be lifesaving (Gould, Moore, Hoyt, et al., 2002).

Control of External Hemorrhage

If a patient is hemorrhaging externally (eg, from a wound), a rapid physical assessment is performed as the patient's clothing is cut away in an attempt to identify the area of hemorrhage. Direct, firm pressure is applied over the bleeding area or the involved artery at a site that is proximal to the wound (Fig. 71-3). Most bleeding can be stopped or at least controlled by application of direct pressure. Otherwise, unchecked arterial bleeding results in death. A firm pressure dressing is applied, and the injured part is elevated to

CHART 71-5

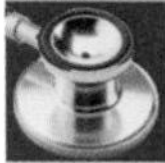

Assessing for Hypovolemic Shock

Be alert for the following signs and symptoms:

- Decreasing arterial pressure
- Increasing pulse rate
- Cold, moist skin
- Delayed capillary refill
- Pallor
- Thirst
- Diaphoresis
- Altered sensorium
- Oliguria
- Metabolic acidosis
- Hyperpnea

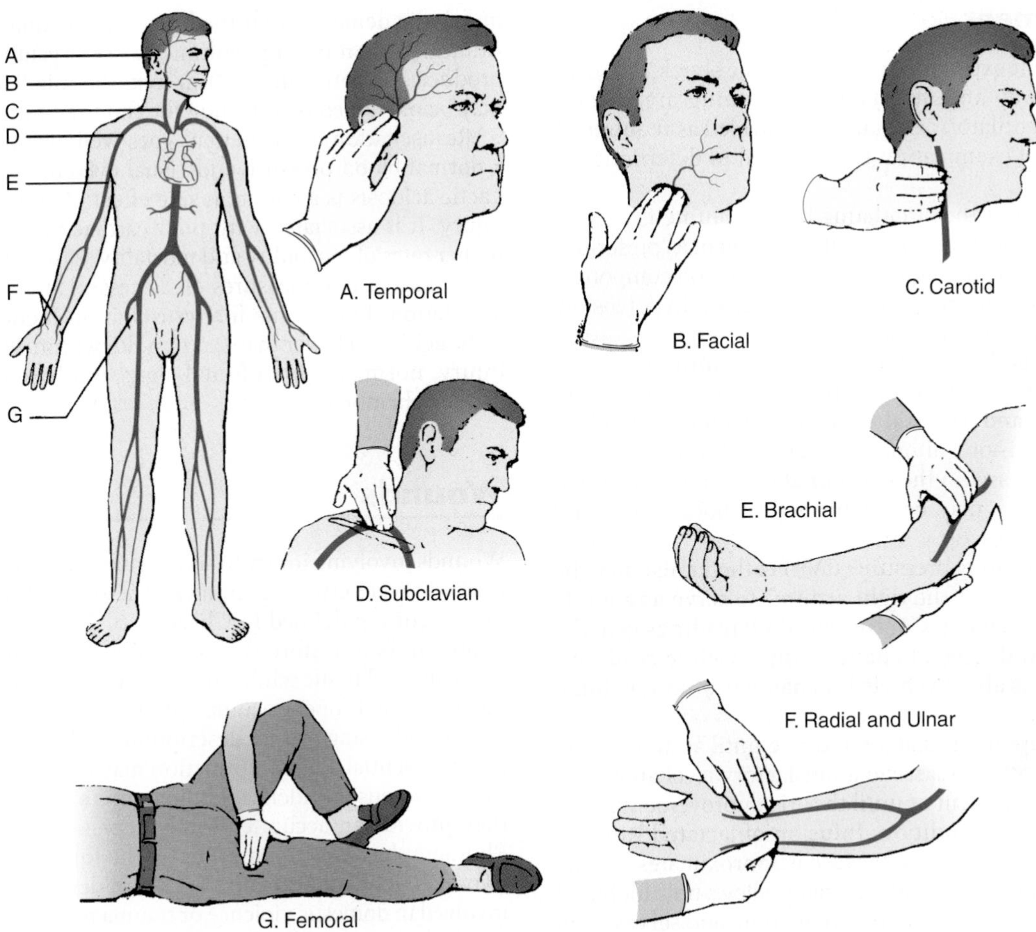

FIGURE 71-3. Pressure points for control of hemorrhage.

stop venous and capillary bleeding if possible. If the injured area is an extremity, the extremity is immobilized to control blood loss.

A tourniquet is applied to an extremity only as a *last resort* when the external hemorrhage cannot be controlled in any other way and immediate surgery is not feasible. Care must be taken when applying a tourniquet because of the risk for loss of the extremity. The tourniquet is applied just proximal to the wound and tied tightly enough to control arterial blood flow. The patient is tagged with a skin-marking pencil or on adhesive tape on the forehead with a "T," stating the location of the tourniquet and the time applied (Lakstein, Blumenfeld, Sokolov, et al., 2003). If there is no arterial bleeding, the tourniquet is removed and a pressure dressing is applied. If the patient has suffered a traumatic amputation with uncontrollable hemorrhage, the tourniquet remains in place until the patient is in the operating room.

Control of Internal Bleeding

If the patient shows no external signs of bleeding but exhibits tachycardia, falling blood pressure, thirst, apprehension, cool and moist skin, or delayed capillary refill, internal hemorrhage is suspected. Typically, packed red blood cells are administered at a rapid rate, and the patient is prepared for more definitive treatment (eg, surgery, pharmacologic therapy). In addition, arterial blood gas specimens are obtained to evaluate pulmonary function and tissue perfusion and to establish baseline hemodynamic parameters, which are then used as an index for determining the amount of fluid replacement the patient can tolerate and the response to therapy. The patient is maintained in the supine position and monitored closely until hemodynamic or circulatory parameters improve, or until he or she is transported to the operating room or intensive care unit.

Hypovolemic Shock

Shock is a condition in which there is loss of effective circulating blood volume. Inadequate organ and tissue perfusion follows, ultimately resulting in cellular metabolic derangements. In any emergency situation, the onset of shock should be anticipated by assessing all injured people immediately. The underlying cause of shock (hypovolemic, cardiogenic, neurogenic, anaphylactic or septic) must be determined. Of these, hypovolemia is the most common cause (see Chapter 14).

Altered tissue perfusion related to failing circulation, impaired gas exchange related to a ventilation–perfusion imbalance, and decreased cardiac output related to decreased circulating blood volume are possible problems associated with hypovolemic shock. Therefore, the goals of treatment are to restore and maintain tissue perfusion and to correct physiologic abnormalities.

Management

For the patient experiencing hypovolemic shock, ensuring a patent airway and maintaining breathing are crucial. Additional ventilatory assistance is provided as required. A rapid physical examination is performed to determine the cause of shock.

Restoration of the circulating blood volume is accomplished with rapid fluid and blood replacement as prescribed based on the patient's response to therapy. Blood component therapy helps optimize cardiac preload, correct hypotension, and maintain tissue perfusion.

Large-gauge IV catheters are inserted into peripheral veins. Two or more catheters are necessary for rapid fluid replacement and reversal of hemodynamic instability. The emphasis is on volume replacement. If it is suspected that a major vessel in the chest or abdomen has been disrupted, IV lines may be established in both upper and lower extremities.

A central venous pressure (CVP) catheter also may be inserted (in or near the right atrium) to serve as a guide for fluid replacement. Continuous CVP readings give the direction and degree of change from baseline readings. The catheter is also a vehicle for emergency fluid volume replacement.

IV fluids are infused at a rapid rate until systolic blood pressure or CVP increases to a satisfactory level above the baseline measurement or until there is improvement in the patient's clinical condition. Infusion of lactated Ringer's solution is useful initially because it approximates plasma electrolyte composition and osmolality, allows time for blood typing and screening, restores circulation, and serves as an adjunct to blood component therapy.

Blood component therapy may also be prescribed, especially if blood loss has been severe or if the patient continues to hemorrhage. Measures to control hemorrhage are instituted because hemorrhage compounds the shock state. Serial hemoglobin and hematocrit values are obtained if continued bleeding is suspected. Also, the patient's legs are elevated slightly to improve cerebral circulation and promote venous return to the heart. However, this position is contraindicated for patients with head injuries. Unnecessary movement is also avoided.

An indwelling urinary catheter is inserted to record urinary output every hour. Urine volume indicates the adequacy of kidney perfusion. However, fluid replacement should not be delayed while monitoring urine output.

Ongoing nursing surveillance of the *total patient* is maintained. Blood pressure, heart and respiratory rates, skin temperature, color, pulse oximetry, neurologic status, CVP, arterial blood gases, ECG recordings, hematocrit, hemoglobin, coagulation profile, electrolytes, and urinary output are monitored serially to assess patient response to treatment. Commonly, a flow sheet is used to document these parameters, providing an analysis of trends rather than single values to reveal improvement or deterioration of the patient's condition.

In addition, the body's defense mechanisms are supported. The patient should be reassured and comforted. Sedation may be necessary to relieve apprehension. Analgesics are used cautiously to relieve pain. Body temperature is maintained within normal limits to prevent increasing metabolic demands that the body may be unable to meet. Administration of large volumes of IV crystalloids, blood products, or both can result in hypothermia. Hypothermia may be prevented by warming the fluids administered.

Resuscitation of the patient goes well beyond achieving a normal blood pressure and visual evidence of perfusion. Lactic acidosis is a common side effect of hemorrhage and injury. It is associated with poor cardiac performance and higher rates of morbidity and mortality. Base deficit and lactic acid are useful measures of successful and complete resuscitation. End points for resuscitation include a serum lactic acid level lower than 2.5 mmol/L within 24 hours after injury, normalization of vital signs and base deficit, and arrest of hemorrhage.

Wounds

Wounds involving injury to soft tissues can vary from minor tears to severe crushing injuries. The types of wounds that may occur are defined in Chart 71-6. The primary goal of treatment is to restore the physical integrity and function of the injured tissue while minimizing scarring and preventing infection. Proper documentation of the characteristics of the wound, using precise descriptions and correct terminology, is essential. Such information may be needed in the future for forensic evidence. Photographs are helpful because they provide an accurate, visible depiction of the wound. Photographs also become important for exigent wounds (wounds that will heal and later be unidentifiable). Patients involved in domestic violence or trauma may need the photographs later to visually describe the extent of injury.

Determining *when* and *how* the wound occurred is important, because a treatment delay increases infection risk. Using aseptic technique, the clinician inspects the wound to determine the extent of damage to underlying structures.

CHART 71-6

Definition of Terms: Wounds

Laceration: skin tear with irregular edges and vein bridging

Avulsion: tearing away of tissue from supporting structures

Abrasion: denuded skin

Ecchymosis/contusion: blood trapped under the surface of the skin

Hematoma: tumorlike mass of blood trapped under the skin

Stab: incision of the skin with well-defined edges, usually caused by a sharp instrument; a stab wound is typically deeper than long

Cut: incision of the skin with well-defined edges, usually longer than deep

Patterned: wound representing the outline of the object (eg, steering wheel) causing the wound

Sensory, motor, and vascular function is evaluated for changes that might indicate complications.

Management

Wound Cleansing

Hair around the wound may be clipped or shaved (only as directed) if it is anticipated that the hairs will interfere with wound closure. Typically, the area around the wound is cleansed with normal saline solution or a polymer agent (eg, Shur-Clens). Antibacterial agents, such as povidone–iodine (Betadine) or hydrogen peroxide, should not be allowed to get deep into the wound without thorough rinsing. These agents are used only for the initial cleansing because they injure exposed and healthy tissue, resulting in further cell injury.

If indicated, the area is infiltrated with a local intradermal anesthetic through the wound margins or by regional block. Patients with soft tissue injuries usually have localized pain at the site of injury. The nurse then assists the physician, nurse practitioner, or physician's assistant in cleaning and débriding the wound.

The wound is irrigated gently and copiously with sterile isotonic saline solution to remove surface dirt. Devitalized tissue and foreign matter are removed because they impede healing and may encourage infection. Any small bleeding vessels are clamped or tied. Alternatively, hemostasis may be achieved with cauterization. After wound treatment, a nonadherent dressing is commonly applied to protect the wound. The dressing may serve as a splint and also as a reminder to the patient that the area is injured.

Primary Closure

The decision to suture a wound depends on the nature of the wound, the time since the injury was sustained, the degree of contamination, and the vascularity of tissues. If primary closure is indicated, the wound is sutured or stapled, usually by the physician, with the patient receiving either local anesthesia or moderate sedation (see Chapter 19). Wound closure begins when subcutaneous fat is brought together loosely with a few sutures to close off the dead space. The subcuticular layer is then closed, and finally the epidermis is closed. Sutures are placed near the wound edge, with the skin edges leveled carefully to promote optimal healing. Instead of sutures, sterile strips of reinforced microporous tape or a bonding agent (skin glue) may be used to close clean, superficial wounds.

Delayed Primary Closure

Delayed primary closure may be indicated if tissue has been lost or there is a high potential for infection.

A thin layer of gauze (to ensure drainage and prevent pooling of exudate), covered by an occlusive dressing, may be used. Other options include split-thickness cadaver allografts or porcine xenografts to simulate the function of epithelium. The wound is splinted in a functional position to prevent motion and decrease the possibility of contracture.

If there are no signs of suppuration (formation of purulent drainage), the wound may be sutured (with the patient receiving a local anesthetic). Use of antibiotics to prevent infection depends on factors such as how the injury occurred, the age of the wound, and the risk of contamination. The site is immobilized and elevated to limit accumulation of fluid in the interstitial spaces of the wound.

Tetanus prophylaxis is administered as prescribed, based on the condition of the wound and the patient's immunization status. If the patient's last tetanus booster was given more than 5 years ago, or if the patient's immunization status is unknown, a tetanus booster must be given. The patient is instructed about signs and symptoms of infection and is instructed to contact the health care provider or clinic if there is sudden or persistent pain, fever or chills, bleeding, rapid swelling, foul odor, drainage, or redness surrounding the wound.

Trauma

Trauma (an unintentional or intentional wound or injury inflicted on the body from a mechanism against which the body cannot protect itself) is the fourth leading cause of death in the United States. Trauma is the leading cause of death in children and in adults younger than 44 years (McQuillan, VonReuden, Hartsock, et al., 2002). The incidence is increasing in adults older than 44 years. Alcohol and drug abuse are often implicated as factors in both blunt and penetrating trauma.

Collection of Forensic Evidence

In assessing and managing any patient with an emergency condition, but especially the patient experiencing trauma, documentation of all that occurs is essential. Included in documentation are descriptions of all wounds, mechanism of injury, time of events, and collection of evidence. In trauma care, the nurse must be exceedingly careful with all potential evidence, handling and documenting it properly.

The basics of care management for patients with traumatic injury include an understanding that trauma in any patient (living or dead) has potential legal or forensic implications if criminal activity is suspected. Hence, proper management from both a medical and forensic perspective is essential.

When clothing is removed from the patient who has experienced trauma, the nurse must be careful not to cut through or disrupt any tears, holes, blood stains, or dirt present on the clothing if criminal activity is suspected. Each piece of clothing should be placed in an individual paper bag. If the clothing is wet, it should be hung to dry. Clothing should not be given to families. Valuables should be placed in the hospital safe or clearly documented as to which family member they were given. If a police officer is present to collect clothing or any other items from the patient, each item is labeled. The transfer of custody to the officer, the officer's name, the date, and the time are documented.

If suicide or homicide is suspected in a deceased trauma patient, the medical examiner examines the body on site or has the body moved to the coroner's office for autopsy. All tubes and lines must remain in place. The patient's hands must be covered with paper bags to protect evidence on the hands or under the fingernails. In the surviving patient, tissue specimens may be swabbed from the hands and nails as potential evidence. Photographs of wounds or clothing are essential and should include a reference ruler in one photo and one without the ruler.

Documentation should also include any statements made by the patient in the patient's own words and surrounded by quotation marks. A chain of evidence is essential. If the patient's case is adjudicated in the future, clear documentation assists the judicial process and helps to identify the activities that occurred in the ED.

Injury Prevention

Any discussion of trauma management must include a discussion of injury prevention. A component of the emergency nurse's daily role is to provide injury prevention information to every patient with whom there is contact, including patients admitted for reasons other than injury. The only way to reduce the incidence of trauma is to prevent the injuries in the first place. Everyone can benefit from injury prevention information. Using the information after leaving the ED or other health care site is the patient's responsibility. However, the information must be provided.

The key to decreasing the incidence of trauma and saving the lives of productive members of society is injury prevention. The emergency nurse should make injury prevention part of daily nursing practice.

There are three components of injury prevention. The first is education. Providing information and materials to help prevent violence and to maintain safety at home and in vehicles is important. Involvement in local injury prevention organizations, nursing organizations, and health fairs promotes wellness and safety. In practice, nursing and other health care professionals should avoid using the word "accident," because trauma events are *preventable* and should be viewed as such rather than as "fate" or "happenstance." Responsibility and accountability must be assigned to traumatic incidents, particularly because of the high rate of trauma recidivism (repeated trauma). People who are at risk for trauma and trauma recidivism should be identified and provided with education and counseling directed toward altering risky behaviors and preventing further trauma.

The second component of injury prevention is legislation. Nurses should be actively involved in safety legislation at the local, state, and federal levels. Such legislation is meant to provide universal safety measures, not to infringe on rights.

The third component is automatic protection. Airbags and automatic safety belts are included in this category. These mechanisms provide for safety without requiring personal intervention.

Multiple Trauma

Multiple trauma is caused by a single catastrophic event that causes life-threatening injuries to at least two distinct organs or organ systems. Mortality in patients with multiple trauma is related to the severity of the injuries and the number of systems and organs involved. Immediately after injury, the body is hypermetabolic, hypercoagulable, and severely stressed.

Care of the patient with multiple injuries requires a team approach, with one person responsible for coordinating the treatment. The nursing staff assumes responsibility for assessing and monitoring the patient, ensuring airway and IV access, administering prescribed medications, collecting laboratory specimens, and documenting activities and the patient's response.

Assessment and Diagnostic Findings

Gross evidence of trauma may be slight or absent. Patients with multiple trauma should be assumed to have a spinal cord injury until it is proven otherwise. The injury regarded as the least significant in appearance may be the most lethal. For example, the pelvis fracture not identified until an x-ray is obtained may be the injury from which the patient is exsanguinating into the pelvic cavity. Another example is a tension pneumothorax that is insidiously increasing in size, eventually compressing both the heart and lungs, while the ED team is focused on repair of external lacerations. An obvious amputation of the arm may have already stopped bleeding from the body's normal response of vasoconstriction, despite being an obvious and devastating injury; meanwhile, the patient may be dying from an internal, less visible, injury.

Management

The goals of treatment are to determine the extent of injuries and to establish priorities of treatment. Any injury interfering with a vital physiologic function (eg, airway, breathing, circulation) is an immediate threat to life and has the highest priority for immediate treatment. Essential life-saving procedures are performed simultaneously by the emergency team. As soon as the patient is resuscitated, clothes are usually cut off, and a rapid physical assessment is performed. Transfer from field management to the ED must be orderly and controlled, with attention given to the verbal report from emergency medical services. Treatment in a level I trauma center is appropriate for patients experiencing major trauma. Treatment priorities are illustrated in Figure 71-4.

Intra-Abdominal Injuries

Intra-abdominal injuries are categorized as penetrating or blunt trauma. *Penetrating* abdominal injuries (ie, gunshot wounds, stab wounds) are serious and usually require surgery. Penetrating abdominal trauma results in a high incidence of injury to hollow organs, particularly the small bowel. The liver is the most frequently injured solid organ. In gunshot wounds, the most important factor is the velocity at which the missile enters the body. High-velocity missiles (bullets) create extensive tissue damage. All abdominal gunshot wounds that cross the peritoneum or are associated with peritoneal signs require surgical exploration. On the other hand, stab wounds may be managed nonoperatively.

Blunt trauma to the abdomen may result from motor vehicle crashes, falls, blows, or explosions. Blunt trauma is commonly associated with extra-abdominal injuries to the

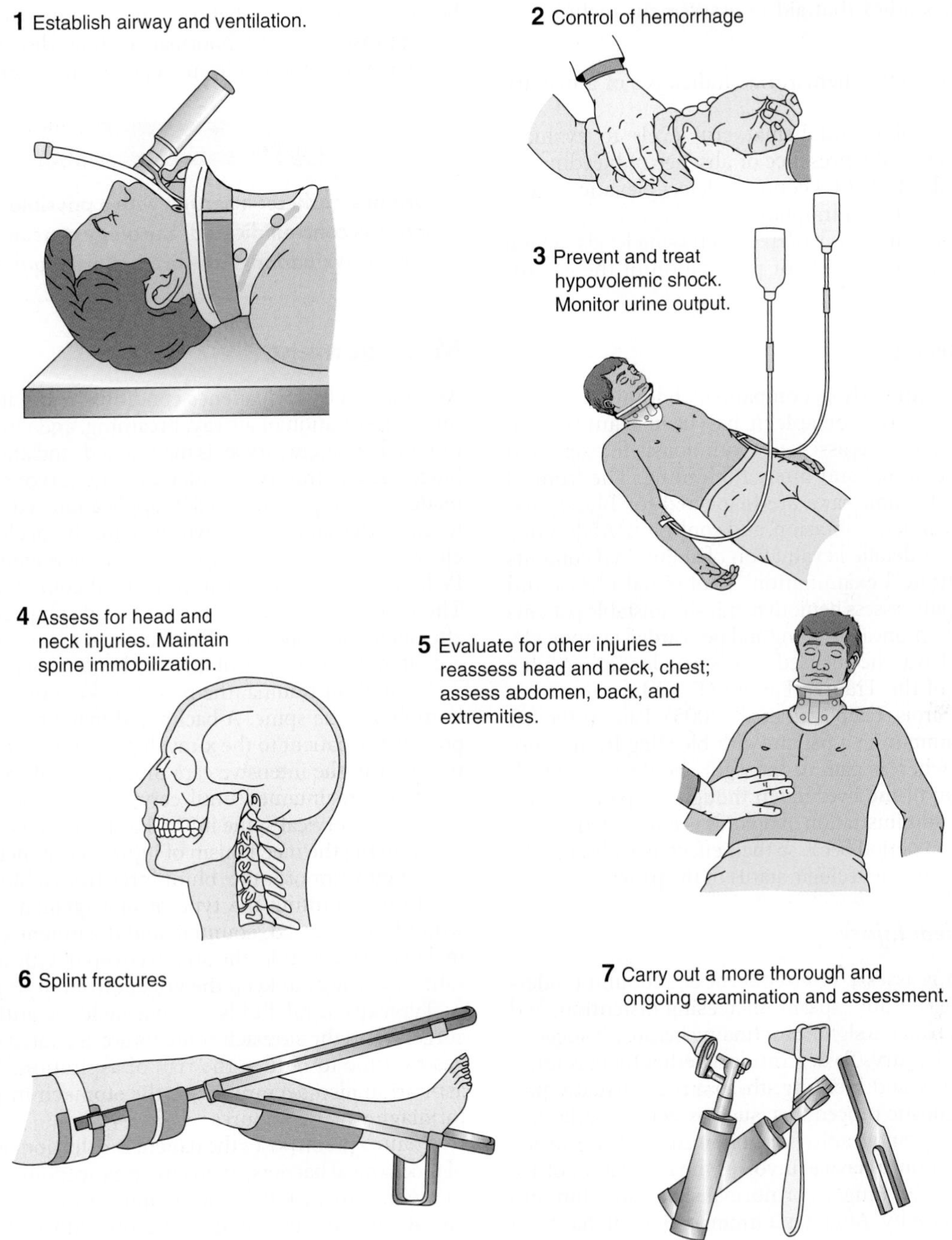
1 Establish airway and ventilation.
2 Control of hemorrhage
3 Prevent and treat hypovolemic shock. Monitor urine output.
4 Assess for head and neck injuries. Maintain spine immobilization.
5 Evaluate for other injuries — reassess head and neck, chest; assess abdomen, back, and extremities.
6 Splint fractures
7 Carry out a more thorough and ongoing examination and assessment.

FIGURE 71-4. Priority management of the patient with multiple injuries.

chest, head, or extremities. Patients with blunt trauma are a challenge because injuries may be difficult to detect. The incidence of delayed and trauma-related complications is greater than for penetrating injuries. This is especially true of blunt injuries involving the liver, kidneys, spleen, or blood vessels, which can lead to massive blood loss into the peritoneal cavity.

Assessment and Diagnostic Findings

As the history of the traumatic event is obtained, the abdomen is inspected for obvious signs of injury, including penetrating injuries, bruises, and abrasions. Abdominal assessment continues with auscultation of bowel sounds to provide baseline data from which changes can be noted. Absence of bowel sounds may be an early sign of intraperitoneal involvement, although stress can also decrease or eliminate bowel sounds. Further abdominal assessment may reveal progressive abdominal distention, involuntary guarding, tenderness, pain, muscular rigidity, or rebound tenderness along with changes in bowel sounds, all of which are signs of peritoneal irritation. Hypotension and signs and symptoms of shock may also be noted. Additionally, the chest and other body systems are assessed for injuries that frequently accompany intra-abdominal injuries.

Laboratory studies that aid in assessment include the following:

- Urinalysis to detect hematuria (indicative of a urinary tract injury)
- Serial hemoglobin and hematocrit levels to evaluate trends reflecting the presence or absence of bleeding
- White blood cell (WBC) count to detect elevation (generally associated with trauma)
- Serum amylase analysis to detect increasing levels, which suggest pancreatic injury or perforation of the gastrointestinal tract

Internal Bleeding

Hemorrhage frequently accompanies abdominal injury, especially if the liver or spleen has been traumatized. Therefore, the patient is assessed continuously for signs and symptoms of external and internal bleeding. The front of the body, flanks, and back are inspected for bluish discoloration, asymmetry, abrasion, and contusion. Abdominal CT scans permit detailed evaluation of abdominal contents and retroperitoneal examination. Abdominal ultrasound studies can rapidly assess hemodynamically unstable patients to detect intraperitoneal bleeding and pericardial tamponade. This is referred to as the Focused Assessment for Sonographic Examination of the Trauma Patient (FAST) examination (Kirkpatrick, Sirois, Laupland, et al., 2005). Pain in the left shoulder is common in a patient with bleeding from a ruptured spleen, whereas pain in the right shoulder can result from laceration of the liver. Even though the patient complains of pain, administration of opioids is minimized during the resuscitation period because their effect may obscure the clinical picture and neurologic status of the patient.

Intraperitoneal Injury

The abdomen is assessed for tenderness, rebound tenderness, guarding, rigidity, spasm, increasing distention, and pain. Referred pain is a significant finding because it suggests intraperitoneal injury. To determine whether there is intraperitoneal injury and bleeding, the patient is usually prepared for diagnostic procedures, such as peritoneal lavage, abdominal ultrasonography, or abdominal CT scanning. **Diagnostic peritoneal lavage** involves the instillation of 1 L of warmed lactated Ringer's or normal saline solution into the abdominal cavity. After a minimum of 400 mL has been returned, a fluid specimen is sent to the laboratory for analysis. Positive laboratory findings include a red blood cell count greater than 100,000/mm^3; a WBC count greater than 500/mm^3; or the presence of bile, feces, or food.

In patients with stab wounds, sinography may be performed to detect peritoneal penetration. In this procedure, a purse-string suture is placed around the wound, and a small catheter is introduced through the wound. A contrast agent is then introduced through the catheter, and x-rays are taken to identify any peritoneal penetration.

Genitourinary Injury

A rectal or vaginal examination is performed to determine any injury to the pelvis, bladder, or intestinal wall. To decompress the bladder and monitor urine output, an indwelling catheter is inserted after a rectal examination has been completed (not before). In the male patient, a high-riding prostate gland (abnormal position) discovered during a rectal examination indicates a potential urethral injury.

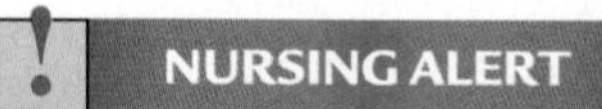

NURSING ALERT

Urethral catheter insertion with a possible urethral injury is contraindicated; a urology consultation and further evaluation of the urethra are required.

Management

As indicated by the patient's condition, resuscitation procedures (restoration of airway, breathing, and circulation) are initiated. A patent airway is maintained, and attempts to stabilize the respiratory, circulatory, and nervous systems are made. Bleeding is controlled by application of direct pressure to any external bleeding wounds and by occlusion of any chest wounds. Circulating blood volume is maintained with IV fluid replacement, including blood component therapy. The patient is monitored for signs and symptoms of shock after an initial response to transfusion therapy, because these are often the first signs of internal hemorrhage.

With blunt trauma, the patient is kept on a stretcher to immobilize the spine. A backboard may be used for transporting the patient to the x-ray department, to the operating room, or to the intensive care unit. Cervical spine immobilization is maintained until cervical x-rays have been obtained and cervical spine injury has been ruled out.

Knowing the mechanism of injury (eg, penetrating force from a gunshot or knife, blunt force from a blow) is essential to determining the type of management needed. All wounds are located, counted, and documented. If abdominal viscera protrude, the area is covered with sterile, moist saline dressings to keep the viscera from drying.

Typically, oral fluids are withheld in anticipation of surgery, and the stomach contents are aspirated with a nasogastric tube to reduce the risk of aspiration. Nasogastric aspiration also decompresses the stomach in preparation for diagnostic procedures.

Trauma predisposes the patient to infection by disruption of mechanical barriers, exposure to exogenous bacteria from the environment at the time of injury, aspiration of vomitus, and diagnostic and therapeutic procedures (nosocomial infection). Tetanus prophylaxis and broad-spectrum antibiotics are administered as prescribed.

Throughout the stay in the ED, the patient's condition is continuously monitored for changes. If there is continuing evidence of shock, blood loss, free air under the diaphragm, evisceration, hematuria, severe head injury, or suspected or known abdominal injury, the patient is rapidly transported to surgery. In most cases, blunt liver and spleen injuries are managed nonsurgically.

Crush Injuries

Crush injuries occur when a person is caught between opposing forces (eg, run over by a moving vehicle, compressed by machinery, crushed between two cars, crushed under a collapsed building).

Assessment and Diagnostic Findings

The patient is observed for the following:

- Hypovolemic shock resulting from extravasation of blood and plasma into injured tissues after compression has been released
- Paralysis of a body part
- Erythema and blistering of skin
- Damaged body part (usually an extremity) appearing swollen, tense, and hard
- Renal dysfunction (prolonged hypotension causes kidney damage and acute renal insufficiency; myoglobinuria secondary to muscle damage can cause acute tubular necrosis and acute renal failure)

Management

In conjunction with maintaining the airway, breathing, and circulation, the patient is observed for acute renal insufficiency. Injury to the back can cause severe kidney damage. Severe muscular damage may cause rhabdomyolysis, a significant release of myoglobin from ischemic skeletal muscle, which can result in acute tubular necrosis. In addition, major soft tissue injuries are splinted early to control bleeding and pain. The serum lactic acid level is monitored; a decrease to less than 2.5 mmol/L is an indication of successful resuscitation (Blow, Magliore, Claridge, et al., 1999).

If an extremity is injured, it is elevated to relieve swelling and pressure. To restore neurovascular function, the physician may perform a **fasciotomy** (surgical incision to the level of the fascia). Medications for pain and anxiety are then administered as prescribed, and the patient is quickly transported to the operating suite for wound débridement and fracture repair. Then, a hyperbaric chamber (if available) may be used for hyperoxygenation of the crushed tissue, if indicated.

Fractures

Immediate appropriate management of a fracture may greatly determine the patient's eventual outcome and may mean the difference between recovery and disability. When the patient is being examined for fracture, the body part is handled gently and as little as possible. Clothing is cut off to visualize the affected body part. Assessment is conducted for pain over or near a bone, swelling (from blood, lymph, and exudate infiltrating the tissue), and circulatory disturbance. The patient is assessed for ecchymosis, tenderness, and crepitation. The nurse must remember that the patient may have multiple fractures accompanied by head, chest, spine, or abdominal injuries.

Management

Immediate attention is given to the patient's general condition. Assessment of airway, breathing, and circulation (which includes pulses in the extremities) is conducted. The patient is also evaluated for neurologic or abdominal injuries before the extremity is treated, unless a pulseless extremity is detected.

If a pulseless extremity is identified, repositioning of the extremity to proper alignment is required. If the pulseless extremity involves a fractured hip or femur, **Hare traction** (a portable in-line traction device) may be applied to assist with alignment. If repositioning is ineffective in restoring the pulse, a rapid total-body assessment must be completed, followed by transfer of the patient to the operating room for arteriography and possible arterial repair.

After the initial evaluation has been completed, all injuries identified are evaluated and treated. The fractured body part is inspected. Using a systematic head-to-toe approach, the clinician inspects the entire body, observing for lacerations, swelling, and deformities, including angulation (bending), shortening, rotation, and asymmetry. All peripheral pulses, especially those distal to the fractured extremity, are palpated. The extremity is also assessed for coolness, blanching, and decreased sensation and motor function, which are indicative of injury to the extremity's neurovascular supply.

A splint is applied before the patient is moved. Splinting immobilizes the joint at a site distal and proximal to the fracture, relieves pain, restores or improves circulation, prevents further tissue injury, and prevents a closed fracture from becoming an open one. To splint an extremity, one hand is placed distal to the fracture and some traction is applied while the other hand is placed beneath the fracture for support. The splints should extend beyond the joints adjacent to the fracture. Upper extremities must be splinted in a functional position. If the fracture is open, a moist, sterile dressing is applied.

After splinting, the vascular status of the extremity is checked by assessing color, temperature, pulse, and blanching of the nail bed. In addition, the patient is assessed for neurovascular compromise if pain or pressure is reported. (See Chapter 69 for a complete description of fracture management.)

Environmental Emergencies

Heat Stroke

Heat stroke is an acute medical emergency caused by failure of the heat-regulating mechanisms of the body. It usually occurs during extended heat waves, especially when they are accompanied by high humidity. People at risk are those not acclimatized to heat, those who are elderly or very young, those unable to care for themselves, those with chronic and debilitating diseases, and those taking certain medications (eg, major tranquilizers, anticholinergics, diuretics, beta-adrenergic blocking agents). Exertional heat stroke occurs in healthy individuals during sports or work activities (eg, exercising in extreme heat and humidity). Hyperthermia results because of inadequate heat loss. This type of heat stroke can also cause death. Strategies used to prevent heat stroke are reviewed in Chart 71-7.

Gerontologic Considerations

Most heat-related deaths occur in the elderly, because their circulatory systems are unable to compensate for stress imposed by heat. Elderly people have a decreased

CHART 71-7

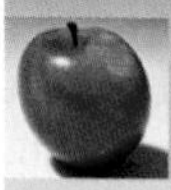

Health Promotion

Preventing Heat Stroke

- Advise the patient to avoid immediate reexposure to high temperatures; hypersensitivity to high temperatures may remain for a considerable time.
- Emphasize the importance of maintaining adequate fluid intake, wearing loose clothing, and reducing activity in hot weather.
- Advise athletes to monitor fluid losses and weight loss during workout activities or exercise and to replace fluids.
- Advise the patient to use a gradual approach to physical conditioning, allowing sufficient time for return to baseline temperature.
- Direct frail elderly patients living in urban settings with high environmental temperatures to places where air conditioning is available (eg, shopping mall, library, church).
- Advise patients to plan outdoor activities to avoid the hottest part of the day (between 10 A.M. and 2 P.M.).

ability to perspire as well as a decreased thirst mechanism to compensate for heat. The risk for heat stroke is greater among the elderly because many elderly people do not drink adequate amounts of fluid, partly because of fear of incontinence. In addition, many elderly people fear being victims of crime, so they tend to keep windows closed, even when the temperature and humidity levels are high.

Assessment and Diagnostic Findings

Heat stroke causes thermal injury at the cellular level, resulting in coagulopathies and widespread damage to the heart, liver, and kidneys. Recent patient history reveals exposure to elevated ambient temperature or excessive exercise during extreme heat. When assessing the patient, the nurse notes the following symptoms: profound central nervous system (CNS) dysfunction (manifested by confusion, delirium, bizarre behavior, coma); elevated body temperature (40.6°C [105°F] or higher); hot, dry skin; and usually anhidrosis (absence of sweating), tachypnea, hypotension, and tachycardia.

Management

The primary goal is to reduce the high temperature as quickly as possible, because mortality is directly related to the duration of hyperthermia. Simultaneous treatment focuses on stabilizing oxygenation using the ABCs (airway, breathing, and circulation) of basic life support.

After the patient's clothing is removed, the core (internal) temperature is reduced to 39°C (102°F) as rapidly as possible. One or more of the following methods may be used as prescribed:

- Cool sheets and towels or continuous sponging with cool water
- Ice applied to the neck, groin, chest, and axillae while spraying with tepid water
- Cooling blankets
- Iced saline lavage of the stomach or colon if the temperature does not decrease
- Immersion of the patient in a cold water bath (if possible)

During cooling procedures, an electric fan is positioned so that it blows on the patient to augment heat dissipation by convection and evaporation. The patient's temperature is constantly monitored with a thermistor placed in the rectum, bladder, or esophagus to evaluate core temperature. Caution is used to avoid hypothermia and to prevent hyperthermia, which may recur spontaneously within 3 to 4 hours.

Throughout treatment, the patient's status is monitored carefully, including vital signs, ECG findings (for possible myocardial ischemia, myocardial infarction, and dysrhythmias), CVP, and level of responsiveness, all of which may change with rapid alterations in body temperature. A seizure may be followed by recurrence of hyperthermia. To meet tissue needs exaggerated by the hypermetabolic condition, 100% oxygen is administered. The patient may require endotracheal intubation and mechanical ventilation to support failing cardiopulmonary systems.

IV infusion therapy of normal saline or lactated Ringer's solution is initiated as directed to replace fluid losses and maintain adequate circulation. Fluids are administered carefully because of the dangers of myocardial injury from high body temperature and poor renal function. Cooling redistributes fluid volume from the periphery to the core.

Urine output is also measured frequently, because acute tubular necrosis may occur as a complication of heat stroke from rhabdomyolysis (myoglobin in the urine). Blood specimens are obtained for serial testing to detect bleeding disorders, such as disseminated intravascular coagulation, and for serial enzyme studies to estimate thermal hypoxic injury to the liver, heart, and muscle tissue. Permanent liver, cardiac, and CNS damage may occur.

Additional supportive care may include dialysis for renal failure, antiseizure agents to control seizures, potassium for hypokalemia, and sodium bicarbonate to correct metabolic acidosis. Benzodiazepines or chlorpromazine may be prescribed to suppress seizure activity. Patient education regarding the prevention of heat stroke (see Chart 71-7) is also important to prevent a recurrence.

Frostbite

Frostbite is trauma from exposure to freezing temperatures and actual freezing of the intracellular fluid and fluids in the intercellular spaces. It results in cellular and vascular damage. Body parts most frequently affected by frostbite include the feet, hands, nose, and ears. Frostbite ranges from first degree (redness and erythema) to fourth degree (full-depth tissue destruction).

Assessment and Diagnostic Findings

A frozen extremity may be hard, cold, and insensitive to touch and may appear white or mottled blue-white. The extent of injury from exposure to cold is not always initially known. The patient history should include environmental temperature, duration of exposure, humidity, and the presence of wet conditions.

Management

The goal of management is to restore normal body temperature. Constrictive clothing and jewelry that could impair circulation are removed. If the lower extremities are involved, the patient should not be allowed to ambulate.

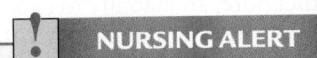

NURSING ALERT

If the patient requires transport, do not initiate rewarming. During transport, rewarming procedures may not be able to be maintained. In addition, any further cooling or freezing experience will cause significant damage to the already frozen body part.

Controlled yet rapid rewarming is instituted. The extremity is usually placed in a 37° to 40°C (98.6° to 104°F) circulating bath for 30- to 40-minute spans. This treatment is repeated until circulation is effectively restored. Early rewarming appears to decrease the amount of ultimate tissue loss. During rewarming, an analgesic for pain is administered as prescribed, because the rewarming process may be very painful. To avoid further mechanical injury, the body part is not handled. Massage is contraindicated.

Once rewarmed, the part is protected from further injury and is elevated to help control swelling. Sterile gauze or cotton is placed between affected fingers or toes to prevent maceration. A foot cradle may be used to prevent contact with bedclothes if the feet are involved. Blebs, which develop 1 hour to a few days after rewarming, are left intact and not ruptured, especially if they are hemorrhagic.

A physical assessment is conducted with rewarming to observe for concomitant injury, such as soft tissue injury, dehydration, alcohol coma, or fat embolism. Problems such as dehydration, hyperkalemia, and hypovolemia, which occur frequently in people with frostbite, are corrected. Risk of infection is also great; therefore, strict aseptic technique is used during dressing changes, and tetanus prophylaxis is administered as indicated. Nonsteroidal anti-inflammatory medication is also prescribed for its anti-inflammatory effects and to control pain.

Additional measures that may be carried out when appropriate include the following:

- Whirlpool bath for the affected extremity to aid circulation and débridement of necrotic tissue to help prevent infection
- Escharotomy (incision through the eschar) to prevent further tissue damage, allow for normal circulation, and permit joint motion
- Fasciotomy to treat compartment syndrome

After rewarming, hourly active motion of the affected digits is encouraged to promote maximal restoration of function and to prevent contractures. Discharge instructions also include encouraging the patient to avoid tobacco, alcohol, and caffeine because of their vasoconstrictive effects, which further reduce the already deficient blood supply to injured tissues.

Hypothermia

Hypothermia is a condition in which the core (internal) temperature is 35°C (95°F) or less as a result of exposure to cold. Hypothermia occurs when a patient loses the ability to maintain body temperature. Urban hypothermia (extreme exposure to cold in an urban setting) is associated with a high mortality rate; elderly people, infants, people with concurrent illnesses, and the homeless are particularly susceptible. Alcohol ingestion increases susceptibility because it causes systemic vasodilation. Trauma victims are also at risk for hypothermia resulting from treatment with cold fluids, unwarmed oxygen, and exposure during examination. The patient may also have frostbite, but the hypothermia takes precedence in treatment.

Assessment and Diagnostic Findings

Hypothermia leads to physiologic changes in all organ systems. There is progressive deterioration, with apathy, poor judgment, ataxia, dysarthria, drowsiness, pulmonary edema, acid–base abnormalities, coagulopathy, and eventual coma. Shivering may be suppressed at a temperature of less than 32.2°C (90°F), because the body's self-warming mechanisms become ineffective. The heartbeat and blood pressure may be so weak that peripheral pulses become undetectable. Cardiac irregularities may also occur. Other physiologic abnormalities include hypoxemia and acidosis.

Management

Management consists of continuous monitoring, rewarming, removal of wet clothing, insulation, and supportive care.

Monitoring

The ABCs of basic life support are a priority. The patient's vital signs, CVP, urine output, arterial blood gas levels, blood chemistry determinations (blood urea nitrogen, creatinine, glucose, electrolytes), and chest x-rays are evaluated frequently. Body temperature is monitored with an esophageal, bladder, or rectal thermistor. Continuous ECG monitoring is performed, because cold-induced myocardial irritability leads to conduction disturbances, especially ventricular fibrillation. An arterial line is inserted and maintained to record blood pressure and to facilitate blood sampling.

Rewarming

Rewarming methods include active core (internal) rewarming and passive external or spontaneous rewarming.

Active core rewarming methods include cardiopulmonary bypass, warm fluid administration, warm humidified oxygen by ventilator, and warmed peritoneal lavage. Core rewarming is recommended for severe hypothermia. Monitoring for ventricular fibrillation as the patient's temperature increases from 31° to 32°C (88° to 90°F) is essential.

Passive external rewarming includes the use of warm blankets or over-the-bed heaters. Passive rewarming of the extremities increases blood flow to the acidotic, anaerobic extremities. The cold blood from peripheral tissues has high lactic acid levels. As this blood returns to the core, it has significant effects on the core temperature and systemic metabolic response and can potentially cause cardiac dysrhythmias and electrolyte disturbances.

Supportive Care

Supportive care during rewarming includes the following as directed:

- External cardiac compression (typically performed only as directed in patients with temperatures higher than 31°C [88°F]).
- Defibrillation of ventricular fibrillation. A patient whose temperature is less than 32°C (90°F) experiences spontaneous ventricular fibrillation if moved or touched. Defibrillation is ineffective in patients with temperatures lower than 31°C (88°F); therefore, the patient must be rewarmed first.
- Mechanical ventilation with positive end-expiratory pressure (PEEP) and heated humidified oxygen to maintain tissue oxygenation
- Administration of warmed IV fluids to correct hypotension and to maintain urine output and core rewarming, as described previously
- Administration of sodium bicarbonate to correct metabolic acidosis if necessary
- Administration of antiarrhythmic medications
- Insertion of an indwelling urinary catheter to monitor urinary output and renal function

Near-Drowning

Near-drowning is defined as survival for at least 24 hours after submersion that caused a respiratory arrest. The most common consequence is hypoxemia. Drowning is the second most common cause of unintentional death in children younger than 14 years. An estimated 7000 drownings and 90,000 near-drownings occur yearly in the United States. More than 140,000 near-drownings occur worldwide.

Factors associated with drowning and near-drowning include alcohol ingestion, inability to swim, diving injuries, hypothermia, and exhaustion. Women usually drown in the ocean or bathtub, whereas men usually drown in rivers, lakes, or ditches (Byard, Houldsworth, James, et al., 2001). Suicide by drowning rarely occurs in pools and rarely involves alcohol. Only 5% of near-drownings are associated with diving injuries (Hwang, Shofer, Durbin, et al., 2003).

Efforts to save the patient should not be abandoned prematurely. Successful resuscitation with full neurologic recovery has occurred in near-drowning patients after prolonged submersion in cold water. This is possible because of a decrease in metabolic demands and/or the diving reflex. The near-drowning process involves the onset of hypoxia, hypercapnia, bradycardia, and dysrhythmias. If there is a violent struggle associated with the near-drowning episode, exercise-induced acidosis and tachypnea can result in aspiration. Hypoxia and acidosis cause eventual apnea and loss of consciousness. When the victim loses consciousness and makes a final effort to breathe, the terminal gasp occurs. Water then moves passively into the airways prior to death.

After resuscitation, hypoxia and acidosis are the primary complications experienced by a person who has nearly drowned; they require immediate intervention in the ED. Resultant pathophysiologic changes and pulmonary injury depend on the type of fluid (fresh or salt water) and the volume aspirated. Fresh water aspiration results in a loss of surfactant and, therefore, an inability to expand the lungs. Salt water aspiration leads to pulmonary edema from the osmotic effects of the salt within the lung. After a person survives submersion, acute respiratory distress syndrome resulting in hypoxia, hypercarbia, and respiratory or metabolic acidosis can occur.

Management

Therapeutic goals include maintaining cerebral perfusion and adequate oxygenation to prevent further damage to vital organs. Immediate cardiopulmonary resuscitation is the factor with the greatest influence on survival. The most important priority in resuscitation is to manage the hypoxia, acidosis, and hypothermia. Prevention and management of hypoxia are accomplished by ensuring an adequate airway and respiration, thus improving ventilation (which helps correct respiratory acidosis) and oxygenation. Arterial blood gases are monitored to evaluate oxygen, carbon dioxide, and bicarbonate levels and pH. These parameters determine the type of ventilatory support needed. Use of endotracheal intubation with PEEP improves oxygenation, prevents aspiration, and corrects intrapulmonary shunting and ventilation–perfusion abnormalities (caused by aspiration of water). If the patient is breathing spontaneously, supplemental oxygen may be administered by mask. However, an endotracheal tube is necessary if the patient does not breathe spontaneously.

Because of submersion, the patient is usually hypothermic. A rectal probe is used to determine the degree of hypothermia. Prescribed rewarming procedures (eg, extracorporeal warming, warmed peritoneal dialysis, inhalation of warm aerosolized oxygen, torso warming) are started during resuscitation. The choice of warming method is determined by the severity and duration of hypothermia and available resources. Intravascular volume expansion and inotropic agents are used to treat hypotension and impaired tissue perfusion. ECG monitoring is initiated, because dysrhythmias frequently occur. An indwelling urinary catheter is inserted to measure urine output. Hypothermia and accompanying metabolic acidosis may compromise renal function. Nasogastric intubation is used to decompress the stomach and to prevent the patient from aspirating gastric contents.

Even if the patient appears healthy, close monitoring continues with serial vital signs, serial arterial blood gas values, ECG monitoring, intracranial pressure assessments, serum electrolyte levels, intake and output, and serial chest x-rays. After a near-drowning, the patient is at risk for complications such as hypoxic or ischemic cerebral injury, acute respiratory distress syndrome, pulmonary damage secondary to aspiration, and life-threatening cardiac arrest.

Decompression Sickness

Decompression sickness, also called "the bends," occurs in patients who have engaged in diving, high-altitude flying, or flying in commercial aircraft within 24 hours after diving. It occurs relatively infrequently, but its effects can be hazardous. Being aware of decompression sickness and assessing the patient properly ensures proper management and results in the least morbidity possible.

Decompression sickness results from nitrogen bubbles trapped in the body. They may occur in joint or muscle spaces, resulting in musculoskeletal pain, numbness, or hypesthesia. More significantly, nitrogen bubbles can become air emboli in the bloodstream and thereby produce stroke, paralysis, or death. Taking a rapid history about the events preceding the symptoms is essential. Recompression is necessary as soon as possible and may necessitate a low-altitude flight to the nearest hyperbaric chamber.

Assessment and Diagnostic Findings

To identify decompression sickness, a detailed history is obtained from the patient or diving buddy. Evidence of rapid ascent, loss of air in the tank, buddy breathing, recent alcohol intake or lack of sleep, or a flight within 24 hours after diving suggests the potential for decompression sickness. Some patients describe a perfect dive yet still have the signs and symptoms of decompression sickness and must be treated as such.

Signs and symptoms include joint or extremity pain, numbness, hypesthesia, and loss of range of motion. Neurologic symptoms mimicking those of a stroke or spinal cord injury could indicate an air embolus. Cardiopulmonary arrest can also occur in severe cases. Because of hypoxia, these patients seldom survive. Any neurologic symptoms should be rapidly assessed. All patients with decompression sickness need rapid transfer to a hyperbaric chamber.

Management

A patent airway and adequate ventilation are established as described previously, and 100% oxygen is administered throughout treatment and transport. A chest x-ray is obtained to identify aspiration, and at least one IV line is started with lactated Ringer's or normal saline solution.

The cardiopulmonary and neurologic systems are supported as needed. If an air embolus is suspected, the head of the bed should be lowered. The patient's wet clothing is removed, and the patient is kept warm. Transfer to the closest hyperbaric chamber for treatment is initiated; to locate the nearest chamber, contact the Divers Alert Network at (919) 684-8111 or http://www.diversalertnetwork.org. If air transport is necessary, low-altitude flight (below 1000 feet) is required. However, the patient who is awake and alert without central neurologic deficits may be able to travel by ground ambulance or by automobile, depending on the severity of symptoms. Throughout treatment, the patient is continually assessed, and changes are documented. If aspiration is suspected, antibiotics and other treatment may be prescribed.

Anaphylactic Reaction

An anaphylactic reaction is an acute systemic hypersensitivity reaction that occurs within seconds or minutes after exposure to certain foreign substances, such as medications (eg, penicillin, iodinated contrast material), and other agents, such as latex, insect stings (eg, bee, wasp, yellow jacket, hornet), or foods (eg, eggs, peanuts). Repeated administration of parenteral or oral therapeutic agents (eg, repeated exposures to penicillin) may also precipitate an anaphylactic reaction when initially only a mild allergic response occurred. Anaphylaxis prevention strategies are given in Chart 71-8.

An anaphylactic reaction is the result of an antigen–antibody interaction in a sensitized person who, as a

CHART 71-8

Nursing Interventions for Preventing Anaphylactic Reactions

- Be aware of the danger of anaphylactic reactions and the early signs of anaphylaxis.
- Ask the patient about previous allergies to medications, foods, stings, latex, pollen, peanuts, nuts from trees, eggs, and so on.
- Before giving a foreign serum or other type of antigenic agent, ask the patient or caregiver whether the agent was received at some earlier time.
- Avoid giving medications to patients with hay fever, asthma, or other allergic disorders unless necessary.
- Avoid giving parenteral medications unless absolutely necessary, because anaphylactic reactions are more likely to occur when the agent is given parenterally.
- Perform a skin test before administration of certain materials known to produce anaphylactic reactions (eg, horse serum). Remember that negative skin test results do not always indicate safety and that skin testing can precipitate anaphylaxis in highly sensitive patients. Have epinephrine, intravenous infusions, and intubation and tracheostomy equipment available as precautionary measures.
- If the patient is an outpatient, keep him or her in the office, hospital, or clinic for at least 30 minutes after injection of any agent. Caution the patient to return if symptoms develop.
- Caution patients who are highly sensitive (eg, to insect bites and stings) to carry kits equipped to treat insect stings (epinephrine). Instruct the patient, family, and significant others in the use of the emergency supplies.
- Encourage patients with allergies to wear medical identification tags or bracelets.

consequence of previous exposure, has developed a special type of antibody (immunoglobulin) that is specific for that particular allergen. The antibody immunoglobulin E (IgE) is responsible for most of the immediate type of human allergic responses. The person becomes sensitive to a particular antigen after production of IgE to that antigen. A second exposure to the same antigen results in a more severe and more rapid response (see Chapter 53).

Anaphylactic reaction produces a wide range of clinical manifestations, especially respiratory symptoms (difficulty breathing and stridor secondary to laryngeal edema), fainting, itching, swelling of mucous membranes, and a sudden decrease in blood pressure secondary to massive vasodilation (Chart 71-9; see Chapters 15 and 53 for additional discussion).

Management

With an anaphylactic reaction, establishing a patent airway and ventilation is essential. (This is performed while another person administers epinephrine.) Early endotracheal intubation is essential to preserve airway patency, and oropharyngeal suction may be necessary to remove excessive secretions. Resuscitative measures are used, especially for patients with stridor and progressive pulmonary edema. If glottal edema occurs, emergent cricothyroidotomy may be necessary to provide an airway.

Simultaneously with airway management, aqueous epinephrine is administered as prescribed to provide rapid relief of the hypersensitivity reaction. Epinephrine may be administered again, if necessary and as prescribed. Judgment is used in choosing one of the following routes of administration:

- Subcutaneous injection for mild, generalized symptoms
- IM injection when the reaction is more severe and progressive, and with the knowledge that vascular collapse will delay absorption of the medication
- IV route (aqueous epinephrine diluted in saline solution and administered *slowly*), used in rare instances in which there is complete loss of consciousness and severe cardiovascular collapse. This method may precipitate cardiac dysrhythmias, so ECG monitoring with a readily available defibrillator is necessary. This method is controversial and is not usually recommended because it can lead to more distress than initially present. An IV infusion of saline solution is initiated to provide for emergency access to a vein and to treat hypotension.

Additional treatments may include the following:

- Antihistamines (eg, diphenhydramine [Benadryl]) to block further histamine binding at target cells
- Aminophylline titrated by IV drip for severe bronchospasm and wheezing refractory to other treatment
- Albuterol (Proventil, Ventolin) inhalers or humidified treatments to decrease bronchoconstriction; crystalloids, colloids, or vasopressors to treat prolonged hypotension
- Isoproterenol (Isuprel) or dopamine (Intropin) for reduced cardiac output; oxygen to enhance tissue perfusion
- IV benzodiazepines (eg, diazepam [Valium]) for control of seizures, and corticosteroids (eg, hydrocortisone [Solu-Cortef]) for prolonged reaction with persistent hypotension or bronchospasm

After the acute symptoms have been treated, the patient is usually admitted to the hospital for observation. The patient should be informed about ways to prevent anaphylactic reactions. See Chapter 53 for further discussion. Chart 71-10 lists strategies to limit exposure to stinging insects.

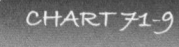

CHART 71-9

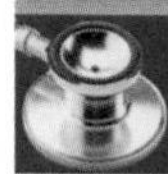

Assessing for Anaphylaxis

Be alert for the following signs and symptoms:

Respiratory Signs

- Nasal congestion
- Itching
- Sneezing and coughing
- Possible respiratory distress that progresses rapidly (caused by bronchospasm or edema of the larynx)
- Chest tightness
- Other respiratory difficulties, such as wheezing, dyspnea, and cyanosis

Skin Manifestations

- Flushing with a sense of warmth and diffuse erythema
- Generalized itching over the entire body (indicates developing general systemic reaction)
- Urticaria (hives)
- Massive facial angioedema possible with accompanying upper respiratory edema

Cardiovascular Manifestations

- Tachycardia or bradycardia
- Peripheral vascular collapse as indicated by
  - Pallor
  - Imperceptible pulse
  - Decreasing blood pressure
  - Circulatory failure, leading to coma and death

Gastrointestinal Problems

- Nausea
- Vomiting
- Colicky abdominal pains
- Diarrhea

Latex Allergy

Another allergic response that emergency nurses frequently treat involves latex. The number of products that contain latex is staggering. Nurses must be aware of latex allergy (health care providers have died from anaphylaxis related to latex allergy) and the potential for patients and staff to react to latex.

There is an increased awareness among manufacturers of the need for products that are latex-free. Latex-free gloves are provided for nurses who have latex allergy or

CHART 71-10

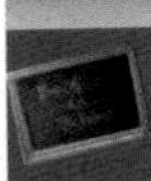

Patient Education

Limiting Exposure to Stinging Insects

To Minimize Your Chances of Being Stung:

- Avoid places where stinging insects congregate, such as camp and picnic sites, and insect feeding areas, such as flower beds, ripe fruit orchards, garbage, and fields of clover.
- Wear covering on the feet, and avoid going barefoot outdoors, because yellow jackets nest and pollinate on the ground.
- Avoid perfumes, scented soaps, and bright colors, which attract bees.
- Keep car windows closed.
- Spray garbage cans with quick-acting insecticide.
- Secure a professional exterminator to dispose of wasp and hornet nests or beehives in the home area.
- Remain motionless if an insect is buzzing around. Motion, especially running, increases the likelihood of being stung.
- If allergic, carry a self-treatment kit containing injectable (Epi-Pen) and inhalant forms of epinephrine, an oral antihistamine, and written instructions. Carry it with you at all times.

If You are Stung, Do the Following:

1. Inject self immediately with epinephrine if allergy is known or allergic response occurs.
2. Remove the stinger with one quick scrape of the fingernail. *Do not* squeeze the venom sac because this may cause injection of additional venom.
3. Clean the area with soapy water, and apply ice.
4. Report to the nearest health care facility for further examination if allergic response or allergy is suspected.

who have signs of allergy, such as itching, redness, or rash associated with use of a latex product. Severe anaphylaxis can occur even on first exposure; therefore, recognition of the signs and symptoms of anaphylaxis is essential. Treatment must be rapid, and the latex product must be removed promptly. See Chapters 19 and 53 for more information about latex allergy.

During triage, assessing allergy risk is one of the most important questions asked. Close attention must be paid to food allergies, especially to strawberries or kiwis, as an indication of significant risk for a latex allergy.

Insect Stings

A person may have an extreme sensitivity to the venoms of insects in the order Hymenoptera (bees, hornets, yellow jackets, fire ants, and wasps). Venom allergy is thought to be an IgE-mediated reaction, and it constitutes an acute emergency. Although stings in any area of the body can trigger anaphylaxis, stings of the head and neck or multiple stings are especially serious.

Clinical manifestations range from generalized urticaria, itching, malaise, and anxiety due to laryngeal edema to severe bronchospasm, shock, and death. Generally, the shorter the time between the sting and the onset of severe symptoms, the worse the prognosis.

Management includes stinger removal if the sting is from a bee because the venom is associated with sacs around the barb of the stinger itself. The stinger is removed with one quick scrape of a fingernail over the site. Wound care with soap and water is sufficient for stings. Scratching is avoided because it results in a histamine response. Ice application reduces swelling and also decreases venom absorption. An oral antihistamine and analgesic will decrease the itching and pain.

In the case of an anaphylactic or severe allergic response, epinephrine (aqueous) is injected subcutaneously (*not* IV) and the injection site is massaged to hasten absorption. The patient is assessed for signs and symptoms of anaphylactic reaction and treated as necessary (see previous discussion and Chapters 15 and 53). Desensitization therapy should be given to people who have had systemic or significant local reactions. Patient and family education is an important measure in preventing exposure to stinging insects (see Chart 71-10).

Snake Bites

Venomous (poisonous) snakes cause 7000 to 8000 bites in the United States each year and result in 5 to 15 deaths (Bowman & Ufberg, 2003). Children between the ages of 1 and 9 years are the most likely victims. The greatest number of bites occur through the daylight hours into early evening during summer months. The most frequent poisonous snake bite occurs from pit vipers (Crotalidae). The most common site is the upper extremity. Of these bites, only 20% to 25% result in **envenomation** (injection of a poisonous material by sting, spine, bite, or other means). Venomous snake bites are medical emergencies.

Nineteen different species of venomous snakes are found in various regions within the United States. Because snake bites are medical emergencies, nurses should be familiar with the types of snakes common to the geographic region in which they practice.

Clinical Manifestations

Snake venom consists primarily of proteins and has a broad range of physiologic effects. It may affect multiple organ systems, especially the neurologic, cardiovascular, and respiratory systems.

Classic clinical signs of envenomation are edema, ecchymosis, and hemorrhagic bullae leading to necrosis at the site of envenomation. Symptoms include lymph node tenderness, nausea, vomiting, numbness, and a metallic taste in the mouth. Without decisive treatment, these clinical manifestations may progress to include fasciculations, hypotension, paresthesias, seizures, and coma.

Management

Initial first aid at the site of the snake bite includes having the person lie down, removing constrictive items such as rings, providing warmth, cleansing the wound, covering the wound with a light sterile dressing, and immobilizing the injured body part below the level of the heart. Airway, breathing, and circulation are the priorities of care. Ice or a tourniquet is *not* applied. Initial evaluation in the ED is performed quickly and includes information about the following:

- Whether the snake was venomous or nonvenomous; if the snake is dead, it should be transported to the ED with the patient for identification. However, caution should be taken when handling the transported snake. Frequently, the patient and family transport the snake in a stunned, not dead, state.
- Where and when the bite occurred and the circumstances of the bite
- Sequence of events, signs and symptoms (fang punctures, pain, edema, and erythema of the bite and nearby tissues)
- Severity of poisonous effects
- Vital signs
- Circumference of the bitten extremity or area at several points; the circumference of the extremity that was bitten is compared with the circumference of the opposite extremity
- Laboratory data (complete blood count, urinalysis, and coagulation studies)

The course and prognosis of snake bite injuries depend on the kind and amount of venom injected, where on the body the bite occurred, and the general health, age, and size of the patient. There is no one specific protocol for treatment of snake bites. Generally, ice, tourniquets, heparin, and corticosteroids are not used during the acute stage. Corticosteroids are contraindicated in the first 6 to 8 hours after the bite because they may depress antibody production and hinder the action of **antivenin** (antitoxin manufactured from the snake venom and used to treat snake bites).

Parenteral fluids may be used to treat hypotension. If vasopressors are used to treat hypotension, their use should be short term. Surgical exploration of the bite is rarely indicated. Typically, the patient is observed closely for at least 6 hours. The patient is *never* left unattended.

Administration of Antivenin (Antitoxin)

Although envenomation is rare, it can occur with snake bites. An assessment of progressive signs and symptoms is essential before considering administration of antivenin, which is most effective if administered within 12 hours after the snake bite. Since 2000, two antivenins have been available, Antivenin Polyvalent (ACP) and Crotalidae Polyvalent Immune Fab Antivenin (FabAV) (Bowman & Ufberg, 2003). The dose depends on the type of snake and the estimated severity of the bite. Indications for antivenin depend on the progression of symptoms, including coagulopathy and systemic reaction. Children may require more antivenin than adults because their smaller bodies are more susceptible to the toxic effects of venom. A skin or eye test should be performed before the initial dose to detect allergy to the antivenin, because as many as 33% of patients who are given ACP (horse serum–derived antivenin) develop hypersensitivity reactions to it. Because even the skin test can cause an anaphylactic reaction, patients should not be tested unless antivenin will be given. If the dose exceeds 10 vials, serum sickness will most likely occur. Serum sickness is a type of hypersensitivity response that results in fever, arthralgias, pruritus, lymphadenopathy, and proteinuria and can progress to neuropathies.

Before administering antivenin and every 15 minutes thereafter, the circumference of the affected part is measured proximally. Premedication with diphenhydramine (Benadryl) or cimetidine (Tagamet) is indicated because these antihistamines may decrease the allergic response to antivenin. Antivenin is administered as an IV infusion whenever possible, although IM administration can be used.

Depending on the severity of the snake bite, the antivenin is diluted in 500 to 1000 mL of normal saline solution; the fluid volume may be reduced for children. The infusion is started slowly, and the rate is increased after 10 minutes if there is no reaction. The total dose should be infused during the first 4 to 6 hours after the bite. The initial dose is repeated until symptoms decrease. After symptoms decrease, the circumference of the affected part should be measured every 30 to 60 minutes for the next 48 hours to detect symptoms of compartment syndrome (swelling, loss of pulse, increased pain, and paresthesias).

FabAV is five times more potent than ACP, with a 20% lower incidence of hypersensitivity as well as a 23% lower incidence of serum sickness (Bowman & Ufberg, 2003). However, FabAV must be administered cautiously to patients receiving anticoagulation therapy. Administration of FabAV may result in a recurring coagulopathy. The dosage and administration of FabAV are different from ACP and should be reviewed carefully prior to administering this medication.

The most common cause of allergic reaction to the antivenin is too-rapid infusion, although about 3% of patients with negative skin test results develop reactions unrelated to infusion rate. Reactions may consist of a feeling of fullness in the face, urticaria, pruritus, malaise, and apprehension. These symptoms may be followed by tachycardia, shortness of breath, hypotension, and shock. In this situation, the infusion should be stopped immediately and IV diphenhydramine (Benadryl) administered. Vasopressors are used for patients in shock, and resuscitation equipment must be on standby while antivenin is infusing.

Poisoning

A poison is any substance that, when ingested, inhaled, absorbed, applied to the skin, or produced within the body in relatively small amounts, injures the body by its chemical action. Poisoning from inhalation and ingestion of toxic materials, both intentional and unintentional, constitutes a major health hazard and an emergency situation. Emergency treatment is initiated with the following goals:

- To remove or inactivate the poison before it is absorbed
- To provide supportive care in maintaining vital organ systems
- To administer a specific antidote to neutralize a specific poison

- To implement treatment that hastens the elimination of the absorbed poison

Ingested (Swallowed) Poisons

Swallowed poisons may be corrosive. **Corrosive poisons** include alkaline and acid agents that can cause tissue destruction after coming into contact with mucous membranes. Alkaline products include lye, drain cleaners, toilet bowl cleaners, bleach, nonphosphate detergents, oven cleaners, and button batteries (batteries used to power watches, calculators, or cameras). Acid products include toilet bowl cleaners, pool cleaners, metal cleaners, rust removers, and battery acid.

Control of the airway, ventilation, and oxygenation are essential. In the absence of cerebral or renal damage, the patient's prognosis depends largely on successful management of respiration and circulation. Measures are instituted to stabilize cardiovascular and other body functions. ECG, vital signs, and neurologic status are monitored closely for changes. Shock may result from the cardiodepressant action of the substance ingested, from venous pooling in the lower extremities, or from reduced circulating blood volume resulting from increased capillary permeability. An indwelling urinary catheter is inserted to monitor renal function. Blood specimens are obtained to determine the concentration of drug or poison.

Efforts are made to determine what substance was ingested; the amount; the time since ingestion; signs and symptoms, such as pain or burning sensations, any evidence of redness or burn in the mouth or throat, pain on swallowing or an inability to swallow, vomiting, or drooling; age and weight of the patient; and pertinent health history.

NURSING ALERT

The area poison control center should be called if an unknown toxic agent has been taken or if it is necessary to identify an antidote for a known toxic agent.

Measures are instituted to remove the toxin or decrease its absorption. The patient who has ingested a corrosive poison is given water or milk to drink for dilution. However, dilution is not attempted if the patient has acute airway edema or obstruction or if there is clinical evidence of esophageal, gastric, or intestinal burn or perforation. The following gastric emptying procedures may be used as prescribed:

- Syrup of ipecac to induce vomiting in the alert patient (*never* use with corrosive poisons)
- Gastric lavage for the obtunded patient (Chart 71-11). Gastric aspirate is saved and sent to the laboratory for testing (toxicology screens).
- Activated charcoal administration if the poison is one that is absorbed by charcoal
- Cathartic, when appropriate

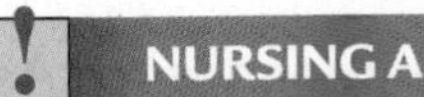

Vomiting is never induced after ingestion of caustic substances (acid or alkaline) or petroleum distillates.

The specific chemical or physiologic antagonist (antidote) is administered as early as possible to reverse or diminish the effects of the toxin. If this measure is ineffective, procedures may be initiated to remove the ingested substance. These procedures include administration of multiple doses of charcoal, diuresis (for substances excreted by the kidneys), dialysis, or hemoperfusion. Hemoperfusion involves detoxification of the blood by processing it through an extracorporeal circuit and an adsorbent cartridge containing charcoal or resin, after which the cleansed blood is returned to the patient.

Throughout detoxification, the patient's vital signs, CVP, and fluid and electrolyte balance are monitored closely. Hypotension and cardiac dysrhythmias are possible. Seizures are also possible because of CNS excitement from the poison or from oxygen deprivation. If the patient complains of pain, analgesics are administered cautiously. Severe pain causes vasomotor collapse and reflex inhibition of normal physiologic functions.

After the patient's condition has stabilized and discharge is imminent, written material should be given to the patient indicating the signs and symptoms of potential problems related to the poison ingested and signs or symptoms requiring evaluation by a physician. If poisoning was determined to be a suicide attempt, a psychiatric consultation should be requested before the patient is discharged. In cases of inadvertent poison ingestion, poison prevention and home poison-proofing instructions should be provided to the patient and family.

Carbon Monoxide Poisoning

Carbon monoxide poisoning may occur as a result of industrial or household incidents or attempted suicide. It is implicated in more deaths than any other toxin except alcohol. Carbon monoxide exerts its toxic effect by binding to circulating hemoglobin and thereby reducing the oxygen-carrying capacity of the blood. Hemoglobin absorbs carbon monoxide 200 times more readily than it absorbs oxygen. Carbon monoxide–bound hemoglobin, called **carboxyhemoglobin**, does not transport oxygen.

Clinical Manifestations

Because the CNS has a critical need for oxygen, CNS symptoms predominate with carbon monoxide toxicity. A person with carbon monoxide poisoning may appear intoxicated (from cerebral hypoxia). Other signs and symptoms include headache, muscular weakness, palpitation, dizziness, and confusion, which can progress rapidly to coma. Skin color, which can range from pink or cherry-red to cyanotic and pale, is not a reliable sign. Pulse oximetry is also not valid, because the hemoglobin is well saturated. It is not saturated

CHART 71-11

Guidelines for Assisting With Gastric Lavage

Gastric lavage is the aspiration of stomach contents and washing out of the stomach by means of a large-bore gastric tube. Gastric lavage is contraindicated after acid or alkali ingestion, in the presence of seizures, or after ingestion of hydrocarbons or petroleum distillates. It is particularly dangerous after ingestion of strong corrosive agents.

Purposes:

- For urgent removal of ingested substance to decrease systemic absorption
- To empty the stomach before endoscopic procedures
- To diagnose gastric hemorrhage and to arrest hemorrhage

Equipment:

Large-bore Levin tubes or large-bore Ewald tube
Large irrigating syringe with adapter
Large plastic funnel with adapter to fit tube
Water-soluble lubricant
Tap water or appropriate antidote (milk, saline solution, sodium bicarbonate solution, fruit juice, activated charcoal)
Container for aspirate; suction apparatus
Nasotracheal or endotracheal tubes with inflatable cuffs
Containers for specimens

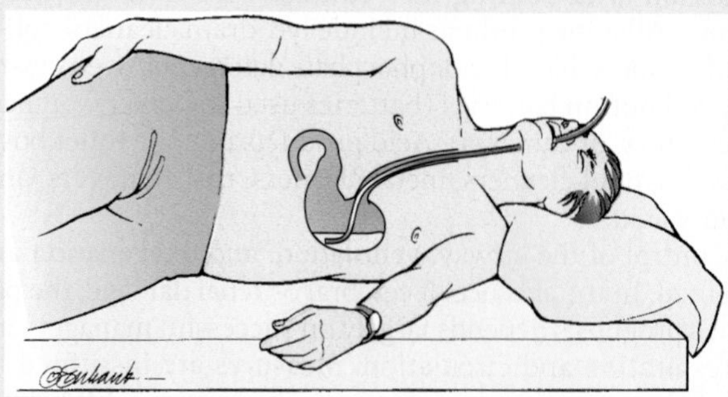

During gastric lavage, the patient is positioned on the left side, which allows the gastric contents to pool and decreases the passage of fluid into the duodenum during lavage.

ACTION	RATIONALE
1. Remove dentures and inspect the oral cavity for loose teeth.	1. This will prevent aspiration of teeth.
2. Measure the distance between the bridge of the nose and the xiphoid process. Mark the tube with indelible pencil or tape.	2. This distance is a rule-of-thumb measurement of the distance the tube must be passed to reach the stomach. This avoids curling and kinking of excess tubing in the stomach.
3. Lubricate the tube with water-soluble lubricant.	3. Lubrication eases insertion of the tube.
4. If comatose, the patient is intubated with a cuffed nasotracheal or endotracheal tube before placement of the nasogastric tube.	4. A cuffed nasotracheal or endotracheal tube decreases the risk of aspiration of gastric contents.
5. Place the patient in a left lateral position with the head lowered about 15 degrees.	5. This position decreases passage of gastric contents into the duodenum during lavage.
6. Pass the tube orally while keeping the patient's head in a neutral position. Pass the tube to the adhesive marking or about 50 cm (20 in). Encourage patient to swallow to assist with passage of the tube. Then lower the head of the stretcher or bed. Have standby suction available.	6. The depth of insertion of the tube varies according to the size of the patient. If the tube enters the trachea instead of the esophagus, the patient will experience coughing, dyspnea, stridor, and cyanosis. Positive confirmation of tube placement is accomplished by x-ray.
7. Aspirate the stomach contents with the syringe attached to the tube before instilling water or an antidote. Save the specimen for analysis. Ensure correct placement before installation.	7. Aspiration is carried out to determine that the tube is in the stomach and to remove the stomach contents. Positive confirmation of tube placement is accomplished by x-ray.
8. Remove the syringe. Attach the funnel to the end of the tube, or use a 50-mL syringe to instill solution in the gastric tube. The volume of fluid placed in the stomach should be small.	8. Overfilling of the stomach may cause regurgitation and aspiration or force the stomach contents through the pylorus.
9. Elevate the funnel above the patient's head and pour 150 to 200 mL of solution into the funnel.	9. Gravity allows the solution to flow into the tube.
10. Lower the funnel and siphon the gastric contents into the container or connect to suction.	10. The fluid should flow in freely and drain by gravity.

CHART 71-11 **Guidelines for Assisting With Gastric Lavage, continued**

NURSING ACTION	RATIONALE
11. Save samples of the first two washings.	11. Keep the first washing sample isolated from other washings for toxicologic analysis.
12. Repeat the lavage procedure until the returns are relatively clear and no particulate matter is seen.	12. This usually requires a total volume of at least 2 L; some clinicians advocate the use of 5 to 20 L.
13. At the completion of lavage:	13.
a. The stomach may be left empty.	a. The stomach is kept empty if no further medications are required.
b. An adsorbent (powder form of activated charcoal mixed with water to form a liquid the consistency of thick soup) may be instilled in the tube and allowed to remain in the stomach.	b. Activated charcoal reduces absorption by adsorbing (attaching to its surface) a wide range of substances; it renders the poison inaccessible to the circulation, thereby reducing its toxicity.
c. A saline cathartic may be instilled in the tube.	c. A cathartic may be given to hasten the elimination of remaining ingested material.
14. Pinch off the tube during removal or maintain suction while the tube is being withdrawn. Keep the patient's head lower than the body.	14. Pinching off the tube prevents aspiration and the initiation of the gag reflex. Keeping the patient's head lower than the body also helps to prevent initiation of the gag reflex.
15. Warn the patient that his stools will turn black from the charcoal.	15. Patient teaching is important to reduce anxiety.

with oxygen, but the pulse oximeter only reads whether or not the hemoglobin is saturated; in this case, it is saturated with carbon monoxide rather than oxygen.

Management

Exposure to carbon monoxide requires immediate treatment. Goals of management are to reverse cerebral and myocardial hypoxia and to hasten elimination of carbon monoxide. Whenever a patient inhales a poison, the following general measures apply:

- Carry the patient to fresh air immediately; open all doors and windows.
- Loosen all tight clothing.
- Initiate cardiopulmonary resuscitation if required; administer 100% oxygen.
- Prevent chilling; wrap the patient in blankets.
- Keep the patient as quiet as possible.
- Do not give alcohol in any form or permit the patient to smoke.

In addition, for the patient with carbon monoxide poisoning, carboxyhemoglobin levels are analyzed on arrival at the ED and before treatment with oxygen if possible. 100% oxygen is administered at atmospheric or preferably hyperbaric pressures to reverse hypoxia and accelerate the elimination of carbon monoxide. Oxygen is administered until the carboxyhemoglobin level is less than 5%. The patient is monitored continuously. Psychoses, spastic paralysis, ataxia, visual disturbances, and deterioration of mental status and behavior may persist after resuscitation and may be symptoms of permanent brain damage.

When unintentional carbon monoxide poisoning occurs, the health department should be contacted so that the dwelling or building in question can be inspected. A psychiatric consultation is warranted if poisoning was determined to be a suicide attempt.

Skin Contamination Poisoning (Chemical Burns)

Skin contamination injuries from exposure to chemicals are challenging because of the large number of possible offending agents with diverse actions and metabolic effects. The severity of a chemical burn is determined by the mechanism of action, the penetrating strength and concentration, and the amount and duration of exposure of the skin to the chemical.

The skin should be drenched immediately with running water from a shower, hose, or faucet, except in the case of lye and white phosphorus, which should be brushed off the skin, dry.

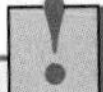

NURSING ALERT

Water should not be applied to burns from lye or white phosphorus because of the potential for an explosion or for deepening of the burn. All evidence of these chemicals should be brushed off the patient before any flushing occurs.

The skin should be flushed with a constant stream of water as the patient's clothing is removed. The skin of health care personnel assisting the patient should be appropriately protected if the burn is extensive or if the agent is significantly toxic or is still present. Prolonged lavage with generous amounts of tepid water is important.

In the meantime, attempts to determine the identity and characteristics of the chemical agent are necessary for future treatment. The standard burn treatment appropriate for the size and location of the wound (antimicrobial treatment, débridement, tetanus prophylaxis as prescribed) is instituted. The patient may require plastic surgery for further wound management. The patient is instructed to have the affected area reexamined at 24 and 72 hours and in 7 days because of the risk of underestimating the extent and depth of these types of injuries.

Food Poisoning

Food poisoning is a sudden illness that occurs after ingestion of contaminated food or drink. Botulism is a serious form of food poisoning that requires continual surveillance. Assessment questions are given in Chart 71-12. For more information about botulism, see Chapter 72.

The key to treatment is determining the source and type of food poisoning. If possible, the suspected food should be brought to the medical facility and a history obtained from the patient or family.

Food, gastric contents, vomitus, serum, and feces are collected for examination. The patient's respirations, blood pressure, level of consciousness, CVP (if indicated), and muscular activity are monitored closely. Measures are instituted to support the respiratory system. Death from respiratory paralysis can occur with botulism, fish poisoning, and other food poisonings.

Because large volumes of electrolytes and water are lost by vomiting and diarrhea, fluid and electrolyte status should be assessed. Severe vomiting produces alkalosis, and severe diarrhea produces acidosis. Hypovolemic shock may also occur from severe fluid and electrolyte losses. The patient is assessed for signs and symptoms of fluid and electrolyte imbalances, including lethargy, rapid pulse rate, fever, oliguria, anuria, hypotension, and delirium. Weight and serum electrolyte levels are obtained for future comparisons.

Measures to control nausea are also important to prevent vomiting, which could exacerbate fluid and electrolyte imbalances. An antiemetic medication is administered parenterally as prescribed if the patient cannot tolerate fluids or medications by mouth. For mild nausea, the patient is encouraged to take sips of weak tea, carbonated drinks, or tap water. After nausea and vomiting subside, clear liquids are usually prescribed for 12 to 24 hours, and the diet is gradually progressed to a low-residue, bland diet.

CHART 71-12

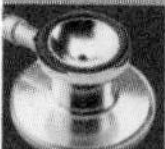

Assessment for Food Poisoning

Use the following questions to elicit information about the circumstances surrounding the possibility of food poisoning:

- How soon after eating did the symptoms occur? (Immediate onset suggests chemical, plant, or animal poisoning.)
- What was eaten in the previous meal? Did the food have an unusual odor or taste? (Most foods causing bacterial poisoning *do not* have unusual odor or taste.)
- Did anyone else become ill from eating the same food?
- Did vomiting occur? What was the appearance of the vomitus?
- Did diarrhea occur? (Diarrhea is usually absent with botulism and with shellfish or other fish poisoning.)
- Are any neurologic symptoms present? (These occur in botulism and in chemical, plant, and animal poisoning.)
- Does the patient have a fever? (Fever is characteristic in salmonella, ingestion of fava beans, and some fish poisoning.)
- What is the patient's appearance?

Substance Abuse

Substance abuse is the misuse of specific substances to alter mood or behavior; drug and alcohol abuse are two examples of substance abuse. Drug abuse is the use of drugs for other than legitimate medical purposes. People who abuse drugs often take a variety of drugs simultaneously (such as alcohol, barbiturates, opioids, and tranquilizers), and the combination may have additive and addictive effects. "Rave" parties are large-scale parties attended by hundreds of teenagers involved in drug use. At these events, one of the most commonly used drugs is 3,4-methylenedioxymethamphetamine (MDMA), or ecstasy, a methamphetamine-based drug that users believe produces a "harmless high." ED nurses should be aware of "rave" parties in their geographic area so they can prepare for a potential influx of patients who abuse this drug. Others may combine ecstasy with sildenafil (Viagra); this drug combination is nicknamed "sextasy." People who abuse IV/injection drugs are at increased risk for HIV infection, acquired immunodeficiency syndrome (AIDS), and hepatitis B and C, and tetanus.

Clinical manifestations vary with the substance used, but the underlying principles of management are essentially the same. Table 71-11, identifies commonly abused drugs, listing their clinical manifestations and therapeutic management. Treatment goals for a patient with a drug overdose are to support the respiratory and cardiovascular functions, to enhance clearance of the agent, and to provide for safety of the patient and staff.

Acute Alcohol Intoxication

Alcohol is a psychotropic drug that affects mood, judgment, behavior, concentration, and consciousness. Many heavy drinkers are young adults or people older than 60 years.

(text continues on page 2548)

TABLE 71-1 Emergency Management of Patients with Drug Overdose

Drug	Clinical Manifestations	Therapeutic Management
Stimulants		
Cocaine Intranasally ("snorting"): inhaled into nostrils through straws By smoking ("freebasing"): cocaine hydrochloride dissolved in ether to yield a pure cocaine alkaloid base (called "crack"); smoking in a small pipe delivers large quantities of cocaine to lungs Intravenously	Cocaine is a central nervous system (CNS) stimulant that can increase heart rate and blood pressure and cause hyperpyrexia, seizures, and ventricular dysrhythmias. It produces intense euphoria, then anxiety, sadness, insomnia, and sexual indifference; cocaine hallucinations with delusions; psychosis with extreme paranoia and ideas of persecution; and hypervigilance. Chronic psychotic symptoms may persist.	1. Ensure airway and ventilation. 2. Control seizures. 3. Monitor cardiovascular effects; have lidocaine and defibrillator available. 4. Treat for hyperthermia. 5. If cocaine was ingested, evacuate stomach contents and use activated charcoal to treat. 6. Refer for psychiatric evaluation and treatment in an inpatient unit that eliminates access to the drug. Include drug rehabilitation counseling.
Opioids		
Heroin Opium or paregoric Morphine, codeine, OxyContin, synthetic derivatives (methadone, meperidine) Fentanyl (Sublimaze)	Acute intoxication (overdose) Pinpoint pupils (may be dilated with severe hypoxia); decreased blood pressure Marked respiratory depression Stupor → coma Fresh needle marks along course of any superficial vein; skin abscesses	1. Support respiratory and cardiovascular functions. 2. Establish an intravenous (IV) line; obtain blood for chemical and toxicologic analysis. Patient may be given bolus of glucose to eliminate possibility of hypoglycemia. 3. Give narcotic antagonist (naloxone hydrochloride [Narcan]) as prescribed to reverse severe respiratory depression and coma. 4. Continue to monitor level of responsiveness and respirations, pulse, and blood pressure. Duration of action of naloxone hydrochloride is shorter than that of heroin; repeated dosages may be necessary. 5. Send urine for analysis; opiates can be detected in urine. 6. Obtain an electrocardiogram. 7. Do not leave patient unattended; he or she may lapse back into coma rapidly. Clinical status may change from minute to minute. Hemodialysis may be indicated for severe drug intoxication. 8. Monitor for pulmonary edema, which is frequently seen in patients who abuse/overdose on narcotics. 9. Refer patient for psychiatric and drug rehabilitation evaluation before discharge.
Barbiturates		
Pentobarbital (Nembutal) Secobarbital (Seconal) Amobarbital (Amytal) Gamma-hydroxybutyrate (GHB, "liquid ecstasy")	Acute intoxication (may mimic alcohol intoxication): • Respiratory depression • Flushed face • Decreased pulse rate; decreased blood pressure • Increasing nystagmus • Depressed deep tendon reflexes • Decreasing mental alertness • Difficulty in speaking • Poor motor coordination • Coma, death GHB: • Sexual disinhibition • Amnesia, myoclonus, agitation • Overdoses when mixed with alcohol	1. Maintain airway and provide respiratory support. 2. Endotracheal intubation or tracheostomy is considered if there is any doubt about the adequacy of airway exchange. a. Check airway frequently. b. Perform suctioning as necessary. 3. Support cardiovascular and respiratory functions; most deaths result from respiratory depression or shock. 4. Start infusion through large-gauge needle or IV catheter to support blood pressure; coma and dehydration result in hypotension and respond to infusion of intravenous fluids with elevation of blood pressure. Sodium bicarbonate may be prescribed to alkalinize urine; it promotes excretion of barbiturates. 5. Evacuate stomach contents or lavage as soon as possible to prevent absorption; repeated doses of activated charcoal may be administered.

continued >

TABLE 71-1 Emergency Management of Patients with Drug Overdose (Continued)

Drug	Clinical Manifestations	Therapeutic Management
		6. Assist with hemodialysis for severely overdosed patient. 7. Maintain neurologic and vital sign flow sheet. 8. Patient awakening from overdose may demonstrate combative behavior. 9. Refer for psychiatric and drug rehabilitation consultation/rehabilitation to evaluate suicide potential and drug abuse.
Inhalants		
Amyl nitrate Freon Propane Trichloroethylene Gasoline Perchloroethylene Toluene	Effects mimic those of alcohol, with dizziness and imbalance: Renal, hepatic, and cardiac toxicity Aplastic anemia Fetal growth retardation Respiratory depression Vasodilation	1. Provide airway support, ventilation, and oxygen. 2. Treat cardiac dysrhythmias and hypotension. 3. Provide advanced cardiac life support (ACLS) as needed. 4. Monitor for profound hypotension when amyl nitrate is combined with MDMA and sildenafil.
Amphetamine-Type Drugs (Pep Pills, "Uppers," "Speed," "Crystal Meth")		
Amphetamine (Benzedrine) Dextroamphetamine (Dexedrine) Methamphetamine (Desoxyn, "speed") 3,4-Methylenedioxymethamphetamine (MDMA) ("ecstasy," "Adam") 3,4-Methylenedioxymethamphetamine (MDEA) ("Eve") 3,4-Methylenedioxyamphetamine (MDA)	Nausea, vomiting, anorexia, palpitations, tachycardia, increased blood pressure, tachypnea, anxiety, nervousness, diaphoresis, mydriasis Repetitive or stereotyped behavior Irritability, insomnia, agitation Visual misperceptions, auditory hallucinations Fearfulness, anxiety, depression, cold, distant hostility, paranoia Hyperactivity, rapid speech, euphoria, hyperalertness Decreased inhibition Seizures, coma, hyperthermia, cardiovascular collapse, rhabdomyolysis MDMA is both a hallucinogenic and stimulant.	1. Provide airway support, ventilation, cardiac monitoring; insert IV line. 2. Employ gastrointestinal (GI) evacuation in cases of oral overdose; activated charcoal, gastric lavage. 3. Keep in calm, cool, quiet environment; elevated temperature potentiates amphetamine toxicity. 4. Use small doses of diazepam (IV) or haloperidol as prescribed for CNS and muscular hyperactivity. 5. Administer appropriate pharmacologic therapy as prescribed for severe hypertension and ventricular dysrhythmias. 6. Treat seizures with benzodiazepines as prescribed. 7. Treat sympathetic stimulation with beta-blocker agents as prescribed. 8. Try to communicate with patient if delusions or hallucinations are present. 9. Place in a protective environment (preferably psychiatric security room with video monitoring) to observe for suicide attempt. 10. Refer for psychiatric and drug rehabilitation evaluation.
Hallucinogens or Psychedelic-Type Drugs		
Lysergic acid diethylamide (LSD) Phencyclidine HCl (PCP, "angel dust") Mescaline, psilocybin Cannabinoids (marijuana) Ketamine ("special K")	Nystagmus Mild hypertension Marked confusion bordering on panic Incoherence, hyperactivity Withdrawn Combative behavior; delirium, mania, self-injury Hallucinations, body image distortion Hypertension, hyperthermia, renal failure Flashback: recurrence of LSD-like state without having taken the drug; may occur weeks or months after drug was taken Ketamine: "out-of-body" experience; increased aggressiveness	*Emergency Management* 1. Evaluate and maintain patient's airway, breathing, and circulation. 2. Determine by urine or serum drug screen whether the patient has ingested hallucinogenic drug or has a toxic psychosis. 3. Try to communicate with and reassure the patient. a. "Talking down" involves understanding the process through which the patient is proceeding and helping him overcome his fears while establishing contact with reality. b. Remind the patient that fear is common with this problem. c. Reassure the patient that he is not losing his mind but is experiencing the effect of drugs and that this will wear off.

TABLE 71-1	Emergency Management of Patients with Drug Overdose (Continued)	
Drug	**Clinical Manifestations**	**Therapeutic Management**
		d. Instruct the patient to keep the eyes open; this reduces the intensity of reaction. e. Reduce sensory stimuli: minimize noise, lights, movement, tactile stimulation. 4. Sedate the patient as prescribed if hyperactivity cannot be controlled; diazepam (Valium) or a barbiturate may be prescribed. 5. Search for evidence of trauma; hallucinogen users have a tendency to "act out" their hallucinations. 6. Manage seizures with benzodiazepines (eg, diazepam [valium]) as necessary. 7. Observe patient closely; patient's behavior may become hazardous. Have safety officers stationed near the patient's room. 8. Monitor for hypertensive crisis if patient has prolonged psychosis due to drug ingestion. 9. Place patient in a protected environment under proper medical supervision to prevent self-inflicted bodily harm. *Management for Phencyclidine Abusers* 1. Place patient in a calm, supportive environment to minimize stimuli; protect from self-injury. 2. Avoid talking down. 3. Do not leave patient unobserved. Treat symptoms as they occur. a. Drug effects are unpredictable and prolonged. b. Symptoms are likely to exacerbate; patient becomes out of control. 4. Refer all patients in this category for psychiatric and drug evaluation/rehabilitation.
Drugs Producing Sedation, Intoxication, or Psychological and Physical Dependence (Nonbarbiturate Sedatives)		
Diazepam (Valium) Chlordiazepoxide (Librium) Oxazepam (Serax) Lorazepam (Ativan) Midazolam (Versed) Flunitrazepam (Rohypnol, "roofies," "date rape drug")	Seizures, coma, circulatory collapse, death Acute intoxication: • Respiratory depression • Decreasing mental alertness • Confusion • Slurred speech, decreased blood pressure • Ataxia • Pulmonary edema • Coma, death Flunitrazepam: • Disinhibition with antegrade amnesia • Weakness and unsteadiness with impaired judgment • Powerlessness	*Management* 1. Endotracheal tube is inserted as a precaution; use assisted ventilation to stabilize and correct respiratory depression. Observe for sudden apnea and laryngeal spasm. 2. Assess for hypotension a. Insert indwelling urinary catheter for comatose patient; decreased urinary volume is an index of reduced renal flow associated with reduced intravascular volume or vascular collapse. b. Start volume expansion with saline or dextrose as prescribed. 3. Evacuate stomach contents; emesis; lavage; activated charcoal; cathartic. 4. Start ECG monitoring. Observe for dysrhythmias. 5. Administer flumazenil (Romazicon), a benzodiazepine antagonist (reversal agent) 6. Refer patient for psychiatric evaluation (potential suicide intent).
Salicylate Poisoning		
Aspirin (present in compound analgesic tablets)	Restlessness, tinnitus, deafness, blurring of vision Hyperpnea, hyperpyrexia, sweating Epigastric pain, vomiting, dehydration Respiratory and metabolic acidosis Disorientation, coma, cardiovascular collapse	1. Treat respiratory depression. 2. Induce gastric emptying by lavage. 3. Give activated charcoal to adsorb aspirin; a cathartic may be administered with charcoal to help ensure intestinal cleansing.

continued >

TABLE 71-1 Emergency Management of Patients with Drug Overdose (Continued)

Drug	Clinical Manifestations	Therapeutic Management
		4. Support patient with IV infusions as prescribed to establish hydration and correct electrolyte imbalances. 5. Enhance elimination of salicylates as directed by forced diuresis, alkalinization of urine, peritoneal dialysis, or hemodialysis, according to severity of intoxication. 6. Monitor serum salicylate level for efficacy of treatment. 7. Administer specific prescribed pharmacologic agent for bleeding and other problems. 8. Refer patient for psychiatric evaluation (potential suicide intent).
Acetaminophen (present in prescription and nonprescription analgesics, antipyretics, and cold remedies)	Lethargy to encephalopathy and death GI upset, diaphoresis Right upper quadrant pain Abnormal liver function tests, prolonged prothrombin time, increased bilirubin Hepatomegaly leading to liver failure	1. Maintain airway 2. Obtain acetaminophen level. Levels ≥ 140 mg/kg are toxic. 3. Laboratory studies—liver function tests, prothrombin time/partial thromboplastin time, complete blood count, blood urea nitrogen, creatinine 4. Administer syrup of ipecac and follow emesis with activated charcoal. 5. Prepare for possible hemodialysis, which clears acetaminophen but does not halt liver damage. 6. Administer *N*-acetylcysteine (NAC, Mucomyst) as soon as possible. NAC replenishes essential liver enzymes and requires a total of 18 doses every 4 hr. Charcoal absorbs NAC; do not administer together. Repeat NAC dose if patient vomits. 7. Refer patient for psychiatric evaluation (potential suicide intent).
Tricyclic Antidepressants (TCA)		
Amitriptyline Doxepin Nortriptyline Imipramine	Dysrhythmia: ventricular fibrillation/tachycardia, tachycardia Hypotension Pulmonary edema, hypoxemia, acidosis Confusion, agitation, coma Visual hallucinations Clonus, hyperactive reflexes, nystagmus, myoclonic jerking Seizures Blurred vision, flushing, hyperthermia	1. Provide airway support, ventilation, cardiac monitoring; insert IV line with normal saline solution. 2. If within 1 hr after overdose, insert a nasogastric tube and instill activated charcoal with sorbitol every 4 hr × 3. 3. Administer a sodium bicarbonate drip to decrease dysrhythmias; the alkaline environment increases the protein binding of the metabolite. 4. Administer vasopressors 5. Use only Class IB antiarrhythmics (eg, lidocaine), as some other types of antiarrhythmics have the same effect as TCA. 6. Manage seizure activity with benzodiazepines (eg, diazepam [valium]) as necessary. 7. Refer patient for psychiatric evaluation for potential suicide intent and evaluation of medication regimen for effectiveness.

*Polydrug use at "rave clubs" frequently involves MDMA, alcohol, amphetamines, LSD, and sometimes dextromethorphan. Terms such as "ecstasy" may refer to flunitrazepam (Rohypnol), GHB, ephedrine, and/or caffeine, in addition to MDMA. The website www.clubdrugs.com provides more information about possible drug abuse and how it may relate to emergency nursing care.

There is a high prevalence of alcoholism among ED patients. Because patients who abuse alcohol return frequently to the ED, they often frustrate and tax the patience of the health care professionals who care for them. Their management requires patience and thoughtful, accurate, long-term treatment.

Alcohol, or ethanol, is a multisystem toxin and CNS depressant that causes drowsiness, impaired coordination, slurring of speech, sudden mood changes, aggression, belligerence, grandiosity, and uninhibited behavior. In excess, it also can cause stupor, coma, and death. Increasingly, underage minors and college students arrive at the ED with alcohol poisoning from binge drinking. Frequently, the result is death.

In the ED, the patient is assessed for head injury, hypoglycemia (which mimics intoxication), and other health problems. Possible nursing diagnoses include ineffective breathing pattern related to CNS depression and risk for violence (self-directed or directed at others) related to severe intoxication from alcohol.

Treatment involves detoxification of the acute poisoning, recovery, and rehabilitation. Commonly, the patient uses mechanisms of denial and defensiveness. The nurse should approach the patient in a nonjudgmental manner, using a firm, consistent, accepting, and reasonable attitude. Speaking in a calm and slow manner is helpful because alcohol interferes with thought processes. If the patient appears intoxicated, hypoxia, hypovolemia, and neurologic impairment must be ruled out before it is assumed that the patient is intoxicated. Typically, a blood specimen is obtained for analysis of the blood alcohol level.

If drowsy, the patient should be allowed to sleep off the state of alcoholic intoxication. During this time, maintenance of a patent airway and observation for symptoms of CNS depression are essential. The patient should be undressed and kept warm with blankets. On the other hand, if the patient is noisy or belligerent, sedation may be necessary. If sedation is used, the patient should be monitored carefully for hypotension and decreased level of consciousness.

In addition, the patient is examined for alcohol withdrawal delirium and also for injuries and organic disease (such as head injury, seizures, pulmonary infections, hypoglycemia, and nutritional deficiencies) that may be masked by alcoholic intoxication. People with alcoholism suffer more injuries than the general population. Also, acute alcohol intoxication is the cause of trauma for many nonalcoholic patients. Pulmonary infections are also more common in patients with alcoholism, resulting from respiratory depression, an impaired defense system, and a tendency toward aspiration of gastric contents. The patient may show little increase in temperature or WBC count. The patient may be hospitalized or admitted to a detoxification center in an effort to examine problems underlying substance abuse.

Alcohol Withdrawal Syndrome/ Delirium Tremens

Alcohol withdrawal syndrome is an acute toxic state that occurs as a result of sudden cessation of alcohol intake after a bout of heavy drinking or, more typically, after prolonged intake of alcohol. Severity of symptoms depends on how much alcohol was ingested and for how long. Delirium tremens may be precipitated by acute injury or infection (pneumonia, pancreatitis, hepatitis) and is the most severe form of alcohol withdrawal syndrome.

Patients with alcohol withdrawal syndrome show signs of anxiety, uncontrollable fear, tremor, irritability, agitation, insomnia, and incontinence. They are talkative and preoccupied and experience visual, tactile, olfactory, and auditory hallucinations that often are terrifying. Autonomic overactivity occurs and is evidenced by tachycardia, dilated pupils, and profuse perspiration. Usually, all vital signs are elevated in the alcoholic toxic state. Delirium tremens is a life-threatening condition and carries a high mortality rate.

The goals of management are to give adequate sedation and support to allow the patient to rest and recover without danger of injury or peripheral vascular collapse. A physical examination is performed to identify preexisting or contributing illnesses or injuries (eg, head injury, pneumonia). A drug history is obtained to elicit information that may facilitate adjustment of any sedative requirements. Baseline blood pressure is determined, because the patient's subsequent treatment may depend on blood pressure changes.

Usually, the patient is sedated as directed with a sufficient dosage of benzodiazepines to establish and maintain sedation, which reduces agitation, prevents exhaustion, prevents seizures, and promotes sleep. The patient should be calm, able to respond, and able to maintain an airway safely on his or her own. A variety of medications and combinations of medications are used (eg, chlordiazepoxide [Librium], lorazepam [Ativan], and clonidine [Catapres]). Haloperidol (Haldol) or droperidol (Inapsine) may be administered for severe acute alcohol withdrawal syndrome. Dosages are adjusted according to the patient's symptoms (agitation, anxiety) and blood pressure response.

The patient is placed in a calm, nonstressful environment (usually a private room) and observed closely. The room remains lighted to minimize the potential for illusions (visual misrepresentations) and hallucinations. Homicidal or suicidal responses may result from hallucinations. Closet and bathroom doors are closed to eliminate shadows. Someone is designated to stay with the patient as much as possible. The presence of another person has a reassuring and calming effect, which helps the patient maintain contact with reality. To orient the patient to reality, any illusions are explained.

NURSING ALERT

Restraints are used as prescribed, if necessary, if the client is aggressive or violent, but only when other alternatives have been unsuccessful. The least restrictive device that will prevent the patient from injuring self or others is used. Caution is taken to ensure that restraints are applied properly and that they are not impairing circulation to any part of the body or interfering with respirations. Restraints must be released according to protocol. Physical observation (eg, skin integrity, circulatory status, respiratory status) is ongoing, and the patient's response is documented.

Fluid losses may result from gastrointestinal losses (vomiting), profuse perspiration, and hyperventilation. In addition, the patient may be dehydrated as a result of alcohol's effect of decreasing antidiuretic hormone. The oral or IV route is used to restore fluid and electrolyte balance.

Temperature, pulse, respiration, and blood pressure are recorded frequently (every 30 minutes in severe forms of delirium) to monitor for peripheral circulatory collapse or hyperthermia (the two most serious complications).

Phenytoin (Dilantin) or other antiseizure medications may be prescribed to prevent repeated withdrawal seizures.

Frequently seen complications include infections (eg, pneumonia), trauma, hepatic failure, hypoglycemia, and cardiovascular problems. Hypoglycemia may accompany alcohol withdrawal, because alcohol depletes liver glycogen stores and impairs gluconeogenesis; many patients with alcoholism also are malnourished. Parenteral dextrose may be prescribed if the liver glycogen level is depleted. Orange juice, Gatorade, or other sources of carbohydrates are given to stabilize the blood glucose level and counteract tremulousness. Supplemental vitamin therapy and a high-protein diet are provided as prescribed to counteract nutritional deficits. The patient should be referred to an alcoholic treatment center for follow-up care and rehabilitation.

Violence, Abuse, and Neglect

Family Violence, Abuse, and Neglect

EDs are often the first place where victims of family violence, abuse, or neglect go to seek help. Each year in the United States, there are 5.3 million cases of domestic violence, and as many as 25% of all women will be in a domestic violence situation sometime during their lives. Of women who experience domestic violence, one study found that 40% sustained a serious physical injury and 44% of those who were murdered experienced a prior domestic violence event in the 2 years that preceded the murder (Centers for Disease Control and Prevention [CDC], 2005). Among women who are pregnant, 4% to 14% suffer physical violence from their intimate partner; 10% to 24% of this population are abused the year before they become pregnant. These statistics are startlingly higher for teenagers, of whom 20% are assaulted while pregnant. The severity of the abuse increases and is associated with battering during pregnancy. Domestic violence is the leading cause of death in young African-American women (Harrell, Toronjo, McLaughlin, et al., 2002).

On average, between 6% and 28% of women seen in the ED have suffered abuse. As many as 6% of these patients are seeking treatment for a complaint related to a recent event. Between 20% and 35% of all ED visits relate to continuous abuse. Young women are most likely to suffer nonlethal violent acts that result in visits to the ED (Moskowitz, Griffith, DiScala, et al., 2001). ED nurses must be aware that men and people with disabilities are also victims of domestic violence and abuse and should include questions to that effect in their evaluations.

Approximately 1 to 2 million elders are abused or neglected annually (Guth & Pachter, 2000). Elder abuse takes many forms, including physical and psychological abuse, neglect, violation of personal rights, and financial abuse (see Chapters 5 and 46).

Clinical Manifestations

When people who have been abused seek treatment, they may present with physical injuries or with health problems such as anxiety, insomnia, or gastrointestinal symptoms that are related to stress. They usually do not identify their abuser.

The possibility of abuse should be investigated whenever a person presents with multiple injuries that are in various stages of healing, when injuries are unexplained, and when the explanation does not fit the physical picture (Chart 71-13). The possibility of neglect should be investigated whenever a dependent person with adequate resources and a designated care provider shows evidence of inattention to hygiene, to nutrition, or to known medical needs (eg, unfilled medication prescriptions, missed appointments with health care providers). In the ED, the most common physical injuries seen are unexplained bruises, lacerations, abrasions, head injuries, or fractures. The most common clinical manifestations of neglect are malnutrition and dehydration.

Assessment and Diagnostic Findings

Nurses in EDs are in an ideal position to provide early detection and interventions for victims of domestic violence. This requires an acute awareness of the signs of possible abuse, maltreatment, and neglect. Nurses must be skilled

CHART 71-13

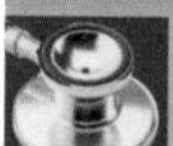

Assessing for Abuse, Maltreatment, and Neglect

The following questions may be helpful when assessing a patient for abuse, maltreatment, and neglect:

- I noticed that you have a number of bruises. Can you tell me how they happened? Has anyone hurt you?
- You seem frightened. Has anyone ever hurt you?
- Sometimes patients tell me that they have been hurt by someone at home or at work. Could this be happening to you?
- Are you afraid of anyone at home or work, or of anyone with whom you come in contact?
- Has anyone failed to help you to take care of yourself when you needed help?
- Has anyone prevented you from seeing friends or other people whom you wish to see?
- Have you signed any papers that you did not understand or did not wish to sign?
- Has anyone forced you to sign papers against your will?
- Has anyone forced you to engage in sexual activities within the past year?
- Has anyone prevented you from using an assistive device (eg, wheelchair, walker) within the past year?
- Has anyone you depend on refused to help you take your medicine, bathe, groom, or eat within the past year?

in interviewing techniques that are likely to elicit accurate information. A careful history is crucial in the screening process. Asking questions in private—away from others—may be helpful in eliciting information about abuse, maltreatment, and neglect.

Whenever evidence leads one to suspect abuse or neglect, an evaluation with careful documentation of descriptions of events and drawings or photos of injuries is important, because the medical record may be used as part of a legal proceeding. Assessment of the patient's general appearance and interactions with significant others, an examination of the entire surface area of the body, and a mental status examination are crucial.

Management

Whenever abuse, maltreatment, or neglect is suspected, the health care worker's primary concern should be the safety and welfare of the patient. Treatment focuses on the consequences of the abuse, violence, or neglect and on prevention of further injury. Protocols of most EDs require that a multidisciplinary approach be used. Nurses, physicians, social workers, and community agencies work collaboratively to develop and implement a plan for meeting the patient's needs.

If the patient is in immediate danger, he or she should be separated from the abusing or neglecting person whenever possible. On the basis of this danger, or on the basis of injuries or neglected medical conditions, hospitalization may be justified until alternative plans are made. However, it must be remembered that third-party payers may not approve hospitalization that is based solely on abuse or neglect. Referral to a shelter may be the most appropriate action, but many shelters are inaccessible to people with mobility limitations.

When abuse or neglect is the result of stress experienced by a caregiver who is no longer able to cope with the burden of caring for an elderly person or a person with chronic disease or a disability, respite services may be necessary. Support groups may be helpful to these caregivers. When mental illness of the abuser or neglecter is responsible for the situation, alternative living arrangements may be required.

Nurses must be mindful that competent adults are free to accept or refuse the help that is offered to them. Some patients insist on remaining in the home environment where the abuse or neglect is occurring. The wishes of patients who are competent and not cognitively impaired should be respected. However, all possible alternatives and available resources should be explored with the patient.

Mandatory reporting laws in most states require health care workers to report *suspected* child or elder abuse to an official agency, usually Adult (or Child) Protective Services. All that is required for reporting is the suspicion of abuse; the health care worker is not required to prove anything. Likewise, health care workers who report suspected abuse are immune from civil or criminal liability if the report is made in good faith. Subsequent home visits resulting from the report of suspected abuse are a part of gathering information about the patient in the home environment. In addition, many states have resource hotlines for use by health care workers and by patients who seek answers to questions about abuse and neglect.

Sexual Assault

The definition of *rape* is forced sexual acts, especially if these acts involve vaginal or anal penetration. Perpetrators and victims may be either male or female. Society is focused on the rights and care of people who have been sexually assaulted, and law enforcement agencies are increasingly sensitive and aggressive in managing these crimes. Rape crisis centers offer support and education and help people who have been sexually assaulted through the subsequent police investigation and courtroom experience.

The manner in which the patient is received and treated in the ED is important to his or her future psychological well-being. Crisis intervention should begin when the patient enters the health care facility. The patient should be seen immediately. Most hospitals have a written protocol that addresses the patient's physical and emotional needs as well as collection of forensic evidence.

In many states, the emergency nurse has the opportunity to become trained as a sexual assault nurse examiner (SANE). Preparing for this role requires specific training in forensic evidence collection, history taking, documentation, and ways to approach the patient and family. Specialized training also includes learning proper photographic methods and the use of colposcopy. Colposcopy facilitates assessment by magnifying tissues and looking for evidence of microtrauma. Evidence is collected through photography, videography, and analysis of specimens. Another tool useful to the SANE is the light-staining microscope, which enables the examiner to identify motile and nonmotile sperm and infectious organisms. This tool saves time and also enhances assessment. The SANE complements the ED staff and can spend more time with both the patient and police officers investigating the incident.

Assessment and Diagnostic Findings

The patient's reaction to rape has been termed *rape trauma syndrome* and is seen as an acute stress reaction to a life-threatening situation. The nurse performing the assessment is aware that the patient may go through several phases of psychological reactions (CDC, 2005; Coker, Amith, Bethea, et al., 2000), which have been described as follows:

- An acute disorganization phase, which may manifest as an expressed state in which shock, disbelief, fear, guilt, humiliation, anger, and other such emotions are encountered or as a controlled state in which feelings are masked or hidden and the victim appears composed
- A phase of denial and unwillingness to talk about the incident, followed by a phase of heightened anxiety, fear, flashbacks, sleep disturbances, hyperalertness, and psychosomatic reactions that is consistent with posttraumatic stress disorder (PTSD)
- A phase of reorganization, in which the incident is put into perspective. Some victims never fully recover and go on to develop chronic stress disorders and phobias.

Management

The goals of management are to give sympathetic support, to reduce the patient's emotional trauma, and to gather available evidence for possible legal proceedings. All of the interventions are aimed at encouraging the patient to gain a sense of control over his or her life.

Throughout the patient's stay in the ED, the patient's privacy and sensitivity must be respected. The patient may exhibit a wide range of emotional reactions, such as hysteria, stoicism, or feelings of being overwhelmed. Support and caring are crucial. The patient should be reassured that anxiety is natural and asked whether a support person may be called. Appropriate support is available from professional and community resources. The Rape Victim Companion Program, if available in the community, can be contacted, and the services of a volunteer can be requested. The patient should never be left alone.

Physical Examination

A written, witnessed informed consent must be obtained from the patient (or parent or guardian if the patient is a minor) for examination, for taking of photographs, and for release of findings to police. A history is obtained only if the patient has not already talked to a police officer, social worker, or crisis intervention worker. The patient should not be asked to repeat the history. Any history of the event that is obtained should be recorded in the patient's own words. The patient is asked whether he or she has bathed, douched, brushed his or her teeth, changed clothes, urinated, or defecated since the attack, because these actions may alter interpretation of subsequent findings. The time of admission, time of examination, date and time of the alleged rape, and the patient's emotional state and general appearance (including any evidence of trauma, such as discoloration, bruises, lacerations, secretions, or torn and bloody clothing) are documented.

For the physical examination, the patient is helped to undress and is draped properly. Each item of clothing is placed in a separate paper bag. Plastic bags are not used because they retain moisture; moisture may promote mold and mildew formation, which can destroy evidence. The bags are labeled and given to appropriate law enforcement authorities.

The patient is examined (from head to toe) for injuries, especially injuries to the head, neck, breast, thighs, back, and buttocks. Body diagrams and photographs aid in documenting the evidence of trauma. The physical examination focuses on the following:

- External evidence of trauma (bruises, contusions, lacerations, stab wounds)
- Dried semen stains (appearing as crusted, flaking areas) on the patient's body or clothes
- Broken fingernails and body tissue and foreign materials under nails (if found, samples are taken)
- Oral examination, including a specimen of saliva and cultures of gum and tooth areas

Pelvic and rectal examinations are also performed. The perineum and other areas are examined with a Wood lamp or other filtered ultraviolet light. Areas that appear fluorescent may indicate semen stains. The color and consistency of any discharge present is noted. A water-moistened rather than a lubricated vaginal speculum is used for the examination. Lubricant contains chemicals that may interfere with later forensic testing of specimens and acid phosphatase determinations. The rectum is examined for signs of trauma, blood, and semen. During the examination, the patient should be advised of the nature and necessity of each procedure and given the rationale for each question asked.

Specimen Collection

During the physical examination, numerous laboratory specimens may be collected, including the following:

- Vaginal aspirate, examined for presence or absence of motile and nonmotile sperm
- Secretions (obtained with a sterile swab) from the vaginal pool for acid phosphatase, blood group antigen of semen, and precipitin test against human sperm and blood
- Separate smears from the oral, vaginal, and anal areas
- Culture of body orifices for gonorrhea
- Blood serum for syphilis and HIV testing and DNA analysis; a sample of serum for syphilis may be frozen and saved for future testing
- Pregnancy test if there is a possibility that the patient may be pregnant
- Any foreign material (leaves, grass, dirt), which is placed in a clean envelope
- Pubic hair samples obtained by combing or trimming. Several pubic hairs with follicles are placed in separate containers and identified as the patient's hairs.

To preserve the chain of evidence, each specimen is labeled with the name of the patient, the date and time of collection, the body area from which the specimen was obtained, and the names of personnel collecting specimens. Then the specimens are given to a designated person (eg, crime laboratory technician), and an itemized receipt is obtained.

Treating Potential Consequences of Rape

After the initial physical examination is completed and specimens have been obtained, any associated injuries are treated as indicated. The patient is given the option of prophylaxis against sexually transmitted disease (STD) (also referred to as sexually transmitted infection [STI]). Ceftriaxone (Rocephin), administered intramuscularly with 1% lidocaine (Xylocaine), may be prescribed as prophylaxis for gonorrhea. Doxycycline (Vibramycin) taken for 10 days may be prescribed as prophylaxis for syphilis and chlamydia.

Antipregnancy measures may be considered if the patient is of childbearing age, is not using contraceptives, and is at high risk in her menstrual cycle. A postcoital contraceptive medication, such as an oral contraceptive medication that contains levonorgestrel and ethinyl estradiol, may be prescribed after a pregnancy test. To promote effectiveness, the contraceptive medication should be administered within 12 to 24 hours and no later than 72 hours after intercourse. The 21-day package rather than the 28-day package is prescribed so that the patient does not take the inert tablets by mistake. An antiemetic may be administered as prescribed to decrease discomfort from side effects. A cleansing douche, mouthwash, and fresh clothing are usually offered.

Follow-Up Care

The patient is informed of counseling services to prevent long-term psychological effects. Counseling services should be made available to both the patient and the family. A referral is made to the Rape Victim Companion Program, if available. Appointments for follow-up surveillance for pregnancy and for STD and HIV testing also are made.

The patient is encouraged to return to his or her previous level of functioning as soon as possible. When leaving the health care facility, the patient should be accompanied by a family member or friend.

Psychiatric Emergencies

A psychiatric emergency is an urgent, serious disturbance of behavior, affect, or thought that makes the patient unable to cope with life situations and interpersonal relationships. A patient presenting with a psychiatric emergency may display overactive or violent, underactive or depressed, or suicidal behaviors.

The most important concern of the ED personnel is determining whether the patient is at risk for injuring self or others. The aim is to try to maintain the patient's self-esteem (and life, if necessary) while providing care. Determining whether the patient is currently under psychiatric care is important so that contact can be made with the therapist or physician who works with the patient.

Overactive Patients

Patients who display disturbed, uncooperative, and paranoid behavior and those who feel anxious and panicky may be prone to assaultive and destructive impulses and abnormal social behavior. Intense nervousness, depression, and crying are evident in some patients. Disturbed and noisy behavior may be exacerbated or compounded by alcohol or drug intoxication.

A reliable source for obtaining an accurate history is needed to identify events leading to the crisis. Past mental illness, hospitalizations, injuries, serious illnesses, use of alcohol or drugs, crises in interpersonal relationships, or intrapsychic conflicts are explored. Because abnormal thoughts and behavior may be manifestations of an underlying physical disorder, such as hypoglycemia, drug or alcohol toxicity, a stroke, a seizure disorder, or head injury, a physical assessment is also performed.

The immediate goal is to gain control of the situation. If the patient is potentially violent, security or local police should be nearby. Restraints are used as a *last* resort and only as prescribed. Approaching the patient with a calm, confident, and firm manner is therapeutic and has a calming effect. Helpful interventions include the following:

- Introduce yourself by name.
- Tell the patient, "I am here to help you."
- Repeat the patient's name from time to time.
- Speak in one-thought sentences and be consistent.
- Give the patient space and time to slow down.
- Show interest in, listen to, and encourage the patient to talk about personal thoughts and feelings.
- Offer appropriate and honest explanations.

A psychotropic agent (eg, one that exerts an effect on the mind) may be prescribed for emergency management of functional psychosis. However, a patient with a personality disorder cannot and should not be treated with psychotropic medications, nor are psychotropic medications used if the patient's behavior results from the use of hallucinogens (eg, lysergic acid diethylamide [LSD]).

Agents such as chlorpromazine (Thorazine) and haloperidol (Haldol) act specifically against psychotic symptoms of thought fragmentation and perceptual and behavioral aberrations. The initial dose depends on the patient's body weight and the severity of the symptoms. After administration of the initial dose, the patient is observed closely to determine the degree of change in psychotic behavior. Subsequent doses depend on the patient's response. Typically, after stabilization, the patient is transferred to an inpatient psychiatric unit or psychiatric outpatient treatment is arranged.

Violent Behavior

Violent and aggressive behavior, usually episodic, is a means of expressing feelings of anger, fear, or hopelessness about a situation. Usually, the patient has a history of outbursts of rage, temper tantrums, or impulsive behavior. People with a tendency for violence frequently lose control when intoxicated with alcohol or drugs. Family members are the most frequent victims of their aggression. Patients with a propensity for violence include those intoxicated by drugs or alcohol; those going through drug or alcohol withdrawal; and those diagnosed with acute paranoid schizophrenic state, acute organic brain syndrome, acute psychosis, paranoid character, borderline personality, or antisocial personality disorders.

The goal of treatment is to bring the violence under control. A specially designated room with at least two exits should be used for the interview. The door of the room should be kept open, and the nurse should remain in clear view of the staff, *staying between the patient and the door.* However, the patient's exit to the door must not be blocked, because the patient may feel trapped and threatened. No objects that could be used as weapons should be in sight, in the room, or carried in with health care personnel. If the interviewer feels anxious or uneasy about the patient's response, security staff, a family member, or another health care worker should be asked to remain in the hall nearby in the event that additional help is needed. The patient should never be left alone, because this may be interpreted as rejection or provide an opportunity for self-harm.

To bring the violence under control, it is crucial to use a calm, noncritical approach while remaining in control of the situation. Sudden movements are avoided. External calm and structure in conjunction with providing the patient some space may help the patient gain control. If the patient is carrying a weapon, the emergency health care provider should ask that it be surrendered. If the patient is unwilling to surrender the weapon, the security staff is called. If necessary, the security staff may seek further assistance from the local police department.

The patient's violent behavior is a crisis situation for the patient and the ED. Crisis intervention, achieved by talking and listening to the patient, is best accomplished by expressing an interest in the patient's well-being while attempting to tune in to the patient and remain firm. The patient's agitated state is acknowledged by statements such as, "I want to work with you to relieve your distress."

The patient is allowed the opportunity to ventilate anger verbally. If the patient is delusional, challenging the patient is avoided. Trying to hear what the patient is saying, conveying an expectation of appropriate behavior, and making the patient aware that help is available are key. The patient should be informed that violent behavior may be frightening to others and that violence is not acceptable. Help that is available in crisis situations (from a clinic or mental health facility) should be described and offered. Often, the offer of protection by hospitalization is welcomed by the patient, who fears losing control or harming self or others. If the patient does not calm down, security personnel or police intervention may be necessary.

If these measures fail to alleviate the patient's tension, medication may be prescribed (rapid sedation with haloperidol, diazepam, or chlorpromazine) to reduce tension, anxiety, and hyperactivity. Restraints must be prescribed by a physician. They are applied with a minimum of force and only when necessary and when other alternatives have been unsuccessful.

NURSING ALERT

The least restrictive device to prevent the patient from injuring self or others is used. Caution is taken to ensure that restraints are applied properly. Restraints should be used with verbal intervention to calm the patient and promote compliance. Appropriate personnel must be available when applying restraints (in such a way that they do not impair circulation to any part of the body or interfere with breathing). Physical observation (eg, skin integrity, circulatory status, respiratory status) is ongoing, and the patient's response is documented.

After combativeness, agitation, and fear have decreased, the patient is referred for further mental health treatment.

Posttraumatic Stress Disorder

PTSD is the development of characteristic symptoms after a psychologically stressful event that is considered outside the range of normal human experience (eg, rape, combat, motor vehicle crash, natural catastrophe, terrorist attack). Symptoms of this disorder include intrusive thoughts and dreams, phobic avoidance reaction (avoidance of activities that arouse recollection of the traumatic event), heightened vigilance, exaggerated startle reaction, generalized anxiety, and societal withdrawal. PTSD may be acute, chronic, or delayed.

Assessment and Diagnostic Findings

Assessment includes an evaluation of the patient's pretrauma history, the trauma itself, and posttrauma functioning. PTSD often presents as multiple readmissions to the ED for minor or recurring complaints without evidence of injury. The patient is allowed to discuss the traumatic event and permitted to grieve.

Management

The goal for the patient is to organize and begin to integrate the experience so that he or she can return to the pretrauma level of functioning as soon as possible. Emergency management focuses on the patient's presenting behaviors. Many interventions are carried out, including crisis intervention strategies, establishing a trusting and sharing relationship, and educating the patient and family about stress management and support services available in the community. Psychiatric support may be useful to the patient.

Underactive or Depressed Patients

In the ED, depression may be seen as the primary condition bringing the patient to the health care facility, or it may be masked by anxiety and somatic complaints. The depressed person has a mood disturbance.

Clinical manifestations may include sadness, apathy, feelings of worthlessness, self-blame, suicidal thoughts, desire to escape, avoidance of simple problems, anorexia and weight loss, decreased interest in sex, sleeplessness, and ceaseless activity or reduction in activity. The agitated depressed patient may exhibit motor restlessness and severe anxiety.

The depressed patient benefits from ventilating personal feelings and should be provided an opportunity to talk about personal problems while emergency health care personnel listen in a calm, unhurried manner. Information about a perceived or real illness or a sudden worsening of depression is an important clue.

Any patient who is depressed may be at risk of suicide. Attempts are made to find out whether the patient has thought about or attempted suicide. Questions such as, "Have you ever thought about taking your own life?" may be helpful. Generally, the patient is relieved to have an opportunity to discuss personal feelings. If the patient is seriously depressed, relatives should be notified. The patient should never be left alone, because suicide is usually committed in solitude.

The patient needs to understand that depression is treatable. Antidepressant and antianxiety agents may be prescribed. Crisis and supportive services in the community, including mental health centers, telephone counseling and referral, suicide prevention centers, group therapy, and marital and family counseling, should be offered to the patient and family. Usually, the patient is referred for psychiatric consultation or to a psychiatric facility.

Suicidal Patients

Attempted suicide is an act that stems from depression (eg, loss of a loved one, loss of body integrity or status, poor self-image) and can be viewed as a cry for help and intervention. Males are at greater risk than females. Others at risk are elderly people; young adults; people who are enduring unusual loss or stress; those who are unemployed, divorced, widowed, or living alone; those showing signs of significant depression (eg, weight loss, sleep disturbances, somatic complaints, suicidal preoccupation); and those with a history of a previous suicide attempt, suicide in the family, or psychiatric illness.

Being aware of people at risk and assessing for specific factors that predispose a person to suicide are key management strategies. Specific signs and symptoms of potential suicide include the following:

- Communication of *suicidal intent*, such as preoccupation with death or talking of someone else's suicide (eg, "I'm tired of living. I've put my affairs in order. I'm better off dead. I'm a burden to my family")
- History of a previous suicide attempt (the risk is much greater in these cases)
- Family history of suicide
- Loss of a parent at an early age
- Specific plan for suicide
- A means to carry out the plan

Emergency management focuses on treating the consequences of the suicide attempt (eg, gunshot wound, drug overdose) and preventing further self-injury. A patient who has made a suicidal gesture may do so again. Crisis intervention is employed to determine suicidal potential, to discover areas of depression and conflict, to find out about the patient's support system, and to determine whether hospitalization or psychiatric referral is necessary. Depending on the patient's potential for suicide, the patient may be admitted to the intensive care unit, referred for follow-up care, or admitted to the psychiatric unit.

Critical Thinking Exercises

1 A young woman arrives at the ED by ambulance after a car crash. She is immobilized on a backboard with a cervical collar and an oxygen mask in place. There is a bruise across her abdomen where the seatbelt was applied. She complains of nausea and abdominal pain. You note no movement of the left chest wall and an angulated right arm. She has no pulses in her lower extremities and cannot move or feel her legs. How would you prioritize the patient's needs? Develop an assessment strategy, identify diagnostic studies that will benefit the patient, and describe the patient's treatment needs.

2 A man was outdoors on his dog sled for the first time this winter. He chose to wear light clothing, expecting warm weather, but neglected to take into account that there were 4 inches of snow on the ground. He spent the day standing on the sled or running in the snow. He now presents to the ED for treatment of frostbite of his feet. His friends have been massaging his feet en route to the ED. The patient insists this makes his feet feel better. Describe how you would respond and the explanation you would give to this patient. How would you proceed with managing this patient's care? Describe the treatment dilemmas for this type of injury.

3 ebp A young woman with a toddler in her arms waits her turn at the triage desk of the ED. The child is crying and rubbing her eyes and face. You overhear the mother telling another patient that the child has eaten strawberries for the first time. While waiting, the child becomes quiet and pale. Analyze this information. What is your immediate response? What is the evidence base for the triage decision that you make for this child?

4 The following five patients present to the triage desk within minutes of each other. How would you prioritize and categorize each of these patients? Which ones need immediate attention? What initial care would you provide at triage?

a. A child with medication-controlled asthma presents with rapid, shallow respirations and cyanosis around the lips and is very anxious. He has been this way for about 20 minutes.

b. A woman who has had a cold for 3 days says she has no primary care physician and must be seen right now because she cannot breathe. Her respirations are normal, pulse oxygenation saturations are 100%, and she has complaints of sinus drainage.

c. A woman was hit by an automobile while she was riding her bike. Instead of calling 911, a friend drove her to the ED. She is complaining of neck pain and tingling in her upper extremities since the injury. She is beginning to have difficulty taking a deep breath.

d. A young boy who was riding his skateboard arrives at the ED with an angulated wrist. Pulses are normal, but the wrist is painful.

e. An elderly woman presents with complaints of 24 hours of vomiting. Her vital signs are normal, but she is diaphoretic and appears weak.

REFERENCES AND SELECTED READINGS

BOOKS

Aelert, B. (2003). *Rapid ACLS on PDA with ACLS quick review study guide* (2nd ed.). St. Louis: Mosby.

American College of Surgeons. (2005). *Advanced trauma life support* (7th ed.). Chicago: Author.

American Heart Association. (2005). *BLS for healthcare providers*. Available online: http://www.americanheart.org. Accessed August 9, 2006.

Auerbach, P. S., Donner, H. S., & Weiss, E. H. (2003). *Field guide to wilderness medicine* (2nd ed.). St. Louis: Mosby.

Berner, A. R. (2005). Triage. In A. Harwood-Nuss (Ed.), *The clinical practice of emergency medicine* (4th ed.). Philadelphia: Lippincott Williams & Wilkins.

Bove, A. A., & Davis, J. C. (1997). *Diving medicine.* Philadelphia: Saunders.

Emergency Nurses Association & Newberry, L. (2003). *Sheehy's emergency nursing* (5th ed). St. Louis: Mosby.

Fultz, J., & Sturt, P. A. (2005). *Mosby's emergency nursing reference* (3rd ed.). St. Louis: Mosby.

Holleran, R. S. (2003). *Air and surface patient transport: Principles and practice* (3rd ed.). St. Louis: Mosby.

Lynch, V. (2006). *Forensic nursing.* St. Louis: C. V. Mosby.

McQuillan, K., VonReuden, K., Hartsock, R., et al. (2002). *Trauma nursing: Resuscitation through rehabilitation* (3rd ed.). Philadelphia: Saunders.

Mohan, D., & Tiwari, G. (2000). *Injury prevention and control.* London: Taylor and Francis.

Porth, C. M. (2005). *Pathophysiology: Concepts of altered health states* (7th ed.). Philadelphia: Lippincott Williams & Wilkins.

JOURNALS

**Asterisks indicate nursing research articles.*

Bierens, J. J., Knape, J. T., & Gelissen, H. P. (2002). Drowning. *Current Opinion in Critical Care, 8*(6), 578–586.

Blow, O., Magliore, L., Claridge, J. A., et al. (1999). The golden hour and the silver day: Detection and correction of occult hypoperfusion within 24 hours improves outcome from major trauma. *Journal of Trauma, 47*(5), 964–969.

Bowman, M. J., & Ufberg, J. W. (2003). From stingers to fangs: Evaluating and managing bites and envenomations. *Trauma Reports, 4*(3), 1–11.

Bright, S., Bradbury, E., McGrane, P., et al. (2002). Injury management in the community. *Emergency Nurse, 10*(7), 28–32.

Byard, R. W., Houldsworth, G., James, R. A., et al. (2001). Characteristic features of suicidal drownings: A 20-year study. *American Journal of Forensic Medicine and Pathology, 22*(2), 134–138.

Campbell, D. J., Sprouse, L. R., Smith, L. A., et al. (2003). Injuries in pediatric patients with seatbelt contusions. *American Surgeon, 69*(12), 1095–1099.

Cassabaum, V. D., & Bourg, P. W. (2002). Emergency nursing update: The ins and outs of renal trauma. *American Journal of Nursing, 102*(9) (suppl), 4–7.

Centers for Disease Control and Prevention (2005). Factsheets. http://www.cdc.gov/ncipc/factsheets/cmfacts.html; Accessed June 29, 2005.

Coker, A. L., Amith, P. H., Bethea, L., et al. (2000). Physical health consequence of physical and psychological intimate partner violence. *Archives of Family Medicine, 9*(5), 45.

Flowers, D. L. (2004). Culturally competent nursing care: A challenge for the 21st century. *Critical Care Nurse, 24*(4), 48–52.

Frakes, M. A., & Evans, T. (2004). Major pelvic fractures. *Critical Care Nurse, 24*(2), 18–32.

Galea, S. (2002). Psychological sequelae of the September 11 terrorist attacks in New York City. *New England Journal of Medicine, 346*(13), 982–987.

Gould, S. A., Moore, E. E., Hoyt, D. B., et al. (2002). The life-sustaining capacity of human polymerized hemoglobin when red cells might be unavailable. *Journal of American College of Surgery, 195*(4), 445–455.

Grossman, M. D., Miller, D., Scaff, D. W., et al. (2002). When is elder old? Effect of preexisting conditions on mortality on geriatric trauma. *Journal of Trauma, 52*(2), 242–246.

Gunnels, D., & Gunnels, M. D. (2003). Snakebite poisoning treatment myths and facts. *Journal of Emergency Nursing, 29*(1), 80–82.

Guth, A. A., & Pachter, H. L. (2000). Domestic violence and the trauma surgeon. *American Journal of Surgery, 179*(2), 134–140.

Harrell, R., Toronjo, C. H., McLaughlin, J., et al. (2002). How geriatricians identify elder abuse and neglect. *American Journal of Medical Sciences, 323*(1), 34–38.

Hwang, V., Shofer, F. S., Durbin, D. R., et al. (2003). Prevalence of traumatic injuries in drowning and near drowning in children and adolescents. *Archives of Pediatrics and Adolescent Medicine, 157*(1), 50–53.

Jacelon, C. S., & Henneman, E. A. (2004). Profiles in dignity: Perspectives on nursing and critically ill older adults. *Critical Care Nurse, 24*(4), 30–35.

Juckett, G., & Hancox, J. G. (2002). Venomous snakebites in the United States: Management review and update. *American Family Physician, 65*(7), 1367–1374.

Kaide, C. G., & Stafford, P. W. (2003). Current strategies for airway management in the trauma patient. *Trauma Reports, 4*(2), 1–11.

Kallenborn, J. C., Gonzalez, K., Crane, N. B., et al. (2004). Cease fire Tampa Bay: A three-tiered approach to firearm injury prevention. *Journal of Trauma Nursing, 11*(1), 6–11.

Kamienski, M. C. (2004). Family-centered care in the ED. *American Journal of Nursing, 104*(1), 59–62.

Kerr, G. W., McGuffie, A. C., & Wilkie, S. (2001). Tricyclic antidepressant overdose: A review. *Emergency Medicine Journal, 18*(4), 236–241.

Kirkpatrick, A. W., Sirois, M., Laupland, K. B., et al. (2005). Prospective evaluation of hand-held focused abdominal sonography for trauma (FAST) in blunt and abdominal trauma. *Canadian Journal of Surgery, 48*(6), 453–460.

Lakstein, D., Blumenfeld, A., Sokolov, T., et al. (2003). Tourniquets for hemorrhage control on the battlefield: A 4-year accumulated experience. *Journal of Trauma, 154*(5), 5221–5225.

Ledray, L. E. (2000). Is the SANE role within the scope of nursing practice? On pelvics, colposcopy, and dispensing of medications. *Journal of Emergency Nursing, 26*(1), 79–81.

*Maclean, S. L., Guzzetta, C. E., White, C., et al. (2003). Family presence during cardiopulmonary resuscitation and invasive procedures: Practices of critical care and emergency nurses. *Journal of Emergency Nursing, 29*(3), 208–221.

McMahon, M. M. (2003). ED triage: Is a five-level triage system best? *American Journal of Nursing, 103*(3), 61–63.

Moskowitz, H., Griffith, J. L., DiScala, C., et al. (2001). Serious injuries and deaths of adolescent girls resulting from interpersonal violence: Characteristics and trends from the United States, 1989–1998. *Archives of Pediatrics and Adolescent Medicine, 155*(8), 903–908.

National Hospital Ambulatory Medical Care Survey. (2003). *2003 Emergency department summary*. Advance Data No. 358. Available online: http://www.cdc.gov/nchs/pressroom/05news/emergencydept.html. Accessed June 26, 2006.

Nayduch, D. A. (1999). Trauma wound management. *Nursing Clinics of North America, 34*(4), 895–906.

Nicholas, J. M., Rix, E. P., Easley, K. A., et al. (2003). Changing patterns in the management of penetrating injuries in patients with penetrating abdominal trauma. *Journal of Trauma, 55*(6), 1096–1108.

O'Neill, P. A., Kirton, O. C., Dresner, L. S., et al. (2004). Analysis of 162 colon injuries in patients with penetrating abdominal trauma. *Journal of Trauma, 56*(2), 304–313.

Ort, J. A. (2002). The sexual assault nurse examiner. *American Journal of Nursing, 102*(9), 24GG–24KK.

Pasero, C. (2003). Pain in the emergency department. *American Journal of Nursing, 103*(7), 73–74.

Pudalek, B. (2002). Geriatric trauma: Special needs for a special population. *AACN Clinical Issues, 13*(1), 61–72.

Rosenthal, R. A., & Kavic, S. M. (2004). Assessment and management of the geriatric patient. *Critical Care Medicine, 32*(4), S92–S105.

Russell Neary, S. (2002). Designer and club drugs: Update for the healthcare provider. Available at: http://www.medscape.com. Accessed June 26, 2006.

Schriver, J. A., Talmadge, R., Chuong, R., et al. (2003). Emergency nursing: Historical, current, and future roles. *Journal of Emergency Nursing, 29*(5), 431–439.

Shinkawa, H., Yasuhara, H., Naka, S., et al. (2004). Characteristic features of abdominal organ injuries associated with gastric rupture in blunt abdominal trauma. *American Journal of Surgery, 187*(3), 394–397.

Stotts, N. A., & Deitrich, C. E. (2004). The challenge to come: The care of older adults. *American Journal of Nursing, 104*(8), 40–47.

Suominen, P., Baillie, C., Korpela, R., et al. (2002). Impact of age, submersion time, and water temperature on outcome in near-drowning. *Resuscitation, 52*(3), 247–254.

Tanabe, P., Gimbel, R., Yarnold, P. R., et al. (2004). The Emergency Severity Index (version 3) 5-level triage systems scores predict ED resource consumption. *Journal of Emergency Nursing, 30*(1), 22–29.

Taylor, M. D., Tracy, J. K., Meyer, W., et al. (2002). Trauma in the elderly: Intensive care unit resource and outcome. *Journal of Trauma, 26*(5), 536–538.

Travers, D. A., Waller, A. E., Bowling, J. M., et al. (2002). Five-level triage system more effective than three-level in tertiary emergency department. *Journal of Emergency Nursing, 28*(5), 395–400.

Uemura, K., Sorimachi, Y., Yashiki, M., et al. (2003). Two fatal cases involving concurrent use of methamphetamine and morphine. *Journal of Forensic Science, 48*(5), 1179–1181.

Warshaw, E. M. (2003). Latex allergy. *SKINmed, 2*(6), 359–366.

Wooten, C., Schultz, P., Sapida, J., et al. (2004). Warming and treatment of mild hypothermia in the trauma resuscitation room: An intervention algorithm. *Journal of Trauma Nursing, 11*(2), 64–66.

Zeglin, D. (2005). Brown recluse spider bites. *American Journal of Nursing, 105*(2), 64–68.

RESOURCES

American College of Surgeons, Committee on Trauma, 633 North Saint Clair Street, Chicago, IL 60611; (800) 621-4111; http://www.facs.org

American Heart Association, 4217 Park Place Ct., Glen Allen, VA 23060; (804) 747-8334; http://www.americanheart.org. Accessed August 10, 2006.

American Trauma Society, 8903 Presidential Pkwy., Ste. 512, Upper Marlboro, MD; http://www.amtrauma.org. Accessed August 10, 2006.

Centers for Disease Control and Prevention, 1600 Clifton Road, NE, Atlanta, GA 30333; (404) 639-3311; http://www.cdc.gov. Accessed August 10, 2006.

Eastern Association for the Surgery of Trauma, P.O. Box 1278, East Northport, NY 11731; (631) 456-9672; http://www.east.org. Accessed August 10, 2006.

Emergency Nurses Association, 915 Lee Street, Des Plaines, IL 60016; (800) 900-9159; http://www.ena.org. Accessed August 10, 2006.

National Safety Council, 1121 Spring Lake Drive, Itasca, IL 60143; (630) 285-1121; http://www.nsc.org. Accessed August 10, 2006.

Society of Trauma Nurses, PMB 300 223 N Guadalupe, Santa Fe, NM 87501; (505) 983-4923; http://traumanursesoc.org. Accessed August 10, 2006.

CHAPTER 72

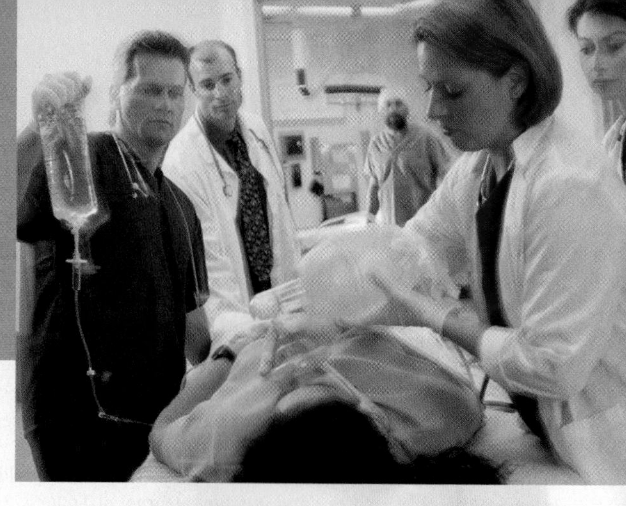

Terrorism, Mass Casualty, and Disaster Nursing

Learning Objectives

On completion of this chapter, the learner will be able to:

1. Identify the necessary components of an emergency operations plan.
2. Discuss how triage in a disaster differs from triage in an emergency.
3. Develop a plan of care for a patient experiencing short- or long-term psychological effects after a disaster.
4. Evaluate the different levels of personal protection and decontamination procedures that may be necessary during an event involving mass casualties or weapons of mass destruction.
5. Describe isolation precautions necessary for bioterrorism agents.
6. Identify the differences among the various chemical agents used in terrorist events, their effects, and the decontamination and treatment procedures that are necessary.
7. Determine the injuries associated with varying levels of radiation or chemical exposure and the associated decontamination processes.

The possibility and reality of mass casualties associated with disasters, terrorism, and biologic warfare are not new to human history; nor is the concept of using **weapons of mass destruction (WMD)**. In fact, the use of WMD dates as far back as the 6th century BCE for biological weapons and the year 436 BCE for chemical weapons (U.S. Army Medical Research Institute of Infectious Disease, 1996; U.S. Army Medical Research Institute of Chemical Defense, 1999). However, geopolitical forces and interests, the "shrinking globe," and the availability of destructive technology have brought the possibility of more terrorist events to our doorstep. Examples include the 1993 bombing of the World Trade Center in New York City; the 1995 Oklahoma City bombing of the Murrah Federal Building; the total destruction of the World Trade Center towers and the damage to the Pentagon on Sept. 11, 2001; and the anthrax exposures that same year. Terrorists have become increasingly sophisticated, organized, and therefore effective. It is no longer a question of *whether* a terrorist event will again lead to mass casualties, but *when* such an event will occur.

In 1999, a government agency called the National Domestic Preparedness Organization was developed to coordinate preparedness in the event of a terrorist attack. The Department of Homeland Security was created after the Sept. 11, 2001, attacks to coordinate federal and state efforts to combat terrorist activity. In 2001 and 2002, all acute care facilities across the nation were asked to present detailed plans to their health departments on how they would handle situations involving WMD.

As distressing as terrorism and warfare are, they are just two of the reasons that health care providers need to plan for mass casualties. Airplane crashes, train crashes, and toxic substance spills are other disasters that can result in casualties and tax the resources of health care facilities and their communities. In addition, natural phenomena such as floods, tornadoes, hurricanes, fires, and earthquakes kill and injure hundreds of thousands of people worldwide each year. Acute care facilities must be prepared for any and all of these disasters. This chapter focuses on disaster preparedness, especially providing information about possible terrorist-sponsored injuries and illnesses that can occur after biologic, chemical, and nuclear or radiation attacks. Information about the process of responding to these emergencies is applicable to other types of mass disasters as well.

CHART 72-1

Disaster Levels

Disasters are often classified by the resultant anticipated necessary response:

Level I: Local emergency response personnel and organizations can contain and effectively manage the disaster and its aftermath.

Level II: Regional efforts and aid from surrounding communities are sufficient to manage the effects of the disaster.

Level III: Local and regional assets are overwhelmed; statewide or federal assistance is required.

Federal, State, and Local Responses to Emergencies

There are many resources available at the federal, state, and local levels to assist in the management of disasters and emergencies. Disasters are often categorized by level to indicate the anticipated level of response (Chart 72-1). A list of local resources with specific instructions about how and when to contact them should be readily available to local disaster planning committees and frequently reviewed by those committees for needed updates. The following are a few of the resources that may be of assistance during a **mass casualty incident** (MCI) or a disaster.

Federal Agencies

Many federal resources can be accessed. The state authorities must request federal assistance with resources through appropriate government channels. A request for federal resources generally is made when local resources have become or are expected to become depleted.

Federal agencies that may provide resources in response to an MCI or a disaster include the Department of Health and Human Services (DHHS), the Department of Justice (DOJ),

Glossary

biological warfare: use of a biological agent, such as anthrax, as a WMD

chemical warfare: use of a chemical agent, such as chlorine, as a WMD

decontamination: process of removing, or rendering harmless, contaminants that have accumulated on personnel, patients, and equipment

mass casualty incident (MCI): situation in which the number of casualties exceeds the number of resources

material safety data sheet (MSDS): provides chemical information to employees and health care providers regarding specific agents; includes chemical name, physical data, chemical ingredients, fire and explosive hazard data, health and reactive data, spill or leak procedures, special protection information, and special precautions. Established under the OSHA Hazard Communication Standard, also known as the Worker's Right to Know.

nuclear warfare: use of nuclear contamination as a WMD

Occupational Safety and Health Association (OSHA): federal agency established for worker safety and protection

personal protective equipment (PPE): equipment beyond standard precautions; may include level A, B, C, and D equipment.

weapons of mass destruction (WMD): weapons used to cause widespread death and destruction and the Department of Homeland Security. Each of these federal departments oversees hundreds of agencies that may respond to MCIs. For example, personnel from the Federal Bureau of Investigation (FBI) (under the DOJ) may be used for scene control and collection of forensic evidence. The Federal Emergency Management Agency (FEMA), which is overseen by the Department of Homeland Security, can activate teams such as the Urban Search and Rescue Teams (USRTs). The DHHS administers the Centers for Disease Control and Prevention (CDC) and the National Disaster Medical System (NDMS). The NDMS has many medical support teams, such as Disaster Medical Assistance Teams (DMATs), Disaster Mortuary Response Teams (DMORTs), Veterinary Medical Assistance Teams (VMATs), and National Medical Response Teams for Weapons of Mass Destruction (NMRTs).

The DMAT organizes voluntary medical personnel who can set up and staff a field hospital; DMATs are located across the country. There are only four NMRTs: the mobile California, North Carolina, and Colorado teams and the Washington, DC team, which is stationary. These specialty teams were developed to respond to situations involving WMD. They consist of specially trained medical and technical personnel. The National Guard Civil Strike Teams (CSTs) are specially trained units that may respond to MCIs or disasters.

Additional federal resources that may be activated include the teams from the CDC. This is the lead federal agency for disease prevention, and it controls activities and provides backup support to state and local health departments. Additional support is available from the American Red Cross, which provides many support systems and shelter as needed.

State and Local Agencies

Some state and local agencies may be branches of the same agencies already listed (eg, local CDC and FBI agencies). Other state and local resources may include the American Red Cross, poison control centers, and other local volunteer organizations. The Metro Medical Response Teams Systems (MMRS) are local teams of health care providers that are located in cities considered possible terrorist targets and are funded for specialty response to WMD. Many state and federal task forces have been developed to assist in the development and improvement of civilian medical response to chemical and biologic terrorism.

Most cities and all states have an Office of Emergency Management (OEM). The OEM coordinates the disaster relief efforts at the state and local levels. The OEM is responsible for providing interagency coordination during an emergency. It maintains a corps of emergency management personnel, including responders, planners, and administrative and support staff.

The Incident Command System

The Incident Command System (ICS) is the local organization that coordinates personnel, facilities, equipment, and communication in any emergency situation. The ICS has a federal mandate and is organized in a template fashion. It becomes the center of operations for organization, planning, and transport of patients in the event of a specific MCI. One person is designated as incident commander and is selected for this role by the local emergency medical system (EMS). The incident commander must be continuously informed of all activities and about any deviation from the established plan (Currance & Bronstein, 1999; Dara, Ashton, Farmer, et al., 2005; Farmer, Jimenez, Talmor, et al., 2003). Other personnel selected to serve with the ICS are likewise solicited and selected by the local EMS. Whereas the ICS is primarily a field structure and process, aspects of it are used at the level of an individual hospital's emergency response plan as well.

Hospital Emergency Preparedness Plans

Health care facilities are required by the Joint Commission on Accreditation of Healthcare Organizations (JCAHO) to create a plan for emergency preparedness and to practice this plan twice a year (JCAHO, 2003). Generally these plans are developed under the Environment of Care Committee or Safety Committee and are overseen by an administrative liaison.

Before the basic emergency operations plan (EOP) can be developed, the planning committee of the health care facility first evaluates characteristics of the community to identify the likely types of natural and manmade disasters that might occur. This evaluative process is the responsibility of the local health care facility and its safety committee, safety officer, or emergency department (ED) manager. This information can be gathered by questioning local law enforcement, fire departments, and emergency medical systems and assessing the patterns of local train traffic, automobile traffic, and flood, earthquake, tornado, or hurricane activity. Consideration is also given to possible mass casualties that could arise because of the community's proximity to chemical plants, nuclear facilities, or military bases. Federal, judicial, or financial buildings, schools, and any places where large groups of people gather can be considered high-risk areas.

The emergency preparedness planning committee must have a realistic understanding of its resources. It must determine, for example, whether the facility has or needs a pharmaceutical stockpile available to treat specific chemical or biological agents (Anteau & Williams, 1997; Stopford, 2000). Another scenario that might be anticipated may include the dispersal of a pulmonary intoxicant or choking agent, which would require that emergency operations planners find out how many ventilators are available within the facility and throughout the greater community. The committee might also outline how staff would triage and assign priority to patients when the number of ventilators is limited. Multiple factors influence a facility's ability to respond effectively to a sudden influx of injured patients, and the committee must anticipate various scenarios to improve its preparedness.

Components of the Emergency Operations Plan

Once the initial assessment is complete, the health care facility develops the EOP. Essential components of the plan are as follows:

- *An activation response:* The EOP activation response of a health care facility defines where, how, and when the response is initiated.
- *An internal/external communication plan:* Communication is critical for all parties involved, including communication to and from the prehospital arena (Dara et al., 2005).
- *A plan for coordinated patient care:* A response is planned for coordinated patient care into and out of the facility, including transfers to other facilities. The site of the disaster can determine where the greater number of patients may self-refer.
- *Security plans:* A coordinated security plan involving facility and community agencies is key to the control of an otherwise chaotic situation.
- *Identification of external resources:* External resources are identified, including local, state, and federal resources and information about how to activate these resources.
- *A plan for people management and traffic flow:* "People management" includes strategies to manage the patients, the public, the media, and personnel. Specific areas are assigned, and a designated person is delegated to manage each of these areas (Anteau & Williams, 1997; Dara et al., 2005).
- *A data management strategy:* A data management plan for every aspect of the disaster will save time at every step. A backup system for charting, tracking, and staffing is developed if the facility has a computer system.
- *Deactivation response:* Deactivation of the response is as important as activation; resources should not be overused. The person who decides when the facility is able to go from the disaster response back to daily activities is clearly identified. Any possible residual effects of a disaster must be considered before this decision is made (Anteau & Williams, 1997).
- *A post-incident response:* Often facilities see increased volumes of patients 3 months or more after an incident. Post-incident response must include a critique and a debriefing for all parties involved, immediately and again at a later date.
- *A plan for practice drills:* Practice drills that include community participation allow for troubleshooting any issues before a real-life incident occurs.
- *Anticipated resources:* Food and water must be available for staff, families, and others who may be at the facility for an extended period.
- *MCI planning:* MCI planning includes such issues as mass fatality and morgue readiness.
- *An educational plan for all of the above:* A strong educational plan for all personnel regarding each step of the plan allows for improved readiness and additional input for fine-tuning of the EOP (Anteau & Williams, 1997; Dara et al., 2005).

The EOP should also include a structure that defines roles for all employees in each emergency situation. The most common structure is the ICS described earlier but applied at the level of the health care facility itself instead of at the site of the disaster. For example, an administrator, possibly the nurse executive, will act as incident commander within the hospital and coordinate all aspects of the implementation of the plan. Other personnel will be designated to perform key roles, such as resource manager or patient disposition coordinator. Such predetermined organization is essential to minimize confusion, ensure that all key operations are directed, and promote a well-coordinated response.

Initiating the Emergency Operations Plan

Notification of a disaster situation to a health care facility varies with each situation. Generally, the notification to the facility comes from outside sources unless the initial incident occurred at the facility. The disaster activation plan should clearly state how the EOP is to be initiated. If communication is functioning, field incident command will give notice of the approximate number of arriving patients, although the number of self-referring patients will not be known.

Identifying Patients and Documenting Patient Information

Patient tracking is a critical component of casualty management. Disaster tags, which are numbered and include triage priority, name, address, age, location and description of injuries, and treatments or medications given, are used to communicate patient information. The tag should be securely placed on the patient and remain with the patient at all times. The tag number and the patient's name are recorded in a disaster log. The log is used by the command center to track patients, assign beds, and provide families with information.

Triage

Triage is the sorting of patients to determine the priority of their health care needs and the proper site for treatment. In nondisaster situations, health care workers assign a high priority and allocate the most resources to those who are the most critically ill. For example, a young adult who has a chest injury and is in full cardiac arrest would receive advanced cardiopulmonary resuscitation, including medications, chest tubes, intravenous (IV) fluids, blood, and possibly even emergency surgery in an effort to restore life. However, in a disaster, when health care providers are faced with a large number of casualties, the fundamental principle guiding resource allocation is to do the greatest good for the greatest number of people. Decisions are based on the likelihood of survival and consumption of available resources. Therefore, this same patient, and others with conditions associated with a high mortality rate, would be assigned a low triage priority in a disaster situation, even if the person is conscious. Although this may sound uncaring, from an ethical standpoint the expenditure of limited resources on people with a low chance of survival, and denial of those resources to others with serious but treatable conditions, cannot be justified.

The triage officer rapidly assesses those injured at the disaster scene. Patients are immediately tagged and transported or given life-saving interventions. One person performs the initial triage while other EMS personnel perform life-saving measures (eg, intubation) and transport patients. Although EMS personnel carry out initial field triage, secondary and continuous triage at all subsequent levels of care is essential.

Staff should control all entrances to the acute care facility so that incoming patients are directed to the triage area first. The triage area may be outside the entry or just at the door of the ED. This allows all patients, including those arriving by medical transport and those who walk in, to be triaged. Some patients already seen in the field may be reclassified in the triage area, based on their current presentation.

Triage categories separate patients according to severity of injury. A special color-coded tagging system is used during an MCI so that the triage category is immediately obvious. There are several triage systems in use across the country, and every nurse should be aware of the system used by his or her facility and community. The North Atlantic Treaty Organization (NATO) triage system is one that is widely used and is presented here. It consists of four colors—red, yellow, green, and black. Each color signifies a different level of priority. Table 72-1 describes each category and gives examples of how different injuries would be classified. (See Chapter 71 for discussion of triage in non-MCI situations.)

Managing Internal Problems

Each facility must determine its supply lists based on its own needs assessment. The Red Cross has developed a basic survival/shelter resource kit. The EOP committee should determine the top 10 critical medications used during normal day-to-day operations and then anticipate which other medications may be required in a disaster or an MCI. For example, the health care facility might plan to have available a stockpile of antidotes (eg, cyanide kits) or antibiotics used in treating biologic agents. Information should be available about stocking or restocking any of the basic and special supplies, how those supplies are requested, and the time required to receive those supplies.

Communicating With the Media and Family

Communication is a key component of disaster management. Communication within the vast team of disaster responders is paramount; however, effective, informative communication with the media and worried family members is also crucial.

MANAGING MEDIA REQUESTS FOR INFORMATION

Although the media have an obligation to report the news and can play a significant positive role in communication, the number of reporters and newscasters and their support teams can be overwhelming, possibly compromising operations and patient confidentiality. A clearly defined process for managing media requests that includes a designated spokesperson, a site for the dissemination of information (away from patient care areas), and a regular schedule for providing updates should be part of the disaster plan.

The disaster plan helps prevent the release of contradictory or inaccurate information. Initial statements should focus on current efforts and what is being done to better understand the scope and impact of the situation. Information about casualties should not be released. Security staff should not allow media personnel access to patient care areas.

CARING FOR FAMILIES

Friends and family members converging on the scene must be cared for by the facility. They may be feeling intense anxiety, shock, or grief and should be provided with information and updates about their loved ones as soon as possible and regularly thereafter. They should not be in the triage or treatment areas, but in a designated area staffed by available social service workers, counselors, therapists, or clergy. Access to this area should be controlled to prevent families

TABLE 72-1 Triage Categories During a Mass Casualty Incident (MCI)

Triage Category	Priority	Color	Typical Conditions
Immediate: Injuries are life-threatening but survivable with minimal intervention. Individuals in this group can progress rapidly to expectant if treatment is delayed.	1	Red	Sucking chest wound, airway obstruction secondary to mechanical cause, shock, hemothorax, tension pneumothorax, asphyxia, unstable chest and abdominal wounds, incomplete amputations, open fractures of long bones, and 2nd/3rd degree burns of 15%–40% total body surface area.
Delayed: Injuries are significant and require medical care, but can wait hours without threat to life or limb. Individuals in this group receive treatment only after immediate casualties are treated.	2	Yellow	Stable abdominal wounds without evidence of significant hemorrhage; soft tissue injuries; maxillofacial wounds without airway compromise; vascular injuries with adequate collateral circulation; genitourinary tract disruption; fractures requiring open reduction, débridement, and external fixation; most eye and CNS injuries.
Minimal: Injuries are minor and treatment can be delayed hours to days. Individuals in this group should be moved away from the main triage area.	3	Green	Upper extremity fractures, minor burns, sprains, small lacerations without significant bleeding, behavioral disorders or psychological disturbances.
Expectant: Injuries are extensive and chances of survival are unlikely even with definitive care. Persons in this group should be separated from other casualties, but not abandoned. Comfort measures should be provided when possible	4	Black	Unresponsive patients with penetrating head wounds, high spinal cord injuries, wounds involving multiple anatomical sites and organs, 2nd/3rd degree burns in excess of 60% of body surface area, seizures or vomiting within 24 hr after radiation exposure, profound shock with multiple injuries, agonal respirations; no pulse, no BP, pupils fixed and dilated.

from being disturbed. Chart 72-2 discusses cultural variables to consider when coping with disaster-related injuries and death.

The Nurse's Role in Disaster Response Plans

The role of the nurse during a disaster varies. The nurse may be asked to perform duties outside his or her area of expertise and may take on responsibilities normally held by physicians or advanced practice nurses. For example, a critical care nurse may intubate a patient or even insert chest tubes. Wound débridement or suturing may be performed by staff registered nurses. A nurse may serve as the triage officer.

Although the exact role of a nurse in disaster management depends on the specific needs of the facility at the time, it should be clear which nurse or physician is in charge of a given patient care area and which procedures each individual nurse may or may not perform. Assistance can be obtained through the incident command center, and nonmedical personnel can provide services where possible. For example, family members can provide nonskilled interventions for their loved ones. Nurses should remember that nursing care in a disaster focuses on essential care from a perspective of what is best for all patients.

New settings and atypical roles for nurses arise during a disaster; for example, the nurse may provide shelter care in a temporary housing area, or bereavement support and assistance with identification of deceased loved ones. People may require crisis intervention, or the nurse may participate in counseling other staff members and in critical incident stress management (CISM). Special care may be warranted for at-risk populations during a disaster (Chart 72-3).

CHART 72-2

Cultural Considerations

Any disaster or mass casualty incident can be expected to involve members of diverse religious, ethnic, and cultural groups or may be targeted at and predominately affect a specific religious or ethnic group. Health care providers likewise include members of all religious, ethnic, and cultural backgrounds and should bear in mind that victims may have:

- Language difficulties that increase fears and frustrations
- Specific religious practices related to medical treatment, hygiene, or diet
- Specific places/times for prayer
- Rituals about handling the dead
- Timing of funeral services

Some religious communities have plans for emergencies and disasters, and local hospitals should integrate these plans to the extent possible into their emergency operations plans.

CHART 72-3

Caring for People with Disabilities During a Disaster

When a disaster occurs, the multiple agencies involved attempt to provide food, water, and shelter to all those affected. People with disabilities have specific needs that require attention. It is recommended that people with disabilities have a personal support network to check on them after a disaster and to provide needed assistance. They should also have a back-up system and an evacuation plan. Agencies need to be aware that service animals are also affected during a disaster and may be brought to shelters with their companions.

Evacuation assistance is imperative for people with disabilities. Directions to personal equipment (eg, communication devices, medications, oxygen) should be available to rescue personnel. In a rapid evacuation, mobility devices, oxygen, suction, and medications will be needed at the shelters. Special efforts to keep those with vision or hearing impairment informed should be implemented. People skilled in sign language are also valuable resources during a disaster. On its website, the American Red Cross provides a handbook for disaster preparedness for people with disabilities: http://www.redcross.org/services/disaster/beprepared/disability/html.

CONSIDERING ETHICAL CONFLICTS

Disasters can present a disparity between the resources of the health care agency and the needs of the victims. This generates ethical dilemmas for nurses and other health care providers. Issues include conflicts related to the following:

- Rationing care
- Futile therapy
- Consent
- Duty
- Confidentiality
- Resuscitation
- Assisted suicide

Nurses may find it difficult to not provide medical care to the dying, or to withhold information to avoid spreading fear and panic. Clinical scenarios that are unimaginable in normal circumstances confront the nurse in extreme instances. Other ethical dilemmas may arise out of health care providers' instinct for self-protection and protection of their families. For example, what should a pregnant nurse do when incoming disaster victims have been exposed to radiation, yet too few nurses are available?

Nurses can plan for the ethical dilemmas they will face during disasters by establishing a framework for evaluating ethical questions before they arise and by identifying and exploring possible responses to difficult clinical situations.

They can consider how the fundamental ethical principles of utilitarianism, beneficence, and justice will influence their decisions and care in disaster response.

MANAGING BEHAVIORAL ISSUES

Although most people pull together and function during a disaster, both people and communities suffer immediate and sometimes long-term psychological trauma. Common responses to disaster include the following:

- Depression
- Anxiety
- Somatization (fatigue, general malaise, headaches, gastrointestinal disturbances, skin rashes)
- Posttraumatic stress disorder
- Substance abuse
- Interpersonal conflicts
- Impaired performance

Factors that influence a person's response to disaster include the degree and nature of the exposure to the disaster, loss of friends and loved ones, existing coping strategies, available resources and support, and the personal meaning attached to the event. Other factors, such as loss of home and valued possessions, extended exposure to danger, and exposure to toxic contamination, also influence response and increase the risk for adjustment problems. Those exposed to the dead and injured, those endangered by the event, the elderly, children, emergency first-responders, and health care personnel caring for victims are considered to be at higher risk of emotional sequelae.

Nurses can assist disaster victims through active listening and providing emotional support, giving information, and referring patients to therapists or social workers. Health care workers must refer people to mental health care services, because experience has shown that few disaster victims seek these services and early intervention minimizes psychological consequences. Nurses can also discourage victims from subjecting themselves to repeated exposure to the event through media replays and news articles, and encourage them to return to normal activities and social roles when appropriate.

Critical Incident Stress Management

Critical Incident Stress Management (CISM) is an approach to preventing and treating the emotional trauma that can affect emergency responders as a consequence of their jobs and that can also occur to anyone involved in a disaster or MCI. CISM is handled by its own teams, which are available to the OEM. There are 350 such teams in the United States. All branches of emergency services have CISM teams, as do the military and many industries (eg, airline industry).

Components of a management plan include education before an incident occurs about critical incident stress and coping strategies; field support (ensuring that staff get adequate rest, food, and fluids, and rotating work loads) during an incident; and defusings, debriefings, demobilization, and follow-up care after the incident.

Defusing is a process by which the person receives education about recognition of stress reactions and management strategies for handling stress. Debriefing is a more complicated intervention; it involves a 2- to 3-hour process during which participants are asked about their emotional reactions to the incident, what symptoms they may be experiencing (eg, flashbacks, difficulty sleeping, intrusive thoughts), and other psychological ramifications. In follow-up, members of the CISM team contact the participants of a debriefing and schedule a follow-up meeting if necessary. People with ongoing stress reactions are referred to mental health specialists.

Preparedness and Response

Recognition and Awareness

Preparedness for terrorism and other disasters as a health care provider includes awareness of the potential for covert use of WMD, self-protection, and early detection, containment, or decontamination of substances and agents that may affect others by secondary exposure. The strength of many toxins, today's mobile society, and long incubation periods for some organisms and diseases can result in an epidemic that can quickly and silently spread across the entire country. For example, there must be awareness that a formerly healthy person with a rapid onset of flu-like symptoms can have an ominous illness, such as anthrax or severe acute respiratory syndrome (SARS), both of which are discussed in more detail later in the chapter.

Health care personnel should have a heightened awareness for trends that may suggest deliberate dispersal of toxic or infectious agents. Some general principles should be considered, such as the following:

- Be aware of an unusual increase in the number of people seeking care for fever, respiratory, or gastrointestinal symptoms.
- Take note of any clusters of patients presenting with the same unusual illness from a single location. For example, clusters can be from a specific geographic location, such as a city, or from a single sporting or entertainment event.
- Be suspicious of a large number of rapidly fatal cases, especially when death occurs within 72 hours after hospital admission.
- Take note of any increase in disease incidence in a normally healthy population. These cases should be reported to the state health department and to the CDC.

If any of these trends are noted, an extensive patient history is taken in an attempt to identify the possible agent involved. This history includes an occupational, work, and environmental assessment in addition to the regular admission history. An exposure history contains, at a minimum, information about current and past exposures to possible hazards and an assessment of the patient's typical day and any deviations in routines. The work history includes, at a minimum, a description of all previous jobs, including short-term, seasonal, and part-time employment and any military service. The environmental history includes assessment of present and previous home locations, water supply, and any hobbies, to name a few factors. The admission history should include such information as recent travel and contact with others who have been ill or have recently died of a fatal illness. This is just a brief review of the extensive history that may need to be obtained to identify an exposure agent. This type of history should become a universal part of admission processes at all health care facilities (Agency for Toxic Substances and Disease Registry, 2001).

Suspicions or findings are reported to the appropriate resources in the facility and to proper authorities in the community. Resources can include the infection control department, **material safety data sheets (MSDS)**, the state health department, the CDC, the local poison control center, and many internet sites (Dara et al., 2005). Reporting furnishes data elements to those agencies responsible for epidemiology and response. Reporting also allows for sharing of information among facilities and jurisdictions and can help determine the source of infections or exposure and prevent further exposures and even deaths.

Personal Protective Equipment

Another component of preparedness and response involves the protection of the health care provider by additional **personal protective equipment (PPE)**. Chemical or biologic agents and radiation are silent killers and are generally colorless and odorless. The purpose of PPE is to shield health care workers from the chemical, physical, biologic, and radiologic hazards that may exist when caring for contaminated patients. The U.S. Environmental Protection Agency (EPA) has divided protective clothing and respiratory protection into the following four categories, level A through level D:

- Level A protection is worn when the highest level of respiratory, skin, eye, and mucous membrane protection is required. This includes a self-contained breathing apparatus (SCBA) and a fully encapsulating, vapor-tight, chemical-resistant suit with chemical-resistant gloves and boots.
- Level B protection requires the highest level of respiratory protection but a lesser level of skin and eye protection than with level A situations. This level of protection includes the SCBA and a chemical-resistant suit (Currance & Bronstein, 1999).
- Level C protection requires the air-purified respirator, which uses filters or sorbent materials to remove harmful substances from the air. A chemical-resistant coverall with splash hood, chemical-resistant gloves, and boots are included in level C protection.
- Level D protection is the typical work uniform.

Level C and level D PPE are the levels most often used in hospital facilities (Currance & Bronstein, 1999).

Protective equipment must be donned before contact with a contaminated patient. The acute care facility's standard precaution PPE (levels D or C) generally is not adequate for protection from a chemically, biologically, or radiologically contaminated patient. The health care provider must use equipment that is capable of providing protection against the agent involved. This may mean using a splash suit along with a full-face positive- or negative-pressure respirator (a filter-type gas mask) or even an SCBA for medical personnel in the field (Currance & Bronstein, 1999; JCAHO, 2003).

No single combination of PPE is capable of protecting against all hazards. Under no circumstances should responders wear any PPE without proper training, practice, and fit testing of respirator masks as necessary.

Decontamination

Decontamination, the process of removing accumulated contaminants, is critical to the health and safety of health care providers by preventing secondary contamination. The decontamination plan should establish procedures and educate employees about decontamination procedures, identify the equipment needed and methods to be used, and establish methods for disposal of contaminated materials (Currance & Bronstein, 1999; Dara et al., 2005).

Although many principles and theories surround decontamination of a patient, authorities agree that, to be effective, decontamination must include a minimum of two steps. The first step is removal of the patient's clothing and jewelry and then rinsing the patient with water. Depending on the type of exposure, this step alone can remove a large amount of the contamination and decrease secondary contamination. The second step consists of a thorough soap-and-water wash and rinse. When patients arrive at the facility after being assessed and treated by a prehospital provider, it should not be assumed that they have been thoroughly decontaminated.

Natural Disasters

Natural disasters may result in mass casualties. Natural disasters can occur anywhere at any time and include events such as tornadoes, hurricanes, floods, avalanches, tidal waves (eg, tsunamis), earthquakes, and volcanic eruptions. In many cases, preparation prior to the natural disaster is the best-laid plan. In the event of a natural disaster, loss of communications, potable water, and electricity are usually the greatest obstacles to a well-coordinated emergency response. Even wireless technology (eg, mobile or cellular phones, computers, other communication devices) may not be functional.

The majority of the immediate casualties are trauma-related. These mass casualties tax the trauma system to its limits to provide triage, transport of patients (in poor weather and road conditions), and management within the trauma centers. Electrocution is also a common injury and can result in death.

Excessive exposure to the natural elements and the need for food and water (by both patients and emergency responders) are critical issues. Without cover (eg, buildings may be unsafe or destroyed) or safe water (eg, water may be either contaminated or unavailable), injuries from exposure to heat, cold, or contaminated food or water can occur. Safety equipment that protects rescue workers from injury, exposure, and potentially dangerous animals (eg, snakes, alligators, spiders) must be readily available. Hypothermia can occur rapidly in workers who are exposed to water at temperatures of 75°F or less. As in all disasters, mental health workers and shelters are needed throughout the community. Veterinary assistance is also essential, because frequently pets are abandoned and injured. In addition, emergency response workers must be prepared to treat the most common ailments experienced after exposure to a specific natural disaster. For instance, pulmonary problems peak with earthquakes and volcanic eruptions due to increased particulate matter in the air. Most volcano-related deaths are from suffocation. After floods or water disasters, waterborne transmission of agents such as *Escherichia coli,* salmonella, shigella, typhoid, leptospirosis, malaria, and tularemia are common and cause widespread disease.

In some instances, early warning systems have assisted in decreasing the number of deaths from tornadoes and hurricanes. When buildings collapse, rapid response to identify and remove trapped victims is the only means of improving survivability. There is a direct relationship between time trapped and survival; if trapped more than 2 to 6 hours, fewer than 50% of people survive. Water-damaged buildings are not safe and require extensive examination before experts can ensure safe occupancy. Larger-scale issues that can cause significant later morbidity and mortality include the absence of water purification, waste removal, removal of human and animal remains, and vector control. Removal or disposal of biologic, chemical, and nuclear agents must also be considered.

Weapons of Terror

Although biologic, chemical, and radiologic events are not everyday events, they can occur at any facility, and every nurse needs to know the basics of caring for affected patients.

Biologic Weapons

Biologic weapons are weapons that spread disease among the general population or the military. Use of biologic weapons dates far back into history, but improved production techniques and genetics engineering have expanded the potential for widespread casualties as a result of biologic weaponry.

Effects of Biologic Weapons

Biologic warfare is a covert method of effecting terrorist objectives. Biologic weapons are easily obtained and easily disseminated and can result in significant mortality and morbidity. The potential use of biologic agents calls for continuous increased surveillance by health departments and an increased index of suspicion by clinicians. Many biologic weapons result in signs and symptoms similar to those of common disease processes.

Biologic agents are delivered in either a liquid or dry state, applied to foods or water, or vaporized for inhalation or direct contact. Vaporization may be accomplished through spray or explosives loaded with the agent. Because of increases in business and pleasure travel by people in industrialized nations, an agent could be released in one city and affect people in other cities thousands of miles away. The vector can be an insect, animal, or person, or there may be direct contact with the agent itself.

The following is a discussion of two of the agents most likely to be used or weaponized. Table 72-2 describes other easily weaponized biologic agents.

Types of Biologic Agents

ANTHRAX

Bacillus anthracis is a naturally occurring gram-positive, encapsulated rod that lives in the soil in the spore state throughout the world. The bacterium sporulates (ie, is liberated) when exposed to air and is infective only in the spore form. Contact with infected animal products (raw meat) or inhalation of the spores results in infection. Cattle and other herbivores are vaccinated against anthrax to prevent transmission through contaminated meat.

It is believed that approximately 8000 to 50,000 spores must be inhaled to put a person at risk (Tasota, Henker, & Hoffman, 2002). As an aerosol, anthrax is odorless and invisible and can travel a great distance before disseminating; hence, the site of release and the site of infection can be miles apart.

Anthrax is recognized as the most likely weaponized biologic agent available. Anthrax has been known as a highly debilitating agent for centuries. It is believed that the plague in 1500 BCE Egypt was caused by anthrax (Spencer, Whitman, & Morton, 2001). In 1979, anthrax was released intentionally in Sverdlosk, Russia, resulting in widespread mortality and morbidity. Anthrax was released with the sarin gas attack in Tokyo, Japan, in 1995; however, the method of release chosen was poorly designed for effect. In 2001, anthrax spores were placed in letters and mailed throughout the United States. The result of this event was 22 inhalation and cutaneous exposures to anthrax and 7 fatalities. Overall, this was a small incidence of exposure; however, as a result, anthrax hoaxes sprung up throughout the country, causing widespread fear (Karwa, Currie, & Kvetan, 2005).

Clinical Manifestations

Anthrax is caused by replicating bacteria that release toxin, resulting in hemorrhage, edema, and necrosis. The incubation period is 1 to 6 days. There are three primary methods of infection: skin contact, inhalation, and gastrointestinal ingestion. Skin lesions (the most common infection) cause edema with pruritus and macule or papule formation, resulting in ulceration with 1- to 3-mm vesicles. A painless eschar develops, which falls off in 1 to 2 weeks.

Ingestion of anthrax results in fever, nausea and vomiting, abdominal pain, bloody diarrhea, and occasionally ascites. If massive diarrhea develops, decreased intravascular volume becomes the primary treatment concern. The bacterium affects the terminal ileum and cecum. Sepsis can occur.

Inhaling anthrax results in the most severe clinical manifestations. Its symptoms mimic those of the flu, and usually treatment is sought only when the second stage of severe respiratory distress occurs. Current antibiotic therapy does not halt the progress of the disease. Inhaled anthrax can incubate for up to 60 days, making it difficult to identify the source of the bacterium. Initial signs and symptoms include cough, headache, fever, vomiting, chills, weakness, mild chest discomfort, dyspnea, and syncope, without rhinorrhea or nasal congestion. Most patients have a brief recovery period followed by the second stage within 1 to 3 days, characterized by fever, severe respiratory distress, stridor, hypoxia, cyanosis, diaphoresis, hypotension, and shock. These patients require optimization of oxygenation, correction of electrolyte imbalances, and ventilatory and hemodynamic support. More than 50% of these patients have hemorrhagic mediastinitis on a chest x-ray (a hallmark sign) (Altman, 2002). The disease can also progress to include meningitis with subarachnoid hemorrhage. Death results approximately 24 to 36 hours after the onset of severe respiratory distress. The mortality rate approaches 100%.

TABLE 72-2 Examples of Biologic Agents That Can Be Used as Weapons

Agent/Organism	Contagion	Decontamination and Protective Equipment	Signs and Symptoms	Treatment (Mortality Rate)
Tularemia—*Francisella tularensis:* gram-negative coccobacillus, one of the most infectious bacteria known	Direct contact with infected animals or aerosolized as a bioterror weapon; bites Not contagious through human-to-human contact	Standard barrier precautions Clothing and linens should be laundered under the usual hospital protocol	*Initial:* Abrupt onset of fever, fatigue, chills, headache, lower backache, malaise, rigor, coryza, dry cough, and sore throat without adenopathy. Nausea and vomiting or diarrhea possible. *As disease progresses:* Sweating, fever, progressive weakness, anorexia, and weight loss demonstrate continued illness. *Mortality secondary to:* pneumonitis (if inhalation is the source) with copious watery or purulent sputum, hemoptysis, respiratory insufficiency, sepsis, and shock.	Streptomycin or gentamicin/aminoglycoside for 10–14 days. Inhalation tularemia must be treated within 48 hours of onset. In mass casualty situations, doxycycline or ciprofloxacin is recommended. For persons exposed to tularemia, tetracycline or doxycycline is recommended for 14 days. (Mortality rate = 2%)
Botulism—*Clostridium botulinum:* Botulinum blocks acetylcholine-containing vesicles from fusing with the terminal membranes of the motor-neuron end-plate, resulting in a flaccid paralysis.	Direct contact Not contagious through human-to-human contact	Any skin exposure to the botulism toxin can be treated with soap and water or a 0.1% hypochlorite solution. Standard precautions are used when treating patients with botulism.	*Gastrointestinal botulism:* abdominal cramps, nausea, vomiting, and diarrhea. *Inhalation botulism:* fever; symmetric descending flaccid paralysis with multiple cranial nerve palsies. Classic signs and symptoms include diplopia, dysphagia, dry mouth, lack of fever, and alert mental status. Other possible symptoms include ptosis of the eyelids, blurred vision, enlarged sluggish pupils, dysarthria, and dysphonia. *Mortality secondary to:* airway obstruction and inadequate tidal volume.	Supportive ventilatory therapy is necessary if respiratory infection occurs. Aminoglycosides and clindamycin are contraindicated because they exacerbate neuromuscular blockage. Equine antitoxin is used to minimize subsequent nerve damage. There is a 2% rate of anaphylaxis to the antitoxin; therefore, diphenhydramine (Benadryl) and epinephrine must be immediately available for use. Supportive care—mechanical ventilation, nutrition, fluids, prevention of complications (Mortality rate = 5%)
Plague—*Yersinia pestis:* nonsporulating gram-negative coccobacillus. The bacterium causes destruction and necrosis of the lymph nodes.	Contagious *Bubonic plague:* transmitted through flea bites with no person-to-person transmission *Pneumonic plague:* transmitted through respiratory droplet contact	Isolation barrier precautions with full face respirators. The patient should wear a mask. Rooms should receive a terminal cleaning. Clothing and linens with body fluids on them should be cleaned with the usual disinfectant. Routine precautions should be used in the case of death.	*Bubonic plague:* Sudden fever and chills, weakness, a swollen and tender lymph node (bubo) in the groin, axilla, or cervical area. The resultant bacteremia progresses to septicemia from the endotoxin and, finally, shock and death. *Primary septicemic plague:* Disseminated intravascular coagulation (DIC), necrosis of small vessels, purpura, and gangrene of the digits and nose (black death). *Pneumonic plague:* Severe bronchospasm, chest pain, dyspnea, cough, and hemoptysis. There is a 100% mortality associated with pneumonic plague if not treated within the first 24 hours.	Streptomycin or gentamicin for 10–14 days. Tetracycline or doxycycline is an acceptable alternative if an aminoglycoside cannot be given. People with close contact exposure (<2 meters) require prophylaxis with doxycycline for 7 days. (Mortality rate = 50%)

Treatment

At present, anthrax is penicillin sensitive; however, strains of penicillin-resistant anthrax are thought to exist. Recommended treatment includes penicillin (Penicillin V), erythromycin (E-mycin, Erythrocin), gentamicin (Garamycin), or doxycycline (Vibramycin). If antibiotic treatment begins within 24 hours after exposure, death can be prevented (Franz & Zajtchuk, 2000). In a mass casualty situation, treatment with ciprofloxacin (Cipro) or doxycycline (Vibramycin) is recommended. Treatment is continued for 60 days. For patients who have been directly exposed to anthrax but have no signs and symptoms of disease, ciprofloxacin (Cipro) or doxycycline (Vibramycin) is used for prophylaxis for 60 days.

Standard precautions are the only precautions necessary to protect the caregiver exposed to a patient infected with anthrax. The patient is not contagious, and the disease cannot spread from person to person. Equipment should be cleaned using standard hospital disinfectant. After death, cremation is recommended because the spores can survive for decades and represent a threat to morticians and forensic medicine personnel.

There is a vaccine for anthrax that has been used in the military; however, it is not yet widely used because it requires multiple time-interval–sensitive boosters and has up to a 48% systemic reaction rate. The federal government is investigating the potential for development of a community-wide vaccine that has fewer side effects and that requires fewer boosters.

SMALLPOX

Smallpox (variola) is classified as a DNA virus. It has an incubation period of approximately 12 days. It is extremely contagious and is spread by direct contact, by contact with clothing or linens, or by droplets from person to person only after the fever has decreased and the rash phase has begun (Karwa et al., 2005). There is an associated 30% case-fatality rate (ie, the likelihood of fatality per case diagnosed). Aerosolization of the virus would result in widespread dissemination.

The World Health Organization declared smallpox eradicated in 1977 and stopped worldwide vaccination in 1980. In the United States, the last child was vaccinated in 1972. Therefore, a large portion of the current population has no immunity to the virus. A smallpox vaccination plan was introduced in 2003 that included a proposal that a designated number of ED staff receive the first vaccinations to ensure that ED staff would be immunized in the event of a smallpox outbreak. The government estimated that 0.1% of those people receiving the vaccine would have serious side effects. Of these, approximately 4% would have life-threatening complications, and 0.1% would die. Mass vaccination is under consideration to eliminate the possibility of the use of smallpox as a biologic weapon.

Smallpox was used as a biowarfare agent as far back as the French and Indian War in 1754–1767, when blankets used by patients with smallpox were sent into the Indian camps, resulting in greater than 50% fatality rates (Inglesby, Henderson, & Bartlett, 1999). In cool temperatures and low humidity, smallpox virus survives for up to 24 hours.

Clinical Manifestations

Signs and symptoms of smallpox infection include high fever, malaise, headache, backache, and prostration. After 1 to 2 days, a maculopapular rash appears, evolving at the same rate, beginning on the face, mouth, pharynx, and forearms (Fig. 72-1). Only then does the rash progress to the trunk and also become vesicular to pustular (Franz & Zajtchuk, 2000). There is a large amount of the virus in the saliva and pustules. Smallpox (variola) is contagious only after the appearance of the rash. There are two forms of smallpox, variola major and variola minor. Variola major is more common and results in a higher fever and more extensive rash. Variola major has a 30% case-fatality rate. Hemorrhagic smallpox, a sub-type of variola major, includes all of the above signs and symptoms plus a dusky erythema and petechiae to frank hemorrhage of the skin and mucous membranes, resulting in death by day 5 or 6.

Treatment

Treatment includes supportive care with antibiotics for any additional infection. The patient must be isolated with the use of transmission precautions. Laundry and biologic wastes should be autoclaved before being washed with hot water and bleach. Standard decontamination of the room is effective. All people who have household or face-to-face contact with the patient after the fever begins should be vaccinated within 4 days to prevent infection and death (Franz & Zajtchuk, 2000). A patient with a temperature of 38°C (101°F) or higher within 17 days after exposure must be placed in isolation. Cremation is preferred for all deaths, because the virus can survive in scabs for up to 13 years.

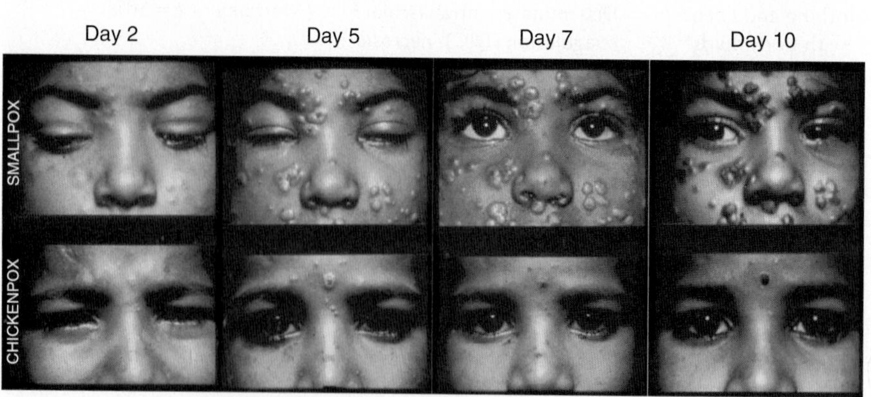

FIGURE 72-1. Comparison of progression of smallpox rash and chicken pox rash. From World Health Organization. (2001). *WHO slide set on the diagnosis of smallpox.* Reproduced by permission of the World Health Organization. Available at: http://www.who.int/emc/diseases/smallpox/slideset/index.htm. Accessed June 26, 2006.

SEVERE ACUTE RESPIRATORY SYNDROME

Not all mass casualty biologic events are terrorist-based. The SARS outbreak in 2003 is a prime example of a non–terrorist-based mass casualty biologic event. The disease started as "atypical" pneumonia in China in February and had spread to 29 countries throughout the world by July. Air travel and worldwide trade have increased the possibility that any contagious disease process may spread rapidly.

SARS is caused by a virus, officially named SARS-CoV. Its incubation period is 2 to 10 days. People at risk include health care workers who have had unprotected exposure to SARS-CoV. See Chapter 70 for further discussion of SARS.

Clinical Manifestations

Early systemic signs are dry cough and shortness of breath with or without other respiratory symptoms. X-ray-confirmed pneumonia or acute respiratory distress syndrome (ARDS; see Chapter 23) is evident at 7 to 10 days, along with fever and respiratory symptoms.

Treatment

Droplet precaution isolation and control of visits to the exposed patient are essential. Treatment is supportive. The overall case-fatality rate is 10%, which increases to more than 50% in patients older than 60 years of age, putting frail, elderly people at risk.

Chemical Weapons

Agents that may be used in **chemical warfare** are overt agents in that the effects are more apparent and occur more quickly than those caused by biologic weapons. Agents are available and well-known, result in major mortality and morbidity, and cause panic and social disruption. There are many agents, including those that affect nerves (sarin, soman), those that affect blood (cyanide), vesicants (lewisite, nitrogen and sulfur mustard, phosgene), heavy metals (arsenic, lead), volatile toxins (benzene, chloroform), pulmonary agents (chlorine), and corrosive acids (nitric acid, sulfuric acid) (Table 72-3). Chlorine, phosgene, and cyanide (including hydrogen cyanide and cyanogen chloride) are widely used in industry and therefore are readily available.

Characteristics of Chemicals

VOLATILITY

Volatility is the tendency for a chemical to become a vapor. The most volatile agents are phosgene and cyanide. Most chemicals are heavier than air, except for hydrogen cyanide. Therefore, in the presence of most chemicals, people should stand up to avoid heavy exposure (because the chemical will sink toward the floor or ground).

PERSISTENCE

Persistence means that the chemical is less likely to vaporize and disperse. More volatile chemicals do not evaporate very quickly. Most industrial chemicals are not very persistent. Weaponized agents (chemicals developed as weapons by the military or terrorists) are more likely than industrial chemicals to penetrate skin and mucous membranes and also cause secondary exposure.

TOXICITY

Toxicity is the potential of an agent to cause injury to the body. The median lethal dose (LD_{50}) is the amount of the

TABLE 72-3 Common Chemical Agents

Agent	Action	Signs and Symptoms	Decontamination and Treatment
Nerve Agents			
Sarin Soman organophosphates	Inhibition of cholinesterase	Increased secretions, gastrointestinal motility, diarrhea, bronchospasm	Soap and water Supportive care Benzodiazepine Pralidoxime Atropine
Blood Agent			
Cyanide	Inhibition of aerobic metabolism	Inhalation—tachypnea, tachycardia, coma, seizures. Can progress to respiratory arrest, respiratory failure, cardiac arrest, death.	Sodium nitrite Sodium thiocyanate Amyl nitrate Hydroxocobalamin
Vesicant Agents			
Lewisite Sulfur mustard Nitrogen mustard Phosgene	Blistering agents	Superficial to partial-thickness burn with vesicles that coalesce	Soap and water Blot; do not rub dry
Pulmonary Agents			
Phosgene Chlorine	Separation of alveoli from capillary bed	Pulmonary edema, bronchospasm	Airway management Ventilatory support Bronchoscopy

chemical that will cause death in 50% of those who are exposed. The median effective dose (ED_{50}) is the amount of the chemical that will cause signs and symptoms in 50% of those who are exposed. The concentration time (CT) is the concentration released multiplied by the time exposed (mg/min). For example, if 1000 mg of a chemical is released and the time a person is exposed to this amount of chemical is 10 minutes, then the concentration time would be 10,000 mg/min.

LATENCY

Latency is the time from absorption to the appearance of symptoms. Sulfur mustards and pulmonary agents have the longest latency, whereas vesicants, nerve agents, and cyanide produce symptoms within seconds.

Limiting Exposure

Evacuation is essential, as is removal of the person's clothing and decontamination as close to the scene as possible and before transport of the exposed person. Soap and water are effective means of decontamination in most cases. Staff involved in decontamination efforts must wear PPE and contain and dispose of the runoff after decontamination procedures.

Types of Chemicals

VESICANTS

Vesicants are chemicals that cause blistering and result in burning, conjunctivitis, bronchitis, pneumonia, hematopoietic suppression, and death. Examples of vesicants include lewisite, phosgene, nitrogen mustard, and sulfur mustard. In World War I and in the Iran–Iraq conflict of 1980–1988, vesicants were used to disable opponents. Vesicants were the primary incapacitating agents, resulting in minimal (less than 5%) death but large numbers of injured (Dara et al., 2005). Liquid sulfur mustard was the most frequently used vesicant in these conflicts. This oily liquid has a garlic odor and a long latent period, and it penetrates the skin if not rapidly removed. The skin damage is irreversible but is seldom fatal (2% to 3% mortality).

Clinical Manifestations

The initial presentation after exposure to a vesicant is similar to that of a large superficial to partial-thickness burn in the warm and moist areas of the body (ie, perineum, axillae, antecubital spaces). There is stinging and erythema for approximately 24 hours, followed by pruritus, painful burning, and small vesicle formation after 2 to 18 hours. These vesicles can coalesce into large, fluid-filled bullae. Lewisite and phosgene result in immediate pain after exposure. Tissue damage occurs within minutes.

If the eye is exposed, there is pain, photophobia, lacrimation, and decreased vision. This progresses to conjunctivitis, blepharospasm, corneal ulcer, and corneal edema.

Respiratory effects are more serious and often are the cause of mortality with vesicant exposure. Purulent fibrinous pseudomembrane discharge leads to obstruction of the airways. Gastrointestinal exposure includes nausea and vomiting, leukopenia, and upper gastrointestinal bleeding.

Treatment

Appropriate decontamination includes soap and water. Scrubbing and the use of hypochlorite solutions should be avoided, because they increase penetration. Once the substance has penetrated, it cannot be removed. Eye exposure requires copious irrigation. For respiratory exposure, intubation and bronchoscopy to remove necrotic tissue are essential. With lewisite exposure, dimercaprol (BAL in oil) is administered IV for systemic toxicity and topically for skin lesions. All persons with sulfur mustard exposures should be monitored for 24 hours for delayed (latent) effects.

NERVE AGENTS

The most toxic agents in existence are the nerve agents such as sarin, soman, tabun, VX, and organophosphates (pesticides). They are inexpensive, effective in small quantities, and easily dispersed. In the liquid form, nerve agents evaporate into a colorless, odorless vapor. Organophosphates are similar in nature to the nerve agents used in warfare and are readily available. Nerve agents can be inhaled or absorbed percutaneously or subcutaneously. These agents bond with acetylcholinesterase, so that acetylcholine is not inactivated; the adverse result is continuous stimulation (hyperstimulation) of the nerve endings. Carbamates, which are insecticides originally extracted from the Calabar bean, are derivatives of carbamic acid; they are nerve agents that specifically inhibit acetylcholinesterase for several hours and then spontaneously become unbound from the acetylcholinesterase. However, organophosphates require the formation of new enzyme (acetylcholinesterase) before nervous system function can be restored.

A very small drop of a nerve agent is enough to result in sweating and twitching at the site of exposure. A larger amount results in more systemic symptoms. Effects can begin anywhere from 30 minutes up to 18 hours after exposure. The more common organophosphates and carbamates (eg, sevin and malathion) that are used in agriculture result in less severe symptoms than do those used in warfare or in terrorist attacks. In an ordinary situation (eg, nonwarfare, nonterrorist attack situation), a patient could arrive at the ED having been unintentionally exposed or intentionally exposed in a suicidal gesture to organophosphates.

Clinical Manifestations

Signs and symptoms of nerve gas exposure are those of cholinergic crisis and include bilateral miosis, visual disturbances, increased gastrointestinal motility, nausea and vomiting, diarrhea, substernal spasm, indigestion, bradycardia and atrioventricular block, bronchoconstriction, laryngeal spasm, weakness, fasciculations, and incontinence. The patient must be examined in a dark area to truly identify miosis. Neurologic responses include insomnia, forgetfulness, impaired judgment, depression, and irritability. A lethal dose results in loss of consciousness, seizures, copious secretions, fasciculations, flaccid muscles, and apnea.

Treatment

Decontamination with copious amounts of soap and water or saline solution for 8 to 20 minutes is essential. The water is blotted off, not wiped off the skin. Fresh 0.5% hypochlorite solution (bleach) can also be used. The airway is maintained, and suctioning is frequently required. Plastic airway equipment will absorb sarin gas, which may result in continued exposure to the agent.

Atropine 2 to 4 mg is administered IV, followed by 2 mg every 3 to 8 minutes for up to 24 hours of treatment.

Alternatively, IV atropine 1 to 2 mg/hr may be administered until clear signs of anticholinergic activity have returned (decreased secretions, tachycardia, and decreased gastrointestinal motility). Another medication that may serve as an antidote is pralidoxime, which allows cholinesterase to become active against acetylcholine. Pralidoxime 1 to 2 g in 100 to 150 mL of normal saline solution is administered over 15 to 30 minutes. Pralidoxime has no effect on secretions and may have any of the following side effects: hypertension, tachycardia, weakness, dizziness, blurred vision, and diplopia.

Diazepam (Valium) or other benzodiazepines should be administered to control seizures, to decrease fasciculations, and to alleviate apprehension and agitation. Military personnel believed to be at risk for chemical attack are provided with Mark I automatic injectors, which contain 2 mg atropine and 600 mg pralidoxime chloride. Diazepam is administered by a partner.

BLOOD AGENTS

Blood agents such as hydrogen cyanide and cyanogen chloride have a direct effect on cellular metabolism, resulting in asphyxiation through alterations in hemoglobin. Cyanide is an agent that has profound systemic effects. It is commonly used in the mining of gold and silver and in the plastics and dye industries. In 1984, the Union Carbide pesticide plant in Bhopal, India, inadvertently released large amounts of cyanide in an industrial disaster, and hundreds of deaths occurred.

A cyanide release is often associated with the odor of bitter almonds. In house fires, cyanide is released during the combustion of plastics, rugs, silk, furniture, and other construction materials. There is a significant correlation between blood cyanide and carbon monoxide levels in patients who survive fires, and in many cases, the cause of death is cyanide poisoning.

Clinical Manifestations

Cyanide can be ingested, inhaled, or absorbed through the skin and mucous membranes. Cyanide is protein-bound and inhibits aerobic metabolism, leading to respiratory muscle failure, respiratory arrest, cardiac arrest, and death. Inhalation of cyanide results in flushing, tachypnea, tachycardia, nonspecific neurologic symptoms, stupor, coma, and seizure preceding respiratory arrest.

Treatment

Rapid administration of amyl nitrate, sodium nitrite, and sodium thiosulfate is essential to the successful management of cyanide exposure. First, the patient is intubated and placed on a ventilator. Next, amyl nitrate pearls are crushed and placed in the ventilator reservoir to induce methemoglobinemia. Cyanide has a 20% to 25% higher affinity for methemoglobin than it does for hemoglobin; it binds methemoglobin to form either cyanomethemoglobin or sulfmethemoglobin. The cyanomethemoglobin is then detoxified in the liver by the enzyme rhodanase. Next, IV sodium nitrite is administered to induce the rapid formation of methemoglobin. Sodium thiosulfate is then administered by IV; it has a higher affinity for cyanide than methemoglobin does and stimulates the conversion of cyanide to sodium thiocyanate, which can be excreted by the kidneys. Although they may be life-saving, these emergency medications do have side effects: sodium nitrite can result in severe hypotension, and thiocyanate can cause vomiting, psychosis, arthralgia, and myalgia.

The production of methemoglobin is contraindicated in patients with smoke inhalation, because they already have decreased oxygen-carrying capacity secondary to the carboxyhemoglobin produced by smoke inhalation. In facilities where a hyperbaric chamber is available, it may be used to provide oxygenation while the previously discussed therapies are initiated. An alternative suggested treatment for cyanide poisoning is hydroxocobalamin (vitamin $B_{12}a$). Hydroxocobalamin binds cyanide to form cyanocobalamin (vitamin B_{12}). It must be administered IV in large doses. Administration of vitamin $B_{12}a$ can result in a transient pink discoloration of mucous membranes, skin, and urine. In high doses, tachycardia and hypertension can occur, but they usually resolve within 48 hours.

PULMONARY AGENTS

Pulmonary agents such as phosgene and chlorine destroy the pulmonary membrane that separates the alveolus from the capillary bed, disrupting alveolar–capillary oxygen transport mechanisms. Capillary leakage results in fluid-filled alveoli. Phosgene and chlorine both vaporize, rapidly causing this pulmonary injury. Phosgene has the odor of fresh-mown hay.

Signs and symptoms include pulmonary edema with shortness of breath, especially during exertion. An initial hacking cough is followed by frothy sputum production. A mask is the only protection required to protect health care personnel. Phosgene does not injure the eyes.

Nuclear Radiation Exposure

The threat of **nuclear warfare** or radiation exposure is very real with the availability of nuclear material and easily concealed simple devices, such as the so-called dirty bomb, for dispersal. A dirty bomb is a conventional explosive (eg, dynamite) that is packaged with radioactive material that scatters when the bomb is detonated. It disperses radioactive material and may be called a radiologic weapon, but is not a nuclear weapon, which uses a complex nuclear fission reaction that is thousands of times more devastating than the dirty bomb.

Sources of radioactive material include not only nuclear weapons but also reactors and simple radioactive samples, such as weapons-grade plutonium or uranium, freshly spent nuclear fuel, or medical supplies (eg, radium, certain cesium isotopes) used in cancer treatments and radiology. Exposure of a large number of people can be accomplished by placing a radioactive sample in a public place. Thousands may be exposed this way; some may be immediately affected, and others may require health monitoring for many years to assess long-term effects.

The effectiveness of these weapons was demonstrated in the devastating results of the bombings of Hiroshima and Nagasaki in World War II. The effects of radiation exposure also were felt by the inhabitants of a small town in Brazil, who in 1987 found and opened a small canister of cesium 137 and rubbed the blue powder on themselves; 249 people were sickened, and 4 died (Jagminas & Suner, 2001). In 1983, a hospital sample was stolen in Mexico, resulting in the release of radioactive material among some scrap metal.

A year later, the radiation contamination was detected when the scrap metal was inadvertently transported to the Los Alamos National Laboratory and triggered a Geiger counter.

On a larger scale, nuclear reactor incidents have occurred in the Chernobyl (1986) and Three Mile Island (1979) nuclear facilities. There were 31 official deaths on the day of the Chernobyl incident, which involved a core meltdown and explosion, releasing radiation throughout the community. The long-term effects of this incident, including increased incidence of thyroid cancers and leukemia, continue to be evaluated. However, nuclear reactor facilities follow very strict security measures and protocols for prevention of core meltdown. These measures decrease the possibility of a radiation incident from a reactor.

Any terrorist-sponsored or unintentional radiation release can be sizeable and may require the entire hospital and prehospital staff to be prepared, recognize signs and symptoms of exposure, and rapidly treat victims without contamination of personnel, visitors, patients, or the facility itself.

Types of Radiation

Atoms consist of protons, neutrons, and electrons. The protons and neutrons are in balance in the nucleus. The protons repel each other, because they are all positively charged. The number of protons is specific for each element in the periodic table. There is a specific ratio of protons and neutrons for each different atom, and the result is element stability. When an element is radioactive, there is an imbalance in the nucleus resulting from an excess of neutrons.

To achieve stability, a radioactive nuclide can eject particles until the most stable number (an even number) of protons and neutrons exists. A proton can become a neutron by ejecting a positron; conversely, a neutron can become a proton by ejecting a negative electron. An alpha particle is released when two protons and two electrons are ejected.

Alpha particles cannot penetrate the skin. A thin layer of paper or clothing is all that is necessary to protect the skin from alpha-radiation. However, this low-level radiation can enter the body through inhalation, ingestion, or injection (open wound). Only localized damage occurs.

Beta particles have the ability to moderately penetrate the skin to the layer in which skin cells are being produced. This high-energy radiation can cause skin damage if the skin is exposed for a prolonged period and can cause injury if beta particles become internal by penetrating the skin.

Gamma-radiation is a short-wavelength electromagnetic energy that is emitted when there is excess core nucleus energy. Gamma particles are penetrating. Therefore, it is difficult to shield against gamma-radiation. X-rays are an example of gamma-radiation. Gamma-radiation often accompanies both alpha- and beta-particle emission.

Measurement and Detection

Radiation is measured in several different units. The *rad* is the basic unit of measurement. A rad is equivalent to 0.01 joule of energy per kilogram of tissue. To determine the damaging effect of the rad, a conversion to the *rem* (Roentgen equivalent man) is necessary. The rem reflects the type of radiation absorbed and the potential for damage. For example, 200,000 mrem results in mild radiation sickness (1 rem = 1000 millirem) (Dara et al., 2005). Typical natural yearly exposure for a person is 360 mrem. Another important concept is *half-life*. The half-life of a radioactive product is the time it takes to lose half of its radioactivity.

Radiation is invisible. The only means of detection is through a device that determines the exposure per minute. There are various devices for this purpose. The Geiger counter (or Geiger-Mueller survey meter) can measure background radiation quickly through detection of gamma- and some beta-radiation. With high-level radiation, the Geiger counter may underestimate exposure. Other devices include the ionization chamber survey meter, alpha monitors, and dose-rate meters. Personal dosimeters are simple tools to identify radiation exposure and are worn by radiology personnel.

Exposure

Exposure is affected by time, distance, and shielding. The longer a person is within the radiation area, the higher the exposure. Also, the larger the amount of radioactive material in the area, the greater the exposure. The farther away the person is from the radiation source, the lower the exposure. Shielding from the radiation source also decreases exposure. One should never touch radioactive materials directly.

Three types of radiation-induced injury can occur: external irradiation, contamination with radioactive materials, and incorporation of radioactive material into body cells, tissues, or organs:

- *External irradiation* exposure occurs when all or part of the body is exposed to radiation that penetrates or passes completely through the body. In this type of exposure, the person is not radioactive and does not require special isolation or decontamination measures. Irradiation does not necessarily constitute a medical emergency.
- *Contamination* occurs when the body is exposed to radioactive gases, liquids, or solids either externally or internally. If internal, the contaminant can be deposited within the body. Contamination requires immediate medical management to prevent incorporation.
- *Incorporation* is the actual uptake of radioactive material into the cells, tissues, and susceptible organs. The organs involved are usually the kidneys, bone, liver, and thyroid.

Sequelae of contamination and incorporation can occur days to years later. The thyroid gland can be largely protected from radiation exposure by administration of stable iodine (potassium iodide, or KI) before or promptly after the intake of radioactive iodine (Dara et al., 2005).

Priorities in the treatment of any type of radiation exposure are always treatment of life-threatening injuries and illnesses first, followed by measures to limit exposure, contamination control, and finally decontamination.

Decontamination

Hospital and countywide disaster plans should be in effect when managing a radiation disaster. Access restriction is essential to prevent contamination of other areas of the hospital. Triage outside the hospital is the most effective means of preventing contamination of the facility itself. Floors are covered to prevent tracking of contaminants throughout the treatment areas. Strict isolation precautions should be in effect. All air ducts and vents must be sealed to prevent spread. Waste is controlled through double-bagging and the use of plastic-lined containers outside of the facility. All radiation-contaminated waste must be disposed in appropriate color-coded yellow and magenta canisters.

Staff are required to wear protective clothing, such as water-resistant gowns, two pairs of gloves, masks, caps, goggles, and booties. Dosimetry devices should be worn by all staff members participating in patient care. The radiation safety officer in the hospital should be notified immediately to assist with surveys (using a radiation survey meter) of the incoming patients and to provide dosimeters to all staff personnel involved in direct care of exposed patients. There is minimal risk to staff if the patients are properly surveyed and decontaminated. The majority of patients can be safely decontaminated with soap and water.

Each patient arriving at the hospital should be first surveyed with the radiation survey meter for external contamination and then directed toward the decontamination area as needed. Decontamination occurs outside of the ED with a shower, collection pool, tarp, and collection containers for patient belongings, as well as soap, towels, and disposable paper gowns for patients. Water runoff needs to be contained. Patients who are uninjured can perform self-decontamination with the use of handheld showers. After the patient has showered, a resurvey is conducted to determine whether the radioactive contaminants have been removed. Additional washings should occur until the patient is free of contamination. It is important to ensure during showers that previously clean areas are not contaminated with runoff from the washed contaminated areas (eg, hair should be washed in a position that protects the body from contamination).

Biologic samples are taken through nasal and throat swabs, and a complete blood count with differential is obtained. Wounds are irrigated and then covered with a water-resistant dressing prior to total body decontamination.

Internal contamination or incorporation requires decontamination through catharsis, gastric lavage with chelating agents (agents that bind with radioactive substances and are then excreted), or both. Samples of urine, feces, and vomitus are surveyed to determine internal contamination levels.

Acute Radiation Syndrome

Acute radiation syndrome (ARS) can occur after exposure to radiation. It is the dose rather than the source that determines whether ARS develops. Factors that determine whether the patient's response to exposure will result in ARS include a high dose (minimum 100 rad) and rate of radiation with total body exposure and penetrating-type radiation. Age, medical history, and genetics also affect the outcome after exposure. The effects follow a predictable course. Table 72-4 identifies the phases of ARS.

Each body system is affected differently in ARS. Systems with cells that rapidly reproduce are the most affected. The effects on the hematopoietic system include decreased numbers of lymphocytes, granulocytes, thrombocytes, and reticulocytes. It is the first system affected and serves as an indicator of the severity of radiation exposure (Dara et al., 2005; Jagminas & Suner, 2001; Jarrett, 2001). A predictor of outcome is the absolute lymphocyte count at 48 hours after exposure. A significant exposure would be indicated by blood lymphocyte counts of 300 to 1200/mm^3 (the normal lymphocyte count is 1500 to 3000/mm^3). Barrier precautions should be implemented to protect the patient from infection. Neutrophils decrease within 1 week, platelets decrease within 2 weeks, and red blood cells decrease within 3 weeks. Hemorrhagic complications, fever, and sepsis are common.

The gastrointestinal system, with its rapidly reproducing cells, is also readily affected by radiation. Doses of radiation required to produce symptoms are approximately 600 rad or higher (Jagminas & Suner, 2001). The gastrointestinal symptoms usually occur at the same time as the changes in the hematopoietic system. Nausea and vomiting occur within 2 hours after exposure. Sepsis, fluid and electrolyte imbalance, and opportunistic infections can occur as complications. An ominous sign is the presence of high fever and bloody diarrhea; these typically appear on day 10 after exposure.

The central nervous system is affected when the dose exceeds 1000 rad (Dara et al., 2005). The symptoms occur when damage to the blood vessels of the brain results in fluid leakage. Signs and symptoms include cerebral edema, nausea, vomiting, headache, and increased intracranial pressure

TABLE 72-4 Phases of Effects of Radiation Exposure

Phase	Time of Occurrence	Signs and Symptoms
Prodromal phase (presenting symptoms)	48–72 hr after exposure	Nausea, vomiting, loss of appetite, diarrhea, fatigue High-dose radiation: fever, respiratory distress, and increased excitability
Latent phase (a symptom-free period)	After resolution of prodromal phase; can last up to 3 wk With high-dose radiation, latent period is shorter	Decreasing lymphocytes, leukocytes, thrombocytes, red blood cells
Illness phase	After latent period phase	Infection, fluid and electrolyte imbalance, bleeding, diarrhea, shock, and altered level of consciousness
Recovery phase	After illness phase	Can take weeks to months for full recovery
OR		
Death	After illness phase	Increased intracranial pressure is a sign of impending death

(ICP). Increased ICP heralds a poor outcome and imminent death. Central nervous system injury with this amount of exposure is irreversible and occurs before hematopoietic or gastrointestinal system symptoms appear. Cardiovascular collapse is usually seen in conjunction with these injuries.

Skin effects can also indicate the dose of radiation exposure. With exposure of 600 to 1000 rad, erythema occurs; it can disappear within hours, and then reappear. The exposed patient must be evaluated hourly for the presence of erythema. With exposures greater than 1000 rad, desquamation (radiation dermatitis) of the skin occurs. Necrosis becomes evident within a few days to months at doses greater than 5000 rad.

Secondary injury can occur when the radiation exposure occurs during a traumatic event such as a blast or burn. Trauma in addition to radiation exposure increases patient mortality. Attention must first be directed toward the primary assessment for trauma. Airway, breathing, circulation, and fracture reduction require immediate attention. All definitive treatments must occur within the first 48 hours. Thereafter, all surgical procedures should be delayed for 2 to 3 months because of the potential for delayed wound healing and the possible development of opportunistic infections several weeks after exposure.

Survival

There are three categories of predicted survival after radiation exposure: probable, possible, and improbable. Triage of victims at the scene, after decontamination, is conducted using the routine system for disaster triage. Presenting signs and symptoms determine the potential for survival and therefore the category of predicted survival during triage.

Probable survivors have either no initial symptoms or only minimal symptoms (eg, nausea and vomiting), or these symptoms resolve within a few hours. These patients should have a complete blood count drawn and may be discharged with instructions to return if any symptoms recur.

Possible survivors present with nausea and vomiting that persists for 24 to 48 hours. They experience a latent period, during which leukopenia, thrombocytopenia, and lymphocytopenia occur. Barrier precautions and protective isolation are implemented if the patient's lymphocyte count is less than 1200/mm^3. Supportive treatment includes administration of blood products, prevention of infection, and provision of enhanced nutrition.

Improbable survivors have received more than 800 rad of total body penetrating irradiation. People in this group demonstrate an acute onset of vomiting, diarrhea, and shock. Any neurologic symptoms suggest a lethal dose of radiation (Jarrett, 2001). These patients still require decontamination to prevent further contamination of the area and of others. Personal protection is essential, because it is virtually impossible to fully decontaminate these patients; all of their internal organs have been irradiated. The survival time is variable; however, death usually ensues swiftly due to shock. If there are no neurologic symptoms, patients may be alert and oriented, similar to a patient with extensive burns. In a mass casualty situation, these patients would be triaged into the black category, where they will receive comfort measures and emotional support. If it is not a mass casualty situation, aggressive fluid and electrolyte therapies are essential.

Critical Thinking Exercises

1 You are the triage nurse at the receiving facility for casualties during a hurricane. Five patients arrive at the same time. Together with the surgeon on duty, you must identify the patients' needs. You are presented with the following five patients: an elderly man with a respiratory rate of 8 breaths/minute, color ashen, status unresponsive, a Glasgow Coma Score (GCS) of 3, and only carotid pulses; a 7-year-old child with a bleeding scalp laceration and a GCS of 8, who needs intubation; the 30-year-old mother of the 7-year-old child, who is crying hysterically and appears to have no pain or visible injuries; a 15-year-old boy who complains of pain in his left leg, with obvious deformity at the calf but good pulses in the foot; and a 65-year-old woman who arrives in a police car holding her right wrist, which is cool, ecchymotic, and painful with good pulses. How would you classify/tag these patients?

Family members, members of the press, and city officials begin arriving at the hospital in large numbers. How should the family members be managed? How should the other people be managed?

2 A patient arrives at the triage desk of the ED complaining of sudden onset of high fever and respiratory flu-like symptoms. What signs and symptoms should you identify if you suspect a biologic warfare agent or contagious process? Which agents cause pneumonia-like signs and symptoms? What precautions should be taken to protect staff? Would you consider the patient's recent travel to Canada an issue?

3 Multiple patients begin arriving at the ED complaining of burning eyes and difficulty breathing. All of these persons work at the railroad yard, where there are frequently tanker trucks transporting chemical agents. What should you do first? Where do you find information about chemical agents and their treatment?

4 ebp You are a member of the Safety Committee at your hospital. The committee is charged with the responsibility of updating the hospital's emergency operations plan (EOP). What types of disasters may occur in and around your facility? There are many essential components of an EOP. What is the evidence base that supports the necessity for a health care facility having such a comprehensive plan? How strong is the evidence and what criteria are used to evaluate the evidence? What plan for triage will be included in the EOP? What types of personal protective equipment (PPE) will you recommend?

REFERENCES AND SELECTED READINGS

BOOKS

Agency for Toxic Substances and Disease Registry. (2001). *Medical management guidelines:* Available online: http://www.atsdr.cdc.gov/atsdrhome.html. Accessed June 26, 2006.

American Red Cross Disaster Services. (2001). *Disaster preparedness for people with disabilities*. Available online: http://www.redcross.org. Accessed June 26, 2006.

Currance, P., & Bronstein, A. C. (1999). *Hazardous materials for EMS: Practices and procedures*. St. Louis: Mosby.

Emergency Management Institute, National Emergency Training Center. (2002). *Mass fatalities incident response course*. Emmitsburg, MD: Federal Emergency Management Agency.

Farmer, J. C., Jimenez, E. J., Talmor, D. S., et al. (2003). *Fundamentals of disaster management*. DesPlaines, IL: Society of Critical Care Medicine.

Jagminas, L., & Suner, S. (2001). *Weapons of terrorism handout*. Baltimore, MD: International Trauma Anesthesia and Critical Care Society.

Sidell, F. R., Patrick, W. C., & Dashiell, T. R. (2000). *Jane's chem-bio handbook*. Alexandria, VA: Jane's Information Group.

U.S. Army Medical Research Institute of Infectious Disease. (1996). *Medical management of biological casualties handbook*. Fort Detrick, MD: U.S. Army.

U.S. Army Medical Research Institute of Chemical Defense. (1999). *Medical management of chemical casualties handbook*. Fort Detrick, MD: Aberdeen Proving Ground.

JOURNALS

**Asterisk indicates nursing research articles.*

Altman, G. B. (2002). Invisible threats. *Nursing Management, 33*(1):43–47.

Anteau, C. M., & Williams, L. A. (1997). The Oklahoma bombing: Lessons learned. *Critical Care Nursing Clinics of North America, 9*(2), 231–236.

Bakken, S. (2002). Biodefense and nursing informatics. *American Journal of Nursing, 102*(9), 79–80.

Bechtel, N. M., Betz, S., Deppe, S. et al. (2004). Update on federal activities related to hospital funding for disaster preparedness. *Journal of Trauma Nursing, 11*(2), 79–83.

Centers for Disease Control and Prevention Strategic Planning Workgroup. (2000). Biological and chemical terrorism: Strategic plan for preparedness and response. *Morbidity and Mortality Weekly Report, 49*, 1–14.

Centers for Disease Control and Prevention. (2004). Severe acute respiratory syndrome (SARS). Available online: http://www.cdc.gov/ncidod/sars. Accessed June 26, 2006.

Cox, E., & Briggs, S. (2004). Disaster nursing: New frontiers for critical care. *Critical Care Nurse, 24*(3), 16–22.

Dara, S. I., Ashton, R. W., Farmer, J. C., et al. (2005). Worldwide disaster medical response. *Critical Care Medicine, 33*(suppl 1), S2–S6.

Davis, K. G., & Aspera, G. (2001). Exposure to liquid sulfur mustard. *Annals of Emergency Medicine, 37*(6), 653–656.

Dennis, D. T., Inglesby, T. V., Henderson, D. A., et al. (2001). Tularemia as a biological weapon. *Journal of American Medical Association, 285*(21), 2763–2773.

Donnellan, C. (2003). Smallpox legislation introduced. *American Journal of Nursing, 103*(4), 29.

Drumm, C., Bruner, J., & Minutillo, A. (2004). Plague comes to New York. *American Journal of Nursing, 104*(8), 61–64.

Franz, D. R., & Zajtchuk, R. (2000). Biological terrorism: Understanding the threat, preparation, and medical response. *Disease-A-Month, 46*(2), 125–192.

Garner, A. (2003) Documentation and tagging of casualties in multiple casualty incidents. *Emergency Medicine, 15*(5), 475–479.

Harrison, T. W. (2003). Radiologic emergency: Protecting schoolchildren and the public. *American Journal of Nursing, 103*(5), 41–49.

Heightman, A. J. (1999). Assault on Columbine. *Journal of Emergency Medical Services, 24*(9), 32–46.

Inglesby, T. V., Dennis, D. T., Henderson, D. A., et al. (2000). Plague as a biological weapon. *Journal of American Medical Association, 283*(17), 2281–2290.

Inglesby, T. V., Henderson, D. A., & Bartlett, J. G. (1999). Anthrax as a biological weapon. *Journal of American Medical Association, 281*(18), 1735–1745.

Jarrett, D. G. (2001). Medical aspects of ionizing radiation weapons. *Military Medicine, 166*(Supp. 12), 6–8.

Joint Commission on Accreditation of Healthcare Organizations. (2003). Healthcare at the Crossroads. Available online: http://www.jcaho.org. Accessed June 26, 2006.

Karwa, M., Currie, B., & Kvetan, V. (2005). Bioterrorism: Preparing for the impossible or the improbable. *Critical Care Medicine, 33*(suppl 1), S75–S95.

Martin, T., & Lobert, S. (2003). Chemical warfare. *Critical Care Nurse, 23*(5), 15–20.

*Martinez Diaz, J. D., & Lopez, M. A. (1999). Voluntary ingestion of organophosphate insecticide by a young farmer. *Journal of Emergency Nursing, 25*(4), 266–268.

Meisenhelder, J. B. (2002). Anniversary responses to terrorism. *American Journal of Nursing, 102*(9), 24AA–24EE.

Middaugh, D. J. (2003). Maintaining management during disaster. *MedSurg Nursing, 12*(2), 125–127.

Reilly, C. M., & Deason, D. (2002). Mass casualty: Plague. *American Journal of Nursing, 102*(11), 47–50.

Sauer, S. W., & Keim, M. E. (2001). Hydroxycobalamin: Improved public health readiness for cyanide disasters. *Annals of Emergency Medicine, 37*(6), 635–641.

*Sebastian, S. V., Styron, S. L., Reize, S. N., et al. (2003). Resiliency of accomplished critical care nurses in a natural disaster. *Critical Care Nurse, 12*(5), 24–37.

Sibley, C. L. (2002). Smallpox vaccination revisited. *American Journal of Nursing, 102*(9), 26–38.

Society of Critical Care Medicine. (2003). Managing exposures to severe SARS. *Critical Connections, 2*(2), 1, 17.

Spencer, D. A., Whitman, K. M., & Morton, P. G. (2001). Inhalational anthrax. *MedSurg Nursing, 10*(2), 308–312.

Stopford, B. M. (2000). Are you prepared? Tips for counter terrorism. *ENA connection, Official Newsletter of the ENA, Emergency Nurses Association, 24*(5), 1, 5–6.

Tasota, F. J., Henker, R. A., & Hoffman, L. A. (2002). Anthrax as a biological weapon: An old disease that poses a new threat. *Critical Care Nurse, 22*(5), 21–34.

Veenema, T. G., & Karam, P. A. (2003). Radiation. *American Journal of Nursing, 103*(5), 32–40.

Yergler, M. (2002). Emergency: Mass casualty. Nerve gas attack. *American Journal of Nursing, 102*(7), 57–60.

RESOURCES

American Red Cross, 431 18th Street NW, Washington, DC 20006; (202) 639-3520; http://redcross.org/services/disaster/beprepared/. Accessed June 26, 2006.

Centers for Disease Control and Prevention, 1600 Clifton Road NE, Atlanta, GA 30333; (404) 639-3311; http://www.cdc.gov. Accessed June 26, 2006.

US Homeland Security; (800) BE-READY; http://www.dhs.gov/dhspublic/theme_home2.jsp. Accessed June 26, 2006.

APPENDIX A

Diagnostic Studies and Interpretation

Test Value Studied

Reference Ranges—Hematology
Reference Ranges—Serum, Plasma and Whole Blood Chemistries
Reference Ranges—Immunodiagnostic Tests
Reference Ranges—Urine Chemistry
Reference Ranges—Cerebrospinal Fluid (CSF)
Miscellaneous Values

Selected Abbreviations Used in Reference Ranges

Conventional Units

kg = kilogram
gm = gram
mg = milligram
μg = microgram
μμg = micromicrogram
ng = nanogram
pg = picogram
dL = 100 milliliters
mL = milliliter
gm = gram
mm^3 = cubic millimeter
fL = femtoliter
mM = millimole
nM = nanomole
mOsm = milliosmole
mm = millimeter
μm = micron or micrometer
mm Hg = millimeters of mercury
U = unit
mU = milliunit
μU = microunit
mEq = milliequivalent
IU = International Unit
mIU = milliInternational Unit

SI Units

g = gram
L = liter
d = day
h = hour
mol = mole
mmol = millimole
μmol = micromole
nmol = nanomole
pmol = picomole

TABLE A-1 Reference Ranges—Hematology*

Determination	Reference Range: Conventional Units	Reference Range: SI Units	Clinical Significance
A_2 hemoglobin	2.0%–3.2% of total hemoglobin	Mass fraction: 0.015–0.035 of total hemoglobin	Increased in certain types of thalassemia
Bleeding time	1.5–9.5 min	1.5–9.5 min	Prolonged in thrombocytopenia, defective platelet function, and aspirin therapy
Factor V assay (pro-accelerin factor)	60%–140%		
Factor VIII assay (antihemophiliac factor)	60%–140%		Deficient in classical hemophilia
Factor IX assay (plasma thromboplastin component)	60%–140%		Deficient in Christmas disease (pseudohemophilia)
Factor X (Stuart factor)	60%–140%		Deficient in Stuart clotting defect
Fibrinogen	200–400 mg/dL	2–4 g/dL	Increased in pregnancy, infections accompanied by leukocytosis, nephrosis Decreased in severe liver disease, abruptio placentae
Fibrin split (degradation) products	<5 μg/mL	<5 μg/mL	Increased in disseminated intravascular coagulation
Fibrinolysins (whole blood clot lysis time)	No lysis in 24 h		Increased activity associated with massive hemorrhage, extensive surgery, transfusion reactions
Partial thromboplastin time (activated)	Lower limit of normal: 20–25 sec; Upper limit of normal: 32–39 sec		Prolonged in deficiency of fibrinogen, factors II, V, VIII, IX, X, XI, and XII, and in heparin therapy
Prothrombin consumption	Lower limit of normal: 10 sec Lower limit of normal: 14 sec		Impaired in deficiency of factors VIII, IX, and X
Prothrombin time	9.5–12 sec		Prolonged by deficiency of factors I, II, V, VII, and X, fat malabsorption, severe liver disease, coumarin anticoagulant therapy.
INR	1.0 2–3 for therapy in atrial fibrillation, deep vein thrombosis, and pulmonary enbolism 2.5–3.5 for therapy in prosthetic heart valves		INR used to standardize the prothrombin time and anticoagulation therapy
Erythrocyte count	Males: 4,600,000–6,200,000/cu mm Females: 4,200,000–5,400,000/cu mm	$4.6–6.2 \times 10^{12}$/L $4.2–5.4 \times 10^{12}$/L	Increased in severe diarrhea and dehydration, polycythemia, acute poisoning, pulmonary fibrosis Decreased in all anemias, in leukemia, and after hemorrhage when blood volume has been restored
Erythrocyte indices			
Mean corpuscular volume (MCV)	84–96 cu μm	84–96 fL	Increased in macrocytic anemias; decreased in microcytic anemia
Mean corpuscular hemoglobin (MCH)	28–33 μμg/cell	28–33 pg	Increased in macrocytic anemias; decreased in microcytic anemia

TABLE A-1 Reference Ranges—Hematology* (Continued)

Determination	Reference Range: Conventional Units	Reference Range: SI Units	Clinical Significance
Mean corpuscular hemoglobin concentration (MCHC)	33%–35%	Concentration fraction: 0.33–0.35	Decreased in severe hypochromic anemia
Reticulocytes	0.5%–1.5% of red cells	Number fraction: 0.005–0.015	Increased with any condition stimulating increase in bone marrow activity (ie, infection, blood loss [acute and chronically following iron therapy in iron deficiency anemia], polycythemia rubra vera) Decreased with any condition depressing bone marrow activity, acute leukemia, late stage of severe anemias
Erythrocyte sedimentation rate (ESR)—Westergren method	Males under 50 yr: <15 mm/h Males over 50 yr: <20 mm/h Females under 50 yr: <25 mm/h Females over 50 yr: <30 mm/h	<15 mm/h <20 mm/h <25 mm/h <30 mm/h	Increased in tissue destruction, whether inflammatory or degenerative; during menstruation and pregnancy; and in acute febrile diseases
Erythrocyte sedimentation ratio—Zeta centrifuge	<50 years: <55% 50–80 years: 40%–60%	Volume fraction: <0.55 0.40–0.60	Significance similar to ESR
Hematocrit	Males: 42%–52% Females: 35%–47%	Volume fraction: 0.42–0.52 Volume fraction: 0.35–0.47	Decreased in severe anemias, anemia of pregnancy, acute massive blood loss Increased in erythrocytosis of any cause, and in dehydration or hemoconcentration associated with shock
Hemoglobin	Males: 13–18 gm/dL Females: 12–16 gm/dL	2.02–2.79 mmol/L 1.86–2.48 mmol/L	Decreased in various anemias, pregnancy, severe or prolonged hemorrhage, and with excessive fluid intake Increased in polycythemia, chronic obstructive pulmonary disease, failure of oxygenation because of congestive heart failure, and normally in people living at high altitudes
Hemoglobin F	Less than 2% of total hemoglobin	Mass fraction: <0.02	Increased in infants and children, and in thalassemia and many anemias
Leukocyte alkaline phosphatase	Score of 15–130 (varies among labs)		Increased in polycythemia vera, myelofibrosis, and infections Decreased in chronic granulocytic leukemia, paroxysmal nocturnal hemoglobinuria, hypoplastic marrow, and viral infections, particularly infectious mononucleosis
Leukocyte count	Total: 4,500–11,000/cu mm	$4.5–11 \times 10^9/L$	Neutrophils increased with acute infections, trauma or surgery, leukemia, malignant disease, necrosis; decreased with viral infections, bone marrow suppression, primary bone marrow disease
Neutrophils	45%–73%	Number fraction: 0.45–0.73	
Eosinophils	0%–4%	Number fraction: 0.00–0.04	
Basophils	0%–1%	Number fraction: 0.00–0.01	

continued >

TABLE A-1 Reference Ranges—Hematology* (Continued)

Determination	Reference Range: *Conventional Units*	Reference Range: *SI Units*	Clinical Significance
Lymphocytes Monocytes	20%–40% 2%–8%	Number fraction: 0.2–0.4 Number fraction: 0.02–0.08	Eosinophils increased in allergy, parasitic disease, collagen disease, subacute infections; decreased with stress, use of some medications (ACTH, epinephrine, thyroxine) Basophils increased with acute leukemia and following surgery or trauma; decreased with allergic reactions, stress, allergy, parasitic disease, use of corticosteroids Lymphocytes increased with infectious mononucleosis, viral and some bacterial infections, hepatitis; decreased with aplastic anemia, SLE, immunodeficiency including AIDS Monocytes increased with viral infections, parasitic disease, collagen and hemolytic disorders; decreased with use of corticosteroids, RA, HIV infection
Platelet count	150,000–450,000/cu mm	$0.15–0.45 \times 10^{12}$/L	Increased in malignancy, myeloproliferative disease, rheumatoid arthritis, and postoperatively; about 50% of patients with unexpected increase of platelet count will be found to have a malignancy Decreased in thrombocytopenic purpura, acute leukemia, aplastic anemia, and during cancer chemotherapy.

*Laboratory values may vary according to the techniques used in different laboratories.

TABLE A-2 Reference Ranges—Serum, Plasma, and Whole Blood Chemistries

Determination	Normal Adult Reference Range		Clinical Significance	
	Conventional Units	*SI Units*	*Increased*	*Decreased*
Acetoacetate	0.2–1.0 mg/dL	19.6–98 μmol/L	Diabetic ketoacidosis Fasting	
Acetone	0.3–2.0 mg/dL	51.6–344.0/μmol/L	Diabetic ketoacidosis Toxemia of pregnancy Carbohydrate-free diet High-fat diet	
Acid, total phosphatase	Males: 2–12 UL Females: 0.3–9.2 UL	Males: 2–12 UL Females: 0.3–9.2 UL	Carcinoma of prostate Advanced Paget's disease Hyperparathyroidism Gaucher's disease	
Acid, phosphatase, prostatic—RIA	2.5–3.37 ng/mL	2.5–3.37 μg/L	Carcinoma of prostate	
Alkaline phosphatase	Adults: 50–120 UL	50–120 UL	Conditions reflecting increased osteoblastic activity of bone Rickets Hyperparathyroidism Hepatic disease Bone disease	
Alkaline phosphatase, thermostable fraction	Hepatic: >25% Combined: 10%–25% Skeletal: <10%			
Adrenocorticotropic hormone (ACTH) (plasma)—RIA*	<50 pg/mL	<50 ng/L	Pituitary-dependent Cushing's syndrome Ectopic ACTH syndrome Primary adrenal atrophy	Adrenocortical tumor Adrenal insufficiency secondary to hypopituitarism
Aldolase	3–8 Sibley-Lehninger U/dL at 37°C	22–59 mU/L at 37°C	Hepatic necrosis Granulocytic leukemia Myocardial infarction Skeletal muscle disease	
Aldosterone (plasma)—RIA	Supine: 3–10 ng/dL Upright: 5–30 ng/dL Adrenal vein: 200–800 ng/dL	0.08–0.30 nmol/L 0.14–0.90 nmol/L 5.54–22.16 nmol/L	Primary aldosteronism Secondary aldosteronism	Addison's disease
Alpha-1-antitrypsin	110–140 mg/dL	1.1–1.4 g/L		Certain forms of chronic lung and liver disease in young adults
Alpha-1-fetoprotein	<15 ng/mL	<15 μg/L	Hepatocarcinoma Metastatic carcinoma of liver Germinal cell carcinoma of the testicle or ovary Fetal neural tube defects—elevation in maternal serum	
Alpha-hydroxybutyric dehydrogenase	<140 U/L	<140 U/L	Myocardial infarction Granulocytic leukemia Hemolytic anemias Muscular dystrophy	
Ammonia (plasma)	15–45 μg/dL (varies with method)	11–32/μmol/L	Severe liver disease Hepatic decompensation	

continued >

TABLE A-2 Reference Ranges—Serum, Plasma, and Whole Blood Chemistries (Continued)

Determination	Normal Adult Reference Range		Clinical Significance	
	Conventional Units	*SI Units*	*Increased*	*Decreased*
Amylase	60–160 Somogyi U/dL	111–296 U/L	Acute pancreatitis Mumps Duodenal ulcer Carcinoma of head of pancreas Prolonged elevation with pseudocyst of pancreas Increased by medications that constrict pancreatic duct sphincters: morphine, codeine, cholinergics	Chronic pancreatitis Pancreatic fibrosis and atrophy Cirrhosis of liver Pregnancy (2nd and 3rd trimesters)
Arsenic	<70 μg/dL; poisoning: 100–150 μg/dL	<0.93–2.6 μmol/L; poisoning: 133–6.65 μmol/L	Intentional or unintentional poisoning Excessive occupational exposure	
Ascorbic acid (vitamin C)	0.4–1.5 mg/dL	23–85 μmol/L	Large doses of ascorbic acid as a prophylactic against the common cold	
ALT (alanine aminotransferase), formerly SGPT	Males: 10–40 U/mL Females: 8–35 U/mL	Males: 0.17–0.68 μkat/L Females: 0.14–0.60 μkat/L	Same conditions as AST (SGOT), but increase is more marked in liver disease than AST (SGOT)	
AST (aspartate aminotransferase), formerly SGOT	Males: 10–40 U/L Females: 15–30 U/L	Males: 0.34–0.68 μkat/L Females: 0.25–0.51 μkat/L	Myocardial infarction Skeletal muscle disease Liver disease	
Bilirubin	Total: 0.3–1.0 mg/dL Direct: 0.1–0.4 mg/dL Indirect: 0.1–0.4 mg/dL	5–17μmol/L 1.7–3.7 μmol/L 3.4–11.2 μmol/L	Hemolytic anemia (indirect) Biliary obstruction and disease Hepatocellular damage (hepatitis) Pernicious anemia Hemolytic disease of newborn	
Blood gases				
Oxygen, arterial (whole blood):				
Partial pressure (PaO_2)	85–95 mm Hg	10.64–12.64 kPa	Polycythemia	Anemia Cardiac or pulmonary disease
Saturation (SaO_2)	95%–99%	Volume fraction: 0.95–0.99		Cardiac decompensation Chronic obstructive lung disease
Carbon dioxide, arterial (whole blood) partial pressure ($PaCO_2$)	35–45 mm Hg	4.66–5.99 kPa	Respiratory acidosis Metabolic alkalosis	Respiratory alkalosis Metabolic acidosis
pH (whole blood, arterial)	7.35–7.45	7.35–7.45	Vomiting Hyperventilation Fever Intestinal obstruction	Uremia Diabetic ketoacidosis Hemorrhage Nephritis

TABLE A-2 Reference Ranges—Serum, Plasma, and Whole Blood Chemistries (Continued)

Determination	Normal Adult Reference Range: Conventional Units	Normal Adult Reference Range: SI Units	Clinical Significance: Increased	Clinical Significance: Decreased
Brain (B-type) natriuretic peptide (BNP)	<100 pg/mL	100 ng/L	Heart failure Cardiac volume overload	
Calcitonin	Basal: <19 pg/mL Stimulation test Males: <350 pg/mL Females: <100 pg/mL	19 ng/L <350 ng/L <100 ng/L	Medullary carcinoma of the thyroid Some nonthyroid tumors Zollinger-Ellison syndrome	
Calcium	8.6–10.2 mg/dL	2.15–2.55 mmol/L	Tumor or hyperplasia of parathyroid Hypervitaminosis D Multiple myeloma Nephritis with uremia Malignant tumors Sarcoidosis Hyperthyroidism Skeletal immobilization Excess calcium intake: milk alkali syndrome	Hypoparathyroidism Diarrhea Celiac disease Vitamin D deficiency Acute pancreatitis Nephrosis After parathyroidectomy
CO_2, venous	Adults: 24–32 mEq/L Infants: 18–24 mEq/L	24–32 mmol/L 18–24 mmol/L	Tetany Respiratory disease Intestinal obstruction Vomiting	Acidosis Nephritis Eclampsia Diarrhea Anesthesia
Catecholamines (plasma)—RIA	Epinephrine: <100 pg/mL Norepinephrine: <400 pg/mL Dopamine: <143 pg/mL	<540 pmol/L <2360 pmol/L <935 pmol/L	Pheochromocytoma	
Ceruloplasmin	20–40 mg/dL	1.26–2.52 μmol/L		Wilson's disease (hepatolenticular degeneration)
Chloride	97–107 mEq/L	97–107 mmol/L	Nephrosis Nephritis Urinary obstruction Cardiac decompensation Anemia	Diabetes mellitus Diarrhea Vomiting Pneumonia Heavy metal poisoning Cushing's syndrome Intestinal obstruction Febrile conditions
Cholesterol	150–200 mg/dL	3.9–5.2 mmol/L	Lipemia Obstructive jaundice Diabetes Hypothyroidism	Pernicious anemia Hemolytic anemia Hyperthyroidism Severe infection Terminal states of debilitating disease
Cholesterol esters	60%–70% of total	Fraction of total cholesterol: 0.6–0.7		The esterified fraction decreases in liver diseases
Cholinesterase	Serum: 0.6–1.6 delta pH Red cells: 0.6–1 delta pH	0.6–1.6 U 0.6–1 U	Nephrosis Exercise	Nerve gas exposure (greater effect on red cell activity) Insecticide poisoning
Chorionic gonadotropin, beta subunit	0–5 IU/L	0–5 IU/L	Pregnancy Hydatidiform mole Choriocarcinoma	Threatened abortion Ectopic pregnancy

continued >

TABLE A-2 Reference Ranges—Serum, Plasma, and Whole Blood Chemistries (Continued)

Determination	Normal Adult Reference Range: Conventional Units	Normal Adult Reference Range: SI Units	Clinical Significance: Increased	Clinical Significance: Decreased
Complement, C_3	80–170 mg/dL	0.8–1.7 g/L	Some inflammatory diseases, acute myocardial infarction, cancer	Acute glomerulonephritis Disseminated lupus erythematosus with renal involvement
Complement, C_4	18–51 mg/dL	180–510 mg/L	Some inflammatory diseases, acute myocardial infarction, cancer	Often decreased in immunologic disease, especially with active systemic lupus erythematosus Hereditary angioneurotic edema
Complement, total (hemolytic)	90%–94% complement	25–70 U/mL	Some inflammatory diseases	Acute glomerulonephritis Epidemic meningitis Subacute bacterial endocarditis
Copper	70–150 µg/dL	11–24 µmol/L	Cirrhosis of liver Pregnancy	Wilson's disease
Cortisol-RIA	8 AM: 5–25/µg/dL 4 PM: 3–16 µg/dL	138–690 nmol/L 83–442 nmol/L	Stress: infectious disease, surgery, burns, etc. Pregnancy Cushing's syndrome Pancreatitis Eclampsia	Addison's disease Anterior pituitary hypofunction
C-peptide reactivity	0.9–4.0 ng/mL	0.9–4.0 µg/L	Insulinoma	Diabetes mellitus
Creatine	0.2–0.8 mg/mL	15.3–61 µmol/L	Pregnancy Skeletal muscle necrosis or atrophy Starvation Hyperthyroidism	
Creatine phosphokinase (CPK)	Males: 50–325 mU/mL Females: 50–250 mU/mL	50–325 U/L 50–250 U/L	Myocardial infarction Skeletal muscle diseases Intramuscular injections Crush syndrome Hypothyroidism Alcohol withdrawal delirium Alcoholic myopathy Cerebrovascular disease	
Creatine kinase (CK) isoenzymes	MM band present (skeletal muscle)- MB band absent (heart muscle)		MB band increased in myocardial infarction, ischemia	
Creatinine	0.7–1.4 mg/dL	62–124 µmol/L	Nephritis Chronic renal disease	
Creatinine clearance	Males: 85–125 mL/min Females: 75–115 mL/min	1.42–2.08 mL/s 1.25–1.92 mL/s		Kidney diseases Kidney diseases
Cryoglobulins, qualitative	Negative		Multiple myeloma Chronic lymphocytic leukemia Lymphosarcoma Systemic lupus erythematosus Rheumatoid arthritis Infective subacute endocarditis Some malignancies Scleroderma	

TABLE A-2 Reference Ranges—Serum, Plasma, and Whole Blood Chemistries (Continued)

Determination	Normal Adult Reference Range: Conventional Units	Normal Adult Reference Range: SI Units	Clinical Significance: Increased	Clinical Significance: Decreased
11-Deoxycortisol	1 µg/dL	<0.029 µmol/L	Hypertensive form of virilizing adrenal hyperplasia due to an 11-β-hydroxylase defect	
Dibucaine number	Normal: 70%–85% inhibition Heterozygote: 50%–65% inhibition Homozygote: 16%–25% inhibition			Important in detecting carriers of abnormal cholinesterase activity who are susceptible to succinylcholine anesthetic shock
Dihydrotestosterone	Males: 50–210 ng/dL Females: none detectable	1.72–7.22 nmol/L		Testicular feminization syndrome
Estradiol—RIA	Females: Follicular: 10–90 pg/mL Midcycle: 100–500 pg/mL Luteal: 50–240 pg/mL Follicular phase: 2–20 ng/dL Midcycle: 12–40 ng/dL Luteal phase: 10-30 ng/dL Postmenopausal: 1–5 ng/dL Males: 0.5–5 ng/dL	 37–370 pmol/L 367–1835 pmol/L 184–881 pmol/L	Pregnancy, ovarian tumor	Ovarian failure
Estriol—RIA	Nonpregnant females: <0.5 ng/mL Pregnant females: 1st trimester: up to 1 ng/mL 2nd trimester: 0.8–7 ng/mL 3rd trimester: 5–25 ng/mL	<1.75 nmol/L Up to 3.5 nmol/L 2.8–24.3 nmol/L 17.4–86.8 nmol/L	Pregnancy	Ovarian failure
Estrogens, total—RIA	Females: cycle days: Day 1–10: 61–394 pg/mL Day 11–20: 122–437 pg/mL Day 21–30: 156–350 pg/mL Males: 40–115 pg/mL	 61–394 ng/L 122–437 ng/L 156–350 ng/L 40–115 ng/L	Pregnancy Measured on a daily basis, can be used to evaluate response of hypo-gonadotrophic, hypo-estrogenic women to human menopausal or pituitary gonadotropin	Fetal distress Ovarian failure
Estrone—RIA	Females: Day 1–10: 4.3–18 ng/dL Day 11–20: 7.5–19.6 ng/dL Day 21–30: 13–20 ng/dL Males: 2.5–7.5 ng/dL	 15.9–66.6 pmol/L 27.8–72.5 pmol/L 48.1–74 pmol/L 9.3–27.8 pmol/L	Pregnancy	Ovarian failure

continued >

TABLE A-2 Reference Ranges—Serum, Plasma, and Whole Blood Chemistries (Continued)

Determination	Normal Adult Reference Range: Conventional Units	SI Units	Clinical Significance: Increased	Decreased
Ferritin—RIA	Males: 20–250 ng/mL Females: 12–250 ng/mL	20–250 μg/L 12–250 μg/L	Nephritis Hemochromatosis Certain neoplastic diseases Acute myelogenous leukemia Multiple myeloma	Iron deficiency
Folic acid—RIA	2.5–20 ng/mL	6–46 nmol/L		Megaloblastic anemias of infancy and pregnancy Inadequate diet Liver disease Malabsorption syndrome Severe hemolytic anemia
Follicle stimulating hormone (FSH)—RIA	Males: 2–10 mIU/mL Females: Follicular phase: 5–20 mIU/mL Peak of middle cycle: 12–30 mIU/mL Luteinic phase: 5–15 mIU/mL Menopausal females: 40–200 mIU/mL	 5–20 IU/L 12–30 IU/L 5–15 IU/L 40–200 IU/L	Menopause and primary ovarian failure	Pituitary failure
Galactose	<5 mg/dL	<0.28 mmol/L		Galactosemia
Gamma glutamyl transpeptidase	Males: 20–30 U/L Females: 1–24 U/L	0.03–0.5/μkat/L 0.02–0.4/μkat/L	Hepatobiliary disease Drug toxicity Myocardial infarction Renal infarction	
Gastrin—RIA	Fasting: 50–155 pg/mL Postprandial: 80–170 pg/mL	 50–155 ng/L 80–170 ng/L	Zollinger-Ellison syndrome Peptic ulceration of the duodenum Pernicious anemia	
Glucose	Fasting: 60–110 mg/dL Postprandial (2 h): 65–140 mg/dL	 3.3–6.05 mmol/L 3.58–7.7 mmol/L	Diabetes mellitus Nephritis Hyperthyroidism Early hyperpituitarism Cerebral lesions Infections Pregnancy Uremia	Hyperinsulinism Hypothyroidism Late hyperpituitarism Pernicious vomiting Addison's disease Extensive hepatic damage
Glucose tolerance (oral)	Features of a normal response: 1. Normal fasting between 60–110 mg/dL 2. No sugar in urine 3. Upper limits of normal: Fasting = 125 1 hour = 190 2 hours = 140 3 hours = 125	 3.3–6.05 mmol/L 6.88 mmol/L 10.45 mmol/L 7.70 mmol/L 6.88 mmol/L	Two-hour value >200 mg/dL (11.1 mmol/L) is diagnostic for diabetes mellitus	Decreased 2- and 3-hour values may occur with hypoglycemia in diabetes mellitus

TABLE A-2 Reference Ranges—Serum, Plasma, and Whole Blood Chemistries (Continued)

Determination	Normal Adult Reference Range		Clinical Significance	
	Conventional Units	*SI Units*	*Increased*	*Decreased*
Glucose-6-phosphate dehydrogenase (red cells)	Screening: Decolorization in 20–100 min Quantitative: 1.86–2.5 IU/mL RBC	 1860–2500 U/L		Drug-induced hemolytic anemia Hemolytic disease of newborn
Glycoprotein (alpha-1-acid)	50–120 mg/dL	0.5–1.2 g/L	Neoplasm Tuberculosis Diabetes mellitus complicated by degenerative vascular disease Pregnancy Rheumatoid arthritis Rheumatic fever Infectious liver disease Lupus erythematosus	
Growth hormone—RIA	Males: 0–4 ng/mL Females: 0–18 ng/mL	0.4 μg/L 0–18 μg/L	Acromegaly	Hypopituitarism
Haptoglobin	30–200 mg/dL	0.3–2.0 g/L	Pregnancy Estrogen therapy Chronic infections Various inflammatory conditions	Hemolytic anemia Hemolytic blood transfusion reaction
Hemoglobin (plasma)	0.5–5 mg/dL	5–50 mg/L	Transfusion reactions Paroxysmal nocturnal hemoglobinuria Intravascular hemolysis	Anemia, pregnancy, chronic renal failure
Glycohemoglobin (GHB, hemoglobin A_{1c}, hemoglobin A1)	Nondiabetics and diabetics with good control: 4.4%–6.4%		Suboptimal glucose control	
Hexosaminidase, total	Controls: 333–375 nM/mL/h	333–375 μmol/L/h	Sandhoff's disease	Tay-Sachs disease and heterozygotes
Hexosaminidase A	Controls: 49%–68% of total Heterozygotes: 26%–45% of total Tay-Sachs disease: 0%–4% of total Diabetics: 39%–59% of total	Fraction of total: 0.49–0.68 0.26–0.45 0–0.04 0.39–0.59		
High-density lipoprotein cholesterol (HDL cholesterol)	Males: 35–70 mg/dL Females: 35 -85 mg/dL	0.91–1.81 mmol/L 0.91–2.20 mmol/L		HDL cholesterol is lower in patients with increased risk for coronary heart disease
17 Hydroxy-progesterone—RIA	Males: 0.5–2.0 ng/mL Females: 0.2–3.0 ng/mL Children: <1.0 ng/mL	1.5–6.0 nmol/L 0.6–9.0 nmol/L <3.0 nmol/L	Congenital adrenal hyperplasia Pregnancy Some cases of adrenal or ovarian adenomas	

continued >

TABLE A-2 Reference Ranges—Serum, Plasma, and Whole Blood Chemistries (Continued)

Determination	Normal Adult Reference Range: Conventional Units	Normal Adult Reference Range: SI Units	Clinical Significance: Increased	Clinical Significance: Decreased
Immunoglobulin A	Adults: 85–385 mg/dL (in children the normals are lower and vary with age)	0.85–3.85 g/L	Gamma A myeloma Wiskott-Aldrich syndrome Autoimmune disease Hepatic cirrhosis	Ataxia telangiectasis Agammaglobulinemia Hypogammaglobulinemia, transient Dysgammaglobulinemia Protein-losing enteropathies
Immunoglobulin D	0–14 mg/dL	0–140 mg/L	IgD multiple myeloma Some patients with chronic infectious diseases	
Immunoglobulin E	100–700 ng/mL	100–700 µg/L	Allergic patients and those with parasitic infections	
Immunoglobulin G	Adults: 565–1765 mg/dL	6.35–14 g/L	IgG myeloma Following hyper-immunization Autoimmune disease states Chronic infections	Congenital and acquired hypogammaglobulinemia IgA myelomas, Waldenström's (IgM) macroglobulinemia Some malabsorption syndromes Extensive protein loss
Immunoglobulin M	Adults: 55–375 mg/dL	0.4–2.8 g/L	Waldenström's macro-globulinemia Parasitic infections Hepatitis	Agammaglobulinemias Some IgG and IgA myelomas Chronic lymphatic leukemia
Insulin—RIA	5–25 µU/mL	0.2–1 µg/L	Insulinoma Acromegaly	Diabetes mellitus
Iron	50–160/µg/dL	9–29 µmol/L	Pernicious anemia Aplastic anemia Hemolytic anemia Hepatitis Hemochromatosis	Iron deficiency anemia
Iron-binding capacity	IBC: 250–350 µg/dL TIBC: 250–475 µg/dL % Saturation: 20–50	45–63 µmol/L 45–85 µmol/L Fraction of total iron-binding capacity: 0.2-0.5	Iron deficiency anemia Acute and chronic blood loss Hepatitis	Chronic infectious diseases Cirrhosis
Isocitric dehydro-genase	50–180 U	0.83–3 UIL	Hepatitis, cirrhosis Obstructive jaundice Metastatic carcinoma of the liver Megaloblastic anemia	
Lactic acid (whole blood)	Venous: 5–15 mg/dL Arterial: 3–11 mg/dL	0.5–1.7 mmol/L 0.36–1.25 mmol/L	Increased muscular activity Congestive heart failure Hemorrhage Shock Lactic acidosis Some febrile infections May be increased in severe liver disease	
Lactic dehydroge-nase (LDH)	90–176 mU/mL	90–176 U/L	Untreated pernicious anemia Myocardial infarction Pulmonary infarction Liver disease	

TABLE A-2 Reference Ranges—Serum, Plasma, and Whole Blood Chemistries (Continued)

Determination	Normal Adult Reference Range: Conventional Units	SI Units	Clinical Significance: Increased	Decreased
*Lactic dehydrogenase isoenzymes Total lactic dehydrogenase	90–176 mU/mL	90–176 U/L	LDH-1 and LDH-2 are increased in myocardial infarction, megaloblastic anemia, and hemolytic anemia	
		Fraction of total LDH:		
LDH-1	22%–36%	0.2–0.36	LDH-4 and LDH-5 are increased in pulmonary infarction, congestive heart failure, and liver disease	
LDH-2	35%–46%	0.35–0.46		
LDH-3	13%–26%	0.13–0.26		
LDH-4	3%–10%	0.03–0.10		
LDH-5	2%–12%	0.02–0.12		
Lead (whole blood)	Up to 40 μg/dL	Up to 2 μmol/L	Lead poisoning	
Leucine aminopeptidase	80–200 U/mL	19.2–48 U/L	Liver or biliary tract diseases Pancreatic disease Metastatic carcinoma of liver and pancreas Biliary obstruction	
†Lipase	<200 U/mL	<200 U/L	Acute and chronic pancreatitis Biliary obstruction Cirrhosis Hepatitis Peptic ulcer	
Lipids, total	400–800 mg/dL	4–8 g/L	Hypothyroidism Diabetes mellitus Nephrosis Glomerulonephritis Hyperlipoproteinemias	Hyperthyroidism
Low-density lipoprotein cholesterol (LDL cholesterol)	mg/dL desirable levels: <160 if no coronary artery disease (CAD) and <2 risk factors <130 if no CAD and 2 or more risk factors <100 if CAD present		LDL cholesterol is higher in patients with increased risk for coronary heart disease	
Luteinizing hormone—RIA	Males: 1.5–9.3 mU/mL Females: Follicular phase: 1.9–12.5 mU/mL Midcycle: 8.7–76.3 mU/mL	 1.5–9.3 U/L 1.9–12.5 U/L 8.7–76.3 U/L	Pituitary tumor Ovarian failure	Pituitary failure
Lysozyme (muramidase)	4.0–15.6 μg/mL	0.28–1.10 μmol/L	Certain types of leukemia (acute monocytic leukemia) Inflammatory states and infections	Acute lymphocytic leukemia
Magnesium	1.3–2.3 mg/dL	0.62–0.95 mmol/L	Excess ingestion of magnesium-containing antacids	Chronic alcoholism Severe renal disease Diarrhea Defective growth
Mercury	<10 μg/L	<50 μmol/L	Mercury poisoning	
Myoglobin	5–70 ng/mL	5–70 μg/mL	Myocardial infarction Myocardial ischemia Rhabdomyolysis Malignant hyperthermia	Rheumatoid arthritis Myasthenia gravis

continued >

TABLE A-2	Reference Ranges—Serum, Plasma, and Whole Blood Chemistries (Continued)			
	Normal Adult Reference Range		**Clinical Significance**	
Determination	***Conventional Units***	***SI Units***	***Increased***	***Decreased***
5′ Nucleotidase	3.2–11.6 IU/L	3.2–11.6 U/L	Hepatobiliary disease	
Osmolality	275–300 mOsm/kg	275–300 mmol/L	Diabetes insipidus, osmotic diuresis	Inappropriate secretion of ADH Addison's disease
Parathyroid hormone	10–65 pg/mL	10–65 ng/L	Hyperparathyroidism, chronic renal failure	Hypoparathyroidism
Phenylalanine	1.2–3.5 mg/dL 1st week 0.7–3.5 mg/dL thereafter	0.07–0.21 mmol/L 0.04–0.21 mmol/L	Phenylketonuria	
Phosphohexose isomerase	20–90 IU/L	20–90 U/L	Malignancy Disease of heart, liver, and skeletal muscles	
Phospholipids	125–300 mg/dL	1.25–3 g/L	Diabetes mellitus Nephritis	
Phosphorus, inorganic	2.5–4.5 mg/dL	0.8–1.45 mmol/L	Chronic nephritis Hypoparathyroidism	
Potassium	3.5–5 mEq/L	3.5–5 mmol/L	Renal Failure Acidosis Cell lysis Tissue breakdown or hemolysis	Hyperparathyroidism Vitamin D deficiency GI losses Diuretic administration
Prealbumin	16.0–35.0 mg/dL	160–350 mg/L	Malnutrition Severe or chronic illness Liver disease	
Progesterone—RIA	Follicular phase: up to 0.8 ng/mL Luteal phase: 10–20 ng/mL End of cycle: <1 ng/mL Pregnant: up to 50 ng/mL in 20th week	2.5 nmol/L 31.8–63.6 nmol/L <3 nmol/L Up to 160 nmol/L	Useful in evaluation of menstrual disorders and infertility and in the evaluation of placental function during pregnancies complicated by toxemia, diabetes mellitus, or threatened miscarriage	
Prolactin—RIA	4–30 ng/mL	4–30 μg/L	Pregnancy Functional or structural disorders of the hypothalamus Pituitary stalk section Pituitary tumors	
Prostate-specific antigen	<4 ng/mL		Prostatic cancer, benign prostatic hyperplasia, prostatitis	
Protein, total Albumin Globulin	6–8 gm/dL 3.5–5.5 g/dL 1.7–3.3 g/dL	60–80 g/L 40–55 g/L 17–33 g/L	Hemoconcentration Shock Globulin fraction increased in multiple myeloma, chronic infection, liver disease	Malnutrition Hemorrhage Loss of plasma from burns Proteinuria
Protein Electrophoresis		35–50 g/L		
Albumin	3.5–5.5 g/dL	40–55 g/L		
Alpha-1 globulin	0.15–0.25 g/dL	1.5–2.5 g/L		
Alpha-2 globulin	0.43–0.75 g/dL	4.3–7.5 g/L		
Beta globulin	0.5–1.0 g/dL	5–10 g/L		
Gamma globulin	0.6–1.3 g/dL	6–13 g/L		

TABLE A-2 Reference Ranges—Serum, Plasma, and Whole Blood Chemistries (Continued)

	Normal Adult Reference Range		Clinical Significance	
Determination	***Conventional Units***	***SI Units***	***Increased***	***Decreased***
Protoporphyrin erythrocyte (whole blood)	Males: 11–45 μg/dL Females: 19–52 μg/dL	0.20–0.80 μmol/L 0.34–0.92 μmol/L	Lead toxicity Erythropoietic porphyria	
Pyridoxine	5–30 ng/mL	20–1.21 nmol/L		A wide spectrum of clinical conditions, such as mental depression, peripheral neuropathy, anemia, neonatal seizures, and reactions to certain drug therapies
Pyruvic acid (whole blood)	0.3–0.9 mg/dL	34–102 μmol/L	Diabetes mellitus Severe thiamine deficiency Acute phase of some infections, possibly secondary to increased glycogenolysis and glycolysis	
Renin (plasma)—RLA	Normal diet: Supine: 0.3–1.9 ng/mL/h Upright: 0.6–3.6 ng/mL/h Low salt diet: Supine: 0.9–4.5 ng/mL/h Upright: 4.1–9.1 ng/mL/h	 0.08–0.52 ng/L/S 0.16–1.00 μg/L/S 0.25–1.25 μg/L/S 1.13–2.53 μg/L/S	Renovascular hypertension Malignant hypertension Untreated Addison's disease Primary salt-losing nephropathy Low-salt diet Diuretic therapy Hemorrhage	Frank primary aldosteronism Increased salt intake Salt-retaining steroid therapy Antidiuretic hormone therapy Blood transfusion
Sodium	135–145 mEq/L	135–145 mmol/L	Hemoconcentration Nephritis Pyloric obstruction	Alkali deficit Addison's disease Myxedema
Sulfate (inorganic)	0.5–1.5 mg/dL	0.05–0.15 mmol/L	Nephritis Nitrogen retention	
Testosterone—RIA	Females: 20–80 ng/dL Males: 240–1200 ng/dL	0.7–2.8 nmol/L 18.3–41.8 nmol/L	Females: Polycystic ovary Virilizing tumors	Males: Orchidectomy for neoplastic disease of the prostate or breast Estrogen therapy Klinefelter's syndrome Hypopituitarism Hypogonadism Hepatic cirrhosis
T_3 (triiodothyronine) uptake	24%–34%	Relative uptake fraction: 0.24–0.34	Hyperthyroidism Thyroxine-binding globulin (TBG) deficiency Androgens and anabolic steroids	Hypothyroidism Pregnancy TBG excess Estrogens and anti-ovulatory drugs
T_3 total circulating—RIA	70–204 ng/dL	1.08–3.14 nmol/L	Pregnancy Hyperthyroidism	Hypothyroidism
T_4 (thyroxine)—RIA	5–11 μg/dL	65–138 nmol/L	Hyperthyroidism Thyroiditis Elevated thyroxine-binding proteins caused by oral contraceptives Pregnancy	Primary and pituitary hypothyroidism Idiopathic involvement Cases of diminished thyroxine-binding proteins caused by androgenic and anabolic steroids Hypoproteinemia Nephrotic syndrome

continued >

TABLE A-2 Reference Ranges—Serum, Plasma, and Whole Blood Chemistries (Continued)

	Normal Adult Reference Range		Clinical Significance	
Determination	***Conventional Units***	***SI Units***	***Increased***	***Decreased***
T_4, free	0.8–2.7 ng/dL	10.3–35 pmol/L	Euthyroid patients with normal free thyroxine levels may have abnormal T3 and T4 levels caused by drug preparations	
Thyroid-stimulating hormone (TSH)—RIA		0.4–4.2 mIU/L	Hypothyroidism	Hyperthyroidism
Thyroid-binding globulin	10–26 µg/dL	100–260/µg/L	Hypothyroidism Pregnancy Estrogen therapy Oral contraceptive use Genetic and idiopathic liver disease	Use of androgens and anabolic steroids Nephrotic syndrome Marked hypoproteinemia
Transferrin	200–380 mg/dL	2.3–3.2 g/L	Pregnancy Iron deficiency anemia due to hemorrhaging Acute hepatitis Polycythemia Oral contraceptive use	Pernicious anemia in relapse Thalassemic and sickle cell anemia Chromatosis Neoplastic and hepatic diseases Malnutrition
Triglycerides	100–200 mg/dL	1.13–3.8 mmol/L	Increased risk for atherosclerosis	
Troponin				
Troponin I	<0.35 ng/mL	<0.35 µg/L	Myocardial infarction	
Troponin T	<0.2 ng/mL	<0.2 µg/L	Rhabdomyolysis Severe crushing injuries	
Tryptophan	1.4–3 mg/dL	68.6–147 nmol/L		Tryptophan-specific malabsorption syndrome
Tyrosine	0.5–4 mg/dL	27.6–220.8 mmol/L	Tyrosinosis	
Urea nitrogen (BUN)	10–20 mg/dL	3.6–7.2 mmol/L	Acute glomerulonephritis Obstructive uropathy Mercury poisoning Nephrotic syndrome	Severe hepatic failure Pregnancy
Uric acid	2.5–8 mg/dL	0.15–0 mmol/L	Gouty arthritis Acute leukemia Lymphomas treated by chemotherapy Toxemia of pregnancy	Defective tubular reabsorption
Viscosity	1.4–1.8 relative to water at 37°C (98.6°F)		Patients with marked increases of the gamma globulins	
Vitamin A	30–120 µg/dL	1.05–4.20 µmol/L	Hypervitaminosis A	Vitamin A deficiency Celiac disease Sprue Obstructive jaundice Giardiasis Parenchymal hepatic disease
Vitamin B_1 (thiamine)	1.6–4 µg/dL	47.4–135.7 nmol/L		Anorexia Beriberi Polyneuropathy Cardiomyopathies

TABLE A-2 Reference Ranges—Serum, Plasma, and Whole Blood Chemistries (Continued)

	Normal Adult Reference Range		Clinical Significance	
Determination	***Conventional Units***	***SI Units***	***Increased***	***Decreased***
Vitamin B_6 (pyridoxal phosphate)	5–30 ng/mL	20–121 nmol/L		Chronic alcoholism Malnutrition Uremia Neonatal seizures Malabsorption, such as celiac syndrome
Vitamin B_{12}—RIA	200–900 pg/mL	148–666 pmol/L	Hepatic cell damage and in association with the myeloproliferative disorders (the highest levels are encountered in myeloid leukemia)	Strict vegetarianism Alcoholism Pernicious anemia Total or partial gastrectomy Ileal resection Sprue and celiac disease Fish tapeworm infestation
Vitamin E	0.5–1.8 mg/dL	12–42 µmol/L		Vitamin E deficiency
Xylose absorption test	2 hr, 30–50 mg/dL	2–3.35 mmol/L		Malabsorption syndrome
Zinc	55–150 µg/dL	7.65–22.95 µmol/L	Coronary artery disease Arteriosclerosis Industrial exposure	Metastatic liver disease Tuberculosis Sprue

*By radioimmunoassay.
†Varies among methods.

TABLE A-3 Reference Ranges—Immunodiagnostic Test

Determination	Normal Value	Clinical Significance
Acetylcholine receptor binding antibody	Negative or <0.03 nmol/L	Considered to be diagnostic for myasthenia gravis in patients with symptoms.
Anti-ds-DNA antibody	<70 U by enzyme-linked immunosorbent assay (ELISA) <1:20 by indirect fluorescence	Valuable in supporting diagnosis or monitoring disease activity and prognosis of systemic lupus erythematosus (SLE).
Antiglomerular basement membrane antibody	Negative or less than 5εUL	Primarily used in the differential diagnosis of glomerular nephritis induced by antiglomerular basement membrane antibodies from other types of glomerular nephritis.
Anti-insulin antibody	<3% binding of labeled beef and pork insulin by patient's serum; or <9 mIU/L	Helpful in determining the best therapeutic agent in diabetics and the cause of allergic manifestations. Also used to identify insulin resistance.
Antinuclear antibody	Negative, <1:40	Increased in SLE, chronic hepatitis, scleroderma, leukemia, and mononucleosis.
Anti-parietal cell antibody	Negative	Helpful in diagnosing chronic gastric disease and differentiating autoimmune pernicious anemia from other megaloblastic anemias.
Antiribonucleoprotein antibody	Negative	Helpful in differential diagnosis of systemic rheumatic disease.
Antiscleroderma antibody	Negative	Highly diagnostic for scleroderma.
Anti-Smith antibody	Negative	Highly diagnostic of SLE.
Anti-SS-A/anti-SS-B antibody	Negative	SS-A antibodies are found in Sjögren's syndrome alone or associated with lupus. SS-B antibodies are associated with primary Sjögren's syndrome.
Antithyroglobulin and antimicrosomal antibodies	<1:100 titer by gelatin or hemagglutination	Presence and concentration is important in evaluation and treatment of various thyroid disorders, such as Hashimoto's thyroiditis and Graves' disease. May indicate previous antoimmune disorders.
CA 15-3 tumor marker	<30 IU/mL	Increased in metastatic breast cancer.
CA 19-9 tumor marker	<37 IU/mL	Increased in pancreatic, hepatobiliary, gastric, and colorectal cancer, gallstones.
CA 125	0–35 IU/mL	Increased in colon, upper gastrointestinal (GI), ovarian, and other gynecologic cancers: pregnancy, peritonitis.
Carcinoembryonic antigen (CEA)—RLK	0–2.5 µg/L (nonsmoker) 0–5/µg/L (smoker)	The repeatedly high incidence of this antigen in cancers of the colon, rectum, pancreas, and stomach suggests that CEA levels may be useful in the therapeutic monitoring of these conditions, but it is not a screening test
Cold agglutinins	Negative or <1:32	Increased in mycoplasma pneumonia, viral illness, mononucleosis, multiple myeloma, scleroderma.
C-reactive protein	<1mg/dL (<10 mg/L)	Increase indicates active inflammation.
High sensitivity assay for C-reactive protein (hs-CRP)	0.2–8.0 mg/L	Cardiovascular disease risk
Cytomegalovirus antibodies (CMV IgG)	Negative: <0.9 units/mL	Positive >1:0 unit/mL if exposed to CMV at any time. Acute and convalescent specimens can help identify acute infection.
Cytomegalovirus antibodies (CMV IgM)	Negative: <0:79 Equivocal: 0:80–1.20	Positive >1:20 usually indicates acute infection. Repeat specimen in 1–2 weeks for equivocal result.
Epstein-Barr virus serology (viral capsid antigen IgG and IgM, early antigen IgG, and nuclear antigen IgG)	Negative: <1:20 or <1:20 for each individual test	Differentiation of acute from chronic or old infection by interpretation of table below.

TABLE A-3 Reference Ranges—Immunodiagnostic Test (Continued)

EBV Interpretation

	VCA-IgG	*VCA-IgM*	*EA-IgG*	*EBV-NA*
Susceptible	–	–	–	–
Acute infection	+	+	±	–
Convalescent phase	+	±	±	+
Chronic or reactivated	+	–	+	±
Old infection	±	–	–	+

Antibody present: +
Antibody absent: –
VCA, viral capsid antigen; EA, early antigen; EBV-NA, Epstein Barr virus-nuclear antigen

Determination	Normal Value	Clinical Significance
Hepatitis A virus antibodies, IgM (HAV-Ab/IgM)	Negative	Positive in acute-stage hepatitis A; develops early in disease.
Hepatitis A virus antibodies, IgG (HAV-Ab/IgG)	Negative	Positive if previous exposure and immunity to hepatitis A.
Hepatitis B surface antigen (HBsAg)	Negative	Positive in acute-stage hepatitis B.
Hepatitis B surface antibody (HBsAb)	Negative	Positive if previous exposure and immunity to hepatitis B.
Hepatitis C virus antibodies	Negative	Positive in exposure to hepatitis C virus; may indicate acute, chronic, or cleared infection.
Hepatitis C virus RNA	Negative	Positive in hepatitis C infection, can be quantitative
Homocysteine	0.54–2.30 mg/L (4–17 μmol/L)	Cardiovascular disease risk Folic acid deficiency Vitamin B_{12} deficiency
Infectious mononucleosis tests (monospot, monotest, heterophile antigen test, Epstein-Barr virus [EBV], antiviral capsid antigen IgM and IgG)	Negative	Positive monospot and monotest are presumptive, positive EBV IgM and IgG indicate acute and recent or past infection, respectively.
Lyme disease titer	Negative, <1:256 by indirect fluorescent antibody method; nonreactive by ELISA	Positive results help diagnose Lyme disease. False positive may occur with high rheumatoid factor titers or syphilis. Positive ELISA confirmed by Western blot test.
Pyroglobulin test	Negative	These abnormal proteins may be associated with myeloma, lymphoma, polycythemia vera, and SLE.
Rheumatoid factor	Negative or less than 40 IU/mL	Elevated in rheumatoid arthritis, lupus endocarditis, tuberculosis, syphilis, sarcoidosis, cancer.
T and B cell lymphocyte surface markers T-helper/T-suppressor ratio	T and B cell lymphocyte surface markers: Percent T cells (CD2) 60–88% Percent helper cells (CD4) 34–67% Percent suppressor cells (CD8) 10–42% Percent B cells (CD19) 3–21% Absolute counts: Lymphocytes 0.66–4.60 thou/mL T cells 644–2201 cells/mL Helper cells 493–1191 cells/mL Suppressor T cells 182–785 cells/mL B cells 92–392 cells/mL Lymphocyte ratio: T_H/T_S ratio > 1	Used to evaluate immune system by identifying the specific cells involved in the immune response. Valuable in diagnosis of lymphocytic leukemia, lymphoma, and immunodeficiency diseases including acquired immunodeficiency syndrome, and in the assessment of patient response to chemotherapy and radiation.

TABLE A-4 Reference Ranges—Urine Chemistry

Determination	Normal Adult Reference Range		Clinical Significance	
	Conventional Units	*SI Units*	*Increased*	*Decreased*
Acetone and acetoacetate	Zero		Diabetic ketoacidosis Starvation	
Aldosterone	With normal salt diet: Normal: 4–20 μg/24 h Renovascular: 10–40 μg/24 h Tumor: 20–100 μg/24 h	 11.1–55.5 nmol/24h 27.7–111 nmol/24 h 55.4–277 nmol/24 h	Primary aldosteronism (adrenocortical tumor) Secondary aldosteronism Salt depletion Potassium loading ACTH in large doses Cardiac failure Cirrhosis with ascites formation Nephrosis Pregnancy	
Alpha amino nitrogen	50–200 mg/24 h	3.6–14.3 nmol/24 h	Leukemia Phenylketonuria Other metabolic diseases	
Amylase	35–260 units excreted per h	6.5–48.1 U/h	Acute pancreatitis	
Arylsulfatase A	>2.4 U/mL			
Bence-Jones protein	None detected		Myeloma	Metachromatic leukodystrophy
Calcium	100–250 mg/24 h	2.5–6.2 mmol/24 h	Hyperparathyroidism Vitamin D intoxication Fanconi's syndrome	Hypoparathyroidism Vitamin D deficiency
Catecholamines	Total: 0–275 μg/24 h Epinephrine: 10%–40% Norepinephrine: 60%–90%	0–275 μg/24 h Fraction total: 0.10–8.4 Fraction total: 0.60–0.90	Pheochromocytoma Neuroblastoma	
Chorionic gonadotrophin, qualitative (pregnancy test)	Negative		Pregnancy Chorionepithelioma Hydatidiform mole	
Copper	15–60 μg/24 h	0.22–0.9 μmol/24 h	Wilson's diseases Cirrhosis Nephrosis	
Coproporphyrin	50–300 μg/24 h	0.075–0.45 μmol/24 h	Poliomyelitis Lead poisoning Porphyria	
Cortisol, free	20–90 μg/24 h	55.2–248.4 nmol/d	Cushing's syndrome	
Creatinine	Males: 1–2 g/24 h Females: 0.8–1.8 g/24 h	8.8–17.7 mmol/24 h 7.1–15.9 mmol/24 h	Muscular dystrophy Fever Carcinoma of liver Pregnancy Hyperthyroidism Myositis	
Creatine	0–270 mg/24 h	0–2.05 mmol/24 h	Typhoid fever Salmonella infections Tetanus	Muscular atrophy Anemia Advanced degeneration of kidneys Leukemia
Creatinine clearance	Males: 85–125 mL/min Females: 75–115 mL/min	1.42–2.08 mL/s 1.25–1.92 mL/s		Renal diseases
Cystine and cysteine	10–100 mg/24 h	0.08–0.83 mmol/24 h	Cystinuria	

TABLE A-4 Reference Ranges—Urine Chemistry (Continued)

	Normal Adult Reference Range		Clinical Significance	
Determination	***Conventional Units***	***SI Units***	***Increased***	***Decreased***
Delta aminolevulinic acid	0–0.54 mg/dL	0–40/µmol/L	Lead poisoning Porphyria hepatica Hepatitis Hepatic carcinoma	
11-Desoxycortisol	20–100 µg/24 h	0.6–2.9/µmol/d	Hypertensive form of virilizing adrenal hyperplasia due to an 11-beta hydroxylase defect	
Estriol (placental)	Weeks of pregnancy 12 16 20 24 28 32 36 40	µm/24 h — mmol/24 h <1 — <3.5 2–7 — 7–24.5 4–9 — 14–32 6–13 — 21–45.5 8–22 — 28–77 12–43 — 42–150 14–45 — 49–158 19–46 — 66.5–160		Decreased values occur with fetal distress of many conditions, including preeclampsia, placental insufficiency, and poorly controlled diabetes mellitus
Estrogens, total (fluorometric)	Females: Onset of menstruation: 4–25 µg/24 h Ovulation peak: 28–100 µg/24 h Luteal peak: 22–105 µg/24 h Menopausal: 1.4–19.6 µg/24 h Males: 5–18 µg/24 h	 4–25 µg/24 h 28–100 µg/24 h 22–105 µg/24 h 1.4–19.6 µg/24 h 5–18 µg/24 h	Hyperestrogenism due to gonadal or adrenal neoplasm	Primary or secondary amenorrhea
Etiocholanolone	Males: 1.9–6 mg/24 h Females: 0.5–4 mg/24 h	6.5–20.6 µmol/24 h 1.7–13.8 µmol/24 h	Adrenogenital syndrome Idiopathic hirsutism	
Follicle-stimulating hormone—RIA	Females: Follicular: 5–20 IU/24 h Luteal: 5–15 IU/24 h Midcycle: 15–60 IU/24 h Menopausal: 50–100 IU/24 h Males: 5–25 IU/24 h	 5–20 IU/d 5–15 IU/d 15–60 IU/d 50–100 IU/d 5–25 IU/d	Menopause and primary ovarian failure	Pituitary failure
Glucose	Negative		Diabetes mellitus Pituitary disorders Increased ICP Lesion in floor of 4th ventricle	
Hemoglobin and myoglobin	Negative		Extensive burns Transfusion of incompatible blood Myoglobin increased in severe crushing injuries to muscles	
Homovanillic acid		<44 µmol/24h	Neuroblastoma	Addison's disease
17-hydroxycorticosteroids	8 mg/24 h 2–10 mg/24 h	5.5–27.5 µmol/d	Cushing's disease	Anterior pituitary hypofunction
5-Hydroxyindoleacetic acid, qualitative	Negative		Malignant carcinoid tumors	

continued >

TABLE A-4 Reference Ranges—Urine Chemistry (Continued)

Determination	Normal Adult Reference Range		Clinical Significance	
	Conventional Units	*SI Units*	*Increased*	*Decreased*
17-ketosteroids, total	Males: 10–22 mg/24 h Females: 6–16 mg/24 h	35–76 μmol/24h 21–55 μmol/24h	Interstitial cell tumor of testes Simple hirsutism, occasionally Adrenal hyperplasia Cushing's syndrome Adrenal cancer, virilism Adrenoblastoma	Thyrotoxicosis Female hypogonadism Diabetes mellitus Hypertension Debilitating disease of mild to moderate severity Eunuchoidism Addison's disease Panhypopituitarism Myxedema Nephrosis
Lead	<125 μg/24 h	<60 μmol/24 h	Lead poisoning	
Luteinizing hormone	Males: 5–18 IU/24 h Females: Follicular phase: 2–25 IU/24 h Ovulatory peak: 30–95 IU/24 h Luteal phase: 2–20 IU/24 h Postmenopausal: 40–110 IU/24 h	 2–25 IU/d 30–95 IU/d 2–20 IU/d 40–110 IU/d	Pituitary tumor Ovarian failure	Failure of pituitary or hypothalamus Anorexia nervosa
Metanephrines, total	<1.4 mg/24 h	<7 μmol/24h	Pheochromocytoma; a few patients with pheochromocytoma may have elevated urinary metanephrines but normal catecholamines and vanillylmandelic acid (VMA)	
Osmolality	250–900 mOsm/kg	250–900 mmol/kg	Useful in the study of electrolyte and water balance	
Oxalate	Up to 45 mg/24 h	Up to 500/μmol/24 h	Primary hyperoxaluria	
Phenylpyruvic acid qualitative	Negative		Phenylketonuria	
Phosphorus, inorganic	0.9–1.3 g/24 h	29–42 mmol/24 h	Hypoparathyroidism Vitamin D intoxication Paget's disease Metastatic neoplasm to bone	Hypoparathyroidism Vitamin D deficiency
Porphobilinogen, qualitative	Negative		Chronic lead poisoning Acute porphyria Liver disease	
Porphobilinogen quantitative	0–1 mg/24 h	0–4.4 μmol/24 h	Acute porphyria Liver disease	
Porphyrins, qualitative	Negative		See porphyrins, quantitative	
Porphyrins, quantitative (coproporphyrin and uroporphyrin)	Coproporphyrin: 50–160 μg/24 h Uroporphyrin: up to 50 μg/24 h	 0.075–0.24 μmol/24h Up to 0.06 μmol/24 h	Porphyria Lead poisoning (only coproporphyrin increased)	

TABLE A-4 Reference Ranges—Urine Chemistry (Continued)

Determination	Normal Adult Reference Range: Conventional Units	Normal Adult Reference Range: SI Units	Clinical Significance: Increased	Clinical Significance: Decreased
Potassium	26–123 mEq/24 h	26–123 mmol/24 h	Hemolysis Chronic renal failure Acidosis Cushing's disease Corpus luteum cysts	Diarrhea Adrenocortical insufficiency
Pregnanediol	Females: Proliferative phase: 0.5–1.5 mg/24 h Luteal phase: 2–7 mg/24 h Menopause: 0.2–1 mg/24 h	 1.6–4.8 μmol/24 h 6–22 μmol/24 h 0.6–3.1 μmol/24 h	When placental tissue remains in the uterus following parturition Some cases of adreno-cortical tumors	Placental dysfunction Threatened abortion Intrauterine death
Pregnancy: Weeks of gestation	mg/24 h	μmol/24 h		
10–12	5–15	15.6–47		
12–18	5–25	15.6–78.0		
18–24	15–33	47.0–103.0		
24–28	20–42	62.4–131.0		
28–32	27–47	84.2–146.6		
Pregnanetriol	Females: 0.1–2.2 mg/24 h Males: 0.4–2.5 mg/24 h	 0.3–6.5 μmol/24 h 1.2–7.5 μmol/24 h	Congenital adrenal androgenic hyper-plasia	
Protein	<150 mg/24 h	<150 mg/24 h	Nephritis Cardiac failure Mercury poisoning Bence-Jones protein in multiple myeloma Febrile states Hematuria	
Sodium	75–200 mEq/24 h	75–200 mmol/24 h	Useful in detecting gross changes in water and salt balance	
Titratable acidity	20–40 mEq/24 h	20–40 mmol/24 h	Metabolic acidosis	Metabolic alkalosis
Urea nitrogen	9–16 gm/24 h	0.32–0.57 mol/L	Excessive protein catabolism	Impaired kidney function
Uric acid	250–750 mg/24 h	1.48–4.43 mmol/24 h	Gout	Nephritis
Urobilinogen	Random urine: <0.25 mg/dL 24-hour urine: up to 4 mg/24 h	<0.42 mol/24 h Up to 6.76 μmol/24 h	Liver and biliary tract disease Hemolytic anemias	Complete or nearly complete biliary obstruction Diarrhea Renal insufficiency
Vanillylmandelic acid (VMA)	0.7–6.8 mg/24 h	3.5–34.3 μmol/24 h	Pheochromocytoma Neuroblastoma Ingestion of coffee, tea, aspirin, bananas, and several different drugs	
Xylose absorption test (5-hour)	16%–33% of ingested xylose	Fraction absorbed: 0.16–0.33		
Zinc	0.15–1.2 mg/24 h	2.3–18.4 μmol/24h		Malabsorption syndromes

TABLE A-5 Reference Ranges—Cerebrospinal Fluid (CSF)

Determination	Normal Adult Reference Range		Clinical Significance	
	Conventional Units	*SI Units*	*Increased*	*Decreased*
Albumin	15–30 mg/dL	150–300 mg/L	Certain neurologic disorders Lesion in the choroid plexus or blockage of the flow of CSF Damage to the blood–brain barrier	
Cell count (white blood cells)	0–5 cells per cu mm	0–5 × 10^6/L	Bacterial meningitis Neurosyphilis Anterior poliomyelitis Encephalitis lethargica	
Chloride	120–130 mEq/L	120–130 mmol/L	Uremia	Acute generalized meningitis Tuberculous meningitis
Glucose	40–80 mg/dL; 50%–80% of blood glucose value	2.75–4.13 mmol/L	Diabetes mellitus Diabetic coma Epidemic encephalitis Uremia	Acute meningitis Tuberculous meningitis Insulin shock Subarachnoid hemorrhage
Glutamine	6–15 mg/dL	0.41–1 mmol/L	Hepatic encephalopathies, including Reye's syndrome Hepatic coma Cirrhosis	
IgG	<5 mg/dL	<50 mg/L	Damage to the blood-brain barrier Multiple sclerosis Neurosyphilis Subacute sclerosing panencephalitis Chronic phases of CNS infections	
Lactic acid	4.5–28.8 mg/dL	0.5–3.2 mmol/L	Bacterial meningitis Hypocapnia Hydrocephalus Brain abscesses Cerebral ischemia Fungal meningitis	
Lactate dehydrogenase	1/10 that of serum level	Activity fraction: 0.1 of serum	CNS disease	
Protein	16–45 mg/dL	150–450 mg/L	Acute meningitis Tubercular meningitis Neurosyphilis Poliomyelitis Guillain-Barré syndrome Subdural hematoma Brain tumor Multiple sclerosis	

TABLE A-6 Miscellaneous Values

Determinations	Normal Value	Clinical Significance: Conventional Units	Clinical Significance: SI Units
Acetaminophen	Zero	Therapeutic level = 10–30 μg/mL	10–30 mg/L
Aminophylline (theophylline)	Zero	Therapeutic level = 10–20/μg/mL	10–20 mg/L
Bromide	Zero	Therapeutic level = 5–50 mg/dL	50–500 mg/L
Carbamazepine	Zero	Therapeutic level = 4–12 μg/mL	34–51 μmol/L
Carbon monoxide	0%–2%	Symptoms with 10%–30% saturation	
Chlordiazepoxide	Zero	Therapeutic level = 0.7–1.0 μg/mL	0.7–1.0 mg/L
Diazepam	Zero	Therapeutic level = 0.2–1.0 μg/mL	0.2–1.0 mg/L
Digitoxin	Zero	Therapeutic level = 18–35 ng/mL	18–35 μg/L
Digoxin	Zero	Therapeutic level = 0.8–2 ng/mL	0.8–2/μg/L
Ethanol	0%–0.01%	Legal intoxication level = 0.1% or above 0.3%–0.4% = marked intoxication 0.4%–0.5% = alcoholic stupor	
Fosphenytoin	Zero	10–20 mg/L	
Gentamicin	Zero	Therapeutic level = 4–10 μg/mL	4–10 mg/L
Lithium	Zero	Therapeutic level = 0.6–1.2 mEq/L	0.6–1.2 mmol/L
Methanol	Zero	May be fatal in concentration as low as 10 mg/dL	100 mg/L
Phenobarbital	Zero	Therapeutic level = 15–40 μg/mL	15–40 mg/L
Phenytoin	Zero	Therapeutic level = 10–20 μg/mL	10–20 mg/L
Primidone	Zero	Therapeutic level = 5–12 μg/mL	5–12 mg/L
Quinidine	Zero	Therapeutic level = 0.2–0.5 mg/dL	2–5 mg/L
Salicylate	Zero	Therapeutic level = 2–25 mg/dL Toxic level = >30 mg/dL	20–250 mg/L 300 mg/L
Vancomycin	Zero	Therapeutic peak 20–40 μg/mL Therapeutic trough 5–10 μg/mL	
Amitriptyline	Zero	Therapeutic level 80–200 ng/mL	289–722 nmol/L
Doxepin	Zero	Therapeutic level 150–250 ng/mL (includes metabolites)	540–900 nmol/L
Imipramine	Zero	Therapeutic level 100–300 ng/mL (includes metabolites)	360–1070 nmol/L
Lidocaine	Zero	Therapeutic level 1.5–5 μg/mL	6.4–21.4 μmol/L
Methotrexate	Zero	Toxic (48 h after high dose) 454 mg/mL	1000 mmol/L
Propranolol	Zero	Therapeutic level 50–100 ng/mL	193–386 nmol/L
Valproic acid	Zero	Therapeutic level 50–100 μg/mL	347–693 μmol/L

References

1. *Jacobs and Demott's Laboratory Test Handbook.* 5th ed. Lexi-Comp. Inc. Hudson (OH), 2001.
2. Traub SL. *Basic Skills in Interpreting Laboratory Data.* 2nd ed. American Society of Health-Systems Pharmacy, Bethesda, 1996.
3. www.bioscientia.de
4. http://www.gpnotebook.co.uk/simplepage.cfm?ID=429195241&linkID=8734
5. www.bloodbook.com/ranges.html
6. http://www.buymedicals.com/MedicalInfo/2-urine.asp
7. http://thailabonline.com/lab-normalrange1.htm
8. Directory of Services and Interpretive Guide. LabCorp. 2001.

APPENDIX B

Understanding Clinical Pathways

Clinical pathways (also called critical pathways) are care plans developed collaboratively by physicians, nurses, physical and occupational therapists, technicians, pharmacists, speech therapists, case managers, and other staff members involved in patient care. Nurses are instrumental in ensuring the successful use of clinical pathways and can best contribute by gaining a thorough understanding of why and how pathways are used.

Understanding and Using Clinical Pathways in Patient Care

Clinical pathways grew out of financial upheaval in the health care industry. They represent a significant change in how patient care is managed. In the past (and currently for many patients), each health care discipline developed its own plan of care and used the patient's medical record as the primary communication tool. Each care provider needed to read the notes of health care providers of other disciplines to get a complete picture of the plan of care and the patient's progress. Although there was probably general agreement about how patient progress would be facilitated and measured, individual steps in the processes of care and outcomes to be achieved were often not identified and communicated. The physician managed the case and most patients remained in the hospital until they required very little care or could be discharged home or transferred to a convalescent center. A hospital stay of 2 to 3 weeks in an acute care facility was not unusual.

Cost and Effects

Although this system worked for decades, it was expensive. The federal government and insurance companies balked at paying these costs when highly skilled care was no longer needed. As a result, the number of days of hospitalization that a patient with a specific diagnosis required was determined. Then insured parties were paid only for that number of days. Decreasing the length of stay was seen as one way to decrease costs and save money. Patients were discharged to home or rehabilitation centers much sooner than before. They were weaker, had relatively fresh incisions, or often could not independently perform even minimal self-care. As hospital stays became shorter, nurses, physicians, consumers, and regulatory agencies expressed concerns about the quality of care. These concerns compelled hospital administrators and clinicians to develop new ways to measure and manage costs, quality, and outcomes. Assessment of how patient care was provided exposed inefficiencies, including lack of face-to-face communication among disciplines. Case management was developed and widely adopted to provide more cost-effective care while saving hundreds of thousands of dollars yearly.

Case Management

Using the case management model, care is planned collaboratively so that important events, such as initiation of physical therapy, home care consultation, or discontinuation of invasive treatments, occur on a schedule that clinicians, through research or experience, have identified as optimum for enhancing recovery. Care is mapped out by day or by other pivotal time intervals, and goals or desired outcomes are specified for each time frame. When the patient has met all the goals, he or she is ready for discharge to home or to the next level of care. Responsibility for monitoring the patient's progress and tracking variance or deviation from the pathway is given to the case manager, who usually (but not always) is a nurse. The tool on which all this information is contained is the clinical pathway. The purposes of a clinical pathway are to

- Promote quality care and improve clinical outcomes
- Standardize important aspects of care
- Reduce unnecessary delays in care
- Reduce costs

Elements of a Clinical Pathway

Clinical pathways are now used in a variety of settings and cover diverse diagnoses and conditions. They are often developed by individual organizations and, although the format varies from institution to institution, clinical pathways have major features in common.

Patient Population

The first important element of the clinical pathway is the patient population (Fig. B-1A). Each pathway clearly specifies those patients who are appropriate for inclusion on the pathway. Pathways tend to cover patient groups in which the treatment and recovery are relatively predictable. Diagnosis-related groups (DRGs) are usually used to identify patients

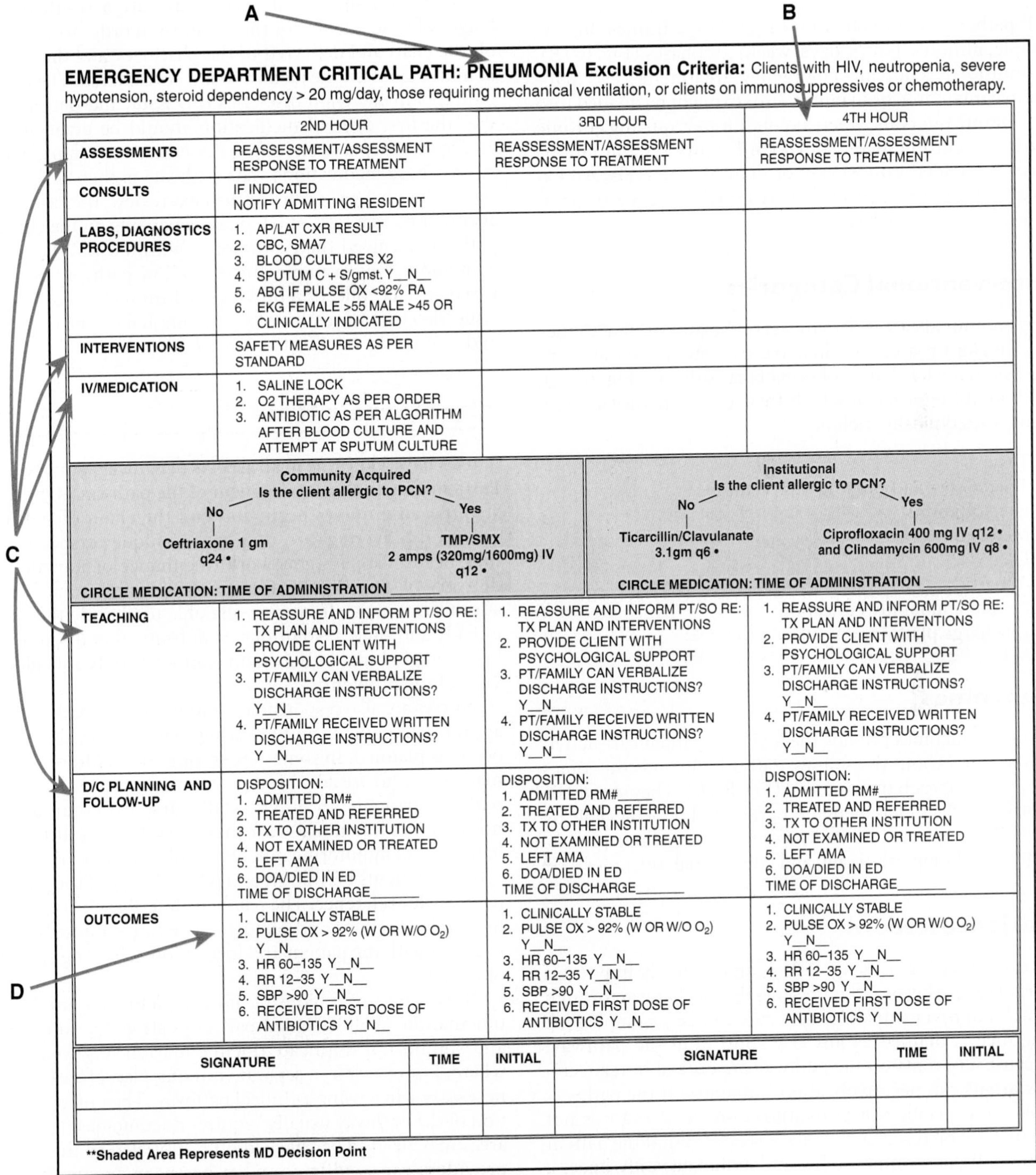

EMERGENCY DEPARTMENT CRITICAL PATH: PNEUMONIA Exclusion Criteria: Clients with HIV, neutropenia, severe hypotension, steroid dependency > 20 mg/day, those requiring mechanical ventilation, or clients on immunosuppressives or chemotherapy.

	2ND HOUR	3RD HOUR	4TH HOUR
ASSESSMENTS	REASSESSMENT/ASSESSMENT RESPONSE TO TREATMENT	REASSESSMENT/ASSESSMENT RESPONSE TO TREATMENT	REASSESSMENT/ASSESSMENT RESPONSE TO TREATMENT
CONSULTS	IF INDICATED NOTIFY ADMITTING RESIDENT		
LABS, DIAGNOSTICS PROCEDURES	1. AP/LAT CXR RESULT 2. CBC, SMA7 3. BLOOD CULTURES X2 4. SPUTUM C + S/gmst. Y__N__ 5. ABG IF PULSE OX <92% RA 6. EKG FEMALE >55 MALE >45 OR CLINICALLY INDICATED		
INTERVENTIONS	SAFETY MEASURES AS PER STANDARD		
IV/MEDICATION	1. SALINE LOCK 2. O2 THERAPY AS PER ORDER 3. ANTIBIOTIC AS PER ALGORITHM AFTER BLOOD CULTURE AND ATTEMPT AT SPUTUM CULTURE		

Community Acquired — Is the client allergic to PCN?
- No: Ceftriaxone 1 gm q24 •
- Yes: TMP/SMX 2 amps (320mg/1600mg) IV q12 •

CIRCLE MEDICATION: TIME OF ADMINISTRATION ______

Institutional — Is the client allergic to PCN?
- No: Ticarcillin/Clavulanate 3.1gm q6 •
- Yes: Ciprofloxacin 400 mg IV q12 • and Clindamycin 600mg IV q8 •

CIRCLE MEDICATION: TIME OF ADMINISTRATION ______

	2ND HOUR	3RD HOUR	4TH HOUR
TEACHING	1. REASSURE AND INFORM PT/SO RE: TX PLAN AND INTERVENTIONS 2. PROVIDE CLIENT WITH PSYCHOLOGICAL SUPPORT 3. PT/FAMILY CAN VERBALIZE DISCHARGE INSTRUCTIONS? Y__N__ 4. PT/FAMILY RECEIVED WRITTEN DISCHARGE INSTRUCTIONS? Y__N__	1. REASSURE AND INFORM PT/SO RE: TX PLAN AND INTERVENTIONS 2. PROVIDE CLIENT WITH PSYCHOLOGICAL SUPPORT 3. PT/FAMILY CAN VERBALIZE DISCHARGE INSTRUCTIONS? Y__N__ 4. PT/FAMILY RECEIVED WRITTEN DISCHARGE INSTRUCTIONS? Y__N__	1. REASSURE AND INFORM PT/SO RE: TX PLAN AND INTERVENTIONS 2. PROVIDE CLIENT WITH PSYCHOLOGICAL SUPPORT 3. PT/FAMILY CAN VERBALIZE DISCHARGE INSTRUCTIONS? Y__N__ 4. PT/FAMILY RECEIVED WRITTEN DISCHARGE INSTRUCTIONS? Y__N__
D/C PLANNING AND FOLLOW-UP	DISPOSITION: 1. ADMITTED RM#_____ 2. TREATED AND REFERRED 3. TX TO OTHER INSTITUTION 4. NOT EXAMINED OR TREATED 5. LEFT AMA 6. DOA/DIED IN ED TIME OF DISCHARGE______	DISPOSITION: 1. ADMITTED RM#_____ 2. TREATED AND REFERRED 3. TX TO OTHER INSTITUTION 4. NOT EXAMINED OR TREATED 5. LEFT AMA 6. DOA/DIED IN ED TIME OF DISCHARGE______	DISPOSITION: 1. ADMITTED RM#_____ 2. TREATED AND REFERRED 3. TX TO OTHER INSTITUTION 4. NOT EXAMINED OR TREATED 5. LEFT AMA 6. DOA/DIED IN ED TIME OF DISCHARGE______
OUTCOMES	1. CLINICALLY STABLE 2. PULSE OX > 92% (W OR W/O O_2) Y__N__ 3. HR 60–135 Y__N__ 4. RR 12–35 Y__N__ 5. SBP >90 Y__N__ 6. RECEIVED FIRST DOSE OF ANTIBIOTICS Y__N__	1. CLINICALLY STABLE 2. PULSE OX > 92% (W OR W/O O_2) Y__N__ 3. HR 60–135 Y__N__ 4. RR 12–35 Y__N__ 5. SBP >90 Y__N__ 6. RECEIVED FIRST DOSE OF ANTIBIOTICS Y__N__	1. CLINICALLY STABLE 2. PULSE OX > 92% (W OR W/O O_2) Y__N__ 3. HR 60–135 Y__N__ 4. RR 12–35 Y__N__ 5. SBP >90 Y__N__ 6. RECEIVED FIRST DOSE OF ANTIBIOTICS Y__N__

SIGNATURE	TIME	INITIAL	SIGNATURE	TIME	INITIAL

**Shaded Area Represents MD Decision Point

FIGURE B-1. Key elements of a clinical pathway. (**A**) Patient population clearly defined. (**B**) Clinically meaningful time frames. (**C**) Interventional categories. (**D**) Outcomes for each time frame should be specific and measurable. Reproduced with permission from Graduate Hospital, Philadelphia, Pennsylvania.

for a specific pathway, but qualifiers may be added. For example, a pathway for community-acquired pneumonia may exclude patients with *Pneumocystis* pneumonia or underlying obstructive pulmonary disease because those patients require highly individualized treatment plans and may not respond as quickly to intervention as patients without these underlying disorders.

Time Frames

All pathways are divided into useful time frames, for example, minutes, hours, days, weeks, or phases (Fig. B-1*B*). Conditions requiring emergency treatment (eg, myocardial infarction, head injury, stroke) might be divided into 15-minute intervals, whereas conditions requiring chronic care (eg, chronic pain, spinal cord injury rehabilitation) may be divided into weekly or monthly intervals. An example of interventions by phases might be seen in post-anesthesia care pathways.

Interventional Categories

Interventional categories consist of the groups of activities that make up a comprehensive treatment plan and are shown in the left-hand column of the pathway (Fig. B-1*C*). Although the order in which they are listed varies, these categories typically include

- Tests
- Treatments and nursing interventions
- Consultations
- Medications
- Diet
- Activity
- Patient and family education
- Discharge planning

Outcomes

Defined outcomes provide the focus for patient care activities for the various disciplines. Pathways include outcomes identified for each time interval (Fig. B-1*D*). They should be realistic, reflect incremental progress, and be achievable by 90% of the population. Pathway outcomes include physiologic, psychological, social, and educational outcomes.

Variance Record

The variance record (Fig. B-2) is an extremely important part of the pathway and represents the mechanism through which improvements in patient care can be accomplished. Variance is defined as any deviation from the pathway. Because all events on the pathway are critical to recovery, deviations can negatively affect outcomes. If the pathway calls for a specific test or treatment on day 2 and it is not carried out on day 2, a variance has occurred. If the patient is to ambulate 3 times a day and ambulates only once, a variance has occurred. The variance and the causes are recorded. Some variance records require a written note; others use code numbers or electronic systems to record variance (see Fig. B-2).

Case managers collect and analyze the variance data to identify trends in patient care and outcomes. For example, a pneumonia pathway may specify that the first dose of antibiotics be given within 3 hours of admission to the hospital (delays in administration of the first dose of an antibiotic are associated with increased morbidity and mortality). The case manager reviews the variance records and determines that only 40% of pneumonia patients are receiving the antibiotic in the specified time frame. Assessment of the issue reveals that delays are a result of the length of time it takes for the medication order to be taken off the chart and delivered to the pharmacy and the length of time it takes for the medication to be delivered. The pneumonia pathway team discusses this issue and determines that the first dose of medication should be given in the emergency department since the emergency department stocks these medications. The pathway is then revised to reflect this change in care. At the next review, the case manager reports that 92% of pneumonia patients on the clinical pathway received their antibiotics within 1 to 2 hours of admission. This example illustrates how pathway use and variance data collection provide the forum for assessing an issue, determining a plan of action, implementing the plan, and evaluating the effectiveness of the plan.

The Nurse's Role

Nurses have a key role in all aspects of clinical pathway use. Participating in the development of the pathway is the first step. Because nurses begin and end the chain of staff involved in delivering care, they have a unique perspective in how health care systems work to enhance or impede the delivery of care. In the above example about antibiotic administration, staff nurses were able to identify the issue quickly and suggest solutions. Staff from other disciplines, being single links in the chain, cannot supply this global view of the problem.

Nurses are also responsible for initiating the pathway for appropriate patients and ensuring that the various events occur as planned. In some care settings or conditions, case managers who are advanced practice nurses closely follow pathway patients; in others, staff nurses or community-based nurses function as case managers. In any setting, enhancing and monitoring outcome achievement is a nursing activity. Patients may be given a printed copy of the patient pathway for reference. The pathway describes the care plan in simple language and pictures. The nurse discusses the pathway with the patient and focuses on achieving specific outcomes.

Nurses are also responsible for completing required documentation. Well-designed pathways strive for simplicity and should not duplicate documentation required elsewhere. For example, a separate nursing plan of care is not necessary when using a clinical pathway. The outcome section of the pathway usually requires documentation; other areas may need to be checked off or initialed so that other providers can readily see what has been accomplished. Documenting variance and initiating steps to address the variance are equally important, as is participating in redesigning care practices to promote the highest quality of cost-effective care.

Clinical Pathway: ____________________
(Department Name)

Patient's Name: ____________________ **MedRecNo:** _ _ _ _ _ _

(Please list each code separately)

Date	Path Day #	Variance Code	Comment / Action Taken
__/__/__			
__/__/__			
__/__/__			
__/__/__			
__/__/__			

A

VARIANCE CODES

Patient's Condition/Problem

A1. Operative
- A1a. Further surgery to control bleeding
- A1b. Further surgery for other reason
- A1c. Perioperative myocardial infarction
- A1d. Tamponade (early or late)
- A1e. Dissection

A2. Infection
- A2a. Sternum, requiring debridement
- A2b. Sternum, superficial (antibiotics and dressings only)
- A2c. Leg
- A2d. Urinary tract infection
- A2e. Sepsis

A3. Neurological
- A3a. Stroke, temporary or permanent deficit
- A3b. Delirium
- A3c. Coma
- A3d. Confusion or agitation

A4. Respiratory
- A4a. Prolonged ventilation
- A4b. Acute respiratory distress syndrome
- A4c. Respiratory failure, reintubation
- A4d. Pneumonia
- A4e. Atelectasis

A5. Renal
- A5a. Renal failure
- A5b. Dialysis

A6. Cardiac
- A6a. Atrial arrhythmia
- A6b. Ventricular arrhythmia
- A6c. Heart block with or without pacemaker implantation
- A6d. Heart failure
- A6e. Cardiac arrest
- A6f. Hemodynamic instability
- A6g. Unable to wean off inotropic agents

A7. Vascular
- A7a. Deep vein thrombosis
- A7b. Limb ischemia

Other Condition/Problem

A8. Other
- A8a. Major gastrointestinal complication requiring surgery (eg, bleeding, perforation, ileus)
- A8b. Minor gastrointestinal complication requiring bowel rest (eg, ileus, nausea, high nasogastric output)
- A8c. Large volume of chest-tube drainage
- A8d. Poor wound healing (ie, significant sterile drainage from leg or chest wound)
- A8e. Pulmonary embolism
- A8f. Anticoagulant complication
- A8g. Thromboembolism
- A8h. Activity intolerance
- A8i. Medication reaction
- A8j. Altered skin integrity

B: Practitioner Related
- B1. Practitioner unavailability
- B2. Transcription error
- B3. Incorrect sequencing of therapy
- B4. Delay in consult or referral
- B5. Incomplete discharge planning
- B6. Delay or cancel test or procedure
- B7. Discharge day delay
- B8. Other

C: Hospital/System
- C1. Bed unavailable (state issue)
- C2. Equipment or supplies not available
- C3. Results not available
- C4. Unable to schedule test, procedure, or therapy
- C5. Case, test, procedure, or therapy delayed
- C6. Preoperative teaching not documented
- C7. Follow-up after discharge not documented

D: Family/Placement
- D1. Extended care not available
- D2. Homecare not available
- D3. Patient or family delaying discharge planning
- D4. Financial issues
- D5. Other

Form used at Westchester County Medical Center for tracking variances from clinical pathway for cardiac surgery (CABG).

B

FIGURE B-2. Variance record. (**A**) Blank pages for recording variance. (**B**) Variance codes. Reproduced with permission from *Critical Care Nurse, 17*(16), December 1997, pp. 29–30.

Pathways in Practice

Several pathways are provided in the following pages to demonstrate the variety of formats the nurse may encounter. Figure B-3 is a pathway used at Thomas Jefferson University Hospital for patients with acute ischemic stroke. The pathway provides clear expected outcomes as well as a variety of checklists identifying all significant and sequential aspects of patient care. Figure B-4 is a pathway used at Yale New Haven Hospital for a patient with acute coronary syndrome with or without percutaneous coronary intervention.

Whatever format is used or condition treated, clinical pathways are documents in transition; they will change as research suggests better treatment strategies and as variance data are analyzed. Nurses' participation in these processes is essential for the successful implementation of clinical pathways and, ultimately, the opportunity to improve patient care.

Acute Ischemic Stroke Critical Pathway Card

	Admission Day / / **Day 0-1 (1st 24 hrs)** **ER to ASU/NICU (or direct to ASU)**	**Day 2** / / **ASU**	**Day 3** / / **ASU/General Floor**
Goals/Outcomes	Identify acute ischemic stroke patient Document time of symptom onset Evaluate for appropriate treatment options and/or clinical trial Avoid Aspiration **NIH Stroke Scale (NIHSS)** ______ **Barthel Index** _____	Neuro status stabilized/improved Avoid medical complications (Aspiration, Fever, Infection) Initial Diagnostic tests results documented Rehab therapies initiated as appropriate **t-PA pts. transferred from NICU to ASU**	Neuro status stabilized/improved Avoid medical complications Diagnostic tests documented Rehab therapies continued as appropriate Pt/Family understands disease process **Transfer from ASU→Floor** Discharge if appropriate **NIHSS** _____ **Barthel Index** _____ (upon dischrg)
Laboratory/ Diagnostic Tests	**STAT CT brain without contrast** **EKG** **CXR** **Carotid Dopplers** **Echocardiogram** **To Consider:** • MRI/MRA • CTA • TCD CBC, PT/PTT SMA-7 SMA-12 ESR RPR UA (if febrile) **To Consider:** • ACLA, LA • ANA, RF • Fibrinogen level • Protein C & S, AT III (if age <55; venous infarct)	Fasting Lipid profile Fasting Homocysteine level Follow up on abnormal tests as needed PTT daily if on heparin PT/INR daily if on warfarin If patient received t-PA: CT brain without contrast **To Consider:** • **MRI/MRA** • CTA • TCD (if VB circulation) • TEE	PTT if on heparin PT/INR if on warfarin Follow-up abnormal tests **To Consider:** • Modified Barum Swallow • SPECT • Angiogram
Assessments/RN Interventions	VS as per Unit/t-PA protocol Neuro check as per Unit/t-PA protocol Cardiac monitoring Continuous Pulse Ox, and titrate O_2 to keep SpO_2 > 95% Bowel/Bladder/Skin assessment Avoid foley cath Compression boots (unless anticoagulated) HOB up 30°/Aspiration Precautions Institute Falls Risk Precautions Barthel Index completed and documented	VS and Neuro checks per Unit protocol Cardiac monitoring Continuous Pulse Ox, and titrate O_2 to keep SpO_2 > 95% Bowel/Bladder/Skin assessment Avoid foley cath Compression boots (unless anticoagulated) HOB up 30°/Aspiration Precautions Pulmonary toilet Turn q2h if pt on bed rest ROM as per Rehab if paralysis exists Hand/foot splint as per Rehab as needed	VS and Neuro checks per Unit protocol Cardiac monitoring (ASU) Continuous Pulse Ox, and titrate O_2 to keep SpO_2 > 95% Bowel/Bladder/Skin assessment Avoid foley cath Compression boots (unless anticoagulated) HOB up 30°/Aspiration Precautions Pulmonary toilet Turn q2h if pt on bed rest ROM as per Rehab, if paralysis exists Hand/foot splint as per Rehab as needed **To Consider:** • D/C cardiace monitor & Pulse Ox & transfer to floor **-or-** • D/C to home
Medications/ Treatments	IV NSS Evaluate admission medications BP meds w/parameters as needed Acetaminophen 650 mg p.o./PR q 4° prn temp > 100° Sliding Scale Insulin as needed Bowel regimen prn **To Consider:** • Antiplatelet treament • IV heparin • t-PA (No ASA, Heparin or Warfarin for 24 hrs.–Refer to t-PA protocol) • Investigational drug (refer to Protocol)	Renew IVF or IV to heplock Reassess BP meds w/parameters as needed Acetaminophen 650 mg p.o./PR q 4° prn temp > 100° Sliding Scale Insulin as needed Bowel regimen prn Continue from Day One as needed Antiplatelet Therapy IV Heparin **To Consider:** • Warfarin if indicated • If pt recieved t-PA, begin antiplatelet treatment or heparin as appropriate • Investigational drug, follow Protocol	Renew IVF, IV to hep lock, or D/C IV Reassess BP meds w/parameters as needed Acetaminophen 650 mg p.o./PR q 4° prn temp > 100° Sliding Scale Insulin and restart diabetic regimen if appropriate Bowel regimen prn Continue as appropriate -Antiplatelet Therapy -IV Heparin → Warfarin If investigational Drug, follow Protocol
Consults	**Notify Case Manager on Admission** **Notify Social Work on Admission** **Consult as Needed:** • Physical Medicine & Rehabilitation (PM&R) • Speech Therapy • Primary MD • Cardiology	**Completion of consults ordered Day 1** **Consult as Needed:** • Home Health • Rehab Coordinator • Neuropsych • Neurosurgery • Vascular Surgery	**Completion of Consults ordered Day 2** GI if feeding tube needed
Activity	Bed rest (HOB up 30°) **-or-** Increase activity as tolerated **To Consider:** • Pt may come off monitor for testing or traveling to Rehab Dept.	Bed rest (HOB up 30°) Increase activity as tolerated **-or-** Increase activity per PM&R	Increase activity as tolerated **-or-** **Pt. seen by PT/OT** Increase activity per PM&R
Nutrition	Nutrition Screen NPO/Aspiration Precautions **-or-** Diet as recommended by Speech	NPO/Aspiration Precautions Advance diet or per Speech/Dietitian recommendations **To Consider:** • Temporary Feeding tube	NPO/Aspiration Precautions Tube feeding per Dietitian recommendations **-or-** Advance diet per Speech/Dietitian Guidelines
Patient/Family Education D/C Planning	Orient to unit routine Educate about disease process Educate about diagnostic tests and meds Discharge Planning Assessment Initiated	Educate about diagnostic tests and meds Discuss discharge care options	Ongoing Stroke Education Start Warfarin teaching as needed **Finalize disp. plans (Home, Rehab, SNF)** **Discharge if appropriate**
Comments			

FIGURE B-3. Clinical pathway for acute ischemic stroke. Courtesy of Thomas Jefferson University Hospital, Philadelphia, PA. Available at www.stroke-site.org.

Acute Ischemic Stroke Critical Pathway Card

	Day 4 / / **ASU/General Floor**	**Day 5-7** / / **ASU/General Floor**	**Post Discharge Care/Home Health**
Goals/Outcomes	Neuro status stabilized/improved Pt transferred to floor Rehab therapies continued as appropriate NIHSS and Barthel Index documented, if patient discharged Discharge if appropriate **NIHSS _____ Barthel Imdex _____ (upon discharge)**	Neuro status stabilized/improved Special diagnostic tests documented Rehab therapies continued as appropriate NIHSS and Barthel Index documented, if patient discharged Discharge if appropriate **NIHSS _____ Barthel Imdex _____ (upon discharge)**	Maintain compliance with meds, diet and risk factor reduction Follow-up with Primary MD/Neurology Absence of recurrent symptoms Return to baseline activity level Recognise Signs & Symptoms and when to call Physician Advance diet accordingly
Laboratory/ Diagnostic Tests	PTT if on heparin PT/INR if on warfarin Follow-up abnormal tests **To Consider:** • Modified Barium Swallow	PTT if on heparin PT/INR if on warfarin	Labs per MD order -PT/INR if on warfarin -CBC q2 weeks x 3 months if on Ticlopidine
Assessments/RN Interventions	VS and Neuro Checks per Unit Protocol Cardiac monitoring (ASU) Continuous Pulse Ox, and titrate O_2 to keep $SpO_2 > 95\%$ Bowel/Bladder/Skin Assessment Avoid foley cath Compresssion boots (unless anticoagulated) HOB up 30°/Aspiration Precautions Turn q2h if pt on bed rest ROM as per Rehab, if paralysis exists Hand/foot splint as per Rehab as needed **To Consider:** • D/C cardiac monitoring & Pulse Ox & transfer to floor **-or-** • D/C to home	VS and Neuro checks per Unit Protocol Cardiac monitoring as needed Continuous Pulse Ox as needed Bowel/Bladder/Skin Assessment Avoid foley cath Compresssion boots (unless anticoagulated) HOB up 30°/Aspiration Precautions Turn q2h if pt on bed rest ROM as per Rehab, if paralysis exists Hand/foot splint as per Rehab as needed	Vital Signs Assess for and educate about recurrent signs and stmptoms of TIA/Stroke Complete Oasis Tool Asses PT/OT/Speech and swallow needs Assess feeding tube functioning Evaluate support systems Bowel/Bladder Training
Medications/ Treatments	IV to hep lock or D/C IV Reassess BP meds and parameters as needed Consider antihypertensive regimen Acetaminophen 650mg p.o./PR q4 prn temp. > 100 Diabetic regimen if appropriate Bowel regimen prn Continue as appropriate -Antiplatelet therapy -IV Heparin Æ Warfarin (D/C heparin when INR 2-3) If Investigational Drug, follow Protocol	IV to hep lock or D/C IV Adjust antihypertensive regimen as needed Adjust diabetic regimen as needed Continue as appropriate -Antiplatelet Therapy -IV Heparin → Warfarin (D/C heparin when INR 2-3) If Investigational Drug, follow Protocol	Review medications Set up med schedule via mediplan or calendar
Consults		Feeding tube placement if needed	Home Health Aid as needed Home PT/OT/Speech as needed Social Work /Registered Dietitian if needed Case Management telephone follow-up
Activity	Increase activity as tolerated **-or-** Increase activity per PM&R	Increase activity as tolerated/as per Rehab guidelines	Encourage increase in activity as tolerated Exercise/Therapy protocols as per PT/OT
Nutrition	Increase tube feedings as tolerated as per Dietitian Guidelines **-or-** Advance diet as tolerated/as per Speech/Dietitian recommendations	NPO for feeding tube placement **-or-** Advance diet as tolerated per Speech/Dietitian recommendations	Reinforce prescribed diet Refer as necessary to Out-Patient Dietitian X5077 Consider Swallow re-eval for removal of feeding tube
Patient/Family Education D/C Planning	Ongoing Stroke Education Warfarin teaching as needed **Finalize disp. plans (Home, Rehab, SNF)** **Discharge if appropriate**	Ongoing Stroke Education Warfarin teaching as needed **D/C instructions based on disposition plans** **Discharge if appropriate**	Reinforce signs/symptoms of stroke and need for urgent intervention Reinforce importance of risk factor reduction and med compliance Reinforce need to stay on meds Encourage pt/family that rehab process continues long after hospital stay and to continue to work towards improvement Advise on the availability of community/ financial/ transportation resources Warfarin teaching as needed
Comments			

FIGURE B-3. (Continued)

UNIT NO.

NAME

ADDRESS

BIRTH DATE:

VISIT NUMBER:

(if handwritten, record name, unit no., birth date, and visit no.)

PERMANENT PART OF MEDICAL RECORD

YALE NEW HAVEN HOSPITAL
CLINICAL PATHWAY

ACUTE CORONARY SYNDROME WITH OR WITHOUT PERCUTANEOUS CORONARY INTERVENTION [F-5021]

DIAGNOSIS: ❑ RO/MI ❑ UNSTABLE ANGINA (USA) ❑ NON ST ELEVATION MI ❑ ST ELEVATION MI (STEMI)

***EXPECTED OUTCOMES - PATIENT IS FREE FROM:**

DATE:	DATE:	DATE:	DATE:	DATE:
Patient Problem	**Patient Problem**	**Patient Problem**	**Patient Problem**	**Patient Problem**
• Myocardial ischemia (angina, ST/ T-wave ECG changes, SOB) • Dysrhythmias • Hypotension / hypertension • Bleeding / hematoma • Hypoxemia (by SpO_2, ABG's) • Heart Failure • Maladaptive coping mechanisms • Education barriers (language, impaired vision or hearing, dementia, developmentally delayed) • Inability to verbalize understanding of: - reportable conditions (CP, etc) - activity limitations - plan of care • Self-care deficit-unable to return home/previous residence	• Myocardial ischemia • Dysrhythmias • Hypotension / hypertension • Bleeding / hematoma • Hypoxemia • Heart Failure • Maladaptive coping mechanisms • Education barriers (language, impaired vision or hearing, dementia, developmentally delayed) • Inability to verbalize understanding of: - reportable conditions - activity limitations - plan of care • Self-care deficit-unable to return home/previous residence	• Myocardial ischemia • Dysrhythmias • Hypotension / hypertension • Bleeding / hematoma • Hypoxemia • Heart Failure • Maladaptive coping mechanisms • Education barriers (language, impaired vision or hearing, dementia, developmentally delayed) • Inability to verbalize understanding of: - reportable conditions - activity limitations - plan of care • Self-care deficit-unable to return home/previous residence	• Myocardial ischemia • Dysrhythmias • Hypotension / hypertension • Bleeding / hematoma • Hypoxemia • Heart Failure • Maladaptive coping mechanisms • Education barriers (language, impaired vision or hearing, dementia, developmentally delayed) • Inability to verbalize understanding of: - reportable conditions - activity limitations - plan of care • Self-care deficit-unable to return home/previous residence	• Myocardial ischemia • Dysrhythmias • Hypotension / hypertension • Bleeding / hematoma • Hypoxemia • Heart Failure • Maladaptive coping mechanisms • Education barriers (language, impaired vision or hearing, dementia, developmentally delayed) • Inability to verbalize understanding of: - reportable conditions - activity limitations - plan of care • Self-care deficit-unable to return home/previous residence
AMI Quality Indicators				
• Aspirin • Beta Blocker • If STEMI - Primary PTCA within 90 minutes	• Aspirin • Beta Blocker	• Aspirin • Beta Blocker	• Aspirin • Beta Blocker	• If LDL > 100 mg/dl - D/C on statin • Discharged on ASA, beta blocker • EF 40%– D/C on ACEI • Complete D/C instructions provided • Smoking cessation advice

* Variance reporting - circle variance, write History and Progress note, individualize Clinical Pathway - If problem cannot be resolved within 8-12 hour shift, add problem to IPOC/NPOC

FIGURE B-4. Clinical pathway for acute coronary syndrome with or without percutaneous coronary intervention. Courtesy of Yale New Haven Hospital, New Haven, CT.

UNIT NO.

NAME

ADDRESS

BIRTH DATE:

VISIT NUMBER:

(if handwritten, record name, unit no., birth date, and visit no.)

PERMANENT PART OF MEDICAL RECORD

YALE NEW HAVEN HOSPITAL
CLINICAL PATHWAY

ACUTE CORONARY SYNDROME WITH OR WITHOUT PERCUTANEOUS CORONARY INTERVENTION [F-5021]

INTERVENTIONS

	DATE: UNIT:	DATE: UNIT:	DATE: UNIT:	DATE: UNIT:	DATE: UNIT:
PATIENT / FAMILY EDUCATION	Initiate GPE: YATAP /SCALES ***Method*** ***Response*** ***Initials***	Initiate GPE: YATAP /SCALES ***Method*** ***Response*** ***Initials***	Initiate GPE: YATAP /SCALES ***Method*** ***Response*** ***Initials***	Initiate GPE: YATAP /SCALES ***Method*** ***Response*** ***Initials***	Initiate GPE: YATAP /SCALES ***Method*** ***Response*** ***Initials***
Key	ventilator	ventilator	ventilator	ventilator	ventilator
Patient Response / Teaching Method	Monitoring equipment	Monitoring equipment	Monitoring equipment	Monitoring equipment	Monitoring equipment
G=Good V=Verbal **F=Fair W=Written**	other:	other:	other:	other:	other:
P=Poor TV = Video **R=Refused**	symptoms to report	symptoms to report	symptoms to report	symptoms to report	symptoms to report
G = complete understanding/ independent in performing skill	plan of care / priority problems	plan of care / priority problems	plan of care / priority problems	plan of care / priority problems	plan of care / priority problems
	diet	diet	diet	diet	diet
F = limited understanding requires reminders/ multiple cues to demonstrate skill	activity	activity	activity	activity	activity
	smoking cessation	smoking cessation	smoking cessation	smoking cessation	smoking cessation
	medications	medications	medications	medications	medications
P = no understanding/ unable to demonstrate skill	weigh / monitor for HF symptoms daily	weigh / monitor for HF symptoms daily	weigh / monitor for HF symptoms daily	weigh / monitor for HF symptoms daily	weigh / monitor for HF symptoms daily
Booklets Distributed:	emotions/coping with illness	emotions/coping with illness	emotions/coping with illness	emotions/coping with illness	emotions/coping with illness
❑ Coumadin **❑ Heart Failure**	risk factors	risk factors	risk factors	risk factors	risk factors
❑ Patient Pathway **❑ Take Care**	tests/procedures	tests/procedures	tests/procedures	tests/procedures	tests/procedures
❑ Stent **❑ Stepping Toward Control** **❑ Straight from the Heart** **❑ Quit Smoking for Life** **❑ Women's Heart Advantage** **❑ Other:**	other:	other:	other:	other:	other:

FIGURE B-4. (Continued)

UNIT NO.

NAME

ADDRESS

BIRTH DATE:

VISIT NUMBER:

(if handwritten, record name, unit no., birth date, and visit no.)

PERMANENT PART OF MEDICAL RECORD

YALE NEW HAVEN HOSPITAL CLINICAL PATHWAY

ACUTE CORONARY SYNDROME WITH OR WITHOUT PERCUTANEOUS CORONARY INTERVENTION [F-5021]

INTERVENTIONS

	DATE: UNIT:	DATE: UNIT:	DATE: UNIT:	DATE: UNIT:	DATE: UNIT:
ASSESSMENT	Cardiac risk factors: ❑ premature family history ❑ tobacco use within year ❑ diabetes ❑ hypertension ❑ hypercholesterolemia ❑ obesity ❑ sedentary Signs and symptoms of: angina/angina equivalent hypoxemia decreased perfusion bleeding maladaptive coping Cardiac rate/rhythm per CMP: Continuous ECG monitoring Hemodynamic parameter, T, RR, lung sound, SpO_2 Other: ____ ____ ____ ❑ PA catheter per NOPM ❑ ABP per NOPM ❑ EF 40% or HF present – I&O weight per SCALES Program ❑ DM - finger sticks ac & hs or as ordered Follow diagnostic and lab data	Cardiac risk factors: ❑ premature family history ❑ tobacco use within year ❑ diabetes ❑ hypertension ❑ hypercholesterolemia ❑ obesity ❑ sedentary Signs and symptoms of: angina/angina equivalent hypoxemia decreased perfusion bleeding maladaptive coping Cardiac rate/rhythm per CMP Hemodynamic parameter, T, RR, lung sound, SpO_2 Other: ____ ____ ____ ❑ EF 40% or HF present – I&O weight per SCALES Program ❑ DM - finger sticks ac & hs or as ordered Follow diagnostic and lab data If discharge-dependent labs drawn, label specimens with special sticker	Signs and symptoms of: angina/angina equivalent hypoxemia decreased perfusion bleeding maladaptive coping Cardiac rate/rhythm per CMP Hemodynamic parameter, T, RR, lung sound, SpO_2 Other: ____ ____ ____ ❑ EF 40% or HF present – I&O weight per SCALES Program ❑ DM - finger sticks ac & hs or as ordered Follow diagnostic and lab data If discharge-dependent labs drawn, label specimens with special sticker	Signs and symptoms of: angina/angina equivalent hypoxemia decreased perfusion bleeding maladaptive coping Cardiac rate/rhythm per CMP Hemodynamic parameter, T, RR, lung sound, SpO_2 Other: ____ ____ ____ ❑ EF 40% or HF present – I&O weight per SCALES Program ❑ DM - finger sticks ac & hs or as ordered Follow diagnostic and lab data If discharge-dependent labs drawn, label specimens with special sticker	Signs and symptoms of: angina/angina equivalent hypoxemia decreased perfusion bleeding maladaptive coping mechanisms D/C continuous ECG monitoring ❑ EF 40% or HF present – I&O weight per SCALES Program ❑ DM - finger sticks ac & hs or as ordered If discharge-dependent labs drawn, label specimens with special sticker
MEDICATIONS	***SAAB (Statin, ASA, ACEI, Beta Blocker) if indicated** Consider: IV GP IIB / IIIA platelet inhibitor, clopidogrel, anticoagulant, nitrate, nicotine replacement tx/bupropion, if tobacco user O_2 via N/C @2L/min IV fluids or IID as ordered	***SAAB if indicated** Consider: IV GP IIB / IIIA platelet inhibitor, clopidogrel, anticoagulant, nitrate, nicotine replacement tx/bupropion, if tobacco user O_2 via N/C @2L/min IV fluids or IID as ordered	***SAAB if indicated** Consider: IV GP IIB / IIIA platelet inhibitor, anticoagulant, nitrate, clopidogrel Consider discontinuing O_2 via N/C @ 2L/min if SPO_2 95% IV fluids or IID as ordered	***SAAB if indicated** Consider: IV GP IIB / IIIA platelet inhibitor, anticoagulant, nitrate, clopidogrel IV fluids or IID as ordered	***SAAB if indicated** **If EF 40% discharge on ACE I; if not prescribed,** document rationale IV fluids or IID as ordered
PAIN **Ischemic pain**	Assess for pain with vital signs & within one hour of an intervention for pain Interventions - CMP: Anginal Symptoms	Assess for pain with vital signs & within one hour of an intervention for pain Interventions - CMP: Anginal Symptoms	Assess for pain with vital signs & within 1 hour of an intervention for pain Interventions - CMP: Anginal Symptoms	Assess for pain with vital signs & within 1 hour of an intervention for pain Interventions - CMP: Anginal Symptoms	Assess for pain with vital signs & within 1 hour of an intervention for pain Interventions - CMP: Anginal Symptoms
Other pain source	Add on to IPOC/NPOC	Add onto IPOC/NPOC	Add onto IPOC/NPOC	Add onto IPOC/NPOC	Add on to IPOC/NPOC

FIGURE B-4. (Continued)

UNIT NO.

NAME

ADDRESS

BIRTH DATE:

VISIT NUMBER:

(if handwritten, record name, unit no., birth date, and visit no.)

PERMANENT PART OF MEDICAL RECORD

YALE NEW HAVEN HOSPITAL
CLINICAL PATHWAY

ACUTE CORONARY SYNDROME WITH OR WITHOUT PERCUTANEOUS CORONARY INTERVENTION [F-5021]

INTERVENTIONS

	DATE: UNIT:	DATE: UNIT:	DATE: UNIT:	DATE: UNIT:	DATE: UNIT:
TESTS / PROCEDURES	Labs: *** Lipid profile,** troponin - draw at: ________ CK, CK/MB every 8 hrs X 3 – draw at: ______ ______ ______ CBC, platelets, lytes, bun/CR, LFTs, PT/PTT CXR, ECG (with RV leads if IWMI) ❑ stress test with imaging ❑ cardiac echo - EF ________% ❑ other: ________ **REFER TO PAGE 5 OF INTERVENTIONS** ❑ cardiac catheterization ❑ PTCA /stent: ________ ❑ brachytherapy	❑ stress test with imaging ❑ cardiac echo - EF ________% ❑ other: ________ **REFER TO PAGE 5 OF INTERVENTIONS** ❑ cardiac catheterization ❑ PTCA /stent: ________ ❑ brachytherapy	❑ stress test with imaging ❑ cardiac echo - EF ________% ❑ other: ________ **REFER TO PAGE 5 OF INTERVENTIONS** ❑ cardiac catheterization ❑ PTCA /stent: ________ ❑ brachytherapy	❑ stress test with imaging ❑ cardiac echo - EF ________% ❑ other: ________ **REFER TO PAGE 5 OF INTERVENTIONS** ❑ cardiac catheterization ❑ PTCA /stent: ________ ❑ brachytherapy	❑ stress test with imaging ❑ cardiac echo - EF ________% ❑ other: ________ **REFER TO PAGE 5 OF INTERVENTIONS** ❑ cardiac catheterization ❑ PTCA /stent: ________ ❑ brachytherapy
ACTIVITY	❑ Bed rest ❑ Bed rest with bedside commode ❑ Bed rest - OOB to bathroom	❑ USA: Advance as tolerated ❑ AMI: Out of bed to chair tid; Ambulate 50 ft, bathroom privileges ❑ Other: ________	❑ USA: Advance as tolerated ❑ AMI: Out of bed to chair as tolerated; Ambulate 100 - 300 ft; Shower sitting - with supervision ❑ Other: ________	❑ USA: Advance as tolerated ❑ AMI: Out of bed to chair as tolerated; Ambulate 100 - 300 ft; Shower sitting - with supervision ❑ Other: ________	❑ USA: Advance as tolerated ❑ AMI: Ambulates 300-400 ft tid/qid ❑ Other: ________
DISCHARGE PROCESS	Identify key contact person and current home care services	Determine self-management needs (home care services, transportation, care provider) If Discharge Day: complete W-10, CR Referral and Written Instructions in CCSS. If AMI, assure quality indicators are addressed	Determine self-management needs If Discharge Day: complete W-10, CR Referral and Written Instructions in CCSS. If AMI, assure quality indicators are addressed	Determine self-management needs If Discharge Day: complete W-10, CR Referral and Written Instructions in CCSS. If AMI, assure quality indicators are addressed	If Discharge Day: complete W-10, CR Referral and Written Instructions in CCSS. If AMI, assure quality indicators are addressed
SIGN OFF **PRINT NAME** **SIGN** **SHIFT**					

FIGURE B-4. (Continued)

UNIT NO.

NAME

ADDRESS

BIRTH DATE:

VISIT NUMBER:

(if handwritten, record name, unit no., birth date, and visit no.)

PERMANENT PART OF MEDICAL RECORD

YALE NEW HAVEN HOSPITAL CLINICAL PATHWAY

ACUTE CORONARY SYNDROME WITH OR WITHOUT PERCUTANEOUS CORONARY INTERVENTION [F-5021]

INTERVENTIONS

	PRE-PROCEDURE DATE:	POST-PROCEDURE DATE:
MEDICATIONS	If allergy to contrast dye, consider prophylactic therapy Consider hydration If creatinine ≥ 1.3 mg/dl, consider acetylcystein 20%- 600 mg bidor 2 days Diabetes: give 1/2 NPH dose, cover with sliding scale; Hold Metformin for 48 hours Hold warfarin ASA PO platelet inhibitor if stent anticipated Discontinue heparin on-call to CV Lab as prescribed	Offer pain medication and sedatives PRN IV hydration Hold Metformin If on warfarin pre-procedure, consider restarting ASA If stent placed - p.o. platelet inhibitor Ensure order written to continue/discontinue heparin; If prescribed begin infusion 4-6 hours after sheath is removed.
TESTS / PROCEDURES		PTCA only: ECG, I&O, CK with MB in AM ________ ❑ Femostop per CCSS orders - Remove @ ________ ❑ ACT prior to sheath removal @ _____ Pull sheaths when ACT ≤ 175 If receiving IIBIIIA platelet inhibitor, draw platelets 4 hours after bolus/infusion initiated - Draw @ ________
ASSESSMENT	Establish baseline lower extremity circulation, movement, sensation (CMS) bilaterally Comfort level or pain with vital signs	Vital signs every 30 minutes X 6, then as needed Monitor CMS of affected extremity and catheter insertion site for bleeding, hematoma every 15 min X 4, every 30 min X2, then every 1 hr Comfort level/pain with vital signs
ACTIVITY		Post cardiac catheterization: Right-sided catheterization - bed rest 4 hours OOB @ ________ Left-sided catheterization - bed rest 6 hours OOB @ ________ Immobolize affected extremity, head of bed <30° If vascular closure device used: ambulate after 1-2 hrs of bed rest or when puncture site stable: OOB @ ________ Post PTCA: bed rest while arterial sheaths in place maintain bed rest 6-8 hours after sheaths removed - OOB @ ________ head of bed <30° If vascular closure devise used: Bed rest x 4hrs then ambulate (see CMP) If IIB IIIA inhibitor infusing - bed rest untill infusion completed
PATIENT / FAMILY EDUCATION Key — **Patient response**: G = good, F = fair, P = poor; **Teaching Method**: V = Verbal, W = Written, TV = Video	**Method** ___ **Response** ___ **Initials** ___ pre-procedure teaching – sensations/experiences ___ ___ ___ other: ________	**Method** ___ **Response** ___ **Initials** ___ activity restrictions post-procedure ___ ___ ___ hold pressure on groin to cough or sneeze ________ call nurse for loss of sensation in extremity below puncture site or bleeding
DIET	If afternoon procedure scheduled - light breakfast, then NPO	Resume diet - encourage PO fluids unless contraindicated

FIGURE B-4. (Continued)

APPENDIX C

Concept Maps

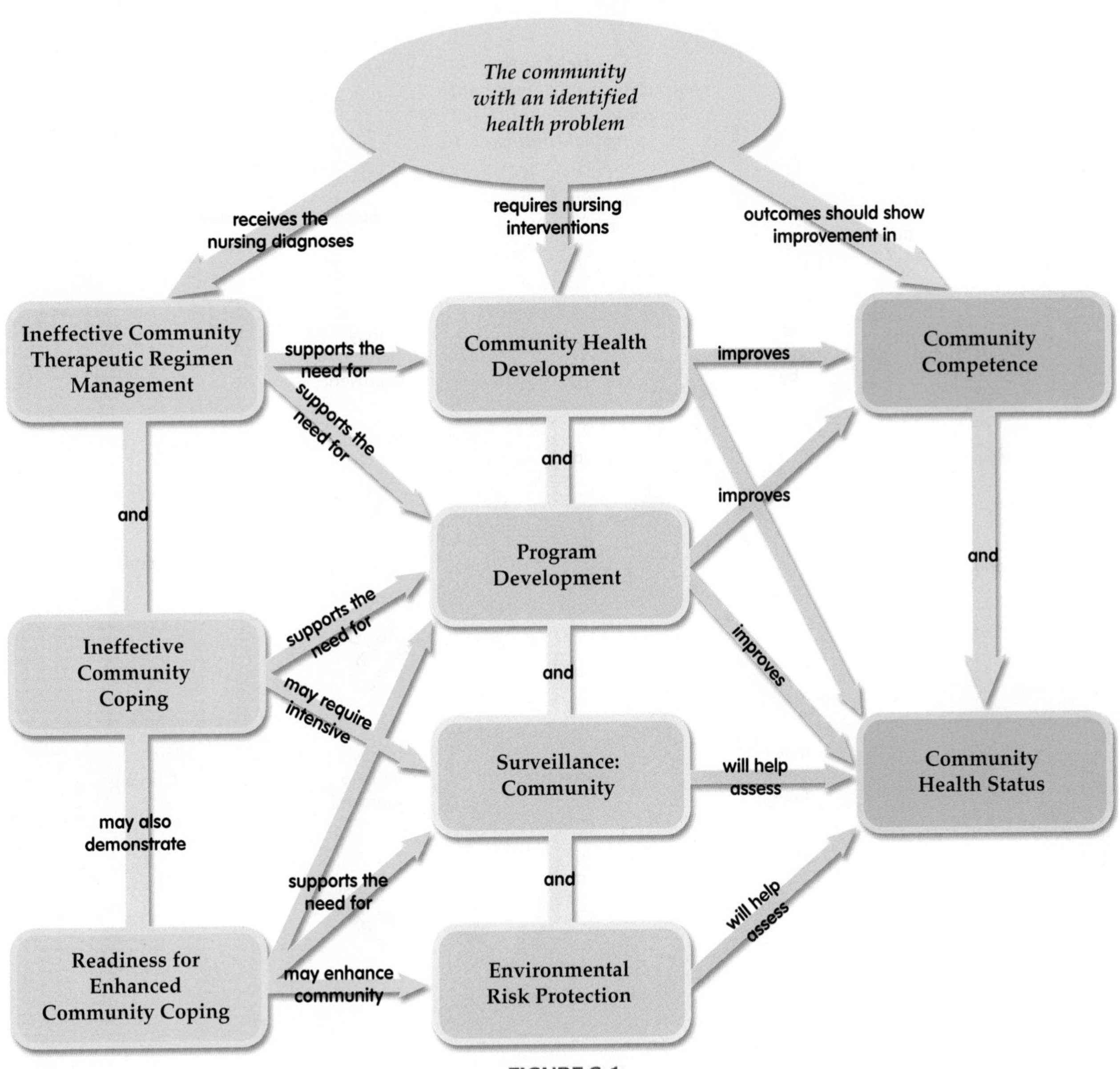
The community with an identified health problem
receives the nursing diagnoses
requires nursing interventions
outcomes should show improvement in
Ineffective Community Therapeutic Regimen Management
supports the need for
Community Health Development
improves
Community Competence
supports the need for
and
improves
and
and
Program Development
and
Ineffective Community Coping
supports the need for
improves
may require intensive
and
Surveillance: Community
will help assess
Community Health Status
may also demonstrate
supports the need for
and
will help assess
Readiness for Enhanced Community Coping
may enhance community
Environmental Risk Protection

FIGURE C-1.

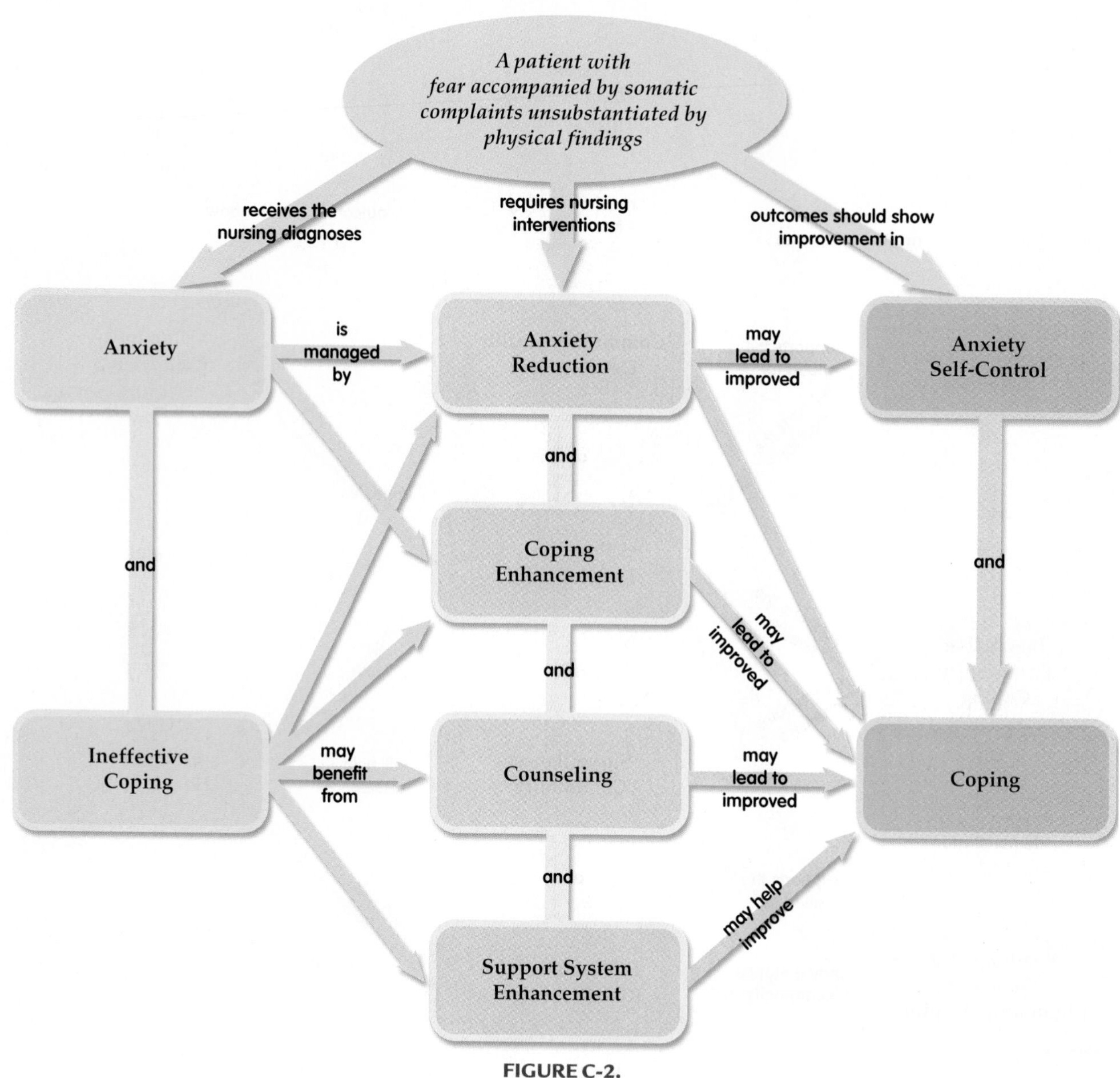
A patient with fear accompanied by somatic complaints unsubstantiated by physical findings
receives the nursing diagnoses
requires nursing interventions
outcomes should show improvement in
Anxiety
is managed by
Anxiety Reduction
may lead to improved
Anxiety Self-Control
and
and
Coping Enhancement
and
may lead to improved
and
Ineffective Coping
may benefit from
Counseling
may lead to improved
Coping
and
may help improve
Support System Enhancement

FIGURE C-2.

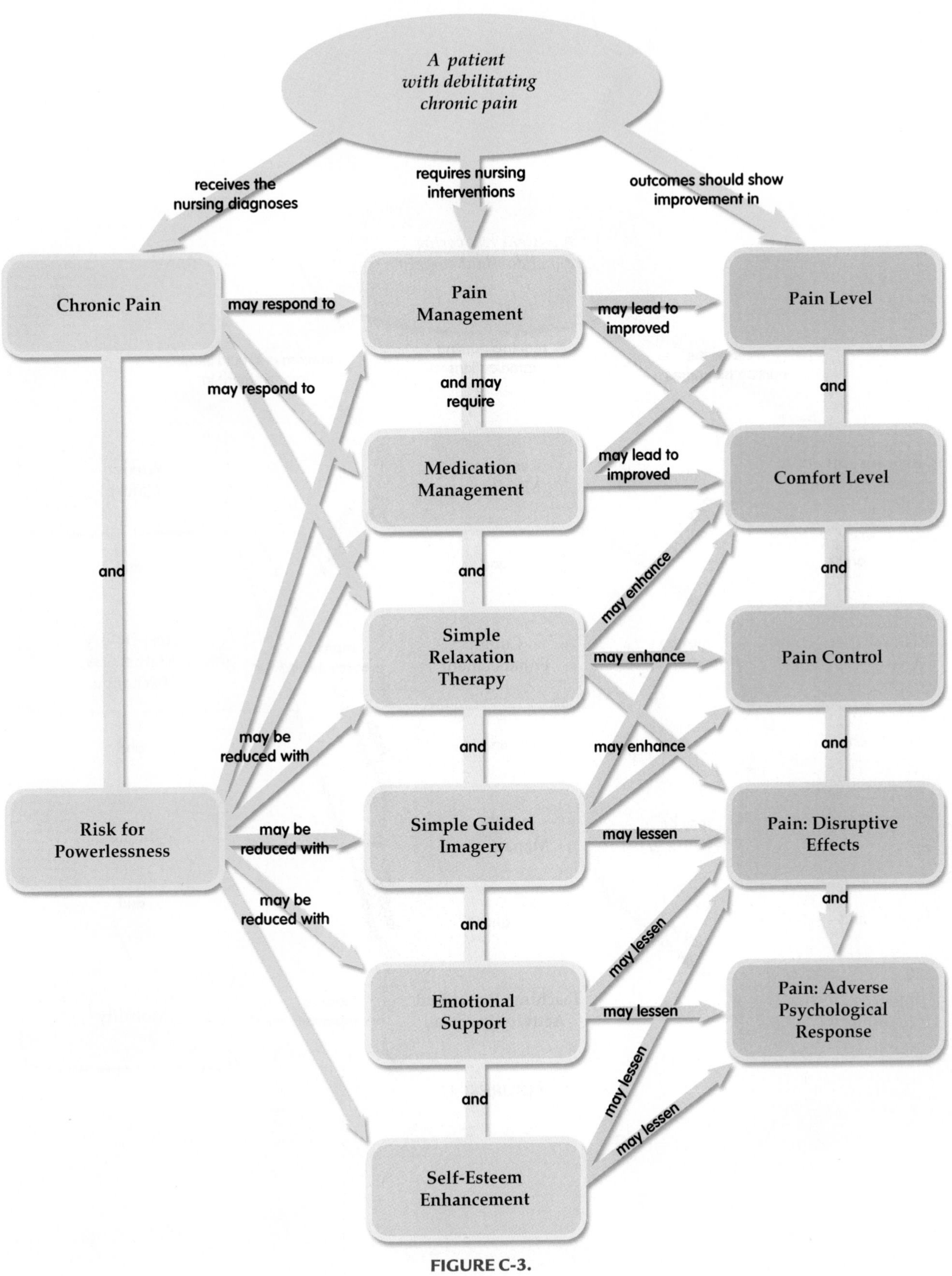
A patient with debilitating chronic pain
receives the nursing diagnoses
requires nursing interventions
outcomes should show improvement in
Chronic Pain
may respond to
may respond to
Pain Management
and may require
Medication Management
and
Simple Relaxation Therapy
and
Simple Guided Imagery
and
Emotional Support
and
Self-Esteem Enhancement
and
Risk for Powerlessness
may be reduced with
may be reduced with
may be reduced with
may lead to improved
may lead to improved
may enhance
may enhance
may enhance
may lessen
may lessen
may lessen
may lessen
may lessen
Pain Level
and
Comfort Level
and
Pain Control
and
Pain: Disruptive Effects
and
Pain: Adverse Psychological Response

FIGURE C-3.

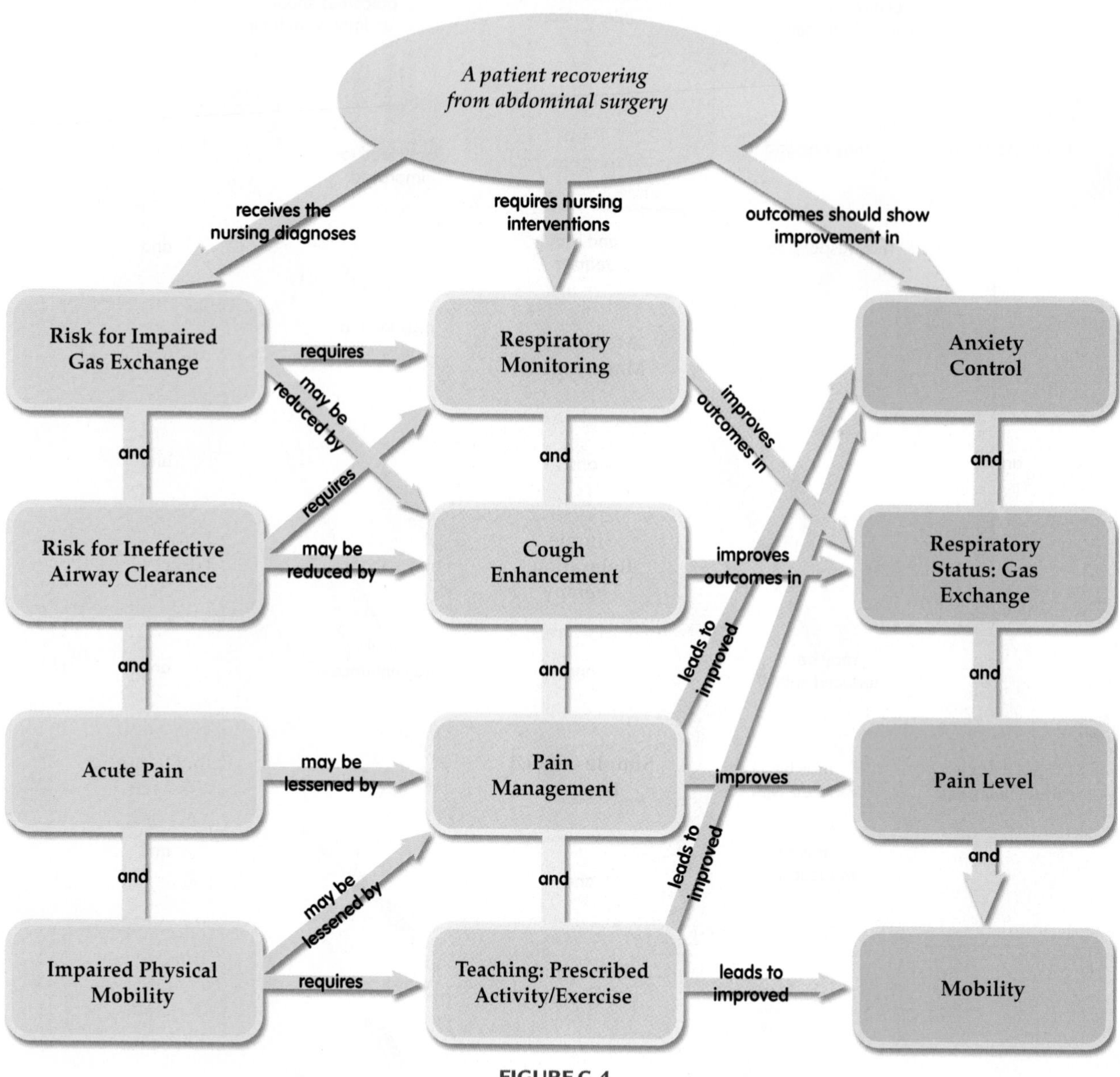
A patient recovering from abdominal surgery
receives the nursing diagnoses
requires nursing interventions
outcomes should show improvement in
Risk for Impaired Gas Exchange
requires
Respiratory Monitoring
Anxiety Control
may be reduced by
improves outcomes in
and
and
and
requires
Risk for Ineffective Airway Clearance
may be reduced by
Cough Enhancement
improves outcomes in
Respiratory Status: Gas Exchange
leads to improved
and
and
and
Acute Pain
may be lessened by
Pain Management
improves
Pain Level
leads to improved
and
and
and
may be lessened by
Impaired Physical Mobility
requires
Teaching: Prescribed Activity/Exercise
leads to improved
Mobility

FIGURE C-4.

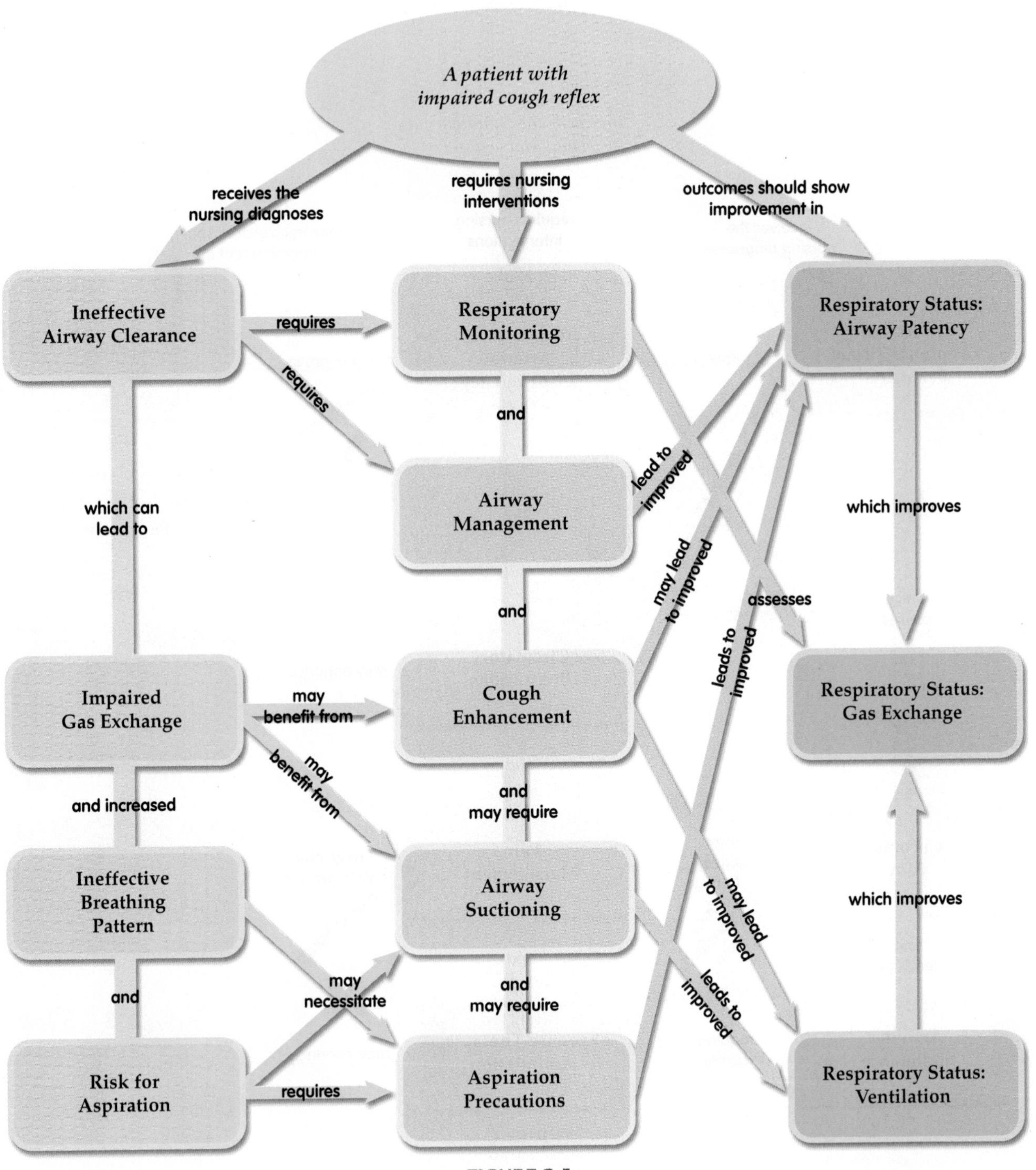
A patient with impaired cough reflex
receives the nursing diagnoses
requires nursing interventions
outcomes should show improvement in
Ineffective Airway Clearance
requires
Respiratory Monitoring
requires
Respiratory Status: Airway Patency
and
lead to improved
Airway Management
which can lead to
which improves
may lead to improved
assesses
and
leads to improved
Impaired Gas Exchange
may benefit from
Cough Enhancement
Respiratory Status: Gas Exchange
may benefit from
and increased
and may require
Ineffective Breathing Pattern
Airway Suctioning
which improves
may lead to improved
and
may necessitate
and may require
leads to improved
Risk for Aspiration
requires
Aspiration Precautions
Respiratory Status: Ventilation

FIGURE C-5.

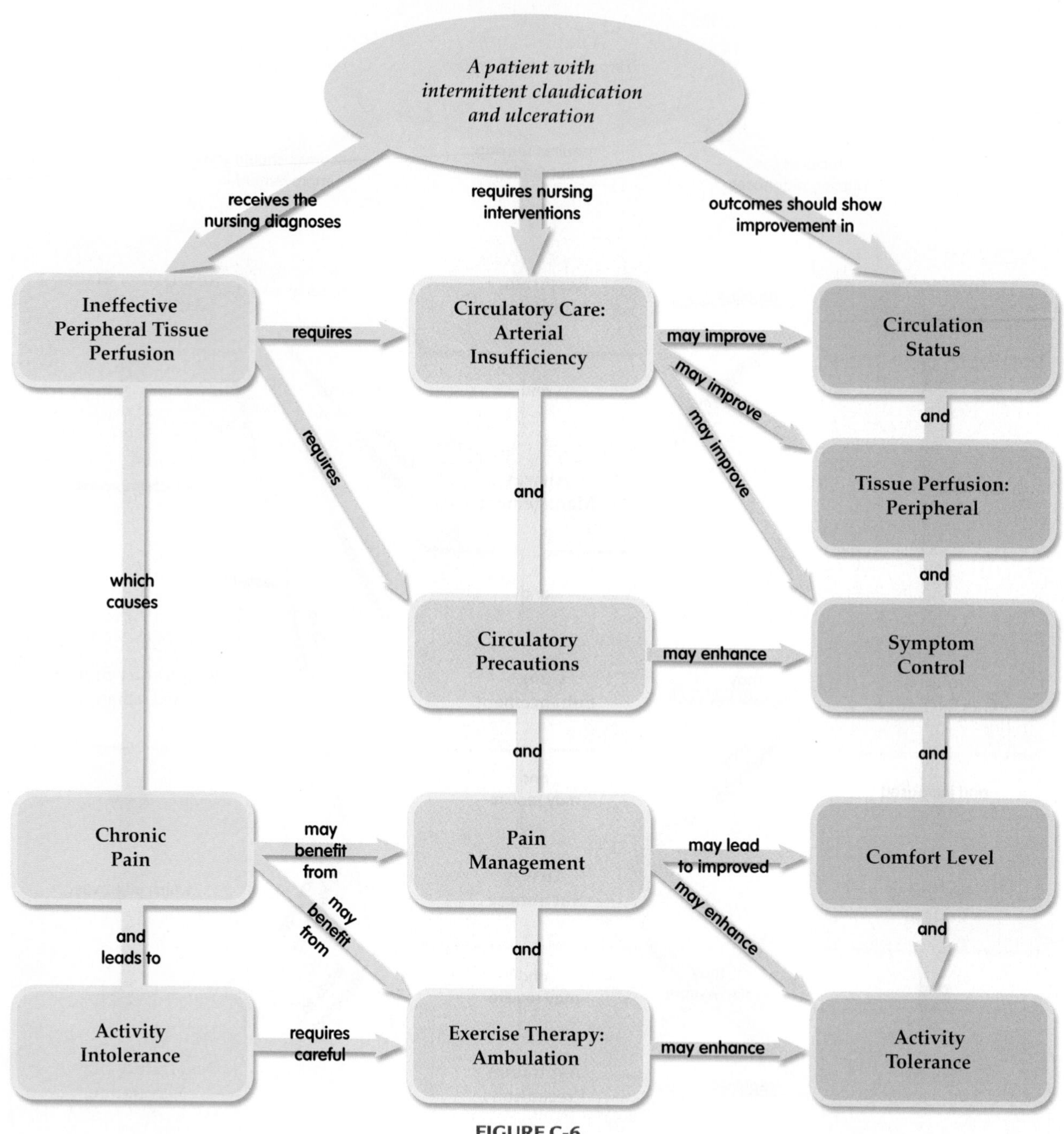
A patient with intermittent claudication and ulceration
receives the nursing diagnoses
requires nursing interventions
outcomes should show improvement in
Ineffective Peripheral Tissue Perfusion
requires
Circulatory Care: Arterial Insufficiency
may improve
Circulation Status
may improve
may improve
and
Tissue Perfusion: Peripheral
requires
and
and
which causes
Circulatory Precautions
may enhance
Symptom Control
and
and
Chronic Pain
may benefit from
Pain Management
may lead to improved
Comfort Level
may benefit from
may enhance
and leads to
and
and
Activity Intolerance
requires careful
Exercise Therapy: Ambulation
may enhance
Activity Tolerance

FIGURE C-6.

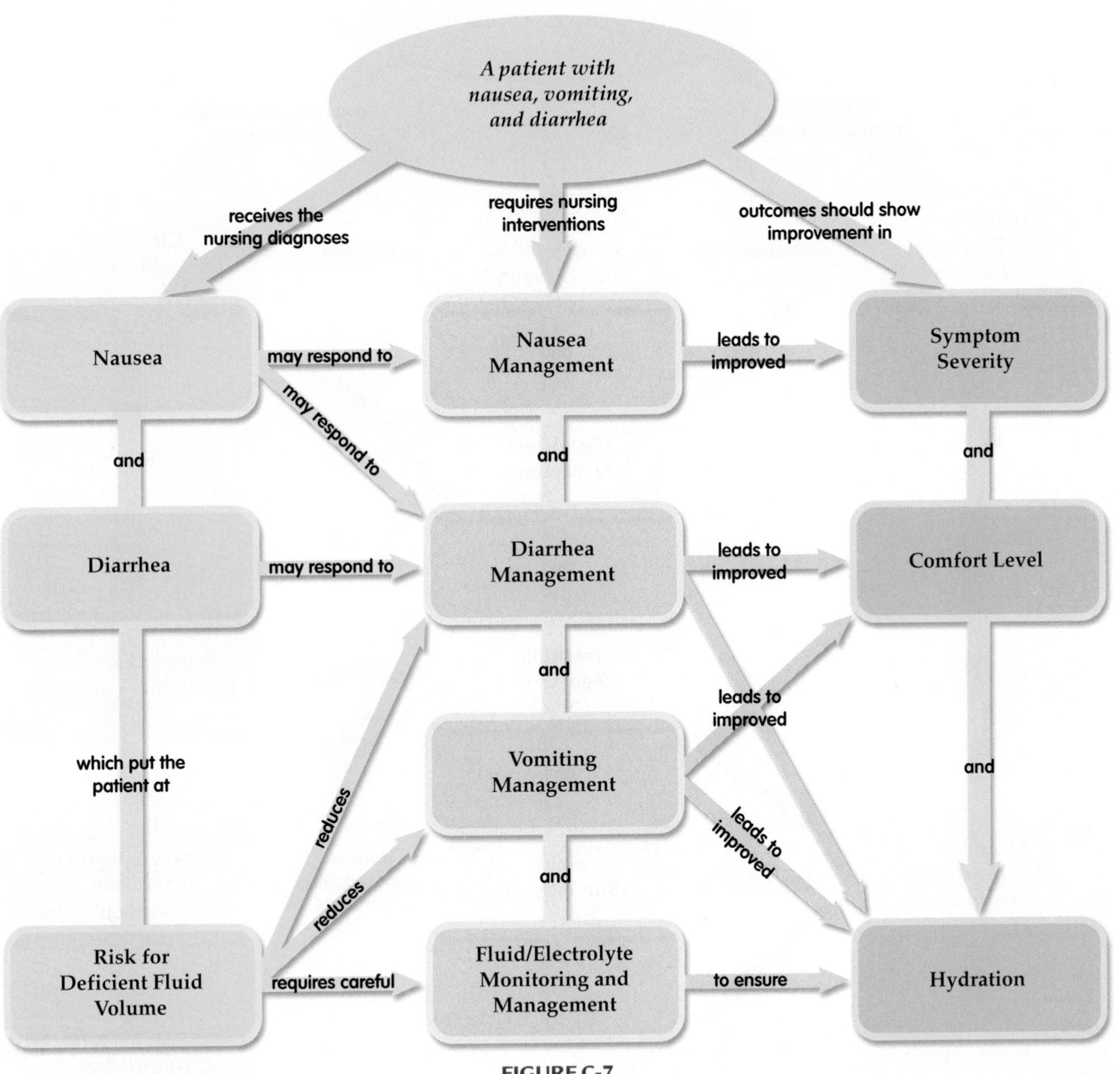
A patient with nausea, vomiting, and diarrhea
receives the nursing diagnoses
requires nursing interventions
outcomes should show improvement in
Nausea
may respond to
Nausea Management
leads to improved
Symptom Severity
may respond to
and
and
and
Diarrhea
may respond to
Diarrhea Management
leads to improved
Comfort Level
and
leads to improved
which put the patient at
Vomiting Management
and
reduces
leads to improved
reduces
and
Risk for Deficient Fluid Volume
requires careful
Fluid/Electrolyte Monitoring and Management
to ensure
Hydration

FIGURE C-7.

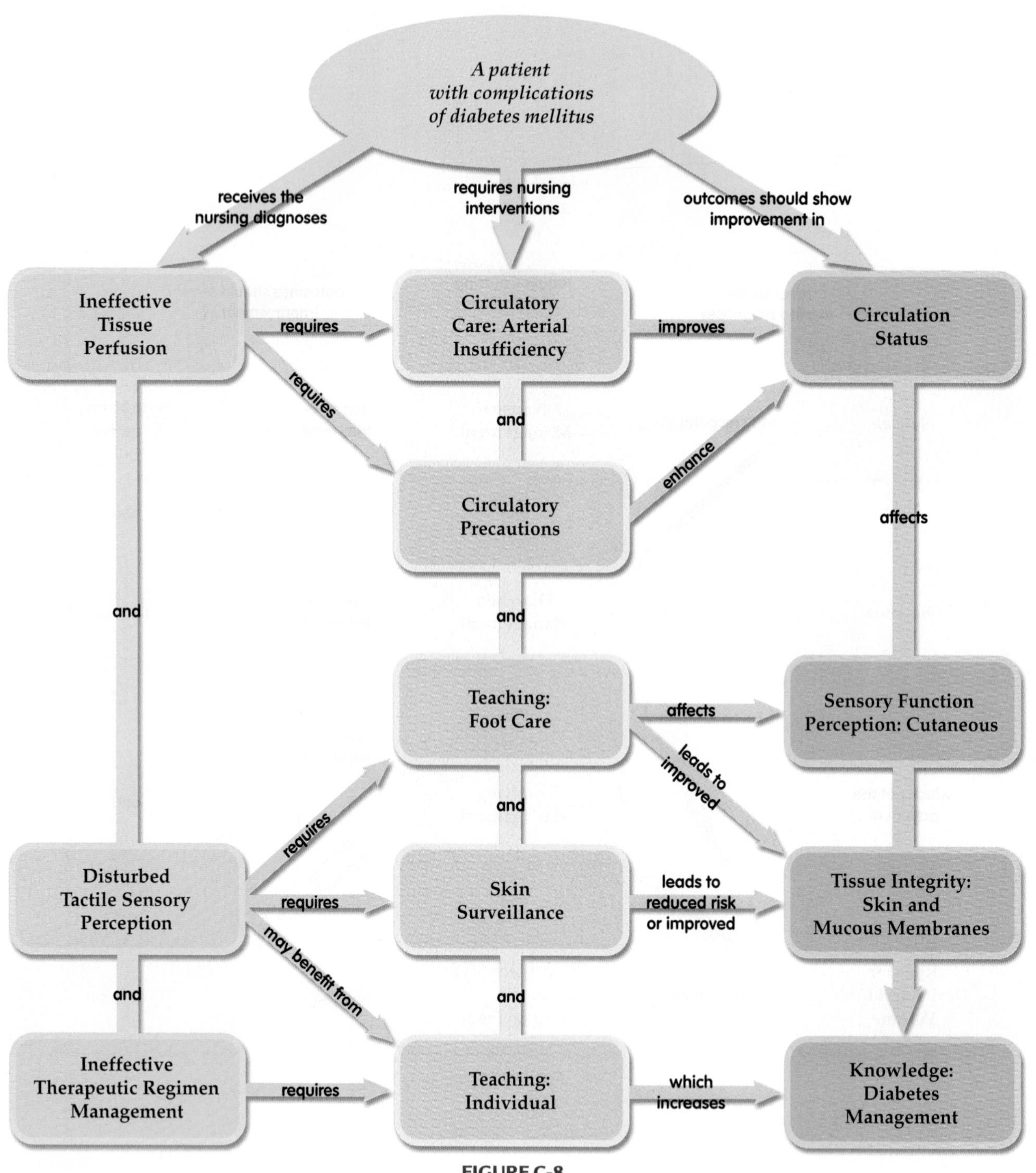
A patient
with complications
of diabetes mellitus
receives the
nursing diagnoses
requires nursing
interventions
outcomes should show
improvement in
Ineffective
Tissue
Perfusion
requires
Circulatory
Care: Arterial
Insufficiency
improves
Circulation
Status
requires
and
enhance
Circulatory
Precautions
affects
and
and
Teaching:
Foot Care
affects
Sensory Function
Perception: Cutaneous
leads to
improved
and
requires
Disturbed
Tactile Sensory
Perception
requires
Skin
Surveillance
leads to
reduced risk
or improved
Tissue Integrity:
Skin and
Mucous Membranes
may benefit from
and
and
Ineffective
Therapeutic Regimen
Management
requires
Teaching:
Individual
which
increases
Knowledge:
Diabetes
Management

FIGURE C-8.

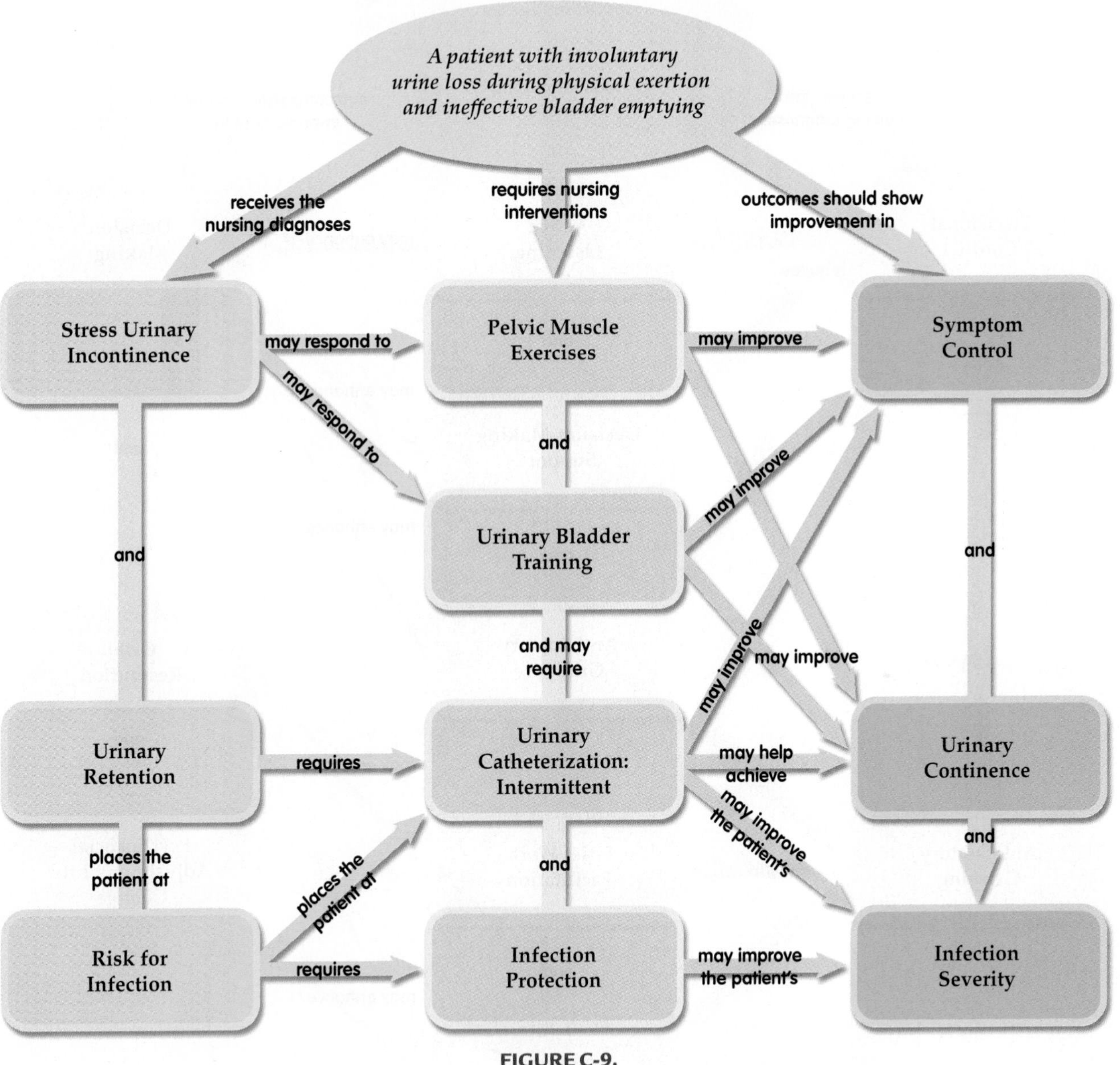
A patient with involuntary urine loss during physical exertion and ineffective bladder emptying
receives the nursing diagnoses
requires nursing interventions
outcomes should show improvement in
Stress Urinary Incontinence
may respond to
Pelvic Muscle Exercises
may improve
Symptom Control
may respond to
and
may improve
Urinary Bladder Training
and
and
and may require
may improve
may improve
Urinary Retention
requires
Urinary Catheterization: Intermittent
may help achieve
Urinary Continence
may improve the patient's
and
places the patient at
places the patient at
and
Risk for Infection
requires
Infection Protection
may improve the patient's
Infection Severity

FIGURE C-9.

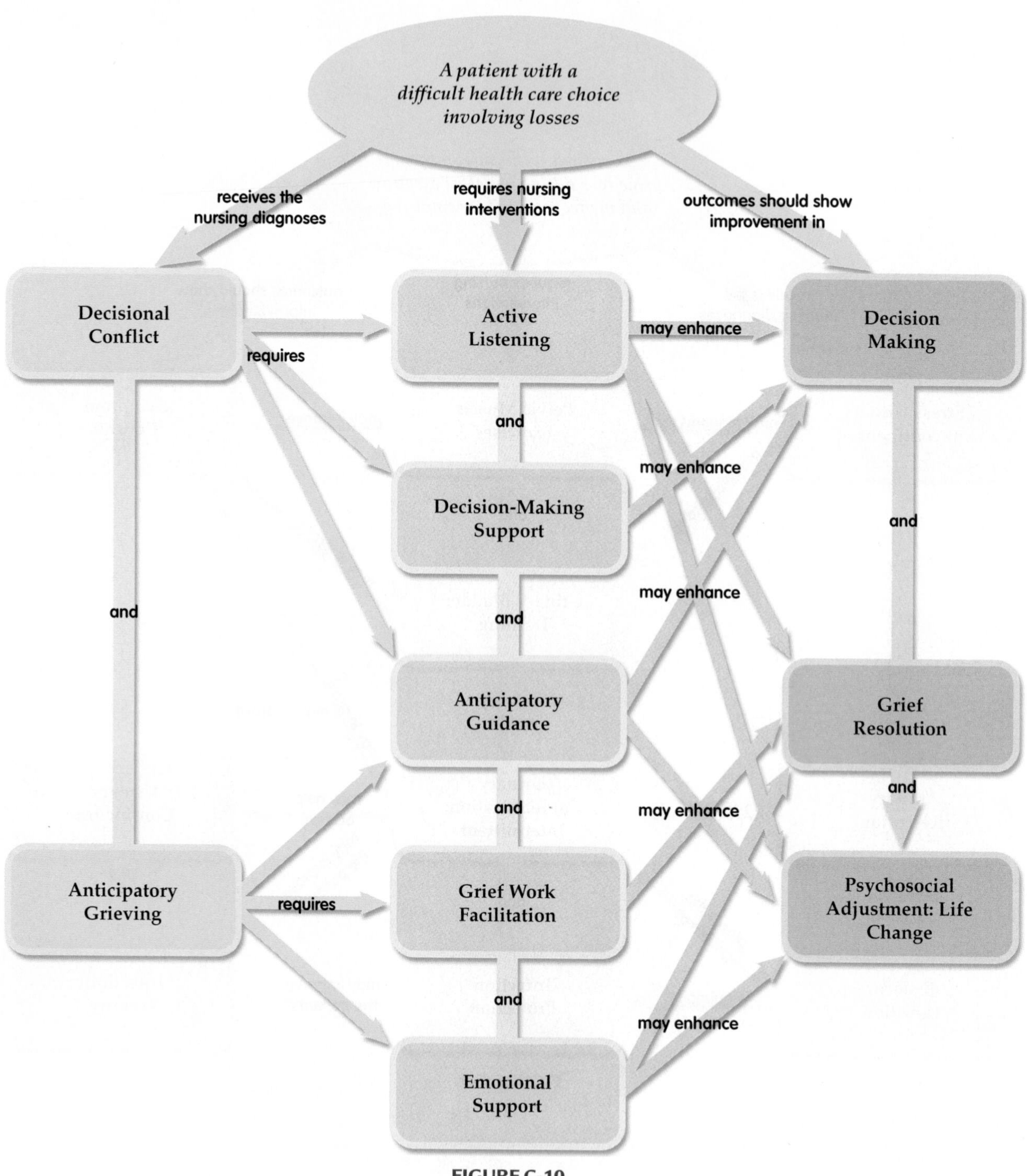
A patient with a difficult health care choice involving losses
receives the nursing diagnoses
requires nursing interventions
outcomes should show improvement in
Decisional Conflict
requires
Active Listening
may enhance
Decision Making
and
Decision-Making Support
may enhance
and
and
may enhance
Anticipatory Guidance
Grief Resolution
and
and
may enhance
Anticipatory Grieving
requires
Grief Work Facilitation
Psychosocial Adjustment: Life Change
and
may enhance
Emotional Support

FIGURE C-10.

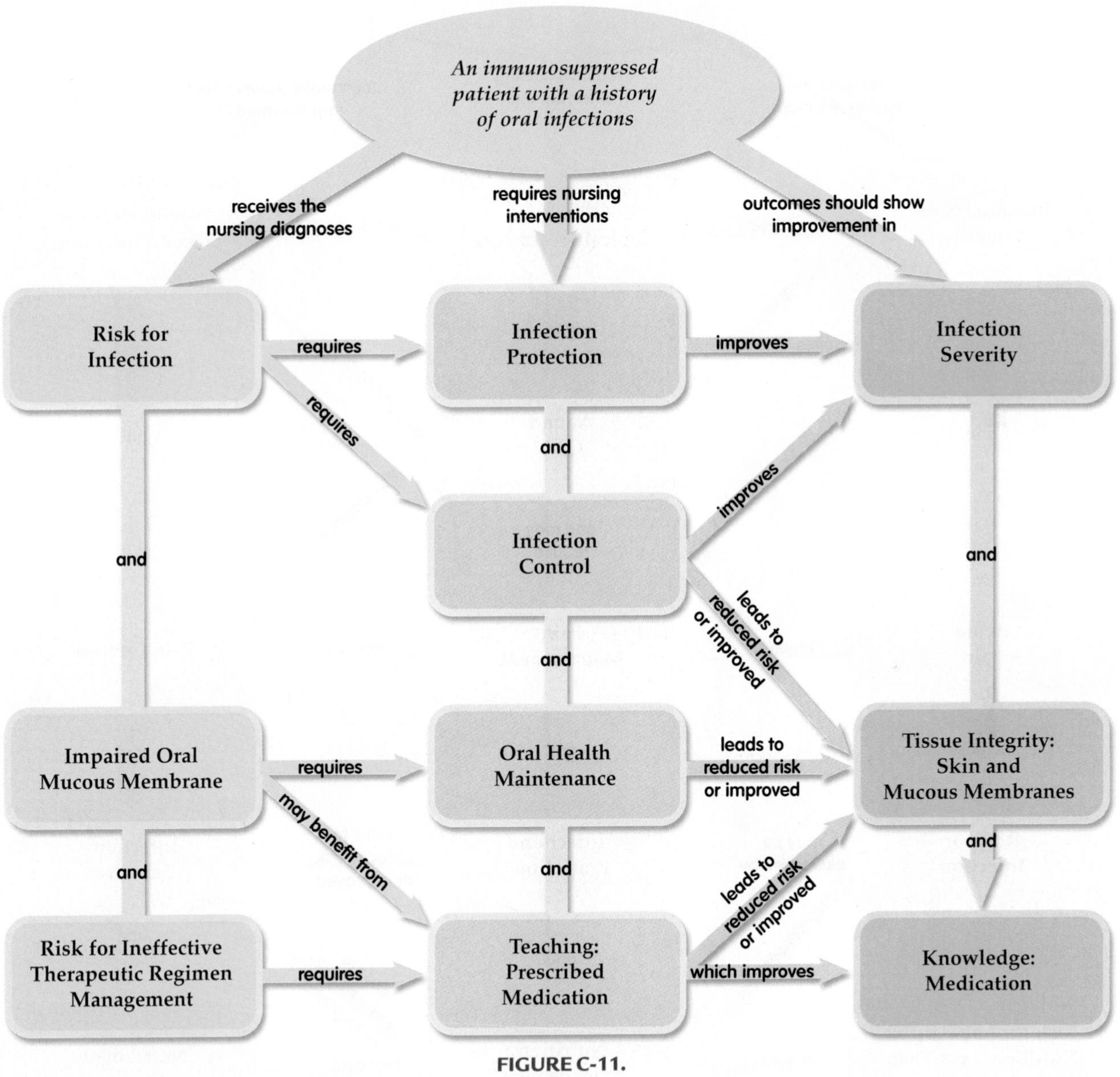

An immunosuppressed patient with a history of oral infections
receives the nursing diagnoses
requires nursing interventions
outcomes should show improvement in
Risk for Infection
requires
Infection Protection
improves
Infection Severity
requires
and
improves
Infection Control
and
and
leads to reduced risk or improved
and
and
Impaired Oral Mucous Membrane
requires
Oral Health Maintenance
leads to reduced risk or improved
Tissue Integrity: Skin and Mucous Membranes
may benefit from
and
and
and
leads to reduced risk or improved
Risk for Ineffective Therapeutic Regimen Management
requires
Teaching: Prescribed Medication
which improves
Knowledge: Medication

FIGURE C-11.

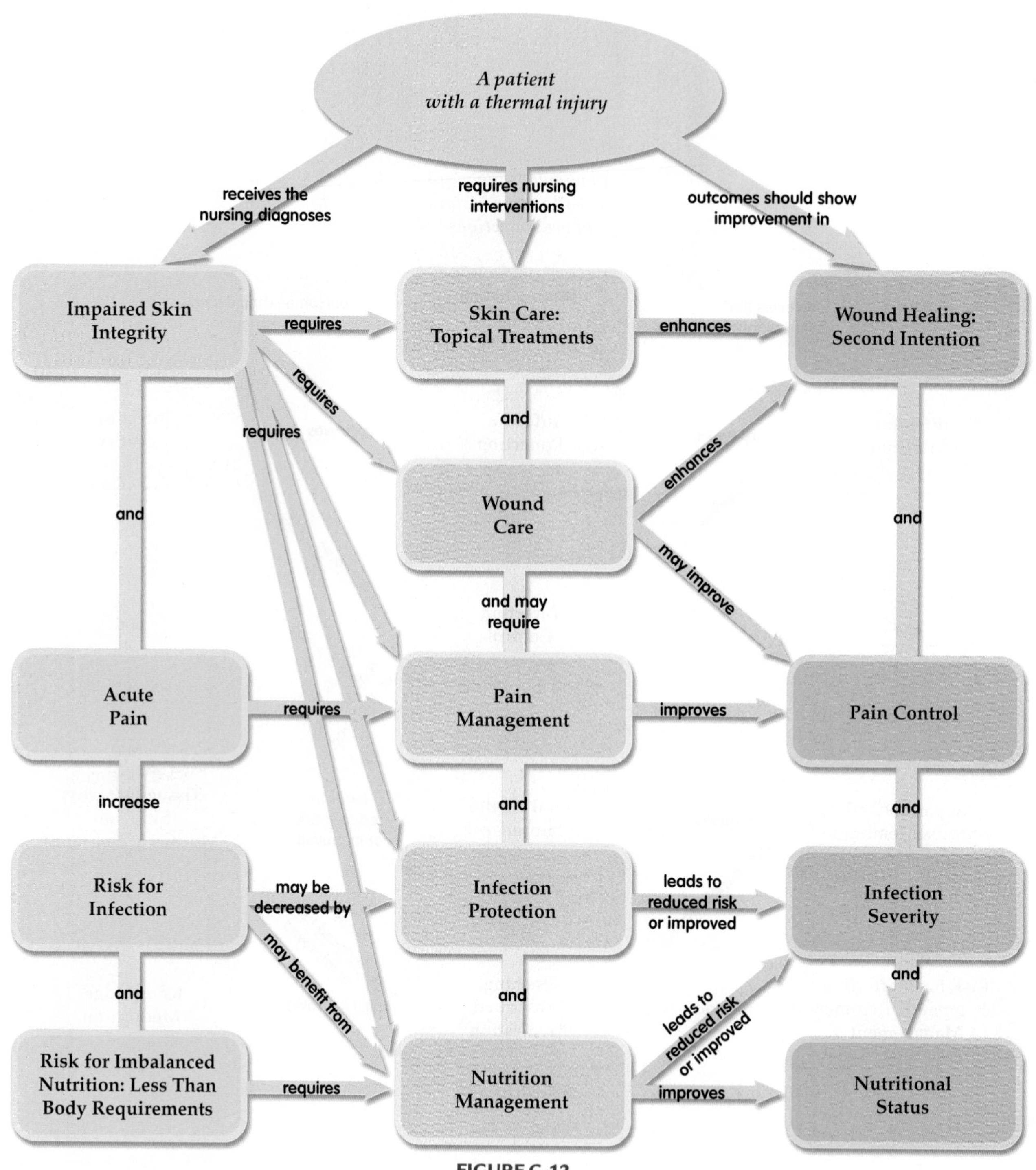
A patient with a thermal injury
receives the nursing diagnoses
requires nursing interventions
outcomes should show improvement in
Impaired Skin Integrity
requires
Skin Care: Topical Treatments
enhances
Wound Healing: Second Intention
requires
requires
and
Wound Care
enhances
and
and
may improve
and may require
Acute Pain
requires
Pain Management
improves
Pain Control
increase
and
and
Risk for Infection
may be decreased by
Infection Protection
leads to reduced risk or improved
Infection Severity
may benefit from
and
and
and
leads to reduced risk or improved
Risk for Imbalanced Nutrition: Less Than Body Requirements
requires
Nutrition Management
improves
Nutritional Status

FIGURE C-12.

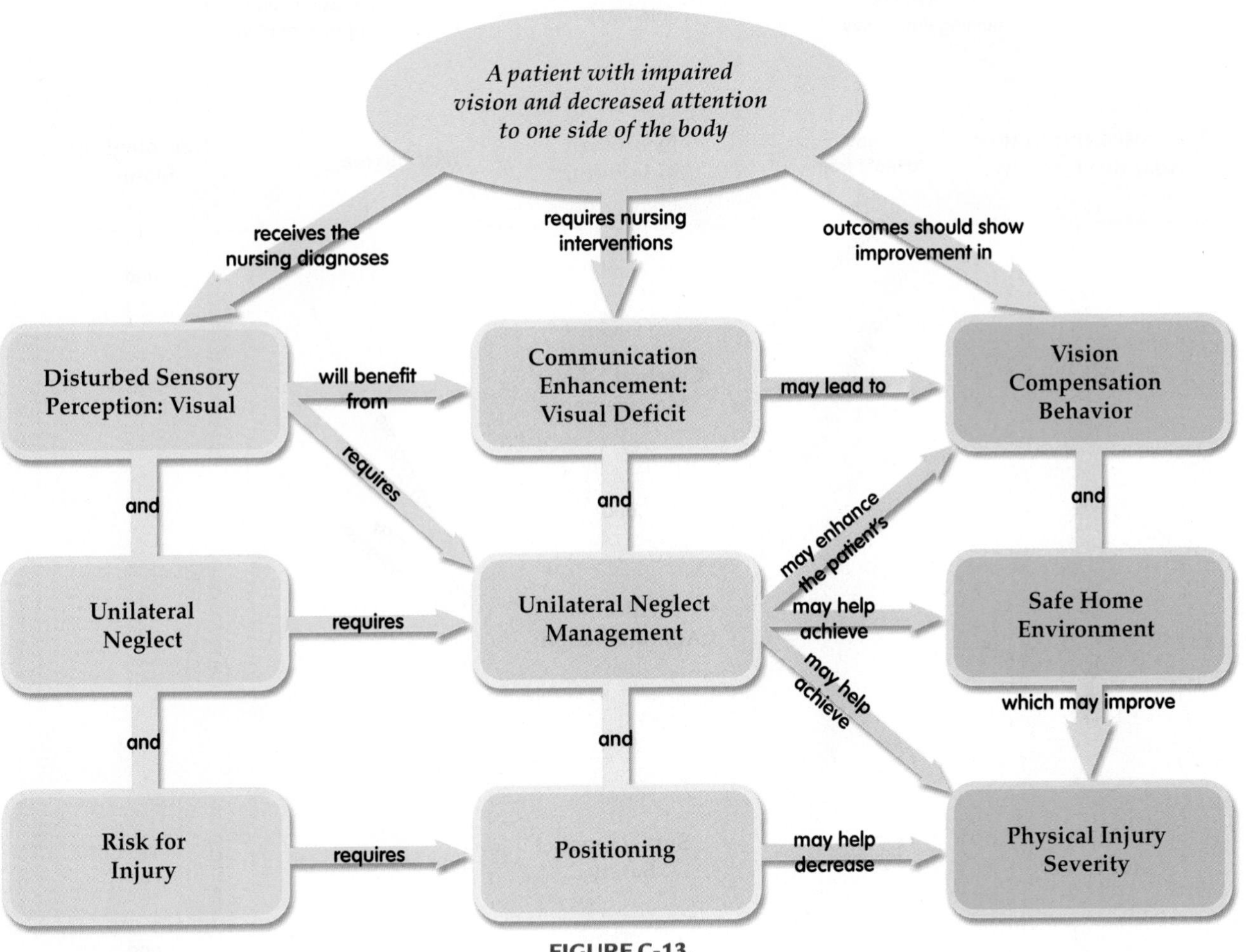

A patient with impaired vision and decreased attention to one side of the body
receives the nursing diagnoses
requires nursing interventions
outcomes should show improvement in
Disturbed Sensory Perception: Visual
will benefit from
Communication Enhancement: Visual Deficit
may lead to
Vision Compensation Behavior
requires
and
and
and
may enhance the patient's
Unilateral Neglect
requires
Unilateral Neglect Management
may help achieve
Safe Home Environment
may help achieve
which may improve
and
and
Risk for Injury
requires
Positioning
may help decrease
Physical Injury Severity

FIGURE C-13.

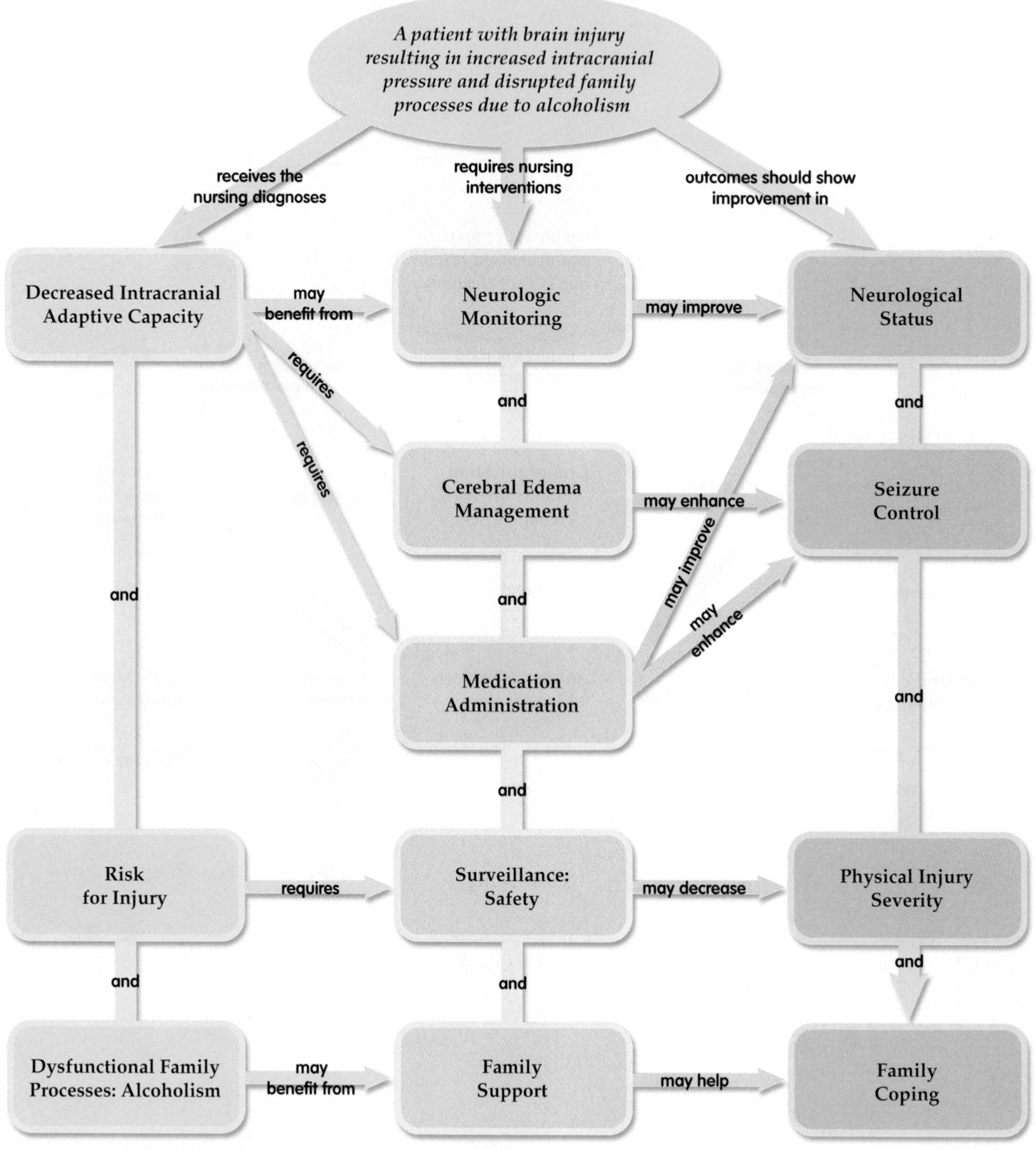

A patient with brain injury resulting in increased intracranial pressure and disrupted family processes due to alcoholism
receives the nursing diagnoses
requires nursing interventions
outcomes should show improvement in
Decreased Intracranial Adaptive Capacity
may benefit from
Neurologic Monitoring
may improve
Neurological Status
requires
requires
and
and
Cerebral Edema Management
may enhance
Seizure Control
may improve
and
and
may enhance
Medication Administration
and
and
Risk for Injury
requires
Surveillance: Safety
may decrease
Physical Injury Severity
and
and
and
Dysfunctional Family Processes: Alcoholism
may benefit from
Family Support
may help
Family Coping

FIGURE C-14.

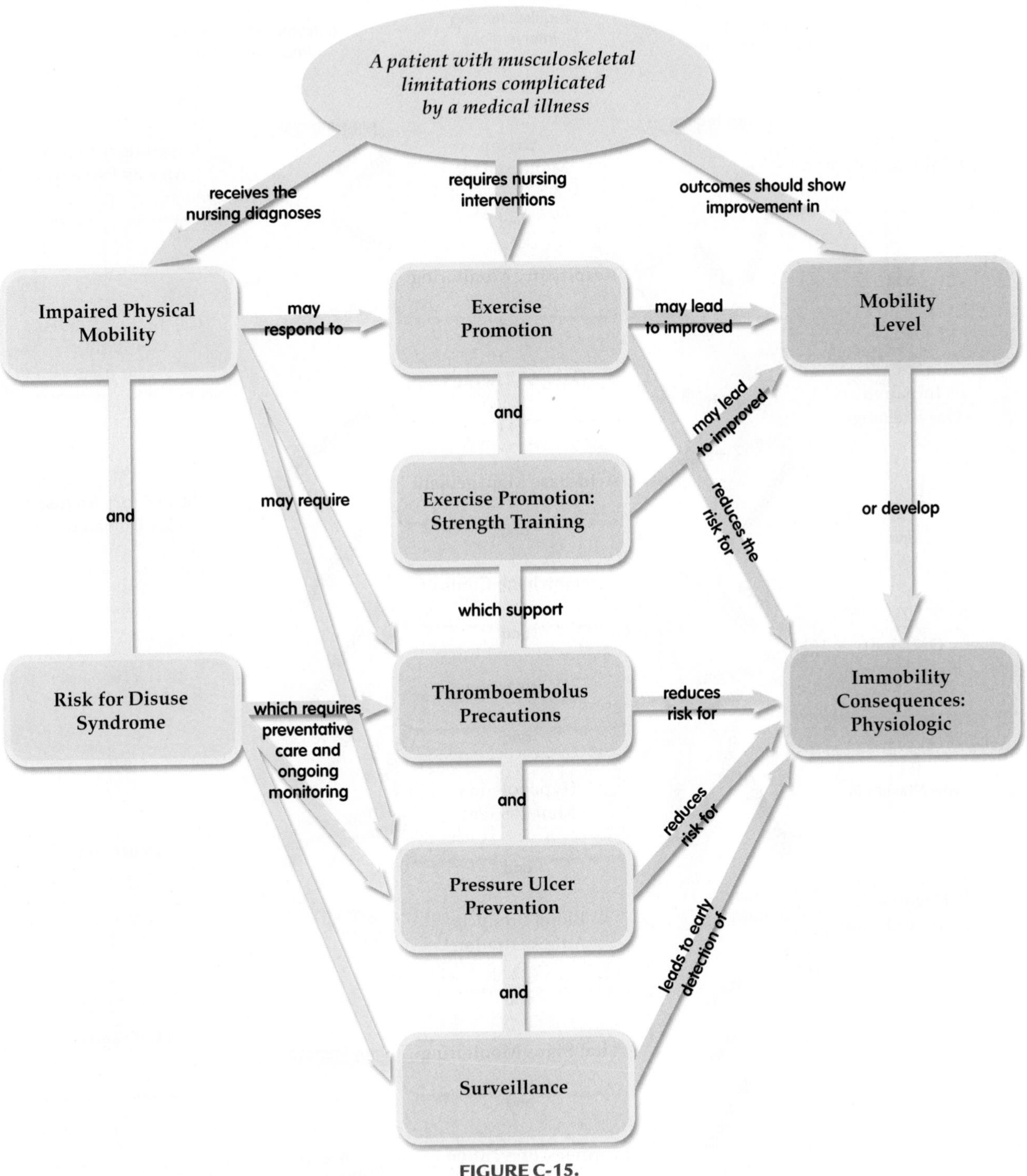

A patient with musculoskeletal limitations complicated by a medical illness
receives the nursing diagnoses
requires nursing interventions
outcomes should show improvement in
Impaired Physical Mobility
may respond to
Exercise Promotion
may lead to improved
Mobility Level
and
may lead to improved
Exercise Promotion: Strength Training
may require
and
reduces the risk for
or develop
which support
Risk for Disuse Syndrome
which requires preventative care and ongoing monitoring
Thromboembolus Precautions
reduces risk for
Immobility Consequences: Physiologic
and
reduces risk for
Pressure Ulcer Prevention
leads to early detection of
and
Surveillance

FIGURE C-15.

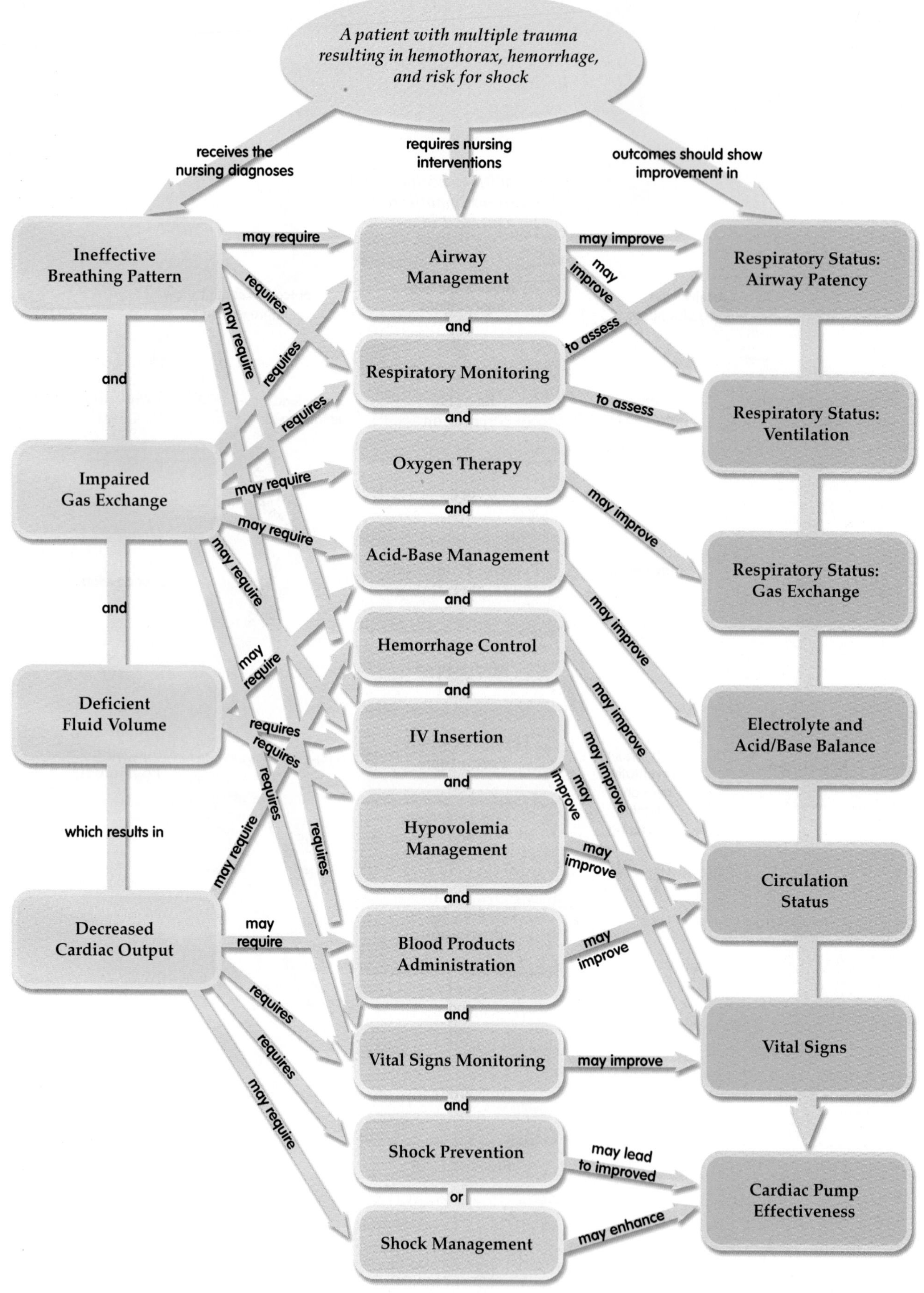

A patient with multiple trauma resulting in hemothorax, hemorrhage, and risk for shock
receives the nursing diagnoses
requires nursing interventions
outcomes should show improvement in
Ineffective Breathing Pattern
and
Impaired Gas Exchange
and
Deficient Fluid Volume
which results in
Decreased Cardiac Output
may require
requires
may require
requires
requires
may require
may require
may require
may require
requires
requires
requires
requires
may require
may require
requires
requires
may require
Airway Management
and
Respiratory Monitoring
and
Oxygen Therapy
and
Acid-Base Management
and
Hemorrhage Control
and
IV Insertion
and
Hypovolemia Management
and
Blood Products Administration
and
Vital Signs Monitoring
and
Shock Prevention
or
Shock Management
may improve
may improve
to assess
to assess
may improve
may improve
may improve
may improve
may improve
may improve
may improve
may improve
may improve
may lead to improved
may enhance
Respiratory Status: Airway Patency
Respiratory Status: Ventilation
Respiratory Status: Gas Exchange
Electrolyte and Acid/Base Balance
Circulation Status
Vital Signs
Cardiac Pump Effectiveness

FIGURE C-16.

Index

Page numbers followed by c indicate charts; those followed by f indicate figures; those followed by t indicate tables.

C

E

F

G

H

M

N

P

U

W

X

Y

Z